Principles and Practice of

SLEEP MEDICINE

Meir Kryger MD, FRCPC
Professor
Department of Pulmonary Critical Care and Sleep Medicine
Yale University
New Haven, Connecticut

Thomas Roth PhD
Director
Sleep Disorders Center
Henry Ford Hospital
Detroit, Michigan

Cathy A. Goldstein MD
Associate Professor
Department of Neurology
University of Michigan
Ann Arbor, Michigan

William C. Dement MD
Lowell W. and Josephine Q. Berry Professor of Psychiatry and Behavioral Sciences
Stanford University School of Medicine
Department of Sleep Sciences & Medicine
Palo Alto, California

Principles and Practice of SLEEP MEDICINE

Seventh Edition

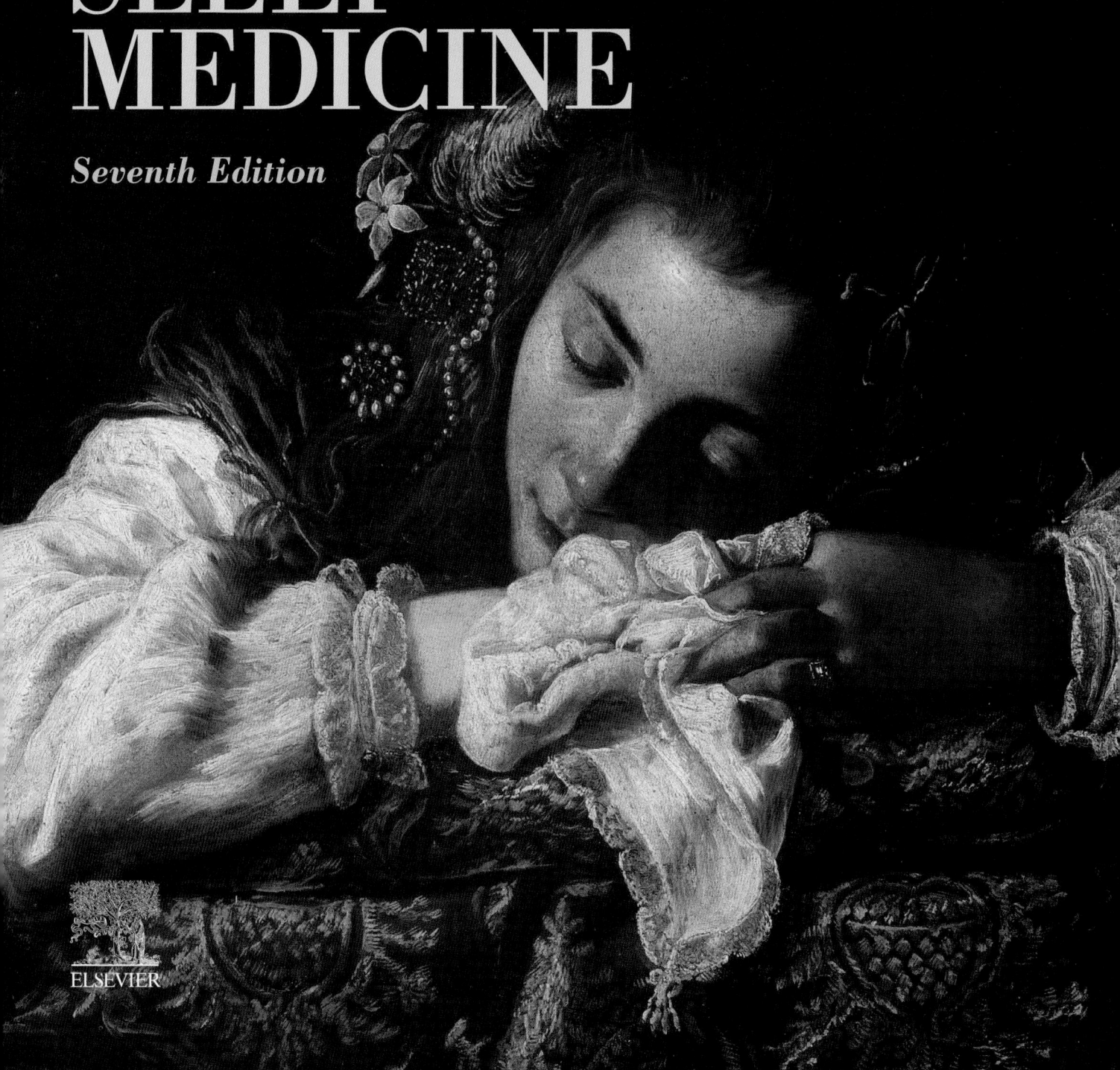

ELSEVIER

ELSEVIER
1600 John F. Kennedy Blvd.
Ste 1600
Philadelphia, PA 19103-2899

PRINCIPLES AND PRACTICE OF SLEEP MEDICINE
ISBN: 978-0-323-66189-8
VOLUME 1 ISBN: 978-0-323-88220-0
VOLUME 2 ISBN: 978-0-323-88221-7

The cover illustration: "Sleeping Girl or Young Woman Sleeping is an oil on canvas painting by an unknown 17th century artist active in Rome, sometimes dated to c.1620 and previously attributed to Theodoor van Loon or Domenico Fetti." Wikipedia.org: https://en.wikipedia.org/wiki/Sleeping_Girl_(17th_century_painting)

Previous editions copyrighted 2017, 2011, 2005, 2000, 1994, and 1989.

ISBN: 978-0-323-66189-8

Senior Acquisitions Editor: Melanie Tucker
Senior Content Development Strategist: Lisa Barnes
Publishing Services Manager: Catherine Jackson
Senior Project Manager: Kate Mannix
Design Direction: Amy Buxton

Printed in India

Last digit is the print number: 9 8 7 6 5 4 3

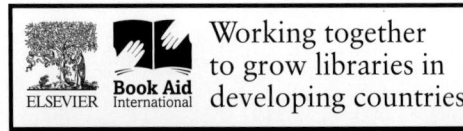

We dedicate this volume to

Barbara Kryger, Jay and Shelley Gold, Emily and Michael Kryger, Steven Kryger and Barr Even

Toni Roth, Daniel and Jeanne Roth, Adam and Carol Roth, Jonathan and Cheyna Roth, Andrea and Justin Leibow

Tadd, Evan, and Cole Hiatt, Larry and Tamara Goldstein, and Carolyn Hiatt

In Memoriam

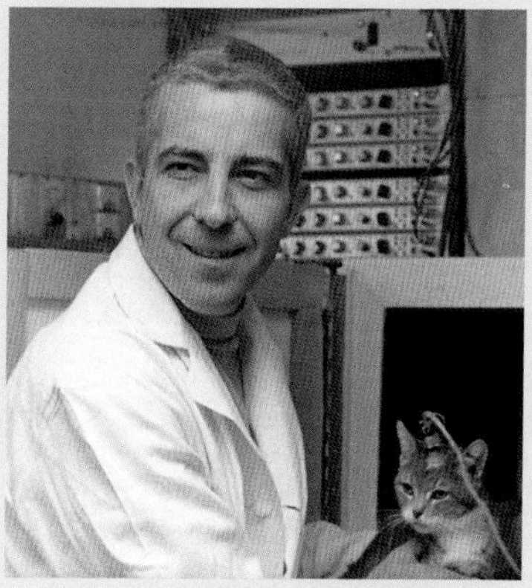

William C. Dement

1928–2020

William C. Dement, the father of sleep medicine, was the inspiration for *Principles and Practice of Sleep Medicine* and was a chief editor starting with the first edition in 1989.

Bill was a brilliant scientist, mentor, teacher, and leader. He did some of the ground-breaking research on rapid eye movement sleep; mentored many of the most productive scientists doing sleep research; taught the most popular course ever at Stanford University, *Sleep and Dreams*; and played a key role in advocating for the importance of sleep to science, governments, and the public. He has affected millions of lives!

I (TR) met Bill for the first time in 1972 when he came to Cincinnati for a CME course on sleep medicine. He invited me to give two lectures and we spent most of the day together. During that day I learned about his intellect, passion for educating the public about sleep medicine, and importantly, his generosity. Over the next 40 years we had many interactions; in every instance they reinforced those initial impressions. It is important recognize that without Bill Dement, the book you are holding would not exist.

I (MK) met Bill for the first time in 1978 at a sleep meeting being held in Stanford. After I gave my presentation (I think I was the only pulmonary trained person in the room) Bill came over to me and said, "My God, you're just a kid." I guess I was. That was the beginning of a beautiful friendship.

In about 1985, we had been discussing and thinking about whether a sleep medicine textbook was needed. We were hesitant to proceed and were actually discouraged by some colleagues who told us there wasn't enough science to warrant a textbook. When presented with the question, Bill said, "You can't have a field without a textbook!" The rest is history. The first edition came out in 1989; it had 730 pages. The sixth edition (2017) was exactly 1000 pages longer. Bill was instrumental in creating the field of sleep medicine. His contributions will never be forgotten. We will miss him.

Meir Kryger Tom Roth Cathy Goldstein

From the Performing Arts

Every Tuesday, Queen Elizabeth II of the United Kingdom (played by Dame Helen Mirren) had a private audience with her Prime Minister in the Private Audience Room on the first floor of Buckingham Palace. This is dramatized in Peter Morgan's play The Audience. *In this scene, Elizabeth is meeting with Prime Minister Gordon Brown.*

Elizabeth: So, back to your weekend, and all this industriousness. Were you up very early?
Brown: Four thirty.
Elizabeth: Oh, dear.
Brown: It's all right. I never sleep much.
Elizabeth: Since when?
Brown: Since always.
Elizabeth: Harold Wilson always used to say, "The main requirement of a Prime Minister is a good night's sleep … and a sense of history." Mrs. Thatcher taught herself to need very little towards the end. But I'm not sure how reassured I am by that. I like the idea of any person with the power to start nuclear war being rested. (*A beat.*) Besides, lack of sleep can have a knock-on effect in other areas.
Brown: Such as?
Elizabeth: One's general sense of health.
A silence.
And happiness.
A silence.
And equilibrium.
Brown looks up. A silence.
I gather there's been some concern …
Brown: About what?
Elizabeth: Your happiness. Don't worry. You wouldn't be the first in your position to feel overwhelmed. Despondent.
She searches for the right word.
Depressed.

From Morgan, Peter. THE AUDIENCE, Faber and Faber, 2013.
Used with permission of Mr. Peter Morgan.

But the tigers come at night
With their voices soft as thunder
As they tear your hope apart
As they turn your dream to shame.

From I Dreamed a Dream, LES MISÉRABLES, with permission, Cameron Mackintosh, producer © 1985 Alain Boublil Music Ltd. Used with permission 1991, CMI.

From Literature

Blessings on him who first invented sleep.—It covers a man all over, thoughts and all, like a cloak.—It is meat for the hungry, drink for the thirsty, heat for the cold, and cold for the hot.—It makes the shepherd equal to the monarch, and the fool to the wise.—There is but one evil in it, and that is that it resembles death, since between a dead man and a sleeping man there is but little difference.

From DON QUIXOTE
By Saavedra M. de Cervantes

"To sleep! To forget!" he said to himself with the serene confidence of a healthy man that if he is tired and sleepy, he will go to sleep at once. And the same instant his head did begin to feel drowsy and he began to drop off into forgetfulness. The waves of the sea of unconsciousness had begun to meet over his head, when all at once—it was as though a violent shock of electricity had passed over him. He started so that he leapt up on the springs of the sofa, and leaning on his arms got in a panic on to his knees. His eyes were wide open as though he had never been asleep. The heaviness in his head and the weariness in his limbs that he had felt a minute before had suddenly gone.

From ANNA KARENINA, Part IV, Chapter XVIII
By Leo Tolstoy

The Body Electric

Every cell in our bodies contains a pore
like a door, which says when to let in
the flood of salt-ions bearing their charge,
but the power in us moves much slower
than the current that rushes into wires
to ignite the lamp by which I undress,
am told to undress by sparks that cross
the gap of a synapse to pass along
the message, *It's time for sleep.* As I pull
back the sheets, ease into bed, I think
if I could only look beneath my skin,
I'd see my body as alive as Hong Kong,
veins of night traffic crawling along
the freeways as tiny faces inside taxis
look up from the glow of their phones,
sensing that someone is watching.

James Crews, Dec. 3, 2020. *New York Times Magazine.* Used with permission of the poet.

Contributors

Ghizlane Aarab, MD
Associate Professor
Department of Oral Kinesiology
The Academic Center for Dentistry
Amsterdam, The Netherlands

Sabra Abbott, MD, PhD
Assistant Professor
Department of Neurology
Center for Circadian and Sleep Medicine
Northwestern University Feinberg School of Medicine
Chicago, Illinois

Shervin Abdollahi, BS
Research Analyst (Contractor)
National Institute of Neurological Disorders and Stroke
Bethesda, Maryland

Philip N. Ainslie, PhD
Professor
Department of Health and Exercise Sciences
The University of British Columbia
Kelowna, British Columbia, Canada

Cathy Alessi, MD
Director
Geriatric Research, Education and Clinical Center
VA Greater Los Angeles Healthcare System;
Professor
Department of Medicine
David Geffen School of Medicine
University of California, Los Angeles
Los Angeles, California

Richard P. Allen, PhD
Professor
Department of Neurology
Johns Hopkins University
Baltimore, Maryland

Fernanda R. Almeida, DDS, MSc, PhD
Associate Professor
Oral Health Sciences
University of British Columbia
Vancouver, British Columbia, Canada

Aurelio Alonso, DDS, MS, PhD
Department of Anesthesiology
Orofacial Pain–Duke Innovative Pain Therapies
Center for Translational Pain Medicine
Duke University
Durham, North Carolina

Neesha Anand, MD
Critical Care Fellow
University of Pittsburgh
Pittsburgh, Pennsylvania

Amy W. Amara, MD
Associate Professor
Department of Neurology
University of Alabama at Birmingham
Birmingham, Alabama

Sonia Ancoli-Israel, PhD
Professor Emeritus
Professor of Research
Department of Psychiatry
University of California, San Diego
La Jolla, California

Anna Anund, PhD
Reserach Director
Department of Human Factors
Swedish National Road and Transport Research Institute;
Associate Professor
Rehabilitation Medicine
Linköping University
Linkoping, Sweden

Taro Arima, DDS, PhD
Lecturer
Division of International Affairs
Graduate School of Dental Medicine
Hokkaido University
Sapporo, Japan

J. Todd Arnedt, PhD
Departments of Psychiatry and Neurology
University of Michigan Medical School
Ann Arbor, Michigan

Isabelle Arnulf, MD, PhD
Sleep Disorders Unit
Pitie-Salpetriere University Hospital
Sorbonne University
Paris, France

Vivian Asare, MD
Assistant Professor
Department of Medicine (Pulmonary, Critical Care, and Sleep Medicine)
Yale University School of Medicine
New Haven, Connecticuit

Lauren Asarnow, PhD
Assistant Professor
Psychiatry
School of Medicine
University of California–San Francisco
San Francisco, California

Hrayr Attarian, MD
Professor
Department of Neurology
Northwestern University
Chicago, Illinois

Alon Y. Avidan, MD, MPH
Director
University of California, Los Angeles Sleep Disorders Center;
Professor
Department of Neurology
University of California, Los Angeles,
Los Angeles, California

Nicoletta Azzi, MD
Sleep Disorders Center
Department of Medicine and Surgery
University of Parma
Parma, Italy

M. Safwan Badr, MD,MBA
Professor
Department of Internal Medicine
The Liborio Tranchida MD Endowed Chair
Wayne State University
Detroit, Michigan

Helen A. Baghdoyan, PhD
Beaman Professor
University of Tennessee
Knoxville, Tennessee;
Joint Faculty, Biosciences Division
Oak Ridge National Laboratory
Oak Ridge, Tennessee

Sébastien Baillieul, MD, PhD
Pneumology-Physiology Department
Grenoble Alpes University Hospital;
INSERM U1300, HP2 Laboratory
Grenoble Alpes University
Grenoble, France

Benjamin Baird, PhD
Wisconsin Institute for Sleep and Consciousness
Department of Psychiatry
University of Wisconsin–Madison
Madison, Wisconsin

Fiona C. Baker, PhD
Director, Center for Health Sciences
SRI International;
Honorary Senior Research Fellow
Brain Function Research Group
School of Physiology
University of the Witwatersrand
Johannesburg, Gauteng, South Africa

Thomas J. Balkin, PhD
Senior Scientist
Behavioral Biology Branch
Walter Reed Army Institute of Research
Silver Spring, Maryland

Siobhan Banks, PhD
Professor
UniSA Justice and Society
University of South Australia
Magill, South Australia

Nicola L. Barclay, BA(Hons), MSc, PhD
Sleep and Circadian Neuroscience Institute (SCNi)
Nuffield Department of Clinical Neurosciences
University of Oxford
Oxford, Great Britain

Steven R. Barczi, MD
Professor of Medicine
Department of Medicine
University of Wisconsin School of Medicine & Public Health;
Director of Clinical Programs
Madison VA Geriatric Research, Education, and Clinical Center
Wm. S. Middleton Veterans Affairs Hospital
Madison, Wisconsin

Mathias Basner, MD, PhD, MSc
Professor of Sleep and Chronobiology in Psychiatry
Unit for Experimental Psychiatry
Division of Sleep and Chronobiology
Department of Psychiatry
Perelman School of Medicine
University of Pennsylvania
Philadelphia, Pennsylvania

Claudio L.A. Bassetti, MD
Professor
Chairman and Head
Neurology Department
Inselspital University Hospital
Bern, Switzerland

Celyne Bastien, PhD
School of Psychology
Laval University
Quebec City, Quebec, Canada

Christian R. Baumann, MD
Department of Neurology
University Hospital Zurich
Zurich, Switzerland

Louise Beattie, PhD
Institute of Health and Wellbeing
University of Glasgow
Glasgow, Great Britain

Bei Bei, DPsych(Clinical), PhD
NHMRC Health Professional Research Fellow
Clinical Psychologist
School of Psychological Sciences
Monash University
Clayton, Victoria, Australia

Gregory Belenky, MD
Research Professor
Sleep and Performance Research Center
Washington State University
Spokane, Washington

Amy Bender, MS, PhD
Adjunct Assistant Professor
Department of Kinesiology
University of Calgary;
Senior Research Scientist
Calgary Counselling Centre
Calgary, Canada

Suzanne M. Bertisch, MD, MPH
Division of Sleep and Circadian Disorders
Brigham and Women's Hospital
Harvard Medical School
Boston, Massachusetts

Carlos Blanco-Centurion, PhD
Department of Psychiatry and Behavioral Sciences
Medical University of South Carolina
Charleston, South Carolina

Benjamin T. Bliska, DDS
Faculty of Dentistry
University of British Columbia
Vancouver, British Columbia, Canada

Konrad E. Bloch, MD
Professor
Respiratory Medicine, Sleep Disorders Center
University Hospital Zurich
Zurich, Switzerland

Bradley F. Boeve, MD
Professor of Neurology
Department of Neurology
Mayo Clinic
Rochester, Minnesota

Patricia Bonnavion, MD
Lab of Neurophysiology
ULB Neuroscience Institute
Université Libre Bruxelles
Brussels, Belgium

Scott B. Boyd, DDS, PhD
Professor of Oral and Maxillofacial Surgery, Retired Faculty
Department of Oral and Maxillofacial Surgery
Vanderbilt University School of Medicine
Nashville, Tennesee

Alessandro Bracci, DDS
Adjunct Professor
Department of Neuroscience
School of Dentistry,
University of Padova
Padova, Italy

Tiffany Braley, MD
Associate Professor of Neurology
Department of Neurology
Multiple Sclerosis and Sleep Disorders Centers
University of Michigan
Ann Arbor, Michigan

Josiane L. Broussard, MD
Assistant Professor
Department of Health and Exercise Science
Colorado State University
Fort Collins, Colorado

Daniel B. Brown, JD
Partner, Taylor English Duma, LLP
Atlanta, Georgia

Luis F. Buenaver, PhD
Assistant Professor of Psychiatry and Neurology
Director, Johns Hopkins Behavioral Sleep Medicine Program
Johns Hopkins University School of Medicine
Baltimore, Maryland

Helen J. Burgess, PhD
Professor
Department of Psychiatry
University of Michigan
Ann Arbor, Michigan

Keith R. Burgess, MBBS, MSc, PhD, FRACP, FRCPC
Clinical Associate Professor
Department of Medicine
University of Sydney
Sydney, Australia

Orfeu M. Buxton, PhD
Professor
Department of Biobehavioral Health
Pennsylvania State University
University Park, Pennsylvania

Daniel J. Buysse, MD
UPMC Professor of Sleep Medicine
Professor of Psychiatry and Clinical and Translational Science
University of Pittsburgh School of Medicine
Pittsburgh, Pennsylvania

Sean W. Cain, PhD
Associate Professor
School of Psychological Sciences
Turner Institute for Brain and Mental Health
Monash University
Clayton, Victictoria, Australia

J. Lynn Caldwell, BS, MA, PhD
Senior Research Psychologist
Naval Medical Research Unit Dayton
Wright-Patterson Air Force Base, Ohio

John A. Caldwell, BS, MA, PHD
Senior Scientist
Fatigue and Sleep Management
Coastal Performance Consulting
Yellow Springs, Ohio

Michael W. Calik, PhD
Assistant Professor
Department of Biobehavioral Nursing Science

Assistant Professor
Center for Sleep and Health Research
University of Illinois Chicago College of Nursing
Chicago, Illinois

Francisco Campos-Rodriguez, MD
Respiratory Department
Hospital Valme
Seville, Andalucía

Craig Canapari, MD
Associate Professor
Department of Pediatrics
Yale University
New Haven, Connecticuit

Michela Canepari, PhD
Department of Humanities, Social and Cultural Enterprises
University of Parma
Parma, Italy

Michelle T. Cao, DO
Clinical Associate Professor
Department of Neurology
Stanford University School of Medicine
Palo Alto, California;
Clinical Associate Professor
Psychiatry and Behavioral Sciences
Stanford University School of Medicine
Redwood City, California

Colleen E. Carney, PhD
Professor
Department of Psychology
Ryerson University
Toronto, Ontario, Canada

Michelle Carr, PhD
Department of Psychiatry
University of Rochester Medical Center
Rochester, New York

Santiago Carrizo, MD
Servicio de Neumología
Hospital Universitario Miguel Servet
Zaragoza, Spain

Mary A. Carskadon, PhD
Professor, Psychiatry and Human Behavior
Alpert Medical School of Brown University;
Director, Chronobiology and Sleep Research
EP Bradley Hospital
Providence, Rhode Island

Diego Z. Carvalho, MD
Assistant Professor
Center for Sleep Medicine
Department of Medicine
Mayo Clinic College of Medicine and Science
Rochester, Minnesota

Anna Castelnovo, MD
Faculty of Biomedical Sciences
Università della Svizzera Italiana
Lugano, Switzerland

Eduardo E. Castrillon, DDS, MSc, PhD
Associate Professor
Section for Orofacial Pain and Jaw Function
Department of Dentistry and Oral Health
Aarhus University
Aarhus, Denmark

Lana M. Chahine, MD
Assistant Professor
Department of Neurology
University of Pittsburgh
Pittsburgh, Pennsylvania

Etienne Challet, PhD
Institute of Cellular and Integrative Neurosciences
Strasbourg, France

Philip Cheng, PhD
Assistant Scientist
Division of Sleep Medicine
Thomas Roth Sleep Disorders and Research Center
Henry Ford Health System
Detroit, Michigan;
Research Assistant Professor
Department of Psychiatry
University of Michigan School of Medicine
Ann Arbor, Michigan

Ronald D. Chervin, MD, MS
Professor of Neurology
Michael S. Aldrich Collegiate Professor of Sleep Medicine
Director, Sleep Disorders Center
University of Michigan Health System
Ann Arbor, Michigan

Soo-Hee Choi, MD, PhD
Associate Professor
Department of Psychiatry
Seoul National University College of Medicine;
Associate Professor
Department of Psychiatry
Seoul National University Hospital
Seoul, Korea

Ian M. Colrain, PhD
President
SRI Biosciences
SRI International
Menlo Park, California;
Professorial Fellow
Melbourne School of Pscyhological Sciences
The University of Melbourne
Parkville, Victoria, Australia

Veda Elisabeth Cost, BA
Research Fellow
National Institute of Neurological Disorders and Stroke
Bethesda, Maryland

Anita P. Courcoulas, MD
Professor of Surgery
Division of Minimally Invasive Bariatric and General Surgery
University of Pittsburgh Medical Center
Pittsburgh, Pennsylvania

Michel A. Cramer Bornemann, MD, DABSM, FAASM
Lead Investigator
Sleep Forensics Associates;
Visiting Professor, Sleep Medicine
Fellowship, Minnesota Regional Sleep Disorders Center
Hennepin County Medical Center
Minneapolis, Minnesota;
Co-Director of Sleep Medicine Services
CentraCare
Saint Cloud, Minnesota

Ashley F. Curtis, PhD
Assistant Professor
Psychiatry
Psychological Sciences
University of Missouri
Columbia, Missouri

Charles A. Czeisler, PhD, MD
Frank Baldino, Jr., Ph.D. Professor of Sleep Medicine
Department of Medicine
Director
Division of Sleep Medicine
Harvard Medical School;
Chief, Division of Sleep and Circadian Disorders
Department Medicine
Brigham and Women's Hospital
Boston, Massachusetts

Michael Czisch, MD
Max Planck Institute of Psychiatry
Munich, Germany

Armando D'Agostino, MD, PhD
Department of Health Sciences
Università degli Studi di Milano
Milan, Italy

O'Neill F. D'Cruz, MD
OD Consulting and Neurological Services, PLLC
Chapel Hill, NC

Steve M. D'Souza, MD
Resident
Eastern Virginia University Medical School
Norfolk, Virginia

Meg Danforth, PhD
Clinical Psychology
Duke University Faculty Practice in Psychology
Durham, North Carolina

Yves Dauvilliers, MD, PhD
Professor
Sleep Unit, Department of Neurology
Gui de Chauliac Hospital
Montpellier, France

Drew Dawson, PhD
Professor
Appleton Institute
Central Queensland University
Wayville, Australia

David de Ángel Solá, MD
Staff Physician
Department of Pediatrics
Yale School of Medicine
New Haven, Connecticut;
Faculty Physician
Department of Neurology
VA Caribbean Healthcare Systems;
Faculty Physician
Department of Pediatrics
San Juan City Hospital
San Juan, Puerto Rico

Luis de Lecea, PhD
Department of Psychiatry and Behavioral Sciences
Stanford University
Palo Alto, California

Massimiliano de Zambotti, PhD
Principle Scientist, Human Sleep Research
Center for Health Sciences
SRI International
Menlo Park, California

Tom Deboer, PhD
Associate Professor
Cell and Chemical Biology
Leiden University Medical Center
Leiden, The Netherlands

Lourdes DelRosso, MD
Associate Professor
Department of Pediatrics
Seattle Children's Hospital
University of Washington
Seattle, Washington

William C. Dement, MD[†]
Lowell W. and Josephine Q. Berry Professor of Psychiatry and Behavioral Sciences
Stanford University School of Medicine
Department of Sleep Sciences & Medicine
Palo Alto, California

Jerome A. Dempsey, PhD
Professor Emeritus
Population Health Sciences;
Director
John Rankin Laboratory of Pulmonary Medicine
University of Wisconsin–Madison
Madison, Wisconsin

Massimiliano DiGiosia, DDS
Orofacial Pain Clinic
Division of Diagnostic Sciences
Adams School of Dentistry
University of North Carolina at Chapel Hill
Chapel Hill, North Carolina

[†]Deceased.

Derk-Jan Dijk, PhD
Professor
Surrey Sleep Research Centre
Department of Clinical and Experimental Medicine
Faculty of Health and Medical Sciences
University of Surrey;
Investigator
Dementia Research Institute Care Research and Technology Centre
Imperial College London
University of Surrey
Guildford, Great Britain

David F. Dinges, MS, MA(H), PhD
Professor and Director, Unit for Experimental Psychiatry
Chief, Division of Sleep and Chronobiology
Department of Psychiatry
Pereleman School of Medicine
University of Pennsylvania
Philadelphia, Pennsylvania

G. William Domhoff, PhD
Distinguished Professor Emeritus and Research Professor in Psychology
Department of Psychology
University of California
Santa Cruz, California

Jillian Dorrian, PhD, MBiostat
Professor and Dean of Research
Behavior-Brain-Body Research Centre
University of South Australia
Adelaide, South Australia

Anthony G. Doufas, MD, PhD
Professor
Department of Anesthesiology, Perioperative and Pain Medicine
Stanford University School of Medicine
Palo Alto, California

Luciano F. Drager, MD, PhD
Associate Professor of Medicine
Department of Internal Medicine
University of Sao Paulo
Sso Paulo, Brazil

Christopher L. Drake, PhD, FAASM, DBSM
Director of Sleep Research
Division of Sleep Medicine
Henry Ford Health System;
Professor
Department of Psychiatry and Behavioral Neuroscience
Wayne State University School of Medicine
Detroit, Michigan

Martin Dresler, PhD
Radboud University Medical Center
Department of Cognitive Neuroscience
Donders Institute for Brain, Cognition, and Behavior
Nijmegen, The Netherlands

Jeanne F. Duffy, MBA, PhD
Division of Sleep and Circadian Disorders
Departments of Medicine and Neurology
Brigham and Women's Hospital;
Division of Sleep Medicine
Harvard Medical School
Boston, Massachusetts

Peter R. Eastwood, PhD
Director, Flinders Health and Medical Research Institute
Dean of Research and Matthew Flinders Fellow
College of Medicine and Public Health
Flinders University
Adelaide, South Australia

Danny J. Eckert, PhD
Professor and Director
Adelaide Institute for Sleep Health
Flinders Health and Medical Research Institute
Flinders University
Bedford Park, South Australia

Jack D. Edinger, PhD
Professor
Department of Medicine
National Jewish Health
Denver, Colorado;
Adjunct Professor
Psychiatry and Behavioral Sciences
Duke University Medical Center
Durham, North Carolina

Bradley A. Edwards, PhD
Department of Physiology
School of Biomedical Sciences and Biomedical Discovery Institute
Monash University
Melbourne, Victoria, Australia

Jason G. Ellis, MD
Northumbria Sleep Research
Faculty of Health and Life Sciences
Northumbria University
Newcastle, United Kingdom

Daniel Erlacher, PhD, MD
Institute of Sport Science
University of Bern
Bern, Switzerland

Gregory Essick, DDS, PhD
Professor
Division of Comprehensive Oral Health
Adams School of Dentistry
University of North Carolina at Chapel Hill
Chapel Hill, North Carolina

Marissa A. Evans, MS
Department of Psychiatry
University of Pittsburgh
Pittsburgh, Pennsylvania

Véronique Fabre, PhD
Neuroscience Paris Seine
INSERM
Sorbonne Université Paris
Paris, France

Francesca Facco, MD
Associate Professor of Medicine
Department of Obstetrics, Gynecology, and Reproductive Sciences
University of Pittsburgh School of Medicine
Pittsburgh, Pennsylvania

Ronnie Fass, MD
Director, Division of Gastroenterology and Hepatology
Department of Medicine
MetroHealth Medical Center;
Professor of Medicine
Case Western Reserve University
Cleveland, Ohio

Luigi Ferini-Strambi, MD
Professor of Neurology
Department of Clinical Neuroscience
Università Vita-Salute San Raffaele
Milano, Italy

Julio Fernandez-Mendoza, PhD, CBSM, DBSM
Associate Professor
Director, Behavioral Sleep Medicine Program
Sleep Research & Treatment Center
Department of Psychiatry and Behavioral Health
Penn State University College of Medicine
Penn State Health Milton S. Hershey Medical Center
Hershey, Pennsylvania

Fabio Ferrarelli, MD, PhD
Associate Professor of Psychiatry
Department of Psychiatry
University of Pittsburgh
Pittsburgh, Pennsylvania

Raffaele Ferri, MD
Sleep Research Centre
Department of Neurology I.C.
Oasi Research Institute - IRCCS
Troina, Italy

Stuart Fogel, PhD
Associate Professor
School of Psychology
University of Ottawa
Ottawa, Ontario, Canada

Jimmy J. Fraigne, PhD
Senior Research Associate
Department of Cell & Systems Biology
University of Toronto
Toronto, Canada

Paul Franken, PhD
Associate Professor
Center for Integrative Genomics
University of Lausanne
Lausanne, Switzerland

Karl A. Franklin, MD, PhD
Assistant Professor
Department of Surgery
Surgical and Preoperative Sciences
Umeå University
Umeå, Sweden

Neil Freedman, MD, FCCP
Head, Division of Pulmonary and Critical Care
Department of Medicine
NorthShore University Healthsystem;
Clinical Professor of Medicine
University of Chicago Pritzker School of Medicine
Chicago, Illinois

Liam Fry, MD, CMD, FACP
Division Chief of Geriatrics and Palliative Medicine
Department of Internal Medicine
University of Texas Dell Medical School;
President
Austin Geriatric Specialists
Austin, Texas

Patrick M. Fuller, MS, PhD
Professor of Neurological Surgery
Vice Chair of Research
University of California, Davis School of Medicine
Sacramento, California

Constance H. Fung, MD, MSHS
Geriatric Research, Education and Clinical Center
VA Greater Los Angeles Healthcare System;
Associate Professor
Department of Medicine
David Geffen School of Medicine
University of California, Los Angeles
Los Angeles, California

Carles Gaig, MD, PhD
Multidisciplinary Sleep Unit
Neurology Department
Hospital Clinic Barcelona
Barcelona, Spain

Philippa H. Gander, PhD, FRSNZ, ONZM
Professor Emeritus
Sleep/Wake Research Centre
Massey University
Wellington, New Zealand

Sheila N. Garland, PhD
Associate Professor
Department of Psychology, Faculty of Science
Discipline of Oncology, Faculty of Medicine
Memorial University
St. John's, Newfoundland, Canada

Philip R. Gehrman, PhD
Associate Professor
Department of Psychiatry
University of Pennsylvania Perelman School of Medicine
Philadelphia, Pennsylvania

Martha U. Gillette, PhD
Alumni Professor
Cell and Developmental Biology
Professor
Beckman Institute for Advanced Science & Technology
Molecular and Integrative Physiology
Director
Neuroscience Program
University of Illinois at Urbana-Champaign
Urbana, Illinois

Kevin S. Gipson, MD, MS
Assistant in Pediatrics
Department of Pediatrics
Massachusetts General Hospital;
Instructor
Harvard Medical School
Boston, Massachusetts

Peter J. Goadsby, MD, PhD, DSc
Department of Neurology
University of California, Los Angeles
Los Angeles, California;
National Institute for Health Research–Wellcome Trust King's Clinical Research Facility
King's College London
London, United Kingdom

Avram R. Gold, MD
Associate Professor of Clinical Medicine
Pulmonary, Critical Care, and Sleep Medicine
Stony Brook University School of Medicine
Stony Brook, New York

Cathy A. Goldstein, MD
Associate Professor of Neurology
Sleep Disorders Center
University of Michigan Health System
Ann Arbor, Michigan

Joshua J. Gooley, PhD
Associate Professor
Program in Neuroscience and Behavioral Disorders
Duke-NUS Medical School
Singapore

Nadia Gosselin, PhD
Associate Professor
Department of Psychology
Université de Montréal;
Researcher
Center for Advanced Research in Sleep Medicine
Hôpital du Sacré-Coeur de Montréal
Montreal, Quebec, Canada

Daniel J. Gottlieb, MD, MPH
Medical Service
VA Boston Healthcare System;
Division of Sleep and Circadian Disorders
Departments of Medicine and Neurology
Brigham and Women's Hospital;
Division of Sleep Medicine
Harvard Medical School
Boston, Massachusetts

R. Curtis Graeber, BA, MA, PhD
Honorary Fellow
Sleep/Wake Research Centre
Massey University
Wellington, New Zealand

Michael A. Grandner, PhD, MTR
Assistant Professor
Department of Psychiatry
University of Arizona
Tucson, Arizona

Harly Greenberg, MD
Professor of Medicine
Northwell Sleep Disorders Center;
Chief, Division of Pulmonary, Critical Care, and Sleep Medicine
Professor of Medicine
Donald and Barbara Zucker School of Medicine at Hofstra-Northwell
New Hyde Park, New York

Alice M. Gregory, BSc, PhD
Professor
Department of Psychology
Goldsmiths
University of London
London, Great Britain

Edith Grosbellet, PhD
Institute of Cellular and Integrative Neurosciences
Strasbourg, France

Ludger Grote, MD, PhD
Professor
Sleep Disorders Center
Department of Respiratory Medicine
Sahlgrenska University Hospital
Gothenburg, Sweden

Ronald Grunstein, MBBS, MD, PhD, FRACP
Professor
Sleep and Circadian Research Group
Woolcock Institute of Medical Research
Sydney, Australia

Christian Guilleminault, MD, BioL[†]
Professor
Department of Psychiatry and Behavioral Sciences
Sleep Medicine Division
Stanford University School of Medicine
Redwood City, California

Andrew Gumley, MD
Institute of Health and Wellbeing
University of Glasgow
Glasgow, United Kingdom

Hannah Gura, BS
Research Fellow
National Institute of Mental Health
Bethesda, Maryland

[†]Deceased.

Monika Haack, MD
Associate Professor of Neurology
Department of Neurology
Beth Israel Deaconess Medical Center
Boston Massachusetts

Martica H. Hall, PhD
Professor
Department of Psychiatry
Clinical and Translational Science
University of Pittsburgh
Pittsburgh, Pennsylvania

Erin C. Hanlon, PhD
Research Associate Professor
Department of Medicine
Section of Pediatric and Adult Endocrinology, Diabetes, and Metabolism
University of Chicago
Chicago, Illinois

Ronald M. Harper, PhD
Distinguished Professor
Department of Neurobiology
David Geffen School of Medicine
Distinguished Professor
Brain Research Institute
University of California at Los Angeles
Los Angeles, California

Krisztina Harsanyi, MD
Assistant Professor
Department of Pediatrics
University of Alabama at Birmingham
Birmingham, Alabama

Eric Heckman, MD
Instructor in Medicine
Division of Pulmonary, Critical Care, and Sleep Medicine
Department of Medicine
Beth Israel Deaconess Medical Center
Harvard Medical School
Boston, Massachusetts

Jan Hedner, MD, PhD
Professor
Sleep and Vigilance Disorders
Department of Internal Medicine
Sahlgrenska University Hospital
Gothenburg, Sweden

Brent E. Heideman, MD
Clinical Felow
Department of Medicine
Division of Allergy, Pulmonary, and Critical Care Medicine
Vanderbilt University Medical Center
Nashville, Tennessee

Raphael Heinzer, MD, MPH
Director
Center for Investigation and Research in Sleep (CIRS)
University Hospital of Lausanne;
Associate Professor
University of Lausanne
Lausanne, Switzerland

Luke A. Henderson, BSc, PhD
Professor
Department of Anatomy and Histology
Brain and Mind Centre
University of Sydney
Sydney, Australia

Rebecca C. Hendrickson, MD, PhD
Northwest Network Mental Illness Research Education and Clinical Center (MIRECC)
Department of Psychiatry and Behavioral Sciences
University of Washington
Seattle, Washington

Alberto Herrero Babiloni, DDS, MS
PhD Candidate
Department of Experimental Medicine
McGill University
CUISS NIM
Montreal, Quebec, Canada

W. Joseph Herring, MD, PhD
Associate Vice President
Clinical Neuroscience
Merck & Co., Inc.
Kenilworth, New Jersey

Elisabeth Hertenstein, MD
University Hospital of Psychiatry and Psychotherapy
University of Bern
Bern, Switzerland

David Hillman, MBBS, FANZCA
Emeritus Physician
Sir Charles Gairdner Hospital;
Clinical Professor
Medical School, Surgery and School of Human Sciences
University of Western Australia
Perth, Australia

Max Hirshkowitz, PhD
Professor (Emeritus)
Department of Medicine
Baylor College of Medicine
Houston, Texas

Aarnoud Hoekema, MD, DMD, PhD
Oral and Maxillofacial Surgery
Tjongerschans Hospital
Heerenveen, The Netherlands;
Department of Oral Kinesiology
Academic Centre for Dentistry Amsterdam
Amsterdam, The Netherlands

Birgit Högl, MD
Head of the Sleep Disorders Clinic
Department of Neurology
Innsbruck Medical University
Innsbruck, Austria

Richard L. Horner, PhD
Professor
Department of Medicine and Department of Physiology
University of Toronto;
Canada Research Chair in Sleep and Respiratory Neurobiology
Toronto, Ontario, Canada

Amanda N. Hudson, BS, MA
Graduate Research Assistant
Sleep and Performance Research Center
Elson S. Floyd College of Medicine
Washington State University
Spokane, Washington

Steven R. Hursh, PhD
President
Institutes for Behavior Resources, Inc.;
Adjunct Professor
Department of Psychiatry and Behavioral Biology
Johns Hopkins University School of Medicine
Baltimore, Maryland

Nelly Huynh, DDS
Faculty of Dental Medicine
Université de Montréal
Montréal, Quebec, Canada

Mari Hysing, MD
Department of Psychosocial Science
University of Bergen
Bergen, Norway

Octavian C. Ioachimescu, MD, PhD, MBA
Section Chief and Medical Director
Sleep Medicine Center
Atlanta VA Clinic
Decatur, Georgia;
Professor of Medicine
Department of Medicine
Division of Pulmonary, Critical Care, and Sleep Medicine
Emory University School of Medicine
Atlanta, Georgia

Mary Ip, MD
Chair and Professor
Department of Medicine
The University of Hong Kong
Hong Kong, China

Alex Iranzo, MD, PhD
Neurologist
Neurology Service
Hospital Clinic de Barcelona
Institut d'Investigació Biomèdiques;
Associate Professor
University of Barcelona
Barcelona, Spain

Bilgay Izci Balserak, PhD
Associate Professor
Department of Biobehavioral Health Science
Center for Sleep and Health Research
University of Illinois College of Nursing
Chicago, Illinois

Chandra L. Jackson, MD
Epidemiology Branch
National Institute of Environmental Health Sciences
National Institutes of Health
Department of Health and Human Services
Research Triangle Park, North Carolina;
Division of Intramural Research
National Institute on Minority Health and Health Disparities
National Institutes of Health
Department of Health and Human Services
Bethesda, Maryland

Shahrokh Javaheri, MD
Professor Emeritus
Department of Pulmonary Critical Care and Sleep
University of Cincinnati
Cincinnati, Ohio;
Adjunct Professor
Department of Cardiology
The Ohio State University
Columbus, Ohio

Sogol Javaheri, MD, MPH, MA
Physician
Department of Sleep Medicine
Brigham and Women's Hospital
Boston, Massachusetts

Peng Jiang, PhD
Research Assistant Professor
Center for Sleep and Circadian Biology
Northwestern University
Evanston, Illinois

Yandong Jiang, MD, PhD
Professor
Department of Anesthesiology
University of Texas, Houston
Health Science Center
Houston, Texas

Hadine Joffe, MD, MSc
Paula A. Johnson Professor of Psychiatry in the Field of Women's Heath
Executive Director of Mary Horrigan Connors Center for Women's Health and Gender Biology
Executive Vice Chair for Academic and Faulty Affairs
Department of Psychiatry
Brigham and Women's Hospital
Harvard Medical School
Boston, Massachusetts

David A. Johnson, MD, MACG, FASGE, MACP
Professor of Medicine and Chief
Department of Internal Medicine
Division of Gastroenterology and Hepatology
Eastern Virginia Medical School
Norfolk, Virginia

Karin Johnson, MD, FAASM, FAAN
Associate Professor
UMMS - Baystate Regional Campus
Neurology at UMMS-Baystate;
Medical Director
Baystate Health Regional Sleep Program
Springfield, Massachusetts

Anne E. Justice, MA, PhD
Assistant Professor of Population Health Sciences
Geisinger Health System
Danville, Pennsylvania

Marc Kaizi-Lutu, BA
Unit for Experimental Psychiatry
Division of Sleep and Chronobiology
Department of Psychiatry
Perelman School of Medicine
University of Pennsylvania
Philadelphia, Pennsylvania

David A. Kalmbach, PhD
Thomas Roth Sleep Disorders & Research Center
Division of Sleep Medicine
Henry Ford Health System
Detroit, Michigan

Elissaios Karageorgiou, MD, PhD
Division Chief
Sleep & Memory Center
Scientific Director
Neurological Institute of Athens
Athens, Greece

Eliot S. Katz, MD
Assistant Professor of Pediatrics
Harvard Medical School;
Division of Pulmonology
Boston Children's Hospital
Boston, Massachusetts

Brendan T. Keenan, MS
Co-Director, Biostatistics Core
Division of Sleep Medicine
Department of Medicine
University of Pennsylvania Perelman School of Medicine
Philadelphia, Pennsylvania

Sharon Keenan, PhD
Director
Department of Sleep Medicine
The School of Sleep Medicine, Inc.
Palo Alto, California

Thomas Kilduff, PhD
Center Director, Center for Neuroscience
Biosciences Division
SRI International
Menlo Park, California

Douglas Kirsch, MD
Medical Director
Department of Sleep Medicine
Professor
Department of Medicine and Neurology
Atrium Health
Charlotte, North Carolina;
Professor
Department of Medicine
University of North Carolina School of Medicine
Chapel Hill, North Carolina

Christopher E. Kline, PhD
Assistant Professor of Health and Physical Activity
Department of Health and Human Development
University of Pittsburgh
Department of Health and Physical Activity
Pittsburgh, Pennsylvania

Melissa P. Knauert, MD, PhD
Assistant Professor
Section of Pulmonary, Critical Care and Sleep Medicine
Department of Internal Medicine
Yale University School of Medicine
New Haven, Connecticuit

Kristen L. Knutson, PhD
Associate Professor
Department of Neurology
Northwestern University
Chicago, Illinois

Abigail L. Koch, MD, MHS
Assistant Chief
Division of Pulmonary Medicine
Miami VA Healthcare System
Miami, Florida

George F. Koob, MD
National Institute on Alcohol Abuse and Alcoholism
National Institutes of Health
Bethesda, Maryland

Sanjeev V. Kothare, MD, FAAN, FAASM
Director, Division of Pediatric Neurology
Department of Pediatrics
Cohen Children's Medical center
New Hyde Park, New York;
Director, Pediatric Neurology Service Line for Northwell Health
Professor of Pediatrics and Neurology
Zucker School of Medicine at Hofstra Northwell
Lake Success, New York

Kyoshi Koyano, DDS, PhD
Professor
Department of Implant and Rehabilitative Dentistry
Faculty of Dental Science
Kyushu University
Fukuoka, Japan

James M. Krueger, PhD, MDHC
Regents Professor
Integrative Physiology and Neuroscience
Washington State University
Spokane, Washington

Meir Kryger, MD, FRCPC
Professor
Pulmonary, Critical Care, and Sleep Medicine
Yale University School of Medicine
New Haven, Connecticuit

Andrew D. Krystal, MD, MS
Ray and Dagmar Dolby Distinguished Professor
Department of Psychiatry
University of California, San Francisco
San Francisco, California

Samuel T. Kuna, MD
Professor of Medicine
Department of Medicine
Perelman School of Medicine at the University of Pennsylvania;
Chief
Sleep Medicine Section
Department of Medicine
Corporal Michael J. Crescenz Veterans Affairs Medical Center
Philadelphia, Pennsylvania

Scott Kutscher, MD
Associate Professor
Department of Sleep Medicine
Stanford University
Redwood City, California

Stephen LaBerge, PhD
Research Associate
Department of Psychology
Stanford University
Palo Alto, California

Annie C. Lajoie, MD
Respirology Fellow
Department of Respirology
Institut Universitaire de Cardiologie et de Pneumologie de Québec
Quebec City, Quebec, Canada

Amanda Lamp, BS, MS, PhD
Research Assistant Professor
Sleep and Performance Research Center
Washington State University
Spokane, Washington

Hans-Peter Landolt, PhD
Human Sleep Psychopharmacology Laboratory
Institute of Pharmacology and Toxicology
Sleep and Health Zürich
University Center of Competence
University of Zürich
Zürich, Switzerland

Jessica Lara-Carrasco, PhD
Clinical Psychologist
Hôpital Maisonneuve-Rosemont
CIUSSS del'Est-de-l'île-de-Montéal
Montreal, Quebec, Canada

Gilles Lavigne, DMD, FRCDI, PhD
Professor
Faculty of Dental Medicine
Université de Montréal
CIUSS NIM and CHUM-Stomatology
Montréal, Quebec, Canada

Michael Lazarus, PhD
International Institute for Integrative Sleep Medicine
University of Tsukuba
Tsukuba, Japan

Han-Hee Lee, MD
Department of Cell and Systems Biology
University of Toronto
Toronto, Ontario, Canada

Guy Leschziner, MBBS, MA, PhD, FRCP
Consultant Neurologist
Sleep Disorders Centre
Guy's and St Thomas' NHS Trust;
Professor of Neurology and Sleep Medicine
Institute of Psychiatry, Psychology, and Neuroscience
King's College London
London, Great Britain

John A. Lesku, PhD
Associate Professor
School of Life Sciences
La Trobe University
Melbourne, Australia

Christopher J. Lettieri, MD
Professor of Medicine
Department of Pulmonary, Critical Care, and Sleep Medicine
Uniformed Services University of the Health Sciences
Bethesda, Maryland

Vicki Li
Project Assistant
Research Institute
California Pacific Medical Center
San Francisco, California

Paul-Antione Libourel, PhD
Neurosciences Reseach Center of Lyon (CRNL)
Team SLEEP
Lyon, France

Melissa C. Lipford, MD
Center for Sleep Medicine
Department of Neurology
Division of Pulmonary and Critical Care Medicine
Mayo Clinic
Rochester, Minnesota

Frank Lobbezoo, DDS, PhD
Professor and Chair
Department of Orofacial Pain and Dysfunction
Academic Centre for Dentistry Amsterdam (ACTA)
Amsterdam, The Netherlands

Geraldo Lorenzi-Filho, MD, PhD
Associate Professor
Department of Cardio-Pulmonology
University of Sao Paulo
Sao Paulo, Brazil

Judette Louis, MD, MPH
James M. Ingram Professor and Chair
Department of Obstetrics and Gynecology
Morsani College of Medicine
University of South Florida
Tampa, Florida

Brendan P. Lucey, MD, MSCI
Associate Professor of Neurology
Sleep Medicine Section Head
Washington University School of Medicine
Saint Louis, Missouri

Ralph Lydic, PhD
Professor
Department of Psychology
University of Tennessee
Knoxville, Tennessee;
Joint Faculty
Biosciences Division
Oak Ridge National Laboratory
Oak Ridge, Tennessee

Madalina Macrea, MD, PhD, MPH
Department of Pulmonary and Sleep Medicine
Salem Veterans Affairs Medical Center
Salem, Virginia;
Associate Professor
University of Virginia
Charlottesville, Virginia

Mary Halsey Maddox, MD
Associate Professor
Department of Pediatrics
University of Alabama at Birmingham
Birmingham, Alabama

Mark W. Mahowald, MD†
Professor of Neurology
University of Minnesota Medical School;
Visiting Professor
Minnesota Regional Sleep Disorders Center
Hennepin County Medical Center
Minneapolis, Minnesota

Atul Malhotra, MD
Professor of Medicine
Peter C. Farrell Presidential Chair in Respiratory Medicine
Department of Pulmonary, Critical Care, and Sleep Medicine
University of Southern California, San Diego;
Research Chief of Pulmonary, Critical Care, and Sleep Medicine
University of California, San Diego School of Medicine
La Jolla, California

Raman K. Malhotra, MD
Associate Professor of Neurology
Washington University School of Medicine
Saint Louis, Missouri

Beth A. Malow, MD, MS
Professor
Department of Neurology and Pediatrics
Director
Sleep Disorders Division
Department of Neurology and Pediatrics
Vanderbilt University Medical Center
Nashville, Tennessee

Rachel Manber, PhD
Professor
Psychiatry and Behavioral Sciences
Stanford University
Palo Alto, California

Daniele Manfredini, DDS, MSc, PhD
Professor
School of Dentistry
University of Siena
Siena, Italy

Jim Mangie, BS
Aeronautical Studies Program Director
Pilot Fatigue Flight Operations Delta Air Lines
Atlanta, Georgia

Edward Manning, MD, PhD
Intensivist, Pulmonologist
Veterans Affairs Connecticut Healthcare System;
Instructor
Pulmonary and Critical Care Medicine
Yale School of Medicine
New Haven, Connecticut

Pierre Maquet, MD, PhD
Sleep and Chronobiology Laboratory
GIGA-Cyclontron Research Center/In Vivo Imaging
University of Liège;
Professor
Department of Neurology
Liège University Hospital
Liège, Belgium

†Deceased.

Jose M. Marin, MD
Head
Respiratory Sleep Disorders Unit
Hospital Universitario Miguel Servet;
Professor of Respiratory Medicine
Department of Medicine
University of Zaragoza
Zaragoza, Spain

Marta Marin-Oto, MD
Respiratory Department
Clinica Universidad de Navarra
Pamplona, Spain

Jennifer L. Martin, PhD
Associate Director for Clinical and Health Services Research
Geriatric Research, Education and Clinical Center
VA Greater Los Angeles Healthcare System;
Professor
Department of Medicine
David Geffen School of Medicine
University of California, Los Angeles
Los Angeles, California

Miguel A. Martínez-Garcia, MD, PhD
Servicio de Neumologia
Hospital Universitario y Politécnico La Fe
Valencia, Spain;
Centro de Investigación Biomédica en Red de Enfermedades Respiratorias (CIBERES)
Madrid, Spain

Kiran Maski, MD, MPH
Associate Professor
Department of Neurology
Boston Children's Hospital
Boston, Massachusetts

Ivy C. Mason, PhD
Postdoctoral Research Fellow
Medical Chronobiology Program
Division of Sleep and Circadian Disorders
Departments of Medicine and Neurology
Brigham and Women's Hospital;
Research Fellow
Division of Sleep Medicine
Department of Medicine
Harvard Medical School
Boston, Massachusetts

Christopher R. McCartney, MD
Professor of Medicine
Department of Medicine
Division of Endocrinology and Metabolism
University of Virginia School of Medicine
Charlottesville, Virginia

Colleen McClung, PhD
Professor
Departments of Psychiatry and Clinical and Translational Science
University of Pittsburgh School of Medicine
Pittsburgh, Pennsylvania

Christina S. McCrae, PHD
Professorr
Department of Psychiatry
University of Missouri-Columbia
Columbia, Missouri

Dennis McGinty, PhD
Adjunct Professor
Department of Psychology
University of California
Research Service
VA Medical Center, GLAHS
Los Angeles, California

Andrew W. McHill, PhD
Research Assistant Professor
Oregon Institute of Occupational Health Sciences
Oregon Health & Science University
Portland, Oregon

Reena Mehra, MD, MS
Professor of Medicine
Sleep Disorders Center, Neurologic Institute
Cleveland Clinic Lerner College of Medicine of Case Western Reserve University;
Respiratory Institute
Department of Molecular Cardiology
Lerner Research Institute
Heart and Vascular Institute
Cleveland, Ohio

Emmanuel Mignot, MD, PhD
Director
Center For Sleep Sciences and Medicine
Stanford University
Palo Alto, California

Katherine E. Miller, PhD
Cpl. Michael J Crescenz VA Medical Center
Philadelphia, Pennsylvania

Brienne Miner, MD, MHS
Assistant Professor
Department of Internal Medicine
Section of Geriatrics
Yale University
New Haven, Connecticut

Jennifer W. Mitchell, PhD
Department of Cell & Developmental Biology
Neuroscience Program
University of Illinois at Urbana-Champaign
Urbana, Illinois

Murray Mittleman, MD, DrPH
Associate Professor
Department of Medicine
Harvard Medical School;
Associate Professor
Department of Epidemiology
Harvard School of Public Health
Boston, Massachusetts

Vahid Mohsenin, MD
Professor (Emeritus)
Department of Medicine
Yale University
New Haven, Connecticuit

Babak Mokhlesi, MD, MSc
J. Bailey Carter Professor of Medicine
Chief, Division of Pulmonary, Critical Care and Sleep Medicine
Co-Director, Rush Lung Center
Department of Internal Medicine
Rush University Medical Center
Chicago, Illinois

Jacques Montplaisir, PhD
Professor
Department of Psychiatry
Université de Montréal;
Center for Advanced Research on Sleep Medicine
CIUSSS du Nord-de-l'Île-de-Montréal
Hôpital du Sacré-Coeur de Montréal
Montreal, Quebec, Canada

Charles M. Morin, PhD
Professor
Department of Psychology
Director
Center for the Study of Sleep Disorders
Canada Research Chair in Sleeping Disorders
Laval University
Quebec City, Quebec, Canada

Mary J. Morrell, PhD
Professor of Sleep and Respiratory Physiology
National Heart and Lung Institute
Imperial College
London, Great Britain

Tanvi H. Mukundan, MD
Program Director, Sleep
Veterans Administration
Portland, Oregon

Erik Musiek, MD, PhD
Associate Professor
Department of Neurology
Washington University School of Medicine
Saint Louis, Missouri

Carlotta Mutti, MD
Sleep Disorders Center
Department of Medicine and Surgery
University of Parma
Parma, Italy

Alexander D. Nesbitt, BM BCh, PhD, FRCP
Consultant Neurologist and Sleep Physician
Sleep Disorders Centre and Department of Neurology
Guy's and St Thomas' NHS Foundation Trust
London, Great Britain

Thomas Nesthus, PhD, FRAeS, FasMA
Engineering Research Psychologist
Aerospace Human Factors Research Division
FAA, Civil Aerospace Medical Institute
Oklahoma City, Oklahoma

Natalie Nevárez, MD
Department of Psychiatry and Behavioral Sciences
Stanford University
Palo Alto, California

Tore Nielsen, PhD
Professor
Department of Psychiatry and Addictology
Université de Montréal;
Director, Dream & Nightmare Laboratory
Center for Advanced Research in Sleep Medicine
CIUSSS du Nord-de-l'Île-de-Montréal (Hôpital du Sacré-Coeur)
Montreal, Quebec, Canada

Christoph Nissen, MD
University Hospital of Psychiatry and Psychotherapy
University of Bern
Bern, Switzerland

Eric A. Nofzinger, MD
Adjunct Professor
Department of Psychiatry
University of Pittsburgh
Pittsburgh, Pennsylvania

Christopher B. O'Brien, BS
Department of Psychology
University of Tennessee
Knoxville, Tennessee

Louise M. O'Brien, PhD, MS
Associate Professor
Division of Sleep Medicine
Associate Professor
Department of Obstetrics & Gynecology
Associate Research Scientist
Oral & Maxillofacial Surgery
University of Michigan
Ann Arbor, Michigan

Bruce O'Hara, PhD
Professor
Department of Biology
University of Kentucky
Lexington, Kentucky

Yo Oishi, PhD
International Institute for Integrative Sleep Medicine
University of Tsukuba
Tsukuba, Japan

Eric J. Olson, MD
Division of Pulmonary and Critical Care Medicine
Center for Sleep Medicine
Mayo Clinic
Rochester, Minnesota

Jason C. Ong, PhD
Associate Professor
Department of Neurology
Center for Circadian and Sleep Medicine
Northwestern University Feinberg School of Medicine
Chicago, Illinois

Mark R. Opp, PhD
Professor and Chair
Integrative Physiology
University of Colorado Boulder
Boulder, Colorado

Edward F. Pace-Schott, PhD
Assistant Professor of Psychiatry
Harvard Medical School
Boston, Massachusetts;
Massachusetts General Hospital
Charlestown, Massachusetts

Allan I. Pack, MB, ChB, PhD, FRCP
John Miclot Professor of Medicine
Division of Sleep Medicine
Department of Medicine
University of Pennsylvania Perelman School of Medicine
Philadelphia, Pennsylvania

John Park, MD
Associate Professor of Medicine
Division of Pulmonary and Critical Care Medicine
Mayo Clinic
Rochester, Minnesota

Liborio Parrino, MD
Professor
Department of Medicine and Surgery
University of Parma
Parma, Italy

Sara Pasha, MBBS
Assistant Professor
Pulmonary, Critical Care, and Sleep Medicine
University of Kentucky
Lexington, Kentucky

Michael Paskow, MPH
Associate Director
Epidemiology, Global Real-World Evidence Generation
Washington, DC

Susheel P. Patil, MD, PhD, ATSF
System Director, UH Sleep Medicine
Section Chief, Sleep Medicine
Division of Pulmonary, Critical Care, and Sleep Medicine
Clinical Associate Professor of Medicine
Case Western Reserve University School of Medicine
Cleveland, Ohio

Alexander Patrician, MSc
Department of Health and Exercise Sciences
The University of British Columbia
Kelowna, British Columbia, Canada

Milena K. Pavlova, MD, FAASM
Medical Director, Faulkner Sleep Testing Center
Department of Neurology
Brigham and Women's Hospital;
Associate Professor of Neurology
Department of Neurology
Harvard Medical School
Boston, Massachusetts

John H. Peever, PhD
Professor
Department of Cell and Systems Biology
University of Toronto
Toronto, Ontario, Canada

Philippe Peigneux, PhD
Full Professor
Neuropsychology and Functional Neuroimaging at Centre for Research in Cognition and Neurosciences
Universite Libre de Bruxelles
Bruxelles, Belgium

Yüksel Peker, MD, PhD
Professor
Department of Pulmonary Medicine
Head of Sleep Medicine Unit
Koç University School of Medicine
Istanbul, Turkey

Rafael Pelayo, MD
Clinical Professor
Sleep Medicine Division
Stanford Univeristy School of Medicine
Stanford, California

Thomas Penzel, MD
Research Director of Sleep Center
Interdisciplinary Sleep Medicine Center
Charité–Universitätsmedizin Berlin
Berlin, Germany

Jean-Louis Pépin, MD, PhD
Pneumology-Physiology Department
Grenoble Alpes University Hospital;
INSERM U1300, HP2 Laboratory
Grenoble Alpes University
Grenoble, France

Michael L. Perlis, PhD
Department of Psychiatry
University of Pennsylvania
Philadelphia, Pennsylvania

Lampros Perogamvros, MD
Department of Medicine
University Hospitals of Geneva
University of Geneva
Geneva, Switzerland

Dominique Petit, PhD
Research Associate
Center for Advanced Research in Sleep Medicine
CIUSSS du Nord-de-l'Île-de-Montréal – Hôpital du Sacré-Coeur de Montréal
Montreal, Quebec, Canada

Megan E. Petrov, PhD
Assistant Professor
College of Nursing and Health Innovation
Arizona State University
Phoenix, Arizona

Dante Picchioni, PhD
Scientist (contractor)
National Institute of Neurological Disorders and Stroke
Bethesda, Maryland

Grace W. Pien, MD, MSCE
Assistant Professor of Medicine
Department of Medicine
Johns Hopkins University School of Medicine
Baltimore, Maryland

Wilfred R. Pigeon, PhD
Professor
Psychiatry & Public Health Sciences
University of Rochester Medical Center
Rochester, New York;
Executive Director
Center of Excellence for Suicide Prevention
U.S. Department of Veterans Affairs
Canandaigua, New York

Margaret A. Pisani, MD, MPH
Associate Professor
Internal Medicine–Pulmonary, Critical Care, and Sleep
Yale University
New Haven, Connecticuit

Melanie Pogach, MD, MMSc
Assistant Professor of Medicine
Tufts University School of Medicine
SEMC/SMG Pulmonary, Critical Care, and Sleep Medicine
Director, Chronic Respiratory Failure Program
St. Elizabeth's Medical Center
Brighton, Massachusetts

Donn Posner, PhD
Department of Psychiatry and Behavioral Science
Stanford University
Palo Alto, California

Ronald Postuma, MD, MSc
Professor
Department of Neurology
McGill University
Montreal, Quebec, Canada

Naresh Punjabi, MD, PhD
Division of Pulmonary and Critical Care Medicine
Department of Medicine
Johns Hopkins University
Baltimore, Maryland

Stacey Dagmar Quo, DDS, MS
School of Dentistry
University of California San Francisco
San Francisco, California

Shadab Rahman, PhD
Instructor in Medicine
Division of Sleep Medicine
Harvard Medical School;
Associate Neuroscientist
Division of Sleep and Circadian Disorders
Departments of Medicine and Neurology
Brigham and Women's Hospital
Boston, Massachusetts

David Raizen, MD, PhD
Associate Professor of Neurology
Perelman School of Medicine
University of Pennsylvania
Philadelphia, Pennsylvania

Preethi Rajan, MD
Division of Pulmonary, Critical Care, and Sleep Medicine
Department of Medicine
Northwell Heath;
Donald and Barbara Zucker School of Medicine at Hofstra-Northwell
New Hyde Park, New York

Shantha Rajaratnam, MD
School of Psychological Sciences
Turner Institute for Brain and Mental Health
Monash University
Melbourne, Victoria, Australia

Kannan Ramar, MD
Center for Sleep Medicine
Division of Pulmonary and Critical Care Medicine
Mayo Clinic
Rochester, Minnesota

Winfried J. Randerath, MD
Department of Clinic of Pneumology
Bethanien Hospital
Institute of Pneumology at the University of Cologne
Solingen, Germany

Karen Raphael, PhD
Professor
Department of Psychiatry and Behavioral Sciences
University of Washington;
Behavioral Sciences Director
Mental Illness Research, Education and Clinical Center
VA Puget Sound Health Care System
Seattle, Washington

Murray Raskind, MD
Professor
Department of Psychiatry and Behavioral Sciences
University of Washington;
Behavioral Sciences Director
Mental Illness Research, Education and Clinical Center
VA Puget Sound Health Care System
Seattle, Washington

Kavita Ratarasarn, MBBS
Associate Professor
Department of Medicine
Medical College of Wisconsin
Milwaukee, Wisconsin

Niels C. Rattenborg, PhD
Group Leader
Avian Sleep
Max Planck Institute for Ornithology
Seewiesen, Germany

Susan Redline, MD, MPH
Peter C. Farrell Professor of Medicine
Department of Medicine
Brigham and Women's Hospital
Beth Israel Deaconess Medical Center;
Department of Medicine
Harvard Medical School
Boston, Massachusetts

Kathryn J. Reid, PhD
Research Professor
Ken and Ruth Davee Department of Neurology
Center for Circadian and Sleep Medicine
Northwestern University Feinberg School of Medicine
Chicago, Illinois

Kathy Richards, PhD, RN, FAAN, FAASM
Research Professor
School of Nursing
University of Texas at Austin
Austin, Texas

Samantha Riedy, PhD, RPSGT
Senior Statistician
Behavioral Biology Branch
Walter Reed Army Institute of Research
Silver Spring, Maryland

Dieter Riemann, PhD
Department of Psychiatry and Psychotherapy
Medical Center–University of Freiburg;
Faculty of Medicine
University of Freiburg
Freiburg, Germany

Timothy Roehrs, PhD
Senior Bioscientist
Division of Sleep Medicine
Thomas Roth Sleep Disorders and Research Center
Henry Ford Health System;
Professor
Department of Psychiatry & Behavioral Neuroscience
Wayne State University
Detroit, Michigan

Thomas Roth, PhD
Director
Division of Sleep Medicine
Thomas Roth Sleep Disorders and Research Center
Henry Ford Hospital
Detroit, Michigan

James A. Rowley, MD
Professor of Medicine
Chief, Pulmonary, Critical Care & Sleep Medicine
Wayne State University School of Medicine
Detroit, Michigan

David B. Rye, MD
Sleep Center
Department of University
Emory University
Atlanta, Georgia

Ashima S. Sahni, MD
Assistant Professor of Clinical Medicine
Division of Pulmonary, Critical Care, Sleep and Allergy
University of Illinois Hospital and Health Science System
Chicago, Illinois

Charles Samuels, MD, CCFP, DABSM
Clinical Assistant Professor
Family Medicine
Adjunct Professor
Faculty of Kinesiology
University of Calgary;
CANMedical Director
Centre for Sleep and Human Performance
Calgary, Alberta, Canada

Anne E. Sanders, MS, PhD, MS
Assistant Professor
Divison of Pediatric and Public Health
Adams School of Dentistry
University of North Carolina at Chapel Hill
Chapel Hill, North Carolina

Clifford B. Saper, MD, PhD
James Jackson Putnam Professor of Neurology and Neuroscience
Harvard Medical School;
Department of Neurology
Beth Israel Deaconess Medical Center
Boston, Massachusetts

Michael J. Sateia, MD, FAASM
Professor of Psychiatry (Sleep Medicine), Emeritus
Geisel School of Medicine at Dartmouth
Hanover, New Hampshire

Josée Savard, PhD
Professor
School of Psychology
Université Laval
CHU de Québec-Université Laval Research Center
Quebec City, Quebec, Canada

Marie-Hélène Savard, PhD
Research Associate
CHU de Québec Cancer Research Center
Québec City, Québec, Canada

Thomas E. Scammell, MD
Professor
Department of Neurology
Beth Israel Deaconess Medical Center;
Professor
Department of Neurology
Boston Children's Hospital;
Professor
Harvard Medical School
Boston, Massachusetts

Matthew T. Scharf, MD, PhD
Assistant Professor
Medical Director, Robert Wood Johnson Sleep Laboratory
Comprehensive Sleep Center
Division of Pulmonary and Critical Care Medicine
Robert Wood University Medical School
Rutgers University
New Brunswick, New Jersey

Steven M. Scharf, MD, PhD
Director
University of Maryland Sleep Disorders Center;
Professor of Medicine
University of Maryland School of Medicine
Baltimore, Maryland

Frank A.J.L. Scheer, PhD, MSc
Professor of Medicine
Department of Medicine
Harvard Medical School;
Director, Medical Chronobiology Program
Department of Medicine and Neurology
Brigham and Women's Hospital
Boston, Massachusetts

Logan Schneider, MD
Staff Neurologist
Stanford/VA Alzhemier's Center
MIRECC Investigator
Department of Psychiatry and Behavioral Sciences
Palo Alto Veteran's Affairs Healthcare System
Palo Alto, California

Michael Schredl, PhD
Head of Research
Sleep Laboratory
Central Institute of Mental Health;
Medical Faculty
Mannheim/Heidelberg University
Mannheim, Germany

Sophie Schwartz, PhD
Professor of Neuroscience
Department of Neurosciences
University of Geneva
Geneva, Switzerland

Paula K. Schweitzer, PhD
Director of Research
Sleep Medicine and Research Center
St. Luke's Hospital
Chesterfield, Missouri

Bernardo Selim, MD
Assistant Professor of Medicine
Section of Pulmonary and Critical Care
Department of Medicine, Sleep Medicine
Mayo Clinic
Rochester, Minnesota

Frédéric Sériès, MD
Centre de pneumologie
Department of Medicine
Institut Universitaire de Cardiologie et de Pneumologie de Québec
Quebec City, Quebec, Canada

Barry J. Sessle, PhD
Professor
Department of Physiology
Neuroscience Platform
University of Toronto
Toronto, Ontario, Canada

Amir Sharafkhaneh, MD, PhD
Professor of Medicine
Department of Medicine
Baylor College of Medicine
Sleep Disorders & Research Center
Medical Care Line
Michael E. DeBaky VA Medical Center
Houston, Texas

Katherine M. Sharkey, MD, PhD
Associate Professor
Department of Medicine
Associate Professor
Psychiatry & Human Behavior
The Warren Alpert Medical School of Brown University
Providence, Rhode Island

Paul J. Shaw, PhD
Professor
Department of Neuroscience
Washington University in St. Louis
St. Louis, Missouri

Ari Shechter, PhD
Assistant Professor of Medical Science
Department of Medicine
Columbia University Medical Center
New York, New York

Stephen H. Sheldon, DO
Professor of Pediatrics and Neurology
Northwestern University Feinberg School of Medicine
Sleep Medicine Center
Division of Pulmonary and Sleep Medicine
Ann & Robert H. Lurie Children's Hospital of Chicago
Chicago, Illinois

Fahmi Shibli, MD
Research Fellow
MetroHealth Medical Center;
Visiting Scholar
Case Western Reserve University
Cleveland, Ohio

Priyattam J. Shiromani, PhD
Professor
Department of Psychiatry
Medical University of South Carolina
Charleston, South Carolina

Tamar Shochat, DSc
Full Professor
Department of Nursing
University of Haifa
Haifa, Israel

Francesca Siclari, MD
Center for Investigation and Research on Sleep
University Hospital Lausanne
Lausanne, Switzerland

Jerome M. Siegel, PhD
Professor of Psychiatry and Biobehavioral Sciences
David Geffen School of Medicine
University of California, Los Angeles;
Chief Neurobiology Research
Veterans Affairs Greater Los Angeles Healthcare System
Los Angeles, California

T. Leigh Signal, Bav, MA (hons), PhD
Lecturer
Sleep/Wake Research Centre
School of Health Sciences
Massey University
Wellington, The Netherlands

Michael H. Silber, MBChB
Professor of Neurology
Center for Sleep Medicine
Department of Neurology
Mayo Clinic College of Medicine
Rochester, Minnesota

Norah Simpson, PhD
Clinical Associate Professor
Psychiatry and Behavioral Sciences
Stanford University School of Medicine
Palo Alto, California

Mini Singh, MBBS
Assistant Professor
Department of Neurology
Medical University of South Carolina
Charleston, South Carolina

Børge Sivertsen, MD
Department of Health Promotion
Norwegian Institute of Public Health
Bergen, Norway

Lillian Skeiky, BS
Graduate Research Assistant
Sleep and Performance Research Center
Elson S. Floyd College of Medicine
Washington State University
Spokane, Washington

Anne C. Skeldon, PhD
Department of Mathematics
Faculty of Engineering and Physcial Sciences
University of Surrey;
UK Dementia Research Institute Care Research and Technology Center
Imperial College London
University of Surrey
Guildford, United Kingdom

Carlyle Smith, MD
Psychology Department
Trent University
Peterborough, Ontario, Canada;
Neuroscience Department
Queens University,
Kingston, Ontario, Canada

Michael T. Smith, PhD
Professor of Psychiatry, Neurology and Nursing
Director, Division of Behavioral Medicine
Johns Hopkins School of Medicine
Baltimore, Maryland

Virend K. Somers, MD, PhD
Alice Sheets Marriot Professor of Medicine
Department of Cardiovascular Medicine
Mayo Clinic
Rochester, Minnesota

Kai Spiegelhalder, MD PhD
Department of Psychiatry and Psychotherapy
Medical Center–University of Freiburg
Faculty of Medicine
University of Freiburg
Freiburg, Germany

Arthur J. Spielman, PhD, FAASM†
Cognitive Neuroscience Doctoral Program
The City College of the City University of New York
Center for Sleep Medicine
Weill Cornell Medical College
New York, New York

Victor I. Spoormaker, PhD, MD
Max Planck Institute of Psychiatry
Munich, Germany

Erik K. St. Louis, MD, MS
Associate Professor
Center for Sleep Medicine
Departments of Neurology and Medicine
Mayo Clinic College of Medicine
Rochester, Minnesota

Robert Stansbury, MD
Associate Professor and Director
WYU Sleep Evaluation Center
Section of Pulmonary, Critical Care, and Sleep Medicine
Department of Medicine
West Virginia University School of Medicine
Morgantown, West Virginia

†Deceased.

Murray B. Stein, MD, MPH
Distinguished Professor
Psychiatry and Public Health
University of California, San Diego
La Jolla, California;
Staff Psychiatrist
Psychiatry Service
Veterans Administration San Diego Healthcare System
San Diego, California

Robert Stickgold, PhD
Professor
Department of Psychiatry
Beth Israel Deaconess Medical Center;
Professor
Department of Psychiatry
Harvard Medical School
Boston, Massachussetts

Katie L. Stone, MA, PhD
Senior Scientist
Research Institute
California Pacific Medical Center
San Francisco, California

Riccardo Stoohs, MD
Director
Sleep Disorders Clinic
Somnolab
Dortmund, Germany

Robyn Stremler, RN, PhD, FAAN
Associate Professor
Lawrence S. Bloomberg Faculty of Nursing
University of Toronto;
Adjunct Scientist
The Hospital for Sick Children
Toronto, Ontario, Canada

Patrick J. Strollo Jr., MD, FACP, FCCP, FAASM
Professor of Medicine and Clinical and Translational Science
Pulmonary, Allergy, and Critical Care Medicine
Vice Chair for Veterans Affairs
Department of Medicine
Vice President, Medical Service Line
VA Pittsburgh Health System
Pittsburgh, Pennsylvania

Shannon S. Sullivan, MD
Clinical Professor
Division of Pediatric Pulmonary, Asthma, and Sleep
Department of Pediatrics
Division of Sleep Medicine
Department of Psychiatry
Stanford University
Palo Alto, California

Peter Svensson, DDS, PhD, Dr.Odont
Professor and Head
Section for Orofacial Pain and Jaw Function
Department of Dentistry and Oral Health
Aarhus University
Aarhus, Denmark

Steven T. Szabo, MD, PhD
Assistant Professor
Psychiatry and Behavioral Sciences
Duke University Medical Center;
Attending Psychiatrist
Mental Health Service Line
Durham Veterans Administration Medical Center
Durham, North Carolina

Ronald Szymusiak, PhD
Adjunct Professor
Department of Medicine
David Geffen School of Medicine
University of California, Los Angeles;
Research Scientist
Research Service
VA Greater Los Angeles Healthcare System
Los Angeles, California

Mehdi Tafti, PhD
Department of Biomedical Sciences
University of Lausanne
Lausanne, Switzerland

Renaud Tamisier, MD, PhD, MBA
Professor of Medicine
Section of Pulmonary and Physiology Medicine
Departmetn of Thorax and Vessel Medicine
Director, Sleep Disorders CCenter
Université Grenoble Alpes
Grenoble, France

Esra Tasali, MD
Associate Professor
Department of Medicine
Section of Pulmonary/Critical Care
University of Chicago
Chicago, Illinois

Daniel J. Taylor, MD, PhD
Professor
Department of Psychology
University of Arizona
Tucson, Arizona

Mihai C. Teodorescu, MD
Associate Professor
Department of Medicine
University of Wisconsin
Madison, Wisconsin

Matthew J.W. Thomas, PhD
Associate Professor
School of Health, Medical, and Applied Sciences
Appleton Institute
Central Queensland University, Australia

Robert Joseph Thomas, MD, MMSc
Associate Professor of Medicine
Division of Pulmonary, Critical Care, and Sleep Medicine
Department of Medicine
Beth Israel Deaconess Medical Center
Harvard Medical School
Boston, Massachusetts

Michael J. Thorpy, MD
Professor of Neurology
The Saul R. Korey Department of Neurology
Albert Einstein College of Medicine at Yeshiva University;
Director
Sleep-Wake Disorders Center
Montefiore Medical Center
Bronx, New York

Lauren A. Tobias, MD
Assistant Professor
Pulmonary, Critical Care, and Sleep Medicine
Yale University School of Medicine
New Haven, Connecticuit

Giulio Tononi, MD, PhD
Professor
Department of Psychiatry
University of Wisconsin
Madison, Wisconsin

Irina Trosman, MD
Attending Physician, Sleep Medicine
Health System Clinician of Pediatrics (Pulmonary Medicine)
Northwestern University Feinberg School of Medicine
Chicago, Illinois

Fred W. Turek, PhD
Charles E.& Emma H. Morrison Professor of Biology
Departments of Neurobiology and Physiology
Director, Center for Sleep and Circadian Biology
Northwestern University
Evanston, Illinois

Raghu Pishka Upender, MD, MBA
Medical Director, Associate Professor
Department of Neurology
Vanderbilt University Medical Center
Nashville, Tennessee

Andrew Vakulin, PhD
FHMRI Sleep Health
Flinders Heath and Medical Research Institute
College of Medicine and Public Health
Flinders University
Adelaide, Austria

Philipp O. Valko, MD
Neurology
University Hospital Zurich
Zurich, Switzerland

Eve Van Cauter, PhD
Frederick H. Rawson Professor
Department of Medicine
Section of Pediatric and Adult Endocrinology, Diabetes, and Metabolism
University of Chicago
Chicago, Illinois

Margo van den Berg, PhD
Lecturer
Sleep/Wake Research Centre
School of Health Sciences
Massey University
Wellington, New Zealand

Hans P.A. Van Dongen, MS, PhD
Professor and Director
Sleep and Performance Research Center
Elson S. Floyd College of Medicine
Washington State University
Spokane, Washington

Eus Van Someren, MD
Netherlands Institute for Neuroscience
Amsterdam, The Netherlands

Olivier M. Vanderveken, MD, PhD
Department of Ear, Nose and Throat, Head and Neck Surgery
Antwerp University Hospital;
Professor
Faculty of Medicine and Health Sciences
University of Antwerp
Antwerp, Belgium

Gilles Vandewalle, PhD
Sleep and Chronobiology Laboratory
GIGA-Cyclontron Research Center/In Vivo Imaging
University of Liège
Liège, Belgium

Andrew W. Varga, MD, PhD
Assistant Professor
Department of Medicine
Icahn School of Medicine at Mount Sinai
New York, New York

Ivan Vargas, PhD
Department of Psychological Science
University of Arkansas
Fayetteville, Arkansas

Bradley V. Vaughn, MD
Professor of Neurology
Department of Neurology
University of North Carolina
Chapel Hill, North Carolina

Øystein Vedaa, PhD
Department Director
Department of Health Promotion
Norwegian Institute of Public Health
Bergen, Norway;
Researcher
Department of Mental Health
Norwegian University of Science and Technology
Trondheim, Norway

Richard L. Verrier, PhD
Associate Professor
Department of Medicine
Harvard Medical School
Beth Israel Deaconess Medical Center
Boston, Massachusetts

Alexandros N. Vgontzas, MD
Professor of Psychiatry
Department of Psychiatry and Behavioral Health
Director, Sleep Research and Treatment Center
Penn State University College of Medicine
Penn State Health Milton S. Hershey Medical Center
Hershey, Pennsylvania

Aurelio Vidal-Ortiz, MD
Laboratory of Sleep Neuroscience
Ralph H. Johnson VA Medical Center
Charleston, South Carolina

Aleksandar Videnovic, MD, MSc
Associate Professor
Department of Neurology
Harvard Medical School/MGH
Boston, Massachusetts

Martha Hotz Vitaterna, PhD
Research Professor
Department of Neurobiology
Deputy Director
Center for Sleep and Circadian Biology
Northwestern University
Evanston, Illinois

Lauren Waggoner, BS, MA, PhD
Fatigue Scientist
Flight Safety, CSSC
Delta Air Lines, Incorporated
Atlanta, Georgia

Arthur S. Walters, MD
Professor of Neurology
Department of Neurology
Vanderbilt University School of Medicine
Nashville, Tennessee

Erin J. Wamsley, PhD
Associate Professor
Department of Psychology
Furman University
Greenville, South Carolina

Paula L. Watson, MD
Assistant Professor
Pulmonary, Critical Care, and Sleep Medicine
Vanderbilt University Medical Center
Nashville, Tennessee

Terri E. Weaver, PhD, RN
Dean and Professor
Biobehavioral Nursing Science
Professor
Division of Pulmonary, Critical Care, Sleep, and Allergy
University of Illinois Chicago College of Medicine
Chicago, Illinois

Gerald L. Weinhouse, MD
Associate Physician
Brigham and Women's Hospital;
Assistant Professor of Medicine
Harvard Medical School
Boston, Massachusetts

Pnina Weiss, MD
Vice Chair of Education
Department of Pediatrics
Yale University School of Medicine
New Haven, Connecticut

Nancy Wesensten, PhD
Air Traffic Organization Safety and Technical Training Safety Services (AJI-15)
Federal Aviation Administration
Washington, DC

Sophie West, MD
Lead
Newcastle Regional Sleep Centre
Newcastle upon Tyne Hospitals National Health Service Trust
Newcastle upon Tyne, United Kingdom

Ephraim Winocur, DMD
Clinical Assistant Professor in Orofacial Pain (ret.)
Section of Function, Dysfunction & Pain in the Stomatognathic System,
Department of Oral Rehabilitation
The Maurice and Gabriela Goldschleger School of Dental Medicine
Tel Aviv University
Tel Aviv, Israel

William Wisden, MA, PhD
Professor
Department of Life Sciences
UK Dementia Research Institute
Imperial College London
London, Great Britain

Lisa F. Wolfe, MD
Associate Professor of Medicine
Division of Pulmonary, Critical Care, and Sleep Medicine
Northwestern University Feinberg School of Medicine
Chicago, Illinois

Christine Won, MD, MS
Associate Professor
Department of Medicine (Pulmonary, Critical Care, and Sleep Medicine)
Yale University School of Medicine;
Medical Director
Yale Centers for Sleep Medicine
New Haven, Connecticuit

Jean Wong, MD, FRCPC
Staff Anesthesiologist
Anesthesia and Pain Management
Toronto Western Hospital;
Staff Anesthesiologist
Department of Anesthesia and Pain Management
Women's College Hospital;
Associate Professor
Department of Anesthesia
University of Toronto
Toronto, Ontario, Canada

Kenneth P. Wright, Jr., PhD
College Professor of Distinction
Department of Integrative Physiology
University of Colorado Boulder
Boulder, Colorado

Lora Wu, PhD
Senior Research Officer
Sleep/Wake Research Centre
Massey University
Wellington, New Zealand

Mark Wu, MD, PhD
Professor
Departments of Neurology, Medicine, and Neuroscience
Johns Hopkins University
Baltimore, Maryland

Don Wykoff, BBA, FRAeS
President Emeritus, Fatigue Working Group
Chair, Flight Time Duty Time Committee
International Federation of Airline Pilots' Associations
Montreal, Quebec, Canada

Lichuan Ye, PhD, RN
Associate Professor
School of Nursing
Bouvé College of Health Sciences
Northeastern University
Boston, University

Magdy Younes, MD, FRCPC, PhD
Distinguished Professor Emeritus
Department of Internal Medicine
University of Manitoba
Winnipeg, Manitoba, Canada

Antonio Zadra, PhD
Professor
Department of Psychology
Université de Montréal;
Researcher
Center for Advanced Research in Sleep Medicine
Hôpital du Sacré-Coeur de Montréal
Montreal, Quebec, Canada

Phyllis C. Zee, MD, PhD
Professor
Department of Neurology
Director, Center for Circadian and Sleep Medicine
Northwestern University Feinberg School of Medicine
Chicago, Illinois

Jamie M. Zeitzer, PhD
Associate Professor
Stanford Center for Sleep Sciences
Stanford University;
Health Science Specialist
Mental Illness Research, Education, and Clinical Center
VA Palo Alto Health Care System
Palo Alto, California

Eric Zhou, PhD
Faculty
Division of Sleep Medicine
Harvard Medical School;
Staff Psychologist
Perini Family Survivors' Center
Dana-Farber Cancer Institute;
Staff Psychology
Department of Neurology
Boston Children's Hospital
Boston, Massachusetts

Andrey V. Zinchuk, MD, MHS
Assistant Professor of Medicine
Section of Pulmonary, Critical Care, and Sleep Medicine
Yale University School of Medicine
New Haven, Connecticut

Ding Zou, MD, PhD
Center for Sleep and Vigilance Disorders
Institute of Medicine
Sahlgrenska Academy
University of Gothenburg
Gothenburg, Sweden

Foreword

Celebrating *PPSM*: Connected, Collaborative, Global

From birth of the first edition in 1989 to the seventh edition in 2021, *Principles and Practice of Sleep Medicine (PPSM)* has been the gold standard of knowledge for this fast-changing discipline. Today, sleep medicine is a well-established medical discipline that stands on a strong foundation of scientific and clinical knowledge, but just a little over 30 years ago (which for some of us, seems like only yesterday), the landscape was quite different. A search of PubMed revealed only about 300 publications matching the term "sleep medicine," compared to nearly 12,000 publications in 2020. The exponential growth in knowledge has fueled the rapid increase in the number of clinical sleep medicine centers and doctoral and postdoctoral training programs in the US and all over the world. Advances in basic and clinical sleep and circadian science continue to open up exciting, innovative approaches to diagnose and treat sleep and circadian disorders, and for defining the role of sleep as a fundamental requirement for the maintenance of health and well-being of people at all stages of life and within the context of health disparities.

It was indeed a "dream come true" when in 2017 the Nobel Prize in Physiology or Medicine was awarded for the discovery of the genetic mechanisms of circadian rhythms. The burgeoning evidence that circadian clocks regulate metabolic, immune, cardiovascular, and neural activity in central and peripheral tissues is gaining attention. Circadian medicine is now an emerging clinical specialty. In the past, there was an artificial separation of circadian and sleep science, but it is increasingly clear that the alignment of these two systems at the molecular, cellular, and system levels is critical for health. The potential of integrating the time domain in medicine has many implications for the future of sleep medicine, and medicine as a whole.

Since the previous edition of *PPSM*, sleep medicine has become even more connected, collaborative, and global. The World Sleep Society, founded in 2016, represents individual members and more than 40 sleep societies in the world. International conferences, courses, and events, such as World Sleep Congress and World Sleep Day, help promote sleep and circadian health, develop training programs for sleep professionals, and foster the development of sleep medicine worldwide. The COVID-19 pandemic highlights that our well-being is deeply interconnected and reinforces the importance of global collaboration to translate scientific discoveries into the clinic and share new perspectives in sleep and circadian medicine. This edition of *PPSM* celebrates the vision and contributions of the pioneers and giants of our field and delivers the most comprehensive state of knowledge of this exciting interdisciplinary field.

Phyllis C. Zee, MD, PhD
Director, Center for Circadian and Sleep Medicine
Northwestern University Feinberg School of Medicine
President-Elect World Sleep Society

Sleep Is Essential to Health

On behalf of the American Academy of Sleep Medicine (AASM) and its more than 11,000 members and accredited sleep centers, we congratulate the editors for completing a new edition of this landmark textbook in this most challenging and difficult time marked by a worldwide pandemic. Each edition of *Principles and Practice of Sleep Medicine* serves as a celebration of how far the field of sleep medicine has come in a relatively short period of time. This latest edition showcases an even greater understanding of the role of sleep and the circadian system in other medical disorders and overall health. As scientists have tirelessly worked to better comprehend sleep and wake physiology, this edition contains sections dedicated to new and exciting pharmacotherapeutics that target novel receptors in the central nervous system to help treat sleep disorders. Although much has changed in content as you turn the pages of this latest edition, which describes the latest findings in areas such as genetics, chronobiology, and consumer sleep monitoring, one constant remains: this textbook serves as the standard reference and guiding light for the field of sleep medicine. Even as the AASM develops innovative training models for sleep medicine physicians, obtaining and reading *Principles and Practice of Sleep Medicine* continues to serve as initiation for our trainees and students as they enter our exciting field, and the textbook remains a reliable companion for the seasoned clinician to reference while taking care of patients with sleep disorders.

At the AASM, we strive to continue the spirit and determination of our founder, and one of the founding editors of this book, Dr. William Dement. Although sleep medicine professionals around the world mourn losing him in 2020, his passion to spread the significance of sleep health has not only emboldened sleep clinicians and scientists to carry on this mission, but it also fostered significant progress in educating our public policy makers and society about the importance of sleep. Recently we have seen the creation of the first ever Sleep Health Caucus in the United States Congress, as well as ongoing progress in legislation to delay school start times, ensuring that our adolescents are better able to achieve sleep health. This textbook plays a central role in supporting the AASM vision that sleep is recognized as essential to health. The AASM and its members look to this textbook to properly care for patients, train our clinicians and scientists, and also allow other specialists to learn about how sleep is essential for the health of their patients.

The textbook represents what we have accomplished as a field thanks to sleep clinicians and scientists, past and present, and perhaps more importantly, it also provides a roadmap for researchers, whose findings will undoubtedly appear in future editions. Completed during a worldwide pandemic, this textbook highlights the resiliency of our many colleagues to continue to explore sleep and circadian science through research, and it is a testimony to the many sleep specialists and clinicians who continue to provide evidence-based, up-to-date clinical care for their patients with sleep disorders while enduring the pandemic. As with many devastating events, growth and progress emerge out of necessity, exemplified in our field through advances such as embracing telemedicine, utilizing home diagnostic testing and monitoring of sleep disorders, and recognizing the prevalence of sleep health disparities. Undoubtedly, adaptation and innovation within sleep medicine will allow us to rise up to future challenges and disruption within the field. The AASM and its members applaud the editors and all of the authors for completing this influential tome amid such obstacles. We thank them for their efforts, which will further the AASM's mission of advancing sleep care and enhancing sleep health to improve lives.

Raman K. Malhotra, MD, FAASM
President, American Academy of Sleep Medicine (2021-2022)
Associate Professor of Neurology, Sleep Medicine Center
Washington University in St. Louis School of Medicine

Acknowledgments

We have been working on *Principles and Practice of Sleep Medicine* for about a third of a century. Thousands of people have been involved in the production of the seven editions. This has been a challenge to produce a volume during a pandemic. Contributors and Elsevier staff worked in the context of lockdowns, isolation, evacuations, while some were caring for hospitalized patients, while others caring for outpatients. As much as we would like to personally thank each person, there is no way that we can thank them all. Some have retired, some have died, and some have made important contributions in the production of the various editions but are unknown to us. This group includes secretaries, copyeditors, artists, designers, people who dealt with the page proofs, internet programmers, and those who physically produced the books.

We would like to acknowledge all the extraordinary Elsevier editors who gave birth to each previous edition of the book. These include Bill Lamsback, Judy Fletcher, Richard Zorab, Cathy Carroll, Todd Hummell, and Dolores Meloni. They fueled the dream that helped establish a new field of medicine.

Many people helped in the preparation of the content of this volume, the seventh edition, including those listed below.

The staff members at Elsevier who helped this book in its seventh journey were Nancy Duffy, Laura Kuehl-Schmidt, Lisa Barnes, Kate Mannix, Melanie Tucker, Amy Buxton, and many others involved in production and design for both the printed volume and the online content.

We also must acknowledge the family members of all the people involved in the book because they indirectly helped produce a work that we believe may have had important positive impact on the lives of thousands, perhaps millions, of people.

Finally, we wish to thank the many hundreds of authors and the magnificent work of the section editors and their deputy editors. All their contributions were so great that they cannot be measured.

Section and Deputy Editors

1E 1989
Mary Carskadon
Michael Chase
Richard Ferber
Christian Guilleminault
Ernest Hartmann
Meir Kryger
Timothy Monk
Anthony Nicholson
Allan Rechtschaffen
Gerald Vogel
Frank Zorick

2E 1994
Michael Aldrich
Mary Carskadon
Michael Chase
J. Christian Gillin
Christian Guilleminault
Ernest Hartmann
Meir Kryger
Anthony Nicholson
Allan Rechtschaffen
Gary Richardson
Thomas Roth
Frank Zorick

3E 2000
Michael Aldrich
Michael Chase
J. Christian Gillin
Christian Guilleminault
Max Hirshkowitz
Mark W. Mahowald
Wallace B. Mendelson
R.T. Pivik
Leon Rosenthal
Mark Sanders
Fred Turek
Frank Zorick

4E 2005
Michael Aldrich
Ruth Benca
J. Christian Gillin
Max Hirshkowitz
Shahrokh Javaheri
Meir Kryger
Mark W. Mahowald
Wallace B. Mendelson
Jacques Montplaiser
John Orem
Timothy Roehrs
Mark Sanders
Robert Stickgold
Fred Turek

5E 2011
Sonia Ancoli-Israel
Gregory Belenky
Ruth Benca
Daniel Buysse
Michael Cramer-Bornemann
Charles George
Max Hirshkowitz
Meir Kryger
Gilles Lavigne
Kathryn Aldrich Lee
Beth A. Malow
Mark W. Mahowald
Wallace B. Mendelson
Jacques Montplaisir
Tore Nielsen
Mark Sanders
Jerome Siegel
Fred Turek

6E 2017
Sonia Ancoli-Israel
Robert Basner
Gregory Belenky
Dan Brown
Daniel Buysse
Jennifer DeWolfe
Max Hirshkowitz
Shahrokh Javaheri
Andrew Krystal
Gilles Lavigne
Kathryn Aldrich Lee
Beth A. Malow
Timothy Roehrs
Thomas Roth
Thomas Scammell
Jerome Siegel
Robert Stickgold
Katie L. Stone
Fred Turek
Bradley V. Vaughn
Erin J. Wamsley
Christine Won

7E 2021
Sabra Abbott
Cathy Alessi
Fiona C. Baker
Bei Bei
Gregory Belenky
Daniel B. Brown
Jennifer Laurel DeWolfe
Christopher L. Drake
Julio Fernandez-Mendoza

Section and Deputy Editors—cont'd		
Constance H. Fung	Eric A. Nofzinger	Renaud Tamisier
Max Hirshkowitz	John Park	Robert Joseph Thomas
Shahrokh Javaheri	Rafael Pelayo	Bradley V. Vaughn
Thomas Kilduff	Samantha Riedy	Erin J. Wamsley
Andrew D. Krystal	Thomas Scammell	Nancy Wesensten
Hans-Peter Landolt	Paul J. Shaw	Lisa F. Wolfe
Gilles Lavigne	Stephen H. Sheldon	Christine Won
Guy Leschziner	Jerome M. Siegel	Kenneth P. Wright, Jr.
Beth A. Malow	Robert Stickgold	Phyllis C. Zee
Jennifer Martin	Erik K. St. Louis	Andrey V. Zinchuk
Kiran Maski	Shannon Sullivan	

Preface

This edition of *PPSM* had a very difficult gestation. It was during the pandemic that washed over our unprotected planet in brutal waves. All our lives were upended and changed. Our beloved friend and co-editor, Bill Dement, died. Most of us knew people infected with COVID or who had died of COVID. We were all deeply concerned that our families and friends might be affected. That was the context of the gestation of the book.

Before the pandemic, Cathy Goldstein had joined the senior editorial team of the book. Section editors and authors had agreed to contribute. Then, in early 2020, contributors in Europe were impacted, followed by contributors from other continents. Some contributors, when contacted, told us they were in the hospital with COVID or had family members with COVID. Many contributors were conscripted to take care of hospitalized patients. Some contributors were banished from their offices with work from home orders and did not have access to the things they needed to complete their chapters. Even the forest fires in California impacted the book, trapping some authors, while others had to evacuate their homes. And at the end of the day, all the contributors produced magnificent chapters.

The book has 22 sections, including a new section on "Transition from Childhood." About 75% of the sections have new editors. The book retains its philosophical underpinnings with content from the diverse disciplines (basic and clinical) with contributors from 4 continents.

While the book was being produced, several contributors from this and previous editions died: Richard Allen, Rosalind Cartwright, Bill Dement, Christian Guilleminault, Mark Mahowald, Art Spielman, and Mario Terzano. Their contributions to medicine will impact the field for generations to come. May their memories be a blessing and an inspiration.

Just as some of the greatest wines come from grapes that survive in the most difficult terrains, we believe that this edition, having weathered a difficult gestation, has produced a volume worthy of the field of sleep medicine and continues the vision outlined over 30 years ago.

Meir Kryger
Cathy Goldstein
Tom Roth

FIRST EDITION PREFACE

Medical disorders related to sleep are obviously not new. Yet the discipline of sleep disorders medicine is in its infancy. There is a large body of knowledge on which to base the discipline of sleep disorder medicine. We hope that this textbook will play a role in the evolution of this field.

Douglas Hofstadter reviewed how ideas and concepts evolve and are transmitted.[1] In 1965, Roger Sperry[2] wrote the following: "Ideas cause ideas and help evolve new ideas. They interact with each other and with other mental forces in the same brain, in neighboring brains, and thanks to global communication, in far distant, foreign brains. And they also interact with the external surroundings to produce *in toto* a burstwise advance in evolution that is far beyond anything to hit the evolutionary scene yet, including the emergence of the living cell." Jacques Monod[3] wrote the following in *Chance and Necessity:* "For a biologist it is tempting to draw a parallel between the evolution of ideas and that of the biosphere. For while the abstract kingdom stands at a yet greater distance above the biosphere than the latter does above the non-living universe, ideas have retained some of the properties of organisms. Like them they tend to perpetuate their structure and to breed; they too can fuse, recombine, segregate their content; indeed they too can evolve, and in this evolution selection must surely play an important role." Hofstadter has called this universe of ideas the ideosphere analogous to the biosphere. The ideosphere's counterpart to the biosphere gene has been called meme by Richard Dawkins.[4] He wrote "just as genes propagate themselves in a gene pool by leaping from body to body via sperm or eggs, so memes propagate themselves in the meme pool by leaping from brain to brain. ... If a scientist hears or reads about a good idea, he passes it on to his colleagues and students. He mentions it in his articles and his lectures. If the idea catches on it can be said to propagate itself spreading from brain to brain ... memes should be regarded as living structures, not just metaphorically but technically."

Thus, this textbook represents an attempt to summarize the body of science and ideas that up to now has been transmitted verbally, in articles, and in a few more specialized books. The memes in this volume are drawn from a variety of disciplines, including psychology, psychiatry, neurology, pharmacology, internal medicine, pediatrics, and basic biological sciences. That a field evolves from multidisciplinary roots certainly has precedents in medicine. The field of infectious diseases has its in microbiology, and its practitioners are expected to know relevant aspects of internal medicine, surgery, gynecology, and pediatrics. Similarly, oncology has its roots in surgery, hematology, and internal medicine, and its practitioners today must also know virology and molecular biology. Patients with sleep problems have in the past 'fallen through the cracks.' It is not uncommon to see a patient with classic narcolepsy who has seen five to ten specialists before a diagnosis is finally made. There is a clinical need for physicians to know about sleep and its disorders.

[1]Hofstadter DR. Chapter 3. In: *Metamagical Themas: Questing for the Essence of Mind and Pattern*. Toronto: Bantam Books; 1986.
[2]Sperry R. Mind, brain, and humanist values. In: Platt JR, editor. *New Views of the Nature of Man*. Chicago: The university of Chicago Press; 1965.
[3]Monod J. *Chance and Necessity*. New York: Vintage Books; 1972.
[4]Dawkins R. *The Selfish Gene*. Oxford: Oxford University Press; 1976. p. 206.

Contents

Section 16 Cardiovascular Disorders 1405

Section 17 Other Medical Disorders 1490

Section 18 Psychiatric Disorders 1565

Section 19 Dentistry and Otorhinolaryngology 1608

Video Contents

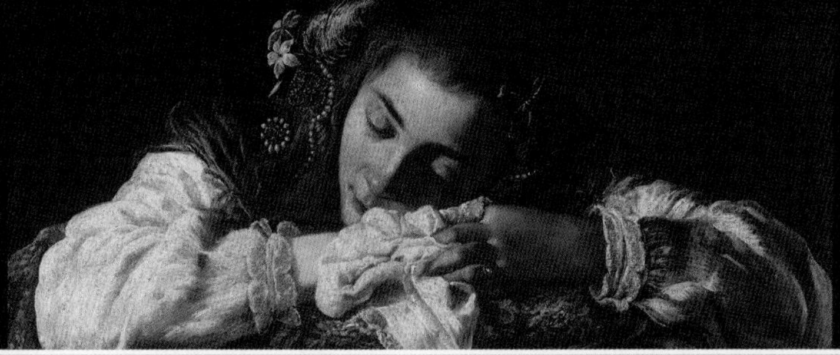

PART I

Principles of Sleep Medicine

Normal Sleep and Its Variants

Section 1

History of Sleep Physiology and Medicine

Chapter 1

Rafael Pelayo; William C. Dement†

Chapter Highlights

- Interest in sleep and dreams has existed since the dawn of humanity. Some of history's greatest figures have attempted to explain the physiologic and psychological bases of sleep and dreaming.
- The modern scientific study of sleep began with the discovery of the electrical activity in the brain. Further progress was marked by the discovery of and distinction between rapid eye movement (REM) and non–REM (NREM) sleep. Identifying sleep pathology eventually led to the creation of sleep clinics.
- Sleep medicine as a medical specialty has existed for just over 50 years. The evolution of the field required clinical research, development of clinical services, training programs, and changes in the insurance industry and public policy that recognized the impact of sleep disorders on society. Perhaps the greatest existential crisis the field has faced is the 2020 COVID-19 viral pandemic.
- The field is still evolving. Sleep impacts almost all aspects of physiology and medicine—new disorders are being discovered, and new treatments are being delivered. As sleep medicine faces new challenges, an understanding of its history can provide researchers with important insights for shaping the future of this discipline.

This chapter's co-author, Dr. William C. Dement, passed away shortly after he finished editing this chapter in 2020. His death was noted by the international community in many tributes (https://science.sciencemag.org/content/369/6503/512.full). His contributions described in this chapter and throughout many parts of this textbook touched all of our lives. Those of us fortunate to have met him will likely remember most the humility, grace, and sense of humor he shared with all.

SLEEP AS A PASSIVE STATE

> Sleep is the intermediate state between wakefulness and death; wakefulness being regarded as the active state of all the animal and intellectual functions, and death as that of their total suspension.[1]

The foregoing is the first sentence of *The Philosophy of Sleep*, a book written by the Scottish physician Robert MacNish in 1830. This sentence exemplifies the overarching historical conceptual dichotomy of sleep research and sleep medicine, which is sleep as a passive process versus sleep as an active process. Until the discovery of rapid eye movements, sleep was universally regarded as an inactive state of the brain. Most experts regarded sleep as the inevitable result of reduced sensory input, with the consequent diminishment of brain activity. Waking up and being awake were considered a reversal of this process, mainly as a result of bombardment of the brain by external stimuli. No real distinction was seen between sleep

†Deceased.

and other states of quiescence such as coma, stupor, intoxication, hypnosis, anesthesia, and hibernation.

The passive-versus-active historical dichotomy also is given great weight by the contemporary investigator J. Allan Hobson.[2] As he noted in his book *Sleep*, published in 1989, "more has been learned about sleep in the past 60 years than in the preceding 6,000." He continued, "In this short period of time, researchers have discovered that sleep is a dynamic behavior. Not simply the absence of waking, sleep is a special activity of the brain, controlled by elaborate and precise mechanisms."[2]

Dreams and dreaming were regarded as transient, fleeting interruptions of this quiescent sleep state. Because dreams seem to occur spontaneously and sometimes in response to environmental stimulation (e.g., the well-known alarm clock dreams), the notion of a stimulus that produces the dream was generalized by postulating internal stimulation from the digestive tract or some other internal source. Some anthropologists have suggested that notions of spirituality and the soul arose from primitive peoples' need to explain how their essence could leave the body temporarily at night in a dream and permanently at death.[3,4] There should be no doubt that dreams influenced the beliefs of primitive cultures.

Sleep-promoting and sleep-inhibiting substances were part of ancient pharmacopeias. It had been observed in antiquity that alcohol would induce a sleep-like state. More than 5000 years ago the opium poppy was cultivated in Mesopotamia. Hippocrates in the fourth century BCE acknowledged its usefulness as a narcotic. Somewhat later, in Ethiopia, coffee consumption was thought to have begun when its power to prevent sleep was recognized. It was cultivated in the Arabian Peninsula in the 15th century, from whence it spread to Europe and later the Americas.

In addition to the reduction of stimulation, other theories were espoused to account for the onset of sleep. Vascular theories were proposed from the notion that the blood left the brain to accumulate in the digestive tract and from the opposite idea that sleep was due to pressure on the brain by blood. Around the end of the 19th century, there were various versions of a "hypnotoxin" hypothesis in which fatigue products accumulated during the day, finally causing sleep, during which they were gradually eliminated. This was an early mirror of current concepts on the role of adenosine accumulation leading to sleepiness. In 1907 Legendre and Pieron showed that blood serum from sleep-deprived dogs could induce sleep in other dogs that were not sleep deprived.[5] The notion of a toxin causing the brain to sleep has gradually given way to the recognition that a number of endogenous "sleep factors" actively induce sleep by specific mechanisms. The search for endogenous sleep-promoting factors goes on today.

In the 1920s the University of Chicago physiologist Nathaniel Kleitman carried out a series of sleep deprivation studies and made the brilliant observation that people who stayed up all night generally were less sleepy and impaired the next morning than in the middle of their sleepless night. Kleitman argued that this observation was incompatible with the notion of a continual buildup of a hypnotoxin in the brain or blood. In the 1939 (first) edition of his comprehensive landmark monograph, *Sleep and Wakefulness*, Kleitman summarized his thinking as follows:

> It is perhaps not sleep that needs to be explained, but wakefulness, and indeed, there may be different kinds of wakefulness at different stages of phylogenetic and ontogenetic development. In spite of sleep being frequently designated as an instinct, or global reaction, an actively initiated process, by excitation or inhibition of cortical or subcortical structures, there is not a single fact about sleep that cannot be equally well interpreted as a let down of the waking activity.[6]

This statement succinctly provides insight into the historical adoption of the yin-yang symbol, ☯, as a symbol of sleep medicine. The yin-yang symbol was part of the official logo of the American Academy of Sleep Medicine until it was changed in 2017.

THE ELECTRICAL ACTIVITY OF THE BRAIN

In 1875 the Scottish physiologist Richard Caton described the electrical rhythms in the brains of rabbits, cats, and monkeys. The centennial of his achievement was commemorated at the 15th annual meeting of the Association for the Psychophysiological Study of Sleep, convening at the site of the discovery, Edinburgh.

Early in the 20th century, Camillo Golgi and Santiago Ramón y Cajal demonstrated that the nervous system was not a mass of fused cells sharing a common cytoplasm but rather a highly intricate network of discrete cells that were able to signal one another. Luigi Galvani discovered that the nerve cells of animals produce electricity, and Emil duBois-Reymond and Hermann von Helmholtz found that nerve cells use their electrical capabilities for signaling information to one another.

It was not until 1928, however, that the German psychiatrist Hans Berger recorded electrical activity of the human brain and clearly demonstrated differences in these rhythms when subjects were awake versus asleep.[7] For the first time, the presence of sleep could be conclusively established without disturbing the sleeper, and more important, sleep could be continuously and quantitatively measured without disturbing the sleeper.

All of the classic major elements of sleep brain wave patterns were described by Loomis, Harvey, Hobart, Davis, and others at Harvard University in a series of influential papers published in 1937, 1938, and 1939.[8-10] Alfred Lee Loomis is a historically interesting figure who also played a pivotal role in World War II. He developed amplifier systems to record sleep, and for reasons that are seemingly lost to history, he coined the term *K-complex*.[11] Blake, Gerard, and Kleitman added to this work from their studies at the University of Chicago. On the human electroencephalogram (EEG), sleep was characterized by high-amplitude slow waves and spindles, whereas wakefulness was characterized by low-amplitude waves and alpha rhythm.[12,13] The image of the sleeping brain completely "turned off" gave way to the image of the sleeping brain engaged in slow, synchronized, "idling" neuronal activity. Although their significance was not widely recognized at the time, these findings constituted some of the most critical developments in sleep research.

Also in the 1930s, a series of investigations by Frederick Bremer seemed to establish conclusively both the passive theory of sleep and the notion that it occurred in response to reduction of stimulation and activity.[14,15] Bremer studied brain wave patterns in two cat preparations. One, which Bremer called "encéphale isolé," was made by cutting a section through the lower part of the medulla. The other, "cerveau isolé," was made by cutting the midbrain just behind the origin of the oculomotor nerves. The first preparation permitted the study of cortical electrical rhythms under the influence of olfactory, visual, auditory, vestibular, and musculocutaneous impulses; in the second preparation, the field was narrowed almost entirely to the influence of olfactory and visual impulses. In the first preparation, the brain continued to show manifestations of wakeful activity alternating with phases of sleep, as indicated by the EEG. In the second preparation, however, the EEG pattern assumed a definite deep sleep character and remained in this condition. Bremer concluded that a functional (reversible, of course) deafferentation of the cerebral cortex occurs in sleep. The cerveau isolé preparation results in a suppression of the incessant influx of nerve impulses, particularly cutaneous and proprioceptive, which are essential for the maintenance of the waking state of the telencephalon. Apparently, olfactory and visual impulses are insufficient to keep the cortex awake. It probably is misleading to assert that physiologists assumed the brain was completely turned off, whatever this metaphor might have meant, because blood flow and, presumably, metabolism continued. However, Bremer and others certainly favored the concept of sleep as a reduction of activity—idling, slow, synchronized, "resting" neuronal activity.

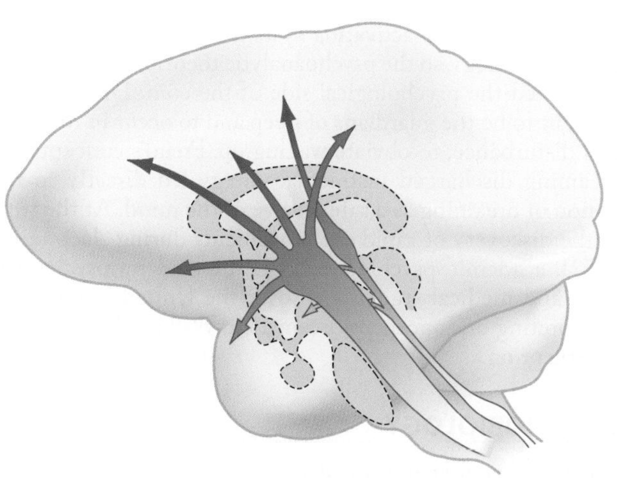

Figure 1.1 Lateral view of the monkey's brain, showing the ascending reticular activating system in the brainstem receiving collaterals from direct afferent paths and projecting primarily to the associational areas of the hemisphere. (Redrawn from Magoun HW: The ascending reticular system and wakefulness. In: Adrian ED, Bremer F, Jasper HH, eds. *Brain mechanisms and consciousness. A symposium organized by the Council for International Organizations of Medical Sciences,* 1954. Courtesy Charles C Thomas, Publisher, Springfield, Illinois.)

THE RETICULAR ACTIVATING SYSTEM

In 1949 one of the most important and influential studies dealing with sleep and wakefulness was published: Moruzzi and Magoun's classic paper *Brain Stem Reticular Formation and Activation of the EEG.*[16] These authors concluded that transitions from sleep to wakefulness or from the less extreme states of relaxation and drowsiness to alertness and attention are all characterized by an apparent breaking up of the synchronization of discharge of the elements of the cerebral cortex, an alteration marked in the EEG by the replacement of high voltage, slow waves with low-voltage fast activity.[16]

High-frequency electrical stimulation with electrodes implanted in the brainstem reticular formation produced EEG activation and behavioral arousal. These findings seemed to indicate that EEG activation, wakefulness, and consciousness were at one end of a continuum, and EEG synchronization, sleep, and lack of consciousness were at the other end.

The demonstration by Starzl and colleagues that sensory collaterals discharge into the reticular formation suggested that a mechanism was present by which sensory stimulation could be transduced into prolonged activation of the brain and sustained wakefulness.[17] Research with chronic lesions in the brainstem reticular formation produced persisting slow waves in the EEG and immobility. The usual animal for this research was the cat, because excellent stereotaxic coordinates of brain structures had become available in this model.[18] The theory of the reticular activating system was an anatomically based passive theory of sleep or an active theory of wakefulness. Figure 1.1 is from the proceedings of a symposium, *Brain Mechanisms and Consciousness,* which was published in 1954 and probably (other than, arguably, Freud's works) was the first genuine neuroscience bestseller.[19]

EARLY OBSERVATIONS OF SLEEP PATHOLOGY

Insomnia has been described since the dawn of recorded history and attributed to many causes, including a recognition of the association between emotional disturbance and sleep disturbance. Important early observations were those of von Economo on "sleeping sickness" and of Pavlov, who observed dogs falling asleep during conditioned reflex experiments.[3] Two early observations about sleep research and sleep medicine stand out. The first is the description in 1880 of narcolepsy by Jean Baptiste Edouard Gélineau, who derived the term from the Greek words *narkosis* ("a benumbing") and *lepsis* ("to overtake"). In France narcolepsy is still referred to as *maladie de Gélineau.* Gélineau was the first to clearly describe the collection of components that constitute the syndrome, although the term *cataplexy* for the emotionally induced muscle weakness was subsequently coined in 1916 by Richard Henneberg.

Obstructive sleep apnea syndrome (OSA), which is certainly the leading sleep disorder of the 20th century, was famously described in 1836, not by a clinician but by the novelist Charles Dickens. In the *Posthumous Papers of the Pickwick Club,* Dickens described Joe, a boy who was obese, a loud snorter, and always sleepy. The novel includes this line: "Come wake up young dropsy!" (*Dropsy* is an old medical term for swelling of soft tissue, so perhaps Dickens is describing right-sided heart failure.) Notably, Joe is praised for his ability to fall asleep instantaneously after drinking alcohol! In addition, Meir Kryger and Peretz Lavie published scholarly accounts of many early references to snoring and conditions that were most certainly manifestations of OSA.[20-22] Professor Pierre Passouant provided an account of the life of Gélineau and his landmark description of the narcolepsy syndrome.[23]

SIGMUND FREUD AND THE INTERPRETATION OF DREAMS

The most widespread interest in sleep was engendered by the theories of Sigmund Freud, specifically about dreams.[24] *The Interpretation of Dreams* was first published in German in 1895 and translated into English in 1913, with several subsequent revisions.[24] Freud wrote about sleep many years before the description of the EEG in humans. Of course, the real interest was in dreaming, with sleep as a necessary concomitant. Freud developed psychoanalysis, the technique of dream interpretation, as part of his therapeutic approach to emotional and mental problems. As the concept of the ascending reticular activating system dominated behavioral neurophysiology, so the psychoanalytic theories about dreams dominated the psychological side of the coin. Dreams were thought to be the guardians of sleep and to occur in response to a disturbance, to obviate waking up. Freud's concept that dreaming discharged instinctual energy led directly to the notion of dreaming as a safety valve of the mind. At the time of the discovery of rapid eye movements during sleep (circa 1952), academic psychiatry was dominated by psychoanalysts, and medical students all over the United States were interpreting one another's dreams. Dr. William Dement was no exception.

CHRONOBIOLOGY

Most, but at first not all, sleep specialists share the opinion that what has been called *chronobiology,* or the study of biologic rhythms, is a legitimate part of sleep research and sleep medicine. This makes the 2017 awarding of the Nobel Prize in Physiology or Medicine to Drs. Jeffery Hall, Michael Rosbash, and Michael Young for "their discoveries of the molecular mechanism controlling the circadian rhythm" a key historical landmark for the sleep field. The 24-hour rhythms in the activities of plants and animals have been recognized for centuries. In 1729 Jean Jacques d'Ortous de Mairan described an experiment in which a heliotrope plant opened its leaves during the day even after it had been moved so that sunlight could not reach it. The plant opened its leaves during the day and folded them for the entire night, even though the environment was constant. This was the first demonstration of the persistence of circadian rhythms in the absence of environmental time cues. Figure 1.2, which represents de Mairan's original experiment, is reproduced from *The Clocks That Time Us,* by Moore-Ede and colleagues.[25]

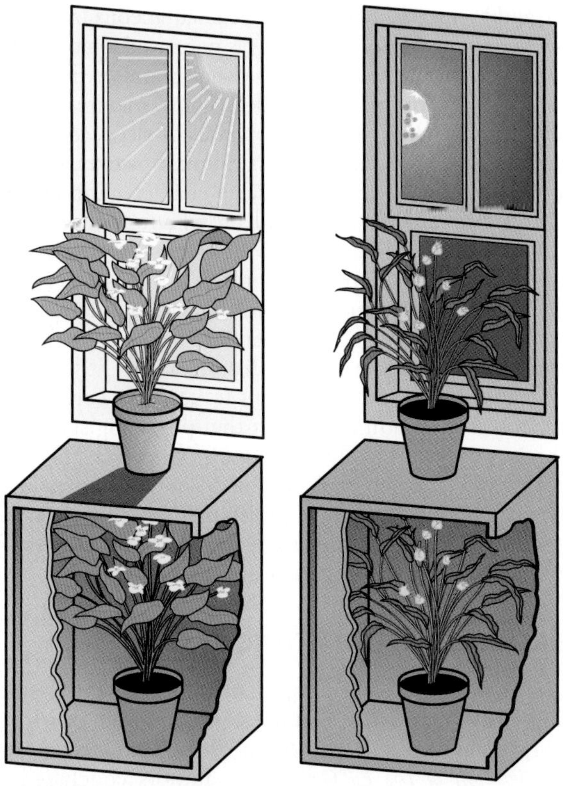

Figure 1.2 Representation of de Mairan's original experiment. When exposed to sunlight during the day (*upper left*), the leaves of the plant were open; during the night (*upper right*), the leaves were folded. De Mairan showed that sunlight was not necessary for these leaf movements by placing the plant in total darkness. Even under these constant conditions, the leaves opened during the day (*lower left*) and folded during the night (*lower right*). (Redrawn from Moore-Ede MC, Sulzman FM, Fuller CA. *The clocks that time us: physiology of the circadian timing system.* Harvard University Press; 1982:7.)

THE DISCOVERY OF RAPID EYE MOVEMENT SLEEP

Nathaniel Kleitman (Figure 1.3; Video 1.1), a professor of physiology at the University of Chicago, had long been interested in cycles of activity and inactivity in infants and in the possibility that this cycle ensured that the infant would have an opportunity to respond to hunger. He postulated that eye motility was a possible measure of "depth" of sleep.[26] In 1951 he assigned the task of observing eye movement to a graduate student named Eugene Aserinsky. Watching the closed eyes of sleeping infants was tedious, and Aserinsky soon found that it was easier to designate successive 5-minute epochs as "periods of motility" if he observed any movement at all, usually a writhing or twitching of the eyelids, versus "periods of no motility." Among the infants studied was his own child. In 1952 William C. Dement, at the time a second-year medical student at the University of Chicago, joined the research effort. The first task he was assigned was looking at the closed eyes of the research subjects, using a flashlight in the dark when electrical potentials were detected in the recording instruments in the adjacent room.

After describing an apparent rhythm in eye motility, Kleitman and Aserinsky decided to look for a similar phenomenon in adults. Again, watching the eyes during the day was tedious,

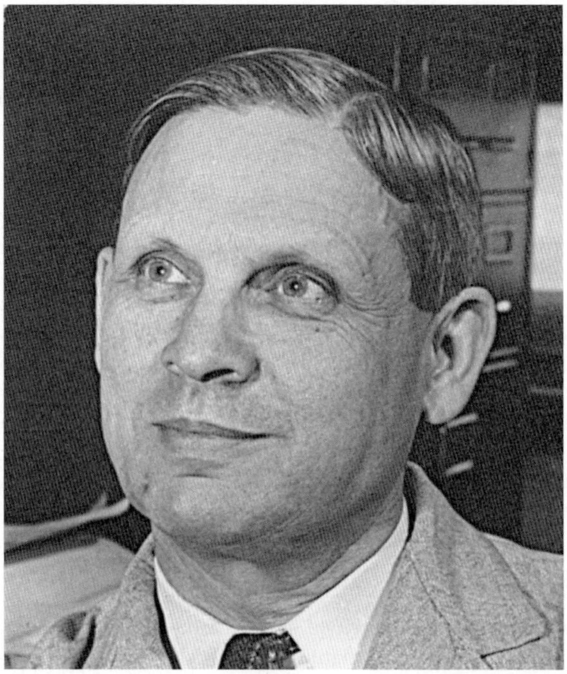

Figure 1.3 Nathaniel Kleitman (circa 1938), Professor of Physiology, University of Chicago School of Medicine.

and at night it was even worse. Casting about, they came upon the method of electrooculography and decided (correctly) that this would be a good way to measure eye motility continuously and would relieve the researcher of the tedium of direct observations. Sometimes in the course of recording electrooculograms (EOGs) during sleep, they saw bursts of electrical potential changes that were quite different from the slow movements at sleep onset.

When they were observing infants, Aserinsky and Kleitman had not differentiated between slow and rapid eye movements. On the EOG, however, the difference between the slow eye movements at sleep onset and the newly discovered rapid motility was obvious. With their presence on the EOG as a signal, however, it was possible to watch the subject's eyes simultaneously, permitting easy detection of the distinct rapid movements of the eyes beneath closed lids.

At this point, Aserinsky and Kleitman made two assumptions:

1. These eye movements represented a "lightening" of sleep.
2. Because the eye movements were associated with irregular respiration and accelerated heart rate, they might represent dreaming.

The basic sleep cycle was not yet identified at this time, primarily because the EOG and other physiologic measures, notably the EEG, were not recorded continuously but rather were "sampled" during a few minutes of each hour or half-hour. The sampling strategy was designed to conserve paper (in the absence of research grants!); moreover, no clear reason to record continuously had been identified. This schedule also made it possible for the researcher to nap between sampling the nocturnal episodes.

Aserinsky and Kleitman initiated a small series of awakenings, both when rapid eye movements were present and when they were not, for the purpose of eliciting dream recall. These workers did not apply sophisticated methods of dream content analysis, but the descriptions of dream content from the two conditions generally were quite different, with awakenings during periods of rapid eye movements often yielding vivid complex stories, in contrast with awakening periods, when rapid eye movements were not present, yielding nothing at all or very sparse accounts. This distinction lead to the hypothesis that rapid eye movements were associated with dreaming. This was, indeed, a breakthrough in sleep research.[27,28] Although Dement participated in this research as a medical student, he was not credited in these early articles. His recollection is that he later coined the abbreviations REM (for rapid eye movement) and NREM (for non–rapid eye movement) to simplify the typing of subsequent manuscripts and publications (Dement, personal communication, 2014). These terms appear for the first time in the literature in a footnote by Dement and Kleitman in 1957.[29]

ALL-NIGHT SLEEP RECORDINGS AND THE BASIC SLEEP CYCLE

The seminal paper by Aserinsky and Kleitman, published in 1953,[27] attracted little attention, and no publications on the subject appeared from any other laboratory until 1959.[30] Staying up at night to study sleep remained an undesirable occupation by any standards. In the early 1950s most previous research on the EEG patterns of sleep, like most approaches to sleep physiology generally, had either equated short periods of sleep with all sleep or relied on infrequent sampling during the night. Obtaining continuous records throughout typical nights of sleep seemed highly extravagant—owing in no small part to the cost of the blocks of special paper required.

However, motivated by the desire to expand and quantify the description of rapid eye movements, Dement and Kleitman did just this: they recorded EEGs over a total of 126 nights with 33 subjects and, by means of a simplified categorization of EEG patterns, scored the paper recordings in their entirety.[31] On examining these 126 records, they found a predictable sequence of patterns, over the course of the night, that had been overlooked in all previous EEG studies of sleep. This sequence has now been observed throughout the world and is referred to as *sleep architecture*. This original description remains essentially unchanged.

Dement and Kleitman found that this cyclic variation of EEG pattern occurred repeatedly throughout the night at intervals of 90 to 100 minutes from the end of one eye movement period to the end of the next. The regular occurrences of REM periods and dreaming strongly suggested that dreams did not occur in response to chance disturbances. At the time of these observations, sleep was still considered to be a single state. Dement and Kleitman characterized the EEG pattern during REM periods as "emergent stage 1," as opposed to "descending stage 1" at the onset of sleep. The percentage of the total sleep time occupied by REM sleep was between 20% and 25%, and the periods of REM sleep tended to be shorter in the early cycles of the night. This pattern of all-night sleep has been seen over and over in normal humans of both sexes, in widely varying environments and cultures, and across the life span.

RAPID EYE MOVEMENT SLEEP IN ANIMALS

The developing knowledge of the nature of REM sleep was in direct opposition to the ascending reticular activating system theory and constituted a paradigmatic crisis. The following observations in humans and animals were crucial:

- Arousal thresholds in humans were much higher during periods of REM sleep associated with a low-amplitude, relatively fast (stage 1) EEG pattern than during similar "light sleep" periods at the onset of sleep.
- Rapid eye movements during sleep were discovered in cats; the concomitant brain wave patterns (low-amplitude, fast) were indistinguishable from those in active wakefulness.[32]
- By discarding the sampling approach and recording continuously in humans, a basic 90-minute cycle of sleep without rapid eye movements, alternating with sleep with rapid eye movements, was discovered.[31]
- Observations of motor activity in both humans and animals revealed the unique occurrence of an active suppression of spinal motor activity and muscle reflexes (paralysis).

Thus, it became obvious that human sleep consisted not of one state but rather of two distinct organismic states, as different from one another as both are from wakefulness. It had to be conceded that sleep could no longer be thought of as a time of brain inactivity and EEG slowing. By 1960 this fundamental change in thinking about the nature of sleep was well established.

It is very difficult now, in the 21st century, to understand and appreciate the exceedingly controversial nature of these findings. The following personal account from Dement[33] illustrates both the power and the danger of scientific dogma:

> I wrote them [the findings] up, but the paper was nearly impossible to publish because it was completely contradictory to the totally dominant neurophysiological theory of the time. The assertion by me that an activated EEG could be associated with unambiguous sleep was considered to be absurd. As it turned out, previous investigators had observed an activated EEG during sleep in cats[28,29] but simply could not believe it and ascribed it to arousing influences during sleep. A colleague who was assisting me was sufficiently skeptical that he preferred I publish the paper as sole author. After four or five rejections, to my everlasting gratitude, Editor-in-Chief Herbert Jasper accepted the paper without revision for publication in *Electroencephalography and Clinical Neurophysiology* [italics added].[33]

Of note, however, many early researchers (Dement included) did not recognize the significance of the absence of muscle potentials during the REM periods in cats. It remained for Michel Jouvet, working in Lyon, France, to insist on the importance of electromyographic suppression in his early papers, the first of which was published in 1959.[30,34] Hodes and Dement began to study the "H-reflex" in humans in 1960, finding complete suppression of reflexes during REM sleep, and Octavio Pompeiano and others in Pisa, Italy, worked out the basic mechanisms of REM atonia in the cat.[35,36]

DUALITY OF SLEEP

Even though the basic REM/NREM sleep cycle was well established, the realization that REM sleep was qualitatively different from that in the remainder of the sleep cycle took years to evolve. Jouvet and colleagues performed an elegant series of investigations on the brainstem mechanisms of sleep that forced the inescapable conclusion that sleep consists of two fundamentally different states.[37] Among their many early contributions were clarification of the role of pontine brainstem systems as the primary anatomic site for REM sleep mechanisms and the clear demonstration that electromyographic activity and muscle tonus are completely suppressed during REM periods and *only* during REM periods. These investigations began in 1958 and were carried out during 1959 and 1960.

It is now well established that atonia is a fundamental characteristic of REM sleep and is mediated by an active and highly specialized neuronal system. The pioneering microelectrode studies of Edward Evarts in cats and monkeys and observations on cerebral blood flow in the cat by Reivich and Kety provided convincing evidence that, during REM sleep, the brain is very active.[38,39] Certain areas of the brain appear to be more active in REM sleep than in wakefulness. By 1960 it was possible to define REM sleep as a completely separate organismic state characterized by cerebral activation, active motor inhibition, and, of course, an association with dreaming. The fundamental duality of REM versus NREM sleep was an established fact.

PRECURSORS OF SLEEP MEDICINE

Sleep research, which emphasized all-night sleep recordings, burgeoned in the 1960s and was the legitimate precursor of sleep medicine and particularly of its core clinical test, polysomnography. Much of the research at that time emphasized studies of dreaming and REM sleep and had its roots in a psychoanalytic approach to mental illness, which strongly implicated dreaming in the psychotic process. After sufficient numbers of all-night sleep recordings had been carried out in humans to demonstrate a highly characteristic "normal" sleep architecture, investigators noted a significantly shortened REM latency in association with endogenous depression.[40] This phenomenon has been intensively investigated ever since. Other important precursors of sleep medicine were the following:

1. Discovery of sleep-onset REM periods (SOREMPs) in patients with narcolepsy
2. Interest in sleep, epilepsy, and abnormal movement—primarily in France
3. Introduction of benzodiazepines and the use of sleep laboratory studies in defining hypnotic drug efficacy

SLEEP-ONSET REM PERIODS AND CATAPLEXY

In 1959 a patient with narcolepsy came to the Mount Sinai Hospital in New York City to see Drs. Charles Fisher and Bill Dement. At Fisher's suggestion, a nocturnal sleep recording was begun. Within seconds after he fell asleep, the patient showed the dramatic and characteristic rapid eye movements and sawtooth waves of REM sleep. The first paper documenting SOREMPs in a specific patient was published in 1960 by Gerald Vogel in Chicago.[41] In a collaborative study between the University of Chicago and the Mount Sinai Hospital, data on nine narcoleptic patients with SOREMPs at night were reported in 1963.[42] Subsequent research showed that sleepy patients who did not have cataplexy did not have SOREMPs, and those with cataplexy always had SOREMPs.[43] For the first time, a clinical role for the polysomnogram as a potential diagnostic tool was being identified! Sleep research was becoming sleep medicine.

THE NARCOLEPSY CLINIC: A FALSE START

In January 1963, after leaving Mount Sinai and moving to Stanford University, Dement was eager to test the hypothesis of an association between cataplexy and SOREMPs. However, not a single narcoleptic patient was located in the San Francisco Bay area. In desperation, the investigators placed a brief "want ad," requesting such subjects, in a daily newspaper, the *San Francisco Chronicle*. More than 100 people responded; approximately 50 of these patients had bona fide narcolepsy and were afflicted with both sleepiness and cataplexy.

The response to the ad was a noteworthy event in the development of sleep disorders medicine. With one or two exceptions, none of the patients with narcolepsy had ever been correctly diagnosed. Responsibility for their clinical management had to be assumed to facilitate their participation in the research. The late Dr. Stephen Mitchell, who had completed his neurology training and was entering a psychiatry residency at Stanford University, joined Dement in creating a narcolepsy clinic in 1964, and soon they were managing well over 100 patients. This program constituted a precursor to the typical sleep disorders clinic, because at least one daytime polygraphic sleep recording was performed in all patients to establish the presence of SOREMPs. Unfortunately, insurance companies declared that sleep recordings in narcoleptic patients were experimental, forcing the closure of the clinic because of insufficient funds.

EUROPEAN INTEREST

In a 1963 symposium held in Paris, organized by Professor H. Fischgold, the proceedings were published as *La Sommeil de Nuit Normal et Pathologique* in 1965.[44] The primary clinical emphasis in this symposium was the documentation of sleep-related epileptic seizures and analyses of a number of related studies on sleepwalking and night terrors. Investigators from France, Italy, Belgium, Germany, and the Netherlands took part. The important role of European sleep scientists in the establishment of clinical sleep medicine is discussed later in this chapter.

BENZODIAZEPINES AND HYPNOTIC EFFICACY STUDIES

Parallel to the discoveries being made in narcolepsy, a renewed interest in the pharmacologic treatment of insomnia was emerging. Benzodiazepines were introduced in 1960 with the marketing of chlordiazepoxide (Librium). This was quickly followed by diazepam (Valium) and the first benzodiazepine introduced specifically as a hypnotic, flurazepam (Dalmane). The first use of the sleep laboratory to evaluate sleeping pills may have been in the 1965 study by Oswald and Priest.[45] An important series of studies establishing the role of the sleep laboratory in the evaluation of hypnotic efficacy was carried out by Anthony Kales and colleagues at the University of California Los Angeles.[46] This group also carried out pioneering studies of patients with hypothyroidism, asthma, Parkinson disease, and somnambulism.[47-50]

THE DISCOVERY OF SLEEP APNEA

The original description of sleep apnea often is attributed to independent publications by Gastaut, Tassinari, and Duron in France and by Jung and Kuhlo in Germany.[51,52] Both of these groups reported their findings in 1965. Earlier work in this area deserves mention (Christian Guilleminault, personal communication, 2014). In a report published in German, a group from Heidelberg University Hospital in 1960 described a patient who had come to the hospital for investigation of recurring morning headaches and was observed to have respiratory pauses during sleep, with recovery breathing associated with a loud snore. A polygraphic recording during a nap was included in the publication.[53] Drachman and Gumnit described evaluation of an obese woman using electroencephalography and blood gas analysis, which identified repetitive stoppage of air exchange despite persistence of thoracoabdominal movements. The patient was placed on a strict diet and after a significant weight loss saw her sleepiness disappear.[54] No further publications in the area of sleep from this group are available, so it appears their work was not appreciated at the time. Peretz Lavie has detailed the historical contributions made by scientists and clinicians around the world in helping to describe and elucidate this disorder.[21]

These important findings were widely ignored in the United States (Video 1.2). The well-known and frequently cited study by Burwell and colleagues—although impressive in a literary sense in its evoking of the somnolent boy Joe from *The Pickwick Papers*—erred badly in evaluating their somnolent obese patients only during waking and in attributing the cause of the somnolence to hypercapnia.[55] The popularity of this paper further reduced the likelihood of discovery of sleep apnea by the pulmonary community. The term *pickwickian* was an instant success as a neologism, and its colorful connotations may have played a role in stimulating interest in this syndrome by the European neurologists who also were interested in sleep.

A small group of French neurologists were in the vanguard of clinical sleep research. Among these was Christian Guilleminault, who was instrumental in later establishing the specialty of clinical sleep medicine at Stanford and throughout the world. Guilleminault also was the first to describe obstructive sleep apnea as a clinical syndrome.[56,57]

One of the collaborators in the French discovery of sleep apnea, C. Alberto Tassinari, joined the Italian neurologist Elio Lugaresi in Bologna in 1970. These clinical investigators, along with Giorgio Coccagna and a host of others, including Guilleminault, over the years performed a crucial series of clinical sleep investigations and, indeed, provided a complete description of the sleep apnea syndrome, including the first observations of the occurrence of sleep apnea in nonobese patients, an account of the cardiovascular correlates, and a clear identification of the importance of snoring and hypersomnolence as diagnostic indicators. These studies are recounted in Lugaresi's book, *Hypersomnia with Periodic Apneas*, published in 1978.[58]

ITALIAN SYMPOSIA

In 1967 Henri Gastaut and Elio Lugaresi (Figure 1.4) organized a symposium, the proceedings of which were published as *The Abnormalities of Sleep in Man*, that encompassed issues across a full range of pathologic sleep in humans.[59] This meeting took place in Bologna, Italy, and the papers presented covered many of what are now major topics in the sleep medicine field: insomnia, sleep apnea, narcolepsy, and periodic leg movements during sleep. It was an epic meeting from the standpoint of the clinical investigation of sleep; the only major issues not represented were clear concepts of clinical practice models and hard data on the high population prevalence of sleep disorders. However, the event that may have finally triggered a serious

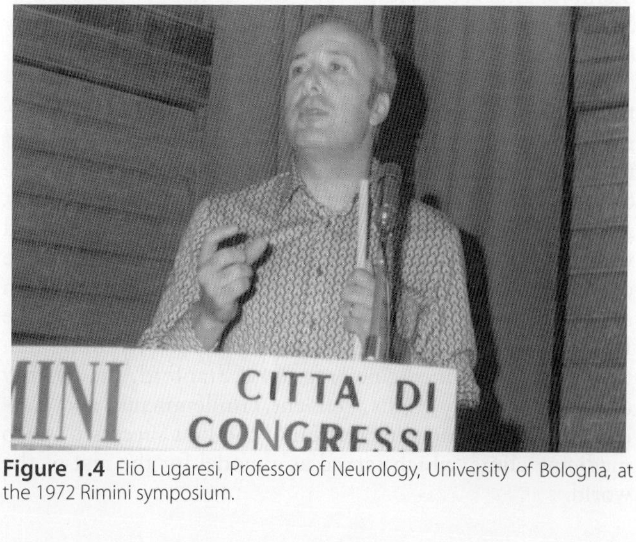

Figure 1.4 Elio Lugaresi, Professor of Neurology, University of Bologna, at the 1972 Rimini symposium.

international interest in sleep apnea syndromes was a symposium organized by Lugaresi in 1972, which took place in Rimini, a small resort on the Adriatic coast.[54]

BIRTH PANGS

Despite all the clinical research, the concept of all-night sleep recordings as a clinical diagnostic test did not emerge for years for several reasons: financial and insurance issues; lack of outpatient facilities; reluctance of nonhospital clinical professionals to work at night; and lack of medical professionals with knowledge about sleep.

Even narcolepsy, which by the early 1970s, was fully characterized as an interesting and disabling clinical syndrome requiring sleep recordings for diagnosis, was not recognized in the larger medical community and was thought to have too low a prevalence to warrant creating a medical subspecialty. A study carried out in 1972 documented a mean of 15 years from onset of the characteristic symptoms of excessive daytime sleepiness and cataplexy to diagnosis and treatment by a clinician. The study also showed that a mean of 5.5 different physicians were consulted without benefit throughout that long interval.[60]

EARLY DEVELOPMENT OF STANFORD SLEEP MEDICINE CLINICAL PRACTICE

Creation of the sleep disorders clinic at Stanford University was in many ways a microcosm of how sleep medicine evolved throughout the world. Dement arrived at Stanford in 1963 to establish a sleep research program. A need for clinical application of the knowledge being acquired soon became obvious. By 1964 subjects in narcolepsy trials also were managed as patients. Patients complaining of insomnia were enrolled in hypnotic efficacy research studies. This arrangement brought the Stanford group into contact with many patients afflicted with insomnia and demolished the notion that a majority of such patients had psychiatric problems. Throughout the second half of the 1960s, as a part of their research, the Stanford group continued to manage patients with narcolepsy and insomnia. As the group's reputation for expertise grew, it began to receive referrals for evaluation from physicians all over the United States. Vincent Zarcone, a psychiatrist, joined this effort to develop the field of clinical sleep medicine at Stanford. In 1970 a sleep clinic was formally established at Stanford. Not surprisingly, the fledging clinic immediately struggled with reimbursement issues.

When the Stanford clinic was opened in 1970, the central role of obstructive sleep apnea as a mechanism of sleep-related pathology was not yet appreciated by this group. It took an international meeting in Bruges, Belgium, for the Stanford group to recognize the importance of this entity. At that meeting, Dr. Zarcone was particularly impressed with Christian Guilleminault, a neurologist with knowledge of sleep apnea who had previously performed sleep research at Stanford with Dr. Steve Hendrickson. As a result of the Bruges meeting, Guilleminault was recruited to strengthen the clinical sleep medicine program at Stanford. The synergy of these three physicians, Dement, Guilleminault, and Zarcone, set in motion the creation of the first successful sleep medicine clinic, which served as a model for the rest of the world.

Starting in 1972, these respiratory and cardiac sensors became a routine part of the all-night diagnostic test. This test was given the permanent name of *polysomnography* in 1974 by Dr. Jerome Holland, a member of the Stanford group. Publicity about narcolepsy and excessive sleepiness resulted in a small flow of referrals to the Stanford sleep clinic, usually with the presumptive diagnosis of narcolepsy. During the first few years, the goal for the Stanford practice was to see at least four new patients per week.

Toward the end of 1972, the basic concepts and formats of sleep disorders medicine were sculpted to the extent that it was possible to offer a daylong course through Stanford University's Division of Postgraduate Medicine. In this course, titled *Sleep Disorders: A New Clinical Discipline*, the topics covered were normal sleep architecture; the diagnosis and treatment of insomnia, with drug-dependent insomnia, pseudoinsomnia, central sleep apnea, and periodic leg movement as diagnostic entities; and the diagnosis and treatment of excessive daytime sleepiness or hypersomnia, with narcolepsy, NREM narcolepsy, and obstructive sleep apnea as diagnostic entities (Figure 1.5).

The cardiovascular complications of severe sleep apnea were alarming and often completely disabling. Unfortunately, the treatment options at this time were limited to often ineffective attempts to lose weight and chronic tracheostomy. The dramatic results of chronic tracheostomy in ameliorating the symptoms and complications of obstructive sleep apnea had been reported by Lugaresi and colleagues in 1970.[61] The notion of using such a treatment, however, was strongly resisted at the time by the medical community. One of the first patients referred to the Stanford sleep clinic for investigation of this severe somnolence and hypertension and who eventually had a tracheostomy was a 10-year-old boy. From the very

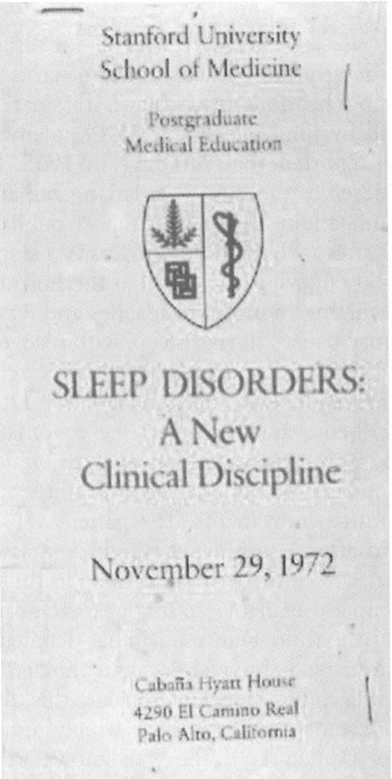

Figure 1.5 First Stanford meeting for the new clinical discipline of sleep medicine.

beginning of the development of clinical sleep medicine, children and adults were treated together. The recognition of polysomnography in California as a reimbursable diagnostic test in 1974 opened the doors for the practice of sleep medicine throughout the nation. In retrospect, it seems clear that the educational effort exerted and resulting policy decisions have undoubtedly saved countless lives and improved the health and well-being of millions of people worldwide.

CLINICAL SIGNIFICANCE OF EXCESSIVE DAYTIME SLEEPINESS

Christian Guilleminault, in a series of studies, had clearly shown that excessive daytime sleepiness was a major clinical complaint in several sleep disorders, as well as a pathologic phenomenon unto itself.[62] It was recognized, however, that methods to quantify this symptom and the underlying condition were not adequate to quantify the treatment outcome. The subjective Stanford Sleepiness Scale, developed by Hoddes and colleagues, did not give reliable results.[63] With the creation of sleep medicine clinics, a new problem emerged: how to objectively quantitate sleepiness.

An early attempt to develop an objective measure of sleepiness was that of Yoss and colleagues, who observed pupil diameter directly by video monitoring and described changes in sleep deprivation and narcolepsy.[64] Subsequently designated *pupillometry,* this technique has not been widely accepted. Dr. Mary Carskadon, while at Stanford, deserves most of the credit for the development of the latter-day standard approach to the measurement of sleepiness, called the Multiple Sleep Latency Test (MSLT).[65] She noted that subjective ratings of sleepiness made before a sleep recording frequently predicted the sleep latency. In the spring of 1976 she undertook to establish sleep latency as an objective measurement of the state of "sleepiness-alertness" by measuring sleep tendency before, during, and after 2 days of total sleep deprivation.[66] The protocol designed for this study has become the standard protocol for the MSLT. The choices of a 20-minute duration of a single test and a 2-hour interval between tests were essentially arbitrary and dictated by the practical demands of that study. This test was then formally applied to the clinical evaluation of sleepiness in patients with narcolepsy and, later, in patients with OSA.[67,68]

Carskadon, along with Sharon Keenan and other colleagues, then undertook a monumental study of sleepiness in children by following them longitudinally across the second decade of life, which is also the decade of highest risk for the development of narcolepsy. Using the new MSLT measure, these investigators found that 10-year-old children were completely alert in the daytime, but by the time the subjects reached sexual maturity, they were no longer fully alert, even though they obtained almost the same amount of sleep at night as they did during the study period. Results of this remarkable decade of work and other studies are summarized in an important review.[69] In an effort spearheaded by Dr. Rafael Pelayo, Stanford University acknowledged the importance of this historic work by installing a permanent plaque in 2012 at the dormitory that housed this research (Figure 1.6).

Early MSLT research established the following important advances in thinking:

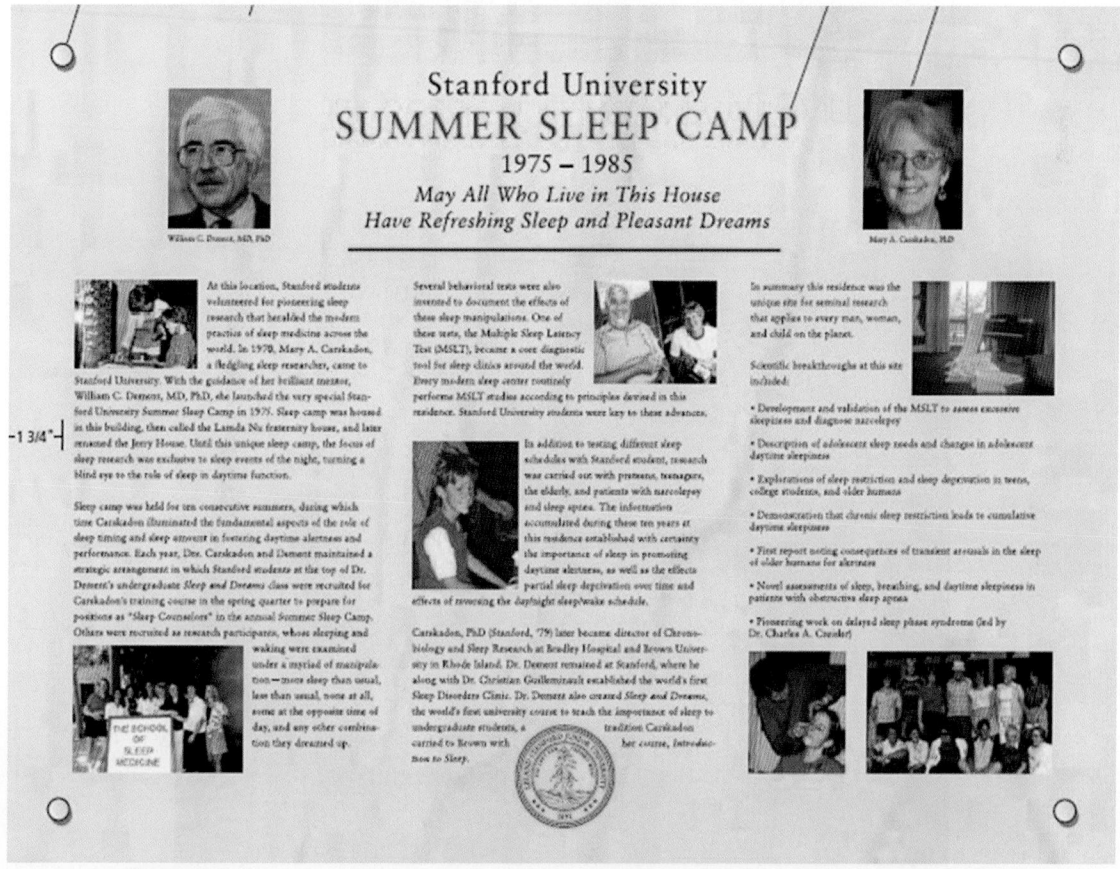

Figure 1.6 Plaque describing Summer Sleep Camp and development of the Multiple Sleep Latency Test.

1. Daytime sleepiness and nighttime sleep are components of an interactive continuum, and the adequacy of nighttime sleep absolutely cannot be understood without a complementary measurement of the level of daytime sleepiness or its antonym, alertness.
2. Excessive sleepiness, also known as impaired alertness, was sleep medicine's most important symptom.

FURTHER DEVELOPMENT OF SLEEP MEDICINE

As the decade of the 1970s drew to a close, the consolidation and formalization of the practice of sleep disorders medicine were largely completed. What is now the American Academy of Sleep Medicine was formed and provided a home for professionals interested in sleep and, particularly, in the diagnosis and treatment of sleep disorders. This body, the Association of Sleep Disorders Centers (ASDC), began with five members in 1975. The organization then was responsible for the initiation of the scientific journal *Sleep*. It fostered the setting of standards through center accreditation and an examination for practitioners by which they were designated "Accredited Clinical Polysomnographers."

Dr. Christian Guilleminault served as the first editor of the journal *Sleep* and remained editor in chief until 1997 (Figure 1.7). He was also the most prolific contributor to the first editions of this textbook. He embodied the way clinical sleep medicine is practiced throughout the world. He passed away in 2019. Dr. William Dement described the importance of Dr. Guilleminault to the sleep field as follows:

> Christian Guilleminault changed the world. When he joined the Stanford Sleep Disorders Clinic with his incredible energy and intellect, he truly put Sleep Disorders Medicine on the map. He was among the first to recognize obstructive sleep apnea and to describe central sleep apnea. He designed protocols for their diagnoses and treatment. I feel extremely fortunate to have had Christian as a colleague and friend. Our collaboration was invaluable to me, both professionally and personally. He tried unsuccessfully to teach me to speak French—that was my fault, not his. He was a beloved supportive mentor to hundreds of new fellows, a founding editor of the journal *Sleep*, and a dedicated clinician who really preferred to score all the records himself. Finally, Christian did more to put Sleep Disorders Medicine on the world stage than anyone else. I feel extremely fortunate that he joined me at Stanford. I will cherish his memory, as should tens of thousands of sleep disorders patients.

The first international symposium on narcolepsy took place in the French Languedoc in the summer of 1975, immediately

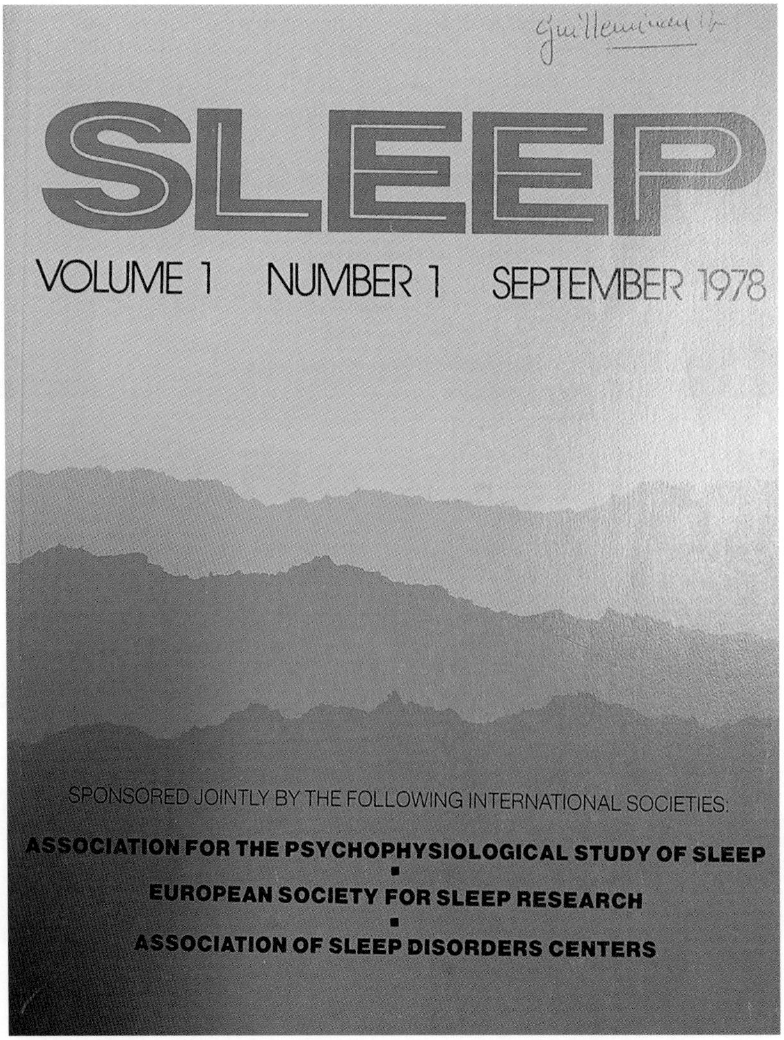

Figure 1.7 Christian Guilleminault's personal copy of first issue of *Sleep*.

after the Second International Congress of the Association for the Physiological Study of Sleep (APSS) in Edinburgh. The APSS meeting, in addition to being scientifically productive, was of landmark significance because it produced the first consensus definition of a specific sleep disorder, drafted, revised, and unanimously endorsed by 65 narcolepsy experts of international reputation.[70] The first sleep disorders patient volunteer organization, the American Narcolepsy Association, also was formed in 1975. The ASDC/APSS Diagnostic Classification of Sleep and Arousal Disorders was published in fall 1979 after 3 years of extraordinary effort by a small group of dedicated persons who made up the "nosology" committee chaired by Dr. Howard Roffwarg.[71] This early nosology was the precursor to the subsequent versions of the International Classification of Sleep Disorders.

Before the 1980s the only effective treatment for severe OSA was chronic tracheostomy. This highly effective but personally undesirable approach was replaced by two new procedures—one surgical, the other mechanical.[72,73] The first was uvulopalatopharyngoplasty (UPPP), which at the time was considered an advance, eventually fell into disfavor because it was both painful and often ineffective. However, UPPP did pave the way for more sophisticated and effective surgical options. The second was the widely used and highly effective continuous positive nasal airway pressure (CPAP) technique introduced by the Australian pulmonologist Colin Sullivan (Video 1.3). The first CPAP machines were very loud and uncomfortable. Fortunately, as the technology improved, CPAP devices entered the medical mainstream. The combination of the high prevalence of OSA and, at the time, newly effective treatments fueled a significant expansion of sleep centers and clinicians. The ramifications of this growth are still being felt today.

The 1980s were capped by the publication of sleep medicine's first textbook, the first edition of *Principles and Practice of Sleep Medicine*.[74] For many years only one medical journal devoted to sleep existed; today, several are in publication, including *Sleep, Journal of Clinical Sleep Medicine, Sleep Health, Journal of Sleep Research, Sleep and Biological Rhythms, Sleep & Breathing, Sleep Medicine, Sleep Medicine Reviews,* and *Sleep Research Online.* Articles about sleep are now routinely published in the major pulmonary, neurology, ear-nose-throat (ENT), pediatric, primary care, and psychiatric journals.

The 1990s saw an acceleration in the acceptance of sleep medicine throughout the world. Nonetheless, adequate sleep medicine services are still not readily available everywhere.[75,76]

In the United States, the National Center on Sleep Disorders Research (NCSDR) was established by statute as part of the National Heart, Lung, and Blood Institute of the National Institutes of Health.[77] The mandate of the NCSDR is to support research, promote educational activities, and coordinate sleep-related activities throughout various branches of the US government. It is perhaps too easy to criticize any government body or to decry insufficient research funding, yet the mere recognition by the federal government of the importance of sleep by establishing the NCSDR is a huge achievement when taken in the perspective of how the sleep field began. This government initiative led to the development of large research projects dealing with various aspects of sleep disorders and the establishment of awards to develop educational materials at all levels of training.

The 1990s also saw the establishment of the National Sleep Foundation, as well as other organizations for patients. This foundation points out to the public the dangers of sleepiness and sponsors the annual National Sleep Awareness Week.

As the internet increases exponentially in size, so does the availability of sleep knowledge for physicians, patients, and the general public. The average person today knows a great deal more about sleep and its disorders than the average person did at the end of the 1980s. It is perhaps unique to the sleep field that the internet, on the one hand, has increased the availability of information on sleep. On the other hand, it seems self-evident that the internet also has accelerated humanity's march toward a sleepless 24-hour society and has increased the pressure for sleep deprivation and poor hygiene, in particular among the young.

THE 21ST CENTURY AND BEYOND

The historical early development of clinical sleep medicine culminated with its acceptance in 2003 by the Accreditation Council on Graduate Medical Education (ACGME) as a formal training program. The field emerged from its embryonic origins to worldwide acceptance in a relatively short period of time, owing in no small part to the great public need for healthier sleep and alertness. The recognition of the importance of sleep as a health and wellness component was exemplified by the appointment of sleep researcher Dr. Mark Rosekind to the National Transportation Safety Board (NTSB) in 2010. For the first time in its history, the NTSB had a trained sleep scientist as a board member (Figure 1.8). The impact of this recognition is likely to be very far-reaching for public safety.

In 2019 California Governor Newsom signed the first law to recognize the importance of sleep for adolescents. Without any external fundraising, a group of volunteers were able to generate support for a bill introduced by state Senator Anthony Portantino that delayed the start of public high schools in the state to be no earlier than 8:30 a.m. This law is serving as a

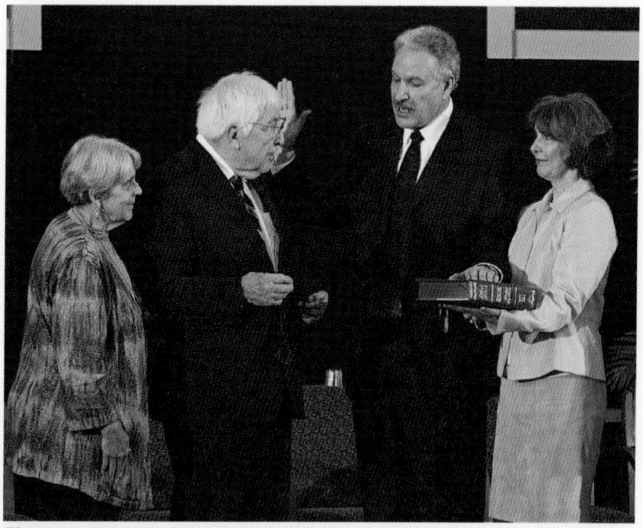

Figure 1.8 Dr. Mark Rosekind is sworn in by Dr. William Dement as the first sleep scientist at the National Transportation Safety Board (NTSB). Drs. Mary Carskadon and Deborah Babcock look on. In 2015 Dr. Rosekind was appointed administrator to the National Highway Traffic Safety Administration. (With permission from Dr. Rosekind and the NTSB.)

model for other states to follow and highlights how far public awareness of sleep has advanced. Dr. William Dement, who played such a vital role in the field, died in 2020.

A new reality is facing the sleep field, which will likely inevitably change the future direction of our field. In 2020 the field of sleep medicine faced perhaps its greatest existential crisis with the outbreak of the worldwide COVID-19 viral pandemic. At the time of this writing, the COVID-19 pandemic was wreaking havoc. It forced us to accelerate the use of home sleep testing (HST) and autotitration positive airway pressure (PAP) devices and the adoption of telemedicine services. The increased use of telemedicine services extended beyond OSA to insomnia and other sleep conditions.

The changes imposed by necessity during the pandemic were expected to produce long-lasting impacts on clinical guidelines, practice patterns, and reimbursement policies. To avoid viral exposure, many sleep laboratories were forced to shut down. Smaller sleep labs faced greater financial pressure as they struggled to provide patient care in a safe environment. With the spreading pandemic, the role of the polysomnography technologist changed with a greater focus on HST. The type of HST utilized was also influenced by the pandemic with a reassessment of equipment and work environment cleaning protocols and a greater reliance on disposable products. Although innovative, disposable HST also produced concerns regarding increased medical waste and cost.

The pandemic forced large, stressed populations to stay indoors and work from home, resulting in changed sleep patterns and sleep problems (see chapter 213). Many patients who recovered from COVID-19 had chronic sleep complaints and fatigue. Because the pandemic coincided with the continued use of consumer technologies that track various health metrics, including sleep, we anticipate that large data sets will emerge that will help us understand how the population's sleep health was affected by social distancing and the stressors of this unprecedented event.

Perhaps in the end, the lessons learned from the COVID-19 pandemic will allow us to do more with less and transform our care to rely more heavily on patient history and outcomes than in laboratory testing.

Sleep medicine has grown tremendously. To put this in perspective, in 1975 the only institutions in the United States offering clinical sleep studies, other than Stanford, were Montefiore Medical Center in New York, Ohio State University, Baylor College in Houston, University of Cincinnati Medical Center, and the University of Pittsburgh Medical School. Now the American Academy of Sleep Medicine (AASM) membership consists of more than 10,000 individuals and accredited member sleep centers. There are more than 2,600 AASM-accredited sleep centers across the United States. As of 2018 close to 6,000 physicians are board certified in sleep medicine in the United States. Sleep medicine and sleep research are increasingly recognized as important throughout the world. The World Sleep Society was founded in 2016 by merging the World Sleep Federation and the World Association of Sleep Medicine. The society has associated professional societies throughout the Americas, Europe, Asia, Australia, and Africa. The society hosts a large biennial meeting, which in 2019 hosted attendees from 77 countries. Worldwide there are an estimated 80 journals covering the sleep field.

From today's vantage point, the greatest challenge for the future is the cost-effective expansion of sleep medicine to provide benefit to the increasing number of patients in society. The management of sleep deprivation and its serious consequences in the workplace, particularly in those industries that depend on sustained operations, continues to require increased attention. Healthy sleep must be a priority for everyone.

The education and training of all health professionals have far to go. This situation was highlighted by the report of the Institute of Medicine.[76] These problems also represent grand opportunities for research. Sleep medicine has come into its own. It has made concern for health a truly 24-hours-a-day enterprise, and it has energized a new effort to reveal the secrets of the healthy and unhealthy sleeping brain.

Looking back at the history of sleep medicine forces the medical profession, and society as a whole, to look forward to the future. The future of sleep research indeed promises to be exciting. Finally answering the ancient questions about the basic functions of sleep and dreaming may be within the grasp of the current generation of young scientists. They would not be poised for these future discoveries if not for the early work described in this chapter.

Many times during its history, the young sleep medicine field seemed to be doomed to fail, yet the huge need to understand sleep and its disorders continued to push it forward (Videos 1.4 and 1.5). Currently, as the field faces new challenges with changes in health care and reimbursement policies, it is easy to be pessimistic about its future. Yet such challenges constitute part of a natural process of change. The forces that have driven the field forward are, if anything, expanding. The population is growing and getting older. Increasingly, people are expected to be alert and productive in a 24-hour society. An increasing role for ambulatory sleep testing and telehealth delivery models are being incorporated. Wearable devices that measure sleep are becoming increasingly popular, not just for medical application but also as part of general health and wellness awareness. Consequently, sleep medicine must continue to adapt to these societal changes. All practitioners in both sleep medicine and sleep research should keep in mind that millions of people have benefited from their work and that billions more still need their help.

We have good reason to remain realistically optimistic about the future of sleep medicine.

CLINICAL PEARL

Recent advances in sleep science, sleep medicine, public policy, and communications will foster an educated public that will know a great deal about sleep and its disorders. Clinicians should expect that their patients may have already learned about their sleep disorders from the information sources that are readily available. They also may have received considerable misinformation from these same sources. Sleep professionals need to know the history of sleep medicine for proper perspective and useful insights as the field evolves.

SUMMARY

Interest in sleep dates to antiquity and has influenced all cultures and religions. Ancient medical texts describe treatments for sleep problems such as insomnia. Just over 100 years ago, sleep was thought of as a passive state. The use of electroencephalography led to the concept of sleep as an active state. The discovery of REM sleep in the 1950s allowed empirical challenge to previously held beliefs. The formal study of sleep disorders using polysomnography progressed in the 1960s. Obstructive sleep apnea was described mostly by researchers based in Europe at that time. Despite a series of false steps, clinical sleep medicine was established at Stanford University in 1970 and shortly thereafter in other institutions. The organization of these groups led to the creation of professional sleep societies and further worldwide growth and recognition of sleep medicine. Sleep medicine was recognized in 2003 by the ACGME as a formal training program. The field continues to evolve. The COVID-19 viral pandemic has forced the sleep field to adapt to a new landscape. As sleep medicine faces new challenges, an appreciation of its historical background can provide practitioners with insights for shaping the future of the discipline.

SELECTED READINGS

Carskadon MA, Dement WC, Mitler MM, et al. Guidelines for the Multiple Sleep Latency Test (MSLT): a standard measure of sleepiness. *Sleep*. 1986;9:519–524.

Dement W, Kleitman N. The relation of eye movements during sleep to dream activity: an objective method for the study of dreaming. *J Exp Psychol*. 1957;53:339–346.

Dement WC, Vaughan CC. *The Promise of Sleep: A Pioneer in Sleep Medicine Explores the Vital Connection Between Health, Happiness, and A Good Night's Sleep*. New York: Delacorte Press; 1999.

Freud S. *The Interpretation of Dreams*. 3rd ed. New York: The Macmillan Company; 1913.

Gastaut H, Lugaresi E, Berti-Ceroni G, Coccagna G. *The Abnormalities of Sleep in Man*. Bologna (Italy): Aulo Gaggi Editore; 1968.

Guilleminault C, Dement WC, Kroc Foundation. *Sleep Apnea Syndromes*. New York: Alan R. Liss; 1978.

Guilleminault C, Dement WC, Passouant P. *Narcolepsy: Proceedings of the First International Symposium on Narcolepsy, July 1975. Montpellier, France*. New York: SP Books, division of Spectrum Publications (distributed by Halstead Press); 1976.

Hobson JA. *Sleep*. New York: Scientific American Library: (distributed by W.H. Freeman); 1989.

Johnson KG, Sullivan SS, Nti A, Rastegar V, Gurubhagavatula I. The impact of the COVID-19 pandemic on sleep medicine practices. *J Clin Sleep Med*. 2021;17(1):79–87.

Kleitman N. *Sleep and Wakefulness*. Rev. and enl. ed. Chicago: University of Chicago Press; 1963.

Mignot EJ. History of narcolepsy at Stanford University. *Immunol Res*. 2014;58:315–339.

Rosekind M. Awakening a nation: a call to action. *Sleep Health*. 2015;1:9–10.

A complete reference list can be found online at ExpertConsult.com.

Chapter 2

Normal Human Sleep: An Overview

Shannon S. Sullivan; Mary A. Carskadon; William C. Dement†; Chandra L. Jackson

Chapter Highlights

- Normal human sleep comprises two states—rapid eye movement (REM) and non–rapid eye movement (NREM) sleep—that alternate cyclically across a sleep episode. State characteristics are well defined: NREM sleep includes a variably synchronous cortical electroencephalogram (EEG; including sleep spindles, K-complexes, and slow waves) associated with low muscle tonus and minimal psychological activity; the REM sleep EEG is desynchronized, muscles are atonic, and dreaming is typical.
- A nightly pattern of sleep in mature humans sleeping on a regular schedule includes several reliable characteristics: Sleep begins in NREM and progresses through deeper NREM stages (stages N2 and N3 using the American Academy of Sleep Medicine Scoring Manual definitions, or stages 2, 3, and 4 using the classic definitions) before the first episode of REM sleep occurs about 80 to 100 minutes later. Thereafter, NREM sleep and REM sleep cycle with a period of about 90 minutes. NREM stages 3 and 4 (or stage N3) concentrate in the early NREM cycles, and REM sleep episodes lengthen across the night.
- Age-related changes in sleep architecture are also predictable: Newborn humans enter REM sleep (called active sleep) before NREM (called quiet sleep) and have a shorter sleep cycle (about 50 minutes); coherent sleep stages emerge as the brain matures during the first year. At birth, active sleep is about 50% of total sleep and declines over the first 2 years to about 20% to 25%. NREM sleep slow waves are not present at birth but emerge in the first 2 years. Slow wave sleep (N3; classically, stages 3 and 4) decreases across adolescence by about 40% from preteen years and continues a slower decline into old age, particularly in men and less so in women. REM sleep as a percentage of total sleep is relatively stable at about 20% to 25% across childhood, adolescence, adulthood, and into old age, except in dementia (see Figure 2.8, *B*).
- Other factors predictably alter sleep, such as previous sleep-wake history (i.e., homeostatic load); phase of the circadian timing system; environmental conditions; medications and substances; genetics[1]; and sleep, medical, and psychiatric disorders.

WHAT IS NORMAL?

Sleep is essential for human life and good sleep supports health. A clear appreciation of the normal characteristics of sleep provides a strong background and template for understanding clinical conditions in which "normal" characteristics are altered, as well as for interpreting certain consequences of sleep disorders. In this chapter, the normal young adult sleep pattern is described as a working baseline pattern. Normative changes associated with aging and other factors are summarized with that background in mind. Several major sleep disorders are highlighted by their differences from the normative pattern, as highlighted in the text that follows.

WHAT CHARACTERISTICS AND MEASURES ARE USED TO DEFINE SLEEP?

According to a simple behavioral definition, sleep is a reversible behavioral state of perceptual disengagement from an unresponsiveness to the environment. It is also true that sleep is a complex amalgam of physiologic and behavioral processes. Sleep is typically (but not necessarily) accompanied by postural recumbence, behavioral quiescence, closed eyes, and all the other indicators commonly associated with sleeping. At times, behaviors typically associated with wake can occur during sleep. These behaviors can include sleepwalking, sleeptalking, teeth grinding, and other physical activities. The converse is also true: in some conditions, intrusions of sleep-related processes may occur when awake: muscle atonia, dream imagery, and even microsleep episodes, for example.

Within sleep, two separate states have been defined on the basis of a constellation of physiologic parameters. These two states of sleep, rapid eye movement (REM) and non–rapid eye movement (NREM), exist in virtually all mammals and birds yet studied, and these states are as distinct from one another as each is from wakefulness. (See Box 2.1 for a discussion of sleep stage nomenclature.)

† Deceased.

Box 2.1 SLEEP MEDICINE METHODOLOGY AND NOMENCLATURE

In 2007 the American Academy of Sleep Medicine (AASM) published a new manual for scoring sleep and associated events. This manual recommends alterations to recording methodology and terminology that the AASM will demand of clinical laboratories in the future. Although specifications of arousal, cardiac, movement, and respiratory rules appear to be value-added to the assessment of sleep-related events, the new rules, terminology, and technical specifications for recording and scoring sleep are not without controversy.

The current chapter uses the traditional terminology and definitions on which most descriptive and experimental research has been based since the 1960s.[68] Thus where the AASM uses the terms *N* for NREM sleep stages and *R* for REM sleep stages, *N1* and *N2* are used instead of stage 1 and stage 2; *N3* is used to indicate the sum of stage 3 and stage 4 (often called *slow wave sleep* in human literature); and *R* is used to name REM sleep. Another change is to the nomenclature for the recording placements. Therefore calling the auricular placements *M1* and *M2* (rather than *A1* and *A2*) is unnecessary and places the sleep electroencephalogram (EEG) recording terminology outside the pale for EEG recording terminology in other disciplines. Although these are somewhat trivial changes, changes in nomenclature can result in confusion when attempting to compare with previous literature and established data sets and are of concern for clinicians and investigators who communicate with other fields.

Of greater concern are changes to the core recording and scoring recommendations that the AASM manual recommends. For example, the recommended scoring montage requires using a frontal (*F3* or *F4*) EEG placement with visual scoring of the recordings, rather than the central (*C3* or *C4*) EEG placements recommended in the standard manual. The rationale for the change is that the frontal placements pick up more slow wave activity during sleep. The consequences, however, are that sleep studies performed and scored with the frontal EEG cannot be compared with normative or clinical data and that the frontal placements also truncate the ability to visualize sleep spindles. Furthermore, developmental changes to the regional EEG preclude the universal assumption that sleep slow wave activity is a frontal event.

Other issues are present in this new AASM approach to human sleep; however, this is not the venue for a complete description of such concerns. In summary, specifications for recording and scoring sleep are not without controversy, and the AASM scoring manual in its current form may not be considered the universal standard for assessing human sleep.[69-74]

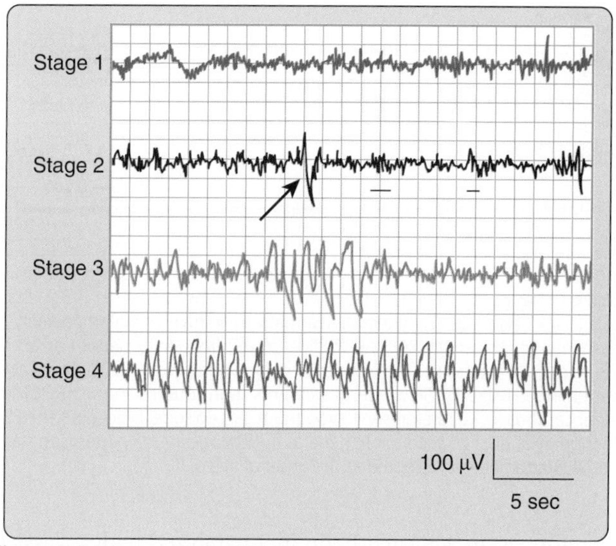

Figure 2.1 The stages of NREM sleep. The four electroencephalogram tracings depicted here are from a 19-year-old female volunteer. Each tracing was recorded from a referential lead (C3/A2) on a Grass Instruments (West Warwick, RI) Model 7D polygraph with a paper speed of 10 mm/sec, time constant of 0.3 seconds, and ½-amplitude, high-frequency setting of 30 Hz. On the second tracing, the *arrow* indicates a K-complex and the *underlining* shows two sleep spindles.

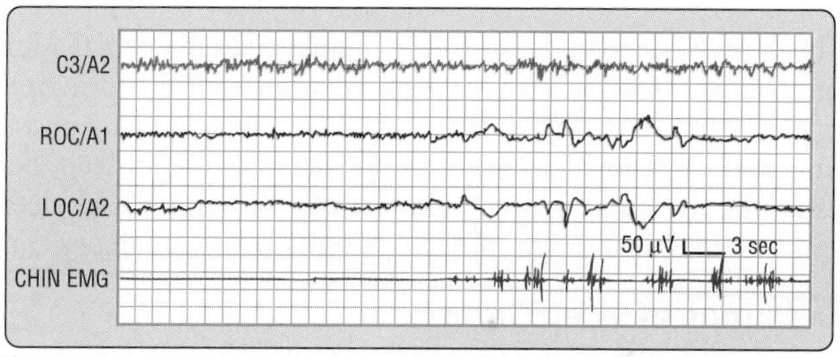

Figure 2.2 Phasic events in human REM sleep. On the *left side* is a burst of several rapid eye movements (out-of-phase deflections in right outer canthus [ROC]/A1 and left outer canthus [LOC]/A2). On the *right side*, there are additional rapid eye movements, as well as twitches on the electromyographic (EMG) lead. The interval between eye movement bursts and twitches illustrates tonic REM sleep.

NREM (pronounced *non-REM*) sleep is conventionally subdivided into four stages defined along one measurement axis, the surface electroencephalogram (EEG). The EEG pattern in NREM sleep is commonly described as synchronous, with such characteristic waveforms as sleep spindles, K-complexes, and high-voltage slow waves (Figure 2.1). The four classical NREM stages (stages 1, 2, 3, and 4) roughly parallel a depth-of-sleep continuum, with arousal thresholds generally lowest in stage 1 and highest in stage 4 sleep. NREM sleep is usually associated with minimal or fragmentary mental activity. A shorthand definition of NREM sleep is a relatively inactive yet actively regulating brain in a movable body.

REM sleep, by contrast, is defined by EEG activation, muscle atonia, and episodic bursts of rapid eye movements. REM sleep usually is not divided into stages, although tonic and phasic types of REM sleep have been identified for research and certain clinical purposes. The distinction of tonic versus phasic is based on short-lived events such as eye movements that tend to occur in clusters separated by episodes of relative quiescence. In cats, REM sleep phasic activity is epitomized by bursts of ponto-geniculo-occipital (PGO) waves, which are accompanied peripherally by rapid eye movements, twitching of distal muscles, middle ear muscle activity, and other phasic events that correspond to the phasic event markers easily measurable in humans. As described in Chapter 8, PGO waves are not usually detectable in humans. Thus the most commonly used marker of REM sleep phasic activity in humans is, of course, the occurrence of rapid eye movements (Figure 2.2); muscle twitches and cardiorespiratory irregularities often accompany the REM bursts. The mental activity of human REM sleep is associated with dreaming, based on vivid dream recall reported after about 80% of arousals from this state of sleep.[2] Inhibition of spinal motor neurons by brainstem mechanisms mediates suppression of postural motor tonus in REM sleep. A shorthand definition of REM sleep,

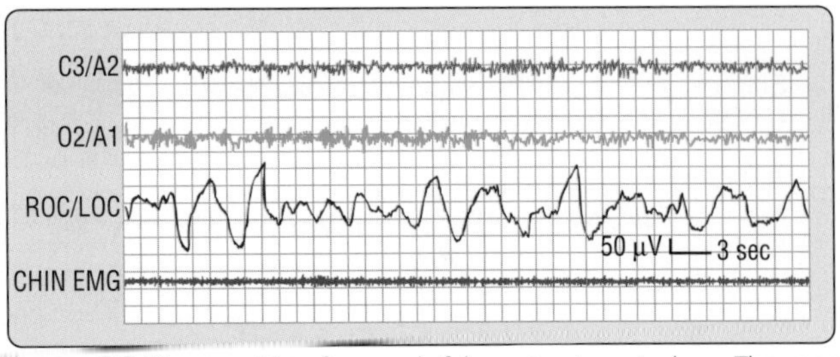

Figure 2.3 The transition from wakefulness to stage 1 sleep. The most marked change is visible on the two electroencephalographic (EEG) channels (C3/A2 and O2/A1), where a clear pattern of rhythmic alpha activity (8 cps) changes to a relatively low-voltage, mixed-frequency pattern at about the middle of the figure. The level of electromyographic (EMG) activity does not change markedly. Slow eye movements (right outer canthus [ROC]/left outer canthus [LOC]) are present throughout this episode, preceding the EEG change by at least 20 seconds. In general, the change in EEG patterns to stage 1 as illustrated here is accepted as the onset of sleep.

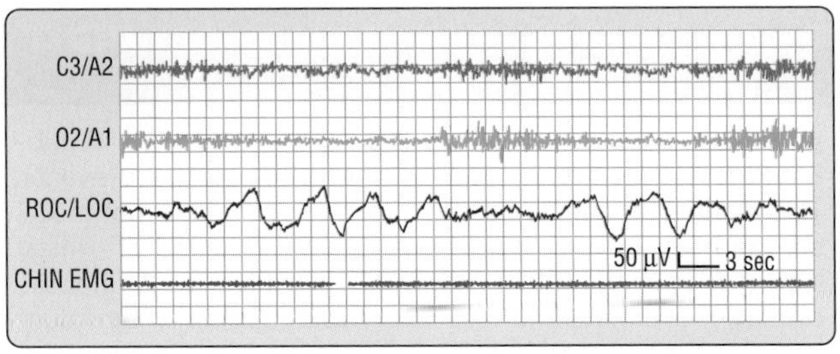

Figure 2.4 A common wake-to-sleep transition pattern. Note that the electroencephalographic pattern changes from wake (rhythmic alpha) to stage 1 (relatively low-voltage, mixed-frequency) sleep twice during this attempt to fall asleep. EMG, Electromyogram; LOC, left outer canthus; ROC, right outer canthus.

therefore, is an activated brain in a paralyzed body. Classical sleep staging relies on visual scoring. More recent advances in computer-assisted techniques such as spectral analysis of surface EEG patterns and intracerebral EEG recordings have revealed additional insights about the characteristics and richness of brain activity in sleep.[3]

SLEEP ONSET

The onset of sleep under normal circumstances in normal adult humans is through NREM sleep. This fundamental principle of normal human sleep reflects a highly reliable finding and is important in considering normal versus pathologic sleep. For example, the abnormal entry into sleep through REM sleep can be a diagnostic sign in adult patients with narcolepsy.

Definition of Sleep Onset

The precise definition of the onset of sleep has been a topic of debate, primarily because there is no single measure that is 100% clear-cut 100% of the time. For example, a change in EEG pattern is not always associated with a person's perception of sleep, yet even when subjects report that they are still awake, clear behavioral changes can indicate the presence of sleep. To begin consideration of this issue, let us examine the three basic polysomnographic measures of sleep and how they change with sleep onset. The electrode placements are described in Chapters 197 and 199.

Electroencephalogram

In the simplest circumstance (Figure 2.3), the EEG changes from a pattern of clear rhythmic alpha (8–13 cycles per second [cps]) activity, particularly in the occipital region, to a relatively low-voltage, mixed-frequency pattern (stage 1 sleep). This EEG change usually occurs seconds to minutes after the start of slow eye movements. With regard to introspection, the onset of a stage 1 EEG pattern may or may not coincide with perceived sleep onset. For this reason, a number of investigators require the presence of specific EEG patterns—the K-complex or sleep spindle (i.e., stage 2 sleep)—to acknowledge sleep onset. Even these stage 2 EEG patterns, however, are not unequivocally associated with perceived sleep.[4] A further complication is that sleep onset often does not occur all at once; instead, there may be a wavering of vigilance before "unequivocal" sleep ensues (Figure 2.4). Thus it is difficult to accept a single variable as marking sleep onset. As Davis and colleagues[5] wrote many years ago (p. 35):

Is "falling asleep" a unitary event? Our observations suggest that it is not. Different functions, such as sensory awareness, memory, self-consciousness, continuity of logical thought, latency of response to a stimulus, and alterations in the pattern of brain potentials all go in parallel in a general way, but there are exceptions to every rule. Nevertheless, a reasonable consensus exists that the EEG change to stage 1, usually heralded or accompanied by slow eye movements, identifies the transition to sleep, provided that another EEG sleep pattern does not intervene. One might not always be able to pinpoint this transition to the millisecond, but it is usually possible to determine the change reliably within several seconds.

Electrooculogram

As sleep approaches, the electrooculogram (EOG) shows slow, possibly asynchronous eye movements (Figure 2.3) that usually disappear within several minutes of the EEG changes described next. Occasionally, the onset of these slow eye movements coincides with a person's perceived sleep onset; more often, subjects report that they are still awake.

Electromyogram

The electromyogram (EMG) may show a gradual diminution of muscle tonus as sleep approaches, but rarely does a discrete EMG change pinpoint sleep onset. Furthermore, the presleep level of the EMG, particularly if the person is relaxed, can be entirely indistinguishable from that of unequivocal sleep (Figure 2.3).

Behavioral Concomitants of Sleep Onset

Given the changes in the EEG that accompany the onset of sleep, what are the behavioral correlates of the wake-to-sleep transition? The following material reviews a few common behavioral concomitants of sleep onset. Keep in mind that, as has been observed since the earliest days of sleep research in the 1930s, "different functions may be depressed in different sequence and to different degrees in different subjects and on different occasions."[3]

Simple Behavioral Response

In the first example, sleepy volunteers sitting at desks were asked to tap two switches alternately at a steady pace. As shown in Figure 2.5, this simple behavior continues after the onset of slow eye movements and may persist for several seconds after the EEG changes to a stage 1 sleep pattern.[6] The behavior

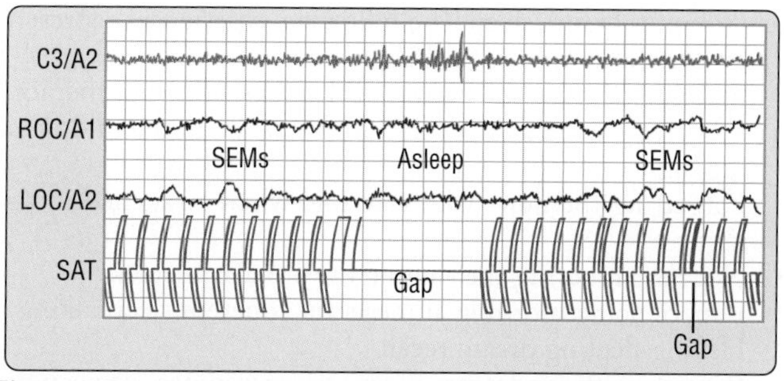

Figure 2.5 Failure to perform a simple behavioral task at the onset of sleep. The volunteer had been deprived of sleep overnight and was required to tap two switches alternately, shown as pen deflections of opposite polarity on the channel labeled SAT. When the electroencephalographic (EEG; C3/A2) pattern changes to stage 1 sleep, the behavior stops, returning when the EEG pattern reverts to wakefulness. LOC, Left outer canthus; ROC, right outer canthus; SEMs, slow eye movements. (From Carskadon MA, Dement WC. Effects of total sleep loss on sleep tendency. *Percept Mot Skills.* 1979;48:495-506.)

then ceases, usually to recur only after the EEG reverts to a waking pattern. This is an example of what one may think of as the simplest kind of *automatic behavior* pattern. That such simple behavior can persist past sleep onset and as one passes in and out of sleep may explain how impaired, drowsy drivers are able to continue down the highway.

Visual Response

A second example of behavioral change at sleep onset derives from an experiment in which a bright light is placed in front of the subject's eyes and the subject is asked to respond when a light flash is seen by pressing a sensitive microswitch taped to the hand.[7] When the EEG pattern is stage 1 or stage 2 sleep, the response is absent more than 85% of the time. When volunteers are queried afterward, they report that they did not see the light flash, not that they saw the flash but the response was inhibited. This is one example of the *perceptual disengagement* from the environment that accompanies sleep onset.

Auditory Response

In another sensory domain, the response to sleep onset is examined with a series of tones played over earphones to a subject who is instructed to respond each time a tone is heard. One study of this phenomenon showed that reaction times became longer in proximity to the onset of stage 1 sleep, and *auditory responses abated* coincident with a change in EEG to unequivocal sleep.[8] For responses in both visual and auditory modalities, the return of the response after its sleep-related disappearance typically requires the resumption of a waking EEG pattern.

Olfactory Response

When sleeping humans are tasked to respond when they smell something, the response depends in part on sleep state and in part on the particular odorant. In contrast to visual responses, one study showed that responses to graded strengths of peppermint (strong trigeminal stimulant usually perceived as pleasant) and pyridine (strong trigeminal stimulant usually perceived as extremely unpleasant) were well maintained during initial stage 1 sleep.[9] As with other modalities, the *olfactory response significantly diminished* in other sleep stages. Peppermint simply was not consciously smelled in stages 2 and 4 NREM sleep nor in REM sleep; pyridine was never smelled in stage 4 sleep, and only occasionally in stage 2 NREM and in REM sleep.[7] On the other hand, a tone successfully aroused the young adult participants in every stage. One conclusion of this report was that the olfactory system of humans is not a good sentinel system during sleep.

Response to Meaningful Stimuli

One should not infer from the preceding studies that the mind becomes an impenetrable barrier to sensory input at the onset of sleep. Indeed, one of the earliest modern studies of arousability during sleep showed that sleeping humans were differentially responsive to auditory stimuli of graded intensity.[10] Another way of illustrating sensory sensitivity is shown in experiments that have assessed discriminant responses during sleep to meaningful versus nonmeaningful stimuli, with meaning supplied in a number of ways and response usually measured as evoked K-complexes or arousal. The following are examples.

- A person tends to have a lower arousal threshold for his or her own name versus someone else's name.[11] In light sleep, for example, one's own name spoken softly will produce an arousal; a similarly applied nonmeaningful stimulus will not. Similarly, a sleeping mother is more likely to hear her own baby's cry than the cry of an unrelated infant.
- Williams and colleagues[12] showed that the likelihood of an appropriate response during sleep was improved when an otherwise nonmeaningful stimulus was made meaningful by linking the absence of response to punishment (a loud siren, flashing light, and the threat of an electric shock).
- Functional magnetic resonance imaging has shown that regional brain activation occurs in response to stimuli during sleep and that different brain regions (middle temporal gyrus and bilateral orbitofrontal cortex) are activated in response to meaningful (person's own name) versus nonmeaningful (beep) stimuli.[13]
- Experimental data suggest the presence of short time windows in sleep during which the brain is open and responsive to external auditory stimuli. This feature is consistent with the observation that even during deep sleep, meaningful auditory events can be detected.[14]

From these examples and others, it seems clear that sensory processing at some level does continue after the onset of sleep.

Hypnic Myoclonia

What other behaviors accompany the onset of sleep? If you awaken and query someone shortly after the stage 1 sleep EEG pattern appears, the person usually reports the mental experience as one of losing a direct train of thought and of experiencing vague and fragmentary imagery, usually visual.[15] Another fairly common sleep-onset experience is hypnic myoclonia, which is experienced as a general or localized muscle contraction very often associated with rather vivid visual imagery. Hypnic myoclonus is not pathologic, although it tends to occur more commonly in association with stress or with unusual or irregular sleep schedules.

The precise nature of hypnic myoclonus is not clearly understood. According to one hypothesis, the onset of sleep in these instances is marked by a dissociation of REM sleep components, wherein a breakthrough of the imagery component of REM sleep (hypnagogic hallucination) occurs in the absence of the REM motor inhibitory component. A response by the individual to the image, therefore, results in a movement or jerk. The increased frequency of these events in association with irregular sleep schedules is consistent with the increased probability of REM sleep occurring at the wake-to-sleep transition under such conditions (see later). Although the usual transition in adult humans is to NREM sleep, REM is the usual portal into sleep in infancy, and may become partially opened under unusual circumstances or in certain sleep disorders such as narcolepsy (see later).

Memory Near Sleep Onset

What happens to memory at the onset of sleep? The transition from wake to sleep tends to produce a memory impairment. One view is that it is as if sleep closes the gate between short-term and long-term memory stores. This phenomenon is best described by the following experiment.[16] During a presleep testing session, word pairs were presented to volunteers over a loudspeaker at 1-minute intervals. The subjects were then awakened either 30 seconds or 10 minutes after the onset of sleep (defined as EEG stage 1) and asked to recall the words presented before sleep onset. As illustrated in Figure 2.6, the 30-second condition was associated with a consistent level of recall from the entire 10 minutes before sleep onset. (Primacy and recency effects are apparent, although not large.) In the 10-minute condition, however, recall paralleled that in the 30-second group for only the 10 to 4 minutes before sleep onset and then fell abruptly from that point until sleep onset.

In the 30-second condition, therefore, both long-term (4–10 minutes) and short-term (0–3 minutes) memory stores remained accessible. In the 10-minute condition, by contrast, words that were in long-term stores (4–10 minutes) before sleep onset were accessible, whereas words that were still in short-term stores (0–3 minutes) at sleep onset were no longer accessible; that is, they had not been consolidated into long-term memory stores. One conclusion of this experiment is that sleep inactivates the transfer of storage from short- to long-term memory. Another interpretation is that encoding of the material before sleep onset is of insufficient strength to allow recall. The precise moment at which this deficit occurs is not known and may be a continuing process, perhaps reflecting anterograde amnesia. Nevertheless, one may infer that if sleep persists for about 10 minutes, memory is lost for the few minutes before sleep. The following experiences represent a few familiar examples of this phenomenon:

- Inability to grasp the instant of sleep onset in your memory
- Forgetting a telephone call that had come in the middle of the night
- Forgetting the news you were told when awakened in the night
- Not remembering the ringing of your alarm clock
- Experiencing morning amnesia for coherent sleeptalking
- Having fleeting dream recall

Patients with syndromes of excessive sleepiness can experience similar memory problems in the daytime if sleep becomes intrusive. Additionally, adequate sleep itself may modify symptoms of memory recall impairment in neurodegenerative conditions, such as preclinical Alzheimer disease, suggesting a complex deeper relationship between sleep and memory.[17]

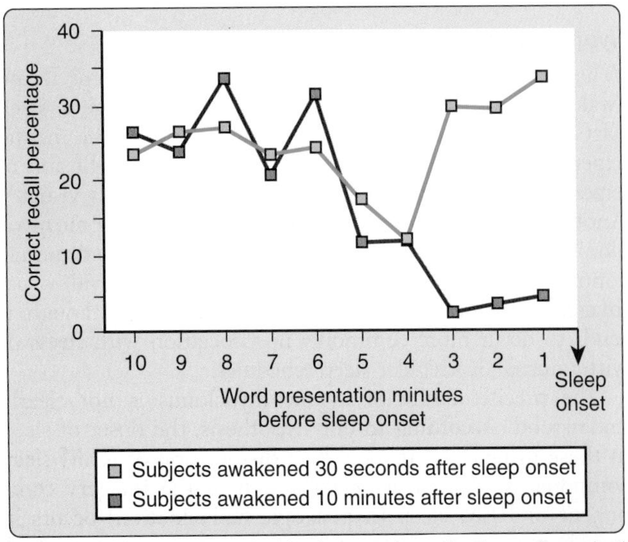

Figure 2.6 Memory is impaired by sleep, as shown by the study results illustrated in this graph. Refer to the text for explanation.

Learning and Sleep

In contrast to this immediate sleep-related "forgetting," the relevance for sleep to human learning—particularly for consolidation of perceptual and motor learning—is of growing interest.[18,19] The importance of this association has also generated some debate and skepticism.[20] Nevertheless, a spate of recent research is awakening renewed interest in the topic, and mechanistic studies explaining the roles of REM and NREM sleep and particular components of the sleep EEG pattern (e.g., sleep spindles) more precisely have shown compelling evidence that sleep plays an important role in learning and memory (see Chapter 29).

PROGRESSION OF SLEEP ACROSS THE NIGHT

Pattern of Sleep in a Healthy Young Adult

The simplest description of sleep begins with the ideal case, the healthy young adult who is sleeping well and on a fixed schedule of about 8 hours per night (Figure 2.7). In general, no consistent male versus female distinctions have been found in the normal pattern of sleep in young adults. In briefest summary, the normal human adult enters sleep through NREM sleep, REM sleep does not occur until 80 minutes or longer thereafter, and NREM sleep and REM sleep alternate through the night, with about a 90-minute cycle (see Chapter 197 for a full description of sleep stages).

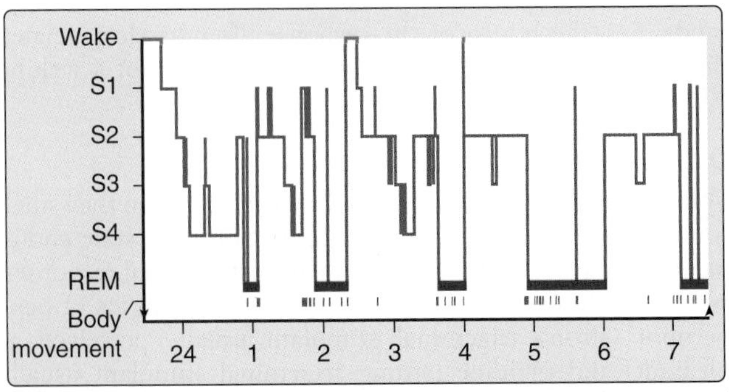

Figure 2.7 The progression of sleep stages across a single night in a normal young adult volunteer is illustrated in this sleep histogram. The text describes the ideal or average pattern. This histogram was drawn on the basis of a continuous overnight recording of electroencephalogram, electrooculogram, and electromyogram in a normal 19-year-old man. The record was assessed in 30-second epochs for the various sleep stages.

First Sleep Cycle

The first cycle of sleep in the normal young adult begins with stage 1 sleep, which usually persists for only a few (1–7) minutes at the onset of sleep. Sleep is easily discontinued during stage 1 by, for example, softly calling a person's name, touching the person lightly, quietly closing a door, and so forth. Thus stage 1 sleep is associated with a low arousal threshold. In addition to its role in the initial wake-to-sleep transition, stage 1 sleep occurs as a transitional stage throughout the night. A common sign of severely disrupted sleep is an increase in the occurrences and percentage of stage 1 sleep.

Stage 2 NREM sleep, signaled by sleep spindles or K-complexes in the EEG (Figure 2.1), follows this brief episode of stage 1 sleep and continues for about 10 to 25 minutes in the first sleep cycle. In stage 2 sleep, a more intense stimulus is required to produce arousal. The same stimulus that produced arousal from stage 1 sleep often results in an evoked K-complex but no awakening in stage 2 sleep.

As stage 2 sleep progresses, high-voltage slow wave activity gradually begins to appear in the EEG. Eventually, this activity meets the criteria[17] for stage 3 NREM sleep, that is, high-voltage (at least 75 μV) slow wave (2 cps) activity accounting for more than 20% but less than 50% of the EEG activity. Stage 3 sleep usually lasts only a few minutes in the first cycle and is transitional to stage 4 as more and more high-voltage slow wave activity occurs. Stage 4 NREM sleep—identified when the high-voltage slow wave activity comprises more than 50% of the record—usually lasts about 20 to 40 minutes in the first cycle of a healthy young adult. An incrementally larger stimulus is usually required to produce an arousal from stage 3 or 4 sleep than from stage 1 or 2 sleep. (Investigators often refer to the combined stages 3 and 4 sleep as slow wave sleep [SWS], delta sleep, or deep sleep, or N3 in the newer nomenclature.)

A series of body movements usually signals an "ascent" to lighter NREM sleep stages. A brief (1- or 2-minute) episode of stage 3 sleep might occur, followed by perhaps 5 to 10 minutes of stage 2 sleep interrupted by body movements preceding the initial REM episode. REM sleep in the first cycle of the night is usually short-lived (under 10 minutes). The arousal threshold in this REM episode is variable, as is true for REM sleep throughout the night. Theories to explain the variable arousal threshold of REM sleep have suggested that at times, the person's selective attention to internal stimuli (i.e., dreaming) precludes a response, or that the arousal stimulus is incorporated into the ongoing dream story rather than producing an awakening. Certain early experiments examining arousal thresholds in cats found highest thresholds in REM sleep, which was then termed *deep sleep* in this species. Although this terminology is still often used in publications about sleep in animals, it should not be confused with human NREM stages 3 and 4 sleep, which is also often called *deep sleep*. In addition, the term *SWS* is sometimes used (as is *synchronized sleep*) as a synonym for all of NREM sleep in other species and is thus distinct from SWS (stages 3 and 4 NREM) in humans.

NREM-REM Cycle

NREM sleep and REM sleep continue to alternate through the night in cyclic fashion. REM sleep episodes usually become longer across the night. Stages 3 and 4 sleep occupy less time in the second cycle and might disappear altogether from later cycles as stage 2 sleep expands to occupy the NREM portion of the cycle. The average length of the first NREM-REM sleep cycle is about 70 to 100 minutes; the average length of the second and later cycles is about 90 to 120 minutes. Across the night, the average period of the NREM-REM cycle is about 90 to 110 minutes. Across the night, stage 1 sleep will account for about 2% to 5%, stage 2 about 45% to 55%, SWS about 10% to 20%, and REM sleep about 20% to 25% of sleep in a healthy young adult.

Distribution of Sleep Stages across the Night

In the young adult, SWS dominates the NREM portion of the sleep cycle toward the beginning of the night (about the first one-third); REM sleep episodes are longest in the last one-third of the night. Brief episodes of wakefulness tend to intrude later in the night, usually near REM sleep transitions, and they usually do not last long enough to be remembered in the morning. The preferential distribution of REM sleep toward the latter portion of the night in normal human adults is linked to a circadian oscillator, which can be gauged by the oscillation of body temperature.[16,21] The preferential distribution of SWS toward the beginning of a sleep episode is not thought to be mediated by circadian processes but shows a marked response to the length of prior wakefulness,[22] thus reflecting the homeostatic sleep system, which is highest at sleep onset and diminishes across the night as sleep pressure wanes or as "recovery" takes place. Thus these aspects of the normal sleep pattern highlight features of the two-process model of sleep as elaborated on in Chapter 38.

Length of Sleep

The length of nocturnal sleep depends on a great number of factors—of which volitional control is among the most significant in humans—and it is thus difficult to characterize a "normal" pattern. Whereas newborns may spend as much as 80% of their day sleeping, and a typical 1-year-old sleeps 10 to 12 hours at night plus two daily naps,[23] most young adults report sleeping about 7.5 hours a night on weekday nights and slightly longer, 8.5 hours, on weekend nights. The variability of these figures from person to person and from night to night, however, is quite high. Sleep length also depends on genetic determinants,[24] and one may think of the volitional determinants (staying up late, waking by alarm, and so on) superimposed on the background of a genetic sleep need. Length of prior waking also affects how much one sleeps, although not in a one-for-one manner. Indeed, the length of sleep is also determined by processes associated with circadian rhythms. Thus *when* one sleeps helps to determine *how long* one sleeps. In addition, as sleep is extended, the amount of REM sleep increases because the occurrence of REM sleep depends on the persistence of sleep into the peak circadian time.

Generalizations about Sleep in the Healthy Young Adult

A number of general statements can be made regarding sleep in the healthy young adult who is living on a conventional sleep-wake schedule and who is without sleep complaints:

- Sleep is entered through NREM sleep.
- NREM sleep and REM sleep alternate with a period near 90 minutes.
- SWS predominates in the first third of the night and is linked to the initiation of sleep and the length of time awake (i.e., sleep homeostasis).

- REM sleep predominates in the last third of the night and is linked to the circadian rhythm of body temperature.
- Wakefulness in sleep usually accounts for less than 5% of the night.
- Stage 1 sleep generally constitutes about 2% to 5% of sleep.
- Stage 2 sleep generally constitutes about 45% to 55% of sleep.
- Stage 3 sleep generally constitutes about 3% to 8% of sleep.
- Stage 4 sleep generally constitutes about 10% to 15% of sleep.
- NREM sleep, therefore, is usually 75% to 80% of sleep.
- REM sleep is usually 20% to 25% of sleep, occurring in four to six discrete episodes.
- Brief arousals may occur during sleep and do not themselves indicate abnormality.

Factors Modifying Sleep Stage Distribution

Age

The strongest and most consistent factor affecting the pattern of sleep stages across the night is age (Figure 2.8). The most marked age-related differences in sleep from the patterns described earlier are found in newborn infants. For the first year of life, the transition from wake to sleep is often accomplished through REM sleep (called *active sleep* in newborns). The cyclic alternation of NREM-REM sleep is present from birth but has a period of about 50 to 60 minutes in the newborn compared with about 90 minutes in the adult. Infants also only gradually acquire a consolidated nocturnal sleep cycle, and the fully developed EEG patterns of the NREM sleep stages are not present at birth but emerge over the first 2 to 6 months of life. When brain structure and function achieve a level that can support high-voltage slow wave EEG activity, NREM stages 3 and 4 sleep become prominent.

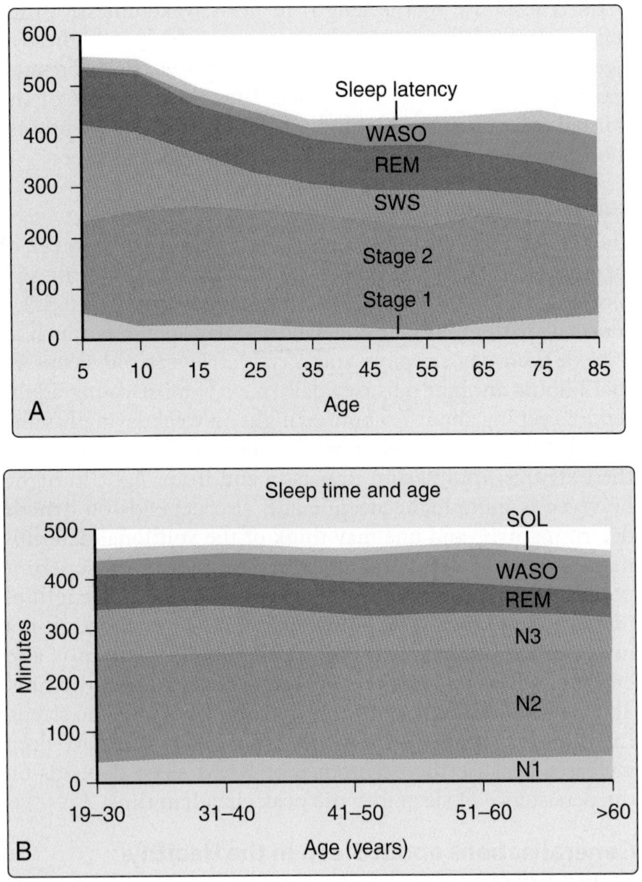

Figure 2.8 Changes in sleep with age. **A,** Time (in minutes) for sleep latency and wake time after sleep onset (WASO) and for REM sleep and NREM sleep stages 1, 2, and slow wave sleep (SWS). Summary values are given for ages 5 to 85 years. **B,** Changes in sleep in adults using the current AASM scoring standards. Time (in minutes) for sleep latency and WASO and for REM sleep and NREM sleep stages N1, N2, and N3. Values are medians. (**A,** From Ohayon M, Carskadon MA, Guilleminault C, et al. Meta-analysis of quantitative sleep parameters from childhood to old age in healthy individuals: developing normative sleep values across the human lifespan. *Sleep.* 2004;27:1255–73; **B,** Data from Mitterling T, Högl B, Schönwald SV, et al. Sleep and respiration in 100 healthy Caucasian sleepers—a polysomnographic study according to American Academy of Sleep Medicine standards. *Sleep.* 2015;38:867-75.)

SWS is maximal in young children and decreases markedly with age. The SWS of young children is both qualitatively and quantitatively different from that of older adults. For example, it is nearly impossible to wake youngsters in the SWS of the night's first sleep cycle. In one study,[25] a 123-dB tone failed to produce any sign of arousal in a group of children whose mean age was 10 years. In addition, children up to midadolescence often "skip" their first REM episode, perhaps because of the quantity and intensity of slow wave activity early in the night. A similar, although less profound qualitative difference distinguishes SWS occurring in the first and later cycles of the night in older humans. A marked quantitative change in SWS occurs across adolescence, when SWS decreases by about 40% during the second decade, even when length of nocturnal sleep remains constant.[26] Feinberg[27] hypothesized that the age-related decline in nocturnal SWS, which parallels loss of cortical synaptic density, is causally related to this cortical resculpting. More recent findings by de Vivo and colleagues in an animal model question that hypothesis.[28] By midadolescence, youngsters no longer typically skip their first REM period, and their sleep resembles that described earlier for young adults. By age 60 years, SWS is quite diminished, particularly in men; women maintain SWS later into life than men.

REM sleep as a percentage of total sleep is maintained well into healthy old age; the absolute amount of REM sleep at night has been correlated with intellectual functioning[29] and declines markedly in the case of organic brain dysfunctions in elderly people.[30]

Arousals during sleep increase markedly with age. Extended wake episodes of which the individual is aware and can report, as well as brief and probably unremembered arousals, increase with aging.[31] The latter type of transient arousals may occur with no known correlate but are often associated with occult sleep disturbances, such as periodic limb movements during sleep (PLMS) and sleep-related respiratory irregularities, which also become more prevalent in later life.[32,33]

Sleep patterns change with advanced age independent of other factors; such changes may include advanced sleep timing, shortened nocturnal sleep duration, increased number of daytime naps, increased number of nocturnal awakenings and time spent awake during the night, and decreased slow wave sleep.[34] Perhaps the most notable finding regarding sleep in elderly people is the profound increase in interindividual variability,[35] which thus precludes generalizations such as those made for young adults.

Prior Sleep History

A person who has experienced sleep loss on one or more nights shows a sleep pattern that favors SWS during recovery (Figure 2.9). Recovery sleep is also usually prolonged

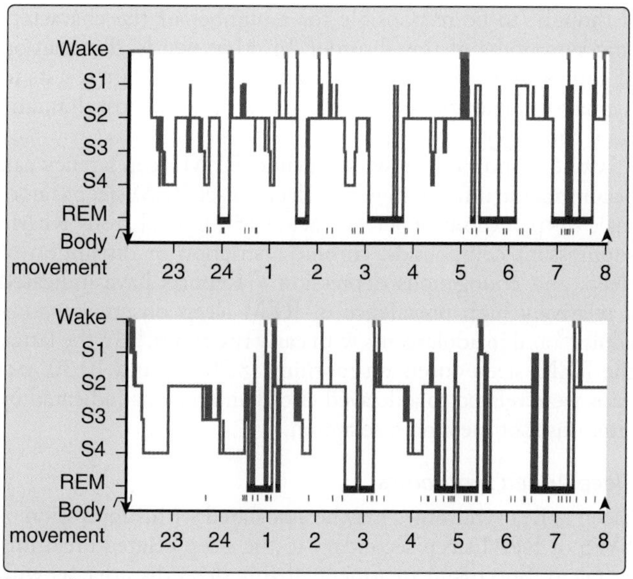

Figure 2.9 The *upper histogram* shows the baseline sleep pattern of a normal 14-year-old female volunteer. The *lower histogram* illustrates the sleep pattern in this volunteer for the first recovery night after 38 hours without sleep. Note that the amount of stage 4 sleep on the lower graph is greater than on baseline and that the first REM sleep episode is markedly delayed.

and deeper—that is, having a higher arousal threshold throughout—than basal sleep. REM sleep tends to show a rebound on the second or subsequent recovery nights after an episode of sleep loss. Therefore with total sleep loss, SWS tends to be preferentially recovered compared with REM sleep, which tends to recover only after the recuperation of SWS. Thus both states of sleep show evidence of homeostatic regulation.

Cases in which a person is differentially deprived of REM or SWS—either operationally, by being awakened each time the sleep pattern occurs, or pharmacologically (see later)—show a preferential rebound of that stage of sleep when natural sleep is resumed. This phenomenon has particular relevance in a clinical setting, in which abrupt withdrawal from a therapeutic regimen may result in misleading diagnostic findings (e.g., sleep-onset REM periods [SOREMPs] as a result of a REM sleep rebound when REM suppressant medication is withdrawn) or could conceivably exacerbate a sleep disorder (e.g., if sleep apneas tend to occur preferentially or with greater intensity in the rebounding type of sleep).

Chronic restriction of nocturnal sleep, an irregular sleep schedule, or frequent disturbance of nocturnal sleep can result in a peculiar distribution of sleep states, most commonly characterized by premature REM sleep, that is, SOREMPs. Such episodes can be associated with hypnagogic hallucinations, sleep paralysis, or an increased incidence of hypnic myoclonia in persons with no organic sleep disorder.

Although not strictly related to prior sleep history, the first night of a laboratory sleep evaluation is commonly associated with more frequent arousals and a disruption of the normal distribution of sleep states, characterized chiefly by a delayed onset of REM sleep.[36] Often this delay takes the form of skipping the first REM episode of the night. In other words, the NREM sleep stages progress in a normal fashion, but the first cycle ends with an episode of stage 1 or a brief arousal instead of the expected brief REM sleep episode. In addition, REM sleep episodes are often disrupted, and the total amount of REM sleep on the first night in the sleep laboratory is also usually reduced from the normal value.

Circadian Rhythms

The circadian phase at which sleep occurs affects the distribution of sleep stages. REM sleep, in particular, occurs with a circadian distribution that peaks in the morning hours coincident with the trough of the core body temperature rhythm.[16,17] Thus, if sleep onset is delayed until the peak REM phase of the circadian rhythm—that is, the early morning—REM sleep tends to predominate and can even occur at the onset of sleep. This reversal of the normal sleep-onset pattern may be seen in a healthy person who acutely undergoes a phase shift, either as a result of a work shift change or as a change resulting from jet travel across a number of time zones. Studies of persons sleeping in environments free of all cues to time show that the timing of sleep onset and the length of sleep occur in association with circadian phase.[37,38] Under these conditions, sleep distribution with reference to the circadian body temperature phase position shows that sleep onset is likeliest to occur on the falling limb of the temperature cycle. A secondary peak of sleep onsets, corresponding to afternoon napping, also occurs; the offset of sleep occurs most often on the rising limb of the circadian body temperature curve.[39]

As with other characteristics of sleep, circadian and other biologic rhythms are affected by age. In infants, coordination of body temperature, cortisol, melatonin, and sleep-wake cycles develop rapidly over the first 6 months of life.[40] While sleep timing and duration in children result from a complex set of cultural. social, family, and environmental factors, by adolescence a delayed pattern of melatonin secretion marking delayed circadian rhythm, as well as a slower build- up of homeostatic sleep pressure during wakefulness is evident.[41] Acknowledgment of this physiologically later sleep onset and later morning awakening has in part driven the debate about school start times for adolescents, with concern that too-early starts may reduce sleep duration, contribute to irregular sleep timing and be associated with negative effects on scholastic performance, health, and safety.[42] Finally, aging is associated with another proposed shift of in timing, commonly experiencing a phase advancement in circadian rhythm leading to sleepiness earlier in the evening and waking up earlier in the morning. This phase advance is seen not only in the sleep-wake cycle, but also in the body temperature rhythm, and in the timing of secretion of melatonin and cortisol. In addition to phase advancement, aging is also associated with a reduction in the amplitude of these circadian rhythms in older adults.

Temperature

Extremes of temperature in the sleeping environment tend to disrupt sleep. REM sleep is commonly more sensitive to temperature-related disruption than is NREM sleep. Accumulated evidence from humans and other species suggests that mammals have only minimal ability to thermoregulate during REM sleep; in other words, the control of body temperature is virtually poikilothermic in REM sleep.[43] This inability to thermoregulate in REM sleep probably affects the response to temperature extremes and suggests that such conditions are less of a problem early during a night than late, when REM sleep tends to predominate. It should be clear, as well, that such responses as sweating or shivering during sleep under ambient temperature extremes occur in NREM sleep and are limited in REM sleep.

Drug and Substance Ingestion

The distribution of sleep states and stages is affected by many common drugs, including those typically prescribed in the treatment of sleep disorders, as well as those not specifically related to the pharmacotherapy of sleep disorders and those used socially or recreationally. Whether changes in sleep stage distribution have any relevance to health, illness, or psychological well-being is unknown; however, particularly in the context of specific sleep disorders that differentially affect one sleep stage or another, such distinctions may be relevant to diagnosis or treatment. A number of generalizations regarding the effects of certain of the more commonly used compounds on sleep stage distribution can be made.

- Benzodiazepines tend to suppress SWS and have no consistent effect on REM sleep.
- Tricyclic antidepressants, monoamine oxidase inhibitors, and certain selective serotonin reuptake inhibitors tend to suppress REM sleep. An increased level of motor activity during sleep occurs with certain of these compounds, leading to a pattern of REM sleep without motor inhibition or an increased incidence of PLMS. Fluoxetine is also associated with rapid eye movements across all sleep stages ("Prozac eyes").
- Withdrawal from drugs that selectively suppress a stage of sleep tends to be associated with a rebound of that sleep stage. Thus acute withdrawal from a benzodiazepine compound is likely to produce an increase of SWS; acute withdrawal from a tricyclic antidepressant or monoamine oxidase inhibitor is likely to produce an increase of REM sleep. In the latter case, this REM rebound could result in abnormal SOREMPs in the absence of an organic sleep disorder, perhaps leading to an incorrect diagnosis of narcolepsy.
- Acute presleep alcohol intake can produce an increase in SWS and suppression of REM sleep early in the night, which can be followed by REM sleep rebound in the latter portion of the night as the alcohol is metabolized. Low doses of alcohol have minimal effects on sleep stages, but they can increase sleepiness in the late evening.[44,45]
- Acute effects of marijuana (tetrahydrocannabinol [THC]) include minimal sleep disruption, characterized by a slight reduction of REM sleep. Chronic ingestion of THC produces a long-term suppression of SWS.[46]

Pathology

Sleep disorders, as well as other nonsleep problems, have an effect on the structure and distribution of sleep. As suggested before, these distinctions appear to be more important in diagnosis and in the consideration of treatments than for any implications about general health or illness resulting from specific sleep stage alterations. A number of common sleep-stage anomalies are associated with sleep disorders. We highlight a few examples in the text that follows; these and others are further detailed in subsequent chapters.

Narcolepsy

Narcolepsy is characterized by an abnormally short delay to REM sleep, marked by SOREMPs. This abnormal sleep-onset pattern occurs with some consistency, but not exclusively; that is, NREM sleep onset can also occur. Thus one diagnostic test consists of several opportunities to fall asleep across a day (see Chapter 207). If REM sleep occurs abnormally on two or more such opportunities, narcolepsy is extremely probable. The occurrence of this abnormal sleep pattern in narcolepsy is thought to be responsible for a number of the characteristic symptoms of this disorder. In other words, dissociation of components of REM sleep into the waking state results in hypnagogic hallucinations, sleep paralysis, and, most dramatically, cataplexy.

Other conditions in which a short REM sleep latency can occur include infancy, in which sleep-onset REM sleep is normal; sleep reversal or jet lag; acute withdrawal from REM-suppressant compounds; chronic restriction or disruption of sleep; and endogenous depression.[47] Reports have indicated a relatively high prevalence of REM sleep onsets in young adults[48] and in adolescents with early rise times.[49] In the latter, the REM sleep onsets on morning (8:30 AM and 10:30 AM) naps were related to a delayed circadian phase as indicated by later onset of melatonin secretion.

Sleep Apnea Syndromes

Sleep apnea syndromes may be associated with suppression of SWS or REM sleep secondary to the sleep-related breathing problem. Successful treatment of this sleep disorder, as with nocturnal continuous positive airway pressure, can produce large rebounds of SWS or REM sleep when first implemented (Figure 2.10).

Movement Disorders and Parasomnias

Unusual events or behaviors in sleep may represent a parasomnia, movement disorder, or other neurologic issue. Some of these, for example rhythmic movements, sleepwalking, REM behavior disorder, or sleep paralysis, emerge characteristically from a certain stage of sleep or certain transitions in sleep-wake. Other conditions, such as restless legs syndrome, are associated with distinct motor findings in sleep such as periodic limb movements, and sleep is marked by increased sleep fragmentation, delayed sleep onset, and increased wake after sleep onset, and decreased sleep duration.[50] The percentages of wake and sleep stage 1 are increased, and sleep stage 2 and REM sleep are decreased in RLS patients. Still other motor phenomena and alterations in sleep architecture may be related to use of medications or substances, as discussed briefly in this chapter. In approaching such sleep-related phenomena, it is important to appreciate both sleep-related predisposing factors and consequences of altered or disturbed sleep.

Sleep Fragmentation

Fragmentation of sleep and increased frequency of arousals occur in association with a number of sleep disorders, as well as with medical disorders involving physical pain or discomfort. Periodic limb movements, sleep apnea syndromes, musculoskeletal conditions, and so forth may be associated with tens to hundreds of arousals each night. Brief arousals are prominent in such conditions as allergic rhinitis,[51,52] juvenile rheumatoid arthritis,[53] and Parkinson disease.[54] In upper airway resistance syndrome,[55] EEG arousals are important markers because the respiratory signs of this syndrome are less obvious than in frank obstructive sleep apnea syndrome, and only subtle indicators may be available.[56] In specific situations, autonomic changes, such as transient changes of blood pressure,[57] can signify arousals; Lofaso and colleagues[58] indicated that autonomic changes are highly correlated with the extent of EEG arousals. Sleep fragmentation may be associated with subcortical events not visible in the cortical EEG signal. These disorders also often involve an increase in the absolute amount of and the proportion of stage 1 sleep.

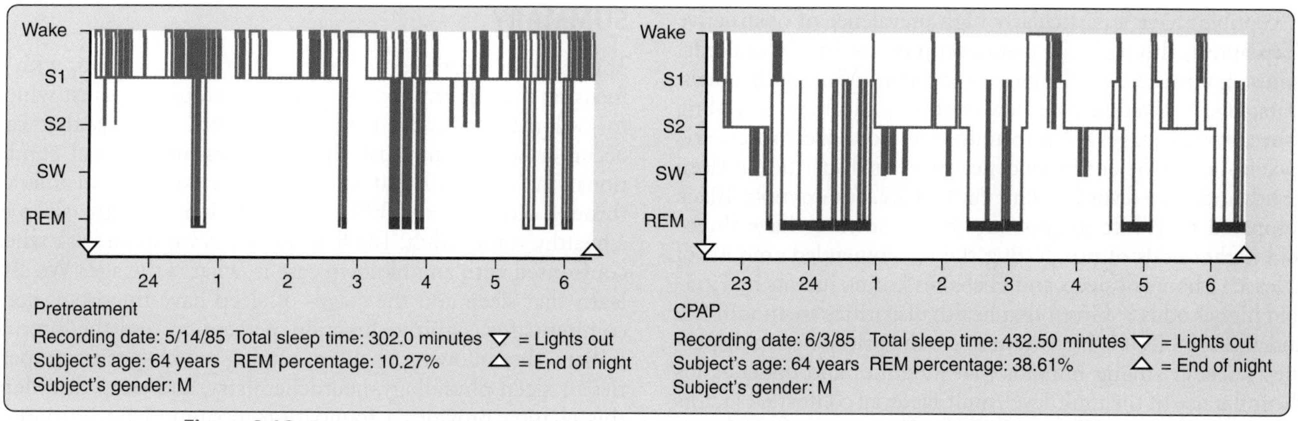

Figure 2.10 These sleep histograms depict the sleep of a 64-year-old male patient with obstructive sleep apnea syndrome. The *left graph* shows the sleep pattern before treatment. Note the absence of slow wave (SW) sleep, the preponderance of stage 1 (S1), and the very frequent disruptions. The *right graph* shows the sleep pattern in this patient during the second night of treatment with continuous positive airway pressure (CPAP). Note that sleep is much deeper (more SW sleep) and more consolidated and that REM sleep in particular is abnormally increased. The pretreatment REM percentage of sleep was only 10%, compared with nearly 40% with treatment. (Data supplied by G. Nino-Murcia, Stanford University Sleep Disorders Center, Stanford, CA.)

SLEEP HEALTH DISPARITIES

Potentially large differences in the modifiable physical and social environments across social identity groups, such as race and ethnicity, likely influence widely observed but poorly understood sleep health disparities. Social conditions and institutions could directly or indirectly affect a person's sleep and biology through the policies and practices that influence where and how a person of a particular social identity group lives in terms of the quality of their residential neighborhood and housing as well as where and how the individual works or acquires education and engages in recreation.

Structural racism, defined as "the totality of ways in which societies foster racial discrimination through mutually reinforcing systems of housing, education, employment, earnings, benefits, credit, media, health care, and criminal justice,"[59] is considered the main, fundamental driver of health disparities and results in marginalized groups having differential access to health promoting resources and greater exposure to health damaging environments that could negatively affect sleep health and circadian alignment. Historical and contemporary examples include racial residential segregation (especially among African Americans or Black individuals), known as redlining and labor market segregation, which contribute to concentrated poverty.[59,60] A higher likelihood of exposure to adverse environments (e.g., pollution from noise, light, and air; psychosocial stress) across the lifespan from conception to death among under resourced, socially disadvantaged groups can more negatively affect the sleep and subsequent health sequelae in these populations through, for instance, more difficulty maintaining biological homeostasis. These factors in the physical and social environments can have downstream consequences on biology, including circadian rhythms, with structural factors such as occupational demands leading to shift work and circadian misalignment, which also differ by social identity. This socioecological perspective illuminates that individual-level human characteristics (including sleep) are shaped by upstream social determinants of health that need to be identified and understood.[61]

A health disparity has been defined as "a health difference that adversely affects defined disadvantaged populations, based on one or more health outcomes."[62] These health outcomes are generally considered preventable and unjust; therefore, social problems caused by environmental factors, as opposed to innate or genetic factors, can lead to observable biological differences. In the USA, socially-disadvantaged groups or populations disproportionately affected by health disparities as designated by the National Institutes of Health include Blacks/African Americans, Hispanics/Latinos, Native Americans/Alaska Natives, Asian Americans, native Hawaiians and other Pacific Islanders, socioeconomically-disadvantaged populations, underserved rural populations, and sexual/gender minorities.[62] Health disparities are present in many nations. Criteria pertaining to health outcomes include higher incidence or prevalence of disease, including earlier onset or more aggressive progression; premature or excessive mortality from specific conditions; greater global burden of disease, such as disability-adjusted life years as measured by population health metrics; poorer health behaviors and clinical outcomes related to the disability-adjusted life years; and worse outcomes on validated self-reported measures that reflect daily functioning or symptoms from specific conditions.[62]

In terms of sleep health disparities that likely result from inopportune exposure to sleep modulators (e.g., psychological stress), a review summarizing the scientific literature in terms of racial/ethnic disparities in sleep health indicates that racial/ethnic minorities are generally less likely than Whites to get the recommended amount of sleep, with the exception of Hispanic/Latinos who were not born in the US.[63-65] Studies have also found lower sleep efficiency across racial/ethnic minority groups in general. Moreover, minorities generally spend less time in slow wave sleep, the most physiologically restorative stage. There tends to be greater variability in sleep timing, a higher likelihood of circadian misalignment, and more daytime sleepiness among racial/ethnic minorities. Black or African American and Asian adults are more likely to report being of a morningness chronotype, which can be influenced by zeitgebers such as social habits. Racial/ethnic minorities are also generally less likely to complain about their sleep despite objective sleep data commonly indicating worse sleep compared to Whites. Furthermore, Blacks or African Americans, Hispanics/Latinos, and Asians (who appear particularly susceptible) have a particularly high prevalence of obstructive sleep apnea, although the condition remains largely underdiagnosed, untreated, and more severe than White individuals. Data, albeit mixed and despite methodological and sampling issues, overall suggest White adults are more likely to experience insomnia. Scientific evidence suggests disparities in sleep health and sleep disorders start early in life. For example, Black compared to White infants have been shown to have threefold higher odds of not getting the recommended amount of at least 12 hours of sleep, and Hispanic/Latino infants had 2.5-fold higher odds.[66] Given that health disparities are modifiable and addressable, it is important to conduct sleep health disparities research among humans that identifies and understands the influence of the multilevel, multifactorial contextual factors on sleep and its downstream biological consequences in hopes of informing effective multi-level interventions.[67] In terms of potential solutions, interventions to improve population health and address health disparities should center efforts around assuring the material and social conditions (especially those known to modulate sleep and circadian rhythms) for optimal health among all individuals regardless of social identity group.

CLINICAL PEARLS

- Sleep architecture norms vary in predictable ways across the lifespan in healthy individuals.
- The clinician should expect to see less slow wave sleep (stages 3 and 4; N3) in older persons, particularly men.
- Clinicians or colleagues might find themselves denying middle-of-the-night communications (nighttime calls) because of memory deficits that occur for events proximal to sleep onset. This issue could be exacerbated by certain medications and might also account for memory deficits in excessively sleepy patients.
- Many medications (even if not prescribed for sleep) can affect sleep stages, and their use or discontinuation alters sleep. For example, REM-suppressing medications can result in a rebound of REM sleep when they are discontinued.
- Certain patients have sleep complaints (insomnia, hypersomnia) that result from attempts to sleep or from being awake at times that are not in synchrony with their circadian phase.
- Patients who wake with events early in the night might have a disorder affecting NREM sleep; patients who wake with events late in the night may have a disorder affecting REM sleep.
- When using sleep restriction to build sleep pressure, treatment will be more effective if sleep is scheduled at the correct circadian phase. The problem of napping in patients with insomnia is that naps diminish the homeostatic drive to sleep.

SUMMARY

This chapter provides an overview of human sleep, with a focus on the healthy young adult as a template against which to evaluate and understand the expected changes that can occur, as well as unusual circumstances and clinical conditions. Thus we find that maturational changes from infancy through old age carry different associations with the sleep of a healthy young adult. The first questions we should ask when confronted with an unknown case is, what is the age? We also learn that sleep and the stages of sleep have important concomitants for cognitive function, perception, and the internal milieu. The following chapters catalog many specific properties of sleep physiology, neurochemistry, and sleep disorders; this chapter provides a foundation to support integration of that detailed information.

SELECTED READINGS

Abel T, Havekes R, Saletin JM, Walker MP. Sleep plasticity and memory from molecules to whole-brain networks. *Curr Biol.* 2013;23:R774–R788.

Berry RB, Brooks R, Gamaldo CE, et al. *For the American Academy of Sleep Medicine.* The AASM manual for the scoring of sleep and associated events: rules, terminology and technical specifications. The AASM Manual for the Scoring of Sleep and Associated Events v2.6. Darien (IL): American Academy of Sleep Medicine; 2020. www.aasmnet.org.

Carskadon M. Sleep in adolescents: the perfect storm. *Pediatr Clin North Am.* 2011;58:637–647.

Eisermann M, Kaminska A, Moutard M-L, et al. Normal EEG in childhood: from neonates to adolescents. *Neurophysiol Clin.* 2013;43:35–65.

Foley D, Ancoli-Israel S, Britz P, Walsh J. Sleep disturbances and chronic disease in older adults: results of the 2003 National Sleep Foundation Sleep in America Survey. *J Psychosom Res.* 2004;56(5):497–502.

Hirshkowitz M, Whiton K, Albert SM, et al. National Sleep Foundation's sleep time duration recommendations: methodology and results summary. *Sleep Health.* 2015;1:40–43.

Jenni O, LeBourgeois M. Understanding sleep-wake behavior and sleep disorders in children: the value of a model. *Curr Opin Psychiatry.* 2005;19:282–287.

Lesku JA, Roth TC, Rattenborg NC, et al. History and future of comparative analyses in sleep research. *Neurosci Biobehav Rev.* 2009;33:1024–1036.

Mitterling T, Högl B, Schönwald SV, et al. Sleep and respiration in 100 healthy Caucasian sleepers—a polysomnographic study according to American Academy of Sleep Medicine standards. *Sleep.* 2015;38:867–875.

Ohayon M, Carskadon MA, Guilleminault C, et al. Meta-analysis of quantitative sleep parameters from childhood to old age in healthy individuals: developing normative sleep values across the human lifespan. *Sleep.* 2004;27:1255–1273.

Roenneberg T, Kuehnle T, Pramstaller PP, et al. A marker for the end of adolescence. *Curr Biol.* 2004;14:R1038–R1039.

A complete reference list can be found online at ExpertConsult.com.

Chapter 3

Normal Aging

Brienne Miner; Brendan P. Lucey

Chapter Highlights

- With normal aging, there are changes to sleep architecture leading to increases in arousals from sleep and decreases in nocturnal total sleep time, as well as changes to circadian rhythmicity. However, while changes to sleep architecture may lead to changes in the timing or consolidation of sleep, short sleep duration (<6 hours) and substantial sleep disturbance should not be considered a normal part of the aging process.
- Napping in the older adult is common and may be associated with both beneficial and adverse health consequences depending on nap timing, characteristics, and overall sleep duration.
- Causes of sleep disturbance in older age are multifactorial and include contributions from increasing medical and psychiatric comorbidity, medication use, and psychosocial and behavioral factors. These factors underpin age as a risk factor for sleep disturbance.
- Considerable differences emerge when comparing the association between sleep and cognitive function in middle-aged versus older adults. While cross-sectional studies of cognitive performance and longitudinal studies of cognitive decline show significant associations of disrupted sleep with poorer cognitive outcomes in middle-aged adults, these associations are weaker or nonsignificant in older adults.

INTRODUCTION

As our population ages, defining how sleep is affected by age is of great importance. Within the United States, the population aged 65 years and older continues to grow more rapidly than the population under age 65, and it is projected that by 2050 over 20% of the population will be over age 65.[1] The ability to discriminate normal from abnormal with respect to sleep in the aging population is an important skill for the sleep medicine specialist. This chapter reviews expected changes to sleep architecture and circadian rhythmicity with age, benefits and risks associated with napping, and causes and consequences of disturbed sleep, especially with respect to cognitive performance and cognitive decline, in the older adult.

SLEEP ARCHITECTURE

Age-related changes in nocturnal sleep architecture have been well summarized by several large meta-analyses of polysomnographic sleep parameters across the human life span.[2-4] Results from the first of these analyses, published by Ohayon and colleagues,[2] found significantly decreased total sleep time, sleep efficiency, and percentage of N3 and rapid eye movement (REM) sleep with increasing age, while sleep-onset latency, wake after sleep onset, and percentage of non–rapid eye movement (NREM) stage 1 (N1) and NREM stage 2 (N2) sleep increased significantly with increasing age. However, the authors noted that although sleep efficiency showed clear age-dependent declines up to and beyond age 90 years, most age-dependent changes in sleep architecture occurred before the age of 60 years, with few changes in NREM stage 3 (N3) sleep, REM sleep, and N1 percentage occurring after that.[2] Some variables (total sleep time, REM) appeared best characterized with a linear decline, whereas others (N3, wake after sleep onset) followed a more exponential course. Sleep latency showed no clear age effect after age 60 years, although it increased up to that point.[2]

More recently, another meta-analysis of polysomnographic parameters in a larger group of healthy adults, published by Boulos and colleagues, has summarized age- and sex-adjusted normative values.[3] Figure 3.1 shows a summary of changes in polysomnographic sleep architecture from ages 18 up to 79 years.[3] Results from this report agree with those of Ohayon and colleagues with respect to age-dependent decreases in total sleep time, sleep efficiency, and increases in sleep-onset latency, N1 percentage, and wake after sleep onset. However, the authors did not find significant age-related changes in N2, N3, and REM percentage (Table 3.1).[3] Additional contributions of the recent meta-analysis include evidence of significant age-dependent increases in the arousal index, apnea-hypopnea index (AHI), and periodic limb movement index, as well as significant decreases in the mean and minimum oxygen saturation (Table 3.2). For example, the mean AHI in persons ages 18 to 34 was 1.6 events per hour, while the mean in persons ages 65 to 79 was 15.5 events per hour.[3] Importantly, the meta-analysis by Boulos and colleagues, as opposed to the study by Ohayon and colleagues, included studies from 2007 through 2016, reflecting modifications to the American Academy of Sleep Medicine (AASM) scoring manual; these emphasized increased agreement when scoring

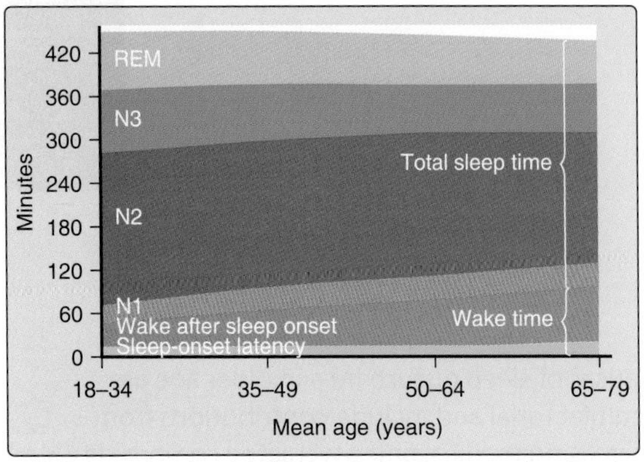

Figure 3.1 Age-related trends for sleep-onset latency, wake after sleep onset, and sleep stages. This sleep ontogeny graph shows age-related decreases in total sleep time and sleep efficiency that are accompanied by increases in wake after sleep onset and sleep-onset latency. (From Boulos MI, Jairam T, Kendzerska T, et al. Normal polysomnography parameters in healthy adults: a systematic review and meta-analysis. *Lancet Respir Med* 2019;7:533–43.)

sleep stages.[5] However, it should be noted that only one study with $n = 10$ males examined parameters in the age group of 80 years and older, substantially limiting the ability to detect differences in this age group.[3] Finally, a third meta-analysis, focused only on REM percentage in samples with and without sleep disorders, noted a cubic trend, with REM apparently increasing after age 75 years and then demonstrating an even steeper drop after age 90 years.[4] REM percentages of 18% to 20% in 75 to 85 year olds were derived from curve smoothing in this meta-analysis.[4]

Changes with age to phasic events of NREM and REM sleep have also been described. In NREM sleep, K-complex and sleep spindle number and density decrease with age.[6] With respect to spindles, there is a progressive decrease in spindle amplitude and duration with a concomitant increase in intra-spindle frequency, findings that are independent of gender.[7,8] The major change in slow wave sleep ascribed to aging has been a decline in delta wave amplitude rather than wavelength (Figure 3.2), which is thought to be due to intracerebral factors, including loss of cortical neurons.[9] The density of eye movements in REM sleep is reduced with aging.[10]

Sex Differences in Sleep Architecture

Sex differences in sleep physiology in older adults may exist, although evidence is mixed.[2,3,11,12] In the most recent meta-analysis of nocturnal sleep architecture using updated AASM scoring criteria (Boulos and colleagues), there were no sex differences found with respect to total sleep time, sleep efficiency, wake after sleep onset, or time in different sleep stages.[3] Men had significantly lower REM latency and mean oxygen saturation and significantly higher arousal index and apnea-hypopnea index than women.

Changes to N3 sleep in older men and women require special mention. In the Sleep Heart Health Study (SHHS), men showed evidence of poorer sleep with aging, most notable with respect to time spent in N3.[11] Large gender differences in N3 percentage were seen at every age in men, while there was no appreciable decline in N3 percentage in aging women.[11] However, meta-analytic data showed no difference in N3 percentage in aging men and women.[2,3] It is important to note that SHHS included persons with a wide variety of medical conditions, including sleep-disordered breathing (SDB).[11] A small study among healthy older men and women may shed light on these discrepancies.[12,13] There were no sex differences in N3 percentage in this study, but substantial differences were found in delta activity, the hallmark of N3 sleep. Delta activity was higher overall in older women, with larger differences in REM than in NREM sleep. However, older men had 50% more delta activity during NREM sleep as well as lower levels of alpha activity.[12] The pattern of lower delta and higher alpha activity during NREM sleep (i.e., alpha-delta sleep) seen in older women has been associated with unrefreshing sleep and may explain their higher prevalence of insomnia symptoms.[12] The authors also found lower sleep-onset release of growth hormone in older women as compared to older men, which may contribute to lower levels of delta activity in NREM sleep in older women.[13]

Arousals and Sleep Fragmentation

Arousal frequency increases steadily with age, from an average of 9.6 events per hour in persons 18 to 34 years old to 18.8 events per hour in persons 65 to 79 years old (Table 3.2).[3] However, healthy older persons may wake up more frequently than younger persons but do not necessarily have greater difficulty falling back to sleep.[14] While brief arousals show a male predominance,[2,3] the influences of age and sex may not be as pronounced as the effects of breathing events.[11] Novel correlates of sleep fragmentation in elderly persons have been noted. For example, beta activity (but not delta activity) in the sleep electroencephalogram correlates strongly with sleep fragmentation regardless of circadian phase.[15] Visually scored arousals in older persons have been shown to be preceded by relatively lower and more temporally limited increments in delta band power relative to similarly scored arousals in middle-aged subjects.[16] Within a population of women and men aged 55 to 100 years, chronologic age was strongly correlated with fragmentation of the rest-activity rhythms measured by actigraphy,[17] the effect being more pronounced in men.

Sleep Duration

The National Sleep Foundation (NSF) recommends 7 to 8 hours of sleep for adults aged 65 years and older.[18] This recommendation is supported by evidence that older adults sleeping anywhere from 6 to 9 hours have better cognition, mental and physical health, and quality of life compared to older adults with shorter or longer sleep durations.[18] Sleep duration is strongly associated with adverse health outcomes, with robust evidence linking both short (less than 6 hours) and long (greater than 9 hours) sleep duration, albeit in cross-sectional analyses, to adverse cardiovascular, metabolic, immunologic, and cognitive outcomes, as well as mortality.[19] Thus the recommended sleep duration is not reduced in older adults, even though the ability to get the recommended amount of sleep may be decreased because of normal changes in sleep architecture.[20] Admittedly, these recommendations refer to nocturnal sleep rather than 24-hour sleep duration. An as yet unanswered question is whether the amount of sleep over a 24-hour period is a better metric for assessing appropriate sleep duration in older adults, particularly since napping increases in prevalence with age.[21]

CIRCADIAN RHYTHMS IN AGING

Circadian rhythms may change over the life span with respect to phase, amplitude, and ability to phase-shift. Aging is often

Table 3.1 Total Sleep Time, Sleep Efficiency, Wake after Sleep Onset, and Duration of Sleep Stages as a Function of Age

This table shows the means with 95% confidence intervals for total sleep time, sleep efficiency, wake after sleep onset, and duration of sleep stages in $n = 5,273$ adults from the 2nd to 10th decades of life according to age, sex, and night of sleep study based on random-effects models.

				Duration of Sleep Stages (percentage of total sleep time)			
	Total Sleep Time (min)	Sleep Efficiency	Wake After Sleep Onset (min)	N1	N2	N3	REM
Total sample	394.6 (388.4–400.8); k = 158	85.7% (84.8–86.6); k = 147	48.2 (43.8–52.6); k = 94	7.9% (7.3–8.5); k = 104	51.4% (50.2–52.6); k = 104	20.4% (19.0–21.8); k = 107	19.0% (18.5–19.6); k = 108
Mean age, years							
18–34	410.6 (404.5–416.6); k = 76	89.0% (88.0–90.0); k = 65	32.1 (28.2–36.1); k = 42	6.0% (5.3–6.7); k = 38	51.3% (49.6–52.9); k = 39	21.4% (20.0–22.8); k = 42	19.8% (18.8–20.8); k = 44
35–49	386.6 (371.4–401.9); k = 32	85.4% (83.7–87.1); k = 35	51.1 (41.1–61.1); k = 22	8.0% (6.9–9.2); k = 23	52.2% (50.6–53.8); k = 24	20.4% (18.5–22.2); k = 23	19.3% (18.2–20.3); k = 24
50–64	372.0 (358.1–85.89); k = 26	83.2% (81.0–85.4); k = 27	64.0 (55.1–72.9); k = 17	8.7% (7.3–10.0); k = 22	52.8% (49.8–55.8); k = 22	18.1% (15.0–21.2); k = 23	18.7% (17.8–19.6); k = 2
65–79	346.0 (326.7–365.4); k = 17	77.5% (73.0–81.9); k = 16	77.1 (57.3–96.9); k = 12	9.3% (7.0–11.6); k = 11	53.3% (50.0–56.7); k = 11	19.9% (17.8–22.1); k = 11	17.7% (16.9–18.5); k = 10
≥80	198.6 (142.5–254.7); k = 1	45.7% (33.7–57.7); k = 1	NA	27.5% (15.0–40.0); k = 1	43.5% (37.8–49.2); k = 1	19.1% (8.3–29.9); k = 1	9.9% (4.4–15.4); k = 1
Sex							
Both	405.2 (398.8–411.7); k = 101	86.7% (85.5–87.8); k = 96	43.3 (37.9–48.8); k = 56	9.7% (8.7–10.6); k = 59	50.6% (48.7–52.5); k = 59	19.5% (17.5–21.4); k = 62	19.2% (18.5–19.9); k = 63
Men only	374.6 (357.3–392.0); k = 30	84.3% (82.0–86.6); k = 27	51.8 (42.1–61.4); k = 20	5.3% (4.5–6.1); k = 23	52.1% (50.2–53.9); k = 24	21.0% (19.5–22.4); k = 24	19.9% (18.5–21.2); k = 24
Women only	356.0 (337.3–374.8); k = 19	84.1% (81.6–86.5); k = 20	55.0 (46.3–63.7); k = 17	4.2% (3.6–4.7); k = 16	55.1% (54.0–56.3); k = 16	22.1% (20.8–23.4); k = 17	18.6% (17.9–19.3); k = 17
Night of sleep study							
First night	371.6 (361.8–381.3); k = 89	84.2% (83.0–85.4); k = 88	52.7 (46.7–58.7); k = 57	7.0% (6.4–7.5); k = 63	52.1% (50.8–53.3); k = 69	20.7% (19.6–21.8); k = 69	18.3% (17.7–18.8); k = 68
Second night or later	419.7 (412.0–427.4); k = 48	89.3% (88.0–90.5); k = 39	37.9 (30.6–45.2); k = 26	6.9% (5.6–8.3); k = 23	48.2% (45.7–50.8); k = 24	22.3% (18.5–26.2); k = 25	21.4% (20.0–22.7); k = 26

Variable k represents the number of control groups combined to reach the pooled estimate. Some studies included more than one control group. NA, No studies available for this variable at this age cutoff; REM, rapid eye movement.

From Boulos MI, Jairam T, Kendzerska T, et al. Normal polysomnography parameters in healthy adults: a systematic review and meta-analysis. *Lancet Respir Med* 2019;7:533–43.

Table 3.2 Sleep-Onset Latency, REM Latency, Arousal Index, AHI, Mean and Minimum SaO_2, and PLMI as a Function of Age

This table shows the means with 95% confidence intervals for sleep-onset latency, REM latency, arousal index, AHI, mean and minimum SaO_2, and PLMI for n = 5,273 adults from the 2nd to 10th decades of life according to age, sex, and night of sleep study based on random-effects models.

	Sleep onset latency (min)	REM latency (min)	Arousal index, events per h	AHI, events per h	Mean SaO_2	Minimum SaO_2	PLMI, events per h
Total sample	15.4 (14.2–16.7); k = 124	97.4 (93.9–100.8); k = 89	12.6 (11.8–13.3); k = 89	2.9 (2.6–3.1); k = 99	95.0% (94.7–95.3); k = 48	89.2% (88.5–89.9); k = 58	2.5 (2.1–2.9); k = 58
Mean age, years							
18–34	14.3 (12.5–16.1); k = 58	96.4 (91.0–101.8); k = 42	9.6 (8.8–10.5); k = 32	1.6 (1.2–2.0); k = 28	96.2% (95.9–96.5); k = 15	91.8% (91.3–92.3); k = 17	1.1 (0.6–1.6); k = 11
35–49	14.4 (12.3–16.6); k = 25	93.4 (88.9–98.0); k = 18	12.5 (10.7–14.2); k = 25	3.1 (2.5–3.7); k = 28	95.3% (94.7–95.8); k = 13	90.5% (89.3–91.7); k = 19	3.1 (1.9–4.3); k = 14
50–64	15.7 (13.7–17.8); k = 19	101.3 (92.8–109.7); k = 14	16.5 (14.9–18.2); k = 19	4.2 (3.6–4.8); k = 28	94.3% (93.9–94.7); k = 11	87.0% (84.7–89.3); k = 12	6.2 (4.1–8.3); k = 15
65–79	19.5 (15.2–23.8); k = 16	99.7 (85.6–113.8); k = 11	18.8 (15.3–22.3); k = 9	15.5 (12.9–18.2); k = 10	93.3% (93.0–93.7); k = 7	84.0% (83.0–85.0); k = 7	8.5 (4.9–12.1); k = 8
≥80	41.4 (14.2–68.6); k = 1	182.0 (118.6–245.4); k = 1	31.6 (15.4–47.8); k = 1	30.3 (12.3–48.3); k = 1	94.2% (92.5–95.9); k = 1	88.0% (84.3–91.7); k =1	14.6 (5.6–23.4); k = 1
Sex							
Both	15.4 (13.7–17.1); k = 76	96.7 (91.9–101.6); k = 44	11.3 (10.3–12.4); k = 47	2.2 (1.9–2.5); k = 54	95.4% (94.8–95.9); k = 14	91.7% (90.9–92.4); k = 21	4.4 (3.4–5.4); k = 26
Men only	14.7 (13.0–16.4); k = 25	92.5 (85.8–99.2); k = 24	14.5 (12.6–16.5); k = 20	5.2 (4.2–6.1); k = 23	94.7% (94.3–95.1); k = 18	87.9% (86.6–89.2); k = 19	2.1 (1.3–3.0); k = 16
Women only	13.5 (11.8–15.1); k = 20	99.5 (95.2–103.9); k = 20	12.7 (11.1–14.4); k = 15	3.1 (2.4–3.8); k = 16	95.0% (94.5–95.6); k = 14	87.6% (86.0–89.3); k = 14	2.1 (1.4–2.8); k = 15
Night of sleep study*							
First night	14.7 (13.3–16.1); k = 68	99.5 (96.1–103.0); k = 49	13.5 (12.5–14.6); k = 62	3.4 (3.1–3.8); k = 72	95.0% (94.7–95.3); k = 40	89.0% (88.1–89.8); k = 49	2.2 (1.8–2.6); k = 45
Second night or later	14.4 (12.3–16.4); k = 41	87.3 (82.4–92.2); k = 28	9.6 (8.0–11.2); k = 14	–	–	–	–

Variable k represents number of control groups combined to reach the pooled estimate; the corresponding number of participants for each estimate is included in the appendix. Some studies included more than one control group.

*Most studies reporting AHI, mean and minimum SaO_2 and PLMI were first-night studies and those remaining predominantly provided average values across the first night and a subsequent night or did not specify the night of study; therefore, night of study was not included as a covariate for those four sleep parameters in the mixed-effects model and the study reported pooled estimates for first-night studies.

AHI, Apnea-hypopnea index; PLMI, periodic limb movement index; REM, rapid eye movement; SaO_2, arterial oxygen saturation.

From Boulos MI, Jairam T, Kendzerska T, et al. Normal polysomnography parameters in healthy adults: a systematic review and meta-analysis. *Lancet Respir Med* 2019;7:533–43.

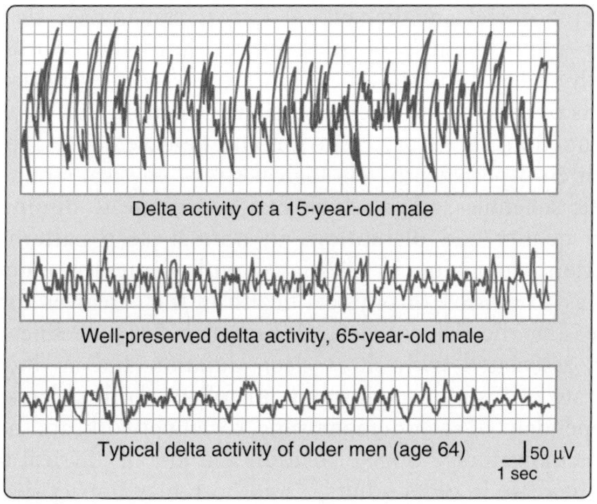

Figure 3.2 Age differences in delta activity. The top tracing shows abundant high-amplitude delta in an adolescent. The middle tracing shows well-preserved delta in an older man. Note the marked decrease in amplitude relative to the adolescent. The bottom tracing is a more typical example of delta activity in an older man. Note the number of waves failing to meet the 75-μV amplitude criterion. (From Zepelin H. Normal age related change in sleep. In: Chase, MH, Weitzman ED, eds. *Sleep Disorders: Basic and Clinical Research.* Spectrum; 1983:431–53.)

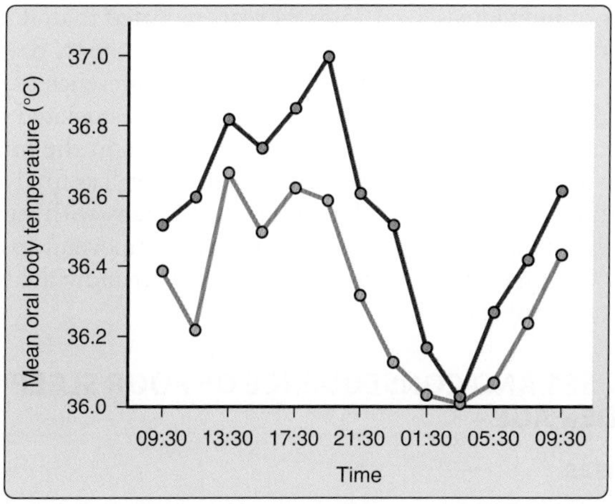

Figure 3.3 Body temperature cycle as a function of age. Oral temperatures in young *(red circles)* and old *(green circles)* subjects, showing decreased amplitude and earlier phase in body temperature cycle as a function of aging. Data were obtained under entrained conditions. (From Richardson GS, Carskadon MA, Orav EJ. Circadian variation of sleep tendency in elderly and young adult subjects. *Sleep*. 1982:5[Suppl 2]:S82–94.)

associated with a phase advance (i.e., a shift in the peak and trough of the circadian rhythm to an earlier time).[22] An age-related phase advance has been demonstrated to affect endogenous rhythms of body temperature and levels of melatonin, cortisol, blood pressure, and white blood cells.[22] With respect to the sleep-wake cycle, a phase advance leads to an earlier onset of sleepiness in the evening and earlier morning awakening.[22] Daytime wakefulness may also be affected by phase advance, with older adults being more alert in the morning and more somnolent in the evening.[23] This advance is not explained by a change in circadian periodicity.[24] The mechanisms contributing to the phase advance are complex and may include interactions between circadian mechanisms (abnormal circadian entrainment, changes in the input or output of the circadian pacemaker, impairment of downstream circadian signals) and impaired homeostatic sleep drive.[24-28]

In older adults, the amplitude of the circadian rhythm may also be affected. A demonstration of this change can be seen when studying body temperature throughout the circadian cycle (Figure 3.3), with older adults demonstrating less of a difference between the peak and trough of body temperature.[29] This decrease in amplitude is more marked in older men than in older women.[22]

Finally, a well-described feature of the aging circadian system is the relative impairment in the ability to phase-shift.[22] This may in part reflect loss of rhythmic function within the suprachiasmatic nucleus.[30] The ability to phase-shift and entrain to light in old age may be particularly impaired because of challenges to the visual system that occur as a part of aging (e.g., cataracts, macular degeneration). In support of this theory, epidemiologic studies have shown that elderly persons with visual impairments were 30% to 60% more likely to have impaired nighttime sleep relative to visually unimpaired elderly subjects.[31] Conversely, older persons who undergo cataract correction via intraocular cataract lens replacement may have improved circadian rhythms, better cognitive performance, and improved sleep.[32] However, even among persons without visual impairment, responsiveness of the circadian system to light exposure may be decreased.[33]

NAPPING

The high prevalence of napping in older age has been established by two landmark studies of sleep and aging, the Established Populations for Epidemiologic Studies of the Elderly (EPESE)[34] and the NSF 2003 Sleep in America Poll.[35] EPESE included 9,282 community-dwelling adults aged 65 and older and found that 25% reported napping.[34] The NSF 2003 Sleep in America Poll confirmed the prevalence of these symptoms, finding that 39% of community-dwelling adults aged 65 to 74 and 46% of adults aged 75 to 84 years reported napping.[35]

Although napping may be prevalent in older age, whether it is harmful or helpful to the health of older adults is less clear. A large body of literature suggests that napping is both a beneficial and potentially protective event in the life of an older person as well as an identifiable risk factor for morbidity and mortality. Napping has been associated with falls,[36] accumulation of beta-amyloid and tau in the brain,[37,38] cognitive decline,[39] depression,[40] nocturia,[41] diabetes,[42] and lower quality of life.[43] Other studies suggest that naps and hypersomnolence portend mortality[44] or ischemic heart disease.[45] On the other hand, evidence continues to accrue that naps may be protective for cardiovascular events[46,47] and improve cognition and daytime function.[48,49]

Reaching a conclusion about the benefits or harms of napping is made difficult by both the lack of comparability across studies with respect to napping frequency or duration and the lack of longitudinal observation studies. In addition, there are the complexities of relying on self-reports to derive estimates of the physiologic tendency of sleep during the daytime hours and the fact that, overarching all other issues, sleeping during the daytime hours in old age is likely to be a multidetermined phenomenon. Whether napping is helpful or harmful probably has to do with the nap characteristics as well as a person's overall sleep duration. In support of this, recently published research found that subjects who napped one to two times per week had lower risk of incident cardiovascular events, while no association was found for more frequent napping or napping duration.[47] Thus failure to account for nap frequency may help explain the discrepant findings regarding the association between napping and cardiovascular risk. Similarly, a study of individuals aged 75 to 94 years reported that, if short nighttime sleep durations were taken into account, daytime naps were protective for mortality, but in the presence of nocturnal sleep longer than 9 hours, naps were associated with increased mortality risk.[50] These studies highlight the importance of accounting for nap characteristics as well as total sleep duration when assessing the association of naps with various health outcomes. In addition, it may also be important to consider the time of day of the nap and whether individuals are habitual nappers.[49]

CAUSES AND CONSEQUENCE OF POOR SLEEP IN OLDER AGE

Causes

The aging process is commonly associated with multiple pathologic processes that can affect sleep, and resulting prevalence rates of insomnia symptoms and daytime sleepiness in epidemiologic studies of older adults are high.[23,51] Insomnia symptoms occur in nearly half of older adults,[34,52,53] while daytime sleepiness is reported by over 20% of older adults.[54]

One of the major issues contributing to sleep problems in older adults is the increasing prevalence of comorbidities.[55] With a rising number of health problems, the likelihood of sleep complaints increases.[35] Particularly relevant are chronic pain conditions, cardiovascular diseases, respiratory conditions, and digestive diseases. In addition to medical comorbidity, the increasing prevalence of psychiatric conditions and primary sleep disorders also contributes to increasing sleep disturbance in older age.[23,51] When persons with such comorbidities are eliminated from consideration, the resulting insomnia prevalence in elderly populations may be only 1% to 3%,[56] reiterating the decreased significance of chronologic age in predicting poor sleep.

Nocturia requires special mention, given its prevalence in older age and association with sleep disruption. In both women and men, the occurrence of nocturia appears to be associated with poor sleep,[57] even when other factors such as pain and medical comorbidity are taken into account. In fact, nocturia may be the single most common factor associated with poor sleep in elderly persons.[57] The duration of the first uninterrupted sleep period, otherwise referred to as the time to first void, has been shown to correlate with nearly all measures of whole-night sleep quality,[58] and lengthening of the first uninterrupted sleep period in a population containing a substantial portion of elderly persons was associated with improvements in many such measures.[59] Effects were independent from age. Additionally, improvements in sleep when nocturnal diuresis is treated have been demonstrated.[60] Nocturia may be a symptom of SDB[61,62] and has been reported to be reduced when SDB is treated with continuous positive airway pressure.[63,64]

Medication and substance use may increase risk for sleep disturbances in older adults. The use of prescription medications, over-the-counter medications, and dietary supplements is on the rise in this age group.[65] Medications can directly impact sleep through multiple mechanisms, including increased daytime drowsiness, activating effects, exacerbation of underlying primary sleep disorders, or disruption of sleep architecture, or by causing sleep-disruptive symptoms.[51]

Similarly, substances such as alcohol, caffeine, and tobacco can disrupt sleep architecture and increase risk for sleep disturbance.[51]

Psychosocial and behavioral factors can impact sleep in older adults because of their associations with worsening health and psychiatric illness.[51] Particularly relevant are the effects of caregiving, loneliness, social isolation, loss of physical function, sedentary behavior, and bereavement. Caregivers often experience psychological stress, physical strain, and erratic schedules, all of which may contribute to diminished sleep quality and disruptions in normal sleep patterns. In addition, caregiving is associated with depressed mood as well as an erosion of physical health in the caregiver, further increasing the risk for sleep disturbance.[66,67] Loneliness has been associated with short sleep duration and an increasing rate of insomnia symptoms in follow-up in older adults independent of sociodemographic, social network, and health status indicators.[68] Social isolation and loss of physical function increase in older adults,[51] and both may impact sleep by contributing to poor sleep hygiene or decreased exposure to environmental cues that entrain circadian rhythms to promote normal sleep-wake cycles.[69] With aging, sedentary behaviors increase and have detrimental effects on sleep.[70,71] Conversely, physical activity interventions may improve subjective and objective measures of sleep in older adults, with recent evidence suggesting that light rather than moderate-to-vigorous physical activity interventions may have more benefit in older adults.[70,71] Finally, bereavement may lead to worsening physical health, mood disorders, substance abuse, and social isolation.[72]

Potential Consequences

Sleep complaints, whether related to insomnia symptoms or drowsiness, have important consequences in older adults. Beyond being distressing for the subject, these symptoms predict poor physical and mental health-related quality of life.[73] In longitudinal studies, insomnia complaints have been associated with detrimental outcomes, including poor self-reported health status, cognitive decline, depression, disability in basic activities of daily living, poorer quality of life, and higher risk of institutionalization.[74,75] Insomnia is also associated with impaired physical function and increased fall risk.[75,76] Daytime drowsiness has also been associated with harmful outcomes in longitudinal studies, including cardiovascular disease, falls, and death.[74] Healthy older adults who have sleep latencies greater than 30 minutes, sleep efficiencies below 80%, or REM sleep percentage below 16% or greater than 25% of total sleep are at increased mortality risk, even after controlling for gender and baseline medical burden.[77]

SLEEP AND COGNITION

An area of emerging interest is whether changes in sleep with aging have ramifications for memory and cognitive changes.[78] With increasing age and disease, there are not only changes in sleep quality (as described earlier) but also declines in memory, attention, executive function, and processing speed.[79] A substantial literature has reported on the short- and long-term effects of poor sleep on cognitive function. Whether poor sleep might contribute to declining cognition and the development of cognitive disorders such as Alzheimer disease is an area of active research.

With respect to short-term effects, significant correlations exist between various sleep measures (self-report, actigraphy, and polysomnography) and performance on cognitive tests in middle-aged and older adults, even after correcting for demographic and health-related confounding variables. In cross-sectional studies, middle-aged adults consistently demonstrate detrimental relationships between cognitive performance and self-reported short sleep, long sleep, difficulty falling asleep, and nighttime awakenings; by contrast, older adults consistently show cross-sectional associations only between cognitive performance and self-reported long sleep duration or delayed sleep-onset latency.[78] Most sleep deprivation studies have shown that sleep deprivation has less of an impact on cognitive performance in older adults than in younger adults.[78,80]

In measurement of cognitive performance before and after a single nap, nap-related benefits to cognitive performance are consistently observed in middle-aged adults.[49] Similar nap-related benefits to cognition also seem to emerge in interventional studies in which participants are asked to attempt to take an afternoon nap every day for a month.[81] However, similar to what has been shown with the sleep deprivation literature, napping interventions focused on older age groups have often failed to result in any cognitive benefits of napping.[82] Pharmacologic enhancement of sleep, specifically defined as increases in spindles[83] and slow wave activity, seems to benefit cognition in young and middle-aged adults[84] but does not greatly benefit older adults.[85]

Several longitudinal studies have connected short and long self-reported sleep at baseline as well as longitudinal changes in sleep duration to subsequent cognitive decline.[86,87] Some large cross-sectional studies have suggested that different aspects of reported lower sleep quality, rather than measured SDB, were most strongly associated with both amnestic and nonamnestic types of mild cognitive impairment.[88] Actigraphy-measured sleep-wake assessments in older adults have tended to implicate wake after sleep onset or sleep efficiency rather than total sleep duration[89] as relevant correlates of impaired cognition. In addition, lower REM sleep quantity and density have been related to cognitive decline in longitudinal studies,[90,91] but whether declining REM sleep causes cognitive functioning to worsen or if age- and disease-related declines in cholinergic neurotransmission drive both decline in REM sleep and cognition remains unclear.

One mechanism by which poor sleep could affect cognitive functioning with advancing age is by reducing the efficiency of sleep-dependent memory consolidation. Animal studies have found reduced hippocampal reactivation of place cells during sleep (i.e., memory "replay").[92] In humans, sleep-dependent memory consolidation also appears to decline steadily across the life span. Memory consolidation effects are larger in middle-aged than in older adults.[93] Aging appears to detrimentally affect both procedural (motor) memory and declarative (episodic or explicit) memory consolidation, and adults in the eighth and ninth decades of life may show no memory consolidation effects at all.[94] Precise coupling of NREM slow waves and spindles is required for memory consolidation. This coupling may be more impaired with aging, particularly if there is atrophy in the medial frontal lobe.[95]

Another potential mechanism connecting poor sleep and cognitive decline involves the hypothesized bi-directional relationship between sleep and Alzheimer disease.[96] Alzheimer disease is defined pathologically by the accumulation of β-amyloid as insoluble extracellular plaque and intracellular tangles of tau proteins that eventually lead to cognitive dysfunction.[97] In humans, self-reported short sleep duration and lower actigraphy-measured sleep efficiency have been associated with higher β-amyloid burden, as measured by positron emission tomography[98] or cerebrospinal fluid (CSF), in cognitively normal individuals.[37] Excessive daytime sleepiness has also been found to predict increased β-amyloid in older adults without dementia.[99] Studies in mice and humans found that sleep deprivation increased soluble β-amyloid and promoted the formation of β-amyloid plaques.[100-102] It has also been shown that sleep disruption leads to the release of soluble tau in both mice and humans and promotes the spread of tau aggregates in mice.[103,104] Further, poorer sleep quality over several days correlates with increased CSF tau.[105] Since tau pathology is associated with the onset of cognitive deficits in Alzheimer disease, these findings add to the mounting evidence of a causal link between disrupted sleep and progression of Alzheimer disease pathology.[106]

CLINICAL PEARLS

- Although sleep disturbance is common in older adults, it is not an inherent part of the aging process and should not be attributed to normal aging.
- In older adults, the etiology of sleep disturbance is often multifactorial, with contributions from medical and psychiatric disease, medication use, and psychosocial and behavioral factors.
- Nocturia is highly prevalent in older age and is the most common factor associated with sleep disturbance in the elderly.
- Napping should never be assumed to be innocuous, nor should sleepiness during the day be attributed unequivocally to underlying disease.
- Poor sleep not only reduces the quality of life of older adults but also portends adverse health consequences.

SUMMARY

Normal aging is associated with changes to sleep architecture that tend to promote awakenings from sleep and decreased nocturnal total sleep time, as well as changes in circadian rhythmicity that affect circadian phase, amplitude, and ability to phase-shift. There is not, however, a decreased need for sleep, and sleep complaints should not be attributed to normal aging. Similarly, napping, while common in older adults, may signal an underlying disorder, particularly if overall sleep duration is long. The etiology of sleep disturbance in older adults is likely to be multifactorial with consequent risks for important aging-related outcomes, including cognitive function, independence, health, and quality of life.

ACKNOWLEDGMENTS

Work on which this chapter is based was supported (in part) by the following: Dr. Miner is supported by the Claude D. Pepper Older Americans Independence Center at Yale School of Medicine (P30AG021342), the American Academy of Sleep Medicine Foundation, a foundation of the American Academy of Sleep Medicine, and the National Institute on Aging T32AG019134. Dr. Lucey is supported by the National Institute on Aging (K76 AG054863).

SELECTED READINGS

Bloom HG, Ahmed I, Alessi CA, et al. Evidence-based recommendations for the assessment and management of sleep disorders in older persons. *J Am Geriatr Soc.* 2009;57:761–789.

Boulos MI, Jairam T, Kendzerska T, Im J, Mekhael A, Murray BJ. Normal polysomnography parameters in healthy adults: a systematic review and meta-analysis. *Lancet Respirat Med.* 2019;7:533–543.

Hirshkowitz M, Whiton K, Albert SM, et al. National Sleep Foundation's sleep time duration recommendations: methodology and results summary. *Sleep Health.* 2015;1:40–43.

Ju Y-E, Lucey BP, Holtzman DM. Sleep and Alzheimer disease pathology-a bidirectional relationship. *Nat Rev Neurol.* 2014;10:115–119.

Ohayon MM, Carskadon MA, Guilleminault C, Vitiello MV. Meta-analysis of quantitative sleep parameters from childhood to old age in healthy individuals: developing normative sleep values across the human lifespan. *Sleep.* 2004;27:1255–1273.

Robbins R, Quan SF, Weaver MD, et al. Examining sleep deficiency and disturbance and their risk for incident dementia and all-cause mortality in older adults across 5 years in the United States. *Aging (Albany NY).* 2021;13(3):3254–3268.

Scullin MK, Bliwise DL. Sleep, cognition, and aging: integrating a half-century of multidisciplinary research. *Perspect Psychol Sci.* 2015;10(1):97–137.

Vanderlinden J, Boen F, van Uffelen JGZ. Effects of physical activity programs on sleep outcomes in older adults: a systematic review. *Int J Behav Nutr Phys Act.* 2020;17:11.

Vaz Fragoso CA, Gill TM. Sleep Complaints in Community-Living Older Persons: A Multifactorial Geriatric Syndrome. *J Am Geriat Soc.* 2007;55:1853–1866.

Watson NF. Sleep duration: a consensus conference. *J Clin Sleep Med.* 2015;11:7–8.

A complete reference list can be found online at ExpertConsult.com.

Chapter 4

Daytime Sleepiness and Alertness

Philip Cheng; Timothy Roehrs; Thomas Roth

Chapter Highlights

- Sleepiness is a multicausal physiologic need state with various neural and neurochemical substrates.
- Determinants of sleepiness include quantity and quality of sleep, circadian rhythms, and pathologies of the central nervous system. Monotony may unmask underlying sleepiness, but it does not cause sleepiness.
- Excessive sleepiness significantly impacts performance and safety and is thus a public health concern.
- Excessive sleepiness can also impair psychosocial functioning and is implicated in psychiatric difficulties.

INTRODUCTION

Scientific and clinical attention to sleepiness arose from the recognition of excessive daytime sleepiness (EDS) as a symptom associated with serious life-threatening medical conditions. In the late 1960s, this symptom—which earlier had been ignored, attributed to lifestyle excesses, viewed as a sign of laziness and malingering, or at best, seen as a sign of narcolepsy—began to be seriously studied by scientist-clinicians. Methods to characterize, detect, and quantify sleepiness were developed. The result has been the growth of scientific literature on the nature of sleepiness and its determinants in clinical populations, selected populations of healthy volunteers, and the general population.[1]

This chapter discusses information regarding the nature and neurobiologic substrates of sleepiness, and the known determinants of sleepiness are described. It also reviews the various methods used to measure sleepiness in the population and in the laboratory; guidelines regarding clinical assessment of sleepiness are offered. Finally, the clinical and public health significance of persistent complaints of sleepiness are discussed.

NATURE OF SLEEPINESS

Sleepiness Is a Physiologic Need State

Sleepiness, according to consensus among sleep researchers and clinicians, is a basic physiologic need state.[2] It may be likened to hunger or thirst, which are physiologic need states that drive individual organisms toward behaviors that fulfill their basic needs for survival. Just as hunger or thirst is modulated with the intake of food and water, sleepiness increases with sleep deprivation or restriction and decreases with accumulation of sleep. However, there are also factors in addition to an organism's daily homeostatic economy that may modulate sleepiness. Just as taste, smell, time-of-day, psychological, and social factors may additionally regulate hunger and thirst, sleep and sleepiness can also be influenced by social (e.g., job, family, and friends) and environmental (e.g., noise, light, and bed) factors.

The physiologic state of sleep need is usually accompanied by the subjective experience of sleepiness and its behavioral indicators (yawning, eye rubbing, head nodding). However, the subjective experiences of sleepiness can be temporarily reduced under conditions of high motivation, excitement, exercise, and competing needs (e.g., hunger, thirst). That is, physiologic sleepiness may not necessarily manifest despite a physiologic sleep need. The expression of mild to moderate sleepiness can be masked by any number of factors that are alerting, including motivation, environment, stress, posture, activity, light, or food intake. For example, studies of sleepiness have shown that average sleep latency can be increased by 6 minutes by altering posture in bed (from lying to sitting) and also by 6 minutes when immediately preceded by a 5-minute walk.[3] However, when physiologic sleepiness is most severe and persistent, the ability to reduce its impact on overt behavior wanes. The likelihood of sleep onset increases, and the intrusion of microsleeps into ongoing behavior occurs. In contrast, a physiologically alert (*sleepiness* and *alertness* are used here as antonyms) person does not experience sleepiness or appear sleepy even in the most soporific situations. Heavy meals, warm rooms, boring lectures, and the monotony of long-distance automobile driving can unmask physiologic sleepiness when it is present, but they do not cause it.

Importantly, when the physiologic state of sleepiness is prolonged and becomes chronic (e.g., regularly sleeping less than one's physiologic sleep need), adaptation to the subjective experience of sleepiness has been shown to occur. This has commonly been observed in the disparities between subjective and objective assessments of sleepiness, even when done with validated scales and procedures. Further, this disparity is typically greatest in the most sleepy individuals,[4,5] who commonly deny feeling sleepiness despite significant objective indicators of sleepiness. Furthermore, clinicians also report anecdotally that sleepy patients who have successfully undergone sleep treatments frequently comment that they had forgotten the experience of complete alertness. In contrast, basally alert individuals demonstrate accuracy in their self-reported sleepiness relative to the increases in electroencephalographic theta activity shown during a simulated driving task after 1 night of acute sleep restriction.[6]

In addition to habituation to the subjective experience of sleepiness, individuals with chronic sleepiness may also perceive themselves to be more alert because of compensatory mechanisms that may mitigate certain cognitive and behavioral effects of sleepiness. Indeed, cognitive and behavioral compensation has been documented after experimental sleep restriction and increased sleepiness, particularly when the sleep loss is mild and accumulates at a slow rate.[7] The absence of a readily apparent behavioral deficiency may serve as feedback and reinforcement of a sense of normalcy, despite the fact that objective measure of sleepiness, such as the Multiple Sleep Latency Test (MSLT), may indicate otherwise.

Sleepiness as a Dimensional Construct

One critical question regarding the nature of sleepiness is whether it is a unidimensional construct (varying only in severity) or multidimensional (varying in etiology and/or chronicity).[8] If it is unidimensional, whether sleepiness and alertness are at opposite poles of the dimension is also an issue. Sleepiness and alertness are commonly used as antonyms, which suggests a unipolar state; however, it is also possible that sleepiness varies in the degree between present to absent and may exist independently from alertness. Additionally, findings from a study of individuals from the general population found that subjective sleepiness was associated with multiple factors, suggesting that it has dimensions beyond simply an increased tendency to fall asleep.[9] Clinical studies have also found that patients often conflate fatigue and sleepiness.[8] Other dimensions cited include rapid eye movement (REM) sleep versus non–rapid eye movement (NREM) sleep, and core versus optional sleepiness.[10] A complete discussion of the heuristic value and evidence to support these distinctions is beyond the scope of this chapter. Nonetheless, the point must be made that these theoretical perspectives may be influenced by different measures, experimental demands, populations studied, and subject or patient motivations (i.e., sensitivity to and capacity to counteract sleepiness).

Evidence Toward Neural Substrates of Sleepiness

Research describing the precise neural substrates of sleepiness are still underway; however, it is understood that sleepiness is a central nervous system (CNS) phenomenon with identifiable neural mechanisms and neurochemical correlates. The neurochemistry of sleepiness-alertness involves critical and complex issues that have not yet been fully untangled (see Chapters 7, 8, and 49 for a complete discussion). First, a basic issue concerns whether sleepiness-alertness has a neural profile that is specific and unique from that associated with the sleep process, per se. Second, it is not clear whether sleepiness and alertness are controlled by separate neurochemicals or by a single substance or system. Third, the relation of the neurochemistry of sleepiness-alertness to circadian mechanisms has not yet been adequately determined. Given the number of questions, it should be of no surprise that these are areas of active research.

Research describing neural activity during sleep deprivation suggests that the phenomenon of sleepiness includes activation of neural mechanisms associated with the sleep process. Indeed, studies examining the neural electrophysiology of sleep deprivation in sleep-deprived organisms have demonstrated the occurrence/intrusion of various electrophysiologic events suggestive of incipient sleep processes during behavioral wakefulness. This includes ventral hippocampal spike activity—characteristic of NREM sleep—during wakefulness after sleep deprivation, with wakefulness defined as the absence of the usual changes in cortical EEG activity indicative of sleep.[11] Human beings deprived of or experiencing restricted sleep also show identifiable microsleep episodes (brief intrusions of EEG indications of sleep) and increased amounts of alpha and theta activity while behaviorally awake.[12] The evidence suggests that sleepiness includes wake state instability, although there appears to be significant individual variation.[13]

An emerging literature of neuroimaging studies, both structural and functional, have implicated a range of brain systems that may be involved in sleepiness. Sleep deprivation in young, healthy volunteers reduced regional cerebral glucose metabolism, as assessed by positron emission tomography, with the greatest reductions in the thalamus, inferior parietal/superior temporal cortices, the prefrontal and anterior cingulate cortices, basal ganglia, and limbic regions of the brain.[14,15] These areas subserve a range of cognitive and emotion regulation processes, including alertness and attention, higher-order analysis, integration of sensory–motor information, as well as affect valence and salience, all of which are impaired during sleepiness and sleep deprivation. Functional neuroimaging research has also shown that sleepiness and its accompanied impairments are associated with increased activity in the default mode network (DMN),[16] which is a distinct network of brain regions most active during wakeful rest and suppressed during goal-directed tasks. Because the DMN is usually deactivated during task performance, the increased DMN activity may represent reduced resources to the motor and attention systems, which then impair performance. Additionally, other studies have also shown reduced functional connectivity within the DMN.[17] In fact, the pattern of reduced connectivity within the DMN associated with sleepiness is similar to the profile of DMN connectivity during NREM sleep,[18] which is consistent with wake state instability and/or intrusions of microsleep. As yet, these imaging data are not conclusive; however, they do suggest identifiable changes in activity in specific brain regions and functions that vary with sleepiness. That said, the nature of the alteration may depend on the behavioral load imposed on the sleepy subject as well as the cause of the sleepiness.

In terms of neurochemistry, studies of sleep and wake mechanisms have implicated histamine, serotonin, orexin, the catecholamines, and acetylcholine in the control of wake, and gamma-aminobutyric acid (GABA) globally in the control of sleep.[19] Indeed, new developments in the histaminergic system have led to the H3 receptor as a recent drug target for daytime sleepiness in narcolepsy and other disorders.[20] Additionally, growing evidence from animal studies suggests that extracellular adenosine is a strong measure of the sleep homeostat, with brain levels of adenosine accumulating in parallel with prolonged wakefulness and declining with sleep.[21] This has been supported with a more recent meta-analysis,[22] which also suggests that the accumulation of adenosine may be particular to the basal forebrain containing a core component of the mechanism for sleep-wake control. More recent research has also examined the effects of more chronic sleep restriction on adenosine and its receptors, with results suggesting significant differences in between acute versus chronic sleep loss[23]; whereas sleepiness associated with acute sleep loss may be mediated by increases in adenosine levels,[24] sleepiness related to chronic sleep loss may be mediated by differences in receptor concentration.[25]

In particular, the hypocretin/orexin system has also received much attention, especially for its role in the pathophysiology of narcolepsy.[26] Orexin peptides are produced in a cluster of neurons located in the lateral hypothalamus that project widely throughout the CNS and heavily innervate regions that promote arousal and suppress REM sleep. Hypocretin/orexin is considered to be a major wake-promoting hypothalamic neuropeptide, and a hypocretin/orexin deficiency related to a loss of hypocretin/orexin neurons has been found in human narcolepsy. Additionally, re-expression of orexin receptors in animal models of narcolepsy rescues wake promotion.[19] Outside of narcolepsy, the interactive role of hypocretin/orexin in the homeostatic control of sleep and sleepiness has yet to be clearly determined (discussed in greater detail in Chapters 8, 49 and 111); however, given its role in wake promotion, a targeted reduction of hypocretin/orexin should result in increased sleepiness and sleep propensity. As such, novel orexin receptor agonists have been developed and approved for use in the United States for insomnia (e.g., suvorexant, lemborexant). These dual orexin receptor antagonists selectively bind to orexin-1 and -2 receptors to downregulate processes that promote wakefulness and have been shown to improve subjective sleep in insomnia acutely in emerging clinical trials.[21,27]

Pharmacologic studies have also provided other interesting hypotheses regarding the neurochemistry of sleepiness-alertness. For example, the benzodiazepines induce sleepiness and facilitate GABA function at the $GABA_A$ receptor complex, thus implicating this important and diffuse inhibitory neurotransmitter.[28] Another example involves histamine, which is considered to be a CNS neurotransmitter and is thought to have CNS-arousing activity.[28] Antihistamines that penetrate the CNS produce sleepiness.[29] A functional neuroimaging study of histamine H_1 receptors in the human brain found that the degree of sleepiness associated with cetirizine (20 mg) was correlated to the degree of H_1 receptor occupancy.[30]

Stimulant drugs suggest several other transmitters and neuromodulators. For example, amphetamines produce psychomotor stimulation and arousal through the blockade of catecholamine.[31] Another class of stimulants, the methylxanthines, which include caffeine and theophylline, are adenosine receptor antagonists. Adenosine, considered the key neurochemical in the homeostatic regulation of sleep, has inhibitory activity on the two major excitatory neurotransmitters acetylcholine and glutamate. It may be a biomarker of sleepiness.[32] On the other hand, some contradictory evidence limits making definitive conclusions.[33-35] The space here is too limited to discuss all the evidence in detail. In conclusion, although it is widely held that sleepiness is a physiologic state, its physiologic substrates are not yet fully defined.

MEASURING AND QUANTIFYING SLEEPINESS

The physiologic state of sleepiness is often accompanied by behavioral signs that are often precursors to a sleep state, including yawning, ptosis (heavy eyelids), reduced activity, lapses in attention, and head nodding. Indeed, before the availability of psychophysiologic measurement tools, sleep/sleepiness was also predominantly determined based on a number of observable principles. These include (1) sleep is a sustained period of behavioral quiescence in a (2) stereotypic posture (e.g., laying horizontally for humans with eyes closed) with (3) an elevated arousal threshold, but is nevertheless (4) rapidly reversible with an adequately strong stimulus. As such behaviors approximating those observations are often used as signs of sleepiness. However, as noted earlier, a number of factors such as motivation, stimulation, and competing needs can reduce the behavioral manifestation and subjective experience of sleepiness.

The various challenges in assessing sleepiness became evident early in research on the daytime consequences of sleep loss. It is clear that sleep loss compromises daytime functions; virtually everyone experiences dysphoria and reduced performance efficiency when not sleeping adequately. But a majority of the tasks used to assess the effects of sleep loss are insensitive.[36] In general, only long and monotonous tasks are reliably sensitive to changes in the quantity and quality of nocturnal sleep. One exception is the 10-minute visual vigilance task, completed repeatedly across the day, during which lapses (response times ≥500 msec) and declines in the best response times are increasingly observed as sleep is lost, either during total deprivation or cumulatively over nights of restricted bedtimes.[37]

In addition to behavioral indicators of sleepiness, individuals can also readily report their subjective level of sleepiness. In various measures of self-reported sleepiness, including factor analytic scales, visual analogue scales, and scales for specific aspects of mood, subjects have shown increased fatigue or sleepiness with acute sleep loss. Among the various subjective measures of sleepiness, the Stanford Sleepiness Scale (SSS) is the best validated and indicates sleepiness in the moment.[38] Yet clinicians have found that chronically sleepy patients may rate themselves alert on the SSS even while they are falling asleep behaviorally.[39] Such scales are state measures that query individuals about how they feel at the present moment. Another approach is to define sleepiness as the likelihood of falling asleep. This is the approach that the Epworth Sleepiness Scale (ESS) takes, asking individuals to rate that likelihood of falling asleep in different circumstances (e.g., while driving, in social conversation, after a meal) and over longer periods of time. The ESS has been validated in clinical populations showing a 74% sensitivity and 50% specificity relative to objective assessments of sleepiness in patients with sleep disorders.[40]

Because behavioral and subjective indicators often underestimate physiologic sleepiness, measurements of sleepiness have emphasized more objective assessments. The standard physiologic measure of sleepiness is the MSLT. Similar to the ESS, it conceptualizes sleepiness as the tendency to fall asleep as operationalized by how quickly a person falls asleep when provided the opportunity. The MSLT has gained wide acceptance within the field of sleep and sleep disorders as the standard method of quantifying sleepiness.[41,42] Using standard polysomnographic techniques, this test measures the latency to fall asleep while lying in a quiet, dark bedroom during five repeated opportunities at 2-hour intervals throughout the day.[42] The MSLT is based on the assumption, as outlined earlier, that sleepiness is a physiologic need state that leads to an increased tendency to fall asleep. The metric typically used to express sleepiness has been average daily sleep latency (i.e., mean of the five tests conducted), but survival analyses have also been successfully used.[43] The reliability and validity of this measure have been documented in a variety of experimental and clinical situations.[44] In contrast to tests of performance, motivation does not seem to reduce the impact of sleep loss as measured by the MSLT. After total sleep deprivation, subjects can compensate for impaired performance, but they cannot stay awake long while in bed in a darkened room, even if they are instructed to do so.[45]

An alternative to the MSLT, suggested by some clinical investigators, is the Maintenance of Wakefulness Test (MWT). Although both are objective measures of sleepiness, the MWT differs from the MSLT in that it assesses ability to maintain wakefulness (against some amount of sleep drive) as opposed to the propensity to fall asleep when given the opportunity. As such, proponents of the MWT have argued that it is more generalizable to circumstances where accidental sleepiness is of interest, such as fitness-for-duty assessments. Although there have historically been variations in how the MWT has been performed, standard guidelines have been published by the American Academy for Sleep Medicine.[42] The guidelines recommend that subjects be comfortably reclined in bed in a dark room and are instructed to try to remain awake.[46] Like the MSLT, the measure of ability to remain awake is the latency to sleep onset. Each trial should last up to 40 minutes or until sleep onset occurs and should be repeated at 2-hour intervals, starting 1½ to 3 hours after habitual wake time (usual start time is around 9:00 a.m. or 10:00 a.m.). As a newer assessment, the MWT has not been as thoroughly tested as the MSLT; however, one study reported similar intertrial correlations for the MSLT (r = 0.609) and the MWT (r = 0.610) in 258 patients with symptoms of daytime sleepiness or sleep apnea,[46] suggesting comparable reliability and internal consistency. Another study reported sensitivity to the therapeutic effects of continuous positive airway pressure (CPAP) in patients with sleep apnea,[47] and several studies reported sensitivity to the therapeutic effects of stimulants in narcolepsy.[48] A study attempted to tease apart the critical factors being measured by the MWT and concluded that, unlike the MSLT, which measures level of sleepiness, the MWT measures the combined effects of level of sleepiness and the degree of arousal as defined by heart rate.[49]

The rationale for the MWT is that clinically the critical issue for patients is how long wakefulness can be maintained. A basic assumption underlying this rationale, however, may not be valid: it assumes that a set of circumstances can be evaluated in the laboratory that will reflect an individual's probability of staying awake in the real world. Such a circumstance is not likely because environment, motivation, circadian phase, and any competing drive states all affect an individual's tendency to remain awake. Stated simply, an individual crossing a congested intersection at midday is more likely to stay awake than an individual driving on an isolated highway in the middle of the night. The MSLT, on the other hand, addresses the question of the individual's risk of falling asleep by establishing a setting to maximize the likelihood of sleep onset: all factors competing with falling asleep are removed from the test situation. Thus the MSLT identifies sleep tendency or clinically identifies maximum risk for the patient. Obviously, the actual risk will vary from individual to individual, from hour to hour, and from environment to environment.

The Future of Sleepiness: Biomarkers

There has been great interest in the field for developing biomarkers of sleepiness to enhance the array of clinical tools that are less cumbersome and more resource and time efficient than existing electrophysiologic and behavioral tests (e.g., MSLT, MWT). Although most have operationalized "biomarkers" as quantifiable molecular and chemical properties of easily accessible biologic samples—such as blood, waste (urine and stool), saliva, and breath—others have used a broader definition of "biomarkers" to include bioinformatics obtained via wearable technologies and other behavioral indicators.[50] Ultimately, the goal for any biomarkers is to enhance the precision, efficiency, and scalability of clinical applications (e.g., diagnostic tools or assessments to monitor treatment response) and population-based research in sleep and circadian health.

Although there are currently no accessible biomarkers on the market, this is a fast-growing area of research with several targets under investigation and in development. Given that sleepiness may be a multidimensional and dynamic construct, many of these targets are technically biomarkers for sleep drive. Indeed, animal models of sleep and sleepiness have identified candidate genes as potential biomarkers for sleepiness as they appear to be expressed with periods of waking that are associated with a homeostatic response.[51-53] Other areas of research have focused on the proteome (i.e., set of proteins encoded by the genome) instead of the genome, apropos to the dynamic nature of sleepiness and sleep drive. Proteins participate in physiologic interactions by responding to differing signals in the cellular environmental; this enables measurement of changes in physiologic states and exponentially increases the complexities of analyses. Finally, in keeping with the rapidly growing industry of mobile and wearable technologies, researchers have also explored the used of bioinformatics as biomarkers of sleepiness. For example, emerging research is validating the use of accelerometer data and light sensors on wrist-worn devices to estimate circadian phase,[54-57] which has implications for predicting patterns in vulnerability to sleepiness, such as windows of circadian low. Additionally, reaction time data, particularly via the psychomotor vigilance test, have also been used to measure risk of performance deficits associated with sleepiness (e.g., fitness-for-duty assessments). Importantly, although reaction time shows high sensitivity to sleep loss and sleepiness, it also suffers from low specificity because it is also affected by a range of other problems such as traumatic brain injuries.[58]

Determinants of Sleepiness

As is with many physiologic need states, there is a certain predictability in their occurrence. As previously discussed, sleepiness clearly arises from deprivation or restriction of sleep; however, sleepiness also ebbs and flows across a 24-hour period. For example, within a conventional 24-hour sleep and wake schedule, maximum sleepiness ordinarily occurs in the middle of the night when the individual is sleeping; consequently, the state of sleepiness typically is not experienced or remembered. Finally, sleepiness may also arise from many medications and pathologies involving the CNS.

Quantity of Sleep

The degree of daytime sleepiness is directly related to the amount of nocturnal sleep. The performance effects of acute and chronic sleep deprivation are discussed in Chapters 5 and 16. Occurrence of both partial and total sleep deprivation for 1 night will acutely increase daytime sleepiness the following day[44]; similarly, modest nightly sleep restriction accumulates over nights to progressively increase daytime sleepiness and performance lapses.[59] However, the speed at which sleep loss is accumulated is critical, as studies have shown adaptation to a slow accumulation of 1 to 2 hours nightly occurs, which then increases the duration of the subsequent recovery process.[60] Increased sleep time in healthy, but sleepy, young adults by extending bedtime beyond the usual 7 to 8 hours per night produces an increase in alertness (i.e., reduction in sleepiness).[61] Further, the pharmacologic extension of sleep time by an average of 1 hour in elderly people produces an increase in mean sleep latency on the MSLT (i.e., increased alertness).[62]

Reduced sleep time explains the excessive sleepiness of several patient and nonpatient groups. For example, a subgroup of sleep clinic patients has been identified whose EDS can be attributed to chronic insufficient sleep.[63] These patients show objectively documented excessive sleepiness, "normal" nocturnal sleep with unusually high sleep efficiency (time asleep–time in bed), and report about 2 hours more sleep on each weekend day than each weekday. Regularizing bedtime and increasing time in bed produces a resolution of their symptoms and normalized MSLT results.[64] The increased sleepiness of healthy young adults also can be attributed to insufficient nocturnal sleep. When the sleepiest 25% of a sample of young adults is given extended time in bed (10 hours) for as long as 5 to 14 consecutive nights, their sleepiness is reduced to a level resembling the general population.[61]

Individual differences in tolerability to sleep loss have been reported.[65] These differences can be attributed to many possible factors. A difference in the basal level of sleepiness at the start of a sleep time manipulation is possible given the range of sleepiness in the general population (Figure 4.1). The basal differences may reflect insufficient nightly sleep relative to one's sleep need.[61] There also may be differences in the sensitivity and responsivity of the sleep homeostat to sleep loss, that is how large a sleep deficit the system can tolerate and how robustly the sleep homeostat produces sleep when detecting deficiency. Finally, genetic differences in sleep need, the set point around which the sleep homeostat regulates daily sleep time, have long been hypothesized, and one study has suggested a gene polymorphism may mediate vulnerability to sleep loss.[66] These all are fertile areas for research.

Quality of Sleep

Daytime sleepiness also relates to the quality and the continuity of a previous night's sleep. One way in which sleep quality may be disturbed is via brief arousals of 3 to 15 seconds' duration. Indeed, sleep in patients with a number of sleep disorders is frequently punctuated by such arousals. These arousals are characterized by bursts of EEG speeding or alpha activity and, occasionally, transient increases in skeletal muscle tone. Standard scoring rules for transient EEG arousals have been developed.[67] A transient arousal is illustrated in Figure 4.2.

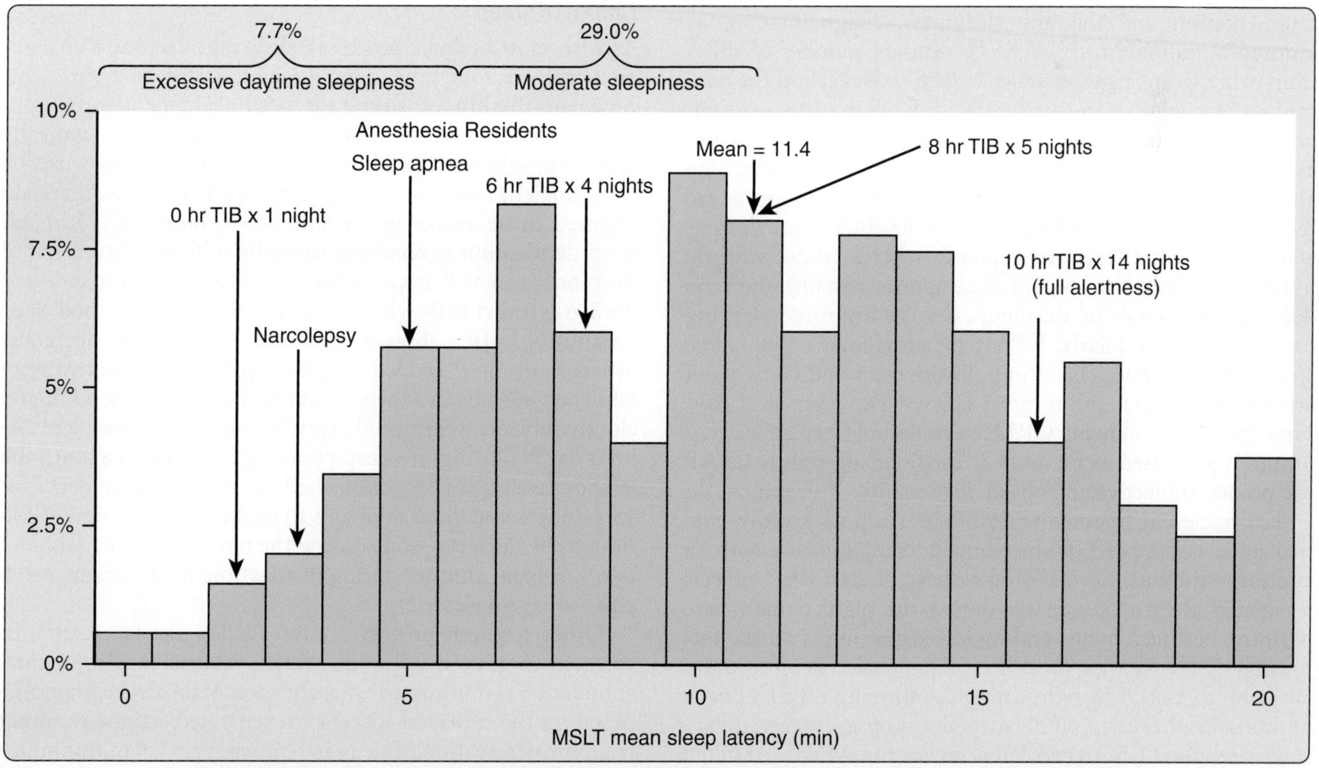

Figure 4.1 The distribution of mean daily sleep latency (minutes) on the Multiple Sleep Latency Test (MSLT) in a subsample (n = 259) recruited (68% response rate) from a large southeastern Michigan random sample (n = 1648) representative of the US population. The population mean is 11.4 minutes, and this is compared with means reported for various patient groups[59,69,70] and the means found in healthy normal individuals after various bedtime manipulations.[22,61] TIB, Time in bed.

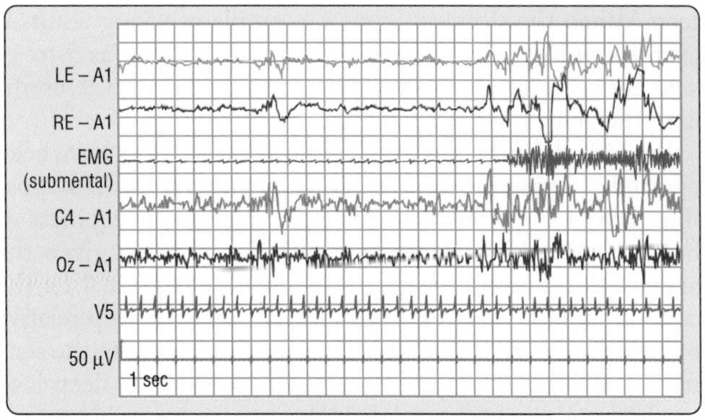

Figure 4.2 A transient arousal (*right side* of figure) fragmenting sleep. The preexistence of sleep is evident by the K-complex at second 9 of the epoch preceding the arousal. C4-A1, Electroencephalogram referenced to A1 from C4 placement; EMG, electromyogram from submental muscle; LE-A1, left electrooculogram referenced to A1; Oz-A1, electroencephalogram referenced to A1 from Oz placement; RE-A1, right electrooculogram referenced to A1; V5, electrocardiogram from V5 placement. (Modified from American Sleep Disorders Association. EEG arousals: scoring rules and examples. *Sleep.* 1992;15:173–84.)

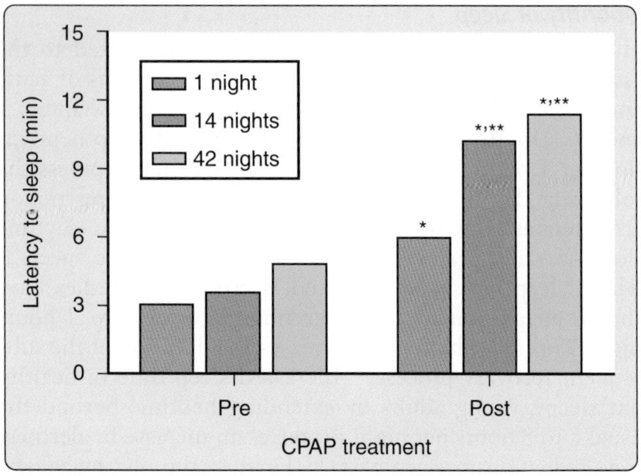

Figure 4.3 Mean daily sleep latency on the Multiple Sleep Latency Test in patients with obstructive sleep apnea syndrome before (pre) and after (post) 1, 14, and 42 nights of continuous positive airway pressure (CPAP) treatment. *$P < .05$; **$P < .01$. (Modified from Lamphere J, Roehrs T, Wittig R, et al. Recovery of alertness after CPAP in apnea. *Chest.* 1989;96:1364–67.)

These arousals typically do not result in awakening by either Rechtschaffen and Kales sleep staging criteria or behavioral indicators, and the arousals recur in some conditions as often as one to four times per minute. The arousing stimulus differs in the various disorders and can be identified in some cases (apneas, leg movements, pain) but not in others. Regardless of etiology, the arousals generally do not result in shortened sleep but rather in fragmented or discontinuous sleep, and this fragmentation produces daytime sleepiness.[68]

Correlational evidence suggests a relation between sleep fragmentation and daytime sleepiness. Fragmentation, as indexed by number of brief EEG arousals, number of shifts from other sleep stages to stage 1 sleep or wake, and the percentage of stage 1 sleep, correlates with EDS in various patient groups.[68] Treatment studies also link sleep fragmentation and excessive sleepiness. Patients with sleep apnea syndrome who are successfully treated by surgery (i.e., number of apneas are reduced) show a reduced frequency of arousals from sleep as well as a reduced level of sleepiness, whereas those who do not benefit from the surgery (i.e., apneas remain) show no decrease in arousals or sleepiness, despite improved sleeping oxygenation.[69] Similarly, CPAP, by providing a pneumatic airway splint, reduces breathing disturbances and consequent arousals from sleep and reverses EDS.[70] The reversal of daytime sleepiness following CPAP treatment of sleep apnea syndrome is presented in Figure 4.3. The hours of nightly CPAP use predict subjective and objective measures of sleepiness.[71]

Experimental fragmentation of the sleep of healthy normal subjects has been produced by inducing arousals with an auditory stimulus. Several studies have shown that subjects awakened at various intervals during the night demonstrate performance decrements and increased sleepiness on the following day.[72] Studies have also fragmented sleep without awakening subjects by terminating the stimulus on EEG signs of arousal rather than on behavioral response. Increased daytime sleepiness (shortened latencies on the MSLT) resulted from nocturnal sleep fragmentation in one study,[73] and in a second study, the recuperative effects (measured as increased latencies on the MSLT) of a nap after sleep deprivation were compromised by fragmenting the sleep on the nap.[74]

One nonclinical population in which sleep fragmentation is an important determinant of excessive sleepiness is the elderly. Many studies have shown that even elderly people without sleep complaints show an increased number of apneas and periodic leg movements during sleep.[75] As noted earlier, the elderly as a group are sleepier than other groups.[4] Furthermore, it has been demonstrated that elderly people with the highest frequency of arousal during sleep have the greatest daytime sleepiness.[76]

Timing of Sleep

As with most biologic processes, sleep and sleepiness changes predictably across time, approximately every 24 hours. This circadian rhythm of sleepiness occurs independently from the homeostatic process, although both processes typically operate synchronously. However, these two processes can be disentangled, such as in night shift work when workers are required to be awake in the middle of the night. Although sleep deprivation is common in night shift workers, signs of sleepiness can still occur when sleep loss is minimized.[77,78] Similarly, individuals who stay awake all night (i.e., total sleep deprivation) often show a temporary reduction in sleepiness by late morning.[79] Indeed, a biphasic pattern of objective sleep tendency was observed when healthy, normal young adult and elderly subjects were tested every 2 hours over a complete 24-hour day.[80] During the sleep period (11:30 p.m. to 8 a.m.) the latency testing was accomplished by awakening subjects for 15 minutes and then allowing them to return to sleep. Two troughs of alertness—one during the nocturnal hours (about 2 to 6 a.m.) and another during the daytime hours (about 2 to 6 p.m.)—were observed.

Other research protocols have yielded similar results. In constant routine studies in which external environmental stimulation is minimized and subjects remain awake, superimposed on the expected increase in self-rated fatigue resulting from the deprivation of sleep is a biphasic circadian rhythmicity of self-rated fatigue similar to that seen for sleep latency.[81] In another constant routine study in which EEG was continuously monitored, a biphasic pattern of "unintentional sleep" was observed.[82] In studies with sleep scheduled at unusual times, the duration of sleep periods has been used as an index of the level of sleepiness. A pronounced circadian variation in sleep duration is found with the termination of sleep periods closely related to the biphasic sleep latency function in the studies cited earlier.[83] If individuals are permitted to nap when they are placed in time-free environments, this biphasic pattern becomes apparent in the form of a midcycle nap.[84]

This circadian rhythm in sleepiness is encompassed within a circadian system in which many biologic processes vary rhythmically over 24 hours. The sleepiness rhythm parallels the circadian variation in body temperature, with shortened latencies occurring in conjunction with temperature troughs.[80] But these two functions, sleep latency and body temperature, are not mirror images of each other; the midday body temperature decline is relatively small compared with that of sleep latency. Further, under free-running conditions, the two functions become dissociated.[85] However, no other biologic rhythm is as closely associated with the circadian rhythm of sleepiness as is body temperature.

Earlier, it was noted that shift workers are unusually sleepy, and jet travelers experience sleepiness acutely in a new time zone. The sleepiness in these two conditions results from the placement of sleep and wakefulness at times that are out of phase with the existing circadian rhythms. Thus not only is daytime sleep shortened and fragmented, but also wakefulness occurs at the peak of sleepiness or trough of alertness. Several studies have shown that pharmacologic extension and consolidation of out-of-phase sleep can improve sleepiness during the wake period[78] (see Chapter 43 for more detail). Yet, the basal circadian rhythm of sleepiness remains, although the overall level of sleepiness has been reduced. In other words, the synchronization of circadian rhythms to the new sleep-wake schedule is not hastened.

CENTRAL NERVOUS SYSTEM DRUGS

Sedating Drug Effects

CNS depressant drugs, as expected, increase sleepiness. Most of these drugs act as agonists at the $GABA_A$ receptor complex. The benzodiazepine hypnotics hasten sleep onset at bedtime and shorten the latency to return to sleep after an awakening during the night (which is their therapeutic purpose), as demonstrated by a number of objective studies.[86] Long-acting benzodiazepines continue to shorten sleep latency on the MSLT the day after bedtime administration.[86] Finally, ethanol administered during the daytime (9 a.m.) reduces sleep latency in a dose-related manner as measured by the MSLT.[87]

Second-generation antiepileptic drugs, including gabapentin, gabatrol, vigabatrin, pregabalin, and others, enhance GABA activity through various mechanisms that directly or indirectly involve the $GABA_A$ receptor.[88] The sedating effects of these various drugs have not been thoroughly documented, but some evidence indicates they do have sedative activity. $GABA_B$ receptor agonists have been investigated as treatments for drug addictions, and the preclinical animal research suggests these drugs may have sedative activity as well.[89]

Antagonists acting at the histamine H_1 receptor also have sedating effects. One of the most commonly reported side effects associated with the use of H_1 antihistamines is daytime sleepiness. Several double-blind, placebo-controlled studies have shown that certain H_1 antihistamines, such as diphenhydramine, increase sleepiness using sleep latency as the objective measure of sleepiness, whereas others, such as terfenadine or loratadine, do not.[90] The difference among these compounds relates to their differential CNS penetration and binding. Other H_1 antihistamines (e.g., tazifylline) are thought to have a greater peripheral compared with central H_1 affinity, and, consequently, effects on daytime sleep latency are found only at relatively high doses.[90]

Many antihypertensives, including beta adrenoreceptor blockers, have been reported to produce sedation during the daytime (although some exceptions exist, such as propranolol).[91] These CNS effects are thought to be related to the differential liposolubility of the various compounds. However, we are unaware of any studies that directly measure the daytime sleepiness produced by beta blockers; the information is derived from reports of side effects. As noted earlier, it is important to differentiate sleepiness from tiredness or fatigue. Patients may be describing tiredness or fatigue resulting from the drugs' peripheral effects (i.e., lowered cardiac output and blood pressure), not sleepiness, a presumed central effect.

Sedative effects of dopaminergic agonists used in treating Parkinson disease have been reported as adverse events in clinical trials and in case reports as "sleep attacks" while driving.[92] It is now clear these "sleep attacks" are not attacks per se, but are the expression of excessive sleepiness. Although the dose-related sedative effect of these drugs has been established, the mechanism by which the sedative effects occur is unknown. The dopaminergic agonists are also known to disrupt and fragment sleep.[93] Thus the excessive sleepiness may be secondary to disturbed sleep or to a combination of disturbed sleep and direct sedative effects.

Alerting Drug Effects

Stimulant drugs reduce sleepiness and increase alertness. The drugs in this group differ in their mechanisms of action. Amphetamine, methylphenidate, and pemoline block dopamine reuptake and to a lesser extent enhance the release of norepinephrine, dopamine, and serotonin. The mechanism of modafinil is not established; some evidence suggests that modafinil has a mechanism distinct from the classical stimulants. Amphetamine, methylphenidate, pemoline, and modafinil are used to treat the EDS associated with narcolepsy, and some have been studied as medications to maintain alertness and vigilance in normal subjects under conditions of sustained sleep loss (e.g., military operations). Studies in patients with narcolepsy using MSLT or MWT have shown improved alertness with amphetamine, methylphenidate, modafinil, and pemoline.[94] There is dispute as to the extent to which the excessive sleepiness of narcoleptics is reversed and the comparative efficacy of the various drugs. In healthy normal persons restricted or deprived of sleep, both amphetamine and methylphenidate increase alertness on the MSLT and improve psychomotor performance.[95,96] Caffeine is an adenosine receptor antagonist. Caffeine, in doses equivalent to one to three cups of coffee, reduced daytime sleepiness on the MSLT in normal subjects after 5 hours of sleep the previous night.[97]

Influence of Basal Sleepiness

The preexisting level of sleepiness-alertness interacts with a drug to influence the drug's behavioral effect. In other words, a drug's effect differs when sleepiness is at its maximum compared with its minimum. As noted previously, the basal level of daytime sleepiness can be altered by restricting or extending time in bed[65]; this in turn alters the usual effects of a stimulating versus a sedating drug. A study showed comparable levels of sleepiness-alertness during the day after 5 hours in bed and morning (9 a.m.) caffeine consumption compared with 11 hours in bed and morning (9 a.m.) ethanol ingestion.[98] Follow-up studies explored the dose relations of ethanol's interaction with basal sleepiness.[99] Dose-related differences in daytime sleepiness following ethanol and 8 hours of sleep were diminished after even 1 night of 5 hours' sleep, although the measured levels of ethanol in breath were consistent day to day. In other words, sleepiness enhanced the sedative effects of ethanol. In contrast, caffeine and methylphenidate produced a similar increase in alertness regardless of the basal level of sleepiness. Clinically, these findings imply, for example, that a sleepy driver with minimal blood ethanol levels may be as dangerous as an alert driver who is legally intoxicated.[99]

The basal state of sleepiness also influences drug-seeking behavior. The likelihood that a healthy individual without a drug abuse history will self-administer methylphenidate is greatly enhanced after 4 hours of sleep the previous night compared with 8 hours of sleep. Although not experimentally demonstrated yet, self-administration of caffeine also may be influenced by basal state of sleepiness, although the habit of caffeine intake also likely has behavioral and social influences. The high volume of caffeine use in the population could relate to the high rate of self-medication for sleepiness because of chronic insufficient sleep in the population.

Central Nervous System Pathologies

Pathology of the CNS is another determinant of daytime sleepiness. The previously noted hypocretin/orexin deficiency is thought to cause excessive sleepiness in patients with narcolepsy.[100] Another sleep disorder associated with excessive sleepiness resulting from an unknown pathology of the CNS is idiopathic CNS hypersomnolence. A report of a series of rigorously diagnosed cases (n = 77) found moderate MSLT scores (8.5 minutes mean latency) relative to narcoleptics (4.1 minutes mean latency).[101] As yet, hypocretin/orexin deficiency has not been shown in this disorder. These two conditions are described in detail in Chapters 111 and 113.

Excessive sleepiness is reported in other neurologic diseases. A study in patients with myotonic dystrophy, type 1, reported excessive sleepiness on the MSLT and reduced cerebrospinal levels of hypocretin/orexin.[102] "Sleep attacks" have been reported in Parkinson disease, and assessment with the MSLT suggests these "attacks" are the expression of EDS.[103] What remains unresolved in the excessive sleepiness of Parkinson disease is the relative contribution of the disease itself, the fragmentation of sleep resulting from periodic leg movement or apnea, and the dopaminergic drugs used in treating Parkinson disease.[104] The previously cited study found no differences in sleepiness as a function of prescribed drug or sleep fragmentation, although further assessment in larger unselected samples is necessary to confirm this finding.

CLINICAL AND PUBLIC HEALTH IMPLICATIONS

Epidemiology of Sleepiness

Prevalence estimates of sleepiness in the population vary widely depending on the definition of sleepiness used and the type of population sampled. Surveys and questionnaires have queried a range of dimensions or expressions of the phenomenology of sleepiness, including the experience of a mood or feeling state of sleepiness; fatigue or tiredness; falling asleep unintentionally; or about struggling to stay awake and fighting sleep onset. Newer developments in the epidemiology of sleepiness have included the use of standardized sleepiness scales and physiologic assessments of sleepiness that measure the behavior of falling asleep, its estimated likely occurrence, or the speed of its actual occurrence. Although the amount of research that focuses on sleepiness in children and adolescents is growing, this chapter addresses only sleepiness in adults.

Many studies have examined sleepiness in samples of convenience or populations at risk for sleepiness (e.g., residents, truck drivers, shift workers). Some studies have focused on epidemiologic samples that are more representative of the larger population. In a study representative of the Finnish population, 11% of women and 7% of men reported daytime sleepiness almost every day.[105] In another survey, representative of a large geographic area in Sweden, 12% of respondents thought their sleep was insufficient.[106] In that survey, insufficient sleep—and not its consequent daytime sleepiness—was the focus of the questions. Two studies representative of the US population used the MSLT to assess sleepiness. Given the necessary time commitment required of participants in MSLT studies, the representative integrity of study results is critically dependent on the recruitment response rate. From a large southeastern Michigan random sample (n = 1648) representative of the US population, a subsample (n = 259) with a 68% response rate was recruited to undergo a nocturnal polysomnogram and MSLT the following day. The prevalence of excessive sleepiness, defined as an MSLT average sleep latency of less than 6 minutes, was 13%.[107] In another probability sample of 6947 Wisconsin state employees, a subsample (n = 632), collected with a 52% response rate, slept at home and then completed a MSLT in the laboratory the next day. Twenty-five percent had an average sleep latency of less than 5 minutes.[43] These two studies also used the ESS to assess sleepiness; in the Michigan study 20% had ESS scores exceeding 10 and in the Wisconsin study 25% had scores exceeding 11. The higher prevalence in the Wisconsin study, despite the more stringent definition of sleepiness (MSLT of 5 versus 6 minutes and ESS of 11 versus 10), could be attributed to an age difference in the samples (51 versus 42 years on average) or the previous night's sleep time and circumstances (habitual at home, on average 7.1 hours versus standard laboratory 8.5 hours). In Figure 4.1 the distribution of sleepiness, defined as average sleep latency on the MSLT, is illustrated for the Michigan population representative sample. The average sleep latency (MSLT) of various clinical samples and experimental sleep time manipulations are provided for comparisons.

Relation of Sleepiness to Behavioral Functioning

Given that the MSLT is a valid and reliable measure of sleepiness, the question arises as to how this measure relates to an individual's capacity to function. Direct correlations of the MSLT with other measures of performance under normal conditions have not been too robust. Several studies have found, however, that when sleepiness is at maximum levels, correlations with performance are high. For example, MSLT scores after sleep deprivation,[108] after administration of sedating antihistamines,[90] and after benzodiazepine administration[109] correlate with measures of performance and even prove to be the most sensitive measure. Studies also have compared levels of sleepiness to the known performance-impairing effects of alcohol.[110] A study relating performance lapses on a vigilance task to the cumulative effects of sleep restriction found a function comparable to that of the MSLT under a similar cumulative sleep restriction[111] (Figure 4.4). The reason many studies have found weak correlations between performance and MSLT at normal or moderate levels of sleepiness is that laboratory performance and MSLT are differentially affected by variables such as age, education, and motivation.

For the most part, the literature relating sleepiness and behavioral functioning has focused on psychomotor and attention behaviors with the major outcomes being response slowing and attentional lapses. These impairments can be attributed to slowed processing of information and microsleeps, that is intrusion of sleep preparatory and sleep-onset behaviors. Research has focused on other behavioral domains not as clearly associated with sleep-mediated behaviors, including decision making and pain sensation. Several studies have shown that increased sleepiness is associated with poor risk-taking decisions.[112] Sleep loss and its associated sleepiness have also been shown to increase pain sensitivity.[113]

Although the patients at sleep disorders centers are not representative of the general population, they do provide some insight regarding the clinical significance of sleepiness. Their sleep-wake histories directly indicate the serious impact excessive sleepiness has on their lives.[114] Nearly half the patients with excessive sleepiness report automobile accidents; half report occupational accidents, some life threatening; and many have lost jobs because of their sleepiness. In addition, sleepiness is considerably disruptive of family life.[115] An elevated automobile accident rate (i.e., sevenfold) among patients with excessive sleepiness has been verified through driving records obtained from motor vehicle agencies.[116]

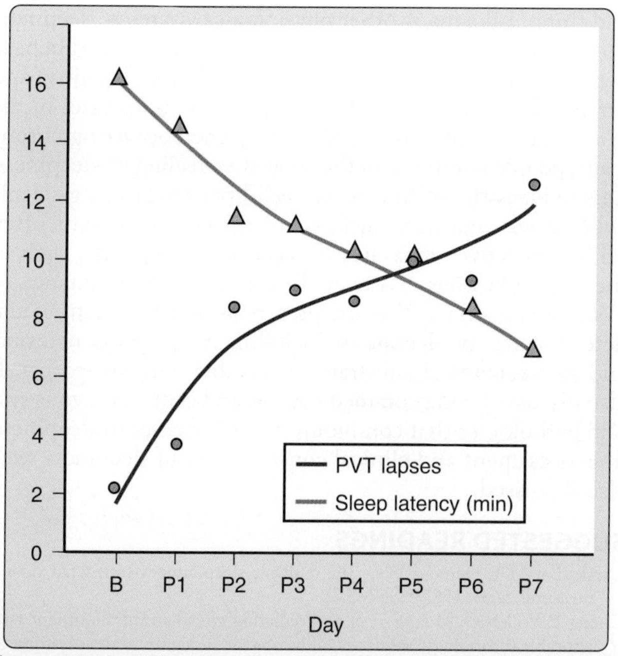

Figure 4.4 Similar functions relating mean daily sleep latency on the Multiple Sleep Latency Test (MSLT) and mean daily lapses on the visual psychomotor vigilance test (PVT) to the cumulative effects of sleep restriction (about 5 hours of bedtime nightly) across 7 consecutive nights (P1 to P7). (Modified from Dinges DF, Pack F, Williams K, et al. Cumulative sleepiness, mood disturbance, and psychomotor vigilance performance decrements during a week of sleep restricted to 4–5 hours per night. *Sleep.* 1997;20:275.)

Population-based information regarding traffic and industrial accidents also suggests a link between sleepiness and life-threatening events. Verified automobile accidents occurred more frequently in a representative sample of people with MSLT scores of 5 minutes or less.[98] The highest rate of automobile accidents occurs in the early morning hours, which is notable because the fewest automobiles are on the road during these hours. Also during these early morning hours, the greatest degree of sleepiness is experienced.[117] Long-haul truck drivers have accidents most frequently (even corrected for hours driving before the accident) during the early morning hours, again when sleepiness reaches its zenith.[118] Increasingly, commercial vehicle accidents have been connected to fatigue and sleepiness in thorough accident investigations.[119]

Workers on the graveyard shift were identified as a particularly sleepy subpopulation. In 24-hour ambulatory EEG recordings of sleep and wakefulness, workers (20% in one study) were found to actually fall asleep during the night shift.[106] Not surprisingly, the poorest job performance consistently occurs on the night shift, and the highest rate of industrial accidents is usually found among workers on this shift.[120] Medical residents are another particularly sleepy subpopulation. In surveys those reporting 5 or fewer hours of sleep per night were more likely to make medical errors and report serious accidents and were two times more likely to be named in medical malpractice suits.[121,122] In a survey of medical housestaff 49% reported falling asleep while driving and 90% of the episodes occurred post-call compared with 13% fall-asleep episodes reported by the medical faculty and 20 of the 70 housestaff were involved in automobile accidents compared to 11 of the 85 faculty.[123]

Cognitive function is also impaired by sleepiness. Adults with various disorders of excessive sleepiness have cognitive and memory problems.[124] The memory deficiencies are not specific to a certain sleep disorder but rather specific to the sleepiness associated with the disorder. When treated adequately, sleepiness is rectified and the memory and cognitive deficits similarly improve.[125] Results of sleep deprivation studies in healthy normal patients support the relation between sleepiness and memory deficiency. Even modest reductions of sleep time are associated with cognitive deficiencies.[126]

Sleepiness also depresses arousability to physiologic challenges: 24-hour sleep deprivation decreases upper airway dilator muscle activity[127] and decreases ventilatory responses to hypercapnia and hypoxia.[128] In a canine model of sleep apnea, periodic disruption of sleep with acoustic stimuli (i.e., sleep fragmentation, in contrast to sleep deprivation) resulted in lengthened response times to airway occlusion, greater oxygen desaturation, increases in inspiratory pressures, and surges in blood pressure.[129] Depressed physiologic responsivity resulting from sleepiness is clinically significant for patients with sleep apnea and other breathing disorders as they are all exacerbated by sleepiness. The emerging data on sleepiness and pain threshold, cited earlier, is also clinically significant in the management of both acute and chronic pain conditions.

Finally, life expectancy data directly link excessive sleep (not specifically sleepiness) and mortality. A 1976 study found that men and women who reported sleeping more than 10 hours a day were about 1.8 times more likely to die prematurely than those sleeping between 7 and 8 hours daily.[130] This survey, however, associated hypersomnia and increased

Table 4.1 Sleeping-Inducing Situations for Patients with Apnea (n = 384 patients)

Situation	Percentage of Patients
Watching television	91
Reading	85
Riding in a car	71
Attending church	57
Visiting friends and relatives	54
Driving	50
Working	43
Waiting for a red light	32

mortality and not necessarily EDS, for which the relation is currently unknown.

Sleepiness in the Clinical Context

Assessing the clinical significance of a patient's complaint of excessive sleepiness can be complex. The assessment depends on two important factors: chronicity and reversibility. Chronicity can be explained simply. Although a healthy normal individual may be acutely sleepy, the patient's sleepiness is persistent and unremitting. As to reversibility, unlike a healthy individual, increased sleep time may not completely or consistently ameliorate a patient's sleepiness. Patients with excessive sleepiness may not complain of sleepiness per se, but rather its consequences: loss of energy, fatigue, lethargy, weariness, lack of initiative, memory lapses, or difficulty concentrating.

To clarify the patient complaint, it is important to focus on soporific situations in which physiologic sleepiness is more likely to be manifest. Such situations may include watching TV, reading, riding in a car, listening to a lecture, or sitting in a warm room. Table 4.1 presents the commonly reported "sleep-inducing" situations for a large sample of patients with sleep apnea syndrome. It is also critical to establish sleep duration and regularity across the week (including both weekdays and weekends), as well as circadian rhythms as a contributor to sleepiness. A history of medical morbidities, medication use, and substance use history may also provide important insights. Once the complaint and the history have been clarified, the clinician should ask the patient about the entire day: morning, midday, and evening. Note that reports of some sleepiness during the midday is part of normative circadian variations of sleepiness. Whenever possible, objective documentation of sleepiness and its severity should be sought. As indicated earlier, the standard and accepted method to document sleepiness objectively is the MSLT.

Guidelines for interpreting the results of the MSLT are available.[41] A number of case series of patients with disorders of excessive sleepiness have been published with accompanying MSLT data for each diagnostic classification.[131] These data provide the clinician with guidelines for evaluating the clinical significance of a given patient's MSLT results. Although these data cannot be considered norms, a scheme for ranking MSLT scores to indicate degree of pathology has been suggested.[47] An average daily MSLT score of 5 minutes or fewer suggests pathologic sleepiness, a score of more than 5 minutes but fewer than 10 minutes is considered a diagnostic gray area, and a score of more than 10 minutes is considered to be in the normal range (Figure 4.1 for MSLT results in the general population). The MSLT is also useful in identifying sleep-onset REM periods, which are common in patients with narcolepsy.[42] The American Academy of Sleep Medicine Standards of Practice Committee has concluded that the MSLT is indicated in the evaluation of patients with suspected narcolepsy.[42] MSLT results, however, must also be evaluated with respect to the conditions under which the testing was conducted. Standards have been published for administering the MSLT, which must be followed to obtain a valid, interpretable result.[41]

CLINICAL PEARL

Sleepiness, when most excessive and persistent, is a signal to the individual to stop operating: it is dangerous and life-threatening to continue without sleep. For the clinician, that signal warns that there may be some underlying pathology or dysfunction that can be successfully treated, or in the very least minimized as to its vital, life-threatening impact.

SUMMARY

Sleepiness is a serious public health and safety concern and is a complex phenomenon. Although sleepiness can be temporarily modulated and/or masked by psychological, social, and environmental factors, excessive daytime sleepiness is highly predictive of impairments to cognition and performance. Indeed, excessive sleepiness has contributed to accidents and fatalities, and thus is of critical importance to occupational health and safety. It is understood as a physiological need state comparable to other biological drives such as hunger and thirst. Like many other physiological systems, sleepiness is determined and regulated by multiple systems and behaviors. This includes history of sleep (duration and quality) and time of day, as well as medication use and pathologies of the central nervous system. Additionally, when occurring chronically, people habituate to the subjective feeling of sleepiness. This reduces the reliability and validity of measuring sleepiness via self-report; as such, standardized assessments often utilize objectives measures of sleep and sleepiness, such as the Multiple Sleep Latency Test and the Maintenance of Wakefulness Test. This chapter reviewed the nature and determinants of sleepiness, including the various neuronal and neurochemical substrates associated with sleepiness. It also discussed common medications and central nervous system pathologies that commonly cause increases in sleepiness. The assessment and clinical consequences of sleepiness were also discussed.

SUGGESTED READINGS

Carskadon MA, Dement WC. The multiple sleep latency test: what does it measure? *Sleep*. 1982;5:S67–S72.

Cheng P, Walch O, Huang Y, et al. Predicting circadian misalignment with wearable technology: validation of wrist-worn actigraphy and photometry in night shift workers. *Sleep*.

Depner C, Cheng P, Devine J, et al. Wearable technologies for developing sleep and circadian biomarkers: a summary of workshop discussions. *Sleep*. 2020;43(2).

Dietmann A, Gallino C, Wenz E, et al. Multiple sleep latency test and polysomnography in patients with central disorders of hypersomnolence. *Sleep Med*. 2021;79:6–10.

Drake CL, Roehrs T, Richardson G, et al. Epidemiology and morbidity of excessive daytime sleepiness. *Sleep*. 2002;25:A91.

Goel N. "Omics" approaches for sleep and circadian rhythm research: biomarkers for identifying differential vulnerability to sleep loss. *Curr Sleep Med Rep*. 2015;1(1):38–46.

Littner MR, Kushida C, Wise M, et al. Practice parameters for clinical use of the Multiple Sleep Latency Test and the Maintenance of Wakefulness Test: An American Academy of Sleep Medicine report. *Sleep*. 2005;28:113–121.

Maski K, Trotti LM, Kotagal S, et al. Treatment of central disorders of hypersomnolence: an American Academy of Sleep Medicine clinical practice guideline. *J Clin Sleep Med*. Published online April, 2021.

Mignot E. A commentary on the neurobiology of the hypocretin/orexin system. *Neuropsychopharmacology*. 2001;25:S5–S13.

Saper CB, Scammell TE. Hypothalamic regulation of sleep and circadian rhythms. *Nature*. 2005;437:1257–1263.

A complete reference list can be found online at ExpertConsult.com.

Chapter
5

Sleep Deprivation

Siobhan Banks; Jill Dorrian; Mathias Basner; Marc Kaizi-Lutu; David F. Dinges

Chapter Highlights

- Approximately 35% of the adult US population report sleeping less than the recommended 7 hours per day.
- Neurobehavioral deficits accumulate across days of sleep restriction to levels equivalent to those found after 1 to 3 nights of total sleep deprivation.
- Neurobehavioral responses to sleep deprivation have been found to be stable and consistent, suggesting they are trait-like and possibly have a genetic component.
- Recovery appears to be affected by the type (acute versus chronic), recovery sleep duration, and the number of days allowed for recovery. Additionally, while individuals may report they feel recovered, their performance may remain impaired, increasing risk for accidents and injury.

INTRODUCTION

Half a century ago, Kleitman first used the phrase "sleep debt" to describe the circumstances in which sleep is lost through delaying sleep-onset time while holding sleep-termination time constant.[1] He described the increased sleepiness and decreased alertness experienced by individuals on such a sleep-wake pattern and proposed that they would be able to reverse these effects by extending their sleep on weekends to "liquidate the debt" (p. 317).[1] More recently, "sleep debt" has been used to refer more generally to the increased pressure for sleep that results from an inadequate amount of physiologically normal sleep. Importantly, both sufficient quality and duration are prerequisite for the recuperative effects of sleep.[2] Sleep deprivation can be acute or chronic. Acute total sleep deprivation refers to wake periods that extend beyond the typical 16 to 18 hours, whereas sleep restriction refers to inadequate sleep per 24 hours for 1 or multiple nights. Sleep restriction occurs frequently and results from a number of factors, including medical conditions (e.g., pain), sleep disorders, work demands (including extended work hours and shift work), and social and domestic responsibilities.[3]

To determine the effects of sleep deprivation on a range of neurobehavioral and physiologic variables, a variety of paradigms have been used, including controlled, restricted time in bed for sleep opportunities in both continuous and distributed schedules (e.g., nocturnal anchor sleep with a daytime nap),[4] gradual reductions in sleep duration over time,[5] selective deprivation of specific sleep stages,[6] and situations in which the time in bed is individualized, such that it is reduced to a percentage of the individual's habitual time in bed.[7]

Epidemiologic studies suggest that habitual short sleep duration is associated with negative health consequences, including obesity,[8] diabetes,[9] hypertension,[10] cardiometabolic risk factors[11] and cardiovascular disease,[12] declines in cognitive function,[13] and all-cause mortality.[14] Importantly, these findings have been observed not only in cross-sectional studies but also in prospective population studies.[14,15] Evidence from experimental studies shows that both acute total sleep deprivation and sleep restriction cause inadequate pancreatic insulin secretion,[16] decreased insulin sensitivity,[17] changes in appetite regulating hormones leptin and ghrelin,[18] an attenuated immune response to vaccination,[19] and increased sympathetic activity and venous endothelial dysfunction in healthy adults.[20] These effects provide biologic plausibility for a causal relationship between short sleep and negative health outcomes, as well as all-cause mortality when considered with the well-documented safety risks of reduced sleep (e.g., the increased risk for motor vehicle crashes).

This chapter reviews the cognitive and neurobehavioral consequences of acute total sleep deprivation and sleep restriction in healthy individuals and the theoretic explanations for these effects.

PREVALENCE OF SLEEP DEPRIVATION

Human sleep need can be defined as the duration of sleep needed to prevent elevated daytime sleepiness and sleep propensity and associated cognitive deficits. Despite the scientifically documented benefits of sufficient sleep for cognitive performance, safety, and health, current representative surveys indicate that 35% to 40% of the adult US population report sleeping less than the usually recommended 7 to 8 hours on weekday nights, and about 15% report sleeping less than 6 hours.[21,22] Importantly, these are self-reported sleep time estimates that have been shown to overestimate actigraphically or polysomnographically measured sleep by up to 1 hour.[23,24] While individual sleep need differs, these statistics suggest that a significant proportion of people are likely obtaining less than their sleep need.

One societal group that commonly may be particularly vulnerable is shift workers. Shift workers currently constitute one out of five working Americans, and this proportion is projected to increase. Shift work includes working evenings, nights, or rotating shifts. Because sleep is often scheduled at an adverse circadian phase, it is often of lower quality and shorter duration.[25] Further, shift workers frequently experience both sleep restriction, across a series of shifts, and acute sleep deprivation, often while transitioning into and out of night shift work.[26]

Indeed, analyses based on the American Time Use Survey indicate that one of the main activities Americans most frequently trade for sleep time is working time. Those working multiple jobs are significantly more likely to be short sleepers, while those self-employed are less likely to be short sleepers compared to private sector employees, likely because of increased flexibility in work start time. In general, sociodemographic characteristics associated with paid work (age 25 to 64, male sex, high income, and employment per se) are consistently associated with short sleep.[27] Other activities traded for sleep include traveling and socializing. Communicating[27] while watching TV or streaming media content is the most frequent activity in the 2 hours pre-bed.[28] Even exercise, a health-promoting activity that also improves sleep quality, was recently shown to compete with sleep for time.[29]

Overall, the prevalence of sleep restriction in the general population is high and is closely linked with working arrangements. Although less is known about the prevalence of acute total sleep deprivation in the population, given the pervasiveness of shift work, including night work, in our 24/7 society, it is likely that the prevalence of acute total sleep deprivation is also increasing.

EFFECTS OF SLEEP DEPRIVATION

Acute Total Sleep Deprivation

The first total sleep deprivation and cognition study was conducted in the late 19th century. Studies at this time involved substantial sleep deprivation periods (36 to 90 hours) and demonstrated that memory and response time were significantly impaired.[30] Over time, hundreds of studies of total sleep loss have found significant cognitive deficits (for review, see Durmer and Dinges[31]). Many facets of waking function are affected by sleep deprivation.

Tasks requiring vigilant attention are particularly adversely affected by sleep deprivation.[32] One of the most sensitive and widely used cognitive tasks in studies of sleep loss is the psychomotor vigilance task (PVT),[33] which is a neurobehavioral performance measure of vigilant attention.[32] Studies have consistently shown that sleep deprivation increases PVT response slowing and lapses,[34] which are thought to reflect microsleeps.[1,35] As sleep deprivation accumulates, microsleeps or brief lapses of a half second can increase to 10 seconds and longer.[1,35,36] It has been suggested that these lapses involve shifts in neuronal activity in frontal, thalamic, and secondary sensory processing areas of the brain.[37] In sleep-deprived subjects, cognitive performance contains lapses of attention that occur unpredictably, and they increase in frequency and duration as a function of the interaction of the length of the sleep deprivation with the endogenous circadian phase of performance testing. This has led to the concept that sleep deprivation results in "wake state instability."[32,34,36,37] This instability appears to involve moment-to-moment fluctuations in the relationship between neurobiologic systems mediating wake maintenance and sleep initiation.[37] State instability manifests in increased failures to respond to stimuli (errors of omission) as well as increased responses in the absence of stimuli (errors of commission).[31,36]

Other aspects of cognition that are impaired by sleep deprivation include cognitive processing speed,[38] constructive thinking,[39] verbal memory[40] and spatial working memory,[41] and memory accuracy.[42] Further, there are increases in subjective sleepiness and increasingly labile mood and emotional processing. In addition, the ability to read positive emotional expressions is reduced, as is the threshold for experiencing stress.[43,44] In contrast, rule-based reasoning, decision-making, and planning tasks appear to be relatively unaffected by sleep loss.[32]

It has been demonstrated that the negative impact of acute total sleep deprivation captured in these laboratory studies is not only measurable but also meaningful. The performance effects of sleep deprivation and alcohol intoxication have been demonstrated to be qualitatively and quantitatively similar.[45] Dawson and Reid[45] found that performance impairment after 17 hours awake was equivalent to that produced by a blood alcohol concentration of 0.05%.

An overarching finding from the studies of total sleep deprivation is that waking function is influenced by a sleep homeostatic process that builds up during wakefulness and declines during sleep in a nonlinear fashion (as measured by slow wave energy or delta power in the non–rapid eye movement sleep electroencephalogram [EEG]) and a circadian process, with near–24-hour periodicity.[46] The combined influences of these factors are described as the two-process model.[47] Since its inception, the two-process model has gained widespread acceptance for its explanation of the timing and structure of sleep. Its use has extended to predictions of waking alertness and neurobehavioral functions in response to different sleep-wake scenarios.[47] This extension of the two-process model was based on observations that as sleep pressure accumulated with increasing time awake, so did waking neurobehavioral or neurocognitive impairment, and as sleep pressure dissipated with time asleep, performance capability improved during the following period of wakefulness. In addition, forced-desynchrony experiments (where day-length was increased to 28 hours under controlled conditions in order to mathematically separate the influence of time awake and time of day; see Chapter 37 for more details) revealed that the sleep homeostatic and circadian processes interacted to create periods of stable wakefulness and consolidated sleep during normal 24-hour days.[48]

The two-process model has been used in the development of tools to model changes in sleep, alertness, and performance on the basis of recent sleep-wake (and/or work) history. In general, these models accurately predict waking performance and self-report responses to total sleep deprivation. However, they often fail to adequately predict sleepiness and cognitive performance responses during sleep restriction.[49] Model extensions have started to deal with these shortcomings.[50]

Sleep Restriction

Our understanding of the effects of sleep restriction have been greatly informed by two large-scale, controlled laboratory studies. These studies identified dose-related effects of short-term sleep restriction on neurobehavioral performance

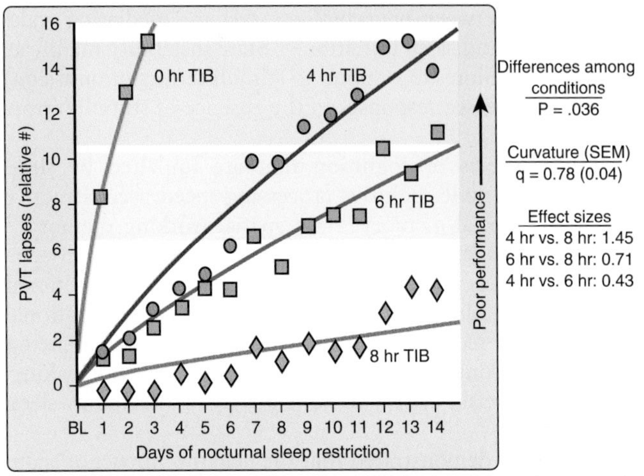

Figure 5.1 Psychomotor vigilance test (PVT) performance lapses under varying doses of daily sleep. Displayed are group averages for subjects in the 8-hour (diamond), 6-hour (light blue square), and 4-hour (circle) sleep period time in bed (TIB) across 14 days and in the 0-hour (light green square) sleep condition across 3 days. Subjects were tested every 2 hours each day; data points represent the daily average (0730 hours to 2330 hours) expressed relative to baseline (BL). The curves through the data points represent statistical nonlinear model–based best-fitting profiles of the response to sleep deprivation for subjects in each of the four experimental conditions. The mean ± SE ranges of neurobehavioral functions for 1 and 2 days of 0 hours of sleep (total sleep deprivation) are shown as light and dark bands, respectively, allowing comparison of the 3-day total sleep deprivation condition and the 14-day sleep restriction conditions. (Redrawn from Van Dongen HPA, Maislin G, Mullington JM, et al. The cumulative cost of additional wakefulness: dose-response effects on neurobehavioral functions and sleep physiology from sleep restriction and total sleep deprivation. *Sleep* 2003;26:117–26.)

measures.[51,52] In one study, truck drivers were randomized to 7 nights of 3, 5, 7, or 9 hours in bed for sleep per night,[52] and the other young adults had their sleep duration confined to 4, 6, or 8 hours in bed per night for 14 nights (Figure 5.1).[51] Individuals in the 3, 4, 5, 6, and 7 hours' time-in-bed groups experienced increases in performance impairment across days of the sleep restriction protocol. Deficits in cognitive functions were observed, including reduced vigilant attention, impaired memory, and slowed mental processing speed.

It also appears that the neurocognitive effects of restricting nocturnal sleep to 6 or 4 hours per night for multiple nights are fundamentally the same as when sleep is split each day into two sleep opportunities.[53] Cognitive performance deficits also accumulate across consecutive days in which restricted sleep occurs during the daytime and wakefulness occurs at night.[54] The primary difference between the nocturnally[51] and diurnally[54] placed restricted sleep periods is that the magnitude of neurobehavioral impairment is significantly greater with daytime sleep.

Collectively, these studies suggest that when time in bed for sleep is restricted to less than 7 hours per night in healthy adults (age 21 to 64 years) for multiple nights, cumulative deficits in a variety of cognitive performance functions can accumulate. Additionally, these deficits can be similar to those seen after 1 or even 2 nights of total sleep deprivation. These findings may suggest that there is a neurobiologic integrator that either accumulates homeostatic sleep drive or the neurobiologic consequences of excess wakefulness.[51,52] No definitive evidence exists yet as to what this neurobiologic integrator might be, but one hypothesis suggests it may involve extracellular adenosine in the basal forebrain.[55]

In contrast to reports of continuing accumulation of cognitive deficits associated with sleep restriction, subjective assessments of sleepiness and alertness demonstrate near-saturating functions across periods of sleep restriction.[51] Self-reported mood, sleepiness, and fatigue do not parallel the continuing decline in cognitive performance associated with nightly restriction of sleep to 7 hours or less.[51] This suggests that individuals may frequently underestimate the impact of sleep deprivation on their performance. Experiments using driving simulators have found similar results.[56]

INDIVIDUAL DIFFERENCES IN RESPONSE TO SLEEP LOSS

While the majority of healthy adults experience sleepiness and related cognitive deficits under conditions of total sleep deprivation or sleep restriction, interindividual variability in the neurobehavioral and physiologic responses is substantial.[1,31,36,57] There are certain individuals who display minimal impairment during sleep loss, some who are moderately affected, and others who are particularly vulnerable (Figure 5.2).[58] Research has not supported the suggestion that differences in vulnerability reflect baseline scores (after adequate rest), nor have studies found that demographic factors such as IQ, habitual sleep amount, or personality account for these differences.[59] Studies investigating whether the same individuals are vulnerable to total sleep deprivation and sleep restriction have yielded mixed results, likely because of small samples and varied methods.[60,61]

Importantly, however, within subjects repeatedly exposed to the same sleep loss intervention, neurobehavioral responses to sleep deprivation have been found to be stable and consistent, suggesting they are trait-like.[62] This seems to be true for both total sleep deprivation and sleep restriction. It has therefore been suggested that these trait-like differences in vulnerability may reflect underlying genetic differences.[59]

DETECTION OF SLEEPINESS

Sleepiness is often defined as the "propensity to fall asleep" and is measured both objectively and subjectively.[63] However, as mentioned previously, studies have shown that self-reported sleepiness ratings do not necessarily mirror changes in performance capability during sleep loss.[64] This highlights the need for brief, objective, and unobtrusive measures of performance capability that can be readily applied under operational conditions.

The measures that best track the subtle changes in performance caused by sleep deprivation are neural state indicators (such as EEG; electrooculogram, EOG; electrocardiogram, ECG; and functional magnetic resonance imaging, fMRI measures) or behavioral indicators of attention stability, such as the PVT.[65] As described previously, the PVT has been shown to be among the most sensitive measures of sleep loss, and it is not confounded by aptitude and learning affects like other performance measures.[32,65] It also reflects performance that has ecological validity (i.e., vigilant attention is needed for learning, safe driving, etc.). The PVT is thus often used as a gold standard measure for the neurobehavioral consequences of sleep loss, against which other fatigue-detection technologies are measured.

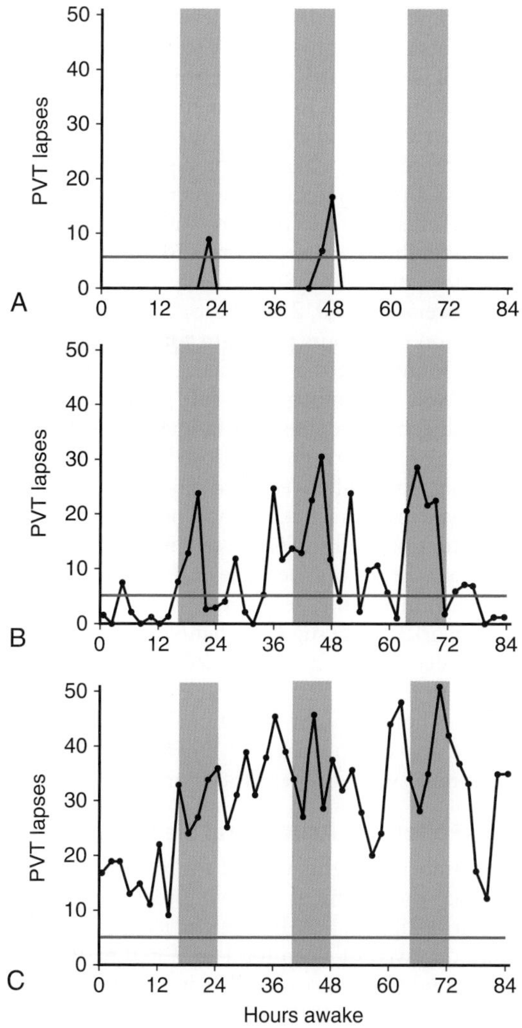

Figure 5.2 Individual differences in the response to sleep deprivation (DF Dinges, unpublished data). The three subjects in panels **A–C** performed a 10-minute psychomotor vigilance task (PVT) every 2 hours during 88 hours of acute total sleep deprivation. *Horizontal line* reflects 5 PVT lapses (number of reaction times >500 ms), and bars indicate the period from 0000 hours to 0800 hours. **A,** A resilient response. **B,** Impacted by sleep deprivation but with daytime improvement. **C,** A vulnerable response to sleep deprivation. These individual differences in the response to sleep deprivation on the PVT were not accounted for by demographic factors, IQ, or sleep need. (Reproduced with permission from Basner M, Rao H, Goel N, Dinges DF. Sleep deprivation and neurobehavioral dynamics. *Curr Opin Neurobiol* 2013;23[5]:854–63.)

Chua and colleagues[66] investigated how well several objective physiologic variables as well as subjective measures of sleepiness correlated with the PVT during 1 night of acute total sleep deprivation. The highest correlations were with the percent of slow eye closures in agreement with several authors who found oculomotor responses to be sensitive to sleep loss and reduced alertness at night.[67,68] Eyelid closure and slow rolling eye movements are part of the initial transition from wake to drowsiness; they are associated with vigilance lapses and have been found to be a sign of drowsiness while driving.[69] Increased slow eye movements attributed to attentional failures have been reported with reduced sleep time in medical residents.[70] Sleep restriction has also been found to decrease saccadic velocity and to increase the latency to pupil constriction in subjects allowed only 3 hours or 5 hours of time in bed for sleep over 7 nights.[71] Other variables that correlated highly with PVT performance included heart rate variability (as indicated by the power spectral density of the ECG RR-interval in the 0.02- to 0.08-Hz range), slow wave brain activity (as indicated by EEG delta power in the 1- to 4.5-Hz range), followed by self-reported measures of sleepiness.[66] The high correlation between heart rate variability and the PVT has been replicated for sleep restriction as well.[72]

SLEEP DEPRIVATION AND BRAIN METABOLISM

Sleep deprivation induces changes in brain metabolism and neural activation that involve distributed networks and connectivity.[2] Early positron emission tomography (PET) sleep deprivation studies found metabolic rate reductions in thalamic, parietal, and prefrontal regions associated with prolonged sleep loss.[52,73] Blood oxygenation level–dependent fMRI studies showed significant declines in regional brain activation during cognitive task performance after 1 night of total sleep deprivation. These changes included reduced fronto-parietal activation during lapses on a visual selective attention task[74] and were mainly observed in vulnerable subjects with larger performance deficits, while resilient subjects demonstrated a trend toward increased parietal activation during performance lapses,[74] suggesting a potential compensatory mechanism after sleep loss. PET studies have observed downregulation of striatal dopamine receptors[75] and increased cerebral serotonin receptor binding with sleep deprivation.[76] This may reflect a complex adaptive response of the brain to sleep deprivation.

Poudel and colleagues[77] used arterial spin-labeled perfusion fMRI to measure resting cerebral blood flow (CBF) changes after 1 night with 4-hour sleep opportunity. Only drowsy participants (established with video of the eyes during the scan) exhibited a significantly reduced fronto-parietal CBF following sleep deprivation, while nondrowsy subjects maintained fronto-parietal CBF and increased CBF in basal forebrain and cingulate regions. These findings support a compensatory mechanism after sleep loss,[77] which may explain some of the variance between those resilient versus those vulnerable to sleep loss. Resting-state functional connectivity fMRI (FC-fMRI) studies have consistently shown an organized mode of resting brain function.[78] Two FC-fMRI studies reported reduced functional connectivity within the default mode network (DMN) and between DMN and its anti-correlated network associated with sleep deprivation,[79] suggesting that functional connectivity of the brain changes as a result of sleep loss. A meta-analysis on the effects of acute total sleep deprivation on the attending brain found decreases in brain activation in the fronto-parietal attention network (prefrontal cortex and intraparietal sulcus) and in the salience network (insula and medial frontal cortex) but increases in thalamic activation (the salience network segregates the most relevant internal and external stimuli to guide behavior). The authors speculate that the latter may reflect a complex interaction between the de-arousing effects of sleep loss and the arousing effects of task performance on thalamic activity.[80]

Sleep Deprivation and Alzheimer Disease

β-Amyloid (Aβ) in the interstitial fluid in the brain has been described as "metabolic waste" and has been implicated in bidirectional relationship between sleep deprivation and Alzheimer disease (AD) pathology.[81,82] Sleep loss increases the concentration of soluble Aβ in the brain, a protein associated with the neuronal atrophy observed in AD, while sleep extension has the opposite effect.[82-85] As Aβ accumulates, increased wakefulness and altered sleep patterns develop.[81] Thus, age-related declines in older adult sleep quality and quantity can contribute to AD.[84] Slow wave sleep, which has a role in both recovery from sleep loss and in memory consolidation, is disrupted by increasing levels of Aβ,[84,86] posing risks to cognitive functions. The sleep-wake cycle also regulates brain interstitial fluid tau in mice and cerebrospinal fluid tau in humans.[87] Slow oscillations (<1-Hz EEG signals) and slow wave spindle coupling activity may be potential biomarkers of increased amyloid beta and tau.[88] Relative only to the risk of AD, a recent systematic review and meta-analysis of six prospective cohort studies found a 63% increased risk of AD with longer sleep duration but no increased risk with shorter sleep duration. The authors cautioned that the findings may reflect other underlying health problems that may contribute to the development of AD.[89]

RECOVERY FROM SLEEP LOSS

An emerging area of research has begun to focus on recovery processes from acute total sleep deprivation and sleep restriction. Results from these studies suggest that the recovery process may be slower and more complex than originally thought. Recovery appears to be affected by the type (acute versus chronic), recovery sleep duration, and the number of days allowed for recovery. Additionally, aspects of neurobehavioral functioning appear to recover at different rates; although individuals may report feeling recovered, their performance may remain impaired, increasing risk for accidents and injury.

Recovery Following Sleep Restriction

Few studies have examined recovery sleep after periods of sleep restriction. Two important sleep restriction studies that also included a short in-laboratory recovery phase were those by Dinges and colleagues[7] and Belenky and colleagues.[52] In the former study, sleep was restricted below habitual sleep duration by 33% (average 4.98, SD 0.57 hours per night) for 7 consecutive nights, after which participants were allowed one or two 10-hour recovery sleeps.[7] In the latter, participants were permitted 3, 5, 7, or 9 hours in bed each night for 7 nights, followed by three 8-hour recovery opportunities.[52] These studies show that either two 10-hour or three 8-hour sleep opportunities were sufficient to recover performance to baseline levels. Although participants felt that their functioning was restored with subjective reports of sleepiness and performance recovering to baseline, subjective measures did not appear to accurately parallel objective measures of neurobehavioral recovery. These findings suggest that more than 2 or 3 nights of extended sleep may be needed to return neurobehavioral functions to baseline levels. This may be especially important in situations in which individuals are not able to choose or extend the length of their recovery sleep period.

Rupp and colleagues[90] manipulated the amount of sleep obtained before a period of sleep restriction in a prophylactic manner, the duration of the recovery period (longer than 3 days), and the length of the recovery sleep opportunity. They also extended the recovery period to five 8-hour sleep opportunities, following a week of sleep restricted to 3 hours in bed each night.[90] Despite the extra recovery nights, performance still failed to return to baseline levels. In the group that extended their sleep prophylactically to 10 hours in bed before the period of sleep restriction, performance declined at a slower rate and recovered to baseline more quickly, suggesting that sleep restriction and recovery vary as function of prior sleep.[90] Therefore sleep extension or supplemental nap sleeps can be used as a prophylactic or countermeasure to lessen the performance effects of sleep deprivation during periods of extended wakefulness or sleep deprivation.

In the first study to systematically investigate different doses of recovery sleep (0, 2, 4, 6, 8, or 10 hours in bed) after sleep restriction of 4 hours per night for 5 nights, Banks and colleagues[38] found that the extended 10-hour recovery sleep opportunity was not enough for full recovery of sustained attention, subjective sleepiness, or fatigue. Importantly, it was observed that each recovery sleep dose had equivalent restorative value (i.e., linear) for sleep and objective sleepiness measures. However, in contrast, recovery of performance outcomes, sustained attention, and subjective sleepiness was exponential, indicating that the restorative value of the recovery sleep doses decreased with increasing sleep time.

Overall, work to date suggests that complete recovery from a period of sleep restriction may necessitate a sleep opportunity of more than 10 hours or more than 3 days if sleep is restricted to 8 hours a night. Additionally, different aspects of performance and neurobehavioral function appear to recover at different rates, with different trajectories.

Recovery Following Acute Total Sleep Deprivation

Both the number of nights needed for recovery and extended recovery sleep opportunities following total sleep deprivation have been investigated.[91,92] In one particular study,[91] participants were deprived of sleep for 1 or 2 nights, followed by 5 consecutive nights for recovery that were either restricted to 6 hours or extended to 9 hours of time in bed. Performance recovered after 1 night of extended sleep following 1 night of sleep deprivation. However, when the period of sleep deprivation was more severe (i.e., 2 nights), cognitive performance remained significantly below baseline even after 5 nights of extended recovery sleep. Neither performance nor subjective sleepiness recovered to baseline when recovery sleep time was 6 hours in bed per night. These studies underscore the importance of not restricting recovery sleep opportunities to less than 6 hours. Indeed, adding just 1 extra hour can significantly increase the rate of recovery from sleep deprivation. It appears that the more severe the sleep loss, the longer the recovery sleep opportunity required.

CLINICAL PEARL

Physicians should be aware that sleep deprivation can be caused by sleep disorders, work schedules, and modern lifestyles. The consequences of sleep deprivation include excessive daytime sleepiness, poor mood, and impaired cognitive performance and driving safety. Further, sleep deprivation appears to play a role in chronic health diseases such as cardiovascular disease, obesity, type 2 diabetes, and Alzheimer disease.

SUMMARY

Sleep is important for healthy functioning, but sleep deprivation is common in many sectors of the community. Sleep

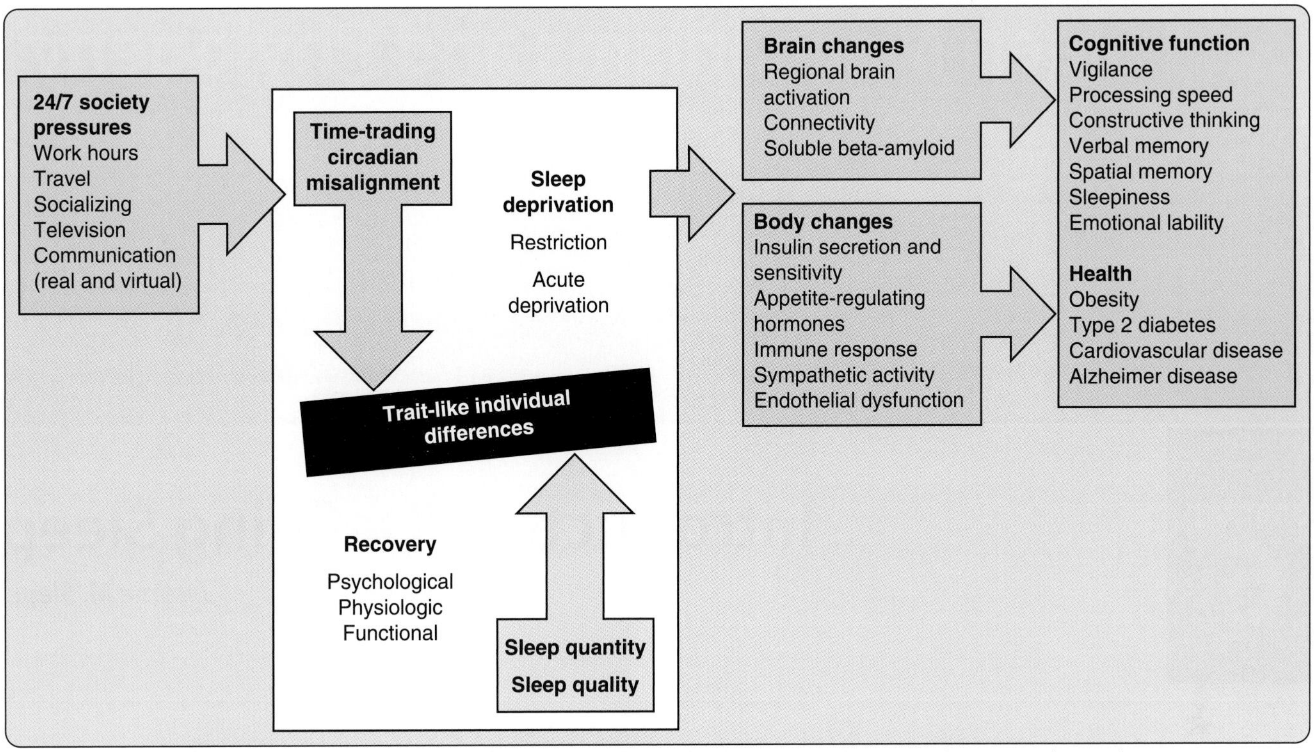

Figure 5.3 Conceptual diagram of the pressures of our 24/7 society that result in time-trading against sleep and circadian misalignment. These cause sleep deprivation, which can be in the form of chronic restricted or acute total sleep deprivation. In contrast, achieving sleep of sufficient quantity and quality assists with recovery of psychological, physiologic, and functional outcomes, all of which are affected differentially by sleep deprivation and have differential recovery trajectories. This balance between sleep deprivation and recovery is modulated by trait-like individual differences in response to sleep deprivation. In turn, sleep deprivation can lead to changes in the brain and body that can negatively impact performance and health outcomes.

deprivation causes a multitude of changes to cognitive and behavioral functioning and increases the risk for chronic diseases such type 2 diabetes, obesity, cardiovascular disease, and AD. There are large individual differences in the cognitive responses to sleep deprivation. These individual differences are stable across multiple exposures and types of sleep loss, suggesting a trait-like (possibly genetic) basis. The negative effects of sleep deprivation can be recovered by extending sleep, but recovery appears to be dependent on the type (acute versus chronic), the recovery sleep duration, and the number of days allowed for recovery (Figure 5.3). Biomathematical models and the development of unobtrusive technologies to detect fatigue while working are ways the deleterious effects of sleep deprivation can be managed in our 24/7 society.

ACKNOWLEDGMENTS

This chapter was written with support from NIH grant R01 NR004281 (DFD) and the National Space Biomedical Research Institute (NSBRI) through NASA cooperative agreement NCC 9-58 (DFD, MB).

SELECTED READINGS

Banks S, Dinges DF. Behavioral and physiological consequences of sleep restriction. *J Clin Sleep Med.* 2007;3(5):519–528.

Banks S, Van Dongen HP, Maislin G, Dinges DF. Neurobehavioral dynamics following chronic sleep restriction: dose-response effects of one night for recovery. *Sleep.* 2010;33(8):1013–1026.

Basner M, Fomberstein KM, Razavi FM, et al. American time use survey: sleep time and its relationship to waking activities. *Sleep.* 2007;30(9):1085–1095.

Belenky G, Wesensten NJ, Thorne DR, et al. Patterns of performance degradation and restoration during sleep restriction and subsequent recovery: a sleep dose-response study. *J Sleep Res.* 2003;12:1–12.

Cappuccio FP, D'Elia L, Strazzullo P, Miller MA. Sleep duration and all-cause mortality: a systematic review and meta-analysis of prospective studies. *Sleep.* 2010;33(5):585–592.

Dorrian J, Rogers NL, Dinges DF. Psychomotor vigilance performance: neurocognitive assay sensitive to sleep loss. In: Kushida C, ed. *Sleep Dep rivation*; 2005.

Satterfield BC, Stucky B, Landolt HP, Van Dongen HPA. Unraveling the genetic underpinnings of sleep deprivation-induced impairments in human cognition. *Prog Brain Res.* 2019;246:127–158.

Lamond N, Jay SM, Dorrian J, Ferguson SA, Jones C, Dawson D. The dynamics of neurobehavioural recovery following sleep loss. *J Sleep Res.* 2007;16(1):33–41.

Liew SC, Aung T. Sleep deprivation and its association with diseases- a review. *Sleep Med.* 2021;77:192–204.

Van Dongen HP, Baynard MD, Maislin G, Dinges DF. Systematic interindividual differences in neurobehavioral impairment from sleep loss: evidence of trait-like differential vulnerability. *Sleep.* 2004;27(3):423–433.

Van Dongen HPA, Maislin G, Mullington JM, Dinges DF. The cumulative cost of additional wakefulness: dose-response effects on neurobehavioral functions and sleep physiology from chronic sleep restriction and total sleep deprivation. *Sleep.* 2003;26(2):117–126.

A complete reference list can be found online at ExpertConsult.com.

Section 2 Sleep Mechanisms and Phylogeny

Chapter 6 Introduction/Defining Sleep

Jerome M. Siegel

A relative seemed to fall asleep at a family gathering, with eyes closed, immobile, and conspicuous uninterrupted snoring. When he was elbowed "awake," he vigorously denied having been asleep. He then proceeded to recite, verbatim, conversations taking place right up to the point he was so rudely "awakened." Clearly it was incorrect to say he was asleep, even though a superficial evaluation might conclude otherwise. Conversely, it is common to fall asleep while watching TV, while a passenger on a long trip, or in a boring situation and to be unaware of this. When told you were asleep, you may deny it, but when quizzed about what you were watching or listening to, there is an undeniable gap in what you remember.

Sleep has historically been distinguished from waking by five criteria: (1) reduced motor activity, (2) decreased response to stimulation, (3) stereotypic postures (e.g., in humans, lying down with eyes closed), (4) relatively easy reversibility (distinguishing it from coma, hibernation, and estivation),[1] (5) homeostatic regulation (i.e., sleep deprivation is followed by sleep rebound). A frequently unstated, but central, attribute of sleep is (6) loss of consciousness of the environment.

It is important to appreciate that these are not binary criteria. At what point is motor activity, responsiveness, or reversibility considered to be reduced? What defines "loss of consciousness"? Is "rebound" always present after reduced sleep and equal to the amount of sleep lost?

How often are these criteria for defining and measuring sleep rigorously applied? In human studies the answer is "rarely." In animal studies the answer is "almost never."

A common practice in studies of mammals is to use electroencephalographic (EEG) activity as the only criterion of sleep, because it appears to correspond to sleep in humans. But this is also not a binary characteristic. Are alpha waves sufficient? Delta waves? Of what signal-to-noise ratio and at what sites within the brain? Clearly EEG is not "sleep determinative" in the case of rapid eye movement (REM) sleep in which the EEG is low-voltage "activated," as in waking, while the behavior is clearly sleep.

Contrary to some folk wisdom, humans are not completely inactive during sleep or even during "deep sleep." Movement is required in both sleep and waking, as is apparent in quadriplegics who cannot move. If they are not moved frequently during sleep and waking periods, bedsores will develop with eventual dire consequences, so nursing care or specially designed beds that frequently change pressure points are necessary. Movement during "sleep" is present even in smaller animals.

While inactivity is relatively easy to document with motion detectors or video, elevated arousal threshold is more difficult to define and measure. Arousal is not simply a response to an intense stimulus. You may not awaken to a thunderstorm, but you may awaken to your baby's faint cries. It is likely that nonhuman animals are similarly able to process sensory inputs during sleep and awaken only to the most salient patterns of noise, light, smell, and so on.

Elevated arousal thresholds must be species specific. If lions and giraffes, which live in the same African ecosystems, had equally elevated sleep arousal thresholds, giraffes would not exist. Adult giraffes must never be as deeply asleep as their predators. Giraffes not only sleep less deeply, but they also sleep less than 4 hours per day, based on observational studies in zoos, making them one of the shortest-sleeping species.[2] Immature giraffes, elephants, and other newborns appear to sleep relatively deeply and longer than adult members of their species, but they are always close enough to their mothers to be defended from predators. Conversely, lions and other predators can benefit from the reduced energy consumption accompanying sleep[3] with greatly elevated arousal thresholds. Individual humans and animals may sleep more or less deeply (i.e., have different arousal thresholds), depending on the sleep environment,[4] their age,[5] and other characteristics.

It has been supposed that lost sleep creates a "sleep debt" that is repaid in a sleep rebound. But in fact rebound is always substantially less than the amount of lost sleep. One of the best-documented periods of human sleep deprivation was an 11-day period of total sleep self-deprivation. This translates to about 80 hours of sleep loss. Day one of recovery sleep produced 14.7 hours of sleep (1.8 hours of REM and 1.9 hours of deep, "stage 4" sleep). Sleep duration was 10.4 hours on the second day and 9.1 hours on the third day. When the next recording was made, 1 week later, the subject had just 7 hours of sleep.[6] In contrast, the major effect of total sleep deprivation in the rat for 11 to 32 days was a striking rebound of REM, not non-REM, sleep.[7] The argument can be made that rebound sleep, although shorter in duration than the sleep "debt," is more "intense," with higher voltage EEG or more rapid eye movements. But since there is no agreement on exactly what the underlying metric of sleep is, the intensity of recovery sleep is difficult to quantify.

Small cetacean (dolphins and whales) marine mammals, such as Commerson's dolphin,[8] are in continuous motion from the moment they are born until the end of their lives. A study of dolphins and of killer whales[9] found similar continuous motion both in calves and in their mothers for weeks to months after birth. During this period, the calves swim in tight formation with their mothers. In the wild, these are times of migration and high danger, and both mother and calf must remain alert. One can assume that brain motor and sensory systems are functioning at high levels, just the opposite of the behavioral definitions of sleep listed previously. Inactive behavior gradually returns to the adult pattern, with no evidence of rebound beyond baseline adult levels. Migrating birds greatly reduce sleep during migration periods without obvious deficits or rebounds.[10,11] Similarly it has been shown that, in certain birds, success in mating behavior is inversely correlated with sleep time during the 3-week mating period.[12,13]

Cetaceans show sleeplike high-voltage EEG in only one hemisphere at a time. Bilateral high-voltage EEG is never seen.[14-19] Cetaceans never show REM sleep. A study that attempted unihemispheric sleep deprivation produced an unclear outcome. A rebound specific to the hemisphere that triggered the deprivation procedure was not seen. Instead the dolphins showed highly asymmetric unihemispheric EEG patterns that were not clearly related to the prior deprivation procedures.[20]

CLINICAL PEARLS

It is frequently said that "all animals sleep" or "all animals with nervous systems sleep." This is incorrect, unless one adopts an extremely fluid definition of sleep.[3] When one makes a statement about sleep in animals, the message transmitted is that these animals sleep "like we do." This implies a period of inactivity, of substantially reduced consciousness and responsiveness, and with homeostatic regulation. Each of these criteria requires further data. These issues get even more difficult when one is studying "sleep" in insects such as drosophila, fish, amphibia, reptiles, or birds. Are we conflating changes in activity with changes in sleep? Without rigorous application of the sleep definition, we need to be more careful with claims of sleep, sleep duration, and sleep depth. We might also profitably highlight quantitative and qualitative individual and species differences in waking versus rest versus sleep patterns and how these may be evolutionarily adaptive.

A complete reference list can be found online at ExpertConsult.com.

Chapter 7

Neural Control of Sleep in Mammals

Dennis McGinty; Ronald Szymusiak

Chapter Highlights

- Mammalian sleep and wake states are regulated by multiple neuronal systems located in the brainstem, diencephalon, and telencephalon. Although the isolated brainstem can generate NREM-like and REM-like states, lesions of several brainstem and forebrain regions in the otherwise intact brain can be associated with altered amounts of NREM and/or REM sleep.
- Arousal and waking are facilitated by chemically distinct neuronal groups localized in the pons, midbrain, the posterior and lateral hypothalamus, and the basal forebrain. Functionally important arousal systems include glutamatergic, histaminergic, orexinergic, serotoninergic, cholinergic, dopaminergic, and noradrenergic neurons.
- Arousal systems have widespread projections that regulate global aspects of arousal, including changes in electroencephalographic, motor, sensory, autonomic, and integrative functions. Arousal systems control the excitability of thalamic and cortical neurons. Reduced activity in arousal systems promotes synchronous discharge of intracortical and thalamocortical circuits that underlie NREM sleep patterns on the electroencephalogram.
- The preoptic anterior hypothalamus—the preoptic area (POA)—contains gamma-aminobutyric acid (GABA)-ergic/galaninergic neurons that exhibit increased activity during NREM and REM sleep and respond to physiologic signals that increase sleep, such as warming, sustained wakefulness, and endogenous sleep factors. POA sleep-active GABAergic neurons project to histaminergic, orexinergic, serotoninergic, and noradrenergic arousal systems and, through coordinated inhibition of these arousal systems, promote transitions from waking to sleep. GABAergic sleep-promoting neurons are also localized in the medullary parafacial zone and exert sleep-related inhibition of wakefulness-promoting glutamatergic neurons in the parabrachial nucleus in the pons.
- Sleep-promoting molecules are related to the multiple functions of sleep: adenosine to resupply brain energy reserves, cytokines to facilitate immune functions, growth hormone–releasing hormone to promote anabolic processes, unfolding protein response signals to prevent protein misfolding, and oxidative stress signaling molecules to prevent oxidative stress–induced cell damage.

DIVERSE BRAIN REGIONS MODULATE WAKING AND NON–RAPID EYE MOVEMENT SLEEP

Isolated Forebrain

The capacity of various brain regions to generate sleep and awake states was first studied by isolating or removing major regions. The physiology of the chronically maintained isolated forebrain, or chronic *cerveau isolé,* preparation has been examined in dogs and cats.[1] Immediately after complete midbrain transections, the isolated forebrain exhibits continuous slow waves and spindles on the electroencephalogram (EEG). Thus structures below the midbrain normally must facilitate awake-like EEG states. By contrast, if a brainstem transection was made at the midpontine level, an activated or wake-like forebrain EEG state predominated immediately after the transection but with some residual episodes of EEG slow wave activity. In this preparation, the forebrain exhibited evidence of classical conditioning and other signs of an integrated waking state.

These studies argue that neuronal groups localized between the midpons and upper midbrain are important for generating a waking (wakefulness)-like state. After 5 to 9 days of recovery, the chronic cerveau isolé rat preparation exhibits a circadian pattern of EEG activation and synchronization.[2] In this preparation, the creation of preoptic area (POA) lesions is followed by a continuously activated EEG pattern. Thus the isolated forebrain can generate a sustained wake-like state, and the POA must play a critical role in initiating the sleep-like EEG state of the isolated forebrain (see later in this chapter). Wake-like and sleep-like EEG states appear to depend on a balance between wake-promoting and sleep-promoting systems. The terms *wake-like* and *sleep-like* are used here because these preparations cannot exhibit the full behavioral spectrum of sleep and wake states.

Diencephalon

Chronic diencephalic cats, in which the neocortex and striatum have been removed, exhibit behavioral waking with persistent locomotion and orientation to auditory stimuli, a quiet sleep-like or non–rapid eye movement (NREM)-like state with typical cat sleeping postures, and a rapid eye movement (REM)-like state, including muscle atonia, rapid eye movements, muscle twitches, and pontine EEG spikes.[3] EEG patterns recorded in the thalamus showed increased amplitude in conjunction with the NREM sleep–like state, although true spindles and slow waves were absent. The thalamic EEG exhibits desynchronization during the REM-like state.

In summary, the neocortex and striatum are not required for any behaviorally defined sleep-wake states, and an NREM-like state occurs in the absence of sleep spindles and slow waves.

Thalamus

Cats subjected to complete thalamectomy continue to exhibit episodes of EEG and behavioral sleep and waking, although spindles are absent on the EEG,[4] and the animals exhibit reductions in both NREM and REM sleep. Fatal familial insomnia[5] is a rare neurodegenerative disease in humans characterized by progressive autonomic hyperactivation, motor disturbances, loss of sleep spindles, and severe NREM sleep insomnia. Neuropathologic examination findings include severe cell loss and gliosis in the anterior medial thalamus, including the dorsomedial nucleus. However, patients with paramedian thalamic stroke with magnetic resonance imaging–verified damage to the dorsomedial and centromedial nuclei present with either severe hypersomnolence or increased daytime sleepiness, not insomnia.[6] In summary, the thalamus plays a critical role in regulating cortical EEG patterns during waking and sleep, and specific regions within this structure appear to have either wake-promoting or hypnogenic functions.

Lower Brainstem

After recovery from the acute effects of the complete midbrain transections in cats (as just described), the lower brainstem can generate rudimentary behavioral waking, an NREM-like state, and a REM-like state.[3] Waking is characterized by crouching, sitting, attempts to walk, dilated pupils, and head orientation to noises. In the first sleep-like state, these cats lie in a random position, pupils exhibit reduced but variable miosis, and eyes exhibit slow and nonconjugate movements. The animals can be aroused by auditory or other stimuli. If this stage is not disturbed, these cats enter another stage characterized by complete pupillary miosis, loss of neck muscle tone, and rapid eye movements, identifying a REM-like state. Additional studies support the hypothesis that the lower brainstem contains sleep-facilitating processes. Low-frequency electrical stimulation of the dorsal medullary reticular formation in the nucleus of the solitary tract produced neocortical EEG synchronization.[7] Lesioning or cooling of this site was followed by EEG activation.[8] Recently, a population of sleep-active neurons has been identified in the rostral medulla of rats and mice, located lateral and dorsal to the facial nerve.[9] Many of these sleep-active medullary neurons express inhibitory neurotransmitters such as gamma-aminobutyric acid (GABA) or glycine. Excitotoxic lesions of the parafacial zone (PZ) are associated with increased waking and decreased NREM sleep.[9]

In summary, widespread structures in the mammalian nervous system, from the neocortex to the lower brainstem, have the capacity to facilitate both sleep-like and waking-like states and to modulate the amounts of sleep.

RETICULAR ACTIVATING SYSTEM AND DELINEATION OF AROUSAL SYSTEMS

The transection studies just described support the concept of a pontomesencephalic wake-promoting or arousal system. No discovery was historically more significant than the description of the reticular activating system (RAS) by Moruzzi and Magoun.[10] Introduction of large lesions of the core of the rostral pontine and mesencephalic tegmentum was followed by persistent somnolence and EEG synchronization, and electrical stimulation of this region induced arousal from sleep. Interruption of sensory pathways did not affect EEG activation. It was hypothesized that cells in the RAS generated forebrain activation and wakefulness.

The concept of the RAS has been superseded by the finding that arousal is facilitated not by a single system but instead by several discrete neuronal groups localized within and adjacent to the pontine and midbrain reticular formation and its extension into the hypothalamus (Figure 7.1). These neuronal systems are differentiated by the expression of enzymes that synthesize specific neurotransmitters and neuromodulators. These include neurons that synthesize serotonin, norepinephrine (noradrenaline), histamine, acetylcholine (ACh), and orexin/hypocretin (herein called orexin). Each of these systems has been studied extensively in the context of the control of specific aspects of waking behaviors. Presented next is a brief overview of each of these *arousal systems,* focusing on their contribution to generalized brain arousal or activation. As background, some general properties of these neuronal systems are summarized in the following list:

1. Arousal is a global process, characterized by concurrent changes in several physiologic systems, including autonomic, motor, endocrine, and sensory systems, as well as in EEG tracings. All the arousal systems share one critical property: their neurons give rise to long, projecting axons with extensive terminal fields that impinge on several regions of the brainstem and forebrain. In this chapter, the emphasis is on the ascending projections from the brainstem and hypothalamus to the diencephalon, limbic system, and neocortex, because these are particularly germane to the generation of cortical arousal. Some arousal systems give rise to descending projections as well, which also are likely to play a role in regulating certain properties of sleep-wake states, such as changes in muscle tone and autonomic function.
2. Arousal systems have been studied by recording the discharge patterns of neurons in "freely moving" animals relative to those in spontaneously occurring wake and sleep states. Increased discharge during arousal or wake states

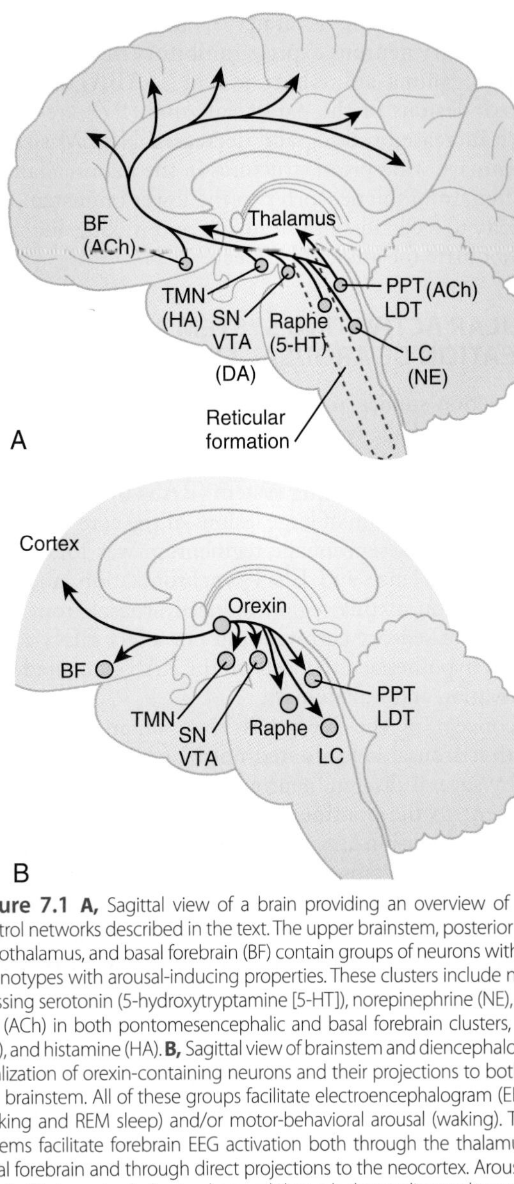

Figure 7.1 A, Sagittal view of a brain providing an overview of the wake-control networks described in the text. The upper brainstem, posterior and lateral hypothalamus, and basal forebrain (BF) contain groups of neurons with identified phenotypes with arousal-inducing properties. These clusters include neurons expressing serotonin (5-hydroxytryptamine [5-HT]), norepinephrine (NE), acetylcholine (ACh) in both pontomesencephalic and basal forebrain clusters, dopamine (DA), and histamine (HA). **B,** Sagittal view of brainstem and diencephalon showing localization of orexin-containing neurons and their projections to both forebrain and brainstem. All of these groups facilitate electroencephalogram (EEG) arousal (waking and REM sleep) and/or motor-behavioral arousal (waking). The arousal systems facilitate forebrain EEG activation both through the thalamus and the basal forebrain and through direct projections to the neocortex. Arousal systems also facilitate motor-behavioral arousal through descending pathways. LC, Locus coeruleus; LDT, lateral dorsal tegmental; PPT, pedunculopontine; SN, substantia nigra; TMN, tuberomammillary nucleus; VTA, ventral tegmental area.

compared with sleep constitutes part of the evidence for an arousal system.

3. The actions of a neurotransmitter on a target neuronal system are determined primarily by the properties of the receptors in the target. The neurotransmitters and neuromodulators underlying arousal systems each act on several distinct receptor types with diverse actions. In addition, postsynaptic effects are regulated by transmitter-specific "reuptake" molecules, which transport the neurotransmitter out of the synaptic space, terminating its action. Pharmacologic actions are usually mediated by actions on specific receptor types or transporters (see examples further on).
4. Chronic lesions of individual arousal systems or genetic knockout of critical molecules have only small or sometimes no effect on sleep-wake patterns (with the exception of orexin knockouts; see later), even though acute manipulations of these same systems have strong effects on sleep-wake. The absence of chronic lesion or knockout effects is likely to be due to the redundancy of the arousal systems such that, over time, deficiency in one system is compensated for by other systems or by changes in receptor sensitivity.
5. Electrophysiologic studies show that the arousal systems normally are activated and deactivated within seconds of a change in behavioral state. Thus effects of acute experimental manipulations of neurotransmitters that mediate arousal, as generated by acute administration of drugs, may best mimic the normal physiologic pattern and be more informative than chronic lesions regarding their function.
6. Optogenetic and chemogenetic methods enable manipulating the excitability of specific cell types in vivo, with high spatial and temporal resolution. Application of these methods are rapidly expanding our understanding of the brain circuits that regulate sleep and arousal.
7. REM sleep is a state associated with behavioral and muscle quiescence and intense cortical EEG arousal. In parallel with these two aspects of REM sleep, arousal systems can be classified into two types: ones that are "off" in the REM state, befitting its sleep-like property, and others that are "on" in the REM state, befitting its wake-like properties. Some arousal-promoting systems (summarized later) also play a role in REM sleep control. Detailed analyses of the control of the role of these systems in REM sleep are presented in Chapter 8.

WAKE-ON/RAPID EYE MOVEMENT–OFF AROUSAL SYSTEMS

Serotonin

Neurons containing serotonin, or 5-hydroxytryptamine (5-HT), are found in the dorsal raphe and median raphe nuclei of the midbrain. These neurons project to virtually all regions of the diencephalon, limbic system, and neocortex. It initially was hypothesized that serotonin might be a sleep-promoting substance,[11] but evidence shows that the immediate effect of serotonin release is arousal (as reviewed by Ursin[12]). Although some heterogeneity is typical, the discharge rates of most dorsal and median raphe neurons are highest during waking and lower during NREM sleep, with minimal discharge in REM sleep. Release of serotonin in the forebrain is highest in waking. Because of the diversity of serotonin receptors (there are at least 14 types), the effects of serotonin on target neurons are complex. Some receptor types are inhibitory, some are excitatory. At least one class of receptors, 5-HT_{2A}, appears to facilitate NREM sleep, because 5-HT_{2A}–knockout mice have reduced non–rapid eye movements.[13] Selective serotonin reuptake inhibitors and serotonin-norepinephrine reuptake inhibitors, which augment the actions of serotonin, are used to treat a variety of medical and psychiatric problems, and some drugs in this class have arousing or alerting properties. 5-HT neurons may mediate CO_2-induced arousals from sleep. Perfusion of CO_2-rich acidified solution into the dorsal raphe evoked arousals from sleep, an effect not seen in the genetic absence of 5-HT neurons or during optogenetic inhibition of 5-HT neurons in the dorsal raphe.[14]

Norepinephrine

Norepinephrine-containing neuronal groups in mammals are found throughout the brainstem, but the primary nucleus giving rise to ascending projections is the locus coeruleus. Norepinephrine neurons in this nucleus project throughout the diencephalon, forebrain, and cerebellum. Most locus coeruleus neurons exhibit regular discharge during waking, reduced discharge during NREM sleep, and near-complete cessation of discharge in REM sleep, a pattern congruent with a role in behavioral arousal.[15] Acute inactivation of the locus coeruleus or introduction of a lesion in the ascending pathway from this nucleus increases slow wave EEG activity during sleep.[16] Optogenetic excitation of norepinephrine neurons in the locus coeruleus are sufficient to promote arousals from sleep.[17] Distinct roles for alpha$_1$, alpha$_2$, and beta norepinephrine receptor types are established. Direct application of alpha$_1$ and beta agonists in POA and adjacent basal forebrain sites induces increased wakefulness (reviewed by Berridge[18]). The arousal-producing effects of psychostimulant drugs such as amphetamines depend partly on induction of increased norepinephrine release and inhibition of norepinephrine reuptake, as well as on enhanced dopamine action (see later in this chapter).

Histamine

Histamine-containing neurons in mammals are discretely localized within the tuberomammillary nucleus (TMN) and adjacent posterior hypothalamus (PH). Histamine neurons project throughout the hypothalamus and forebrain, including to the neocortex, as well as to the brainstem and spinal cord (reviewed by Haas and colleagues[19]). Administration of histamine type 1 (H_1) receptor antagonists (antihistamines) that penetrate the blood-brain barrier can result in sedative effects.[19] Transient inactivation of the TMN region results in increased NREM sleep.[20] Histamine neurons exhibit regular discharge during waking, greatly reduced discharge during NREM sleep, and cessation of discharge in REM sleep.[21] Optogenetic inhibition of histamine neurons promotes REM sleep.[22] Histamine neurons express H_3-type inhibitory autoreceptors and therefore can be inhibited by histamine. Administration of an antagonist H_3 receptor causes disinhibition of histamine neurons and increased waking.[23]

Orexin (Hypocretin)

The loss of orexin neurons is known to underlie the human disease narcolepsy, the major symptoms of which are cataplexy and excessive sleepiness.[24,25] Orexin-containing neurons are localized within the midlateral hypothalamus, and like other arousal systems, they give rise to projections to several brain regions, including the brainstem.[26] Among the targets of orexin terminals are other arousal-promoting neurons including histamine, 5-HT, norepinephrine, neurons, as well as dopamine neurons in the ventral tegmental area (VTA) and cholinergic neurons in the brainstem and basal forebrain. Orexin-containing neurons are active in waking and exhibit very low rates of discharge in both NREM and REM sleep.[27,28] Local administration of orexin in several brain sites induces arousal.[29] Optogenetic excitation of orexin neurons promotes transitions from NREM sleep to wakefulness.[30] Locus coeruleus neuronal activity appears to be critical for orexin-induced awakenings from sleep, as coincident optogenetic inhibition of norepinephrine neurons suppresses the ability of photostimulation of orexin neurons to evoke arousals from sleep.[31]

WAKE-ON/RAPID EYE MOVEMENT–ON AROUSAL SYSTEMS

Acetylcholine

ACh-containing neurons are localized within two regions: the dorsolateral pontomesencephalic reticular formation, including the pedunculopontine tegmental and laterodorsal tegmental nuclei, and the basal forebrain (BF).[32] The pontomesencephalic ACh neuronal group projects to the thalamus, hypothalamus, and basal forebrain; the basal forebrain group projects to the limbic system and neocortex. Neurons in both groups exhibit higher rates of discharge in both waking and REM sleep than in NREM sleep,[33-35] and release of ACh also is increased in these states.[36] Optogenetic stimulation of BF ACh neurons induces cortical activation and arousal from NREM sleep.[35,37]

Dopamine

Dopamine-containing neurons are localized primarily within the substantia nigra and the adjacent VTA of the midbrain and the basal and medial hypothalamus.[38] Release of dopamine in the frontal cortex is higher during wakefulness than during sleep.[39] Dopamine is inactivated primarily through reuptake by the dopamine transporter. Stimulant drugs such as amphetamines and modafinil act primarily through dopamine receptors, particularly by binding to and suppressing the dopamine transporter, reducing reuptake.[40] The degeneration of the nigrostriatal dopamine system is a neuropathologic basis of Parkinson disease, which can be accompanied by excessive daytime sleepiness.[41]

In vivo calcium imaging of dopaminergic neurons in the VTA demonstrates that these neurons exhibit the highest activity levels in waking and REM sleep compared to NREM sleep.[42] Optogenetic excitation of VTA dopamine neurons promotes wakefulness, and inhibition of these neurons evokes sleep preparatory behaviors and sleep. An additional population of dopamine-containing wake-active neurons is localized in the rat ventral periaqueductal gray (PAG) and dorsal raphe, and destruction of dopaminergic neurons in this region with 6-hydroxy-dopamine increases daily sleep time by 20%.[43] Activity of PAG dopamine neurons is elevated during waking versus sleep.[43,44] Optogenetic activation of PAG dopamine neurons promotes waking, and optogenetic inhibition promotes sleep.[44]

Glutamate

Glutamate is the most widespread excitatory neurotransmitter of the brain. Glutamate-containing neurons are found throughout the brain, including in the core of the pontine and midbrain reticular formation.[45] Extracellular levels of glutamate in the cortex and in the hypothalamus are elevated during waking and REM sleep, compared with NREM sleep.[46,47] Arousal is increased by application of glutamate to many sites.[48] Its actions are mediated by receptors controlling membrane ion flux, including the *N*-methyl-D-aspartate (NMDA) receptor and "metabotrophic" receptors controlling intracellular processes. Humans may be exposed to systemic NMDA receptor antagonists in the form of anesthetics (e.g., ketamine) or recreational drugs (e.g., phencyclidine). The effects are dosage dependent: low dosages produce arousal, and high dosages produce sedation. In rats, exposure to NMDA antagonists induces a potent long-lasting enhancement of NREM slow wave activity.[49]

SLEEP-PROMOTING MECHANISMS

As noted in the foregoing review of evidence for multiple neurochemically specific arousal systems, the activity of each of these neuronal groups is reduced during NREM sleep. In most groups, the reduction in neuronal discharge precedes EEG changes that herald sleep onset. How is the process of sleep onset orchestrated?

Rostral Hypothalamic Sleep-Promoting System

Sleep-Active Neurons in the Preoptic Area

More than 70 years ago, von Economo postulated a POA sleep-promoting area on the basis of his observation that postmortem examinations in patients with encephalitis who had severe insomnia showed inflammatory lesions in this area of the brain.[50] Patients with hypersomnia had lesions in the vicinity of the PH. To von Economo, these observations suggested the concept of opposing hypothalamic sleep-promoting and wake-promoting systems. In rats, symmetric bilateral transections of the POA resulted in complete sleeplessness, and symmetric bilateral transections of the PH caused continuous sleep.[51] Rats that underwent both POA and PH transections exhibited continuous sleep, as with PH transections alone. This was interpreted as showing that the POA normally inhibits the PH wake-promoting region. The PH wake-promoting system can now be understood as the rostral extension of arousal-promoting systems and pathways summarized earlier.

The existence of a sleep-promoting mechanism in the POA has been confirmed by a variety of methods. Bilateral lesions of the POA with diameters of 1 to 2 mm in rats and cats induce partial sleep loss. Larger bilateral lesions (3 to 5 mm in diameter) that extend into the adjacent basal forebrain are associated with more severe insomnia (as described in our review of this work[52]). After introduction of POA lesions that result in partial sleep loss, residual sleep is characterized by reduced slow wave (delta) EEG activity.[53] Because delta activity is recognized as a marker of enhanced sleep drive, this finding suggests that POA output contributes to the regulation of sleep drive.

The identification of sleep-active POA neurons has been advanced by the application of the c-Fos immunostaining method.[54] Rapid expression of the proto-oncogene *c-fos* has been identified as a marker of neuronal activation in many brain sites and in multiple cell types.[55] Thus c-Fos immunostaining permits functional mapping of neurons, identifying neurons that were activated in the preceding 30 to 60 minutes. After sustained sleep, but not waking, a discrete cluster of neurons exhibiting c-Fos is found in the ventrolateral preoptic area (VLPO).[54] The VLPO is located at the base of the brain, lateral to the optic chiasm. Sleep-related Fos immunoreactive neurons are also localized within the rostral and caudal median preoptic nucleus (MnPN).[56] Examples of c-Fos immunostaining and the correlations between c-Fos counts and sleep amounts are shown in Figure 7.2.

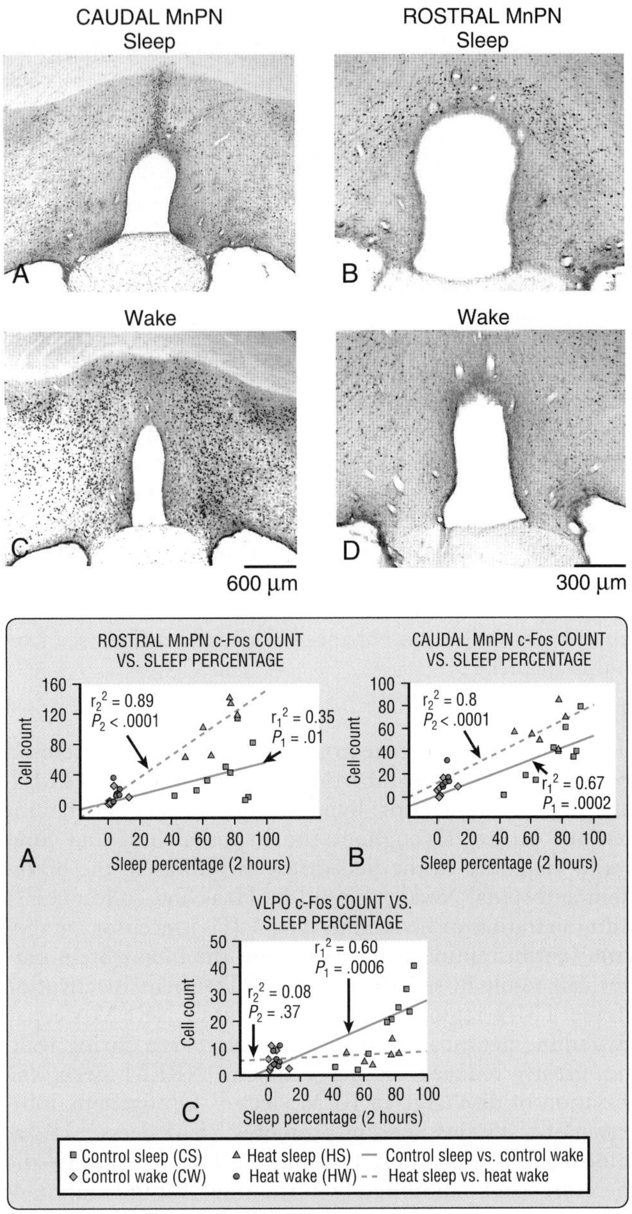

Figure 7.2 *Upper panel:* Examples of c-Fos immunostaining of preoptic area (POA) neuronal nuclei, identified by *dark spots* after either sustained spontaneous sleep or wakefulness. c-Fos immunostaining is a marker of neuronal activation and is a method for mapping the localization of sleep-active neurons in the brain. After sleep, increased staining was seen in the midline **(A)** or around the top of the third ventricle **(B)** relative to the wake samples **(C** and **D).** These sites correspond to the caudal and rostral median preoptic nucleus (MnPN). Similar results were seen in the ventrolateral preoptic area (VLPO). In other POA sites, c-Fos immunostaining was seen after both waking and sleep. *Lower panel:* Regression functions and correlations relating c-Fos counts and sleep amounts before sacrifice among individual animals. In all sites, significant correlations were found between sleep amounts and c-Fos counts at a normal ambient temperature. Groups of animals were studied in both normal and warm ambient temperatures. In a warm ambient temperature, c-Fos counts after sleep and correlations between counts and sleep amounts were increased in MnPN sites **(A** and **B),** but they were suppressed in the VLPO **(C).** (From Gong H, Szymusiak R, King J, et al. Sleep-related c-Fos expression in the preoptic hypothalamus: effects of ambient warming. *Am J Physiol Regul Integr Comp Physiol* 2000;279:R2079–88.)

The VLPO and the MnPN contain a high density of neurons with sleep-related discharge.[57,58] Most sleep-active neurons in these nuclei are more activated during both NREM and REM sleep than in awake states (Figure 7.3). VLPO neurons typically exhibit increases in activity during

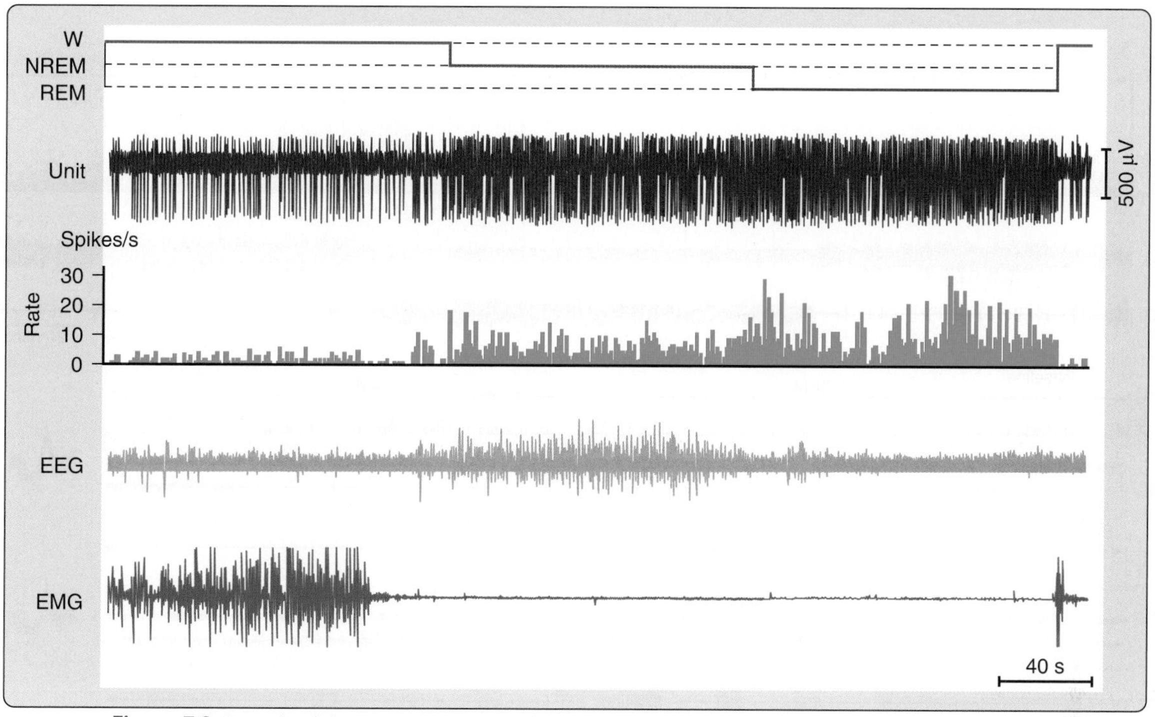

Figure 7.3 Example of sleep-active neurons in the median preoptic nucleus (MnPN). Shown is a continuous recording of discharge of an MnPN neuron during a wake (W)-NREM-REM cycle (*top*). Discharge rate increased at the onset of sleep, as indicated by the increased amplitude of the electroencephalogram (EEG). Discharge rate increased further in association with REM sleep (*right*). Such sleep-active neurons constituted a majority of those encountered in the MnPN and the ventrolateral preoptic area (VLPO). The presence of sleep-active neurons is one critical piece of evidence for the importance of a brain region in the facilitation of sleep. EMG, Electromyogram. (From Suntsova N, Szymusiak R, Alam MN, et al. Sleep-waking discharge patterns of median preoptic nucleus neurons in rats. *J Physiol* 2002;543:665–77.)

spontaneous transitions between waking and sleep and display a progressive increase in discharge rate from light to deep NREM sleep.

VLPO and MnPN sleep regulatory neurons are dynamically responsive to changes in homeostatic sleep pressure induced by sleep deprivation. In the MnPN, c-Fos expression in GABAergic neurons is increased after a brief (2- to 3-hour) period of sleep deprivation, even if no opportunity for recovery sleep is permitted.[59] Fos expression in GABAergic VLPO neurons is increased during recovery sleep subsequent to sleep deprivation. When the neuronal discharge of individual sleep-active neurons in the MnPN and VLPO is continuously recorded across baseline sleep-wake, sleep deprivation, and recovery sleep, dynamic responses to changing homeostatic sleep pressure are evident[60] (Figure 7.4). MnPN and VLPO neurons identified as sleep-active during spontaneous baseline sleep exhibit progressive increases in waking discharge rate during sleep deprivation that are correlated with behavioral indices of sleep pressure (Figure 7.4). NREM sleep–related discharge is elevated in comparison with baseline NREM sleep early in the recovery period and then declines in association with the reduction in EEG delta power.[60] Thus sleep-active neurons in the MnPN/VLPO are involved in orchestrating spontaneous wake-sleep transitions (see further in this chapter) and function as components of the neuronal circuits that mediate homeostatic responses to sustained wakefulness.

How do POA sleep-active neurons initiate and sustain sleep? VLPO neurons that exhibit c-Fos immunoreactivity during sleep express glutamic acid decarboxylase, the synthetic enzyme of the *inhibitory* neurotransmitter GABA. They also express the inhibitory neuropeptide galanin.[61] A majority of MnPN neurons that exhibit sleep-related Fos-immunoreactivity also express glutamic acid decarboxylase.[62] VLPO neurons project to histamine neurons in the TMN.[61] Additional projections of the VLPO include the midbrain dorsal raphe and the locus coeruleus. The MnPN also projects to both the dorsal raphe and locus coeruleus.[63] Both MnPN and VLPO project to the perifornical lateral hypothalamic area, where orexin neurons are located.[63] Thus discharge of VLPO and MnPN GABAergic neurons during sleep is expected to release GABA at these sites. Indeed, GABA release is increased during NREM sleep and further increased in REM sleep in the PH, doral raphe, and locus coeruleus.[64-66] Sleep-active neurons in VLPO and MnPN exhibit discharge-rate-change profiles across the wake-NREM-REM cycle that are reciprocal to those of wake-promoting histamine, 5-HT, norepinephrine, and orexin neurons (Figure 7.5). Optogenetic activation of GABAergic neurons in the POA that project to the TMN promotes sleep.[67] Chemogenetic excitation of galanin-expressing neurons in the POA promotes sleep and restores sleep in an animal model of insomnia.[68] These findings support a hypothesis that POA sleep-active neurons, through release of GABA and or galanin, inhibit multiple arousal systems.

GABAergic neurons in the VLPO region are inhibited by 5-HT and norepinephrine.[69] MnPN neurons are inhibited by norepinephrine.[70] Wake-active GABAergic neurons in the lateral hypothalamus project to and inhibit VLPO galanin sleep-promoting neurons.[71] Thus POA sleep-active neurons inhibit arousal systems, and arousal systems inhibit POA sleep-active neurons. These mutually inhibitory processes are hypothesized

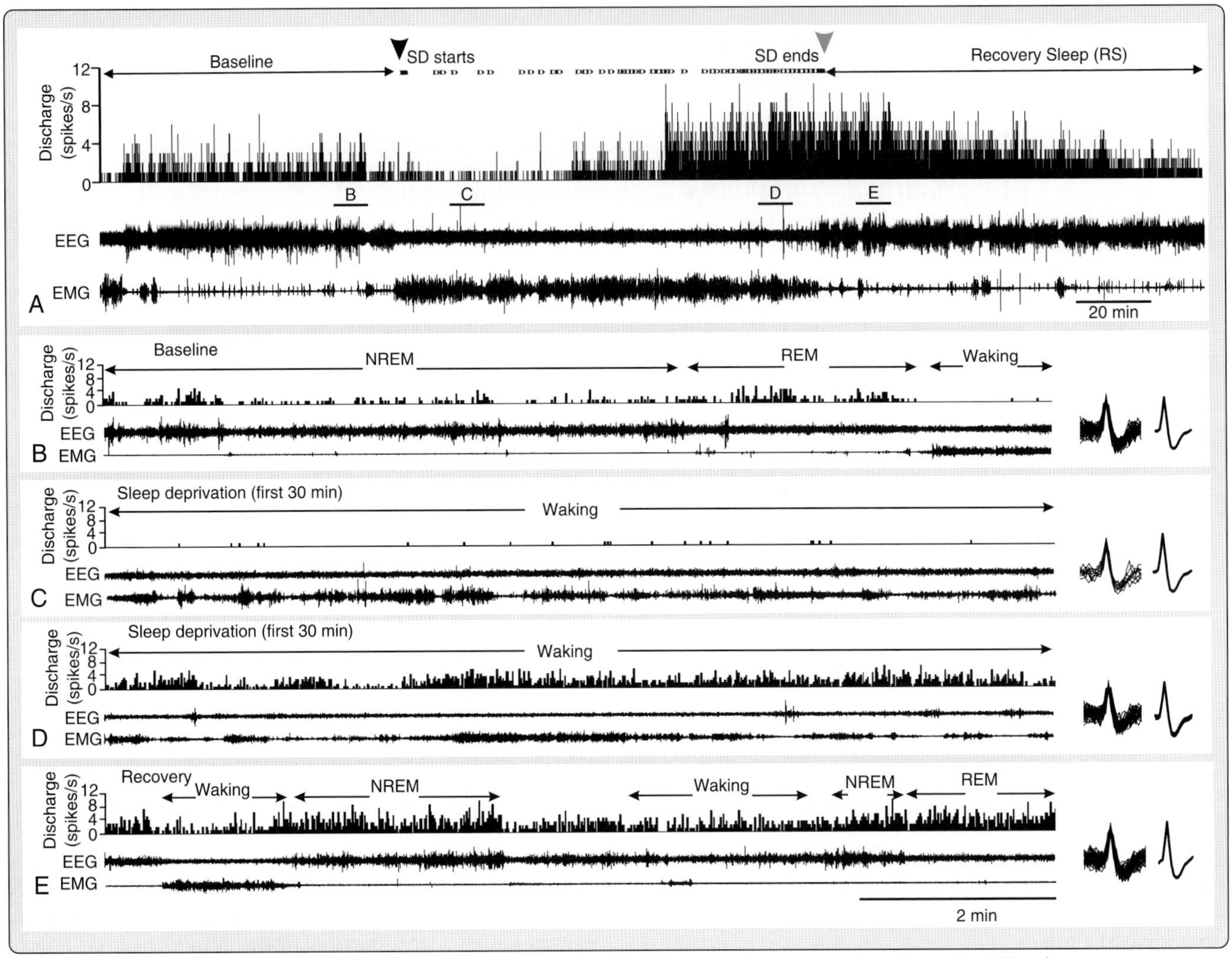

Figure 7.4 Responses of the median preoptic nucleus (MnPN) sleep-active neuron to sleep deprivation (SD) and during recovery sleep (RS). **A,** *From top to bottom:* discharge rate histogram (spikes/s), cortical electroencephalogram (EEG), and neck muscle electromyogram (EMG) recordings during baseline, SD, and RS. *Black* and *gray arrowheads* at the top indicate start and end of SD, respectively. The *dots* between the *arrows* indicate times when the animal began to fall sleep and the experimenter intervened to maintain wakefulness. **B** through **E,** Expansion of areas labeled in **A,** showing 10 minutes of recording during baseline **(B),** the first 30 minutes of SD **(C),** the last 30 minutes of SD **(D),** and early RS **(E).** The waveforms at the right of **B** to **E** are superimposed, and averaged action potentials recorded the 10 minutes shown in each figure, demonstrating stability of unit recording across all three experimental conditions. During the baseline period, the cell exhibited elevated discharge rates during NREM and REM sleep compared with waking **(B).** At the start of SD, only infrequent interventions were required to keep the animal awake (**A,** *top trace*), and discharge rate of the cell was uniformly low at less than 1 spikes/second **(C).** As homeostatic sleep pressure increased with continuing SD, as evidenced by the increasing number of interventions required to maintain wakefulness **(A),** the discharge rate of the cell increased. By the end of 2 hours of SD, the waking discharge rates were approximately double that during baseline sleep (**B** and **D**). Discharge of the cell remained elevated in comparison with baseline during early RS (**B** and **E**) but returned to baseline levels after 2 hours of unrestricted sleep **(A).** (From Alam MA, Kumar S, McGinty D, et al. Neuronal activity in the preoptic hypothalamus during sleep deprivation and recovery sleep. *J Neurophysiol* 2014;111:287–99.)

to underlie a bi-stable sleep-wake switch (Figure 7.5).[72] Activation of arousal systems inhibits sleep-active neurons, thereby removing inhibition of arousal systems and facilitating stable episodes of waking. In turn, activation of sleep-promoting neurons would inhibit arousal-related neurons, thereby disinhibiting sleep-promoting neurons and promoting consolidated sleep episodes. This model provides a mechanism for the stabilization of both sleep and waking states.

Medullary Sleep-Promoting Neurons: The Parafacial Zone

GABAergic/glycinergic medullary neurons in the region of the PZ, located lateral and dorsal to the facial nerve, have sleep regulatory functions. PZ neurons in mice express c-Fos after sleep but not after waking.[9] Neurons with sleep-related discharge are found in the PZ of rats.[73] Cell-specific lesions of the PZ in mice cause significant sleep loss as does disruption of PZ GABAergic/glycinergic neurotransmission.[9] The primary circuit through which PZ neurons promote sleep involve monosynaptic projection to the pontine parabrachial nucleus. Neurons in the parabrachial nucleus are glutamatergic and project to cortically projecting neurons in the basal forebrain.[74] At the wake-sleep transition, PZ neurons evoke GABA-mediated inhibition of parabrachial neurons, which results in disfacilitation of basal forebrain neurons that promote cortical activation.[74] The discharge patterns of PZ sleep-active neurons during wake-sleep transitions and stable sleep

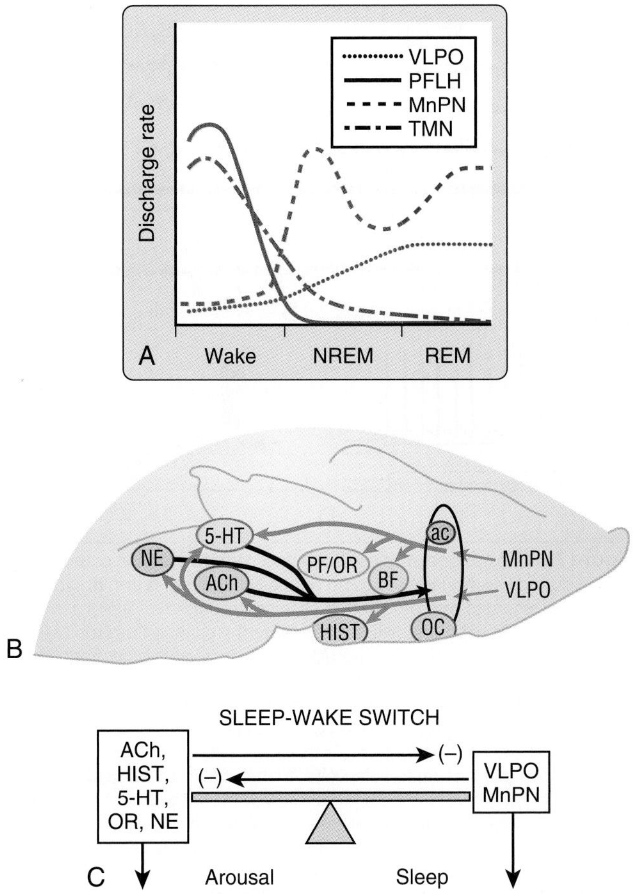

Figure 7.5 Interactions of the preoptic area (POA) sleep-promoting neuronal system with arousal systems that can account for the orchestration of the sleep process. **A,** The neuronal discharge rates across the wake-NREM-REM cycle of sleep-active neurons from the ventrolateral preoptic area (VLPO) and the median preoptic nucleus (MnPN), and from arousal-related (wake-active) neurons in the perifornical lateral hypothalamus (PFLH) and tuberomammillary nucleus (TMN). These neuronal groups generally have reciprocal discharge patterns, although MnPN and VLPO neurons exhibit peak activity at different times during NREM episodes. The wake-active, NREM-diminished, REM-off discharge pattern shown for TMN and a subgroup of PFLH neurons also is characteristic of putative serotoninergic neurons of the dorsal raphe nucleus (DR) and putative noradrenergic neurons of the locus coeruleus (see also **C**). **B,** Sagittal section of the diencephalon and upper brainstem of the rat showing anatomic interconnections of MnPN and VLPO neurons with arousal-related neuronal groups. The MnPN and VLPO distribute projections to sites of arousal-related activity including the (1) basal forebrain (BF), (2) PFLH, which includes orexin-containing neurons PF/OR, (3) histamine (HIST)-containing neurons of the TMN, (4) pontomesencephalic acetylcholine (ACh)-containing neurons, (5) pontomesencephalic serotonin (5 hydroxytryptamine [5-HT])-containing neurons, and (6) noradrenergic (norepinephrine [NE]-containing) neurons of the pons, particularly the locus coeruleus (LC). 5-HT, NE, and ACh arousal-related neurons provide inhibitory feedback to sleep-active neurons. The arousal-related neuronal groups also have widespread additional ascending and descending projections that control state-related functions throughout the brain. AC, Anterior commissure; OC, optic chiasm. **C,** Wakefulness and sleep are each facilitated by several neurotransmitters and neuromodulators. ACh-, 5-HT-, NE-, histamine (HA)-, and glutamate -expressing neurons directly activate thalamocortical and cortical neurons as well as hypothalamic and basal forebrain nuclei to promote waking. Orexin (OR) neurons facilitate arousal through direct effects and through excitation of ACh, 5-HT, NE, and HA neurons. Sleep-promoting neurons expressed in the POA are gamma-aminobutyric acid (GABA)-ergic and act by inhibiting wake-promoting neurons. Other sleep-promoting molecules, adenosine (AD), endoplasmic reticulum stress signaling molecules, growth hormone–releasing hormone, certain cytokines, and signals of oxidative stress such as oxidized glutathione (GSSG) (see text), are thought to act indirectly, by either facilitating sleep-active neurons or inhibiting wake-promoting neurons, or both in the case of AD. Subsets of wake-promoting neurons and sleep-promoting neurons are mutually inhibitory. Accordingly, if one system is more strongly activated, the opposing system is inhibited, with consequent reduced feedback inhibition of the initiating neurons, thereby facilitating sleep-wake state stability, as in an electrical "flip-flop" switch. The circadian clock in the suprachiasmatic nucleus regulates the timing of sleep by exciting arousal systems during the active phase of the day and by exciting or disinhibiting sleep-promoting neurons during the rest phase. Because of the redundancy of both wake-promoting and sleep-promoting systems, deficiency of any one system may have only small effects on the amount of sleep but may reduce the stability of sleep. ac, Anterior commissure. (Modified from McGinty D, Szymusiak R. Hypothalamic regulation of sleep and arousal. *Front Biosci* 2003;8:1074–83.)

are similar to those of VLPO and MnPN neurons,[73] suggesting that medullary and preoptic sleep-promoting systems act in a complementary manner.

Sleep Regulatory Functions of Melanin-Concentrating Hormone Neurons

Neurons expressing the inhibitory peptide melanin-concentrating hormone (MCH) are located in the PH, where they are intermingled with orexin neurons (reviewed by Bittencourt[75]). A majority of MCH neurons also express the inhibitory neurotransmitter GABA. MCH groups include a medial cluster found adjacent to the third ventricle, a perifornical cluster, a far lateral cluster located medial to the internal capsule and extending to the zona incerta, and a more posterior-medial group localized in the supramammillary region.[75] MCH neurons have anatomic interconnectivity with hypothalamic and brainstem nuclei implicated in sleep-wake regulation.[75,76]

Intracerebroventricular injection of MCH increases NREM and REM sleep, identifying a potential sleep-regulatory role for the peptide.[77] Subsequent work pointed to a role for MCH neurons in REM sleep control. Increased c-Fos immunoreactivity was observed in MCH neurons during REM-enriched sleep after 72 hours of REM sleep deprivation.[78] REM sleep–related c-Fos expression was found in MCH neurons with descending projections to critical brainstem nuclei implicated in REM sleep control.[79] Identified MCH neurons located in the lateral hypothalamus, recorded in head-restrained rats, discharge at higher rates during REM sleep relative waking and NREM sleep,[80] consistent with a hypothesized REM sleep regulatory role. Targeted optogenetic excitation of MCH neurons during NREM sleep was found to promote transitions to REM sleep,[81,82] whereas stimulation at REM sleep onset prolonged REM bout durations.[81] Release of GABA by MCH neurons in response to optogenetic stimulation may be responsible for REM sleep effects.[81] Optogenetic silencing of MCH neurons had no effect on REM sleep measures,[82] indicating that activation of MCH neurons is sufficient but not necessary to promote REM sleep from a background of NREM sleep.

Other selective genetic manipulations of MCH neuronal function point to a key role for these neurons in the control of sleep onset and NREM sleep. Continuous optogenetic excitation of MCH neurons (by light pulses delivered for 1 minute every 5 minutes at 10 Hz) at the start of the dark (active) phase in mice reduced sleep latency, decreased the duration of waking episodes by 50%, and increased NREM and REM sleep time.[83] In the human brain, MCH release, as measured in the amygdala, is maximal at sleep onset.[84] Widespread conditional ablation of the MCH neuronal population by cell-specific expression of diphtheria toxin A increased wakefulness and decreased NREM sleep without affecting REM sleep.[82] Collectively, the findings suggest a heterogeneity of MCH neuronal function, with some neurons interacting with circuits that control REM sleep and another population of MCH neurons functioning to promote NREM sleep onset and maintenance.

Cortical Sleep-Active Neurons

A population of cortical GABAergic interneurons specifically activated during sleep has been described.[85] In addition to GABA, these neurons colocalize immunoreactivity for neuronal nitric oxide synthase (nNOS) and the substance P receptor, NK1.[86,87] Expression of c-Fos immunoreactivity in these neurons is correlated with time spent in NREM sleep and with NREM EEG delta power. Fos expression during recovery sleep is proportional to the duration of previous time awake, suggesting that sleep-active cortical nNOS neurons are inhibited during waking and activated in response to homeostatic sleep pressure.[86,87] Waking inhibition may be mediated by synaptic input from basal forebrain cholinergic neurons and from monoaminergic inputs arising from the TMN, dorsal raphe nucleus, and locus coeruleus.[86] It is unclear if activation during sleep is due to disinhibition caused by sleep-related silencing of subcortical input, or if sleep-related excitation from neuronal and/or neuromodulatory sources (e.g., adenosine, cytokines) also is involved.

Although sleep-active cortical nNOS neurons are found in multiple cortical areas in rats and mice, the density of these neurons is low. These cortical neurons appear to be a subset of type II nNOS interneurons—that is, those with the largest cell bodies, which are a source of cortico-cortical and other long-range projections (as reviewed by Wisor and colleagues[87]). In keeping with this anatomic feature, sleep-active nNOS neurons are well suited to organize synchronous discharge across large ensembles of cortical neurons that are characteristic of deep NREM sleep. These neurons may be a component of local cortical circuits responsible for use-dependent augmentation of EEG slow wave activity.[87-89] The differential functional roles of GABA versus nitric oxide sulfate (NOS) signaling by cortical sleep active neurons are unknown.

THALAMIC-CORTICAL INTERACTIONS AND GENERATION OF THE SLEEP ELECTROENCEPHALOGRAM

Changes in cortical EEG patterns usually are the defining feature of NREM sleep in mammals. Briefly reviewed here are thalamocortical mechanisms underlying NREM sleep EEG patterns and how modulation of thalamocortical circuits by arousal and sleep regulatory neuronal systems has an impact on key features of the sleep EEG.

Thalamocortical circuits exhibit two fundamentally different modes of operation across the sleep-wake cycle: a state of tonic activation, or desynchrony, during waking and REM sleep and a state of rhythmic, synchronized activity that is characteristic of NREM sleep.[90] The two functional modes of thalamocortical activity are evident at the level of single neurons. During waking and REM sleep, thalamocortical neurons exhibit tonic firing of single action potentials (Figure 7.6, *A*) that are modulated by the levels of excitatory input from thalamic afferents, including specific sensory afferents.[90,91] During NREM sleep, relay neurons discharge in high-frequency bursts of action potentials, followed by long pauses (Figure 7.6, *B*).

These two modes of action potential generation reflect the expression of intrinsic properties of thalamocortical neurons, and a specialized, voltage-sensitive Ca^{2+} current plays a critical role.[92] This Ca^{2+} current, known as the low-threshold or transient Ca^{2+} current (I_t), is inactivated (nonfunctional) when

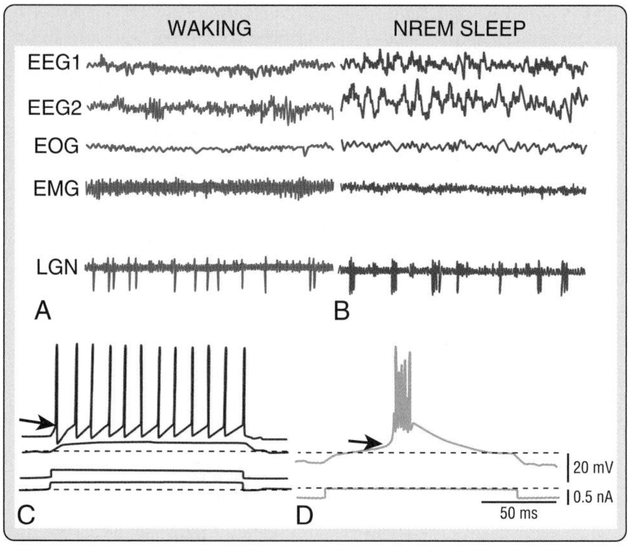

Figure 7.6 Thalamic neurons exhibit distinct patterns of action potential generation during waking/REM sleep and during NREM sleep. **A** and **B,** Typical extracellularly recorded discharge patterns of a neuron in the cat lateral geniculate nucleus during waking and NREM sleep. Note the change from tonic, single-spike firing during the awake state **(A)** to high-frequency-burst firing during NREM sleep **(B).** Tonic versus burst firing reflects intrinsic, voltage-dependent properties of thalamic neurons. These discharge patterns can be recorded in neurons from isolated slices of thalamus. **C** and **D,** In vitro intracellular recordings of a relay neuron from guinea pig thalamus. In **C,** direct current (DC) injections and recordings of intracellular voltage labeled 3 and 4 are shown. Spontaneous resting potential for the cell is indicated by the *dashed line.* A depolarizing current step delivered at resting potential (>–65 mV) evokes a tonic depolarizing response in the neuron that is subthreshold for action potential generation. When membrane potential is rendered more positive by DC injection, the same depolarizing step evokes tonic generation of fast action potentials (*arrow*) that persist for the duration of the depolarizing pulse. In **D,** the neuron has been hyperpolarized below resting potential (<–65 mV) by negative DC injection, and the low threshold Ca^{2+} current (I_t) is activated. When a depolarizing pulse is applied on the background of hyperpolarization, a slow Ca^{2+} spike is evoked (*arrow*), and it is crowned by a high-frequency burst of fast Na^+ action potentials. I_t is inactivated in response to the Ca^{2+}-mediated depolarization, and membrane potential sags toward the hyperpolarized level despite the continuance of the depolarizing current step. EOG, Electrooculogram; LGN, lateral geniculate nucleus. (**A** and **B** modified from McCarley RW, Benoit O, Barrionuevo G. Lateral geniculate nucleus unitary discharge during sleep and waking: state- and rate-specific effects. *J Neurophysiol* 1983;50:798–818. **C** and **D** modified from Jahnsen H, Llinas R. Electrophysiological properties of guinea-pig thalamic neurons: an in vitro study. *J Physiol* 1984;349:205–26.)

the membrane potential of thalamic relay neurons is relatively depolarized (less negative than −65 mV). Thus, when depolarizing input is delivered to a relay neuron that is resting at this level of membrane polarization, the cell responds with tonic single-spike firing (Figure 7.6, *C*). When relay neurons are hyperpolarized (membrane potential more negative than −65 mV), I_t becomes activated, and depolarizing input evokes a slow Ca^{2+}-mediated depolarization (100 to 200 milliseconds in duration) that is crowned by a burst of three to eight fast Na^+-mediated action potentials (Figure 7.6, *D*). There is a pause in the generation of fast action potentials after the burst, because I_t is self-inactivated by the Ca^{2+}-mediated depolarization, and membrane potential falls below the threshold for action potential generation and is restored back to the resting, hyperpolarized state (Figure 7.6, *D*). The properties of I_t equip thalamocortical neurons with the ability to generate action potentials in two different modes: (1) tonic firing when stimulated from a relatively depolarized resting state and (2) burst-pause firing from a hyperpolarized resting state.[90,91]

The major NREM sleep EEG rhythms—spindles, delta waves, and slow oscillations—all arise through a combination of intrinsic neuronal properties (e.g., I_t) and the synaptic organization of cortical and thalamic circuits.[93] A schematic of the core circuitry responsible for the generation of sleep rhythms in the EEG is shown in Figure 7.7. Thalamocortical relay neurons receive excitatory input from sensory neurons and from several of the brainstem arousal systems that function to promote depolarization and tonic firing in relay cells during waking. During waking, this excitation is faithfully conveyed by ascending thalamocortical axons to the functionally relevant area of cortex for processing and integration. Thalamic relay neurons also send a collateral projection to the adjacent portion of the thalamic reticular nucleus (RE), which is a thin band of neurons that surrounds most thalamic relay nuclei. RE neurons are GABAergic, and they send an inhibitory projection back to relay neurons. These reciprocal connections between relay and RE neurons are thought to be important for aspects of waking thalamic function.

The final critical piece of the basic circuitry for consideration is the feedback projection from layer VI pyramidal cells in the cortex to both thalamic relay neurons and RE neurons. Corticothalamic projections are topographically organized so that each cortical column has connectivity with the same relay neurons from which they derive thalamic inputs and with the corresponding sector of the RE. In this anatomic/functional scheme, a key feature is the central location of RE neurons, which receive copies of thalamocortical and corticothalamic activity and send an inhibitory projection back to the relay neurons. Although corticothalamic projections have excitatory effects on their postsynaptic targets in the thalamus, corticothalamic inputs to the RE are so powerful that the net response evoked in relay neurons by cortical stimulation often is inhibition.[93]

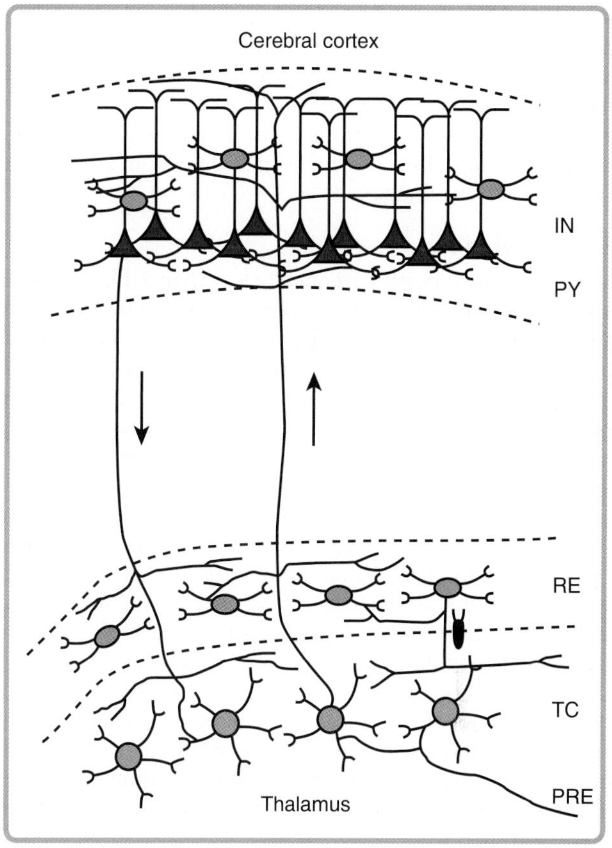

Figure 7.7 Schematic representation of thalamic and cortical cell types involved in the generation of sleep electroencephalogram rhythms and of the synaptic connectivity among the cell types. Four cell types are shown: thalamocortical relay (TC) cells, thalamic reticular nucleus (RE) neurons, cortical pyramidal (PY) cells, and cortical interneurons (IN). TC cells receive excitatory inputs from prethalamic afferent fibers (PRE) arising from specific sensory systems and from cholinergic and monoaminergic arousal systems located in the brainstem and posterior hypothalamus. Activity in sensory systems is relayed to the appropriate cortical area by ascending thalamocortical axons (*up arrow*). TC neurons also send an axon collateral that makes synaptic contact with RE neurons. RE neurons are GABAergic, and they send an inhibitory projection back to TC neurons (*down arrow*). Corticothalamic feedback is mediated by layer VI, PY neurons that project back to the same relay neurons from which they derive thalamic input, and they send an axon collateral to RE neurons. Corticothalamic projections are excitatory on both RE and TC cells, but cortical stimulation can evoke net inhibitory effects on TC neurons because of activation of GABAergic RE neurons. (From Destexhe A, Sejnowski TJ. Interactions between membrane conductances underlying thalamocortical slow-wave oscillations. *Physiol Rev* 2003;83:1401–53.)

Sleep Spindles

In humans, EEG spindles are waxing and waning, nearly sinusoidal waves with a frequency profile of 10 to 15 Hz. Spindles are generated in the thalamus, as evidenced by the fact that thalamectomy eliminates spindles in the sleep EEG.[4] At the level of the thalamus, spindles are generated by an interplay between neurons in the RE and the relay nuclei.[90,91,93] RE neurons also possess I_t calcium channels and exhibit high-frequency-burst firing from a hyperpolarized background. A high-frequency burst in RE neurons will produce strong inhibitory postsynaptic potentials (IPSPs) in relay neurons that are followed by rebound slow Ca^{2+} spikes and a high-frequency burst. This burst of firing in the relay neuron is conveyed back to the RE, evoking an excitatory postsynaptic potential that triggers a calcium spike and a burst in RE neurons. In thalamic slices in which connectivity between the RE and the adjacent relay nuclei is preserved, this disynaptic circuit can generate spontaneous spindle-like oscillations that can propagate across the slice.[91] In the intact brain, the spindle oscillation in the thalamus is conveyed to the cortex by the pattern of burst firing in thalamic relay neurons.[93,94] However, relay of specific sensory information through the thalamus to the cortex is severely compromised during spindle oscillations because of the combination of disfacilitation of relay neurons resulting from loss of excitatory input from arousal systems and the rhythmic IPSPs evoked by RE input. This sensory deafferentation of the cortex is believed to play an important role in maintaining NREM sleep continuity. Although the spindle oscillation originates in the thalamus, cortical feedback to the thalamus and cortico-cortical connections are important in synchronizing the occurrence of spindles over widespread thalamic and cortical areas.[93,94] Phasic activation of layer VI pyramidal neurons excites neurons in the RE and synchronizes IPSP–rebound burst sequences in thalamic relay neurons with cortical activity.

Delta Waves

The delta oscillation of NREM sleep appears to have both cortical and thalamic components. This dual origin is evidenced by the fact that cortical delta activity in the 1- to 4-Hz range persists after complete thalamectomy[4] and by the demonstration that isolated thalamic relay neurons can generate a spontaneous clock-like delta oscillation resulting from the interplay of I_t and a hyperpolarization-activated cation current known as the h-current.[95] In the intact, sleeping brain, both sources of delta oscillation contribute to the frequency content of the cortical EEG. As discussed previously for spindles, corticothalamic and cortico-cortical connections function to synchronize delta oscillations over widespread cortical areas.

Slow Oscillations

Slow oscillations (with a frequency less than 1 Hz) are a key aspect of the sleep EEG because they coordinate the occurrence of other synchronous EEG events (e.g., delta waves, spindles, and K-complexes). Slow oscillations are thought to be primarily of cortical origin. They are absent from the thalamus in chronic decorticate animals and are present in the cortex after thalamectomy as well as in isolated cortical slices.[93,94] It has been recently reported that cortical deafferentation causes an acute suppression of slow oscillations that recovers over time, indicating a thalamic contribution (as reviewed by David and Schmiedt[96]). Underneath the slow oscillations, fluctuations occur between two states of activity in nearly all cortical neurons.[95,97] "Up" states are characterized by depolarization and generation of trains of action potentials. Up states occur simultaneously in all cell types, including interneurons, and both fast excitatory and IPSP are characteristic of cortical neuronal activity during this state. Up states are followed by a prolonged period of hyperpolarization and quiescence, referred to as "down" states (Figure 7.8).

Generation of up states occurs through recurrent excitation in local cortical circuits and depends on excitatory transmission through α-amino-3-hydroxy-5-methyl-4-isoxazole propionic acid and NMDA receptors.[98] Transitions from up to down states involve a combination of activation of outward K^+ currents and disfacilitation resulting from depression of excitatory synapses.[98,99] Discharge of layer IV corticothalamic projection neurons during up phases can synchronize IPSPs in thalamic relay neurons through activation of RE neurons, causing the expression of EEG spindles and delta activity of thalamic origin on the background of the slow oscillation. Slow oscillations organize the synchronization and propagation of cortical delta activity through cortico-cortical connections. Frequency spectra of the human NREM sleep EEG reflect this dynamic, with prominent spectral peaks in the delta (1 to 4 Hz) and slow oscillation (less than 1 Hz) frequency ranges.[100]

Because they orchestrate the temporal and spatial coherence of rhythmic oscillations in thalamocortical circuits, slow oscillations are thought to be important in promoting the functional sensory deafferentation of the cortex during sleep, which in turn enhances sleep continuity and sleep depth. The transitions between up and down states in cortical neurons have been hypothesized to underlie changes in synaptic plasticity, or synaptic strength, during sleep and to contribute to sleep-dependent changes in learning and memory.[101]

Spindle and delta oscillations are blocked by stimulation of the rostral brainstem, which activates cholinergic, monoaminergic, orexinergic, and glutamatergic inputs to the thalamus. Activity of cholinergic and monoaminergic neurons facilitates thalamic *depolarization* through inhibition of potassium channels.[102] Accordingly, *inhibition* of these arousal systems facilitates hyperpolarization of thalamic neurons, permitting the activation of voltage-dependent membrane currents underlying spindles and slow waves.

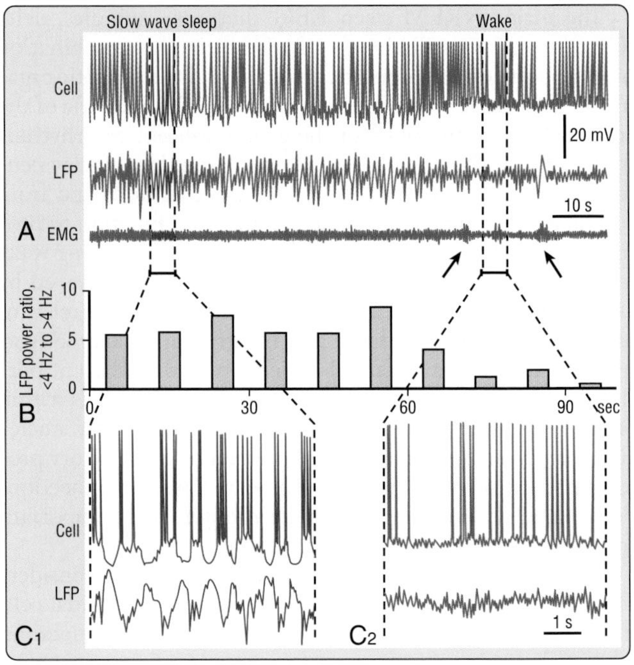

Figure 7.8 Slow oscillations in local cortical field potentials (LFPs) and in the membrane potential of a cortical neuron during NREM sleep. **A,** Simultaneous intracellular, LFP, and electromyogram (EMG) recording during sleep and wakefulness. The animal is in NREM sleep at the beginning of the recording, with a transition to waking after approximately 70 seconds (*arrows* indicate EMG activation). Action potentials are truncated in the intracellular recording. **B,** Levels of delta power in the LFP are higher during NREM sleep than during waking. Plotted are 10-second bins of the ratio of spectral power (<4 Hz/>4 Hz) recorded in the LFP. **C,** Intracellular activity and LFP recording from **A** shown at expanded time scale. Note clear fluctuations of the membrane potential between depolarized (up) and hyperpolarized (down) states during slow wave (NREM) sleep (**C_1**) in association with the slow oscillation (<1 Hz) in the LFP. During wakefulness (**C_2**), cell is tonically depolarized, and no sustained episodes of hyperpolarization are present. (From Mukovski M, Chauvette S, Timofeev I, Volgushev M. Detection of active and silent states in neocortical neurons from the field potential signal during slow-wave sleep. *Cereb Cortex* 2007;17:400–14.)

INTEGRATION OF CIRCADIAN RHYTHMS AND SLEEP

The suprachiasmatic nucleus (SCN) of the POA generates the signals that bring about the circadian patterns of sleep-waking.[103] Direct projections from the SCN to areas of the POA implicated in sleep regulation are sparse, but multisynaptic pathways by which SCN signals can control sleep-active neurons have been described. Introduction of lesions of a primary SCN projection target, the subparaventricular zone (SPVZ), like those of the SCN itself, eliminates circadian rhythms of sleep-waking.[104] The SPVZ projects directly to the MnPN and indirectly to the VLPO, MnPN, and other POA regions through the dorsomedial hypothalamic nucleus.[105,106] Lesions of the dorsomedial hypothalamic nucleus disrupt the circadian distribution of sleep-waking states in rats. In diurnal animals, activity of SCN neurons could inhibit sleep-promoting neurons during the light phase and facilitate sleep-promoting neurons in the dark phase, with the reciprocal pattern occurring in nocturnal animals.

SLEEP-PROMOTING NEUROCHEMICAL AGENTS

Conceptions of sleep control based on neuronal circuitry, as outlined earlier, are deficient in that they do not provide explanations for quantitative features of sleep or sleep homeostasis. The control of neuronal activity by neurochemical mechanisms, including the release of GABA, occurs in a time frame of seconds. Sleep regulation and homeostasis operate within a time frame of hours to days, not seconds. In addition, a complete description should account for biologic variations in sleep such as the high daily sleep quotas in some species,[107] higher sleep quotas in infants, sleep facilitation after body heating, and increased sleep propensity during acute infection. The investigation of biochemical mechanisms with sustained actions is needed to address these issues. Presented next is a brief overview of this approach, focusing on neurochemical agents with sleep-promoting properties. (Details of the biochemical mechanisms of sleep-wake regulation are available in a review by Obal and Krueger.[108])

Adenosine

Adenosine is recognized as an inhibitory neuromodulator in the central nervous system, whose role in sleep is suggested by the potent arousal-producing effects of caffeine, an antagonist of adenosine A_1 and A_{2A} receptors. Adenosine and its analogues were found to promote sleep after systemic administration by intraperitoneal injection, intracerebroventricular administration, and intra-POA microinjection and after administration by microdialysis in the basal forebrain (reviewed by McCarley[109]). In the basal forebrain and, to a lesser extent, in the neocortex, adenosine recovered through microdialysis increases during sustained waking in cats. No increase is found in thalamus or brainstem sites. Application in the basal forebrain of an antisense oligonucleotide to the adenosine A_1 receptor messenger RNA (mRNA), which blocks synthesis of receptor protein, slightly reduced spontaneous sleep but strongly reduced rebound after sleep deprivation.[110] Adenosine A_1 agonists delivered using microdialysis adjacent to basal forebrain neurons inhibited wake-active neurons during both waking and sleep.[111] One hypothesis is that the effects of adenosine on sleep-waking are mediated by basal forebrain cholinergic neurons through A_1 receptors.[109] Adenosine could act at multiple sites. Adenosine A_{2A} receptors also are present in restricted brain regions and seem to mediate some sleep-promoting effects of adenosine. Administration of A_{2A} agonist by either intracerebroventricular infusion or infusion into the subarachnoid space ventral to the POA increases sleep amounts and increases c-Fos expression in GABAergic neurons in the MnPN and VLPO.[112] Knockdown of A_{2A} receptors in the shell of the nucleus accumbens significantly attenuates the alerting effects of caffeine.[113]

Brain adenosine levels rise when adenosine triphosphate (ATP) production is reduced; under these conditions, inhibition of neuronal activity is neuroprotective. Astrocytes as well as neurons are potential sources of adenosine. Genetically inhibiting the release of gliotransmitters, including ATP, by astrocytes diminishes homeostatic responses to sleep deprivation.[114] It has been proposed that increased adenosine is a signal of reduced brain energy reserves that develop during waking and that sleep is induced as an energy-restorative state.[115] With respect to the brain energy restorative concept, some but not all studies show reduced cerebral glycogen, an energy-supply substrate, after sleep deprivation.[116] Functional evidence that brain energy supply is compromised after sleep deprivation is lacking. This absence of evidence is a critical gap in the theory. Of course, adenosine could be a sleep-promoting signal based on functions other than energy supply limitation.

Proinflammatory Cytokines

Several proinflammatory cytokines have sleep-promoting properties. Summarized next is work on a well-studied and prototypical molecule, interleukin (IL)-1. When administered intravenously, intraperitoneally, or into the lateral ventricles, IL-1 increases sleep, particularly NREM sleep (as reviewed by Krueger and colleagues[117]). Basic findings have been confirmed in several species. REM sleep usually is inhibited by IL-1. Additional evidence supports a hypothesis that IL-1 modulates spontaneous sleep. Administration of agents that block IL-1 reduces sleep. In rats, IL-1 mRNA is increased in the brain during the light phase, when rat sleep is maximal. Sleep deprivation also increases IL-1 mRNA in the brain.

Increased sleep associated with peripheral infection also may be mediated by responses to circulating IL-1, either through vagal afferents or by induction of central IL-1 or other hypnogenic signals. POA sleep-active neurons are activated by local application of IL-1, and wake-active neurons are inhibited.[118] IL-1 fulfills several criteria for a sleep-promoting signal, and it is likely to be important in facilitating sleep during infection.

Prostaglandin D_2

Administration of prostaglandin D_2 (PGD_2) by intracerebroventricular infusion or by microinjection into the POA increases sleep, but the most potent site for administration is the subarachnoid space ventral to the POA and basal forebrain (reviewed by Huang and colleagues[119]). Sleep induced by PGD_2 administration is indistinguishable from normal sleep based on EEG analysis. The enzyme required for PGD_2 synthesis, lipocalin-PGD synthase (L-PGDS), is enriched in the arachnoid membrane and choroid plexus, but the receptor (the D-type prostanoid receptor) is localized in the leptomeninges under the basal forebrain and the TMN. L-PGDS–knockout mice experienced normal baseline sleep, but unlike the control animals, they exhibited no rebound increase in NREM sleep after sleep deprivation. The PGD_2 concentration was higher in the cerebrospinal fluid during NREM sleep than in wakefulness and was higher in the light phase in the rat (when sleep amounts are high). Sleep deprivation increased the PGD_2 concentration in the cerebrospinal fluid. On this basis, it was proposed that PGD_2 plays a central role in sleep homeostasis. The hypnogenic action of PGD_2 is hypothesized to be mediated by adenosine release acting on an adenosine A_{2A} receptor. Administration of A_{2A} antagonists blocked the effects of PGD_2. A functional basis for the role of PGD_2 in sleep homeostasis or its primary localization in the meninges has not been identified.

Growth Hormone–Releasing Hormone

Growth hormone–releasing hormone (GHRH) is known primarily for its role in stimulating the release of growth hormone (GH). A surge in GH release occurs early in the major circadian sleep period in humans, specifically during the earliest N3 or N4 NREM sleep episodes. GHRH is a peptide with a restricted localization in neurons in the hypothalamic arcuate nucleus and in the adjacent ventromedial and periventricular nuclei. Neurons in the latter locations are thought to be the source of projections to the POA and basal forebrain. GHRH promotes NREM sleep after intraventricular, intravenous, intranasal, or intraperitoneal administration or after direct microinjection into the POA (as reviewed by Obal and Krueger[120]). Blockade of GHRH by administration of a competitive antagonist reduces baseline sleep and rebound sleep after short-term sleep deprivation. Mutant mice with GHRH signaling abnormalities have lower amounts of NREM sleep. GHRH stimulates cultured GABAergic hypothalamic neurons; these may constitute the GHRH target in the sleep-promoting circuit.[121] Intracerebroventricular infusion of GHRH activates c-Fos expression in GABAergic neurons in the MnPN and VLPO, whereas intracerebroventricular infusion of a competitive GHRH antagonist suppresses c-Fos in these neurons.[122] It has been suggested that GHRH may elicit sleep onset in conjunction with release of GH as a coordinated process for augmenting protein synthesis and protecting proteins from degradation during the fasting associated with sleep. In the brain, protein synthesis increases during sleep, and inhibition of protein synthesis augments sleep.[123] GHRH is proposed to be one element of a multiple-element sleep-promoting system.[108]

Endoplasmic Reticular Stress

Brain protein synthesis is increased during sleep. The endoplasmic reticulum (ER) is a large cellular organelle that houses the machinery that synthesizes and folds new proteins on instructions from mRNA, including proteins needed for neuronal growth, repair, and plasticity. The capacity of the ER, particularly with respect to the process of new protein folding, is limited, and overloading can contribute to cell death. The ER generates a set of signals to prevent overloading, called the unfolding protein response (UPR), which temporarily inhibits new protein synthesis. UPR signals are induced by sleep deprivation.[124] Studies in both *Drosophila*[125] and rats[126] suggest that UPR signals also can facilitate sleep. Neuronal damage from long-term sleep deprivation has been linked to the failure of protection by the UPR.[127]

Sleep as Detoxification or Protection from Oxidative Stress

Reactive oxygen species (ROS) include superoxide anion (O_2^-), hydrogen peroxide (H_2O_2), hydroxyl radical (OH^-), nitric oxide (NO), and peroxynitrite ($OONO^-$). These molecules are generated during oxidation reactions or reactions between O_2^- and H_2O_2 or NO. ROS normally are reduced by constitutive antioxidants such as oxidized glutathione (GSSR), endogenous glutathione (GSH), and different forms of superoxide dismutase (SOD). Oxidative damage ensues when antioxidant mechanisms fail to adequately scavenge ROS, resulting in generation of oxidized lipids identified by malondialdehyde (MDA), oxidized proteins (carbonyl proteins), and oxidized nucleic acids identified by 8-hydroxy-deoxy-guanosine.

GSSR was identified as one of four sleep-promoting substances in brain tissue extracted from sleep-deprived rats.[128] Infusion of GSSR into the lateral ventricle of rats during the dark phase increases both NREM and REM sleep (as reviewed by Ikeda and colleagues). GSH levels were lower in the hypothalamus of rats after 96 hours of sleep deprivation in studies using the platform-over-water method. Lobo[129] sleep deprivation for 5 to 11 days using the disk-over-water method reduces cytosolic SOD as well as glutathione peroxidase in the hippocampus and brainstem.[130] Also in rats, 4 days of sleep deprivation using the platform-over-water method reduced GSH and increased MDA in the hippocampus,[131] and 72 hours of sleep deprivation using the same method reduced GSH in whole-hippocampus and neocortex samples.[132] In mice, 48 or 72 hours of sleep deprivation using the platform-over-water method increased MDA levels in whole-hippocampus samples.[133] These studies suggest that by reducing antioxidant availability, sleep deprivation can increase the risk of oxidative damage and that sleep is protective against actions of ROS. The possibility that sleep deprivation could cause neuronal damage was suggested by a finding that supraoptic nucleus neurons exhibited signs of subcellular damage after exposure to sleep deprivation.[134] Supraoptic nucleus neurons may be sensitive to sleep deprivation because of their high rate of protein synthesis.[134] In mice, after only 8 hours of sleep deprivation, locus coeruleus neurons were found to lose antioxidant expression and expression of a key regulator of responses to metabolic stress, Sirt3.[135] Locus coeruleus neurons were reduced in number by 30%.

What are the signaling molecules related to oxidative stress that increase as a function of sustained wakefulness and can promote sleep? In addition to GSH, as summarized previously, a probable signal is NO, which can be a response to glutamatergic stimulation, to cytokines and inflammation, and to oxidative stress.[136] Activity of an NO-synthetic enzyme, cytosolic NOS, was increased during the dark phase in rats, most strongly in the hypothalamus (as reviewed by Gautier-Sauvigne and colleagues[137]), and NO metabolites are increased during waking and decreased during sleep.[138] Intracerebroventricular or intravenous administration of an NOS inhibitor strongly reduced sleep in rabbits and rats and suppressed NREM sleep response to sleep deprivation. Administration of NO donors increased sleep. NO inhibits oxidative phosphorylation and may stimulate the production of adenosine. NO production could therefore be a mediator of several sleep factors.

ROS may play a role in the underlying pathology of obstructive sleep apnea. Affected patients exhibit signs of increased oxidative stress, including increased O_2^- production by neutrophils, monocytes, and granulocytes derived from patients. OSA patients exhibit elevated levels of vascular endothelial growth factor that normally is induced by ROS. These changes were reversed by treatment with continuous positive airway pressure. On the basis of these and several additional findings, it has been proposed that the increased cardiovascular disease in patients with obstructive sleep apnea results from oxidative damage to vascular walls. Oxidative stress is hypothesized to play a central role in other forms of vascular disease and in neurodegenerative disease. It is important to recognize that adenosine, ROS, glutamate, and NO have brief lives in the synaptic space—no more than a few seconds. If these molecules regulate sleep, they must have sustained release, or they may regulate the gene expression to generate sustained downstream effects. These mechanisms are the subject of current investigations.

Sleep-promoting molecules are clearly related to the multiple functions of sleep: adenosine to resupply brain energy reserves, cytokines to facilitate immune functions, GHRH to promote anabolic processes, UPR signals to prevent protein misfolding, and GSSR and NO to prevent oxidative stress–induced cell damage.

CLINICAL PEARLS

- Sleep is reduced in the presence of a wide variety of localized brain lesions; this correlation may account for the association of insomnia with various neuropathologic conditions.
- Degeneration of the hypothalamic wake-promoting cell type that expresses the neuropeptide orexin is known to underlie narcolepsy.
- Identification of certain sleep-promoting molecules strongly suggests that sleep serves to restore brain energy reserves, facilitate immune functions, promote macromolecule synthesis, prevent protein misfolding, and curtail oxidative stress–induced cell damage.

SUMMARY

Progress has been achieved in the elucidation of the neural circuitry underlying the facilitation of sleep and the orchestration of NREM sleep, as well as the facilitation of arousal. Wake and arousal are facilitated by several chemically distinct neuronal groups, including groups synthesizing and releasing acetylcholine, serotonin, norepinephrine, dopamine, histamine, orexin/hypocretin, and glutamate. These neuronal groups distribute axons and axon terminals throughout the brain, providing a basis for concurrent changes in physiology associated with arousal. At the center of the sleep-promoting circuitry is the POA of the hypothalamus. The POA sleep-promoting circuitry has reciprocal inhibitory connections with several arousal-promoting systems. A balance between the activities of sleep-promoting and arousal-promoting neuronal systems determines sleep-waking state. The circadian clock in the SCN has both direct and multisynaptic connections with wake and sleep regulatory neurons, providing a neurologic basis for generation of the daily rhythm of sleep-waking. Both sleep-promoting and arousal-promoting neuronal groups are modulated by a host of processes, including sensory, autonomic, endocrine, metabolic, and behavioral influences, accounting for the sensitivity of sleep to a wide range of centrally acting drugs and behavioral manipulations.

The long-term regulation of sleep—sleep homeostasis—is the subject of competing and still incomplete hypotheses. Long-term sleep homeostasis may reflect the actions of several neurochemical processes that express "sleep factors." Some of these sleep factors, including adenosine, PGD_2, IL-1β, and GHRH, are known to act directly on the POA or adjacent basal forebrain neuronal targets. Sleep factors have been linked to distinct functional models of sleep homeostasis, including brain energy supply (adenosine); control of protein synthesis (GHRH and UPR signaling); local sleep, immune protection, and temperature elevation (IL-1); and protection against oxidative or glutamatergic stress (NO, antioxidant enzymes). All of these factors may be involved in sleep homeostasis, but the relative importance of each factor for daily sleep has yet to be established.

ACKNOWLEDGMENT

Work on which this chapter is based was supported by the Medical Research Service of the Department of Veterans Affairs.

SELECTED READINGS

Destexhe A, Sejnowski TJ. Interactions between membrane conductances underlying thalamocortical slow-wave oscillations. *Physiol Rev.* 2003;83:1401–1453.

Donlea JM, Alam MN, Szymusiak R. Neuronal substrates of sleep homeostasis: lessons from flies, rats and mice. *Curr Opinion Neurobiol.* 2017;44:228–235.

Eban-Rothschild A, Applebaum L, de Lecea L. Neuronal mechanisms of sleep/wake regulation. *Neuropharmacol.* 2018;43:937–952.

Haas HL, Sergeeva O, Selbach O. Histamine in the nervous system. *Physiol Rev.* 2008;88:1183–1241.

Huang Z-L, Urade Y, Hayaishi O. Prostaglandins and adenosine in the regulation of sleep and wakefulness. *Curr Opin Pharmacol.* 2007;7:33–38.

Kilduff T, Cauli B, Gerashchenko D. Activation of cortical interneurons during sleep: an anatomical link to homeostatic sleep regulation? *Trends Neurosci.* 2011;34:10–19.

McGinty D, Szymusiak R. Hypothalamic regulation of sleep and arousal. *Front Biosci.* 2003;8:1074–1083.

Mondino A, Hambrecht-Wiedbusch VS, Li D, et al. Glutamatergic neurons in the preoptic hypothalamus promote wakefulness, destabilize NREM sleep, suppress REM sleep, and regulate cortical dynamics. *J Neurosci.* 2021;41(15):3462–3478.

Obal Jr F, Krueger JM. Biochemical regulation of non-rapid-eye-movement sleep. *Front Biosci.* 2003;8:520–550.

Obal Jr F, Krueger JM. GHRH and sleep. *Sleep Med Rev.* 2004;8:367–377.

Scammell TE, Arrigoni E, Lipton JO. Neural circuitry of wakefulness and sleep. *Neuron.* 2017;93:747–765.

Scammell TE, Judeson AC, Franks NP, et al. Histamine: neural circuits and new medications. *Sleep.* 2019;42(1):zsy183. https://doi.org/10.1093/sleep/zsy183.

A complete reference list can be found online at ExpertConsult.com.

Chapter 8

Rapid Eye Movement Sleep Control and Function

Jerome M. Siegel

Chapter Highlights

- Rapid eye movement (REM) sleep was first identified by its most obvious behavior: rapid eye movements during sleep. In most adult mammals the electroencephalogram (EEG) of the neocortex is low in voltage during REM sleep, as it is in waking. In contrast, the echidna and platypus, monotreme mammals, have high-voltage EEG during REM sleep. This is also the case in most very young mammals—including human babies. The hippocampus has regular high-voltage theta waves throughout REM sleep in adult placental mammals.
- The key brain structure for generating REM sleep is the brainstem, particularly the pons and adjacent portions of the caudal midbrain. The isolated brainstem can generate REM sleep, including rapid eye movements, spike potentials linked to eye movements, called ponto-geniculo-occipital (PGO) waves (most easily observed in cats), autonomic variability and muscle tone suppression (atonia). The structures rostral to the caudal midbrain-pontine brainstem, including the hypothalamus, cannot generate the forebrain aspects of REM sleep, such as PGO waves or rapid eye movements, and are not necessary for brainstem REM sleep phenomena. The brainstem and the hypothalamus contain cells that are maximally active in REM sleep, called REM-on cells, and cells that are minimally active in REM sleep, called REM-off cells. Subgroups of REM-on cells use the transmitter gamma-aminobutyric acid (GABA), acetylcholine, glutamate, or glycine. Subgroups of REM-off cells use the transmitters norepinephrine, epinephrine, serotonin, histamine, and GABA.
- Destruction of large regions within the midbrain and pons can prevent the occurrence of REM sleep. More limited damage to portions of the brainstem can cause abnormalities in certain aspects of REM sleep. Of particular interest are manipulations that affect the regulation of muscle tone within REM sleep. Early animal work found that lesions of several regions in the pons and medulla can cause REM sleep to occur without the normal loss of muscle tone. In REM sleep without atonia, animals exhibit locomotor activity, appear to attack imaginary objects, and execute other motor programs during a state that otherwise resembles REM sleep. Subsequent work found a similar syndrome in humans, which has been termed the REM sleep behavior disorder. Stimulation of portions of the REM sleep–controlling area of the pons can produce a loss of muscle tone in antigravity and respiratory musculature during waking, without eliciting all aspects of REM sleep.
- Narcolepsy is characterized by abnormalities in the regulation of REM sleep. Most cases of human narcolepsy are caused by a loss of hypocretin, or orexin, neurons. Hypocretin neurons, which are located in the hypothalamus, contribute to the regulation of the activity of norepinephrine, serotonin, histamine, acetylcholine, glutamate, and GABA cell groups. Hypocretin neurons have potent effects on alertness and motor control and are normally activated in relation to particular, generally positive emotions in humans as well as in animals.

INTRODUCTION

Rapid eye movement (REM) sleep was discovered by Aserinsky and Kleitman in 1953.[1] They reported that REM sleep was characterized by the periodic recurrence of rapid eye movements, linked to a dramatic reduction in the amplitude of the electroencephalogram (EEG) from the higher-voltage activity of the prior non–rapid eye movement (NREM) sleep period. They found that the EEG of REM sleep closely resembled the EEG of alert waking and that subjects who were awakened from REM sleep reported vivid dreams. Dement identified a similar state of low voltage EEG with eye movements in cats.[2] Jouvet repeated this observation, finding, in addition, a loss of muscle tone ("atonia") in REM

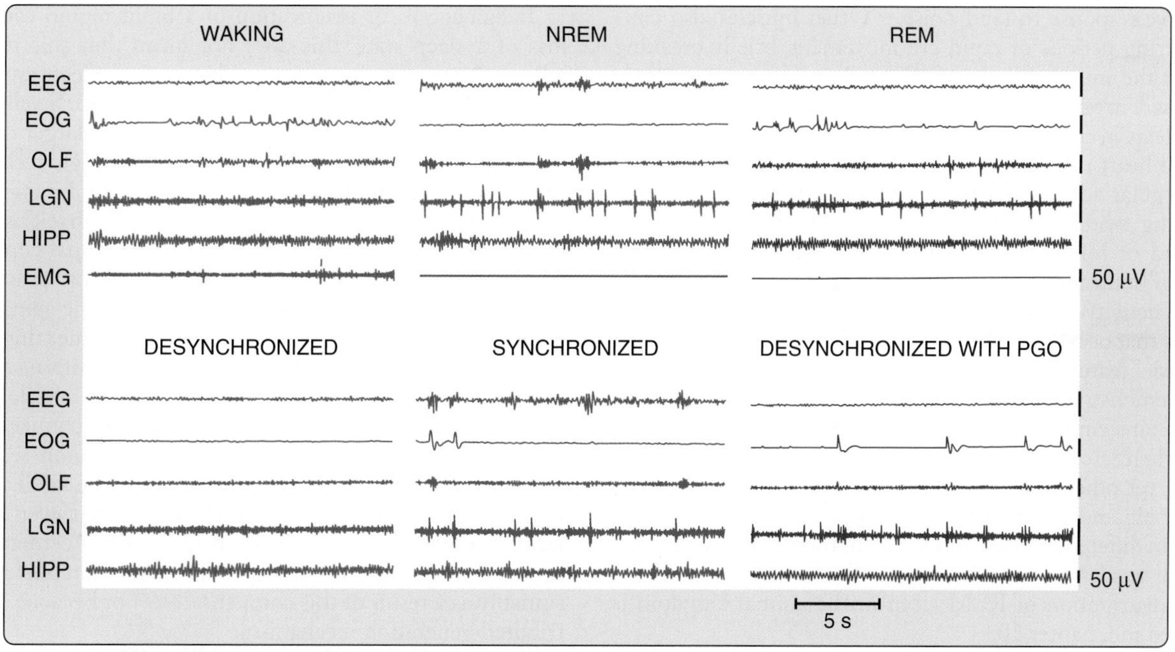

Figure 8.1 *Top*, Polygraph tracings of states seen in the intact cat. *Bottom*, Examples of states seen in the forebrain 4 days after transection at the pontomedullary junction. The medulla is not necessary for REM sleep nor for NREM sleep occurrence in cortical or pontine and midbrain regions. EEG, Sensorimotor electroencephalogram; EMG, dorsal neck electromyogram; EOG, electrooculogram; HIPP, hippocampus; LGN, lateral geniculate nucleus; OLF, olfactory bulb; PGO, ponto-geniculo-occipital.

sleep. He used the name "paradoxical sleep" to refer to this state. The "paradox" was that the EEG resembled that of waking, while behaviorally the animal remained asleep and unresponsive.[3-5] Subsequent authors have described this state as "activated" sleep, or "dream" sleep. More recent work in humans has shown that mental activity can be present in NREM sleep but has supported the original finding linking our most vivid dreams to the REM sleep state. Lesions of parietal cortex and certain other regions prevent dreaming in humans, even in individuals continuing to show normal REM sleep as judged by cortical EEG, suppression of muscle tone, and rapid eye movements.[6] Children younger than age 6, who have larger amounts of REM sleep than adults, do not typically report dream mentation, perhaps because these cortical regions have not yet developed.[7] The physiologic signs of REM sleep in both the platypus, the animal showing the most REM sleep,[8] and the related monotreme, the short-nosed echidna,[9] are largely restricted to the brainstem, in contrast to their propagation to the forebrain, producing low-voltage–activated forebrain EEG in adult placental and marsupial mammals. These findings make it questionable whether all or any nonhuman mammals that have REM sleep, all of which have cortical regions whose structure differs from that of adult humans, have dream mentation.[10]

This chapter reviews (1) the defining characteristics of REM sleep, including its physiology and neurochemistry; (2) the techniques used to investigate the mechanisms generating REM sleep; (3) the mechanisms responsible for the suppression of muscle tone during REM sleep and the pathologic effects of the disruption of these mechanisms; (4) narcolepsy and its link to mechanisms involved in REM sleep control and especially to the peptide hypocretin; and (5) the functions of REM sleep.

THE CHARACTERISTICS OF RAPID EYE MOVEMENT SLEEP

The principal electrical signs of REM sleep include a reduction in forebrain EEG amplitude, particularly in the power of its lower-frequency components (Figure 8.1, *top*). REM sleep is also characterized by a suppression of muscle tone (called atonia), visible in the electromyogram (EMG). Erections tend to occur in males.[11] Thermoregulation (e.g., sweating and shivering) largely ceases in most animals, and body temperatures drift toward environmental temperatures, as in reptiles.[12] Pupils constrict, reflecting a parasympathetic dominance in the control of the iris.[13] These changes that are present throughout the REM sleep period have been termed "tonic" features.

Also visible are electrical potentials that can be most easily recorded in the lateral geniculate nucleus of the cat.[14] These potentials originate in the pons, appear after a few milliseconds in the lateral geniculate nucleus, and can be observed with further delay in the occipital cortex, leading to the name ponto-geniculo-occipital (PGO) spikes. They occur as large-amplitude, isolated potentials 30 or more seconds before the onset of REM sleep as defined by EEG and EMG criteria. After REM sleep begins, these potentials arrive in bursts of 3 to 10 waves, usually correlated with rapid eye movements. PGO-linked potentials can also be recorded in the motor nuclei of the extraocular muscles, where they trigger the rapid eye movements of REM sleep. They are also present in thalamic nuclei other than the geniculate and in neocortical regions other than the occipital cortex.[15] PGO-like activity can also be recorded in other species.[16-21]

In humans, rapid eye movements are loosely correlated with contractions of the middle ear muscles of the sort that accompany speech generation and that are part of the protective response to loud noise.[22] Other muscles also contract during periods of rapid eye movement, briefly breaking through the muscle atonia of REM sleep. There are periods of marked irregularity in respiratory and heart rates during REM sleep, in contrast to NREM sleep, during which respiration and heart rate are regular. No single pacemaker for all of this irregular activity has been identified. Rather, the signals producing twitches of the peripheral or middle ear muscles may lead or follow PGO spikes and rapid eye movements. Bursts of brainstem neuronal activity may likewise lead or follow the activity of any particular recorded muscle.[23-26] These changes that occur episodically in REM sleep have been called its "phasic" features.

As demonstrated later in this chapter, certain manipulations of the brainstem can eliminate only the phasic events of REM sleep, whereas others can cause the phasic events to occur in waking; yet other manipulations can affect tonic components. These tonic and phasic features are also expressed to varying extents in different species, and not all of these features are present in all species that have been judged to have REM sleep.[27]

The distribution of REM sleep in the animal kingdom is discussed in Chapter 10.

RAPID EYE MOVEMENT GENERATION MECHANISMS

Technical Considerations

The identification of sleep-generating mechanisms can be achieved by **inactivation** or destruction of particular brain regions or neurons, by the **activation** of populations of neurons, or by **observation of** the activity of neurons or measurement of the release of neurotransmitters. Each approach has its advantages and limitations.

Inactivation of Neurons by Lesions, Inhibition, Antisense Administration, or Genetic Manipulation, Including Optogenetic Inhibition

More has been learned about brain function and about sleep control from brain damage caused by stroke, injury, or infection in patients and by experimentally induced brain lesions in animals than by any other technique. However, some basic principles must be borne in mind when interpreting such data.

Brain lesions can result from ischemia, pressure, trauma, and degenerative or metabolic changes. In animals, experimental lesions are most commonly induced by aspiration, transection of the neuraxis, electrolysis, local heating by radio frequency currents, or by the injection of cytotoxins. The latter include substances such as *N*-methyl-D-aspartate (NMDA) and kainite, which cause cell death by excitotoxicity, and targeted cytotoxins such as saporin coupled to a particular ligand, which will kill only cells containing receptors for that ligand. Cytotoxic techniques have the considerable advantage of sparing axons passing through the region of damage, so deficits will be attributable to the loss of local neurons rather than interruption of these axons. Injection of inhibitory neurotransmitters, such as muscimol allow reversible inactivation of neurons in the injection region. Designer receptors exclusively activated by designer drugs can also be used to inactivate or activate groups of neurons. Viral vectors or transgenic mouse models can be used to express the receptors in the desired populations, which can then be manipulated by the locally or systemically applied designer drug.

If damage to or inactivation of a brain region causes the loss of a sleep state, this does not mean that this region is where a "center" for the state resides. Lesion effects are usually maximal immediately after the lesion is created. Swelling and circulatory disruption make the functional loss larger than will be apparent from standard postmortem histologic techniques. The loss of one brain region can also disrupt functions that are organized elsewhere. For example, "spinal shock" is a well-known phenomenon in which severing the spinal cord's connection to more rostral brain regions causes a loss of functions known to be mediated by circuits intrinsic to the spinal cord.

On the other hand, with the passage of time, this sort of denervation-induced shock dissipates. In addition, adaptive changes occur that allow other regions to take over lost functions. This is mediated by sprouting of new connections to compensate for the loss. A striking phenomenon seen after placement of lesions aimed at identifying the brain regions responsible for REM and NREM sleep is that even massive lesions targeted at putative sleep-generating "centers" often produce only a transient disruption or reduction of sleep, presumably as a result of this compensation[28] or because of a distributed generation mechanism.

A particularly useful approach to the understanding of REM sleep generation has been the transection technique. In this approach, the brain is cut at the spinomedullary junction, at various brainstem levels, or at forebrain levels by passing a knife across the coronal plane of the neuraxis. Regions rostral to the cut may be left in situ or may be removed. It may seem that such a manipulation would completely prevent sleep phenomena from appearing on either side of this cut. However, to a surprising extent this is not the case. As we will review later in this chapter, REM sleep reappears within hours after some of these lesions. When both parts of the brain remain, signs of REM sleep usually appear on only one side of the cut. This kind of positive evidence is much more easily interpreted than loss of function after small lesions, because one can with certainty state that the removed regions are not essential for the signs of REM sleep that persist.

It is increasingly possible to acquire mutant mice in which any one, or several, of more than 20,000 genes are inactivated. Investigation of three mutants[29-32] led to major insights into the etiology of human narcolepsy.[33-35] Techniques for the postnatal inactivation of genes permit investigation of gene deletions without the developmental effect of these deletions. They can also be used for investigation of the effects of gene inactivation within particular brain regions. A similar inactivation can be achieved by localized microinjections of antisense. Many if not most such mutants can be expected to have some sleep phenotype, such as increases or decreases in total sleep or REM sleep time, altered sleep rebound, altered responses of sleep to environmental variables, and altered changes in sleep with to development and aging. The same interpretive constraints long appreciated in lesion studies apply to the interpretation of manipulations that inactivate genes or prevent gene expression, with the additional possibility of direct effects of genetic manipulation on tissues outside the brain.

Activation of Neurons by Electrical or Chemical Stimulation, Gene Activation, Insertion of mRNAs, or Optogenetic Stimulation

Sites identified by lesion or anatomic studies can be stimulated to identify their roles in sleep control. Older studies used electrical stimulation and were successful in identifying the medial medulla as a region mediating the suppression of muscle tone[36-38] and basal forebrain as a site capable of triggering sleep.[39] Electrical stimulation is an obviously a physiologic technique, involving the forced depolarization of neuronal membranes by ion flow at a frequency set by the stimulation device, rather than by the patterned afferent impulses that normally control neuronal discharge. For this reason, it has been supplanted for many purposes by administration of neurotransmitter agonists, either by direct microinjection or by diffusion from a microdialysis membrane that is placed in the target area and perfused with high concentrations of agonists, and most recently by optogenetic activation.

Responses produced by such agonist administration do not necessarily demonstrate a normal role for the applied ligand. For example, many transmitter agonists and antagonists have been administered to the pontine regions thought to trigger REM sleep. In some cases this administration has increased REM sleep. But the logical conclusion from this is that cells in the region of infusion have receptors for the ligand and have connections to REM sleep–generating mechanisms. Under normal conditions, these receptors may not have a role in triggering the state. Only by showing that the administration duplicates the normal pattern of release of the ligand in this area, and that blockade of the activated receptors prevents normal REM sleep, can a reasonable suspicion be raised that a part of the normal REM sleep control pathway has been identified.

Because it is far easier to inject a substance than to collect and quantify physiologically released ligands, there have been many studies implying that various substances are critical for REM sleep control based solely on microinjection. These results must be interpreted with caution. For example, hypocretin is known to depolarize virtually all neuronal types. It should therefore not be surprising to find that hypocretin microinjection into arousal systems such as the locus coeruleus produces arousal,[40] that microinjection of hypocretin into sites known to control feeding increases food intake,[41] that injection into regions known to contain cells that are waking active increase waking,[42] that injection into regions known to contain cells selectively active in REM sleep will increase the occurrence of this state,[43,44] that injection into regions known to facilitate muscle tone will increase tone, that identical injections into regions known to suppress tone will decrease tone,[45] and that intracerebroventricular injection of hypocretin can increase water intake[46] and can activate other periventricular systems.[43] Such types of findings do not by themselves demonstrate a role for hypocretin (or any other neurotransmitter) in the observed behavior. It is necessary to obtain data on the effects of inactivation of, for example, hypocretin or hypocretin receptors and to record evidence that indicates activity of hypocretin neurons at the appropriate times before seriously entertaining such conclusions.

Genetic manipulations enable activation of neurons or nonneuronal cells of a particular type. A recent example of a genetic approach is the insertion of a light-sensitive ion channel into hypocretin cells using a lentivirus. Fiberoptic delivery of light could then be used to activate just these cells and determine the effect on sleep-waking transitions.[47]

Observation of Neuronal Activity

Recording the activity of single neurons in vivo can provide a powerful insight into the precise time course of neuronal discharge. Unit activity can be combined with other techniques to make it even more useful. For example, electrical stimulation of potential target areas can be used to antidromically identify the axonal projections of the recorded cell. Intracellular or "juxtacellular"[48] labeling of neurons with dyes, with subsequent immunolabeling of their transmitter can be used to determine the neurotransmitter phenotype of the recorded cell. Calcium imaging can be used to observe activity of particular cell phenotypes in vivo.[49] Combined dialysis and unit recording or iontophoresis of neurotransmitter from multiple barrel recording and stimulating micropipettes can be used to determine the transmitter response of the recorded cell, although one cannot easily determine if the effects seen are the direct result of responses in the recorded cell or are mediated by adjacent cells projecting to the recorded cell. Such distinctions can be made in in vitro studies of slices of brain tissue by blocking synaptic transmission or by physically dissociating studied cells; however, in the latter case their role in sleep may not be easily determined.

Although the role of a neuron in fast, synaptically mediated events happening in just a few milliseconds can be traced by inspection of neuronal discharge and comparison of that discharge with the timing of motor or sensory events, such an approach may be misleading when applied to the analysis of sleep state generation. The sleep cycle consists of a gradual coordinated change in EEG, EMG, and other phenomena over a period of seconds to minutes, as waking turns into NREM sleep and then as NREM sleep is transformed into REM sleep.

Despite this mismatch of time courses, the "tonic latency," a measure of how long before REM sleep-onset activity in a recorded cell changes, has been computed in some studies. Neurons purported to show a "significant" change in activity many seconds or even minutes prior to REM sleep onset have been reported. However, such a measure is of little utility because at the neuronal level, the activity of key cell groups can best be seen as curvilinear over the sleep cycle, rather than changing abruptly in the way that activity follows discrete sensory stimulation. A major determinant of the tonic latency computed as defined earlier, is the level of "noise" or variability in the cell's discharge, which affects the difficulty of detecting a significant underlying change in rate in a cell population. It is therefore not surprising that cell groups designated as "executive neurons" for REM sleep control on the basis of their tonic latencies were later found to have no essential role in the generation of REM sleep.[50-52] The more appropriate comparison of the unit activity cycle to state control is to compare two different cell types to see what the phase relation of the peaks or troughs of their activity is under similar conditions. This kind of study is difficult, involving the simultaneous long-term recording of multiple cells, and is rarely performed. Even in this case, a phase lead does not by itself prove that the "lead" neuron is driving activity seen in the "following" neuron, but it does indicate that the reverse is not the case. However, awakening is a process that can be studied in this way, since it can be elicited by external stimuli and appears to be preceded by abrupt changes in the activity of many neuronal groups.[53] A major advantage of electrical neuronal recording approaches in the intact animal to understanding sleep and other behavioral processes is their high level of temporal resolution.

Observation of the normal pattern of neurotransmitter release and neuronal activity can help determine the neurochemical correlates of sleep states. The natural release of neurotransmitters can be most easily determined by placing a tubular dialysis membrane 1 to 5 mm in length in the area of interest and circulating artificial cerebrospinal fluid through it. Neurotransmitters released outside the membrane will diffuse through the membrane and can be collected. Each sample is collected at intervals typically ranging from 2 to 10 minutes. The collected dialysates can be analyzed by chromatography, radioimmunoassay, mass spectroscopy, or other means. The temporal resolution of this technique is typically approximately a few minutes for each sample.[54-56]

Unit recording and dialysis approaches require a sharp research focus on a particular neurotransmitter or neuronal group. In contrast, histologic approaches can be used to measure the activity of the entire brain at cellular levels of resolution. The most popular such approach in animal studies labels the activation of immediate early genes. These genes are expressed in the nucleus, when a neuron is highly active and their expression is an early step in the activation of other downstream genes mobilizing the response of the cell to activation. Activation of these genes can be detected by immunohistochemistry, most commonly by staining for the production of the Fos protein or the mRNA used to synthesize this protein.[57] Neurons can be double labeled to determine the transmitter they express, allowing investigators to determine, for example, whether histaminergic neurons in the posterior hypothalamus were activated in a particular sleep or waking state. Metabolic labels such as 2-deoxyglucose can also provide an indication of which neurons are active.[57,58] Similar techniques using radioactive ligands in positron emission tomography (PET) studies can be used in living humans or animals. In vivo measurements of blood flow can be made throughout the brain with functional magnetic resonance imaging (fMRI). All of these techniques have in common their ability to make anatomically driven discoveries of brain regions that are active in particular states, independent of specific hypotheses, thus leading to major advances in understanding. However, another common feature of these types of "recording" techniques is their very poor temporal and spatial resolutions in comparison to neuronal recording approaches. Fos activation can take 20 minutes or more. PET takes a similar amount of time and fMRI can observe events lasting on the order of 1 to 15 seconds. It is uncertain if areas active during a particular state caused the state or were activated because of the state.

Summary of Technical Considerations

Clearly there is no perfect technique for determining the neuronal substrates of sleep states. Ideally all three approaches should be used in concert to reach conclusions. The next sections explore the major findings derived from lesion, stimulation, and recording studies of REM sleep control mechanisms.

Transection Studies

The most radical types of lesion studies are those that slice through the brainstem, severing the connections between regions rostral and caudal to the cut. Sherrington[59] discovered that animals in which the forebrain is removed after transecting the neuraxis in the coronal plane at the rostral border of the superior colliculus showed tonic excitation of the "antigravity muscles" or extensors (Figure 8.2, level A). This "decerebrate rigidity" was visible as soon as anesthesia was discontinued. Bard reported in 1958 that animals with decerebrate rigidity would show periodic limb relaxation.[60] Actually, Bard was observing the periodic muscle atonia of REM sleep.

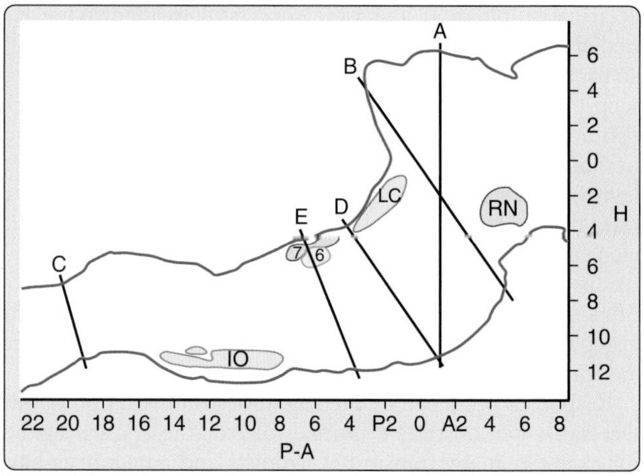

Figure 8.2 Outline of a sagittal section of the brainstem of the cat drawn from level L = 1.6 of the Berman atlas, indicating the level of key brainstem transection studies. 6, Abducens nucleus; 7, genu of the facial nerve; IO, inferior olive; LC, locus coeruleus; RN, red nucleus. H (horizontal) and P-A (posterior-anterior) scales are drawn from the atlas of the cat brain. (Berman AL. *The brain stem of the cat.* University of Wisconsin Press; 1968.)

After the discovery of REM sleep in the cat,[2] Jouvet found that this state was normally accompanied by the reduction or elimination of muscle tone in the neck muscles, termed "atonia."[4] Jouvet then examined the decerebrate cat preparation used by Sherrington and Bard, now adding measures of muscle tone, eye movement, and EEG. It may have seemed that, considering its association with dreaming, REM sleep is generated in the forebrain, but Jouvet found something quite different. When he recorded in the forebrain after separating the forebrain from the brainstem at the midbrain level (Figure 8.2, level A or B), he found no clear signs of REM sleep. In the first few days after transection, the EEG in the forebrain was always high voltage, but when low-voltage activity appeared, the PGO spikes that help identify REM sleep in the intact cat were absent from the thalamic structures, particularly the lateral geniculate where they can be most easily recorded. Thus it appeared that the isolated forebrain had slow wave sleep (SWS) states and possibly waking, but no clear evidence of REM sleep. In contrast, the midbrain and brainstem behind the cut showed clear evidence of REM sleep. Muscle atonia appeared with a regular periodicity and duration, similar to that of the intact cat's REM sleep periods. This atonia was accompanied by PGO spikes with a similar morphology to those seen in the intact animal. The pupils were highly constricted during atonic periods, as in REM sleep in the intact cat.

An interesting feature of REM sleep in the decerebrate animal is that its frequency and duration varied with the temperature of the animal. In the decerebrate animal, the forebrain thermoregulatory mechanisms are disconnected from their brainstem effectors. Shivering and panting do not occur at the relatively small temperature shifts that trigger them in the intact animal. For this reason, if the body temperature is not maintained by external heating or cooling, it will tend to drift toward room temperature. Jouvet, Arnulf, and colleagues[61,62] found that if body temperature was maintained at a normal

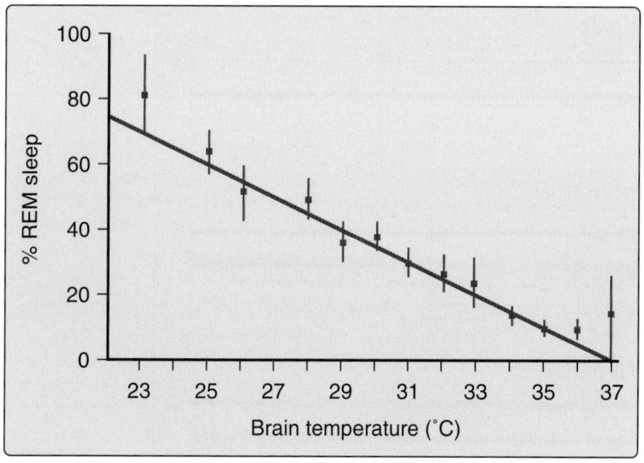

Figure 8.3 Relation between brain temperature and REM sleep amount in the brainstem of the cat whose neuraxis is severed at the junction between the pons and midbrain. Allowing temperature to fall induces a nearly continuous REM sleep state. In the intact animal, NREM sleep is associated with a fall in brain temperature, and REM sleep is associated with a brain temperature rise,[233] suggesting that REM sleep in the brainstem regulates brain temperature across the sleep period. (From Jouvet M, Buda C, Sastre JP. Hypothermia induces a quasi-permanent paradoxical sleep state in pontine cats. In Malan A, Canguilhem B, eds. *Living in the cold.* John Libbey Eurotext, 1989:487–97.)

level, little or no REM sleep appeared (Figure 8.3). But if temperature was allowed to fall, REM sleep amounts increased to levels well above those seen in the intact animal. This suggests that REM sleep facilitatory mechanisms are on balance less impaired by reduced temperature than are REM sleep inhibitory mechanisms. Another way of looking at this phenomenon is that brainstem mechanisms are set to respond to low temperatures by triggering REM sleep, perhaps to stimulate the brainstem, and that high brainstem temperatures inhibit REM sleep. It is unclear whether this mechanism is operative in the intact animal, where temperature shifts are within a narrower range. See the section The Functions of Rapid Eye Movement Sleep at the end of this chapter.

A further localization of the REM sleep control mechanisms can be achieved by examining the sleep of humans or animals in which the brainstem-spinal cord connection has been severed (Figure 8.2, level C). In this case, normal REM sleep in all its manifestations, except for spinally mediated atonia, is present.[63] Thus we can conclude that the region between the caudal medulla and rostral midbrain is sufficient to generate REM sleep.

This approach can be continued by separating the caudal pons from the medulla (Figure 8.2, level D or E). In such animals no atonia is present in musculature controlled by the spinal cord, even though electrical or chemical stimulation of the medial medulla in the decerebrate animal suppresses muscle tone.[64] Furthermore neuronal activity in the medulla does not resemble that seen across the REM-NREM sleep cycle, with neuronal discharge very regular for periods of many hours, in contrast to the periodic rate modulation that is linked to the phasic events of REM sleep in the intact animal[65] (Figure 8.4). This demonstrates that the medulla and spinal cord together, although they may contain circuitry whose activation can suppress muscle tone, are not sufficient to generate this aspect of REM sleep when disconnected from the pons and more rostral brainstem structures.

In contrast, the regions rostral to this cut show aspects of REM sleep[66] (Figure 8.1, *bottom,* and Figure 8.5). In these regions we can see the progression from isolated to grouped PGO spikes and the accompanying reduction in PGO spike amplitude that occurs in the pre-REM sleep period and the REM sleep periods in the intact animal. We also see increased forebrain unit activity, with neuronal unit spike bursts in conjunction with PGO spikes, just as in REM sleep.[65,67]

To summarize, this work shows that when pontine regions are connected to the medulla, atonia, rapid eye movements, and the associated unit activity of REM sleep occur, whereas the medulla and spinal cord together, disconnected from the pons, are not sufficient to generate these aspects of REM sleep. When the pons is connected to the forebrain, forebrain aspects of REM sleep are seen, but the forebrain without attached pons does not generate these aspects of REM sleep. Further confirmation of the importance of the pons and caudal midbrain comes from the studies of Matsuzaki and colleagues.[68] They found that when two cuts were placed, one at the junction of the midbrain and pons and the other at the junction of the pons and medulla, one could see periods of PGO spikes in the isolated pons, but no signs of REM sleep in structures rostral or caudal to the pontine "island."

These transection studies demonstrate, by positive evidence, that the pons is sufficient to generate the pontine signs of REM sleep, that is, the periodic pattern of PGO spikes and irregular neuronal activity that characterizes "phasic" REM sleep. A likely conclusion is that the pons is the crucial region for the generation of REM sleep. This chapter later addresses in more detail the structures within this region that synthesize the core elements of REM sleep.

However, it is also clear that the pons alone does not generate all the phenomena of REM sleep. Atonia requires the activation of motor inhibitory systems in the medulla.[69] In the intact animal, forebrain mechanisms interact with pontine mechanisms to regulate the amplitude and periodicity of PGO spikes,[70] which in turn are linked to the twitches and rapid eye movements of REM sleep. It is evident from cases of human REM sleep behavior disorder that the motor activity expressed in dreams is linked to the imagery of the dream.[71] An extrapolation to dream imagery in normal humans may lead to this hypothesis: because the structure of REM sleep results from an interaction of forebrain and brainstem mechanisms, the dream itself is not just passively driven from the brainstem but rather represents the result of a dynamic interaction between forebrain and brainstem structures.

Localized Lesion Studies

The transection studies point to a relatively small portion of the brainstem, the pons and caudal midbrain, as critical for REM sleep generation. Further specification of the core regions can be achieved by destroying portions of the pons in an otherwise intact animal and seeing which areas are necessary and which are unnecessary for REM sleep generation. An early systematic study by Carli and Zanchetti in the cat[72] and other subsequent studies emphasized that lesions of locus coeruleus[73] and the dorsal raphe[74] nuclei or of simultaneous lesions of locus coeruleus, forebrain cholinergic neurons, and histamine neurons[28] do not block REM sleep. Carli and Zanchetti concluded that lesions that destroyed the region ventral to the locus coeruleus, called the "nucleus reticularis

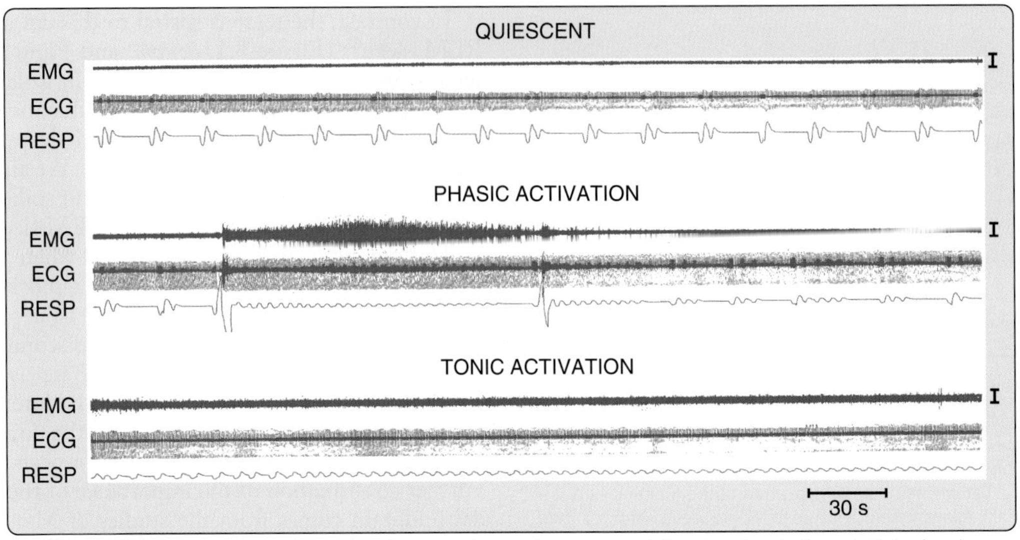

Figure 8.4 States seen caudal to chronic transection at the pontomedullary junction in the cat. Note the absence of periods of atonia. ECG, Electrocardiogram; EMG, electromyogram; RESP, thoracic strain gauge. Calibration, 50 μV. (From Siegel JM, Tomaszewski KS, Nienhuis R. Behavioral states in the chronic medullary and mid-pontine cat. *Electroencephalogr Clin Neurophysiol* 1986;63:274–88.)

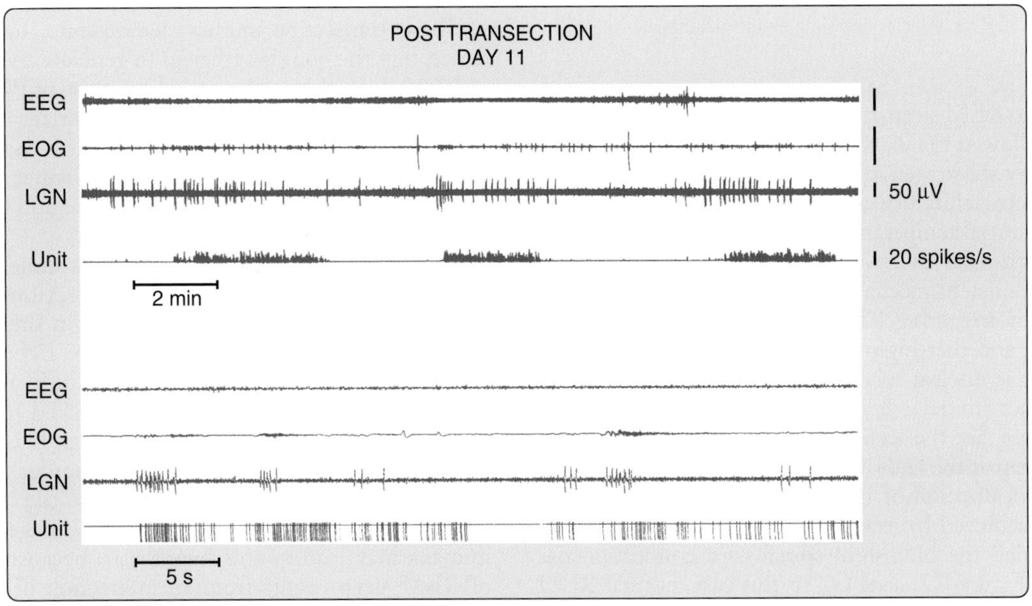

Figure 8.5 States seen rostral to chronic transection at the pontomedullary junction in the cat. Note the presence of ponto-geniculo-occipital (PGO) spikes and associated increases in unit activity triggered by the pons. Midbrain unit: electroencephalogram (EEG), electrooculogram (EOG), and lateral geniculate nucleus (LGN) activity rostral to chronic transections at the pontomedullary junction. In the *upper portion* of the figure, the unit channel displays the output of an integrating digital counter resetting at 1-sec intervals. In the *lower portion,* one pulse is produced for each spike by a window discriminator. (From Siegel JM. Pontomedullary interactions in the generation of REM sleep. In McGinty DJ, Drucker-Colin R, Morrison A, et al, eds. *Brain mechanisms of sleep.* Raven Press; 1985:157–74.)

pontis oralis" or the "subcoeruleus region," produced a massive decrease in the amount of REM sleep. (Different maps of the brainstem use different nomenclatures to identify similar or identical regions. Thus this region or closely adjacent regions have been called the sublaterodorsal or medial parabrachial pons.) In their studies, Carli and Zanchetti used the electrolytic lesion technique, in which a current is passed, depositing metal that kills cells and axons of passage. As cytotoxic techniques that allowed poisoning of cell bodies without the damage to axons of passage came into use, these initial conclusions were confirmed and refined. It was shown that neurons in medial pontine regions, including the "giant cell" region, were not important in REM sleep control[69,75,76] because near total destruction of these cells was followed by normal amounts of REM sleep as soon as anesthesia dissipated.[51,77] However, lesions of the subcoeruleus and adjacent regions with cytotoxins did cause a prolonged reduction in the amount of REM sleep. According to one study, the extent of this loss was proportional to the percentage of cholinergic cells lost in the subcoeruleus and adjacent regions of the brainstem of the cat.[78] In rats, lesion or inactivation of the same region below the locus coeruleus (called the sublaterodorsal nucleus in the terminology of Swanson[79]) has been found to reduce REM sleep.[80]

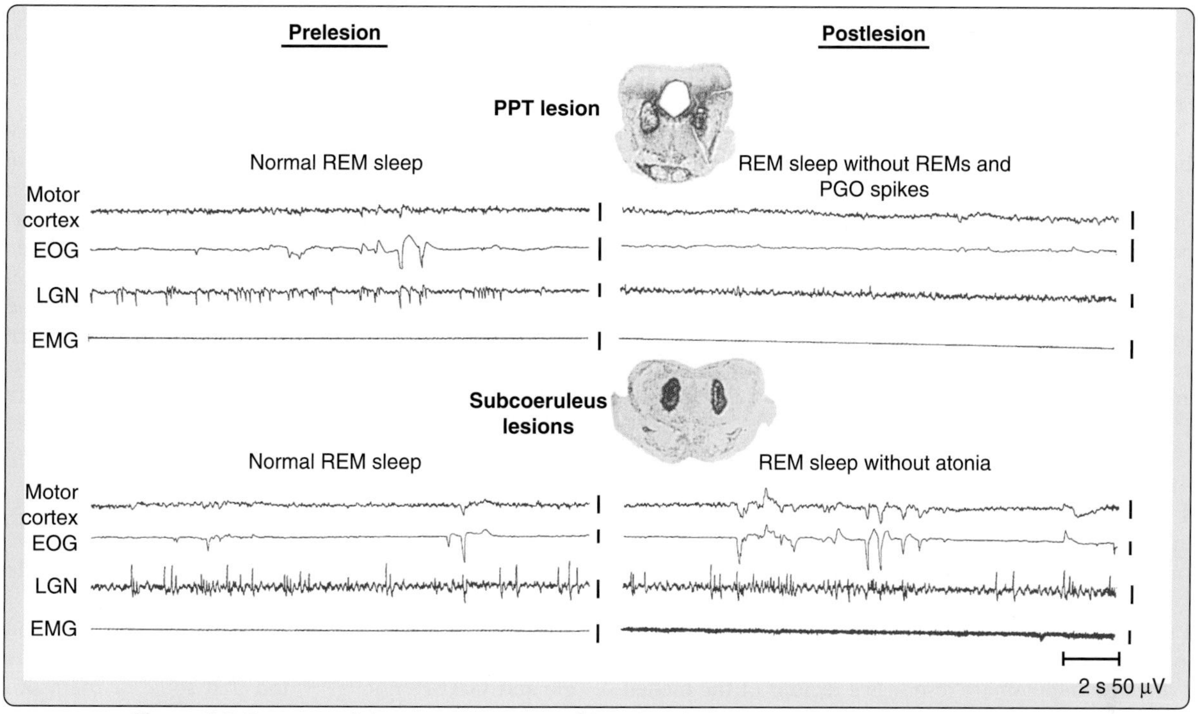

Figure 8.6 Disruption of phasic or tonic aspects of REM sleep by lesions. Twenty-second polygraph tracings of REM sleep before and after lesions, together with a coronal section through the center of the pontine lesions. Electroencephalogram voltage reduction of REM sleep (recorded from motor cortex) was present after both lesions. *Top*, Radiofrequency lesions of the pedunculopontine region diminished ponto-geniculo-occipital (PGO) spikes and eye movement bursts during REM sleep. *Bottom*, Lesions in the region ventral to the locus coeruleus produced REM sleep without atonia without any diminution of PGO spike or REM frequency. EMG, Electromyogram; EOG, electrooculogram; LGN, lateral geniculate nucleus; PPT, pedunculopontine tegmentum. (Reprinted from Brain Research, vol 571, Shouse MN, Siegel JM, Pontine regulation of REM sleep components in cats: integrity of the pedunculopontine tegmentum [PPT] is important for phasic events but unnecessary for atonia during REM sleep, 50–63, Copyright 1992, with permission from Elsevier Science.)

Although large lesions may eliminate all aspects of REM sleep, small, bilaterally symmetrical lesions within the pons can eliminate specific aspects of REM sleep. Lesions of lateral pontine structures allow muscle atonia during REM sleep. However, PGO spikes and the associated rapid eye movements are absent when lesions include the region surrounding the superior cerebellar peduncle of the cat[81] (Figure 8.6, *top*). This points to the role of this lateral region in the generation of PGO waves and the associated phasic activity of REM sleep.

Small lesions confined to portions of the subcoeruleus regions identified as critical for REM sleep by Carli and Zanchetti, or to the medial medulla[69] result in a very unusual syndrome. After NREM sleep, these animals enter REM sleep, as indicated by lack of responsiveness to the environment, PGO spikes, EEG desynchrony, and pupil constriction. However, they lack the muscle atonia that normally characterizes this state[5,82] (Figure 8.6, *bottom*). During "REM sleep without atonia" these cats appear to act out dreams, attacking objects that are not visible, exhibiting unusual affective behaviors and ataxic locomotion. When they are awakened, normal behavior resumes. More recent studies have demonstrated that lesions of a system extending from the ventral midbrain to the medial medulla can cause REM sleep without atonia and that activation of this system can suppress muscle tone.[69,83-85]

This subcoeruleus region is under the control of midbrain regions. A midbrain region located just beneath and lateral to the periaqueductal gray (and called the dorsocaudal central tegmental field in the cat) appears to inhibit REM sleep by inhibiting the critical "REM-on" subcoeruleus neurons. Muscimol, a gamma-aminobutyric acid ionotropic receptor Family A ($GABA_A$) receptor agonist, injected into this midbrain region silences these cells and increases REM sleep, presumably by blocking the inhibition.[86] The same phenomena have been observed when muscimol is injected into the corresponding region of guinea pig[87] and the rat.[88] (In the rat this midbrain region has been called the deep mesencephalic nucleus.) The midbrain region of the deep mesencephalic nucleus is the heart of the classic reticular activating system, shown to induce waking when electrically stimulated[89] and coma when lesioned.[90]

Increasing the levels of GABA in the subcoeruleus region (also called the pontine oralis nucleus in the rat and cat) produces an increase in waking, rather than the increase in REM sleep seen with GABA injection into the midbrain regions indicated previously.[91,92] This is another reminder that, despite the sleep inducing effect of systemic administration of GABAergic hypnotic medications (such as benzodiazepines), local manipulation shows that the effect of GABA on sleep and waking states varies across brain regions. Blocking GABA in the subcoeruleus has been reported to increase REM sleep in the cat.[93]

Stimulation Studies

The first study showing that stimulation could elicit REM sleep was carried out by George and colleagues.[94] They found that application of the acetylcholine agonist carbachol to specific regions of the pons ventral to the locus coeruleus could elicit REM sleep in the cat. An impressive proof that a unique REM sleep–generation mechanism was being activated was the long duration of the elicited REM sleep periods, which could last hours. Microinjection of acetylcholine into this region in the decerebrate cat produces an immediate suppression of decerebrate rigidity. Later studies showed that, depending on the exact site, either REM sleep or just atonia in a waking state could be triggered by such stimulation.[95-97] When stimulation was applied to the lateral regions whose lesion blocked PGO waves, continuous PGO spikes were generated even though the animal was not always behaviorally asleep.

Increased REM sleep has been reported in the rat after microinjection of cholinergic agonists into the subcoeruleus region,[98-100] although this effect is not as robust as it is in the cat.[101]

The first study demonstrating a role for glutamate in the control of REM sleep was done in the cat. We found that a profound suppression of muscle tone could be elicited by the injection of glutamate into the subcoeruleus region or into the ventral medullary region.[64,102,103] Further work has demonstrated that the pontine cells in this inhibitory region receiving cholinergic input use glutamate as their transmitter and project directly to glutamate responsive regions of the medial medulla.[102,104-111]

Work in the rat has emphasized the strong triggering of REM sleep by glutamatergic excitation of this region.[80,112] Glutamatergic excitation of this region in the cat also increases REM sleep,[113] suggesting that both cholinergic and glutamatergic mechanisms are intimately involved in the triggering of REM sleep. However, there does appear to be a species difference in the relative potency of the effect of microinjection of these two neurotransmitters.

Neuronal Activity, Transmitter Release

The transection, lesion, and stimulation studies all point to the same regions of the pons and caudal midbrain as the critical region for the generation of the state of REM sleep as a whole, and smaller subregions in the brainstem and forebrain in the control of its individual components. The pons contains a variety of cells differing in their neurotransmitter, receptors, and axonal projections. Unit recording techniques allow an analysis of the interplay between these cell groups and their targets to further refine our dissection of REM sleep mechanisms.

Medial Brainstem Reticular Formation

Most cells within the medial brainstem reticular formation are maximally active in waking, greatly reduce the discharge rate in NREM sleep, and increase the discharge rate back to waking levels in REM sleep.[23,24,76,114,115] Discharge is most regular in NREM sleep and is relatively irregular in both waking and REM sleep. The similarity of the waking and REM sleep discharge pattern suggests a similar role of these cells in both states. Indeed, most of these cells have been shown to be active in waking in relation to specific lateralized movements of the head, neck, tongue, face, or limbs. For example, a cell may discharge only with extension of the ipsilateral forelimb or abduction of the tongue. The twitches that are normally visible in facial and limb musculature during REM sleep and the phenomenon of REM sleep without atonia suggest that these cells command movements that are blocked by the muscle tone suppression of REM sleep. A lesion in these cells has little or no effect on REM sleep duration or periodicity[51,52] but does dramatically prevent movements of the head and neck in waking.[116]

Cholinergic Cell Groups

Cholinergic cell groups have an important role in REM sleep control in the cat. As was pointed out earlier, microinjection of cholinergic agonists into the pons of the cat reliably triggers long REM sleep periods that can last for minutes or hours. Microdialysis studies show that pontine acetylcholine release is greatly increased during natural REM sleep when compared to either NREM sleep or waking.[117] Recordings of neuronal activity within the cholinergic cell population demonstrate the substrates of this release. Certain cholinergic cells are maximally active in REM sleep (REM-on cells). Others are active in both waking and REM sleep.[118,119] Presumably the REM-on cholinergic cells project to the acetylcholine responsive region in the subcoeruleus area.[120]

Cells with Activity Selective for REM Sleep

Cells with activity selective for REM sleep can be identified within the subcoeruleus area in both cats[121] and rats.[88] Anatomic studies using Fos labeling and tract tracing and unit recording studies indicate that these neurons are glutamatergic and GABAergic[122-128] and that some of them project to the ventral medullary region involved in the triggering of the muscle atonia of REM sleep.*

Monoamine-Containing Cells

Monoamine-containing cells have a very different discharge profile. Most if not all noradrenergic[134,135] and serotonergic[136] cells of the midbrain and pontine brainstem and histaminergic[137] cells of the posterior hypothalamus are continuously active during waking, decrease their activity during NREM sleep, and further reduce or cease activity during REM sleep (Figure 8.7). As was pointed out earlier, these cell groups are not critical for REM sleep generation, but it is likely that they modulate the expression of REM sleep. The cessation of discharge in monoaminergic cells during REM sleep appears to be caused by the release of GABA onto these cells,[138-141] presumably by REM sleep-active GABAergic brainstem neurons.[26,49,142-145] Administration of a GABA agonist to the raphe cell group increases REM sleep duration,[139] demonstrating a modulatory role for this cell group in REM sleep control. Some studies indicate that dopamine cells do not change discharge across sleep states.[56,146,147] Other work suggests that there is increased release of dopamine in REM sleep,[148,149] decreased release in REM sleep,[150] or selective waking activity in these neurons.[151] These findings may reflect the heterogeneity of firing of different dopamine cell groups and presynaptic control of release in dopamine terminals.

Other Cholinergic Cells in Lateral Pontine Regions

Other cholinergic cells in lateral pontine regions discharge in bursts before each ipsilateral PGO wave.[152,153] These cells may therefore participate in the triggering of these waves. We know that PGO waves are tonically inhibited in waking by serotonin input.[154-156] Therefore it is likely that certain groups of cholinergic cells receive direct or perhaps indirect serotonergic inhibition in waking and that the decrease of this inhibition in NREM sleep and REM sleep facilitates PGO wave and REM sleep generation.

*References 64, 80, 88, 102, 104–106, 129–133.

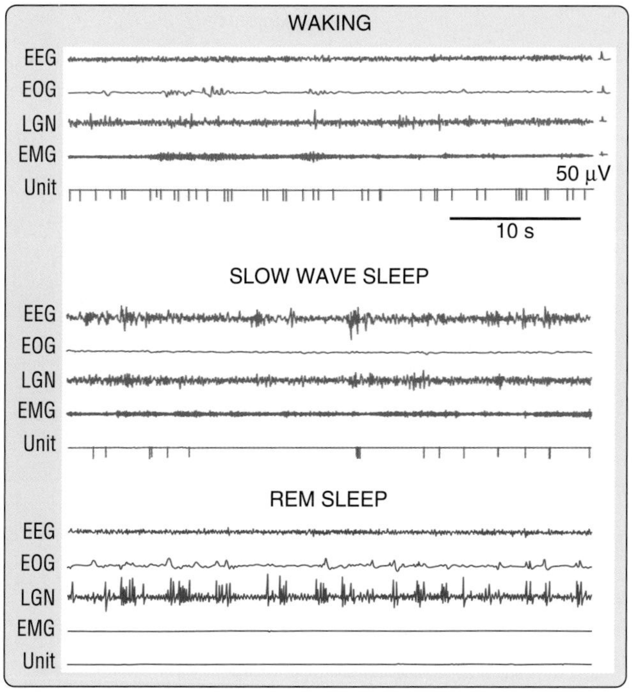

Figure 8.7 Activity of a "REM–off" cell recorded in the locus coeruleus. EEG, Sensorimotor electroencephalogram; EMG, neck electromyogram; EOG, eye movements; LGN, lateral geniculate activity; Unit, pulses triggered by locus coeruleus cell.

Fos Labeling

A more global mapping of neurons active in REM sleep can be achieved by using the Fos labeling to identify neurons active within the 20-minute (or longer) period before sacrifice. Quattrochi and colleagues demonstrated that microinjections of the cholinergic agonist carbachol that triggered episodes of continuous PGO waves in waking activated neurons within the laterodorsal and pedunculopontine nuclei. Destruction of these nuclei blocks these waves.[156-158]

More extensive Fos mapping has been done to identify neurons activated during REM sleep in the rat. Verret and colleagues[159] found that only a few cholinergic neurons from the laterodorsal and pedunculopontine tegmental nuclei were Fos-labeled after REM sleep. In contrast, a large number of noncholinergic Fos-labeled cells were observed in the laterodorsal tegmental nucleus, subcoeruleus region, and lateral, ventrolateral, and dorsal periaqueductal grey of the midbrain. In addition, other regions outside of the brainstem regions critical for REM sleep control were labeled. These included the alpha and ventral gigantocellular reticular nuclei of the medulla, dorsal, and lateral paragigantocellular reticular[160] nuclei and the nucleus raphe obscurus. Half of the cells in the latter nucleus were cholinergic, suggesting that these neurons may be a source of acetylcholine during REM sleep. In a second study, an effort was made to identify the source of the GABAergic input thought to cause the cessation of discharge in locus coeruleus cells during REM sleep.[140] Verret and colleagues[103] found that the dorsal and lateral paragigantocellular reticular nuclei of the medulla and regions of the periaqueductal gray of the midbrain, regions with large percentages of GABAergic cells, are active in REM sleep. Maloney and colleagues[142] found GABAergic cells adjacent to the locus coeruleus that expressed Fos during periods of high REM sleep. Because the critical phenomena of REM sleep do not appear to require the medulla, it seems likely that the periaqueductal gray GABAergic neurons and GABAergic neurons adjacent to locus coeruleus and raphe nuclei are sufficient to suppress the activity of noradrenergic and serotonergic neurons,[139,161] although medullary neurons may participate in the intact animal.

Fos mapping has also been used to identify forebrain regions likely to control REM sleep. The preoptic region, important in NREM sleep control (see Chapter 7) contains neurons that express Fos maximally in REM sleep–deprived animals, suggesting that these neurons may be related to the triggering or duration of REM sleep by brainstem systems.[162] Fos studies also indicate that melanin-concentrating hormone neurons, which are located in the hypothalamus, express Fos during periods with large amounts of REM sleep and that intracerebroventricular administration of melanin-concentrating hormone increases the amount of subsequent REM sleep.[163,164] These results suggest that melanin-concentrating hormone neurons are an additional source of forebrain modulation of REM sleep. However, our study in humans showed maximal melanin-concentrating hormone release at sleep onset, not during the period of maximal REM sleep.[165]

Certainly, the identity of the cells involved in triggering and controlling REM sleep is not easily determined. The Fos studies do not necessarily identify all the cells active during REM sleep, only those of a phenotype that allows them to express Fos during the tested manipulations. Certain cell types do not readily express Fos even when very active. In other words, cells not expressing Fos during periods of REM sleep may be involved and may even have a critical role in REM sleep control. Conversely, cells expressing Fos because of their activity during REM sleep may be responding to the motor and autonomic changes characteristic of this state, rather than causing these changes. With neuronal activity recording, the identification of the cells responsible for starting the process of REM sleep triggering cannot easily be determined without a complete profile of discharge across the sleep cycle and a direct comparison of candidate cell groups, for the reasons reviewed earlier. Finally, recording from neurons in head-restrained animals, while easier than in freely moving animals, can be misleading because it can lower the activity of movement related cells in waking, making them appear to be selectively active in REM sleep.[50] Nevertheless by comparing the results of multiple recording and stimulation techniques, with those of lesions we gather evidence that helps identify the brainstem and forebrain neuronal groups that are the best candidates for controlling the REM sleep state.

CONTROL OF MUSCLE TONE

Abnormalities of muscle tone control underlie many sleep disorders. During REM sleep, central motor systems are highly active, whereas motoneurons are hyperpolarized.[166] The normal suppression of tone in the tongue and laryngeal muscles in REM sleep is a major contributing factor in sleep apnea. The failure of muscle tone suppression in REM sleep causes REM sleep behavior disorder.[167] Triggering of the REM sleep muscle tone control mechanism in waking is responsible for cataplexy.[168]

Early work using intracellular recording and microiontophoresis showed that motoneuron hyperpolarization during

REM sleep was accompanied by the release of glycine onto motoneurons.[166,169] Microdialysis sampling showed that both GABA and glycine are released onto motoneurons during atonia induced by carbachol in the cat.[55] This release occurs in spinal ventral horn motoneurons as well as in hypoglossal motoneurons. The glycinergic inhibition during a carbachol-elicited REM sleep–like state was investigated with immunohistochemistry and found to be due to the activation of glycinergic neurons in the nucleus reticularis gigantocellularis and nucleus magnocellularis in the rostro-ventral medulla and the ventral portion of the nucleus paramedianus reticularis,[169] regions whose activation has been shown to suppress muscle tone in the unanesthetized decerebrate animal.[102] A second population of glycinergic neurons is located in the caudal medulla adjacent to the nucleus ambiguus; these neurons may be responsible for the REM sleep–related inhibition of motoneurons that innervate the muscles of the larynx and pharynx.

In related work it has been shown that norepinephrine and serotonin release onto motoneurons is decreased during atonia.[170] Because these monoamines are known to excite motoneurons and GABA and glycine are known to inhibit motoneurons, it appears that the coordinated activity of these cell groups produces motoneuron hyperpolarization and hence atonia in REM sleep by a combination of inhibition and disfacilitation.

The inhibitory and facilitatory systems are strongly and reciprocally linked. Electrical stimulation of the pontine inhibitory area (PIA located in the subcoeruleus region[102]) produces muscle tone suppression. Even though the PIA is within a few millimeters of the noradrenergic locus coeruleus, electrical stimulation in the PIA that suppresses muscle tone will always cause a cessation of activity in the noradrenergic neurons of the locus coeruleus and other facilitatory cell groups.[171] Cells that are maximally active in REM sleep ("REM-on" cells) are present in the PIA and also in the region of the medial medulla that receives PIA projections (Figure 8.8).

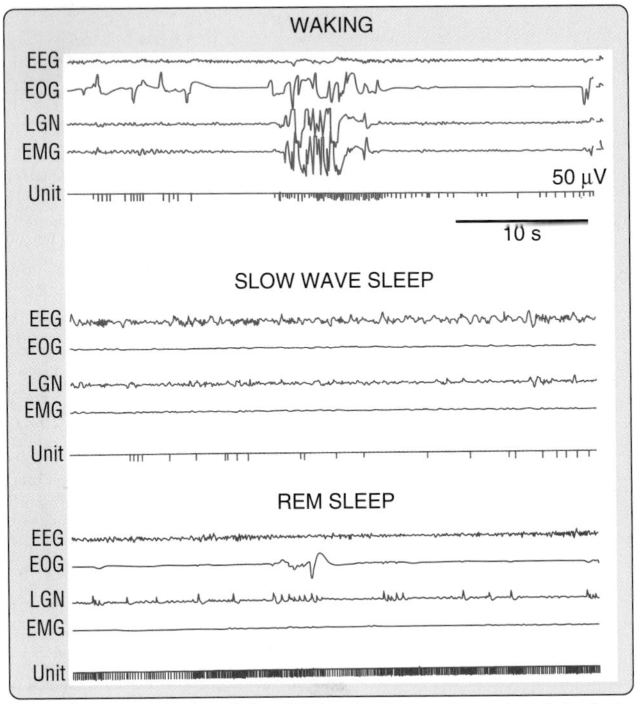

Figure 8.8 Activity of medullary "REM–on" cell. Note the tonic activity during REM sleep. In waking, activity is generally absent even during vigorous movement. However, some activity is seen during movements involving head lowering and postural relaxation. EEG, Sensorimotor electroencephalogram; EMG, neck electromyogram; EOG, eye movements; LGN, lateral geniculate activity; Unit, pulses triggered by REM-on cell.

The release of GABA and glycine onto motoneurons during REM sleep atonia is most likely mediated by a pathway from the PIA to the medial medulla.[105,106] The pontine region triggering this release is not only sensitive to acetylcholine but also responsive to glutamate[104] (Figure 8.9).[102] The medullary region with descending projections to motoneurons can be subdivided into a rostral portion responding to glutamate and a caudal portion responding to acetylcholine[64,172] (Figure 8.9). The medullary interaction with pontine structures is critical for muscle tone suppression, because inactivation of pontine regions greatly reduces the suppressive effects of medullary stimulation on muscle tone.[173,174] This ascending pathway from the medulla to the pons may mediate the inhibition of locus coeruleus during atonia and may also help recruit other active inhibitory mechanisms. Thus damage anywhere in the medial pontomedullary region can block muscle atonia by interrupting ascending and descending portions of the pontomedullary inhibitory system, as can muscimol injection into the pons,[173] again indicating that the pons is a key component of the circuit producing motor inhibition.

The studies reviewed previously focused largely on ventral horn and hypoglossal motoneurons. However, the control of jaw muscles is also a critical clinical issue. The success of jaw appliances indicates that reduced jaw muscle activity can contribute to closure of the airway in sleep apnea. Jaw muscle relaxation is a common initial sign of cataplexy, and tonic muscle activation underlies bruxism.

Investigation of the control of masseter motor neurons allows analysis of the regulation of muscle tone on one side of the face, while using the other side as a control for changes in behavioral state caused by application of neurotransmitter agonist and antagonists.[175] Using this model, researchers determined that tonic glycine release reduces muscle tone in both waking and NREM sleep. However, blockade of glycine receptors did not prevent the suppression of muscle tone in REM sleep. In a similar manner, blockade of GABA receptors alone or in combination with glycine receptors increased tone in waking and NREM sleep but did not prevent the suppression of masseter tone[176] or of genioglossus tone in REM sleep.[177] However, both of these manipulations increased phasic masseter muscle activity in REM sleep.

Further studies showed that a blockade of glutamate receptors reduces the normal enhancement of muscle tone in waking relative to the level in NREM sleep. Glutamate also contributes to the phasic motor activity during REM sleep. However, reduction in glutamate alone is not sufficient to account for the suppression of muscle tone in REM sleep, because stimulation of NMDA and non-NMDA glutamate receptors does not appear to restore muscle tone in REM sleep.[178]

A study in the anesthetized rat suggested that activation of norepinephrine receptors, in combination with the activation of glutamate receptors, was sufficient to potently increase muscle tone in the masseter muscles.[110] A study of the hypoglossal motor nucleus in the unanesthetized rat concluded that the suppression of muscle tone in REM sleep was mediated to a large extent by a reduction in norepinephrine release, but not

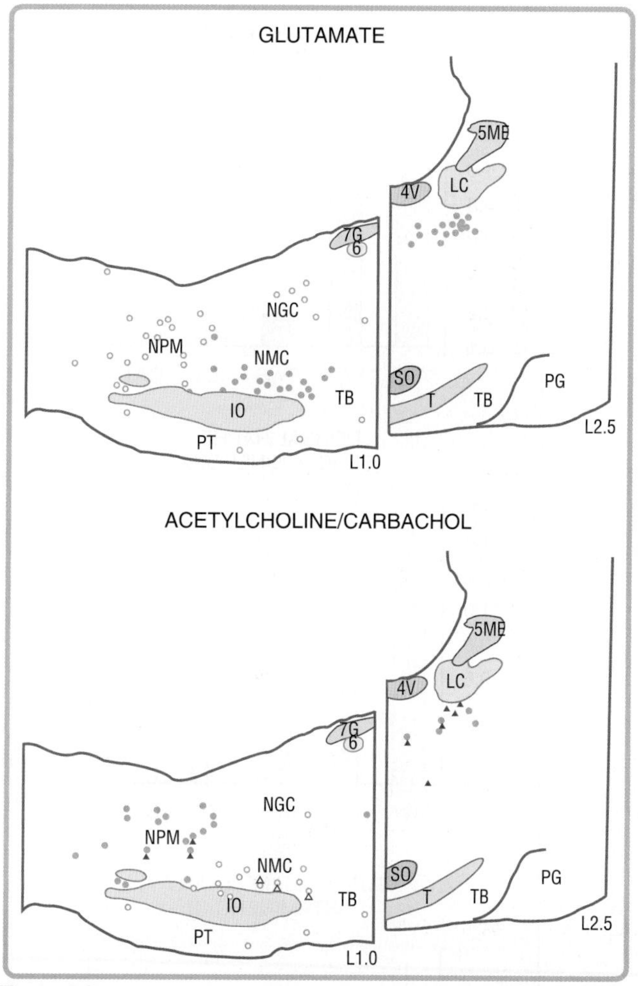

Figure 8.9 Sagittal map of pontomedullary inhibitory areas. Electrical stimulation produced atonia at all the points mapped. All electrically defined inhibitory sites were microinjected with glutamate or cholinergic agonists. *Filled symbols* represent points at which microinjections decreased muscle tone (to less than 30% of baseline values or to complete atonia). *Open circles* indicate points at which injections increased or produced no change in baseline values. Glutamate injections are shown at the top, acetylcholine (ACh) and carbachol (Carb) injections at the bottom. At the bottom, *circles* and *triangles* represent ACh and Carb injections, respectively. 4V, fourth ventricle; 5ME, mesencephalic trigeminal tract; 6, abducens nucleus; 7G, genu of the facial nerve; IO, inferior olivary nucleus; LC, locus coeruleus nucleus, NGC, nucleus gigantocellularis; NMC, nucleus magnocellularis; NPM, nucleus paramedianus; PG, pontine gray; PT, pyramid tract; SO, superior olivary nucleus; T, nucleus of the trapezoid body; TB, trapezoid body. (From Lai YY, Siegel JM. Medullary regions mediating atonia. *J Neurosci.* 1988;8:4790–6.)

by reduced serotonin release.[179] Thus this work, in the context of prior microdialysis analysis of transmitter release, suggests that the reduction of norepinephrine release may be a key factor regulating muscle tone, along with the earlier-described changes in amino acid release. These conclusions are consistent with prior work indicating that cataplexy was linked to a reduction in the activity of noradrenergic neurons (see later in this chapter).[180] Although the current literature suggests that trigeminal, hypoglossal, and ventral horn motoneurons are subjected to similar neurochemical control across the sleep cycle, direct comparison of these systems has not been made. It is likely that some aspects of control may differ across systems as well as species.

The role of reduced serotonin release in the suppression of muscle tone has been investigated in the hypoglossal nucleus of the rat. It was found that the modulation of genioglossus activity across natural sleep-wake states was not greatly affected by endogenous input from serotonergic neurons, although prior studies in vagotomized and anesthetized rats had shown an effect of serotonin on muscle tone under these aphysiologic conditions.[181-183]

In contrast to the norepinephrine, serotonin, and histamine cell groups, it was reported that mesencephalic dopaminergic neurons do not appear to alter their discharge rate across the sleep cycle.[146] Dopamine release in the amygdala measured by dialysis does not significantly vary across the sleep cycle.[184] In disagreement with this finding, a Fos study indicated that dopaminergic neurons within the ventral portion of the mesencephalic tegmentum were activated during periods of increased REM sleep.[185] A unit recording study indicated that dopaminergic neurons in the ventral tegmental area of the midbrain show maximal burst firing in both waking and REM sleep.[148] Other work using the Fos labeling technique identified a wake active dopaminergic cell population in the ventral periaqueductal gray.[151] In dialysis measurements of dopamine release, we have seen reduced dopamine release in the dorsal horn of the spinal cord during the REM sleep–like state triggered by carbachol. We did not see such a decrease in the ventral horn or hypoglossal nucleus.[170] These data suggest either heterogeneity in the behavior of sleep cycle activity of dopaminergic neurons or presynaptic control of dopamine release independent of action potentials in the cell somas.

Figure 8.10 illustrates some of the anatomic and neurochemical substrates of the brainstem generation of REM sleep.

NARCOLEPSY AND HYPOCRETIN

Narcolepsy has long been characterized as a disease of the REM sleep mechanism. Patients with narcolepsy often have REM sleep within 5 minutes of sleep onset, in contrast to normal individuals who rarely show such "sleep-onset REM sleep." Most narcoleptics experience cataplexy,[186] a sudden loss of muscle tone with the same reflex suppression that is seen in REM sleep. High-amplitude theta activity in the hippocampus, characteristic of REM sleep, is also prominent in cataplexy as observed in dogs.[180] Further evidence for links between narcolepsy and REM sleep comes from studies of neuronal activity during cataplexy. Many of the same cell populations in the pons and medulla that are tonically active only during REM sleep in neurologically normal become active during cataplexy in patients with narcolepsy, including cells in the medial medullary inhibitory region that are selectively active in relation to the atonia of REM sleep.[25,168] Likewise, cells in the locus coeruleus, which cease discharge only in REM sleep in normal animals, invariably cease discharge in cataplexy.[187] However, just as cataplexy differs behaviorally from REM sleep in its maintenance of consciousness, not all neuronal aspects of REM sleep are present during cataplexy. As was noted previously, in the normal animal, noradrenergic, serotonergic, and histaminergic cells are tonically active in waking, reduce discharge in nonREM sleep, and cease discharge in REM sleep.[180,187] However, unlike noradrenergic cells, serotonergic cells do not cease discharge during cataplexy, only reducing discharge to quiet waking levels. Histaminergic cells actually increase discharge in cataplexy relative to quiet waking levels (Figure 8.11).[188] These findings allow us

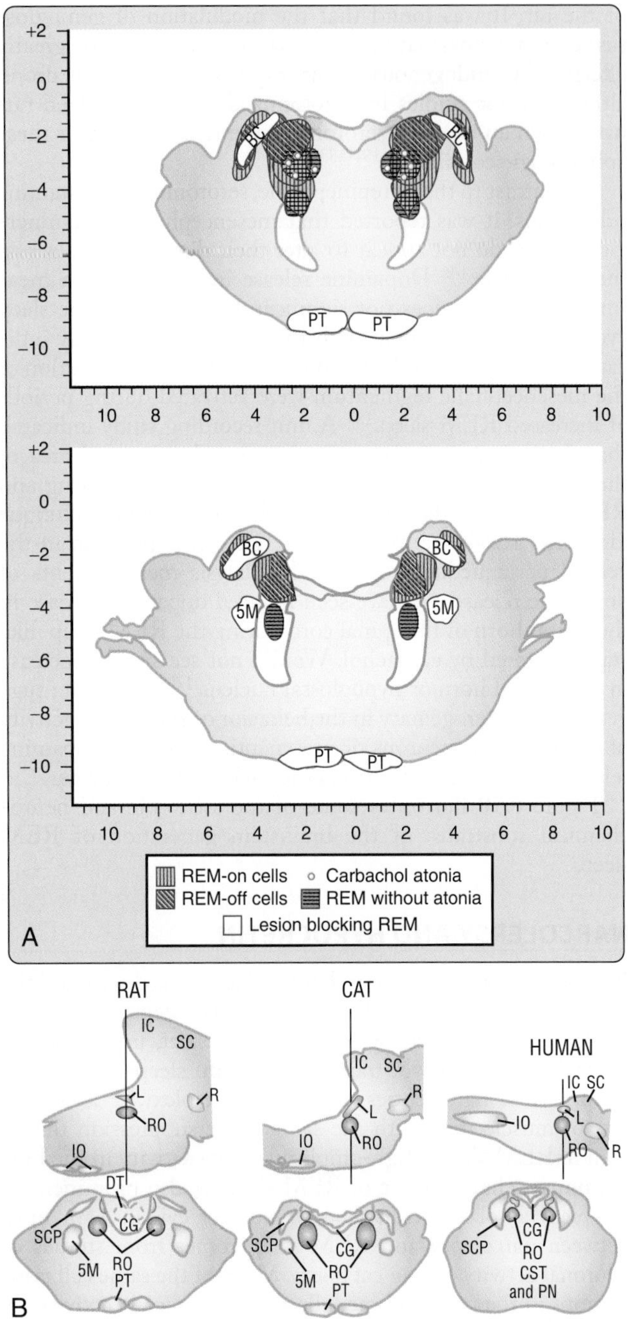

Figure 8.10 **A** and **B,** Anatomic relation of "REM–on" and "REM–off" cells, carbachol-induced atonia sites, lesions blocking atonia but not preventing REM sleep, and lesions completely blocking REM sleep. B shows anatomic locations of REM on areas in cats rat and projected location in human in sagittal and coronal views. 5M, Motor nucleus of the trigeminal nerve; BC, brachium conjunctivum; CG, central 8-gray; CST, corticospinal tract; DT, dorsal tegmental; IO, inferior olive; L, locus coeruleus; PN, pontine nuclei; PT, pyramidal tract; R, red nucleus; RO, reticularis oralis nucleus; SC, superior colliculus; SCP, superior cerebellar peduncle (brachium conjunctivum). (From Siegel JM, Rogawski MA. A function for REM sleep: regulation of noradrenergic receptor sensitivity. *Brain Res.* 1988;13:213–33; Siegel JM. The stuff dreams are made of: anatomical substrates of REM sleep. *Nature Neurosci.* 2006;9:721–2, 2006.)

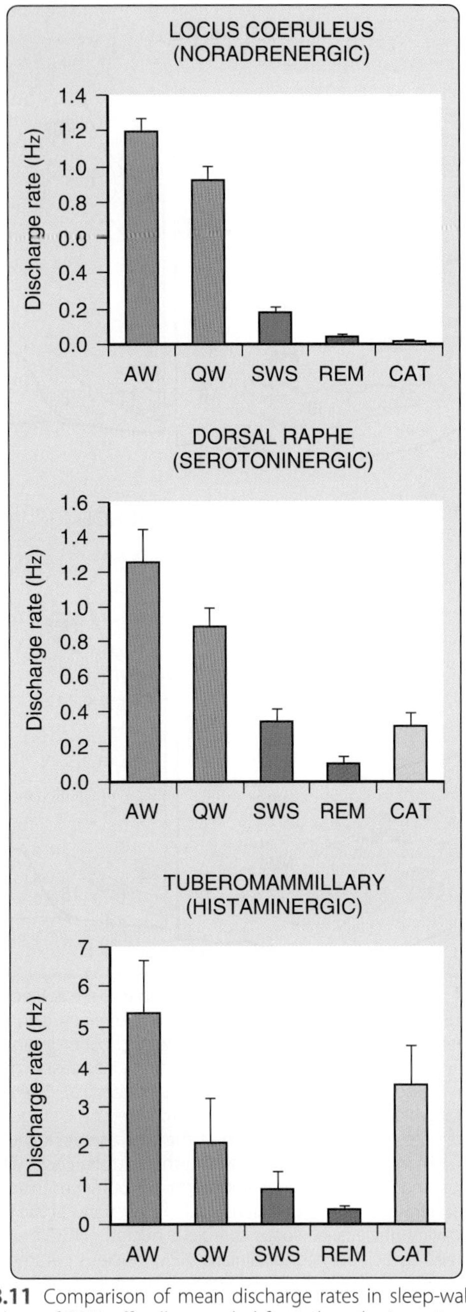

Figure 8.11 Comparison of mean discharge rates in sleep-waking states and cataplexy of REM-off cells recorded from three brain regions. Posterior hypothalamic histaminergic neurons remain active, whereas dorsal raphe serotonergic neurons reduced discharge, and locus coeruleus noradrenergic neurons cease discharge during cataplexy (CAT). All of these cell types were active in waking, reduced discharge in NREM sleep, and were silent or nearly silent in REM sleep. AW, Active waking; QW, quiet waking; REM, REM sleep; SWS, slow wave (NREM) sleep. (From John J, Wu MF, Boehmer LB, Siegel JM. Cataplexy-active neurons in the posterior hypothalamus: implications for the role of histamine in sleep and waking behavior. *Neuron.* 2004;42:619–34.)

to identify some of the cellular substrates of cataplexy. Medullary inhibition and noradrenergic disfacilitation are linked to cataplexy's loss of muscle tone. In contrast, the maintained activity of histamine neurons is a likely substrate for the maintenance of consciousness during cataplexy that distinguishes cataplexy from REM sleep. Thus the study of neuronal activity in the narcoleptic animal provides an insight into both narcolepsy and the normal role of these cell groups in maintaining consciousness and muscle tone.

In 2001 researchers discovered that most human narcolepsy was caused by a loss of hypothalamic cells containing the peptide hypocretin (Figure 8.12).[34,35] We determined that, on average, 90% of these cells are lost in human patients with narcolepsy. Subsequently, it was discovered that a lesser reduction in the number of hypocretin cells was seen in Parkinson

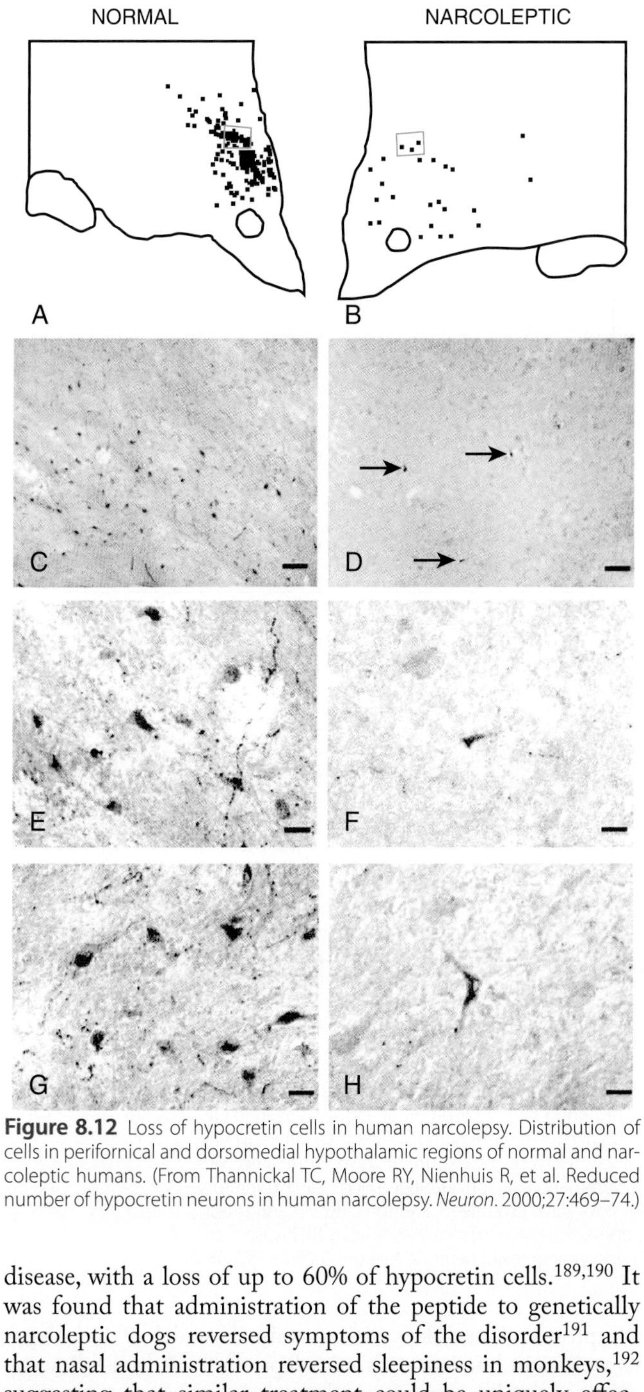

Figure 8.12 Loss of hypocretin cells in human narcolepsy. Distribution of cells in perifornical and dorsomedial hypothalamic regions of normal and narcoleptic humans. (From Thannickal TC, Moore RY, Nienhuis R, et al. Reduced number of hypocretin neurons in human narcolepsy. *Neuron.* 2000;27:469–74.)

disease, with a loss of up to 60% of hypocretin cells.[189,190] It was found that administration of the peptide to genetically narcoleptic dogs reversed symptoms of the disorder[191] and that nasal administration reversed sleepiness in monkeys,[192] suggesting that similar treatment could be uniquely effective for narcolepsy and perhaps for other disorders characterized by sleepiness.[193-195] More recently we found that human patients with narcolepsy have a greater than 65% increase in the number of detectable histamine cells.[196,197] It has been speculated that since this change is not seen in any of four different animal genetic models of narcolepsy, this increase may be related to the presumed immune activation that causes human narcolepsy.[196]

Researchers determined that, in normal animals, identified hypocretin neurons discharge at their highest rates during active waking[48,198] (Figure 8.13). This discharge was reduced or absent during aversive waking situations, even if the EEG indicated high levels of alertness.[48] The hypocretin level in normal dogs is nearly doubled when they are let out into a yard to play with other dogs. However, when these same dogs run at maximal speed on a treadmill, hypocretin levels are unchanged, demonstrating that motor activity and associated changes in respiratory rate, heart rate, and body temperature do not by themselves determine the release of hypocretin. Studies of hypocretin release in the cat[199] are also consistent with this hypothesis. Hypocretin cells send ascending projections to cortical and basal forebrain regions, in addition to their descending projection to locus coeruleus and other brainstem regions. In the absence of hypocretin-mediated facilitation of forebrain arousal centers, waking periods are truncated, resulting in the sleepiness of narcolepsy.[200]

The functions of hypocretin have been investigated in knockout animals that do not have the peptide and in their wild-type littermates, using operant reinforcement tasks. Hypocretin knockout mice are deficient in the performance of bar presses to secure food or water reinforcement. However, they do not differ from their normal littermates in their performance when trained to bar press to avoid foot shock. Periods of poor performance on the positive reinforcement tasks are characterized by EEG deactivation.[201] This deficit is restricted to the light phase, suggesting that hypocretin neurons mediate the arousing and mood-elevating effects of light,[201] effects that are central to an understanding of depression. Fos labeling of normal littermates showed that the positive reinforcement task used in this study is characterized by activation of hypocretin neurons. However, hypocretin neurons are not activated in the negative reinforcement task or during the same positively motivated task in the dark phase, despite high levels of EEG activation, indicating that non-hypocretin systems mediate arousal during these behaviors.

The conclusions of these animal studies were extended in the first study of hypocretin release within the human brain. It was found that hypocretin levels are maximal during positive emotion, social interaction, and anger, factors that induce cataplexy in humans with narcolepsy. This is consistent with the hypothesis that release of hypocretin facilitates motor activity during emotionally charged activities of the sort that trigger cataplexy in narcoleptics.[200,202,203] Even neurologically normal individuals experience weakness at these times, seen in the "doubling over" that often accompanies laughter or the weakness that can result from other sudden-onset, strong emotions. In the absence of the hypocretin-mediated motor facilitation of locus coeruleus and other brainstem regions, muscle tone is lost at these times. In contrast, the release in humans of melanin-concentrating hormone, a peptide produced by neurons intermixed in the hypothalamus with the hypocretin neurons, is minimal during social interaction but is increased after eating. Both peptides are at minimal levels during periods of postoperative pain despite high levels of arousal. Melanin-concentrating hormone levels increase at sleep onset, consistent with a role in sleep induction,[204] whereas hypocretin-1 levels increase at wake onset, consistent with a role in wake induction. Levels of these two peptides in humans are not simply linked to arousal but rather to specific emotions and state transitions[165] (Figure 8.14).

The findings that hypocretin is released and hypocretin neurons are active only during arousal linked to certain emotions suggest a new approach to the understanding of arousal systems. Hypocretin is clearly related to arousal linked to certain, generally positive emotions. Other arousal systems must mediate arousal during aversive situations. An analysis of the

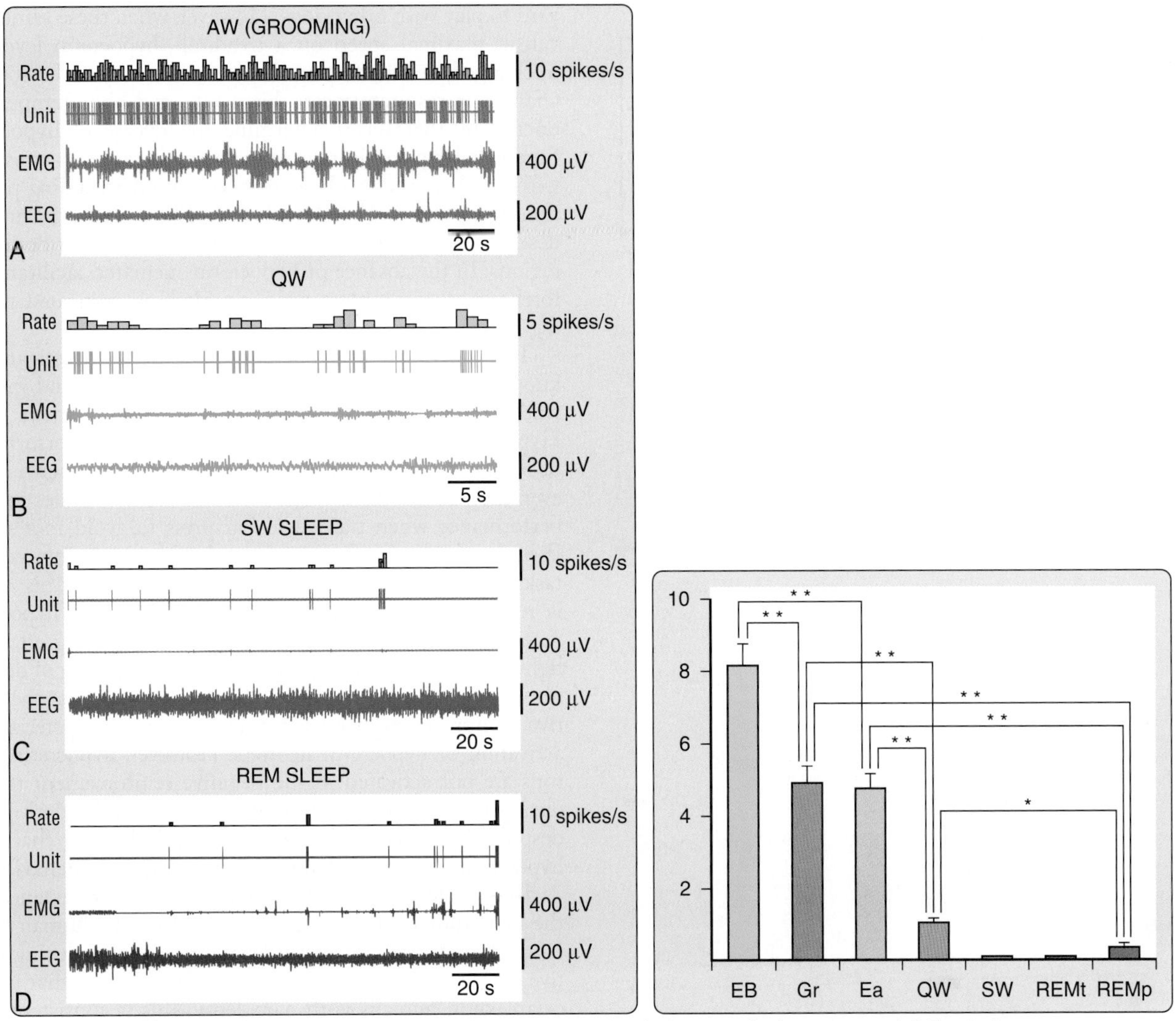

Figure 8.13 Firing rate of hypocretin cells in waking and sleep behaviors in freely moving rats. *Left,* The discharge pattern of a representative hypocretin neuron across the sleep-waking cycle in the freely moving rat. **A,** High firing rates are seen during AW (active waking-grooming). **B,** Reduced firing rate or cessation of activity is seen in QW (quiet waking) and drowsiness. **C,** A further decrease or cessation of firing is seen during SW sleep. **D,** Minimal firing rate is seen during the tonic phase of REM sleep. Brief hematocrit (Hcrt) cell discharge bursts are correlated with muscle twitches during the phasic events of REM sleep. *Right,* Summary data from identified Hcrt cells: exploratory behavior (EB), grooming (Gr), eating (Ea), quiet waking (QW), slow wave (SW) sleep, and tonic (REMt) and phasic (REMp) sleep. Maximal discharge is seen during exploration-approach behavior. (From Mileykovskiy BY, Kiyashchenko LI, Siegel JM. Behavioral correlates of activity in identified hypocretin [orexin] neurons. *Neuron.* 2005;46:787–98.)

differential activation of arousal systems as a function of emotion, light level, and other variables may provide important clinical and basic science insights into the unique roles of each arousal system.

Continued work with human narcolepsy requires brains of human "controls" to determine the correlates of narcolepsy. My research team encountered what we thought would be a control human brain, but when we counted its hypocretin neurons, we were startled to discover that the brain had 54% more than the average in control brains. The hypocretin neurons were substantially smaller than in other human "control" brains. We discovered that this individual was a heroin addict. We then acquired additional brains of opiate addicts and discovered the same pattern. We conducted studies in mice and found that chronic, but not acute, morphine administration produced the same changes seen in human opiate addicts and that chronic opiate administration could reduce or eliminate symptoms of narcolepsy in an animal model of narcolepsy as well as in humans with narcolepsy.[32,205,206] In a follow-up study, a similar increase in the number of hypocretin neurons was found in cocaine-addicted rats, suggesting that this change in hypocretin neurons is a more general correlate of addiction.

Hypocretin appears to act largely by modulating the release of amino acid neurotransmitters.[207] Systemic injection of hypocretin causes a release of glutamate in certain hypocretin-innervated regions, producing a potent postsynaptic excitation.[175,208] In other regions it facilitates GABA release, producing postsynaptic inhibition.[199,209] The loss of these competing inhibitory and facilitatory influences in narcolepsy appears to leave brain motor regulatory and arousal systems less stable than the tightly regulated balance that can be maintained in the presence of hypocretin (Figure 8.15). According to this hypothesis, this loss of stability is the underlying

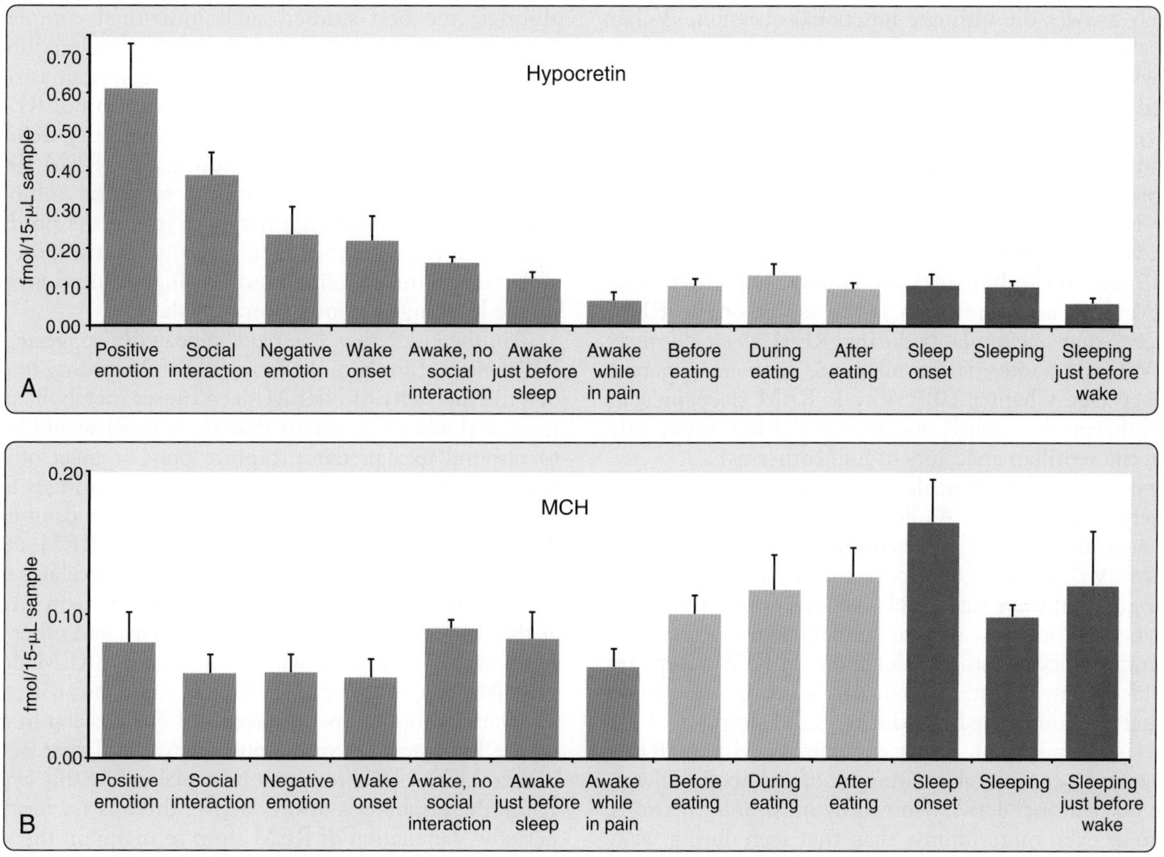

Figure 8.14 Hypocretin (Hcrt) and melanin-concentrating hormone (MCH) levels across waking and sleep activities in humans. **A,** Maximal Hcrt levels in waking are seen during positive emotions, social interactions, and awakening; minimal levels are seen before sleep and in alert waking, while reporting pain. Changes during and after eating are smaller than those during monitored non–eating-related activities. Waking values in *shades of green*, sleep values in *shades of blue*. Awake indicates samples in which subjects were awake but were not exhibiting social interaction or reporting emotion. **B,** Maximal MCH levels are seen at sleep onset and after eating. Minimal levels are seen during wake onset, social interaction, and pain. Error bars represent ±s.e.m. (From Blouin AM, Fried I, Wilson CL, et al. Human hypocretin and melanin-concentrating hormone levels are linked to emotion and social interaction. *Nat Commun*. 2013;4:1547. doi:10.1038/ncomms2461.:1547)

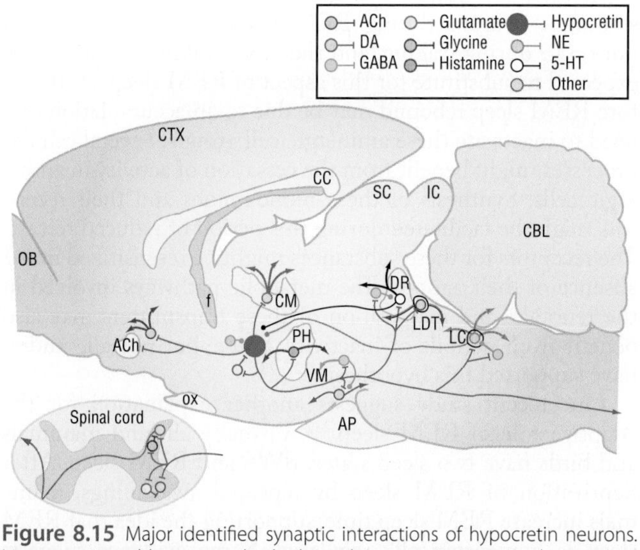

Figure 8.15 Major identified synaptic interactions of hypocretin neurons. Lines terminated by perpendicular lines denote excitation; circular terminations indicate inhibition. 5-HT, 5-hydroxytryptamine; ACh, acetylcholine; AP, anterior pituitary; CBL, cerebellum; CC, corpus callosum; CM, centromedian nucleus of the thalamus; CTX, cortex; DA, dopamine; DR, dorsal raphe; f, fornix; GABA, gamma-aminobutyric acid; IC, inferior colliculus; LC, locus coeruleus; LDT, laterodorsal tegmental and pedunculopontine; NE, norepinephrine; OB, olfactory bulb; OX, optic chiasm; PH, posterior hypothalamus; SC, superior colliculus; VM, ventral midbrain.

cause of narcolepsy, with the result being inappropriate loss of muscle tone in waking and inappropriate increases of muscle tone during sleep, resulting in a striking increased incidence of REM sleep behavior disorder in humans with narcolepsy. In the same manner, although a principal symptom of narcolepsy is intrusions of sleep into the waking period, individuals with narcolepsy sleep poorly at night, with frequent awakenings.[210-212] In other words, those with narcolepsy are not simply weaker and sleepier than normals. Rather, their muscle tone and sleep-waking state regulation is less stable than that in neurologically normal individuals as a result of the loss of hypocretin function.

THE FUNCTIONS OF RAPID EYE MOVEMENT SLEEP

Research into the control of REM sleep turns into a seemingly infinite regression, with REM-on cells inhibited by REM-off cells, which in turn may be inhibited by other REM-on cells. It is very difficult to identify the sequence in which these cell groups are normally activated because the axonal condition and synaptic delays could not be more than a few milliseconds between these cell groups, yet REM sleep onset occurs over a period of minutes in humans and cats and at least 30 or more seconds in the rat. It also does not completely answer the ultimate functional question, "What is REM sleep for?" Answering this question requires determining what, if any, physiologic process is altered over REM sleep periods. Is some toxin excreted[213] or some protein synthesized? If so, how do we account for the widely varying durations of the typical REM sleep? In humans, REM sleep typically lasts from 5 to 30 minutes, whereas in mice it typically lasts 90 seconds.[214] What can be accomplished in 90 seconds in the mouse but requires an average of approximately 15 minutes in humans? The biologic need that initiates REM sleep is unknown, as is the source or the REM sleep "debt" that accumulates during REM sleep deprivation.[215] Why do some marine mammals have no apparent REM sleep (see Chapter 10)? Why is REM sleep present in homeotherms (i.e., birds and mammals) but apparently absent in the reptilian ancestors of homeotherms?

Great progress has been made in localizing the mechanisms that generate REM sleep. As described previously, many of the key neurotransmitters and neurons involved are known. The discovery of the role of hypocretin in narcolepsy serves as a reminder that there may still be key cell groups that must be identified before we can gain fundamental insights into the generation mechanism and functions of REM sleep. Yet despite this caveat, a substantial amount is already understood about what goes on in the brain during REM sleep.

What is clear is that increased brain activity in REM sleep consumes considerable amounts of metabolic energy. The intense neuronal activity shown by most brain neurons, similar to or even more intense than that seen during waking, extracts a price in terms of energy consumption and "wear and tear" on the brain. It is unlikely that such a state would have produced a Darwinian advantage and remained so ubiquitous among mammals if it did not have benefits compensating for its obvious costs. But what might these benefits be?

One idea that has received much media attention is that REM sleep has an important role in memory consolidation. However, the evidence for this is poor.[216] Although early animal work suggested that REM sleep deprivation interfered with learning, subsequent studies showed that it was the stress of the REM sleep–deprivation procedure rather than the REM sleep loss itself that was critical.[217] A leading proponent of a sleep and memory consolidation relationship has concluded that sleep has no role in the consolidation of declarative memory,[218] which would exclude a role for sleep in rote memory, language memory, and conceptual memory, leaving only the possibility of a role in procedural memory, the sort of memory required for learning to ride a bicycle or play a musical instrument. However, studies supporting a role for sleep in the consolidation of human procedural learning have made contradictory claims about similar learning tasks, with some concluding that REM but not NREM sleep is important, others stating just the reverse, yet still others claiming that both sleep states are essential.[216] Millions of humans have taken monoamine oxidase inhibitors or tricyclic antidepressants, often for 10 to 20 years. These drugs profoundly depress or in many cases completely eliminate all detectable aspects of REM sleep.[216,219] However, there is not a single report of memory deficits attributable to such treatment. Likewise, well-studied individuals with permanent loss of REM sleep resulting from pontine damage show normal learning abilities; the best-studied such individual completed law school after his injury[220] and was the puzzle editor of his city newspaper. Humans with multiple system atrophy can have a complete loss of SWS and disruption of REM sleep without manifesting any substantial memory deficit.[221] A recent well-controlled study showed that REM sleep suppression with selective serotonin reuptake inhibitors or serotonin-norepinephrine reuptake inhibitors produced no significant decrement in memory consolidation on any task and even produced a small but significant improvement in a motor learning (i.e., procedural) task.[219]

Another idea that has been repeatedly suggested is that REM sleep stimulates the brain.[222-224] According to this theory, the inactivity of NREM sleep causes metabolic processes to slow down to an extent that the animal would be unable to respond to a predator, capture prey, or meet other challenges upon awakening. This would leave mammals functioning like reptiles, with slow response after periods of inactivity. This hypothesis explains the appearance of REM sleep after NREM sleep under most conditions. It also explains the well-documented increased proportion of sleep time in REM sleep as the sleep period nears its end in humans and other animals. Humans are more alert when aroused from REM sleep than NREM sleep, as are rats,[225] which is consistent with this idea. The very low amounts or absence of REM sleep in dolphins whose brainstem is continuously active and that never have bilateral EEG synchrony can be explained by this hypothesis. If one hemisphere is always active, there is no need for the periodic stimulation of REM sleep to maintain the ability to respond rapidly. However, the brain stimulation hypothesis of REM sleep function does not explain why waking cannot substitute for REM sleep in terrestrial mammals. REM sleep–deprived individuals have a REM sleep rebound even if they are kept in an active waking state for extended periods, although this may be a result of stress rather than REM sleep loss.[217]

One phenomenon that may explain REM sleep rebound is the cessation of activity of histamine, norepinephrine, and serotonin neurons during REM sleep. This cessation does not occur during waking, and therefore waking would not be expected to substitute for this aspect of REM sleep.[226] Therefore REM sleep rebound may be due to an accumulation of a need to inactivate these aminergic cell groups. Several cellular processes might benefit from the cessation of activity in aminergic cells. Synthesis of these monoamines and their receptors might be facilitated during this period of reduced release. The receptors for these substances might be resensitized in the absence of their agonist. The metabolic pathways involved in the reuptake and inactivation of these transmitters may also benefit from periods of inactivity. Some, but not all, studies have supported this hypothesis.[227-231]

Our recent study suggests another explanation for the adaptive role of REM sleep.[232] Virtually all land mammals and birds have two sleep states: SWS and REM sleep. After deprivation of REM sleep by repeated awakenings, mammals increase REM sleep time, supporting the idea that REM sleep is homeostatically regulated. Some evidence suggests that periods of REM sleep deprivation for a week or more cause physiologic dysfunction and eventual death. However, separating the effects of REM sleep loss from the accompanying NREM sleep loss and the stress of repeated awakening is difficult. The northern fur seal (*Callorhinus ursinus*) is

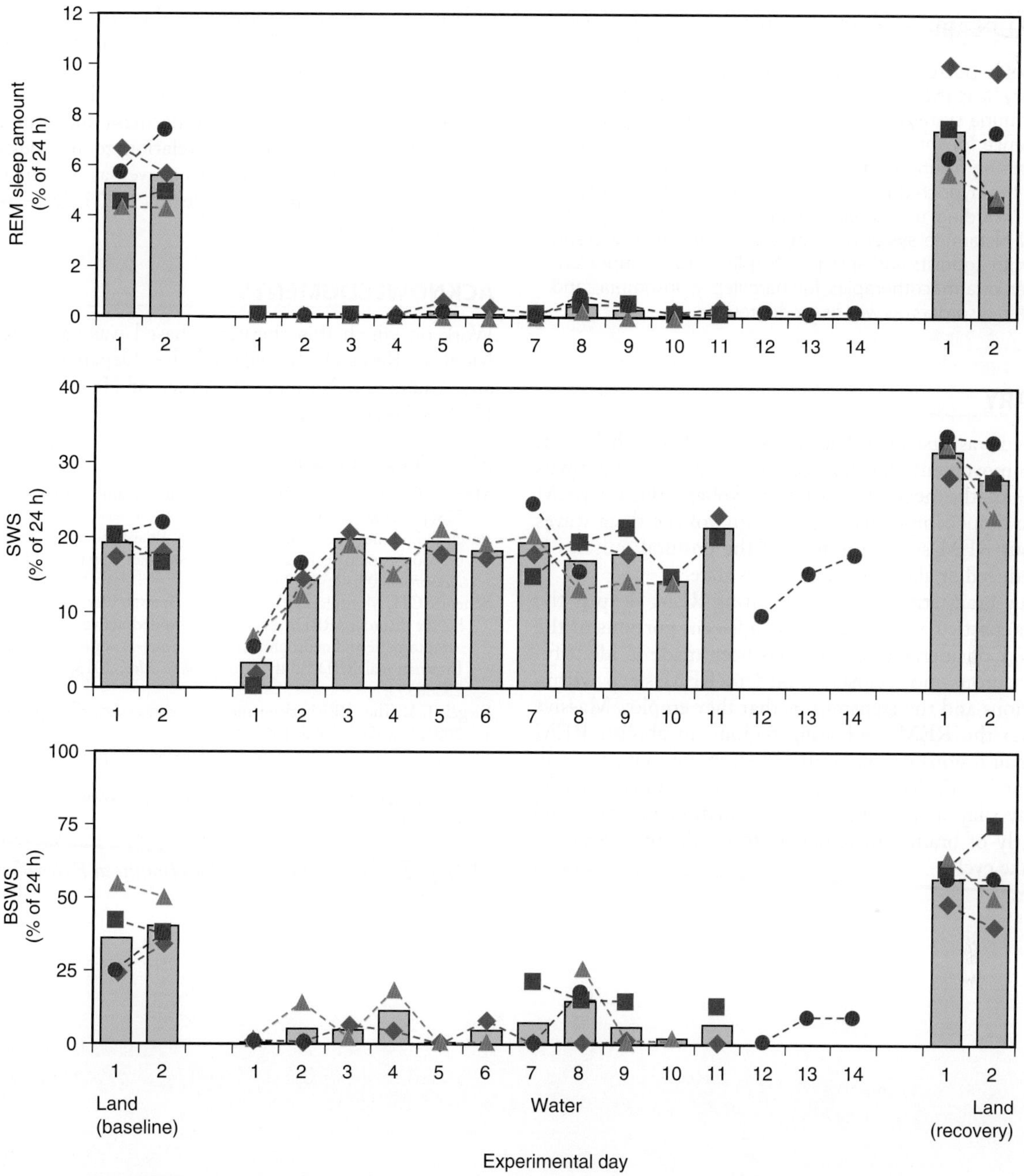

Figure 8.16 REM sleep is suppressed when fur seals are in seawater for 14 days, with little or no rebound when returned to baseline conditions "Land." When in water, bilateral NREM sleep is suppressed, as in the dolphin, which never has bilateral NREM sleep. Dolphins also never have REM sleep (see Chapter 10). Fur seals spend at least 7 months a year in water. Unilateral slow wave sleep (SWS) persists in water also as in the dolphin. The *colored lines and symbols* mark individual seals, and the *light green bars* indicate the average values. BSWS, Bilateral slow wave sleep. (See Oleg I, Lyamin PO, Kosenko, SMet al. Fur seals suppress REM sleep for very long periods without subsequent rebound. *Current Biology*. 18;28(12):2000-2005.e2.)

a semiaquatic mammal. It can sleep on land and in seawater. The fur seal is unique in showing both the bilateral SWS seen in most mammals and the asymmetric sleep previously reported in cetaceans. We find that when the fur seal stays in seawater, where it spends most of its life, it goes without or greatly reduces REM sleep for days or weeks (Figure 8.16). After this nearly complete elimination of REM, it displays minimal or no REM rebound upon returning to baseline conditions. It is well established that brain temperature decreases in NREM sleep and increases in REM sleep.[232,233] Our data are consistent with the hypothesis that REM sleep, by the increase in brainstem neuronal activity described earlier, may reverse the reduced brain temperature and metabolic effects of bilateral NREM sleep, a state that is greatly reduced when the fur seal is in the seawater,[232] rather than REM sleep being directly homeostatically regulated. This can explain the absence of REM sleep in the dolphin and other cetaceans that never have bilateral NREM sleep and its increasing proportion as the end of the sleep period approaches in humans and other mammals.

CLINICAL PEARL

The loss of hypocretin neurons is responsible for most human narcolepsy. It is thought that this cell loss may be the result of an immune system attack on these neurons, but convincing evidence for this is lacking. Administration of hypocretin is a promising future avenue for the treatment of narcolepsy. Because the hypocretin system has potent effects on arousal systems including the norepinephrine, serotonin, acetylcholine, and histamine systems, manipulation of the hypocretin system with agonists and antagonists is likely to be important in further pharmacotherapies for narcolepsy, insomnia, and other sleep disorders, as well as for depression.

SUMMARY

REM sleep was first identified by its most obvious behavior: rapid eye movements during sleep. In most adult mammals the EEG of the neocortex is low in voltage during REM sleep. The hippocampus has regular high-voltage theta waves throughout REM sleep. The tone of the postural muscles is greatly reduced or abolished during this state.

The key brain structure for generating REM sleep is the brainstem, particularly the pons and adjacent portions of the midbrain. Considerable progress has been made in identifying the neurons most closely linked to REM sleep within these regions and the transmitters that they employ. Massive damage to the REM-generating region can abolish REM sleep. Small lesions can cause REM sleep without atonia in animals or REM sleep behavior disorder in humans. REM sleep may play a key role in the regulation of brain and particularly of brainstem temperature regulation across the sleep-wake cycle.

Narcolepsy is characterized by abnormalities in the regulation of REM sleep. Most cases of human narcolepsy are caused by a loss of hypocretin (orexin) neurons, a cell group whose somas are localized in the hypothalamus. Hypocretin neurons have potent effects on alertness and motor control and are normally activated in relation to particular, generally positive emotions in humans as well as in animals. In the absence of this cell group, cataplexy, a REM sleep–like loss of muscle tone, occurs.

ACKNOWLEDGMENTS

Work on which this chapter is based was supported by the Medical Research Service of the Department of Veterans Affairs and National Institutes of Health (NIH) grants HL148574 and DA034748.

SELECTED READINGS

Manger PR, Siegel JM. Do all mammals dream? *J Comp Neurol.* 2020;528(17):3198–3204.

Rasch B, Pommer J, Diekelmann S, Born J. Pharmacological REM sleep suppression paradoxically improves rather than impairs skill memory. *Nat Neurosci.* 2009;12:396–397.

Schenck CH, Montplaisir JY, Frauscher B, et al. Oertel W· REM Sleep behavior disorder (RBD): devising controlled active treatment studies for symptomatic and neuroprotective therapy—A consensus statement by the International RBD Study Group. *Sleep Med.* 2013;14:795–806. PMID: 23886593.

Siegel JM. The REM sleep-memory consolidation hypothesis. *Science.* 2001;294(5544):1058–1063.

Siegel JM. Clues to the functions of mammalian sleep. *Nature.* 2005;437:1264–1271.

Further relevant literature can be found at http://www.semel.ucla.edu/sleep-research.

A complete reference list can be found online at ExpertConsult.com.

Chapter 9

Deep-Brain Imaging of Brain Neurons and Glia during Sleep

Priyattam J. Shiromani; Aurelio Vidal-Ortiz; Carlos Blanco-Centurion

Chapter Highlights

- In the influenza pandemic of 1918, von Economo identified specific brain regions regulating sleep and wake. Since then there has been a progressive use of better tools that have defined the circuitry underlying sleep and wake.
- New tools have validated existing data, corrected errors, and made new discoveries to advance science. The brain is a challenge, but new tools can disentangle the brain network.
- The newest tool is a miniature microscope that provides an unprecedented view of activity of glia and neurons in freely behaving mice. The data from deep-brain imaging of brain cells identifies activity at the cellular level in normal versus diseased brains and in response to specific hypnotics.

One goal of neuroscience is to pinpoint the neurons responsible for specific behaviors, because by identifying specific circuits, it will then be possible to correct abnormal behavior. In the area of sleep neurobiology, this involves identifying neurons responsible for waking and non–rapid eye movement (NREM) and rapid eye movement (REM) sleep. Researchers have used conventional neuroscience tools, such as transections, lesions, cell recordings, c-FOS, and track-tracing methodologies, to identify neuronal populations regulating waking and NREM, and REM sleep. These studies have helped derive a first-order circuit map of neurons involved in regulating sleep and wake (Figure 9.1). However, conventional tools have fundamental limitations and can only accomplish so much to answer key questions. To disentangle brain circuits that regulate specific behaviors, such as sleep, requires new technology. In the last 10 years, new genetically engineered tools have been developed, and we refer the reader to a review paper by Shiromani and Peever that described these tools and how they could be used to identify the circuit underlying sleep.[1]

This chapter focuses on live-cell imaging of cells, a method that makes it possible to image activity of individual neurons and glia deep within the brains of freely behaving animals. The method enables real-time monitoring of activity of individual neurons and glia across conditions and over many days to months. From the dataset, it is possible to map the activity of the cells and to test hypotheses regarding normal versus abnormal activity in the network. The network map can be used to identify abnormal activity and normal network traffic restored by repairing defective nodes in the circuit using the gene transfer approach or with optogenetic stimulation.

THE DEEP-BRAIN IMAGING METHOD

Currently, the electroencephalogram (EEG) is used to record activity of the brain, and the EEG machine still represents the cornerstone of all sleep laboratories. However, the EEG measures activity at the cortical surface but does not reveal anything about activity in individual cells at the subcortical levels. A new method has been developed that images activity of individual cells deep within the brains of freely behaving mice and rats.[2] The images are captured with a miniature single-photon microscope (Inscopix.com, Palo Alto, California), also referred to as a miniscope, that sits atop the animal's head (Figure 9.2). The miniscope connects to a microendoscope that penetrates the brain. The microendoscope is a glass lens, referred to as a GRIN lens (Gradient-Index; ThorLabs, Newton, New Jersey), that focuses the images of the underlying cells onto the miniscope. The miniscope captures changes in intracellular levels of calcium ions (Ca^{2+}).[3,4] Special genetically tagged sensors, referred to as green fluorescent-calmodulin protein-s (GCaMPs), fluoresce as a function of the rise in intracellular Ca^{2+} levels, and the miniscope is able to capture the change in fluorescence. At rest the cells containing the GCaMP will exhibit a basal fluorescent signal. However, when a cell (astrocyte or neuron) is excited, there is an increase in the levels of Ca^{2+} inside the cells, causing an increase in the intensity of the fluorescence. The change in intensity of the fluorescent signal can be empirically determined (df/f) and reflects the activity of the cell.[5] It has been established that the fluorescence is linked to depolarization of the neuron.[8] In our studies we have confirmed that Ca^{2+} fluorescence is directly linked to action potentials.[6] New genetically encoded Ca^{2+} indicators

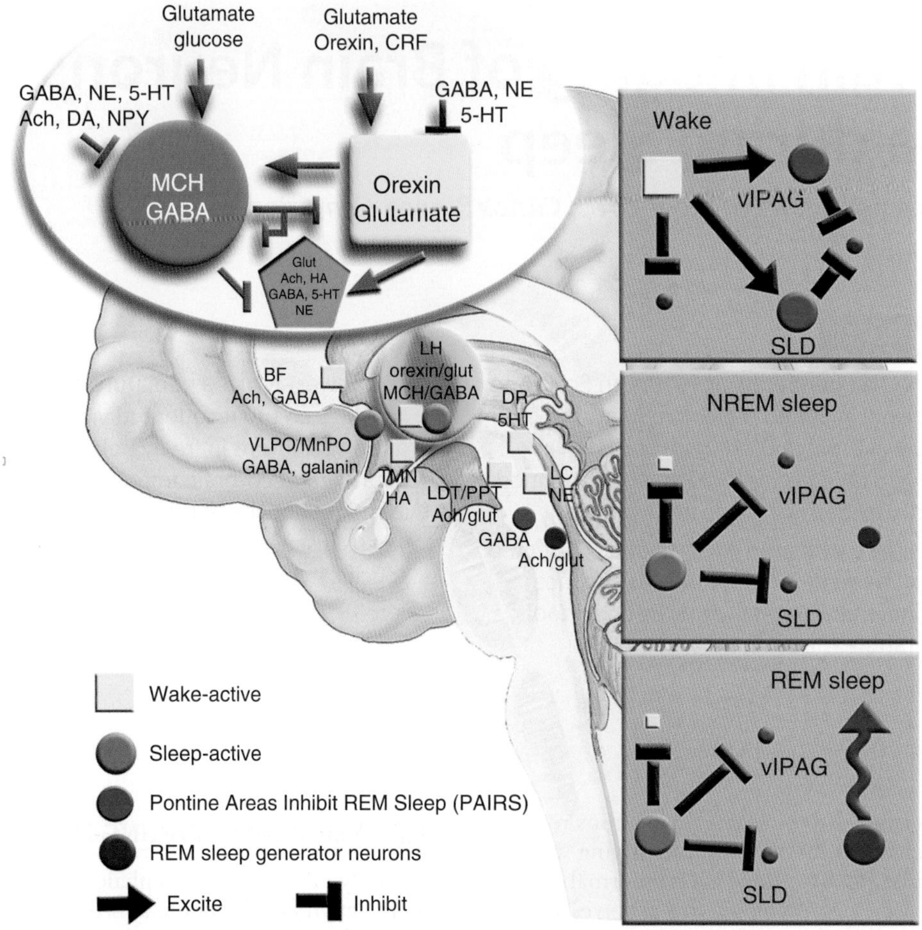

Figure 9.1 A distributed network of neurons regulating waking, NREM and REM sleep derived from lesion, electrophysiology and c-FOS studies. *New tools can further refine the model.* Ach, Acetylcholine; BF, basal forebrain; CRF, corticotrophin releasing factor; DA, dopamine; DR, dorsal raphe; GABA, gamma-aminobutyric acid; glut, glutamate; HA, histamine; 5-HT, serotonin; LC, locus coeruleus; LDT, laterodorsal tegmental; LH, lateral hypothalamus; MnPO, median preoptic area; NE, norepinephrine; NPY, neuropeptide Y; NREM, non–rapid eye movement; PPT, pedunculopontine; REM, rapid eye movement; SLD, sublateral dorsal nucleus; TMN, tuberomammillary nucleus; vlPAG, ventral lateral periaqueductal grey; VLPO, ventrolateral preoptic.

are available from commercial vendors to measure Ca^{2+} influx in astrocytes[7] and neurons.[8]

To image a specific phenotype of neurons or glia, adeno-associated virus-DJ (AAVDJ)-EF1a-DIO-GCaMP6m is injected into the target site in the brains of mice that express cycle recombinase (Cre) (Figure 9.3). Mice that express the Cre in specific phenotypes of neurons or glia are available (Jax.org). The mice are anesthetized (isofluorane: 2% to 3% continuous gas) and placed in a stereotaxic instrument. The AAV particles are slowly injected into the target site with a microliter syringe (usually 0.2-to 1-μL volume). A GRIN lens is inserted at the microinjection site and the baseplate cemented onto the skull. At this time EEG and electromyogram electrodes are attached to the skull, and the entire assembly is secured with dental cement (see reference 6 for details). The mice are returned to their home cages and allowed to recover for 21 days from the surgery. This time period also enables the GCaMP6 to be expressed in the Cre-positive cells at the injection site, and the cells begin to fluoresce as a function of the change in intracellular levels of Ca^{2+}.[8]

A typical experiment begins with a 3-day adaptation period that allows the animals to acclimate to the sleep recording cables and the miniscope. During the adaptation period, the focusing on the miniscope is adjusted to obtain the sharpest images of the fluorescence in the somata. The focal plane can be adjusted up to 300 μm by manually turning the miniscope. In the newest model, the focusing is motorized (Inscopix.com). The position of the miniscope that gives the sharpest images is noted, and all imaging for that mouse is done at that position. It is possible to adjust the focal plane so that other neurons become visible. This makes it possible to image many more neurons along the dorsal-ventral focal plane. An experimental session consists of recording sleep and fluorescence images through a number of wake and NREM cycles. The images can be recorded while the animal is engaged in various tasks (feeding, grooming, locomotor activity) over a period of days. Thus the same neurons can be imaged longitudinally, allowing for pre-postexperiments. Upon completion of the experimental paradigm, postmortem histology is done to confirm the presence of the

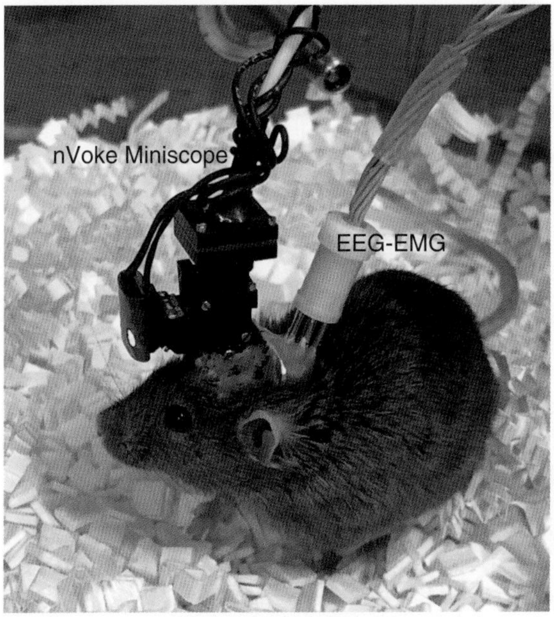

Figure 9.2 A mouse with an implanted nVoke miniscope (Inscopix.com) and electrodes to record sleep. A single-photon minimicroscope weighing 2 g can be securely attached to the skull along with electrodes to record sleep. The miniscope images the activity of individual neurons or glia deep within the brains of freely behaving mice, allowing investigators to determine network activity of specific neurons or glia during sleep-wake states. EEG, electroencephalogram; EMG, electromyogram.

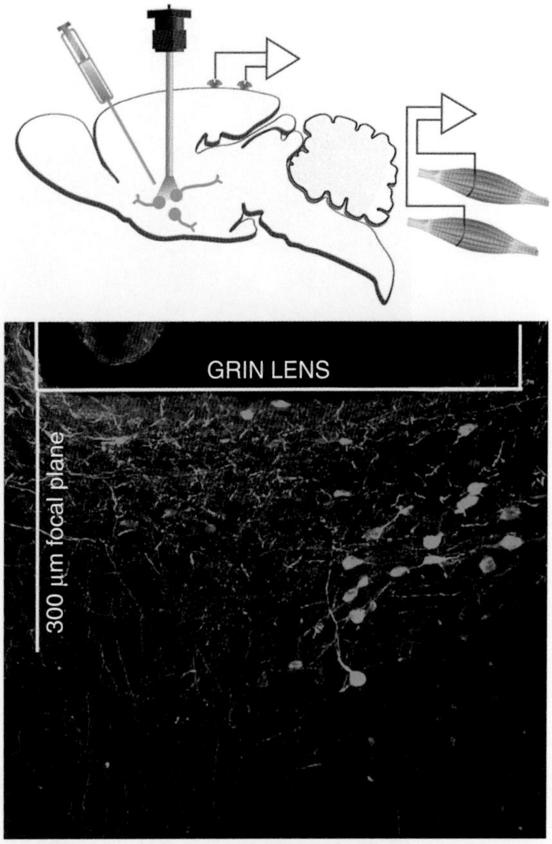

Figure 9.3 Neurons containing the calcium indicator, green fluorescence calmodulin protein-6 (GCaMP6), relative to the focal plane of the GRIN lens. The *top* figure schematically depicts that a microinjection of adenoassociated virus-DJ (AAVDJ)-EF1a-DIO-GCaMP6m is made to express GCaMP6 in cells that are cycle recombinase positive. At the same time, a GRIN lens (600-μm diameter) is inserted into the brain along with electrodes to record the electroencephalogram and electromyogram. Three weeks after injection, a miniscope is attached to image the fluorescence associated with the intracellular changes in calcium. *Bottom* figure is the postmortem histology depicting many GCaMP6-containing neurons below the lens.

GCaMP6-containing neurons within the focal plane of the GRIN lens (Figure 9.3).

The data consists of video images captured by the miniscope, and it is stored on high-capacity storage disks (typically 1-terabyte solid-state drives). A high-end computer workstation with a powerful video graphics processor is necessary to analyze the video images. The data processing is done offline using specialized software (Mosaic) supplied by Inscopix, the vendor of the miniscopes. Mosaic is compatible with MathLab (MathWorks Natick, Massachusetts), and it allows the data to be exported so that it can be integrated with the sleep data (Neuroexplorer.com, Colorado Springs, Colorado).

Next, we summarize the sequential stages of data analysis. The raw image file is downsampled (antialiasing; 2×), fixed for defective pixels, row noise, and isolated dropped frames, if any. The clean images are then corrected for motion artifacts resulting from the animal's respiration (along the *x* and *y* axes). If a miniscope is not attached properly, then there will be severe motion artifacts, and it is best to discard the data. The motion-corrected images are further cleaned with a band-pass filter, and then a reference fluorescence (F0) frame is determined. All of the frames in the dataset are compared against the reference frame by principal component analysis (PCA), followed by an independent component analysis (ICA). The PCA-ICA yields a defined region of interest (ROI) representing fluorescent cells. If a ROI clearly indicates that it represents two adjacent cells, topographic segregation of Ca^{2+} signals is achieved by manually drawing the respective ROI. We emphasize that it is necessary to obtain clear fluorescent signals at the time of data collection, and this can be done by focusing the miniscope. The investigator will have to conduct preliminary studies to identify the concentration and volume of AAV-GCaMP that yields the clearest signal. Inscopix (Inscopix.com) is now providing GRIN lenses with the AAV-GCaMP coated onto the lens.

The change in fluorescence (ΔF) is computed as follows: ΔF = current fluorescence (F) at pixel (*x*, *y*) minus F0 at pixel (*x*, *y*) divided by F0 at pixel (*x*, *y*). The dataset is normalized (Z scores), and the change in fluorescence in individual ROIs is plotted over time (usually in seconds) and correlated with sleep or other behaviors. Figure 9.4 summarizes the final product of the data analysis. The ROI representing the neurons are clearly visible within the field of view of the GRIN lens (Figure 9.4, *A* and *C*). The change in fluorescence in each ROI can be tracked and plotted along with the sleep-wake states (Figure 9.4, *B* and *D*).

The same set of cells can be tracked during different conditions or treatments, which allows investigators to determine the activity of the cell over many days to months. Indeed, this a major advantage of live imaging. Electrophysiology can record activity of single neurons, but it is extremely labor intensive, slow, and it cannot selectively identify the exact phenotype of the recorded neuron. On the other hand, with live-cell imaging a researcher can now "watch" the activity of individual and populations of neurons of known phenotypic origin and rapidly determine its role in behavior. This

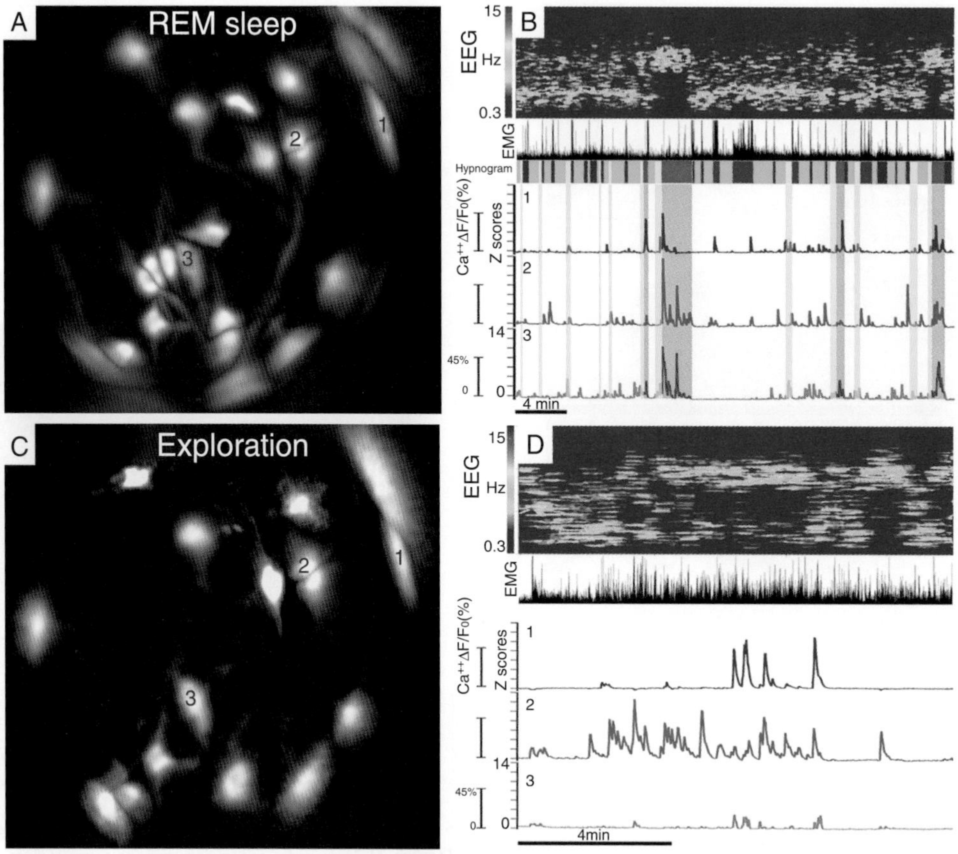

Figure 9.4 Calcium fluorescence in individual melanin-concentrating hormone (MCH) neurons. **(A)** and **(C)** depict the same field of view of the GRIN lens with fluorescence (Δ*F/F0*) in somata and processes extracted automatically by principle component analysis-independent component analysis (PCA-ICA) analysis. We have labeled the three neurons (labeled 1, 2, and 3) whose Ca^{2+} fluorescence is plotted in **(B)** and **(D). (A)** depicts green fluorescent calmodulin protein-6s (GCaMP6s) fluorescence (Δ*F/F0*) in MCH neurons during REM sleep. Ca^{2+} imaging was performed simultaneously with recording of cortical EEG and EMG activity in the nuchal muscles. Behavioral video recordings were obtained and examined to identify behaviors such as walking, eating, grooming, or eating. Activity in the EEG (depicted as power spectra, 0.3 to 15 Hz) and the EMG is used to identify wake, NREM, and REM sleep states (labeled as hypnogram). The traces depict the change in fluorescence *(ΔF/F0)* during wake–sleep bouts of the three neurons identified in **A.** In each neuron, the *ΔF/F0* (expressed as a Z-score) varies with the wake-sleep state of the animal, with peak fluorescence associated with REM sleep. The hypnogram categorizes the sleep-wake states in the following colors: *purple,* active wake; *blue,* quiet wake; *green,* NREM sleep; *yellow,* pre-REM sleep; *red,* REM sleep. **C** is the same field of view as in **(A),** but this image shows the PCA-ICA extracted neurons (ΔF/F0) while the mouse was engaged in exploring novel objects placed in its home cage. This image shows that some neurons that were evident in REM sleep **(A)** were also activated during exploratory behavior. However, some neurons in **(A)** were not evident during exploratory behavior, indicating selective activation of these neurons during REM sleep **(A).** Thirty percent of the neurons were activated during REM sleep but not during exploratory behavior, indicating that a subset of MCH neurons is selectively active in REM sleep. **D,** GCaMP6s fluorescence in MCH neurons while exploring novel objects. The traces are from the same neurons represented in REM sleep **(A).** EEG, Electroencephalogram; EMG, electromyogram; NREM, non–rapid eye movement; REM, rapid eye movement. (For further details, see Blanco-Centurion and colleagues.[6])

method was used to settle the question of the activity pattern of neurons containing melanin-concentrating hormone (MCH).[6] An electrophysiologic study in head-restrained rats had sampled activity of MCH neurons and concluded that the neurons were active only during REM sleep.[9] This result remained unchallenged until we used the deep-brain imaging method and found that 70% of the MCH neurons were also active during periods of exploratory behavior during waking.[6] Another study confirmed the results.[10] Activity of glutamatergic (Vglut2-IRES-Cre mice),[11] gamma-aminobutyric acid (GABA) (gad2-IRES-Cre mice),[12,13] galanin,[14] and neurotensin[15] neurons has been imaged during sleep.[16] Glia are also being imaged during sleep (laboratory of Marcos G. Frank[16a]). With the deep-brain imaging method, hitherto unknown neuronal populations regulating sleep have been identified.[17]

CALCIUM IMAGING IDENTIFIES NETWORK ACTIVATION

The group at University California-Berkeley was the first to use the deep-brain imaging method to monitor activity of neurons during sleep (see reference 17, for example). We were next and imaged the MCH neurons.[6] In contrast to others, we see the utility of brain imaging as a tool to identify network activation of specific circuits (Figure 9.5). By monitoring network activity in specific regions, it is possible to determine the pattern

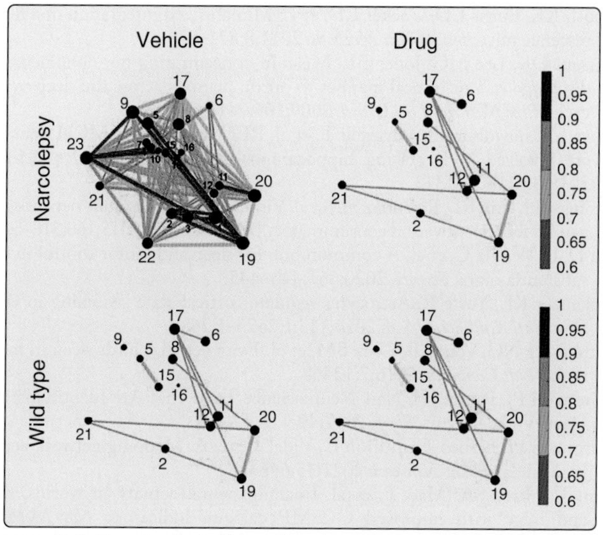

Figure 9.5 Hypothetical effect of a drug on network activity of sleep-inducing neurons in a mouse model of narcolepsy. The *circles* represent neurons that increase Ca^{2+} fluorescence during sleep. The size of the *circles* and the *lines* between the neurons identifies the strength of the fluorescence between pairs of neurons. In narcolepsy (vehicle) the sleep network has a hyperactive pattern of activity that leads to sleep fragmentation and narcoleptic behavior. The drug reduces network activity so that it is similar to that seen in normal wild-type animals.

of activity as the sleep-inducing signal propagates across the brain. Such a brain activity map is essential to understanding how the brain shifts between states of consciousness and what causes sleep disorders. As noted earlier, a distributed network of neurons has been found to generate waking, NREM sleep, and REM sleep. The chemical signature and connectivity of these neurons is also known. The next step is to determine the time course of a signal between these neuronal populations. This will yield a temporal and spatial map of signaling across the brain as the waking brain falls asleep. Which population is affected first? Which population is the last to receive the sleep signal? What is the temporal response of specific sleep versus wake neurons to the stimulation and to the emergence of sleep? What is the temporal response between glia and neurons? Such information is necessary to identify circuits and nodes that are key to sleep. These can then be targeted with hypnotics to facilitate sleep.

During the Ebola virus crisis, cell-phone data and activity on social networking sites was used to derive temporal and spatial maps of spread of disease. Indeed, in the current COVID-19 pandemic, cell-phone signals are used to track individuals and the spread of disease. We believe that for the first time it is possible to derive point-to-point activity maps of the brain as it falls asleep. Activity in small networks can differentiate patients in a minimally conscious state compared to a vegetative state/unresponsive wakefulness syndrome.[18,19] In other words, functional activity in small networks can identify normal versus diseased brains. Most important, pharmacotherapeutics should be able to repair the network and normalize function (Figure 9.5). For decades, pharmaceuticals have corrected cardiac, epileptiform, and other electrical activities in small networks. However, in the area of sleep disorders medicine, there is no data on the effect of pharmacotherapeutics on activity of small sleep networks, even though there are several drugs that are U.S. Food and Drug Administration approved for treatment of narcolepsy.[20] There is a growing impetus to demonstrate effects of these drugs at the cellular level, first in animal models and then in humans. We argue that any drug demonstrating that it normalizes cellular network activity and function will gain advantage.

The deep-brain imaging approach empowers researchers with the ability to identify activity in neural circuits during identified behaviors. For example, this approach is being used to deconstruct the activity of specific neurons during cataplexy. Activity of GABA (identified with the vesicular GABA transporter in vGAT-Cre mice) neurons in the amygdala was imaged in narcoleptic orexin-knockout mice, and it was found that some GABA neurons became active just before the onset of cataplexy.[21] This indicates hyperactivity in a subset of amygdala neurons just before cataplexy. The activity of these neurons can be blocked to show that it also blocks cataplexy. Activity of the MCH neurons in the hypothalamus was found to be unchanged, indicating that these neurons are not triggering the cataplexy.[21a]

It is important to recognize that microendoscopy, like electrophysiology, is a tool that provides descriptive data, and other methods, such as optogenetics or chemogenetics, have to be used to mechanistically drive the circuit to cause the behavioral change. The limitation of the calcium imaging method is that it does not reveal rate or pattern of activity of the imaged neurons. For instance, it cannot reveal whether the imaged neurons fired as single spikes or in clusters. It also lacks millisecond precision that is necessary to identify the time course and sequence of events linked to specific behaviors. The GCaMP6m fluorescence may quench, which makes it necessary to capture the images for short time periods at a given time. However, these limitations are likely to be resolved with faster cameras and more stable dyes.

FUTURE DIRECTIONS

Miniaturized electronic amplifiers and battery-powered devices have made it possible to identify sleep in birds during long periods of flight.[22] A miniature microscope can finally answer questions that have proved to be challenging. The newer miniscopes, referred to as nVoke (Inscopix.com), allow investigators to optogenetically stimulate a cell and image response in the neighboring cell(s). Such a miniscope can stimulate neurons and image activity of adjacent glia, or vice versa, thereby determining how juxtacellular cells influence each other in freely behaving animals. Microendoscopy can also be used to determine with certainty that REM sleep exists in reptiles or that REM sleep is also unihemispheric, like NREM sleep. This can be done quite easily by imaging activity of conserved phenotype of neurons, for example, hypocretin or MCH neurons, to determine whether their activity is directly correlated with REM sleep as in mice.

CLINICAL PEARL

Miniature microscopes have made it possible to monitor activity of cellular circuits regulating specific behaviors, including sleep. Functional activity in small networks can determine normal versus diseased brain, or identify sleep in less sentient species. If network activity is abnormal, pharmacotherapeutics should be able to repair the network and normalize function. Drugs that normalize cellular network activity and function will gain advantage.

SUMMARY

Conventional neuroscience tools, such as lesions, cell recordings, c-Fos, and track-tracing methodologies, have been instrumental in identifying the complex and intermingled populations of sleep- and arousal-promoting neurons that orchestrate and generate wakefulness and NREM and REM sleep. The challenge is to observe activity of specific neurons during specific behaviors. This is now feasible because of the development of a miniature microscope that can peer deep into the brains of freely behaving animals. For the first time, sleep neurobiologists can witness dynamic activation of specific neurons during sleep and identify activity in specific networks in normal versus diseased brains.

ACKNOWLEDGMENT

Priyattam J. Shiromani was supported in part by the Department of Veterans Affairs, Veterans Health Administration, Office of Research Development (BLR&D), and National Institutes of Health grants NS052287 and NS079940.

SELECTED READINGS

Blanco-Centurion C, Luo S, Spergel DJ, et al. Dynamic network activation of hypothalamic MCH neurons in REM sleep and exploratory behavior. *J Neurosci*. 2019;39:4986–4998.

Chen TW, Wardill TJ, Sun Y, et al. Ultrasensitive fluorescent proteins for imaging neuronal activity. *Nature*. 2013;499:295–300.

Flusberg BA, Nimmerjahn A, Cocker ED, et al. High-speed, miniaturized fluorescence microscopy in freely moving mice. *Nat Methods*. 2008;5:935–938.

Ghosh KK, Burns LD, Cocker ED, et al. Miniaturized integration of a fluorescence microscope. *Nat Methods*. 2011;8:871–878.

Hassani OK, Lee MG, Jones BE. Melanin-concentrating hormone neurons discharge in a reciprocal manner to orexin neurons across the sleep-wake cycle. *Proc Natl Acad Sci U S A*. 2009;106:2418–2422.

Izawa S, Chowdhury S, Miyazaki T, et al. REM sleep-active MCH neurons are involved in forgetting hippocampus-dependent memories. *Science*. 2019;365:1308–1313.

Jennings JH, Ung RL, Resendez SL, et al. Visualizing hypothalamic network dynamics for appetitive and consummatory behaviors. *Cell*. 2015;160:516–527.

Liu D, Li W, Ma C, et al. A common hub for sleep and motor control in the substantia nigra. *Science*. 2020;367:440–445.

Poskanzer KE, Yuste R. Astrocytes regulate cortical state switching in vivo. *Proc Natl Acad Sci. U S A*. 2016;113:E2675–E2684.

Rattenborg NC, Voirin B, Cruz SM, et al. Evidence that birds sleep in mid-flight. *Nat Commun*. 2016;7:12468.

Shiromani PJ, Peever JH. New Neuroscience Tools That Are Identifying the Sleep-Wake Circuit. *Sleep*. 2017;40.

Shiromani PJ, Blanco-Centurion C, Vidal-Ortiz A. Mapping network activity in sleep. *Front Neurosci*. 2021;15:646468.

Tian L, Hires SA, Mao T, et al. Imaging neural activity in worms, flies and mice with improved GCaMP calcium indicators. *Nat Methods*. 2009;6:875–881.

Vanini G, Torterolo P. Sleep-wake neurobiology. *Adv Exp Med Biol*. 2021;1297:65-82.

Weber F, Hoang Do JP, Chung S, et al. Regulation of REM and non-REM sleep by periaqueductal GABAergic neurons. *Nat Commun*. 2018;9:354.

Xu M, Chung S, Zhang S, et al. Basal forebrain circuit for sleep-wake control. *Nat Neurosci*. 2015;18:1641–1647.

A complete reference list can be found online at ExpertConsult.com.

Chapter 10

Evolution of Mammalian Sleep

Jerome M. Siegel

Chapter Highlights

- In most adult animals, sleep is incompatible with mating and feeding. Animals seem to be vulnerable to predation during sleep. Why has evolution preserved this state? I conclude that the presence of sleep in nearly all animals and the enormous variation in sleep time across species is best explained as an adaptation to ecological and energy demands.
- Sleep is not a "maladaptive state" that needs to be explained by undiscovered functions (which nevertheless undoubtedly exist). Genetic success is closely linked to the efficient use of resources and to the avoidance of risk. Thus inactivity can reduce injury, and safe sleeping sites reduce predation. Sleep greatly reduces brain and body energy consumption. In the wild, most animals are hungry and are seeking food most of the time they are awake. If ample food is available, the population of a species quickly expands until again faced with food scarcity, a phenomenon that is illustrated by the great increase in the human population in the past century. A "small" energy saving every day produces a big evolutionary advantage.
- Conversely, if food is available but is time consuming to acquire, it is advantageous for animals to reduce sleep time. Similarly, it is advantageous to reduce or eliminate sleep to allow migration and respond to other needs. Many examples of extended periods of elimination or sleep reduction without "rebound" have been documented.
- Many have assumed that predation risk is increased during sleep; that is, that more animals are killed per hour during sleep than during waking. However, there is scant evidence to support this contention. Most animals seek safe sleeping sites, often underground, in trees or in groups that provide communal protection. Those large herbivores that cannot find safe sleeping sites appear to have smaller amounts of sleep and sleep less deeply. Large animals that are not at risk for predation, such as big cats and bears, can sleep for long periods, often in unprotected sites, and appear to sleep deeply.
- Much has been made of mathematical analyses comparing reported sleep time across species with other aspects of comparative each species. For example, total sleep time or REM sleep time is compared with body weight, brain-body weight ratio, and lifespan. The available sleep parameters generally come from studies of animals in controlled environments in laboratories or zoos. Such analyses have been undermined by recent work showing that sleep time varies substantially with season, temperature, migration, age, and breeding phase. Conversely, the constant temperature conditions, complete lack of predatory risk, and ad libitum food and water availability in captivity are almost never experienced in the wild and undoubtedly are major factors controlling the evolution of sleep. A complete understanding of sleep evolution requires analyses of sleep under the actual conditions in which each species evolved and continues to live. Fortunately, advances in electronics now make such studies more practical and will lead to a better understanding of the evolutionary determinants of sleep.
- "Natural" human sleep, as observed in human hunter-gatherers, does not commence at sunset, is not normally interrupted by extended waking periods, is somewhat shorter in duration than that in industrial societies, and shows a nearly 1-hour difference between summer and winter. Napping is not a regular feature of hunter-gatherer sleep, and insomnia is rare.

ADAPTIVE INACTIVITY

Sleep should be viewed in the context of other forms of "adaptive inactivity." Most forms of life have evolved mechanisms that permit the reduction of metabolic activity for long periods of time when conditions are not optimal. In animals, this usually includes a reduction or cessation of movement and sensory response. The development of dormant states was an essential step in the evolution of life and continues to be essential for the preservation of many organisms. Many species have evolved seasonal dormancy or hibernation patterns that allow them to anticipate periods that are not optimal for survival and propagation. In other species dormancy is triggered by environmental conditions. Many organisms spend most of their lifespan in dormancy, becoming active only when conditions are optimal. A continuum of states of adaptive inactivity can be seen across living organisms including plants, unicellular and multicellular animals, and animals with and without nervous systems.[1]

In the plant kingdom, seeds are often dormant until the correct season, heat, moisture, and pH conditions are present. One documented example of this was a lotus seed that produced a healthy tree after a 1300-year period of dormancy.[2] Another was a 2000-year-old date palm seed that produced a viable sapling.[3] Some forms of vegetation can germinate only after fires that may come decades apart. These include the giant sequoias native to the US southwest. Most deciduous trees and plants have seasonal periods of dormancy during which they cease photosynthesis, a process called abscission.

A tiny colony of yeast trapped inside a Lebanese weevil covered in ancient Burmese amber for up to 45 million years has been reported to have been brought back to life and used to brew a modern beer.[4] Rotifers, a group of small multicellular organisms, have extended dormant periods lasting from days to months in response to environmental stresses, including lack of water or food.[5,6] Parasites can become dormant within an animal's tissues for years, emerging during periods when the immune system is compromised.[7] Some invertebrate parasites have extended dormant periods, defending themselves by forming a protective cyst.[8] Insect dormancy or diapause can be seasonal, lasting several months, and anecdotal reports indicate that, under some conditions, can last for several years to as long as a century.[9] This can occur in an embryological, larval, pupal, or adult stage. During diapause insects are potentially vulnerable to predation, as are some sleeping animals. Passive defense strategies are employed, such as entering dormancy underground or in hidden recesses, having hard shells, and tenacious attachment to substrates. Land snails and slugs can secrete a mucus membrane for protection and enter a dormant state.[10]

Reptiles and amphibia that live in lakes that either freeze or dry seasonally and snakes that live in environments with periods of cold or extreme heat have the ability to enter dormant states. These may occur just during the cool portion of the circadian cycle or may extend for months in winter.[11] Estivation is a form of dormancy that occurs during warm periods. It allows reptiles, amphibia, fish, and insects[12-16] to emerge with the first rains from what had been a dry, apparently lifeless environment.

In the mammalian class, a continuum of states ranging from dormancy to continuous activity can be seen. Small animals that cannot migrate long distances and live in temperate or frigid environments often survive the winter by hibernating. Some bats, many species of rodents, marsupials, and insectivores hibernate. This condition is entered from, and generally terminates in, non–rapid eye movement (NREM) sleep. During hibernation, body temperature can be reduced to below 10° C to as low as −3° C (with antifreeze protection).[17,18] Animals are quite difficult to arouse during hibernation, with full arousal taking as long as 2 hours. Consequently, hibernators are vulnerable to predation and survive hibernation by seeking protected sites. Torpor[17] is another form of dormancy that can be entered by mammals and birds daily. Torpor is entered and exited through NREM sleep and can recur in a circadian rhythm or can last for weeks or months. Animals in shallow torpor are less difficult to arouse than hibernating animals but are still unable to respond quickly when stimulated. Some other mammals such as bears have extended periods of sleep in the winter during which their metabolic rate and body temperature are reduced by 4° to 5° C,[19] but they remain more responsive than animals in torpor.

Sleep can be seen as a form of adaptive inactivity lying on this continuum. What is most remarkable about sleep is not the unresponsiveness or vulnerability it creates but rather its ability to reduce activity and body and brain metabolism, but still allow a high level of responsiveness relative to the states of dormancy described earlier in this chapter. The often cited example of a parent arousing at a baby's whimper but sleeping through a thunderstorm illustrates the ability of the sleeping human brain to continuously process sensory signals during the sleep period and trigger complete awakening to significant stimuli within a few hundred milliseconds. This capacity is retained despite the great reduction in brain energy consumption achieved in sleep relative to quiet waking.[20,21]

Adolescent humans are less responsive than adults to stimuli presented during sleep, as anyone who has raised teenagers can attest. This may have been selected for by evolution, because protection from predators is provided by older members of the family group who also tend to the nocturnal needs of infants. The inactivity of children benefits the group by reducing their relatively large portion of the family's food needs and diverting food energy to growth.

Some animals that live in climates with seasonal reduction in food or light availability or a periodic increase in threat from predators have evolved migration to survive. Many species of birds do this, as do certain species of marine mammals (see the section Marine Mammals). Although some may maintain circadian rhythms of activity during migration, others remain continuously active for weeks or months. Some vertebrates do not ever appear to meet the behavioral criteria for sleep, remaining responsive, or responsive and active, throughout their lifetime.[22]

Humans with a complaint of "insomnia" are typically not sleepy during the day, despite a reduced (or in many cases normal) duration of nighttime sleep. They may be viewed as falling closer to migrating animals or short-sleeping animals, in contrast to humans with sleep disturbed by sleep deprivation, sleep apnea, or pain, who are sleepy during the day.[23] Conversely, many individuals with hypersomnia appear to need more sleep and sleep more deeply, rather than being the victims of a shallow or disrupted sleep that is compensated for by extended sleep time. Perhaps these individuals may be expressing genes and a behavior that was highly adaptive for reducing energy consumption.

QUANTITATIVE ANALYSES OF THE CORRELATES OF SLEEP DURATION IN MAMMALS

Mathematically inclined researchers have attempted to correlate the data that have been collected on sleep duration in mammals with physiologic and behavioral variables in order to develop hypotheses as to the function of sleep. However, the data these studies are based on are not ideal. Only approximately 80 mammalian species have been studied with sufficient measurements to determine the amounts of rapid eye movement (REM) and NREM sleep over the 24-hour period. These are by no means a random sample of the more than 5000 mammalian species. Rather they are species that are viable and available for study in laboratories or in some instances for noninvasive (and less accurate) studies in zoos. In laboratories, animal subjects for sleep studies are typically fed ad libitum; are at relatively invariant, thermoneutral, temperatures; and are on artificial (usually 12-12) light-dark cycles. These environments differ greatly from those in which animals evolved. Digital recording and storage technologies now exist that will enable the collection of polygraphic data on animals in their natural environments.[24] An excellent example is a 2018 study by Davimes and colleagues of the Arabian oryx under natural conditions. This animal shows a major seasonal difference in sleep duration (6.7 hours in winter and 3.8 hours in summer), and the circadian timing of its sleep differs greatly across the seasons.[25] Such "natural" observations are necessary to determine the variation in sleep times caused by hunger, response to temperature changes, predation, and the other variables that have driven evolution. Very few animals whose sleep has been studied have been tested for arousal threshold, the nature and extent of sleep rebound, and other aspects of sleep whose variation across species would contribute to an understanding of sleep evolution and function. In humans, we know that sleep depth, as assessed by either arousal threshold or electroencephalogram (EEG) amplitude, increases after sleep deprivation. Can sleep time be profitably compared across animals without incorporating information on sleep depth[26]?

One of the earliest studies comparing REM and NREM sleep durations with physiologic variables found that sleep duration was inversely correlated with body mass.[27,28] Our subsequent analysis found that this relationship applied only to herbivores, not to carnivores or omnivores.[29] This study also showed that, as a group, carnivores slept more than omnivores, who in turn slept more than herbivores (Figure 10.1). In an early study, a significant negative correlation was found

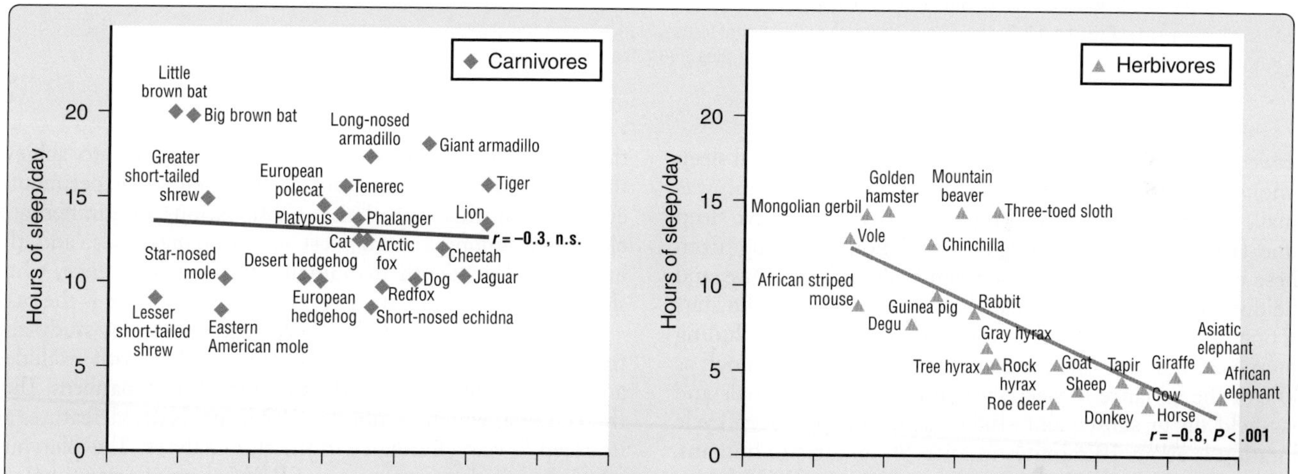

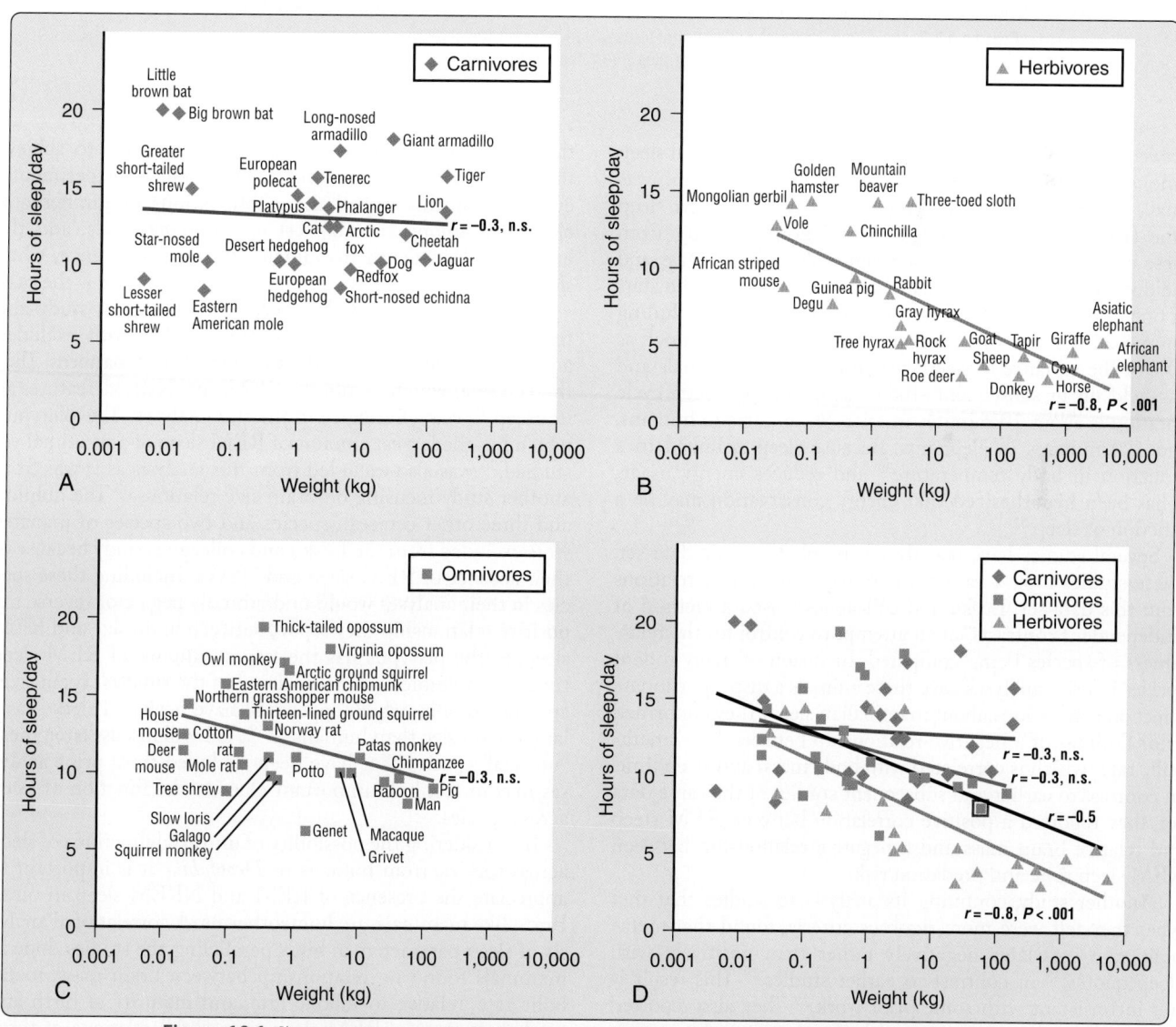

Figure 10.1 Sleep time in mammals. **A,** Carnivores are shown in dark red; **B,** herbivores are in green; and **C,** omnivores are in gray. Sleep times in carnivores, omnivores, and herbivores differ significantly, with carnivore sleep amounts significantly greater than those of herbivores. Sleep amount is an inverse function of body mass over all terrestrial mammals *(black line)*. This function accounts for approximately 25% of the interspecies variance **(D)** in reported sleep amounts. Herbivores are responsible for this relation because body mass and sleep time were significantly and inversely correlated in herbivores but were not in carnivores or omnivores. (From Siegel JM. Clues to the functions of mammalian sleep. *Nature* 2005;437:1264–1271.)

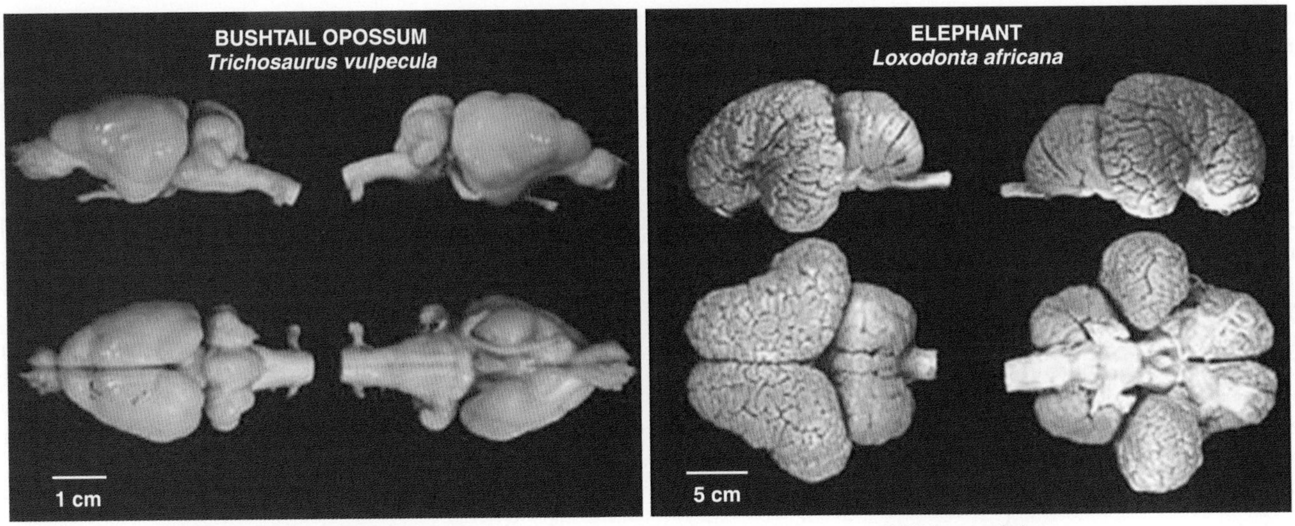

Figure 10.2 Sleep amount is not proportional to the relative size of the cerebral cortex or to the degree of encephalization, as illustrated by these two examples. (From Siegel JM. Clues to the functions of mammalian sleep. *Nature* 2005;437:1264–1271.)

between brain weight and REM sleep time (but not total sleep time). It should be emphasized that this latter correlation was small, accounting for only 4% of the variance in REM sleep time (Figure 10.2). The largest correlation emerging from these early studies was that between body or brain mass and the duration of the sleep cycle, that is the time from the start of one REM sleep period to the start of the next, excluding interposed waking. This correlation accounted for as much as 80% of the variance in sleep cycle time between animals and has held up in subsequent studies in mammals. Sleep cycle duration is about 10 minutes in mice, 90 minutes in humans, and 120 minutes in elephants. Because sleep is linked to a reduction in body temperature[30] and reduces energy usage, it has been hypothesized that energy conservation may be a function of sleep.[31]

Several studies have reanalyzed the phylogenetic data set. These studies took a variety of strategies to extract relations from this data set. Lesku and colleagues[32] used a method of "independent contrasts" in an attempt to control for the relatedness of species being compared. Inclusion of many rodent species in prior analyses gave these animals a disproportionate effect on conclusions about mammalian sleep. They confirmed prior findings of a negative relationship between basal metabolic rate (which is correlated with body mass) and sleep time. In contrast to earlier and subsequent studies of the same data set, they reported a positive correlation between REM sleep and relative brain mass and a negative relationship between REM sleep time and predation risk.

Another study, confining its analysis to studies that met what they felt were more rigorous criteria, found that metabolic rate correlates negatively rather than positively with sleep quotas,[33] in contrast to earlier studies.[28] This result is not inconsistent with some prior work.[29] They also reported that neither adult nor neonatal brain mass correlates positively with adult REM or NREM sleep times, differing from earlier studies.[28,33] They find, in agreement with prior analyses, that animals with high predation risk sleep less.[29,34] In keeping with the concept that there is some fixed need for an unknown function preformed only during sleep, they propose that short-sleeping species sleep more intensely to achieve this function in less time, but they present no experimental evidence for this hypothesis. Observations of giraffes and elephants, among the shortest sleeping mammals, and the increased sleep depth in humans during adolescence, when sleep duration is high, suggests that just the reverse is the case.

A notable feature of the Lesku and colleagues study and the Capellini and colleagues studies is that both excluded animals that they concluded had unusual sleep patterns. Thus the echidna, which combines REM and NREM features in its sleep,[35] was eliminated from the analyses. The platypus, which has the largest amount of REM sleep of any animal yet studied,[36] was also excluded from this analysis as it was from another study focusing on brain size relations.[37] The dolphin and three other cetacean species and two species of manatee were excluded from the Lesku and colleagues study because of their absence of REM sleep and USWs. Including these species in their analyses would undoubtedly negate or reverse the positive relationship they report between brain size and REM sleep, as the platypus has the largest amount of REM sleep time of any studied animal and one of the smallest brain sizes and the dolphin, which appears to have no REM sleep, has a larger brain size than humans.[38,39] As I will discuss later, these "unusual" species that have been excluded from prior analyses may in fact hold important clues to the function of sleep across species.

In considering the possibility of universal functions of sleep across species, from humans to *Drosophila*, it is important to appreciate the presence of REM and NREM sleep in birds. Birds, like mammals, are homeotherms. A correlational analysis of sleep parameters in birds paralleling the studies done in mammals found no relationship between brain mass, metabolic rate, relative metabolic rate, and maturity at birth and total sleep time or REM sleep time.[40] All relations of these parameters were found to be "markedly nonsignificant." The only significant relation found was a negative correlation between predation risk and NREM sleep time (but not REM sleep time), in contrast to the relation reported earlier in this chapter in mammals between predation risk and REM sleep time (but not NREM sleep time). This lone significant relation explained only 27% of the variance in avian NREM sleep time.

To summarize, a variety of correlation studies, most done under laboratory or zoo conditions, reach disparate and often opposite conclusions about the physiologic and functional correlates of sleep time. It should be emphasized that with the exception of the strong relationship between sleep cycle length and brain and body mass, all of the "significant" correlations reported explain only a small portion of the variance in sleep parameters, throwing into question whether the correlational approach is getting at the core issues of sleep function. Despite similar genetics, anatomy, cognitive abilities, and physiologic functioning, closely related mammalian species can have very different sleep parameters and distantly related species can have very similar sleep parameters. Many such examples exist despite the relatively small number of species in which REM and NREM sleep time have been determined (Figure 10.3). For example, the guinea pig and baboon have the same daily amounts of REM and NREM sleep.[41]

THE DIVERSITY OF SLEEP

On the assumption that sleep satisfies an unknown yet universal function in all animals, some work has been carried out on animals whose genetics and neuroanatomy are better

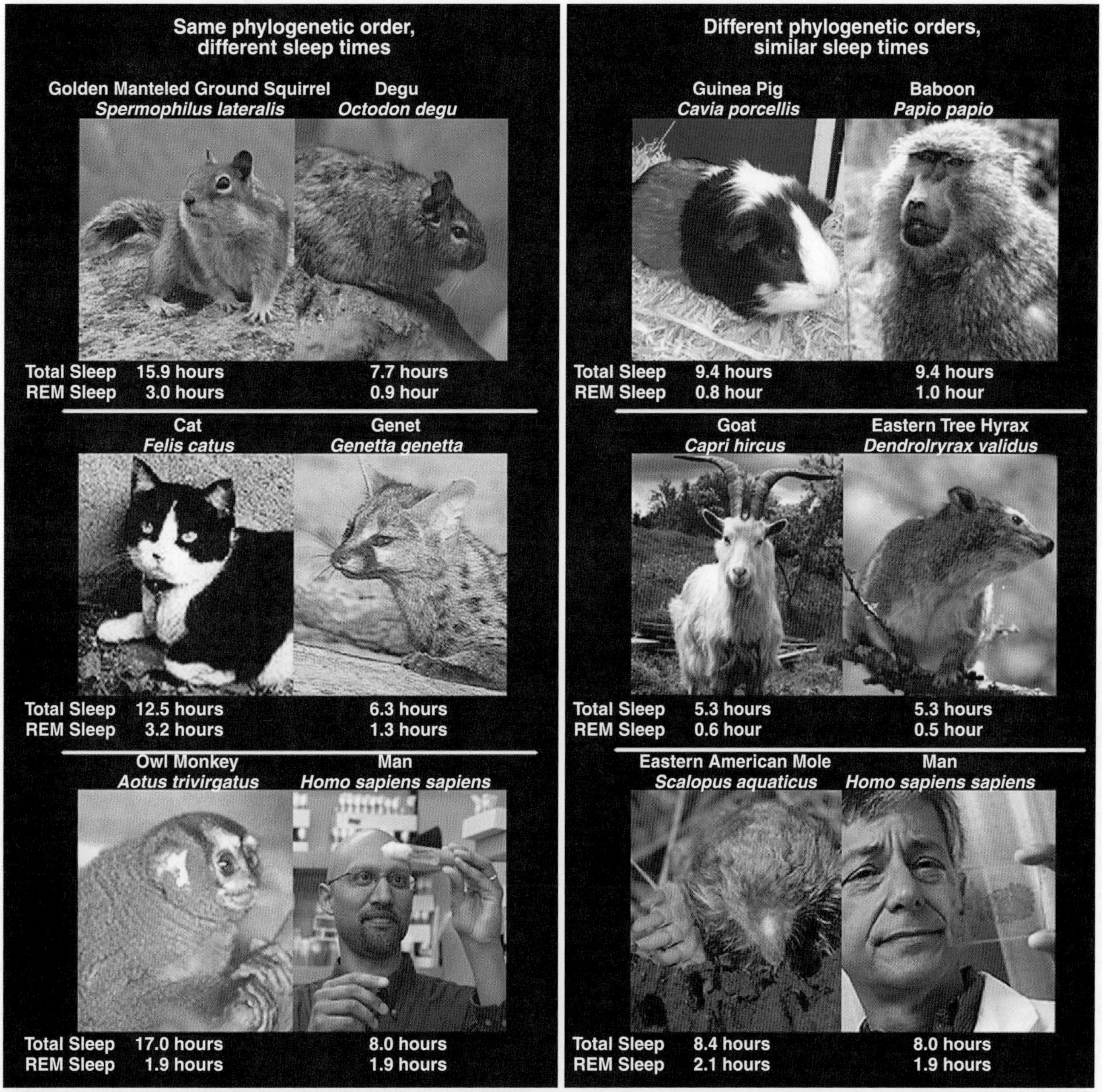
Same phylogenetic order, different sleep times
Golden Manteled Ground Squirrel
Spermophilus lateralis
Degu
Octodon degu
Total Sleep 15.9 hours
REM Sleep 3.0 hours
7.7 hours
0.9 hour
Cat
Felis catus
Genet
Genetta genetta
Total Sleep 12.5 hours
REM Sleep 3.2 hours
6.3 hours
1.3 hours
Owl Monkey
Aotus trivirgatus
Man
Homo sapiens sapiens
Total Sleep 17.0 hours
REM Sleep 1.9 hours
8.0 hours
1.9 hours
Different phylogenetic orders, similar sleep times
Guinea Pig
Cavia porcellis
Baboon
Papio papio
Total Sleep 9.4 hours
REM Sleep 0.8 hour
9.4 hours
1.0 hour
Goat
Capri hircus
Eastern Tree Hyrax
Dendrolryrax validus
Total Sleep 5.3 hours
REM Sleep 0.6 hour
5.3 hours
0.5 hour
Eastern American Mole
Scalopus aquaticus
Man
Homo sapiens sapiens
Total Sleep 8.4 hours
REM Sleep 2.1 hours
8.0 hours
1.9 hours

Figure 10.3 Mammalian phylogenetic order is not strongly correlated with sleep parameters. On the left are three pairs of animals that are in the same order but have very different sleep parameters. On the right are three pairs of animals from different orders with similar sleep amounts. Mammalian sleep times are not strongly correlated with phylogenetic order. (From Allada R, Siegel JM. Unearthing the phylogenetic roots of sleep. *Curr Biol.* 2008;18:R670–R679.)

understood and more easily manipulated than those of mammals. Much of this work has focused on the fruit fly, *Drosophila melanogaster*. These animals appear to meet the behavioral definition of sleep. Their response threshold is elevated during periods of immobility, but they will rapidly "awaken" when sufficiently intense stimuli are applied. They make up for "sleep" deprivation with a partial rebound of inactivity when left undisturbed. However, major differences between the physiology and anatomy of these organisms and those of mammals make it difficult to transfer insights gleaned from studies of *Drosophila* sleep to human sleep. The *Drosophila* brain does not resemble the vertebrate brain. Hypocretin, a major sleep regulating transmitter in mammals, does not exist in *Drosophila*.[41] *Drosophila* are not homeotherms, whereas thermoregulation has been closely linked to fundamental aspects of mammalian sleep[29,30,43] and they do not have REM sleep. Two studies have shown that *Drosophila* sleep and sleep rebound is markedly impaired by genetic alteration of a potassium current that regulates neuronal membrane excitability.[44,45] Regulation of potassium currents may be a core function of sleep or it simply may affect the excitability of circuits regulating activity and quiescence, just as such currents affect seizure susceptibility.[46,47]

A 2019 paper by Leung and colleagues claimed to detect a REM sleep-like state in larval zebrafish.[48] However, there have been no reports or REM sleep in adult zebrafish, or in any other fish species, to my knowledge. Arousal thresholds and homeostatic regulation were not demonstrated in larval zebrafish, so it is not clear that the described state is sleep, much less REM sleep. *Caenorhabditis elegans,* a roundworm with a nervous system much simpler than that of *Drosophila*, has also been investigated for sleep-like behavior.[49] *C. elegans* reaches adulthood in 60 hours and has periods of inactivity during this maturation called "lethargus" occurring before each of the four molts it undergoes before reaching maturity. Stimulation of *C. elegans* during the lethargus period produced a small but significant decrease in activity during the remainder of the lethargus period, but did not delay the subsequent period of activity or increase quiescence overall, phenomena that differ from the effects of sleep deprivation in mammals. It is not clear if adult *C. elegans* shows sleep behavior.[50]

Fundamental species differences in the physiology and neurochemistry of sleep have been identified even within the mammalian line. Although there are many similarities, the EEG aspects of sleep also differ considerably between humans, rats, mice, and cats, the most studied species.[51-53] Human stage 4 NREM sleep (N3 in the newer nomenclature) is linked to growth hormone secretion. However, in dogs, growth hormone secretion normally occurs in waking, not sleep.[54] Melatonin release is maximal during sleep in diurnal animals but is maximal in waking in nocturnal animals.[55] Erections have been shown to be present during REM sleep in humans and rats[56]; however the armadillo has erections only in NREM sleep.[57] Dolphins do not have REM sleep. Blood flow and metabolism differ dramatically between neocortical regions in adult human REM sleep,[58] although most animal sleep deprivation and sleep metabolic studies treat the neocortex as a unit.

Animal Dreaming?

Lesions of the parietal cortex and certain other regions eliminate dreaming recall in humans, even in individuals that continue to show normal REM sleep as judged by cortical EEG, rapid eye movements, and suppression of muscle tone.[59] Humans before age 6 do not generally report dream mentation, perhaps because these cortical regions have not yet developed.[60] These findings make it questionable whether nonhuman mammals that have REM sleep, all of which have cortical regions whose structure differs from that of adult humans, have dream mentation. We have reviewed data on REM and NREM sleep duration in mammals in the context of species differences in the anatomy of structures linked to REM sleep control.[61] We speculated on the possibility that certain species dream, emphasizing that we cannot know whether animals dream, regardless of whether or not they have REM sleep. But what we know about the physiology of sleep in different species suggests that some, such as cats and dogs, may dream, whereas others, such as cetaceans (whales and dolphins—animals that have the largest brains on our planet) are very unlikely to dream.

Elephants and Sloths

The sleep of elephants is of great interest. They are the largest land mammals, with the largest brain of any land mammal and one of the longest mammalian life spans. They have social structures and behaviors that rival those of primates in their complexity. In the wild they travel daily to find optimal resources of grasses, plants, bushes, fruit, twigs, and roots to eat. Typically the matriarch will lead the herd. She has to navigate to regions where the herd has not fed recently, a prodigious task and one consistent with the aphorism that "an elephant never forgets." Current theories postulating a strong relation of sleep to cognitive factors, life span, and health might suggest longer sleep durations in elephants than in animals with less social structure and lesser memory requirements. Yet studies of elephants in captivity had concluded that Asiatic elephants sleep only 4 to 6.5 hours a day.[62] Similar results were reported in a second study of captive elephants.[63] In our recent study we recorded from two wild African elephants in Botswana for 35-day periods. Satellite tracking revealed that they traveled as far as 45 km/day, averaging 15 km/day. We monitored sleep behavior by recording periods where the trunk was not moving, indicative of rest or sleep periods. We found that average rest periods were 2 hours per day. Even if all of these quiescent periods are sleep the amount is far lower than sleep times in captivity and are the lowest of any mammal (Figure 10.4), a challenge for theories that sleep duration is linked to cognitive or social structure factors. But from a behavioral standpoint it should not be too surprising that elephants in captivity, which have a bale of hay tossed into their enclosure in the morning, sleep more than elephants that have to walk 15 km a day on average to acquire food; that is elephants in zoos rest or sleep more because they do not need to be active. A similar phenomenon is seen when comparing sloths in captivity to those in the wild. Sloths in the wild sleep much *less* than sloths in captivity.[24,64] More species need to be examined in natural environments to determine whether this is a common or universal pattern. But our results in human hunter-gatherers (see the section Humans) suggest that humans living in the environment and with the lifestyle in which our species evolved also have lower sleep durations than humans in industrialized societies, notwithstanding the common assumption that industrial society and its electric lights have greatly reduced human sleep time below its "natural" level.

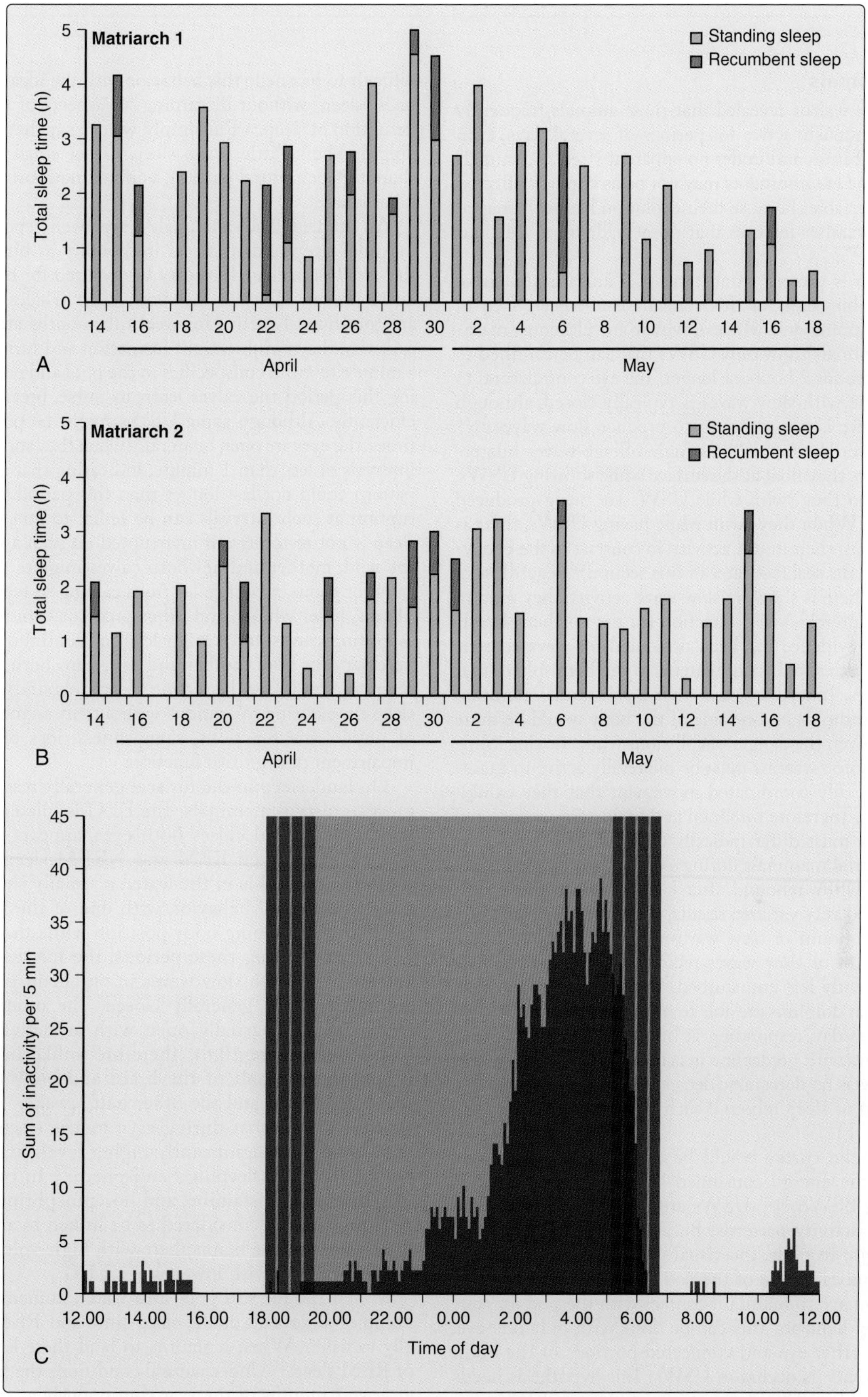

Figure 10.4 Sleep times, episodes, and timing in the elephant. **A,B,** Bar graphs representing total sleep time on each day through the 35-day recording period for each elephant. **A,** Matriarch 1; **B,** Matriarch 2. Note that on certain days no sleep was observed. The bars also represent the amount of time spent in standing sleep (blue) and in recumbent sleep (purple), although recumbent sleep did not occur on each day. **C,** Graph illustrating the average count of inactivity/sleep episodes for any given 5-minute period scored over the 35-day recording period and combining the data from both elephants. Note the clearly nocturnal pattern of inactivity, with little inactivity occurring during the daytime. The vast majority of sleep episodes occurred in the early morning during the hours of 02:00 and 06:00. The gray region represents the period between sunset (ss) and sunrise (sr). h, hour. (Gravett et al, 2017 Elephant.)

Marine Mammals

A study of the walrus revealed that these animals frequently become continuously active for periods of several days, even when fed ad libitum and under no apparent stress.[65] Animals living in marine environments may not be as strongly affected by circadian variables because their evolution has been shaped by tidal and weather features that do not adhere to 24-hour cycles.

REM sleep is present in all terrestrial animals that have been studied, but signs of this state have not been seen in cetaceans (dolphins and whales), which are placental mammals. These animals show only USWs that can be confined to one hemisphere for 2 hours or longer. The eye contralateral to the hemisphere with slow waves is typically closed, although covering the eye is not sufficient to produce slow waves.[36,66] Cetaceans never show persistent high-voltage waves bilaterally. Sometimes they float at the surface while showing USWs. However, often they swim while USWs are being produced (Figure 10.5). When they swim while having USWs, there is no asymmetry in their motor activity, in contrast to the behavior seen in the fur seal (see later in this section). Regardless of which hemisphere is showing slow wave activity, they tend to circle in a counterclockwise direction (in the northern hemisphere[67]). No evidence has been presented for elevated sensory response thresholds contralateral to the hemisphere that has slow waves. Indeed it seems that a substantial elevation of sensory thresholds on one side of the body would be quite maladaptive given the danger of collisions while moving. Similarly, brain motor systems must be bilaterally active to maintain the bilaterally coordinated movement that they exhibit during USWs. Therefore forebrain and brainstem sensory and motor activity must differ radically during USWs from that seen in terrestrial mammals during sleep (Chapter 8[68,69]). The one study of USW rebound after USW deprivation in dolphins produced very variable results, with little or no relation between the amount of slow waves lost in each hemisphere and the amount of slow waves recovered when the animals were subsequently left undisturbed.[70] In two other studies it was shown that dolphins are able to maintain continuous vigilance 24 hours/day, responding at 30-second intervals, for 5 and for 15 days with no decline in accuracy. At the end of this period there was no detectable decrease of activity or evidence of inattention or sleep rebound such as might have been expected.[22,71,72]

USWs in the cortex would be expected to save nearly one-half of the energy consumed by the forebrain that is saved during BSWS.[20,21] USWs are well suited to the dolphins' group activity patterns. Because dolphins and other cetaceans swim in pods, the visual world can be monitored by dolphins on each side of the pod and the remaining dolphins merely have to maintain contact with the pod. In routine "cruising" behavior this can be done with only one eye, allowing the other eye and connected portions of the brain to reduce activity as occurs in USWs. This hypothesis needs to be explored by EEG observations of groups of cetaceans in the wild.

In some smaller cetaceans, such as the harbor porpoise[73] and Commerson's dolphin,[74] motor activity is essentially continuous from birth to death; that is they never float or sink to the bottom and remain still. They move rapidly, and it is evident that they must have accurate sensory and motor performance and associated brain activation to avoid collisions. It is difficult to reconcile this behavior with the idea that all mammals "sleep" without discarding all aspects of the behavioral definition of sleep.[22] Put simply, we can say that Commerson's dolphin shows little or no sleep. Other small dolphins may share this behavioral pattern, as do all newborn dolphins and killer whales.

All studied land mammals have been reported to show maximal sleep and maximal immobility at birth, leading to the conclusion that sleep may be required for brain and body development. However, newborn killer whales and dolphins are continuously active for weeks to months after birth.[75] In captivity, they swim in tight formation and turn several times a minute to avoid conspecifics in the pool and pool walls. During this period the calves learn to nurse, breathe, and swim efficiently. Although some USWs might be present at these times, the eyes are open bilaterally when they surface at average intervals of less than 1 minute, indicating that any slow wave pattern could not last longer than this period.[75] Sleep interruption at such intervals can be lethal to rats,[76] and human sleep is not restorative if interrupted on such a schedule.[77] In the wild, mother and newborn calves migrate together, typically for thousands of miles from calving to feeding grounds. Sharks, killer whales, and other predatory animals target the migrating calves and a high level of continuous alertness is necessary for both mother and calf. Thus both cetaceans and migrating birds (see the section Sleep Rebound) greatly reduce sleep time during migrations without any sign of degradation of physiologic functions, sluggishness, loss of alertness, or impairment of cognitive function.

On land, sleep in the fur seal generally resembles that in most terrestrial mammals. The EEG is bilaterally synchronized, the animal closes both eyes, appears unresponsive, and cycles between REM and NREM sleep. In contrast, when the fur seal is in the water, it usually shows an asymmetric pattern of behavior, with one of the flippers being active in maintaining body position while the other flipper is inactive. During these periods, the fur seal has a high-voltage EEG with slow waves in one hemisphere with the contralateral eye generally closed. The other eye is generally open or partially open with an activated, waking-like EEG (Figure 10.6). Therefore unlike in the dolphin, it appears that half of the brain and body may in some sense be "asleep" and the other half "awake." Microdialysis studies showed that during asymmetric sleep, the waking hemisphere has significantly higher levels of acetylcholine release than the sleeping hemisphere.[78] In contrast, levels of serotonin,[79] histamine, and norepinephrine,[80] transmitters traditionally considered to be linked to arousal, do not differ between the hemisphere with high-voltage EEG and the hemisphere with low-voltage EEG.

When the fur seal goes into water, unihemispheric sleep occupies almost all of the sleep time and REM sleep virtually vanishes. When it returns to land there is no "rebound" of REM sleep.[81] Under natural conditions the fur seal spends at least 7 months of the year continuously at sea. The results in the fur seal reinforce the idea that the apparent absence of REM sleep in the dolphin is not a problem of the state being difficult to detect in cetaceans. Rather it appears that REM is linked to bilateral NREM sleep. In the absence of bilateral NREM, REM does not occur. I will deal with the issue of why this occurs, which bears directly on the issue of the function of REM sleep, in Chapter 8.

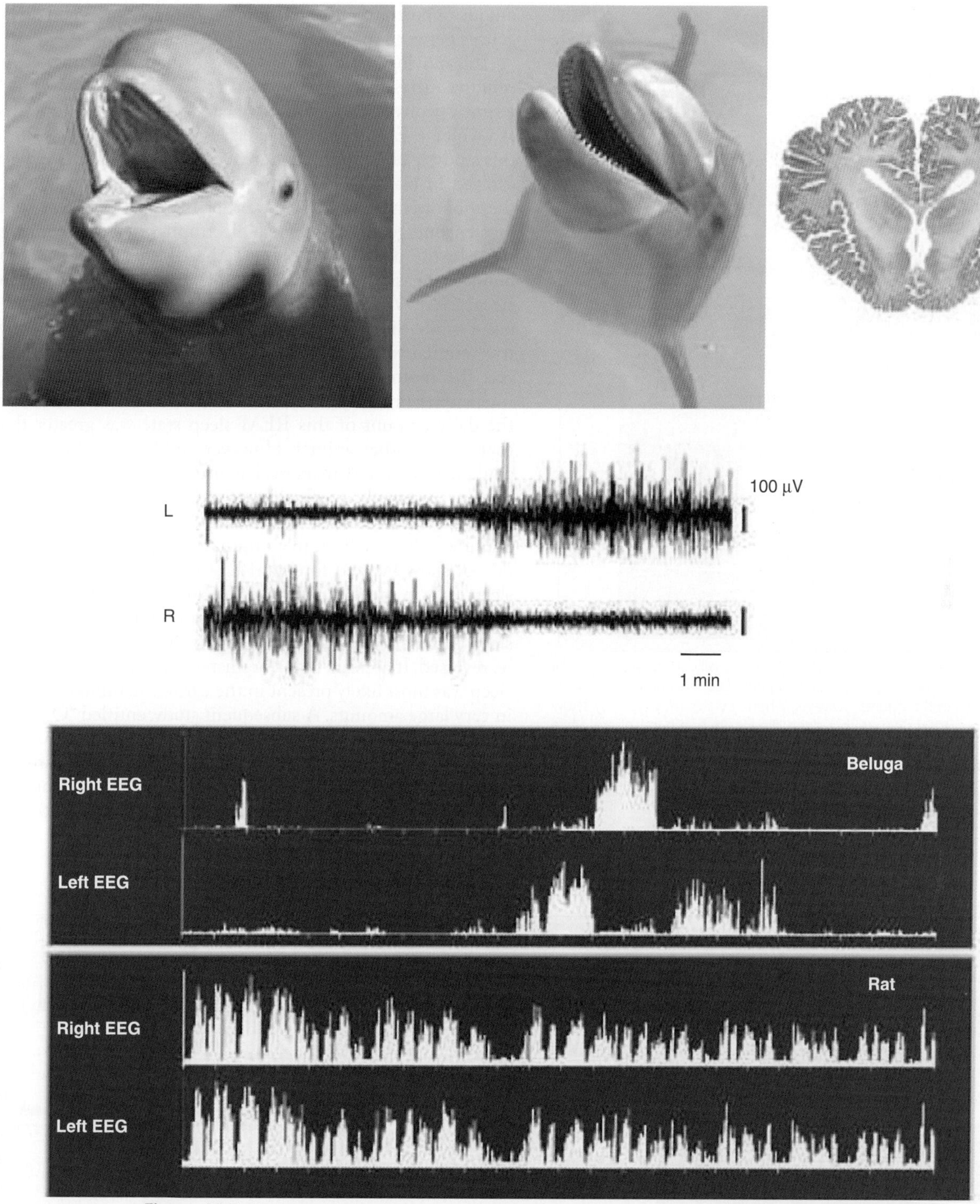

Figure 10.5 Cetacean sleep: unihemispheric slow waves in cetaceans. *Top*, Photos of immature beluga (*left*), adult dolphin and section of adult dolphin brain. Electroencephalogram (EEG) of adult cetaceans, represented here by the beluga, during sleep are shown. All species of cetacean so far recorded have unihemispheric slow waves. *Top traces* show left and right EEG activity. The spectral plots show 1-to 3-Hz power in the two hemispheres over a 12-hour period. The pattern in the cetaceans contrasts with the bilateral pattern of slow waves seen under normal conditions in all terrestrial mammals, represented here by the rat (*bottom traces*). (From Siegel JM. Clues to the functions of mammalian sleep. *Nature* 2005;437:1264–1271.)

Monotremes

The mammalian class can be subdivided into three subclasses: placentals, marsupials, and monotremes. There are just three extant monotreme species, the short-beaked and long-beaked echidna and the platypus. Fossil and genetic evidence indicates that the monotreme line diverged from the other mammalian lines about 150 million years ago and that both echidna species are derived from a platypus-like ancestor.[82-85] Although monotremes are distinctly mammalian, they do display a number of reptilian features, making study of their physiology a

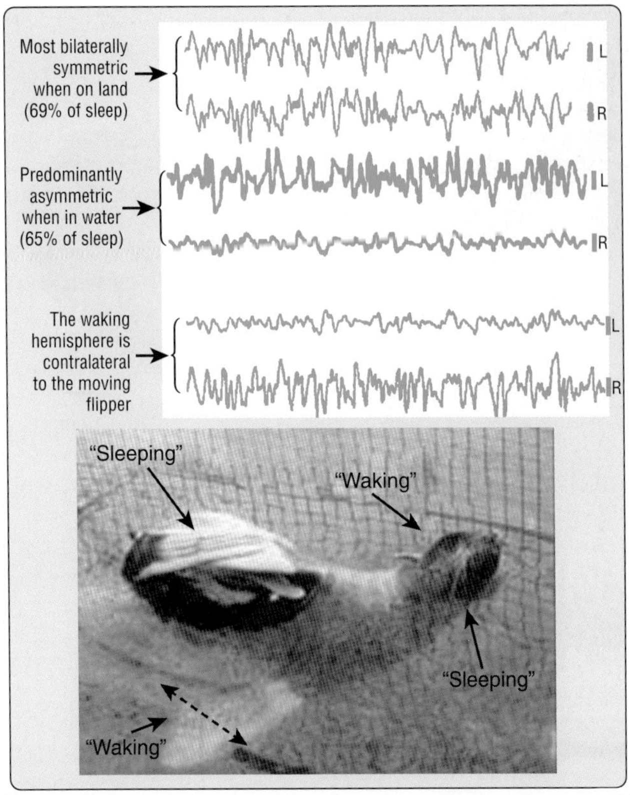

Figure 10.6 Fur seal sleep. On land fur seals usually sleep like terrestrial mammals, with bilateral electroencephalogram (EEG) synchrony and REM sleep (not shown in the figure). However, when in water they typically show asymmetric slow wave sleep with a sleep-like EEG in one hemisphere while the other hemisphere has a waking-like EEG. Unlike the dolphin, the asymmetric EEG of the fur seal is accompanied by asymmetric posture and motor activity with the flipper contralateral to the hemisphere with low-voltage activity used to maintain the animal's position in the water while the other flipper and its controlling hemisphere "sleep."

unique opportunity to determine the commonalties and divergences between mammalian and reptilian physiology.[83,86,87]

This phylogenetic history led to an early study of the echidna to test the hypothesis that REM sleep was a more recently evolved sleep state. No clear evidence of the forebrain low-voltage EEG that characterizes REM sleep was seen in this study, leading to the tentative conclusion that REM sleep evolved in placentals and marsupials after the divergence of the monotreme line from the other mammals.[88] These findings encouraged us to perform electrophysiological studies of sleep in the platypus. We found that the platypus had pronounced phasic motor activity typical of that seen in REM sleep[89] (see Video 10.1). This intense motor activity could occur while the forebrain EEG exhibited high-voltage activity,[36] similar to the phenomena seen in the echidna. Not only was the motor activity during sleep equal to or greater in intensity than that seen in REM sleep in other animals, but the daily amount of this REM sleep state was greater than that in any other animal. However, unlike the condition in adult placental and marsupial mammals, the signs of REM sleep were largely confined to the brainstem (Figures 10.7 and 10.8). This bears some resemblance to the sleep of most mammals that are born in an immature (altricial) state, which do not show marked forebrain EEG activation during REM sleep early in life. The tentative conclusion reached in the initial studies of the echidna, that the monotremes had no REM sleep and that REM sleep was a recently evolved state, had to be reversed. It appears that a brainstem manifestation of REM sleep was most likely present in the earliest mammals, perhaps in very large amounts. A subsequent study, entitled "Ostriches sleep like platypuses,"[90] found a similar pattern of REM sleep in the ostrich, considered to be a relatively "primitive" bird.[90] It may be the brainstem quiescence of NREM sleep along with the cortical EEG desynchrony (i.e., low-voltage "activated"

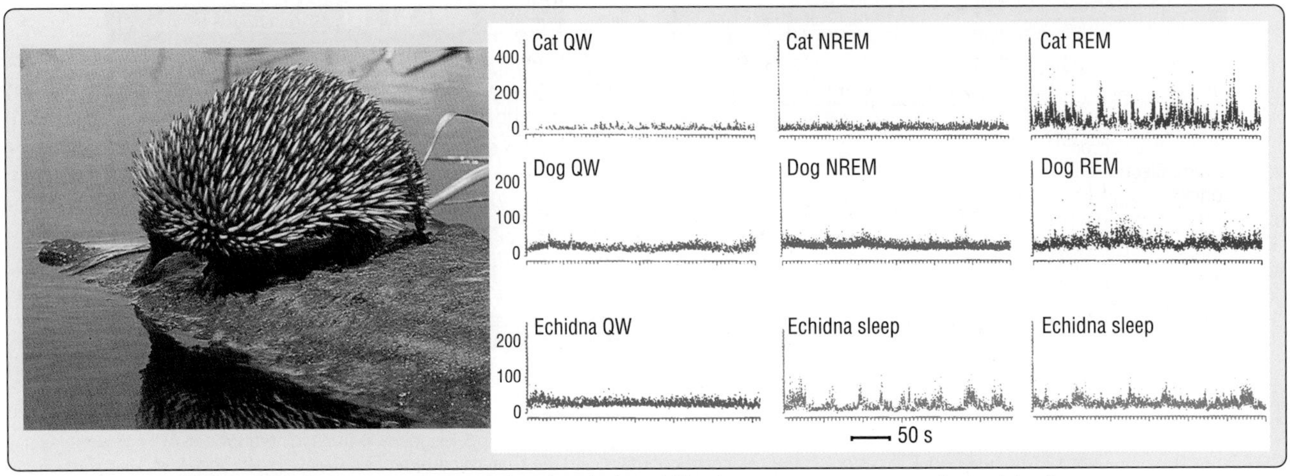

Figure 10.7 Brainstem activation during sleep in the echidna. Instantaneous compressed rate plots of representative units recorded in nucleus reticularis pontis oralis of the cat, dog, and echidna. Each point represents the discharge rate for the previous interspike interval. In cat quiet waking (QW) and NREM sleep, the discharge rate is low and relatively regular. The rate increases and becomes highly variable during REM sleep. A similar pattern can be seen in a unit recorded in the dog. In the echidna, sleep is characterized by variable unit discharge rates as is seen in REM sleep, but this occurs while the cortex is showing high-voltage activity. (From Siegel JM, Manger P, Nienhuis R, Fahringer HM, Pettigrew J. The echidna *Tachyglossus aculeatus* combines REM and nonREM aspects in a single sleep state: implications for the evolution of sleep. *J. Neurosci.* 1996;16:3500–3506.)

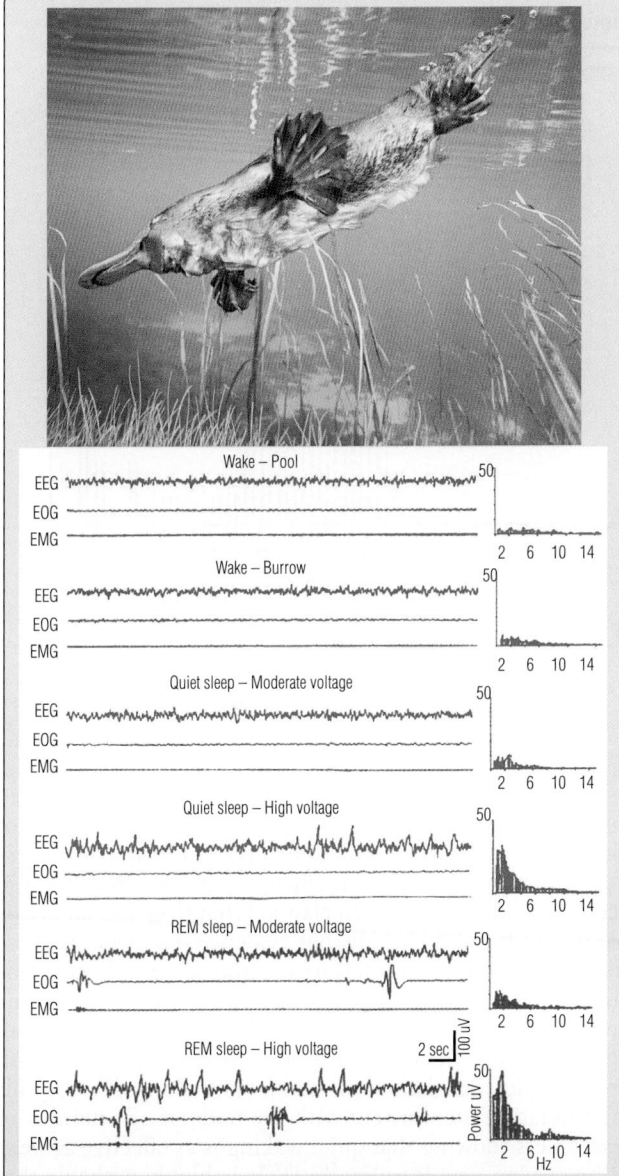

Figure 10.8 Brainstem REM sleep state in the platypus. Rapid eye movements and twitches can occur while the forebrain is showing a slow wave activity pattern. Electroencephalogram (EEG), electrooculogram (EOG), and electromyogram (EMG) power spectra of samples shown of sleep-wake states in the platypus. (From Siegel JM, Manger PR, Nienhuis R, Fahringer HM, Shalita T, Pettigrew JD. Sleep in the platypus. *Neuroscience* 1999;91:391-400.)

pattern) of REM sleep that are the most recently evolved aspects of sleep in the mammalian line.

Humans

The considerations reviewed earlier in this chapter and the great difference between sleep durations seen in elephants and sloths in captivity versus the same species "in the wild" made us wonder how humans slept before the industrial age. It has been commonly thought that electric lights have shortened sleep time in industrial populations and that this shortening may have had negative health consequences in humans. Therefore we undertook a study of three human hunter-gatherer populations, one in the Kalahari Desert of Namibia, one in equatorial Tanzania, and one in the Bolivian Amazon.[91-93] We found that, contrary to what had been assumed by many, the hunter-gatherers almost never go to sleep at sunset, have total sleep durations that are somewhat shorter than those in industrial populations, seldom nap, and usually sleep in a single uninterrupted nightly block[92] (Figure 10.9).

There has long been controversy concerning whether there was any seasonal difference in human sleep, with the consensus view being that here was little if any such difference.[94,95] We therefore examined this issue in hunter-gatherer populations in Namibia and Bolivia, located 20 and 15 degrees latitude south of the equator. We found a nearly 1-hour greater sleep duration in the winter than in the summer. This is a far larger difference than has ever been seen in industrial populations. It remains to be determined whether light or temperature conditions are the principal determinants of this difference.

In contrast to the 10% to 30% insomnia rates that appear to be universal in industrial populations, fewer than 5% of hunter-gatherers report having any difficulty getting to sleep or staying asleep. Similarly, in our more than 1165 days of recording we did not see any individuals who consistently showed reduced sleep during the nighttime sleep period. One possibility we are investigating is that exposure to the daily temperature rhythm, largely eliminated in industrial societies, may be a key to the normal regulation of sleep onset and continuity, and to the near absence of insomnia in hunter-gatherer populations. Obesity is extremely rare among hunter-gatherers[91-93] and in general cardiovascular health is far better than in industrial populations.[96] This reality is sometimes obfuscated by the high childhood death rate, largely resulting from the lack of vaccinations, which reduces average life span.

Sleep Rebound

Sleep rebound,[97] the increased sleep after a period of deprivation, is not always seen. In dolphins and killer whales mentioned earlier in this chapter, a near total abolition of "sleep-like behavior" for periods of several weeks during migration is followed by a slow increase back to baseline levels with no rebound above baseline. The same phenomenon is seen in migrating white sparrows.[98] Humans with mania greatly reduce sleep time for extended periods and there is no persuasive evidence for progressive degradation of performance or physiologic function during the manic period, despite the emotional pathology, or of sleep rebound after this period. Zebrafish can be completely deprived of sleep for an extended period by placing them in continuous light but show no rebound when returned to a 12-12 light-dark cycle.[99] On the other hand, when they are deprived by repetitive tactile stimulation they do show rebound, suggesting that the deprivation procedure, rather than the sleep loss, underlies the rebound. Stressing rats by restraint can produce increased REM sleep even when no sleep has been lost. This is mediated by the release of pituitary hormones.[100,101] It is possible that in some species other aspects of rebound are driven by changes in hormonal release linked to sleep deprivation[1] rather than by some intrinsic property of sleep.

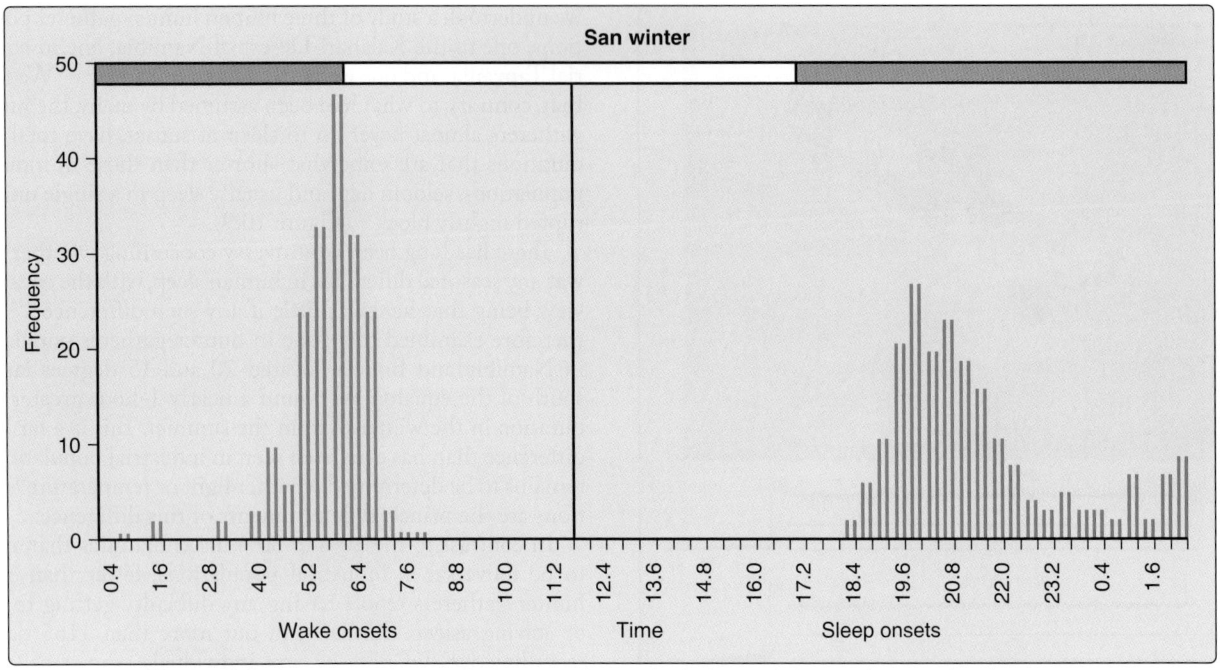

Figure 10.9 Sleep averaged over 10 San hunter-gatherer individuals recorded in Namibia. Note that sleep onset occurs on average more than 3 hours after sunset and is relatively irregular. Wake onset is much more regular occurring before and after dawn. (Yetish, G, Kaplan H, Gurven M, et al. Natural sleep and its seasonal variations in three pre-industrial societies. *Curr Biol.* 2015;25(21):2862–2868.)

CLINICAL PEARL

Although sleep and sleep stages differ in amount between species, human sleep does not appear to be qualitatively unique. This factor makes animal models suitable for the investigation of many aspects of pharmacology and pathology.

SUMMARY

Sleep can be seen as an adaptive state, benefiting animals by increasing the efficiency of their activity. Sleep does this by suppressing activity at times that have maximal predator risk and permitting activity at times of maximal food and prey availability. It also increases efficiency by decreasing brain and body metabolism. However, unlike the dormant states employed in plants, simple multicellular organisms, and ectothermic organisms and the hibernation and torpor employed in some mammals and birds, sleep allows rapid arousal for tending to infants and responding to environmental changes. Many organisms can reduce sleep for long periods of time without rebound during periods of migration.

The big brown bat, currently documented as having the longest sleep time of any mammal, specializes in eating mosquitoes and moths that are active from dusk to early evening. The big brown bat typically is awake only about 4 hours a day.[29] This waking is synchronized to the period when flies are active. It is not likely that this short waking period can be best explained by the need for some time-consuming unknown process that occurs only during sleep and requires 20 hours to complete. It can be more easily explained by the ecological specializations of this bat. Similarly "sleep" in ectothermic animals is most likely determined by temperature and other environmental variables, rather than any information processing or physiologic maintenance requirement.

Many vital processes occur in both waking and sleep including recovery of muscles from exertion, control of blood flow, respiration, growth of various organs, and digestion. Some may occur more efficiently in sleep but can also occur in waking. It has been claimed that sleep has an essential role in learning, but further evidence has disputed these claims. It appears that interference from the nearly continuous learning in the waking state, rather than some unique process in sleep, accounts for the difference between recall of processes learned before a sleep period compared with processes learned before an extended waking period. This interpretation is consistent with the findings of a number of researchers showing that quiet waking is as effective as sleep in preserving new learning.[102-107] It is highly probable that some functions have migrated into or out of sleep in various animals. Neurogenesis,[106] synaptic downscaling,[107] immune system activation, and reversal of oxidative stress may be accomplished in sleep in mammals. It remains to be seen if these or any other vital functions can be performed only in sleep. However, this review of the phylogenetic literature suggests that such functions cannot explain the variation of sleep amounts and the evident flexibility of sleep physiology within and between animals. Viewing sleep as a period of well-timed adaptive inactivity that regulates behavior and reduces energy consumption, can better explain this variation.

ACKNOWLEDGMENTS

Work on which this chapter is based was supported by RO1 HL148574 and DA034748. Dr. Siegel is the recipient of a Senior Research Career Scientist Award 1IK6BX005245 from the Department of Veterans Affairs.

SELECTED READINGS

Kendall-Bar JM, Vyssotski AL, Mukametov LM, Siegel JM, Lyamin OI. Eye state assymetry during aquatic unihemispheric slow wave sleep in northern fur seals (Callorhinus ursinus). *PloSONe*. 2019;14(5):e0217205.

Lyamin OI, Siegel JM, Nazarenko EA, Rozhnov VV. Sleep in the lesser mouse deer (Tragulus kanchil). *Sleep*. 2021 (in press).

Lyamin OI, Kibalnikov AS, Siegel JM. Sleep in ostrich chicks (Struthio camelus). *Sleep*. 2021;44:1–14.

Manger P, Siegel JM. Do all mammals dream? *J Compar Neurol*. 2020;528(17):3198–3204.

Schmidt MH. The energy allocation function of sleep: a unifying theory of sleep, torpor, and continuous wakefulness. *Neurosci Biobehav Rev*. 2014;47:122–153.

Siegel JM. Clues to the functions of mammalian sleep. *Nature*. 2005;437:1264–1271.

Siegel JM. Do all animals sleep? *Trends Neurosci*. 2008;31:208–213. PMCID: 18328577.

Siegel JM. Sleep viewed as a state of adaptive inactivity. *Nat Rev Neurosci*. 2009;10:747–753. PMID: 19654581.

Siegel JM. Memory consolidation is similar in waking and sleep. *Curr Sleep Med Reports*. 2021.

Further relevant literature can be found at http://www.semel.ucla.edu/sleep-research.

See discussion of the evolution and diversity of sleep at http://thesciencenetwork.org/programs/sleep-2009/jerome-siegel.

A complete reference list can be found online at ExpertConsult.com.

Chapter 11

Sleep in Nonmammalian Vertebrates

Niels C. Rattenborg; John A. Lesku; Paul-Antoine Libourel

Chapter Highlights

- Despite being distantly related to mammals, birds exhibit sleep states similar to mammalian non–rapid eye movement (NREM) and rapid eye movement (REM) sleep. Avian NREM sleep is characterized by propagating slow waves that are homeostatically regulated in a local, use-dependent manner, as in mammals. However, some of the NREM sleep brain oscillations implicated in processing hippocampal memories in mammals have not been found in birds.
- As in mammals, avian REM sleep is characterized by electroencephalographic (EEG) activation, diminished thermoregulatory responses, rapid eye movements, and recovery following deprivation, as well as its preponderance early in development. However, unlike mammals, reductions in muscle tone are posture dependent and largely restricted to the muscles supporting the head. Birds experience hundreds of short REM sleep episodes every day.
- NREM and REM sleep either evolved independently in mammals and birds or were inherited from their common ancestor. Studies of reptiles, amphibians, and fish have not yet provided a straightforward answer to this question, largely because of unexpected diversity in the way sleep manifests in reptiles and few studies of amphibians and fish. Notably, sleep states comparable (in part) to NREM and REM sleep in mammals and birds have been found in only some species of reptiles.
- Recent EEG-based studies of birds in the wild have revealed an unprecedented ability to perform adaptively in challenging real-world ecologic circumstances, despite forgoing large amounts of sleep.

Insight into the mechanisms and functions of sleep in humans can be gained through examining sleep across the animal kingdom. Research on animals employs either model-based or comparative-based approaches. Model-based approaches aim to gain insight into human sleep through examining animals with mammalian-like sleep that are amenable to experimental manipulation. The utility of a model species is often viewed as limited by the degree to which its sleep mimics that of humans. By contrast, comparative-based research gives equal emphasis to similarities and differences across *all* taxonomic groups in an attempt to reveal overarching principles that may remain obscure using a narrower approach.[1,2] In addition, this comparative approach can reveal adaptations in unusual animals that inspire new perspectives on sleep in humans. For instance, the recent discovery that poor sleep on our first night in a new environment (i.e., "the first-night effect") is attributable to lighter sleep in parts of the left hemisphere[3] was inspired by ecologically based research on sleep in ducks.[4,5]

In this chapter, we summarize comparative sleep research focused on avian and nonavian reptiles (the latter hereafter referred to as *reptiles*) and amphibians. We also discuss one recent study on zebrafish that has direct bearing on the evolution of sleep states in vertebrates. The evolutionary relationships between these groups are summarized in Box 11.1, and the comparative neuroanatomy of vertebrates, as it relates to the later discussions, is reviewed in Box 11.2.

AVIAN SLEEP

Sleep States

Birds exhibit two sleep states in many respects similar to mammalian rapid eye movement (REM) and non–rapid eye movement (NREM) sleep (Figure 11.1). Wakefulness and NREM sleep, also called slow wave sleep (SWS), are distinguished primarily by the presence of high-amplitude, slow waves with a peak frequency around 2 Hz in electroencephalography (EEG)[6-12] and intra-"cortical" local field potential (LFP) recordings of the hyperpallium (primary visual cortex; Box 11.2) during NREM sleep (Figure 11.2).[13] Although intracellular recordings have not been reported during natural sleep in birds, under anesthesia, pallial neurons show slow oscillations between hyperpolarized "down states" without action potentials and depolarized "up states" with action potentials[14] similar to those described in mammals during anesthesia and natural NREM sleep.[15] The few recordings from birds suggest that the frequency of the oscillation may be higher (1–2 Hz) than in mammals (<1 Hz). During NREM sleep in pigeons (*Columba livia*), LFP slow waves usually originate within and propagate through the hyperpallial regions that receive visual input via the thalamic lateral geniculate nucleus (Figure 11.2).[13] As propagating slow waves have been described in humans and other mammals,[16] they are a fundamental property of NREM sleep.

BOX 11.1 EVOLUTIONARY RELATIONSHIPS OF VERTEBRATES

Our interpretation of the evolution of sleep states in vertebrates depends on an accurate understanding of their phylogenetic relationship. Mammals, birds, and reptiles last shared a common ancestor as recently as 320 million years ago (mya).[135] Although the exact identity of this ancestor is unknown, paleontologists refer to it as the "stem amniote" because the production of amniotic eggs distinguishes mammals, birds, and reptiles from amphibians and fish, which produce anamniotic eggs. The stem amniote, a reptile-like (reptiliomorph) animal, gave rise to two lineages: the synapsids, leading to the evolution of mammals (monotremes, marsupials, and eutherians [formerly placentals], and the sauropsids, giving rise to reptiles, a lineage that includes birds.

Within mammals, monotremes and therian mammals (marsupials and eutherians) diverged 166 mya. Among the living reptilian groups, birds are most closely related to crocodilians,[136] both being members of a group called Archosauria. Fossil evidence indicates that within Archosauria, birds evolved from flightless, feathered theropod dinosaurs more than 150 mya.[137] Living birds include two groups, the Palaeognathae (large flightless ostriches, emus, rheas and cassowaries, the much smaller flightless kiwis, and volant tinamous) and Neognathae (all other birds), which diverged 72 mya.[138] Within Palaeognathae, flightlessness secondarily evolved several times, with only tinamous retaining the ancestral ability to fly.[101]

Contrary to the early view that turtles represented the most basal type of reptiles, recent genetic data indicate that turtles are more closely related to Archosaurs.[139] Instead, Lepidosaurs (lizards and snakes) represent an early split from the lineage that gave rise to turtles and Archosaurs. Finally, amphibians and amniotes last shared a common ancestor 338 mya, and the last common ancestor shared between tetrapods (amphibians and amniotes) and zebrafish, an emerging species in comparative sleep research, lived 430 mya.

Finally, it is important to note that all animals alive today have undergone evolution for the same amount of time.[140] When fish and the ancestor to tetrapods split 430 mya, both lineages continued to evolve. It is also important to recognize that the phenotypes of extant species reflect a mosaic of primitive, derived, convergently evolved, and evolutionarily lost traits.[2,98,101,141,142] Consequently, conclusions about the evolution of sleep drawn from a single species can be misguided by idiosyncrasies of that species' evolutionary history.[40,106] To distinguish between possible evolutionary scenarios and truly identify primitive and derived sleep phenotypes, several species within all taxonomic groups must be examined whenever possible. Only then will we be able to tease apart the evolution of sleep and the functional implications of its diversity.

Despite these similarities, thalamocortical spindles, a prominent feature of mammalian NREM sleep, have not been detected in EEG recordings in birds.[13,17-26] Early reports of spindles proved to be artefacts from intermittent high-frequency oscillations of the eyes occurring during NREM sleep, REM sleep, and wakefulness[27] (Figure 11.1), which are thought to keep the poorly vascularized avian retina oxygenated.[28] Recently, van der Meij and colleagues used intracerebral LFP recordings of the hyperpallium and thalamus to determine whether spindles might have been missed in the previous (epidural) EEG recordings; however, spindles were not detected.[13]

Hippocampal activity during NREM sleep also appears to differ between mammals and birds. In mammals, the hippocampus exhibits sharp-wave ripples (SWRs), large bursts of synchronous activity, which occur during NREM sleep, as well as while grooming, feeding, and pauses in ambulation in rodents.[29] The few studies that examined hippocampal activity in birds did not report SWRs during wakefulness nor NREM sleep.[22]

As with NREM sleep, avian REM sleep (Figure 11.1, *B*) shares many features with mammalian REM sleep. Avian REM sleep is characterized by EEG activation similar to that occurring during wakefulness.[30,31] However, in contrast to mammals, a hippocampal theta oscillation has not been observed during REM sleep in birds.[10,21-23,25,30-35] EEG activation during avian REM sleep is associated with rapid eye movements and twitches of the bill, wings (unpublished data), head, and body,[19,23,36-38] closure of the eyes (if they were open during preceding NREM sleep),[a] and elevated arousal thresholds when compared with NREM sleep.[25,26,37,41] Changes in respiratory and heart rates between NREM and REM sleep vary considerably among the species examined.[25,42,43]

Behaviorally, REM sleep is typically accompanied by head drops.[b] Drooping of the wings[34] and swaying[11] and tipping of the body[23] have also been observed in standing birds. The behavior of the head depends (in part) on its position at the start of a REM sleep episode: when it is facing forward and unsupported it drops, whereas when the head is turned backward, resting on the bird's shoulder, it may slide off the shoulder or not move at all.[19,24,42] When the head is fully supported on the back, it remains still during REM sleep.[42] Despite the head drops reported in several species, the neck electromyogram (EMG) shows either no change from preceding NREM sleep or only partial reductions (hypotonia) in muscle tone.[c] Mammal-like atonia has been observed only in domestic geese (*Anser anser domesticus*).[42] As in other birds, when geese enter REM sleep with the head facing forward and unsupported, it drops and the neck EMG shows hypotonia or no change; however, mammal-like atonia occurs when the head is fully supported on the back (Figure 11.3).[42] As the duration of REM sleep episodes does not depend on head position,[42] this posture-dependent difference in neck muscle tone is due to other factors. In many species, rather than dropping unabated, the head drops in a slow and controlled manner, often interrupted by pauses.[d] In addition, slow raising of the head can also occur during REM sleep.[11,50] This, and the posture-dependent differences in tone observed in geese, suggest that competitive processes are acting on the neck musculature, one driving reduced tone, and one seemingly limiting or controlling the drop of the unsupported head.[42] Finally, the fact that the head can drop, even when the single EMG recording shows no reduction in activity,[e] indicates that the methods previously used to measure neck muscle tone fail to reflect the full dynamics of muscle tone regulation in birds.

Unlike mammals, birds can engage in REM sleep while standing, even while balancing on one foot. Contrary to the long-held idea that birds rely on a passive locking mechanism in their feet and legs to stand during sleep, recent work in common starlings (*Sturnus vulgaris*) suggests that they need

[a]References 10, 11, 23, 26, 32, 39, 40.
[b]References 8, 11, 12, 25, 26, 35, 36, 38-41, 44-47.
[c]References 17, 20, 24-26, 30, 32, 39, 40, 47-49.
[d]References 17, 18, 20, 26, 47, 50.
[e]References 20, 23, 25, 26, 35, 45.

BOX 11.2 COMPARATIVE NEUROANATOMY

Interpreting the similarities and differences between sleep in vertebrates requires an understanding of brain evolution. Many of the subcortical nuclei that regulate sleep and wakefulness are conserved between zebrafish and mammals.[143] By contrast, the organization of forebrain pallial neurons has diversified during vertebrate evolution.[135] Although sauropsids lack the six-layered neocortex found in mammals, their forebrains contain homologous pallial neurons organized in a different manner. Based on gene expression profiles and connectomics, amniotes share three general types of pallial neurons: input neurons that receive projections from the thalamus, intratelencephalic projecting neurons, and output neurons that project from the pallium to other brain regions.[135,144]

It is currently debated whether most pallial neurons in sauropsids are homologous to mammalian neocortical neurons, or if only some sectors of their pallia are homologous to the neocortex and others to the pallial claustrum and amygdala.[144-147] This is due (in part) to the manner in which the pallial neurons are organized. The embryonic dorsal pallium, which forms much of the neocortex in mammals, gives rise to the dorsal cortex in reptiles, a three-layered laminar structure.[148] In birds, the dorsal cortex present in their reptilian ancestors evolved into the hyperpallium, or Wulst, a bulge on the dorsal surface of the brain composed of several nuclei stacked one on top of the other.[135,145,146,148] Unlike the reptilian dorsal cortex and the mammalian neocortex, the hyperpallium lacks pyramidal neurons with apical dendrites extending across the layers and toward the surface of the brain; instead, the avian pallium comprises stellate neurons. Although the hyperpallium is involved in processing visual, somatosensory, and olfactory information, most of this region is dedicated to processing visual input from the thalamic lateral geniculate nucleus and therefore is considered functionally homologous to the mammalian primary visual cortex (V1).[148]

In addition to the differences in pallial cytoarchitecture in the dorsal pallium, sauropsids have a brain region called the dorsal ventricular ridge (DVR), a large nuclear structure protruding medially into the lateral ventricle that is not present in mammals, amphibians, or fish.[135] It is still actively debated whether the DVR is homologous to portions of the neocortex or to the claustrum and pallial amygdala. The transcriptomic profiles of DVR neurons have been interpreted as supporting both hypotheses to varying degrees.[135,144,145,149-152] Embryological studies indicate that the DVR develops from the lateral and ventral pallia, regions that give rise to the claustrum and pallial portions of the amygdala in mammals.[147] By contrast, connectomics suggest homology between the DVR and neocortex, with subpopulations of the neurons corresponding to specific layers[152] or, more generally, to specific neuron types (i.e., input, intratelencephalic, and output) in the neocortex.[135,145]

Regardless of which scenario is correct, there is a general consensus that the DVR is involved in performing functions similar to those handled by the neocortex. Although the crocodilian DVR has subregions similar to those making up the avian DVR (mesopallium, nidopallium, and endopallium),[145,153] the DVR reaches its largest size in birds, in which it has been most extensively studied.[154,155] In birds, the independent evolution of large brains comparable in relative size to those in mammals,[156] is due, in large part, to expansion of the DVR.[153,157] Remarkably, the density of neurons in the avian pallium, which mostly comprises the DVR, actually exceeds that of primates with similar-sized brains.[158] The DVR includes primary and secondary sensory (visual and auditory) areas, as well as high-order association regions involved in performing complex cognitive processes, including those performed by the mammalian prefrontal cortex.[154,155,159] Indeed, despite lacking the laminar arrangement of neurons, the avian brain generates complex behaviors in some cases comparable with those performed by primates, including the manufacture and use of tools.[1,154]

to actively maintain some muscle tone to stay upright.[51] Consequently, during REM sleep birds sustain tone in the muscles required to balance while standing,[47] as well as those that actively hold the other foot up. Taken together with the data from geese described previously, this suggests that in contrast to the centralized, largely global regulation of skeletal muscle atonia observed during mammalian REM sleep,[52] muscle tone during avian REM sleep is regulated in a local manner.

Episodes of REM sleep are very short in birds. For 23 species from 9 orders, REM sleep bouts last 11.5 ± 7.8 seconds (mean ± SD). However, the species with the six highest values (mean 22.7 ± 7.1 seconds) originate from one research group. When these unreplicated values are excluded, the mean drops to just 7.6 ± 2.1 seconds.

Transitional States

Quantifying the exact time spent in NREM and REM sleep poses several challenges. This is largely due to the fact that birds engage in hundreds of transitions between states every day. Given that transitional states by definition contain features of the state being exited and the state being entered, they are prone to subjectivity during scoring.

Transitional states have been scored using various approaches. Drowsiness is a poorly defined and inconsistently used behavioral state typically characterized by frequent blinking of the eyes and small head movements occurring in conjunction with slow wave activity (SWA) intermediate between unequivocal wakefulness and NREM sleep and/or SWA rapidly fluctuating between waking and NREM sleep levels.* One study also defined a short-lasting intermediate sleep state with spectral features between wakefulness and NREM sleep or NREM and REM sleep that occurred during transitions between states, including REM sleep.[9] Similar transitional states are common in birds because of the daily occurrence of hundreds of short bouts of REM sleep.† How these transitional epochs are handled undoubtedly has a large influence on the amount of REM sleep scored.[17] Given these scoring issues, comparative studies based on data from multiple species and laboratories[6,9,55] should be interpreted with caution.

Eye States

Birds rarely close their eyes while awake. However, some species exhibit levels of EEG SWA (typically, 0.5–4.5 Hz spectral power) comparable with NREM sleep during extended periods of immobility with their eyes partially or fully open,[11,23,26,32,39] a state also observed in some mammalian species.[56] This state has been variably categorized as quiet wakefulness, drowsiness,[7] or NREM sleep,[10,39] in some cases

*References 7, 8, 17, 25, 41, 44, 48.
†References 9, 17-20, 23, 26, 32, 35, 39, 53, 54.

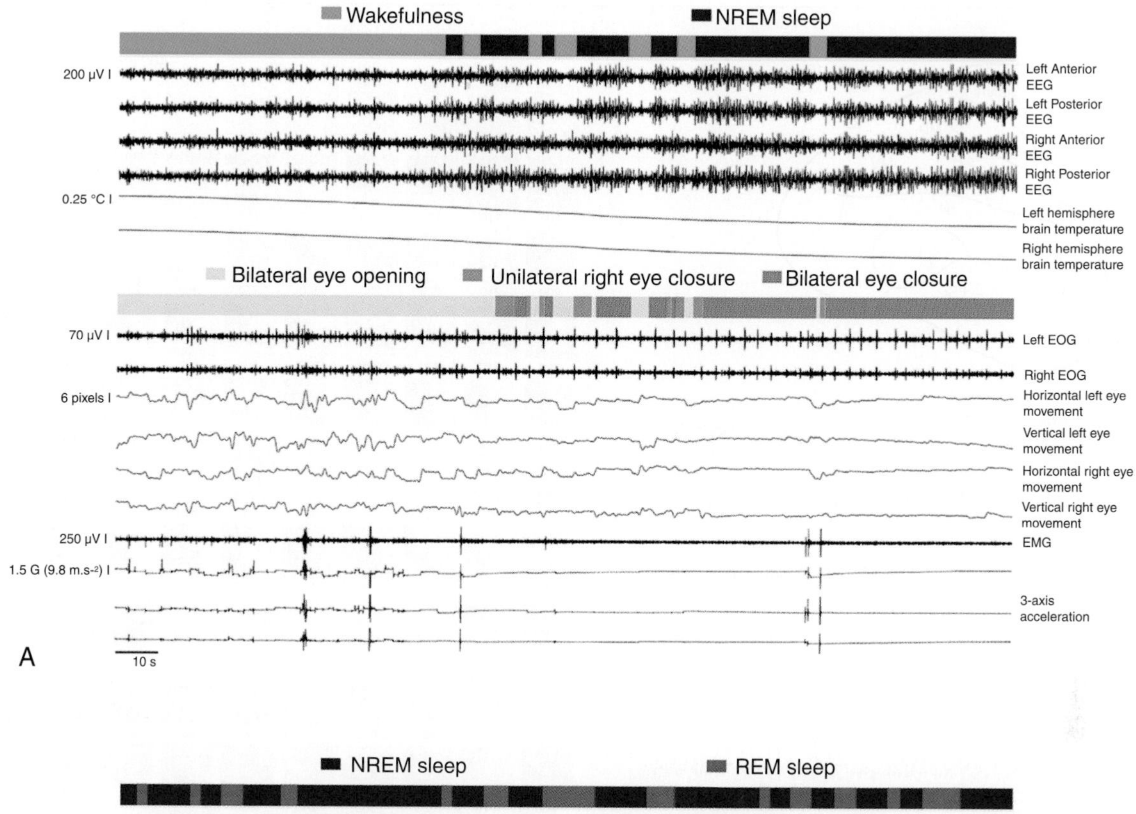

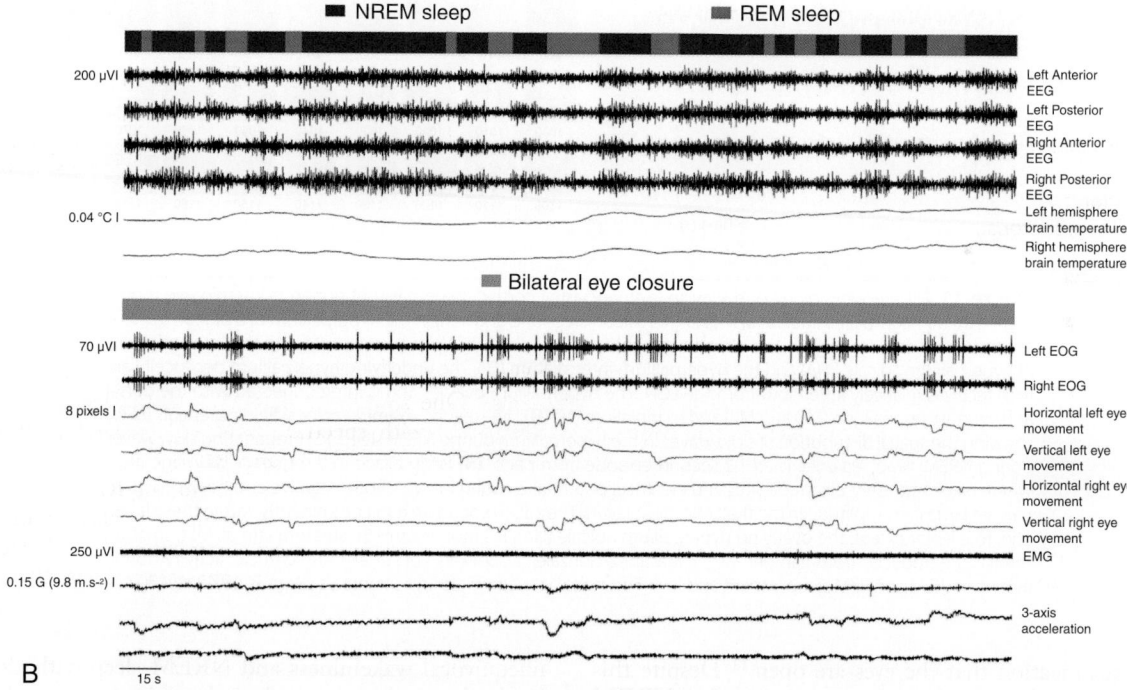

Figure 11.1 Avian sleep states. **(A)** Transition from wakefulness to non-rapid eye movement (NREM) sleep, and **(B)** alternations between NREM and rapid eye movement (REM) sleep in a pigeon. *Top bar,* Hypnogram showing wakefulness (*green*), NREM sleep (*blue*), and REM sleep (*red*); electroencephalogram (EEG) recorded from the anterior and posterior hyperpallia of the left (L) and right (R) hemispheres; brain temperature recorded from the L and R hyperpallia; eye state, both open (*light grey*), both closed (*dark grey*), and left open and right closed (*orange*); electrooculogram (EOG) recorded from the L and R eyes band-pass filtered (25–39 Hz) to show occurrence of high-frequency eye oscillations present in all states; L and R eye movements along horizontal and vertical axes defined relative to the plain of eyelid closure calculated from pupillometry (positive increases in signal values represent rostral and dorsal movements, respectively); neck electromyogram (EMG); head movements along three axes recorded with an accelerometer. Trace duration: A = 210 s and B = 320 s. (From Gianina Ungurean, unpublished data.)

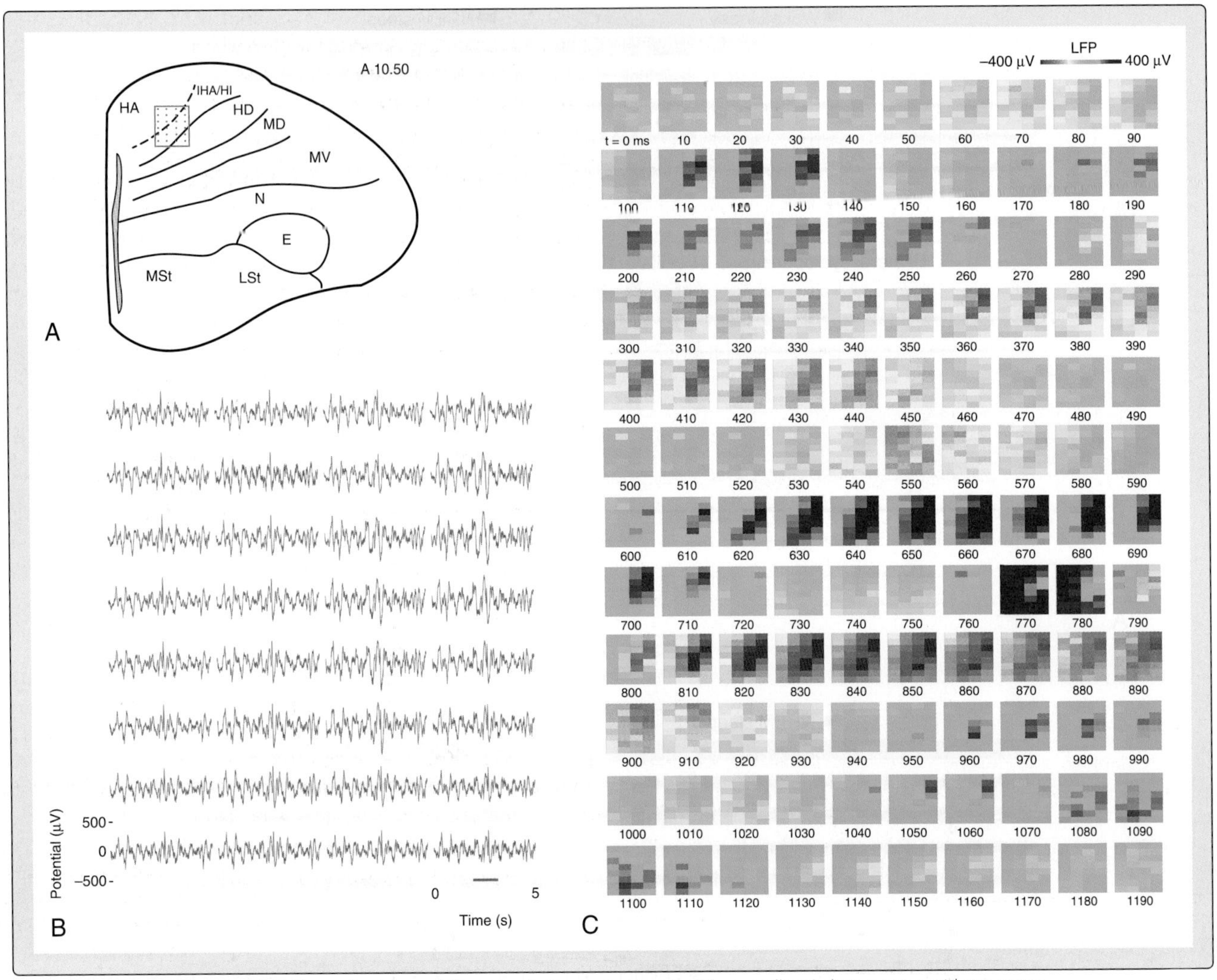

Figure 11.2 Neurophysiology of the avian "primary visual cortex" (hyperpallium) during non-rapid eye movement (NREM) sleep. **(A)** Position of a 32-channel silicon electrode grid (*red*) in the hyperpallium of a pigeon (*medial, left* and *dorsal, top*). Input from the avian lateral geniculate nucleus (LGN) projects primarily to the interstitial part of hyperpallium apicale (*IHA*) and the hyperpallium intercalatum (*HI*). The underlying hyperpallium densocellulare (*HD*) receives relatively little input from the LGN. The hyperpallium overlies and is interconnected with the dorsal and ventral mesopallium (*MD* and *MV*) and nidopallium (*N*). **(B)** Five-second example of local field potentials (LFPs) showing the spatial distribution of slow waves in the hyperpallium during NREM sleep. **(C)** Propagating slow waves during NREM sleep: *red underlined* 1.2-second episode from panel **(B)** is visualized in a sequence of image plots where pixels represent electrode sites and electrical potential is coded in color. Both negative and positive potentials are largest in amplitude in the thalamic input layers. They also propagate most prominently within these layers and, to a lesser extent, the overlying hyperpallium apicale (HA). E, Entopallium; LSt, striatum lateral; MSt, striatum medial. (Reproduced from van der Meij J, Martinez-Gonzalez D, Beckers GJL, et al. Intra-"cortical" activity during avian non-REM and REM sleep: variant and invariant traits between birds and mammals. *Sleep*. 2019;42:zsy230.)

with the qualification that the eyes are open.[11] Despite this awake-like behavior, these slow waves appear to reflect NREM sleep because they often terminate with a transition to REM sleep characterized by closure of both eyes, behavioral signs of reduced muscle tone, and EEG activation.[11,24,26,32] By keeping their eyes open while exhibiting EEG slow waves, birds may be able to maintain some responsiveness to threatening visual stimuli in the environment while still obtaining some of the benefits of NREM sleep.

A trade-off between visual vigilance and NREM sleep processes is suggested by birds sleeping with only one eye open. Many birds often engage in unilateral eye closure, a behavior associated with high levels of SWA in the hemisphere contralateral to the closed eye, and SWA levels intermediate between unequivocal wakefulness and NREM sleep with closed eyes in the hemisphere contralateral to the open eye.[4,5,9,21,57-61] This state has been referred to as asymmetric SWS (ASWS) or unihemispheric SWS (USWS).[61] Birds are able to switch between bihemispheric SWS (BSWS) with both eyes closed and ASWS with one eye open in response to ecologic demands for wakefulness.[4,5] In mallards (*Anas platyrhynchos*), when compared with individuals flanked by other birds, the ratio of SWS with one versus both eyes closed increases when the birds are positioned at the edge of a group.[4,5] Moreover, when sleeping with one eye open, mallards at the edge direct the open eye away from the other birds, as if watching for approaching predators. This, and the finding that the open eye is responsive to threatening visual stimuli, suggests that sleeping with one

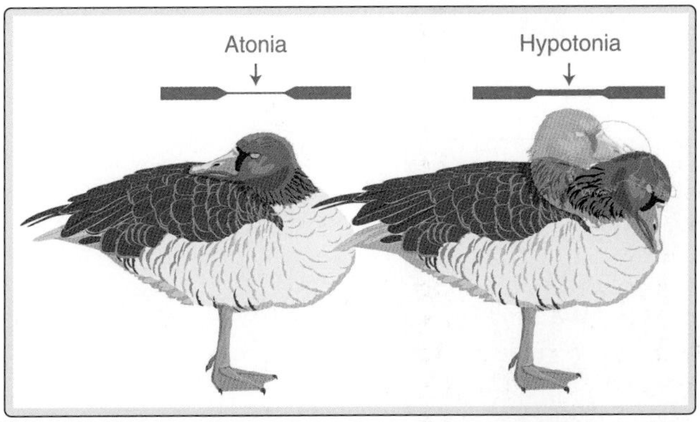

Figure 11.3 Posture-dependent regulation of muscle tone during rapid eye movement (REM) sleep in geese. Like many other birds, geese can engage in REM sleep while balancing on one foot. The head can face backward, supported on the bird's back (*left bird*) or forward and unsupported (*right bird*). When the head is supported, it usually remains still, and the neck electromyogram (EMG) shows atonia. By contrast, when the head is unsupported, it drops in a controlled manner and the neck EMG shows hypotonia. Birds only occasionally show behavioral signs of reduced tone in the muscles involved in holding the wings against the body and balancing on one foot. (Illustration by Damond Kyllo based on Dewasmes G, Cohen-Adad F, Koubi H, et al. Polygraphic and behavioral study of sleep in geese: existence of nuchal atonia during paradoxical sleep. *Physiol Behav.* 1985;35:67–73.)

eye open reflects a visually based anti-predator strategy.[4,5,60,62] (Reptiles also keep one eye open and on the lookout in risky situations, although the neural correlates of this behavior have not been systematically investigated.[59,63-65]) The fact that mallards at the edge of the group only open one eye, rather than both, suggests that a trade-off exists between visual vigilance and processes linked to EEG SWA. Consequently, NREM sleep with both eyes open may reflect a similar strategy used when threats are perceived in all directions.

NREM Sleep Regulation

In mammals, the level of EEG SWA during NREM sleep increases as a function of time spent awake and decreases as a function of time spent in NREM sleep. This relationship, and the positive correlation between SWA and arousal thresholds,[66] suggest that SWA reflects homeostatically regulated processes occurring during NREM sleep. Although a direct link between the level of NREM sleep SWA and arousal thresholds has not been determined in birds (but see the work by Szymczak and colleagues[43]), the temporal pattern of SWA suggests that NREM sleep is more intense early in the night in diurnal songbirds.[8,43,44] In pigeons, however, changes in NREM sleep SWA across the night are either absent[7,11,67]or weak,[10] possibly because of their propensity to take frequent naps across the day.[67] Although pigeons that are sleep deprived by gentle handling for 24 hours did not show an increase in SWA during recovery NREM sleep,[11] depriving them of daytime naps for 8 hours resulted in a significant increase in SWA during recovery sleep at night.[10] An increase in NREM sleep SWA was also observed after 4 to 8 hours of nighttime sleep deprivation in songbirds,[8,68] suggesting that this is a general feature of avian sleep.[69]

Berger and Phillips[7] reported that constant light suppressed sleep greatly in pigeons for up to 74 days but failed to cause an increase in SWA when the birds were switched to constant dim light. However, when quantified irrespective of scored sleep state, SWA in pigeons kept in constant light was maintained at 94.5% of the level occurring during the 12:12 light:dark schedule.[7,8,10] Consequently, it is perhaps not surprising that SWA did not increase in dim light.

Local NREM Sleep Homeostasis

Lesku and colleagues used unilateral visual stimulation and total sleep deprivation to determine whether NREM sleep-related SWA is homeostatically regulated in a local, use-dependent manner in birds (Figure 11.4).[70] In contrast to the symmetric increase in SWA observed after sleep deprivation without asymmetric visual stimulation,[10] a pronounced asymmetry in SWA was evident during recovery NREM sleep with the hyperpallium previously visually stimulated showing a large increase in SWA, and the visually deprived hyperpallium showing no change in SWA. As in humans,[71,72] the former likely reflects a homeostatic response to extended time awake and taxing brain use, whereas the latter probably reflects the summation of factors with opposing effects on SWA: increased time awake increasing SWA and decreased visual input decreasing SWA. Importantly, this asymmetry was restricted to the visual hyperpallium, underscoring the specific link between visual stimulation and local SWA homeostasis.

REM Sleep Homeostasis

Sleep-depriving pigeons for 8 or 24 hours caused a significant increase in REM sleep.[10,11] However, this occurred during the second half of the night after 8 hours of daytime sleep deprivation, and during the first half of the night after 24 hours of sleep deprivation. A similar relationship between the duration of sleep deprivation and the timing of REM sleep during recovery sleep has also been described in rats.[73] REM sleep homeostasis has also been demonstrated in response to changes in housing conditions that likely influence the birds' perceived risk of predation.[67] Finally, as in rats, pigeons deprived of sleep using a modified version of the disk-over-water method also show a large rebound in REM sleep.[74] Interestingly, however, for the variables measured, pigeons did not develop signs of the sleep deprivation syndrome described in rats using the disk-over-water method.[75]

Sleep Architecture

Birds from diverse orders exhibit sleep architecture similar to mammals. In many diurnal birds, NREM sleep, as a proportion of sleep time, declines and REM sleep increases across the night, largely because of an increase in the number of REM sleep episodes* and, in some species, their duration.[9,10,40] However, this pattern is not a universal finding in diurnal birds.[35,76,77] In nocturnal barn owls (*Tyto alba pratincola*), the number and duration of REM sleep episodes increase across the daylight hours.[78]

The duration of the "sleep cycle" between episodes of NREM and REM sleep has not been systematically quantified in birds. Although REM sleep becomes more prevalent later in the major sleep phase in several species, the interval between individual episodes is highly variable. Qualitatively, this arises from the fact that birds alternate between periods of sleep with infrequent and frequent episodes of REM sleep.[44]

Sleep Ontogeny

In most mammals examined electrophysiologically, the time spent sleeping, particularly in REM sleep, is high early in life

*References 9, 10, 17-19, 24, 40, 44, 49.

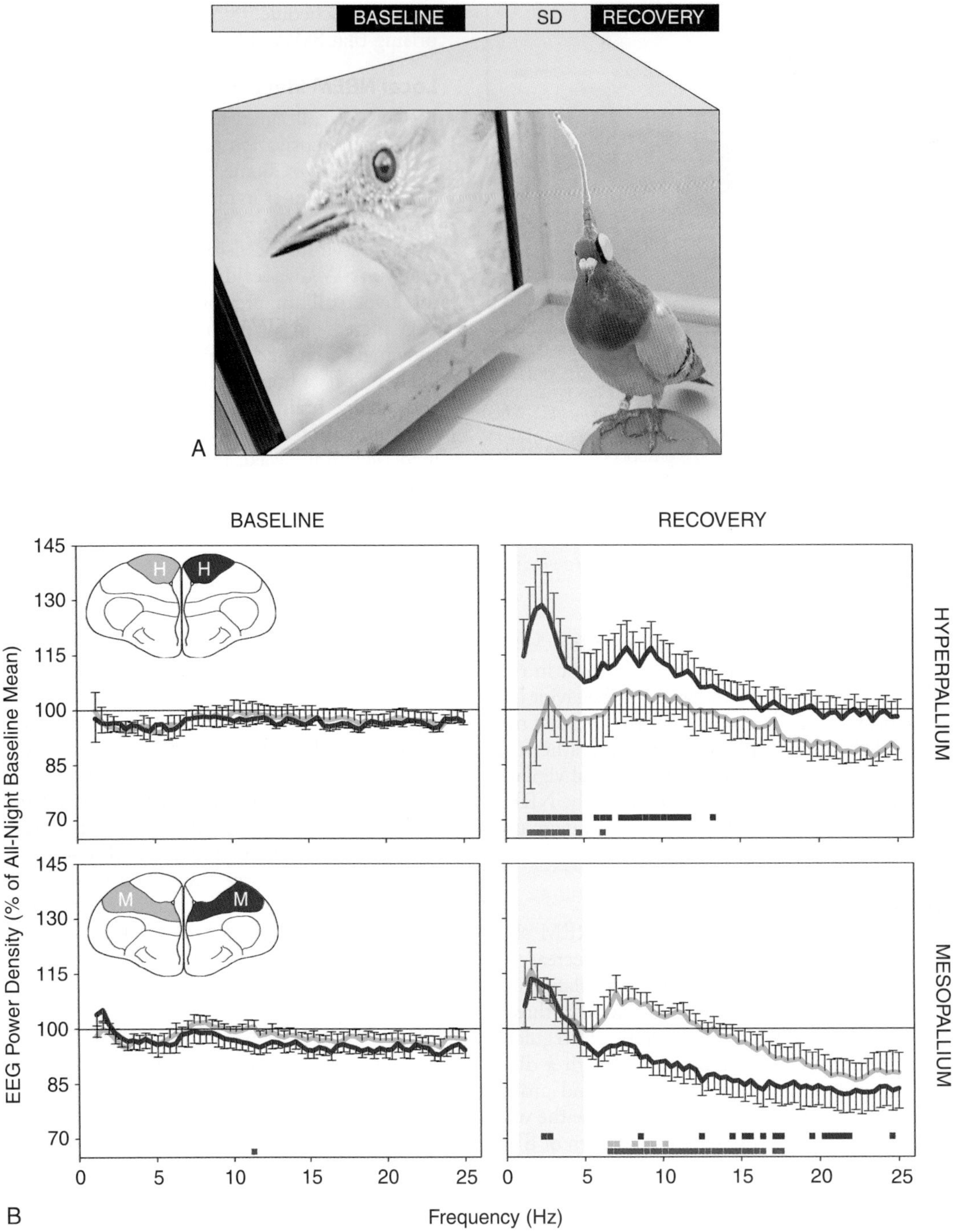

Figure 11.4 Local sleep homeostasis in the avian brain. **(A)** Experimental design: a 12-hour baseline night, 8-hour period of bihemispheric sleep deprivation (SD) with unilateral visual stimulation and a 12-hour recovery night. Photograph shows the experimental environment during the treatment. **(B)** Normalized spectral power density (0.78–25.00 Hz) during non-rapid eye movement sleep for the first quarter of the baseline and recovery nights for the stimulated (*dark blue*) and visually deprived (*light blue*) hyperpallia and mesopallia. Data are presented as mean ± standard error. *Colored squares* at the bottom of each recovery night plot reflect a significant pairwise comparison between the baseline and recovery night of the stimulated (*dark blue*) and visually deprived (*light blue*) hyperpallia; *red squares* denote a significant asymmetry between the left and right brain region during recovery sleep. Although the experimental treatment induced interhemispheric asymmetries across a wide range of frequencies, slow wave activity (*yellow shading*) in the hyperpallium showed the largest asymmetry. *Insets*, Frontal view of a transverse section through the cerebrum of a pigeon highlighting the hyperpallium (H) and mesopallium (M). (Courtesy of Axel Griesch.)

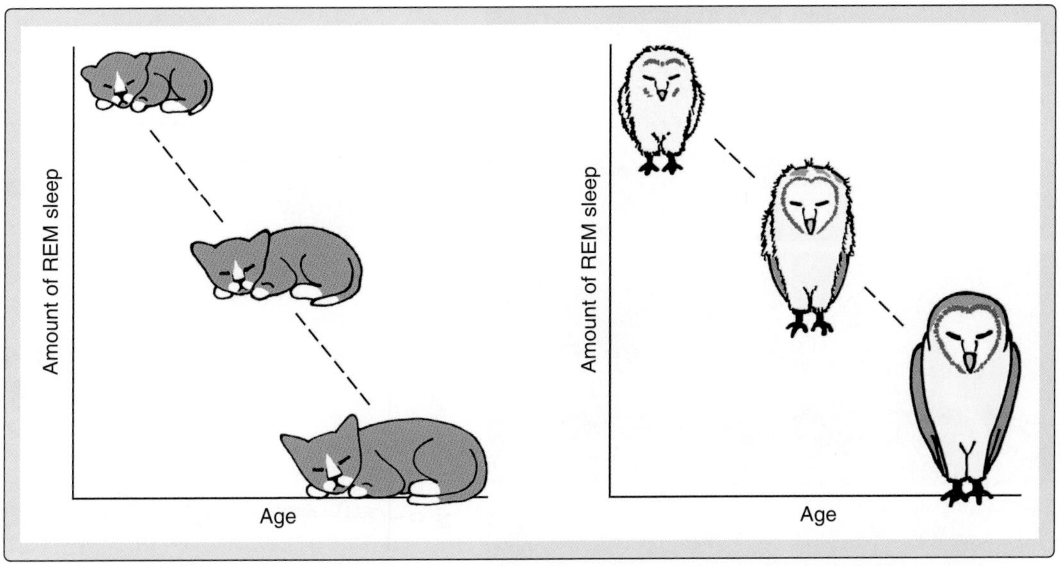

Figure 11.5 Mammalian-like rapid eye movement (REM) sleep ontogeny in barn owls. In both altricial mammals, such as cats, and altricial barn owls, REM sleep as a proportion of recording and sleep times is high early in life and progressively declines to adult levels.[12] The figure conveys the general pattern and not absolute values. (Courtesty of Ninon Ballerstädt.)

and then gradually declines to adult levels[79] (see Scriba and colleagues[12]). Until recently it had been unclear whether REM sleep also declines with age in young birds (see the review by Scriba and colleagues[12]). Sleep ontogeny was recently examined in barn owls (*Tyto alba guttata*) in the wild.[12] REM sleep expressed as a percent of total recording or sleep time declined with age (Figure 11.5), suggesting that, as in mammals, REM sleep is involved in brain maturation.

Temperature and Photoperiod

Mammals and birds, both homeotherms, show similar changes in thermoregulation across states. Although birds pant or shiver during NREM sleep when thermally challenged, these thermoregulatory behaviors diminish when they enter REM sleep.[12,80,81] As in many mammals,[82] brain temperature in birds declines and increases during NREM and REM sleep, respectively (Figure 11.1, *B*).[83]

Adaptive Sleeplessness

Pectoral sandpipers (*Calidris melanotos*) reproduce in the Arctic Circle under continuous daylight during a 3-week breeding season. The males are polygynous and as such their reproductive success is determined by their ability to mate with as many females as possible. Conversely, a female must choose the best quality male to sire her only clutch of the year. Consequently, competition among males for access to choosy fertile females is intense. Males establish and defend territories against rival males and display to females with aerial and ground displays (Figure 11.6, *A*, *B*), which precede copulation when performed effectively.

The biologic drive to sleep on a daily basis is so strong that humans will fall asleep even in life-threatening situations, such as while driving a car. Moreover, sleep restriction and fragmentation impair waking performance in humans[84-87] and other animals,[88] suggesting that sleep performs restorative processes that maintain adaptive brain function.[84,89,90] Thus were it not for a biologic drive for sleep, and the dependence of waking performance on prior sleep, male pectoral sandpipers would be able to secure mates around the clock. Accordingly, in this highly competitive environment, sexual selection has favored males with an ability to perform well on the tasks leading up to mating while getting little sleep. Using actigraphy and EEG/EMG recordings in the wild, Lesku and colleagues determined that some males had a remarkable ability to sleep very little for several weeks.[91] In the most extreme case, a male was active more than 95% of the time for 19 days. In addition, the little sleep some males obtained was highly fragmented, and although these males attempted to compensate for lost sleep by sleeping more intensely (i.e., higher SWA), they nevertheless maintained a large sleep debt. Surprisingly, however, these males were best able to convince choosy females to mate with them and ultimately sired the most offspring (Figure 11.6, *B*), indicating that their waking performance was not impaired in any meaningful way. Importantly, these findings indicate that impaired performance is not an evolutionarily inescapable outcome of sleep restriction and fragmentation.[91]

Migration

Normally diurnal songbirds switch to flying at night during migration.[92] In response to an endogenous circannual rhythm, captive songbirds exhibit nocturnal migratory restlessness (*Zugunruhe*), consisting of hopping and wing flapping, during the spring and fall, when their conspecifics in the wild would be migrating.[92] Captive songbirds exhibiting nocturnal migratory restlessness reduce the time spent sleeping at night by two-thirds but may compensate (in part) for lost nighttime sleep by increasing the time spent drowsy or napping in the day.[44,50,57]

Recently, sleep behavior and physiology were examined in garden warblers (*Sylvia borin*) caught at a migratory stopover site immediately after crossing the Mediterranean Sea.[93] Interestingly, at night, birds with low body fat, body mass, and muscle mass spent more time sleeping, were more likely to assume a heat-retaining sleep posture with the head tucked in the feathers, and had a lower metabolic rate during sleep but were less responsive to a sound simulating an approaching

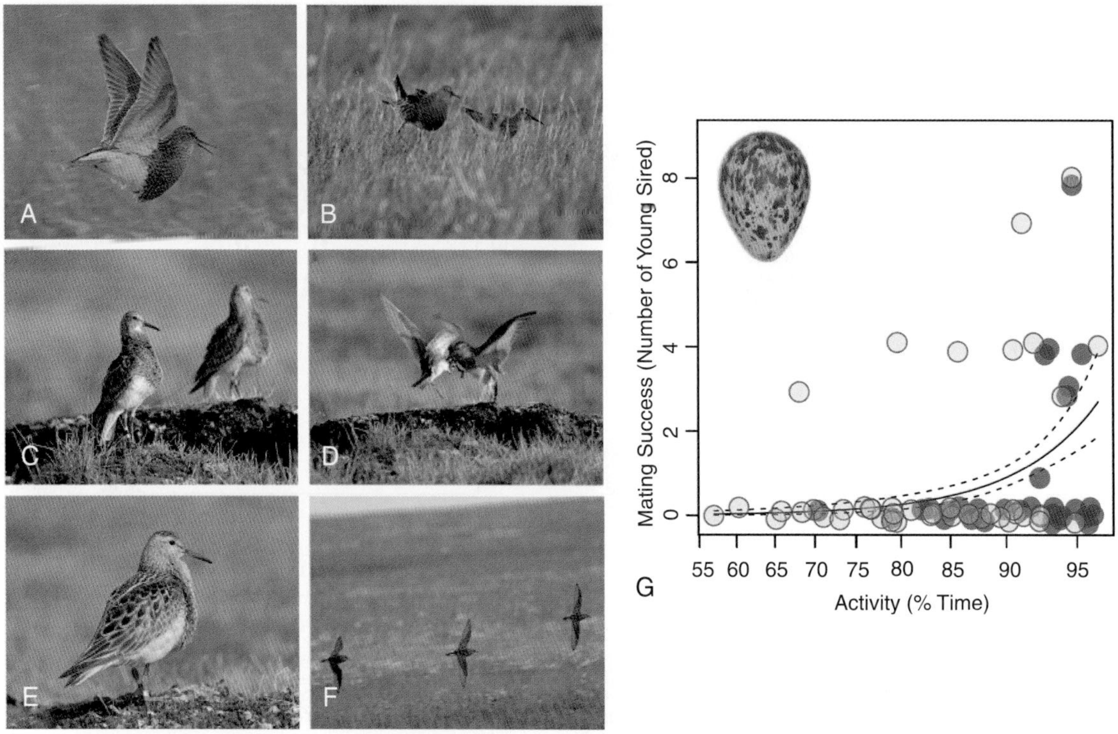

Figure 11.6 Adaptive sleep loss in polygynous male pectoral sandpipers. Male pectoral sandpipers engaging in various behaviors during an intense period of male–male competition for territories and females. Male displaying in flight **(A)**. Male displaying to a female (smaller bird) on the ground **(B)**. Territorial displays between two males **(C)** leading to a physical fight **(D)**. A male standing vigilant for intruding males, available females, and predators **(E)**. Males engaged in an aerial chase **(F)**. The graph **(G)** shows the positive relationship (*fitted line*, with the dotted lines showing the 95% confidence intervals) between time spent active (awake) and the number of young sired for 2 years (*light and dark grey circles* reflect raw data). *Inset,* A pectoral sandpiper egg. (A-D, F: Courtesy of Wolfgang Forstmeier, Max Planck Institute for Ornithology. E: Courtesy of B.K.)

predator than birds in better physical condition. In addition, birds in better condition exhibited more migratory restlessness,[93] suggesting that they would have continued their migration that night in the wild.[92] Collectively, these findings indicate that birds in poor condition invest in deep nocturnal sleep at the expense of antipredatory vigilance, to conserve energy and, possibly, recover sleep lost during the adverse environmental conditions (e.g., difficult foraging or prolonged flights) that caused their poor physical condition.

Sleep in Flight

In contrast to most migrating songbirds, which have opportunities to land and sleep each day, recent advances in tracking and actigraphy have confirmed that several other types of birds fly nonstop for periods lasting several days to months (reviewed in Rattenborg[94]). For example, great frigatebirds (*Fregata minor*) spend up to 2 months foraging over the ocean[95] but cannot land on the water without becoming waterlogged, and therefore fly continuously.[95] Given the universal need for daily sleep,[89] it has been assumed that these birds sleep in flight.[94]

By deploying EEG data loggers on great frigatebirds, Rattenborg and colleagues established for the first time that sleep can occur in flight (Figure 11.7, *A*).[96] Sleep occurred primarily during the first hours of the night while the birds were soaring in circles, to the left or right, on rising air masses, but never during flapping flight (Figure 11.7, *B*). NREM sleep was categorized as BSWS or ASWS based on the degree of interhemispheric asymmetry in EEG SWA; USWS was a subcategory of ASWS with an asymmetry exceeding the threshold used to define USWS in marine mammals.[97] Most SWS was ASWS, with nearly half of it consisting of USWS; however, BSWS also occurred in flight. Although episodes of sleep lasted on average just 12 seconds (versus 52 seconds on land), bouts of USWS, ASWS, and BSWS occasionally lasted for several minutes. The accelerometry recordings revealed that when sleeping deeper (based on SWA) with the left hemisphere, the birds circled to the left and when sleeping deeper with the right hemisphere they circled to the right (Figure 11.7, *B* and *C*). Interestingly, interhemispheric asymmetries in gamma (30 to 80 Hz) showed the opposite relationship with turning direction (Figure 11.7, *C*). Given that each hyperpallium primarily receives input from the contralateral eye, and gamma has been implicated in visual processing, this suggests that the birds kept the eye facing into the turn open (Figure 11.7, *D*), possibly to avoid collisions with other birds. Finally, in addition to engaging in BSWS, frigatebirds also exhibited REM sleep in flight. During bouts of SWS, brief periods of EEG activation occurred in conjunction with accelerometry signals indicative of head dropping similar to that observed during REM sleep on land.

Surprisingly, during their 6-day flights, frigatebirds only slept on average for 42 minutes per day, whereas after landing they slept over 12 hours each day. The low amount of sleep in flight suggests that frigatebirds face unexpected demands for attention at night that usually exceed that afforded by ASWS or USWS. In addition to sleeping more, in longer bouts, and more symmetrically, during all types of SWS, sleep intensity

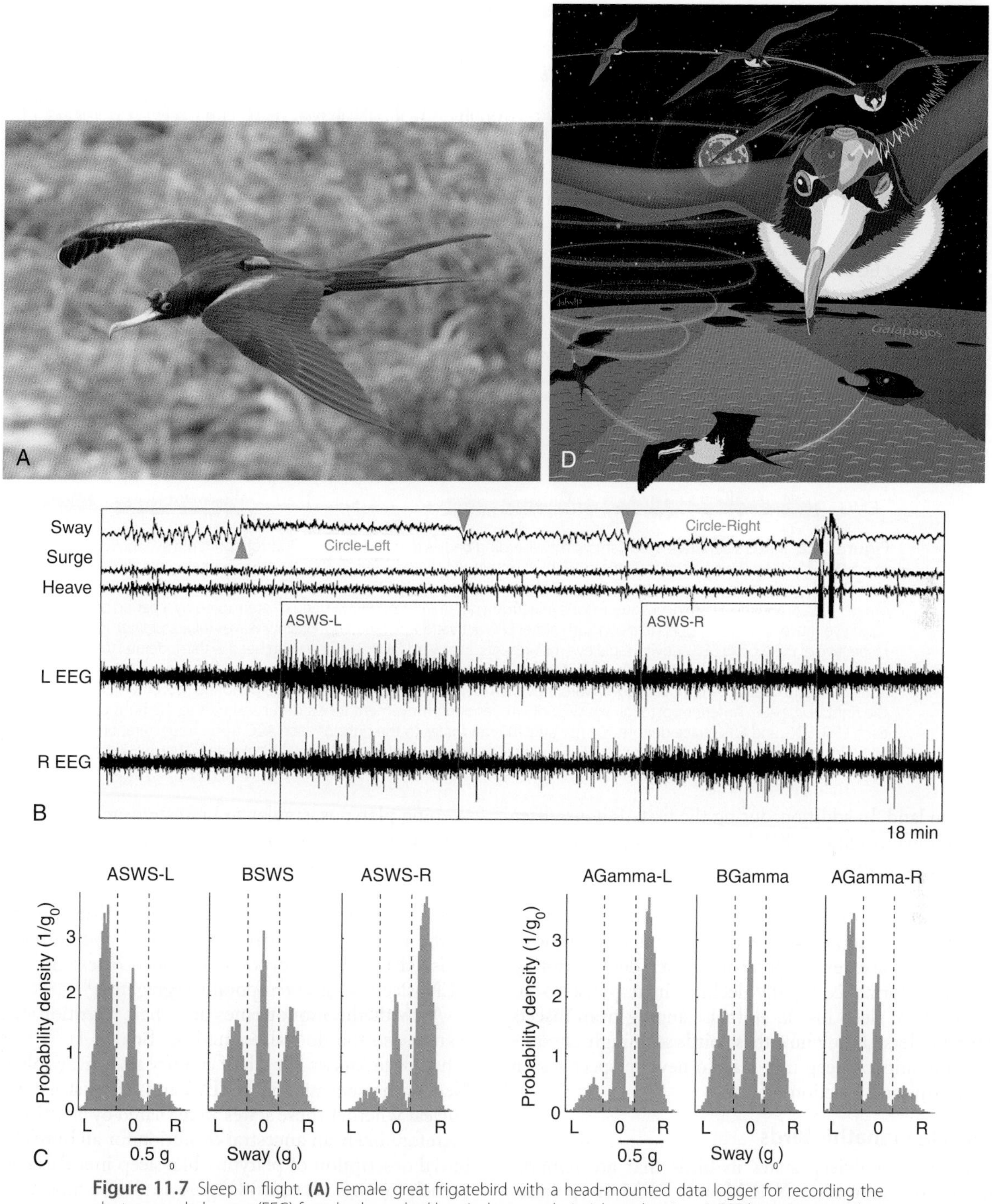

Figure 11.7 Sleep in flight. **(A)** Female great frigatebird with a head-mounted data logger for recording the electroencephalogram (EEG) from both cerebral hemispheres and triaxial acceleration. A GPS logger mounted on the back recorded position and altitude. **(B)** EEG and accelerometry (sway, surge, and heave) recordings from a frigatebird sleeping while circling in rising air currents. When the bird circled to the left (as indicated by centripetal acceleration detected in the sway axis), it showed asymmetric slow wave sleep (ASWS) with the left hemisphere sleeping deeper (larger slow waves) than the right (asymmetric slow wave sleep, left; ASWS-L), and when the bird circled to the right, the right hemisphere slept deeper than the left (asymmetric slow wave sleep, right; ASWS-R); during the other recording segments the bird was awake. **(C)** The relationship between interhemispheric asymmetries in slow wave activity (SWA; 0.75–4.5 Hz) and gamma activity (30–80 Hz) during slow wave sleep (SWS) for all birds combined. During ASWS, the birds usually circled toward the side with greater SWA and lower gamma activity. By contrast, during bihemispheric SWS (BSWS) without asymmetries in SWA or gamma (bihemispheric gamma; BGamma), the birds showed no preference for circling in one particular direction. SWS with greater gamma in the left (asymmetric gamma, left; AGamma-L) or right (asymmetric gamma, right; AGamma-R) hemisphere. **(D)** Illustration showing a bird circling to the right while sleeping with the right hemisphere. Although the birds' eye state is not known, based on studies from other birds, the EEG asymmetries suggest that the frigatebirds kept the eye connected to the more awake (lower SWA and higher gamma) hemisphere open and facing the direction of the turn. (**A** photo by Bryson Voirin. **D** illustration by Damond Kyllo. Panels [A to C] reproduced from Rattenborg NC, Voirin B, Cruz SM, et al. Evidence that birds sleep in mid-flight. *Nat Commun.* 2016;7:12468.)

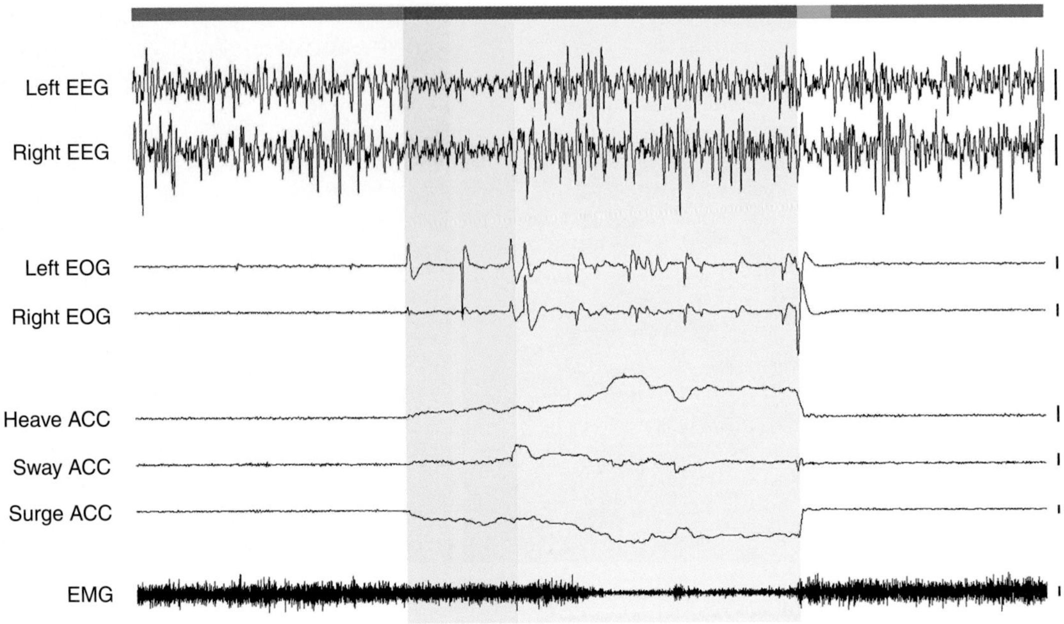

Figure 11.8 Mixed sleep state in an ostrich. The recording begins and ends with periods of non-rapid eye movement (NREM) sleep (*blue bar*) characterized by high amplitude, slow waves in the electroencephalogram (EEG), absence of rapid eye movements (measured via electrooculogram [EOG]), absence of head movements (accelerometer [ACC]), and moderate neck muscle tone (electromyogram [EMG]). NREM sleep is interrupted by a period of rapid eye movement (REM) sleep (*red bar*) with either EEG activation (*red shading*) or slow waves (*blue shading*). Irrespective of the type of EEG activity, rapid eye movements, a forward falling and swaying head with moderate-to-low muscle tone occurred invariably during REM sleep in the ostrich. *Heave ACC,* Movement along the dorsoventral axis with an upward slope denoting downward movement. *Sway ACC,* Lateral axis with up denoting movement to the right. *Surge ACC,* Anterior-posterior axis with down denoting movement forward. Vertical bars to the right of each EEG, EOG, and EMG trace denote 100 mV and 100 mg-forces to the right of each ACC trace. Trace duration: 60 s. (Reproduced from Lesku JA, Meyer LC, Fuller A, et al. Ostriches sleep like platypuses. *PLoS One.* 2011;6:e23203.)

was higher on land. In addition, during the first 10 hours after landing, a gradual decline in SWA occurred, suggesting that the birds were compensating (at least in part) for sleep lost in flight.

The small amount of sleep exhibited by female great frigatebirds in flight and some male pectoral sandpipers is difficult to reconcile with the extensive body of research demonstrating that waking performance rapidly declines in response to far shorter periods of sleep loss in animals ranging from insects to humans. Understanding how these birds seemingly circumvent large amounts of sleep may lead to new perspectives on the mechanisms and functions of sleep.

Sleep in Palaeognathic Birds

The presence of two sleep states in birds that are remarkably similar to mammalian NREM and REM sleep raises the question as to how these similarities arose. Although the fossilization of hard anatomical structures allows paleontologists to trace how bones have changed over evolutionary time, scientists can only infer the evolution of sleep states by studying living animals as proxies for extinct ones. Notably, modern-day monotremes are mammals yet lay eggs like reptiles. Because these animals retain some "primitive" traits thought to be present in the common ancestor to all mammals, including egg-laying, monotremes are often viewed as a window into the biology of early mammals.[98] Studies of sleeping monotremes, such as the platypus (*Ornithorhynchus anatinus*), may therefore provide clues to the evolutionary origins of mammalian NREM and REM sleep. Siegel and colleagues recorded eye movements and twitches of the head and bill in sleeping platypus, similar to brainstem-generated REM sleep phenomena in marsupial and eutherian mammals; however, the EEG did not show REM sleep-like activation but instead showed NREM sleep-like slow waves.[99] The presence of this mixed state in monotremes suggests that with the appearance of the lineage giving rise to marsupial and eutherian mammals, REM sleep incorporated the neocortex and NREM and REM sleep became temporally segregated.[100]

As with the monotremes and their retention of ancestral features, so too do Palaeognathae (Box 11.1).[98,101] Although it had been known for a half century that invariably species of Neognathae engaged in NREM and REM sleep, it remained unclear whether these states were shared by all living birds and therefore likely an ancestral condition for all birds. Despite an initial description of platypus-like sleep in a Palaeognath, the ostrich (*Struthio camelus*) (Figure 11.8),[39] a more recent study on another Palaeognath, the elegant crested tinamou (*Eudromia elegans*), showed behavioral and electrophysiologic sleep states typical of Neognathae.[40] Given that the small, flighted tinamous may better represent early birds (Box 11.1), that were also small and flighted, they may also better represent the form of sleep states in the most recent common ancestor to all birds than the large, flightless ostrich. Consequently, the evolutionary pattern proposed for mammals may not apply to birds.[40]

REPTILES, AMPHIBIANS, AND FISH

The similarities between sleep in mammals and birds reflect either inheritance from a common ancestor (stem amniote) with similar states or a case of convergent evolution.[25] Although we cannot tell for certain how the stem amniote slept, in theory, we can infer how it slept through examining sleep in living reptiles, amphibians, and fish. Unfortunately, this seemingly straightforward approach has been confounded by the diversity of findings reported in the few reptiles, amphibians, and fish examined (reviewed in Libourel and Herrel,[64] Eiland and colleagues,[102] Hartse,[103] and Kelly and colleagues[104]). Reports include no behavioral nor electrophysiologic signs of sleep, signs of one NREM sleep-like state, two types of sleep suggestive of NREM and REM sleep, or electrophysiologic states that are not readily relatable to either NREM or REM sleep. Our ability to interpret this diversity is hindered by uncertainty over its source. In addition to interspecific differences in sleep, the animals' age, variation in neural architecture, electrode type and placement, housing conditions and habituation, temperature effects on the poikilotherm EEG, and the method used to assess arousal thresholds (when conducted) may all contribute to the variation across studies. In most cases, the lack of replication by independent laboratories further complicates matters. Without knowing the extent to which this variation reflects true interspecific differences, it is impossible to reconstruct the evolution of sleep states in vertebrates.

Two recent studies of lizards, using state-of-the-art methods, suggest that some of this variation reflects interspecific differences in the neural correlates of sleep behavior. Shein-Idelson and colleagues recorded the bearded dragon lizard (*Pogona vitticeps*) at night using high-density electrode arrays placed in the dorsal cortex and dorsal ventricular ridge (DVR; Box 11.2).[105] During behavioral sleep, the DVR recordings revealed two electrophysiologic patterns that alternated approximately every 80 seconds with equal time spent in each state. The first was characterized by high-amplitude sharp waves, similar (in part) to those previously reported in some studies of lizards, turtles, and crocodilians.[64,103] The second was characterized by DVR activity similar to that occurring during wakefulness and eye movements occurring more frequently than during the first sleep state. Based on these findings, the authors proposed that these states are homologous to NREM and REM sleep in mammals and birds.

Importantly, Libourel and colleagues replicated these findings in the bearded dragon, but not in another species of lizard, the Argentine tegu (*Salvator merianae*), despite recording from the same brain region (Figure 11.9).[106] Two sleep states, named S1 and S2, were identified in tegus. S1 was also characterized by high-amplitude sharp waves, but the amplitude was lower, the duration was shorter, and they occurred far less often than in dragons. As in earlier reptile studies,[64,103] high-amplitude sharp waves increased in number after sleep deprivation. The second sleep state (S2) was associated with isolated eye movements, but the LFP was characterized by a 15-Hz oscillation not found during wakefulness. Nonetheless, this oscillation was suppressed by a selective serotonin reuptake inhibitor, a category of drugs that suppresses REM sleep in mammals and birds.[107] Interestingly, the sleep architecture of tegus more closely resembled that of birds than dragons, in that short bouts of REM-like S2 occurred hundreds of times a night. Finally, in both species, no twitches occurred during putative REM sleep. Despite the differences in phenotype, these two studies suggest that two sleep states, in some respects, similar to NREM and REM sleep are present in at least some reptiles.

In contrast to the few early electrophysiologic investigations of adult fish (reviewed in Hartse[103] and Kelly and colleagues[104]), a recent study suggests that two sleep states may exist in young zebrafish (*Danio rerio*). Leung and colleagues used larval zebrafish, genetically modified to fluoresce, to image whole brain activity, eye movements, heart rate, and trunk muscle activity.[108] The fish were recorded restrained in agar at night during (I) spontaneous wake and sleep, (II) sleep following sleep deprivation, and (III) after being treated with drugs known to induce NREM and REM sleep in mammals. Two types of sleep called slow bursting sleep (SBS) and propagating wave sleep (PWS) were identified. SBS was characterized by synchronous bursts of activity punctuated by periods of neuronal silence in the dorsal pallium that were most pronounced following sleep deprivation or the administration of hypnotic drugs. During spontaneous sleep, the onset of PWS was characterized by a wave of trunk muscle contraction lasting 10 to 15 seconds and a burst of neural activity lasting 5 minutes that propagated throughout the neuroaxis. After the burst of neural activity, activity across the neuroaxis was suppressed below waking levels for 20 minutes. A similar state was induced by drugs that induce REM sleep in mammals, although the temporal sequence of events differed considerably from that during spontaneous PWS. Finally, although the eyes moved freely during wakefulness, rapid eye movements were not detected during spontaneous PWS.

The synchronous bursts of cortical activity during SBS bear some similarity to the bursts of activity associated with slow waves during mammalian and avian NREM sleep, although the frequency is much slower in zebrafish. And, in general terms, the widespread activation of the neuroaxis during PWS is similar to the activation of the neuroaxis occurring during mammalian REM sleep. However, the long muscle contraction at the onset of PWS is unlike the brief, intermittent twitches that characterize REM sleep in mammals and birds. The absence of eye movements, a finding also reported in a behavioral study of adult zebrafish,[109] is also inconsistent with the proposed relationship between PWS and REM sleep. In addition, the prolonged period of suppressed neural activity following the wave of activity is unexpected if this state is homologous to REM sleep.

The recent studies on dragons, tegus, and zebrafish have important implications for interpreting the confusing research on sleep in poikilothermic vertebrates. Notably, the differences between two species of lizards recorded using the same methodology in the same laboratory suggest that at least some of the variability reported in the earlier literature reflects real interspecific differences in sleep. Further research on poikilothermic vertebrates, using modern methods, is clearly needed to characterize the ancestral sleep state(s) present in the stem amniote, as well as the functional implications of sleep's diverse expression in poikilotherms.

FUNCTIONAL IMPLICATIONS

Relatively few studies have examined the functional aspects of sleep in nonmammalian vertebrates. Early on, the fact that unequivocal NREM and REM sleep had been found only in mammals and birds, both homeotherms, led to the proposal that NREM sleep, in particular, evolved to conserve energy.[110] The lower metabolic rate during NREM sleep[111] and its continuity with hypometabolic states, such as torpor and

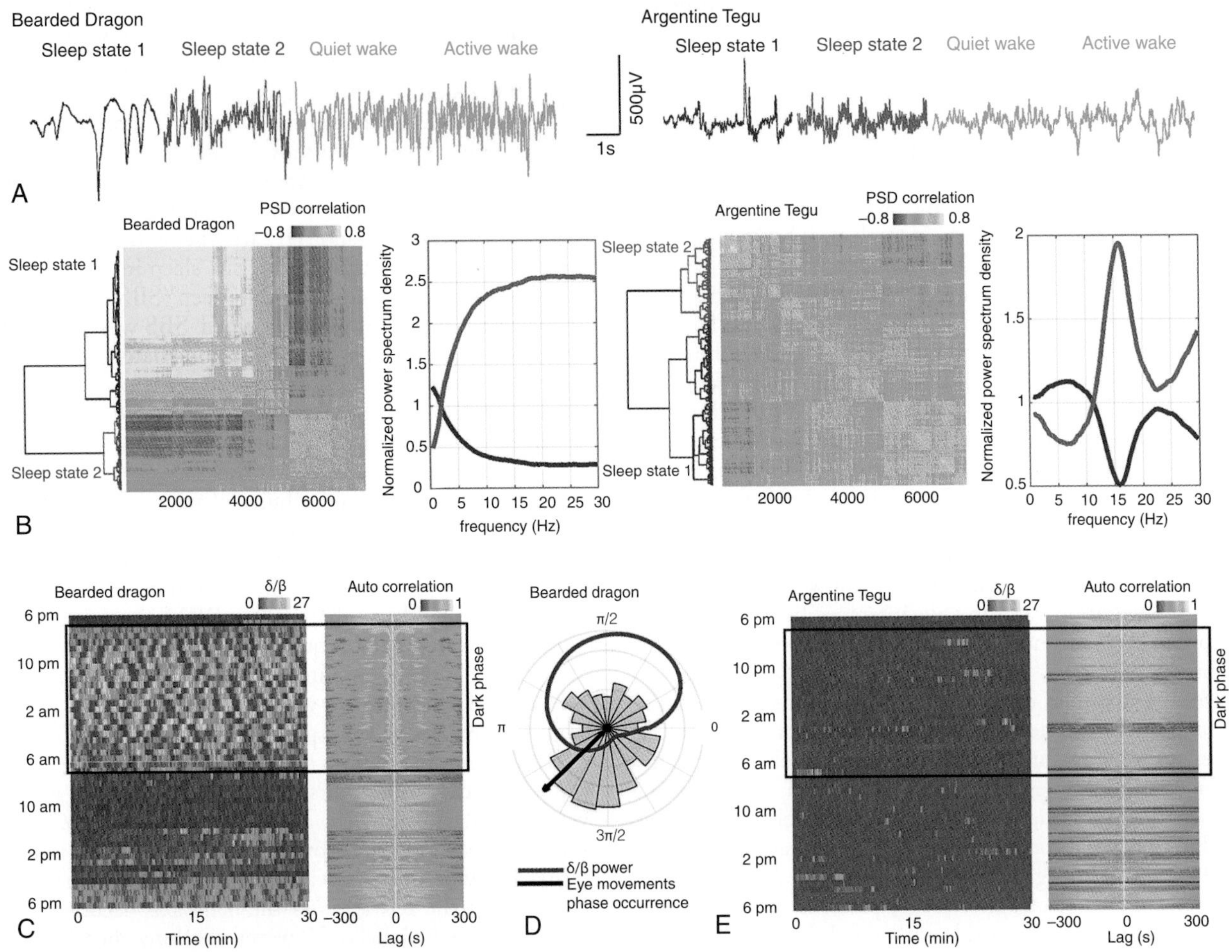

Figure 11.9 Sleep states in lizards. **(A)** Local field potential (LFP) recorded from the dorsal ventricular ridge of a bearded dragon (*left*) and Argentine tegu (*right*) during sleep state 1 (S1, sharing similarities with mammalian non-rapid eye movement sleep) in *blue*, sleep state 2 (S2, sharing similarities with mammalian rapid eye movement sleep) in *red*, and quiet and active wake in *green*. **(B)** Plots for each species (dragon, *left*; tegu, *right*), show a dendrogram (*left*) and correlation map (*middle*) obtained from the hierarchic clustering of the distance between the correlation of each LFP 3-second window power spectrum density (*PSD*). To the right of each correlation map are the normalized mean power spectra of the two clusters computed for one animal representing the two distinct sleep states identified, S1 in *blue* and S2 in *red*. The comparison of the normalized power spectra of each state reveals a frequency profile that is clearly different between the two species, with desynchronized activity (composed of all the frequencies higher than 5 Hz) for the bearded dragon during S2 and a power spectrum mainly composed of 15-Hz oscillations for S2 in the tegu. **(C)** The band power ratio (δ [0.5–4 Hz]/β [11–30 Hz]) computed as in Shein-Idelson and colleagues[105] for the bearded dragon. Each horizontal segment represents 30 minutes of the computed ratio. The value of the ratio is color coded from 0 (*blue*) to 27 (*yellow*). The figure from the *top* to the *bottom* represents the evolution of the ratio over 24 hours, with the *dark rectangle* indicating the dark phase. On the right, the normalized autocorrelation map of the ratio is illustrated. Both figures reveal a rhythmic alternance with a period of around 90 seconds across episodes, with δ frequencies (*yellow*) and episodes with β (*blue*) during the dark phase, when the animal is lying on the floor with the eyes closed. **(D)** The distribution of the eye movements within each δ–β cycle; the mean phase is represented with a *black arrow*. The *red line* is the mean δ/β power ratio across the δ–β cycle. **(E)** Same as **(C),** but for the Argentine tegu. The figure reveals no clear cycle in the δ/β power ratio over 24 hours. (Reproduced from Libourel PA, Barrillot B, Arthaud S, et al. Partial homologies between sleep states in lizards, mammals, and birds suggest a complex evolution of sleep states in amniotes. *PLoS Biol.* 2018;16:e2005982.)

hibernation,[112] contributed to this hypothesis. More recently, Schmidt proposed that the primary energy savings resulting from sleep is not simply due to the reduction in metabolic rate, but rather arises from the more efficient allocation of energy to specific processes during specific states.[113] In mammals and birds, REM sleep with its suppressed thermoregulatory responses, may allow energy usually allocated to thermoregulation to be reallocated toward other processes without incurring additional energetic costs.[82,113] Although the presence of NREM and REM sleep-like states in some poikilothermic reptiles suggests that these states may not be exclusively linked to homeothermic animals, engaging in two sleep states may still conserve energy in poikilothermic animals if performing the associated functions during temporally segregated states is more efficient.[113]

Along with many other lines of evidence, the fact that some marine mammals and birds sleep unihemispherically during continuous activity (rather than dispensing with sleep altogether)[96,97] suggests that sleep performs functions that specifically benefit the brain. Research on sleep's role in maintaining adaptive brain performance has primarily focused on mammals. Brain-related functions fall into two general categories: (1) maintenance and restoration and (2) synaptic dynamics involved in memory consolidation.[114] As in the mammalian neocortex, transcripts that encode proteins involved in cellular maintenance are expressed in the forebrain of sleeping birds.[115] Also, the local, use-dependent regulation of NREM sleep SWA suggests that SWA is involved in, or correlated with, restorative processes occurring in the brain in response to prior waking activation.[70] In addition, as in mammals,[116] sleep has been implicated in various forms of memory processing, including imprinting in chicken chicks,[117,118] song learning in zebra finches,[119,120] and memory consolidation in starlings.[121] However, little work has linked sleep-dependent memory processing to specific sleep states or brain oscillations in birds.

In mammals, several studies suggest that the brain oscillations occurring during sleep are actively involved in processing information.[16,90,116,122-125] In particular, a prominent model suggests that neocortical slow waves, thalamocortical spindles, and hippocampal SWRs form a system of interacting oscillations involved in gradually integrating information initially stored in the hippocampus into existing information in the neocortex for long-term storage, via a process of memory reactivation during sleep.[116] Direct connections from the hippocampus to the medial prefrontal cortex (PFC) play an important role in this systems-level memory consolidation.[126,127] However, unlike the mammalian hippocampus, which receives input from most high-order neocortical association areas contributing to a memory via the entorhinal cortex, most comparable regions in the avian DVR do not provide input to the hippocampus.[22,128] Moreover, anatomic or functional connections between the hippocampus and nidopallium caudolateral (NCL)—the avian analogue of the mammalian PFC—have not been found in birds.[22,128,129] Furthermore, although the avian hippocampus is involved in storing spatial memories, there is no evidence of hippocampal memories transferring to other brain regions in birds.[22] Consequently, it is perhaps not surprising that some of the oscillations (spindles and SWRs) implicated in transferring hippocampal memories during mammalian NREM sleep have not been found in birds.[13,22]

Even though there is reason to think that hippocampal memories are not processed at a systems level during avian sleep, propagating slow waves could be involved in transferring memories between other brain regions.[13,16,117,130] In addition, the local, use-dependent regulation of slow waves may also be involved in processing information locally in avian and mammalian brains.[70,71] Local slow waves might strengthen synapses and thereby memories stored in the respective region, while weakening unimportant synapses that would otherwise introduce noise into the system and increase its energetic demands.[90]

In contrast to its role in mammals and birds, sleep's potential role in processing information in reptiles has not been examined. Attempts to infer how the reptilian brain may process information are complicated by the fact that the electrophysiologic correlates of sleep vary across studies and species. Nonetheless, the high-amplitude sharp wave, an electrophysiologic correlate of sleep in several reptilian species, has recently received attention with regard to memory processing. Recordings from the dorsal cortex and DVR revealed high-amplitude sharp waves in a variety of reptiles; although their incidence, duration, and morphology vary across studies and species.[64,106] Hartse[103] noted the similarity between reptilian sharp waves and sharp waves recorded from the mammalian hippocampus during NREM sleep. More recently, Shein-Idelson and colleagues[105] also noted this similarity between these electrophysiologic events. In addition, they also detected high-frequency (>70 Hz) oscillations during sharp waves that they relate to the ripple component of mammalian hippocampal SWRs. However, it is unclear whether these sharp waves reflect the same phenomenon as mammalian hippocampal SWRs or a variant of the slow oscillation that gives rise to slow waves in mammals and birds,[13,15,131] as fast (80–200 Hz) ripple-like activity also occurs during the up state of the neocortical slow oscillation.[132] Regardless of which interpretation is correct, reptilian sharp waves are likely to be involved in memory reactivation, as it is thought to occur during both mammalian SWRs *and* slow oscillation up states.[132]

The function of avian REM sleep and REM sleep-like states in reptiles remains unclear. As in mammals, the high amount of REM sleep in developing owls suggests a common role in brain development. However, the apparent absence of a hippocampal theta oscillation suggests that processes linked to this oscillation in mammals[122] occur either via different mechanisms or not at all in birds. In reptiles, the various ways in which REM sleep-like states manifest (or do not) makes it difficult to generalize about the functional implications of these findings. Even within lizards, the reptilian group with the most reports of REM sleep-like states, the neural signatures, vary widely.[106] Further research is clearly needed to understand the mechanisms and functional implications of this unexpected, yet potentially informative, diversity. Additional research is also needed to understand why REM sleep has not been demonstrated in several studies of reptiles. Was REM sleep missed in some species? If not, was it evolutionarily lost, or did REM sleep evolve independently multiple times in mammals, birds, and some reptiles? If REM sleep is really only present in some reptiles, further comparisons of reptilian species with and without REM sleep may provide clues to its functions. Hints of a REM sleep-like state in cuttlefish (*Sepia officinalis*),[133] members of an invertebrate group (cephalopod molluscs) renowned for their complex cognitive abilities, but not in sea slugs (gastropod molluscs),[134] raises the intriguing possibility that REM sleep has evolved many times, even in invertebrates, during the course of evolution.

CLINICAL PEARL

Comparative research on animals from diverse taxonomic groups can influence our understanding of sleep in humans. Research on birds can provide new perspectives on the "first night effect," motor control during sleep, the functions of brain oscillations, and neurobehavioral performance during prolonged wakefulness. The recent discovery of REM sleep-like states in some reptiles provides a new opportunity to investigate the functions of this mysterious state.

SUMMARY

Despite last sharing a common ancestor over 300 million years ago, birds exhibit two states that are in many, but not all, respects similar to mammalian NREM and REM sleep.

Through studying reptiles, amphibians, and fish, researchers have attempted to determine whether these states were present in the last common ancestor to mammals and birds or evolved independently in each lineage via convergent evolution. However, in contrast to mammals and birds, wherein the two states are similar across most of the species examined within each group, the results have been highly variable in poikilothermic vertebrates. These include no behavioral or electrophysiologic signs of sleep, signs of one NREM sleep-like state, two types of sleep suggestive of NREM and REM sleep, or electrophysiologic states that are not readily comparable to either NREM or REM sleep. Recent studies suggest that at least some of this variability reflects true interspecific differences in the electrophysiologic correlates of sleep. This diversity thwarts attempts to draw simple conclusions regarding the evolution of NREM and REM sleep. Nonetheless, it may serve as a rich resource for investigating the mechanisms and functions of sleep-related brain activity.

SELECTED READINGS

Aulsebrook AE, Johnsson RD, Lesku JA. Light, sleep and performance in diurnal birds. *Clocks Sleep*. 2021;3(1):115–131.

Dave AS, Margoliash D. Song replay during sleep and computational rules for sensorimotor vocal learning. *Science*. 2000;290:812–816.

Derégnaucourt S, Mitra PP, Fehér O, et al. How sleep affects the developmental learning of bird song. *Nature*. 2005;433:710–716.

Dewasmes G, Cohen-Adad F, Koubi H, et al. Polygraphic and behavioral study of sleep in geese: existence of nuchal atonia during paradoxical sleep. *Physiol Behav*. 1985;35:67–73.

Jones S, Pfister-Genskow M, Benca RM, et al. Molecular correlates of sleep and wakefulness in the brain of the white-crowned sparrow. *J Neurochem*. 2008;105:46–62.

Lesku JA, Rattenborg NC, Valcu M, et al. Adaptive sleep loss in polygynous pectoral sandpipers. *Science*. 2012;337:1654–1658.

Lesku JA, Vyssotski AL, Martinez-Gonzalez D, et al. Local sleep homeostasis in the avian brain: convergence of sleep function in mammals and birds? *Proc Biol Sci*. 2011;278:2419–2428.

Leung LC, Wang GX, Madelaine R, et al. Neural signatures of sleep in zebrafish. *Nature*. 2019;571:198–204.

Libourel PA, Barrillot B, Arthaud S, et al. Partial homologies between sleep states in lizards, mammals, and birds suggest a complex evolution of sleep states in amniotes. *PLoS Biol*. 2018;16:e2005982.

Lyamin OI, Kibalnikov AS, Siegel JM. Sleep in ostrich chicks *(Struthio camelus)*. *Sleep*. 2021;44(5):zsaa259.

Rattenborg NC, Voirin B, Cruz SM, et al. Evidence that birds sleep in mid-flight. *Nat Commun*. 2016;7:12468.

Scriba MF, Ducrest AL, Henry I, et al. Linking melanism to brain development: expression of a melanism-related gene in barn owl feather follicles covaries with sleep ontogeny. *Front Zool*. 2013;10:42.

Tisdale RK, Lesku JA, Beckers GJL, et al. Bird-like propagating brain activity in anesthetized Nile crocodiles. *Sleep*. 2018;41:zsy105.

van der Meij J, Martinez-Gonzalez D, Beckers GJL, et al. Intra-"cortical" activity during avian non-REM and REM sleep: variant and invariant traits between birds and mammals. *Sleep*. 2019;42:zsy230.

van Hasselt SJ, Mekenkamp GJ, Komdeur J, et al. Seasonal variation in sleep homeostasis in migratory geese: a rebound of NREM sleep following sleep deprivation in summer but not in winter. *Sleep*. 2021;44(4):zsaa244.

Yamazaki R, Toda H, Libourel PA, Hayashi Y, Vogt KE, Sakurai T. Evolutionary origin of distinct NREM and REM sleep. *Front Psychol*. 2020;11:567618.

A complete reference list can be found online at ExpertConsult.com.

Section 3

Genetics and Genomic Basis of Sleep

Chapter 12

Introduction: Genetics and Genomics of Sleep

Paul Shaw

The inclusion of *Genetics and Genomics of Sleep* in this volume signifies that the genetic control of the sleep-wake cycle has become an active area for sleep research, both for characterizing regulatory mechanisms underlying the control of the sleep-wake cycle and for elucidating the function(s) of sleep. The first Nobel Prize in the sleep field recognized the importance of the intersection of sleep, circadian physiology, and genetics. The inclusion of the term "genomics" in the title of this section confirms that many sleep researchers have embarked on a systemwide genomic approach for investigating this interplay of genes and gene networks regulating the multiple phenotypes or traits that constitute the sleep-wake cycle and the interplay with disease states. Indeed, as genetic and genomic approaches are being used for the study of sleep in diverse species from flies to mice to humans (see Chapters 14 to 16), the evolutionary significance of the many functions of sleep that have evolved over time is becoming a tractable subject for research, as many investigators are bringing the tools of genetics and genomics to the sleep field. The complexity of the sleep-wake phenotypes and the difficulty in collecting phenotypic data on a large enough number of animals or humans to begin to unravel genetic mechanisms have been partly responsible for why few comprehensive attempts have been made to identify "sleep genes" beyond the circadian clock genes regulating the timing of sleep (see Chapter 13).

The focus on genetic and genomic approaches to sleep is predicated in large part on the notion that the mechanisms of sleep regulation are conserved from simple organisms highly amenable to genetic analysis, such as the fruit fly and zebrafish, to conventional rodent models and even to humans (see Chapters 15 to 17). The best example of such evolutionary conservation comes from the discovery of the core circadian clock genes that regulate the diurnal sleep-wake cycle, as well as most, if not all, 24-hour behavioral, physiologic, and cellular rhythms. These core clock genes were first identified in fruit flies, employing mutagenesis and the screening of thousands of flies for mutant phenotypes, and eventually led to the finding the same genes in mice and humans. Indeed, similar screens in rodents leveraging the simplicity and ease of monitoring a representative "output rhythm" of the central circadian clock from literally thousands of rodents in a single laboratory, such as the precise rhythm of locomotor activity or wheel running in rodents, was also a major factor in uncovering conserved molecular transcriptional-translational feedback loops that give rise to 24-hour output signals (see Chapter 27). The discovery of the core clock genes controlling the timing of sleep-wake cycles represents one of the great triumphs of behavioral genetics and serves as a road map to uncover the mechanisms of sleep homeostasis. The 2017 Nobel Prize in Physiology or Medicine was awarded jointly to Jeffrey C. Hall, Michael Rosbash, and Michael W. Young to recognize their discoveries of molecular mechanisms that control the circadian rhythm.

In addition, substantial evidence has now accumulated demonstrating that deletion or mutations in many canonical circadian clock genes can lead to fundamental changes in other sleep-wake traits, including the amount of sleep and the response to sleep deprivation.[1] The finding that different alleles of a core circadian gene, *per,* first identified in flies, can affect the homeostatic response to sleep deprivation and/or the amount of slow wave sleep (Chapter 16) argues that uncovering sleep genes in flies will lead directly to changes in sleep-wake traits in mammals. As discussed in Chapter 15, on sleep genetics in rodents, one can argue that many circadian clock genes are also "sleep genes." As noted by Dijk and

Landolt (Chapter 16), sleep is a rich phenotype that can be broken down into a wide variety of sleep-wake traits based on the electroencephalogram and electromyogram. Furthermore, the "genetic landscape" for regulating multiple sleep-wake traits clearly is going to involve hundreds of genes and integrated molecular neurobiologic networks.[2,3] Although early work by Valtex and colleagues using inbred strains of mice[4] and early human twin studies[5] provided considerable evidence of a strong genetic basis for some sleep-wake traits, little has been done to unravel the complex network of genetic interactions that must underlie this universal behavior in mammals. The fact that the environment and the subject's own volition also can have major effects on sleep-wake traits, particularly sleep duration, also makes it difficult to uncover the underlying genetic control mechanisms. Indeed, although a large number of genome-wide association studies in humans have identified multiple genetic loci and genes involved in the regulation of a wide variety of physiologic systems and disease states, only recently has this approach been used to uncover sleep-wake genes (Chapters 16 and 17). Franken and colleagues pioneered the use of quantitative trait loci in recombinant inbred mouse strains, which has led to the identification of a small number of genes that are associated with specific sleep-wake properties[6] (see Chapter 13). More recently, the first attempt to record sleep in a large genetically segregating population of mice revealed considerable complexity to the genetic landscape for multiple sleep-wake traits.[2,3] Uncovering these loci and elucidating how gene-environment interactions contribute to different sleep-wake states are expected to not only reveal the molecular events underlying the sleep-wake cycle but also identify new targets for drug discovery. New therapies based on the genetic control of sleep may be particularly important for treating both genetically and environmentally based disorders of sleep (Chapter 17).[7]

SELECTED READINGS

Casale CE, Goel N. Genetic markers of differential vulnerability to sleep loss in adults. *Genes (Basel)*. 2021;12(9):1317.

Kocevska D, Barclay NL, Bramer WM, Gehrman PR, Van Someren EJW. Heritability of sleep duration and quality: a systematic review and meta-analysis. *Sleep Med Rev*. 2021;59:101448.

Rosbash, M. Nobel Lecture. The Circadian Clock, Transcriptional Feedback and the Regulation of Gene Expression. https://www.nobelprize.org/prizes/medicine/2017/rosbash/lecture/.

Shafer OT, Keene AC. The Regulation of Drosophila Sleep. *Curr Biol*. 2021;31(1):R38–R49. https://doi.org/10.1016/j.cub.2020.10.082.

Webb JM, Fu YH. Recent advances in sleep genetics. *Curr Opin Neurobiol*. 2021;69:19–24. https://doi.org/10.1016/j.conb.2020.11.012.

A complete reference list can be found online at ExpertConsult.com.

Chapter 13

Genetics and Genomics of Circadian Clocks

Martha Hotz Vitaterna; Fred W. Turek; Peng Jiang

Chapter Highlights

- Circadian (near-24-hour) rhythms can be produced by individual mammalian cells in a self-sustaining manner. These rhythmic patterns result from coordinated daily oscillations in the transcription and translation of key clock component genes. The positive elements CLOCK and BMAL1 regulate transcription of the negative elements of *Per* and *Cry* genes, forming the core feedback loop of the timekeeping mechanism.
- Interactions between these genes and their products, as well as other proteins, tune the clock and link it to other cellular pathways. The genetic clock also regulates a tissue-specific circadian program of gene expression.
- In addition to the transcriptome, rhythms in other layers of -omes, such as the epigenome, proteome, phosphoproteome, as well as "genomes beyond our own"—the microbiome, are being explored, adding to a more complete picture of the circadian clock network.

INTRODUCTION

Over the past three decades, remarkable progress has been made in elucidating the molecular substrates that underlie the generation of 24-hour rhythms in mammals. A major finding that has arisen over the past decade is that most cells and tissues of the body contain and express the core 24-hour molecular clock mechanism. Although normally coordinated, individual tissues and cells are capable of producing sustained rhythms in isolation. These rhythms result from oscillatory expression of a core set of interrelated circadian genes. This chapter describes the genes expressed in cells of the hypothalamic suprachiasmatic nucleus (SCN) and other oscillators and our understanding of the roles they play in this daily rhythmicity. In addition, in view of the homology of mammalian clock genes with those in the fly, where appropriate, a discussion of the discovery of fly and mammalian genes is provided.

THE MAMMALIAN CELLULAR CIRCADIAN CLOCK

Several lines of evidence pointed to the SCN as the site of the master circadian pacemaker, beginning in the 1970s. Destruction of the SCN abolishes circadian oscillations in the plasma concentration of cortisol[1] and in locomotion and drinking.[2] These oscillations are independent of inputs from the eye,[1] although an autonomous circadian clock had been demonstrated to exist within the eye that controls, among other functions, the shedding of rod outer segment disks.[3] Normal circadian rhythms can be restored to an SCN-lesioned animal by transplantation of fetal SCN tissue but not by transplantation of fetal tissue from other regions of the brain.[4] Transplantation into an SCN-lesioned animal of fetal tissue from the SCN of a circadian mutant animal confers the short period of the donor,[5] indicating that the properties of the rhythm are determined by the SCN rather than other tissues or brain regions. Thus several lines of evidence point to the SCN as the site driving or controlling circadian behavior for mammals.

More recent studies of rhythms in gene expression indicated that persistent rhythms can be observed in tissues throughout the organism, even in tissue explants kept in culture for extended periods of time.[6,7] The phase of these peripheral tissue rhythms differs from that of the SCN but nonetheless appears coordinated by the SCN. In SCN-lesioned animals, these peripheral rhythms persist but no longer exhibit the consistent phase seen in intact animals.[7] Some environmental manipulations, such as temperature cycles or restricted feeding can alter the phase of peripheral rhythms.[8,9] In addition, studies confirm the presence of oscillations in gene expression throughout the body, with different phases in different tissues.[10–13] Loss of many of these rhythms is reported with SCN lesions. However, it is important to note that these studies cannot discriminate between a loss of rhythmicity by individual cells and a loss of synchronicity among the cells. Thus the roles of the SCN and of the peripheral oscillators in the mammalian circadian system continue to be defined.

CIRCADIAN CLOCK PROPERTIES AND CLOCK GENES

Nearly half a century ago, the formal properties of the circadian "clock" function had been well defined. Included among the 16 "empirical generalizations about circadian rhythms" defined by Colin Pittendrigh[14] were that circadian rhythms are ubiquitous in living systems; they are endogenous; they are innate; they are not learned from nor impressed by the environment; they occur autonomously at both cell and whole-organism levels of organization; the free-running period of circadian rhythms are so slightly temperature dependent that it is proper to emphasize its near-independence of temperature; and they are surprisingly intractable to chemical perturbation. These observations already suggest what we now know to be the case: A cell-autonomous program of gene expression makes up the mammalian circadian "clock" that produces these rhythms.

How do individual cells generate rhythmic activity with a period of about 1 day? Many pacemaker neurons generate oscillatory activity, such as rhythmic patterns of action potentials, and these relatively rapid oscillations can be explained by the concerted action of a small number of ion channels. However, the much slower oscillations of the individual SCN neurons are not likely to involve the same mechanisms. Pittendrigh's observation that circadian rhythms are not sped up or slowed down by changes in temperature, and that they are relatively impervious to chemical perturbations, would similarly argue against such a neuronal mechanism underlying the generation of 24-hour oscillations. In fact, the finding that nonneuronal tissues (Pittendrigh's cell autonomy) can produce sustained circadian rhythms, as well as the prevalence of circadian rhythms in plants and unicellular organisms (Pittendrigh's ubiquity), would argue against a neural process underlying circadian rhythm generation.

Indeed, it appears that the synthesis of proteins by each oscillatory cell is central to the mechanism for the generation of 24-hour rhythms. The initial evidence for this is that application of protein synthesis inhibitors in the region of the SCN shifts the circadian phase of activity of animals by an amount and in a direction that depends upon the time at which the inhibition is imposed.[15,16] A similar shift in the phase of vasopressin release from explanted SCN also results from inhibition of protein synthesis.[17] Thus gene expression is central to the generation of circadian oscillations.

As will be discussed in detail in the following, gene expression profile studies, in which expression levels are sampled at regular time points in constant darkness (DD; free-running conditions) focusing on the SCN and on peripheral tissues, reveal that approximately one-third of the transcriptome is rhythmically expressed, even in peripheral tissues.[18–21] Reporter gene constructs combining genes known to be rhythmically expressed with luciferase (thus allowing visualization of expression in culture via converting luciferin to light-emitting oxyluciferin) demonstrated in rats and in mice that peripheral tissues are capable of self-sustained rhythms.[6,7] With so many genes exhibiting circadian expression, and competent oscillators present in such a variety of tissues, one cannot assume that either rhythmic expression or expression in the SCN is valid criterion for a "clock gene." Identification of which genes are central to the generation and maintenance of circadian cycles thus represents a challenge.

A potential solution to the challenge of identification of clock genes (vs. clock-controlled genes) is to refocus attention on the formal properties of the circadian system. Arnold Eskin and others promoted this conceptual framework in the late 1970s by characterizing rhythm properties as arising from the input pathway, the clock itself, or the output pathway[22] (Figure 13.1). As articulated for pharmacologic approaches (but equally valid for genetic ones), manipulations that produce phase-dependent shifts in the rhythm (a phase response curve), or changes in the phase response curve or the free-running period are likely to be affecting the clock, or at least, not affecting an output process.[23] Applying this logic, a genetic perturbation that alters the free-running period in DD, the phase response curve to light pulses, or the persistence of rhythmicity in constant conditions may be likely to be a perturbation in a clock gene, although no one alteration alone is necessarily a clock change (vs. input or output).

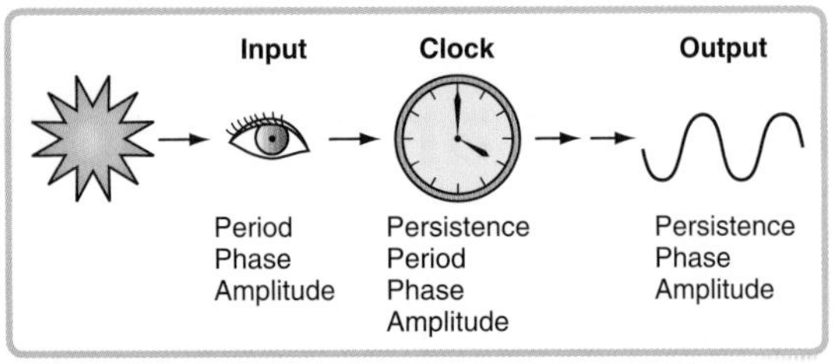

Figure 13.1 Classical view of circadian system and circadian clock properties. At minimum, the circadian clock system would have an input pathway by which entraining signals are received (light is illustrated), a clock mechanism, and output pathways. No single property of observed circadian rhythms is necessarily determined by the clock mechanism; these properties may be affected by changes in the input or output. However, when a mutation is observed to affect multiple properties of circadian rhythms, then that genetic change may most parsimoniously be attributed to a change in the clock mechanism itself.

Zatz and others[2425] proposed more restrictive criteria: Null mutations should abolish rhythmicity; the gene's protein product level or activity should oscillate and be reset by light pulses; changes in amount or activity should result in phase shifts; and prevention of oscillation of protein levels/activity should result in loss of rhythmicity.[24] In the parlance of the field, these criteria would define a "state variable"—a rate-limiting element that itself defines the phase of the core oscillation. A self-sustaining clock would require at least two state variables,[26] although more are clearly possible. To date, no single gene in the mammalian system has satisfied all the criteria for a state variable. Indeed, a hallmark of the mammalian circadian clock seems to be the multiple homologues of many genes that appear to play related but nonredundant roles. It may thus be that "state variable" status is actually shared by related groups of genes in the mammalian system.

POSITIVE ELEMENTS

Clock

In the early 1990s, no genes in mammals had been identified as even possible candidate circadian clock genes, leading us to undertake mutagenesis and screening in mice in an effort to identify mammalian circadian clock genes. For this, we used the C57BL/6J mouse strain, in which wild-type mice show robust entrainment to a light-dark cycle and have a circadian period between 23.6 and 23.8 hours under free-running conditions in DD. In a screen for mutations of more than 300 progeny of mutagen-treated mice, we found one animal that had a free-running period of about 24.8 hours, more than six standard deviations longer than the mean.[27] In the homozygous condition, this mutation results in a dramatic lengthening of the period to about 28 hours, which is usually followed by the eventual loss of circadian rhythmicity (i.e., arrhythmicity) after about 1 to 3 weeks in DD. The affected gene was mapped to mouse chromosome 5 and named *Clock*.[27,28] We cloned the *Clock* gene by a combination of genetic rescue and positional cloning techniques. *Clock/Clock* mutant mice were phenotypically rescued by a bacterial artificial chromosome transgene that contained the *Clock* gene, allowing for functional identification of the gene.[29] The *Clock* gene encodes a transcriptional regulatory protein having a basic helix-loop-helix (bHLH) DNA-binding domain, a PAS dimerization domain, and a Q-rich transactivation domain. The mutant form of the CLOCK protein (CLOCK Δ19) lacks a portion of the activation domain found in wild-type protein, and thus, although it is capable of protein dimerization, transcriptional activation is diminished or lost. The PAS domain is so named because of the genes originally identified with this protein dimerization domain: *per*, *ARNT* and *sim*. *Clock* messenger ribonucleic acid (mRNA) is expressed in the SCN and other tissues, but it has not been found to oscillate in a circadian fashion.[30]

Bmal1

The presence of the PAS dimerization domain in CLOCK protein suggested that it may form a heterodimer similar to that of PER and the protein product of another *Drosophila* clock gene, TIM.[31] A screen for potential partners for the CLOCK protein using the yeast two-hybrid system revealed that a protein of unknown function, BMAL1 (Brain and Muscle ARNT-Like 1), was able to dimerize with the CLOCK protein.[32] Creation of mice harboring a null allele of *Bmal1* (also referred to as *MOP3*) demonstrated the critical role of this gene in circadian rhythm generation. These mutant mice, although displaying light-dark responsive differences in activity level, become arrhythmic immediately upon release in DD.

Recently, additional actions of the CLOCK:BMAL1 heterodimer have become clear. Although *Clock* mRNA does not oscillate, its protein's nuclear versus cytoplasmic localization does.[33] By studying the intracellular localization of CLOCK and BMAL1 in fibroblasts of mouse embryos with mutations in different clock genes and ectopically expressing the proteins, it was found that nuclear accumulation of CLOCK was dependent on formation of the CLOCK:BMAL1 dimer, as was phosphorylation of the complex and its degradation.[33] Other PAS domain–containing proteins failed to affect the localization of CLOCK, indicating that these posttranslational events are specific to the CLOCK:BMAL dimer.

NEGATIVE ELEMENTS

The *Period* Genes

The first identified gene (defined as a "mendelian" gene, as opposed to a sequenced, cloned gene) that encodes a clock component, *period*, denoted with the symbol *per*, was discovered in 1971 in *Drosophila* by using a forward genetic approach consisting of chemically inducing random mutations in the genome and detecting those mutations that affect circadian rhythms by screening the progeny of the mutagenized individuals for altered rhythmicity.[34] This approach has the advantage that no assumptions are made about the nature of the genes or gene products involved, but it is based on the presumption that there exist genes that, when mutated, will alter rhythms in a detectable manner. At the time, this presumption of the existence of genes that regulate a complex behavior was considered radical but has proven to have been a field-defining moment.

Initially, three alleles of the *per* gene were identified by the process of mutagenesis and screening. Flies carrying these alleles had either no apparent rhythm in eclosion (emergence from the pupal case) or locomotion, or had either long (e.g., 29 hours) or short periods (e.g., 19 hours) for the rhythms of eclosion and locomotor activity.[34] It is important to note that the finding of three alleles with three different phenotypes made it possible to have confidence in the conclusion that the *per* gene encodes a protein that is a clock component. Had only an arrhythmic mutant been found, then the alternative explanation could be proposed that the lack of circadian behavior was secondary to another primary defect that did not lie in a clock component. It also should be noted that the approach of mutagenesis and screening has also been successful in identifying circadian clock genes in other organisms, such as *Neurospora crassa*,[35] plants,[36] and cyanobacteria.[37] However, a discussion of these important findings is outside the scope of this chapter.

Confirmation of the importance of the *per* gene as a central circadian clock component was the rescue of the mutant phenotype after introduction of the wild-type allele of the *per* gene into mutant flies.[38,39] The level of the mRNA transcript encoded by the *per* gene was shown to oscillate in a circadian fashion[40] as a result of transcriptional regulation,[41] and the levels of the PER protein were shown to lag the *per* mRNA levels.[42] In fact, shifts in the circadian phase can be evoked by the induction of PER protein under the control of a noncircadian promoter.[43] Thus many lines of evidence indicate that the *per* gene encodes a protein that is a clock component. Three orthologues of the *per* gene, *Per1*, *Per2*, and *Per3*, have now been identified in the mouse, and the levels of their mRNA have also been shown to oscillate with a circadian period.[44–48]

After the identification of CLOCK:BMAL1 dimerization, the ability of this heterodimer to regulate transcription was tested using a reporter construct based on the upstream regulatory elements of the *per* gene. The *per* gene of *Drosophila* contains an upstream regulatory element, the "clock control region," within which is contained a sequence needed for positive regulation of transcription, the E-box element (CACGTG).[49] CLOCK-BMAL1 heterodimers were found to activate transcription of the *mPer* gene in a process that requires binding to the E-box element.[32] However, CLOCK-Δ19 mutant protein was not able to activate transcription, consistent with the finding that exon 19, which is skipped in *Clock* mutant animals,[30] is necessary for transactivation. Thus CLOCK protein interacts with the regulatory regions of the *per* gene to allow transcription of the *per* mRNA and eventual translation of PER protein. A similar activation of transcription of the *tim* gene by the CLOCK-BMAL1 heterodimer also occurs in flies.[50] However, this positive regulation alone will not produce an oscillation in *per* mRNA levels, which is known to be responsible for the oscillation in PER protein levels.[41] Findings that the *Clock* mutation dramatically decreases *per* genes' expression also confirms the positive regulation of CLOCK:BMAL1 on *per* transcription in situ[51,52] Mice with null mutations of *Per1*, *Per2*, or *Per3* alone display altered circadian periods,[53,54] whereas mice with both *Per1* and *Per2* null mutations lose rhythmicity. *Per3* null mutant mice exhibit only a subtle alteration in rhythmicity, and *Per1/Per3* or *Per2/Per3* double mutants are not substantially distinct from the *Per1* or *Per2* single mutants. These findings suggest there may be some compensation of function among the different mammalian *per* genes, and raise the question of the significance of *Per3* for the generation of mammalian circadian rhythms.

Cryptochromes

Cryptochromes are blue light–responsive flavoprotein photopigments related to photolyases, so named because their function was cryptic when first identified. In mammals, two cryptochrome genes, *Cry1* and *Cry2,* have been identified and were found to be highly expressed in the ganglion cells, the inner nuclear layer of the retina, and the SCN,[55] and their mRNA expression levels oscillate in these tissues. Targeted mutant mice lacking *Cry2* exhibit a lengthened circadian period, whereas mice lacking *Cry1* have a shortened circadian period; mice with both mutations have immediate loss of rhythmicity upon transfer to DD.[56–58] Thus, like the mammalian *period* genes, the *cryptochrome* genes appear to have both distinct (given their opposite effects on circadian period) and compensatory (given that either gene can sustain rhythmicity in the absence of the other) functions.

Because of their expression pattern, the *cryptochromes* were thought to be the long-unidentified mammalian circadian photoreceptors (see later), and thus light responses were examined in characterizing the null mutants. *Cry2* mutant mice exhibit altered phase-shifting responses to light pulses.[56] *Cry1/Cry2* double mutants exhibit impaired light induction of *Per1* in the SCN, whereas light induction of *Per2* in double mutants remains.[57,59] Neither *Per1* nor *Per2* exhibits persistent oscillations in expression in the SCN, in constant conditions in *Cry1/Cry2* double mutants.[57,59] Thus, although the *cryptochromes* are not the mammalian circadian photoreceptor, they do appear to play a central role in the generation of circadian signals.

Further evidence for a central clock function is the finding that the *cryptochromes* appear to share a number of regulatory features with the *period* genes. In *Clock* mutant mice, the mRNA levels of *Cry1* and *Cry2* are reduced in the SCN and in skeletal muscle,[60] suggesting that the *cryptochromes* also are induced by CLOCK:BMAL1 transactivation. Using mammalian (NIH 3T3 or COS7) cell lines, CRY1 and CRY2 were found by coimmunoprecipitation to interact with PER1, PER2, and PER3, leading to nuclear localization of the CRY:PER dimer, as indicated by cotransfection assays with epitope-tagged proteins.[60] Luciferase assays indicate that CRY:CRY or CRY:PER complexes were capable of inhibiting CLOCK:BMAL1 transactivation of *mPer1* or vasopressin transcription.[60] Thus the CRYs and the PERs are capable of a negative feedback function, inhibiting CLOCK:BMAL1-induced transcription.

MODULATORS AND OTHER COMPONENTS OF THE CLOCK

Timeless

How is the level of the PER protein regulated by the circadian clock? The first hint came from the identification of the *timeless* gene *tim*, which when mutated produces abnormal circadian rhythms in *Drosophila*.[61] The levels of the mRNA encoded by the *tim* gene oscillate with a time course that is indistinguishable from those of *per* mRNA.[62] The levels of the TIM protein lag behind those of *tim* mRNA by several hours,[63] similar to the finding with *per* mRNA and PER protein. The PER and TIM proteins form heterodimers[64] that are transported to the nucleus.[65] The finding that the heterodimer is transported to the nucleus suggested that it might be involved in the regulation of transcription of the *per* or *tim* genes. Indeed, recent experiments have shown that the transcription of the *per* and *tim* genes is repressed by the PER-TIM protein heterodimer.[50] This finding is very important because it demonstrates that the production of mRNA encoded by a clock component gene, the delayed accumulation of the encoded protein, and later feedback to the clock gene's promoter in the nucleus are able to explain the basic features of the circadian clock in *Drosophila*.

However, PER-TIM interactions are not sufficient, and the basic mechanism does not become clear until one adds interactions with other clock genes. In experiments using a luciferase reporter assay, the luminescent luciferase protein was expressed under the control of the promoter regions of the *Drosophila per* and *tim* genes. It was found that the fly homologue of *Clock*[66] was capable of driving expression of luciferase[50] in cells that have high endogenous levels of the *Drosophila* homologue of BMAL1, CYC (*cycle*). The effect of the PER-TIM heterodimer on the ability of the CLOCK-CYC heterodimer to drive the transcription of the *per* and *tim* genes was tested by cotransfecting the encoding genes into the cells that expressed the luciferase reporter gene. Indeed, it was found that the expression of both the *per* and *tim* genes were reduced by their own protein products. This negative feedback has recently been found for a mammalian heterodimer consisting of homologues of the TIMELESS and PER1 proteins.[67]

Whether the mammalian *tim* homologue identified[67,68] actually represents an orthologous gene has been called into question.[69] This issue has been difficult to resolve, as gene targeting to create a null mutant resulted in early embryonic lethality. Differences in results obtained by different groups examining the oscillation of *Tim* expression could result from both a full-length and a truncated protein being expressed, with only the full-length form oscillating.[70] Using antisense oligodeoxynucleotides directed against *Timeless* in rat SCN slice preparation results in a disruption of neuronal oscillations in vitro, suggesting a role in rhythmicity may exist.[70] However, true functional homology of *Timeless* in mammals remains to be demonstrated.

Casein Kinase 1

The *tau* mutation of the hamster arose spontaneously in a laboratory stock.[71] The mutation is semidominant and shortens the period from 24 to 22 hours in heterozygotes and 20 hours in homozygotes. This mutation has been of great importance for several reasons.[1] The mutation predated the *Clock* mutation and demonstrated that single-gene mutations could profoundly alter the circadian clock in mammals, just as in flies and *Neurospora*.[2] *Tau* mutants display several other physiologic phenotypes, such as alteration of the responses of males to photoperiod length[72] and effects of the estrous cycles in females,[73] which gave further insights into the importance of the circadian clock for other biologic cycles.[3] The evidence that the SCN is indeed the site of the master circadian oscillator (see earlier) was demonstrated unequivocally using transplantation of the SCN that used the *tau* mutation. These manipulations also gave rise to the evidence necessary to conclude that the *tau* mutation encodes a protein that is a clock component. Unfortunately, the genetic tools needed for cloning this important and interesting gene were not available for the hamster, and thus its molecular identity could not be determined by conventional genetic mapping/positional cloning approaches.

Lowrey and colleagues[74] were able to identify a genomic region of conserved synteny (a grouping of genes together on a chromosome), in hamsters, mice, and humans, that encompassed the *tau* mutation. *Tau* was thus identified as being a mutation in the *Casein Kinase 1 epsilon* (*CK1ε*) gene, the mammalian orthologue of the *Drosophila doubletime* gene. Sequencing of the gene identified a point mutation, which leads to altered enzyme dynamics and an autophosphorylation state. In vitro assays demonstrated that CKε can phosphorylate PER proteins and that the *tau* mutant enzyme is deficient in this ability. Thus CK1ε may lead to degradation of PERs, slowing the accumulation of PER in the nucleus and thus repression of CLOCK:BMAL1. *Casein Kinase 1 delta* (*CK1δ*) has also been implicated in mammalian circadian rhythmicity.[75–78]

Rev-erb alpha and *ROR*

Although the negative feedback of PER and CRY proteins on their own CLOCK:BMAL1-induced transcription constitutes a form of negative feedback, and may be sufficient to explain the oscillations in expression of *Per* and *Cry* genes, the rhythmic expression of *Bmal1* with an opposite phase is not explained by this feedback. What regulatory elements produce the rhythmic transcription of *Bmal1*, with an antiphase relationship to the *Pers*? *Rev-erb alpha*, an orphan nuclear receptor, may act as the missing link. Its promoter region contains three E-boxes, and transcription is thus positively regulated by CLOCK and BMAL1.[79] Its transcription is negatively regulated by PER and CRYs and is at a minimum when mPER2 is at a maximum, and it is constitutively expressed at intermediate levels in *Cry1/Cry2* or *Per1/Per2* double knockouts. REV-ERBα protein appears to drive the circadian oscillation in *Bmal1* transcription: The *Bmal1* promoter includes two RORE sequences (enhancer sequences that recognize members of the REV-ERB and ROR orphan nuclear receptor families), and *Bmal1* expression is drastically reduced in *Rev-erb alpha* null mutants.[79] Thus *Rev-erb alpha* may act to link the positive and negative regulatory signals of other clock genes to the transcription of *Bmal1*. Given the importance of orphan nuclear receptors in regulating cellular metabolic properties,[80] interaction with circadian clock genes may, at the molecular level, form the links between circadian clocks and metabolic regulation, with important implications for health and disease. Such molecular links between circadian clocks and cellular metabolism also include a clock-metabolism feedback loop. CLOCK:BMAL1 activity is suppressed by a nicotinamide adenine dinucleotide $(NAD)^+$-dependent deacetylase, sirtuin 1 (SIRT1), which is in turn regulated by the circadian control of NAD^+ biosynthesis.[81–84] See Chapter 41 for more details.

Rev-erb alpha also contributes to the differences between the phase of *Cry1* mRNA rhythms relative to other clock genes whose transcription is enhanced by CLOCK:BMAL binding to E-boxes. The *Cry1* gene has three candidate REV-ERB/ROR binding sites[85]; in vitro assays indicate that REV-ERBα binds to two of these sites. Luciferase reporter assays indicate that REV-ERBα protein can inhibit transcription of *Cry1* through binding at these two sites. REV-ERBβ also appears to share some functional redundancy with REV-ERBα.[86]

Fbxl3 and *Fbxl21*

In addition to *Rev-erb* modulation of Cry (described earlier), other genes appear to modulate the activity of the cryptochromes. The *Overtime* mutation in mice was identified in a mutagenesis screen based on a lengthened free-running circadian period.[87] The responsible mutation was ultimately identified as being in a known gene encoding the F-box protein *Fbxl3*, but a gene previously unknown to be involved in circadian rhythmicity. *Fbxl3*^{OVTM} mutants appear to be functionally comparable to null mutants. FBXL3 protein leads to degradation of CRY1, whereas the OVTM mutant protein is less effective in this capacity. Thus the period lengthening may be a direct result of a delay in degradation of CRY, effectively preventing the core cycle from restarting. Recently, the closely related protein FBXL21[88] has been found to function in a similar manner.[89,90]

NPAS2

NPAS2 (neuronal PAS family member 2) shares the closest homology with CLOCK of all identified bHLH-PAS family members. Null mutants of this gene have altered circadian activity patterns, notably the absence of a "siesta" in later subjective night, but no dramatic alterations in circadian free-running period or persistence.[91] However, when null mutants of the *Clock* gene had less dramatic phenotypes than the Δ19 mutant,[92] the role of NPAS2 was reexamined. In the absence of functioning CLOCK, NPAS2 appears to be able to partially compensate.[93]

Dec1 and *Dec2*

Like other clock genes, *Dec1* and *Dec2* are bHLH transcription factors that bind to E-boxes. DEC1 and DEC2 have been found to inhibit transactivation of Per by CLOCK and BMAL1.[94] DEC1 and DEC2 form dimers.[95] The inhibition of CLOCK and BMAL1 transactivation may be related to interactions with BMAL1 but can also be attributed to binding to (and thus possibly competition for) E-boxes.[96]

Recently two human allelic variants in *Dec2* have been linked with total sleep time.[97,98] This functional relationship between *Dec2* and the amount of sleep has been confirmed in transgenic mice expressing one of the human *Dec2* alleles.[97]

Other Regulators of the Clock

The discovery of the core molecular machinery of the circadian clock has allowed identification of additional regulators of the circadian clock by characterizing proteins that interact with known clock components. For example, an RNA- and DNA-binding protein, NONO, and a subunit of histone methyltransferase complexes, WDR5, were identified as interacting proteins and modulators of PER1. Knockdown of *NONO* using RNA interference (RNAi) in mammalian cells and a *NONO* mutant in flies both disrupt circadian rhythms.[99] Another study later shows that NONO and PER1 are involved in the regulation of circadian gating of cell cycles via controlling the circadian expression of a cell cycle checkpoint gene, *p16-Ink4A*.[100] Similarly, RACK1 (receptor for activated C kinase 1) and PKCα (protein kinase C alpha) were found interacting with BMAL1 and modulating CLOCK-BMAL1 transcriptional activity. Knockdown of either PKCα or RACK1 by RNAi shortens circadian period.[101] Clock modulators identified by studying proteins interacting with known clock components also include E3 ligases Arf-bp1 and Pam, which are involved in the regulation of the degradation of REV-ERBα.[102]

Furthermore, high-throughput screening studies using a combination of luciferase reporter assays in cell-based systems and large-scale RNAi libraries have also identified many other genes that modulate the circadian oscillation of core clock genes. One study focused on known and predicted kinases, as well as phosphatases and F-box proteins, and identified 22 kinases, 7 phosphatases (or regulatory subunits), and 6 F-box proteins as potential components of the clock.[103] Among those, casein kinase 2 (CK2) was shown to phosphorylate PER2 and regulate its nuclear accumulation and stability. Using a similar RNAi screening approach, Zhang and colleagues[104] searched the entire genome and identified more than 200 candidates that strongly affected the circadian period or amplitude when knocked down. Protein interaction network analysis suggests that most of these identified candidates are directly or indirectly connected with the core clock components, suggesting that large-scale and complex interactions among the molecular clockworks are likely to be involved in the regulation of circadian timing.

Finally, along with the accumulation of "-omic" (i.e., genomic, proteomic, interactomic, metabolomic, etc.) datasets, it recently became possible to predict clock components using "in silico" approaches. The first computer-assisted study to identify clock components was performed by Anafi and colleagues.[105] The authors collected a number of genome-wide datasets and established metrics that describe key features of core clock components, including (1) 24-hour oscillatory expression, (2) components affecting circadian rhythms when mutated or knocked down, (3) interaction with other core clock proteins, (4) ubiquity expressed in multiple tissues, and (5) conservation between vertebrates and flies. Although these clock features are not absolute, the core clock metrics allowed the authors to use a machine learning algorithm to identify genes that share similar metrics with known core clock genes. The top identified genes include many that have already been implicated in the circadian clockwork. In addition, a previously uncharacterized gene, *Gene Model 129* (*Gm129*), was also among the top candidate clock genes, and the authors renamed it *Chrono*, for *c*omputationally *h*ighlighted *r*epressor *o*f the *n*etwork *o*scillator. Validation experiments show that *Gm129* expression exhibits strong circadian rhythms in liver, heart, and adipose tissue. GM129 protein interacts with the C-terminus of BMAL1 and suppresses CLOCK/BMAL1 transcriptional activity. Finally, free-running periods of the mice are lengthened in *Gm129* knockout mice. Of interest, the role of *Gm129* in the circadian clockwork was also independently discovered using conventional biochemical approaches,[106] at roughly the same time of this in silico–assisted study. With the rapid growth of bioinformatics techniques and databases, it can be expected that computational approaches will greatly complement traditional biochemical approaches, contributing to a full understanding of the circadian clock network.

It is important to note that many regulators of the clock are also key regulators in other cellular processes, including metabolism and redox homeostasis (such as *Rev-erb alpha* and *Sirt1*), cell cycle (such as *NONO*), cell signaling (such as *PKCα*), and many others. The interactions between clock and other cellular pathways are further supported by results from large-scale RNAi screen studies, as pathway analysis suggests the identified clock modulators are overrepresented for genes involved in the insulin and hedgehog signaling, the cell cycle, and the folate metabolism.[104] Many of these pathways and key regulators that influence the circadian clock are themselves regulated by the clock. Taken together, these findings suggest that the molecular clock machinery is hardwired to diverse cellular processes and pathways, providing a basis for functional coordination of multiple pathways by the circadian clock.

OUTPUT REGULATION

Transcriptional Output of the Clock

As described earlier, the core clock components form a transcriptional and translational feedback loop that produces a program of oscillatory gene expression involving roughly one-third of the transcriptome. Many efforts have been devoted to understanding the details of how circadian transcriptome is regulated by the clock. Bioinformatics analyses of promoter regions of oscillatory genes in multiple tissues suggest enrichment of classical enhancer elements, such as E-box and D-box.[107,108] Many of the clock-controlled, E-box–containing genes are themselves transcription factors, which are thought to be important for expanding the repertoire of clock-regulated transcription to a wide range of genes. Of interest, bioinformatics studies have also suggested that rather than a single E-box, an arrangement of two closely spaced (6 to 7 base pairs apart) E-box–like elements, namely E1 and E2 elements, are critical for robust oscillations in many of the clock-regulated genes in both flies and mice.[109,110] Using chromatin immunoprecipitation (CHIP), combined with deep sequencing (CHIP-seq), one study characterized direct DNA-binding targets of BMAL1 in mouse liver.[111] A total of 2049 BMAL1 target binding sites were identified, 60% of which exhibited rhythmic binding. Sequence analysis suggests that 13% of the BMAL1 binding sites consist of a pair of E1-E2 elements, and these E1-E2 sites are associated with more robust rhythmic BMAL1 binding, whereas a single E-box alone is sufficient for rhythmic CLOCK:BMAL1 binding.[111] Another study used CHIP-seq and compared the binding targets of seven clock components, including CLOCK, BMAL1, NAPS2, PER1, PER2, CRY1, and CRY2, in mouse liver.[112] Remarkably, although more than 1400 target sites were found common for CLOCK, BMAL1, PER1, PER2, CRY1, and CRY2, distinct target profiles were apparent for each of these core clock components. Although targets of all clock components are commonly enriched with E-boxes, sites that are specifically bound by PER2, CRY1, or CRY2 show a reduction in E-boxes and an enrichment for nuclear hormone receptors, consistent with known partnerships between the negative elements of the clock and nuclear receptors.[113,114] Finally, it is interesting to note that E-box elements can be occupied by other transcription factors. For example, USF1, a suppressor of the *Clock*$^{\Delta 19}$ mutant phenotype, competes with CLOCK:BMAL1 for E1 sites, modulating the circadian transcriptome.[115]

Many other mechanisms are likely to be involved in the regulation of the circadian transcriptome. For example, multiple lines of evidence have supported a role of rhythmic histone modification and chromatin remodeling in the regulation of circadian transcription. P300, a histone acetyltransferase, immunoprecipitates together with CLOCK in liver nuclear preparations, with a peak at Circadian Time (CT) 6 and minimum at CT 18.[85] P300 enhances CLOCK:BMAL1-mediated transcription of reporter gene, and this increase in expression is inhibited by CRY1 and CRY2, suggesting a potential mechanisms by which CRY proteins can preclude CLOCK:BMAL1 transactivation of target genes. It has also been demonstrated that CLOCK protein itself can also function as a histone acetyltransferase, and the acetyltransferase activity is critical for transcriptional activation of clock genes and rescue of circadian rhythmicity in *Clock*$^{\Delta 19}$ mutant cells.[116] Indeed, genome-wide circadian chromatin modifications have been extensively describe in a number of studies.[111,117,118] Remarkably, the binding of CLOCK:BAML1 to target DNA promotes removal of nucleosomes, which leads to chromatin opening at the binding site, allowing for rhythmic binding of other transcription factors.[119] Finally, a recent study has reported clock-controlled long-range interactions and chromosomal organization, suggesting a genomic environment that is coordinated with the rhythmic gene expression.[120]

In addition to direct transcriptional activation and chromatin remodeling, posttranscriptional mechanisms are likely to be involved in shaping output programs of the clock. By separating intronic and exonic signals in whole genome RNA-seq data, Koike and colleagues[112] were able to infer the oscillatory patterns of pre-mRNA from total mRNA. Of interest, genes that exhibited both exonic and intronic cycling signals account for only 22% of the exonic cycling genes and 30% of the intronic cycling genes, suggesting that de novo transcription only contributes to a relatively small portion of circadian program of the transcriptome. Similar results were observed by comparing rhythmic expression pattern of nascent and total mRNA using RNA-seq in both mice and flies,[121,122] indicating significant contributions of posttranscriptional mechanisms in regulating circadian transcriptome.

A complex profile of rhythmic gene expression arises from clock-dependent transcriptional, epigenetic, and posttranscriptional regulations. Early microarray studies have suggested that up to a third of the expressed genes exhibit circadian oscillations.[18–21] More recent studies with higher temporal resolutions have added a great amount of details to the overall picture of the circadian transcriptome, including transcripts that exhibited clock-controlled harmonic oscillations (i.e., 12-hour and 4-hour rhythms)[123] and rhythmically expressed noncoding regulatory RNAs.[118,124] Of interest, only a small fraction of rhythmically expressed genes are commonly found in the SCN and liver,[20] in the liver and heart,[21] as well as in liver and skeletal muscle[125] (Figure 13.2). Adding together all oscillatory genes from all the tissues that have been examined so far, a total of 43% of protein-coding genes oscillate in the body.[124] At least in flies, a tissue-specific program of circadian gene expression is correlated with a tissue-specific preference in cis-regulatory motifs of genes that are bound by CLOCK and other partner transcription factors.[126] Gene ontology suggests that rhythmically expressed genes are involved in diverse pathways and cellular functions. In addition, the tissue specificity of circadian gene expression are tightly related to the specific functions of the tissue. For example, genes cycling in the SCN include those involved in protein/neuropeptide synthesis, processing, and degradation, as well as genes known to be important for circadian locomotor activity, whereas genes cycling in the liver are involved in nutrient metabolisms and regulation of metabolic intermediates.[20] Nonetheless, expression of genes involved in essential cell functions, such as redox homeostasis, appear to be under circadian regulation across

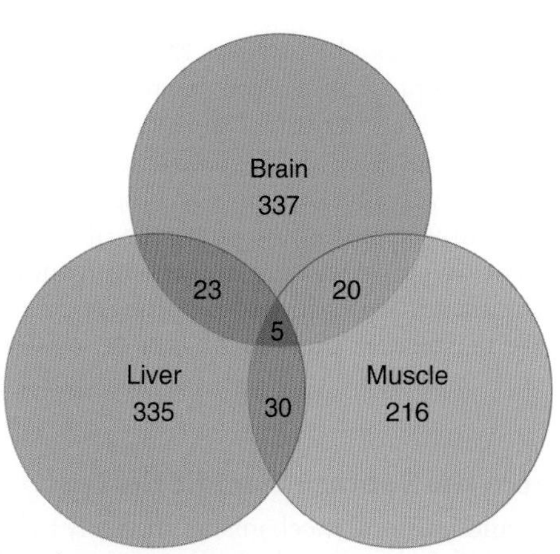

Figure 13.2 Rhythmic gene expression varies among cells and tissues. Gene expression profiling studies[124,184] have revealed that up to a third of genes expressed in any given tissue may do so rhythmically. Although the core circadian clock genes comprising the transcription-translation feedback loop are rhythmically expressed in all tissues, and some common regulatory elements may be expressed in multiple tissues, the vast majority of these rhythmic transcripts are specific to the cell type and functions of the particular tissue. The contribution of various regulatory mechanisms in determining the tissue specificity remains to be determined. (Data from Miller BH, McDearmon EL, Panda S, et al. Circadian and CLOCK-controlled regulation of the mouse transcriptome and cell proliferation. *Proc Natl Acad Sci U S A*. 2007;104(9):3342–47; McCarthy JJ, Andrews JL, McDearmon EL, et al. Identification of the circadian transcriptome in adult mouse skeletal muscle. *Physiol Genomics*. 2007;31(1):86–95; Hogenesch, JB, Panda S, Kay S, et al. Circadian transcriptional output in the SCN and liver of the mouse. *Novartis Found Symp*. 2003;253:171–180; discussion 52–5, 102-9, 180–3 passim.)

different tissues. Remarkably, a recent study suggests that the targets of best-selling drugs and World Health Organization essential medicines are highly enriched with oscillating genes.[124] This finding has significant clinical implications, as the treatment outcome drugs with short half-lives could potentially be improved by circadian-timed administration.

It is important to note that the oscillatory gene expression pattern observed outside of the SCN is driven by both local cell-automatous clock machineries and system cues originated from the SCN. Using an inducible hepatocyte-specific *Rev-erb alpha* transgene, Kornmann and colleagues[127] were able to arrest the liver clock by suppressing *Bmal1* expression upon activation of the transgene. Of interest, 10% of the liver circadian transcriptome, including the transcript of core clock gene *Per2*, remained cycling when the hepatocyte clock was arrested. Circadian expression of these genes are thus attributed to the output signals from the master clock, including direct neural and humoral signals from the SCN and indirect cues, such as those associated with clock-controlled sleep-wake, feed-fast, and body temperature rhythms. In particular, sleep-wake affects the expression of a large number of genes,[128,129] and large-scale interactions between circadian- and sleep/wake-related genes have been recently documented[130,131] (for a detailed discussion, see Chapter 15). Of note, when animals are sleep deprived at different times of the day so that the amount of sleep debt and homeostatic drive is similar across the sampling time points, diurnal rhythms in the whole-brain transcriptome and the forebrain synaptic proteasome are largely diminished,[132,133] suggesting these rhythmic patterns are predominantly driven by sleep-wake rhythms rather than the SCN clock. Similarly, by manipulating the time of food availability, a study found feeding rhythm is responsible for 70% of the rhythmically expressed genes in the liver.[134] Recent studies also suggest that the circadian transcriptome can be reprogrammed by environmental conditions. For example, compared to normal chow-feeding, feeding with a high-fat diet suppressed cycling of more than 1000 genes, including those involved in insulin signaling, in the liver while eliciting rhythmic expression of hundreds of other genes.[135] In addition, of the genes cycling under both conditions, 66% exhibited significant shifts in circadian phase. These findings suggest that the circadian program of gene expression is highly plastic to environmental conditions and associated functional challenges.

Output from the Suprachiasmatic Nucleus

Both neural and humoral mechanisms are likely to be involved in the output of the master clock. The molecular clock controls a firing rhythm in SCN neurons, and the SCN neurons project to many other brain areas.[136] On the other hand, encapsulated SCN grafts are capable of rescuing the circadian locomotor activity in SCN-lesion animals,[137] suggesting that secreted factors are also involved in SCN output. To date, a few proteins, such as prokineticin 2 (PK2), transforming growth factor-α (TGF-α), cardiomyotrophin-like cytokine (CLC), and vasoactive intestinal polypeptide (VIP) have been implicated in the SCN humoral outputs.

PK2 is rhythmically expressed in the SCN,[138] and infusion of PK2 into the cerebral ventricles inhibits locomotor activity. Mice with a null mutation in the *PK2* gene exhibit dramatically reduced levels of activity[139] with reduced circadian amplitude. These mice also exhibit attenuated the rebound in non–rapid eye movement sleep, rapid eye movement sleep, and delta power after sleep deprivation.[140]

The peptide TGF-α (transforming growth factor-α) was identified in a screen for SCN factors that might inhibit locomotor activity; when infused into the third ventricle, this peptide inhibits locomotor activity. Mice with targeted mutations of the epidermal growth factor (EGF) receptor (the receptor likely to bind TGF-α) also display disruption of activity rhythms.[141] These effects are attributable to actions on the EGF receptors.

Mice that lack the peptide receptor VPAC2 show abnormal entrainment and disrupted rhythms, indicating that VIP signaling in the SCN may be necessary for normal expression and coordination of rhythms.[142]

CLC also is expressed in the SCN in a rhythmic manner in vasopressin neurons. Infusion of CLC into the third ventricle (near the SCN) dramatically inhibits locomotor activity, whereas infusion of antibodies to the CLC receptor increases activity.[143]

INPUT REGULATION

The circadian rhythms of many humans who are blind, with no conscious perception of light, are nevertheless able to be entrained by light.[144] This intriguing observation led to studies of the circadian light input pathway and the photoreceptors and photopigments in mammals.

In mice with mutations that result in degeneration of rods[145] or both rods and cones,[146] light entrainment of the circadian rhythm was preserved.[147] However, the eye must be the site of the light-entraining pathways in mammals because enucleated mammals are not capable of light entrainment.[145] Indeed, a morphologically distinct set of retinal ganglion cells projects to the SCN via the retinohypothalamic tract.[148] Ablation of the SCN abolishes circadian rhythmicity, and ablation of the retinohypothalamic tract abolishes light entrainment.[149] Thus the light signal responsible for light entrainment enters the SCN via a unique axonal pathway from the eye.

Melanopsin, a member of the opsin family of photopigments, was first found in the inner retina[150] and later found to be expressed in the somata and dendrites of retinal ganglion cells of the retinohypothalamic tract.[151] Neurons that contribute axons to the retinohypothalamic tract were found to express the marker pituitary adenylate cyclase-activating polypeptide (PACAP)[151]; when PACAP was used as a marker for rat retinohypothalamic tract neurons, every PACAP-positive neuron was found to express melanopsin, and every melanopsin positive neuron was PACAP positive.[151]

Further evidence confirming the role of melanopsin as the phase-shifting pigment has come from genetically engineered mice in which the gene encoding melanopsin was disrupted.[152,153] Two behavioral measures of circadian rhythm responses to light were altered in these mice: The phase-shifting response to a discrete light pulse was of lesser amplitude in the knockout mice than in wild-type mice, and the free-running periods of the knockout mice were lengthened less by exposure to constant light than the periods of wild-type mice. Hence it appears that melanopsin represents a primary photopigment, with other photopigments also having input to the circadian system.

The *Rab3a* gene was identified in a mutagenesis screen (*earlybird*) based on an advanced phase angle of entrainment and shortened circadian period. Null mutant mice display a similar phenotype.[154] Further, both the *Rab3a* null and *earlybird* mutants exhibit alterations in the homeostatic response to sleep deprivation[154] and alterations in emotional behavior.[155]

NONCANONICAL OSCILLATOR

It is interesting to note that recent studies have identified a transcription-independent oscillator. In human mature red blood cells, with the nucleus and thus the transcriptional-translational clock absent, the hyperoxidation of peroxiredoxins shows a sustained circadian rhythm that is entrainable and temperature compensated.[156] The redox rhythms of peroxiredoxins appear to be highly conserved between eukaryotes and prokaryotes[157,158] and can also be observed in the mitochondria.[159] Prior studies of rhythms of redox state had indicated that nicotinamide adenine dinucleotide phosphate (NADP) and SIRTs could connect mitochondrial function and the canonical clock, allowing for mutual regulation.[81–84,160] These findings thus raise an intriguing hypothesis that the transcription-independent redox rhythms of peroxiredoxins may represent an ancient form of circadian oscillators. This redox oscillator may be influenced by the transcriptional-translational clock, because the peroxiredoxin redox rhythm in cultured mouse embryonic fibroblasts was disrupted by ablating *Cry1* and *Cry2*,[156] although the in vivo peroxiredoxin rhythm in mouse liver was largely unaffected by deletion of *Bmal1*.[161] The functional output of this redox oscillator is unclear. Of interest, in mice lacking *Bmal1* and kept in DD, rhythms remained in the transcriptome, proteome, and phosphoproteome, although the pattern of these rhythms and the involved genes/proteins are distinct from those in the wild-type animals.[161] In bioinformatics analyses, transcription factors that may regulate the rhythmic gene expression in the absence of *Bmal1* can be linked to peroxiredoxins and canonical clock via other circadian redox regulators, such as *Sirt1*.[161] Future studies are needed to elucidate the functional significance of the peroxiredoxin redox oscillation and its relationship with the canonical transcriptional-translational clock. These studies are also expected to unveil the evolutional history of circadian time keeping.

POSSIBLE MICROBIAL CLOCKS IN THE GASTROINTESTINAL TRACT

A new forefront of genomic studies of the circadian clock concerns genomes beyond our own. The gut microbiome, which refers to the genomes of the microbial flora living in the mammalian gastrointestinal tract, interacts with the host genome and plays important roles in host metabolic, immune, and neurobehavioral functions. The composition of the gut microbiome is altered by genetic and environmental disturbances in the host circadian rhythms.[162–165] This interaction is bidirectional, as circadian oscillations in the peripheral transcriptome, including the rhythmic expression of clock genes, are altered germ-free animals.[166–168] Of note, diurnal rhythms in the relative abundance of gut microbes have been observed.[164–166,169] It is thus of interest to understand whether these rhythms are passively driven by host rhythms (e.g., feeding, metabolism, and body temperature) or at least, in part, generated endogenously within each bacterial cell and entrained by host rhythms. At least in one gut bacterium, *Enterobacter aerogenes* express a circadian rhythm in swarming and motility when cultured under constant conditions.[170] The transcription of *MotA*, a gene encoding the a flagellar stator component in this bacterium, display endogenous, entrainable, and temperature-compensated rhythms,[170,171] suggesting the existence of a bacterial circadian clock. The molecular identity of this bacterial clock is unknown, and it is unclear whether it shares similarity with the circadian clock in cyanobacteria. These questions, together with the relationship between the gut bacterial clocks and host clocks, are important topics for future studies.

CONCLUSIONS

The core circadian oscillator is autonomous to individual neurons of the SCN and is the result of the daily oscillation in the levels of several clock component proteins. The basis for this oscillation in mammals, as in other organisms, lies in rhythmic feedback regulation of transcription of the genes encoding these proteins. The levels of the PER and CRY proteins alter the rate of transcription of their own genes. This alteration is achieved by inhibition of the enhancement of transcription that results from binding of the CLOCK-BMAL1 heterodimer to the E-box element of the promoter region of the *Per* and *Cry* genes. Additional interactions between circadian clock proteins may slow the time course of this feedback, achieving the near-24-hour interval: The phosphorylation of PER by CK1ε may lead to its degradation, and the association with BMAL1 appears needed for CLOCK to be present in the nucleus. Rhythmic transcription of *Bmal1* appears to result from regulation via REV-ERBα, itself regulated by E-box elements. Finally, it appears that rhythms in histone acetylation contribute to the circadian expression pattern of some core circadian genes. Additional genes have been identified based on altered circadian rhythms in mutants, although the roles of these genes in the circadian system remain to be determined.

It is of interest that the majority of the core genes have been identified in mice or in flies by forward genetics, in which mutations were induced in the genome randomly, and those mutations which specifically affect the circadian oscillator were identified with carefully crafted circadian phenotypic screens. Now that these clock component proteins have been identified, it will be easier to find the proteins that serve the input and output pathways of the circadian oscillator and to identify the components that are out of order in disease states that affect circadian rhythms. Furthermore, as great advances have been made in genomic, proteomic, and metabolomic techniques, studies have been integrating and depicting the circadian program at a multiscale level.[172–177] These studies will eventually facilitate a comprehensive understanding of how the clock is coupled with other cellular and physiologic functions. It is fortuitous that the unraveling of the molecular basis for circadian rhythmicity is occurring at a time when the general public is becoming aware of the importance of normal circadian timekeeping for human health, safety, performance, and productivity.

REMAINING QUESTION: HOW MANY LEVELS OF GENETIC REGULATION OF CLOCKS EXIST?

The developing picture of the molecular genetic clock is becoming many-layered and complex. At its core is a transcriptional-translational feedback loop of CLOCK:BMAL1 and PER:CRY. This loop interacts intimately with a cellular metabolism loop, via redox state, NAD, and SIRT. The genetic circadian clock regulates rhythms of gene expression via direct transcriptional regulation, via histone acetylation/deacetylation, chromatin modifications, and possibly other modifications. These modifications may be tissue specific but can be influenced by the SCN.[178] Rhythms/behaviors (driven by the SCN), such as melatonin levels,[179] body temperature,[180] feeding,[181] or sleep,[131,182] can also influence gene expression rhythms in the periphery. It thus seems that the so-called "cell-autonomous" genetic circadian clock is subjected to a wide array of modulators, ranging from the intracellular to nutritional, endocrine, and behavioral. How cell autonomous is our clock? Whether such disruptions in physiology and behavior are due to altered circadian information from the SCN, or are due to local tissue specific changes in the molecular circadian clock, requires further study. Reconstituting a functional circadian clock specifically in the liver of *Bmal1* knockout animals (i.e., liver-specific rescue of *Bmal1*) is associated with rhythmic patterns in the hepatic transcriptome and metabolome that are only partially in agreement with those in the wild-type animals.[183] Regardless of the mechanisms, such results point to a very central role of circadian clock genes in regulating biochemical, metabolic, and physiologic processes at many different levels of organization.

CLINICAL PEARL

Our understanding of the genetic and genomic basis of the circadian clock has evolved rapidly from a handful of core clock genes to multilayered molecular circadian programs with tissue specificity. The timings of these circadian programs are intricately coordinated across tissues by the SCN clock and behavioral and environmental cues, and disruptions in such coordination are involved in many adverse health conditions in humans, such as metabolic disorders and cancer. Timing of the circadian program also has important implications for the efficacy and safety of U.S. Food and Drug Administration–approved therapeutics, as the targets or metabolizing enzymes of roughly half of these drugs are circadian regulated, at least at the mRNA level. Since the discovery of core clock genes and the characterization of the transcriptional-translational feedback loop, the core molecular mechanism of the circadian clock has been and will continue to be used as a blueprint for biomedical researchers to understand the clinical significance of circadian timing, and the insights are accumulating to enable a new frontier of medicine: circadian medicine.

SUMMARY

The cell-autonomous circadian clock found in all mammalian cells and tissues has, at its core, a feedback loop of transcription and translation of a key set of "clock genes." Identification of clock genes has been guided by examining the effects of gene alterations on clock properties. A substantial proportion of expressed genes exhibit circadian variation; however, distinct cell types appear to have their own unique sets of "clock-controlled genes," whereas the core clock genes remain the same. The clock-controlled genes are involved in diverse cellular functions, suggesting important implications for health and diseases. The transcription-translation feedback loop is subject to regulation at multiple levels, including histone, chromatin, and posttranscriptional modifications. Signals from the SCN of the hypothalamus and from behavioral states, such as sleep-wake or feed-fast, also can influence clocks in peripheral tissues.

ACKNOWLEDGMENT

Preparation of this manuscript was in part supported by National Institutes of Health grant PO1 AG 11412.

SELECTED READINGS

Baggs JE, Hogenesch JB. Genomics and systems approaches in the mammalian circadian clock. *Curr Opin Genet Dev.* 2010;20(6):581–587.

Bass J. Circadian topology of metabolism. *Nature.* 2012;491:348–356.

Bedont JL, Blackshaw S. Constructing the suprachiasmatic nucleus: a watchmaker's perspective on the central clockworks. *Front Syst Neurosci.* 2015;9:74.

Buhr ED, Takahashi JS. Molecular components of the mammalian circadian clock. *Handb Exp Pharmacol.* 2013;217:3–27.

Jiang P, Turek FW. Timing of meals: when is as critical as what and how much? *Am J Physiol Endocrinol Metab.* 2017;312(5):E369–E380.

Laing EE, et al. Exploiting human and mouse transcriptomic data: identification of circadian genes and pathways influencing health. *BioEssays.* 2015;37:544–556.

Mauvoisin D, Dayon L, Gachon F, Kussmann M. Proteomics and circadian rhythms: it's all about signaling!. *Proteomics.* 2015;15:310–317.

Pácha J, Balounová K, Soták M. Circadian regulation of transporter expression and implications for drug disposition. *Expert Opin Drug Metab Toxicol* 2021;17(4):425-439.

Rosbash M. Circadian rhythms and the transcriptional feedback loop (Nobel Lecture)*. *Angew Chem Int Ed Engl* 2021;60(16):8650-8666.

Ruben MD, Smith DF, FitzGerald GA, Hogenesch JB. Dosing time matters. *Science.* 2019;365:547–549.

A complete reference list can be found online at ExpertConsult.com.

Chapter 14

Genetics and Genomic Basis of Sleep in Simple Model Organisms

Mark Wu; David Raizen

Chapter Highlights

- The availability of simpler animal model systems, such as worms, flies, and fish, has greatly facilitated the genetic analysis of sleep.
- These simpler animal models exhibit the defining features of sleep, including reversible behavioral quiescence, reduced responsiveness to sensory stimuli, and homeostatic regulation.
- Genetic studies in these simpler models have revealed both circuit and molecular pathways involved in sleep regulation, including many that are shared with mammals.

The complexity of sleep in mammals has led to examining related phenomena in simpler organisms that harbor technical advantages not present in mammalian models. These systems include the fruit fly *Drosophila melanogaster*, the roundworm *Caenorhabditis elegans*, and the zebrafish, *Danio rerio*, which have been used for genetic studies for over 100 years, 50 years, and 30 years, respectively. Remarkably, mammalian homologues of fruit fly, roundworm, and zebrafish genes have been found to function in a manner similar to that observed in these simple systems. Most human disease genes have clear fly, worm, and fish homologues. In view of this genetic similarity, it is not surprising that these animals exhibit many of the defining features of sleep, including reversible quiescence that is timed by an internal clock, reduced responsiveness to sensory stimuli, and homeostatic regulation. Furthermore, preliminary indications are that even the genetic and pharmacologic underpinnings of sleep are conserved among these simple systems and mammals. Topics addressed in this chapter include use of the *Drosophila* model for sleep studies and the unique features of the zebrafish *D. rerio* and the nematode *C. elegans* to study sleep. Insights derived from these model organisms could prove to be important in elucidating the genetic basis of human sleep and, ultimately, answering the question of why organisms sleep.

In contrast with studies of naturally occurring genetic variation in humans, it is possible to induce mutations in animal models to test whether a given gene is important for sleep. One strategy to investigate the molecular basis of complex behaviors such as sleep is termed *classical* or *forward genetics*.[1] Here, a population of animals are randomly mutagenized using deoxyribonucleic acid (DNA)-altering chemicals or mobile DNA transposable elements. The mutagenized population is then screened for a mutant phenotype of interest, such as altered sleep. Molecular genetics techniques are then applied to identify the mutant gene responsible for the mutant phenotype. Thus forward genetics can be used to establish causal relationships between the function of individual genes and phenotypes. Forward genetics is unbiased in the sense that it does not require previous knowledge about the genetic basis of the phenotype of interest. Given the infant state of our knowledge about sleep, forward genetic approaches are powerful approaches for studying sleep. By contrast, *reverse genetics* starts with a disrupted gene in search of a phenotype. The finding of a gene can provide insight into biochemical and cellular pathways that are important for sleep, perhaps even providing novel diagnostic tests or targets for drug development for sleep disorders.

DROSOPHILA AS A MODEL SYSTEM FOR GENETICS

The fruit fly *D. melanogaster* (Figure 14.1) has been a workhorse for genetic studies since the pioneering work of Thomas Morgan in the early 20th century.[2] A major advantage of *Drosophila* over mammalian model systems is the ability to grow and handle large numbers of animals relatively easily and cheaply.[1] A single female can produce hundreds of offspring. In addition, fruit flies have a short generation time, approximately 10 to 12 days from fertilized egg to fertile adult at room temperature. Because of these traits, *Drosophila* has proven powerful for high-throughput screening of mutants with altered phenotypes. The facility of genetic mapping, gene disruption using transposable elements (mobile DNA), and whole genome sequencing allows rapid identification of mutant genes responsible for mutant phenotypes.[3] Remarkably, the mammalian versions (i.e., homologues) of *Drosophila* genes have been found to function in a manner similar to that for their *Drosophila* counterparts. Indeed, entire signaling pathways are often shared between *Drosophila* and their mammalian counterparts.[4-6]

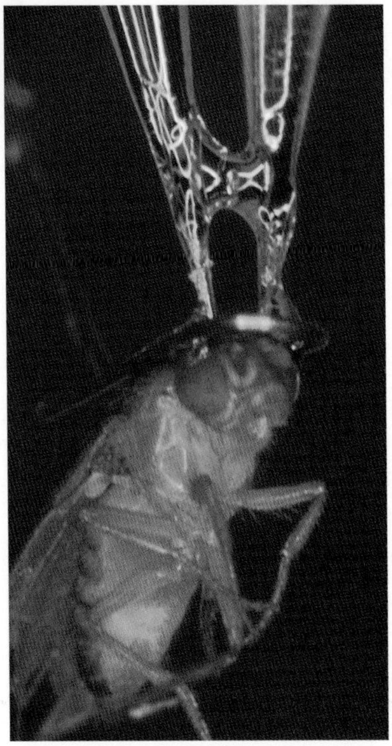

Figure 14.1 *Drosophila*, a genetic model organism. Shown is a fruit fly attached to a tether with recording electrodes implanted for measurement of electrical correlates for behavioral states. (Courtesy B. Van Swinderen.)

The conservation between flies and mammals extends to the nervous system. Although flies have six orders of magnitude fewer neurons than humans do (10^5 versus 10^{11}), the fly and human genomes are similar in gene number (approximately 14,000 and 22,000, respectively), with differences largely the result of gene duplication.[7] The fly brain uses comparable neuronal machinery, including neurotransmitters, ion channels, receptors, and signal transduction pathways.

DROSOPHILA AS A MODEL FOR STUDIES OF SLEEP

Studies of *Drosophila* sleep have been predicated on a small but noteworthy literature examining sleep-like states in other invertebrate models such as mollusks[8] and other insects including cockroaches[9] and honey bees.[10,11] These classical descriptions of sleep behavior formed the basis for pursuing similar studies in *Drosophila.*

Sleep in the fruit fly typically is measured behaviorally using the *Drosophila* Activity Monitoring (DAM) system (developed by Trikinetics Inc., Waltham, Massachusetts) (Figure 14.2), which allows for high-throughput analyses. Single flies are placed into a small transparent glass tube, plugged on one end by agar food and the other end by a porous cap, allowing air passage. Each tube is placed into a monitor that contains a series of 32 infrared emitter-detector pairs, one for each tube. An awake fly will move back and forth in the tube, periodically breaking the infrared beam. Independent methods indicate a close correlation between infrared beam breaks and overall activity. A 5-minute period of inactivity (i.e., no beam breaks) has been found to be a reliable indicator of sleep. Video-based monitoring also has been coupled to measurements of beam breaks to provide higher spatial resolution analysis of fly sleep behavior.[12,13] The use of consolidated inactivity to measure sleep in flies is conceptually similar to the use of actigraphy to measure sleep in humans.[14]

Fruit flies exhibit many of the defining features of sleep. They exhibit extended periods of behavioral quiescence that can last for hours, with most quiescence bouts lasting more than 30 minutes.[12] Sleeping flies, like sleeping humans, exhibit reduced responsiveness to sensory stimuli.[12,15-18] Indeed, *Drosophila* sleep studies do not solely rely on measures of spontaneous movement but also assess responsiveness to sensory stimuli. Arousal threshold is assayed by application of a stimulus and measuring a behavioral response, typically induction of locomotor activity. During periods of extended immobility, flies are less likely to respond to a range of sensory stimuli, including social, mechanical, vibratory, thermal, and visual.[12,16,19,20] Although this responsiveness typically is measured behaviorally, it also can be uncoupled from movement using electrophysiologic measures.[21] The typical fly demonstrates an increase in arousal threshold, reaching a plateau after 5 minutes.[16,20] The 5-minute criterion for fly sleep is largely based on this observation. More recent analysis suggests that like mammals, flies exhibit deeper stages of sleep, characterized by more elevated arousal thresholds after 10 minutes or more of inactivity.[22] Nonetheless, quiet wakefulness can be distinguished from sleep by assessing arousal threshold.

Importantly, fly sleep is under homeostatic regulation—that is, flies deprived of sleep will exhibit increases in sleep duration and intensity (the latter as measured by sleep bout length or arousal threshold) the following day. Flies typically are deprived of sleep mechanically using automated devices or by tapping the flies by hand[12,16,20,23] (Figure 14.2). Sleep rebound is not observed, or is much less evident, if similar deprivation protocols are applied to flies that are already awake, arguing against nonspecific stress effects of mechanical disruption.[12,16,20] Continuous sleep deprivation ultimately results in premature death,[23] as it does in some mammals.[24] Thus sleep is essential for life in the fly.

Likely because of differences in brain structure, fly brains do not undergo the global synchronous changes in neural activity seen as slow waves on the electroencephalogram (EEG) found in mammalian sleep.[19] That said, emerging data suggest that the use of newer imaging techniques may reveal the presence of slow oscillations in specific sleep circuits, as discussed later in this chapter.[25] Flies do exhibit electrical correlates of sleep, providing behavior-independent state markers. Electrical recordings from the center of the *Drosophila* brain of a tethered fly that can still move its legs[19] (Figure 14.1) show local field potentials (LFPs), which reflect activity of the neuronal population near the electrode. There is a general correlation between spike-like potentials recorded from the central brain and waking leg movement. Exposure of the tethered fly to a rotating stripe results in LFPs in the 20- to 30-Hz frequency, reflecting attention to the stimulus, but these LFPs are reduced when the fly is asleep.[21] Periods of poor correlation between LFPs and movement are associated with increased arousal threshold and precede behavioral quiescence.[21] As discussed in the following, more recent work suggests that different fly sleep states are associated with distinct electrophysiologic signatures, such as broad reductions in neuronal activity or specific oscillatory activity.[21a,b] These approaches demonstrate that differences in arousal states can be characterized electrophysiologically as they can in mammals. Differences between

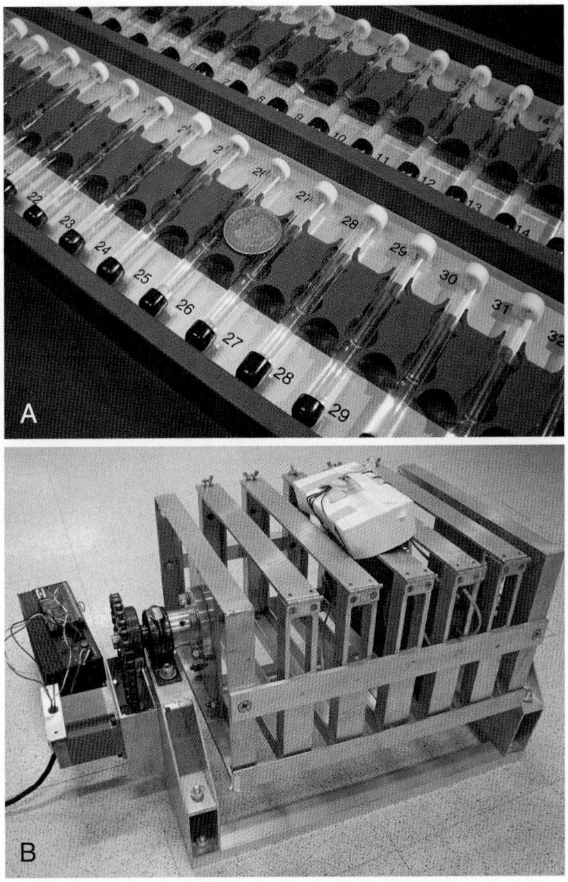

Figure 14.2 The *Drosophila* Activity Monitoring (DAM) system and rotating sleep-depriving box. **A,** The DAM system. A US dime (diameter ≅ 1.5 cm) is shown for scale, placed over the location of the infrared emitter/detectors. **B,** *Drosophila* sleep deprivation apparatus. A DAM monitor can be placed into a slot, and then the box is rotated randomly to disrupt fly sleep. (Courtesy B. Chung.)

fly and mammalian neuroanatomy are likely to account for the differing electrical manifestations of sleep even if the underlying molecular and cellular mechanisms are similar.

Like humans, flies display age-related changes in sleep architecture. Directly after emergence from the pupal case, young flies exhibit increased amounts and depth of sleep, as in their mammalian counterparts.[16,26] With increasing age, sleep becomes more fragmented and less consolidated.[27] In addition, drugs that increase oxidative stress can induce changes that mimic these effects.[27] Thus the fruit fly has the potential to become a valuable model for the analysis of aging effects on sleep.

Mammalian sleep enhances various aspects of memory consolidation.[28] Similarly, flies also display sleep loss–related deficits in learning and memory. For example, flies normally are attracted to light (i.e., display positive phototaxis) but can learn to avoid light (i.e., display negative phototaxis) after simultaneous exposure to light with aversive stimuli. After reduced sleep, flies show poor learning of this association.[29] In another learning paradigm, well-rested male flies learn to stop courting females that have already mated and continue to do so for 24 hours. In contrast, flies that are sleep deprived after training fail to retain this memory.[30] Finally, waking experience, in particular, social experience, can increase subsequent sleep amount, suggesting that learning itself affects

Table 14.1 *Drosophila* Clock Genes and Their Highly Conserved Mammalian Homologues

Drosophila	Mammals
Period	*Period 1, 2, 3*
Timeless	*Timeless*
Clock	*Clock, NPAS2*
Cycle	*Bmal1*
Doubletime	*CK1δ/ε*
CK2	*CK2*
Cryptochrome	*Cryptochrome 1, 2*
Clockwork orange	*Dec1, 2*
Slimb	*β-TRCP*

sleep need.[30] Taken together, these data suggest a reciprocal relationship between sleep-wake regulation and plasticity and memory in *Drosophila,* as is proposed for mammals.

DROSOPHILA CIRCADIAN BEHAVIOR REVEALS CONSERVED MECHANISMS BETWEEN FLIES AND HUMANS

The best case for the argument that *Drosophila* genetics will illuminate the genetics of human sleep has emerged from studies of circadian behavior. As in most organisms, sleep is under temporal control of a circadian clock in *Drosophila.*[12,16] Forward genetic screens played a crucial role in unraveling the nature of the molecular clock. The first-identified fly circadian mutants displayed short- and long-period rhythms in constant conditions and phase-advanced and delayed activity in light-dark conditions, analogous to human advanced and delayed sleep phase syndromes.[31,32] Cloning of the genes responsible for these fly phenotypes led to breakthroughs in the understanding of the core biochemical mechanisms of circadian timing, culminating in the 2017 Nobel Prize in Physiology or Medicine.[33] Although circadian clocks often have been viewed solely as timekeepers, both circadian genes and their accompanying neural circuits extensively regulate sleep-wake, perhaps independent of their timing functions (see later in this chapter). Thus a deeper molecular understanding of the circadian system should provide insights into the control mechanisms for sleep.

Most aspects of the fly molecular clockwork are conserved with mammals, including humans (Table 14.1).[34,35] People affected by familial advanced sleep phase syndrome exhibit an advanced phase of sleep-wake rhythms and shortened circadian period that is inherited in a dominant manner.[32] Mutations in the human *PER2* and *CK1delta* genes, orthologues of fly circadian genes *period* and *doubletime,* respectively, are responsible for the advanced sleep phase in some families.[36,37] These data provide argument that the basic architecture and core components of circadian clocks can be traced back to the shared ancestor of flies and humans hundreds of millions of years ago. In view of the close association of circadian with sleep behavior, the basic mechanisms of sleep homeostasis too are presumably conserved with flies. Thus approaches used in the study of circadian timing may also help elucidate the processes underlying sleep and sleep homeostasis.

CELLULAR AND MOLECULAR BASIS OF *DROSOPHILA* SLEEP

Substantial progress has been made in identifying discrete molecular and neural circuits that convey signals to time sleep and wake behavior. Presented next is an overview of the neural circuits that contribute to sleep-wake behavior, along with the genes that regulate sleep. The emerging picture is that the molecular mechanisms governing *Drosophila* sleep may be shared with mammals.

Specific Neural Circuits Important for Sleep-Wake Regulation

A theme of mammalian sleep studies is the notion that discrete neural circuits regulate brain-wide sleep and wake states in a top-down manner. In flies too, distinct neural circuits regulate sleep. A number of anatomically defined loci have been implicated in sleep-wake regulation: the mushroom bodies (MBs), the ellipsoid body (EB) ring, the dorsal fan-shaped body (dFB), the pars intercerebralis (PI), and the circadian pacemaker neurons—the small and large ventral lateral neurons (sLNv and lLNv)—and the dorsal neuron 1 cluster (DN1) (Figure 14.3). In addition to these loci, other circuits have been defined according to their neurotransmitter (e.g., dopamine). These circuits are discussed later in this chapter. To discover novel circuits involved in sleep regulation, an approach akin to forward genetics has been employed; instead of screening for genes conferring phenotypes, researchers screen for circuits regulating particular behavioral phenotypes.

A cornerstone of this approach is the binary GAL4/upstream activating sequence (UAS) system.[38,39] In one parental strain, the yeast transcription factor GAL4 is placed under the control of a tissue-specific promoter. In the second parental strain, the UAS, bearing GAL4-binding sites, is fused to an effector gene of interest. In the progeny of these two strains, the effector gene is expressed in the distribution specified by the tissue- or circuit-specific promoter driving GAL4. A plethora of GAL4 lines are available that provide a nearly limitless display of temporal and spatial expression patterns.

In addition to the multitude of GAL4 lines, UAS effector lines have been generated to alter specific cellular properties such as membrane excitability or synaptic transmission. A number of cellular effectors have been successfully utilized for *Drosophila* sleep studies. One tool that has been used to conditionally block synaptic transmission is the UAS-driven *shibire*^{1} (*shi*^{1}) transgene.[40] This transgene encodes a multimeric guanosine triphosphatase (GTPase) required for vesicle scission, a process that is in turn required for synaptic vesicle recycling and hence the maintenance of fast synaptic transmission. UAS-driven expression of the *shi*^{1} allele in a wild-type neuron blocks synaptic transmission at an elevated temperature (e.g., 29° C) but not at a low temperature (e.g., 21° C). Using the GAL4/UAS system, it is possible to manipulate synaptic transmission in discrete neural circuits in a live-behaving animal, with temperature acting as a remote control, and then assay the behavioral consequences of circuit modulation. Tools to manipulate cellular excitability also have been developed and applied using ectopically expressed constitutive and conditionally active ion channels that can activate or silence neuronal activity. For example, light-gated channel rhodopsin ion channels ("optogenetics") and the thermosensitive TrpA1 channel ("thermogenetics") have been used to increase cellular excitability.[41,42] Conversely, a variety of engineered potassium channels have been employed to silence neurons.[43,44]

The use of these transgenic tools in combination with various GAL4 drivers led to the discovery of a sleep regulatory role for the MBs, a bilateral neuropil known for its role in learning and memory.[45-47] The MBs are functionally analogous to the mammalian cerebral cortex and hippocampus.[48,49] Conditional inhibition of the MBs using *shi*^{ts1} as well as chemical ablation reduces overall sleep levels.[46,47] Flies with impaired or absent MBs have a reduced life span, suggesting that the sleep reduction has important consequences.[46] Using different MB-GAL4 lines that can be activated in adult flies[50,51] to drive activating and silencing molecular tools demonstrates that other parts of the MBs promote wakefulness. Therefore different parts of the MB play opposing roles in sleep regulation. Sleep and memory functions are promoted by the same MB neurons, demonstrating a functional connection between sleep and memory.

As mentioned previously, one of the defining features of sleep is that it is under homeostatic control. That is, sleep loss leads to an increase in the drive to sleep. The mechanisms by which this occurs remain unclear, but most research has traditionally centered on somnogenic molecules whose levels rise with greater sleep need.[52] This focus is due, in large part, to classic work by Ishimori and Pieron in the early 20th century, which showed that the cerebrospinal fluid extracted from sleep-deprived animals could induce sleep when injected into awake animals.[53] However, the short half-lives (e.g., minutes) of these somnogenic molecules suggest that additional mechanisms are involved in the generation of sleep drive, which can last for hours. Recently, a subset of EB neurons has been proposed to encode sleep drive in *Drosophila*.[54] The EB is a neuropil that integrates information from sensorimotor processes as well as the internal state to regulate various behaviors.[55] The mechanism by which activation of these EB sleep-drive neurons induces persistent sleep appears to involve structural plastic changes that modulate synaptic transmission.[54] Interestingly, the use of functional imaging approaches has revealed slow wave oscillations in these EB sleep drive neurons and shown that the power of these oscillations increases with greater sleep need.[25] Thus slow wave oscillations associated with sleep, which have been traditionally studied in mammals and birds,[56] may be more broadly conserved across the animal kingdom.[25,57,58] Another group of neurons that can induce persistent sleep behavior after their activation comprise a subset of peripheral neurons that project to the brain.[59] Because there is growing evidence in mice and humans that sensory inputs can modulate sleep behavior,[60-62,62a,b] this line of research may reveal peripheral processes that regulate the homeostatic mechanisms controlling sleep. Beyond neurons, emerging data also implicate astrocytes (a subtype of glial cell) in sensing need and regulating sleep homeostasis.[62c-e] Similar findings have been made in mice, suggesting that these processes are broadly conserved.[62f-h]

Decades of research in mammals have led to the identification of discrete sleep and arousal centers in the brain.[63] For example, the gamma-aminobutyric acid (GABA)-ergic ventrolateral preoptic nucleus (VLPO) located in the anterior hypothalamus promotes sleep, whereas monoaminergic and acetylcholinergic nuclei in the brainstem and posterior hypothalamus enhance wakefulness.[63] In *Drosophila*, the dFB is a defined sleep center because activation of dFB neurons using TrpA1 induces sleep during activation (Figure 14.3),[64] and sleep deprivation in flies enhances dFB neuron excitability.[66,67] The dFB neurons appear to function downstream of the EB sleep drive neurons to promote sleep[54] but also participate in a recurrent circuit, whereby they signal back to the EB sleep

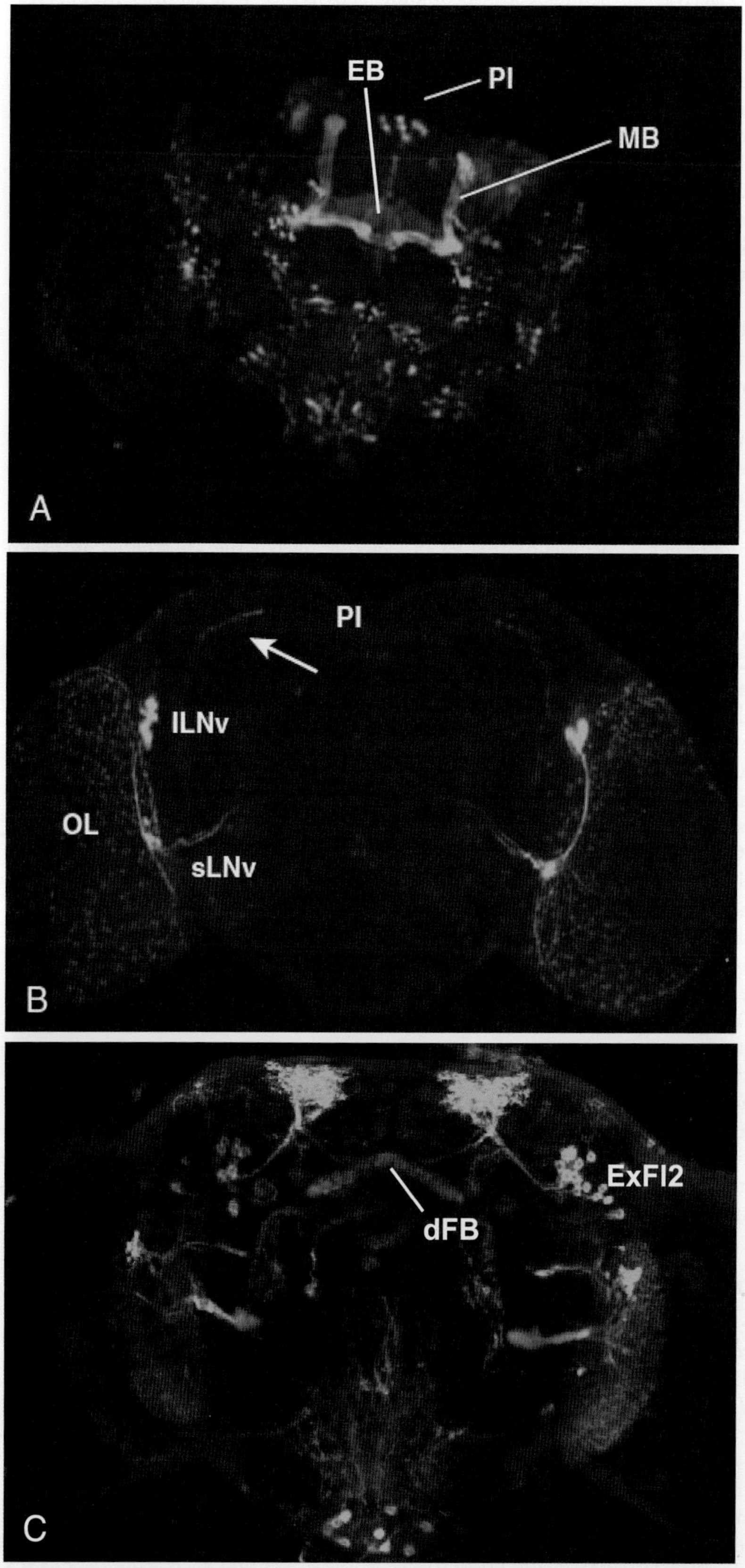

Figure 14.3 Neuroanatomy of *Drosophila* sleep-wake circuits. **A,** The sleep regulatory mushroom bodies (MBs), ellipsoid body (EB), and pars intercerebralis (PI) neurons are labeled with green fluorescent protein (GFP). **B,** Large and small ventral lateral neurons (lLNv and sLNv, respectively) labeled with GFP. The arousal-promoting large subset of neurons send projections to the ipsilateral and contralateral sLNv and optic lobes (OL). sLNv sends projections to the PI (*arrow*). **C,** The sleep-promoting ExFl2 neurons are labeled with GFP. The ExFl2 neurons send projections to the terminal dorsal fan-shaped body structure (dFB) in the central complex.

drive neurons. This feedback loop may directly reduce sleep drive when sleep is induced.[68] Recent work has examined the neurophysiologic brain states of flies following dFB activation. In one study using electrophysiological field recordings, 7-10 Hz oscillatory activity was observed.[21a] Another study used Ca^{2+} imaging to compare the activity of broad neuronal populations during natural sleep with that induced by the dFB neurons. Spontaneous sleep was associated with a general decrease in neuronal activity. Interestingly, the sleep state seen with activation of dFB neurons resembled a paradoxical "wake-like" state, during which the fly is poorly responsive to the environment.[21b] These findings suggest that dFB-induced sleep is a distinct stage of sleep, and the functions of these different sleep sub-states is an important area of future research.

Another sleep regulatory locus is the PI, which serves neuroendocrine functions similar to those of the mammalian hypothalamus.[69] Reductions in epidermal growth factor (EGF) function in the PI result in reduced sleep.[70] Importantly, EGF family members likely serve similar functions in promoting sleep in *C. elegans*[71] and mammals,[72,73] suggesting an ancient sleep function for EGF. As discussed further on, specific PI neurons act downstream of monoaminergic circuits to promote arousal.[74] In addition, the PI may be a direct target of circadian pacemaker neurons.

In addition to sleep-wake circuits in the MBs, EB, dFB, and PI, circadian clock neurons also regulate wakefulness and sleep (Figure 14.3). The *Drosophila* clock circuit comprises approximately 150 neurons,[75] which together are analogous to the mammalian circadian pacemaker, the suprachiasmatic nucleus. Within this network are the two subgroups of LNv neurons mentioned earlier, the large (lLNv) and small (sLNv) clusters, which have opposite roles in regulating sleep. The lLNv promote arousal, whereas the sLNv induce sleep.[76-79] Activity of arousal-promoting lLNv is inhibited by GABA,[78] a relationship that is reminiscent of a similar organization of mammalian sleep circuits.[80] The sLNv, in turn, enhance sleep by inhibiting the lLNv cells through the action of short neuropeptide F (sNPF) (which is functionally related to mammalian neuropeptide Y [NPY]).[79] Downstream of the LNv are a group of dorsal clock networks, called the DN1. Activation of different subsets of these neurons induces wakefulness or sleep depending on the target of their projections.[81-85] One projection from the DN1 innervates a region of the PI, and this pathway promotes arousal,[81,85] whereas another projection regulates the activity of EB ring neurons and promotes sleep.[83,84] These studies demonstrate that distinct clock subcircuits can promote wake or sleep, implying that similar principles may apply to the mammalian suprachiasmatic nucleus.

Arousal Neurotransmitters: Monoaminergic Arousal Pathways

A number of different neurotransmitters and neuromodulators have been shown to play important roles in sleep regulation. Whereas the anatomic organization of the *Drosophila* brain is different from that in mammals, flies use a similar system of neurotransmitters and receptors. In flies, as in mammals, monoamines play key roles in sleep-wake regulation, suggesting that the nervous system of the common ancestor of flies and mammals used similar arousal transmitters.

The monoamine most strongly linked to arousal in *Drosophila* is dopamine. Flies with mutations of the dopamine transporter gene *fumin* have dramatically reduced sleep.[86,87] The psychostimulant methamphetamine, which increases dopaminergic neurotransmission, also reduces sleep.[88] When awake, flies with enhanced dopamine neurotransmission display increased spontaneous locomotor activity as well as hyperresponsiveness to mechanosensory stimuli, suggesting that these flies are hyperaroused.[86-88] In addition, although its mechanism of action remains unclear, the wake-promoting drug modafinil may operate by enhancing dopaminergic neurotransmission.[89] Importantly, modafinil has similar wake-promoting properties in *Drosophila*.[90]

In mammals, the predominant model for how sleep and wake circuits intersect involves mutually inhibitory interactions, promoting fast switching between bistable states.[63] Of interest, in flies, arousal-promoting dopaminergic neurons project to and inhibit the sleep-promoting dFB circuit.[91,92] This dopaminergic signaling switches the dFB neurons from an active to a stable electrically silent state by modulating various voltage-gated and voltage-independent potassium channels.[67] This dopaminergic (DA-dFB) circuit also plays a critical role in age-dependent effects on sleep. This circuit is hypoactive when flies are young (0 to 1 day old), resulting in more sleep that is deeper in quality.[26] Finally, the DA-dFB circuit also is involved in mediating the effects of a volatile anesthetic on arousal in flies,[93] which parallels the finding in mice of increased activation of the VLPO circuit by volatile anesthetics.[94] Taken together, these data indicate that dopamine is an important transmitter for arousal and cognitive function in *Drosophila*.

Two other monoaminergic transmitters implicated in fly arousal are octopamine and histamine. Octopamine is considered the functional homologue of mammalian norepinephrine. Reduced octopamine synthesis or reduced octopamine neuron activity results in increased sleep.[95] Specific wake-promoting octopamine cells send projections to the PI circuit discussed earlier, and octopamine inhibits the function of a Ca^{2+}-dependent potassium channel and increases cyclic adenosine monophosphate (cAMP) signaling in these PI neurons to promote wakefulness.[74] Histamine has been implicated principally by pharmacology-based studies. The histamine H_1 receptor antagonist hydroxyzine induces sleep and reduces sleep latency in flies,[16] suggesting conserved functions for histamine. A small-molecule screen performed in adult flies identified reserpine, which is an inhibitor of vesicular monoamine transporter (VMAT), as causing an increase in sleep.[96] In light of the fact that the function of VMAT is to load monoaminergic neurotransmitters in vesicles, these data further reinforce the importance of monoamines in promoting arousal in flies. However, not all monoamines are arousal-promoting in *Drosophila*, as serotonin appears to be sleep promoting.[97] Nonetheless, the role for monoamines in promoting arousal in mammals is largely preserved in *Drosophila*.

Sleep Neurotransmitters: Gamma-aminobutyric Acid and Adenosine Sleep Pathways

A crucial neurotransmitter for sleep promotion in both flies and mammals is the inhibitory neurotransmitter GABA. Most hypnotics used clinically act at ionotropic GABA receptors, promoting GABAergic neurotransmission.[98] Silencing of GABAergic neurons reduces sleep in flies, a finding consistent with a sleep-promoting role.[99] In *Drosophila*, a mutation in a $GABA_A$ receptor subunit gene is responsible for resistance to the dieldrin insecticide; hence its name, *resistant to DieLdrin* (*Rdl*). These receptors rapidly desensitize on GABA activation, and this process is reduced in insecticide-resistant *Rdl* mutants, prolonging GABA-activated currents.[99] In these *Rdl* mutants, the latency to sleep after lights-off is increased, an observation consistent with an important role for GABA in promoting sleep onset in *Drosophila.*[99] *Rdl* may promote sleep onset in part by reducing the activity of PDF arousal-promoting neurons (see earlier; Figure 14.3).[78,100,101]

Adenosine is thought to play a key role in sleep homeostasis in mammals.[102] Adenosine also has been implicated in the promotion of sleep in *Drosophila.* Adenosine, a metabolic product of adenosine triphosphate, acts through G protein–coupled receptors.[102] In mammals, the stimulant effects of caffeine are thought to operate by antagonizing adenosine receptors.[103] Flies fed caffeine exhibit reduced sleep, whereas flies administered cyclohexyladenosine, an adenosine agonist, exhibit increased sleep.[12,16] However, caffeine may function differently in flies versus mammals. Besides antagonizing adenosine signaling, caffeine, like other methylxanthines, is a nonselective inhibitor of phosphodiesterase activity.[103] Deletion of the single adenosine receptor identified in the fly genome did not block the wake-promoting effects of caffeine, suggesting that this drug promotes wakefulness by another mechanism.[104] Instead, reduction of neuronal protein kinase A (PKA) activity largely suppressed the effects of caffeine on sleep,[104] suggesting that, at least in flies, wake-promoting effects of caffeine are explained by its effect on cAMP levels.

GENETICS AND PHARMACOLOGY OF SLEEP: WHICH MOLECULES REGULATE SLEEP?

A key power of the *Drosophila* system lies in the ability to identify novel genes important for sleep. One strategy is to manipulate the function of genes and assay the consequences on sleep. Traditional pharmacologic approaches have complemented genetics to identify pathways whose function is important for sleep. The discovery of novel sleep genes in *Drosophila* using genetics has relied on a combination of candidate gene approaches and classical forward genetics. In addition, the molecular identification of quantitative trait loci contributing to sleep using inbred strains also has identified numerous candidate sleep genes.[105] Unbiased forward genetic screens are especially powerful because they tend to identify the strongest contributors to a process among thousands of mutagenized candidates. Not surprisingly, identified genes play a role in various aspects of neural function, including genes involved in the circadian system, neurotransmitter/neuromodulator signaling, stress and immune responses, cellular excitability, and signal transduction. These findings suggest that many sleep pathways are conserved between flies and mammals and support the notion that studies in *Drosophila* should yield insights into the molecular basis of sleep in more complex systems.

Circadian Clock Pathway

As in many species, sleep is under the control of a circadian clock in *Drosophila.*[12,16] Mutations in the core clock transcription factors Clock (Clk) and cycle (cyc) result in reduced sleep.[101,106] However, in certain arrhythmic mutants, such as per^{01}, sleep homeostasis is intact, suggesting that the circadian process is molecularly distinct from the homeostatic process of sleep regulation as previously proposed.[12,16] Clock gene effects on sleep may be mediated by the PDF neuropeptide through its function in the arousal promoting lLNv[77,78] (Figure 14.3).

Although a detailed molecular understanding of the nature of the core circadian oscillator has emerged, the mechanisms by which this core clock regulates sleep remain poorly understood. A molecule named Wide Awake (WAKE) is a likely candidate for a key clock output molecule that regulates the timing of sleep onset.[101] WAKE exhibits cycling expression in the lLNv clock, peaking in the evening, when it acts to silence these arousal-promoting cells by upregulating $GABA_A$ receptors. Conversely, the degradation of $GABA_A$ receptors in lLNv clock is also regulated by the circadian clock. Levels of the E3 ubiquitin ligase Fbxl4 peak in the morning, leading to proteasome-mediated degradation of $GABA_A$ receptors and enabling increased activity of this arousal circuit at that time.[107]

Dopamine Pathways

BTB protein-protein interaction motifs also have been implicated as a genetic contributor to restless legs syndrome (RLS). Loss of the *Drosophila* homologue of the RLS gene *BTBD9* (*dBTBD9*) results in fragmented sleep and increased locomotor activity, which parallels the clinical disorder.[108] The dBTBD9 protein appears to function in dopaminergic neurons and is important to maintain dopamine levels consistent with the established role for dopamine in RLS.[108] These data provide support for using *Drosophila* to model human sleep disorders.

Stress and Immune Pathways

Immune-related cytokines are important regulators of sleep in mammals.[109] The innate immune response also regulates sleep in *Drosophila.* Activity of the immune system master regulator nuclear factor-kappa B, Relish, is upregulated in response to sleep deprivation.[110] Decreased Relish function in the fat bodies, a key immune response tissue in *Drosophila,* results in reduced sleep.[110] An antimicrobial peptide called NEMURI was identified in a forward genetic screen in *Drosophila* to strongly induce sleep.[111] This finding suggests that immune-related molecules serving as circulating "somnogens" may be an evolutionarily conserved mechanism for conveying sleep need.[109,111]

Although the function(s) of sleep remain debated, one proposed function is that sleep protects against oxidative stress, by enhancing clearance of reactive oxygen species (ROS).[112] Recent work in *Drosophila* supports a bidirectional relationship between oxidative stress and sleep.[113] Short-sleeping mutants are sensitive to oxidative stress, whereas flies with increased sleep are resistant. Reducing oxidative stress by increasing expression of antioxidant genes results in decreased sleep, suggesting that ROS may be a signal for increased sleep need.[113] Interestingly, sleep loss has been shown to increase oxidative stress in the sleep-promoting dFB neurons, which alters the activity of specific voltage-gated potassium channels. These changes lead to an increase in dFB neuron firing and promote sleep, providing a circuit mechanism by which ROS directly regulates sleep.[114] While many of these studies have focused on the role of ROS in neurons, there is intriguing evidence that the lethality triggered by sleep loss is driven by ROS accumulation in non-neuronal gut cells.[114a] These findings serve as a reminder that the functions of sleep reach beyond the nervous system. Another putative function of sleep is the clearance of "waste" generated by neurons, which was first described in mice.[114b] Strikingly, there is a potential parallel in flies, where rhythmic pumping of the proboscis (the elongated mouthpart in many insects) during sleep promotes waste clearance.[114c]

Endoplasmic reticulum (ER) stress responses also may participate in regulating sleep after sleep deprivation. The ER chaperone BiP, which is upregulated as part of the ER stress response, increases expression after sleep deprivation,[16,115] and the amount of rebound sleep after sleep deprivation is dependent on BiP levels.[115] BiP is upregulated as part of the unfolded protein response (UPR), which is activated when unfolded proteins accumulate in the ER. The UPR is itself upregulated in mammals subjected to sleep deprivation.[116] These data suggest that the UPR response and subsequent BiP activation may occur as a consequence of extended wakefulness and support a potential role for ER stress pathways in sleep homeostasis.

Membrane Excitability

A role for membrane excitability in sleep regulation is evident from studies using engineered heterologous ion channels that regulate membrane excitability (see earlier); however, these studies leave open the question of which specific channels normally underlie sleep function. Studies in *Drosophila* have highlighted the function of the voltage-gated potassium channel Shaker (Sh). The *Sh* mutant was discovered several decades ago as a mutant whose legs shake under ether anesthesia.[117] Positional cloning of this mutant led to the identification of the first voltage-gated potassium channel and subsequently several similar channels in mammals, highlighting the similarity in fly and mammalian nervous system components.[118-120]

Independent, unbiased mutagenesis screens identified mutants in the Sh potassium channel and a novel Sh regulator, called Sleepless (SSS), that exhibit dramatically reduced sleep amounts, with loss of as much as 80% of total sleep in an *sss* mutant.[121,122] The gene *sss* encodes a glycosylphosphatidyl-linked membrane protein,[122] and strikingly it was found that SSS directly regulates the levels, localization, and function of Sh channels.[123] In addition, mutants of an Sh regulatory subunit, *Hyperkinetic*, also exhibit a reduced sleep phenotype.[124] The function of Sh in sleep is highly conserved as genetic inactivation of mammalian Sh orthologues also results in reduced sleep.[125,126] In humans, severe insomnia is a prominent complaint of persons with Morvan syndrome and other autoimmune disorders characterized by antibodies to voltage-gated potassium channels.[127,128]

Signal Transduction

Components of the cAMP signaling pathway play conserved roles in sleep regulation. Various neurotransmitters act at cell surface G protein–coupled receptors to activate intracellular signal transduction cascades via metabotropic receptors (e.g., dopamine). Activation of G protein–coupled receptors such as dopamine receptors leads to modulation of adenylate cyclase activity, which in turn regulates cAMP levels. Cyclic AMP activates PKA, which phosphorylates a number of targets, including the transcription factor CREB (cAMP response element–binding protein). Mutants with increased PKA activity have increased wakefulness, whereas mutants with decreased cAMP levels generally exhibit reduced wakefulness.[47,129] Furthermore, CREB activity is linked to sleep homeostasis. A cAMP response element (CRE) reporter gene is upregulated in response to sleep deprivation, and reduced CREB activity results in an elevated sleep rebound.[129] In addition to a wake-promoting role for this pathway in *Drosophila*, the cAMP pathway serves similar functions in both nematodes and mice.[130,131] Many of the mutations that affect the cAMP pathway were originally isolated in unbiased genetic screens for mutations that disrupt learning and memory. Thus signaling important for sleep and memory may intersect at cAMP pathways.

In mammals, acetylcholinergic signaling, originating from the lateral dorsal and pedunculopontine tegmental nuclei, promotes wakefulness as well as rapid eye movement (REM) sleep. In flies, nicotinic acetylcholine receptors play a role in the sleep homeostatic output pathway. The *redeye* (*rye*) gene, which encodes a nicotinic acetylcholine receptor alpha subunit,[132] is required for normal sleep amounts in flies. Rye protein levels increase with greater sleep need, suggesting that Rye acts as a sleep homeostatic output molecule. At present, however, the circuits that Rye regulate remain unclear.

Summary: *Drosophila*

The fruit fly *D. melanogaster* is now well established as a genetic model organism for studying sleep. The track record of *Drosophila* genetics in unraveling the molecular mechanisms underlying the circadian clock supports the idea that this approach will yield key insights into sleep as well. The neural circuitry regulating sleep in flies remains less well characterized than in mammals, where these circuits have been studied for more than 50 years. In view of the ever-expanding technological resources available in fly model systems, however, rapid progress in delineating the circuits regulating sleep-wake is expected. Reflecting the intersection of sleep with multiple biologic processes, a number of pathways and genes have been identified that affect sleep. A current challenge is to integrate these findings to determine how these molecules fit into the context of specific circuits in the regulation and function of sleep.

NEWER GENETIC MODEL SYSTEMS FOR STUDYING SLEEP

The success of the fruit fly as a model for sleep and circadian research has in part motivated the development of other genetically tractable animal models for studying sleep. Discussed next are two such models: the zebrafish *D. rerio* (Figure 14.4) and the nematode worm *C. elegans* (Figure 14.5).

Zebrafish as a Vertebrate Model System for Genetics

In the 1970s George Streisinger and colleagues laid the groundwork for the use of the zebrafish *D. rerio* as a model system for the genetic analysis of vertebrate development.[133] Zebrafish are particularly well suited for these studies owing to their small size (approximately 0.5 cm for larvae and 2.5 cm for adults), ease of maintaining large collections, rapid development, and transparent body during embryonic and larval stages, which facilitates visualization of internal structures. After hatching, zebrafish spend approximately 1 month in a larval stage and can live up to 2 to 3 years as adults. Zebrafish mating pairs can yield hundreds of progeny, but one relative disadvantage is that their generation time approaches 3 months, which is similar to that for mice and much longer than that for flies (approximately 10 days) or worms (approximately 3 days).

Large-scale chemical mutagenesis screens for developmental mutants have been carried out in zebrafish,[134-136] illustrating their suitability for forward genetics approaches. In addition, generating transgenic zebrafish is routine. One disadvantage for genetic analysis is that the genome of zebrafish is relatively large, and there are often more members of a given gene family than in mammals, which can complicate analysis of loss of function mutant phenotypes.[137,138]

One major advantage of zebrafish as a model system is that, as a vertebrate, the anatomy and molecular organization of its nervous system is, compared to invertebrate model systems, more similar to those in humans.[139-141] While similar to mammals, the nervous system of zebrafish is smaller (~100,000 neurons in larval fish) and simpler. For comparison, mice have approximately 5,000 hypocretin/orexin (Hcrt/Orx)

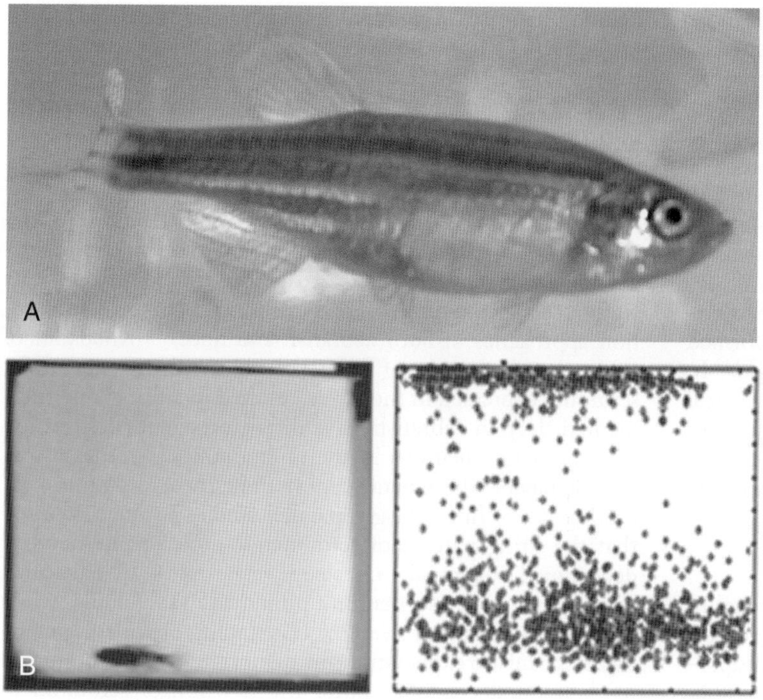

Figure 14.4 Zebrafish, an emerging genetic model organism to study sleep. The zebrafish, *Danio rerio,* is a relatively new genetic model organism for studying sleep in a vertebrate. **A,** An adult zebrafish. Zebrafish typically grow to approximately 1 inch long. **B,** *Left,* An adult zebrafish sleeping with a drooping caudal fin. *Right,* Preference for the top or bottom of the tank during sleep; *dots* represent location of sleep bouts. (**A,** Courtesy S. Liu. **B,** From Yokogawa T, Marin W, Faraco J, et al. Characterization of sleep in zebrafish and insomnia in hypocretin receptor mutants. *PLoS Biol* 2007;5:e277.)

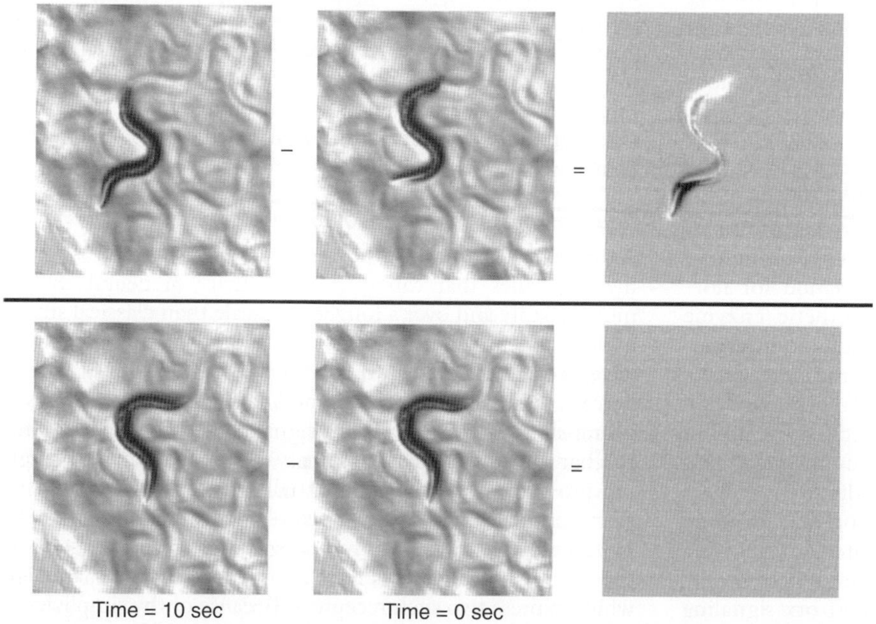

Figure 14.5 *Caenorhabditis elegans* lethargus as a model for studying sleep. Lethargus is a quiescent developmental stage in the roundworm *C. elegans,* which shares behavioral, molecular, and genetic characteristics with sleep in other animals. Behavioral quiescence in worms is measured using a frame subtraction method, as shown. *Dark pixels* indicate where the animal has moved to, and *white pixels* show where the animal has moved from. (From Macmillan Publishers Ltd: Raizen DM, Zimmerman JE, Maycock MH, et al. Lethargus is a Caenorhabditis elegans sleep-like state. *Nature* 2008;451:569–72; with permission, copyright 2008.)

neurons, whereas larval zebrafish have approximately 10 such neurons.[142-144] Another advantage of zebrafish models is the ease of performing large-scale drug screens in these animals, which can then be used to inform mechanisms of drug action, to dissect molecular pathways underlying a behavior of interest, and to discover novel pharmaceuticals.[145,146]

Zebrafish as a Model System for Studying Sleep

Like fruit flies and humans, zebrafish are diurnal, with higher locomotor activity during the day than at night. In contrast, the other vertebrate genetic model organism commonly used in sleep research— the house mouse—is nocturnal. Sleep in zebrafish has been characterized during two developmental stages: larval and adult stage.[139,140,143,147,148] As in fruit flies and roundworms, zebrafish sleep is defined by behavioral criteria.[139,140] Zebrafish exhibit periods of quiescence under circadian control, during which they are less responsive to external stimuli. This behavior is under homeostatic control and is associated with postural changes. To measure sleep in zebrafish, video tracking is employed; using changes in arousal threshold as criteria, immobility for 1 minute or 6 seconds is used to identify a minimum bout of sleep in larvae and adults, respectively. Sleep amount in zebrafish changes throughout the life span—sleep amounts are higher in larval fish than in adults.[149] Most studies of zebrafish sleep have utilized larvae, because their sleep behavior can be characterized within approximately 1 week after hatching and their transparency allows for powerful imaging approaches (see later in this chapter).

Zebrafish sleep behavior is under circadian control, as indicated by its variation throughout the day in the absence of environmental cues. Molecular components of the core circadian oscillator are well conserved in zebrafish.[150] However, it is unclear whether zebrafish have a suprachiasmatic nucleus, and even if present, it may not have the central importance in organizing rhythms as in mammals. Instead, because zebrafish are largely transparent and have many light-entrainable cells throughout their body,[151,152] there may not be a need for a single master clock.

Zebrafish sleep also is under homeostatic control. To examine these phenotypes, sleep deprivation typically is performed using mechanical perturbation or mild electric shock.[147,148] In larval zebrafish, sleep deprivation induced using mechanical vibration results in "rebound sleep" (i.e., reduced locomotor behavior associated with an increase in arousal threshold).[147] However, homeostatic regulation may not be as pronounced in adult zebrafish.[139,148]

Signaling Mechanisms Regulating Sleep in Zebrafish

As discussed earlier, a number of monoaminergic and cholinergic cell groups in the brainstem and hypothalamus promote wakefulness in mammals. A majority of these groups—namely, the tuberomammillary nucleus (histamine), the raphe nucleus (serotonin), and locus ceruleus (norepinephrine)—are well conserved in zebrafish.[153] In terms of sleep-promoting centers, zebrafish have a cluster of galanin-expressing neurons in the preoptic area, which is analogous to VLPO in mammals.[154] In addition, zebrafish sleep is regulated by various neuropeptides, including hcrt/orx, the hormone melatonin, and the EGF signaling pathway.

Neurotransmitters Regulating Sleep and Wakefulness

Norepinephrine is a classical neuromodulator that promotes wakefulness in mammals.[155] While pharmacologic data have been consistent in supporting an arousal function for norepinephrine, genetic knockout of its biosynthetic enzyme (dopamine β-hydroxylase, DBH) in mice results in inconsistent effects on sleep-wake states.[155-157] On the other hand, using optogenetic approaches (expression of light-gated ion channels in specific neural circuits)[158] to activate or inhibit noradrenergic neurons in the locus coeruleus in mice leads to increases and decreases in wakefulness duration, respectively.[159] To further investigate the role of norepinephrine in sleep-wake states, *dbh* mutants were generated in zebrafish, which revealed a substantial increase in sleep behavior.[160] Moreover, the wake-promoting effects of hcrt/orx signaling are suppressed in these mutants.[160] These studies support a physiologic role for endogenous norepinephrine in promoting wakefulness and mediating hypocretin-dependent arousal.

Histamine is another wake-promoting mammalian neurotransmitter.[161] Interestingly, mice lacking histidine decarboxylase (HDC), the biosynthetic enzyme for histamine, exhibit mild defects in baseline sleep, although these animals do have difficulty arousing to novel stimuli.[162,163] Similarly, in zebrafish, predicted null mutations in *hdc* and multiple histamine receptors (alone or in combination) do not cause significant sleep phenotypes.[164] Some of the differences between the phenotypes resulting from constitutive genetic deletion versus acute pharmacologic or circuit manipulations may result from compensation in the former situation. As an example, acute inhibition of the histaminergic tuberomammillary neurons increases non–rapid eye movement (NREM) sleep in mice, but chronic loss of histamine in these neurons has little effect on sleep.[165] Still, chronic loss of norepinephrine, but not histamine, in zebrafish leads to a substantial increase in sleep, suggesting that factors beyond developmental compensation may account for the difference between these two phenotypes.[160,164]

Among neuromodulators proposed to function in the ascending arousal system,[166] the function of serotonin is arguably the most controversial.[167] To address this controversy, one study utilized pharmacologic, genetic, and circuit manipulation approaches in both zebrafish and mice.[168] Knockout of tryptophan hydroxylase (TPH2), the biosynthetic enzyme for serotonin expressed in the raphe, resulted in reduced and fragmented sleep in zebrafish. In addition, optogenetic activation of serotonergic neurons in the raphe induced an increase in sleep behavior. These data support a role for serotonin in promoting sleep. Interestingly, parallel studies in mice revealed that the firing pattern of serotonergic dorsal raphe neurons determined its impact on sleep-wake states. In particular, burst firing of these neurons promoted wakefulness, while tonic firing enhanced sleep.[168] This finding provides a potential mechanistic explanation for distinct roles of serotonin in modulating sleep-wake states. The function of serotonin in sleep-wake regulation was also previously addressed in *Drosophila*, and this work supported a sleep-promoting role for serotonin.[97,169] Together, these studies suggest that a simple view of serotonin as strictly wake-promoting is likely to be incorrect. In general, studies in zebrafish have supported the importance of neuromodulatory neurotransmitters in regulating sleep and wakefulness and have clarified specific mechanisms by which they act in these processes.

Neuropeptidergic Control of Sleep-Wake States

Neuropeptides are an important class of modulatory signaling molecules that can tune the activity of neural circuits more broadly and over a longer timescale than classical small-molecule neurotransmitters.[170] A number of neuropeptides have been implicated in regulating sleep-wake states,[171] and here we discuss neuropeptides modulating sleep-wake states in zebrafish. Impairment of Hcrt signaling is the key pathogenic mechanism underlying narcolepsy. As in mammals, a single pre-pro-Hcrt protein is differentially cleaved to yield two distinct peptides, Hcrt-1 (i.e., orexin-A) and Hcrt-2 (orexin-B) in zebrafish. However, only a single Hcrt receptor exists in the zebrafish proteome (HcrtR2), in contrast with mammals, which express two such receptors. Because of the simplicity of the zebrafish nervous system, the number of Hcrt neurons is substantially smaller (approximately 10 per brain hemisphere in larvae and 50 per hemisphere in adults). In larvae, these cells are located in the lateral hypothalamus[142] and have been shown to send extensive projections to multiple arousal centers, including noradrenergic cells of the LC.[143,144] Consistent with this observation, Hcrt2 is broadly expressed and found in monoaminergic arousal centers.[143]

To address the function of Hcrt in zebrafish, Hcrt prepropeptide was overexpressed in larval zebrafish using an inducible heat-shock promoter, which led to an increase in wakefulness and arousal.[143] Inducible ablation of Hcrt neurons in larval zebrafish increases daytime sleep and the number of sleep-wake transitions, supporting the notion that Hcrt promotes wakefulness and sleep-wake stability.[172] Moreover, as discussed later, monitoring Hcrt neuronal activity in vivo reveals that these neurons are active during periods of robust locomotor activity, when larvae presumably are highly aroused.[173] By contrast, a null mutation in the only fish Hcrt receptor (Hcrt2) results in sleep fragmentation, consistent with loss of hcrt signaling in mice.[174] However, a surprising reduction in total nighttime sleep time was observed in these mutant fish.[148] Differences in the results of the two studies may be explained by inducible (hs:hcrt) versus constitutive (HcrtR2 null) manipulations and by analysis of larvae in one study (hs:hcrt) and adults in the other (HcrtR2 null). Overall, these studies suggest significant conservation of the neuronal circuitry and function of Hcrt between zebrafish and mammals and point toward the promise of the zebrafish system in unraveling molecular and cellular mechanisms that regulate this pathway.

The VLPO is a major sleep-promoting region in mammals. Most of the sleep-active neurons in this region express galanin, an inhibitory neuropeptide,[175] and activation of galanin-expressing neurons in this region can strongly induce sleep in mice.[176] Recent work in zebrafish has implicated galanin in the homeostatic regulation of sleep.[154] Prior studies have suggested that sleep need is driven by increases in neuronal activity, since activation of specific brain regions results in local increases in slow-wave sleep.[177,178] Thus, to uncouple sleep need from waking experience, the investigators exposed awake fish to drugs that increase neuronal activity. Animals with elevated neuronal activity showed a sleep rebound, and galanin neurons in the fish's preoptic area are active during this pharmacologically induced rebound sleep. While fish lacking galanin exhibit a mild reduction in baseline sleep duration, they show a strong reduction in pharmacologically induced rebound sleep.[154] These data provide an example of how sleep need can be disentangled from duration of wakefulness and demonstrate an important role for galanin in the homeostatic sleep response.

Galanin has also been identified as an output mechanism by which the neuropeptide prokineticin 2 (Prok2) inhibits the wake-promoting effects of light.[179] Prok2 was previously implicated in mice as a circadian output molecule regulating locomotion and/or sleep.[180-182] In zebrafish, overexpression of Prok2 results in increased sleep during the day but reduced sleep during the night, and these different effects on sleep are dependent on light, not circadian time.[179] *prok2* mutants have reduced sleep during the day under light/dark conditions, but not in constant darkness. Overexpression of Prok2 upregulates galanin expression, but only in the presence of light. Together, these data support a model whereby Prok2 upregulates galanin to suppress light-dependent arousal.

As mentioned previously, the zebrafish system is amenable to large-scale forward genetic screens because of the large numbers of progeny that are generated. Because the fish genome often contains multiple paralogues with overlapping functions, mutations in single genes can have small or no effects. In contrast to such loss-of-function approaches, a gain-of-function overexpression approach circumvents issues of redundancy in fish and typically shows stronger phenotypes. Such a gain-of-function large-scale screen has led to the identification of multiple neuropeptides regulating sleep-wake. These include neuromedin U,[183] which is wake promoting, and neuropeptide Y,[184] neuropeptide VF (NPVF),[185] and the aforementioned galanin,[154,179] which are all sleep promoting.

Neuromedin U promotes arousal and acts via corticotropin-releasing hormone (CRH)-dependent signaling.[183] In contrast, neuropeptide Y, which has previously been suggested to regulate sleep in mammals, induces sleep in zebrafish and does so by inhibiting noradrenergic signaling.[184] RF amide neuropeptides have been previously described to regulate sleep in flies and worms,[79,186-188] but NPVF is the first example of this class of neuropeptides doing so in a vertebrate.[185] In summary, a growing number of neuropeptides, including Hcrt/Orx, have been implicated in regulating sleep-wake in zebrafish. Future studies will continue to elucidate how these neuropeptides and their diverse downstream signaling mechanisms are coordinated to modulate different aspects of sleep behavior.

Melatonin Promotes Sleep

In mammals, melatonin is produced by the pineal gland and is released at night in both diurnal and nocturnal animals. Similarly, melatonin is secreted by the pineal gland of zebrafish under circadian control, with higher circulating levels at night. Also, as in mammals, direct projections from Hcrt neurons to the pineal gland have been identified in zebrafish, suggesting that the melatonin/pineal gland system can be modulated by noncircadian circuits.[189] However, unlike in mammals, where circadian release of melatonin is driven by the suprachiasmatic nucleus, in zebrafish, the pineal gland is thought to function as an independent circadian oscillator able to generate rhythmic melatonin release.[190,191] This distinction may reflect anatomic differences, whereby the pineal gland can be directly entrained by light in zebrafish, whereas it is not subject to direct light exposure in mammals. In zebrafish, melatonin has significant sleep-promoting effects. Administration of melatonin to larval zebrafish during the daytime leads to a marked increase in sleep time.[147] These effects appear to be more pronounced than those seen in humans, in whom sleep time is only mildly increased with administration of melatonin.[192-194] However, this difference may reflect administration of melatonin during the night done in a majority of studies, when sufficient levels of melatonin are already present.[192] Indeed, if melatonin is administered to humans during the daytime, significant increases in sleepiness can be observed.[195] These studies in zebrafish highlight the role of melatonin as a sleep-promoting factor, which is regulated by circadian timing mechanisms. Of interest, melatonin does not promote sleep in nocturnal rodents,[196,197] and commonly used laboratory mouse strains (e.g., C57BL/6 and 129/Sv) do not synthesize melatonin.[198] Thus zebrafish may be a better model organism than mice for studying the effects of melatonin on sleep.

Epidermal Growth Factor Signaling Is a Conserved Pathway Promoting Sleep

Over the past 10 to 15 years, the development of technologies driving genome-wide association studies (GWAS) and next-generation sequencing has produced an explosion of data regarding variants and mutations in human genomes. Understanding the functional relevance of these variants is one of the key challenges of the postgenomic era. Organisms such as zebrafish are well suited for modeling these genomic variants and characterizing their effects on the relevant phenotype or behavior. A recent study in zebrafish provides an example of this approach. Studies in flies and worms have demonstrated a role for EGF signaling in enhancing sleep.[70,71] A similar role has recently been reported in zebrafish; overexpression of an EGFR ligand, transforming growth factor α (TGFα), increases sleep, while genetic knockout of TGFα reduces sleep.[199] EGF activates expression of the sleep-promoting neuropeptide NPVF in fish, demonstrating remarkable conservation with EGFêRFamide signaling in *C. elegans*.[200] Importantly, analysis of GWAS data available in the large UK Biobank cohort revealed that variants in EGF-signaling–related genes (*ERBB* and *KSR2*) in humans are associated with increased daytime sleepiness and/or greater sleep duration.[199] Thus EGF regulation of sleep is likely conserved across the animal kingdom, from worms, flies, fish, and humans, and this observation underscores the utility of using nonmammalian organisms for studying sleep.

Pharmacology Regulating Sleep

As is the case for other genetic model organisms for sleep, including mice and fruit flies, zebrafish sleep is responsive to sleep- and wake-promoting drugs. GABA receptor agonists such as diazepam and pentobarbital promote sleep,[139] whereas modafinil promotes wakefulness.[201] However, a clear strength of the zebrafish system is the ease of performing drug-feeding assays in a high-throughput manner. Drugs can be added to the water, and because zebrafish larvae are approximately 0.4 mm long, individual animals can be monitored in 96-well plates.[202] Furthermore, zebrafish larvae readily take up small molecules and lack a functional blood-brain barrier.[146] A large-scale screen of approximately 4,000 compounds was carried out for sleep-wake phenotypes in zebrafish larvae.[146] This study found conservation of known molecular pathways regulating sleep in other animals, such as monoamines, GABA, adenosine, and Shaker-type potassium channels. Moreover, novel roles for ether-a-go-go–related gene potassium channels and L-type calcium channels in sleep-wake regulation were identified. In addition to studying well-described drugs, such an approach in fish has the potential to reveal mechanisms of action for compounds that are poorly characterized.[146]

Imaging Approaches to Study Sleep and Neural Circuit Function in Zebrafish

The transparency of zebrafish embryos and larvae facilitates live imaging approaches in intact animals. Coupled with their useful genetic traits and their relatively simple neural networks, zebrafish hold tremendous potential for the analysis of long-term in vivo imaging as well for systems neuroscience. A growing body of evidence suggests that synaptic structure is regulated by circadian- and sleep-dependent processes.[203-207] For example, the *Drosophila* PDF$^+$ sLNv exhibit circadian-dependent changes in their terminal projections.[208,209] To address this issue in larval zebrafish, two-photon imaging of the same Hcrt neurons was performed over a 24-hour period. An increase in synaptic terminal number of Hcrt neurons projecting to the pineal gland was observed during the daytime, suggesting that Hcrt synaptic terminal structure is under circadian control.[210]

Besides neuronal structure, investigations into the function of neural circuits have been revolutionized by the use of the genetically encoded neuronal activity reporters, including GCaMP, which measures Ca^{2+} levels.[211] For example, zebrafish researchers have used GCaMP to monitor dynamics of brainwide circuit function underlying optomotor behavior.[212] One drawback for the use of GCaMP for studying sleep-wake circuits is that the blue light used for excitation can affect behavior, so experiments using this tool should employ either 2-photon imaging or Ca^{2+} reporters with red excitation spectra. Bioluminescence approaches, which do not require fluorophore excitation and can measure neuronal activity over a time scale of minutes to hours, can be used to measure neuronal activity in vivo in freely behaving zebrafish. To examine Hcrt neuron activity in freely behaving zebrafish larvae, the Ca^{2+}-activated bioluminescent reporter green fluorescent protein (GFP)-apoAequorin was expressed in these neurons. The activity of these neurons, as assessed by total neuroluminescence, was continuously measured and found to be increased during periods of arousal,[173] similar to results obtained in rodents.[213,214] At present, these bioluminescence techniques lack the spatial resolution to distinguish changes in activity in distinct cells. However, the use of genetically encoded reporters should allow researchers to probe brainwide dynamics of sleep-wake circuits in zebrafish, yielding information about how these networks function and interact under different circadian and sleep homeostatic conditions.

Recently, in vivo imaging was used in zebrafish to characterize sleep, beyond traditional behavioral criteria often used in nonmammalian organisms.[58] Zebrafish larvae expressing GCaMP in the dorsal pallium, which is analogous to the mammalian neocortex, were immobilized and imaged. Strikingly, synchronous bursts of neuronal activity interspersed with periods of silence were observed during presumptive sleep. During these sleep states, fluorescence-based imaging revealed a decrease in heart rate and muscle tone similar to that observed during mammalian and avian NREM sleep. The pattern of neuronal activity is reminiscent of the alternation of "on" and "off" states that underlie generation of slow waves seen on EEG in mammals,[215] leading to the provocative suggestion that slow oscillatory neuronal activity during sleep is conserved across hundreds of millions of years of evolution. However, as mentioned previously, because blue light used to excite GCaMP can affect fish behavior, it will be helpful to validate these findings using alternative imaging approaches.

Summary: Zebrafish

The zebrafish *D. rerio* has a well-established history as a powerful genetic model system for the study of vertebrate development and has more recently been utilized to study sleep. Advantages of this system include (1) the ability to study the molecular and cellular mechanisms underlying sleep in a diurnal vertebrate animal with a relatively simple nervous system; (2) a higher degree of conservation with mammals of neuroanatomic structures and sleep-related neuropeptides and hormones; (3) the ability to perform high-throughput behavioral assays; (4) transparency of early stage zebrafish, which facilitates in vivo neuronal imaging; and (5) the ease of performing large-scale drug screens. Disadvantages include (1) a long generation time; (2) a relative dearth of genetic/genomic tools, at least in comparison to *Drosophila* and *C. elegans*; and (3) a relatively large genome, with a significant number of paralogues, which can complicate genetic analysis of loss-of-function phenotypes. The emerging body of work in the zebrafish sleep field has substantially contributed to the growing consensus of broad conservation of the molecular and cellular mechanisms regulating sleep across species, including humans. Future studies will continue to exploit the special strengths of this system, including the power of large-scale genetic or drug screens and the ability to perform in vivo imaging of the neural networks regulating sleep at a systems level.

CAENORHABDITIS ELEGANS AS A MODEL SYSTEM FOR GENETICS

The nematode *C. elegans*, which offers powerful genetic tools similar to flies, offers additional advantages for the study of sleep. Adult animals are approximately 1 mm long, so large quantities (up to 10,000) can be cultivated in a single Petri dish. They have a simple nervous system, comprising only 302 neurons, permitting a highly reductionist approach to studying neural function.[216] The small size of the worm has permitted the identification of all neuronal connections at the ultrastructural level.[217] This connectome is a great boon for researchers studying how neural circuits regulate behavior in worms. Like zebrafish, *C. elegans* is transparent and therefore highly amenable to manipulations and recording of physiologic neural activity. Adult *C. elegans* have a short generation time of about 3 days, allowing for rapid genetic manipulations.

C. elegans sleep during a developmental stage called lethargus,[130] as well as during the adult stage, in response to sickness or extreme starvation[218-220] or after a feast.[220,221] As described next, studying quiescent behavior in worms can reveal shared mechanisms underlying sleep and identify novel genetic mechanisms.

CAENORHABDITIS ELEGANS AS A MODEL SYSTEM FOR STUDYING SLEEP

As discussed previously, behavioral criteria have been used to define sleep in small nonmammalian animal models.[222] On the surface, worms do not meet the criterion of "behavioral quiescence under circadian control."[223] That is, these worms have not been reported to display daily cycling of behavioral quiescence. It has long been appreciated, however, that the *C. elegans* nematode exhibits consolidated episodes of behavioral quiescence during larval development.[224] There is a stage termed "lethargus" that precedes each larval molt, in which the animals do not feed and move very little. An important clue linking lethargus to sleep was the finding that the Period homologue in worms, *lin-42*, did not exhibit a daily cycling rhythm as seen in other animals but rather showed episodic expression, coordinated with the timing of lethargus.[225] Moreover, loss of *lin-42* causes arrhythmic timing of molting and lethargus behavior.[226] Lethargus is thus a behaviorally quiescent state under control of a molecule best known for its role in regulating the circadian clock. Quiescence during lethargus meets all other behavioral criteria for sleep.[130] First, during lethargus, worms assume a specific quiescent posture with reduced body curvature.[227] Second, quiescent animals during lethargus are less responsive to weak stimuli but respond normally to strong stimuli, that is, they exhibit an increased arousal threshold.[130,228,229] Third, depriving *C. elegans* of lethargus behavior leads to an increased drive for this behavior, indicating that it is under homeostatic control.[130,230,231] The duration of quiescent bouts is greater in the early part of a lethargus period[227] and is influenced by duration of active bouts.[230] As is the case for rats and flies,[23,24] complete deprivation of lethargus sleep-like behavior is associated with lethality in worms.[232,233] Finally, molecular pathways that modulate sleep in other organisms do so also in worms.[71,234] Because lethargus is associated with molting, an important point is that this immobility is fully reversible to strong stimulation and therefore not simply because of physical constraints related to the molting process.[130,227]

As in the study of zebrafish sleep, measurement of lethargus quiescence in worms uses high-resolution video analysis. These studies have focused on the lethargus state occurring during the first larval stage and the fourth larval stage. A popular method for automatic detection of quiescent bouts is the digital subtraction of temporally adjacent video fra mes,[13,130,235] although some features of wake behavior remain best appreciated by direct observations of the animals.[235a] Lethargus lasts 2 to 3 hours, and within this period, hundreds of bouts of quiescence, each lasting approximately 30 seconds and seen predominantly during the early part of this stage, are interspersed with bouts of activity. Whereas sleep measurements in fruit flies and zebrafish use a specified duration of inactivity as the minimum bout length for sleep, worm researchers report total quiescence (or fraction of time spent quiescent) without using a quiescence minimum threshold. This is because quiescent bouts tend to be too short for accurate arousal threshold measurements.

In addition to lethargus, which is often referred to as developmentally timed sleep (DTS), worms also sleep when sick,[218] similar to mammals[236] and flies,[110] which also sleep during sickness. Exposures that result in sickness include heat shock, cold shock, osmotic shock, and ultraviolet irradiation.[218,237] Because these exposures have in common the generation of proteotoxic or genotoxic stress (collectively, cellular stress), the behavior during sickness is often termed stress- or sickness-induced sleep (SIS).[238] Like DTS, SIS is a reversible quiescent behavior associated with reduced responsiveness, although homeostatic regulation of SIS has not yet been reported. Finally, worms have been noted to have periods of immobility when cultivated for several hours in the absence of food[219,220] or when re-fed after prolonged starvation.[221]

While the absence of diurnal sleep rhythms in adult animals limits the types of questions one could address using *C. elegans*, the power to perform genetic and neural circuit analyses is unrivaled in worms and makes this system a compelling one to address aspects of conserved quiescent behaviors and phylogenetically ancient functions of sleep.

Sleep-Wake Circuitry in *Caenorhabditis elegans*

The smallness of the *C. elegans* nervous system has facilitated identification of sleep-regulating neurons. Whole-brain imaging with genetically encoded Ca^{2+} indicators has shown that excitability of nearly all *C. elegans* neurons is reduced during sleep.[239] Only two to three neurons show elevated activity during sleep. The best characterized of these is a single interneuron called RIS.[239,240] The RIS neuron exhibits increased cytoplasmic Ca^{2+} when the animal is quiescent (during all types of quiescence), and optogenetically activating the RIS neuron confers quiescent behavior anachronistically.[240] Finally, removal of the RIS neuron or inhibition of its activity results in defective sleep behavior.[220,240]

Another well-characterized somnogenic neuron is called ALA. ALA is a second-order interneuron that is required for SIS but probably not for DTS.[187,218] ALA (like RIS) is activated by EGF signaling when the animal is sick[218,241] and releases a cocktail of neuropeptides[186,187] to inhibit a distributed network of wake-promoting neurons. These neuropeptides are encoded by the genes *flp-13, flp-24*, and *nlp-8*, each of which alone has only a small effect on ALA-induced quiescent behavior but collectively are fully required for this quiescence.[186] Overexpression of these three neuropeptide-encoding genes affects subprograms of sleep behavior such as feeding quiescence, body movement quiescence, nose movement quiescence, defecation quiescence, and elevated arousal threshold.[186] This analysis in the simple worm suggests that, in other animals too, subsets of sleep behavior are regulated by different neurochemical and neural circuits.

The peptides encoded by *flp-11*, *flp-13*, and *flp-24* belong to a class of neuropeptides characterized by an amidated C-terminus arginine-phenylalanine (RFamide) motif. RFamides are found throughout phylogeny from jellyfish to humans.[242] Remarkably, nematode-derived FLP-13 causes reduced activity in the vertebrate zebrafish.[185] Moreover, a FLP-13 orthologue called NPVF, whose expression is restricted to a small population of neurons in the hypothalamus, plays a strong role in the regulation of fish sleep.[185] Just as FLP-13 levels and release are regulated by EGF signaling in worms[186,187] so is NPVF in fish.[199] As in worms and fish, RFamide neuropeptides[243] and EGF signaling[70,244] also promote sleep in *Drosophila*. These findings demonstrate striking molecular conservation of sleep-signaling pathways and provide strong support for the notion that the *C. elegans* system can be used to discover fundamental and conserved mechanisms of sleep.

Shared Molecular Mechanisms between Lethargus and Sleep in Other Animals

In addition to the conserved role of RFamide peptides described previously, other shared sleep-wake signaling pathways have been identified in worms. For example, the *C. elegans* orthologues of 20 fly sleep-regulating genes also regulate worm sleep during lethargus.[234] Dopamine signaling promotes wakefulness in worms just as it does in flies and mammals,[234] and *C. elegans* PDF-1 promotes arousal, similar to fly PDF.[245] Finally, melatonin promotes sleep in *C. elegans* as it does in vertebrates.[245a] These studies and others support the notion that the developmental lethargus stage is analogous to a sleep state in other animals.

Protein Kinase Signaling Can Promote or Inhibit Sleep-like States

Three protein kinases have been implicated in regulating lethargus behavior in worms. The cyclic guanine monophosphate (cGMP)-dependent protein kinase (PKG) promotes behavioral quiescence, whereas the cAMP protein kinase (i.e., PKA) inhibits quiescence. Loss of *egl-4*, a worm PKG, results in decreased quiescence,[130,221,246,247] whereas a gain-of-function mutation causes elevated quiescence,[130,246] suggesting that PKG signaling promotes sleep; similar observations were subsequently made in flies.[130,248] In mice, reduced PKG activity is associated with decreased power in the delta band of the EEG, suggesting a reduced drive to sleep.[249] *egl*-4 functions in worm sensory neurons[130] by dampening sensory input,[250] suggesting that it regulates sensory gating during sleep. By contrast, PKA signaling promotes wakefulness in worms, flies, and mice.[47,129,131] In worms, increasing PKA activity through a loss-of-function mutation in the PKA regulatory subunit *kin-2* or a gain-of-function mutation in the adenylyl cyclase *acy-1* reduces the amount of quiescent behavior during lethargus.[227,251,252] Finally, KIN-29, which is a homolog of the murine sleep-promoting protein kinase SIK3, is required for the metabolic regulation of *C. elegans* sleep.[252a]

Gating of Sensory Stimuli Is an Important Mechanism Regulating Behavioral Quiescence

An important mechanism involved in regulating sleep is "sensory gating." In mammals, the thalamus is thought to gate sensory input, such that sensory information is processed at a subcortical level during sleep and wakefulness.[253] Sensory gating would protect sleep continuity as stimuli from minor noises would be filtered out and not reach the cortex to disturb sleep. Studying lethargus in the nematode *C. elegans* has provided insights into the mechanisms underlying sensory gating. For instance, the effects of Egl-4/PKG and Notch signaling on lethargus depend on their function in sensory neurons,[130,247] and activity of sensory neurons is inhibited during lethargus. For example, the ALM mechanosensory neuron exhibits Ca^{2+} transients in response to gentle mechanical stimulation, and these Ca^{2+} transients are substantially reduced in amplitude during lethargus.[228] Another sensory neuron type that exhibits state-dependent changes during lethargus is the ASH neuron, which responds to aversive mechanical and olfactory stimuli.[229] ASH sensory neurons demonstrate reduced activation after exposure to aversive chemical stimuli during the lethargus state.[229] In addition to modulation of sensory neuron activity during lethargus, the activity of interneurons becomes asynchronous, and synchronizing the activity of these neurons promotes arousal.[229]

An additional example of a sensory gating mechanism regulating lethargus is the PDF-1 neuropeptide. During lethargus, release of PDF is inhibited by NPR-1,[245] a neuropeptide receptor similar to the NPY receptor in mammals. Outside of lethargus, PDF-1 acts on its receptor PDFR-1 in mechanosensory neurons to enhance their sensitivity to touch stimuli, thus promoting arousal. PDFR-1 is required for the increased touch-evoked Ca^{2+} transients in these neurons in *npr-1* mutants.[245] Collectively, these data suggest that NPR-1 inhibits PDF-1/PDFR-1 signaling during lethargus, which dampens the response of sensory neurons to external stimuli. Such sensory gating mechanisms would promote sleep by inhibiting its interruption by external stimuli.

Mechanisms of Sleep Homeostasis in C. elegans

Like other animals, sleep in *C. elegans* is under homeostatic control. Unlike the case of *Drosophila*, which show rebound quiescence at times of day that they are typically awake, worms show only deeper and more consolidated sleep after extended wakefulness.[130] This sleep homeostatic response requires the stress-responsive FOXO transcription factor DAF-16,[232,233,254] suggesting that cellular stress responses are engaged during sleep deprivation in worms, as they are in other animals.[16,255] The observation of a homeostatic response to sleep deprivation suggests that sleep is serving a vital function for the worm that cannot be easily bypassed. Indeed, animals lacking DAF-16/FOXO often die in response to mechanical stimulation during lethargus,[232,233] and animals with a defective ALA neuron show accelerated mortality and poor repair of cellular homeostasis after a heat shock stressor.[218,256] Interestingly, sleepless animals that have defective RIS neurons display a striking accelerated-aging phenotype when cultivated under conditions of chronic metabolic stress where they are deprived of food.[220] Taken together, these studies demonstrate that in worms, as in other animals, sleep is important for health and is homeostatically protected.

Table 14.2 Comparison of the Relative Strengths of Worms, Flies, Zebrafish, and Mice as Genetic Model Organisms for the Study of Sleep

Organism	Throughput	Simple Nervous System	Temporal Niche	Genetic Toolkit	Relevance to Human Physiology	Special Features
C. elegans	++++	++++	-	++++	+	Connectome, imaging
Drosophila	+++	++	Diurnal	++++	++	Circadian mechanisms
Zebrafish	++	+	Diurnal	++	+++	Imaging, drug screens
Mouse	+	-	Nocturnal	++	++++	Electroencephalogram

-, Not applicable; + fair; ++, good; +++, strong; ++++, very strong.

Summary: *Caenorhabditis elegans*

The advantages of using *C. elegans* to study sleep include the powerful molecular genetic techniques, as well as the simple nervous system with a fully defined wiring diagram for its 302 neurons. In support of the hypothesis that lethargus behavior is sleep, a number of signaling mechanisms known to regulate sleep in other animals also regulate lethargus in *C. elegans*. The degree to which cellular and molecular mechanisms of worm sleep generalize to other animals remains to be determined. The potential disadvantages of *C. elegans* for sleep research relate to some of its unique properties, such as its association with the molt and its apparent lack of circadian regulation. Therefore it is possible that sleep in *C. elegans*, which do not have prominent 24-hour behavioral and physiologic rhythms and live only 2 to 3 weeks, may not serve the same functions as in other organisms. In view of current knowledge on this topic, however, it is likely that many genetic and molecular pathways underlying sleep will be conserved in worms; in future investigations, the major strengths of this system will be the identification of novel molecules and how they act within a precisely defined neural circuit to regulate sleep.

CLINICAL PEARL

Chronic sleep loss can lead to adverse health consequences. Indeed, sleep deprivation in the fruit fly and worm leads to premature death.

SUMMARY

Over the past 20 years, the fruit fly model of sleep has been validated as an important model for the study of sleep. The fly has many of the core features of sleep in common with mammalian systems. Many features of *Drosophila* sleep are independent of changes in spontaneous movement and include elevated arousal threshold, homeostatic regulation, electrophysiologic correlates, and conserved responses to sleep-wake regulatory drugs. In addition, genetic screens have identified shared genes/pathways of sleep control with their mammalian brethren. Zebrafish and *C. elegans* have more recently joined the fruit fly as established nonmammalian genetic model organisms for dissecting the molecular and cellular mechanisms underlying sleep, and each system has particular advantages for such study (Table 14.2). Future work exploiting the power of genetics in these model organisms promises to reveal the underlying molecular and cellular mechanisms of sleep regulation and ultimately provide some clues to the function of sleep.

ACKNOWLEDGMENTS

We thank Ravi Allada for writing and David Prober for comments on a previous version of this chapter.

SELECTED READINGS

Allada R, Chung BY. Circadian organization of behavior and physiology in drosophila. *Annu Rev Physiol.* 2010;72:605–624.

Axelrod S, Saez L, Young MW. Studying circadian rhythm and sleep using genetic screens in Drosophila. *Methods Enzymol.* 2015;551:3–27.

Chiu CN, Prober DA. Regulation of zebrafish sleep and arousal states: current and prospective approaches. *Front Neural Circuits.* 2013;7:1–14.

Cirelli C. Genetic and molecular regulation of sleep: from fruit flies to humans. *Nat Rev Neurosci.* 2009;10:549–560.

Gandhi AV, Mosser EA, Oikonomou G, Prober DA. Melatonin is required for the circadian regulation of sleep. *Neuron.* 2015;85(6):1193–1199.

Nelson MD, Raizen DM. A sleep state during *C. elegans* development. *Curr Opin Neurobiol.* 2013;23:824–830.

Sehgal A, Mignot E. Genetics of sleep and sleep disorders. *Cell.* 2011;147:207.

Shafer OT, Keene AC. The regulation of Drosophila sleep. *Curr Biol.* 2021;31(1):R38–R49.

A complete reference list can be found online at ExpertConsult.com.

Chapter 15

Genetic and Genomic Basis of Sleep in Rodents

Peng Jiang; Bruce O'Hara; Fred W. Turek; Paul Franken

Chapter Highlights

- Sleep, the genome, and the brain are all well conserved across mammalian orders. Rodents, and especially the house mouse, *Mus musculus*, offer the ability to dissect the role of genes in multiple pathways, including those that influence or underlie sleep-wake regulation.
- Results from a variety of genetic approaches in mice and humans provided confirmatory evidence of five important classes of molecular networks that serve as substrates of sleep function and regulation; namely neurotransmission, synaptic plasticity, circadian rhythms, inflammation, and energy metabolism.
- Aided by computational tools integrating multilevel genetic and genomic data within and across species, systems genetics brought new insights into the central and peripheral signaling pathways affected by sleep loss.

INTRODUCTION

Sleep is a complex, multifaceted behavioral state. A comprehensive description of one's sleep characteristics requires the quantification of many interrelated phenotypes. Despite the complexity, sleep phenotypes are among the highest heritable traits, making genetics and genomics important tools to identify the molecular machinery underlying sleep and to uncover the cellular processes involved in the functions of this fascinating behavioral state. Over the past two decades, many genetic and genomic studies have linked a large number of genes to the manifestation, regulation, and functions of sleep. Although the exact functions and the underlying molecular mechanisms of sleep remain to be fully defined, a few general "themes" start to emerge via functional categorization of the growing number of sleep-related genes. These emerging themes are consistent with a few popular hypotheses regarding sleep and include many restorative functions, such as balancing energy expenditure, tuning synaptic functions, modulating inflammatory signaling, and maintaining the appropriate cellular load of macromolecules, to name a few. This is consistent with the fact that sleep is homeostatically regulated, and genes involved in the regulatory processes of these restorative functions are often found to influence sleep homeostasis. Furthermore, the breadth of sleep-related genes and biologic processes highlights the profound roles of sleep in performance, health, and well-being. From this point of view, studies of the genetic and genomic basis of sleep not only add to our understanding of sleep regulation and function but also provide mechanistic insights into the detrimental consequences of insufficient or disordered sleep as well as sleep disturbances associated with a wide spectrum of diseases. The latter is indeed a key frontier of sleep medicine.

At this time, rodents, especially mice, represent the best animal models for genetic and genomic studies of sleep, thanks to the rich genetic resources that have already been established, including many genetically modified mouse lines and collections of mouse strains with diverse genetic makeups. Given the similarities in physiology and genetics across eutherian mammals, it is likely that genes influencing sleep traits in mice also influence sleep traits in humans. As in humans and many other mammals, sleep in mice manifests in two physiologically and functionally distinct stages, non–rapid eye movement (NREM) sleep and rapid eye movement (REM) sleep, which can be clearly distinguished by the patterns of electrical activity in the cerebral cortex recorded using electroencephalography (EEG). To capture a full picture of sleep architecture, studies often employ dozens of measures to describe each sleep-wake stage, such as the amount of time spent in the stage, the degree of consolidation or fragmentation, characteristics of stage transitions, and the EEG spectral composition (or the power of various frequency bands). It is often also of interest to study the dynamics and distribution of sleep measures over the 24-hour day and the homeostatic changes in sleep after sleep loss. For example, the dynamics of the power of EEG delta waves (1 to 4 Hz) during NREM sleep is often a phenotype of interest in studies involving sleep-wake regulation, as it is a widely used marker of sleep homeostatic pressure and correlates tightly with the amount of prior wakefulness.

While sleep measures in both humans and mice are sensitive to environmental stimuli and change considerably during early development and aging, they are genetically regulated, as indicated by studies of twins in humans[1-3] and mouse inbred strains[4-11] (Figure 15.1). A recent analysis of more than 240 sleep phenotypes in mice reported high narrow-sense heritabilities

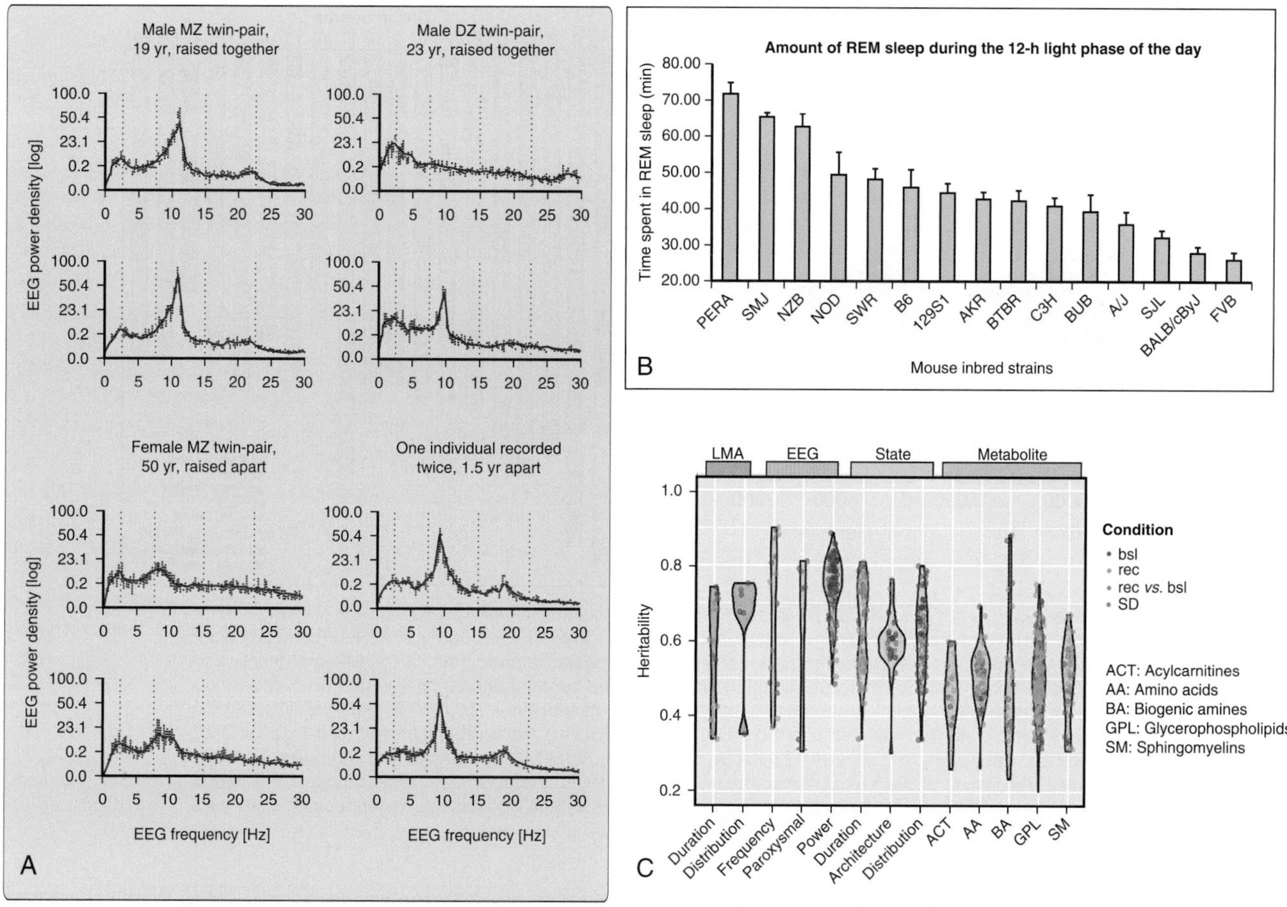

Figure 15.1 Sleep-wake phenotypes are highly heritable. **A,** As one example, the spectral composition of the waking electroencephalogram (EEG) is under strong genetic control, and twin studies identified heritabilities of up to 90%, indicating that 90% in the variance of the phenotype can be accounted for by additive genetic factors. Note the higher similarity in monozygotic (MZ) versus dizygotic (DZ) twins even when raised apart. MZ twins are nearly as similar as the same subject recorded on two different occasions. **B,** As another example, the amount of REM sleep during the 12-hour light phase of the day varies dramatically across mouse inbred strains under the same environmental conditions. The genetic makeup is identical in mice from the same strain but highly diverse across strains. **C,** Narrow-sense heritability (h^2) for locomotor activity (LMA), EEG, behavioral state, and metabolite phenotypes measured under conditions of undisrupted baseline sleep (bsl), sleep deprivations (SD), and recovery sleep (rec). (**A,** From Stassen HH, Lykken DT, Propping P, Bomben G. Genetic determination of the human EEG. Survey of recent results on twins reared together and apart. *Hum Genet* 1988;80:165-76. **C,** From Diessler S, Jan M, Emmenegger Y, et al. A systems genetics resource and analysis of sleep regulation in the mouse. *PLoS Biol* 2018;16:e2005750, licensed under CC BY 4.0.)

(h^2; i.e., the proportion of phenotypic variance attributed to additive genetic effects), with the median heritability found at 0.68.[12] Despite such high heritabilities of sleep traits, the underlying genetic basis is complex. Each sleep phenotype is typically linked to many genes and thus should be considered as a quantitative and polygenic trait. While many sleep phenotypes are tightly correlated with each other and linked to overlapping sets of genes, many others appear to be independent traits with distinct inheritance patterns. Given this complexity in sleep phenotypes and their inheritance, it is important to recognize that a full understanding of the genetic and genomic basis of sleep requires not only identifying sets of genes, each underlying a specific aspect of sleep, but also elucidating how they interact with each other in large networks, linking the functions and regulations of sleep to other aspects of physiology.

Toward this goal, sleep studies using new genetic and genomic tools and resources have added to our understanding of molecular machinery involved in sleep architecture and function, identified new neuronal populations and brain regions involved in the regulation of sleep, and uncovered mechanisms underlying sleep disorders and disease-related sleep aberrations. In this chapter, we first introduce the genetic and genomic tools and resources that have been used in the study of sleep, highlighting the advantages and limitations of using these tools to understand sleep. We then discuss the insights gained from the genetic and genomics studies of sleep. While we do not attempt to provide a complete catalogue of genes that have been linked to sleep, we discuss a few functional categories of sleep-related genes in the context of hypothesized functions of sleep. Finally, we discuss future studies needed for a more complete understanding of the molecular underpinnings of sleep as well as how such molecular machinery interacts with other biologic functions and pathophysiologic conditions.

GENETIC AND GENOMIC APPROACHES IN SLEEP RESEARCH

Genetic studies associate allelic variations of genes to phenotypic variations. This is typically done using two general strategies. One could study the phenotypic difference in a

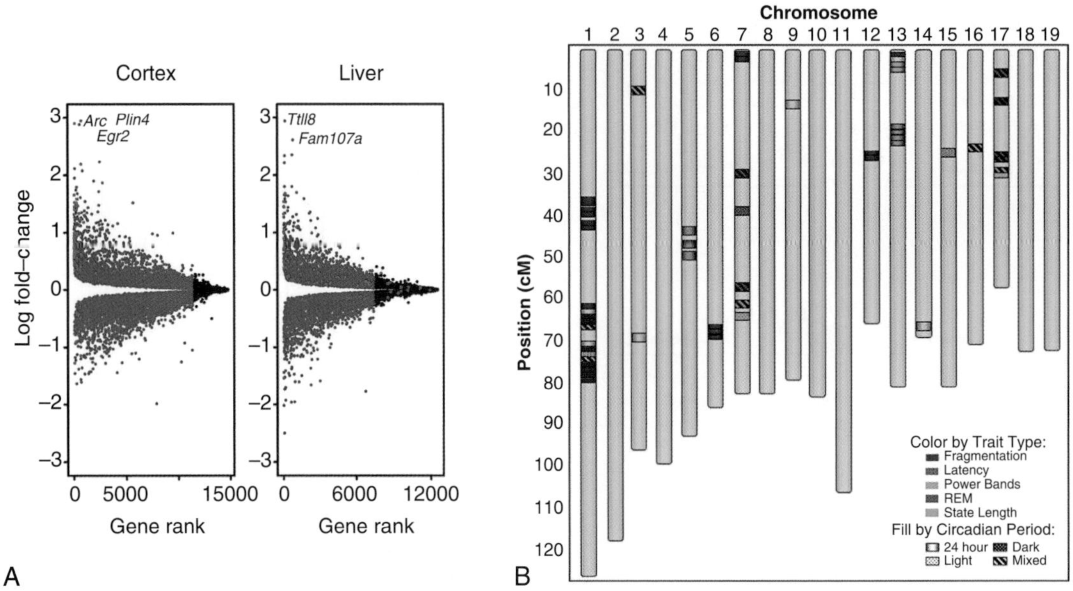

Figure 15.2 Sleep is polygenic. **A,** Sleep deprivation (SD) induces overwhelming transcriptomic changes in the cerebral cortex and liver, measured in a large population of BXD/RwwJ RI mice. Each gene is represented by a *dot, colored red* if the differential expression of the gene is significant (false discovery rate < 0.05). *Blue dots* denote a set of 78 genes considered core molecular components of the sleep homeostatic response in the cortex, as their differential expression has been consistently observed under spontaneous waking, after SD, and after SD in adrenalectomized mice.[41] **B,** The quantitative trait loci (QTL) landscape of sleep/wake phenotypes studied in a population of C57BL/6J × (BALB/cByJ × C57BL/6J) N2 mice. (**A,** From Diessler S, Jan M, Emmenegger Y, et al. A systems genetics resource and analysis of sleep regulation in the mouse. *PLoS Biol* 2018;16:e2005750, licensed under CC BY 4.0. **B,** From Winrow CJ, Williams DL, Kasarskis A, et al. Uncovering the genetic landscape for multiple sleep-wake traits. *PLoS ONE* 2009;4:e5161, licensed under CC BY 4.0.)

population and map the genomic loci of the possible causal alleles, a strategy known as forward genetics. Alternatively, one could introduce mutant alleles, particularly null alleles (i.e., gene knockouts), into specific target genes and study the phenotypic changes, known as reverse genetics. In addition, studies also associate the variations or dynamics of gene products, such as levels of mRNA, protein, and/or phosphoprotein (or other posttranslational modifications), to the variations and dynamics of phenotypes. Such studies are now often done at an "-omic" scale (e.g., transcriptomics, proteomics, and phosphoproteomics), falling into a broadly defined field of functional genomics. Variants or combinations of these approaches, each with advantages and limitations, applied to sleep research over the last two decades, have uncovered a large number of genes associated with various aspects of sleep.

Transcriptomics and Other Functional Genomics Approaches

The investigation of variations in gene expression patterns between sleep and wake began with a targeted investigation of single genes of interest, later used microarrays, and now uses ribonucleic acid (RNA)-sequencing to elucidate global changes in the transcriptome in the brain and other tissues to identify genes with no prior assumptions about their functional involvement in sleep. These studies typically compare animals subjected to sleep deprivation (SD) to those left undisturbed during a period when rats and mice normally spend most of the time asleep (e.g., during the light phase of the day, particularly the first few hours) so that the differences can be evaluated at the same time of the day to control the effects of circadian timing on gene expression. Early microarray studies in rodents have suggested that roughly 5% to 20% of the transcriptome in a given brain region varied after SD.[13-15] While these early studies used relatively small numbers of animals, a recent study analyzed a few dozens of samples pooled from more than 200 mice, allowing for sufficient statistical power to detect even small changes in gene expression. These researchers reported 78% of all expressed genes were differentially expressed after SD in the cerebral cortex (Figure 15.2,*A*).[12] These overwhelming changes in the cortical transcriptome suggest that the functional configurations of the brain may be fundamentally altered by loss of sleep. In addition, SD also induces extensive gene differential expression in mouse liver (Figure 15.2,*A*)[12,16] and human peripheral blood,[17] suggesting the functional impact of sleep-wake is not limited to the brain, consistent with the widely documented detrimental effects of sleep disturbances on physical, not just mental, health. Detailed patterns of gene differential expression, especially the genes showing a relatively large magnitude of changes, varied across different regions of the brain.[13-15] A study that used high-throughput in situ hybridization in combination with microarray analysis of laser-microdissected samples has further demonstrated the anatomically specific gene expression signatures of SD.[18] Future studies are expected to take advantage of the rapid evolution of technologies, such as those combining in situ transcriptomics and single-cell RNA sequencing,[19] to elucidate a comprehensive and detailed transcriptomic atlas that links gene expression to the functions and activities of specific neuronal populations in sleep and wake.

Of note, transcript-level changes do not always translate to changes in the abundance of proteins, although large-scale studies have suggested moderate correlations between the levels of transcripts and corresponding proteins.[20-22] While the proteomics technology is still at an early stage and is insufficient to evaluate the entire proteome, a few proteomics studies have been done and associated the impact of SD to largely the same functional pathways as those in transcriptomic studies.[23-25] In addition to the abundance of proteins, functionally significant changes in gene products also involve posttranslational protein modifications, such as phosphorylation, which alters the activity of proteins. Recent phosphoproteomics studies have revealed profound sleep-wake–dependent variations in the phosphorylation of proteins, especially those located in synapses.[26,27] Finally, recent studies have reported SD-associated changes in the expression of non–protein-coding transcripts such as microRNAs.[28] By the silencing and destabilization of mRNAs, microRNAs are involved in the posttranscriptional regulations of gene expression, through which sleep-wake could alter the transcriptome. Interestingly, intracerebroventricular injection of a specific inhibitor of a sleep-wake–dependent microRNA, miR-138, reduced total amount of sleep and NREM delta power, suggesting that some microRNAs are also involved in sleep regulation.[29]

Importantly, transcriptomic/proteomic profiling studies provide only a snapshot of the relative abundance of the transcripts or proteins after some time of (mostly) asleep or awake. Interpretations of the findings from these profiling studies thus must be cautious regarding how cellular functions and processes may be influenced by sleep-wake behavioral state as reflected by the differences in the abundance of gene products. For example, when the mRNA levels of a group of genes are higher during wake compared with sleep, it is unclear whether wake employs the cellular functions associated with these genes by activating their transcription or sleep suppresses these functions by shutting down gene transcription or posttranscriptionally silencing the genes. Incorporating multiple time points during SD and recovery sleep can partially address this issue by showing whether the expression of the genes is increased or decreased during the time course of being awake or asleep,[15,16] but it is still insufficient to infer the underlying processes leading to the observed differences in abundance. Combining transcriptomics data with epigenomic analysis, such as the assessment of open chromatin areas or profiling DNA methylation and hydroxymethylation, has been used to provide mechanistic insights into how sleep-wake states influence global transcription.[30,31] Also, profiling translating mRNA associated with ribosome can provide a proxy of protein synthesis activities, and expressing tagged ribosomal components in particular cell populations allows for cell-type–specific translational profiling of affinity-purified samples. Using this approach, a recent study uncovered translating mRNAs differentially associated with sleep and wake (SD or spontaneous wake at the opposite circadian phase) in astrocytes.[32] Future studies using these techniques are expected to reveal more mechanistic insights into how cellular functions in various cell populations are regulated by sleep and wake on an "-omics" scale.

Another issue regarding the study of differences in the abundance of gene products between sleep and wake is the dynamics of the underlying processes. Transitions between NREM sleep, REM sleep, and wake occur within seconds. Also, sleep in mice is much less consolidated than in humans, and mice typically switch between sleep and wake more than 100 times throughout the 24-hour light-dark cycle with a median sleep bout duration of only 2 to 5 minutes. Only rapid molecular responses, such as protein phosphorylation, appear to be fast enough to correspond to the dynamics of sleep and wake, particularly in mice. Other processes, such as induction or suppression of transcription or translation, take a longer time, even hours, to produce functionally significant changes in abundance. Thus the abundance of transcripts or proteins is unlikely to be related to the molecular events of behavioral state transitions. Rather, they may reflect the cumulative impact of prior sleep-wake history on cellular functions. The accumulation or depletion of some gene products on various timescales during a particular behavioral state may impose limitations to the continuation of the behavioral state and thus influence the propensity or probability of state transitions. Future studies are needed to evaluate the detailed dynamics of various types of gene products during sleep and wake and elucidate the functional significance of such dynamics. Interestingly, a recent study suggested that SD induces transcriptomic changes with complex dynamics, including delayed or long-lasting changes well beyond the recovery of sleep phenotypes.[30] Further investigations are thus needed to examine whether such "after-effects" are related to long-lasting physiologic changes associated with SD (particularly chronic SD), such as disrupted energy metabolism, which is insufficiently alleviated by recovery sleep in humans,[33,34] as well as a change in sleep homeostatic set point (i.e., allostasis).[35-37]

A final note for studying SD-associated molecular changes is that SD procedures are generally stressful. The increase in glucocorticoids and other stress-related changes after SD may represent a confounding factor for understanding the effects of sleep-wake states. It is arguable whether wakefulness itself is stressful. In humans, plasma cortisol levels are elevated after voluntary prolonged wakefulness.[38] Higher cortisol levels and hypothalamic-pituitary-adrenal reactivity have also been reported in patients with insomnia.[39] Aside from sleep loss (voluntary or pathologic), however, cortisol levels exhibit a circadian rhythm that is primarily driven by the circadian clock, not sleep-wake.[40] Therefore prolonged waking, even voluntary, may be different from normal waking. Also, SD in rodents may be associated with additional handling stress. One study tried to address this issue by examining SD-associated transcriptomic changes in the forebrain of adrenalectomized (ADX) and sham-lesioned mice.[41] ADX led to reduced amplitudes of the SD-induced changes in gene expression. However, the estimated fold-changes in gene expression induced by SD in ADX mice were highly correlated with those in sham mice, suggesting that stress (or at least the stress hormone) amplifies, rather than fundamentally alters, the effects of sleep and wake on the transcriptomic organization. Nevertheless, a set of 78 genes whose differential expression can be detected after SD in sham animals, after SD in ADX animals, and after a period of spontaneous waking may represent a core molecular component of sleep homeostasis.[41]

Reverse Genetics

While studying the abundance changes of gene products is widely used to infer the impact of sleep-wake on the activities of genes and their related cellular processes, to understand how these processes influence sleep and wake often requires the study of the functional consequences of gene allelic variations. With an a priori hypothesis, reverse genetics approaches are used to manipulate a set of target genes and evaluate changes in sleep-wake phenotypes. Advanced reverse genetic approaches manipulate target genes in an inducible and/or cell-type–specific fashion, providing mechanistic insights into the functions of sleep-regulating genes and elucidating the role of specific neuronal populations in sleep-wake control. Particularly, recent efforts using genetically engineered controllable ion channels (i.e., optogenetic and chemogenetic approaches) have mapped many sleep-wake–regulatory neural circuits.[42] Because the goal of optogenetic and chemogenetic studies is to uncover sleep-regulating circuitry rather than genes, we will not discuss these studies in this chapter; the findings from these studies are highlighted in Chapter 7.

While most reverse genetic studies target only a few genes of interest, an extended variant of the reverse genetic approach screens a large number of mutant mouse lines in an unbiased fashion without a priori hypotheses. The first large-scale screening study takes advantage of the mouse gene knockout lines generated in the International Mouse Phenotyping Consortium[43] and a noninvasive piezoelectric system[44] that allowed high-throughput sleep phenotyping in thousands of animals.[45] This study unbiasedly screened 343 single-gene knockout lines and identified 122 genes influencing at least one sleep phenotype, such as the amount of sleep and sleep bout length during light or dark phase of the day. Such a strikingly high "hit rate" (~36%) speaks to the polygenic nature of sleep and the complexity of its underlying molecular machinery. Although expanding the application of such a screening approach to the whole genome is challenged by the efficiency of generating gene knockout lines in mice using traditional homologous-recombination-based techniques, genome-wide screening studies can benefit from rapidly evolving new technologies, such as clustered regularly interspaced short palindromic repeats (CRISPR), which can generate targeted mutations more efficiently. A small-scale proof-of-concept study has used the CRISPR-Cas9 system and screened all seven genes that encode the *N*-methyl-D-aspartate (NMDA) receptor family members and found *Nr3a* as a short-sleeper gene.[46] Subsequent studies used the same approach and identified sleep-influencing genes from the acetylcholine receptor family and those involved in Ca^{2+}-dependent hyperpolarization.[47,48] In addition to scaling up to genome-wide screens, future reverse genetic screens can also benefit from the flexibility of CRISPR to generate and test a range of mutant alleles, in addition to the null allele, which may not produce a mutant phenotype because of compensation by paralogous genes.

Mutagenesis Screens

In contrary to the reverse genetic approach, forward genetics does not target a specific gene, but rather screens a genetically diverse population and searches through the genome to link genotypic variations at various loci to the phenotypic variations. Genetic variations can be introduced randomly into the genome chemically by injection of mutation-inducing agents (e.g., *N*-ethyl-N-nitrosourea [ENU] in mice) or genetically using transposons. The mutations occurring in the Germline are passed on to the progeny, allowing for the phenotypic screening for animals with large changes in phenotypes (i.e., phenodeviants). Phenodeviants will then be outcrossed to wild-type animals of a different strain. The progeny are genotyped throughout the genome at regular intervals using polymorphic markers so that the genomic locus of the mutation can be mapped by tracking the genetic markers that are closely co-segregated with the mutant phenotype. This approach, known as the mutagenesis screen, has been proven to be a very powerful tool in the closely related field of circadian rhythms, because it had remarkable successes in identifying the core components of the circadian clocks in multiple organisms. The applications of mutagenesis screens in sleep research, however, have not led to similar breakthroughs, even though a few sleep-regulating genes have been identified using this approach in fruit flies (*Drosophila melanogaster*)[49-51] and, recently, in mice.[52,53] The first report of this large-scale mutagenesis screen in mice described two sleep-regulating mutations, including one in the *Sik3* (*salt-inducible kinase 3*) gene, which increases NREM sleep amount and elevated sleep homeostatic drive, and another one in *Nalcn* (*Na^+ leak channel, nonselective*), which reduces the amount of REM sleep.[52] Continuation of this endeavor has led to the identification of *Cacna1a* (*Ca^{2+} voltage-gated channel subunit $\alpha 1$ A*), which influences the daily amount of wakefulness.[53]

The mutagenesis approach has many important advantages. In addition to providing a genome-wide search for new sleep-regulating genes without a priori hypotheses, mutagenesis screens often produce functionally more interesting mutant alleles than the null allele, which may be compensated. This is particularly the case for studies using a "dominant screen" approach, in which the F1 progeny of the mutagenized and wild-type animals (i.e., heterozygous mice) are phenotypically screened for phenodeviants, leading to the identification of (semi-) dominant gain-of-function alleles.

However, there are two major drawbacks of using ENU mutagenesis screens to study the genetics of sleep in mice. The first is the mutation bias associated with the use of ENU. A recent large-scale whole-exome sequencing analysis of ENU mutagenized mice found that the distribution of mutations was biased toward open chromatin areas, hence limiting the coverage of inheritable mutations to potentially as low as a few percent of the genome that is accessible in the Germline.[54] Although it is not clear whether the inaccessible regions cover predominantly noncoding regions of the genome, and additional studies are needed to further characterize the bias of ENU mutagenesis, findings from this study raise an alarming limitation of the current mutagenesis screen approach in mice, which requires the ENU-induced mutations to be passed on through the Germline.

The other major drawback of sleep mutagenesis screens is low efficiency. The previously mentioned sleep mutagenesis screen in mice has lasted for years and has screened more than 10,000 mice to allow the identification of 57 phenodeviants.[53] Only 14 of the 57 phenodeviants show robust inheritance in their N2 progeny (~100 mice per phenodeviant pedigree) so that the genomic location of the mutations can be mapped. These sleep-influencing mutations have been mapped to 10 loci, 4 of which had been resolved to causal genes by mid-2019.[53] Despite multiple optimizations of the procedure, such as the use of genetically close-related substrains of mice to facilitate genetic mapping and the use of whole-exome sequencing to expedite the identification of causal variants, efficiency bottlenecks exist in the occurrence of sleep phenodeviants (estimated at ~5 phenodeviants per 1,000 mice screened) and the robustness of inheritance in the sleep phenodeviant pedigrees (~25% pedigrees).[53] This efficiency is lower than many other dominant ENU mutagenesis screens in mice,[55-64] including the discovery of *Clock* in a screen of only 304 mice for circadian clock mutants.[55]

A key contributing factor to this low efficiency is likely the polygenic nature of quantitative sleep traits. Although the number of mutations induced by ENU depends on the dosage and mouse strain, a few thousand mutations per genome are typically expected.[65] Most of the mutations are expected to cause only small perturbations to the functions of nearby genes, but collectively they may substantially influence sleep phenotypes and cause large variations in the mapping population. Consequently, only a small number of animals can emerge as phenodeviants, and the identified phenodeviants may harbor multiple causal mutations in multiple genes, which are passed on to different offspring mice, leading to diluted effects and difficulties in inheritance confirmation and genetic mapping.[53] In addition, since many genes interact in pathways to influence sleep, a mutation that causes large deficits in function of a gene may not lead to significant changes in the pathway-level functions because of compensatory changes in the expression or activities of other genes in the pathway, an effect known as genetic buffering,[66] which adds to the difficulties in the identification of phenodeviants and causal mutations. Given these challenges, even though a few interesting sleep-regulatory genes have been identified through mutagenesis screens, more efficient and less-biased approaches are favorable for the comprehensive elucidation of the genetic landscape of sleep. Finally, in addition to these major drawbacks, it is also worth noting that the induced mutations, while useful for identifying genes involved in the regulation of sleep, provide limited insights into the variations and heritability of complex traits in the general population.

Quantitative Trait Loci Analysis

Without chemical mutagens, mutations occur naturally at a low rate. In some "lucky" cases, animals barring a spontaneous mutation show noticeable abnormality, and the underlying gene can be mapped in a similar way as in a mutagenesis screen. These include the identification of casein kinase I-ε (encoded by *Csnk1e*) as a circadian clock regulator by mapping the spontaneous *tau* mutation in hamsters[67] as well as the discovery of the wake-promoting hypocretin (also known as orexin; encoded by *Hcrt*) signaling by analyzing a pedigree of narcoleptic dogs.[68] More recently, a few rare mutations that influence the amount of sleep in humans have been identified in families of short sleepers and confirmed using transgenic mice bearing the mutant form of the human gene,[69-72] which are discussed later in this chapter.

Aside from these large-effect mutations, most of the naturally occurring mutations found in the general population produce only moderate to small quantitative effects. The accumulation of these naturally occurring genetic variations determines the heritability of complex traits and allows for mapping of genomic loci that underlie quantitative traits. This approach, referred to as quantitative trait loci (QTL) analysis, evaluates many small-effect genetic variations throughout the genome in a single population[73-76] and is particularly suited for the study of sleep, which is highly heritable and polygenic. Several studies have used this approach and demonstrated a complex genetic landscape, uncovering dozens or even hundreds of loci that influence different aspects of sleep-wake regulation in mice (Figure 15.2, *B*).[12,77,78]

QTL analyses in mice typically are performed in segregating populations that are generated by crossing different inbred lines, such as intercrosses, backcrosses, recombinant inbred (RI) strains, or heterogeneous stocks (e.g., outbred mice derived from breeding multiple inbred strains together). Mapping the genomic location of a QTL is similar to mapping causal mutations in the mutagenesis screens and is based on tracking polymorphic genetic markers that co-segregate with higher or lower phenotypic values because of genetic linkage to the causal genetic variant. The main challenge of the QTL approach, though, is the difficulties in identifying the underlying causal genetic variant of a QTL. The resolution of genetic mapping is limited by the number of combinations accumulated in the mapping population, which breaks the linkage between the causal variant and distal genetic markers, leaving only the genetic markers more closely located to the causal variant still in linkage. Genetic mapping using a few hundred mice in an intercross or backcross typically yields a candidate region of 10 to 60 Mb, harboring hundreds of genes. Unlike mutagenesis screens, in which the causal variant is a novel allele induced by chemicals and thus can be identified by exon-sequencing of the candidate region, QTL analysis often requires assistance from additional genetic mapping resources, such as collections of related inbred strains, advanced RI panels, and congenic mouse lines, to narrow down the candidate genomic, before candidate causal genes can be identified.

Despite this difficulty, several sleep QTL studies have successfully identified candidate genes. Examples include the identification of *Acads* (*short-chain acyl-coenzyme A dehydrogenase*) underlying a QTL that influences the peak frequency of the REM-characteristic theta (~5 to 9 Hz) oscillations[79] as well as the identification of *Rarb* (*retinoic acid receptor beta*) underlying a QTL that influences EEG synchronization during sleep.[80] Verification of the identified candidate genes, however, remains challenging, as exemplified by the identification and characterization of *Homer1a* as a sleep regulatory gene. *Homer1a* is a short splicing variant of the *Homer1* gene and encodes a negative regulator of the full-length HOMER1 protein, which is involved in postsynaptic density scaffolding proteins for group 1 metabotropic glutamate receptors. In an analysis of a panel of RI mice originated from C57BL/6J and DBA/2J strains (i.e., the BXD RI panel), a QTL influencing the homeostatic rebound of EEG delta power after SD[11] was mapped to chromosome 13, and subsequent bioinformatic and gene expression analyses identified *Homer1a* as the candidate gene.[16,81] However, knockout of *Homer1a*, without disturbing the full-length *Homer1* transcript, does not affect homeostatic EEG responses after SD.[82] Instead, this study argues for a role of *Homer1a* in sustaining long bouts of wakefulness.[82] It is possible that the allelic difference between C57BL/6J and DBA/2J in *Homer1a* indeed influences homeostatic EEG activity after SD, while its role is somehow compensated by other functionally related genes (such as splicing variants of other *Homer* genes) in the *Homer1a* knockout mice. Future studies are needed to test this hypothesis using precise genetic manipulations, such as gene knock-in or CRISPR-based approaches, to generate mice bearing the DBA/2J haplotype in *Homer1a* on an otherwise C57BL/6J genetic background (or vice versa). It is also possible that genetic variations of other genes in the QTL region are responsible for the observed effect, despite the role of *Homer1a* in other aspects of sleep regulation and functions.

New genetic mapping panels in mice are under development and are expected to augment QTL analysis to uncover the genetic basis of sleep-wake traits. For example, a large panel of RI strains, known as the Collaborative Cross (CC), is being developed in a consortium effort.[83] CC strains are generated from eight genetically diverse strains, capturing as much as 89% of genetic variance in mice,[84] which will allow for a more complete description of the genetic landscape of sleep regulation. Also, the resolution of QTL mapping using the full panel of approximately 1,000 CC lines is expected to be less than 100 kb, an interval in most cases small enough to resolve a single candidate gene.[85] This new genetic resource, even though still under development, has already proven useful for sleep research. A study of the pre-CC mice (incomplete-inbred CC mice) has mapped a QTL affecting the time of peak activity after SD to a 530-kb region on chromosome 9, which harbors only three genes, including *Ntm* (neurotrimin), *Snx19* (sorting nexin 19), and a microRNA gene.[86] To date, roughly 100 CC lines are reaching a complete inbred state and can be readily distributed. However, the development of additional CC RI lines appears to be slow, because of an unusually high extinction rate during inbreeding.[87] This difficulty has in part promoted the development of a related genetic resource, known as the Diversity Outbred (OD) mice, which were generated by randomized outcrossing of pre-CC line.[88] Because of the continued accumulation of recombination through generations of outcrossing, mapping resolution in OD mice is expected to be even higher than CC mice. Genetic studies of circadian and sleep-wake phenotypes in OD mice are currently underway.[89]

A variant of QTL analysis can be performed in an outbred population without knowing the pedigree. An outbred population can be viewed as the descendants from a limited number of common ancestors, like the OD mice, although the ancestry of OD mice is known. Most genetic loci in an outbred population do not appear to be linked to each other, a phenomenon known as linkage equilibrium, the result of shuffling of the ancestor haplotypes by recombination events through generations. However, genotypic associations exist between closely located genetic loci (i.e., linkage disequilibrium), allowing for the inference of a nearby causal variant via the association between genetic marker genotype and phenotypic values. This approach, termed genome-wide association study (GWAS), is widely used to search for genetic underpinnings of diseases in humans, including sleep disorders, such as restless legs syndrome.[90,91] In addition to binary phenotypes (i.e., disease vs. healthy control), quantitative estimates of sleep duration and other sleep characteristics inferred from self-reports or wrist actimetry have been analyzed using GWAS. To date, a dozen such studies have been done in large cohorts of human subjects, ranging from thousands to over a million subjects, and have reported hundreds of sleep-influencing loci,[92-103] although collectively they may only account for a small fraction of phenotypic variance in the general population.[103] These findings again highlight the complexity of the genetic underpinning of sleep-wake regulation. Future studies are expected to take advantage of the fast-evolving wearable sensor technologies and more accurate sleep-inferring algorithms to reduce noise in sleep phenotypic data, thereby enhancing the efficiency and reproducibility of sleep GWAS in humans. Sleep GWAS have also been performed in mice. As part of a larger phenotyping pipeline, sleep phenotypes have been analyzed using the high-throughput piezoelectric system in a large cohort (n = 1,577) of Swiss Webster outbred mice.[104] Five sleep-influencing loci were reported, and two of those, which influence sleep fragmentation, were resolved to single-gene candidates, *Ppargc1a* (*Peroxisome Proliferator-activated receptor γ coactivator 1 α*) and *Unc13c* (*Unc-13 homolog c*), both involved in synaptic transmission. Together, these studies in mice and humans have demonstrated GWAS and QTL analysis as efficient tools to uncover the genetic landscape of sleep. However, in addition to the challenges of verifying the candidate genes, the identification of a large number of small-effect genetic variants also imposes a challenge for the understanding of how these alleles and genes function in a normal physiologic context to regulate sleep and wake. These challenges can be partially addressed by an extension of the QTL analysis, systems genetics.

Systems Genetics

Systems genetics approaches incorporate the abundance of gene products as intermediate phenotypes in QTL analyses to describe how the effects of genetic variations propagate through interacting molecular networks and eventually lead to phenotypic variations. The first advantage of systems genetics approaches is that it adds to the ability to identify QTL candidate genes with high confidence. For example, a large-scale QTL study has identified 52 sleep-regulating QTL, including one influencing the amount of REM sleep, number of REM sleep bouts, and wake amount.[77] By incorporating transcriptomics data in three brain regions (frontal cortex, hypothalamus, and thalamus/midbrain), a subsequent study found that this REM-regulating QTL is tightly linked to an expression QTL (eQTL) that regulates the expression of *Ntsr1*, which encodes a receptor for neurotensin,[105] a neuropeptide tightly linked to the dopaminergic system and implicated in several psychiatric disorders. Knockout of *Ntsr1* in mice confirmed its role in regulating REM sleep, particularly during the night.[105] Similarly, in another follow-up study of the previously mentioned QTL analysis, a sophisticated statistical method, called causal inference test,[106] was used to delineate the information flow between genotype, expression, and phenotype and identify candidate causal genes underlying the sleep-regulating QTL.[107] A subset of the candidate causal genes was then selected for pharmacologic validation, as they encode receptors and ion channels for which pharmacologic agents were readily available. Treating animals with antagonists and/or agonists of these selected receptors and channels indeed affected aspects of the sleep-wake cycle that were consistent with the predictions from the causal inference test.[108] More recently, a systems genetics study used the BXD/RwwJ RI lines (i.e., a recent expansion of the original BXD RI panel) and accessed comprehensive sleep-wake phenome, cortical and liver transcriptome, as well as plasma metabolome under undisturbed baseline conditions and after SD.[12] Through integrated analysis of multiomics data, this study highlighted a role of genes involved in the trafficking of α-amino-3-hydroxy-5-methyl-4-isoxazolepropionic acid (AMPA)-type glutamate receptors and fatty acid turnover in homeostatic responses to sleep loss,[12] which are discussed further in the context of hypothesized sleep functions later in this chapter.

The second advantage of the systems genetic approaches is that it can be used to delineate interactions between genes and thus provide an inference of the molecular pathways through which genetic variations affect complex phenotypes. Transcriptomic profiling in genetically diverse populations allows the modeling of coordinated gene expression and gene regulatory relationships as gene networks. Using this approach, recent studies have analyzed two intercrosses of mice (C57BL/6J × A/J F2 and C57BL/6J × 129S1/SvImJ F2), reconstructed gene networks in several brain regions, and correlated the summarized network-level gene expression with various categories of sleep phenotypes.[78,109] The identified sleep-associated gene networks were enriched with genes involved in specific cellular functions and/or resembling particular cell types, allowing inference of biologic processes involved in different aspects of sleep regulation and functions. Also, these two studies extensively phenotyped affective and cognitive neurobehaviors, enabling the elucidation of the transcriptomic basis of the extensive interactions between sleep-wake and affective/cognitive functions. Interestingly, almost all sleep-associated gene networks also were associated with at least one affective/cognitive phenotype, while only a handful of candidate causal genes were found to be pleiotropically linked to phenotypes of different neurobehavioral domains, suggesting that the network-level analysis is more efficient in uncovering the molecular underpinnings of the role of sleep in other brain functions.[78]

Finally, the comprehensive genetic, molecular, and phenotypic data collected in systems genetics studies provide rich resources that enable the integration of disease-relevant data to understand the relationships between dysfunctional sleep and disease pathophysiology. For example, in the previously mentioned study of C57BL/6J × A/J F2 mice, the sleep- and affect-associated gene networks identified in the striatum were used to query the human GWAS catalogue for genes associated with neuropsychiatric disorders. Interestingly, genes implicated in neuropsychiatric disorders by GWAS were enriched in a network that consists of genes associated with mitochondrial and synaptic functions and whose gene expression was correlated with anxiety-related behaviors and stress-induced changes in REM sleep and are more likely to be located in the most upstream regulator position of this network.[78] This finding thus provides intriguing biologic contexts to the GWAS findings by describing how genetic variations contribute to the risks of neuropsychiatric disorders via influencing gene network level involved in specific cellular and neurobehavioral functions.

In a follow-up study, striatal gene networks associated with sleep and affective/cognitive behavior in the C57BL/6J × A/J F2 mice were integrated with transcriptomics data relevant to Parkinson disease, leading to the identification of a gene network whose expression in the F2 mice was correlated with phenotypes related to sleep fragmentation, the most common type of sleep disturbance reported in patients with Parkinson disease.[110] This network consists of genes regulated by the circadian clock and involved in chromatin organization. Further analysis has suggested that it functions in the striatal medium spiny neurons and responds to dopamine, providing mechanistic insights into the emergence of sleep dysfunctions in Parkinson disease. This finding also implicated a role of striatal medium spiny neurons in sleep regulation, consistent with the implications from a recent integrative analysis of sleep GWAS data with tissue-specific eQTL data in humans.[103] Indeed, recent studies using optogenetic approaches start to reveal the functions of basal ganglia motor-control circuits in sleep-wake control.[111] Studies are currently underway to understand the sleep-regulatory function of striatal medium spiny neurons and how this function is disturbed in Parkinson disease.

As a final example, sleep-related gene networks identified in the C57BL/6J × 129S1/SvImJ F2 mice have also been used in integrative analyses to understand the sleep disturbances under pathologic conditions. Combining these networks with transcriptomics datasets collected in mice after SD and those in patients with major depressive disorder (MDD) has identified three gene networks in the cerebral cortex whose network-level gene expression was altered in MDD in the opposite directions to their expression changes induced by SD (Figure 15.3, *A*).[109] Loss of sleep is a key risk factor and a core symptom of MDD, although acute SD is used clinically to induce antidepressant effects in patients with MDD. This complex interaction between sleep and MDD has led to the hypothesis that an impaired sleep homeostat is at the core of MDD: the sleep homeostatic pressure accumulates during wake at a much slower rate in MDD patients, leading to sleep loss, but when it is forced to a high level after SD, improvement in the mood regulation can be achieved.[112] Therefore the identification of the networks that were oppositely perturbed by MDD and SD suggests plausible molecular correlates for the impaired sleep homeostat in MDD.

Taken together, the systems approach is a powerful tool not only for the identification of sleep-regulatory genes but also for the understanding of molecular processes and pathways involved in sleep and its functions and dysfunctions in health and disease. Although sleep systems genetic studies to date have focused primarily on transcriptomic networks, future studies are expected to expand such applications to incorporate multiomics data (e.g., transcriptome, proteome, phosphoproteome, and metabolome) across multiple tissues and cell types for a more comprehensive elucidation of sleep regulatory mechanisms and functions.

INSIGHTS FROM GENETIC AND GENOMIC STUDIES OF SLEEP

As the number of genes implicated by genetic and genomic studies continues to grow, it starts to become clear that cellular functions of sleep-related genes generally fall into a few general categories that are consistent with some of the hypotheses regarding sleep functions and regulations. In this section of the chapter, we discuss how the functions of sleep-related genes are related to these theories of sleep, with an attempt to provide some perspective into the possible components of the molecular machinery underlying sleep.

Neurotransmission, Ion Channels, and Neuronal Activity

Many neurotransmitters and neuromodulator systems are involved in the regulation of sleep and wake. Consistently, sleep is altered by perturbing genes involved in the metabolism and signaling cascade of various neurotransmitters and neuromodulators. Most of these systems function as switches to regulate the transitions between behavioral states in well-defined neural circuits. Genetic dysfunctions in these systems often lead to a reduced amount or fragmentation of a behavioral state resulting from difficulties in initiating or maintaining the behavioral state. Most notably, CRISPR-Cas9–mediated double-deletion of muscarinic acetylcholine receptors *Chrm1* and *Chrm3* almost completely eliminates REM sleep,[47] suggesting an essential role of *Chrm1* and *Chrm3* in REM sleep or at least the EEG/EMG

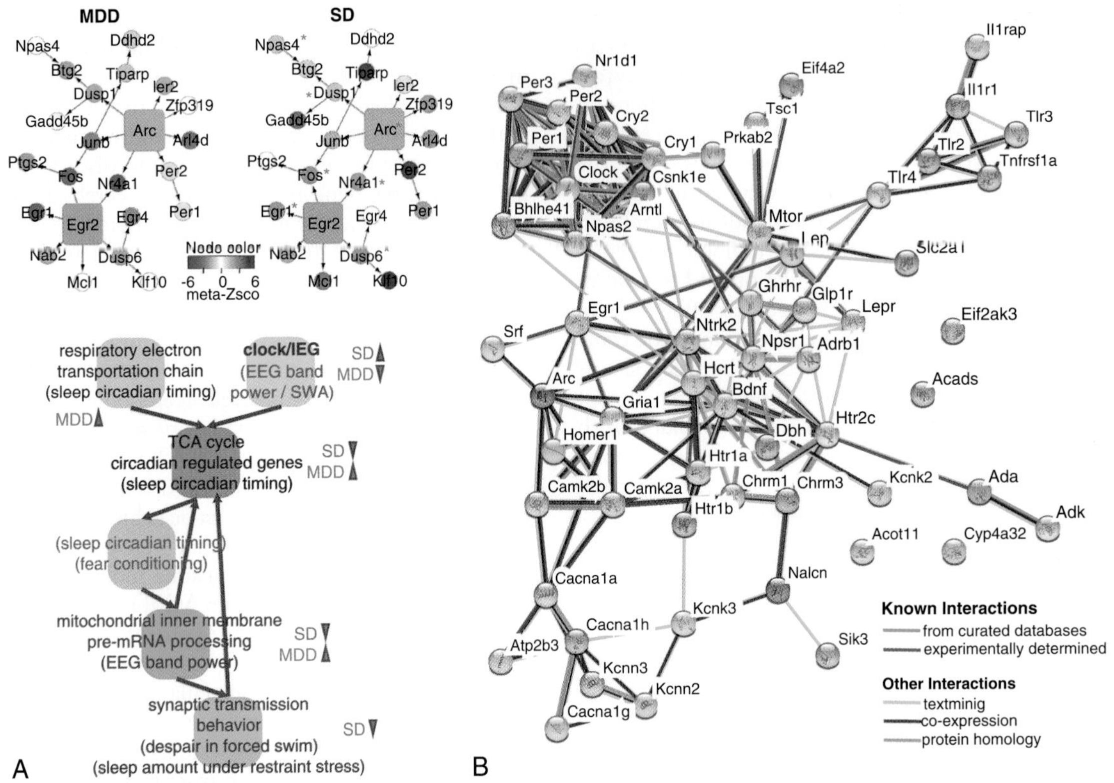

Figure 15.3 Sleep-related genes can be assembled into interactive networks. **A,** *Upper panel:* A circadian clock and immediate-early gene (IEG) network in the cerebral cortex is oppositely altered by major depressive disorder (MDD) and sleep deprivation (SD). Network edges denote gene regulatory relationships predicted by Bayesian network reconstruction using eQTL as causal anchors. Genes are colored according to expression changes determined by meta-analyses of MDD and SD datasets. *Lower panel:* The clock/IEG network (i.e., the network in the upper panel) is upstream of other SD-affected gene networks. Networks (denoted by *colored squares*) are labeled with its gene ontology and top associated phenotypes (*in parentheses*) measured in a population of C57BL/6J × 129S1/SvlmJ F2 mice. Directions of SD-/MDD-induced expression changes are denoted by up-/down-pointing triangles. Regulatory edges were determined by summarization of gene-gene regulations and confirmed by transcription regulatory information curated from databases. A green asterisk (*) next to a gene label indicates the gene belongs to a set of 78 genes considered core molecular components of the sleep homeostatic response in the cortex, as their differential expression has been consistently observed under spontaneous waking, after SD, and after SD in adrenalectomized mice.[41] **B,** A demonstration of interactions among sleep-related genes that are highlighted in the second part of this chapter. The network is constructed and visualized using the STRING database. While functional clusters (e.g., circadian clock, inflammation, metabolism, neurotransmission and excitability, and synaptic plasticity) of genes can be seen because of extensive interactions within the functional cluster, interactions among genes of different functional groups are also widely observed. (**A,** Modified from Scarpa JR, Jiang P, Gao VD, et al. Cross-species systems analysis identifies gene networks differentially altered by sleep loss and depression. *Sci Adv* 2018;4:eaat1294, licensed under CC BY 4.0.)

manifestation characteristic of REM sleep. This finding is striking, since other genes identified so far influence sleep-wake quantitatively but do not preclude a behavioral state. *Chrm1/Chrm3* double-knock mice thus present an intriguing model for the study of fundamental functions of REM sleep, as it is distinct from the selective REM sleep deprivation (RSD) model, in which animals are disturbed to wake up once they enter REM sleep.

A few neuromodulators also appear to regulate sleep homeostatic drive across different brain regions. One such neuromodulator is norepinephrine, which is produced by neurons including those in the locus coeruleus, a key wake-promoting brain region. The wake-promoting function of norepinephrine is mediated through the adrenergic receptors or adrenoceptors, various subtypes of which are expressed in many different regions of the brain. For instance, *Adrb1* (*Adrenoceptor β1*) is expressed in a group of wake-promoting neurons in the dorsal pons, and a dominant mutation in *Adrb1* that promotes wakefulness and the activity of the *Adrb1+* neurons has been identified recently in a human pedigree of short sleepers.[70] Interestingly, pharmacologic depletion of norepinephrine in the brain led to an attenuated homeostatic elevation of NREM delta power after SD, although the SD-induced NREM sleep rebound was grossly intact.[113] Mice lacking norepinephrine and epinephrine because of deletion of *Dbh* (*dopamine β-hydroxylase*), the gene required for norepinephrine synthesis, show 2 hours of increase in the daily amount of NREM sleep at the cost of wake and REM sleep, elevated NREM delta power with abolished diurnal rhythmicity, and impairment of SD-induced NREM sleep rebound.[114] Hence, although detailed results differ between genetic and pharmacologic depletion of NE, both suggest a role of norepinephrine signaling in sleep homeostasis in addition to wake-promoting. Future studies are needed to dissect the specific functions of adrenoceptor subtypes and corresponding neuronal populations that are involved in the norepinephrine-associated sleep homeostatic regulation.

Another neuromodulator that is involved in sleep homeostasis is adenosine, which generally inhibits the activity of neurons that express adenosine receptors and promotes sleep. The extracellular levels of adenosine rise locally after SD,[115,116] paralleled with increased neuronal metabolic activity,[117] and the elevated levels of adenosine and its inhibitory effects on neuronal activity are thought to be an important component of sleep homeostasis.[118] Interestingly, a polymorphism in adenosine deaminase (encoded by *Ada*), which reduces adenosine to inosine, influences the duration and intensity of slow wave sleep (i.e., delta-dominated deep NREM sleep) as well as subjective sleepiness during prolonged wakefulness.[119,120] Tissue-specific knockout of *Adora1*, the gene encoding the adenosine A_1 receptor, in the brain or forebrain glutamatergic neurons attenuates SD-induced increase of NREM delta power.[121,122] Glia-specific deletion of *Adk* (*adenosine kinase*), a gene encoding the enzyme that clears adenosine by converting it to adenosine monophosphate (AMP), results in a slower decay of delta power after its elevation during wake.[121] These findings thus suggest a neuron-glia axis in sleep homeostasis via regulating local adenosine signaling.

As a third example, serotonin signaling appears to be involved in both NREM and REM sleep regulation and homeostasis. Mice lacking the serotonin-2C receptors (encoded by *Hrt2c* gene) show decreased NREM sleep under baseline conditions but an augmented elevation of NREM delta power during recovery sleep after SD,[123] while mice lacking the serotonin-1A or -1B receptors (encoded by *Htr1a/1b* genes) display increased REM sleep under baseline conditions but no REM sleep rebound after RSD.[124,125]

Furthermore, genetic studies of hypocretin, a wake-promoting neuromodulator not directly involved in the homeostatic regulation of sleep, have also led to interesting insights into sleep homeostasis. The role of hypocretin neurons in sleep-wake regulation was discovered through the studies of narcolepsy, a sleep disorder characterized by an extreme tendency to abruptly fall asleep, via a combination of forward genetics in dogs,[68] mouse knockouts,[126] human pathology and pathophysiology,[127,128] and earlier, the use of gene expression analysis and rat neuroanatomy.[129] Although the hypocretin system is thought to primarily stabilize sleep-wake state and deletion of the *Hcrt* gene in mice does not alter the homeostatic responses to SD,[130] a recent study found that spontaneous waking in *Hcrt* knockout mice fails to induce a delta power reflective of prior waking duration because of impaired maintenance of wake theta (6.0 to 9.5 Hz) and fast-gamma (55 to 80 Hz) activity,[131] an EEG feature typically correlated with explorative behavior. When actively awake, particularly during SD, theta/gamma activity was fully implemented in the knockout mice, leading to a normal accumulation of sleep homeostatic pressure. Through detailed analysis and modeling, this study further suggests that theta-dominated wake, rather than overall wake, drives sleep homeostatic pressure.

In addition to neurotransmitter/neuromodulator-related genes, genes encoding ion channels have also been implicated in sleep-wake regulation. As mentioned previously, chemically induced point mutations in *Nalcn*, a voltage-independent non-selective cation channel, and *Cacna1a*, a voltage-dependent calcium channel, dramatically reduced time spent in REM sleep and wakefulness, respectively.[52,53] Expression of hyperpolarization-promoting ion channel genes, such as *Kcnk2* (*K^+ channel subfamily K member 2*; also known as *Trek-1*) and *Kcnk3* (also known as *Task-1*), is higher during sleep compared to wake.[13] In addition, a recent study modeled the burst-firing pattern of cortical and thalamic neurons during slow wave sleep by simplifying neuron networks to a self-interacting "averaged neuron" and predicted that Ca^{2+}-dependent hyperpolarization is crucial for the oscillations of bursting and silent phases, synchronization of which across cortical neurons give rise to delta wave.[48] Consistent with this prediction, CRISPR-Cas9-mediated deletion of Ca^{2+}-dependent K^+ channels (*Kcnn2* and *Kcnn3*), voltage-gated Ca^{2+} channels (*Cacna1g* and *Cacna1h*), or Ca^{2+}/calmodulin-dependent kinases (*Camk2a* and *Camk2b*, which regulate the conductance of KCNNs) decrease sleep duration, while deleting plasma membrane Ca^{2+} ATPase (*Atp2b3*) increases sleep duration.[48] Observations further in line with this prediction include decreased sleep duration resulting from pharmacologically inhibiting or genetically deleting NMDA receptors.[46,48] Together, these observations highlight the importance of regulating membrane excitability in the manifestation of different behavioral states.

A key question remaining is how sleep regulatory signals, especially homeostatic signals, communicate with these ion channels to regulate membrane excitability. At least in the fruit flies, this process involves membrane-associated proteins that regulate ion channel activities. *Shaker*, a gene identified in a mutagenesis screen,[49] encodes the pore-forming alpha-subunit of a voltage-gated K^+ channel that controls membrane repolarization.[132] Null alleles of *Shaker* in flies or its mammalian homologues in mice reduce the total sleep time without altering the circadian timing of sleep or the homeostatic response to SD.[49,133] The expression levels, brain localization, and channel activity of *Shaker* are regulated by *sleepless*,[50,134] a gene encoding a glycosylphosphatidylinositol-anchored protein with no known mammalian homologue. Like *Shaker*, null alleles of *sleepless* also greatly reduce the amount of sleep. However, flies carrying a *sleepless* mutation that only results in a partial loss of its protein function exhibit essentially a normal amount of baseline sleep but a pronounced reduction in the homeostatic rebound after SD.[50] Thus *sleepless* may be important for linking sleep homeostatic pressure to membrane excitability.

The distinct neuronal excitability and firing patterns between sleep and wake are tightly linked to the marked difference in the expression of immediate-early genes (IEGs), whose expression is rapidly induced by a wide range of stimuli, including excitation of neurons. Most brain regions are more active during wake than sleep and thus show higher levels of expression of IEGs during wake.[135-137] The study of IEG expression as a neuronal activity marker across different brain regions has also assisted the identification and characterization of brain regions that are active during sleep, such as cortical nNOS (neuronal nitric oxide synthase)–expressing neurons[138,139] and ventrolateral preoptic area (VLPO) in the anterior hypothalamus.[140] More recent studies have identified a few additional wake-active neuronal populations, and a detailed discussion of these circuits and their functions in sleep-wake regulation is presented in Chapter 7.

A remaining key question, however, is how distinct neuronal activities during sleep and wake are linked to the molecular events underlying the diverse functions associated with specific behavioral states. One of such links may involve the IEGs. Many of the IEGs encode transcription factors, which are involved in diverse cellular processes.[141] Therefore their activation during wake may function as a "master switch" that reprograms the transcriptome to allow activation of genes involved in the cellular functions needed during wake and/or signaling cascades leading to the buildup of sleep homeostatic pressure. Consistent with this hypothesis, by combined analysis of transcriptomic data and genome accessibility, *Srf* (*serum response factor*), an IEG, was predicted as a key transcriptional regulator shaping the pattern and dynamics of transcriptomic responses to SD, including the responses of other IEGs and circadian clock genes.[30] Also, a gene network consisting of IEGs and clock genes showed elevated gene expression after SD and were found to be at the upstream of other SD-altered gene networks in the global transcriptomic regulatory network (Figure 15.3, *A*).[109] Genes of these downstream SD-altered networks are indeed involved in some key aspects of the hypothesized cellular functions of sleep, such as regulations of mitochondrial and synaptic functions, which are discussed later in this chapter. How these typically sleep-associated functions are performed in the sleep-active brain regions (e.g., VLPO and cortical nNOS neurons), however, remains an intriguing topic for future studies.

Synaptic Plasticity

A prominent difference between sleep and wake in the brain transcriptome involves synaptic plasticity-related genes,[13-16] although their differential expression pattern across brain regions is highly complex.[18] Transcript-level changes in synaptic plasticity-related genes are consistent with the observation that SD alters the DNA methylation of these genes in the genome.[31] These observations, together with findings from electrophysiologic and imaging studies, strongly support the hypothesis that regulation and facilitation of synaptic plasticity is one of the key functions of sleep. One of such hypotheses, referred to as the synaptic homeostasis hypothesis (SHY), states that exposure to new information during wake leads to an overall potentiation and strengthening of synapses, which are renormalized, resulting in a net downscaling of synaptic strength and an improved signal-to-noise ratio, during sleep when the brain is offline and the synaptic connections can be "sampled" systematically to select weak synapses to downscale and strong synapses to leave unaffected or even upscale.[142] This hypothesis provides an elegant conceptual framework regarding the function and homeostasis of slow wave sleep and can accommodate many experimental observations, especially those in the cerebral cortex, the brain region that displays NREM delta waves. However, alternative hypotheses have been proposed and differ from SHY mainly in the cellular processes that are involved in the function of sleep in synaptic plasticity. Most notably, a hypothesis that builds on the synaptic tagging and capture (STC) theory of memory consolidation proposes that sleep is the preferred time for memory consolidation by capturing plasticity-related products (PRPs) to synapses that have been tagged or primed by learning during wake, as a way to solidify changes in synaptic strength (both strengthening and weakening).[143] The STC-based hypothesis does not predict a net up- or downscaling after sleep and thus is more flexible and can easily accommodate the observations of an overall strengthening of synapses after sleep under certain conditions, particularly in relevant neural circuits involved in processing prior experience during wake.[143] Despite their discrepancies, both hypotheses imply that the synaptic processes during wake contribute to the accumulation of sleep pressure and the synaptic processes during sleep contribute to the dissipation of sleep pressure. A prediction drawn from this implication is that genes involved in these sleep-wake–associated synaptic processes also regulate sleep homeostasis. Observations from a few genetic studies suggest that it is likely the case.

One class of such genes includes *Homer1a*, *Bdnf* (brain-derived neurotrophic factor) and *Arc* (activity-regulated cytoskeleton-associated protein), which belong to a subgroup of IEGs called effector IEGs. Like other IEGs, the expression of effector IEGs is associated with neuronal activity and is generally higher after SD across many brain regions that are active during wake and low during sleep. As discussed earlier in this chapter, *Homer1a* was identified as a candidate gene of a QTL that was linked to NREM delta power rebound after SD,[16,81] although the loss of *Homer1a* does not alter sleep homeostasis[82] and although this QTL was not replicated in the extended BXD/RwwJ RI panel, perhaps because of a low minor allele frequency.[12] A recent study has shown that downscaling of glutamatergic excitatory synapses during sleep requires the recruitment of HOMER1A protein to the postsynaptic density, a process induced by the adenosinergic sleep-promoting signals and inhibited by the norepinephrinergic wake-promoting signals.[144] Another effector IEG, *Bdnf*, encodes a neurotrophin whose role in neural development and plasticity (particularly long-term potentiation) has been extensively characterized.[145,146] In rats, the induction of BDNF by an enriched environment during wake was correlated with an increase in NREM delta power during subsequent sleep.[147] Unilateral microinjection of BDNF in the cerebral cortex followed by novel experience induces an augmented EEG delta power during subsequent NREM sleep specifically in the injected hemisphere.[148] Conversely, local reduction of NREM delta power can result from unilateral microinjection of polyclonal anti-BDNF antibody or an inhibitor of TrkB (tropomyosin receptor kinase B, a BDNF receptor) during prior wakefulness.[148] Consistently, a functional Val66Met polymorphism in the human BDNF leads to a reduction in the activity-dependent secretion of the mature peptide and is associated with less deep (i.e., stage 4) NREM sleep and reduced EEG delta power.[149] However, intracerebroventricular injections of BDNF without exposure to novelty in rats and rabbits only induced more NREM sleep with no enhancement or even a reduction of NREM delta power.[150] Deletion of a truncated isoform and negative regulator of TrkB in mice or a 50% reduction in the BDNF protein levels in heterozygous *Bdnf* null rats did not alter NREM sleep amount nor EEG delta power.[151,152] These discrepancies may point to the importance of exposure to novelty and learning during wake in BDNF-related NREM homeostatic process: the neuronal activity-dependent release of BDNF coupled with learning rather than the base-level BDNF signaling is involved in the regulation of NREM sleep, a hypothesis that warrants further investigation.

A third effector IEG, *Arc*, plays a profound role in synaptic plasticity.[153] For example, synaptic ARC protein promotes internalization of AMPA receptors and long-term depression,[154] while translocation of ARC into the nucleus is necessary for the suppression of *Gria1* (*Glutamate ionotropic receptor AMPA type subunit 1;* also known as *GluA1)* transcription and homeostatic downscaling of AMPA receptor transmission,[155] implying a transcriptional co-factor function of

ARC. Incidentally, *Arc* was found to be a key upstream regulator in the previously mentioned IEG gene network that shows upregulated gene expression after SD and is upstream of other SD-affected gene networks in the mouse cerebral cortex (Figure 15.3, *A*).[109] This regulatory network model reconstructed using systems genetic analysis is in agreement with the experimental observation that ARC coimmunoprecipitates with CREB-binding protein,[155] a key regulator of CREB (cAMP response element-binding protein)–mediated activity-dependent transcription of IEGs. Strikingly, SD-induced homeostatic responses are blunted in *Arc* knockout mice at the behavioral (e.g., NREM sleep rebound), electrophysiologic (e.g., accumulated delta energy during recovery NREM sleep), and molecular (e.g., elevated GRIA1 and its phosphorylation at synapses, induction of IEG transcription, and suppression of *Gria1* expression) levels.[156] Given these observations, *Arc* is well poised as a versatile hub linking sleep homeostasis and synaptic plasticity.

In addition to effector IEGs, recent studies suggest that phosphorylation of synaptic proteins is likely another key molecular process linking sleep homeostasis and synaptic plasticity. Phosphorylation of proteins in the synaptoneurosomes shows diurnal fluctuations that are primarily driven by sleep and wake.[27] The oscillating synaptic phosphoproteins included many kinases, including SIK3,[27] a gain-of-function allele of which (i.e., $Sik3^{Sleepy}$) causes a constitutively high NREM pressure.[52] Phosphoproteomic profiling in the brain of sleep-deprived and $Sik3^{Sleepy}$ mice has identified 80 synaptic sleep-need-index phosphoproteins (SNIPPs), whose phosphorylation state correlates with sleep homeostatic pressure.[26] SIK3 preferentially interacts with these SNIPPs, which are involved in diverse synaptic plasticity processes, such as neurotransmitter release, GTPase regulation, actin/microtubule modulation, and scaffolding. A subset of the SNIPPs is also known to alter sleep-wake. Together, these observations suggest that the phosphorylation of synaptic proteins may be an important component of the molecular mechanisms underlying synaptic plasticity-related sleep homeostatic processes.

An intriguing relationship between sleep homeostasis and memory consolidation has been observed in transgenic mice bearing a mutant form of the human *Npsr1* (*neuropeptide S receptor 1*) gene that is identified in a family of short sleepers.[69] This mutation leads to hypersensitivity to neuropeptide S in neurons expressing *Npsr1* and causes reduced sleep time, elevated but quickly dissipated NREM delta power after spontaneous wake or SD, and a largely intact rebound of NREM sleep time after SD. Despite the short sleep time, mice bearing this mutation show normal contextual memory consolidation and are resistant to the SD-induced impairment in memory consolidation. Given the role of neuropeptide S in enhancing memory consolidation,[157] it is tempting to speculate that this gain-of-function mutation in *Npsr1* enables some memory consolidation processes to occur during wake without the offline state of sleep, while other unaffected functions of sleep constitute the need for sleep in the transgenic *Npsr1* mutant mice.

A key area that requires further study to understand the relationships between sleep and synaptic plasticity regards REM sleep. The molecular and genetic evidence discussed above as well as the synaptic plasticity-related sleep function hypotheses primarily consider NREM sleep, although REM sleep also plays important roles in memory consolidation.[158-160] Notably, recent data suggest that REM sleep selectively prunes as well as strengthens new synapses of layer 5 pyramidal neurons in the mouse motor cortex during development and motor learning.[161] In addition, the regulation of REM sleep appears to include both a "short-term" component regulating NREM-REM sleep transitions and a "long-term" homeostatic component determining the overall amount of REM sleep.[162] It is thus important to understand how NREM and REM sleep split and coordinate the tasks of plastic processes during sleep and how such state-specific but coordinated molecular events are related to the regulations of NREM-REM sleep cycles and REM homeostasis. These molecular events may once again involve IEGs. For example, expression of *Egr1* (*Early growth response protein 1*; aka. *zif-268*) is typically high during wake and low during NREM and REM sleep, but when rats were exposed to a novel enriched environment during waking, reactivation of *Egr1* transcription during subsequent REM sleep was observed in the hippocampus and cerebral cortex.[163] Similarly, cortical reactivation *Egr1* transcription during REM sleep can also result from the induction of hippocampal long-term potentiation during prior waking.[164] Furthermore, in rats, BDNF protein levels are elevated in brainstem REM sleep–regulatory areas after RSD and were positively correlated with EEG delta power during the RSD period and the number of REM sleep episodes during the subsequent recovery sleep.[165] *Bdnf* heterozygous null rats show dramatically reduced REM sleep and increased REM sleep latency, although a rebound of REM sleep is still present after RSD.[152] Similarly, mice lacking TrkB.T1, a negative regulator of BDNF signaling, show increased REM sleep amount and reduced REM sleep latency.[151] These findings suggest that BDNF is also involved in REM sleep regulation, particularly the hypothesized short-term process interacting with NREM sleep, in addition to its role in NREM sleep. More studies are needed to further elucidate the genetic and molecular mechanisms underlying REM homeostasis and the function of REM sleep in synaptic plasticity.

Macromolecule and Energy Metabolism

The hypothesized functions of sleep also include the restoration of certain molecules that are perhaps depleted during wake. This hypothesis is strongly supported by gene expression profiling studies, which suggest that sleep may be a preferred time for the biosynthesis of macromolecules.[13,15,166] For example, mRNA levels of positive regulators of protein synthesis, such as *Eif4a2* (*eukaryotic translation initiation factor 4A2*) in the cerebral cortex and *mTOR* (*mammalian target of rapamycin*) in the hippocampus, are high during sleep and low during wake.[13,166] Conversely, negative regulators of protein synthesis, such as *Eif2ak3* (*eukaryotic translation initiation factor 2A kinase 3,* also known as *PEK*), are expressed at a lower level during sleep compared to wake.[13] Wake is also associated with higher levels of phosphorylation and presumably also the activity of AMP-activated protein kinase (AMPK), an inhibitor of protein synthesis.[26,167] These findings are consistent with earlier protein work using 14C-Leu autoradiography in both rats and monkeys, which showed the rate of labeled leucine incorporation in the brain was positively correlated with the occurrence of slow wave sleep.[168,169] Furthermore, sleep disturbances resulting from disrupted mTOR signaling have been observed in mice deficient of *Tsc1* (*Tuberous sclerosis complex 1*), which encodes an inhibitor of mTOR-dependent promotion of protein synthesis.[170] These mice show reduced REM sleep and blunted diurnal sleep-wake rhythms, which are effectively treated by rapamycin. Together, these observations suggest the exciting possibility that one function of sleep might be the restoration of proteins through increased synthesis. In addition to protein synthesis, restorative functions of sleep may include lipid synthesis (e.g., cholesterol) and transport, heme and porphyrin synthesis, as well as the production of mitochondrial components (e.g., enzymes for oxidative phosphorylation and the citric cycle), since genes involved in these cellular functions are also upregulated during sleep.[15]

What could be the biologic significance of allocating macromolecule biosynthesis to sleep? It is possible that a high level of neuronal activity and signaling events during wake impose cellular stress in neurons, causing damages in functional cellular components, organelles, and protein complexes. Even though the transcription and translation of genes involved in unfolded protein response are rapidly activated after wake,[13,15,171] this cellular protective mechanism may not be sufficient to offset the cellular stress. Replenishing damaged cellular components during wake while the cellular stress is high may be maladaptive; therefore sleep and the associated offline state are preferred for allocating restorative processes. Also, protein synthesis–dependent synaptic plasticity is critical to memory consolidation, and thus the elevated protein synthesis during sleep may be a requirement for consolidating changes in the synapses that are temporarily modulated and tagged during wake.[143] Particularly, inhibition of mTOR-dependent protein synthesis during sleep blocks the consolidation of synaptic strengthening,[172] and enhancement of the same pathway rescues SD-induced memory impairment.[173] Finally, allocating macromolecules biosynthesis may be an adaptive process for energy balance. Maintaining membrane excitability and synaptic processes during wake is energy expensive (e.g., requiring ATP-dependent transportation of Na^+ and K^+), and it is thus adaptive to allocate other energy-costly processes, such as macromolecule synthesis and transport as well as mitochondrial restoration, to sleep.

Regulation of energy metabolism is indeed a key hypothesized function of sleep. Notably, brain energy expenditure is lower during NREM sleep and higher during wake and REM sleep, although the difference is relatively small (e.g., ~15%). It has been hypothesized that a function of sleep is to replenish energy. For example, ATP and AMP levels are thought to influence the balance of the adenosine metabolic pathway, and higher energy demands during wake lead to a decreased ATP:AMP ratio and elevated extracellular levels of adenosine, which, as discussed previously, facilitate sleep.[174,175] However, the dynamics of cellular energy molecules during sleep and wake are complex, and their exact metabolic processes need further investigation.[176,177] More recently, it has been proposed that sleep may not simply conserve or replenish energy but rather allocates different types of energy-intensive processes for the overall fitness.[178] A possible molecular basis may involve AMPK, a key cellular energy sensor that is regulated by AMP:ATP and ADP:ATP ratios, and upon activation by phosphorylation promotes glucose uptake and inhibits protein and lipid biosynthesis.[179,180] Thus sleep-wake–dependent AMPK phosphorylation[26,167] may function as a switch between differential metabolic programs associated with sleep and wake. Interestingly, perturbations of this energy regulatory pathway lead to altered sleep-wake patterns. Injections of an inhibitor or an activator of AMPK into the mouse brain respectively suppress or enhance NREM delta power.[181] Neuronal specific knockdown of the *Drosophila* ortholog of *Prkab2*, which encodes the beta subunit of AMPK, leads to fragmented sleep, reduction in sleep time, and suppressed sleep rebound after SD.[182] AMPK also promotes the transcription and inhibits the endocytosis of glucose transporter GLUT1 (encoded by *Slc2a1*),[183] whose mRNA levels are high during wake and low during sleep.[13] Mice heterozygous for a missense mutation in GLUT1 show reduced NREM sleep and increased wake.[184] These data suggest that regulation of energy metabolism not only is a function of sleep but also is required for normal sleep-wake patterns.

Importantly, the interaction between sleep and cellular metabolism is likely not limited to the brain but rather a multisystem phenomenon. Repeated insufficient sleep leads to decreased insulin sensitivity and is associated with risk of diabetes, obesity, and hepatic steatosis in humans.[185] In mice under fasting conditions, SD induces glucose intolerance accompanied by disrupted fatty acid metabolism as indicated by metabolomic and transcriptomic profiling in the liver.[186] Interestingly, systems genetic studies have identified a few metabolic genes whose expression in the liver rather than the brain was linked to sleep phenotypes. For instance, the expression of *Glp1r* in the liver, not the frontal cortex, hypothalamus, or thalamus, was found to mediate the causal effect of a QTL regulating the amount of NREM sleep and wake amount.[108] *Glp1r* encodes the receptor of glucagon-like peptide 1, a hormone that inhibits appetite and lowers blood glucose, and peripheral administrations of GLP1R agonists promote light sleep at the costs of wake and slow wave sleep.[108] This finding is consistent with observations in mice deficient of leptin or leptin receptors (i.e., $Lep^{ob/ob}$ and $Lepr^{db/db}$ mice, respectively), which are obese and diabetic and show profound changes in sleep, including fragmented sleep, reduced sleep-wake rhythmicity, increased NREM sleep, and suppressed homeostatic responses to SD.[187,188] In addition, a hepatic eQTL of *Acot11* (*acyl-coenzyme A thioesterase 11*), a gene involved in fatty acid metabolism, was colocalized with a QTL linked to the amount and dynamic of NREM sleep rebound after SD, and *Acot11* knockout mice show blunted NREM sleep rebound specifically during the second half of the dark period after SD.[12] Finally, *Cyp4a32*, a gene that is not expressed in the brain and encodes a cytochrome 450 liver enzyme catalyzing the omega-hydroxylation of fatty acids, was identified as a candidate gene underlying a QTL linked to the peak frequency of theta waves during REM sleep,[12] consistent with a previous QTL study that identified *Acads*, a gene involved in beta-oxidation of fatty acids, in regulating the speed of REM theta oscillations.[79] It is worth noting that the pharmacologic and genetic manipulations used in these studies are not peripheral tissue specific, and further studies are needed to understand the contributions of central and peripheral (or systemic) influence of metabolism on sleep-wake regulation as well as the underlying mechanisms. Nevertheless, the links between peripheral gene expression and sleep under genetic or behavioral perturbations argue that sleep function and regulation are likely to involve multiple organ systems beyond the brain.

Inflammation

Another systemic level process that is linked to the function and regulation of sleep is inflammation. It has long been documented that chronic insufficient sleep is associated with impaired immune functions and that sleep is often enhanced during infections.[189] Central and peripheral levels of proinflammatory signals are elevated by loss of sleep.[190,191] Consistently, gene expression profiling in peripheral blood after repeated sleep loss in humans suggested a more proinflammatory, activated state of leukocytes.[192] Interestingly, proinflammatory signals also appear to promote sleep. Evidence of this can be traced back to the early 1980s, when the sleep-promoting "factor S," isolated from the cerebral spinal fluid and brains of sleep-deprived animals, turned out to likely have an origin of bacterial cell wall peptidoglycan.[193,194]

Since then, many proinflammatory agents, and more recently, genes involved in the proinflammatory pathway have been tested for a somnogenic role. Most notably, two proinflammatory cytokines, interleukin (IL)-1β and tumor necrosis factor (TNF)-α, have been studied extensively and appear to be particularly important.[189] In mice deficient of type 1 IL-1β receptor, type 1 TNF-α receptor, or both (encoded by *Il1r1* and *Tnfrsf1a*, respectively), the amount of daily NREM sleep is reduced.[195-197] The *Il1r1*/*Tnfrsf1a* double knockout mice also show a shorter period of NREM sleep rebound but a longer period of elevated EEG delta power after SD.[197] Impaired NREM homeostasis also has been observed in mice lacking the neuronal-specific isoform of the *Il1rap* gene, which encodes the IL-1 receptor accessory protein, a component of the IL-1 receptor complex.[198] Furthermore, IL-1 and TNF-α signaling also mediate the sleep-promoting effects of infections, as influenza infection-induced sleep responses are altered in mice deficient of the neuronal-specific isoform of *Il1rap* or in *Tnfrsf1a*/*b* double-knockout animals.[198,199] The induction of proinflammatory cytokines during infections is regulated by Toll-like receptors (TLRs), which play a key role in the innate immune system by recognizing microbe-derived molecules. Mice deficient of *Tlr4* or both *Tlr2* and *Tlr4* genes show reduced NREM sleep, and infection-induced augmented sleep is attenuated by knocking out *Tlr3*.[200-202]

Importantly, while these inflammatory cytokines have been shown to directly act in the brain to regulate sleep,[189-191] peripheral cytokines can elicit proinflammatory signals in the CNS by acting on the vagus nerve.[203] Also, the bidirectional exchange of central and peripheral cytokines may occur through the meningeal lymphatic system and the glymphatic system.[204,205] Furthermore, there is likely crosstalk between sleep-interacting immune functions and other sleep-interacting systemic functions, such as metabolism. Incidentally, influenza A virus infection induces a decline in NREM sleep in mice bearing a mutation in the growth hormone-releasing hormone (GHRH) receptor (i.e., $Ghrhr^{lit/lit}$ mice), as opposed to an increase of NREM sleep in wild-type animals.[206] GHRH has been well characterized for its sleep-promoting role, which is independent of the release of growth hormone and is thought to synchronize anabolic activities under favorable physiologic conditions associated with sleep.[207] Similarly, high-fat diet-induced glucose intolerance and insulin resistance are absent in mice deficient for both *Tlr2* and *Tlr4*.[200] It has been hypothesized that inflammation-promoted sleep (particularly NREM sleep) during infections is adaptive as it supports anabolic processes and generation of fever in an energy-balanced manner that is beneficial for recovery and ultimately survival.[189] More broadly, the genetic and molecular links between sleep and inflammation may be a systemic level mechanism underlying the impact of sleep on overall health and well-being. Consistent with this point of view, the association between short sleep and increased mortality in the elderly may be attributed to the levels of proinflammatory markers.[208]

Circadian Clock Genes

Another class of genes that are involved in the multisystem function and regulation of sleep is the circadian clock genes. In the suprachiasmatic nucleus (SCN) of the hypothalamus, a translational and transcriptional feedback loop of clock genes, including the positive regulators, *Clock* and *Arntl* (also known as *Bmal1*), and the negative regulators, *Per1*/*2*/*3* and *Cry1*/*2*, generates the circadian rhythms of numerous molecular, physiologic, and behavioral processes, including the sleep-wake cycles (see Chapter 13). Over the past two decades, the role of circadian clock genes in regulating other aspects of sleep, including sleep homeostasis, and the timing of sleep, has been established.

Clock gene expression in the SCN is intrinsically rhythmic and can be entrained to the external light-dark cycle because of rapid induction of clock gene *Per1* and *Per2* transcription by signal cascades elicited upon photoreception in the eye. However, in other regions of the brain, particularly the cerebral cortex, *Per1* and *Per2* expression appears to be coupled with sleep and wake cycles and is rapidly elevated during wake.[13,41,109,209,210] Similarly, the diurnal oscillations of *Clock* and *Npas2* (a paralog of *Clock*) mRNA levels in the cerebral cortex are also primarily driven by sleep-wake.[30] All core clock genes and many clock-regulator genes (e.g., *Csnk1e*, *Bhlhe41*, and *Nr1d1*) in both mice and humans have been found to influence noncircadian sleep-wake phenotypes, including the amount of NREM or REM sleep as well as their homeostatic response to SD.[72,211-219] These accumulating findings strongly argue that the circadian clock machinery regulates not only the timing but also the amount and homeostasis of sleep.

A few mechanisms may be involved in the role of clock genes in noncircadian sleep-wake regulation. First, the influence of disrupted clock genes on the amount of sleep may be related to a deficient SCN clock. The SCN innervates multiple sleep-wake regulatory areas of the brain, and ablations of the SCN lead to changes in the amount of sleep in a species-dependent manner, in addition to the loss of rhythmicity of sleep-wake.[220] Also, as a set of transcriptional regulators, clock genes are expressed in other areas of the brain and throughout the body, and they may regulate the sleep-wake regulatory signaling pathways in relevant brain regions. For example, a missense mutation in a circadian clock regulator gene, *Bhlhe41* (also known as *Dec2*), causes a reduced amount of sleep in humans and mice,[72] and this effect is mediated at least in part by regulating the transcription of *Hcrt* in hypothalamic *Hcrt*+ neurons.[221]

Furthermore, the transcriptional output program of the clock is linked to diverse cellular functions, the most notable of which include metabolism. The involvement of the circadian clock in metabolism has been extensively studied at the whole organism level and across multiple tissues (for a review, see Jiang and Turek[222]). Therefore it has been hypothesized that a key cellular process and mechanism underlying the role of the clock in sleep homeostatic regulation involves clock-controlled metabolism throughout the body.[223] Strikingly, through tissue-specific knockout and rescue of *Arntl*, a recent study shows that *Arntl* in the skeletal muscle, not the brain, influences NREM sleep amount and SD-induced homeostatic rebound in NREM sleep and EEG delta power, while the diurnal rhythmicity in sleep is regulated by *Arntl* in the brain.[224] Although further studies are needed to understand how *Arntl* function in the skeletal muscle regulates sleep, findings from this study clearly demonstrate the peripheral impact on sleep, a biologic process regulated primarily by the brain. The skeletal muscle is a major glucose user in the body, and loss of *Arntl* leads to glucose intolerance and nonfasting hyperglycemia.[225] Thus systemic glucose homeostasis may be a key intermediate linking the function of the circadian clock in the skeletal muscle and NREM sleep amount and homeostasis. Finally, there are significant crosslinks among the circadian clock, metabolism, and inflammation, such as those involving the circadian gene *Nr1d1* (also known as *Rev-erbα*),[226-228] which encodes a nuclear receptor-type transcription repressor that functions in a "stabilizing loop" of the circadian clock and as a circadian "gatekeeper" of metabolic and inflammatory processes. Expression of *Nr1d1* is decreased after SD,[41] and loss of *Nr1d1* leads to advanced timing of sleep as well as a slower increase of homeostatic sleep need during wakefulness, which is then reflective by fragmented sleep and reduced EEG delta power during subsequent sleep.[219] While future studies are needed to understand how the circadian clock regulates sleep through complex interactions with other cellular and systemic functions, the deep involvement of the clock machinery in a wide range of biologic processes may allow it to be an interesting integrator to regulate the timing, amount, and homeostatic drive of sleep, based on "summed" information of cellular and systemic states.

DISCUSSIONS AND OUTLOOK

Genetic and functional genomic studies have revealed a polygenic nature of sleep. Despite decades of research, the blueprint of the genetic and molecular basis of sleep is undoubtedly still incomplete. Major challenges for future studies include not only the efficient identification of a large number of new genes and alleles that are linked to sleep but also the elucidation of the interactions among these genes, their products, and interventions such as SD. This information must be assembled into molecular pathways so that genetic and genomic findings can be turned into insights and eventually knowledge of sleep mechanisms. To achieve this task, tools to mine and integrate the many available databases and infer causality in multiomic networks are becoming increasingly important, and better-performing tools are being actively developed (e.g., see Sing and colleagues[229] and Argelaguet and colleagues[230]).

As discussed in this chapter, sleep-related genes can be grouped into a few broadly defined categories that are consistent with popular hypotheses regarding the fundamental functions of sleep. While the categorization presented in this chapter may be simplistic, components of the complex sleep machinery become increasingly apparent. Importantly, new or even surprising functions of sleep may come into view and may be linked to additional sets of genes or those that have already been associated with other aspects of sleep. For example, recent studies suggest that clearance of metabolic waste and toxic misfolded proteins in the brain is driven by sleep, particularly delta waves, via regulating the glymphatic passage and cerebrospinal fluid oscillations.[204,231-233] Whether these processes are genetically regulated and whether the underlying molecular processes also influence sleep itself are intriguing topics for future studies. It is nonetheless worth noting that the expression of genes involved in membrane trafficking is higher during sleep and the expression of heat-shock proteins (chaperons) is higher during wake.[13,15,171] It is thus interesting to understand whether and how these processes are coordinated to respond to an accumulation of unfolded/misfolded proteins during wake and expel them during sleep. Also, while sleep-wake–dependent changes in the expression of cytoskeleton organization genes[15] are often thought as related to neural plasticity, these changes may also be associated with sleep-wake–associated alterations in extracellular space. Interestingly, sleep-wake–dependent expression of genes involved in extracellular matrix and cytoskeleton also are observed in astrocytes.[32]

It is important to emphasize that the individual aspects of sleep functions and regulations are likely interrelated at the genetic and molecular levels (Figure 15.3, *B*). This is expected to become more apparent as new genes are being added to the blueprint of the sleep machinery. A key question in the field of sleep genetics is whether there is a set of "master" sleep genes that are upstream of other sleep-regulatory genes and essential for the manifestation and core functions of sleep, as analogous to the core clock genes in generating circadian rhythms. As discussed earlier in this chapter, a clock/IEG network appeared to be at the upstream of other sleep-associated gene networks (Figure 15.3, *A*).[109] Also, an IEG, *Srf*, has been predicted as a transcriptional regulator driving immediate transcriptomic response to SD.[30] However, as such inference was based mainly on transcriptomic variations, it is perhaps not surprising that transcription factors with diverse regulatory targets, such as clock genes and IEGs, were identified as the most upstream regulators. When additional layers of "-omics" data, especially those reflective of faster processes (e.g., protein modification), are included, it is possible that the overall structure of the global network switches from a more centralized network to a more decentralized or even distributed network, in which no single set of genes is the master regulator. A decentralized network avoids a single point of failure and thus may be more adaptive as the underlying machinery for essential and multifaceted functions such as sleep. This is consistent with the fact that the genetic variants with large sleep-regulating effects are rare.

These large-effect genes may represent local hubs of subnetworks that are specialized for certain aspects of sleep functions. While it can be expected that, along with continuing advances in the technical capabilities of multiscale molecular profiling and computational modeling, extensive network models will be reconstructed to capture the interactions among sleep regulatory genes and molecules. The main challenge for future studies is to efficiently validate the reconstructed network models. Perhaps with new developments in CRISPR-based technologies that allow for multiplexed gene editing,[234] it will soon become possible to evaluate gene network-level functions by manipulating many genes simultaneously.

Furthermore, the field of neuroscience has been advancing in understanding the functions of neural circuits and networks. Future genetic and genomic studies could embrace these exciting developments by incorporating not only cell-type–specific or single-cell transcriptomics but also large-scale imaging data of neural network connectivity, the density of synapses, and neuronal activities as intermediate phenotypes for comprehensive causal modeling.

Another future direction of genetic and genomic studies regards gene-environment interactions. As mentioned earlier in this chapter, environmental exposure during wake modulates subsequent sleep and may impact the observation of the functions of genes in sleep regulation. It is thus important to consider gene-environmental interactions in future studies. In a broader sense, since the function of sleep appears to be so diverse, genetic and genomic studies of sleep before, during, and after the engagement of other biologic functions in response to environmental stimuli, such as memory tasks, metabolic challenges, infections, and many others, provide unique opportunities to more comprehensively depict the gene networks linking sleep regulation to functions. Furthermore, a special type of environment that needed to be incorporated into future research comes from the inside of the body—the gut microbiome. Accumulating studies have demonstrated an important role of the gut microbial community in host metabolic, immune, and neurobehavioral functions. Although with some debate,[235,236] repeated sleep disturbances appear to alter the gut microbial composition,[237-239] and prebiotic diets that alter the gut microbiome have been shown to modulate sleep.[240,241] Through extensive interactions with the environment and host metabolic and immune pathways, the gut microbes may alter the penetrance of host genetic variants.[242] Therefore studies of the microbiome, the "genome beyond our own," need to an integrated component of future genetic and genomic studies of sleep.

While extensive research is still needed to identify more sleep regulatory genes as well as to elucidate the complex relationships among the identified genes to draw a more complete blueprint of the sleep machinery, the potential reward is immense. A comprehensive understanding of the molecular machinery of sleep ultimately may not only allow for the understanding and treatment of sleep disorders and other diseases/disorders associated with disrupted sleep (e.g., almost all neurologic/neuropsychiatric disorders and many non–nervous system disorders, including obesity, diabetes, and cardiovascular disease) but also may provide insights into and solutions for sleep hygiene–related socioeconomic issues prevalent in our modern sleep-deprived societies.

CLINICAL PEARL

An understanding of the genes and gene alleles that influence sleep and wake quality and the susceptibility to sleep loss may suggest novel targets or approaches to improve sleep and wake as well as for the treatment of sleep disorders. As in other areas of medicine, allelic differences in these genes may suggest different treatments for different individuals with the same disorder because the pathophysiology may be distinct. Rodent studies using molecular, forward, and reverse genetic approaches, in combination with human studies, are likely to lead to novel insights into the regulation and function of sleep, which can then be translated into improved treatments for sleep-wake disorders as well as for other mental and physical disorders associated with disrupted sleep.

SUMMARY

Sleep is a complex behavior that is strongly influenced by genetic factors that are specific to each of sleep's many facets. In this two-part chapter we gave an overview of the progress made in identifying the genes and gene pathways underlying sleep, with some emphasis on the homeostatic aspect of sleep regulation using the mouse as a model species. In the first part, we present the advances in the techniques and approaches researchers use to unveil the relevant genes and their products. Of these approaches, systems genetics, which integrates multilevel information (from genome to inter alia, transcriptome, proteome, metabolome, and microbiome, to phenome) obtained in genetic reference populations, seems the way forward as much has been learned on the central and peripheral pathways involved and how these are perturbed by sleep loss. The second part highlights five focus areas in sleep research pertinent to sleep function and regulation that insights gained from both mice and human genetic studies helped solidify. An understanding of the molecular machinery regulating sleep will help not only with the treatment of sleep disorders but also with the many disorders associated with disrupted sleep, including depression and metabolic syndrome.

ACKNOWLEDGMENT

This work was in part supported by the Office of Naval Research MURI Grant #N00014-15-1-2809 (PJ and FWT).

SELECTED READINGS

Diessler S, Jan M, Emmenegger Y, et al. A systems genetics resource and analysis of sleep regulation in the mouse. *PLoS Biol.* 2018;16:e2005750.

Franken P. A role for clock genes in sleep homeostasis. *Curr Opin Neurobiol.* 2013;23:864–872.

Jan M, O'Hara BF, Franken P. Recent advances in understanding the genetics of sleep. *F1000Res.* 2020;9:F1000 Faculty Rev-214, 2020.

Jiang P, Scarpa JR, Fitzpatrick K, et al. A systems approach identifies networks and genes linking sleep and stress: implications for neuropsychiatric disorders. *Cell reports.* 2015;11:835–848.

Scarpa JR, Jiang P, Gao VD, et al. Cross-species systems analysis identifies gene networks differentially altered by sleep loss and depression. *Sci Adv.* 2018;4:eaat1294.

A complete reference list can be found online at ExpertConsult.com.

Chapter 16

Genetics and Genomic Basis of Sleep in Healthy Humans

Hans-Peter Landolt; Derk-Jan Dijk

Chapter Highlights

- Distinct characteristics of human sleep are regulated by different molecular and genetic mechanisms with different degrees of heritability.
- Understanding the genetic and molecular mechanisms controlling the circadian system have progressed over the last decades, yet the genes regulating sleep homeostasis still remain poorly understood.
- The sleep electroencephalogram is one of the most heritable traits in humans. Elucidating the underlying genes may reveal novel sleep functions.
- Several proposed genetic associations with distinct characteristics of sleep and sleep regulatory processes await independent replication and confirmation in dedicated experimental protocols and high-quality data sets.
- The effects of genetic variants often cross boundaries between sleep and wakefulness and circadian and homeostatic aspects of sleep-wake regulation.

EVIDENCE FOR TRAIT-LIKE AND GENOTYPE-DEPENDENT DIFFERENCES IN DIURNAL PREFERENCE, SLEEP TIMING, SLEEP EEG, SLEEP ARCHITECTURE, AND SLEEP DURATION

Many aspects of sleep and sleep-wake regulation are highly variable among individuals yet highly stable within individuals. Uncovering genetic factors contributing to these trait-like individual differences in healthy human sleep constitutes one of the promising avenues to foster our understanding of the neurobiology of sleep in health and disease. This chapter summarizes the current evidence for genotype-dependent differences in timing, duration, and structure of sleep, as well as the sleep electroencephalogram (EEG) in healthy individuals. We also review how these differences may relate to the homeostatic and circadian regulation of sleep, yet we do not discuss here the sleep characteristics that differ between the sexes and ethnic groups.

The manifestation and regulation of sleep and the sleep EEG reflect different aspects of complex behaviors. Each of these aspects is likely to be under the control of multiple genes, which may interact and are also influenced by the environment and other factors such as age. In humans, our current knowledge about the genes that contribute to the trait-like, individual "circadian" and "sleep" phenotypes is still limited, although a considerable number of genes that contribute to circadian rhythmicity have been discovered in animals.

Different techniques for the genetic dissection of normal human sleep are currently available. The first is to examine the effect of candidate genes, for which evidence exists that they are implicated in sleep and sleep-wake regulation. With this method, individuals with distinct genotypes of known genetic polymorphisms are prospectively studied in the sleep laboratory. This approach precludes discovery of novel "sleep genes" but may help understand the consequences of these polymorphism for sleep-wake physiology. By contrast, studying familial pedigrees with extreme phenotypes and genome-wide association (GWA) studies can lead to the identification of novel "sleep genes" and the discovery of novel sleep-wake regulatory pathways. Family pedigrees can be highly informative in discovering rare mutations that are likely to be missed in GWA studies, which typically reveal genomic regions modifying subtle aspects of sleep-wake phenotypes in large population samples. Weaknesses and strengths of these strategies to advance the understanding of the genetics underlying normal sleep were recently discussed in detail.[1]

Large interindividual differences are observed in preferred time of day for completion of distinct cognitive tasks, sleep timing, sleep EEG, sleep structure, and sleep duration. For some of these variables the magnitude of interindividual differences exceeds by far the size of the effects of manipulations of sleep-wake regulatory processes, such as sleep deprivation.[2] Genes contribute to each of these phenotypes, and a moderate to high degree of heritability, that is the percentage of variance explained by overall genetic effects, has been demonstrated for these variables. In the following sections, we discuss genetic variants for which convergent evidence indicates that they contribute to genotype-dependent differences in diurnal preference or sleep timing, sleep EEG, as well as sleep structure and duration (summarized in Table 16.1).

GENES CONTRIBUTING TO HUMAN MORNINGNESS/EVENINGNESS AND TIMING OF SLEEP

Candidate Genes

The timing of the peaks and troughs of daytime alertness and the timing of nocturnal sleep (i.e., diurnal preference)

Table 16.1 Evidence for Genes to Contribute to Individual Differences in Diurnal and Sleep Phenotypes in Healthy Humans

Gene Family	Chromosomal Location	Gene	Diurnal Preference/ Sleep Timing	FASPS	Sleep EEG/ Sleep Architecture	Sleep Duration/ FNSS	Sleep Homeostasis
Clock mechanisms	4q12	*CLOCK*	░			░	
	17p13.1	*PER1*	■				
	2q37.3	*PER2*	■	■	░		░
	1p36.23	*PER3*	■	■	■		░
	1q25.3	*RGS16*	■				
	7q22.1	*FBXL13*	■				
	12p12.1	*BHLHE41*			■	■	░
Transcription factors	2q14.1	*PAX8*				■	
	2p16.1	*VRK2*				■	
	2p14	*MEIS1*				■	
	11p14.1	*BDNF*			░		░
Receptors	6p12.1	*HCRTR2*	■				
	7p14.3	*NPSR1*				■	
	10q25.3	*ADRB1*				■	
	11q23.2	*DRD2*				■	■
Transporter enzymes	5p15.33	*DAT1*				■	■
	1p31.1	*AK5*	■				
	20q13.11	*ADA*			■		░
	22q11.1	*COMT*			■		

Gene: National Center for Biotechnology Information (NCBI) gene symbol. *ADRB1*, Adrenoceptor beta 1; *AK5*, adenylate kinase 5; *BDNF*, brain-derived neurotrophic factor; *BHLHE41*, basic helix-loop-helix family member E41; *CLOCK*, circadian locomotor output cycles protein kaput; *DAT1*, dopamine transporter; *DRD2*, dopamine receptor D2; *FBXL13*, F-box and leucine-rich repeat protein 13; *HCRTR2*, hypocretin receptor 2; *MEIS1*, homeobox protein Meis1; *NPSR1*, neuropeptide S receptor 1; *PAX8*, paired-box gene 8; *PER1-3*, period circadian regulators 1 to 3; *RGS16*, regulator of G protein signaling 16; *VRK2*, vaccinia related kinase 2.
ADA, Adenosine deaminase; *COMT*, catecholamine *O*-methyl transferase; EEG, electroencephalogram; FASPS, familial advanced sleep phase syndrome; FNSS, familial natural short sleep.
■ Convergent evidence from multiple studies or genetic approaches.
░ Independent replication/confirmation missing or partly inconsistent findings.

are highly variable among healthy individuals.[3] Some of us go to sleep when others wake up. Self-rating scales such as the Horne-Östberg morningness-eveningness Questionnaire (MEQ) and the Munich Chronotype Questionnaire show normal distribution along an "eveningness–morningness" axis,[4-6] indicating the contribution of additive, small effects of multiple genes in combination with the environment. Studies in large numbers of monozygotic (MZ) and dizygotic (DZ) twin pairs and population- and family-based cohorts revealed roughly 50% heritability for diurnal preference[7] and 22% to 25% for habitual bedtime.[8]

Morningness/eveningness and timing of sleep are thought to be determined in part by characteristics of the central circadian oscillator, and associations between the intrinsic period and/or phase marker of this oscillator and diurnal preference have been reported.[9-12] These oscillators consist at the molecular level of a network of interlocked transcriptional/translational feedback loops, which involve several clock-related genes including the transcription regulators *CLOCK*, *BMAL1*, *PER1-3*, *CRY1-2*, and other genes. This knowledge has provided an obvious rational basis for the search for associations between these genes and morningness/eveningness and altered sleep timing.

The effect of a single-nucleotide polymorphism (SNP) in the 3′-untranslated region (UTR) of the human "Circadian locomotor output cycles kaput" gene (*CLOCK*) located on chromosome 4 on diurnal preference was first studied in middle-aged adults. This SNP may affect stability and half-life of messenger RNA,[13] and thus alter the protein level that is finally translated. Katzenberg and colleagues[14] reported that homozygous carriers of the 3111C allele have increased evening preference for mental activities and sleep, with delays ranging from 10 to 44 minutes compared with individuals carrying the 3111T allele. A similar association with diurnal preference was found in a Japanese population, and MEQ scores were significantly correlated with sleep onset time and wake time.[15] By contrast, studies in healthy European and Brazilian samples failed to confirm an association between genetic variation in *CLOCK* and diurnal preference.[16,17]

Mouse *Per1* and *Per2* are involved in maintaining circadian rhythmicity,[18] and possible associations between variation in these genes and diurnal preference were also investigated in humans. Screening for missense mutations and functional or synonymous polymorphisms in promoter, 5′- and 3′-UTR and coding regions of the period-1 gene (*PER1*) in volunteers with extreme diurnal preference and patients with delayed sleep phase syndrome (DSPS) remained initially unsuccessful. By contrast, the distribution of the C and T alleles of a silent polymorphism in exon 18 was found to differ between extreme morning and evening types.[19] More specifically, the frequency of the 2434C allele was roughly double in subjects with extreme morning preference (24%) compared with subjects with extreme evening preference (12%). This polymorphism may be linked to another functional polymorphism or directly affect *PER1* expression at the translational level.[19] In a candidate gene association study with replication, a polymorphism in *PER1* (single-nucleotide polymorphism identification number: rs7221412) was found to be associated with sleep timing based on actigraphy.[20]

A missense mutation in the human period-2 gene (*PER2*) currently provides the most striking example of a direct link between genetic variation in a clock gene and changed circadian rhythms. Linkage analyses in families afflicted with familial advanced sleep phase syndrome (FASPS) revealed associations with functional polymorphisms of *PER2* that cause altered amino acid sequences within the casein kinase 1 delta/epsilon (CK1δ/ε) binding region of PER2, which is thought to play an important role in phosphorylation of the protein and the stability of the molecular clock.[21-23] The subsequent engineering of a transgenic mouse model expressing the human FASPS mutation provided further evidence that PER2 is an important part of the molecular machinery regulating circadian rhythm in humans.[24] In accordance with this notion, a C111G polymorphism located in the 5′-UTR of *PER2* modulates diurnal preference in healthy volunteers.[25] The 111G allele is more prevalent in subjects with extreme morning preference (14%) than in individuals with extreme evening preference (3%). Computer simulation predicted that the 111G allele has a different secondary RNA structure than the 111C allele and that the two transcripts may be differently translated.[25]

Although findings in mice suggest that Per3 primarily has functions outside the central circadian clock,[18,26] association studies have linked different variants of the human period-3 gene (*PER3*) to diurnal preference. First, a variable-number-tandem-repeat (VNTR) polymorphism was found to modulate morning and evening preference. More specifically, a 54-nucleotide sequence located in a coding region of this gene on human chromosome 1 is either repeated in four or five units. This difference may alter the dynamics in PER3 protein phosphorylation. The longer five-repeat allele was repeatedly associated with morning preference, and the shorter four-repeat allele with evening preference.[27] More recently, SNP rs228697 of *PER3*, which is associated with a proline to alanine amino acid substitution, was reported to be associated with diurnal preference in a sample of 925 healthy Japanese controls.[28] Thus the major C allele was more prevalent in morning types and the minor G allele was more common in evening types. In addition, in 966 young adults in Britain, a significant association between SNP rs10462020 of *PER3* and diurnal preference was reported such that G/G individuals had an increased morning preference compared with T/G and T/T individuals.[29] In this study also an association between a polymorphism (rs922270) in *BMAL* (*ARNTL2*) and diurnal preference was found. Finally, two rare missense variants in *PER3* (rs150812083 and rs139315125) were identified in a family afflicted by FASPS.[30] When engineered into transgenic mice, these polymorphisms delayed the phase and lengthened the period in circadian wheel-running rhythms. Findings at the molecular level suggested that these variants decrease PER3 protein stability and reduce the stabilizing effect of PER3 on PER1 and PER2.[30]

Genome-Wide Association Studies

In the Framingham Heart Study 100K Project,[8] phenotypic and genetic analyses were conducted in 749 subjects and revealed a heritability estimate for habitual bedtime of 22%. Although such a low sample size provides only limited power for a GWA study, this early work suggested that the nonsynonymous polymorphism rs324981 of the gene *NPSR1* (neuropeptide S receptor 1) modulates questionnaire-derived usual bedtime. This polymorphism is located in a coding region of *NPSR1* and leads to a gain-of-function mutation that strongly increases the sensitivity of the receptor protein for its ligand, neuropeptide S (NPS).[31] Although further analyses of a larger sample of the Framingham Offspring Cohort and an independent candidate gene study employing actigraphy-derived sleep estimates in 393 older participants[32] did not confirm the prior result, more recent work indicates that human sleep patterns are indeed influenced by the NPS system. Nevertheless, sleep duration rather than bedtime appears to be affected by functional genetic variation of *NPSR1* (see later).[32,33]

Multiple GWA studies in large samples were recently conducted and more than 350 genetic loci were suggested to associate with variations in chronotype. Collectively, these studies suggest that the chronotype loci affect sleep timing but not the quality and duration of sleep.[34,35] Some of the chronotype associated loci include variants in the genes *PER2* and *PER3*, already known from family studies to be causative in familial advanced or delayed sleep phase. By contrast, other variations such as *KC1δ* and *TIMELESS* suggested to cause familial sleep-wake phase disorders, were not identified through GWA studies. Although many loci have not been replicated in independent GWA cohorts, it is noteworthy that four large studies consistently identified loci near the genes coding for PER2, FBXL13 (F-box and leucine-rich repeat protein 13), RGS16 (regulator of G protein signaling 16), and AK5 proteins (adenylate kinase 5).[35-38] The genes *PER2*, *FBXL13*, and *RGS16* have known roles in the circadian system. In addition, polymorphisms in the gene encoding hypocretin receptor type-2 (*HCRTR2*) were consistently found in three GWA studies to associate with morning chronotype.[34,36,37] It is well established that the hypocretin system plays an important role in regulating sleep-wake states and causes narcolepsy when it is deficient.

THE SLEEP EEG IS AMONG THE MOST HERITABLE TRAITS IN HUMANS

Studies relying on quantitative measures of amplitude and prevalence of EEG oscillations with distinct frequencies strongly suggest that the waking and sleep EEG are highly heritable traits in humans. All-night sleep EEG spectra derived from multiple recordings in healthy individuals show large interindividual variation and high intraindividual stability.[39] Buckelmüller and colleagues[40] recorded in eight young men two pairs of baseline nights separated by 4 weeks. Although the spectra in non–rapid eye movement (NREM) sleep differed largely among the individuals, the absolute power values and the shape of each subject's spectra were impressively

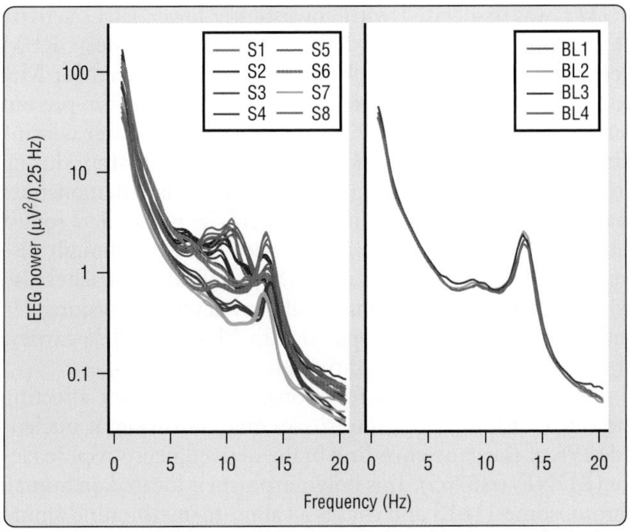

Figure 16.1 High *inter*individual variation *(left)* and high *intra*individual stability *(right)* in all-night electroencephalogram (EEG) power spectra in NREM sleep in 32 baseline nights of eight young men (S1–S8). The largest interindividual variation is observed in theta, alpha, and sigma frequencies (~5–15 Hz). The spectra of all 4 baseline nights (BL1–BL4) of one individual (S8) are virtually superimposable. (Adapted and modified from Buckelmüller J, Landolt HP, Stassen HH, Achermann P. Trait-like individual differences in the human sleep electroencephalogram. *Neuroscience*. 2006;138:351-6.)

constant across all nights (Figure 16.1). The largest differences among the subjects were present in the theta, alpha, and sigma (~5–15 Hz) ranges. Hierarchical cluster analysis of Euclidean distances based on spectral values as feature vectors demonstrated that all four nights of each individual segregated into the same single cluster.[40] Similar results were obtained in rapid eye movement (REM) sleep, and by other researchers in men and women of older age.[39] These data strongly suggest that the sleep EEG contains systematic and stable interindividual differences, which are at least in part genetically determined.

This notion is further supported by twin studies investigating the heritability of the sleep EEG. Ambrosius and colleagues[41] quantified the sleep EEG profiles in 35 pairs of MZ twins (17 male pairs, 18 female pairs; age range: 17–43 years) and 14 pairs of DZ twins (7 male pairs, 7 female pairs; age range: 18–26 years). Stable and robust interindividual differences in a broad range of the NREM sleep EEG were observed. Furthermore, intraclass correlation coefficients (ICCs) of spectral power were significantly higher in MZ twins than in DZ twins.[41] The ICC reflects within-pair similarity of twin pairs. In frequencies between 0.75 and 13.75 Hz, the ICC equaled roughly 0.8 in MZ twins and roughly 0.6 in DZ twins. The differences between MC and DC twin pairs appeared most pronounced in theta and alpha (4.75–11.75 Hz) frequencies.

De Gennaro and colleagues[42] also conducted a twin study to test the hypothesis that the EEG in NREM sleep reflects a genetically determined, individual "fingerprint." They recorded baseline and recovery sleep after sleep deprivation in 10 MZ and 10 DZ twin pairs (mean age: 24.6 ± 2.4 years; 5 male and 5 female pairs in each group) and observed highest variability in the 8 to 16 Hz range. In this frequency band, group similarity as quantified by an ICC procedure was more than double in MZ pairs (ICC = 0.934; 95% confidence intervals: 0.911–0.965) than in DZ pairs (ICC = 0.459; 95% confidence intervals: 0.371–0.546). This difference suggested 95.9% heritability independently of sleep pressure.[42] As such, the sleep EEG qualifies as one of the most heritable traits known so far, matched only by heritability estimates for distinct brain characteristics such as cortical gray matter distribution.[43] It is likely that trait characteristics of rhythmic brain oscillations during sleep, for example, sleep spindles, and distinct neuroanatomic features are interrelated.[43a]

In conclusion, striking evidence suggests that the sleep EEG is a highly heritable trait, yet the underlying genetic determinants remain largely unknown. Collectively, the findings demonstrate that genetic variation of various cells, molecules, and signaling pathways can profoundly modulate sleep EEG and other sleep phenotypes. Although a coherent picture on the core genes regulating specific aspects of the sleep EEG has not yet emerged, the effects of allelic variants within selected genes and pathways that have been replicated in independent studies will be briefly discussed in the following paragraphs.

GENES CONTRIBUTING TO THE SLEEP EEG

Circadian Clock Genes

A wealth of studies in genetically modified mice and flies demonstrates that circadian clock genes are strong determinants of major characteristics of the sleep EEG.[43] The aforementioned VNTR polymorphism of *PER3* (rs57875989) is the most intensively studied "clock gene" variant in healthy humans.[27] Apart from its effect on diurnal preference, this polymorphism also modulates the sleep EEG in NREM sleep, as well as in REM sleep. Compared with individuals with the *PER3*$^{4/4}$ genotype, young adult homozygous carriers of the long-repeat allele (*PER3*$^{5/5}$ genotype) exhibited higher EEG activity in the delta range (1–2 Hz) in NREM sleep and in the theta/alpha range (7–10 Hz) in REM sleep.[44] Partly similar observations were made in healthy older individuals between 55 and 75 years of age.[45]

Variants in other clock associated genes, rs6753456 located in the upstream promoter region of *PER2* and missense mutation c.1086C>T (p.Tyr362His) of *BHLHE41* (basic helix-loop-helix family member e41; formerly known as *DEC2*), were also proposed to associate with altered delta frequency activity in NREM sleep and EEG response to sleep deprivation.[46,47] These findings support the mutual interdependence between the circadian system and sleep homeostasis at the genetic level (see Genetic Basis of Sleep-Wake Regulation: Interaction Between Circadian and Homoestatic Systems).

Adenosinergic Neuromodulation

The neuromodulator adenosine is released in activity-dependent manner, and genes encoding adenosine-metabolizing enzymes and adenosine receptors are thought to play a major role in regulating the quality of sleep and wakefulness in animals and humans.[48,49] Adenosine kinase and adenosine deaminase (ADA) importantly contribute to the regulation of extracellular adenosine levels.[50] Genetic studies in mice suggest that both enzymes are involved in sleep-wake homeostasis.[51,52] In humans, the *ADA* gene is located on chromosome 20q13.11 and encodes two electrophoretic variants of ADA, referred to as ADA*1 and ADA*2 (rs73598374). The ADA*2 variant results from a guanine-to-adenine transition at nucleotide 22, which is translated into an asparagine-to-aspartic acid amino acid substitution at codon 8 (D8N). The heterozygous ADA*1-2 (G/A) genotype shows reduced catalytic activity of ADA compared with homozygous individuals carrying the ADA*1 (G/G genotype) variant. Rétey and colleagues[53] observed that this polymorphism affects the spectral composition of the sleep EEG. More specifically, EEG delta activity in NREM sleep (0.25–5.5 Hz) and REM sleep (2.0–2.25 and 3.5–4.75 Hz) was higher in the G/A genotype than in the G/G genotype. Inspired by studies in inbred mice showing that the genomic region encoding *Ada* modifies the rate at which sleep need accumulates during wakefulness,[51] it was then examined whether individuals with G/A and G/G genotypes respond differently to sleep deprivation. In accordance with the original study, delta (0.75–1.5 Hz) activity in NREM sleep was elevated in the G/A genotype compared with the G/G genotype in both baseline and recovery nights.[54] The genotype-dependent EEG alterations, however, were not restricted to the low-delta range in NREM sleep, but also included a pronounced increase in theta/alpha frequencies (~6–12 Hz) in NREM sleep, REM sleep, and wakefulness. Importantly, an independent study in a large epidemiologic sample confirmed that A-allele carriers have higher delta power in NREM sleep and increased theta power in NREM and REM sleep compared with homozygous G/G genotype carriers.[55]

Adenosine contributes to sleep-wake regulation by binding to high-affinity A_1 and A_{2A} receptors, which are differently expressed in different brain areas.[49] No study yet has investigated the possible effects of variants of the A_1 receptor gene on the human sleep EEG. By contrast, a small study suggested that the common variation rs5751876 of the adenosine A_{2A} receptor gene (*ADORA2A*) located on chromosome 22q11.2 affects the EEG in NREM and REM sleep. This polymorphism is linked to a 2592C>T_{ins} polymorphism in the 3′-UTR of *ADORA2A* and may modulate receptor protein expression. In a case-control study, Rétey and colleagues observed that EEG activity in the approximately 7- to 10-Hz range was invariably higher in all vigilance states in subjects with the C/C genotype of rs5751876 than in subjects with the T/T genotype.[53] Although not relying on polysomnographic (PSG) measures, larger studies confirmed an effect of rs5751876 on sleep quality, suggesting increased time awake (as estimated from wrist-actigraphy) and more frequent sleep complaints in C allele homozygotes compared with T allele carriers.[56,57]

Signaling Pathways

Accumulating evidence suggests a previously unrecognized, important contribution of dopaminergic neurotransmission to sleep-wake regulation. Cerebral dopaminergic signaling in humans is controlled primarily by the dopamine transporter (DAT) in the striatum and by catecholamine *O*-methyl transferase (COMT) in the prefrontal cortex. The COMT enzyme plays a major role in the metabolic degradation of brain catecholamines, including dopamine. The gene encoding COMT is located on human chromosome 22q11.2, in proximity to *ADORA2A*. Human *COMT* contains a common functional 544G>A variation that alters the amino acid sequence of COMT protein at codon 158 from valine (Val) to methionine (Met).[58] Individuals homozygous for the Val allele show higher COMT activity and lower dopaminergic signaling in prefrontal cortex than Met/Met homozygotes.[59,60] Sleep variables and the sleep EEG response to extended wakefulness do not differ between male carriers of Val/Val and Met/Met genotypes.[61-63] By contrast, the Val158Met polymorphism of *COMT* was associated with consistently lower EEG activity in the upper-alpha (11–13 Hz) range in NREM sleep, REM sleep, and wakefulness in Val/Val compared with Met/Met homozygotes.[64] The difference in NREM sleep was present before and after sleep deprivation and persisted after administration of the wake-promoting compound modafinil during prolonged wakefulness (Figure 16.2). These data demonstrate that a functional variation of the *COMT* gene predicts robust interindividual differences in the sleep EEG. Although discrepant reports with different methodological approaches also exist,[65] reduced alpha/sigma oscillatory activity in waking[66,67] and sleep[63] in Val/Val compared with Met/Met allele carriers of *COMT* rs4680 were confirmed in recent studies.

Another example of a functional genetic variant affecting the sleep EEG is a guanine-to-adenine transition at nucleotide 196 of the gene encoding brain-derived neurotrophic factor (BDNF) (rs6265). This polymorphism is located on human chromosome 11p13 and causes a valine-to-methionine amino acid substitution at codon 66 of the pro-BDNF sequence. In vitro studies suggest that the presence of a Met allele reduces intracellular trafficking and activity-dependent secretion of mature BDNF protein.[68] This polymorphism is typically associated with reduced performance on cognitive tasks that are also affected by sleep deprivation. Sleep and the sleep EEG were first investigated in case-control fashion in 11 carriers of the Val/Met genotype and 11 prospectively matched Val/Val homozygotes. It was found that the Val66Met polymorphism of *BDNF* not only reduced response accuracy on a verbal 2-back working memory task but also modulated the spectral composition of the EEG in frequency- and vigilance state–specific manner.[69] In baseline and recovery nights after sleep deprivation, EEG delta, theta, and alpha activity was lower in NREM and REM sleep in Met allele carriers compared with Val/Val homozygotes. Although the effect size of the genotype-dependent differences was probably overestimated in the small first study, the effect of *BDNF* rs6265 on brain alpha oscillations was since corroborated in a large and ethnically diverse population-based epidemiologic sample during sleep[70] and in more than 100 surgical patients during desflurane-induced general anesthesia.[71] Further supporting and extending these findings, BDNF Met allele carriers appear to be more vulnerable to the effects of sleep deprivation, such that these individuals take longer than the Val/Val genotype when inhibiting a prepotent response on an executive function task, particularly during the biologic night[72] (Figure 16.3).

GENES CONTRIBUTING TO SLEEP ARCHITECTURE

Many PSG-based variables characterizing sleep architecture demonstrate large variation among individuals and high stability within individuals.[2,40] For example, the ICC coefficients to estimate the intraindividual stability of a given sleep variable across different conditions, that is baseline versus sleep deprivation, was reported to be 0.73 for slow wave sleep (SWS) and 0.48 for REM sleep.[2] This observation suggests the presence of trait-like, interindividual differences in physiologic sleep variables, apart from the EEG. These variables may also have a genetic basis. Indeed, twin studies show striking similarity and concordance in visually defined sleep variables in MZ twins, yet not in DZ twins. Already the first PSG sleep studies in MZ twins revealed almost complete concordance in the temporal sequence of sleep stages.[73] Subsequent work showed

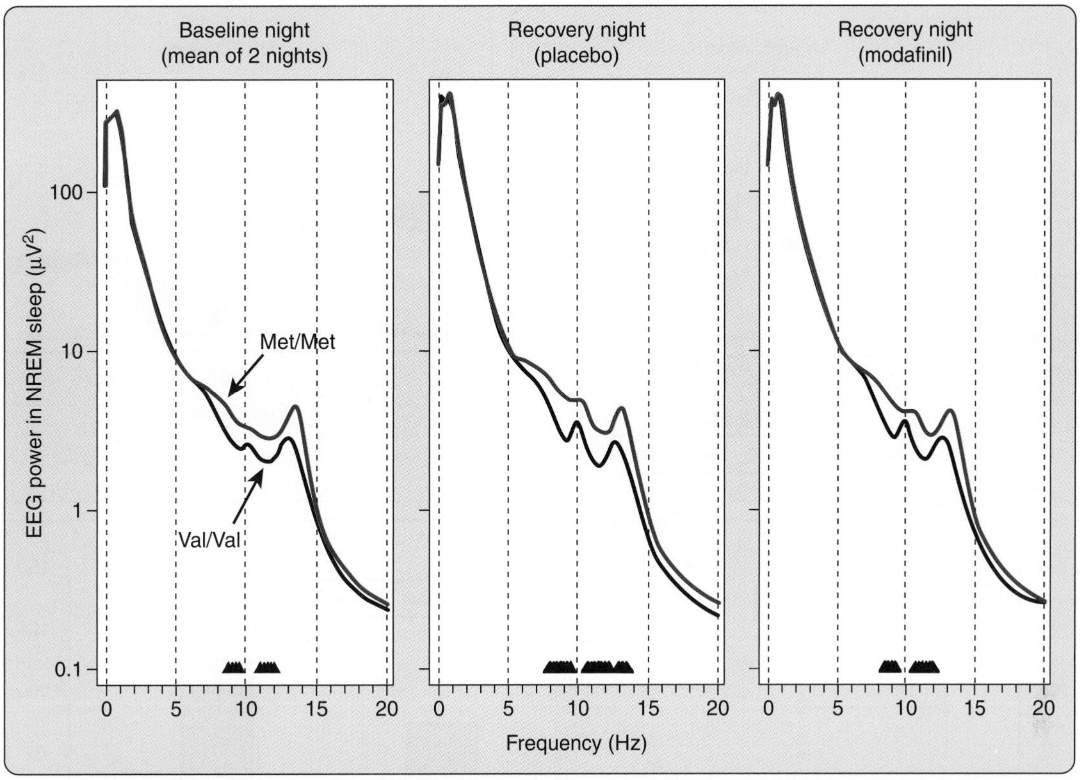

Figure 16.2 The Val158Met polymorphism (rs4680) of the gene-encoding catecholamine O-methyl transferase (COMT) modulates electroencephalogram (EEG) alpha activity in NREM sleep (all-night power spectra of stages 2–4). *Black triangles* at the bottom of the panels indicate frequency bins, which differ significantly between Val/Val ($n = 10$, *black lines*) and Met/Met ($n = 12$, *red lines*) genotypes ($P < .05$, unpaired, two-tailed *t*-tests). The frequency-specific effect of the genetic variation is robust against the effects of prolonged wakefulness and the stimulant modafinil. (Data replotted from Bodenmann S, Rusterholz T, Durr R, et al. The functional Val158Met Polymorphism of COMT Predicts interindividual differences in brain alpha oscillations in young men. *J Neurosci.* 2009;29:10855-62.)

that particularly those variables that most reliably reflect sleep need are under tight genetic control. Apart from total sleep time, these variables include the duration of NREM sleep stages, especially SWS, and the density of rapid eye movements in REM sleep.[74-76] Linkowski[75] estimated that heritability of markers of sleep homeostasis is up to 90% (REM density). Nevertheless, quantifying the heritability of the sleep homeostatic process will require quantification of the change in these putative markers of sleep homeostasis in response to sleep deprivation. Such experiments have been conducted in mice,[51] but not yet in humans. Interestingly, accumulating deficits on a psychomotor vigilance task during an extended wakefulness resulted in a broad sense heritability estimate of approximately 0.83%.[77]

Slow Wave Sleep

A few studies have conducted PSG assessments in defined genotypes. Young homozygous carriers of the long-repeat, *PER3*$^{5/5}$ allele of *PER3* were found to fall asleep more rapidly and have more SWS (particularly stage 4 sleep) compared with homozygous four-repeat individuals.[44,78] A difference in SWS, albeit less pronounced, was also observed in older people.[45]

Not only genetic variation in *PER3*, but also the polymorphism rs6753456 of *PER2* may modulate SWS in healthy humans. Although no confirmation is currently available, carriers of the variant allele may exhibit 20 minutes less SWS than noncarriers.[47] Other visually scored sleep variables did not differ between the genotypes.

Referring to polymorphism rs73598374 of *ADA*, healthy carriers of the ADA*2 allele (G/A genotype) consistently showed more SWS than subjects with the G/G genotype.[53,54] All other sleep variables were similar in both *ADA* genotypes.

Finally, the effect of the rs6265 (Val66Met) polymorphism of *BDNF* on the sleep EEG also had a counterpart in sleep architecture. In baseline and recovery nights, Val/Val allele carriers spent roughly 20 minutes more time in deep stage 4 sleep than the Val/Met genotypes. By contrast, superficial stage 2 sleep was reduced compared with the Met allele carriers.[69]

Taken together, functional variation in the genes encoding *PER3*, *PER2*, *ADA*, and *BDNF* not only modulate the spectral characteristics of the sleep EEG but also sleep architecture.

Genome-Wide Association Studies

Because of the prohibitively high time and cost investments required to conduct GWA studies of classic EEG- and PSG-derived sleep phenotypes in large human samples under controlled conditions, no such studies are currently available.

GENES CONTRIBUTING TO HABITUAL SLEEP DURATION

Habitual sleep duration shows large variation among healthy individuals, and the physiologic sleep and circadian determinants of habitual short and long sleepers have been studied in small groups of individuals. The temporal profiles of nocturnal melatonin and cortisol levels, body temperature, and sleepiness

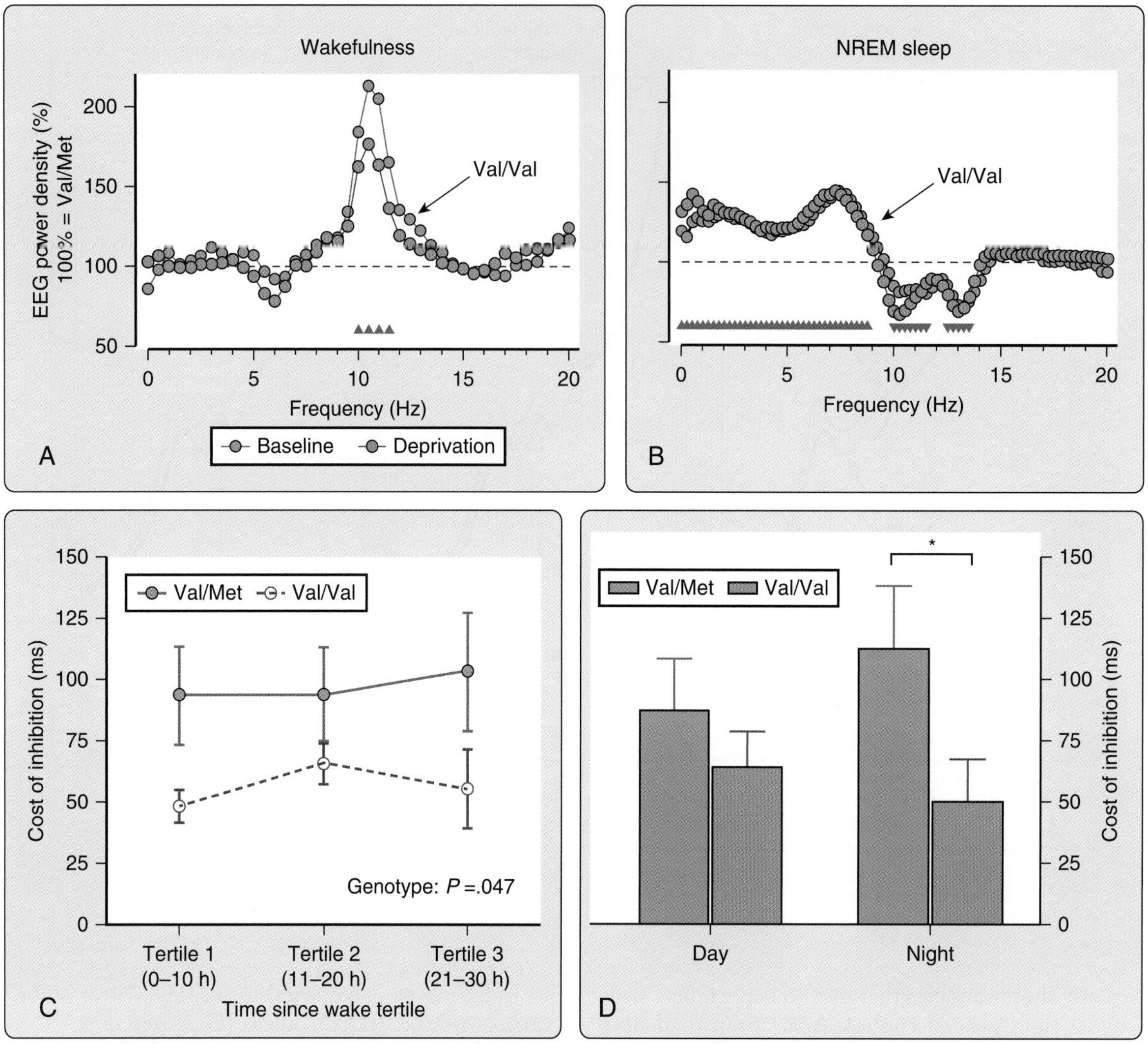

Figure 16.3 The Val66Met polymorphism (rs6265) of the gene-encoding, brain-derived neurotrophic factor (BDNF) affects the EEG in wakefulness and NREM sleep in state-specific manner, as well as cognitive performance during sleep deprivation. **(A** and **B)** Absolute power values in individuals carrying the Val/Val genotype (n = 11) were expressed as a percentage of the corresponding value of individuals with the Val/Met genotype (n = 11; *horizontal dashed lines* at 100%). Wakefulness: Relative electroencephalogram (EEG) power spectra in wakefulness on day 1 (baseline) and day 2 (deprivation). NREM sleep: Relative EEG power spectra in baseline and recovery nights. *Triangles* at the bottom of the panels indicate frequency bins in which power differed significantly between Val/Val and Val/Met genotypes. **(C)** Inhibition score on the Stroop Color Naming Task in Val/Val (n = 18) and Val/Met (n = 12) genotypes for each tertile of 30 hours of extended wakefulness. **(D)** During the biologic night, the Val/Met genotype responded slower when inhibiting a prepotent response then the Val/Val genotype (* $P < .03$). (**C,** Data replotted from Bachmann V, Klein C, Bodenmann S, et al. The BDNF Val66Met polymorphism modulates sleep intensity: EEG frequency- and state-specificity. *Sleep.* 2012;35:335–44. **D,** Data replotted from Grant LK, Cain SW, Chang AM, Saxena R, Czeisler CA, Anderson C. Impaired cognitive flexibility during sleep deprivation among carriers of the brain derived neurotrophic factor [BDNF Val66Met allele. *Behav Brain Res.* 2018;338:51-5.)

under constant environmental conditions and in the absence of sleep suggest that the circadian pacemaker programs a longer biologic night in long sleepers than in short sleepers.[79] Individual differences in this program may contribute to the large variation in habitual sleep duration, which shows a normal distribution in large populations.[6] Such a distribution is consistent with the presence and influence of multiple, low-penetrance polymorphisms. Indeed, there are currently no known genes in either animals or humans for which a loss-of-function mutation precludes any sleep.[1] Twin and GWA studies reported a moderate heritability estimate of 38% (95% confidence intervals: 16%, 56%) for sleep duration. The high heterogeneity of the estimates suggests that important moderators such as participants' age and environmental factors affect the heritability of sleep duration.[80]

Circadian Clock Genes

A first candidate gene study investigated possible associations between sleep duration as assessed with the Munich Chronotype Questionnaire and 194 clock gene variants in a European population (n = 283).[81] One *CLOCK* variant located on chromosome 4, rs12649507, significantly associated with self-reported sleep duration in the original discovery sample, in a replication sample (n = 1011), as well as in the meta-analysis of the two populations ($P < .009$). PSG data collected in three large independent cohorts of European ancestry providing greater than 99% power to confirm the original observation, revealed no support for a significant association of *CLOCK* variants with sleep duration.[82] Interestingly, however, evidence from almost 15,000 participants in nine European cohorts indicated that rs12649507 may modify the relationships between short sleep duration and obesity by affecting polyunsaturated fatty acid intake.[83]

Familial natural short sleep (FNSS) has been defined as a stable trait among physiologic short sleepers requiring only 4 to 6.5 hours of sleep per night without symptoms of daytime sleepiness or cognitive impairments.[84] A candidate gene study in such a rare family revealed that a point mutation in exon 5 of the gene *BHLHE41* leads to reduced sleep duration.[85] Due to this missense mutation (c.1151C>G), proline is replaced by arginine at amino acid position 384 (p.Pro384Arg), which reduces the activity of the transcriptional repressor, BHLHE41.[86] Reduced activity of this transcription factor increases expression of the wakefulness-promoting neuropeptides hypocretin 1 and 2. Confirming the causal role of this variant in regulating sleep length, knocking-in the human mutation into mice and *Drosophila* reduced sleep duration in the transgenic animals.[85] Based on this original study, other variants of the *BHLHE41* gene were searched for by DNA sequencing in two larger cohorts ($n = 417$) of healthy volunteers and two other rare variants in the same exon of *BHLHE41* were found.[46] The phenotypic data reported in three carriers of the nonsynonymous variant c.1151C>A (p.Pro384Gln) and in one DZ twin pair discordant for the functional c.1086C>T (p.Tyr362His) polymorphism suggested that variants that alter the suppression of *CLOCK/BMAL1* activation lead to short sleep, whereas a polymorphism that does not affect this suppression has no effect on sleep duration.[46]

Neurotransmitter Receptors and Transporters

Another causative mutation in an FNSS family was recently identified in the gene encoding the adrenergic β_1 receptor (*ADRB1*).[87] This receptor is highly expressed in brain regions such as the dorsal pons that are active in wakefulness and REM sleep. Activation of *ADRB1* positive neurons can lead to wakefulness, and neuronal activity is affected by the identified mutation. The mutation decreases protein stability and reduces the potency of receptor agonists in vitro. Engineering the human variant into mice lead to short sleep behavior of the mutated animals, albeit less pronounced compared with the human phenotype.[87]

As mentioned previously in this chapter, a genetic association study suggested that the gain-of-function mutation rs324981 (N107I) of the *NPSR1* gene reduced habitual sleep length.[32] More specifically, homozygous carriers of the minor T allele exhibited slightly shorter (~20 min) actigraphy-derived sleep than A/A allele carriers. Intriguingly, a mutation (Y206H) in the same gene was recently identified in another FNSS family to cause a much stronger phenotype (>2 hours shorter sleep).[33] The N107 and Y206 residues are both located at the extracellular domains of the G protein–coupled NPS receptor and may increase ligand affinity or agonist efficacy.[31,33] Interestingly, introduction of a homologous Y206H mutation into mice produced a short sleep phenotype similar to human FNSS.[33] These convergent data support the conclusion that mutations that increase the sensitivity of NPS activation cause a short sleep trait in affected individuals.

The effect of 27 common SNPs from 20 different candidate genes on self-reported habitual sleep duration was recently evaluated in two large European cohorts.[88] All SNPs were suggested in previous studies to associate with various sleep phenotypes. They included a common VNTR polymorphism (rs28363170) of the gene *DAT1* (also known as *SLC6A3* [solute carrier family 6 member 3]) encoding the DAT. This polymorphism affects *DAT1* expression[89] and DAT availability in the human striatum.[90] In an exploratory study, this polymorphism was previously associated with subjective sleepiness yet not with actigraphy-based sleep duration.[91] Rhodes and colleagues[88] confirmed the lack of association with sleep length. Nevertheless, these authors found a strong link between another variant of *DAT1*, rs464049, and self-reported sleep duration in 111,975 middle-aged individuals.[88] This finding was successfully replicated in a follow-up study of an additional 261,870 participants in the UK Biobank. These consistent results support a role for DAT in sleep-wake regulation that is consistent with various animal models.

Further evidence for a link between the striatal dopamine system and sleep-wake regulation comes from two variants of the *DRD2* gene encoding the dopamine D_2 receptor. More specifically, the rs17601612 and rs11214607 polymorphisms appear to strongly associate with reported sleep duration.[88] The same two variants were already linked to sleep duration in a prior GWA study in 25,000 individuals of different ethnic descents (see Genome-Wide Association Studies). Although each minor allele of the *DAT1* and *DRD2* polymorphisms conferred only a 1-minute change in reported sleep duration, the findings were statistically highly consistent. They could indicate that variants of these genes slightly modulate the intrinsic need for sleep or the functional consequences of sleep deprivation. Indeed, although focusing on other *DAT1* (rs28363170) and *DRD2* (rs6277) polymorphisms, controlled laboratory experiments confirmed that functional variation in these genomic regions can alter the neurophysiologic and behavioral consequences of prolonged wakefulness.[92-95] Biologic follow-up studies of these associations are warranted to reveal novel insights into the molecular processes underlying sleep-wake regulation in humans.

Genome-Wide Association Studies

In accordance with this notion, Cade and colleagues[96] investigated the effects of approximately 50,000 SNPs on self-reported habitual sleep length in 25,000 individuals of different ethnic descents and identified the polymorphisms rs17601612 and rs11214607 of *DRD2* to influence sleep duration. These findings corroborate a role for the dopamine D_2 receptor in sleep-wake regulation. They support the conclusion that genetic loci enriched in pathways, including striatal development and dopamine signaling, associate with accelerometer-based sleep duration.[34]

Recent GWA studies of self-reported sleep duration analyzed data of increasingly large samples, some of which including far more than 100,000 individuals.[34,35] In the largest cohort so far, consisting of more than 446,000 participants in the UK Biobank, 78 genome-wide significant loci associated with self-reported habitual sleep length.[35] Although these loci explained only 0.7% of the variance and each affected allele exerted an average change of only approximately 1 minute in sleep duration, the 5% participants carrying the most sleep duration increasing alleles reported approximately 22 minutes longer sleep duration compared with the 5% carrying the fewest.[35] This effect size is comparable to other common factors recognized to influence sleep duration.

The strongest associations with self-reported sleep duration included variants at or near the *PAX8* (paired box gene 8) and *VRK2* (vaccinia related kinase 2) genes on human chromosome 2. These associations are consistent with previous work in smaller samples of European ancestry.[38,97] PAX8 is a thyroid-specific transcription factor and VRK2 is a serine/threonine kinase important in several signal transduction cascades. Importantly, the effect of these genomic regions for habitual sleep length was confirmed in smaller (sub)samples of participants by objective estimates of sleep duration with motion-detecting actigraphy devices.[35,98]

An additional genomic locus on chromosome 2 that was consistently found to contribute to self-reported and accelerometer-based estimates of sleep duration includes the gene encoding MEIS1 (homeobox protein Meis1).[35,98] This protein acts as a transcriptional regulator for nervous system development and medium spiny neuron activity in the striatum. Interestingly, the *MEIS1* locus had already emerged from the first human GWA study of sleep, as a risk locus for restless legs syndrome (RLS).[99] The overlap between sleep duration and sleep-related movements may reflect the use of a sleep measuring device relying on motor activity, shared etiology, or pleiotropy of the *MEIS1* gene effects. Pleiotropy is very common between sleep and neurologic phenotypes.[100]

GENETIC BASIS OF SLEEP-WAKE REGULATION: INTERACTION BETWEEN CIRCADIAN AND HOMEOSTATIC SYSTEMS

Many of the traits and genes described previously in this chapter concern sleep-wake characteristics as assessed under baseline conditions. How these alterations in sleep characteristics relate to sleep-wake regulation and how they may lead to functional consequences remains largely unexplored. The available data, however, already indicate that the effects cross boundaries between sleep and wakefulness, and homeostatic and circadian aspects of sleep-wake regulation. For example, polymorphisms of *PER3*, *ADA*, and *DAT1* genes affect the EEG in NREM sleep, REM sleep, and wakefulness. To investigate whether these changes reflect changes in EEG generating mechanisms with or without a relation to sleep regulatory processes requires these processes to be challenged, for example, by sleep deprivation. Although it was previously demonstrated that individuals differ in their behavioral response to sleep loss and that this vulnerability is a trait-like, heritable characteristic,[77] the degree of heritability of neurophysiologic markers of sleep homeostasis in humans is unknown.

Circadian Clock Genes

Comparing the effects of sleep deprivation to $PER3^{4/4}$ individuals revealed that the increase in theta activity in the EEG during wakefulness was more rapid in carriers of the $PER3^{5/5}$ genotype.[44] In addition, in recovery sleep after total sleep deprivation, REM sleep was reduced in $PER3^{5/5}$ individuals. Finally, some data suggested that the increase in slow wave energy after sleep restriction was slightly higher in adults carrying the $PER3^{5/5}$ genotype than in $PER3^{4/5}$ and $PER3^{4/4}$ allele carriers,[101] and also the decline of cognitive performance during prolonged wakefulness and after sleep restriction differed as a function of the *PER3* genotype.[102-104] The differential susceptibility to the negative effects of sleep loss on waking performance was particularly pronounced in the second half of the circadian night and on tasks of executive functioning.[102] One interpretation of these data is that the VNTR polymorphism in *PER3* affects the dynamics of the homeostatic process, which then through its interaction with the circadian regulation of performance leads to differential sleep ability and vulnerability to the negative effects of sleep loss.[102,105] The data suggest a contribution of *PER3* to individual tolerance to shift work and jetlag, which become more and more prevalent in society.

A 6-hour sleep deprivation in mice carrying the Pro384Arg mutation of *BHLHE41* resulted in a smaller rebound in both NREM sleep and REM sleep and a smaller relative increase in EEG delta power compared with control mice.[85] A functional variant (c.1086C>T) at another locus of the same exon was studied in a DZ twin pair. The carrier of the variant allele produced fewer lapses of attention during prolonged waking and exhibited less recovery sleep than the no-variant carrier, suggesting that BHLHE41 functioning contributes to the homeostatic regulation of sleep.[46] In a functional assay in vitro, the variant reduced the ability of BHLHE41 to suppress CLOCK/BMAL1 and NPAS2/BMAL1 transactivation.

Adenosinergic Neuromodulation

Based on the observation that a genomic region including *Ada* modifies the rate at which NREM sleep need accumulates in mice,[51] it was investigated in humans whether carriers of G/A and G/G genotypes of *ADA* respond differently to sleep deprivation.[54,106] Bachmann and colleagues systematically studied attention, learning, memory, executive functioning, and self-reported sleep duration in 245 healthy adults. The heterozygous carriers of the variant allele (G/A genotype, $n = 29$) performed significantly worse on the d2 attention task than the G/G homozygotes ($n = 191$). To test whether this difference reflected elevated sleep pressure, sleep and sleep EEG before and after sleep deprivation were recorded in two prospectively matched groups of 11 G/A and 11 G/G genotypes. Corroborating two independent earlier studies,[53,55] EEG delta activity and slow wave sleep were higher in G/A than in G/G genotype. In addition, sustained attention (d2 and psychomotor vigilance tasks) and vigor were reduced, while EEG alpha oscillations in waking, as well as sleepiness, fatigue, and α-amylase activity in saliva (a proposed biomarker of sleep drive), were increased throughout prolonged wakefulness.[54] These convergent behavioral, neurophysiologic, subjective, and biochemical data demonstrated that genetically reduced ADA activity is associated with elevated sleep pressure. By contrast, the dynamics of the homeostatic response to sleep deprivation were not affected by *ADA* genotype.[54,106] Thus the data suggest an elevated level in overt NREM sleep propensity in the G/A genotype compared with G/G homozygotes, which may be due to elevated adenosinergic tone at the synapse because of genetically reduced ADA activity.

Dopaminergic Neuromodulation

Consistent with an important role for striatal dopaminergic neurotransmission in sleep homeostasis, the sleep deprivation–induced increase in SWS; EEG delta activity; and number, amplitude, and slope of low-frequency (0.5–2.0 Hz) oscillations in NREM sleep was larger in the homozygous 10R/10R genotype than in 9R allele carriers of the functional 3′-UTR VNTR polymorphism of the gene *DAT1* (*SLC6A3*).[92] Given that the 10R allele homozygotes have 15% to 20 % reduced DAT availability compared with 9R allele carriers,[90] the human data nicely converge with evidence from transgenic animals.[107,108] They indicate that the homeostatic response to sleep deprivation is more pronounced in 10R/10R than in 9R allele carriers of *DAT1*. In addition, the functional c.957C>T polymorphism of *DRD2* modulate both EEG and distinct behavioral markers of elevated sleep need and the effects of caffeine and modafinil on these markers.[93,95] The consistent findings support the notion that striatal medium spiny neurons, which coexpress high densities of adenosine A_{2A} and dopamine D_2 receptors, mediate the consequences of sleep loss. These neurons have major projections to the ventral pallidum and may contribute to sleep-wake regulation by modulating the ascending arousal pathways and the thalamus. Systematic human pharmacogenetic dissection of adenosinergic-dopaminergic signaling pathways in regulating markers of sleep need support this conclusion.[109]

CONCLUSION

Sleep and wakefulness are complex behaviors, and so are the genetic influences on sleep and sleep-related functions. Polymorphic variations in many genes were suggested to affect several characteristics of sleep, yet only a few genes were replicated in multiple studies. The genes for which evidence across different genetic approaches and successful independent replication is available are highlighted in this overview. The most consistent genes include circadian clock mechanisms (*PER1-3*, *RGS16*, *FBXL13*) that modulate diurnal preference and sleep timing, as well as different transcription regulators encoded by chromosome 2 (*PAX8*, *VRK2*, *MEIS1*) that contribute to the large interindividual variance in habitual sleep duration. Although some of the evolving genetic systems and pathways have established roles in regulating circadian clock functions (e.g., *PER2*) and sleep-wake mechanisms (e.g., adenosinergic neurotransmission), the effect of other genetic variants (e.g., *DAT1*, *DRD2*) advanced our understanding of individual differences in normal sleep-wake behavior.

For most genetic loci, much more work is needed to elucidate the biologic pathways relevant for the observed variation in circadian and/or sleep phenotypes. For example, it is unlikely, or will be very rare, that a causal link between a single gene variant and sleep-related phenotypes will be identified. Furthermore, it can be expected that the biologic work-up of genomic associations from GWA studies will not always lead to the closest gene as causative for the observed phenotype. Combined approaches, including intermediate phenotypes such as genome, transcriptome, proteome, metabolome, inflammasome, biome, and others, are necessary to follow the flow of information from the genome to the phenome. In animal studies of sleep regulation such systems genetic approaches were already implemented.[110] These approaches can reveal the interactions among sets of traits, networks of genes, and the developmental and environmental factors determining healthy sleep-wake phenotypes. In other words, groups of phenotypes (biologic systems) as emerging from a complex web of interacting networks and undergoing multiple genetic and environmental influences need to be simultaneously considered. These novel approaches challenge the simplified notion of causality as starting with the genotype. Public databases such as the UK Biobank and 23andMe are amassing incredible amounts and varieties of information. Nevertheless, to elucidate genetic, epigenetic, and environmental determinants of healthy sleep, new approaches are needed, in which the same individuals are followed through time and exhaustively characterized using the available -omics and deep sleep-wake phenotyping techniques, such as proposed for systems medicine.[111]

CLINICAL PEARL

The first "sleep" GWA study was a case-control study for the sleep-related disorder RLS,[99] which is clinically treated with dopamine D_2 receptor agonists. Functional follow-up studies, including the use of mouse models, demonstrated that the transcription factor homeobox protein Meis1 (MEIS1) confers an increased risk for RLS. In large cohorts of the general population, the genomic locus of *MEIS1* on chromosome 2 was consistently found to modulate self-reported and accelerometer-based estimates of sleep duration.[35,98] MEIS1 acts as a transcriptional regulator for nervous system development and medium spiny neuron activity in the striatum. Together with deep sleep-wake phenotyping in candidate-gene and pharmacogenetic studies in healthy humans,[109] the findings of these complementary genetic approaches now converge to support a new role for striatal dopaminergic mechanisms in regulating sleep-wake phenotypes in health and disease.

SUMMARY

Sleep is a very rich phenotype, and many aspects of sleep differ considerably in the population of healthy individuals (even when only a very narrow age range is considered). Interindividual variation in sleep timing (diurnal preference); sleep duration; sleep structure; and the EEG in NREM sleep, REM sleep, and wakefulness have all been shown to have a genetic basis. The response to challenges of sleep regulatory processes such as sleep deprivation and circadian misalignment has also been shown to vary between individuals. Some of the polymorphic variations in genes contributing to variation in sleep characteristics have now been identified. The most consistent variants include genes associated with circadian clock mechanisms (e.g., *CLOCK*, *PER1-3*, *BHLHE41*), adenosinergic (*ADA*) and monoaminergic (e.g., *DAT1*, *DRD2*, *ADRB1*) neurotransmission, as well as transcription-regulating pathways (e.g., *PAX8*, *VRK2*, *MEIS1*). For some of these genes, so far only associations with one aspect of sleep have been reported (e.g., *HCRTR2* and sleep timing). Variations in other genes have been shown to affect multiple aspects of sleep and wakefulness, as well as the response to sleep loss or pharmacologic interventions. For example, *PER3*, *ADA*, and *BDNF* affect the EEG and performance during prolonged waking, whereas *DAT1*, *DRD2*, and *ADORA2A* modulate EEG and response to stimulants such as caffeine and modafinil. Apart from a few genes identified in familial pedigrees with extreme phenotypes (e.g., *NPSR1* in a family with natural short sleep), the currently known polymorphic variations explain only a small part of the variation in healthy human sleep phenotypes. Deep phenotyping approaches covering the EEG in all three vigilance states, sleep structure, and homeostatic aspects of sleep-wake regulation will be needed to provide further insights into intertwined and widespread consequences of genetic variants for healthy human sleep.

ACKNOWLEDGMENTS

The authors' research has been supported by the Swiss National Science Foundation, the University Center of Competence Sleep & Health Zurich, the Clinical Research Priority Program "Sleep & Health" of the University of Zurich, the Zurich Center for Integrative Human Physiology, the Neuroscience Center Zurich, and several private foundations (to HPL), and Biotechnology and Biological Sciences Research Council, Wellcome Trust, the Airforce Office of Scientific Research, the Higher Education Funding Council for England and a Wolfson-Royal Society Award (to DJD).

SELECTED READINGS

Archer SN, Schmidt C, Vandewalle G, Dijk DJ. Phenotyping of PER3 variants reveals widespread effects on circadian preference, sleep regulation, and health. *Sleep Med Rev*. 2018;40:109–126.

Ashbrook LH, Krystal AD, Fu YH, Ptacek LJ. Genetics of the human circadian clock and sleep homeostat. *Neuropsychopharmacol*. 2020;45:45–54.

Elgart M, Redline S, Sofer T. Machine and deep learning in molecular and genetic aspects of sleep research. *Neurotherapeutics*. 2021;18(1):228–243.

Garfield V. Sleep duration: a review of genome-wide association studies (GWAS) in adults from 2007 to 2020. *Sleep Med Rev*. 2021;56:101413.

Jan M, O'Hara BF, Franken P. Recent advances in understanding the genetics of sleep. *F1000Research*. 2020;9.

Landolt HP, Holst SC, Valomon A. Clinical and experimental human sleep-wake pharmacogenetics. *Handb Exp Pharmacol*. 2019;253:207–241.

Madrid-Valero JJ, Rubio-Aparicio M, Gregory AM, Sanchez-Meca J, Ordonana JR. Twin studies of subjective sleep quality and sleep duration, and their behavioral correlates: systematic review and meta analysis of heritability estimates. *Neurosci Biobehav Rev*. 2020;109:78–89.

Price ND, Magis AT, Earls JC. A wellness study of 108 individuals using personal, dense, dynamic data clouds. *Nat Biotechnol*. 2017;35:747–756.

Satterfield BC, Stucky B, Landolt HP, Van Dongen HPA. Unraveling the genetic underpinnings of sleep deprivation-induced impairments in human cognition. *Prog Brain Res*. 2019;246:127–158.

Shi G, Wu D, Ptacek LJ, Fu YH. Human genetics and sleep behavior. *Curr Opin Neurobiol*. 2017;44:43–49.

Veatch OJ, Keenan BR, Gehrman PR, Malow BA, Pack AI. Pleiotropic genetic effects influencing sleep and neurological disorders. *Lancet Neurol*. 2017;16:158–170.

Wulff K, Porcheret K, Cussans E, Foster RG. *Curr Opin Genet Dev*. 2009;19:237–246.

A complete reference list can be found online at ExpertConsult.com.

Chapter 17

Genetics and Genomic Basis of Sleep Disorders in Humans

Allan I. Pack; Brendan T. Keenan; Philip R. Gehrman; Anne E. Justice

Chapter Highlights

- Genetic studies in humans, using constantly evolving methods, have led to the understanding that there are genetic risk factors for sleep disorders.
- Genome-wide association studies have shown that there are genetic determinants of variability in sleep duration, chronotype, and response to sleep deprivation.
- Genetic studies in narcolepsy show that human leukocyte antigen (HLA) variants confer increased risk and protection. In addition, variants in T-cell alpha receptors support the autoimmune basis of the disorder.
- Genetic studies of restless leg syndrome identify genes and novel pathways (e.g., *MEIS1* and *BTBD9*), whose roles must be identified.
- Genetic studies of sleep breathing disorders identify genes and novel pathways (e.g., *PHOX2B*, *LPAR1*, and *IL18R1*/*IL18RAP*).
- Variations in clock-associated genes affect not only timing of sleep but also sleep duration and response to sleep deprivation.

APPROACHES TO IDENTIFYING GENETIC VARIANTS IN HUMANS

The overwhelming majority of biologic traits and disorders in humans have a genetic component as part of their etiology. Many recent studies have shown that sleep and disorders of sleep are no exception. The role of genetic factors in human disease has been studied for decades, progressing from classical heritability and linkage studies to more focused candidate gene analyses, then to genome-wide analyses. Genome-wide analyses have been made possible by the sequencing of the human genome, which has led to scientific advances in array-based genotyping technologies and, more recently, whole exome and whole genome sequencing analyses, as well as typing of genome-wide epigenetic modifications. Using these technologies, biomedical research has made great progress in understanding the genetic architecture and molecular pathways underlying human disease.[1,2] However, there is still opportunity for further discoveries,[1,2] particularly for sleep disorders. Only a small number of validated genetic risk variants have been discovered for sleep-related traits. There are several reasons for this lack of discovery, including inadequate sample sizes, heterogeneity in phenotypes, and many pathways to disease. The appendix at the end of this chapter reviews the methodology used in genetics research. Understanding this methodology—in particular, the appropriate thresholds for statistical significance, importance of independent replication, and necessity of functional validation—is crucial for proper interpretation of the current genetic literature on sleep and sleep disorders. Thus the reader may want to review this appendix before embarking on the following sections, which describe current genetic evidence for specific sleep-related disorders and phenotypes.

GENETICS OF SLEEP DURATION

The duration of sleep in individuals varies substantially in the general population. In the Finnish population 14.5% of the population have a sleep duration less than 7 to 8 hours on average, whereas 13.5% have longer duration.[3] In the United States there is a much larger percentage of the population with short sleep, with around 35% sleeping less than 6 hours per night on average. Although much of this short sleep is behaviorally induced (e.g., secondary to commitments of modern life), there is also a genetic component. Classical twin studies analyzing the differences in sleep duration in monozygotic and dizygotic twins give heritability estimates of 31% to 44% for sleep duration.[4-6]

Common and rare variants associated with sleep duration have been described. A number of genome-wide association studies (GWAS) have been reported. An initial GWAS, based on the Framingham cohort, used a relatively small sample (n = 738) and evaluated 70,987 single nucleotide polymorphisms (SNPs). No genome-wide significant associations with sleep duration were identified. The most significant association was with sleepiness assessed by the Epworth Sleepiness Scale and an SNP in the intron of *PDE4D*, which encodes a cAMP-specific phosphodiesterase, a plausible biologic candidate.[7]

Another GWAS study with a larger number of subjects (n = 42,517; all of European ancestry) found a genome-wide significant association in the discovery phase[8] with an intronic variant in *ABCC9*. This gene encodes one of the 17 transmembrane domains of the pore-forming subunit of an adenosine triphosphate (ATP)–sensitive potassium channel (K_{ATP}). However, the association with this variant and sleep duration was not significant in the replication phase. Subsequent GWAS have also failed to demonstrate this association.[9,10]

Moreover, a study specifically designed to confirm the association described by Allebrandt and colleagues[8] failed to replicate this finding.[11] There was, however, a significant association with another variant in *ABCC9* and depression symptoms.[11]

Although it seems highly unlikely that this variant of *ABCC9* explains variation in sleep duration in human populations, Allebrandt and colleagues[8] did further examine the role of this gene in sleep-wake control. They used a *Drosophila* model expressing an RNAi in neurons to knock down the expression of a *Drosophila* homologue of the gene. The study revealed reduced sleep amounts at night in the *ABCC9* knockdowns, particularly in the early part of the night, but not during the day. Thus this channel likely does play a role in sleep-wake control, and further investigation is warranted.

A larger GWAS was reported from the CHARGE consortium.[10] The study used data from 18 community-based cohorts that had information on self-reported sleep duration and had genotyped their subjects (n = 47,180). This large sample size led to not only genome-wide significant associations but also, for the first time, associations that were replicated in independent samples. The most strongly associated locus that was found was located on chromosome 2 between two genes: *PAX8* (paired box protein Pax-8) and *CBWD2* (cobalamin synthase W domain-containing protein 2). *PAX8* has been replicated in other more recent GWAS.[12-14] *PAX8* is a transcription factor involved in thyroid development, but potentially more broadly. *CBWD* has unknown function but is widely expressed in brain. The initial association was found in individuals of European ancestry but was replicated in an independent sample of Blacks (n = 4771). The causative variant remains to be identified.

Additional GWAS have also recently been conducted to assess variants associated with sleep duration.[12-16] These are based on the highly productive UK Biobank. Two major approaches have been used. First, studies have used self-reported sleep duration from simple questionnaires.[12-15] Second, studies have examined objective phenotypes from accelerometers available in a subset of subjects.[14-16] Although accelerometry initially was planned to assess activity levels, studies comparing data from the accelerometer to full polysomnography (PSG) allowed an algorithm to be developed to estimate objectively sleep duration.[17] These GWAS have looked for associations with not only sleep duration but also other sleep traits, including excessive sleepiness. We describe the results for both later.

As described previously, self-report studies have consistently shown an association with a variant of *PAX8*.[12-14] This has been replicated in the UK Biobank and the CHARGE Consortium.[10] In addition to a role in thyroid development,[18] *PAX8* is expressed in many cancers.[19] The genes in which expression is altered by variants in *PAX8* with respect to sleep duration are unknown, and ultimately the effect of this variant on sleep duration is small. The other gene that has been consistently identified in studies of self-reported sleep duration is *VRK2* (*vaccinia-related kinase 2*).[12,14] Variants for this gene have also been associated with multiple psychiatric and neurologic disorders, including schizophrenia, major depressive illness, and genetic generalized epilepsy.[20]

Studies with accelerometer-defined sleep duration, not surprisingly, reveal a richer set of associated genes given the known problems with self-reported sleep duration. Heritability estimates of objectively measured sleep duration (19.0% [95% confidence interval, CI: 18.2% to 19.8%]) are higher than for self-reported sleep (8.8% [8.6%, 9.0%]).[16] Both GWAS of objectively measured sleep identified associations with variants in the *DPYD*, *LOC101928419*, *MEIS1*, and *PAX8* genes. Variants in other genes were identified in one of the studies,[15,16] including for *BTBD9* and *ANK1*. Given that both *MEIS1* and *BTBD9* are associated with restless legs syndrome (RLS; see later), it is conceivable that there is a considerable amount of unrecognized RLS in the subjects in the UK Biobank sample. This remains an open question.

Findings on genetic variants associated with sleep duration have led to development of a polygenic risk score (PRS), a single score that summarizes the estimated genetic risk of an individual for a trait.[21] Studies with the PRS were done in the large electronic health record (EHR) biobank in the Partners BioBank.[21] Data were available on self-report sleep duration and prevalence of specific diseases from the EHR. The PRS explained, however, only 1.4% of the phenotypic variance in sleep duration. On the other hand, the PRS was associated with congestive heart failure, obesity, hypertension, RLS, and insomnia.[21] Clearly, research has a long way to go, and it is unclear whether the identified genes are actually causal for specific conditions that result in short sleep.

GWAS of excessive sleepiness have also been conducted based on subjects in the UK Biobank.[22] These analyses are based on the response to a single question: how likely are you to doze off or fall asleep during the daytime when you do not mean to (e.g., when working, reading, or driving)? Forty-two variants were identified that associated with this phenotype. There was enrichment for genes that are expressed in brain tissue and in neuronal transmission pathways.[22] Not surprisingly, associations were attenuated at several loci after adjustment for the presence of known sleep disorders. There was some limited evidence of replication of individual associations in other cohort studies. A PRS was developed, but it did not replicate in two other cohorts.

These studies show the potential of the large-scale GWAS approach. However, to fully realize this potential there must be more in-depth assessment of phenotypes and better characterization of whether individuals have specific underlying sleep disorders. Wearable technologies that are rapidly being developed to assess sleep patterns and disorders have great potential in this regard. Collins and Varmus advocated use of wearables for phenotyping as part of the developing Precision Medicine Initiative in the United States.[23]

Rare variants affecting sleep duration have also been described.[24,25] The seminal study of He and colleagues[24] is based on only two subjects who slept from around 10:00 p.m. to 4:00 a.m. (i.e., 6 hours) without evidence of daytime impairment. He and colleagues sequenced all clock and clock-associated genes in these subjects. They found a mutation in exon 5 of *BHLEH41* (*class E basic helix-loop-helix protein 41*), also known as *DEC2*, at the amino acid position 384. The mutation results in a proline being replaced by an arginine at this locus. To assess the functional role of this variant, He and colleagues knocked this mutation into *Drosophila* and mice and showed it resulted in less sleep, that is, shortened sleep duration. Moreover, in mice with this mutation there was a marked reduction in recovery sleep after sleep deprivation compared with wild-type controls.

Given that genes that exhibit rare mutations with large effects may show multiple such mutations, that is, they are "hot spots," it is not unreasonable to suspect that other rare variants of *DEC2* may affect sleep duration and response to sleep loss. Pellegrino and colleagues[25] addressed this question and sequenced *DEC2* in two human samples, that is, a previous twin study[26] and a study of chronic partial sleep deprivation.[27] Two new mutations in *DEC2* were identified. One was at a different location in the same exon as that discovered by He and colleagues.[24] It also resulted in an amino acid change. This occurred in one member of a dizygotic twin pair. The twin with the mutation slept 2 hours less per day than the twin partner and had substantially fewer performance lapses during prolonged sleep deprivation. The other mutation was at the same site as that described by He and colleagues[24] and was found in three unrelated individuals in the cohort who had chronic partial sleep deprivation. There was, however, no obvious effect of this variant on sleep duration.

To further investigate why some variants of *DEC2* had effects on sleep duration while others did not, Pellegrino and colleagues knocked these different mutations into a cell-based system that used a PER2:luciferase reporter to assess rhythmic changes in expression of PER2.[25] Both the variant described by He and colleagues[24] and that in the twin (see previously) resulted in reduced ability of DEC2 to suppress CLOCK/BMAL1 transactivation; that is, they had clear functional consequences. In contrast, the mutation found in the three unrelated individuals had no such functional effect. This is likely the reason that there is no effect on sleep duration in these individuals. Random mutagenesis of exon 5 in *DEC2* found a number of other mutations that reduced the ability of DEC2 to suppress CLOCK/BMAL1 transactivation. Whether these mutations also occur in human populations remains to be determined. It seems likely, however, that other variants of *DEC2* will be identified that result in short sleep.

THE ROLE OF VARIABLE NUMBER OF TANDEM REPEATS

Perhaps the most studied gene variant with respect to its role in normal sleep-wake behavior is a 54-nucleotide variable number of tandem repeats (VNTR) in exon 18 of the *PER3* gene (see review by Dijk and Archer[28]). This polymorphism is found only in primates.[29,30] The number of repeats varies from 2 to 11 in different primate species.[30] Humans can be homozygous for four ($PER3^{4/4}$) or five ($PER3^{5/5}$) repeats, or heterozygous ($PER3^{4/5}$). In populations of European ancestry, about 10% are $PER3^{5/5}$, 50% are $PER3^{4/4}$, and 40% $PER3^{4/5}$ heterozygotes.[31] In New Guinea, the prevalence of these different genotypes is reversed.[31] Thus this is a common polymorphism with likely a small effect, and large samples with independent replications are needed to be sure of a real associations. Studies in this area have, however, had very small sample sizes, around 20 individuals. Power has been increased by selectively recruiting individuals based on genotype, thereby enriching the sample studied for the less common $PER3^{5/5}$ genotype. Even with this, the studies remain underpowered. This issue of power likely contributes to the varying results in the literature. Moreover, this polymorphism has been associated with a large number of different phenotypes (Table 17.1), further inflating the likelihood of finding spurious associations.

The initial claim for this polymorphism was related to diurnal preference. The $PER3^{5/5}$ genotype was found to be

Table 17.1 Positive Associations Reported in Humans for the Tandem Repeat Polymorphism in *PER3*

Phenotype	Reference
Diurnal preference	Archer SN, Robilliard DL, Skene DJ, et al. A length polymorphism in the circadian clock gene Per3 is linked to delayed sleep phase syndrome and extreme diurnal preference. *Sleep.* 2003;26:413–5.
Changes in EEG spectra during extended wakefulness	Viola AU, Archer SN, James LM, et al. PER3 polymorphism predicts sleep structure and waking performance. *Curr Biol.* 2007;17:613–8.
Changes in cognitive performance during extended wakefulness	Groeger JA, Viola AU, Lo JC, et al. Early morning executive functioning during sleep deprivation is compromised by a PERIOD3 polymorphism. *Sleep.* 2008;31:1159–67.
Sympathovagal heart rate balance during baseline and recovery sleep	Viola AU, James LM, Archer SN, et al. PER3 polymorphism and cardiac autonomic control: effects of sleep debt and circadian phase. *Am J Physiol Heart Circ Physiol.* 2008;295:H2156–163.
Changes in fMRI assessed brain response to an executive task in a period without sleep	Vandewalle G, Archer SN, Wuillaume C, et al. Functional magnetic resonance imaging-assessed brain responses during an executive task depend on interaction of sleep homeostasis, circadian phase, and PER3 genotype. *J Neurosci.* 2009;29:7948–56.
Alerting response to light	Chellappa SL, Viola AU, Schmidt C, et al. Human melatonin and alerting response to blue-enriched light depend on a polymorphism in the clock gene PER3. *J Clin Endocrinol Metab.* 2012;97:E433–7.
Suppression of melatonin secretion with blue light	Chellappa SL, Viola AU, Schmidt C, et al. Human melatonin and alerting response to blue-enriched light depend on a polymorphism in the clock gene PER3. *J Clin Endocrinol Metab.* 2012;97:E433–7.
Insomnia severity in alcohol dependence	Brower KJ, Wojnar M, Sliwerska E, et al. PER3 polymorphism and insomnia severity in alcohol dependence. *Sleep.* 2012;35:571–7.
Salivary cortisol secretion	Wirth M, Burch J, Violanti J, et al. Association of the Period3 clock gene length polymorphism with salivary cortisol secretion among police officers. *Neuro Endocrinol Lett.* 2013;34:27–37.
Sleep ability	Maire M, Reichert CF, Gabel V, et al. Sleep ability mediates individual differences in the vulnerability to sleep loss: evidence from a PER3 polymorphism. *Cortex.* 2014;52:47–59.

of higher prevalence in morning types and very low in individuals with delayed sleep phase syndrome.[32] The strength of the association with diurnal preference attenuates with age.[33] The association with diurnal preference, but not delayed sleep phase, was replicated in Brazil.[34] Association with diurnal preference has also been found in South Africa,[35] but not in Colombia[36] nor in Norway.[37] The latter negative study cannot be attributed to age because it was conducted in Norwegian university students.

Following these initial observations, a more in-depth phenotyping study was done in a small sample of $PER3^{5/5}$ homozygotes (n = 10) and $PER3^{4/4}$ homozygotes (n = 14).[38] No difference was found in circadian behavior, including the timing of the onset of melatonin secretion. Instead, the major differences between genotypes were in sleep and wake behavior, particularly during sleep deprivation. Compared to those with the $PER3^{4/4}$ genotype, individuals with the $PER3^{5/5}$ genotype showed larger rise in theta power during constant wakefulness and worse performance on a battery of tests during extended wakefulness. The $PER3^{5/5}$ homozygotes performed particularly poorly during the biologic night. Moreover, those with $PER3^{5/5}$ had stronger inhibition of rapid eye movement (REM) sleep during recovery sleep after sleep deprivation. A subsequent report highlighted that the PER3 polymorphism affects the impact of sleep deprivation on performance in the early morning hours.[39] There are, however, again negative studies (see work by Kuna and colleagues,[26] Barclay and Ellis,[40] and Goel and colleagues[41]). The best direct evidence that this VNTR polymorphism in *PER3* directly affects sleep homeostasis comes from elegant studies in mice.[42] Hasan and colleagues[42] created mice on a C57BL/6 background, in which they knocked in the humanized $PER3^{4/4}$ or $PER3^{5/5}$. The phenotypes of these mice were assessed and compared with wild-type. There was no difference in baseline sleep-wake or circadian behavior. There was, however, a difference in the response to sleep deprivation. The increase in EEG delta power, a measure of sleep homeostasis, with sleep loss was greater in the $PER^{5/5}$ mice compared with the other genotypes, and these mice more fully compensated for the effects of sleep deprivation. Changes in gene expression with sleep loss in cortex and hypothalamus were also different between genotypes.

These results in mice are compatible with the positive human studies. Ultimately, translation of these findings to humans will require much larger samples, replication data, and careful phenotyping. Currently, the jury is still out as to the importance of this polymorphism in the human population.

CHRONOTYPE AND CIRCADIAN RHYTHM SLEEP DISORDERS

Chronotype and circadian rhythm sleep disorders (CRSDs) would be logical candidates for genetic studies given the tremendous success in identifying the components of the molecular circadian clock intrinsic to all cells. The molecular circadian clock consists of an autoregulatory negative feedback loop involving the *Period (PER1, PER2,* and *PER3*) and *Cryptochrome* (*CRY1* and *CRY2*) genes.[43] Other genes involved in the molecular generation of circadian rhythms include *casein kinase 1δ* and *1ε* (*CK1δ* and *CK1ε*), *CLOCK, NPAS1, NPAS2, DEC2, BMAL1,* and *BMAL2*. With respect to chronotype, several twin and family studies have estimated the heritability of the broader trait of morningness and eveningness, rather than examining CRSDs. Most of these studies assessed chronotype with the Horne-Ostberg Morningness-Eveningness Questionnaire (MEQ).[44] Using twin data, the heritability of chronotype was estimated to be 54% in the United States[45] and 44% in the Netherlands.[46] Family-based studies of Hutterites[47] and in the Amazon[48] estimated lower heritability, with h^2 estimates of 14% and 23%, respectively. Taken together, results suggest that chronotype is a moderately heritable trait, with genetic factors potentially explaining as high as 50% of the variability within populations. The heritability of CRSDs is currently unknown.

There have been a few reports of extended families with high rates of CRSDs, primarily advanced sleep phase syndrome (ASPS). In the first such report, three family members with very strong advanced sleep phase based on clinical history and objective markers were found to have a shorter intrinsic period of their endogenous rhythm.[49] In other families, it has been possible to identify specific genetic variants that segregate with ASPS. A serine to glycine mutation in the casein kinase epsilon binding region of *PER2* was reported in one study,[50] although there was no evidence of this mutation in two ASPS pedigrees in Japan. In another pedigree, a missense mutation in the *CKIδ* gene was identified as the causal variant.[51] Of note in this study, the gene was studied in transgenic *Drosophila* and mice, with the model systems showing opposing phenotypes of longer and shorter circadian period, respectively. This demonstrates the power of using model systems in combination with human studies to better isolate causal variants and their mechanisms of action.

Several studies have used a candidate gene approach and examined the association between circadian genes and either chronotype or CRSDs. Studies have examined the association between eveningness and the 3111C allele of the *CLOCK* gene, with some,[52,53] but not all,[54-56] finding a significant association. Morningness has been found to be associated with polymorphisms in the clock genes, *PER1* and *PER2*, in other studies.[57,58] Associations have been found between delayed sleep phase syndrome and the PER3 VNTR polymorphism[32,34,59] (for further discussion, see earlier) and 3111C allele of the *CLOCK* gene.[52] Lastly, polymorphisms in the *PER3* and *ARNTL2* genes were associated with chronotype in a sample of 966 British adults.[60] The results of these studies are therefore mixed, which is likely due to the relatively small sample sizes (n < 450). However, the overall patterns suggest that, not surprisingly, circadian genes play an important role in the determination of chronotype. Too few studies have been conducted in CRSDs to draw any firm conclusions.

Recently, there have been three separate GWAS to assess gene variants associated with chronotype[61-63] (see the review by Kalmbach and colleagues[64]). These GWAS were based on limited questionnaire data from either the 23andMe cohort or the UK Biobank. 23andMe is a commercial program for individuals interested in their own genotype data, whereas the UK Biobank is a large enterprise funded by the Wellcome Foundation. Data from the UK Biobank are made available to interested investigators. There are differences between studies in how they defined chronotype and analysis procedures. As a result, the two studies from the UK Biobank do not report identical results.[62,63] The questionnaires were not full chronotype instruments, such as the Horne-Ostberg,[44] but rather individuals typically were asked to define whether they believed they are a morning person, night person, or neither.

Despite the lack of depth in phenotype information, a large number of genome-wide significant associations were identified. All 3 GWAS reported associations with chronotype for *PER2*, *RGS16*, *FBXL3*, and *AK5*. Two of these genes—*PER2* and *RGS16*—are known to play a role in the circadian clock. Five additional genes were shown to be associated in two of the three studies, including *HCRTR2*, which encodes the hypocretin (orexin) receptor 2; *HTR6*, the receptor 6 for serotonin; *TNRC6B*, a gene that belongs to a family of genes involved in microRNA gene silencing; *APH1A*, which encodes for a subunit of the V-secretion complex that clears the amyloid-β system protein; and *ERC2*, which encodes for a member of a family of proteins that regulates neurotransmitter release. Another 19 loci were identified in only one of the three studies (see the table in the article by Kalmbach and colleagues[64]).

GENETICS OF INSOMNIA

There are few studies on the genetics of insomnia. In part, this may reflect uncertainty as to the appropriate phenotype. Insomnia as a clinical diagnosis is defined as difficulty initiating or maintaining sleep that is associated with significant distress or daytime consequences. As such, a phenotype for genetic studies could rely on self-reported insomnia symptoms on a questionnaire such as the Insomnia Severity Index.[65] Alternatively, phenotypes could be based on quantitative parameters such as sleep latency or wakefulness after sleep onset from sleep diaries. Another approach would be to use objective assessment of sleep using actigraphy or PSG to generate quantitative parameters. There is intuitive appeal to using objective assessment given that it avoids the cognitive biases associated with self-reports and considering that EEG-based parameters are some of the most heritable traits that have been measured.[66] A limitation of the objective assessment of insomnia is that there is often a discrepancy between these measures and self-reports of sleep in patients with insomnia. Subjects with insomnia complaints who are short sleepers have worse outcomes than those with insomnia but normal sleep duration,[67] suggesting the importance of considering both objective and subjective data.

A number of family and twin studies using self-reported measures of insomnia traits have demonstrated moderate heritability. In one of the only studies of childhood-onset insomnia, Hauri and colleagues found that patients whose insomnia began in childhood reported a positive family history of sleep complaints at a higher rate (55%) than those with adult-onset insomnia (39%).[68] In a larger cohort study[69] there was no significant difference in positive family history of insomnia in those categorized as good sleepers and those having symptoms of insomnia or meeting criteria for a full insomnia syndrome (32.7%, 36.7%, and 38.1%, respectively). Significant differences were found only when the good sleepers were separated into those with and without a personal history of insomnia, where those without a personal history had a significantly lower rate of family history (29.0%) than those with a past history (48.9%). Several twin studies have examined the heritability of insomnia-related traits such as sleep latency and sleep quality. A study conducted in the Australian twin registry of 1792 monozygotic and 2101 dizygotic twin pairs included several questions related to sleep quality, disturbance, and overall patterns.[4] Additive genetic influences were found for sleep quality ($h^2 = 0.32$), initial insomnia ($h^2 = 0.32$), sleep latency ($h^2 = 0.44$ for men and 0.32 for women), "anxious insomnia" ($h^2 = 0.36$), and "depressed insomnia" ($h^2 = 0.33$). In a study of twin pairs from the Vietnam Era Twin Registry,[70] similar heritability estimates were observed for trouble falling asleep ($h^2 = 0.28$), trouble staying asleep ($h^2 = 0.42$), waking up several times per night ($h^2 = 0.26$), waking up feeling tired and worn out ($h^2 = 0.21$), and a composite sleep score ($h^2 = 0.28$). Thus data suggest self-reported insomnia traits are moderately heritable, with 30% to 40% of the variance attributable to additive genetic factors.

There are three recent GWAS looking for associations with insomnia.[13,71,72] In these studies, insomnia is defined based on limited questionnaire data. All studies are based on the UK Biobank,[13,71,72] with one study also including data from 23andMe.[72] In the UK Biobank sample, the identification of insomnia was based on a single question about trouble sleeping and how frequently this occurred.

The largest study in the UK Biobank only[71] identified 57 loci using data from 453,379 individuals. However, these 57 associations explained only 1% of phenotypic variance. Association with *MEIS1* was identified, confirming the result of an earlier study using the UK Biobank data in a much smaller sample.[13] Replication of the finding with *MEIS1* was found with independent samples from the HUNT population study and from a case (physician-diagnosed insomnia) cohort study using data from the Partners Biobank. A PRS was developed and was associated with insomnia in the HUNT study and in the Partners Biobank. The associations were, however, not strong (ORs of 1.015 and 1.017, respectively).

The largest genetic study of insomnia[72] was based on the UK Biobank ($n = 386{,}533$) and 23andMe ($n = 944{,}477$). Thus the study included more than 1.0 million subjects (1,331,010). In total, 202 loci that could be mapped to 956 genes were identified. However, with these extensive data, only 2.6% of the variance was explained. This, in part, reflects the high statistical power to detect very small (and perhaps clinically nonsignificant) effects with such a large sample. Among those genes implicated in this study, both *MEIS1* and *BTBDP9* were found to be associated, perhaps reflecting previously identified associations with RLS (see later in this section).

Investigators in this study[72] also examined where in the brain the implicated genes were expressed using data from available expression databases. Four brain regions showed significant enrichment for genes identified in the analysis: overall central cortex, Broadman area 9 of the frontal cortex, anterior cingulate cortex, and the cerebellar hemisphere. Whether neurons in these brain regions play an important role in insomnia remains to be determined.

There is an overlap between genes associated with insomnia and psychiatric traits.[72] The strongest correlations were with depression symptoms followed by anxiety disorder, major depression, and neuroticism. It is unclear as to the basis of this correlation but worth noting that insomnia is a risk factor for other neuropsychiatric conditions, such as depression. Alternatively, this correlation may be explained by pleiotropy, that is, the same gene variant leads directly to an increased risk of insomnia and other neuropsychiatric disorders. It is likely that genetic pleiotropy explains the higher rate of sleep abnormalities in a number of neurologic and psychiatric conditions.[73]

It is remarkable how much progress has been made given the relative lack of in-depth phenotypic information; studies have essentially relied on the response to a single question.

This is, however, only a beginning. We need to determine whether these population-based approaches can be extrapolated to subjects with insomnia who present clinically. There is a need for complimentary strategies based on actual patients with the disorder and for more in-depth phenotyping. We know that insomnia is a heterogeneous disorder.[67] Thus the issue of genetic heterogeneity must be addressed, that is, are there subsets of subjects with different phenotypic profiles and unique patterns of genetic risk.

GENETICS OF NARCOLEPSY

It has been known since 1984, following a study in Japan, that narcolepsy is associated with specific HLA antigens.[74] HLA antigens are expressed in immune cells and are involved in presenting foreign peptides to receptors on T cells. In Japanese and those of European descent, the risk allele for narcolepsy is *DQB1*0602*, which occurs on a haplotype with *DQA1*0102*.[75] There are differences in Blacks,[76] where the DQB1 alleles are found with distinct DRB1 haplotypes—*DRB1*1503*, *DRB1*1501*, *DRB1*1101* and *DRB1*0806*.[77,78] The association between *DQB1*0602* and narcolepsy is particularly strong in cases of narcolepsy with cataplexy, compared to cases without cataplexy.[79] Data from the European Narcolepsy study showed a very high association in multiple European countries between narcolepsy with cataplexy and *DQB1*0602*, with a large aggregate odds ratio (OR) of 251 (Table 17.2).[80] This may be the result of a clearer definition of cases.

There are also protective HLA class II haplotypes for narcolepsy.[81] These were demonstrated in a GWAS in European individuals with a case-control design and in an independent replication sample. After identification of a protective variant near *HLA-DQA2*, analysis revealed that cases almost never carried a trans-*DRB1*1301-DQB1*0603* haplotype (OR = 0.02, $P < 6 \times 10^{-14}$). The magnitude of these effects is such that studying HLA antigen profiles in suspected cases of narcolepsy could have clinical utility. This remains to be assessed.

Although it is clear that the presence of specific *HLA-DQB1** alleles confer substantial risk or protection for narcolepsy with cataplexy,[80,81] Ollila and colleagues presented the idea that HLA typing of *HLA-DQA1**, in addition to *HLA-DQB1**, to better characterize the specific haplotypes and possible heterodimers, may be an important next step in understanding this relationship.[82] They propose an allele competition model, in which the risk conferred by specific *DQB1** alleles is modified based on the specific *DQA1** alleles present, because of the differences in binding affinity between specific *DQA1** and *DQB1** alleles. For example, although patients homozygous for the *DQA1*01:02~DQB1*06:02* haplotype have the highest risk of narcolepsy, patients with only one *DQA1*01:02~DQB1*06:02* haplotype may have either moderately increased risk (OR = 1.0 – 1.5) if they have *DQA1*01:02* and a *DQB1*05/06* allele that is not *DQB1*06:02* at the other chromosome, or be protected from narcolepsy (OR = 0.5) if they carry a *DQA1*01* allele that is not *DQA1*01:02* on the other chromosome. Although preliminary data support these assertions, the validity of the allele competition model hypothesis has been questioned.[83] Regardless, it remains clear that HLA-DQ alleles are strongly associated with narcolepsy.

Although there is a very strong association between narcolepsy with cataplexy and *DQB1*0602*, this is also a common variant in many individuals without narcolepsy. The frequency varies by ancestry, with 12% of Japanese and 38% of Blacks carrying the variant.[75] Thus having this variant, even if homozygous, is not sufficient to develop narcolepsy. There are two possible explanations. First, narcolepsy could be a complex disorder with multiple associated gene variants other than *DQB1*0602*. Second, the presence of *DQB1*0602* could make individuals more susceptible to as yet largely unidentified environmental causes. These are not mutually exclusive possibilities.

To address the former, Hallmayer and colleagues performed an innovative GWAS (Figure 17.1).[84] They assembled multiple cohorts of cases with narcolepsy and cataplexy of different ethnicities. All individuals were positive for *DQB1*0602*. This design removes the *DQB1*0602* effect, which would overwhelm other signals, allowing other potential gene variants to be identified. With this strategy they identified three significantly associated SNPs within the T-cell receptor alpha (*TRCA*) locus. The highest association had an OR of 1.87 ($P = 1.9 \times 10^{-12}$). These associations were replicated in independent White samples and Asians from Japan and Korea. There was a similar, nonsignificant trend in the Black sample. This may be an issue of sample size, since this was the smallest sample studied. This association has already been replicated in other studies—in the European narcolepsy study[80] and in China.[85]

Table 17.2 Association in European Countries with DQB1*0602 in Cases with Narcolepsy and Cataplexy

Country (case, control)	Case-DQB1+ N (%)	Control-DQB1+ N (%)	OR	*P*
DE (232, 296)	227 (97.84)	72 (24.3.2)	141.24	9.71E-26
CH (66, 473)	65 (98.48)	102 (21.56)	236.42	7.01E-8
NL (323,469)	318 (98.45)	114 (24.31)	198.05	3.62E-30
PL (63, 197)	63 (100)	44 (22.33)	438.08	2.65E-09
FR (341, 499)	335 (98.24)	94 (18.84)	240.56	1.18R-37
IT (66, 433)	64 (96.97)	30 (6.93)	429.87	3.21E-16
Mantel-Haenszel (meta-analysis)	1,198 (98.36)	626 (17.68)	251.12	1.04-120

CH, Switzerland; DE, Germany; FR, France; IT, Italy; NL, Netherlands; PL, Poland; OR, odds ratio.
The frequency of DQB1*0602 in cases and controls with OR for increased risk and the *P* value for the association are shown.
From Tafti M, Hor H, Dauvilliers Y, et al. DQB1 locus alone explains most of the risk and protection in narcolepsy with cataplexy in Europe. *Sleep*. 2014;37(1):19–25, with permission.

This association with the *TRCA* locus was also replicated in a study using an "immune-chip" to evaluate variants relevant to the immune system.[86] This study also identified two other associations, one in *cathepsin H* and one in *tumor necrosis factor (ligand) super-family member 4* (*TNFSF4*). This led the author to propose that antigen presentation to T-cell receptor is a key part of the pathogenesis of narcolepsy (Figure 17.2).

Another GWAS study in narcolepsy with cataplexy has identified a SNP in the 3′ untranslated region of the *purinergic receptor subtype P2Y$_{11}$* gene (*P2RY11*).[87] The variant has an OR of 1.28 (95% CI = 1.19 to 1.39; $P = 6.1 \times 10^{-10}$). It seems that this variant may also play a role in the immune system.

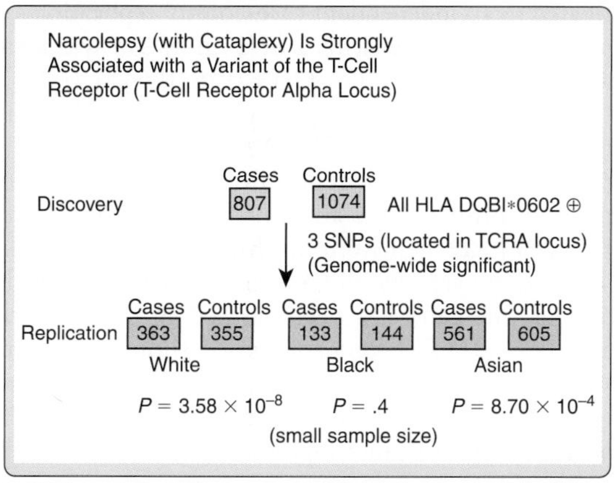

Figure 17.1 Design of the genome-wide association study in narcolepsy with cataplexy that identified the role of variants in the T-cell receptor alpha locus. All cases and controls in the study were positive for HLA DQB1*0602. There was an initial discovery phase followed by three replication samples in different ethnic groups. The variants were found replicated in Whites and Asians, but not in Blacks. There was, however, a much smaller sample of Blacks that may explain this failure to replicate. (From Hallmayer J, Faraco J, Lin L, et al. Narcolepsy is strongly associated with the T-cell alpha receptor locus. *Nat Genet.* 2009;41:708–11.)

The variant is associated with substantial reduced expression of P2RY11 in CD^{4+} T lymphocytes and natural killer cells. Thus narcolepsy is a complex disorder, but all variants recognized as of this writing are likely to affect the immune system. This has led to a strengthening of the idea that narcolepsy is a very specific autoimmune disorder.

As in other areas, there are also rare variants with large effects that can lead to narcolepsy. These typically align with syndromes that include narcolepsy. One syndrome is autosomal dominant cerebellar ataxia, deafness, and narcolepsy. Symptoms typically develop at 30 to 40 years of age. Narcolepsy and deafness typically appear before ataxia. Exome sequencing in three individuals identified rare mutations in the *DNA methyltransferase gene* (*DNMT1*).[88] This enzyme is responsible for maintaining methylation patterns in development. It is expressed in immune cells and is required for the differentiation of CD^{4+} cells into T regulatory cells. Another variant of this gene was described in a single Brazilian patient.[89]

Another rare variant in *myelin oligodendrocyte glycoprotein* (*MOG*) in a family with narcolepsy and cataplexy has been described.[90] This discovery was based on a linkage study of a single large family with 12 affected individuals. Exome sequencing identified a rare mutation in the second exon of the gene. This mutation was present in all affected individuals but absent in all unaffected family members and in 775 unrelated control subjects.

There are likely other rare variants conferring risk for narcolepsy and studies with exome sequencing and whole genome sequencing are in progress. Exome sequencing in 18 families with at least two affected individuals with narcolepsy and cataplexy have shown that there are nonsynonymous mutations in the second exon of the *P2RY11* gene.[91] Reduced P2RY11 signaling plays an important role in the development of narcolepsy with cataplexy.[91]

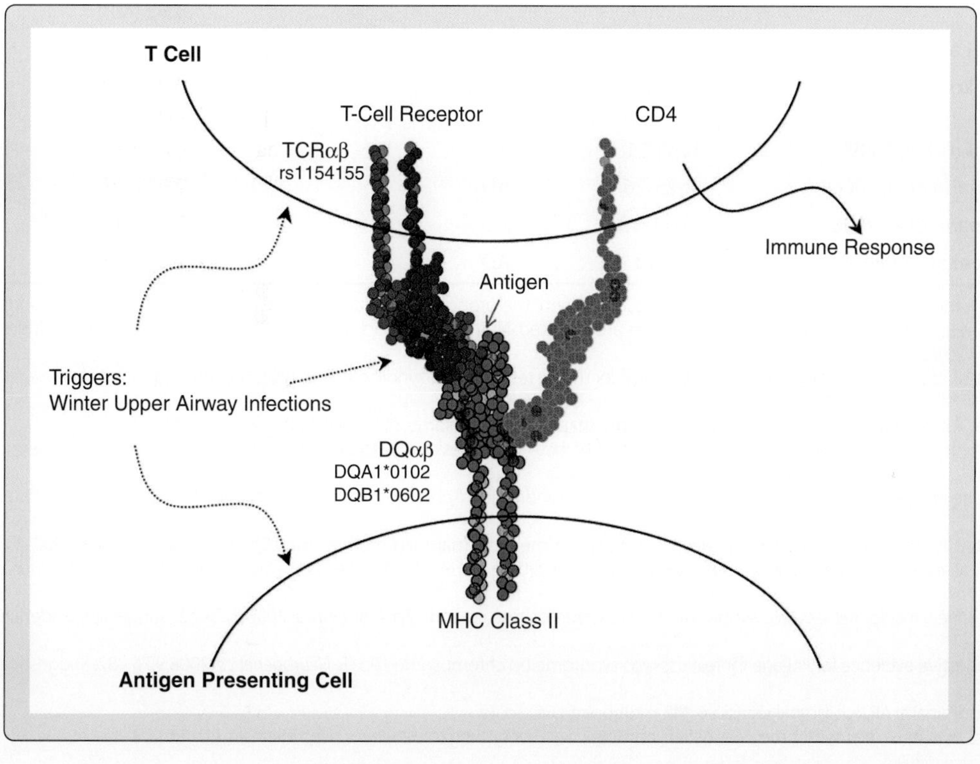

Figure 17.2 The pathogenesis of narcolepsy is likely autoimmune. Variants of human leukocyte antigens confer risk or protection for narcolepsy. In addition, variants of the T-cell receptor alpha locus confer risk. These variants are suspected to make individuals susceptible to an environmental challenge, such as upper airway infections. (From Faraco J, Mignot E. Genetics of narcolepsy. *Sleep Med Clin.* 2011;6:217–28 with permission.)

Overall, the information on genetic risk for narcolepsy supports the autoimmune hypothesis as to the pathogenesis of narcolepsy. Support for this hypothesis comes from studies that show that CD^{4+} T cells in blood of patients with narcolepsy respond to hypocretin (orexin) in vitro.[92] (See the review by Szabo and colleagues.[93])

GENETICS OF RESTLESS LEGS SYNDROME

One of the major accomplishments in the modern genetic era of elucidating gene variants for a sleep disorder are the discoveries related to RLS. That this occurred where the primary phenotype is based on a questionnaire is particularly notable. That the key gene variants have now been replicated in multiple studies should put to rest the debate by critics as to whether this is a real disorder. This accomplishment was based on a solid base of defining diagnostic criteria.[94]

Genetic research in this area was initially stimulated by the findings of a large proportion of patients with RLS who had positive family histories.[95-97] Twin studies confirmed heritability.[98-100] Complex segregation analyses studied the mode of inheritance in German families with RLS.[101] For early age of onset of RLS, that is, before 30 years of age, the pattern of inheritance was best described by an autosomal dominant model with a single major gene. A similar study in the United States came to the same conclusion.[102]

Since family aggregation was so high in RLS, this led to using linkage analyses within large family pedigrees. This was done in different parts of the world, including French Canada, northern Italy, North America, and southern Tyrol. These studies resulted in a number of different regions with strong evidence of linkage that were genome-wide significant (RLS-1 to RLS-5; Table 17.3). However, until case-control association analyses of SNPs in these linkage regions were performed, linkage studies on their own did not identify specific gene variants.

The first linkage region to be investigated in this way was RLS-1 on chromosome 12.[103] Case-control association analysis was conducted with 1536 SNPs in this region in the discovery phase, with 24 of the most significantly associated SNPs being investigated in an independent case-control replication sample. A significant association with a SNP in *nNOS* was identified that was protective (OR [95% CI] = 0.76 [0.64, 0.91]).[103]

A similar strategy was used to evaluate the RLS-3 region on chromosome 9, with 3270 SNPs in the discovery phase and 8 in the independent replication sample.[104] Two different SNPs in introns of the *protein tyrosine phosphatase receptor type delta* (*PTPRD*) gene were shown to associate significantly with RLS. There are two independent association signals. The function of this gene has been studied in mouse knockout models.[105,106] *PTPRD* knockout mice show impairment in long-term potentiation in memory formation and abnormal axon targeting to motoneurons during development.[105,106] It is conceivable that this developmental role could underlie the

Table 17.3 Linkage Regions Identified in Studies of Restless Legs Syndrome (RLS) in Families

Locus (OMIM)	Reference	Chromosomal Location	Inheritance Mode	Parametric LOD Score
RLS-1	Desautels et al, 2001[a]	12a22-23.3	AR pseudo dominant	3.42 (2P) 3.59 (MP)
RLS-2	Bonati et al, 2003[b]	14q13-22	AD	2.23 (2P)
RLS-3	Chen et al, 2004[c]	9p24-22	AD	3.77 (2P) 3.91 (MP)
RLS-4	Pichler et al, 2006[d]	2q33	AD	4.1 (2P)
RLS-5	Levchenko et al, 2006[e]	20p13	AD	3.34 (2P) 3.86 (MP)
--	Levchenko et al, 2009[f]	16p12.1	AD	3.5 (MP)
--	Winkelmann et al, 2006[g]	4q25-26	AD	2.92 (MP)
--	Winkelmann et al, 2006[g]	17p11-13	AD	2.83 (MP)
--	Kemlink et al, 2008[h]	12p13	AD	2.61 (MP)

The linkage regions for RLS are given with their chromosomal position by chromosome band, the proposed inheritance mode, and the logarithm of the odds (LOD) scores from parametric linkage analysis. Both two-point and multipoint scores are reported. Numbering of loci has been indicated as listed in Online Mendelian Inheritance in Man (OMIM), January 2010.

[a]Desautels A, Turecki G, Montplaisir J, et al. Identification of a major susceptibility locus for restless legs syndrome on chromosome 12q. *Am J Hum Genet.* 2001;69:1266–70.

[b]Bonati MT, Ferini-Strambi L, Aridon P, et al. Autosomal dominant restless legs syndrome maps on chromosome 14q. *Brain.* 2003;126:1485–92.

[c]Chen S, Ondo WG, Rao S, et al. Genomewide linkage scan identifies a novel susceptibility locus for restless leg syndrome on chromosome 9p. *Am J Hum Genet.* 3004:74(5):876–885.

[d]Pichler I, Marroni F, Volpato CB, et al. Linkage analysis identifies a novel locus for restless legs syndrome on chromosome 2q in a South Tyrolean population isolate. *Am J Hum Genet.* 2006;79:716–23.

[e]Levchenko A, Provost S, Montplaisir JY, et al. A novel autosomal dominant restless legs syndrome locus maps to chromosome 20p13. *Neurology.* 2006;67:900–1.

[f]Levchenko A, Montplaisir JY, Asselin G, et al. Autosomal-dominant locus for Restless Legs Syndrome in French-Canadians on chromosome 16p12.1. *Mov Disord.* 2009;24:40–50.

[g]Winkelmann J, Lichtner P, Kemlink D, et al. New loci for restless legs syndrome map to chromosome 4q and 17p. *Mov Disord.* 2006;21:S412. Suggestive evidence only.

[h]Kemlink D, Plazzi G, Vetrugno R, et al. Suggestive evidence for linkage for restless legs syndrome on chromosome 19p13. *Neurogenetics.* 2008;9:75 –82. Suggestive evidence only.

2P, Two-point LOD score; AD, Autosomal-dominant; AR, autosomal recessive; MP, multipoint LOD score.

From Schormair B, Winkelmann J. Genetics of restless legs syndrome: Mendelian, complex, and everything in between. *Sleep Med Clin.* 2011;6:203–15.

role of this gene in RLS. An independent replication of this association has been reported.[107]

Although linkage studies have led to new insights, the seminal event in RLS genetics was the essentially simultaneous publication of two independent successful GWAS in 2007.[108,109] These studies implicated three genetic loci, including the genes *MESI1* (chromosome 2), *BTBD9* (chromosome 6), and *MAP2K5/SKOR1* (chromosome 15). Both these initial GWAS and subsequent replication studies provide additional information on potential mechanisms and gene-specific associations.

The first GWAS was conducted in Germans and French Canadians[108] and used a questionnaire-based case definition. The study employed a discovery phase with two independent case-control samples for replication (see Figure 17.3 for study design). It identified associations in three different loci: two intronic SNPs in *MEIS1* on chromosome 2; five intronic SNPs in *BTBD9* on chromosome 6; and seven intronic or intergenic SNPs on chromosome 15 in the *MAP2K5* gene and the adjacent *SKOR1* gene.

The other GWAS, conducted primarily in Iceland,[109] used a discovery sample in Iceland and two independent replication case-control samples—one in Iceland and one in the United States. These investigators used a different phenotyping strategy based on actigraphy of the legs to measure the frequency of periodic limb movements over several nights of recording. They found an association with the same SNP for *BTBD9* as the study in Germans and French Canadians. This association was only found in cases with periodic limb movements and not in cases with only sensory symptoms, suggesting the *BTBD9* variant likely contributes to the motor manifestations of RLS.

The discovered associations of *MEIS1* and *BTBD9* have been confirmed in one study,[110] and all three identified loci have been confirmed in others.[111-113] Association with risk for RLS has also been demonstrated with several variants in the *MAP2K5/SKOR1* loci in another study.[114] In a secondary form of RLS that occurs in patients with end-stage renal disease, variants of *BTBD9* and *MEIS1* were again associated with RLS, but not variants in *MAP2K5/SKOR1*.[115]

Both *MEIS1*[116] and *SKOR1*[117] play a role in organismal development, suggesting a potential shared pathway. Interestingly, the SNP in *BTBD9* was associated with ferritin levels in the GWAS in Iceland. It has long been known that alterations in iron metabolism can play a role in the pathogenesis of RLS (see the review by Earley and colleagues[118]), supporting a potential mechanism. However, *BTBD9* has not been implicated as a gene determining iron metabolism in other studies.[119] Moreover, studies looking for an association of RLS with genes known to affect iron metabolism have been negative.[120]

A recent meta-analysis using data from four GWAS identified 13 new risk loci for RLS and confirmed six previously identified loci.[121] Identified pathways were involved in neurodevelopment and genes were linked to axon guidance, synapse formation, and neuronal specification.[121] The strongest association was again for variants in *MEIS1*.

Although these findings are exciting, the identified variants account for only around 3% of the heritability of RLS.[122] This, unfortunately, is not unusual for complex traits.[123] The reasons for "missing heritability" include the role of rare variants. Rare variants can be identified by deep resequencing of relevant genes, including exome sequencing or whole genome sequencing. Efforts to use these approaches to investigate the genetics of RLS have begun but are still in their infancy. One study has shown that individuals

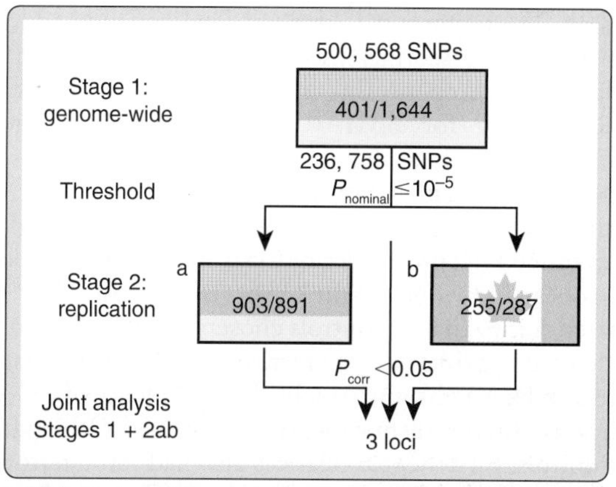

Figure 17.3 Design of the seminal genome-wide association study (GWAS) on restless legs syndrome. The stage 1 discovery phase involved assessing a large number of single-nucleotide polymorphisms (SNPs) in 431 cases and 1644 controls. The few SNPs that were nominally significant at $P < 10^{-5}$ (they were not genome-wide significant) were assessed in two replication samples: one had 903 cases and 891 controls, while the other had 255 cases and 287 controls. The SNPs that were significant in the replication samples were then assessed in a joint analysis across all three samples. (From Winkelmann J, Schormair B, Lichtner P, et al. Genome-wide association study of restless legs syndrome identifies common variants in three genomic regions. *Nat Genet.* 2007;39:1000–6 with permission.)

with RLS have an excess of rare variants of *MEIS1* compared with controls.[124] In particular, there is an excess of loss-of-function alleles in cases with RLS.[124] Application of exome sequencing has also begun.[125] A variant of *PCDHA3* in a family with RLS that was absent in 500 controls suggests a functional role. This gene encodes protocadherin-alpha 3, a member of the protocadherin gene family. It is expressed in neurons and is present at synaptic junctions, where it plays a role in neural cell-cell interaction.[126] Recently, studies using next generation sequencing in 84 candidate genes also found there was a differential burden of low frequency rare variants in patients with RLS compared with controls.[127]

Thus there is little doubt that a search for rare variants with new sequencing technology will continue in RLS, as will studies of copy number variation and altered methylation patterns. Given the large number of carefully assembled case-control and family-based cohorts, we can look forward to further exciting developments in this area. For helpful reviews on genetics of RLS, see the articles by Jimenez-Jimenez and colleagues[128] and Winkelmann and colleagues.[129] For review of the role of *MEIS1* in RLS, see the work by Salminen and colleagues.[130]

GENETICS OF OBSTRUCTIVE SLEEP APNEA

Obstructive sleep apnea (OSA) is a common condition.[131] The major risk factor in middle-aged adults is obesity.[131] With increasing obesity rates in the United States, the prevalence of this condition is increasing.[132] It has long been known that OSA aggregates in families. The initial finding that OSA has likely a major genetic component came from a study of a single family with a high prevalence of OSA.[133] Subsequently, it was shown that symptoms of OSA such as habitual snoring, excessive sleepiness, snorting, gasping, and witnessed apneas also aggregate in families.[134]

These observations led to studies of family members that included measurement of apneas and hypopneas during sleep. Such studies were conducted in the United States,[135,136] Israel,[137] Scotland,[138] and Iceland.[139] Because obesity, a major risk factor for OSA, is itself heritable,[140-143] whether family aggregation of OSA is simply due to obesity had to be addressed. The important Cleveland Family Study addressed this issue and assessed increased relative risk of OSA in first-degree family members. This increased risk was not affected after controlling for BMI.[135] Thus family aggregation is unlikely to be simply explained by obesity.

Obesity as an explanation for family aggregation of OSA was more definitively addressed by Mathur and Douglas.[138] They examined the prevalence of OSA in first-degree relatives of less obese individuals with OSA (BMI < 30 kg/m^2) and compared this to that in controls chosen at random from a list of patients in a primary care practice. Controls were matched for age, gender, height, and weight. The prevalence of OSA was significantly higher in first-degree relatives of OSA patients than controls. First-degree relatives also had more retroposed mandibles and maxillae than controls.[138] Thus, in these less obese cases, subtle differences in craniofacial structure likely played the key role, suggesting genes for craniofacial structure could be involved. (See the review of these early studies on genetics of OSA by Redline and Tishler.[144])

Although familial aggregation has been known for two decades, there has been limited progress in identifying relevant gene variants. Studies in this area have been particularly problematic. Early family-based linkage studies were underpowered, did not find genome-wide significant linkages, and did not employ fine mapping to confirm the peak and narrow the linkage region.[145-147] Candidate gene studies examining multiple candidates did not employ any replication samples[148] and have been massively underpowered for small effects expected for common variants[149] (e.g., OR ~1.2; Figure 17.4). Meta-analyses reveal that most claimed candidate gene variants, including *APOE-ε4*, show no association.[149,150] The one exception is the 308 tumor necrosis factor-α (*TNF-α*) promoter polymorphism. This variant affects gene transcription.[151] Association with this SNP and OSA has been identified in European populations[152] and in Indians.[153] However, it seems unlikely that this gene variant actually contributes to the risk of OSA. In the pediatric population with OSA, excessive sleepiness is more pronounced in patients with OSA with this SNP than in those patients without the SNP.[154] Thus this SNP may contribute to one of the key recognized consequences of OSA, making patients with this variant more likely to seek evaluation and be diagnosed. This concept adds additional difficulty to determining the gene variants conferring risk for OSA.

Evidence of a relevant gene variant comes from a study that used subjects that were part of the Cleveland Family Study and the Sleep Heart Health Study.[155] They used a custom candidate gene array with 45,237 SNPs from more than 2000 candidate genes chosen because of their potential relevance to heart, lung, blood, and sleep disorders.[156] Replication samples for subjects of European ancestry came from the Western Australia Sleep Health Study and for Blacks from the Cleveland Sleep Apnea Study and Case Transdisciplinary Research in Energetics and Cancer Colon Polyp Study.

In Blacks, one SNP in the intronic region of the *lysophosphatidic acid receptor I* (*LPAR1*) gene showed a genome-wide association with log transformed apnea-hypopnea index (AHI). Using AHI as a quantitative phenotype is challenging given the

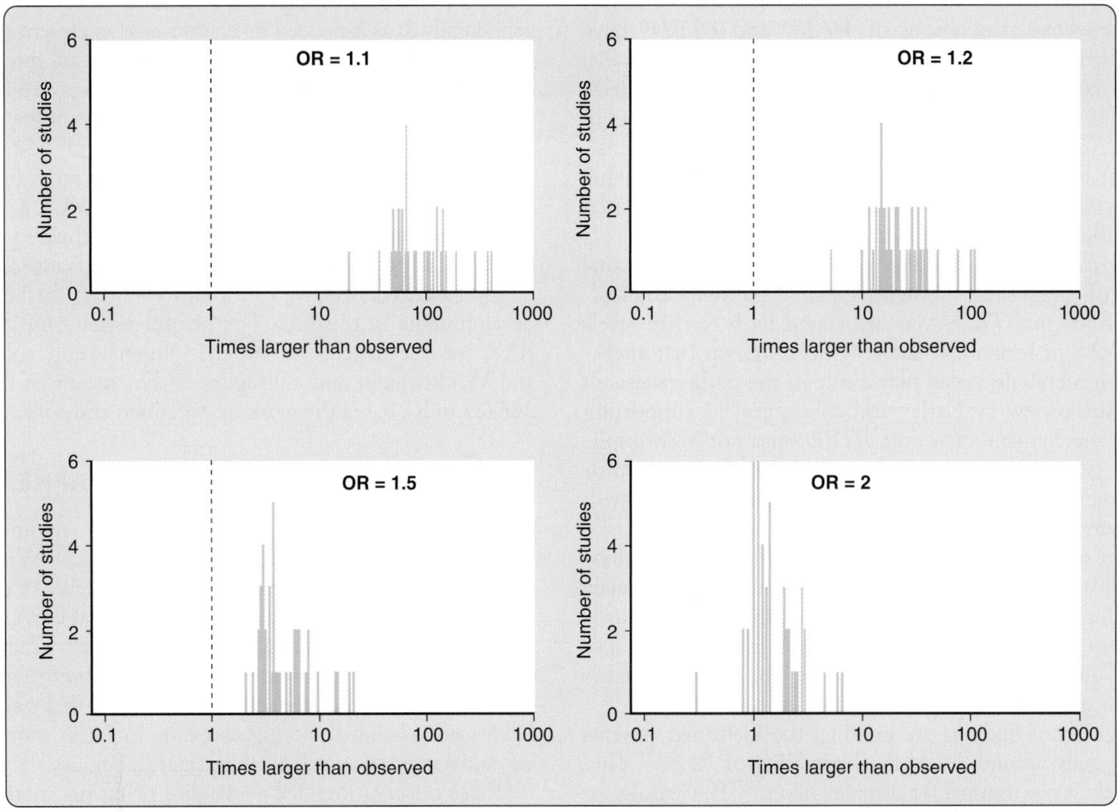

Figure 17.4 Calculation of how much larger candidate gene studies for obstructive sleep apnea would be needed to identify odds ratios (OR) of 1.1 (*top left panel*), 1.2 (*top right panel*), 1.5 (*bottom left panel*), and 2.0 (*bottom right panel*). Common variants typically result in low OR, such as 1.2. As can be seen for this OR, studies would have to be between 10 and 100 times larger than was used in the original studies. The majority of studies are underpowered to even detect an OR of 2.0, an effect typically not found with common variants. (From Varvarigou V, Dahabreh IJ, Malhotra A, et al. A review of genetic association studies of obstructive sleep apnea: field synopsis and meta-analysis. *Sleep.* 2011;34:1461–8 with permission.)

known night-to-night variability in the measure.[157] This association was greater in the nonobese compared with obese subjects. The association with OSA status was confirmed in Blacks in a replication sample. In European samples, this SNP also showed evidence of association to an apnea phenotype ($P = 0.01$) and a trend for association with log AHI ($P = 0.06$). *LPAR1* is thought to play a proinflammatory role.[158,159] It is also expressed in developing cerebral cortex.[160] A mouse knockout of the gene results in changes in behavior as well as craniofacial abnormalities.[161] Thus the connection with OSA may be due to either neural differences in airway control or craniofacial alterations.

In this investigation of studies of cohorts of European ancestry, no SNP met criteria for a statistically significant association with log AHI. One SNP in the intronic region of the *prostaglandin receptor 2* gene was significantly associated with OSA. There was some evidence of association in the replication sample.

That genetic studies of OSA have had such limited success is not only related to the poor study designs; this is also an extremely challenging area. There are multiple pathways contributing to OSA risk or protection (Figure 17.5), each with many likely associated variants.

As discussed, a major risk factor for OSA is obesity. Is it well accepted that genetic predisposition contributes to obesity, as supported by more than 1000 identified independent associations with obesity, BMI, and other adiposity-related traits from numerous GWAS.[162-165] These obesity-related loci highlight the importance of genes acting on appetite regulation in the central nervous system in overall obesity and genes related to adipogenesis, angiogenesis, lipid biology, and insulin resistance for traits related to body fat distribution.[162-168] Yet the role of these genes in OSA has not been determined. It may, moreover, not simply be obesity, but rather a particular distribution of fat that contributes to OSA risk. Novel imaging studies reveal that there is a difference in volume of fat in the tongue between cases with OSA and controls even after controlling for differences in overall BMI.[169] Subjects with OSA who lose weight show improvements in severity of OSA (AHI) and in volume of tongue fat determined by Dixon imaging.[170] Mediation analysis shows that approximately 30% of the effect of weight loss on AHI improvement is explained by reductions in tongue fat.[170] There are gene variants associated with other specific distributions of fat, for example, pericardial fat.[171] Determining whether tongue fat is a unique fat distribution and whether genetic variants influence tongue fat is an area of opportunity.

The volume of soft tissue structures also likely contributes to the genetics of OSA. The volume of key upper airway soft tissues that confer risk for OSA are heritable.[172] Specifically, data suggest a heritability estimate of 25.6% for the volume of the lateral pharyngeal walls, 37.8% for tongue volume, and 41.3% for total volume of upper airway soft tissue structures. This is not simply related to obesity, because after controlling for total neck fat volume, heritability estimates either stay the same or increase.

Soft tissue structures are not the only relevant anatomic risk factors, so too are craniofacial structures. Although several differences in craniofacial structures have been demonstrated between OSA cases and controls, the most robust finding is reduced mandibular length in OSA cases, as revealed by meta-analyses.[173] Heritability of craniofacial dimensions by cephalometric analysis has been shown.[174,175] This heritability has been supported by three-dimensional analysis with MRI.[176] Mandibular length and mandibular width are both heritable. Investigating the gene variants associated with these different structural quantitative traits is an area of opportunity.

These various structural risk factors play a unique role in different ethnic groups. An elegant study comparing Whites in Sydney, Australia, to Chinese from Hong Kong with the same degree of OSA found that the Whites were more obese and had a larger tongue volume.[177] Craniofacial dimensions played a larger role in Chinese, with more restriction of the craniofacial base.[177] These ethnic-specific differences are also supported by a recent study comparing Icelandic and Chinese patients with OSA using MRI.[178] Thus the relative role of different genetically determined pathways to OSA varies by ethnic group.

There are, however, not only structural risk factors for OSA but also physiologic.[179] Key physiologic variables include overall loop gain, arousal threshold, and airway muscle responsiveness. Among these, overall loop gain is important.[179,180] There are individuals with OSA who do not have particularly collapsible airways but do have high loop gain.[179] The main determinant of loop gain is ventilatory response to hypoxia and hypercapnia. The hypoxic response is also a highly heritable trait, as revealed by studies in twins.[181] Gene variants determining the hypoxic response have, however, not been identified. Thus this is another potential genetic contribution to OSA.

As with other sleep disorders, there have been recent GWAS to identify risk variants associated with OSA.[182-184] There are insufficient data in the UK Biobank to do this, and

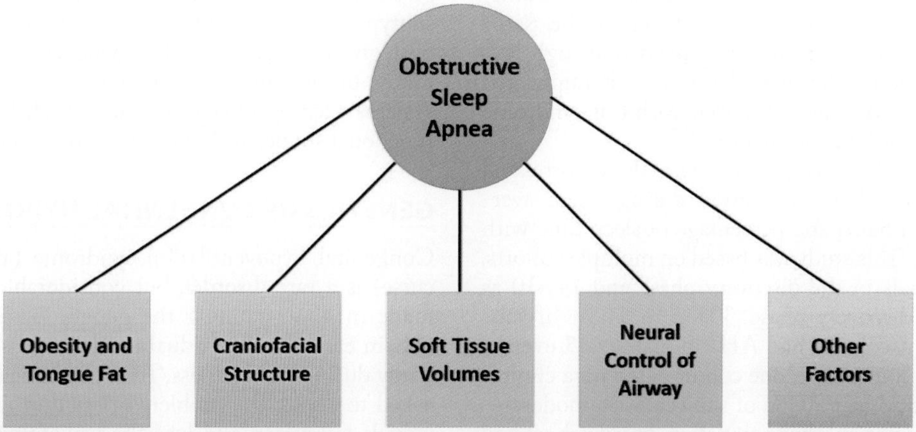

Figure 17.5 Multiple pathways to obstructive sleep apnea (OSA). Each is likely to have many and unique genetic variants involved. These multiple pathways make finding gene variants conferring risk for or protection against obstructive sleep apnea challenging.

these studies have largely been on population-based studies in the United States that were originally established to identify risks for cardiovascular disease but now include overnight sleep studies. The fact that OSA is associated with obesity and a large number of other comorbidities (e.g., hypertension) represents a major challenge for case-control GWAS in OSA. Often, identified genetic variants are related to obesity and associated with underlying comorbidities, making finding signals unique to OSA difficult. As a result, the approaches used in GWAS for OSA have focused largely on quantitative trait analysis of measures of OSA severity determined from the overnight sleep study. Studies based on the Cleveland Family Study showed that AHI, average nocturnal O_2 saturation, percentage of sleep time with SaO_2 < 90%, and average duration of respiratory events are heritable.[185] Thus these variables have been used in quantitative trait analyses. Although a number of these GWAS have been performed, there is surprisingly little replication from study to study. The basis for this lack of replication is unclear, but it means that results must be interpreted with caution.

The first major GWAS for OSA-related traits was based on Hispanic/Latino Americans.[186] Two novel loci were found to be genome-wide significant in quantitative trait analyses with AHI as the phenotype. One locus spanned several genes, including *GPR83*, *LINC01171/C11ORF97*, and *MRE11A*. A significant association with event duration was also found on chromosome 6q21 in a genomic region that spanned two pseudogenes (*CCDC162P* and *C6ORF183/LOC100996694*). There was, unfortunately, no replication. The results of this study highlight one of the challenges of this approach. Although subjects came from three different cohort studies, almost all subjects included came from the Hispanic Community Health Study/Study of Latinos (HCHS/SOL). Subjects in this cohort had very little OSA, with a median (interquartile range) AHI of only 1.97 (0.42, 6.62) events/hour. Thus quantitative trait analyses are mainly evaluating genetic associations with AHI in the normal/mild range.

Other GWAS have used different cohorts. Seven cohorts were included in a multi-ethnic GWAS.[183] Findings were replicated in other cohorts, with the main replication cohort being an independent physiologic study of only 67 individuals. Non–rapid eye movement (NREM) AHI and REM AHI were studied separately, and analyses were performed in male and female subjects separately. A genome-wide association was found for NREM AHI in men. This was not significantly associated in women. The SNPs identified were in the *RAI1* gene, which encodes a protein that is expressed at high levels in neurons. Haploinsufficiency of this gene is implicated in Smith-Magenis syndrome.[187] Subjects with this syndrome have multiple craniofacial abnormalities.[187]

GWAS have also been conducted with three correlated measures of oxyhemoglobin saturation during sleep: average SaO_2, minimum SaO_2 and percentage of sleep time with SaO_2 below 90%.[182] This study was based on multiple cohorts, with 8326 individuals in the discovery phase and 14,410 as replication. In the discovery phase, 30.0% to 54.8% of subjects in the different cohorts had AHI of at least 15 events/hour. In the replication sample, one cohort based on a clinical sleep study population had 70.9% of subjects with moderate-to-severe OSA, whereas another population-based cohort had only 11.7%.

Genome-wide significant associations were identified with minimum SaO_2 in the *IL18R1* region and with average SaO_2 in the *HK1* region. HK1 is the rate-limiting enzyme in the glycolysis pathway, and its activity is regulated by hypoxia inducible factor 1a.[182,188] The *IL18R1* gene encodes a receptor subunit of the IL18 receptor. The biologic mechanism for this role of IL18 receptor is unclear. It is known that IL18 regulates expression of HIF1A.[189]

The same investigative team has employed an admixture mapping strategy.[190] This is an approach that can be applied to recently admixed populations whose ancestors came from different isolated continents. The technique is taking advantage of the different ancestry. It has been used extensively to identify genetic risks for asthma.[191] Associations were sought for four measures: AHI, event duration, and two measures of hypoxia (average, % time < 90% SaO_2). Novel variants in *FECH* (ferrochelatase) were found to be significantly associated with AHI and percent time with SaO_2 below 90%. These associations were replicated in independent cohorts. FECH is the last enzyme of the heme biosynthesis pathway.[190] It is largely expressed in blood.

As in other areas, studies are moving beyond genotype data from SNP arrays. A study with whole genome sequencing data has recently been reported (although not yet peer reviewed).[184] The study is based on the same cohorts used in the earlier GWAS and was part of the TOPMed program of the National Heart, Lung, and Blood Institute. Associations were again sought for the various metrics from the overnight sleep study that may have been shown to be heritable,[185] with analyses performed overall and stratified by sex. Results were presented for gene-based tests and single variants. For gene-based analysis, four significantly associated genes were reported in analysis of multiple populations. One gene, *ARMCX3*, is expressed at high levels in the central nervous system and plays a role in neuronal development.[192] In single-variant analysis, variants in *IL18RAP* were associated with average event desaturation and minimum SaO_2. This is consistent with findings from an earlier GWAS.[182]

Thus, although progress is being made in study of genetics of OSA, progress is extremely slow. Apart from the variant in the *IL18R1/IL18RAP* locus, there has been no replication in follow-up studies. As with insomnia, there are challenges. First, it is unclear if individuals with sleep-disordered breathing in community-based samples are reflective of subjects who present clinically.[193] There is also likely to be genetic heterogeneity given the different pathways to disease and the different clinical subtypes.[194] This will require novel analytic approaches. Moreover, given the nature of the phenotype, it seems unlikely that follow-up functional studies can be done in high-throughput systems such as *Drosophila* and zebrafish. Instead, follow-up functional studies will likely have to be done in mice.

GENETICS OF CONGENITAL HYPOVENTILATION

Congenital hypoventilation syndrome (also called Ondine's curse) is a rare disorder, but considerable progress has been made in understanding the genetic basis. It typically presents in early life. Individuals with this disorder ventilate normally during wakefulness. They can increase ventilation when asked to do so. The problem arises during sleep. When individuals fall asleep and lose the wakefulness drive to breathe, they hypoventilate. The problem is in their CO_2-dependent ventilatory system. They have very low or absent ventilatory responses to hypercapnia. This hypoventilation can be major, with marked elevations in pCO_2. Hence they require assisted ventilation during sleep. This is typically done by creating a tracheostomy early in life with positive pressure ventilation through the tracheostomy during sleep (see the review by Healy and Marcus[195]).

The relevant gene is *PHOX2B*. This is a transcription factor involved in the development of the autonomic nervous system. The role of this gene in this condition was identified in 2003 by Amiel and colleagues.[196] Mice that have the mutation of the gene most frequently found in humans with the disease do not respond to hypercapnia and die in the early postnatal period.[197]

In humans, the most common mutation is expression of polyalanine repeats in exon 3 of the gene.[196] The upper limit of normal for the number of repeats is 20.[196] Most mutations occur de novo, that is, there is no family history.[198] There are rare cases that are autosomal dominant and up to 25% of cases show somatic mosaicism, that is, the mutation is found in some, but not all, cells in the parents of cases.[199] Ninety-two percent (92%) of cases with this condition have expansion of the polyalanine repeats (25 to 33 repeats).[200] There are case reports of individual cases with 25 repeats who presented as adults.[201] There is a case report of an individual with a more typical mutation who also presented as an adult.[202]

Patients with this disorder who do not have increased polyalanine repeats in exon 3 most commonly have other mutations in *PHOX2B*.[198,203] Patients with congenital hypoventilation syndrome have an increased rate of Hirschsprung disease and tumors of neural crest origin.[203] These associated conditions are more common in patients who have different mutations in *PHOX1B* compared with those with increased polyalanine repeats.[203] For a helpful review, see the work of Bishara and colleagues.[204]

CLINICAL PEARLS

- Clinicians should be aware of the relevance of sample size (power) and of importance of independent replication in assessing literature on gene variants for sleep and its disorders.
- There are many common gene variants with small effects as well as rare variants with large effects that contribute to risk for, and protection against, sleep disorders.
- There have been successful genetic studies in narcolepsy (HLA antigens, e.g., *DQB1*0602*), restless legs syndrome (*MEIS1* and *BTBD9*), and congenital hypoventilation syndrome (*PHOX2B*).
- Variants of the clock-associated gene, *DEC2*, affect duration of sleep and response to sleep deprivation. Their functional role is confirmed by studies in model systems.
- Genetic studies of sleep and circadian phenotypes that leverage large-scale data resources, such as the UK Biobank and 23andMe, are rapidly emerging. In-depth phenotyping and replication studies are still needed.

SUMMARY

There has been a rapid development of methods to identify gene variants conferring risk for or protection against sleep disorders. It is important to understand the importance of study design, sample size, and replication in genetics research. Studies ranging from linkage analysis and candidate gene association analysis in small samples to large-scale GWAS using self-reported phenotypes have suggested a number of possible genotype-phenotype associations. However, much of the published literature on genetics of sleep disorders does not meet the criteria required for firm conclusions to be reached. (For a full description of the different methodologies, see the Appendix.)

There have been important discoveries in narcolepsy, RLS, and congenital hypoventilation syndrome. For the latter, genotyping and identifying the causative mutation is now part of routine clinical care. For narcolepsy and RLS, the genetic variants identified have not yet altered current clinical practice. The findings in narcolepsy, in particular with respect to the role of different HLA antigens, do suggest that studying these variants in individual patients could have a clinical role. This remains to be determined. This is not the case for RLS, because the variants identified explain so little of the heritability. The current key value of the results in this area is identification of novel genes and implicated pathways. The question now is, what do these genes do? This opens up entirely new opportunities to understand the fundamental pathogenesis of sleep disorders and develop novel targets for therapeutic intervention. One example of this is the gene *BTBD9*, which has been found to be associated with RLS in multiple studies. The approach to begin to identify its function is to study animal models in which expression of the gene is altered. For *BTBD9*, this has been done both in *Drosophila* and mice. A knockout of *BTBD9* in mice led to phenotypic differences.[205] Knockout mice had enhanced long-term potentiation in hippocampus and enhanced cued and contextual fear conditioning. Thus *BTBD9* is involved in synaptic plasticity. Sleep was not studied in these mice. Studies in *Drosophila* link *BTBD9* more directly to the function of dopamine neurons and to iron metabolism.[206] Flies with loss of function of *BTBD9* have fragmented sleep. Knockdown of *BTBD9* only in dopaminergic neurons using RNAi leads to the same phenotype. Flies with loss of *BTBD9* had lower dopamine levels in the brain, and agonists of dopamine that are used to treat RLS in humans reverses the sleep fragmentation phenotype in *Drosophila*. The connection to iron comes from studies in cell culture. Specifically, overexpression of *BTBD9* leads to reduction in iron-responsive element-binding protein with a resultant increase in ferritin levels. The connection between dopamine neuronal function and iron metabolism has not been investigated.

These functional studies are a start. Ultimately, we need to understand the role of these newly identified gene variants and whether they represent potential targets for future drug development. There are databases that indicate whether a gene that is identified is a "druggable" target. Thus we are at the early stages of this exciting journey and much remains to be discovered.

APPENDIX

The following gives a brief overview of the potential approaches to genetic studies relevant for sleep disorders.

Heritability Estimation

Heritability analyses are the first step in understanding the genetic underpinnings of disease. They establish whether there is a relationship between genetic risk factors and a disease phenotype by estimating the amount of disease variability explained by genetic variants. Heritability can be defined broadly as the proportion of phenotypic variability that is attributable to genetic factors; higher estimates suggest a larger influence of genetics on the variability of a given trait in the population. There exist numerous techniques for estimating heritability, ranging from utilizing phenotype information from twins[207] or family pedigree data[208,209] to more recently developed statistical techniques for estimating heritability based on genome-wide genotyped data on unrelated individuals.[210] It is important to remember that heritability is only an estimate for the specific population included in a study. There is not one true heritability for a given disorder or trait. Instead, the heritability can vary over time as environments change, and it can vary by geography, ethnic groups, or age groups (see the work by Visscher and colleagues for a review of heritability concepts[210]).

Estimating the heritability of a given trait using twin or family data does not require specific measurement of genetic variants. Rather, these methods are based on the principle that people who are more genetically related to each other should be more phenotypically similar. For binary traits such as sleep disorders, one can measure the recurrence risk in relatives. That is, given a family member has been diagnosed with a disorder, what is the risk in their family members of having the same disorder. This recurrence risk can be compared with disease risk in the general population to estimate familial aggregation.

More recently established techniques allow for estimation of heritability in unrelated individuals by simultaneously examining the association between a given trait and all genetic polymorphisms.[210-213] These techniques have been used and extended to capture more accurately the amount of variability we can expect to explain through genome-wide association analyses.

Heritability has been estimated for sleep-related disorders and intermediate phenotypes, including sleep duration,[4-6] chronotype,[45-48] restless legs syndrome,[98-100] insomnia,[4,68-70] parasomnia,[214] OSA,[133-139] and key OSA-related traits such as craniofacial structures,[176] upper airway soft tissue volumes,[172] ventilatory responses to hypoxia, and hypercapnia.[181] Heart rate response to arousal has also been shown to be heritable.[215] One of the most heritable behavioral traits is the spectral characteristics of the EEG during sleep.[66] Despite observing heritability estimates over 50% for some of these traits, the genetic variants discovered typically explain less than 5% of the known overall variability in any given phenotype, or roughly 10% of the estimated heritability. Finding the causes of this "missing heritability" is an ongoing area of research, and methods for determining heritability of a given phenotype continue to develop (see the reviews by Lander,[1] Altshuler and colleagues,[2] Manolio and colleagues,[123] Maher,[216] and Eichler and colleagues[217]). Explanations for "missing heritability" include a large number of common variants with small effects, multiple rare variants with large effects, insufficient tagging of causal variants in current genotyping platforms, gene-gene and gene-environment interactive effects, and the role of other types of genetic variations such as copy number variants and epigenetic modification.

Linkage Analysis

Once a trait has been shown to be heritable, the next obvious question is, "Which genes or regions are associated with

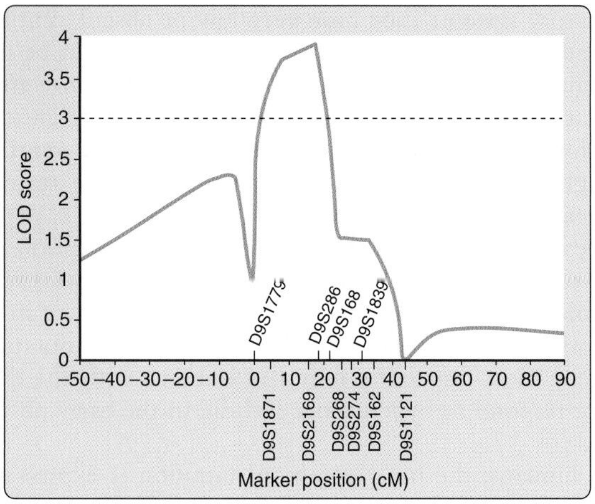

Figure 17.6 Example of identifying a region by linkage analysis. Marker location is on X-axis, and log-odds (LOD) score is on Y-axis. When a significant linkage is found with equally spaced polymorphic markers across the genome (*dashed line* represents threshold for genome-wide significance linkage), LOD scores for additional markers in region (see annotations on X-axis) are calculated. As shown, this results in narrowing the genomic region and leads to increased LOD scores. In this example, there is little doubt that there is a variant conferring risk for resetless legs syndrome in this region. (From Chen S, Ondo WG, Rao S, et al. Genomewide linkage scan identifies a novel susceptibility locus for restless legs syndrome on chromosome 9p. *Am J Hum Genet.* 2004;74:876–85, with permission.)

the phenotype?" One strategy for answering this question is to perform a genetic linkage analysis.[218-224] At their most basic level, linkage studies compare chromosomal regions between affected and unaffected individuals to identify those DNA segments that are more commonly shared between affected relatives,[219,220] which are expected to contain disease-related genetic factors. The approach does not involve initial assessment of genes, but rather use of multiple polymorphic genetic markers, such as microsatellites or SNPs, spread across the genome. Then the maximum likelihood log-odds (LOD score) is calculated as a function of marker location. Once a marker location with a high LOD score is identified, the genomic region can be narrowed and the linkage validated by determining LOD scores for an additional set of markers that are specific to this region—fine mapping (see example, Figure 17.6). This strategy has been successfully employed in studying the genetic risk factors for RLS[103] (Table 17.3).

Because linkage analysis performs multiple computations across the genome, false associations may occur by chance. Generally accepted thresholds for statistical significance level have been developed depending on the mapping method and model of inheritance.[219] These thresholds include a LOD score of at least 3.3 for genome-wide significant linkage (corresponding to a $P = 4.9 \times 10^{-5}$) for families and slightly higher thresholds of LOD of at least 3.6 in sib-pair studies. Following the identification of a genomic region with significant linkage, fine-mapping analysis—examining specific genetic markers within the identified region—is an important next step to narrow genomic regions and identify specific variants associated with the phenotype of interest.

Linkage studies have been around for decades, and one of the most successful examples in sleep-related diseases is the identification of five linkage regions for RLS, that is, *RLS-1* through *RLS-5* (Table 17.3).[225-229] This was based on studies of several large family pedigrees with RLS in different parts of the world. Subsequent fine-mapping analyses identified specific variants of interest,[103] leading to new insights into RLS genetics. In contrast, early linkage analyses for OSA in Europeans and Blacks have led to results that have not been replicated.[145-147] These studies reported linkage with most LOD scores not reaching statistical significance and did not complete any fine mapping.[145-147] Thus these early studies were underpowered for robust effects. It seems unlikely that linkage approaches alone will lead to identification of genomic regions harboring risk to OSA.

Candidate Gene Studies

A more direct approach to discovering important genes and genetic variants is by association studies using a candidate gene approach. These studies can use unrelated individuals (e.g., cases and controls), as well as families. One can use targeted genotyping to examine the association between variants within or near a priori hypothesized genes of interest and a given phenotype that may come from linkage analyses and GWAS (see following) or from existing knowledge about the biologic mechanisms. Also, as fewer association tests are conducted compared with genome-wide linkage and association studies with a high multiple testing burden, a less stringent significance threshold is required to maintain a lower error rate.[220,230,231] Using strong functional hypotheses is an important aspect for candidate gene studies, as false positive may be common.[220,230,232] However, candidate gene studies involve a priori assumptions about which genetic regions are most likely to be associated with a phenotype and thus may be limited by the amount of information currently known.

At their most basic level, association studies using candidate genes are no different than typical epidemiologic studies examining the relationship between nongenetic risk factors and a phenotype of interest. Standard statistical modeling can be used to assess the association between the alleles and the phenotype of interest.

Compared to linkage analysis, candidate gene studies have been shown to have stronger statistical power for complex disease traits.[230,233] However, as with many types of association analyses, initial candidate gene studies are prone to overestimates of the true association (also referred to as "winner's curse").[234-236] Another important consideration is population stratification, which occurs when differences in disease prevalence and allele frequency between populations of different ancestry result in apparent associations, even when none exist, when combining samples from multiple ancestries.[237-243] Approaches to correct for population stratification, which are applicable to both candidate gene studies and GWAS, have been discussed in detail.[237,240-243] This potential for confounding, coupled with small sample sizes and the large number of gene associations that are not replicated in independent datasets, has led to considerable debate about the utility and interpretation of results.[220,230,231,234-236,244] This is highlighted for candidate gene studies in OSA that were markedly underpowered to detect expected effects (Figure 17.4).

By design, candidate gene studies focus primarily on variants in the coding regions of genes. However, it is becoming increasingly apparent that common genetic variation found outside of protein-coding genes contributes to the etiology of disease.[245] Our understanding of noncoding functional areas of the genome has improved dramatically in the past few years, and it is no longer sufficient to focus solely on variants in the exome. This may in part explain the limited success of candidate gene studies in identifying well-replicated sleep-associated genes and variants.

Genome-Wide Association Studies

The completion of the Human Genome Project, and the subsequent mapping and sequencing projects that characterized genetic variation among individuals, dramatically increased our ability to perform genetic association studies.[1,246-252] Rather than relying on the identification of broad regions through linkage, or restricting our focus to hypothesized candidate genes, genome-wide genotyping allows for an unbiased and "hypothesis-free" examination of the relationship between a given trait and individual genetic variants throughout the genome. Using GWAS, thousands of genetic loci have now been associated with complex traits, as detailed by the National Human Genome Research Institute-European Bioinformatics Institute (NHGRI-EBI) GWAS Catalog (available at https://www.ebi.ac.uk/gwas/).[253-255] GWAS analyses often require large samples; however, recent GWAS with respect to sleep have shown that discoveries can be made with limited phenotype data, as discussed earlier in this chapter. Important considerations include interpretation of results, appropriate significance thresholds, and the need for well-designed studies with replication and consideration of ancestral population structure.

Much of the primary focus of current studies examining the association between genetic variants and disease has been on SNPs. This is because SNPs, which are different among individuals in the DNA sequence at one nucleotide among individuals, are the most frequent form of genetic variation. Owing to the block-like structure of the genome, where genomic regions that are close together tend to be transmitted together, referred to as linkage disequilibrium (LD), genotyping one SNP can provide information on genetic variation at many nearby SNPs. Initial publications suggested that approximately 500,000 common polymorphisms provided power to capture 90% of the variability in the genome.[2,256] Thus most GWAS rely on a subset of genetic variants using microarray-based genotyping methods.[257] This sparse genetic information can then be used to impute missing genotype information by using reference human genome sequences, including the Human Genome Project,[1,249-252] the International HapMap Project,[247,248] the 1000 Genomes Project,[246] the Haplotype Reference Consortium (HRC),[258] and the Trans-Omics for Precision Medicine (TOPMed) project.[259]

After genetic data have been collected, performing a GWAS involves conducting individual regression models assessing the relationship between each SNP and the phenotype. In these models, SNPs may be coded additively with respect to the number of copies of the allele of interest, or one can assume a dominant or recessive genotype effect. Because of the large number of tests resulting from all SNPs being examined individually, a multiple test correction is necessary to determine statistical significance and protect against false-positive associations. A P value less than 5×10^{-8} is typically required to claim genome-wide significance, reflecting a Bonferroni correction for 1 million independent tests.[2,232,260,261] As the number of genetic variants included in analyses continues to increase, stricter criteria will become necessary.

Although reaching statistical significance is important, determining a robust genetic association requires a critical review of initial studies and replication analyses. The

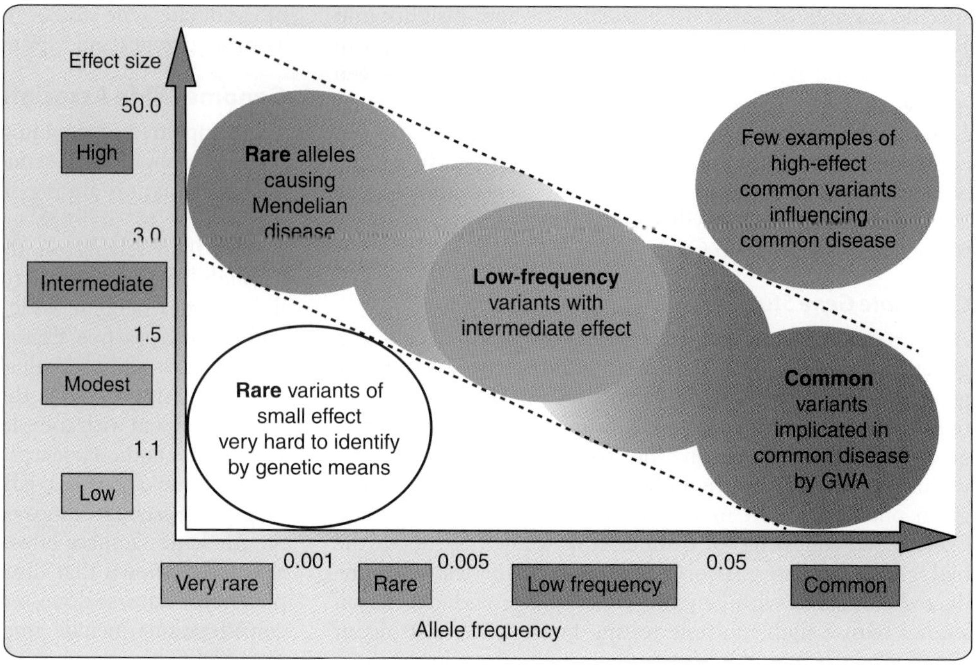

Figure 17.7 Relationship between allele frequency of variant (X-axis) and effect size of variant. Common variants at *bottom right* of figure have frequency in population of more than 5% but have smaller effect in controls. Variants to *left* are rare but have large effects. GWA, Genome-wide association. (From Manolio TA, Collins FS, Cox NJ, et al. Finding the missing heritability of complex diseases. *Nature.* 2009;461:747–53 with permission.)

NCI-NHGRI Working Group on Replication in Association Studies has published an excellent review on the interpretation, validity, replication, and publication of genotype-phenotype associations.[232] Criteria for establishing the validity of initial association reports include sufficient sample size, power to detect reasonable effects, appropriate correction for multiple tests, consistent results for any similar phenotypes and population subsets, standard and well-described quality control methods applied to genotypes, assessment of potential confounding by population stratification, similar associations between the most highly associated SNP and those in linkage disequilibrium, and reported results from replication studies (even if these are null).[232]

Despite the established heritability, GWAS for sleep-related traits have led to mixed results. Briefly, there have been notable successes using GWAS to understand genetic influences on RLS and narcolepsy. For other traits, including chronotype,[61-64] sleep duration,[12-16] and insomnia,[13,71,72] the development and availability of large-scale genetic resources with phenotypic information, such as the UK Biobank and 23andMe, have led to a recent influx of GWAS analyses. However, these studies have identified gene variants using mainly self-reported phenotypes. These traits may have significant differences when compared with results from objective data, because subjective assessment of sleep is a "noisy" phenotype that requires a very large number of subjects.

Another important consideration for interpreting GWAS results is that the results do not necessarily identify the causative gene or variant, as other genes or variants in LD with the SNP identified could actually be causative. Thus it is best to take the view that a GWAS gives evidence supporting a given locus or genetic region. New approaches are evolving to define all likely causative genes based on findings for a specific locus in a GWAS.[262] Once possible causative genes are identified, their functional role can be studied by evaluating phenotypes of interest in model organisms or tissues in which the genes are altered at the site of interest, or animals are created with loss and gain of function of the gene. For sleep and circadian rhythm, we are in the fortunate position that both of these phenotypes can now be assessed in model systems that are very high throughput, that is, *Drosophila* and zebrafish.

Rare Variant Analysis

Although GWAS analyses have increased our understanding of the genetic architecture underlying disease, analyses of genetic variants obtained through genotyping chips are typically restricted to common and low-frequency SNPs. Analysis approaches distinguish between common polymorphisms (occurring with >5% frequency in the population), which are likely to confer smaller effect sizes, and low frequency (<5% frequency) or rare polymorphisms (<1% frequency), which may lead to larger effects, but are more difficult to discover (Figure 17.7).

Rare variants may be analyzed in family or twin studies, as well as in identified extreme phenotypes, by examining the shared occurrence of rare variants in a particular region within individuals with the same phenotype.[263,264] Rare variants may also be examined in unrelated individuals with more recently established techniques.[263,265-272] Information about variants of this frequency is typically obtained via deep-imputation or sequencing analyses.[273] Although early studies evaluating rare variants proposed that the large effects, combined with extreme phenotyping designs, would allow identification of important variants in even small samples, more recent publications indicate that large samples sizes are still required.[274]

Individual variant tests examining the associations between the outcomes of interest and rare variants, as is done with common variants, may result in unstable effect estimates and are typically underpowered as a result of fewer copies of alleles being present in a study population. Instead, rare variants can be analyzed using a variety of established techniques, including meta-analysis across multiple studies or by collapsing all relevant variants across genes or regions of interest.[265-272] Because of the instability of standard error estimates for rare variants, other test statistics are used in rare variant analysis, such as the score test and Firth test.[275] The Firth test has been shown to have the best combination of type I error and statistical power characteristics for joint analysis of rare frequency variants.[275] However, the score test is preferable in meta-analysis of rare variant association tests for a number of reasons, including more stable P values, faster computation,[276,277] the best balance between power and controlling type I error rate,[275] and maintaining power in situations with case-control imbalance within or across studies (a large concern when examining rare variants in rare diseases).[277,278]

For rare variants, we can often assume that changes in a particular gene or region produce a similar effect on a biologic function, and ultimately alter the phenotype. Therefore it is possible to aggregate variants within a gene or region into a single score, thus creating multiple "copies" for testing associations. Most aggregate tests can be classified as burden-type tests or variance component tests.[279] The burden test is most powerful when the rare variants have effects going in the same direction (i.e., all harmful or all protective), whereas variance component kernel-based association methods (e.g., SKAT) are more powerful when a region contains rare variants that are both harmful and protective. The SKAT-O test combines both tests as special cases and is optimal across multiple scenarios.[266,267] In addition to basing these tests on specific chromosomal regions, tests can consider only rare variants predicted to have a significant impact on the function of a protein by altering the amino acid composition or regulating gene activity (i.e., through expression). Functional prediction scores can also be incorporated into rare variant tests.[265,280] Restricting only to these functional variants can increase power for detecting rare variant association through elimination of neutral nonfunctional variants.

Current and Future Directions: Sequencing, Copy Number Variation, and Epigenetics

Although sleep-related literature has focused mainly on heritability, linkage, and candidate gene or GWAS analyses, emerging areas of focus in genetic research include whole exome and whole genome sequencing, study of copy number variation (CNV), and whole genome epigenetic effects. Emerging sequencing technologies have resulted in the ability of researchers and clinicians to sequence large regions of the genome at lower cost. When coupled with emerging bioinformatics techniques for variant calling, whole exome and whole genome sequencing provide accurate identification of all genetic variation within protein coding genes or the entire genome, respectively.[273,281,282] Accurate variant identification through sequencing allows for the identification of important variants, including de novo mutations, that is, variants that have not been inherited from parents.[273,282]

Research has focused on relationships between single nucleotide variation and phenotypic variability. However, two additional types of genetic variation may account for some of the missing heritability in current research. The first, CNV, is defined as structural variations in DNA that are greater than 1 kilobase in size, including deletions, insertions, and duplications.[283-285] In contrast to SNPs, in which only a single base is changed in the DNA sequence, CNVs lead to the removal or duplication of large numbers of bases, including in some circumstances whole genes or groups of genes. Hence there is reason to believe that CNVs can have large effects on phenotypes. Because they can have large effects on development and functioning, individual CNVs are often very rare, and therefore associations can be hard to detect. For this reason, many studies have focused on evaluating whether there is an overall enrichment in the number of CNVs in cases when compared with controls. One study found an enrichment of rare large (<1% frequency and >100 kb long) CNVs in Japanese narcoleptic patients when compared with controls,[286] implicating the region near the *PARK2* gene as harboring CNVs associated with narcolepsy. Given their impact upon behavioral traits,[287-289] analysis of the role of CNVs in sleep disorders is likely to prove fruitful in the future.

In addition to CNV, state-of-the-art genetic research has begun examining the impact of epigenetics,[290-293] or heritable modifications in gene function or activity that do not involve alterations in the underlying DNA sequence. One of the most studied forms of epigenetic modification is that of DNA methylation, which involves the addition of methyl (CH3) groups at cytosine-guanine (CpG) dinucleotides that typically repress regional gene expression.[294] Although methylation patterns are heritable, DNA methylation is also subject to modification through the environment and behaviors, such as diet,[295] smoking,[296] physical activity,[297] and sleep patterns.[298-300] Because of their role in gene expression, alterations in epigenetic patterns are a mechanism by which these and other environmental factors may modify genetic susceptibility to disease.[301,302] Epigenetic modification is expected to play an important role in disease given its ability to regulate and modify gene expression within specific cell types.[290,303] Although the field continues to advance, recent progress includes the use of genome-wide characterizations of DNA methylation, resulting in the first epigenome-wide association studies (EWAS), which have recently been published for a number of traits, including BMI.[304-306]

As methodologies for analyzing these data continue to develop, and prices for sequencing continue to decrease, research in these emerging genetic areas will further our current understanding of the genetic architecture that underlies complex diseases. Given the known heritability of many sleep and circadian traits and disorders in humans, this will be a major opportunity for sleep research.

SELECTED READINGS

Bishara J, Keens TG, Perez IA. The genetics of congenital central hypoventilation syndrome: clinical implications. *Appl Clin Genet.* 2018;11:135–144.

Bush WS, Moore JH. Genome-wide association studies. *PLoS Comput Biol.* 2012;8(12):e1002822.

Chanock SJ, Manolio T, Boehnke M, et al. Replicating genotype-phenotype associations. *Nature.* 2007;447(7145):655–660.

Collins FS, Varmus H. A new initiative on precision medicine. *N Engl J Med.* 2015;372(9):793–795.

Elgart M, Redline S, Sofer T. Machine and deep learning in molecular and genetic aspects of sleep research. *Neurotherapeutics.* 2021;18(1):228–243.

Freeman AA, Rye DB. The molecular basis of restless legs syndrome. *Curr Opin Neurobiol.* 2013;23:895–900.

Hallmayer J, Faraco J, Lin L, et al. Narcolepsy is strongly associated with the T-cell receptor alpha locus. *Nat Genet.* 2009;41:708–711.

He Y, Jones CR, Fujiki N, et al. The transcriptional repressor DEC2 regulates sleep length in mammals. *Science.* 2009;325:866–870.

Jansen PR, Watanabe K, Stringer S, et al. Genome-wide analysis of insomnia in 1,331,010 individuals identifies new risk loci and functional pathways. *Nat Genet.* 2019;51(3):394–403.

Jones SE, van Hees VT, Mazzotti DR, et al. Genetic studies of accelerometer-based sleep measures yield new insights into human sleep behaviour. *Nat Commun.* 2019;10(1):1585.

Kalmbach DA, Schneider LD, Cheung J, et al. Genetic basis of chronotype in humans: insights from three landmark GWAS. *Sleep.* 2017;40(2).

Kosmicki JA, Churchhouse CL, Rivas MA, Neale B. Discovery of rare variants for complex phenotypes. *Hum Genet.* 2016;135(6):625–634.
Lane JM, Liang J, Vlasac I, et al. Genome-wide association analyses of sleep disturbance traits identify new loci and highlight shared genetics with neuropsychiatric and metabolic traits. *Nat Genet.* 2017;49(2):274–281.
Manolio TA, Collins FS, Cox NJ, et al. Finding the missing heritability of complex diseases. *Nature.* 2009;461:747–753.
Szabo ST, Thorpy MJ, Mayer G, Peever JH, Kilduff TS. Neurobiological and immunogenetic aspects of narcolepsy: Implications for pharmacotherapy. *Sleep Med Rev.* 2019;43:23–36.
Tafti M, Hor H, Dauvilliers Y, et al. DQB1 locus alone explains most of the risk and protection in narcolepsy with cataplexy in Europe. *Sleep.* 2014;37:19–25.
Toh KL, Jones CR, He Y, et al. An hPer2 phosphorylation site mutation in familial advanced sleep phase syndrome. *Science.* 2001;291:1040–1043.
Varvarigou V, Dahabreh IJ, Malhotra A, et al. A review of genetic association studies of obstructive sleep apnea: field synopsis and meta-analysis. *Sleep.* 2011;34:1461–1468.

A complete reference list can be found online at ExpertConsult.com.

Section 4

Physiology in Sleep

Chapter 18

Introduction to Physiology in Sleep

Kenneth P. Wright, Jr.; Renaud Tamisier

Chapter Highlights

Studying and reading about physiology in sleep explores the essence of sleep research and medicine. Understanding of physiology leads to an understanding of pathophysiology. For clinicians, this knowledge is the backbone needed to diagnose and manage the wide spectrum of diseases that are related to sleep. This section covers all aspects of sleep physiology. Insights from the essential mechanisms of sleep to pathways leading to sleep disorders are presented by the most outstanding researchers and clinicians. These authors explain in a clear and precise manner the most elaborate concepts, allowing all readers to benefit from their knowledge.

Sleep medicine is a relatively new discipline that encompasses a wide spectrum of disorders from neurologic to respiratory disease. Sleep, on the other hand, is a physiologic state that could be altered by environments, such as altitude or temperature, but is also impaired when organs or physiologic functions are compromised. To this extent, physiology in sleep brings insights to researchers and clinicians to help them understand the different processes and pathways involved in sleep disorders.

In this section, 14 chapters cover this knowledge, which is so important for those who are willing to embrace the specialized concepts that are fundamental in research and clinical practice in sleep. The first 6 chapters give us an up-to-date view of the basic physiologic notions, from anatomic neurophysiology to upper airway physiology (see Chapters 19 to 24). Sleep is a particularly vulnerable time for respiratory control stability. Many of the potential compensatory inputs to breathing are markedly diminished or absent during this physiologic state. In accordance, regardless of the underlying cause, abnormality in one or more of the components that are important contributors to respiratory control can cause sleep-disordered breathing. The resulting sleep-related respiratory instability depends on the extent to which the respiratory control system is impaired. The understanding of respiratory and cardiovascular physiology (see Chapters 21 and 23) and their interactions (see Chapter 20) are reviewed, showing how specifically sleep interacts with cardiovascular and respiratory functions but also how cardiovascular and respiratory coupling must be considered when willing to translate these into clinical practice. These chapters are indeed an endless resource for clinicians and researchers. Finally, the chapter on central neural control of respiratory neurons and motoneurons during sleep gives an overview of central processing of motoneurons during sleep, including effects of drugs, and opens a new area of treatment for sleep disorders (see Chapter 22). Physiologic phenotyping will be useful in the personalized treatment of sleep breathing disorders as described in Chapter 129.

The second part of this section is more related to how the environment or other physiologic states may interfere with sleep and sleep physiology. Therefore sleep physiology is reinvented at high altitude or with the effect of body temperature and hibernation (see Chapters 25 and 28). Four chapters are dedicated to the interaction between major physiologic functions and sleep. Endocrine function, memory, sensory, and motor processing are indeed tightly linked with neurologic pathways and the function of sleep (see Chapters 27, 29, and 30).

The last three chapters of this section relate to local and use-dependent aspects of sleep (see Chapter 31) and how disease states may affect sleep and host defense (see Chapter 26) and traumatic brain injury (see Chapter 32). The chapter on local sleep is entirely new and offers the challenge of bringing highly specialized concepts from molecular biology and electrophysiology to neurologic physiology in explaining how this hypothesis provides further understanding to previously unexplained sleep anomalies, such as sleepwalking, sleep inertia, poor performance during prolonged waking, insomnia, and other disassociated states.

Now the challenge will be to choose from where to start.

Chapter 19

What Neuroimaging Reveals about the Brain Areas Generating, Maintaining, and Regulating Sleep

Gilles Vandewalle; Pierre Maquet

Chapter Highlights

- The development of neuroimaging techniques has made it possible to characterize regional cerebral function in humans under a variety of sleep-related conditions. These techniques have been used to characterize brain activity throughout the sleep-wake cycle in normal human subjects.
- Regional brain activity during sleep is segregated and integrated within cortical and subcortical areas differently than during wakefulness.
- Regional brain activity is influenced by incoming stimuli, by previous waking experience, and by the circadian system.
- Functional neuroimaging identified the neural correlates of sleep-wake regulation by homeostatic sleep pressure, circadian rhythms, and the non-image-forming effects of light.
- Finally, functional imaging of patients with sleep disorders and in response to treatment interventions indicated reliable changes in neural systems across the sleep-wake cycle.

Functional neuroimaging consists of all techniques that can generate images of brain activity. In humans such techniques usually include single photon emission computed tomography (SPECT), positron emission tomography (PET), functional magnetic resonance imaging (fMRI), optical imaging, diffusion-weighted imaging (DWI), and, to a lesser extent, multichannel electroencephalography (EEG) and magnetoencephalography (MEG). Each technique has its own advantages and drawbacks in terms of spatial and temporal resolutions, accessibility, safety, and cost. For instance, EEG and MEG record brain oscillations with an excellent temporal resolution (usually on the order of a few milliseconds), but given the limited number of sensors positioned outside the brain volume, their localizing capacity is limited and methods modeling the electric or magnetic sources of the signal remain suboptimal. MEG and EEG can therefore provide limited information about the brain correlates of sleep-related mechanisms. By contrast, SPECT, PET, and MRI provide excellent spatial resolution (≈0.5 mm to a few millimeters), but they are based on the measure of hemodynamic or metabolic parameters, which reduces their temporal resolution from approximately 1 second to many minutes.

In accordance, a comprehensive understanding of brain substrates subtending sleep functions will require human brain function during sleep and wakefulness to be characterized using as many techniques as possible, while keeping up with the constant flow of technical innovation. For instance, the recent advent of ultra–high-field MRI at 7 tesla or higher, quantitative MRI, and diffusion-weighted MRI (DWI) open a totally new scale with direct observation at the submillimeter scale (0.02 to 1 mm) and inferences about microscopic properties (<0.02 mm [e.g., myelin content, neurite density]).[1,2] Likewise, pioneer PET developments with high sensitivity, requiring much lower ionization and short acquisitions time (<1 second), will undoubtedly open new perspectives for sleep research in years to come.[3]

This chapter summarizes the main advances made using functional neuroimaging in the current understanding of human sleep and its intimate relationships with waking performance and cognition, both in normal healthy sleepers and in patients with sleep disorders. These advances are considered in the context of five main topics: the characterization of regional brain activity during normal human sleep, the regional brain function in conditions of increased sleep pressure, the neural correlates of the regulation of sleep-wake cycle by the circadian system, and the nonclassical photoreception system, and finally, the clinical applications for the management of sleep disorders.

FUNCTIONAL SEGREGATION AND INTEGRATION DURING NORMAL HUMAN SLEEP

Preclinical research has identified the basic circuits in the brain that are responsible for promoting arousal.[4] In general, reduction in activity in these systems is essential for generating and maintaining sleep. A major component of this network is the brainstem reticular core, a diffuse network of predominantly glutamatergic long-projecting neurons and a smaller collection of presumed local circuit gamma-aminobutyric acid (GABA) neurons. Additional components include a collection of nuclei in the brainstem tegmentum, mostly dorsal to the reticular formation, that includes cholinergic and monoaminergic (serotoninergic, noradrenergic, and dopaminergic) neurons. These nuclei send rostral projections that are parallel to and are interconnected with those of the brainstem reticular core. Cholinergic nuclei also are clustered rostrally in the basal forebrain, including septal nuclei and the diagonal band of Broca. The reticular nucleus of the thalamus, which surrounds a large part of the diencephalic structure, also plays a role in sleep initiation and maintenance, as well as in sleep phasic activity.

Research has focused on a significant role for the hypothalamus in arousal and in regulating transitions between sleep and waking states. Specifically, the tuberomamillary histaminergic neurons and the perifornical hypocretin neurons in the posterior hypothalamus have extensive interconnections and interactions with the basic arousal systems (for more information, see Chapters 7 and 8). Activity changes in these primary regulating areas result in profound modifications in activity patterns in thalamocortical circuits, including inhibitory reticular nucleus activity, and in associated structures, such as basal ganglia or cerebellum. A primary aim of functional imaging studies has been to characterize this reorganization of regional brain function during normal human sleep and the responses to external stimuli as well as the influence of previous waking experience on regional brain activity during sleep. The results of these studies, summarized in Table 19.1, are detailed next (Figure 19.1).

Non–Rapid Eye Movement Sleep

Neurophysiologic recordings in sleeping animals indicate that during non–rapid eye movement (NREM) sleep, the neural activity of the brain is shaped by a slow rhythm (<1 Hz), characterized by a fundamental oscillation of membrane potential made up of a depolarizing phase, associated with important neuronal firing ("up" state), followed by a hyperpolarizing phase during which cortical neurons remain silent for a few hundred milliseconds ("down" state).[5,6] The slow oscillation occurs synchronously in large neuronal populations in such a way that it can be reflected on EEG recordings as high-amplitude, low-frequency waves.[5,7–9] The slow rhythm entrains and is entrained by other sleep oscillations in a coalescence of multiple rhythms.[7,10] Among the latter, spindles are associated with burst firing in thalamocortical populations. They arise from a cyclic inhibition of thalamocortical neurons by reticular thalamic neurons, which are activated by cholinergic neurons of the basal forebrain (BF) and brainstem and which elicits postinhibitory rebound spike bursts in thalamocortical cells, which in turn entrain cortical populations in spindle oscillations.[10,11]

At the macroscopic systems level, the measure of brain metabolism or hemodynamics by PET usually requires the integration of the brain activity over extended time periods (from tens of seconds for $H_2{}^{15}O$-PET to 45 minutes for F-18 fluorodeoxyglucose [^{18}F-FDG] PET), resulting in the averaging of brain activity over the up and down states described earlier. In consequence, NREM sleep has systematically been associated with lower brain energy metabolism than that seen in wakefulness.[12] Relative to wakefulness, cerebral glucose and oxygen metabolism, as well as cerebral blood flow, is decreased by 5% to 10% during stage 2 sleep[13,14] and by 25% to 40% during slow wave sleep (SWS)—that is, stage 3 NREM sleep (see also Chapter 20).[15–17] These global findings were confirmed using EEG in MRI concomitant with arterial spin labeling (ASL) measurements, which also allows the measurement of absolute cerebral blood flow (but with a much better temporal resolution, as whole brain volume acquisition takes ≈10 seconds).[18]

Both PET and MRI ASL indicate that these decreases are not homogeneous but show a reproducible regional distribution. It is thought that brain areas with a high proportion of neurons committed in synchronous sleep oscillations are likely to have the lowest regional activity.[12] During light NREM sleep, cerebral blood flow decreases in the pons and thalamic nuclei, as well as in frontal and parietal areas, but is maintained in the midbrain.[19] Consistent with the implication of thalamic nuclei in the generation of spindles, thalamic blood flow during stage 2 sleep decreases in proportion to the power density within the sigma frequency range (12 to 15 Hz).[20] During SWS the most consistent decreases were observed in areas playing a permissive or active role in generating NREM sleep and its characteristic oscillations. These areas are the dorsal pons and mesencephalon, thalami, basal forebrain, and hypothalamus. The topography of the decreases in cortical blood flow during NREM sleep also is very reproducible and encompasses the prefrontal cortex, anterior cingulate cortex, precuneus, and mesial aspect of the temporal lobe. MRI ASL further revealed that the cerebral blood flow decrease associated with NREM sleep in all areas reported earlier (i.e., in the cortex, diencephalon, and pons) was proportional to the power density in the lower frequency band of the EEG, usually referred to as *slow wave activity* (SWA),[18] which has proved to be a very useful and popular parameter because it best quantifies the dissipation of homeostatic sleep pressure during NREM sleep.[21] EEG combined with MRI ASL also reveals that the occipital pole and parahippocampal gyrus seem to be characterized by an increased cerebral blood flow relative to pre–sleep-wake and in proportion to SWA (positive correlation),[18] potentially due to dream-like activity, basic sensory processing, and/or memory processes (for the parahippocampus). Furthermore, cerebral blood flow during wakefulness immediately after sleep is lower than wakefulness preceding sleep in most of the areas undergoing decreased blood flow during sleep, potentially constituting a correlate of the so-called sleep inertia[18] together with their previously identified progressive reactivation and functional reorganization.[22]

The mechanisms that produce changes in regional blood flow are unclear, but a tight relationship is therefore present between slow wave amount and/or intensity and cerebral blood flow, even though no causal/directional inferences has been proposed. The frontal and parietal polymodal associative cortices are among the most active brain structures during wakefulness.[12] In consequence, homeostatic sleep pressure locally accrued during a normal waking day is thought to be particularly important in these cortical areas, resulting during NREM sleep in a considerable amount of local slow waves, with a substantial decrease in local energy metabolism.[12] Significant decreases in blood flow also were unexpectedly observed in the cerebellum and basal ganglia. It is currently not known whether these changes in blood flow indicate that these two areas have a role in generating and maintaining

Table 19.1 Summary of the Modifications in Global and Regional Hemodynamic or Metabolic Parameters during NREM and REM Sleep

	Deep NREM Sleep					REM Sleep			
	Kety-Schmidt[a]		PET		fMRI	Kety-Schmidt		PET	
Area	*Oxygen Metabolism*	*Blood Flow*	*Glucose Metabolism*	*Blood Flow*	*BOLD Signal*	*Oxygen Metabolism*	*Blood Flow*	*Glucose Metabolism*	*Blood Flow*
Global Changes									
	↓ relative to W and REM sleep	↓ relative to W and REM sleep	↓ relative to W and REM sleep	↓ relative to W and REM sleep		≅ W	≅ W	≅ W	≅ W
Regional Changes									
Lateral frontal				↓ relative to W	↑ in response to slow waves				↓ relative to W
Medial prefrontal (including orbitofrontal)					↑ in response to slow waves			↑ relative to W	
Lateral parietal				↓ relative to W					↓ relative to W
Medial parietal (including precuneus)				↓ relative to W	↑ in response to slow waves				↓ relative to W
Temporo-occipital			↑ relative to W					↑ relative to W	
Anterior cingulate cortex									↑ relative to W or SWS
Medial temporal lobe (hippocampus, parahippocampus)					↑ in response to slow waves				↑ relative to W or SWS
Medial temporal lobe (amygdala)									↑ relative to W or SWS
Thalamus				↓ relative to W					↑ relative to W or SWS
Basal ganglia				↓ relative to W					
Pons, midbrain				↓ relative to W	↑ in response to slow waves				
Cerebellum				↓ relative to W	↑ in response to slow waves				

[a]Kety-Schmidt: A method for measuring organ blood flow, first applied to the brain in 1944 by C.F. Schmidt and S.S. Kety. A chemically inert indicator gas is equilibrated with the tissue of the organ of interest, and the rate of disappearance from the organ is measured. Blood flow is calculated on the assumption that the tissue and venous blood concentrations of the indicator gas are in diffusion equilibrium at all blood flow rates and that the rate of disappearance of the indicator from the tissue is a function of how much of the indicator is in the tissue at any time; the rate of disappearance is assumed to be exponential.

≅, Approximately the same activity; ↓, decrease; ↑, increase; BOLD, blood oxygen level–dependent; fMRI, functional magnetic resonance imaging; NREM, non–rapid eye movement; PET, positron emission tomography; REM, rapid eye movement; SWS, slow wave sleep; W, wakefulness.

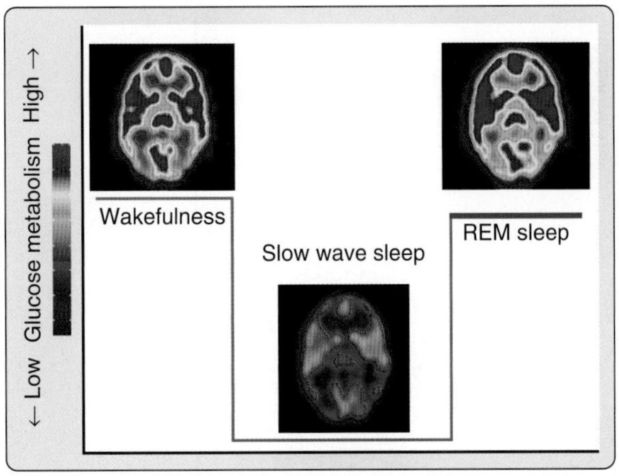

Figure 19.1 Schematic representation of the variations in global cerebral glucose metabolism in resting wakefulness, slow wave sleep, and rapid eye movement (REM) sleep. The images represent the cerebral glucose metabolism measured in a single subject during three different sessions with fluorodeoxyglucose F-18 positron emission tomography. Functional images are displayed at the same brain level and use the same color scale. Similar rates of brain glucose metabolism are measured during wakefulness and REM sleep. Brain glucose metabolism is significantly decreased during slow wave sleep relative to that in both wakefulness and REM sleep. (Modified from Maquet P, Dive D, Salmon E, et al. Cerebral glucose utilization during sleep-wake cycle in man determined by positron emission tomography and [^{18}F]2-fluoro-2-deoxy-d-glucose method. *Brain Res.* 1990;513:136–43.)

cortical oscillations or if they are merely entrained by the cortical slow rhythm.

Advances in event-related EEG and fMRI have allowed a finer-grained characterization of brain activities associated with transient events, such as spindles[23] or slow waves.[24] In humans, some evidence suggests the occurrence of two different types of spindles during sleep, slow and fast EEG spindles, which differ by their scalp topography and some aspects of their regulation.[25] Both spindle types trigger significant activity in the thalami, the anterior cingulate and insular cortices, and the superior temporal gyri.[23] Beyond the common activation pattern, slow spindles (frequencies of 11 to 13 Hz) are associated with increased activity in the superior frontal gyrus. By contrast, fast spindles (13 to 15 Hz) recruit a set of cortical regions involved in sensorimotor processing and recruit the mesial frontal cortex and hippocampus.

During SWS, the largest waves (>140 μV) have been taken as realizations of the slow oscillation (<1 Hz), whereas small slow waves (75 to 140 μV) were deemed to correspond to the delta rhythms.[26,27] Transient increases in brain activity associated with slow (>140 μV) and delta EEG waves (75 to 140 μV) can be detected in the pontine tegmentum (in an area encompassing the locus coeruleus), midbrain, and cerebellum, as well as in several cortical areas, including the inferior frontal, medial prefrontal, precuneus, and posterior cingulate parahippocampal gyrus,[24] areas that have been shown to be current sources underpinning human slow waves.[28]

Compared with baseline activity, slow waves are associated with significant activity in the parahippocampal gyrus, cerebellum, and brainstem, whereas delta waves are related to frontal responses.[24] These findings show that NREM sleep is not a state of brain quiescence but is an active state during which neural activity is consistently synchronized by sleep oscillations (spindles, slow rhythm) in specific cerebral regions. Electrophysiology and computational evidence from the cortex and thalamus indicates that the tonic firing pattern and fluctuations of the membrane potential during slow oscillation up states are similar to those characteristic of the waking state, suggesting that the up state is a ubiquitous feature of neuronal dynamics in corticothalamic networks, reproducing a "micro" wake-like state that facilitates neuronal interactions.[29]

EEG-fMRI is also proposed to refine the characterization of sleep stages. Uninstructed data-driven temporal analyses of fMRI data lead to the isolation of different states, or periods of time of quasi-stationary activity, across 90 regions of interest (ROIs) covering the entire brain and recorded while awake, trying to fall asleep, and while asleep.[30] These states are most prominently associated with wakefulness, N2, or N3 and clustered into a group of states preferentially switching between one another. State and clusters are primarily associated with decrease or increased activity in specific subsets of ROIs. SWS is characterized by more stable states (less switching between states and less states), whereas N1 is very heterogeneous in terms of oscillation composition and is therefore difficult to characterize in terms of stationary states associated with it, indicating that N1 remains the most vaguely defined sleep stage within polysomnography, with the highest disagreement between human visual scores. This novel approach reveals a higher complexity of brain activity than given through traditional sleep scoring, but it is unknown yet whether this high complexity allows a more refined understanding of the functions of sleep. Increased mean activation in the default mode network seems to be associated with the switch from wakefulness states to the NREM sleep-states cluster. This comes on top of event-related fMRI demonstration of a partial overlap between the regional activity pattern related to SWS waves and the default mode network, which could therefore play a key role for sleep initiation and for the brain responses synchronized by the slow oscillation during NREM sleep[24] (Figure 19.2).

Processing of External Stimuli during Non-Rapid Eye Movement Sleep

To date, only a few neuroimaging studies have investigated the human brain correlates of external stimuli processing during sleep, and their results are controversial. In sedated young children, examined with fMRI, visual stimulation elicited a paradoxical decrease in response in the anterior medial occipital cortex.[31] Although the neurobiologic significance of this enigmatic finding remains elusive, it has been replicated in naturally sleeping adults during SWS, using fMRI and PET.[32] This response pattern does not seem to be specific to visual stimulations because it also is observed when auditory stimuli are delivered during NREM sleep.[33]

In sharp contrast with these results, other data suggest that the brain still processes auditory stimuli up to cortical areas during NREM sleep.[34] Significant responses to auditory stimuli were detected in bilateral auditory cortex, thalamus, and caudate nuclei during wakefulness and light NREM sleep. In addition, the left amygdala and the left prefrontal cortex are recruited by stimuli of particular affective significance for the individual subject. It appears, however, that sound processing during sleep is altered or absent in higher cortical areas during sleep spindles and during the negative going phase of the slow oscillation.[35] Opposed to this, when sounds are associated with the positive going phase of a slow oscillation, the responses are elicited in distant frontal areas. It seems therefore that sensory information processing during NREM sleep

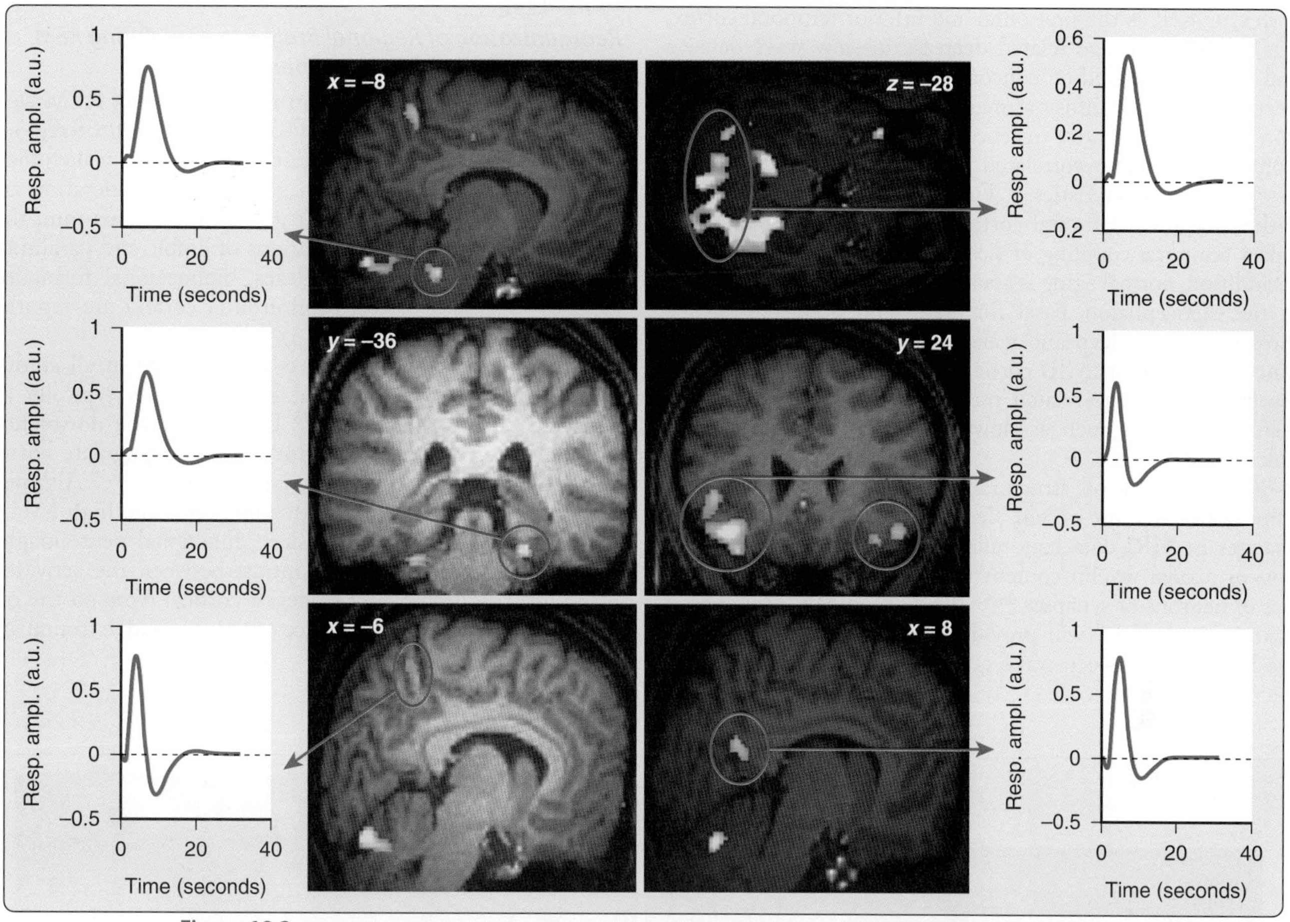

Figure 19.2 Brain regions activated in relation to slow oscillations (both high-amplitude slow waves and delta waves) as observed with combined electroencephalography and functional magnetic resonance imaging. *Structural images—center panels,* Significant responses are associated with both slow and delta waves. Functional results are displayed on an individual image (display at $P < .001$, uncorrected) at different levels of the *x, y,* and *z* axes as indicated for each section. *Side panels (left* and *right),* time course (in seconds) of fitted response amplitudes (in arbitrary units [a.u.]) during slow waves or delta waves in the corresponding circled brain area. All responses consisted in regional increases of brain activity. From *left to right* and then *top to bottom*: pontine tegmentum, cerebellum; right parahippocampal gyrus, inferior frontal gyrus; precuneus, posterior cingulate cortex. Ampl., Amplitude. (Modified from Dang-Vu TT, Schabus M, Desseilles M, et al. Spontaneous neural activity during human slow wave sleep. *Proc Natl Acad Sci U S A.* 2008;105:15160–5.)

is constrained by fundamental brain oscillatory modes (slow oscillations and spindles), which results in a complex interplay between spontaneous and induced brain activity. These distortions of sensory information may functionally isolate the cortex from the environment and provide unique conditions favorable for off-line memory processing. (More information on how the brain processes sensory input during sleep can be found in Chapter 30.)

Increasing attention has also been given to memory reactivation during sleep through sensory stimulations associated with learned material during sleep, which seems to be effective under certain circumstances.[36,37] When delivered during sleep while fMRI data are recorded (without concomitant EEG), olfactory stimulation associated with pairs of objects in an object-location memory task during the preceding period wakefulness triggers activation of the hippocampus.[38] Similarly, presentation during sleep of odor cues associated with an object-location memory task during wakefulness increases activation levels in the ventromedial prefrontal cortex, involved in memory recall, that significantly correlates with postsleep memory performance.[39] This further reinforces the idea that sleep is an active state and that the regional brain processing of stimulation from the external world can participate in complex processes even during sleep. (See the following and Chapter 29 for more information on off-line memory processing).

Age-Related Changes in Non–Rapid Eye Movement Sleep

Changes in sleep and wakefulness regulation are hallmarks of the aging process. As early as the fifth decade of life, sleep becomes shorter, more fragmented, and presents fewer slow waves, putatively reflecting a reduced buildup and dissipation of sleep need. Sleep also occurs earlier during the 24-hour day, likely because of an advance in the circadian timing system in aging. (More information on age-related changes in sleep can be found in Chapters 3 and 42).[40,41]

Despite these well-accepted common changes, little information, if any, has been gathered about the brain areas whose activity may underlie age-related changes in sleep in humans. Brain structural correlates have been reported, however. For instance, in healthy older individuals, MRI-based cortical thinning of several portions of the insular and cingulate cortex, as well as the prefrontal and inferior temporal cortex, was linked to an age-related decrease in slow wave density and amplitude, based on concomitant EEG measures during sleep.[42] Likewise, diffusion imaging indicated that modification in the white matter tracts connecting the thalamus to the frontal cortex were correlated to age-related modifications in spindle characteristics.[43] Furthermore, selective atrophy within the medial frontal cortex in older adults predicted a looser temporal coupling of sleep slow waves and spindles.[44] In addition, normal aging is associated with structural changes in the diencephalon, basal forebrain, and brainstem structures regulating sleep and wakefulness.[45] However, whether functional PET or fMRI cortical or subcortical measures are associated with age-related modification of transient EEG features of sleep, such as slow oscillations and spindles, is unknown.

Interpretation of structural brain changes are further complicated by the recent demonstration that age-related changes in MRI data may reflect modifications in neuronal iron or axonal myelin content rather than reflecting a mere loss of neurons or synapses.[46,47] The development of unbiased quantitative MRI[48] will provide important tools to address the link between sleep-wake quality and brain structure and microstructure.

REM Sleep

Reorganization of Regional Brain Function during REM Sleep: Relation with Dream Characteristics

The level of energy metabolism recorded during REM sleep is similar to waking levels.[16,17] The distribution of regional brain activity, however, significantly differs from wakefulness. In addition to areas known to participate in generation and maintenance of REM sleep (e.g., pontine tegmentum, thalamic nuclei), significant activations of limbic and paralimbic areas (e.g., amygdaloid complexes, hippocampal formation, anterior cingulate cortex, orbitofrontal cortex) are reported during REM sleep (Figure 19.3).[15,49,50]

Although this observation is not reported in all studies, posterior cortices in temporal occipital areas typically are activated during REM sleep.[15] By contrast, the dorsolateral prefrontal cortex, parietal cortex, posterior cingulate cortex, and precuneus are the least active brain regions.[15,50] Although early animal studies had already mentioned the high level of limbic activity during REM sleep, functional neuroimaging in humans highlighted the contrast between the activation of limbic, paralimbic, and posterior cortical areas on the one hand and the relative quiescence of the associative frontal and parietal cortices on the other.

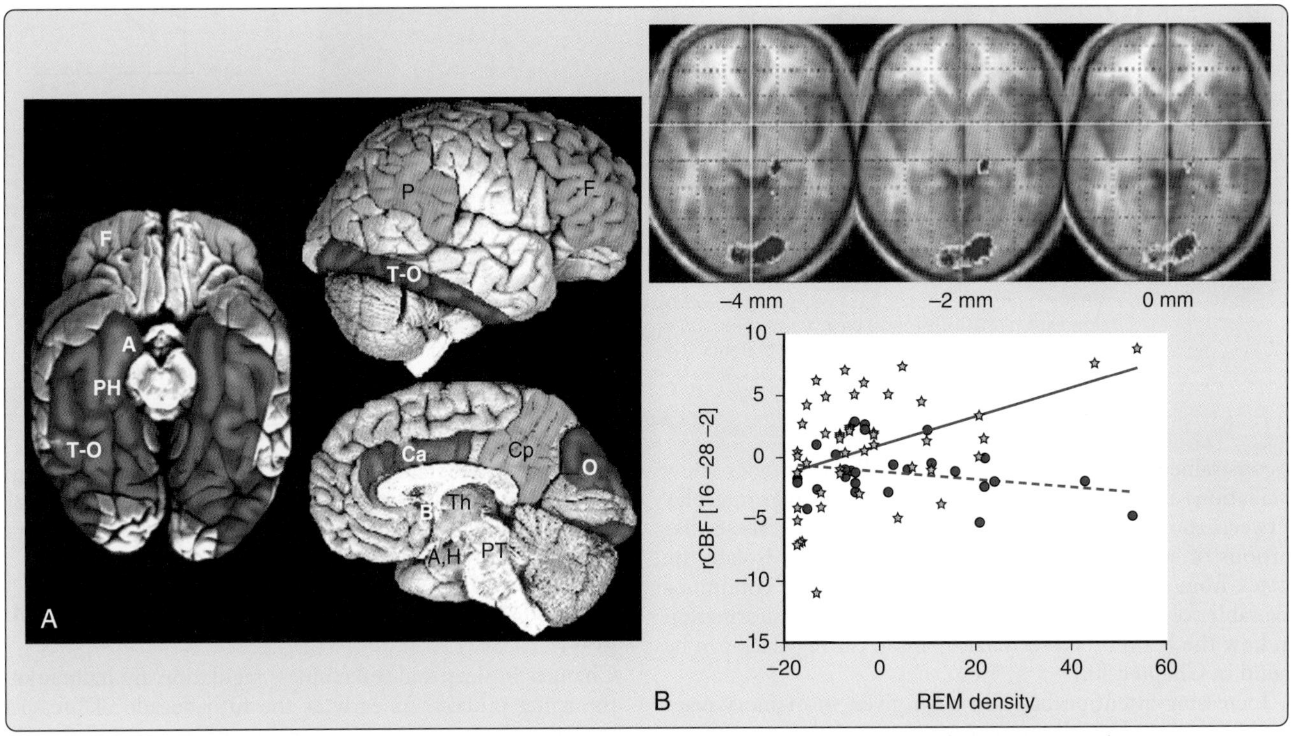

Figure 19.3 A, Schematic representation of the relative increases and decreases in neural activity associated with rapid eye movement (REM) sleep as observed with positron emission tomography. **B,** *Top,* Cerebral areas more active in relation to rapid eye movements during paradoxical sleep than during awake states. Transverse sections are from 24 to 0 mm from the bicommissural plane. The functional data are displayed at $P < .001$ uncorrected, superimposed on the average magnetic resonance imaging scan of the brain of sleeping subjects, coregistered to the same reference space. *Bottom,* Plot of the adjusted regional cerebral blood flow (rCBF) in arbitrary units in the right geniculate body in relation to the REM counts. The geniculate cerebral blood flow is correlated more strongly with the REM counts during REM sleep (*red circles*) than during wake (*green stars*). A,H, Amygdala and hippocampus; B, basal forebrain; Ca, anterior cingulate gyrus; Cp, posterior cingulate gyrus and precuneus; F, prefrontal cortex; H, hypothalamus; M, motor cortex; P, parietal supramarginal cortex; PH, parahippocampal gyrus; PT, pontine tegmentum; O, occipital-lateral cortex; Th, thalamus; T-O, temporooccipital extrastriate cortex. (**A,** Modified from Schwartz S, Maquet P. Sleep imaging and the neuro-psychological assessment of dreams. *Trends Cogn Sci.* 2002;6:23–30; **B,** modified from Peigneux P, Laureys S, Fuchs S, et al. Generation of rapid eye movements during paradoxical sleep in humans. *Neuroimage.* 2001;14:701–8.)

Regional functional integration is also modified during REM sleep relative to wakefulness. For instance, the functional interactions between striate and extra-striate cortices, which are positive during wakefulness, become negative during REM sleep.[51] Likewise, the functional connectivity between the amygdala and temporal occipital areas is tighter during REM sleep than during resting wakefulness.[52]

The organization of human brain function during REM sleep somehow relates to some of the characteristics of dreaming activity.[50,53] The perceptual aspects of dreams would be related to the activation of posterior (occipital and temporal) cortices, whereas emotional features in dreams would be related to the activation of amygdalar complexes, orbitofrontal cortex, and anterior cingulate cortex. The recruitment of mesiotemporal areas would account for the memory content commonly observed in dreams. The relative hypoactivation of the prefrontal cortex might help to explain the alteration in logical reasoning, working memory, episodic memory, and executive functions characterizing dream reports collected from experimentally induced REM sleep awakenings. Activation of the anterior cingulate cortex and surrounding mesial prefrontal cortex has been described, in studies on waking cognitive neuroscience, to be related to self-referential cognition and to the monitoring of performance. Activation of these structures within REM sleep might represent a role for REM sleep in the internal monitoring of aspects of the self, especially those having emotional significance, in keeping with the activation of other related limbic and paralimbic structures.[54] (More information on the neurobiology of dreaming can be found in Chapters 57 and 58).

Brain Imaging and Other Characteristic Features of REM Sleep

REMs constitute a prominent feature of REM sleep. Cerebral mechanisms underpinning the generation of spontaneous ocular movements differ between REM sleep and wakefulness in humans. Regional cerebral blood flow changes in the lateral geniculate bodies and in the striate cortex are significantly more correlated with ocular movement density during REM sleep than during wakefulness,[55] a pattern that was later confirmed using fMRI.[56] This pattern of activity is reminiscent of ponto-geniculo-occipital waves, that is, prominent phasic bioelectrical potentials associated with eye movements that occur in isolation or in bursts just before and during REM sleep and are most easily recorded in cats and rats in the mesopontine tegmentum, the lateral geniculate bodies, and the occipital cortex.[57]

Another important feature in REM sleep is the instability in autonomic regulation and especially in cardiovascular regulation. During awake states, the right insula is involved in cardiovascular regulation,[58] but during REM sleep, the variability in heart rate is related to the activity in the right amygdaloid complex.[59] The functional connectivity between the amygdala and the insular cortex, two brain areas involved in cardiovascular regulation, differ significantly in REM sleep compared with wakefulness.[59] These results suggest a functional reorganization of central cardiovascular regulation during REM sleep (see also Chapter 20).

Experience-Dependent Modifications of Regional Brain Function during NREM and REM Sleep

Waking experience substantially influences regional brain activity during subsequent sleep. For instance, the blood flow of the hippocampus and parahippocampal gyrus during NREM sleep is increased in subjects who were navigating a virtual town (by means of a computer software program) during the previous waking period, compared with naïve participants.[60] The level of hippocampal activity expressed during SWS positively correlates with the improvement of performance in route retrieval the next day, suggesting that hippocampal activity during NREM sleep is related to subsequent "off-line" processing of spatial memory.[60] Similarly, a large response in the fusiform gyrus is observed in the presence of fast spindles after a declarative memory task for sequences of face.[61] Of importance, the task also recruits the fusiform gyrus both during encoding before sleep and during successful recall after sleep, and the overnight increase in fusiform gyrus activation from encoding to recall correlated with recall performance. These findings support that hippocampus and cortical reactivation during sleep of brain regions involved in previous declarative learning promotes consolidation of memory traces and learning performance improvement.

Aside from declarative memory, several brain areas activated during the execution of a serial reaction time task during wakefulness (brainstem, thalamus, and occipital, parietal and premotor areas) are significantly more active during REM sleep in subjects previously trained on the task than in non-trained subjects.[62] These increased activations during REM sleep were further suggested to be associated with significant changes in brain functional connectivity.[63] In addition, after learning a finger tapping task, the neural representation of the task during training is weakened during NREM sleep to the progressive benefit of the neural representation of the task that is assessed the next day.[64] Collectively, these results support the hypothesis that the memory of a motor sequence is further processed and reorganized during NREM and REM sleep in humans (Figure 19.4). (More information about the role of sleep in memory consolidation and the changes taking place during aging both for declarative and procedural memory can be found in Chapter 29.)

BRAIN IMAGING OF HUMAN SLEEP DEPRIVATION

Sleep generation and maintenance are strongly affected by the homeostatic sleep drive. In accordance, an understanding of the neural correlates of the awake brain during sleep deprivation, which is more prone to errors because of the increased homeostatic sleep drive and wrong alignment with the circadian signal, can be expected to provide additional clues about the mechanism associated with sleep functions and the detection and prevention of accidents due to sleep loss. (More information on the consequences of sleep deprivation on brain functioning during wakefulness can be found in Chapters 5, 37, and 38).

One study[65] assessed regional cerebral metabolism using the ^{18}F-FDG PET method in healthy subjects before and after 32 hours of sleep deprivation. The investigators noted prominent decreases in metabolism in the thalamus, basal ganglia, temporal lobes, and cerebellum and increases in visual cortex. Another study[66] described the effects of 24, 48, and 72 hours of sleep deprivation on waking regional cerebral metabolism assessed using ^{18}F-FDG PET, as well as alertness and cognitive performance. Sleep deprivation was associated with global declines in absolute cerebral metabolism. Regionally, these declines were most notable in the thalamus and

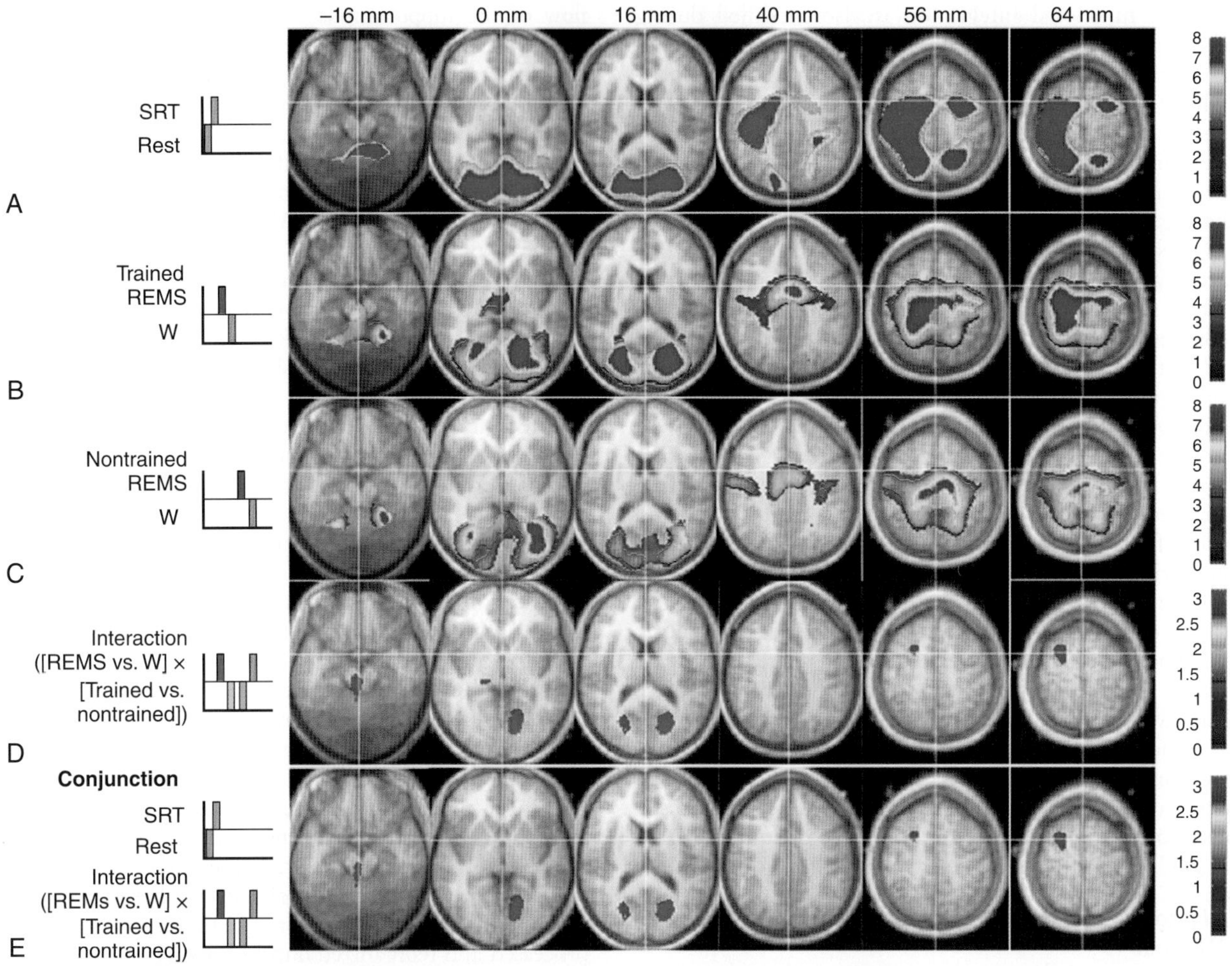

Figure 19.4 Influence of previous waking experience, in this case a procedural motor learning sequence, on the distribution of regional brain activity during subsequent rapid eye movement (REM) sleep. Statistical parametric maps of different contrasts are displayed at six different brain levels (from 16 mm below to 64 mm above the bicommissural plane), superimposed on the average (coregistered and normalized) magnetic resonance imaging scan of the brain in sleeping subjects. All maps were thresholded at $P < .001$ (uncorrected), except for **A,** which was thresholded at corrected voxel level ($P < .05$). **A,** Brain regions activated during performance of a serial reaction time (SRT) task during wakefulness (SRT-rest). **B,** Brain regions activated during REM sleep (REM sleep–wakefulness) in subjects previously trained to the SRT task. **C,** Brain regions activated during REM sleep (REM sleep–wakefulness) in nontrained subjects. **D,** Brain regions activated more in trained subjects than in nontrained subjects during REM sleep—that is, the intersection of the condition (REM sleep vs. wakefulness) by group (trained vs. nontrained). **E,** Brain regions that were both recruited during the execution of motor tasks and more activated in trained than in nontrained subjects scanned during REM sleep—that is, the conjunction of SRT-rest with the condition (REM sleep vs. wakefulness) by group (trained vs. nontrained). W, Wakefulness. (Modified from Maquet P, Laureys S, Peigneux P, et al. Experience-dependent changes in cerebral activation during human REM sleep. *Nat Neurosci.* 2000;3:831–6.)

frontoparietal cortex in agreement with the observation that the effects of sleep deprivation on SWS and on spontaneous EEG activity during wakefulness are greatest in frontal EEG leads.

Many fMRI studies compared well-rested versus sleep-deprived brains while engaged in sustained attention or executive tasks. Reduced fronto-parietal response to a sustained attention task is observed after a night of sleep deprivation.[67,68] Moreover, vigilance failures (lapses) are associated with reduced activation within these cortical areas and in the thalamus.[69,70] Beyond abnormal brain activations, vigilance and sustained attention decline during sleep deprivation appears to be related to modifications in the cross-talk between brain areas. This is indicated by changes in spontaneous (i.e., task free) functional connectivity, showing reduced within-network connectivity (or integration) in the default mode and dorsal/ventral attention networks (including many frontal and parietal regions), and in reduced segregation between these networks.[71–74] Furthermore, effective connectivity within the cingulate cortex decreases after sleep deprivation and predicts subsequent worse performance to a sustained attention task.[75]

After sleep deprivation, the most consistent decreases in responses to working memory tasks are observed in posterior (parietal, occipital, temporal) cortices, in addition to frontal areas.[76–79] By contrast, albeit not always detected,[79] response increases, which could be seen as compensating for the detrimental effects of sleep deprivation (see next section), are typically reported in thalamic nuclei, anterior cingulate cortex, and prefrontal areas.[66,76,77,79,80] Moreover, these regionally specific response patterns appear to differentiate vulnerable from more resilient participants to sleep deprivation when engaged in a working memory task. Thus the decrease in parietal activation after sleep deprivation has been proposed as a physiologic marker of vulnerability to sleep deprivation for working memory.[81] By contrast, sleep deprivation–induced increases in ventral prefrontal cortex are typically reported in the less vulnerable individuals.[82]

BRAIN IMAGING AND NEURAL CORRELATES OF ENDOGENOUS SLEEP-WAKE CYCLE REGULATION

The timing of sleep and wake episodes is regulated by the interaction between the homeostatic sleep pressure and an intrinsic circadian oscillation.[83] (See Chapters 36 to 38 for more information on sleep and wakefulness regulation.) It is therefore essential to assess function of the awake brain at different circadian phases and under different sleep-wake histories. Using ^{18}F-FDG PET, a relative increase in regional glucose metabolism is detected in the evening compared to the morning in a large cluster of midline and brainstem structures (but see Shannon et al.,[84] where no changes were detected). More specifically, changes are localized in the pontine and midbrain reticular formation, midbrain raphe, locus coeruleus, and posterior hypothalamus. Of note, evening wakefulness is associated with decreased relative metabolism in posterior cortical regions.

Using fMRI resting-state data, changes in functional connectivity between the medial temporal lobe (MTL) and the rest of the brain are detected between morning and evening measurements.[84] In the morning, bilateral MTL regions appear to be mainly functionally connected to local areas, whereas their connectivity spread cortically in the evening, in a set of regions important for memory consolidation. This finding could support the progressive potentiation of experience-dependent change during the day. They may also plead for a circadian modulation of MTL connectivity.

Also using fMRI, a handful of studies capitalized on interindividual differences in sleep-wakefulness regulation to assess the impact of sleep homeostasis and circadian factors on regional brain function. Executive responses to a working memory task were investigated during a normal sleep-wake cycle and during sleep loss in a population of young healthy volunteers stratified according to homozygosity for a variable-number (4 or 5) of tandem-repeat polymorphisms in the coding region of the clock gene *PERIOD3 (PER3)*.[85] Homozygosity to the long allele (5/5) is associated with faster buildup of sleep homeostasis and increased vulnerability to sleep loss.[86] In the less vulnerable genotype (4/4), no changes are observed in brain responses during the normal sleep-wake cycle. During sleep loss, these subjects recruit supplemental anterior frontal and temporal regions in addition to the thalamus pulvinar while executive function is maintained. By contrast, in the vulnerable genotype (5/5), activation in a posterior prefrontal area is already reduced in comparing evening to morning responses during a normal sleep-wake cycle. Furthermore, in the morning after a night of sleep loss, widespread reductions in activation in prefrontal, temporal, parietal, and occipital areas are observed in this genotype. Such differences occurred in the absence of genotype-dependent differences in circadian phase. These findings clearly showed that the allocation of prefrontal resources is constrained by sleep pressure and circadian phase.

Cerebral correlates of sustained attention in persons categorized as extreme early- and late-chronotype individuals were assessed in the morning and in the evening (1.5 and 10.5 hours, respectively, after preferred waking time).[87] Early and late chronotypes are known to differ in terms of circadian phase, but early-morning types also are known to accrue a larger homeostatic sleep pressure during wakefulness than is seen in evening types.[88] Brain responses associated with sustained attention differ between chronotypes in the thalamus and areas compatible with the locus coeruleus and suprachiasmatic area. Remarkably, sustained attention-related activity in the suprachiasmatic region in the evening is negatively related to the SWA recorded during the subsequent first sleep cycle. This finding suggested that the activity profile of the suprachiasmatic nucleus (SCN) master clock acting on the cerebral correlates of sustained attention inherently depends on the status of the sleep homeostat. In other words, during the evening hours, whereas evening types can benefit from the increasing circadian alertness signal to achieve optimal performance levels, morning types have to fight against a disproportionally increasing homeostatic sleep pressure and are therefore less able to profit from the beneficial circadian alertness signal, which is also "advanced" and decreases earlier, to accomplish sustained attention performance.

This finding is partially replicated when considering conflict processing.[89] Cognitive interference is crucial for maintaining a coherent stream of thought and thus represents a cognitive aspect required for behaving suitably in many daily live functions.[90] The neural bases of interference processing in chronotypes was assessed with the Stroop paradigm. Within this framework, chronotypes differ in daily fluctuations of interference-related cortical responses.[89] More precisely, interference-related hemodynamic responses are maintained or even increased in evening types from the subjective morning to the subjective evening in a set of brain areas playing a pivotal role in successful cognitive inhibition, whereas they decrease in morning types under the same conditions. Similar to the sustained attention context, during the evening hours, interference activity in a posterior hypothalamic region correlates in a chronotype-specific manner with SWA at the beginning of the night, speaking again in favor of a differential expression of subcortical-driven wake-promoting signals throughout a normal waking day. Note that the cluster of activation is located more posterior than the anterior hypothalamic area detected during a sustained attention task and may correspond to the posterior-lateral hypothalamus reported to show a decrease in gray matter concentration in narcoleptic patients.[91]

When considering working memory and executive function, extreme chronotypes again present different sensitivities to changes in circadian phase and sleep need.[92] In the evening hours, evening types exhibit higher thalamic activity than morning types for high working memory load. Conversely, morning-type individuals exhibit higher activity associated with high working memory load in the dorsolateral prefrontal cortex during the morning session. This is somewhat reminiscent of the finding reported earlier in individuals characterized by different *PER3* genotypes.[85] Demanding optimal performance for an executive task may be favored by a temporary increase in thalamic-related arousal levels in evening types in the evening or in $PER3^{4/4}$ genotypes in the morning after sleep loss. Concomitantly, performance in the morning hours in morning types may be supported by increased strategic or attentional recruitment of prefrontal areas, whereas

$PER3^{5/5}$ genotype individuals, who seem to undergo a fast buildup of sleep need, as a morning chronotype, are not able to maintain such prefrontal activity in the evening.

Rather than relying on interindividual differences, two recent studies emphasized the influence of the circadian system and of sleep homeostasis on wakefulness brain function by increasing the sampling rate of the fMRI assessments over the 24-hour cycle. The first one is a within-subject crossover design, including two distinct sets of five fMRI sessions spread over a 40-hour period, during which participants performed a sustained attention task.[93] These 40 hours could consist of total sleep deprivation, where sleep need increases progressively as a function of prior wake duration, or in a "multiple nap protocol," including 10 alternating cycles of 160 minutes of scheduled wakefulness and 80 minutes of scheduled sleep, where sleep need remains low. When sleep deprived, thalamic activation associated with sustained attention parallels the time course of subjective sleepiness, with high values at night and troughs on the subsequent day. Thalamic activity further correlates with a composite value representing the amplitude of the circadian signal promoting wake and sleep. In contrast, task-related cortical activation decreased when sleepiness increased as a consequence of higher sleep debt, that is, during the night and thereafter during the following day. Under low sleep pressure, no significant association between brain responses and subjective sleepiness was detected. These findings further emphasize that the two processes regulating sleep and wakefulness affect brain function mostly when sleep pressure is high and do so differently for cortical areas, which undergo decreased activation and may reflect more closely cognitive outputs, and subcortical brain activity, which may integrate sleep need and the circadian signal and counterbalance the cortical decrease.

A full representation of the dual impact of the two processes at the regional brain level requires, however, more fMRI assessments. A second study included 12 fMRI sessions, during which participants performed a sustained attention task, spread over a 42-hour sleep-deprivation protocol, as well as a 13th session after recovery sleep.[94] Results reveal that a large part of the cortex undergoes circadian fluctuations, but the phase of the rhythm varies across brain regions, with maximum responses occurring overall earlier in occipital and allocortical areas (amygdala and cingulate cortex) than in multimodal association areas (precuneus, temporal cortex, and prefrontal areas). The study further reveals that subcortical areas (midbrain, cerebellum, basal ganglia, and thalamus) show strong circadian modulation, that is, they follow melatonin secretion profile but show no or little effect of sleep debt (Figure 19.5). In contrast, and reminiscent of the study detailed in the preceding paragraph, a negative effect of sleep debt is observed in a large set of cortical areas that span high-order association cortices of the frontal, parietal, insular, and cingulate cortices, as well as visual and sensorimotor cortices. Their response pattern show a decrease in response to elapsed time awake, with a return to baseline levels after recovery sleep. It appears that the respective influence of sleep debt and circadian rhythmicity is more balanced in posterior cortical areas, whereas sleep debt exerts a disproportionately larger influence in more anterior associative areas. This differential regulation of regional brain responses might explain the supposedly "compensatory" responses repeatedly reported in thalamic areas during sleep loss. However, these strong thalamic responses might merely indicate a dependency of cortical and subcortical response amplitude on the circadian phase. This last study demonstrates the relative contributions of circadian rhythmicity and homeostatic sleep pressure to regionally specific (i.e., local) brain function.

BRAIN IMAGING OF THE NON–IMAGE-FORMING IMPACT OF LIGHT ON SLEEP AND WAKEFULNESS REGULATION

The activity of the SCN, the master circadian clock, is influenced by external temporal markers (zeitgebers), the most important of which is light. In addition to vision, light profoundly affects human physiology and modulates sleep-wake cycles, body temperature, endocrine functions, alertness, and performance.[95] Animal and human studies demonstrated that a *non–image-forming* or *nonvisual* photoreception system mediates these effects, which include the synchronization of the circadian system, suppression of melatonin, regulation of sleep, and improvements in alertness and cognition. This photoreception system recruits the classical retinal photoreceptors (rods and cones) and intrinsically photosensitive retinal ganglion cells expressing melanopsin, which is a photopigment maximally sensitive to blue wavelength light (≈480 nm), such that the light sensitivity of retinal ganglion cell expressing it is biased toward short-wavelength light.[96] The retinal ganglion cells expressing melanopsin project to numerous nuclei of the brainstem, hypothalamus, thalamus, and cortical structures; such anatomic connectivity suggests that the non-image-forming system can influence many brain functions.

A series of experiments characterized the impact of light on wakefulness quality and detailed light-induced modulation of ongoing cortical and subcortical activity while performing various cognitive challenges, first using polychromatic light (vs. darkness) and then monochromatic light geared toward melanopsin-expressing ganglion cells (vs. other wavelengths-favoring cones responses). Polychromatic bright white light (>7000 lux) enhances responses to attentional tasks in subcortical (hypothalamus and thalamus) and cortical areas, both during the night and during daytime.[97,98] These effects depend mostly on the blue content of polychromatic light, as monochromatic blue (470 nm) light was reported to enhance brain responses to a working memory task in areas such as the thalamus and association cortices.[99] Blue light impact on the later brain responses seems to outlast the exposure; at least, when exposure duration is set to 30 minutes.[100] When light exposure is reduced to less than a minute, the most striking difference is that the significant modulations of brain activity seems to be mostly confined to subcortical areas, such as the pulvinar (thalamus), hypothalamus, and brainstem, and limbic areas, such as the amygdala. This would be compatible with a scenario where light first affects the areas where melanopsin ganglion cells or the SCN project, which are areas involved in alertness, attention, and sleep regulation.[95,101] Aside from the impact of light on attention and executive function, light also affects the brain's processing of emotional stimulation in the amygdala and hypothalamus, an effect that may underlie part of the long-term impact of light on mood—the positive impact of light therapy and the negative impact of lack of light in winter.[102]

It also appears that these immediate effects of ambient light on cognition in turn depend on circadian phase, homeostatic

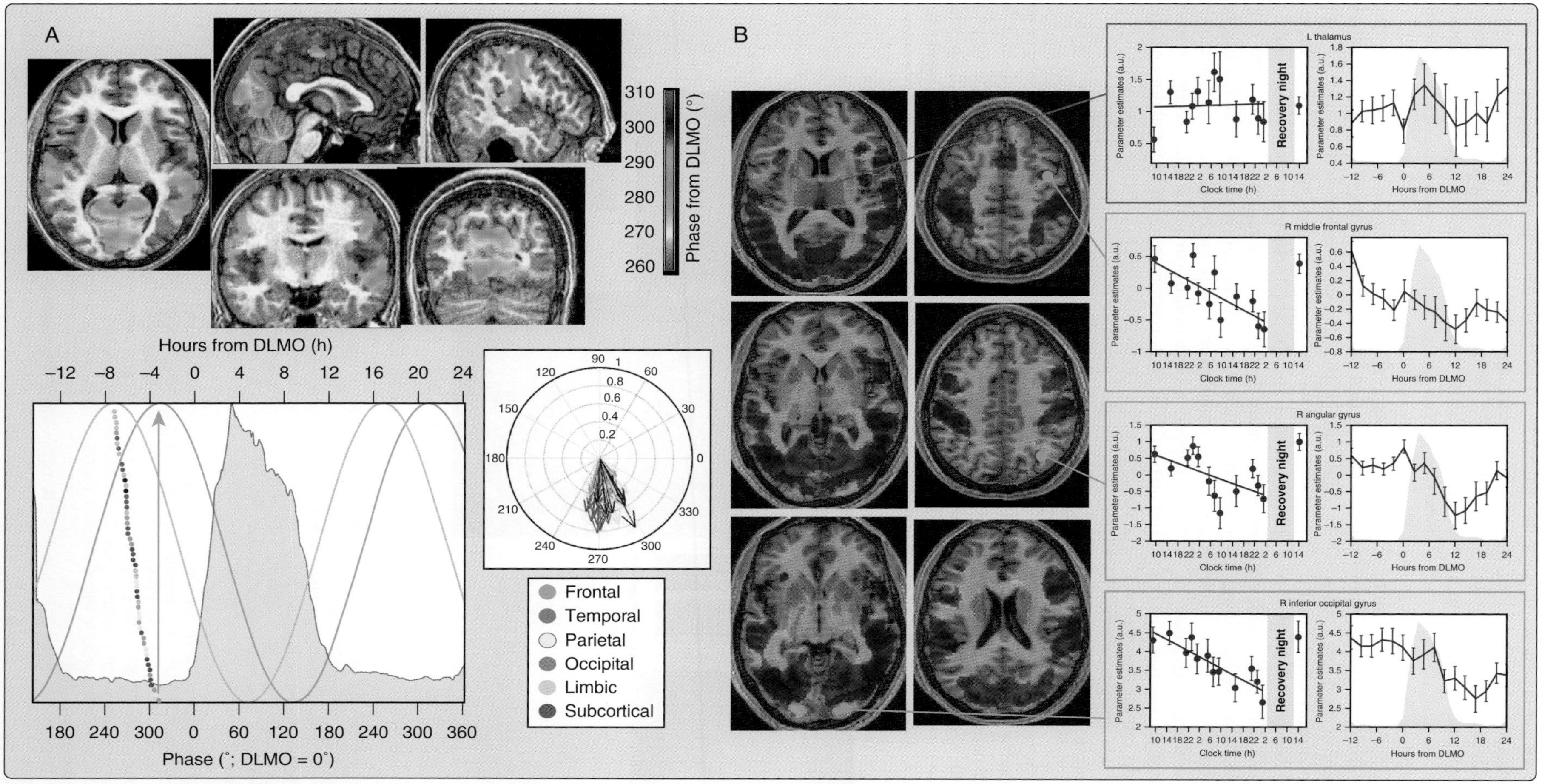

Figure 19.5 Dual impact of the circadian system and of sleep homeostasis on cognitive brain responses. **A,** *Top,* Circadian phase map of brain responses to the psychomotor vigilance task, which probes sustained attention, as inferred using sine-wave-like regressor with fixed 24-hour period ($P < .05$, false discovery rate over the whole brain). The local response phase is displayed according to the color scale (°, onset of melatonin secretion corresponding to dim light melatonin onset (DLMO) = 0°) and overlaid over an individual normalized T1 magnetic resonance (MR) scan. Coordinates are in millimeters along *z, y,* and *x* axes. *Bottom left,* Predicted time courses of 24-hour period responses expressed as phase and approximate hours from DLMO. Mean melatonin profile is shown in *gray.* Sine waves illustrate the earliest (*beige,* amygdala) and latest (*green,* inferior frontal gyrus) response timing. Between these two extreme phases, the *staggered dots* correspond to the timing of significant regional peak responses. These responses were grouped in six different areas according to the color code. *Bottom right,* Polar representation of response phases (°, DLMO = 0°) of the different brain regions. **B,** *Left,* Changes in psychomotor vigilance task brain responses during 42 hours of sustained wakefulness and after recovery sleep. Images show significant effects of homeostatic sleep pressure (*blue*) and circadian rhythmicity (*red*) and their interaction (*green*) displayed at $P < .05$ (family-wise error correction for multiple comparisons—whole brain) over an individual normalized T1-weighted MR scan. *Right,* Two different representations of representative time courses of brain responses, which were significant for sleep debt (*blue border*), circadian (*red border*), or the interaction (*green border*) contrasts. Irrespective of the contrast, beta estimates are plotted against clock time (*left panels:* linear regression is computed with respect to time awake during the sleep deprivation period) and time relative to DLMO (*right panels:* mean melatonin levels are shown in *gray*). *Right panels, second row,* recovery night as is row 1, 3, and 4. Note that all cortical areas show a dual impact of the circadian system and sleep homeostasis with a gradient from frontal regions, mostly sleep homeostasis dependent, to occipital regions, showing a significant dual impact. Subcortical region appears mostly influenced by the circadian system. a.u., Arbitrary units. (Modified from Muto V, Jaspar M, Meyer C, et al. Local modulation of human brain responses by circadian rhythmicity and sleep debt. *Science.* 2016; 353:687–90)

sleep pressure, and genotype.[103] An fMRI study shows that in a genotype reported to be more vulnerable to sleep loss (*PER3*$^{5/5}$), exposure to as little as 1 minute of blue light in the morning, after sleep deprivation, increases responses in a left thalamo-fronto-parietal circuit. By contrast, no impact of ambient light was observed during sleep loss in the genotype reported to be less vulnerable to sleep (*PER3*$^{4/4}$). These results support the view that the impact of light on cognitive brain function is especially present in challenging conditions, when endogenous alerting mechanisms are not already active. Finally, fMRI studies in aging, which is associated with alteration in the regulation of sleep and wakefulness and with a reduction in pupil size and lens transmission, respectively, through senile miosis and lens yellowing, reduces the impact of light on ongoing nonvisual cognitive brain activity.[104] Inclusion of individuals who had lens replacement after cataract surgery suggests that the reduced impact of light impact does depend on lens transmission as no differences are observed between the individuals with clear lenses and control individuals with partly yellowed lens.[105]

Collectively, these findings show that light, and especially blue light, not only can influence the timing of sleep and wake cycles (see Chapter xx for more information on the phase-shifting impact of light on the circadian system) but can also profoundly and swiftly influence regional brain function. The underlying mechanism is more likely to be a modulation of the activity in subcortical structures promoting alertness (e.g., anterior hypothalamus, mesopontine tegmentum, thalamus) (Figure 19.6).[95] It is likely that, to trigger the same effect in older individuals, the exposure has to be adapted, either in terms of higher intensity or blue wavelength composition. All these effects of light are most likely heavily dependent on melanopsin-expressing retinal ganglion cells. An fMRI study indeed shows that blue light affects ongoing cognitive activity in blind individuals, who, despite complete absence of visual perception, retain melatonin suppression by light at night, very likely because they retain melanopsin-expressing ganglion cells[106] (Figure 19.6). Furthermore, variations in light compositions, which stimulate melanopsin cells while keeping rod and cones stimulation mostly unchanged (using "metameric light), triggers modulation of cortical activity while performing no particular task except fixating on a central dot on a dark screen.[107]

FUNCTIONAL NEUROIMAGING IN SLEEP DISORDERS: THE CASE OF INSOMNIA

Although an overview of all neuroimaging studies in the full spectrum of all sleep disorders would be beyond the scope of this chapter, it bears mentioning that extensive studies exist in circadian rhythm disorders, narcolepsy and the hypersomnia disorders, sleep-related breathing disorders, parasomnias,

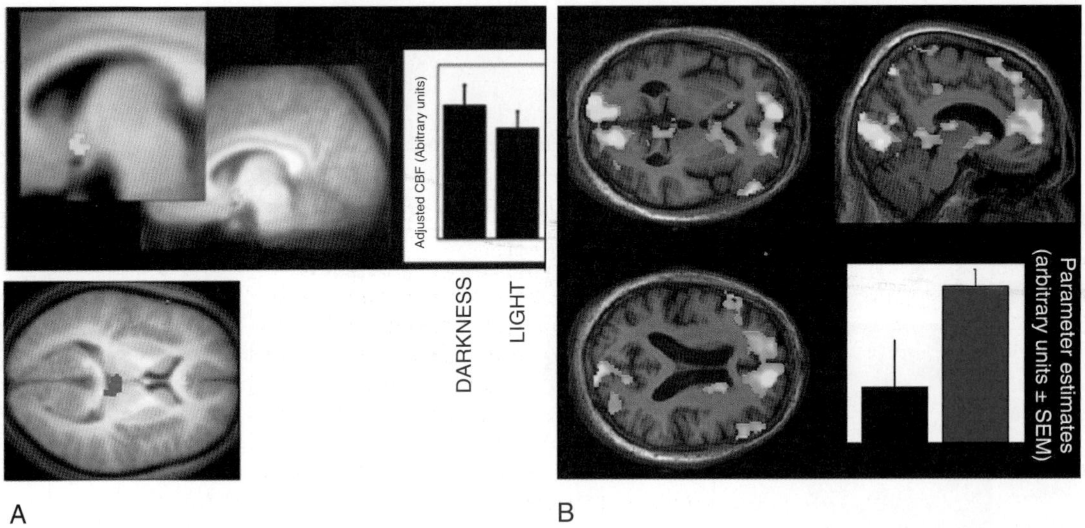

Figure 19.6 **A,** *Top,* Effects on regional brain activity of exposure to bright white light during the night, as assessed with positron emission tomography. Regional cerebral blood flow (rCBF) was measured in subjects attending to auditory stimuli in near darkness after light exposures (>8000 lux) or after complete darkness. The suprachiasmatic area shows a significant decrease in blood flow in proportion to the duration of the previous exposure to light. The inset shows the corresponding adjusted blood flow after darkness or after light exposure. *Bottom,* Effects on regional brain activity of exposure to bright white light during the day as assessed with functional magnetic resonance imaging. Regional BOLD signal was measured in subjects attending to auditory stimuli in near darkness after light exposures (>7000 lux) or after complete darkness. The thalamus pulvinar shows an increased BOLD response after light as compared to after darkness. **B,** Impact of light in totally blind individuals retaining non-image-forming photoreception. Blind individuals were alternatively exposed to monochromatic blue light (9.7×10^{14} photons/cm^2/sec) or maintained in darkness while performing an auditory cognitive task. Brain areas showing significant increases in activity under blue light exposure while performing the task, compared with darkness, are overlaid over the mean structural image of the participants. Inset shows one example of activity estimates (arbitrary unit ± SEM) in a region showing significant differences between blue light and darkness episodes ($P < .05$, corrected). BOLD, Blood oxygen level–dependent; SEM, standard error of the mean. (**A,** *Top,* Modified from Perrin F, Peigneux P, Fuchs S, et al. Nonvisual responses to light exposure in the human brain during the circadian night. *Curr Biol.* 2004;14:1842–6; **A,** *Bottom,* modified from Vandewalle G, Balteau E, Phillips C, et al. Daytime light exposure dynamically enhances brain responses. *Curr Biol.* 2006;16:1616–21; **B,** modified from Vandewalle G, Collignon O, Hull JT, et al. Blue light stimulates cognitive brain activity in visually blind individuals. *J Cogn Neurosci.* 2013;25:2072–85.)

restless legs syndrome, and periodic limb movement disorder, as well as neuroimaging studies reporting the effects of various treatments for sleep disorders on brain function. These findings have been reviewed in more extensive detail in the textbook *Neuroimaging of Sleep and Sleep Disorders*, by Nofzinger, Maquet, and Thorpy (2013), listed in the Selected Readings section of this chapter.

Alterations in the sleep EEG are not always found in persons with subjective complaints of insomnia. Consistently reported impairments include fragmented sleep, hyperarousal, rumination, and emotional and executive dysfunction.[108] For instance, people with insomnia have been shown to have elevated temperature and muscle tone at sleep onset, elevated heart rate and elevated sympathovagal tone in heart rate variability, and positive correlations between wake times after sleep onset and urinary norepinephrine and dopamine metabolites.[109,110] The hyperarousal of insomnia is supported by higher rates of self-reported ruminations and intrusive thoughts among insomniac patients (see also Chapters 89 to 100).

An emerging body of evidence exists showing specific regional brain alterations despite the relative absence of EEG sleep signs of the disorder. Human sleep neuroimaging studies in insomniac subjects support the involvement of basic arousal networks in disturbances in NREM sleep. Insomniacs show a smaller decrease than for healthy subjects in relative PET glucose metabolism imaging from waking to NREM sleep in the brainstem reticular core and in the hypothalamus, supporting the concept that persistent activity in this basic arousal network may be responsible for the impaired objective and subjective sleep in insomniac patients (Figure 19.7).[111] In addition, insomniac persons show a smaller relative decrease than healthy subjects in metabolism from waking to NREM sleep in the insular cortex, amygdala, hippocampus, anterior cingulate, and medial prefrontal cortices, suggesting that persistent overactivity in a limbic or paralimbic level of the arousal system contributes to the nonrestorative sleep in insomnia patients.[111] fMRI further indicates that patients with insomnia are characterized by reduced recruitment of the head of the left caudate nucleus during executive functioning at wake, whereas individual differences in caudate recruitment are associated with hyperarousal severity.[112] Input from a projecting orbitofrontal area with reduced gray matter density seems to contribute to altered caudate recruitment in patients with insomnia. Attenuated caudate recruitment persisted after successful treatment of insomnia, warranting evaluation as a potential vulnerability trait. Of interest, a similar selective reduction in caudate recruitment could be elicited in healthy individuals by SWS fragmentation, providing a model to facilitate investigation of the causes and consequences of insomnia.[112]

The significant epidemiologic overlap documented between insomnia and disorders of emotion has oriented some of the research on insomnia. REM sleep, which is related to activation of emotion and mood limbic and anterior paralimbic structures, and is altered in depression (with more REM sleep), appears to be relatively restless in insomnia. Restless REM sleep may reflect a process that interferes with the overnight resolution of distress, which, if repeated and accumulated, may promote the development of chronic hyperarousal, rumination, and unresolved distress. In support of this, restless REM sleep in healthy individuals impeded overnight amygdala adaptation to emotion processing in proportion to the total duration of consolidated REM sleep.[113] In addition, abnormal limbic response, particularly in the dorsal anterior cingulate cortex, are detected in insomnia patients reliving shameful experiences from the past, while this response is not present in normal sleepers.[114] Further limbic involvement in insomnia comes from a report that more severe insomnia and worse sleep quality is detected in people with a stronger functional connectivity between the bilateral hippocampus and the left middle frontal gyrus, which may contribute to rumination.[115]

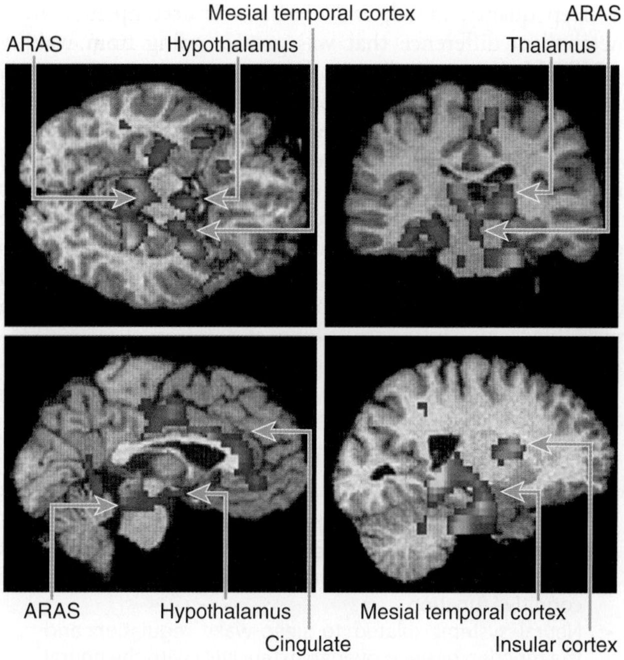

Figure 19.7 Brain structures that do not show decreased metabolic rate from waking to sleep in insomniacs. All regions shown reach statistical significance at the $P < .05$ corrected in relation to healthy sleeper control subjects. ARAS, Ascending reticular activating system. (From Nofzinger EA, Buysse DJ, Germain A, et al. Functional neuroimaging evidence for hyperarousal in insomnia. *Am J Psychiatry.* 2004;161:2126–31.)

In apparent contradiction to the hyperarousal hypothesis of insomnia, patients with insomnia show a consistent pattern of hypoperfusion across large parts of the brain, according to whole-brain SPECT recordings during sleep.[116] Likewise, insomniac patients present hypoactivation of the medial and inferior prefrontal cortical areas during the completion of a category task and a letter-fluency task. Inconsistencies across insomnia studies is further pointed out in a meta-analysis that finds no significant convergent evidence for the combination of structural atrophy and functional disturbances across carefully selected studies.[117] The difficulty in characterizing and understanding insomnia, as well as treating it, is likely related to the heterogeneity of insomnia patients. This will be further emphasized in following sections, but insomnia is indeed likely composed of different subtypes, potentially five, according to the level of distress, reactivity, and sensitivity to reward.[108] These subtypes remain to be carefully distinguished from one another to envisage adapted treatments.

In terms of interventions, the action of sedative-hypnotics may be primarily on basic arousal systems. Brain imaging analyses of data acquired in eight subjects suggest that the beneficial impact of 2 weeks of treatment with eszopiclone, a nonbenzodiazepine cyclopyrrolone, on subjective perception of sleep quality, mood, and alertness is accompanied by a metabolism difference that was greater going from waking to NREM sleep, including in the pontine reticular formation and ascending into the midbrain, subthalamic nucleus, and thalamus, as well as in prefrontal, temporal, parietal, and cingulate structures.[118] Nonmedicated interventions are essential insomnia treatments. Cognitive behavioral therapy stands as the current best approach to relief insomnia symptoms in the long term. fMRI shows that this type of intervention reverses prefrontal cortex abnormal activity during category task and a letter-fluency task, suggesting that insomnia interferes in a reversible fashion with activation of the prefrontal cortical system during daytime task performance.[119]

CLINICAL PEARLS

- Brain imaging technology has helped the field of sleep medicine explore more precisely the relation between sleep-wake and sleep disturbances and their relation to cognitive function.
- Neural systems related to sleep-wake regulation and the function of sleep overlap extensively with the neural systems involved in essential aspects of waking cognitive and emotional behavior.
- Disruptions in sleep in patients with sleep disorders can therefore be associated with alterations in these neural systems, and, in turn, altered sleep leads to changes in these neural systems and impair waking behavior.

SUMMARY

The application of functional neuroimaging methods to the study of sleep in health and diseases in human subjects has provided unique insights into the neural mechanisms of sleep generation and maintenance. In many instances these studies provide secondary support for those mechanisms that have been discovered in preclinical research. They also have shed light on the involvement and interaction of broad neural networks operating at the subcortical and cortical levels in a defined and regular manner to produce the final experience of sleep in humans. Brain imaging studies are contributing to the understanding of how wake and sleep networks can behave pathologically to produce various sleep disorders and to the identification of those cases in which specific treatments, either pharmacologic or behavioral, can reverse these abnormalities.

ACKNOWLEDGMENTS

Past and current research of Gilles Vandewalle and Pierre Maquet were/are conducted with the help of grants from the Belgian Fonds National de la Recherche Scientifique (FNRS), Fondation Médicale Reine Elisabeth (FMRE), Research Fund of the University of Liège, Wallonia-Brussel Federation Action de Recherche Concertée, Walloon Excellence in Life Science and Biotechnology (WELBIO), Alzheimer Research Foundation (Belgium), and Canadian Institutes of Health Research.

SELECTED READINGS

Chee MWL, Zhou J. *Functional Connectivity and the Sleep-Deprived Brain. Progress in Brain Research*. 1st ed. Vol. 246. Elsevier; 2019.

Gaggioni G, Maquet P, Schmidt C, et al. Neuroimaging, cognition, light and circadian rhythms. *Front Syst Neurosci*. 2014;8:126.

Ma N, Dinges DF, Basner M, Rao H. How acute total sleep loss affects the attending brain: a meta-analysis of neuroimaging studies. *Sleep*. 2015;38:233–240.

Marshall L, Cross N, Binder S, Dang-Vu TT. Brain rhythms during sleep and memory consolidation: neurobiological insights. *Physiology (Bethesda, Md)*. 2020;35(1):4–15.

Muto V, Jaspar M, Meyer C, et al. Local modulation of human brain responses by circadian rhythmicity and sleep debt. *Science.)*. 2016;353(6300):687–690.

Nofzinger EA, Maquet P, Thorpy M. *Neuroimaging of Sleep and Sleep Disorders*. Cambridge (UK): Cambridge University Press; 2013.

Rué-Queralt J, Stevner A, Tagliazucchi E, et al. Decoding brain states on the intrinsic manifold of human brain dynamics across wakefulness and sleep. *Commun Biol*. 2021;4(1):854.

A complete reference list can be found online at ExpertConsult.com.

Chapter 20

Cardiovascular Physiology and Coupling with Respiration: Central and Autonomic Regulation

Ronald M. Harper; Luke A. Henderson; Richard L. Verrier

Chapter Highlights

- Sleep states contribute to substantial variability in heart rate and coronary artery flow, mediated by pronounced activation and deactivation of parasympathetic and sympathetic components of the autonomic nervous system. Surges in both components of the autonomic nervous system concurrent with electroencephalographic phasic activity during rapid eye movement sleep can significantly alter heart rate and coronary flow, potentially compromising individuals with heart disease or sleep-disordered breathing.
- Sleep-disordered breathing results in significant changes in brain tissue, including cell and axonal loss and glial alterations indicative of injury. The changes appear in neural structures that serve essential autonomic, hormonal, cognitive, affective, and motor control functions; involve nuclei that are origins of neurotransmitter systems, as well as important medullary cardiovascular sites; and are often lateralized.
- The specificity and asymmetry of injury to autonomic regulatory areas, which include autonomic cortical sites as well as hypothalamic and medullary regions, result in marked functional consequences expressed as hypertension, potential for cardiac arrhythmia, and altered cerebral perfusion.
- Several syndromes, including those of sudden infant death (SIDS), sudden unexpected death in epilepsy (SUDEP), and sudden unexplained nocturnal death syndrome (SUNDS) appear to have sleep-related disturbed autonomic regulation as their basis.

INTRODUCTION

Because of the close neurohumoral coupling between central structures and cardiorespiratory function, a dynamic coordination exists between heart rhythm, arterial blood pressure, coronary artery blood flow, and ventilation. Non–rapid eye movement (NREM) sleep is associated with relative autonomic stability and functional coordination between respiration, pumping action of the heart, and maintenance of arterial blood pressure. During rapid eye movement (REM) sleep, surges in cardiac-bound sympathetic and parasympathetic activity provoke accelerations and pauses in heart rhythm, respectively. These surges occur in association with alterations on the electroencephalogram (EEG) indicative of phasic central nervous system activation in REM sleep, so-called phasic REM sleep. Whereas autonomic nervous system perturbations are well tolerated in normal individuals, patients with heart disease or sleep-disordered breathing may be at heightened risk for cardiac events, especially because of the exaggerated sympathetic tone of REM sleep. Autonomic regulation is often compromised by injury to central autonomic regulatory sites in obstructive sleep apnea (OSA) and heart failure, resulting in preferentially lateralized high sympathetic nerve output and inappropriate responses to momentary challenges. In patients with severely compromised hearts, NREM sleep is associated with the potential for onset of hypotension, which can in turn impair blood flow through stenotic coronary vessels. During a typical night's sleep, a broad spectrum of autonomic patterns unfolds that provides both respite and stress to the cardiovascular system. These effects result from natural, carefully orchestrated changes in central nervous system physiology, as the brain periodically reexcites during REM sleep from the relative tranquility of NREM sleep.

This chapter surveys central and autonomic nervous system mechanisms that regulate cardiovascular function during sleep and identifies some dysfunctions that can arise in patients with underlying pathologic conditions. Particular attention is focused on cardiac electrical stability and coronary artery blood flow, because disturbances in these factors of cardiovascular function can trigger life-threatening cardiac arrhythmias and myocardial ischemia and infarction in patients with heart disease. Attention also is directed toward central mechanisms underlying the high sympathetic tone found in conditions associated with sleep-disordered breathing, including OSA and heart failure, and with cardiovascular function in infants, particularly because nocturnal regulatory perturbations of these systems may be an important factor in sudden infant death syndrome (SIDS). The importance of these issues to public health is underscored by the annual toll of nocturnal, sleep-related cardiac events, which account for an estimated 20% of myocardial infarctions (approximately 250,000/year) and for 15% of sudden cardiac deaths (47,500/year) in the United States.[1] For detailed reports and discussion of clinical findings, see Chapters 144 and 145. Interventions against pathologic respiratory and cardiovascular issues during sleep in a noninvasive manner are currently the object of a range of peripheral neuromodulatory procedures. Such approaches, which include enhancing parasympathetic tone or triggering timely breathing patterns, may address concerns of breathing and cardiovascular interactions not managed well by current positive air pressure therapy.

SLEEP STATE CONTROL OF CARDIOVASCULAR FUNCTION

The first NREM sleep cycle, from sleep onset, is characterized by a period of relative autonomic stability, with vagus nerve dominance and heightened baroreceptor gain. During NREM sleep, a near-sinusoidal modulation of heart rate variation occurs from coupling of respiratory and cardiorespiratory brain centers, resulting in what is termed "normal respiratory sinus arrhythmia" (Figure 20.1). During inspiration, heart rate accelerates to accommodate increased venous return, increasing cardiac output, followed by progressive heart rate slowing during expiration. This normal sinus variability in heart rate, particularly during NREM sleep, is generally indicative of cardiac health, whereas absence of intrinsic variability has been associated with cardiac pathology and advancing age.[2] The reflexive cardiovascular changes during breathing, manifested as cyclic heart rate variation, also have a converse relationship observed as transient elevation of arterial blood pressure, which results in slowing, cessation, or diminution of breathing efforts. This cascade of reflex adaptations is enhanced during sleep,[3] when even small reductions in arterial blood pressure increase respiratory rates.[4,5] These breathing pauses and increased rates serve as compensatory mechanisms to normalize arterial blood pressure. Reduced breathing variation and absence of normal breathing pauses, as well as declines in respiration-induced heart rate variation, are characteristic of infants who later succumb to SIDS[6] and may hint at failing compensatory mechanisms in the syndrome. Reduced heart rate variability appears in infants afflicted with congenital central hypoventilation syndrome, a condition characterized by reduced drive to breathe during sleep and compromised autonomic regulation, with high sympathetic tone.[7] Exaggerated heart rate variation appears in children with OSA, coincident with the enhanced bradycardia/tachycardia of apnea, but with lower sinus arrhythmia.[8] Patients with heart failure, who typically exhibit high levels of sympathetic tone, also have diminished respiratory function–related heart rate variation.[9] Thus the common denominator of cardiac risk associated with decreased heart rate variability appears to be enhanced sympathetic activity, together with reduced vagus nerve function.

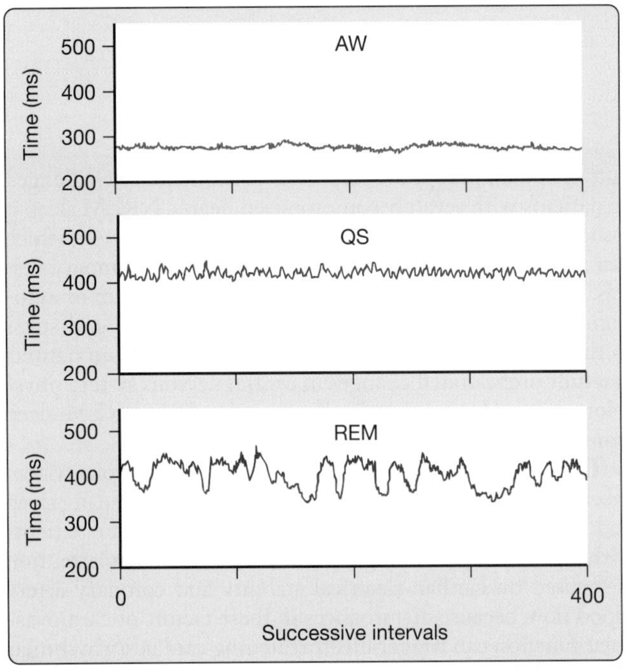

Figure 20.1 The x-axis represents successive heartbeats and the intervals between heartbeats from a healthy 4-month-old infant during quiet sleep (QS), REM sleep, and wakefulness (AW). The y-axis represents time (in milliseconds) between those heartbeats. Note the rapid modulation of intervals during quiet sleep contributed by respiratory variation. Also evident are lower-frequency modulation during REM sleep and epochs of sustained rapid rate during wakefulness.

Sympathetic nerve activity appears to be relatively stable during NREM sleep, and its cardiovascular input is reduced by more than half from wakefulness to stage N3 of NREM sleep.[10] In general, the autonomic stability of NREM sleep, with hypotension, bradycardia, reduced cardiac output, and systemic vascular resistance, provides a relatively salutary neurohumoral background when the heart has an opportunity for metabolic restoration.[11] The bradycardias appear to result mainly from increased vagus nerve activity, whereas the hypotension is primarily attributable to reduced sympathetic vasomotor tone.[12] During NREM-to-REM sleep transitions, vagus nerve activity bursts may result in pauses in heart rhythm and frank asystole.[13] REM sleep is initiated at approximately 90-minute intervals and, in subserving brain neurochemical functions and behavioral adaptations, can disrupt cardiorespiratory homeostasis.[14]

The brain's increased excitability during REM sleep can result in major surges in cardiac sympathetic nerve activity to the coronary vessels. Baroreceptor gain is reduced. Heart rate fluctuates strikingly, with marked tachycardia and bradycardia episodes.[15,16] Cardiac efferent vagus nerve tone is generally suppressed during REM sleep,[11] and the highly irregular breathing patterns can lead to lower oxygen levels, particularly in patients with pulmonary or cardiac disease.[14] Neurons serving the principal diaphragmatic respiratory muscles are spared the generalized inhibition,[17] although accessory and upper airway muscles diminish activity.[18] (See also Chapter 22.) The REM atonia is especially marked in infant thoracic and abdominal muscles,[19] leading to the potential for dangerously low residual tidal volumes from the resulting increased thoracic wall compliance when the rib cage is not yet calcified. During sleep apnea, loss of central respiratory activity and/or airway obstruction may occur several hundred times each night, with dire consequences for neural structures from the resulting intermittent hypoxia.

CARDIORESPIRATORY INTERACTIONS

Central Mechanisms

Integration of cardiorespiratory function during sleep is achieved at several neuraxis levels. Several pontine and supra-pontine as well as cerebellar mechanisms can alter cardiorespiratory patterns during sleep and waking, and cerebral cortex sites play major roles, especially in modulating sympathetic and parasympathetic outflow and breathing effort. Regional pontine roles in REM sleep activation have been documented by imaging studies of REM sleep, which also show preferential activation of limbic and paralimbic regions in REM sleep, compared with waking or with NREM sleep.[20-22] The pontine and medullary raphe nuclei contain serotoninergic neurons exerting significant roles in vascular control and heart rate[23]; the raphe is damaged in OSA and heart failure (Figure 20.2),[24-26] probably resulting from altered perfusion and intermittent hypoxia accompanying sleep-impaired breathing

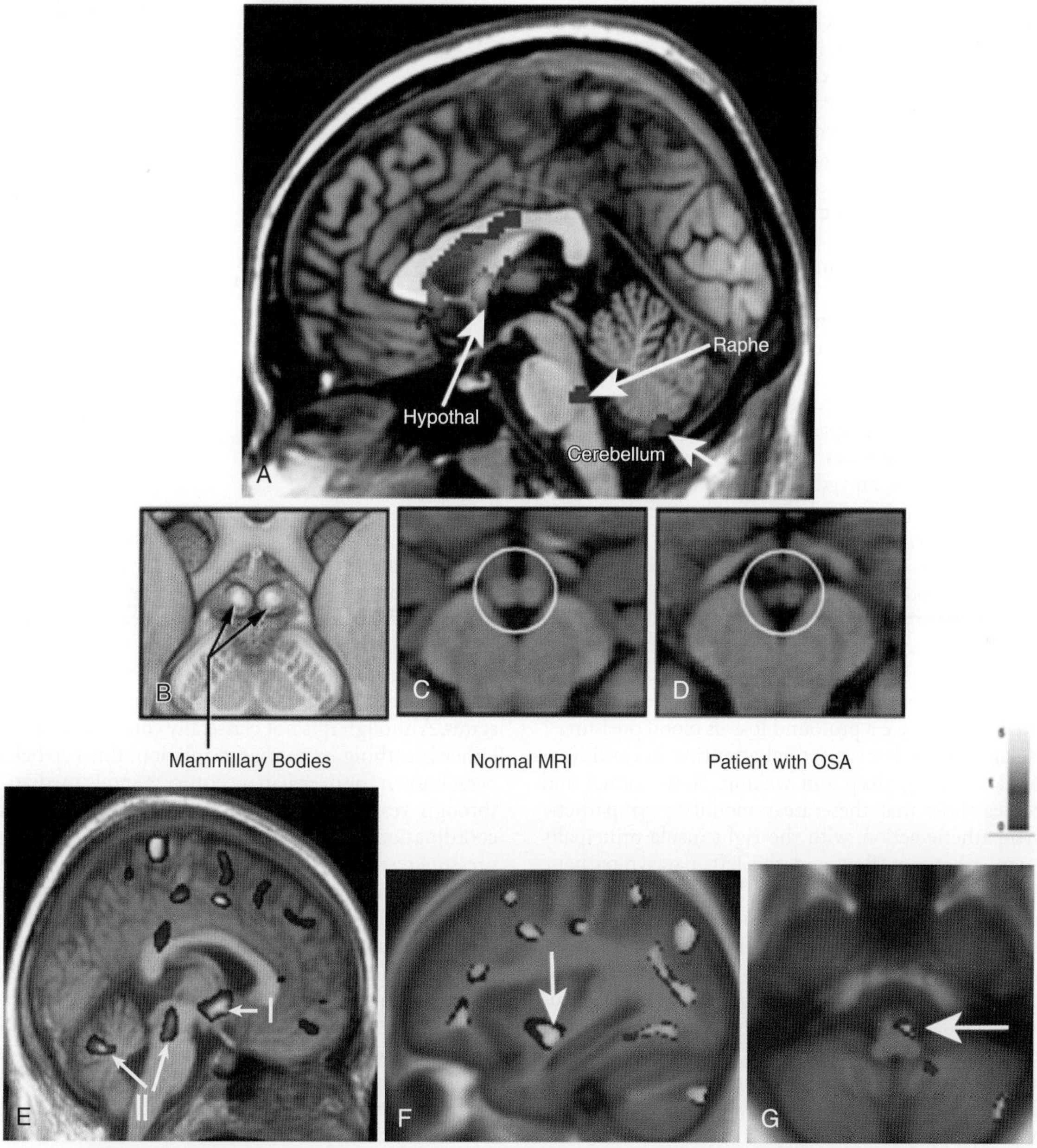

Figure 20.2 **A,** Midline view demonstrating injury in pontine raphe, cerebellum, and hypothalamus of patients with heart failure, as detected by T2 relaxometry procedures. Pontine raphe (*arrow*), fibers of the fornix, hypothalamus, and cerebellum show injury. **B** through **D,** Mammillary body volume loss in obstructive sleep apnea (OSA). **B,** Cartoon of mammillary bodies. **C** and **D,** T1-weighted magnetic resonance imaging images. **C,** Control subject mammillary bodies. **D,** Mammillary bodies in patient with OSA. **E,** Mean diffusivity scans, hypothalamic (I) and cerebellar and midbrain (II) injury in OSA. **F,** Mean diffusivity scans, insula (*arrow*) injury in OSA. **G,** Mean diffusivity scans, ventrolateral medullary injury (*arrow*) in OSA. (Data from Woo MA, Kumar R, Macey PM, et al. Brain injury in autonomic, emotional, and cognitive regulatory areas in patients with heart failure. J Cardiac Fail 2009;15:214–23; Kumar R, Birrer BV, Macey PM, et al. Reduced mammillary body volume in patients with obstructive sleep apnea. Neurosci Lett 2008;438:330–4; Kumar R, Chavez AS, Macey PM, et al. Altered global and regional brain mean diffusivity in patients with obstructive sleep apnea. J Neurosci Res 2012;90:2043–52. Drawing by Acerland International.)

in these conditions.[24,26-28] Furthermore, the region of the rostral ventrolateral medulla (RVLM), which contains almost all sympathetic premotor neurons in the brain, displays significant damage in both OSA and heart failure[26,27,29] (Figure 20.2). The nucleus of the solitary tract integrates baroreceptor and other sensory signals, relaying information to the region of the caudal ventrolateral medulla (CVLM), which in turn projects to the RVLM and then to the spinal cord intermediolateral column for sympathetic outflow. The human RVLM and CVLM are dorsally displaced relative to usual anatomic descriptions in rodents, and their resting signal fluctuations are correlated with spontaneous bursts of muscle sympathetic nerve discharge.[30] Furthermore, in OSA, multiple brain structures are damaged from hypoxia and other processes; this injury especially appears in the raphe and RVLM,[25,26,31-33] and the extent of damage in both structures is strongly correlated to the ongoing increases in muscle sympathetic nerve activity.[34]

In addition to brainstem sites, the ventral medial frontal, cingulate, and insular cortices, along with portions of the hippocampal formation, mammillary bodies, and hypothalamic structures, participate in cardiorespiratory patterning, autonomic control, cognitive and affective functions; all of these structures (Figure 20.2) are injured in OSA.[25,26,31-33] The amygdala central nucleus projects extensively to the parabrachial pons, the nucleus tractus solitarii (NTS), the dorsal motor nucleus, and the periaqueductal gray (PAG), all areas exerting significant influences on breathing and cardiac action.[35] Portions of the amygdala, cingulate, hippocampus, and frontal and insular cortices help mediate transient arterial blood pressure changes elicited by cold pressor or Valsalva challenges.[36,37] Injury to those areas may contribute to the impaired dynamic blood pressure control and chronic hypertension in OSA. Injury to hypotension-mediating areas cannot be overlooked, since sudden unexpected death can occur in OSA and is a serious concern during sleep in sudden unexpected death in epilepsy (SUDEP)[38]; activation of the subgenu cingulate can induce a profound loss of blood pressure.[39]

The insular cortices deserve special attention in cardiovascular regulation during sleep and waking. Both animal and human studies show that these areas modulate sympathetic and parasympathetic action, with the right insula principally affecting sympathetic outflow and the left, parasympathetic action,[40] although both sides interact.[41] The right anterior insula modulates baroreflex action,[41] and a lateralized and anterior-posterior topography of functional magnetic resonance imaging (fMRI) signals emerges to different autonomic (Valsalva, hand grip, or cold pressor) challenges.[42] The insular functional topographic organization has implications for sleep, heart failure, and stroke fields, because the right insula is preferentially damaged in OSA and heart failure[24,26,31,43,44] (Figure 20.3, *A*) and can be vascularly compromised from middle cerebral artery stroke. Heart failure and OSA are accompanied by enhanced sympathetic nerve discharge and hypertension, possibly from injury to the anterior insula and its baroreflex modulation roles. This insular damage is accompanied by impaired amplitude and timing of fMRI signals to autonomic challenges and an inability to mount appropriate heart rate responses.[45-48] A unilateral seizure focus in the insula could exert profound influences on arterial blood pressure and heart rate,[49] which might include exaggerated sympathetic drive from right-sided foci, leading to circumstances that may contribute to SUDEP.[50,51] The ventral medial frontal and cingulate cortices also exert major roles in vagal and sympathetic control, respectively.[52-55] The cortical influences on subcortical sites carry significant import for cardiorespiratory control.

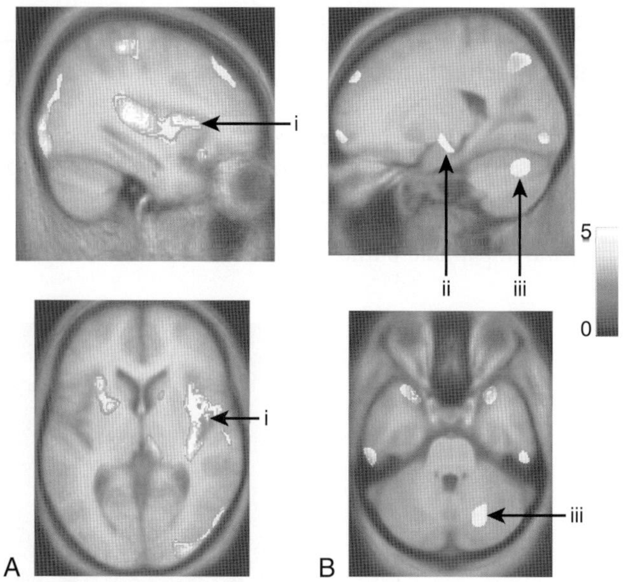

Figure 20.3 Areas of gray matter loss (*arrows*) within the insula (i) of patients with heart failure (n = 9) **(A),** and in the hippocampal region (ii) and cerebellum (iii) of patients with obstructive sleep apnea (OSA) (n = 21) **(B).** Gray matter loss was calculated from structural magnetic resonance imaging scans relative to those obtained in control subjects. The 0 to 5 scale represents *t* values; all *light areas* are significant ($P < .05$). (**A,** From Woo MA, Macey PM, Fonarow GC, et al. Regional brain gray matter loss in heart failure. *J Appl Physiol* 2003; 95:677–84; **B,** From Macey PM, Henderson LA, Macey KE, et al. Brain morphology associated with obstructive sleep apnea. *Am J Resp Crit Care Med* 2002;166:1382–7.)

The cerebellum is especially important for regulating cardiovascular and respiratory control in both sleep and waking states. Although it is not classically considered a component of either breathing or cardiac regulation, this cerebellar role has been known for over half a century[56] and is mediated partially through vestibular/cerebellar mechanisms in blood pressure coordination.[57] Vestibular mechanisms modify arterial blood pressure responses to rapid postural changes, a process familiar to orthostatic hypotensive individuals who suffer syncope on rising rapidly from the horizontal position. Lesions of feline cerebellar fastigial nuclei result in ineffective compensatory responses to hypotension[58] with ensuing death. The deep cerebellar nuclei also participate in termination of apnea, serving a "rescue" role for survival.[59] Significant gray matter loss occurs in the cerebellar cortex and deep nuclei in patients with heart failure[43] (Figure 20.3, *B*), with OSA,[44] and who succumb to SUDEP[60] and probably contributes to aberrant cardiovascular control in these syndromes. Abnormal cerebellar development or cerebellar insult contributions to cardiorespiratory disturbances, and especially to OSA, are well described.[61-63]

Cardiorespiratory Homeostasis

An important consideration in preserving circulatory homeostasis during sleep is coordination of control over two systems: the respiratory system, essential for oxygen exchange, and the cardiovascular system, for blood transport. The coordination of two motor systems, one for somatic musculature (i.e., diaphragmatic, intercostal, abdominal, and upper airway musculature) and the other for autonomic regulation (to the heart and vasculature), is a formidable task during sleep and is particularly challenging in patients with diseased respiratory or cardiovascular systems, especially in apnea or heart failure, or in infants, whose developing control systems may become compromised. Respiratory neuron activity varies greatly between sleep states, as does heart rhythm regularity. Tachycardia, polypnea, sweating, and dramatic elevations in arterial blood pressure secondary to intense autonomic activity occur primarily during REM sleep.

Maintaining perfusion of vital organs through adequate arterial blood pressure control is essential for cardiorespiratory homeostasis. Respiratory mechanisms are recruited to support cardiovascular action by assisting venous return and by reflexly altering cardiac rate. REM sleep induces a near-paralysis of accessory respiratory muscles, including upper airway musculature, and diminishes descending forebrain influences on brainstem vasculature and motor control regions.[64,65] This reorganization during REM sleep may interfere with compensatory breathing mechanisms that assist arterial blood pressure management and may lead to removal of protective forebrain influences on hypotension or hypertension. The significant interaction between breathing and arterial blood pressure appears in the partial normalization of blood pressure by delivery of continuous positive airway pressure (CPAP) in patients with apnea-induced hypertension.[66]

Arterial blood pressure control during sleep is of interest in examining mechanisms of failure in SIDS. Several reports indicate that the fatal sequence in SIDS may originate with a cardiac rhythm failure.[67] Specifically, an arrhythmia, or bradycardia and hypotension, rather than an initial breathing cessation, characterizes the final event.[68,69] Antecedent tachycardia may be present for up to 3 days. The terminal events in SIDS appear to parallel the two stages of shock—namely, an initial sympathoexcitation followed by a sudden, centrally triggered sympathoinhibition and bradycardia, leading to a life-threatening fall in arterial blood pressure. Some monitored SIDS cases show a near-total loss of arterial blood pressure within a minute of onset of the fatal event. Because SIDS deaths occur largely during sleep, some interaction of state and compensatory mechanisms is suspected. The prone sleeping position enhances the risk for SIDS, which may derive from the vestibular and cerebellar contributions to arterial blood pressure control[57] described earlier. Because vestibular and cerebellar mechanisms assist mediation of arterial blood pressure to postural changes, static stimuli, such as those from the prone position, can directly modify cardiovascular responses to blood pressure challenges.[70-73] Sleep effects on vestibular systems must be considered in examination of arterial blood pressure control mechanisms.

The cerebellar role in blood pressure maintenance, recovery from apnea, and cardiovascular and respiratory coordination suggests means to normalize that role in compromised conditions. Activation of cerebellar structures by electrical or optical stimulation has long been known to suppress seizures, modify blood pressure, and normalize breathing patterns.[59,74] The cerebellum can be activated readily by noninvasive proprioceptive stimulation, and that principle has been used to reduce central apnea, periodic breathing, and bradycardia in infants with apnea of prematurity.[75]

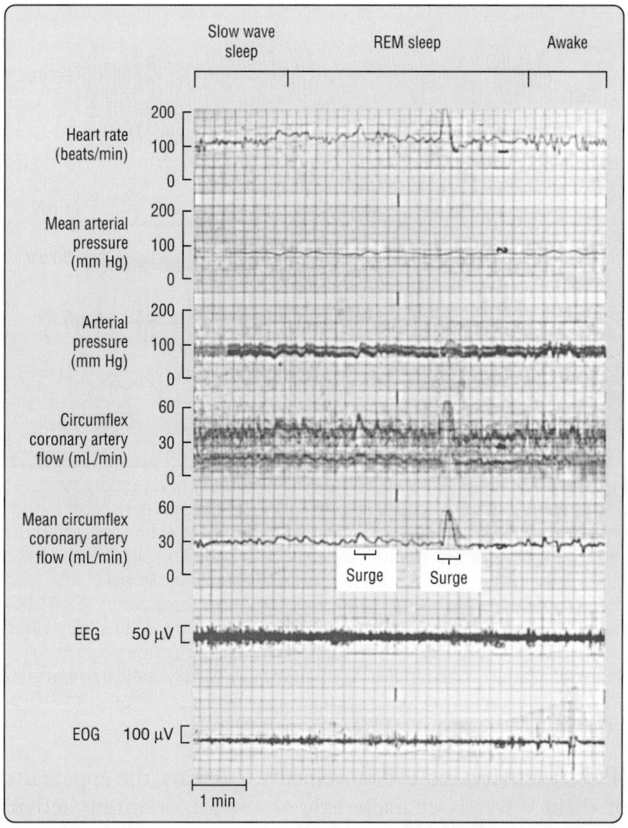

Figure 20.4 Effects of NREM sleep (slow wave sleep), REM sleep, and quiet wakefulness on heart rate, phasic and mean arterial blood pressure, phasic and mean left circumflex coronary flow, electroencephalogram (EEG), and electrooculogram (EOG) in the dog. Sleep spindles are evident during NREM sleep, eye movements during REM sleep, and gross eye movements on awakening. Surges in heart rate and coronary flow occur during REM sleep. (From Kirby DA, Verrier RL. Differential effects of sleep stage on coronary hemodynamic function. *Am J Physiol* 1989; 256:H1378–83.)

SLEEP STATE–DEPENDENT CHANGES IN HEART RHYTHM

Recent evidence indicates that the pronounced changes in heart rate occurring during REM sleep and transitions between sleep states are attributable to distinct mechanisms associated with specific brain sites, rather than representing a continuum of autonomic change.

Heart Rate Surges

Several investigators have reported REM sleep–induced increases in heart rate in experimental animals.[12,15,76-79] Accelerations consisting of an abrupt, although transitory, 35% to 37% increase in rate that are concentrated during phasic REM sleep were observed in canines (Figure 20.4).[76] These marked heart rate surges are accompanied by a rise in mean arterial blood pressure and are followed by a heart rate deceleration that is apparently baroreceptor mediated. Because the sequence is completely abolished by interruption of sympathetic neural input to the heart,[76-78] the acceleration does not appear to be dependent on withdrawal of parasympathetic nerve activity.[15,78]

REM sleep state–dependent heart rate surges also have been observed in felines. The rate accelerations are linked to central nervous system activation as reflected in a concomitant increase in hippocampal theta frequency, ponto-geniculo-occipital

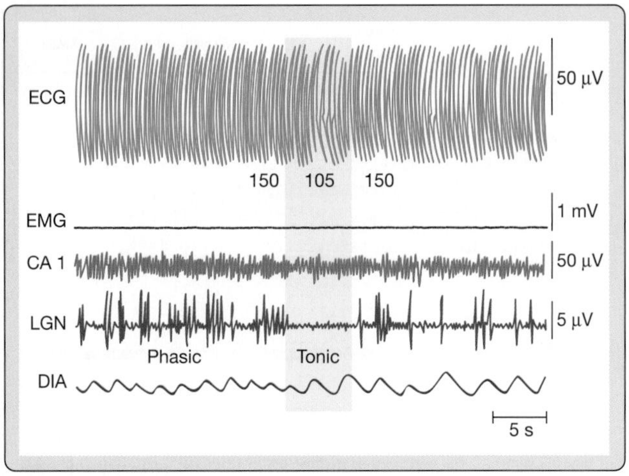

Figure 20.5 Representative polygraphic recording of a primary heart rate deceleration during tonic REM sleep. During this deceleration, heart rate decreased by 30% from 150 to 105 beats/min. The deceleration occurred during a period devoid of ponto-geniculo-occipital (PGO) spikes in the lateral geniculate nucleus (LGN) or theta rhythm in the hippocampal (CA 1) leads. The abrupt decreases in amplitude of hippocampal theta waves (CA 1), PGO waves (LGN), and respiratory rate (DIA) are typical of transitions from phasic to tonic REM sleep. ECG, Electrocardiogram; EMG, electromyogram. (From Verrier RL, Lau RT, Wallooppillai U, et al. Primary vagally mediated decelerations in heart rate during tonic rapid eye movement sleep in cats. *Am J Physiol* 1998;43:R1136–41.)

(PGO) activity, and eye movements.[79] In cats, the appearance of theta waves is characteristic of arousal, orienting activity, alertness, and REM sleep.[79-83] The surges are abolished by cardioselective beta-adrenergic receptor blockade with atenolol, suggesting, as in canines, that the peripheral effect is attributable to bursting of cardiac sympathetic efferent fiber activity, which directly affects heart rate. The main difference in rate responses between the two species is that in dogs, the rate acceleration is accompanied within seconds by a baroreflex-mediated deceleration. The precise basis for these differences in the pattern of heart rate responses is unclear, but a plausible explanation is that the canine studies were performed in beagles, dogs that are bred for intense physical activity, a factor known to augment baroreceptor responsiveness.

Heart Rhythm Pauses

A complementary finding to centrally mediated heart rate surges is the observation in cats of an abrupt heart rhythm deceleration that occurs predominantly during tonic REM sleep and is not associated with any preceding or subsequent heart rate or arterial blood pressure change (Figure 20.5).[84] The vagus nerve involvement appears to be directly initiated by central influences, as no antecedent or subsequent change in resting heart rate or arterial blood pressure occurs. The primary involvement of central nervous system activation is shown by the consistent, antecedent, abrupt cessation of PGO activity and the concomitant interruption of hippocampal theta rhythm. In normal human volunteers, Taylor and colleagues[85] observed heart rate decelerations during REM sleep that preceded eye movement bursts by 3 seconds and suggested that the phenomenon reflects an orienting response at dreaming onset. The processes underlying the central nervous system changes accompanying the tonic REM sleep–induced increase in vagus nerve tone, suppressing sinus node activity, remain unknown. Notwithstanding extensive studies of the physiologic and anatomic bases for PGO activity, little is known about its conductivity and functional relationship to heart rhythm control during sleep.

The most likely basis for the abrupt deceleration in heart rate during tonic REM sleep is a centrally induced decline in sympathetic nerve activity or enhanced vagus nerve tone or both in combination. In felines, cardioselective beta$_1$-adrenergic receptor blockade with atenolol did not affect the incidence or magnitude of decelerations, but muscarinic blockade with glycopyrrolate completely abolished the phenomenon. These observations suggest that the tonic REM sleep–induced decelerations are primarily mediated by cardiac vagus nerve efferent fiber activity. It is well known that enhanced vagus nerve activity can abruptly and markedly affect the sinus node firing rate.[86] Because beta-adrenergic receptor blockade exerted no effect on the frequency or magnitude of decelerations, it does not appear that withdrawal of cardiac sympathetic tone is an important factor in the observed rate changes. Respiratory interplay is not an essential component of the deceleration, inasmuch as the phenomenon often occurs in the absence of a temporal association with inspiratory effort.

This primary heart rate pause phenomenon appears to be distinct from baroreceptor-mediated reductions in heart rate that almost invariably follow accelerations in rate and elevation of arterial blood pressure (Figure 20.6).[13] This second group of heart rhythm pauses was observed in canines and occurs mainly during the transition from slow wave sleep to desynchronized sleep and more frequently during phasic than tonic REM sleep. These pauses persist for 1 to 8 seconds and are followed by dramatic increases in coronary blood flow averaging 30% and ranging up to 84% that are independent of metabolic activity of the heart as reflected in the heart rate–blood pressure product. An intense burst of vagus nerve activity appears to produce the phenomenon, because the pauses develop against a background of marked respiratory sinus arrhythmia with varying degrees of heart block (with nonconducted P waves) and with low heart rate. Moreover, the heart rhythm pauses could be reproduced by electrical stimulation of the vagus nerve. Guilleminault and colleagues[87] documented similar pauses in healthy young adults.

CORONARY ARTERY BLOOD FLOW REGULATION DURING SLEEP

Striking changes in coronary blood flow occur during REM and sleep state transitions.[13,76-78,88] Vatner and colleagues[88] studied the effects of the sleep-wake cycle on coronary artery function in baboons. During the nocturnal period, when the animals were judged to be asleep by behavioral indicators, coronary blood flow increased sporadically by as much as 100%. The periodic oscillations in blood flow were not associated with alterations in heart rate or arterial blood pressure and occurred while the animals remained motionless with eyes closed. Because the baboons were not instrumented for electroencephalographic recordings, no information was obtained regarding sleep stage, nor was the mechanism for the coronary blood flow surge defined.

Concomitant with the heart rate surges of REM sleep found in canines,[76-78] as described earlier, were remarkable episodic surges in coronary blood flow with corresponding declines in coronary vascular resistance. These phenomena occurred predominantly during periods of REM sleep marked by intense eye movement phasic activity.[78] No significant

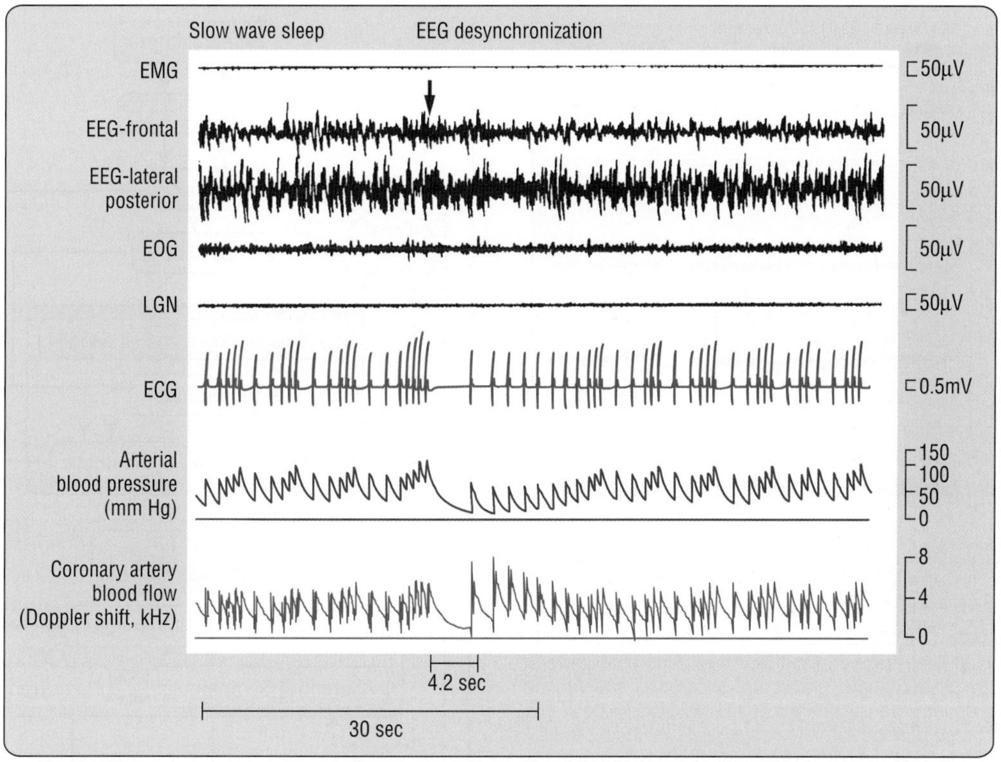

Figure 20.6 Coronary blood flow (CBF) surge during deep NREM sleep interrupted by electroencephalographic desynchronization. This response pattern is common and appears to represent a brief, low-grade arousal. The 4.2-second pause in heart rhythm was followed by a brief increase of 46% in average peak CBF and a decrease of 49% in the heart rate–systolic blood pressure product. ECG, Electrocardiogram; EEG, electroencephalogram; EMG, electromyogram; EOG, electrooculogram; LGN, lateral geniculate nucleus field potential recordings; SWS, slow wave sleep. (From Dickerson LW, Huang AH, Nearing BD, et al. Primary coronary vasodilation associated with pauses in heart rhythm during sleep. *Am J Physiol* 1993;264:R186–96.)

changes in mean arterial blood pressure were seen. Heart rate was elevated during the coronary flow surges, suggesting increased cardiac metabolic activity as the basis for the coronary vasodilation. In fact, the close coupling between rate-pressure product, an index of metabolic demand, and the magnitude of the flow surges indicates that the surges do not constitute a state of myocardial hyperperfusion. These surges in coronary blood flow appear to result from enhanced adrenergic discharge, because they were abolished by bilateral stellectomy and not from nonspecific effects of somatic activity or respiratory fluctuations.

During severe experimental coronary artery stenosis (with baseline flow reduced by 60%) in canines, phasic decreases in coronary arterial blood flow, rather than increases, were observed during REM sleep coincident with these heart rate surges (Figure 20.7).[77] An increase in adrenergic discharge could lead to a coronary blood flow decrement by at least two possible mechanisms. The first is by stimulation of alpha-adrenergic receptors on the coronary vascular smooth muscle. Such an effect, however, could be only transitory, because alpha-adrenergic stimulation results in brief (10 to 15 seconds) coronary constriction even during sympathetic nerve stimulation in anesthetized animals[89] or during intense arousal associated with aversive behavioral conditioning.[90] The second possible mechanism is mechanical: a decrease in diastolic coronary perfusion time caused by the surges in heart rate. In support of this explanation, a strong correlation (r^2 = 0.96) was found between the magnitude of the increase in heart rate and the decrease in coronary blood flow.[77] The link between REM-induced changes in heart rate and the occurrence of myocardial ischemia in patients with advanced coronary artery disease was reported by Nowlin and colleagues.[91] Furthermore, nocturnal myocardial ischemia carries significant potential to affect coronary function and cardiac electrical stability in patients with ischemic heart disease, because it has been linked to myocardial infarctions, 20% of which occur at night, and arrhythmias (Chapter 144).

IMPACT OF SLEEP ON ARRHYTHMOGENESIS

Central Nervous System Sites Influencing Cardiac Electrical Stability

Extensive investigation of central nervous system–induced cardiac arrhythmias has provided evidence that triggering of arrhythmias by the central nervous system not only is the consequence of intense activation of the autonomic nervous system but is also a function of the specific neural pattern elicited. Regulation of cardiac neural activity is highly integrated and is achieved by circuitry at multiple levels (Figure 20.8).[92] Higher brain centers operate through elaborate pathways within the hypothalamus, modulated by cortical influences and by medullary cardiovascular regulatory sites. Baroreceptor mechanisms have long been recognized as integral to autonomic control of the cardiovascular system, as evidenced by heart rate variability and baroreceptor sensitivity testing in both cardiac patients and normal subjects. While the basic circuitry responsible for the baroreflex lies in the medulla, this circuitry can be modulated by various higher centers including the midbrain (PAG)

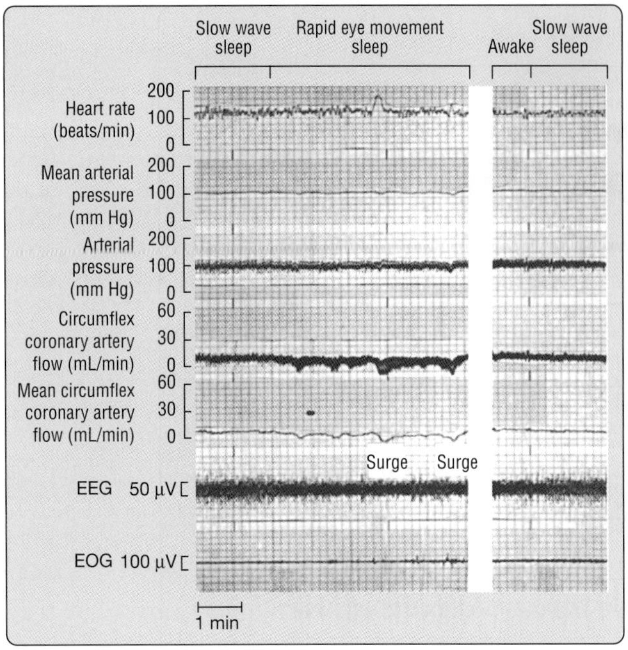

Figure 20.7 Effects of sleep stage on heart rate, mean and phasic arterial blood pressure, and mean and phasic left circumflex coronary artery blood flow in a typical dog during coronary artery stenosis. Note phasic decreases in coronary flow occurring during heart rate surges while the dog is in REM sleep, with a characteristic lower-amplitude, higher-frequency pattern in the electroencephalogram (EEG). The electrooculogram (EOG) tracing indicates the presence of eye movements during REM but not slow wave sleep. (From Kirby DA, Verrier RL. Differential effects of sleep stage on coronary hemodynamic function during stenosis. *Physiol Behav* 1989;45:1017–20.)

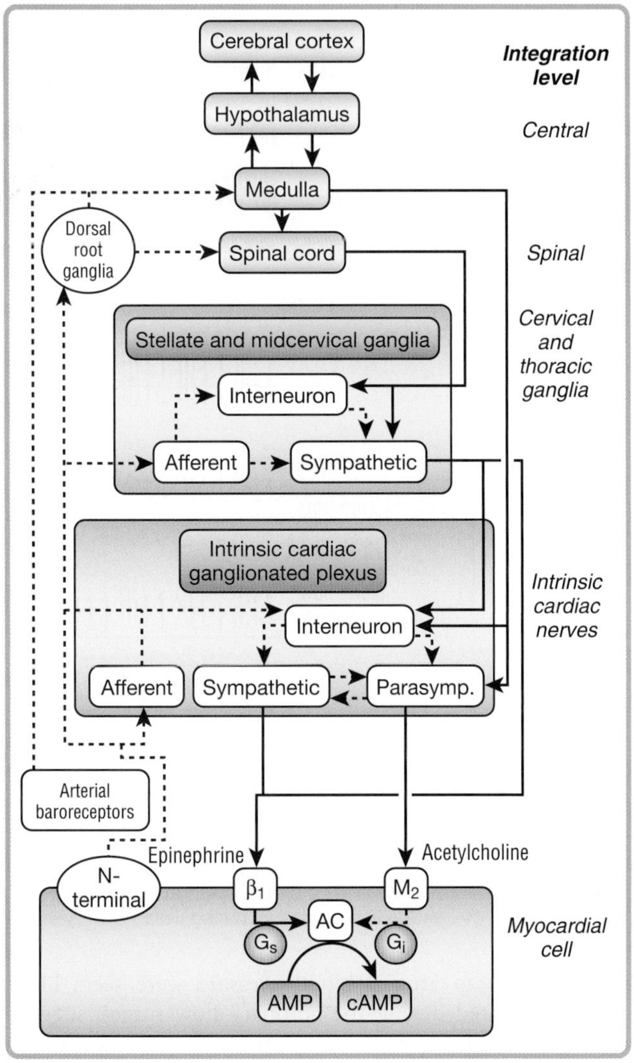

Figure 20.8 Synthesis of new and present views on levels of integration important in neural control of cardiac electrical activity during sleep. More traditional concepts focused on afferent tracts (*dashed lines*) arising from myocardial nerve terminals and reflex receptors (e.g., baroreceptors) that are integrated centrally within hypothalamic and medullary cardiostimulatory and cardioinhibitory brain centers and on central modulation of sympathetic and parasympathetic outflow (*solid lines*) with little intermediary processing at the level of the spinal cord and within cervical and thoracic ganglia. More recent views incorporate additional levels of intricate processing within the extraspinal cervical and thoracic ganglia and within the cardiac ganglionic plexus, where interneurons are envisioned to provide new levels of noncentral integration. Release of neurotransmitters from postganglionic sympathetic neurons is believed to enhance excitation in the sinoatrial node and myocardial cells through norepinephrine binding to beta$_1$-adrenergic receptors, which enhance adenyl cyclase (AC) activity through intermediary stimulatory G proteins (G_s). Increased parasympathectomy outflow enhances postganglionic release and binding of acetylcholine to muscarinic (M_2) receptors and, through coupled inhibitory G proteins (G_i), inhibits cyclic adenosine monophosphate (cAMP) production. cAMP alters electrogenesis and pacemaking activity by affecting the activity of specific membrane sodium, potassium, and calcium channels. (From Lathrop DA, Spooner PM. On the neural connection. *J Cardiovasc Electrophysiol* 2001;12:841–4, with permission.)

matter, hypothalamus, and the insular cortex,[41] as well as locally by intrinsic cardiac nerves and fat on the heart itself.

The phenomenon of electrical remodeling is attributable to nerve growth and degeneration. At the level of the myocardial cell, autonomic receptors influence G proteins to control ionic channels, pumps, and exchangers. The influence of the vagus nerve on ventricular electrical properties is contingent on the level of sympathetic tone, a phenomenon referred to as accentuated antagonism. The underlying mechanism is that acetylcholine, released by vagus nerve activation, exerts its opposing effects by presynaptic inhibition of norepinephrine release from sympathetic nerve endings and through an antagonism of second messenger formation at the cardiac receptor level.[93] Thus the balance in cardiac input from either limb of the autonomic nervous system and their interactions must be considered. Another important concept is that triggering of arrhythmias by central nervous system activity also may depend on several intermediary mechanisms. These include direct effects of neurotransmitters on the myocardium and its specialized conducting system and changes in myocardial perfusion resulting from alterations in coronary vasomotor tone, enhanced platelet aggregability, or both. The net influence on the heart thus depends on a complex interplay between the specific neural pattern elicited and the underlying cardiac pathology.

More than 100 years ago, Levy[94] demonstrated that ventricular tachyarrhythmias can be elicited in normal animals by stimulating specific areas in the brain, a finding subsequently confirmed in several species. Hockman and colleagues,[95] using stereotactic techniques, demonstrated that cerebral stimulation and hypothalamic activation evoked a spectrum of ventricular arrhythmias. Stimulation of the posterior hypothalamus causes a ten fold increase in the incidence of ventricular fibrillation elicited by experimental occlusion of the coronary artery.[96] This enhanced vulnerability was linked to increased sympathetic nerve activity, because beta-adrenergic receptor blockade, but not vagotomy, prevented it. These findings are consistent with clinical reports that cerebrovascular disease (particularly intracranial hemorrhage) can elicit significant cardiac repolarization abnormalities and life-threatening arrhythmias.[97,98] Cryogenic blockade of the thalamic gating mechanism or its output from the frontal cortex to the brainstem[99] and of the amygdala[100] delayed or prevented the occurrence of ventricular fibrillation during stress in pigs.

There is also strong evidence correlating chronic emotional stress to the development of cardiovascular diseases, including hypertension, ischemic heart disease, and cardiac arrhythmias, and the findings that acute stressors can evoke sudden cardiac dysfunction and death.[101-105] Importantly, emotional stress is able to precipitate ectopic beats in patients with coronary artery disease or other structural heart disease and even in individuals with no demonstrable or detectable cardiac deficits.[106,107] It is now recognized that cardiorespiratory responses to psychological stressors are likely mediated by the dorsomedial hypothalamus (DMH), which projects directly to the paraventricular hypothalamus for the release of cortisol as well as to brainstem sites such as the PAG, RVLM, raphe, and NTS for the neural control of cardiorespiratory function.[108] Furthermore, asymmetric autonomic output from the DMH and the PAG to the heart during emotional stress has been proposed as a causal factor that can precipitate cardiac arrhythmias.[109-112] Indeed, a positive relationship exists between right midbrain activity and pro-arrhythmic abnormalities in ventricular repolarization during mental stress,[113] and activation of the right DMH evokes more ectopic beats than activation of the left DMH.[114] In addition to the potential for cardiac arrhythmias to occur during hypothalamic stimulation, they can also ensue immediately on cessation of diencephalic or hypothalamic stimulation, the appearance of which requires intact vagi and stellate ganglia.[115,116] The likely electrophysiologic basis for such post–central nervous system stimulation arrhythmias is the loss of rate overdrive suppression of ectopic activity. This phenomenon occurs when the vagus nerve regains its activity after cessation of centrally induced adrenergic stimulation. Accordingly, the enhanced automaticity induced by adrenergic stimulation of ventricular pacemakers is exposed when vagus nerve tone is restored and slows the sinus rate.[116] Although these arrhythmias, including ventricular tachycardia, may be dramatic in appearance, they rarely degenerate into ventricular fibrillation.[117] This proarrhythmic effect of dual autonomic activation has been erroneously interpreted as profibrillatory.

The antiarrhythmic influence of beta-adrenergic receptor blockade may result in part from blockade of central beta-adrenergic receptors. Parker and colleagues[118] determined that intracerebroventricular administration of subsystemic doses of L-propranolol (but not D-propranolol) significantly reduced the incidence of ventricular fibrillation during combined left anterior descending coronary artery occlusion and behavioral stress in pigs. In a surprising turn, intravenous administration of even a relatively high dose of L-propranolol was ineffectual. The latter result may relate in part to a species dependence; unlike canines, pigs do not show a suppression of ischemia-induced arrhythmias in response to beta-adrenergic receptor blockade.[119] It has been proposed that the centrally mediated protective effect of beta-adrenergic receptor blockade results from a decrease in sympathetic nerve activity and in plasma norepinephrine concentration.[118,120,121] Of importance, whereas central actions of beta-adrenergic receptor blockers may play an important role in reducing susceptibility to ventricular fibrillation during acute myocardial ischemia, they are unlikely to constitute the sole mechanism because beta-adrenergic receptor blockers prevent the profibrillatory effect of direct stimulation of peripheral sympathetic structures such as the stellate ganglia.[122] Of note, all three of the beta-adrenergic receptor blockers that have long-term effects on mortality in cardiac patients (propranolol, metoprolol, and carvedilol) are lipophilic[123] and therefore cross the blood-brain barrier readily to affect sleep structure, with significant perturbations of sleep continuity.[124]

Autonomic Factors in Arrhythmogenesis during Sleep

NREM sleep generally is salutary with respect to ventricular arrhythmogenesis, as indicated both by extensive studies of neurocardiac interactions and by clinical experience. Activation of the vagus nerve reduces heart rate, increases cardiac electrical stability, and reduces rate-pressure product, an indicator of cardiac metabolic activity, to improve the supply-demand relationship in stenotic coronary artery segments. In the setting of severe coronary disease or acute myocardial infarction, however, hypotension during NREM sleep can lead to myocardial ischemia as a consequence of inadequate coronary perfusion pressure, thereby provoking arrhythmias and myocardial infarction.[11,125] The abrupt increases in vagus nerve tone that can occur during periods of REM sleep or sleep state transitions can result in significant pauses in heart rhythm, bradyarrhythmias, and, potentially, triggered activity, a mechanism of the lethal cardiac arrhythmia torsades de pointes. Patients with the long QT syndrome who have the type 3 phenotype are more prone to experience arrhythmogenic levels of T-wave alternans[126] and torsades de pointes at night rather than during stress or exercise.[70] Tonic control of the vagus nerves over the caliber of the epicardial coronary vessels[127] could be an important factor in dynamic regulation of coronary resistance as a function of the sleep-wake cycle. An important question is whether tonic vagus nerve activity exerts a protective or a deleterious influence on myocardial perfusion and arrhythmogenesis in individuals with atherosclerotic disease. In these patients, nocturnal surges in vagus nerve activity could precipitate myocardial ischemia and arrhythmias as a result of coronary vasoconstriction rather than dilation in atherosclerotic segments because of impaired release of endothelium-derived relaxing factor.[128]

Because of the attendant surges in sympathetic nerve activity and heart rate, REM sleep has the potential to trigger ventricular arrhythmias.[129,130] The striking variability of heart rate and breathing pattern can exert a significant impact on cardiovascular functioning, as is evident in the development of ischemia and arrhythmias in patients whose myocardium is compromised. Indeed, the only clinical studies in which sleep staging has been employed have identified REM as the state in which arrhythmias occurred.[11,131,132] The increased sympathetic nerve activity that occurs at REM sleep onset[10] provides a potent stimulus for ventricular tachyarrhythmias because of the arrhythmogenic influence of neurally released catecholamines. Sympathetic nerve activation by stimulation of central[94-96,115,116] or peripheral adrenergic structures,[122,133] infusion of catecholamines,[134] or imposition of behavioral stress[135,136] can increase cardiac vulnerability in the normal and the ischemic heart. These profibrillatory influences are substantially blunted by beta-adrenergic receptor blockade.[135] A wide variety of supraventricular arrhythmias also can be induced by autonomic activation.[117]

Enhanced sympathetic nerve activity increases cardiac vulnerability in the normal and in the ischemic heart by complex mechanisms. The major indirect effects include an impaired oxygen supply-demand ratio resulting from increased cardiac metabolic activity and coronary vasoconstriction, particularly in vessels with injured endothelium and in the context of altered preload and afterload. The direct profibrillatory effects on cardiac electrophysiologic function are attributable to derangements in impulse formation or conduction, or both.[117] Increased levels of catecholamines activate beta-adrenergic receptors, which in turn alter adenylate cyclase activity and intracellular calcium flux. These actions are likely mediated by the cyclic nucleotide and protein kinase regulatory cascade, which can alter spatial heterogeneity of calcium transients and consequently increase dispersion of repolarization. The net influence is an increased susceptibility to ventricular fibrillation.[90,137,138] Conversely, reduction of cardiac sympathetic drive by stellectomy has proved to be antifibrillatory.

Notwithstanding the evidence that autonomic factors can significantly alter susceptibility to arrhythmias, the observation that the heart rate surges of REM sleep are conducive to myocardial ischemia, and the epidemiologic data in humans on the extent of sleep-induced cardiac events,[1] very little information is available on the effects of myocardial infarction during sleep. Ventricular ectopic activity, but not ventricular fibrillation, emerges during NREM sleep in pigs after myocardial infarction.[139] This pattern may be attributable to slowing of heart rate and increased vagus nerve activity during NREM sleep, conditions that can inhibit the normal overdrive suppression of ventricular rhythms by sinoatrial node pacemaker activity and result in firing of latent ventricular pacemakers and triggered activity. Snisarenko[140] found significant elevations in heart rate in both the acute (4 to 10 days) and subacute (3 to 12 months) periods after myocardial infarction in a feline model. In the acute period, these effects were accompanied by increased wakefulness, decreased heart rate variability, and severely disordered sleep. In the intervening weeks, sleep quality recovered fully until, in the subacute period, beta-adrenergic receptor blockade with propranolol led to renewed, pronounced disturbances in sleep structure, with increased wakefulness, reduction in REM sleep, and prolongation of stages N1 and N2 of NREM sleep. Snisarenko attributed these results to reflex activation of adrenergic, noradrenergic, and dopaminergic nerves in several brain structures after coronary artery ligation.[140]

CURRENT TREATMENT REGIMENS FOR SLEEP-RELATED CARDIOVASCULAR EVENTS

Sleep-disordered breathing syndromes such as OSA have long been associated with significantly increased muscle sympathetic nerve activity during both sleep and waking,[34,66,141-146] leading to hypertension and increased cardiovascular morbidity,[147,148] including myocardial infarction.[149] The standard treatment option for OSA is CPAP, which maintains airway patency and prevents apneas and their associated surges in blood pressure, heart rate, and sympathetic activity. CPAP therapy can reverse the elevated sympathetic drive as well as altered brain activity and structure in areas such as the RVLM and raphe nuclei (Figure 20.9).[29,66,150,151] While CPAP therapy effectively reverses the elevated sympathetic nerve activity associated with OSA, there is debate about whether it reverses the elevated blood pressure. A recent meta-analysis that included 32 randomized controlled trials reported that CPAP therapy was associated with a mean reduction in daytime blood pressure of approximately 2 to 3 mm Hg, with greater effects in those individuals with more severe OSA.[152] While this effect on blood pressure is modest, it has been suggested that CPAP therapy might reduce overall cardiovascular risk by reducing the large blood pressure spikes that occur during sleep apnea/hypopnea episodes without altering resting blood pressure significantly.[153] Stabilization of cardiovascular patterns during apnea using noninvasive neuromodulatory procedures might be a useful target for adults as it has been for neonates.[75]

Heart failure is also associated with increased muscle sympathetic activity[154,155] and altered resting heart rate variability,[9] as well as with biochemical,[156] volumetric,[43] and diffusivity[157] changes in brain regions that regulate autonomic activity such as the insula, RVLM, and medullary raphe nuclei. Elevated muscle sympathetic activity in heart failure is associated with the existence of sleep-disordered breathing, including both obstructive and central sleep apnea syndromes,[158] which is itself associated with increased mortality and cardiac events.[159,160] Furthermore, CPAP therapy is successful in reducing blood pressure and sympathetic activity in heart failure patients with either apnea syndrome.[161,162] While CPAP in central sleep apnea does not trigger inspiration, it improves oxygen stores and reduces apnea frequency and norepinephrine levels and increases nocturnal oxygen saturation and ejection fraction.[163] Although how CPAP reduces sympathetic drive in heart failure patients is unknown, given the effects of CPAP in OSA patients without heart failure, CPAP may restore the structure and function of autonomic-related brain regions, such as the insula and RVLM.

While CPAP is the standard treatment for individuals with OSA, adaptive servo-ventilation has been developed more recently to treat primarily central sleep apnea. Although this therapy also relies on delivering positive airway pressure, it adjusts its settings according to breathing effort to maintain steady minute ventilation and low-grade positive end-expiratory pressure. Recent studies suggest that adaptive servo-ventilation reduces indices of cardiac and muscle sympathetic activity in heart failure patients.[164-166] Although the use of adaptive servo-ventilation was considered advantageous for reducing the deleterious symptoms in all individuals with central apnea, more recently it has become clear that there are some individuals in whom this therapy is not recommended. Servo-ventilation is associated with an increased risk of cardiac mortality in heart failure patients, an ejection fraction ≤45%, and moderate or severe central sleep apnea.[167] Thus, while adaptive servo-ventilation can be used to reduce damage caused by apneas and lessen cardiovascular risk in some individuals, in others, such positive pressure procedures are ill advised, and alternative therapies are needed. This is especially the case since long-term compliance with these procedures is poor.[168]

In addition to positive airway pressure interventions for obstructive and central sleep apnea, other alternative treatment regimens are being developed, particularly for neonates

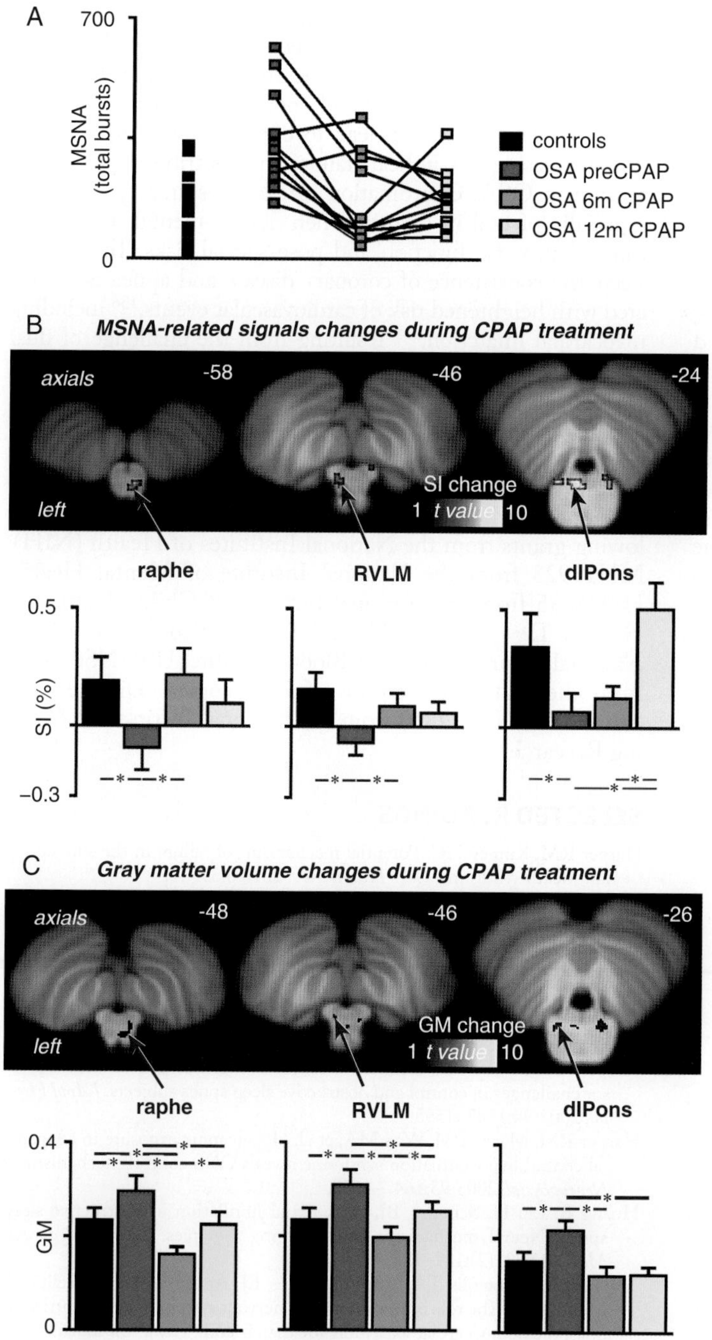

Figure 20.9 Effects of continuous positive airway pressure (CPAP) therapy on muscle sympathetic activity (MSNA), MSNA-coupled brainstem activity, and regional brainstem volume. **A,** Resting MSNA levels in controls (*black*) and obstructive sleep apnea (OSA) patients prior to (*red*) and following 6 months (*orange*) and 12 months (*yellow*) of CPAP therapy. Note the reduction in resting MNSA following CPAP. **B,** Changes in MSNA-coupled functional magnetic resonance imaging (fMRI) signal intensity (SI) in the same control and OSA subjects. Note that CPAP therapy restores MSNA-coupled activity to control levels in the medullary raphe, rostral ventrolateral medulla (RVLM), and dorsolateral pons (dlPons). Locations in Montreal Neurological Institute space are indicated at the top right of each slice. **C,** Changes in regional gray matter (GM) volume in the same control and OSA subjects. Again, note that CPAP therapy restores GM volume to control levels in the raphe, RVLM, and dlPons. *$P < .05$. (Modified from Henderson LA, Fatouleh RH, Lundblad LC, et al. Effects of 12 months of continuous positive airway pressure on sympathetic activity related brainstem function and structure in obstructive sleep apnea. *Front Neurosci* 2016;10:90 with permission from the authors.)

in whom a danger for injury in underdeveloped lungs exists or for patients with periodic breathing in whom circulation timing, with disrupted interactions between blood flow and chemosensing for breathing, is an underlying problem. One approach to overcome usual chemoreceptor drive and cardiovascular actions is to recruit drives to breathing other than from temperature and chemical stimuli, which, by reflexive action, may normalize cardiovascular action. That approach has been demonstrated by using exaggerated proprioceptive activation to "trick" the brain into enhancing breathing drive by simulating limb movement,[75] an approach that also assists cardiovascular processes.

Therapies such as implantable nerve stimulators are being developed to activate either diaphragmatic or upper airway muscles directly. Implantable phrenic nerve stimulators are currently available to treat central sleep apnea by eliciting smooth diaphragmatic contractions similar to normal respiration during sleep. These nerve stimulators are well tolerated and effective at reducing the severity of central sleep apnea, although whether they also improve autonomic function[169,170] is unclear; the procedure is frequently used for congenital central hypoventilation,[171] an intervention that must be carefully pressure retitrated to protect against upper airway obstruction. To avoid upper airway collapse directly, stimulation of the hypoglossal nerve, which innervates the principal upper airway dilator, the genioglossus, and other upper airway muscles, has also been used[169,172]; these nerve stimulation interventions require invasive surgery.

Direct stimulation of the vagus nerve can worsen sleep-disordered breathing. This therapy has been used for over

20 years to control refractory epilepsy and can reduce seizures by up to 50% in adults and 90% in pediatric patients.[173,174] However, vagus nerve stimulation can significantly increase apneic events and should be used with care.[175,176] Of course, vagus nerve stimulation alters parasympathetic flow to the heart and also activates brainstem autonomic regulatory regions such as the NTS. This places the vagus nerve in a position to alter sympathetic/parasympathetic balance and improve autonomic function, and indeed vagus nerve stimulation improves outcomes in individuals with heart failure.[177] The glossopharyngeal nerve is also involved in autonomic control, transmitting baroreceptor information to the NTS and carotid sinus, and direct stimulation of this cranial nerve may aid in the treatment of sleep-disordered breathing. Further research exploring the effects of glossopharyngeal and other cranial nerve stimulators on sleep-disordered breathing and its sequelae are needed.

There are multiple options in addition to positive air pressure to support ventilation in sleep-disordered breathing; the problem is to choose a timely approach that will provide both upper airway and diaphragmatic drive (remembering that the upper airway dilation must precede diaphragmatic descent) and concurrently to provide cardiovascular support, considering that brain structures mediating sympathetic action are often damaged in sleep-disordered breathing cases.

CLINICAL PEARLS

- REM sleep is characterized by surges in sympathetic and vagus nerve activity, which are well tolerated in normal individuals but may result in cardiac arrhythmias, myocardial ischemia, and myocardial infarction in those with heart disease.
- During NREM sleep, systemic blood pressure may fall, potentially reducing flow through stenotic coronary vessels to precipitate myocardial ischemia or infarction.
- Sleep-disordered breathing induces significant injury in brain autonomic regulatory areas.
- There is an increased prevalence of atrial fibrillation in obstructive sleep apnea.
- In essence, sleep constitutes an autonomic stress test for the heart, and nighttime monitoring of cardiorespiratory function is of considerable diagnostic value.[136]

SUMMARY

Sleep states exert a major impact on cardiorespiratory function as a direct consequence of the significant variations in brain states that occur in the normal cycling between NREM and REM sleep. Dynamic fluctuations in central nervous system variables influence heart rhythm, arterial blood pressure, coronary artery blood flow, and ventilation. Whereas REM sleep–induced surges in sympathetic and parasympathetic nerve activity, with accompanying significant surges and pauses in heart rhythm are well tolerated in normal people, patients with heart disease may be at heightened risk for life-threatening arrhythmias and myocardial ischemia and infarction.[91,130] During NREM sleep in the severely compromised heart, a potential for hypotension exists that can impair blood flow through stenotic coronary vessels to trigger myocardial ischemia or infarction.[11] Cumulative damage incurred as a consequence of sleep-disordered breathing, heart failure, or stroke to the central brain areas that regulate autonomic activity and coordinate upper airway and diaphragmatic action can lead to enhanced sympathetic outflow, increasing risk in heart failure and contributing to hypertension in OSA. Coordination of cardiorespiratory control is especially pivotal in infancy, when developmental immaturity can compromise function and pose special risks. Throughout sleep, the coexistence of coronary disease and apnea is associated with heightened risk of cardiovascular events,[136] including myocardial infarction,[149] resulting from the challenge of dual control of the respiratory and cardiovascular systems.

We thank Sandra S. Verrier for her editorial contributions.

ACKNOWLEDGMENTS

Work on which this chapter is based was supported by the following grants from the National Institutes of Health (NIH): MH13923 from the National Institute of Mental Health, HD22695 from the National Institute of Child Health and Human Development, HL22418 and HL60296 from the National Heart, Lung, and Blood Institute, U01-NS090407 from the National Institute of Neurological Diseases and Stroke, and NR012810 from the National Institute of Nursing Research.

SELECTED READINGS

Harper RM, Kinney HC. Potential mechanisms of failure in the sudden infant death syndrome. *Curr Pediatr Rev*. 2010;6:39–47.

Harper RM, Kumar R, Macey PM, et al. Functional neuroanatomy and sleep-disordered breathing: implications for autonomic regulation. *Anat Rec. (Hoboken)*. 2012;295:1385–1395.

Harper RM, Kumar R, Macey PM, et al. Affective brain areas and sleep-disordered breathing. *Prog Brain Res*. 2014;209:275–293.

Harper RM, Kumar R, Ogren JA, et al. Sleep-disordered breathing: effects on brain structure and function. *Respir Physiol Neurobiol*. 2013;188:383–391.

Harper RM, Macey PM, Henderson LA, et al. fMRI responses to cold pressor challenges in control and obstructive sleep apnea subjects. *J Appl Physiol*. 2003;94:1583–1595.

Harper RM, Macey PM, Woo MA, et al. Hypercapnic exposure in congenital central hypoventilation syndrome reveals CNS control mechanisms. *J Neurophysiol*. 2005;93:1647–1658.

Huang B, Liu H, Scherlag BJ, et al. Atrial fibrillation in obstructive sleep apnea: Neural mechanisms and emerging therapies. *Trends Cardiovasc Med*. 2021;31(2):127–132.

Manolis AA, Manolis TA, Apostolopoulos EJ, Apostolaki NE, Melita H, Manolis AS. The role of the autonomic nervous system in cardiac arrhythmias: the neuro-cardiac axis, more foe than friend? *Trends Cardiovasc Med*. 2020;S1050–1738(20)30066–9.

Mansukhani MP, Wang S, Somers VK. Chemoreflex physiology and implications for sleep apnoea: insights from studies in humans. *Exp Physiol*. 2015;100:130–135.

Ogren JA, Macey PM, Kumar R, et al. Impaired cerebellar and limbic responses to the Valsalva maneuver in heart failure. *Cerebellum*. 2012;11:931–938.

Rucinski C, Winbo A, Marcondes L, et al. A population-based registry of patients with inherited cardiac conditions and resuscitated cardiac arrest. *J Am Coll Cardiol*. 2020;75(21):2698–2707.

Woo MA, Palomares JA, Macey PM, et al. Global and regional brain mean diffusivity changes in patients with heart failure. *J Neurosci Res*. 2015;93:678–685.

A complete reference list can be found online at ExpertConsult.com.

Chapter 21

Cardiovascular Physiology: Autonomic Control in Health and in Sleep Disorders

Sébastien Baillieul; Virend K. Somers; Jean-Louis Pépin

Chapter Highlights

- Autonomic control of the circulation is pivotal in ensuring an adequate cardiac output to the vital organs through continuous and rapid adjustments of heart rate (HR), arterial blood pressure (BP), and redistribution of blood flow. In the longer term, neural circulatory control appears to be coupled with the circadian rhythm, the sleep-wake cycle, and ultradian rhythms, including rapid eye movement (REM) and non–rapid eye movement (NREM) sleep processes.
- The cardiovascular autonomic nervous system's primary role is to ensure an adequate cardiac output to the vital organs through continuous and rapid adjustments of heart rate (HR), arterial blood pressure (BP), and redistribution of blood flow.
- HR and BP have a diurnal rhythm characterized by a significant reduction during nighttime hours. This physiologic pattern can be altered by sleep insufficiency and sleep disorders, with important implications for cardiovascular health.
- During non-rapid eye movement (NREM) sleep, there is an increase in cardiovagal drive and a reduction in cardiac and peripheral sympathetic activity. Baroreflex gain is heightened in response to BP increments rather than decrements during NREM sleep to ensure the maintenance of stable low BP and HR during NREM sleep. By contrast, rapid eye movement (REM) sleep is a state of autonomic instability, dominated by remarkable fluctuations between parasympathetic and sympathetic influences.
- Sleep loss, alterations in sleep quality, and sleep disorders are associated with persistence of high sympathetic activity during the night and reduction in physiologic nocturnal BP dipping. These effects lead to sustained sympathetic activation with increased BP during the succeeding days.

OVERVIEW

Autonomic circulatory control operates via parasympathetic neurons to the heart and by sympathetic neuronal efferents to the heart, blood vessels, kidneys, and adrenal medulla.[1] Parasympathetic stimulation of the heart, through the activation of cardiac muscarinic receptors, results in bradycardia, whereas sympathetic stimulation of the heart, through activation of beta$_1$-adrenergic receptors, results in tachycardia and increased contractility. Sympathetic activation in the vascular bed induces vasoconstriction, by stimulating alpha$_1$ adrenoreceptors, and vasodilation, by stimulating beta$_2$ adrenoreceptors. Several reflexes, including the arterial baroreflex, cardiopulmonary reflexes, and chemoreflexes, also are important in the rapid adjustments of circulation that occur in association with postural changes, hypoxemia, temperature changes, and sleep. Heart rate (HR) and blood pressure (BP) have a diurnal rhythm characterized by a significant reduction during nighttime hours, secondary to changes in activity and posture, as well as sleep and circadian influences. This physiologic pattern can be altered by sleep insufficiency and sleep disorders, with important implications for cardiovascular health.

The cardiovascular autonomic nervous system works to maintain homeostasis through precise control of numerous hemodynamic variables, including HR, arterial BP, and peripheral blood flow, on a beat-by-beat basis. Neural circulatory control is intimately linked to sleep and circadian physiology, as demonstrated by the disrupted autonomic control that accompanies sleep disruption, for example, with sleep loss and sleep apnea. On the other hand, whether primary alterations in autonomic function may translate into sleep disturbances also must be considered.

This chapter begins with a general overview of autonomic cardiovascular regulation and of its central and peripheral controllers, followed by a description of the methods used to explore cardiovascular neural control during sleep in humans and their advantages and limitations. The chapter continues with an outline of some of the current knowledge of neural circulatory control during normal sleep and changes that may occur as a consequence of sleep deprivation, alterations in sleep quality, sleep apnea, and autonomic dysfunction such as may occur in diabetes.

THE CARDIOVASCULAR AUTONOMIC NERVOUS SYSTEM: DEFINITION AND FUNCTIONS

The cardiovascular autonomic nervous system is a highly integrated network that controls visceral functions, which on a short timescale (seconds to hours), adjusts the circulation in keeping with behavior, the environment, and emotions. Its primary role is to ensure an adequate cardiac output to the vital organs through continuous and rapid adjustments of HR, arterial BP, and redistribution of blood flow. In the longer term, this neural circulatory regulation appears to be coupled with the circadian rhythm, the sleep-wake cycle, and some ultradian rhythms, including rapid eye movement (REM) and non–rapid eye movement (NREM) sleep processes, as well as hormones implicated in long-term BP regulation.

Neural control of the circulation operates via parasympathetic neurons to the heart, and sympathetic neuronal efferents to the heart, blood vessels, kidneys, and adrenal medulla. Parasympathetic stimulation of the cardiovascular system is mediated primarily via the vagus nerve through the activation of muscarinic receptors; it results in bradycardia. Sympathetic stimulation of the heart acts through activation of $beta_1$ adrenoreceptors at the sinoatrial node (the cardiac pacemaker) and in the myocardium (the cardiac muscle) and results in tachycardia and increased contractility. Sympathetic activation in the vascular bed induces vasoconstriction by stimulating $alpha_1$ adrenoreceptors (in the skin and splanchnic districts) and vasodilation by stimulating $beta_2$ adrenoreceptors (in the heart and skeletal muscles). Parasympathetic and sympathetic efferent activity to the heart may also modulate cardiac electrophysiologic properties that can be relevant to the genesis of several types of arrhythmias, particularly in the presence of a pro-arrhythmic substrate.

Central organization of the autonomic nervous system and its relationship with sleep-modulating mechanisms are detailed in Chapter 20. Briefly, autonomic impulses to the vasculature and heart originate from the vasomotor center in the brainstem, located bilaterally in the reticular substance of the medulla and pons. The vasomotor center is in turn modulated by higher nervous system regions in the pons, mesencephalon, and diencephalon, including the hypothalamus and many portions of the cerebral cortex. Several cardiovascular reflexes are also important in the rapid adjustments of BP occurring in association with postural changes, hypoxemia, exercise, and moderate temperature changes and may also be implicated in cardiovascular changes observed during sleep. These include the arterial baroreflex, cardiopulmonary reflexes, and chemoreflexes. The renin-angiotensin-aldosterone system, vasopressin, and other vasoactive mechanisms may also contribute to cardiovascular regulation during sleep. More information on the interaction between cardiovascular disorders and sleep can be found in Section 15 of this book, Cardiovascular Disorders.

Arterial Baroreflex

The arterial baroreflex is an important regulator of BP in the short term.[2] The baroreceptors are sensory receptors in the aortic arch and carotid sinuses that relay in the medullary regions of the brain. Changes in arterial baroreceptor afferent discharge trigger reflex adjustments that buffer or oppose the changes in BP. For instance, increments in BP stretch the receptors, resulting in heightened afferent traffic to the brainstem neuronal network. This inhibits efferent sympathetic outflow to cardiac and vascular smooth muscle and increases parasympathetic cardiac tone, resulting in slowing of HR, reduction in contractility, and reduced peripheral vasoconstriction with subsequent compensatory decreases in BP. A decrease in BP has opposite effects and elicits reflex tachycardia, increased contractility, and peripheral vasoconstriction with subsequent compensatory increases in BP.

Cardiopulmonary Reflexes

Cardiopulmonary reflexes are triggered by the stimulation of low-pressure receptors located in the atria, ventricles, and pulmonary arteries. Cardiopulmonary receptors are volume receptors that serve to mitigate changes in BP in response to changes in blood volume. The firing pattern of these receptors parallels the pressure changes within the cardiac chambers or vessels and helps to regulate blood volume. Cardiopulmonary reflex activation results in peripheral vasodilation, reduction in sympathetic outflow to the kidney, and activation of the posterior pituitary gland to inhibit the release of antidiuretic hormone, resulting in increased urine excretion.

Arterial and cardiopulmonary reflexes are implicated in BP regulation during postural changes. Assumption of the upright position produces a caudal shift in blood volume and acutely reduces stroke volume and BP. The circulatory adjustment to this orthostatic stress is rapid and is characterized by reflex increases in HR and peripheral vascular resistance, followed by enhanced secretion of antidiuretic hormone and activation of the renin-angiotensin system. Recumbency, as occurs during sleep, produces an increased volume load in the cardiac chambers and elicits the opposite effects.

Chemoreflexes

The chemoreflexes mediate the ventilatory response to hypoxia and hypercapnia and exert important cardiovascular effects.[3] The peripheral arterial chemoreceptors, the most important of which are located in the carotid bodies, respond primarily to changes in the partial pressure of oxygen. Hypoxemic stimulation elicits an increase in respiratory muscle output, inducing hyperventilation, and an increase in sympathetic outflow to peripheral blood vessels, resulting in vasoconstriction. Hyperventilation in turn activates pulmonary stretch receptors, which buffer the increases in sympathetic and vagal outflow, thereby maintaining homeostasis under normal conditions. During apnea, when hyperventilation is absent or prevented, vasoconstriction is potentiated and occurs simultaneously with activation of the cardiac vagal drive, resulting in bradycardia. This is collectively termed the "diving reflex," a protective mechanism that helps preserve blood flow to the heart and brain while limiting cardiac oxygen demand.[4,5]

The central chemoreceptors are located in the brainstem and respond to changes in pH mediated primarily by carbon dioxide tension. Stimulation of central chemoreceptors by hypercapnia also elicits sympathetic and respiratory activation, but without the cardiovagal effects seen with hypoxemia.[3]

MEASURES TO EXPLORE AUTONOMIC CHANGES DURING SLEEP AND THEIR PHYSIOLOGIC SIGNIFICANCE

Heart Rate, Arterial Blood Pressure, and Their Variability

RR interval, the time elapsed between two successive R waves of the QRS signal on the electrocardiogram (and its reciprocal, the HR), is a function of intrinsic properties of the sinus node as well as autonomic influences. BP is a function of vascular resistance (an expression of arterial constriction or dilation) and cardiac output (the blood volume being pumped by the heart in 1 minute), which is a function of HR, cardiac contractility, and diastolic blood volume, all components controlled in part by the autonomic nervous system.

Autonomic cardiovascular regulation can be investigated through the quantification of average HR and BP as assessed in steady conditions (e.g., wakefulness and sleep) or in their responses to endogenous or exogenous challenges (e.g., changes in posture, response to respiratory changes, and arousal from sleep).

Both HR and BP exhibit spontaneous fluctuations, which can be described by the standard deviation around the mean or by their rhythmic and nonrhythmic characteristics. When described by the standard deviation over 24-hour ambulatory recordings, high variability of the RR interval is a recognized index of the ability of the cardiovascular system to cope with environmental challenge.[6] On the contrary, heightened BP variability is found to accompany aging and hypertension.[7] Among the various cyclic components that characterize 24-hour HR and BP variability, those occurring from daytime wakefulness to nighttime sleep have received great attention. Specifically, HR and BP physiologically decrease during night hours.[8] This diurnal pattern is evident in ambulatory subjects, and even in recumbent subjects maintaining the sleep-wake cycle.[9] The contribution of circadian versus noncircadian factors and how these may be modified in sleep disorders are discussed later.

RR and BP also manifest short-term oscillations, in a frequency range between 0 and 0.5 Hz, which appear to be under the influence of intrinsic autonomic rhythms and of respiratory inputs. Spectral analysis of RR and BP variability provides an estimate on how power (i.e., variance) of the signal is distributed as a function of frequency. Indeed, RR and BP variability appear to be organized in three major components: the high-frequency (HF) respiratory band (>0.15 Hz), the low-frequency (LF) band (around 0.1 Hz), and the very low–frequency (VLF) band (0.003–0.039 Hz) (Figure 21.1 and Table 21.1).[10] The HF components of RR variability primarily reflect the respiration-driven modulation of sinus rhythm, evident as sinus arrhythmia, and have been used as an index of tonic vagal drive. Nonneural mechanical mechanisms, linked to respiratory fluctuations in cardiac transmural pressure, atrial stretch, and venous return, are also determinants of HF power and may become especially important after cardiac denervation such as heart transplantation.[11] The LF rhythm, which appears to have a widespread neural genesis,[12] reflects in part the sympathetic modulation of the heart[13] as well as the baroreflex responsiveness to the beat-to-beat variations in arterial BP,[14] but can also be modulated

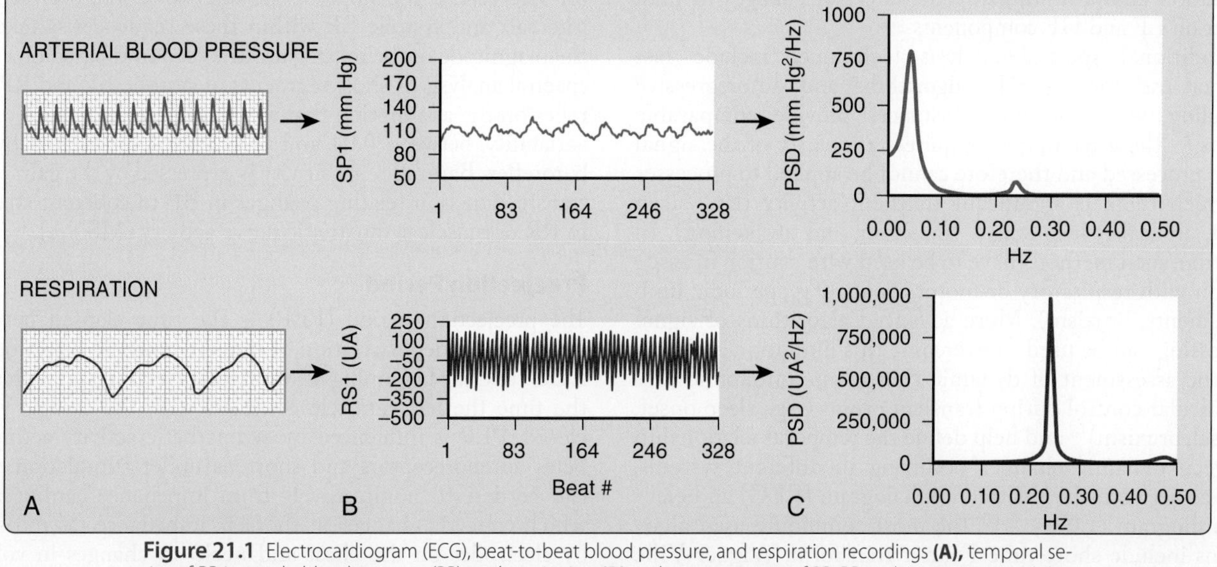

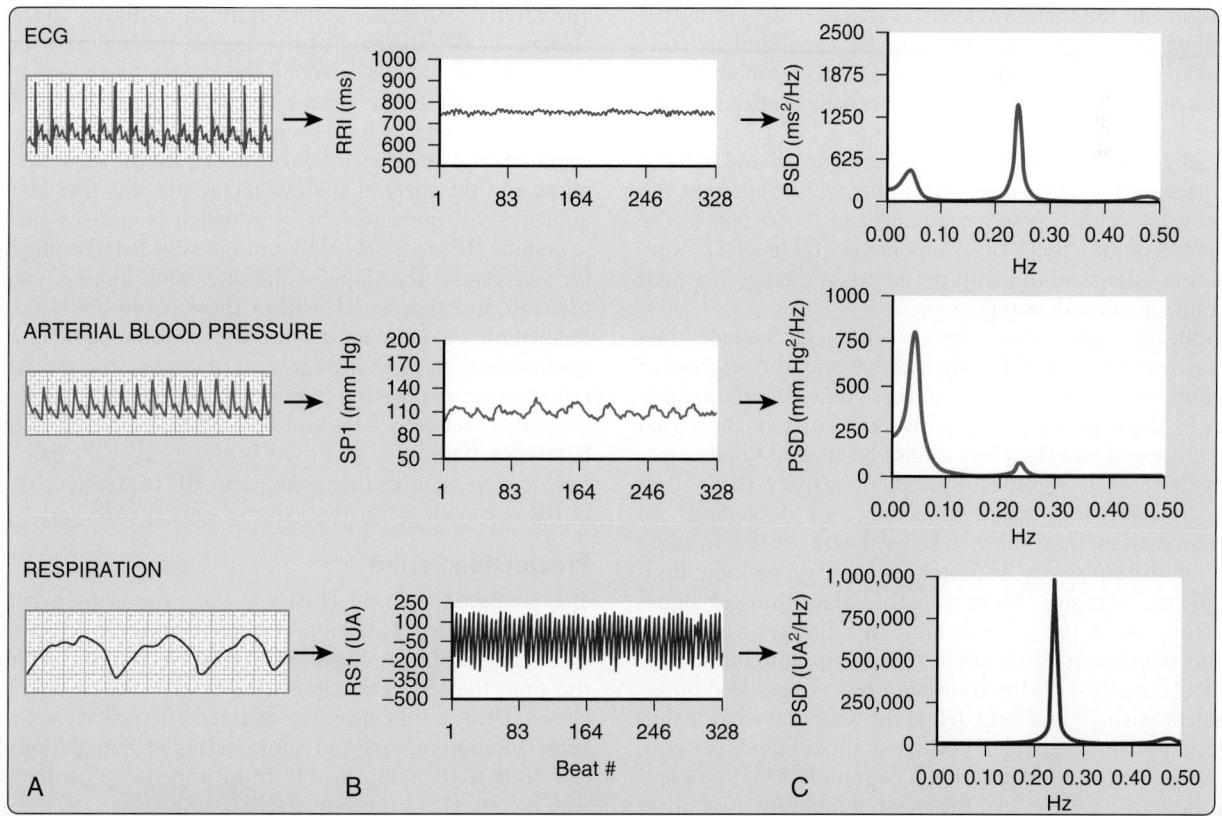

Figure 21.1 Electrocardiogram (ECG), beat-to-beat blood pressure, and respiration recordings **(A)**, temporal series of RR intervals, blood pressure (BP), and respiration **(B)** and power spectra of RR, BP, and respiration variability **(C)** in a single healthy subject. PSD, Power spectral density; RRI, RR intervals; RS1, Respiratory signal; SP1, Systolic pressure; UA, Arbitrary units.

Table 21.1 Spectral Components of RR Interval Variability in the Short Term[a]

Variable	Units	Description Analysis of Short-Term Recordings (5 min)	Frequency Range
Total power	ms^2	The variance of RR intervals over the temporal series analyzed	Approximately ≤0.4 Hz
VLF	ms^2	Power in the VLF range	≤0.04 Hz
LF	ms^2	Power in the LF range	0.04–0.15 Hz
LF norm	%	LF power in normalized units: LF/(Total power – VLF) × 100	
HF	ms^2	Power in HF range	0.15–0.4 Hz
HF norm	%	HF power in normalized units: HF/(Total power – VLF) × 100	
LF/HF		Ratio: LF (ms^2)/HF (ms^2)	

HF, High frequency; LF, low frequency; VLF, very low frequency.

by low-frequency or irregular breathing patterns. Importantly, LF components in respiration confound the interpretation of the LF component of cardiovascular variability in helping to understand the autonomic characteristics of cardiovascular control. Therefore, in any assessment of the relative contributions of the LF and HF components to any particular physiologic state or disease condition, it is crucial to ensure that the respiratory pattern is limited to the HF component. The LF/HF ratio is used to provide an index of the balance of the sympathovagal influence on the sinus node,[15] providing measurements are obtained in strictly controlled conditions. Finally, the VLF has been hypothesized to reflect thermoregulation and the renin-angiotensin system.[16] Regarding BP variability, LF components in systolic BP variability are considered an index of efferent sympathetic vascular modulation, whereas the HF components reflect mechanical effects of respiration on BP changes.[13] Measurements of HF, LF, and VLF are usually made in absolute values (ms), but LF and HF are often presented in normalized units (nu), which represent the relative value of each power component in proportion to the total power minus the VLF components (Table 21.1). Normalization allows minimizing the effect of changes in total power on LF and HF components.

Traditional spectral analysis techniques include fast Fourier transform (FFT) algorithms and autoregressive modeling, which in most instances provide comparable results.[17] These techniques require stationarity of the signal being processed and therefore cannot be applied to processes in which there is significant transient activity (e.g., sleep onset, arousals, sleep stages transition, and awakening). In addition, such methods have to be used with caution in association with respiratory or motor events (e.g., periodic limb movements, bruxism). More advanced algorithms of signal processing can be used to overcome this limitation and permit the assessment of dynamic changes in autonomic cardiovascular control during transient events (e.g., sleep onset, arousal, bruxism)[18] and help define the temporal relationship between dynamic changes occurring in different systems, such as between the electroencephalogram (EEG) and electrocardiogram (ECG).[19,20] The most commonly used algorithms include short-time Fourier transform, Wigner-Ville distribution, time variant autoregressive models, wavelets, and wavelet-packets.[18]

Finally, in addition to the periodic oscillatory behavior observed in RR interval and arterial BP, a less specific variability occurs with nonperiodic behavior, which can be described by methods based on nonlinear system theory ("chaos theory and fractal analysis").[21] The physiologic basis for this nonharmonic beat-to-beat behavior, which extends over a wide time range (seconds to hours), is still unsettled, although it has been proposed that it is under higher central modulation.[22] The application of this type of analysis to sleep cardiovascular physiology is still limited.

Baroreflex Sensitivity

The arterial baroreflex is important in buffering short-term changes in BP. The gain of the arterial baroreflex, or baroreflex sensitivity, is measured by the degree of change in HR or sympathetic traffic for a given unit change in BP.[23] Two techniques primarily have been used in sleep research to assess spontaneous baroreflex modulation of HR: the sequence technique and the spectral analysis technique. The first identifies sequences of consecutive beats in which progressive increases in systolic BP are followed by a progressive lengthening in RR (or vice versa). The slope of the regression line between RR intervals and systolic BP within these sequences is taken as the magnitude of the reflex gain. The second is based on cross-spectral analysis of short segments of systolic BP and RR and relies on the assumption that a certain frequency band of RR variability, between 0.04 and 0.35 Hz, is modulated by the baroreflex. Baroreflex sensitivity is expressed by the gain of the transfer function relating changes in BP to coherent changes in RR or muscle sympathetic nerve activity (MSNA).

Preejection Period

The preejection period (PEP) is the time elapsed between the electrical depolarization of the left ventricle (QRS on the ECG) and the beginning of ventricular ejection and represents the time the left ventricle contracts with the cardiac valves closed. PEP is influenced by sympathetic activity acting via $beta_1$ adrenoreceptors and shortens under stimulation. PEP can be derived noninvasively from impedance cardiography, which converts changes in thoracic impedance (as measured by electrodes on the chest and neck) to changes in volume over time and allows tracking of volumetric changes such as those occurring during the cardiac cycle. This method has been applied, although not intensively, to assess cardiac sympathetic influences in steady state conditions during sleep.[24,25] The application to transient sympathetic responses is unfortunately limited because errors can occur in interpretation in the presence of BP increases, which can induce a lengthening of PEP (instead of the expected shortening) because of the longer time required to overcome the external pressure.

Microneurographic Recording of Sympathetic Nerve Activity

Microneurography provides direct information on sympathetic vasomotor and sudomotor activity to muscle and skin. Muscle sympathetic nerve activity (MSNA), usually measured at the peroneal nerve, induces vasoconstriction and is modulated by the baroreflex.[26] MSNA also increases in response to hypoxic and hypercapnic chemoreceptor stimulation.[2] Skin sympathetic nerve activity reflects thermoregulatory output related to sudomotor and vasomotor activity and is affected by emotional stimuli but not by the baroreflex.

While microneurography provides a direct measure of peripheral sympathetic drive, it is invasive and technically demanding for both operator and patient. In addition, the information provided is limited to regional sympathetic neural activity. Given the heterogeneity of system-specific innervations, MSNA and skin sympathetic nerve activity assessments may not necessarily reflect global sympathetic tone.

Peripheral Arterial Tone and Pulse Transit Time

Peripheral arterial tone (PAT), as measured from the finger, provides an indirect index of sympathetic vasoconstrictory mechanisms directed to the peripheral vascular bed. It is based on measurement of the pulsatile volume changes in the vascular bed at the fingertip, which decreases secondary to sympathetically mediated alpha-adrenergic vasoconstriction. Accordingly, PAT amplitude declined less in patients with sleep apnea at end-apnea and arousal after administering the alpha-adrenergic blocker phentolamine.[27] PAT does not provide absolute values. Only within-subject changes in pulse wave analysis during a limited time interval can be evaluated but may be sufficient to assess PAT attenuation related with respiratory events and microarousals.[28] PAT is noninvasive, can be monitored continuously during sleep, and has been proposed as a measure of the autonomic changes occurring with arousal in adults and children.[29-31] PAT, in combination with actigraphy and oxymetry, has been used in the diagnosis of sleep apnea. REM sleep is associated with increased and hugely variable sympathetic tone. High sympathetic tone corresponds on the PAT signal to a sustained attenuation that has been reported to help identify REM sleep.[32] Moreover, episodic vasoconstriction associated with the occurrence of rapid eye movements is superimposed on this attenuation. Differences in amplitude of the PAT signal and its variability during REM sleep in comparison with NREM sleep have been reported, and an automatic REM scoring algorithm has been developed and validated with the PAT device to score REM.[33]

Pulse transit time (PTT, see also Chapter 167) refers to the time it takes a pulse wave to travel between two arterial sites.[34] In practice, in a noninvasive estimate of PTT, the R wave in the ECG is generally used to indicate the starting point of the measure and the peripheral waveform (assessed by photoplethysmography at the finger) to indicate the end of the measure. PTT is sensitive to moment-to-moment sympathetic neural activity and shortens when BP increases and lengthens when BP falls. Importantly, PTT encompasses several physiologic components difficult to control for, and intersubject comparison is not recommended. Only intraindividual relative PTT changes from a baseline condition (over several readings) are instead recommended. Like PAT, PTT can also be monitored continuously and has been used in the assessment of sympathetic responses to arousals[29,30] and respiratory events, especially in children.[35,36] During REM sleep, variations in sympathetic activity are spontaneously very high and therefore the PTT baseline is highly variable. Thus the recognition of true microarousals during REM sleep is less specific than in other sleep stages. The heart and large vessels are located in the thoracic cavity and are thus affected by variations in thoracic volume and pressure. During inspiration, the volume of the thoracic cavity increases, reducing intrathoracic pressure, which in turn reduces the compression of the heart and large vessels (vena cava and aorta), decreasing BP and slowing PTT. The opposite is true for expiration. As the intrathoracic pressure increases, the heart is compressed, BP increases, and PTT quickens. PTT may serve as a noninvasive marker of respiratory effort, especially when defining certain respiratory events (hypopneas, respiratory effort–related arousals, and central events).[37,38]

Systemic Catecholamines

Measurement of plasma catecholamines (epinephrine and norepinephrine) provides an estimate of global sympathetic activity. However, blood norepinephrine reflects only a small percentage (8% to 10%) of neurotransmitter release during sympathetic activation. Moreover, the relatively rapid clearance of catecholamines from the bloodstream may limit the ability to detect transient changes in sympathetic activity. Consequently, only frequent sampling through sleep may detect changes related to the sleep-wake cycle and sleep stages.[39] The measure of urinary excretion of catecholamines and their metabolites is a simpler approach to provide an estimate of the cumulative catecholamine secretion over time and has been used widely in the clinical and sleep research settings. Urinary catecholamine excretion is strictly dependent on renal function. Therefore a correction of excreted catecholamine for indices of renal function (urinary creatinine) is recommended.

SLEEP-RELATED CARDIOVASCULAR AUTONOMIC CHANGES

Day-Night Changes in Neural Circulatory Control

HR and BP physiologically decrease during nighttime as compared to daytime in ambulant subjects as well as in subjects kept in the supine position for 24 hours.[9] Specifically, the normal 24-hour BP pattern consists of a 10% or greater systolic BP reduction during sleep compared to daytime, a reduction that is commonly referred to as "dipping." Posture and activity strongly influence HR and BP during the day,[40] whereas posture and sleep affect HR and BP at night.[9] However, the nocturnal sleep-related cardiovascular dipping is evident even in subjects who maintain the supine position for 24 hours,[9] underscoring the importance of sleep in inducing decreases in nighttime HR and BP. Studies investigating the autonomic changes associated with the wake-sleep cycle noted that indices of parasympathetic function, such as RR interval and HF components of RR variability, begin to change as early as

2 hours before sleep onset,[24] whereas indices of cardiac and peripheral sympathetic activity such as LF/HF ratio, preejection period, MSNA, and catecholamines start to decrease only after sleep onset and continue to decrease with the deepening of sleep.[24,26,39] Morning awakening induces a stepwise activation of the sympathoadrenal system, with increased HR, BP, and plasma catecholamines, with further increases occurring with postural change and physical activity.[24,41]

Studies conducting 24 hours of sleep deprivation in supine conditions showed that the nocturnal fall of HR and cardiovagal indices is still present, whereas the fall in nocturnal BP and PEP prolongation (i.e., decreased sympathetic activity) are blunted.[24,42] Therefore it may be that HR and parasympathetic mechanisms are largely under circadian influences and might be implicated in mechanisms preparatory to sleep, whereas sympathetic drive to the heart and vessels is mainly linked to the sleep-wake cycle. There is increasing evidence that the mean nocturnal BP level is a major predictor of cardiovascular morbidity and mortality irrespective of the 24-hour BP levels.[43] Any deterioration in sleep quality or quantity may be associated with an increase in nocturnal BP, which could participate in the development or poor control of hypertension.[44]

Physiologic Responses to NREM and REM Sleep

In healthy subjects, autonomic cardiovascular regulation varies considerably with sleep stage, and different autonomic patterns dominate in NREM versus REM sleep. As NREM sleep progresses from stages 1 to 3, RR, respiratory-mediated HF components of RR variability, and PEP increase, whereas BP, LF components in systolic BP variability, and MSNA significantly decrease compared to wakefulness. These changes suggest an increase in cardiovagal drive and a reduction in cardiac and peripheral sympathetic activity[9,26,45] (Figure 21.2). Baroreflex sensitivity appears also to be increased during

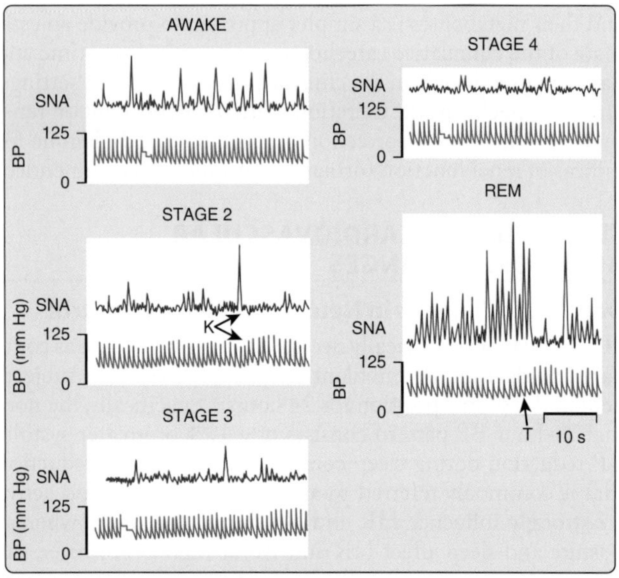

Figure 21.2 Recordings of sympathetic nerve activity (SNA) and mean blood pressure (BP) in a single subject while awake and while in stages 2, 3, 4, and REM sleep. SNA and BP gradually decrease with the deepening of non-REM sleep. Heart rate, BP, and BP variability increase during REM sleep, together with a profound increase in the frequency and amplitude in SNA. (Reprinted from Somers VK, Dyken ME, Mark AL, Abboud FM. Sympathetic-nerve activity during sleep in normal subjects. *N Engl J Med* 1993;328[5]:303–7, with permission of the publisher.)

NREM sleep compared with that of wakefulness.[46] However, the response is variable. Namely, compared with that of wakefulness, baroreflex gain is heightened in response to BP increments rather than decrements during NREM sleep. This mechanism probably serves to ensure the maintenance of stable low BP and HR during NREM sleep.

In contrast, REM sleep is a state of autonomic instability, dominated by remarkable fluctuations between parasympathetic and sympathetic influences, which produce sudden and abrupt changes in HR and BP.[47] The average HR and BP are higher during REM than in NREM sleep, as is sympathetic neural vasomotor drive.[26] The cardiovascular excitation of REM sleep is also reflected by a significant increase of the low-frequency components (LF, ~0.1 Hz) and a shift of the LF/HF ratio toward sympathetic predominance.[9]

RR Variability and Electroencephalographic Coupling

Studies assessing the overnight relationship between RR variability and EEG profiles showed the dynamic of RR variability is closely related to the dynamic of EEG, reflecting the depth of sleep. The presence of an ultradian 80- to 120-minute rhythm in the normalized LF, with high levels during REM sleep and low levels during slow wave sleep, has been described.[48] These oscillations were strikingly coupled in a "mirror-image" to the overnight oscillations in delta wave activity, which reflect sleep deepening and lightening. Similarly, it was reported that normalized HF components of RR variability were coherent with all EEG spectral bands, with a maximum gain (ratio HF amplitude/EEG amplitude was higher) for delta activity and minimum (i.e., HF was lower) with beta activity.[49] The two oscillations were coupled with a phase-shift of several minutes, with cardiac changes preceding the EEG changes. Although the mechanisms underlying this coupling are not known, it has been hypothesized that there might be a central generator synchronizing the oscillatory process in autonomic and sleep modulation, in which cardiovascular function may anticipate sleep-stage changes.[48]

Autonomic Responses Associated with Arousal from Sleep and from Periodic Leg Movements

Arousals

Electrocortical arousal from sleep (i.e., EEG desynchronization with appearance of low-voltage, high-frequency EEG), spontaneous, provoked by an exogenous stimuli, or in the context of sleep-disordered breathing, is associated with sympathetic neural surges, leading to transient increases in HR, BP, and MSNA[50-52]; abrupt PTT dips; and PAT attenuations. The typical cardiac response is biphasic with tachycardia lasting 4 to 5 seconds followed by bradycardia, with HR increasing prior to cortical arousals. With use of time-variant analysis, it appears that the surge in sympathoexcitation as represented by LF components of RR variability and BP variability remains substantially elevated above baseline long after the HR, BP, and MSNA return to baseline values.[19] This can be particularly relevant in conditions characterized by frequent arousals across the night, conceivably leading to a sustained sympathetic influence on the cardiovascular system. In sleep apnea, an association between repetitive attenuations in PAT during sleep and office BP has been reported independently of age, sex, and body mass index (BMI).[53] These results suggest that nocturnal sympathetic activity may represent a direct stimulus to chronically elevated BP in humans, even in the daytime.

Auditory stimuli during sleep may result in autonomic and respiratory modifications, even in the absence of overt EEG activation (the so-called "autonomic arousal"), or in association with an EEG pattern different from conventional arousal, such as K-complexes or bursts of delta waves not followed by EEG desynchronization (the so-called "subcortical arousal").[51,52] These observations imply that there is a range of partial arousal responses implicating autonomic responses with EEG manifestations different from classical arousals and even without any EEG response. The different EEG patterns and the associated cardiac responses indicate a hierarchical spectrum of increasing strength from the weaker high-amplitude delta burst to a stronger low-voltage alpha rhythm[52] (Figure 21.3).

Periodic Leg Movements during Sleep

Periodic leg movements (PLM) are described as a repetitive rhythmic extension of the big toe and dorsiflexion of the ankle, with occasional flexion at the knee and hip. PLM can occur during wakefulness as well as during sleep (PLMS). PLMS occur frequently in several sleep disorders (such as restless legs syndrome [RLS], narcolepsy, REM sleep behavior disorder, and sleep apnea) and in patients with congestive heart failure[54] but are also seen in healthy, asymptomatic subjects, especially with advancing age.[55] In the context of sleep apnea, PLMS may coexist with (and are often difficult to distinguish from) respiratory-related leg movements, which are part of the arousal response at the end of airway obstruction (in obstructive sleep apnea [OSA]) or at the peak of ventilation (in central sleep apnea). Approximately 30% of PLMS are associated with cortical arousal, whereas more than 60% are associated with K-complexes or bursts of delta waves.[56]

What causes PLMS is still unknown. However, studies of cardiovascular changes associated with PLMS and their temporal relationship with EEG events are providing new insights into the physiologic mechanisms of PLMS. A stereotyped autonomic response accompanies PLMS, consisting of a rapid rise in HR and arterial BP[56,57] followed by a significant and rapid bradycardia and a return of BP to baseline values (Figure 21.4). Such cardiovascular changes are present whether the PLMS are associated with arousals or not. However, the magnitude of the cardiovascular response is greater when PLMS are associated with cortical arousals. In addition, the amplitude of cardiovascular responses of PLMS is greater during sleep than that associated with spontaneous or simulated PLMS during wakefulness. These observations suggest that the intensity of cardiovascular responses observed with PLMS is related to the degree of central brain activation (brainstem to cortical activation) that accompanies PLMS and much less to the somatomotor response (i.e., not a classical sensory motor reflex).

Studies assessing the temporal relationship between the leg motor event and autonomic and cortical activation consistently reported that changes in HR and EEG activity precede by several seconds the leg movement.[56,58] Specifically, HR and EEG delta waves rise first, followed by motor activity and eventually progressive activation of faster EEG frequencies (i.e., in the alpha, beta, and sigma frequencies). A recent study assessing the dynamic time course of RR variability changes and EEG changes in association with PLMS confirmed the LF components of RR variability to be the first physiologic change to occur, followed by EEG changes in delta frequencies, and thereafter the leg movement with or without faster EEG frequencies.[20] These data corroborate an original hypothesis suggesting the presence of an integrative hierarchy of the arousal response primarily involving the autonomic responses with sympathoexcitation, then progressing toward EEG synchronization (represented by bursts of delta waves), and finally EEG desynchronization (arousal) and eventually awakening.[56] In this view, leg movements are part of the same periodic activation process that is responsible for cardiovascular and EEG changes during sleep.[58]

The clinical significance of PLMS has been a subject of debate. RLS is characterized by dysesthesia and leg restlessness occurring predominantly at night during periods of immobility. RLS is associated in 80% of the cases with PLMS. PLMS and RLS have been found to be associated with an increase in cardiovascular risk,[59] and PLMS has been

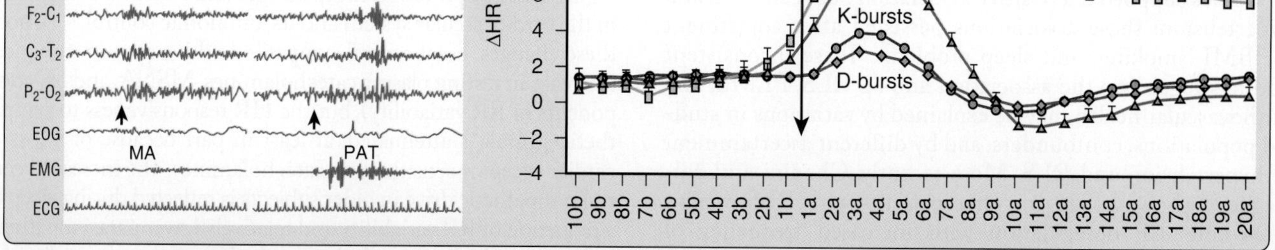

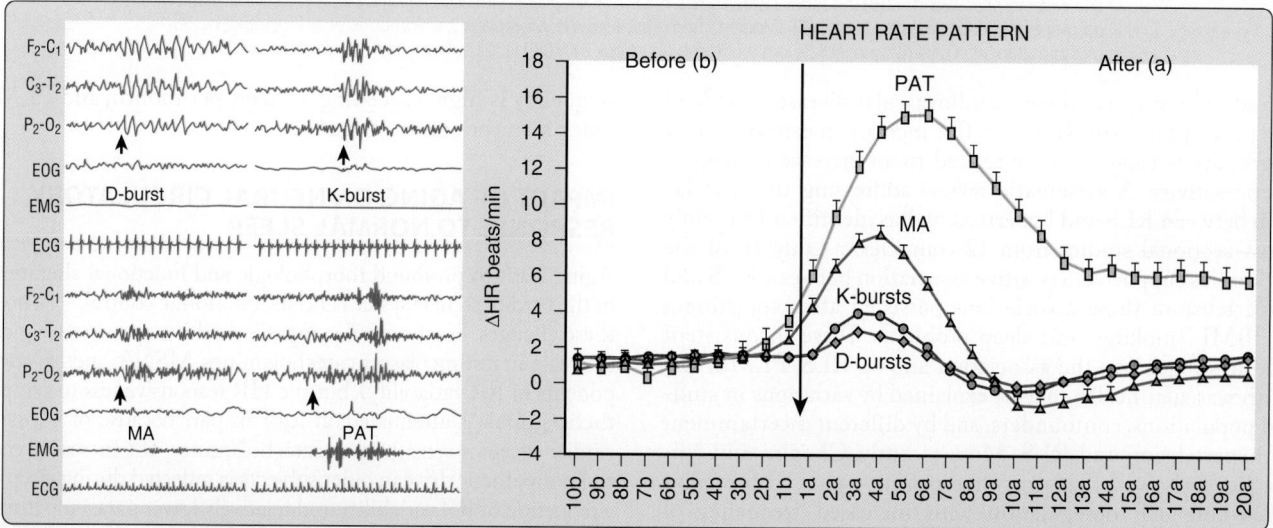

Figure 21.3 Heart rate response in association with different patterns of electroencephalogram activation. (Modified from Sforza E, Jouny C, Ibanez V. Cardiac activation during arousal in humans: further evidence for hierarchy in the arousal response. *Clin Neurophysiol* 2000;111[9]:1611–1619, with permission of the publisher.)

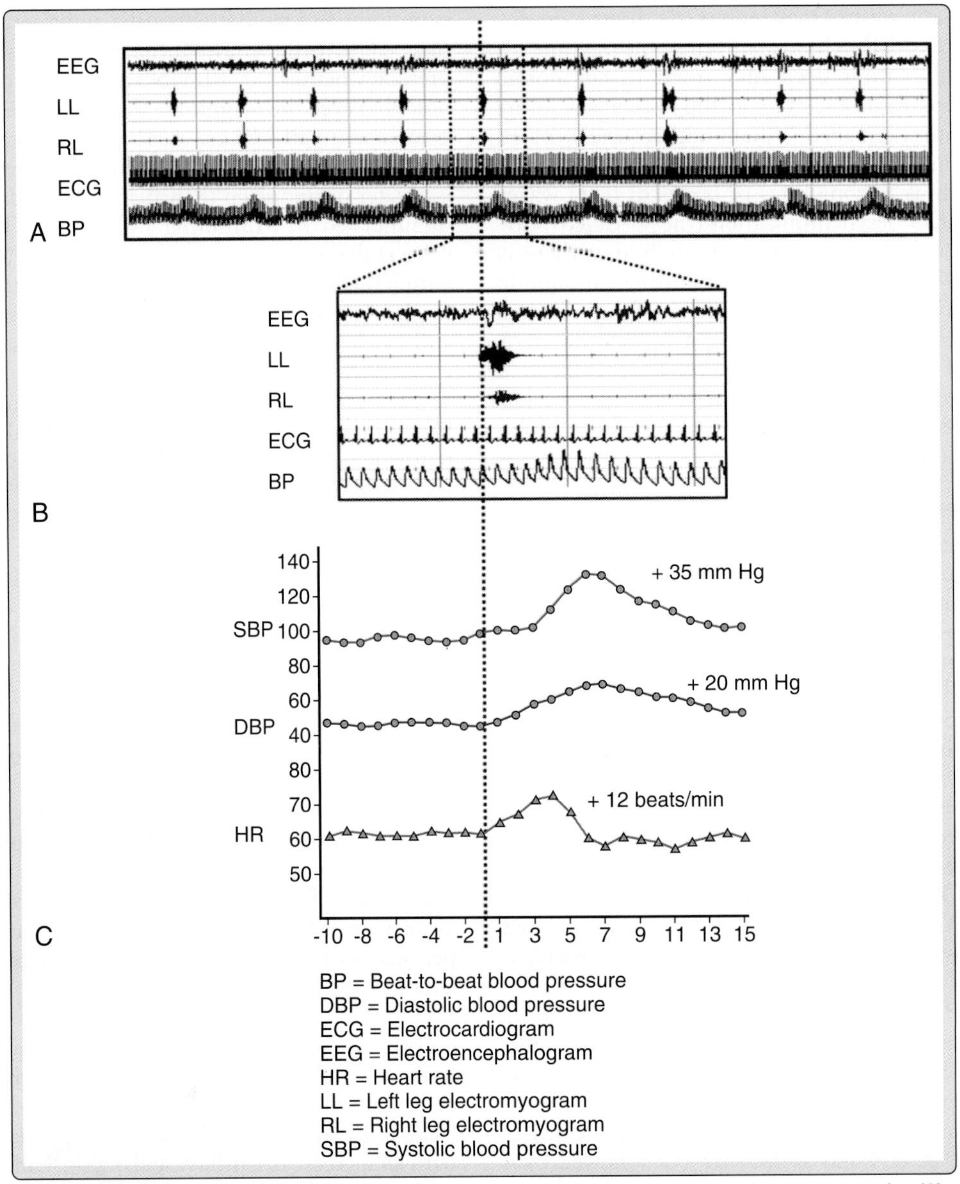

Figure 21.4 Electrocardiogram, beat-to-beat blood pressure, and polysomnographic recording in a compact window **(A),** and wider temporal window **(B)** in a subject with restless legs syndrome. Significant heart rate and blood pressure increases accompany periodic leg movements **(C)**. (Modified from Pennestri MH, Montplaisir J, Colombo R, et al. Nocturnal blood pressure changes in patients with restless legs syndrome. *Neurology* 2007;68[15]:1213–8, with permission of the publisher.)

found to be associated with cardiovascular disease outside of the association with RLS.[60-62] This increase in cardiovascular morbidity is thought to be related to an increase in sympathetic activity. A systematic review addressing the association between RLS and hypertension has identified 17 mainly cross-sectional studies from 12 countries.[63] Only 10 of the 17 studies supported a positive association between RLS and hypertension; these associations persisted after adjustment for BMI, smoking, and sleep problems. These inconsistent findings regarding the association among RLS, PLMS, and cardiovascular health may be explained by variations in studied populations, confounders, and by different ascertainment of hypertension and RLS. More recently, Chenini and colleagues[64] showed that drug-free patients with RLS exhibit a 24-hour BP deregulation with increased frequency of systolic nondipping profiles compared to matched-healthy controls. Collectively, these studies indicate that RLS might be positively related to hypertension when RLS symptom frequency is high, exceeding 15 days per month, and PLMS index is in the severe range.[65]

IMPACT OF AGING ON NEURAL CIRCULATORY RESPONSE TO NORMAL SLEEP

Aging leads to profound morphologic and functional alterations in the cardiovascular system and its autonomic control.[66] Among these changes, basal central sympathetic drive appears enhanced (increase in resting plasma catecholamines, MSNA, and LF components of RR variability), but the HR responsiveness to sympathetic stimuli is attenuated, at least in part because of a loss of cardiac receptor sensitivity to catecholamines. The increased central sympathetic drive in older subjects is reflected during sleep by a reduction of RR variability and relatively lower parasympathetic influences, which appear linked to the loss of slow wave sleep.[67]

The cardiac response to EEG arousals and PLMS is also modified by age. Specifically, the HR increments are attenuated and bradycardia is less profound in older as compared to younger subjects.[68,69] The attenuated tachycardia can be part of the general age-related attenuation in the cardiac response to sympathetic stimuli, whereas impairment in baroreflex mechanisms, encountered in older individuals, could be a factor implicated in the blunted bradycardia.

EFFECTS OF DISORDERED SLEEP AND PRIMARY AUTONOMIC DYSFUNCTION ON DAY-NIGHT AUTONOMIC CHANGES

Effects of Sleep Loss and Sleep Disorders on Nighttime Blood Pressure

As mentioned previously, HR and BP physiologically decrease during nighttime as compared to daytime, a reduction commonly referred to as "dipping." The persistence of high nighttime systolic BP and lack of systolic BP dipping are clinically important and have been linked to precursors of atherosclerosis, including inflammation and endothelial dysfunction.[70] Lack of systolic dipping[71] and, more recently, lack of HR dipping,[72] have been associated with increased cardiovascular mortality, after correction of several confounding variables, including daytime values. Sleep loss and sleep disturbances have been invoked as some of the potential factors underlying these abnormalities.[44] Controlled studies show that during partial sleep deprivation/restriction (allowing 4 hours of sleep) nighttime BP and catecholamine levels remain high while nighttime nocturnal wakefulness is maintained and then decrease normally in association with subsequent sleep.[73,74] In the same studies, the morning surge in BP and catecholamines appears more pronounced after sleep deprivation than in control conditions, particularly in hypertensive subjects.[73,74] A study in male workers showed that, relative to a normal working day allowing 8 hours of sleep, working overtime and sleeping 4 hours induced higher daytime BP on the following day, accompanied by higher LF components of HR variability and increased urinary excretion of norepinephrine.[75] Hence it appears that sleep loss (1) is associated with persistence of high sympathetic activity and attenuates physiologic nocturnal BP dipping, as long as nocturnal wakefulness is maintained; (2) may enhance sympathetic activation during morning awakening; and (3) induces sustained sympathetic activation with increased BP during the following day.

In different cohorts of normotensive and hypertensive subjects without sleep disorders, absence of BP dipping was associated with indices of poor and fragmented sleep, including longer wake-time after sleep onset and higher arousal frequency.[76,77] Increased nighttime BP has been reported in subjects with moderate to severe OSA,[78] the degree of BP alteration being proportional to the severity of sleep apnea.

Several mechanisms have been proposed to explain the absence of BP dipping and the enhanced cardiovascular risk inherent with a higher nighttime BP. Added to the factors previously mentioned (i.e., high sympathetic tone, decreased baroreflex sensitivity), increased salt sensitivity has been proposed as promoting high BP during sleep by promoting natriuresis.[79] This may be of interest in the impact of OSA as a risk factor for kidney dysfunction.[80,81]

Insomnia

According to the American Academy of Sleep Medicine, insomnia is clinically defined by a difficulty falling asleep, difficulty staying asleep, early morning awakenings, or a nonrestorative or nonrefreshing sleep. Sleep fragmentation and the decrease in slow wave sleep may induce a decrease in parasympathetic tone during sleep, and an unbalanced sympathovagal tone that may be a plausible hypothesis for the increased risk of cardiovascular disease and the high prevalence of hypertension in patients suffering from insomnia with objective impairment of sleep structure. Recent studies have used polysomnography to show that insomnia with objective short sleep duration is associated with a significant risk of hypertension. First, with use of 24-hour beat-to-beat BP recordings concurrently with polysomnography, it has been reported that normotensive subjects with chronic insomnia had higher nighttime systolic BP and blunted day-to-night systolic BP dipping compared to aged-matched good sleepers.[82] Vgontzas and colleagues[83] have demonstrated that insomnia was associated with prevalent hypertension only when insomnia was associated with objectively measured short sleep duration. The prevalence of hypertension increased 3.5-fold when sleep duration was between 5 and 6 hours and 5.1-fold when sleep duration was below 5 hours/night. Accordingly, chronic insomnia with short sleep duration (less than 6 hours slept during polysomnography) was associated with an increased risk for incident hypertension (odds ratio 3.8) in a general population sample of 786 adults of the Penn State cohort without hypertension at baseline and followed over 7.5 years.[84]

Narcolepsy-Cataplexy

There are two clinical types of narcolepsy, type 1 and type 2. In both types, the main symptom is excessive daytime sleepiness, which is associated with cataplexy (sudden loss of muscle tone usually induced by a strong emotion) only in type 1 narcolepsy. In both types, sleep-wake cycles are disrupted by the frequent occurrence of REM sleep–onset episodes during daytime sleep and by numerous awakenings during nocturnal sleep.[85] Type 1 narcolepsy (T1N) is characterized by a marked decrease in the number of hypocretin neurons in the paraventricular nucleus, which are known to play a role in central autonomic and cardiovascular regulation.[86,87] There are only few cardiovascular studies in human narcolepsy, even though narcolepsy is classically associated with obesity, type 2 diabetes, and metabolic syndrome, comorbidities leading to an increased cardiovascular risk. Recently, a study described the 24-hour ambulatory blood pressure measurement pattern of drug-free patients with narcolepsy compared to control subjects.[88] A "nondipping status" was found in one-third of patients with T1N versus in only 4.8% of controls. Nondipping of diastolic BP was strongly associated with narcolepsy by an odds ratio up to twelvefold, with a significant association with the percentage of REM sleep even after adjustment for confounders. Grimaldi and colleagues[89] demonstrated that systolic BP during nighttime REM sleep was increased in narcolepsy. T1N is therefore a unique example of increased nocturnal BP mainly during REM sleep. However, considering that patients having narcolepsy will be treated with psychostimulants for the rest of their lives, a therapy that has direct impact on both the autonomic and cardiovascular systems, preliminary studies demonstrating the effects of T1N on the dipping pattern of BP might have important clinical implications. Thus further studies addressing longitudinal associations between T1N and hypertension as well as further mechanistic studies are clearly warranted.

Loss of Diurnal Variation in Autonomic Function in Diabetes Mellitus: What Comes First?

Cardiovascular autonomic neuropathy is a serious complication of diabetes mellitus. It results from damage to autonomic fibers involved in HR and BP control, in the presence of impaired glucose metabolism.[90] In subjects with insulin-independent diabetes (or type 2 diabetes) the 24-hour periodicity of HR and RR variability is lost, with attenuated sympathetic control in the daytime and blunted parasympathetic function during the night.[91] In subjects with different degrees of glucose abnormalities without overt diabetes, RR variability and its spectral components appear similar to controls in the daytime but are significantly altered during sleep, with strikingly higher normalized LF and lower HF, proportional to the degree of insulin resistance.[92] Insulin resistance (a state in which there is a reduced biologic effect of insulin) and sympathetic overactivity are known to be linked and possibly potentiate each other, with insulin increasing sympathetic activity and neuroadrenergic mechanisms acting to increase plasma glucose availability and to reduce peripheral insulin sensitivity. These data suggest that a primary alteration in the autonomic nervous system may occur during sleep in these subjects before overt diabetes is evident and may be linked to the level of insulin resistance. However, one study also observed that selectively altered nighttime autonomic function was also present in nondiabetic offspring of parents with type 2 diabetes, whether or not they had insulin resistance.[93] This suggests that nighttime impaired parasympathetic mechanisms, possibly of genetic origin, may precede metabolic abnormalities.

Type 2 diabetes is a complex disease that derives from the interaction of environmental factors on a background of a genetic susceptibility. Chronic sleep debt, either because of sleep restriction or sleep apnea, has been shown to be one factor that can alter glucose handling[94] and increases the likelihood of developing type 2 diabetes.[95] Little is known about the relationship and interactions between these sleep disturbances and early autonomic dysfunction in subjects with differing severities of glucose abnormalities and their healthy offspring. Patients with type 1 diabetes who presented with a nondipping pattern of their nighttime BP had shorter sleep duration than those who presented with a physiologic nocturnal dip of BP.[96,97]

SYMPATHETIC ACTIVATION IN OBSTRUCTIVE SLEEP APNEA

The sympathetic nervous system appears to play a key role in the cardiac pathophysiology of sleep apnea (see also Section 15).[98,99] OSA is rarely present in the absence of other cardiometabolic risk factors or conditions. Obesity, high lipid levels,[100] hypertension, and diabetes are all associated with high autonomic cardiovascular tone.[101]

Even when OSA patients are awake, breathing normally, and in the absence of any overt cardiovascular disease such as hypertension or heart failure, they have evidence for impaired sympathetic cardiovascular regulation. Specifically they have high levels of muscle sympathetic nerve activity, increased catecholamines, faster HRs, and attenuated HR variability.[102] Furthermore, even though they are normotensive, they have excessive BP variability.[103] In the setting of apnea, the inhibitory effect of the thoracic afferents is absent, thus resulting in further potentiation of sympathetic activation. The consequent vasoconstriction results in marked surges in BP, as noted earlier. Sympathetic activity abruptly ceases at onset of breathing because of the inhibitory effect of the thoracic afferents (Figure 21.5).[104]

In a minority of OSA patients, the diving reflex, noted earlier, is activated. Therefore these patients may have marked

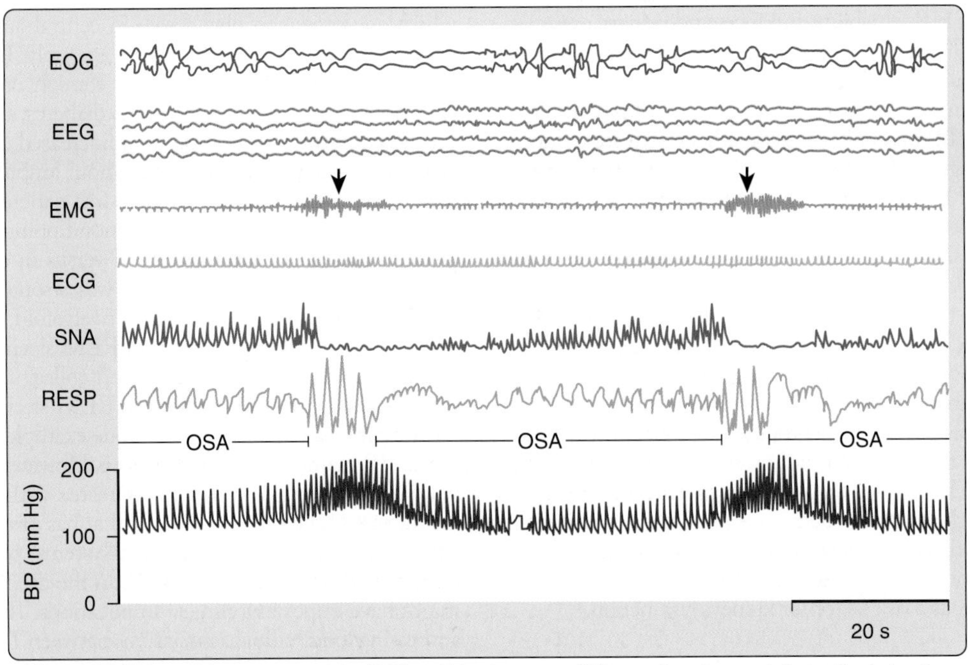

Figure 21.5 Sympathetic nerve activity (SNA) and blood pressure (BP) recordings in association with obstructive sleep apnea (OSA). SNA increases progressively during the apnea because of the activation of the peripheral and central chemoreflexes by hypoxemia and hypercapnia. The consequent vasoconstriction results in marked surges in BP, which reaches a peak during the hyperventilation. SNA abruptly ceases at onset of breathing as a result of the inhibitory effect of the thoracic afferents. ECG, Electrocardiogram; EEG, electroencephalogram; EMG, electromyogram; EOG, electrooculogram; RESP, respiration. (Reprinted from Somers VK, Dyken ME, Clary MP, Abboud FM. Sympathetic neural mechanisms in obstructive sleep apnea. *J Clin Invest* 1995;96[4]:1897–904.)

bradyarrhythmias in association with the obstructive apnea, even though they do not have any intrinsic conduction system abnormality.[5] The bradycardia is secondary to cardiac vagal activation because of the combination of hypoxia and apnea. These acute responses to obstructive apnea may predispose to longer term abnormalities in cardiac and vascular structure and function.

Several mechanisms have been proposed that could link OSA to cardiovascular diseases resulting from the recurrent nocturnal cycles of hypoxia/reoxygenation.[105] These promote oxidative stress and low-grade inflammation, which are the initiators of a pathophysiologic cascade leading first to sympathetic overactivity. The high vascular sympathetic tone exhibited by OSA patients results in elevated systemic resistance and hence elevated BP. Impaired arterial vasodilatory capacity may contribute to elevation of BP and lead to vascular disease. Animal models of chronic intermittent hypoxia (CIH) alone or with the other stimuli that characterize OSA (i.e., respiratory effort, asphyxia, and arousal from sleep) show elevated BP during the non-CIH portion of the day. These data suggest that the BP elevation results first from sympathetic activation. This requires an intact chemoreflex loop. It has also been demonstrated that in OSA, arterial baroreflex gain is decreased. Although animal models have advanced our understanding, there are specific aspects of human physiology that may not be adequately represented. Therefore models of intermittent hypoxia in healthy humans have been developed that induce unstable ventilation and sleep fragmentation similar to those observed in OSA patients. Healthy humans exposed to 1 or 2 weeks of CIH exhibit an increase in both hypoxic and hypercapnic ventilatory responses, confirming that augmentation of carotid chemoreflex function participates in inducing sustained sympathetic overactivity. After 2 weeks of CIH exposure, MSNA is increased and baroreflex control of sympathetic outflow declines. Consequently, CIH significantly increased daytime ambulatory BP after 2 weeks of exposure (8 mm Hg systolic and 5 mm Hg diastolic)[106] (Figure 21.6).

CLINICAL PEARL

The autonomic nervous system is the mediator of central-cardiovascular interactions occurring during sleep, and its normal function appears to be important in preserving health. Despite the recognized methodologic limitations (technically demanding and cautious interpretation of outcomes of interest as described in Table 21.1), broadening sleep polygraphic monitoring to include heart rate and BP recordings may contribute to a better understanding of the physiology and pathology of sleep-related cardiovascular autonomic modulation. They may provide an avenue for innovation in the management of many medical conditions or disorders that are related to sleep (e.g., hypertension, diabetes, metabolic syndrome, periodic limb movements, and sleep-disordered breathing).

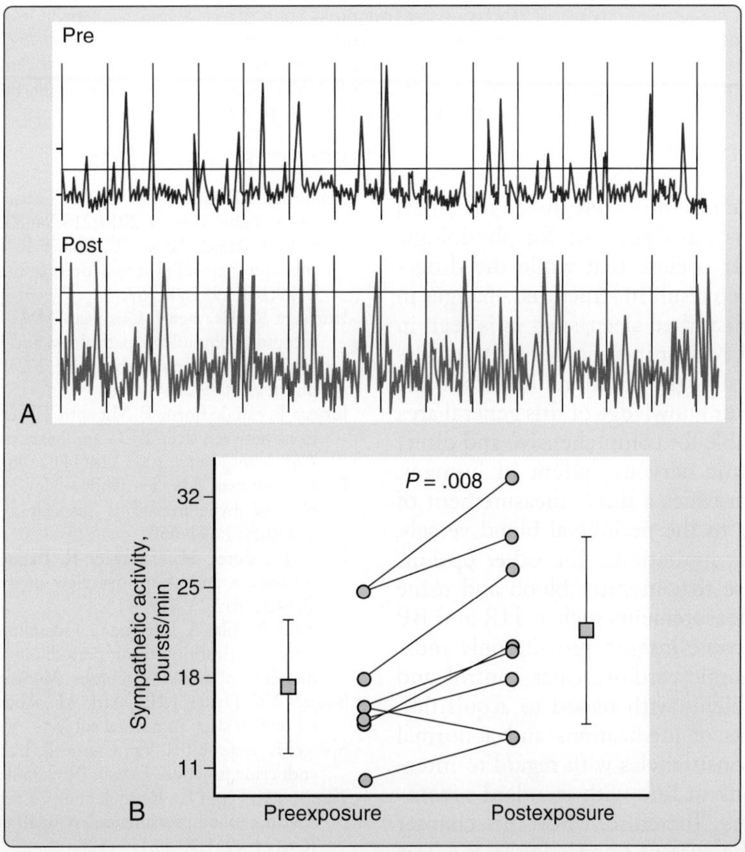

Figure 21.6 Intermittent hypoxia elevates daytime blood pressure and sympathetic activity in healthy humans. **A,** Representative neurograms of muscle sympathetic nerve activity (MSNA) during supine rest while breathing room air before (Pre) and after (Post) 2 weeks of intermittent hypoxia (IH) exposure. **B,** MSNA increased across the exposure (17.2±5.1 versus 21.7±7.3 bursts/min; *P P* = .008) thus reflecting sympathoactivation.

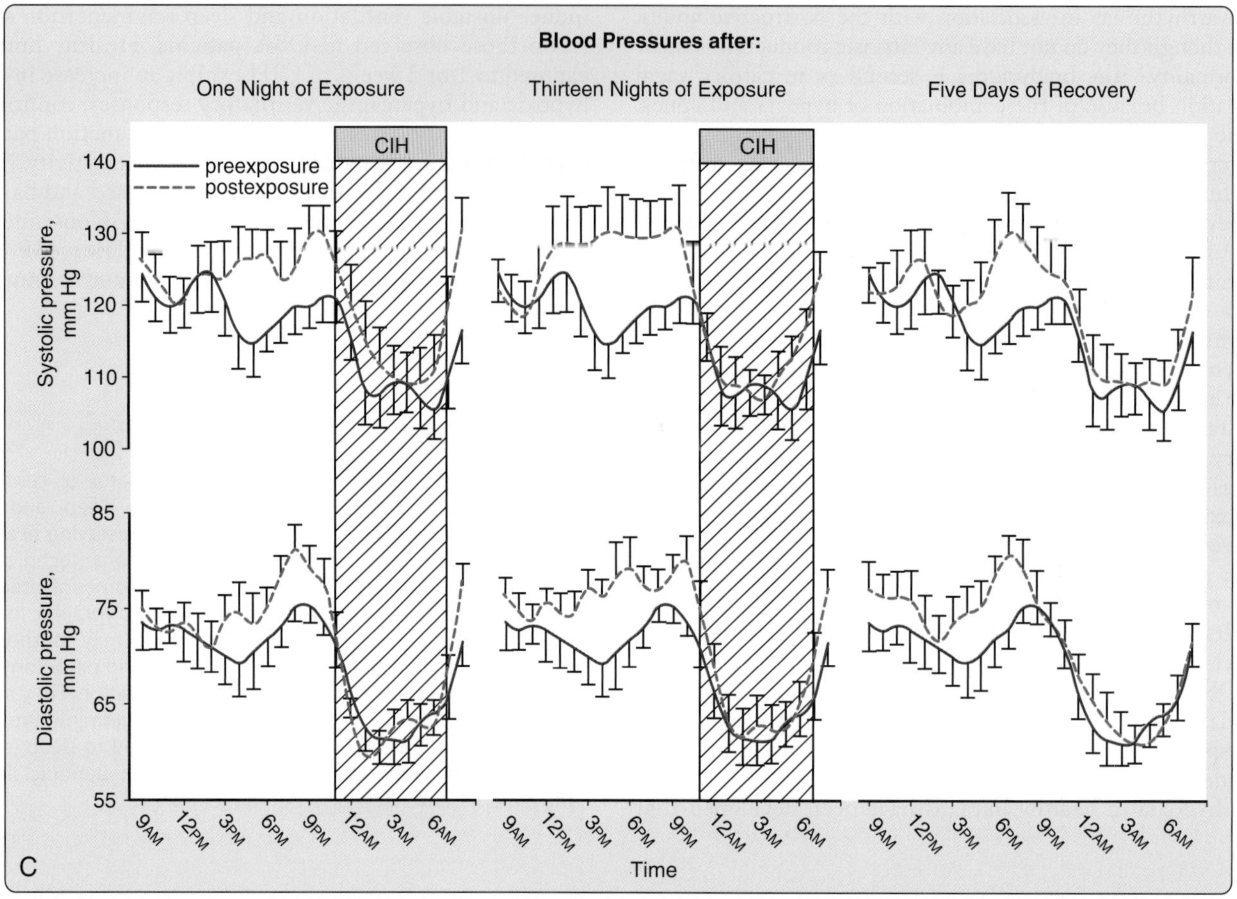

Figure 21.6, cont'd C, Hour-by-hour systolic and diastolic blood pressures during 24 hours of monitoring in healthy humans. Data are presented after 1 night, 13 nights, and recovery from exposure to chronic intermittent hypoxia (CIH) as compared to preexposure values. *Solid red line,* preexposure; *dotted green line,* postexposure. CIH significantly increased daytime ambulatory blood pressure after a single night of exposure (3 mm Hg for mean and diastolic) and further increased daytime pressures after 2 weeks of exposure (8 mm Hg systolic and 5 mm Hg diastolic). (Modified from Tamisier R, Pepin JL, Remy J, et al. 14 nights of intermittent hypoxia elevate daytime blood pressure and sympathetic activity in healthy humans. *Eur Respir J* 2011;37[1]:119–28.)

SUMMARY

The autonomic nervous system is intimately linked to central neural state changes. This is especially true for physiologic sleep and sleep disorders. It is clear that while the different stages of physiologic sleep result in structured changes in neural circulatory control, disturbed sleep, such as is seen in patients with OSA, with PLMS, or in sleep deprivation, disrupts the sleep-related physiologic variations in autonomic regulation of HR and BP. Our knowledge of this general area is limited by the tools available for comprehensive and direct assessment of the autonomic nervous system in humans. While microneurography provides a direct measurement of sympathetic neural activity to the peripheral blood vessels, this measurement itself has limitations. The other options available are primarily those that monitor blood and urine levels of catecholamines. Measurements such as HR and BP variability, while allowing some insight, provide only indirect information on autonomic cardiovascular control and are limited because of problems with regard to acquisition of data, confounding effects of medications and abnormal breathing patterns, and inconsistencies with regard to interpretation. Rigorous methods in line with standard recommendations[10] are mandatory. Therefore, while this chapter seeks to address some of the current knowledge in the area of neural circulatory control during normal and disordered sleep, the available data are limited in part because of methodologic shortcomings and because of the obvious difficulties inherent in nighttime studies of sleep physiology in humans.

SELECTED READINGS

Benarroch EE. Control of the cardiovascular and respiratory systems during sleep. *Auton Neurosci.* 2019;218:54–63.

Daly MD, Angell-James JE, Elsner R. Role of carotid-body chemoreceptors and their reflex interactions in bradycardia and cardiac arrest. *Lancet.* 1979;1(8119):764–767.

Iturriaga R, Alcayaga J, Chapleau MW, Somers VK. Carotid body chemoreceptors: physiology, pathology, and implications for health and disease [published online ahead of print, 2021 Feb 11]. *Physiol Rev.* 2021;10.1152/physrev.00039.2019.

Jurysta F, van de Borne P, Migeotte PF, et al. A study of the dynamic interactions between sleep EEG and heart rate variability in healthy young men. *Clin Neurophysiol.* 2003;114(11):2146–2155.

Li Y, Vgontzas AN, Fernandez-Mendoza J, et al. Insomnia with physiological hyperarousal is associated with hypertension. *Hypertension.* 2015;65(3):644–650.

Pepin JL, Borel AL, Tamisier R, Baguet JP, Levy P, Dauvilliers Y. Hypertension and sleep: overview of a tight relationship. *Sleep Med Rev.* 2014;18(6):509–519.

Sforza E, Nicolas A, Lavigne G, Gosselin A, Petit D, Montplaisir J. EEG and cardiac activation during periodic leg movements in sleep: support for a hierarchy of arousal responses. *Neurology.* 1999;52(4):786–791.

Somers VK, Dyken ME, Mark AL, Abboud FM. Sympathetic-nerve activity during sleep in normal subjects. *N Engl J Med.* 1993;328(5):303–307.

Spiegel K, Leproult R, Van Cauter E. Impact of sleep debt on metabolic and endocrine function. *Lancet.* 1999;354(9188):1435–1439.

Tamisier R, Pépin JL, Rémy J, et al. 14 nights of intermittent hypoxia elevate daytime blood pressure and sympathetic activity in healthy humans. *Eur Respir J.* 2011;37(1):119–128.

Tamisier R, Weiss JW, Pépin JL. Sleep biology updates: Hemodynamic and autonomic control in sleep disorders. *Metabolism.* 2018;84:3–10.

A complete reference list can be found online at ExpertConsult.com.

Chapter 22

Respiratory Physiology: Central Neural Control of Respiratory Neurons and Motoneurons during Sleep

Richard L. Horner

Chapter Highlights

- The *wakefulness stimulus* to breathing, and its withdrawal in sleep, is an enduring principle in respiratory medicine because it is the root mechanism for determining the effects of sleep on breathing. The neural basis for this wakefulness stimulus is identified.
- Central to understanding breathing in sleep has been delineation of the neurobiology of sleep, its impact on central respiratory neurons and motoneurons, and the important role of tonic excitatory (nonrespiratory) drives in contributing to the overall level of excitability in the respiratory system across sleep-wake states.
- Significant developments include identifying the neural basis for the suppression of pharyngeal muscle activity in sleep, especially rapid eye movement (REM) sleep. Mechanisms of genioglossus muscle suppression in sleep include withdrawal of excitatory inputs from wakefulness-dependent cell groups and active inhibition. This understanding has led to initial success with pharmacotherapy for obstructive sleep apnea.
- Mechanisms of respiratory rhythm generation and factors influencing motor excitability are both essential for the manifestation of effective breathing across sleep-wake states. The neurodepressive effects of commonly administered drugs such as opioids and sedative-hypnotics acting at critical sites in the respiratory network can explain the sometimes-severe respiratory depression that can occur during sleep with use of such agents.

RESPIRATORY NEUROBIOLOGY: BASIC OVERVIEW

Medullary Respiratory Neurons and Motoneurons

Bilateral columns of neurons in the medulla show activity patterns that vary in phase with some component of the respiratory cycle. The dorsal respiratory group (DRG) is located in the dorsomedial medulla, specifically in the ventrolateral nucleus of the solitary tract, and contains predominantly inspiratory neurons[1,2] (Figure 22.1). The DRG and the other subnuclei of the solitary tract also are the primary projection sites for vagal afferents from the lung and for afferents from the carotid and aortic chemoreceptors and baroreceptors, which exert important reflex influences on breathing. These projections indicate that the nuclei of the solitary tract, including the DRG, are key sites of integration of sensory information from the lung, as well as information regarding the prevailing levels of arterial P_{CO_2}, P_{O_2}, pH, and systemic blood pressure. The ventral respiratory group (VRG) extends from the facial nucleus to the first cervical segment of the spinal cord and contains both inspiratory and expiratory neurons (Figure 22.1).[1,2] The nucleus ambiguus also consists of a rostral to caudal column of neurons expressing respiratory-related activity, with subregions containing motoneurons that innervate the muscles of the larynx and pharynx that are not considered part of the VRG per se.[3] In addition to the nucleus ambiguus, from rostral to caudal, the VRG is composed of Bötzinger complex (expiratory) neurons, pre-Bötzinger complex (inspiratory) neurons, rostral retroambigualis (predominantly inspiratory) neurons, and caudal retroambigualis (predominantly expiratory) neurons (Figure 22.1).[1,2]

The VRG and DRG contain both bulbospinal respiratory pre-motoneurons (i.e., neurons that project to spinal motoneurons, which in turn innervate the respective respiratory pump and abdominal muscles of breathing) and propriobulbar neurons (i.e., neurons that project to, and influence the activity of, other medullary respiratory neurons but themselves do not project to motoneurons per se) (Figure 22.1).[1,2] The hypoglossal, trigeminal, and facial motor nuclei also innervate muscles important to pharyngeal motor control and the maintenance of upper airway patency[3] (Figure 22.1). Expression of respiratory-related activity is not restricted, however, to neurons of the DRG, VRG, and cranial motoneurons innervating the pharyngeal and laryngeal muscles. For example, neurons

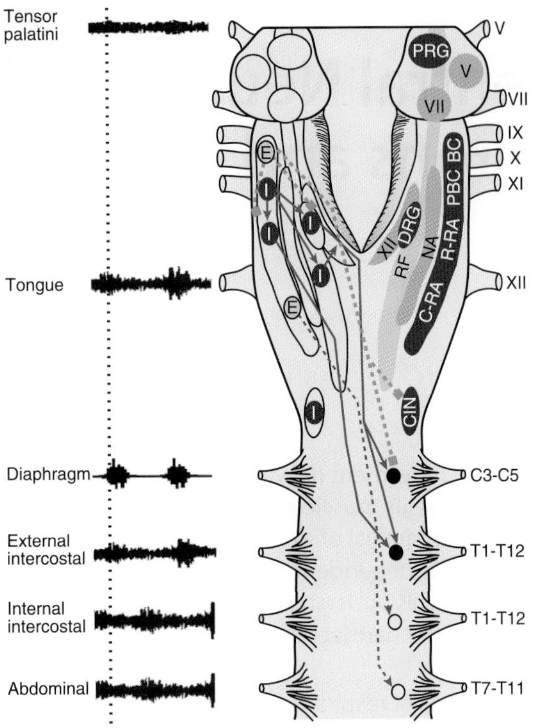

Figure 22.1 Ventral view of the brainstem (with cerebellum removed) showing the main aggregates of respiratory neurons in the dorsal and ventral respiratory groups (DRG and VRG, respectively). The locations of expiratory (E) and inspiratory (I) neurons in the Bötzinger complex (BC), pre-Bötzinger complex (PBC), rostral retroambigualis (R-RA), and caudal retroambigualis (C-RA) are shown. The locations of cervical inspiratory neurons (CIN) and respiratory-related neurons in the lateral reticular formation (RF) projecting to the hypoglossal motor nucleus (XII) also are shown. The projections of inspiratory and expiratory neurons are depicted as *solid* and *dashed lines,* respectively, whereas excitatory and inhibitory synaptic connections are depicted by *arrowhead* and *square symbols,* respectively. The electromyographic activities of various inspiratory-related (e.g., tongue, diaphragm, external intercostal) and expiratory (e.g., internal intercostal, abdominal) muscles are shown. Note that the level of respiratory-related and tonic activities varies for different muscles, with some muscles such as the tensor palatini expressing mainly tonic activity. The onset of muscle activity with respect to the diaphragm is shown by the *dashed line.* The rootlets of cranial nerves V, VII, IX, X, XI, and XII and the cervical (C) and thoracic (T) segments of the spinal cord also are shown, as are the motor nuclei of cranial nerves XII, VII, and V. The locations of the pontine respiratory group (PRG) and the nucleus ambiguus (NA) are shown, although their projections are not included for clarity. See text for further details.

expressing respiratory-related activity in the pons, such as the pontine respiratory group (PRG) in Figure 22.1, are thought to play an important role in shaping the activity of medullary respiratory neurons during breathing.[4]

Pre-Bötzinger Complex

Pre-Bötzinger complex neurons have pacemaker-like properties that are thought to be important to the generation of the basic respiratory rhythm and to the expression of rhythmic neuronal activity elsewhere in the respiratory network[5,6] (Figure 22.1). Respiratory rhythm–generating pre-Bötzinger complex neurons coexpress μ opioid and neurokinin-1 receptors (i.e., the receptors for substance P), which slow and increase respiratory rate, respectively.[6] The development of uncoordinated (ataxic) diaphragm breathing after introduction of lesions of neurokinin-1–expressing pre-Bötzinger complex neurons in animal studies, with this abnormal breathing first appearing in sleep,[7] suggests that pre-Bötzinger complex neurons contribute significantly to normal breathing in vivo. First identified and characterized in rodents, and subsequently in other mammalian species, the pre-Bötzinger complex also has been identified in humans.[8,9] Loss of pre-Bötzinger complex neurons may predispose affected persons to abnormal or ataxic breathing and to central apneas in sleep, such as with aging and in neurodegenerative brainstem diseases.[6,9]

The presence of μ opioid receptors on pre-Bötzinger complex neurons may explain a significant component of the clinically important phenomenon of respiratory rate depression with opioid drugs.[10] The respiratory slowing and central apneas produced by systemically applied opioids are prevented by local application of the μ opioid receptor antagonist naloxone to the pre-Bötzinger complex, showing that this region of medulla is a critical (although not likely the only) site mediating opioid-induced respiratory rate depression.[10] Moreover, deep non–rapid eye movement (NREM) sleep and general anesthesia are the most vulnerable states for respiratory rate depression produced by opioids at the pre-Bötzinger complex.[10] This observation has significant clinical relevance regarding the potential hazards of administering opioids, for example, in the perioperative setting and when a patient is asleep. The key point here is that opioid (and other respiratory-depressive) agents may be deemed well tolerated in the initially alert patient but, when the stimulating effects of wakefulness are withdrawn during sleep, the patient may suffer major respiratory depression (i.e., "crash").

Neuronal Connections

The anatomic connections between the neurons that make up the essential respiratory network (i.e., respiratory propriobulbar neurons, pre-motoneurons, and motoneurons), and the membrane properties of these cells, are ultimately responsible for the two key components of overall respiratory activity: (1) the generation of respiratory rhythm and (2) the shaping of the central respiratory drive potentials that activate respiratory motoneurons (pattern generation). An analysis of the mechanisms involved in the generation of the basic respiratory rhythm is outside the scope of this chapter; excellent summaries of the concepts underlying pacemaker models (whereby respiratory rhythm is *intrinsic* to some cells, which then drive others in the respiratory network), network models (whereby respiratory rhythm is *dependent* on the inhibitory and excitatory synaptic connections between neurons, and the tonic excitation is derived from both the respiratory chemoreceptors and brainstem reticular neurons), and hybrid models are available in referenced sources.[1,3,6]

The tonic drive to the respiratory system arising from the respiratory chemoreceptors includes both the peripheral and central chemoreceptors, the latter including neurons at the ventral medullary surface such as the retrotrapezoid nucleus, as well as inputs from CO_2-activated sleep state–dependent neurons of the aminergic arousal system (e.g., serotonin and noradrenergic neurons; see the following section).[11] Additional aspects of the organization of the central respiratory network are particularly relevant to understanding the effects of sleep on respiratory neurons and motoneurons; these concepts are discussed briefly next.

During inspiration the central respiratory drive potential is transmitted to phrenic and intercostal motoneurons via monosynaptic connections from inspiratory pre-motoneurons of the DRG and VRG[1] (Figure 22.1). Bötzinger complex expiratory neurons have widespread inhibitory connections throughout the brainstem and spinal cord, and these neurons inhibit inspiratory pre-motoneurons and motoneurons during expiration (Figure 22.1). Caudal retroambigualis neurons also increase the excitability of spinal expiratory motoneurons in expiration (Figure 22.1), although this excitation does not necessarily reach the threshold to manifest as expiratory muscle activity.

Of physiologic and clinical relevance, these fundamental aspects of the neural control of spinal respiratory motoneuron activity appear to be different from those for the mechanisms controlling the activity of pharyngeal motoneurons. For example, animal studies show that the source of inspiratory drive to hypoglossal motoneurons (predominantly from reticular neurons lateral to the hypoglossal motor nucleus [lateral tegmental field]) is different from the source of drive to phrenic motoneurons (from bulbospinal VRG and DRG neurons [Figure 22.1]).[1] Of importance, brainstem reticular neurons provide a significant source of tonic drive to the respiratory system, with this drive particularly affected in sleep.[3]

Further differences in the functional control of pharyngeal and diaphragm muscles are shown by the observation that, unlike phrenic motoneurons, hypoglossal motoneurons are not actively inhibited in expiration.[1] Accordingly, the activity of the genioglossus muscle in expiration is simply a manifestation of the prevailing tonic inputs. The practical implication of this circuitry is that the overall activation of hypoglossal motoneurons during breathing is, by an inspiratory drive, added to a continuous tonic drive, which persists in expiration when the inspiratory activation is withdrawn. Moreover, this tonic drive to the pharyngeal muscles, which contributes to baseline airway size and stiffness, is most prominent in wakefulness but withdrawn in sleep, resulting in an upper airspace that is more vulnerable to collapse and that plays an important role in the emergence of obstructed breathing episodes during sleep. Stimulation of the hypoglossal nerve has been developed as a treatment modality.[12]

Characterization and quantification of this tonic *wakefulness stimulus* have been performed for the pharyngeal muscles in humans.[13] A more detailed analysis of the neural mechanisms controlling the activity of respiratory neurons and motoneurons follows a brief overview of the brain mechanisms modulating the states of wakefulness, NREM sleep, and rapid eye movement (REM) sleep.

SLEEP NEUROBIOLOGY: BASIC OVERVIEW

Although a more detailed discussion of arousal and sleep state regulation is provided in Section 2 of this book, some details are key to the control of respiratory neurons and motoneurons in sleep. Accordingly, a brief overview of the neurobiology of sleep and wakefulness-generating systems is presented next.

Wakefulness

Figure 22.2 shows some of the main neuronal groups contributing to the ascending arousal system from the brainstem that promotes wakefulness. This ascending arousal system includes the cholinergic laterodorsal and pedunculopontine tegmental nuclei that promote cortical activation by way of excitatory thalamocortical projections.[14] The ascending arousal system also incorporates the aminergic arousal system that originates from brainstem neuronal groups principally containing serotonin (dorsal raphe nuclei), norepinephrine (locus coeruleus), histamine (tuberomammillary nucleus), and dopamine (ventral periaqueductal gray). Orexin neurons from the perifornical region of the hypothalamus and cholinergic neurons from the basal forebrain also contribute to this ascending arousal system.[14] Overall, multiple neuronal systems contribute to cortical arousal and wakefulness. These neuronal systems also are positioned to influence respiratory neurons and motoneurons by way of their anatomic projections to the pons, medulla, and spinal cord (Figure 22.2).

NREM Sleep

Sleep is actively generated by neurons in the ventrolateral preoptic area, anterior hypothalamus, and basal forebrain (Figure 22.2).[14] These neurons become active in NREM sleep, an effect influenced by the thermal stimulus that accompanies the circadian rhythm–mediated decline in body temperature at normal bedtime.[15] This circadian-mediated decline in body temperature is mediated by a change in the set point of hypothalamic temperature-regulating neurons, which initially leads to a relative "warm stimulus" because body temperature is at first higher than the new set point—that is, before heat loss occurs. This warm stimulus activates NREM sleep-active hypothalamic neurons and so promotes sleep onset. This effect of internal body temperature on sleep is distinct from the influences of ambient environmental temperature on sleep regulation. Activation of ventrolateral preoptic neurons leads to a direct suppression of cortical arousal, this by way of ascending inhibitory cortical projections. Ventrolateral preoptic neurons also promote sleep through descending inhibition of the aforementioned brainstem arousal neurons through release of gamma-aminobutyric acid (GABA) and galanin.[15,16] This effect of GABA explains the sedative-hypnotic effects of barbiturates, benzodiazepines, imidazopyridine compounds, and alcohol, as well as some general anesthetics, all of which enhance GABA-mediated neuronal inhibition through interactions with binding sites on the $GABA_A$ receptor.[17] $GABA_A$ receptors also are strongly implicated in respiratory control and are present throughout the respiratory network,[18] excessive stimulation of which can promote respiratory depression.[19] In summary, sleep onset is triggered by increased GABAergic neuronal activity, and this is accompanied by a massed and coordinated withdrawal of activity of brainstem arousal neurons comprising serotonergic, noradrenergic, histaminergic, and cholinergic neurons. With the widespread projections of these sleep state–dependent neuronal groups, these changes in neuronal activity in sleep also are positioned to influence respiratory neurons and motoneurons (Figure 22.2).[20]

REM Sleep

Decreased serotonergic and noradrenergic activity preceding and during REM sleep withdraws inhibition of the laterodorsal and pedunculopontine tegmental nuclei.[14,16] This effect leads to increased acetylcholine release into the pontine reticular formation and facilitation of transitions into REM sleep[21,22] and stability of the REM sleep state.[23,24] However, the endogenous release of acetylcholine into this region does not seem necessary to the primary generation of the REM sleep state per se (see later in this chapter).[23,24] Nevertheless, exogenous application of cholinergic agonists or acetylcholinesterase inhibitors (to increase acetylcholine) into the same region of the pons is used to mimic this release experimentally in animal studies, that is, the "carbachol model" of REM sleep.[21,22] A significant component of the motor suppression of REM sleep is mediated by descending pathways involving

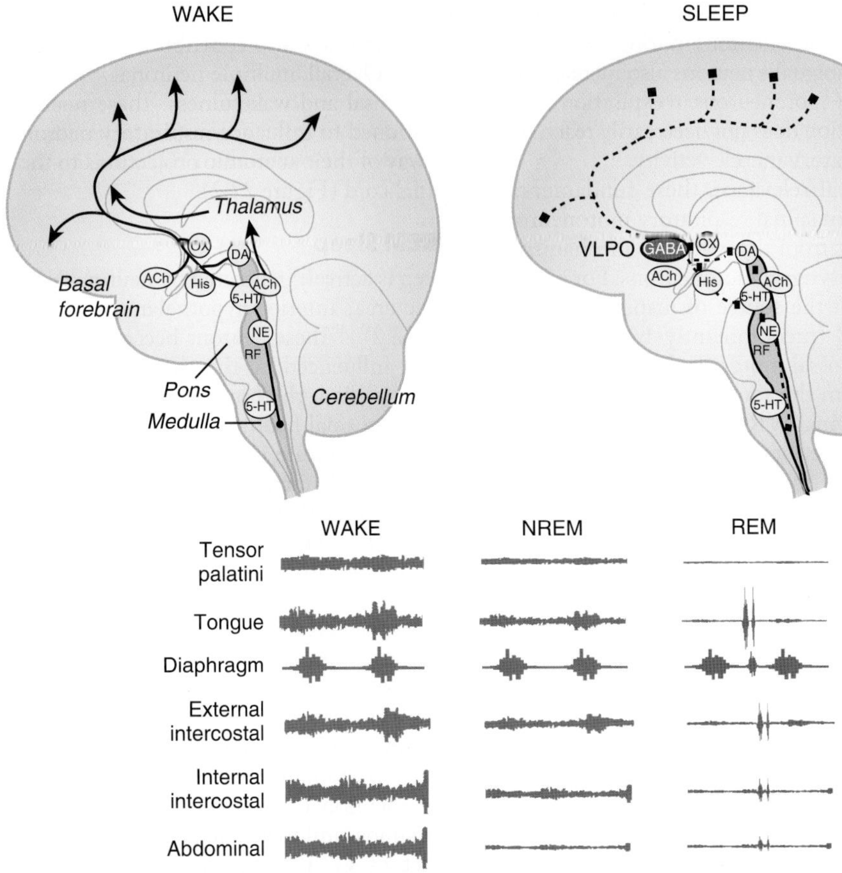

Figure 22.2 Sagittal section of the brain showing the main wake- and sleep-generating neural systems. In wakefulness, acetylcholine (ACh), orexin (OX), histamine (His), dopamine (DA), 5-hydroxytryptamine (5-HT), and norepinephrine (NE) containing neurons contribute to brain arousal (depicted as *black lines* with *arrows*). This ascending arousal system is inhibited in sleep by GABA-containing neurons from ventrolateral preoptic (VLPO) neurons (inhibitory projections shown by *dashed lines* and ■ symbols). By their anatomic projections to the pons, medulla, and spinal cord, these wake- and sleep-promoting neuronal systems also are positioned to influence respiratory neurons and motoneurons (Figure 22.1). However, whether the influences of the different arousal-related neurons is excitatory or inhibitory will depend on the receptor subtypes activated (this uncertainty is depicted by the symbol ● in the medulla). Overall, these changes in neuronal activities across sleep-wake states, and their impact on respiratory neurons and motoneurons, mediate the stereotypical changes in the tonic and respiratory components of activity for different respiratory muscles and their different susceptibilities to motor suppression in sleep. See text and referenced sources[20,21] for further details. GABA, Gamma-aminobutyric acid; RF, reticular formation. (Modified from Saper CB, Scammell TE, Lu J. Hypothalamic regulation of sleep and circadian rhythms. *Nature.* 2005;437:1257–63.)

activation of ventral medullary reticular relay neurons[25] that are inhibitory to spinal motoneurons via release of glycine.[26]

Despite the strong association and interactions between pontine aminergic and cholinergic neurons in facilitating REM sleep, more recent evidence has implicated a glutamatergic-GABAergic mechanism as key to the primary generation of the REM sleep state per se.[27,28] In addition to the critical contribution of different neural circuits and neuronal interactions to the generation of REM sleep, another difference between the aminergic-cholinergic and the glutamatergic-GABAergic mechanisms of REM sleep generation is that the motor atonia is produced by another pathway that does not require a relay in the ventral medullary region.[28] Rather, in the glutamatergic-GABAergic mechanism of REM sleep induction, the REM sleep-active pontine neurons are thought to lead to suppression of spinal motoneuron activity by way of long glutamatergic projections to the ventral horn of the spinal cord, which then activate local glycinergic interneurons to inhibit motor activity.[28] These inhibitory mechanisms are thought to be involved in the strong inhibition of spinal intercostal motoneurons in REM sleep. Recent findings identifying the mechanism of upper airway motor inhibition in REM sleep are discussed later in this chapter (see the section Inhibitory Influences across Sleep-Wake States). Reviews are available for additional details and further discussion.[29,30]

In summary, a number of neural systems exhibit changes in activity across sleep-wake states and project to respiratory neurons and motoneurons. Inasmuch as motoneurons are the final common output pathway for the influence of the central nervous system on motor activity, this chapter initially focuses on the control of respiratory motoneurons across sleep-wake states before addressing the control of the central respiratory neurons that ultimately drive breathing by those motoneurons.

CONTROL OF RESPIRATORY MOTONEURONS

A characteristic and defining feature of mammalian motor activity is that postural muscle tone is highest in wakefulness, decreased in NREM sleep, and minimal in REM sleep, with the hypotonia of REM sleep punctuated by occasional muscle twitches that are associated with vigorous eye movements and "phasic" REM sleep events.[26] Whether *respiratory* muscle activity is affected in the same way as postural muscle activity across sleep-wake states is somewhat complicated by the interaction of the primary influence of sleep state (e.g., producing suppression of muscle tone) and any subsequent respiratory response (e.g., to compensate for any hypoventilation). On balance, however, the overall stereotyped pattern of suppression of postural muscle activity across sleep-wake states also typically occurs in respiratory muscles, with the degree of sleep state–dependent modulation most readily apparent in those muscles that combine respiratory *and* nonrespiratory (e.g., postural and/or behavioral) functions such as the intercostal and pharyngeal muscles.[31] In these respiratory muscles, decreases in activity typically occur immediately at sleep onset,[31] indicating a primary suppressant effect of sleep neural mechanisms on the activity of respiratory motoneurons—that is, before any compensatory increase in activity takes place in response to altered blood gases, mechanical loads, or sleep-disordered breathing. In contrast with those respiratory muscles with both respiratory and nonrespiratory functions, the diaphragm has an almost solely respiratory function and undergoes lesser suppression of activity in NREM sleep and is largely spared the motor inhibition of REM sleep (Figure 22.2).[32] Other chapters in this section provide more detail regarding clinical aspects of the control of breathing and upper airway function during sleep, whereas this chapter describes the fundamental mechanisms underlying these effects of sleep on the respiratory system.

DETERMINANTS OF RESPIRATORY MOTONEURON ACTIVITY

Tonic and Respiratory-Related Inputs to Respiratory Motoneurons

The changes in muscle tone across sleep-wake states ultimately result from the impact of sleep neural mechanisms on the electrical properties and membrane potential of individual motoneurons located in the respective motor pools in the central nervous system. In turn, the excitability of individual motoneurons changes across sleep-wake states because of varying degrees of excitatory and inhibitory inputs to those motoneurons from sleep-wake–related regions in the brain, and from neurons activated during specific behaviors such as purposeful motor acts in wakefulness.[20] At each individual motoneuron, therefore, the relative strengths of, and balance between, time-varying excitatory and inhibitory inputs ultimately determine net motor output, with neural activity being generated when the membrane potential rises above threshold for the production of action potentials (Figure 22.3). In addition to the excitatory and inhibitory *nonrespiratory* inputs to a motoneuron that alter membrane potential across sleep-wake states, a respiratory motoneuron also receives additional inputs (excitatory and inhibitory) that alter membrane excitability and neural activity in phase with the inspiratory or expiratory phases of the respiratory cycle. In short, a respiratory motoneuron resembles a postural motoneuron in its control and organizational principles, except that it receives an additional rhythmic drive related to respiration—that is, the central respiratory drive potential. Figure 22.3 highlights the fact that the electromyographic activity recorded in a given respiratory muscle is dependent on the overall sum of the respiratory *and* nonrespiratory (i.e., tonic) inputs to the motoneurons innervating that muscle.

Recognition of the importance of *both* the tonic and respiratory-related inputs to a motoneuron in determining overall motor output is necessary to any interpretation of the changes in respiratory muscle activity observed across sleep-wake states. Indeed, periods of hypoventilation, apparent central apnea, and even the sporadic respiratory muscle activations that occur during REM sleep all can result from *independent* effects of sleep neural processes on the tonic and/or respiratory-related inputs to a respiratory motoneuron (Figure 22.3, *A* to *E*). For example, the apparent absence of activity recorded in a respiratory muscle cannot be taken as evidence that the controlling circuitry is inactive; that is, an apparent apnea may not be truly due to a "central" cessation of respiratory drive. Indeed, a simple withdrawal of tonic drive in sleep may be sufficient to take a population of (e.g., otherwise respiratory-related) motoneurons close to, or below, the threshold for the generation of motor activity, such that any excitatory respiratory inputs to the motoneurons are subthreshold for the generation of action potentials and therefore are not revealed as respiratory muscle activity (Figure 22.3, *C*).

In summary, nonrespiratory tonic drives exert important influences on the resting membrane potential of respiratory motoneurons, thereby significantly modulating the excitability of motoneurons in response to the incoming central respiratory drive potential. This significant effect of nonrespiratory tonic drives on the activity of respiratory motoneurons has clear physiologic relevance: when identified experimentally, the tonic drive to respiratory motoneurons typically is reduced from wakefulness to NREM sleep, with consequent important contributions to sleep-related reductions in respiratory muscle activity leading to hypoventilation (Figure 22.3, *A* and *B*).[33,34] Tonic drive to respiratory motoneurons can also be further reduced in REM sleep, although time-varying fluctuations in this tonic drive can produce transient increases or decreases in respiratory muscle activity and contribute to changes in lung ventilation in REM sleep by a mechanism independent of effects on the respiratory-related inputs (Figure 22.3, *E*). Indeed, the presence of endogenous excitatory inputs to respiratory motoneurons in REM sleep (i.e., unrelated to breathing per se and akin to the mechanisms producing phasic muscle twitches in limb muscles) can produce sporadic activation of respiratory muscle and contribute to the expression of rapid and irregular breathing in REM sleep (Figure 22.3, *E*), even in the presence of low CO_2 levels that are otherwise sufficient to produce central apnea in NREM sleep.[33,34]

Electrical Properties of Motoneurons

The electrical properties of the motoneuron membrane also significantly affect the responses of that motoneuron to a given synaptic input. For example, reduced motoneuron responses to an incoming respiratory drive potential can be due not only to the aforementioned effects of reduced tonic drives and consequent membrane hyperpolarization (Figure 22.3) but also to the electrical resistance of the motoneuron membrane itself. The input resistance of a membrane is defined as its voltage response to a given synaptic current, with a decrease in input resistance resulting in less membrane depolarization for a given synaptic drive—that is, a decrease

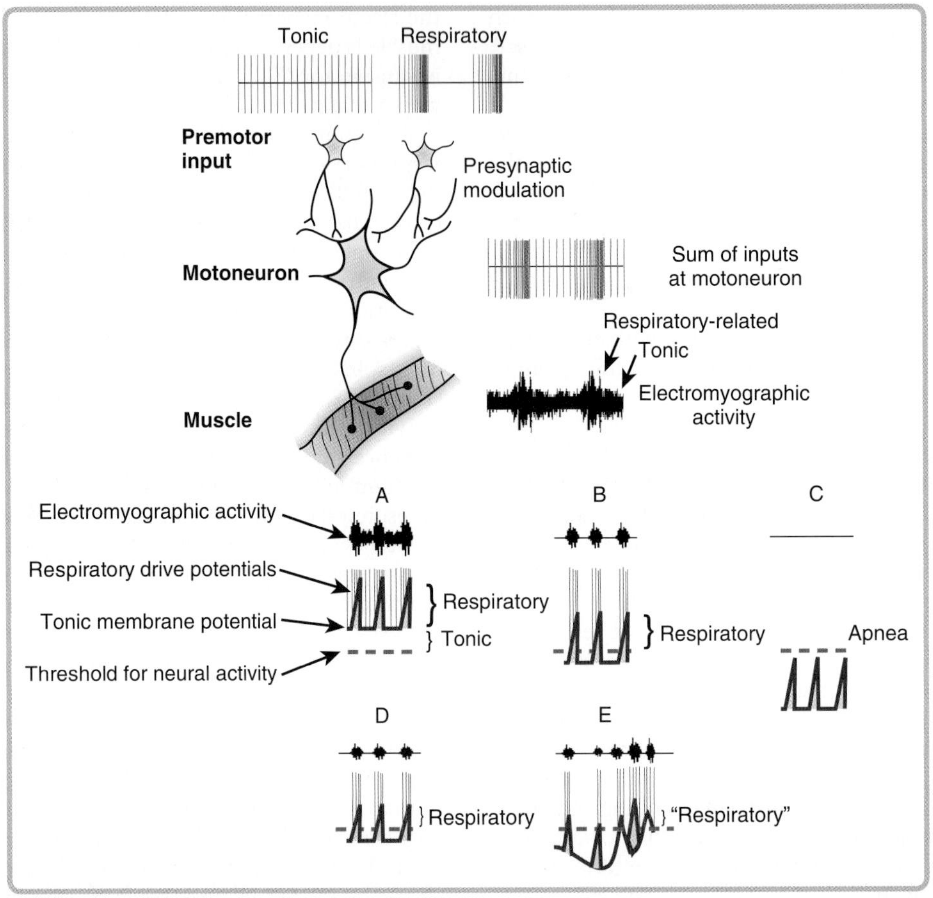

Figure 22.3 Schema depicting how converging tonic (e.g., postural, nonrespiratory) and respiratory inputs to a motoneuron summate to produce the tonic and respiratory components of electromyographic activity. These premotor tonic and respiratory inputs can be excitatory or inhibitory, but here they are shown as excitatory for simplicity. Diagrams **A** to **E** further show how changes in the tonic and respiratory components of respiratory muscle activity can result from *independent* changes in either tonic drives affecting tonic membrane potential (**A, B, C,** and **E**) (such as may occur on transition from wakefulness to NREM and REM sleep) or the magnitude of the respiratory drive potential (**B** versus **D**) (such as may occur in NREM and REM sleep compared with wakefulness). Changes in respiratory drive potential at the motoneuron can result from decreases in the input from respiratory neurons, presynaptic modulation of that input, and/or changes in input resistance of the motoneuron membrane per se (see text for further details). In the examples shown in **A** to **E,** respiratory drive is indicated as three depolarizing potentials, each associated with the generation of motoneuron action potentials when the membrane potential exceeds threshold (*dashed line*). Diagram E also shows that time-varying alterations in membrane potential, as occur in REM sleep, for example, can produce respiratory muscle activation unrelated to the prevailing respiratory input. Thus, from peripheral measurements of diaphragm activity or airflow, there appear to be five "breaths," although only three respiratory drive potentials are generated by the central respiratory oscillator.

in cell excitability (Figure 22.3). This electrical property of excitable membranes has clear physiologic relevance because a large (~44%) decrease in input resistance of motoneurons occurs in REM sleep compared with NREM sleep and wakefulness.[26] In addition, transient fluctuations in input resistance occur throughout REM sleep episodes, such as the decreased input resistance of somatic motoneurons that occurs in temporal association with the phasic events of REM sleep. Such an effect is likely to contribute to the periods of marked suppression of inspiratory upper airway muscle activity in humans during phasic REM sleep compared with tonic REM sleep.[35]

In summary, a decrease in motoneuron input resistance in REM sleep, especially in association with eye movements, can contribute to decreased motor outflow to the pharyngeal and respiratory pump muscles, leading to periods of increased upper airway resistance and hypoventilation. Moreover, such decreases in respiratory motoneuron activity can occur *despite* the persistence of a continuing, and even heightened, activity of the central respiratory neurons that innervate those motoneurons in REM sleep (Figure 22.4) (see the later section Control of Respiratory Neurons).[3,34] This observation highlights that a powerful inhibition and/or disfacilitation (i.e., withdrawal of excitation) must be taking place at respiratory motoneurons to explain the periods of reduced motor *output* despite continuing, and even heightened, *inputs* from respiratory neurons in REM sleep (Figure 22.4).[3,36,37]

Presynaptic Modulation

The control of respiratory motoneuron activity by changes in sleep state–dependent neuromodulators and/or inputs from respiratory neurons often emphasizes the postsynaptic effects of released neurotransmitters (see earlier). Such postsynaptic

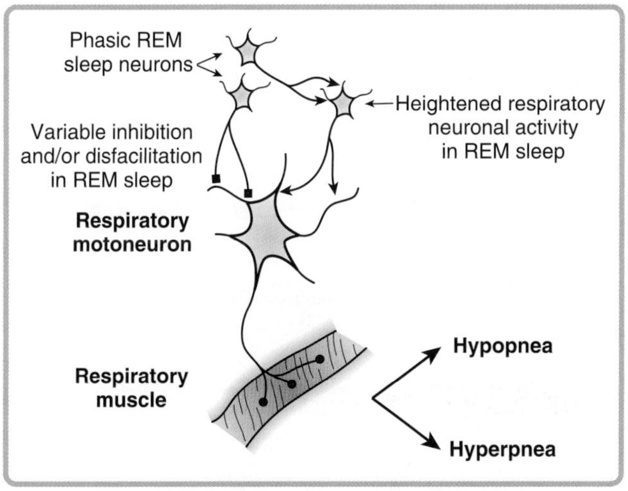

Figure 22.4 Schema depicting how respiratory motoneurons receive competing excitatory (*arrowheads*) and inhibitory (■) drives in REM sleep, the balance of which leads to time-varying increases and decreases in respiratory rate and amplitude, which manifest as hyperpnea and hypopnea, respectively. Additional factors that contribute to this variable lung ventilation in REM sleep are the similar competing excitatory and inhibitory influences at (1) pharyngeal motoneurons in REM sleep that lead to time-varying alterations in upper airway size and resistance, and (2) chest wall and abdominal muscles[26] that modulate resting lung volume and compliance of the chest wall. (Modified from Orem J. Neuronal mechanisms of respiration in REM sleep. *Sleep.* 1980;3:251–67.)

effects do not fully account for the control of motoneuron activity, however, because presynaptic modulation of the prevailing inputs also is important in motor control (Figure 22.3). For example, inhibitory inputs arriving at a nerve terminal before the subsequent arrival of a descending excitatory drive can lead to marked reductions in the release of excitatory neurotransmitters, so leading to the suppression of motoneuron activity. Such presynaptic modulation of neuronal activity is thought to be significant for information processing in neurons innervated by several converging pathways, as is the case for the organization of respiratory motoneurons (Figure 22.3). Accordingly, under specific behaviors, some inputs can be selectively suppressed, whereas others are left unaffected. This presynaptic modulation of specific inputs allows for selective control of motoneuron excitability, an effect that could not be achieved by a generalized postsynaptic modulation that affects the whole cell. This differential control has particular relevance in the control of motoneurons with dual respiratory and nonrespiratory functions, such as hypoglossal motoneurons innervating the genioglossus muscle of the tongue. In hypoglossal motoneurons, the presynaptic inhibition of the incoming central respiratory drive potentials allows for the switching of motor output appropriate for other behaviors such as swallowing, sucking, or speech, without the interference of respiration.[38]

Tonic and Respiratory-Related Activity in Respiratory Muscle

Some respiratory muscles exhibit more respiratory-related activity than others, whereas other muscles are more tonically active and exhibit little respiratory-related activity (Figures 22.1 and 22.2). For example, the genioglossus muscle of the tongue shows both tonic and respiratory-related activity, with the decreased activity of this muscle during sleep strongly linked to the pathogenesis of obstructive sleep apnea.[39] Similarly, the different intercostal muscles show various degrees of respiratory-related and tonic activities related to both the respiratory and postural functions of these muscles, with the expression of this respiratory-related versus tonic activity related to specific anatomic location in the chest wall and ongoing behaviors.[32,40] Suppression of intercostal muscle activity in REM sleep is thought to increase the compliance of the chest wall and to contribute to decreased functional residual capacity, effects that can in turn contribute to hypoventilation, especially in infants because of their already highly compliant chest wall.[32] In contrast with these muscles with respiratory-related activity, the tensor palatini muscle of the soft palate displays mostly tonic activity, which decreases with progression from wakefulness to NREM and REM sleep. The tonic activity in the tensor palatini is thought to enhance stiffness in the segment of the upper airway at the level of the soft palate, a consistent site of airway closure in obstructive sleep apnea.[4] Accordingly, decreases in tonic tensor palatini muscle activity from wakefulness to sleep (Figure 22.2) contribute to increased upper airway resistance and the predisposition to airway occlusion in sleep, with this effect of sleep predominantly affecting breathing by an effect on the tonic (nonrespiratory) inputs to these motoneurons, which receive little or no respiratory input at rest. Ultimately, whether some muscles exhibit respiratory-related activity at rest depends on both the "strength" of the input from respiratory neurons compared with the tonic drives (see Figure 22.5 and the later section Control of Respiratory Neurons)[3] and the degree of suppression of the respiratory activity by vagal afferents related to lung volume.[4]

NEUROMODULATION OF RESPIRATORY MOTONEURONS ACROSS SLEEP-WAKE STATES

Studies addressing the neurochemical basis for the modulation of respiratory motor activity across natural sleep-wake states, in vivo, have been confined largely to the hypoglossal and trigeminal motor nuclei.[21,26,30,41] This focus on pharyngeal motoneurons is clinically relevant in elucidating the pathogenesis of obstructive sleep apnea, with airway obstructions occurring behind the tongue both at the level of the soft palate and below.[4] In contrast with this focus on pharyngeal motoneurons, similar studies investigating the control of intercostal and phrenic motoneurons in naturally sleeping animals are lacking. Nevertheless, studies of spinal motoneurons have provided important information regarding the control of postural motoneurons across sleep-wake states.[26] Because intercostal motoneurons perform both postural and respiratory functions, the mechanisms identified at primary postural motoneurons are likely to have close similarities to the mechanisms controlling the nonrespiratory (postural) component of intercostal motor activity. A focus on the control of motoneurons innervating the muscles of the respiratory pump also is relevant within the scope of this chapter because significant hypoventilation can occur in sleep, especially REM sleep, in patients with restrictive lung diseases (e.g., kyphoscoliosis, obesity hypoventilation) and neuromuscular weakness (e.g., postpolio syndrome, muscular dystrophy, amyotrophic lateral sclerosis, partial diaphragm paralysis).[42] Summarized next are the major findings from animal studies addressing the sleep state–dependent modulation of respiratory motor activity. These data derive in large part from studies at the hypoglossal

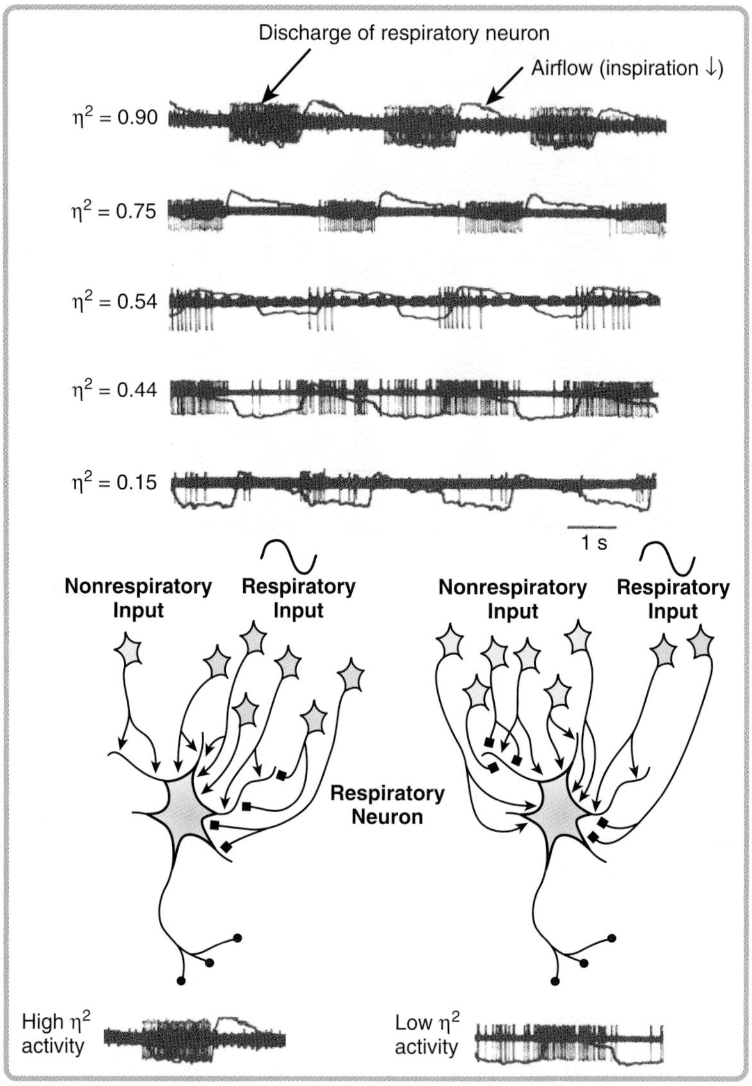

Figure 22.5 Five different medullary respiratory neurons recorded in intact cats in NREM sleep. These neurons vary in the strength of their relationship to breathing, an effect that is quantified by the η^2 statistic with values ranging from 0 (weak relationship) to 1.0 (strong relationship). High η^2 cells are considered to be more strongly influenced by respiratory inputs than nonrespiratory inputs and vice versa for low η^2 cells. (Modified from Orem J, Kubin L. Respiratory physiology: central neural control. In: Kryger MH, Roth T, Dement WC, eds. *Principles and Practice of Sleep Medicine.* 3rd ed. WB Saunders; 2000.)

motor nucleus, a model motor pool with dual respiratory and nonrespiratory functions.[20,30]

Excitatory Influences across Sleep-Wake States

The concept of a tonic drive activating respiratory muscle in wakefulness but not in sleep (i.e., the wakefulness stimulus for breathing) has been an important and enduring notion in respiratory medicine,[3,32] not least because it is useful in understanding sleep effects on breathing and in elucidating the pathogenesis of sleep-related breathing disorders. Neurons of the aminergic arousal system provide an important source of tonic drive to the respiratory system (Figure 22.2).[3,20,21] Serotonin- and norepinephrine-containing neurons have been of particular attention experimentally because these neurons send excitatory projections to respiratory motoneurons, and because these neurons show their highest activity in wakefulness, reduced activity in NREM sleep, and minimal activity in REM sleep—a pattern that may contribute to reduced respiratory muscle activity in sleep through withdrawal of excitation.[3,20,21]

Animal studies show that an endogenous noradrenergic drive to the hypoglossal motor nucleus contributes to both the respiratory and tonic components of genioglossus muscle activation in wakefulness, and the residual expression of respiratory-related activity that persists in NREM sleep as the tonic drive is withdrawn.[43] Moreover, this noradrenergic contribution to genioglossus muscle tone was shown to be minimal in REM sleep, thereby explaining, at least in part, the periods of genioglossus muscle hypotonia during REM sleep.[43,44] The identification of an endogenous excitatory noradrenergic drive that contributes to genioglossus muscle activation in wakefulness, but is withdrawn in sleep, is particularly significant because since the first clinical description of obstructive sleep apnea, this was the first identification of a neural drive contributing to the sleep state–dependent activity of a muscle that is central to this disorder. The location of the central noradrenergic neurons that may provide this drive to hypoglossal and other respiratory motoneurons is reviewed elsewhere.[20] As noted previously, with the widespread projections of brainstem aminergic neurons, they also are positioned to provide an endogenous input to other respiratory neurons and motoneurons and thereby influence respiratory pump muscle activity and ventilation across sleep-wake states.[45,46] Additional data also point to a role for endogenous glutamatergic inputs in the tonic excitatory drive that increases pharyngeal muscle activity in wakefulness, the withdrawal of which contributes to reduced activity in sleep.[20,47,48] In contrast with these functionally active tonic inputs, endogenous levels of serotonin at the hypoglossal motor nucleus contribute less to the changes in genioglossus muscle activity in sleeping animals.[20] Whether this minimal influence of endogenous serotonin on genioglossus muscle activity also applies to humans remains to be determined. If so, it may explain (at least in part) the lack of clinically significant effects of selective serotonin reuptake inhibitors on pharyngeal muscle activity and obstructive sleep apnea severity in patients receiving these drugs.[20,49-51]

Local application of serotonergic, noradrenergic, and glutamatergic agonists to the hypoglossal or trigeminal motor nuclei produces robust motor activation in wakefulness and NREM sleep.[20,48] These observations provide "proof of principle" for the notion that it may be possible to develop pharmacologic strategies to increase respiratory muscle activity in sleep—for example, as a potential treatment for obstructive sleep apnea. Of importance, however, a major component of the motor activation observed in response to these agonists in NREM sleep is overcome in REM sleep.[20,48] An important practical implication of this differential modulation of pharyngeal motor responses to otherwise potent excitatory neuromodulators between NREM and REM sleep has been recognized. For example, even if it is possible to effectively target pharyngeal motoneurons with directed pharmacologic manipulations, such as for treatment for obstructive sleep apnea, then different strategies may be required to produce sustained pharyngeal muscle activation throughout both the NREM *and* REM sleep stages, because the neurobiology of motor control is fundamentally different between these two states.[20,52] A recent breakthrough in obstructive sleep apnea pharmacotherapy by targeting such mechanisms is discussed in a later section (see the section Mechanisms Operating across Sleep-Wake States and Potential for Obstructive Sleep Apnea Pharmacotherapy).

Inhibitory Influences across Sleep-Wake States

Glycine and GABA are the main inhibitory neurotransmitters in the central nervous system. Glycine and $GABA_A$ receptor stimulation at the hypoglossal motor nucleus in vivo produces the expected depression of genioglossus muscle activity, whereas antagonism of these receptors increases genioglossus activity across all sleep-wake states.[20,29,30] The augmentation of respiratory-related motor activity across *all* sleep-wake states with application of antagonists for these inhibitory neurotransmitters fits best with the notion of a continuous background (i.e., tonic) inhibitory tone that constrains the rhythmic activation via gain modulation.[53] Moreover, any motor-activating effects observed with glycine and GABA receptor blockade at the cranial motor pools are trivial and, of note, are of *smallest* magnitude in REM sleep compared with wakefulness and NREM sleep. These findings, observed at both the hypoglossal[54,55] and trigeminal[41,56] motor pools, suggest that inhibition by glycine and GABA should not be viewed as a significant mediator of pharyngeal motor inhibition in REM sleep, because the inhibitory tone is present across all sleep-wake states and is weakest of all in REM sleep (see referenced sources[29,30,57] for further details, and see discussion in subsequent paragraphs of this subsection of the strong inhibitory (cholinergic) mechanism that operates at the hypoglossal motor pool in REM sleep).

Nevertheless, the tonic inhibitory effects of GABA at respiratory neurons[18] and motoneurons[20] are clinically relevant in view of the widespread use of sedative-hypnotic drugs. For example, benzodiazepine and imidazopyridine drugs commonly are prescribed as sedative-hypnotics (e.g., lorazepam and zolpidem, respectively), and both of these classes of sedatives promote sleep by enhancing GABA-mediated neuronal inhibition through interactions with binding sites on $GABA_A$ receptors.[17] The presence of lorazepam and zolpidem at the hypoglossal motor nucleus also leads to inhibition of genioglossus muscle activity.[20] This inhibitory effect of sedative-hypnotics at respiratory motor nuclei may underlie a component of the respiratory depression observed clinically with *excessive* $GABA_A$ receptor stimulation and the potential predisposition to obstructive sleep apnea in some persons taking sedative-hypnotics in combination with other $GABA_A$ receptor–modulating neurodepressive drugs such as alcohol and certain general anesthetics.[19]

Large inhibitory glycinergic potentials appear to play an important role in the inhibition of spinal motoneuron activity in REM sleep,[26] and this probably explains the inhibition of intercostal respiratory muscle activity in this sleep state.[32] As discussed previously, however, glycine and $GABA_A$ receptor antagonism at the hypoglossal[54,55] and trigeminal[41,56] motoneuron pools fails to reverse the profound *tonic* suppression of genioglossus or masseter muscle activity in REM sleep, although in both cases this antagonism increases the amount and/or magnitude of the sporadic *phasic* motor activations in REM sleep.[20,41] These increases in phasic motor activity during REM sleep with glycine and $GABA_A$ receptor antagonism point to a functional role for *sporadic* inhibitory neurotransmission in the modulation of hypoglossal and trigeminal motor excitability,[20,41] and such inhibitory potentials have been recorded at hypoglossal motoneurons in REM sleep.[58] Based on the findings described here, however, this inhibitory glycinergic and GABAergic mechanism appears not to be as profound as the inhibition demonstrated at spinal motoneurons.[26]

Indeed, the mechanism of hypoglossal motor suppression in REM sleep appears to be different from that for spinal motoneurons. A cholinergic (muscarinic) receptor mechanism linked to G protein–coupled inwardly rectifying potassium (GIRK) channels mediates the strong inhibition of the tongue musculature in REM sleep.[57] This inhibition is strong enough to counteract the inspiratory excitatory drive to hypoglossal motoneurons that originates from the respiratory network (Figure 22.1), such that respiratory motor activation of the tongue musculature can be abolished during REM sleep even during strong respiratory stimulation with hypercapnia.[59] Moreover, unlike glycine and $GABA_A$ receptor blockade at the hypoglossal motor pool, blockade of this cholinergic-GIRK channel mechanism is capable of reversing the REM sleep–induced hypoglossal motor suppression and of restoring respiratory genioglossus activity throughout REM sleep.[29,57,60]

The degree of suppression observed in a variety of *respiratory pump* muscles in REM sleep appears to be strongly correlated with the muscle spindle density of these different muscles.[40] The diaphragm has few, if any, spindles and little inhibition in REM sleep, whereas different intercostal muscles (especially the external inspiratory intercostals) have significant numbers of muscle spindles and profound suppression of activity in REM sleep, with variation in the degree of suppression in accordance with muscle spindle density.[32,40] Of clinical relevance, *acute* diaphragm paralysis leads to increased reliance on the intercostal and accessory muscles to maintain effective lung ventilation, but this compensation is lost in REM sleep, when the motoneurons innervating these muscles with dual respiratory and postural functions are inhibited.[61] Of interest, however, patients with *chronic* bilateral diaphragm paralysis are able to recruit nondiaphragmatic inspiratory muscle activity during REM sleep, thereby lessening any attendant hypoventilation. This compensation suggests that the central nervous system in these patients is able to functionally reorganize the drives controlling the accessory respiratory muscles such that activity is less suppressed by REM sleep mechanisms in the long term.[62,63]

Mechanisms Operating across Sleep-Wake States and Potential for Obstructive Sleep Apnea Pharmacotherapy

Current information from experiments in sleeping animals indicates that reduced excitation, largely through withdrawal of endogenous noradrenergic and glutamatergic inputs, is principally responsible for reductions in pharyngeal muscle tone from wakefulness to NREM and REM sleep.[20,21,48] By comparison, an endogenous serotonergic drive plays a lesser role.[20] Increased inhibitory neurotransmission mediated by glycine and GABA also contributes to suppression of pharyngeal motor activity in REM sleep, but the contribution of this mechanism appears to be much less than expected[20,21,29,48] from studies at spinal motoneurons.[26] Rather, a cholinergic-GIRK channel inhibitory mechanism operates at the hypoglossal motor pool, with the largest inhibitory influence of this mechanism seen in REM sleep and minimal or no effects in waking or NREM sleep.[29,30,57] This mechanism is the major cause of inhibition of the tongue musculature in REM sleep.[29,30,57] By contrast, glycine and GABA exert a continuous background (i.e., tonic) inhibitory tone that is present across all sleep-wake states, with constraint of hypoglossal respiratory motor outflow by this tone through gain modulation. Augmentation of this tonic inhibitory GABA tone with commonly administered neurodepressive drugs may lead to further suppression of pharyngeal muscle activity and precipitation of upper airway obstructions in susceptible persons, such as those with anatomically narrow upper airways who already are prone to experience obstructive sleep apnea.

Currently there is no pharmacotherapy for obstructive sleep apnea, but there is no known a priori physiologic reason that there should not be one.[52] Identification of key neuromodulators and the effects of their manipulation to increase tongue motor tone during sleep is a necessary first step for such potential pharmacotherapy.[52] A recent screen also led to the identification of targets of high strategic interest for activating motor output to the tongue musculature during sleep.[52] Moreover, important recent clinical data identify that there is significant potential for obstructive sleep apnea pharmacotherapy using a combination of atomoxetine (a noradrenaline reuptake inhibitor) and oxybutynin (a muscarinic receptor antagonist).[51,64] Atomoxetine was selected[51,64] because it may boost the aforementioned endogenous excitatory noradrenergic drive to pharyngeal motoneurons,[43] whereas oxybutynin was selected[51,64] because it may block the strong muscarinic-receptor mediated cholinergic inhibition of pharyngeal motoneurons that occurs in REM sleep.[57]

Future studies will establish potential for clinical efficacy in a larger number of patients for the observed improvements in obstructive sleep apnea severity (as judged by apnea-hypopnea index), oxygen desaturation, and genioglossus muscle responsiveness to esophageal pressure swings, as well as the mechanism and sites of action of these drugs in mediating these effects.[51,64] It is important to stress, however, that pharmacotherapy may not cure or eliminate obstructive sleep apnea per se but may still be a useful adjunct to improve the effectiveness of, and adherence to, other treatment mainstays such as continuous positive airway pressure by reducing the required effective therapeutic pressures.

CONTROL OF RESPIRATORY NEURONS

Varying Strength of the Relationship between Respiratory Neurons and Breathing

Studies by John Orem and colleagues in sleeping animals led to the fundamental concepts that still best explain the neural basis for the effects of sleep on breathing, including the nature of the wakefulness stimulus, and the rapid and irregular breathing pattern of REM sleep.[3] Key to this achievement was development of a statistical approach to quantify the consistency and strength of the respiratory-related component of a neuron's activity as related to its overall discharge. The strength of this relationship was quantified by the *eta-squared statistic* (η^2), with η^2 values ranging from 1.0 (strongest relationship) to 0 (i.e., weakest relationship).[3] Of importance, different brainstem respiratory neurons vary in the strength of their relationship to the inspiratory or expiratory phase of the breathing cycle (Figure 22.5).

The interpretation and physiologic meaning of the η^2 value for any given respiratory neuron are best explained in the following quote from Orem, for whom cells with high η^2 values were "quintessentially respiratory … protected from nonrespiratory distortions, perhaps because of rigid sequences of excitatory and inhibitory postsynaptic potentials that preclude activity that is not strictly respiratory."[3] By comparison, the activity of "low η^2-valued cells is the apparent result of mixtures of inputs that have respiratory and nonrespiratory forms."[3] Figure 22.5 further illustrates this concept by showing that the degree of respiratory-related activity of a given respiratory neuron (i.e., its η^2 value) depends on the balance of the respiratory *and* nonrespiratory inputs to that neuron. This is an important concept because respiratory neurons with different η^2 values are differentially affected by sleep-wake state.

Respiratory Neuron Activity in NREM Sleep

The notion that the degree of respiratory-related activity of a particular respiratory neuron depends on the balance of its respiratory and nonrespiratory inputs assumes significant physiologic and clinical relevance with the following experimental observations, made across the sleep-wake cycle:

- Neurons with low η^2 activity—that is, those that are less influenced by the respiratory oscillator but are strongly influenced by nonrespiratory tonic drives—are *most* affected by the transition from wakefulness to NREM sleep, such that their activity can even cease during sleep.
- Neurons with high η^2 activity—that is, those that presumably are strongly coupled to, and controlled by, the respiratory oscillator—are *least* affected by the transition from wakefulness to NREM sleep.

These observations and findings are illustrated in Figure 22.6.[3]

Of note, those respiratory neurons with low η^2 values that become inactive in sleep are not ceasing their activity simply because these neurons lose their respiratory input. That idea is discounted because experimental reexcitation of those low η^2

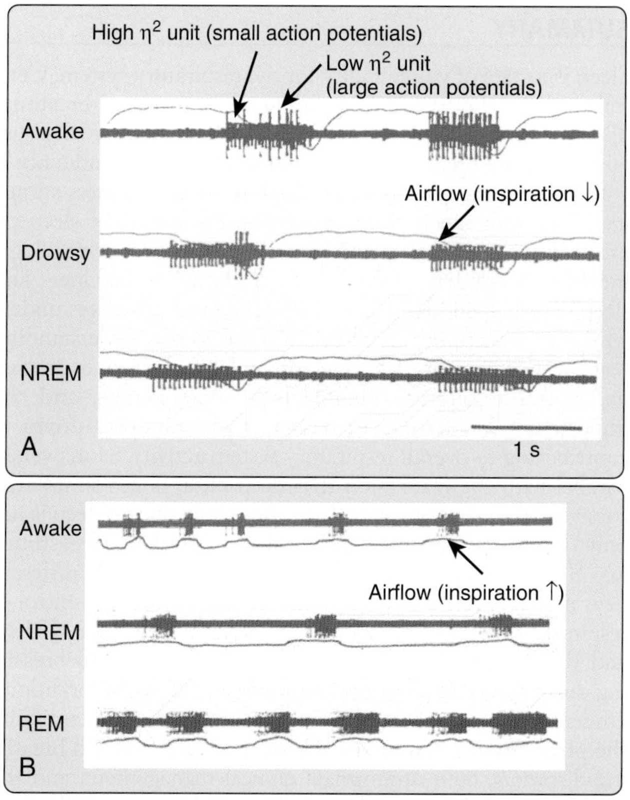

Figure 22.6 **A,** The activity of high η^2 medullary respiratory neurons is little affected by NREM sleep, whereas the activity of low η^2 cells is significantly suppressed in NREM sleep. This differential effect of NREM sleep on these different classes of respiratory neurons is thought to be due to the particular sensitivity of the tonic nonrespiratory inputs to changes in sleep-wake state, which is the basis of the so-called wakefulness stimulus for breathing. **B,** Electromyographic tracings showing increased and advanced activity of a late inspiratory neuron in REM sleep. (Modified from Orem J, Kubin L. Respiratory physiology: central neural control. In: Kryger MH, Roth T, Dement WC, eds. *Principles and Practice of Sleep Medicine.* 3rd ed. WB Saunders; 2000.)

respiratory neurons that become silenced during NREM sleep restores their rhythmic respiratory activity. This finding shows that the respiratory-related input persists onto those inactive low η^2 respiratory neurons in NREM sleep but that this respiratory signal was subthreshold and therefore did not show itself as motor activation (see Figure 22.3, *C,* for comparison and explanation of this principle).[3,65] The major principle here, well articulated by Orem, is that the magnitude of the "effect of sleep on a respiratory neuron is proportional to the amount of nonrespiratory activity in the activity of that neuron," such that the "wakefulness stimulus to breathing is nonrespiratory in form and affects some respiratory neurons more than others."[3] This principle underscores the key importance of tonic drives in the expression of both tonic *and* respiratory neuronal activities.

Respiratory Neuron Activity in REM Sleep

REM sleep is characterized by (1) overall depression of the ventilatory responses to hypercapnia and hypoxia[32]; (2) periods of profound suppression of motor activity in respiratory muscles (e.g., intercostal and pharyngeal)[20,21] and nonrespiratory (i.e., postural) muscles[26]; and (3) occasional periods of slowing of respiratory rate. Periods of sporadic respiratory slowing in REM sleep are associated with increased release of acetylcholine into the pontine reticular formation.[22] It is not correct, however, to consider REM sleep as a state of *overall* depression of central respiratory neurons because, as for most cells in the central nervous system, the activity of brainstem respiratory neurons typically is *greater* in REM sleep than in NREM sleep.[3] As an example, late-inspiratory neurons have increased and advanced activity in REM sleep; that is, cells that discharge in the latter part of inspiration in NREM sleep can be active throughout inspiration in REM sleep (Figure 22.6).[3]

A large degree of variability has been observed in the discharge pattern of respiratory neurons in REM sleep; this variability is associated with tonic and phasic REM sleep events.[3] For example, increased medullary respiratory neuronal activity is associated with increased occurrence of ponto-geniculo-occipital waves, these waves being a defining feature of phasic REM sleep events. This finding suggests that the activity of respiratory neurons in REM sleep is strongly influenced by processes and activities that are peculiar to the neurobiology of the REM sleep state per se, rather than being an intrinsic component of the respiratory network.[3] This notion of significant influences on respiratory network activity by nonrespiratory inputs has similarities to the major influence of tonic drives discussed previously in the context of the wakefulness stimulus to breathing. Together, these concepts highlight that the activity levels of central respiratory neurons and motoneurons are determined by the interaction of their component nonrespiratory *and* respiratory inputs. The component nonrespiratory inputs have major influences on overall respiratory activity and are particularly sensitive to changes in sleep-wake state.

As discussed previously for respiratory motoneurons, this effect of REM sleep in activating central respiratory neurons can lead to periods of increased respiratory rate and respiratory muscle activity. Of importance, and as mentioned, these periods of increased respiratory network activity in REM sleep are intimately related to the neural substrate for the REM sleep state per se. As a consequence, they also are largely *unrelated* to processes of respiratory control, including homeostatic feedback regulation and responses to prevailing blood gas tensions.[3,33,34] This increased activity of central respiratory neurons in REM sleep also is likely to be responsible for producing the periods of increased respiratory rate and higher respiratory muscle activity at times when the normally time-varying inhibition of respiratory motoneurons is briefly weakened or withdrawn (Figures 22.3 and 22.4). REM sleep can lead to periods of heightened diaphragm activity unrelated to prevailing blood gas tensions; this has particular relevance for the clinical observation that hypocapnic central apneas most commonly occur in NREM sleep but can be absent in REM sleep, when breathing is characteristically erratic.[66,67] Figure 22.4 illustrates how this balance of excitatory and inhibitory influences at respiratory motoneurons can underlie the highly variable respiratory activity in REM sleep, including periods of respiratory depression despite activation of central respiratory neurons.

Neuromodulation of Respiratory Neurons across Sleep-Wake States

Unlike the studies performed at respiratory motor pools,[20,21] no studies have been conducted to identify or otherwise characterize the neurochemicals that may mediate the control of respiratory neurons in vivo as a function of sleep-wake states. Nevertheless, it is a reasonable working hypothesis that the neuronal groups involved in the modulation of respiratory motoneurons across sleep-wake states also are likely to affect respiratory neurons. Accordingly, influences from brainstem reticular neurons (probably glutamatergic) are positioned to provide a source of tonic drive to respiratory neurons, with alteration of this influence from wakefulness to NREM and REM sleep.[3,20,21,48] Brainstem reticular neurons generally show decreased activity in NREM sleep compared with wakefulness, and increased activity in REM sleep[3,25]—a pattern similar to the changes in respiratory neuron activity discussed earlier. Electrical stimulation of reticular neurons in the midbrain converts the activity of several respiratory motor nerves or muscles from a sleep-like pattern to one more like wakefulness.[3] One key source of the tonic (nonrespiratory) input to medullary respiratory neurons in the awake state (i.e., the wakefulness stimulus) is thought to arise from brainstem reticular neurons.[3] The source or sources of the drives activating central respiratory neurons in REM sleep, however, have not been determined.

Neurons of the aminergic arousal system (serotonergic, histaminergic, and noradrenergic), and other sleep state–dependent neuronal groups, also are positioned to provide a source of tonic (i.e., nonrespiratory) drive to respiratory neurons across sleep-wake states. However, whether these tonic drives would be excitatory or inhibitory to respiratory neurons depends on the receptor subtypes activated, and on the pre- or postsynaptic location of these receptors (Figures 22.2 and 22.3). This lack of knowledge of the sleep state–dependent neuromodulation of respiratory neurons can be addressed by further research, which also may identify specific pharmacologic approaches that can preserve respiratory neuron activity in sleep and in states of drug-induced brain sedation, so as to minimize respiratory depression. The various brain structures that exert behavioral control of the respiratory system also should be considered as a source of the wakefulness stimulus for breathing.[3] However, it is unknown if this collection of inputs shares the same neurochemicals as the aforementioned inputs from the brainstem reticular neurons and sleep state–dependent neuronal systems.

CLINICAL PEARL

The withdrawal of the wakefulness stimulus to breathing at the transition from wakefulness to sleep is the principal mechanism underlying the major clinical sleep-related breathing disorders. Current evidence identifies neurons of the aminergic arousal system and reticular neurons as providing the key components of this wakefulness stimulus. Withdrawal of this tonic excitatory drive to the muscles of the upper airway is thought to underlie the normal sleep-related increase in upper airway resistance and the hypoventilation, flow limitation, and obstructive sleep apnea observed in susceptible persons (e.g., those with already anatomically narrow upper airways). Stimulation of branches of the hypoglossal nerve has emerged as a therapeutic option in obstructive sleep apnea. Patients with restrictive lung diseases and neuromuscular weakness rely, to various degrees, on the activation of nondiaphragmatic respiratory muscles to help maintain adequate ventilation in the awake state, but this compensation can be reduced or absent in sleep, leading to severe hypoventilation, as the essential tonic excitatory drive that is present in wakefulness is withdrawn. REM sleep mechanisms also lead to inhibition of respiratory motoneurons, thereby explaining the typically increased severity of abnormal breathing events in REM sleep compared with NREM sleep. There is a potential predisposition to obstructive sleep apnea in some persons taking sedative-hypnotics in combination with other $GABA_A$ receptor–modulating neurodepressive drugs such as alcohol and certain general anesthetics.

SUMMARY

Sleep is a state of vulnerability for the respiratory system. Central to the pathogenesis of a variety of sleep-related breathing disorders is the presence of the *wakefulness stimulus* that sustains adequate breathing in wakefulness but whose influence is withdrawn in sleep. This withdrawal of the wakefulness stimulus is the root mechanism underlying the effects of sleep on breathing. Significant developments in the neurophysiologic mechanisms underpinning breathing during wakefulness and sleep have helped identify the neurochemical substrates underlying this wakefulness stimulus. Central to this understanding have been delineation of the neurobiology of sleep, its impact on central respiratory neurons and motoneurons, and the important role of tonic excitatory (nonrespiratory) drives in contributing to overall respiratory system activity. Moreover, in parallel with the realization that sleep onset is not simply the passive withdrawal of wakefulness, breathing during sleep is not only due to the passive withdrawal of the wakefulness stimulus. NREM sleep and REM sleep are fundamentally different neurobiologic states that exert distinct effects on the control of respiratory neurons and motoneurons. Accordingly, the NREM and REM sleep modes pose different problems with breathing during sleep in people with different pathologic conditions. Understanding these mechanisms is necessary for identifying the physiologic basis for the spectrum of sleep-related breathing disorders, their appropriate clinical management, and the potential for new and/or adjunct therapies.

ACKNOWLEDGMENTS

Work on which this chapter is based was supported in part by the Canadian Institutes of Health Research, the Ontario Thoracic Society, and the Canada Foundation for Innovation and the Ontario Research and Development Challenge Fund.

SELECTED READINGS

Fuller PM, Saper CB, Lu J. The pontine REM switch: past and present. *J Physiol.* 2007;584:735–741.

Grace KP, Hughes SW, Horner RL. Identification of the mechanism mediating genioglossus muscle suppression in REM sleep. *Am J Respir Crit Care Med.* 2013;187:311–319.

Horner RL, Grace KP, Wellman A. A resource of potential drug targets and strategic decision-making for obstructive sleep apnoea pharmacotherapy. *Respirology.* 2017;22:861–873.

Horner RL, Hughes SW, Malhotra A. State-dependent and reflex drives to the upper airway: basic physiology with clinical implications. *J Appl Physiol.* 2014;116:325–336.

Luppi PH, Gervasoni D, Verret L, et al. Paradoxical (REM) sleep genesis: the switch from an aminergic-cholinergic to a GABAergic-glutamatergic hypothesis. *J Physiol (Paris).* 2006;100:271–283.

McGinty D, Szymusiak R. The sleep-wake switch: a neuronal alarm clock. *Nat Med.* 2000;6:510–511.

Nguyen G, Postnova S. Progress in modelling of brain dynamics during anaesthesia and the role of sleep-wake circuitry [published online ahead of print, 2021 Jan 5]. *Biochem Pharmacol.* 2021;114388.

Saper CB, Scammell TE, Lu J. Hypothalamic regulation of sleep and circadian rhythms. *Nature.* 2005;437:1257–1263.

Taranto-Montemurro L, Messineo L, Sands SA, et al. The combination of atomoxetine and oxybutynin greatly reduces obstructive sleep apnea severity: a randomized, placebo-controlled, double-blind crossover trial. *Am J Respir Crit Care Med.* 2019;199:1267–1276.

Taranto-Montemurro L, Messineo L, Wellman A. Targeting endotypic traits with medications for the pharmacological treatment of obstructive sleep apnea. A review of the current literature. *J Clin Med.* 2019;8:1846.

A complete reference list can be found online at ExpertConsult.com.

Chapter 23

Respiratory Physiology: Understanding the Control of Ventilation

Danny J. Eckert

Chapter Highlights

- In the absence of respiratory disease, we give little thought to our breathing. Yet it is clearly fundamental to survival.
- Multiple inputs can regulate the rate and depth in which we breathe. These are regulated by feedforward and feedback mechanisms that control blood gas levels within relatively narrow limits to maintain homeostasis.
- Our capacity to alter our breathing is substantial. When metabolic demand decreases during sleep, we can tolerate very low levels of ventilation. However, the major changes that occur to the control of breathing during sleep can cause breathing disruption.
- How ventilation is controlled may affect the pathophysiology of a patient with a sleep breathing disorder and may predict outcome of therapy.
- This chapter outlines the key neuroanatomic inputs to breathing, describes the changes that occur in the control of breathing during sleep, including differences between men and women, and briefly highlights how abnormal control of ventilation can contribute to sleep-disordered breathing.

OVERVIEW OF THE CONTROL OF BREATHING

Breathing is controlled via highly effective feedforward and feedback mechanisms. Conceptually, the functional organization consists of three key elements: (1) brainstem neurons responsible for respiratory pattern generation (*central control*), (2) respiratory muscles that generate force to move airflow in and out of the lungs (*effectors*), and (3) multiple inputs that relay respiratory sensory information (*sensors*) to brainstem respiratory control centers to allow for adjustments according to the prevailing physiologic conditions (Figure 23.1). Breakdown or damage to any one of these components can lead to breathing abnormalities. However, during wakefulness, there are multiple additional inputs that can be activated to maintain breathing and blood gas levels within acceptable levels despite damage to key elements that underlie the control of breathing. For example, there is greater cortical contribution to breathing in healthy older adults and those with chronic obstructive pulmonary disease compared to healthy young people.[1] Accordingly, breathing problems often only emerge (or worsen) during sleep when wakefulness compensatory mechanisms are either downregulated or absent. Control of breathing may affect the pathophysiology in patients with a sleep breathing disorder and may predict outcome of therapy (see Chapter 129).

This chapter outlines the key components that underpin the control of breathing and highlights the major changes that occur during sleep. This chapter is a synthesis of many elements described in Chapters 20, 22, 24, and 25, plus Section 14 on Sleep Breathing Disorders with a perspective of applying the information toward a more comprehensive understanding of breathing and sleep disturbances in humans.

CENTRAL CONTROL OF BREATHING

The precise neuroanatomic locations that contribute to respiratory pattern generation within the brainstem are incompletely understood. The central respiratory control network involves both inspiratory and expiratory neurons. A brief summary of some of the key brainstem sites and their interconnections, based primarily upon animal work, is outlined below.

Central respiratory control and rhythmicity occur within the pons and medulla. Within the medulla, the dorsal and ventral respiratory groups are particularly important (Figure 23.2). The **dorsal respiratory group** contains the nucleus tractus solitaries (nTS). The nTS is a key cardiorespiratory sensory integration site. Afferent information from phrenic, vagus, and peripheral chemoreceptors (via glossopharyngeal nerve) arrive at the nTS. The nTS has numerous outputs to important control-of-breathing centers including to the nearby retrotrapezoid nucleus[2-4] (see Chapters 20 and 22). The ventrolateral region of the nTS is believed to be particularly important for inspiratory-related activity. There are also major projections to other key respiratory control centers within the ventral respiratory group. However, it is not known if there is direct output to respiratory motoneurons.

The pre-Bötzinger complex forms part of the **ventral respiratory group** (Figure 23.2). The pre-Bötzinger complex is believed to be the major putative respiratory pacemaker.[5] This stems from findings that show persistence of respiratory rhythmicity within these cells in minimal slice preparations.[6] In support of the importance of this region to respiratory control, the pre-Bötzinger complex has multiple projections to other known respiratory control sites within the brainstem.[7] Adjacent to the pre-Bötzinger is the Bötzinger complex. This area plays an active role during expiration by inhibiting respiratory motor neurons to modulate the overall motor output. The rostral ventral respiratory group also includes inspiratory premotor neurons such as those located in the nucleus ambiguus. The nucleus ambiguus provides respiratory motor output to the larynx and pharynx via the vagi. The nucleus retroambiguus may also contribute to respiratory rhythm generation.[8,9]

While respiratory rhythm generation neurons predominantly reside within the medulla, the **pontine respiratory group** (previously referred to as the pneumotaxic center) can also importantly contribute to central respiratory control[10,11] (Figure 23.2). The pontine respiratory group includes the nucleus parabrachialis medialis containing expiratory active neurons. The parabrachialis lateralis and the Kölliker-Fuse (upper pons) contain inspiratory neurons. Pontine respiratory group activation can decrease inspiratory activity within the dorsal respiratory group leading to a decrease in inspiratory time. This "inspiratory-expiratory phase transition" can increase breathing frequency.

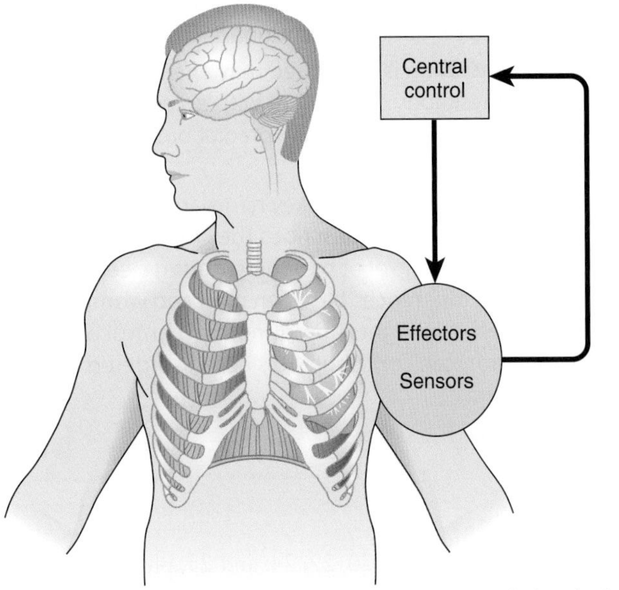

Figure 23.1 Control of breathing overview. Breathing is controlled via feedforward and feedback mechanisms involving central control, effectors, and sensors. Refer to text for further details.

CHEMICAL CONTROL OF BREATHING

Chemical control is the most important regulator of breathing in healthy people during quiet breathing. This is true during both wakefulness and sleep. All cells can modify their activity in response to extreme changes in the chemical environment. However, certain cells are highly sensitive to quite minor changes. These chemically sensitive areas can regulate the control of breathing directly or have projections to central control-of-breathing sites. Accordingly, these groups of cells known as chemoreceptors are fundamentally important to the control of breathing.

Peripheral versus Central

Chemoreceptors are located peripherally and centrally (Figure 23.3). The main peripheral chemoreceptors lie at the bifurcation of the common carotid arteries. The carotid bodies have long been known to respond to changes in oxygen, carbon dioxide, and hydrogen ions.[12] Detection of these stimuli can alter breathing quickly (within one to two breaths). In addition, recent findings show that the carotid bodies respond to a wide range of other stimuli, including potassium, noradrenaline, temperature, glucose, insulin, and immune-related cytokines.[12,13]

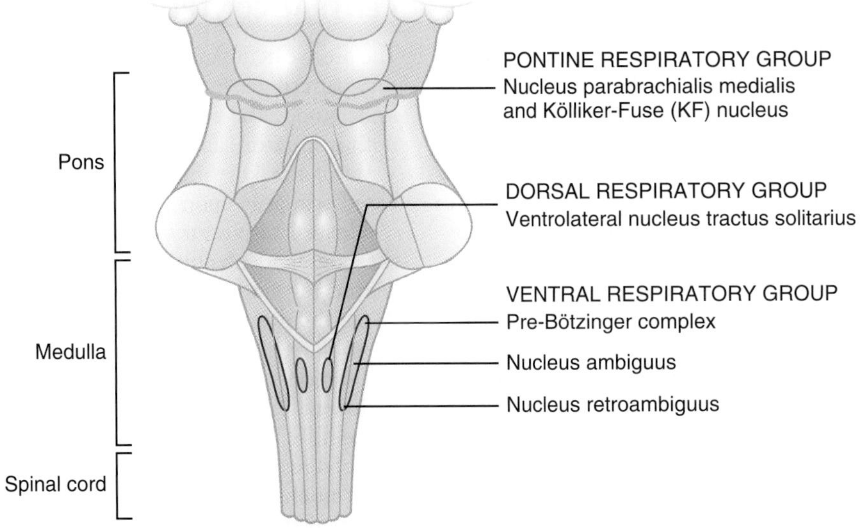

Figure 23.2 Central control of breathing. Major regions involved in the central control of breathing lie within the pontine respiratory group (nucleus parabrachialis medialis and Kölliker-Fuse), the ventral respiratory group (pre-Bötzinger complex, nucleus ambiguous and nucleus retroambiguus), and the dorsal respiratory group (ventrolateral nucleus tractus solitaries). Refer to text for further details. (From Eckert DJ, Roca D, Yim-Yeh S, Malhotra A. Control of breathing. In: Kryger M, ed. *Atlas of Clinical Sleep Medicine*. Vol 2. 2nd ed. Elsevier Saunders; 2014:45–52.)

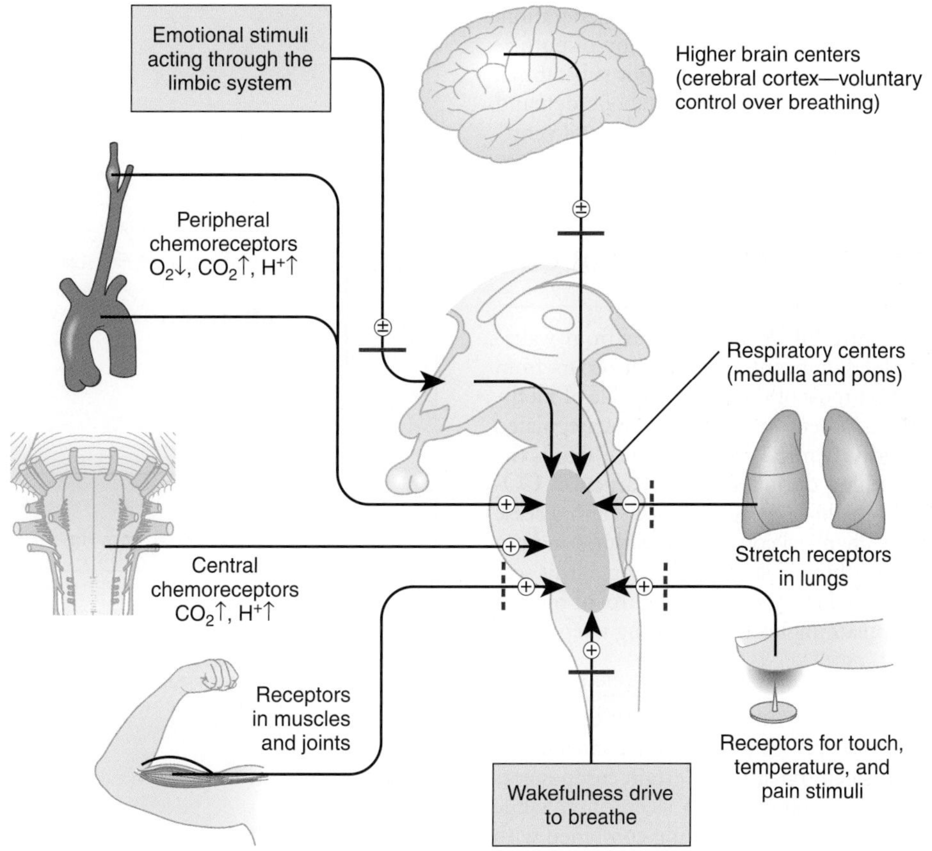

Figure 23.3 Inputs to breathing. Schematic of the multiple inputs that are capable of regulating breathing. During sleep many of these inputs are either substantially diminished (*dashed red lines*) or absent (*solid red lines*). Thus, the predominant inputs to breathing during sleep are the chemoreceptors, which are also downregulated and affected by state. *Note:* For simplicity, voluntary control of breathing is shown to act via the respiratory centers. However, it is not known if this is the case or whether voluntary control acts directly upon the respiratory motoneurons. Refer to text for further details. (Modified from Kehlmann GB, Eckert DJ. Central sleep apnea due to a medical condition not Cheyne Stokes. In: Kushida CA, ed. *Encyclopedia of Sleep.* Vol 1. 1st ed. Elsevier; 2013:244–52; Eckert DJ, Roca D, Yim-Yeh S, Malhotra A. Control of breathing. In: Kryger M, ed. *Atlas of Clinical Sleep Medicine.* Vol 2. 2nd ed. Elsevier Saunders; 2014:45–52.)

Repetitive exposure to hypoxia can cause plasticity within the carotid bodies.[13] The changes that occur can contribute to disease pathology, including increased propensity for breathing instability during sleep.[12,13] In addition to the carotid bodies, the nearby aortic bodies are also capable of responding to changes in oxygen and other chemical stimuli. Although the peripheral chemoreceptors are important for moment-to-moment modulation of breathing, the most powerful input to breathing during quiet wakefulness is from the central chemoreceptors.

Located on the ventral surface of the medulla, adjacent to the ventral respiratory group, is the retrotrapezoid nucleus. This region is particularly important for central chemoreception.[14,15] The retrotrapezoid nucleus has major projections to key respiratory control centers, including to the nTS within the dorsal respiratory group.[2,3] The central chemoreceptors respond to pCO_2 via changes in the pH of the extracellular fluid. CO_2 diffuses across the blood-brain barrier to increase hydrogen ion concentration in the cerebrospinal fluid. Thus, compared to the relatively fast-responding peripheral chemoreceptors, central chemoreceptors can take up to a minute to respond to changes in chemical stimuli. As discussed later, chemoreceptor response delays are critically important in mediating cyclic breathing instability during sleep.[16-18]

Although the peripheral and central chemoreceptors are anatomically distinct and have different response characteristics, recent findings indicate complex interconnectivity.[12,13,19,20] Specifically, the activity of the central chemoreceptors is critically dependent on the activity of the peripheral chemoreceptors and vice versa. This link has been described as a "hyperadditive model."[12,13,19,20]

OTHER INPUTS TO BREATHING

In addition to input from the chemoreceptors, there are other important inputs and sensors that can contribute to the rate and depth at which we breathe (Figure 23.3). Receptors in the limb muscles and joints can respond to movement to increase minute ventilation. Similarly, when receptors responsible for touch, temperature, and pain are stimulated, breathing increases. There is also an independent stimulus to breathing known as the wakefulness drive to breathe.[21] Conversely, overinflation or excess lung stretch can inhibit minute ventilation via the Hering-Breuer reflex.[22] Other inputs can either stimulate or inhibit breathing. These include limbic system input in response to emotional stimuli or cortical control.[1] It remains uncertain, however, if voluntary override of breathing acts indirectly via changes in central respiratory pattern generation, directly via phrenic motoneurons, or a combination of both.[23] Nonetheless, our capacity to alter our breathing is substantial. As highlighted later in the chapter, when metabolic demand decreases during sleep, we can tolerate very low levels of ventilation (less than 5 L/min). Conversely, during intense exercise, ventilation can increase to over 200 L/min.

STATE-RELATED CHANGES IN THE CONTROL OF BREATHING

Major changes in the control of breathing occur from wakefulness to sleep. The most significant change that occurs from wakefulness to sleep is that most of the inputs capable of modifying breathing are either absent or markedly downregulated (Figure 23.3). Accordingly, chemical control of breathing is the dominant driver of breathing during sleep. In particular, CO_2 is a critical mediator of breathing during sleep. Certain disease states adversely affect the chemical control of breathing and can cause sleep-disordered breathing in susceptible people. This section outlines key state-related changes in the control of breathing that underlie cyclic breathing instability during sleep.

Sleep Onset

Respiratory control is inherently unstable during the transition from wakefulness to sleep.[24] Several factors contribute to respiratory instability at sleep transition. Certain components of respiratory control change rapidly with sleep onset while others require more time. Mismatch in timing combined with downregulation in important respiratory control mechanisms underlie breathing disturbances during the sleep-onset period. Indeed, brief breathing stoppages at sleep onset are very common, even in otherwise healthy people.

Mechanistically, the wakefulness drive to breathe and behavioral influences cease with sleep onset.[25] Movement and excitatory input to breathe from other external sensors become minimal or absent. Chemosensitivity also decreases[26] (Figures 23.3 and 23.4). Accordingly, respiratory pump muscle activity is reduced and minute ventilation decreases.[27] There is also an abrupt reduction in upper airway muscle tone and protective reflexes with sleep onset.[27-31] These changes contribute to increased upper airway resistance.[29] The timing and magnitude of these changes vary between individuals. Rapid withdrawal of excitatory drive to breathe in and of itself can cause respiratory events resulting from the delay required to elicit a compensatory response from the chemoreceptors.[32] Sleep apnea patients appear to be more prone to major reductions in the wakefulness drive to breathe compared to healthy controls.[33] Thus, sleep onset affects all components of respiratory control and can cause major "state instability."

Stable Sleep

The downregulation or absence of most excitatory inputs to breathing that occurs with sleep onset remains during stable sleep. Respiratory load compensation is also reduced during stable sleep compared to wakefulness.[34] Thus, minute ventilation decreases during stable sleep as compared to the wakefulness level, and chemical input dominates the control of breathing. However, downregulation in chemosensitivity is not isolated to the sleep-onset period. Ventilatory responses to hypoxia are reduced during N2 and slow wave sleep (N3) compared to wakefulness such that major reductions in oxygen are required to stimulate breathing during sleep (Figure 23.4).[35-37] Accordingly, CO_2 is the main regulator

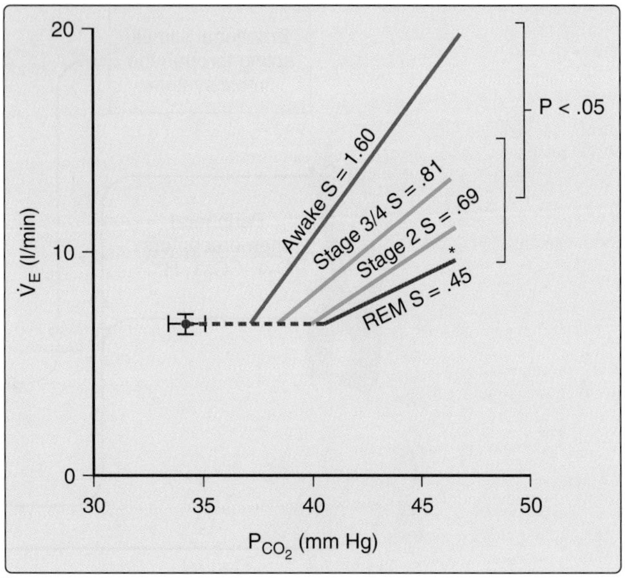

Figure 23.4 Mean minute ventilation/$PETco_2$ relationships for all 12 subjects indicating the mean ± SEM resting minute ventilation/CO_2 point in the awake state. The hypercapnic ventilatory response is reduced in Stages 2 and 3/4 compared with that in wakefulness and is further decreased in REM sleep. $\dot{V}_E$, Expired ventilation; *, $p < .05$ REM different from Stage 2 and 3/4 sleep. (From Douglas NJ, White DP, Weil JV, et al. Hypercapnic ventilatory response in sleeping adults. *Am Rev Resp Dis.* 1982;126[5]:758–62.)

of breathing during sleep. However, ventilatory responses to hypercapnia are also reduced during sleep compared to wakefulness, albeit to a lesser extent than in hypoxia.[38] Consequently, we can tolerate lower levels of minute ventilation and higher levels of CO_2 during sleep compared to wakefulness. Typically, depending on the prevailing metabolic conditions, minute ventilation is reduced by 1 to 2 L/min, and partial pressure of carbon dioxide in the blood ($PaCO_2$) increases by 3 to 8 mm Hg during stable sleep compared to wakefulness[39] (Figure 23.5, *A*).

In the absence of respiratory disease, breathing is quite regular during stable non–rapid eye movement (NREM) sleep. However, rapid eye movement (REM) sleep is characterized by breathing irregularity. Many regions within the medulla that contribute to central control-of-breathing have increased activation during REM compared to NREM sleep.[40] In humans, breathing frequency increases, and major variations in breath-to-breath tidal volume occur. Active eye movements during REM sleep are associated with inhibition of upper airway dilator muscle activity and tidal volume.[34,41] Protective upper airway reflexes are also inhibited.[42] Thus, obstructive apnea is common during REM sleep.

Brief Awakenings (Arousal from Sleep)

Brief cortical arousals from sleep lasting less than 15 seconds occur between 10 to 20 times per hour in healthy individuals. Arousal frequency increases with age.[43] Arousals can occur spontaneously or with a sleep disorder such as sleep apnea or periodic leg movement disorder. Historically, arousals were believed to be essential for reopening the upper airway during obstructive breathing events.[44] Indeed, arousal can be beneficial in certain circumstances to rapidly resolve blood gas disturbances and alleviate the increased work of breathing during flow-limited breathing.[45] However, although the initial arousals associated with physiologic changes may be beneficial for

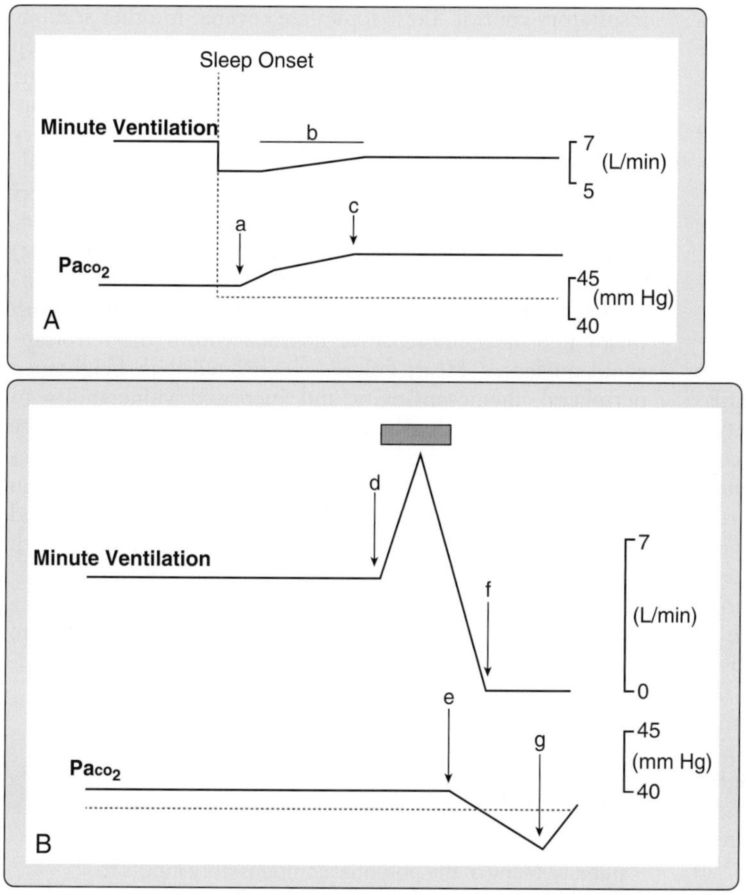

Figure 23.5 Sleep state changes to the control of breathing. **A,** Schema showing typical changes in minute ventilation and $PaCO_2$ from wakefulness to sleep. At sleep onset (*dashed vertical line*), there is a rapid reduction in minute ventilation (from 7 to 5 L/min). There is delay between the reduction in ventilation and changes in $Paco_2$ (sleep onset to point *a*). As CO_2 rises, upper airway muscles may be recruited and minute ventilation may increase somewhat (period *b*) until a new eucapnic sleeping ventilation (5.5 L/min) and $Paco_2$ (45 mm Hg) are reached (point *c*). The *horizontal red line* represents the theoretical apnea threshold (in this case, 39 mm Hg). **B,** Schematic representation of a central apnea following an arousal from sleep. At point *d*, a brief arousal from sleep occurs (arousal duration represented by the *grey box*). Hyperventilation occurs in association with reintroduction of wakefulness stimuli (ventilatory response to arousal). The hyperventilation lowers $PaCO_2$. However, a delay between the change in ventilation and the change in $PaCO_2$ is present (point *d* to point *e*). As the patient returns to sleep, the reduction in $PaCO_2$, caused by the ventilatory response to arousal, falls below the apnea threshold (which, in this example, is very close to the eucapnic sleeping $PaCO_2$ level), and apnea occurs (point *f*). The apnea leads to an increase in $PaCO_2$ until either an arousal occurs and the cycle is repeated, or the apnea threshold is crossed and breathing resumes. Refer to text for further details. (From Kehlmann GB, Eckert DJ. Central sleep apnea due to a medical condition not Cheyne Stokes. In: Kushida CA, ed. *Encyclopedia of Sleep*. Vol 1. 1st ed. Elsevier; 2013:244–52.)

respiratory homeostasis, the rapid switch from sleep to wakefulness and the subsequent resumption of sleep can be highly destabilizing for respiratory control.[45] The extent to which arousals destabilize breathing and contribute to central or obstructive breathing events is dependent on two key features: (1) an individual's threshold for arousal (*the arousal threshold*) and (2) the ventilatory response to arousal.

Arousal Threshold

Whether an arousal occurs spontaneously, because of a periodic leg movement, or in association with a respiratory disturbance, an individual who wakes up easily (*low arousal threshold*) may be susceptible to sleep-state breathing instability. Specifically, a predisposition to sleep-onset breathing instability and a low arousal threshold may cause repetitive breathing disturbances as the individual oscillates between wakefulness and sleep.[16] Approximately one-third of people with obstructive sleep apnea or more in certain patient populations (e.g., non-obese people with sleep apnea) arouse to modest levels of respiratory stimuli (negative airway pressure less than 15 cm H_2O).[45-47] This is likely to contribute to their sleep-disordered breathing.[45] Increasing the arousal threshold in patients with a low respiratory arousal threshold can stabilize breathing.[48] Indeed, although the precise mechanisms remain uncertain, the arousal threshold and upper airway muscle activity increase in deeper stages of sleep, and sleep-disordered breathing severity decreases.[49-51] However, it is not known if deeper stages of sleep are intrinsically more stable in terms of respiratory control or if breathing stability allows sleep to deepen.

Ventilatory Response to Arousal

In much the same way that rapid changes in respiratory control occur during sleep onset, arousal from sleep causes a rapid change in the homeostatic control of breathing. As highlighted, during stable sleep we can tolerate lower levels of minute ventilation and higher levels of CO_2 compared to wakefulness (approximately 3 to 8 mm Hg higher). With arousal, the wakefulness chemical control of breathing is reinstated and the increased levels of CO_2 that were tolerated during sleep suddenly become excessive. Upper airway motoneurons are activated, and sleep-related upper airway resistance is rapidly resolved.[52] The wakefulness drive to breathe is also reintroduced. Accordingly, arousal from sleep is associated with a rapid increase in breathing. The magnitude of the ventilatory response to arousal is dependent on the integrative effects of each of the previously mentioned factors and may be further augmented by an independent wakefulness reflex.[53] Indeed, the magnitude of the ventilatory response to arousal varies substantially between individuals.[54] As outlined later, upon the resumption of sleep, the prior ventilatory response to arousal can drive $PaCO_2$ levels below a critical level known as the apnea threshold[55] (see the following section and Figure 23.5*B*).

APNEA THRESHOLD

There are multiple compensatory mechanisms that oppose breathing cessation even during major reductions in $Paco_2$ during wakefulness (Figure 23.3). However, during sleep this is not the case. Specifically, if $Paco_2$ falls below a critical level during sleep, breathing ceases. The apnea threshold ranges between 2 and 6 mm Hg below the stable sleep $Paco_2$ level. Thus, the apnea threshold is similar to the wakefulness $Paco_2$ level[56,57] (see the 2005 journal article by Dempsey[58] for details). The difference between the wakefulness $Paco_2$ level and the apnea threshold is often termed the "CO_2 reserve." The reduction in $Paco_2$ required to cause apnea is importantly dependent on the peripheral chemoreceptors.[59] Schematic examples outlining important state-related changes in the control of breathing are displayed in Figure 23.5.

Loop Gain

As outlined in this chapter, there are multiple inputs that contribute to the control of breathing. Loop gain is one approach to conceptualize and quantify the overall sensitivity of the ventilatory control system (see also Chapters 22 and 25 for respiration in high altitude). Specifically, the gain of the ventilatory control feedback loop can be quantified as the ratio of a ventilatory response to a ventilatory disturbance.[16,60] Loop gain comprises three major elements: (1) plant gain (*the efficiency of breathing to remove CO_2, which is determined by the properties of the lungs, blood, and body tissues*), (2) mixing and circulation delays (*the time required for a change in alveolar CO_2 to mix with the blood in the heart and the arteries before reaching the chemoreceptors*), and (3) controller gain (*the sensitivity of the chemoreceptors*). Given that CO_2 is the predominant modifier of ventilatory control during sleep, determining the loop gain during sleep provides important insight into the overall sensitivity of the ventilatory control system and allows for comparisons to be made among individuals and patient groups. Accordingly, techniques have been developed to quantify the steady state loop gain during sleep.[61-63] If certain elements that contribute to loop gain are abnormal (e.g., plant or controller gains), breathing instability can occur. Circulation delay is an integral component of breathing instability: without it, cyclic breathing would not occur. However, although increasing circulation delay increases the length and duration of breathing instability, increased circulation delay alone does not cause breathing instability.

Sex Differences

Sleep-disordered breathing is more common in men than in women. Respiratory control differences between the sexes may contribute to this difference, at least in part. Progesterone is a respiratory stimulant, and sleep-disordered breathing is more common in women following menopause. However, although ventilatory responses to CO_2 and hypoxia vary throughout the menstrual cycle, ventilatory responses during sleep to chemical stimuli do not appear to be systematically different between the sexes.[64,65] Consistent with these earlier observations, overall steady state loop gain is not different between men and women.[66,67] However, in accordance with increased vulnerability to breathing instability, important differences in breathing during sleep onset, the ventilatory response to arousal, and the apnea threshold have been observed between men and women.[24,68-70] Whether men have systematically lower arousal thresholds remains unclear. Such differences may explain sex-related phenotypes in sleep apnea patients; females have lower loop gain, less airway collapsibility, and lower arousal threshold in NREM sleep than males.[71]

CLINICAL MANIFESTATIONS

Altered respiratory control can contribute to various forms of sleep-disordered breathing. There are many causes of abnormal respiratory control. These topics are covered in other sections of this book (Chapters 65 and 66, and Section 14, Sleep Breathing Disorders) and have been the focus of comprehensive reviews.[16-18,72-74] Briefly, an abnormality in one or more of the components that importantly contribute to respiratory control as outlined in this chapter can cause breathing instability during sleep. Damage to central respiratory control centers or drugs that impair its function (e.g., certain brain tumors, Chiari type I malformation, multiple sclerosis, and morphine) can directly affect central respiratory control.[16-18,75-77] Congenital central hypoventilation syndrome is associated with major loss of chemosensitive neurons within the retrotrapezoid nucleus.[17] Heart failure is associated with heightened peripheral chemosensitivity and increased vulnerability to crossing the apnea threshold. Conversely, patients with obesity hypoventilation syndrome have blunted ventilatory responses to chemical stimuli and experience sustained hypoventilation and major blood gas disturbances during sleep. Thus, high and low loop gain can be problematic and can contribute to both obstructive and central breathing instability during sleep.[72] Indeed, approximately one-third of obstructive sleep apnea patients have abnormally high loop gain, which is likely to importantly contribute to the pathogenesis of their obstructive apnea.[46,78]

CLINICAL PEARL

Sleep is a particularly vulnerable time for respiratory control stability. Many of the potential compensatory inputs to breathing are markedly diminished or absent during sleep. Accordingly, regardless of the underlying cause, abnormality in one or more of the components that importantly contribute to respiratory control can cause or worsen sleep-disordered breathing. The ensuing sleep-related breathing instability depends on the extent to which the respiratory control system is altered and which components of the respiratory control system are involved.

SUMMARY AND CONCLUSIONS

Understanding the control of ventilation provides important insight into the causes of various forms of sleep-disordered breathing. Ventilatory control is regulated via highly effective feedforward and feedback mechanisms that control blood gas levels within relatively narrow limits to maintain homeostasis. There are multiple inputs that regulate ventilatory control. While these processes are predominantly under autonomic control, we can also modulate our breathing voluntarily.

The dorsal, ventral, and pontine respiratory groups are key regions within the medulla and pons responsible for central respiratory control. Central (e.g., retrotrapezoid nucleus) and peripheral (e.g., carotid bodies) chemoreceptors provide essential sensory information to modify breathing. Other sensory systems can also provide input to alter the rate and depth in which we breathe. However, most are either downregulated or absent during sleep. Accordingly, the chemical control of breathing (in particular CO_2) is the dominant input to ventilatory control during sleep. Sleep onset is particularly destabilizing for ventilatory control stability. Arousal from sleep and high loop gain can lead to marked fluctuations in CO_2

and breathing cessation during sleep if the apnea threshold is crossed. Abnormalities in one or more of the components that contribute to ventilatory control can contribute to both central and obstructive breathing events during sleep.

ACKNOWLEDGMENT

Danny J. Eckert is supported by a Senior Research Fellowship from the National Health and Medical Research Council of Australia (1116942) and an Investigator Grant (1196261). The author has no conflicts to declare in relation to the topic of this manuscript.

SELECTED READINGS

Chowdhuri S, Badr MS. Control of Ventilation in Health and Disease. *Chest.* 2017;151:917–929.

Coughlin K, Davies GM, Gillespie MB. Phenotypes of Obstructive Sleep Apnea. *Otolaryngol Clin North Am.* 2020;53(3):329–338. https://doi.org/10.1016/j.otc.2020.02.010.

Dempsey JA, Smith CA, Blain GM, Xie A, Gong Y, Teodorescu M. Role of central/peripheral chemoreceptors and their interdependence in the pathophysiology of sleep apnea. *Adv Exp Med Biol.* 2012;758:343–349.

Dempsey JA, Smith CA. Pathophysiology of human ventilatory control. *Eur Respir J.* 2014;44:495–512.

Dempsey JA. Crossing the apnoeic threshold: causes and consequences. *Exp Physiol.* 2005;90:13–24.

Eckert DJ, Jordan AS, Merchia P, Malhotra A. Central sleep apnea: pathophysiology and treatment. *Chest.* 2007;131:595–607.

Eckert DJ, Roca D, Yim-Yeh S, Malhotra A. Control of Breathing. In: Kryger M, ed. *Atlas of Clinical Sleep Medicine.* 2nd ed. Vol 2. Philadelphia: Elsevier Saunders; 2014:45–52.

Finnsson E, Ólafsdóttir GH, Loftsdóttir DL, et al. A scalable method of determining physiological endotypes of sleep apnea from a polysomnographic sleep study. *Sleep.* 2021;44(1):zsaa168. doi:10.1093/sleep/zsaa168.

Guyenet PG, Stornetta RL, Souza G, Abbott SBG, Shi Y, Bayliss DA. The Retrotrapezoid Nucleus: Central Chemoreceptor and Regulator of Breathing Automaticity. *Trends Neurosci.* 2019;42:807–824.

Javaheri S, Dempsey JA. Central sleep apnea. *Compr Physiol.* 2013;3:141–163.

Khoo MC, Kronauer RE, Strohl KP, Slutsky AS. Factors inducing periodic breathing in humans: a general model. *J Appl Physiol.* 1982;53:644–659.

Kumar P, Prabhakar NR. Peripheral chemoreceptors: function and plasticity of the carotid body. *Compr Physiol.* 2012;2:141–219.

Won CHJ, Reid M, Sofer T, et al. Sex differences in obstructive sleep apnea phenotypes, the multi-ethnic study of atherosclerosis. *Sleep.* 2020;43(5):zsz274. https://doi.org/10.1093/sleep/zsz274.

A complete reference list can be found online at ExpertConsult.com.

Chapter 24

Physiology of Upper and Lower Airways

Annie C. Lajoie; Raphael Heinzer; Frédéric Sériès

Chapter Highlights

- Sleep has an impact on ventilation and gas exchange mediated through an increase in airway resistance and a decrease in lung volume and thoracopulmonary compliance.
- Upper airway stability can be altered during sleep, especially during the rapid eye movement (REM) stage.
- When upper airway anatomy is compromised, these sleep-related effects can trigger obstructive disordered breathing.
- Evaluation of the location and pattern of collapse of the upper airway during sleep has emerged as an important tool in predicting response to hypoglossal nerve stimulation therapy of obstructive sleep apnea.

Some of the earliest clinical investigations in sleep-disordered breathing recognized that abnormal upper airway physiology played a critical role.[1] One dimension in phenotyping patients with these disorders is to evaluate the upper airway to help make management decisions (see Chapter 129).[2] Thus an understanding of the normal and abnormal function of the upper airway is paramount.

The main purpose of breathing is to provide oxygen to all tissues of the body and to eliminate carbon dioxide resulting from cell metabolism. This is achieved through continuous gas exchange between inspired and exhaled air and the blood in the pulmonary circulation. After blood coming from the right side of the heart has been loaded with oxygen, it passes to the left side of the heart, which sends it to every part of the body through the arterial system. Different organs then take up oxygen from the arterial blood and remove carbon dioxide. Blood loaded with carbon dioxide travels through the venous system to reach the pulmonary circulation, where carbon dioxide passively diffuses through the alveolocapillary membrane into the airway, whence it is exhaled. Survival depends on the integrity of this physiologic process, and death can occur if respiratory function stops for more than a few minutes. Maintenance of normal arterial blood gases involves several physiologic systems—control of breathing, thoracopulmonary mechanics, circulatory components, and blood transport—that are intimately linked to one another. This chapter considers only the mechanical properties of the chest and the upper and lower airways, which influence ventilation during sleep (Box 24.1).

ANATOMY AND PHYSIOLOGY

The upper airway, which includes the nasal cavities, pharynx, and larynx, moistens and warms inspired air and conducts it to the trachea and lungs. Although breathing is possible through either the nose or the mouth, nasal breathing is the physiologic breathing route allowing for humidification and filtration of inspired air. Upper airway muscles, which help maintain upper airway patency, are also involved in phonation and swallowing. A very subtle regulation of vocal cord tension also allows humans to speak and sing during exhalation. It is hypothesized that the evolution of speech, which requires substantial mobility of the pharynx, led to a loss of the rigid support of the upper airway, which makes it more collapsible in humans than in most mammals. The lower airway includes the trachea and the lungs (bronchi and alveoli). Thin blood vessels lining the alveoli, the capillaries, allow gas exchange between inspired air and blood.

The rib cage provides protection for the lungs and allows them to change volume from a minimum of approximately 1.5 L to a maximum of 6 to 8 L, depending on the height, sex, and ethnicity of the person.[3] The ribs articulate with the transverse processes of the thoracic vertebrae and have flexible anterior cartilaginous connections with the sternum. The inner aspects of each hemithorax are lined with parietal pleura, and the lungs are covered by thin visceral pleura. The virtual space between the visceral and the parietal pleura contains a few milliliters of lubricating fluid, which allows these layers to slide against each other easily during ventilation. Owing to the proximity of the esophagus to the pleural tissue, the esophageal pressure varies in parallel with the changes in pleural pressure and often is used to quantify respiratory efforts.

Respiratory Muscles

The diaphragm is the main muscle of respiration. It is a dome-shaped muscle that separates the thoracic and abdominal cavities. The diaphragm is innervated by the phrenic nerves. During inspiration, the neural outflow coming from the central respiratory centers leads to diaphragm contraction; the shortening of those muscle fibers flattens the diaphragm, with consequent loss of its dome shape, thereby increasing

BOX 24.1 SOME DEFINITIONS USED IN RESPIRATORY MECHANICS

Chest or Lung Compliance
Change in volume per change in pressure: $\Delta V/\Delta P$

Minute Ventilation
Tidal volume times respiratory rate: $V_T \times RR$

Laminar Flow
Change in pressure per resistance: $\Delta P/R$

Turbulent Flow
Pressure drop along the airway is proportional to flow and its square values: $\Delta P \propto aV + bV^2$ (V is air flow, and a and b are constants)

intrathoracic volume. Intercostal muscles also can increase the intrathoracic volume by elevating ribs and increasing the anteroposterior diameter of the thorax (Figure 24.1). Accessory breathing muscles such as the scalene or sternocleidomastoid muscles are not active during normal breathing, but they can be recruited during an effort or in the presence of thoracopulmonary disorders.

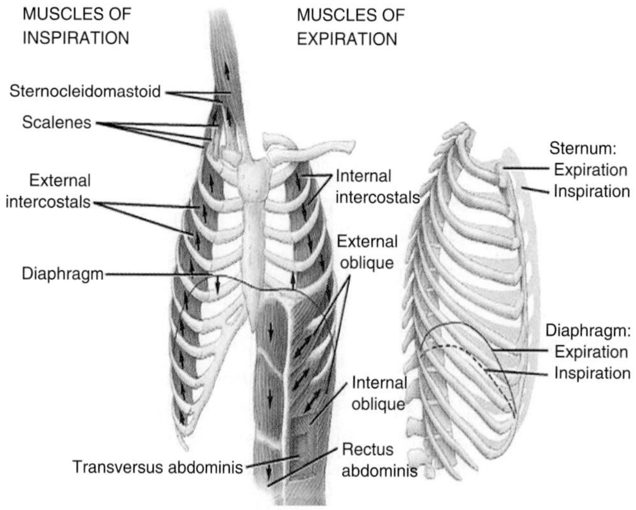

Figure 24.1 Drawing of inspiratory and expiratory muscles from abdomen to neck. The main inspiratory muscles include the diaphragm and external intercostal muscles. Accessory inspiratory muscles include the scalene and sternocleidomastoid muscles. Expiration usually is a passive process. However, internal intercostals and abdominal muscles are recruited during forced expiration. (Reproduced from Netter FH. *Atlas of Human Anatomy.* Saunders; 2006.)

Elastic Forces and Lung Volumes

An isolated lung (not surrounded by the thoracic cage) will tend to contract until it eventually collapses, owing to the large amount of elastic fibers inside the lung tissue. The lung is thus submitted to a constant recoil force. By contrast, the isolated thoracic cage tends to expand to a volume approximately 1 L more than its natural, in vivo, resting position. In a relaxed subject with an open airway and no airflow, the inward elastic recoil of the lungs will be balanced by the outward resting force coming from the thoracic cage. *Lung compliance* or *distensibility* is defined as the change in lung volume per unit change in transmural pressure gradient:

$$\text{Compliance} = \Delta V / \Delta P$$

where V is volume and P is pressure.

The lung volume in the natural resting end-expiratory position is called the *functional residual capacity* (FRC). *Total lung capacity* (TLC) is reached when the thoracic cage and lungs are fully expanded (maximal inspiratory effort). *Residual volume* (RV) represents the volume remaining in the lungs at the end of a forced expiration. *Vital capacity* (VC) is the maximum amount of air that can be expelled after the lungs have been fully inflated. *Tidal volume* (V_T) is the volume of air inspired or expired during each quiet breathing cycle (Figure 24.2). The typical V_T value is 500 mL, but it can dramatically increase during exercise. Only approximately two-thirds of inspired air participates in oxygen and carbon dioxide exchange, because the volume corresponding to upper airway, trachea, and bronchi does not contribute to gas exchange; this area is the *dead space* of the respiratory tract.[3]

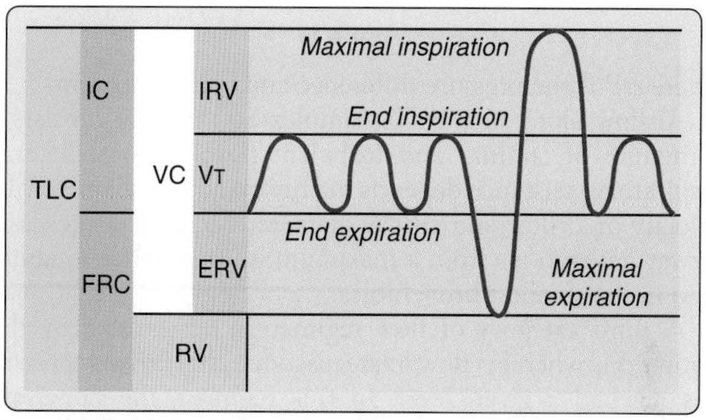

Figure 24.2 Schematic illustration of the static lung volumes determined by a spirometer in which airflow velocity does not play a role. Lung capacity is estimated by the sum of two or more lung volume subdivisions. ERV, Expiratory reserve volume; FRC, functional residual capacity; IC, inspiratory capacity; IRV, inspiratory reserve volume; RV, residual volume; TLC, total lung capacity; VC, vital capacity; V_T, tidal volume. (Reproduced with permission from American Association for Respiratory Care. AARC clinical practice guideline: static lung volumes: 2001 revision & update. *Respir Care.* 2001;46:531–9.)

Breathing Cycle and Minute Ventilation

Air always flows from an area of higher pressure to one of lower pressure to achieve equilibrium. The pressure inside the pleural space is generated by the forces developed during inspiration and expiration and is proportional to the amount of respiratory effort. The pleural pressure represents the driving pressure. During inspiration, the diaphragm and intercostal muscles contract and the pressure inside the thorax decreases below the atmospheric pressure (negative transpulmonary pressure gradient). This gradient is responsible for air movement from the nose (atmosphere) to the tracheobronchial tree down to the alveoli. During expiration, the inspiratory muscles relax, making resting expiration a passive phenomenon. However, during active expiration (volitional or during exercise), the contraction of abdominal and external intercostal muscles enhances the changes in intrathoracic pressure. This causes an abrupt increase in pleural pressure to a less-negative value, with a corresponding rise in alveolar pressure by the same amount. These changes generate a positive pressure gradient from the alveoli to the mouth, which is responsible for exhalation. Lung and chest volume decrease as air flows out, causing lung recoil pressure to fall until a new equilibrium is reached at FRC.

The respiratory rate, or breathing frequency, represents the number of breaths per minute. Average respiratory rate in a healthy adult subject at rest is approximately 12 (range, 10 to 18) breaths/min. Minute ventilation ($\dot{V}$) can be calculated using the following equation:

$$\dot{V} = RR \times V_T$$

where RR is the respiratory rate and V_T is the tidal volume. During quiet breathing, the minute ventilation is approximately 6 L/min but can rise up to 180 L/min during exercise.

Resistance

Different profiles of airflow may be observed inside the airways, depending on airway anatomy (in accordance with the specific division of the tracheobronchial tree) and mechanical properties (caliber, shape, collapsibility) of the airway structures and on the amount of driving pressure. With a constant laminar flow regimen, the resistance is directly proportional to the pressure gradient along the tube:

$$Flow = \Delta P/R$$

where ΔP is the pressure difference and R is the resistance. Airflow is described as *turbulent* when the pressure drop along the airway is proportional to flow and its square values:

$$\Delta P \propto aV + bV^2$$

where ΔP is the pressure difference and V is the airflow.

Airflow along airways is complex and usually consists of a mixture of laminar and turbulent flow. In normal lungs, respiratory resistance depends mainly on airway diameter. The velocity of airflow and airway diameter decrease in successive airway generations from a maximum in the trachea to almost zero in the smallest bronchioles.

A third category of flow regimen is represented by flow limitation, whereby flow plateaus once the driving pressure has reached a given level. In this regimen, the flow value depends on the difference between intraluminal and extraluminal pressures, as well as on the compliance of the airway. Flow limitation can occur during expiration when the pressure generated by expiratory forces increases intraluminal pressure and induces an external compression of the airway walls at the same time. This pattern of flow is, however, more likely to be seen during inspiration at the level of the upper airway. Upper airway resistance depends on nasal and pharyngeal anatomy, position of the vocal cords, and lung volume (see later in this chapter).

EFFECTS OF BODY POSITION AND OBESITY ON LUNG VOLUMES

In an awake, normal, and healthy subject, a reduction in FRC and TLC is observed in the supine position in comparison with the upright position, both in adults[4] and in children.[5] This reduction is thought to be due to an increase in intrathoracic blood volume or to the gravitational effect of abdominal contents pushing the relaxed diaphragm into a more rostral position.[6] The change in diaphragm position reduces its ability to contract, as suggested by a decreased maximal inspiratory pressure in the supine posture relative to that in the upright and sitting positions.[7] Moreover, this restrictive defect in lung volume increases the work of breathing and deteriorates gas exchange by decreasing the ventilation-perfusion ratio in the dependent parts of the lungs. Decreased lung volume also can increase upper airway resistance by reducing the caudal traction of the mediastinum and trachea on the pharyngeal walls, making them more collapsible during inspiration (as discussed later in the chapter).[8]

In obese subjects, a restrictive defect in lung volume is also observed in the sitting position.[9,10] A further small decrease of 70 to 80 mL from approximately 2.4 L (for an average-sized man) in FRC and TLC occurs when obese subjects lie supine.[4] In view of the effects of abdominal volume on lung function in sitting obese subjects, a greater reduction in lung volume with adoption of the supine position compared with that in lean persons might be expected. However, a lesser decline in FRC and TLC in obese subjects in the supine position has been documented.[4,6] One possible explanation is that in sitting obese subjects, the diaphragm is already shifted in a more rostral position and cannot move much farther in the supine position. Two experimental studies also suggest a possible protective or adaptive mechanism against large changes in end-expiratory lung volume during wakefulness[11] and sleep.[12]

Maximal minute ventilation, expiratory reserve volume, FVC, and, to a lesser extent, forced expiratory volume in 1 second (FEV_1) also are affected by obesity.[13] The estimated reduction of forced vital capacity (FVC) is 17.4 mL/kg weight gain for men and 10.6 mL/kg weight gain for women.[14] Men show more impairment of FVC with weight gain than women, possibly because of differential patterns of fat deposition: waist circumference is negatively associated with FVC and FEV_1. On average, a 1-cm increase in waist circumference was associated with a 13-mL reduction in FVC.[15] All of these effects observed with change from the upright to the supine position and in obese persons may contribute to the exacerbation of respiratory disturbances in the presence of sleep-disordered breathing, as described Chapters 137 and 138.

EFFECTS OF SLEEP ON LUNG VOLUME

A modest but significant decrease in FRC occurs during sleep in most healthy subjects. FRC decreases by approximately 200 mL in stage 2 non–rapid eye movement (NREM) sleep and by 300 mL during slow wave sleep (SWS) and rapid eye movement (REM) sleep when measured with a helium dilution technique, in comparison with normal FRC obtained with the subject awake (approximately 2.4 L for an average-size man).[16] When plethysmography is used to measure differences in lung volume, a 440- to 500-mL decrease in lung volume has been reported in NREM sleep (stages 2 to SWS), with a similar decrease in REM sleep.[17] Possible mechanisms of the decrease in FRC during sleep are rostral displacement of the diaphragm secondary to diaphragmatic hypotonia, alteration of the respiratory timing from the central generator of breathing, decrease in lung compliance, decrease in thoracic compliance, and central pooling of blood.

A reduction in V_T by approximately 6% to 15% has been reported during NREM sleep (stages N2 and SWS), with a further decrease during REM sleep (approximately 25% lower than during wakefulness).[18,19] Minute ventilation is significantly lower during all NREM sleep stages compared with wakefulness and decreases further during REM sleep, especially during phasic REM sleep (approximately 84% of the level during wakefulness)[18] (Figure 24.3). The decrease is presumably due to

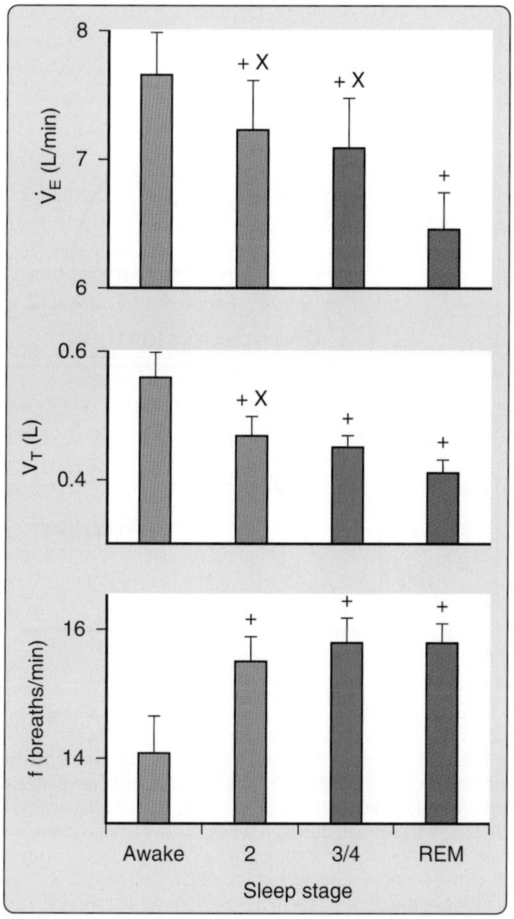

Figure 24.3 Effects of sleep on ventilation and lung volumes. Minute ventilation ($\dot{V}E$), tidal volume (VT), and breathing frequency (f) during wakefulness and different sleep stages are illustrated. $\dot{V}E$ is reduced during NREM sleep, with a further reduction in REM sleep. +, *P* value <0.05 versus awake; +X, *P* value < 0.05 versus REM sleep. (Reproduced with permission from Douglas NJ, White DP, Pickett CK, et al. Respiration during sleep in normal man. *Thorax.* 1982;37:840–4.)

a faster and shallower breathing pattern in all sleep stages with a lower VT, especially during REM sleep. This explanation is, however, controversial, because another study showed no significant change in VT between wakefulness and any sleep stage and suggested that the decrease in minute ventilation (8% in NREM sleep and 4% in REM sleep) is due to a decrease in respiratory rate.[20] Nevertheless, most studies agree that during NREM sleep, the rib cage's contribution to VT increases in association with an approximately 34% increase in the activity of intercostal muscles.[20] There is thus an apparent contradiction between the increase in electromyogram activity of thoracic muscles and a decrease in minute ventilation. A possible explanation is that even though muscle activity increases, the actual negative thoracic pressure decreases because of a decrease in the efficiency of muscle contraction during NREM sleep.[21] During REM sleep, the relative contribution of the rib cage and abdomen is not significantly different from that during wakefulness.[22] Age and sex do not seem to significantly alter sleep-related changes in lung volume.

EFFECTS OF SLEEP ON BREATHING PATTERN AND BLOOD GASES

During NREM sleep, the decrease in minute ventilation induces a drop in Pao_2 of 3 to 9 mm Hg and an increase in $Paco_2$ and $PACO_2$ levels ranging from 2 to 4 mm Hg.[23] During stable NREM sleep, the breathing pattern usually is regular. However, periodic breathing with waxing and waning ventilation commonly is observed at sleep onset (unstable NREM sleep).[23,24] Complete cessation of breathing for more than 10 seconds with respiratory effort (obstructive sleep apnea) or without respiratory effort (central sleep apnea) can occur at this time even in healthy persons. In these circumstances, the transient periodic breathing seems to be due to an unstable ventilatory feedback loop (loop gain). A low arousal threshold during this stage also can induce instability in the sleep-wake cycle and contribute to unstable breathing. Because of the higher CO_2 set point during sleep, arousals are associated with a sudden increase in ventilation, which will then decrease CO_2 level. If the CO_2 level is below the apnea threshold (below which the central respiratory drive is abolished) when sleep resumes, an apneic event will occur with breathing resumption when the CO_2 level again reaches the sleep set point. The magnitude and the breathing fluctuation depend on several factors such as chemoreceptor sensitivity (controller gain), lung-to-chemoreceptor circulation delay, and the efficiency of the respiratory system in inducing changes in CO_2 level (plant gain).[25,26]

During REM sleep, ventilation is notably variable in both amplitude and frequency. This heterogeneity seems to be directly related to the intensity of phasic activity, as indicated by bursts of eye movements. Specifically, phasic REM activity, characterized by a high density of rapid eye movements and muscle twitches, seems to have an inhibitory influence on ventilation.[18] Overall alveolar ventilation tends to fall by approximately 20% compared with wakefulness, mainly because of a fall in VT.[22]

Upper Airway

Among the mechanical determinants of ventilation just summarized, the upper airway plays a unique role because its mechanical properties are dramatically affected by sleep.

The airway can be divided into intrathoracic and extrathoracic components. These include the upper part of the trachea, the larynx, and the different pharyngeal (nasopharynx, velopharynx, orophrarynx, hypopharynx) segments. The upper airway corresponds to the pharyngeal and laryngeal structures. The airway should remain open throughout the respiratory cycle. The intrathoracic, tracheal, and laryngeal airway structures are supported by cartilaginous structures that prevent them from collapsing during tidal breathing in normal persons. Pharyngeal airways do not have such rigid support and are prone to close in conditions of imbalance between the forces that tend to dilate or close them.

From a mechanical standpoint, the upper airway behaves as a Starling resistor, in which the pharyngeal airway represents the collapsible segment and is situated between two noncollapsible structures (larynx and nasopharynx). The flow pattern depends on the forces applied inside and outside the collapsible segment. The transmural pressure gradient is the net pressure difference between all of these opposite forces. The collapsing forces are represented by the negative inspiratory transmural pressure gradient and the pressure applied by upper airway tissue (Figure 24.4). The contraction of upper airway stabilizing muscles (upper airway dilators) is the main dilating force, the other being represented by tracheal traction (Figure 24.5). Therefore the amount and timing of the

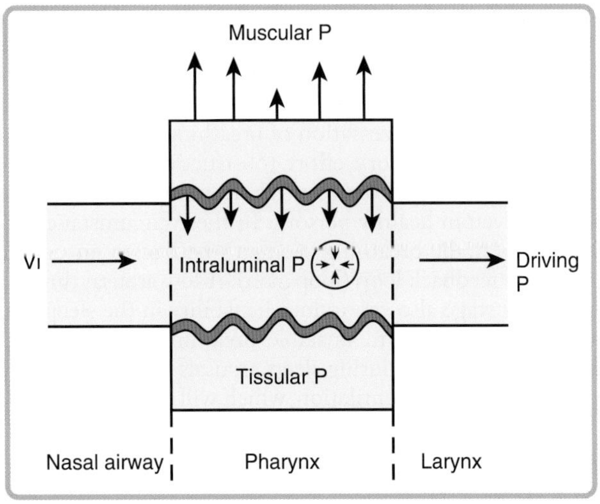

Figure 24.4 Schematic representation of the upper airway (UA) and of the forces applied to the pharyngeal airway. The muscular pressure represents the dilating force coming from the tonic and phasic activity of UA dilator muscles. The intraluminal pressure and the tissue pressure both tend to occlude the UA. P, Pressure; Vi, inspiratory flow volume.

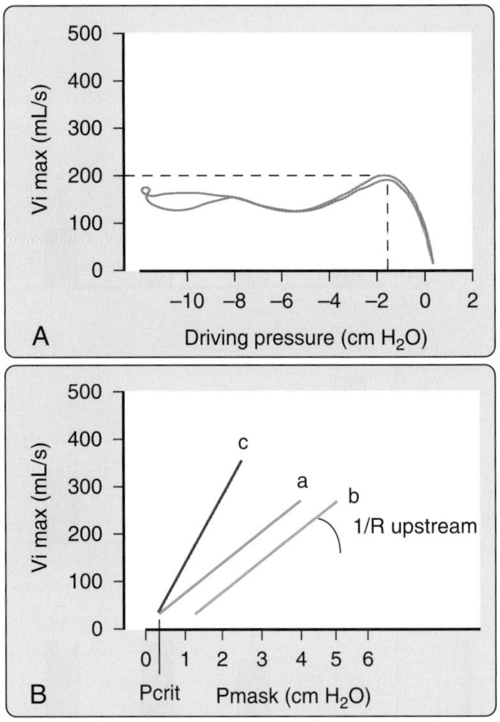

Figure 24.5 **A,** A representative example of the relationship between the respiratory flow over the driving pressure during a flow-limited breath. The instantaneous flow value reaches a maximum value and then plateaus despite the continuous decrease in driving pressure. **B,** Typical relationship between flow and upstream pressure during a series of flow-limited breaths (slope *a*). An increase in the instability of the upper airway will be accompanied by a right shift of the flow-pressure curve (slope b). A decrease in upstream resistance will increase the slope of the flow-pressure curve (slope c). Pcrit, Critical pressure; Pmask, mask pressure; 1/R upstream, reciprocal of upstream resistance; Vi max, maximal inspiratory flow.

neuromuscular activation process of upper airway stabilizing muscles and the mechanical properties of upper airway tissues play a pivotal role in determining upper airway stability.

According to the Starling resistance model,[27] inspiratory flow increases with rising inspiratory efforts (driving pressure) up to a maximal value and then plateaus independently of respiratory efforts (Figure 24.5, *A*). These features of the flow-pressure relationship characterize a flow limitation regimen. The steepness of the initial rise in flow depends on the resistance upstream and downstream of the collapsing site. The pressure at which flow begins to plateau depends on upper airway mechanical properties. The critical pressure (Pcrit) represents the pressure at which the dilating forces cannot overcome the collapsing ones, leading to upper airway closure. The changes in maximal inspiratory flow with modifying upstream pressure can be used to determine Pcrit and resistance upstream to the collapsing site. A linear positive relationship between these variables can be shown (Figure 24.5, *B*). The slope of the relationship corresponds to the reciprocal of upstream resistance, and the pressure at which flow is zero represents Pcrit. In a given subject, an increase in the propensity for the upper airway to occlude translates the flow-pressure relationship to the right, without changes in slope (i.e., slope a to slope b), making the Pcrit value more positive. In the situation of a decrease in upstream resistance, the steepness of the slope will rise (greater changes in flow occur with changing upstream pressure), but the Pcrit value will remain unchanged (i.e., slope a to slope c on Figure 24.5, *B*).

Collapsing Forces

The negative intrathoracic pressure generated by diaphragmatic contraction is transmitted to the whole airway, from the alveoli to the nose, to create inspiratory flow. At the pharyngeal level, the difference between intraluminal and peritissue pressures (transmural pressure) represents a suction force that tends to dynamically close the upper airway. According to the Bernoulli principle, the pressure along the walls of a tube drops with the increase in its velocity, making the intraluminal pressure decrease (become more negative) with increasing inspiratory flow. Changes in flow from a laminar to a turbulent pattern increase air velocity near airway walls, which will further reduce intraluminal pressure. The pattern of collapse is also affected by location in the upper airway. Most commonly the pattern of collapse at the retropalatal level is concentric, while at the hypopharyngeal level, lateral wall collapse occurs most commonly.[28] Evaluation of the location and pattern of collapse has emerged as an important tool in predicting response to hypoglossal nerve stimulation therapy of obstructive sleep apnea.[29]

The weight of upper airway tissue (including that resulting from an enlarged tongue) significantly influences upper airway stability.[30] On the other hand, negative pressure applied around the neck significantly unloads the upper airway,[31] and resection of upper airway tissue improves Pcrit in patients with sleep apnea.[32]

Fluid shift, occurring when the patient assumes a supine position after prolonged standing, also contributes to airway collapsibility as a result of rostral redistribution of fluid from the legs toward the neck and chest.[33] The resulting upper airway edema increases the neck circumference and reduces the cross-sectional diameter of the pharynx, thus predisposing to greater airway collapsibility. The phenomenon has been described in the nonobese individual and seems to be an important determinant of obstructive sleep apnea in patients with fluid-retaining conditions, such as in chronic heart or kidney diseases.[34]

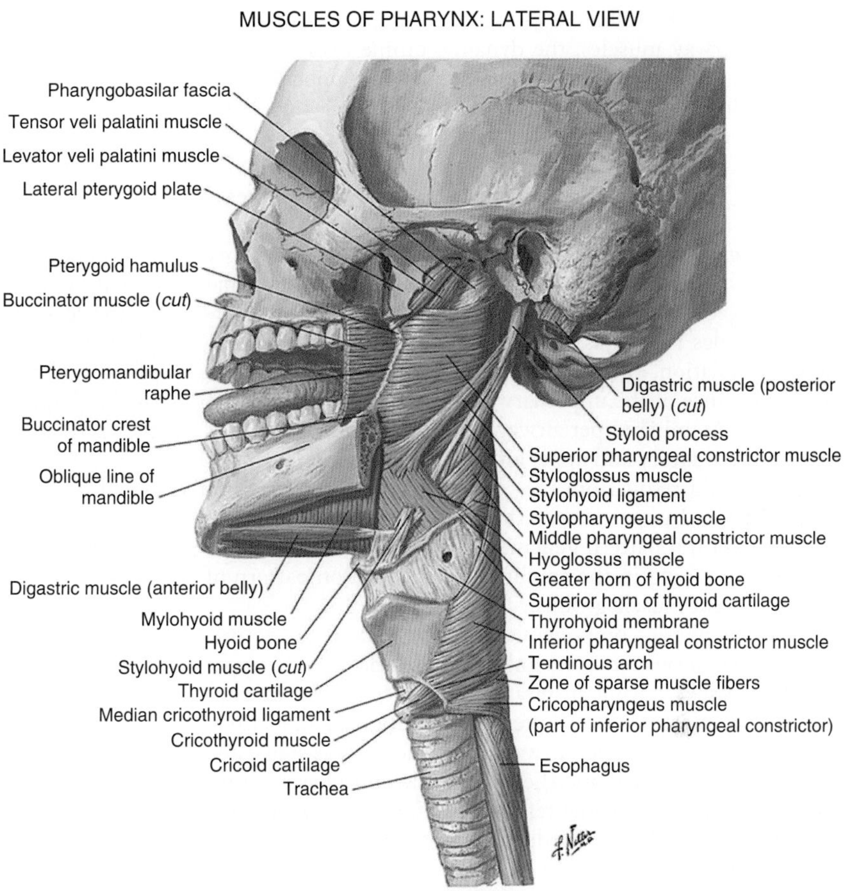

Figure 24.6 Drawing of upper airway muscles. (Reproduced from Netter FH. *Atlas of Human Anatomy.* Saunders; 2006.)

Dilating Forces

Contraction of inspiratory muscles—diaphragm, intercostals, and accessory muscles—leads to lung inflation. The downward movement of the diaphragm produces a longitudinal traction of the bronchi and of the trachea. This traction is transmitted to the upper airway, where it contributes to unloading of that region.[8] From a dynamic perspective, tracheal traction improves upper airway stability by unfolding upper airway soft tissue and by decreasing extraluminal airway pressure.[35]

Numerous upper airway stabilizing muscles (such as the genioglossus, levator palatini, tensor palatini, geniohyoid, musculus uvulae, and palatopharyngeus) contribute to the maintenance of upper airway patency (Figure 24.6). Activation of masseter and pterygoid muscles also may contribute to stabilizing the upper airway by their influence on the position of the mouth and the mandible.[36] The activation profile of the upper airway muscles is characterized by their tonic activity and the respiratory-related and afferent reflex–mediated phasic activities.[37] This last factor is an important determinant of activity of the upper airway muscles, the negative pressure developed inside the upper airway having a positive feedback on muscle activity through activation of tensoreceptor and mechanoreceptor pathways.[38]

Tonic activity contributes to the maintenance of the upper airway aperture, its obligatory fall during sleep leading to a reduction in upper airway volume.[39] Inspiratory phasic activity has an automatic component that is linked with the central respiratory activity through projections of premotor inspiratory neurons to the hypoglossal motor nucleus (as detailed in Chapters 22 and 23.)[39]

Neuromodulators—serotonin, norepinephrine, glutamate, thyrotropin-releasing hormone, and substance P—play a key and complex role in the activity of upper airway muscles.[40] In lean animals, resting tonic and phasic activities of the genioglossus muscles mainly depend on endogenous norepinephrine, rather than serotonin drive on hypoglossal motor nucleus, but these neuromodulators have similar stimulating effects.[41]

However, the influence of the serotonin drive on upper airway stabilizing muscle activity may be enhanced if upper airway patency is compromised, as demonstrated by the detrimental effects of serotonin antagonists (ritanserine) on upper airway caliber and stability, and on the occurrence on breathing abnormalities in animal models of obstructive sleep apnea.[42] Such changes in the balance of the norepinephrine-serotonin drive could result from facilitating hypoglossal nerve activities induced by intermittent hypoxia,[43,44] or from the relative vulnerability of norepinephrine and serotonin neurons to intermittent severe hypoxia.[44] Stimulation of peripheral chemoreceptors by intermittent hypoxia can lead to a prolonged rise in minute ventilation (long-term facilitation)[45] and a decrease in upper airway resistance.[46] These ventilatory and upper airway facilitation effects are thought to be mediated by the serotonin-driven changes in activity of the phrenic and hypoglossal nerves through plasticity.[43,47] In humans, post-hypoxia upper airway facilitation is observed during sleep in conditions of flow-limited breathing (as in snorers and persons with sleep apnea)[46,48] but is not observed during wakefulness[49-51] unless periodic desaturation is associated with hypercapnia.[52]

Apart from the influence of the extent of phasic activation of upper airway muscles, the dynamic profile of this phasic activity plays a key role in the maintenance of upper airway patency. Phasic activation of upper airway muscles precedes and reaches its peak value earlier than that of respiratory muscles.[53] Phasic activity and the preactivation delay increase with increasing central respiratory activity[53,54] and with decreasing upper airway pressure.[55] This activation pattern decreases upper airway resistance and prevents upper airway inspiratory collapse. The occurrence of upper airway obstruction in normal awake subjects when this preactivation of upper airway stabilizing muscles is lost (as with diaphragmatic pacing, phrenic nerve stimulation, or iron lung ventilation)[56] further supports the importance of the upper airway muscle preactivation pattern in maintaining upper airway patency. The link that exists between ventilatory and upper airway stability (see later in this chapter) could result from the common activation process of respiratory and upper airway stabilizing muscles originating from the central pattern generator that would be responsible for the fine tuning in the amplitude and activation pattern of these different muscle groups.

Another phasic component comes from the reflex activation of upper airway muscles linked with the decrease in upper airway pressure during inspiration.[55] Upper airway mechanoreceptor afferents contribute to modulation of the different components of upper airway muscle activity, as suggested by the effects of local anesthesia on tonic and phasic activities[57] and on genioglossus reflex–mediated negative pressure response.[58] Accordingly, modulating any of these components of the upper airway muscle activation profile can have an influence on upper airway patency[59] and stability.[60-62]

EFFECTS OF SLEEP ON UPPER AIRWAY MUSCLE ACTIVITY

The loss of wakefulness stimulus contributes to the sleep-induced decrease in upper airway muscle activity.[63] Tonic and phasic upper airway activities are significantly altered during sleep.[37,64,65] The impact of sleep on the activation profile of upper airway muscles differs among the various muscles. The tensor palatini has a tonic activity, but the genioglossus, palatoglossus, and levator palatini demonstrate phasic activities. These activity levels are higher during wakefulness, but only tensor palatini activity consistently falls at sleep onset.[66] The decrease in tensor palatini activity correlates with the sleep-induced rise in upper airway resistance, and a compensatory rise occurs in genioglossus activity.[66]

The tensor palatini and genioglossus muscles strongly differ in their response to negative airway pressure during both wakefulness and sleep,[67] with no correlation being found between tensor palatini activity and driving pressure. Even if tensor palatini and genioglossus activities are governed by different efferent motor fibers (trigeminal motor nucleus versus hypoglossal motor nucleus), both activities depend on central neuromodulator drive.[68,69] The preferential decrease in upper airway muscle tonic activity observed during sleep[70] may relate to decrease in central excitatory drive to upper airway motor nuclei stemming from the loss of the awake corticomotor-stimulating drive and from a decrease in the stimulating effects of neuromodulators.[41,71-73] Sleep also may compromise upper airway stability by altering the pattern of preactivation of upper airway muscles.[74] The loss of such preactivation is associated with the rise in upper airway resistance and upper airway closure. The reappearance of alpha activity on the electroencephalogram restores the normal preactivation pattern with a parallel drop in upper airway resistance and ventilatory resumption.

The neuromuscular activation processes of upper airway and respiratory muscles are closely linked. Tidal inspiration has a facilitating effect—increase in amplitude and reduction in latency of motor response—on diaphragm bulbospinal activity, which is enhanced during sleep. This can be attributed to the loss of a wakefulness-related tonic depolarization of phrenic motor neurons with secondary unmasking of the role of the bulbospinal command on the corticomotor excitability of the diaphragm. It is not known how sleep interacts with the facilitating effect of inspiration on upper airway muscle excitability.[75] On the other hand, some evidence indicates that breathing instability during sleep may promote upper airway closure.

Obstructive breathing disorders are mainly observed during stages N1 and N2 of NREM and REM sleep, when ventilation is physiologically unstable, and less often during slow wave sleep, when breathing amplitude and frequency are particularly regular.[76] Breathing remains unstable (periodic) after relief of upper airway obstruction with tracheostomy in patients with obstructive sleep apnea.[77] This finding may explain the development of complex sleep in patients first started on continuous positive airway pressure.[78] In normal sleeping subjects, the induction of periodic breathing can lead to partial upper airway obstruction.[79] Ventilatory stimulation with CO_2 decreases the occurrence of obstructed breaths in patients afflicted with sleep apnea.[80] In patients with a moderate increase in upper airway collapsibility, the frequency of obstructive sleep-disordered breathing correlates with the degree of breathing instability.[81]

FACTORS INFLUENCING STABILIZING AND COLLAPSING FORCES

For a given amount of upper airway neuromuscular outflow, the net mechanical effect of the neuromuscular activation process depends on the mechanical effectiveness of the contraction of upper airway stabilizing muscles.[82] Such function depends on factors such as the shape and dimensions of the upper airway. In fact, the amount of phasic activity required to maintain a given upper airway cross-sectional area increases when the upper airway axis converts from a transverse to an anteroposterior orientation.[83,84] Lung volumes influence upper airway dimension, as demonstrated by the decrease in pharyngeal cross-sectional area and the increase in upper airway resistance and collapsibility when lung volume decreases from TLC to RV.[85-87] Upper airway dimension also varies throughout the respiratory cycle, being maximal at the beginning of expiration and minimal at end expiration.[88] Vascular tone also interacts with upper airway collapsibility through its effect on upper airway dimension; the decrease in vascular tone or increase in vascular content decreases upper airway caliber but not upper airway collapsibility.[89] In these physiologic situations, various factors as described can interact with upper airway patency to favor obstruction of the upper airway if upper airway stability is already compromised (i.e., with a highly compliant upper airway).

The mechanical conditions that prevail during muscle contraction also determine the force the involved muscles can develop. The suctioning effect of negative intraluminal pressure can result in a lengthening of upper airway muscles during inspiration (eccentric contraction)[90] that interferes with their ability to dilate the upper airway and leads to upper airway muscle fatigue and structural damage.[91-93] The characteristics of the soft tissues surrounding the upper airway muscles also influence the ability of these muscles to improve upper airway patency, the increase in tissue stiffness impeding the transmission of the dilating force to the upper airway structure.[94]

CONCLUSIONS

Numerous factors are involved in the regulation of normal breathing, including a predominant role of different muscles such as respiratory and upper airway muscles as well as the mechanical conditions that determine the effectiveness of their contraction. Sleep can interfere with several determinants of normal ventilation such as ventilatory control, skeletal muscle activity, and lung volumes. Therefore, because of the influence of thoracopulmonary mechanics on upper airway patency and the close link between respiratory and upper airway muscles, sleep also has a strong impact on upper airway aperture and mechanical properties. Careful delineation of sleep-related changes in respiratory physiology is key to improving our knowledge of sleep-disordered breathing, because these principles are involved in all nocturnal breathing disturbances: hypoventilation, periodic breathing, central apnea, and upper airway closure.

CLINICAL PEARL

Numerous factors contribute to ventilation and mechanical properties of the thoracopulmonary system. Because sleep interacts with several of these factors, it has an impact on ventilation and gas exchange through its effect on airway resistance, thoracopulmonary compliance, and lung volumes. As a consequence of its effect on upper airway muscle control and chest mechanics, sleep has a strong influence on upper airway stability. Accordingly, persons with compromised upper airway anatomy are at increased risk for development of obstructive, sleep-induced, disordered breathing, especially during the transition between wakefulness and sleep. Relieving obstruction in such patients may lead to complex sleep apnea.

SUMMARY

The respiratory system can be divided into two compartments, the upper and lower airways. The mechanics of both compartments are strongly influenced by sleep. Lung volume, rib cage muscle activity, and minute ventilation tend to decrease during sleep, as does the activity of upper airway stabilizing muscles. The upper airway also plays a critical role in determining ventilation and breathing pattern during sleep. Its patency is influenced not only by pharyngeal and orofacial muscle activity, but also by thoracopulmonary mechanics. Sleep therefore has a strong impact on upper airway aperture and mechanical properties. Even though obesity and susceptible pharyngeal anatomy are important contributors to the development of sleep-induced disordered breathing, sleep plays a key role in generating upper airway instability and therefore in determining the underlying pathophysiology.

SELECTED READINGS

Deacon NL, Catcheside PG. The role of high loop gain induced by intermittent hypoxia in the pathophysiology of obstructive sleep apnoea. *Sleep Med Rev*. 2015;22:3–14.

Dempsey JA, Veasey SC, Morgan BJ, O'Donnell CP. Pathophysiology of sleep apnea. *Physiol Rev*. 2010;90:47–112.

Gederi E, Nemati S, Edwards B, et al. Model-based estimation of loop gain using spontaneous breathing: a validation study. *Respir Physiol Neurobiol*. 2014;201:84–92.

Giannadaki K, Schiza S, Vavougios B, et al. Small airways' function in obstructive sleep apnea-hypopnea syndrome [published online ahead of print, 2020 Aug 26]. *Pulmonology*. 2020;S2531-0437(20)30122–7.

Heinzer RC, Stanchina ML, Malhotra A, et al. Lung volume and continuous positive airway pressure requirements in obstructive sleep apnea. *Am J Respir Crit Care Med*. 2005;172(1):114–117.

Horner RL, Hughes SW, Malhotra A. State-dependent and reflex drives to the upper airway: basic physiology with clinical implications. *J Appl Physiol*. 2014;116:325–336.

Osman AM, Carberry JC, Burke PGR, Toson B, Grunstein RR, Eckert DJ. Upper airway collapsibility measured using a simple wakefulness test closely relates to the pharyngeal critical closing pressure during sleep in obstructive sleep apnea. *Sleep*. 2019;42(7):zsz080. https://doi.org/10.1093/sleep/zsz080.

Series F, Cormier Y, Desmeules M. Influence of passive changes of lung volume on upper airways. *J Appl Physiol*. 1990;68(5):2159–2164.

Stanchina M, Robinson K, Corrao W, et al. Clinical use of loop gain measures to determine continuous positive airway pressure efficacy in patients with complex sleep apnea. A pilot study. *Ann Am Thorac Soc*. 2015;12(9):1351–1357.

Stradling JR, Chadwick GA, Frew AJ. Changes in ventilation and its components in normal subjects during sleep. *Thorax*. 1985;40(5):364–370.

Trinder J, Whitworth F, Kay A, Wilkin P. Respiratory instability during sleep onset. *J Appl Physiol*. 1992;73(6):2462–249.

White DP, Younes MK. Obstructive sleep apnea. *Compr Physiol*. 2012;2:2541–2594.

A complete reference list can be found online at ExpertConsult.com.

Chapter 25

Respiratory Physiology: Sleep at High Altitude

Alexander Patrician; Keith R. Burgess; Philip N. Ainslie

Chapter Highlights

- Ventilatory acclimatization to altitude involves cellular and neurochemical reorganization in the chemoreceptors and central nervous system.
- Sleep at high altitude is disturbed by various factors, including a change of sleep environment, snoring, and insomnia.
- Periodic breathing during sleep, however, probably causes the most disturbances and occurs in a majority of people above 3500 meters.
- The extent of periodic breathing during sleep at high altitude intensifies with duration and severity of exposure and is explained, in part, by elevations in loop gain—an engineering term used to measure/describe the propensity for a system governed by feedback loops to develop unstable behavior.
- Because periodic breathing may elevate—rather than reduce—mean arterial oxygen saturation (Sao_2) during sleep, this may represent an adaptive rather than a maladaptive response to altitude.
- Although new mechanical and pharmacologic management techniques are emerging, an oral acetazolamide regimen remains, so far, to be the most effective and practical means to reduce periodic breathing in high altitude.

INTRODUCTION

All those who have been to high altitudes can attest that sleeping is initially impaired in this environment. This ubiquitous problem affects skiers and trekkers alike who sleep at altitudes of 2500 to 3000 meters, as well as the well-acclimatized climber who spends time at higher altitudes. Common complaints include difficulty falling asleep, frequent awakenings, and persistent feelings of fatigue upon awakening in the morning. In addition to the physical discomforts from cold or unsatisfactory bedding and the noise of other people's snoring, vivid dreams, racing thoughts, and feelings of suffocation upon awakening are other common experiences for many people. Underlying these subjective complaints are important changes in sleep physiology, including changes in sleep architecture and the control of breathing. Alterations in the latter frequently lead to periodic breathing, a major contributor to altered sleep quality at high altitude, which has been recognized as a problem since the 19th century. This common problem, which can cause severe degrees of hypoxemia following apneic periods at extreme altitudes,[1] may be one of the factors that influences tolerance to very great altitudes and sheds light.

This chapter considers in detail the physiology of sleep at high altitude, including sleep architecture, control of breathing, and periodic breathing, and points out the potential influence of adaptation on sleep at high altitude by focusing on periodic breathing, or the lack thereof, in high-altitude natives (i.e., populations with generational exposure and adaptational characteristics to high altitude). Consideration is also given to pharmacologic and nonpharmacologic measures to improve sleep quality in this environment as well as changes that may occur in children and patients with sleep-disordered breathing at sea level who travel to higher elevations. The material considered here overlaps that of Chapter 141: the control of ventilation has important influences on breathing patterns during sleep at high altitude.

HISTORICAL PERSPECTIVE

Sleep Quality

Decrements to sleep quality were among some of the first anecdotal reports of sleep at high altitude. Joseph Barcroft described his sleep during his glass case experiment[5] at Cambridge, UK, as "very light and fitful with incessant dreams… the quality of sleep in most cases was of inferior order…the night seemed long and we woke unrefreshed."[6] Barcroft's impression of sleep at high altitude being abnormal and associated with an increased frequency of awakenings and a feeling of being less refreshed in the morning has been confirmed in more recent studies at high altitude.[7,8]

Periodic Breathing

Various references to an uneven pattern of breathing during sleep at altitudes greater than 2500 meters were made during the 19th century. English physicist John Tyndall, an ardent

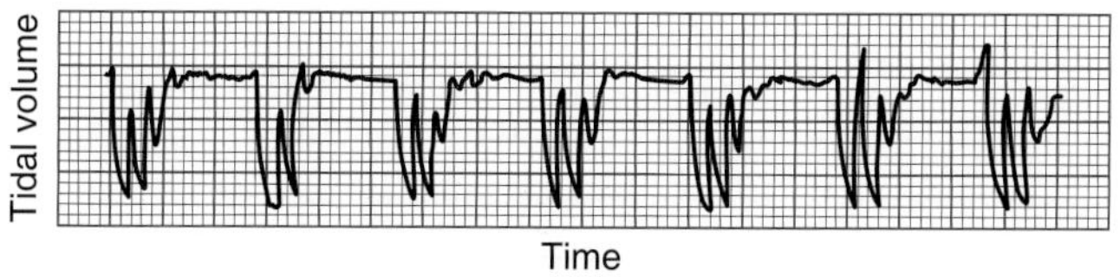

Figure 25.1 Periodic breathing during sleep in the Regina Margherita Hut (at 4559 meters in the Italian Alps). (Modified from Mosso A. *Life of Man on the High Alps*. London; 1898.)

mountaineer, who, during his first ascent of Mount Blanc in 1857 became very fatigued and laid down to rest. He subsequently wrote, "I stretched myself upon a composite couch of snow and granite, and immediately fell asleep. My friend, however, soon aroused me. 'You quite frightened me,' he said, 'I listened for some minutes and have not heard you breathe once.'" This breathing pattern, of "Stokes character," was again noted by Egli-Sinclair in 1893 in an article on mountain sickness.[9] He was referring to the breathing pattern known as Cheyne-Stokes breathing, which was described by Irish physicians William Stokes[10] and John Cheyne.[11] Despite the common term Cheyne-Stokes breathing, it was mentioned in 1973 by Michael Ward[12] that the phenomenon was first described by John Hunter in 1781.[13]

The first extensive studies of periodic breathing during sleep at high altitude were first performed by Angelo Mosso[14] in 1886 (Figure 25.1). Using a level resting on the chest to measure breathing movements, he showed that in his brother (Ugolino Mosso) periods of apnea lasted 12 seconds. Follow-up observations revealed that the waxing and waning of breathing movements were interspaced by the shorter periods of apnea.[14] These observations were also confirmed by other investigators a few decades later.[15]

CHARACTERISTICS OF SLEEP DURING HIGH-ALTITUDE ASCENT

Upon acute exposure to hypobaric hypoxia (i.e., the reduction in arterial oxygen content due to a reduction in barometic pressure and a lower partial pressure of inspired oxygen), sleep is negatively impacted by an increase in frequency of arousals, changes to sleep state, and control of breathing. These changes are outlined in the following sections.

Increased Frequency of Arousals

People at high altitude often report that they wake more frequently during the night than at sea level. This phenomenon has been confirmed in several careful studies[7,8,16,17] using continuous recordings of the electroencephalogram (EEG), electromyography (EMG), and eye movements, during which arousal was recognized by the occurrence of EMG activation, eye movements, and alpha wave activity on the EEG. For example, in one study at an altitude of 4300 meters, there were on average 36 arousals per night compared with 20 at sea level.[17] Some investigators believe that the arousals are caused in some way by periodic breathing and/or that more frequent arousals coincide with a higher strength of periodic breathing. Some evidence suggests that arousals are more frequent when the strength of periodic breathing is high. It is easy to imagine that the strenuous muscular activity required to generate large breaths after a prolonged period of apnea could contribute to an arousal. Indeed, this may be associated with the air hunger caused by long apneic periods during periodic breathing. However, since arousals also occur in individuals who do not develop periodic breathing, periodic breathing cannot be solely responsible for the increased frequency of arousals at high altitude.[7,18]

Changes in Sleep State

Multiple EEG studies have provided objective evidence of changes in sleep architecture at high altitude that support subjective conclusions that sleep at high altitude is often of poor quality, and not as refreshing as sleep at sea level. One of the earliest studies in this regard was performed by Joern and colleagues,[19] who evaluated changes in sleep architecture near the South Pole, where the barometric pressure is reduced because of the actual altitude and also the very high latitude. They reported a near absence of sleep stages 3 and 4 coupled with an approximately 50% reduction in rapid eye movement (REM) sleep. Although the light–dark cycle was atypical compared to other sleep settings, their findings have been confirmed at more moderate latitudes.

Several years later, Reite and colleagues[7] studied sleep patterns in six subjects following a rapid ascent to Pikes Peak (4300 meters). The authors found a similar shift from deeper to lighter sleep stages and a great reduction in REM sleep. Periodic breathing was common but disappeared during REM sleep. The changes in the pattern of sleep and respiration were greatest on the first night at high altitude and then declined thereafter.

Subsequent studies have generally confirmed the findings that time spent in light sleep (stages 1 and 2 of non–rapid eye movement [NREM] sleep) is increased, while the time spent in deep sleep (stages 3 and 4 of NREM sleep using the previous classification) is decreased. The data regarding the time spent in REM sleep has been conflicting, however, with some animal studies reporting that it is virtually abolished[20,21] and other studies reporting either a decrease[22,23] or no change in the time spent in this stage.[8,24-26]

With respect to altered sleeping patterns, there are similarities between the behavior of sleep-deprived subjects and people at high altitude whose brains are affected by hypoxia. In both instances, mental activities that are "mechanical" in nature, such as tabulating a set of data, can be accurately accomplished, whereas activities that require problem solving and initiative are seriously affected. It may be that some of the impairment of central nervous system function in individuals living at high altitude can be ascribed to the poor quality of sleep, but the direct effects of hypoxia on the brain also clearly play a role, as reviewed by West.[27]

Changes in Control of Breathing

The control of breathing during sleep at sea level has been discussed in earlier chapters (see Chapters 22 and 23). Few studies have examined the impact of high altitude on the hypercapnic and hypoxic ventilatory responses during sleep (see the section Periodic Breathing and Hypoxic Ventilatory Response). One of the few studies on this issue[28] monitored hypercapnic ventilatory responses (HCVR) in six healthy men on nights 1, 4, and 7 at 4300 meters and found that the response was diminished to similar degrees seen at sea level during both NREM and REM sleep. They also observed that minute ventilation fell from wakefulness to NREM and REM sleep with the bulk of the decrease being attributable to a decrease in tidal volume. Minute ventilation did increase over time at altitude, largely because of increases in respiratory rate. Alterations in cerebral blood flow (CBF) have also been proposed to alter the control

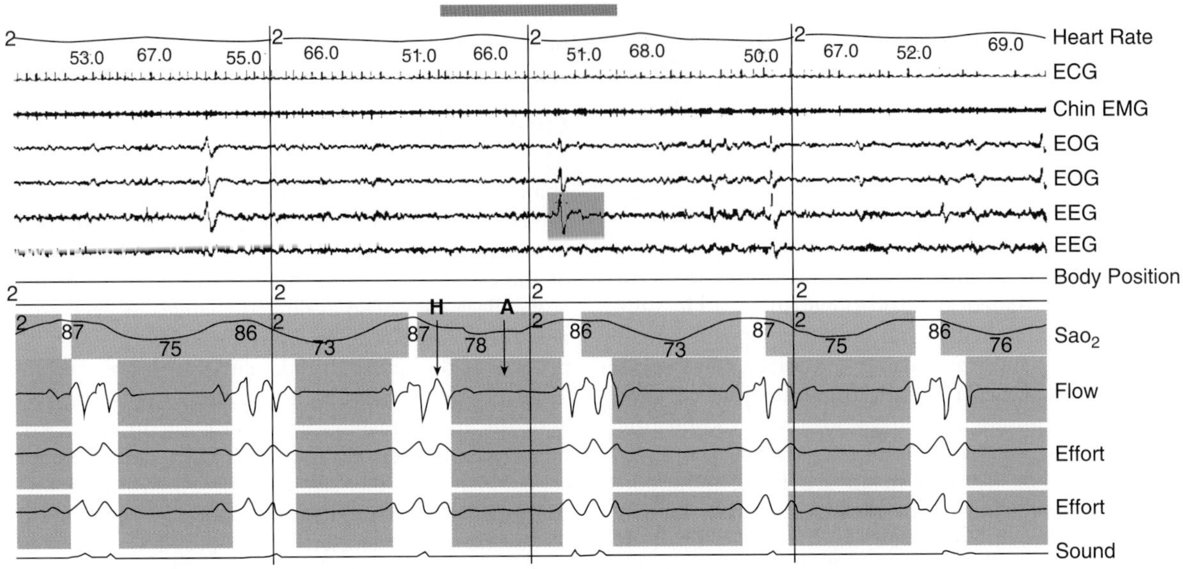

Figure 25.2 A 2-minute epoch from a polysomnogram recorded from one subject during sleep at 5050 meters showing central sleep apnea (CSA). *Arrows*: H indicates the period of hyperpnea, and A, the period of apnea. Arterial oxygen saturation (Sao_2) reading shows periods of desaturation. Nasal airflow was measured using a pressure-transduced nasal cannula. Respiratory effort was measured by means of piezoelectric bands. ECG, Electrocardiogram; EEG, electroencephalogram; EMG, electromyogram; EOG, electrooculogram. (Modified from Ainslie PN, Lucas SJE, Burgess KR. Breathing and sleep at high altitude. *Respir Physiol Neurobiol*. 188(3):233–256, 2013.)

of breathing (see the section Role of Cerebral Blood Flow in Breathing Stability at Altitude).

PERIODIC BREATHING

Characteristics

The common pattern of periodic breathing has now been confirmed in many studies carried out at various altitudes from sea level up to 8050 meters.[15,25,29,30] A typical pattern recorded at an altitude of 5050 meters in a well-acclimatized lowlander using modern equipment is shown in Figure 25.2 (as described in a review by Ainslie and colleagues[31]). Note that the tidal volume (i.e., flow) waxed and waned during each burst of breathing, with apneic periods of about 8 seconds, with periodic breathing cycling every 15 to 25 seconds. Arterial oxygen saturation as measured by pulse oximeter (Spo_2) fluctuated with the same frequency as the periodic breathing, which also mirrors large swings in blood pressure that also drive oscillations in CBF (Figure 25.3, *middle* and *right panels*). Although there are phase differences between the resumption of breathing and swings in Spo_2, the Spo_2 nadir is actually occurring at approximately the end of the apneic period. These cyclical fluctuations in Spo_2 can likely be accounted for being on the steep part of the oxygen dissociation curve and by the related circulation time from the lung capillaries to the finger where the oxygen saturation was measured. For example, in the study of nocturnal periodic breathing carried out at an altitude of 6300 meters, Spo_2 varied from a minimal value of 64.5% to a maximum of 74.5%, with a mean of 68.8%, for at least 50% of total sleep time.[1] Heart rate was measured from the electrocardiogram and showed marked fluctuations with the same frequency as the periodic breathing. Likely reflective of some cardiopulmonary baroreflex mechanisms, the highest heart rate appeared at the end of the burst of ventilation.

Beyond the fact that periodic breathing is common among lowlanders who ascend to high altitude, there are several important features of this phenomenon, which will be discussed further.

Percentage of Time Spent Periodic Breathing

Another important feature is that the percentage of time occupied by periodic breathing increases with altitude. For example, Waggener and colleagues reported that periodic breathing with apnea occupied 24% of the time asleep at 2440 meters, and that the percentage increased to 40% at 4270 meters.[32] This increase in proportion of time is consistent with a theoretical model discussed later in this chapter (see the section Mechanism of Periodic Breathing)[33] and has been documented previously.[25,31,34,35]

Periodic Breathing and Sleep Staging

Multiple studies have shown that periodic breathing is very common during NREM sleep at high altitude and may even occur during the drowsy period that precedes sleep onset.[7,29] It typically does not occur during REM sleep at moderate altitudes, although periodically may still occur during REM sleep at high elevations, a phenomenon that has been reviewed elsewhere.[18,31] Coincidentally, at least when examined at sea level, the apneic threshold (i.e., the transient reduction in $Paco_2$ that causes an apnea) that resides within 2 to 5 mm Hg $PaCO_2$ below normal awake levels in healthy subjects in NREM is not readily demonstrable in phasic REM.[36] The ventilatory response above eupnea to added carbon dioxide (CO_2) is also blunted in NREM (versus wakefulness) in part because of a truly reduced CO_2 chemoreceptor sensitivity[37]; there is also a loss of tonic neural motor input to pharyngeal dilator muscles resulting in increased upper airway resistance.[38] Transient arousal at apnea termination temporarily restores this tonic input and reduces airway resistance, thereby contributing to ventilatory overshoot prior to sleep restoration. Similarly, in REM sleep ventilatory responsiveness to CO_2 above eupnea is reduced in slope and shows an almost random tidal volume

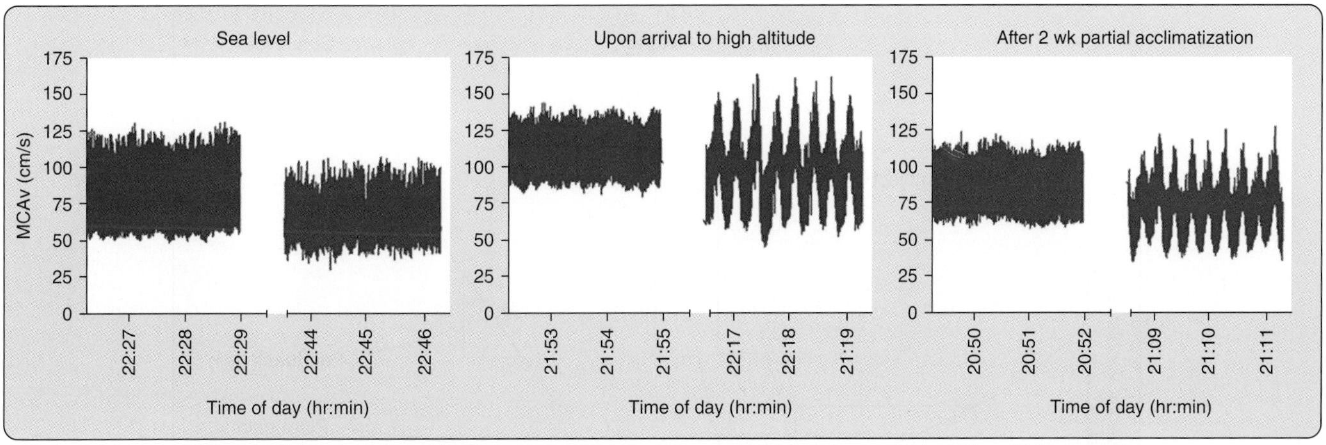

Figure 25.3 A typical profile of the observed changes in cerebral blood flow, as indexed by middle cerebral artery blood velocity (MCAv), before sleep onset (*left-hand trace*), and during stage 2 sleep (*right-hand trace*) at sea level, then on arrival, and after 2 weeks at high altitude, as recorded in one participant. Note the elevation in MCAv on arrival, compared with that after 2 weeks of acclimatization. (Modified from Burgess KR, Lucas SJ, Shepherd KL, et al. Worsening of central sleep apnea at high altitude—a role for cerebrovascular function. *J Appl Physiol.* 2013;114:1021–8.)

and/or diaphragmatic EMG responses to increasing Pa_{CO_2} (with or without coincident airway occlusion), rather than an orderly dose-response as in quiet wakefulness or NREM sleep.[39] These carefully conducted laboratory studies at sea level must be extrapolated to high altitudes in future research.

Periodic Breathing Cycle Length

Early evidence indicated that cycle length of the apnea (when corrected for the individual strength of ventilatory response) decreases with increasing altitude with a mean cycle length of 20 seconds at 3350 meters and 18 seconds at 4300 meters,[32] whereas data from the American Medical Research Expedition to Everest (AMREE)[30] reported a mean cycle period of 19 seconds in well-acclimatized lowlanders at 5400 meters. More evidence is necessary to confirm whether cycle length decreases or remains constant, but a summary of the studies conducted at high altitude illustrates that cycle lengths remain somewhat stable, or even decrease, with increasing high altitude and duration of exposure (see the section Persistence of Periodic Breathing over Time at High Altitude).

Mechanism of Periodic Breathing

The mechanisms causing periodic breathing are discussed in a general context in earlier chapters (see Chapters 22 to 24). An altitude-specific focus also has been covered in a subsequent chapter (see Chapter 141), but a brief review of the likely changes experienced at high altitude and the implications for periodic breathing is warranted here.

The principal reason for the occurrence of apnea and periodic breathing during sleep in hypoxic environments is believed to be elevations in controller or feedback gain—often termed "control theory," as evidenced by the steep increase in the CO_2 response slope above and below eupnea and the greatly narrowed CO_2 reserve.[31,40] Control theory can be used to better understand the central mechanisms responsible for periodic breathing.[33,41] For example, control systems are marked by two key features: a "disturbance" (e.g., a change in alveolar ventilation) followed by a "corrective action," which tends to suppress the disturbance. In the case of an increase in alveolar ventilation (caused by a sigh, for example) the corrective action would be a lowering of P_{CO_2}, which would tend to reduce ventilation by its action on central and peripheral chemoreceptors and thus constitute negative feedback.

Sustained oscillatory behavior will occur in such a system when two requirements are met. First, the magnitude of the corrective action must exceed that of the disturbance, this ratio being known as the loop gain. Second, the corrective action must be presented 180 degrees out of phase with the disturbance so that what would otherwise inhibit the change in ventilation now augments it. This sustained oscillatory behavior occurs when the loop gain exceeds unity at a phase difference of 180 degrees. Control theory predicts that the higher the loop gain at a phase angle of 180 degrees, the more likely periodic breathing is to occur, the more marked the pattern of periodic breathing, and the shorter the cycle length of the periodic breathing.

The main factor increasing loop gain in acclimatized lowlanders at high altitude is the increased chemoreceptor gain, particularly the response to severe hypoxia. However, as described in detail elsewhere,[42] it should be noted that loop gain of the chemoreceptor control system is a product of two gains: (1) the controller gain (i.e., the ventilatory reflex gain ($[\Delta V_E/\Delta CO_2]$) and (2) the plant gain (i.e., the effectiveness of alveolar ventilation in imparting changes in blood gases $[\Delta CO_2/\Delta V_E]$). Although poorly understood, especially in humans, another gain—called the mixing gain—may also influence breathing stability. The mixing gain is known as the effectiveness of CBF in imparting changes at the level of the central chemoreceptors ($\Delta CO_2/\Delta CBF$). Another important factor that has been postulated to influence ventilatory stability and thus periodic breathing is the post-stimulus short-term potentiation, or what was initially called the "ventilatory afterdischarge."[43] Although these concepts have been described in detail with sleep apnea,[42] an update is provided on the likely changes experienced at high altitude and the implications for periodic breathing.

The transient cessation of the medullary respiratory pattern generator neurons requires an unmasking of a sensitized apneic threshold in NREM sleep, as induced by a transient ventilatory overshoot involving both mild to moderate hypocapnia plus augmented tidal volumes. In cats and rats, carotid body denervation studies demonstrate that the carotid bodies

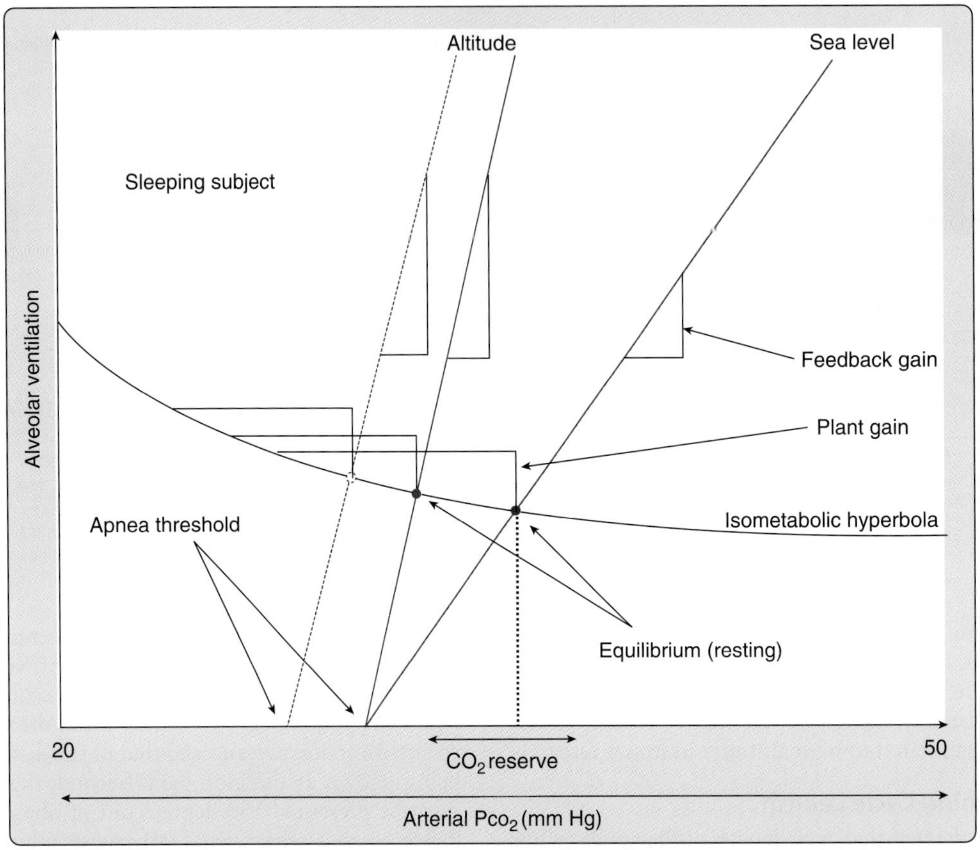

Figure 25.4 Illustration of the relationship between alveolar ventilation and alveolar P_{CO_2} at a fixed CO_2 production (e.g., 250 mL/min). Ascent to altitude increases the chemoreflex slope (*solid blue line*) but does not necessarily change the apnea threshold; the increase in slope moves the equilibrium to an increased ventilation and lower P_{CO_2}, thereby decreasing plant gain. This effect—chronic hyperventilation induced by the high altitude and subsequent reductions in plant gain—indicates that a greater transient increase in alveolar ventilation (V_A) and corresponding reduction in Pa_{CO_2} is required to reach the apneic threshold than would be the case under conditions of normocapnia. Therefore this reduction in plant gain acts to stabilize breathing. Should the apnea threshold also be decreased with acclimatization at altitude (*dotted blue line*), then ventilation increases and P_{CO_2} decreases, and plant gain is further decreased. For a given background Pa_{CO_2}, alterations in the slope of the change in V_E per change in Pa_{CO_2} relationship below eupnea would alter the CO_2 reserve (i.e., the amount of reduction in Pa_{CO_2} required to cause apnea). Changing the slope of the ventilatory response to CO_2 above eupnea would alter susceptibility for transient ventilatory overshoots. Although at altitude the chronic hyperventilation-induced hypocapnia may be "protective" against apnea and breathing instability through reductions in plant gain, the other chemoreceptor (e.g., controller gain) and nonchemoreceptor (e.g., increased pulmonary pressures, behavioral drives, awake-to-sleep transitions, locomotion feedback/forward stimuli) factors may contribute, potentially negating this response. (Modified from Ainslie PN, Lucas SJ, Burgess KR. Breathing and sleep at high altitude. *Respir Physiol Neurobiol.* 2013;188:233–56.)

are required for sensing the low Pa_{CO_2} and causing ventilatory instability and cyclic apneas.[42,44] However, hypocapnia induced at the level of *both* peripheral and central chemoreceptors is required to elicit apnea.[45,46] Vagal blockade in sleeping animals also shows that inhibitory feedback from lung stretch accompanying transient increases in tidal volume contributes to the apnea following a ventilatory overshoot.[47] These inhibitory effects on breathing are opposed by excitatory central short-term potentiation mechanisms that preserve ventilatory drive immediately following ventilatory overshoots while awake but apparently not during NREM sleep.[48,49] Two additional mechanisms to enhance postapneic ventilatory overshoots include (a) apneas are commonly prolonged until Pa_{CO_2} rises above its normal preapneic, eupneic level[50] and (b) transient arousals at end apnea are common and will enhance the magnitude of the transient ventilatory overshoot response to chemoreceptor stimulation.

These mechanisms underlie a sleep-induced apnea, but the repeated, cyclic occurrence of transient ventilatory undershoots (apneas/hypopneas) and overshoots requires that subjects' respiratory control system "loop gain" be elevated. The principal component to the high loop gain is a high chemosensitivity to CO_2 both above and below the level of eupneic ventilation. This high gain means that both ventilatory undershoots in response to a transient hypocapnia and ventilatory overshoots in response to a combination of apneic-induced hypoxemic and hypercapnic chemoreceptor stimuli are excessive, thereby precipitating the continued breathing periodicity.[40,51] The concept of loop gain and its two main principal components, controller (CO_2 chemosensitivity or $\Delta V_E/\Delta Pa_{CO_2}$ slope) and plant gain (or $\Delta Pa_{CO_2}/\Delta V_E$), are illustrated in Figure 25.4.[52]

Loop gain is increased in hypoxia or at high altitude because chemoreceptor CO_2 sensitivity is increased more than controller gain is reduced. Thus the apneic threshold resides within 1 to 2 mm Hg of the eupneic Pa_{CO_2} during NREM sleep, ensuring a significant ventilatory undershoot with even small levels of transient hypocapnia. In addition, the ventilatory overshoot at apnea terminations are amplified because of the synergistic stimulatory effects on carotid chemoreceptors of hypoxemia plus hypercapnia (i.e., asphyxia).[53] Chemoreceptor sensory inputs drive both medullary rhythm-generating neurons as well as arousal-producing cortical neurons.[29,51] These combined oscillating powerful drives and inhibitors to breathing likely explain, respectively, the abrupt large ventilatory overshoots at apnea termination and abrupt ventilatory undershoots at end hyperpnea in hypoxic environments, resulting in the cluster-type breathing pattern (Figure 25.2).

Periodic Breathing and Hypoxic Ventilatory Response

If elevations in controller gain are the principal precipitating mechanism for periodic breathing, then, other things being equal, persons with the highest hypoxic and hypercapnia ventilatory responses should have more severe periodic breathing. Although many studies cite the classic Lahiri study[30] to provide evidence of the correlation of hypoxic ventilatory response (HVR) and periodic breathing, this relationship was largely created by the inclusion of a Sherpa group with a blunted HVR. Upon examination, no obvious relationship was found between HVR and periodic breathing within the so-called lowlander population. This absence of a relationship was further confirmed, albeit in a subgroup (n = 5), at 6300 and 8050 meters.[1] These findings are consistent with those of Masuyama and colleagues, where two of nine mountaineers did not develop central sleep apnea (CSA) at altitude despite normal values for HVR.[54] More recently, absence of a relationship between HVR and periodic breathing at 5050 meters has been reported.[26] By contrast, at 4400 meters in a small sample size (n = 4), it was shown that the respiratory stimulant almitrine doubled the HVR and elevated periodic breathing compared with acetazolamide or placebo.[55] Nevertheless, the known blunted HVR and diminished periodic breathing in Sherpas[30] lend support to a role for HVR in periodic breathing. A number of potential explanations exist for these discrepant and variable findings, including evidence that the hypoxic and CO_2 response are not always similar above and below eupnea[40]; differences in awake versus sleep respiratory control; variable acid-base status; and methodologic differences (e.g., chemoreflex testing and hence inclusion of CBF using steady state or rebreathing methods, natural versus simulated altitude, or other means). At least on the basis of rebreathing measures in humans at high altitude,[56-58] it is not clear if actual wakefulness chemoreflex gain differs above and below resting equilibrium. Collectively, these findings highlight the multifactorial complexity of characterizing and studying periodic breathing at high altitude.

Sex Differences in Periodic Breathing

Interestingly, sex may influence the extent of periodic breathing (as indexed by the apnea-hypopnea index [AHI]) at high altitude. For example, in contrast to males, females demonstrate less hypopnea at 2000 meters[59] and have a reduced AHI at 5400 meters[60] and simulated altitudes of 3500, 4500, and 5500 meters.[61] Additionally, in a study conducted at 4559 meters, men were shown to have a greater severity of periodic breathing during sleep when compared to females at altitude, which was attributed to their increased hypoxic chemosensitivity.[62] Nevertheless, acetazolamide counteracted the occurrence of periodic breathing at altitude in both sexes, modifying the apneic threshold and improving oxygenation.[62] A detailed description of sex differences during sleep are discussed in a general context in later chapters (see Chapters 183 to 189).

Other Factors Influencing Periodic Breathing

Periodic breathing in hypoxia occurs in breath "clusters," with tidal volume increasing from zero to three to four times control levels, almost instantaneously following each apneic interval. This pattern has been suggested to reflect the presence of a transient arousal state at apnea termination that would further augment the responsiveness of the respiratory control system and produce the sudden ventilatory overshoot.[63] Another possible influence on periodic breathing is a direct influence of brain hypoxia.[42] Other evidence, also based on findings in animals,[64,65] supports the notion that breathing instability may also involve pulmonary J receptors. These receptors are stimulated by pulmonary congestion/lung edema at high altitude and evoke reflex inhibition of ventilation, which prolongs the apnea. Additionally, acute pulmonary hypertension (as reflected in elevations in left atrial pressure by 5.7 mm Hg in the well-controlled animal model) during sleep results in a narrowed CO_2 reserve and thus predisposes affected subjects to exhibit apneas/unstable breathing.[66] It seems likely that the periodic breathing-induced oscillations in CBF also act to destabilize breathing by provoking large swings in brain tissue pH and hence central chemoreflex stimulation and inhibition. Although clear evidence for these complex pathways at high altitude is still lacking, it is known that at sea level, periodic breathing during sleep is more pronounced in patients with pulmonary hypertension than in those without.[67]

ACCLIMATIZATION

As summarized perfectly by Houston and Riley in 1947, "Acclimatization to high altitude consists of a series of integrated adaptations which tend to restore the tissue oxygen pressure towards normal sea level values in spite of lowered oxygen pressure of the atmosphere."[68] This acclimatization process has two major components: ventilatory adaptation to hypoxia and the renal excretion of bicarbonate, allowing further ventilatory adaptation. Detailed reviews on this topic are available.[31,69,70]

In brief, acute exposure to high altitude results in the following sequence of physiologic events: (1) Initial changes consist of a decrease in the alveolar partial pressure of oxygen (Po_2) and, correspondingly, in the partial pressure of arterial oxygen (Pao_2). (2) This decrease in oxygen tension results in stimulation of the peripheral chemoreceptors (predominantly at the carotid sinus), with a resultant increase in ventilation. (3) This initial increase in ventilation (the hypoxic ventilatory response) decreases Pco_2 and increases Po_2 in the alveolar gas according to the alveolar ventilation and gas equations. (4) The decrease in arterial Pco_2 (and consequent increase in arterial pH—defining conditions of respiratory alkalosis) acts to inhibit the peripheral chemoreceptor. In addition, because CO_2 is freely diffusible across the blood-brain barrier, a decrease in cerebrospinal fluid CO_2 occurs, thereby raising cerebrospinal fluid and brain extracellular fluid pH, causing inhibition at the central chemoreceptors. (5) Finally, both of these effects act to return ventilation back toward sea level values. Over a period of hours to days at high altitude, however, the body compensates for the respiratory alkalosis by increasing bicarbonate excretion in the kidney and increasing bicarbonate removal from the extracellular fluid by the choroid plexus. (6) Thus the inhibition at the central and peripheral chemoreceptors is removed and the ventilation once again increases. A direct influence of hypoxia on the central nervous system also may act to drive these progressive elevations in ventilation (reviewed in Ainslie and colleagues[31]). As shown

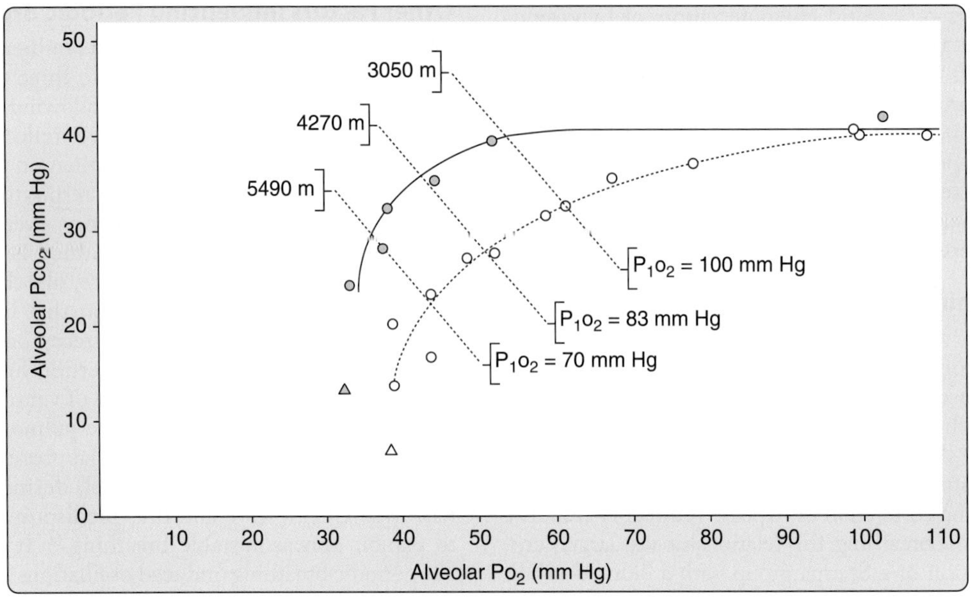

Figure 25.5 Effect of altitude acclimatization on alveolar gas composition. *Blue symbols* represent unacclimatized data. *Open (white) symbols* represent acclimatized data. Iso-altitude lines were determined using the ideal alveolar gas equation and an assumed respiratory exchange ratio of 0.85. (Data from Rahn H, Otis AB. Man's respiratory response during and after acclimatization to high altitude. *Am J Physiol.* 1949;157:445–559; West JB, Hackett PH, Maret KH, et al. Pulmonary gas exchange on the summit of Mount Everest. *J Appl Physiol.* 1983;55:678–87; Malconian MK, Rock PB, Reeves JT, et al. Operation Everest II: gas tensions in expired air and arterial blood at extreme altitude. *Aviat Space Environ Med.* 1993;64:37–42; and Wagner PD, Sutton JR, Reeves JT, et al. Operation Everest II: pulmonary gas exchange during a simulated ascent of Mt. Everest. *J Appl Physiol.* 1987;63:2348–59.)

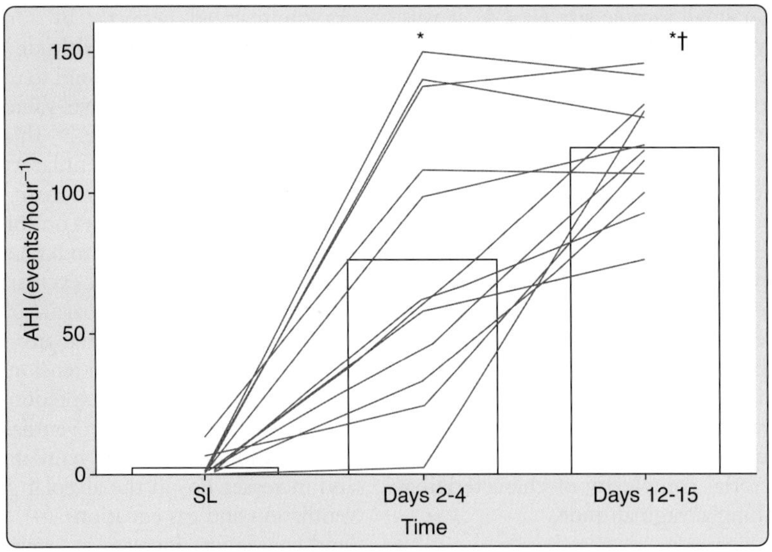

Figure 25.6 Increase in apnea-hypopnea index (AHI) with time at 5050 meters. *Lines* represent individual subjects. *Asterisks* and *dagger* indicate level of statistical significance, such that * ≤0.01, † ≤0.01. SL, Sea level. (Modified from Burgess KR, Lucas SJ, Shepherd KL, et al. Worsening of central sleep apnea at high altitude–a role for cerebrovascular function. J Appl Physiol. 2013;114:1021–8.)

in Figure 25.5, acclimatization at high altitude is reflected in reductions in $PaCO_2$ and an increase in PaO_2. Although these changes tend to mitigate the deleterious effects of the hypoxic environment, it should be noted that restoration of PaO_2 back to sea level values can never occur.

Periodic Breathing Changes with Both Magnitude and Duration of Hypoxic Stimulus

It was originally considered that the amount of periodic breathing in sleep is greatly reduced over time in normobaric hypoxia.[18,29,71] However, at least at high altitude, evidence derived using full polysomnography shows the opposite—that periodic breathing intensifies over time (12 to 15 days) at a given altitude in all subjects[26] (Figure 25.6).

Additionally, as highlighted in Figure 25.7, it is clear that periodic breathing increases proportionally with altitude, and as illustrated in Figure 25.8, a small but progressive decrease occurs in the average duration of the apnea-hypopnea events at altitude. Because the development of CSA is almost exclusive to NREM sleep (especially during stage 1 and 2), collectively, this information allows determination of the theoretical ceiling of CSA at high altitude. Naturally, this limit would

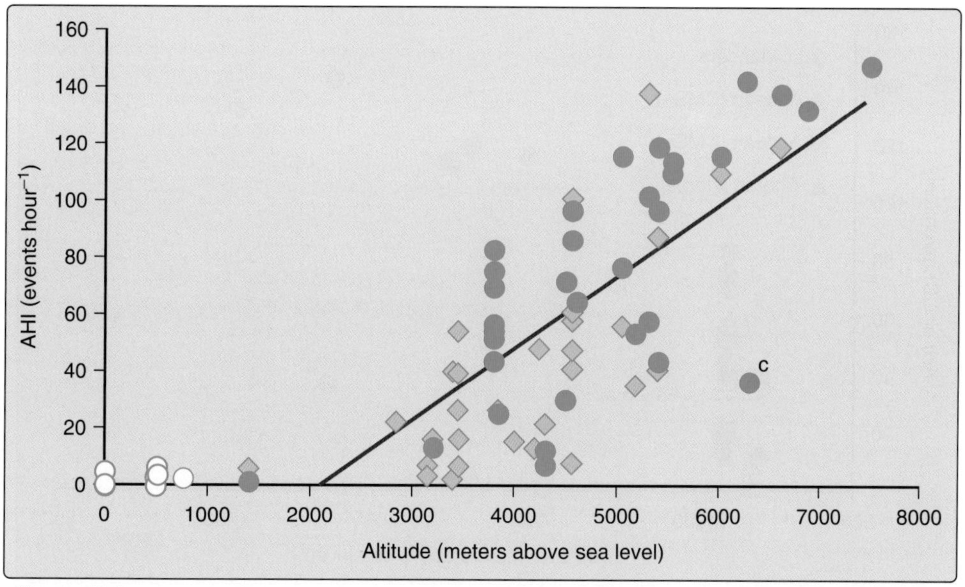

Figure 25.7 Relationship between altitude and apnea-hypopnea index (AHI). Each point refers to a specific time-point of a study (*open circle,* baseline; *solid diamond,* acute exposure [i.e., up to 2 days at specified altitude]; *solid circle,* prolonged exposure [i.e., greater than 2 days at specified altitude]), and the *pink solid line* denotes the regression between time points. C, Calculated AHI based on individual data of the ratio of number of periodic breathing cycles over study duration, multiplied by 60. (The figure compiles results from multiple studies.*)

* References 1,8,24,26,28,30,34,35,60,62,72,87,97,130,142,145-152.

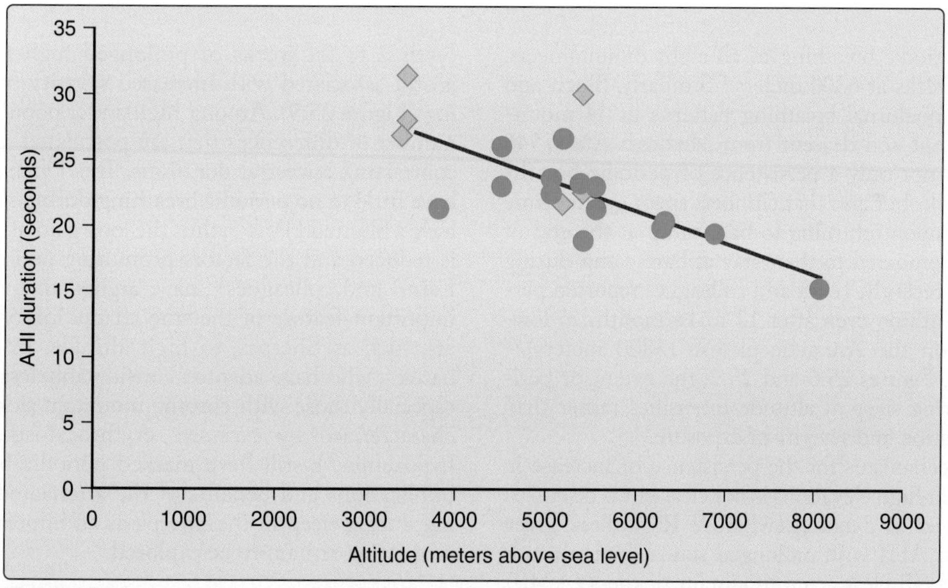

Figure 25.8 Relationship between altitude and apnea-hypopnea duration. Each point refers to a specific time point of a study (*solid diamond,* acute exposure [i.e., up to 2 days at specified altitude]; *solid circle,* prolonged exposure [i.e., greater than 2 days at specified altitude]), and the *pink solid line* denotes the regression between time points. (The figure compiles results from multiple studies.*)

* References 1,24,34,35,54,60,87,142.

vary depending on individual differences in cycle duration and percentage of time in REM sleep. Nevertheless, on the basis of this information, it is possible to ascertain when apnea-hypopnea cycling has reached the maximal theoretical value. At this point, which may occur with acclimatization, these calculations are important, because they indicate that the development of CSA becomes independent of key factors affecting its severity (e.g., controller gain, apneic threshold, and cerebrovascular influences).

Persistence of Periodic Breathing over Time at High Altitude

A prominent feature of prolonged exposure to high altitude is the persistence of periodic breathing. West and colleagues

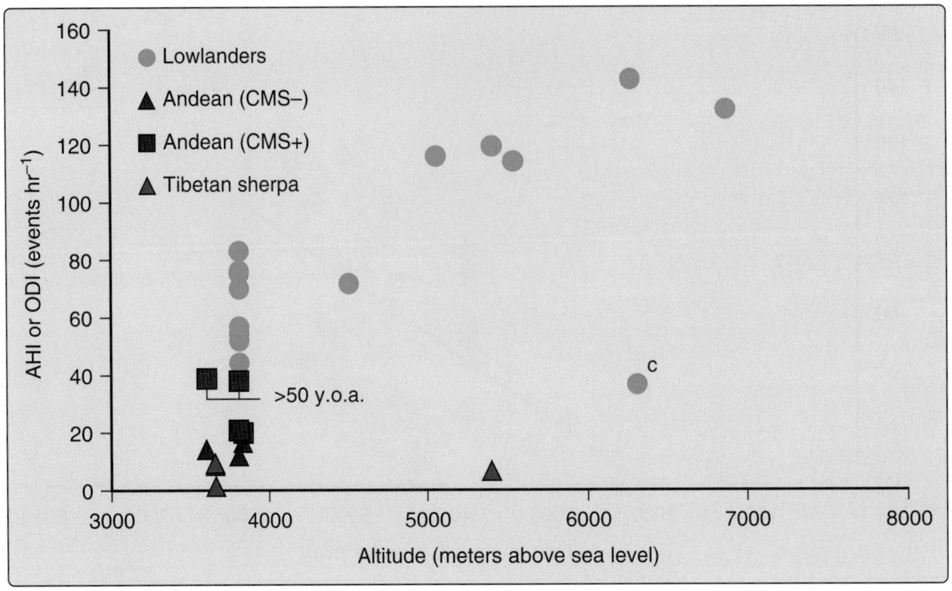

Figure 25.9 Summary of partially acclimatized lowlanders (≥2 weeks) and high-altitude native populations. C, Calculated AHI based on individual data of the ratio of number of periodic breathing cycles over study duration, multiplied by 60. CMS, chronic mountain sickness; y.o.a., years of age. Lowlander studies: [30]*n* = 7 after >32 nights at 5400 meters; [1]*n* = 8 after 17 days at 6300 meters and 3–5 weeks at ≥5400 meters; [24]*n* = 3 after 3 weeks at 3800 meters; [34]*n* = 24–32 ~2–3 weeks at altitudes from 4497–6865 meters; [87]*n* = 12 after ~2 weeks at 5050 meters; [26]*n* = 12 after ~2 weeks at 5050 meters; [72]*n* = 7 after 6–24 weeks at 3800 meters). High-altitude native studies: [153]Andean (*n* = 6 CMS–; *n* = 14 CMS+); [79]Andean (*n* = 12 CMS–; *n* = 23 CMS+); [154]Andean (*n* = 171 CMS–, *n* = 8 CMS+); [30]Sherpa (*n* = 6); [78]Sherpa (*n* = 11); [75]Sherpa (*n* = 61).

showed obvious periodic breathing in all eight mountaineers, even after several weeks at 6300 meters.[1] Similarly, Bloch and colleagues studied nocturnal breathing patterns in 34 mountaineers during ascent and descent from Muztagh Ata (7546 meters) and found not only a persistence of periodic breathing over several weeks but also that climbers spent greater time periodic breathing upon returning to base camp at the end of their climb when compared to their stay at base camp during the ascent.[34] More recently, Tellez and colleagues reported persistent periodic breathing even after 12 to 14 months in lowlanders stationed on the Antarctic plateau (3800 meters).[72] As summarized in Figures 25.6 and 25.7, the extent of periodic breathing during sleep at altitude intensifies rather than improves with duration and severity of exposure.

The putative mechanisms for the persistence or increase in periodic breathing at high elevations is not clear but is discussed further and reviewed in detail elsewhere.[31] Regardless, given that the increase in AHI with prolonged stay at high altitude coincides with generally less acute mountain sickness (AMS), and that periodic breathing may elevate rather than reduce mean Sao_2 during sleep suggests that periodic breathing may represent an adaptive rather than maladaptive response.

Periodic Breathing in High-Altitude Populations

Native populations of the Tibetan plateau and Andean highlands have both descended from approximately 25,000 years and 11,000 years, respectively, of high-altitude ancestry. Both populations have had time for natural selection of traits to offset the unavoidable environmental stress of severe lifelong exposure to high altitude, and the physiologic and genetic consequences of this environmental stress have been elegantly reviewed.[73,74] These populations exhibit minimal periodic breathing at high altitude, which in contrast to lowlanders (with 2 to 24 weeks of prolonged high-altitude exposure), is still associated with increased severity of periodic breathing (Figure 25.9). Among highlander populations, there are a number of differences that are postulated to stem from their contrasting ancestral durations. The Tibetan Sherpa tend to have little to no periodic breathing during sleep[30,75] and often have a blunted HVR[76]; thus the loop gain of the control system is reduced and the factors promoting periodicity are weak.[30] Lahiri and colleagues[30] have argued that this represents an important feature of the true adaptation of native highlanders, such as Sherpas, to high altitude. In contrast, Andean natives, who have adapted considerably less than the Sherpa, especially those with chronic mountain sickness (a condition characterized by excessive erythrocytosis and accentuated hypoxemia[77]), still have marked periodic breathing.[78,79] The implications and benefits of the attenuated periodic breathing during sleep in the Sherpa as an important phenotype of adaptation remain to be explored.

A ROLE OF CEREBRAL BLOOD FLOW IN BREATHING STABILITY AT ALTITUDE

The supportive evidence for a putative role of CBF and reactivity on breathing stability is now clear. First, pharmacologic blunting of CBF and its reactivity to CO_2 leads to elevations in controller gain, reduced CO_2 reserve, and subsequent increased susceptibility to onset of apnea and breathing instability during sleep.[80] These changes also are evident during wakefulness.[81] Moreover, acute elevations in CBF velocity and reactivity to $Paco_2$, induced by intravenous acetazolamide, have been demonstrated to be related to improvements in breathing stability at high altitude during wakefulness[82] and sleep.[83] In support, modeling studies have shown that, theoretically, doubling of cerebrovascular reactivity to CO_2 leads to a marked dampening of respiratory oscillations in conditions of sleep at high altitude.[84] Conversely, when cerebrovascular reactivity to CO_2 was halved, a simple sigh was sufficient to transform the stable breathing pattern into a periodic breathing pattern—consequently, restoring reactivity leads to a restored stability.[84] Thus CBF and its related CO_2 reactivity, through its influence on central chemosensitivity, provide an important mechanism in the pathophysiology of CSA (Figure 25.10).

As mentioned earlier, CBF is elevated on a person's initial arrival to high altitude. This elevated CBF aims to restore O_2 delivery in light of reduced arterial oxygen content[85] but also likely provides a protective effect from CSA.[86] In 11 subjects at 5050 meters, an increase in CBF facilitated an increased removal of locally produced CO_2 from the central chemoreceptors, causing a reduction in hypercapnic ventilatory response and, consequently, reduced loop gain.[86] After partial acclimatization, CBF and its reactivity decline, resulting in a further increase in HCVR and universally severe CSA at altitude[26]—changes ultimately mediated by elevations in controller gain[87] and reduced CO_2 reserve.

The stimulation of the central chemoreceptors is from the CO_2 that is actually produced in the surrounding brain. Arterial blood flow to the brain washes the CO_2 away from the chemoreceptors. This means that CBF during sleep may be very important in ventilatory control. In the absence of the wakefulness drive to breathe, marked oscillations in CBF occur as a consequence of the periodic breathing, similar in nature to that reported in patients who experience sleep apnea at sea level.[88,89] Previous studies[26,90] demonstrated a relation between the decline in CBF from awake to NREM sleep, albeit being only a modest predictor of CSA. Of interest, the relation was stronger after 2 weeks at high altitude, when absolute perfusion was lower (both awake and during sleep), further supporting the idea that reduced [H^+] washout within the brain enhances chemoreceptor activation. Moreover, in view of the link between breathing pattern and CBF,[91,92] these oscillations in CBF are likely to be important in the pathophysiology of periodic breathing. Indeed, regardless of the causation of the first apneic episode, that is, whether alterations in basal CBF[93] or in cerebral or arterial Pco_2[94-96] (or a combination of these and other factors) start the apnea cycle, the large swings in CBF that ensue seem likely to exacerbate the under- and overshooting of the ventilatory drive that characterizes the CSA disorder.[42]

The potential role for alterations in CBF during sleep at high altitude in the control of breathing has been further supported by the results of artificially increasing and reducing CBF during sleep by the use of medications. In a group of 12 healthy volunteers at 5050 meters, the administration of

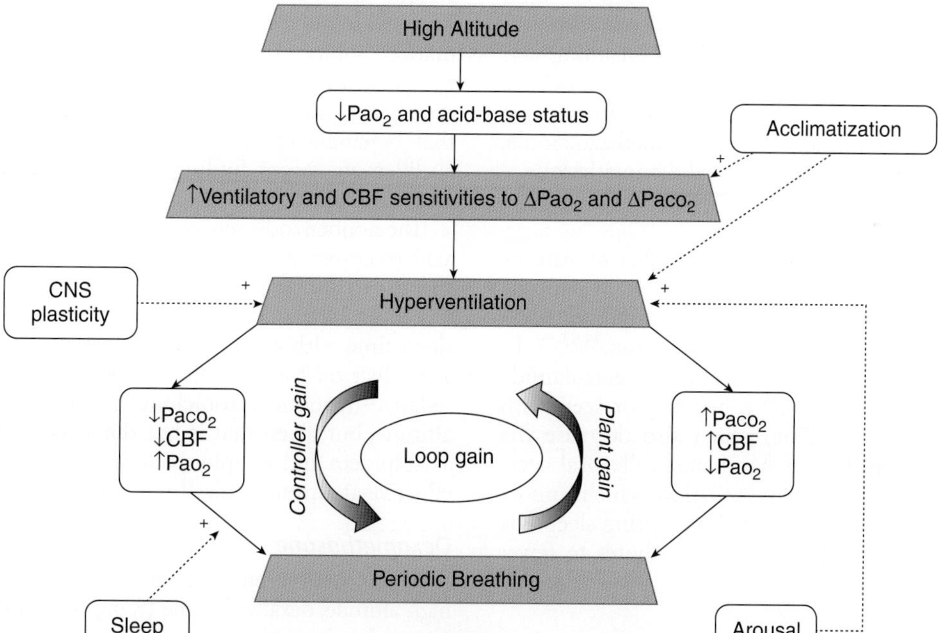

Figure 25.10 Schematic diagram showing various mechanisms by which high-altitude exposure leads to the development of periodic breathing during sleep. Initial effects of high-altitude exposure include a reduction in the partial pressure of arterial oxygen (Pao_2) and acid-base adjustments. These changes lead to alterations in chemoreflex control and cerebrovascular responses to changes in arterial blood gases. Overall, these complex cellular and neurochemical changes in chemoreflexes, acid-base status, and the central nervous system (CNS) lead to hyperventilation. Acclimatization, at least in lowlanders, magnifies these changes. Elevations in loop gain outweigh the improvements in plant gain caused by the chronic hypocapnia, leading to periodic breathing. Sleep and arousals lead to greater breathing instability. Apnea, which is associated with an increase in $Paco_2$ and decrease in Pao_2 (and/or arousal), restimulates the peripheral chemoreceptors and consequently ventilation. These changes in blood gases also lead to marked alterations in cerebral blood flow (CBF) (Figure 25.3), which in turn may result in a sudden elevation (with reduced CBF) or reduction (with increased CBF) in brainstem pH. (Modified from Ainslie PN, Duffin J. Integration of cerebrovascular CO_2 reactivity and chemoreflex control of breathing: mechanisms of regulation, measurement, and interpretation. *Am J Physiol Regul Integr Comp Physiol.* 2009;296:R1473–95.)

100 mg oral indomethacin, which reduced CBF by approximately 23%, increased the severity of CSA by 16%.[83] The HCVR also increased by 66%, suggesting that the reduction in CBF may have caused the increase in HCVR, which in turn increased the severity of CSA. Conversely, the administration of intravenous acetazolamide, which increased CBF by 28% without changing acid-base balance in the short term, reduced the severity of CSA by approximately 47%.[83] These results are consistent with modeling studies and suggest that CBF, through its influence on the central chemoreceptors, support ventilation at rest and stabilize breathing during sleep at altitude.

IMPROVING SLEEP AT HIGH ALTITUDE

Since there is a strong relationship between absolute altitude and severity of CSA (Figure 25.7), the obvious treatment would be to reverse that process and descend. If this is not desired nor practical, there are a number of options to reduce periodic breathing that can be broadly divided into two broad categories: pharmacologic and nonpharmacologic interventions, with the latter category including medical gases and devices. The evidence of effectiveness of these treatment approaches is considered in the next sections.

Pharmacologic Interventions

Given the contribution of periodic breathing to poor sleep quality following ascent, there has been considerable interest in the use of medications to decrease periodic breathing and improve sleep quality at high altitude. A number of studies have used pharmacologic manipulation at high altitude to improve periodic breathing, including acetazolamide, methazolamide, theophylline, various sedative-hypnotics, and dexamethasone.

Acetazolamide

Oral acetazolamide has been shown by a number of authors to effectively suppress the amount of time spent in periodic breathing (by 50%–80% during sleep) and improves arterial oxygen saturation at high altitude saturation.[55,97-99] In addition to the effects on periodic breathing, acetazolamide decreases the incidence of AMS,[98] a benefit not seen with other agents such as theophylline, which also decrease the incidence of periodic breathing.[97] Mechanistically, oral acetazolamide elicits steady state hyperventilation, which importantly reduces loop gain, stabilizes breathing during sleep (via a reduction in periodic breathing), and contributes to fewer arousals.[99-101]

Methazolamide

Methazolamide is an analogue of acetazolamide, and as such after 3 days of oral administration, methazolamide causes a metabolic acidosis and shifts the ventilatory CO_2 response curve leftward without reducing O_2 sensitivity.[102] Interestingly, methazolamide appears to be associated with less neuromuscular fatigue when compared to acetazolamide[103]; however, the implications of this on sleep have yet to be investigated.

Theophylline

Theophylline has respiratory stimulant properties and has been shown to reduce the extent of periodic breathing and reduce the magnitude of oxygen desaturation during sleep.[97] However, the medication has a narrow therapeutic window and the potential for significant toxicity and, as a result, is a far less useful option than acetazolamide or the other agents discussed in this section.

Diphenhydramine

Although it is a commonly used sleep aid at sea level, diphenhydramine has never been researched for the purpose of examining its use with sleep at high altitude. Because it has the potential for lingering sedation the day following nocturnal use, it is not a great option for improving sleep in people who need to perform highly technical or risky activities the following day.

Sedative-Hypnotics

Part of the disruption to sleep at high altitude is the insomnia (both sleep onset and sleep maintenance) resulting from repeated arousals and awakenings from the hyperpneic phase of periodic breathing. Theoretically, sedative medications could suppress ventilatory responsiveness and potentially lead to worsened arterial oxygen saturation during sleep, which may also impair sleep quality and exacerbate AMS. However, several placebo-controlled studies performed in the field, evaluating hypnotic medications, have reported improvements in subjective and objective measures of sleep quality with 10 mg of benzodiazepine temazepam.[104-106] Röggla and colleagues did report an increased P_{CO_2} and decreased P_{O_2} measured from earlobe blood during temazepam use, but these assessments were made only 1 hour following administration in unacclimatized subjects and may not reflect the utility and safety of the medication over an entire night of sleep or with a longer duration of stay at high altitude.[106] Although data indicate that benzodiazepines can reduce CSA by reducing arousals,[105] more recent findings indicate that this role has been overemphasized.[26]

The nonbenzodiazepine hypnotics or gamma-aminobutyric acid receptor agents, zolpidem and zaleplon, have also been shown to improve sleep quality and sleep architecture, including increased slow wave and stage IV sleep and total sleep time, although there is no evidence these agents have any effect on the incidence of periodic breathing.[107-110] The sedative-hypnotic eszopiclone has not been studied at high altitude, but given that it has the same mechanism of action as zolpidem and zaleplon, one would expect it to be safe and effective at altitude as well.[111]

Dexamethasone

Although not typically seen as an option for improving sleep at high altitude, dexamethasone (8 mg twice a day, started prior to ascent) has been shown to prevent severe hypoxemia and sleep disturbances in high-altitude pulmonary edema (HAPE)-susceptible individuals at 4559 meters, whereas use 24 hours after arrival at 4559 meters increases oxygenation and deep sleep.[112]

Although it is unknown if dexamethasone is effective in non–HAPE-susceptible individuals, it also has been reported that, in lowlanders with chronic obstructive pulmonary disease traveling to 3100 meters, dexamethasone (4 mg twice daily) starting 24 hours prior to ascent and continued after arrival improved nocturnal oxygen saturation, periodic breathing, and subjective sleep quality.[113]

The optimal doses of the various sleep aids remain unclear, as do the utility and safety of combination therapy or the relative efficacy of the various agents when used as monotherapy.[111]

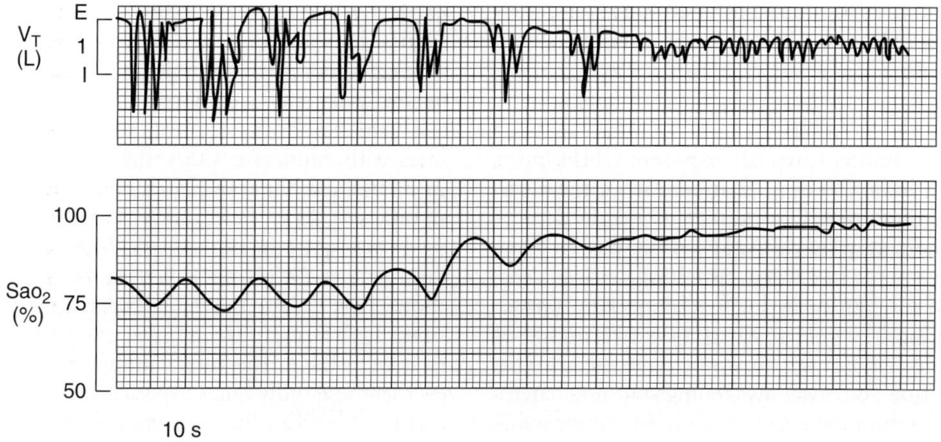

Figure 25.11 Polygraphic tracing. The effect of oxygen on periodic breathing and arterial oxygen saturation during sleep at 5400 meters. As oxygen arterial saturation increases, periodic breathing is replaced by shallow and continuous breathing.[30] E, Expiration; I, inspiration. (Modified from Lahiri S, Maret K, Sherpa MG. Dependence of high altitude sleep apnea on ventilatory sensitivity to hypoxia. *Respir Physiol.* 1983;52:281–301.)

Nonpharmacologic Interventions

Medical Gases

Lahiri and colleagues have shown clearly the curative effects of supplemental oxygen therapy on a subject with sustained CSA at 5300 meters (Figure 25.11).[30] Upon rapid restoration of normal Sa_{O_2} via increased $F_{I}O_2$, periodic breathing continues with prolonged apneic periods until hyperventilation is gradually reduced and Pa_{CO_2} returns to normal.

Stabilizing effects of small additions of $F_{I}CO_2$ have also been reported to have a comparable effect.[29] The mechanism is probably via stabilization of the carotid bodies and hence blunting the transient changes in Pa_{CO_2} during the hyperpnea phase of the CSA.

Adding oxygen to the ventilation of a room also shows promise as a way of combating the hypoxia of high altitude, particularly for people who commute to high altitude to work.[114] Luks and colleagues carried out a randomized, double-blind trial at an altitude of 3800 meters to determine whether oxygen enrichment of room air to an $F_{I}O_2$ of 0.24 at night improved sleep quality and performance and well-being the following day. Following sleep in the oxygen-enriched environment, subjects had higher arterial oxygen saturation and fewer apneas and spent significantly less time in periodic breathing with apneas compared to sleep in ambient air.[115] Sleeping in the oxygen-enriched environment also improved subjective assessments of sleep quality and AMS scores upon awakening, but no changes were noted during performance on psychometric testing. Using a similar study protocol, Barash and colleagues also noted improvements in sleep architecture during oxygen-enriched sleep including greater time in slow wave sleep.[116] McElroy and colleagues confirmed these finding in a subsequent study and suggested the elevation in arterial oxygen saturation was likely due to a lower incidence of subclinical pulmonary edema rather than an effect of room oxygen enrichment on ventilatory control, as no changes were observed in hypoxic or hypercapnic ventilatory responses between the different treatments.[117] Most recreational skiers and trekkers do not travel to the altitudes described in these studies but still report significant sleep disturbances at lower elevations between 2000 and 3000 meters. Oxygen enrichment of room air is feasible for resorts at such elevations[118] and can be expected to greatly improve the quality of sleep.

Devices

Recently a number of devices have shown potential to treat periodic breathing at altitude, including bilevel positive airway pressure (PAP), a simple addition of dead space via a modified facemask, and expiratory resistance.

PAP administered via servo ventilator or continuous positive airway pressure (CPAP) was not consistently effective in reducing CSA in hypoxia in otherwise healthy volunteers[119] or individuals with obstructive sleep apnea (OSA).[120] In contrast, Johnson and colleagues documented improvements in nocturnal oxygen saturation and AMS scores in normal individuals sleeping at 3800 meters with noninvasive positive pressure ventilation but did not make any objective or subjective measurements of sleep quality.[121] At least in laboratory studies in normoxic hypoxia, adding 1 to 2 mm Hg Pa_{CO_2} (via increased $F_{I}CO_2$) is sufficient to completely eliminate periodic breathing via reduced plant gain.[29,122]

The simple addition of a 500-mL dead space also has been shown to improve sleep in some subjects at 3500 meters.[123] This study was conducted in 12 unacclimatized persons using full polysomnography. In random order, half of the night was spent with a 500-mL increase in dead space through a custom-designed full face mask and the other half without it. Although the dead space had no effect on individuals with AHI less than 30 events/hour, it did lead to marked reductions in AHI (from 70 to down to 30 events/hour) and oxygen desaturation index (from 73 to 43). Thus a 500-mL increase in dead space through a fitted mask may improve nocturnal breathing in those with severe altitude-induced sleep-disordered breathing.[123] Similar to the aforementioned studies that have used elevations in $F_{I}CO_2$ to improve periodic breathing, the mechanism via elevations in dead space is likely through the stabilizing influence of elevations in Pa_{CO_2} on the CO_2 reserve.

Expiratory resistance, typically using a one-way lever system to allow normal inhalation but restricting flow through a narrowed orifice, has shown improvements in the level of hypoxemia and in treating and preventing AMS.[124,125] Likely related to elevated Pa_{CO_2}, a recent laboratory study reported an AHI reduction of approximately 50% during sleep in subjects who wore an expiratory resistance mask containing a small amount of dead space when compared to a sham device.[126]

However, when evaluated in the field, upon acute ascent to 4300 meters, a mask of slightly altered design did not yield an improvement in AHI.[127]

Intermittent Hypoxic Strategies

Various forms of intermittent hypoxic exposure (IHE) prior to a planned ascent have also been considered as a means to improve sleep at high altitude. Exposure to the equivalent of 4300 meters for 3 hours/day over a 7-day period was not associated with improvements in oxygen saturation during sleep, sleep quality, or sleep quantity during a subsequent exposure to the same elevation,[128] while seven consecutive nights of sleep in normobaric hypoxia led to improvements in mean sleep oxygen saturation and fewer awakenings but no changes in the number of desaturation events or duration of wakefulness upon subsequent exposure to a terrestrial altitude of 4300 meters.[129] The time spent in periodic breathing was not examined in either study. One reason for the lack of clear benefit from IHE may relate to the fact that IHE enhances ventilatory acclimatization and, as a result, may worsen the loop gain phenomenon that contributes to the periodic breathing problems that play a large role in poor sleep quality. Another challenge with the literature on IHE is the significant variability in protocols for hypoxic exposure between studies, which makes it challenging to compare results across studies and understand which regimen provides the optimal approach.

ARE THESE TREATMENT MEASURES NECESSARY?

Although there are pharmacologic and nonpharmacologic measures that decrease periodic breathing and improve sleep quality, it is worth asking whether such measures are really necessary. As noted previously, sleep quality improves over time at high altitude despite persistence of periodic breathing.[130] In addition, there is no clear evidence that poor sleep or periodic breathing predispose to complications at high altitude including acute altitude illness, evident by the elimination of "sleep quality" as a metric, from the Lake Louise AMS scoring questionnaire.[131] For these reasons, one could make the argument that the benefits of these interventions do not outweigh the risks of medicinal side effects nor the logistic challenges of traveling to high altitude with the medical gases or devices mentioned previously. Interestingly, however, it was recently reported that stabilizing breathing at 3800 meters (via adaptive seroventilation) or increasing oxygenation (via supplemental oxygen) during sleep can reduce feelings of fatigue and confusion, but that daytime hypoxia may play a larger role in other cognitive impairments reported at high altitude.[132] Therefore it would seem that in some individuals, such as those who must perform complex technical work the following day, might still benefit from these interventions, whereas for the majority of travelers, poor sleep may simply be a self-limited nuisance that does not warrant aggressive preventive measures.

CONSIDERATIONS WHEN TRAVELING TO HIGH ALTITUDE

Obstructive Sleep Apnea

In addition to the issues described previously, it is useful to consider what happens to sleep at high altitude in those individuals with known sleep disorders at sea level. A question of particular importance is whether those with OSA will experience the same or fewer obstructive events during a high-altitude sojourn when not using CPAP compared to what they normally experience at home. Burgess and colleagues reported a fall in the obstructive respiratory disturbance index in five men with moderate OSA (baseline apnea hypopnea index 25.5±14.4 per hour) at 2750 meters that was accompanied by a significant rise in the central respiratory distress index.[133] This study was done in normobaric hypoxia; however, subsequent field studies involving exposure to hypobaric hypoxia have shown that despite the fall in barometric pressure and air density at high altitude, the number of obstructive events remained relatively stable. The total number of apneas increased, however, as these individuals experienced a large number of central events.[134,135] The increase in the AHI was not only associated with lower nocturnal oxygen saturation but also impaired tracking performance during simulated driving at high altitude compared to lower elevation, increased systolic blood pressure, and increased cardiac arrhythmias.[134,135] These latter two findings are likely related to increased sympathetic stimulation from the increased arousals and exaggerated hypoxemia.

Because obstructive events continue following ascent, it is reasonable for individuals with OSA to bring their CPAP machine with them to high altitude provided they have access to electrical power. The increasing availability of lightweight, battery-powered, portable CPAP machines has the potential to increase the range of situations in which CPAP can be used in this environment.[136] Consideration can also be given to adding acetazolamide to auto-CPAP, as the combination of interventions decreased the number of central apnea and the total apnea hypopnea index and improved nocturnal oxygen saturation when compared to auto-titrating CPAP alone.[120]

One issue that warrants consideration when planning for CPAP use at high altitude is whether the barometric pressure changes at high altitude affect CPAP machine performance and, in particular, their ability to deliver the intended pressure. Whereas older machines lacked pressure-compensating features that affected their ability to compensate for changes in barometric pressure,[137] more recent devices are capable of doing so. Patz and colleagues, for example, used recent-generation, auto-titrating CPAP devices to track CPAP requirements in seven high-altitude residents traveling to lower elevation and found no significant changes in the pressures used to prevent obstructive events between low and high elevation.[138] Product information provided by manufacturers indicates that pressure compensation is effective to altitudes of about 8,000 to 8500 feet, which happens to correspond to the maximum allowable altitude for commercial aircraft at cruising altitude, but a case report suggests that some devices may still deliver the intended pressure at altitudes as high as approximately 13,000 feet (3900 meters).[136]

Children

It is not uncommon for children to travel to high altitude. As such, it is important to be conscious of how children respond to high altitude and whether acute or long-term exposure affects their development, especially given that neural development, myelination, metabolic demands, and increased cerebral utilization of glucose is poorly understood in the pediatric brain.[139] This section focuses on sleep at high altitude in children, but a more comprehensive guide into children at high altitude has been published elsewhere.[140,141]

Acutely, children typically present with similar physiologic responses to hypoxia as adults, but interestingly, have less periodic breathing.[142,143] Kohler and colleagues performed respiratory inductive plethysmography in children (9 to 12 years) and their fathers at 3450 meters and showed children had, during two consecutive nights, 26% and 13% less periodic breathing compared to their fathers, which was attributed to a lower apneic threshold for CO_2. Actual age of the child may also contribute to responsiveness to hypoxia, with infants being more susceptible to cerebral tissue oxygen desaturation (measured via near-infrared spectroscopy).[144]

It is pertinent to note that children are as likely to suffer from altitude illnesses as adults,[140,141] which is especially important in young children who are unable to voice their symptoms. Therefore, in children unable to voice/portray distress, it should be assumed that they are suffering from altitude illness unless there are clear signs of an alternative diagnosis.[141]

CLINICAL PEARL

At high altitudes, for example, above 3500 meters, the most common cause of disturbed sleep in sojourners is periodic breathing resulting from the associated hypoxia. Surprisingly, the severity of periodic breathing increases over time, for at least 1 month at the same altitude, during acclimatization. Established treatments, apart from descent to a lower altitude, include regular oral acetazolamide, which reduces CSA severity (as well as improves Pao_2, thereby decreasing the symptoms of AMS), and hypnotic medications, which reduce sleep disturbance from arousals.

SUMMARY

Sleep at high altitude is disturbed by various factors, including a change of sleep environment, snoring, and insomnia; however, periodic breathing during sleep probably causes the most disturbances and occurs in almost everyone above 5000 meters. Over days or weeks at altitude, ventilatory acclimatization involves cellular and neurochemical reorganization in the peripheral chemoreceptors and central nervous system. The extent of periodic breathing during sleep at altitude intensifies with duration and severity of exposure—this increase is explained in part by elevations in loop gain. Although new mechanical and pharmacologic management techniques are emerging, oral acetazolamide remains the most effective and practical means to reduce periodic breathing. Use of benzodiazepine and other hypnotic agents appear to be a safe way to improve sleep quality at very high altitudes; however, recommendations should be given with caution, as they may also have some impacts on decision processing and vigilance. Dexamethasone is a proven treatment for AMS (and associated sleep disturbance) but probably has no other effect on sleep quality.

SELECTED READINGS

Ainslie PN, Lucas SJ, Burgess KR. Breathing and sleep at high altitude. *Respir Physiol Neurobiol.* 2013;188(3):233–256.

Andrews G, Ainslie PN, Shepherd K, et al. The effect of partial acclimatization to high altitude on loop gain and central sleep apnea severity. *Respirology.* 2012;17(5):835–840.

Burgess KR, Johnson PL, Edwards N. Central and obstructive sleep apnoea during ascent to high altitude. *Respirology.* 2004;9(2):222–229.

Burgess KR, Lucas SJ, Shepherd K, et al. Influence of cerebral blood flow on central sleep apnea at high altitude. *Sleep.* 2014;37(10):1679–1687.

Dekker MCJ, Wilson MH, Howlett WP. Mountain neurology. *Pract Neurol.* 2019;19(5):404–411. https://doi.org/10.1136/practneurol-2017-001783.

Dempsey JA. Crossing the apnoeic threshold: causes and consequences. *Exp Physiol.* 2005;90(1):13–24.

Hackett PH, Roach RC, Harrison GL, et al. Respiratory stimulants and sleep periodic breathing at high altitude. Almitrine versus acetazolamide. *Am Rev Respir Dis.* 1987;135(4):896–898.

Hoiland RL, Howe CA, Coombs GB, Ainslie PN. Ventilatory and cerebrovascular regulation and integration at high-altitude. *Clin Auton Res.* 2018;28:423–435.

Lahiri S, Maret K, Sherpa MG. Dependence of high altitude sleep apnea on ventilatory sensitivity to hypoxia. *Respir Physiol.* 1983;52(3):281–301.

Nickol AH, Leverment J, Richards P, et al. Temazepam at high altitude reduces periodic breathing without impairing next-day performance: a randomized cross-over double-blind study. *J Sleep Res.* 2006;15(4):445–454.

Rexhaj E, Rimoldi SF, Pratali L, et al. Sleep-disordered breathing and vascular function in patients with chronic mountain sickness and healthy high-altitude dwellers. *Chest.* 2016;149(4):991–998.

Simonson TS. Altitude adaptation: a glimpse through various lenses. *High Alt Med Biol.* 2015;16:125–137.

Swenson ER, Leatham KL, Roach RC, et al. Renal carbonic anhydrase inhibition reduces high altitude sleep periodic breathing. *Respir Physiol.* 1991;86(3):333–343.

White DP, Gleeson K, Pickett CK, et al. Altitude acclimatization: influence on periodic breathing and chemoresponsiveness during sleep. *J Appl Physiol.* 1987;63(1):401–412.

Xie AL, Skatrud JB, Barczi SR, et al. Influence of cerebral blood flow on breathing stability. *J Appl Physiol.* 2009;106(3):850–856.

A complete reference list can be found online at ExpertConsult.com.

Chapter 26

Sleep and Host Defense

Mark R. Opp; Monika Haack; James M. Krueger

Chapter Highlights

- Sleep is altered during sickness; this has been known for millennia. Yet systematic and controlled studies aimed at elucidating the extent to which sleep is altered in response to immune challenge have only been conducted during the last 30 years.
- Substances historically viewed as components of the innate immune system are now known to be involved in the regulation or modulation of physiologic sleep-wake behavior in the absence of immune challenge. Changes in sleep during immune challenge are actively driven and result from amplification of these physiologic mechanisms.
- Although the precise changes in sleep-wake behavior depend on the pathogen, route of infection, timing of infection, host species, and other factors, altered sleep during immune challenge is generally characterized by periods of increased non–rapid eye movement (NREM) sleep, increased delta power during NREM sleep, and suppressed rapid eye movement sleep. Infection-induced alterations in sleep are often accompanied by fever or hypothermia.
- Altered sleep has been studied in humans during pathologies and/or infections with pathogens, including human immunodeficiency virus/acquired immunodeficiency syndrome, rhinovirus (common cold), streptococci, trypanosomes, prions, and sepsis. Laboratory animal models include sepsis, influenza and other viruses (gamma herpesvirus, vesicular stomatitis virus, rabies, feline immunodeficiency virus), several bacterial species, trypanosomes, and several prion diseases.
- Mechanisms that link sleep to innate immunity involve a biochemical brain network composed of cytokines, chemokines, growth factors, transcription factors, neurotransmitters, enzymes, and their receptors. Each of these substances and receptors is present in neurons, although interactions with glia are critical for host defense responses to immune challenge. Redundancy, feed-forward, and feedback loops are characteristic of this biochemical network. These attributes provide stability and flexibility to the organismal response to immune challenge.

INTRODUCTION

Most individuals have experienced the lethargy, malaise, and desire to sleep that may occur at the onset of infection. Further, most have been admonished to "get plenty of rest, or you will get sick." Conventional wisdom and personal experience suggest a connection between sleep and host defense systems; our sleep is perceptively different when sick, and insufficient sleep may predispose to getting sick. These beliefs are not new. Indeed, Hippocrates, Aristotle, and many of our predecessors acknowledged such a relationship. But only within the past 30 years have modern science and medicine systematically investigated relationships between sleep and host defense systems. This chapter is organized around four main themes related to sleep and host defense. They are (1) the acute phase response and host defense; (2) infection-induced alterations in sleep; (3) effects of sleep loss on immune function; and (4) mechanisms linking sleep and immunity. Finally, in the Clinical Pearl box, we briefly present sleep as a recuperative process during sickness.

THE ACUTE PHASE RESPONSE AND HOST DEFENSE

Rapidly after infection or trauma or during some malignant conditions, a complex response involving many cell types and peripheral organs is evoked that is collectively referred to as the acute phase response (APR). Markers of the APR include changes in serum concentrations of acute phase proteins. Measurement of acute phase proteins, such as C-reactive protein (CRP), for example, is useful in clinical practice because they indicate inflammation. In addition to changes in serum concentrations of acute phase proteins, the APR includes physiologic changes such as fever and increased vascular permeability and other metabolic and pathologic changes. A major theme of this chapter is that altered sleep as a host defense also is part of the APR to inflammatory challenge. Altered sleep during inflammatory challenge is actively driven by multiple mediators and systems, many of which are shared with other facets of the APR.

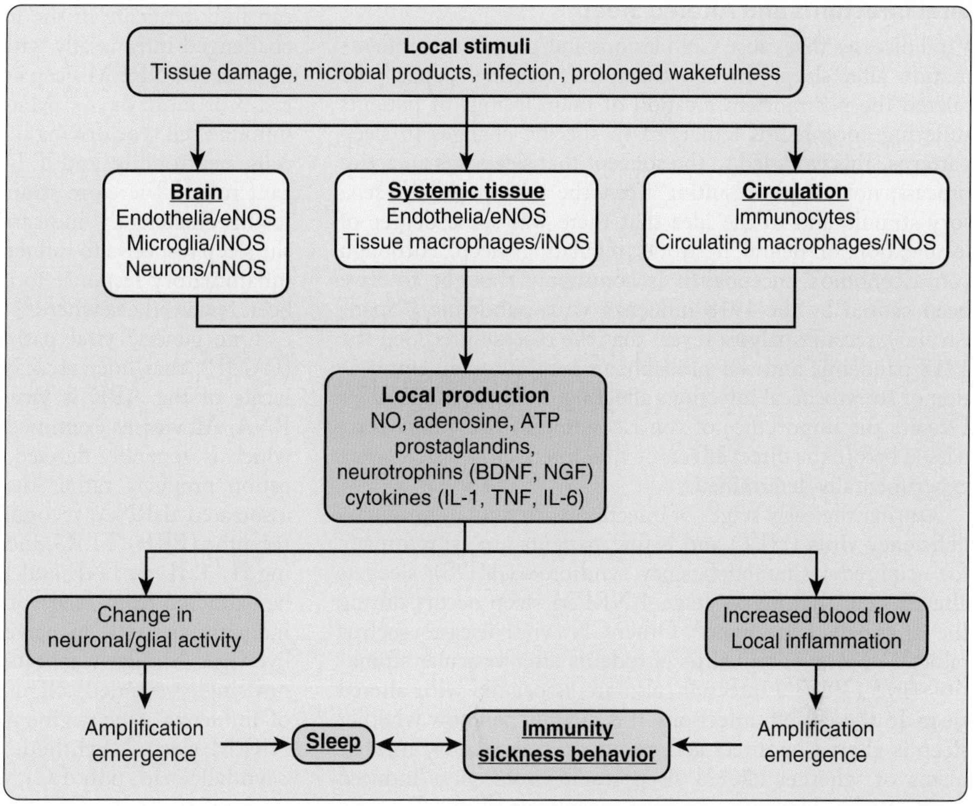

Figure 26.1 Multiple cell types from various tissue compartments (*yellow boxes*) contribute to sleep and host defense responses to microbial and tissue damage challenges (*green box*). The sleep and inflammatory responses are mediated by a common set of regulatory molecules whose production/release is modified in response to local stimuli, which enhance cell activity, for example, action potentials in neurons (*brown boxes*). These regulatory molecules are vasodilators and through that action contribute to local inflammation. These molecules are also sleep regulatory substances via their production and actions in brain. Local actions as they increase in number and merge and amplify higher order levels of tissue organization leading to emergent whole animal processes (e.g., sleep). Local actions provide some degree of compartmentalization of sleep and inflammatory actions. However, these responses remain influential upon each other (*lower blue boxes*). Such actions are likely responsible for the low-grade inflammation associated with certain sleep pathologies such as sleep apnea. ATP, Adenosine triphosphate; eNOS, endothelial nitricoxide synthase; IL, interleukin; iNOS, inducible nitric oxide synthase; NO, nitric oxide; TNF, tumor necrosis factor.

Recent advances in our knowledge of central nervous system (CNS) innate immunity provide a framework for understanding many of the shared mechanisms underlying the APR in general, and the specific alterations in sleep that occur during immune challenge. The APR is a critical innate immune response[1] that follows any inflammatory challenge, such as an infection or traumatic injury. Inflammatory challenges that are localized (e.g., a minor cut or splinter) may activate a low-level APR that manifests as redness at the site of injury and may not be perceived by the subject. But with increased injury severity, or response to an infectious challenge, the full systemic APR develops. The APR to infection by invading pathogens develops within a matter of hours, and the subject feels sick. In the case of infections, the function of the APR is to alert the host to the invasion and mobilize systemic protective responses, isolate and destroy invading pathogens, and remove tissue debris. The systemic inflammatory response activates the brain, liver, and bone marrow to react in a stereotypic manner. The APR includes physiologic and behavioral responses (e.g., fever, excess sleep, anorexia), as well as biochemical responses (e.g., CRP, serum amyloid A, mannose binding protein). Increased secretion of a broad array of endocrine hormones, including the stress hormones, also occurs. This complex of responses leads to host protective behaviors (such as social withdrawal),[2] physiologic responses (such as fever, which can increase efficiency of the immune response and inhibit growth of some microorganisms),[3,4] and immune responses (such as mobilization of leukocytes and natural killer [NK] cells).[1] Hormonal changes (such as prolactin regulation of antimicrobial nitric oxide levels)[5] and biochemical changes (such as potentiation of microbial phagocytosis)[6] also contribute to host defense. Although physical barriers (skin, mucosa) are the first line of defense, the APR is the first responder of host defense and is the trigger for acquired immunity, mediated by specific antibodies, and cytotoxic T lymphocytes.[7]

A major class of proteins, cytokines, initiates the APR. Cytokines are generally associated with immune cells, but they are made by most cell types. More than 100 of these intercellular signaling molecules have been identified, and the complexity of their interactions rivals that of the CNS. Cytokines induce their own production and the production of other cytokines, and they form biochemical cascades characterized by much redundancy. Cytokines are classified into two major groups, type I cytokines that promote inflammation (proinflammatory) and type II cytokines that suppress it (antiinflammatory).[8] Three proinflammatory cytokines appear to be primary triggers of the APR. These early responder cytokines are interleukin-1β (IL-1β), tumor necrosis factor-α (TNF-α), and IL-6, each of which is implicated in the regulation/modulation of sleep. The class II cytokines include interferon (IFN)-α, IFN-β, IL-4, and IL-10. These cytokines damp the APR and may also modulate sleep responses; for example, IL-4 and IL-10 inhibit spontaneous non–rapid eye movement (NREM) sleep. Cytokines can act in an autocrine, juxtacrine, paracrine, or endocrine manner to activate numerous APRs via such effectors as nitric oxide, adenosine, and prostaglandins (Figure 26.1).

INFECTION-INDUCED ALTERATIONS IN SLEEP

The impact of infection on sleep has been determined for viral, bacterial, and fungal pathogens; prion-related diseases; and protozoan parasites. Most studies have used virus and bacteria as the infectious agent, and so in this chapter we focus primarily on altered sleep in response to these pathogens.

Viral Infections and Altered Sleep

Viral diseases that cause CNS lesions and/or systemic inflammation alter sleep.[9] In von Economo's seminal paper,[10] he related the postmortem location of brain lesions of patients suffering encephalitis lethargica to specific changes in sleep patterns. This work led to the concept that sleep was an active process, not simply resulting from the withdrawal of sensory stimuli, and to the idea that there was some degree of localization of neural networks regulating sleep. Although von Economo's encephalitis is commonly thought to have been caused by the 1918 influenza virus pandemic ("Spanish flu"), recent analyses reveal that the disease preceded the 1918 pandemic and was probably an autoimmune complication of streptococcal infections affecting the basal ganglia.[11,12] Despite the importance of von Economo's work, many years passed before the direct effects of viral infections on sleep were experimentally determined.

During the early stages of infection with human immunodeficiency virus (HIV) and before patients are symptomatic for acquired immunodeficiency syndrome (AIDS), sleep is altered such that excess stage 4 NREM sleep occurs during the latter half of the night.[13] Other CNS viral diseases, such as rabies[14] or viral encephalitis in rodents after vesicular stomatitis virus (VSV[15]) infection, also are associated with altered sleep. In these CNS infections, it is difficult to know whether sleep is altered by direct actions on sleep regulatory mechanisms or whether altered sleep results from virus-induced brain lesions. However, cytokine messenger ribonucleic acid (mRNA) translation and toll-like receptor (TLR) signaling pathways are altered before VSV neuroinvasion, suggesting that at least some viruses modulate sleep regulatory systems in the absence of overt pathology.[16]

One model that has been used frequently to determine effects of viral infections on sleep is influenza. Influenza virus localizes to the respiratory tract and the olfactory bulb during the early stage of disease and does not cause brain lesions. In addition, influenza infections pose tremendous public health burdens because of the hundreds of thousands of lives lost each year and the threat of pandemics. Smith and colleagues[17] report that low doses of influenza in humans increase sleep and cognitive dysfunction; these symptoms appear after low viral doses that fail to induce the better known characteristics of the APR, such as a fever. However, in that study indices of behavior, not polysomnography, were used. Drake and colleagues[18] demonstrated in healthy human volunteers that infection with rhinovirus 23 disrupts sleep and impairs cognitive performance. (Rhinoviruses are the predominant cause of the "common cold.") In naturally occurring respiratory infections, individuals had subjectively and objectively disturbed sleep during the symptomatic phase of the infection, while spending a longer time in bed and had increased total sleep time.[19] In rabbits, intravenous injections of influenza virus are also associated with large increases in NREM sleep and suppressed rapid eye movement (REM) sleep, even though the virus does not replicate in this species.[9] Studies in mice infected with influenza virus demonstrate profound changes in sleep through the course of disease progression.[20-22] Changes in sleep of mice during influenza infection share some features of sleep responses to bacterial infections (described later). As a preclinical model, influenza infection of mice is clinically relevant because mouse-adapted strains of this virus can be introduced into the respiratory tract and can fully replicate in the lungs, causing a severe APR. Mice challenged intranasally with influenza virus display profound increases in NREM sleep and inhibition of REM sleep, which last 3 or more days.[20] Macrophages appear to be the critical immune cell type driving increased NREM sleep, whereas NK cells, neutrophils, and T lymphocytes do not play a significant role.[23] There are strain differences in responses of mice to this challenge,[24] indicating a genetic component affecting the sleep response to influenza virus. Genetic regulation of the inflammatory response to influenza in mice and humans has been reviewed elsewhere.[25]

One generic viral pathogen-associated molecule pattern (PAMP) that increases NREM sleep and initiates other facets of the APR is virus-associated double-stranded (ds) RNA. All viruses examined produce virus-associated dsRNA, which is generally derived from the annealing of viral replication products rather than from the virus itself.[26] Virus-associated dsRNA, recognized by the pathogen recognition receptor (PRR) TLR3, induces numerous cytokines, including IL-1, IL-6, TNF, and IFN. Virus-associated dsRNA can be extracted from lungs of infected mice[27] and is capable of inducing an APR in naïve rabbits that is similar to that of live virus. Similarly, rabbits given short double-stranded (but not single-stranded) oligomers that correspond to a portion of influenza gene segment 3 also exhibit large increases in NREM sleep.[28] Synthetic dsRNA (polyriboinosinic:polyrib ocytidylic acid; poly I:C), when inoculated into the lungs of mice primed with IFN-α, induces an APR that is virtually identical to that after influenza virus.[26] Influenza virus is a single-stranded negative-sense RNA virus; during replication the positive-sense strand is synthesized, and double-stranded influenza RNA forms. In contrast, severe acute respiratory syndrome coronavirus 2 (SARS-CoV-2), the virus that causes coronavirus disease 2019 (COVID-19), is a single-stranded positive-sense RNA virus[29]; during its intracellular replication, double-stranded viral RNA is also expected to form and be biologically active. It is not known, as of this writing, whether SARS-CoV-2 dsRNA in lungs and/or olfactory bulbs is responsible for potential sleep responses or anosmia. Regardless, these observations suggest that virus-associated dsRNA is sufficient to initiate the APR.

It is apparent that, in severe cases of COVID-19, plasma inflammatory mediators are elevated, including IL-1β, TNF-α, and IFN-γ, among others.[29] Based upon plasma concentrations in severe cases, TNF-α may be among mediators that contribute to, or indicate, disease severity.[30] One of the PRRs that coronaviruses activate is TLR7, which subsequently initiates a signaling cascade that upregulates type I IFN and other inflammatory cytokines.[29]

Interferons play a major role in viral symptoms. Knockout (KO) mice have been widely used to better understand the role of specific cytokines or hormones in host defense. Mice genetically deficient for the receptor that binds both IFN-α and IFN-β (the type I receptor) respond to poly I:C with altered sleep and a hypothermic response that is similar to that seen in infected wild-type mice. However, in influenza-infected IFN-receptor KO mice, the APR occurs earlier,[31] suggesting that type I IFNs may modulate the APR, presumably by regulating proinflammatory cytokine production. Influenza-infected IFN-receptor KO mice are less ill later in the infection and recover sooner.[31] Sleep-modulatory cytokines, in addition to IFNs, likely mediate the sleep responses to influenza virus. For example, although the duration of altered NREM and REM sleep is the same in both strains after viral challenge, mice deficient in the 55-kD and 75-kD TNF receptors manifest reduced electroencephalogram (EEG) delta power, a measure of sleep intensity, whereas in wild-type control mice, delta power increases.[32] IL-1 signaling in brain requires a brain-specific receptor accessory protein.[33] Mice lacking the IL-1 receptor brain-specific accessory protein have higher morbidity and mortality after influenza inoculation, and they sleep less during the infection than do wild-type mice.

Mice and rats with natural mutations of the growth hormone–releasing hormone (GHRH) receptor express a dwarf phenotype and altered spontaneous NREM sleep.[34] The GHRH receptor is a candidate protein for regulating NREM sleep increases in response to influenza virus.[35] Dwarf mice with nonfunctional GHRH receptors (called lit/lit mice) fail to respond to influenza virus with increased NREM sleep or EEG delta power.[36] Instead, infected lit/lit mice manifest a pathologic state with EEG slow waves, enhanced muscle tone, and increased mortality.[36] Such results indicate that single genes can substantially modify sleep responses to infectious challenge. Importantly, results from lit/lit mice also demonstrate that the sleep responses forming part of the APR correlate with survival.

Influenza virus is a frequently used model for APR studies, in part because it was assumed that the virus does not invade the brain or lead to the complications associated with the use of neurovirulent viruses. Recent studies, however, demonstrate that the strain of influenza most commonly employed in preclinical studies rapidly invades the olfactory bulb of the mouse brain after intranasal inoculation.[37] The virus activates microglia in the outer layer of the olfactory bulb and upregulates IL-1 and TNF at times that correspond to the postinfection time period when the systemic APR begins. The same mechanisms may be true for other viruses. For example, cytokine mRNA transcription is detected in mouse olfactory bulb within hours after intranasal inoculation with VSV.[16] Collectively, these studies suggest that cytokines made in the olfactory bulb impact the CNS components of the APR to some viruses, including sleep responses.

Bacterial Challenge

Altered sleep is also observed after bacterial infection. Indeed, results obtained after inoculating rabbits with the gram-positive bacteria *Staphylococcus aureus* were the first to suggest that NREM sleep responses were part of the APR.[38] In those experiments, rabbits were given *S. aureus* intravenously to induce septicemia; within a few hours of the inoculation NREM sleep was twice the amount as during comparable periods after control inoculation. Associated with the increase in NREM sleep were increases in amplitude of EEG slow waves. EEG slow wave (0.5 to 4.0 Hz) amplitudes are thought to indicate the intensity of NREM sleep. This initial phase of increased duration and intensity of NREM sleep lasted about 20 hours; it was followed by a more prolonged phase of decreased NREM sleep and decreased EEG slow wave amplitudes.[38] During both phases of the NREM sleep changes, REM sleep is inhibited and animals are febrile. Other changes characteristic of the APR (e.g., fibrinogenemia and neutrophilia) occurred concurrently with the changes in sleep.[38] In subsequent studies in which gram-negative bacteria and other routes of administration were used, a similar general pattern of biphasic NREM sleep responses and REM sleep inhibition was observed.[39] However, the timing of sleep responses depends upon the bacterial species and the route of administration. For example, after intravenous administration of *Escherichia coli*, NREM sleep responses are rapid in onset, but increased NREM sleep lasts only 4 to 6 hours. The subsequent phase of reduced NREM sleep and reduced amplitude of EEG slow waves is sustained for relatively long periods. In contrast, if the gram-negative bacterium *Pasteurella multocida* (a natural respiratory pathogen in rabbits) is given intranasally, a different time course of sleep responses is observed. In this case, the increased NREM sleep responses occur after a longer latency, and the magnitude of the increases in NREM sleep is less than the effects of this pathogen given by other routes of administration.

The intestinal lumen of mammals contains large amounts of many different bacteria species. Bacteria translocate into the intestinal lymphatics under normal conditions. Of importance to this discussion, intestinal permeability is altered after sleep deprivation, resulting in increased release of bacterial products into the lymphatics. Local lymph node macrophages phagocytose and digest these bacterial products,[40] releasing PAMPs that can trigger sleep responses. This mechanism operates at a low basal rate under normal conditions and is amplified during systemic inflammation. The phagocytosis by macrophages of bacterial products is also likely to be involved in sleep responses induced by sleep deprivation and excess food intake. A role for gut bacteria in sleep modulation is also evidenced by observations that reducing bacterial populations in the intestine is associated with reduced sleep.[41]

Another bacterial product that is involved in sleep responses to gram-negative bacteria is the lipopolysaccharide (LPS) component of cell wall endotoxin. LPS is the dominant PAMP associated with endotoxin, and it binds to TLR4. LPS has been intensively studied in animal models[42] and humans volunteers[43] with respect to effects on sleep. LPS alters sleep in humans and nonhuman animals.[44,45] Healthy human volunteers injected with LPS manifest sleep changes, fever, cytokine expression, and hormonal changes[43] somewhat similar to those seen in animals. However, the impact of LPS on the human EEG differs from those observed in rabbits or rats, and in humans it requires a higher LPS dose to increase NREM sleep than it does to suppress REM sleep.

Most experimental studies of bacterial infections and sleep have used inoculation of a single pathogen species as the infectious challenge. The gut microbiome, however, is polymicrobial, and many infections result from invasion by multiple pathogen species. Such is true in sepsis, during which polymicrobial infections routinely occur. Clinical studies demonstrate EEG anomalies in patients who become septic.[46] The etiology of sepsis is complex, and sepsis may result from many different kinds of insult. As a consequence, several preclinical models have been developed to study sepsis. Although each model used has strengths and limitations, the model currently considered to be the gold standard is cecal ligation and puncture (CLP[47]). CLP produces a polymicrobial infection that is considered clinically relevant because of its time course, because it reproduces the dynamic changes in cardiac function observed in human patients, and because there is a progressive release of inflammatory mediators. The severity of the ensuing infection is readily titrated in this model. Sleep is altered during the acute phase of CLP sepsis in rats, which occurs from 1 to 4 days after sepsis induction.[48] During this period, NREM and REM sleep of rats increases during the dark period (the normal active period for nocturnal rodents), whereas these sleep phases are reduced during the light period (the inactive period for nocturnal rodents). These changes in sleep coincide with increased cytokine mRNA and protein in brain.[49] Of interest, effects of sepsis on body temperature and activity rhythms persist long after the animal has recovered and is no longer at risk of dying.[49] These observations suggest that sepsis alters brain function and are in agreement with observations that patients surviving sepsis often suffer severe and debilitating cognitive impairment.

In summary, infectious challenge is associated with profound changes in sleep. As mentioned in the overview of the APR, PRRs such as the TLR and NLR receptor families detect the various PAMPs capable of altering sleep. Detection of PAMPS by the innate immune system explains, in part, why diverse microbial pathogens activate stereotypic host defense responses such as fever, anorexia, and altered sleep. Microbe-induced alterations in sleep, like the other components of the APR, are adaptive.[50]

EFFECTS OF SLEEP LOSS ON IMMUNE FUNCTION

Sleep is altered during immune challenge, yet whether sleep loss alters immune function has been more difficult to demonstrate. There are multiple systems associated with immunity, each with a myriad of mediators and modulators. There are positive and negative feedback control mechanisms that interact in complex ways. This complexity of the immune system makes it difficult to determine what measurement(s) one should use to assess immune function. From a functional perspective, the most important question is whether sleep loss renders the animal or human more vulnerable to infection, tumor formation, or systemic inflammatory diseases. (We already know that sleep loss renders an individual more vulnerable to accidental injury.) Although few studies have been conducted within the context of sleep, some suggest relationships between sleep and functional immune outcomes. For example, among 12 mammalian species sampled, those with longer daily sleep times have the greatest number of white blood cells and are least susceptible to parasites.[51] Susceptibility to infection has been used as an end point in some studies of human subjects.

Results from studies of laboratory animal subjected to short-term sleep deprivation are consistent with most human studies. Toth and colleagues[52] challenged rabbits with *E. coli* before or after 4 hours of sleep deprivation. They concluded that sleep deprivation failed to exacerbate *E. coli*–induced clinical illness, although the combination of sleep deprivation and bacterial infection altered some facets of sleep responses as compared with either manipulation alone.[52] Furthermore, mice immunized against influenza virus and then re-challenged with influenza just before sleep deprivation fail to clear the virus from their lungs.[53] However, in a similar study,[54] sleep loss failed to alter preexisting mucosal and humoral immunity in either young or senescent mice. The variation in the effects of sleep loss on outcomes in mice subjected to influenza virus is likely due to differences in the sleep deprivation protocols, end points analyzed, and influenza models employed. Little research has focused on sleep deprivation and clinical responses to bacteria, but mortality is greater in mice in which sleep is disrupted after they are made septic by CLP.[55] Collectively, these studies suggest that acute sleep loss impairs or alters host defense.

The effects of long-term sleep loss on host defense in laboratory rodents are more striking. If rats obtain only about 20% of their normal sleep when deprived by the disk-over-water method,[56] they die after a period of 2 to 3 weeks.[57] Yoked control rats, which manage to maintain about 80% of their normal sleep during the protocol period, survive. The experimental rats, but not the yoked controls, develop septicemia.[57] Bacteria cultured from the blood are primarily facultative anaerobes indigenous to the host and environment. These results demonstrate that, using this method, innate host defenses in the rat are compromised by long-term sleep loss. These results suggest that prolonged sleep loss likely amplifies the normally occurring process of gut permeability to bacteria and bacterial products.

Sleep disruption may induce low-grade inflammation or may render the animal more susceptible to inflammatory challenge. We recently demonstrated that disrupting daytime sleep of mice for prolonged periods (9 days) exacerbates febrile responses to LPS.[58] The exacerbated febrile response to LPS under the conditions of this study may be due to sleep disruption per se, because no other parameters measured (corticosterone, food or water intake, body weight) differed substantially from either home cage control animals or animals housed on the sleep disruption device but allowed ad libitum sleep.

In contrast to animal studies, experiments using in vivo challenges with bacteria or viruses are rare in humans. Investigations mainly focus on sleep loss–induced changes of leukocyte numbers in blood (e.g., monocytes, neutrophils, T cells), immune cell activity and proliferation (e.g., NK cells, lymphocyte proliferation, T regulatory function), and cytokine and cytokine receptor levels in blood or production by stimulated immune cells (see the comprehensive review by Besedovsky and colleagues[59]). With respect to cytokine responses, for example, acute total sleep deprivation increased levels of IL-1b and IL-1ra in the blood circulation of healthy volunteers.[60] In studies using models mimicking common patterns of sleep restriction (generally restricted to 4 hours of sleep/night), IL-1b and IL-6 production by stimulated peripheral blood mononuclear cells,[61] expression of TNF, and IL-6 by stimulated monocytes[62] and in the blood circulation[63] increased. Furthermore, the IL-2/IL-4 ratio was reduced by several days of sleep restriction, indicating a shift toward a Th2 cytokine balance.[64] In a recent study using a model that mimics common patterns of recurrent sleep restriction with intermittent recovery sleep over 3 weeks, monocytic expression of IL-6 progressively increased with ongoing exposure to sleep restriction[65] and did not fully recover after a night of full sleep. Although these immune measures do not directly indicate an impact on host defense, cytokines, such as IFN, IL-1, and TNF, are well known for their role as immunomodulators, and their perturbation deteriorates tumor and pathogen defense in the long term (see the review by Frasca and colleagues[66]).

There are several reports that show in healthy volunteers that plasma levels of cytokines are related to the sleep-wake cycle. Such relationships were first described by demonstrating that plasma IL-1–like activity was related to the onset of slow wave sleep.[67] Plasma concentrations of TNF vary in phase with EEG slow wave amplitudes.[68] There is also a temporal relationship between sleep of healthy human volunteers and IL-1 activity.[69] Several clinical conditions associated with sleepiness, such as sleep apnea, chronic fatigue syndrome, chronic insomnia, preeclampsia, postdialysis fatigue, psychoses, rheumatoid arthritis (RA), and AIDS, are associated with enhanced plasma levels of TNF and other cytokines.[70] Only those sleep apnea patients showing elevated TNF activity experience fatigue.[71]

Other facets of the immune response are also linked to sleep. About 40 years ago, altered antigen uptake after sleep deprivation was reported.[72] Studies carried out in the 1970s also showed a decrease in lymphocyte DNA synthesis after 48 hours of sleep deprivation and a decrease in phagocytosis after 72 hours of sleep deprivation.[73,74] Sleep deprivation also induces changes in mitogen responses. Circulating immune complexes fall during sleep and rise again just before an individual gets out of bed. In mice sleep deprivation reduces IgG catabolism, resulting in elevated IgG levels. In contrast, one study failed to show an effect of sleep deprivation on spleen cell counts, lymphocyte proliferation, or plaque-forming cell responses to antigens in rats.[55,75] In a comprehensive study of human volunteers, 64 hours of sleep deprivation reduced CD4, CD16, CD56, and CD57 lymphocytes after 1 night of sleep loss, although the number of CD56 and CD57 lymphocytes increased after 2 nights of sleep loss.[76] Another group also showed that a night of sustained wakefulness reduced counts of all lymphocyte subsets measured.[77]

Sleep and sleep loss are associated with changes in NK cell activity. NK cell activity is reduced in patients with insomnia[78] and decreases after partial night sleep restriction.[79,80] In contrast, NK cell activity increases after 64-hour total sleep deprivation.[76] Circulating NK cell activity, as well as NK cell activity in a variety of tissue compartments, may be sensitive to sleep, although the exact nature of relationships between NK cell activity and sleep likely depends upon the specific experimental conditions used to elucidate them.

In summary, determination of sleep deprivation effects on immune function may be confounded by stress and other coincident physiologic responses in animals. Concurrent physiologic changes (other than stress) also complicate sleep deprivation studies in humans. Sleep deprivation protocols are not standardized in animal or human studies, making comparison of results across studies difficult. The lack of standardized sleep deprivation protocols is just one among many factors contributing to the often disparate results reported.

MECHANISMS LINKING SLEEP AND IMMUNITY

Substantial evidence now suggests that IL-1 and TNF are involved in physiologic sleep regulation.[70,81] Furthermore, IL-1 and TNF mRNA and protein change during pathologies characterized by altered sleep. Sleep deprivation is associated with enhanced sleepiness, sleep rebound, sensitivity to kindling and pain stimuli, cognitive and memory impairments, performance impairments, depression, and fatigue. Exogenous administration of IL-1 or TNF induces these sleep loss–associated symptoms.[42,70] Further, chronic sleep loss–associated pathologies such as metabolic syndrome, chronic inflammation, and cardiovascular disease are also characterized by changes in IL-1 and TNF activity,[42,70] and in some cases these pathologies are attenuated if these cytokines are inhibited.[82-84] Clinically available inhibitors of either IL-1 (e.g., the IL-1–receptor antagonist, anakinra) or TNF (e.g., the TNF-α soluble receptor, etanercept) alleviate fatigue and excess sleepiness in humans with pathologies such as sleep apnea or RA.[82,83,85] The IL-1-receptor antagonist and TNF soluble receptor are normal gene products found in blood and brain, and their concentrations are altered by sleep.[42]

In addition to being immunocyte products, whose production is amplified by viral and bacterial components, IL-1 and TNF are also found in the normal brain.[42,70] IL-1 and TNF mRNA have diurnal rhythms in brain with the highest values being associated with periods of maximum sleep. TNF protein also has a sleep-associated diurnal rhythm in several brain areas, and IL-1 in cerebrospinal fluid varies with the sleep-wake cycle.[86] Cortical expression of TNF is enhanced by afferent nerve activity,[87] and IL-1 and TNF expression are enhanced in culture when neurons are stimulated,[88] which may be part of the process that is responsible for local use-dependent sleep.[42]

Administration of either IL-1 or TNF promotes NREM sleep.[42,44,70] The increase in NREM sleep after either IL-1 or TNF administration is physiologic in the sense that sleep remains episodic and readily reversible if animals are disturbed. Further, IL-1 or TNF enhances NREM sleep intensity, as measured by the amplitude of EEG delta waves. The effects of IL-1 on sleep depend upon dose and the time of day it is given.[89,90] IL-1 and TNF inhibit the binding of the BMAL/CLOCK complex in the suprachiasmatic nucleus[91]; this action may be responsible for the differential effects of these cytokines at different times of the day. Finally, knockout strains of mice that lack the type I IL-1 receptor,[92] the 55 kD TNF receptor,[93] or both of these receptors[94] sleep less than control strains.

NREM sleep increases after sleep deprivation, excessive food intake, or acute mild increases in ambient temperature. The somnogenic actions of each of these manipulations are associated with enhanced production of either IL-1 or TNF. After sleep deprivation, circulating IL-1 increases, brain levels of IL-1 mRNA increase, and the NREM sleep rebound that would normally occur after sleep deprivation is greatly attenuated if either IL-1 or TNF is blocked using antibodies or soluble receptors.[95]

IL-1 and TNF act within a biochemical network (Figure 26.2). For example, IL-1 and TNF stimulate nuclear factor kappa B (NFκB) production. NFκB is a DNA-binding protein involved in transcription. Other sleep-altering cytokines, such as acidic fibroblast growth factor, epidermal growth factor, and nerve growth factor also stimulate NFκB production. NFκB promotes IL-1 and TNF production and thus forms a positive feedback loop. Sleep deprivation is associated with the activation of NFκB in the cerebral cortex, basal forebrain cholinergic neurons, and the lateral hypothalamus. Activation of NFκB also promotes IL-2, IL-6, IL-8, IL-15, and IL-18 production, each of which promotes sleep in rats.[42,44,70]

The mechanisms by which sleep regulatory substances (SRSs) are regulated and induce sleep are beginning to be understood. TNF and IL-1 neuronal expression is enhanced in response to afferent nerve activity. For instance, excessive stimulation of rat facial whiskers for 2 hours enhances IL-1 and TNF immunoreactivity in the cortical layers of the somatosensory cortical columns that receive the enhanced afferent input.[87]

What is it about neuronal activity or wakefulness that causes the enhanced SRS activity? Neuronal activity manifests

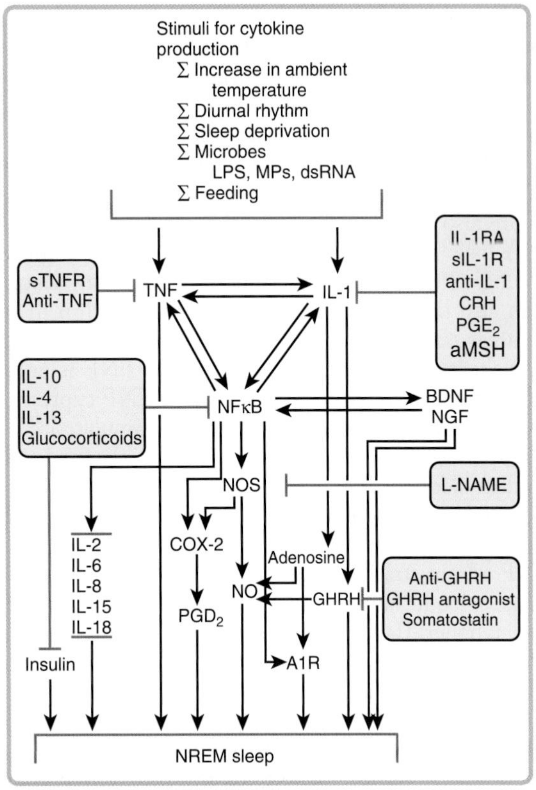

Figure 26.2 Interleukin (IL)-1β and tumor necrosis factor (TNF)-α are part of a brain biochemical network that regulates physiologic sleep and links multiple facets of innate immunity to sleep regulation. Much is known about mechanisms by which IL-1 and TNF directly or indirectly regulate/modulate non–rapid eye movement (NREM) sleep. Less is known about mechanisms of action for the rapid eye movement (REM) sleep–suppressing effects of immune challenge. Current knowledge of the biochemical network that translates information about environmental perturbation into host responses that actively drive changes in sleep-wake behavior is much more complicated than depicted, and sites of action are not indicated (but see the work by Imeri and Opp[50]). This biochemical cascade included cytokines, chemokines (not included), growth factors, transcription factors, neurotransmitters, enzymes, and their receptors. Because the network is redundant and parallel, inhibition of any single component does not result in complete sleep loss, nor does it block altered sleep in response to immune challenge. Such redundant pathways provide stability to the sleep regulatory system and alternative mechanisms by which sleep-promoting or sleep-inhibitory stimuli may affect sleep. Substances in boxes inhibit NREM sleep and inhibit either the production of, or the actions of, substances in downstream pathways. The receptor and intracellular signaling systems for all these substances are found in neurons. Also not depicted in this schema are interactions of components of this biochemical network with glial cells. Gliotransmission is implicated in the modulation of physiologic sleep and is likely to play a critical role in brain responses to immune challenge that result in altered sleep-wake behavior (see the work by Ingiosi and colleagues[97] and Porkka-Heiskanen). → indicates stimulation or upregulation; ⊥ indicates inhibition or downregulation. BDNF, brain-derived neurotrophic factor; CRH, corticotropin-releasing hormone; GHRH, growht hormone-releasint hormone; MSH, melanocyte stimulating hormone; NGF, nerve growth factor; PGD, prostaglandin.

as presynaptic and postsynaptic events that act in both the short and long term. Neuronal activity in presynaptic neurons results in the release of transmitters and adenosine triphosphate (ATP).[96] In turn, some of that ATP is converted to adenosine and some ATP acts on purine P2X7 receptors on glia to release TNF and IL-1.[42,97] ATP also acts to release cytokines in immunocytes.[98] The extracellular adenosine derived from ATP interacts with neurons via the adenosine A_1 receptor (A1AR). The TNF released in response to ATP activates NFκB in postsynaptic and presynaptic neurons.[42] NFκB enhances the A1AR, thereby rendering the cell more sensitive to adenosine. NFκB also enhances production of a subunit of the α-amino-3-hydroxy-5-methyl-4-isoxazolepropionic acid (AMPA) receptor gluR1 mRNA. The time courses of enhanced mRNA for receptors or ligands are much slower than the direct actions of adenosine or TNF; the subsequent production of protein offers a way for the brain to keep track of prior neuronal network activity and translate that activity into a greater sleep propensity. The various time courses of action of the neurotransmitters (milliseconds), the conversions of ATP to adenosine and its actions (seconds), and the actions of ATP-induced release of cytokines and their subsequent effects on gene expression (minutes to hours) provide a mechanism for activity-dependent oscillations of neuronal assembly sleep.[99]

There is a growing literature demonstrating direct effects of IL-1 and TNF on neural substrates implicated in the regulation of sleep. Some of these mechanisms include interactions with classical neurotransmitters such as glutamate, serotonin, acetylcholine, gamma-aminobutyric acid, histamine, and dopamine.[100] For example, IL-1 increases serotonergic activity in brain regions implicated in sleep regulation,[101] and an intact serotonergic system is required for the full effects of IL-1 on sleep to manifest.[102,103] IL-1 inhibits discharge rates of serotonergic[104,105] and cholinergic[106] neurons in the brainstem. Within the hypothalamus, IL-1 increases c-Fos[107] and inhibits wake-active neurons.[108] TNF promotes sleep if microinjected into the anterior hypothalamus, while injection of a soluble TNF receptor into this area reduces sleep.[109] TNF also alters sleep if injected into the locus coeruleus,[110] effects likely related to interactions with alpha$_2$-adrenergic receptive mechanisms and norepinephrine release.[111] Interestingly, TNF or IL-1, if applied locally onto the surface of the cerebral cortex unilaterally, enhances EEG delta activity on the side to which it is applied but not the contralateral side.[112,113] Conversely, application of the TNF soluble receptor unilaterally onto the cortex of sleep-deprived rats attenuates sleep loss–induced EEG delta activity on the side injected but not on the opposite side. Further, unilateral application of a TNF siRNA (inhibits TNF) reduces spontaneous cortical TNF expression and EEG slow wave activity on the ipsilateral side.[114] These latter studies suggest that TNF acts locally within the cortex (in addition to its somnogenic actions in the hypothalamus) to enhance EEG synchronization and possibly sleep intensity. In fact, application of TNF directly to the cortex of intact mice[87] or to co-cultures of neurons and glia[88] increases the probability that a sleep-like state will manifest in local circuits.

CLINICAL ASPECTS AND IMPLICATIONS

Effects of Sleep on Infection Risk and Vaccination Responses

In controlled experimental settings, acute short and/or disturbed sleep affects a wide array of immune cells, mediators, and functions.[115] Such immune changes also occur in more chronic forms of short or disturbed sleep, such as observed in insomnia disorder or shift work. It is thought that these changes increase infection and other disease risks over time, but the exact mechanisms remain unknown. Some studies investigated the effects of sleep on more clinical outcomes, such as infection risk or vaccination responses, which is discussed in the following sections.

Sleep and Infection Risk

In rodents, sleep can affect the outcome of bacterial or parasitic infections, such that the survival rates decrease or increase with reducing or prolonging sleep duration, respectively.[116,117] Human studies focus on the association between sleep and infection risk, rather than infection outcome (i.e., survival). Using an experimental model of upper respiratory infection induced by a rhinovirus, participants who reported to sleep less than 7 hours/night the week before the experimental infection were almost three times more likely to develop a clinical cold.[118] This finding was replicated in a study that objectively measured sleep duration using actigraphy.[119] With respect to naturally occurring infections, pneumonia risk in a large cohort of nurses increased by almost 40% (adjusted odds ratio [OR] of 1.39) in women sleeping less than 5 hours.[120] Respiratory infection risk, including influenza and pneumonia, increased by about 50% (adjusted OR of 1.51) in a large cohort of adults sleeping less than 5 hours compared with those sleeping 7 hours.[121] A recent study focused on the effect of sleep disturbances, rather than sleep duration, found that self-reported insomnia symptoms in an adult population were prospectively associated with respiratory tract infections as assessed through daily infection diaries.[122] Influenza and pneumonia are among the top 10 leading causes of death in the United States[123] (https://www.cdc.gov/nchs/fastats/leading-causes-of-death.htm), and current research findings suggest that adequate sleep can help to prevent airway and other infections, possibly including infections with SARS-CoV-2. Although not yet documented, the lack of sleep in emergency and critical care health providers is expected to aggravate respiratory distress and other symptoms associated with COVID-19.

Sleep and Vaccination Responses

Vaccinations are effective only when the antigenic challenge (the vaccination) induces a sufficient antibody response (acquired immunity) such that, upon subsequent exposure to the same or similar pathogen, there is an effective immune memory. Some individuals do not respond to vaccination with an antibody response sufficient to confer protection, and factors contributing to "nonresponders" are not well understood. The effects of sleep duration on subsequent antibody responses to vaccines in humans are experimentally studied. Total sleep deprivation of a single night or sleep restriction over several nights before or after vaccinations against hepatitis A, hepatitis B, or influenza strains reduces antibody responses.[124-127] Across studies, antibody responses are on average reduced by half, and the duration of the sleep deprivation–induced reduction in the antibody response varies across studies. In some studies, the effect disappeared at 4 weeks after vaccination, while in another study, the effect was still present at 1 year after the initial vaccination (see the review by Bsedovsky and colleagues[115]). One study investigated the effects of habitual sleep duration on the magnitude of the antibody response after a standard three-vaccination series against hepatitis B.[128] Shorter sleep duration (as assessed objectively with actigraphy) in the days surrounding the first vaccination is associated with lower secondary antibody levels. When sleep duration was categorized into less than 6 hours, 6 to 7 hours, and greater than 7 hours of sleep/night, each hour of less sleep is associated with a reduction of the antibody response by about 50%. Of importance, sleeping less than 6 hours translated into a significant risk of being unprotected against the virus, as assessed 6 months after the final vaccination. The mechanisms underlying the beneficial effect of sleep on infection risk or vaccination responses is not understood, but elevations of inflammatory mediators, as frequently observed in response to short or disturbed sleep, is associated with a decreased ability to mount adaptive immune responses.[129] Collectively, these aforementioned studies suggest that adequate sleep can help to prevent and/or lower the risk of airway and other infections and support optimal antibody responses to vaccinations.

Sleep Disturbances in Chronic Infectious and Inflammatory Diseases: Effects of Pharmacologic and Nonpharmacologic Interventions

Sleep disturbances are increasingly common in the general population, with 30% of the population reporting symptoms of insomnia (e.g., difficulties falling or staying asleep) and 6% meeting diagnostic criteria for insomnia disorder (see the review by Ohayon[130]). Insomnia or symptoms of insomnia are even more common in medical populations with chronic infectious or inflammatory diseases. These include patients infected with the human immunodeficiency virus,[131] hepatitis C virus,[132] or Epstein-Barr virus,[133] and patients with inflammatory diseases, such as inflammatory bowel diseases (IBD),[134] RA,[135] systemic lupus erythematosus,[136] Sjögren syndrome,[137] and other chronic diseases with an inflammatory involvement, such as osteoarthritis or migraines (see the review by Bjurstrom and colleagues[138]). The high comorbidity between chronic infectious or inflammatory diseases with sleep disturbances is not surprising given the bidirectional sleep-immune relationship. Consequently, physiologic sleep regulation will likely fail when inflammatory mediators are constantly dysregulated, and, in turn, sleep disturbances may negatively affect the underlying immunopathologic process, thus feeding into a vicious circle. Interventions that target either immune dysregulation or sleep disturbances are likely to have a beneficial outcome on both sleep and the immunopathologic process.

Pharmacologic Interventions Targeting Inflammation

Antiinflammatory therapies are often used to treat several chronic inflammatory diseases, including RA or IBD. In RA, about 50% of patients experience sleep disturbances,[135] and PSG-derived sleep is characterized by indices of disturbed sleep, such as increased alpha-EEG intrusions, increased nocturnal wake time, or frequent sleep stage transitions (see the review by Bjurstrom and colleagues[138]). The immunopathology of RA is reasonably well understood and involves inappropriate production of various cytokines, in particular TNF, which was one of the first cytokines validated as a therapeutic target for RA.[139] Downregulation of increased TNF production may also have direct effects on sleep given TNF's sleep-regulatory properties (see the review by Rockstrom and colleagues[140]). Indeed, anti-TNF therapy improves subjective and objective measures of sleep in RA patients; anti-TNF infusion treatment in patients with active disease reduced sleep-onset latency, increased sleep efficiency,[141] and reduced wake time at night.[142] These sleep improvements were not associated with a reduction in joint pain in the morning after infusion treatment, suggesting that the effect on sleep may independently result from the inhibition of TNF actions in the CNS.[87] Similarly, treatment of RA patients with active disease with an IL-6 receptor inhibitor (tocilizumab) improves self-reported sleep quality and daytime sleepiness. The observed sleep improvement could not be explained by a reduction in disease activity, again suggesting a direct effect of cytokines on sleep regulation that is independent of disease activity.[143] Administration of the antiinflammatory agents anti-integrin (vedolizumab) or anti-TNF (infliximab or adalimumab) also improved sleep quality in patients with IBD within 6 weeks of therapy initiation.[144] These limited findings suggest that pharmacologically reducing TNF production or blocking IL-6 actions in rheumatic diseases or IBD may have a direct effect on sleep regulation, rather than just being the result of improved disease activity, such as pain.

Nonpharmacologic Sleep Interventions

Sleep hygiene (i.e., good sleep habits), mindfulness, and relaxation training are effective strategies to improve sleep quality in populations reporting poor sleep health (see review by Murawski and colleagues[145]). In clinical populations meeting diagnostic criteria for insomnia disorder, cognitive behavioral therapy for insomnia (CBT-I) is the first-line treatment[146] and outperforms pharmacologic treatment with respect to long-term benefits.[147] A few studies have assessed the immunologic effects of CBT-I. In adults diagnosed with insomnia disorder, CBT-I has been shown to lower systemic levels of the acute phase protein CRP. This reduction was associated with the remission of insomnia and sustained at 16 months posttreatment.[148] CBT-I additionally reduced cellular expression levels of TNF and IL-6 by monocytes, downregulated gene transcripts involved in inflammation (e.g., TNF, IL-6, IL-1β), while upregulating genes involved in interferon and antibody responses (e.g., CD19, MX-1).[149] These immune effects suggest that CBT-I in adults suffering from insomnia disorder reduce both insomnia symptoms and inflammation. There is very little knowledge on the effects of CBT-I in medical populations with chronic infectious or inflammatory conditions, although insomnia symptoms are very common in these populations. In adults with osteoarthritis comorbid with insomnia, CBT-I is reported to improve sleep and disease activity[150,151] and results in less serum IL-6 reactivity to a physiologic challenge (cold pressor test) in adults showing an improvement in sleep compared with those without.[152]

Although more research is needed in this area, findings suggest an avenue by which improving either sleep or immunopathologic processes can have a beneficial effect on both sleep and immune outcomes.

Sleep and Postsurgical Outcomes

Sleep patterns in postoperative periods can be severely disrupted with a suppression of both slow wave and REM sleep.[153] Sleep quantity and quality after surgery are influenced by a multitude of factors, including hospital-related environmental factors (e.g., noise, light), interruptions in sleep resulting from nurse checks or other medical interventions, the extent of surgical tissue injury, the magnitude of the surgical stress response (i.e., autonomic, neuroendocrine and inflammatory responses to surgical trauma), the effectiveness of the analgesics, and pain, which is one of the cardinal signs of an inflammatory response to infection or tissue injury.[154] Sleep disturbances induce hyperalgesia and thereby have the potential to amplify pain in the postsurgical phase.[155] A recent meta-analytical review on the effects of pharmacologic sleep interventions (zolpidem or melatonin) administered in the perioperative phase reported an improvement of pain control in the postoperative period, as indicated by a decrease in pain reports and the use of analgesics.[156] It is currently unknown whether pharmacologically induced sleep improvements mediate the beneficial effect on pain control, or whether pharmacologic agents exert a direct effect on pain control mechanisms, independent of their sleep-promoting effect.

Sleep disturbances are also an issue in the presurgical period. Presurgical short or disturbed sleep contribute to poorer postsurgical outcomes. In patients with coronary artery bypass graft surgery, self-reported sleep complaints in the month before surgery were associated with greater physical symptoms and sensory pain in the 2 months after surgery, indicative of a poorer physical recovery.[157] In breast cancer patients receiving mastectomy surgery, poor sleep quality before surgery predicted higher incidence of severe postoperative pain and fever and higher demands of analgesics in the first postoperative 24 hours.[158] Using a surgical incision model in rats, acute sleep deprivation the night before surgery caused a marked increase in mechanical hypersensitivity after surgery and prolonged postoperative recovery time.[159] Increasing sleep time before surgery has clinical benefit on postsurgical outcomes. Thus habitually short-sleeping patients scheduled to undergo joint replacement surgery were asked to extend their time in bed by 2 hours the week before surgery. This bed time extension resulted in an increase of actigraphy-monitored sleep time by 1 hour per night in the preoperative period, which resulted in less daily pain and less opiate use in the postoperative period compared with patients who stayed on their habitual bed time.[160] With respect to mechanisms underlying the association between preoperative sleep disturbances and poorer postsurgical pain control, dysregulation of inflammatory pathways have been suggested, including mediators involved in both sleep and pain control, such as IL-1, IL-6, and TNF.[156] Whether sleep disturbance–induced inflammatory dysregulations could potentially affect the magnitude of the surgical stress response to tissue damage, which is associated with a host of postoperative outcomes,[161] warrants further investigations. In summary, obtaining good quantity and quality sleep the night *before* surgery may serve as an interventional target in the management of surgical pain.

Contrary to the detrimental effects of short or disturbed sleep on postsurgical outcomes, there is limited evidence suggesting that sleep deprivation can also have a beneficial influence in certain clinical models. Using a skin allotransplant model, a prolonged allograft survival has been reported after acute sleep deprivation and chronic sleep restriction in rats, which was accompanied by a reduced number of graft-infiltrating CD4 T cells.[162] Using an ischemic stroke model, several studies have shown that sleep deprivation before stroke improves outcomes (e.g., less ischemic brain damage), whereas sleep deprivation after stroke is harmful (see the review by Pincherle and colleagues[163]). One explanation is that if sleep loss occurs before stroke, increased entry of microbial products (e.g., peptidoglycans) from blood into the brain site of stroke damage is priming the brain as such products do in the immune system. Overall, much research is needed to investigate whether there are certain clinical situations in which controlled sleep deprivation outweighs the overall detrimental consequences of short or disturbed sleep.

To conclude, sleep can affect infection risk, vaccination outcomes, chronic infectious or inflammatory pathologies, postsurgical outcomes, as well as many other immune-related pathologies that have not been discussed here, such as allergic diseases or tumor-related immune responses.[164,165] These findings indicate a beneficial effect of sleep improving interventions in numerous clinical settings.

CLINICAL PEARL

Although physicians routinely prescribe bed rest to aid in recuperation from infections and other maladies, as yet there is little direct evidence that sleep aids in recuperation. Such studies are difficult to perform because the recovery from an infection, for instance, is influenced by the baseline severity of the infection (i.e., differences in exposure or innate resistance that determine the replication level and clearance of the invading microbe) as well as by what the patient does during the infection. Physicians will continue to prescribe bed rest, and often this is just what the patient wishes to do. It seems likely that such advice is beneficial, as enhanced sleep is part of the adaptive APR. The only evidence of which we are aware that is relevant to this issue is consistent with the concept that sleep aids in recuperation; after infectious challenge, animals that have robust NREM sleep responses have a higher probability of survival than animals that fail to exhibit NREM sleep responses.[166] Although strictly correlative, these data suggest that sleep does indeed facilitate recovery. Perhaps our grandmothers' folk wisdom pertaining to the preventative and curative attributes of sleep and sickness is correct, although much additional research is needed before we know whether this admonishment has a biologic basis.

SUMMARY

Sleepiness, like fever, is commonly experienced at the onset of an infection or other cause of systemic inflammation. Changes in sleep in response to microbes appear to be one facet of the APR. Typically, soon after infectious challenge, time spent in NREM sleep increases and REM sleep is suppressed. The exact time course of sleep responses depends upon the infectious agent, the route of administration, and the time of day the infectious challenge is given.

There is a common perception that sleep loss renders one vulnerable to infection. Some studies demonstrate that sleep loss impairs acquired immunity, and many studies have shown that sleep deprivation alters selected aspects of the innate immune response. A few studies have combined sleep deprivation with infectious challenge. After mild sleep deprivation, several immune system parameters (such as NK cell activity) change, and resistance to a viral challenge is decreased in individuals who spontaneously sleep less. Studies have not yet been done to determine the effects of sleep deprivation on recovery from an infection.

The molecular mechanisms responsible for the changes in sleep associated with infection appear to be an amplification of a physiologic sleep regulatory biochemical cascade. Sleep regulatory mechanisms and the immune system share regulatory molecules. The best characterized are IL-1 and TNF, which are involved in physiologic NREM sleep regulation. IL-1 and TNF are key players in the development of the APR induced by infectious agents. During the initial response to infectious challenge, these proinflammatory cytokines are upregulated, leading to the acute phase sleep response. *This chain of events includes well-known immune response modifiers such as prostaglandins, nitric oxide, and adenosine. Each of these substances, and their receptors, is a normal constituent of the brain, and each is involved in physiologic sleep regulation.*

ACKNOWLEDGMENTS

During the writing of this chapter, the authors were supported, in part, by grants from the National Institutes of Health, NS25378 (JMK), HL136310 (MH), and AG064465 (MRO) and by the W. M. Keck Foundation (JMK).

SELECTED READINGS

Besedovsky L, Lange T, Haack M. The sleep-immune crosstalk in health and disease. *Physiol Rev*. 2019;99:1325–1380.

Besedovsky L, Ngo HVV, Dimitrov S, Gassenmaier C, Lehmann R, Born J. Auditory closed-loop stimulation of EEG slow oscillations strengthens sleep and signs of its immune-supportive function. *Nat Com*. 2017;8: Article Number 1984.

Chen Y, Zhao A, Xia Y, et al. In the big picture of COVID-19 pandemic: what can sleep do. *Sleep Med*. 2020;72:109–110.

Imeri L, Opp MR. How (and why) the immune system makes us sleep. *Nat Rev Neurosci*. 2009;10:199–210.

Ingiosi AM, Opp MR, Krueger JM. Sleep and immune function: glial contributions and consequences of aging. *Curr Opin Neurobiol*. 2013;23:806–811.

Irwin M. Sleep and inflammation: partners is sickness and in health. *Nat Rev Immunol*. 2019;19:702–715.

Irwin MR, Opp MR. Sleep Health: reciprocal regulation of sleep and innate immunity. *Neuropsychopharmacol*. 2017;42:129–155.

Lange T, Born J, Westermann J. Sleep matters: CD4+ T cell memory formation and the central nervous system. *Trends Immunol*. 2019;40:674–686.

Lange T, Dimitrov S, Born J. Effects of sleep and circadian rhythm on the human immune system. *Ann N Y Acad Sci*. 2010;1193:48–59.

Liu PY, Irwin MR, Krueger JM, Gaddameedhi S, Van Dongen HPA. Night shift schedule alters endogenous regulation of circulating cytokines. *Neurobiol Sleep Circadian Rhythms*. 2021;10:100063.

McCusker RH, Kelley KW. Immune-neural connections: how the immune system's response to infectious agents influences behavior. *J Exp Biol*. 2013;216:84–98.

Motivala SJ. Sleep and inflammation: psychoneuroimmunology in the context of cardiovascular disease. *Ann Behav Med*. 2011;42:141–152.

Preston BT, Capellini I, McNamara P, et al. Parasite resistance and the adaptive significance of sleep. *BMC Evol Biol*. 2009;9:7.

Zielinski MR, Krueger JM. Sleep and innate immunity. *Front Biosci (Schol Ed)*. 2011;3:632–642.

A complete reference list can be found online at ExpertConsult.com.

Chapter 27

Endocrine Physiology in Relation to Sleep and Sleep Disturbances

Erin C. Hanlon; Eve Van Cauter; Esra Tasali; Josiane L. Broussard

Chapter Highlights

- Sleep and circadian rhythmicity both modulate endocrine and metabolic function and affect activity of the hypothalamic-pituitary axes, carbohydrate metabolism, appetite regulation, bone metabolism, and the hormonal control of blood pressure and body-fluid balance.
- There is increasing evidence for strong and intricate interactions between sleep-wake regulation, the circadian system, and metabolism. The relative effect of sleep versus that of circadian timing cannot be dissociated, but their relative importance for endocrine function seems to vary from axis to axis.
- Sleep curtailment has become an endemic behavior in modern society. Current evidence from well-controlled laboratory studies suggests that insufficient sleep duration has deleterious effects on endocrine function, glucose metabolism, and appetite regulation and increases the risk of obesity and type 2 diabetes.
- There is emerging evidence to indicate that behavioral sleep extension in chronic short sleepers may have beneficial metabolic effects and facilitate adherence to a weight loss program.
- Accurate assessments of metabolic status and endocrine function should not be limited to the "morning after an overnight fast" window. Information about sleep duration and quality during the night before testing and about habitual sleep-wake behavior should be collected routinely and taken into account in the interpretation of diagnostic and follow-up tests.

INTRODUCTION

This chapter reviews the effects of sleep and sleep disturbances on the endocrine system, the effect of reduced sleep duration and quality on hormonal and metabolic function, and the emerging evidence for a beneficial effect of behavioral sleep extension on the risk of obesity and type 2 diabetes. For a detailed review of associations between sleep disorders and endocrine disease, the reader is referred to Chapter 155. This chapter is divided into three main sections. We start with a review of the interactions between sleep and endocrine release in the hypothalamic-pituitary axes and the roles of sleep in carbohydrate metabolism, appetite regulation, bone metabolism, and hormonal control of body-fluid balance in healthy adults. Table 27.1 provides basic information about the hormones that are discussed in this chapter. We then summarize the growing body of experimental evidence linking insufficient sleep duration with alterations of endocrine and metabolic function. We end with a review of the emerging evidence of beneficial metabolic effects of sleep extension in chronic short sleepers.

MODULATION OF ENDOCRINE FUNCTION BY SLEEP-WAKE HOMEOSTASIS AND CIRCADIAN RHYTHMICITY

Overview of Physiologic Pathways

In healthy adults, reproducible changes of essentially all hormonal and metabolic variables occur during sleep and around wake-sleep and sleep-wake transitions. These daily events partly reflect the interaction of central circadian rhythmicity and sleep-wake homeostasis. Pathways by which the central nervous system control of circadian rhythmicity and sleep-wake homeostasis affects peripheral endocrine function and metabolism include the modulation of the activity of the hypothalamic releasing and inhibiting factors, the autonomous nervous system control of endocrine and metabolic activity, and the 24-hour periodicity of circulating glucocorticoids and melatonin. The daily variation of circulating glucocorticoid is perhaps the largest and most robust circadian rhythm of all blood constituents in mammals. Glucocorticoid receptors are ubiquitous in both brain and peripheral tissues and mediate the multiple actions of glucocorticoids on immunity, inflammation, metabolism, cognitive function, mood, growth, reproduction, cardiovascular function, and the stress response. The functional significance of the wide daily variation of circulating cortisol levels as a major synchronizer of the multioscillatory human circadian timing system has only begun to be understood.[1] The 24-hour rhythm of melatonin levels plays a similar role of internal synchronizer, but probably entrains fewer peripheral oscillators because melatonin receptors are not as widely distributed. Chapters 40 and 51 address the role of melatonin as a synchronizing agent and as a metabolic regulator.

To differentiate between effects of circadian rhythmicity and those depending on the sleep-wake homeostat,

Table 27.1 Origin and Main Action of Hormones

Hormone	Main Secreting Organ/Cells	Primary Action in Adults
Growth hormone (GH)	Pituitary gland/somatotropic cells	Anabolic hormone that regulates body composition
Prolactin (PRL)	Pituitary gland/lactotropic cells	Stimulates lactation in women; pleiotropic actions, including positive immune modulator
Adrenocorticotropic hormone (ACTH)	Pituitary gland/adrenocorticotropic cells	Stimulates release of cortisol from adrenal cortex
Thyroid-stimulating hormone (TSH)	Pituitary gland/thyrotropic cells	Stimulates the release of thyroid hormones from the thyroid gland
Luteinizing hormone (LH)	Pituitary gland/gonadotropic cells	Stimulates ovarian release of estradiol and progesterone (in females) and testicular release of testosterone (in males)
Follicle-stimulating hormone (FSH)	Pituitary gland/gonadotropic cells	Stimulates follicular growth (in females) and sperm production (in males)
Cortisol	Adrenal cortex	Mediates stress response and gluconeogenesis
Epinephrine	Adrenal medulla	Mediates stress response; increases heart rate, muscle strength, blood pressure, and glucose metabolism
Testosterone	Gonads	Anabolic and virilizing hormone, stimulates sperm development
Estradiol	Ovaries	Stimulates follicular growth and maturation
Triiodothyronine (T_3) and thyroxine (T_4)	Thyroid/follicular cells	Regulate metabolism
Insulin	Pancreas/beta cells	Regulates blood glucose levels
Glucagon	Pancreas/alpha cells	Increases glucose and fatty acids in circulation, increases energy expenditure
Pancreatic polypeptide (PP)	Pancreas/PP cells	Satiety factor affecting the secretion of other pancreatic hormones
Leptin	Adipose tissue	Satiety hormone regulating energy balance
Ghrelin	Mainly stomach cells	Hunger hormone regulating energy balance
Peptide tyrosine-tyrosine (PYY)	Intestine (ileum and colon)	Anorexigenic peptide
Glucagon-like peptide 1 (GLP-1)	Intestine (ileum and colon)	Satiety peptide, affects gastrointestinal motility, inhibits glucagon secretion, stimulates insulin secretion
Gastric inhibitory polypeptide (GIP)	Intestine (duodenum and jejunum)	Stimulates insulin secretion and glucagon secretion
Melatonin	Pineal gland	Hormone of the dark that transmits photic information to the circadian clock

researchers have used experimental strategies that take advantage of the fact that rhythms primarily under the control of the central circadian pacemaker take several days to adjust to a large sudden shift of sleep-wake and light-dark cycles (e.g., occur in jet lag and shift work). Such strategies allow for the effects of circadian modulation to be observed in the absence of sleep and for the effects of sleep to be observed at a variety of circadian times. Figure 27.1 illustrates mean profiles of hormonal and glucose concentrations, and of insulin-secretion rates (ISRs) observed in healthy subjects who were studied before and during an abrupt 12-hour delay of the sleep-wake and dark-light cycles. To eliminate the effects of dietary intake, fasting, and postural changes, the participants remained recumbent throughout the study, and the meals were replaced by intravenous glucose infusion at a constant rate.[2] As shown in Figure 27.1, this drastic manipulation of sleep had only modest effects on the wave shape of the cortisol profile, in sharp contrast with the immediate shift of the growth hormone (GH) and prolactin (PRL) rhythms that followed the shift of the sleep-wake cycle. The temporal organization of thyroid-stimulating hormone (TSH) secretion appeared to be under dual control by circadian and sleep-dependent processes. Indeed, the evening elevation of TSH levels occurred well before sleep onset, reflecting the circadian phase. During sleep, an inhibitory process prevents TSH concentrations from rising further. Consequently, in

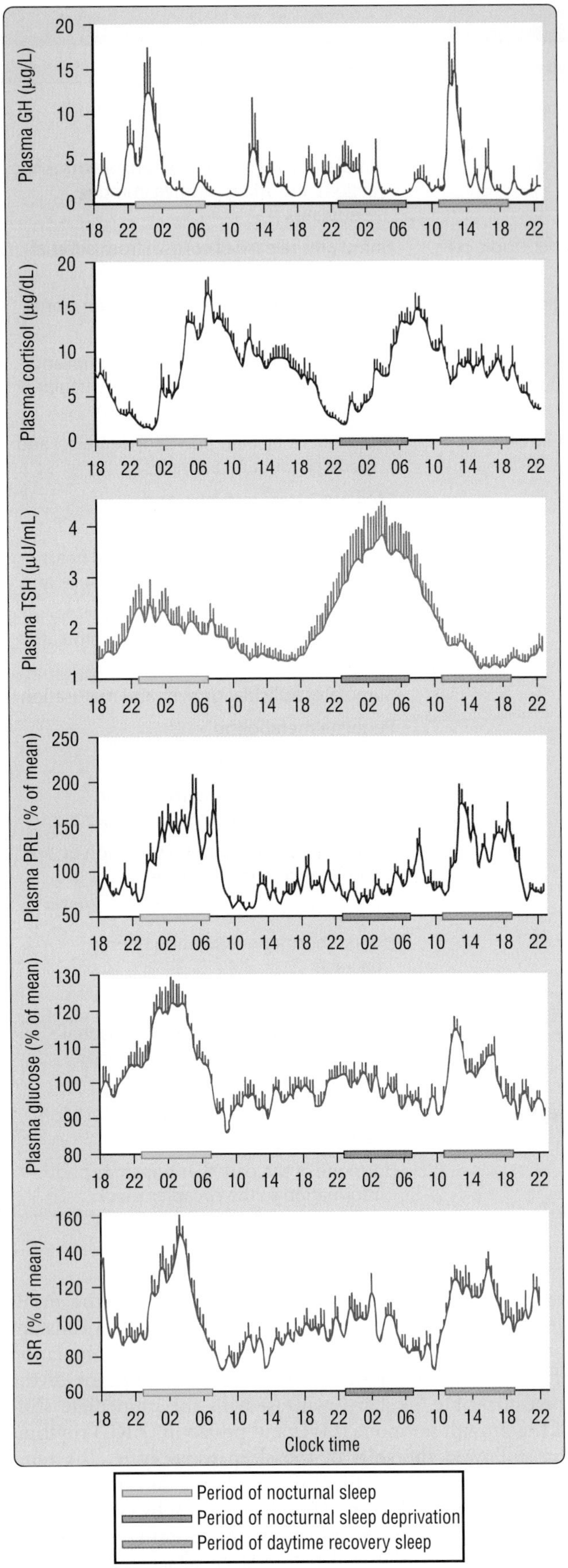

Figure 27.1 *From top to bottom:* Mean 24-hour profiles of plasma growth hormone (GH), cortisol, thyrotropin (TSH), prolactin (PRL), glucose, and insulin-secretion rates (ISR) in a group of 8 healthy young men (20–27 years old) studied during a 53-hour period including 8 hours of nocturnal sleep (*blue horizontal bar*), 28 hours of sleep deprivation (*red bar*), and 8 hours of daytime sleep (*orange bar*). The *vertical bars* on the tracings represent the standard error of the mean (SEM) at each time point. The *blue bars* represent the sleep periods. The *red bars* represent the period of nocturnal sleep deprivation. The *orange bars* represent the period of daytime sleep. Caloric intake was exclusively under the form of a constant glucose infusion. Shifted sleep was associated with an immediate shift of GH and PRL release. In contrast, the secretory profiles of cortisol and TSH remained synchronized to circadian time. Both sleep-dependent and circadian inputs can be recognized in the profiles of glucose and ISR. (Modified from Van Cauter E, Spiegel K. Circadian and sleep control of endocrine secretions. In: Turek FW, Zee PC, editors. *Neurobiology of sleep and circadian rhythms.* New York: Marcel Dekker; 1999; and Van Cauter E, et al. Modulation of glucose regulation and insulin secretion by sleep and circadian rhythmicity. *J Clin Invest.* 1991;88:934-942.)

the absence of sleep, the nocturnal TSH elevation is markedly amplified. Both sleep and time of day clearly modulated glucose levels and ISRs. Nocturnal elevations of glucose and ISRs occurred even when the subjects were sleep deprived, and recovery sleep at an abnormal circadian time was also associated with an elevation of glucose and ISR. Of note, altered patterns in glucose levels and ISRs reflect changes in glucose utilization because exogenous glucose infusion largely inhibits endogenous glucose production. Figure 27.1 illustrates that the relative importance of the sleep-wake cycle versus circadian rhythmicity varies greatly from one endocrine axis to another.

The Growth Hormone Axis

Pituitary release of GH is stimulated by hypothalamic growth hormone–releasing hormone (GHRH) and inhibited by somatostatin. In addition, the acylated form of ghrelin, a peptide produced predominantly by the stomach, is a potent endogenous stimulus of GH secretion.[3] There is a combined and probably synergistic role of GHRH stimulation, elevated nocturnal ghrelin levels, and decreased somatostatinergic tone in the control of GH secretion during sleep. Although sleep clearly involves major stimulatory effects on GH secretion, there is substantial evidence to indicate that the hormones of the somatotropic axis, including GHRH, ghrelin, and GH itself, appear to exert in turn effects on sleep regulation.[4,5] In healthy adults, the 24-hour profile of GH levels consists of stable low levels abruptly interrupted by bursts of secretion. The most reproducible GH pulse occurs shortly after sleep onset. In men, the sleep-onset GH pulse is generally the largest, and often the only secretory pulse observed over the 24-hour span. In women, daytime GH pulses are more frequent, and the postsleep onset pulse, although present, does not account for the majority of the 24-hour secretory output. A presleep pulse is often detected. Sleep onset elicits a pulse in GH secretion whether sleep is advanced, delayed, or interrupted and reinitiated. The mean GH secretion profile shown in Figure 27.1 illustrates the maintenance of the relationship between sleep onset and GH release when sleep is acutely delayed. There is a consistent relationship between the appearance of delta waves in the electroencephalogram (EEG) and elevated GH concentrations, and maximal GH release occurs within minutes of the onset of slow wave sleep (SWS).[6] In healthy young men, there is a quantitative correlation between the amount of GH secreted during the sleep-onset pulse and the duration of the SWS episode. Pharmacologic stimulation of SWS increases GH secretion.[7-9] Sedative hypnotics that do not increase slow wave activity, such as the commonly used benzodiazepines and imidazopyridines, do not increase nocturnal GH release. The robust relationship between sleep onset and GH release is consistent with a synchronization between anabolic processes in the body and a state in which behavioral rest occurs and cerebral glucose uptake is at its lowest point.[10] There is evidence to indicate that stimulation of nocturnal GH release and of SWS reflect, to a large extent, synchronous activity of at least two populations of hypothalamic GHRH neurons.[10] Sleep-onset GH secretion appears to be primarily regulated by GHRH stimulation occurring during a period of decreased somatostatin inhibition of somatotropic activity.[11,12] In addition, ghrelin may play a role in causing increased GH secretion during sleep due the postdinner rebound of its circulating levels.[13] The upper panel of Figure 27.1 shows that GH secretion is increased during sleep independently of the circadian time when sleep occurs and that sleep deprivation results in a drastic reduction of GH release. After a night of total sleep deprivation, GH release is increased during the daytime such that the total 24-hour secretion is not significantly affected.[14] This daytime secretion could reflect an elevation of ghrelin levels, which has been observed in multiple experimental studies of partial or total sleep deprivation.[15-17] Significant rises in GH secretion may also occur before the onset of sleep. These presleep GH pulses could reflect the presence of a sleep debt because they have been consistently observed after recurrent experimental sleep restriction.[18-21] The short-term negative feedback inhibition exerted by GH on its own secretion may then inhibit or reduce the GH pulse during the first slow wave period. Awakenings interrupting sleep have an inhibitory effect on GH release.[22] Thus sleep fragmentation generally decreases nocturnal GH secretion.

The Corticotropic Axis

Activity of the corticotropic axis—a neuroendocrine system associated with the stress response and behavioral activation—may be measured peripherally through plasma levels of the pituitary adrenocorticotropic hormone (ACTH) and of cortisol, the adrenal hormone directly controlled by ACTH stimulation. The plasma levels of these hormones peak in the early morning and decline throughout the daytime, reaching concentrations near the lower limit of most assays in the late evening and early part of the sleep period. Although the rhythm of ACTH reflects a circadian variation in corticotropin-releasing hormone (CRH) activity, itself under control by the central circadian pacemaker, a peripheral clock in the adrenals enhances the rhythm of glucocorticoid release, one of the largest and most robust rhythms in humans.[23,24] In addition, there is evidence for a direct multisynaptic pathway connecting the suprachiasmatic nucleus to the adrenals.[25] Sleep is normally initiated when corticotropic activity is quiescent. Reactivation of ACTH and cortisol secretion occurs abruptly a few hours before the usual waking time.

The mean cortisol secretion profile shown in Figure 27.1 illustrates the remarkable persistence of this diurnal variation even in the presence of a drastic manipulation of the sleep-wake cycle. Nonetheless, modulatory effects of sleep or wake have been clearly demonstrated. Indeed, sleep onset is reliably associated with a short-term inhibition of cortisol secretion. Under normal conditions, because cortisol secretion is already quiescent in the late evening, this inhibitory effect of sleep, which is temporally associated with slow wave sleep,[26-28] prolongs the quiescent period. Conversely, awakening at the end of the sleep period is consistently followed by a pulse of cortisol secretion, often referred to as the "cortisol awakening response."[29]

During sleep deprivation, the rapid effects of sleep onset and sleep offset on corticotropic activity are obviously absent, and, as may be seen in Figure 27.1, the nadir of cortisol level is slightly higher than during nocturnal sleep (because of the absence of the inhibitory effects of the first hours of sleep), and the morning maximal peak is slightly lower (because of the absence of the stimulating effects of morning awakening). Overall, the amplitude of the rhythm is reduced by about 15% during sleep deprivation compared with normal conditions. In addition to the immediate modulatory effects of sleep-wake transitions on cortisol levels, nocturnal sleep deprivation, even partial, results in an elevation of cortisol levels on the following evening.[30]

The Thyroid Axis

Daytime levels of plasma TSH are low and relatively stable until the initiation of a rapid elevation in the early evening resulting in maximal concentrations around the beginning of the sleep period.[31,32] Then, TSH levels decline progressively, and daytime values resume shortly after morning awakening. The first 24 hours of the study illustrated in Figure 27.1 are typical of the TSH rhythm. The nocturnal rise of TSH occurs well before the time of sleep onset and is dependent on circadian timing.[32] A marked effect of sleep on TSH secretion may be seen during sleep deprivation, when nocturnal TSH secretion may be increased by as much as 200%. Sleep thus exerts an inhibitory influence on TSH secretions, and sleep deprivation removes this inhibition. Interestingly, when sleep occurs during daytime hours, TSH secretion is not suppressed significantly below normal daytime levels, indicating once again the interaction between the effects of circadian time and sleep. When the depth of sleep at the habitual time is increased by prior sleep deprivation, the nocturnal TSH rise is more markedly inhibited, suggesting that SWS is probably the primary determinant of the sleep-associated fall.[32] Awakenings interrupting nocturnal sleep appear to disinhibit TSH release and are consistently associated with a short-term TSH elevation. Circadian and sleep-related variations in thyroid hormones have not been consistently observed, probably because these hormones have long half-lives and are bound to serum proteins. However, under conditions of sleep deprivation, the increased amplitude of the TSH rhythm may result in a detectable increase in plasma triiodothyronine (T_3) levels that parallels the nocturnal TSH rise.[33] If sleep deprivation is continued for a second night, the nocturnal rise of TSH is markedly diminished compared with the first night.[33,34] It is likely that after the first night of sleep deprivation, the elevated thyroid hormone levels, which persist during the daytime period because of the aforementioned prolonged half-life of these hormones, limit the subsequent nocturnal TSH rise via a negative feedback. A study of 64 hours of sleep deprivation suggested that prolonged sleep loss is associated with an upregulation of the thyroid axis, with lower levels of TSH and higher levels of thyroid hormones.[35]

Prolactin Secretion

Under normal conditions, PRL levels undergo a major nocturnal elevation starting shortly after sleep onset and culminating around midsleep. In adults of both sexes, the nocturnal maximum of PRL is about twofold higher than mean daytime levels.[33] Morning awakenings and awakenings interrupting sleep are both consistently associated with a rapid inhibition of PRL secretion.[33] Studies of the PRL profile during daytime naps or after shifts of the sleep period have consistently demonstrated that sleep onset, irrespective of the time of day, has a stimulatory effect on PRL release. This is well illustrated by the profiles shown in Figure 27.1, in which elevated PRL levels occur both during nocturnal sleep and daytime recovery sleep, whereas the nocturnal period of sleep deprivation was not associated with an increase in PRL concentrations. However, a small nocturnal rise of PRL may still be detectable during sleep deprivation, likely reflecting a circadian effect.[36-38] A close temporal association between increased PRL secretion and slow wave activity is apparent.[39] However, in contrast to the quantitative correlation between slow wave activity and GH release that exists in men, no such "dose-response" relationship has been demonstrated for PRL in either men or women.

Commonly used hypnotics, such as triazolam and zolpidem, may cause a transient increase in the nocturnal PRL rise, resulting in concentrations near the pathologic range for part of the night.[40,41] In contrast to PRL, neither triazolam nor zolpidem has any effect on the 24-hour profiles of cortisol, melatonin, or GH.[40,41] A single bedtime dose of sodium oxybate results in a concomitant increase of PRL release and SWS in both normal subjects and narcoleptic patients.[42]

The Gonadal Axis

The relationship between sleep and the 24-hour patterns of gonadotropin release and gonadal steroid levels varies according to age and sex (for review, see Copinschi and Challet[33]). Before puberty, luteinizing hormone (LH) and follicle-stimulating hormone (FSH) are secreted in a pulsatile pattern, and an augmentation of pulsatile activity is associated with sleep onset in a majority of both girls and boys. The increased amplitude of gonadotropin release during sleep is one of the hallmarks of puberty. Simultaneous frequent sampling of LH levels during polysomnography has revealed that during puberty, the majority of LH pulses that occur after sleep onset are preceded by SWS. Even when SWS is fragmented experimentally by acoustic stimuli, the accumulation of SWS remains a predictor of the occurrence of an LH pulse.[43,44] Thus SWS appears play a pivotal role in sexual maturation during the pubertal transition.

During the transition from puberty to adulthood, major sex differences in the temporal organization of gonadal hormone secretion become apparent. In males the amplitude of daytime LH pulses increases, and in adults the day-night variation of plasma LH levels is dampened or even undetectable. During sleep, the majority of LH pulses are initiated during non–rapid eye movement (NREM) sleep, similar to that occurring during puberty.[45] Despite the low amplitude of the nocturnal increase in gonadotropin release, a marked diurnal rhythm in circulating testosterone levels is present, with minimal levels in the late evening, a robust rise after sleep onset, and maximal levels in the early morning.[46,47] The nocturnal rise of testosterone appears temporally linked to the duration of the first NREM period.[48] A robust rise may also be observed during daytime sleep, suggesting that sleep, irrespective of time of day, stimulates gonadal hormone release.[49] Experimental sleep fragmentation in young men results in attenuation of the nocturnal rise of testosterone.[50] Androgen concentrations in young adults decline significantly during periods of total sleep deprivation and recover promptly after sleep is restored.[49,51] The importance of sleep for androgen release has been confirmed in several experimental studies of partial sleep restriction. For a review of the bidirectional interactions between sleep disorders and the male reproductive axis in disease states, the reader is referred to Chapter 155.

In adult menstruating women, diurnal profiles of FSH, LH, estradiol, and progesterone exhibit episodic pulses throughout the 24-hour span.[33] The 24-hour variation in plasma LH is markedly modulated by the menstrual cycle.[52,53] In the early follicular phase, LH pulses are large and infrequent, and a marked slowing of the frequency of secretory pulses occurs during sleep, suggestive of inhibitory effect of sleep on pulsatile GnRH release. Awakenings interrupting sleep are usually associated with a pulse of LH concentration.[54] In the midfollicular phase, pulse amplitude is decreased, pulse frequency is increased, and the frequency modulation of LH pulsatility by sleep is less apparent. Pulse amplitude increases again by the late follicular phase. In the early luteal phase, pulse amplitude is markedly increased, pulse frequency is decreased, and nocturnal slowing of pulsatility is again evident. In the mid and late luteal phases, pulse amplitude and frequency are decreased and there is no modulation by sleep.

Glucose Regulation

The consolidation of human sleep in a single 7- to 9-hour period implies that an extended period of fast must be maintained overnight. Despite the prolonged fasting condition, glucose levels remain relatively stable across the night. In contrast, if subjects are awake and fasting in a recumbent position, glucose levels fall by an average of 0.5 to 1.0 mmol/L (±10–20 mg/dL) over a 12-hour period.[55] Thus a number of mechanisms that operate during nocturnal sleep must intervene to maintain stable glucose levels during the overnight fast. The lower panels of Figure 27.1 show profiles of blood glucose and ISRs observed under conditions of constant glucose infusion, a condition inhibiting endogenous glucose production. Thus changes in plasma glucose levels mainly reflect changes in glucose utilization. A marked decrease in glucose tolerance is apparent during nighttime, as well as daytime sleep. A smaller elevation of glucose and insulin also occurs during nocturnal sleep deprivation, indicating an effect of circadian-dependent mechanisms. Recovery sleep is associated with a robust increase in glucose and insulin, owing to sleep-onset GH release. During nocturnal sleep, the overall increase in plasma glucose during infusion ranged from 20% to 30%, despite the maintenance of rigorously constant rates of caloric intake. Maximal levels are reached around the middle of the sleep period. During the later part of the night, glucose tolerance begins to improve, and glucose levels progressively decrease toward morning values. The mechanisms underlying these robust variations in set-point of glucose regulation across nocturnal sleep are different in early sleep and late sleep. It is estimated that about two thirds of the fall in whole-body glucose utilization during early sleep is due to a decrease in brain glucose metabolism[56] related to the predominance of SWS, which is associated with a 30% to 40% reduction in cerebral glucose metabolism compared with the waking state.[57] The remainder of the fall would then reflect decreased peripheral use, including diminished muscle tone and rapid hyperglycemic effects of the sleep-onset GH pulse. Furthermore, the nocturnal elevation of melatonin levels could contribute to the nocturnal decrease in glucose tolerance.[58] Toward the end of the sleep period, glucose levels and insulin secretion return to presleep values, partially because of the increase in wake and rapid eye movement (REM) stages.[59] Indeed, glucose use during REM sleep and wake is higher than during NREM sleep.[57] In addition, an increase in insulin sensitivity due to a delayed effect of low cortisol levels during the evening and early part of the night may lower glucose levels.[60]

Hunger and Appetite

Sleep plays an important role in energy balance. In rodents, food shortage or starvation results in decreased sleep[61] and, conversely, total sleep deprivation leads to marked hyperphagia.[62] The identification of hypothalamic excitatory neuropeptides, referred to as hypocretins or orexins, that have potent wake-promoting effects and stimulate food intake has provided a molecular basis for the interactions between the regulation of feeding and sleeping.[63,64] Orexin-containing neurons are active during wake and quiescent during sleep. Orexin activity is inhibited by leptin, a satiety hormone released by adipose tissue, and stimulated by ghrelin, an appetite-promoting hormone secreted by stomach cells. Multiple peptides and nonpeptide signals derived from the gut, fat, and other tissues participate in the control of hunger and satiety and there is experimental evidence that some of them can be influenced by sleep.[65-67] Figure 27.2 shows representative individual profiles of multiple metabolic signals that present consistent temporal variations across the 24-hour cycle reflecting the effect of the feeding-fasting schedule, the sleep-wake cycle, and circadian timing. The participants received three identical high-carbohydrate meals while undergoing frequent blood sampling and polysomnography. The top three panels on the left illustrate the profiles of insulin, amylin, and pancreatic polypeptide (PP), three distinct peptides secreted simultaneously by different pancreatic cell types in response to the postprandial glucose increase. Amylin is cosecreted with insulin from the pancreatic beta cells and acts as a satiety agent.[68,69] PP is secreted by the F cells and, similar to amylin, slows the transit of food through the gut and promotes satiety. Infusion of PP in lean subjects reduces food intake[70] and PP levels are reduced in obesity.[70,71] It can be seen in the PP profile illustrated in Figure 27.2 that the PP response to meal presentation is biphasic, with the first phase referred to as "cephalic" because it occurs very shortly after meal presentation, before the food enters the stomach and before the rise in circulating glucose levels.[72] The cephalic PP response involves vagal stimulation by oronasal signals. The lower left panels of Figure 27.2 show that the intake of carbohydrate-rich meals stimulates the release of two peptides originating from intestinal cells, glucagon-like peptide-1 (GLP-1; lower intestinal L cells) and glucose-dependent insulinotropic peptide (GIP; upper intestinal K cells). GLP-1 and GIP are referred to as the "incretin" hormones because they enhance insulin secretion and are rapidly released in response to meal intake.[73,74] Agonists of GLP-1 and GIP are widely used classes of antidiabetic drugs. Agonists of GLP-1 also reduce appetite and promote weight loss. Contrasting with the coordinated postprandial release of insulin, amylin, PP, GLP-1, and GIP after the maintenance of stable low levels during the overnight fast, the profiles shown on the right side of Figure 27.2 appear modulated by factors other than the responses to meal intake. Ghrelin, a potent hunger hormone, is released by stomach cells.[75] Daytime profiles of plasma ghrelin levels are primarily regulated by the schedule of food intake: levels drop sharply after each meal intake and rebound in parallel with increased hunger until the initiation of the following meal.[76] During sleep, ghrelin levels first increase, partly driven by the postdinner rebound but then decrease steadily through the sleep period, consistent with the need to suppress hunger while sleeping.[13] The 24-hour profile of peptide tyrosine-tyrosine (PYY), released by the L cells of the lower intestine and colon and an appetite suppressant, in a reverse relationship to that of ghrelin with short-term increases following food ingestion and a steady decrease in the evening and first half of the sleep period. The lower three panels of the right side of Figure 27.2 show the 24-hour profiles of the circulating levels of free fatty acids (FFAs; released from triglyceride stores in adipocytes), leptin (a satiety hormone released by the adipocytes) and the endocannabinoid (eCB) 2-arachidonylglycerol (2-AG, a stimulant of hedonic food intake). These three circulating metabolic signals display large amplitude variations across the 24-hour cycle that are not primarily driven by the alternation of feeding and fasting. The nocturnal rise in FFAs is partly dependent on sleep, because it is in large part dependent on the lipolytic effects of sleep-onset GH secretion, an event tightly linked with the first episode of SWS.[21] Circulating leptin concentrations in humans peak before midsleep and then decline until midmorning. Leptin levels then increase in response to accumulated caloric intake during the daytime.[77] These changes in leptin levels have been associated with reciprocal changes in hunger. The nocturnal elevation of leptin has been thought to suppress the hunger during the overnight fast. Although daytime food intake plays a major role in the progressive rise of leptin from morning to evening,[77] a study using continuous enteral nutrition to eliminate the effect of meal intake showed the persistence of a sleep-related leptin elevation, although the amplitude was lower

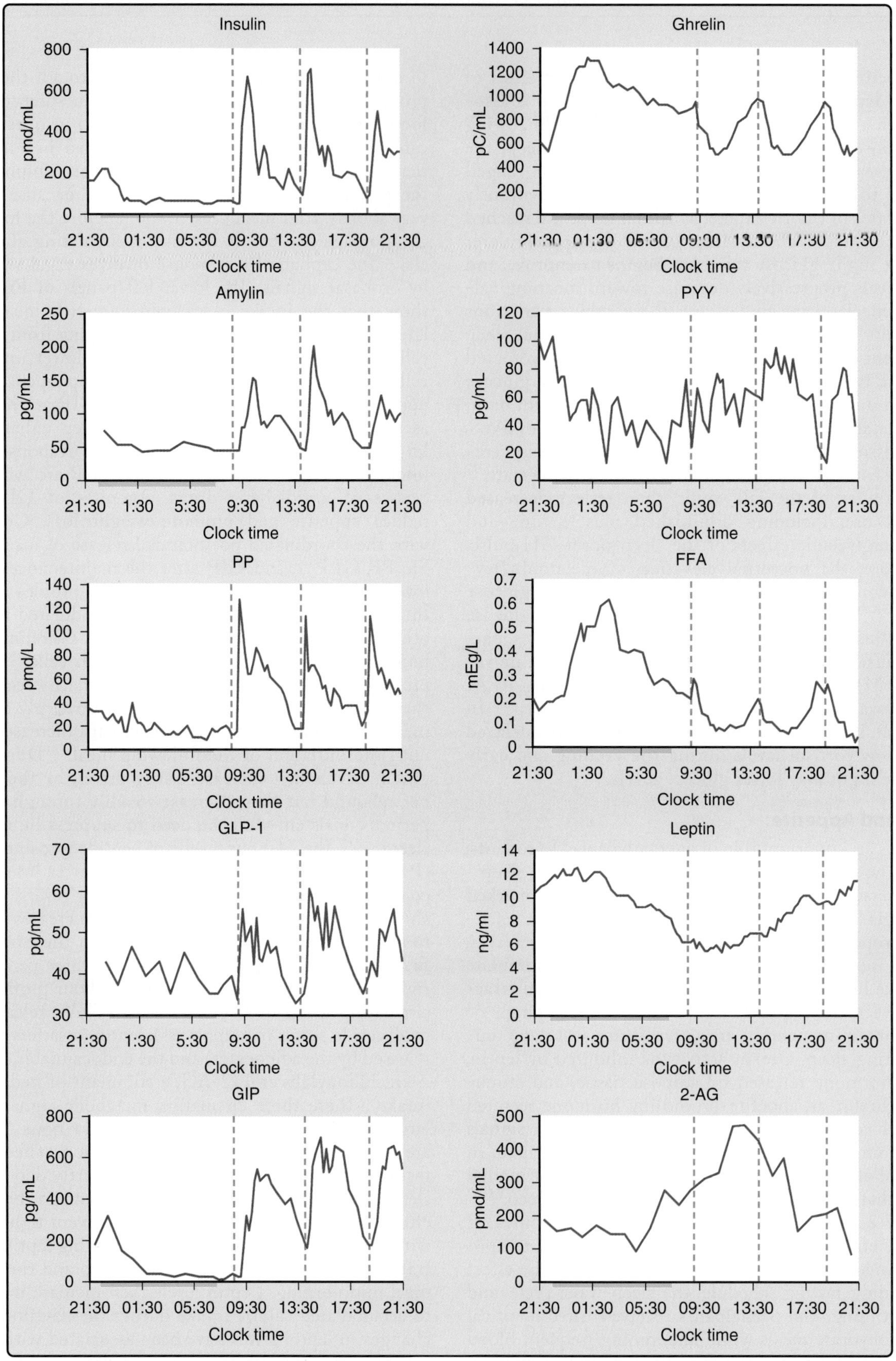

Figure 27.2 Typical individual 24-hour profiles of circulating metabolic signals measured simultaneously in healthy, young, lean men who were studied in the Clinical Research Center at the University of Chicago where they received three identical high-carbohydrate meals (9:00 A.M., 2:00 P.M.,7:00 P.M.) while undergoing frequent blood sampling and polysomnography. The panels on the left illustrate the profiles of insulin, amylin, and pancreatic polypeptide (PP), three distinct peptides secreted by different pancreatic cell types, and of two peptides originating from intestinal cells, glucagon-like peptide-1 (GLP-1; lower intestinal L cells), and glucose-dependent insulinotropic peptide (GIP; upper intestinal K cells). These five hormones are all rapidly released in response to the postprandial glucose elevations. The panels on the right illustrate the profiles of ghrelin (from stomach cells), peptide tyrosine-tyrosine (PYY; from the lower intestine), leptin (from adipocytes), free fatty acids (FFAs; from adipocytes), and 2-arachidonylglycerol (2-AG; an endocannabinoid released by multiple tissues). These five circulating metabolic signals display large amplitude variations across the 24-hour cycle that are not primarily driven by the alternation of feeding and fasting and are partly dependent on sleep. Time in bed is denoted by the *black bars*. The *vertical dotted lines* denote the time of presentation of identical high-carbohydrate meals. (Unpublished data from the Sleep, Metabolism and Health Center at the University of Chicago.)

than during normal eating conditions.[78] Prolonged total sleep deprivation results in a decrease in the amplitude of the leptin diurnal variation.[79] Lastly, as shown in Figure 27.2, a robust 24-hour variation of the circulating levels of the most abundant eCB ligand 2-AG has been recently demonstrated.[80] The specific origin of peripheral concentrations of eCBs remains unclear but that they could be derived from the multiple tissues in which the enzymatic machinery to synthesize eCBs are located, including but not limited to, brain, gut, muscle, pancreas, and adipose tissue.[81,82] The eCB system is composed of the cannabinoid receptors, CB1 and CB2; the endogenous ligands of these receptors, including 2-AG and anandamide (AEA); and the enzymes responsible for the biosynthesis and degradation of the eCBs. The eCB system is involved in the control of feeding, body weight, and peripheral metabolism and has been the target of efforts to develop antiobesity drugs. Hedonic eating, defined as eating for pleasure rather than to fulfill an energy need, has been shown to be associated with enhanced plasma 2-AG, as well as ghrelin levels.[83,84] Thus the more than threefold increase in 2-AG levels from midsleep to midday suggests that the hedonic drive to eat increases from early morning to reach a peak around habitual lunchtime. The 24-hour profile of AEA concentrations is markedly different from that of 2-AG,[85] suggesting a differential effect of sleep regulation and the circadian system on these two components of the eCB system.

Water and Electrolyte Balance during Sleep

Water and salt homeostasis is under the combined control of vasopressin, a hormone released by the posterior pituitary, the renin-angiotensin-aldosterone system, and the atrial natriuretic peptide. Urine flow and electrolyte excretion are higher during the day than during the night, and this variation partly reflects circadian modulation. In addition to this 24-hour rhythm, urine flow and osmolarity oscillate with the REM-NREM cycle. REM sleep is associated with decreasing urine flow and increasing osmolarity. Vasopressin release is pulsatile but without apparent relationship to sleep stages.[86] Levels of atrial natriuretic peptide are relatively stable and do not show fluctuations related to the sleep-wake or REM-NREM cycle.[87] Whether the levels of plasma atrial natriuretic peptide exhibit a circadian variation is still a matter of controversy.[87] Figure 27.3 illustrates the 24-hour rhythm of plasma renin activity (PRA) in an individual studied during a normal sleep-wake cycle and after a shift of the sleep period.[88] The initiation of sleep, irrespective of time of day, is associated with a robust increase in PRA. In contrast, the nocturnal elevation of PRA does not occur when the subject is sleep deprived (lower panel of Figure 27.3). A well-documented study[89] has delineated the mechanisms responsible for the elevation of PRA during sleep. The initial event is a reduction in sympathetic tone, followed by a decrease in mean arterial blood pressure and an increase in slow wave activity. The rise in PRA becomes evident a few minutes after the increase in slow wave activity. During REM sleep, sympathetic activity increases, whereas renin and slow wave activity decrease and blood pressure becomes highly variable. This pattern of changes in PRA during sleep drives the nocturnal profile of aldosterone levels (reviewed in[90]). Acute total sleep deprivation eliminates the nocturnal PRA rise, dampens the nighttime elevation of plasma aldosterone, and increases natriuresis.[90] A close relationship between the beginning of REM episodes and decreased activity has been consistently observed for both PRA and aldosterone.[90] This relationship was confirmed in studies with selective REM-sleep deprivation in healthy subjects[91] and increases in PRA parallel increases in slow wave EEG activity.[90,91]

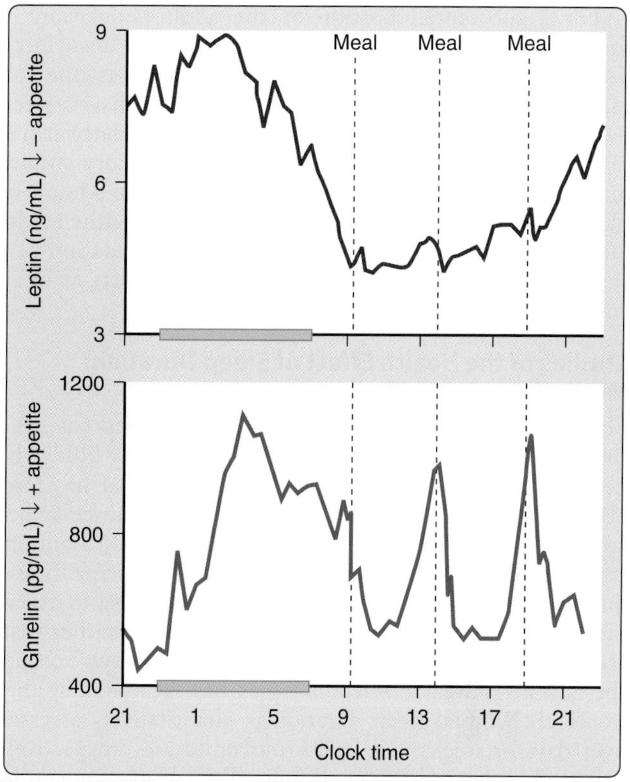

Figure 27.3 The 24-hour profiles of plasma renin activity sampled at 10-minute intervals in a healthy subject. **A,** Nocturnal sleep from 11:00 P.M. to 7:00 A.M. **B,** Daytime sleep from 7:00 A.M. to 3:00 P.M. after a night of total sleep deprivation. The temporal distribution of stages wake (W); REM; 1, 2, 3, and 4 are shown above the hormonal values. The oscillations of plasma renin activity are synchronized to the REM-NREM cycle during sleep. (From Brandenberger G, , et al. Twenty-four hour profiles of plasma renin activity in relation to the sleep-wake cycle. *J Hypertens.* 1994;12:277-283.)

RECURRENT SLEEP RESTRICTION: IMPACT ON ENDOCRINE RELEASE, METABOLIC FUNCTION, AND ENERGY INTAKE

Insufficient Sleep: A Very Common Condition in Contemporary Society

In 2015 a panel of experts issued a consensus statement recommending a sleep duration of "at least 7 hours per night on a regular basis" to promote optimal health in adults.[92] In stark contrast to this recommendation, a 2014 Survey of the Centers for Disease Control and Prevention revealed that the percentage of the adult population reporting usually sleeping less than 7 hours per night varied from state to state, from 28.5% to 44.5%.[93] An analysis of 324,242 US adults aged 18 years or older showed that between 1985 and 2012 the age-adjusted percentage of individuals sleeping 6 hours or less increased by 31%.[94] A more recent analysis found that this proportion of adults has further increased after 2012.[95]

For a substantial portion of the adult population in industrialized countries, the cumulative sleep loss for a 5-day workweek may correspond to as much as one full night of sleep deprivation. Younger adults who have a sleep need as high as 9 hours per night may be particularly at risk of accumulating a sleep debt.[92] Indeed, laboratory studies of bedtime extension provided evidence that 7 to 8 hours of habitual sleep do not meet the sleep need of healthy adults 30 years old or younger, resulting in the accumulation of a sleep debt even in the absence of obvious efforts at sleep curtailment.[96-99]

Studies of the Health Effect of Sleep Duration: Methodology and Challenges

Since 2000, the health effect of insufficient sleep has been the topic of an abundance of literature, rightfully filling the need for a rigorous scientific evaluation of what has long been a neglected aspect of human behavior. Three major approaches have been used. First, well-controlled laboratory studies are necessarily limited in number of participants and duration of the intervention but have the potential to examine physiologic variables over the 24-hour cycle rather than at a single time point and to reveal causal pathways. Second, the advent of wearable technologies has facilitated studies in which habitual sleep duration is quantitatively assessed over days or weeks and health outcomes are prospectively collected under real-life conditions. The sample size can be much larger than for studies confined to the laboratory but there is a need to control statistically for potential confounders. Lastly, self-reported sleep duration, with its biases and inaccuracies, is most frequently the independent variable in large prospective epidemiologic cohorts examining the effect of sleep time on biomedical outcomes. The large sample size allows for the exploration of the roles of demographic and social factors on the relationship between sleep behavior and health markers.

These three approaches have been complementary and the emerging body of evidence has been quite consistent in showing multiple adverse health consequences of insufficient sleep. Comparing studies of sleep restriction from different laboratories, however, remains challenging, owing to differences in time in bed; number of days of intervention; timing of the restricted sleep period; participant demographics; dietary, activity, and lighting conditions; and methods used to enforce wakefulness. The issue of whether there is a "dose-response" relationship between the severity of a specific disturbance and the magnitude of the "sleep debt" remains unresolved. The translation of the findings of laboratory studies to real-life conditions is challenging because in the laboratory, the sleep debt is accumulated day after day while in real life, multiple days of insufficient sleep are generally followed by at least 1 day of extended bedtimes. Whereas epidemiologic studies have fairly consistently observed significant adverse effects of habitual sleep duration of 6 hours or less, which would correspond to a sleep debt of 5 to 10 hours over a 5-day period for a healthy adult, laboratory studies have generally used a more severe daily bedtime restriction in order to accumulate a substantial sleep debt more rapidly and limit the duration of the intervention. Lastly, restricting bedtime involves extending the duration of indoor light exposure, potentially affecting the circadian system. Despite all of these limitations, the findings of laboratory, population, and epidemiologic studies have generally been convergent when similar outcome measures have been used.

Here, we review the hormonal and metabolic findings of laboratory studies that manipulated sleep duration, either by restriction or by extension, for at least two consecutive nights in healthy adults under controlled conditions. The metabolic and endocrine effect of acute total sleep deprivation, necessarily a short-term condition, has been previously contrasted to that of recurrent sleep restriction[99] and will not be considered.

Endocrine and Metabolic Effect of Mild versus Severe Sleep Restriction

In an effort to address the issue of *amount of accumulated sleep debt* versus *qualitative and quantitative hormonal and metabolic disturbances*, we will compare two separate laboratory studies completed at the University of Chicago and attempt to provide responses to important questions. What are the early versus delayed consequences of repeated sleep restriction? Is there a "dose-response" relationship between the total accumulated sleep debt and the magnitude of endocrine and metabolic disturbances? Can this comparison provide mechanistic insights? In these two studies, the participants had similar demographics, the data were collected in the same environment under similar dietary and light-dark conditions, recording and analytical methods were nearly identical, and the timing of restricted bedtime was similarly centered on the timing of midsleep under habitual conditions. The left panels of Figure 27.4 summarize some of the hormonal and metabolic findings of the first "sleep debt study,"[100] which examined the effect of 6 days of bedtime restriction to 4 hours per night compared with 6 days of bedtime extension to 12 hours per night in 11 healthy young men.[20,101] Each subject served as his own control. Sleep extension followed sleep restriction. Blood sampling for 24 hours started after the fifth night in the bedtime restriction condition and after the sixth night in the bedtime extension condition. From top to bottom, the 24-hour profiles of GH, cortisol, TSH, glucose, insulin, and leptin are presented for both bedtime conditions. In this study, by the time the first blood sample was collected in the restriction condition, the participants had received 48 hours less sleep opportunity than in the 12-hour bedtime condition when they had obtained on average 10 hours 9 minutes ± 15 minutes of sleep per night. In the comparative analysis that follows, we will refer to this study as "Severe sleep restriction." The right panels of Figure 27.4 illustrate the 24-hour profiles of the same 6 blood constituents in 19 healthy young men who participated in a randomized controlled study examining the effect of 4 nights of bedtime restricted to 4.5-hour versus 4 nights of 8.5-hour bedtimes.[17,21] Blood sampling for 24 hours started after the second night in both bedtime conditions. In this study, by the time the first blood sample was collected in the restriction condition, the participants had received 16 hours less sleep opportunity than in the 8.5-hour condition. Relative to the "Severe sleep restriction" study, we will refer to this study as "Mild sleep restriction."

The qualitative comparison of the profiles in Figure 27.4 can be summarized as follows:

1. After both mild and severe restriction, the temporal organization of nocturnal GH release was altered such that a

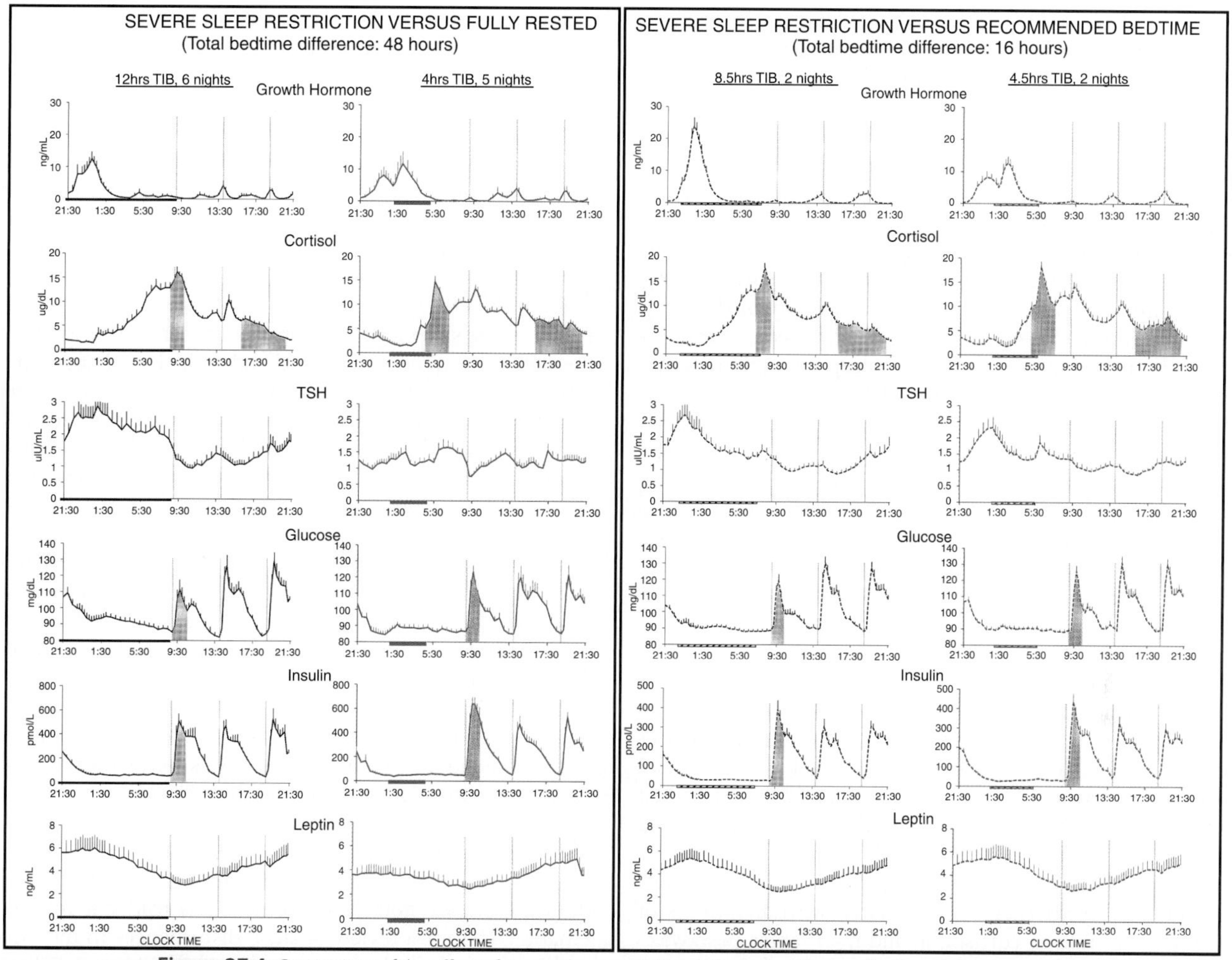

Figure 27.4 Comparison of the effect of severe sleep restriction (*left panels;* 48 hours of reduced sleep opportunity between fully rested state [shown in *black*] and sleep-restricted state [shown in *red*]; $n = 11$ men) versus mild sleep restriction (*right panels;* 16 hours of reduced sleep opportunity between recommended bedtimes [shown in *black*] and sleep restriction [shown in *red*]; $n = 19$ men) on the 24-hour profiles of growth hormone, cortisol, thyroid-stimulating hormone (TSH), glucose, insulin, and leptin in healthy young men. *Horizontal solid bars* represent the bedtime period. On the cortisol profiles, the *shaded areas* show the increase in evening cortisol levels and in the postawakening cortisol pulse. On the glucose and insulin profiles, the *shaded areas* show the response to the morning meal. (Data sources[18,21,22,113,114]. TSH data in the mild sleep restriction panels have not been previously published.)

GH pulse occurred consistently before sleep onset, preceding the usual postsleep onset pulse. The physiologic consequences of the extended GH release include a stimulation of the nocturnal release of free fatty acids.[21]

2. The overall waveshape of the cortisol profile was preserved irrespective of the sleep condition. The amplitude of the postawakening cortisol response was increased roughly twofold after mild restriction but more than threefold after severe restriction. Evening levels (4:00–9:00 P.M.) levels nearly doubled after severe sleep restriction but were minimally affected after mild sleep restriction.
3. Mean 24-hour levels of TSH declined markedly after 6 days of 4-hour bedtimes but were not significantly decreased by 2 days of 4.5-hour bedtimes.
4. The glucose response to breakfast was increased in both sleep restriction conditions, but this effect was larger when the sleep debt was larger. The increase in postbreakfast glucose response under both sleep restriction conditions occurred despite slightly higher insulin responses, indicating the presence of insulin resistance.
5. Overall leptin levels were not affected after a mild sleep debt, but declined markedly in the presence of a large sleep debt accumulated over 6 days.

This comparison reveals that the splitting of the nocturnal GH pulse, the increase in the postawakening cortisol response, and reduced morning glucose tolerance associated with insulin resistance are disturbances that appear early on when a sleep debt accumulates but become more pronounced when sleep loss continues. In contrast, significant reductions in TSH and leptin levels, two major regulators of energy balance, become apparent only in the presence of a much larger sleep debt. In what follows, we discuss possible mechanistic pathways underlying the effect of sleep restriction for the main endocrine axes and for glucose and appetite regulation.

Pituitary and Pituitary-Dependent Hormones

Sleep-Dependent Hormones: GH and Prolactin

There is scant information on the effect of sleep restriction on the two pituitary hormones that are most dependent on sleep for their release, GH and prolactin, because sampling across day and night is crucial to evaluate the integrity of these pituitary axes. Regarding GH, we are not aware of data other than those shown in the upper panels of Figure 27.4.[20,21] Even mild amounts of sleep restriction result in the splitting of nocturnal GH release in a presleep and a postsleep pulse. Reflecting the well-known negative feedback of GH on its own release, in the presence of a sleep debt, sleep-onset GH release is negatively correlated to the amount of presleep secretion.[20] The splitting of nocturnal GH release in two pulses results in an increase in the duration of active nighttime release during the nighttime, similar irrespective of the severity of the sleep debt (on average, +52 minutes in the mild sleep restriction study and +47 minutes in the severe sleep restriction study). Mechanisms leading to the release of GH before sleep onset have not been explored. A modest sleep-independent circadian input to nocturnal GH release, mediated by decreased somatostatin inhibition, is possible. Ghrelin levels have been measured in the mild sleep restriction study[17,21] but, during the presleep period, were essentially superimposable to those observed under normal sleep conditions. Thus a role for ghrelin in the appearance of a presleep GH pulse in the presence of a sleep debt is unlikely.

The Corticotropic Axis

Sleep restriction generally results in increased activity of the stress-responsive corticotropic axis. In a randomized crossover design study comparing levels of plasma ACTH and cortisol across the waking period after 2 nights of 10 hours in bed versus 2 nights of 4 hours in bed, overall levels of ACTH and cortisol were elevated by 30% and 20%, respectively, in the short sleep condition.[102] In the data shown in Figure 27.4, recurrent sleep restriction was associated with alterations of the 24-hour profile of cortisol, including a larger postawakening pulse and elevated levels in the late afternoon and evening. The elevation of evening cortisol levels, reflecting a shorter period of quiescence of the axis, was much larger after severe, than after mild, sleep restriction. Several studies that have assessed the profile of plasma or saliva cortisol levels across the daytime period in individuals submitted to 2 to 7 days of sleep restriction by 4 to 5 hours per night have similarly observed an elevation of cortisol concentrations in the late afternoon or evening.[102-104] Thus insufficient sleep may dampen the circadian rhythm of cortisol, a major internal synchronizer of central and peripheral clocks.[1] A recent study[105] has examined whether the relative hypercortisolism occurring in the late afternoon and evening in individuals subjected to sleep restriction is associated with alterations in the ACTH-cortisol response to corticotropin-releasing hormone (CRH) stimulation. To this effect, an intravenous injection of CRH was administered at 6:00 P.M. under both sleep conditions. Sleep restriction was associated with a reduction of the overall ACTH and cortisol responses to evening CRH stimulation, and a reduced reactivity and slower recovery of the cortisol response. This study thus showed that insufficient sleep may be associated with a blunting of the pituitary-adrenal response to CRH, a pivotal element of the neuroendocrine response to stress, and a reduced resilience of the adrenal gland to recover from stimulation. Contrasting with the reduced responsiveness of the corticotropic axis in the evening, the cortisol awakening response (CAR), a rapid cortisol rise starting right after morning awakening that may continue for about 1 hour,[106] is amplified in the presence of a sleep debt. The data shown in Figure 27.4 strongly suggest that this effect is greater with increasing amounts of sleep restriction. Prolonged awakenings (roughly ≥5 minutes) interrupting sleep are almost systematically associated with a cortisol pulse. In the case of sleep restriction, the CAR may represent a more severe stress response than under normal sleep conditions, as the participant usually needs to be awakened by an alarm system or by an investigator. The CAR phenomenon appears to occur at all circadian times.[106]

The Thyrotropic Axis

In the severe sleep restriction study (left panels of Figure 27.4), the state of sleep debt was associated with clear changes in thyrotropic function.[100] The nocturnal TSH rise was dampened and thyroid hormone levels were higher in the sleep debt state. Previous studies have demonstrated that total sleep deprivation is initially associated with a marked increase in TSH secretion (Figure 27.1), which becomes smaller when sleep deprivation continues, presumably because of negative feedback effects from slowly rising levels of thyroid hormones. Similar mechanisms are likely to underlie the alterations in thyrotropic function after recurrent sleep restriction. Findings of elevations in free thyroxine (T_4) index and in levels of free triiodothyronine (T_3) and free T_4 in subjects submitted to sleep restriction or total sleep deprivation are consistent with this hypothesis.[100,101,107,108] In middle-aged overweight adults exposed to 14 days of moderate sleep restriction, TSH and free T_4 levels were lower after sleep restriction compared with normal sleep.[109]

The Pituitary-Gonadal Axis

There is a paucity of studies examining the effect of sleep duration on sex steroids in women. The reader is referred to Chapter 155 for a review of sleep disturbances in menopause and in the polycystic ovary syndrome. Evidence implicating an adverse effect of insufficient sleep on the gonadal axis has been obtained for testosterone levels in men. One week of partial sleep restriction (5 hours in bed) in healthy young men resulted in a 10% to 15% decrease in afternoon and evening testosterone levels compared with a well-rested condition of 10 hours in bed.[110] This decrease in testosterone levels was noted to translate into an effect of 15 to 20 years of aging.[110] A similar trend was observed in a study of 5 nights of sleep restriction to 4 hours in bed.[104] In a study examining morning testosterone levels after 1 night of total sleep deprivation or after sleep restricted to the first 4.5 hours of the night, testosterone levels were also reduced by about 20%.[111] Lastly, a recent analysis of the National Health and Nutrition Examination Survey epidemiologic study including 2295 men 16 years of age and older (median age 46 years) examined testosterone levels in relation to self-reported sleep duration.[112] Multivariate regression analysis revealed testosterone levels decreased by 5.85 ng/dL/h of sleep loss ($P < .01$) while the effect of age was only 0.49 ng/dL/yr. Of note, this epidemiologic analysis is cross-sectional and therefore does not provide evidence for a causal relationship. Taken together, these findings suggest that obtaining an estimation of habitual sleep duration, as well as sleep duration during the night before testosterone testing may be important in the diagnosis of androgen deficiency. Because prescriptions for exogenous testosterone replacement for complaints of low energy, fatigue, and reduced libido in adult men have increased dramatically in since 2010, the possibility that partial sleep restriction, a condition that can produce these symptoms, may be involved in producing or exacerbating the condition should be considered.

Glucose Metabolism

In the study of severe sleep restriction (left panels of Figure 27.4), the difference in peak postbreakfast glucose levels between the sleep debt and fully rested conditions (i.e., ±15 mg/dL) is consistent with the development of impaired glucose tolerance.[100] Intravenous glucose tolerance testing which was performed in this study after the sixth night of 4-hour bedtimes confirmed the clinical significance of this deterioration in glucose tolerance.[100] Reduced glucose tolerance was found to be the combined consequence of a decrease in glucose effectiveness, a measure of non–insulin-dependent glucose use, and of a reduction in the acute insulin response to glucose despite decreased insulin sensitivity. The product of insulin sensitivity and acute insulin response to glucose, known as the Disposition Index, a validated marker of diabetes risk, was decreased by nearly 40% in the state of sleep debt, reaching levels typical of populations with an elevated diabetes risk.[113] Of note, the effect of recurrent sleep restriction was seen only in the responses to the meal and intravenous challenge, while fasting levels were unchanged. Glucose tolerance to the morning meal and to intravenous glucose was similarly reduced in the study of mild sleep restriction but to a lesser extent, consistent with a dose-response relationship.[21]

To date, there have been at least 15 well-controlled studies addressing the effects of sleep restriction on glucose metabolism.[21,100,103,104,114-124] All but two[115,122] observed a decrease in glucose tolerance in the state of sleep debt. In the laboratory studies, the duration of sleep restriction ranged from 2 to 14 nights, with 4 to 5.5 hours in bed. Figure 27.5 summarizes the findings of the 8 laboratory studies that used intravenous testing to assess insulin sensitivity, involving a total of 95 subjects. A reduction in insulin sensitivity was found in all 8 studies, ranging from 17.5% to 39%.[21,100,103,114,117,118,123,124] The largest reduction in insulin sensitivity (SI) was observed in a study in which testing in the sleep restricted condition was scheduled roughly 1 hour after wake-up time, at a time when melatonin levels were still elevated.[123] This morning circadian misalignment likely contributed to the robust decline in SI. Two studies have examined the effect of a reduction in sleep quality, rather than duration, on glucose metabolism using intravenous testing.[125,126] They both reported a decrease in SI (Figure 27.5).

A variety of mechanisms have been proposed to explain the development of insulin resistance in response to a sleep debt. In a randomized crossover study[127] comparing 4 days of 4.5 hours in bed versus 8.5 hours in bed, biopsies of subcutaneous abdominal fat were obtained from 7 participants at the end of each sleep condition. Adipocytes were exposed in vitro to incremental insulin concentrations to examine the ability of insulin to stimulate the phosphorylation of Akt, a crucial step in the insulin-signaling pathway. The insulin concentration needed to achieve the half-maximal phosphorylation of Akt response was nearly threefold higher when subjects had restricted sleep, indicating that sleep is an important modulator of insulin action in this peripheral tissue. This 2012 study[127] was the first to address molecular mechanisms involved in the reduction in systemic insulin sensitivity after recurrent sleep restriction. Using the same randomized crossover protocol, the authors went on to report that the reduction in total body insulin sensitivity was significantly associated with an increase in fasting FFAs.[21] Although this correlation does not

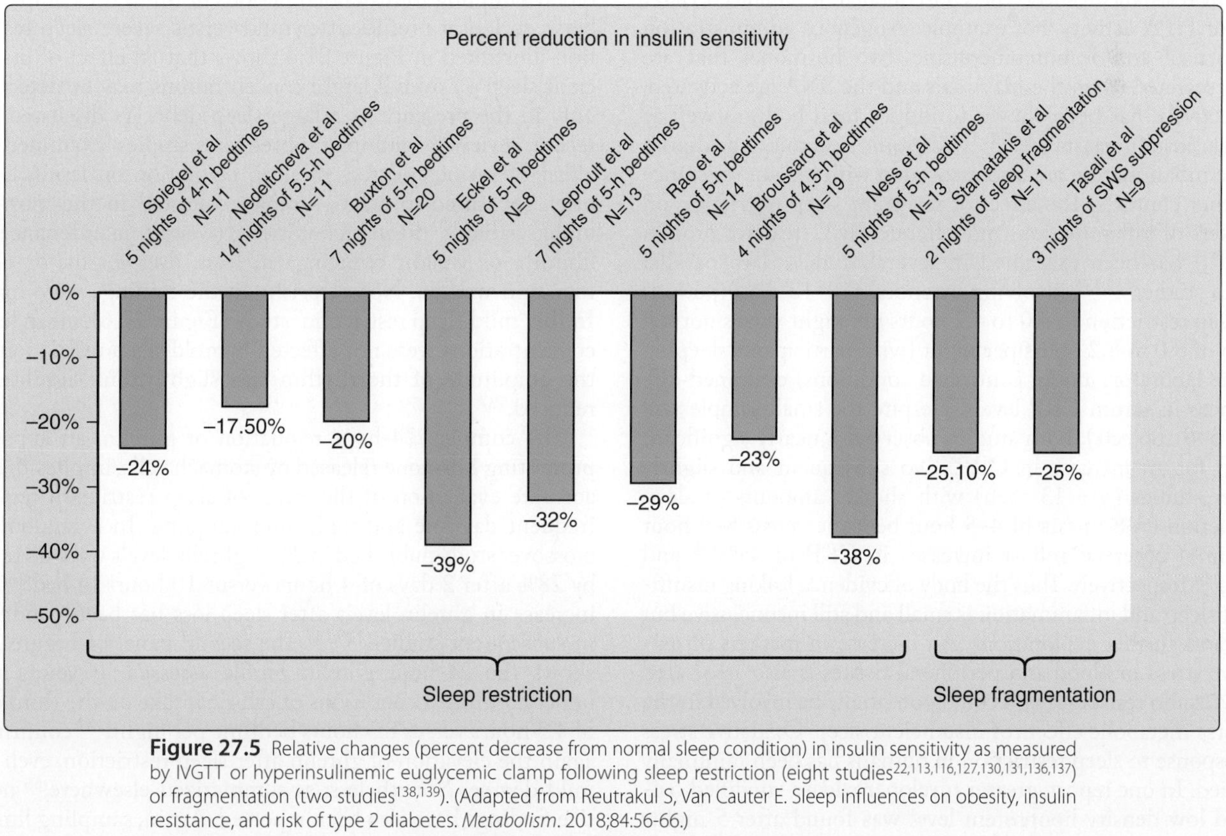

Figure 27.5 Relative changes (percent decrease from normal sleep condition) in insulin sensitivity as measured by IVGTT or hyperinsulinemic euglycemic clamp following sleep restriction (eight studies[22,113,116,127,130,131,136,137]) or fragmentation (two studies[138,139]). (Adapted from Reutrakul S, Van Cauter E. Sleep influences on obesity, insulin resistance, and risk of type 2 diabetes. *Metabolism*. 2018;84:56-66.)

demonstrate a direct causal link, acute elevations in circulating FFA concentrations have been associated with insulin resistance in healthy subjects in multiple previous studies.[128,129] Thus adipose tissue dysfunction after insufficient sleep may contribute to the decline in whole body insulin sensitivity via increased lipolysis and elevated FFAs in plasma. In 2015 a well-documented randomized crossover study[117] used the hyperinsulinemic euglycemic clamp method to make indirect assessments of muscle-specific insulin sensitivity and hepatic insulin sensitivity (measured by stable isotope techniques) in 14 participants who underwent 2 admissions each, one with 5 nights of bedtime restricted to 4 hours and one with 5 nights of normal 8-hour bedtimes. Muscle insulin sensitivity decreased by 29% after sleep restriction whereas hepatic insulin sensitivity (estimated as endogenous glucose production) did not change significantly, although gluconeogenesis increased.[117] An increase in nocturnal lipolysis in the sleep restriction condition was evidenced on the basis of a robust elevation of fasting FFA levels, similar to the observations of Broussard and colleagues.[21] The authors proposed that elevated FFA levels are partially responsible for the decrease in peripheral sensitivity and modulation of hepatic metabolism (i.e., increase in gluconeogenesis without increase in endogenous glucose production).[117] Hypothetically, the combined outputs of these three studies[21,117,127] suggest a tentative pathway linking the central alteration in sleep-wake homeostasis, to an alteration of the temporal organization of GH secretion, to elevated morning FFA concentrations, leading to reduced insulin sensitivity in adipose tissue and muscle. Increased activity of the hypothalamic-pituitary-adrenal (HPA) axis and of sympathetic nervous activity (SNA) both occur after insufficient sleep[100-104,118] and could also be involved in the reductions in whole body and cellular insulin sensitivity. Indeed, insulin resistance can be the consequence of enhanced SNA and/or HPA activity. For example, exogenous administration of cortisol and/or norepinephrine, two hormones that are hypersecreted when the HPA axis and the SNA are activated, respectively, has been shown to induce total body, as well as cellular insulin resistance.[130-132] Chronic systemic and adipose tissue inflammation are also associated with insulin resistance in other contexts. The effect of recurrent sleep restriction on markers of inflammation (most frequently C-reactive protein [CRP]) has been examined in several studies. Two parallel group studies[133,134] involving extended (10–12 days) periods of sleep restriction to 4.0 to 4.2 hours per night versus normal sleep of 8.0 to 8.2 hours per night (with participants sleeping in the laboratory under controlled conditions) examined differences in serum CRP levels. Despite the small sample size (n = 5–9 subjects), both studies observed a nearly significant trend for an increase in CRP. Two subsequent and slightly larger studies (n = 13 each) with shorter amounts of sleep restriction (5–8 nights of 4–5 hour bedtime versus 8–9 hour bedtime) observed robust increases in CRP of 45%[135] and 64%,[114] respectively. Thus the body of evidence linking insufficient sleep and inflammation is small and still inconclusive but warrants further explorations. An increase in markers of oxidative stress in blood and peripheral tissues is also associated with insulin resistance and could potentially be involved in the adverse metabolic effects of insufficient sleep. Oxidative stress in response to sleep restriction in humans has been minimally studied. In one report, greater myeloperoxidase-modified oxidized low density lipoprotein level was found after 5 nights of sleep restriction to 5 hours per night in healthy men.[136] Finally, additional mechanisms that may play a role in metabolic impairments include reduced brain glucose utilization and circadian misalignment. Both of these alterations have the potential to result in elevated blood glucose levels and consequent insulin resistance. In conclusion, there are undoubtedly multiple mechanisms acting in parallel or in synergy to impair glucose metabolism after sleep restriction.

Neuroendocrine Control of Appetite

Figure 27.6 illustrates the 24-hour profiles of five circulating signals that have been each implicated in the control of appetite and were assessed on the third day of sleep restricted to 4.5 versus 8.5 hours under well-controlled dietary intake and stable weight in nonobese adults.[80,85,137] This randomized crossover study is independent of the mild sleep restriction study illustrated in Figure 27.4 but followed a similar protocol. Leptin, a satiety signal originating from adipose tissue, was the first to be examined in the context of sleep curtailment. The first two studies linking insufficient sleep with a dysregulation of the satiety hormone leptin were published in 2003.[79,138] Both involved severe sleep restriction, the first by limiting bedtime to 4 hours for 7 consecutive days and the other by submitting the participants to 88 hours (i.e., >3 full days) of continuous wakefulness. Both indicated that leptin levels and amplitude of diurnal variation were reduced after sleep loss. These early findings were confirmed and extended in the severe sleep restriction study illustrated on the left side of Figure 27.4.[101] The reduction in mean leptin levels ranged between 20% and 30%, suggesting that sleep restriction may alter the ability of leptin to accurately signal energy balance. The finding was confirmed in a subsequent randomized crossover study[16] that also assessed leptin levels using frequent blood sampling for extended periods of time. The comparison between leptin profiles after mild versus severe sleep restriction illustrated in Figure 27.4 shows that an effect of insufficient sleep on overall leptin concentrations may be detectable only in the presence of a large sleep debt. As discussed in a recent review,[66] multiple subsequent studies examined the effect of various degrees of sleep restriction on leptin levels, often measured in a few samples collected in the morning, under variable dietary conditions (weight maintenance, ad libitum, or weight reducing) in lean, overweight, or obese men and women. Not surprisingly, the findings were mixed. In the "mild sleep restriction" study (Figure 27.6), mean leptin concentrations were not affected by mild sleep restriction but the amplitude of the rhythm was slightly, but significantly reduced.[137]

The complex 24-hour regulation of ghrelin, an appetite-promoting hormone released by stomach cells, implies that an accurate evaluation of the effect of sleep restriction requires frequent daytime and nighttime sampling. In a randomized crossover study published in 2004, ghrelin levels were increased by 28% after 2 days of 4 hours versus 10 hours in bed.[16] This increase in ghrelin levels after sleep loss has been confirmed in subsequent studies.[115,139] The second panel of Figure 27.6 shows the 24-hour ghrelin profile assessed in young men under controlled conditions of caloric intake on the third days of 4.5 hours versus 8.5 hours bedtime per night,[137] confirming again the elevation of ghrelin after sleep restriction, even to a mild degree. Nonetheless, as summarized elsewhere,[66] negative findings have also been reported. Again, sampling limited

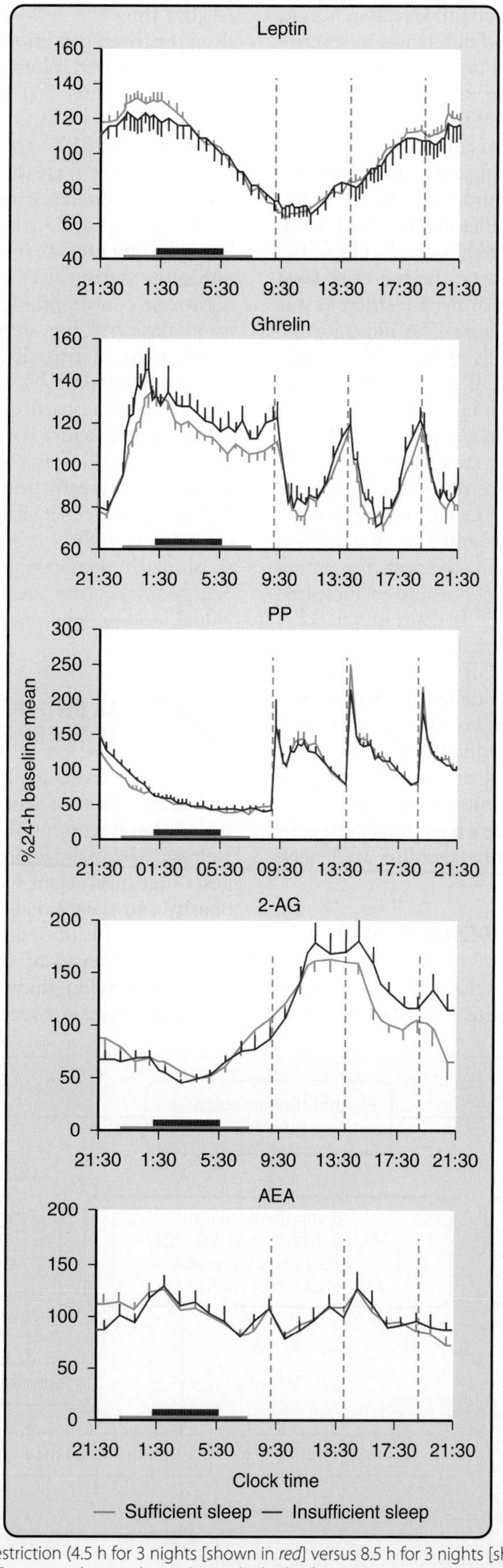

Figure 27.6 Impact of experimental sleep restriction (4.5 h for 3 nights [shown in *red*] versus 8.5 h for 3 nights [shown in *red*]) on the mean 24-hour profiles of blood levels of hormones regulating appetite. *From top to bottom:* leptin (satiety); ghrelin (hunger), pancreatic polypeptide (PP; satiety), and the endocannabinoids 2-arachidonylglycerol (2-AG) and AEA (hedonic drive for food). The data were obtained in a single laboratory study involving 14 young nonobese adults who received a weight-maintenance diet consisting of three identical carbohydrate meals. *Vertical lines* at each time point represent the standard error of the mean (SEM). *Vertical dotted lines* denote timing of meal intake. Note that in the case of leptin and 2-AG, an effect of sleep restriction would not have been detected if sampling had been limited to early morning hours. (Data sources[82,87,152]. The PP data have not been previously published.)

to the morning period, uncontrolled food intake, differences in demographics of study participants, and differences in severity of sleep restriction may all be involved in the discrepant findings. Given the mixed results regarding studies of the effect of sleep restriction on leptin and ghrelin, it is not surprising that two recent meta-analyses found no overall significant effects of sleep restriction on ghrelin or leptin, and noted high heterogeneity among studies.[65,140] The third panel from the top in Figure 27.6 shows the 24-hour profiles of PP in both sleep conditions. PP is a satiety factor secreted by the F cells of the pancreas that promotes satiety by slowing the transit of food through the gut. No significant effect of sleep restriction was detected. The two lower panels of Figure 27.6 illustrate the profiles of the two most studied ligands of the eCB receptor, 2-AG and AEA. Activation of the eCB receptor system has long been recognized as a powerful stimulant of appetite. The ligand 2-AG is the most abundant in peripheral blood and binds to the CB1 receptor, a target of antiobesity drugs. The profiles shown in Figure 27.6 demonstrate the existence of marked differences in regulation of 2-AG and AEA across the 24-hour span.[85,137] Sleep restriction resulted in an amplified 2-AG rhythm with a delayed and augmented peak, suggesting that an alteration in eCB tone may contribute to increased hedonic eating in a state of sleep debt.[137] In contrast, the AEA profile was not affected by sleep restriction, suggesting distinct regulatory pathways of the two eCBs and indicating that time of day needs to be controlled to delineate their relative roles.[85] GLP-1 and PYY are two gut hormones that inhibit appetite and have been rarely examined in subjects submitted to sleep restriction. After 4 days of 4-hour sleep, afternoon GLP-1 levels were lower in women but not in men,[115] suggesting that this pathway may promote overeating in response to insufficient sleep in women. Results regarding PYY have been inconsistent.[66]

Effect of Insufficient Sleep on Hunger and Food Intake

We identified 11 studies of sleep restriction for 2 days or more that assessed subjective hunger or appetite.[16,104,116,124,137,141-146] All but three[104,116,141] reported an increase in hunger in the sleep restricted condition compared with normal sleep. Eleven studies compared caloric intake during sleep restriction versus normal sleep and seven of them observed an increase in caloric intake in the state of sleep debt (listed in[66]). A meta-analysis published in 2019[65] concluded that sleep restriction results in a significant increase in subjective hunger on a 100-mm scale (mean difference = +13.4, $P < .001$) and in excess caloric intake averaging 253 kcal/day ($P = 0.011$). Several studies have documented that food consumption patterns become unhealthy during sleep restriction, including late evening or nighttime consumption,[147,148] more snacking,[17,147] and more fat intake.[148,149] In a study of healthy adults ($n = 19$) who each participated in two sleep restriction experiments (5 nights of 4-hour bedtime[150]), separated by at least 60 days, it was noted that male participants exhibited consistent changes in caloric intake across both exposures to sleep restriction (correlation of 0.69). Late-night (10:00 P.M. to 4:00 A.M.) food intake varied greatly from one participant to the other but was highly reproducible within participants across both exposures (correlation: 0.86) for both men and women. A recent analysis similarly demonstrated large interindividual variations in energy intake after sleep restriction and suggested that individual food preferences, often ignored, may play a role in this variability.[151]

BENEFICIAL ENDOCRINE AND METABOLIC EFFETCS OF SLEEP RECOVERY OR EXTENSION

The body of evidence regarding the adverse metabolic and endocrine effects of experimental sleep restriction reviewed in the section Recurrent Sleep Restriction: Impact on Endocrine Release, Metabolic Function, and Energy Intake strongly suggests that insufficient habitual sleep may increase the risk of obesity and type 2 diabetes. Figure 27.7 illustrates the pathways linking insufficient sleep with these two highly prevalent metabolic diseases of contemporary society. Epidemiologic evidence from longitudinal cohorts has consistently concluded that short sleep is associated with a significant risk of weight

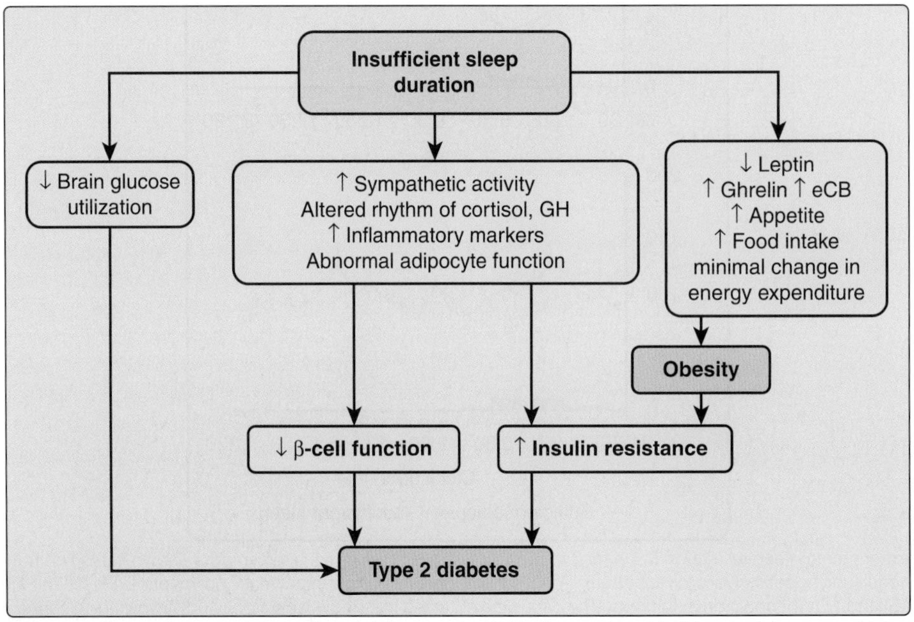

Figure 27.7 Pathways linking insufficient sleep to obesity risk and diabetes risk. eCB, Endocannabinoid; GH, growth hormone. (Adapted from Reutrakul S, Van Cauter, E. Sleep influences on obesity, insulin resistance, and risk of type 2 diabetes. *Metabolism*. 2018;84:56-66.)

gain and obesity, as well as of incident diabetes. Systematic reviews and meta-analyses published since 2010 have summarized the data.[152-157] The relative risk of developing obesity associated with insufficient sleep has been estimated at 1.45 (95% confidence interval [CI]: 1.25–1.67) in a 2014 study,[153] 1.38 (95% CI: 1.25–1.67) in a 2017 study,[156] with consistent findings in the most recent study.[157] For diabetes risk, the relative risk of incident diabetes associated with short sleep (5–≤6 hours) was first estimated in 2014 at 1.28 (95% CI: 1.03,1.60).[152] Another meta-analysis concluded that the lowest risk of incident diabetes was associated with a sleep duration of 7 to 8 hours, and increases by 9% per hour of sleep curtailment.[154] Comparing the risk of short sleep to traditional risk factors for diabetes[155] revealed that the relative risk for sleeping 5 hours or less was 1.48 (95% CI: 1.25,1.76) and for 6 hours was 1.18 (1.10,1.26), in the same range or greater than physical inactivity, a well-established risk factor.

The pathways illustrated in Figure 27.7 represent a simplification of the multiple physiologic mechanisms by which chronic sleep restriction, a behavior probably unique to the human among all mammalian species, affects metabolism. The take home message from this schematic representation is that it is unlikely that a pharmacologic approach targeting one of these pathways could prevent or even mitigate the effect of a chronic sleep debt. Therefore behavioral interventions to increase habitual sleep duration in individuals with chronic short sleep could provide a simple, low-cost approach to prevent metabolic dysfunction by promoting weight maintenance or facilitate weight loss, as well as by reducing the burden of insulin resistance on the beta cell and therefore the risk of diabetes. The extent and amount of recovery sleep required to reverse the metabolic consequences of insufficient sleep is an emerging area of investigation. A few short-term laboratory studies have examined a few days of bedtime extension after recurrent sleep restriction to determine whether metabolic deficits could be corrected. Even more challenging is the question of whether chronic insufficient sleep, which affects 30% to 45% of Americans today, is a behavior that can be modified to obtain beneficial effects not only on hormones and metabolism but also on other aspects of health and well-being.

The 1999 "sleep debt study"[100] allowed for the examination of subjective sleepiness, morning and afternoon cardiac sympathovagal balance (from analyses of heart rate variability), evening levels of free cortisol (from saliva samples), 24-hour plasma leptin profiles and morning glucose responses under three bedtime conditions: 8-hour (3 day), 4-hour (6 days), and 12-hour (6 days).[101] During the first night with a 12-hour bedtime, the subjects achieved a total sleep time slightly longer than 10 hours whereas by the sixth night, their total sleep time averaged 9 hours 43 minutes. Considering the data collected at the end of each condition, there was a dose-response relationship between total sleep time and each of the assessed variables, with optimal values at the end of sleep extension. This analysis showed not only that recovery was possible but also that the recommended 8-hour bedtimes represent a form of mild sleep restriction for young men. Real-life conditions rarely permit such a long extension of bedtimes for nearly 1 week. Eckel and colleagues[123] assessed both intravenous and oral insulin sensitivity in subjects who were sleep restricted to 5 hours for 5 days and then given a sleep opportunity of 9 hours for 5 days. Oral insulin sensitivity returned to baseline after 3 days with 9 hours in bed while intravenous insulin sensitivity did not, even after 5 days of 9 hours in bed. With respect to recovery sleep from a milder experimental sleep loss, a 2016 study[158] showed that 2 nights of recovery sleep (12-hour followed by 10-hour) after 4 nights of sleep restriction to 4.5 hours per night were sufficient to return insulin sensitivity to baseline levels. In contrast, a more recent study involving 3 baseline nights (10 hours in bed), followed by 5 nights of 5-hour bedtime and 2 recovery nights (10 hours in bed) showed that the reduction of insulin sensitivity in the state of sleep debt was not fully corrected after recovery sleep,[159] perhaps because the debt was larger and recovery sleep shorter than in the previous study. However, the response of nonesterified fatty acid to intravenous glucose injection and to ingestion of a high-fat dinner normalized after recovery sleep.[124,159] Lastly, results from a study of simulated weekend recovery sleep compared the impact of a 8-day period of sleep restriction to 5 hours per night to an 8-day period including 5 days with 5-hour bedtimes, followed by 2 days of ad libitum sleep simulating a weekend, followed by 1 more day of 5-hour bedtimes.[160] At the end of the two conditions, reductions in insulin sensitivity relative to baseline and postdinner increases in energy intake relative to baseline were similar. Thus extended bedtimes during the weekend may not prevent metabolic dysregulation associated with weeklong insufficient sleep. In sum, five studies of recovery sleep after short-term sleep restriction suggest that recovery is possible but unlikely under normal living conditions.

The potential benefits of sleep extension on glucose homeostasis in habitual short sleepers who chronically curtail bedtimes remain unclear. The first attempt involved 125 obese habitual short sleepers. Although the protocol was marred by a Hawthorne effect, spontaneous home sleep extension for a median duration of 81 days was associated with an improvement in insulin resistance and a reduction in the prevalence rates of abnormal fasting glucose and metabolic syndrome.[161,162] One more recent study examined the effects of home sleep extension on glucose metabolism in healthy volunteers (n = 16) who were chronic short sleepers during work days but could extend sleep time during nonworkdays, indicating that they did not suffer from insomnia.[163] After 6 weeks of sleep extension (average increase: 44 minutes/day), there was a robust correlation between the increase in actigraphy-based sleep duration and the improvement in fasting insulin sensitivity. In another study, 10 overweight young adults reporting habitual sleep duration 6.5 hours or less were studied in their home environments.[164] Habitual bedtimes for 1 week were followed by bedtimes extended to 8.5 hours for 2 weeks, resulting in an increase in sleep duration averaging 1.6 hours. Sleep extension was associated with a 14% decrease in overall appetite and a 62% decrease in desire for sweet and salty foods. Further, sleep extension to 10 hours per night for only 3 nights in healthy young men who regularly curtail their sleep to 6 hours during the week but "catch up" on sleep during the weekend was found to improve in oral glucose tolerance.[165] Lastly, a study of 19 Thai adults who reported sleeping 6 hours or less per night and were crossed over from 2 weeks of habitual sleep to 2 weeks of sleep extension was published in 2019.[166] Oral glucose tolerance testing was conducted at the end of each condition. Sleep duration by actigraphy during normal sleep conditions averaged 5 hours 19 minutes and the participants extended their sleep by only 36 minutes on average. Glucose tolerance was not ameliorated by sleep "extension" in these short sleepers. In the subset of participants who extended sleep to more than 6 hours (n = 8), insulin resistance decreased and insulin release increased. The study showed the challenges of sleep extension in chronic short sleepers but the results were encouraging when compliance was obtained. In sum, there is a small, but consistent, body of evidence suggestive of a beneficial role of optimizing habitual sleep duration to reduce the risk of obesity and diabetes in chronic short sleepers. Larger and longer studies are needed to extend and confirm the findings.

CLINICAL PEARL

Endocrine function and metabolism vary greatly across the 24-hour day. This is true for the vast majority of hormones and markers of metabolism. A large number of experimental and epidemiologic studies have demonstrated that insufficient sleep affects multiple pathways that lead to glucose intolerance and diabetes, as well as weight gain and obesity. Conversely, there is emerging evidence to indicate that sleep extension in habitual short sleepers is feasible and may have metabolically beneficial consequences. Clinicians should systematically obtain information about sleep duration, quality, and regularity when evaluating endocrine status and risk and severity of metabolic disease. Randomized clinical trials of interventions to prevent or treat obesity and/or diabetes should examine habitual sleep duration as potential modulators of the response.

SUMMARY

This chapter reviews the interactions between sleep and endocrine release in the hypothalamic-pituitary axes and the roles of sleep in carbohydrate metabolism, appetite regulation, bone metabolism, and hormonal control of body-fluid balance in healthy adults. Understanding the complexity of the endocrine system as a major signaling network has greatly increased since 2010. It has been recognized that most, if not all, endocrine cells are capable of circadian time-keeping and are influenced by the timing, duration, and quality of sleep. Yet the vast majority of clinical testing and research studies on hormones and metabolism continues to be scheduled at a single time of day and to ignore the sleep and circadian history of the subjects. Furthermore, despite the increased understanding of the ubiquitous role of sleep in endocrine and metabolic regulation, at least 30% of the US adult population reports sleeping less than 6 hours. Since the publication of the 6th edition of this volume, the scientific community has vigorously pursued studies that demonstrate the serious adverse hormonal and metabolic consequences of insufficient sleep. A major focus of this chapter is to summarize the findings and their implications. An exciting aspect of progress in recent years is the identification of beneficial health effects of sleep extension in habitual short sleepers.

SELECTED READINGS

Abdelmaksoud AA, Salah NY, Ali ZM, Rashed HR, Abido AY. Disturbed sleep quality and architecture in adolescents with type 1 diabetes mellitus: Relation to glycemic control, vascular complications and insulin sensitivity. *Diabetes Res Clin Pract*. 2021;174:108774.

Broussard JL, et al. Sleep restriction increases free fatty acids in healthy men. *Diabetologia*. 2015;58(4):791–798.

Chen P, Baylin A, Lee J, et al. The association between sleep duration and sleep timing and insulin resistance among adolescents in Mexico City. *J Adolesc Health*. 2021;69(1):57–63.

Depner CM, et al. Ad libitum weekend recovery sleep fails to prevent metabolic dysregulation during a repeating pattern of insufficient sleep and weekend recovery sleep. *Curr Biol*. 2019;29(6):957–967.e4.

Fritz J, Phillips AJK, Hunt LC, et al. Cross-sectional and prospective associations between sleep regularity and metabolic health in the Hispanic Community Health Study/Study of Latinos. *Sleep*. 2021;44(4):zsaa218.

Guyon A, et al. Effects of insufficient sleep on pituitary-adrenocortical response to crh stimulation in healthy men. *Sleep*. 2017;40(6).

Hanlon EC. Impact of circadian rhythmicity and sleep restriction on circulating endocannabinoid (eCB) N-arachidonoylethanolamine (anandamide). *Psychoneuroendocrinology*. 2020;111:104471.

Ikegami K, et al. Interconnection between circadian clocks and thyroid function. *Nat Rev Endocrinol*. 2019;15(10):590–600.

Itani O, et al. Short sleep duration and health outcomes: a systematic review, meta-analysis, and meta-regression. *Sleep Med*. 2017;32:246–256.

Kothari V, Cardona Z, Chirakalwasan N, Anothaisintawee T, Reutrakul S. Sleep interventions and glucose metabolism: systematic review and meta-analysis. *Sleep Med*. 2021;78:24–35.

Leproult R, et al. Beneficial impact of sleep extension on fasting insulin sensitivity in adults with habitual sleep restriction. *Sleep*. 2015;38(5):707–715.

Mokhlesi B, Temple KA, Tjaden AH, et al. The association of sleep disturbances with glycemia and obesity in youth at risk for or with recently diagnosed type 2 diabetes. *Pediatr Diabetes*. 2019;20(8):1056–1063.

Ness KM, et al. Two nights of recovery sleep restores the dynamic lipemic response, but not the reduction of insulin sensitivity, induced by five nights of sleep restriction. *Am J Physiol Regul Integr Comp Physiol*. 2019;316(6):R697–R703.

Patel P, et al. Impaired sleep is associated with low testosterone in US adult males: results from the National Health and Nutrition Examination Survey. *World J Urol*. 2019;37(7):1449–1453.

Reutrakul S, Van Cauter E. Sleep influences on obesity, insulin resistance, and risk of type 2 diabetes. *Metabolism*. 2018;84:56–66.

Spaeth AM, Dinges DF, Goel N. Phenotypic vulnerability of energy balance responses to sleep loss in healthy adults. *Sci Rep*. 2015;5:14920.

Swanson CM, et al. Bone turnover markers after sleep restriction and circadian disruption: a mechanism for sleep-related bone loss in humans. *J Clin Endocrinol Metab*. 2017;102(10):3722–3730.

A complete reference list can be found online at ExpertConsult.com.

Chapter 28

Thermoregulation in Sleep and Hibernation

Eus Van Someren; Tom Deboer

Chapter Highlights

- Despite the long-term awareness that thermoregulation and sleep are intimately coupled, there is still a lack of knowledge about the crucial mechanisms.
- This chapter describes normal sleep in humans in relation to circadian regulation of core body temperature. Based on this correlation, human and animal experimental intervention studies changing ambient temperature or sleep pressure are described to gain information about more causative mechanisms. Thermal interventions might play a role in treatment of insomnia.
- In addition to sleep, the torpid state in animals is described. Because this state is entered through normal sleep, it may be a valuable model to further investigate the relationship between thermoregulation and sleep.

The thermoregulatory system and the sleep regulatory system are both driven independently by two interacting physiologic principles, homeostasis and circadian regulation.[1] The chapter is divided into three main sections: (1) a brief introduction into the circadian regulation of core body temperature (CBT); (2) the interaction of sleep and thermoregulatory mechanisms; and (3) hibernation, a special condition displayed by a limited number of mammalian species.

Animals increase survival by residing in a safe sleeping site and have used sleep to maximize energy savings by reducing body and brain energy consumption and to conduct a variety of recuperative processes.[2,3] Knowledge about thermophysiology and its relation to sleep leads to the hope that temperature-related interventions can alleviate sleep disturbances and be helpful to cure certain aspects of sleep and alertness problems in the general population. Although a great deal is known about the variability in rest and sleep states and thermophysiology across the animal kingdom,[2,3] to limit the scope of this chapter, we focus on findings from humans and rodents.

CIRCADIAN REGULATION OF CORE BODY TEMPERATURE

More than 50 years ago, Aschoff[4] showed that the human body consists of two thermophysiologic compartments: the heat-producing, homeothermic core and the heat-loss-regulating, poikilothermic shell. The size of the latter is largely dependent on environmental temperature. In a warm environment, the shell is small; in a cool environment, it is large and thus acts as a buffer to protect the core from dangerous cooling. All peripheral tissues, such as fat, the skin, and in particular the skeletal muscles of the legs and arms, can contribute substantially to the size of the shell, provided that peripheral blood flow is low. Therefore rates of blood flow through muscles and skin are the main determinants of shell size variability and hence of peripheral insulation. The distal skin regions, in particular fingers and toes, are the main thermoeffectors to lose core body heat because they possess the physical and physiologic properties to best serve the function of heat loss. They have ideal surface shapes (round, small radius) for good heat transfer to the environment; the surface-to-volume coefficient increases from proximal to distal skin sites. The distal skin temperatures therefore provide a good measure of the shell size.

CBT comprises the temperature of the brain and the abdominal cavity, including inner organs (e.g., liver, heart, kidney).[4] The average core temperature of mammals is about 38° C; examples of the lower and upper side are 36.5° C for elephants and about 39.7° C for goats. Behavioral and physiologic processes keep CBT within a narrow range across a broad environmental temperature range. A detailed description of the thermoregulatory system can be found elsewhere.[5]

CBT is regulated by independent thermoeffector loops, each with their own afferents and efferents.[6] Coordination between the loops is achieved through their common controlled variable, CBT, for which the thermoeffector thresholds are subject to circadian modulation.[7] Circadian rhythms in mammals are generated by the self-sustaining central pacemaker localized in the suprachiasmatic nuclei (SCN) of the hypothalamus. Postmortem studies confirmed that also in humans the temperature rhythm critically involves the SCN.[8] Even an immature SCN, as is found in premature neonates, often already shows the capacity to generate an endogenous temperature rhythm.[9] Diurnal temperature (and other) rhythms are usually entrained to the 24-hour solar day, mainly by the synchronizer light.[10] The SCN is also involved in the immediate effects of light on body temperature.[11]

A rostral projection from the SCN to the preoptic anterior hypothalamus (POAH) conveys the circadian signal to the thermoregulatory system.[10] The regulation of CBT results from the concerted action of homeostatic and circadian processes. In humans, the daily decline of CBT in the evening results from a regulated decline in the thermoregulatory thresholds of heat production and heat loss; the inverse happens in the morning. When heat production surpasses heat loss, body heat content increases, and vice versa.

Depending on environmental temperature, about 70% to 90% of body heat content is located in the body core. Therefore changes in CBT reflect to a great extent changes in body heat content. Heat production and heat loss change with activities such as muscular exertion and fluid and food intake. Such activities commonly occur at specific phases of the circadian cycle and can therefore contribute to the measured temperature cycle.[11] The constant routine (CR) protocol was developed to study the temperature rhythm in humans under artificial conditions that minimize certain phase-specific contributions.[12] With this protocol it was shown that the time course of heat production precedes heat loss and that CBT varies as an intermediate resultant.[12] Heat production and heat loss are separated not only in time but also in space in the body.[4] Under resting conditions, about 70% of heat production depends on the metabolic activity of inner organs, whereas body heat loss is initiated by heat redistribution from the core to the shell through blood flow to the distal skin regions.[4] Thermoregulatory distal skin blood flow is regulated by the autonomic nervous system by constriction or dilation of arteriovenous anastomoses. These are shunts between arterioles and venules exclusively found in nonhairy distal skin regions such as the toes and fingers.[4] When they are open, warm blood flows rapidly and directly from arterioles to the dermal venous plexus, enabling an efficient heat exchange from the core to the distal skin. The distal-proximal skin temperature gradient (DPG) therefore provides a selective measure of distal skin blood flow and hence body heat loss through the extremities.[4] Sympathetic nerve activity seems to be crucial for peripheral vasoconstriction, but the exact neural process by which this regulation is achieved is still a matter of debate.[13]

Under the artificial CR conditions that minimize certain phase-specific behavioral and physiologic contributions to temperature, the time course of distal skin temperatures (hands and feet) exhibits an inverse circadian rhythm in comparison with CBT, with a phase advance of about 100 minutes[12] (i.e., in the evening, distal skin temperatures rise before CBT declines).[12] The amplitude of these distal skin temperature rhythms is about three times larger than that of CBT.[12,14] In contrast, temperatures of proximal skin regions (e.g., thigh, infraclavicular region, stomach, forehead) change in parallel with CBT, and the amplitudes are of similar magnitude.[12,14] Curves obtained during CR protocols have been suggested to represent the "true unmasked" circadian rhythm. However, the curves and their phase relationships have been studied in one specific type of artificial CR only: where people are kept supine and inactive continuously. It may well be that the findings do not generalize to artificial CR conditions where people are kept active, sitting, or standing continuously. CR may also solve some issues while introducing other ones by trying to study a complex system after blocking part of the processes that are normally connected. Findings should be interpreted with caution because the approach may result in finding opposite conditioned compensatory responses that emerge in the absence of a normally connected process. Another example of possible profound problems due to the disruption of otherwise connected processes is the massive alteration in gene expression profiles after enforced sleeping and/or waking at the wrong time of day,[15] as is common in both CR and ultrashort sleep-wake rhythm paradigms.

Nocturnal secretion of the pineal hormone melatonin, which is under control of the SCN, plays a crucial role in the evening decrease in CBT.[16] Administration of melatonin in the afternoon, when endogenous melatonin levels are low, provokes exactly the same thermophysiologic effects as observed naturally in the evening.[16] Whether melatonin induces distal vasodilation in humans by acting directly on blood vessel receptors, indirectly through modulation of sympathetic nerve activity, or both, remains to be determined.[16] In addition, both subjective ratings of sleepiness and the level of activity in the electroencephalogram (EEG) theta and alpha rhythms as an objective outcome of the sleep-wake state are increased.[16] Moreover, it is noteworthy that rise in melatonin secretion in the evening belongs to a well-orchestrated circadian physiologic regulation controlled by the SCN, simultaneously lowering CBT, increasing sleepiness, and facilitating sleep onset.

COVARIATION OF SLEEP AND THERMOPHYSIOLOGIC VARIABLES

In the following subsections, two lines of evidence are presented to clarify the relationship between sleep and thermoregulatory systems: at baseline thermal comfort condition and under various different conditions, such as circadian, temperature, and sleep pressure changes. Furthermore, research has provided insights into the relationship between thermoregulation and sleep on the basis of neuroanatomic studies showing significant interaction of the two systems.

Body Temperature around Sleep Onset

The overt diurnal profiles of body temperatures reflect a complex system of circadian thermoregulatory changes and behaviors, including sleep, posture, activity, food intake, and light exposure. A change from standing to supine body position induces a redistribution of blood, together with heat, from the core to the periphery, thereby increasing skin temperatures, decreasing CBT, and increasing sleepiness.[17] The postural change resulting from the behavior of lying down thus significantly contributes to the observed CBT decline from before, to after, sleep onset. The temporal relationship among thermophysiologic variables, heart rate, subjective ratings of sleepiness, and salivary melatonin secretion around habitual bedtime and for the following sleep episode under CR conditions is summarized in Figure 28.1. The only thing that changed during this protocol was that the low-intensity lights (<10 lux) were switched off at time = 0 with the implicit permission to fall asleep. Before lights off, the previously described endogenous pattern of CBT downregulation is already visible. In the evening, heart rate (an indirect measure of intrasubject variation of heat production) declines first, followed by heat loss and finally by a decrease in CBT. Subjective ratings of sleepiness increase in parallel with DPG and salivary melatonin levels. The proximal skin temperature exhibits a similar pattern as CBT, but only during the artificial CR condition of enforced

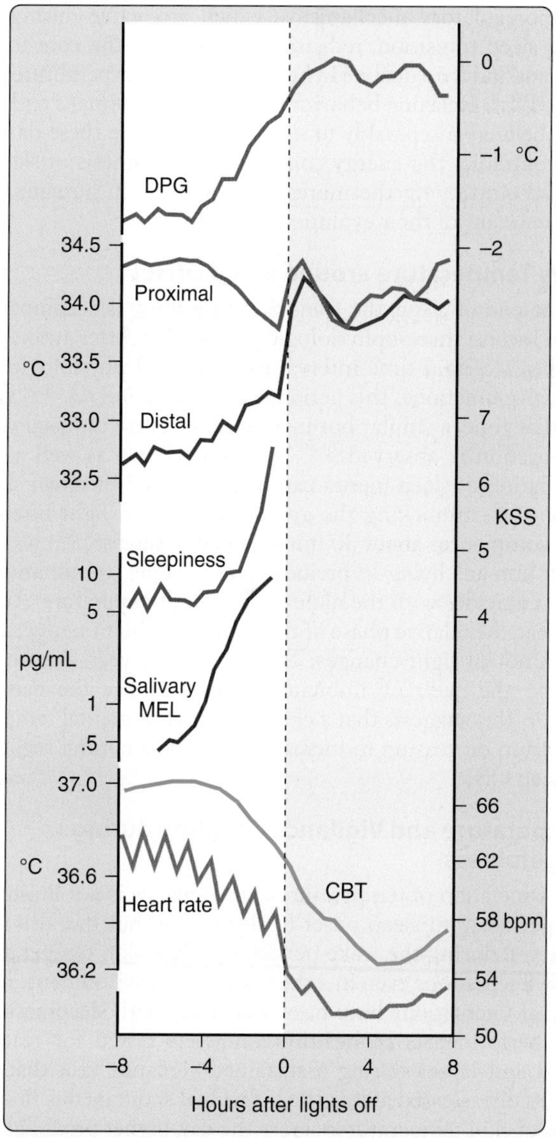

Figure 28.1 Time course of heart rate and core body temperature (CBT) (see lower traces) and changes in salivary melatonin concentration, sleepiness ratings, distal and proximal skin temperatures, and the distal-proximal skin temperature gradient (DPG) in a baseline 7.5-hour constant routine followed by a 7.5-hour sleep period, *yellow area*. Continuously measured data are plotted in 30-minute bins. Mean values of *n* = 18 male subjects. Subjective ratings of sleepiness: KSS, Karolinska sleepiness scale; MEL, melatonin; heart rate, bpm. *Note:* Distal and proximal skin temperatures exhibit inverse time course before lights off but are nearly indistinguishable approximately 1 hour later. Heart rate reflects the study protocol rhythm of one hourly food and water intake before lights off and declined sharply thereafter. Mean sleep-onset latency: 12 ± 4 minutes. (Modified from Kräuchi K, Cajochen C, Werth E, Wirz-Justice A. Functional link between distal vasodilation and sleep-onset latency? *Am J Physiol Regul Integr Comp Physiol.* 2000;278:R741–8.)

inactivity and a supine posture. In strong contrast, in everyday life the proximal skin temperature is in fact one or even more degrees higher during the sleep period than it is during wakefulness.[18-20] Immediately after lights off and before sleep stage 2, the distal and proximal skin temperature increase and heart rate declines.[21] In addition, an increase in sweating is often observed, depending on CBT.[22]

The typical increase in distal skin temperature, as shown in Figure 28.1, is caused by redistribution of heat from the core to the shell. Similar findings at sleep onset have been described in the lower legs.[23] CBT also exhibited a slight but significant acceleration in the decrease rate after lights off,[4,24] leading to approximately 0.3°C lower CBT values during sleep compared with quiet wakefulness.[25] In contrast to the fast changes in skin temperature, the decline in CBT is slow, which can be explained by a reduction in cardiac output during sleep initiation, impeding a faster heat loss during the sleep episode under thermoneutral conditions.[21] The magnitude of the decrease in CBT is negatively correlated with environmental temperature.[26] A DPG of 0°C indicates that during sleep the thermoregulatory shell has disappeared, resembling a state similar to that of the human body in the awake state in a warm environment (e.g., 35°C).[4] Heat redistribution from the core to the shell is completed within approximately 1 hour after lights off. Such a completely relaxed one-compartment body, when thermophysiologic core and shell are fused, is prone to fast cooling when sleep occurs in a cool environment. Under normal conditions, CBT is protected because humans and animals try to occupy a sleep berth in a comfortable thermal environment.[27] When humans initiate sleep outside the natural temporal niche, for instance, by taking an afternoon nap, similar thermophysiologic changes occur right after lights off and before the initiation of sleep stage 2.[28] There are subjects, a majority of whom are women, who are prone to cold hands and feet and therefore to having a large shell.[29,30] These subjects show alteration in some of the macrostructure variables of sleep such as a significant prolonged sleep-onset latency to stage 2 (SOL2).[29,30] In fact, it has been shown that subjects with sleep-onset insomnia respond well to a mild heating with reduced thermoregulatory heat loss from their fingers.[31] Within this context, it has been shown that wrist skin temperature best predicts thermal sensation, especially in women, and therefore seems useful as a physiologic parameter to determine thermoregulatory behavior,[32] such as using thermophysiologic remedies (e.g., bed socks).[23]

Body Temperature during Sleep

In humans, the temperature minimum normally occurs between 04:00 and 06:00 a.m.[33] Studies carried out to describe changes in thermophysiologic variables show that changes in CBT and proximal and distal skin temperature related to the non–rapid eye movement (NREM)–rapid eye movement (REM) sleep cycle are very small.[34,35] Heart rate is clearly increased shortly before and during REM sleep relative to NREM sleep, which is, however, reflected only in a minor, if any, increase in energy expenditure during REM sleep relative to slow wave sleep (SWS), but not relative to stage 1 or 2 sleep.[36-39] Extensive studies on thermophysiologic alterations regarding the NREM/REM sleep cycle concluded that changes in brain heat production are practically not relevant for changes in brain temperature.[40] To our knowledge, only one human study recorded brain temperature together with sleep EEG data, but no significant systematic changes regarding the NREM/REM sleep cycle were found.[41]

One of the advantages of animal research is the parallel recording of body and brain temperature together with sleep-wake and EEG recordings. In small mammals (rabbit, rat, Djungarian hamster), NREM sleep is associated with a decrease in brain temperature, whereas REM sleep and waking are associated with an increase[42,43] (Figure 28.2).

In an elegant study performed in the rat, it was shown that heat is redistributed across the body when vigilance states

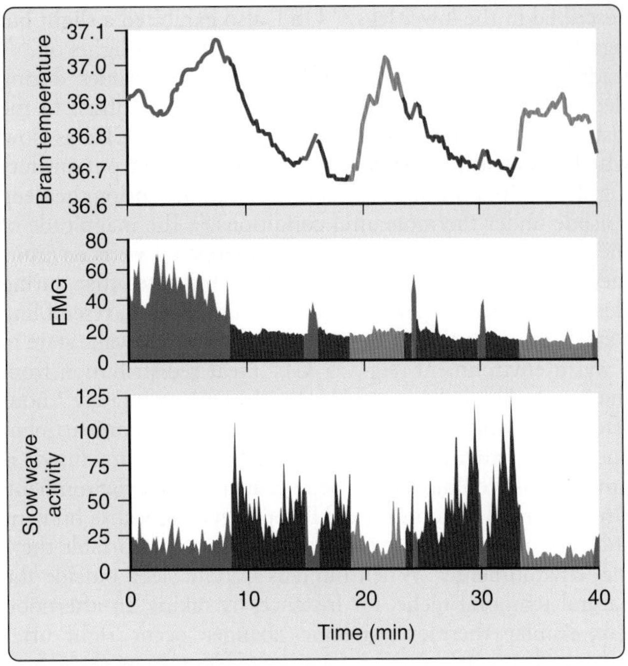

Figure 28.2 A 40-minute record of brain temperature measured at the parietal cortex, integrated electromyogram (EMG) activity from the neck muscles, and electroencephalogram (EEG) slow wave activity (SWA; mean EEG power density between 0.75 and 4.0 Hz) of a Djungarian hamster (*Phodopus sungorus*). *Blue*, Waking; *red*, NREM sleep; *green*, REM sleep. Values are plotted for 8-second epochs. Note the decrease of brain temperature at the entrance into NREM sleep and the increase during REM sleep and waking.

change.[44] At the initiation of NREM sleep, the brain and intraperitoneal temperature decrease, whereas the tail skin temperature increase. The opposite occurs at the transition from NREM sleep to wake. At transitions from NREM to REM sleep, brain temperature rises slightly, whereas intraperitoneal and tail temperature do not change. These data are in accordance with those obtained in humans. Heat is redistributed from the core to the shell at the onset of sleep. Humans thermoregulate by vasodilation and vasoconstriction of blood vessels within the skin of extremities; in rats similar changes are observed in the tail. The main difference lies in the timing of the redistribution of heat relative to the onset of sleep and waking. In humans, changes are visible several hours before sleep onset; in the rat the same changes occur at the immediate onset of sleep. This difference is probably related to the smaller body size and to the shorter and repetitive ultradian sleep-wake pattern in the rat, which renders a time lag of several hours to be nonfunctional.

Applying a CR in rodents is not possible. However, on the basis of the relationship between brain temperature and vigilance states, it was possible to subtract the influence of vigilance state changes on brain temperature, rendering a mathematic CR.[45] This study concluded that, in the rat, about 90% of the variance in brain temperature is caused by changes in vigilance. The vigilance state–related changes in brain temperature are independent of the functioning of the circadian clock because they remained intact after removing the SCN.[46]

Taken together, there are robust thermoregulatory effects induced by lying down and the preparatory relaxing sleep behavior; however, the NREM/REM sleep cycle seems to have minor thermoregulatory associations in humans. The thermoregulatory mechanisms, which are active during the wake-sleep transition, redistribute heat from the core to the shell and induce a decline in heart rate, energy expenditure,[36,47] and CBT.[35] Relaxing behavior before sleep in humans and animals belongs inseparably to sleep, and therefore these data do not contradict the energy conservation hypothesis of sleep.[48] The accompanying thermoregulatory effects in humans may be a remnant of their evolutionary past.[48]

Body Temperature around Sleep Offset

At the end of sleep, the transition to waking is accompanied by an inverse thermophysiologic pattern.[28,49] After awakening it takes a certain time interval to recover all physiologic and cognitive functions. This period is called *sleep inertia*.[28,49] During that time, a similar but inverse time course in distal vasoconstriction is observed.[28,49] This time course as well as the dissipation of sleep inertia can be accelerated by dawn simulation (i.e., mimicking the gradual increase in light intensity that commences about 30 minutes before sunrise).[50]

In humans living in preindustrial societies, termination of sleep coincides with the nadir of ambient temperature. Across the year, the relative phase of the nadir of ambient temperature and ambient light changes. Throughout the year, sleep offset follows the nadir of ambient temperature, not the nadir of light.[51] This suggests that a change in environmental temperature from decreasing to increasing may be a natural regulator of sleep offset.

Temperature and Vigilance Coupling during Wakefulness

The association of temperature with vigilance is not limited to the period from sleep onset to sleep offset but has also been observed during the wake period. Daytime skin temperatures show fluctuations even in a thermoneutral environment. These normal fluctuations have been associated with sleepiness and task performance. In healthy volunteers tested for reaction speed and lapses during a sustained vigilance task that was repeatedly assessed across the individual spontaneous fluctuations of skin temperatures across the day, higher proximal skin temperature in particular was associated with slower responses and more lapses.[52] In patients with narcolepsy, again particularly higher proximal temperature was associated with a faster sleep onset.[53] Although CBT does not show the relatively fast fluctuations that can be observed in skin temperature, people perform best around the peak plateau of the 24-hour CBT and fall asleep easiest while their CBT declines.[54,55]

Indirect Correlated Temperature and Sleep Manipulation Studies

Indirect manipulation studies showed that similar thermophysiologic effects seen during sleep initiation can be observed after administration of benzodiazepines, without falling asleep.[50] This is also the case with relaxation techniques such as yoga, autosuggestion of warmth, autogenic training, and meditation.[4,56-58] These techniques induce a reduction in muscular and cutaneous sympathetic nerve activity, which leads to increased distal skin temperature and to a reduction in heart rate, energy expenditure, and CBT.[56,57] After caffeine administration inverse effects were induced with elevated CBT, distal vasoconstriction, disturbed daytime recovery sleep, and prolonged sleep-onset latency after night sleep deprivation.[59] Therefore distal vasodilation followed by a drop in CBT appears to be a thermophysiologic event, which is primarily related to relaxation occurring before sleep onset,[60] and the opposite is true for vasoconstriction. Direct manipulation studies, altering core or skin temperature to evaluate effects on vigilance, are described later in this chapter.

Changed Circadian Conditions

It has been observed that subjects living under normal conditions choose their bedtime (lights off) at the maximal rate of decrease in their CBT rhythm.[61] However, when subjects are living on self-selected sleep-wake schedules in a time-free environment, bedtime is phase-delayed close to the CBT minimum, which is an indication that the sleep-wake cycle and the circadian rhythm of CBT are separate but usually entrained (synchronized) oscillatory systems.[62] Unfortunately, neither direct nor indirect measurements of heat loss and heat production were carried out in parallel in these time-free environment studies. Therefore it is possible that CBT is not the crucial variable for sleep induction, but rather one of its determinants (i.e., heat loss). The duration of sleep episodes was maximum when initiated at the time when CBT reached its maximum, and at the opposite, minimal sleep lengths occurred when sleep was initiated during the rising phase of the CBT rhythm.[63] Because heat loss seems to be closely linked to sleep initiation, it may be speculated that the circadian rhythm of heat loss is phase-delayed under free-run conditions.

Under most experimental conditions, REM sleep propensity exhibits a strong circadian pattern with a peak about 1 to 2 hours after the circadian minimum of CBT.[35,63] There is also a reproducible and robust circadian rhythm in SOL2, which is closely related to the circadian CBT rhythm and thermoregulatory effects described previously.[33] In forced desynchrony studies (i.e., living on a scheduled 28-hour day, including a 9.3-/18.7-hour sleep-wake cycle), it was shown that SOL2 is longest at the circadian phase where CBT reaches its maximum, that is, 1.5 hours before CBT starts to decline and melatonin secretion rises.[63] At this circadian phase, named the *wake-maintenance zone*,[64] inner heat conduction is lowest as indicated by the largest difference between CBT and distal skin temperature and the largest negative DPG values. Thereafter, SOL2 declines rapidly and is minimal around the time when CBT reaches its circadian trough, when inner heat conduction is largest (distal skin temperature is highest and the difference between CBT and distal skin temperature is lowest). However, it remains to be determined whether thermal interventions, for instance, lower leg warming, at the wake-maintenance zone will be successful in reducing SOL2, as was shown for melatonin administration.[65]

Taken together, self-selected sleep timing, SOL2, REM sleep latency, REM sleep propensity, and sleep duration are closely associated with CBT. Even though these variables are not fully in phase with CBT, it is possible that one of the determinants of CBT (e.g., heat production, heat loss) is directly interrelated with sleep. It still remains to be established whether these rhythms are independently governed by the SCN or causally linked directly to measured thermophysiologic outcomes. These correlative findings lead to the question, how is sleep affected by thermoregulatory challenges?

INTERVENTION STUDIES IN HUMANS

Direct Temperature Manipulation Effect on Sleep in Humans

Direct temperature manipulation studies have evaluated whether changes in core and skin temperature are merely correlated to features of sleep and alertness or rather causally involved. Several studies applied heat loads and observed how altered CBT correlated with changes in vigilance. Other studies hypothesized that imposed skin temperature changes within the comfortable range may have causal effects, supposedly mediated by projections of cutaneous thermoreceptors to brain structures involved in the regulation of sleep and arousal.[66]

Thermal interventions, applied either passively or actively by physical exercise, can induce significant changes in skin temperatures and CBT,[35,47,63,67,68] while some dedicated interventions managed to alter more specifically proximal or distal skin temperature without affecting CBT.[69-72] The intensity of a thermal intervention is crucial, as are the skin region selected and the time of application. During sleep only passive thermal loads can be applied. It has been shown that sleep reduces the thresholds and gains of the autonomic temperature defense mechanisms and expands the interthreshold zone (the temperature range for activation of metabolic heat production or evaporative heat loss).[63,69,73] These threshold changes are modest in SWS but much stronger in REM sleep (Box 28.1).[63,68] As a consequence, CBT and skin temperatures

BOX 28.1 DOES THERMOREGULATION STOP DURING REM SLEEP?

There are several lines of evidence supporting the notion that thermoregulation is limited or absent during REM sleep.

- Warming the environment within the thermoneutral zone (from the low end to the high end) can increase REM sleep duration by twofold,[158,159] which suggests that REM sleep mainly occurs when thermoregulatory corrections are minimally needed.
- Within the thermoneutral zone, thermoregulatory sweating is absent during REM sleep,[160–162] and above the thermoneutral zone, the threshold for sweating is largely increased during REM sleep.[163] Below the lower end of the thermoneutral zone, or when hypothalamic brain temperature is artificially lowered, thermoregulatory responses are virtually absent during REM sleep.[164] During REM sleep, thermoregulation is inhibited and body temperature depends on ambient temperature; therefore, REM sleep has even been referred to as a poikilothermic state.[165]
- The modulation of these thermoregulatory responses by the vigilance states was also observed at the level of the preoptic-anterior hypothalamus. The number of thermosensitive neurons as well as the thermosensitivity of the individual neurons is reduced during NREM sleep compared with waking, and most neurons become insensitive to temperature changes during REM sleep.[166,167]
- Research with melanin-concentrating hormone (MCH) receptor knockouts and optogenetic stimulation of MCH neurons suggests that the MCH system plays a role in the dynamics of changes in REM sleep under influence of changing ambient temperatures.[168] However, the concomitant loss of thermoregulatory control is still poorly understood.

are more sensitive to changes in environmental temperature during sleep. Maximal total sleep time (TST) is found in the thermoneutral zone (the range of ambient temperature at which temperature regulation is achieved solely by vasomotor responses), and REM sleep was shown to be more vulnerable to thermal interventions than SWS.[63,68] Too-intense thermal interventions induce arousals and awakenings, which in turn can induce thermophysiologic effects, such as elevating CBT.[68] When a thermal load is applied repeatedly, the thermoregulatory system can adapt and the effects on sleep are changed; for example, the arousing effects of cold or warmth are reduced. Indigenous Australians in the Central Australian desert and nomadic Sami people in Arctic Finland were experiencing comparable degrees of cold exposure during the night, and both showed lower thermoregulatory thresholds for shivering before modern ambient thermoregulatory technology arrived.[74,75] As a consequence, in these subjects CBT was more reduced during sleep, and undisturbed sleep occurred at a lower environmental temperature. Among limitations in actual knowledge is the fact that too many modalities of thermal interventions on sleep are understudied and, in addition, the effect of thermal interventions on sleep may differ between normal and sleep-disturbed subjects.

Changing Ambient Temperature

Ambient temperature, especially in combination with high humidity, is important for both the quantity and quality of sleep.[68] When sleep occurs in a warm environmental temperature (31 to 38° C), duration of wakefulness increases and duration of both REM and NREM sleep decreases.[47,63,67,68] Also, cold exposure (21° C) induces more awakenings, less time in sleep stage 2, and less TST but does not affect the duration of the other sleep stages. Marked thermoregulatory effects were induced under such manipulations.[47] The decrease in CBT observed during the night episode was larger at 21° C compared with the thermoneutral 29° C condition. With cold exposure, forehead temperature and oxygen consumption during REM sleep increased, and feet temperature decreased, compared with SWS. Therefore cold-exposed humans may not exhibit a complete inhibition of thermoregulation during REM sleep as has been observed in small mammals (Box 28.1).

When ambient temperature was gradually decreased during sleep, an earlier CBT nadir and an advanced peak for REM sleep propensity were obtained.[76] Duration of deep sleep stages increased when the normal nocturnal decrease of CBT was augmented by a constant and mild reduction in ambient temperature, despite decreased sleep efficiency.[76] Similarly, after a 2° C reduction in ambient temperature during sleep, it was observed that the increase in SWS occurred simultaneously with the rise in slow wave activity (SWA; EEG power density approximately 1 to 4 Hz) without any change in sleep efficiency or reduced amount of REM sleep.[77] The thermal manipulation reduced not only leg skin temperature but also CBT and heart rate. Taken together, the augmentation of heat loss leading to reduced CBT during sleep seems to be the crucial variable for increased SWS. This knowledge is now applied in experiments using high heat capacity mattresses to gradually cool the subjects and possibly make them sleep more deeply.[78,79]

Changing Body Heat Content before Sleep

In humans, body heat content and hence CBT can also be effectively manipulated by body immersion in warm or cold baths. For instance, as a result of rapid conductive heat loss in a cold bath, CBT decreases faster compared with the drop observed in air at the same temperature. Rewarming of the cool shell after cool bathing leads to a characteristic after-drop in CBT.[80] Several studies showed effects of positive heat load on sleep,[47,67,68] but no study examined effects on sleep after a cold bath. In general, passive body heating (40 to 43° C for 30 to 90 minutes with a CBT increase of 1.4 to 2.6° C) has a positive effect on many aspects of sleep in healthy young adults and in older and sleep-disturbed subjects. It was found that warm bathing in the evening shortened sleep-onset latency, enhanced SWS duration, and sometimes reduced REM sleep duration. The increase in SWS, however, is not dependent on a reduction in REM sleep. At present, it cannot be determined which thermophysiologic correlate represents the causal factor to increase SWS and reduce sleep latency. Nevertheless, heat load before sleep seems to increase the duration of SWS. Bathing performed in the morning or early afternoon had no effect on sleep architecture.[47,67] In principle, actual levels of CBT at sleep onset or the decline in CBT afterward could be related to the amount of SWS after warm bathing.[47,67] Additionally, hot bathing during the evening resulted in a later CBT minimum. The delay correlated with the concomitant increase in SWS.[81] All these CBT characteristics could be correlated because directly after a positive heat load the velocity of CBT decline is larger, the CBT level is elevated before sleep onset, and the overt CBT nadir during sleep may be delayed. However, phase shifting effects of passive heat loads in humans have not been studied systematically. Variables other than CBT, such as skin temperature, may play a role. The available findings are inconsistent because of the diversity in study designs and methodology and the low statistical power of many studies. In a study in which hot full-body and hot foot bathing were performed 35 minutes before lights off,[82] CBT increased by about 1° C only during full-body bathing. Both conditions, however, increased mean skin temperatures and reduced sleep-onset latency and movement during subsequent sleep. These findings indicate that elevated skin temperature, not change in CBT, is crucial for a rapid onset of sleep, which is supported by specific skin temperature manipulations as will be discussed later.[71,83]

Older sleep-disturbed subjects responded to hot foot bathing with slightly reduced sleep-onset latency to stage 1 (SOL1) and significantly decreased wakefulness in the second NREM sleep period.[84] In these older subjects not only DPG but also CBT were elevated after hot foot bathing during the first hour of sleep. However, the same authors reported later that warming the feet may improve sleep only for those who have cold feet.[85]

Intense exercise is a manipulation that can also raise CBT. Subsequently, CBT declines as a result of the thermoregulatory heat loss drive through increased vasodilation and sweating. A number of reproducible changes on sleep have been identified after exercise in the evening: shortened sleep-onset latency, increased TST and SWS, longer REM sleep-onset latency, and less REM sleep.[86,87] Exercise exhibits negative effects on sleep when performed close to sleep onset. The optimal temporal positioning of physical activity is thought to be 4 to 8 hours before bedtime.[87] Chronic exercise studies have not provided much stringent evidence of a sleep-promoting effect. Conversely, with reduced exercise load in trained athletes, SWS and REM sleep-onset latency were reduced and REM sleep duration and sleep-onset latency were increased.[88] Taken together, after intense exercise, sleep appears to commence faster and is deeper.

Changing Skin Temperature during Sleep

Of clinical relevance are the data describing that REM sleep duration and TST are reduced when electric heat blankets are used throughout the night,[89] suggesting that heat load exerted through the blanket is too strong an intervention and disturbs rather than supports sleep. In a series of experiments with a thermal suit, the effects of small changes in skin temperatures of only 0.4 to 2° C within the thermal comfort zone, without significantly altering CBT, were investigated on several sleep parameters.[83] It was demonstrated that intermittent elevation, particularly in skin temperature during the sleep episode, suppressed nocturnal awakenings and deepened sleep in young and older healthy subjects, as well as in patients with insomnia or narcolepsy.[71,83] Notably, the manipulations were mild and temporary, therefore not affecting CBT. It remains to be demonstrated whether the effects could be sustained all night, given the adverse effect on sleep that can be expected if manipulations increase CBT.

It has been proposed that the solution could be a closed-loop feedback–controlled manipulation of skin temperature to increase no more than required to trigger maximal skin blood flow. Such a manipulation would promote heat loss to the environment without the risk of "injecting" heat from the environment back into the bloodstream that would occur at higher skin manipulation temperatures and increase CBT.[66] Nevertheless, the findings emphasize the importance of skin temperatures, primarily of the proximal skin (including the trunk) and have been replicated across young and older subjects, in people suffering from insomnia or narcolepsy,[70,83] Moreover, the altered thermal perception in people with insomnia as revealed with a dedicated questionnaire[90] impedes normal sleep onset.[72] Finally, a causal contribution of skin temperature changes to vigilance changes is further supported by daytime manipulation studies, again indicating vigilance reducing and sleep-promoting effects of mild skin warming across young and old participants and across health and disease.[69,71,91,92]

In conclusion, warm skin temperatures, induced either by endogenous circadian heat loss regulation in the evening, homeostatic downregulation of CBT after passive and active heat load, or selective skin warming, predisposes to a rapid onset of sleep, to deeper sleep and to worse sustained attention. Further studies must investigate the optimal time interval between thermal intervention and bedtime and which physiologic mechanisms are involved in the observed effects. It is possible that thermal afferents affect neuronal activity in brain regions involved in vigilance regulation.[19]

Changing Sleep Pressure

Results of studies on the effects of sleep deprivation on the thermoregulatory system may differ depending on whether they used CR protocols or regular office or clinical conditions. A CR protocol that kept people in a supine posture suggested that 40 hours of sleep deprivation does not change CBT, distal and proximal skin temperatures, heart rate, and energy expenditure despite the huge increase in sleepiness.[12] A similar CR study that included regularly scheduled naps to reduce sleep pressure also found no alterations. The lack of effects in supine CR conditions were surprising given the common notion of feeling chilly after sleep deprivation. Also, earlier animal work showed, for example, an increased firing rate of hypothalamic warm-sensitive neurons,[93,94] a reduced ability to retain body heat,[95] and consequently a steep drop in CBT with prolonged sleep deprivation.[96] There are effects of sleep deprivation on thermophysiology in paradigms that do not impose a continuous supine posture. In people assessed in a sitting posture, sleep deprivation induced a marked dissociation of thermoregulatory skin temperature gradient fluctuations, indicative of attenuated heat loss from the hands co-occurring with enhanced heat loss from the feet.[97] The findings suggest that sleep deprivation affects the coordination between skin blood flow fluctuations and the baroreceptor-mediated cardiovascular regulation that prevents venous pooling of blood in the lower limbs when there is the orthostatic challenge of an upright posture. These effects would not be detectable when imposing a semi-supine posture as is common in CR paradigms.

INTERVENTION STUDIES IN RODENTS

Changing Temperature

In the rat, a general decrease in the daily percentage of REM sleep occurs when ambient temperature decreased,[44,98] indicating that REM sleep is very sensitive to changes in temperature and incompatible with low ambient temperature. Djungarian hamsters enter REM sleep more easily when brain temperature is relatively low,[99] but probably also in this species REM will disappear first when ambient temperature is lowered. In this context, low ambient temperatures are applied as a REM sleep deprivation tool to investigate REM sleep regulatory mechanisms.[100,101]

In general, the impression exists that increasing ambient temperature increases sleep pressure. In rats, when ambient temperature was increased to 33 to 35° C for 3 hours, resulting in a brain temperature of approximately 40° C, subsequent NREM sleep displayed more slow waves than in sleep-matched controls.[102] The amount of REM sleep did not change compared with controls, and brain temperature was significantly decreased in the first 5 hours of recovery. Under these conditions, animals slept less during the heating compared with baseline, indicating that too-high ambient temperatures override sleep demand.

In two separate experiments in rats in which ambient temperature was increased to 30 to 32° C for 24 hours, well above the upper threshold of the thermoneutral zone, which, in rats, is approximately 28° C,[103] cortical brain temperature was significantly increased by 0.3 to 1.0° C but hypothalamic temperature did not change.[104,105] This treatment resulted in one case in increased NREM sleep and in both experiments in an increase in SWA in NREM sleep in the dark period. These data indicate that changes in sleep can be induced by increasing ambient temperature without changing hypothalamic temperature.

Another approach is heating the POAH, increasing hypothalamic brain temperature locally, without changing ambient temperature. This approach resulted in increased SWA and NREM sleep during 1 hour of warming (1.0° C above baseline) in cats.[106] One hour of cooling (2.0° C below baseline) did not elicit a response. The data suggest that an acute increase in ambient or brain temperature (0.3 to 1.0° C) can increase NREM sleep and possibly increase the occurrence of slow waves in the NREM sleep EEG.

Changing Sleep Pressure

During sleep deprivation, brain temperature is higher compared with baseline, and subsequent recovery is characterized by a decrease in brain temperature below baseline and an increase in NREM sleep and in SWA in NREM sleep.[43,105,107,108] This result was interpreted as a heat load incurred during the sleep deprivation that was subsequently recovered by increasing NREM sleep and SWA.[93] One of the clear results obtained from these experiments is a negative correlation between the amount of NREM sleep and the level of brain temperature.[99,107] There is no significant correlation, however, between SWA in NREM sleep and brain temperature,[99,107] ruling out the possibility that the depth of sleep determines brain temperature directly. Moreover, in Djungarian hamsters, well adapted to a short winter photoperiod with a brain temperature 1° C below summer photoperiod brain temperature, recovery sleep after sleep deprivation is accompanied by an increase in brain temperature.[99] This is in contrast to the same species under a long photoperiod, during which sleep deprivation is followed by a decrease in brain temperature.[43,99] A correlation between SWA and brain temperature, combining these data, supported the notion that brain temperature after sleep deprivation is set to the same temperature in both conditions,[99] suggesting that there may be an optimal temperature for high-amplitude slow waves in NREM sleep during recovery.

Two experiments in rats in which ambient temperature was raised to 32° C during a sleep deprivation of 2.5 hours[105] or 3 hours[108] did not result in similar outcomes. Short-lasting increases in SWA and NREM sleep were observed after a 2.5-hour sleep deprivation[105] but not after a 3-hour sleep deprivation.[108] In contrast, a short-lasting increase in REM sleep was observed after a 3-hour sleep deprivation[108] but not after a 2.5-hour sleep deprivation.[105] It may be questionable whether consistent results can be obtained in the rat with these short sleep deprivation durations. Probably a more systematic approach of scanning different ambient temperatures with longer sleep deprivations is needed to resolve these differences.

Brain Temperature, Electroencephalogram, and Thermosensitive Neurons

The EEG is influenced by changes in brain temperature as well. From analysis of the EEG of the Djungarian hamster during spontaneous entrance into the hypothermic state of torpor (see the section Hibernation) and from experiments in which rats, cats, or humans were cooled, it was found that the amplitude and frequency of the EEG changes when brain temperature decreases. The amplitude becomes smaller, and prominent frequencies in the EEG slow down with decreasing temperature.[109] The slowing down of the EEG was confirmed in rats in which hypothermia was induced pharmacologically by inhibiting neurons in the central nervous pathways for thermoregulatory cold defense.[110] This relation between EEG frequency and brain temperature was shown to follow a Q_{10} of approximately 2.5,[111] which means that the frequency became 2.5 times slower when brain temperature decreased by 10° C. Under the influence of euthermic changes this effect is relatively small, but it can be significant even for frequencies below 5 Hz.[109] Faster frequencies such as the theta rhythm (6 to 9 Hz) in rodents[109,112] and frequencies above 10 Hz[109,112] are significantly influenced by these daily changes in brain temperature.

Measuring the electrical activity of neurons in the POAH revealed the activity of two distinct types of neurons that either increase or decrease firing rate when brain temperature increases. The latter are called *cold-sensitive neurons,* whereas the first group is called *warm sensitive*. A biochemical process (i.e., neuronal firing) that slows down when temperature is increased is unique, and therefore cold-sensitive neurons, when observed, can be considered to be genuine. In contrast, a biochemical process that speeds up when temperature is increased is normal. Such a process was theoretically explained at the end of the 19th century.[109] Many processes, ranging from the firing rate of SCN neurons[113] to the frequency of prominent EEG waves,[109,114] to muscle contraction,[115] double or triple when temperature is increased by 10° C ($2 < Q_{10} < 3$).

To identify warm-sensitive neurons, two criteria are applied in the literature. The first determines that an increase in firing rate must be more than double when temperature is increased by 10° C ($Q_{10} > 2$).[116] The second says that the increase in firing rate must be more than 0.8 impulses per second per 1° C of warming.[117] Both definitions are insufficient. The criterion of a Q_{10} above 2 ignores the fact that most biochemical processes have a Q_{10} somewhere between 2 and 3. Therefore a Q_{10} of at least 3 must be reached before one can be relatively sure that the change in firing rate can be distinguished from the passive biochemical response of the temperature-insensitive neurons. With the second criterion, fast firing neurons have a relatively large chance of being included even when they follow the passive biochemical Q_{10} rule of doubling firing rate when temperature is increased by 10° C. Nevertheless, there are genuine warm-sensitive neurons in the POAH[118] and other brain areas, such as the diagonal band.[119]

The firing rate of warm- and cold-sensitive neurons in the POAH is known to be vigilance state dependent. Most warm-sensitive neurons increase their activity at the onset of NREM sleep. On the other hand, most cold-sensitive neurons are more active during waking.[118,119] Those results emphasize the importance of combining electrophysiology with polysomnographic recordings to be able to disentangle the vigilance state–related changes in firing rate from temperature-related changes.[120] Noradrenergic afferents from sleep-wake regulatory centers such as the locus coeruleus and the lateral tegmental system are also involved in the change in firing rate observed in the POAH.[121] The changes in firing rate of the ensemble of neurons are thought to shape the sleep-wake response to thermoregulatory demands encountered by the animal.

HIBERNATION

The hypothermic state observed during the hibernation season may be a valuable model to investigate the relationship between thermoregulation and sleep and may generate relevant data to the understanding of human physiology. Most hibernating mammals are small and weigh between 10 and 1000 g.[122] During the hibernation season these animals spend a considerable amount of time in a torpid state with body temperature below euthermia (i.e., below 30 to 32° C). This sustained hypothermic state is entered voluntarily and can be terminated by the animal. Body temperature can drop by more than 35° C,[123] and the metabolic rate is only a fraction of that during normothermia.[124]

In hibernators the torpid state can last for several days or weeks. A group of smaller mammals with body weights between 5 and 50 g display daily torpor in which body temperature is dropped for a couple of hours during the rest phase but returns to euthermia during the active phase.[122] Both hibernation and daily torpor result in substantial energy savings[125,126] and are therefore considered to be adaptive mechanisms that permit the conservation of energy during unfavorable environmental conditions.

Whether circadian rhythms continue during hibernation is unclear. In hibernating ground squirrels, rest-activity rhythms only slowly reappeared a couple of days after termination of torpor bouts, and this correlated with the number of vasopressin-containing neurons in the SCN.[127] Also, sleep-wake distribution in hibernating ground squirrels did not show a circadian modulation.[128] In contrast, responses to, for instance, sleep deprivation, temperature changes, and other homeostatic regulatory processes are still functioning.[129-133] Under certain circumstances a small circadian modulation of body temperature can be observed during hibernation[134]; however, one can conclude that the contribution of the circadian clock is reduced, whereas homeostatic regulation seems to be virtually identical to its regulation outside the hibernation season.

Thermoregulation and Metabolic Rate Reduction

The mechanism by which the animals reach the reduction in metabolic rate is still controversial. The traditional view was that metabolic rate falls as body temperature decreases at torpor entry. The Q_{10} of metabolic rate between euthermia and torpor is often close to 2, which is typical for biochemical processes.[109] Therefore the reduction in metabolic rate seems to be explained solely by the temperature effect on biochemical processes in the body.[135,136]

However, Q_{10} values above 3 for metabolic rate have been observed during torpor entry and during torpor at relatively high temperatures. It was therefore proposed that an additional physiologic inhibition must be involved in the reduction of metabolic rate.[137,138] Metabolic rate is downregulated before torpor entry, and the decrease in body temperature is the consequence and not the cause of the metabolic rate reduction.[139-141] As an alternative hypothesis it was proposed that metabolic rate is a function of the difference between ambient temperature and body temperature, similar to that during euthermia.[139] Because this difference is generally very small during torpor, metabolic rate is equally reduced.

Inhibition of metabolic rate during torpor may be caused by reduced pH, which slows down metabolic processes.[142] In hibernating ground squirrels the respiratory quotient drops during entrance into torpor and rises during subsequent arousal, suggesting CO_2 storage, which may result in decreased pH. In contrast, in Djungarian hamsters, who display daily torpor, respiratory quotient increases during entrance into torpor and decreases before emergence from torpor. Changes in enzyme activity are other candidates for metabolic rate reduction. Mitochondrial respiration is reduced by 50% during torpor in hibernating ground squirrels compared with euthermic individuals.

The previous data support the notion that the mechanism of metabolic rate reduction differs between hibernators and animals that use daily torpor.[142] The reduction in metabolic rate in animals who display daily torpor seems to be largely determined by the decrease in body temperature, whereas hibernators may apply some kind of extra reduction in metabolic rate.[143]

For some essential but unknown reason, deep torpor in hibernators is interrupted on a regular basis by short (<24 hours) euthermic periods.[144,145] Above 0° C body temperature, torpor bout length correlates negatively with ambient temperature,[146] and metabolic rate solely depends on ambient temperature and therefore body temperature. The timing of the euthermic period (also called *arousal*) correlates with the ambient temperature and the metabolic rate of the animal during the preceding hibernation bout. The arousal is probably not induced by a process accumulating in the course of a multiday torpor bout but that there exists a separate arousal process of which the onset is more susceptible at higher body or ambient temperatures.[147] Although the mechanism of the arousal is not known, it appears to be totally endogenous in its origin.

The question of the reason for the arousal is important. The function of hibernation is clearly energy conservation, and energy expenditure during the hibernation season is reduced to less than 15% of the energy the animals would have spent if they remained euthermic throughout the winter season.[124] However, there is still room for improvement because the energy costs of the periodic arousals constitute 64% to 90% of the total energy expenditure during the hibernation season.[124,148,149] It has been proposed that arousals are required to eliminate metabolic waste products, to replenish blood glucose levels, or to restore cellular electrolyte balance. All these hypotheses have not survived critical experimental testing.[150] Based on EEG observations it was proposed that animals terminate torpor and return to euthermia to restore a sleep debt.[151,152] NREM sleep was deepest at the beginning of a euthermic period, and most of the euthermic period was spent in sleep. The putative restorative function of NREM sleep was thought to be incompatible with torpor.

Torpor and Sleep

Animals in torpor appear to be sleeping. They remain in their nest in a sleep-like posture with elevated arousal thresholds. Based on several behavioral and physiologic findings, it is generally accepted that torpor has evolved as an extension of sleep. When the animals enter torpor, analysis of the EEG shows that rodents are mainly in NREM sleep and that REM sleep is reduced or not present.[153,154] Recordings of neuronal activity in the hypothalamus of hibernators with brain temperatures of 10 to 20° C indicate that these animals keep alternating between long NREM sleep bouts and short waking bouts.[155] Below 10° C it is not possible to determine vigilance states with electrophysiologic methods.[147] These findings supported the hypothesis that NREM sleep is an adaptive behavior for energy conservation, which function is strengthened during torpor.[126,148,156]

However, when the animals subsequently emerge from torpor, they immediately enter deep NREM sleep, irrespective of whether the animals emerge from deep hibernation[151,152] or daily torpor.[154] This observation suggests that, during deep torpor, the function of sleep cannot be fulfilled completely and animals have to return to euthermia to recover from a sleep deprivation incurred during the hypothermic state. Initially, the hypothesis was confirmed in the Djungarian hamster by combining daily torpor with sleep deprivation experiments.[129] In contrast, similar experiments in hibernating ground squirrels resulted in rejection of the sleep deprivation hypothesis.[131,132] After recovering from pharmacologically induced hypothermia in rats, the increase in deep sleep was also observed.[110] An analysis of the shape of the slow waves in the NREM sleep EEG following torpor in the Djungarian hamster suggests that the processes taking place during this sleep may differ from the processes in sleep after sleep deprivation.[157] This would mean that the sleep after torpor has a different function than the sleep after sleep deprivation, but that still some kind of recovery takes place. This recovery may involve recovery of lost synaptic connections during the previous torpor period.

Still, there appear to be fundamental differences between animals that display daily torpor and hibernating animals that display multiple-day torpor bouts. The mechanisms of metabolic rate reduction seems to differ.[142] Another fundamental difference between the two groups of animals is the effect of torpor on subsequent sleep. In hibernating animals who display deep torpor similar to ground squirrels or hamsters, regulation of temperature and sleep seems to be reduced to a level that currently cannot be measured reliably. In contrast, animals who display daily torpor appear to make use of the same processes, although applied in an extreme way, which reduces body temperature at the onset of sleep in humans. This latter similarity may provide an opportunity to investigate the relationship between sleep and body temperature with much larger variability.

CLINICAL PEARL

Humans with cold hands and feet are predisposed to difficulties initiating sleep. Better knowledge about sleep thermophysiology may help to develop evidence-based thermal interventions to alleviate sleep disturbances and to manage certain aspects of sleep and alertness problems in the general population. Therefore, to assess dysfunctional thermoregulation, clinicians can use objective skin temperature measurements (e.g., wrist and instep seem promising sites for gender-related cold sensation assessment in relation to sleep) in conjunction with patient self-reports about thermal discomfort (e.g., sensation of cold hands and feet) to diagnose, monitor, and advise patients on their sleep disturbances or thermal discomfort–related complaints.

SUMMARY

The human sleep-wake cycle is tightly coupled to the circadian time course of CBT. The evening increase in heat loss through distal skin regions and reduction in heat production is associated with sleepiness and the ease of falling asleep. After sleep initiation, ultradian NREM/REM sleep cycle fluctuations seem to have minor thermoregulatory functions, especially in humans. Sleep deprivation–induced increases in homeostatic sleep pressure may not affect the thermoregulatory system in supine conditions, while effects emerge in upright conditions.

The POAH integrates input from brain areas involved in circadian, temperature, and sleep-wake regulation and in turn influences vigilance states and body temperature in response to that input. Experimental data show that mild skin warming, supposedly impinging on the POAH, can increase sleep propensity, sleep consolidation, and the duration of SWS.

In animals, the torpid state may be a valuable model to investigate the relationship between thermoregulation and sleep. During daily torpor, similar physiologic processes occur as during normal entrance into sleep, but this is observed in a more extreme way, providing an excellent opportunity to investigate these processes in more detail.

SELECTED READINGS

Colbert RW, Holley CT, Stone LH, et al. The recovery of hibernating hearts lies on a spectrum: from bears in nature to patients with coronary artery disease. *J Cardiovasc Transl Res.* 2015;8(4):244–252.

Deboer T. Brain temperature dependent changes in the electroencephalogram power spectrum of humans and animals. *J Sleep Res.* 1998;7(4):254–262.

Dijk DJ, Czeisler CA. Contribution of the circadian pacemaker and the sleep homeostat to sleep propensity, sleep structure, electroencephalographic slow waves, and sleep spindle activity in humans. *J Neurosci.* 1995;15(5 Pt 1):3526–3538.

Geiser F. Metabolic rate and body temperature reduction during hibernation and daily torpor. *Annu Rev Physiol.* 2004;66:239–274.

Giroud S, Habold C, Nespolo RF. The torpid state: recent advances in metabolic adaptations and protective mechanisms. *Front Physiol.* 2021;11:623665. Published 2021 Jan 20.

Harding EC, Franks NP, Wisden W. Sleep and thermoregulation. *Curr Opin Physiol.* 2020;15:7–13.

Horne JA. Why sleep? *Biologist.* 2002;49(5):213–216.

Jacquot CM, Schellen L, Kingma BR, et al. Influence of thermophysiology on thermal behavior: the essentials of categorization. *Physiol Behav.* 2014;128:180–187.

Kräuchi K. The thermophysiological cascade leading to sleep initiation in relation to phase of entrainment. *Sleep Med Rev.* 2007;11(6):439–451.

Krauchi K, Deboer T. The interrelationship between sleep regulation and thermoregulation. *Front Biosci. (Landmark Ed).* 2010;15:604–625.

Mekjavic IB, Eiken O. Contribution of thermal and nonthermal factors to the regulation of body temperature in humans. *J Appl Physiol.* 2006;100:2065–2072.

Parmeggiani PL. REM sleep related increase in brain temperature: a physiologic problem. *Arch Ital Biol.* 2007;145:13–21.

Siegel JM. Do all animal sleep? *Trends Neurosci.* 2008;31:208–213.

Van Someren EJW. Mechanisms and functions of coupling between sleep and temperature rhythms. *Prog Brain Res.* 2006;153:309–324.

A complete reference list can be found online at ExpertConsult.com.

Chapter 29

Memory Processing in Relation to Sleep

Stuart Fogel; Carlyle Smith; Philippe Peigneux

Chapter Highlights

- Sleep is an opportune time for the optimal transformation and strengthening of newly acquired memories to take place. This process is thought to unfold in part through reactivation of the new memory trace, ultimately resulting in a more resilient, more easily retrieved, integrated, and lasting long-term memory.
- Sleep stages and specific sleep features (e.g., brain oscillatory activity, slow waves, spindles) variously contribute to memory consolidation processes, including synaptic plasticity, long-term potentiation, reactivation, and enhanced functional connectivity. Features such as spindles are also electrophysiologic markers of cognitive abilities.
- Disturbed and reduced sleep affect cognitive functions, especially learning and memory. By contrast, enhancing sleep can restore sleep-related memory deficits.

SUMMARY

Although each of us empirically recognizes the utmost importance of sleep for the quality of our everyday life, the functions of sleep have long remained shrouded in mystery. Beyond its putative physiologic functions, there is now growing evidence that sleep plays a prominent role in brain plasticity and memory consolidation processes. According to this proposal, memory traces formed during a learning episode are not immediately stored in their ultimate form. Rather, they initially remain in a labile, fragile state during which they can be easily disrupted or interrupted. Over time and during sleep, memory traces subsequently undergo a series of transformations during which they will be consolidated and fully integrated into long-term memory. In this chapter, we present experimental data that provide support for the hypothesis that sleep exerts a promoting effect on plastic processes of memory consolidation. Several sources of support for this hypothesis are described in this chapter, including: (1) studies assessing the effects of post-training sleep deprivation on memory consolidation and on the reorganization of the neural substrates of long-term memories; (2) the effects of learning on post-training sleep and re-expression of behavior-specific neural patterns during post-training sleep; and (3) the effects of within-sleep stimulation on sleep patterns and overnight memories. Despite advances that have refined our understanding of the relationships between sleep and cognitive processes, the underlying mechanisms still remain to be fully elucidated. Further steps are now required to understand how sleep disorders and pathologies accompanied by sleep disturbances affect cognitive functions, and especially learning and memory consolidation in humans, eventually leading to remedial interventions.

INTRODUCTION

In 1867 Hervey de Saint Denys reported a series of ingenious experiments showing that experienced events are incorporated into our dreams, in which they can be combined to create original associations between "memory images" of the past.[1] Hence he opposed the widely held idea that sleep may be a sudden drop in a state of cognitive "non-being," in which our resting brain is disconnected. On the contrary, he claimed that "... sleep without dreams cannot exist, just as wake without mentation does not exist." Besides dreaming activity, however, already addressed in this book (see Part VII), we know that the sleeping brain houses a great variety of cognitive processes, including, to name a few, the ongoing processing of external stimuli, the revival of past experiences, and the consolidation of new information into long-term memory. Interestingly, recognition that persistence of mental activity in the sleeper may be an integral part of the physiologic processes that support memory consolidation only arose in the last quarter of the 20th century. It is now widely accepted that the sleeping brain is highly active and dynamic, but until recently it was not well understood to what end this particular activity may serve beyond the initiation and maintenance of sleep itself.

This chapter introduces issues surrounding the role that sleep may play in memory consolidation, focusing on studies in humans. It must be kept in mind that memory is not a unitary phenomenon, both from cognitive and neurophysiologic perspectives. Rather, memory should be seen as a generic concept for information storage, encompassing a series of specific subdomains. Consequently, the interaction between the multidimensional states of sleep and distinctive memory systems makes it logical that not all sleep manipulations will affect performance to the same extent, depending on the nature

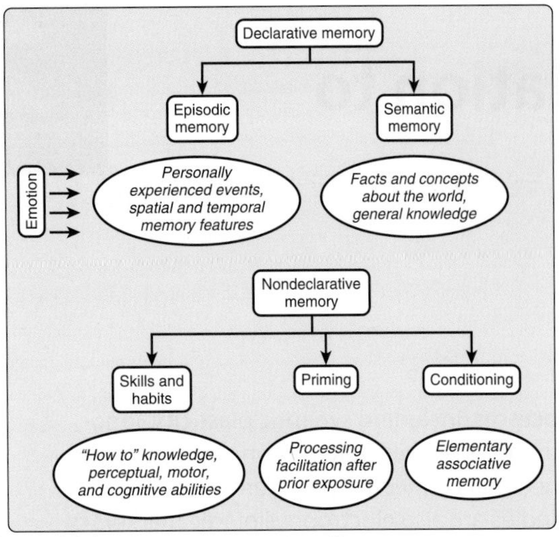

Figure 29.1 Schematic organization of long-term memory systems.

and demands of the memory task. The relationship between consolidation of newly formed memories and sleep is a crucial issue because memory is at the root of most of our daily behaviors, such as simple skill acquisition (e.g., typewriting), sophisticated operational procedures (e.g., using computer-based systems), or keeping track of personal events and relationships, but is also an integral component of mental health therapeutic interventions.[2]

MEMORY SYSTEMS AND MEMORY CONSOLIDATION

Long-term memories in humans, primarily delineated between declarative and nondeclarative memories (Figure 29.1), are supported by distinct neuroanatomic substrates. Declarative memory is distinct in that information is easily accessible to verbal description and that encoding and/or retrieval is usually carried out explicitly (i.e., the subject is aware that the stored information exists and is being accessed). Distinctive features of nondeclarative memories, on the other hand, are less easily accessible to verbal description and can be acquired and reexpressed implicitly (i.e., without conscious knowledge or awareness of encoding or retrieval). Nondeclarative memory also includes skills, habits, priming, conditioning, and even some forms of problem solving.

Newly acquired information is not immediately stored at the time of learning in its final form. Rather, memories undergo a series of transformations over time periods ranging from hours to days, even years, during which they will be gradually incorporated into preexisting mnemonic representations[3,4] and will be subjected to forgetting[5] or reconsolidation.[6] This dynamic longitudinal process refers to the concept of memory consolidation, which can be defined as the time-dependent process that transforms labile memory traces into more permanent and/or enhanced forms.[7]

In this framework, scientific evidence suggests that sleep and associated processes of brain plasticity[8] are important players in time-dependent processes of memory consolidation, acting as key constituents in the chain of transformations that help integrate information for the long term. Furthermore, these studies have suggested that the electroencephalogram (EEG) features of sleep and the respective sleep states that they characterize may have distinct memory-related functions. These findings have been interpreted in two different but nonexclusive manners. According to the "dual-process hypothesis," rapid eye movement (REM) and non–rapid eye movement (NREM) sleep act differently on memory traces, depending on the memory system or process to which they belong. For instance, it was proposed that slow wave sleep (SWS) facilitates consolidation of declarative and spatial memories, whereas REM sleep facilitates consolidation of nondeclarative memories[9] (but see an alternative interpretation of sleep and declarative memory consistent with Tulving's serial, parallel, independent (SPI) model[10] or an alternative explanation of the relationship between sleep states and nondeclarative memory[11]). Another model hypothesized that memory processing during sleep takes place in a sequential manner, whereby particular transitions from one sleep state to another each handle particular aspects of memory consolidation.[12] Both approaches assume that it is sleep on the first posttraining night that is most important for memory consolidation. Notwithstanding, it would be inappropriate to claim that only sleep may achieve the necessary conditions to consolidate novel memories in the nervous system, as both sleep-like cognitive and neural processes of memory consolidation have also been observed during wakefulness.[13,14] Although there is a wealth of support for the notion that sleep is an opportune time for consolidation processes to take place and may even actively enhance consolidation, thereby affording a preferential benefit to memory strengthening, the precise nature of the relationship between online (i.e., during actual learning) and wake- and sleep-offline (i.e., post-learning) consolidation processes remains to be fully disentangled.

MAIN METHODS FOR STUDYING THE ROLE OF SLEEP FOR MEMORY CONSOLIDATION

Three broad classes of experimental approaches have been used to test the hypothesis that sleep exerts a favorable or promoting effect on memory consolidation: (1) effects of posttraining sleep deprivation on memory consolidation and on the reorganization of the neural substrates of long-term memories, (2) effects of learning on posttraining sleep and reexpression of behavior-specific neural patterns during posttraining sleep, and (3) effects of within-sleep stimulation on sleep patterns and overnight memories.

Posttraining Sleep Deprivation

The earliest type of investigation probed the putatively detrimental effect of sleep deprivation on the night after learning, based upon the assumption that memory performance over the long term will be better if participants are allowed to sleep after learning, compared with sleep-deprived subjects. This is in essence a "lesion technique," whereby sleep (or part of sleep) is removed or disturbed, and the resulting deficits are observed relative to well-rested controls. In classical experimental procedures, subjects learn new material. Afterward, some participants are allowed to sleep normally, whereas others (1) do not sleep at all (total sleep deprivation), (2) are awakened at the onset of occurrences of the sleep stage under study (selective sleep deprivation), (3) are kept awake during the period of the night in which the sleep stage is predominant (partial sleep deprivation), or (4) have a shortened sleep duration (sleep restriction). Finally, pre- and postnight memory measures are compared between sleeping and sleep-deprived subgroups either the next day or several days later. This approach first was used more than 80 years ago[15] and revealed that the normal forgetting curve for newly learned verbal material is significantly dampened by the presence of an intermediate period of sleep, an effect interpreted by the authors as a mere protective role of sleep against "interference, inhibition, or obliteration of the old by the new."[15]

The hypothesis of a purely passive role for sleep in memory processes has been challenged by selective sleep deprivation studies attributing a specific role to REM sleep in memory storage and consolidation both in human and animal species.[16] Also, it was demonstrated that memory over an interval with relatively high amounts of SWS was superior to memory over an interval with relatively high amounts of REM sleep.[17] This seemingly apparent contradiction was resolved later with the demonstration that recall of paired-associate lists was significantly better after sleep than wakefulness in the SWS-rich first part of the night only, whereas consolidation of mirror-tracing skills specifically benefited from sleep in the REM-rich second part of the night.[9] Other experimental manipulations inferred a specific role for stage 2 sleep, particularly in the second part of the night for the consolidation of motor memories.[18] Hence sleep deprivation studies have suggested that all stages of human sleep (REM, SWS, and stage 2 sleep) might be actively involved in distinctive ways in learning and memory consolidation processes.[19,20]

Neuroimaging approaches have demonstrated (a) that sleep deprivation during the posttraining night eventually impedes the reorganization and optimization of the cerebral activity subtending delayed retrieval of consolidated memories during wakefulness,[21,22] and (b) that sleep-dependent changes in memory-related brain activity patterns may be present even in cases in which similarity in behavioral performance between posttraining sleep conditions suggests an absence of sleep-related effect on memory.[23,24] The latter further indicates that long-term memory performance can be achieved using different cerebral strategies initiated as a function of the status of sleep during the posttraining night.

Posttraining Sleep Modifications

EEG studies have demonstrated that both the architecture of sleep and distinctive features of sleep stages can be affected by prior learning experience. For instance, postlearning sleep modifications have been observed by looking at absolute or proportional (i.e., relative to total sleep time) increases in the duration of REM sleep,[19,25] stage 2 sleep,[26,27] and SWS[25] episodes. Other studies have reported increased density of rapid eye movements[28,29] and stage 2 spindle activity,[30-34] as well as increases in REM sleep theta power.[27] Many found relationships between quantitative parameters of sleep and overnight performance improvements[25,30,31,34-37] or levels of performance at the end of learning,[38] suggesting a close link between changes in sleep physiology and memory consolidation. In support of the sequential double-step hypothesis described previously, other studies demonstrated relationships between performance changes and the organization of NREM/REM sleep cycles.[39,40] Hence, these investigations, mostly based on noninvasive electrophysiologic techniques, have consistently demonstrated that prior learning during the day influences the physiology of sleep.

Noninvasive neuroimaging studies, initially using positron emission tomography (PET) measurements and, more recently, functional magnetic resonance imaging (fMRI) and magnetoencephalography (MEG) studies have provided evidence that neural activity occurring during memory task practice in learning-related cerebral structures can be re-expressed or continued both during REM[41,42] and NREM[43] stages of sleep as well as during posttraining wakefulness.[13] Recent advances in simultaneous EEG-fMRI recordings enabled investigating functional activations in brain regions associated with sleep EEG features. These studies showed that activity in brain regions active during learning and then during subsequent sleep are preferentially strengthened and transformed,[44] and that this memory trace reactivation is time-locked to phasic events, such as sleep spindles.[45,46] These data are in close agreement with intracerebral recording studies in animals, which demonstrated neuronal reactivation during sleep,[47,48] although these seminal animal studies did not seek to establish a link to memory consolidation or behavioral relevance of this reactivation per se. In this context, human neuroimaging data showed that experience-dependent reactivations of local—hippocampal—activity during SWS are correlated to overnight gains in memory performance after spatial navigation.[43] Conversely, levels of implicit procedural learning achieved prior to sleep correlated with the amplitude of reactivation in cortical areas during REM sleep,[42] during which connectivity patterns between learning-related areas were additionally reinforced.[49] fMRI studies also revealed reactivation of hippocampal activity time locked to sleep spindles following both declarative[45] and procedural[46] learning. Moreover, procedural learning-dependent reactivation recruited other task-relevant structures and strengthened communication within a network of brain regions recruited during learning, including the putamen,[44] the extent of which correlated with overnight improvement. Taken together, human reactivation studies suggest that there is neuronal replay of previous experience during sleep and that posttraining sleep activity in brain areas involved during the learning episode represent a neural signature of memory-related cognitive processes, possibly linked with phasic sleep events such as spindles. An alternate but not exclusive hypothesis is that learning during wake induces local synaptic changes, which themselves induce local changes in slow wave activity (SWA), the main marker of sleep homeostasis, and that these changes are ultimately beneficial to imprint novel memories.[50,51]

Within-Sleep Stimulations

Demonstrating an active, and potentially causal, role for sleep in memory consolidation processes, several studies employing targeted memory reactivation (TMR) paradigms have established that stimulations within the posttraining sleep period may enhance performance as compared to a normal, unmodified posttraining night.[52-55] Indeed, presentation of nonawakening auditory stimulations during REM sleep after Morse code learning[52] or re-presentation during REM sleep of sounds heard in background while learning a complex logic task[53] increased overnight memory performance. Importantly, the effect was only present when auditory stimulations were displayed in coincidence with the bursts of rapid eye movements that reflect phasic ponto-geniculo-occipital (PGO) activity in humans, further suggesting that the characteristics of sleep are important markers, and perhaps even tied to cellular mechanisms of memory consolidation processes but reflected at a macroscopic level. Likewise, presentation during SWS of odors that were used as contextual cues during the learning episode triggers hippocampal responses and improves overnight retention of declarative memories but not procedural memories.[55] A similar approach was used during postlearning stage 2 sleep, which was found to enhance consolidation for procedural memories.[56] Thus targeted reactivation of memory traces is not merely an epiphenomenon of sleep but rather is highly specific to the previously learned task. Indeed, in subjects trained to produce two musical melodies by following sequences of movements, motor sequence accuracy was significantly more enhanced for the melody that was replayed during sleep,[57] and improvement correlated with the amount of posttraining SWS and sleep spindles. Also, the effect of TMR was found specific to the verbal material cued again during sleep,[58] and the size of the beneficial impact of TMR during NREM sleep was actually associated with the amount of ensuing REM sleep,[59] thus supporting the idea of a continuous and possibly differential processing of information across NREM/REM sleep stages.[12] The association with spindles was reinforced, showing that presentation of learning-related stimuli during NREM sleep actually leads to increased sleep spindle activity and consolidation, but that spindle activity is suppressed upon presentation on a second stimulation within 1.3 seconds of the first one, with no related overnight consolidation effects.[60,61] Likewise, transcranial direct current stimulation that modulates excitability in cortical areas improves declarative memory when applied during SWS,[62] especially when application of oscillating potentials at about 0.75 Hz induced slow oscillation-like potential fields that mimic the slow oscillations (SOs) of deep NREM sleep.[54]

Most recently, brain oscillations have been precisely targeted and enhanced using closed-loop auditory stimulation in an effort to enhance memory processing during sleep. Unlike TMR, closed-loop stimulation employs nonmeaningful but rhythmic acoustic stimuli to enhance specific sleep oscillations, such as SOs[63] and sleep spindles.[64] Remarkably, these studies showed that it is possible to enhance slow oscillatory frequencies and the related spindle activity using precisely timed auditory stimuli, resulting in enhancement of declarative memory performance as compared to controls. Remarkably, at least one study showed that new simple stimulus-reaction associations can be created during sleep.[65] Finally, artificially maintaining high levels of cortisol feedback and cholinergic tone during SWS impairs hippocampus-dependent declarative memory formation,[66,67] suggesting that the natural shift in central nervous system cholinergic tone from high levels during acquisition-related wakefulness periods to minimal levels during SWS optimizes declarative memory consolidation.[68] Conversely, preventing natural increases in cortisol during REM sleep periods appears to enhance amygdala-dependent emotional memory.[67] Notably, subsequent research found that artificially maintaining a high cholinergic tone during SWS does not alter the beneficial impact of TMR during this sleep stage,[69] suggesting that the mechanisms subtending spontaneous and cued (i.e., TMR) memory reactivation during sleep are partially distinct.

Other emerging noninvasive brain stimulation techniques such as TMS and transcranial direct current stimulation (tDCS) have been used to boost neuronal activity (e.g., enhance slow waves) or to stimulate brain regions to strengthen the memory of recently acquired information. For example, using tDCS to enhance SOs during postlearning sleep has been shown to result in a subsequent memory benefit.[54,62] However, because of varying methodologic approaches, it remains unclear what types of memory may benefit from noninvasive brain stimulation, what stages of sleep are ideal targets, and what the underlying physiologic mechanisms are.

These studies have demonstrated beneficial (or detrimental) effects of various stimulations and manipulations within the posttraining sleep periods on overnight gains in performance and therefore have provided further evidence that sleep does not merely play a passive role in memory processing by protecting novel memories from interference. Rather, the studies support the hypothesis that sleep acts in a complex manner in providing optimal conditions for the consolidation of novel memories in the nervous system.

SLEEP AND DECLARATIVE MEMORY

As described previously, long-term declarative memory comprises (1) semantic and (2) episodic memory components. Experimental data indicate that the role of sleep in consolidating these two memory components may be dissociated to a certain extent and that (3) emotional variables play a modulatory role in episodic memory consolidation. These aspects are covered in the following section.

Semantic Memory

Few studies have looked at the role of sleep for consolidation of semantic information per se, although evoked-related potentials studies have demonstrated that semantic processing of externally presented stimuli is possible during REM and stage 2 sleep, but not during SWS.[70–72] Also, it has been shown that semantic priming (i.e., the facilitating processing effect resulting from prior presentation of semantically related material) qualitatively differs upon awakening from stage 2 and REM sleep stages.[73] Sleep also enhances the creation of semantically related false memories (i.e., "theme words" associated with lists of semantically related words[74]; but see the article by Fenn and colleagues[75] for an alternative view). Furthermore, both accurate and illusory recollections have been associated with increased hippocampal activity after sleep, although behavioral effects were similar.[76] Despite evidence for residual semantic processing, attempts to create novel semantic associations using direct auditory stimulation during sleep have been unsuccessful,[77] but see the research by Züst and colleagues.[78] One possible explanation for this is that the transfer of novel information from hippocampus-dependent episodic memory stores to neocortical semantic, decontextualized memory representations is a gradual, slow process that may take years to complete.[79] Therefore initial encoding, posttraining sleep periods, and retrieval that are temporally close are usually not best suited to segregate the semantic component of memory from other constituents. One promising approach used to address this issue[80] is to investigate the integration of novel words that were either part of densely or sparsely populated networks of semantic memory. Results showed that sleep spindles and SWA (0.5 to 4 Hz) increased more after learning sparsely than densely semantically integrated words, suggesting the involvement of these NREM sleep parameters in the integration of new information into existing semantic networks.

In this respect, a few neuroimaging studies have investigated the cerebral correlates of declarative memory retrieval after extended periods of time up to 6 months using a paired-associates list of words[22] or pictures of landscapes.[81] Although these experiments were not specifically designed to probe whether the memorized material was "semanticized" at the time of retesting, neuroimaging results clearly indicated a transfer from activity in hippocampal locations, observed early after learning, toward activity in medial prefrontal cortical (mPFC) sites recorded 6 months later during memory retrieval.[22,81] Furthermore, total sleep deprivation on the postlearning night hindered this gradual process of consolidation. Indeed, 6 months after learning verbal material, memory retrieval more strongly activated the mPFC when initial encoding was followed by a night of sleep than by sleep deprivation, suggesting that sleep leads to long-lasting changes in the representation of memories at the neuroanatomic level.[22] These results may be consistent with the hypothesis that sleep exerts an effect on the gradual semantic integration of the learned material. Notably, the time delay needed to integrate and consolidate novel information in verbal memory might be dependent of the developmental phase. There is evidence for a rapid hippocampal-neocortical transfer of verbal information after a single nap in prepubertal children,[82] probably linked to the high amount and density of SWA at this developmental phase.

Episodic Memory

The effect of sleep on episodic memory has been extensively studied using a series of declarative memory paradigms. Among these, most studies using partial behavioral[9,22,83] or pharmacologic[66] sleep deprivation have consistently found that SWS, or at least the first half of the night of sleep, which is rich in SWS, is beneficial for the consolidation of novel declarative memories, particularly when the to-be-remembered material is of future importance.[84] Moreover, the benefit of sleep to episodic recall is greater for young as compared to older subjects and correlated with sleep duration,[85] and long-term forgetting is correlated with sleep disruptions in this population.[86] It suggests that age-related changes in sleep contribute to deterioration of episodic memory with age. Additionally, consolidation of declarative learning was linked to increased spindle activity during posttraining stage 2 sleep,[30,31,34,36,37] as well as to the alteration of SWS[87] and spindles[88] in schizophrenia. Spindles are strong candidates to subserve memory consolidation processes during NREM sleep because they are thought to support neural plasticity.[89] In addition, declarative learning abilities have been linked with increased spindle activity during stage 2 sleep[35] and periodic arousal fluctuations during NREM sleep[90] in healthy subjects. Conversely, declarative memory deficits are associated with decreased sleep spindle activity in Alzheimer disease patients[91] and NREM sleep duration and number of cycles in patients with chronic nonrestorative sleep.[92] Others have reported that overnight performance gains on declarative verbal memory primarily depend on preserved organization of sleep cycles (i.e., sleep continuity) rather than on the integrity of a specific sleep stage per se.[40] Also, REM sleep deprivation was found to specifically impair recall of spatial and temporal features of memories, as well as the subject's confidence in its own remembering.[93] These parameters are considered as genuine components of episodic memory, as opposed to general recall, which may partially rely on semantic, decontextualized memories.[10] Accordingly, it has been reported that consolidation during sleep enhances explicit recollection in recognition memory[94] and strengthens the original temporal sequence structure for lists of triplet words.[95] Taken together, these studies provide compelling evidence that sleep is important for the formation of novel episodic experiences and the preservation, integration, and recollection of episodic memory. When sleep is adversely affected with age, by psychiatric and neurodegenerative conditions, or more simply by sleep disruption or deprivation, episodic memory is impaired.

Emotion in Episodic Memory

Emotion can be seen as an important contextual cue in retention of episodic memories. Notwithstanding, emotional material was found better recalled after REM than NREM sleep[96] and altered after sleep deprivation,[97] although more for the emotional content than the context of the information.[98] Others have found emotional memories preserved, or at least less disrupted than neutral memories after total sleep deprivation.[67] These latter results suggest that consolidation of emotional memories also occurs efficiently during wake periods, an effect that may be explained by the important ecological value of rapidly acquiring emotional stimulus-response associations. Moreover, a lack of behavioral effect does not guarantee that sleep was without any consequence on memory consolidation processes, since the underlying patterns of brain activity at retrieval were effectively altered by sleep deprivation on the posttraining night.[23,99,100]

From another perspective, mood-dependent memory effects (i.e., better recall for neutral material in the same than in a different mood during learning) were attenuated when tested after 3 days of normal sleep, but not when sleep deprivation took place on the postlearning night.[101] However, mood-dependent memory effects were equally preserved after 4 hours of sleep dominated either by NREM or REM sleep[102] or after a night of sleep,[103] suggesting that emotional decontextualization of neutral memories takes place over several nights of sleep, the process being initiated on the first posttraining night. Further studies are needed to ascertain whether this effect is specifically emotional or merely related to contextual information in general.[104]

SLEEP AND NONDECLARATIVE MEMORIES

As previously mentioned, memory abilities aggregated under the nondeclarative category comprise various heterogeneous subtypes. These may be relatively independent both from cognitive and neuroanatomic standpoints but are collectively considered procedures for "how" to perform various tasks, which are often divorced from explicit knowledge of the experiences in which these skills were acquired. Skills and habits, which refer to the gradual acquisition of novel perceptual, motor, and cognitive abilities through repeated practice (e.g., discriminating figures, playing piano, riding a bicycle, or detecting environmental regularities), have been the most widely investigated in relation to sleep. In this respect, numerous studies have found that posttraining sleep boosts acquisition levels on nonverbal motor,[105-107] perceptual,[108-110] and perceptual-motor[18,49,51] procedural learning tasks. Sleep was also shown to reinforce proactive interference effects in motor learning in children,[111] a population in whom procedural memory effects are typically not observed using direct measures.[112] Additionally, a few studies have found that pharmacologic enhancement (e.g., using non-benzodiazepine hypnotics) of sleep spindles restores sleep-dependent motor memory consolidation in schizophrenia.[113] Also, sleep particularly enhances procedural memory performance in brain damaged individuals[114] but not in patients suffering from degenerative Parkinson disease.[115] Age-related changes in sleep spindles may also underlie age-related reduction in striatal activation and the related deficits in motor memory consolidation.[116] In the following section we further describe the role of sleep on perceptual, motor, perceptual-motor learning, and priming.

Sleep and Perceptual Learning

Sleep has been implicated in the development of visual discrimination abilities. Most studies have used the texture discrimination task,[117] in which learning is retinotopic, that is, specific to the trained visual quadrant,[110,118,119] and improvement was initially linked to REM sleep.[117] Overnight improvement was then found to be a direct function of both the amount of SWS in the first quarter of the night and the amount of REM sleep in the last quarter of the night,[25] suggesting that SWS prompts memory formation, which is possibly, but not necessarily, consolidated during REM sleep. There is further evidence of the complementary role of sleep in the offline (i.e., occurring outside of actual practice) processes of consolidation for visual perceptual learning. Indeed, others have found that repeated practice on the task within the same day does not lead to any improvement and can even result in performance deterioration for the trained visual quadrant, unless there is an intervening sleep episode.[109] But most important, they demonstrated that the duration of the sleep episode and its constituent phases are crucial in this process as 30-minute daytime naps merely discontinued performance deterioration over repeated sessions,[109] 60-minute naps reverted performance to its original level,[109] and 90-minute naps yielded improvement in discrimination performance.[118] The main difference was more time spent in NREM sleep in the 60-minute versus the 30-minute nap and the occurrence of REM sleep in the 90-minute nap. Other studies confirm the importance of posttraining sleep in the consolidation of coarse visual discrimination[120] as well as the effect of visual adaptation paradigms on subsequent sleep parameters,[121] thus demonstrating the importance of both REM and NREM sleep states for consolidation of procedural abilities in the visual system.

Interestingly, visual perceptual skill performance transfer to the untrained eye also tends to generalize to the untrained visual quadrant following sleep, suggesting that sleep contributes in the generalization of perceptual skill learning beyond the primary visual cortex.[122] However, sleep-dependent improvements cannot yet be fully generalized across modalities as contradictory results have been reported in the auditory domain.[123,124] Looking at more sophisticated auditory discrimination abilities, however, it has been shown that integration of newly learned spoken word forms, which must be discriminated from similar-sounding entries during auditory word recognition, requires an incubation-like period containing sleep.[125]

Sleep and Motor Learning

Studies of time-dependent evolution of motor learning found that posttraining sleep significantly enhances performance in the absence of further practice, as compared to the same amount of time-elapsed wake.[32,106,107] However, contrary to the observations made using perceptual visual discrimination tasks described in the prior section, it cannot be claimed here that posttraining time spent awake prevents the formation of long-term motor memories as performance merely stabilizes at the level achieved at the end of learning and does not deteriorate, but rather modestly improves over repeated practice sessions. Still, a transitory boost in performance is observed 5 to 30 minutes after the end of learning[126]; that disappears if tested without an intermediate sleep period more than 4 hours later.[32,126] Interestingly, performance improvement over the 5- to 30-minute boost predicts performance levels after a night of sleep.[126] This precocious posttraining period appears important for the initial stabilization of motor memories[13]; it has been shown that learning another sequence during that time can interfere with the initial sequence, unless a nap is allowed.[127] When a night of sleep occurs after initial training, offline gains in performance and increased activation in the putamen are observed using fMRI 12 hours later, as compared to an equivalent period of wake.[116,128] Sleep spindle density, particularly for fast frequency (~13 to 15 Hz) spindles at parietal regions, is correlated with both sleep-dependent behavioral changes[129] and neural changes.[130] With age, the beneficial impact of sleep on motor sequence consolidation is reduced, along with an age-related reduction in the activation of the putamen, in turn correlated with spindle density.[116] Noteworthy, a role of sleep for motor memory consolidation extends beyond a genuine motor component as training-related changes in sleep architecture are observed after practice of a sequence of finger movements but not after random key presses.[105] As well, sleep is important in the acquisition of new and complex motor patterns such as trampolining[131,132] but not after the familiar and well-known motor activities of soccer or dancing.[132] These latter results were in line with the demonstration that sleep provides maximal benefit for motor-skill procedures that proved to be most difficult during learning.[133] Motor learning–related changes in posttraining sleep parameters were mostly observed during stage 2 sleep,[33,106] although others have reported links with REM sleep[132] or both SWS and REM sleep, resulting in a lengthening of the ultradian sleep cycle.[131] Taken together, these results suggest that sleep may strengthen the initially labile memory trace formed during learning, possibly via a reactivation process.

Neuroimaging studies have shown that the striatum and motor cortical regions are recruited during motor sequence learning,[134–136] and striatal activity is enhanced when a retention interval contains sleep versus wake.[128] The extent of the increase in activation is associated with the features of sleep spindles (e.g., amplitude).[130] Thus spindles might be markers of consolidation that unfold during sleep. This hypothesis was directly tested using combined EEG-fMRI during sleep following acquisition of a motor sequence task.[44,46,137] Over a period of nocturnal sleep, the network of brain regions that were recruited during the initial performance of a motor skills task was transformed to recruit the putamen more strongly and became less reliant on motor cortical regions, consistent with the notion that sleep facilitates the automation of performance. Interestingly, the strength of functional communication within this consolidated network was increased only after a period of sleep, whereby functional connectivity in the putamen increased progressively with sleep but not wake.[44,137] In addition, sleep spindle activity in the same brain regions that were active during practice correlated with overnight improvement in performance and the change in functional connectivity. Moreover, spindles were associated with activation in striatal regions, suggesting that different types of spindles may consolidate different aspects of the memory trace. Further studies are needed to delineate precisely the role and benefit of sleep on various types of motor learning and the neurophysiologic mechanisms involved.

Sleep and Perceptual-Motor Learning

The motor learning tasks described previously have definite features. They are self-initiated, and acquisition is initially carried out in an explicit, almost declarative manner as the motor sequence of movements to be generated is already known and can even be verbalized. In this respect, motor procedural learning reflects the optimization of predefined motor forms, possibly created with the contribution of episodic memory processes. By contrast, perceptual-motor procedural learning entails a motor performance triggered by external stimulations, but the organization of the material to be learned is not necessarily obvious to the subject, although it affects their performance. These features should allow us to distinguish the role of sleep for consolidation of covertly versus overtly formed memories.

It was initially found that performance improvement on the pursuit rotor task was blocked by total sleep deprivation and sleep deprivation of the second part of the night, but not by selective REM sleep deprivation.[18] Task improvement was also associated with increased sleep spindle activity,[38,138] together suggesting that consolidation of motor adaptive memories is mostly dependent on stage 2 sleep. fMRI additionally showed that posttraining total sleep deprivation hampered both performance improvement and the reorganization of brain activity on a visuomotor pursuit task with hidden regularities in the target's trajectory.[21] However, mirror-tracing skills were reported to improve more during the late part of the night[9] and to be associated with REM sleep increases in well-performing individuals,[27] suggesting that this latter task may rather be REM-sleep dependent. Still, performance improvement on mirror tracing was also found to occur after naps dominated by stage 2 sleep[139] and to correlate with stage 2 sleep spindle activity. This apparent discrepancy between sleep stages and task associations within the perceptual-motor learning domain might be explained by differences in initial skill levels of participants. Indeed, an association was reported between performance improvement on the pursuit rotor task and stage 2 spindle activity in highly skilled subjects, whereas a similar relationship was established with REM sleep density in lower skilled subjects,[38] in line with the proposal that motor skills tasks involving REM and stage 2 sleep might be dependent on two separate, but overlapping, neural systems.[29]

This interpretation may be consistent with neuroimaging data that have established a relationship between posttraining REM sleep activity and the consolidation of higher-order perceptual-motor cognitive skills. Indeed, subcortical and neocortical areas already activated during practice on a probabilistic sequence learning task[134] (i.e., a paradigm of implicit sequence learning) were reactivated during posttraining REM sleep in subjects previously trained to the task.[41,42,49] It was further demonstrated that these reactivations were not merely activity dependent but specifically occurred as a result of the fact that a rules-based sequence was implicitly learned during prior practice,[42] supporting the possibility that REM sleep is deeply involved in the reprocessing and optimization of the high-order information contained in the material to be learned (as in the mirror tracing task, and Tower of Hanoi). Most recently, it has been shown that the acquisition of expertise on such higher-order information benefits from sleep and that NREM sleep might "fine-tune" the motor skills required to perform and learn the underlying strategy.[29,38,140] Indeed, one study showed that sleep, but not wake, facilitates the application of a newly acquired cognitive strategy to a more complex problem but not the motor movements involved in acquiring the strategy itself.[141]

These results appear to contradict the previously mentioned findings of REM-sleep dependency for high-order probabilistic sequence learning in which learning was undoubtedly implicit.[42,134] However, one overlooked difference between these studies and those claiming a sleep-dependency exclusively for explicit sequential material is that the latter have used deterministic, repeated sequences, whereas the probabilistic sequences used in the former studies are much more ambiguous. Accordingly, neural responses to unpredictable elements in the probabilistic SRT were attenuated over sleep, suggesting better integration of the learned structure.[24] It is therefore possible that sleep (and especially REM sleep) mostly supports the consolidation of implicitly acquired complex relationships. This interpretation may be in line with the proposal that different aspects of a procedural memory are processed separately during consolidation. For example, the movement sequence in itself (e.g., a repeated, deterministic sequence) improves over daytime wakefulness periods independently of sleep, whereas its goal (e.g., the complex, abstract rules for items succession in a probabilistic sequence) improves after a night of sleep.[142] Further studies tried disentangling motor learning from cognitively complex strategies involved in higher-order sequences of movements, as well as deterministic sequences of motor movements. Specifically, mounting evidence suggests that the benefit of sleep for procedural motor skills would occur only if the task is learned explicitly, in other words, with conscious awareness. Thus, when the sequence is learned implicitly, performance would not benefit following a night of sleep over and above an equivalent period of wakefulness,[24,42,143] although this remains to be thoroughly investigated. In terms of higher-order cognitive strategies that are acquired through motor skills practice, there is also mounting evidence to suggest that sleep and only sleep would enhance performance for motor skills that require the acquisition of a novel cognitive strategy.[140,141] Interestingly, when compared directly to a condition that involves the same sequence of movements but where access to information needed to learn the strategy is not available, sleep preferentially enhances memory for the cognitive strategy per se, but not the implicit motor skills used to acquire the strategy. Moreover, it appears that for this type of procedural skill learning, both stage 2 and REM sleep are involved in the mastery of the cognitive strategy.[140] These issues remain to be further investigated to determine the exact conditions in which sleep is beneficial to postlearning consolidation processes for motor learning.

Sleep and Priming

Perceptual priming refers to the facilitation or bias in the processing of a stimulus as a function of a recent encounter with that stimulus.[144] The few studies that have investigated a role for sleep in consolidating the memory representations subtending priming[83,145] have yielded discrepant results.[145,146] Studies have found that intervening deprivation of sleep, especially REM sleep, alters priming effects in word stem completion[83] and face processing[146,147] and enhances reactivity for emotional pictures.[148] However, another study failed to disclose sleep-dependent effects using better controlled tachistoscopic identification of drawings,[145] and total sleep deprivation was found to affect priming-like performance in the right hemisphere only, suggesting interhemispheric differences in sleep-dependent processes of memory consolidation.[146]

SLEEP-DEPENDENT MECHANISMS OF BRAIN PLASTICITY AND MEMORY CONSOLIDATION

In this section, we provide an overview of specific mechanisms viewed as particularly important to support sleep stage–related processes of brain plasticity and memory consolidation: (1) PGO waves, (2) hippocampal rhythms, and (3) sleep spindles.

Ponto-geniculo-occipital Waves

PGO waves are prominent phasic bioelectrical potentials closely related to rapid eye movements occurring in isolation or in bursts during the transition from NREM to REM sleep or during REM sleep itself. In humans, intracerebral recordings in epileptic patients,[149] noninvasive PET,[150] fMRI,[151] and MEG[152] scanning in healthy volunteers indicate that the rapid eye movements observed during REM sleep are generated by mechanisms similar or identical to PGO waves in animals. Most importantly, animal data indicate that PGO activity during REM sleep is associated with learning and memory consolidation,[153] suggesting that activation of this generator during REM sleep may represent one of the natural physiologic processes of memory, possibly through the synchronization of fast oscillations that would convey experience-dependent information in thalamocortical and intracortical circuits.[154]

Despite evidence from animal studies, a direct demonstration of the association between PGO activity and memory consolidation during REM sleep in humans has yet to be done. Nonetheless, the hypothesis is supported by studies showing an increase in the density of rapid eye movements during REM sleep after procedural learning[29,155] and intensive learning periods,[28] and by correlations between declarative memory performance[156] or retention levels after learning a Morse code[157] and rapid eye movements during posttraining REM sleep.[157] Also, presenting sounds in the background while learning a complex logic task at wake enhanced next morning performance when the same sounds were presented again during REM sleep. Most interestingly, however, enhancement was found only when sounds were coincident with the bursts of posttraining rapid eye movements that reflect PGO activity,[53] further suggesting its association with memory consolidation processes. Also, it has been proposed that during human phasic REM sleep, propagation of PGO activity in the parahippocampal/hippocampal areas is linked with verbal learning performance and mnemonic retention values.[158]

Hippocampal Rhythms

The theta rhythm (i.e., regular sinusoidal oscillations in the frequency range of 4 to 7 Hz recorded in the hippocampal EEG) constitutes a prominent signature of REM sleep in mammals including humans.[159] Theta represents the "on-line" state of the hippocampus, believed to be critical for temporal coding/decoding of active neuronal ensembles and the modification of synaptic weights.[159] Additionally, population synchrony of pyramidal cells is maximal during quiet wakefulness and SWS, associated with sharp waves (i.e., sharp waves of SWS are the consequence of synchronous discharge of bursting CA3 pyramidal neurons) and fast ripples (140 to 200 Hz). Sharp waves and ripples during SWS constitute good candidates to induce neuronal plasticity.[160] Hence the alternation between both REM sleep/active wake theta activity and SWS/quiet wakefulness sharp waves and ripples could contribute to brain plasticity. According to the two-stage model of memory formation,[160] neocortical information activates the entorhinal input, which will cause synaptic changes to occur in the hippocampal CA3 system during learning associated with active waking and REM sleep theta rhythmic activity in the hippocampus. In the subsequent non-theta state (i.e., SWS but also possibly quiet wakefulness), previously activated neurons are reactivated during sharp waves bursts, and the memory representation transiently stored in the CA3 region can be transferred to neocortical targets for the long term.

Also, animal[161] and human studies have shown increases in theta rhythms during REM sleep following learning in declarative memory tasks,[27] as well as correlations between theta during REM sleep and memory facilitation for emotional tasks.[162] Human brain imaging studies have demonstrated after spatial navigation in a virtual town the experience-dependent reactivation of hippocampal activity during SWS, but not during REM sleep.[43] Additionally, intracerebral recordings in humans suggest that slow EEG frequencies in the hippocampus during NREM sleep contribute to the consolidation of spatial memories.[163] Similarly, an odor-cued activation in hippocampus-related memory areas was observed during SWS,[55] eventually leading to overnight performance improvement. These studies also found long-term transfer of hippocampal memories toward neocortical stores,[22,81] an effect disturbed by sleep deprivation on the posttraining night.[22] In parallel, neuroimaging data have suggested the offline persistence of memory-related cerebral activity during active wakefulness and its dynamic evolution in the hippocampus.[13] Although this model is well supported by the previously mentioned data and may account for the offline processing of declarative material, the fact that reactivations have been observed both during posttraining REM sleep[41,42] and wakefulness[13] after procedural, non-hippocampal learning suggests that other routes for consolidation exist, which should likewise be investigated.

Sleep Spindles, Slow Waves, and Hippocampal Ripples

Although spindles occur most frequently in stage 2, they also appear to a lesser extent in SWS but are obscured by delta activity. Spindles are considered to be due to the intrinsic properties and to the connectivity patterns of the thalamic neurons and are regulated by SOs.[164] Spindle generation seems an ideal mechanism for neural plasticity.[89] Therefore spindles may play an important role in the processes of memory consolidation during sleep. Accordingly, several studies have reported links between the consolidation of verbal declarative memory and increases in spindle density during nocturnal and diurnal sleep that follows learning.[30,31,35,36] Verbal memory association with spindle density increased in the left frontocentral scalp location at night, whereas memory for faces did not elicit this effect.[36] Similarly, postlearning increases are observed during daytime napping in low sigma frequency spectral power (11.25 to 13.75 Hz), particularly in the left frontal scalp region. Additionally, these increases are positively correlated with learning performance for difficult word associations, but not easy word associations,[31] and the integration of new verbal learning with existing knowledge is correlated with sleep spindles.[165]

Recent studies have attempted to causally manipulate spindles to investigate memory enhancement processes. One such study observed that increasing sleep spindle density improved verbal memory.[113] A functional neuroimaging investigation found hippocampal reactivation during sleep after declarative learning, time-locked to the onset of sleep spindles, modulated by spindle amplitude, and correlated with memory performance.[45,166] It suggests that spindles are actively involved in memory consolidation, possibly via repeated reactivation of the newly formed memory. This process may also drive communication between brain regions, resulting in a transformation of the memory trace, whereby it becomes increasingly reliant on brain regions that support automization of performance (e.g., the striatum). Moreover, SOs group faster frequencies including spindles (see the review by Steriade[164]). Recent studies provided potential insight into the functional significance of these phase-amplitude interactions for memory consolidation.[167,168] Specifically, the up state of the SO is coupled to spindles following learning. These two temporally related events may work together, whereby spindles may induce synaptic strengthening.[169] By contrast, SWA may be involved in synaptic downscaling,[170] a necessary operation for the optimization of newly formed memories. In addition to the cross-frequency coupling of slow waves and spindles, higher-frequency bursts of hippocampal activity (100 to 200 Hz), or "ripples," are also temporally coupled to spindles.[171,172] This coordination between neocortical spindles and hippocampal ripples has been suggested as a putative mechanism of hippocampal-neocortical information transfer.[171] Finally, further studies demonstrated the necessity for a silent and undisturbed plastic period during sleep after cueing in a TMR procedure to achieve successful reactivation and the ensuing gain in memory consolidation.[60,61] Indeed, the presentation of a conditioned stimulus was repeatedly shown to elicit increased sigma (spindle)-related activity, however, the presentation of a second auditory stimulation within a 1300-msec range period both disrupts sigma activity and cancels the beneficial effect of cueing on memory. Taken together, these studies suggest that sleep spindles are important for the overnight consolidation of declarative memories and that the occurrence of sleep spindles in brain structures recruited during initial learning contributes to the reactivation and consolidation processes along with the coordinated activity of cortical SOs and hippocampal ripples.

Similarly for procedural memory, posttraining stage 2 sleep deprivation impaired memory for a perceptual-motor task,[18] and the amount of stage 2 sleep correlated with learning progress on the finger-tapping task.[106] Also, intensive training on perceptual-motor learning tasks results in marked increases in number and density of spindles during subsequent stage 2 sleep[27] as well as an increase in average spindle duration.[27] Posttraining increases in slow sigma power (12 to 14 Hz) have been observed in frontal and occipital regions with no changes in high-frequency sigma.[27] Napping studies using the same task provided similar results: subjects who take naps regularly showed positive correlations between postnap performance and stage 2 spindle density.[173] In this case, low-frequency spindle activity (12 to 14 Hz) was correlated with performance at frontal sites, whereas high-frequency spindle activity (14 to 16 Hz) was correlated with performance at central and parietal sites. Moreover, subjects who did not nap on a regular basis did not benefit from the nap.[173] In another study using a longer (60- to 90-minute) nap after motor performance for the finger tapping task, it was found that subjects with the most significant increases in motor performance also had the largest increases in stage 2 sleep, with a significant correlation between spindle density and postnap performance that was confined to the learning hemisphere.[32] Finally, a marked increase in stage 2 spindle densities was observed after acquisition of the finger tapping task, but not after a control motor task, indicating that the changes were not due to general motor activity.[105] Neuroimaging studies also revealed that, similar to declarative memory, activation time-locked to sleep spindles in brain regions (e.g., hippocampus, putamen) recruited during practice of a motor procedural task was correlated with overnight gains in performance.[46] The fact that spindles have been related to consolidation both for declarative and nondeclarative memories indicates their prominent role in sleep-dependent memory processes, although it remains to be investigated if spindles subserve the same process across declarative and procedural memory.

Finally, spindle oscillations may not act in isolation, as they are grouped and regulated by slow waves[174] that are thought important for memory consolidation and synaptic plasticity, as discussed previously. Indeed, experience-dependent regional increases in delta activity have been observed during NREM sleep,[51] suggesting the existence of local homeostatic mechanisms for memory consolidation.[170] Furthermore, coherence was found to increase after learning in the depolarizing phase of the SOs below the 1-Hz frequency.[174] Conversely, tDCS that may contribute to modulation of cortical excitability was found to improve the overnight retention of declarative memories when applied during NREM sleep at a slow rhythm whose frequency (<1 Hz) approximates SOs.[54] Further, reducing SWA during NREM sleep with tDCS reduces verbal declarative memory retention,[175] suggesting a causal relationship between slow waves and declarative memory. Taken together, available data suggest that SOs during NREM sleep may play a facilitating role in neuronal plasticity and the ongoing transformations and consolidation of memory traces, either in concert with spindles, or perhaps contributing in some unique way to memory consolidation processes. Further study is required to better dissociate the unique roles that these two interrelated aspects of NREM sleep may have for memory consolidation.

SLEEP AND INTELLECTUAL ABILITIES

Trait-like interindividual differences in cognitive strengths and weaknesses are often described in terms of "intelligence" and can be described as a subset of factors consisting of distinct cognitive domains and skills (e.g., fluid intelligence and crystallized intelligence).[176] The sleep spindle is the only known spontaneous neural oscillation that has been identified as an electrophysiologic marker of cognitive abilities and aptitudes that are typically assessed by intelligence quotient (IQ) tests (see the review by Fogel and Smith[138]). Spindles have even been suggested as one of possibly many "electrophysiologic fingerprints," because they are remarkably stable from night to night but vary considerably from one individual to another.[177]

Interindividual differences in spindle characteristics are related to the capacity for reasoning, that is, the ability to identify complex patterns and relationships, the use of logic, existing knowledge, skills, and experience to solve novel problems.[33,178-180] Moreover, the relationship between spindles and cognitive abilities seems to be predominantly specific to the capacity for reasoning and not verbal abilities or short-term memory[181,182] and to be independent of other related factors such as sleep quality and circadian chronotype.[183] However, the neuroanatomic and neurophysiologic mechanisms that mediate the relationship between spindles and cognitive abilities remain largely unknown. Interestingly, a large subset of the brain regions recruited during spindle activity are known to support reasoning abilities. It has been recently shown that the neural activation patterns time-locked with spindles correlate with reasoning but not verbal or short-term memory abilities.[181] Moreover, functional connectivity of the cortical-striatal circuitry and the thalamocortical circuitry were related to reasoning abilities, but not short-term memory or verbal abilities.[182] Taken together, available evidence suggests that spindles may serve as an electrophysiologic marker of brain efficiency and activations in brain regions that support the ability to employ reasoning to solve problems and apply logic in novel situations.

CONCLUSIONS

Although elusive at times, studies supporting the proposal that sleep is an integral component in the off-line processes that subtend memory consolidation have now substantially flourished. Still, when compared to other domains of cognition, the field obviously remains underdeveloped. Indeed, there is an urgent need of replication and validation of studies to confirm or disprove a series of hypotheses regarding the type of memories that can benefit from sleep and in which circumstances it can occur. Furthermore, the mechanisms that support these processes remain to be fully elucidated and/or fully understood. And most importantly, it remains for us to understand how sleep disorders and the numerous pathologies accompanied by sleep disturbances affect cognitive processes and especially learning and memory in humans.

CLINICAL PEARL

In the long term, patients with inadequate REM sleep may be expected to experience more difficulty learning novel cognitive procedures than same-age individuals with healthy sleep. Patients exhibiting little or impaired SWS may be impaired in declarative learning (e.g., in memorizing large amounts of factual material). Those with specific stage 2 sleep disturbances (e.g., reduced spindles) may be expected to have trouble refining and performing reasonably simple motor skill tasks and exhibit declarative memory deficits. These sleep state abnormalities may serve as markers and perhaps even therapeutic targets of cognitive deficits in psychiatric and neurologic conditions. Finally, those patients with poor sleep quality or pathologies affecting all sleep stages would be expected to have deteriorated long-term memory performance pervasively on all types of memory. As sleep is only a part of memory consolidation processes, however, these deficits may manifest in a subtle manner and be compensated to a certain extent by alternate consolidation strategies taking place either at wake or during sleep.

SELECTED READINGS

Cowan E, Liu A, Henin S, Kothare S, Devinsky O, Davachi L. Sleep spindles promote the restructuring of memory representations in ventromedial prefrontal cortex through enhanced hippocampal-cortical functional connectivity. *J Neurosci.* 2020;40(9):1909–1919.

Feld GB, Born J. Neurochemical mechanisms for memory processing during sleep: basic findings in humans and neuropsychiatric implications. *Neuropsychopharmacology.* 2020;45(1):31–44.

Fernandez LMJ, Lüthi A. Sleep spindles: mechanisms and functions. *Physiol Rev.* 2020;100(2):805–868. https://doi.org/10.1152/physrev.00042.2018.

Fogel S, Smith C. The function of the sleep spindle: a physiological index of intelligence and a mechanism for sleep-dependent memory consolidation. *Neurosci Biobehav Rev.* 2011;35:1154–1165.

Maquet P, Smith C, Stickgold R, eds. *Sleep and Brain Plasticity.* Oxford: Oxford University Press; 2003.

Peigneux P, Urbain C, Schmitz R. Sleep and the brain. In: Espie C, Morin C, eds. New-York: Oxford University Press; 2011:11–37.

Rasch B, Born J. About sleep's role in memory. *Physiol Rev.* 2013;93:681–766.

Urbain C, Galer S, Van Bogaert P, et al. Pathophysiology of sleep-dependent memory consolidation processes in children. *Int J Psychophysiol.* 2013;89:273–283.

A complete reference list can be found online at ExpertConsult.com.

Chapter 30

Sensory and Motor Processing during Sleep and Wakefulness

John H. Peever; Han-Hee Lee; Barry J. Sessle

Chapter Highlights

- Sensory and motor processing are reduced during sleep, and their integration is differentially affected during different sleep states. For example, respiratory reflexes are reduced during non–rapid eye movement (NREM) sleep but are virtually abolished during rapid eye movement (REM) sleep. Such observations suggest that discrete NREM and REM sleep mechanisms modulate and control sensory and motor processes in a sleep state–dependent manner.
- Changes in sensory processing during sleep affect the somatosensory pathways that transduce and relay nociceptive signals to and within the central nervous system. Sensory mechanisms are affected by sleep, and sleep is in turn affected by nociceptive processes. The interaction between pain and sleep is common in patients suffering from chronic pain states, such as pain related to cancer or temporomandibular disorders.
- Abnormal sensory and motor functions during sleep underlie common sleep disorders. For example, reduced chemical control of breathing during sleep plays a role in congenital central hypoventilation syndrome, and pathologic motor control during REM sleep underlies REM sleep behavior disorder. Abnormal motor control and sensory processes also are associated with periodic limb movement disorder, sleep bruxism, narcolepsy, and sleep apnea.

Sleep has a profound impact on the mechanisms by which the central nervous system (CNS) transduces and expresses sensory and motor commands. Transmission of sensory information to the CNS is markedly attenuated during sleep, which enables sleep continuity; in certain circumstances, however, some sensory inputs, such as pain, may influence sleep patterns. Sleep mechanisms not only modulate the pathways that relay sensory commands to the CNS but also affect the manner in which regulatory brain centers, such as the thalamocortical circuits, relay afferent inflow to appropriate sensory and motor control centers, including somatic motoneurons. The neurocircuits that generate sleep-wake states also affect the fundamental integration and expression of sensorimotor processes.

This chapter focuses on three main topics: (1) pathways and mechanisms of sensory processes, especially those related to pain; (2) the integration of sensory and motor processes; and (3) respiratory reflexes. Each of these is considered during both sleep and wakefulness. Also discussed is how sleep influences the central processing of nociceptive information and how pain itself may affect sleep. Although all sensory and motor systems are affected by sleep, a primary focus in this context is on how sleep affects the sensorimotor processes related to reflex functions, including spinal reflexes and jaw reflexes, as well as the respiratory responses to chemical (e.g., carbon dioxide [CO_2]) and mechanical stimuli (e.g., airway pressure). The clinical correlates of these features and underlying processes are also presented because an appreciation of these physiologic systems is important for the clinician to realize that sleep-related changes in sensory-motor processing and their integration have a direct impact on human health and disease and can underlie common and serious sleep-related disorders.

MODULATION OF SENSORY PROCESSES DURING SLEEP AND WAKEFULNESS

Sensory Pathways and Mechanisms

The body's peripheral tissues, such as skin, mucosa, teeth, muscles, and joints, are supplied by small-, medium-, and large-diameter primary afferent nerve fibers. Most of the medium-diameter (A-delta) and large-diameter (A-beta) afferents are myelinated and terminate in the tissues as sense organs (receptors) detecting tactile or proprioceptive stimuli applied to the tissues. However, some of the A-delta afferents, along with unmyelinated C-fiber afferents, terminate in the tissues as free nerve endings; some of these function as thermoreceptors responding to warming or cooling stimuli, but many of them instead act as nociceptors, that is, they are the sense organs that respond to noxious stimulation of the peripheral tissues. The activation of ion channels and membrane receptors on the nociceptive afferent terminals may

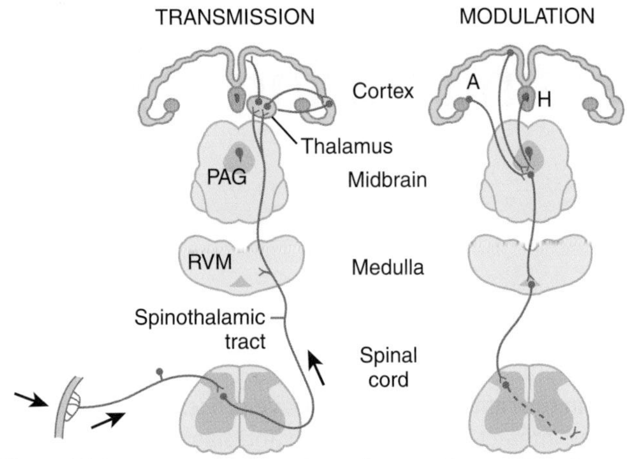

Figure 30.1 Major nociceptive pathways from spinal tissues. This schematic shows the ascending and descending pathways that transmit and modulate nociceptive signals from spinally innervated tissues. Nociceptive afferents synapse onto spinothalamic neurons in the spinal dorsal horn, which in turn relay afferent signals to the thalamus and then to the cortex (e.g., anterior and posterior cingulate cortex). Ascending spinothalamic neuronal inputs also are modulated by descending pathways located in higher brain centers, such as the cortex, amygdala (A), and hypothalamus (H). Such descending pathways converge in the periaqueductal gray (PAG) and then in the rostral ventral medulla (RVM) before synapsing onto spinothalamic neurons. (From Price DD. *Psychological Mechanisms of Pain and Analgesia.* IASP Press; 1999:250–71.)

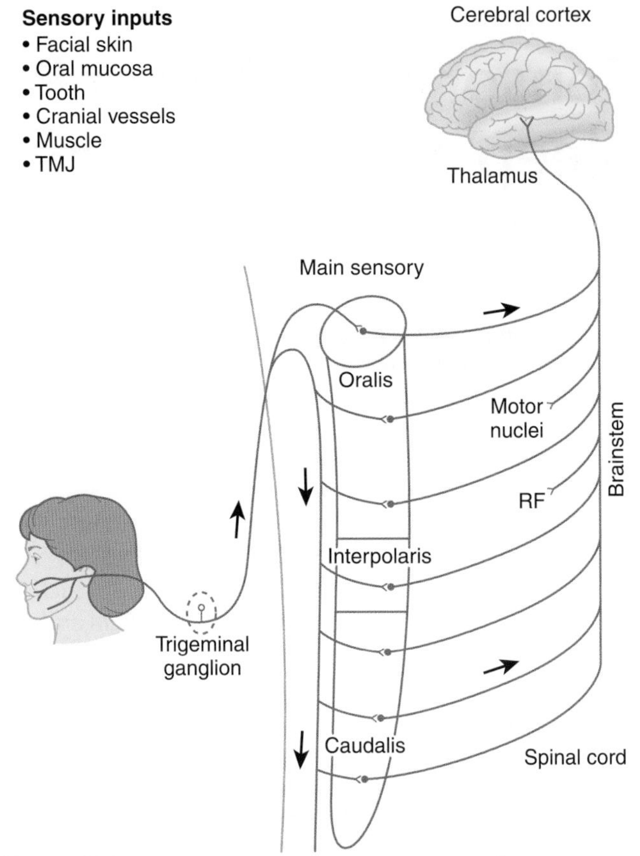

Figure 30.2 Major somatosensory pathway from the face and mouth. Trigeminal primary afferents project by way of the trigeminal ganglion to second-order neurons in the trigeminal brainstem sensory nuclear complex. These neurons may project to neurons in higher levels of the brain (e.g., thalamus) or in brainstem regions, such as cranial motor pools or the reticular formation (RF). *Not shown* are the projections of some cervical nerves and cranial nerve VII, X, and XII afferents to the trigeminal complex and the projection of many VII, IX, and X afferents to the solitary tract nucleus. TMJ, Temporomandibular joint. (From Sessle BJ. Acute and chronic craniofacial pain: brainstem mechanisms of nociceptive transmission and neuroplasticity, and their clinical correlates. *Crit Rev Oral Biol Med.* 2000;11:57–91.)

result in the elicitation of action potentials in the A delta or C-fiber afferents, and these action potentials are conducted along the afferents into the CNS and thereby provide the brain with sensory-discriminative information about the location, quality, intensity, and duration of the noxious stimulus.[1–8]

After tissue injury or inflammation, a prolonged increase in excitability of the nociceptors frequently occurs, and they become more responsive to noxious stimulation or even start responding to stimuli that normally are innocuous. This "peripheral sensitization" may contribute to the hyperalgesia (increased sensitivity to a stimulus that is normally painful) and allodynia (pain resulting from a stimulus that normally does not provoke pain) that occur in certain pain conditions. Numerous chemical mediators are involved in peripheral sensitization and in the activation of nociceptors by noxious stimuli.[1,9–11]

The primary afferents in spinal nerves activated by tactile or proprioceptive stimulation of tissues of the limbs, trunk, and neck project to the spinal cord, where they synapse on and activate second-order nonnociceptive neurons (e.g., low-threshold mechanoreceptive [LTM] neurons) predominantly located in the spinal dorsal horn and the dorsal column nuclei.[7,8] Analogous trigeminal (V) afferents innervating orofacial tissues terminate at all levels of the trigeminal brainstem sensory nuclear complex (V-BSNC). This structure is subdivided into the main or principal sensory nucleus and the spinal tract nucleus.[6,12,13] Subnucleus caudalis, the most caudal component is the V-BSNC, has many anatomic and physiologic features analogous to those of the spinal dorsal horn and is nowadays often referred to as the medullary dorsal horn.[11,12] Spinal and V primary afferents carrying thermoreceptive or nociceptive information terminate, respectively, in the spinal dorsal horn (Figure 30.1) and subnucleus caudalis (Figure 30.2), and through their release of excitatory neurotransmitters or neuromodulators (e.g., glutamate and substance P) can activate nociceptive neurons that are of two main types: nociceptive-specific (NS) neurons, which are excited only by noxious stimuli (e.g., pinch, heat) applied to a localized receptive field in peripheral tissues (e.g., skin), and wide-dynamic-range (WDR) neurons, which are excited by nonnoxious (e.g., tactile) stimuli and by noxious stimuli.[8,11,12]

Some NS and WDR neurons in the spinal dorsal horn and subnucleus caudalis are activated only by noxious stimulation of superficial (e.g., cutaneous) tissues and possess encoding properties, suggesting that they are critical neural elements for the detection and discrimination of superficial pain. However, nociceptive information from deep tissues (e.g., muscle, joint, viscera) is processed predominantly by nociceptive spinal dorsal horn or caudalis neurons that receive extensive convergent afferent inputs from these tissues and from skin. These convergence patterns appear to underlie the CNS mechanisms contributing to deep pain and also may explain the poor localization, spread, and referral of pain that is typical of pain conditions involving deep tissues.

Neuroplastic changes can be manifested in caudalis and spinal dorsal horn nociceptive neurons as a result of nociceptive afferent inputs evoked by injury or inflammation.[8,11,12] This neuroplasticity results from the release from the nociceptive afferent terminals of neurochemicals (e.g., glutamate) that induce a cascade of intracellular events in the nociceptive neurons by acting on ion channels or membrane receptors on the neurons. These events can result in an increase in nociceptive neuronal excitability, reflecting a "central sensitization" of the nociceptive neurons. Central sensitization has been documented in both acute and chronic pain models and involves nonneuronal (i.e., glial cell) and neural processes. The neuroplastic alterations underlying central sensitization represent mechanisms that, along with peripheral sensitization (discussed previously), can explain the allodynia and hyperalgesia, as well as pain spread and referral that characterize several pain conditions.

The solitary tract nucleus (NTS) is another brainstem region receiving primary afferent inputs, in this case from respiratory and alimentary tract afferents, taste afferents, and cardiovascular, chemoreceptor, and baroreceptor afferents. The NTS plays an important role in autonomic (e.g., respiratory, cardiovascular) functions, taste, and reflexes evoked by stimuli applied to the respiratory and alimentary tracts (e.g., cough, swallow).

Some neurons in the spinal dorsal horn, dorsal column nuclei, NTS, and the V-BSNC give rise to axons that ramify within that structure and serve to modulate the activity of other neurons. Nevertheless, many neurons in these structures project to other spinal cord or brainstem regions, including the reticular formation, periaqueductal grey (PAG), raphe nuclei, and spinal ventral horn or cranial nerve motor nuclei. Such connections provide the central circuitry underlying autonomic and muscle reflex responses to peripheral stimuli or provide sensory inputs to neurons in some of these structures that contribute to descending modulatory systems (discussed later) by which noxious stimulation may influence sleep and consciousness.[14,15]

Many neurons in the spinal dorsal horn, dorsal column nuclei, NTS, and V-BSNC also (or instead) project to the contralateral thalamus (Figures 30.1 and 30.2). The main thalamic regions receiving and relaying this sensory information are the ventrobasal complex (or ventroposterior nucleus in the primate), medial thalamus, and posterior nuclear group.[7,11,16,17] These thalamic regions contain LTM, thermoreceptive, NS, and WDR neurons, some of which project to the overlying somatosensory cerebral cortex, where their relayed signals are processed to provide for the detection and localization of tactile, nonnoxious thermal, and noxious stimuli. In the case of pain, such spatiotemporal encoding through this thalamic-somatosensory cortical circuitry is thought to be crucial for the sensory-discriminative dimension of pain. By contrast, the spatiotemporal encoding properties of most nociceptive neurons in the medial thalamic nuclei and posterior nuclear group and their connections to areas such as the anterior cingulate cortex are more suggestive of a role in the motivational or affective dimensions of pain.[18,19] It also is noteworthy that neurons at brain higher levels (e.g., somatosensory thalamus, sensorimotor cortex) also are subject to neuroplastic changes reflecting central sensitization.

Modulation of Sensory Processes, Including Those Related to Pain

The thalamocortical transfer and processing of sensory information is subject to modulation or "gating" as a result of facilitatory and inhibitory processes exerted by local neural circuits or inputs to the thalamus and cortex from other CNS regions, such as the reticular formation.[1,20–23] These gating processes are especially apparent during changes in behavioral state and consciousness. During non–rapid eye movement (NREM) sleep, for example, there is marked attenuation of the sensory information flow from the thalamus; this likely serves to maintain sleep continuity. In contrast, flow is still very evident or even increased during wakefulness in order that arousal and cognition are maintained.

Nonetheless, modification of somatosensory transmission also can occur at spinal and brainstem levels and, in addition, may be operational in various degrees during different behavioral states and indeed may contribute to specific features of these states—for example, the hypotonia of rapid eye movement (REM) sleep. These modulatory mechanisms may involve neural circuits within the spinal dorsal horn, V-BSNC, and NTS and adjacent regions, as well as inputs from primary afferents and descending inputs from reticular formation, raphe nuclei, locus coeruleus (LC), and the cerebral cortex, to name a few. Various neurochemicals are used by these circuits and inputs, including gamma-aminobutyric acid (GABA), norepinephrine, 5-hydroxytryptamine (5-HT), and opioids.

In the case of nociceptive transmission, the variety of inputs and interconnections in spinal dorsal horn and subnucleus caudalis noted earlier provide the basis for considerable interaction between the various afferent inputs derived from peripheral tissues (e.g., so-called segmental or afferent inhibition) or from intrinsic brain regions (e.g., descending inhibition).[11] Examples are the interneuronal system within the substantia gelatinosa of the spinal dorsal horn and subnucleus caudalis, and the descending inputs to these structures from the PAG/raphe nuclei, reticular formation, cerebral cortex, and several other brain centers (Figure 30.1). Several neurochemicals, including GABA, 5-HT, norepinephrine, dopamine, hypocretin, cholecystokinin, prolactin, melatonin, and opioids (e.g., enkephalins), provide a neurochemical substrate by which many of the afferent and descending inputs can exert their modulatory actions on nociceptive transmission. Of note, many of these neurochemicals and descending influences also are involved in sleep mechanisms.[20,21] Inhibitory influences exerted by many of these inputs on nociceptive neurons have been implicated as intrinsic mechanisms contributing to the analgesic effects of several procedures used to control pain, including deep brain stimulation, acupuncture, and opiate-related (e.g., morphine) and 5-HT agonist (e.g., amitriptyline) drugs. Some have, instead, a role in facilitating nociceptive transmission (e.g., in the central sensitization process noted earlier).[8,11,12]

Processing Related to Pain during Sleep and Wakefulness

As noted previously, sensory transmission through the spinal cord and brainstem, as well as the thalamus and cerebral cortex, may be modulated during sleep and thereby may contribute, for example, to the decreased responsiveness to external stimuli during NREM sleep to favor sleep continuity. The modulatory influences on nociceptive neurons of behavioral factors, including state of alertness, attention, and distraction, are just some examples in which the higher brain centers involved in these states give rise to descending influences operating at these levels and thereby contribute to the influence of these behavioral factors on pain. Unfortunately, although much has been learned independently about pain and sleep, investigation of how sleep affects pain and vice versa has been limited, especially in the case of interactions between chronic pain and sleep (see Chapter 156).[14]

Sensory processing, including that related to pain, is reduced in sleep states compared with wakefulness, but the underlying processes are still unclear. However, it has been shown that somatosensory transmission through several ascending pathways originating in the spinal dorsal horn is tonically diminished during REM sleep. Apparently, the gating process is quite complex during REM sleep because modulation of somatosensory transmission may be different between phasic and tonic REM sleep.[24] Other evidence of complex gating during NREM sleep includes findings that sensory transmission through some ascending tracts may be attenuated in some stages of NREM sleep and that this is reflected in reduced thalamic and cortical activity in these sta ges.[21,22,24–26] The modulation of spinal sensory transmission during REM sleep appears to involve presynaptic inhibition and postsynaptic inhibitory mechanisms,[24] supporting earlier findings that presynaptic regulatory processes are important in REM sleep and contribute to the reduction in motor activity during this sleep phase (discussed later). In addition, the presynaptic inhibitory processes in the spinal cord use GABA, and the postsynaptic inhibition uses glycine. Several other neurochemicals released from neurons in higher brain centers also have been implicated in the sleep-dependent modulation of spinal cord neurons or their thalamic targets; these include 5-HT, norepinephrine, acetylcholine, and hypocretin.[14,21,24–26]

A complex gating mechanism also has been documented in the rostral components of the V-BSNC that is state-dependent; for example, the activity of many rostral V-BSNC neurons and their responses to sensory inputs, including those evoked by noxious (tooth pulp) stimuli, may be presynaptically and postsynaptically inhibited during REM sleep through, respectively, GABA and glycine-based modulatory processes.[14,21,24–26] Comparable investigations, however, have not been made in more caudal V-BSNC nociceptive (e.g., caudalis) neurons, which as noted previously have many features analogous to those of spinal dorsal horn nociceptive neurons and play crucial roles in trigeminal nociceptive transmission; thus, if and how sleep stages affect their properties constitute an important area of future study. Of note, the state-dependent processes on spinal and V-BSNC nociceptive transmission that have been revealed have been studied only in acute sleep models, and it is unclear what neural modulatory processes are involved in the more clinically challenging sleep-pain interactions that may occur in chronic pain conditions (discussed later). Furthermore, if nociceptive afferents inputs do reach cortical levels and result in the conscious feeling of pain, then sleep may be disrupted to alert the subject to the noxious event.

Clinical Correlates

When healthy subjects are sleeping in conditions favoring good sleep quality (e.g., a quiet, comfortable environment), low-intensity stimuli may have little or no effect on sleep quality, whereas a loud noise or a sudden pain attack during sleep can produce awakening that may potentially trigger anxiety or concern that impedes subsequent sleep.[14,27] Nonetheless, several other factors in addition to pain can influence sleep quality (e.g., past experiences, psychological variables, anxiety, mood, life style, health status, and any concomitant pain-sleep interactions).

Patients with pain may experience long delays in falling asleep, as well as sleep-stage shifts, frequent sleep arousals, and undesirable body movements; furthermore, some analgesic drugs (e.g., opioids) may affect sleep patterns (see Chapter 52).[14] Insomnia is a feature of about one-third of patients with chronic pain,[28,29] and although the majority of patients with chronic pain report that pain occurred before or at the onset of poor sleep, suggesting that pain may have a direct effect on sleep quality, studies using experimental noxious stimuli have revealed only minor sleep disturbance in healthy subjects.[30,31] However, these studies have elicited acute pain, and it remains unclear the mechanisms by which chronic pain may negatively influence sleep quality. Nonetheless, as noted earlier, chronic pain can be associated with neuroplastic changes in spinal dorsal horn, V-BSNC, and thalamocortical relays, so these or other pain-related changes may potentially have effects on sleep; however, how these changes influence the brainstem and thalamocortical circuits involved in sleep is largely unknown.[14,21]

The reverse situation, that poor sleep might be a significant cause of pain, also is unclear. According to some reports, experimental sleep deprivation or fragmentation can lead to pain, and restoration of sleep quality (continuity and duration) can reduce this pain in humans.[32] Likewise, in animals, sleep restriction leads to a reduction in nociceptive threshold during wakefulness that is reversed once sleep is restored.[33] Some studies, however, suggest that other factors (e.g., fatigue, mood changes, cognitive impairment) may be involved,[33] thereby raising doubts about whether poor sleep is indeed a dominant or a pathognomonic cause of pain. Changes in the respiratory system may also play a role. For example, sleep apnea and sleep-disordered breathing may influence pain, as exemplified by findings that almost 30% of patients with pain associated with temporomandibular disorders (TMDs) also have obstructive sleep apnea (OSA), and signs and symptoms of OSA are associated with increased odds for first onset TMD.[34,35]

Thus the interactions between sleep and pain are very complex, and many factors can influence the interactions. It does seem nonetheless that poor-quality sleep can exacerbate pain and that chronic pain in particular can disrupt sleep in many patients, perhaps after a "circular" pattern whereby the chronic pain patient has a night of poor sleep followed by a day of exacerbated pain that is then followed by a night of poor sleep. In contrast, acute pain might influence sleep, but its disruptive effect on sleep is usually transitory, and if the acute pain is dealt with effectively, sleep will soon return to normal; such a pattern suggests a "linear" relationship between pain and sleep.[14]

MODULATION OF SENSORIMOTOR PROCESSES DURING SLEEP AND WAKEFULNESS

Sleep mechanisms markedly affect sensorimotor functions. Sleep not only suppresses basal muscle tone but also attenuates and, in some cases, even abolishes motor reflexes (see the section Specific Reflexes). Sensory and motor processes and their integration are also differentially affected by prevailing behavioral states. For example, during wakefulness, chemical and mechanical stimulation of laryngeal tissues evokes coughing; during sleep, however, the same stimulus elicits only a brief expiration. Such observations suggest not only that sensorimotor processes are suppressed by sleep but also that sleep mechanisms per se control the integration and expression of sensorimotor processes.

Sensorimotor Pathways and Mechanisms

The afferent inputs that provide access to the spinal cord, brainstem, thalamus, and cerebral cortex are involved not only in perceptual processes but also in sensorimotor integration and control.[5,13,36,37] The neuromuscular system is reflexively influenced by receptors that signal pain, touch, joint position, and muscle stretch or tension. In the case of muscles of the trunk, neck, and limbs, afferents from spinally innervated tissues enter the dorsal root and project into the spinal cord, where they can excite or inhibit motoneurons that innervate skeletal muscles. Motoneurons that innervate craniofacial muscles (e.g., jaw, soft palate, laryngeal, tongue) reside in motoneuron pools in the brainstem, most notably the trigeminal, facial, ambiguus, and hypoglossal nuclei.

One source of afferent input that reflexively influences motoneurons is derived from the muscle spindle, a stretch-sensitive receptor signaling muscle length. The group Ia primary afferents innervating muscle spindles monosynaptically excite motoneurons to produce contraction of the stretched muscle. This monosynaptic circuitry is the neural substrate for the H-reflex and jaw-closing reflex. Muscle spindle afferents are a fundamental motor control mechanism in limb, neck, and trunk muscles; however, because there are insignificant numbers of muscle afferents in most craniofacial muscles (e.g., anterior digastric, facial, pharyngolaryngeal muscles), other receptor systems, such as the receptors in tooth-supporting tissues and in the pharyngeal and laryngeal mucosa, play a significant role in the control of these muscles.[5,13,36]

Some afferent inputs trigger either excitatory or inhibitory reflexes by affecting the activity of interneurons, which are located in the spinal dorsal horn, V-BSNC, or NTS, or within motor pools per se. Both interneurons and motoneurons also are modulated by the descending neural systems that regulate somatosensory transmission, such as the reticular formation, PAG, limbic system, lateral hypothalamus (LH), basal ganglia, LC, red nucleus, cerebellum, and sensorimotor cerebral cortex.[11,36,37] Some of these systems also are involved in the initiation and guidance of movements such as the sensorimotor cortex, which contributes to the learning of novel sensorimotor skills through neuroplastic changes in sensory and motor representations in the sensorimotor cortex. Others are involved in the control and guidance of movements and their integration with other sensorimotor functions (e.g., basal ganglia; spinal or brainstem pattern generators for locomotion, chewing, or swallowing) and yet others in the regulation of sleep-wake states per se (e.g., PAG, lateral pontine tegmentum, LH).[38]

Processing of Somatic Reflexes during Sleep and Wakefulness

Sleep influences the processing of sensory-motor responses, such as the withdrawal reflex, jaw-closing reflex, jaw-opening reflex, and other H-reflexes. Because changes in somatic reflex responses are linked to movement disorders, such as periodic limb movement disorder (PLMD) and restless legs syndrome (RLS),[39,40] it is important to consider how such reflexes normally are affected by sleep and to identify mechanisms by which these reflexes are modulated during sleep, as reviewed next. Also discussed is how H-reflexes are affected during periods of cataplexy because such changes provide valuable insight into understanding how brain function is affected by narcolepsy.

The withdrawal reflex (also known as the flexion reflex) is a polysynaptic multisegmental spinal reflex that triggers withdrawal (flexion) of the stimulated limb. It functions to remove the affected limb from potentially noxious stimuli that could cause tissue damage. The withdrawal reflex is composed of two excitatory responses. The first component, termed *RII,* is considered a tactile response and is characterized by muscle activation (e.g., biceps femoris muscle) that occurs 40 to 60 milliseconds after nerve stimulation (e.g., sural nerve). The second component, termed *RIII,* occurs 85 to 120 milliseconds after stimulation and is considered a nociceptive polysynaptic reflex.[41] The first and second components probably represent, respectively, the activation of A-beta and A-delta cutaneous afferent fibers. Because a robust correlation has been found between the RIII threshold and subjective pain thresholds, the primary focus here is on the effects of sleep on this component of the reflex.

Sleep has a marked impact on the expression of the withdrawal reflex in humans. Compared with wakefulness, a significant increase in the stimulus intensity is required to activate the reflex during both NREM and REM sleep.[42] The polysynaptic jaw-opening reflex (a reflex analogous to the limb withdrawal reflex) also is suppressed during NREM sleep in monkeys; reduced trigeminal motoneuron excitability is one factor that may cause suppression of this reflex during NREM sleep.[15,43,44] Although stimulus thresholds are elevated during sleep, the withdrawal reflex, like other somatic reflexes, is most reliably activated and most stable during NREM sleep. An increase in the latency to the RIII component also is observed during both NREM and REM sleep,[42] suggesting that sleep reduces nociceptive reflex excitability and acts to filter sensory inputs to preserve sleep continuity. However, there is an increase in both the magnitude and duration of the RIII reflex during REM sleep. This second finding is paradoxical because monosynaptic reflexes are maximally suppressed during this state,[45] and somatic motoneurons are hyperpolarized during REM sleep in cats.[46] The mechanism(s) underlying RIII reflex facilitation during REM sleep are unknown.

Unlike the RIII nociceptive component, the RII tactile reflex is absent during sleep.[42] This observation is physiologically important because it suggests that sleep differentially affects the individual components of the sensory pathways that mediate this two-part reflex, which implies that sleep mechanisms do not affect all physiologic systems equally. This concept is of clinical relevance because it suggests that sleep suppresses tactile responses (i.e., RII), which if activated by body repositioning, for example, could cause unwanted arousal, whereas nociceptive reflexes (i.e., RIII) and their motor component remain active during sleep. Preservation of this protective reflex would therefore ensure that painful stimuli elicit appropriate motor responses and, if necessary, arousal from sleep.

Sleep also has powerful effects on the expression of monosynaptic reflexes, such as the masseteric jaw-closing reflex and the classic H-reflex. In humans a progressive reduction in the magnitude of the H-reflex amplitude is seen during stages 1 to 4 of NREM sleep, along with a near-complete

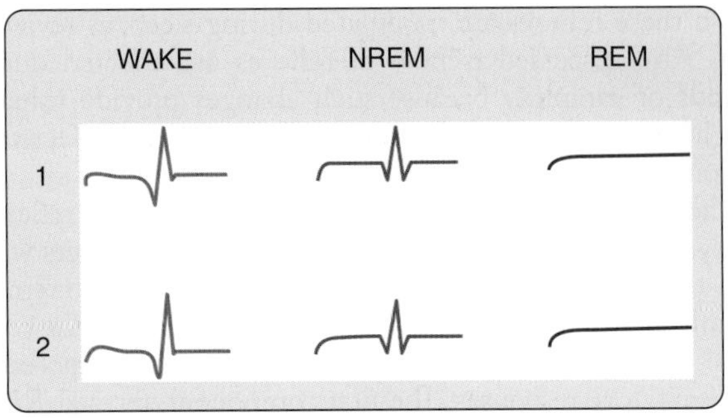

Figure 30.3 Magnitude of the H-reflex during sleep and wakefulness. The H-reflex of the calf muscle was triggered by electrical stimulation of the tibial nerve in a 22-year-old man during wakefulness (WAKE), non–rapid eye movement (NREM) sleep, and rapid eye movement (REM) sleep, with reflex responses obtained on two separate measurements (1 and 2). Relative to that in wakefulness, the H-reflex is depressed in NREM sleep and abolished in REM sleep. (From Shimizu A, Yamada Y, Yamamoto Y, et al. Pathways of descending influence on H reflex during sleep. *Electroencephalogr Clin Neurophysiol.* 1966;20:337–47.)

loss of the reflex during REM sleep[45] (Figure 30.3). Animal studies also show that the stimulus intensity needed to trigger the masseteric reflex is increased in sleep and that reflex responses are reduced during NREM sleep, minimal during tonic REM sleep, and maximally suppressed during periods of active REM sleep (i.e., during rapid eye movements). Because trigeminal motoneurons, which ultimately mediate the masseteric reflex, are inhibited by GABA and glycine during both NREM and REM sleep,[43] such inhibitory mechanisms may act to shunt the excitatory afferent inputs onto motoneurons during sleep. The available evidence, however, suggests that presynaptic inhibition of Ia afferents onto spinal motoneurons also may function to suppress monosynaptic spinal reflexes during REM sleep.[47] Therefore descending inhibitory inputs acting on both motoneurons and Ia afferents contribute to reduce monosynaptic reflexes during sleep.

Clinical Correlates

Sleep Bruxism

Sleep bruxism, classified as a sleep-related movement disorder, is characterized by tooth grinding and jaw clenching that can lead to destruction of teeth or dental restorations and cause jaw and head pain (see Chapters 169 and 170).[14,48,49] It occurs in 8% to 10% of the adult population and is characterized by rhythmic episodes of involuntary jaw muscle activity occurring primarily during NREM sleep and less frequently in REM sleep.[50] Although the etiology and pathophysiology of sleep bruxism are not fully understood, abnormal sensorimotor processing within the CNS level, rather than an abnormal processing of peripheral sensory feedback (e.g., from the teeth), is recognized to underlie the genesis of sleep bruxism.[14,15]

Brainstem structures (e.g., reticular formation, LC, raphe nuclei) that influence sleep-wake control and sensorimotor processes also influence the mechanisms underlying sleep bruxism, and involve many of the same neurochemicals (e.g., 5-HT, GABA, acetylcholine, dopamine). In addition, the rhythmic movements appear secondary to CNS events related to "arousals," with increases in autonomic (cardiac and respiratory) and brain activity reflecting reactivation of the reticular formation arousal system preceding the movements.[14,48] The activity of noradrenergic cells in the LC also may contribute to the pathogenesis of sleep bruxism (see Chapter 169).

Descending cortical pathways, producing rhythmic masticatory movements during wakefulness, also may be involved in bruxism. Findings comparing cortically induced jaw movements in the awake and sleep states of primates indicate that cortical influences are suppressed during NREM sleep.[15] These findings suggest that corticobulbar excitatory influences are deactivated during sleep to preserve sleep continuity, providing indirect support for the importance of brainstem structures in the genesis of sleep bruxism.

Periodic Limb Movement Disorder and Restless Legs Syndrome

Abnormal sensorimotor processing contributes to both RLS and PLMD. For example, marked hyperexcitability of both monosynaptic and polysynaptic reflexes is a feature of these two disorders.[39] The threshold required to activate the withdrawal reflex is lower, and the response magnitude is larger during sleep in patients with RLS and PLMD than in healthy control subjects.[39] Changes in the response attributes of the soleus H-reflex in patients with RLS and PLMD also are seen—specifically, an increased late facilitation and a decreased late inhibition of the reflex response.[52] Reduced inhibition of either spinal motoneurons or presynaptic mechanisms may underlie the facilitation of motor responses and could explain why patients with RLS and PLMD exhibit hyperexcitability of spinal reflexes.[51,53] Brain imaging studies show changes in thalamic, cerebellar, and pontine activity in both patient populations,[51,54,55] suggesting that these regions may affect spinal reflex activity and hence contribute to RLS and PLMD.

Narcolepsy

Cataplexy is characterized by a sudden loss of skeletal muscle tone (i.e., atonia) despite maintenance of consciousness, and it is a pathognomonic symptom of narcolepsy.[56] It generally is triggered by strong positive emotions (see Chapters 111 and 112). Because motor atonia is a defining feature of both cataplexy and REM sleep, similar neurocircuits may mediate both motor phenomena. In human and canine narcolepsy, the atonia of cataplexy can last from several seconds to several minutes.[57] In both dogs and humans the monosynaptic H-reflex is either absent or minimal during cataplectic attacks.[58] This observation demonstrates that the loss of "wakefulness drive," which has been proposed to cause loss of muscle tone in sleep,[59] does not mediate motor suppression during cataplexy because wakefulness is preserved during this state. Loss of excitatory noradrenergic drives onto motoneurons may mediate the loss of muscle tone and the H-reflex during cataplexy because noradrenergic cells in the LC project to motoneurons, and they cease firing during cataplectic attacks in narcoleptic dogs[60] (Figure 30.4). Furthermore, because LC neurons reduce their discharge activity in NREM sleep and virtually stop firing during REM sleep,[60] loss of noradrenergic drives onto motoneurons also may explain why motor reflexes and muscle tone are reduced in NREM and REM sleep.[61]

RESPIRATORY REFLEXES DURING SLEEP AND WAKEFULNESS

Sleep not only affects the processing of spinal and craniofacial sensorimotor activities but also changes how the respiratory system responds to both mechanical and chemical stimuli (see Chapters 22 to 24). The focus of this section is

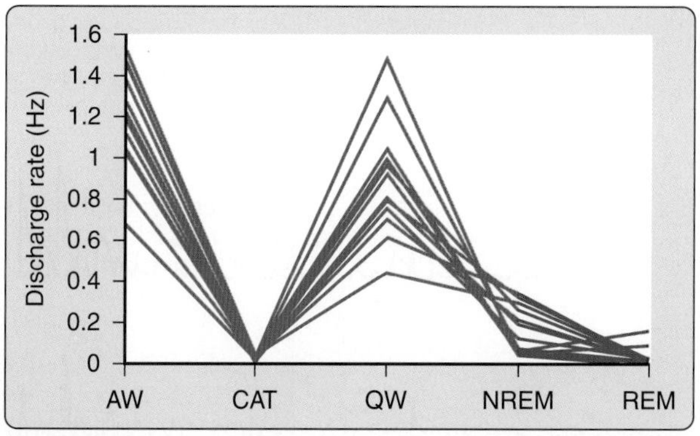

Figure 30.4 Discharge activity of putative noradrenergic cells in the locus coeruleus of narcoleptic dogs during wakefulness, sleep, and cataplexy. The discharge rate for locus coeruleus neurons is tightly correlated with behavioral state. Cell activity is maximal during active and quiet wakefulness (AW and QW, respectively), reduced during non–rapid eye movement (NREM) sleep, and minimal or absent when motor hypotonia/atonia is present, that is, during rapid eye movement (REM) sleep and cataplexy (CAT). (From Wu MF, Gulyani SA, Yau E, et al. Locus coeruleus neurons: cessation of activity during cataplexy. *Neuroscience.* 1999;91:1389–99.)

on sensory-motor integration in upper airway and craniofacial muscles because sleep-dependent changes in these reflexes can cause respiratory instability during sleep. Airway reflexes, including coughing, swallowing, laryngeal closure, apnea, and the negative-pressure reflex, function to protect the airway from inhalation of inappropriate substances and to preserve airway patency during vulnerable periods, such as during anesthesia and sleep. A multitude of afferent nerve endings in the upper alimentary and airway mucosa and muscles that detect changes in muscle tone, pressure, airflow, temperature, and chemical status (e.g., acidic fluids) are able to respond to and thus trigger appropriate respiratory reflexes. Presented next is a summary of how two important airway reflexes are affected by sleep; the potential mechanisms underlying state-dependent regulation of such reflexes are then reviewed.

Specific Reflexes

Airway Negative-Pressure Reflex

One of the most clinically relevant reflexes is the airway response to negative pressure. The airway negative-pressure reflex is characterized by increased upper airway muscle tone in response to the negative suction pressures generated by diaphragmatic contraction. During normal breathing, the reflex is inactive because airway pressure is below the stimulus threshold required to trigger it; however, during sleep, particularly REM sleep, reductions in airway muscle tone cause airway narrowing and increased resistance, which increases negative pressure, and this triggers the pressure reflex. The primary function of the negative-pressure response is to increase upper airway muscle tone when airway pressures threaten to occlude the airspace. This reflex response plays an important role in OSA.

The negative-pressure reflex is typified by short-latency activation of a variety of craniofacial and pharyngeal muscles (e.g., tensor palatini and genioglossus) when airway pressure drops below a variable threshold. Studies using resistive loading, which approximates the effects of sleep on airway pressure, show that the negative-pressure reflex is reduced in sleep and indeed often is absent, except in the presence of hypercapnia or hypoxia.[62] Studies in both animals and humans show that the magnitude of pharyngeal dilator activation is reduced during NREM sleep and further reduced during REM sleep[63] (Figure 30.5).

The mechanisms mediating the airway negative-pressure reflex are not fully understood (see Chapter 24). Changes in pressure probably are detected by mechanoreceptors located within both airway mucosa and airway muscles themselves; whether both mechanisms operate at all levels of the airway is unknown. Trigeminal nerve afferents play a particularly important role in detecting upper airway pressure changes because not only do they respond to pressure changes, but the pressure reflex also is diminished when regions of the airspace innervated by trigeminal afferents are locally anesthetized.[64] Reductions in the negative-pressure reflex during sleep could be mediated, at least in part, by changes in the excitability of trigeminal pathways. Neuronal activity in the rostral V-BSNC is reduced during REM sleep[23]; because some of these neurons relay their excitatory signals to the respiratory centers and motoneurons that trigger reflex expression, reductions in their activity could function to reduce reflex responses in sleep, particularly during REM sleep.

Changes in airway pressure also are detected by mechanoreceptors supplied by the superior laryngeal nerve; such afferent signals are relayed to the NTS before reaching respiratory centers. Because excitatory (e.g., serotonergic raphe neurons, hypocretin cells) and inhibitory (GABAergic in the ventrolateral preoptic nucleus) components of the sleep-generating circuitry also project to and synapse onto NTS neurons, reduced excitation and increased inhibition of NTS neurons could act to reduce the negative-pressure reflex during sleep.[38] In addition, GABAergic and glycinergic inhibition of upper airway motoneurons during NREM and REM sleep[43] may function to shunt the excitatory signals arising from pressure afferents; this effect also would limit the expression of the negative-pressure reflex during sleep.

Laryngeal and Bronchopulmonary Reflexes

Chemoreceptors in the nose, mouth, pharynx, larynx, and lower airways (e.g., trachea) detect various chemical stimuli that elicit protective upper airway reflexes. Stimulation of the larynx with acidic liquids or mechanical forces causes the laryngeal reflex, which during wakefulness in adults triggers swallowing or coughing. During NREM and REM sleep, however, the laryngeal reflex is not simply suppressed (and the stimulus threshold increased); it is transformed into a fundamentally different motor response. Compared with the waking reflex, which triggers coughing, laryngeal stimulation during sleep often initiates apnea and bradycardia[65] (Figure 30.6). Activation of bronchopulmonary receptors also elicits different respiratory motor responses during waking and sleep. Mechanical activation of the bronchopulmonary receptors that detect changes in airflow and/or lung stretch triggers the cough reflex during wakefulness but elicits reflexive apnea during both NREM and REM sleep.[66] Such an observation implies that sleep circuits inhibit the expression of these reflex responses or that activation of wake-generating circuits is required to trigger these reflexes.

The mechanisms responsible for reversing laryngeal and bronchopulmonary reflexes during sleep have not been determined. This type of response reversal, however, previously has been identified and studied in other motor pathways. During wakefulness, auditory stimuli (e.g., sudden loud noises) or skeletal muscle stimulation (e.g., muscle stretch) cause

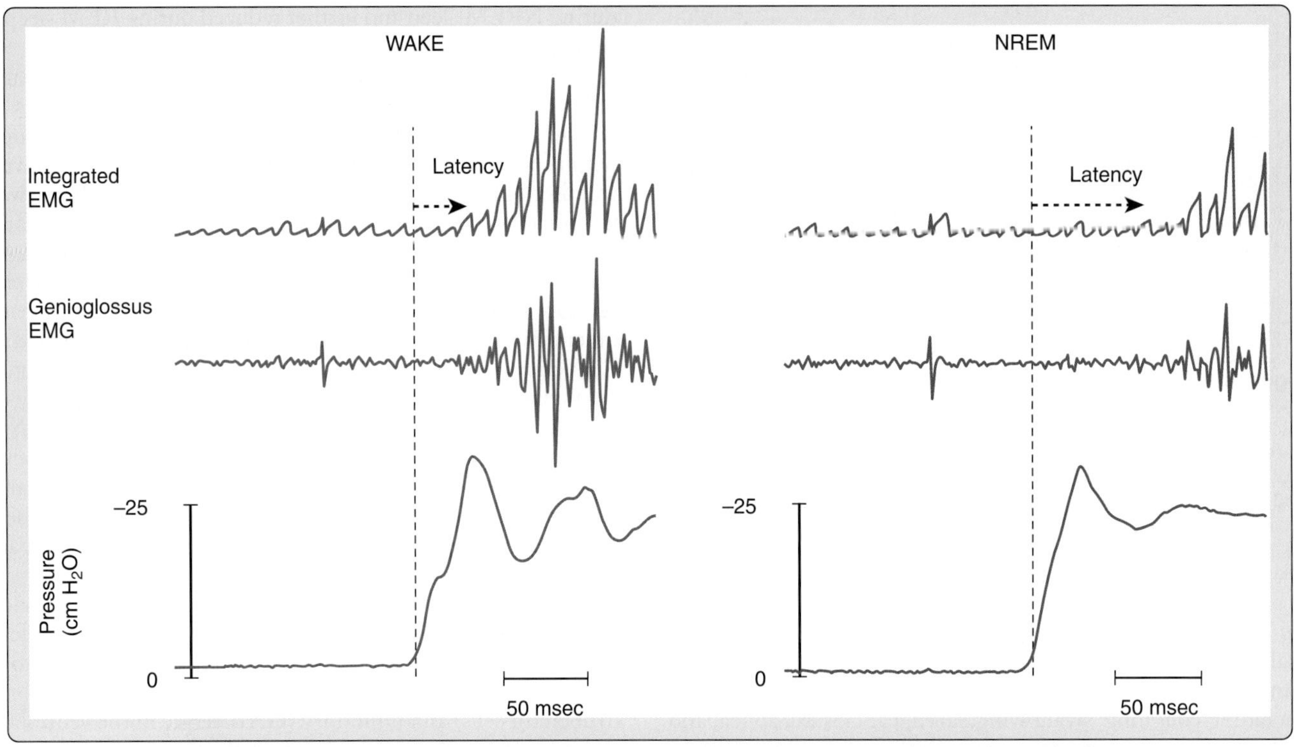

Figure 30.5 The airway negative-pressure reflex is suppressed during sleep as seen in this typical example of an electromyogram (EMG) recorded in a human subject during wakefulness and sleep. *Top two traces,* Integrated and raw EMG activity recorded from the genioglossus muscle; *bottom trace,* changes in airway pressure. During waking, negative airway pressure (−25 cm H_2O) triggers a short latency activation of genioglossus muscle tone; during non–rapid eye movement (NREM) sleep, however, the reflex magnitude is suppressed, and a significant increase in response latency is evident. ECG, Electrocardiogram; EEG, electroencephalogram. (From Horner RL, Innes JA, Morrell MJ, et al. The effect of sleep on reflex genioglossus muscle activation by stimuli of negative airway pressure in humans. *J Physiol.* 1994;476:141–51.)

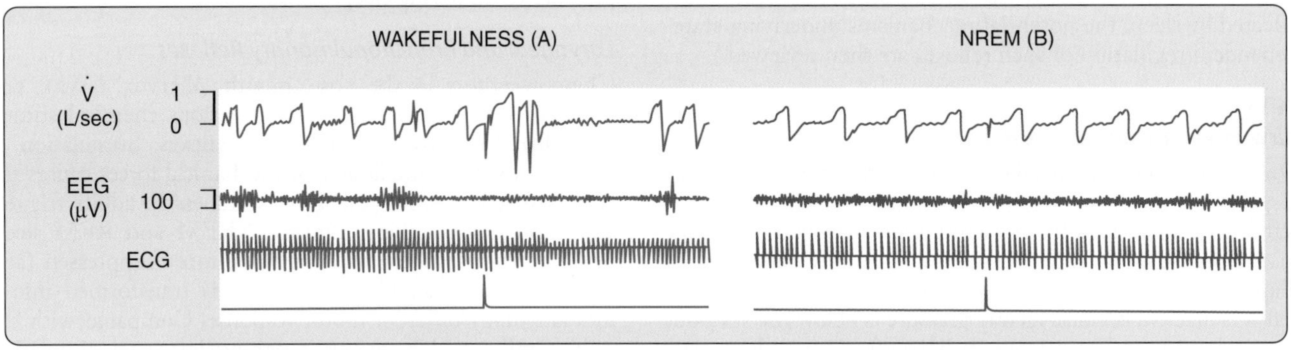

Figure 30.6 Laryngeal stimulation triggers the cough reflex during wakefulness but not during sleep, as seen in this example depicting the effects of such stimulation on respiratory activity during wakefulness **(A)** and sleep **(B)** in a dog. Airflow ($\dot{V}$) data are tracked on the *top trace,* with inspirations shown as upward spikes and expirations as downward spikes. The *upper middle trace* is the concomitant EEG; the *lower middle trace* is heart rate on the ECG).The *bottom trace* indicates when water was injected into the larynx. Injection of 0.2 mL of water into the laryngeal region of the trachea caused immediate expiration followed by the cough reflex **(A)**. Injection of the same volume of water during NREM sleep produced only a brief expiration; it did not trigger the cough reflex **(B)**. ECG, Electrocardiogram; EEG, electroencephalogram; $\dot{V}$, ventilation. (From Sullivan CE, Murphy E, Kozar LF, et al. Waking and ventilatory responses to laryngeal stimulation in sleeping dogs. *J Appl Physiol.* 1978;45:681–9.)

reflexive activation of somatic motoneurons with subsequent facilitation of skeletal muscle tone; during REM sleep, however, identical stimuli, albeit at greater intensities, cause the opposite effect, that is, motoneuron inhibition and reduced muscle tone. This type of state-dependent response reversal is mediated, at least in part, by the pontomesencephalic reticular formation (PMRF) that participates in sleep-wake regulation.[67] Stimulation of the PMRF causes excitatory postsynaptic potentials (i.e., excitation) in trigeminal motoneurons when the jaw-closing masseteric reflex is evoked during waking, but PMRF stimulation during REM sleep triggers inhibitory postsynaptic potentials (i.e., inhibition) in motoneurons and reduced masseteric reflex output.[67] The PMRF may therefore function to gate sensory-motor reflexes during different sleep-wake states; during wakefulness, it allows sensory stimuli to produce appropriate motor facilitation, such as coughing, whereas during sleep, when motor activation could elicit inappropriate arousals, such stimuli trigger motor inhibition (e.g., apnea). Whether this type of response reversal underlies state-dependent changes in laryngeal and bronchopulmonary reflexes is unknown.

Processing of Chemoreflexes during Sleep and Wakefulness

During wakefulness, respiratory control mechanisms are acutely sensitive to changes in blood and tissue CO_2 levels, with subtle increases in CO_2 levels causing potent increases in ventilation. However, sleep has profound effects on the respiratory sensitivity to CO_2, which influences the control of breathing during sleep. During sleep, ventilation decreases even though CO_2 levels increase. The decrease in ventilation is paradoxical in that increased CO_2 levels trigger potent increases in ventilation during waking. These changes are of physiologic importance because during waking, an increase of 1 mm Hg in the partial pressure of CO_2 (Pco_2) causes a 20% to 30% increase in ventilation; during sleep, however, CO_2 levels can increase by 2 to 6 mm Hg without affecting breathing. Therefore during sleep there is a change in the relationship between ventilation and the mechanisms that detect CO_2 levels; this change reflects the fact that sleep dramatically affects the processing of respiratory chemoreflexes.

The hypercapnic ventilatory response undergoes two important changes during sleep. First, the Pco_2 threshold that normally triggers increased ventilation during wakefulness is significantly increased during sleep. This sleep-related change indicates that higher CO_2 levels are required to increase ventilation during sleep, which could partially explain why ventilation decreases below waking levels during NREM sleep. Second, the sensitivity of the ventilatory response to CO_2 during sleep is significantly reduced from that in awake states. For example, decreases of 25% to 75% have been reported in the hypercapnic ventilatory response during NREM sleep compared with waking.

REM sleep also has a profound impact on the ventilatory sensitivity to CO_2. Compared with NREM sleep, there is a further reduction in the hypercapnic ventilatory response during REM sleep. In fact, CO_2 sensitivity often is suppressed to such a degree that high levels of CO_2 have negligible effects on breathing during REM sleep. In dogs, even high levels of CO_2 have minimal effects on breathing, and despite potent CO_2 stimulation, the irregular breathing patterns (e.g., rapid fluctuations in tidal volume and breathing frequency) that predominate during REM sleep still persist.[68] This is a notable observation because such levels of CO_2 normally would cause breathing to become deep and regular during waking and NREM sleep. The persistence of irregular breathing during REM sleep indicates that REM phenomena override the sensory control of breathing.

CO_2 sensitivity is different during tonic (i.e., no eye movements) versus phasic (i.e., eye movements) REM sleep. Compared with either waking or NREM sleep, the ventilatory response to CO_2 is potently suppressed during periods of phasic REM sleep. By contrast, the CO_2 response during tonic REM sleep is no different than during NREM sleep; however, CO_2 sensitivity remains below waking levels during this state.[69] This important observation underscores the fact that CO_2 sensitivity is differentially affected by NREM and REM sleep and also is subject to intrastate variability. Such findings suggest that behavioral states have a marked impact on the sensory mechanisms by which the CNS detects and responds to changes in CO_2.

Sleep also affects the manner by which different respiratory muscles respond to CO_2. In both humans and animals, hypercapnia causes marked increases in both diaphragmatic and upper airway (e.g., the genioglossus muscle) muscle activity; compared with waking, however, a marked reduction in levels of muscle activity is seen during both NREM and REM sleep. Although hypercapnia increases diaphragmatic muscle tone during NREM and REM sleep, the sensitivity of genioglossus upper airway muscle tone is severely blunted during REM sleep.[70] Therefore, although hypercapnia can trigger increased diaphragm activity in REM sleep, it has comparatively minimal effects on recruiting upper airway muscles whose activation is required for keeping the airspace open and for overcoming OSA (see the following section Clinical Correlates).

Sleep-dependent suppression of respiratory muscle function could limit the expression of the hypercapnic ventilatory response. Although respiratory muscle tone is reduced in NREM sleep, it is unlikely that this change explains reduced CO_2 sensitivity because hypercapnic exposure during this state increases ventilation and respiratory muscle tone (e.g., diaphragm and genioglossus) to within waking levels. During REM sleep, however, upper airway muscle tone is minimal and virtually unresponsive to hypercapnia; these effects could mask the ventilatory response to CO_2. Bypassing the upper airway by means of chronic tracheotomy can prevent the stereotypic loss of the ventilatory responses to CO_2 during REM sleep in cats,[71] which suggests that loss of upper airway muscle tone is, at least in part, responsible for the suppression of CO_2 sensitivity during REM sleep. Nevertheless, it is unlikely that REM sleep muscle atonia fully accounts for suppression of the hypercapnic ventilatory response because CO_2 responses are minimal or absent during phasic REM sleep, when skeletal muscles are transiently activated, and CO_2 responses are present during tonic REM sleep, when skeletal muscle tone is lowest.[69]

Two mechanisms by which the nervous system detects changes in CO_2 levels are recognized. First, sensory cells (glomus cells) in the carotid body chemoreceptors respond to changes in arterial Pco_2 (and O_2). It is unknown how this sensing mechanism contributes to sleep-related changes in CO_2 sensitivity; however, because glomus cells relay their afferent signals to the brain via the NTS, sleep mechanisms that affect the activity of NTS neurons presumably could affect CO_2 sensitivity. Second, intrinsic CO_2-sensing mechanisms also are located within the brain itself. These CO_2 sensors, termed *central chemoreceptors,* consist of neurons that respond to local tissue changes in CO_2, which in turn trigger ventilation. The primary areas that detect changes in CO_2 are the NTS, LC, raphe nuclei, and retrotrapezoid nucleus (RTN).[72,73] Hypocretin/orexin neurons in the LH, which form part of the neurocircuitry underlying arousal, also respond to and detect changes in CO_2. Focal acidification (i.e., increased CO_2) of hypocretin neurons causes them to depolarize and increase their firing frequency.[74] Genetic deletion of hypocretin neurons reduces the ventilatory response to CO_2 in awake mice and promotes respiratory instability during NREM and REM sleep,[75] suggesting that hypocretin neurons act as central CO_2 sensors that function to maintain normal respiratory reflexes during both sleep and waking.[73]

Animal research demonstrates that some CO_2 sensors are able to detect changes in CO_2 only during waking, whereas others are able to detect CO_2 changes *only* during sleep. For example, local increases in CO_2 within the RTN activates breathing only during waking; the same stimulus has no effect on breathing during sleep[72] (Figure 30.7). Although CO_2 stimulation of the NTS triggers increased ventilation during both waking and sleep, the response is significantly larger during waking than in sleep. Therefore the RTN and NTS could serve as the primary CO_2 sensors during wakefulness; loss of their CO_2 sensitivity during sleep may explain why the hypercapnic ventilatory response is suppressed during sleep. Although CO_2 sensitivity is reduced in sleep, it is not abolished; therefore other CO_2 sensors must continue to monitor tissue CO_2 levels during sleep. The serotoninergic raphe nucleus is one potential candidate because local increases in CO_2 levels in this brain region increase breathing only during sleep; it does not affect breathing during wakefulness (Figure 30.7).[72] The raphe nucleus may therefore be the primary CO_2 sensor during sleep. This concept is supported by the fact that mice lacking functional serotonin neurons have abnormal arousal responses to CO_2 stimulation during sleep.

The neurocircuits that regulate sleep may also influence the ability of CO_2 sensors to transmit their excitatory drives to respiratory centers, thus limiting the expression of the hypercapnic ventilatory response during sleep. For example, because monoaminergic (e.g., noradrenergic in the LC; Figure 30.4) and hypocretin neurons reduce their discharge activity during sleep, and because these neurons also project to CO_2 sensors (e.g., RTN), then reduced excitatory drive from these sites would limit the ability of CO_2 sensors to relay their afferent signals to respiratory motor pools and to the respiratory centers that trigger the CO_2 response.[76,77] Conversely, increased inhibitory drives from the GABAergic neurons in the ventrolateral and median preoptic nuclei that regulate NREM sleep could function to suppress CO_2 sensitivity during this state because such inhibitory regions also project to CO_2 sensors and respiratory centers. Therefore both reduced excitation and increased inhibition during sleep may curtail CO_2-sensing mechanisms such that the hypercapnic ventilatory response is reduced in sleep.

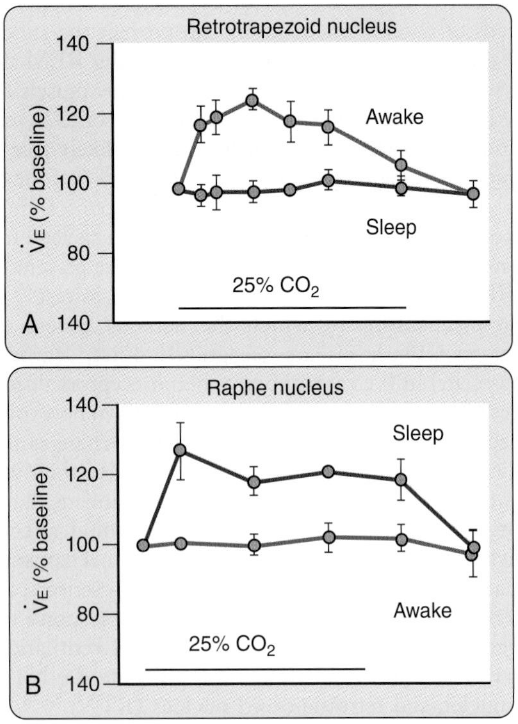

Figure 30.7 Some carbon dioxide (CO_2) sensors function only during wakefulness, whereas others function only during sleep. **A** and **B,** Plots of data for changes in expired total ventilation ($\dot{V}_E$) triggered by activation of CO_2 sensors in the retrotrapezoid nucleus (RTN) **(A)** or raphe nucleus **(B)** during wakefulness (*green line*) and sleep (*red line*) in behaving rats. To activate CO_2 sensors, 25% CO_2 (in saline) was perfused directly into either the RTN or raphe nuclei; this CO_2 concentration has physiologically relevant effects on CO_2 sensors. Activation of CO_2 sensors in the RTN increases ventilation only during waking; it has no effect during sleep (see **A**). Conversely, activation of CO_2 sensors in the raphe nucleus increases ventilation only during sleep; ventilation is unaffected during wakefulness (see **B**). (From Nattie EE. Central chemosensitivity, sleep, and wakefulness. *Respir Physiol.* 2001;129:257–68.)

Clinical Correlates

Although breathing continues without respite during wakefulness, it becomes fragile during sleep, and in approximately 2% to 5% of the adult population, it is punctuated by transient apneic episodes, which can manifest clinically as sleep-disordered breathing (see the section Sleep Breathing Disorders). OSA is the most common and serious respiratory-related sleep disorder. Its prevalence is growing in keeping with its recognized link with obesity and the current obesity epidemic. A defining feature of OSA is that it occurs exclusively during sleep; patients with OSA breathe normally while awake but not while asleep. Changes in both chemical and mechanical processing during sleep account for the drastic changes in respiratory control that contribute to OSA. Reduced upper airway muscle tone during sleep, particularly REM sleep, is the primary cause of OSA; it causes either airway narrowing or complete airway obstruction, both of which lead to hypoventilation and subsequent asphyxia. Under waking conditions, these respiratory stimuli (i.e., airway narrowing and asphyxia) trigger an increase in upper airway muscle tone, which reopens the airspace by activating both the negative-pressure reflex and the hypercapnic ventilatory responses. Because these reflexes are suppressed during sleep, however, they are only partially reactivated, so airway muscle tone does not cause airway reopening. In accordance, the airway remains occluded, and asphyxia worsens until it finally triggers awakening from sleep. Although wakefulness reinstates and reactivates the respiratory reflexes that increase muscle tone and thus causes airway reopening, it also causes hyperventilation, which in turn leads to hypocapnia. Hypocapnia then reflexively triggers a brief apneic episode, coincident with reentrance into sleep; this timing is problematic because sleep reduces the sensitivity of the mechanoreflexes and chemoreflexes needed to overcome apnea. Therefore apnea continues until the accompanying asphyxia produces arousal from sleep. This vicious circle occurs repeatedly throughout the night and underlies the sleep fragmentation, excessive daytime sleepiness, and related comorbid conditions (e.g., hypertension) that typify OSA.

CIRCUIT MECHANISMS THAT INDUCE AROUSAL IN RESPONSE TO PAIN AND HYPERCAPNIA DURING SLEEP

As outlined earlier, sleep influences the sensory systems and the processing of both pain and respiratory responses to hypercapnia. But the sensory systems also influence sleep stability.

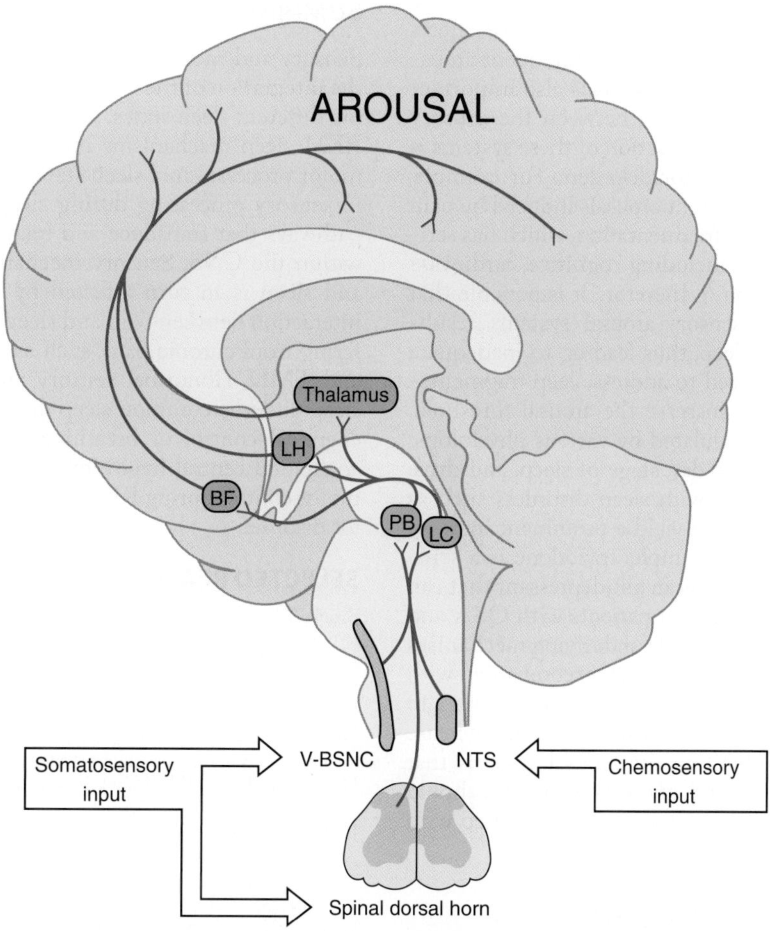

Figure 30.8 Circuits underlying arousal responses to somatosensory and chemosensory information during sleep. Sensory information encoding for pain and hypercapnia are processed from the trigeminal brainstem sensory nuclear complex (V-BSNC)/spinal dorsal horn and solitary tract nucleus (NTS), respectively. This sensory information is then relayed through the parabrachial (PB) nucleus and locus coeruleus (LC), which serve as a hub that distributes the sensory information to various nuclei of the arousal system, including the lateral hypothalamus (LH), thalamus, and basal forebrain (BF). Through this sensory-arousal pathway, suprathreshold sensory input, such as pain and hypercapnia, can stimulate the arousal system and promote arousal during sleep.

The focus of this final section is to outline how suprathreshold sensory stimuli, such as those related to pain and hypercapnia, trigger arousal during sleep. The body's sensory systems communicate directly with arousal systems that stabilize (or destabilize) sleep. For example, the parabrachial nucleus (PB), located in the dorsal pons, has been identified as a site where sensory-arousal communication takes place (Fig. 30.8).[14,78,79] It is well documented that the sensory information encoding for both pain and hypercapnia from the trigeminal nucleus and spinal dorsal horn and the NTS converge within the PB.[79,80] These sensory inputs increase the activity of the PB neurons, which subsequently triggers an arousal response from sleep by sending excitatory signals to wake-promoting nuclei, such as the basal forebrain (BF), LH, and thalamus.[81–83] A recent study has shown that the suppression of glutamate-releasing neurons in the PB during sleep significantly delays the arousal response to hypercapnia.[78] In addition to the PB, the LC, located caudal to the PB, shares a similar function. Noradrenaline-releasing LC neurons, which densely innervate arousal systems, induce rapid arousal when activated by sensory stimuli (see Fig. 30.8).[84,85] For example, LC neurons are highly responsive to different sensory stimuli, such as those related to pain, hypercapnia, and sound, which makes the LC an optimal site for sensory processing.[86,87] A recent study demonstrated that the suppression of the LC neurons during sleep significantly attenuates the arousal response induced by auditory stimuli.[88] This study confirmed that the LC, in addition to the PB, is a hub for relaying sensory signals to arousal circuits during sleep. The modification of the sensory-arousal system also occurs in other brain centers. For example, studies have shown that the suppression of the BF and LH, which receive ascending afferents from both the PB and LC, or the RTN, which sends ascending afferents to the PB, can also attenuate the arousal response induced by hypercapnia.[78,89,90] Together, these findings demonstrate the connectivity between sensory and arousal systems, and how these systems function together to influence sleep stability.

Clinical Correlates

Detection of sensory stimuli during sleep may serve to promote arousal from sleep and, as such, function as a protective mechanism against external threats, such as predation and natural hazards during sleep. However, overstimulation of sensory systems by environmental conditions, such as traffic sounds, ambient light, and air pollution, has negative effects on sleep maintenance by causing repeated and frequent arousals, thus resulting in sleep fragmentation. It is also important to recognize that inappropriate gating between the sensory and arousal systems and/or hyperactivation of these systems is associated with certain sensorimotor disorders. For example, in both RLS and OSA, the recurrent arousals induced by pain or hypercapnia may cause sleep fragmentation, which has serious physiologic consequences, including cognitive, cardiovascular, and immune dysfunction.[91] Therefore it is possible that chronic overstimulation of sensory-arousal systems results in repetitive waking during sleep, thus leading to inadequate sleep. A common approach used to address sleep fragmentation in these conditions is to increase the arousal threshold. Arousal thresholds can be modulated by various physiologic factors, such as age, time of the day, stage of sleep, and drive to sleep,[92–94] but when dealing with sleep disorders such as OSA, medications can be used to yield a prominent increase in the arousal threshold.[95] For example, trazodone is a serotonin antagonist commonly used as an antidepressant that can also increase the arousal threshold in patients with OSA and improve sleep quality.[95,96] However, its underlying mechanism remains unclear, and various side effects are accompanied with its usage.[97] Therefore further investigations are required to develop better therapeutic agents that can sufficiently increase the arousal threshold by inhibiting the arousal systems that receive input from sensory stimuli, and such strategies should improve the treatment of sleep fragmentation associated with OSA, RLS, and insomnia.[78]

CLINICAL PEARL

Determining how sleep controls sensory and motor processes is of notable importance in sleep medicine because some sleep disorders result from disturbances in sensory or motor control. As indicated by the available evidence, nociceptive transmission in the CNS is affected by sleep, and acute pain causes some sleep disturbance, but the extent and mechanisms by which chronic pain influences sleep, and vice versa, are largely unexplored. Clinicians need to be mindful that, although there is some evidence suggesting a circular relationship between chronic pain and poor sleep in many patients, there is no simple relationship between chronic pain and sleep quality that holds for every patient because a number of factors can influence the sleep-pain interactions. Abnormalities in motor control during sleep underlie most of the major sleep disorders, including OSA, narcolepsy-cataplexy, RLS, PLMD, and sleep bruxism. Identifying the underlying mechanisms of motor regulation during sleep is a prerequisite for developing more rational treatments for such sleep disorders.

SUMMARY

Sensory and motor processing are reduced during sleep, and the integration of these processes is differentially affected during different sleep states, suggesting that discrete NREM and REM sleep mechanisms modulate and control sensory and motor processes in a sleep state–dependent manner. Changes in sensory processing during sleep affect the somatosensory pathways that transduce and relay nociceptive signals to and within the CNS. Sensory mechanisms are affected by sleep, and sleep is in turn affected by nociceptive processes. The interaction between pain and sleep is common in patients suffering from chronic pain, such as that associated with cancer and TMD. Abnormal sensory and motor functions during sleep underlie common sleep disorders. For example, reduced chemical control of breathing during sleep plays a role in congenital central hypoventilation syndrome, and pathologic motor control during REM sleep underlies REM sleep behavior disorder.

SELECTED READINGS

Brooks PL, Peever JH. Glycinergic and GABA(A)-mediated inhibition of somatic motoneurons does not mediate rapid eye movement sleep motor atonia. *J Neurosci.* 2008;28:3535–3545.

Burke PG, Kanbar R, Basting TM, et al. State-dependent control of breathing by the retrotrapezoid nucleus. *J Physiol.* 2015;593:2909–2926.

Dauvilliers Y, Siegel JM, Lopez R, et al. Cataplexy—clinical aspects, pathophysiology and management strategy. *Nat Rev Neurol.* 2014;10:386–395.

Horner RL, Peever JH. Brain Circuitry Controlling Sleep and Wakefulness. *Continuum (Minneap Minn).* 2017;23(4, Sleep Neurology):955–972.

Lavigne G, Khoury S, Laverdure-Dupont D, et al. Tools and methodological issues in the investigation of sleep and pain interactions. In: Lavigne G, Sessle BJ, Choinière M, Soja PJ, eds. *Sleep and Pain.* Seattle: IASP Press; 2007:235–263.

Lavigne GJ, Sessle BJ. The neurobiology of orofacial pain and sleep and their interactions. *J Dent Res.* 2016;95:1109–1116.

Lee H, Peever J. Neuroscience: an arousal circuit that senses danger in sleep. *Curr Biol.* 2020;30(12):R708–R709.

Massimini M, Ferrarelli F, Huber R, et al. Breakdown of cortical effective connectivity during sleep. *Science.* 2005;309:2228–2232.

Peever J, Fuller PM. The Biology of REM Sleep. *Curr Biol.* 2017;27(22):R1237–R1248.

Soja PJ. Modulation of prethalamic sensory inflow during sleep versus wakefulness. In: Lavigne G, Sessle BJ, Choinière M, Soja PJ, eds. *Sleep and Pain.* Seattle: IASP Press; 2007:45–76.

Sullivan CE, Murphy E, Kozar LF, Phillipson EA. Waking and ventilatory responses to laryngeal stimulation in sleeping dogs. *J Appl Physiol.* 1978;45:681–689.

Sullivan CE, Murphy E, Kozar LF, Phillipson EA. Ventilatory responses to CO_2 and lung inflation in tonic versus phasic REM sleep. *J Appl Physiol.* 1979;47:1305–1310.

A complete reference list can be found online at ExpertConsult.com.

Chapter 31

Local and Use-Dependent Aspects of Sleep

James Krueger; Mehdi Tafti

Chapter Highlights

- Variations in localized sleep intensity, as determined by electroencephalogram (EEG) slow wave power, are dependent upon prior awake activity.
- Unilateral application of sleep-promoting substances to the surface of the cortex enhances sleep intensity ipsilaterally, while inhibition of those substances decreases EEG slow wave power. Further, unilateral sleep states occur in marine mammals and some birds.
- Individual cortical columns oscillate between wake-like and sleep-like states with the percentage of columns in the wake-like state being high during whole animal waking and conversely with a high percentage of columns being in a sleep-like state during whole animal sleep states.
- Performance errors during a specific learned task dependent upon single cortical column activity are experimentally correlated with sleep- and wake-like states of the individual column.
- Co-cultures of dispersed neurons and glia manifest sleep- and wake-like states, as determined by neuron burstiness, synchrony of electrical activity, slow wave (0.25 to 3.5 Hz) power, gene expression patterns, sleep homeostasis, and spontaneously reversibility. Further, such cultures enter a deeper sleep-like state if treated with sleep regulatory substances and display more time in the wake-like state if excitatory amino acids or peptides are applied.
- Collectively these data indicate that small neuronal/glial networks are the minimum component of brains capable of sleep-like states and that the brain can simultaneously express sleep and wake states. This hypothesis provides fuller understanding to previously unexplained sleep anomalies such as sleepwalking, sleep inertia, poor performance during prolonged waking, insomnia, and other disassociated states.

INTRODUCTION

History

The simultaneous occurrence of sleep and wake states, such as that occurring during sleepwalking, has been evident to lay individuals for eons. Thus sleepwalkers appear to be asleep because they can be awakened and yet sometimes they can walk and navigate around objects as if awake. More recently the characterization of sleep inertia indicates that, upon awakening, it takes considerable time for cognitive performance to maximize, suggesting that parts of the brain are remaining in a sleep-like state. Conversely, with prolonged wakefulness, cognitive and behavioral performances deteriorate, suggesting that some of the small networks involved in carrying out the task are falling into sleep-like states.[1] Neurologists have also long recognized that unusual clinical observations (e.g., rapid eye movement [REM] sleep) in a patient with a behavior disorder, may be explained by state dissociations.[2] Thus sleepwalking, sleep inertia, deteriorating performance with prolonged waking, and disassociated states represent anomalies to the paradigm viewing sleep as an all-or-nothing, whole-brain phenomenon.

Retrospective reinterpretation of experimental evidence reinforces the concept that parts of the brain can be asleep while other parts are awake. For example, as early as 1949 waxing and waning of slow potentials, which we now know are associated with sleep states, were observed in isolated cortical islands lacking thalamic input yet retaining their blood flow.[3] After mid-pontine transection of the brain, the forebrain seems to oscillate between wake-like states and high-amplitude electroencephalogram (EEG) slow wave sleep (hereafter called non–rapid eye movement sleep, or NREM sleep) while posterior to the transection waxing and waning of REM sleep occur.[4] Slow stimulation of many areas of the cortex induces transient synchronization of the EEG that outlasts the period of stimulation. Indeed, Jouvet posited that if one used slow waves to define sleep, then the "entire encephalon has hypogenic properties."[5] Although Jouvet rejected this hypothesis, it likely is the initial recognition that sleep may be fundamentally a local process.

Dolphin unilateral NREM sleep determined using EEG measurements is a direct demonstration that sleep and wake states occur simultaneously within a brain.[6] Dolphins do not exhibit NREM sleep in both cerebral hemispheres simultaneously, and they also lack REM sleep altogether. Further, unihemispheric sleep deprivation leads to NREM sleep rebound in the ipsilateral cortex but not in the non–sleep-deprived cortex.[7] This work has been extended to other marine mammals and to birds.[8]

There is substantial evidence that specific subcortical areas are involved in sleep regulation. However, it remains to be demonstrated that any of them are required for sleep expression. Thus, despite millions of poststroke clinical cases occurring in numerous parts of the brain and many experimental brain lesions to sleep regulatory areas, not a single postlesion human/animal has failed to sleep, albeit not always normally. For example, if rabbits are given large anterior hypothalamic lesions (a sleep regulatory area), duration of NREM sleep and REM sleep is greatly reduced. However, in the immediate postlesion period they remain responsive to sleep-inducing substances. Further, after a week or more of recovery, duration of spontaneous sleep returns toward prelesion values.[9] This experiment confirms the earlier work of von Economo,[10] confirmed by many others, showing that the anterior hypothalamus is involved in the active regulation of sleep. However, it also suggests, as did the stimulation data reviewed by Jouvet,[5] that multiple sites are capable of initiating sleep.

The work cited thus far led to the hypothesis that "sleep is basically use-dependent instead of simply wake-dependent; it explains why certain structures seem to be important for sleep regulation while their lesions will not elicit permanent insomnia. It suggests that sleep can be initiated at the local neuronal group level."[11] Within the past 28 years, this theory has been extended and clarified, and much experimental data have been generated in support of it. The remainder of this chapter summarizes those advances.

Definitions

There are several mental, behavioral, physiologic, and biochemical measures that correlate with sleep. Because there is no single measurement that is always indicative of when sleep is occurring, experimentally and clinically, two or more measures are usually used to characterize sleep (Box 31.1). Some of these characteristics are whole-brain or body properties, and whether those are useful to use as criteria for the identification of local sleep is debatable. Thus, for example, reduced locomotor activity is often used as a surrogate measure of sleep in fruit fly sleep studies. However, mammals severely infected with influenza virus are often motionless yet, as judged by their EEG, are awake. Similarly, sleepwalkers can walk yet simultaneously appear to be asleep as judged by mentation upon awakening. Regardless, many defining characteristics of sleep (red type in Box 31.1) occur locally in parts of the brain and even in vitro. For example, the EEG power in the rat visual cortex is higher during daylight hours followed by lower power at night. In contrast, the somatosensory cortex, which receives input from facial whiskers that rats use to navigate during the night, has higher EEG slow wave power during the night compared to the day.[12] Such results link a characteristic sleep EEG, the high slow wave amplitude, to local use dependency.

BOX 31.1 DEFINITIONAL CHARACTERISTICS OF SLEEP

- Reduced responsiveness to afferent input
- Reduced locomotor activity
- Distinct sleep postures
- Mentation quality
- Circadian rhythm linked
- Characteristic developmental patterns
- Spontaneously reversible
- Characteristic electroencephalogram wave forms
- Homeostatic regulation
- Characteristic neuronal firing patterns (e.g., burst/pause firing)
- Characteristic gene expression patterns
- Induced by sleep regulatory substances or suppressed by wake neuromodulators

The defining biologic characteristics of sleep are discussed in multiple chapters in this book. For whole animal sleep, characteristics include all those listed in this box. The list does not include all defining characteristics of sleep (e.g., changes in respiratory and cardiac frequency) and some that are specific to REM sleep vs. NREM sleep (e.g., variable respiratory and heart rates, compromised thermoregulation). The characteristics demonstrated thus far for local sleep in vivo are those in red. If a characteristic has also been demonstrated in vitro, it is underlined in addition. References for those in red are provided throughout this chapter.

LOCAL SLEEP PHENOTYPES

Local Electroencephalogram Slow Wave Power Is Dependent upon Waking Activity

The EEG slow wave power is often used as a measure of sleep intensity, for example, NREM delta wave sleep (old stage 4). Sleep intensity is identified by the occurrence of high-voltage slow waves and requires a more intense stimulus to awaken the subject than do stages 1, 2, or REM sleep. Localized EEG slow waves can be measured in multiple species, including humans, cats, rats, mice, chickens, and pigeons. If a localized area is disproportionately stimulated during waking, EEG delta power in that area is enhanced during subsequent NREM sleep.[12-18] Indeed, the first experimental test of the idea that sleep is a local use-dependent phenomenon used a hand vibrator to stimulate the contralateral somatosensory cortex for prolonged periods. In subsequent NREM sleep, EEG slow wave power was greater on the side that received enhanced afferent input.[19] As indicated, that finding has been replicated many times in multiple species. An eloquent demonstration that localized EEG slow wave power is quantitatively dependent upon afferent input was the demonstration that EEG slow wave power during NREM sleep was reduced in the somatosensory cortex if the subject's arm was immobilized during a 10-hour waking before sleep onset.[20] Such findings suggest that sleep intensity is dependent upon waking activity and is localized to the areas activated or inhibited.

Many additional human studies used transcranial magnetic stimulation to enhance local brain activity during waking and were followed by measurement of subsequent EEG slow wave power during sleep. These studies reached a similar conclusion: localized sleep intensity is dependent upon prior waking activity.[21,22] Further, functional magnetic resonance and positron emission tomography techniques have been used to similar ends. Thus such studies indicate that changes in localized cerebral blood flow or metabolism alter subsequent localized sleep.[23,24] Mechanistically, multiple sleep regulatory substances produced in the brain are vasodilators (Figure 31.1).

Experimental Manipulation of Unilateral Slow Wave Power and Sleep in Cortical Columns

To emphasize the sleep-linked roles of use-dependent molecules and their local origins, how they affect either sleep or sleep biomarkers at various levels of tissue organization is now

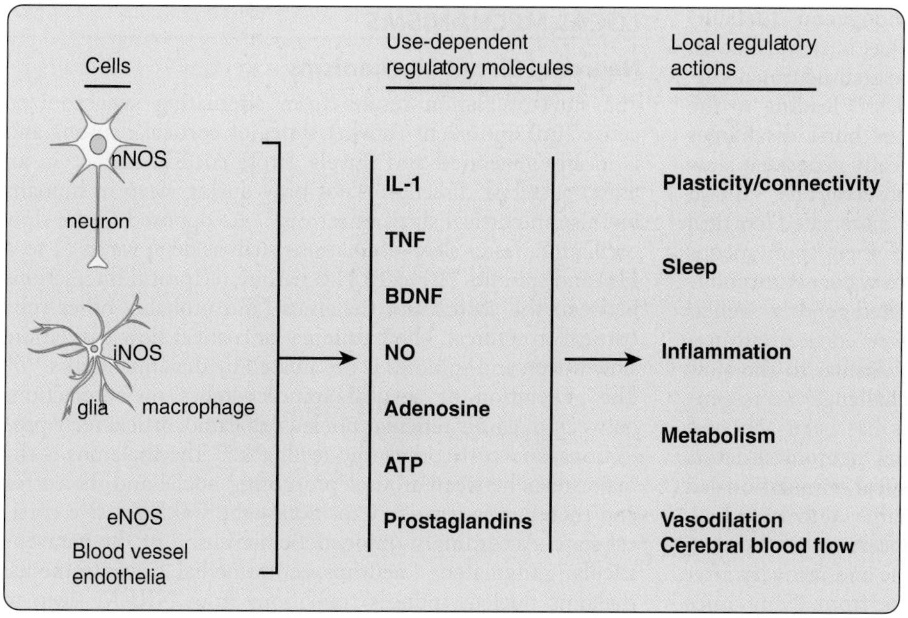

Figure 31.1 Brain cell types produce multiple sleep regulatory molecules in response to local cell use. These molecules initiate local events (*right*) that can emerge at higher levels of organization to alter multiple behaviors including sleep. ATP, Adenosine triphosphate; BDNF, brain-derived neurotrophic factor; eNOS, endothelial NOS; IL-1βb, interleukin-1β; iNOS, inducible NOS; nNOS, neuronal nitric oxide synthase; NO, nitric oxide; TNF-α, tumor necrosis factor α.

presented. At the whole animal level, exogenously administered interleukin-1β (IL-1), tumor necrosis factor-α (TNF-α), growth hormone–releasing hormone, and brain-derived neurotrophic factor (BDNF) enhance sleep if given intracerebroventricularly or if injected into hypothalamic sleep regulatory areas, and all are well-characterized sleep regulatory molecules.[21,25] Unilateral localized injections of these substances onto the surface of the cortex enhances EEG slow wave power ipsilaterally, suggesting a deeper state of sleep at the injected side.[26-29] Conversely, inhibition of these substances reduces unilateral EEG slow wave power.[28,30,31] Cortical application of these substances also affects the cortical expression of each other.[32] Collectively, these experiments suggest, as evidenced by amplitudes of EEG slow waves, that locally acting sleep regulatory substances influence cortical sleep states unilaterally.

Within visual cortical receptive fields, the patterns of neurons becoming silent in monkeys performing a visual task as they fall asleep provide convincing evidence of local sleep and that it is regulated in a precise manner. Thus, as the behaving monkeys are falling asleep, some of the neurons stop firing; those neurons in the outer edges of the receptive field being engaged by the task are the first to stop firing. As sleep progresses into deeper stages and animals stop performing the visual task, neurons near the center of the engaged receptive field stop firing as well. Pigarev and colleagues concluded that this pattern of localized asynchronous development of sleep indicated that sleep is initiated as a localized process.[33]

Smaller local cortical networks, such as individual cortical columns, oscillate between wake-like and sleep-like states, as determined by their amplitudes of evoked response potentials (ERPs). When the subject is awake, ERPs are smaller in amplitude compared to ERPs occurring during sleep.[34-36] During waking periods, most of the cortical columns are in a wake-like state. In contrast, during whole animal sleep, most of the columns are in the sleep-like state. Individual columns also exhibit sleep homeostasis. Thus the longer an individual column is in the wake-like state, the higher the probability it will enter a sleep-like state. Further, individual cortical column state affects behavior. Thus Rector and colleagues[23] trained rats to lick a sweet solution in response to a facial whisker stimulation. If the somatosensory cortical column that received the whisker afferent input was in the wake-like state, the rat did not make performance mistakes. In contrast, if the column was in the sleep-like state, errors of commission and omission were made. Such results indicate that small local circuits in vivo oscillate between sleep and wake states. Local application of TNF to cortical columns induces higher ERP amplitudes, suggesting that sleep regulatory substances act at the local level to initiate sleep.[37] Further, because TNF and other sleep regulatory substances (Figure 31.1) are cell activity–dependent and prolonged wakefulness is associated with longer cell activation, the results also have implications for the poor performance outcomes in sleep-deprived subjects.[1] That in vivo cortical expression of IL-1, TNF, and BDNF upregulate with enhanced afferent input[38,39] and induce local sleep-like states suggests the local states and these molecules are driving the local enhancements of EEG slow wave power associated with enhanced localized activity during prior waking, as described previously.

Sleep In Vitro

As outlined previously, the definition of sleep as a whole organism behavior is insufficient to account for several network, cellular, and molecular aspects. To determine the minimal network capable of sleep, multiple other approaches are needed. We have proposed that sleep might be a default property of any simple neural network, which is modified by multiple other networks distributed throughout a complex nervous system. In vitro models (neural cultures, organotypic cultures, or slices) have long been used in the field of neuroscience with significant contributions to our understanding of basic mechanisms of central nervous system functions (e.g., long-term potentiation in hippocampal slices). More recently, human neurodevelopmental, neurodegenerative, and neuropsychiatric disorders are being modeled in vitro, either in rodent-derived primary neuronal cultures or human-derived neuronal induced pluripotent stem cells.[40-43]

In vitro evidence of the burst-pause neuronal discharge, characteristic of slow wave sleep, was first demonstrated using dissociated rat cortical cultures.[44] This endogenous (default) discharge activity of neuronal networks has been verified in both organotypic explants[45,46] and dissociated neuronal cultures on multi-electrode arrays (MEAs),[47,48] leading to the proposal by Corner that the spontaneous burst discharges recorded in vitro are the basis of intrinsically generated slow wave sleep in vivo.[49] To extend these observations, Hinard and colleagues used mouse embryonic dissociated cortical cultures grown on MEAs and recorded their spontaneous discharge activity. The cellular responses to wake neuromodulators and the expression of plasticity-related genes as well as metabolic changes were measured.[50] Since cortical cultures invariably develop a burst-pause activity similar to the slow oscillation (<1 Hz) of NREM sleep, the challenge was to generate "wake-like" discharge activity. This has been achieved by applying a cocktail of known waking neuromodulators at physiologic concentrations. The chemical stimulation led to a desynchronized "wake-like" discharge activity, which was followed 24 hours later by the reappearance of the slow oscillation. Comparisons between baseline and recovery after in vitro stimulation with cortical tissues from living mice either at baseline or after sleep deprivation revealed a surprising similarity in terms of gene expression and metabolic changes.[50] This study and others, by using different techniques, convincingly demonstrated that the sleep-like state recorded in vitro is an emergent network property of mature neuron-glia cultures.[51,52]

In a parallel and complementary work by Jewett and colleagues, cultured cortical neurons and glia were stimulated by electrical, TNF, and optogenetic techniques.[51] Detailed analysis revealed that electrical stimulation led to the loss of synchronous burst-pause activity, which showed a homeostatic rebound (as measured by the slow wave power density) a day later, and this homeostatic response was stimulus pattern dependent.[51] On the contrary, addition of TNF to the cultures enhanced burstiness and synchrony, suggesting a deeper sleep-like state. The effects of IL-1, another sleep-promoting agent, was also investigated in the in vitro model of sleep.[53] Cultures from wild-type mice treated, whereas IL-1 showed enhanced slow wave activity, whereas cultures using cells from neuron-specific IL-1 accessory protein receptor knockout mice had delayed maturation in their spontaneous discharge activity, and delta activity following IL-1 treatment was not enhanced.[53] In another study, the homeostatic regulation of discharge activity in vitro was also demonstrated by neuromodulator stimulation at three different concentrations (mimicking different duration of enforced wakefulness in vivo).[54] The evidence that the emergent burst-pause network activity in vitro is identical to the slow oscillation (<1 Hz) of NREM sleep was confirmed by both local field potentials (LFP) and intracellular recordings.[55,56] Collectively, the in vitro work summarized previously is consistent with the hypothesis that small neuronal/glial networks manifest sleep-wake states that share properties similar to those of localized sleep within the cortex and whole animal sleep. One of the most important findings of in vitro studies is that continuous stimulation of neural networks cannot prevent the reemergence of the sleep-like state,[50,55] strongly confirming that the network stimulation (either by electrical or excitatory neuromodulators in vitro or by wakefulness in living animals) activates homeostatic processes to reestablish the default state sleep.

LOCAL MECHANISMS

Neuronal Circuit Mechanisms

The slow oscillation results from alternating synchronized active (up) and silent (down) states of cortical neurons and is locally generated and travels across cortical surface in an anteroposterior direction[57] not only during sleep in humans but also in cortical slices of ferrets.[58] As opposed to the slow oscillation, faster sleep oscillations such as delta waves (1 to 4 Hz) and spindles (10 to 15 Hz) require reciprocal interactions between the cortex and thalamus (and probably other subcortical structures). The frequency of cortical slow oscillation, slow waves, and spindles is modulated by thalamic inputs.[59,60] The generation of cortical spindles relies on interactions between thalamic reticular nucleus, thalamocortical relay projections, and corticothalamic feedback.[61] The thalamus is the major relay between arousal-promoting nuclei and the cortex and therefore is necessary to induce the waking active cortical state. Accordingly, optogenetic activation of the paraventricular glutamatergic neurons, centromedial, or ventromedial thalamic nucleus induces transitions from NREM sleep to wakefulness.[60,62,63]

So far, only the slow oscillation, as the characteristic feature of NREM sleep, was revealed in cultures of cortical and hippocampal neurons. Whether other sleep features can be recapitulated in vitro in thalamocortical co-cultures is under investigation. It is also not known if subcortical networks show locally similar or other features of sleep in vitro. The fact that the NREM sleep-like state is a default state even in species without a complex brain such as *C. elegans* strongly suggests that sleep is an emergent property of any neural network.[64] The enigma remains as to whether, similar to NREM sleep features, periodic desynchronization of cortical networks and associated muscle atonia and eye movements of REM sleep can also occur locally.

Local Use-Dependent Mechanisms Are Shared by Multiple Brain Processes Linked to Sleep

There are several linked brain physiologic processes that local cell use initiates. These include sleep, cerebral blood flow, inflammation, plasticity, and metabolism. Multiple molecules are produced and secreted in response to cell use, including nitric oxide (NO), adenosine triphosphate, adenosine, prostaglandins, IL-1, and TNF (Figure 31.1). These molecules dilate cerebral vessels, influence brain plasticity, and promote local inflammation and sleep.[23-25] Although all these processes are initiated by local events, the resultant changes manifest as emergent properties of higher, more complex levels of organization. For example, changes in local circuit plasticity may result in a new memory, or localized inflammation can lead to whole animal behavior, including sleep. Individual effector mechanisms for each process are, to a degree, compartmentalized partially because of the different cell types affected by local cell activation (e.g., neurons versus macrophages). Further, the higher-order emergent processes provide feedback in the forms of behavior, temperature, various dynamic electrochemical potentials, and so on to modify the initial cell-activation events. The mechanisms responsible for the higher-order emergent events begin at the cellular level and then diverge as the locally induced events merge, integrate, synchronize, and amplify into larger events as they climb up organizational levels.

BOX 31.2 MECHANISTIC HYPOTHESIS AND IMPLICATIONS FOR LOCAL USE-DEPENDENT SLEEP

Step 1: Cell activity (i.e., metabolism and electrical activity) induces synthesis and release of local sleep regulatory substances (SRS) (Figure 31.1) (*sleep is initiated locally*)
Step 2: SRS production is thus activity dependent (*sleep is homeostatically driven*)
Step 3: SRSs act locally to alter receptive, hence electrical, properties of nearby neurons and thus alter input-output relationships of the network within which they are found (*sleep is targeted to previously active networks*)
Step 4: The altered input-output network relationships reflect a functional state change (*sleep is local*)
Step 5: Sleep-like states in small local circuits synchronize with each other leading to organism state changes (*organism sleep is a network emergent property*)[a]
Step 6: Sleep regulatory circuits coordinate the individual network (e.g., cortical columns) functional states into organism sleep architecture (*sleep is adapted to the organism niche*)
Step 7: SRSs act on multiple levels of the neural axis to promote sleep (*sleep mechanisms are ubiquitous and evolutionarily ancient*)

[a]For a discussion of spontaneous synchronization, see Strogatz S. *Sync: The Emerging Science of Spontaneous Order.* Hyperion; 2003. For a mathematical model see Roy S, Krueger JM, Rector DM, Wan Y. Network models for activity-dependent sleep regulation. *J Theor Biol.* 2008;253:462–8.

However, regulation of sleep, inflammation, plasticity, cerebral blood flow, and metabolism are very difficult to separate experimentally from each other because of common local molecular initiating events. Thus among proposed sleep functions are plasticity, inflammation, metabolism, and cerebral blood flow. Further, most of the molecules mentioned also affect appetite, body temperature, and mood; it is proposed that modulation of these brain processes are also sleep functions. Thus, although it is understandable why these sleep functions have been proposed, the primordial sleep function must explain why reduced responsiveness to environmental cues (e.g., altered consciousness) is required.[65] As previously argued, circuit use–dependent plasticity/connectivity provides exceptional evolutionary fitness. Yet plasticity/connectivity involves changing local circuits, resulting in changes in circuit outputs to a given input. Thus the circuit output during waking is adaptive, presumed because the animal is alive, yet waking activity is causing the circuit to change via the actions of use-dependent molecules and thereby alters output to a given input. During such times, it would be advantageous if the animal were not behaving; unconsciousness would ensure such a reduced responsiveness state (i.e., sleep). Other proposed sleep functions could be accomplished with less risk without altering behavior. However, the synchrony of all the proposed use-dependent sleep functions within the rest phase would provide even greater evolutionary fitness.

Local to Global Hypotheses and Implications

Local events involved in the initiation of local network states eventually will manifest as whole organism sleep. The steps involved and their implications for sleep are briefly outlined in Box 31.2 (see the red type). There remains much work to fill in the details, especially determination of the timing of individual events and their relationship to the emergence and characterization of the various levels of organization involved (e.g., cellular–small networks–large networks–whole brain). In this chapter we focused on developing the hypothesis that small networks, whether in vivo or in vitro, display sleep-like properties.

CLINICAL PEARL

The use-dependent biochemical mechanisms responsible for local sleep are involved in multiple additional biologic processes, such as inflammation, cerebral blood flow, metabolism, and neuroplasticity. Sleep pathologies are likely to affect these processes. Further, localized sleep occurring during waking is likely linked to multiple clinical observations, such as insomnia, sleep inertia, dissociated states, poor performance, and excessive sleepiness. Finally, the local cerebral circuits involved in the perception of wakefulness remain active during sleep, and wakefulness may be perceived even though the patient is asleep as judged by other criteria, such as occurs during insomnia.[23,66,67]

SUMMARY

Ample historic evidence suggests that parts of the brain can be asleep while other parts are awake (e.g., sleepwalking, sleep inertia, dolphin unilateral sleep). Small networks, whether in vivo or in vitro, exhibit sleep-like properties, and that sleep within these networks is initiated by local cell activity has been hypothesized. Many, perhaps all, sleep regulatory molecules are locally synthesized in response to cell activity. Experimentally, local cortical sleep intensity can be increased or decreased by prior local activation or inhibition, respectively, whether achieved by enhanced or reduced localized afferent input, or by treatment with sleep regulatory substances or their inhibitors. Cortical columns oscillate between sleep- and wake-like states; behavior dependent upon a single cortical column is disturbed if the column is in the sleep-like state. Neuronal/glial co-cultures have a default sleep-like state, and their stimulation, electrically or chemically, is followed by enhanced expression of sleep regulatory substances and rebound sleep-like state indicating sleep homeostasis. The in vitro sleep-like state, like whole animal sleep, is also characterized by neuronal burstiness, synchrony of slow potentials, sleep-associated gene expression, and spontaneous reversibility. We conclude that small neuronal/glial networks constitute a minimal part of the brain capable of sleep states and that sleep-like states are the default state dependent upon prior cell use. This proposition provides greater explanatory parsimony of dissociated brain states, poor behavioral performance, insomnia, sleep-inertia, and other sleep anomalies and pathologies.

ACKNOWLEDGMENTS

This work was supported in part by grants from The National Institutes of Health (USA) (Grant NS025378) and the W. M. Keck Foundation (to JMK) and by The Swiss National Science Foundation (Grant 173126 to MT).

SELECTED READINGS

Bandarabadi M, Vassalli A, Tafti M. Sleep as a default state of cortical and subcortical networks. *Curr Opin Physiol.* 2020;15:60–67.

Hinard V, Mikhail C, Pradervand S, et al. Key electrophysiological, molecular, and metabolic signatures of sleep and wakefulness revealed in primary cortical cultures. *J Neurosci.* 2012;32:12506–12517.
Huber R, Ghilardi MF, Massimini M, et al. Arm immobilization causes cortical plastic changes and locally decreases sleep slow wave activity. *Nat Neurosci.* 2006;9:1169–1176.
Jewett KA, Taishi P, Sengupta P, Roy S, Davis CJ, Krueger JM. Tumor necrosis factor enhances the sleep-like state and electrical stimulation induces a wake-like state in co-cultures of neurons and glia. *Eur J Neurosci.* 2015;42:2078–2090.
Jubera-García E, Gevers W, Van Opstal F. Local build-up of sleep pressure could trigger mind wandering: Evidence from sleep, circadian and mind wandering research [published online ahead of print, 2021 Feb 18]. *Biochem Pharmacol.* 2021;114478.
Krueger JM, Obál Jr F. A neuronal group theory of sleep function. *J Sleep Res.* 1993;2:63–69.
Krueger JM, Rector DM, Roy S, Van Dongen HPA, Belenky G, Panksepp J. Sleep as a fundamental property of neuronal assemblies. *Nat Rev Neurosci.* 2008;9:910–919.
Krueger JM, Huang Y, Rector DM, Buysee DJ Sleep. A synchrony of cell activity-driven small network states. *Eur J Neurosci.* 2013;38:2199–2209.
Mahowald MW, Schenck CH. Dissociated states of wakefulness and sleep. *Neurology.* 1992;42(7 suppl 6):44–52.
Rattenborg NC, Lima SL, Lesku JA. Sleep locally, act globally. *Neuroscientist.* 2012;18:533–546.
Rector DM, Topchiy IA, Carter KM, Rojas MJ. Local functional state differences between rat cortical columns. *Brain Res.* 2005;1047:45–55.
Saberi-Moghadam S, Simi A, Setareh H, Mikhail C, Tafti M. In vitro cortical network firing is homeostatically regulated: a model for sleep regulation. *Sci Rep.* 2018;8:6297.

A complete reference list can be found online at ExpertConsult.com.

Chapter 32

Pathophysiology of Sleep-Wake Disturbances after Traumatic Brain Injury

Nadia Gosselin; Christian R. Baumann

Chapter Highlights

- Sleep-wake disturbances (SWDs), particularly fatigue, excessive daytime sleepiness, and pleiosomnia (an increased sleep need per 24 hours), are very common after traumatic brain injury (TBI), but their pathophysiology is poorly understood.
- The bulk of animal studies consistently show that TBI leads to modification in sleep-wake patterns, which suggests that the TBI itself causes a proportion of SWDs.
- Posttraumatic brain dysfunction results in impaired neurotransmitter signaling, changes in gene expression, altered circadian rhythms, cerebral hypometabolism, neuroinflammation, and hypopituitarism; all have been identified as potential contributors to the emergence and persistence of posttraumatic SWDs.
- Other factors that may occur in association with TBI in humans are pain and psychiatric comorbidities, which can independently affect sleep-wake pattern after TBI. Prolonged use of sedatives/analgesics and psychoactive medication is associated with increased SWDs.
- The role of sleep in cognition, neuroplasticity, and neurogenesis is now well recognized, but increasing evidence suggests that sleep and its abnormalities after TBI influence recovery on both a clinical and a neuropathologic level. Improving the current understanding of factors involved in posttraumatic SWDs could lead to more specific and efficient interventions in this clinical population. Whether SWDs have the potential to explain the increased risk of dementia after TBI is an emerging question.

Traumatic brain injury (TBI) is the leading cause of death and disability among young adults in industrialized countries.[1] Incidence is estimated at up to 600 per 100,000 in the general population, and a majority of victims are young men entering their most productive years. TBI often results in short- and long-term impairments that interfere with the return to normal life. Fatigue, excessive daytime sleepiness, pleiosomnia (an increased sleep need per 24 hours), and insomnia are among the most persistent and the most disabling symptoms after TBI. Chronic sleep-wake disturbances (SWDs) are reported by at least 50% of patients with TBI, but despite their high prevalence, the emergence and evolution of SWDs are still poorly understood and probably involve interaction among multiple causal factors.

This chapter is organized into three main sections: (1) an introduction to the diagnosis and the pathophysiology of TBI; (2) a survey of recent animal models that were developed to characterize posttraumatic sleep-wake patterns; and (3) an update on human neuropathology data giving insights into potential pathophysiologic causes, physiologic factors, and influences of comorbid conditions that may contribute to SWD onset or maintenance. Other important sleep-wake disorders associated with TBI, not covered in this chapter, include insomnia, narcolepsy, sleep-disordered breathing, and sleep-related movement disorders; these are discussed elsewhere in this volume.

INTRODUCTION TO TRAUMATIC BRAIN INJURY

TBI is an alteration in brain function or other evidence of brain pathology caused by an external force.[2] In turn, alteration in brain function is defined as one of the following signs: any period of decreased level of consciousness, any loss of memory for events immediately before (retrograde amnesia) or after the injury (posttraumatic amnesia), neurologic deficits (e.g., weakness, loss of balance, change in vision, aphasia), or any alteration in mental state at the time of the injury (e.g., confusion, disorientation). Other evidence of brain pathology may include visual, neuroradiologic, or laboratory confirmation of damage to the brain. The diagnosis of TBI involves a severity assessment.[3] In general, *mild TBI* is characterized by a short loss of consciousness (<30 minutes), an initial Glasgow Coma Scale (GCS) score between 13 and 15, and a short period of posttraumatic amnesia (<24 hours). *Moderate TBI* typically is associated with a loss of consciousness of 30 minutes to 24 hours, a GCS score between 9 and 12, and posttraumatic amnesia lasting 1 to 14 days. *Severe TBI* generally is characterized by a loss of consciousness of more than 24 hours, a GCS score between 3 and 8, and posttraumatic amnesia persisting for several weeks.

Pathophysiology of Traumatic Brain Injury

Cerebral damage after TBI results from primary and secondary insults.[4] *Primary insults* result when the application of biomechanical forces causes local lesions (i.e., skull fracture, intracranial hematoma, lacerations, and contusions) or diffuse axonal injury. *Secondary insults* occur in the hours or days after the initial trauma as a consequence of neuronal hypoxia caused by several dysfunctions that alter the cerebral oxygen and glucose supplies.[5] Intracranial hypertension is the most common form of secondary insult. Both primary and secondary insults lead to neurochemical changes, such as an increase in extracellular excitatory amino acids (glutamate and aspartate),[6] which provokes excessive intracellular calcium influx, leading to free radical production, mitochondrial dysfunction, apoptosis, and inflammatory response.

Brain computed tomography scan is performed in patients who present with TBI, particularly those with moderate or severe TBI, and is considered a good clinical tool for detecting focal lesions[7] that are mostly localized in the ventral and polar frontal regions and in the anterior temporal lobes.[8] However, TBI often is associated with diffuse axonal injury, which is difficult to quantify with computed tomography. Rapid acceleration-deceleration of the brain generates traumatic shearing forces, ultimately leading to diffuse axonal injury. Diffusion tensor imaging, which allows the measurement of microstructural white matter integrity, shows white matter injuries in the corpus callosum and the internal capsule, as well as a global white matter loss, within 2 weeks after TBI, that are mostly attributed to axonal swelling.[9,10] Neuroimaging findings in the acute stage of TBI are extremely variable from one patient to another in terms of severity and localization of lesions, with mild TBI generally causing no acute white matter lesions.[11]

TBI also may lead to permanent pathologic modifications of brain structures, which can explain some of the neuropsychiatric and cognitive dysfunctions observed in this population. In patients with chronic TBI, loss of gray matter may be observed, particularly in the hippocampus, but also in the frontal and temporal cortex, the thalamus, the basal forebrain, the anterior cingulate, the caudate nucleus, and the insula.[12,13] This long-term decrease in gray matter density is more severe in patients with lower initial GCS score or in those who presented with intracranial hypertension in the intensive care unit (ICU).[14] In more severely affected patients, white matter degeneration can be observed in all of the major fiber tracts, including the corpus callosum, the cingulum, the superior and inferior longitudinal fasciculus, the uncinate fasciculus, and the brainstem.[15] In general, more severe disruptions in cortico-cortical and cortical-subcortical pathways correlate with poorer cognitive functioning.

Traumatic Brain Injury and Neurodegenerative Diseases

Several studies have shown that TBI may later be followed by the development of a neurodegenerative disease; TBI increases the risk of developing Alzheimer's disease or another dementia later in life by 50%, with more severe TBI associated with greater risk.[16] Healthy axons contain amyloid precursor protein in high concentrations, and amyloid precursor protein markedly accumulates in damaged axons, most likely through impaired axonal transport, which in general leads to the production and accumulation of toxic proteins and peptides, including amyloid-beta plaques and neurofibrillary tangles after TBI.[17]

In many people with TBI, a presumed underlying pathologic process involves multiple lifetime traumatic injuries, particularly among contact sports athletes. Repetitive acceleration and deceleration forces directed to the brain may cause chronic traumatic encephalopathy, which is associated with dementia and amyloid-beta deposition, either as diffuse or neuritic plaques, but the underlying pathophysiology is still not fully understood.[18,19] Also, increased levels of α-synuclein protein, which is known to play an important role in the development of Parkinson's disease and other neurodegenerative disorders, have been detected in brain tissue samples from persons with a history of TBI.[20] Using patient self-report measures and clinical interviews, one study showed that repetitive TBI increases the severity of posttraumatic insomnia.[21] In view of the probable role of TBI in the development of later neurodegenerative disease, it is not surprising that such injuries are reported to have chronic and long-term impact on brain functioning, including sleep-wake and circadian regulation.

Behavioral and Cognitive Consequences of Traumatic Brain Injury

After moderate and severe TBI, an alteration in the level of consciousness, followed by a period of delirium, confusion, agitation, and posttraumatic amnesia, generally is apparent when patients are in the awakening stage in the ICU. Neurobehavioral impairments, such as impulsivity, irritability, disinhibition, mutism, and apathy, can be observed.[22] The extent of functional and cognitive deficits observed in the postacute period is highly variable among patients with TBI and depends on several factors, such as brain injury severity, location of focal lesions, severity of diffuse axonal injury, duration of posttraumatic amnesia, age, level of education, and preexisting conditions. Despite the variability of cognitive dysfunction, certain deficits are common, including arousal and alertness impairments, reduced information processing speed, impaired memory, executive dysfunctions, impaired language, and reduced self-awareness. Unfortunately, these impairments persist for longer than 1 year in 50% of patients with moderate or severe TBI and may also be observed in chronic mild TBI, and these impairments may lead to dependency in activities of daily living and problems with return to work or school.[23]

Biomarkers of Outcome after Traumatic Brain Injury

Several TBI studies have searched for sensitive and reliable markers of short- and long-term neurologic and functional outcome. The first group of studies supports the concept that genetic factors influence functional outcome after TBI. Among the most studied polymorphisms in the TBI population is the apolipoprotein (APOE) ε4 allele, which was associated with poor outcome at 6 months after injury and with greater risk of later cognitive decline.[24] Preliminary evidence also suggests that functional polymorphisms of the brain-derived neurotropic factor (BDNF) and the catechol-*O*-methyl transferase

(COMT) genes, which are involved, respectively, in brain plasticity regulation and dopamine modulation, influence cognitive recovery after TBI.[25,26] BDNF polymorphisms contribute to the regulation of slow wave sleep oscillations and hence non–rapid eye movement (NREM) sleep intensity in humans.[27] Moreover, preliminary evidence suggest that BDNF Val/Met polymorphisms moderate the link between sleep quality and cognition,[28] which reinforces the relevance of studying BNDF to understand interindividual variability in post-TBI SWDs and their consequences. Other potential genetic biomarkers may be related to circadian disorders. For instance, the expression of bone morphogenetic protein-6 coincides with melatonin levels.[29]

The second group of studies investigated proteomic markers of outcome. The serum level of the S100B protein is among the most extensively studied marker in the TBI patient population.[30] It is known to predict unfavorable outcome in severe TBI and also is sensitive and specific for intracranial lesions in mild TBI,[31] but changes in S100B serum concentration are not specific for TBI and can be observed in several other conditions, such as infection and with orthopedic injuries. Glial fibrillary acid protein (GFAP) is a protein specifically expressed in astrocytes and is a well-known marker of central nervous system pathology. In a study that included 94 patients with mild TBI, GFAP serum level at admission predicted return to work and functional outcome.[32] A study in mice 4 weeks after TBI suggested that GFAP expression and microglial cell activation are increased in the reticular thalamic nucleus preceding sleep disturbance.[33] No sufficient evidence, however, is available on how these proteins might affect sleep-wake behavior after TBI.

PATHOPHYSIOLOGY OF POSTTRAUMATIC SLEEP-WAKE DISTURBANCES

Surveyed in this section are recent animal models that were specifically developed to improve the current understanding of posttraumatic sleep-wake patterns. Also reviewed are potential pathophysiologic causes, physiologic factors, and influences of comorbid conditions that may contribute to SWD onset or maintenance. Figure 32.1 presents an integrative model of potential contributors to posttraumatic SWD.

Experimental Models of Traumatic Brain Injury and Studies of Sleep-Wake Behavior in Animals

Fluid Percussion

After craniotomy in mice, an insult is inflicted by application of a fluid pressure pulse to the dura,[34] which leads to bilateral cortical alterations and other physiologic changes that have been interpreted as a model for human TBI.[35] *Midline fluid percussion injury* led to a marked increase in sleep within the first 6 hours after trauma.[34] In a subsequent study and by applying the same methods, these investigators could not identify persistent SWD 2 to 5 weeks after injury.[36] On the other hand, when applying repetitive TBI at a 3-hour interval, which disrupts posttraumatic sleep, the same group observed more severe functional and histopathologic consequences then when applying the second TBI at a 9-hour interval.[37]

Lateral fluid percussion injury is reproducible and recapitulates many injuries observed in humans.[38] Electroencephalogram (EEG)/electromyogram (EMG) recordings after lateral fluid percussion injury found that TBI persistently impairs the ability to sustain wakefulness.[39] The brain-injured mice exhibited more wake to NREM, NREM to wake, and rapid eye movement (REM) to wake transitions in comparison with sham injury control animals, indicating a higher fragmentation of behavioral states.

A study in mice that suffered from lateral fluid percussion injury and in humans with mild TBI found, in both cases, higher theta:alpha amplitude ratios and more EEG slow waves during wakefulness than in control subjects, with a significant correlation between less EEG global coherence and more severe of postconcussive symptoms.[40] These findings from mice and humans might suggest that quantity and coherence of slow waves might represent a biomarker for the prognosis of mild TBI.

Controlled Cortical Impact Model

One study performing EEG/EMG recordings within the first 3 days after controlled cortical impact injury in mice reported a reduction in wakefulness and shorter wake bouts during the active period after trauma but not in control animals.[41] This TBI model leads to diffuse axonal injury and other pathologic alterations in subcortical areas, cerebellar structures, midbrain, and brainstem.

Weight Drop Model

A closed-head mouse TBI model, using a weight drop system in adult mice, showed that mild TBI decreased long bouts of wakefulness in the first 24 hours after injury,[42] similar to findings reported independently by other studies,[41] suggesting an altered capacity to sustain wakefulness after TBI. In addition, some studies adopted a closed-impact acceleration TBI rodent model with a physical hit to the skull with subsequent acceleration-deceleration mechanisms, which also allowed for EEG/EMG recordings.[43,44] Briefly summarized, a blow from a falling metal rod onto the exposed rat skull, which is placed on a thick foam pad, led to acceleration mechanisms similar to those in human TBI, with subsequent widespread histopathologic changes, including diffuse axonal injury, particularly in the corpus callosum, midbrain, cerebral and cerebellar peduncules, and brainstem.[35] Rats that were subjected to TBI exhibited an increase in NREM sleep at 1 month after injury, and sleep was less fragmented.[44]

Repeated Traumatic Brain Injury

Repeated TBI has been shown to have different and accentuated effects on brain health and long-term outcomes compared to one-time injuries. A mouse model was used, whereby a series of six concussive impacts were delivered daily for 7 days. This model allowed the comparison of groups of single-injury and sham-injury control animals.[45] EEG/EMG was recorded at 1 month after injury for a period of 24 hours; animals in the single- and repetitive-TBI groups exhibited a reduction in NREM sleep, more NREM sleep fragmentation, and an increase in wake time compared to control animals. Moreover, EEG spectral analysis during NREM sleep demonstrated reduced power for very low frequencies (1 to 2 Hz) and increased power in the theta band in single- and repetitive-TBI groups compared with the control group. Still needed are larger studies to support these animal observations that repeated trauma leads to a higher SWD burden, not only in relation to insomnia but also in association with other SWDs.

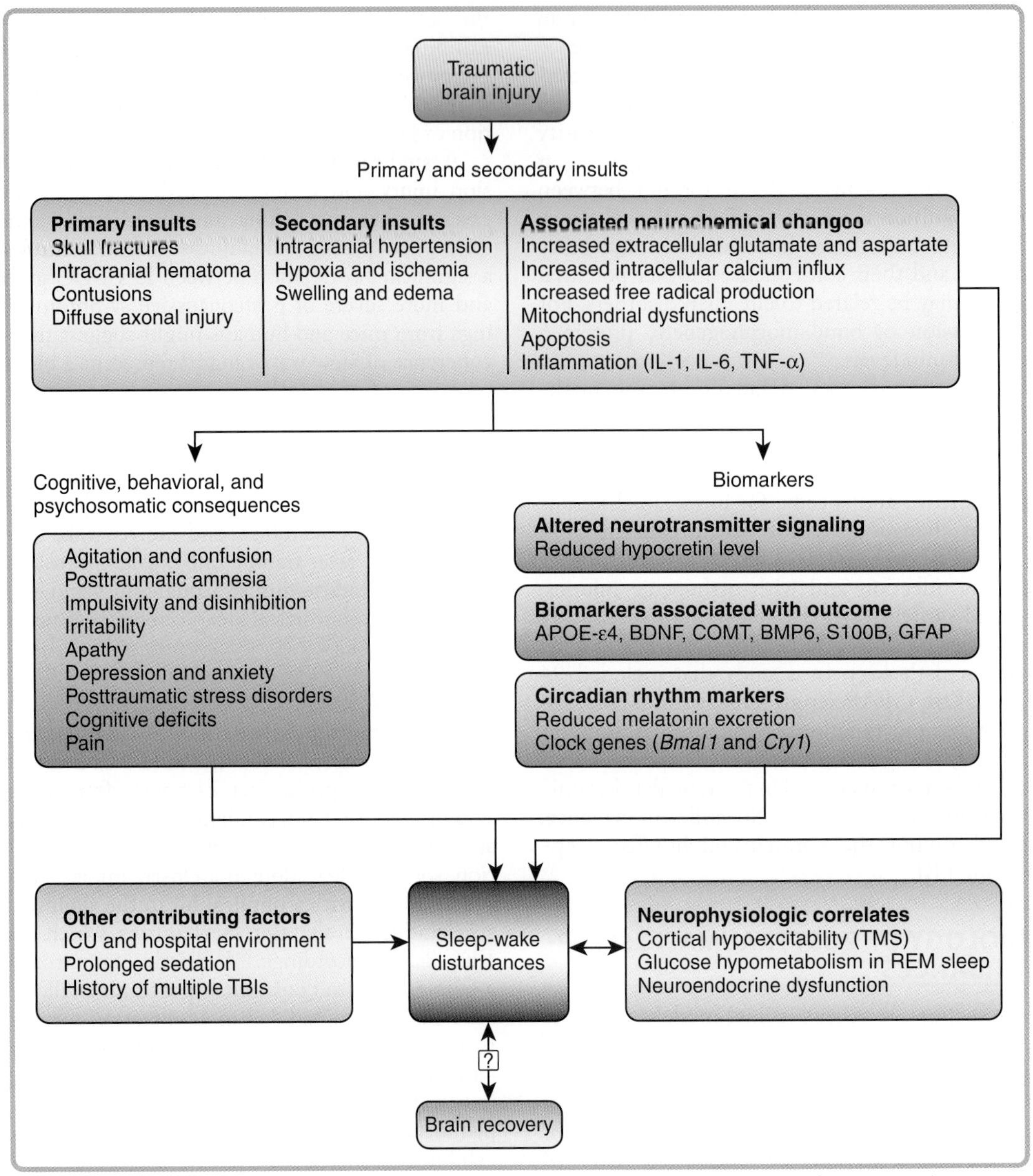

Figure 32.1 Integrative model of potential contributors to sleep-wake disturbance (SWD) after traumatic brain injury (TBI). All potential contributors to SWD after mild, moderate, or severe TBI are included. TBI causes primary and secondary insults that may directly influence sleep-wake patterns, but these injuries also have cognitive, behavioral, and/or psychosomatic consequences known to increase the risk of SWD. Several biomarkers have been associated with outcome, and an increased risk of SWD has been identified for certain of these markers. Other significant contributing factors are environment, medication, and history of multiple TBIs. SWDs have been associated with physiologic changes in patients with TBI, more specifically, cortical hypoexcitability, reduced glucose metabolism in rapid eye movement (REM) sleep, and neuroendocrine dysfunction. Posttraumatic SWDs possibly influence brain recovery after TBI. APOE, Apolipoprotein; BDNF, brain-derived neurotrophic factor; BMP6, bone morphogenetic protein-6; COMT, catechol-*O*-methyl transferase; GFAP, glial fibrillary acidic protein; ICU, intensive care unit; IL, interleukin; S100B, S100 calcium-binding protein B; TMS, transcranial magnetic stimulation; TNF-α, tumor necrosis factor-α.

Another group delivered mild repeated injury by applying a closed-skull impact TBI mouse model.[46] Three consecutive mild TBIs blocked the effect of enriched environment on REM sleep, that is, decreased the REM-enhancing effect of enriched environment, which is conceptualized to improve functional recovery after TBI. This effect should be further evaluated as it might have important implications for rehabilitation of TBI patients.

In conclusion, different models of rodent TBI have been used to examine posttraumatic SWD, both behaviorally and by means of EEG/EMG recordings. This heterogeneity of applied methods probably is responsible for the somewhat inconclusive results so far. Nevertheless, most studies found an increased amount of sleep and a reduction of the capability to maintain wakefulness not only in the first few days, but also in the 2 to 4 weeks after TBI. Issues to be investigated in the future include whether this observed increase in sleep after TBI is a mere reaction to the trauma and consecutive disturbed signaling within sleep-wake modulating pathways or whether sleep is critical for recovery.

Inflammation Mediators from Animal Studies

Mediators of inflammation that are secreted as a result of TBI are important potential contributors to SWD. The acute inflammatory response occurring after TBI is characterized by an increase in interleukin 1 (IL-1), IL-6, and tumor necrosis factor-α (TNF-α). Proinflammatory cytokines IL-1β and TNF-α are known to increase sleepiness, prolong duration of slow wave sleep, and increase EEG delta power.[47] TNF-α also is known to inhibit melatonin synthesis and hypocretin (orexin) activity in rats,[48,49] which can have a significant impact on sleep and wakefulness. One murine study has suggested an association between proinflammatory cytokine IL-1β level and increasing sleep duration in the hours after a mild TBI.[34] The investigators argued that increased sleep in their TBI mice may result from the inflammatory response associated with the secondary injury, but this association needs to be confirmed in future studies.

More recently, the same group tested whether novel TNF receptor inhibitors not only impact posttraumatic sleep but also improve functional recovery after murine TBI.[37] The authors found that treated mice slept significantly less than vehicle-treated animals, and one inhibitor restored cognitive, sensorimotor, and neurologic functions. Whether it is altered sleep or neuroinflammatory response that impacts functional TBI outcome, however, must be elucidated by further studies.

Impaired Neurotransmitter Signaling in Animal Models of Traumatic Brain Injury

Brain structures, especially the hypothalamic, midbrain, and brainstem networks that are involved in sleep, wake, and circadian rhythmicity, can be impaired or damaged in a proportion of patients with TBI, potentially explaining some forms of SWD observed in this population. In this line of thought, consecutive impairment of neurotransmitter signaling would contribute to altered regulation of behavioral states.

Some studies performed intracerebral microdialysis after controlled cortical impact in mice and found that hypothalamic hypocretin levels were depressed.[41] Furthermore, the associations between hypocretin levels and wakefulness were diminished. Abnormal hypocretin dynamics were not associated with acute loss of hypocretin neurons but with hypothalamic astrogliosis. Lim and colleagues,[39] who performed fluid percussion injury in mice (see earlier), measured c-Fos protein in the lateral hypothalamus, where the hypocretin neurons reside. Mice with TBI exhibited significantly decreased hypocretin neuronal activation during wakefulness but, again, normal hypocretin neuron numbers, suggesting that nonfatal injury in these animals primarily affects hypocretin physiology rather than marked cell loss. In this study, dietary branch-chain amino-acid supplementation, precursors to de novo glutamate and gamma-aminobutyric acid synthesis, restored hypocretin neuronal activity and sleep-wake regulation. In a subsequent study, the same group found evidence that TBI decreases relative glutamate density in presynaptic terminals making axodendritic contacts in hypothalamic and cortical structures, which suggests that TBI compromises hypocretin neuronal function via decreased glutamate density.[50]

In addition, one study investigated the immunoreactivity of hypocretin-1 receptors after murine TBI, and the authors found transiently increased immunoreactivity in the surrounding penumbra of the injury.[51] Last but not least, one group assessed posttraumatic sleep in hypocretin-knockout and wild-type animals and observed more NREM sleep and other sleep alterations after moderate TBI only in the wild-type animals, which lost about one-quarter of hypocretin neurons.[52] Again, all of these results suggest that hypocretin and its receptors may play an important role in sleep-wake behavioral abnormalities after TBI, but the exact nature of dysfunctional hypocretin signaling and its pathophysiologic impact remain elusive thus far.

Additional observations in post-TBI rats point toward a critical role of the histamine system in pathologic sleep-wake behavior after trauma.[44] Stereologic cell counts in these animals revealed fewer histaminergic neurons in the tuberomammillary nucleus, and the number of histamine-producing neurons was inversely correlated with the total amount of sleep per 24-hour period. These findings might be among the first initiatives for delineating the mechanisms behind sleep disturbances after TBI.

Impaired Neurotransmitter Signaling in Human Traumatic Brain Injury

For obvious reasons, human data on neurotransmitter signaling after TBI are sparse. The first hint toward dysfunctional hypocretin signaling after TBI appeared in the supplementary data of a publication on hypocretin levels in neurologic disorders, showing pathologically decreased hypocretin levels in the cerebrospinal fluid (CSF) of some brain-injured patients.[53] A systematic approach in prospectively assessed CSF from patients with TBI within the first 4 days after trauma confirmed a massive decrease in hypocretin levels similar to that in narcolepsy patients.[54] Several months later, however, hypocretin levels mostly had recovered to normal (Figure 32.2).[55] Altogether, these CSF-based results suggested that impaired signaling of wake-promoting hypocretin neurons may at least contribute to decreased arousal after TBI.

A pilot study in four deceased patients with fatal TBI reported a significant 27% loss of hypocretin neurons in the hypothalamus.[56] Similarly, in 12 brains from patients who

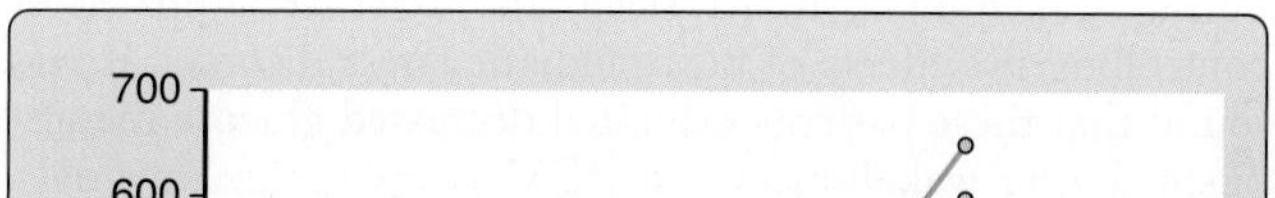

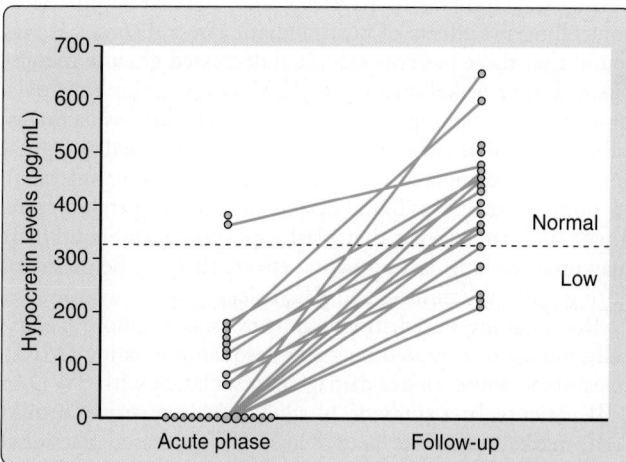

Figure 32.2 Cerebrospinal fluid hypocretin (orexin) levels in subjects with traumatic brain injury. Levels were measured 1 to 4 days after trauma (acute phase; $n = 27$) and 6 months later (follow-up; $n = 21$). Lines connect hypocretin values from the same patient ($n = 15$). Many patients had undetectable levels in the acute phase (plotted as 0). In all patients, levels recovered toward normal, but in some patients, they remained low. (From Baumann CR, Werth E, Stocker R, et al. Sleep-wake disturbances 6 months after traumatic brain injury: a prospective study. *Brain.* 2007;130:1873–83.)

died of fatal TBI, a significant 21% loss of hypothalamic hypocretin neurons was documented.[57] The most marked cell loss (41%), however, involved the wake-maintaining histamine-producing neurons in the tuberomammillary nucleus. Wake-promoting neurons in the brainstem are less severely affected than hypothalamic neurons.[58] Again, these data suggest that damage to a susceptible and exposed posterior hypothalamic area might be involved in the SWD we often see after TBI.

Cortical Hypoexcitability and Transcranial Magnetic Stimulation

As suggested earlier, lesions to midbrain or brainstem structures presumably could lead to posttraumatic SWDs. One group of investigators used transcranial magnetic stimulation (TMS) in humans to determine whether SWDs after trauma are linked to pathologic excitability of the cerebral cortex.[59] The study included patients with TBI demonstrating excessive daytime sleepiness, fatigue, or increased sleep need and appropriate control subjects. Only in those patients with objective excessive daytime sleepiness (as confirmed by the Multiple Sleep Latency Test) were correlates of cortical hypoexcitability found. The investigators concluded that this finding on a cortical level might reflect the deficiency of the excitatory hypocretin system. In fact, earlier functional imaging studies showed that brain perfusion abnormalities, as assessed by single-photon emission computed tomography, are present predominantly in the midbrain structures and less so in cortical areas.[60]

Neuroimaging of Sleep

Functional neuroimaging comprises noninvasive techniques that allow exploring patterns of brain activation during wakefulness and sleep in humans. Although some studies that included normal control subjects and used functional neuroimaging during sleep were published in past years, only one study was performed in persons with mild TBI.[61] That study included five consecutive in-laboratory polysomnographic (PSG) recordings in 14 military veterans with a history of blast exposure and/or mild TBI (42.6 ± 26.9 months after injury) using ^{18}F-fluorodeoxyglucose positron emission tomography during wakefulness, REM sleep, and NREM sleep. After controlling for effects of posttraumatic stress disorder, it was found that these patients exhibited decreased glucose metabolism during wakefulness and REM sleep in the amygdala, hippocampus, parahippocampal gyrus, thalamus, insula uncus, culmen, visual association cortex, and midline medial frontal cortex when compared with control subjects (other veterans). Hypometabolism was found despite normal sleep architecture. These findings suggest that blast exposure and/or mild TBI may produce long-lasting neural effects that can be observed during both wakefulness and REM sleep.

Recent studies used structural neuroimaging, more specifically, diffusion-weighted magnetic resonance imaging (MRI), to estimate white matter damage in association with SWD in TBI patients. In a study of 34 adults within a year of a mild TBI, markers of white matter loss (i.e., decreased fractional anisotropy and increased mean, radial, and/or axial diffusivities) in multiple tracts were associated with worse subjective sleep quality and depression symptoms.[62] Regarding objective sleep measures and considering that white matter loss is the signature hallmark of more severe TBI, how white matter loss impacts sleep microarchitecture, most notably NREM sleep oscillations (sleep spindles and slow waves), is intriguing. In fact, preliminary evidence shows that white matter characteristics predict NREM sleep oscillation density and morphology in healthy control subjects.[63,64] In studies by Sanchez and colleagues,[15,65] they tested 23 patients with moderate to severe TBI and 27 control subjects with MRI and PSG. They surprisingly found that massive white matter loss in the thalamocortical tracts does not prevent the generation of normal spindles in patients with TBI. Moreover, TBI and control subjects did not differ in terms of slow wave density and morphology. However, they observed that greater white matter damage was strongly associated with larger slow waves in N2 and N3 sleep and with steeper negative-to-positive slow wave slopes, a marker of neuronal synchrony. White matter damage was also associated with reported fatigue and higher slow wave activity power, probably reflecting higher homeostatic sleep pressure.

Circadian Rhythms

One factor potentially contributing to SWDs is the presence of alteration in the circadian timing system. Irregular circadian rhythms are known to be translated into increased daytime sleep, reduced nocturnal sleep, and fragmented sleep.[66] Circadian disruption may occur when the main biologic clock of the hypothalamus is not synchronized to the 24-hour day and/or when it produces a circadian signal too weak to entrain the peripheral clocks of the brain and body. Short (acute phase) and long-term studies were conducted after TBI, and it is obvious that the paucity of literature necessitates caution in interpreting the following data.

Circadian Studies in Acute Traumatic Brain Injury

Only a few studies have investigated melatonin, cortisol, and body temperature rhythms, three well-known markers of circadian rhythms, in sedated patients with TBI while they were hospitalized in ICUs. In a study performed in 3 patients with TBI and 8 patients with other acute neurologic injuries, an absence of circadian rhythms was found for plasmatic melatonin, plasmatic cortisol, and body temperature.[67] When results were compared with those from critically ill patients without neurologic injury, alteration in circadian rhythms was greater in patients with brain lesions. These results suggest that brain injuries are in part responsible for altered circadian rhythms seen in ICUs. In another study, reduction in serum melatonin concentration was observed in addition to irregular circadian cycles in 8 sedated patients with TBI, and these alterations were correlated with brain injury severity.[68] Using microdialysis, an absence of cortisol circadian rhythm also was found in 10 patients with severe TBI under analgosedation.[69] Among mechanisms that may explain the absence of circadian rhythms in critically ill brain-injured patients is a cerebral lesion in the suprachiasmatic nucleus, because this region is known as the master clock that synchronizes most endogenous circadian rhythms.[70] Other possible causes include an altered pattern of light exposure, such as with too little contrast between day and nighttime light exposure,[71] hypoxia,[72] and anesthesia/sedation.

Circadian Studies in Postacute Traumatic Brain Injury

An absence of 24-hour sleep-wake cycle has been documented with actigraphy in patients hospitalized for a moderate to severe TBI.[73] This absence of a circadian cycle was specifically observed in patients with TBI and not in control patients, that is, non-TBI patients with severe orthopedic injuries, hospitalized in the same environment, which suggests a role of TBI in flattened circadian cycling.[74] The most obvious suspect for this absence of circadian sleep-wake cycle is the circadian clock, which is responsible for the elevated melatonin production at the beginning of the night. In a study performed in an intermediate care unit, on average 18.3 days postinjury, actigraphic sleep-wake cycle and urinary melatonin circadian rhythm (measured hourly for 26 consecutive hours) were evaluated in 17 nonsedated patients with TBI compared to 14 non-TBI patients with orthopedic injuries.[74] Nocturnal 6-sulfatoxymelatonin excretion was similar in the two groups, with a significant increased nighttime concentration beyond daytime concentration peaks. Despite the presence of melatonin circadian rhythm, TBI patients exhibited a nonconsolidated sleep-wake cycle, whereas those with non-TBI orthopedic injuries had a clear 24-hour sleep-wake cycle. These results suggest that a nonconsolidated sleep-wake cycle in the postacute stage of TBI is not due to an absence of melatonin-production circadian rhythm. However, the absence of circadian sleep-wake cycle could be due to post-TBI melatonin receptors, as one study using controlled cortical impact in rats showed that MT1 and MT2 receptors—a major target for melatonin therapy—were reduced in the frontal cortex and the hippocampus.[75]

Circadian Studies in Chronic Traumatic Brain Injury

Several case studies reported circadian rhythm disturbances associated with chronic TBI (see Chapter 43 for more details), and two studies specifically investigated salivary dim-light melatonin onset in patients with chronic TBI. The first study reported no group difference in the timing of nighttime melatonin onset, but a high variability among the subjects was noted.[76] A second study conducted by the same investigators found lower levels of evening melatonin production in patients with mild to severe TBI than in control subjects, but again, no changes were found for dim-light melatonin onset (Figure 32.3).[77] Because saliva melatonin concentration was

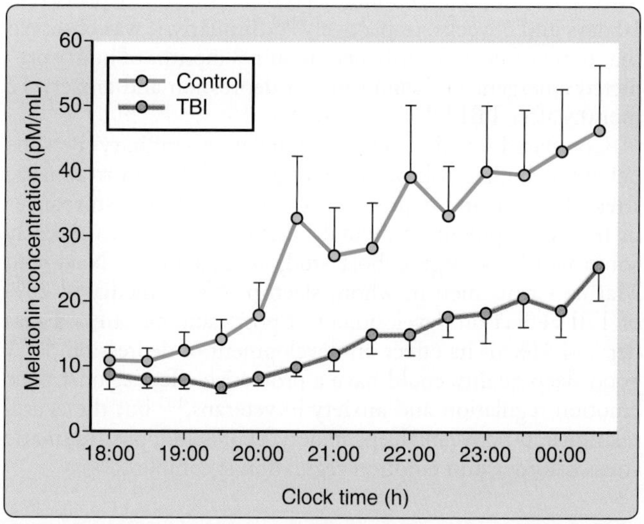

Figure 32.3 Nighttime salivary melatonin levels in patients with traumatic brain injury (TBI) and control subjects. Salivary melatonin levels of TBI (*orange*) and control group (*green*) from 6:00 p.m. to 12:30 a.m. Data are presented as mean ± standard error. Salivary samples were collected every half hour. The TBI group had lower melatonin concentrations across the sampling period compared with the control group. (From Shekleton JA, Parcell DL, Redman JR, et al. Sleep disturbance and melatonin levels following traumatic brain injury. *Neurology.* 2010;74:1732–8.)

measured only for 6.5 consecutive hours during the evening (i.e., from 6:00 p.m. to 12:30 a.m.), in this latter study, it was not possible to determine whether a phase delay of melatonin secretion could explain the reduced melatonin production in the TBI group.

Clock Genes

It has been hypothesized that circadian rhythm disruption after TBI is mediated by changes in expression of clock genes in the suprachiasmatic nucleus and hippocampus. It was found that in rats with fluid percussion-induced TBI, compared with sham-operated ones, that the circadian expression of two key clock genes (i.e., *Bmal1* and *Cry1*) was altered in both the suprachiasmatic nucleus and the hippocampus.[78] In this study, altered daily rhythm of locomotor activity coincided with the deregulation of clock genes. The investigators suggested that a disturbance in the transcriptional-translation feedback loops that modulate circadian timing could be induced by TBI. Recently, one preliminary study has explored circadian clock gene expression levels in patients with mild TBI with and without sleep disorders.[79] The authors found that patients with sleep-wake disorders had lower and/or abnormal messenger RNA (mRNA) melatonin, *Clock* gene, and *Per2* gene circadian expression but normal *Bmal1* gene expression.

Neuroendocrine Dysfunctions

Neuroendocrine dysfunctions, mostly hypopituitarism, are common in patients after TBI. The prevalence is estimated at 15% to 68% in the acute phase of TBI, with the highest prevalence among persons with moderate and severe TBI, but tends to decrease over the first year after the injury.[80] Chronic hypopituitarism may lead to growth hormone and gonadotropin deficiency and to hypothyroidism. These alterations in neuroendocrine functioning are important to consider in the pathophysiology of SWD after a TBI because bidirectional interactions between hormonal secretion and sleep are well documented.[81] Among the most important hormonal disturbances in this context is the growth hormone deficiency, which was found to be closely associated with increased slow wave sleep and EEG delta power but with worsened subjective sleep quality and sleepiness. To date, few studies have investigated neuroendocrine changes in relation to sleep alterations and fatigue after TBI, and only preliminary evidence exists for a role of hypopituitarism and SWD or fatigue in the TBI population. In one study, patients with TBI reporting fatigue exhibited an overall higher prevalence of growth hormone deficiency than patients not reporting fatigue.[82] In another study, however, no correlation was observed between abnormal endocrine function and fatigue in a sample of 119 patients with TBI tested at least 1 year after injury.[83] In these two studies, sleep was assessed with questionnaires, and no objective measures of sleep were performed. Further studies are indicated to investigate whether neuroendocrine dysfunctions among patients with TBI explain not only subjective evaluation of sleep quality but also abnormal PSG findings in this population.

Effects of Prolonged Sedation and Psychoactive Medication

Sedative and analgesic agents are commonly administered to patients with severe TBI admitted to the ICU for prolonged periods regardless of the patient's specific circadian rhythm.

These agents are used to prevent agitation, facilitate mechanical ventilation, and reduce pain, and they also may improve intracranial pressure and cerebral perfusion. Still not clear, however, is whether sedation and analgesia share the restorative properties of sleep, since they show clear differences in both behavioral and electrophysiologic (EEG) expression. Some studies have shown that prolonged sedation with propofol does not result in sleep deprivation. After a 12-hour infusion of propofol followed by withdrawal, rats did not show the typical increase in slow wave activity that occurs in response to sleep deprivation.[84] Controversial results, however, were reported for isoflurane anesthesia and its recovery effect.[85,86] In any case, sedation and analgesia have adverse effects on circadian rhythms, particularly when these agents are not administered during the circadian time for sleep—that is, when they are given during the day, they impair the sleep-wake cycle mechanism more potently than when they are administered during the night.[87] How sedative and analgesic agents interact with an injured brain to promote the development of sleep and circadian rhythm disorders is still not well understood, but one study showed no correlation between the cumulative dose of sedatives and analgesics received in the ICU and SWD in the postacute stage of TBI recovery.[88] For more information on mechanism and effects of opioid analgesia on sleep, see Chapter 52.

A large proportion of TBI survivors uses psychoactive medication in the long term, and whether or not these patients should be excluded from sleep studies is a matter of debate. In fact, medication itself can modify sleep characteristics, but medication use can also be a consequences of sleep disturbances and/or more complex TBI. In an actimetry study of 34 patients with chronic moderate to severe TBI who were compared to 34 control subjects, longer total sleep time was found for TBI patients using psychoactive medications, whereas no changes in total sleep time were observed in patients who did not use medication when compared to control subjects.[89] Although this study cannot conclude to a causal role of medication in the sleep patterns observed, it highlights the importance of documenting medications used in TBI studies.

Pain

A case-control study showed that pain is prevalent after TBI and strongly associated with insomnia.[90] Anxiety, depression, and pain influence sleep quality; however, only anxiety and pain seem to explain 32% of the variance in the sleep-quality assessments.[91] Conversely, after multiple stepwise analyses controlling for many factors, another study reported that depression mainly accounts for the poor sleep quality complaints as assessed by the Pittsburgh Sleep Quality Index.[92] Such discrepancy in findings is not surprising because chronic pain is multifactorial; it is a frequent comorbid accompaniment of TBI and is reported to be independent of posttraumatic stress disorder and depression in brain-injured patients.[93] The interaction between pain and mood on the one hand and long-term outcome on the other deserve studies with larger sample sizes, taking into account the heterogeneity of the population under investigation.

In view of the probable impact of pain on sleep quality, one group of researchers aimed to identify how pain affects sleep quality and quantity, as well as sleep microstructure, using actimetry and quantitative EEG analysis.[92,94] Compared to TBI patients not afflicted by pain, those with pain showed longer total sleep time, more frequent naps, increased rapid EEG frequency bands (9 to 50 Hz) mostly during REM sleep, and increased beta bands (16 to 30 Hz) in NREM sleep. Whether the changes in sleep microarchitecture can explain a possible increased sleep need is unknown. Moreover, the specificity of this phenomenon remains to be demonstrated because intrusion of fast EEG activity in sleep of TBI patients with pain is not an exclusive phenomenon. Such differences also might reflect altered nociceptive processing at the central nervous system level, exacerbation of hypervigilance, and presleep cognitive arousal, as seen in the sleep of chronic pain patients.

Psychiatric Comorbid Illness

Approximately 65% of patients with TBI suffer from at least one psychiatric disorder, with depression, anxiety, and posttraumatic stress disorders being among the most common.[95] The associations between these psychiatric disorders and sleep disturbances, mostly insomnia, have been well described in the non-TBI population.[96] In agreement with this strong association, SWDs are included among the diagnostic features of major depressive disorder, generalized anxiety disorder, and posttraumatic stress disorder.[97]

For instance, most studies that investigated the prevalence of comorbid SWDs and psychiatric syndromes among patients with TBI consistently found a higher burden of psychiatric disorders among those with sleep complaints than among those without sleep complaints. For example, in two different cohort studies of chronic TBI, depression and anxiety symptoms were found to be among the variables that significantly contributed to the prediction of an insomnia syndrome.[98,99]

Still poorly understood, however, is how psychiatric disorders interact with TBI in the emergence and/or the persistence of SWDs. Some studies point to the predictive role of SWDs in the emergence of mental health problems. One retrospective study in 443 patients with mild TBI showed that reporting sleep complaints at 10 days after injury is associated with a 9.9- and 6.3-fold increased risk of feeling depressed at 10 days and 6 weeks, respectively.[100] Similarly, it was observed that onset of sleep disturbances within 3 months of injury predicted emergence of symptoms of depression and anxiety 12 months after TBI.[101]

Compared to the general population, military personnel are at higher risk of presenting mild TBI, posttraumatic stress disorder, and depression. The role of sleep disturbances in the development of mental health problems was recently confirmed by a large cohort study of 29,640 US Navy and Marine Corps men in whom sleep problems mediated 26% of TBI's effect on development of posttraumatic stress disorder and 41% of its effect on development of depression.[102] A good sleep quality could have a protective effect against poor emotion regulation and anxiety in veterans,[103] but the causal relationship between sleep, anxiety, depression, posttraumatic stress disorder, and emotion regulation is complex.

SLEEP AND BRAIN RECOVERY: BASIC AND ANIMAL STUDIES

The role of sleep in memory and structural plasticity is now well recognized.[104,105] Sleep optimizes the consolidation of memory by strengthening new synapses and has been shown to have a crucial role in neurogenesis. Indeed, chronic sleep deprivation or fragmentation (>3 days) in rodents was associated with a 30% to 80% reduction in hippocampal cell proliferation and with a decrease in the percentage of cells that mature and develop into adult neurons.[106,107] To address the question as to whether sleep abnormalities in the acute phase after TBI influence recovery, on both a clinical and a neuropathologic level, an animal study investigated impact of acute 6-hour sleep disruption after TBI in adult mice, and no effect on recovery of neurologic and cognitive functions was found.[108] This study suggests that short-duration sleep disruption after relatively mild TBI does not affect functional outcome. Other studies, however, found that 24 hours of sleep deprivation in rats before TBI results in faster recovery.[109] Also, 24 hours of sleep deprivation after TBI was reported to reduce morphologic damage and to improve behavioral recovery in rats.[110] Whether or not these associations have something to do with deep sleep-rich recovery sleep remains elusive.

In this line, recent evidence suggests that slow wave activity enhancement with either pharmacologic sleep induction or partial sleep deprivation with strong rebound sleep in the first days after weight-drop-induced TBI in rats improved functional recovery and histologic outcome, that is, by reducing diffuse axonal injury with deepened sleep.[111] In an animal study, the reverse association between sleep disruption and recovery was also found.[42] Genes associated with sleep regulation and neuronal plasticity were investigated in adult mice with mild TBI before and after two consecutive 6-hour periods of sleep deprivation during the light period of the day-night cycle. Quantification of mRNA levels was performed in the cerebral cortex and the hippocampus, and in a region incorporating the thalamus and the hypothalamus. In the hippocampus, sleep deprivation decreased the expression of *Arc* and *EfnA3* only in mice with mild TBI. In the thalamus-hypothalamus, sleep deprivation decreased *Homer1a* only in mice with mild TBI. These results point to an accentuated effect of sleep deprivation on sleep- or plasticity-related genes after mild TBI.

SLEEP AND BRAIN RECOVERY: HUMAN AND CLINICAL STUDIES

Extrapolation of the significance of these findings to human TBI suggests that chronically restricted or disrupted sleep in persons with TBI should reduce learning abilities, cerebral plasticity, and generation of new neurons in their brain, particularly in the hippocampus. This association is particularly important in the context of brain injury, where recovery is dependent specifically on new learning, cerebral plasticity, and neurogenesis. A study applying multimodal brain imaging techniques found that local changes in network structure important for improved behavioral outcomes, such as language and visuomotor function, are paralleled with recovery of synchronization of sleep spindling activity, suggesting a role for sleep and EEG synchronization for functional remodeling.[112] Similarly, in a pediatric cohort, sleep-related disturbances also significantly correlated with reductions in functional connectivity between these brain regions as measured by MRI techniques.[113]

In humans, SWDs have been associated with worse functional outcome in the acute stage of TBI, whereby consolidated sleep-wake cycle predicted resolution of posttraumatic amnesia length and functional recovery at hospital discharge.[114,115] In 238 patients followed for 6 months after TBI, another group found that patients who reported poor sleep were at risk for impeded recovery with poor global functioning.[116] Moreover, in a TBI inpatient rehabilitation unit, patients with agitation had worse sleep efficiency and total sleep time.[117] Considering these observations, the next step is to explore the temporal causal link between improvement in sleep and improvement in cognition and behavior. In a study on 30 hospitalized patients in the acute stage of moderate to severe TBI, cross-correlation between cognition/consciousness level and sleep consolidation showed that the best-fit lag was 0, suggesting that improvement in cognition/consciousness occurs in parallel with improvement in sleep consolidation and that they may all be driven by a general brain recovery.[88] In the chronic stage of moderate and severe TBI, however, improving sleep was associated with subsequent improvement in cognitive functioning.[118] Thus monitoring sleep after TBI could serve as a strategy to identify patients with poor prognoses and allow for early intervention to improve functional outcomes.

Another pilot study has already exploited the possibility to improve sleep after TBI by nonpharmacologic means and found a combination of sleep hygiene with 30 minutes blue light treatment in the morning to be successful to improve actigraphy measures of sleep.[119] In addition, a randomized, double-blinded, placebo-controlled trial in 32 adults with recent mild TBI applied blue light versus amber placebo light in the morning (30 minutes over 6 weeks) and observed phase-advanced sleep timing, reduced daytime sleepiness, improved executive functioning, greater thalamo-cortical functional connectivity, and increased axonal integrity of these pathways.[120] Altogether, and despite contradictory results in the literature, the possibility remains that some aspects of sleep may potentially influence recovery after TBI, and the challenge is to define the mechanism and how such an improvement would be mediated.

SLEEP, TRAUMATIC BRAIN INJURY, AND NEURODEGENERATION: IS THERE A KEY ROLE OF THE PUTATIVE GLYMPHATIC SYSTEM?

TBI has been associated to increased risk of Alzheimer's disease and chronic traumatic encephalopathy (see earlier). Given that it is now well recognized that chronic sleep disturbances are potential contributors for cognitive decline and dementia,[121] the question as to whether SWD caused by TBI could represent a key mechanism linking TBI to dementia is intriguing.

Despite ultimate proof for the existence and significance of the so-called glymphatic system is still lacking, this concept gained much attention over the past years. This putative system of CSF and brain interstitial fluid exchange across the perivascular space has been termed the *glymphatic system* and is conceptualized to clear interstitial solutes from the brain into the bloodstream, in a pulsative manner and primarily during deep sleep.[122] Recent discoveries showed that sleep favors CSF and brain interstitial fluid exchange across the perivascular space, the glymphatic system, to clear metabolic waste, including beta-amyloid peptides.[123] Preliminary results showed that enlarged perivascular space, a possible marker of impaired glymphatic system, is associated with shorter total sleep time and worse sleep efficiency in a small group of adults with history of TBI.[122] Recently, it has been hypothesized that posttraumatic SWD may impair the clearance of neuropeptides involved in the pathogenesis of posttraumatic headaches and thus contribute to the otherwise poorly understood headaches after TBI.[124] Future studies are needed to clarify how the interaction between sleep disturbances and the glymphatic system could increase the risk of dementia or even posttraumatic headaches in individuals with TBI.

CLINICAL PEARLS

- Both traumatic brain injury (TBI) and comorbid conditions, such as pain and psychiatric disorders, are potential causes of posttraumatic sleep-wake disturbance (SWD) in the acute and chronic phases of injury.
- Acute SWD may adversely influence brain recovery after TBI and contribute to comorbid posttraumatic symptoms.
- Identifying mechanisms associated with the pathogenesis of posttraumatic SWD and factors that contribute to their persistence could lead to improved management in the chronic phase.

SUMMARY

Fatigue, excessive daytime sleepiness, and pleiosomnia are common SWDs after TBI. Recently developed animal models have conferred new understanding of posttraumatic SWD; the translation of animal findings to human TBI suggests that specific factors are associated with the pathophysiology of TBI and contribute to emergence of SWDs. Consistent with animal models, an important decrease in hypocretin occurs in acute human TBI, which is reversed in the months after the injury. Prolonged use of sedative and analgesic agents in the ICU, altered circadian timing, comorbid pain, anxiety, depression, posttraumatic stress disorder, and psychoactive medication are among the factors associated with the emergence and/or persistence of SWD after a TBI. How acute sleep disturbances and sleep disruption improve or impede brain recovery after TBI needs further investigation, but interesting preliminary observations suggest a role for an accentuated effect of sleep deprivation on sleep and/or genes involved in neuroplasticity after TBI. The differences observed between acute and chronic phases suggest that studies should be conducted within a longer time frame to elucidate TBI and SWD pathophysiology and derive best-management strategies.

SELECTED READINGS

Baumann CR, Bassetti CL, Valko PO, et al. Loss of hypocretin (orexin) neurons with traumatic brain injury. *Ann Neurol.* 2009;66(4):555–559.

Baumann CR, Werth E, Stocker R, et al. Sleep-wake disturbances 6 months after traumatic brain injury: a prospective study. *Brain.* 2007;130(Pt 7):1873–1883.

Duclos C, Dumont M, Arbour C, et al. Parallel recovery of consciousness and sleep in acute traumatic brain injury. *Neurology.* 2017;88(3):268–275.

Gilbert KS, Kark SM, Gehrman P, Bogdanova Y. Sleep disturbances, TBI and PTSD: implications for treatment and recovery. *Clin Psychol Rev.* 2015;40:195–212.

Nardone R, Bergmann J, Kunz A, et al. Cortical excitability changes in patients with sleep-wake disturbances after traumatic brain injury. *J Neurotrauma.* 2011;28:1165–1171.

Paredes I, Navarro B, Lagares A. Sleep disorders in traumatic brain injury. *Neurocirugia (Astur : Engl Ed).* 2021;32(4):178–187.

Rowe RK, Striz M, Bachstetter AD, et al. Diffuse brain injury induces acute post-traumatic sleep. *PLoS One.* 2014;9:e82507.

Sabir M, Gaudreault PO, Freyburger M, et al. Impact of traumatic brain injury on sleep structure, electrocorticographic activity and transcriptome in mice. *Brain Behav Immun.* 2015;47:118–130.

Sanchez E, El-Khatib H, Arbour C, et al. Brain white matter damage and its association with neuronal synchrony during sleep. *Brain.* 2019;142(3):674–687.

Shekleton JA, Parcell DL, Redman JR, et al. Sleep disturbance and melatonin levels following traumatic brain injury. *Neurology.* 2010;74(21):1732–1738.

Stocker RPJ, Cieply MA, Paul B, et al. Combat-related blast exposure and traumatic brain injury influence brain glucose metabolism during REM sleep in military veterans. *Neuroimage.* 2014;99:207–214.

A complete reference list can be found online at ExpertConsult.com.

Chronobiology

Section 5

Introduction

Chapter 33

Phyllis C. Zee; Sabra Abbott

Circadian rhythms encompass the multiple near-24-hour oscillations in physiology and behavior observed across nearly all terrestrial species, allowing an organism to appropriately time activity in relation to our 24-hour environment. Although the chapters in this section focus primarily on the mammalian circadian system, circadian rhythms are ubiquitous from bacteria to plants to insects to humans. An important milestone in circadian science occurred in 2017 when the Nobel prize was awarded to Jeffrey Hall, Michael Rosbash, and Michael Young for their discovery of the molecular mechanisms controlling circadian rhythms in *Drosophila* spp. in 1984.[1] The discovery that biologic clocks use oscillating proteins in feedback loops to generate self-sustaining, near-24-hour rhythms in nearly all tissues has fueled rapid discoveries of the essential role of circadian rhythms for health and disease beyond their obvious effect on sleep and wake functions. However, as highlighted in Chapter 34, the master clock of the circadian system, located in the suprachiasmatic nucleus, coordinates rhythmic information from the environment and behavior with internal rhythmic biologic processes.

Two chapters in this section deal with the circadian clock system, focusing on the anatomy of the neuronal clock system in mammals (Chapter 35) and the physiology of the mammalian circadian clock system (Chapter 36). Chapters that review the molecular and genetic bases for the circadian clock core machinery, which has been highly conserved at least from insects to mammals, are included in Section 3 of this volume. Chapters 37 and 38 involve discussions from different vantage points about how the circadian clock system is highly integrated with the sleep-wake regulatory system. Chapter 39 focuses on how the circadian clock and sleep homeostatic regulatory systems independently and interactively regulate the expression of neurobehavioral performance.

In the now-classic, two-process model of Borbely and colleagues, the timing of sleep and wake is a function of a homeostatic process that defines sleep need as being dependent on the previous amount of sleep and wake (process S) and the circadian clock (process C) that modulates the timing and propensity of sleep[2] (Chapters 37 and 38). However, as noted by Buxton and Czeisler, the interactions between the circadian pacemaker and sleep homeostat should not be underestimated; there is great difficulty in separating these two processes functionally. In addition, recent genetic and anatomic findings (Chapter 35) also tend to “blur” the distinction between the homeostatic and circadian inputs in the regulation of the sleep-wake cycle. Although the two-process model has guided and will continue to guide our understanding of sleep regulation mechanisms, understanding the interactions between circadian, homeostatic, metabolic, and perhaps other physiologic processes that underlie the complex regulation of the sleep-wake cycle will be be necessary to explain how disruption of these processes can have such broad health consequences.

Misalignment and/or decreased amplitude of circadian rhythms results in either disturbed timing of sleep and wake activity or fragmented sleep and wake bouts throughout the 24-hour day. Thus sleep disturbances are the most common clinical presenting symptoms of circadian disorders. The final chapter in this section (Chapter 43) reviews sleep and wake disorders resulting from a disruption of the circadian system. Circadian rhythm sleep-wake disorders (CRSWDs) are still underrecognized in clinical medicine, and there is limited understanding of their underlying pathophysiology. In addition to sleep and wake disturbances, alterations in the timing of the phase relationship between the central and peripheral internal rhythms, peripheral rhythms with one another, and internal rhythms with the external environment can result in adverse health outcomes and accidents. The chapter also discusses evaluation and treatment approaches for CRSWDs.

There is mounting evidence that disruption of circadian rhythms and sleep is associated with increased risk for poor mental and physical health. However, only in the last few years have animal models begun to emerge that elucidate the importance of internal circadian synchronization for the health and well-being of the organism and for the molecular events that are disrupted at the level of cells and tissues (Chapter 40). Indeed, there is considerable emerging evidence that disruption of the circadian clock can exacerbate and perhaps modify the expression of a variety of physical and mental disorders, as reviewed in Chapters 41 and 42. The rapid advance of our understanding of the essential role of circadian rhythms in health and expression of disease indicates a need to incorporate the time domain in medicine and a future for the emerging area of circadian medicine.

SELECTED READINGS

Abbott SM, Zee PC. Circadian Rhythms: Implications for Health and Disease. *Neurol Clin*. 2019;37(3):601–613.

A full reference list is available online at ExpertConsult.com.

Chapter 34

Master Circadian Clock and Master Circadian Rhythm

Phyllis C. Zee; Fred W. Turek

Chapter Highlights

- Consolidation of sleep and wake times to certain parts of the 24-hour cycle evolved over time to maximize survivability of the species. In mammals, the suprachiasmatic nucleus is the top biologic clock regulating the timing of sleep and wake, therefore influencing the expression and coordination of a myriad of other essential biologic processes.
- At the molecular, cellular, and systems levels, circadian clocks regulate sleep-wake homeostasis, metabolic and immune functions, and neuronal activity, which are important determinants of sleep duration and timing.
- The sleep-wake regulatory system is highly integrated with the circadian clock system, so when circadian dysregulation is combined with sleep deficiency, the adverse consequences on mental and physical health are even more pronounced than with short sleep duration alone.

One of the distinguishing characteristics of sleep in animals as diverse as insects, fish, and mammals is the timing of sleep and wake, which for the majority of species is confined to certain times of the day or night.[1] As detailed in a number of chapters in this section, the master biologic clock regulating the timing of sleep and wake in mammals also regulates most, if not all, near-24-hour (circadian) behavioral, physiologic, and biochemical rhythms. In mammals, this master circadian clock is located in the bilaterally paired suprachiasmatic nucleus (SCN) of the anterior hypothalamus.[2] It has recently been discovered that many tissues and organs can generate circadian rhythms in vitro, and their rhythmicity is therefore independent of the SCN.[3] However, the SCN remains at the top of the hierarchy of the mammalian circadian clock system: many central brain rhythms outside of the SCN, as well as rhythms in peripheral tissues, are normally synchronized by 24-hour behavioral rhythms under the control of the SCN.

Indeed, one could argue that the sleep-wake cycle represents the "master circadian rhythm"; the SCN control of this rhythm in turn, via neural and humoral signals, coordinates the timing and expression of a multitude of downstream rhythms. Although the expression of many 24-hour rhythms may be primarily under the control of the circadian clock in the SCN, the expression of many rhythms is largely dependent on whether the organism is asleep or awake, regardless of the circadian clock time.[4] Undoubtedly, the expression of most rhythms at the behavioral, physiologic, and biochemical levels is regulated by the integration of inputs from the circadian clock and the sleep-wake state of the animal. Indeed, it can be argued that the overall temporal organization of an organism represents an integrated coordinated effect of environmental and behavioral signals, such as light, physical activity and feeding, circadian clock inputs, and the sleep-wake state of the organism. Thus the circadian and sleep-wake control centers have evolved together to ensure that the timing of internal events relative to one another and to the external environment is coordinated in such a fashion to maximize the survival of the species.

Of particular note regarding the "downstream" rhythms regulated by the circadian clock is the feeding rhythm, which of course is highly dependent on the sleep-wake cycle since animals normally do not eat when asleep. In the last few years, a number of studies have demonstrated that the timing of food intake can regulate the expression of circadian clock genes in many peripheral tissues, which in turn control the 24-hour rhythm in the expression of many clock-controlled genes (perhaps as many as 10% to 50% of all genes expressed in a given tissue).[5] The many interactions between the systems regulating circadian, sleep, and energy balance, from molecular to behavioral rhythms, have led to much interest in the importance of these linkages to obesity, diabetes, and cardiometabolic disorders.[6]

The need to "rest" and the need to adjust to the daily changes in the physical environment because of celestial mechanics certainly represented two Darwinian pressures that guided the evolution of living organisms since life appeared on the earth. (At an earlier time in the history of the earth, the solar day is thought to have been 18 hours. With the change to the current 24-hour day occurring over millions of years, there was plenty of time for clock genes to be altered so that the molecular circadian cycle stayed in synchrony with the solar day.) As detailed in the rest of this chapter, the early linkage for the need to rest, and to rest at a specific phase of the daily external environment, may have resulted in the circadian clock and sleep-wake cycle evolving together and being integrated with one another at many different levels of organization, including integration with the complex behavioral, cellular, and behavioral events associated with metabolism and the regulation of energy inputs and outputs.

INTEGRATION OF THE CIRCADIAN CLOCK AND SLEEP-WAKE SYSTEMS

Many chapters in this section involve discussions from different vantage points about how the circadian clock system is highly integrated with the sleep-wake regulatory system at a number of levels of biologic organization, from the molecular to the behavioral as well as with respect to the neural circuitry in the brain. This new understanding of a cohesive system involving the regulation of sleep and circadian rhythms, in parallel with increased knowledge of the complex relationship between the circadian and sleep-wake systems, has been a revolution in our understanding of the importance of synchronized sleep and circadian rhythms for the health and well-being of the organism. There is now considerable evidence that disruption in the normal organization of 24-hour rhythms, in conjunction with fragmented and decreased sleep, can exacerbate and perhaps even initiate a cascade of biologic changes that cause a variety of mental and physical disorders.[2,6] It is noteworthy that many pre-existing health problems, particularly in underserved populations, have been linked to increased morbidity and mortality in patients affected by the COVID-19 pandemic; many of these pre-existing health conditions (e.g., hypertension, obesity, diabetes) have been linked to poor sleep and/or disrupted rhythms.

The circadian and sleep fields are closely related. What were once considered two different areas of biomedical research have now come together in elucidating how the circadian and sleep homeostatic processes that underlie the complex regulation of sleep are integrated and how a breakdown in this integration, because of either physical or socially induced causes, can impact health and disease.

In the two-process model originally proposed by Borbely and colleagues, the electroencephalographic slow wave activity in non–rapid eye movement (NREM) sleep serves as an indicator of sleep homeostasis either under baseline or after sleep deprivation conditions. Although there is substantial evidence to indicate that "sleep homeostasis," as defined by the slow wave activity during NREM sleep, is independent mechanistically from the circadian clock, much less is known about how the two processes actually contribute to the overall "sleep need" of the organism or what role the circadian clock may play in other homeostatically regulated sleep functions. Indeed, the finding that different alleles in the *per* gene in humans are associated with differences in slow wave sleep emphasizes how closely linked the circadian clock and the homeostatic process are in regulating sleep (see Section 3). Similarly, mutations and/or knock out of core circadian genes that make up the molecular clock are now known to influence many sleep properties beyond just the timing of sleep.[7]

REGULATING SLEEP AMOUNT: A HOMEOSTATIC AND A CIRCADIAN INPUT

Many sleep and wake traits are under homeostatic control. That is, the longer one is awake or deprived of specific sleep stages (e.g., rapid eye movement [REM] sleep deprivation), the greater will be the drive to recover the lost sleep or sleep stage. However, this may be true only after short periods of sleep deprivation because during continuous chronic partial sleep deprivations in rodents, there is a loss of the homeostatic recovery sleep increase, as the sleep-wake system appears to change from a homeostatic to an allostatic response system.[8,9] In addition, the different phases of normal sleep and wake are under circadian control; the clock is doing more than saying "wake up" or "go to sleep" at specific times of day.

An unanswered question is, what actually regulates the amount of sleep? Or put another way, what are the relative contributions of the homeostatic and circadian processes to the actual amount of time a given animal is awake and interacting with the external world or asleep and avoiding the external world? Studies in laboratory, zoo, and wild animals reveal that total sleep time may be unrelated to taxonomic classification, and as noted by Siegel,[10] "the range of sleep amount of different primates extensively overlaps that of rodents which overlaps that of carnivores, and so on across many orders of mammals." Total sleep time is correlated in a global sense to body size; for example, the opossum sleeps 18 hours, the ferret sleeps 14.4 hours, the cat sleeps 12.5 hours, the dog sleeps 10.1 hours, humans sleep 8 hours, and the elephant sleeps 3 hours.[10] Although on a global level, body size (and associated metabolic rate) is inversely related to total sleep time, there appear to be other factors regulating sleep duration, as indicated by the fact that the smaller mouse sleeps about the same amount as the larger rat.[11,12] Indeed, there is considerable variability in sleep amount among strains of mice; strains of mice that are of similar size and of the same species can show total sleep time differences up to as much as 2.5 hours.[12]

In the evolution of life on Earth, there has been great pressure for organisms to adapt their lifestyle to the external world and to coordinate the internal temporal environment, to maximize the chances of survival, and to pass on their genetic material to the next generation. Total sleep time could be expected to be part of the survival strategy to ensure that animals are engaged as well as disengaged with the external environment at the appropriate times of day and night. Similarly, as noted at the beginning of this chapter, the sleep-wake cycle can be considered the master circadian rhythm, as the expression of so many behavioral and physiologic rhythms is tied to the sleep-wake/activity-rest cycle. Thus the total amount and timing of sleep and wake may have evolved in individual species, in part, to create an internal temporal framework, in conjunction with the circadian clock, to maximize survival and reproduction fitness.

The fact that the master circadian clock also plays a major role in determining the pressure to sleep or the ability to stay awake has mechanistic implications on various neural, genetic, and molecular levels as well as potentially important therapeutic implications for applying novel circadian-based approaches for the treatment of sleep-wake disorders that go beyond the classical circadian rhythm sleep-wake disorders.

CLINICAL PEARL

Our 24/7 society has led humans to be the only animal species that routinely ignores its biologic clock: we are often awake when the clock is telling us to be asleep. Both the chronic disruption of circadian organization and chronic insufficient sleep have been associated with a wide range of mental and physical disorders. Modern medicine is only beginning to recognize that the treatment of many disorders of human health may need to take into account circadian medicine to improve overall 24-hour temporal organization between and within the central nervous system and peripheral tissues.

SUMMARY

Recent discoveries, including that the SCN is the master mammalian biologic clock, help us more fully understand the significant relationship between sleep-wake mechanisms and circadian clocks in organisms. These systems have evolved over millions of years to maximize survival of species. As our understanding of this complex relationship grows, we are also able to see how disruptions of these two integrated processes adversely affect the health and may contribute to the many chronic diseases we see in modern society.

ACKNOWLEDGMENTS

The authors recognize support from the National Institutes of Health: National Heart, Lung, and Blood Institute (HL140580-03, HL141881-02, HL007909-21), National Institute on Aging (AG011412-20), and Northwestern University Feinberg School of Medicine Center for Circadian and Sleep Medicine.

SELECTED READINGS

Feillet C, van der Horst GT, et al. Coupling between the circadian clock and cell cycle oscillators: implication for healthy cells and malignant growth. *Front Neurol.* 2015;6. 96.

Finger AM, Kramer A. Mammalian circadian systems: Organization and modern life challenges. *Acta Physiol (Oxf).* 2021;231(3):e13548.

Fuhr L, Abreu M, Pett P, Relógio A. Circadian systems biology: when time matters. *Comput Struct Biotechnol J.* 2015;13:417–426.

Van Drunen R, Eckel-Mahan K. Circadian rhythms of the hypothalamus: from function to physiology. *Clocks Sleep.* 2021;3(1):189–226. Published 2021 Feb 25.

A complete reference list can be found online at ExpertConsult.com.

Chapter 35

Anatomy of the Mammalian Circadian System

Joshua J. Gooley; Patrick M. Fuller; Clifford B. Saper

Chapter Highlights

- Circadian rhythms in mammals, including sleep-wake cycles, are endogenously driven by the suprachiasmatic nucleus (SCN) in the anterior hypothalamus.
- The SCN is a master clock that transmits circadian output signals to effector systems to temporally coordinate behavioral and physiologic rhythms with daily changes in the environment.
- The near-24-hour rhythm of neuronal activity in the SCN is normally entrained to the 24-hour light-dark cycle defined by the earth's rotation. Light information is transmitted to the SCN from specialized retinal ganglion cells that contain the photopigment melanopsin. Upon activation by light, retinal axons release glutamate and pituitary adenylate cyclase–activating polypeptide onto SCN neurons. Clock cells in the SCN also receive input from the intergeniculate leaflet in the thalamus, the median raphe nucleus, and the ventral tegmental area, all of which play a modulatory role in regulating circadian rhythms.
- The primary neuronal pathway underlying the circadian regulation of sleep-wake cycles involves a dense SCN efferent projection to the adjacent subparaventricular zone, followed by a secondary projection to the dorsomedial hypothalamic nucleus, which projects to other brain regions critical for regulating sleep and wakefulness. The SCN also projects directly and indirectly to the paraventricular hypothalamic nucleus to regulate corticosteroid secretion and synthesis of the hormone melatonin. In addition to regulating circadian cycles of behavior and endocrine function, the SCN plays a hierarchical role in coordinating the timing and function of clocks located in peripheral tissues.
- Understanding the cellular, circuit, and synaptic basis of circadian rhythms is important for developing therapies to improve the quality of sleep-wake cycles, especially in persons with circadian rhythm sleep disorders. This chapter describes the intrinsic organization, inputs, and outputs of the circadian clock in the SCN, with emphasis on the neuronal circuitry and neurotransmitters underlying circadian control of sleep-wake and rest-activity cycles.

INTRODUCTION

Most animals show a pronounced daily rhythm of rest-activity that is synchronized with the solar day. To a large degree, the timing of these rhythms is determined by the circadian ("about a day") system. Although circadian rhythms persist even in the absence of periodic environmental cues, they are normally entrained by the light-dark cycle and feeding schedules. The primary role of the circadian system is to ensure that behavioral and physiologic rhythms are temporally coordinated with daily changes in the environment. By providing an internal representation of day and night, the circadian system anticipates the rising and setting of the sun, hence allowing animals to appropriately time sleep and foraging behavior. The circadian system therefore facilitates adaptation to daily environmental cycles to maintain energy balance, which is thought to increase survival and reproductive fitness. This chapter reviews the organization of the circadian system and the anatomic basis for circadian regulation of sleep-wake cycles and endocrine function.

THE MASTER CIRCADIAN CLOCK IN THE SUPRACHIASMATIC NUCLEUS

The master circadian clock for behavioral rhythms, including the sleep-wake cycle, is located in the suprachiasmatic nucleus (SCN).[1] The SCN is situated in the anterior hypothalamus immediately dorsal to the optic chiasm and lateral to the third ventricle (Figure 35.1, *A*). The circadian rhythm of neural activity in the SCN is generated at the cellular level by a transcriptional-translational-posttranslational molecular feedback mechanism. If the molecular clock is rendered dysfunctional, patterns of rest-activity exhibit irregular and non-24-hour cycles. Similarly, lesions of the SCN or its efferent

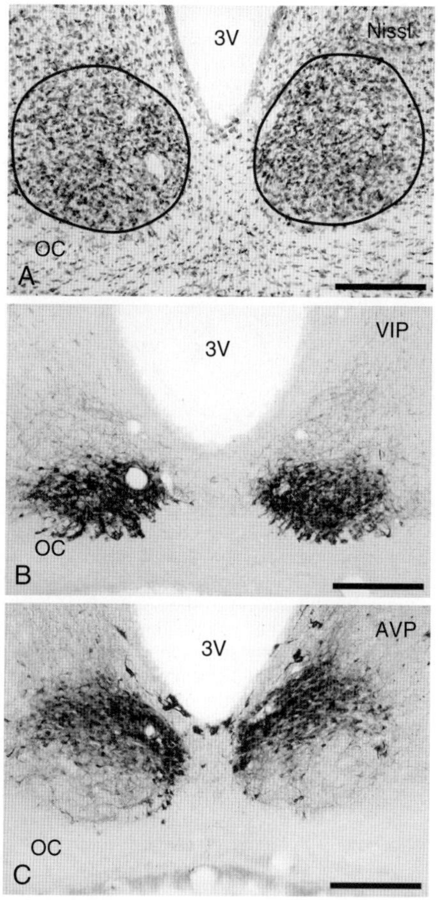

Figure 35.1 The suprachiasmatic nucleus (SCN) is composed of ventrolateral (SCNvl) and dorsomedial (SCNdm) subdivisions. **A,** In Nissl-stained coronal sections in rats, the SCN can be identified by its tightly compacted small-diameter neurons located immediately dorsal to the optic chiasm and lateral to the third ventricle. **B,** VIP-immunoreactive perikarya are found in the SCNvl. **C,** AVP-immunoreactive cell bodies are found in the SCNdm. 3V, Third ventricle; AVP, arginine vasopressin; OC, optic chiasm; VIP, vasoactive intestinal polypeptide. Scale bars equal 200 μm.

projections abolish behavioral and endocrine rhythms, demonstrating a critical role for the SCN clock in generating circadian rhythms, including sleep.

Based on neurotransmitter phenotype and afferent-efferent connections, the SCN has historically been divided into ventrolateral and dorsomedial components, commonly referred to as the core and shell, respectively.[2] The core contains many vasoactive intestinal polypeptide (VIP)–containing neurons (Figure 35.1, *B*), whereas the shell contains a large population of arginine vasopressin (AVP)–containing neurons (Figure 35.1, *C*). In studies of the SCN, the boundaries of the core and shell are often defined by the distribution of VIP and AVP immunoreactivity, as these cell groups are conserved in the SCN of rodents, monkeys, and humans. While SCN neurons differ in their neuropeptide content, by comparison, the fast inhibitory neurotransmitter gamma-aminobutyric acid (GABA), its receptors, and the vesicular GABA transporter (Vgat, which is required for packaging and synaptic release of GABA) are heavily expressed throughout both SCN subdivisions, and these are contained in most, if not all, SCN neurons.[3] The core of the SCN in rodents also contains many neurons that express gastrin-releasing peptide (GRP) and smaller numbers expressing neurotensin (NT). In humans, an extensive population of NT-immunoreactive cells are found throughout the SCN,[4] and neuropeptide Y (NPY)–containing neurons are located predominantly in the central part of the nucleus, where they overlap with the distribution of VIP-immunoreactive cells. Smaller subpopulations of neurons containing angiotensin II, enkephalin (ENK), somatostatin, neuromedin S, and substance P have also been described in the SCN, but there are species-specific differences in the abundance and distribution of these neurotransmitters.[4-6] Therefore, although the human SCN is functionally homologous to the SCN of other mammals, the relative contributions and combinations of SCN neurotransmitters that regulate circadian rhythms appear to vary across species. The SCN also contains a considerable population of astrocytes, and while their role in circadian timekeeping is incompletely understood, studies have clearly demonstrated a capacity for SCN astrocytes to modulate SCN neuronal function, likely via release of various gliotransmitters.[7]

The SCN is functionally subdivided such that VIP and GRP neurons in the SCN core receive dense innervation by retinal axons, whereas fewer synaptic contacts are made on AVP neurons in the internal shell region.[8,9] VIP-immunoreactive neurons project heavily to both subdivisions within the SCN, overlapping with the distribution of VPAC2 receptor (also known as VIP receptor type 2), whereas GRP receptors are found primarily in the SCN shell. A functional role for VIP and GRP in transmitting photic information in the SCN is supported by studies demonstrating that microinjection of either VIP or GRP into the SCN region induces phase resetting of rest-activity rhythms similar to the effects of light[10] and that SCN VIP neurons are acutely responsive to light in vivo.[11,12] Conversely, co-application of VIP and GRP receptor antagonists in the SCN region attenuates circadian light responses.[13] Behavioral circadian rhythms in enucleated mice can also be entrained by optogenetic stimulation of VIP neurons in the SCN.[14] The finding that VIP knockout mice and VPAC2-receptor knockout mice have profoundly weakened or arrhythmic locomotor activity rhythms in constant darkness[15,16] is further evidence for a role of VIP signaling in coordinating the activity rhythm of SCN neurons.[17,18] Additionally, selective, genetically driven disruption of the molecular clock or cell-type–specific ablation of SCN VIP neurons produces similar arrhythmic locomotor rhythms in constant darkness,[11] whereas selective chemogenetic manipulation of SCN VIP neurons can acutely modulate locomotor activity levels, heart rate, and circulating corticosterone levels in mice.[11,14,19] It also has been recently revealed that at least a subset of VIP/GRP SCN neurons harbor androgen receptors. Given well-described androgenic effects on the SCN clock,[20] VIP/GRP SCN neurons may mediate the effects of nonphotic, androgenic input on pacemaker function. If so, and given the established role of VIP and GRP in mediating photic input to the SCN, it is tempting to speculate that SCN VIP/GRP neurons may play a unique role in integrating photic and nonphotic sensory flow to the SCN clock. Since the previous edition of this chapter was written, a subset of SCN neurons expressing the neuropeptide neuromedin S (NMS) has been revealed and shown to be necessary—via genetically driven and selective disruption of their molecular clock—for the generation of coherent daily rhythms in behavior.[5] NMS itself is not necessary for proper SCN function. The SCN NMS cell population is large, comprising approximately 40%

of all SCN neurons, spans portions of both the SCN core and shell, and encompasses most but not all neurons expressing AVP and VIP.

Despite the abundance of AVP and its receptors (V1a and V1b) in the SCN shell, as well as robust circadian gene expression of AVP in the SCN, AVP signaling was not historically viewed as playing an important role in generating the SCN rhythm or for output of rest-activity cycles. Consistent with this notion, AVP-deficient rats show normal behavioral circadian rhythms, and injection of AVP or V1 receptor antagonists into the SCN region does not alter the phase or period of locomotor activity.[21] Nonetheless, double knockout mice for the V1a and V1b receptors are resistant to jet lag compared to wild-type mice and can rapidly adapt to a large shift in the timing of the light-dark cycle.[22] More recent genetically targeted work has shown that selective disruption of the molecular clock within AVP neurons lengthens the free-running period and enhances re-entrainment to light,[23,24] supporting the view that AVP SCN neurons are involved in regulating the coupling of SCN neurons (i.e., interneuronal coupling) and hence play a fundamental role in sculpting circadian behavioral rhythms.

The output of SCN neurons is thought to be principally inhibitory, based on the observation that most clock cells contain GABA. Histologic and functional studies indicate that GABA acts on both ionotropic GABAA receptors and metabotropic GABAB receptors in the SCN. In hypothalamic brain slices, GABAA receptor agonists inhibit neuronal and metabolic activity of SCN neurons,[25,26] and the GABAB receptor agonist baclofen inhibits optic nerve–stimulated field potentials.[27] Consistent with these findings, light-induced phase shifts of locomotor activity are blocked by a single injection of either GABAA or GABAB receptor agonists.[28] By comparison, repeated injections of a GABAA receptor agonist in the SCN over several hours mimics the resetting effects of light, whereas prolonged application of a GABAA receptor antagonist attenuates the phase-resetting effects of light on behavior.[29] The effects of GABAergic signaling on circadian responses may therefore depend on the time course of neurotransmitter release. In dissociated cell culture, daily administration of GABA synchronizes SCN neuronal electrical rhythms,[30] suggesting that GABAergic signaling might also play a role in coordinating the circadian phase of individual SCN cellular oscillators.

SUPRACHIASMATIC NUCLEUS INPUTS

The endogenous circadian rhythm of neuronal activity in the SCN is close to, but not exactly, 24 hours. To entrain to the imposed solar day length, the SCN clock must therefore be reset daily by extrinsic time cues, most notably the light-dark cycle. Light activation of SCN neurons triggers calcium-dependent intracellular signaling cascades that lead to resetting of the molecular clock. The SCN rhythm can be further tuned by nonphotic inputs in order to coordinate behavioral and physiologic patterns with diurnal changes in the environment. The SCN core receives dense input from the retina, the intergeniculate leaflet (IGL), and the midbrain raphe nuclei,[31] whereas the SCN shell primarily receives projections from other hypothalamic areas, the basal forebrain, the limbic cortex, the septal area, and the brainstem (Figure 35.2, *A*).[32] In the following sections, we discuss some of the major pathways that regulate the timing of the SCN neural activity rhythm.

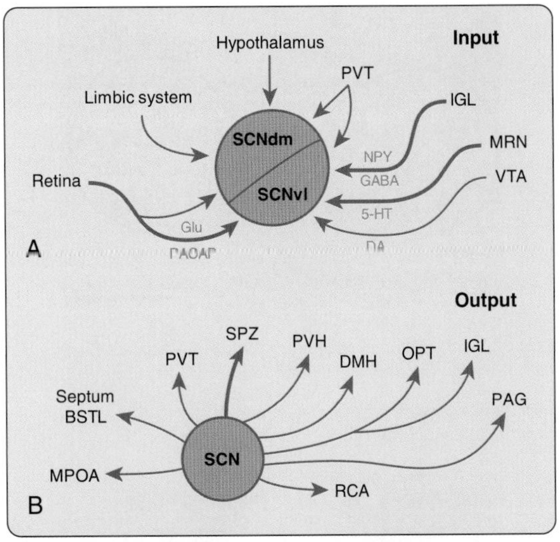

Figure 35.2 Afferent and efferent projections of the suprachiasmatic nucleus (SCN). **A,** SCN afferent projections terminate differentially in the ventrolateral (SCNvl) and dorsomedial (SCNdm) subdivisions. Neurotransmitters contained in these projections are shown next to the arrows. **B,** SCN efferent projections are primarily confined to the hypothalamus. 5-HT, 5-Hydroxytryptamine (serotonin); BSTL, bed nucleus of the stria terminalis; DA, dopamine; DMH, dorsomedial hypothalamic nucleus; GABA, gamma-aminobutyric acid; Glu, glutamate; IGL, intergeniculate leaflet; MPOA, medial preoptic area; MRN, median raphe nucleus; NPY, neuropeptide Y; OPT, olivary pretectal nucleus; PACAP, pituitary adenylate cyclase–activating polypeptide; PAG, periaqueductal gray matter; PVH, paraventricular hypothalamic nucleus; PVT, paraventricular thalamic nucleus; RCA, retrochiasmatic area; SCNdm, dorsomedial suprachiasmatic nucleus (shell); SCNvl, ventrolateral suprachiasmatic nucleus (core); SPZ, subparaventricular zone; VTA, ventral tegmental area.

Retina

The retinohypothalamic tract (RHT) projects bilaterally to the SCN (Figure 35.3, *A*). The RHT sends its densest projection to the SCN core, where VIP-immunoreactive cells are located, but smaller numbers of RHT axons also reach the SCN shell, subparaventricular zone (SPZ), and other hypothalamic areas. These retinal projections originate from intrinsically photosensitive retinal ganglion cells (ipRGCs) that contain the photopigment melanopsin (OPN4),[33,34] which is preferentially sensitive to short-wavelength (blue) light.[35,36] In mice, there are currently six known types of OPN4 ganglion cells (M1 to M6), which differ in their morphology, intraretinal connections, physiologic responses to light, phototransduction cascade, and behavioral functions.[37] In humans and macaques, there are two distinct populations of OPN4 ganglion cells based on their dendritic stratification near the inner or outer border of the inner plexiform layer.[38,39] In human organ donor retinas, three different functional ipRGC subtypes have been described, which differ in their sensitivities and temporal responses to light.[40] Additional studies are needed to understand how diversity in response characteristics of OPN4 ganglion cells may influence SCN neural activity and circadian behavior.

In mice, M1 ganglion cells project densely to the SCN and are thought to be principally responsible for photic circadian entrainment.[37] M2 ganglion cells also innervate the SCN, but their role in circadian light responses has not been directly characterized. The M1 ganglion cells project not only to the SCN but also to other brain areas that are involved in nonvisual photoreception, including the ventrolateral preoptic nucleus (VLPO), which is a sleep-promoting area in the

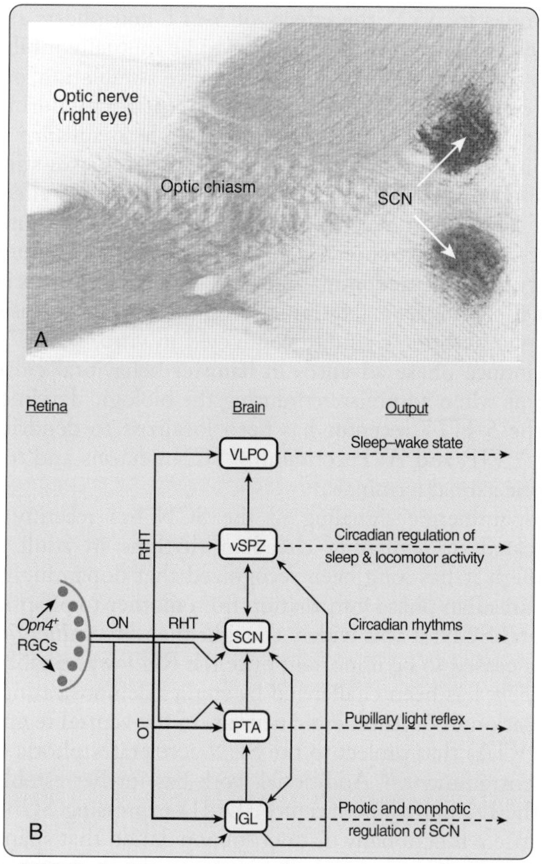

Figure 35.3 Retinal input to the circadian timing system from melanopsin-expressing retinal ganglion cells. **A,** Following intraocular injection of cholera toxin B subunit into the left eye, anterogradely labeled axons project bilaterally to the SCN of rats, as shown in a horizontal section through the optic chiasm. **B,** Melanopsin-expressing retinal ganglion cells project to brain areas involved in processing nonvisual information, including the SCN and IGL. The *branched arrows* from melanopsin cells indicate collateralized projections to the SCN and PTA, and to the SCN and IGL. *Long dashed arrows* indicate physiologic and behavioral outputs of the targeted retinorecipient brain areas. Direct projections between brain areas are shown, but indirect projections are not shown for reasons of clarity. IGL, Intergeniculate leaflet; Opn4+ RGCs, melanopsin-positive retinal ganglion cells; ON, optic nerve; OT, optic tract; PTA, pretectal area; RHT, retinohypothalamic tract; SCN, suprachiasmatic nucleus; VLPO, ventrolateral preoptic nucleus; vSPZ, ventral subparaventricular zone. (**B** from Gooley JJ, Lu J, Fischer D, et al. A broad role for melanopsin in nonvisual photoreception. *J Neurosci.* 2003;23:7093–106. Copyright 2003 by the Society for Neuroscience.)

anterior hypothalamus; the SPZ, which is important for circadian regulation of sleep (discussed later); the olivary pretectal nucleus (OPT), which is part of the afferent pathway mediating the pupillary light reflex; and the IGL, which plays a role in modulating circadian rhythms (Figure 35.3, *B*).[36,41] Recent genetic tracing studies have shown that individual M1 ganglion cells innervate the SCN bilaterally and send axons collaterally to other brain areas involved in sleep-wake regulation.[8] These observations suggest that photic input from OPN4-expressing retinal ganglion cells (RGCs) can modulate sleep and circadian rhythms via multiple routes.

Although OPN4-expressing RGCs are intrinsically photosensitive, they also receive light information from rod and cone photoreceptors in the outer retina.[35,42] Despite these additional inputs, even in the absence of rod and cone function, ipRGCs are able to mediate circadian responses to light, as demonstrated in blind humans and sightless mice with rod and cone damage but intact function of the inner retina.[43,44] In addition, even in normally sighted individuals, phase shifting and melatonin suppression are most sensitive to blue light[45,46] in the range of the peak stimulus for melanopsin, indicating that it plays an important role in circadian photoreception. OPN4-deficient mice with intact rod-cone function show moderate deficits in circadian light resetting, but these animals can still entrain to light-dark cycles, suggesting that visual photoreceptors and melanopsin play overlapping roles in circadian photoreception. Consistent with these findings, spectral responses of the circadian system in humans suggest involvement of rod-cone photoreceptors and OPN4, although the relative contribution of these photoreceptor types appears to depend on the irradiance and duration of exposure to light.[47] Based on studies in mice, circadian responses to light are only eliminated when rod-cone and OPN4 signaling pathways are disrupted simultaneously, or if OPN4-expressing RGCs are genetically ablated.[48,49] Hence, ipRGCs appear to function as a necessary conduit for light information to reach the circadian clock in the SCN. This organizational scheme enables ipRGCs to respond to light stimuli over a wide range of irradiances (from dim scotopic light levels to bright photopic light levels)[50] and may support the integration of cone-derived chromatic signals in the SCN to ensure stable circadian-driven behavior under real-world conditions in which light intensity may not be a reliable indicator of time of day (e.g., as a result of weather-related changes in light levels).[51]

Several lines of evidence suggest that photic information is conveyed to the SCN via the release of excitatory amino acids such as glutamate from RHT terminals. Optic nerve stimulation induces the release of glutamate and aspartate in the SCN in brain slice preparations,[52] and glutamate mimics the effects of optic nerve stimulation on the circadian rhythm of SCN neuronal activity in vitro.[53] Microinjection of *N*-methyl-D-aspartate (NMDA) into the SCN region in vivo also mimics the phase-shifting effects of light on rest-activity rhythms.[54] Receptor subunits from the NMDA-, α-amino-3-hydroxyl-5-methyl-4-isoxazole-propionic acid (AMPA)–, and kainate-preferring classes of ionotropic glutamate receptors are found in the SCN, in addition to subunits from metabotropic glutamate receptors.[55] Glutamate transmission from ipRGCs is necessary for normal circadian responses to light, as shown in mice in which vesicular glutamate transport is selectively disrupted in OPN4 cells.[56,57] These mice can still entrain to bright light intensities, however, suggesting that other neurotransmitters that may be released only at higher firing intensity can signal light information to the SCN. The ipRGCs that give rise to the RHT also express pituitary adenylate cyclase–activating polypeptide (PACAP),[58] which colocalizes with glutamate at RHT terminals. PACAP binds the PACAP-type 1 (PAC1) receptor and VPAC2 receptor with equal affinity, both of which are expressed in the SCN. Mice deficient in PACAP or PAC1 receptors show abnormal circadian resetting but can nonetheless entrain to light-dark cycles,[59] suggesting that PACAP signaling plays a partially redundant role with glutamate in photic circadian entrainment. Recently, it was shown that a subset of OPN4 cells releases GABA onto SCN neurons, and disrupting GABA synthesis in these cells results in more robust photic circadian entrainment under dim lighting conditions.[60] These findings suggest that GABAergic ipRGCs may dampen SCN light responses and contribute to the relative insensitivity of circadian resetting at low light levels.

Intergeniculate Leaflet

In rodents, the IGL is a thin cellular layer sandwiched between the dorsal and ventral subdivisions of the lateral geniculate nucleus (LGN) of the thalamus. The IGL projects heavily to the SCN core via the geniculohypothalamic tract (GHT).[61] The IGL receives dense bilateral projections from OPN4-expressing RGCs, the IGL itself, and the retrochiasmatic area (RCA), as well as smaller projections from the SCN, locus coeruleus, midbrain raphe nuclei, and brainstem cholinergic nuclei. Unlike the dorsal LGN, which is viewed primarily as a relay in image-formation visual processes, the IGL has a well-established role in circadian rhythm regulation.[62] Lesions of the IGL result in a broad array of circadian phenotypes, including slowing the rate of re-entrainment following a shift in the photoperiod, blocking the circadian period lengthening effect of constant light, and eliminating the circadian resetting induced by introducing a running wheel into an animal's cage.[63] Based on these findings, the IGL is thought to transmit both photic and nonphotic information to the circadian clock. However, animals with lesions placed in the region of the IGL are clearly able to entrain to light-dark cycles, indicating that the IGL is not necessary for photic circadian entrainment and rhythm generation, but instead plays a modulatory role.

Most IGL neurons contain the inhibitory neurotransmitter GABA, and the IGL is also characterized by large populations of NPY- and ENK-containing neurons.[64] In rodents, NPY-containing neurons in the IGL project heavily to the SCN core region and form synapses on VIP-containing neurons. The effects of NPY and photic stimuli on the circadian pacemaker appear to be mutually inhibitory. Consistent with the effects of NPY on SCN electrical activity in hypothalamic slices, microinjection of NPY into the SCN region induces a phase advance in locomotor activity when administered during the biologic daytime, and NPY-induced phase shifts are attenuated by glutamate or light.[63] Conversely, glutamate-induced phase shifts in SCN electrical activity or light-induced phase shifts in locomotor activity are inhibited by NPY. Pharmacologic studies suggest that NPY attenuates light-induced phase shifts via Y1 and/or Y5 receptors,[65] whereas the Y2 receptor mediates phase resetting of the locomotor activity rhythm.[66] Optogenetic activation of GABAergic IGL neurons also suppresses SCN responses to light, demonstrating that the GHT plays an important role in modulating circadian light responses.[67]

Midbrain Nuclei

The SCN receives a dense serotoninergic input from neurons in the median raphe nucleus (MRN) and relatively sparse input from neurons in the dorsal raphe nucleus (DRN).[68] Serotonin (5-HT)-immunoreactive axonal terminals in the SCN overlap extensively with the terminal fields of the RHT and GHT, forming synapses with VIP-containing neurons. In contrast to the MRN, the DRN projects to the IGL and to the SPZ immediately dorsal to the SCN, with few fibers to the SCN itself. The midbrain raphe nuclei are not required for photic circadian entrainment nor for maintaining circadian rhythmicity, but 5-HT modulates photic and nonphotic input to the circadian clock. Lesions of the midbrain raphe nuclei have been reported to phase advance locomotor activity onset, lengthen the active phase, induce deficits in rhythmicity in constant light, and reduce the amplitude or precision of circadian rhythms.[69]

Similar to NPY, the effects of 5-HT and photic stimuli on the circadian pacemaker appear to be mutually inhibitory. Phase shifts induced by light, optic nerve stimulation, or glutamate are attenuated by administration of 5-HT during the biologic night, whereas 5-HT–induced phase advance shifts are inhibited by glutamate agonists or optic chiasm stimulation.[70] The 5-HT1B receptor mediates inhibitory effects of 5-HT on light-induced phase shifts,[71] and electron microscopic studies have shown that 5-HT1B receptor immunoreactivity is found predominantly in presynaptic terminals in the SCN, including axonal terminals from the RHT.[72] Consistent with pharmacologic studies conducted in vitro, 5-HT7 agonists induce phase advances in hamster behavioral circadian rhythms when administered during the biologic daytime,[73,74] and the 5-HT7 receptor has been localized to dendrites of GABA, VIP, and AVP-containing SCN neurons and to presynaptic axonal terminals.[72]

Dopaminergic signaling in the SCN has recently been implicated in regulating circadian rhythms in adult mice. Although it has long been recognized that dopamine transmits circadian phase information from mother to offspring in the fetal SCN, it was widely thought that dopaminergic signaling ceased to be important once the RHT was established. This view has been challenged by studies demonstrating that stimulation of dopaminergic neurons in the ventral tegmental area (VTA) that project to the SCN accelerates photic circadian entrainment.[75] Additional work has further established that the D1 dopamine receptor (Drd1)-expressing SCN cells comprise a functionally distinct subpopulation that spans elements of both core and shell. Similar to the SCN NMS cell population, the Drd1 cell population is large, comprising 50% to 60% of all SCN neurons, including most SCN VIP cells and approximately 50% of AVP cells.[76] Selectively activating Drd1-expressing neurons in the SCN resets behavioral circadian rhythms similar to the effects of light,[75,77] whereas knocking out these receptors slows the rate of re-entrainment to a shift in the light-dark cycle. The firing rate of neurons containing D1 receptor corresponds with the magnitude of circadian resetting,[77] suggesting that dopaminergic signaling may play an important role in the modulating phase of the SCN neural rhythm.

SUPRACHIASMATIC NUCLEUS OUTPUTS

Considering the important role that the SCN plays in regulating circadian behavior and physiology, the number and density of SCN efferent pathways are surprisingly limited (Figure 35.2, *B*).[78,79] The SCN projects rostrally to limbic structures, including the lateral septum and the bed nucleus of the stria terminalis (BSTL), and to the medial preoptic area (MPOA) and VLPO. The SCN sends projections dorsally to the midline thalamus, including the paraventricular thalamic nucleus (PVT) and the paratenial thalamic nuclei, and dorsocaudally to the SPZ, the paraventricular hypothalamic nucleus (PVH), and the dorsomedial hypothalamic nucleus (DMH). A caudal projection from the SCN terminates in the RCA, and some fibers branch toward the supraoptic nucleus and the lateral hypothalamic area (LHA). The SCN also sends a minor projection laterally to the IGL and small posterior projections to the OPT and central gray matter. Based on retrograde tracing studies in rats, the SCN shell projects more strongly to the MPOA, DMH, and BSTL, whereas the SCN core projects more strongly to the lateral septum and tuberal hypothalamus.[78,80] Both SCN subdivisions project strongly to the SPZ and midline thalamus. In monkeys, VIP-immunoreactive axons from the SCN project rostrally into the MPOA and dorsally into the SPZ and anterior hypothalamic area ventral to the PVH, and small numbers of terminals also are observed in the PVH, LHA, and PVT. A dense VIP-containing projection extends caudally into the RCA, and some fibers continue into the capsule of the ventromedial hypothalamic nucleus, DMH, and dorsal hypothalamic area. In humans, VIP-containing SCN neurons project most heavily into the region just dorsal to the SCN and extending to the area just ventral to the PVH, corresponding to the SPZ in rodents.[4] Similar to monkeys, the SCN in humans sends a dense VIP-immunoreactive projection caudally into the RCA. Together, these studies demonstrate that the SCN projects extensively to other hypothalamic regions, and the pattern of projections is generally conserved across mammalian species.

Sleep-Wake Rhythm

The densest output from the SCN is to the SPZ, which is located immediately dorsal to the SCN and extends dorsocaudally ventral to the PVH.[79] Tracing studies have shown that the SCN core projects more strongly to the lateral SPZ, whereas the SCN shell projects more densely to the medial SPZ.[80] Consistent with these results, AVP-immunoreactive axonal terminals are found medially in the SPZ, whereas VIP-containing terminals are found more laterally. The SPZ innervates similar targets as the SCN but in much greater density, suggesting that the SPZ amplifies circadian output from the SCN. Cell-specific lesions of the SPZ eliminate circadian rhythms of sleep, locomotor activity, and core body temperature, suggesting that the SPZ is part of the primary neuronal pathway mediating the output of SCN-generated circadian rhythms.[81] Lesions in the ventral part of the SPZ abolish circadian rhythms of sleep and locomotor activity while having lesser effects on the body temperature rhythm, whereas lesions in the dorsal SPZ reduce the body temperature rhythm while having minimal effects on rhythms of wake-sleep or locomotor activity. The ventral SPZ, in turn, sends a strong projection caudally to the DMH while the dorsal SPZ projects more extensively to the VMH.[82] Cell-specific lesions of the DMH eliminate circadian rhythms of sleep-wake, locomotor activity, feeding, and plasma corticosteroids but not body temperature or plasma melatonin,[83] whereas deletion of Vgat in the more dorsal SPZ reduces circadian rhythms of aggressive behavior.[84] Hence, the major neuronal pathway mediating the SCN-generated circadian rhythm of sleep is through a first-order projection to the SPZ, followed by a second-order projection to the DMH. Functional, polysynaptic connectivity between SCN VIP neurons and downstream DMH and VMH neurons has been recently demonstrated using channelrhodopsin-assisted circuit mapping in ex vivo brain slices.[11,84]

As might be expected, the DMH projects heavily to brain areas involved in regulating sleep and wakefulness. For example, the DMH sends a primarily GABAergic projection to the VLPO. Sleep-promoting neurons in the VLPO contain the neurotransmitters GABA and galanin[85] and promote sleep via inhibitory projections to the ascending arousal systems.[86,87] Although the SCN and SPZ also send minor projections directly to the VLPO, the projection originating from the DMH is one of the largest inputs to the VLPO.[88]

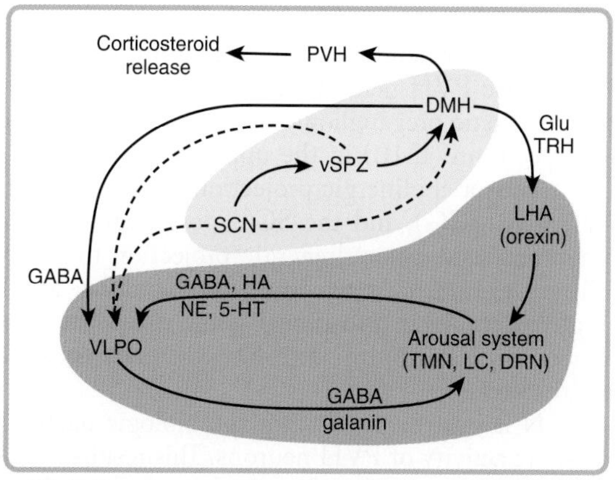

Figure 35.4 Circadian regulation of sleep-wake. The neuronal pathway that regulates circadian sleep-wake cycles (SCN to vSPZ to DMH, indicated in beige) directly interacts with arousal- and sleep-promoting brain regions (indicated in *light* reddish brown), providing a putative pathway for the circadian regulation of sleep-wake. *Solid arrows* indicate prominent neuronal projections, and *dashed arrows* indicate relatively small projections. Neurotransmitters contained in these projections are shown next to the *arrows*. 5-HT, 5-Hydroxytryptamine (serotonin); DMH, dorsomedial hypothalamic nucleus; DRN, dorsal raphe nucleus; GABA, gamma-aminobutyric acid; Glu, glutamate; HA, histamine; LC, locus coeruleus; LHA, lateral hypothalamic area; NE, norepinephrine; PVH, paraventricular hypothalamic nucleus; SCN, suprachiasmatic nucleus; TMN, tuberomammillary nucleus; TRH, thyrotropin-releasing hormone; VLPO, ventrolateral preoptic nucleus; vSPZ, ventral subparaventricular zone.

The DMH also sends a primarily glutamatergic projection to the lateral hypothalamus, which contains wake-promoting neurons, including orexin-expressing neurons.[83] In summary, the DMH receives circadian input from the SCN (including SCN VIP neurons) and the SPZ and projects to the VLPO and LHA, defining a putative pathway for the circadian regulation of sleep and wakefulness (Figure 35.4).

The relay of SCN circadian signals in the SPZ and then the DMH might allow for modification of circadian rhythms by other inputs such as food availability, external temperature, or social cues. Consistent with this hypothesis, the DMH has been shown to play an important role in circadian adaptation to restricted feeding.[89-91] Mice with genetic ablation of orexin neurons also show blunted behavioral adaptation to restricted feeding cycles,[92] suggesting that the outflow pathway from the DMH to orexin neurons might be important for integrating photic and nonphotic information in order to establish a pattern of sleep-wake behavior that is most adaptive for survival. Other signaling molecules implicated in food entrainment include dopamine, ghrelin, and melanocortin, further suggesting that neural pathways involved in circadian rhythms, feeding behavior, and/or energy balance overlap extensively in the hypothalamus. Recent findings suggest that entrainment to light and feeding schedules may also converge at the SCN. Inhibition of NPY-containing IGL neurons that project to the SCN decreases food anticipatory activity to time-restricted feeding, and this circuit requires normal retinal innervation of the SCN during early development.[93]

Circadian Regulation of Melatonin and Cortisol

Under normally entrained conditions, release of melatonin usually begins a few hours before a person's bedtime. Plasma melatonin levels are highest in the middle of the night and then decrease before usual wake time. The SCN is required for the circadian synthesis and release of melatonin by the pineal gland.[94] A subset of SCN neurons projects directly to dorsal parvocellular neurons in the autonomic subdivision of the PVH. These PVH neurons send an excitatory projection to the sympathetic preganglionic neurons in the intermediolateral cell column (IML) in the upper thoracic spinal cord. The IML sends a cholinergic projection to the superior cervical ganglion (SCG), and the SCG postganglionic sympathetic neurons send a noradrenergic projection to the pineal gland. The release of noradrenaline activates alpha- and beta-adrenergic receptors in the pineal gland that stimulate the production of melatonin by controlling the enzyme serotonin *N*-acetyltransferase.

The SCN is most active during the biologic daytime and inhibits tonic activity of PVH neurons. This results in a lower firing rate in the remainder of the pathway, effectively inhibiting melatonin synthesis. Therefore melatonin is produced during the biologic night, when SCN activity is low; this is a common feature of both diurnal and nocturnal animals. Exposure to light during the biologic night activates SCN neurons via the RHT, resulting in the inhibition of melatonin synthesis through the aforementioned pathway. Similar to circadian light resetting of the melatonin rhythm, light-induced suppression of melatonin synthesis is mediated by OPN4-expressing RGCs.[49]

Melatonin can also provide direct feedback to the circadian system via melatonin receptors (MT1 and MT2) located in the SCN. Melatonin acutely inhibits SCN electrical activity, and this response is mediated by the MT1 receptor.[95] The locomotor activity rhythm of rats can be entrained by periodic administration of melatonin as long as the SCN remains intact,[96] suggesting that melatonin-receptor signaling in the SCN is required for melatonin-induced entrainment. Melatonin-induced phase shifts persist in MT1- or MT2-receptor knockout mice, suggesting that melatonin receptor subtypes play an overlapping role in this response.[95,97] In humans, daily administration of melatonin can entrain the circadian system of blind persons,[98,99] indicating that melatonin elicits phase shifts of the human circadian clock and can be used to treat circadian rhythm sleep disorders even in the absence of photoreception.

Early lesion studies of the SCN showed loss of the circadian rhythm of adrenal corticosterone, the major glucocorticoid in rodents. In humans, the circadian rhythm of cortisol rises sharply before the waking period, presumably to promote a general state of readiness in anticipation of the myriad stressors and metabolic demands associated with the active phase. SCN neurons project directly and indirectly to the DMH, which sends glutamatergic efferents to the PVH and is critical for expression of the corticosteroid rhythm.[83] Corticotropin-releasing hormone (CRH)-containing neurons in the PVH project to the median eminence, where CRH is released into the portal circulation and activates the release of adrenocorticotropic hormone (ACTH) from the anterior pituitary gland. The SCN-driven release of ACTH into the blood results in rhythmic induction of corticosteroid secretion from the adrenal gland.

Diffusible Suprachiasmatic Nucleus Output Signals

In SCN-lesioned hosts, transplantation of fetal SCN grafts into the third ventricle restores a low-amplitude circadian rest-activity rhythm with the period of the donor animal.[100] In contrast, photic entrainment, reproductive responses to photoperiod, estrous cycles, and corticosteroid and melatonin rhythms are not restored by SCN transplants. Polymer-encapsulated SCN transplants that prevent neuronal communication between host and donor tissue reinstate low levels of locomotor activity rhythms in SCN-lesioned hosts, suggesting that a diffusible factor can partially reconstitute the rest-activity cycle.[101] The distance of SCN transplants from the normal site of the SCN is an important factor for the recovery of the locomotor rhythm, indicating that a diffusible factor acts locally in a paracrine fashion. Candidate diffusible mediators have been identified in the SCN that might regulate the output of circadian behavioral rhythms, including transforming growth factor (TGF)-α, cardiotrophin-like cytokine, and prokineticin 2 (PK2). PK2 is a clock-controlled gene that is rhythmically expressed in the SCN, and PK2 null mice show attenuated circadian rhythms of sleep-wake, body temperature, and glucocorticoids.[102] Consistent with a role for PK2 as an SCN output factor, PK2 receptor has been described in many SCN output regions, including the PVH, DMH, PVT, paratenial nucleus, lateral septum, and the SCN itself.[103] Additionally, PK2-receptor knockout mice show reduced circadian expression of rest-activity and body temperature rhythms.[104]

SYNCHRONIZATION OF CENTRAL AND PERIPHERAL OSCILLATORS

The circadian system is thought to be hierarchically organized. The SCN contains a master clock for regulating behavioral rhythms, but circadian clocks are also found in tissues throughout the body. The molecular clock mechanism is preserved across different cell types, and circadian expression of clock genes has been demonstrated in nearly all tissues studied, as well as in many sites in the brain.[105] Notably, damage to SCN neurons causes peripheral clocks to fall out of synchrony, even though individual cells in peripheral tissues can continue to generate circadian rhythms of gene transcription.[106] Under most conditions, the SCN entrains peripheral clocks to ensure coordinated changes in physiology that are appropriately timed to the rest-activity cycle. The pathways by which the SCN entrains clocks in peripheral tissues is not fully understood, but there is evidence that shifts in temperature can reset peripheral, but not SCN, clocks.[107] Thus, by controlling the daily cycle of body temperature, the SCN would reset clocks throughout the body and keep them in synchrony.

Other aspects of physiology that are directly regulated by the SCN may also contribute to tissue circadian phase. For example, glucocorticoid signaling activates clock gene expression and influences the rate of entrainment of peripheral clocks to feeding cycles.[108,109] The phase of peripheral clocks can become uncoupled from the SCN pacemaker in animals that are given daily restricted access to food, as shown for circadian gene expression in tissues such as the liver, kidney, and heart.[110,111] Entrainment of peripheral clocks by feeding cycles can potentially occur through nutrient-sensing pathways, as proteins involved in metabolism and energy balance (e.g., sirtuin 1 and AMP-activated protein kinase) interact with core clock proteins and affect their function.[112] The dietary composition and timing of meals can also affect the molecular clock and clock-controlled metabolic function.[113] This has potential clinical implications for shift workers or other persons who regularly consume meals during the biologic night.

CLINICAL PEARL

The SCN is an internal body clock that allows daily scheduling of sleep and wakefulness, feeding, corticosteroid secretion, and other bodily functions during a normal light-dark cycle. This cycle can be modified by light exposure or by administration of melatonin, which resets the body clock, but feeding schedules can also reset the daily activity cycle by acting on circuits that are downstream of the clock. Thus, in patients with difficulty adjusting to shift work, jet lag, or other disruptions of their schedules, in addition to adjusting light exposure and taking melatonin, it is usually possible to adjust to a new schedule more quickly if the mealtimes, social interactions, and sleep-activity schedule of the new environment are adopted as soon as possible.

SUMMARY

The circadian system plays an integral role in coordinating behavioral and physiologic rhythms. Under normally entrained conditions, exposure to light activates OPN4-expressing RGCs, which transmit light information to the core region of the SCN by releasing glutamate and PACAP. The effects of light on SCN neuronal activity are modulated by input from NPY- and GABA-containing neurons in the IGL, serotoninergic input from the MRN, and dopaminergic input from the VTA. The solar day-night cycle entrains the master clock in the SCN, which is responsible for generating circadian patterns of behavior. The SCN regulates the circadian sleep-wake rhythm via a primary projection to the SPZ followed by a secondary projection to the DMH. The DMH, in turn, projects to brain areas critical for promoting sleep or wakefulness. A direct projection from the SCN to the PVH mediates rhythmic control of melatonin secretion from the pineal gland, and an indirect projection from the SCN to the PVH via the DMH is critical for the circadian release of corticosteroids. Although SCN neuronal projections are required for photic entrainment and circadian control of endocrine rhythms, SCN-diffusible factors are sufficient to support a weak circadian rest-activity rhythm. The SCN also coordinates the timing of peripheral clocks, which respond to SCN-directed circadian changes in temperature, glucocorticoids, and nutrient-sensing pathways. Through the aforementioned pathways, the circadian system ensures that sleep and other biologic rhythms are timed appropriately with daily changes in the environment.

SELECTED READINGS

Berson DM, Dunn FA, Takao M. Phototransduction by retinal ganglion cells that set the circadian clock. *Science*. 2002;295:1070–1073.

Chou TC, Scammell TE, Gooley JJ, Gaus SE, Saper CB, Lu J. Critical role of dorsomedial hypothalamic nucleus in a wide range of behavioral circadian rhythms. *J Neurosci*. 2003;23:10691–10702.

de Assis LVM, Oster H. The circadian clock and metabolic homeostasis: entangled networks [published online ahead of print, 2021 Mar 8]. *Cell Mol Life Sci*. 2021;10.1007/s00018-021-03800-2.

Leak RK, Moore RY. Topographic organization of suprachiasmatic nucleus projection neurons. *J Comp Neurol*. 2001;433:312–334.

Moore RY, Weis R, Moga MM. Efferent projections of the intergeniculate leaflet and the ventral lateral geniculate nucleus in the rat. *J Comp Neurol*. 2000;420:398–418.

Panda S, Antoch MP, Miller BH, et al. Coordinated transcription of key pathways in the mouse by the circadian clock. *Cell*. 2002;109:307–320.

Patton AP, Hastings MH. The suprachiasmatic nucleus. *Curr Biol*. 2018;28:R816–R822.

Paul S, Brown TM. Direct effects of the light environment on daily neuroendocrine control. *J Endocrinol*. 2019;243:R1–R18.

Saper CB, Lu J, Chou TC, Gooley J. The hypothalamic integrator for circadian rhythms. *Trends Neurosci*. 2005;28:152–157.

Sondereker KB, Stabio ME, Renna J. Crosstalk: the diversity of melanopsin ganglion cell types has begun to challenge the canonical divide between image-forming and non-image-forming vision. *J Comp Neurol*. 2020;528:2044–2067.

Van Drunen R, Eckel-Mahan K. Circadian Rhythms of the hypothalamus: from function to physiology. *Clocks Sleep*. 2021;3(1):189–226.

Yamazaki S, Numano R, Abe M, et al. Resetting central and peripheral circadian oscillators in transgenic rats. *Science*. 2000;288:682–685.

A complete reference list can be found online at ExpertConsult.com.

Chapter 36

Physiology of the Mammalian Circadian System

Jennifer W. Mitchell; Martha U. Gillette

Chapter Highlights

- The *suprachiasmatic nucleus (SCN)* of the anterior hypothalamus is the master circadian pacemaker for the expression of circadian rhythms. The SCN coordinates these approximately 24-hour rhythms throughout the brain and body and adjusts them to environmental changes. The SCN is highly peptidergic, exhibiting well-defined patterns of regional expression of neuropeptides.
- The *circadian timekeeping system* orchestrates and integrates body rhythms. This system has three components: (1) *the central circadian clock in the SCN* that generates a near–24-hour time base, which it adjusts when it receives signals reporting desynchronization, (2) *input pathways* that transmit information about environmental and body state, and (3) *output pathways* that disseminate information about the timing status of the SCN and mediate the daily expression of rhythms of behavior and physiology.
- Circadian rhythms emerge from *transcriptional/translational feedback loops* comprising a limited number of circadian clock genes and their protein products. Although rhythmic clock gene expression was first identified in the SCN, subsequent work found similar molecular clocks in cells and tissues throughout the body. Nevertheless, coherence of rhythms within a tissue decays in the absence of the SCN, whereas SCN tissue is tightly coupled, even in tissue explants.
- The circadian pacemaker is *entrained by environmental light-dark cycles* and other salient periodic events. Light entrainment depends upon intrinsically photosensitive retinal ganglion cells that express the blue-light photopigment, melanopsin, and that give rise to the retino-hypothalamic tract, terminating in the SCN and certain other nonvisual brain areas. The SCN restricts its own sensitivity to inputs to discrete temporal windows throughout the circadian day-night cycle.
- The mammalian circadian master pacemaker in the SCN synchronizes and coordinates downstream circadian clocks distributed throughout the brain and body. Internal desynchronization or failure of internal entrainment to the environment appears to be both a cause and an effect of disease-related pathophysiology. Thus, the balance between health and disease is strongly dependent on the proper coordination within and between central and peripheral circadian oscillating systems.

AN INTERNAL CLOCK FOR OPTIMAL FUNCTION

Physiologic modulation at the neural level relies on the ability of neurons to respond to salient stimuli. Among the most relevant stimuli for life on Earth are the alternating environmental states of day and night. Day-night changes in metabolism, physiology, and behavior are orchestrated by an endogenous time-keeping system that oscillates with a circadian (*circa*, about, and *dies*, a day) period. Behavioral outputs change significantly so that some behaviors occur in the day, others occur at night, and some are expressed at dawn and dusk.

Internal daily oscillations are a result of adaptation to this major environmental variable: the ever-changing cycle of day and night. Early organisms that optimized cycles of behavior to these changes held a competitive advantage—they could predict environmental state changes. Behaviors that anticipated rather than only reacted to rhythmic environmental changes offer significant benefits. Adaptation to these needs occurred through the emergence of a circadian system capable of optimizing behavioral, physiologic, and metabolic processes with respect to this light-dark cycle. The circadian system organizes body systems so that they occur in 24-hour rhythms. Uninterrupted, this circadian rhythm persists in the absence of exogenous timing cues, such as light, food availability, or social cues.

Outputs of these circadian rhythms can be used as a marker of circadian phases. Patterning of the sleep-wake cycle as well as core body temperature are often used as markers

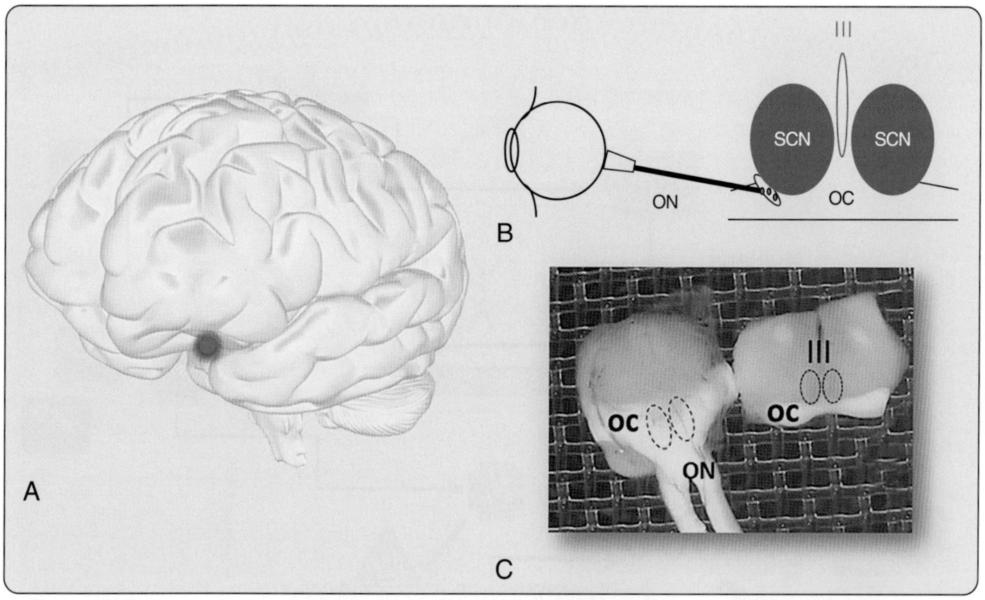

Figure 36.1 Anatomy of the suprachiasmatic nucleus (SCN), site of the master circadian clock. **(A)** The human SCN is located in the mediobasal hypothalamus, as indicated by the *red dot*. **(B)** The SCN receives light information from intrinsically photosensitive retinal ganglion cells via the retinohypothalamic tract of the optic nerve (*ON*). Light provides the primary timing cue to the SCN. The paired SCNs are nestled above the optic chiasm (*OC*) on either side of the third ventricle (III). **(C)** Two orientations of rat hypothalamic brain slices; the SCN is demarcated by *dashed ovals*. The horizontal brain slice (*left*) preserves the ONs, whereas in the coronal slice (*right*) of the SCN is identified by its medial position embedded in the OC directly lateral to the third ventricle (*III*) and the ventral displacement of the area of the ON bordering the paired nuclei.

of circadian phase. In addition, numerous endogenous hormones oscillate with a predictable phase relationship to day and night (reviewed by Van Cauter[1]). Hormonal rhythms can be complex, as the circadian pacemaker, homeostatic state of the organism (activity level, sleep, and feeding), and the pulsatile nature of secretion can affect their oscillations. Nevertheless, clear diurnal patterns of secretion have been reported. Plasma melatonin,[2] growth hormone,[3] prolactin,[4] thyrotropin-releasing hormone,[5] luteinizing hormone,[6] and leptin[7-9] all are elevated during the night. Conversely, adrenocorticotropic hormone and cortisol peak during the day.[10,11] These oscillations in hormone secretion are clock regulated; they continue in a constant environment. Overall, circadian rhythmicity appears to be present at virtually every level of function studied.

This chapter focuses on the neurobiology of circadian timekeeping, describing what is known about the master pacemaker for circadian rhythmicity; the generation of circadian time-keeping via expression of transcription-translation feedback loops; roles of neural activity; how various biologic systems can provide input to the endogenous biologic timing; and how the pacemaker can, in turn, influence the physiology and behavior of the individual. We discuss how the circadian system can adapt to a changing environment by resetting the circadian clock in response to a variety of inputs, including changes in light, activity, and the sleep-wake cycle.

SUPRACHIASMATIC NUCLEI AS PACEMAKER

In mammals, circadian rhythms are regulated by the suprachiasmatic nucleus (SCN), a paired set of brain nuclei located at the base of the hypothalamus, directly above the optic chiasm (Figure 36.1). Each nucleus contains approximately 10,000 cells.[12] The SCN acts as the central pacemaker, coordinating circadian rhythms throughout the brain and body. Lesioning the SCN disrupts rhythmicity in corticosterone levels, drinking, and wheel-running behavior.[13,14] This provided the initial evidence that the central pacemaker for the mammalian clock lay within the SCN. Transplanting fetal SCN tissue in situ or into the third ventricle of animals in which the SCN had been lesioned demonstrated that restoring the SCN could restore rhythmicity.[15,16] Furthermore, when fetal SCN tissue from a wild-type hamster was implanted into the third ventricle of a hamster with a genetic alteration that shortened the free-running period, the new free-running period resembled that of the SCN donor rather than the host animal. Hence, not only is the SCN necessary for generating rhythms, but also the period of this rhythmicity is an intrinsic property of the SCN cells—the presence of SCN is sufficient to drive the animal's peripheral rhythms.[17,18]

The circadian timekeeping system can be categorized into three major components: (1) a central clock mechanism that generates circadian rhythms, (2) input pathways that synchronize the clock, and (3) output pathways that regulate the daily expressions of behavior and physiology. This simple three-part model has provided a solid foundation for our understanding of circadian timekeeping.

GENERATION OF CIRCADIAN RHYTHM

Molecular Basis for Rhythm Generation

The nature of the biologic substrates of circadian timekeeping that could generate a time base as lengthy as 24 hours was for many years a mystery. Many creative and talented scientists pursued numerous approaches in an array of organisms before timekeeping was proven to be embedded in the

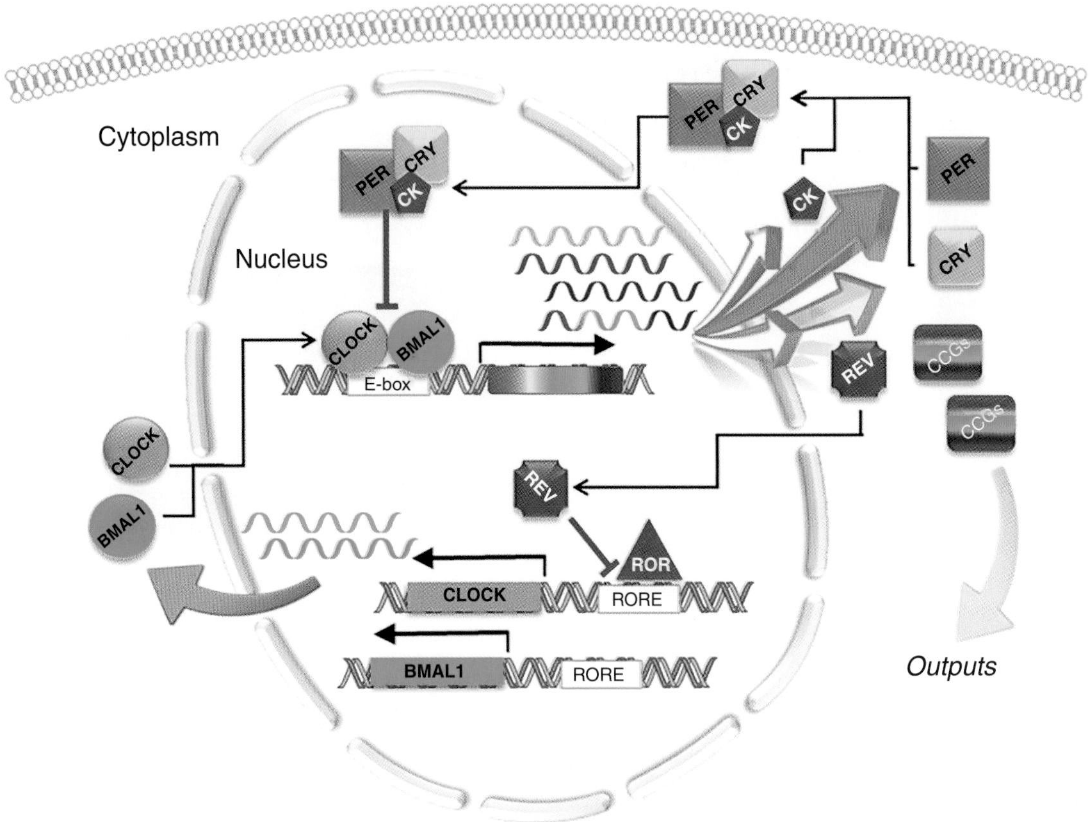

Figure 36.2 Transcriptional/translational feedback loops (TTLs) of the mammalian circadian clock. BMAL1 and CLOCK, the key positive elements of the core circadian clock, heterodimerize and activate transcription of the *Per* and *Cry* genes by binding to the E-box elements in their promoter regions. Their translational products, PER and CRY proteins, heterodimerize in the cytoplasm and then translocate to the nucleus where they interact with the BMAL1/CLOCK complex to inhibit their own transcription. A secondary autoregulatory feedback loop involves retinoic acid receptor-related orphan receptor element (RORE)-mediated transcription, which retinoic acid receptor-related orphan receptor (ROR) activates and REV-ERB represses. Additionally, this TTL-based clock mechanism also controls rhythmic expression of numerous clock-controlled genes (CCGs), which perform biochemical or physiologic roles that vary with circadian timing.

genome. Timekeeping was found to be an emergent property of a negative transcription-translation feedback loop of highly conserved "clock genes." Key elements of proof are based on elegant experiments in mutagenized fruit flies, *Drosophila*. Altering a single gene, *Period,* changes the period of rhythms of locomotory activity permanently. The 2017 Nobel Prize in Physiology or Medicine was awarded to three chronobiologists, Jeffrey Hall, Michael Rosbash, and Michael Young, for their discovery of molecular mechanisms controlling circadian rhythms. This work along with the discovery that single, dispersed mammalian cells can exhibit circadian rhythms,[19] established the important molecular processes within single cells that generate a near 24-hour rhythm.

The approximately 24-hour rhythm emerges from a feedback cycle involving a set of core clock genes, their messenger RNAs (mRNAs), and proteins.[20-22] This cycle involves of a set of interconnected positive and negative feedback loops, and their regulatory elements (Figure 36.2). The core molecular feedback loop in mammals includes positive elements, *Clock* and *Bmal1,* which are transcribed into mRNA, translated into proteins that heterodimerize in the cytoplasm, and then translocate into the nucleus. The proteins CLOCK and BMAL1 are members of a family of transcription factors containing the basic helix-loop-helix (bHLH)-PAS motif by which they bind E-box enhancer sequences of gene promoters.[23-25] This enables them to activate transcription of their own genes, as well as activating transcription of negative regulatory elements. The negative elements, which include the *Period (Per) homologs (Per1, Per2, Per3)*, and the *Cryptochrome (Cry) homologs (Cry1, Cry2)* and *Rev-erb*α, are then transcribed and translated. Proteins of the negative elements also associate in complexes and translocate to the nucleus, where they feed back to inhibit transcription of the positive elements.[20-22]

In addition to the core molecular feedback loop, there is an additional interlocking loop involving *Bmal1*. *Bmal1* is regulated by a retinoic acid receptor–related orphan receptor (ROR) enhancer site located upstream of the *Bmal1* gene; ROR binding activates gene expression, while REV-ERBα binding inhibits transcription.[26] REV-ERBα is regulated by an E-box enhancer located upstream of its transcription start site, resulting in an expression pattern that subsequently puts expression of *Bmal1* completely out of phase with the negative elements of the core molecular feedback loop.[27] These feedback loops are further affected by regulatory enzymes, including casein kinase 1 epsilon (CKIε) and glycogen synthase kinase (GSK),[28-30] and small intracellular regulatory molecules, such as calcium and cyclic adenosine monophosphate (cAMP) with established roles in signal transduction.[31,32] The cycle of these feedback loops takes approximately 24 hours to complete.

Beyond this sequence of interactions, the molecular clockwork modulates and is modulated by cellular redox state. The BMAL1/CLOCK heterodimer regulates the expression of nicotinamide phosphoribosyltransferase, a rate-limiting enzyme in the nicotinamide adenosine dinucleotide (NAD+) salvage pathway. This relationship is the driving force for rhythmic levels of NAD+, which in turn activate NAD+-dependent histone deacetylases, sirtuin 1 (SIRT1), and SIRT3.[33,34] SIRT1, an important element of metabolic control, displays circadian oscillatory activity and alters PER2 stability and CLOCK function.[33,35] SIRT1 is localized in the mitochondrial matrix, where it mediates the deacetylation of metabolic enzymes.[32,36,37] Additional bHLH transcription factors, *Dec1 (Bhlhe40/Stra13/Sharp2)* and *Dec2 (Bhlhe41/Sharp1)*, can repress their own transcription by directly binding to the BMAL1 protein as well as occupying E-Box enhancer sequences and, thus, inhibiting transcription of other clock-controlled genes.[38,39]

A number of mutations in the genes of the circadian molecular feedback loop result in alterations in circadian phenotypes. A dominant-negative form of the *clock* gene causes lengthening and gradual loss of rhythms under continuous dark (DD) conditions.[40] However, loss of *clock* in null mutants results in shortening of circadian rhythms,[41] likely because of the substitution of the NPAS2 protein for CLOCK in its complex with BMAL1.[42] There is an immediate loss of rhythmicity with null mutation of BMAL.[43] Disruption of *Per1* or *Per2* genes results in a shortened period. $Cry1^{-/-}$ mice have a shorter period length, and $Cry2^{-/-}$ mice have a significantly longer period length, but both maintain rhythmic behavior.[44,45] These observations indicate that the molecular clockwork is extremely sensitive to alterations in its elements.

Electrical and Redox Rhythms

The SCN expresses additional intrinsic rhythmic properties, including a circadian rhythm in spontaneous electrical activity. When the SCN is isolated by knife-cut from inputs from the rest of the brain[46] or in a brain slice in vitro,[47] circadian rhythms of neuronal firing continue. This property is essential to the function of the circadian timing system,[48-50] peaking in midday in both diurnal and nocturnal mammals. The neurons of the SCN exhibit limited electrical activity during the night.[51,52] Underlying this change in action potential generation is a day/night rhythm in resting membrane potential. The resting membrane potential of SCN neurons is most depolarized and thus more likely to reach threshold for an action potential, during midday and most hyperpolarized in the early night.[52] Differences in membrane potential and ionic conductances between day and night persist even in the absence of synaptic activity.[53] To maintain oscillations in spontaneous activity in the absence of synaptic input, the intrinsic currents must change intrinsically to alter the membrane potential over the day-night cycle.

A potential regulator of intrinsic currents is cellular redox state. Redox state, the potential of molecular substrates to receive or donate electrons, is the manifestation of cellular metabolic state. Near 24-hour oscillations of redox state in the SCN have been identified. They revealed that cellular metabolic state could modulate neuronal excitability via modification of redox-sensitive K+ channels.[52,54] Interestingly, imposed changes in redox state cause immediate changes in excitability.[55] Thus, unlike the transcriptional-translational relationship of changes in the molecular clock to SCN physiology, redox modulation is tightly coupled to neuronal excitability.[54]

Reciprocal interaction between redox state, the molecular clock, and neuronal excitability has been proposed.[52,55]

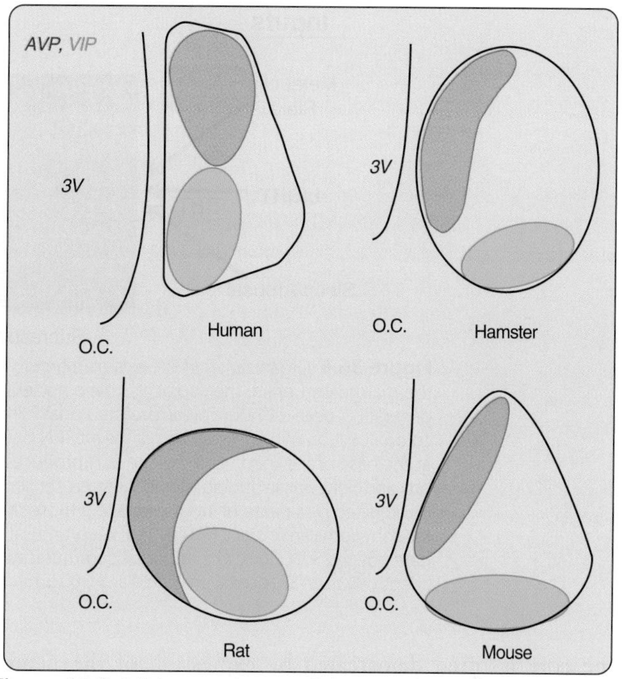

Figure 36.3 Cellular organization of the suprachiasmatic nucleus (SCN). Patterns of neuropeptide immunoreactivity reveal that the SCN has distinct regions of neuropeptide content. Localizations of vasoactive intestinal polypeptide (VIP) and arginine vasopressin (AVP) are salient and highly conserved features across species. The ventrolateral core (*blue*) and a dorsomedial shell (*orange*), both densely packed with somata of small neurons (8–12 μm in diameter), are marked by VIP and AVP, respectively. Light signals from the eyes are conveyed to the ventral core by the retinohypothalamic tract (RHT). The majority of output projections from the SCN originate from the dorsomedial shell. (Modified from Abrahamson EE, Moore RY. Suprachiasmatic nucleus in the mouse: retinal innervation, intrinsic organization and efferent projections. *Brain Res.* 2001;916:172–91; Antle MC, Silver R. Orchestrating time: arrangements of the brain circadian clock. *Trends Neurosci.* 2005;28:145–51; Moore RY, Speh JC, Leak RK. Suprachiasmatic nucleus organization. *Cell Tissue Res.* 2002;309:89–98; Hofman MA. The human circadian clock and aging. *Chronobiol Int.* 2000;17:45–259.)

Reduced forms of the redox cofactors NAD(H) and NADP(H) enhance the DNA-binding activity of the core clock proteins BMAL1 and CLOCK, whereas their oxidized forms inhibit it.[56] Even minute changes in cellular redox state can affect binding activity of these circadian transcriptional activators.

The probable linkage between gene expression, redox state, and electrical activity is further supported by the association of clock-gene expression with intracellular signaling pathways regulating neuronal membrane potential and firing rate. Reciprocally, at the cell membrane, these ionic currents may be necessary for self-sustainment of the molecular clock and could influence the molecular clock via similar intracellular signals.[57]

FUNCTIONAL ARCHITECTURE

More than 300 neuropeptides have been identified in the SCN by mass spectrometry.[58-61] The SCN can be subdivided into two regions based on distribution of neuropeptides: the ventrolateral core region and a dorsomedial shell region (Figure 36.3). The core region receives external input and acts as an integrator, communicating phase-resetting information to the rest of the SCN. The neurons of the core exhibit low amplitude rhythms that are susceptible to clock-resetting cues.[62,63]

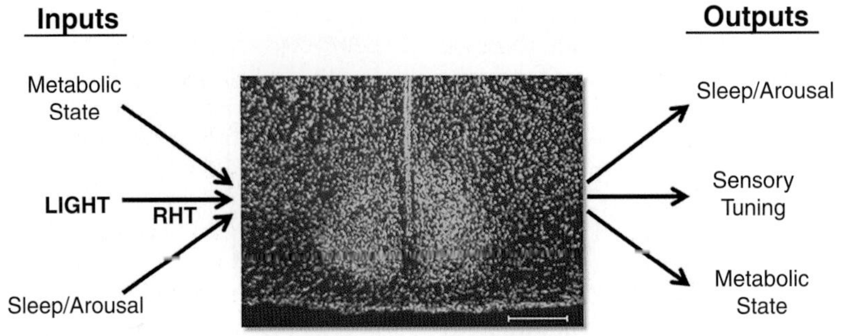

Figure 36.4 Organization of the circadian timing system. Circadian rhythms are orchestrated by a single site in the mammalian brain, the suprachiasmatic nucleus (SCN). The SCN is an endogenous oscillator, spontaneously generating near–24-hour rhythms of neuronal firing rate, output signals, and sensitivity to incoming signals. A coronal section of the medial part of the rat SCN is seen here as two brightly staining clusters of Nissl-positive cells at the base of the third ventricle. The SCN produces output signals that coordinate circadian rhythms of physiology and behavior, including metabolic state, sensory tuning, and sleep and arousal. Phasing of the SCN clock can be adjusted by a range of inputs, including those that communicate metabolic state, environmental light (via the retinohypothalamic tract [RHT]), and sleep/arousal states. Windows of sensitivity to phase-resetting signals are gated by the SCN clock so that signals communicating loss of desynchronization with day-night or output targets adaptively reset SCN clock phasing. Bar = 300 μm.

The core is often demarcated by expression of the neuropeptide vasoactive intestinal peptide (VIP). It also contains neurons that express gamma-aminobutyric acid (GABA) and calretinin. Neurons of a central region, often integrated into the core region, express gastrin-releasing peptide (GRP) colocalized with GABA, and the little SAAS neuropeptide.[12,64-67] The shell region generates robust circadian oscillations in neural activity, neuropeptide release, and *cfos* and *Per* gene expression.[68-71] It comprises larger neurons that express arginine vasopressin (AVP), met-enkephalin, angiotensin II, prokineticin 2 (PK2), and GABA.[12,65,66] There are topographic connections between all regions of the nucleus, as well as bilateral communication between the two nuclei of the animal.[72]

Although the human SCN is larger and less compact than in rodents, its peptidergic organization is similar (Figure 36.3). The dorsal and medial regions contain neurophysin/vasopressin neurons. The central region contains calbindin, synaptophysin, and VIP neurons, whereas the ventral and rostral regions contain synaptophysin, calbindin, and substance P.[73]

Inputs

The SCN is positioned in the mediobasal hypothalamus directly above the optic chiasm, where axons of the optic nerve cross over, which enables stereoscopic vision. The paired nuclei lie adjacent to the walls of the third ventricle (Figures 36.1 and 36.4). Thus the SCN is central to hypothalamic nuclei that control homeostatic physiology and behavior. In addition, the SCN receives inputs and sends outputs to many more distant brain regions; for a more detailed presentation of the anatomy of this system, see Chapter 35. The SCN performs a central integrating role, receiving input via projections that communicate temporal state beyond the SCN (Figure 36.4). This role complements SCN's timekeeping function and enables appropriate alignment of the circadian clock to brain, body, behavioral, and environmental states.

Retinohypothalamic Tract

The primary cue in establishing entrainment to the world is environmental light. Light signals are communicated from the eye to the SCN via a direct projection from the retina, the retinohypothalamic tract (RHT). The RHT is both necessary and sufficient for photic entrainment,[74,75] as disruption of the RHT results in an inability to respond to resetting light signals[76,77] and RHT stimulation can mimic light-resetting cues.[67,78] A subpopulation of retinal ganglion cells is intrinsically photosensitive (ipRGCs), a property conferred by their expression of the blue-light photopigment, melanopsin.[79] These melanopsin-containing retinal ganglion cells are photosensitive at wavelengths that are most effective for circadian resetting.[80] Terminals of melanopsin-positive retinal ganglion cells co-localize glutamate (GLU) and pituitary adenylate cyclase-activating polypeptide (PACAP),[81] the neurotransmitters of the RHT.[82,83]

Melanopsin-containing retinal ganglion cells are distinct from those giving rise to the primary visual pathway.[84] Animals lacking visual photoreceptors (rods and cones), both hereditarily retinal-degenerate strains of mice[85] and genetically modified mice that lack rods and cones,[86] still exhibit normal circadian responses to light. There is redundancy in the circadian photoreception system in the retina. Circadian entrainment is maintained in mice lacking the gene for melanopsin.[87,88] Only when both classical and melanopsin-based photoreception are eliminated is entrainment abolished.[79,89,90]

Intergeniculate Leaflet of the Thalamus

The RHT sends projections to the thalamic intergeniculate leaflet (IGL), which sends projections to the SCN through the geniculohypothalamic tract (GHT). Neurons of the GHT express neuropeptide Y (NPY) and GABA. Retinal signals are conveyed to the IGL, in part by bifurcating axons of the ipRGCs of the RHT.[91] The IGL/GHT provides an indirect, auxiliary pathway by which photic information reaches the SCN. Disruption of the GHT does not prevent entrainment,[92] yet it can result in subtle modifications in the response to light-shifting effects on circadian phase and period.[93,94] The IGL has been suggested to be involved in a more refined photic entrainment as in seasonally altered daylengths or dim nighttime illumination.[95,96]

The IGL also plays a role in in the nonphotic regulation of the circadian system by arousal-related stimuli. IGL lesions abolish phase-shifting effects of novelty-induced wheel-running[97,98] and benzodiazepine administration in hamsters.[76,99,100] Lesion of the IGL results in shortening of the intrinsic circadian period (*tau*)[101] and interferes with the entrainment effect of scheduled daily treadmill activity in mice.[102] IGL neurons are sensitive to metabolic signals and the GHT may mediate the effects of such signals on the SCN pacemaker.[103,104] This is noteworthy because NPY contributes to integrating metabolic and appetite-related signals within other hypothalamic circuits.[4] Orexins/hypocretins modulate the activity of neurons in the IGL.[105] NPY is believed to be involved in activity-induced phase shifts during the daytime in nocturnal animals but also appears to be able to modulate light-induced phase shifts.[106-108]

Raphe

The SCN receives direct serotonergic input from the median raphe, and indirectly via a raphe-to-IGL pathway.[32,109-112] Serotonergic projections to the SCN and IGL have been implicated in (1) modulation of photic effects on the circadian pacemaker during the subjective night[113] and (2) mediation of nonphotic effects on the pacemaker during subjective day.[114] Serotonin depletion results in photic phase shifting that is potentiated, while effects of nonphotic phase-shifting stimuli are impaired.[115,116] Conversely, elevating serotonin, either by electrical stimulation of the serotonergic raphe or injecting serotonergic agonists onto the SCN, inhibits photic phase shifting during subjective night and evokes nonphotic phase shifting during subjective day.[111,117-119]

The SCN may influence the regulation of sleep-wake states by communicating its circadian signal through indirect pathways to the raphe nuclei.[120] Projections from the dorsal and median raphe may convey feedback information to the SCN regarding the vigilance state of the animal. Such reciprocal interactions between the circadian and sleep-wake regulatory systems may contribute to the stable yet adaptive rhythmicity of daily sleep-wake cycles.

Evidence suggests that differential effects of serotonin on the SCN are mediated through different 5-hydroxytryptamine (5-HT) receptors with distinct localizations. Facilitatory effects are mediated by 5-HT1A/7 receptors within the SCN,[117,119] while serotonergic inhibition of light-induced phase-shifts acts through 5-HT1B receptors located presynaptically on RHT terminals.[121,122] Whereas light itself has little phase-shifting effect during mid-subjective day, light at night can block the phase-shifting effects of a serotonin agonist.[123] This suggests that nonphotic and photic (glutamatergic) serotonergic inputs to the SCN are mutually inhibitory.

Brainstem and Basal Forebrain

Cholinergic projections to the SCN originate both in the brainstem and basal forebrain in brain nuclei with identified roles in sleep and arousal[124] and were demonstrated to also be present in diurnal animals.[125] Within the brainstem, these cholinergic projections arise from three nuclei. The parabigeminal nucleus is considered a satellite region of the superior colliculus, which appears to play a role in generating target-location information as part of saccadic eye movements.[126] The laterodorsal tegmental (LDTg) and pedunculopontine tegmental (PPTg) nuclei both are important for regulating the sleep-wake cycle.[127] In the basal forebrain, the substantia innominata within the nucleus basalis magnocellularis (NBM) contributes to arousal and focused attention.[128] Unlike the RHT, IGL, and raphe projections described earlier, which generally form overlapping terminal fields in the SCN core, these afferents preferentially project onto the SCN shell.[129,130] The LDTg, PPTg, and NBM are interconnected, and all play roles in regulating the sleep and arousal states of the animal. Stimulation of the LDTg or PPTg releases acetylcholine (ACh) onto the SCN and adjusts behavioral rhythms in a time-of-day dependent manner.[131] These observations suggest that the cholinergic inputs to the SCN may provide a signal regarding the sleep and arousal states of the animal, providing a link between the sleep-wake cycle and circadian rhythms.

Notably, the SCN receives input from approximately 35 areas identified by retrograde tracing and summarized in Morin.[132] Additional sleep-wake input to the SCN may come from the tuberomammillary nucleus.[133] Histamine is a regulator of the sleep-wake cycle, primarily providing a signal of wakefulness. Noradrenergic projections from the locus coeruleus (LC) may provide afferent inputs to the circadian system. The extent of the potential input from these additional monosynaptic and multisynaptic projections onto the SCN allows for an enormous capacity for modulation by a wide range of stimuli.[132]

Outputs

Although circadian physiology influences almost every aspect of physiology and behavior, target sites of SCN efferent projections are relatively small and local, primarily at the level of the hypothalamus. These targets are well-established relays to the autonomic and neuroendocrine systems as well as to structures regulating affective, sensory, and motor processes.[134-136] Neurons from the ventral regions of the SCN project to the lateral region of the hypothalamic subparaventricular zone (sPVHz), the perisuprachiasmatic area, and the ventral tuberal area. The dorsal region of the SCN projects to multiple hypothalamic sites: the medial preoptic area (MPOA), medial sPVHz, dorsal parvocellular paraventricular nucleus (dPVN), and the dorsal medial hypothalamus (DMH).[137] Targets of efferents to the dPVN include endocrine, autonomic, and intermediate neurons, thereby allowing integration of a number of hypothalamic signals.[135] SCN efferents emerge from both the core and shell subnuclei and release both neurotransmitters and peptides, including GABA, GLU, and AVP.

In addition to neuronal efferents, the SCN regulates certain rhythmic processes through diffusible paracrine signals. The presence of a diffusible SCN output signal was first suggested by the finding that complete surgical isolation of the SCN within a “hypothalamic island” abolished SCN-dependent neuroendocrine responses but allowed for persisting locomotor activity rhythms in the same animals.[138] Although this surprising finding conflicted with prior studies suggesting that the ability of SCN transplants to restore rhythmicity in SCN-lesioned hosts depended on anatomic integration with the host brain,[139-141] evidence that transplantation of SCN tissue encapsulated within semipermeable capsules could restore locomotor rhythms provided strong confirmation of the paracrine hypothesis.[18] Several diffusible candidate molecules now have been implicated as circadian output signals, including PK2, tumor necrosis factor-α, and AVP.[138]

Many SCN projection sites are regulators of sleep and arousal. The DMH projections are especially interesting, as many of these neurons appear to project to neurons containing hypocretin/orexin, a peptide well known for its role in arousal.[142,143] In addition, evidence exists for a multisynaptic pathway between the SCN and LC, an important arousal center in the brain, mediated by orexin,[144] with the DMH as a relay.[145] A minor set of SCN efferents project to the ventrolateral preoptic nucleus, a region that, if lesioned, produces prolonged reduction in sleep duration and amplitude.[146] The SCN projects to the paraventricular thalamic (PVT) nucleus and IGL of the thalamus. Both nuclei project back to the SCN. The PVT loop is proposed to provide assessment of sleep/arousal states and SCN modulation, whereas the IGL loop is thought to provide the SCN with information from higher, integrative visual centers.[93,147,148] The PVN acts as a relay between the SCN and the amygdala, which may provide a link between the circadian system and affective states.[149] Overall, the SCN is uniquely situated within a network that enables close interaction with brain regions controlling sleep and arousal states.

CIRCADIAN RESETTING

Timekeeping is a cellular process.[150,151] The expression of independently phased circadian firing rhythms from individual neurons dissociated from neonatal rat SCN cultured on an electrode array provides compelling evidence for the cellular nature of the clock.[152] It follows, then, that the properties gating sensitivity of the circadian clock within the SCN to resetting stimuli and phase resetting must be cellular. The range of responses of the clock must be restricted so that activation of select signaling pathways can occur only at the appropriate time in the circadian cycle.[32,153-155] How does the SCN clock temporally regulate its own responsiveness of specific signaling pathways?

In an attempt to define and understand the underlying control mechanisms subserving clock-gated windows of sensitivity, the SCN under constant conditions was exposed either in vivo or in vitro to treatments that activate elements of specific signaling pathways. Treatments were administered at various discrete points in the circadian cycle, and effects on the time-of-peak in subsequent intrinsic rhythms, such as neuronal activity or clock gene activity, were assessed. If the time-of-peak appears earlier during cycle(s) after treatment compared with controls, the phase of the rhythm is advanced. If the time-of-peak appears later than in controls, then the phase is delayed by the treatment. Assessing the changing relationship between the circadian time of treatment and its effect on phasing of an oscillation can generate a phase-response curve (Figure 36.5). This relationship graphically presents the temporal pattern of SCN sensitivity to activation of specific signaling pathways and, in fact, defines the window of sensitivity to phase resetting via this pathway. Timing of the peak activity after experimental reagents are administered at specific circadian times is compared with the time-of-peak activity in media-treated controls. The permanence of the phase shift is examined by evaluating the time of the peak in the oscillation of activity over the days after a treatment.

Temporal domains identified as sensitive to phase resetting via specific first and second messenger pathways coincide with discrete portions of the circadian cycle. Based on these temporal windows of sensitivities, the circadian cycle can be divided into several temporal states, or domains, of the clock: day, night, dusk, and dawn.[153,154] These studies not only contribute to defining the properties of the clock's temporal domains but also emphasize the complexity of control that the clock exerts over signal integration and phase-resetting within the SCN. These properties have been incorporated into clock-gated regulatory pathways. Each is discussed in the context of the clock domain that is regulated.

Subjective day and night are distinct with respect to their sensitivities and response characteristics under constant environmental conditions. Each correlates with specific neurotransmitter systems that impinge upon this hypothalamic site as evidenced by a large body of neuroanatomic studies.[156] This permits speculation regarding the function of pathways that gain access to and regulate the biologic clock at different points in the circadian cycle. We now consider, in turn, the major identified domains of clock sensitivity (Figure 36.6).

CIRCADIAN CLOCK REGULATORS

Daytime

A number of neurotransmitters and neuropeptides are important in resetting circadian rhythms during the daytime, including 5-HT, PACAP, NPY, and GABA. The majority of these experiments were performed in nocturnal rodents, so daytime is defined as the time during which the lights are on, and/or the model rodent is inactive. As a result, the functional context of this regulation appears tied to arousal-induced resetting, often referred to as nonphotic resetting.[157,158] Nonphotic signals cover a wide variety of phenomena, including sleep deprivation, dark pulses during the light period, and activity associated with exposure to a novel wheel or cage. The unifying factor in nonphotic signals is that they involve arousal during a time when the animal would normally be inactive.

Serotonin, or 5-HT, is believed to play a role in nonphotic, activity-induced phase shifts during the daytime. Increasing 5-HT in the SCN during the *subjective day* of an animal free running in a constant environment induces an advance in peak electrical firing rate in vitro or onset of wheel running in vivo.[111,159] 5-HT levels in the SCN are increased in vivo by electrical stimulation of the dorsal or median raphe.[111,160] Forced wheel running or sleep deprivation during the day also increases 5-HT in the SCN,[161,162] which suggests a role for 5-HT in nonphotic phase shifting. However, depleting 5-HT from raphe projections does not prevent this nonphotic daytime shift,[163] and serotonergic antagonists are not able to attenuate this phase shift,[164] providing mixed evidence for the role of 5-HT. This suggests modulation by additional messengers, possibly neuropeptides.

A second daytime modulator of the SCN clock is PACAP. PACAP is not intrinsic to the SCN but instead is released from synapses of the RHT, where it colocalizes with GLU.[165] Levels of PACAP oscillate throughout the day in SCN samples, which include synaptic terminals of the RHT, but not in other brain regions.[166] If PACAP alone is applied to the SCN brain slice in micromolar quantities, it elicits an advance in peak neuronal firing during the day but has little effect during the night.[81] In vivo findings, however, conflict with this, as attempts to block or remove PACAP's contribution to clock-resetting at night have generated phenotypes that differ in their responses to light or GLU.[167-170] These data suggest that

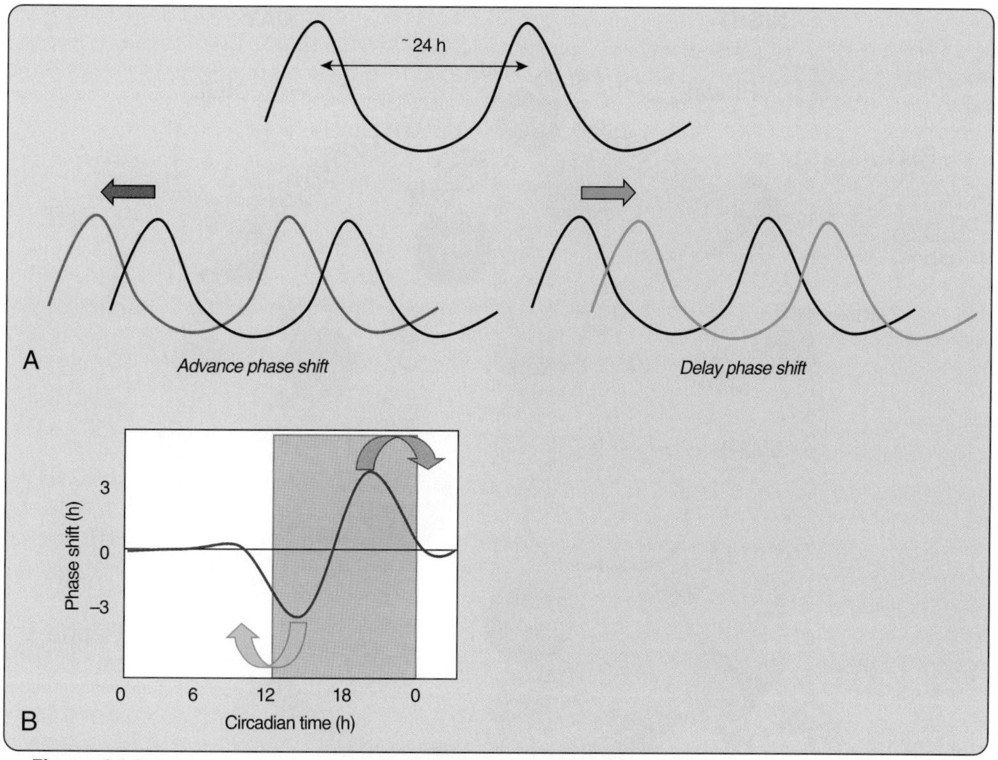

Figure 36.5 Schematic of phase resetting of circadian rhythms. **(A)** Circadian rhythms can be studied as a reportable, endogenous rhythm of approximately 24 hours. The period of the rhythm is measured at an identifiable, reproducible point, which in this example is the time of peak in the neuronal activity rhythm (*top*). A phase advance (*in orange*) occurs when phasing of the rhythm, measured here as the peak activity, appears earlier than in controls (*lower left*). Conversely, a phase delay (*in green*) results from a stimulus that causes the rhythm, again measured at the peak, to occur later than in controls (*lower right*). **(B)** The phase-response curve graphically relates the response to a stimulus with the time it was encountered (under constant conditions where the clock is free-running). This example plots the response in the suprachiasmatic nucleus neuronal firing rhythm to glutamate, the excitatory neurotransmitter of the optic nerve, or in wheel-running of rats to a pulse of light.[82] Notice that there is a temporal change in the sensitivity to light or glutamate. During subjective daytime under these constant conditions, the stimuli have no effect of phasing of the rhythm. Indeed, the circadian system is synchronized to the environment when it senses light during daytime. Within the nighttime domain, in grey, these stimuli can activate downstream signaling targets during restricted periods of sensitivity. This gating of sensitivity/responsiveness results in a phase delay in early subjective night (negative deflection) and a phase advance in late subjective night (positive deflection), respectively.

further study of PACAP's effects on the clock in the context of GLU signaling during the day is warranted.

A third daytime regulator of the clock, NPY, appears to play a dual role in the SCN, resetting the circadian clock both during the daytime and at night. NPY is released from the GHT, the projection from the IGL to the SCN. When NPY is applied during the daytime either to an SCN brain slice in vitro[106] or directly to the SCN in vivo,[171,172] it induces a phase advance. Additional in vivo studies stimulated the IGL, presumably inducing the release of NPY at the SCN. These stimulations also produced advances in wheel-running behavior during the daytime.[173] Interestingly, exposing an animal to light[174] and applying GLU to the brain slice[175] were both capable of blocking the response to daytime application of NPY. The addition of the $GABA_A$ antagonist bicuculline can inhibit the action of NPY,[176] suggesting that the effects of NPY are linked to GABAergic signaling.

A common feature of daytime signaling pathways is their ability to act via cAMP. In the hypothalamic brain slice, cAMP or cAMP analogues applied during the daytime induce phase-advances in the circadian clock, whereas at night they have little effect.[51,177] In addition, endogenous cAMP is high during late day and late night,[178] suggesting a role for cAMP in the transition periods between day and night. It can be hypothesized that by increasing cAMP, these daytime resetting signals are moving the animal to a state that resembles late day, thus resetting the clock to that time.

Dawn and Dusk

The primary resetting signal associated with dawn and dusk is melatonin. This "hormone of darkness" is produced at night in the absence of light, providing a means by which the animal can measure night-length. Photoperiod is an important measure for animals, such as hamster and sheep, that are seasonally reproductive. Melatonin is produced by the pineal gland, and in lower vertebrates, such as fish, lizards, and some birds, the pineal, rather than the SCN, is the primary regulator of circadian rhythms. However, in mammals this timekeeping mechanism has moved to the SCN, as demonstrated by the fact that removal of the pineal does not significantly disrupt circadian rhythms of rats.[179]

Although the pineal is not necessary for maintenance of mammalian circadian rhythms, it is possible to entrain free-running rats with daily injections of melatonin. Entrainment appears to work best if the melatonin injections are timed to occur shortly before the onset of the animal's active period. This entrainment appears to be working through the SCN, as

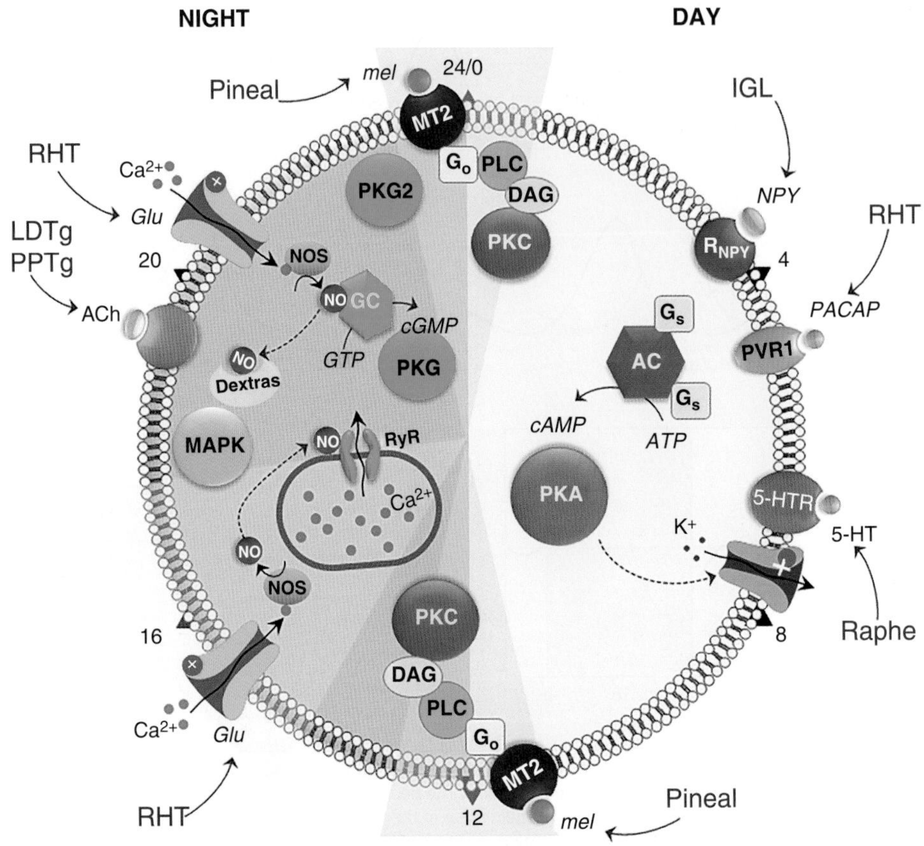

Figure 36.6 Temporally restricted sensitivity of the suprachiasmatic nucleus (SCN) to activation of discrete pathways with distinct effects on clock phasing. Schematic representation of the 24-hour circadian cycle comprising four major time domains (daytime, dawn/dusk, early night, and late night) with respect to temporal sensitivities of the SCN to various signaling pathways. The circadian clock controls the opening and closing of the windows of sensitivity to activation of these pathways so they are temporally relevant and thus convey a signal that is imbued with temporal information. AC, Adenylate cyclase; ACh, acetylcholine; cGMP, cyclic guanosine monophosphte; DAG, diacylglyceride; G_o, G-protein o; G_s, G-protein stimulating AC; GC, guanylate cyclase; GTP, guanosine 5′-triphosphate; 5-HT, 5-hydroxytryptamine/serotonin; IGL, intergeniculate leaflet of the thalamus; LDTg/PPTg, laterodorsal tegmentum and pediculopontine tegmentum of the brainstem; MAPK, mitogen-activated protein kinase; mel, melatonin; MT2, melatonin receptor type 2; NO, nitric oxide; NOS, nitric oxide synthase; NPY, neuropeptide Y; PKA, cAMP-dependent protein kinase; PKC, protein kinase C; PKG, cGMP-dependent protein kinase; PLC, phospholipase C; PVR1, PACAP/VIP receptor type 1; RHT, retinohypothalamic tract; RyR, ryanodine receptor.

lesioning the SCN, but not the pineal, abolishes the ability of a rat to entrain to melatonin injections.[180]

Evidence that melatonin can entrain circadian rhythms led to a number of studies looking at the direct effect of melatonin on the SCN. Melatonin application immediately before dusk in rat or hamster tissue in vitro decreases SCN metabolic or neuronal activity, measured by 2-deoxy-[1-^{14}C]glucose (2-DG) uptake or neuronal firing rate.[181-183] Additionally, melatonin applied to SCN brain slices at either dawn or dusk advances the peak in neuronal firing. Melatonin is ineffective when applied at other times of day.[184,185] This resetting pattern is reproduced by direct activation of protein kinase C (PKC) and can be blocked by inhibitors of PKC, suggesting that PKC is a downstream component of this resetting pathway.[185] In addition, phase-resetting effects of melatonin are inhibited by antagonists specific for the MT-2 type melatonin receptor.[186] In humans, circadian sensitivity to melatonin also occurs at dawn and dusk, but the effect is to advance the circadian system at dusk and to delay it at dawn, in antiphase to the effects of light at night.

Nighttime

In the nighttime domain, there are two known key neurotransmitters, GLU and acetylcholine (ACh), as well as a number of modulatory substances associated with these signals. As was discussed previously, considerable evidence supports GLU as the neurochemical signal transmitting photic stimuli from the retina to the SCN. Cholinergic innervation of the SCN comes from brainstem regions involved in sleep regulation and from the basal forebrain.[131,187,188]

The GLU signaling pathway is similar to many of the pathways that already have been discussed in that it resets the circadian clock at a discrete time of day and in a specific direction. The GLU signaling pathway can either advance or delay the clock, depending on what time of day the signal is presented.[82,189] The GLU resetting pathway has been demonstrated both in vitro and in vivo to be mediated through an

N-methyl-D-aspartate (NMDA) receptor–mediated rise in intracellular Ca^{2+}, followed by nitric oxide synthase activation and production of nitric oxide (NO).[82,190-193] Downstream, the early and late night pathways diverge. During the early night, GLU induces delays in the circadian clock through ryanodine receptor (RyR)-mediated Ca^{2+}-induced Ca^{2+}-release.[194] GLU exposure during the late night, however, advances the circadian clock through a cyclic guanosine monophosphate/protein kinase G (cGMP/PKG) signaling cascade followed by cAMP response element-binding (CREB) protein-activated transcription.[194-196]

Although GLU alone is capable of resetting circadian rhythms, there are many substances that modulate this resetting. These can be divided into two categories: those that decrease the amplitude of the phase-resetting effect of GLU during both the early and late night, which include NPY and GABA,[107,159] and those that have differing effects on GLU-induced phase shifts, depending on what time of night they are applied.

This second category of time-dependent modulators includes 5-HT and PACAP. If animals are depleted of 5-HT, they show increased phase delays in response to light.[197,198] Co-application of a PACAP antagonist, however, either in vitro or in vivo, decreases the phase delay in early night, and when applied during late night, increases the amplitude of the phase advance in both rat and hamster.[199,200] When PACAP is administered in conjunction with GLU in early night, it increases the amplitude of delay, but in late night it decreases the phase advance. This is similar to the effects seen after application of cAMP analogues to the hypothalamic brain slice, suggesting that the effects of PACAP may be mediated via a cAMP pathway.[200,201]

The role of ACh in resetting circadian rhythms has been unclear, with much of the confusion arising from the fact that its effects vary depending on the site of application. The first evidence that ACh may play a role in resetting the circadian clock was discovered when Zatz and Brownstein examined whether pharmacologic manipulation could affect circadian rhythms.[202] They found that injections of the ACh agonist carbachol into the lateral ventricle of Sprague-Dawley rats at CT 15 caused phase delays that were similar to, but not as large as, the phase delays produced by light.[202] Carbachol injections into the lateral ventricle were also later repeated in mice[203] and hamsters,[204] where it was found that administration of carbachol during early night caused phase delays, whereas late night administration caused phase advances.

This pattern of sensitivity and responses is similar to that previously demonstrated in response to light or GLU. Support for the involvement of ACh in the light response came from studies looking at ACh levels in the rat SCN using a radioimmunoassay.[205] Using this technique, no significant oscillation in ACh levels was found under constant conditions, but light pulses administered at CT 14 were found to increase ACh levels in the SCN. However, only one time-point was examined, so it is not known whether this increase was simply a response to exposure to light or if there was actually a circadian pattern to the light-stimulated release. The implication of these studies was that ACh could be the primary neurotransmitter providing the signal of light to the clock.

However, significant evidence began to emerge, indicating that ACh was unlikely to be the primary signal of light. First, whereas it had previously been determined that the RHT transmitted the signal of light from the eye to the SCN, it was found that choline acetyltransferase was not present in this projection.[206] This made it anatomically unlikely that ACh was the primary neurotransmitter involved in this signal.

Additional evidence against ACh being the signal of light came from experiments that found intracerebroventricular (*icv*) injections of hemicholinium, which significantly depletes ACh stores in the brain, did not block the ability of the animal to phase shift in response to light.[207] There was also evidence that injecting NMDA receptor antagonists could block carbachol-induced phase shifts, suggesting that although ACh may play a role in the light response, it must be upstream of a glutamatergic signal.[208] Finally, Liu and Gillette,[209] using extracellular recording in vitro, found that microdrop applications of carbachol directly to the SCN caused only phase advances, regardless of whether the carbachol was applied early or late in the night.

In an attempt to explain these contradicting data, it was hypothesized that the dual response pattern of the SCN to cholinergic stimulation was a result of the location of stimulation. Note that in the initial in vivo studies, carbachol was injected into the lateral or third ventricle, where the drug could have diffuse effects, while in the in vitro studies carbachol was applied in microdrops directly to the SCN. If the in vivo experiments were performed by injecting carbachol directly into the SCN rather than into the ventricle, a phase response pattern similar to that observed in the in vitro experiments using microdrop applications resulted.[187] This suggests that ACh has at least two different effects on the circadian clock, depending upon the site of application. There is an indirect response, working through ventricular pathways, that is likely an upstream of a glutamatergic signal, and a direct response in the SCN that is mediated by the M_1AChR.[210] Based on the anatomic studies tracing cholinergic projections to the SCN that originate in the LDTg and PPTg, the current hypothesis is that this cholinergic signal may be involved in linking sleep and wakefulness with circadian cycles.[124]

COUPLING OF CENTRAL AND PERIPHERAL CLOCKS

Because circadian clocks are fundamental components of cells, it follows that there are myriad individual oscillating clocks in the body. In an intact organism, these clocks are aligned so that each individual tissue maintains a stable phase relationship to the SCN so that clock genes are expressed at the same time each day. When the SCN is removed or the phase is shifted, cells of various tissues maintain their individual circadian rhythms, but they quickly fall out of phase with each other.[211-213] This indicates a hierarchic relationship in which the SCN is the master regulator that synchronizes and aligns the rest of the body's clocks. Many studies of the coupling of extra-SCN clocks to the central pacemaker have been undertaken; several examples are highlighted in the following discussion.

Early SCN-isolation studies established the SCN's role as the master clock necessary for orchestrating the rest of the body clocks. These studies also hint at the various means by which the SCN exerts control over peripheral structures. When the SCN is surgically isolated from the rest of the hypothalamus in rats, oscillations in serum corticosterone levels continue, while locomotor rhythms are lost.[214] Additionally, surgical cuts between the SCN and PVN abolish reproductive rhythms in hamsters, but rhythmic locomotor activity is maintained in hamsters[215,216] and rats.[217] These findings provided early evidence for both synaptic coupling of SCN to output tissues, as well as the possibility that humoral signals entrain peripheral tissues. This idea was furthered by transplantation studies in which an encapsulated fetal SCN is transplanted into an animal with SCN lesions.[18] Fenestrations in the encapsulating polymer were too small to permit neurite passage, and, indeed, no neural connectivity to the recipient brain could be found. The transplant restored locomotor, feeding, drinking, body temperature, and sleep-wake, but not endocrine, rhythms to the lesioned animal. Clearly, some non-SCN rhythms require physical connections and some do not.

Many brain regions are coupled to the SCN by synaptic connections. Anatomic studies have shown SCN projections that extend to several hypothalamic nuclei, including the organum vasculosum of lamina terminalis (OVLT), MPOA, and PVN, forming direct synapses with gonadotropin-releasing hormone and corticotropin-releasing hormone neurons in these regions.[218-220] Additionally, the neuronal networks connecting the SCN to the IGL and PVT of the thalamus mediate with bi-directional communication between the SCN and these sleep/arousal modulatory regions.[93,147,148]

The SCN is one of many regulators of sympathetic and parasympathetic autonomic signals to peripheral organs. Anatomic studies using retrograde tracers injected into peripheral organs, such as liver, adrenal gland, pancreas, and adipose tissue, reveal a multisynaptic pathway connecting these tissues to autonomic centers in the spinal cord, brainstem, PVN, DMH, SCN, and other hypothalamic regions.[221-224] Tracing of either sympathetic or parasympathetic tracts identifies SCN neurons in overlapping areas of the nucleus, however these neurons seem to be involved in signaling to one or the other of these pathways.[222,223] Light from the external environment can affect these two pathways through SCN-mediated control. For example, exposure of rats to light at night results in increased sympathetic activity and suppressed parasympathetic activity. When the SCN is abolished, this effect is lost.[225] Also, heart rate decreases after light exposure at night in a nocturnal rodent, whereas SCN-lesioned animals do not exhibit this response.[226] Thus the SCN plays a role in modulating autonomic signals to the periphery, but it works in concert with many other regions of the brain, including those regulating body temperature, metabolism, reproductive state, and other physiologic functions.

A growing body of evidence supports a role for humoral signaling in coupling of rhythms between the SCN and other regions. In brain-slice cultures containing PVN tissue, an electrical rhythm emerges in the PVN only after co-culture with an SCN brain slice. The lack of neuronal connections between the two slices in vitro strongly supports a diffusible factor as mediator of the electrical oscillation of the PVN.[227] Additionally, parabiosis experiments connecting the circulatory system of an intact mouse to that of an SCN-lesioned mouse indicate that diffusible signals from the intact animal can entrain peripheral organs (liver and kidney) in the lesioned recipient.[228] Co-culturing SCN tissue with peripheral cells or tissue induces rhythms in these cells that follow the SCN under culture conditions that prevent synaptic connections.[229-231]

These studies indicate that diffusible signals can modulate rhythms between the brain and body. Neuropeptides are abundant in the SCN[59] and are good candidates for humoral signals. As described previously, major neuropeptides found in the SCN include VIP, GRP, little SAAS, and AVP, among others. These peptides are released from the SCN in a circadian fashion,[58,65,71] and each has been implicated in a physiologic role in some aspect of circadian biology.[65,67,71,232-238] Identification of the diffusible signals that couple other tissues to the SCN is currently the subject of intense study, with high therapeutic potential.

Another role for diffusible factors from the SCN may be to provide a signal inhibitory to behavioral activity. Two candidate factors for communicating such signals include transforming growth factor-α (TGF-α) and prokineticin 2 (PK2). Under normal conditions, TGF-α peptide is expressed rhythmically in the SCN with a peak during the animal's inactive period, and a trough during the active period. When infused continuously into the cerebral ventricles, TGF-α fully inhibits locomotor activity. Conversely, mice lacking the cognate receptor, epidermal growth factor (EGF) receptor, are unable to respond to TGF-α and show an excessive amount of daytime activity.[239] PK2 also is expressed rhythmically in the SCN, again showing peak expression during the animal's inactive period, and can inhibit locomotor activity when infused continuously.[240] This suggests a role for output signals from the SCN in promoting an inactive state that would be permissive for sleep.

Some tissues appear to require both synaptic and humoral signals to synchronize to the SCN. When autonomic innervation to the liver is severed, plasma insulin and corticosterone levels remain rhythmic, but plasma glucose levels do not.[241] However, liver tissue from an SCN-lesioned mouse with surgical parabiosis with an intact animal recovers and continues to maintain rhythmicity from that point onward.[228] This suggests that control of liver timing requires both neural and diffusible signals that coordinate separate physiologic functions. Dissecting the intricacies of circadian regulation among peripheral tissues requires careful study.

Coupling of the SCN to peripheral targets, regardless of the manner of this connection, has important implications for health. This interaction allows for synchronization of internal systems to environmental light signals, both on a day-by-day basis and to adjust the animal to seasonal changes. Modern human activities, such as shift work and transcontinental flight, result in significant desynchronization of the central internal clock and various body tissues. This circadian disarray can have significant negative consequences for human health, including increased risks of various cancers, reproductive health, stroke, metabolic syndrome, cardiovascular disease,[242-244] and overall mortality in older individuals.[245]

HEALTH AND DISEASE

Disturbance of the circadian timing system is linked to adverse health effects associated with a loss of synchronization between central and peripheral oscillations. Estimates suggest 10% to 20% of the entire genome displays rhythmic expression in any given tissue or organ,[246,247] and this provides a link to the circadian system to health and disease.[248] A number of core clock elements play critical roles in human sleep disorders. For example, inherited forms of advanced sleep-wake phase disorder are associated with a mutation in the *Per2* gene that alters a normal phosphorylation site of CKIδ/ε[249] or with a mutation in CKIδ.[250] Delayed sleep-wake phase disorder, which is prevalent in almost 10% of the population,[251,252] has been found to be associated with specific polymorphisms of PER3,[32,253,254] CRY1,[255] and a missense variant of PER2.[256] PER3 expression patterns in human leukocytes correlate with sleep-wake timing, particularly in those individuals with a preference for morningness.[257] Further, morningness or eveningness preferences have been associated with polymorphisms of the human *Clock* gene.[32,258,259]

A number of clock gene mutations in rodents have demonstrated adverse physiologic effects. *Clock*$^{\Delta 19}$ mice are moderately more susceptible to cancer and display a marked metabolic phenotype involving obesity, dyslipidemia, hepatic steatosis, and hyperglycemia.[260,261] Interestingly, the *Clock*$^{-/-}$ mice (mice deficient in the *Clock* gene because of targeted gene knockout) do not exhibit the same phenotype as the mice with a partial deletion, *Clock*$^{\Delta 19}$. *Clock*$^{-/-}$ mice have a reduced life span, age-related cataract development, and increased risk for dermatitis.[41,42,262] Differences between *Clock*$^{\Delta 19}$ and *Clock*$^{-/-}$ mouse models likely arise from the fact that the *Clock*$^{\Delta 19}$ mice have a dominant negative mutation in CLOCK, whereas *Clock*$^{-/-}$ are deficient of CLOCK altogether and may experience compensation from upregulation of NPAS2.

Humans often voluntarily override signals from their circadian clock and disconnect their sleep-wake and feeding cycles from their external environment. Under such circumstances, irregular phase relationships are expressed between rhythmic process (such as sleep-wake behaviors and feeding-fasting states) and the circadian clock. Although the internal desynchronizes that occur with jet lag and shift work may be the most dramatic, they are not the only examples of real-world circadian disruption. Widespread occurrence of social jet lag resulting from social overstimulation, work schedules, and the use of artificial lighting may occur in people living under relatively stable entrained conditions. Indeed, many phase-shift their sleep and feeding times they when return to the workdays after free-running according to their clock-time during weekends and holidays.[263] In sum, our around-the-clock society and our interaction with it tend to oppose human evolutionary selection toward diurnality, often with negative health consequences.

CONCLUSION

Circadian rhythms, the near–24-hour oscillations in brain and body functions such as core body temperature, hormone release, and the sleep-wake cycle are embedded in the physiology of cells and tissues. The master pacemaker regulating these rhythms, the SCN, is optimally situated in the hypothalamus to receive input about environmental light, sleep-wake state, and activity status. The SCN alters its phasing in response to changes in environmental conditions and internal states. This change in SCN state, in turn, alters the timing of output signals that regulate the timing of rest/activity and behavioral cycles.

The core mechanisms of timekeeping are encoded in transcription/translation feedback loops of evolutionarily conserved clock genes. The molecular clockwork comprises both positive and negative elements, coupled with other intracellular elements associated with signaling events. Proteins encoded by clock genes are targets of molecular tools to further study clocks in diverse tissues and to treat desynchronized conditions.[264] They are revealing how the SCN synchronizes these various body clocks to environmental cycles and imposed work schedules, and what changes with disease. Circadian-rhythm sleep phenotypes as well as sleep disorders correlate with abnormalities in the genes regulating circadian rhythms. Why internal desynchrony of peripheral tissues with the SCN has negative consequences for human health and longevity remains unknown. New research is necessary for discovering therapeutic mechanisms for timing disorders of the SCN and peripheral clocks as well as treatments that resynchronize the molecular clockworks in health and disease.

CLINICAL PEARL

Circadian rhythms emerge from molecular clockworks that bear the tremendous genetic diversity of the human family and are present throughout the human body. This genetic diversity, as well as contemporary lifestyles, can lead to circadian dysregulation that initiates or exacerbates chronic and acute disease. Dysregulation of the circadian system is linked to increased risk of metabolic, cardiovascular, immunologic, and neurologic disorders, and, notably, disruption of sleep-wake cycles. Light occurring at inappropriate times during the dark phase of the circadian cycle as well as alteration in neurotransmitters and small-molecule profiles can alter sleep-wake patterns, leading to decrements in overall health. Coordination of circadian rhythms, both internally and with respect to the environment or disease state, is necessary for robust health and longevity.

SUMMARY

The SCN of the hypothalamus is the master pacemaker for the mammalian circadian system. The many coupled cellular oscillators within the SCN generate rhythmicity through dynamic, cell-based, transcriptional/translational feedback loops. These molecular feedback loops are formed of positive and negative transcriptional elements that regulate the clock genes that encode them. The activity of the core molecular loop interacting with cellular redox state generates circadian rhythms in SCN electrical activity and neurotransmitter and neuropeptide release, resulting in the transmission of circadian timing signals to downstream oscillators throughout the brain and body. The circadian pacemaker is entrained by environmental light-dark cycles as well as other rhythmic stimuli by restricting its own sensitivity to various entraining signals to discrete temporal windows throughout the circadian cycle. The circadian system regulates the timing of sleep and wakefulness, and disorders can arise within this system. Good health, well-being, and longevity depend on robust internal synchronization both within and between tissues throughout the brain and the body.

ACKNOWLEDGMENTS

The authors recognize present and past support from the National Institutes of Health: National Heart, Lung, and Blood Institute (HL67007, HL86870, HL92571, HL159948), National Institute of Neurological Diseases and Stroke (NS22155, NS35859), National Institute of Mental Health (MH85220, MH101655, MH109062, and MH 117377), and National Institute of Drug Abuse (P30 DA018310), from the National Science Foundation (CHE 0526692, IOS 0818555, IOS CBET-0939511, IOS 1354913, DGE 1735252), the Air Force Office of Scientific Research (NL-0205), and the University of Illinois Research Board.

SELECTED READINGS

Abbott SM, Zee PC. Circadian Rhythms: Implications for Health and Disease. *Neurol Clin*. 2019;37:601–613.

Antle MC, Silver R. Orchestrating time: arrangements of the brain circadian clock. *Trends Neurosci*. 2005;28:145–251.

Colwell CS. Linking neural activity and molecular oscillations in the SCN. *Nat Rev Neurosci*. 2010;12:553–569.

Ding JM, Chen D, Weber ET, et al. Resetting the biological clock: mediation of nocturnal circadian shifts by glutamate and NO. *Science*. 1994;266:1713–1717.

Gandhi AV, Mosser EA, Oikonomou G, Prober DA. Melatonin is required for the circadian regulation of sleep. *Neuron*. 2015;85:1193–1199.

Golombek DA, Rosenstein RE. Physiology of circadian entrainment. *Physiol Rev*. 2010;90:1063–1102.

Iyer R, Wang TA, Gillette MU. Circadian gating of neuronal functionality: a basis for iterative metaplasticity. In, 'Sleep and Circadian Rhythms in Plasticity and Memory,' edited by J Gerstner, HC Heller, S Aton. *Front Syst Neurosci*. 2014;8:164:34.

Ko CH, Takahashi JS. Molecular components of the mammalian circadian clock. *Hum Mol Genet*. 2006;15:R271–R277.

Morin LP. Neuroanatomy of the extended circadian rhythm system. *Exp Neurol*. 2013;243:4–20.

Silver R, LeSauter J, Tresco PA, Lehman MN. A diffusible coupling signal from the transplanted suprachiasmatic nucleus controlling circadian locomotor rhythms. *Nature*. 1996;382:810–813.

Wang TA, Yu YV, Govindaiah G, et al. Circadian rhythm of redox state regulates excitability in suprachiasmatic nucleus neurons. *Science*. 2012;337:839–842.

Welsh DK, Takahashi JS, Kay SA. Suprachiasmatic nucleus: cell autonomy and network properties. *Annu Rev Physiol*. 2010;72:551–577.

A complete reference list can be found online at ExpertConsult.com.

Chapter 37

Human Circadian Timing System and Sleep-Wake Regulation

Charles A. Czeisler; Orfeu M. Buxton

Chapter Highlights

- The circadian pacemaker (or biologic clock) confers endogenous rhythmicity with a period just slightly greater than 24 hours, persists in the absence of periodic changes in the external environment, and has timing or phase relative to the time of day that is genetically determined and influenced by environmental synchronizers.
- Under appropriate conditions, melatonin, body temperature, and many other physiologic processes can be used to assess circadian phase or biologic clock time.
- Although environmental light-dark schedules are the primary circadian synchronizer, other nonphotic stimuli such as exercise can shift circadian phase.
- The circadian pacemaker interacts with sleep-wake regulatory processes to influence many physiologic variables: hormone levels, autonomic nervous system activity, neurobehavioral performance, and the propensity for and timing and internal structure of sleep. Environmental, social, behavioral, and genetic factors; pharmacologic agents; and age influence most elements of this system.
- This chapter emphasizes, for the benefit of the student and the practitioner, the complexity of interactions of the circadian pacemaker and the sleep homeostat in regulating physiology, with important implications for health, performance, and clinical practice.

Circadian oscillations (or biologic clocks) are phylogenetically ubiquitous, found in species from prokaryotes to humans. Circadian clocks have several defining characteristics: endogenous rhythmicity that persists independent of periodic changes in the external environment, a near-24–hour period (*circadian* from Latin *circa* meaning "about" and *dies* meaning "day"), and the capacity for environmental input to modify or reset the timing or phase of the rhythm.[1,2] We provide an overview of the human circadian timing system and describe how this system interacts with sleep-wake regulatory processes to influence physiologic variables, including hormone levels, autonomic nervous system activity, neurobehavioral performance, and the propensity for, timing, and internal structure of sleep. We consider the influence of episodic and daily recurring behaviors, including sleep itself, on these physiologic variables relative to that of the endogenous circadian pacemaker.

IDENTIFYING THE MAMMALIAN CIRCADIAN PACEMAKER

In mammals, the suprachiasmatic nucleus (SCN) in the anterior hypothalamus is the central neural pacemaker of the circadian timing system. On the basis of careful patient histories characterized by disruptions of sleep-wake timing (e.g., insomnia, reversal of the sleep-wake schedule), Fulton and Bailey[3] postulated in 1929 that a region in the anterior hypothalamus appeared to regulate not the occurrence of sleep but its timing within the 24-hour day. In 1972 the SCN was identified as the site of the mammalian circadian pacemaker.[4,5] Physiologic studies show that multiple distributed circadian oscillators drive daily rhythms in peripheral systems.[6] Molecular research confirms the presence of peripheral clocks that use the same molecular machinery as the central circadian pacemaker in the SCN. Pacemakers like the SCN convey internal synchrony to these distributed oscillators.

INFLUENCE OF SLEEP AND CIRCADIAN RHYTHMS ON HUMAN PHYSIOLOGY

The discovery of the SCN's role as a central circadian pacemaker set the stage for understanding how it drives prominent circadian rhythms in a wide array of physiologic functions in humans synchronized to the 24-hour day and on a normal sleep-wake schedule (Figure 37.1, *left column of panels*).[7] Core body temperature is lowest and melatonin levels (not shown) are highest[8] during night sleep. Cortisol is low at habitual sleep onset but high at habitual morning wake time. When these endogenous circadian rhythms are entrained or synchronized to the 24-hour day, the temporal profile of each of these parameters exhibits a characteristic fingerprint that results from a combination of drives, from the timing of the sleep-wake state to the endogenous circadian pacemaker, and responses evoked by other factors such as posture, mood, exercise, and environmental lighting.[8]

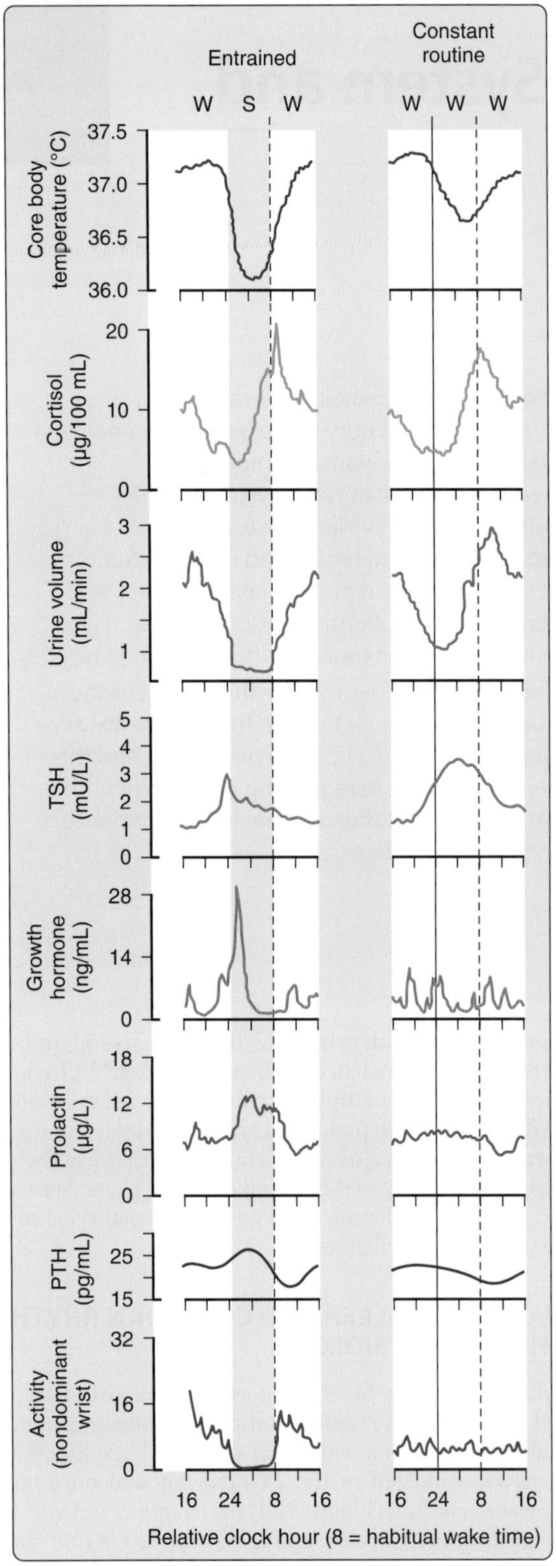

Figure 37.1 Comparison of temporal profiles of an array of physiologic and behavioral variables from participants studied under baseline conditions while maintaining a regular schedule of nocturnal sleep (S) (*yellow shaded area*) and daytime wake (W) at their habitual times (*left column of panels*) compared with profiles from participants under constant-routine conditions while maintaining a schedule of continuous wake in a semirecumbent posture (*right column of panels*). The *vertical dashed line* indicates habitual wake-up time during the week before the study, when participants were required to maintain a regular sleep-wake schedule. All data are from normal young men, 18 to 30 years old, studied under similar conditions. For a given variable, data in the *left panel* are from the same participants as data in the *right panel*; however, not all variables were monitored in the same participants. PTH, Parathyroid hormone; TSH, thyroid-stimulating hormone. (TSH data reproduced with permission from Allan JS, Czeisler CA. Persistence of the circadian thyrotropin rhythm under constant conditions and after light-induced shifts of circadian phase. *J Clin Endocrinol Metab.* 1994;79:508–12, copyright The Endocrine Society. Prolactin data reproduced with permission from Waldstreicher J, Duffy JF, Brown EN, et al. Gender differences in the temporal organization of prolactin [PRL] secretion: evidence for a sleep-independent circadian rhythm of circulating PRL levels—a Clinical Research Center study. *J Clin Endocrinol Metab.* 1996;81:1483–7, copyright The Endocrine Society. PTH data reproduced with permission from El Hajj Fuleihan G, Klerman EB, Brown EN, et al. Parathyroid hormone circadian rhythm is truly endogenous. *J Clin Endocrinol Metab.* 1997;82:281–6, copyright The Endocrine Society.)

To characterize the circadian pacemaker–driven component of a diurnal temporal profile from the effects of sleep-wake state, behavior, posture, and periodic environmental stimuli, the constant-routine protocol originally proposed by Mills and colleagues has been extended[9]; participants typically undergo continuous enforced wakefulness throughout day and night in a constant posture at a constant level of minimal physical activity and in constant, relatively dim, ambient illumination.[10] Under such conditions, the temporal profiles of many physiologic variables are significantly altered, and the components of these rhythms that are driven by the endogenous circadian pacemaker can be separated from those that reflect changes in the sleep-wake state, posture, or periodic external environment. Given the influence of posture[11] and the minimal influence of sleep[12] on the endogenous circadian melatonin rhythm, we have sometimes used a constant posture protocol in which participants are maintained in a constant semirecumbent posture, in constant dim light, but are allowed to sleep at night so that endogenous circadian melatonin phase can be assessed.

Body temperature declines during sleep,[13-15] as illustrated by the profile of core body temperature recorded during a normal sleep-wake schedule and on a constant routine (Figure 37.1, *right column of panels*). Sleep and changes in posture, light intensity, and activity level generate a drop in body temperature relative to wake.[6,15-19] This sleep episode–induced drop in body temperature combines with the circadian-driven decline in body temperature during the biologic night to yield a larger apparent amplitude than that of the endogenous circadian component alone (as measured on constant routine). Urine volume exhibits a robust oscillation under constant-routine conditions that is also influenced by sleep-wake state.[20]

Rhythmicity in some variables appears nearly independent of sleep-wake state. The temporal pattern of the hormone melatonin is relatively unchanged whether a participant is asleep or awake all night on a constant routine, although significant age-dependent effects of sleep and sleep deprivation on melatonin amplitude have been quantified.[12] Posture is reported to somewhat influence circulating melatonin concentrations.[11] Because the endogenous circadian cortisol rhythm is usually at its nadir at the time of habitual sleep onset, the overall profile of cortisol is relatively unchanged whether a person sleeps on a habitual schedule or remains awake all night, although cortisol levels will be elevated if the person continues to remain awake throughout the following afternoon and evening.[21] However, suppression of plasma cortisol concentrations by deep slow wave sleep is evident whenever sleep onset occurs at the crest of the cortisol rhythm rather than at the nadir.[22]

Several other hormones are sensitive to the sleep-wake state. Sleep opposes the circadian rhythm–regulating thyroid-stimulating hormone (TSH), inhibiting TSH release during the peak of the endogenous circadian TSH rhythm, which would otherwise occur in the middle of the night.[23-25] Under entrained conditions, nocturnal TSH secretion is blunted by the timing of sleep, such that TSH levels are highest just before sleep onset and continue to be suppressed during the remainder of the sleep episode. This inhibitory effect of sleep on TSH secretion has been closely associated with slow wave sleep[26] and with relative delta power in the sleep electroencephalogram (EEG).[27] Growth hormone, prolactin, and parathyroid hormone levels demonstrate a prominent sleep-dependent increase.[25] For growth hormone, a major sleep-related secretory episode is associated with slow wave sleep[28] and with relative delta power of the sleep EEG,[29] although such associations for prolactin, which remains elevated throughout the sleep episode, are controversial.[30] Interestingly, growth hormone levels blunted by acute sleep deprivation at night are increased during wakefulness the following day in sleep-deprived participants, compensating for the blunting of the major sleep-related pulse, such that average 24-hour levels are similar.[31] After restricting sleep to 4 hours per night from 1:00 to 5:00 a.m. for 1 week, growth hormone levels were maintained by the combination of a presleep, circadian-related secretory episode, together with a somewhat diminished sleep-related response.[32]

Leptin levels exhibit circadian rhythmicity, although the typical day-night pattern is reflected in the interaction of circadian rhythmicity with energy intake and expenditure[33] and sleep duration.[34] Ghrelin levels exhibit a day-night variation related to energy intake, related to the presence of sleep[35] and to sleep duration.[36]

Ultradian variations in the release of renin from the kidney—a key factor in blood pressure control—are closely linked to the timing of the rapid eye movement (REM) and non–rapid eye movement (NREM) sleep cycle,[37] an association evident even among patients with disturbed sleep, whose plasma renin profiles reflect pathologic changes in sleep structure. Increased relative delta power in the sleep EEG is associated with increased levels of plasma renin activity, whereas decreased slow wave activity is associated with a decrease.[38]

Even in the absence of sleep, prolactin and parathyroid hormone also have an endogenous circadian component that is lowest a few hours after habitual wake-up time,[25] and GH responses to exogenous growth hormone–releasing hormone exhibit a circadian rhythm.[39]

Effects of the interaction between sleep-dependent and circadian factors on these hormones can be important when the sleep-wake schedule is not synchronized with the circadian pacemaker. Shift workers who remain awake throughout the first night shift, for example, will secrete more TSH compared with that released at night under normal sleep-wake conditions during entrainment, because of the absence of sleep-related suppression of TSH during the nocturnal peak of endogenous TSH secretory drive (Figure 37.1); such increased secretion is not reversed during subsequent daytime sleep because the endogenous circadian rhythm of TSH secretion is already very low at that time. On the other hand, these workers would be deprived of their normally higher levels of growth hormone, prolactin, and parathyroid hormone during the waking night, although the sleep-related release of these hormones will recur during subsequent daytime sleep. Such alterations of the profiles of a variety of hormones have been documented in laboratory studies of night-shift workers.[40] In a laboratory simulation of circadian misalignment, participants exhibited increased leptin and increased glucose (despite increased insulin) and misalignment of the endogenous circadian rhythm of cortisol secretion with respect to the inverted sleep-wake schedule, along with the expected reduction in sleep efficiency.[41]

The circadian pacemaker significantly influences a variety of neurobehavioral and cognitive functions.[42-45] Under the conditions of the constant routine, participants display a circadian variation in short-term memory, cognitive performance, and alertness that is tightly coupled to the timing of the body temperature rhythm (Figure 37.2).[46] During a constant routine, these cognitive functions tend to be at their nadir shortly after habitual wake-up time because of an interaction between sleep loss and the circadian rhythms of performance.

Effects of Light on Human Circadian Rhythms

The light-dark cycle is the primary environmental signal that synchronizes circadian systems in a wide array of species, including humans.[7,47] Nonvisual or non–image-forming retinal photoreception provides input to the circadian system, the pupillary light reflex, and other systems. Direct retinal input travels through the retinohypothalamic tract, a monosynaptic pathway by which information about the environmental light-dark cycle reaches the SCN. Postmortem studies reveal that the human brain contains the same key structural elements—the SCN and retinohypothalamic tract—as that of other mammals.[48] Neuropathologic studies associate damage to these structures with abnormalities in the timing of the sleep-wake cycle and other circadian rhythms.[49-51]

Studies in rodents and humans have shown that the three-cone system and rods, the visual photoreceptors, are not required for transmitting light signals to the circadian system.[7] A distinct set of ganglion cells in the inner retinal layer that project to the SCN are intrinsically photosensitive. Only the ganglion cells that project from retina to SCN selectively contain the vitamin A–based photopigment melanopsin.[52] Blue and short-wavelength green light (about 450 to 500 nm), which matches the sensitivity peak of melanopsin, is the most potent in shifting circadian phase in animals[53,54] and for melatonin suppression and phase-shifting responses in humans.[55] Both daytime and nighttime retinal exposure to such monochromatic blue (460 nm) light significantly improves reaction time, reduces attentional failures, and improves EEG correlates of alertness.[56] The magnitude and duration of the alerting effect of light at night depends on illuminance history and appears to be subject to sensitization and adaptation. The alerting response to light is greater and lasts longer when the light exposure occurred after prior exposure to dim light (1 lux) compared with ordinary indoor light (90 lux).[57] Within this specific set of intrinsically photosensitive retinal ganglion cells, melanopsin is the active photopigment. Rods and cones that synapse onto melanopsin-containing ganglion cells also participate, creating redundancy in circadian photoreception.[58]

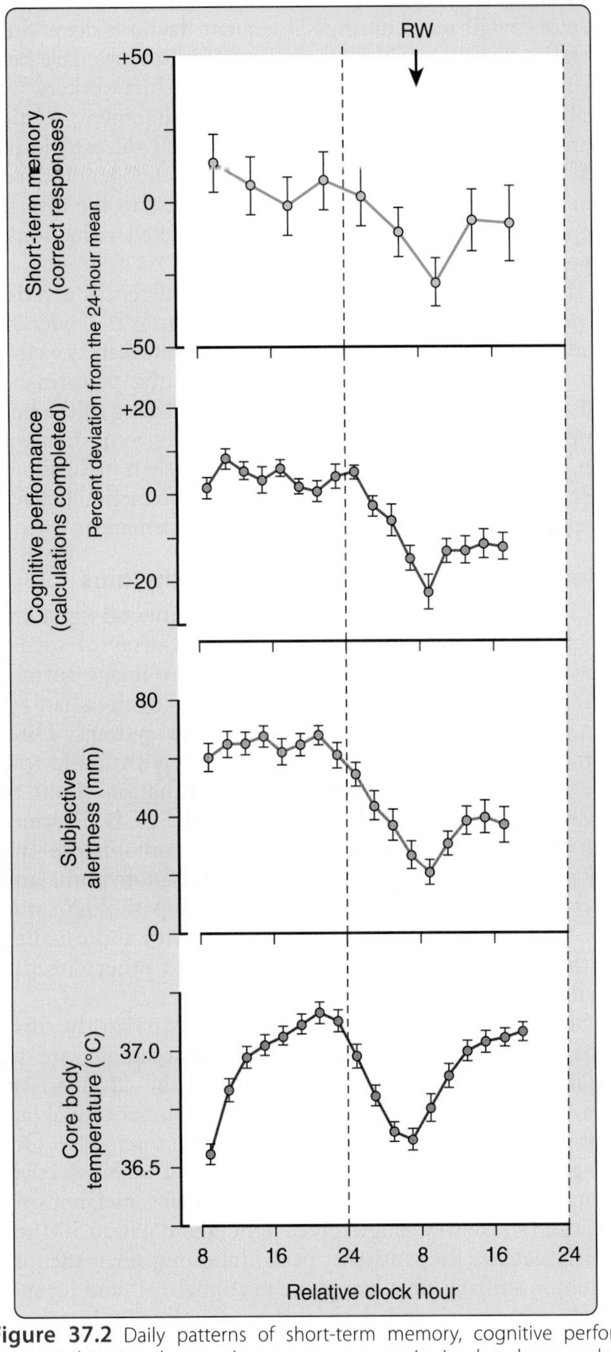

Figure 37.2 Daily patterns of short-term memory, cognitive performance, subjective alertness (mm on a non-numeric visual analogue scale), and core body temperature (°C) averaged across 18 participants during a 36-hour constant routine. Data collection times are normalized with respect to each participant's regular wake-up time (RW) (assigned a reference value of 8:00 a.m. and indicated by the *downward arrow*). The extent to which memory and performance scores deviated from the participant's 24-hour mean is averaged across participants. Data are expressed as percentages by which these absolute deviations differed from the participants' overall 24-hour mean score (assigned a reference value of zero). Each point is the centered mean (± SEM) of all determinations made across a 2-hour interval for performance, alertness, and temperature and across a 4-hour interval for short-term memory. (Reproduced with permission from Johnson MP, Duffy JF, Dijk D-J, et al. Short-term memory, alertness and performance: a reappraisal of their relationship to body temperature. *J Sleep Res.* 1992;1:24–9.)

Photic Suppression of Melatonin Secretion

A neural output pathway of the SCN passes through the intermediolateral cell column of the upper thoracic spinal cord to the superior cervical ganglion that provides sympathetic input into the pineal gland. The absence of melatonin secretion in patients who have cervical spinal cord injury is due to disruptions of this neural pathway to the pineal gland[59] and is associated with decreased sleep efficiency.[60] The neural pathway from the SCN to the pineal provides for the regulation of the pineal output of melatonin by the SCN, including inhibition of melatonin release by retinal light exposure through a retinohypothalamic pathway[61] that can be used as an assay for the functional input of light into the circadian system.[62,63]

Preservation of light-induced melatonin suppression in otherwise totally blind people suffering from severe damage to the outer retina[63,64] led to the discovery that a distinct visual system mediates photic entrainment.[65,66] The nocturnal increase in melatonin is illustrated in Figure 37.3 (*upper panel*) for a normally sighted participant on a constant routine.[63] During a second peak of melatonin in the next night, a bright light stimulus induced an acute suppression of melatonin levels, which returned to elevated nighttime levels after light exposure was terminated. In the lower panel, bright light still suppresses melatonin even in a totally blind participant with no conscious light perception and a negative electroretinogram. The loss of conscious light perception does not necessarily indicate the loss of photic input to the circadian timing system,[63] although that is the case in most blind individuals without light perception. Two distinct visual systems exist: one for visual perception and a separate non–image-forming visual system. The non–image-forming system synchronizes the circadian pacemaker in the SCN, provides alerting input to the sleep switch in the ventrolateral preoptic area, suppresses melatonin secretion, and mediates of the pupillary light reflex.[52,67] Even in blind individuals, non–image-forming photoreception through intrinsically photosensitive retinal ganglion cells can trigger some awareness for light, which stimulates higher cognitive brain activity, independent of vision and in the absence of functional impact from the rods and cones; also, it can engage supplemental brain areas to perform an ongoing cognitive process.[51,68]

In natural-light–only conditions, the internal circadian clock is synchronized to solar time with melatonin onset near sunset and melatonin offset before wake time and after sunrise, at a significantly earlier circadian phase.[69] In contrast, evening reading from an electronic tablet that emits short-wavelength–enriched visible light delays endogenous circadian melatonin phase and the timing of REM sleep and increases evening alertness, sleep latency, and morning sleepiness compared with reading a printed book.[70] Taken together, these findings suggest that artificial light between dusk and dawn alters physiology through the non–image-forming visual system by shifting circadian phase, inhibiting sleep-promoting neurons, activating arousal-promoting orexin neurons in the hypothalamus, and suppressing melatonin. These effects of nocturnal artificial light in turn mask sleepiness, transiently increase alertness, and directly interfere with sleep, leading to chronic sleep deficiency.[71]

Human Phase-Response Curves to Light

In circadian biology, the phase-response curve (PRC) is used to characterize the synchronizing effects of light on a circadian pacemaker.[1,10,72,73] To construct a photic PRC, discrete light

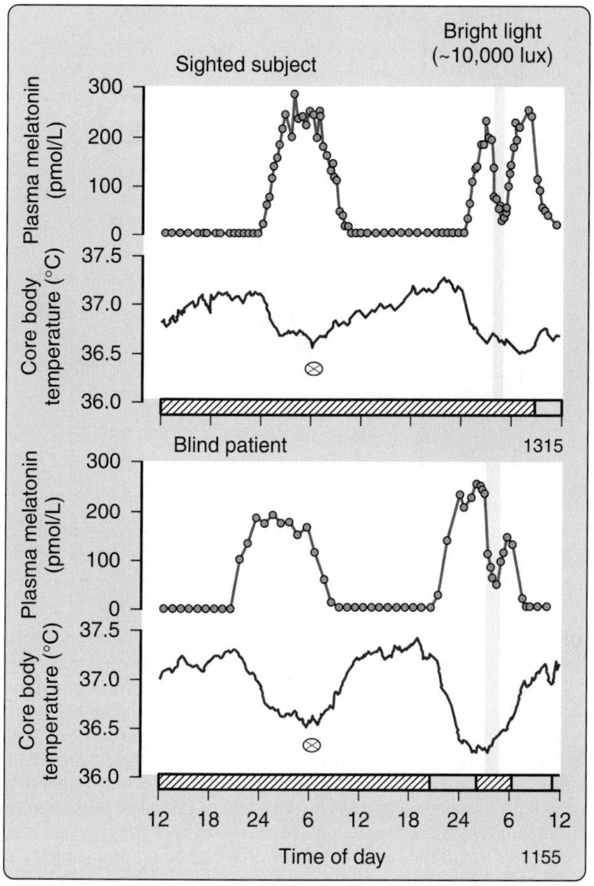

Figure 37.3 Melatonin-suppression test in a healthy sighted participant (*upper panel*) and a blind participant (*lower panel*). In each, plasma melatonin (*upper green traces*) and temperature (*lower red traces*) were measured repeatedly during a constant routine (*hatched bar*) and subsequent episode(s) of sleep (*solid blue bars*). The light intensity was approximately 10 to 15 lux during the constant routines, less than approximately 0.02 lux during the sleep episodes, and approximately 10,000 lux during 90 to 100 minutes of exposure to bright light (*open columns*) 22 to 23 hours after the initial fitted temperature minimum (*encircled Xs*). In both participants plasma melatonin concentrations decreased markedly in response to bright light and increased after the return to dim light. (Reproduced with permission from Czeisler CA, Shanahan TL, Klerman EB, et al. Suppression of melatonin secretion in some blind patients by exposure to bright light. *N Engl J Med.* 1995;332:6–11.)

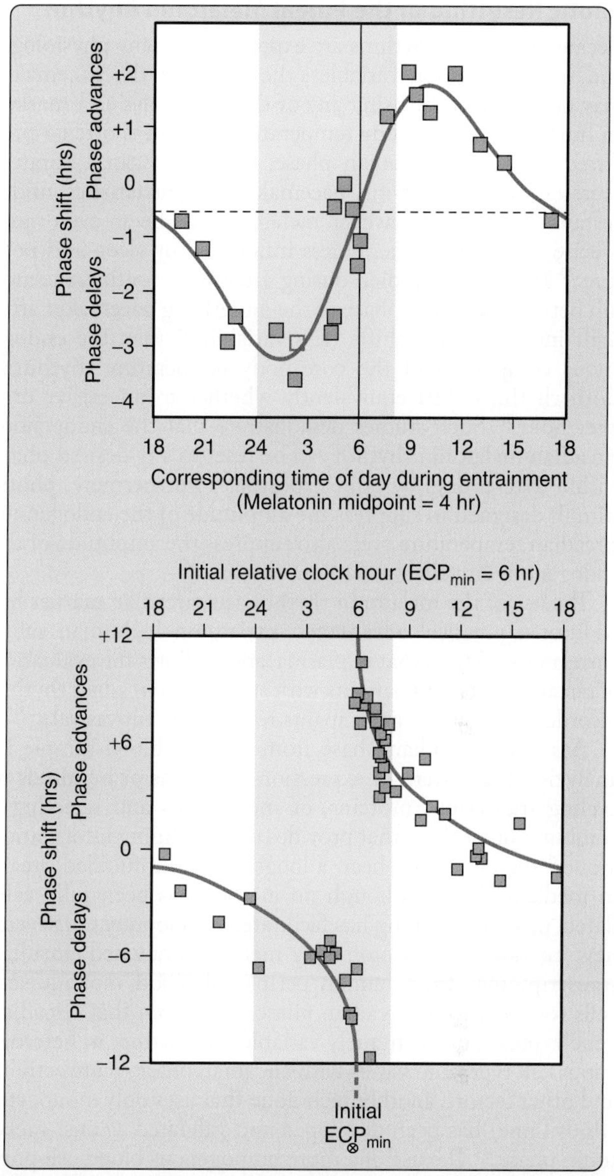

Figure 37.4 Circadian phase-dependent resetting of the human circadian system in response to light. A 1-pulse phase response curve to single 6.7-hour light pulses (top panel) and 3-pulse phase response curve to light (bottom panel) and in human participants. Phase shift in hours is plotted for a light pulse centered at different times relative to the initial endogenous circadian phase of the timing of melatonin secretion (top panel) or core body temperature (bottom panel). By convention, phase advances to an earlier time are depicted as positive numbers, and phase delays as negative numbers. (Reproduced with permission from Khalsa SB, Jewett ME, Cajochen C, Czeisler CA. A phase response curve to single bright light pulses in human subjects. *J Physiol* 2003;549:945–52. Reproduced with permission Czeisler et al., *Science* 1989.)

stimuli are applied systematically over the entire circadian cycle, and the magnitudes of light-induced phase shifts are plotted as a function of circadian phase at which the organism is exposed to the stimuli. In humans, measurement of the phase of endogenous circadian rhythms on a constant routine has been used to estimate both the initial circadian phase of the pacemaker before a stimulus and the final circadian phase after a stimulus, with the difference representing the phase shift.

All circadian systems exhibit a characteristic photic PRC, in which the largest light-induced phase shifts are generated in the biologic night. Phase delays are generated in response to light stimuli late in the biologic day and early in the biologic night, and phase advances are generated from stimuli in the late biologic night and early biologic day.[1] Figure 37.4 illustrates the PRC to a single pulse of light in humans. In humans, phase delays were observed in response to single, 1-hour and 6.7-hour bright light pulses applied before the minimum of the core body temperature cycle, which occurs on average about 2.3 hours before habitual wake-up time. Phase advances were observed when such light pulses were applied after the core body temperature nadir. The resultant human PRCs to single light pulses[74,75] exhibit the classic patterns of light PRCs in many organisms,[1,73] including phase advances and delays, and suggest that appropriate light intensities can shift the phase of the human pacemaker in morning and late afternoon or evening as well as at night. This has important clinical implications, such as use of phototherapy to reset circadian phase in delayed or advanced sleep-wake phase disorder.

Photic Resetting of the Pineal Melatonin Rhythm

Because circadian rhythms are expressed in many physiologic and neurobehavioral variables, the phase of the pacemaker may be estimated by using any of these variables as a marker. In humans, the core body temperature rhythm is often a preferred marker of circadian phase, because it can accurately represent the underlying pacemaker's characteristics under certain conditions. However, melatonin can be an even more precise circadian marker,[76] less influenced by sleep and posture.[77] In humans studied during a constant routine, melatonin better reflects the phase of the underlying pacemaker after light-induced phase shifts (less variability) than the endogenous component of the core body temperature rhythm.[77] Both rhythms shift equivalently whether to an earlier or a later hour.[76] Such studies demonstrate that the endogenous circadian melatonin rhythm can be reset to any desired phase within 2 to 3 days by light exposure.[76] Furthermore, photic stimuli designed to suppress the amplitude of the endogenous circadian temperature cycle also suppress the amplitude of the endogenous circadian melatonin rhythm.[76]

The use of the melatonin rhythm as a circadian marker has additional practical advantages: melatonin in human saliva correlates well with that in plasma, and it allows the evaluation of circadian phase in patients with suspected circadian rhythm disorders or research participants relatively noninvasively.[78]

Assessing circadian phase from a single blood sample by analyzing the pattern of expression of dozens or hundreds of cycling transcripts, proteins, or metabolites and selecting a combination of them that provides unique timing information around the clock "has been a longstanding unfulfilled dream in medicine."[79-81] Although no method has been fully validated, machine learning has facilitated development of several new methods.[82] Two promising methods evaluated circadian transcriptomes from human peripheral blood mononuclear cells for estimating circadian phase.[83,84] Given that circadian gene expression is extremely variable and distinct in heterogenous cell types and varies with circadian phase, acute activity, and other factors, another technique that uses only monocytes (BodyTime) has been developed and validated against melatonin phase.[85] The use of a more homogenous blood cell population with a high-amplitude circadian clock may be more robust in the face of acute activity and other factors.[85] Future work is needed to expand the accuracy of the measurement of circadian phase in near real-time in a variety of patient populations and real-world contexts.

Human Dose-Response Curve to Circadian Phase-Resetting Effects of Light

In addition to dependence on wavelength and circadian phase, the degree of light-induced phase shift also depends on light stimulus intensity and consecutive days of exposure. Three consecutive daily pulses of light can generate a larger phase shift than a single light pulse. This intensity relationship also applies to brightness or illuminance level of light to which the retina is exposed. After a 6.5-hour, single bright light stimulus of different intensities, at a circadian phase known to generate a phase delay, an increase in resetting response is seen at 50 lux, with maximal slope at 100 lux and maximal shifts by about 550 lux (Figure 37.5).

The observation that ordinary room lighting of about 100 lux with only 1% of the intensity induces 50% of the resetting response to a 10,000 lux stimulus has important implications.

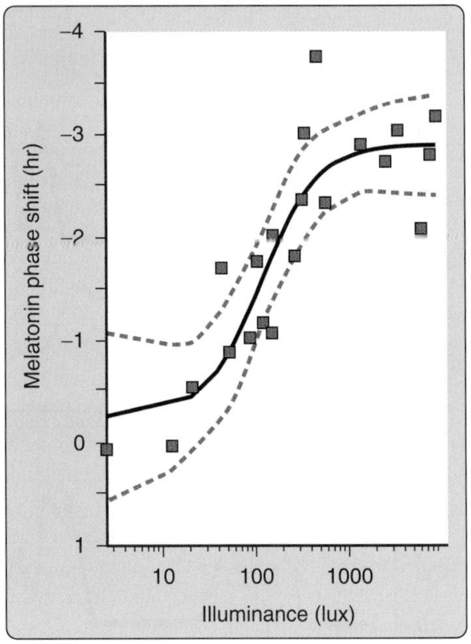

Figure 37.5 Illuminance-response curve of the phase-shifting effect of light on the human circadian pacemaker. Shifts in phase of the melatonin rhythm following the 6.5-hour light pulses, as assessed 1 day after the photic stimulus, are fit with a four-parameter logistic model, using a nonlinear least-squares analysis, that predicts an inflection point of the curve (i.e., sensitivity of the system) at approximately 120 lux; phase shifts saturate at approximately 550 lux. Data from individual participants represented by *closed boxes*, model by *solid line*, and 95% confidence intervals by *dashed lines*. (Modified with permission from Zeitzer JM, Dijk D-J, Kronauer RE, et al. Sensitivity of the human circadian pacemaker to nocturnal light: melatonin phase resetting and suppression. *J Physiol [Lond]*. 2000;526:695–702.)

We are exposed to bright light for a relatively short time each day,[86,87] but in modern industrialized societies we are exposed to ordinary indoor room light for many hours, a predominance of exposure that may have a greater impact on our circadian system than a few minutes of exposure to bright light. Phase-resetting and melatonin suppression responses to the resetting effects of evening light exposure are dose dependent and nonlinear; shorter light exposures (only 12 minutes long) more efficiently phase-shift the clock, suppress melatonin, and induce alertness than longer durations of retinal light exposure.[88]

Figure 37.6 illustrates the influence of the circadian pacemaker and the sleep-wake state on physiologic variables and the influence of light input through the eye to the circadian pacemaker. The feedback loop from the sleep-wake state to the eye represents the effects of exposure to the environmental light cycle because the sleeping state in humans is usually associated with eyelid closure and self-selected exposure to darkness, achieved by drawing window shades and switching off artificial light sources, whereas the waking state in humans is usually associated with opening of the eyelids and exposing the retina to light through self-selected use of artificial light or exposure to outdoor light during waking hours. Under a strict sleep-wake and light exposure schedule, the pacemaker's timing is consistent from day to day. However, whenever sleep is initiated late or terminated early, or a waking episode occurs within a sleep episode, the associated light exposure can reset the pacemaker. This association between waking and light exposure and the fact that low light intensity has a significant resetting effect on the pacemaker have practical relevance

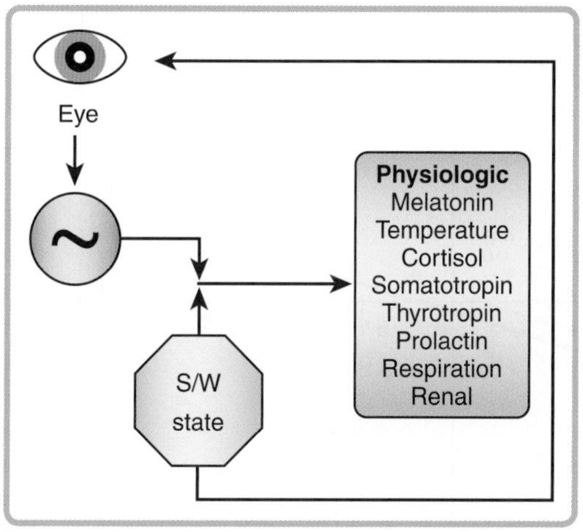

Figure 37.6 Schema illustrating influence of the circadian pacemaker (*circle with oscillator symbol*) and sleep-wake state (*octagon*) on several physiologic variables. Under normal conditions, the circadian pacemaker and sleep-wake state each influence these variables; relative contribution and nature of interaction (i.e., synergistic or oppositional) of each depends on the variable observed. Also illustrated are the influences of environmental illumination on the human circadian clock through the eye and of the sleep-wake state in determining timing of this illumination through behavioral action (i.e., switching off artificial indoor room lights, drawing bedroom window shades at bedtime, eyelid closure during sleep, and eyelid opening during waking).

for routine sleep-wake scheduling and for understanding the influence of sleep disruption, which is often associated with light exposure, on circadian phase.

Nonphotic Circadian Phase Resetting and Reentrainment

Nonphotic input to the human circadian system is less well characterized than photic input. Results of early studies, which focused on social cues such as gong sounds or regularly scheduled performance tests, meals, and bedtimes,[89] were confounded by limitations of phase measures used and self-selected lighting conditions. Exposure of healthy young men to nocturnal exercise of 1 to 3 hours' duration resulted in phase delays in nocturnal melatonin the following day.[90,91] Early evening 1-hour high-intensity exercise (at approximately 6:30 p.m.) elicited *phase advances* significantly different from the phase delays in response to morning, afternoon, and nocturnal exercise and in no-exercise participants (Figure 37.7). In a study of the facilitation of reentrainment to a delay-shifted sleep-wake episode in extremely dim light (to control for ambient light during exercise), exercise during the biologic night produced phase delays compared with no exercise.[91] Thus appropriately timed nonphotic stimuli such as exercise or other forms of arousal can facilitate adaptation to acute changes in light-dark cycle.

That appropriately timed exposure to exercise also results in phase advances and is demonstrated by partial entrainment to a 23.5-hour light-dark and sleep-wake schedule in healthy volunteers exercising at moderate intensity twice daily (midday and late afternoon) over 2 weeks.[92] Participants exercising daily in late afternoon exhibited partial entrainment, advancing on average 10 minutes per day more than nonexercising controls, consistent with phase-advancing effects of late afternoon exercise on the human circadian clock. Given the slightly greater than 24-hour endogenous circadian period of humans and the net daily phase advance required for stable entrainment, evening exercise, particularly repeated daily exposure, could result in daily phase advances leading to nonphotic entrainment of the human circadian system if the timing and intensity of the exercise were optimized.

INVESTIGATING CIRCADIAN AND SLEEP-WAKE DEPENDENT MODULATION

The Kleitman Protocol

Separation from 24-Hour Environmental and Behavioral Cues

Nathaniel Kleitman was the first investigator to study human circadian rhythms in the absence of periodic 24-hour cues in the external environment (Figure 37.8).[42] Core body temperature records from one of his two participants in Mammoth Cave, Kentucky, in 1938, who underwent a 28-hour imposed sleep-wake schedule, were compared with laboratory data collected at the University of Chicago from the same participant living on a 24-hour routine[42] (shown in Figure 37.9). On a 24-hour schedule, there were seven cycles of the body temperature rhythm, as one would expect over the course of a 1-week recording. The week with an imposed 28-hour schedule also has seven cycles of body temperature rhythm, but only six sleep-wake cycles (Figure 37.9, *upper panel*). Despite the confounding effect of sleep on core body temperature, this experimental protocol still separated the influence of timing of the sleep-wake schedule from that of the circadian pacemaker—at least in this participant.

This imposed desynchrony between sleep-wake schedule and output of the circadian pacemaker driving the temperature rhythm occurs when the non–24-hour sleep-wake schedule is outside the range of entrainment or range of capture of the circadian system. This protocol, termed the *forced-desynchrony* protocol, is useful in evaluating the influence of the circadian pacemaker on many physiologic variables because it allows separation of the confounding effect of the sleep-wake schedule from the output of the endogenous circadian pacemaker.[19,42,93] Figure 37.10 illustrates a raster plot of a forced-desynchrony experiment incorporating core body temperature and wake data for a participant living on a 28-hour day in a laboratory shielded from external time cues.[94] The waking episodes in this protocol are 18 hours, 40 minutes, followed by sleep episodes of 9 hours, 20 minutes. Core body temperature exhibited a period of 24.3 hours in this participant and was therefore desynchronized from both the 24-hour day and the timing of the imposed 28-hour sleep-wake schedule.

Separating Circadian Modulation and Sleep-Wake Modulation

The constant-routine protocol does not permit complete and unconfounded separation of the circadian and homeostatic influences on neurobehavioral and physiologic variables. However, in the Kleitman forced-desynchrony protocol, sleep and wake are distributed much more evenly over the entire circadian cycle during the course of the experiment. It is thus possible to average data over either successive circadian cycles or successive sleep-wake episodes to separate these components. Averaging isolates the circadian profile of the variable of interest by removing the contribution of the confounding sleep-wake contribution in the averaging process. Conversely, the temporal contribution of the sleep-wake profile can be isolated from the confounding circadian influence. This averaging

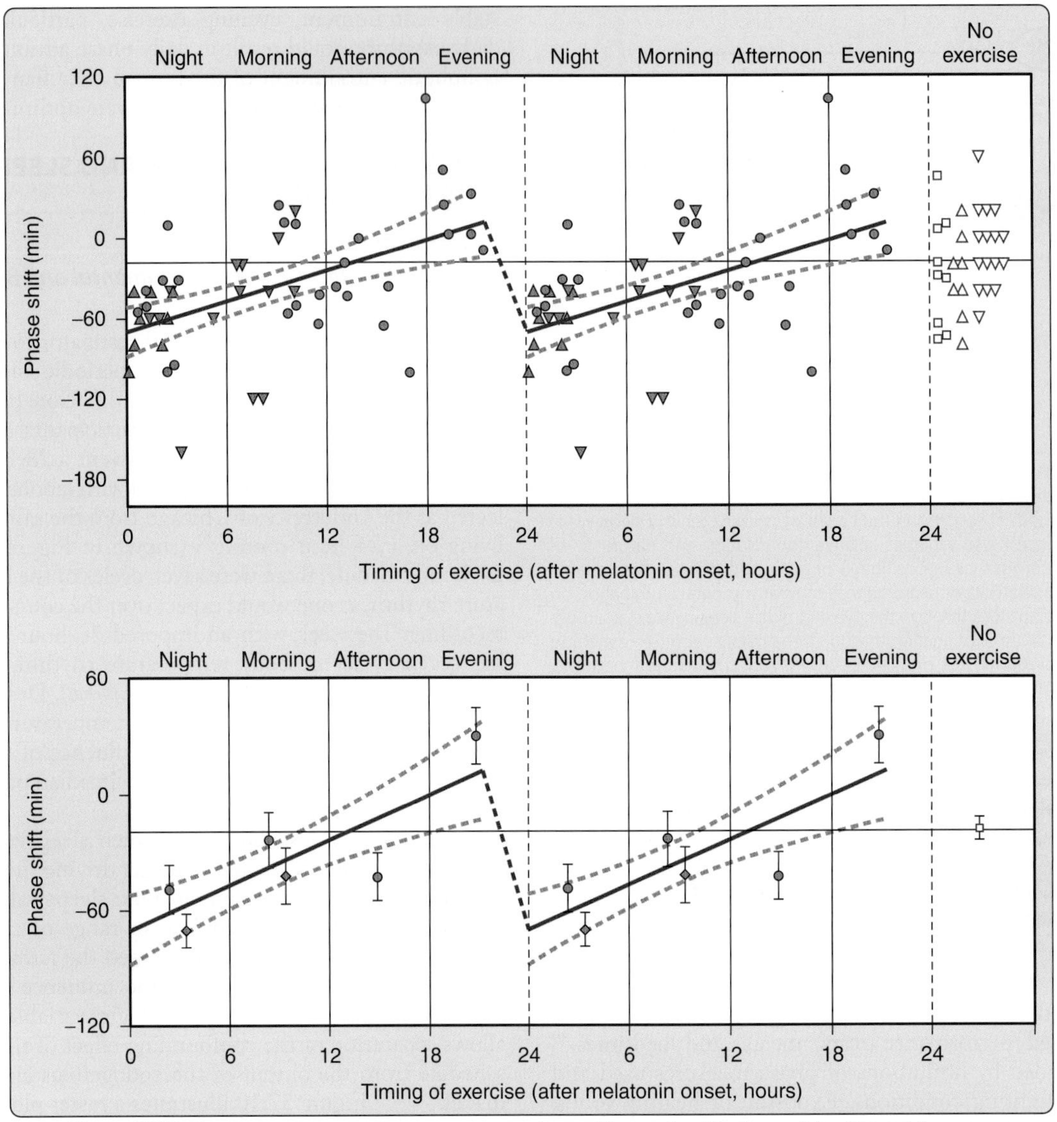

Figure 37.7 Phase-response curves in response to exercise at different circadian times of day. Phase delays were observed in response to nocturnal exercise; phase advances were observed in response to exercise during late afternoon or early evening. *Closed circles* indicate phase shifts in response to high-intensity, 1-hour nocturnal exercise and daytime exercise. *Upward* and *downward triangles* (*top panel*) and *diamonds* (*bottom panel*) indicate phase shifts in response to low-intensity, 3-hour exercise sessions. The *line* indicates a significant relationship between phase shifts and circadian time of exercise (r^2 = 0.28, P = .0003; slope significantly different from zero). *Dashed curves* indicate 95% confidence intervals of slope of line. (Reproduced with permission from Buxton OM, Lee CW, L'Hermite-Balériaux M, et al. Exercise elicits phase shifts and acute alterations of melatonin levels that vary with circadian phase. *Am J Physiol.* 2003;284:R714–24. Copyright 2003 American Physiological Society.)

process is similar to that of cortical evoked potential recordings that effectively subtract background noise not temporally related to the evoked response.

Neurobehavioral Functions

To understand and predict the time course of neurobehavioral function, we must recognize the influence of the sleep-wake state on what is termed a *sleep homeostat*[19] driving neurobehavioral functions, as is apparent when we examine these variables during a longer course of sleep deprivation when more than one circadian cycle has elapsed.[46] The cyclic influence of the circadian pacemaker on alertness and performance is superimposed on an overall decline in function during the experiment, as described in models incorporating both homeostatic and circadian influences in the regulation of sleep and wake.[95,96] The rate of this performance decline increases sharply under conditions of chronic sleep restriction.

In a 20-hour forced-desynchrony protocol, the temporal profiles of cognitive performance and subjective sleepiness as a function of both circadian phase and time into the scheduled waking day[97] (Figure 37.11) suggest that the overall magnitudes of circadian and wake-dependent drives are similar during a typical waking day. From the timing of circadian and sleep-dependent profiles, we can qualitatively reconstruct their separate contributions to maintenance of alertness and performance over a normal waking day (Figure 37.11). In the first half of the day after wake time, there is little homeostatic sleep drive because it was discharged by the prior sleep episode, so both alertness and cognitive performance are high. In the latter half of the waking episode, when homeostatic sleep drive

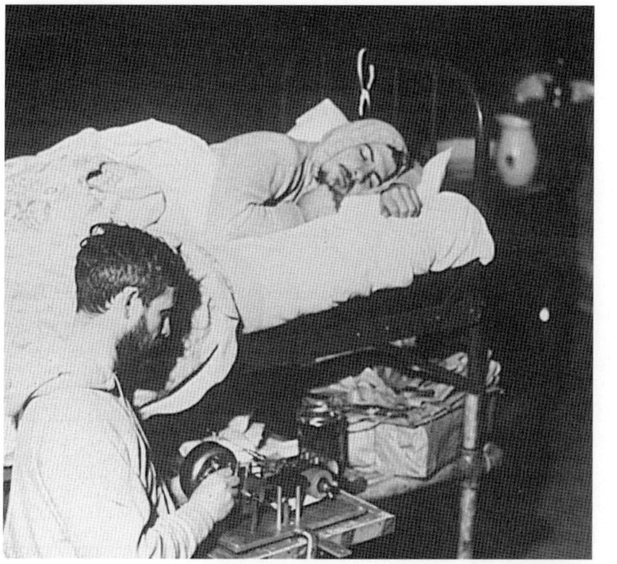

Figure 37.8 Professor Nathaniel Kleitman (*left*) attends to experimental equipment while fellow research participant Bruce Richardson lies in bed deep within Mammoth Cave in Kentucky where, for the first time, human participants were studied while shielded from periodic environmental changes on Earth's surface. The two pioneers lived on an imposed 28-hour sleep-wake schedule in these quarters from June 4 to July 6, 1938, in an effort to approximate uniform environmental and behavioral conditions, free from the influence of Earth's 24-hour day. In a 60-foot wide chamber free from any external environmental sounds, the temperature remained at 54°F (±1°), humidity approached complete vapor saturation, and darkness was absolute when the artificial light used during waking hours was shut off. The Mammoth Cave Hotel provided daily meals, which were consumed on awakening and after the 7th and 13th hour of each 19-hour waking day. (Photo courtesy of National Park Service, Mammoth Cave National Park, Mammoth, Kentucky; description adapted from Kleitman N. *Sleep and Wakefulness*. Chicago: University of Chicago Press; 1963:178–9.)

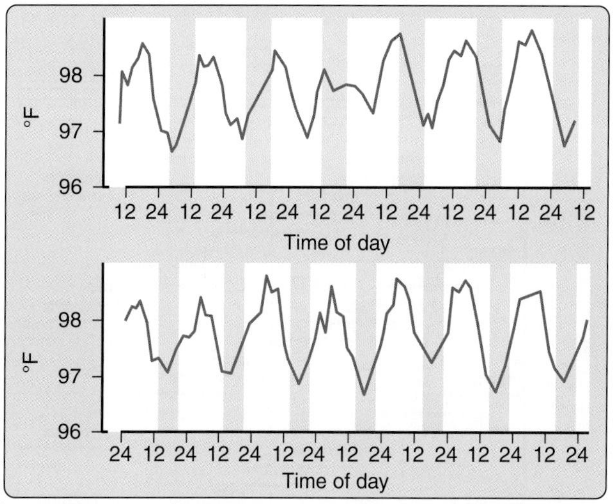

Figure 37.9 Weekly body temperature rhythms of a participant under two different routines of sleep and wake. *Top*, Data from participant K on a 28-hour daily routine of 19 hours' wake and 9 hours' sleep during Professor Kleitman's historic forced-desynchrony protocol (Figure 37.8). Data based on last 3 weeks in Mammoth Cave. *Bottom*, Laboratory data recorded at the University of Chicago from participant K on his customary daily 24-hour routine of 17 hours' wake and 7 hours' sleep. *Shaded areas* indicate time in bed attempting to sleep. Data are from the 5 weeks after the 24-hour routine of living. Each weekly record shows seven body temperature waves, within minima in *shaded areas* on the customary 24-hour routine but not on the artificial 28-hour sleep-wake schedule. This participant's endogenous circadian temperature cycle maintained a near–24-hour oscillation, despite the scheduled 28-hour length of his sleep-wake cycle. Temperature data from participant R (not shown) appeared to adapt to the non–24-hour routine, something not observed in more recent forced-desynchrony studies. Interindividual differences in the strength of endogenous versus evoked components of the body temperature rhythm may account for what appeared to be circadian adaptation during forced desynchrony in participant R of Kleitman's pioneering experiment. (Figure and parts of legend adapted with permission from Kleitman N. *Sleep and Wakefulness*. Chicago: University of Chicago Press; 1963. Copyright 1963 by the University of Chicago.)

would otherwise cause alertness and cognitive performance to decline, the circadian drive rises and opposes that decline, thereby sustaining a high, stable level of alertness throughout the normal waking day. Performance in the 3 hours before the onset of melatonin secretion (i.e., the wake maintenance zone) is significantly improved compared with performance during a 3-hour block earlier in the biologic day, despite a longer time awake. This effect is greater after extended wakefulness (i.e., on day 2 of a circadian rhythm), when homeostatic sleep pressure is high. The wake maintenance zone may therefore contribute to sleep-onset insomnia complaints when sleep timing is highly variable.[98] Remarkably, neurobehavioral performance, as measured by reaction time, can be preserved during this circadian wake maintenance zone even under conditions of chronic sleep restriction.[99]

Sleep and Wake

Similar dynamics apply for reconstructing the respective circadian and homeostatic contributions to sleep and wakefulness. The raster plot of the forced-desynchrony experiment (Figure 37.10) shows that almost all wakefulness within a scheduled sleep episode occurs when the participant's sleep episode is not in phase with the body temperature nadir,[94] an observation first quantified by Kleitman from his Mammoth Cave data.[42] Averaging polysomnographically recorded sleep data from free-running participants on a self-selected cycle and in an environment free of time cues yields the data in Figure 37.12, showing the temporal profiles of sleep parameters as a function of circadian phase.[100] The circadian contribution to REM sleep timing is robust and exhibits a maximum centered just after the core body temperature nadir.

Figure 37.13 depicts sleep-dependent changes in the propensity for wake as a function of the circadian phase at which a sleep episode is initiated.[19] Under entrained conditions, a consolidated bout of sleep is maintained with minimal wake during the scheduled sleep episode by initiating the sleep episode at the end of the wake maintenance zone. However, when sleep is initiated in the early morning hours (as in a shift worker after the first night shift), a high percentage of time is spent in wake during the latter half of this intended sleep episode. During entrained conditions, homeostatic drive for sleep is greatest after an extended bout of wake at sleep onset and facilitates sleep in the first half of the night. In the latter half of the sleep episode, as the homeostatic drive declines, the circadian drive for sleep becomes greater, thus maintaining elevated sleep drive through the end of the sleep episode. These two components interact to facilitate consolidated sleep throughout the night.[19,94]

The three-dimensional representation in Figure 37.14 combines the temporal profiles of circadian and sleep-dependent drives to illustrate their respective contributions in maintaining wake.[19,94] A maximum in sleepiness quantified by slow rolling eye movements occurs at the endogenous circadian temperature nadir, which corresponds to occurring

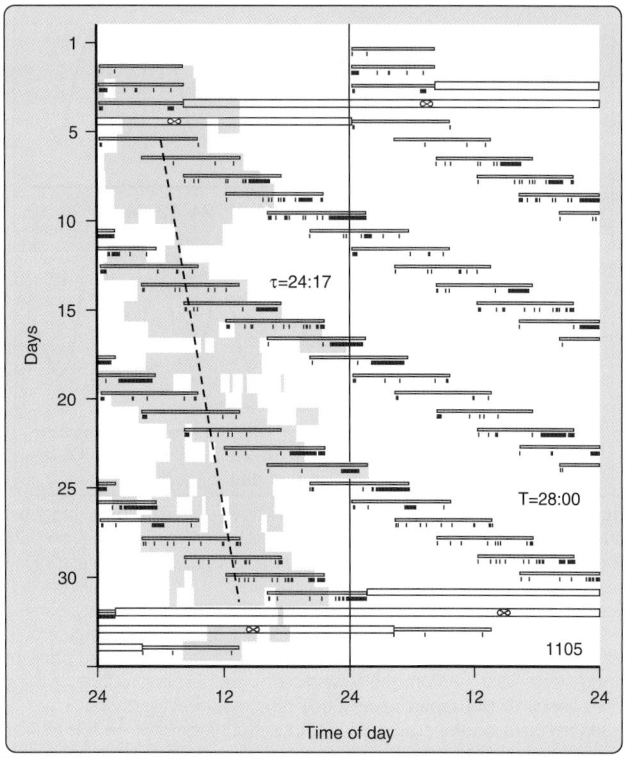

Figure 37.10 Double plot of a 28-hour forced-desynchrony protocol. Successive days are plotted next to and beneath each other. Scheduled sleep episodes are indicated by *narrow open bars*, polysomnographically determined wake within each sleep episode is indicated by *red tick marks* below the *narrow open bars*, and intervals during which core body temperature was below mean are indicated by the *blue area*. Intrinsic temperature cycle of 24.3 hours from this participant's data was estimated by nonparametric spectral analysis of core body temperature data during the forced-desynchrony part of the protocol. The *broken line* indicates the phase of circadian temperature rhythm minimum. The *encircled* X indicates the minimum of endogenous circadian rhythm of core body temperature unmasked by the 40-hour constant-routine protocol (*narrow open bars*). (Reproduced with permission from Dijk D-J, Czeisler CA. Paradoxical timing of the circadian rhythm of sleep propensity serves to consolidate sleep and wakefulness in humans. *Neurosci Lett.* 1994;166:63–8.)

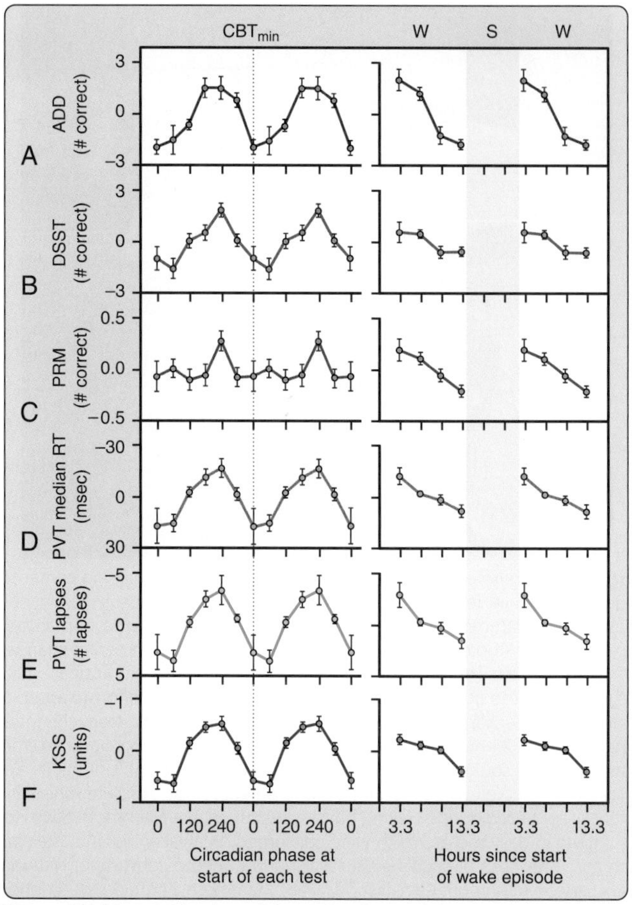

Figure 37.11 Double plots of the main effects of the circadian phase relative to the minimum of core body temperature CBT$_{min}$ (*left panels*) and duration of scheduled wake (*right panels*: *w*, wake; *s*, sleep) on neurobehavioral measures. Plotted points show deviation from mean values during forced desynchrony and standard errors of the mean (SEMs). For all panels, values plotted lower in the panel represent impairment of that measure. Addition Task (ADD) **(A)**, Digit Symbol Substitution Task (DSST) **(B)**, and Probed Recall Memory (PRM) **(C)** scores were derived from total correct responses. Psychomotor Vigilance Task (PVT) results represent median reaction time **(D)** and total lapses (**E,** reaction times >500 msec). Karolinska Sleepiness Scale (KSS) scores **(F)** represent responses on this 1-9 Likert-type scale; higher scores represent greater sleepiness. (Reproduced with permission from Wyatt JK, Ritz-De Cecco A, Czeisler CA, Dijk DJ. Circadian temperature and melatonin rhythms, sleep, and neurobehavioral function in humans living on a 20-h day. *Am J Physiol.* 1999;277:R1152–63.)

just before the habitual wake time. The sleep-dependent contribution exhibits an increasing profile over the wake episode, with the greatest propensity of slow rolling eye movements after 14 hours of wakefulness. The magnitude of the circadian rhythms of sleepiness and performance increases with increasing homeostatic sleep drive. Thus, when increasing homeostatic sleep pressure combines with an adverse circadian phase, the drive for sleep is so great that slow eye movements and lapses of attention often intrude involuntarily during wake. The performance impairment is an order of magnitude more severe when extended wakefulness coincides with an adverse circadian phase under conditions of chronic sleep restriction.[99]

The circadian and sleep-wake modulation of sleep-wake propensity and neurobehavioral function are illustrated schematically in Figure 37.15. Experimental evidence indicates that a simple additive model cannot account for variations in alertness and cognitive performance data.[44,46,101] In fact, when averaged across all circadian phases, relatively little circadian variation occurs in waking neurobehavioral measures in the first few hours of wakefulness, when homeostatic sleep drive is low, and the circadian contribution increases as a function of number of hours awake, suggesting that homeostatic and circadian drives are not independent and further suggesting a nonadditive interaction between homeostatic and circadian systems that drive alertness and cognitive performance.[102] Furthermore, the buildup of the homeostatic drive in response to acute sleep deprivation is distinct from the response to chronic sleep loss.[99]

Internal Sleep Structure

REM sleep propensity varies with circadian phase.[19,100,103] Studies with nap opportunities evenly distributed throughout day and night every 1.5 to 3 hours first established the REM sleep propensity rhythm in a protocol that did not involve concomitant variations in prior wake length.[100,104,105] REM sleep latency, the rate of REM sleep accumulation, REM sleep episode duration, and REM sleep propensity were then shown to vary with phase of the endogenous circadian temperature cycle in free-running participants whose self-selected

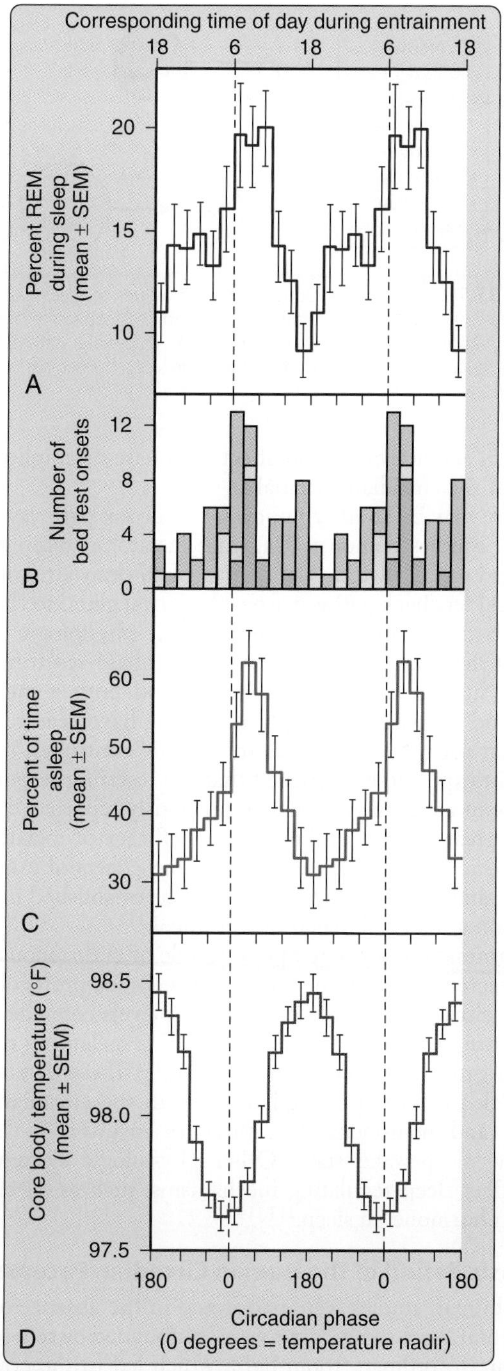

Figure 37.12 Variations in occurrence and internal organization of sleep with circadian temperature cycle phase (94 days of data from four participants). **A,** Percent of REM during sleep; **C,** Percent of time asleep; **D,** Core body temperature. In panel **B,** REM sleep episodes that occurred within 10 minutes after bed rest onset are indicated by *green* areas; those in which REM sleep episodes occurred within 30 minutes after bed rest onset are indicated by *peach* areas. (Reproduced with permission from Czeisler CA, Zimmerman JC, Ronda JM, Moore-Ede MC, et al. Timing of REM sleep is coupled to the circadian rhythm of body temperature in man. *Sleep.* 1980;2:329–46.)

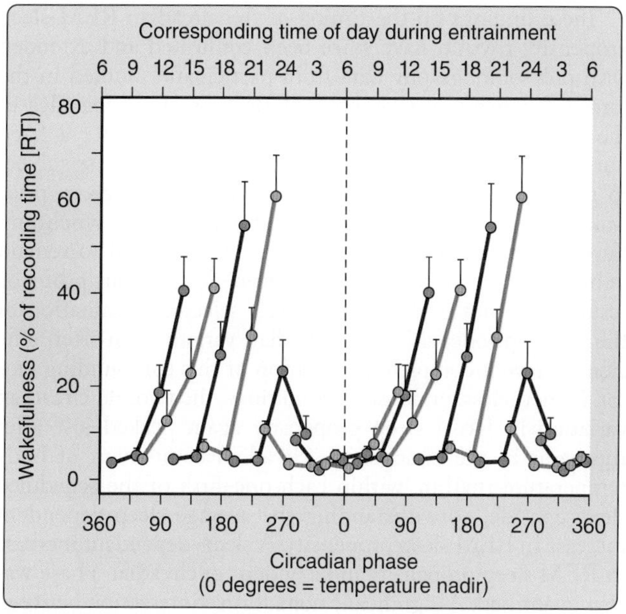

Figure 37.13 Wakefulness during scheduled sleep episodes (expressed as percentage of recording time) as a function of circadian temperature phase. Sleep episodes were assigned to twelve 30-degree bins based on circadian phase at lights out. (Modified with permission from Dijk D-J, Czeisler CA. Contribution of the circadian pacemaker and the sleep homeostat to sleep propensity, sleep structure, electroencephalographic slow waves, and sleep spindle activity in humans. *J Neurosci.* 1995;15:3526–38.)

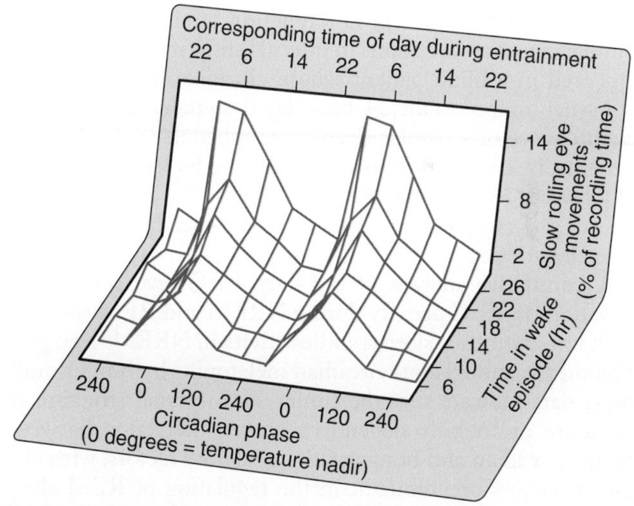

Figure 37.14 Quasi three-dimensional plot of slow rolling eye movements (SREMs) within scheduled wake episodes relative to circadian phase and time elapsed since start of wake episode. Data were assigned to twelve 30-degree circadian-phase bins and six 112-minute time-since-start-of-wake-episode bins. Each point represents SREMs expressed as percentage of recording time in a bin. (Modified with permission from Cajochen C, Wyatt JK, Bonikowska M, et al. Non-linear interaction between circadian and homeostatic modulation of slow eye movements during wakefulness in humans. *J Sleep Res.* 2000;9:58.)

rest-activity cycle spontaneously desynchronized from the timing of the endogenous circadian temperature cycle (Figure 37.12).[100,106] The peak of the endogenous circadian rhythm in REM sleep propensity in these participants was just after the nadir of the endogenous component of the circadian temperature cycle, coincident with the circadian peak of sleepiness and sleep propensity (Figures 37.11 to 37.14).[100,106] During such spontaneous desynchrony, free-running participants who chose to go to bed near the peak of the REM sleep propensity rhythm usually exhibited sleep-onset REM sleep episodes,[100,106] an otherwise rare phenomenon normally diagnostic of narcolepsy. Under these conditions, the density of rapid eye movements per minute of REM sleep exhibits a sleep-dependent variation apparently dissociated from the REM sleep propensity rhythm itself.[107]

These findings on the timing of the circadian REM sleep propensity rhythm have since been confirmed and extended with polysomnography data from participants studied in the forced-desynchrony protocol.[19,94] Because sleep episodes in the forced-desynchrony protocol always begin after a fixed duration of enforced wakefulness, the results were less subject to the confounding effects of systematic variations in prior wake durations characteristic of spontaneous desynchrony. Furthermore, because participants were scheduled to remain in bed for a fixed interval on the forced-desynchrony protocol, results were not confounded by self-selected termination of the sleep episode, although circadian variations in sleep efficiency prevent complete elimination of this confounding factor. Nonetheless, under such conditions, the twofold circadian variation in REM sleep propensity again peaked just after the nadir in the endogenous circadian component of body temperature rhythm, within each one-fifth of the scheduled sleep episode, notwithstanding the average sleep-dependent increase in REM sleep propensity. A sleep-dependent increase in REM sleep propensity independent of circadian phase was also quantified. A significant nonadditive interaction between circadian phase and time since the start of the sleep episode was found from the REM sleep data collected during forced desynchrony.[19]

With the forced-desynchrony protocol, significant and substantial circadian and sleep-dependent variations in NREM sleep propensity were also observed, whereas the robust sleep-dependent decline in slow wave activity was associated with only a small but statistically significant variation of slow wave activity as a function of circadian phase.[19] Similar circadian variations in internal sleep structure are documented in a blind patient whose circadian pacemaker was not synchronized to the 24-hour day, despite his decades-long maintenance of a regular sleep-wake schedule.[108] Such blind patients, in essence, live in society on the biologic equivalent of a forced-desynchrony protocol, because the 24-hour day is outside the range of entrainment of the circadian pacemaker in such patients.

Quantitative analysis of the sleep EEG reveals circadian variations in EEG activity during NREM and REM sleep,[109] with low-frequency sleep spindle activity in NREM sleep paralleling the endogenous circadian melatonin rhythm. Overall, these data indicate that the timing and internal structure of sleep are profoundly dependent on an interaction between robust circadian and homeostatic regulatory factors, with circadian factors predominant in the regulation of REM sleep and with sleep-dependent factors predominant in the regulation of slow wave sleep.

Potential Feedback Pathways

As is typical of physiologic regulatory systems, feedback pathways play a significant role in this system. The neurobehavioral variables influenced by the circadian pacemaker and the sleep homeostat can influence the sleep-wake state through the influence of wake and sleep propensity on determination of sleep and wake times. For example, a sleep episode is more likely to be initiated after a rise in sleep propensity to a high level during an extended waking episode, and a sleep episode is more likely to be terminated after a decline in sleep propensity to a low level over the course of a sleep episode. This influence on behavior, in turn, influences the level of the sleep homeostat and, because of associated changes in light exposure and activity, it can affect the phase or amplitude (or both) of the circadian pacemaker.

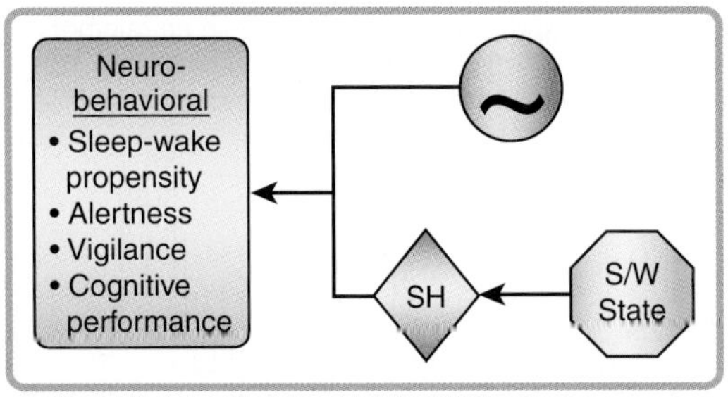

Figure 37.15 Schema illustrating combined influence of circadian clock and sleep-wake state on neurobehavioral variables (sleep-wake propensity, alertness, vigilance, and cognitive performance). Sleep-wake state (S/W state) influence is illustrated by an intermediary of the sleep homeostat (*SH in blue diamond*).

There may be another important feedback pathway in this system. Studies demonstrating that melatonin receptors can be found on cells within the human SCN draw attention to a potential feedback pathway from the pineal gland to the SCN through circulating melatonin. Several physiologic studies suggest that exogenous melatonin has a phase-resetting effect on the human circadian pacemaker, and both a melatonin PRC and dose-dependent phase shifting have been reported. The first such study that has thoroughly controlled for retinal light exposure has revealed that the resetting responses to melatonin are even greater than previously reported.[110] There is also great interest in the potential efficacy of melatonin as a hypnotic because the sleep-promoting effects of exogenous melatonin depend on circadian phase, as established in young adults on a forced-desynchrony protocol.[111]

Examination of the temporal profile of endogenous melatonin secretion during the forced-desynchrony protocol shows a daily circadian increase in melatonin levels coincident with a decrease in wake (Figure 37.16).[109] This melatonin rise may open a gate that allows sleep to occur.[112] These data suggest feedback from the pineal gland to both the circadian pacemaker and neurobehavioral variables involved in regulating the sleep-wake state. Other physiologic systems may also affect sleep-regulating mechanisms, such as an effect of growth hormone on sleep.[113,114]

Intrinsic Period of the Human Circadian Pacemaker

Early human studies were performed in the absence of environmental synchronizers but were confounded by self-selected exposure to ordinary room light, which led to the erroneous conclusion that the average period of the human circadian pacemaker was 25 hours.[47,93] Participants were permitted to illuminate their living quarters while awake and switch off lighting while asleep because these experiments were predicated on the incorrect belief that ordinary room light had no resetting effect on the human circadian system.[115,116] Thus results of these studies were systematically compromised by this retinal light exposure.[47,93] Recognition of this confounding effect led to the use of Kleitman's forced-desynchrony protocol to assess the intrinsic period of the human circadian pacemaker.[47,93,117]

Subsequent studies using the Kleitman forced-desynchrony protocol have controlled the intensity of background illumination and timing of exposure to the light-dark cycle.[47,93] With this forced-desynchrony protocol in participants living

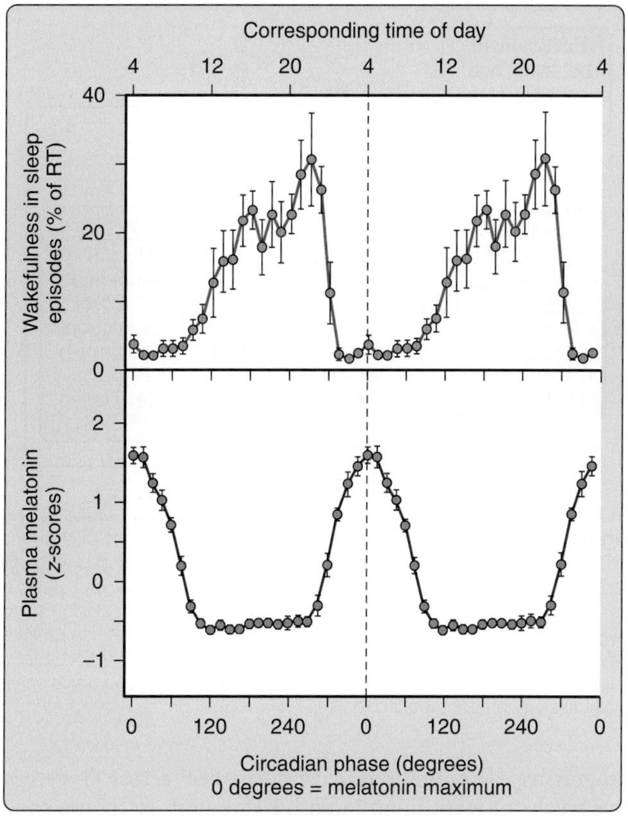

Figure 37.16 Phase relationships between endogenous circadian rhythms of wakefulness and plasma melatonin were assessed during a forced-desynchrony protocol. Data were plotted against the circadian phase of the plasma melatonin rhythm (0 degrees on the lower abscissa scale corresponds to fitted melatonin maximum). To compare with entrained conditions, the upper abscissa scale indicates the approximate clock time corresponding to circadian melatonin rhythm during the first day of the forced-desynchrony protocol (i.e., immediately on release from entrainment). Plasma melatonin data are expressed as *z*-scores to correct for interindividual differences in mean values. Wakefulness is expressed as a percentage of recording time (RT). Data are double plotted (i.e., all data plotted left of the *dashed vertical line* are repeated to the right of the *vertical line*). (Modified from Dijk D-J, Shanahan TL, Duffy JF, et al. Variation of electroencephalographic activity during non–rapid eye movement and rapid eye movement sleep with phase of circadian melatonin rhythm in humans. *J Physiol [Lond]*. 1997;505[3]:851–8.)

in dim light (about 10 to 15 lux) on either a 28-hour or a 20-hour schedule, the average intrinsic period of the circadian pacemaker is estimated to be much closer to 24 hours than 25 hours. The intrinsic circadian period averages 24.15 hours in healthy adults and is shorter in women (24.1 + 0.2 hours) than in men (24.2 + 0.2 hours)[117,118] (Figure 37.17). This holds true for all of the circadian markers tested—core body temperature, melatonin, and cortisol—and is consistent with results of other studies under a variety of protocols.[119-122] The average intrinsic period of the human circadian pacemaker is significantly shorter in women [24.09 ± 0.2 hour (24 hours, 5 minutes ± 12 minutes)] than in men [24.19 ± 0.2 hours (24 hours, 11 minutes ± 12 minutes)].[118] Entrainment studies have functionally confirmed the intrinsic circadian period in humans to be near 24 hours because a weak stimulus (candlelight during the scheduled day and sleep in darkness during the scheduled night) can entrain most people to a light-dark cycle with an imposed period of 24.0 hours but not an imposed period of 23.5 or 24.6 hours.[123]

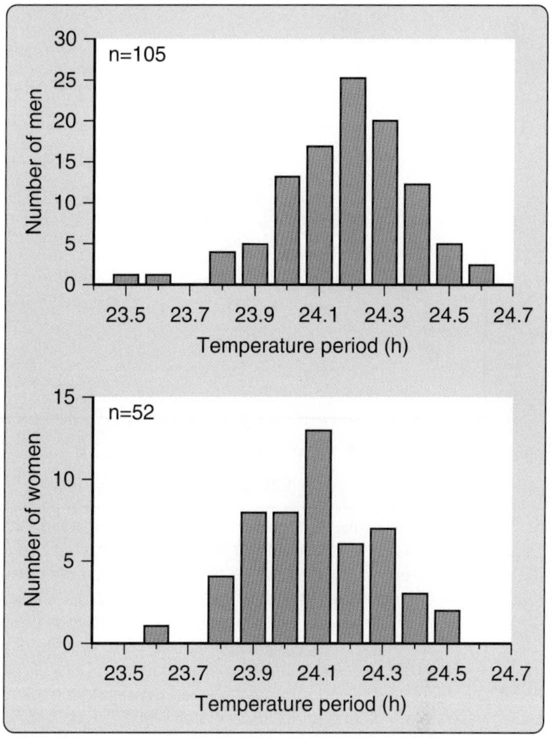

Figure 37.17 Histogram of intrinsic circadian period estimates derived from male and female participants. Intrinsic circadian period (t) estimates of male participants (top panel) and female participants (bottom panel). Each participant's estimated intrinsic circadian period is reported as the estimated period from his or her melatonin rhythms. (Reproduced with permission from Duffy et al, 2011 PNAS.)

AGING AND CIRCADIAN SLEEP-WAKE REGULATION

Aging also has a pervasive influence on many aspects of the circadian and sleep-wake regulating system.[124-130] The prevalence of disrupted sleep complaints is much greater in older than in younger people. In fact, 57% of people in the United States older than 65 years complain of at least one chronic sleep problem, 43% complain of difficulty initiating or maintaining sleep, and 19% complain of awakening too early in the morning.[131] Key to examining this question is the extent to which the circadian pacemaker or the sleep homeostat is involved in these age-related changes.

On average, the circadian clock is set to an earlier hour, and the amplitude of some endogenous circadian rhythms is lower in older people than it is in young adults (Figure 37.18).[126,132] However, the intrinsic circadian period does not shorten with age in healthy humans.[117,118,133] Importantly, young participants can sleep over a much wider range of circadian phases than older people, who awaken spontaneously at an earlier internal circadian phase.[132,134] Because older people usually awaken at an earlier circadian phase, they are typically exposed to light at an earlier hour; this earlier light exposure, which will reset the circadian pacemaker to an earlier hour, likely accounts for the earlier average entrained circadian phase observed in older people.[132] Remarkably, older participants are much less vulnerable to the adverse effect of sleep loss and misalignment of circadian phase on neurobehavioral performance.[135] At the same time, a polymorphism near the *PER1* clock gene is associated with the timing of activity rhythms and with the time of death, such that rs7221412GG

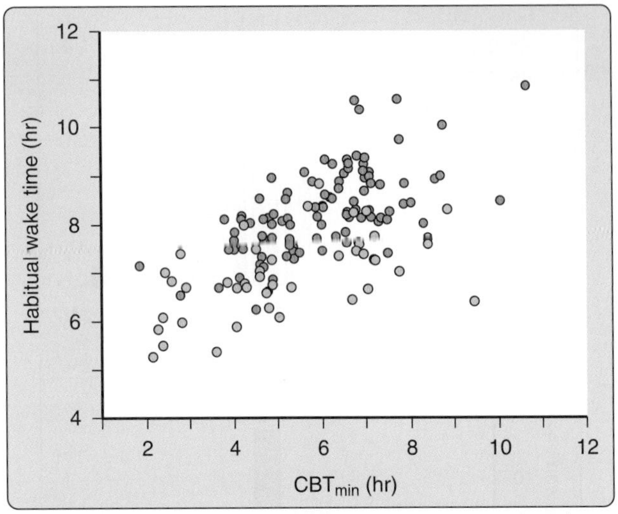

Figure 37.18 Habitual wake time versus endogenous circadian phase of young and older adults. Symbols represent average self-reported wake time from the pre-study week versus the phase of core body temperature minimum (CBT_{min}) for each participant. *Yellow circles* indicate older participants ($n = 44$); *green circles* indicate young participants ($n = 101$). Between-groups relationship is significant (slope of older participants, 0.266 ± 0.06; slope of young participants, 0.471 ±0.05). (Reproduced with permission from Duffy JF, Dijk D-J, Klerman EB, Czeisler CA. Later endogenous circadian temperature nadir relative to an earlier wake time in older people. *Am J Physiol.* 1998;275:R1478–87.)

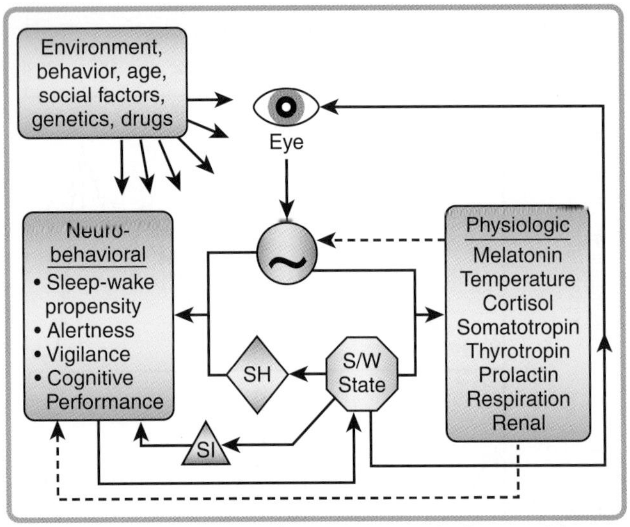

Figure 37.19 Overall schema illustrating potential influence of the circadian clock on neurobehavioral and physiologic variables and of physiologic variables (e.g., melatonin, body temperature) on neurobehavioral variables or circadian clock (*dashed arrows*), feedback influence of variables on sleep-wake state (S/W State) (*solid arrow*), influence of sleep-wake state on variables through sleep homeostat (SH) and sleep inertia (SI) (*solid arrows*). Global influence of environment, behavior, age, social factors, genetics, and drugs on virtually all elements contributing to sleep-wake regulation are also represented.

individuals have a mean time of death nearly 7 hours later than rs7221412AA/AG individuals.[136]

INFLUENCE OF SOCIAL AND WORK-RELATED FACTORS

The self-selection of sleep and wake times in humans is another important factor in the sleep-wake regulatory system. Although circadian and homeostatic drives for sleep influence the choice of sleep and wake times through a feedback pathway, social factors (e.g., child care, school and work responsibilities, entertainment, social interaction) and environmental factors (e.g., noise, artificial light, alarm clocks) often override those biologic determinants. In contrast, animal behavior exhibits activity and sleep predictable enough to be used as markers of the biologic time of day. Humans, especially since the advent of alarm clocks and artificial lighting, can and do override the signals from the circadian and sleep-wake regulating system and freely decide to stay awake later than they otherwise would or wake up earlier than they would spontaneously because of job or school requirements or recreational and social events. Thus modern humans may be more sleep deprived than their ancestors.[137]

The long-term consequences of this relatively recent trend in industrialized society are unknown. Yet the modern consolidated sleep episode is significantly different from that under more naturalistic conditions in which sleep episode duration was determined by longer length of darkness in the natural winter environment.[69,137,138] The most conspicuous example of this self-selection is rotating shift work, when people choose to work in direct opposition to the modulation of circadian and homeostatic regulatory systems, resulting in internal temporal dissociation, fragmented sleep, and impaired wake. This does have consequences. Resident physicians working extended-duration work shifts (24 to 30 hours) every third day showed progressive deterioration in performance across 3 successive weeks of work in an intensive care unit. Response times deteriorated with time on shift and cumulatively, demonstrating chronic sleep deficiency with each successive extended-duration work shift.[139] Prolonged exposure to prolonged sleep restriction with concurrent circadian disruption in controlled laboratory conditions decreases resting metabolic rate and increases plasma glucose concentrations after a meal, an effect resulting from inadequate pancreatic insulin secretion, suggesting that prolonged sleep restriction with concurrent circadian disruption alters metabolism and could increase the risk for obesity and diabetes.[140] Therefore, in any realistic model of the human circadian and sleep-wake regulatory system used to manage performance and prevent disease, such environmental and societal influences must be recognized.

We can assemble an overall system schema and incorporate the feedback pathway of neurobehavioral variables on sleep-wake state and the putative feedback pathways from melatonin and other physiologic variables onto the circadian pacemaker and neurobehavioral function (Figure 37.19). This schema incorporates the global influence of environmental, social, behavioral, genetic, pharmacologic, and age as factors influencing all elements of this system, together with the decrements in neurobehavioral performance and alertness that immediately follow the sleep-to-wake transition, a phenomenon called *sleep inertia*. The time course of sleep inertia has been shown to persist for up to 2 hours after a long sleep episode, and it is most profound within the first few minutes after awakening.[141,142] Although the final schema incorporates much of what is known about the roles of the circadian pacemaker and sleep homeostat in regulating sleep, it is not intended to completely represent all factors involved in the regulation of sleep, which is beyond the scope of this chapter. Nevertheless, its strength is its use in understanding the interplay between circadian and homeostatic drives and perhaps as a framework for initiating future scientific inquiry.

CLINICAL PEARL

Disruption of the circadian timing system by shift work, travel across time zones, and the activities of our round-the-clock society has an adverse effect on many physiologic variables, including hormones, glucose, metabolism, autonomic nervous system activity, the immune system, inflammation, neurobehavioral performance, and the propensity for, timing, and internal structure of sleep. This disruption can result in patient complaints of insomnia or excessive daytime sleepiness and can impair overall health.

SUMMARY

The circadian pacemaker interacts with sleep-wake regulatory processes to influence many physiologic variables: hormone levels, autonomic nervous system activity, neurobehavioral performance, and the propensity for and timing and internal structure of sleep. Environmental, social, behavioral, and genetic factors; pharmacologic agents; and age influence most elements of this system. Under ordinary circumstances, when people sleep at night in darkness and are awake in daylight, it is difficult to distinguish the relative contributions of the sleep homeostat and that of the circadian pacemaker to a given recurrent daily characteristic, symptom, or disorder of sleep or wakefulness (e.g., narcolepsy, delayed sleep phase syndrome). A pathologic event, such as a nocturnal seizure that occurs the same time each night, may be driven by the circadian pacemaker, the sleep homeostat, a specific sleep stage, or some combination of these processes. It is currently possible, although difficult, to experimentally dissociate these factors for research purposes (e.g., using the forced-desynchrony protocol in humans or suprachiasmatic lesions in animals). Clinically feasible techniques, such as measurement of dim-light salivary melatonin onset, can provide useful information about circadian phase.[143] Continued basic and clinical research is needed to assess the impact of the complex interaction of sleep and circadian rhythmicity on sleep disorders, such as insomnia, and overall health and well-being.

SELECTED READINGS

Anderson C, Sullivan JP, Flynn-Evans EE, et al. Deterioration of neurobehavioral performance in resident physicians during repeated exposure to extended duration work shifts. *Sleep.* 2012;35(8):1137–1146.

Buxton OM, Cain SW, O'Connor SP, et al. Adverse metabolic consequences in humans of prolonged sleep restriction combined with circadian disruption. *Sci Transl Med.* 2012;4(129):129–143.

Chang AM, Aeschbach D, Duffy JF, Czeisler CA. Evening use of light-emitting eReaders negatively affects sleep, circadian timing, and next-morning alertness. *Proc Natl Acad Sci U S A.* 2015;112(4):1232–1237.

Czeisler CA. Perspective: casting light on sleep deficiency. *Nature.* 2013;497(7450):S13.

Dijk DJ, Czeisler CA. Paradoxical timing of the circadian rhythm of sleep propensity serves to consolidate sleep and wakefulness in humans. *Neurosci Lett.* 1994;166(1):63–68.

McHill AW, Sano A, Hilditch CJ, et al. Robust stability of melatonin circadian phase, sleep metrics, and chronotype across months in young adults living in real-world settings. *J Pineal Res.* 2021;70(3):e12720.

Scheer FA, Hilton MF, Mantzoros CS, Shea SA. Adverse metabolic and cardiovascular consequences of circadian misalignment. *Proc Natl Acad Sci U S A.* 2009;106(11):4453–4458.

Smith-Coggins R, Broderick KB, Marco CA. Night shifts in emergency medicine: the American Board of Emergency Medicine longitudinal study of emergency physicians. *J Emerg Med.* 2014;47(3):372–378.

Wright Jr KP, McHill AW, Birks BR, et al. Entrainment of the human circadian clock to the natural light-dark cycle. *Curr Biol.* 2013;23(16):1554–1558.

A complete reference list can be found online at ExpertConsult.com.

Chapter 38

Sleep Homeostasis and Models of Sleep Regulation

Derk-Jan Dijk; Anne C. Skeldon

Chapter Highlights

- Homeostasis refers to regulatory processes that maintain physiologic systems in a stable state. The role of sleep in maintaining homeostasis and the extent to which sleep is under homeostatic control has been investigated by describing the phenomenology of sleep and by sleep deprivation experiments in which sleep duration is curtailed acutely, repeatedly, or in experiments in which specific aspects of sleep, such as rapid eye movement (REM) sleep or slow wave sleep (SWS), are restricted.
- During baseline sleep, slow waves in non–rapid eye movement (NREM) sleep decay in the course of sleep, and sleep spindle activity and REM sleep duration increase. These time courses and the time course of slow waves, in particular, are thought to reflect the completion of sleep-associated recovery processes.
- The first sign of a deviation from the homeostatic set point for sufficient sleep is an increase in sleepiness, that is, an increase in the drive to initiate sleep, as expected for a motivated behavior. Total and selective sleep deprivation experiments show that sleep duration, REM sleep, and slow wave sleep are all under precise homeostatic control. The expression of this homeostatic control is often curtailed by circadian processes or social factors.
- The homeostatic regulation of sleep interacts with the circadian regulation of sleep to shape the daily sleep-wake cycle and its structure such that the sleep recovery process is timed to preferentially occur during the biological night.
- Homeostatic regulation of slow wave activity (SWA) has been conjectured to play a key role in the sleep-associated recovery process. The dynamics of SWA have been captured in quantitative models and combined with the circadian regulation of sleep in the two-process model of sleep regulation. Other models have incorporated the alternation of NREM and REM sleep as well as the synchronization of the circadian oscillator to the 24-hour day by the light-dark cycle.
- The concept of, and mathematical models for, an interaction of sleep homeostasis and circadian rhythmicity has been successfully applied to explain a variety of sleep phenotypes ranging from polyphasic sleep in infants, later sleep in adolescents, and earlier and shorter sleep in older people. Models in which the homeostatic and circadian regulation of sleep are combined with the effect of light on circadian timing provide a quantitative understanding of the effects of access to electric light.
- Even though slow waves respond in a predictable manner to variations in sleep-wake history, local- and frequency-dependent differences in their time course challenge the notion of one single sleep homeostatic process. Aspects of sleep beyond SWA, such as REM sleep and total sleep duration, as well as sleep propensity, should be considered as relevant markers of sleep homeostasis. Models for the homeostatic and circadian regulation of sleep are yet to incorporate the homeostatic regulation of REM sleep, provide a quantitative account of sleep continuity, or provide an account of how sleep homeostatic processes map onto the effects of chronic sleep loss on waking performance and individual differences therein.
- Current and future models of the homeostatic and circadian regulation of sleep will inspire new experiments, provide new insights into sleep phenotypes in health and disease, and guide the development of new interventions to treat sleep timing disorders.

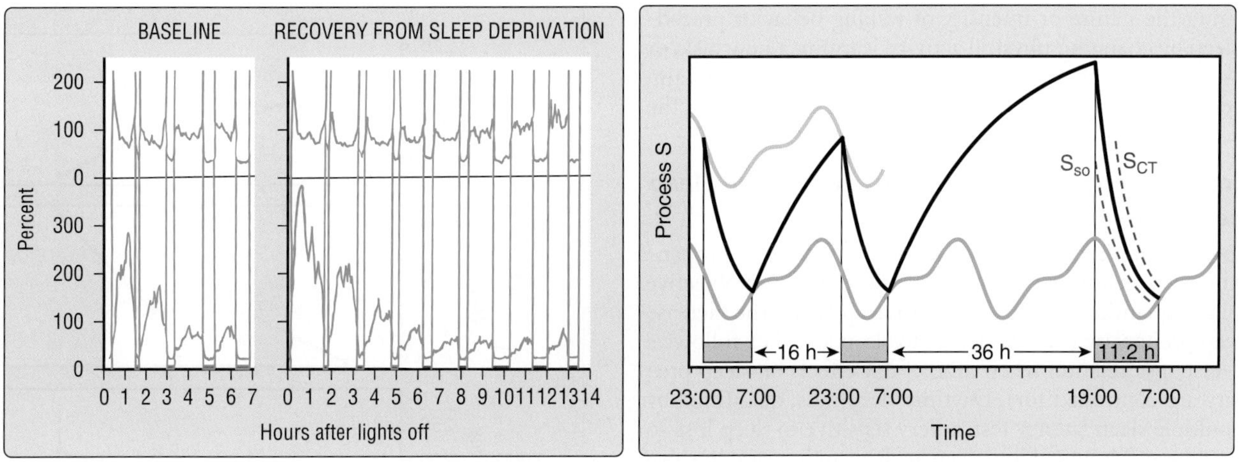

A B

Figure 38.1 **A,** Time course of slow wave activity (SWA; EEG power in the 0.75–4.5 Hz band; *lower curves*) and activity in the spindle frequency range (13.25–15.0 Hz; *upper curves*) recorded during baseline nocturnal sleep initiated at 11 p.m. and after 36 hours of wakefulness with recovery sleep initiated at 7 p.m. The timing of REM sleep episodes is delimited by *vertical lines* and *black bars* above the horizontal axis. **B,** Simulation of process S and the sleep and wake thresholds of the two-process model during a normal 8-hour sleep: 16-hour wakefulness cycle followed by a period of 36 hours of wakefulness (sleep deprivation) with recovery sleep initiated at 7 p.m. $S_{SO,}$ Time course of Process S during baseline plotted at the time of sleep onset during recovery. $S_{CT,}$ Time course of Process S during baseline plotted at the time of sleep onset during baseline. Please note that the time course of the data (panel **A**) shows that the time course of S and SWA is linked to sleep onset and not to clock time. (Reanalysis of data from Dijk DJ, Brunner DP, Borbély AA. Time course of EEG power density during long sleep in humans. *Am J Physiol.* 1990; 258:R650–61 by D. Aeschbach.)

HOMEOSTASIS

Homeostasis refers to the ability of an organism to maintain an internal biologic equilibrium through regulatory mechanisms.[1] Homeostasis can be demonstrated by driving the system away from a state of equilibrium and then monitoring the response of the system. The concept of homeostasis has been applied to sleep and incorporated in models for sleep regulation.[2]

Salient Sleep Phenomena and Homeostasis

Sleep has several important features, and the phenomenology of their dynamics during a nocturnal sleep episode may provide clues to their regulation and function. In the course of a nocturnal sleep episode, the duration of rapid eye movement (REM) sleep increases, while the duration of non–rapid eye movement (NREM) sleep episodes becomes shorter.[3,4] The duration of this ultradian NREM-REM cycle is rather constant with a period of approximately 70 to 100 minutes in adult humans. Brain activity within each NREM episode displays a typical time course: electroencephalography (EEG) slow waves, often quantified by spectral analysis and referred to as slow wave activity (SWA; EEG power density in the 0.75- to 4.5-Hz range) or period-amplitude analysis, increases for most of the NREM episode to then rapidly decline to low levels in REM sleep.[5,6] Superimposed on this ultradian pattern is a global decrease of SWA in the course of a nocturnal sleep episode, which, in standard sleep scoring, is reflected in the time course of slow wave sleep (SWS) and was described more than 80 years ago.[7] This dominance of SWA at the beginning of sleep, and its subsequent dissipation in the course of sleep, is often considered as evidence that SWA is closely related to a sleep-associated recovery process. Sleep spindle activity increases at the beginning of each NREM episode, is somewhat lower when SWA activity is high in the middle and second part of the NREM episode, and then rises again before it suddenly drops to low levels when REM sleep is initiated. Over the course of a nocturnal sleep episode, sleep spindle activity increases (Figure 38.1).[5,6]

Here we first present the experimental evidence for homeostatic regulation of some of sleep's essential features and in particular the regulation of SWA is presented. Next we describe how circadian rhythmicity affects these features and how homeostatic regulation interacts with circadian rhythmicity are described. Finally, we present conceptual and mathematical models for the homeostatic, circadian, and ultradian regulation of sleep.

Approaches to Investigate Sleep Homeostasis

Homeostatic regulation of sleep has been investigated primarily by depriving participants, be it humans or animals, from sleep. Here we focus mainly on human studies. Sleep deprivation can be "total," that is, 1 night without any sleep, or partial (e.g., 6 or 5, or 4 hours of sleep rather than 8 hours). Partial sleep deprivation may be imposed for 1 or several nights. Investigation of the homeostatic regulation of sleep can be extended to the substates of sleep, that is, NREM and REM sleep in selective sleep deprivation paradigms. REM sleep can be greatly reduced by awakening participants as soon as they enter REM sleep. This intervention is effective because reentry into sleep is primarily through NREM sleep. For the same reason, selective deprivation of NREM sleep is not possible. But it is feasible to deprive participants from sleep dominated by slow waves, that is, by not allowing SWA to fully develop within a NREM episode. This can be achieved by delivering acoustic or other stimuli that suppress slow waves without inducing wakefulness. Sleep fragmentation by administration of stimuli that trigger brief awakenings or arousals is another approach that may trigger homeostatic responses. Finally, sleep homeostatic mechanisms have been investigated by changing the nature or intensity of waking behavior preceding sleep by changing physical activity, learning a new task, or exposure to a novel environment. These latter approaches aim to identify which aspects of waking behavior contribute to the need for sleep.

Effects of Sleep Deprivation on Key Features of Sleep

Propensity to Initiate Sleep

Sleep deprivation leads to an increase in the drive or propensity for sleep as indexed by subjective sleepiness and objective sleepiness quantified by the latency to sleep onset. The increase in sleep propensity is proportional to sleep lost (i.e., follows a dose-response relation when time of day effects on sleep propensity are controlled for). Daytime sleepiness, quantified by the multiple sleep latency test, is very sensitive to sleep loss so that as few as 2 hours of lost sleep leads to an increase in sleep propensity, and repeated partial sleep deprivation leads to a progressive increase in sleep propensity.[8-11] In real-world studies the spontaneous night-to-night variation in sleep duration is associated with variation in self-reported sleepiness.[12] Sleep loss increases the drive for sleep, and sleepiness is an early and sensitive measure of insufficient sleep (Figure 38.2).

Sleep Duration

When sleep is initiated after total sleep deprivation, the duration of this recovery sleep is generally longer than normal, as expected for a variable under homeostatic control.

However, the duration of recovery sleep is much shorter than what one would predict if all lost sleep were recovered. Often cited examples include Randy Gardner's 11-day sleep deprivation "record,"[12a] which was followed by "two recovery sleep periods which were less than 15 and 11 hours long." In a sleep deprivation experiment, which was the basis of the two-process model (2-PM) of sleep regulation, sleep duration after 40 hours of wakefulness was only 20 minutes longer than baseline.[13] In other sleep deprivation experiments only 10% to 20% of lost sleep time was recovered. When sleep deprivation is induced by delaying the onset of sleep and recovery sleep is scheduled to occur during the daytime, recovery sleep duration may even be shorter than baseline.[14]

In many laboratory experiments the duration of recovery sleep is constrained by the design of the experiment (e.g., recording period was initiated at habitual bedtime limited to 8 hours). Studies in which constraints on recovery are minimized by using enforced bed rest periods after sleep deprivation demonstrate dose-response relations between sleep time recovered and sleep time lost. When participants are sleep deprived for 1 night, 71.6% of lost sleep time is recovered (Figure 38.2).[11,15]

Long-term studies of extended sleep opportunity provide additional evidence for homeostatic regulation of sleep duration.[16,17] In such studies, total sleep time is initially above the levels obtained during the participants' normal routine. After several days sleep duration levels off to approximately 8.9 hours per 24 hours in young adults. The interpretation of these data is that many people carry a sleep debt. When they are given ample sleep opportunity, that sleep debt is paid off by increasing sleep duration, but it takes several days for this homeostatic response to be completed.[18]

REM Sleep Duration

When the opportunity to recover from total sleep deprivation is not restricted by the experimental design, 82% of lost

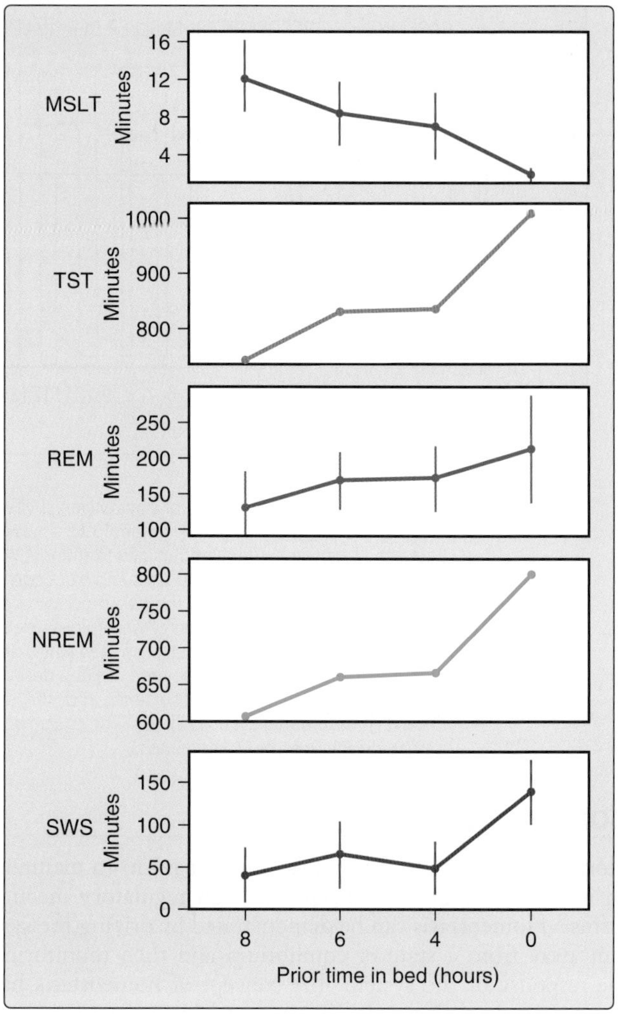

Figure 38.2 Effects of sleep loss (0, 8, 6, 4 hours) on subsequent sleep and sleepiness. In each participant, response to sleep loss was assessed twice; once to assess effects on the multiple sleep latency test (MLST) and once to assess effects on sleep duration and structure (i.e., total sleep time [TST]; rapid-eye movement sleep [REM]; non-rapid-eye movement sleep [NREM], slow wave sleep [SWS]). For the latter assessment, participants were "forced" to stay in bed for 24 hours. Note dose-response relations for all sleep parameters. (Based on data published in Rosenthal L, Roehrs TA, Rosen A, Roth T. Level of sleepiness and total sleep time following various time in bed conditions. *Sleep.* 1993;16:226–32.)

REM sleep is recovered, compared with 72% of recovery for total sleep time. The duration of REM sleep in recovery sleep is linearly related to the number of REM sleep minutes lost[15] (Figure 38.2). Repeated partial sleep deprivation experiments, which lead to a substantial loss of REM sleep, also provide evidence for homeostatic regulation of REM sleep such that during recovery sleep REM sleep duration and REM sleep expressed as a percentage of total sleep time is greater.[19,20] Further evidence for homeostatic regulation of REM sleep is derived from selective REM sleep deprivation experiments. REM sleep deprivation leads to an increase in REM sleep during subsequent recovery sleep.[21,22] The increase in REM sleep duration can be observed within a single sleep episode when REM sleep is suppressed only in the initial part of sleep.[23]

One salient feature of REM sleep deprivation experiments is that the number of awakenings required for preventing REM sleep increases in the course of a REM sleep deprivation night and across REM sleep deprivation nights. The increase in the number of required awakenings during REM sleep deprivation is interpreted as an increase in the drive for REM sleep.

Evidence for the homeostatic regulation of REM sleep is even stronger in rodents.[24] In rats and mice, almost all of lost REM sleep will be recovered, provided the period during which the recovery is monitored is sufficiently long (e.g., 24 hours or longer). The memory for an incurred REM sleep deficit can be carried over a period in which REM sleep is suppressed such that a physiologically induced REM sleep deficit acquired before suppression of REM sleep by antidepressants is fully recovered after the pharmacologic suppression has worn off.[25]

One particular question about the homeostatic regulation of REM sleep is, "Does REM sleep need increase during wakefulness, during NREM sleep, or both?" The current evidence favors the last option.

NREM Duration

In experiments in which there is opportunity for homeostasis for NREM time to be expressed and homeostatic regulation for total sleep time is observed, NREM time also displays a homeostatic response. In the first 24 hours of recovery, 69% of NREM time was reported to be recovered[15] (Figure 38.2).

Slow Wave Sleep and Slow Wave Activity within NREM Sleep

In humans the continuous NREM sleep process is subdivided into stages—N1, N2, and N3; N3 (or stage 3 and 4 in older sleep scoring schemes) is also referred to as SWS. Slow waves are abundant in N3 but are also present in N2. Slow waves have been quantified by various signal analysis approaches that can assess the amplitude, number, or intensity of slow waves.[26] SWA, derived from spectral analysis of the EEG based on the Fourier transform, is another frequently used measure.[13] When participants undergo total sleep deprivation and the recovery sleep opportunity is not restricted, all manually quantified SWS time lost is recovered; this recovery is completed early in the recovery period.[15] When the recovery period is restricted to the duration of baseline sleep, recovery sleep is enriched with SWS (i.e., there are more minutes of SWS). Slow waves quantified as SWA or number or amplitude of delta waves are enhanced.[13,27,28] Thus the spectral composition of the EEG in NREM sleep changes such that SWA increases after total sleep deprivation, even though time in NREM does not markedly change. This increase is, however, short lasting (Figure 38.1). Similar observations have been made in rodents.[29,30]

In humans, naps occurring progressively later in the day contain more SWS and SWA.[31,32] This, together with the observation that SWA declines in the course of sleep, is consistent with the notions that (1) the drive for slow waves builds progressively during wakefulness and then dissipates during sleep and that (2) slow wave measures are a marker for a homeostatic process. This concept is further supported by the observation that after a nap during the day, and in particular naps in the late afternoon, less SWA is observed in the subsequent nocturnal sleep episode[33,34] (Figure 38.3).

Suppression of SWA in the initial part of sleep, without inducing wakefulness, is followed by a rebound of SWA in the undisturbed remaining part of the sleep episode.[35,36] When

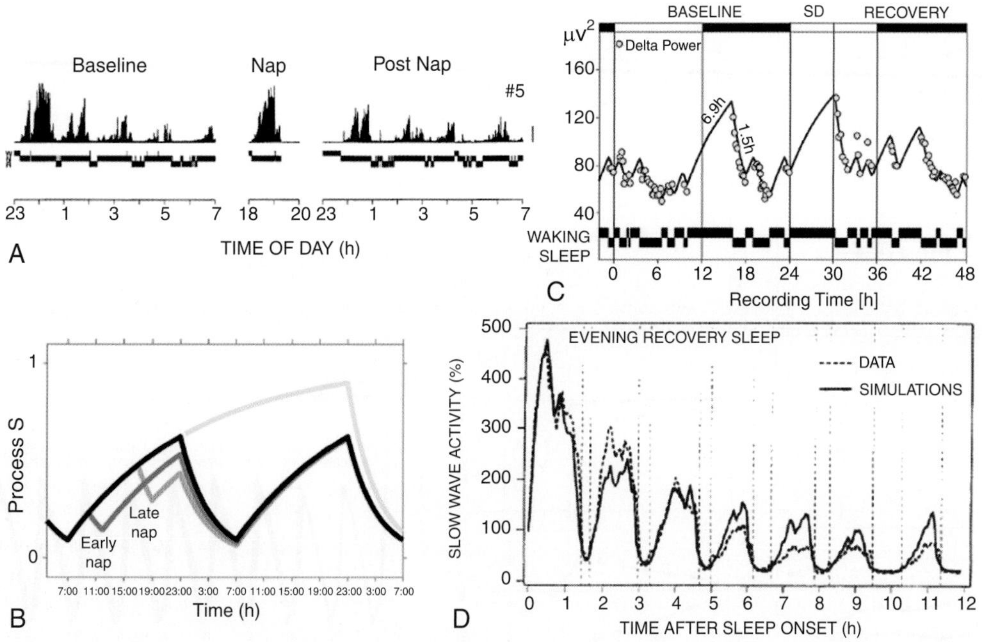

Figure 38.3 A, Slow wave activity (SWA) during baseline sleep, an early evening nap and sleep after the nap in a single human participant. SWA in an evening nap is at levels similar to the beginning of a nocturnal sleep episode. SWA in nocturnal sleep after the nap is much lower than during baseline. Please note the longer sleep latency in the postnap sleep episode. **B,** Simulation of the time course of Process S during a 16-hour wake 8-hour sleep cycle (*black line*) during a 40-hour sleep deprivation (*grey line*) and during and after an early nap or a late nap. After a late nap S is much lower than baseline and also lower than after an early nap. **C,** Time course of SWA, here referred to as delta activity (*yellow*), in a single mouse. SWA during sleep is higher after longer spontaneous wake episodes (e.g., during the dark period) and after sleep deprivation. This time course can be simulated (*blue line*) by exponential saturation functions during wakefulness (time constant 6.9 hours) and an exponentially declining function (time constant 1.5 hours). **D,** Simulation of the ultradian time course of SWA during recovery sleep from 36 hours of sleep deprivation (Figure 38.1). (A: Data from Werth E, Dijk DJ, Achermann P, Borbély AA. Dynamics of the sleep EEG after an early evening nap: experimental data and simulations. *Am J Physiol.* 1996;271:R501–10; C: data from Franken P, Chollet D, Taft M. The homeostatic regulation of sleep need is under genetic control. *J Neurosci.* 2001;21[8]:2610–21; D: data from Achermann P, Dijk DJ, Brunner DP, Borbély AA. A model of human sleep homeostasis based on EEG slow wave activity: quantitative comparison of data and simulations. *Brain Res Bull.* 1993;31:97–113.)

SWS/SWA disruption is continued for the entire sleep episode or continued for 2 or more consecutive nights, SWS/SWA during the next undisturbed recovery night is above baseline.[37,38] This implies that SWA is more than just a marker but actually is related to the core of the homeostatic process controlling slow wave propensity.

In some settings, SWA may relate to the drive or propensity to initiate sleep. In nocturnal sleep episodes after a late afternoon nap, the latency to sleep onset is longer than at baseline.[33] When SWA is suppressed during a nocturnal sleep episode, sleep propensity during the subsequent waking day is greater.[39] These findings support the notions that SWA is related to sleep propensity and that SWA is involved in a sleep-associated recovery process.

The changes in SWA in response to time awake and time asleep have been interpreted as an increase in the "intensity" of sleep; these led to the view that lost sleep can be made up, at least in part, by an increase in its intensity.[40]

Partial sleep deprivation always removes the last part of a sleep episode and therefore primarily leads to a loss of light NREM sleep (N1, N2), that is, NREM sleep with little SWA, SWS, and REM sleep. Loss of SWA is also limited but more pronounced than loss of SWS because N2 also contains SWA.

During and after partial sleep deprivation SWS and SWA are only marginally increased or not increased at all[20,41] (Figure 38.4). Despite the absent or small increase of SWA after repeated partial sleep deprivation, daytime sleep propensity is noticeably augmented, and waking performance deteriorates progressively and dissociates from SWS and SWA.[10,20,42]

Thus SWA in NREM sleep exhibits a very predictable relation with sleep-wake history even within a "physiologic" range of wake durations typical in everyday life in both humans and rodents. This time course may, however, not parallel the functional capacity of the waking brain.

Local Occurrence and Local Homeostatic Regulation of Slow Wave Activity

Traditionally, sleep regulation and sleep homeostasis were considered global brain processes. However, slow waves can occur locally in both humans and rodents, and this may imply local sleep and local sleep homeostasis.[43,44] In the context of sleep regulation these phenomena have been linked to a "use dependency" hypothesis.[45] According to this concept, a neural network that is used intensively during wakefulness will build up a higher sleep need, be more likely to fall asleep, and sleep more intensely than a network that is used less extensively during wakefulness.[46]

Sleep Spindle Activity

Sleep spindles are a prominent hallmark of NREM sleep, and total sleep deprivation will lead to a loss of sleep spindles. Sleep spindle activity or EEG activity in the frequency range of sleep spindles after total or repeated partial sleep deprivation is not enhanced. In fact, in experiments in which the duration of recovery sleep was limited, the density of sleep spindles and sleep spindle activity are reduced.[5] Although on the basis of these sleep deprivation experiments one may conclude that sleep spindles are not under homeostatic regulation,

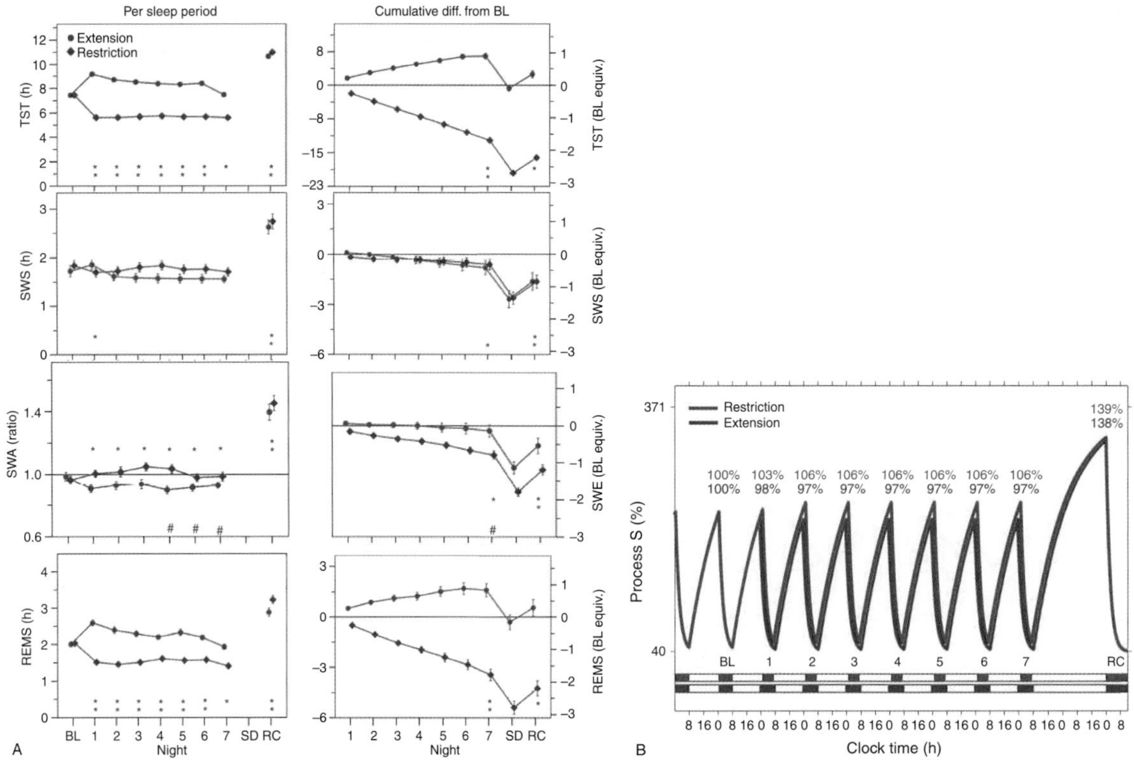

Figure 38.4 Effects of 7 nights of sleep restriction (6 hours' time in bed [TIB]) and sleep extension (10 hours' TIB) and subsequent total sleep deprivation (39 to 41 hours' wakefulness) on total sleep time (TST), slow wave sleep (SWS), slow wave activity (SWA), and REM sleep (REMS). Data are presented per sleep period and as cumulative difference from baseline and expressed in hours, ratio of baseline, and baseline equivalents. BL, Baseline. SWE = SWA × NREM time. *: significant difference from baseline; # significant difference from simulation. (Modified from Skorucak J, Arbon EL, Dijk DJ, Achermann P. Response to chronic sleep restriction, extension, and subsequent total sleep deprivation in humans: adaptation or preserved sleep homeostasis? *Sleep.* 2018;41[7].)

sleep spindle activity increases in the course of a nocturnal sleep episode. This could be interpreted as a sleep-dependent (homeostatic) regulation of spindles such that when the recovery process nears its completion, sleep spindles are abundant.

The NREM-REM Cycle

Whereas sleep deprivation, whether total, partial, or selective, leads to changes in SWA and REM time, there is little evidence in either humans or rodents that any of these interventions fundamentally affect the periodicity of the alternation between NREM and REM sleep. However, reducing sleep pressure through, for example, a nap, may shorten the latency to REM onset.[33] In the course of the night or after sleep deprivation the time spent in NREM and REM sleep alters, but the periodic process that drives the alternation of the NREM-REM cycles is not markedly perturbed by homeostatic manipulations. The NREM-REM cycle is initiated at sleep onset and is not a continuation of a basic-rest activity cycle, which continues during wakefulness and sleep. The cycle is reset by awakenings, provided that they are sufficiently long.

This implies that the homeostatic regulation of SWA and REM duration occurs within the constraints of the periodic NREM-REM cycle.

CIRCADIAN RHYTHMICITY AND THE REGULATION OF PHYSIOLOGY AND BEHAVIOR

The concept of homeostasis has been very successful in guiding research on the mechanisms governing the regulation of physiology and behavior, but unexpected periodic changes in behavior and physiology challenged the view that it was the only regulatory process.

Sleep for a long time has been viewed as an exclusively homeostatically regulated system, but several observations challenge a simple homeostatic model.[47] For example, the correlation between the duration of sleep or rest and the duration of the prior wake or activity period is negative rather than positive, as would be expected based on a homeostatic mechanism.

Although circadian regulation, which, for example, curtails the duration of recovery sleep after extended wakefulness, may at first seem to challenge homeostatic regulation, it can be reconciled with this concept. Homeostasis as observed in sleep deprivation experiments can be described as reactive homeostasis (i.e., an adaptive response to an unanticipated perturbation brought about by unexpected events). By contrast, circadian rhythmicity can be conceptualized as predictive homeostasis (i.e., preparing the organism for challenges of homeostasis by environmental factors, which predictably reoccur within a 24-hour period and are driven by the Earth's rotation around its axis and the 24-hour societal day-night cycle).[48] Circadian rhythmicity can be seen to function as an adaptive mechanism by which homeostatic responses are gated to the appropriate time of day.

Key Characteristic of the Circadian Regulation of Sleep

The most fundamental description of the circadian regulation of human sleep timing and duration was obtained in experiments conducted in the second half of the 20th century, in which participants were studied in isolation from the external world, including the natural light-dark cycle and time cues such as clocks.[49,50] The participants were free to select when to sleep. Under these conditions the sleep-wake cycle persists but is no longer synchronized to the 24-hour day. In most participants sleep duration is similar to normal, but sleep onset drifted progressively later. This demonstrates the existence of an internal oscillatory process with a period that deviates from 24 hours and is now estimated to be 24 hours and 9 minutes with a standard deviation of 12 minutes.[51]

Under normal conditions this oscillator is synchronized to the 24-hour day by the light-dark cycle. The timing of the endogenous clock relative to the 24-hour day depends on the strength of the light-dark cycle and the intrinsic period of the individual circadian pacemaker.[52] In time isolation studies, several participants display a sleep-wake cycle with a period that is on average much, much longer, and in some individuals shorter, than 24 hours, while at the same time core body temperature and urine production continue to oscillate with a period close to 24 hours. This phenomenon is referred to as spontaneous (internal) desynchrony. These observations suggest that the sleep-wake cycle represents an oscillatory process that is, to some extent, separable from the circadian oscillator driving rhythms in other physiologic variables. These observations led to models in which the sleep-wake cycle was governed by two oscillatory processes.

During spontaneous desynchrony the duration and structure of sleep episodes are to a significant extent determined by the circadian phase at which sleep episodes are initiated rather than by the duration of wakefulness. Sleep duration is shortest when it is initiated near the nadir of core body temperature. Sleep is rarely initiated at some phases of the core body temperature rhythm, and this phase is referred to as the wake maintenance zone.[53] Propensity for REM sleep is strongly modulated by circadian phase such that sleep is enriched for REM sleep when it occurs just after the nadir of the core body temperature rhythm (i.e., close to habitual wake time). SWS declines in all sleep episodes independent of circadian phase.[54]

Separation and Comparison of Homeostatic and Circadian Influence on Sleep

Under the assumption that sleep is governed by two oscillatory processes (i.e., the two processes of sleep, or the sleep homeostat and circadian rhythmicity), it becomes pertinent to quantify their separate contributions. Quantification of the separate contribution of sleep homeostasis (S) and circadian rhythmicity (C) requires that a large range of homeostatic sleep pressure values and circadian phase values are available. During a normal sleep-wake cycle the circadian and homeostatic process change simultaneously, and only very few of all possible combinations of circadian phase and time awake or time asleep are realized. In forced-desynchrony experiments sleep timing is not spontaneous, but participants are "forced" to a sleep-wake cycle with noncircadian periods such as 20 or 28 hours. When these experiments are conducted in dim light, the central circadian pacemaker driving the rhythms of many physiologic variables, including core body temperature, cortisol, and melatonin oscillates at its near 24-hour intrinsic period, and sleep and wake now occur at all circadian phases[55,56] (Figure 38.5).

In forced desynchrony protocols a large range of combinations of S and C are realized. By assigning an S and C value to the repeated assessments of sleep, EEG, alertness, sleepiness, or performance, we can now separate the circadian and sleep-wake dependent influences and document their interaction.

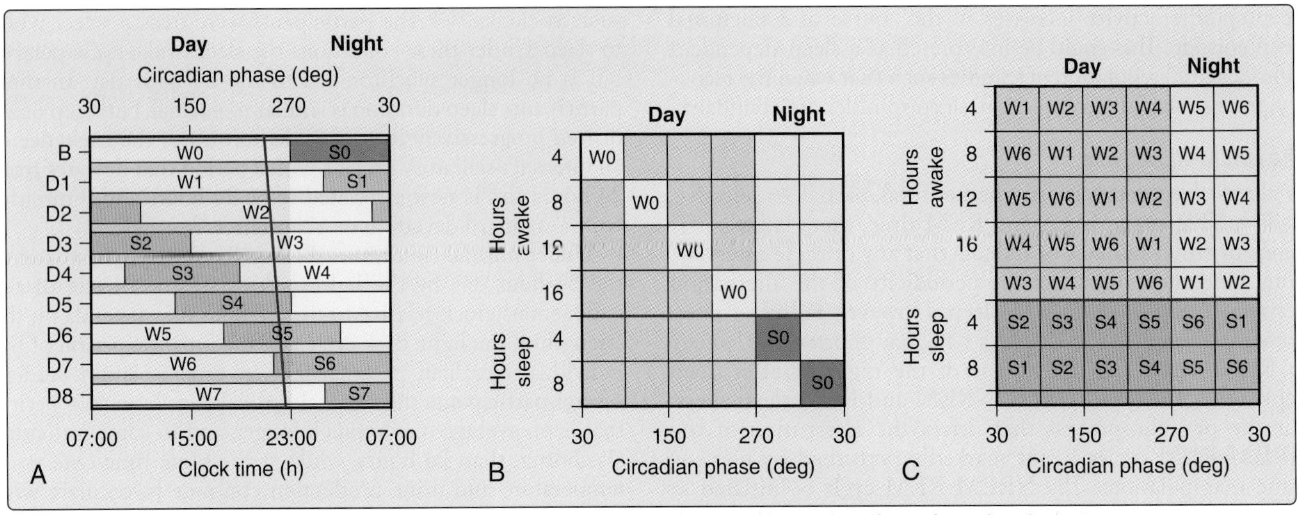

Figure 38.5 The forced desynchrony protocol is designed to separate out the effects of circadian rhythmicity and sleep homeostasis by imposing a sleep-wake cycle that is either shorter or longer than 24 hours. A typical forced desynchrony protocol for a sleep-wake cycle of 28 hours is illustrated in **(A)** for an individual with a habitual wake time of 7:00 and bedtime of 23:00. After one 24-hour baseline period of one wake episode (W0) of 16 hours and one sleep episode (S0) of 8 hours, there follows at least 7 days in which wake is extended to 18 hours, 40 minutes (labeled W1 to W7), and sleep is extended to 9 hours, 20 minutes (labeled S1 to S7). This maintains a wake-sleep ratio of 2:1. During baseline, wake occurs during the subjective day and sleep occurs during the subjective night and are entrained to the 24-hour day-night cycle so only occur at selected circadian phases. This is illustrated in **(B),** where baseline wake/sleep are represented by the diagonal light-/dark-colored squares. The forced desynchrony protocol results in wake and sleep episodes that occur at all circadian phases, as shown in **(C).** Circadian phase is expressed here as circadian degrees relative to the core body temperature nadir (0 degrees).

Quantification of the circadian aspects of sleep regulation in these forced desynchrony experiments confirmed and extended the findings from spontaneous desynchrony studies.[57,58] In particular it was found that sleep propensity is lowest just before the onset of nocturnal melatonin secretion (i.e., close to the time of habitual sleep onset), and highest just after the nadir of core body temperature (i.e., close to habitual wake time). The circadian pacemaker promotes wakefulness during the biological day when body temperature rises and plasma melatonin levels are low, and the strongest circadian drive for wakefulness occurs in the wake maintenance zone, which under entrained conditions is located in the evening hours just before the onset of nocturnal melatonin secretion (Figure 38.6). The circadian pacemaker promotes sleep during the biological night and most strongly so near the temperature nadir, which under normal conditions occurs in the early morning hours at approximately 5 to 6 a.m. This paradoxical timing of the circadian sleep propensity rhythm serves to consolidate sleep and wakefulness.[59] However, when the sleep-wake cycle is displaced, such as in night shift work, and sleep now occurs during the daytime, it will be short and fragmented.

None of these analyses provide evidence for an increase in circadian sleep propensity in the afternoon (the siesta phase).

Circadian regulation of sleep is not limited to propensity and sleep structure. Circadian regulation of EEG activity during sleep is prominent for sleep spindle activity and observed for alpha activity in REM sleep.[60] SWA and characteristics of slow wave, such as their slope, decline in the course of sleep episodes initiated at all circadian phases but are also, to some extent, modulated by circadian phase[57] (Figure 38.6).

Body temperature is affected by the circadian cycle and the sleep-wake cycle; REM sleep is under circadian control but also becomes progressively disinhibited as sleep progresses. Spindle activity increases with time asleep and is promoted by circadian process in the beginning of the biological night (Figure 38.6). Detailed analyses of the EEG during NREM, REM, and wakefulness illustrate the predominance of sleep-wake influence on low frequency activity, such as slow wave and theta activity, and predominance of circadian influences on sleep spindle activity and alpha activity.[60,61]

Interaction of Homeostasis and Circadian Rhythmicity: Effects on Amplitude of Overt Circadian Rhythmicity

Analyses of the propensity to wake up as a simultaneous function of time awake and circadian phase show how the circadian amplitude to wake up is dependent on sleep pressure. When sleep pressure is high, the circadian amplitude of the propensity to wake up is small, but this amplitude grows as homeostatic sleep pressure dissipates. A similar dependency of overt circadian amplitude on homeostatic sleep pressure is present for a range of variables, including REM sleep expressed as a percentage of total sleep time, sleep spindle activity, and SWA.[55] This implies that the homeostatic and circadian processes do not simply add up but that they interact (nonadditive). This nonadditive interaction extends to aspects of the waking brain, such as the EEG during wakefulness and performance.[62] Thus the circadian deterioration of waking performance during the biological night is only modest when sleep pressure is low, but very substantial when sleep pressure is high. This has important implications for the assessment of risks associated with shift work. For example, working at 6 a.m. in the morning is relatively safe when the worker has been awake for only a few hours and homeostatic sleep pressure is low but dangerous when the worker has been awake for 20 hours and therefore homeostatic sleep pressure is high.

The interaction of acute time awake and circadian phase also interacts with accumulated chronic sleep debt as demonstrated in an extensive experiment in which chronic sleep

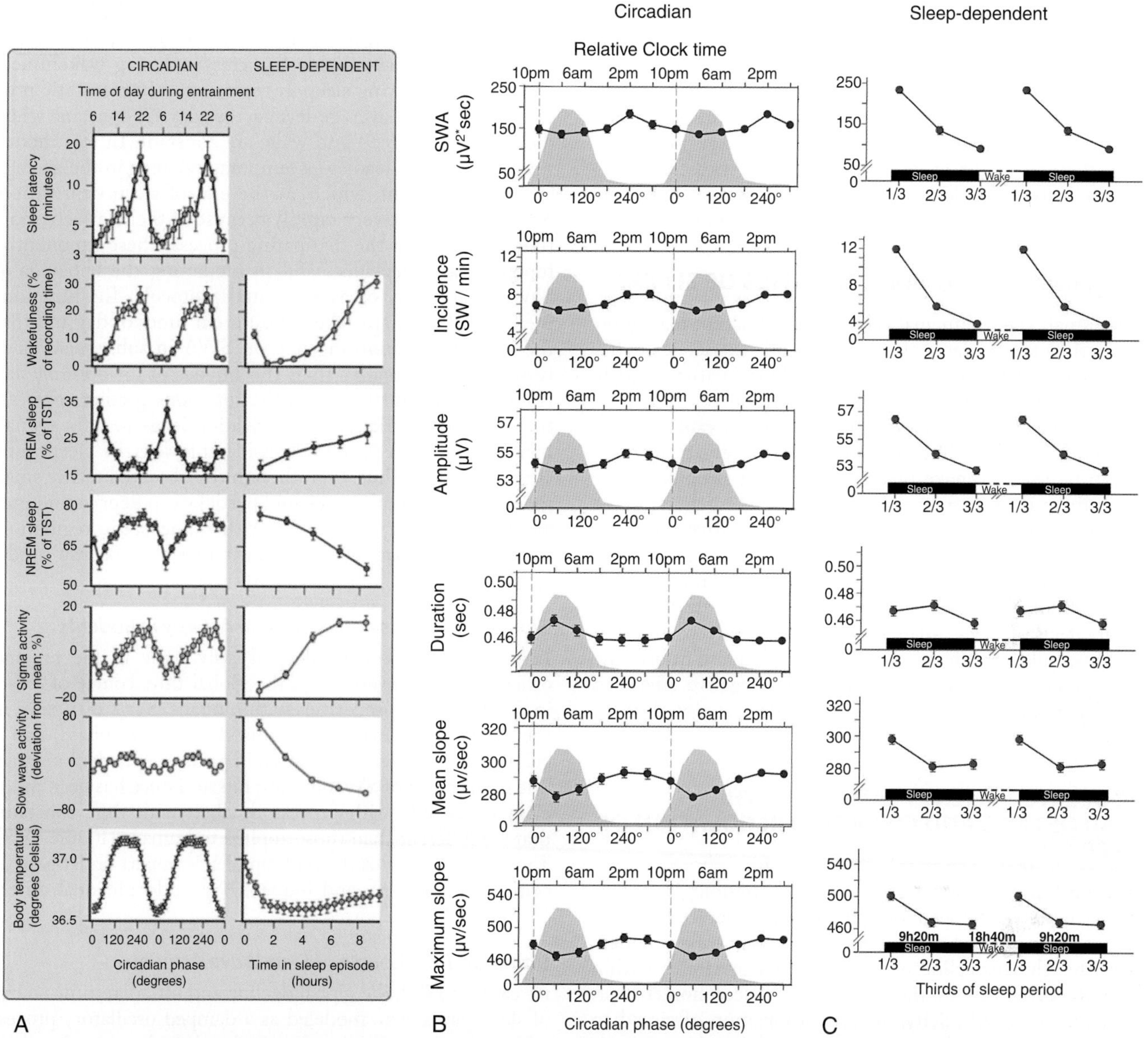

Figure 38.6 Circadian and sleep-dependent aspects of sleep structure and slow wave (SW) characteristics. **(A)** Circadian and sleep-dependent or homeostatic factors in sleep regulation. The main effects of circadian phase and sleep homeostasis on sleep were analyzed by aligning the data relative to the circadian component of the body temperature cycle (*left panels*) or the beginning of the sleep opportunity (*right panels*). Slow wave activity (SWA) shows weak circadian and strong sleep-dependent modulation; sigma (sleep spindle) activity shows strong circadian and sleep-dependent modulation. NREM sleep percentage shows equal circadian and sleep-dependent components. REM sleep percentage shows a marked circadian maximum just after the temperature nadir and sleep-dependent increase (disinhibition). Wakefulness in scheduled sleep episodes shows that the circadian drive for wakefulness is a maximum of 7 to 9 hours before temperature nadir, which is 1 to 3 hours before habitual bedtime; there is a strong wake-dependent increase. Sleep latency shows strong circadian modulation; the longest sleep latencies occur 7 to 9 hours before the body temperature nadir, and the shortest sleep latencies occur at the body temperature nadir. TST, Total sleep time. Circadian **(B)** and sleep-dependent **(C)** regulation of SWA, incidence of slow waves, amplitude of slow waves, duration of slow waves, and the mean and maximum slope of slow waves during a 28-hour forced desynchrony protocol. Data are plotted relative to the onset of melatonin (= 0 degrees). Please note circadian regulation of sleep wave characteristic with higher values during the biologic day (i.e., when melatonin is low) for SWA, incidence, amplitude, and slopes but lower values for their duration. (A: modified from Dijk DJ, Czeisler CA. Contribution of the circadian pacemaker and the sleep homeostat to sleep propensity, sleep structure, electroencephalographic slow waves and sleep spindle activity in humans. *J Neurosci.* 1995;15:3526–38; B: modified from Dijk DJ, Czeisler CA. Paradoxical timing of the circadian rhythm of sleep propensity serves to consolidate sleep and wakefulness in humans. *Neurosci Lett.* 1994;166:63–8; Lazar AS, Lazar ZI, Dijk DJ. Circadian regulation of slow waves in human sleep: Topographical aspects. *Neuroimage.* 2015;116:123–34.)

restriction was combined with forced desynchrony.[63] This interaction is such that at the beginning of a waking day, effects of chronic sleep restriction are minor, as if the immediately preceding sleep is of sufficient duration to complete recovery. However, as the waking period progresses, the latent effects of sleep restriction emerge and become very prominent when the end of the wake period coincides with the circadian night. Thus the sleep homeostatic process has a profound impact on the overt amplitude of circadian rhythmicity.

WHY MODEL KEY CHARACTERISTICS OF SLEEP?

Conceptual and mathematical models of sleep regulation summarize accumulated knowledge and extract essential principles underlying empirical facts. Quantitative models also test whether our understanding of phenomena as formulated in conceptual frameworks is sufficient to explain these phenomena quantitatively. Quantitative mathematical models can be used to make predictions even in sleep scenarios where there is no current data, facilitating the generation of testable hypotheses and the design of quantitative interventions. Ultimately, models for sleep regulation should help us to understand sleep phenotypes, treat sleep disturbances, and design physical and social environments to maximize the beneficial effects of sleep. Quantitative models on sleep, circadian rhythms, and their effects on waking function also inform the development of policies to minimize the negative effects of insufficient and mistimed sleep such as associated with work schedules.

MODELING SALIENT FEATURES OF THE HOMEOSTATIC AND CIRCADIAN REGULATION OF SLEEP

Here we consider mathematical or neurophysiologic models that have been developed for only a few key characteristics of sleep: the timing and duration of sleep, the processes underlying the global decline of SWA and its dynamics within NREM sleep episodes, the interaction of sleep homeostasis and circadian rhythmicity, the synchronization of circadian clocks by light, as well as the interaction of sleep homeostasis and the alternation between NREM and REM sleep.

Modeling Slow Wave Activity

Global Time Course of Slow Wave Activity in Humans as an Indicator of a Homeostatic Process

The global dissipation of SWA during sleep and its buildup during wakefulness have been modeled by fitting functions to baseline and recovery from total sleep deprivation data.[13,27,64] Dissipation is estimated to be exponential, and the buildup can be described as an exponential saturating curve. SWA is a measure related to the square of the amplitude of slow waves. This implies that if amplitude changes linearly with time asleep, power will change exponentially.

Implications of the exponential, rather than linear, functions are that the pressure for SWA builds up very fast at the beginning of a wake episode, and this increase becomes progressively smaller with longer time awake. Likewise, the dissipation of SWA is very fast at the beginning of a sleep episode, and then this dissipation proceeds at a slower rate. SWA reaches asymptotic levels at the end of long sleep episodes (Figure 38.1). The functions describing the time course of global SWA are hypothesized to reflect Process S (sometimes referred to as sleep pressure, or H, for homeostat), in which the variable S increases during wakefulness and dissipates during sleep. It represents a homeostatic process such that its average level across days is constant when the duration of sleep and wake are constant. In this model, sleep deprivation leads to a temporary change in the average level of sleep debt, which, at the end of sleep deprivation, reverts to baseline very rapidly because of the relatively short time constants of the dissipating process. These exponential functions are very successful in predicting the behavior of SWA in a variety of experimental protocols. The functions predict SWA in naps taken at different times of day and that the impact of a morning nap on SWA in subsequent nocturnal sleep is smaller than the impact of an evening nap (Figure 38.3). Furthermore, the functions predict correctly that repeated partial sleep deprivation leads to only a small increase in SWA despite considerable loss of sleep time (Figure 38.4).[20] Thus, even though the observed rather small increase in SWA after repeated partial sleep deprivation may at first glance be at variance with homeostatic regulation, they are consistent with a quantitative homeostatic model of SWA.

Global Time Course of Slow Wave Activity in Rodents

In contrast to humans, sleep is polyphasic in the rat and other rodents. Nevertheless, the global time course of SWA in the rat shows similarities with humans. SWA dissipates in the course of the major sleep episode (the light phase) and is enhanced after sleep deprivation in a dose-dependent manner. The time course of SWA in both rats and mice has been modeled successfully with process S, albeit with time constants that are different than those applied to humans (Figure 38.3). The time constant of the buildup of S is in part under genetic control in animals[65] and humans,[66,67] and individual differences have been reported.[68]

Ultradian Time Course of Slow Wave Activity

As early as 1972, the global decline and ultradian time course of slow waves were modeled as a damped oscillatory process with parameters that were posited to be related to the dissipation of sleep need.[69] More recently, the dynamics of SWA within a NREM episode have been modeled using an extension of the model for the global time course of SWA.[70] In this ultradian model, S denotes the global time course of SWA and is assumed to always increase during REM sleep and wake and decrease during NREM sleep. SWA denotes the short-term dynamics and increases during REM sleep and wakefulness. During NREM, the rise rate of SWA initially is determined by S, and S declines in proportion to SWA produced. For quantitative comparison with data, the timing of the onset and offset of REM sleep is determined from the experiment.

This model successfully reproduces the time course of SWA during very long recovery sleep episodes initiated in the evening (Figure 38.3), as well as the occurrence of high levels of SWA at the very end of very long extended baseline sleep episodes, which terminate in the late morning.[71] This model of the ultradian dynamics of SWA has some resemblance to models based on the synaptic homeostasis hypothesis for the function of sleep (see later) and neurophysiologic models, which emphasize the impact of neuromodulators on the synchronization of the EEG in the various vigilance states.[72] The maximum level of SWA within an NREM episode is determined by a homeostatically regulated process such as synaptic strength, but the dynamics of the EEG are determined by the neuromodulator environment, which varies across the NREM-REM cycle (Figure 38.7).

Challenges for Models Linking Slow Wave Activity to Sleep Homeostasis

Although SWA and its time course are often considered quantitative indicators of the sleep homeostatic process, there are a number of challenges to this view.

Analyses of the topography of the dissipation of SWA have shown that the time constants of the decay of SWA vary across brain regions.[73-75] This implies that various brain networks may display a differential sleep need/sleep pressure and fall asleep and recover at different rates. Analyses of the time course of oscillations within the low-frequency range show that the time constants for the decay during sleep and buildup during wakefulness are frequency dependent.[31,76] SWA power density in the 0.75- to 4.5-Hz range is the modeled range, but other frequencies such as those representing the slow oscillation (<1 Hz) or theta activity have time constants for the buildup during wakefulness and dissipation during sleep very different from the time constants of SWA. Even within the 0.74- to 4.5-Hz range the time constants are not identical. Thus the frequency range included in the quantitative description of the homeostatic process affects the parameters of the observed dynamics. This heterogeneity of slow waves and differential response to sleep manipulations has been documented by quantitative evaluation of slow waves by spectral analysis and other approaches. The very low frequency slow waves, which may represent the slow oscillation to which important functions have been attributed, do not increase after sleep deprivation, and the decline in the course of a sleep episode appears to be more linear rather than exponential as has been observed for slow waves with a higher frequency.[76,77]

Changes in the homeostatic process are thought to be reflected primarily in changes in SWA in response to sleep manipulations rather than in the absolute values of SWA and individual differences therein.[75] This emphasis on changes in SWA implies that characterization of the homeostatic process always requires a "manipulation." In fact, because the functions describing the process are nonlinear, at least three data points are needed to estimate parameters, and one simple sleep deprivation cannot be used to make inferences about the homeostatic process.

The model based on the dynamics of SWA has also been taken to reflect the dynamics of other aspects of sleep regulation and brain function, such as sleep propensity, alertness, and psychomotor vigilance performance. Comparison of the time course of performance decrements observed in partial sleep deprivation experiments indicate that the time course of SWA can dissociate from the time course of performance deficits, in particular tasks probing vigilant attention.[10,20,42,78] This implies that not all recovery processes during sleep are adequately represented by the time constants derived from the time course of SWA.

Models of SWA assume the dynamics of SWA are independent of circadian phase. However, initial values of SWA and characteristics of slow waves such as their slope and amplitude are, in fact, to some extent modulated by circadian phase[55,57] (Figure 38.6).

In summary, models for SWA are only models for SWA, but within that restricted context, the models perform very well.

Combining the Model for Slow Wave Activity Homeostasis with the Circadian Regulation of Sleep: The Two-Process Model of Sleep Regulation

The 2-PM of sleep regulation is a very influential model that can reproduce a wide range of experimental observations and has inspired many new experiments.[40,79,80] The 2-PM unifies observations that support homeostatic regulation of sleep with observations that also indicate circadian regulation of sleep and observations that sleep timing appears to be governed by two oscillatory processes. In essence the model posits that sleep timing is governed by a homeostatic process, or hourglass oscillator, driven by sleep wake behavior and that the points at which the hourglass turns are determined by thresholds that are modulated by a circadian oscillator.

Qualitative versions of the 2-PM were developed by Alexander Borbély to explain observations on sleep and SWA in sleep deprivation experiments in rats.[81]

Subsequent qualitative and quantitative versions of the 2-PM were developed for human sleep timing by Borbély, Daan, and Beersma.[40,80] Data sets that played a central role in the development of the 2-PM for human sleep timing were studies describing the effects of sleep deprivation on SWA, a study describing the duration of sleep in a protocol in which sleep onset was delayed by 4, 8, 12, 16, 20, and 24 hours, and subsequent recovery sleep was terminated by spontaneous awakening,[14] as well as spontaneous desynchrony studies conducted in Germany by Aschoff, Wever, and Zulley.[82]

Purely homeostatic models of sleep timing would suggest that sleep duration increases with time awake, and purely circadian models for sleep timing would predict a fixed end point of sleep (i.e., awakening) independent of time awake (Figure 38.8). The combination of the two processes predicts a waveform in which with increasing wake extension there is initially a reduction of recovery sleep duration, followed by a sudden increase in sleep duration followed by a subsequent decline, as observed in the empirical data. A model in which a homeostatic process oscillates between two thresholds that are modulated by circadian phase can replicate this fundamental phenomenon (Figure 38.8). Key parameters of the model are the buildup and dissipation of process S with time constants based on SWA. The amplitude and waveform of the thresholds were chosen to match sleep duration data from the delayed sleep study. The average level of the thresholds relative to the 0-1 scale of the Process S were chosen to account for the average sleep duration.

In the original formulation the model did not adequately describe sleep duration around the wake maintenance zone and did not match observations on sleep duration and sleep propensity in forced desynchrony experiments. In current versions of the model as shown in Figure 38.8, the wake- and sleep-onset thresholds are skewed to the right. The timing of the maximum values of these thresholds reflects the wake maintenance zone which, under entrained conditions, coincides with the evening hours. At this circadian phase the circadian process strongly opposes the homeostatic process and thereby allows the individual to be awake and alert despite high homeostatic sleep drive. One interpretation of the functional benefits of the phase relationship between the homeostatic and circadian process, which is such that we normally

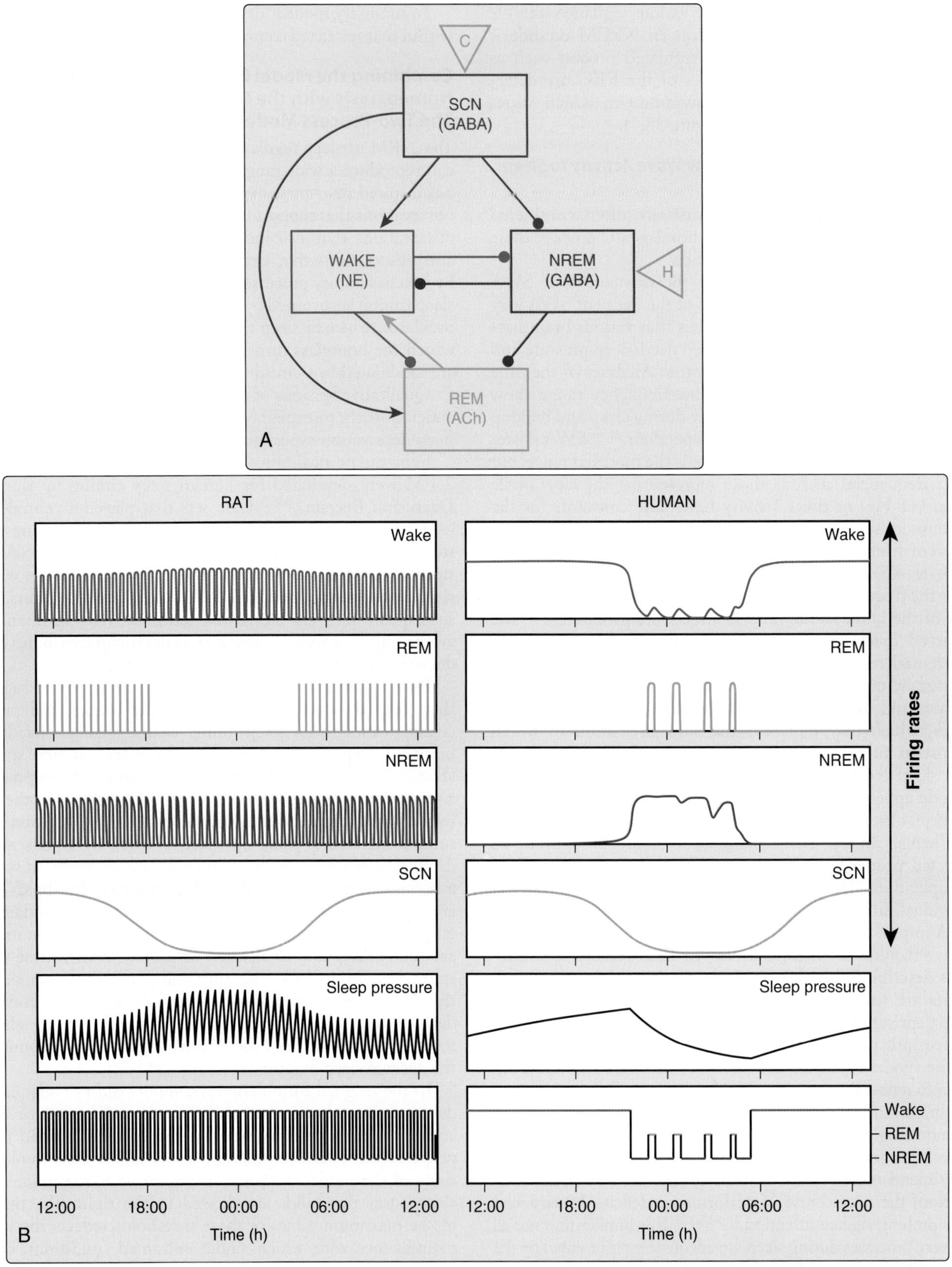

Figure 38.7 Models that describe the interaction of neuronal populations that promote wake and NREM and REM sleep have been constructed. One such model is shown in **(A).** Simulating such models results in the time course of the firing rates of the different neuronal populations, sleep pressure, and circadian rhythmicity and predictions for the timing of the three vigilant states: wake, NREM, and REM. **(B)** By varying the time constants associated with the different processes and the strength of the connections between the different neuronal populations, the time course of both rat (*left side*) and human (*right side*), NREM, and REM sleep can be simulated. ACh, Acetylcholine; C, circadian input; GABA, gamma-aminobutyric acid; H, homeostatic sleep pressure; NE, norepinephrine; SCN, suprachiasmatic nucleii. (Parameters for these simulations were provided by V. Booth and C.G. Diniz-Behn). (Mathematical model from Booth V, Xique I, Diniz-Behn CG. One-dimensional map for the circadian modulation of sleep in a sleep-wake regulatory network model for human sleep. *J Appl Dyn Syst.* 2017;16:1089–112.)

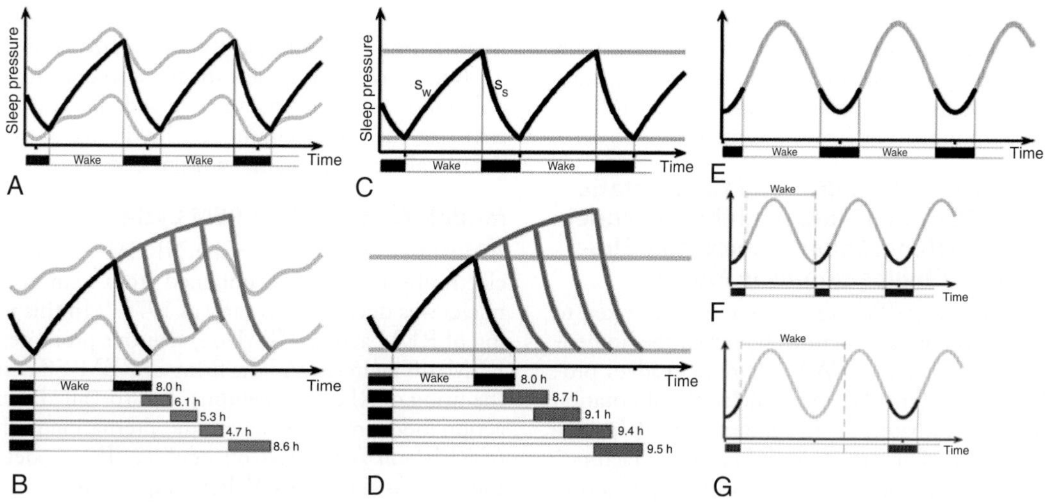

Figure 38.8 Sleep-wake regulation models: two-process, homeostatic, and circadian models. In **(A)** the two-process model is shown. Sleep pressure increases during time awake (S_W) and decreases during sleep (S_S) as shown in *black*. Switching between wake and sleep occurs at thresholds modulated by a 24-hour periodic signal, here modeled as the sum of a sine wave with period of 24 hours and one of 12 hours (*grey*). Timing of sleep is indicated by the *black horizontal bars*. **(B)** A simulation replicating the data published in Akerstedt and Gillberg.[14] The duration of recovery sleep becomes successively shorter than baseline when time awake is increased from 16 h up to 28 h by delaying sleep by increments of 4 h. Only when time awake is increased to 32 h is an increase in sleep duration observed (similar simulations were published in Borbély[44] and Daan et al.[80]) **(C)** and **(D)** illustrate that a model based on sleep homeostasis alone cannot explain the data since increasing time awake results in increasing duration of recovery sleep. Similarly, a model based solely on circadian rhythmicity, shown in **(E)** and **(F)** and **(G),** also cannot replicate the observations. Within this circadian model, sleep is constrained to occur only within a band of circadian phases **(E),** so although extending wake up to 32 hours does curtail the duration of subsequent recovery sleep **(F),** longer sleep durations mean that an entire sleep episode is missed. Consequently, it would predict that after 32 hours of wake, no sleep would occur until a further 16 hours had elapsed. In addition, sleep duration could not exceed baseline duration.

wake up close to the minimum drive for sleep and go to sleep shortly after the maximum drive for wakefulness, is that it supports consolidation of the sleep-wake cycle. The model can be viewed as an opposing process system, as proposed by Dale Edgar.[83] This interpretation is consistent with observations that a lesion of the suprachiasmatic nucleus (SCN) leads to fragmentation of the sleep-wake cycle with a uniform distribution of sleep and wakefulness across the 24-hour cycle. In the squirrel monkey, an SCN lesion also leads to a marked increase in total sleep time per 24 hours, which has been interpreted to imply that the wake-promoting effect of the circadian process during the daytime is stronger than the sleep-promoting signal at night.

Models for Circadian Rhythmicity and Entrainment by Light

In the 2-PM, circadian rhythmicity was modeled by thresholds modulated by a circadian pacemaker, but entrainment of the circadian pacemaker to the 24-hour light-dark cycle was not accounted for. This implies that the 2-PM can model sleep timing relative to circadian phase markers but not relative to clock time or the light-dark cycle.

Most models of circadian rhythmicity have focused on explaining how circadian rhythms in messenger RNA (mRNA) can occur from molecular interactions, focusing on the transcription-translation feedback loops consisting of core clock genes. Networks of oscillators have subsequently been used to show how the 10,000 or so individual neurons in the SCN can produce coherent circadian rhythms. Fewer models have focused on how light affects the timing of the human circadian pacemaker and entrainment, the aspect that is most relevant for understanding sleep timing. Within this latter context, the most widely used models are those originating from Kronauer and colleagues.[84-87] A number of different variants have been used, but all share some common characteristics. In all cases, they model the circadian oscillator as a van der Pol oscillator, one of the simplest possible ways of modeling a self-sustaining oscillation. In the absence of light, this oscillator is parameterized to produce oscillations with a period of 24.2 hours. The effect of light on the circadian system is modeled by process L. Process L consists of a caricature of the photoreceptive system and generates a signal that feeds into the circadian oscillator. The photoreceptive system is modeled by a single differential equation representing the fraction of activated photoreceptors. When lights are turned on, the photoreceptors activate with a characteristic time constant that is dependent on the light intensity raised to a power (variously 1/3, 0.5, 0.6) and the fraction of available photoreceptors. When lights are turned off, they deactivate with a (different) characteristic time constant. The signal to the circadian oscillator is proportional to the rate of activation of the photoreceptors and modulated by circadian phase. Together this results in a system in which light in the first few minutes of a light pulse has more effect than light later in a light pulse and the difference between 100 and 200 lux is much more significant than the difference between 1000 and 1100 lux. The original model was parameterized to closely match data from laboratory experiments of the phase-shifting effects of light.

It predates the discovery of the separate contributions of the five photoreceptors in the human retina (rods, short, medium long wavelength sensitive cones and the melanopsin expressing retinal ganglion cells[88]) but has been used successfully to model circadian entrainment by light in humans.

Combining Light Input, Circadian and Homeostatic Regulation and a Neuronal Mutual Inhibition Model for Sleep-Wake Switching: Saper's Conceptual Flip-Flop Model and the Phillips-Robinson Model

The two processes in the 2-PM are to some extent linked to physiologic process and brain structures such that the homeostatic process is linked to EEG SWA and the circadian process to the SCN. Neuroscientists have modeled the alternation between vigilance states based on the interaction of specific brain nuclei and included homeostatic and circadian factors.

A conceptual neuronal model of sleep-wake regulation in which sleep-promoting neurons, primarily located in the ventrolateral preoptic nucleus, and wake-promoting neurons in the ascending arousal system play a central role was proposed by Saper and colleagues.[89] This conceptual model posits inhibitory pathways between sleep- and wake-promoting neurons such that the firing of sleep-promoting neurons inhibits the firing of wake-promoting neurons and vice versa. This mutual inhibition between sleep- and wake-promoting neurons leads to consolidated sleep and wake states. The timing of switching between states was hypothesized as driven by sleep homeostasis and circadian inputs from the SCN.

The Phillips-Robinson (PR) model translates this conceptual model into a quantitative mathematical model, consisting of two coupled first-order differential equations, describing the mean cell-body potentials resulting from firing of wake-promoting and sleep-promoting neurons, respectively.[90,91] Mutual inhibition is included, and the system is driven from sleep to wake via a homeostatic component that increases during wake and decreases during sleep and an oscillatory, circadian component, in early versions modeled as a sinusoid. The PR model was parametrized to reproduce sleep duration accurately for adult human sleep and results in consolidated periods of sleep and wake with transitions between states that happen on the time scale of seconds.

Mathematically, formally considering time scales that are long compared with seconds (e.g., hours), it has been shown that the PR model is equivalent to the 2-PM. This is of value because it enables the thresholds of the 2-PM to be interpreted physiologically. For example, increasing input to sleep-promoting neurons is equivalent to lowering both thresholds simultaneously and results in longer sleep durations.[92] Increasing input to wake-promoting neurons raises both thresholds and increases the rate of accumulation of homeostatic sleep pressure. Consequently, short-term increases in inputs to wake-promoting neurons result in delays to sleep onset. But the homeostatic, use-dependent, effect means that increased inputs to wake-promoting neurons result in sleep homeostasis, increasing more rapidly during wake, ultimately resulting in longer sleep duration.

Later versions of the PR model replace the simple sinusoid description of the circadian rhythm with Kronauer's model. Importantly, this then enables a quantitative analysis of the effects of light on sleep timing. Furthermore, it recognizes that not only does the circadian rhythm drive the sleep-wake cycle but also the sleep-wake cycle drives circadian rhythmicity by gating light input to the SCN. This gating effect, which is often ignored in models for the circadian regulation of the polyphasic rest-activity cycles in rodents, contributes significantly to the understanding of the timing of the monophasic sleep-wake cycle in humans (Figure 38.9).

Models for the NREM-REM Cycle

A quantitative model for the NREM-REM cycle based on electrophysiologic data obtained from neurons in brainstem nuclei was developed as early as 1975.[93] In this model, the firing of REM active (REM-on) neurons promotes the firing of REM-off neurons, and the firing of REM-off neurons inhibits the firing of REM-on neurons. This so-called reciprocal interaction model results in a periodic alternation in the firing rates of REM-on and REM-off neurons. The model is essentially the same as the Lotka-Volterra equations for modeling oscillations in the abundance of predator and prey. Subsequently many more brain areas have been implicated in the regulation of REM and NREM sleep, and several computational models for the NREM-REM cycle have been developed.[94]

A Three-State (W, N, R) Neuronal Model with Sleep Homeostasis and Circadian Rhythmicity

The original McCarley-Hobson reciprocal interaction model only considered the two sleep states.[95] Booth and Diniz-Behn developed a number of physiology-based models consisting of wake-promoting neurons, NREM-promoting neurons, and REM-promoting neurons.[96-98] The NREM and wake-promoting neurons are mutually inhibitory, thereby forming a flip-flop switch. NREM neurons exert an inhibitory influence on REM neurons, and so do wake active neurons. REM active neurons provide an excitatory influence on wake active neurons. Circadian rhythmicity acting via the SCN exerts an activating influence on wake active neurons and REM active neurons. Homeostatic sleep drive acts on the NREM active nuclei (Figure 38.7). The resulting model then enables the simulation of the time course of the firing rates of the different nuclei and can produce a monophasic sleep-wake cycle and an ultradian alternation of NREM and REM sleep. The firing rate of wake active neurons increases at the end of each REM episode, and this may reflect the larger likelihood of waking up from REM sleep compared with NREM sleep. The firing rate of NREM active neurons during sleep is lowest at the beginning of each NREM episode, and as homeostatic sleep pressure dissipates in the course of sleep, the low firing rate becomes lower and lower. Later versions of the model also account for the effect of light on the circadian pacemaker by incorporating Kronauer's model. However, no provision for REM sleep homeostasis is made.

Changing the time constants for the homeostatic process and the firing rate response dynamics and adjusting some of the weights for the postsynaptic effects of neurotransmitter concentrations transform a monophasic sleep-wake cycle characteristic of adult humans to a polyphasic sleep-wake cycle as observed in rodents. Changing the direction of the projection from the SCN to the wake and to the NREM populations changes the model from diurnal to nocturnal. Changing the parameters can reduce the period of the NREM-REM period from approximately 90 minutes in humans to shorter periods such as observed in rodents (Figure 38.7).

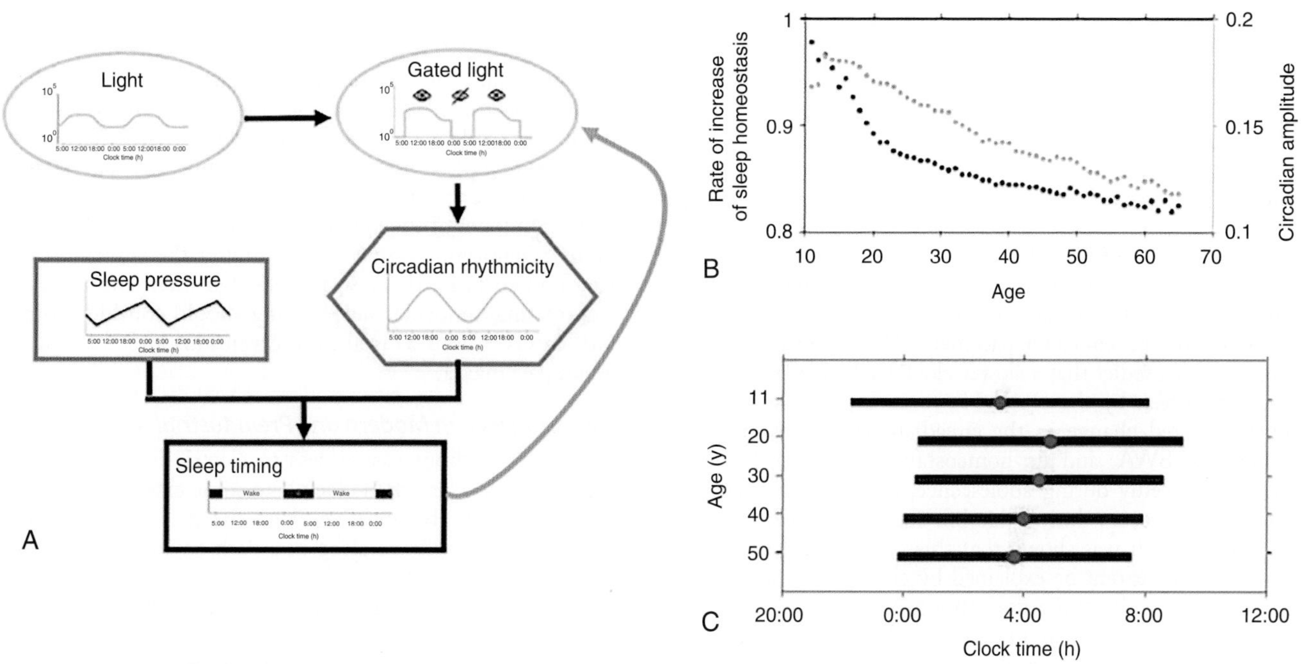

Figure 38.9 The two-process model describes the relative timing of sleep and circadian rhythmicity and does not directly relate sleep and circadian timing to clock time and the external world. Mathematical models that combine light as an external zeitgeber to a simple model of circadian rhythmicity have been constructed and accurately describe human phase response to light interventions. Coupling such a light/circadian model to the two-process model or to the Phillips-Robinson model, as shown schematically in **(A)** then makes it possible to construct a mathematical model that can describe the timing of sleep and circadian rhythmicity with respect to clock time. Varying parameters in a physiologically plausible manner **(B)**, enables the accurate simulation of data for mean sleep duration and timing from pre-teen to retirement **(C)**, where the *black bars* indicate sleep timing and the *red dots* mark the midpoint of sleep). (A: Representation of the model in Phillips AJ, Chen PY, Robinson PA. Probing the mechanisms of chronotype using quantitative modeling. *J Biol Rhythms*. 2010;25:217–27. (B) and (C) are based on Skeldon AC, Derks G, Dijk DJ. Modelling changes in sleep timing and duration across the lifespan: Changes in circadian rhythmicity or sleep homeostasis? *Sleep Med Rev*. 2016;28:96–107. The simulations accurately match sleep duration and timing in Roenneberg T, Kuehnle T, Pramstaller PP, Ricken J, Havel M, Guth A, Merrow M . A marker for the end of adolescence. *Curr Biol*. 2014;14:R1038–9, Roenneberg T, Chronobiology: the human sleep project. *Nature*. 2013;498:427–428)

APPLICATION OF CONCEPTS AND MODELS FOR THE HOMEOSTATIC AND CIRCADIAN REGULATION OF SLEEP

The utility of concepts and models relates in part to the range of phenomena to which they can be applied. The concept of the homeostatic and circadian regulation has provided new insights into sleep phenomena and in particular those that relate to sleep timing.

Desynchrony

Internal Desynchrony

Models have successfully captured the desynchronization of the sleep-wake cycle and circadian rhythmicity as seen in social isolation experiments. Both early results from the 2-PM and later results using the PR model show that desynchrony can result by decreasing the amplitude of the circadian input. Alternatively, with the PR model, it was shown that increasing the drive to wake-promoting neurons, which 2-PM terms is equivalent to raising the mean level of the thresholds, was an alternative explanation for the data.[99,100]

Forced Desynchrony

The main phenomena observed during forced desynchrony such as dependency of sleep duration on circadian phase, the decline of SWA during sleep independent of circadian phase, and the interaction between sleep homeostasis and circadian rhythmicity can be simulated by 2-PM.

Sleep Duration

Short and Long Sleepers

Within a given age group some people may sleep short, whereas others sleep long. Long sleepers have in general less SWA than short sleepers, but the dynamics of the homeostatic process are similar in long versus short sleepers. In the 2-PM and related models this difference in sleep duration can be demonstrated by lowering the average level of the circadian thresholds, which in essence reduces the circadian-generated drive for wake and therefore also the mean sleep pressure. This is consistent with observations that long sleepers live on a lower average sleep pressure level than short sleepers.[101] Similar explanations may be invoked for the hypersomnia observed in some mental health disorders such as schizophrenia.

Polyphasic Sleep in Infants and Small Mammals

In adult humans the sleep-wake cycle is consolidated with a major sleep episode at night. In many small mammals and in human infants the sleep-wake cycle is polyphasic. This polyphasic pattern could be related to an immature or absent circadian system or lack of connections between a competent circadian pacemaker and sleep executive neuronal centers. Model simulations show that such a polyphasic pattern can be generated in a system with an adult-like circadian system, but an altered homeostatic process such that the rate at which sleep need increases is faster in infants than in adults.[80,92,102]

Sleep Timing

Models that include the effect of light on the circadian pacemaker give a way to link clock-time to timing in the 2-PM.

Sleep Timing in Adolescents

Sleep timing in adolescents is later than in children and in adults. This has often been attributed to changes in the intrinsic period of the circadian pacemaker.[103] Circadian entrainment models predict that a slower clock leads to a later timing of events driven by the clock. However, little evidence for a puberty-related change in the circadian period has emerged in humans. SWA, and its homeostatic regulation, however, changes markedly during adolescence, reflecting the synaptic pruning that occurs during this life stage.[104-106] With use of the PR model, it was shown that this change in sleep timing may to a large extent be explained by changes in the homeostatic process without the assumption of an altered circadian period.[107] These results are in part related to the gating of light input to the circadian pacemaker by the sleep-wake cycle. Thus, even though little evidence has emerged that light sensitivity per se is altered in adolescence, the changes in the homeostatic process mean that adolescents can stay awake for longer than younger children. With access to electric light, this then leads to more light exposure in the evening, typically the point in the circadian cycle where light leads to a phase delay of the clock.

Sleep Timing in Aging

Healthy older people wake up earlier and have less SWA, and sleep duration is reduced. Whereas the earlier sleep timing with aging has been hypothesized to be related to an age-dependent reduction in the period of the circadian pacemaker, no evidence for such an age-related change in the period of the human circadian clock has emerged.[108] Likewise, age-related differences in the sensitivity to light, which could affect the phase of entrainment, have also not been consistently reported.[109] Several studies have demonstrated that older healthy people are less impaired by total sleep deprivation and repeated partial sleep deprivation.[110] The interaction between sleep homeostasis and circadian rhythmicity has been compared in young and older participants. With aging the circadian regulation of sleep is not fundamentally changed, although the strength of the sleep-promoting signal in the morning hours may be weaker. However, because homeostatic drive is diminished with aging, the circadian wake-promoting signal during the biological day makes it difficult for healthy older people to sleep during the day: it is not easy to sleep in when you are older.[56]

These data and the reduced sleepiness in older people[38] are consistent with a reduced need for sleep and a reduced buildup of homeostatic sleep drive in older people. Computer simulations in which parameters of the homeostatic process are changed replicate the empirical observations, and these extend to the reduced ability of older people to consolidate sleep during the daytime.[107]

Diurnal Preference

Early and late sleepers can be found in any age group. This phenotype has been associated with differences in intrinsic period of the circadian process such that early sleepers have a faster clock.[111,112] This, however, is not the only difference in the homeostatic and circadian regulation of sleep. Early sleepers also have more SWA and a steeper decline of SWA during the sleep episode.[113,114] The PR model has successfully shown that the same phenotype can be the result of either circadian or homeostatic effects.[115]

A main tenet of the application of the 2-PM to these sleep timing phenotypes is that they highlight the contribution of sleep homeostasis. This also implies that interventions aimed at correcting abnormal sleep timing should consider homeostatic interventions as well as interventions aimed at the circadian pacemaker.

Timing of Sleep in Modern and Preindustrial Societies

In societies without easy access to electric light, light input into the human circadian clock is to some extent gated by the sleep-wake cycle because we close our eyes when we go to sleep and may prefer to sleep in a dark environment. In preindustrial societies, this gating effect is small because sleep tends to be aligned with the natural light-dark cycle.[116]

A characteristic of modern societies is access to electric light and later sleep timing relative to the natural light-dark cycle.[117,118] This is most likely and at least in part because their citizens can at will extend the photoperiod and reduce the scotoperiod. The light-dark cycle to which we are exposed is then to a larger extent driven by the sleep-wake cycle. Self-selection of light exposure in the evening will reduce sleepiness, delay bedtime and circadian phase. Consequently, due to the homeostatic regulation of sleep wake time will also delay unless sleep is terminated by the alarm clock.

To model how the light environment affects our circadian rhythms and sleep timing requires light regulation of circadian rhythmicity to be integrated with the homeostatic and circadian regulation of sleep. Later versions of the PR model provide this integration and have been used to explore issues related to electric light, school start times, social jet lag, and the effect of daylight savings time on human sleep and circadian rhythms[119] (Figure 38.10).

These simulations demonstrate the potential of mathematical models for the interaction of physiologic processes, environmental factors, and social constraints. Social constraints are in part driven by societal demands and may be altered by changes in government policies. These modeling approaches can be used to design interventions that are theory driven and can help to predict the consequences of policies. For example, when we take into account that most humans spend more than 90% of their time indoors, the quality and intensity of light becomes critical for entrainment of the clock. Simulations show that if people are not awakened by an alarm clock, many of us would no longer be synchronized to the 24-hour day, and in most of us the timing of wake time and bedtime would drift progressively later. This is because in approximately 75% of people the intrinsic period of the circadian pacemaker is longer than 24 hours. According to model simulations keeping the lights on in the evening will further delay circadian rhythms. This effect is not observed in models that do not account for the gating of light input by the sleep-wake cycle and the homeostatic contribution to sleep propensity.

Simulations with the integrated model suggest that interventions such as reducing exposure to evening light are more effective than delaying school start times in enabling

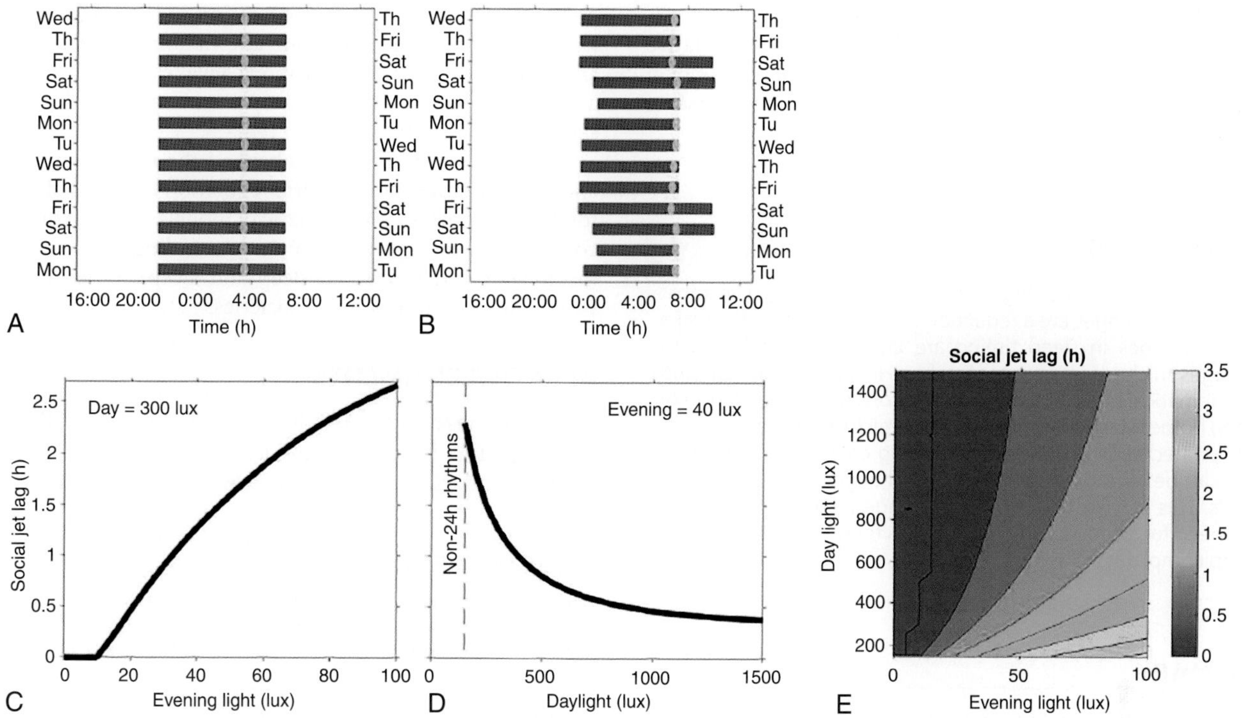

Figure 38.10 We are able to override the physiologic cues that we need to sleep and stay awake even when we are tired. This ability to control when we are awake according to social constraints has been modeled and makes it possible to untangle the three timescales of importance for understanding sleep in society: internal biologic (circadian) time, the timing of the environmental light-dark cycle, the timing of social constraints. In such models it is seen that appropriately timed light that is bright enough during the biologic day and dim enough in the biologic evening results in early wake times **(A).** With light that is less intense during the day or brighter in the evening, spontaneous wake time is later and conflicts with social schedules **(B),** resulting in social jet lag. The dependence on social jet lag, here measured as the difference between wake time on Saturday and wake time during the working week, is shown in **(C)** and on daylight for a fixed level of evening light is shown in **(D).** Because it is the relative balance between light during the day and evening light that is important, in **(E)** the social jet lag for a range of evening and daylight levels is shown. (Simulations based on Skeldon AC, Phillips AJ, Dijk DJ. The effects of self-selected light-dark cycles and social constraints on human sleep and circadian timing: a modelling approach. *Sci Rep.* 2017;7:45158. https://doi.org/10.1038/srep45158)

adolescents to get up on time to attend. This prediction obviously does not address which of the two interventions is most likely to be adhered to or which one is most popular.

These model simulations are based on state-of-the-art understanding of entrainment and sleep regulation, provide arguments to be considered, suggest experiments and interventions that can be tested, and thereby demonstrate the utility of quantitative models for the homeostatic and circadian regulation of sleep.

OUTLOOK

Models for the homeostatic and circadian regulation are, in the first instance, models for the timing of sleep after sleep displacement and sleep deprivation and not for recovery functions attributed to sleep. Within these models there has been an emphasis on the homeostatic regulation of slow waves and homeostasis of REM sleep, and sleep duration has been largely ignored. Quantitative versions of the circadian and homeostatic sleep timing models have been useful in furthering our understanding of sleep phenotypes not only in humans and rodents but also in drosophila. The qualitative concept that most behavioral, physiologic, and molecular variables are influenced by both sleep-wake dependent (i.e., homeostatic factors) and circadian factors has been proven to be a very productive framework. The homeostatic-circadian framework has been applied to molecular processes. For example, circadian and sleep contributions have been identified for the blood transcriptome, and these findings may lead to new markers for sleep debt and circadian status.[120-122] The concept of sleep-wake dependent and circadian regulation has been applied well beyond sleep timing and sleep. It has been successfully applied to waking performance and fatigue and is the basis of tools that evaluate shift-work schedules. Mismatches between empirical data and predictions of quantitative models have pointed to key areas of a lack of quantitative understanding (e.g., how repeated partial sleep loss is so much different from effects of acute sleep deprivation). The conceptual framework clarifies that the detrimental effects of shift work can be mitigated by managing sleep pressure (e.g., the work by Isherwood and colleagues[123]).

Incorporating quantitative models of the effects of light on the circadian process enables simulations of sleep timing in real-world situations and has informed the understanding of phenomena such as social jet lag and discussions around societal issues such as school start time and daylight saving time. These integrated models hold promise for the design of interventions to correct sleep timing abnormalities such as observed in circadian rhythm sleep disorders, insomnia, schizophrenia, bipolar disorder, and dementia.

Key areas for future models to address are the homeostatic regulation of REM sleep, sleep continuity, ability to capture day-to-day variability and individual differences in the sleep-wake cycle, modeling NREM/REM in greater quantitative depth, better quantification of the impact of sleep debt on physical and cognitive performance, and the time course of recovery.

CLINICAL PEARL

Sleep changes with aging, even in healthy aging. The most noticeable changes are a reduction in SWS and an earlier wake time. Changes in sleep timing are commonly attributed to changes in the circadian pacemaker. However, empirical and mathematical model-based investigations of the interaction of sleep homeostasis and circadian rhythmicity indicate that most age-related changes in sleep, including changes in sleep timing, can be attributed to age-related changes in sleep homeostasis. This can be interpreted as an age-related reduction in the need for sleep and has implications for the management of sleep complaints in aging.

SUMMARY

Sleep is assumed to serve important recovery functions for the brain and body, and sleep duration and sleep structure are therefore expected to be accurately regulated. Homeostatic regulation of sleep duration and sleep structure has been investigated by total, repeated partial, or sleep stage–specific deprivation experiments. Sleep loss invariably leads to an increase in the drive to initiate sleep. Lost NREM and REM time, and thereby total sleep time, are often not completely recovered because of circadian and protocol constraints. Accurate homeostatic regulation of REM and NREM time is observed when recovery is imposed or recorded over longer periods of time.

EEG SWA responds to variations in the duration of wakefulness and sleep according to exponential saturating and declining functions, respectively. In accordance with these functions, chronic sleep restriction only results in a marginal increase in SWA despite considerable loss of sleep time and associated increase in sleep propensity and deterioration of waking performance.

The homeostatic regulation of SWA has been combined with the circadian regulation of sleep propensity in the 2-PM of sleep regulation. This model predicts the time course of SWA in many experimental protocols as well as sleep timing in sleep displacement experiments.

The concept of homeostatic and circadian regulation has been applied to a wide range of phenomena, such as internal and forced desynchrony and sleep timing across the life span. Other mathematical models, which have incorporated the effects of light on the circadian process and the effects of sleep on light input to the circadian process, have provided new insights into phenomena such as social jet lag and the role of evening light on sleep timing. Further mathematical models, in part based on the identification of specific neuronal populations involved in the generation of the vigilance states, also incorporate the ultradian alternation between NREM and REM sleep and the transition to wake. In all these models and their explanation of specific phenomena, sleep homeostasis plays an important role.

Sleep homeostasis extends beyond the regulation of SWA and incorporating homeostatic regulation of REM sleep, and total sleep time in mathematical models may further their contribution to a quantitative understanding of the effects of insufficient and misplaced sleep and sleep timing disorders, which are common in many societies.

ACKNOWLEDGMENTS

This work was supported by the UK Dementia Research Institute, The Biotechnology Biological Sciences Research Council, and the Engineering and Physical Sciences Research Council.

SELECTED READINGS

Achermann P, Borbély AA. Low-frequency (< 1 Hz) oscillations in the human sleep electroencephalogram. *Neurosci.* 1997;81(1):213–222.

Booth V, Diniz Behn CG. Physiologically-based modeling of sleep-wake regulatory networks. *Math Biosci.* 2014;250:54–68.

Borbély AA. A two process model of sleep regulation. *Hum Neurobiol.* 1982;1(3):195–204.

Borbély AA, Daan S, Wirz-Justice A, Deboer T. The two-process model of sleep regulation: a reappraisal. *J Sleep Res.* 2016;25(2):131–143.

Daan S, Beersma DG, Borbély AA. Timing of human sleep: recovery process gated by a circadian pacemaker. *Am J Physiol.* 1984;246(2 Pt 2):R161–R183.

Dijk DJ, Czeisler CA. Contribution of the circadian pacemaker and the sleep homeostat to sleep propensity, sleep structure, electroencephalographic slow waves, and sleep spindle activity in humans. *J Neurosci.* 1995;15(5 Pt1):3526–3538.

Hubbard J, Gent TC, Hoekstra MMB, et al. Rapid fast-delta decay following prolonged wakefulness marks a phase of wake-inertia in NREM sleep. *Nat Commun.* 2020;11(1):3130.

Lazar AS, Lazar ZI, Dijk DJ. Circadian regulation of slow waves in human sleep: topographical aspects. *Neuroimage.* 2015;116:123–134.

Nir Y, Staba RJ, Andrillon T, et al. Regional slow waves and spindles in human sleep. *Neuron.* 2011;70(1):153–169.

Ocampo-Garcés A, Bassi A, Brunetti E, Estrada J, Vivaldi EA. REM sleep dependent short-term and long-term hourglass processes in the ultradian organization and recovery of REM sleep in the rat. *Sleep.* 2020;43(8):zsaa023.

Phillips AJ, Chen PY, Robinson PA. Probing the mechanisms of chronotype using quantitative modeling. *J Biol Rhythms.* 2010;25:217–227.

Shochat T, Santhi N, Herer P, Dijk DJ, Skeldon AC. Sleepiness is a signal to go to bed: data and model simulations [published online ahead of print, 2021 May 15]. *Sleep.* 2021;zsab123.

Skeldon AC, Derks G, Dijk DJ. Modelling changes in sleep timing and duration across the lifespan: Changes in circadian rhythmicity or sleep homeostasis? *Sleep Med Rev.* 2016;28:96–107.

Skeldon AC, Phillips AJ, Dijk DJ. The effects of self-selected light-dark cycles and social constraints on human sleep and circadian timing: a modelling approach. *Sci Rep.* 2017;7:45158.

Tononi G, Cirelli C. Sleep and the price of plasticity: from synaptic and cellular homeostasis to memory consolidation and integration. *Neuron.* 2014;81(1):12–34.

A complete reference list can be found online at ExpertConsult.com.

Chapter 39

Circadian Rhythms in Sleepiness, Alertness, and Performance

Lillian Skeiky; Amanda N. Hudson; Hans P.A. Van Dongen

Chapter Highlights

- Alertness and performance vary across the day, driven by the circadian rhythm of the biologic clock. We tend to be less alert in the early morning and late at night, but changes in alertness and performance over time also depend on the circumstances.
- A variety of other factors (e.g., activity, posture, caffeine intake) influence the pattern of circadian rhythmicity as observed in alertness and performance measures. Investigating the effect of the biologic clock requires careful control over these so-called masking effects.
- Temporal patterns of alertness and performance also reflect the interaction of the circadian process with a homeostatic process regulating sleep. Accounting for this homeostatic process is critical for understanding and predicting the occurrence of performance deficits across the 24 hours of the day.

The timing and duration of wakefulness and sleep are modulated by an endogenous, circadian regulating system, the biologic clock, located in the suprachiasmatic nuclei of the anterior hypothalamus. However, the impact of the biologic clock goes beyond compelling the body to fall asleep and to wake up again. The biologic clock also modulates hour-to-hour waking behavior, as reflected in alertness and performance, generating circadian rhythmicity in almost all neurobehavioral variables investigated.

Before a discussion of circadian rhythmicity in waking neurobehavioral functions, a brief description of some variables capturing aspects of waking functioning is important, because different definitions can be found in the literature.[1-3] Here we use the term *sleepiness* for subjective reports of sleepiness or the desire to sleep. In operational settings the term *fatigue* is often used instead[4] (but in this chapter, the term is not used). By *alertness* we mean the antonym of sleepiness (although these terms have been differentiated[5]) and the ability to sustain attention. *Performance* refers to cognitive functioning on tasks ranging from psychomotor vigilance and working memory tests to logical reasoning and decision-making tasks. These concepts may be discussed collectively as *neurobehavioral functioning*.

The term *sleepiness* captures the link between alertness and performance during wakefulness on the one hand and sleep on the other hand. The interaction of circadian rhythmicity with sleep and wakefulness in determining sleepiness, alertness, and performance is described in the second part of this chapter. Sleep propensity[6,7] is not covered in this chapter; the focus here is on effortful cognitive performance and the associated subjective states.

CIRCADIAN RHYTHMS

Self-Report Measures of Sleepiness and Alertness

Many different techniques are available for the measurement of circadian rhythmicity in neurobehavioral variables, including a wide array of self-report measures of sleepiness and alertness. These include a variety of visual analogue scales (VAS)[8] to measure subjective assessments on a continuum: Likert-type rating scales such as the Stanford Sleepiness Scale[9] and the Karolinska Sleepiness Scale,[10] and adjective checklists such as the Profile of Mood States.[11] Despite structural differences among these scales, self-report measures of sleepiness and alertness tend to be highly correlated over time. They have been used to index circadian rhythmicity through repeated administration across the day.[12-14]

Subjective measures of sleepiness and alertness are subject to numerous confounding influences, which can "mask" their circadian rhythmicity. *Masking* refers to the evoked effects of noncircadian factors on measurements of circadian rhythmicity. The context in which such measurements are taken (i.e., the environmental and experimental conditions) is a major source of masking effects.[15] Masking can alter or obscure a circadian rhythm or create the appearance of a circadian rhythm where there is none. Masking factors affecting sleepiness and alertness may include, but are not limited to, demand characteristics of the experiment,[16] distractions by environmental stimuli and noise,[17] boredom and motivational factors,[18-20] stimulation,[21] stress,[22] food intake,[23,24] posture and activity,[25,26] ambient temperature,[19] ambient lighting conditions,[27,28] and drug intake (e.g., caffeine).[29,30]

Physical, mental, and social activities can be masking factors for circadian rhythms in subjective sleepiness and alertness as well. For example, subjects report feeling less alert after performing a challenging cognitive task than before performing said task.[31] In general, prior activity can influence subjective estimates, and it can interact with circadian effects if not properly controlled when measuring rhythmicity in subjective states. Sleep and wakefulness can also be considered masking factors when measuring circadian rhythmicity in neurobehavioral variables. Sleep and sleep loss have significant effects on alertness and performance, as discussed in the second part of this chapter.

A variety of factors may also affect the biologic clock itself, changing its timing through phase advances or delays. Such factors are called *zeitgebers* (time givers or time cues) and include light exposure, exercise, social cues, food intake, and sleep. Under most circumstances, light exposure is the most prominent zeitgeber[32-37]—especially blue light,[38,39] even if it is relatively dim.[40] Light exposure also has an acute (non-zeitgeber) alerting effect, which may further modify circadian rhythms in sleepiness and alertness.[41-43] However, the impact of these factors typically varies depending on the timing of exposure relative to the circadian cycle of the biologic clock, making it difficult to account for them. As such, it is important to control zeitgebers in studies designed to measure circadian rhythms in neurobehavioral variables.

Cognitive Performance

Rather than relying on subjective measures of neurobehavioral functioning, many studies of circadian rhythms have used objective performance measures. For example, studies have employed search-and-detection tasks and simple and choice reaction time tasks[44,45] to obtain objective measures of circadian variation in cognitive performance. In many tasks, the speed and/or accuracy of responses to a series of stimuli are analyzed. The sensitivity of the performance metrics in such tasks depends on speed-accuracy trade-offs (which in turn depend on the demand characteristics of the experiment), task duration, stimulus density (number of stimuli presented per unit time), and whether the task is subject paced versus experimenter or computer paced.[46-48]

A wide range of performance outputs have been considered, including signal detection,[49] simple sorting,[50] logical reasoning,[51] memory access,[52] meter reading accuracy,[53] and school performance.[54] Furthermore, a number of subcomponents of cognition and cognitive processes involved in task performance can be distinguished, such as sensory input, stimulus encoding, working memory updating, and motor response.[55,56] A variety of tasks have been used to study circadian variation in these different aspects of performance. Some studies concluded that different tasks[57,58] and different task outcomes[59,60] may yield different peak phases of circadian rhythmicity. This has led to speculation that there are many different circadian rhythms and multiple different clock mechanisms controlling them.[61,62]

Under strictly controlled laboratory conditions, however, most of the intertask differences disappear.[63,64] As illustrated in Figure 39.1, it can generally be stated that under such conditions, the circadian rhythms of neurobehavioral performance variables covary with subjective sleepiness. Furthermore, these rhythms reflect the circadian rhythm of core body temperature (CBT), a conventional marker of the biologic clock. High and low CBT roughly correspond to good and poor performance, respectively.[64-67] That being said, there is a phase difference such that neurobehavioral variables exhibit their average minimum approximately between 3.0 and 4.5 hours after the time of the body temperature minimum.

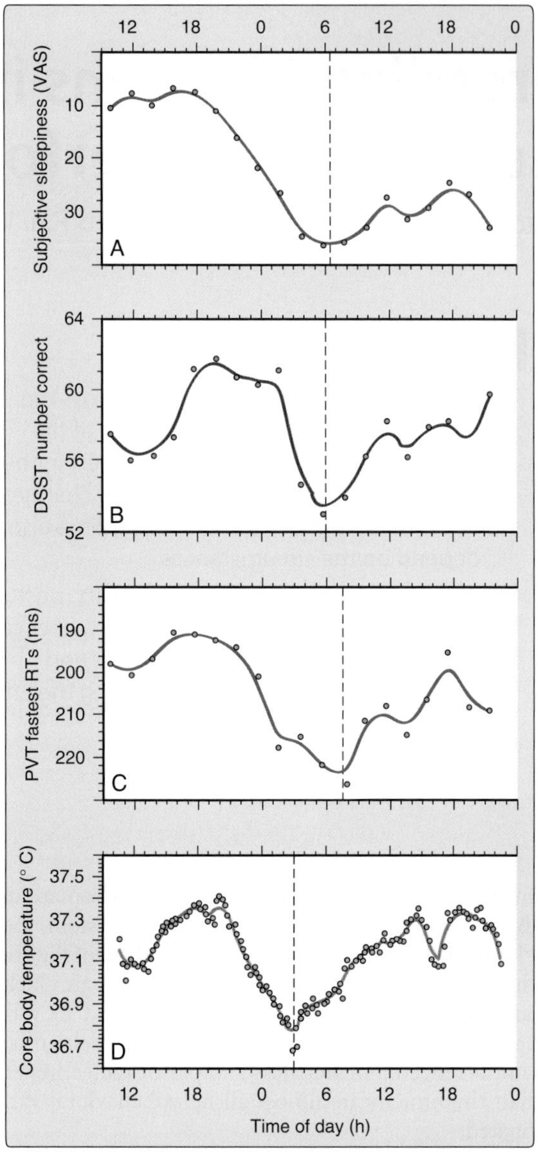

Figure 39.1 Covariation of circadian changes in neurobehavioral variables and core body temperature. **A,** Subjective sleepiness (scale reversed) as assessed by visual analogue scale (VAS).[8] **B,** Cognitive performance as assessed by the digit symbol substitution task (DSST).[153,186,187] **C,** The 10% fastest reaction times (RTs; scale reversed) as assessed by the psychomotor vigilance test (PVT).[140] **D,** Core body temperature as assessed using a rectal probe. Data shown are the mean values from five subjects who remained awake in dim light, in bed, and in a constant routine protocol for 36 consecutive hours. A smoothing function was fitted to each of the variables to highlight the temporal profiles. The circadian trough in each variable is marked by a *vertical broken line.*

This phase delay contradicts the common belief that alertness and performance are worst at the body temperature minimum. Although body temperature predominantly reflects the endogenous biologic clock, neurobehavioral functions are also affected by homeostatic pressure for sleep, which builds up over time awake (as discussed in the second part of this chapter) and contributes to the phase delay. Thus neurobehavioral

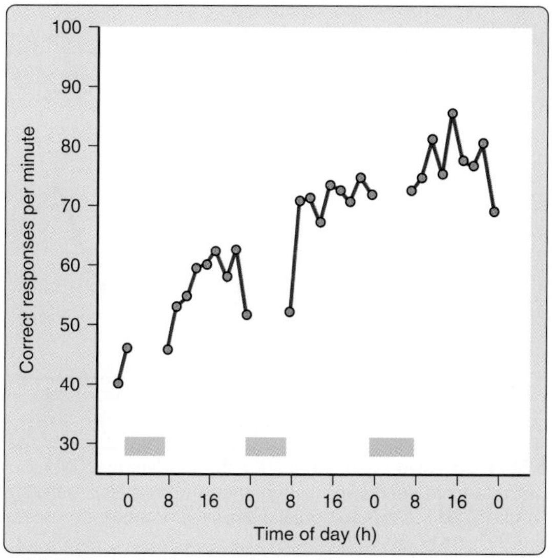

Figure 39.2 Practice effect on the serial addition-subtraction test. Data shown are mean cognitive throughput (correct responses per minute) of 29 subjects tested every 2 hours from 7:30 a.m. until 11:30 p.m. each day over a 3-day period. In the serial addition-subtraction test, subjects are presented with a rapid sequence of two single digits (0–9) followed by an operator (+ or –). They are instructed to enter only the least-significant single digit of the algebraic sum, unless the result is negative, in which case 10 is to be added to the answer first.[188] The *solid bars* indicate 8-hour sleep periods (from 11:30 p.m. until 7:30 a.m.).

functions generally show a circadian decline at night, as is observed in CBT, but they continue their decline after CBT begins to rise, making the subsequent 2- to 6-hour period (approximately 6 a.m. to 10 a.m.) a zone of maximum vulnerability to degraded alertness and performance failure.

The assessment of circadian rhythmicity in cognitive performance tends to be more complicated than the assessment of subjective sleepiness and alertness.[68] For some tasks, subjects may change their performance strategy over time.[69] Or their effort to maintain good performance may change over time, which can be especially notable if subjects are informed about their results during a performance task (i.e., performance feedback).[70] Differences among people in aptitude for a task may also confound the assessment of circadian rhythmicity in cognitive performance. Within-subject study designs and analysis strategies can be useful to circumvent this issue.

Another complicating factor for the assessment of circadian rhythmicity in cognitive performance is the practice effect (or learning curve). This is illustrated in Figure 39.2, which shows substantial improvements in performance on a serial addition-subtraction task across 3 consecutive days (notice the doubling of mean correct responses within 30 test bouts). This practice effect dominates the performance profile, masking circadian changes within days. The practice effect contaminates most cognitive performance tasks and is difficult to dissociate from the circadian rhythm in performance. This problem may be circumvented by training subjects to asymptotic performance levels before attempting to assess circadian rhythmicity in cognitive performance, although a highly practiced task may not measure the same aspects of neurobehavioral functioning as more novel tasks.[71,72]

Most of the variables that mask circadian rhythmicity in subjective estimates of sleepiness and alertness (e.g., demand characteristics, distractions, motivation, posture, ambient temperature, lighting conditions; see earlier) may also mask circadian variation in performance. The effects of masking include distortion of the magnitude of circadian variation, shifting of the timing of observed circadian rhythmicity, and changes in the shape of the circadian profile; even total concealment of the circadian rhythm is possible (Figure 39.2, where sleep prevents measurement of nocturnal performance and the practice effect obscures circadian variation in diurnal performance). Thus it is challenging to extract meaningful information about the amplitude (magnitude) and phase (timing) of the circadian rhythm in performance measures without understanding the masking effects that influence these variables.

Physiologic Measures

The circadian rhythm in cognitive performance reflects functional changes in the brain over time of day. Evoked or event-related potentials (ERPs)—waves (peaks and troughs) in the electroencephalogram (EEG) produced by the brain in response to a stimulus—have been used to measure alertness and cognitive performance. Typically, many ERP measurements are needed (i.e., many stimuli must be presented) to average out the background EEG. Therefore ERPs are usually recorded during repetitive search-and-detect and reaction time tasks. Diurnal changes in the amplitude and the location of ERP waves have been interpreted as reflecting circadian variations in alertness.[73,74] Hemispheric differences have been detected,[75] suggesting separate circadian rhythms for the left and right hemispheres. However, the interpretation of ERP data is complicated by masking from a variety of sources.[76]

Changes in background EEG during wakefulness have also been associated with circadian variation in alertness. Despite difficulties in the recording and analysis of the waking EEG,[77,78] the amounts of theta and alpha activity (i.e., EEG activity in the frequency bands from 4 to 8 Hz and from 8 to 12 Hz, respectively) in the resting EEG (with eyes held either open or closed to avoid artifacts from blinking) have been related to alertness level.[79-81]

EEG has also been used to measure sleep-onset latency (SOL)—a measure of sleep propensity—at various times of day. Examples of SOL tests include the Multiple Sleep Latency Test (MSLT)[6] and the Maintenance of Wakefulness Test (MWT).[82] SOL tests are covered in other chapters in this volume.

Ocular features and behaviors such as slow eyelid closures and slow-rolling eye movements have been found to be systematically related to sleepiness.[10,83-90] Pupil diameter is related to autonomic tone, which covaries with sleep pressure.[91] Therefore pupillometry may also yield estimates of sleepiness,[92] but only if environmental light and other sources of error variance are strictly controlled. The various ocular measures of sleepiness have been investigated primarily under conditions of considerable sleep loss, when the observed effects are more pronounced than across the circadian cycle. The same applies for cardiovascular measures that have been found to correlate with sleepiness, such as heart rate variability.[93,94] Whether ocular and cardiovascular measures can be employed reliably for detecting circadian fluctuations in sleepiness remains to be determined.

Interindividual Differences

Interindividual differences in circadian phase[95] and amplitude[96] are reported throughout the literature. Interindividual differences in the intrinsic, free-running circadian period have also been reported,[97] although under normal, entrained circumstances the circadian period equals 24 hours,[98] and differences in the intrinsic period manifest as phase differences.[99,100] In part, interindividual differences in circadian variables have been linked to development[101,102]—with a marked phase delay during adolescence,[103] which is an important facet of the ongoing debate about school start times for optimal academic performance[104,105]—and advanced aging.[106-109] Genetic factors also play a role.[110,111]

Morningness-eveningness—the tendency to be an early "lark" or a late "owl"—is a well-known, phenotypic aspect of interindividual variation in circadian rhythmicity.[112] Morningness-eveningness is commonly measured with questionnaires that ask about a person's preferred timing of sleep and daily activities.[113,114] Laboratory studies have shown that morning- and evening-type individuals differ in the phase (timing) of the endogenous circadian rhythms in CBT[95] and circulating levels of melatonin.[115] This difference is echoed in the timing of their sleep[116] and the diurnal course of their neurobehavioral functioning[117,118]—some people are more alert and perform better in the morning hours, whereas others are at their best later in the day.[119]

In some individuals, there appears to be an afternoon dip in the circadian profiles of CBT and neurobehavioral variables,[119,120] which is referred to as the midafternoon, siesta, postprandial, or postlunch dip. This phenomenon has been observed in both field studies[53] and controlled laboratory experiments[121] and is thought to be endogenous and independent of food intake. Epidemiologic analyses of human performance (e.g., road accident rates across the 24 hours of the day[122]) seem to support the existence of a midafternoon dip (Figure 39.3). However, proper interpretation of such data requires accounting for temporal variation in exposure, that is, differential amounts of activity contributed by varying numbers of people over time,[123] which is complicated. More direct evidence for the existence of a midafternoon dip in some individuals comes from studies on sleep propensity[124,125] and on the natural timing of daytime naps.[126] This suggests that interindividual differences in sleep-wake parameters may play a role.

CIRCADIAN RHYTHMICITY VERSUS SLEEP-WAKE CYCLES

Sleep Deprivation

Considerable research effort has been devoted to unmasking circadian rhythms, that is, eliminating sources of extraneous variance to expose the endogenous circadian rhythms in variables of interest, including alertness and cognitive performance. The constant routine procedure[127,128] is generally regarded as the gold standard for measuring unmasked circadian rhythms. By keeping subjects awake with a fixed posture in a constant laboratory environment for at least 24 hours, researchers can record circadian rhythms in a variety of physiologic and neurobehavioral variables without confounds. For CBT and melatonin in particular, the circadian rhythm is believed to be free of masking effects when measured under constant routine.

The elimination of sleep (i.e., sleep deprivation) and the stimulation required to sustain wakefulness constitute masking factors for neurobehavioral variables. In constant routine

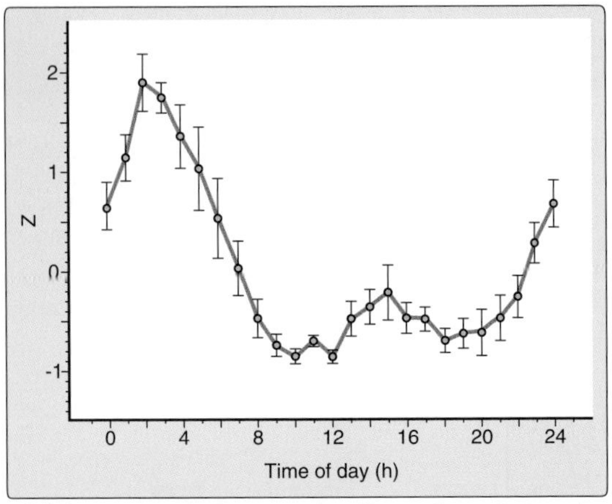

Figure 39.3 Circadian rhythm in road traffic accident risk. Data shown are mean (with standard error) over six published studies after Z transformation. (From Folkard S. Black times: temporal determinants of transport safety. *Accid Anal Prev.* 1997;29:417–30, with permission.)

experiments, these masking effects are evident in both subjective and objective measures of alertness.[95,129] Figure 39.1 shows the somewhat increased sleepiness and reduced cognitive performance following 30 hours of sustained wakefulness under constant routine compared with the values of these variables 24 hours earlier (at the same circadian time but without sleep deprivation).

Typically, superimposed on the circadian rhythm in a neurobehavioral variable, there is a progressive change across time spent awake.[130,131] When total sleep deprivation is continued for several days (whether in a constant routine procedure or an experimental design involving ambulation), the detrimental effects on alertness and performance increase. Although circadian rhythmicity can thus be exposed,[132] it is overlaid by a continuing change reflecting a buildup of pressure for sleep.[133]

This is illustrated in Figure 39.4, which shows lapses of attention on a psychomotor vigilance test (PVT)[134] during a 16-hour baseline day and a 64-hour period of total sleep deprivation. As seen in the figure, lapses on the PVT are relatively rare during the baseline day and during the first 16 hours of the sleep deprivation period, both of which fall on the diurnal portion of the circadian cycle and have little pressure for sleep. However, after the first 16 hours of the sleep deprivation period, lapses are clearly evident, indicating a substantial increase in neurobehavioral dysfunction. There is a steady rise in lapses across days, modulated by a pronounced circadian rhythm—the combined effect roughly takes the form of a staircase function.

Neurobehavioral functions that show circadian variation also appear to respond to sleep loss, and vice versa. The interaction of the circadian rhythm with the effect of sleep deprivation, which is nonlinear,[135,136] makes it difficult to dissociate the two effects in constant routine and sleep deprivation experiments (although it is possible by focusing on interindividual differences[137]). However, a reasonable separation of the two effects can be achieved with other experimental designs, as discussed later.

It is noteworthy that performance impairment during the circadian trough and while sleep deprived is associated with increased moment-to-moment variability (i.e., increased instability) in brain functioning,[138,139] of which lapses on the PVT are a sensitive measure.[140] As posited in the state

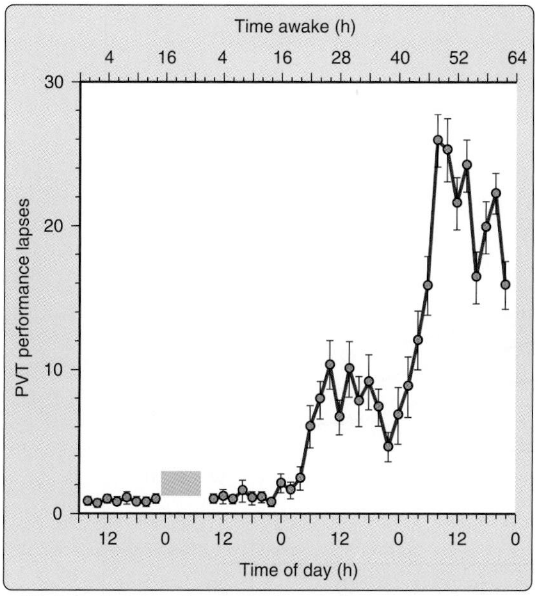

Figure 39.4 Performance lapses on the psychomotor vigilance test (PVT) during a 16-hour baseline day and a 64-hour period of sleep deprivation. Data shown are mean (with standard error) number of lapses (reaction times longer than 500 ms) for 24 subjects tested every 2 hours on the 10-minute PVT. This simple reaction time task requires subjects to respond as quickly as possible to a stimulus that appears on a display at random intervals of 2 to 10 seconds.[140] The *solid bar* indicates an 8-hour sleep period (from 11:30 p.m. until 7:30 a.m.) between the baseline day and the sleep deprivation period.

instability hypothesis, this moment-to-moment variability may be caused by sleep-initiating mechanisms interfering with sustained wakefulness, making cognitive performance unstable and dependent on compensatory mechanisms such as increased effort to perform.[141] Furthermore, according to local sleep theory,[142] the instability may occur specifically in brain networks involved in performance of the cognitive task at hand.[143,144] This network specificity may explain, in part, why the particular effects of sleep deprivation on neurobehavioral functioning appear to depend on the distinct cognitive processes required for the task being performed.[145,146]

Sleep-Wake Regulation

The observed superposition of circadian modulation of alertness and performance on monotonic change during sleep deprivation (Figure 39.4) has prompted efforts to mathematically model the regulatory processes involved. The two-process model of sleep regulation has been applied to describe the temporal profiles of sleep[147,148] as well as waking alertness and performance.[148,149] The model consists of a homeostatic process (process S) and a circadian process (process C), which combine to determine the onset and offset of sleep. The two processes together also drive waking neurobehavioral functioning.

The homeostatic process represents a drive for sleep that increases during wakefulness and decreases during sleep. When the "homeostat" increases above a certain threshold, sleep is triggered; when it decreases below another threshold, wakefulness is invoked. The circadian process represents daily oscillatory modulation of the two thresholds.[147] An alternative (but equivalent) view is that the circadian process promotes wakefulness to counteract the homeostatic drive for sleep.[150,151] The two-process model is discussed more extensively in another chapter in this volume.

The circadian and homeostatic processes interact to determine waking neurobehavioral functions.[131,135,152] This is clearly seen in prolonged sleep deprivation experiments (Figure 39.4). For both alertness and performance, sleep and sleep loss are not only masking factors but also dynamic biologic forces that interact with the circadian system.

Under conditions of chronic sleep restriction—that is, daily curtailment of sleep (rather than total sleep deprivation)—there is a progressive buildup of pressure for sleep across days that is not predicted by the two-process model.[153] It has been hypothesized that this reflects allostatic adjustment of the set point of the homeostatic process.[154] The buildup of sleep pressure across days notwithstanding, the circadian process partially protects the afternoon and early evening from neurobehavioral impairment,[155] as illustrated in Figure 39.5 (see also Figure 39.1). The period when this is most noticeable, a window of several hours preceding habitual bedtime, is known as the "forbidden zone for sleep"[156] or "wake maintenance zone."[157]

Forced Desynchrony and Ultradian Days

The forced desynchrony protocol[151,158,159] is an experimental procedure designed to dissociate the effects of the circadian and homeostatic processes. In this protocol, a subject is housed in an environmentally and temporally isolated laboratory in which the sleep-wake cycle is scheduled to deviate substantially from the normal 24-hour day (e.g., 20-hour and 28-hour sleep-wake cycles). The biologic clock is unable to synchronize to such a schedule. The subject therefore experiences two distinct influences simultaneously: the schedule of predetermined sleep and wake times controlling the homeostatic process and the rhythm of the subject's unsynchronized, free-running circadian process.

Neurobehavioral variables can be recorded during the subject's waking periods within this experimental design. By folding the data over either the free-running circadian cycle or the imposed sleep-wake cycle, the influence of the other cycle can be averaged out. This allows the effects of the circadian and homeostatic processes on the recorded variables to be separated. As expected, forced desynchrony studies have found that both the circadian and homeostatic processes influence alertness and performance. The interaction of the two processes appears to be oppositional during natural diurnal wake periods (from about 7 a.m. until 11 p.m.) such that a relatively stable level of alertness and performance can be maintained throughout the day.[151] This explains why studies of alertness and performance tend to find little temporal variation during the waking portion of a normal day (Figure 39.4).

Another way to dissociate the circadian and homeostatic processes is through study designs with very short (i.e., ultradian) sleep-wake cycles. Such paradigms seek to redistribute the opportunities for sleep and wakefulness across the natural 24-hour day to sample waking behavior across the circadian cycle without significantly curtailing the total amount of sleep. Studies have been done with a 7-minute/13-minute sleep-wake schedule,[7] which alternately allows subjects to sleep for 7 minutes and forces them to stay awake for 13 minutes; with a 90-minute day schedule,[160] which alternately permits subjects to sleep for 30 minutes and forces them to stay awake for 60 minutes; and with a 3-hour ultrashort sleep-wake schedule,[161] which alternates 1 hour of sleep and 2 hours of wake periods.

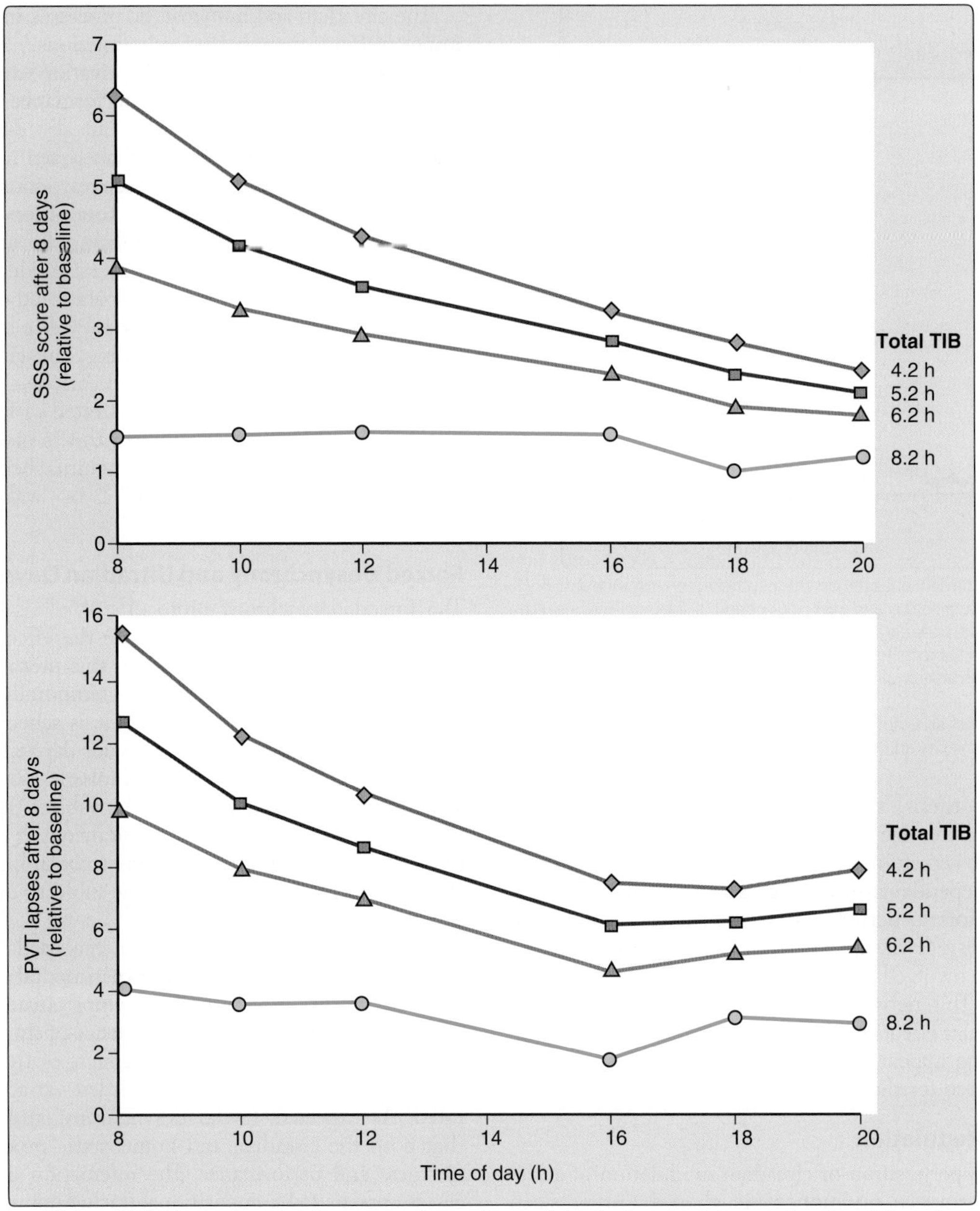

Figure 39.5 Sleepiness and performance under conditions of chronic sleep restriction as a function of time of day. Data shown are mean subjective sleepiness score on the Stanford Sleepiness Scale[9] (SSS; *top panel*) and mean number of lapses (reaction times longer than 500 ms) on the 10-minute psychomotor vigilance test (PVT)[140] (*bottom panel*) after 8 days of nocturnal sleep restriction with or without a daytime nap. Total time in bed (TIB) per day was 4.2 hours, 5.2 hours, 6.2 hours (sleep restriction conditions), or 8.2 hours (control condition); 90 subjects were each randomized to one of these conditions. (From Mollicone DJ, Van Dongen HPA, Rogers NL, et al. Time of day effects on neurobehavioral performance during chronic sleep restriction. *Aviat Space Environ Med.* 2010;81:735–44, with permission.)

With respect to objective measures, studies with very short sleep-wake cycles have focused primarily on sleep propensity. However, cognitive performance was assessed in an experiment using the 7-/13-minute sleep-wake schedule and in an experiment employing the 3-hour ultrashort sleep-wake schedule. Robust circadian rhythms emerged for response times on a choice reaction time task[162] and on an abbreviated (5-minute) version of the PVT.[161]

Subjective sleepiness scores were recorded in the 7-minute/13-minute sleep-wake schedule,[163] the 90-minute day schedule,[160] and the 3-hour ultrashort sleep-wake schedule,[161] all of which yielded clear circadian rhythms. However, after a 24-hour period of 7-minute/13-minute sleep-wake cycles (but not after 24 hours on the schedules with 90-minute or 3-hour cycles), the level of subjective sleepiness was elevated compared to the initial level 24 hours earlier. This suggests that across 24 hours of the 7-minute/13-minute sleep-wake schedule, the recovery potential of the sleep obtained—which itself is modulated by the circadian process—may have been insufficient.

All things considered, the separation of circadian and homeostatic influences on neurobehavioral variables presents a conceptual, experimental, and mathematical problem. The interaction of the two processes has been found to be

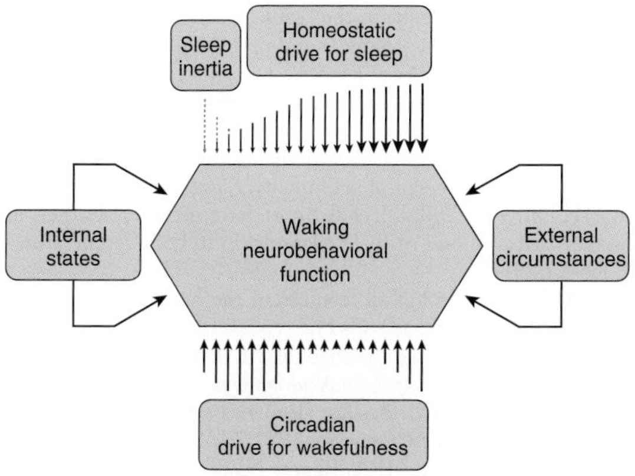

Figure 39.6 Schematic representation of the conceptual interplay of circadian and homeostatic processes and other factors in the regulation of neurobehavioral functioning. Sleep inertia and the homeostatic process degrade performance. Sleep inertia dissipates rapidly after awakening, whereas the homeostatic drive for sleep builds up progressively over time awake. The circadian process provides an oscillatory countereffect by promoting wakefulness during the day and withdrawing the effect at night. A wide range of internal states and external circumstances modulate waking neurobehavioral functions. Their effects are typically transient and may improve or degrade neurobehavioral functioning in interaction with the homeostatic and circadian processes.[4,31]

nonlinear.[135,136] It is therefore difficult, if not impossible, to quantify the relative importance of the two influences on neurobehavioral functions, even in forced desynchrony and ultradian day experiments. Moreover, the relative contributions of the two processes may vary across different experimental conditions[63,135] and among subjects.[137,164]

Sleep inertia is yet another problem that may interfere with the assessment of alertness and performance in circadian studies and with the dissociation of the circadian and homeostatic processes. Sleep inertia refers to the feeling of disorientation, grogginess, tendency to return to sleep, and cognitive performance impairment experienced immediately after awakening.[165] Sleep inertia may affect alertness and performance on every artificial day of a forced desynchrony study or ultradian sleep-wake cycle study. The circadian and homeostatic processes appear to interact with sleep inertia,[166-170] thereby varying the impact of sleep inertia across the artificial days in these study designs and making it difficult to account for its effects.

Circadian Regulation of Alertness and Performance in Context

Figure 39.6 shows a conceptual schematic of how the circadian drive for wakefulness, the homeostatic drive for sleep, the sleep inertia effect, and various internal states and external circumstances simultaneously affect neurobehavioral functioning.

As illustrated in the upper part of the figure, wakefulness typically begins with rapidly dissipating sleep inertia, which suppresses neurobehavioral functioning for a brief period after awakening. The homeostatic drive for sleep accumulates throughout wakefulness and progressively downregulates neurobehavioral performance and alertness. Unlike the circadian process, which is limited in amplitude, the homeostatic drive for sleep may accumulate far beyond the levels typically encountered in a 24-hour day (indicated in Figure 39.6 by the increasing density of downward arrows).

In opposition to these suppressing influences on performance and alertness is the endogenous circadian rhythm of the biologic clock, as illustrated in the bottom part of the figure. The circadian process modulates performance and alertness by promoting wakefulness. The improvement in waking neurobehavioral functions by the circadian drive for wakefulness is an oscillatory process, which periodically involves robust opposition to the homeostatic process alternated with withdrawal of the circadian drive.

Modulators of neurobehavioral functions other than the sleep and circadian drives are subsumed in Figure 39.6 under the broad categories of internal states and external circumstances. These may include wake-promoting factors—endogenous (e.g., anxiety) or exogenous (e.g., caffeine intake)—that counteract the homeostatic drive for sleep. They may also include sleep-promoting factors—endogenous (e.g., immune response–induced) or exogenous (e.g., rhythmic motion)—that oppose the circadian drive for wakefulness, either directly or indirectly by exposing the homeostatic drive for sleep.

The neurobiologic substrates of these exogenous and endogenous factors are diverse. Although common in the real world, they are considered masking factors in most laboratory experiments. However, with regard to the regulation of alertness and performance, they cannot be regarded as mere confounds that should be eliminated or controlled. Although the effects of internal states and external circumstances tend to be transient, they are an integral part of the regulation of neurobehavioral functions and the interaction of individuals with their environment.[112]

Understanding the complexity of circadian rhythmicity in neurobehavioral functions is important when the sleep-wake rhythm is misaligned, as during night and shift work schedules,[171-174] or when the circadian rhythm is misaligned, as is the case after transmeridian flights.[175,176] In such situations, the circadian and homeostatic processes are not properly synchronized, and their interaction degrades alertness and performance. This problem is compounded when sleep is lost chronically,[153,177-179] putting individuals at increased risk of accidents.[180-183] The emerging field of *fatigue risk management* is concerned with addressing these issues based on the biologic and behavioral principles described in this chapter.[184,185]

CLINICAL PEARL

Clinicians should recognize that 24-hour profiles of alertness and performance combine the effects of endogenous circadian rhythmicity, homeostatic regulation of sleep, sleep inertia, and a variety of endogenous and exogenous "masking" influences. Distinguishing these factors and accounting for interindividual differences is important for diagnosis and treatment of sleep disorders involving excessive daytime sleepiness and/or circadian dysregulation.[3]

SUMMARY

The biologic clock drives circadian rhythms and regulates changes in behavior over the 24 hours of the day. There are circadian rhythms in almost all variables describing alertness and performance. People tend to be less alert in the early morning and late at night, but it also depends on the circumstances.

A variety of factors (e.g., activity, posture, light exposure) can mask circadian rhythms. Even with masking influences experimentally controlled, measurements of the endogenous circadian rhythmicity in alertness and performance still reflect the interaction of the biologic clock with the homeostatic regulation of sleep. It has been argued that certain masking factors (e.g., sensory stimulation, body movement) are an integral part of the mechanisms regulating waking neurobehavioral functions. Accounting for their interactions with the biologic clock helps to explain or predict the occurrence of cognitive performance deficits across the circadian cycle.

SELECTED READINGS

Daan S, Beersma DGM, Borbély AA. Timing of human sleep: recovery process gated by a circadian pacemaker. *Am J Physiol.* 1984;246:R161–R178.

Dijk DJ, Czeisler CA. Paradoxical timing of the circadian rhythm of sleep propensity serves to consolidate sleep and wakefulness in humans. *Neurosci Lett.* 1994;166:63–68.

Duffy JF, Czeisler CA. Age-related change in the relationship between circadian period, circadian phase, and diurnal preference in humans. *Neurosci Lett.* 2001;318:117–120.

Ferris M, Bowles KA, Bray M, et. al. The impact of shift work schedules on PVT performance in naturalistic settings: a systematic review [published online ahead of print, 2021 Mar 11]. *Int Arch Occup Environ Health.* 2021;10.1007/s00420-021-01668-0.

Folkard S, Åkerstedt T. Trends in the risk of accidents and injuries and their implications for models of fatigue and performance. *Aviat Space Environ Med.* 2004;75:A161–A167.

Horne JA, Brass CG, Pettitt AN. Circadian performance differences between morning and evening types. *Ergonomics.* 1980;23:29–36.

Johns MW. Sleep propensity varies with behaviour and the situation in which it is measured: the concept of somnificity. *J Sleep Res.* 2002;11:61–67.

Johnson MP, Duffy JF, Dijk DJ, et al. Short-term memory, alertness and performance: a reappraisal of their relationship to body temperature. *J Sleep Res.* 1992;1:24–29.

Kerkhof GA. Inter-individual differences in the human circadian system: a review. *Biol Psychol.* 1985;20:83–112.

Lavie P. Ultrashort sleep-waking schedule. III. "Gates" and "forbidden zones" for sleep. *Electroencephalogr Clin Neurophysiol.* 1986;63:414–425.

Minors DS, Waterhouse JM. Anchor sleep as a synchronizer of rhythms on abnormal routines. *Int J Chronobiol.* 1981;7:165–188.

Mollicone DJ, Van Dongen HPA, Rogers NL, et al. Time of day effects on neurobehavioral performance during chronic sleep restriction. *Aviat Space Environ Med.* 2010;81:735–744.

Taillard J, Sagaspe P, Philip P, Bioulac S. Sleep timing, chronotype and social jetlag: Impact on cognitive abilities and psychiatric disorders [published online ahead of print, 2021 Feb 2]. *Biochem Pharmacol.* 2021;114438.

Van Dongen HPA, Dinges DF. Sleep, circadian rhythms, and psychomotor vigilance. *Clin Sports Med.* 2005;24:237–249.

A complete reference list can be found online at ExpertConsult.com.

Chapter 40

Central and Peripheral Circadian Clocks

Edith Grosbellet; Etienne Challet

Chapter Highlights

- The master clock in the suprachiasmatic nucleus (SCN) controls the sleep-wake cycle and hormonal rhythms, as well as a multitude of other circadian rhythms.
- The SCN clock conducts the multitude of brain and peripheral clocks to ensure circadian temporal organization and its adjustment to the daily variations of the environment.
- Rhythmic signals from the SCN couple the master clock to secondary brain and peripheral clocks through behavioral, nervous, and neurohumoral pathways. Endocrine rhythms (e.g., pineal melatonin and adrenal glucocorticoids) distribute internal temporal messages within the body.
- Light perceived by the retina is the most potent synchronizer of the master clock in the SCN, whereas most brain and peripheral clocks can be shifted as a function of mealtime as well as the timing of sleep.
- Circadian clocks and intracellular metabolism are tightly and reciprocally connected.

THE MASTER CIRCADIAN CLOCK

Self-Sustained Oscillations

In mammals, the master clock is located in the suprachiasmatic nucleus (SCN) of the hypothalamus (Figure 40.1). The SCN controls most circadian rhythms in behavior (e.g., sleep-wake cycle) and physiology (e.g., hormonal rhythms). The SCN consists of a heterogeneous population of neuronal and glial cells distributed in two anatomic subdivisions: a ventral "core" region, receiving retinal input, and a dorsal "shell" region, receiving dense input from the core.[1] When physically isolated, either in vitro or in vivo, the SCN generates pronounced circadian rhythms of electrical activity.[2,3] Neuronal firing and chemical and electrical (gap junctions) synapses are required for circadian coupling within the SCN in vivo.[1] The molecular clock machinery involves 24-hour oscillations of core clock components called *clock genes* (Figure 40.1).[4,5] The SCN clock machinery also modulates the expression of numerous clock-controlled genes (e.g., vasopressin), which constitute circadian outputs that provide either local or distributed timing signals.[6]

Photic Entrainment of the Master Clock

The daily synchronization of a self-sustained oscillator by an external signal (zeitgeber) is called *entrainment*. The most potent synchronizer of the master clock is light perceived by the retina. Light intensity is detected in the retina by classical photoreceptors, namely rods and cones, and by intrinsically photosensitive ganglion cells containing the photopigment melanopsin, which is highly responsive to blue light.[7] The axons of these ganglion cells constitute the retinohypothalamic tract and project monosynaptically to the SCN core.[8] A few other structures can also convey indirect light information to the SCN, such as the intergeniculate leaflets (IGLs) of the thalamus and the basal forebrain nuclei.[9,10] In response to light, glutamate and pituitary adenylate cyclase–activating polypeptide (PACAP) released from retinohypothalamic terminals bind to their receptors expressed in ventral SCN neurons.[11] This downstream signaling induces acute expression of clock genes *Per1* and *Per2*, in addition to several immediate early response genes such as *c-fos*,[12-14] which are induced by light only at night (i.e., during the photosensitive phase of the SCN). Because only the SCN core receives photic inputs, synchronization of the shell to light is mediated through core-to-shell projections involving gamma-aminobutyric acid (GABA), nitric oxide, and vasoactive intestinal polypeptide (VIP) signaling.[11,15,16]

In addition to its phase-shifting effects, light also modulates daily rhythmicity by direct, clock-independent responses to light. For example, bright light at night has an immediate inhibitory effect on physical activity and promotes sleep in nocturnal rodents, whereas it enhances alertness and sustained attention in (diurnal) humans.[17,18] Furthermore, light at night inhibits melatonin secretion.[19] Light also influences other peripheral functions, such as heart rate, blood glucose, and glucocorticoids.[20-23] These direct effects of light could be conveyed successively by the SCN clock, the subparaventricular hypothalamic region, and the sympathetic nervous system.[20,22] Because melanopsin-containing ganglion cells project to several brain targets beyond the SCN, such as the subparaventricular hypothalamic zone,[8] light cues can also bypass the SCN and reach directly this hypothalamic region, which could, in turn, relay photic signals to peripheral organs through the sympathetic pathways. This alternative mechanism is supported by the properties of light-induced release of glucocorticoids.[23]

Nonphotic Phase-Shifting of the Master Clock

Even if the light is the most important zeitgeber, the environment provides numerous other temporal cycling cues (e.g., temperature, food availability, social interactions) called

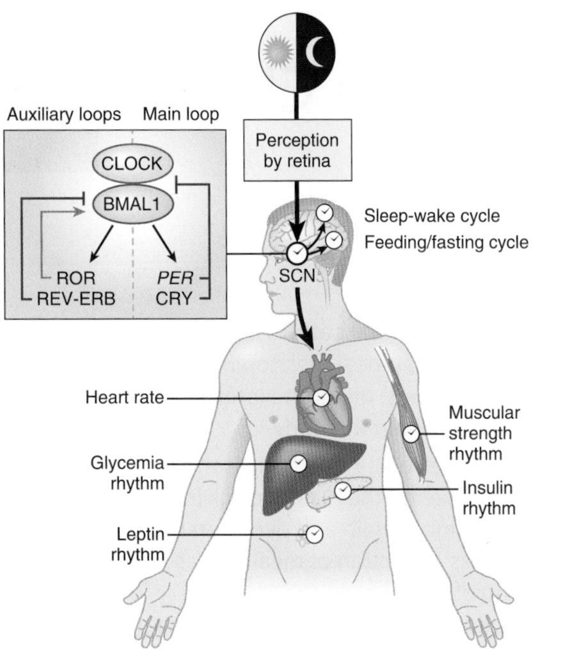

Figure 40.1 Hierarchical organization of the circadian system. The master clock located in the suprachiasmatic nucleus (SCN) synchronizes a network of brain and peripheral clocks, leading to circadian rhythms of physiologic, metabolic, and hormonal parameters. The molecular clockwork relies on transcriptional-translational feedback loops. The main loop involves CLOCK-BMAL1 stimulating the transcription of *Per* and *Cry* genes, which in turn inhibit the transcriptional activity of CLOCK-BMAL1. In the auxiliary loops, after stimulation of their transcription by CLOCK-BMAL1, ROR, and REV-ERB stimulate and inhibit the transcription of *Bmal1*, respectively. The auxiliary loops help stabilize the 24-hour oscillations of clock proteins. BMAL1, Brain-muscle-arnt-like protein; CLOCK, circadian locomotor output cycles kaput; CRY, cryptochrome; *PER*, period; REV-ERB, reverse viral erythroblastis oncogene product; ROR, retinoic acid receptor-related orphan nuclear receptor.

nonphotic synchronizers. One of the best-studied nonphotic factors is exercise, voluntary or forced. Transient hyperactivity or arousal in nocturnal rodents typically causes phase advances of their locomotor activity rhythm if it occurs during the subjective day, corresponding to their normal resting period.[24-26] In humans, exercise in evening and late night leads to phase advances and delays, respectively.[27] Metabolic cues serve as other nonphotic signals that could affect or entrain the SCN clock (see later in chapter). Two input pathways are mainly considered to transmit nonphotic messages to the SCN: the geniculohypothalamic fibers from the IGLs and the serotonergic input from the midbrain raphe nuclei, also projecting to the IGLs.[9,28] Stimulation of neuropeptide Y or serotonin receptors in the SCN of nocturnal rodents activates kinase-mediated phosphorylation events,[29,30] leading to a reduction in *Per1* and *Per2* messenger RNA (mRNA) levels.[31,32] Injections of antisense oligonucleotides against *Per1* in the SCN region produce nonphotic-like phase advances of the rest-activity rhythm.[33] Most nonphotic and photic stimuli interact with one another, usually in opposite directions.[34] The IGLs, which receive both photic and nonphotic cues, may be involved in integrating these conflicting signals before they reach the SCN.[9] Other input pathways implicated in arousal-induced phase-shifts of the SCN clock arise from cholinergic cells in basal forebrain[35] and from orexigenic neurons in the lateral hypothalamus.[36]

Outputs from the Master Clock

The SCN clock, which controls peripheral rhythms, is considered a conductor within the multioscillatory circadian network. Rhythmic signals from the SCN are distributed to the brain and the entire body by two main pathways: (1) release of neurotransmitters and neuropeptides from terminals of SCN efferents, a pathway critical for controlling hormonal rhythms[37] and (2) a neurohumoral pathway involving secretion of diffusible output signals regulating preferentially the rest-activity rhythm.[38] The SCNs project most densely to the medial hypothalamus, in particular to the subparaventricular zone. These SCN neuronal efferents are mainly GABAergic, although also glutamatergic and neuropeptidergic.[39] The second possible mode of transmission for circadian cues from the SCN is the secretion of molecules into the extracellular space and cerebrospinal fluid. The existence of such a neurohumoral pathway was first supported by the fact that SCN grafts, encapsulated to prevent axonal growth and sprouting, are still capable of restoring behavioral rhythmicity in otherwise arrhythmic SCN-lesioned rodents.[38] Thus the rest-activity rhythm is thought to be regulated preferentially by diffusible output signals such as transforming growth factor-alpha, prokineticin 2, and cardiotropin-like cytokine.[40-42] These three molecules contribute to the suppression of locomotor activity, although possible stimulatory factors have not yet been identified.

BRAIN AND PERIPHERAL CIRCADIAN CLOCKS

Extra-Suprachiasmatic Nucleus Brain Clocks

The core clock mechanism described in the SCN is present in almost all brain regions and peripheral (i.e., outside the brain) tissues studied so far.[43,44] Many brain areas exhibit daily oscillations of clock genes.[45,46] Retina and olfactory bulbs are the only extra-SCN clocks with very strong oscillatory capacities that have been identified so far.[47,48] Other brain areas, such as the arcuate nucleus and dorsomedial hypothalamic nucleus, two structures of the mediobasal hypothalamus involved in feeding and energy metabolism, are capable of self-sustained oscillations for several cycles when isolated in vitro. Cells of these oscillators exhibit independent circadian rhythms but are weakly coupled, and their synchronization requires daily inputs.[49,50] Strikingly, the timing of clock gene oscillations and rhythm of electrical activity in the secondary brain clocks of nocturnal rodents differ from the SCN in most cases. In the SCN, electrical activity and *Per1* expression peak during (subjective) daytime, whereas the corresponding peaks occur at night (i.e., during the active period) in extra-SCN oscillators.[49,51] In sharp contrast, the bed nucleus of stria terminalis, a basal forebrain structure modulating a wide range of physiologic and motivational processes, displays electrical activity in phase with the SCN, suggesting a strong coupling between the two structures.[51] Furthermore, several brain structures, such as the ventromedial hypothalamic nucleus, display a daily rhythmicity dependent on timed inputs because these structures become arrhythmic as soon as they are isolated in vitro.[50] Of note, the core clock mechanisms in brain oscillators seem very close to those identified in the SCN. In the forebrain, however, neuronal PAS domain-containing protein 2 (NPAS2) replaces the transcription factor CLOCK (for Circadian Locomotor Output Cycles Kaput) as a partner of

BMAL1 (for for Brain and Muscle Aryl-hydrocarbon receptor nuclear translocator-Like protein 1) in the positive loop of the molecular clockwork.[52]

Clocks in Peripheral Tissues

Around 10% of a tissue's transcriptome has a circadian pattern of expression.[53,54] Most peripheral cells contain the molecular clock machinery.[55,56] Bioluminescent constructs have allowed for real-time visualization of oscillations in clock genes, both in vitro and in vivo.[43,44,57] Peripheral clocks, such as liver explants, can generate a number of circadian cycles of *Per2*-luciferase expression.[44] With in vivo conditions, the SCN participates in the phase coherence between hepatocytes.[58] Cultured fibroblasts have been an in vitro model of choice to study the molecular regulation of the circadian clocks.[55,56] Similar to the master clock, cultured fibroblasts are resilient to large changes in temperature and overall transcription rates.[59] Activation of a multitude of intracellular pathways affects their clockwork.[60] Cultured fibroblasts do not generate metabolic rhythmicity as assessed by 2-deoxyglucose uptake, in spite of synchronized oscillations of clock genes. Sustained oscillations of 2-deoxyglucose uptake, however, can be produced in fibroblasts if they are cocultured (without physical contact) with immortalized SCN cells.[61]

In the liver, clock-controlled genes encode key enzymes involved in hepatic metabolism of fatty acids, cholesterol, bile acids, amino acids, and xenobiotics.[62-94] Specific inactivation of *Bmal1* in the livers of mice (L-*Bmal1*$^{-/-}$) disrupts rhythmic expression of glucose regulatory genes and glucose metabolism, including circulating glucose levels. L-*Bmal1*$^{-/-}$ mice are mildly hypoglycemic during the resting phase, suggesting that the hepatic clock drives a daily rhythm of hepatic glucose export counterbalancing the brain-driven fasting-feeding cycle.[65]

The adipose tissue also exhibits robust oscillations of core clock components, controlling the circadian expression of many transcription factors.[66,67] The lipoprotein lipase displays a rhythmic activity in adipose tissue, suggesting that the adipose clock is somehow involved in lipid metabolism.[68] Moreover, the adipose tissue secretes several hormones termed adipokines, including leptin and adiponectin, involved in the regulation of energy balance. Several adipokine genes show a rhythmic expression in mouse adipose tissue.[66] Circulating levels of leptin display clear diurnal variations in both rodents and humans.[69-71] Moreover, leptin secretion was shown to be rhythmic in cultured adipocytes, suggesting that rhythmic synthesis or secretion of this adipokine may be under the control of the adipose clock.[72]

Altogether the results show that peripheral cells, such as fibroblasts, hepatocytes, or adipocytes, fulfill the usual criteria to consider them as peripheral cellular clocks. In most peripheral tissues, however, neighboring cellular clocks fail to maintain phase coherence, in contrast to the strong intercellular coupling in the SCN. Another functional difference with the SCN is the fact that CLOCK is indispensable for circadian gene expression in peripheral tissues, at least the liver and lung.[73] Moreover, there can be specific differences in the characteristics of the clockwork according to the cell type.[74]

Intestinal microbiota contains circadian clocks that influence the host circadian system through local and distal (i.e., systemic) interactions. Notably, the intestinal and hepatic clocks are markedly affected by changes in gut microbial composition and rhythmicity.[75-77] Conversely, defective clocks and circadian desynchronization of the host lead to intestinal dysbiosis associated with impaired microbial rhythmicity.[78,79]

Molecular Links between Core Clock Components and Metabolism

Several transcriptional networks connect the core clock mechanisms with intracellular metabolic pathways. These interactions involve, among others, a number of nuclear receptors, including reverse viral erythroblastis oncogene products (REV-ERBs) and retinoic acid receptor-related orphan receptors (RORs) (i.e., circadian components defining auxiliary loops in the clock mechanism) and peroxisome proliferator–activated receptors (PPARs), which are transcription factors activated by fatty acids. In the skeletal muscle, RORα directly regulates genes involved in fatty acid metabolism.[80] Moreover, REV-ERBα plays a pivotal role at the interface between the liver clock and lipid metabolism.[81] REV-ERBα also plays a pivotal role in the daily variations of fuel utilization.[82] *Pparα* is rhythmically expressed in tissues with high rates of fatty acid oxidation, such as the muscles, heart, or liver, and is strongly involved in lipoprotein and lipid metabolism.[83] *Pparα* is a clock-controlled gene whose activation involves CLOCK and BMAL1, which in turn can activate *Bmal1* transcription.[84,85] Thus PPARα provides a close link between circadian clocks and lipid metabolism in peripheral tissues, in particular in the liver. Additionally, a critical role has been demonstrated for PGC-1α, a coactivator of PPAR (PPAR coactivator-1α), which stimulates *Bmal1* expression through coactivation of RORs. Because PGC-1α is a metabolic regulator sensitive to various signals including nutritional status and temperature, it could be a key component in the coupling of metabolism to circadian clocks.[86] Furthermore, lipidomic profiling in adipose tissue indicates that PER2 is implicated in normal lipid metabolism. This effect is mediated by PPARγ, a major regulator of adipogenesis and lipid metabolism in adipose tissue, whose transcriptional activity is directly repressed by PER2.[87]

Interactions between the circadian clocks and cellular metabolism also involve cellular energy sensors such as sirtuin1 (SIRT1) and adenosine monophosphate (AMP)-activated protein kinase (AMPK). SIRT1 catalyzes NAD^+-dependent deacetylation of various substrates. By deacetylating histones, SIRT1 participates in chromatin condensation and thus epigenetic silencing. SIRT1 also contributes to multiple metabolic pathways and plays a crucial role in the life span extension associated with calorie restriction, in part through the SCN clock.[88] SIRT1 influences the transcription of several clock genes and promotes deacetylation and degradation of PER2, thus modulating the timing of the core clock loops.[89,90] Inhibition of SIRT1 leads to circadian disturbances and to the acetylation of BMAL1 and histone H3, both substrates of the acetylase function of CLOCK.[90]

Besides SIRT1, AMPK is another important metabolic fuel gauge, sensing changes in the intracellular AMP/adenosine triphosphate (ATP) ratio. AMPK integrates nutritional and hormonal signals in peripheral tissues and the hypothalamus, where it mediates cellular effects of adipokines (e.g., leptin) in regulating glucose and lipid homeostasis. Like SIRT1, AMPK responds to low energy levels.[91] In mouse skeletal muscle, AMPK enhances SIRT1 activity by increasing cellular NAD^+ levels, resulting in the deacetylation and modulation of the activity of SIRT1 targets, such as PGC-1α,[92] which in turn affects the circadian clock. AMPK also has direct actions on the clock machinery. AMPK phosphorylates not only the clock protein CRY1 but also casein kinase1ε, leading to subsequent degradation of PER2 and phase-shifts of peripheral oscillations.[93,94]

The connections between the cellular metabolism and the clockwork have been intensively investigated in peripheral tissues. Although much less is known, close mechanisms may be found in central extra-SCN oscillators. In particular, AMPK is a potent regulator of energy balance within the hypothalamus.[91] AMPK signaling is a likely route through which circadian and feeding signals are integrated in the hypothalamus.[95]

COUPLING BETWEEN CENTRAL AND PERIPHERAL CLOCKS

Entrainment of Peripheral Clocks by Nervous Outputs of the Suprachiasmatic Nucleus

It is now well established that the SCN clock controls timing in peripheral organs through the sympathetic pathways.[39,96] To illustrate this, the liver and the white adipose tissue have been chosen as two representative examples in this section. The liver plays a pivotal role in glycemic regulation as a site of glucose uptake and a major source of glucose production.[97] The daily rhythmicity of plasma glucose, peaking before activity onset in rats, is not a passive response to food intake.[98] A functional liver clock is important for glucose metabolism[65] but is not sufficient because SCN-lesioned rats lose their daily rhythmicity of blood glucose.[98] Retrograde tracing studies from the liver revealed projections through both sympathetic and parasympathetic components of the autonomous nervous system to third-order neurons in the SCN. Moreover, the glucose rhythm can be abolished by inactivation of either the sympathetic or parasympathetic inputs, underlying the importance of balanced inputs from the autonomous nervous system. Rhythmic GABAergic input from the SCN is considered to inhibit the sympathetic and parasympathetic preautonomic neurons of the paraventricular nucleus (PVN) of the hypothalamus, predominantly during the day. By contrast, glutamatergic projections from the SCN stimulate sympathetic preautonomic neurons of the PVN. Thus the entrainment of circadian glucose rhythm is performed by the SCN, fine-tuning the balance between both branches of the autonomous nervous system that innervate the liver clock.[97] Moreover, hypothalamic expression of orexin exhibits a diurnal rhythm entrained by GABAergic inputs from the SCN. Besides its role in behavioral activation, orexin is also a key regulator of plasma glucose in rats, modulating in particular the daily peak at dusk through the sympathetic nervous system.[99]

The rich innervation of adipose tissue by sympathetic fibers is well known, and their activation enhances lipolysis. Parasympathetic innervation of white adipose tissue has been shown more recently.[100] As for the liver, the SCN controls both branches of the autonomous nervous system that innervate adipose tissues, thus modulating circadian rhythmicity of metabolic and endocrine outputs of the adipose clock. For instance, activity of the hormone-sensitive lipase exhibits a daily rhythmicity that is modified by adipose denervation.[100] Moreover, the leptin rhythm is under the control of both the local adipose and SCN clocks because lesions of the SCN abolish the daily rhythm of plasma leptin in rats.[69,72] Through modulation of the autonomic innervations of liver and adipose clocks, the SCN therefore controls circadian rhythmicity of metabolites (carbohydrates and lipids) and metabolic hormones (e.g., leptin). Some peripheral clocks, however, do not respond directly to nervous cues, and rhythmic hormones (glucocorticoids and melatonin) may additionally transmit timing signals from the SCN to a variety of peripheral organs that express glucocorticoid or melatonin receptors.

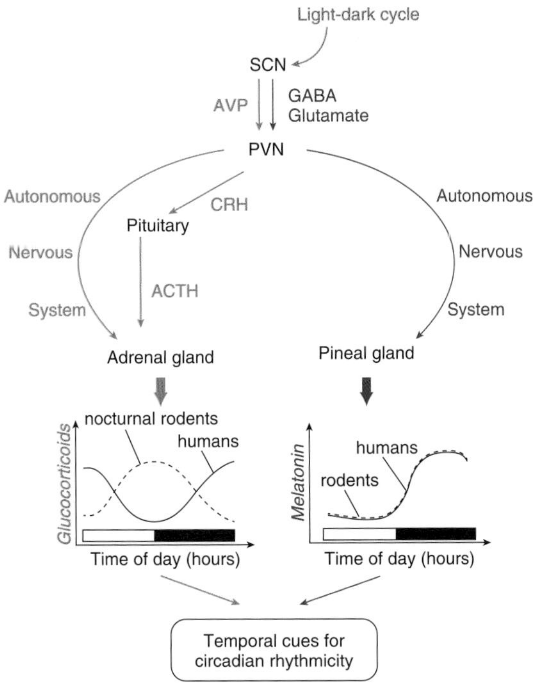

Figure 40.2 Rhythmic secretion of adrenal glucocorticoids and pineal melatonin is driven by the suprachiasmatic nucleus (SCN) and acts in turn as temporal cues for circadian rhythmicity. ACTH, Adrenocorticotropic hormone; AVP, arginine-vasopressin; CRH, corticotropin-releasing hormone; GABA, gamma-aminobutyric acid; PVN, paraventricular nucleus.

Entrainment of Peripheral Clocks by Suprachiasmatic Nucleus–Controlled Hormonal Outputs

Melatonin and glucocorticoids are two hormones with time-giving properties because their rhythmic release is tightly controlled by the SCN through nervous pathways, and when released, these endocrine messages can in turn affect or even entrain peripheral clocks (Figure 40.2).

Melatonin synthesized in the pineal gland is best known as a transducer of the photoperiodic information into neuroendocrine changes through the duration of its nocturnal peak.[101,102] The daily high-amplitude rhythm of melatonin also has a circadian role. Melatonin synthesized from tryptophan is always secreted during the dark phase in both nocturnal and diurnal mammals.[103] The release of melatonin is driven by the SCN clock through a multisynaptic pathway, including the PVN, the intermediolateral cell column of the spinal cord, and the superior cervical ganglions that send sympathetic fibers, which release noradrenalin in the vicinity of the pinealocytes. This noradrenergic release triggers the nocturnal synthesis of melatonin.[104] The daily rhythm of nocturnal melatonin provides temporal signals to a multitude of tissues expressing melatonin receptors, including peripheral organs and the SCN themselves. In isolated adipocytes, rhythmic melatonin mimicking a biologic night triggers expression of clock genes, such as *Per1* and *Clock*, and stimulates a lipogenic response.[105] Melatonin modulates clock gene expression in adrenal explants.[106] Furthermore, in the pars tuberalis of the adenohypophysis, rhythmic oscillations of clock genes (i.e., *Cry1* and *Per1*) are driven by the daily rhythm of melatonin.[107]

The nocturnal rhythm of endogenous melatonin is a reliable phase marker of the SCN clock because it is relatively impervious to most internal and external disturbances, except bright light exposure at night, which immediately inhibits its synthesis, therefore blunting its temporal message.[19]

Glucocorticoids (corticosterone in rats and mice; cortisol in humans) show a strong daily rhythm, peaking systematically at about wake-up time (dawn and dusk in nocturnal rodents and humans, respectively). This daily peak results from the adrenal clock, which is controlled by SCN cues through the hypothalamic-pituitary-adrenal axis and sympathetic fibers, the latter modulating the sensitivity of the adrenal glands to adrenocorticotropic hormone (ACTH).[108-111] The glucocorticoid nuclear receptors are expressed in most cell types in periphery and the brain, with the notable exception of adult SCN cells.[112] Dexamethasone, a glucocorticoid receptor agonist, activates *Per1* expression and synchronizes rat fibroblasts in vitro. Moreover, dexamethasone produces in vivo phase-shifts of peripheral clocks (e.g., liver, kidney, and heart), but not of the SCN clock.[113] Activity of glucocorticoid receptors is directly modulated by the clockwork because their transcription can be repressed by cryptochrome proteins (CRYs) and they can be acetylated by CLOCK.[114,115] In extra-SCN brain structures, such as the bed nucleus of stria terminalis and central amygdala, oscillations of the clock protein PER2 disappear after adrenalectomy and are restored by rhythmic supply of corticosterone through drinking water.[116] In midbrain raphe nuclei that do not express clock genes, rhythmic corticosterone also drives the daily rhythm of tryptophan hydroxylase mRNA, a limiting enzyme for synthesis of serotonin.[117] Thus daily variations of circadian glucocorticoids possess resetting and time-giving properties for central and peripheral structures.

However, the circadian rhythm of glucocorticoids can be blunted or markedly modified by environmental conditions, including stressful events, light, and feeding. Acute stress leads to ACTH-induced release of glucocorticoids that is not necessarily in phase with the circadian pattern.[109] Also, light exposure at night induces *Per1* gene expression in the adrenal gland and corticosterone release by activation of sympathetic fibers independently of hypothalamic-pituitary-adrenal axis.[22] In addition, restricted feeding triggers an anticipatory rise in circulating glucocorticoids before food access. This anticipatory peak is ACTH independent and distinct from the circadian rhythm of glucocorticoids controlled by the SCN clock.[118] Therefore circulating glucocorticoids can influence circadian clocks by conveying various temporal signals, only some of them being strictly dependent on the SCN.

Feedback of Peripheral Hormonal Signals to the Suprachiasmatic Nucleus

The presence of both MT1 and MT2 receptors in the SCN suggests that melatonin may have feedback effects on the master clock.[119] Daily injections or perfusions of supraphysiologic doses of melatonin entrain the free-running activity of rats in constant darkness, when injections occur at the subjective dusk.[120,121] In vitro application of melatonin on cultured SCN explants induces two distinct effects. First, melatonin acutely inhibits neuronal firing.[122] Second, melatonin shifts the circadian rhythm of electrical activity of SCN neurons in a time-dependent manner.[123] The acute inhibitory effect seems to be mediated by MT1 receptors, whereas the phase-resetting effect may rely on MT2 receptor signaling.[124-125]

Glucocorticoids are not expected to feed back directly to the SCN because their receptors are not expressed in sizeable amount within adult SCN cells.[112] Furthermore, the glucocorticoid agonist dexamethasone can induce phase-shifts of clock gene expression in peripheral clocks but not in SCN neurons.[113] However, glucocorticoids modulate the daily synchronization of the SCN to light, as evidenced by faster reentrainment to a new light-dark cycle in adrenalectomized rodents.[126,127] The indirect feedback of glucocorticoids to the SCN is thought to be mediated through serotonergic projections from midbrain raphe.[126] Such a feedback would prevent uncoordinated resetting of the circadian system (e.g., in response to sporadic light exposure) and thus serves as a protection from zeitgeber noise.[127] Together, melatonin and glucocorticoid rhythms appear to stabilize the functioning of the circadian system.

ADJUSTING CLOCKS WITH FEEDING

Extra-Suprachiasmatic Clocks Are Entrained by Feeding Time

Among the different ways used by the SCN to synchronize peripheral clocks, the feeding rhythm is a strong zeitgeber for many tissues. In normal conditions, food intake takes place during the active period. Restricted feeding in nocturnal rodents (i.e., when food access is limited to few hours during daytime, a time when nocturnal rodents usually rest) inverts the phase of gene expression in peripheral organs within about a week, thereby uncoupling peripheral clocks from the SCN that remain phase-locked to the light-dark cycle.[128,129] The synchronization velocity is tissue specific. Indeed, food-induced phase resetting proceeds faster in liver than in kidney, heart, or pancreas, with large phase-shifts within 2 days of altered feeding schedule. Furthermore, there are peripheral clocks, such as the submaxillary salivary glands, that fail to entrain to restricted feeding (Figure 40.3).[96]

In the brain, food restriction entrains the activity of a number of, but not all, oscillating structures outside the SCN. For example, the multineuronal activity in the lateral hypothalamus of rats under restricted feeding shows a peak entrained to the time of feeding.[130] Moreover, daily patterns of *Per1* and *Per2* mRNA in the cerebral cortex, striatum, and PVN from mice entrained to restricted feeding also show a phase-shift with peaks around mealtime, as opposed to the nocturnal peaks of expression in animals fed *ad libitum*.[45,46] Other structures, such as the hippocampus, display small or no phase-change in patterns of clock gene expression.[45] Nevertheless, these data suggest that most secondary clocks within and outside of the brain are affected by restricted feeding schedules.

Under restriction feeding, several behavioral and physiologic functions become entrained to the availability of food. More specifically, body temperature and plasma corticosterone rise before food access in phase with behavioral activation, called *food-anticipatory activity*, thought to be the laboratory equivalent of food-seeking behavior in the wild. This rhythmic bout of activity is still expressed in SCN-lesioned animals and is considered a behavioral output of a food-entrainable clock, sometimes called the "food clock."[131,132] The precise location of the food clock (outside the SCN) and its mechanisms have been the subject of much debate and controversy. Most experimental arguments support the current view that the food clock is a network of

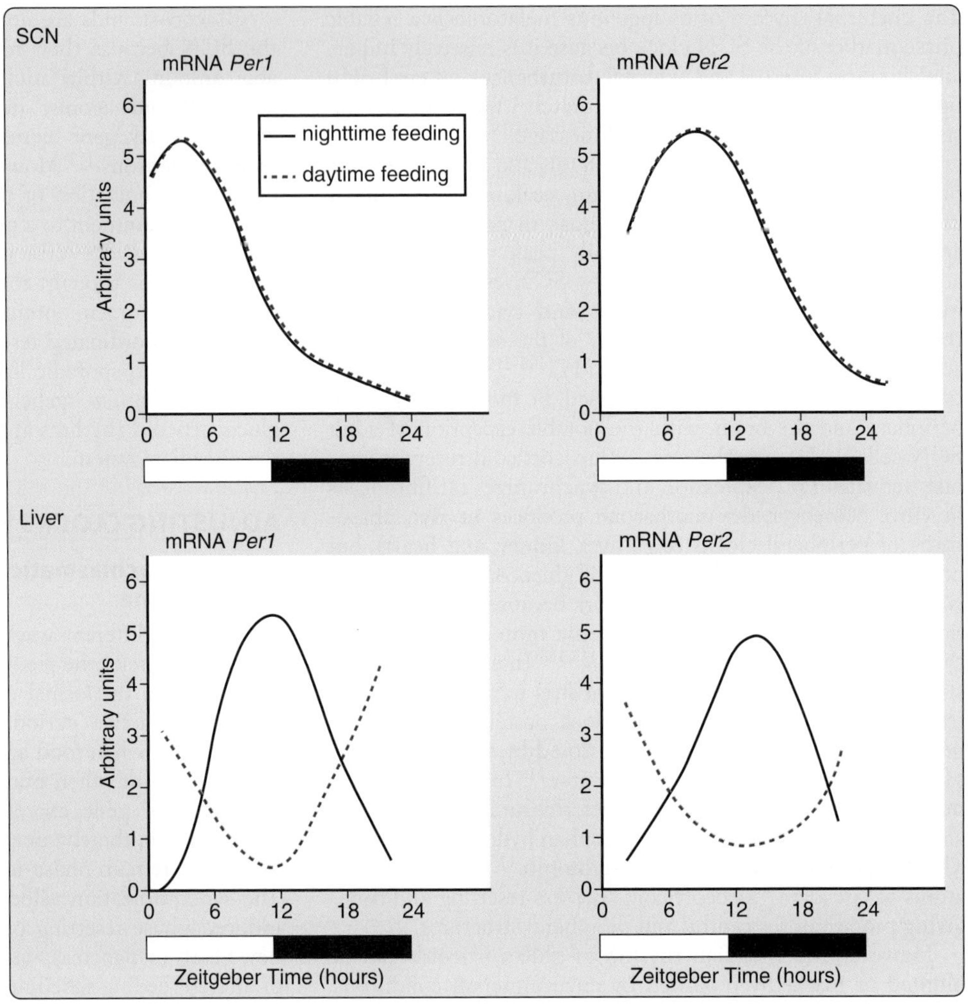

Figure 40.3 Daily expression of *Per1* and *Per2* in the liver and in the suprachiasmatic nucleus (SCN) of mice fed at nighttime (*solid lines*) or at daytime (*dotted lines*). Zeitgeber time 0 is defined as time of lights on. Feeding time affects daily rhythmicity of clock gene expression in peripheral clocks but not in the SCN. Timed changes in food intake can thus lead to an uncoupling of peripheral oscillators from the master clock. (Data from Damiola F, Le Minh N, Preitner N, et al. Restricted feeding uncouples circadian oscillators in peripheral tissues from the central pacemaker in the suprachiasmatic nucleus. *Genes Dev.* 2000;14:2950–61.)

coupled neural structures, likely involving mediobasal hypothalamic nuclei and metabolic brainstem structures, which interact together to provide timing and behavioral entrainment of feeding.[132,133]

Possible Mechanisms of Entrainment of Extra-Suprachiasmatic Nucleus Clocks by Food

The nature of signals that arise from feeding and that entrain peripheral clocks has been an area of intense investigation. Feeding cues include a number of parameters, including food absorption, postprandial increase in temperature, secretion of metabolic hormones, food-derived metabolites, and changes in the energetic status of cells.

Variations in temperature are known to entrain behavioral rhythms of heterotherms, such as *Drosophila* spp.[134] Moreover, temperature fluctuations mimicking body temperature rhythms sustain previously induced oscillations in cultured rat fibroblasts. Inverted environmental temperature cycles in vivo reverse circadian rhythms of clock genes (*Per2* and *Cry1*) in the mouse liver without affecting the SCN.[135] Thus diet-induced thermogenesis during the postprandial period could be an entraining pathway from feeding-fasting cycle in homeothermic organisms. The mechanisms of entrainment by temperature involve heat-shock factor 1 (HSF1), as revealed in vitro.[136,137] Hepatic HSF1 exhibits a highly rhythmic activity, which drives the expression of heat-shock proteins in liver.[138] Therefore HSF1 could be a key component linking temperature fluctuations and the phase of molecular clocks.

Anorexigenic (insulin) and orexigenic hormones (ghrelin) may participate in the entrainment of peripheral clocks by feeding. On one hand, insulin that rises in the plasma during the postprandial period causes an acute induction of *Per1* mRNA levels in cultured rat fibroblasts.[60] Moreover, insulin triggers upregulation of *Per2* mRNA and downregulation of *Rev-erbα* mRNA in the liver, thus mimicking the effects of refeeding after fasting.[139] The insulin-dependent phase-shifts of peripheral clocks involve phosphoinositide 3-kinase (PI3K)- and mitogen-activated protein kinases (MPAK)-mediated signaling pathways.[140] Feeding-induced insulin secretion may thus be a critical step in feeding-induced entrainment of peripheral clocks.[141] On the other hand, released ghrelin from the stomach during fasting is thought to signal hunger state to the brain. Cerebral activation of ghrelin signaling has been implicated in food-anticipatory activity that the animals express prior to timed food access.[142,143]

Another hormone linked to meal entrainment is corticosterone. An anticipatory rise of plasma corticosterone is induced by restricted feeding schedules,[144] and corticosterone is known to entrain peripheral clocks (see earlier).[113] However, corticosterone injections fail to mimic the phase-shifting effects of feeding in rats.[129] Gene expression rhythms in the liver of adrenalectomized or glucocorticoid receptor-deficient mice are still entrained by restricted feeding. Glucocorticoid signaling may actually provide resetting cues conflicting with feeding synchronizers because food-induced phase-shifts of the liver are actually faster in the absence of glucocorticoids.[145] The net effect of these synchronizing interactions depends on the tissue because the liver clock appears to be more sensitive to feeding cues, whereas the lung and kidney clocks are more easily reset by glucocorticoids.[146]

Fascinatingly, the application of glucose in the culture medium of rat fibroblasts causes a downregulation of *Per1* and *Per2* mRNA levels and induces rhythmic expression patterns of numerous genes, including transcription factors. The decrease of *Per1* and *Per2* mRNA levels by glucose seems indirect and mediated by glucose metabolism (i.e., involving transcriptional regulators) rather than by glucose.[147] Many nuclear receptors, such as PPARs (transcription factors activated by fatty acids), contribute to the daily variations of lipid and glucose metabolism. In addition to their role of mediators of metabolism, PPARs interact with clock components (see earlier).[85] Thus both plasma fatty acids and glucose, two major circulating metabolites, are potential mediators by which food-related cues entrain peripheral clocks.

As mentioned earlier, intestinal microbiota and its diurnal rhythmicity influence the host circadian clocks. Among other systemic signals, microbiota-derived short-chain fatty acids modulate phase adjustment by feeding cues of peripheral clocks, such as liver and kidney.[148]

Another possibility for feeding entrainment is that clock proteins, such as CLOCK (or its paralog NPAS2), BMAL1, or PERs, sense directly food-related signals. These proteins all contain PAS domain, which detects redox state (i.e., the reduced or oxidized environment within the cell), reflecting the energy status. Redox signals are transduced by PAS domains, which modulate the functional state of the protein.[149] The reduced forms of the nicotinamide adenine dinucleotide, NADH and NADPH, activate DNA binding of CLOCK (or NPAS2)/BMAL1, whereas the oxidized forms, NAD^+ and $NADP^+$, inhibit DNA binding. NAD(P)H/$NAD(P)^+$ ratio is closely tied to mitochondrial activity, and the switch between activation and inhibition of DNA binding is very sensitive, providing a rapid mechanism that could convey changes in fuel availability to the cellular clocks.[52] Therefore, even if feeding can be viewed as a dominant entraining factor for peripheral clocks, the underlying mechanisms are complex because multiple signals appear to be involved at different levels of the circadian system.

Effects of Nutritional Cues on the Master Clock

Although most peripheral clocks are highly sensitive to the synchronizing effects of feeding time and food-related cues, the SCN clock seems impervious to them, provided that animals are exposed to a light-dark cycle and ingest enough daily energy.[128,129] However, the SCN can respond to nutritional cues under specific caloric conditions. Indeed, rats under a light-dark cycle and entrained to timed hypocaloric feeding display phase-advances of daily rhythms of locomotor activity, body temperature, and pineal melatonin.[150] Entrainment to light-dark cycle is also altered in mice submitted to a timed calorie restriction. In addition to the phase-advanced rest-activity (i.e., nocturnal mice becoming partially diurnal), expression of clock proteins and the clock-controlled factor *Vasopressin* is phase-advanced in the SCN, and the circadian responses of the SCN to light are altered.[151,152] In addition, circadian phase-shift responses to light are reduced in animals under low glucose availability.[153] Furthermore, glucose availability modifies firing rate of glucose-sensitive SCN neurons through ATP-sensitive K^+ channels.[154] Altogether these results challenge the idea that the SCN is impervious to any nutritional cues. Notably, the reward aspect of food also seems important because in mice housed in constant dark conditions, the SCN entrain to rhythmic access to palatable food (chocolate) given in addition to regular food pellets available *ad libitum*.[155]

Little is known about the pathways conveying metabolic signals to the SCN. Timed calorie restriction may directly change the redox status of SCN cells, as in peripheral clocks (see previous paragraph), and affect subsequently the SCN molecular clockwork. Self-sustained redox cycles have been identified in the SCN cells, where they regulate neuronal activity.[156] In addition, feeding-related hormones such as insulin, ghrelin, and leptin, whose receptors are present in metabolic hypothalamus (i.e., nuclei of hypothalamus involved in the regulation of energy balance), are possible candidates for conveying metabolic information to the SCN, most likely through detection in the mediobasal hypothalamus.[141,157] Moreover, orexigenic and anorexigenic neurons in the hypothalamus that control feeding behavior respond to fluctuations in circulating nutrient (e.g., glucose, fatty acid, amino acid) levels that reflect the nutritional status.[158] Because the SCN receives numerous projections from various hypothalamic nuclei, the metabolic region of the hypothalamus could integrate and transmit information from circulating feeding-related hormones and nutrients to the SCN.[159,160]

CONCLUSIONS

This overview of the central and peripheral clocks shows the hierarchic organization of the mammalian circadian system at the top of which is the SCN. Because light is the most potent synchronizer of this master clock, a proper temporal organization is normally achieved under a light-dark cycle. When synchronized to light, the SCN controls behavioral (i.e., sleep-wake and feeding-fasting cycles) and physiologic rhythms (e.g., body temperature and plasma melatonin and glucocorticoids) that will, in turn, reinforce the robustness of daily rhythmicity by sending internal timing cues. Forced or voluntary feeding limited to the usual rest period is a potent timer of peripheral oscillations that disturbs internal coupling between the various clocks, depending on their sensitivities to meal resetting. As a consequence of the close connections between cellular clocks and intracellular metabolism, genetic clock disruptions affect metabolism in rodents. Moreover, chronic alterations in the main zeitgebers of the circadian system, such as bright light exposure during the subjective night (chronic jet lag, shift work) and mealtimes, lead to circadian desynchronization with detrimental consequences on metabolic health.

CLINICAL PEARL

As a consequence of the reciprocal connections between circadian clocks and intracellular metabolism, situations of circadian misalignment, such as night-eating syndrome, shift work, and chronic jet lag, disrupt sleep homeostasis and increase metabolic risk factors, including obesity, impaired glucose tolerance, and hypertension.

SUMMARY

The master clock, located in the SCN of the hypothalamus, synchronizes a multitude of brain and peripheral clocks. These clocks allow organisms, tissues, and cells to anticipate ongoing changes and optimize the efficiency of a given function at the expected time of daily occurrence. Brain and peripheral clocks also segregate incompatible behaviors (e.g., sleep and feeding) and chemically incompatible reactions (e.g., hepatic gluconeogenesis and glycolysis), respectively. Rhythmic signals from the SCN couple the master clock to secondary brain and peripheral clocks through behavioral, nervous, and neurohumoral pathways. Endocrine rhythms (i.e., pineal melatonin and adrenal glucocorticoids) distribute internal temporal messages within the body.

Light perceived by the retina is the most potent synchronizer of the master clock in the SCN. A few other stimuli, different from light, called nonphotic cues (e.g., exercise, arousal), can phase-shift the SCN, especially when the photic synchronizer is weak or absent. Clocks in peripheral tissues share many molecular properties with the SCN. Besides the stronger intercellular coupling in the SCN, another functional difference is the high sensitivity of most brain and peripheral clocks to the synchronizing effects of feeding as opposed to the relative resistance of the SCN. Cellular clocks and intracellular metabolism are tightly and reciprocally connected. The putative mechanisms by which food-related cues can reset peripheral timing are discussed. Even if the SCN is not shifted by mealtime, metabolic cues can affect SCN clockwork and modulate its synchronization to light.

SELECTED READINGS

Bechtold DA, Loudon AS. Hypothalamic clocks and rhythms in feeding behaviour. *Trends Neurosci.* 2013;36:74–82.

Bedont JL, Blackshaw S. Constructing the suprachiasmatic nucleus: a watchmaker's perspective on the central clockworks. *Front Syst Neurosci.* 2015;9:74.

Challet E. The circadian regulation of food intake. *Nat Rev Endocrinol.* 2019;5:393–405.

Dibner C, Schibler U, Albrecht U. The mammalian circadian timing system: organization and coordination of central and peripheral clocks. *Annu Rev Physiol.* 2010;72:517–549.

Dickmeis T. Glucocorticoids and the circadian clock. *J Endocrinol.* 2009;200:3–22.

Gerhart-Hines Z, Lazar MA. Circadian metabolism in the light of evolution. *Endocr Rev.* 2015;36:289–304.

Golombek DA, Rosenstein RE. Physiology of circadian entrainment. *Physiol Rev.* 2010;90:1063–1102.

Guilding C, Hughes AT, Brown TM, Namvar S, Piggins HD. A riot of rhythms: neuronal and glial circadian oscillators in the mediobasal hypothalamus. *Mol Brain.* 2009;2:28.

Kalsbeek A, Yi CX, La Fleur SE, Fliers E. The hypothalamic clock and its control of glucose homeostasis. *Trends Endocrinol Metab.* 2010;21:402–410.

Mistlberger RE. Neurobiology of food anticipatory circadian rhythms. *Physiol Behav.* 2011;104:535–545.

Oster H, Challet E, Ott V, et al. The functional and clinical significance of the 24-hour rhythm of circulating glucocorticoids. *Endocr. Rev.* 2017;38:3–45.

Panda S, Antoch MP, Miller BH, et al. Coordinated transcription of key pathways in the mouse by the circadian clock. *Cell.* 2002;109:307–320.

Pevet P, Challet E. Melatonin: both master clock output and internal time-giver in the circadian clocks network. *J Physiol Paris.* 2011;105:170–182.

Sinturel F, Petrenko V, Dibner C. Circadian clocks make metabolism run. *J Mol Biol.* 2020;432 (12):3680–3699.

Tsang AH, Barclay JL, Oster H. Interactions between endocrine and circadian systems. *J Mol Endocrinol.* 2014;52:R1–R16.

A complete reference list can be found online at ExpertConsult.com.

Chapter 41

Circadian Dysregulation and Cardiometabolic and Immune Health

Ivy C. Mason; Andrew W. McHill; Kenneth P. Wright, Jr.; Frank A.J.L. Scheer

Chapter Highlights

- Circadian rhythms are a vital component of human health, and their dysregulation has been shown to contribute to adverse changes in cardiovascular, metabolic, and immune function.
- The most common form of circadian dysregulation in modern society is the misalignment of environmental and/or behavioral rhythms with the endogenous circadian system resulting from factors such as shift work, (social) jet lag, light at night, or late-night eating. Such conditions may also lead to a mismatch of circadian clock function at the cellular or systems level in the central clock or peripheral tissues. Evidence indicates that such circadian misalignment increases the risk of adverse health outcomes.
- Given the high prevalence of disorders relating to cardiometabolic and immune function, understanding circadian contributions to these disorders and investigating approaches to enhance circadian function have high potential for clinical translation and positive effects on human health outcomes.

INTRODUCTION

This chapter reviews the circadian control of cardiovascular (CV), metabolic, and immune function and the effects of circadian disruptions (such as those induced by shift work, jet lag, social jet lag, daylight saving time, light at night, and adverse meal timing) on these functions and disease outcomes.

Circadian is a term derived from the Latin phrase *circa dies*, meaning "about a day." It describes endogenous biologic rhythms with a period of approximately 24 hours (Box 41.1). The fact that a circadian rhythm is self-sustained, that is, persists independently of environmental and behavioral cues, sets it apart from a "diurnal" rhythm (also known as a nycthemeral rhythm), which may be driven, in part, by an endogenous circadian rhythm and/or, in part, by exogenous environmental and behavioral rhythms. Environmental rhythms include the light-dark cycle, while behavioral rhythms include the sleep-wake and fasting-eating cycles.

Circadian alignment, depicted in Figure 41.1, *A*, occurs when electrical and natural light-dark cycles (environmental), sleep-wake and fasting-eating cycles (behavioral), and peripheral oscillators are properly aligned with the central clock. Disruptions to circadian alignment, leading to a form of circadian dysregulation (desynchronization or misalignment of these rhythms) can result in adverse health outcomes. Circadian misalignment can occur between the central clock and environmental (i.e., environmental misalignment) or behavioral (i.e., behavioral misalignment) rhythms or between the central clock and peripheral clocks (i.e., internal misalignment) (Figure 41.1, *B* and *C*, and Figure 41.2). Circadian misalignment can be caused by external or internal factors and can lead to myriad acute and chronic consequences (Figure 41.2). While disturbance of clock function is another type of circadian dysregulation (Figure 41.2), this chapter focuses mainly on circadian misalignment as it pertains to cardiometabolic and immune health.

Behaviors that can lead to circadian misalignment (e.g., shift work, [social] jet lag, light at night, or late-night eating) are common in modern industrialized society. The availability of electrical light exposure combined with social and work demands often lead to environments and behaviors that are mismatched with circadian rhythms.[1] Shift work, in which 20% of the US workforce is engaged[2] (night shift, rotating shift, early morning shift, or other schedules besides regular day/evening shift), often leads to circadian misalignment (Figure 41.1, *B*) as does jet lag (Figure 41.1, *C*) with travel across time zones.[3]

The increased prevalence of these modern lifestyle factors that are disruptive to the circadian system has occurred concurrently with the rapid increase in prevalence of disease and health issues relating to CV, metabolic, and immune function. For instance, diagnosed cases of type 2 diabetes mellitus (T2DM) have grown exponentially in the past few decades,[4,5] alongside a high prevalence of obesity.[6] There is evidence, as discussed in the following sections of this chapter, that these cardiometabolic and immune functions and their health/disease consequences are, in part, under circadian control and affected by circadian misalignment (Figure 41.3). Given the prevalence of disorders relating to cardiometabolic and immune health, investigating how circadian misalignment contributes to these adverse health outcomes may aid in developing novel treatment strategies and thus has high potential for clinical translation.

There are many types of studies that are used to investigate how circadian misalignment influences cardiometabolic

Box 41.1 GLOSSARY OF CIRCADIAN RHYTHM TERMINOLOGY

- **Biologic day:** The circadian phase during which endogenous circulating melatonin concentrations are low (or when the individual is habitually exposed to light)
- **Biologic night:** The circadian phase during which endogenous circulating melatonin concentrations are high (or when the individual is habitually exposed to darkness)
- **Chronobiology:** An area of biology concerned with biologic events that cycle over time
- **Chronotherapy**: The timing of therapies (i.e., medications) to match the optimal circadian phase of action
- **Circadian rhythm:** Term derived from the Latin phrase *circa dies*, meaning "about a day"; endogenous biologic rhythm with a period of approximately 24 hours that is self-sustaining and thus persists independent of environmental (e.g., light-dark, warm-cold) and behavioral (e.g., sleep-wake, fasting-eating cycles) influences
- **Constant routine:** Experimental protocol in which participants are kept in a semi-recumbent posture and given isoenergetic snacks at regular intervals during extended wakefulness in a time-free, dim-light environment; designed to remove 24-hour cycling in all environmental and behavioral inputs, thus enabling measurement of endogenous circadian rhythms, thus independent from those masking effects
- **Diurnal, nycthemeral, or day-night rhythm:** A rhythm that may be driven partly by an endogenous circadian rhythm and/or partly by environmental and behavioral rhythms, such as the sleep-wake, fasting-eating, and light-dark cycles; the external rhythms mask the endogenous rhythm, making it difficult to distinguish the contributions of each to the day-night rhythm
- **Entrainment:** Synchronization of one cyclic pattern to another cyclic pattern at a stable phase angle (e.g., synchronization of the circadian system to the light-dark cycle)
- **Forced desynchrony:** Experimental protocol in which participants are studied in time-free conditions under dim light during a recurrent short or long sleep-wake cycle (e.g., 20-hour or 28-hour days, including fasting-eating, rest-activity, and postural cycles of the same period); disentangles the effect of the circadian system from the effects of behavioral and environmental changes and allows for measurements of biologic processes in response to behavioral/environmental cycles across all circadian phases, including investigation of alignment/misalignment
- **Jet lag:** Symptoms experienced resulting from transient misalignment of biologic rhythms with the local light-dark cycle associated with rapid eastward or westward travel between time zones
- **Masking:** Obscuring of endogenous rhythm by behavioral or environmental conditions that induce acute effects on the measure of interest
- **Misalignment:** The incorrect timing of a rhythm in relation to another rhythm
- **Period:** Cycle length, or the time it takes to cycle from one circadian phase to the same phase again
- **Phase:** Time within a cycle when an event occurs (e.g., minimum, maximum)
- **Night shift work:** shift(s) in which part or all of the shift(s) includes working during the biologic night
- **Social jet lag:** Symptoms experienced due to variations in timing of behaviors (such as sleep and physical activity) between work and work-free days
- ***Zeitgeber*:** A German word meaning "time-giver"; a time cue that can entrain rhythms

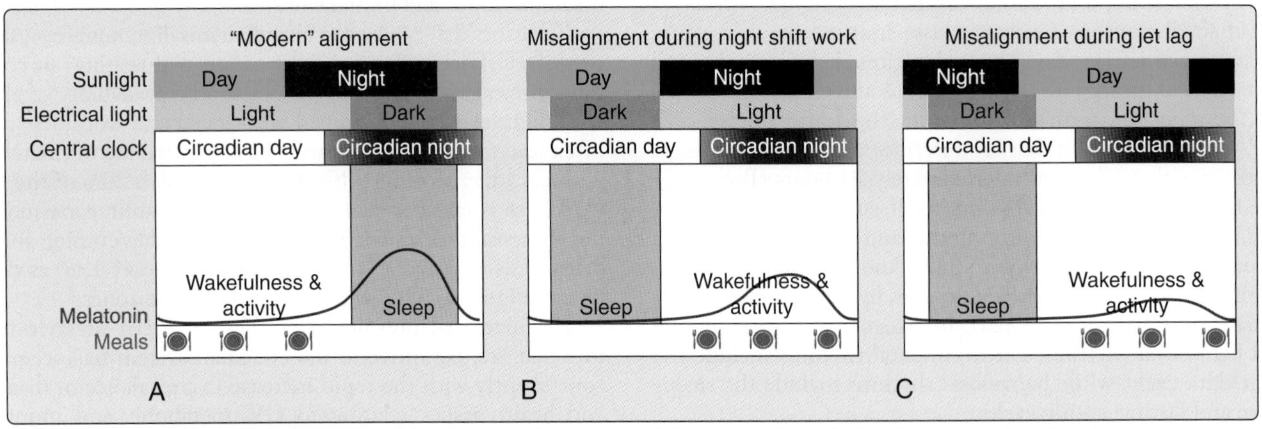

Figure 41.1 Comparison of the alignment of environmental, circadian, and behavioral rhythms in a modern diurnal lifestyle **(A),** during night-shift work **(B),** and during jet lag **(C).** Environmental light exposure patterns are determined by sunlight (although this is shielded when indoors) and electrical light. Sunlight is shown as varying by day (*dark teal bar*) and night (*black bar*); electrical light is shown as varying by light (*light teal bar*) or dark (*grey bar*). Endogenous circadian rhythms are illustrated by the central clock and profiles of melatonin, varying by circadian day (when there is no circadian drive for melatonin production and melatonin levels are low; *white background*) and circadian night (when there is circadian drive for melatonin production and melatonin levels are high; *graded gray background*). The *fuschia curve* represents endogenous melatonin levels across the wake and sleep episodes, with behavioral rhythms shown as the episodes of wakefulness and activity (*white background*) and sleep (*grey background*) episodes and eating patterns (meals illustrated by the plate with knife and fork). In the modern lifestyle **(A),** there is relative alignment between the daylight, electrical light, circadian day, wake period, and meal timing, although generally hours delayed compared with the solar day ("midnight" for many at the start of their sleep episode). The melatonin curve shows a robust rhythm and is aligned to the environmental and behavioral rhythms. Acutely, during shift work **(B),** the wake period and (often) meal ingestion occur during circadian night, with electrical lighting in place of sunlight. With this acute misalignment, there is dampened rhythm of melatonin because of electrical light suppression. Jet lag occurs in response to rapid shifts in time zone **(C).** While the sunlight and electrical light align with the wake period and meal ingestion in this scenario (if following the local social schedule), they are inverted to the circadian day-night pattern, and the melatonin profile is dampened. (Modified from Mason IC, Qian J, Adler GK, Scheer FA. Impact of circadian disruption on glucose metabolism: implications for type 2 diabetes. *Diabetologia.* 2020;63[3]:462–72.)

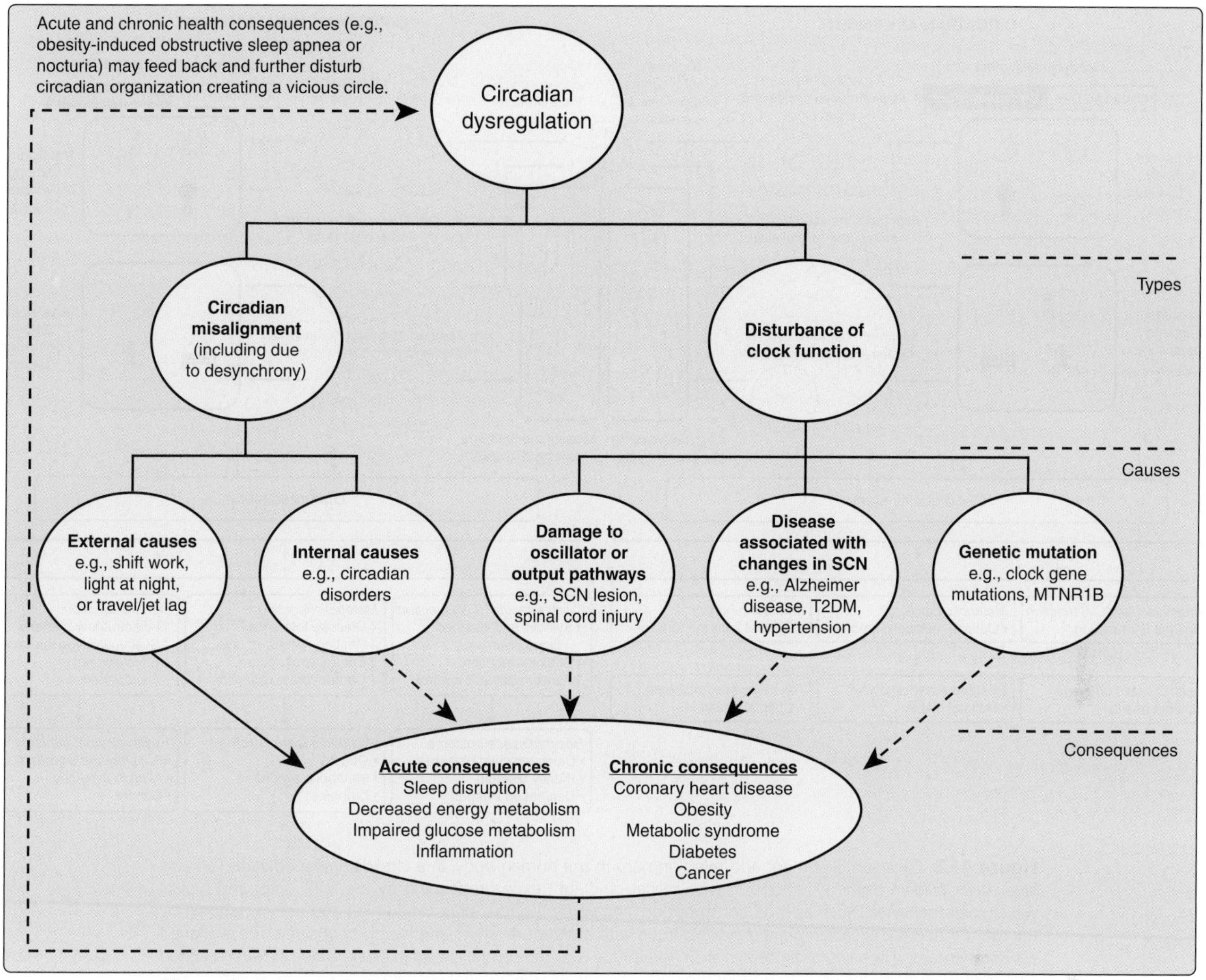

Figure 41.2 Examples of different types of circadian dysregulation, their causes, and potential acute and chronic health consequences. *Dotted arrows* point to hypothesized acute and chronic consequences and feedback. Note that the types or causes are not absolute or mutually exclusive (e.g., certain circadian disorders may be due to blindness or genetic mutations, but may also be due to environmental or behavioral factors). (Modified from Rüger M, Scheer FAJL. Effects of circadian disruption on the cardiometabolic system. *Rev Endocr Metab Disord.* 2009;10[4]:245–60.)

and immune function and disease. Environmental and behavioral rhythms typically mask the endogenous circadian component, and thus stringent circadian protocols are required to tease out circadian contributions to an observed daily rhythm. Studies on the effects of circadian disruption in a real-world setting can also have confounds such as differences in socioeconomic status, access to and consumption of healthy foods, workload, and so on, between those with circadian disruptions (such as shift workers) and those without (such as non-shift workers). Many of the epidemiologic/observational studies of circadian disruption are furthermore based mostly on correlation, although they are able to compile data over longer durations of time and in a large population. Some controlled experimental studies of circadian misalignment have been used to isolate the contributions of circadian misalignment and demonstrate causality, although they are necessarily short in duration given their intensive nature. It therefore becomes imperative to consider both epidemiologic and experimental approaches; the combination of results from both types of studies provides converging evidence toward elucidating the contributions of circadian rhythms and circadian disruptions to cardiometabolic and immune health outcomes.

CARDIOVASCULAR HEALTH

Circadian System and Cardiovascular Health

The interplay and alignment between the endogenous circadian timing system and CV physiology are thought to be necessary for optimal CV health. CV disease is the leading cause of death in the United States,[7] and, although CV events can happen at all hours of the day, there is a clear daily pattern with increased risk of sudden cardiac death, myocardial infarction, stroke, and ventricular arrhythmias in the morning hours (approximately 6 a.m. to noon).[8,8a,b] While the exact cause for this early morning pattern is unknown, considerable in-laboratory work has been dedicated to uncovering basic physiologic circadian mechanisms that may contribute to the increased risk. Using a Forced Desynchrony protocol, designed to evenly spread out the influence of sleep and behaviors on physiology across the 24-hour day and thus desynchronize these sleep and behavioral factors from circadian rhythms, underlying circadian patterns in CV biomarkers that peak in the morning hours have been elucidated. These biomarkers include plasma cortisol,[9] cardiac vagal modulation,[9] platelet aggregability[11] and the prothrombotic plasminogen activator inhibitor-1 (PAI-1),[12] with large endogenous circadian rhythms that peak at approximately 6 a.m. to

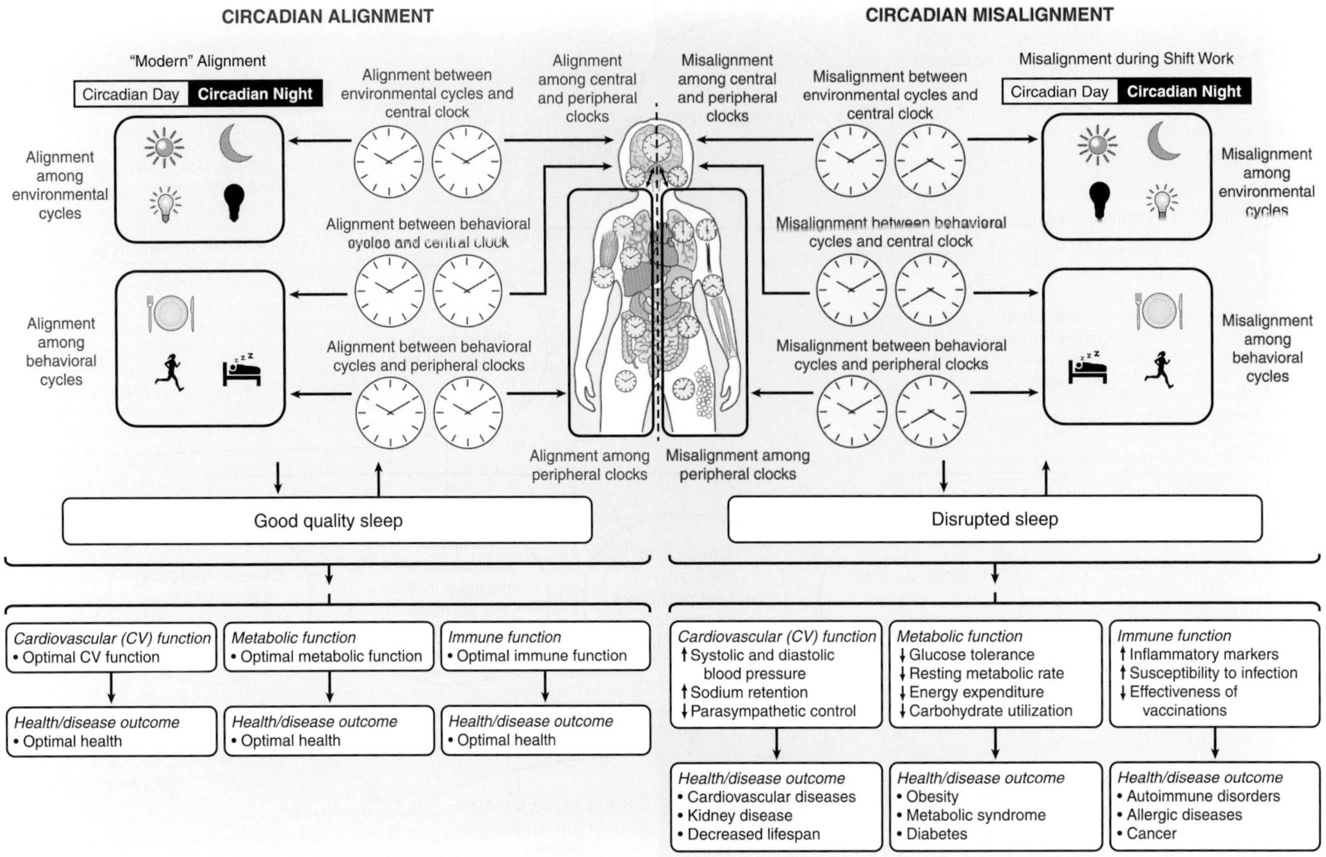

Figure 41.3 Circadian alignment and misalignment in the human body. In a circadian aligned state (*left side, blue*), the circadian day is synchronized with our electric light exposure (shown by the light bulb) and typical wakefulness behaviors, such as food consumption (shown by the fork, plate, and knife) and activity (shown by the runner), and the circadian night is synchronized with ambient darkness and inactivity or sleep. These aligned environmental and behavioral exposures are in synchrony with the central circadian clock, which in turn is aligned with peripheral clocks located throughout the body. This circadian alignment allows for sleep (shown by the sleeping person in the bed) to be commenced at the ideal time, and together, circadian alignment and healthy sleep promote optimal cardiometabolic and immune function and health. In a circadian misaligned state (*right side, red*), the circadian day consists of limited exposure to light and with increased exposure during the circadian night. The circadian night is also often accompanied by food consumption and activity and the main sleep episode during the circadian day. This misalignment between environmental and behavioral exposures, at times when the circadian system is not promoting these behaviors, creates a misalignment between the central clock that is most strongly synchronized with light exposure, and peripheral clocks that seem most strongly synchronized to behavioral exposures (although there is still limited evidence in humans). Additionally, this circadian misalignment will disturb sleep during the circadian day, and together, these factors result in acutely impaired cardiometabolic function and are correlated with chronically poorer health and eventual disease.

noon. These assessments of circadian control are remarkably similar when using a forced desynchrony protocol with either a 20-hour or 28-hour sleep-wake cycle, or a completely different circadian protocol, the constant routine protocol, in which research participants are kept awake, in semi-recumbent posture while at rest, with equally spaced, isocaloric snacks, and in dim light, showing that these rhythms are not an artifact of the circadian protocol and that these circadian rhythms are robust.[13] Moreover, the time of day in which a CV event occurs in mice may have an impact on the ability of the myocardial tissue to tolerate the event,[14] likely driven by circadian alterations in cellular fate.[15-17]

One key CV biomarker that also follows a robust circadian pattern under different conditions of controlled laboratory settings is blood pressure, although it does not peak in the early morning hours in healthy individuals.[9,13] Both systolic and diastolic blood pressure peak in the circadian evening hours, with peak-to-trough amplitudes ranging between 3 and 6 mm Hg, and with the largest reactivity of blood pressure increase to standardized exercise in the circadian evening and slowest blood pressure recovery occurring in the circadian morning.[9,13,18] One potential mechanism for this rhythm in blood pressure could be, in part, changes in blood volume as regulated by the kidneys.[19,20] Several of the kidney's physiologic functions exhibit a diurnal pattern (i.e., the combined effect of endogenous circadian rhythmicity and behaviors, such as eating) to anticipate the metabolic and physiologic workload expected of the kidney throughout a 24-hour day.[21] Other factors relevant to kidney function and blood pressure, such as aldosterone secretion and the renin-angiotensin-aldosterone system, have been shown to demonstrate circadian rhythmicity[16] with peaks in the morning hours. Additionally, alterations in vascular function may also contribute to the observed circadian rhythm in blood pressure,[22] as vascular endothelial function has been shown to display a circadian rhythm with its lowest levels across the circadian night and into the morning hours.[23]

Work schedules, lifestyles, and environmental exposures that are prone to induce circadian disruption are associated with detriments to CV health.[8b] For example, individuals that participate in overnight or rotating shift work are shown to have up to a 40% increased risk for CV disease as compared with their daytime working counterparts,[25,26] potentially driven in part by increased inflammatory markers, such as C-reactive protein.[27,28] Moreover, the longer an individual engages in shift work, the greater their risk for CV disease,[29,30] while the discontinuation of working shift work ameliorates the risk.[30] In less drastic examples of circadian misalignment, smaller and/or more transient misalignments, such as would occur with the changing of time zones or a delay in our internal clock from a weekend of extended evening electrical light exposure, also have stark consequences. For example, humans are more likely to experience sudden cardiac death on Monday morning as compared to any other day of the week[31,32] or myocardial infarction in the days after spring daylight saving time (1-hour advance in external clock time) than the weeks preceding the time change, although the effect of daylight saving time may be modest and may no longer hold true in stratified analyses by gender or age.[33,34] Remarkably, even geographic differences within a time zone have wide-ranging health consequences; those living further westward, and thus receiving morning light at a later clock time, have a lower life expectancy than those living more eastward,[35] and even subtle misalignment within a single geographic time zone can increase the risk of CV diseases.[36] Although these examples are primarily correlative and endogenous circadian phase is not assessed, they provide epidemiologic evidence for the impact of circadian disruption on CV health and disease.

In the laboratory, animal models have provided a glimpse of what may occur during chronic circadian misalignment if an individual is in an already vulnerable health state.[37] In a seminal study, chronically shifting light-dark cycles to induce circadian misalignment resulted in an 11% decrease in median life span in cardiomyopathic Syrian hamsters.[38] Similarly, simulating jet lag in older mice by repeatedly advancing their light exposure by 6 hours every 7 days resulted in a 36% decrease in survival rate as compared with those that did not shift their schedules.[39] Moreover, altering the light-dark (LD) cycle length in mice, and thereby inducing circadian misalignment, results in prolonged QT intervals of cardiac repolarization,[37] which has potential for severe cardiac problems to arise such as ventricular arrhythmias and sudden cardiac death.

In humans, highly controlled in-laboratory protocols simulating typical night-shift work schedules have provided potential mechanisms for increased CV risk during circadian misalignment. An 8-day simulated shift-work protocol and an 8-day day-shift protocol in a randomized, crossover design revealed that acute circadian misalignment increased both 24-hour systolic and diastolic blood pressure, primarily through increases in sleeping blood pressure, and decreased parasympathetic control, along with increasing blood biomarkers of inflammatory stress (e.g., resistin, interleukin-6 [IL-6], tumor necrosis factor-α [TNF-α], and C-reactive protein).[40] The increase in blood pressure and C-reactive protein resulting from experimental circadian misalignment under controlled laboratory conditions in a randomized-crossover study was also observed in chronic shift workers, supporting its relevance in this population.[41] (A more detailed description of the effects of circadian misalignment on inflammatory markers can be found later in the chapter.) In a 6-day simulated shift-work protocol designed to examine how circadian misalignment may affect circulating proteins involved with CV health results indicated that, in response to simulated shift work, many proteins associated with heart disease were found to be altered by circadian misalignment.[42] Circadian desynchronization may also increase the development of major risk factors for chronic kidney disease, such as tubular dilation, proteinuria, and cellular apoptosis, which could in turn affect CV health as observed in hamsters.[43] Using the somewhat naturalistic experiment simulating the Martian day (24 hours, 40 minutes), a within-participant prospective study found that participants on a fixed sodium diet for up to 205 days had increased 24-hour urinary aldosterone excretion with associated increased sodium retention in the days that included a night shift and increased blood pressure the morning after a shift work as compared with days without night-shift work.[44]

METABOLIC HEALTH

Circadian System and Energy Metabolism

The circadian timing system and metabolic processes are intimately coupled. At the cellular level, simple processes such as the conversion from Adenosine diphosphate (ADP) to adenosine triphosphate (ATP) follow a rhythm that is synchronized to the sun's light-dark cycle.[45] In more complex systems, rate-limiting enzymes that are vital for many metabolic processes are under circadian control.[46] Likely, these changes in metabolism across the day aid in the prediction of nutrient availability and metabolic needs associated with eating/wakefulness/activity and fasting/sleep/inactivity.[47] Indeed, human resting metabolic rate studied within controlled laboratory settings displays a circadian variation, with a peak in energy expenditure during the daytime/evening hours and a trough during the nighttime/early morning hours.[48-50] This observed rhythm in energy expenditure also matches the endogenous circadian rhythm for self-reported feelings of hunger and appetite,[51,52] further demonstrating the tight relationship between the circadian system and energy metabolism.

As with CV health, misalignment between endogenous circadian rhythms and eating/wakefulness/activity behaviors results in significant detriments to metabolic health. Epidemiologically, chronic shift workers can again serve as a model population to examine the impact of circadian misalignment on metabolic health, recognizing the potential limitations of confounders, mediators, and reversed causality. Overall obesity and abdominal obesity rates are approximately 25% to 45% higher in shift workers than their day working counterparts,[53,54] and shift workers are at an approximately 60% to 70% higher risk for having three metabolic risk factors (obesity, hypertension, and high triglycerides).[53] Also in conditions less extreme than shift work, daily circadian misalignment is associated with poorer metabolic health. For example, individuals that have a larger mismatch in the timing of their sleep midpoint between work and free days (i.e., social jet lag) are more likely to be obese.[55] Cross-sectional data suggest that for every additional hour of social jet lag an individual is experiencing, there is a 1.3 increased odds of that person having metabolic syndrome.[56] Moreover, eating during the night, an example of probable misalignment of a daily behavior with the circadian timing system, has also been shown to affect metabolic health.[57,58] Findings from cross-sectional studies show relationships between the later timing of food consumption and weight gain[59] and higher body mass index.[60] In a longitudinal observational study, individuals who ate their lunch at a later time of day lost significantly less weight than those who ate earlier in the day during a weight loss intervention program.[61] In relation to a physiologic circadian marker, eating a higher percentage of calories closer to and after the timing of melatonin onset, denoting the start of an individual's biologic night, is associated with higher body mass and body fat composition in college students.[62,63] Conversely, experimentally shortening an individual's daily eating duration and thus typically restricting the timing of calories to only the daytime hours[62] reduces weight[64,65] and improves glucose tolerance.[66] Likewise, providing a meal in the morning, as opposed to a nutrient-equivalent meal in the evening, increases lipid oxidation.[67] Implementing a time-restricted eating protocol, such that daily calories can only be consumed before 3 p.m., improves cardiometabolic health in the absence of weight loss.[68] Moreover, the relationship between the timing of food intake with obesity may differ depending on an individual's morning or evening chronotype (i.e., preference of timing of activities and/or behaviors), such that increased caloric intake in the morning in individuals with an earlier chronotype is associated with lower body weight and increased caloric intake in the evening in those with later chronotypes is associated with higher body weight.[69] Furthermore, a targeted metabolomics study with a 24-hour constant routine that followed a 3-day simulated night-shift schedule found that 95% of metabolites with 24-hour rhythmicity had rhythms driven by behavioral time cues rather than the central circadian clock; furthermore, most of these circulating metabolites and metabolic pathways related to the liver, pancreas, and digestive tract.[70]

Animal models have allowed for examination of the consequences of long-term circadian misalignment and metabolic health. In mice, imposing strict restrictions on the timing in which they are given food can have drastic metabolic effects. Allowing mice to eat a high-fat diet only during their biologic day (the rest phase in nocturnal rodents), and thereby inducing a circadian misalignment between the fasting-feeding and the light-dark cycles, rapidly increases body mass as compared with mice eating at the correct biologic time (nighttime), without a significant difference in caloric intake or locomotor activity.[71] Simulating "night-shift work" in mice by shifting their activity patterns to the biologic day (light phase, when these nocturnal rodents are typically mostly inactive), but providing chow during only the biologic day or night to tease apart the impact of food versus wakefulness/activity on cardiometabolic health, researchers found that shifting the chow to the biologic day (inverted eating) increases abdominal obesity with no difference in chow intake.[72] Restricting food intake to the active phase while continuing to maintain a night-shift schedule abolished these abdominal obesity differences.[72] Exposing mice to constant light across 24 hours, and thereby inducing circadian dysregulation in the form of a blunted rhythm amplitude of the in vivo multiunit firing rate in the suprachiasmatic nucleus, results in increases in body mass without increased caloric intake or decreased activity,[73] and the increases observed in this condition occur more rapidly than in mice fed a high-fat diet.[74] However, restricting the timing of food to only the active phase, despite keeping mice in constant dim-lighting conditions, prevents the increases in body mass, suggesting that the adverse metabolic effect of constant light on body weight is mediated by a blunting of the fasting-feeding cycle.[73] Moreover, lesioning the central clock in mice to abolish rhythmicity results in a small weight gain and increased fat mass.[75]

Human studies have found alterations in energy metabolism in response to circadian desynchronization and misalignment. A forced desynchrony protocol that was designed to distribute all meals and behaviors evenly across the 24-hour day showed that resting metabolic rate was approximately 8% lower after circadian misalignment and sleep restriction as compared with baseline circadian alignment and adequate sleep.[76] In another study, a 6-day simulated shift-work protocol using a whole-room indirect calorimeter to measure 24-hour energy expenditure studied participants during daytime wakefulness and nighttime sleep followed by 3 days of daytime sleep and nighttime wakefulness while having participants maintain a constant bedrest posture and eating identical daily meals. Simulated shift work decreased 24-hour energy expenditure by approximately 3% to 4% as compared with the day shift, with approximately 12% to 16% decreases in energy expenditure occurring during the participant's daytime sleep opportunities.[77] In that same study, the diet-induced thermogenesis (DIT), or the energy expended in response to a meal, decreased by approximately 4% of the energy content of the meal when it was consumed at approximately 2230 hours relative to the same meal content at approximately 1830 hours.[77] A randomized, crossover trial with two 8-day in-laboratory protocols including a simulated 12-hour slam-shifted night-shift protocol (in which the rapid inversion of shifts from simulated day to simulated night shift occurred abruptly) and a normally aligned protocol compared the early-phase DIT after standardized mixed meals and showed that DIT was twice as large during the circadian morning as compared with the circadian evening. Even though DIT contributes only to approximately 10% of the 24-hour caloric expenditure, these results indicate that circadian control of DIT may provide a mechanism that may help explain the differential effects of time of eating on energy balance and body weight control.[78] Additionally, protocols examining substrate utilization have found decreases in carbohydrate utilization during circadian misalignment,[77,79,80] which could contribute to weight gain over time. Furthermore, a recent metabolomics study investigated effects of a simulated night-shift work protocol on the 24-hour variation of metabolic processes.[81] Results indicated that approximately 75% of rhythmic metabolite profiles were primarily influenced by the behavioral cycle (e.g., fast-eat and sleep-wake) rather than by the endogenous circadian clock, thereby leading to a state of misalignment relative to the endogenous circadian system. Interestingly, there were high levels of interindividual variability with some participants showing metabolite rhythms that adjusted to the shift, while other participants showed no adjustment.

Circadian System and Glucose Metabolism

Proper glycemic control is vital for micro[82] and macro[83] vascular health. Inability to adequately control blood glucose levels may result in CV complications that could lead to death.[84,85] In epidemiologic studies, a high-risk time for poor glycemic control is during the early morning hours (5 a.m. to 9 a.m.)[86] when individuals experience the "dawn phenomenon," a surge in blood glucose production and decrease in insulin sensitivity,[87] requiring up to a 50% increase in insulin requirement[86] and often resulting in hyperglycemia.[86,88] These observations are partly driven by an underlying endogenous circadian control of glucose and insulin, with levels of those hormones peaking in the circadian morning hours.[89]

Disrupting the circadian system has both long-term and acute effects on glucose metabolism.[90,91] For example, individuals working rotating shift work have higher odds of having type 2 diabetes as compared with their daytime working counterparts.[92] Moreover, this risk for type 2 diabetes is higher when combined with unhealthy lifestyle behaviors such as smoking or low physical activity.[93,94] Furthermore, these impacts on glucose metabolism may have long-lasting effects. In a cohort of retired shift workers who worked irregular shifts for more than 10 years, the odds of current diagnosis of diabetes was up to 10% higher than those working day shifts, and individuals working shift work more than 20 years had increased odds of up to 16%.[95] However, the association of shift work with diabetes risk is often confounded by other health factors, such as obesity risk and lifestyle factors (described previously),[96] and thus laboratory work is needed to understand the direct impact of circadian misalignment on glucose metabolism.

Often, circadian misalignment is accompanied by disrupted sleep, which makes the impact of sleep disruption versus circadian misalignment difficult to discern. We know from highly controlled in-laboratory studies that when combining sleep restriction with circadian disruption, postprandial glucose is impaired in wake of a decrease in insulin production.[76] Moreover, when individuals were scheduled to be awake and eat 12 hours out of phase from their habitual timing, there is a 6% increase in glucose concentration in tandem with a 22% increase in insulin.[97] Using an innovative 11-day protocol that included participants randomized to sleep restriction and circadian alignment or sleep restriction and circadian misalignment, researchers were able to systematically identify the impact of sleep restriction and circadian misalignment, independently. They found that during the circadian misaligned state in male participants, the impact of sleep restriction with circadian misalignment on insulin sensitivity was almost twice that of sleep restriction without circadian misalignment.[98] Further teasing apart the impact of behaviors (e.g., breakfast versus dinner), circadian phase (e.g., time of day), and circadian misalignment (e.g., 12-hour invert of schedules), it has been shown that an evening circadian phase and circadian misalignment have independent adverse effect on glucose metabolism, working through differing mechanisms (reduced beta cell function versus reduced insulin sensitivity, respectively),[99,100] and is relevant in chronic shift workers.[101] The adverse effect of circadian misalignment, while testing during the circadian night, on insulin sensitivity was confirmed by euglycemic hyperinsulinemic clamp and shown to be driven mostly by reduced skeletal muscle nonoxidative glucose disposal.[102]

While there are many signals by which the circadian system may change glucose control, including circadian control of peripheral oscillators (e.g., in metabolic tissues), cortisol and autonomic nervous system output to, e.g., pancreas and liver,[102a] the hormone melatonin also appears to play a key role. Elevated levels of the pineal hormone melatonin may lead to decreased glucose tolerance when eating during the circadian night or after exogenous melatonin intake.[103] Melatonin typically increases in levels approximately 2 hours before habitual sleep onset and decreases after habitual wake time.[104] During circadian misalignment, impaired glucose tolerance may be in part due to eating at times when endogenous melatonin concentrations are elevated.[97,101,105,106] Furthermore, during sleep restriction, when individuals awaken early in the morning, when melatonin is high, to consume a meal, the concentrations of melatonin are significantly associated with decreases in insulin sensitivity.[105] This mechanism is supported by findings from placebo-controlled studies showing that exogenous melatonin administration causes impairment of glucose tolerance,[107,108] especially in carriers of the common T2DM-risk variant in the melatonin receptor 1b (*MTNR1B*) gene.[109] Furthermore, in a randomized, crossover trial, experimentally postponing the evening dinner to a time of elevated circulating melatonin concentrations worsens glucose tolerance, especially in these *MTNR1B* risk carriers.[110-113] Interestingly, carriers of this *MTNR1B* risk variant also have an extended duration of elevated melatonin in the morning,[114] which could increase the risk of impaired glucose tolerance during morning food consumption when melatonin is elevated as observed in the laboratory.[105]

IMMUNE HEALTH

Immune health relies on a defense system consisting of various tissues, cells, and proteins that protect the body from pathogens, infection, and disease. The immune response is generally divided into the innate and adaptive responses, although there can be overlap between the constituents of the two responses. The innate response consists of nonspecific responses to pathogens such as barriers (e.g., skin, mucosa), phagocytosis, and antimicrobial and inflammatory molecules, whereas the adaptive response consists of specific responses of antigen recognition and antibody production. Various components of both the innate and adaptive immune system have been shown to exhibit daily rhythms.[115-118] For instance, human peripheral blood mononuclear cells (PBMCs), which include many immune cell types such as lymphocytes and monocytes, have circadian clock genes *(hPer1, hPer2, hPer3,* and *hDec1)* that are expressed in a circadian manner with the peak levels occurring in the morning and afternoon during the habitual time of activity.[119] Some of these clock genes *(hPer1* and *hPer2)* in PBMCs were altered after 2 days of simulated night-shift work in a time-free laboratory study.[120] Similarly, with real-world circadian disruption, policemen exposed to night-shift work have higher levels of total white blood cells, neutrophils, lymphocytes, and monocytes, indicating disruption of the immune system during common circadian misalignment.[121] Additionally, there is evidence that time of day of exposure influences susceptibility to infection, effectiveness of vaccinations, and symptom severity in immune diseases such as rheumatoid arthritis,[117] which is further discussed at the end of this section. The link between endogenous circadian biology and the immune response provides possibilities for translational applications to optimize and improve immune health. Accordingly, there has been much interest in and progress toward understanding the role of circadian rhythms and timing in immune health as detailed in a 2020 National Institutes of Health workshop report.[122]

Innate Immune Response

Innate immunity refers to the nonspecific first line defense mechanism that plays a role immediately or within hours of the detection of pathogens. The mounting of the innate immune response includes several cascading physiologic processes. For example, circulating monocytes mature into macrophages, which then can phagocytize pathogens and secrete signaling molecules such as cytokines (e.g., TNF, interleukin-1 [IL-1], IL-6, IL-8, and IL-12) and chemokines. Such signaling molecules can promote inflammatory processes and act as chemoattractants. Neutrophils are often the first innate cells to respond at the site of infection, and natural killer (NK) cells are part of immune response host-rejection against infection and tumors/cancer.

Evidence suggests that innate immune functions such as infection response, inflammation and stress response are impacted by time of day and are potentially circadian regulated.[123,124] Findings from rodent studies indicate that time of day affects infection; specifically, virus replication in mice infected at the start of the day, which is when nocturnal animals start their resting phase, is 10 times greater than in mice infected 10 hours into the day, which is when they are transitioning to their active phase.[125] Strikingly, when the same experiment was conducted on mice lacking the clock gene *Bmal1*, thereby inducing loss of circadian rhythmicity, there were high levels of virus replication regardless of the time of day that infection occurred.[125] This suggests that susceptibility to infection, and possibly treatment, may be circadian phase dependent. Similarly, it has been demonstrated that circadian clock genes BMAL1 and REV-ERBα are involved in the hepatitis C virus life cycle and genetic knockouts of *Bmal1* and overexpression of REV-ERB inhibits the replication of hepatitis C virus and related flaviviruses dengue and Zika.[126] Furthermore, findings from rodent studies show that natural killer (NK) cells have 24-hour oscillations in expression level of clock genes in constant darkness,[127] and more than 8% of the macrophage transcriptome oscillates in a circadian manner with rhythms in TNF-α and IL-6 secretion from the spleen.[128]

In healthy humans, diurnal rhythms of immune cell counts (of granulocytes such as neutrophils) have been shown, with the amplitude of diurnal rhythmicity reduced with sleep deprivation (29-hour wakefulness).[129] Teasing apart behavioral/environmental and circadian contributions, an in-laboratory study of 13 healthy human participants studied under a 48-hour baseline and 40 to 50 hours of a constant routine protocol assessed ex vivo lipopolysaccharide stimulation of whole blood and found 24-hour rhythms in proinflammatory cytokines and chemokines during baseline (monocyte chemotactic protein, granulocyte-macrophage colony-stimulating factor, and IL-8) and during constant routine (monocyte chemotactic protein, granulocyte-macrophage colony-stimulating factor, IL-8, and TNF-α).[130] This provides evidence of endogenous circadian regulation in cytokine and chemokine immune response and, by extension, that there may be adverse effects of circadian misalignment on innate immune function.

There has indeed been epidemiologic and observational work showing associations between night work and elevated inflammatory markers such as IL-6 and C-reactive protein (CRP).[131,132] Similarly, an experimental rodent study of four consecutive weekly 6-hour phase-advances in light-dark schedule resulted in increased proinflammatory cytokines.[133] Likewise, findings from an in-laboratory chronic circadian misalignment protocol (i.e., non-entrainment) and simulated night-shift protocol showed that circadian misalignment significantly increased TNF-α, IL-10, and CRP in humans,[40,134] including in chronic shift workers.[41] On the other hand, simulated night-shift work for 3 days in the laboratory with 9 humans showed a shift in cytokine rhythm but not in rhythms of monocytes and lymphocytes, indicating a mismatch or desynchronization of rhythmic immune parameters.[135] In another simulated night-shift work protocol, 73% of transcripts remained rhythmic but had dampened amplitude; out of 24 transcripts that shifted with night-shift work, 7 were related to NK cells that kill tumors and virally infected cells.[136] This is similar to rodent studies showing that circadian disruption altered circadian expression of clock genes and suppressed circadian expression of NK function of killing tumor cells, leading to lung cancer growth.[137]

Adaptive Immune Response

Adaptive immune response refers to defense mechanisms that respond to specific antigens. As the antigen must be identified (by T lymphocyte cells) and the relevant cells (B lymphocyte cells, dendritic cells) for the response to be called to action, this response takes place on a longer time scale and is the second line of defense after the innate immune response. Adaptive immunity also includes learned immunity mechanisms (conducted by a subset of B and T lymphocytes that differentiate into memory cells) that make future responses to the same antigen more rapid.

While initial work has highlighted the effect of the circadian system on the first line of defense of the innate immune response, more recent work has made it increasingly apparent that the circadian system may also play a role in the later stage adaptive immune response,[138] although the role of circadian rhythms in the adaptive immune response is recognized as a high-priority knowledge gap area.[122] Among the first hints of possible circadian contributions to the adaptive immune response were seen in a study that took 24-hour blood samples in six men and six women and showed diurnal variations in lymphocyte counts, with peaks at 10 p.m. or 3 a.m. and minimum at 8 a.m. or 11 a.m.[139] Human blood counts of B and T cells are generally found to be higher at night, decline in the morning, and remain low during the day,[140] and T cells from human blood have been shown to display rhythms in clock gene expression across the day.[141] Rodent work has also shown a time-of-day dependence in lymphocyte proliferation[142] and that lymphocyte migration occurs in a circadian manner,[143] which may help to explain why time of day of immunizations influences success of the adaptive immune response. Given the circadian contribution to the cellular components of adaptive immunity, effective activation of the adaptive immune response with vaccinations may also be under regulation by the circadian system. Several studies have reported that T and B cell responses to vaccinations may vary with time of day,[144-148] although elucidation of optimal timing remains to be determined as the time of day of inoculation varies with different vaccines and different animal models.

Research on circadian misalignment provides further evidence that the circadian system plays a role in the adaptive immune response. Mice exposed to chronic jet lag protocols, thereby subjected to long-term circadian misalignment, suffer from early mortality, in part because of changes in immune system pathways, including an increase in T cells and B cells, chronic inflammation, and immune disease in the liver and kidneys.[149] Genetic studies have shown a critical time-specific role for lymphocyte BMAL1 in adaptive immunity: disruption of T cells in mice has also been shown to result in loss of oscillations in lymphocyte migration,[143] while conditional *Bmal1* ablation did not alter T-cell and B-cell lymphocyte differentiation, suggesting that this adaptive immune response is not affected by the cell-intrinsic circadian clock but rather by extrinsic circadian factors influencing multiple cell types.[150] In humans, in-laboratory circadian misalignment via mistimed food and sleep (daytime food with nighttime sleep versus daytime sleep with nighttime food) has been shown to alter adaptive immune function proteins, interferons, that increase antigen presentation.[42] Another human study that used the forced desynchrony protocol showed that mistimed sleep led to reduced rhythmic transcripts in the human blood transcriptome and had impacts on T-cell differentiation and B-cell receptor signaling pathways.[151]

Immune Disease Models

Abnormalities in the immune response can lead to immunodeficiencies, autoimmune disorders, and allergic diseases.[152] While the adaptive immune response is a critical component of protecting the body against pathogens, it can also give rise to autoimmunity, in which an abnormal host immune response is activated against itself. The cause of such autoimmune disorders is largely unknown[153]; however, symptoms associated with several autoimmune disorders have shown circadian influences.

Multiple sclerosis is the most common immune disorder to affect the central nervous system,[154] with the disease mediated by T cells that mount an immune response against myelin, leading to demyelination of the neurons in the brain and spinal cord.[155] This immune response against myelin leads to the activation of other immune processes that include breakdown of the blood–brain barrier and cytokine release.[155] Lower melatonin levels have also been reported to be associated with higher levels of fatigue and longer duration of relapsing-remitting multiple sclerosis,[156] and lower levels of melatonin have also been posited as the reason the disease shows seasonal cycles, with relapses occurring more often in spring and summer.[157] In addition to seasonal variations, fatigue symptoms in patients with multiple sclerosis also appear to have faster buildup across the day, with more severe increase in fatigue earlier in the afternoon and evening when compared with control participants.[158] Furthermore, multiple sclerosis has been tied to possible circadian disruption and sleep loss stemming from shift work; incidence of multiple sclerosis has been shown to be higher in those conducting shift work in multiple studies including rotating shift work nurses,[159] and is more pronounced in those who start shift work earlier in life.[160,161]

Rheumatoid arthritis causes inflammation and damage to the joints. As with multiple sclerosis, patients exhibit variability in symptom severity across the day, with higher reports of joint pain and stiffness in the morning[162] that is correlated with increased levels of proinflammatory cytokines and longer duration of elevated morning IL-6 and TNF-α.[163-165]

Inflammatory bowel diseases (IBD), which cause inflammation of the gastrointestinal tract, have been linked to possible behaviors conducive to circadian disruptions. IBD severity is correlated with poor sleep quality, later chronotype, social jet lag, and inconsistent breakfast or dinner times.[166]

Allergic diseases such as asthma also stem from immune responses to which the circadian system may contribute. Asthma is a pulmonary inflammatory disease that causes airway narrowing and heightened responsiveness, with inflammation caused by allergens (such as pollen or dust mites) activating proinflammatory cytokines.[167] Symptoms of asthma are reported to show daily variations, with exacerbated symptoms overnight and in the early morning, possibly resulting from heightened numbers of macrophages, neutrophils, and T cells at those times.[168-170] Recently, we have shown that pulmonary function, airway resistance, and symptom-driven rescue inhaler use by patients with asthma is under robust influence of the endogenous circadian system, as shown consistently by using both the constant routine protocol and the forced desynchrony protocol.[170a]

CLINICAL IMPLICATIONS

As described in this chapter, proper alignment of the circadian system with daily activities and behaviors is paramount to optimal physiologic functioning and health. Importantly, by understanding how underlying endogenous rhythms interact with daily behaviors, interventions and public health campaigns can be geared toward targeting certain aspects of circadian timing to improve health (i.e., "chronotherapy"). For example, a prospective end point trial reported that hypertensive patients routinely taking their antihypertensive medications at night, as compared with patients taking their medication in the morning upon awakening, have a 45% decreased risk of a major CV event.[171] Similarly, nighttime ingestion of hypertension medication has been reported to significantly reduce risk of developing chronic kidney disease.[172] Likewise, glucocorticoid treatment for rheumatoid arthritis with low-dose nighttime-release prednisone at approximately 3 a.m. has been shown to be optimal for providing relief from symptoms, improving functional status, and slowing progression of the disease.[164,173] Furthermore, a transcriptomic analysis of mouse organs to uncover the role of the circadian clock in coding genes found that not only do approximately half of the coding genes in the body follow circadian rhythmicity in transcription but also that the majority of top-selling drugs on the market have circadian gene targets.[174] Taken together, these findings suggest that by targeting the circadian timing of drug administration, the effectiveness of the drug may be increased with implications for potentially reducing dosage and/or decreasing side effects of the drug.[175] This hypothesis has been illustrated in an examination of 24-hour hospital operational rhythms and the timing of orders and first-dosing administration. An observational study designed to determine the peak timing of when orders for drugs are placed and administered found that the ordering of drugs peak with hospital rounding practices, with a 2-hour delay in first-dose timing, and that these timing practices may have detrimental effects to patients' health.[176] Using the antihypertensive medication hydralazine as an example, they found that administration of the drug during the night, and not during typical rounding hours, resulted in up to a 4% reduction in blood pressure as compared with when administered in the typical morning hours.[176] In line with targeting the circadian timing of drug administration is targeting the timing of vaccinations. Several studies have reported that the adaptive immune response of T cells and B cells to vaccinations may vary with time of day,[144-148] although optimal timing of inoculation remains to be determined and may vary by vaccine type. Mechanistic explorations into the effectiveness of vaccinations based on timing include recent work that showed that the circadian clock of CD8 T cells modulates early response to vaccination.[148] Furthermore, the differential effects of time of day of infection and virus replication demonstrated in herpes and flu could also play a role in effectiveness of vaccines based on timing.[125] In addition to medication timing, improving the timing of behavioral and environmental interventions, based on not just *what* we do, but also *when* we sleep, eat,[176a] exercise, are exposed to light, and perform surgeries[17] may lead to improved evidence-based therapeutic regimens for optimizing prevention, maintenance, and—hopefully even—treatment of chronic diseases. Last, recent work has shown the potential value and feasibility of biomarkers for circadian phase and circadian misalignment to guide such timing, which may provide objective measures by which chronotherapies could be implemented in the future (reviewed in the articles by Anderson and colleagues[177,178]).

FUTURE PERSPECTIVES AND CONCLUSIONS

There is increasing evidence showing contributions of the circadian system to cardiometabolic and immune function as well as evidence linking circadian misalignment to poor cardiometabolic and immune outcomes and disease. Knowledge of the processes by which circadian systems and circadian misalignment play a role in these functions provides us with the tools to understand the associated diseases and provide clinical applications such as chronotherapy. Current study designs used to investigate these points, such as epidemiologic and experimental protocols, should be interpreted with their strengths and limitations in mind, namely the long-term nature of certain designs with possible potential confounds (including but not limited to undiagnosed comorbidities, lifestyle factors, access to and consumption of healthy foods, workload, and so on) and the shorter duration, but with experimental design and thus the ability to test causality and mechanism, respectively. With the emergence of highly controlled methods to study circadian rhythms and with the increased recognition of the importance of incorporating circadian measurements into research studies of cardiometabolic and immune health, it is likely that research gaps in these fields will soon be filled and can be extended to the sleep and circadian medicinal fields. Areas for future investigation include further disentanglement of circadian from behavioral/environmental contributions, chronotherapy and circadian optimization of health through meal timing, light-dark exposure patterns, and timing of other daily behaviors (i.e., activity).

CLINICAL PEARLS

- Circadian rhythms are increasingly recognized as an important contributor to human health, and thus circadian misalignment is also increasingly being recognized as a key contributor to disease risk.
- Taking circadian timing and alignment into account is a critical component for the CV, metabolic, and immune health care of patients.
- Circadian interventions, or chronotherapy, are beginning to show promising potential to mitigate and alleviate adverse health symptoms, decrease risk of disease, and improve treatment results.

SUMMARY

Circadian rhythms play a vital role in human health, and circadian misalignment contributes to adverse impacts on CV, metabolic, and immune function. Misalignment of environmental and/or behavioral rhythms with the endogenous circadian system can occur via common modern lifestyle behaviors such as shift work, travel (jet lag), social jet lag, light exposure at night, or late-night eating. Such misalignment is thought to increase the risk of adverse health outcomes and may be related to the high prevalence of disorders relating to cardiometabolic and immune function. Increased understanding of the circadian contributions to these health measures can lead to approaches to enhance circadian function, thereby providing translational applications to clinical sleep and circadian medical care.

DISCLOSURES

I.C.M. reports during the writing of this review receiving support from the American Heart Association (AHA postdoctoral fellowship #19POST34380188). A.M. reports during the writing of this review receiving support from the NIH (K01HL146992). K.P.W. reports during the writing of this review being a board member of the Sleep Research Society; chair of the American Academy of Sleep Medicine Clinical Practice Guideline for the Treatment of Adults with Shift Work Disorder and Jet Lag Disorder Workgroup; receiving research support from the NIH, the Office of Naval Research, the PAC-12 conference, and consulting for Circadian Therapeutics, LTD, Circadian Biotherapies, Inc. Philips Respironics, and the US Army Medical Research and Materiel Command-Walter Reed Army Institute of Research outside the submitted work. F.A.J.L.S. reports during the writing of this review being a board member of the Sleep Research Society; and receiving research support from the NIH.

SELECTED READINGS

Baxter M, Ray DW. Circadian rhythms in innate immunity and stress responses. *Immunology*. 2019.

Chellappa SL, Jingyi Q, Vujovic N, et al. Daytime eating prevents internal circadian misalignment and glucose intolerance in night work. *Sci Adv.* In press.

Chellappa SL, Vujovic N, Williams JS, Scheer F. Impact of circadian disruption on cardiovascular function and disease. *Trends Endocrinol Metab.* 2019;30:767–779.

Depner CM, Melanson EL, McHill AW, Wright Jr KP. Mistimed food intake and sleep alters 24-hour time-of-day patterns of the human plasma proteome. *Proc Natl Acad Sci U S A.* 2018;115. E5390-e9.

Downton P, JO Early, Gibbs JE. Circadian rhythms in adaptive immunity. *Immunology*. 2019.

Mason IC, Qian J, Adler GK, Scheer F. Impact of circadian disruption on glucose metabolism: implications for type 2 diabetes. *Diabetologia.* 2020;63:462–472.

Morris CJ, Purvis TE, Hu K, Scheer FA. Circadian misalignment increases cardiovascular disease risk factors in humans. *Proc Natl Acad Sci U S A.* 2016;113:E1402–E1411.

Morris CJ, Purvis TE, Mistretta J, Scheer FA. Effects of the internal circadian system and circadian misalignment on glucose tolerance in chronic shift workers. *J Clin Endocrinol Metab.* 2016:jc20153924.

Ruben MD, Smith DF, FitzGerald GA, Hogenesch JB. Dosing time matters. *Science.* 2019;365:547–549.

Scheiermann C, Gibbs J, Ince L, Loudon A. Clocking into immunity. *Nat Rev Immunol.* 2018;18:423–437.

Sutton EF, Beyl R, Early KS, Cefalu WT, Ravussin E, Peterson CM. Early time-restricted feeding improves insulin sensitivity, blood pressure, and oxidative stress even without weight loss in men with prediabetes. *Cell Metab.* 2018;27:1212–12121. e3.

Wehrens SMT, Christou S, Isherwood C, et al. Meal timing regulates the human circadian system. *Current biology*. 2017;27:1768–1775. e3.

Wright Jr KP, Drake AL, Frey DJ, et al. Influence of sleep deprivation and circadian misalignment on cortisol, inflammatory markers, and cytokine balance. *Brain Behav Immun.* 2015;47:24–34.

A complete reference list can be found online at ExpertConsult.com.

Chapter 42

Circadian Dysregulation in Brain Aging and Neuropsychiatric Health

Colleen McClung; Aleksandar Videnovic; Erik Musiek

Chapter Highlights

- Circadian rhythm disruption, often accompanied by sleep disturbance, is a common symptom of normal aging and numerous age-related neurodegenerative diseases, including Parkinson disease and Alzheimer disease. Fragmentation of rhythms in activity is the most common finding in aging and these conditions.
- Psychiatric diseases are also associated with prominent circadian disruption. These vary depending on the disease and can be present in patients of all ages.
- Emerging data suggest disruption of the molecular clock in these conditions and implicate circadian dysfunction as a possible contributor to disease pathogenesis.

INTRODUCTION

The circadian system serves to couple cellular function, physiology, and behavior with the light-dark cycles of the earth. Circadian clocks are found in most plants and animals on the earth and allow organisms to predict and adapt to the daily changes in the environment. The circadian system has been proven vital for organismal health. Disruption of circadian function in animals, altered by either light exposure or genetic manipulation of clock gene, can exacerbate a variety of pathologic conditions. Moreover, circadian dysfunction in humans, as can occur in the setting of shift work, sleep disorders, jet lag, or simply the realities of modern life, has been implicated as a risk factor for numerous chronic diseases, ranging from diabetes to cancer.[1] This chapter discusses the evidence supporting a role for circadian rhythm dysfunction in psychiatric and neurodegenerative diseases, conditions that exert enormous burdens on society and for which there are few effective therapies.

The cellular and molecular basis of the circadian clock has been described in other chapters. Briefly, the master circadian clock resides in the suprachiasmatic nucleus (SCN) of the hypothalamus, which receives direct input from the retina to coordinate its activity to the external light-dark cycle. Cells of the SCN, as well as most cells of the body, express a set of conserved circadian clock proteins, which form a transcription-translational feedback loop that can maintain near-24-hour oscillations in transcription and cellular activity.[2] These clock proteins include the positive transcriptional limb consistent of BMAL1 (also known as ARNTL), CLOCK, and NPAS2, and the negative feedback limb consisting of PERIOD1 to PERIOD3, CRYPTOCHROME 1 and 2, and REV-ERBα/β protein.[2] The SCN serves to synchronize cellular peripheral clocks in organs throughout the body (including the rest of the brain) to maintain optimal function.

Circadian behavioral rhythms are commonly assessed by monitoring patterns in movement throughout the course of many days, using either wheel-running caged rodents or wristwatch actigraphy for humans.[3] Circadian rhythms can be quantified in humans and mice by monitoring other parameters, such as temperature, blood pressure, hormone levels (such as cortisol or melatonin), or even clock gene expression in blood samples or other tissues. Because exposure to light can induce changes in behavior in animals independently of the circadian clock, true circadian studies are carried out under constant lighting conditions, usually dim light. While this is feasible with lab animals, it is very difficult with humans, particularly when assessing circadian rhythms in disease populations. Thus a caveat of much of the data pertaining to circadian function in human aging and neuropsychiatric disease is that they are obtained under normal environmental light-dark conditions. It is also notable that the SCN regulates the timing of sleep, with SCN lesioning or BMAL1 deletion in rodents leading to fragmented sleep with no clear night-day differentiation.[4,5] Thus circadian effects on sleep timing and consolidation are difficult to disentangle from effects related to other aspects of clock dysfunction.

CIRCADIAN DYSFUNCTION IN AGING

Aging is well known to impact the circadian system. Fragmentation of circadian activity rhythms is observed in older humans, usually manifested as increases in both daytime napping and nocturnal awakenings.[6,7] There is also a shift in circadian phase in older people, as they tend to go to sleep and awaken earlier.[8] Studies in human postmortem brains find that there is a general loss of normal molecular rhythms in prefrontal cortical regions with aging; however, there appears to be a gain of rhythmicity in a separate set of genes, which may be compensatory.[9] Studies in aged mice show a pronounced loss of amplitude in neuronal firing, as well as more subtle disorganization and blunting of rhythms in clock gene expression, in the SCN.[10,11] Decreased amplitude in clock gene expression rhythms is also observed in peripheral organs from aged mice, including heart and liver, although it is unclear if this is due to impaired signals from the SCN or altered local clock function. Secretion of melatonin, a hormone that is directly controlled by the circadian system and regulates sleep timing, also declines with age, which may impact sleep timing in the elderly.[12-14] Other factors, including poor light exposure, cataracts, physical disability limiting activity, and limited social interaction may also contribute to age-related declines in rhythmic activity. Thus disrupted circadian function occurs with aging and may therefore contribute to age-related diseases.

Circadian Dysfunction in Alzheimer Disease

Alzheimer disease (AD) is the most common cause of dementia in older adults and affects more than 10% of the population above the age of 65. AD is characterized clinically by slowly progressive cognitive impairment, which usually begins as short-term memory loss then progresses to involve other domains. The pathologic hallmarks of AD include extracellular amyloid plaques, which accumulate many years before cognitive symptom onset and contain aggregated forms of amyloid-β peptide (Aβ) as well as neurofibrillary tangles, which are intracellular accumulations of aggregated tau protein and more closely correlate temporally and spatially with neurodegeneration and cognitive decline.

Circadian Rhythm Disruption in Patients with Alzheimer Disease

Individuals with symptomatic AD dementia exhibit a variety of changes in circadian function, including rhythm fragmentation and phase delay.[15] Rhythm fragmentation, which often manifests as increased napping during the day and restlessness during the night, is commonly observed in both older people and patients with AD dementia. It has also been observed in the presymptomatic phase of the disease, when biomarkers of brain amyloid plaque and neurofibrillary tangle pathology are positive but no cognitive symptoms are yet apparent.[16-19] Thus circadian fragmentation in AD appears very early in the disease course and may represent an exacerbation of a condition that occurs in normal aging. Phase delay, which manifests as a peak in activity later than normal in the day, has only been observed in symptomatic patients with AD and has been hypothesized as a possible contributor to the phenomenon of "sundowning," in which patients with dementia frequently become more confused and agitated in the late afternoon and evening.[20,21] Modest circadian abnormalities can also be observed in some mouse models of AD, in particular those that accumulate both Aβ and tau pathology, although the exact nature of the changes does not seem to be consistent across mouse lines.[22,23]

Mechanism Driving Circadian Dysfunction in Alzheimer Disease

The mechanisms driving circadian dysfunction in aging and AD are not fully understood, although several pathologic studies point to degeneration of the SCN as a possible culprit. Postmortem assessment reveals significantly decreased numbers of two critical neuronal populations, vasoactive intestinal peptide (VIP)–expressing and arginine vasopressin (AVP)–expressing neurons, in the SCN in patients with AD and has associated these changes with accumulation of tau pathology in that region.[15,24-26] Premortem circadian behavioral rhythm changes were correlated with the degree of loss of VIP-ergic neurons in the SCN on postmortem analysis in both aged individuals and patients with AD.[27] Decoupling of SCN input to the pineal gland, which produces melatonin, is also observed in AD, as both pineal gland clock gene expression and melatonin production are dysregulated in the disease.[13,14] Peripheral clock dysfunction may also play a role in AD. A study using fibroblasts derived from patients with AD showed abnormal methylation of the BMAL1 promoter in AD, leading to dysrhythmic clock gene expression, although the upstream causes of these epigenetic changes are unknown.[28] Furthermore, Aβ has been reported to induce the degradation of BMAL1 protein by multiple mechanisms in cells and mice, and incubation of SCN slices with Aβ can alter clock gene rhythms, suggesting a possible direct effect of Aβ on the core clock.[22,29] Finally, patients with AD may have loss of melanopsin-containing retinal ganglion cells, specialized neurons that conduct light information from the retina to the SCN.[30] Loss of these cells could impair the responsiveness of the SCN to changes in environmental light levels. Thus AD appears to disrupt circadian system function at multiple levels, although the exact mechanisms are not fully understood.

The impact of circadian dysfunction on the pathogenesis and symptomatology of AD also is poorly understood. The circadian system regulates sleep timing, and a variety of sleep disturbances, including difficulty sleeping at night with increased daytime sleep, are observed in AD.[31] Sleep deprivation can directly drive both amyloid plaque deposition[32] and tau pathology[33,34] in mouse models and can acutely increase cerebrospinal fluid levels of Aβ and tau in humans,[33,35] suggesting that circadian disruption could exacerbate Aβ and tau pathology through its effect on sleep. Sleep also appears to regulate extracellular fluid flow in the brain, potentially mediating clearance of Aβ and other toxic substances via multiple mechanisms.[36,37] However, core clock genes exert sleep-independent effects on neuroinflammation and oxidative stress in the mouse brain.[38] Accordingly, mice lacking BMAL1, which have fragmented sleep rhythms but no sleep deprivation, exhibit accelerated amyloid plaque deposition.[39] Thus sleep-independent effects of the circadian system on AD pathogenesis are possible and are the topic of ongoing study.

Therapy for Circadian Rhythm Disorders in Alzheimer Disease

Symptomatically, circadian rhythm disruption in patients with AD is a major cause of morbidity and institutionalization and is thus an area of concerted effort for therapy development. Numerous efforts have been made to treat circadian dysfunction in patients with dementia with light therapy, melatonin, or combinations of the two. These studies have yielded mixed results.[40-43] Morning light (2500 lux) and evening melatonin (5 mg) improved circadian function and decreased daytime sleep in patients with AD, with no effect on nighttime sleep.[40] Combined treatment with bright light exposure during the day (1000 lux) and melatonin therapy at bedtime (2.5 mg) yielded slight improvement in measures of cognition and mood, with more substantial improvement in evening agitation.[42] However, melatonin alone worsened mood, suggesting that combination therapy was important.

In summary, considerable human and animal data suggest a bidirectional relationship between circadian function and AD, as AD is associated with significant circadian dysfunction,

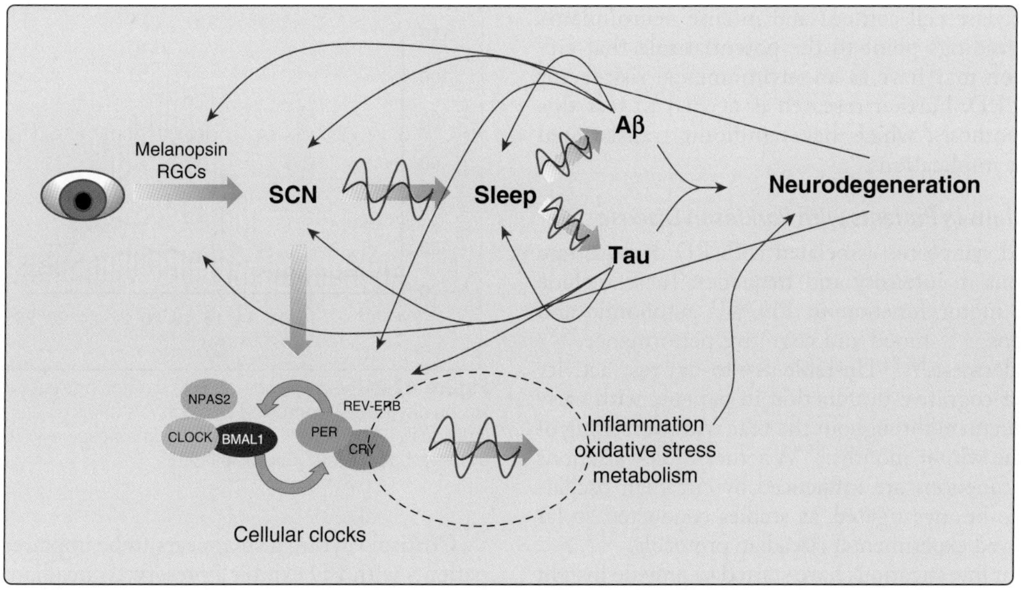

Figure 42.1 Schematic of circadian mechanisms in neurodegenerative diseases. The suprachiasmatic nucleus (SCN) integrates light input from the retina and then generates circadian rhythms in sleep-wake and other physiologic processes, as well as synchronizing cellular clocks. Sleep-wake rhythms regulate levels of Aβ and tau proteins. In the setting of aging or neurodegenerative diseases (*red lines*), blunting of SCN-generated rhythms could disrupt Aβ and tau metabolism and disrupt cellular clocks, which promote inflammation and oxidative stress. RGCs, Retinal ganglion cells.

whereas circadian and sleep disruption appear to drive pathology in early AD (Figure 42.1). Further study is needed to understand how to better optimize circadian function to alleviate symptoms of AD and to potentially reduce AD risk.

Circadian Dysfunction in Parkinson Disease

Parkinson disease (PD) is the second most common neurodegenerative disorder. Nonmotor symptoms (NMSs) affect up to 98% of patients with PD.[44] Disruption of the sleep-wake cycle is among the most common NMS in PD.[45] Alterations of the circadian system are increasingly being recognized as an etiology for disrupted sleep, alertness, and other manifestations of PD.

Dopamine and the Circadian System

Dopaminergic neurotransmission lies at the core of PD and is relevant in all three major components of the circadian system: its input, the pacemaker (SCN), and the output. The existence of diurnal variation in dopamine (DA) and some of its metabolites has been known for many years.[46,47] Striatal DA levels[48-50] and clock genes[51,52] also exhibit periodic variations. In the retina DA plays an important role in the modulation of circadian retinal input.[53] Specifically, DA is involved in light adaptation and the rhythmic expression of melanopsin and clock genes. DA also modulates light input to the SCN from the retina.[53] Further, rhythmic dopaminergic activity may also regulate the activity of the SCN.[54,55] Dopaminergic activity can also be considered an output of the SCN, since evidence points to the primary role of SCN in circadian variations of DA.[54] Dopaminergic input is required for proper modulation of the clock gene *PER2* in the dorsal striatum.[50] Moreover, functional loss of rhythmicity induced by bright constant light[51] or SCN lesions[55] disrupts DA and tyrosine hydroxylase rhythms and reward-related behaviors such as interval timing. Circadian genes within dopaminergic neurons also directly regulate DA synthesis and DA neuron activity.[56-58] Within striatal regions, circadian transcription factors (NPAS2 in particular) also directly regulate expression of DA receptors.[59] In summary, DA exhibits a two-way interaction with the circadian system at several levels.

Circadian Disruption in Parkinsonism: Lessons from Animal Models

Disruption of circadian rhythms has been well documented in animal models of parkinsonism.

1-methyl-4-phenyl-1,2,3,6-tetrahydropyridine (MPTP)-treated dogs exhibit blunted circadian oscillations in renal parameters, including urine volume, creatinine, and several hormones.[60-62] The 6-hydroxy dopamine (6-OHDA) models exhibit disruptions in circadian rhythms of locomotion, temperature, and heart rate.[63] Some of these abnormalities are partially reversible by levodopa (L-DOPA) administration.[63] Circadian changes have been also documented in rotenone-induced neurodegeneration, including changes in serotonergic transmission and clock genes expression.[64] α-Synuclein transgenic mice exhibit accelerated fragmentation of rest-activity and reductions in neuronal activity in the SCN.[65] In a mouse model of parkinsonism that involves deactivation of a mitochondrial transcription factor, MitoPark, diurnal patterns of rest/activity rhythms are altered.[66] Collectively, these basic investigations provide support for the concept of alterations of the circadian system in parkinsonism.

Neurodegenerative processes intrinsic to PD contribute to the disruption of sleep-wake and circadian rhythms, as major anatomic networks that regulate these rhythms become affected as the neurodegeneration progresses. Conversely, emerging studies suggest that circadian disruption may influence this neurodegenerative process as well, although the evidence supporting this relationship is less clear at this point. Preexposure to circadian disruption in mice treated with MPTP results in an exacerbation of motor deficits and a significant reduction in the capability of acquiring motor skills.[67] These changes are associated with a greater loss of tyrosine hydroxylase cell content and intense neuroinflammation. These findings point to the potential role that circadian disruption may have as an environmental risk factor for developing PD. Further research is needed to test this interesting hypothesis, which has significant translational and therapeutic implications.

Circadian Rhythms in Patients with Parkinson Disease

Many signs and symptoms associated with PD demonstrate diurnal variations in intensity and frequency. These include fluctuations of motor function in PD,[68-71] autonomic and sensory functions,[72-77] mood and cognitive performance,[78,79] and sleep and alertness.[80-83] Unstable day-to-day rest-activity rhythms predict cognitive dysfunction in patients with early PD.[84] NMSs fluctuate throughout the year, with worsening of symptoms in the winter months.[85] Whether these variations in physiologic functions are influenced by circadian oscillations remains to be investigated, as studies conducted so far have not employed experimental circadian protocols.

Several recent investigations have started to provide insight into the neuropathology that may underlie circadian symptoms in patients with PD. Retinal neuropathology in PD encompasses degeneration of dopaminergic amacrine cells and retinal ganglion cells.[86] The number of melanopsin-containing retinal ganglion cells as well as their branches and terminals is significantly reduced in patients with PD compared with controls.[87,88] Further, α-synuclein deposition is present in the retina of patients with PD.[88,89] Similarly, postmortem examination of the pineal gland and the SCN in patients who suffered from PD reveals deposits of α-synuclein.[90] Further studies are needed for understanding the neuroanatomic basis of circadian dysregulation in PD.

Markers of endogenous circadian rhythmicity, such as melatonin, cortisol, and core body temperature, have been investigated in the PD population. The amplitude of melatonin rhythm is significantly lower in patients with moderate PD compared with age-matched controls.[91] Those patients with excessive daytime sleepiness have significantly lower amplitudes of their melatonin rhythm compared to those with good alertness (Figure 42.2). This low amplitude of melatonin rhythms points to a weak alerting circadian signal, which may contribute to the excessive daytime sleepiness frequently reported by patients with PD. Similar changes in the amplitude of melatonin rhythms have been observed in early stages of PD.[92] Bolitho and colleagues demonstrated prolongation of the phase angle of entrainment of melatonin rhythm in medicated patients with PD compared to the unmedicated group and controls with PD.[93] These observations provide the rationale to suggest an uncoupling of circadian timing and sleep-wake regulation, possibly related to dopaminergic therapy.

Time-related variations in the expression of core clock genes in patients with PD have been reported. The relative abundance of the clock gene *Bmal1* is significantly lower during the night in a small group of patients with PD. Expression levels of *Bmal1* in patients correlate with PD severity as assessed by the Unified Parkinson Disease Rating Scale (UPDRS).[94] A lack of time-dependent variation in *Bmal1* expression in patients with PD was recently confirmed in another study.[92] These studies have laid out the groundwork for future clinical investigations related to molecular regulation of circadian timekeeping in PD and other neurodegenerative disorders.

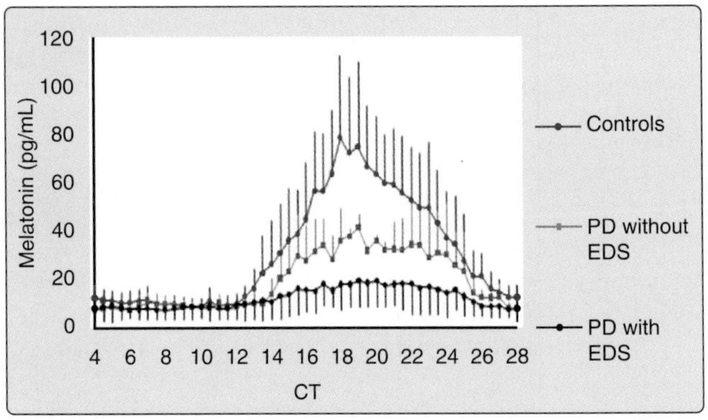

Figure 42.2 The amplitude of daily melatonin release is decreased in Parkinson disease (PD) compared with controls, and a greater decrease is seen in individuals with PD with excessive daytime sleepiness (EDS) compared with those without EDS. CT, Circadian time.

Cortisol rhythm also appears to be impaired in PD. While patients with PD exhibit a preserved circadian rhythm of cortisol, the amount of cortisol secreted is elevated in early PD.[92] However, somatotrophic, thyrotrophic, and lactotrophic axes appear to be intact in early stage PD.[95] Adipokines are endocrine factors released by fat cells and have an important role in feeding, body weight regulation, and metabolism. Because patients with PD frequently experience weight loss, a recent study by Aziz and colleagues focused on the circadian aspects of adipokines in PD, specifically leptin, adiponectin, and resistin, revealing no differences in the levels between patients with PD and controls.[96] A significant decrease in the core body temperature mesor and amplitude has been reported in PD.[97]

Circadian-Based Treatment Approaches in Parkinson Disease

As a consequence of their overall sedentary lifestyle, patients with PD are likely to be exposed to lower intensities of bright light, the most potent synchronizer of the circadian system. Age-related changes may further limit retinal light exposure. Degeneration and impairment of retinal ganglion cells in PD may contribute to decreased sensitivity to light and consequently aberrant melanopsin-mediated responses. Collectively, these factors strongly point to the possibility that patients with PD may benefit from light therapy. Several studies have assessed the safety and therapeutic efficacy of light therapy in patients with PD.[98-103] Results of these investigations revealed benefits to sleep, other nonmotor manifestations, and even some motor symptoms such as rigidity and bradykinesia. Several unresolved questions related to the utility of light therapy in PD remain. These include the optimization of several aspects related to the dose of light therapy and its mechanism of action in PD.

Regular physical activity has been accepted as an important lifestyle modification that reduces the burden of PD symptoms and perhaps may influence the biology of PD-specific neurodegeneration. The use of timed physical activity as a nonphotic zeitgeber that may improve synchronization of circadian system, however, has not been systematically examined in patients with PD. Another chronotherapeutic, melatonin, has a potential role in alleviating sleep-wake cycle disturbances in PD,[104,105] although its effects as a modulator of the circadian system have not been explored in studies published to date. Future studies should focus on optimizing the protocols as well as the parameters of light exposure and other circadian-based approaches geared toward improving symptoms and quality of life and even slowing down disease progression in patients with PD.[106]

CIRCADIAN RHYTHMS, SLEEP, AND PSYCHIATRIC DISEASE

Disruptions to the sleep-wake cycle are a cardinal feature of nearly all psychiatric disorders and are typically one of the core diagnostic criteria used by psychiatrists for diagnosis. The exact phenotype can be variable: for example, some subjects with depression experience insomnia, early morning awakening, and too little sleep, whereas others sleep too much, often missing work or other activities. Fragmented or disrupted circadian rhythm and sleep patterns are also common in psychiatric disorders as is a late or delayed chronotype (i.e., preference for activity during the night). Moreover, environmentally induced changes to the normal sleep-wake schedule can exacerbate symptoms and precipitate episodes. In later sections we highlight some of the associations between circadian phenotypes and specific psychiatric disorders, as well as chronobiology-based treatments.

Development and Childhood: Focus on Autism Spectrum Disorders

Sleep disturbances and circadian disruptions are associated with several neurodevelopmental disorders, including autism spectrum disorders (ASDs). Sleep problems are very often found in children diagnosed with ASD. The most common complaints are delay in sleep onset (insomnia) and issues with sleep maintenance, resulting in overall reduced sleep duration.[107] Night wakings of 2 to 3 hours are common in children with ASD.[108,109] While some of these sleep problems could be behavioral, circadian rhythm abnormalities have also been measured in children with ASD. These include irregular sleep-wake patterns, early morning wakening or sleep-onset delay, and free-running rhythms.[110] Genetic studies have suggested an association between polymorphisms in several core circadian genes with ASD.[111-113] Several studies have also found abnormalities in the regulation of melatonin levels in children with ASD. The most consistent finding in ASD is significantly lower levels of evening melatonin.[114-117] Importantly, low levels of melatonin correlate with severity of autism symptoms.[114] Moreover, studies have found that unaffected parents of children with ASD also have lower melatonin levels, suggesting that this effect may be genetic.[117] One hypothesis is that circadian rhythm disruptions in children with ASD are the result of mutations in genes involved in melatonin synthesis *(ASMT)*[117] and that melatonin, along with the clock genes, are important in the underlying changes in synaptic transmission seen in ASD.[118] In addition to its role as a circadian entraining molecule, melatonin acts as a potent antioxidant. One possibility is that a reduction of melatonin during development leads to a buildup of oxidative stress, which is harmful to the developing nervous system.[119] This would increase the risk for ASD and other neurodevelopmental disorders.

Melatonin therapy is often used by clinicians to treat the sleep disturbances seen in children with ASD. A recent study assessed the impact of prolonged-release melatonin (2 to 5 mg) on 125 children with ASD in whom sleep failed to improve with behavioral interventions alone.[120] The authors found that, after 13 weeks of this double-blind study, the melatonin treatment was associated with an increase in sleep by nearly 1 hour (57.5 minutes) compared to only 9 minutes with placebo. They also found that sleep latency decreased by 40 minutes and that 68.9% of participants had a clinically meaningful response with very few side effects. It will be interesting in future studies to determine if other chronotherapies are affective in managing the symptoms of ASD.

Other genetic studies have found significant associations between ASD and synaptic proteins in the SHANK family, which act as scaffold-organizing factors in the postsynaptic density of excitatory synapses.[122] Furthermore, SHANK3 protein levels in mice oscillate in the hippocampus and striatum over the light-dark cycle and correlate with changes in serum melatonin.[123] In addition, levels of SHANK3α expression show patterns in the thalamus, cortex, and striatum that associate with diurnal rhythms in activity levels.[123] These studies suggest that there may be an association between deficits in circadian rhythms and changes in synaptic proteins that are strongly linked to ASD.

Adolescence: A Time of Developmental and Environmental Risk

Adolescence is a particularly vulnerable time for the emergence of psychiatric and addictive disorders. In addition to the neurobiologic changes occurring during adolescence, hormonal and other biologic changes associated with puberty lead to an evolutionarily conserved shift in circadian rhythms in which preferred sleep and wake times become later. This shift is more prominent in boys than in girls, but it occurs in both sexes.[124] This shift in rhythms is also seen in measures of melatonin onset, which gradually become later during puberty.[125,126] During adulthood, most people show a shift back toward the earlier chronotypes observed in childhood, making adolescence a unique time in which the late chronotype prevails. Teenagers are exposed to a number of social and environmental factors that weaken, shift, or misalign their natural rhythms. These include very early high school start times, increased social interactions with peers, highly caffeinated energy drink consumption, nicotine exposure, and the use of electronic devices at night. To compound these effects, prepubertal and midpubertal kids are biologically more sensitive to the melatonin-suppressing effects of light at night than older adolescents or adults are.[127] Thus the current lifestyle of many teenagers creates a perpetual state of circadian misalignment known as "social jet lag": they wake up for school early 5 days a week but stay up late, often using illuminated electronic devices, and then sleep in on weekends.[128,129] The shift to later sleep times on weekends is equivalent in some teens to traveling from San Francisco to New York City—and back again—each week, significantly disrupting normal biologic rhythms throughout the brain and body. Because of these changes and other factors, the typical adolescent is chronically sleep deprived.[130] A recent study published by the Centers for Disease Control and Prevention[130a] showed that less than 10% of teenagers get the 8 to 10 hours of sleep a night recommended by the American Academy of Pediatrics. In fact, the American Academy of Pediatrics has labeled insufficient sleep in this population as a public health epidemic that increases risk for substance abuse, along with other problems such as depression, obesity, and suicide.[131-133] Studies have found that even a single night of sleep deprivation in healthy adolescents leads to an increase in activity in the ventral striatum and reduced deactivation in the medial prefrontal cortex during the receipt of monetary reward relative to the same task after normal sleep conditions.[134] However, this response is variable, and although most adolescents experience some form of sleep/circadian disruption, not all go on to have psychiatric disorders. This raises the possibility that individual, biologically driven sleep/circadian phenotypes, or gene-by-environment interactions, mediate increased susceptibility to these diseases.

Mood and Anxiety Disorders

Depression, bipolar disorder, and anxiety disorders are associated with very disrupted sleep-wake cycles. Symptoms often become worse with environmental sleep-wake or light disruption. In fact, one of the most common mood disorders affecting approximately 2% to 5% of the population in temperate climates is seasonal affective disorder (SAD), a syndrome in which depressive symptoms occur only in the winter months when there are shorter days and a later dawn.[135,136] Delayed rhythms during adolescence and early adulthood strongly associate with depression and severity of mood symptoms.[137,138] Furthermore, more recent work has found that circadian rhythm disruptions in high-risk adolescents predict worse prognosis and symptoms in several longitudinal studies.[139,140] Together, these findings suggest that sleep and circadian disruptions (both biologic and environmental) have a role in the precipitation of disorder symptoms and vulnerability to mood disorders. Biologic circadian rhythm and sleep abnormalities have been described for decades in patients with mood disorders.[141,142] These include disrupted rhythms in sleep/activity, body temperature, plasma cortisol, norepinephrine, thyroid-stimulating hormone, melatonin, pulse, and blood pressure.[143] Interestingly, these rhythms usually return to normal with antidepressant or mood stabilizer treatment and patient recovery. A study of the human postmortem brain[144] found that the amplitude in diurnal rhythms in a number of rhythmic mRNA transcripts was significantly altered in several brain regions from individuals with major depression when compared to healthy controls. The abnormalities in the brains of subjects with depression included shifted gene expression peak timing and disrupted phase relationships between individual circadian genes in several reward-related brain regions, including the hippocampus, amygdala, and ventral striatum.[144] This suggests that there are fundamental molecular rhythm disruptions across brain regions that contribute to depression. Furthermore, genetic circadian disorders such as familial advanced sleep-wake phase disorder or delayed sleep-wake phase disorder are both often comorbid with depression and anxiety.[145-147] As with other psychiatric disorders, individuals who are genetically predisposed toward an evening chronotype are more likely to develop mood disorders.[148-150]

Multiple human genetic studies (including some genome-wide association studies) have identified single-nucleotide polymorphisms or other disruptions in core circadian genes that associate significantly with mood disorders, in particular SAD and bipolar disorder.[151-153] Polymorphisms in *ARNTL* (i.e., *BMAL1*) have been linked to bipolar disorder through convergent functional genomic approaches and are suggested by the International Society for Bipolar Disorders Biomarkers Task Force to be one of four genes with variants that serve as potential biomarkers for the disease.[154] In addition to the effects on sleep, recent studies have determined that the circadian system is intricately involved in the molecular and cellular control of virtually all processes that are hypothesized to underlie mood disorders.[155]

Multiple theories have been put forth over the years to try to explain the development of mood disorders which involve multiple systems and regions of the brain. These include (but are not limited to) mitochondrial or metabolic dysfunction, neuroinflammation, monoamine imbalance, disrupted neurogenesis, and hypothalamic-pituitary-adrenal axis dysregulation, all of which are regulated by the molecular clock. Furthermore, animal studies find that the circadian genes contribute in a fundamental way to neuronal synchronization across multiple brain regions and to the regulation of neuronal circuitry that controls mood and anxiety.[156-159] It seems clear that a combination of biologic and environmental factors contribute to changes in mood, and the diagnosis of mood disorders continues to grow. One contributing factor is likely to be our modern lifestyle, which includes increased exposure to artificial light at night, shift work, less sleep or fragmented sleep patterns, travel across time zones, and reduced exposure to daytime sunlight. These environmental disruptions to the biologic clock are particularly deleterious for vulnerable individuals (i.e., those with mutations in one or more clock-associated genes). Animal studies have also found that exposure to chronic stress disrupts the circadian clock in the SCN and that the severity of disruption correlates directly with increased anxiety- and depression-related behavior.[160] Light exposure at night, constant light, or constant dark also increases depressive and anxiety-like behavior in rodent models.[161]

Given the cyclic nature of bipolar disorder with extreme changes in sleep-wake patterns, many researchers have speculated that circadian abnormalities underlie its development and are a core component of the disorder.[162-164] Furthermore, it is common for symptoms to be seasonal, in that subjects are more likely to have depressive symptoms in the winter and manic symptoms during the summer.[163,165,166] In many subjects with bipolar disorder, manic or depressive episodes are precipitated by disruptions to their normal sleep-wake cycle.[167] For these subjects, shift work or jobs with erratic work schedules can be severely detrimental. Mood episodes can also be brought on by periods of stress, which disrupt natural sleep-wake rhythms. The social zeitgeber theory[168] proposes that in vulnerable individuals, life stress affects sleep-wake and social rhythms, leading to circadian clock disruption and subsequent depressive or manic episodes.[169] It has been hypothesized that many individuals with bipolar disorder have a molecular clock that is unable to properly adapt to changes in the environment, and this underlies the precipitation of these episodes.[169] Dramatic mood-stabilizing effects in patients with bipolar disorder can be obtained through strict regulation of the sleep-wake cycle via a cognitive behavioral approach known as interpersonal and social rhythm therapy (IPSRT).[167] This therapy allows patients to track their time awake, time to first interactions, meals, and sleep with the goal of maintaining a very rigid and regular sleep-wake and social schedule. Other treatments for depression, SAD, and bipolar disorders in adults have been developed to amplify, phase advance, or delay circadian rhythms. These include bright light therapy for depression, acute sleep deprivation, dark therapy for mania, and therapeutic melatonin agonists (such as agomelatine).[170-173] Moreover, antidepressant and mood-stabilizing medications such as lithium, valproic acid, and selective serotonin reuptake inhibitors have dramatic effects on the amplification and timing of gene expression rhythms that may, at least in part, underlie their therapeutic efficacy.[174-176] Furthermore, a recent study found that the rapid and lasting antidepressant effects of low-dose ketamine can be predicted based on circadian rhythm measures prior to treatment and on how well ketamine strengthens low-amplitude rhythms, suggesting that the therapeutic effects are directly related to the strengthening of the circadian system.[177] Thus rhythm alignment and amplification is emerging as an important therapeutic approach to helping prevent or treat psychiatric disorders.

The International Society on Bipolar Disorders recently published a systematic review of and practice recommendations for chronotherapy and chronobiology.[178] This task force generally concluded that (1) the acute antidepressant efficacy of bright light therapy was supported; (2) adjunctive dark therapy for bipolar mania is also generally supported as was IPSRT for mood stabilization and improved sleep; (3) data on melatonergic agonists were limited and showed some conflicting evidence. Overall, chronotherapies were generally safe and well tolerated. Such chronotherapy for these disorders, however, must be personalized based on the particular needs of the individual. For example, subjects with depression are more responsive to morning light therapy combined with wake therapy and sleep-time stabilization if they are evening chronotypes and have a positive diurnal variation in mood with the best mood in the evening.[179] In contrast, subjects with bipolar depression respond best to midday light therapy, as morning light therapy can induce manic episodes.[180] In addition to amplifying rhythms, lithium treatments lengthen the period in *Drosophila* spp., nonhuman primates, rodents, and humans.[181-185] Interestingly, patients with bipolar disorder who have an abnormally fast clock respond positively to lithium treatment, whereas the patients who begin with an abnormally slow clock generally do not respond favorably to lithium treatment.[148,162,186] These actions of lithium on the free-running period appear to be SCN dependent[187] and again suggest a personalized medicine approach to chronotherapy is needed.

Schizophrenia

Schizophrenia (SCZ) is a psychiatric disease associated with positive (i.e., psychosis-related symptoms), negative (i.e., affect-related symptoms), and cognitive symptoms. Significant disruptions in diurnal rhythmicity of activity patterns, cortisol and melatonin profiles, and body temperature rhythms are commonly associated with SCZ. For example, actigraphy measurements in subjects with SCZ found that a subset of subjects with SCZ free run, similar to people who are completely blind with non-24-hour disorder, suggesting their rhythms are not able to entrain to the light-dark cycle, while other subjects showed highly disorganized and fragmented rhythms.[188] Furthermore, a study that measured circadian gene expression in blood samples and cultured fibroblasts from subjects with SCZ found a loss of rhythmicity and decreased expression of circadian genes compared to controls.[189] Several studies have identified differential gene expression in numerous transcripts in human cortical regions in the postmortem brains of subjects with SCZ. The most consistent results include reduced expression of genes associated with GABAergic transmission and mitochondrial function and increased expression of transcripts associated with neuroimmune function.[190-194] Using a time-of-death analysis similar to the depression study discussed previously, researchers discovered that subjects with SCZ not only have a loss in rhythmicity in most normally rhythmic transcripts but also have a very different set of transcripts with 24-hour rhythmicity in the dorsolateral prefrontal cortex compared with control subjects.[195] The top pathways identified in transcripts that have 24-hour rhythms only in subjects with SCZ are associated with mitochondrial function, and nearly all of them appear to peak during the day and trough during the night. Interestingly, these novel rhythms drive differential expression patterns of many genes that have long been implicated in SCZ (i.e., *BDNF* and GABAergic-related transcripts), suggesting that the change in molecular rhythmicity is responsible for the difference in expression of these genes. These altered rhythms in neurotransmission and mitochondrial-related transcripts may either drive, or be a marker of, significant diurnal differences in neuronal activity in the prefrontal cortex in subjects with SCZ.

Human genetic studies (mostly candidate gene studies) have identified variants in circadian genes that associate with SCZ; however, these have not been identified in more recent, large-scale studies performed by groups such as the Psychiatric Genomics Consortium. An analysis of 21 different circadian genes in 1527 subjects identified an association between *NPAS2* and SCZ.[196] In a genome-wide association study analysis of a United Kingdom biobank, a genetic correlation was also found between longer sleep duration and SCZ risk.[197] Therefore circadian and sleep gene variation may be important in SCZ but are only one contribution; there are hundreds of genes that contribute small amounts of risk.

Both human and animal experimental work suggest that the interplay between sleep and circadian function and DA is important in the generation and maintenance of psychosis.[198] In particular, both animal and human data suggest that sleep disruption increases DA release and sensitivity. Furthermore, elevated DA disrupts sleep and circadian rhythms.[198] Thus the current literature suggests that circadian rhythms, DA dysregulation, and psychosis are intricately linked, and, as already mentioned, several animal studies have found that circadian genes directly control nearly all aspects of dopaminergic transmission, including DA synthesis, uptake, and receptor activity.[199,200] More work must be done, however, to determine if specific chronobiologic approaches will be useful in the treatment of SCZ.

CONCLUSIONS

Circadian rhythm and sleep disruption are key features of several neurodegenerative diseases, including AD and PD, as well as many psychiatric disorders. The exact mechanisms underlying these phenotypes remain uncertain; however, they likely involve a combination of genetic disruptions to molecular pathways regulating rhythms and sleep, paired with environmental sleep-wake disruption (Figure 42.3). Disruption of the circadian clock exerts a wide array of effects on different aspects of disease pathogenesis, and preclinical data suggest that clock disruption could contribute to disease pathogenesis through multiple pathways. The molecular clock is thus a potential therapeutic target for these disorders. Although existing therapeutic strategies have largely involved light exposure, melatonin, or sleep-inducing agents, future treatments will have to be tailored to the specific disease process and individual patient, as

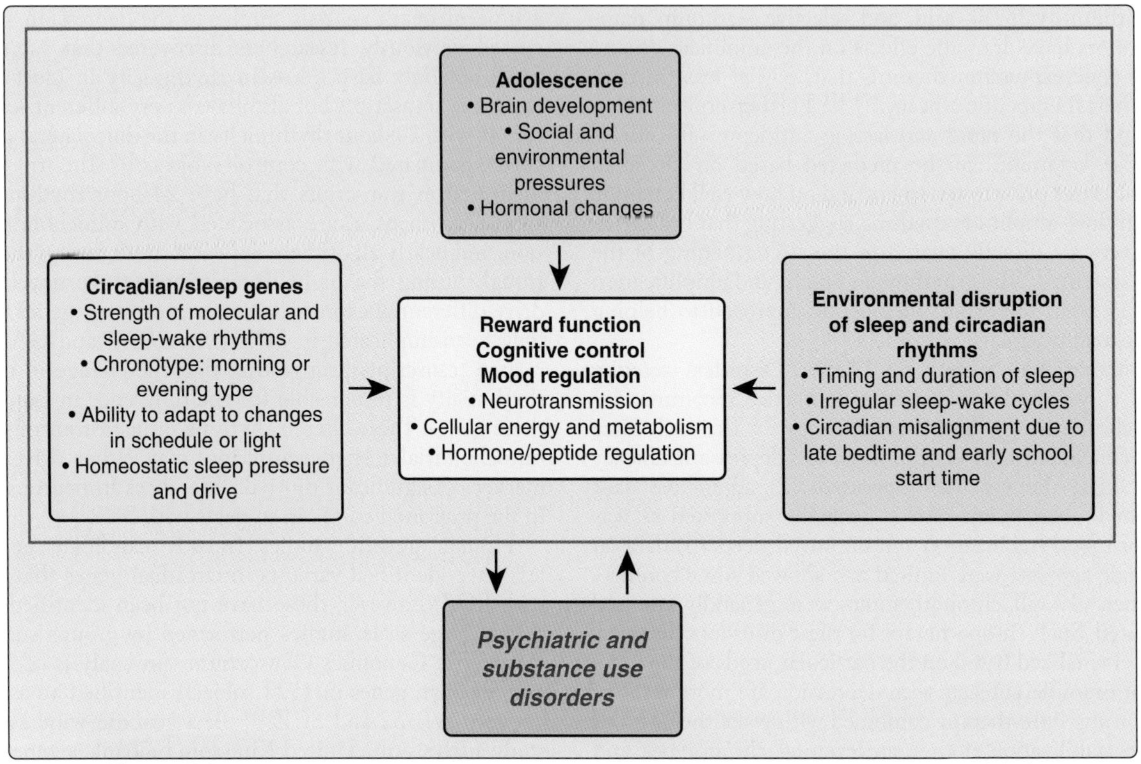

Figure 42.3 Circadian mechanisms in psychiatric disorders. Circadian clock genes/proteins, environmental clock disturbance, and adolescent brain development all interact with reward, cognitive, and mood centers to influence psychiatric disease.

there is a large degree of variability between diseases and within patient groups in terms of phase advances, phase delays, insomnia, fragmentation, and so on. As more specific biomarkers are developed to pinpoint specific sleep and circadian abnormalities within patient populations with neurodegenerative diseases and psychiatric disorders, this will provide better guidance regarding the appropriate treatment options.

CLINICAL PEARL

Screening for sleep disturbances and circadian disruption in patients with neurodegenerative and psychiatric conditions in the clinic is important: treatment of these symptoms may improve function. Treatment of sleep and circadian disturbances in older adults and in patients with dementia is difficult and must rely on nonsedating medications.

SUMMARY

Disruption of circadian rhythms and the molecular circadian clock is a hallmark of many neurodegenerative disorders and psychiatric diseases. Emerging evidence suggests that impaired circadian function occurs early in many of these diseases and may contribute to disease pathogenesis. Degeneration of the master clock in the SCN may drive rhythm fragmentation in AD, which may in turn promote protein aggregation and inflammation. Dopaminergic neurodegeneration in PD may lead to circadian disturbances, causing sleep-wake and behavioral disturbances. Circadian disruption can be both a cause and an effect in several psychiatric disorders, emphasizing the bidirectional relationship between circadian disturbance and brain dysfunction.

SELECTED READINGS

Fifel K, Videnovic A. Circadian and sleep dysfunctions in neurodegenerative disorders-an update. *Front Neurosci*. 2021;14:627330. Published 2021 Jan 18.

Frank E, Soreca I, Swartz HA, Fagiolini AM, et al. The role of Interpersonal and social rhythm therapy in improving occupational functioning in patientes with bipolar I disorder. *Am J Psychiatry*. 2008;165:1559–1565.

Hatfield CF, Herbert J, van Someren EJ, Hodges JR, Hastings MH. Disrupted daily activity/rest cycles in relation to daily cortisol rhythms of home-dwelling patients with early Alzheimer's dementia. *Brain*. 2004;127:1061–1074.

Kang JE, Lim MM, Bateman RJ, et al. Amyloid-beta dynamics are regulated by orexin and the sleep-wake cycle. *Science*. 2009;326:1005–1007.

Li JZ, et al. Circadian patterns of gene expression in the human brain and disruption in major depressive disorder. *Proc Natl Acad Sci U S A*. 2013;110:8850–9955.

Lucey BP, Hicks TJ, McLeland JS, et al. Effect of sleep on overnight CSF amyloid-beta kinetics. *Ann Neurol*. 2017.

Melke J, et al. Abnormal melatonin synthesis in autism spectrum disorders. *Mol Psychiatry*. 2008;13:90–98.

Roenneberg T, et al. A marker for the end of adolescence. *Curr Biol*. 2004;14:R1038–R1039.

Wang JL, Lim AS, Chiang WY, et al. Suprachiasmatic neuron numbers and rest-activity circadian rhythms in older humans. *Ann Neurol*. 2015;78:317–322.

Wulff K, Dijk D-J, Middleton B, Foster RG, Joyce EM. Sleep and circadian rhythm disruption in schizophrenia. *Br J Psychiatry*. 2012;200:308–316.

Xie L, Kang H, Xu Q, et al. Sleep drives metabolite clearance from the adult brain. *Science*. 2013;342:373–377.

A complete reference list can be found online at ExpertConsult.com.

Chapter 43

Circadian Disorders of the Sleep-Wake Cycle

Sabra Abbott; Kathryn J. Reid; Phyllis C. Zee

Chapter Highlights

- Circadian rhythms are regulated by a complex network, including the suprachiasmatic nucleus in the hypothalamus and molecular clocks throughout the body.
- Circadian rhythm sleep-wake disorders can result from (1) changes in the light-dark cycle in relation to the internal clock, (2) changes in the internal clock in relation to the light-dark cycle, and (3) dysfunction in the clock mechanisms.
- Circadian rhythm sleep-wake disorders can be treated with a combination of behavioral interventions and carefully timed light and melatonin.
- Selection of optimal treatment paradigms can benefit by determining the phase of the circadian clock.

The sleep-wake cycle is generated by a complex interaction of endogenous circadian and sleep homeostatic (need for sleep increases as a function of prior wakefulness) processes, as well as social and environmental factors. Physiologic sleepiness and alertness not only vary with prior waking duration but also exhibit circadian variation. In humans, daily variation in physiologic sleep tendency reveals a biphasic circadian rhythm of wake and sleep propensity,[1,2] with a midday increase in sleep tendency occurring at about 2 p.m. to 4 p.m. followed by a robust decrease in sleep tendency and increase in alertness that lasts through the early to middle evening hours. A primary role of the circadian clock is to promote wakefulness during the day and thus also to facilitate the consolidation of sleep during the nighttime hours.[1,3-5] In humans, this interaction between circadian and homeostatic processes results in approximately 16 hours of wakefulness and 8 hours of nocturnal sleep.

The timing and duration of the sleep-wake cycle depend on the synchronization of the endogenous circadian clock with the external physical light-dark (LD) cycle, as well as social or professional demands. Circadian rhythm sleep-wake disorders (CRSWDs) arise when there is either disruption of this internal timing mechanism or a misalignment between the timing of the circadian clock and the 24-hour social and physical environments. In this chapter, the nomenclature and diagnostic criteria for CRSWD and its subtypes are based on the criteria published in the *International Classification of Sleep Disorders,* third edition. These dyssynchronous states fall into three categories: (1) the terrestrial LD cycle may change relative to circadian timekeeping (shift work and jet lag), (2) circadian timekeeping may change relative to the terrestrial LD cycle (delayed sleep-wake phase disorder [DSWPD], advanced sleep-wake phase disorder [ASWPD], or non-24-hour sleep-wake rhythm disorder [N24SWD]), or (3) dysfunction in clock mechanisms (irregular sleep-wake rhythm disorder [ISWRD]). The first category occurs in the presence of a normal circadian timekeeping system and is generally self-limited or resolves with environmental change. The second category is believed to occur because of chronic alteration in the circadian system, resulting in the inability of the circadian pacemaker to achieve a conventional phase relation with the external world. The third is primarily due to dysfunction of the central clock or its afferent-efferent pathways. This chapter focuses on the second and third groups of disorders. Because circadian variation in wakefulness and sleep propensity is the most apparent of the many behavioral and physiologic outputs of the circadian pacemaker, it is not surprising that the most apparent circadian rhythm disorders to be recognized involve the sleep-wake cycle.[6]

Disruptions in the timing of sleep and wakefulness are often associated with symptoms of difficulty falling or staying asleep at the desired times or excessive sleepiness that causes patients to seek medical attention. Thus, in clinical practice, CRSWD is often underrecognized yet should be considered in the differential diagnosis of any patient presenting with symptoms of insomnia or hypersomnia. A multimodal treatment approach of behavioral or pharmacologic strategies aimed to improve circadian function and alignment of circadian rhythms to the 24-hour environment is often necessary to consolidate sleep and improve daytime function in patients with CRSWD. Growing knowledge about how the circadian system responds to photic as well as to nonphotic entraining agents is increasing the number of practical therapies that can be used in "real-life" clinical settings.

REGULATION AND ENTRAINMENT OF CIRCADIAN RHYTHMS

The suprachiasmatic nucleus (SCN), in the anterior hypothalamus, is the central pacemaker responsible for the generation of circadian rhythmicity in mammals.[7] Animals and humans removed from the external LD cycle and other time cues (zeitgebers) exhibit a self-sustaining cycle of sleep and wakefulness as well as many other physiologic and hormonal rhythms.

The endogenous frequency of this cycle of oscillation or free-running period is largely genetically determined.[8] The basic molecular mechanism by which SCN neurons generate and maintain a self-sustaining rhythm is through an autoregulatory feedback loop in which oscillating circadian gene products regulate their own expression through a complex system of transcription, translation, and posttranslational processes.[9] In the mouse[10] and hamster,[11] genes have been identified that lengthen[10] and shorten[11,12] the free-running period. The mammalian circadian period is generally slightly longer than 24 hours in diurnal animals and slightly shorter than 24 hours in nocturnal animals. In humans, the average circadian period has been estimated to be approximately 24.18 hours[13] and must therefore be synchronized or entrained on a regular basis to the 24-hour terrestrial day by external influences.

Entrainment by Light

Light is the major external time cue in mammals. Light reaches the SCN by afferent projections from the retina through the retinohypothalamic tract.[7] Evidence indicates that the primary circadian photoreceptors are the melanopsin-containing retinal ganglion cells, which in turn send photic information through projections to the SCN.[14,15]

Although circadian rhythms can be entrained to LD cycles that are not exactly 24 hours in duration, entrainment is restricted to cycles with periods that are "close" to 24 hours in duration.[16] The range of entrainment can vary from species to species and is dependent on the experimental conditions (e.g., intensity of LD cycle, whether period of LD cycle is changed gradually or rapidly), but in general, animals do not entrain readily to LD cycles that are more than a few hours shorter or longer than the period of the endogenous circadian rhythm. If the period of the LD cycle is too short or too long for entrainment to occur, the circadian rhythm will free-run, following the period of the endogenous pacemaker rather than the external environment.

One of the most widely used methods to examine how the LD cycle influences the circadian system has been to expose animals and humans maintained in constant conditions to pulses of light. The effects of the light pulse on a phase reference point of a circadian rhythm (e.g., onset of melatonin, minimum of body temperature) in subsequent cycles is then determined. The direction and magnitude of the phase shifts are strongly dependent on the circadian time at which the light pulse occurs. A phase response curve (PRC) is a plot of the magnitude and direction of the time shift induced by an environmental perturbation as a function of the circadian time at which the perturbation is given. Light pulses presented near the onset of the subjective night (part of the circadian cycle that occurs during the dark or nighttime) delay circadian rhythms, whereas light pulses presented in the late subjective night or early subjective day (part of the circadian cycle that occurs during the light or daytime) phase-advance circadian rhythms. Extensive studies have demonstrated that the LD cycle can entrain circadian rhythms and that bright light can be used to manipulate human rhythms under a variety of experimental conditions.[17,18] Although bright light (intensities approximating sunlight) is a very strong and reliable entraining agent for the circadian system,[18] there is evidence that lower intensities, such as those encountered in ordinary room lighting[19] or emitted from electronic devices such as e-readers, computers, or cell phones[20] and even very short pulses (milliseconds) of light,[21,22] can affect the timing of human circadian rhythms. In humans, both light-induced phase shifts and melatonin suppression are most sensitive to short-wavelength light of approximately 460 nm.[23,24] There is also evidence that light-induced phase shifts and melatonin suppression might be functionally independent of each other, such that the degree of phase shift is not equivalent to the degree of melatonin suppression.[25] These discoveries provide exciting avenues for the development of novel light therapies to treat CRSWDs.

Entrainment by Nonphotic Signals

The role of activity and social cues as synchronizing agents for the human circadian system has been recognized since the early 1970s. Studies by Aschoff and colleagues showed that scheduled bedtimes, mealtimes, and various timed social cues were able to entrain circadian rhythms.[26] More recent studies indicate that sleep and social schedules may also phase-shift the circadian clock.[27] In addition, physical exercise during the night can produce a phase delay in human circadian rhythms,[28,29] whereas exercise during the morning can accelerate entrainment following a phase advance in the sleep-wake cycle.[30] These findings indicate that scheduled social and physical activity programs may also be useful strategies for the treatment of CRSWDs.

Melatonin

Melatonin is an important modulator of circadian rhythms[31] and alters the timing of circadian rhythms in animals[32] and humans.[33] The circadian rhythm of melatonin production and release is controlled by the SCN through an indirect pathway, a noradrenergic synapse from the superior cervical ganglion to the pineal gland.[34] The PRC for melatonin in humans indicates that administration of exogenous melatonin to humans in the early evening advances the phase of circadian rhythms, whereas administration in the early morning delays the phase, with the strongest phase-shifting effects of exogenous melatonin occurring during the evening, just preceding the increase in endogenous melatonin levels.[35-37] In addition to its phase-resetting properties, evidence supports a role for melatonin in sleep modulation by increasing evening sleep propensity and reducing core body temperature.[31] Melatonin has been shown to decrease the firing rate of SCN neurons,[38] and it has been proposed that, by its inhibition of SCN firing, the increase of melatonin in the evening creates a sleep-permissive state.

The potential importance of melatonin for regulating the sleep-wake cycle has led to interest in its use for treatment of insomnia and CRSWDs. Indeed, there is good evidence that melatonin may be effective for entraining circadian rhythms in blind people with non-24-hour sleep-wake cycles[39] and phase-advancing circadian rhythms in people with DSWPD.[40] Another potential use for melatonin has been to maintain consolidation of sleep during the early morning hours in elderly people.[41]

Given the importance of melatonin as a modulator of circadian rhythms and its relationship with sleep, the timing of melatonin secretion is a useful marker of the timing of the circadian clock.[42] Furthermore, the degree of mismatch between the timing of melatonin secretion and sleep-wake timing and regularity may be an indicator of the underlying reason for the sleep-wake disturbance.[43]

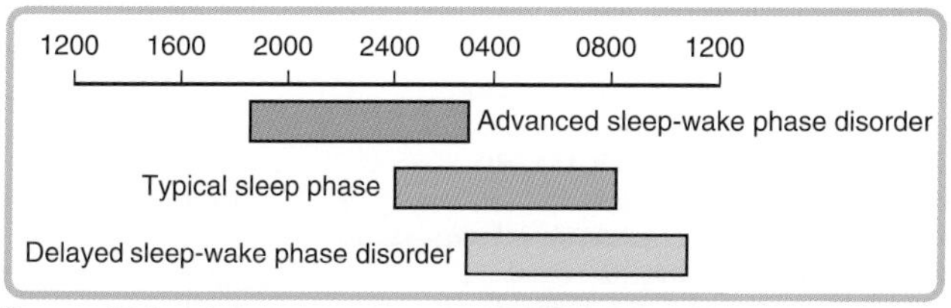

Figure 43.1 Schematic representation of the temporal distribution of sleep and wake in patients with circadian rhythm sleep disorders. Patients with advanced sleep-wake phase disorder typically complain of evening sleepiness and either early morning awakening or sleep disruption. Patients with delayed sleep-wake phase disorder complain of difficulty initiating sleep, usually before 2 a.m., and have difficulty awakening in the morning.

DELAYED SLEEP-WAKE PHASE DISORDER, DELAYED SLEEP PHASE TYPE, DELAYED SLEEP PHASE SYNDROME

Clinical Features

DSWPD is characterized by sleep onset and wake times that are usually delayed more than 2 hours and often up to 3 to 6 hours relative to conventional sleep-wake times (Figure 43.1). The typical patient finds it difficult to initiate sleep before 2 to 6 a.m. and, when free of societal constraints, prefers wake times of 10 a.m. to 1 p.m. Sleep itself is reported to be normal for age.[44,45] These symptoms are chronic, usually lasting at least 3 months, and often of many years' duration. The clinical picture may be similar to sleep-onset insomnia. Patients are unable to advance their sleep times despite repeated attempts and may report a history of prolonged sedative-hypnotic drug use, bedtime use of alcohol, behavioral interventions, or psychotherapy.[46] Patients often report feeling most alert in the late evening and score highly as evening types on a morningness-eveningness scale.[47] Enforced "conventional" wake times may result in chronically insufficient sleep and excessive daytime sleepiness. Sleepiness is greatest in the morning and lessens as the circadian drive for wakefulness peaks in the late afternoon. In adolescents the syndrome may be associated with daytime irritability and poor school performance,[48] whereas in adulthood, the syndrome may be associated with impaired job performance and associated financial difficulty, as well as marital problems.[49] DSWPD may be mistaken for depression, in which the sleep-wake cycle may also be delayed (or advanced). Several studies, generally from psychiatric clinics, have emphasized an association of DSWPD with mood, obsessive-compulsive symptoms, and personality disorders.[49-52]

Epidemiology

DSWPD has been reported as young as preadolescence and beyond 60 years of age.[49] Although the actual prevalence of DSWPD in the general population is not well characterized, evidence from one population-based study indicates a prevalence of 0.17%.[53] DSWPD is reported to be more common in adolescents and young adults, with a reported prevalence of 3.3% to 7%,[54-56] whereas in middle-aged adults, the prevalence may be one-tenth of that, or 0.7%.[57] In a group of New Zealand adults the prevalence was found to be 1.51% to 8.90%, depending on the definition used.[58] In a sleep disorders clinic, 6.7%[45] to 16%[50] of patients seen for a primary complaint of insomnia were determined to have DSWPD. There are no known sex differences in prevalence.

Pathogenesis

It has been pointed out that the tendency for late sleeping is not simply a function of the circadian drive for wakefulness interacting with the sleep homeostat but is analogous to eating or other behaviors that are mandated by physiology but overlaid by varying individual emotional, social, and medical states.[50] Although the exact cause of DSWPD is not known, there have been several mechanisms proposed, including both behavioral and physiologic factors. Behavioral preference may play a major role in some cases of DSWPD, particularly when bedtimes and rise times are not enforced. In fact, a study of 182 patients with clinical features of DSWPD demonstrated that 43% of those patients did not exhibit significant delays in the timing of melatonin onset, despite having delayed sleep-wake timing, suggesting a "non-circadian" cohort of patients with DSWPD.[59]

In adolescence the biologic delay in the timing of circadian rhythms[60] is likely exacerbated by late evening activities, such as doing homework, watching TV, and using the internet.[61] Other factors may include use of caffeine to combat sleepiness during normal waking hours. Staying up late and waking up late in the morning or afternoon may result in an abnormal relationship between the endogenous circadian rhythm and the sleep homeostatic process that regulates sleep and wakefulness. Evidence also shows that under certain conditions (a background of dim light), ambient artificial light (as low as 100 lux) at night may be of sufficient intensity to affect circadian timing.[19] Therefore light exposure later in the evening may also perpetuate and exacerbate the phase delay. Furthermore, late wake times will delay exposure to light in the morning and may prevent active advancement of the circadian clock, allowing it to drift to a new phase relation with external clock time. In addition, late bedtimes result in a decrease in the amount of phase advance that occurs in response to morning light, so even if patients with DSWPD do wake up on time, staying up later at night makes it more likely that they will delay over time.[62] Studies in adolescents with subclinical DSWPD have found that simply following a fixed advanced sleep-wake schedule can result in significant advances in salivary melatonin rhythms,[63] suggesting a strong behavioral component.

For many individuals with DSWPD, however, symptoms often persist despite attempts to structure sleep and wake times, resulting in severe social or professional consequences[46,64,65] and suggesting that behavioral factors alone do not fully explain this disorder. There is considerable evidence that DSWPD is the result of alterations in the endogenous circadian system. For example, many physiologic markers of circadian phase persist in a delayed pattern despite enforced sleep-wake times.[46] There is also evidence that some individuals with DSWPD have a hypersensitivity to nighttime suppression of melatonin and circadian phase delays produced by evening bright light exposure.[66,67] Furthermore, the pupillary response to light may be a marker of "circadian" versus "noncircadian" DSWPD.[68] Reduced sensitivity of the oscillator to photic entrainment (i.e., a reduction in the amplitude of the advance portion of the PRC to light) has also been hypothesized, as has a prolonged free-running period length of the circadian cycle.[46,69-72] DSWPD has also been reported after minor traumatic brain injury.[73] Furthermore, the duration and timing of environmental light and dark exposure may play a role in the expression of the DSWPD phenotype.

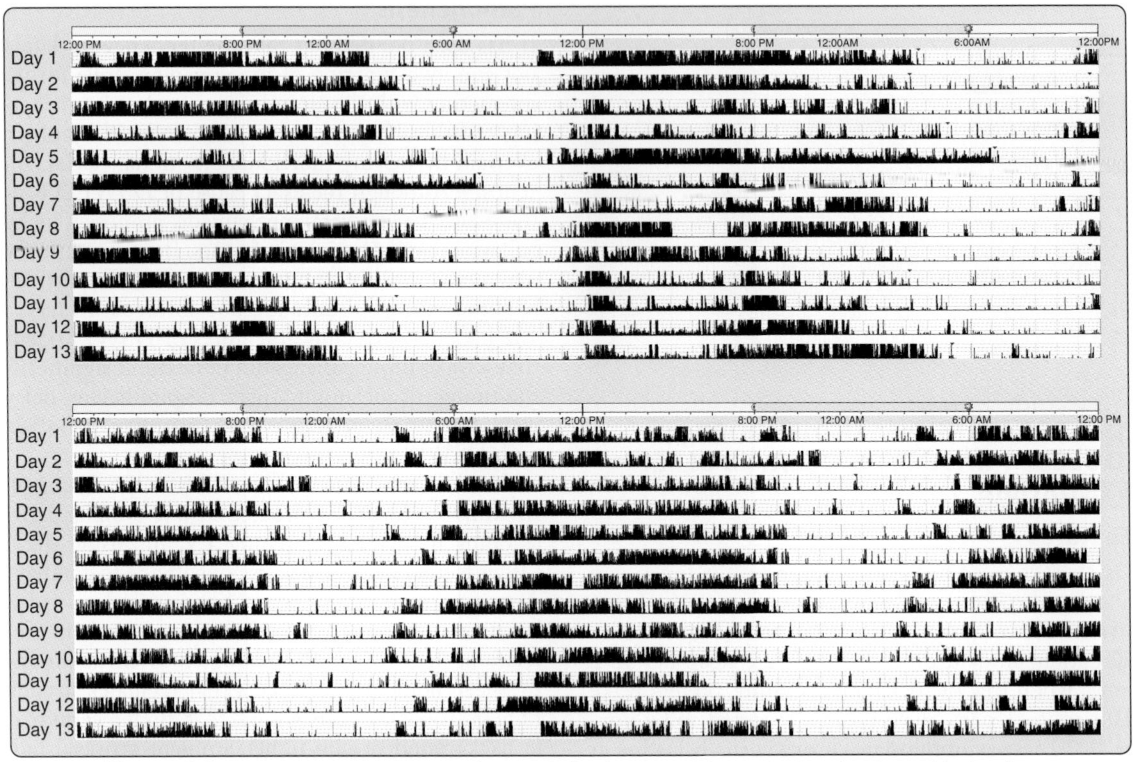

Figure 43.2 Representative rest-activity cycles recorded with wrist-activity monitoring of patients with circadian rhythm sleep disorders. The *black bars* indicate activity levels recorded at the nondominant wrist. Delayed sleep-wake phase disorder with sleep-onset times of approximately 3 a.m. to 4 a.m. and wake time of noon (*top panel*). Advanced sleep-wake phase disorder with sleep onset between 8 a.m. and 10 p.m. and wake time of 4 to 5 a.m. (*bottom panel*).

For instance, the prevalence of DSWPD may be increased at extreme latitudes.[74] Interestingly, individuals with DSWPD do not exhibit an increase in evening light exposure prior to bedtime[75] but do have a decrease in light exposure during the daytime.[76]

There is also evidence for a genetic basis to DSWPD. In some cases the syndrome may be familial, presenting with an autosomal dominant mode of inheritance.[49,77] Further support for a genetic basis for DSWPD derives from reports of polymorphisms in circadian genes such as *hPer3*, arylalkylamine *N*-acetyltransferase, human leukocyte antigen DR1, and *Clock* that are associated with diurnal preference and DSWPD.[78-82] More recently two familial cohorts of DSWPD have been identified, one with a mutation in *hCry1*,[83] and the other with a mutation in *hPer2*.[84]

Although it is commonly accepted that DSWPD is predominantly a result of alterations of circadian timing, there is evidence that alterations in the homeostatic regulation of sleep may play an important role as well.[85,86] Polysomnography (PSG) recordings of sleep in both adults and adolescents with DSWPD have shown that sleep architecture is not disrupted after the initiation of sleep when subjects are allowed to sleep until their desired wake times,[48,49,87,88] although individuals with DSWPD have been shown to have increased difficulty awakening from rapid eye movement (REM) sleep compared with controls.[89] Following 24 hours of sleep deprivation, subjects with DSWPD, compared with controls, show a decreased ability to compensate for sleep loss during the subjective day and the first hours of subjective night.[85,90] Therefore it is likely that both alterations in circadian timing and impaired sleep recovery contribute to symptoms of insomnia and excessive sleepiness in DSWPD.

Diagnosis

The diagnosis of DSWPD is usually made on the basis of the patient's history of chronic or recurrent symptoms of insomnia resulting from a stable delay in the timing of the major sleep and wake period.[91] The sleep disturbance is associated with impairment of social, occupational, or other areas of functioning. In addition, sleep log or actigraphy monitoring should be performed for at least 7 days, but preferably 14 days, to demonstrate a stable delay in the timing of the habitual sleep period. Actigraphy is a practical tool for assessing sleep-wake cycles relative to clock time and has become more widely available clinically[92] (Figure 43.2). A morningness-eveningness questionnaire, such as the Horne-Östberg[47] or the Munich Chronotype[93] Questionnaire, may be useful in confirming the patient's circadian preference but is not required to make the diagnosis.[94,95]

To make the diagnosis, medical, mental, or sleep disorders that may cause alterations in the sleep-wake cycle, insomnia, or excessive sleepiness should be excluded or be adequately treated. In adolescents, social maladjustment, family dysfunction, school avoidance, and affective disorders should be considered in the differential diagnosis. Nocturnal PSG is not necessary to establish the diagnosis but should be performed when another primary sleep disorder such as sleep apnea or parasomnia is suspected. When performed during conventional sleep laboratory hours, PSG often shows a prolonged sleep-onset latency as well as prolonged REM latency and

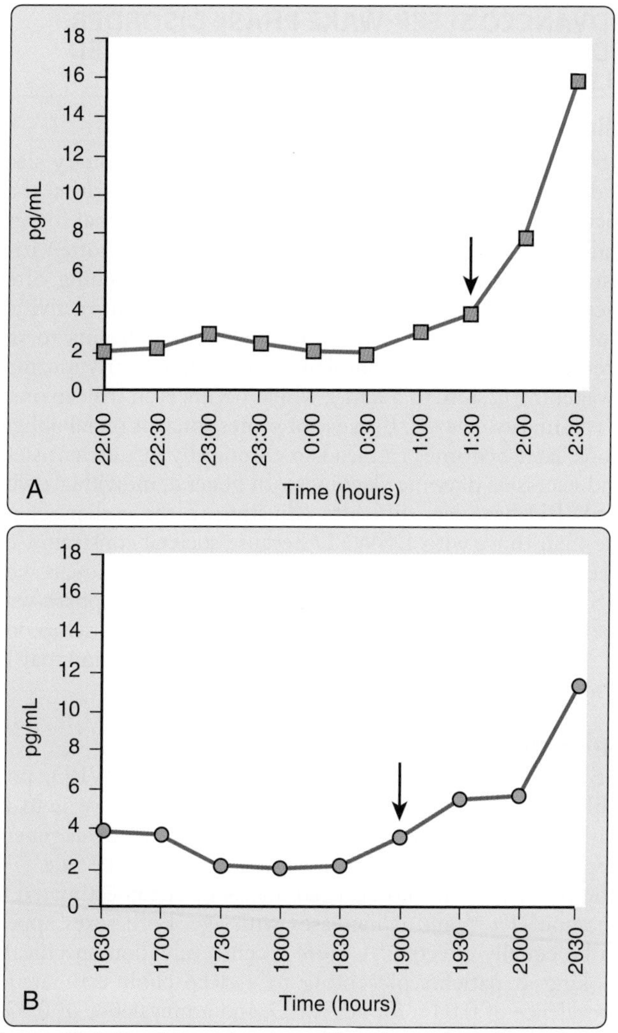

Figure 43.3 Dim light melatonin profiles of an individual with delayed sleep-wake phase disorder with a dim light melatonin onset (DLMO) at 1:30 a.m. (**A**) and an individual with advanced sleep-wake phase disorder with a DLMO at 7 p.m. (**B**). The *arrow* indicates the DLMO calculated as 2 standard deviations above the mean of baseline.

may sometimes, in conjunction with an antecedent sleep log, be a clue to the diagnosis.

The use of other physiologic markers of circadian timing, such as continuous recording of body temperature[96] or dim light melatonin onset (DLMO),[97] may also aid in determining the phase relation of circadian and terrestrial time, although routine clinical availability remains limited. DLMO is probably the most useful marker for circadian pacemaker output.[98,99] Individuals with DSWPD usually have DLMO times that occur after 10 p.m.[97,100,101] (Figure 43.3). Determination of DLMO can be made by measurements of melatonin from plasma or saliva. Commercially available salivary determination of DLMO for clinical use may be feasible in the near future.

Treatment

The goal of therapy is to align the timing of the circadian clock with the desired 24-hour LD cycle. Adherence to good sleep hygiene principles and identification and treatment of comorbid medical and psychiatric disorders are essential components in the management of DSWPD. In addition, light therapy and pharmacologic agents such as melatonin have been shown to be useful treatments for patients with DSWPD.

Light

As described earlier, light plays a major role in resetting the human circadian pacemaker.[17,18,102] Therapy with bright light in the morning (the advance portion of the human PRC) should advance the phase of circadian rhythms in DSWPD.[103,104] The human PRC to a single 3-hour bright light pulse suggests that a light pulse given slightly before the time of body temperature minimum will result in a maximal phase delay, whereas a pulse given slightly after the minimum will cause a maximal phase advance (each about 2 hours).[102] When light pulses over three successive cycles are used, larger shifts (4 to 7 hours) can be produced. Because body temperature minimum is not routinely measured clinically, light therapy is usually timed using sleep logs to estimate the patient's endogenous circadian phase. A light pulse of 1 to 2 hours' duration and between 2500 and 10,000 lux is usually administered toward the end of the sleep-wake cycle. Because the portion of the PRC at which the greatest phase advance can be achieved occurs during sleeping hours, light is usually given immediately on awakening in the morning, which results in a smaller phase advance. It should be noted, however, that in severely delayed individuals the sleep-wake cycle may not necessarily correlate with circadian phase; therefore early morning light could in theory be inadvertently given on the delay portion of the PRC, worsening the problem. Regestein and Pavlova reported a patient who slept later after exposure to light at 6 a.m.[50] Another factor that may limit the practicality of bright light treatment is that many individuals with DSWPD may find it difficult to wake in time for administration of bright light therapy.[50]

Although a number of reports of successful application of bright light therapy in DSWPD exist,[105-108] large, randomized, placebo-controlled studies to determine the intensity, duration, and overall effectiveness are still needed. Rosenthal and colleagues found that 2 hours of bright light exposure (2500 lux) in the morning, together with light restriction in the evening, successfully phase-advanced (by 1.4 hours) circadian rhythms of core body temperature and multiple sleep latencies in 20 patients chosen prospectively after meeting clinical criteria for DSWPD.[108] In contrast, a retrospective report from a referral sleep clinic found that only 7 of 20 patients with DSWPD treated with bright light alone were able to entrain reliably to a desired sleep schedule.

In addition to timed morning light exposure during the phase advance portion of the PRC, timed light avoidance during the phase delay portion of the PRC may also be an effective treatment strategy. In a small open-label trial, wearing blue light–blocking glasses in the evening resulted in an average phase advance of just over 1 hour,[109] suggesting that careful attention to overall light scheduling throughout the day may be an important treatment strategy.

Melatonin

Administration of exogenous melatonin also shifts the phase of the endogenous circadian clock. It should be noted that the PRC for melatonin is nearly opposite the PRC for light exposure: melatonin delays circadian rhythms when administered in the morning and advances them when administered in the afternoon or early evening.[35,37] The physiologic (phase-shifting) dose of melatonin is approximately 0.1 to 0.5 mg or one-tenth to one-fiftieth of most commercially available preparations.[110] Side effects of melatonin at these dose ranges are minimal, although sedative effects occur at higher (5- to 80-mg) doses.

In a randomized, double-blind, placebo-controlled crossover study of eight patients with DSWPD, 5 mg of melatonin administered at 10 p.m. resulted in a phase advance in all subjects with a mean advance of sleep onset time of 82 minutes and of wake time of 117 minutes.[111] On stopping melatonin, all patients reverted to their previous sleep-wake cycle within 2 to 3 days. A study to determine the optimal timing and dose of melatonin to treat DSWPD indicated that melatonin given about 6 hours before the DLMO resulted in the largest phase advance and that there was no significant difference in the effect of either a 0.3-mg or 3-mg dose.[112] A more recent PRC specifically examining the effects of lower doses of melatonin (0.5 mg) demonstrated maximal phase advances when administered 2 to 4 hours before DLMO.[113] In the largest placebo-controlled clinical trial for DSWPD to date, 116 patients with DSWPD were randomized to either placebo or 0.5 mg of melatonin taken 1 hour prior to their desired bedtime. After 4 weeks of following this schedule, those receiving melatonin fell asleep, on average, 34 minutes earlier than the placebo group.[114] Melatonin has also been used successfully in several recent studies in children or adolescents with a combination of delayed sleep phase and other comorbid conditions such as attention deficit disorder and neurodevelopmental disabilities.[115-117]

Although several studies have demonstrated the potential effectiveness of melatonin administered in the evening,* the relatively small number of clinical studies, together with the variability in dose and time of administration, have been limiting factors in the development of a standardized approach for treatment with melatonin. However, while the ideal timing and dose of melatonin are still being determined, the most recent practice parameters established by the American Academy of Sleep Medicine do recommend the use of timed melatonin for the treatment of DSWPD in adults, adolescents, and children.[120]

Several studies have evaluated the use of a combination of bright light and melatonin. A combination of bright light on awakening and melatonin, 3 mg taken 8 hours before bedtime, resulted in significantly larger advances (1.04 hours) than either melatonin (0.72 hours) or light (0.31 hours) alone.[121] Using a combination of bright light (10,000 lux) for 30 to 45 minutes on awakening in conjunction with 3 mg of melatonin taken 8 hours before sleep midpoint resulted in significant improvement in daytime sleepiness, fatigue, and cognitive functioning.[122]

In summary, the clinical approach to a patient with DSWPD should initially include assessment of circadian sleep phase by sleep diary or actigraphy measures for a period of at least 7 days but ideally 14 days.[92,94] Behavioral interventions such as a structured sleep-wake schedule, good sleep hygiene practices, and avoidance of exposure to bright light in the evening should be prescribed for all patients.[94] In addition, exposure to bright light in the morning (1 to 2 hours in duration, beginning shortly after awakening) and/or administration of melatonin in the evening (5 to 6 hours before habitual sleep time) can advance the timing of the sleep-wake cycle. It is important to note that melatonin has not been approved by the U.S. Food and Drug Administration for this indication.

*References 40, 111, 112, 116, 118, 119.

ADVANCED SLEEP-WAKE PHASE DISORDER, ADVANCED SLEEP PHASE TYPE, ADVANCED SLEEP PHASE SYNDROME

Clinical Features

ASWPD is characterized by habitual and involuntary sleep and wake times that are usually more than 2 hours earlier than societal averages (Figure 43.1). Sleep itself is normal for age. Individuals frequently complain of persistent and often irresistible sleepiness in the late afternoon or early evening, often preventing their participation in desired evening activities. Because their circadian drive for wakefulness begins to rise prematurely, they may complain of involuntary early morning awakening (2 a.m. to 5 a.m.), which occurs even if sleep onset is voluntarily delayed. Because of professional or social obligations, later bedtimes can lead to chronically insufficient sleep and excessive daytime sleepiness. In general, individuals with ASWPD have less difficulty adjusting to the earlier schedule than those with DSWPD because societal constraints on sleep time are less rigid than on wake time. Individuals with ASWPD may gravitate to professions that are in phase with their endogenous circadian clock. Because of the symptoms of early morning awakening, a diagnosis of depression may be erroneously made.

Epidemiology

ASWPD is less frequently reported than DSWPD, possibly because affected individuals may not perceive it to be pathologic. The actual prevalence of ASWPD in the general population is unknown but has been thought to be rare.[53,123] The prevalence in middle-aged adults has been estimated to be about 1%,[57] and it increases with age. Both sexes appear to be equally affected. A more recent evaluation specifically looking at patients presenting to a sleep clinic estimated a prevalence of 0.04% for ASWPD, and a prevalence of 0.33% for advanced sleep phase (without symptoms related to their sleep-wake timing).[124]

Pathogenesis

As with DSWPD, the etiology of ASWPD is not well understood, although several hypotheses have been proposed. An abnormal PRC to light exhibiting an increased area under the advance portion of the curve could in theory result in a persistent phase advance. ASWPD may also be the result of a shortened endogenous period. Evidence of a shortened free-running period of less than 24 hours has been demonstrated in a 66-year-old woman with advanced sleep and wake times with intact or even enhanced responsiveness to photic entrainment[17] and in a single member of a familial case of ASWPD.[125] In addition, several studies of adults born prematurely have demonstrated significant advances in the sleep-wake cycle in preterm infants with low birth weight.[126,127]

Several familial cases of ASWPD have been reported in the literature.[125,128-133] These families show a clear autosomal-dominant mode of inheritance of ASWPD. Genetic analysis of these familial cases indicates that there is heterogeneity of this disorder between and even within large families. Gene polymorphisms have been identified in the circadian clock gene *hPer2* in a large family with advanced sleep phase,[134] and a missense mutation in CKI-δ has also been reported.[135] More recently familial ASWPD has also been associated with mutations in *hPer3*,[132] *Cry2*,[131] and *Timeless*.[133]

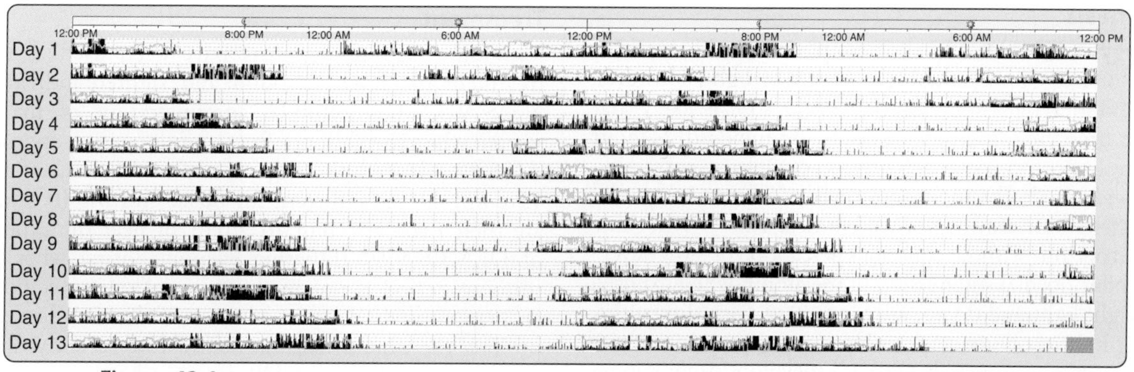

Figure 43.4 Rest-activity cycles recorded with wrist-activity monitoring of a sighted individual with non-24-hour sleep-wake disorder. The *black bars* indicate activity levels recorded at the nondominant wrist. Note that sleep onset is later on each consecutive day and that sleep is initiated from anytime between 5 p.m. and 1 a.m. for the 13 days represented in this actogram.

Diagnosis

A diagnosis of ASWPD is made primarily on the basis of the clinical history. Individuals have a chronic or recurrent complaint of difficulty staying awake until the desired time in the evening and inability to remain asleep until the desired and socially acceptable time for awakening. The sleep disturbance is associated with impairment of social, occupational, or other areas of functioning.[91] When allowed to choose their preferred schedule, patients will exhibit normal sleep quality and duration for age and maintain an advanced but stable phase of entrainment to the 24-hour day. Sleep log or actigraphy monitoring for at least 7 days and preferably 14 days should be performed to confirm a stable advance in the timing of the habitual sleep period.[91] The use of actigraphy, if available, is frequently helpful (Figure 43.2).

Other medical, mental, or sleep disorders may cause alterations in the sleep-wake cycle. Insomnia or excessive sleepiness should be excluded or adequately treated. Major affective disorders should be carefully excluded. PSG is not required for the diagnosis, but in some patients, it may be necessary to evaluate for sleep-disordered breathing, periodic limb movements, or other causes of sleep disruption. PSG should ideally be performed during the patient's normal sleep period. If it is carried out at conventional laboratory hours, a shortened or normal sleep-onset latency, early REM sleep, and early wake time may be seen. Therefore it is important to consider depression, narcolepsy, or other disorders in the differential diagnosis.[123,136]

When the diagnosis is in question, additional physiologic measures of circadian timing, such as continuous ambulatory monitoring of body temperature or collection of salivary melatonin samples to determine DLMO (Figure 43.3) may be clinically useful to confirm the advance in circadian phase. Patients with ASWPD have been reported to have a DLMO[128,129] and core body temperature minimum[125] that are advanced several hours compared with controls. A morningness-eveningness scale, such as the Horne-Östberg or Munich Chronotype Questionnaire to gauge the patient's best time of performance is also useful.[47,137]

Treatment

There are several therapeutic approaches used to treat ASWPD, each with practical limitations. A chronotherapeutic approach—advancing bedtime by 3 hours every 2 days until the desired bedtime was reached—has been reported,[123] although relapse occurred quickly.[136] Bright light therapy during the delay portion of the PRC (early evening) is usually tried, although data on its efficacy in ASWPD are limited. Bright light from 7 p.m. to 9 p.m. in elderly subjects with sleep maintenance complaints resulted in a phase delay and reduced awakenings.[138] The recent practice parameters established by the American Academy of Sleep Medicine suggest using bright light as a treatment option for ASWPD.[120]

Melatonin given in the early morning, usually on awakening, could in theory result in a phase delay according to data from the PRC to melatonin.[35,110] However, evidence for its effectiveness or safety in the treatment of patients with ASWPD is generally lacking.[95,139] It should be noted that the sedating effects of melatonin, which can be variable in patients, may limit its usefulness in this regard.

NON-24-HOUR SLEEP-WAKE DISORDER, FREE-RUNNING DISORDER, NONENTRAINED TYPE, HYPERNYCHTHEMERAL SYNDROME

Clinical Features

N24SWD is thought to be the result of a circadian pacemaker that lacks a stable phase relation to the 24-hour LD cycle. Because most individuals must maintain a regular sleep-wake schedule, the clinical picture is that of periodically recurring problems with sleep initiation, sleep maintenance, and waking as the circadian cycle of wakefulness and sleep propensity moves in and out of synchrony with a fixed sleep period time.[140] Without social constraints, sleep onset and wake times are often successively delayed each day (Figure 43.4). This is analogous to the free-running state created when all zeitgebers are removed.[141,142] Because the duration and quality of sleep depend on when it occurs in relation to the circadian cycle,[3] phase "jumps" between two physiologically permissive periods for sustained sleep can be observed.[143-145]

Epidemiology

N24SWD is rare in sighted people, occurring most often in totally blind individuals[140,142,146-149] with estimates ranging from 18% to 50% of those who are totally blind[148,150] and 13% of those who are almost blind.[151] Cases of N24SWD have also been reported in sighted individuals.[141,152-154]

Pathogenesis

The etiology of N24SWD in blind people is most likely either reduction or loss of the entraining effects of light. However, not all blind individuals develop N24SWD, so it is likely that nonphotic time cues, such as an externally imposed 24-hour sleep-wake cycle and social activity, are capable of entraining some individuals.[140] The melatonin rhythm may be damped[155] or nonexistent[156] or may be normal but delayed.[141,147] In some cases, blind persons without conscious perception of light nevertheless exhibit normal suppression of melatonin when exposed to very bright light and do not appear to have sleep difficulties, suggesting intact non–image-forming visual perception of circadian light cues, presumably through melanopsin-containing retinal ganglion cells.[157] Coexistent cognitive impairment, which could make it difficult to process social time cues, may contribute to symptoms in some individuals.[146]

The etiology of N24SWD in sighted individuals is unknown. It has been postulated that sighted individuals may have a reduced sensitivity to the phase-resetting effects of light[141] and may have an increased incidence of psychiatric conditions[153] such as depression or certain personality disorders, which could precipitate the development of the syndrome by changing or removing social time cues.[141,158] In addition, several studies have demonstrated that the intrinsic period of sighted individuals with N24SWD was significantly longer than in controls.[71,72,159]

Nonentrained sleep-wake cycles have developed after chronotherapy for apparent delayed sleep phase type,[141,160] prompting the proposal that such therapy could prolong the free-running period to the point at which it becomes nonentrainable to a 24-hour LD cycle.[160] However, free-running periods, which are too short (<23 hours) or too long (>27 hours)[18] for stable entrainment to a 24-hour cycle, have never been demonstrated in humans. Because persons with DSWPD tend to receive more light exposure in the delay (evening) portion of their PRCs than during the advance portion (early morning), progressive phase delays may sometimes be observed and mistaken for a nonentrained pattern.[6,141]

Diagnosis

The diagnosis of N24SWD is made primarily by a clinical history of insomnia or excessive sleepiness related to abnormal synchronization between the 24-hour LD cycle and the endogenous circadian rhythm of sleep and wake propensity.[91] The pattern of sleep and wake times typically delay each day with a period longer than 24 hours. The pattern is present for at least 1 month and can be confirmed by sleep diary or actigraphy for at least 7 days (but preferably longer) to establish the progressive daily drift in the timing of sleep and wake times (Figure 42.4). Close analysis of the sleep-wake cycle may reveal two distinct sleep-wake cycle periods, alternation between which can be manifested by phase jumps.[144,145] The sleep disturbance should be accompanied by impairment of social, occupational, or other areas of functioning.

It is important to exclude or adequately treat other medical, mental, or sleep disorders that may cause alterations in the sleep-wake cycle, insomnia, or excessive sleepiness. If the diagnosis is in question, PSG may be useful to evaluate for other types of sleep disorders. PSG, when performed at the appropriate circadian time, is usually normal.[141] Overriding behavioral factors predisposing to irregular sleep-wake cycles (substance abuse, dementia, personality, or affective disorders) should also be considered in the evaluation.

Treatment

Melatonin receptor agonists have been used as the initial treatment of choice in blind and sighted individuals with N24SWD.* For example, administration of melatonin is started when the patient's free-running period approaches the normal or desired phase (i.e., sleep-onset times of 10 p.m. to 11 p.m.). Doses sufficient for phase shifting (0.1 to 0.5 mg) are then given at 8 p.m. to 9 p.m. or near the expected time of DLMO.[141,149] Initiating evening dosing when the free-running period is not in the "normal" phase could result in an inappropriate delay or advance of the circadian phase and prolong the time to entrainment. More recently the melatonin agonist tasimelteon (20 mg) has been approved for use in the treatment of N24SWD, given in a similar manner as melatonin at a fixed time every night, with approximately 20% of patients demonstrating entrainment after 1 month of usage.[165] Common side effects include sedation, headache, elevated liver enzymes, and nightmares.

In sighted patients with N24SWD, additional treatments may also be considered. Bright light entrainment is an option in sighted individuals or in blind individuals who exhibit intact photic suppression of melatonin.[166] Entrainment by nonphotic stimuli (e.g., structured social cues) alone has not been successful; however, an approach based on the use of both photic and nonphotic zeitgebers may be effective.[154] The recent practice parameters established by the American Academy of Sleep Medicine recommend the use of timed melatonin in blind individuals with N24SWD but do not provide any recommendations for sighted N24SWD.[120]

IRREGULAR SLEEP-WAKE RHYTHM DISORDER, IRREGULAR SLEEP-WAKE TYPE, IRREGULAR SLEEP-WAKE DISORDER

Clinical Features

ISWRD is characterized by the absence of a well-defined circadian sleep-wake cycle. There is typically no major sleep period. Rather, patients present with three or more sleep episodes of varying length during a 24-hour period. Diagnosis of this disorder requires a complaint of insomnia or excessive sleepiness associated with multiple irregular sleep bouts or naps during a 24-hour period.[91] Despite irregular and fragmented sleep periods, the total sleep time per 24-hour period is usually normal for age.

Epidemiology

The prevalence of ISWRD in the general population is unknown, but it is estimated to be rare.[167] There is no evidence of sex differences. ISWRD is most commonly seen in association with age-related comorbid neurologic disorders such as dementia and Alzheimer disease.[95] It is also seen in patients with brain injury and in children with cognitive impairment and neurodevelopmental disorders.[168]

Pathogenesis

ISWRD is thought to result from dysfunction of the central processes responsible for the generation of circadian rhythms[169,170] receiving circadian timing inputs[171] or reduced exposure to bright light and regular social schedules. A recent case report demonstrated decreased amplitude of core body temperature rhythmicity in two individuals with ISWRD.[172]

*References 33, 141, 142, 146, 147, 149, 161-164.

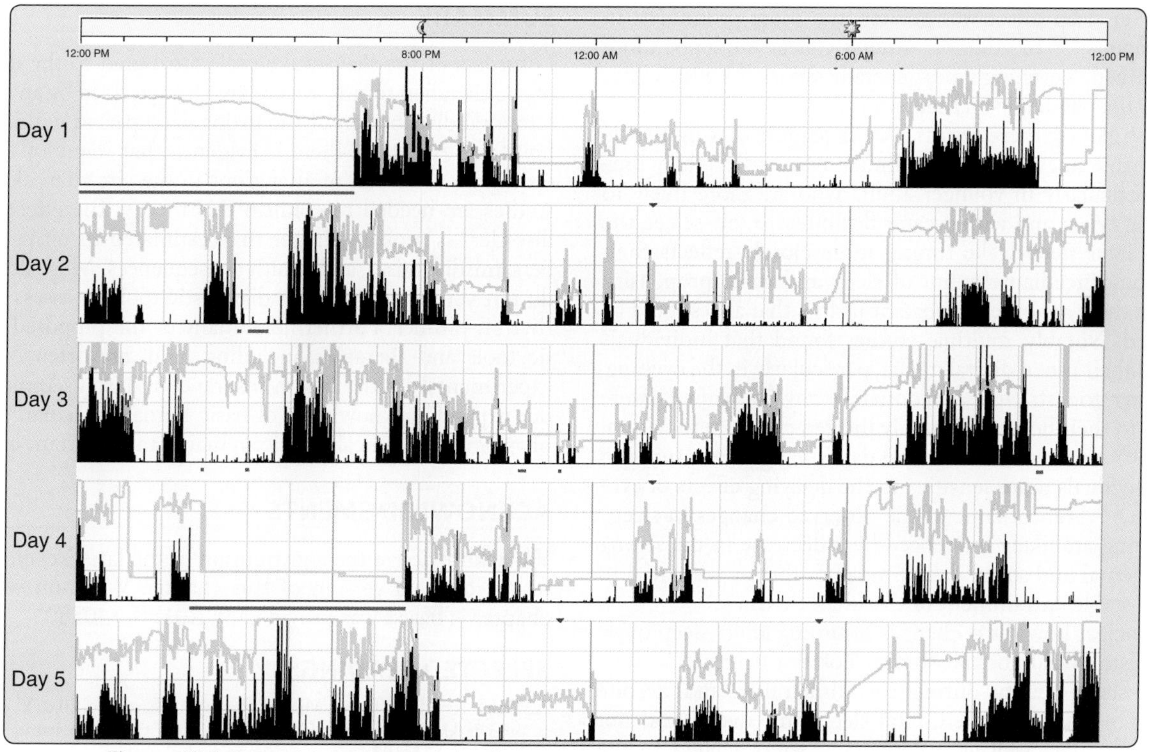

Figure 43.5 Rest-activity cycle recorded with wrist-activity monitoring of an older adult with irregular sleep-wake rhythm disorder. The *black bars* indicate activity levels, and the *yellow bars* indicate the level of ambient light exposure recorded at the nondominant wrist. Note the lack of a discernible circadian sleep and wake rhythm. Sleep is characterized by nocturnal fragmentation and multiple short periods of sleep and wake across the entire 24-hour day.

In institutionalized elderly patients and those with dementia, these factors are thought to contribute to the development and maintenance of irregular sleep-wake patterns.[173,174] Even with controls in place for the level of dementia, lower daytime light levels have been associated with an increase in nighttime awakenings.[175] Evidence suggests that both dysfunction of circadian regulation and reduced exposure to environmental signals are likely involved in the etiology of irregular or arrhythmic sleep and wake patterns.

Diagnosis

In addition to a clinical history, continuous monitoring of sleep and wake activity with actigraphy or a sleep log (completed by the patient or caretaker) for a minimum of 2 weeks is useful diagnostically. Actigraphic recordings show disturbed or low-amplitude circadian rhythm and loss of the normal diurnal sleep-wake pattern with at least three distinct sleep periods per 24 hours (Figure 43.5). This disturbed sleep-wake pattern should be associated with a chronic complaint of insomnia (usually sleep maintenance) and excessive daytime sleepiness. ISWRD should be distinguished from poor sleep hygiene and voluntary maintenance of irregular sleep schedules as seen with shift work.[91]

Treatment

Clinical management aims to improve the amplitude of circadian rhythms and their alignment with the external environment. Increasing exposure to synchronizing agents, such as bright light,[176-179] and structured social and physical activities[180] have been used to consolidate sleep-wake cycles. Several randomized controlled studies using mixed-modality therapies have shown increases in the robustness of the rest-activity rhythm and reductions in nighttime awakening following treatments that include increasing light levels, increasing light in combination with evening melatonin administration, implementing measures to keep nursing home residents out of bed during the day, structuring physical activity, instituting a bedtime routine, and taking measures to reduce nighttime noise and light in residents' rooms.[181-184]

Evening melatonin administration has been used successfully to improve disturbed sleep-wake patterns in children with mental disability.[185-187] In this population melatonin is recommended as a treatment option in the recent practice parameters established by the American Academy of Sleep Medicine; however, melatonin monotherapy is not recommended for the treatment of ISWRD in adults with dementia.[120] Despite the potential utility of both behavioral and pharmacologic interventions, treatment may be difficult and outcomes variable.

CIRCADIAN RHYTHMS IN SITU: INSIGHT FROM THE COVID-19 PANDEMIC

The COVID-19 pandemic brought unprecedented and dramatic changes to school, work, and social schedules. Implementation of shelter-in-place orders during the height of the pandemic had a significant impact on sleep-wake timing in populations all around the world, with large sectors of the population abruptly shifting to working or studying from home, or suddenly becoming unemployed. In parallel with the relaxation of regularly timed structured activities, there were notable changes in sleep-wake timing. Studies using self-reported sleep logs or activity trackers consistently demonstrated later sleep-wake timing and mid-sleep time, as well as a decrease in social jet lag.[188-193] Although both sleep onset and offset were later, the delay in sleep offset was greater, and more prominent in younger adults.[194] In addition, among college students, those who identified as evening types generally reported a positive net impact of the pandemic on their sleep.[189]

At first glance, these results would suggest that as a society, pre-pandemic sleep-wake timing was earlier than preferred, particularly in younger adults who are more likely to be evening types, and with greater flexibility to self-select, the observed later sleep-wake timing more closely reflects their endogenous circadian rhythm of sleep and wake propensity. However, there are other important factors that also should be considered. Notably, multiple studies found that individuals increased their use of digital media, particularly in the evening, and during the strictest lockdowns many individuals were confined to their homes, with only limited exposure to natural light.[195,196] Limited morning and daytime light exposure can make individuals more sensitive to the delaying effects of evening light.[197] Hence, some of the observed changes in sleep-wake timing are likely influenced by a decrease in the strong environmental and social daily time cues that are essential to maintain stable entrainment of circadian rhythms.[193]

It is unclear how these changes in timing affect sleep quality. Interestingly, almost all studies noted a decrease in self-reported sleep quality during this timeframe, and despite spending more time in bed, total sleep time overall did not increase.[190,194] As well as experiencing stress related to the pandemic and associated job loss, many individuals experienced social isolation and general anxiety in response to social distancing measures, so other factors besides timing likely contribute to overall sleep quality.

As societies begin to navigate the post-pandemic work and school environment, it will be important to take into account both the positive and negative impacts of the increased flexibility associated with remote work and learning on sleep-wake timing and quality. Although little is known about the impact of the pandemic specifically on individuals with CRSWDs, these considerations are relevant to the management of patients with CRSWDs, in which appropriately timed, structured light-dark exposure and social and physical activities are important components of treatment.

CLINICAL PEARLS

CRSWDs should be considered in the differential diagnosis of patients presenting with symptoms of insomnia or excessive sleepiness. Furthermore, CRSWDs, such as DSWPD, may be comorbid with other types of sleep disorders, making the diagnosis and treatment even more challenging. Effective management of CRSWD relies upon as accurate a measure of circadian timing as possible. Sleep-onset time (determined by sleep diary or actigraphy) can be useful to determine circadian phase (DLMO occurs approximately 2 hours before sleep onset) in the clinical setting.

Behavioral interventions such as sleep hygiene, particularly enforcement of stable sleep and wake times, exposure to light at the correct time of the day, and avoidance of exposure at the wrong time of the day compose the basic approach for all patients. For the treatment of DSWPD and N24SWD, the use of melatonin may be useful (see specific sections for details). However, the use of melatonin for the treatment of CRSWD has not been approved by the U.S. Food and Drug Administration, and vascular and endocrine adverse effects must be taken into account, particularly in patients who are at increased risk.

SUMMARY

Disorders of the sleep-wake cycle attributed to the disruption of the circadian timing system are characterized by an abnormal temporal distribution of the major sleep period within the 24-hour day. Although there is evidence that many of these disorders are the result of alterations in the circadian clock, more studies are needed to confirm this theory. The effect of these disorders is probably larger than estimated in terms of numbers, misdiagnoses, and health consequences. Most sleep clinics do not yet provide specific diagnostic tools to assess circadian rhythm profiles. Furthermore, many of the proposed diagnostic tools and therapies, including light, are often considered experimental by the health insurance industry. Application of our expanding knowledge of basic human circadian and sleep physiology to clinical practice remains an important challenge.

ACKNOWLEDGMENTS

We acknowledge the contribution of the late Steven K. Baker to the original version of this chapter. Work on which this chapter is based was provided by R01HL140580.

SELECTED READINGS

AMHSI Research Team, Milken Research Team, Roitblat Y, et al. Owls and larks do not exist: COVID-19 quarantine sleep habits. *Sleep Med.* 2021;77:177–183.

Burgess HJ, Revell VL, Eastman CI. A three pulse phase response curve to three milligrams of melatonin in humans. *J Physiol.* 2008;586(2):639–647.

Czeisler CA, Allan JS, Strogatz SH, et al. Bright light resets the human circadian pacemaker independent of the timing of the sleep-wake cycle. *Science.* 1986;233:667–671.

Flynn-Evans EE, Tabandeh H, Skene DJ, Lockley SW. Circadian rhythm disorders and melatonin production in 127 blind women with and without light perception. *J Biol Rhythms.* 2014;29:215–224.

Freedman MS, Lucas RJ, Soni B, et al. Regulation of mammalian circadian behavior by non-rod, non-cone, ocular photoreceptors. *Science.* 1999;284:502–504.

Gandhi AV, Mosser EA, Oikonomou G, Prober DA. Melatonin is required for the circadian regulation of sleep. *Neuron.* 2015;85:1193–1199.

Jones CR, Campbell SS, Zone SE, et al. Familial advanced sleep-phase syndrome: a short-period circadian rhythm variant in humans. *Nat Med.* 1999;5:1062–1065.

Kitamura S, Hida A, Enomoto M, et al. Intrinsic circadian period of sighted patients with circadian rhythm sleep disorder, free-running type. *Biol Psychiatry.* 2013;73(1):63–69.

Minors DS, Waterhouse JM, Wirz-Justice A. A human phase-response curve to light. *Neurosci Lett.* 1991;133(1):36–40.

Morgenthaler TI, Lee-Chiong T, Alessi C, et al. Practice parameters for the clinical evaluation and treatment of circadian rhythm sleep disorders: an American Academy of Sleep Medicine report. *Sleep.* 2007;30:1445–1459.

Neubauer DN. Tasimelteon for the treatment of non-24-hour sleep-wake disorder. *Drugs Today (Barc).* 2015;51:29–35.

Sack RL, Auckley D, Auger RR, et al. Circadian rhythm sleep disorders: part II, advanced sleep phase disorder, delayed sleep phase disorder, free-running disorder, and irregular sleep-wake rhythm. An American Academy of Sleep Medicine review. *Sleep.* 2007;30:1484–1501.

Sack RL, Lewy AJ, Blood ML, et al. Melatonin administration to blind people: Phase advances and entrainment. *J Biol Rhythms.* 1991;6:249–261.

Sinha M, Pande B, Sinha R. Impact of COVID-19 lockdown on sleep-wake schedule and associated lifestyle related behavior: a national survey. *J Public Health Res.* 2020;9(3):1826.

Wilhelmsen-Langeland A, Saxvig IW, Pallesen S, et al. A randomized controlled trial with bright light and melatonin for the treatment of delayed sleep phase disorder: effects on subjective and objective sleepiness and cognitive function. *J Biol Rhythms.* 2013;28:306–321.

Zhou J, Hsiao FC, Shi X, et al. Chronotype and depressive symptoms: a moderated mediation model of sleep quality and resilience in the 1st-year college students. *J Clin Psychol.* 2021;77(1):340–355.

A complete reference list can be found online at ExpertConsult.com.

Section 6

Pharmacology

Chapter 44

Introduction

Thomas Kilduff; Andrew D. Krystal; Thomas Roth

A major revision seen in this edition of *Kryger's Principles and Practice of Sleep Medicine* is in the section Pharmacology. In previous editions this section was organized by broad categories of medication therapeutic use (hypnotics, wake promoting medications, medications used for other purposes that have sleep/wake side-effects). The current section is organized by the individual neurotransmitter systems that regulate sleep/wake function. This change was made to incorporate both basic science and clinical research advancing the understanding of the basic pharmacologic regulation of sleep/wake function and to provide better delineation of the mechanisms and associated properties of medications that have therapeutic and adverse effects on sleep and waking. In terms of the latter, it addresses the challenge that medications used for different purposes and of different types may share an effect on a particular neurotransmitter system. For example, there are medications that are of interest for insomnia treatment and treatment of disorders of excessive daytime sleepiness that impact hypocretin/orexin receptors. The current organization prevents more than one chapter addressing each of the important sleep/wake neurotransmitter systems. This change in organization will also provide a better characterization of medications currently in development and potential targets for future drug development.

The neurotransmitter systems covered in this section include adenosine (see Chapter 45), catecholamines (see Chapter 46), GABA (see Chapter 47), histamine (see Chapter 48), hypocretin/orexin (see Chapter 49), serotonin (see Chapter 50), melatonin (see Chapter 51), and opioids (see Chapter 52). In addition, a chapter was included on drugs used for purposes other than treatment of sleep disorders that have adverse effects on sleep or wakefulness (see Chapter 53). There is evidence that neuromodulators other than those covered in this chapter may impact sleep/wake function. However, at the time of writing there was insufficient data documenting their having significant impacts on sleep/wake function to merit inclusion. As new research emerges, it is expected that the list of neurotransmitter systems covered in this section will grow.

Additional content on clinical pharmacology is now to be found in the sections on individual disorders. Chapters 98, 99, and 100 discuss the various pharmacologic approaches to treat insomnia. The treatment of narcolepsy is found in the chapter on narcolepsy (see Chapter 112) and restless legs syndrome (see Chapter 121). Chapter 133 addresses the various approaches to treat sleep apnea syndromes with medication.

Chapter 45

Adenosinergic Control of Sleep

Michael Lazarus; Yo Oishi; Hans-Peter Landolt

Chapter Highlights

- Adenosine is an endogenous purine ribonucleoside found in all mammalian tissues that modulates a variety of important synaptic processes and signaling pathways in the central nervous system. Adenosine affects sleep-wake patterns via adenosine A_1 or A_{2A} receptors in various brain areas. Emerging evidence suggests that activating A_{2A} receptors suppresses arousal, thereby promoting sleep. Activation of A_1 receptors, on the other hand, mediates sleep need and the response to sleep deprivation. Both receptor types are considered to be critically involved in sleep functions.
- Caffeine is a psychoactive compound with arousal effects that is widely consumed throughout the world in dietary products such as coffee, tea, soft drinks, energy drinks, and chocolate. Some nonprescription medications such as pain-relievers and cold remedies also contain caffeine. At the doses commonly consumed by humans, caffeine antagonizes the actions of adenosine at both A_1 and A_{2A} receptors. The arousal effect of caffeine is mediated by A_{2A} receptors in the nucleus accumbens.
- The mesolimbic dopamine pathway between the ventral tegmental area and nucleus accumbens links motivation with sleep-wake regulation, which may explain why people often feel sleepy when bored. Psychiatric disorders such as schizophrenia, attention-deficit/hyper-activity disorder, and addiction are strongly linked to pathologic deviations in the mesolimbic system and are commonly accompanied by sleep abnormalities. Mesolimbic dopamine-adenosine interactions may constitute an important molecular mechanism underlying the sleep alterations associated with psychiatric disorders.

INTRODUCTION

Approximately one-third of human life is spent in sleep, yet the functions of sleep remain elusive. In non–rapid eye-movement (NREM) sleep, cortical neuronal activity alternates between periods of firing and periods of silence known as the ON and OFF states. These states, which are widely synchronized across neurons, are represented by slow wave activity (SWA) in the electroencephalogram (EEG). SWA is a slow oscillatory neocortical activity (traditionally defined as a spectral power ranging from 0.5–4.5 Hz) that intensifies with prolonged wakefulness and diminishes across consecutive NREM sleep episodes (stage N3 sleep in humans and NREM sleep in animals, which is sometimes referred to as slow wave sleep [SWS]). SWA is widely used as a marker of mammalian sleep homeostasis. The buildup and decay rates of SWA can be altered in mammals by extreme sleep loss, as well as by pharmacologic or genetic manipulations, especially those affecting adenosine systems in the central nervous system (CNS). The adenosine system is involved in gating SWS-SWA expression by modulating the arousal level, which may alter sleep homeostasis and function.[1]

Adenosine is a purine nucleoside comprising an adenine attached to a β-D-ribofuranose moiety and is the key building block in adenosine triphosphate (ATP), adenosine diphosphate (ADP), and adenosine monophosphate (AMP). Adenosine derivatives have important roles in biochemical processes, such as energy transfer as ATP and ADP and intracellular signal transduction as cyclic AMP (cAMP). Adenosine regulates cellular activity by acting on four evolutionarily well-conserved metabotropic receptors, the purinergic G protein–coupled adenosine receptors referred to as A_1R, $A_{2A}R$, $A_{2B}R$, and A_3R. Although adenosine is released from nerve endings, it is not considered a neurotransmitter or a typical neuromodulator because its levels can be increased by various processes in all cell types and in all cell parts. Since the discovery of the somnogenic effect of adenosine in 1954,[2] it has been classified as a sleep substance.

PHYSIOLOGY OF ADENOSINE

Regulation of Adenosine Levels

Adenosine is formed by 5′-nucleotidase–mediated hydrolysis of AMP or from *S*-adenosylhomocysteine (SAH) by SAH hydrolase.[3,4] SAH also acts to trap adenosine in the presence of excess L-homocysteine. The constant presence of finite cellular concentrations of adenosine is ensured by the bidirectionality of the actions of SAH hydrolase in the cell. It remains unclear, however, whether SAH hydrolase is involved in generating adenosine in the brain.[5]

Extracellular adenosine can also be formed by converting ATP to adenosine via ADP and AMP (Figure 45.1). ATP is released

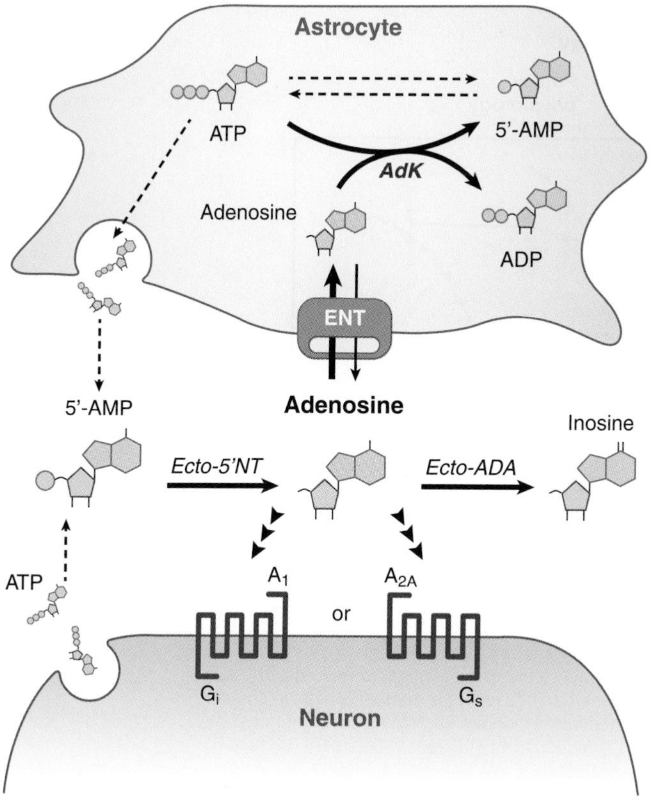

Figure 45.1 Control of the adenosine concentration by the metabolic state of astrocytes. Adenosine taken up by astrocytes is rapidly phosphorylated to 5'-AMP by adenosine kinase (AdK), an enzyme expressed predominantly in glia in the adult CNS. AdK effectively controls the intracellular adenosine concentration by catalyzing the transfer of a phosphate group from ATP to adenosine to produce ADP and AMP. As a result, the rate of adenosine metabolism is reflected by the [ATP]/[ADP][AMP] ratio, linking the rate of adenosine metabolism to the metabolic state of the cell. Equilibrative nucleoside transporters (ENT) bidirectionally regulate the concentration of adenosine available to pre- and postsynaptic A_1R and $A_{2A}R$. ADA, Adenosine deaminase; 5'-NT, 5'-nucleotidase.

from various cell types through multiple mechanisms including co-release from storage vesicles together with other hormones as a neurotransmitter, a "kiss-and-run" mechanism,[6] lysosome exocytosis,[7] controlled release through pannexin hemichannels,[8,9] release from inflammatory cells or vascular endothelia through connexin hemichannels and channels such as $P2X_7$ receptors,[10-12] and uncontrolled leakage from necrotic cells.[13]

Extracellular ATP and ADP are broken down to AMP via several ecto-enzymes, such as CD39.[14] In the brain, AMP is broken down to adenosine exclusively by ecto-5'-nucleotidase, which is also known as CD73.[15-17] Under pathologic conditions, such as cortical seizures, adenosine-mediated synaptic depression is independent of CD73 activity and not a consequence of astrocytic (or neuronal) ATP release. Instead, it is due to the activation of postsynaptic neurons, which leads to the release of adenosine. This mechanism constitutes an autonomic feedback signal that suppresses excitatory transmission during prolonged activity.[16] Under physiologic conditions, such as those involved in the regulation of sleep and wakefulness, adenosine may also be generated in a similar CD73-independent manner.

High adenosine levels are reduced by the actions of adenosine deaminase (ADA) or by being taken up by cells and rapidly phosphorylated to AMP by adenosine kinase (AdK). AdK also effectively controls the intracellular adenosine concentration (Figure 45.1).[18-20] Importantly, AdK binds a molecule of ATP and adenosine and catalyzes the transfer of a phosphate group from ATP to adenosine to produce ADP and AMP. Thus the rate of adenosine metabolism is reflected by the [ATP]/[ADP][AMP] ratio, which links the rate of adenosine metabolism to the metabolic state of the cell. In the adult CNS, AdK expression occurs predominantly in the glia,[21] and thus the concentration of adenosine is controlled by the metabolic state of the glia.

Bidirectional equilibrative nucleoside transporters regulate the concentration of adenosine available to adenosine receptors at the cell surface.[20,22] Therefore adenosine levels are dependent on both the formation and removal of extracellular adenosine. Whereas extracellular adenosine levels are low under basal conditions (30–300 nM),[23] under more extreme conditions such as mild hypoxia or strenuous exercise, they may exceed 1 μM and can reach up to several tens of micromolar concentrations in severely traumatic situations, including local ischemia.[4]

Adenosine Receptors

Extracellular adenosine reacts with one of the four adenosine receptors: A_1R, $A_{2A}R$, $A_{2B}R$, and A_3R.[24] When these receptors are expressed at the same level (~200,000 receptors/cell), adenosine appears to be equally potent at adenosine A_1R, $A_{2A}R$, and A_3R, and the levels of adenosine occurring under basal physiologic conditions are sufficient to activate these receptors (Figure 45.2). Activation of $A_{2B}R$ requires higher concentrations of adenosine. The potency of an agonist such as adenosine on its receptor depends on the number of receptors available; that is in the presence of only a few receptors, higher adenosine concentrations are required to exert an effect. Both A_1R and $A_{2A}R$ are more highly expressed in the brain than $A_{2B}R$ and A_3R,[19] and may be primarily involved in sleep-wake regulation. The roles of A_1R and $A_{2A}R$ in sleep-wake regulation have been extensively investigated by pharmacologic and genetic tools (cf. the section Adenosine and Sleep), whereas the involvement of $A_{2B}R$ and A_3R has not been reported.

INTERVENTIONS TARGETING ADENOSINE RECEPTORS

Receptor Antagonists (Including Caffeine)

Selective pharmacologic tools are crucial for assessing the in vivo actions of adenosine receptors. Over the past 20 years, medicinal chemistry has generated agonists and antagonists with high affinity (K_d values in the low nanomolar range) and selectivity (>100- to 200-fold over other adenosine receptor subtypes) for the human variants of each of the four adenosine receptors. Most of the known adenosine receptor agonists are derivatives of purine nucleosides, either adenosine or xanthosine, while adenosine receptor antagonists have diverse structures.[25] Many $A_{2A}R$-selective antagonists have been developed from different structural classes, including 8-(3-chlorostyryl) caffeine, MSX-2 (and its water-soluble prodrug MSX-3), ZM 241385, SCH-58261, and KW-6002. In addition, radioactive, and fluorescent or radiolabeled ligands of adenosine receptors (e.g., the A_1R ligand ^{18}F-8-cyclopentyl-3-[3-fluoropropyl]-1-propylxanthine or the $A_{2A}R$ ligand ^{11}C-Preladenant) have also been introduced for drug screening and monitoring of in vivo receptor occupancy in humans.[26,27]

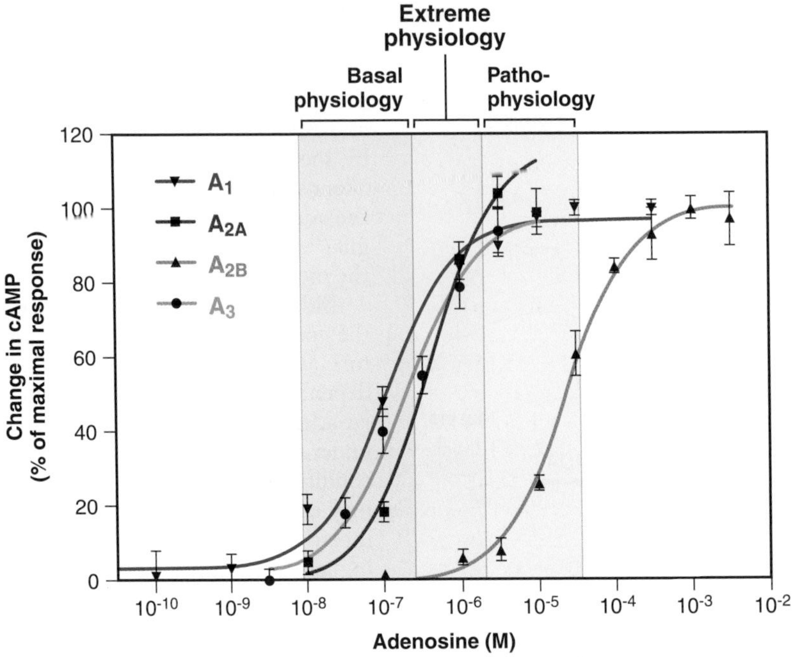

Figure 45.2 Schematic illustration of the ability of adenosine to activate the four adenosine receptors. The A_1Rs, A_{2A}Rs, and A_3Rs are activated by basal levels of adenosine at sites where the receptor number is high. In contrast, A_{2B}Rs are mostly activated under pathologic conditions. (Adapted from Fredholm BB. Adenosine, an endogenous distress signal, modulates tissue damage and repair. *Cell Death Differ.* 2007;14:1315–23.)

Caffeine is a classic nonselective adenosine receptor antagonist, although it is rather weakly potent at adenosine receptors (K_i = 10 μM). At doses commonly consumed by humans, caffeine produces its arousal effect by partial (25%–50%) and nonselective (similar affinity for both A_1R and A_{2A}R) blockade of adenosine receptors.[28] Caffeine is metabolized to paraxanthine and theophylline,[29] which are more potent inhibitors of A_1R and A_{2A}R than caffeine. Therefore eliminating caffeine does not predict the elimination of adenosine receptor blockade or the effects of subsequent caffeine administration.

Receptor Knockouts and Other Transgenic Techniques

Genetic knockout (KO) models for all four G protein–coupled adenosine receptors have been generated by targeted deletion of critical exons.[30-32] These adenosine receptor KO models have provided insight into the physiologic function of modulation of the sleep-wake cycle by overcoming the limitations of pharmacologic agents with partial specificity and by targeting the adenosine receptor in defined cellular populations. For example, A_{2A}R KO models can be used to overcome concerns about the partial specificity of A_{2A}R antagonists (particularly after focal injection at relatively high concentrations) and have convincingly demonstrated that the sleep-promoting effect of A_{2A}R agonists and the caffeine-induced arousal effect are mediated by A_{2A}R and not by A_1R.[33] Global A_1R and A_{2A}R KO approaches, however, are limited by confounding developmental effects and the lack of cell-type specificity.[30] To overcome these limitations, the Cre-*loxP* system has been used to produce conditional KO of adenosine receptor genes in defined brain regions (e.g., forebrain versus striatum) and cell-type (e.g., neurons versus astrocytes; for review see Wei and colleagues[31]). Brain region–specific deletion of A_{2A}R has been achieved in the forebrain and striatum.[34-36] Local deletion of A_1R in hippocampal CA1 or CA3 neurons and A_{2A}R in the nucleus accumbens (NAc) has also been achieved by local injection of adeno-associated viral (AAV) vectors containing the *cre* transgene into the brains of mice carrying *loxP*-flanked A_1R or A_{2A}R genes.[37,38] Conditional KO strategies that allow for a temporal and regional specificity have uncovered previously underappreciated functions of adenosine receptors in the basal ganglia for controlling the sleep-wake cycle (see detailed discussion in the section Effects of A_{2A}R Activation and Control of Arousal). In addition, the application of AAV carrying short-hairpin RNA targeted to produce site-specific silencing of the A_{2A}R gene in rats demonstrated that the arousal effect of caffeine is mediated by A_{2A}R in the shell of the NAc.[38] The recent development of optogenetics-based specific local modulation of neuronal activity using genetically engineered optical switches (e.g., channelrhodopsin)[39-41] or chemogenetics to study G-protein signaling in freely behaving animals by the directed molecular evolution of designer receptors exclusively activated by designer drugs (DREADDs)[42,43] has contributed to a more detailed understanding of the brain circuits underlying the sleep-wake cycle.[44] A probe for selective optogenetic control of A_{2A}R signaling (optoA_{2A}R) has also been developed.[45]

ADENOSINE AND SLEEP

Association Between Adenosine Levels and Sleep

ATP depletion is positively correlated with increases in extracellular adenosine levels,[46] and both are positively associated with sleep.[47,48] Adenosine levels may thus represent a state of relative energy deficiency. During spontaneous sleep-wake behavior in cats and rats, adenosine levels in several brain regions are higher during SWS than during wakefulness.[47,49] Moreover, in vivo microdialysis studies in cats revealed that adenosine concentrations increase twofold in the basal forebrain (BF) during a prolonged 6-hour period of wakefulness compared with adenosine concentrations at the beginning of sleep deprivation.

These studies, however, have some limitations. Adenosine levels rapidly change in tissues during sampling and therefore, to preserve the in vivo adenosine levels, tissue samples must be frozen within 1 second. Such rapid inactivation is difficult to achieve, however, even with focused microwave techniques; hence, measurement of regional adenosine brain levels by sampling tissue is highly problematic. Microdialysis studies have the limitation of recovery time necessary to overcome the tissue damage that occurs when inserting the microdialysis probe.[23,50,51] Furthermore, if the probe is allowed to remain in the tissue too long, it becomes covered with glial cells, which hampers the exchange of purines.[51] Thus the reported adenosine levels that occur in sleep and wakefulness should be cautiously interpreted. A series of genetically encoded G protein–coupled receptor activation–based (GRAB) sensors led to a breakthrough for the in vivo quantification of dynamic changes in neurotransmitters and neuromodulators.[52,53] Studies in which extracellular ATP or adenosine are measured using GRAB sensors based on purinergic receptors are currently being developed to study possible associations between ATP/adenosine levels and sleep-wake patterns.[53a]

Under more chronic sleep deprivation protocols, the increases in adenosine concentrations during prolonged waking are no longer observed,[54] suggesting that an altered adenosine response may mark a shift from a homeostatic response to an allostatic response due to the chronic sleep restriction.

Although it has been more than 60 years since the discovery that adenosine is involved in sleep, the mammalian brain cell types mediating the sleep-promoting effects of adenosine remain unclear. Extracellular adenosine concentrations are decreased in genetically engineered mice in which ATP release is nonspecifically blocked in astrocytes by selective expression of a dominant negative SNARE domain.[55] Although these mice exhibit the same amounts of wakefulness, SWS, and REM sleep as wild-type mice, they have reduced SWA and recovery sleep after sleep deprivation.[56] Reducing AdK in astrocytes, which increases the adenosine tone, is sufficient to increase SWS-SWA and sleep consolidation, reduce the decrease in SWA across the light phase, and slow the decay of SWS-SWA within an average SWS episode, whereas selectively reducing AdK in neurons has no effect.[57] These observations suggest that adenosine mediates the sleep deprivation-induced homeostatic sleep response. Although the control of extracellular adenosine modulating sleep need involves glial metabolism mediated by AdK,[57] the source of the released adenosine is controversial. Some adenosine may originate from astrocytes and the majority may originate from neurons, but direct proof is lacking and thus the exact source of adenosine is unknown.

Radulovacki and colleagues extensively investigated the effects of adenosine on wakefulness and found that increasing the levels of adenosine in the CNS of rats by systemic administration of the ADA inhibitor deoxycoformycin leads to increases in REM sleep and SWS.[58] In addition, a functional genetic variant that reduces ADA enzymatic activity in humans increases the sleep EEG-defined sleep depth and subjective sleepiness and impairs neurobehavioral performance in rested and sleep-deprived states.[59-62] Oishi and colleagues[18] reported that focal administration of the ADA inhibitor coformycin into the rat tuberomammillary nucleus (TMN), where ADA is dominantly expressed, increases SWS, further supporting a role for adenosine and ADA in sleep-wake regulation.

Although adenosine is thought to promote sleep by acting through A_1R or $A_{2A}R$, the relative contributions of these receptor subtypes to sleep induction remain controversial.[63,64] Indirect evidence provided by comparing the effects of caffeine, the A_1R antagonist 8-cyclopentyltheophylline, and the nonselective $A_1R/A_{2A}R$ antagonist alloxazine on sleep in rats[65] may partially support the popular notion that A_1R are more important for sleep-wake regulation than $A_{2A}R$. However, this classic approach and related studies have serious limitations, particularly with respect to interpretation of the pharmacologic data. For example, it is difficult to compare different receptor antagonists because of differences in solubility, blood-brain barrier permeability, and neuropharmacodynamic characteristics. Most importantly, the pharmacologic agents typically have nonspecific or off-target effects, especially at higher concentrations. Moreover, the diffuse expression patterns of inhibitory A_1R in the brain may have obscured possible brain region-specific roles of adenosine in sleep-wake regulation.[66-69] Indeed, the advent of genetically engineered systems, including transgenic animals and recombinant viral vectors, as well as convergent findings in humans, have convincingly established a pivotal role of $A_{2A}R$ in regulating sleep and wakefulness.[70-72]

Effects of A_1 Receptors and Sleep Homeostasis

It is thought that adenosine acting at A_1R facilitates sleep because nonselective and selective A_1R agonists increase sleep and SWA,[73-75] whereas A_1R antagonists decrease sleep and SWA.[65,76-78] Furthermore, A_1R antagonism within the BF reduces the homeostatic sleep and SWA responses following acute sleep deprivation.[79]

Conditional KO of A_1R predominantly affecting forebrain glutamatergic neurons prevents the increase in SWA induced by sleep deprivation, indicating that A_1Rs are necessary for normal sleep homeostasis.[80] Conversely, in mixed background mice with constitutive A_1R KO, the normal sleep homeostatic response, on the basis of the slow wave energy in NREM sleep (i.e., total SWA during NREM sleep), is maintained.[81] Moreover, acute application of a selective A_1R antagonist blocks the sleep deprivation–induced rebound in SWS-SWA in wild-type animals, whereas the same intervention is ineffective in constitutive A_1R KO mice under the same conditions.[81] These findings suggest that compensatory mechanisms are present in mice with constitutive KO that are not present in mice with conditional KO. Sleep facilitation via A_1R occurs by inhibiting wake-active neurons in several brain areas including the brainstem and forebrain regions of the cholinergic arousal system (mesopontine tegmentum[48] and BF,[82,83] respectively) and the lateral hypothalamus containing hypocretin/orexin neurons (Figure 45.3, *A* and *B*).[84] Administration of a selective A_1R agonist into the TMN decreases histamine in the frontal cortex and increases sleep and SWA,[18] suggesting that adenosine also inhibits the activity of this wake-promoting neurotransmitter system. An additional mechanism by which adenosine facilitates sleep through A_1R is the disinhibition of sleep-active neurons in the ventrolateral preoptic (VLPO) area and anterior hypothalamic area (Figure 45.3, *B*).[85,86]

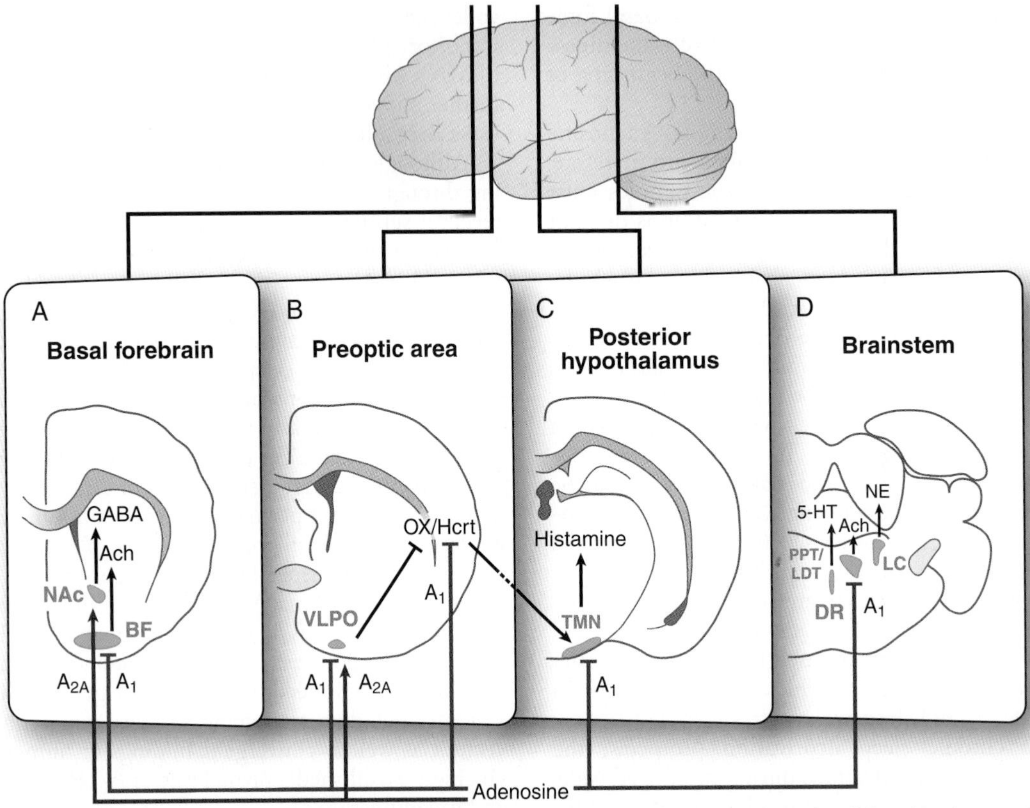

Figure 45.3 Circuit basis of sleep-wake regulation. **A,** Acting through the A_1R, adenosine inhibits the release of acetylcholine from the basal forebrain (BF) cholinergic neurons, thereby promoting slow-wave sleep. **B–D**, A flip–flop switching mechanism involving mutually inhibitory interactions between sleep-promoting neurons in the ventrolateral preoptic area (VLPO) and wake-promoting neurons in the hypothalamus (i.e., histaminergic tuberomammillary nucleus [TMN]) and brainstem (i.e., noradrenergic locus coeruleus [LC], serotonergic dorsal raphe nucleus [DR], and cholinergic laterodorsal tegmental nucleus [LDT]). The flip-flop switch between the VLPO and hypothalamus and brainstem is stabilized by orexin/hypocretin (OX/Hcrt) inputs from the lateral hypothalamus (LHA). Adenosine acts as an endogenous somnogen and promotes sleep via inhibitory A_1 receptors (A_1) in the basal forebrain, VLPO, LHA, and TMN, as well as excitatory A_{2A} receptors (A_{2A}) in the nucleus accumbens (NAc) and VLPO. Ach, Acetylcholine; GABA, gamma-aminobutyric acid; 5-HT, 5-hydroxytryptamin (serotonin); NE, norepinephrine.

Finally, A_1Rs mediate homeostatic sleep pressure based on astrocytic gliotransmission[56] and as part of a glial-neuronal circuit.[57] Sleep deprivation increases the expression of A_1R in both humans and rodents,[87,88] with expression levels normalizing after recovery sleep in humans.[89]

As mentioned previously in this chapter, the change in EEG power within the SWA frequency range after extended wakefulness is the primary indicator of homeostatically regulated sleep need. SWA reflects both the number of cells firing at SWA frequencies, which is an intrinsic feature of thalamocortical neurons,[90,91] and the synchronicity of firing across neurons, which is a circuit effect involving cortical neurons, thalamocortical neurons, and reticular nucleus of the thalamus neurons.[92] Activating A_1R influences SWA by both direct and indirect mechanisms. The direct mechanism is based on presynaptic inhibition of cortical and thalamic neurons, which results in relative functional deafferentation along with an A_1R-induced increase in whole cell, G protein–coupled inwardly rectifying potassium channel conductance and decreased hyperpolarization-activated currents, such that adenosine enhances slow oscillations in thalamocortical neurons.[93] The indirect mechanism is a reduction in cholinergic tone by A_1R-mediated inhibition of cholinergic arousal neurons.[47,48] Acetylcholine inhibits slow oscillations in thalamocortical neurons.[94-96] Thus the reduction of cholinergic tone is permissive for expressing SWA.

Effects of A_{2A}R Activation and Control of Arousal

Infusion of the selective A_{2A}R agonist CGS 21680 into the subarachnoid space below the ventral surface of the rostral BF in rats or into the lateral ventricle of mice robustly increases SWS and REM sleep.[97,98] In in vivo microdialysis experiments, infusing CGS 21680 into the BF dose-dependently decreases histamine release in the frontal cortex and medial preoptic area and increases the release of gamma-aminobutyric acid (GABA) in the TMN but not in the frontal cortex.[99] Infusion of the GABA antagonist picrotoxin into the TMN attenuates the CGS 21680-induced inhibition of histamine release, suggesting that the A_{2A}R agonist induces sleep by inhibiting the histaminergic system through increasing the release of GABA in the TMN. Intracellular recordings of VLPO neurons in rat brain slices demonstrated that two distinct types of VLPO neurons exist in terms of their responses to monoamines, acetylcholine, and adenosine receptor agonists.[100] The VLPO neurons are inhibited by noradrenaline, acetylcholine, and an A_1R agonist, whereas serotonin inhibits type 1 neurons, but excites type 2 neurons. An $A_{2A}R$ agonist postsynaptically excites type 2, but not type 1, neurons. These findings suggest that type 2 neurons are involved in initiating sleep, whereas type 1 neurons may contribute to sleep consolidation because they are activated only in the absence of inhibitory effects from wake-inducing systems.

Administration of CGS 21680 into the rostral BF, however, produces c-Fos expression not only in the VLPO, but also within the NAc shell and the medial portion of the olfactory tubercle.[101,102] Direct infusion of the $A_{2A}R$ agonist into the NAc induces SWS that corresponds to approximately 75% of the sleep amount measured when the $A_{2A}R$ agonist is infused into the subarachnoid space.[101] This observation may indicate that activation of $A_{2A}R$ within or close to the NAc induces sleep (Figure 45.3, *A*). Caffeine enhances wakefulness by acting as an antagonist for both A_1R and $A_{2A}R$ subtypes. At doses commonly consumed by humans, caffeine partially (25%–50%) and nonselectively (similar affinity for both A_1R and $A_{2A}R$) blocks adenosine receptors.[28] Experiments using mice with global genetic A_1R and $A_{2A}R$ KO revealed that $A_{2A}Rs$, but not A_1Rs, mediate the wakefulness-inducing effect of caffeine,[33] while single-nucleotide polymorphisms of the $A_{2A}R$ gene confer sensitivity to caffeine and sleep deprivation.[103] The specific role of $A_{2A}R$ in the striatum was investigated in conditional $A_{2A}R$ KO mice based on the Cre/*lox* technology and local infection with AAV carrying short-hairpin RNA of the $A_{2A}R$ to silence $A_{2A}R$ expression. Selective deletion of $A_{2A}R$ in the NAc shell blocks caffeine-induced wakefulness.[38]

For caffeine to be effective as an $A_{2A}R$ antagonist, adenosine must tonically activate excitatory $A_{2A}R$ within the NAc shell. This activation likely occurs in the NAc shell because $A_{2A}R$ are abundantly expressed throughout the striatum, including the NAc shell and sufficient levels of adenosine are available under basal conditions.[104,105] A recent study showed that chemogenetic or optogenetic activation of NAc $A_{2A}R$ core neurons projecting to the ventral pallidum in the BF strongly induces SWS, whereas chemogenetic inhibition of these neurons prevents sleep induction but does not affect homeostatic sleep rebound.[106,107] Interestingly, motivational stimuli suppress sleep and inhibit the activity of ventral pallidum-projecting NAc $A_{2A}R$-expressing neurons. The sleep-gating ability of the NAc indirect pathway may explain the tendency to fall asleep in boring situations. Another recent study revealed that adenosine is a plausible candidate molecule for activating NAc core $A_{2A}R$-expressing neurons to induce SWS because elevated adenosine levels in the NAc core promote SWS via $A_{2A}R$.[108] The medium spiny GABAergic neurons in the NAc can be divided into two groups that respond differentially to stimulation by dopamine or adenosine. Direct pathway neurons express excitatory dopamine D_1 receptors and inhibitory adenosine A_1R, whereas neurons of the indirect pathway express inhibitory dopamine D_2 receptors and excitatory $A_{2A}R$. Dopamine produced by neurons in the ventral tegmental area has a key role in processing rewarding, aversive, or cognitive signals,[109-111] and projections from ventral tegmental area dopaminergic neurons to the NAc, commonly known as the mesolimbic pathway, constitute a well-characterized reward circuit in the brain.[112,113]

Dysfunction of the striatum leads to devastating motor disorders, including Parkinson disease, highlighting the central function of the striatum in the control of movement.[114] Up to 90% of patients with Parkinson disease exhibit severe sleep disturbances, which is one of the most frequent nonmotor symptoms.[115] Dysfunction of the striatum may also contribute to sleep disturbances in patients with Parkinson disease. Ablation of the striatum in cats and rats decreases sleep,[116,117] and chemogenetic activation of $A_{2A}R$-expressing neurons in the striatum induces sleep in a topographically organized manner.[118] Thus activation of $A_{2A}R$-expressing neurons in the rostral, centromedial, and centrolateral striatum increases sleep, whereas activation of $A_{2A}R$-expressing neurons in the caudal striatum does not promote sleep.

Although $A_{2A}R$ appear to primarily regulate SWS, a few studies suggest that $A_{2A}R$ are also involved in the control of REM sleep. REM sleep is increased when CGS 21680 is infused into the medial pontine reticular formation area.[119] A recent study found that blocking $A_{2A}R$- or $A_{2A}R$-expressing neurons in the olfactory bulb of rodents increases REM sleep, suggesting that the olfactory bulb is a key site for adenosine/$A_{2A}R$-mediated regulation of REM sleep.[120] Because olfactory dysfunction can be ameliorated by an $A_{2A}R$ antagonist, e.g., caffeine or ZM 241385,[121] it is possible that REM sleep is linked to the perception of odors in the olfactory bulb. Interestingly, the ability to smell is reduced in patients with REM sleep behavior disorders.[122]

A Model of Adenosinergic Sleep-Wake Regulation: Gating of Sleep Homeostasis by Arousal

Increasing knowledge of the molecular and circuit bases of sleep-wake regulation has elucidated new roles of adenosine receptors in modulating different aspects of sleep.[1] For example, $A_{2A}Rs$ appear to promote sleep by suppressing arousal whereas A_1Rs mediate sleep need and the response to sleep deprivation. These receptors may thus play complementary, crucial roles in sleep function. In light of the dissociable effects of adenosine for gating sleep and mediating sleep need at the receptor level, it is plausible that the sleep state is regulated by arousal when an organism must consolidate wakefulness in response to environmental changes. A typical example is motivated behavior that efficiently reduces sleep of all stages and promotes arousal by activating mesolimbic dopaminergic systems, whereas the wake state is attenuated in the absence of motivating stimuli by activating $A_{2A}R$ in the NAc.[106,123] The circadian and hypothalamic feeding systems have indirect influences by driving internally generated arousal, e.g., increasing motivation to forage according to the circadian phase. Thus in the absence of motivating/external arousing stimuli, the loss of the arousing influence of the circadian system (the sleep phase) may be sufficient to allow the transition from wakefulness to sleep. On the other hand, sleep is necessary for SWS-SWA to facilitate the expression of sleep need and for the resolution of sleep debt, a process in which A_1Rs play a crucial role.[57]

Although these conclusions are based on findings from rodent studies, the pharmacogenetic dissection of adenosinergic-dopaminergic pathways in humans suggests that $A_{2A}Rs$ also contribute to the regulation of neurophysiologic markers of sleep homeostasis.[124] Species-specific differences in the expression of the different adenosine receptor subclasses may contribute to the partly discrepant findings. Thus studies to elucidate the distinct roles of adenosine receptor subtypes for sleep initiation and the homeostatic regulation of sleep need in humans are warranted (see later). The recent advent of selective $A_{2A}R$ antagonists and radioligands to noninvasively quantify $A_{2A}R$ availability with positron emission tomography[27] may provide invaluable tools to tackle these questions.

EFFECTS OF ADENOSINE RECEPTOR TARGETING AGENTS IN HUMANS AND ANIMALS

Effects of Natural Compounds on Sleep and Wakefulness via Adenosine Receptors

Although no approved drugs targeting adenosine receptors are currently available, a variety of natural compounds promote sleep by activating adenosine receptors. In support of the role of $A_{2A}R$ in promoting sleep, Japanese sake yeast supplementation improves the quality of sleep in humans, whereas pretreatment with the $A_{2A}R$ antagonist ZM 241385 abolishes sake yeast-induced SWS in mice.[125] Because sake yeast, but not other *Saccharomyces cerevisiae* yeasts (e.g., baker's and brewer's yeast), contains a large amount of *S*-adenosyl-L-methionine and the *S*-adenosyl-L-methionine metabolite methylthioadenosine, the sleep-inducing effect of sake yeast is likely due to the activation of $A_{2A}R$ by *S*-adenosyl-L-methionine or methylthioadenosine.[126]

In contrast, paeoniflorin, a principal active component from the root of *Paeonia lactiflora,* shortens sleep latency and increases the amount of SWS exclusively by activating A_1R, a conclusion based on the finding that the effects of paeoniflorin can be blocked by treatment with a selective A_1R antagonist and are absent in A_1R KO mice.[127] In addition, paeoniflorin significantly increases the mechanical pain threshold, prolongs thermal pain latency, and increases SWS in mice with partial sciatic nerve ligation, a mouse neuropathic pain model characterized by persistent pain and insomnia.[128] Therefore the A_1R-mediated analgesic and hypnotic effects of paeoniflorin may be of potential use for the treatment of neuropathic pain and associated insomnia.

Moreover, N^6-(4-hydroxybenzyl) adenine riboside isolated from *Gastrodia elata* has hypnotic effects in mice[129] and may dose-dependently increase SWS via mechanisms that involve A_1R and $A_{2A}R$. Finally, cordycepin (3-deoxyadenosine), an adenosine analogue isolated from *Cordyceps* fungi, promotes SWS in rats, but it remains unclear whether the sleep-inducing effect is, in fact, mediated by adenosine receptor activation.[130]

Effects of Caffeine in Humans and Possible Roles of More Selective Adenosine Receptor Drugs

The findings described previously in this chapter linking adenosine to sleep were obtained from animal experiments, but evidence suggests that this link also holds true in humans. This is largely based on the well-known effects of caffeine on sleep. Caffeine is the most widely consumed psychoactive compound in the world and is found in coffee, tea, soft drinks, energy drinks, and chocolate, as well as in some pain relievers and cold remedies. Worldwide, the average caffeine consumption is estimated to be just under 80 mg/day, although the average intake of caffeine in countries such as Sweden and Finland is in the range of 400 mg/day,[28] most likely due to long, gloomy, and depressing winters.

Caffeine is widely consumed to promote wakefulness and counteract fatigue in doses at which adenosine receptor antagonism is the dominant effect. In some individuals, however, caffeine consumption at normal levels leads to anxiety and panic attacks[131,132]; this is more common at higher doses. One study found that people with polymorphisms at the $A_{2A}R$ gene are at risk of experiencing increased anxiety when consuming caffeine-containing products.[133] Distinct $A_{2A}R$ polymorphisms also consistently modulate the objective and subjective effects of caffeine on sleep quality, sleep architecture, and the sleep EEG.[103,134,135]

Whether caffeine affects circadian rhythm and thereby alters the timing of sleep is currently a matter of debate. Recent work suggests that caffeine alters the phase of the mammalian circadian clock. In one study, caffeine delayed the human circadian melatonin rhythm by blocking A_1R and chronic caffeine treatment lengthened the circadian period of molecular oscillations in human osteosarcoma U2OS cells expressing clock gene luciferase reporters.[136] Furthermore, application of pharmacologic tools and small-interfering RNA knockdown revealed that the effect of caffeine on molecular oscillations is attenuated by perturbation of A_1R signaling, but not ryanodine receptor or phosphodiesterase activity. These findings point to a possible molecular mechanism for the clinical observation in humans that 200 mg caffeine intake 3 hours before bedtime may induce a roughly 40-minute phase delay in the circadian melatonin rhythm, as suggested by a double-blind, placebo-controlled, approximately 49-day long, within-subject study. Nevertheless, no change in the circadian time courses of melatonin or cortisol was found after chronic intake of 3 × 150 mg caffeine per day for 9 days, an intake pattern that is common in many European countries.[137] These divergent findings may indicate that acute and chronic caffeine intake differentially affect circadian rhythms. Contrasting effects after acute and chronic (2 weeks) caffeine consumption were also observed on running wheel activity, vigilance states, and sleep EEG in mice.[138] The available evidence in mice suggests that rather than disturbing sleep, chronic caffeine consumption increases the light sensitivity of the mouse circadian clock[139] and enhances the light-dark amplitude of vigilance states, as well as sleep pressure, possibly by adaptive changes in adenosine receptor expression and extracellular adenosine levels.[138]

Consistent with the notion that the arousal effect of caffeine in mice is exclusively mediated by $A_{2A}R$, emerging evidence supports the modulation of the sleep-wake cycle by $A_{2A}R$ antagonists. For example, the newly developed dual adenosine $A_{2A}R/A_1R$ antagonist JNJ-40255293 dose-dependently enhances wakefulness in rats.[140] Moreover, since the clinical approval in 2013 of the $A_{2A}R$ antagonist istradefylline (also known as KW-6002) for motor improvement in patients with Parkinson disease in Japan, a report of four patients indicated that evening treatment with this antagonist reduces sleep duration in the evening and increases daytime sleepiness.[141] Thus selective $A_{2A}R$ antagonists may have considerable potential as eugeroics (wakefulness-enhancing drugs) while avoiding some of the $A_{2A}R$-independent side effects of caffeine (such as anxiety) or negative effects of other psychostimulants, including dependence.

Adenosine receptor stimulation should also be considered as a potential treatment approach for insomnia. Insomnia is a sleep disorder that affects millions of people around the world and frequently co-occurs with a wide range of psychiatric disorders.[142-144] Although $A_{2A}R$ agonists strongly induce sleep, classical $A_{2A}R$ agonists have adverse cardiovascular effects and cannot be used clinically to treat sleep disorders. Moreover, the development of adenosine analogues to treat

CNS disorders, including insomnia, is hampered by the poor transport of these drugs across the blood-brain barrier. In mice, a small blood-brain barrier permeable monocarboxylate was recently found to induce sleep by enhancing $A_{2A}R$ signaling in the brain but, surprisingly, did not exhibit the typical unwanted cardiovascular effects of $A_{2A}R$ agonists.[145] Therefore molecules that allosterically enhance $A_{2A}R$ signaling may be developed to help people with insomnia to more easily fall asleep. Such compounds may also show potential for the treatment of neuropsychiatric symptoms. Similarly, molecules that enhance A_1R signaling may enhance sleep efficiency.

CLINICAL PEARL

The mesolimbic dopamine system consisting of the ventral tegmental area and the NAc plays a central role in motivation. Recent findings demonstrate that the ventral tegmental area and NAc also contribute to sleep-wake regulation, which may explain why people feel sleepy when bored. Psychiatric disorders such as schizophrenia, attention-deficit/hyperactivity disorder (ADHD), and addiction, all of which are commonly accompanied by sleep/wake disturbances, are strongly linked to pathologic deviations in the mesolimbic system. For example, excessive daytime sleepiness is observed in children with ADHD, the most frequently diagnosed mental disorder in children, with a prevalence of 4% to 5%. Children with ADHD who are prevented from being active, a self-stimulatory behavior that may be exhibited to avoid feeling bored and to stay awake, often respond by daydreaming and napping.[146] Adenosine receptor antagonists may be beneficial to improve certain impairments in children with ADHD.[147-149]

SUMMARY

Adenosine is a well-known endogenous sleep substance that affects normal sleep-wake patterns through several mechanisms and in various brain locations via A_1R or $A_{2A}R$. Many cells and processes contribute to modulating the extracellular concentration of adenosine at neuronal A_1R or $A_{2A}R$. Current evidence accumulated mainly from rodent studies suggests that A_1R and $A_{2A}R$ are differentially involved in regulating sleep. Activation of $A_{2A}R$ in the brain promotes sleep, that is these receptors provide sleep gating by activating NAc neurons, whereas activation of A_1R modulates the homeostatic aspects of sleep-wake regulation; that is these receptors are essential for the expression and resolution of sleep need. Activation of A_1R also facilitates sleep by inhibiting wake-active neurons in several brain areas, including cholinergic brainstem and basal forebrain neurons, the lateral hypothalamus containing hypocretin/orexin neurons, and the TMN containing histamine neurons, and disinhibition of sleep-active neurons in the VLPO and anterior hypothalamic areas. The development of selective modulators of A_1R and $A_{2A}R$ for use in clinical studies and radioligands for molecular brain imaging may help elucidate the distinct roles of these receptor subclasses in sleep-wake regulation in humans.

SELECTED READINGS

Bjorness TE, Dale N, Mettlach G, et al. An adenosine-mediated glial-neuronal circuit for homeostatic sleep. *J Neurosci.* 2016;36:3709–3721.

Clark I, Landolt HP. Coffee, caffeine, and sleep: a systematic review of epidemiological studies and randomized controlled trials. *Sleep Med Rev.* 2017;31:70–78.

Dijk DJ, Landolt HP. Sleep physiology, circadian rhythms, waking performance and the development of sleep-wake therapeutics. *Handb Exp Pharmacol.* 2019;253:441–481.

Garcia-Gil M, Camici M, Allegrini S, Pesi R, Tozzi MG. Metabolic aspects of adenosine functions in the brain. *Front Pharmacol.* 2021;12:672182. Published 2021 May 14.

Halassa MM, Florian C, Fellin T, et al. Astrocytic modulation of sleep homeostasis and cognitive consequences of sleep loss. *Neuron.* 2009;61:213–219.

Korkutata M, Saitoh T, Cherasse Y, et al. Enhancing endogenous adenosine A_{2A} receptor signaling induces slow-wave sleep without affecting body temperature and cardiovascular function. *Neuropharmacology.* 2019;144:122–132.

Lazarus M, Shen H-Y, Cherasse Y, et al. Arousal effect of caffeine depends on adenosine A_{2A} receptors in the shell of the nNucleus accumbens. *J Neurosci.* 2011;31:10067–10075.

Lazarus M, Huang Z-L, Lu J, Urade Y, Chen J-F. How do the basal ganglia regulate sleep–wake behavior? *Trends Neurosci.* 2012;35:723–732.

Lazarus M, Chen JF, Huang ZL, Urade Y, Fredholm BB. Adenosine and sleep. *Handb Exp Pharmacol.* 2019;253:359–381.

Lazarus M, Oishi Y, Bjorness TE, Greene RW. Gating and the need for sleep:dissociable effects of adenosine A1 and A2A receptors. *Front Neurosci.* 2019;13:740.

Oishi Y, Xu Q, Wang L, et al. Slow-wave sleep is controlled by a subset of nucleus accumbens core neurons in mice. *Nat Commun.* 2017;8:734.

Oishi Y, Lazarus M. The control of sleep and wakefulness by mesolimbic dopamine systems. *Neuroscience Res.* 2017;118:66–73.

Peng W, Wu Z, Song K, Zhang S, Li Y, Xu M. Regulation of sleep homeostasis mediator adenosine by basal forebrain glutamatergic neurons. *Science.* 2020;369(6508):eabb0556.

Rétey JV, Adam M, Khatami R, et al. A genetic variation in the adenosine A2A receptor gene (ADORA2A) contributes to individual sensitivity to caffeine effects on sleep. *Clin Pharmacol Ther.* 2007;81:692–698.

A complete reference list can be found online at ExpertConsult.com.

Chapter 46

Catecholamines

Jimmy J. Fraigne; Rebecca C. Hendrickson; Murray Raskind; John H. Peever

Chapter Highlights

- Activity of noradrenergic neurons varies across the sleep-wake cycle. For example, the discharge activity of noradrenergic neurons in the locus coeruleus is highest in waking, reduced in non–rapid eye movement sleep, and minimal or absent during rapid eye movement sleep. This observation suggests that the noradrenergic system contributes to the control of sleep and waking states and that disturbances in this system's activity could impair normal sleep-wake function.
- Common wake-promoting drugs such as modafinil recruit the dopamine system to induce wakefulness, and lesions of some dopamine nuclei (e.g., ventral periaqueductal gray) suppress wakefulness by promoting sleep. These observations suggest that the dopamine system contributes to sleep-wake control and that impairments of dopamine system function could underlie abnormal sleep-wake regulation.
- Disturbances in the activity of both noradrenergic and dopaminergic systems are associated with sleep disorders such as narcolepsy and restless legs syndrome and contribute to sleep abnormalities in posttraumatic stress disorder and Parkinson disease. Pharmacologic compounds that target noradrenergic and dopaminergic system activity are useful in the treatment of sleep disturbances in these disorders.

Catecholamines are monoamine neurotransmitters that are highly conserved throughout the animal kingdom. The main catecholamines in the central nervous system (CNS) are noradrenaline (NA) and dopamine, which have been implicated in arousal and waking behavior since the 1960s. Work in the past decade has provided new insights into their roles in arousal, as well as in mechanisms underlying several sleep disorders. In this chapter, we describe the distribution of catecholamine-releasing neurons, their connection with other brain nuclei, and their activity through the sleep-wake cycle and show the role that they play in sleep-wake regulation and function. Finally, we highlight how disruption of catecholamine system activity contributes to disorders such as posttraumatic stress disorder (PTSD), Parkinson disease (PD), narcolepsy, and periodic leg movements (PLMs).

THE ROLE OF NORADRENALINE IN SLEEP-WAKE REGULATION

Understanding the noradrenergic mechanisms responsible for the generation and maintenance of sleep has been complicated by the complexity of the systems involved, the redundancy of the involved mechanisms,[1,2] and the diversity of sleep structures between species commonly studied in research.[1,3] Despite these challenges, a number of core mechanisms that orchestrate and maintain sleep have been identified, and NA release from the locus coeruleus (LC) and smaller brainstem reticular formation noradrenergic neurons plays a major role in several of them[4] (Figure 46.1).

Locus Coeruleus Activity and Noradrenaline Release during Sleep Versus Wake

The role of NA in the sleep-wake cycle has long been both intriguing and at times confusing to researchers and, to this day, is often described in somewhat contradictory terms. This inconsistency is apparent beginning even with the very basic question of how LC activity and noradrenergic signaling change during different stages of sleep versus wake. Some publications state bluntly that the firing of LC neurons "slows during NREM sleep and ceases prior to and during REM sleep,"[1] while others emphasize the evidence for some level of preserved noradrenergic transmission[5]—a distinction that may be important for understanding the origin of inappropriately persistent or pathologically increased brain noradrenergic and peripheral sympathetic nervous system (SNS) activation during rapid eye movement (REM) sleep.[6]

The first electrophysiologic recordings of putative LC neurons during natural sleep were obtained in the 1970s, and the idea that the cessation of activity by noradrenergic neurons could be a part of the mechanism of REM sleep was introduced. Initially, these experiments were done in cats in which the noradrenergic neurons of the LC and the cholinergic neurons of the mesopontine tegmentum are intermingled, making precise identification of the individual neurons recorded difficult. These studies identified a subpopulation of peri-LC neurons whose firing rates decreased somewhat as the animal moved from wake to non–rapid eye movement (NREM) sleep and then decreased further as the animal transitioned from NREM to REM sleep.[7,8] This was, however, only a subpopulation of recorded neurons. For example, in the frequently cited

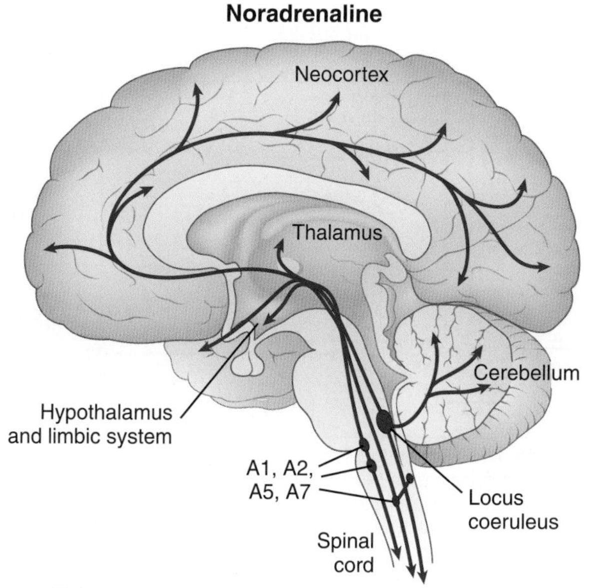

Figure 46.1 Schematic of human central nervous system (CNS) noradrenergic projections. The majority of CNS noradrenergic neurons originate from the locus coeruleus in the dorsal pons. Together with noradrenergic neurons originating from smaller brainstem nuclei termed A1, A2, A5, and A7, they project diffusely to all CNS areas, including neighborhood brainstem regions, hypothalamus and limbic brain, neocortex, cerebellum, and spinal cord. This CNS noradrenergic system modulates arousal, sleep-wake, and attention to novel stimuli.

publication by Hobson and colleagues, they identified only 13 of 21 LC and nearby cells whose firing rates decreased during sleep. Within this subset of cells, the average firing rates decreased from 4 Hz during wake to 3.5 Hz during NREM sleep, then decreased to 0.25 Hz during REM sleep.

The frequently cited view that LC neurons shut off entirely during REM sleep is based on results from work by Aston-Jones and Bloom in rats, an animal in which the LC is more precisely anatomically defined than in the cat and is without intermixed nonadrenergic cells. In their 1981 publication,[9] they recorded both single-unit and multiunit activity from LC neurons in 117 freely behaving rats and categorized the responses by sleep stage. During REM sleep LC neurons were "virtually silent," with the mean firing rates dropping from 2.15 Hz in stage 1 sleep, 1.4 Hz in stage 2 sleep, 0.68 Hz in stage 3 sleep, 0.22 in stage 4 sleep, and 0.2 Hz in REM sleep. It should be noted, however, that recordings of REM sleep were obtained from only nine neurons, which did not evenly span the LC. These same experiments also provided evidence of topographic differences in the firing rates of LC neurons. The firing observed was restricted to a subset of cells with edge-specific locations. In addition, the authors make no mention of the presence of phasic activity within REM periods other than noting that the action potentials that were recorded from LC neurons during REM sleep "usually were associated with phasic movements of burst of EMG activity." Thus these results do not represent total silence of LC neurons during REM and, perhaps more importantly, do not rule out the possibility that a subset of LC neurons may retain higher levels of activity during this time—a possibility that may be particularly relevant during periods of phasic REM activity.

Several research groups have sought to clarify this situation further by using microdialysis to measure NA concentrations in the amygdala[10,11] and LC[11] in both cats[11] and rats.[10] Their results have been consistent with clear decreases in NA levels between wake and NREM sleep and between NREM and REM sleep, but with the lowest levels recorded still representing approximately 15% of the waking concentrations in the cat and approximately 60% in the rat, a finding since cited as evidence for some persistent noradrenergic activity even during REM sleep.[5] One challenge with interpreting these experiments, however, is that in both studies, the dialysate was collected in 5-minute segments, but sleep-state periods in the animals were not generally stable for this length of time. The criterion for the NA concentration in a particular dialysate sample corresponding to a "REM sleep" period was that at least 80% of the 5-minute period be counted as REM sleep in the cat studies and 50% in the rat studies. Thus the recorded levels are likely to be overestimates of the true NA concentrations during REM sleep.

There are other possible explanations for persistent NA in cerebrospinal fluid (CSF) dialysate during REM sleep. Even if LC neurons are nearly silenced during REM sleep, other noradrenergic nuclei may show a different pattern of activity. Alternatively, NA can also be released by nonexocytotic mechanisms.[12]

Functional Role of Noradrenaline in the Regulation of Sleep-Wake and Sleep Architecture

Substantially decreased CNS NA during NREM and REM sleep indicated early on that the noradrenergic system supports wakefulness. Additional wake- and alertness-promoting systems include the dopaminergic system (discussed later), the cholinergic systems (both in the basal forebrain (BF) and the mesopontine tegmentum [LDT/PPT]), the serotonergic dorsal raphe nuclei (DRN), histamine release from the tuberomammillary nucleus (TMN), and orexin released by lateral hypothalamic neurons. These systems—constituting the reticular activating system (RAS)—are highly interconnected and frequently reinforce each other's activation.

The role of NA in this interaction of systems is threefold. First, NA supports alertness by both direct cortical projections (primarily via alpha$_1$-adrenergic receptors [α1ARs] but also through postsynaptic alpha$_2$ and beta receptors; Figure 46.2) and through activation of other wake- and alertness-promoting regions, including thalamic relay neurons, serotonergic DRN neurons, cortically projecting cholinergic BF neurons, the histaminergic TMN, and a wake-active subset of PPT cells.[1,13,14] Although these activating functions are generally effected primarily by alpha$_1$ receptors, the activation of the TMN is actually through postsynaptic α2AR-mediated inhibition of GABAergic interneurons that inhibit histamine release.[1] In addition, NA promotes wakefulness by inhibiting regions involved in the generation of sleep, including the sleep-active hypothalamic regions of the ventrolateral preoptic nucleus (VLPO)[1,15] and median preoptic nuclei, and the REM-active brainstem cholinergic neurons of the LDT/PPT through postsynaptic alpha$_2$ receptors[13,16,17] (Figure 46.3). Last, NA has been found to interrupt the generation of NREM-type slow oscillations in both hippocampus and cortex via inhibition of slow calcium-dependent afterhyperpolarizations, although there is evidence for this being mediated by either beta receptors[1,18] or alpha$_1$ receptors[19] in different locations.

NA also participates in the regulation and generation of specific features of NREM and REM sleep architecture. REM sleep is characterized by diffuse cortical activation driven by

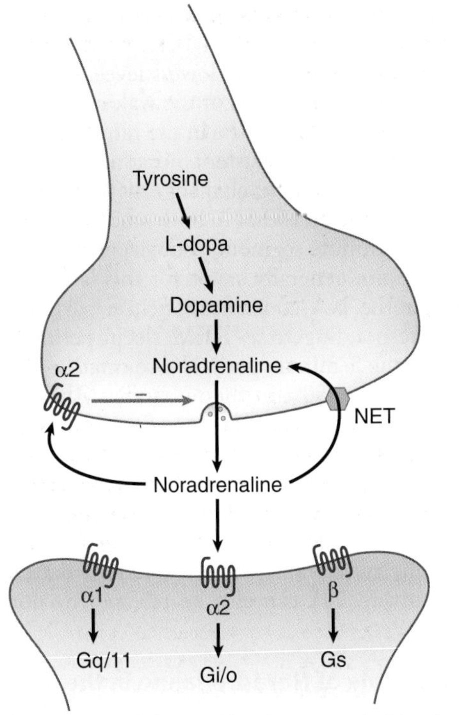

Figure 46.2 Schematic of CNS noradrenergic synapse. Noradrenaline released into the synaptic space stimulates postsynaptic G protein-coupled α_1- and β-adrenergic receptors to propagate downstream signaling (i.e., through Gq/11, Gi, and Gs pathways). Presynaptic α_2 inhibitory autoreceptors reduce noradrenaline release when stimulated. There also are some postsynaptic α_2 receptors involved in downstream signaling. The presynaptic norepinephrine transporter (NET) helps clear noradrenaline from the synapse by reuptake into the presynaptic neuron.

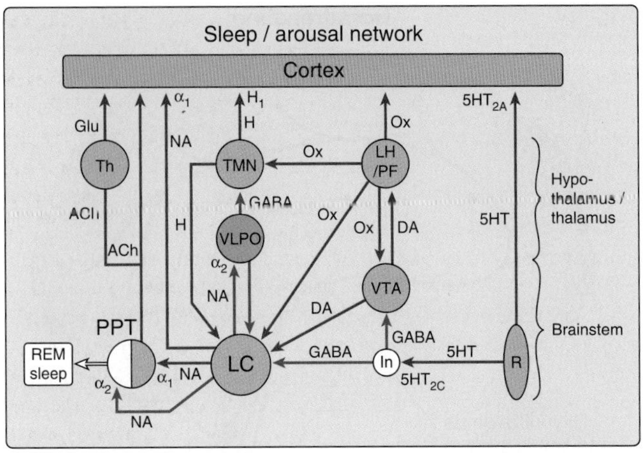

Figure 46.3 Role of the locus coeruleus in the sleep and arousal network. Multiple wakefulness-promoting nuclei (*brown*) exert an activating effect on the cerebral cortex, modulated by sleep-promoting nuclei (*red*) and GABAergic interneurons (*white*). The locus coeruleus (LC) contributes to wakefulness via multiple mechanisms: by releasing noradrenaline broadly in the cortex, by stimulating the wakefulness-promoting neurons of the pedunculopontine tegmental nucleus (PPT), and by inhibiting sleep-promoting neurons within the ventrolateral preoptic nucleus (VLPO) and PPT. Other major wakefulness-promoting nuclei include the ventral tegmental area (VTA), which acts largely via activation of the LC, and the lateral hypothalamic/perifornical area (LH/PF), which acts primarily via activation of the tuberomammillary nucleus (TMN) and the LC. The LC is inhibited by GABAergic interneurons in the VTA and the region surrounding the LC, which are driven by excitatory 5-HT_{2C} receptors. This wakefulness-inhibiting effect of serotonin from the raphe nuclei (R) modulates the primarily wakefulness-promoting effects of serotonin directly on cortex. In the diagram, excitatory connections are indicated by *red arrows*, inhibitory connections by *blue arrows*. Neurotransmitters and receptors: 5-HT: serotonin (excitatory receptors 5-HT_{2A} and 5-HT_{2C}); Ach: acetylcholine; DA: dopamine; Glu: glutamate; H: histamine (excitatory receptor H1); NA: noradrenaline (excitatory α_1-adrenoceptor and inhibitory α_2-adrenoceptor); Ox: orexin. (From Samuels ER, Szabadi E. Functional neuroanatomy of the noradrenergic locus coeruleus: Its roles in the regulation of arousal and autonomic function. Part II: Physiological and pharmacological manipulations and pathological alterations of locus coeruleus activity in humans. *Curr Neuropharmacol.* 2008;6:254–85 with permission from Bentham Science Publishers.)

cholinergic signaling from brainstem LDT/PPT to the BF and then to the cortex, and by reduced serotonergic and noradrenergic inputs.[1,20,21] Synchronized electrical field potentials that move from the pons through the lateral geniculate nucleus and to the occipital cortex (ponto-geniculo-occiptal [PGO] waves) begin to emerge as single waves during the transition into REM sleep and then occur intermittently in lower amplitude bursts throughout REM sleep. PGO waves are closely correlated with the rapid eye movements of REM sleep and are thought to be related to the strong visual component of REM sleep dream content. The circuitry responsible for the generation and regulation of PGO waves involves a small area near the LDT/PPT that is termed the subcoeruleus in cats and the sublaterodorsal tegmental nucleus (SLD) in rats. The lateral area of this region contains neurons with burst firing patterns correlated with PGO waves.[1,6] These bursts appear driven by cholinergic input[22] from the LDT/PPT,[23] a process that has been demonstrated to be inhibited by serotonergic activity[23] and may be similarly inhibited by LC activity.

The SLD is important in the generation of REM atonia (loss of skeletal muscle tone).[1,6] Caudally projecting, predominantly glutamatergic SLD neurons promote REM atonia through the excitation of GABAergic and glycinergic neurons in the medullary ventral gigantocellular nucleus and locally in the spinal cord. These REM-active SLD neurons receive direct noradrenergic inhibition via $alpha_2$ receptors.[24] Evidence supports a parallel importance of decreased serotonergic and noradrenergic excitatory[25] input directly onto primary motor neurons in the generation of REM atonia. This model is supported by both the increase in REM sleep behavior disorder (RBD) observed in individuals taking serotonergic medications, and by the abrupt shut-off of LC neurons time-locked to REM-like cataplectic attacks in narcoleptic dogs.[1,26]

Thus there are two ways that decreased noradrenergic tone during REM sleep leads to atonia: (1) an $alpha_2$ receptor–mediated disinhibition of pontine REM-active regions that facilitate GABAergic inhibition of primary motor neurons and (2) an $alpha_1$ receptor–mediated mechanism through disfacilitation of motor neurons because of the decreased noradrenergic tone of REM sleep.

Role of Noradrenaline in the Regulation of Autonomic Nervous System Functioning during Sleep

Parasympathetic tone increases upon sleep entry and further increases as NREM sleep deepens.[27,28] This pattern is reflected in progressively decreased mean blood pressure, heart rate, and muscle sympathetic nerve activity (MSNA) throughout these stages.[27] These shifts likely result from both an increase in parasympathetic and a simultaneous drop in sympathetic activity.[28] In REM sleep, this pattern reverses with mean MSNA increasing substantially above its waking baseline, and blood pressure (BP) and heart rate returning to levels similar to waking.[27] In contrast to waking, however, brief surges in BP during REM are accompanied by abrupt cessation of sympathetic-nerve discharge,[27] while the cardiac pre-ejection period (PEP), a marker of sympathetic tone, increases.[29]

Changes in autonomic nervous system function retain a temporal complexity that is at least partially independent of sleep stage but linked to cortical electroencephalography (EEG). As noted previously, phasic activity during REM sleep is often accompanied by surges of significantly increased BP but abrupt drops in MSNA. Phasic activity during REM sleep generally involves bursts of rapid eye movements and brief periods of muscle activity restoration (often referred to as "REM twitches"). This implies that the peripheral autonomic changes are occurring in coordination with centrally generated events. Similarly, it has been observed that K complexes in stage 2 NREM sleep are consistently associated with momentary increases in MSNA and BP.[27,28] In addition, studies have found cyclic changes in heart rate variability, suggestive of increased sympathetic predominance during the periodic arousals associated with the centrally defined cyclic alternating pattern[28] that can be recognized in the EEG during NREM sleep.[30] These examples of the connections between central events and autonomic nervous system changes, especially SNS changes, strongly suggest that these events are the result of central regulation.

Impact of Altered Noradrenergic Transmission on Sleep Physiology

The previous description of the role of NA in sleep-wake regulation supports a number of predictions regarding the impact of perturbations in this system on observed sleep-wake cycles, whether those perturbations result from pharmacologic, pathophysiologic, or environmental changes. Given the role of NA in promoting excitation of every major wake-promoting region of the RAS, as well as its direct activating actions on the neocortex, one would expect that persistently elevated NA signaling would result in increased total time awake, both through delayed entry into sleep and increased interruptions of sleep regardless of stage. Given the particularly prominent inhibitory interactions between the REM-active regions and the LC, one would expect a particularly high likelihood of REM sleep disruption, such as decreased total time in REM sleep, decreased entries into REM sleep, and shorter REM sleep durations with persistent noradrenergic signaling. The potential role of NA in preventing slow wave oscillations in the hypothalamus and neocortex would also be expected to interfere with the generation, maintenance, and/or depth of NREM sleep.

Effects of Electrical or Behavioral Modulations of Noradrenergic Signaling on Sleep

Animal models have been used to test these types of predictions for both the direct expected effects of increased NA release and for the impact of various types of stress (presumably accompanied by increased noradrenergic signaling) on sleep. When the LC was directly stimulated using bilaterally implanted electrodes, sleep-wake cycles showed significantly increased wake time and decreased total REM time via decreased frequency of REM episodes.[31] The period of decreased REM duration was followed by several days of both increased duration and frequency of REM, a finding that highlights the likelihood of a complex temporal course of consequences of even a brief period of increased NA.

Experiments assessing the impact of various stress paradigms on animal sleep are numerous[32] and have had often highly inconsistent results. The most common results have been increased latency to REM, decreased total REM, either decreased REM frequency or increased REM frequency but of significantly briefer REM episodes, and increased PGO waves.[32-34] However, immobilization-type stress or "milder" stress paradigms have at times reported increased REM or SWS,[32,35] including findings that the magnitude of this increase in REM and SWS after immobilization stress is reduced when the LC is lesioned.[32,36] Interestingly, a single shock-training fear conditioning paradigm was able to cause either an increase or a decrease in REM on the night of the training paradigm, depending on whether the rat slept in the same cage in which the shock-training had been done.[37] This finding raises the possibility that the effect of a stressful experience on sleep may depend strongly on cues regarding whether the animal is still in danger versus safe during the following sleep periods. Thus these experimental results are partially in line with the predictions listed previously but highlight the important differences between types of trauma exposure and the context in which sleep is recorded.

Effects of Pharmacologic Manipulations of Noradrenergic Signaling on Sleep in Animal Models

Assessments of alpha$_1$ receptor agonism have primarily been carried out using the alpha$_1$ receptor agonist methoxamine and have generally resulted in decreased total sleep and total REM sleep[38] in dogs,[39] cats,[40,41] and rats.[42] In some studies, it also resulted in decreased SWS.[39,42] Although α2ARs are primarily thought of as presynaptic inhibitory autoreceptors that reduce NA release—a model that would lead one to expect that alpha$_2$ agonists should have the opposite effects of alpha$_1$ agonists—studies of alpha$_2$ agonists, including clonidine and xylazine, have also primarily demonstrated decreased REM sleep[38] including in rats[43] and cats[44] as well as decreased SWS,[43,44] suggesting a more complex role for α2ARs in sleep physiology than simply modulation of NA release.

Beta receptor antagonism decreased REM sleep time, decreased SWS, and increased wakefulness.[38,45] These studies suggest that beta antagonism affects SWS in general and could even affect interactions between SWS and memory consolidation. There is also evidence that the CNS-penetrant beta-receptor antagonist propranolol may interrupt nonexocytotic release of NA from nerve terminals,[46] an effect that could play a role in the sleep changes after traumatic stress. These observations are supported by studies suggesting that prolonged wakefulness can result in LC neuronal loss, potentially accompanied by compensation by remaining neurons in a manner that increases susceptibility to inappropriate NA release via nonexocytotic mechanisms.[47]

The effects of alpha$_1$ receptor antagonists in general, and prazosin in particular, have been explored more frequently but with perhaps even more complex results. In general, they led to an increase in total REM time,[38,48] but these effects were sometimes noted to be on an inverse U-shaped curve, with the highest doses producing the opposite effect,[41,48,49] while others found either a decrease or a variable effect in both rats[42] and cats.[40] Although the inverse U-shaped curve was initially proposed to be related to systemic cardiovascular effects,[41] the notably inconsistent effects among animals even when the drug was injected directly into the dorsal pontine tegmentum makes this less likely[40] and instead raises the possibility that the effect depends more on the individual animal's baseline noradrenergic transmission pattern. Another possible explanation is the ability of prazosin to antagonize alpha$_2$ receptors of the B and C subtypes (α_2B, α_2C).[50] Although presynaptic and somatodendritic autoreceptors are thought to be primarily α_2A/D subtypes, there is evidence for a functional component potentially being due to α_2C signaling.[51] It is possible that at higher doses, prazosin causes some amount of alpha$_2$ autoreceptor antagonism, resulting in increased NA release that can then cause REM disruption via α_2A/D-mediated inhibition of REM-active regions.

Effects of Pharmacologic Manipulations of Noradrenergic Signaling on Sleep Physiology in Humans

A number of studies of the effects of these pharmacologic agents have been conducted in humans. The first study found that the alpha$_1$ antagonist thymoxamine, administered by intravenous infusion, induced an increase in the duration of REM episodes.[52] The first study to assess the effect of the alpha$_1$ antagonist prazosin administered orally on sleep in subjects with civilian trauma PTSD was a small crossover randomized controlled trial (RCT).[53] In addition to significant improvement in overall PTSD with prazosin, this study found a significant 94-minute increase in total sleep time (280 ± 105 to 374 ± 86 min) as well as increased REM sleep time and mean REM period duration when subjects were on prazosin as compared with placebo.

In another prazosin trial, military veterans with chronic sleep disturbance and nightmares were randomized to prazosin, psychotherapy, or placebo.[54] Subjective sleep latency was decreased in the prazosin and psychotherapy groups as compared with the placebo group; however, percentage of REM sleep, percentage of SWS, and REM sleep density were all unchanged in both groups. Overall, these results did not support the expected outcomes of increased REM sleep and/or SWS. One possible interpretation of these results compared with those of the previous study is that prazosin may have the largest effect on total sleep, and perhaps REM sleep only increases in individuals with a higher severity of baseline sleep disruption.[55]

Preserved noradrenergic tone during REM sleep is a possible mechanism for the increase in motor behaviors during sleep observed in subjects with PTSD or a history of severe trauma. Mysliwiec and colleagues described four soldiers with combat trauma exposure and distressing nighttime behaviors.[56] They characterized these soldiers using polysomnography (PSG), as well as their clinical response to prazosin. Nighttime symptoms included sleep talking and yelling, thrashing, night sweats, and aggressive behaviors. All four individuals had REM sleep without atonia. In one individual, PSG captured a nightmare event during which loud vocalizations, body movements, tachypnea, and tachycardia occurred. Increased autonomic activation during nighttime sleep disruption is consistent with changes in autonomic regulation during sleep observed in subjects with PTSD and contrasts with the decreased cardiac autonomic activation seen during spontaneous body movements in RBD.[57] Mysliwiec and colleagues noted that in their clinical experience, clonazepam, the treatment of choice for traditional RBD, was largely ineffective in this trauma-related syndrome (for which they have proposed the name "trauma-related sleep disorder"). In contrast, prazosin was helpful for all four of these soldiers, resulting in complete resolution of the motor and behavioral symptoms at 4 to 5 mg at bedtime for two of them. These findings are consistent with the suggestion that increased large muscle movement during REM sleep after severe trauma may reflect increased noradrenergic tone that can be suppressed or eliminated with a CNS-penetrant alpha$_1$ antagonist.

A frequently observed response of human subjects or patients to pharmacologic manipulation of noradrenergic neurotransmission is the increased rate and intensification of preexisting nightmares in individuals who take beta blockers (e.g., propranolol).[58,59] Polysomnography in subjects taking beta blockers known to be CNS penetrant (pindolol, propranolol, and metoprolol) or partially CNS penetrant (atenolol) have reported either a trend or a significant increase in wake time after sleep onset, but primarily decreased REM sleep time and increased REM sleep latency; this is particularly seen with pindolol, a medication known to also have direct sympathomimetic properties.[60,61]

There are, at present, two commonly proposed mechanisms for the increased awakenings from sleep seen with beta blockers. First, beta$_1$ receptor activation has been found to stimulate melatonin release from the pineal gland,[62] an effect further potentiated by alpha$_1$ receptor agonism,[63] a mechanism consistent with the finding of a correlation between increased melatonin secretion and the experience of nightmares on beta blockers.[64] A second potential explanation is that many beta blockers also have cross-reactivity with serotonin (5-HT) receptors and may interrupt sleep via this pathway. The impact of different beta blockers on sleep has been suggested to be most closely associated with occupancy rates at beta$_2$ and 5-HT receptors rather than with beta$_1$ receptor occupancy.[65] The explanation for increased nightmares remains unclear but could be due to an increased recall of dream content secondary to the increased frequency of awakenings.[59] Finally, there is no obvious mechanism by which beta blockade would potentiate nightmares in those who already suffer from them, but, from our own clinical experience, beta blockade is well tolerated once the nightmares are reduced or eliminated with alpha$_1$-receptor blockade.

EFFECTS OF ALTERED NORADRENERGIC TRANSMISSION ON SLEEP FUNCTION

Memory Formation, Emotional Memory Consolidation, and Sleep

The interactions between memory consolidation and affective memory modulation during sleep are an extremely active area of research,[34] and a review of this area is far outside the scope of this work; the interested reader is directed to recent reviews from different perspectives.[34,66-70] Nonetheless, we briefly review the major theories regarding possible interactions, highlighting how they have begun to be tested translationally and the role of noradrenergic signaling in these theories.

In addition to the general evidence that memory, emotion, and sleep are connected, there is evidence that sleep disruptions either before a traumatic experience, immediately after the experience, and/or during the expected period of recovery may be tightly linked to the development of PTSD.[71,72] This has prompted significant theorizing regarding the potential causal relationships between different forms of sleep disruption and subsequent impacts on fear memory consolidation, generalization, extinction, and reactivity. The details of these relationships, however, have proved to be highly complex. In brief, several studies found that (1) REM sleep promotes consolidation of emotional memories but decreases the affective coloring of the memory,[73,74] (2) REM sleep promotes consolidation of emotional memories, including the affective strength and tone,[75] (3) REM sleep consolidates emotional memories with no effect on affective tone,[76,77] or (4) slow wave sleep promotes consolidation of emotional memories, particularly those required for fear extinction.[34,78-80]

Some experimental results appear to be related to factors that interact with memory consolidation and affect modulation during sleep, including the potential confounding factor of circadian rhythm independently of sleep itself.[81] The type of memory may also significantly affect how consolidation occurs during sleep, with hippocampal-dependent memories being significantly more tied to slow wave sleep than non–hippocampal-dependent memories.[82,83] There is increasing evidence that hippocampal modulation of amygdala activation is a necessary mechanism for discriminating which environments are dangerous and inhibiting learned fear responses in the presence of safety cues.[84] This is in opposition to the overgeneralization of fear learning seen in PTSD[85] and prompts the possibility that this aspect of memory consolidation may be particularly relevant to the pathophysiology of PTSD.

There have also been suggestions that that the ability of sleep to modulate the affective intensity of a memory is related to not only the amount of REM sleep but also the more subtle characteristics of REM sleep structure as quantified by EEG. Specifically, it has been found that the degree of emotional memory depotentiation experienced by individuals after a period of sleep is inversely related to the strength of γ-frequency EEG activity during their period of REM sleep.[73,74] As γ-frequency EEG activity has been suggested as a potential indirect measure of central adrenergic signaling,[73] this idea is consistent with the idea that either sleep deprivation *or* inappropriately elevated noradrenergic signaling during slow wave and REM sleep after trauma could lead to persistently high arousal symptoms such as those seen in PTSD. In addition, it suggests that pharmacologic blockade of this inappropriately high noradrenergic signaling (e.g., by the alpha$_1$ antagonist prazosin) may restore the ability of sleep to depotentiate affective responsivity to traumatic memories.[68] In contrast, several studies suggest that delaying, restricting, or preventing sleep immediately after a traumatic event may actually decrease the long-term affective intensity of the memory.[86,87]

Potential Role of Noradrenergic Signaling in Regulating Brain Glymphatic Clearance during Sleep

Several years ago, a new, paravascular pathway for CSF flow through the parenchyma of the brain (the "glymphatic system") was identified that significantly contributes to the clearance of interstitial solutes. These include beta-amyloid and tau,[88,89] the most prominent pathologic proteins in Alzheimer disease. Intriguingly, the rate of clearance through this pathway increased substantially during both sleep and anesthesia.[89,90] These effects may result from the decrease in noradrenergic signaling during these states, as they can be replicated by noradrenergic blockade at the alpha$_1$ receptor.[90]

A strong candidate for the mechanism underlying this regulation appears to be via the astrocytic processes that surround cerebral microvessels and receive the central noradrenergic innervation of these vessels.[91,92] Although these processes express both beta and alpha$_1$ receptors,[93,94] it is the alpha$_1$ receptors that have been found to regulate the coordinated calcium signaling[95] posited to control the aquaporin-4 water channels that underlie the glymphatic flow in the paravascular clearing pathway.[96] How alterations in glymphatic clearance of extracellular neurotoxic material relate to the development of clinical disorders such as Alzheimer's disease, and how such alterations relate to changes in total sleep time and noradrenergic signaling during sleep, are under ongoing investigations.[97,98]

Posttraumatic Stress Disorder Sleep Disturbance and Trauma Nightmares: Therapeutic Response to Prazosin

Increased noradrenergic signaling appears to contribute to PTSD sleep disturbance pathophysiology in a substantial subgroup of persons meeting diagnostic criteria for this disorder.[99,100] Inappropriately high noradrenergic signaling, particularly during REM and other sleep stages, is a likely contributory mechanism for the distressed awakenings and the realistic and frightening trauma content nightmares that are hallmarks of this disorder.[101] PTSD is biologically complex and clinically heterogeneous.[102] This led to the proposal of a "noradrenergic" subtype of PTSD, for whom distressed awakenings from frightening trauma nightmares as well as terrifying daytime flashbacks and hyperarousal symptoms are accompanied by both increased SNS and central noradrenergic activity.[55,103] Manifestations include sweating, tachycardia, anxiety, increased vigilance, and higher blood pressure than is typical for an individual's demographic group. This noradrenergic PTSD subtype appears particularly prevalent among military veterans who have sustained periods of intense life-threatening combat operations, and perhaps others for whom periods of sustained vigilance or threat were punctuated by periods of acutely elevated traumatic stress.

A rational and feasible therapeutic approach for the noradrenergic PTSD subtype is pharmacologic antagonism of postsynaptic adrenoreceptors with available drugs originally developed as antihypertensives. Although noradrenergic stimulation at both the alpha$_1$ and beta postsynaptic adrenoreceptors produces arousal,[4] the propensity of propranolol and other beta receptor antagonists to intensify dreams (see previously) favored an initial alpha$_1$ antagonist therapeutic approach. Prazosin is the most lipid soluble and therefore most CNS penetrant of available alpha$_1$ antagonists and has been demonstrated to decrease CNS noradrenergic signaling when administered peripherally.[104] Since the first case series suggesting prazosin benefit for PTSD trauma nightmares and sleep disruption in Vietnam veterans who had experienced intense combat,[105] six of seven "prazosin for PTSD" RCTs (six in combat veterans) have demonstrated prazosin's efficacy for improving sleep quality and reducing trauma nightmares and daytime hyperarousal symptoms.[53,106-110] Doxazosin is a long-acting alpha$_1$ antagonist that also appears to be CNS penetrant. Case reports suggest potential benefit of doxazosin for PTSD as well.[111] The only placebo-controlled trial, a brief underpowered crossover study in eight veterans, failed to demonstrate efficacy on the primary PTSD outcome measure, the total Clinician Administered PTSD Scale (CAPS) score but found a trend level benefit for the hyperarousal symptom cluster that includes sleep disturbance.[112]

Higher Pretreatment Blood Pressure in Young Active-Duty Soldiers with Posttraumatic Stress Disorder Predicts Therapeutic Response to Prazosin

In a prazosin RCT for PTSD in active-duty US soldiers recently returned from combat deployments in Iraq and Afghanistan, prazosin substantially improved sleep quality and reduced trauma nightmares and overall PTSD symptoms.[108] However, as with all psychopharmacologic treatments for any behavioral disorder, therapeutic response to prazosin varied among soldiers. Two-thirds of those randomized to prazosin meaningfully improved, whereas one-third did not. There were no differences in prazosin dose achieved or baseline behavior rating scores between prazosin responders and nonresponders. One possible explanation for the observed differential therapeutic response to prazosin is that responders had elevated activation of CNS $alpha_1$ receptors, the presumed pharmacologic target of prazosin. Although CNS $alpha_1$ activation cannot be quantified directly in living humans, blood pressure is an easily accessible biologic parameter regulated by noradrenergic activation of $alpha_1$ receptors at peripheral arterioles that likely reflects noradrenergic activation status of CNS $alpha_1$ receptors.[113] It was hypothesized that higher pretreatment BP would predict therapeutic response in the prazosin group (but not the placebo group).[103] This hypothesis was supported: each 10-mm Hg higher baseline standing systolic BP increment resulted in an additional 14-point reduction in total CAPS score. Much of this improvement was accounted for by improved sleep and reduction of trauma nightmares, consistent with $alpha_1$ activation contributing to the pathophysiology of sleep disruption and trauma nightmares in this "noradrenergic" subgroup (Figure 46.4).

THE ROLE OF DOPAMINE IN SLEEP-WAKE CONTROL

The role of the dopamine system in motivation,[114-116] motor coordination,[117-119] reward,[120-122] and memory[123-125] has been well characterized; however, until recently[126-129] the role of dopamine neurons in the regulation of sleep-wake behavior has been overlooked. While other catecholamine neurons (i.e., NA neurons) are located in the lower part of the brainstem,[130] dopamine neurons are distributed through the midbrain (A8-A10), hypothalamus (A11-A14), olfactory bulb (A15-16), and retina (A17). The ventral tegmental area (VTA, A10) and its dorsocaudal extension located in the ventral periaqueductal gray (vPAG, A10dc), as well as the substantia nigra (SN, A9) are the main source of dopamine released in the brain and have all been implicated in the regulation of sleep[131,132] (Figure 46.5).

The effect of dopamine in the CNS is mediated through five subtypes of G protein–coupled receptors, dopamine receptors D1 through D5. Whereas D1 and D5 are linked to Gs, which increases the activity of cyclic adenosine monophosphate (cAMP) and leads to neuronal depolarization, the D2-D4 subtypes are linked to Gi/o, inhibit cAMP, and lead to hyperpolarization[133-135] (Figure 46.6). This section describes (1) the evidence that the dopamine system plays a major role in triggering wakefulness, (2) how wake-promoting compounds manipulate the dopamine system, (3) what are the mechanisms and circuits through which this catecholaminergic system functions, and (4) how disturbances and dysregulations of this system are implicated in disorders such as narcolepsy, PD, and restless legs syndrome (RLS).

Wake-Promoting Drugs Depend on the Dopamine System to Exert Their Effects

The strongest evidence that dopamine plays an important role in regulating sleep-wake behavior is that the most widely used wake-promoting drugs depend on a functional dopamine system.[136,137] The action of dopamine is tightly regulated by the ability of presynaptic terminals of dopamine-containing neurons to reuptake neurotransmitters through dopamine transporters (DAT). Cocaine, amphetamine, and modafinil[138,139] are wake-promoting compounds that have been used to sustain arousal[137,140] and to treat patients with debilitating daytime sleepiness.[137,141] Since early studies, it has been hypothesized that these compounds act to stimulate arousal and alertness by directly blocking DAT to prevent reuptake of dopamine from the synaptic cleft, thereby increasing the amount of dopamine in the synapse, which will then saturate postsynaptic D1 and D2 receptors[142] (Figure 46.6).

The affinity of both cocaine and amphetamine for the DAT directly correlates with an increase in wake in both normal and narcoleptic dogs.[143,144] DAT blockers, but not blockade of other noradrenergic transporters, increase wakefulness.[144] In addition, the use of both amphetamine and modafinil to induce wake remains effective even when the LC, the main source of NA in the brain, is lesioned.[145] This highlights the importance of the dopamine system in drug-induced arousal.

The use of DAT knockout mice further revealed the necessity for an intact dopamine system to mediate the effect of wake-promoting substances. DAT knockout mice have decreased NREM sleep duration and increased wakefulness similar to what is seen with DAT inhibitors.[138] These mice tend to be easily stimulated by novel objects and spend more time wheel-running and exploring their environment compared with control mice.[146] Moreover, amphetamine and modafinil fail to further increase locomotion or increase wake duration despite an intact noradrenergic system.[138] Thus wake-promoting drugs require the dopamine system to function. Finally, wake-promoting drugs also require intact dopamine receptors for their effects since D2 receptor knockout mice spend more time asleep[147] and the wake-promoting effect of modafinil in these mice is strongly reduced.[148]

Effect of Dopamine Agonists and Antagonists on Arousal and Sleep

D1 and D2 receptors are the most prominently expressed dopamine receptors in the CNS and constitute the main effectors of the dopamine system[149] (Figure 46.6). Agonists and antagonists of these receptors have been used to elucidate the importance of dopamine in sleep-wake control.

D1 receptors are postsynaptic and lead to depolarization of the targeted neurons. Activation of the D1 receptor pathway with D1 agonists leads to increased arousal. For example, systemic administration of D1 receptor agonists such as SKF38393 and A68930 led to an increase in the amount of time spent in wake and reduced both NREM and REM sleep in a dose-dependent manner.[150-152] Both of these D1 agonists led to strong desynchronization of EEG activity, and the wake periods induced by these compounds was accompanied by active motor behavior, predominantly grooming.[149-154] The effect of these D1 agonists can be partially attenuated or fully prevented by the use of D1 receptor antagonists such as SCH23390, while D2 receptor antagonists had no effect.[155] Conversely, systemic application of SCH23390 (D1 antagonist) increased both NREM and REM sleep while decreasing wake.[150,155-157]

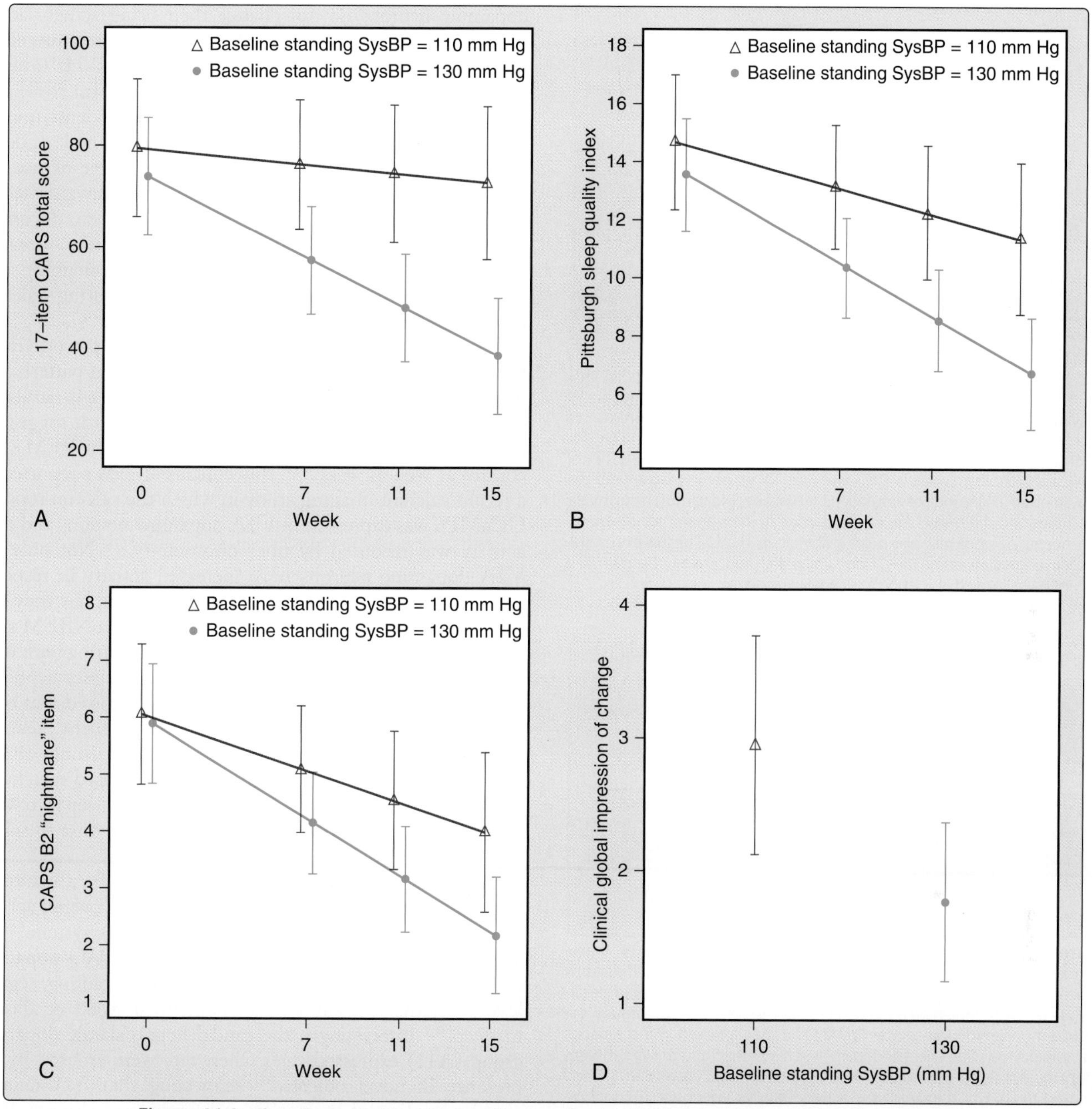

Figure 46.4 Effect of prazosin on posttraumatic stress disorder (PTSD) symptoms is modulated by standing blood pressure before treatment. In a randomized controlled trial of prazosin for PTSD in active-duty soldiers, the effect of prazosin on all major outcome measures was strongly related to standing systolic blood pressure (SysBP) measured at entry into the clinical trial. Shown are the results of linear mixed-effects models for outcome measures in the prazosin treatment arm, as a function of SysBP. The impact of prazosin on overall PTSD symptoms (as measured by the Clinician Administered PTSD Scale [CAPS] for DSM-IV) **(A)**; overall sleep quality (as measured by the Pittsburgh Sleep Quality Index, **(B)**; higher scores represent increased symptom burden), the "nightmare" item from the CAPS for DSM-IV **(C)**, and the clinical global impression of change **(D)** are all seen to be significantly larger in individuals with a higher baseline SysBP. Note that the use of liner mixed-effects models allowed the results to be adjusted for the covariates of sex and current use of any antidepressant, but constrained the results for the three time-varying items (A through C) to a linear slope, which should not be taken to indicate that the effect of prazosin on symptoms was necessarily linear over the course of the trial. Error bars indicate 95% confidence intervals. For full details, see original publication. (Reprinted with permission from the American Journal of Psychiatry [Copyright ©2013]. American Psychiatric Association. All rights reserved.)

D2 receptor mechanisms are slightly less straightforward because D2 receptors are located both presynaptically, where they act as autoreceptors regulating the activity of dopamine-containing neurons, and on the postsynaptic side of synaptic cleft. This leads to a biphasic effect of D2 agonists (e.g., apomorphine, quinpirole, and bromocriptine), with low doses activating autoreceptors and causing both NREM and REM sleep, increased delta power and decreased locomotion, whereas high doses activate postsynaptic D2 receptors, causing arousal and decreases in NREM and REM sleep. In addition, the specific D2 autoreceptor agonist, (-)3-PPP, induced sleep and suppressed locomotion when systemically administered in

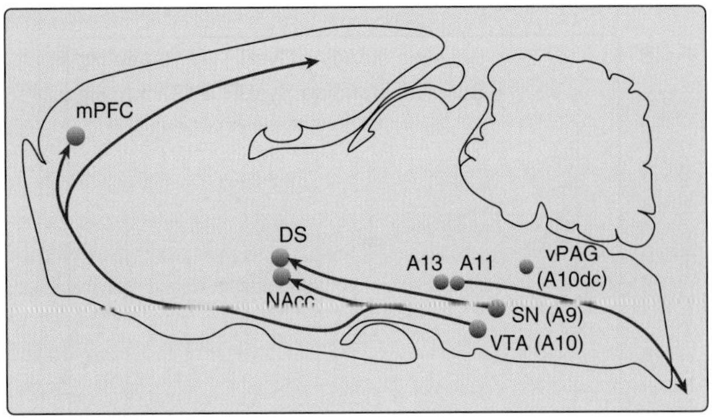

Figure 46.5 Dopamine neurons involved in sleep-wake control. Dopamine neurons are distributed through the midbrain (A8-A10), hypothalamus (A11-A14), olfactory bulb (A15-16), and retina (A17). The ventral tegmental area (VTA, A10) and its dorsocaudal extension located in the ventral periaqueductal gray (vPAG, A10dc), as well as the substantia nigra (SN, A9), are the main sources of dopamine released in the brain and have all been implicated in the regulation of sleep. The VTA neurons synapse onto the nucleus accumbens (NAcc) and medial prefrontal cortex (mPFC), while the SN neurons synapse onto the dorsal striatum (DS) to induce arousal. A11 (caudal hypothalamus) neurons are wake-active and the main source of dopamine in the spinal cord, while A13 (zona incerta) neurons may play a role in REM sleep. The A12 (arcuate nucleus), A14 (periventricular), and A15-A17 dopamine cell groups are not shown and have not been studied in relation to sleep-wake control.

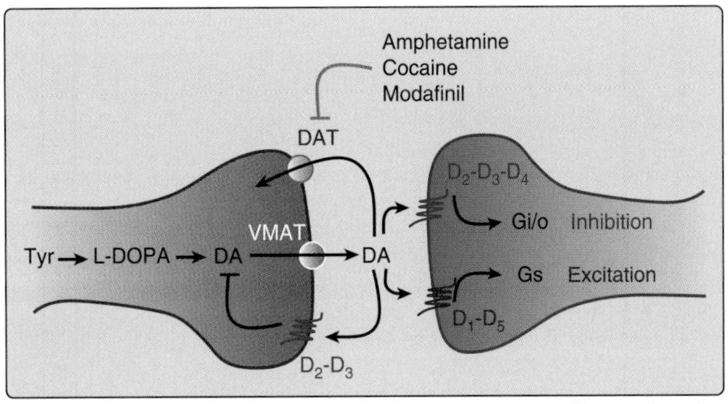

Figure 46.6 Dopamine synaptic mechanisms and effects of wake-promoting drugs. Dopamine is synthesized from tyrosine (Tyr) and L-dopa by the action of two enzymes, tyrosine hydroxylase (TH) and amino acid decarboxylase (AADC). Dopamine is transported into synaptic vesicles through the vesicular monoamine transporter (VMAT) and then released in the synaptic cleft via exocytosis. The effect of dopamine is mediated through five subtypes of dopamine receptors, D1 to D5. These are G-coupled receptors with D1 and D5 linked to Gs, which increase the activity of cyclic adenosine monophosphate (cAMP) and lead to neuronal depolarization (i.e., excitation), whereas the D2-D4 receptors are linked to Gi/o, inhibit cAMP, and lead to hyperpolarization (i.e., inhibition). The action of dopamine is tightly regulated by the ability of presynaptic terminals of dopamine-containing neurons to reuptake neurotransmitters through dopamine transporters (DAT). Cocaine, amphetamine, and modafinil are wake-promoting compounds that act to stimulate arousal and alertness by directly blocking the DAT to prevent reuptake of dopamine from the synaptic cleft, thereby increasing the amount of dopamine in the synapse, which will then saturate both D1- and D2-like dopamine receptors postsynaptically. Inhibitory D2-D3 receptors are located on the presynaptic side as autoreceptors and regulate the activity of dopamine neurons.

rats.[158] This evidence illustrates that both D1 and D2-mediated mechanisms play a fine-tuning role in sleep-wake regulation.

Activity Pattern of Dopamine Neurons

Despite the strong effects of dopamine agonists and wake-promoting compounds affecting dopamine reuptake, the role of the dopamine system has been underappreciated because early single-unit recordings had shown that both SN and VTA dopamine neurons do not change their firing activity across the sleep-wake cycle.[159,160] Midbrain dopamine neurons either fire in a slow tonic manner between 0.5 and 10 Hz (average 4.5 Hz) or in 15- to 30-Hz bursts (average 20 Hz).[161,162] This activity pattern is highly conserved and seen in rodents, nonhuman primates, and zebrafish.[123,162,163] The burst mode of dopamine neurons correlates with increased dopamine release and has been strongly associated with locomotion, reward mechanisms, and motivation.[164-166] The link between dopamine neuron bursting and waking behavior such as locomotion and reward led to the assumption that dopamine-containing neurons are more involved in behaviors occurring during wakefulness rather than the control over the state itself.[167]

However, this assumption has recently been put into question. VTA dopamine neurons change their firing pattern during REM sleep to exhibit bursting activity that is similar to what is observed under locomotion and reward, suggesting that VTA dopamine neurons may play a role in REM sleep control as well as wake.[162] This conclusion was supported by a recent calcium imaging study in which the calcium reporter GCaMP6 was expressed in VTA dopamine neurons and their activity was recorded by fiber photometry.[126] Not only did VTA dopamine neurons have increased activity in response to salient cues such as food and novel objects, but they also showed increased activity at the transition from NREM sleep to wake or REM sleep, as well as high activity during both wake and REM sleep.[126] Similarly, Cho and colleagues expressed GCaMP6 in vPAG dopamine neurons and showed that these neurons increase their activity in response to salient cues such as a mating partner, chocolate, and aversive footshock.[128] The activity of vPAG dopamine neurons also increased specifically at the transition from NREM sleep and REM sleep into wake, suggesting a role of these cells not only in response to salient stimuli but also in sleep-wake control.[128]

Expression of the immediate-early gene *c-fos*, a marker of neuronal activity, has been used to observe the overall activity of dopamine neurons throughout the nervous system.[168-170] These studies revealed that SN, VTA, and vPAG dopamine groups almost never exhibited *c-fos* immunostaining, regardless of whether the animal was maintained awake or allowed to sleep.[169] Interestingly, the caudal hypothalamic dopamine group (A11) expressed *c-fos* when rats were aroused by the presence of novel objects,[169] suggesting that A11 neurons may be implicated in specific wake processes (Figure 46.5). Finally, vPAG dopamine neurons have greater *c-fos* expression in awake compared with sleeping animals.[171] Despite the early unit recordings studies, both *c-fos* expression and calcium imaging have shown that dopamine neurons in several distinct groups change their activity with vigilance and behavioral states, suggesting that they play an active role in either controlling the timing of the state itself and/or in behaviors that occur specifically during wakefulness.

Dopamine Release across the Sleep-Wake Cycle

VTA neurons project to the cerebral cortex (mesocortical pathway), the hypothalamus and thalamus (mesodiencephalic pathway), and the dorsal raphe, medial raphe, LC, pontine tegmentum, reticular formation, and cerebellum (mesorhombencephalic pathway).[172] However, the strongest projection from VTA neurons synapses onto the nucleus accumbens (NAcc) and basal forebrain (mesolimbic pathway) neurons[172] (Figure 46.5). Microdialysis studies show increased dopamine release during wake and REM

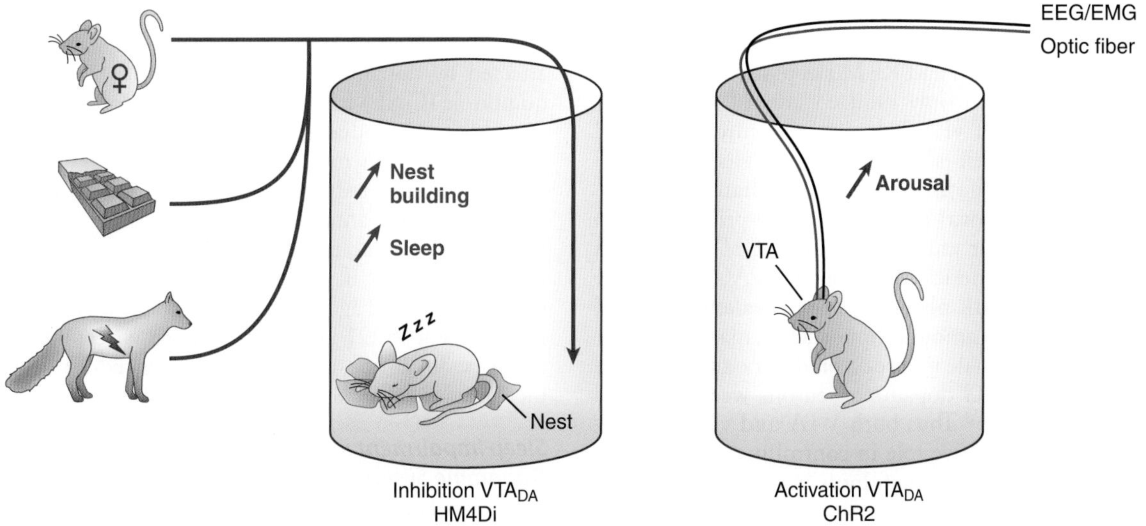

Figure 46.7 Manipulation of ventral tegmental area (VTA) neurons reveals their function in inducing arousal and controlling wake behavior. Eban-Rotschild and colleagues[126] have shown that chemogenetic inhibition (i.e., activation of hM4Di by clozapine-N-oxide [CNO]) of VTA dopamine neurons increased both NREM and REM sleep, even when animals were presented with arousing stimuli such as food, mating partner, or predator odor.[126] Interestingly, the inhibition of VTA dopamine neurons not only promoted sleep but also induced a complex sleep preparatory behavior (i.e., nesting). In addition, they showed that light-activated VTA dopamine neurons induced arousal from sleep and promoted wakefulness even after 4 hours of sleep deprivation. This light-induced arousal was observed not only when VTA dopamine cell bodies were activated but also when light activated the release of dopamine from VTA fibers in the nucleus accumbens (NAcc).

sleep in the NAcc and medial prefrontal cortex (mPFC),[173,174] whereas voltammetry recordings showed that striatal dopamine release is higher during wakefulness than in sleep.[175,176] It has been hypothesized that the NAcc is a sleep-promoting region and that release of dopamine from the VTA silences NAcc neurons. Injection of amphetamine in the NAcc induced arousal,[136,177,178] while the effect of modafinil was blocked by lesions of this striatal nucleus.[179,180] The NAcc strongly expresses D2 dopamine receptors and injection of a D2 receptor agonist induced wake, whereas a D2 receptor antagonist increased sleep.[181]

SN dopamine neurons mainly project to the dorsal striatum[182] (Figure 46.5). This targeted area has also been implicated in promoting wake as lesions in the area leads to a decrease or disruption of wakefulness.[183-185] As mentioned previously, microdialysis and voltammetry have been used to detect dopamine release; however, these tools lack the temporal resolution necessary to understand the role of dopamine release in state transitions. Recently, a novel fluorescent dopamine sensor (dLight1.1) has been used to track the level of dopamine release in the striatum throughout the sleep-wake cycle.[129] This sensor is based on a mutated D1 receptor that emits green fluorescence when bound to dopamine without activating the D1 cellular downstream pathway. Using fiber photometry, dopamine levels were found to be highest in wake, lower in NREM sleep, and lowest in REM sleep.[129] Dopamine levels also rise at the transition from NREM sleep to wake and increase significantly in response to salient cues and the injection of modafinil.[129] The systematic use of this approach should help identify how dopamine release at the level of all projections of both VTA and SN neurons affects sleep-wake regulation.

Manipulation of Dopamine Neuron Activity Reveals Dopamine Neuron Function in Arousal and Waking Behavior

Methodological advances in the past 10 years have made possible the ability to reversibly control the activity of discrete and specific neuronal populations with millisecond time resolution (i.e., optogenetics) or for longer periods of time (minutes to hours) (i.e., chemogenetics) in freely behaving animals.[186-189] These new techniques helped reveal a clear function for dopamine cell groups. Optogenetic activation of VTA dopamine neurons induced arousal from sleep and promoted wakefulness even after 4 hours of sleep deprivation.[126] Arousal was observed not only when VTA dopamine cell bodies were activated but also when light activated the release of dopamine from VTA fibers in the NAcc.[126] Chemogenetic inhibition of VTA dopamine neurons increased both NREM and REM sleep even when mice were presented with arousing stimuli such as food, a mating partner, or predator odor. Of particular interest: the inhibition of VTA dopamine neurons not only promoted sleep but also induced a complex sleep preparatory behavior (i.e., nesting)[126] (Figure 46.7).

Other studies showed that chemogenetic activation of VTA dopamine neurons and not SN dopamine neurons triggered wake and increased its duration through a D2 receptor-mediated mechanism.[127] However, chemogenetic inhibition and selective cell lesioning of VTA dopamine neurons by diphtheria toxin had no effect on sleep-wake regulation.[127] GABA-releasing neurons in the VTA were shown to play a critical role in regulating wakefulness under normal conditions by regulating dopamine receptor mechanisms.[190] The contradictory results of these studies have been tentatively explained by technical differences (e.g., the use of TH-Cre versus DAT-Cre mice).[191] Nevertheless, a finer dissection of the subpopulations of dopamine VTA neurons based on their projection profiles or anatomic location may elucidate the range of functions that dopamine VTA neurons play in the regulation of wakefulness and its related behaviors.

The function of vPAG dopamine neurons was also investigated using optogenetics and chemogenetics.[128] Cho and colleagues expressed channelrhodopsin in these cells and drove their activity either tonically (i.e., continuous 2-Hz stimulation) or phasically (i.e., ten 30-Hz stimulations every 5 seconds) for 2-minute trials.[128] Phasic activation led mice to transition from NREM and REM sleep into wakefulness, whereas tonic activation only induced arousal from REM sleep. The activation of vPAG dopamine neurons induced arousal from sleep even after 4 hours of sleep deprivation.[128] This wake-promoting effect was mediated by dopamine release as arousal was prevented by the prior injection of D1 and D2 receptor antagonists (i.e., SCH-23390 and eticlopride). Chemogenetic inhibition of vPAG dopamine neurons during the dark phase decreased wakefulness and increased NREM sleep amount. Importantly, male mice presented with either a female mouse or predator odor remained asleep when their vPAG dopamine neurons were inhibited by injection of CNO.[128] Thus both VTA and vPAG dopamine neurons play an active role in controlling arousal from sleep as well as sustaining wakefulness in response to motivating stimuli.

Dopamine and Clinical Correlates

Dysregulation of the dopamine system has been implicated in several sleep disorders or disorders that present sleep abnormalities as symptoms, as illustrated by the following three examples. Narcolepsy, a sleep disorder caused by the loss of orexin/hypocretin neurons and characterized by excessive daytime sleepiness (EDS),[192-194] is also characterized by a dysregulation of dopamine transmission[195] that is partially relieved by drugs affecting dopamine pathways.[196-198] The loss of SN dopamine neurons underlies the debilitating motor symptoms of PD,[199,200] and patients suffering from this disorder often present with sleep-wake dysregulation.[199,201,202] Finally, a dysfunction of dopamine transmission contributes to the pathobiology of RLS and PLMs.[203,204]

Dopamine Impairment in Narcolepsy

Narcolepsy is an autoimmune neurodegenerative disorder characterized by EDS, cataplexy, short-onset REM sleep, sleep paralysis, and sleep hallucination.[205] Since the end of the 1990s, we know that the root cause of narcolepsy is the progressive loss of orexin/hypocretin neurons located in the hypothalamus.[193,206,207] The loss of this wake-promoting neurotransmitter leads to a cascade of downstream effects implicating several wake-promoting circuits including dopamine.[208] Dopamine levels in CSF of patients with narcolepsy is lower than in healthy controls,[209] and dopamine binding to D2 (but not D1) receptors is increased in narcoleptics.[195,210]

One of the most debilitating symptoms of narcolepsy is the inability of patients to stay awake (i.e., EDS). This sleepiness strongly affects their day-to-day lives as they often need to take naps, fall asleep in the middle of a conversation, and are prevented from driving because this may lead to fatal accidents. Because wakefulness maintenance is affected, dysregulation of the dopamine system is suspected, which is supported by the fact that the most potent treatment for EDS in narcolepsy is modafinil.[211-216] Amphetamines were used before the development of modafinil to treat narcolepsy[217,218]; however, the low risk of abuse potential of modafinil made it the treatment of choice.

The other narcoleptic symptom affecting the day-to-day life of patients with narcolepsy is cataplexy, which is defined as the sudden loss of muscle tone during normal wakefulness.[205] This dissociative state, characterized by the intrusion of REM sleep muscle atonia during normal waking behavior, is also affected by dopamine compounds.[192,208,219] The D2 agonist quinpirole (QNP) triggers cataplexy in Doberman narcoleptic dogs.[220,221] Microdialysis infusion of QNP into the VTA, SN, and A11 leads to worsening of cataplexy.[221-223] The D2 antagonist raclopride reduces cataplexy, whereas the D1 agonist (SKF38393), D1 antagonist (SCH23390), and DAT inhibitor (bupropion) had no effect on cataplexy.[144,222,224] Quinpirole in the VTA but not in the SN increased drowsiness.[221] In narcoleptic mice, D2 agonists worsen cataplexy while D2 antagonists prevent it; D1 antagonists increase sleepiness, while D1 agonists, dopamine, and amphetamines reduce sleepiness and increase wake.[208]

Sleep Impairment in Parkinson Disease and the Role of the Dopamine System

PD is a neurodegenerative disease that is characterized by the loss of dopamine cells in the SN.[200] This loss underlies the severe motor impairments that define the disease (i.e., tremor, bradykinesia, rigidity, and gating and postural difficulties). However, PD is also characterized by several sleep disturbances such as insomnia, EDS, RBD, RLS, and PLMs.[199,202,225,226]

The mechanism through which PD develops has been clearly identified.[227-229] Progressive aggregation of the pathologic form of the protein α-synuclein (α-syn) into Lewy bodies and neurites leads to neuronal cell death. According to Braak's hypothesis, pathologic α-syn progresses from the gut and the olfactory tract to the brainstem and eventually moves rostrally to the midbrain, where the SN dopamine neurons are located.[229,230] PD pathobiology is divided into several progressive stages. Stage 1 includes premotor symptoms such as constipation and loss of olfaction, stage 2 includes symptoms resulting from the degeneration of brainstem structures such as RBD, and stage 3 includes degeneration of dopamine neurons leading to motor symptoms.[202]

The first and strongest prodromal sleep symptom of PD is RBD.[231-233] This disorder is defined as the loss of motor atonia during REM sleep, and approximately 90% of patients with RBD are diagnosed with PD during the following 10 to 15 years.[26,192] It is thought that this symptom is due to the degeneration of the SLD and the ventral medulla (vM), two structures that form the circuit that controls motor atonia during REM sleep.[219,234,235] Imaging studies in patients with idiopathic RBD and patients with PD and RBD show specific loss of neuronal activity in both the SLD and the vM,[26,236] and postmortem studies show inclusions of pathologic α-syn in these regions.[232,237] However, this symptom precedes the impairment of midbrain dopamine cells. Eventually, patients with PD develop insomnia and EDS that may in part be due to the deficiency of the dopamine system. Patients with PD exhibit impaired sleep quality, sleep fragmentation, a decrease in slow wave sleep (i.e., NREM sleep), an increased latency to enter REM sleep, and increased PLMs.[225,238-241]

Multiple animal models of PD (i.e., MPTP, 6-OHDA, rotenone) induced by lesioning dopamine SN neurons recapitulate the sleep impairments seen in patients with PD.[183,184,242-247] In brief, lesions of SN dopamine neurons decrease NREM and REM sleep, increase sleep fragmentation during their inactive phase (i.e., insomnia), and sleep during their active phase (i.e., excessive daytime sleepiness). These findings support the idea that loss of dopamine neurons in PD underlies sleep abnormalities as well as motor symptoms. A recent study induced overexpression of α-syn in dopamine SN neurons, which led to aggregation in Lewy bodies and neurites, cell death, and the development of motor impairments.[248] This is a relevant pathophysiologic model of PD, as it mimics the progressive nature of the disease.[229] In this study, animals also had impaired sleep regulation, decreased REM sleep, and increased sleep fragmentation.[248]

Finally, patients with PD often experience RLS with or without PLMs (10% to 25% of patients).[201] This syndrome is characterized by uncomfortable sensations in the lower limbs at night that are transiently relieved by movements. Because this happens at night, it causes severe sleep disruption and fragmentation. RLS is thought to be due to a decrease in iron stores in the striatum and SN, which may affect dopamine synaptic transmission (see later).

Altered Dopamine Transmission Contributes to Restless Legs Syndrome and Periodic Leg Movements during Sleep

RLS affects 5% to 10% of the population and is considered a disorder of hyperarousability that leads to decreased sleep duration.[249] Patients describe an uncomfortable feeling of restlessness in the legs at night that leads to the urge to move. RLS is often (approximately 80% of the time) accompanied with actual movement of the legs as PLMs.[250] This syndrome may be due to the hyperexcitability of the cortical-striatal-thalamic circuit. Imaging studies (i.e., functional magnetic resonance imaging) showed increased activity in thalamus, striatum, and frontal cortex in people with RLS compared with people without RLS.[251]

One of the root causes of RLS is CNS iron deficiency.[204] Patients with RLS show decreased levels of ferritin in CSF,[252] and imaging studies demonstrate a specific reduction in the SN.[204] An iron-deficient diet in rats induces RLS symptoms with an increase in wake duration specifically at the end of the dark period, increased motor activity, decreased sleep efficiency, and alteration of the dopamine system.[204]

Imaging studies in patients with RLS revealed that an increase in dopamine synthesis and release, and decreased dopamine reuptake and D2 receptor mechanisms, may explain the hyperexcitability that characterizes this disorder.[204,253,254] Positron emission tomography (PET) scans showed an increase in activity of tyrosine hydroxylase (TH), the main enzyme necessary for the synthesis of dopamine, a decrease in expression of DAT at the level of the synaptic membrane, and decrease in D2 receptor expression in the striatum.[204,254,255] Dopamine released at the level of the spinal cord has also been implicated in the disease mechanism.[256] The source of dopamine in the spinal cord only comes from dopamine-containing neurons of the A11 region (i.e., caudal hypothalamus).[257,258] It has been suggested that loss of the inhibitory D2 receptor mechanism may explain the hyperexcitability in RLS. This could be due to lesions of A11 dopamine neurons[256]; however, patients with RLS do not show any sign of A11 cell loss.[259] In addition, activation of these neurons leads to increased locomotion.[260] This increased activity could be due to recruitment of D1 receptor excitatory pathways,[261] as D2 receptor levels are decreased in RLS.

CLINICAL PEARL

Determining the role of how catecholamines control sleep and wakefulness is of notable importance in sleep medicine because several neurologic and neuropsychiatric disorders stem from imbalances in noradrenergic and dopaminergic regulation. As indicated by the available evidence, increases in noradrenergic signaling are a contributing factor in sleep disturbances in some patients with PTSD. Therefore a feasible therapeutic approach for treating patients with PTSD is antagonism of noradrenergic signaling pathways. However, clinicians need to be mindful that PTSD is biologically complex and clinically heterogeneous and, as such, a single treatment approach is unrealistic. Identifying mechanisms of noradrenergic dysfunction in PTSD and how NA regulates sleep and wakefulness is therefore a prerequisite for developing more rational treatments for PTSD.

SUMMARY

Catecholamines are intimately involved in the control of both sleep and wakefulness. Research over the past decade has provided valuable insight into the roles that both NA and dopamine systems play in the control of arousal states and their potential involvement in sleep disorders. In this chapter, we highlighted some of the known and potential mechanisms by which catecholamine-releasing neurons and drugs that modulate their activity and their receptors regulate sleep-wake states. We also highlighted how disturbances in catecholamine-signaling pathways contribute to sleep and waking disorders such as PTSD, PD, narcolepsy, RLS, and PLM disorder. We suggest that identifying mechanisms of noradrenergic and dopaminergic dysfunction is an important avenue for developing rational drug-based treatments for these disorders.

SELECTED READINGS

Brown RE, Basheer R, McKenna JT, et al. Control of sleep and wakefulness. *Physiol Rev.* 2012;92:1087–1187.

Burgess CR, Tse G, Gillis L, et al. Dopaminergic regulation of sleep and cataplexy in a murine model of narcolepsy. *Sleep.* 2010;33:1295–1304.

Dauvilliers Y, Siegel JM, Lopez R, et al. Cataplexy–clinical aspects, pathophysiology and management strategy. *Nat Rev Neurol.* 2014;10:386–395.

Germain A, Buysse DJ, Nofzinger E. Sleep-specific mechanisms underlying posttraumatic stress disorder: integrative review and neurobiological hypotheses. *Sleep Med Rev.* 2008;12:185–195.

Herrera-Solis A, Herrera-Morales W, Nunez-Jaramillo L, Arias-Carrion O. Dopaminergic modulation of sleep-wake states. *CNS Neurol Disord Drug Targets.* 2017;16(4):380–386.

Raskind MA, Dobie DJ, Kanter ED, et al. Peskind, The alpha1-adrenergic antagonist prazosin ameliorates combat trauma nightmares in veterans with posttraumatic stress disorder: a report of 4 cases. *J Clin Psychiatry.* 2000;61:129–133.

Torontali ZA, Fraigne JJ, Sanghera P, et al. The Sublaterodorsal tegmental nucleus functions to couple brain state and motor activity during REM sleep and wakefulness. *Current Biol: CB.* 2019;29:3803–3813. e3805.

Wisor JP, Nishino S, Sora I, et al. Edgar, dopaminergic role in stimulant-induced wakefulness. *J Neurosci.* 2001;21:1787–1794.

A complete reference list can be found online at ExpertConsult.com.

Chapter 47

GABA: Its Metabolism, Receptors, and the Drugs for Treating Insomnias and Hypersomnias

David B. Rye; William Wisden

Chapter Highlights

- Gamma-aminobutyric acid (GABA) and its receptors are among the most studied targets for pharmacologics that influence vigilance states.
- $GABA_A$ receptors are expressed on nodal points of brain circuits that initiate and sustain sleep.
- GABA agonists and modulators that allosterically enhance $GABA_A$ receptors induce sleep, whereas antagonists and negative allosteric modulators promote wakefulness.
- Natural/endogenous and synthetic/exogenous compounds that modulate GABA availability and $GABA_A$ receptors are legion and, to the observant clinician, a reminder that GABA modulates a multitude and diversity of human behaviors.
- Leveraging this clinical experience and expanding knowledge of GABA's biology will point the way to novel treatments for disorders of the wake-sleep continuum.

GABA RECEPTOR ACTIVATION CAUSES NEURONAL INHIBITION

Sleep and wake are orchestrated by distributed neural networks and diverse signaling molecules.[1-4] Principal among these molecules is gamma-aminobutyric acid (GABA), which acts at ionic receptors ($GABA_ARs$), which are mostly located in synapses,[5] and metabotropic ($GABA_B$) receptors, which are mostly extrasynaptic.[6] Specialized GABA neurons promote sleep in both mammals and insects,[3,7,8] suggesting a strongly conserved function. GABA reduces the excitability of neurons either by increasing the flow of chloride ions into neurons via the $GABA_A$ receptors and directly causing hyperpolarization or, in the case of $GABA_B$ receptors, by triggering changes in second messengers (e.g., reducing cyclic adenosine monophosphate [cAMP] levels), causing in turn changes in kinase and phosphatase activity and thereby promoting the opening of certain potassium channels or inhibition of voltage-gated calcium channels.[9] $GABA_A$ receptor signaling works on the millisecond time scale; $GABA_B$ receptors signal on a scale of minutes.[9] Looking at this another way, GABAergic inhibition consists of two forms: fast synaptic inhibition through activation of synaptic $GABA_AR$ and slow inhibition through activation of extrasynaptic $GABA_AR$ and extrasynaptic $GABA_B$ receptors. In contrast to a short, spatially restricted action of phasic or synaptic inhibition, the slow inhibition mediates a prolonged and more continuous action in inhibitory signaling.[10] Both forms of inhibition, fast and slow, work together to set the overall activity level of nervous systems.

Drugs designed to enhance $GABA_AR$ function have a long history of clinical use for anesthesia and promoting sleep.[6,11,12] Drugs that are agonists and antagonists at the $GABA_B$ receptors are fewer but also have specialized applications in promoting sleep. Because small changes in GABA-mediated inhibition impart robust effects upon neuronal excitability, a wide range of compounds that modify GABA's availability and $GABA_A$ receptor sensitivity are relied upon clinically for anesthesia, to prevent seizures, and for the treatment of neuropsychiatric disorders affecting the sleep-wake continuum.[13]

GABA is required for the operation of all central brain and spinal cord circuitry. GABA neurons are ubiquitous in the brain, both as short-range interneurons, involved in local circuit modulation, as is often found in the neocortex and hippocampus,[14] and in long-range projections, which connect disparate brain regions with one another.[15] Some of these GABA long-range projections can induce non–rapid eye movement (NREM) sleep.[16-18] Consequently, $GABA_A$ and $GABA_B$ receptors are present in all regions of the brain and probably on all types of neurons and supporting elements such as astrocytes. Additionally, GABA can itself be coreleased with other transmitters—sometimes these are inhibitory peptides (e.g. somatostatin, neuropeptide Y, and galanin),[18] but GABA can also be coreleased with excitatory transmitters, such as glutamate, histamine, or acetylcholine[19-21] and also with gaseous transmitters such as nitric oxide.[22] This dual transmitter release is presumed to give neural circuits more processing capacity.

Using GABA agonist and positive $GABA_A$ receptor modulator drugs that promote NREM-like sleep or sedation comes with many side effects because the whole brain is affected by these drugs. Some of the GABA allosteric modulators are more powerful than others. Propofol, a selective positive allosteric modulator (PAM) at $GABA_A$ receptors, is so effective that although light doses of this drug induce an NREM-like sleep (sedation), higher doses administered intravenously potently suppress neuronal activity, including, in the worst-case scenario, brainstem neurons that drive respiration. Hence, under the supervision of an anesthetist, propofol is used for inducing and maintaining general anesthesia where the electroencephalogram (EEG) is essentially flat rather than displaying the delta waves characteristic of NREM sleep and the patient is unconscious, but not because they exhibit the physiological signatures of behavioral sleep.[11] This shows the continuum of effects along the wake–sleep–sedation–general anesthesia axis produced by potentiating the actions of GABA at $GABA_A$ receptors.

THE DISCOVERY OF THE GABAERGIC SYSTEM AND THE FIRST GABAERGIC SLEEPING MEDICATIONS

The history of GABA's discovery is inextricably interwoven with the evolution of neuroscience and the disciplines of neurology, psychiatry, and anesthesia in the 20th century, in addition to the subspecialty of sleep medicine. Noteworthy is the empirical manner in which expediency and serendipity in clinical practice have compelled mechanistic understanding. The first several decades of the 20th century ushered in the neuron doctrine. A logical extension of this doctrine was acknowledgment that neuropsychiatric disorders had an organic basis rooted in disturbances in communication between the fundamental building blocks of the nervous system, namely, nerve cells (i.e., neurons). These disorders being common, chronic, and disabling, collectively they posed a formidable burden to society and the fuel that ignited and sustained clinical and scientific inquiry. Knowledge of the biology responsible for balancing excitation and inhibition of the elements comprising the nervous system held out the promise of remedies for a panoply of human conditions. Principal among these was epilepsy, whose clinical spectrum—as elaborated upon by the Victorian neurologist Sir William Gowers in his influential 1903 book *The Borderland of Epilepsy*—shared alterations of consciousness and "some sleep symptoms" with vasovagal fainting, migraine, vertigo, and notably, narcolepsy in addition to hypersomnia.[23] Additional reinforcement to deciphering the neural networks and molecules underlying consciousness states were advances in general anesthesia rendered necessary by the rapid expansion of surgical procedures in this era.

Although nerve-mediated inhibition had been demonstrated in invertebrate preparations, the neurotransmitter(s) responsible remained a mystery until the discovery of GABA in 1950.[24] The mammalian brain was found to contain high GABA concentrations (viz., 1 mg/gram weight) compared with other organs, suggesting a unique role in modulating the function of the central nervous system (CNS).[25] An essential criterion for GABA's finally attaining classical neurotransmitter status was that its physiologic effects could be blocked or reversed specifically,[24] and in GABA's instance, this standard was fulfilled by picrotoxin—a poisonous compound first extracted from plants in 1812. Picrotoxin is—as are most GABA antagonists that mimic it—an analeptic (i.e., a cardiorespiratory *and* a CNS stimulant) that is proconvulsant (i.e., it provokes seizures) when present in sufficient amounts. The first GABAergic compound that gained widespread clinical use was an antagonist of GABA, namely, pentylenetetrazol (PTZ). Its discovery in the 1920s and subsequent medicinal uses were precisely because of its picrotoxin-like analeptic qualities. This predated GABA's discovery and mechanistic understanding by many decades, with PTZ's in vivo potency now known to correlate most strongly with its in vitro affinity for the picrotoxin binding site on receptors that mediate GABA's cellular effects.[26]

Thus the first drugs found to work on the GABA system for clinical use were the opposite of sleeping medications. The clinical use of PTZ notably predated the discovery and widespread use of amphetamines as analeptics in the 1930s and of barbiturates to counteract behavioral arousal—by what eventually came to be revealed was a result of their GABA-promoting effects. In the ensuing decades, PTZ, marketed under a variety of names (e.g., Cardiazol and Metrazol), found widespread use in clinical practice and experimental drug discovery. As a proconvulsant, PTZ replaced insulin shock therapy for psychiatric disorders for a time, whereas in the post–World War II era, it was marketed primarily for parenteral use to stimulate cardiorespiratory function[27] and, for many decades thereafter, aided in diagnosing epilepsy.[28] Clinical use extended to reversal of barbiturate overdoses and hastening recovery of respiration and consciousness from anesthesia.[29]

PTZ became extensively relied upon to screen drugs for anticonvulsant, antianxiety, sedating, "taming," and muscle "relaxation" properties in a variety of mammals, including nonhuman primates and humans. Compounds exhibiting such features were highly clinically desirable and, in the late 1950s, found to be common to the benzodiazepine (BZD) family of molecules because of advances in medical chemistry,[30] as well as to serendipity.[31] Only 2 to 3 years elapsed between initial pharmacologic testing and market introduction of chlordiazepoxide (Librium) and diazepam (Valium) in the early 1960s. Their efficacies—along with other novel psychotropics—proved monumental in shifting psychiatric practice from hospitals to the community and addressed enormous unmet clinical needs. By the early 1970s, Valium had become the best-selling drug in the United States and no fewer than five additional BZDs had been developed. Insights into the mechanisms underlying BZD's behavioral effects followed rapidly as a result of methodological advances in electrophysiology and molecular biology.[13,24,32]

GABA SYNTHESIS AND METABOLISM

GABA is a four-carbon, nonproteogenic amino acid.[33] The enzymes and transporters participating in its synthesis and recycling reinforce GABA's duality as a metabolite in cellular respiration *and* as a neurotransmitter key to maintaining balance in neuronal networks.[33] In order to make a "GABAergic" neuron, the cell must have a means of synthesizing GABA, requiring specialist enzymes and, once synthesized, have a means to package the GABA molecule into vesicles, which requires a transporter protein.

The GABA shunt is a closed loop that affords production and conservation of GABA (Figure 47.1). Glucose is the principal precursor for GABA production in vivo, although pyruvate and other amino acids can act as precursors. The first step in the GABA shunt is the transamination of α-ketoglutarate formed from glucose metabolism in the tricarboxylic acid (TCA) cycle by GABA 4-aminobutyrate aminotransferase (GABA-T), which is localized in the mitochondrial matrix, into l-glutamic acid/glutamate.[33] Cytosolic 65 and 67 kilodalton isoforms of glutamate decarboxylase (GAD), encoded by distinct genes *Gad2* and *Gad1,* respectively, expressed in GABAergic neurons (but not glutamatergic neurons) then catalyze the irreversible decarboxylation of glutamate to form GABA.[34,35] GABA-T can also be considered a degradative enzyme that catabolizes GABA to succinic semialdehyde (SSA) in the mitochondrial matrix followed by its oxidation to succinate by the concerted actions of GABA-T and succinic semialdehyde dehydrogenase (SSADH). Succinate then reenters the TCA cycle, completing the loop.

A potentially abundant source of GABA unique to primate brains is homocarnosine, an intracellular and extracellular dipeptide of GABA and histidine that accounts for 30% to 40% of the adult human brain's total GABA.[36] Although threefold to sixfold more abundant in adults than in infants and highly concentrated (0.3–1.6 mM) in GABAergic neurons with long-projecting axons as opposed to interneurons, little is known about the regulation of homocarnosine's synthesis, degradation by carnosine dipeptidase 1 (CNDP1) (Figure 47.1), and its potential contribution to GABA-mediated neural inhibition.

In axon terminals of presynaptic inhibitory GABAergic neurons, GABA is packaged into vesicles for synaptic release by way of the vesicular GABA transporter (vGAT), encoded by the solute carrier family 32 member 1 (*SLC32A1*) gene.[37] There are also suggested to be noncanonical ways by which neurons that express GAD, but not the vesicular transporter, can release GABA. For example, certain types of dopamine neurons leverage the vesicular monoamine transporter (vMAT) to package GABA into vesicles.[38] These cells do not seem to make their own GABA, but rather scavenge it from the surroundings, and then locally rerelease it.[38] But this is the exception and not the rule; most neurons that use GABA synthesize it themselves using GAD and then package it into synaptic vesicles via the vGAT.

Once released into the synaptic cleft, GABA's actions are terminated by high-affinity sodium- and chloride-dependent reuptake by way of the GABA transporter in presynaptic GABA neurons (GAT-1; encoded by the *SLC6A1* gene) and local

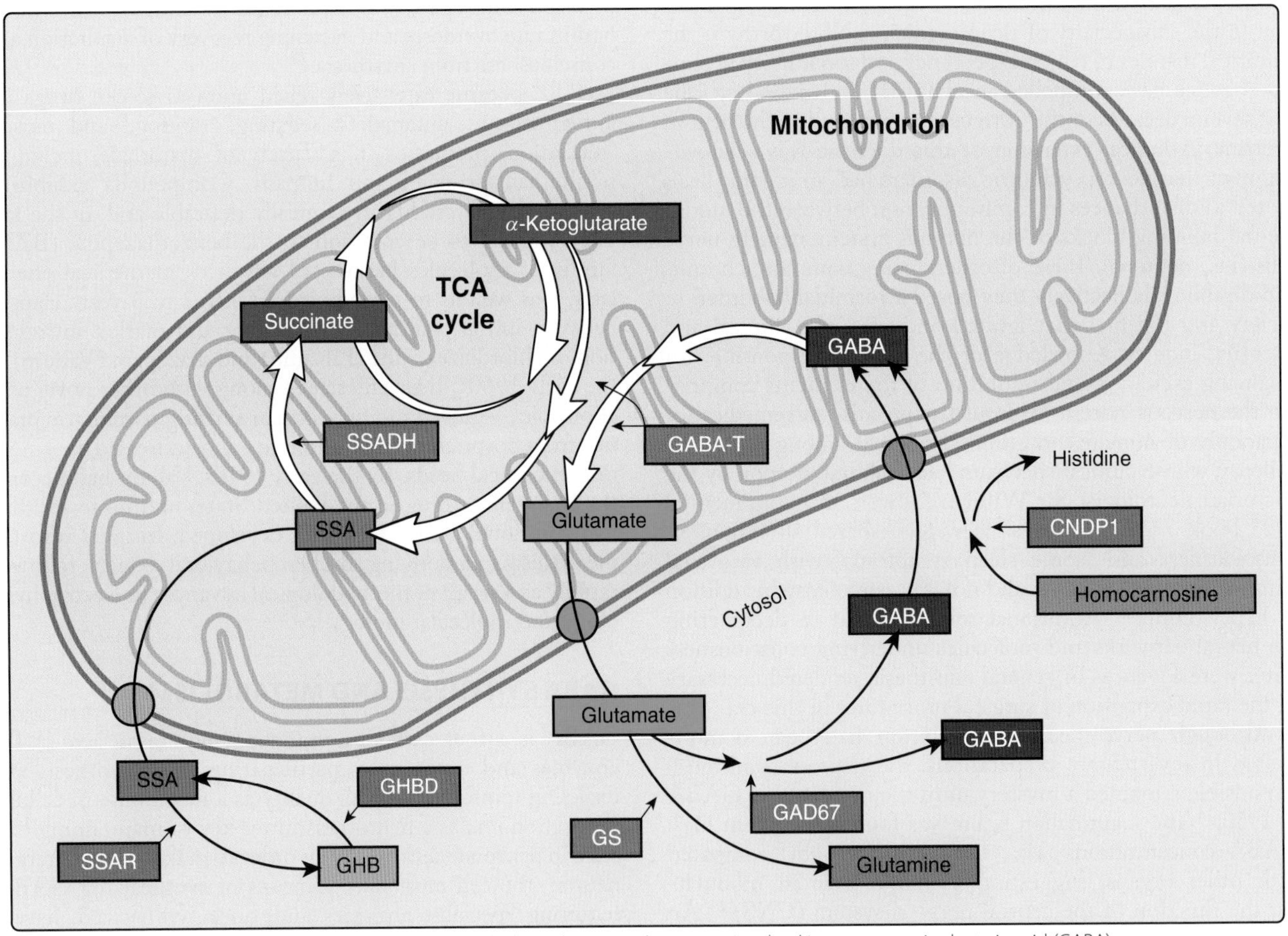

Figure 47.1 Schematic of the metabolic pathways and enzymes involved in gamma-aminobutyric acid (GABA) synthesis (see text for more details). GABA is synthesized in the cytosol from glutamate by the 65 and 67 kilodalton isoforms of the enzyme glutamate decarboxylase (GAD). A lesser-known and little-studied source accounting for nearly one-third of GABA in the primate brain derives from carnosine dipeptidase 1 (CNDP1)–mediated cleavage of homocarnosine. GABA then enters the mitochondrion, whereupon it is catalyzed by GABA-transaminase (GABA-T) to succinate semialdehyde (SSA). The vast majority of SSA is irreversibly oxidized by succinate semialdehyde dehydrogenase (SSADH) to succinate, which, by entering the tricarboxylic acid (TCA) cycle, effectively conserves GABA by allowing for reformation of its immediate precursor glutamate. Alternatively, GABA can be metabolized to gamma-hydroxybutyrate (GHB) by succinic semialdehyde reductase (SSAR). GABA can be recovered from GHB via its conversion back to SSA by cytosolic GHB dehydrogenase (GHBD). Unique to astrocytes is the enzyme glutamine synthetase (GS), which is critical to an intercellular shuttle that ensures an adequate supply of glutamate to GABAergic neurons in the form of glutamine (see also Figure 47.2).

astrocytes (GAT-3; encoded by the *SLC6A11* gene). GABA taken back up into nerve terminals can then be repackaged into vesicles for reutilization, but GABA in astrocytes is destined for metabolization to SSA and cannot be resynthesized in the glial compartment because astrocytes do not contain GAD. Ultimately, GABA is recovered in astrocytes by a circuitous route involving the TCA cycle referred to as the *glutamate/GABA-glutamine shuttle.*[39] Astrocytic GABA is converted to glutamate, which is then aminated to form glutamine by the enzyme glutamine synthetase (GS) that is present only in astrocytes (Figure 47.2). Glutamine is transferred, in turn, from astrocytes to neurons, where it is transformed back to glutamate by phosphate-activated glutaminase,[40] thereby replenishing excitatory and inhibitory neurotransmitter pools. Glutamine's efflux from the astrocytic compartment and neuronal uptake occur through members of the sodium-coupled neutral amino acid transporter (SNAT; *SLC38* gene) family, namely, the isoforms SNAT3 and SNAT5, and SNAT1 and SNAT2, respectively.

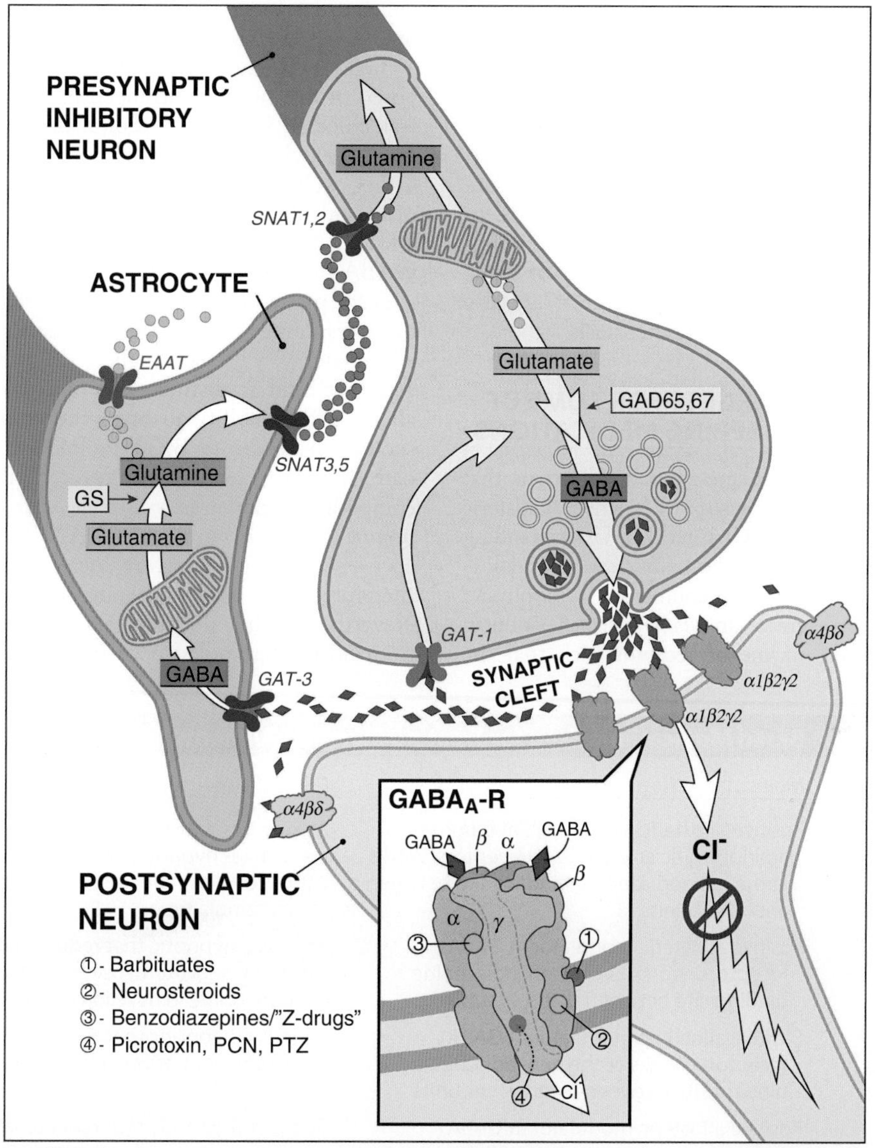

Figure 47.2 Illustration of the triumvirate of structures (i.e., presynaptic and postsynaptic neural elements and astrocytes) and molecular machinery governing gamma-aminobutyric acid (GABA) homeostasis and signaling at a canonical GABAergic synapse (see text for additional details). GABA released into the synapse *(red diamonds)* is shown here engaging $GABA_A$ receptors ($GABA_A$-R) that function as ligand-gated chloride channels. Receptors composed of α_1, β_2, and γ_2 subunits are the most abundant pentameric combination in the brain and responsible for fast, phasic inhibition, whereas extrasynaptic α_4, β, and δ receptors mediate a persistent, tonic inhibition of neural activity. Different combinations of subunits and synaptic trafficking and regional brain differences in expression of $GABA_A$Rs confer unique functional and behavioral properties. $GABA_A$-R subtypes differ in affinities not only for GABA but also for endogenous and exogenous compounds. These compounds, through their binding to unique sites of the receptor complex (1–3) or chloride channel pore (4), can allosterically activate, deactivate, or desensitize $GABA_A$-Rs. The actions of GABA are terminated by its reuptake by way of the GABA transporter in presynaptic GABA neurons (GAT-1) and local astrocytes (GAT-3). The former mechanism allows for vesicular repackaging and reutilization of GABA, whereas astrocytes convert GABA to glutamate. Extracellular glutamate taken up by way of excitatory amino acid transporters (EAATs) is an additional source for astrocytes. Amination of glutamate to form glutamine by the enzyme glutamine synthetase (GS) is critical in replenishing excitatory and inhibitory neurotransmitter pools because of glutamine's efflux from astrocytes and uptake by neurons via sodium-coupled neutral amino acid transporter isoforms SNAT3 and SNAT5, and SNAT1 and SNAT2, respectively. PCN, Penicillin; PTZ, pentylenetetrazol.

The GABA shunt and glutamate/GABA-glutamine shuttle are critical to balancing the needs for cellular energy originating in the TCA cycle with the state of synaptic excitability. The relative importance of the GABA shunt is substantial. The TCA cycle in GABAergic neurons alone, for example, has been estimated to account for one-third of the whole brain's yield of energy derived from TCA cycle activity.[41] Local astrocytes and excitatory glutamatergic synapses are critical to GABA homeostasis.

Several enzymes necessary for sustaining GABA homeostasis are differentially distributed among neurons and astrocytes. Besides GS, neurons lack pyruvate carboxylase, whose role in catalyzing the first step in gluconeogenesis (i.e., pyruvate oxidation) links glycolysis to the TCA cycle. Thus neurons cannot synthesize the neurotransmitters glutamate and GABA from glucose de novo. This highlights their reliance upon astrocytes as a source for precursors that replenish TCA-cycle intermediates required for glutamate (from α-ketoglutarate) and GABA (from glutamate) synthesis. In short, astrocytes are glutamate producers for neurons[42]; thus reuptake of synaptic glutamate by astrocytes by way of excitatory amino acid transporters (EAATs) (Figure 47.2) also proves critical to GABA synthesis and homeostasis.

GABA$_A$ RECEPTORS ARE TARGETS FOR SOME OF THE MOST IMPORTANT SLEEPING MEDICATIONS

Most of our current sleeping and anesthetic medications that work on GABA$_A$ receptors are what are termed "allosteric modulators" (Table 47.1; see also Chapter 53). Understanding allostery is essential to appreciate how many sleeping medications work. Allostery is a universal phenomenon in biophysics whereby a small molecule—termed an *allosteric ligand*—induces a structural change in an enzyme or receptor such that the receptor/protein site where, for example, the neurotransmitter binds, becomes more or less active. Allostery was originally postulated and understood for the manner by which metabolites regulate transcription factors in bacteria (the *lac* operon)[43] and then, for the neuroscience field, through studies on the nicotinic acetylcholine receptor.[44] The nicotinic receptor has been referred to as the prototypical "allosteric machine,"[44] but this description applies even more so to GABA$_A$ receptors. Even before the GABA$_A$ receptor was purified and cloned, it was understood that this was a richly allosteric protein complex with multiple sites at which drugs, independent of the GABA binding site, increased or decreased GABA's binding to the receptor complex.[45-48]

GABA$_A$Rs are heteromeric membrane proteins composed of five subunits arranged in a pentamer around a central chloride ion pore.[49] Some drugs, including picrotoxin and PTZ, block the channel pore (see inset of Figure 47.2). Other well-known drugs are GABA agonists or antagonists and bind at the GABA site, including muscimol and THIP/gaboxadol (agonists) and bicuculline (an antagonist). GABA$_A$ receptor complexes have a large number of binding sites for many important classes of drugs such as BZDs, barbiturates, some steroids, and anesthetics such as propofol and etomidate.[11,48,50-53] All of these drugs are allosteric modulators that bind at distinct sites on the receptor complex and alter GABA's ability to open the chloride channel. PAMs, such as diazepam (a BZD), zolpidem, propofol, and etomidate, increase GABA's efficacy to differing extents. Other compounds, known as *inverse agonists at the allosteric sites* or *negative allosteric modulators* (NAMs), decrease GABA's efficacy—such drugs therefore increase excitability and would therefore not be used as sleeping medications or in anesthesia. Nevertheless, they do have specific clinical uses, for example, to treat hypersomnolence, when patients need to be woken up

Table 47.1 GABAergic-Based Medications Used for Treating Sleeping Ailments (Insomnia or Hypersomnia)

Drug	Molecular Action	Clinical Use
Benzodiazepines (e.g., diazepam [Valium]; clonazepam [Klonopin])	Positive allosteric modulators at gamma-aminobutyric acid (GABA)$_A$ receptors. Works at the benzodiazepine binding site between α and γ$_2$ subunits.	Anxiolytics, muscle relaxants, anticonvulsants, and sedative- hypnotics with longer duration of effect (≥6–20 hr half-life). Used often to treat many parasomnia types.
Zolpidem (an imidazopyridine)	Positive allosteric modulator at GABA$_A$ receptors. Works at the benzodiazepine binding site between α and γ$_2$ subunits	Sedative-hypnotic that reduces latency to sleep. Meant for short-term use (several weeks) and is intermediate in duration of action (2–4 hr half-life).
Zaleplon (a pyrazolopyrimidine)	Positive allosteric modulator at GABA$_A$ receptors. Works at the benzodiazepine binding site between α and γ$_2$ subunits.	Sedative-hypnotic that reduces latency to sleep with very short duration of action (≈1 hr half-life).
Zopiclone (a cyclopyrrolone)	Positive allosteric modulator at GABA$_A$ receptors. Works at the benzodiazepine binding site between α and γ$_2$ subunits.	Sedative-hypnotic that reduces latency to sleep with longer duration of action (6–8 hr half-life).
Flumazenil (Ro 15-1788)	A competitive antagonist at the benzodiazepine binding site of GABA$_A$ receptors and partial agonist at higher concentrations.	Treating excessive daytime sleepiness and hypersomnia in nonhypocretin-deficient central disorders of hypersomnolence. Extremely short half-life limits bioavailability, requiring compounded formulations.
Clarithromycin (a macrolide antibiotic)	A negative allosteric modulator at GABA$_A$ receptors.	Treating excessive daytime sleepiness and hypersomnia in nonhypocretin-deficient central disorders of hypersomnolence. Commonly used to treat lung and ear/nose/throat infections and bacterial overgrowth of the stomach.
GHB (gamma-hydroxybutyrate)	Unclear mechanism of action. Agonist at GABA$_B$ receptors and other targets. Can be metabolically converted to GABA (Figure 47.1).	Reduces daytime sleepiness and cataplexy in narcolepsy. Dosed at sleep onset and several hours later. Several hours half-life.

(see later). For example, some antibiotics such as clarithromycin are NAMs at $GABA_A$ receptors and increase wakefulness (see the Endogenous $GABA_A$ Receptor Ligands for Treating Hypersomnolence section).[54] Antagonists such as flumazenil (Ro 15-1788) block the action of agonists and inverse agonists at the benzodiazepine binding site, but by themselves, have little ability to change GABA's efficacy.[50,51]

The genes encoding $GABA_A$ receptor subunits are in the same superfamily as those encoding the nicotinic acetylcholine, glycine, and 5-hydroxytryptamine (serotonin; 5-HT)$_3$ receptor subunits, but in a different gene superfamily from that encoding mammalian ionotropic glutamate receptor subunits. Over the years, much knowledge has been gleaned about how the $GABA_A$ receptor works in principle from studying the nicotinic acetylcholine receptor.[55] Binding of two molecules of GABA to the extracellular part of the receptor complex triggers a conformational change in the receptor such that the chloride channel opens and chloride ions flow down their electrochemical gradient into the cell, making the intracellular compartment of the neuron more negative and less likely to fire an action potential. In mammals, there are six α subunits, three β subunits, three γ subunits, a δ subunit, and ε and θ subunits, all encoded by distinct genes.[6,56] These genes are differentially transcribed throughout the immense diversity of neurons,[57-59] and the subunits assemble with complex rules that are still being discovered.[60] Because of the large number of subunit combinations, the number of subtypes of the $GABA_A$ receptor in the brain is unknown.[57] The α_1, β, γ_2 subunit combination is the most abundant type of $GABA_A$ receptor, followed by receptors with α2 and α3 subunits and β and γ2 subunits.[61] The differential roles of the three β subunits are unknown.

Recently the atomic structure was determined for the α1β3γ2 $GABA_A$ receptor subtype.[49,62] The structures of all other $GABA_A$ receptor complexes are expected to be similar. The excitement surrounding the revelation of these new structural details is that we can now see with great detail which amino acids and elements within the receptor subunits comprise the different allosteric modulator binding domains. As illustrated in the inset to Figure 47.2, GABA (and other GABA agonists) bind at the interfaces between the α and β subunits.[62] PAMs such as zolpidem and diazepam bind at the interface between the α and γ2 subunits.[49] Other allosteric drugs, such as neurosteroids and propofol, bind elsewhere in the receptor in various parts of the transmembrane domains.[63,64]

Z DRUGS

All drugs that potentiate GABA receptor function are likely to be sedatives,[65,66] even if there are more or less unwelcome side effects. BZDs used to be the main drugs prescribed to hasten sleep onset and to maintain sleep. The newer "Z drugs" (e.g., zolpidem, zopiclone, eszopiclone, and zaleplon—all in different chemical classes—for example, zolpidem is an imidazopyridine) introduced in the late 1980s through the millennium and still in widespread clinical use are PAMs at the $GABA_A$ receptor BZD binding site (Table 47.1). They are much less potent anxiolytics, muscle relaxants, and anticonvulsants compared with BZDs. These drugs all induce an NREM-like sleep as measured by the EEG, respiratory depression, and muscle relaxation.[66] BZDs and the Z drugs all require $GABA_A$ receptors that contain a γ2 subunit[67,68] and bind at the interface between the α and γ2 subunits[51,69] (Figure 47.3). As mentioned previously, these drugs allosterically potentiate the chloride current activated by GABA by altering the biophysics of the receptor complex (Figure 47.3).

BZDs and the Z drugs all reduce the latency to NREM sleep, increase sleep continuity, tend to increase total sleep time, delay the onset of rapid eye movement (REM) sleep and decrease its amount, and subtly change the power characteristics of the EEG spectrum so that it does not quite resemble natural NREM sleep (BZD/Z drug–induced NREM sleep has lower EEG power), and on occasion, contribute to undesirable residual effects (e.g., sedation, cognitive impairment, and amnesia).[12,65] Thus the sleep induced by BZDs and Z drugs is not quite the same as natural NREM sleep and is probably best described as "NREM-like." A reduction in EEG power in NREM sleep in the delta frequency range has been interpreted by some to suggest that the sleep is less "deep" relative to natural sleep or that the sleep is less restorative. Z drugs also increase spindle frequency in the EEG.[12,70]

Among the Z drugs, zolpidem is highly popular for treating primary insomnia[66,71] (Table 47.1). Compared with most BZDs, zolpidem is preferred, given its faster onset of action, more rapid degradation, and clearance, which renders it less prone to daytime carry-over effects, and fewer "off-target" side effects because of its specificity for fewer $GABA_A$ receptor subtypes (viz., zolpidem preferentially potentiates the α1βγ2, α2βγ2, α3βγ2 subunit-containing receptors)[67,68,72] (Figure 47.3). Although zolpidem is often described as an α1-selective ligand, it is also active in vitro at α2- and α3-containing receptors[67,68] at concentrations typically achieved with standard dosing (e.g., zolpidem will also target the α2βγ2 and α3βγ2 $GABA_A$ receptors). Indeed, transgenic mice engineered with a point mutation that renders the α1 subunit unable to bind zolpidem can still be sedated by zolpidem,[73] suggesting that zolpidem is also active at the α2- and α3-containing $GABA_A$ receptors to affect sleep. In fact, some wake-promoting neurons, such as the histamine neurons in the hypothalamus, express both α1βγ2 and α2βγ2 receptors, and consequently, zolpidem is thought to increase the inhibitory GABAergic input onto histamine neurons (among many other targets) to help induce NREM sleep[72] (Figure 47.3). Nevertheless, although $GABA_A$ receptors occur in many brain regions and thus affect most aspects of brain function, sleep usually ensues quickly after zolpidem ingestion before any side effects because of the inhibition of other brain circuits can become manifest.

All of the BZDs and Z drugs may lead to the development of tolerance and dependence and tend to cause rebound insomnia if they are discontinued abruptly.[12] It has been hypothesized that rebound insomnia results from downregulation of $GABA_A$ receptors on sleep-promoting neurons because of chronic use.[4]

NEW IMPROVED SLEEPING MEDICATIONS THAT WORK ON SPECIFIC $GABA_A$ RECEPTOR SUBTYPES?

The medications that work on $GABA_A$ receptors to induce sleep, or indeed, to induce any other desired effect, were discovered by serendipity and without a priori knowledge of $GABA_A$ receptor structure or function.[31,65] For years, it has been hoped that drugs could be developed that are specific for $GABA_A$ receptors of a unique subunit composition and function. Theoretically, this would mean more selective medications for treating sleep onset versus sleep maintenance insomnia or for treating anxiety or pain without causing

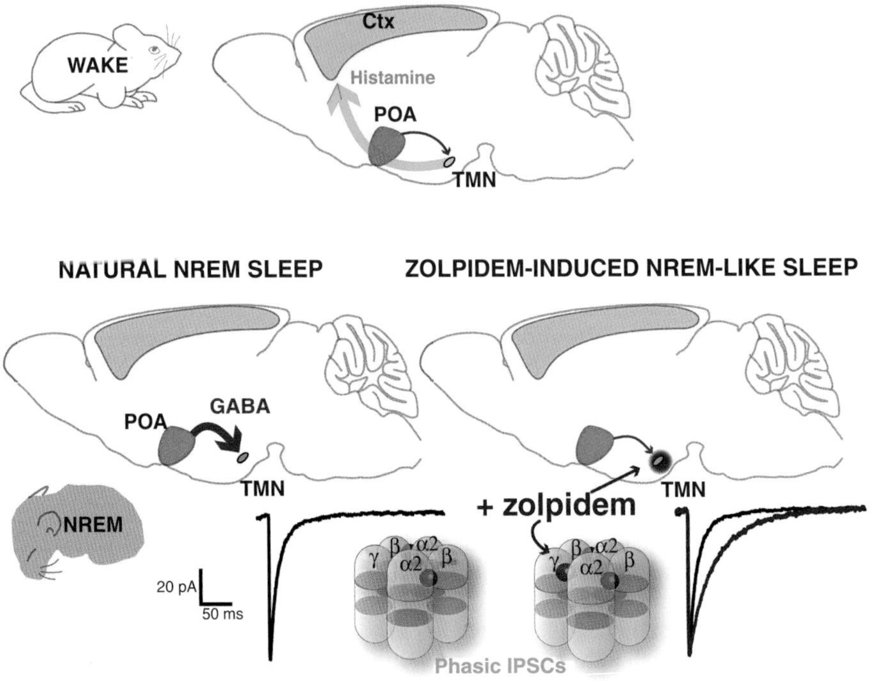

Figure 47.3 Schematic of how sleep medications such as zolpidem that act at gamma-aminobutyric acid $(GABA)_A$ receptors reduce the activity of wake-promoting neurons, such as histamine neurons, and induce a NREM-like state. The concept is shown here for mice but is expected to be the same in humans. In the awake state, wake-active and wake-promoting neurons, such as histamine neurons in the posterior hypothalamus *(TMN area)*, release histamine via their ascending axons widely in the brain, for example, into the neocortex. Other neurons such as noradrenaline and the orexin/hypocretin neurons *(not shown here)* would also be similarly active and wake-promoting. During NREM sleep, GABA-projecting neurons in the preoptic area of the hypothalamus (POA) are active and release GABA via long-range projections onto histamine neurons in the TMN and onto the orexin and other wake-promoting neurons[2] *(thick red arrow)*. As a result of this inhibition, histamine neurons fire less, or not at all, and levels of the wake-promoting modulator histamine decline in the neocortex and other regions. Even during wake, however, there is a small active GABA component from the POA onto the histamine neurons *(thin red arrow)*, and this weak GABA drive is exploited by zolpidem. Zolpidem, a positive allosteric modulator at $GABA_A$ receptors, is not active unless GABA is bound to the receptor. On ingestion of zolpidem, the drug acts to potentiate the GABA drive onto, for example, histamine neurons and effectively mimics the natural situation of increased GABA drive during NREM sleep. The $GABA_A$ receptors with their five subunits, in this case 2, are shown schematically. GABA *(orange spheres)* binds at the interface between the subunits; two molecules bind each receptor. Binding causes a shape change in the receptor, and Cl^- ions flow through the channel into the cell to hyperpolarize it. This is shown as the black hyperpolarizing trace on the bottom left. This trace was recorded from with an electrode placed on the histamine neurons, a technique known as patch-clamping.[72] In the presence of zolpidem *(purple spheres)*, which binds between the subunits, GABA can open the chloride channel more effectively and more chloride ions can flow through the $GABA_A$ receptor into the cell *(purple trace)*, a phenomenon known as allosteric potentiation. Ctx, Neocortex; IPSCs, inhibitory postsynaptic currents; TMN, tuberomammillary nucleus. (Modified from Brickley SG, Franks NP, Wisden W. Modulation of GABA-A receptor function and sleep. *Current Opinion in Physiology*. 2018;2:51-47.).

sedation.[74] However, this dream has not materialized to date. In seminal studies carried out nearly 20 years ago, for example, α1,2,3and 5 subunit point mutation (i.e., "knock-in") mice suggested that different α subunits in αβγ2 combinations conferred some behavioral specificity compared with the diversity of behaviors affected by BZDs.[75,76] Based on this work, a segregation of distinct behaviors elicited by potentiating BZDs with different $GABA_A$ receptor subtypes was posited: selectively potentiating α1-containing receptors mediated sedation (as assessed by lack of movement) and anterograde amnesia,[75,77] whereas potentiating α2- and α5-containing ones produced anxiolysis.[76,78] These studies were replete with interpretative confounds, at least from a sleep/sedation point of view. One problem was that without the benefit of simultaneous EEG assessments, the tools employed were insufficient to differentiate sedation from akinesia, abulia, or quiet wakefulness and, conversely, anxiolysis from drowsiness. A second complication was that these constructs ignored the consideration that $GABA_A$ receptor subtypes might be coexpressed in the same neurons.[72] We now know that there is no example of the expression of a single $GABA_A$ receptor subtype within an anatomically and functionally defined circuit. It is even less likely that this would be the case in larger neural networks. Nevertheless, pharmacologists will soon be in a position, based on structural knowledge of the receptor, to design drugs that work on specific αβγ2 $GABA_A$ receptor complexes.[62,74]

In addition to the genes that encode the αβγ2 type receptors, there are some more rarely expressed $GABA_A$ receptor subunit genes: γ1, γ3, δ, ε, and θ.[6] These subunits may take the place of the γ2 subunits in the $GABA_A$ receptor pentamer and pair up with particular α and β subunits. So, for example, the δ subunit pairs with the α4 and β2 subunit in thalamic neurons. The γ subunits have binding sites for proteins that ensure trafficking of the $GABA_A$ receptor to the synaptic cleft to allow for more efficient inhibition, whereas the δ subunit lacks synapse-anchoring signals so that receptors containing δ subunits tend to localize extrasynaptically, where they mediate tonic inhibition (Figure 47.2).

The α4β8 receptors were found to be uniquely activated by a direct GABA agonist, THIP (later rebranded as gaboxadol). This drug had been around for decades and has been tested in many types of ailments. In early trials, patients reported side effects of sleep and, indeed, only at a rather late stage did researchers note that it produced robust increases in NREM sleep. This drug was thus investigated as a promising new sleeping medication,[6,79] but was abandoned at a late stage in human clinical trials because of a lack of consistent results.[80]

Other than gaboxadol, the field is left with considering whether to develop drugs for the $GABA_A$ receptors that contain the γ1, ε, and θ subunits. Intriguingly, these subunits are expressed rather selectively in hypothalamic and brainstem circuits,[6,81,82] some of which are well-established to regulate arousal (e.g., locus coeruleus). However, there seems to be little enthusiasm to investigate these rare types of the $GABA_A$ receptor. Nevertheless, the receptors may be present on key nodal points of circuitry where arousal-promoting neurons project widely throughout the brain and thus influence many brain regions, such that potentiating these receptors on such nodal neurons could have large influences on vigilance state.[72,83,84] Because the receptors with γ1, ε, and θ subunits are rarely expressed beyond the hypothalamus and brainstem, any drugs might have fewer side effects.

ENDOGENOUS $GABA_A$ RECEPTOR LIGANDS FOR TREATING HYPERSOMNOLENCE

When the BZ binding site was first identified,[85] the nearly coincidental discovery that enkephalins and endorphins were naturally occurring substrates for opioid receptor binding sites in the CNS gave birth to a notion that endogenous ligands could bind to $GABA_A$ receptors and affect their function.[86] Such hypothetical ligands have been termed *endozepines*.[87,88] Nowadays, however, the best established endogenous allosteric ligands for $GABA_A$ receptors with clinical and therapeutic implications are not BZDs, but steroids.[48,52,53] Pregnanolone and allopregnanolone, in particular, have been recognized for some time to have potent sedative, anesthetic, and anticonvulsant properties that reflect preferential actions at extrasynaptic $GABA_A$Rs containing δ subunits that mediate tonic inhibition, are more sensitive to GABA, and exhibit slower ion channel kinetics and weaker desensitization[89,90] (Figure 47.2). Neurosteroid-related potentiation of phasic inhibition also occurs and is conveyed by their binding to a transmembrane domain in the α subunits.[91] Other neurosteroids minimally affect intrinsic GABA signaling, but are able to inhibit neurosteroid PAMs.

Given the diversity in $GABA_A$ receptor subunit composition, differential expression in different brain regions, and dual PAM and NAM effects, the relevance of exogenous and circulating steroid hormones and neurosteroids synthesized within the brain to clinical sleep medicine remains ill defined. Nonetheless, brexanolone (allopregnanolone) has received US Food and Drug Administration (FDA) approval for postpartum depression, and indications for its wider use in the treatment of mood disorders and anxiety are being explored.[90] Excessive sleepiness is not an unexpected adverse effect, given brexanolone's mechanism of action, but details of its effects upon sleep and sleep architecture are unknown. Endogenous modulation of $GABA_A$ receptors in the thalamus is detectable in brain slice preparations depleted of allopregnanolone by focal application of the 5α-reductase inhibitor finasteride[92]; however, the physiologic effects differ among thalamic regions. A similarly motivated study exploring finasteride's effects upon profiles of thalamocortical activity in humans failed to observe hypothesized changes in sleep microarchitecture (e.g., spindle frequency and EEG power spectrum).[93]

Considerable mechanistic insights into two additional naturally occurring molecules that modulate $GABA_A$ receptor currents have been advanced. Both molecules have been referred to as endozepines because of their close association with pharmacologic or behavioral features of the BZD-binding site on $GABA_A$ receptors.[87] Closer inspection, however, reveals that the term "endozepines" for these molecules is not entirely deserved. The first molecule is a large peptide expressed in neurons and astrocytes whose original name is an accurate descriptor (viz., diazepam binding inhibitor [DBI]).[94,95] Behaviors associated with exogenous administration of DBI or its peptide fragments promote a heightened state of neural excitability, as might be expected from a NAM as opposed to an endozepine. The majority of evidence confirms that cleavage products of DBI are predominantly NAMs at $GABA_A$ receptors, whereas PAM actions, as might be expected of a genuine endozepine, have been more difficult to demonstrate.[88] DBI can exhibit opposing effects at $GABA_A$ receptors expressed in functionally distinct divisions of the thalamus.[96] DBI released from astrocytes, for example, can enhance $GABA_A$ receptor currents through α3βγ2type-$GABA_A$ receptors on reticular thalamic neurons[96]—an effect attenuated by flumazenil, a competitive antagonist at the BZD-binding domain. DBI has since been discovered to be identical to acyl-CoA binding protein (ACBP), a highly conserved, 90–amino acid protein that binds and traffics medium- and long-chain acyl-CoA esters. Interestingly, ACBP release is stimulated by hunger and is orexigenic, suggesting that its systemic behavioral effects are more in line with a state of wakefulness, which is not at all expected if it were genuinely BZD-like.[97]

A second endozepine-like molecule has been implicated in the cause of central disorders of hypersomnolence wherein daytime sleepiness persists despite prodigious amounts of nonrestorative sleep that can be unyielding to wake-promoting drugs that the FDA has approved to treat narcolepsy type 1. Cerebrospinal fluid (CSF) from many of these patients reveals evidence for a small peptide that acts as a PAM in enhancing GABA's action at a variety of αβ2γ2 receptors.[98,99] This bioactivity is reversed in vitro by flumazenil, suggesting that it is predicated on the integrity of the canonical $GABA_A$ receptor BZD-binding domain. Yet modest enhancement is still present in $GABA_A$ receptors genetically engineered to be insensitive to BZDs, and CSF does not competitively displace BZDs from human brain tissue as might be expected of a genuine "endozepine." These observations, nonetheless, compelled an unblinded proof-of-principle study that documented improvement in subjective and objective measures of vigilance in a small group of patients challenged with intravenous flumazenil.[98] These observations prompted reformulation of flumazenil for wider open-label use in this patient population for which it has proved beneficial.[100] The beneficial effects of flumazenil appear unique to this patient population and may reflect antagonism of an endozepine-like substance because it is not alerting in nonsleepy controls,[101] and flumazenil lacks major intrinsic pharmacologic or behavioral activity per se.[102] Flumazenil, for example, has modest wake promotion—and inhibits slow-wave sleep—with sleep deprivation[103-105] and after intravenous delivery during normal NREM sleep,[106] suggesting that $GABA_A$ receptors and related intrinsic signaling factors interact with sleep homeostatic mechanisms in yet-to-be-determined ways.

Scant attention has been paid to the strategy of increasing neuronal excitability by targeting $GABA_A$ receptors with the intent of improving vigilance, reversing hypersomnolence/sleep, or hastening recovery from anesthesia. Alternative strategies favor enhancement of monoaminergic signaling in part out of familiarity, as well as for fear that $GABA_A$ receptor antagonism might present a narrow therapeutic window fraught with potentially serious adverse events such as anxiety, insomnia, hypomania, delirium, and seizures. Nonetheless, there is an untapped potential for leveraging $GABA_A$ receptor antagonism as a means to treat hypersomnolence.[107] A single case whose profound hypersomnia that resolved with daily flumazenil use, for example, experienced a dramatic metamorphosis to insomnia upon being prescribed the macrolide antibiotic clarithromycin for an intercurrent bronchitis. This iatrogenic effect of clarithromycin suggested its agonistic interaction with flumazenil, thereby magnifying flumazenil's genuine therapeutic benefit (Table 47.1). Clarithromycin contributes to hyperexcitability in single neurons because it is a dose-dependent NAM of $GABA_A$ receptors,[54] which in this clinical scenario, seemingly potentiated flumazenil's blockade of a putative endozepine-like peptide. Among commonly prescribed antibiotics, clarithromycin has one of the highest reported rates of insomnia, and it has long been associated with agitation, mania, and delirium[108] (Clarithromycin Prescribing Information [FDA]. www.accessdata.fda.gov/drugsatfda_docs/label/2013/050662s052lbl.pdf). Taken together, this knowledge informed open-label and placebo-controlled[109] studies demonstrating clarithromycin's effectiveness in treating refractory hypersomnolence (Table 47.1), and its more limited effects in ameliorating the disabling periodic hypersomnia that is the core feature of Kleine-Levin syndrome (KLS).[110,111]

There are a number of unique classes of antibiotics and other drugs whose off-target effects include acting as NAMs or antagonists at $GABA_A$ receptors. Notable examples include fluoroquinolone antibiotics (which act as NAMs),[112,113] penicillin and PTZ (which act as noncompetitive antagonists that block the $GABA_A$ receptor channel pore; Figure 47.2),[114] and the hemostatic agent tranexamic acid (a competitive antagonist).[115] Heightened arousal states accompanying routine use of fluoroquinolones were so notable upon their introduction, particularly when coadministered with nonsteroidal antiinflammatory drugs, that it yielded a negative study of ciprofloxacin's potential benefits upon subjective and objective (electroencephalographic, evoked potential, and reaction time) metrics of arousal in a small number of healthy controls.[116] Inclusion of PTZ on the World Anti-Doping Agency list of performance-enhancing stimulants[117] and its activating effects upon the EEG in narcolepsy type 1 speak further to the potential benefits of $GABA_A$ receptor antagonism in hypersomnolence disorders.[118]

One final research avenue to consider in treating hypersomnias with GABA signaling is that a small number of GABA pathways are selectively wake-promoting, and such pathways could be artificially stimulated, at least in principle. In particular, GABA neurons in the lateral hypothalamus send projections to inhibitory GABA neurons in the reticular thalamus and sleep-promoting GABAergic neurons in the preoptic hypothalamus.[119,120] Disinhibition occurs when a GABAergic neuron inhibits a postsynaptic GABA cell, with the net effect being excitation. Activation of the relevant GABAergic neurons in the lateral hypothalamus specifically promotes awakening from NREM sleep and even activates the neocortex during general anesthesia.[119,120]

$GABA_B$ RECEPTORS AND GAMMA-HYDROXYBUTYRATE: REDUCING DAYTIME SLEEPINESS AND CATAPLEXY IN NARCOLEPSY

$GABA_B$ receptors are essential for brain function. These receptors are G-protein–coupled metabotropic receptors whose actions are conveyed by second messenger cascades.[9,121] Their activation therefore produces a chronic form of inhibition (tonic inhibition) that is functionally similar to that produced by the $GABA_A$ receptors. The $GABA_B$ receptors are located on both presynaptic terminals, serving as inhibitory autoreceptors and heteroreceptors to reduce GABA or other neurotransmitter release, in addition to many locations outside the synapse. $GABA_B$ receptor activation opens various potassium channels and inhibits voltage-gated calcium channels. Unlike synaptic $GABA_A$ receptors, which faithfully transmit signals conveying temporal details, $GABA_B$ receptor signaling is not temporally locked to GABA release—the receptors set the overall level of excitability at the network level. Mice engineered to lack $GABA_B$ receptors have severe epilepsy and fragmented sleep.[122] In the fruit fly *Drosophila,* $GABA_B$ receptors also help maintain sleep.[7]

$GABA_B$ receptors have little molecular diversity—there are only two subtypes of receptor, equally widely expressed in the brain.[9] Consequently, for $GABA_B$ receptor drugs, there is probably little promise of useful drugs that will only induce sleep—there will always be many side effects with $GABA_B$ drugs. Nevertheless, $GABA_B$ drugs still have specialist applications in neurology. The most well-known $GABA_B$ agonist is baclofen, used for treating muscle spasticity. A side effect of baclofen is sleepiness. There is also interest in one of the molecules involved in GABA metabolism, gamma-hydroxybutyrate (GHB), that could be an agonist at $GABA_B$ receptors.[123]

As discussed earlier, there is an alternative to the GABA shunt for GABA degradation whereby succinic semialdehyde reductase (SSAR) mediates synthesis of GHB[124] (Figure 47.1). Whereas a neuromodulatory function for endogenous GHB remains unclear, exogenous delivery, depending on dose, induces general anesthesia, increases NREM sleep, and ameliorates daytime sleepiness and cataplexy in narcolepsy.[125] GHB is simultaneously a metabolite of, and potential precursor for, GABA in that it can be converted back to SSA via GHB dehydrogenase (GHBD) (Figure 47.1). Because this conversion proceeds at a several log-fold lower rate than the rapidity at which SSA is oxidized to succinate, factors that regulate these enzymes will, in turn, influence endogenous levels of GHB and the magnitude and duration of exogenous GHB-related behaviors.[126]

Unfortunately, there remains a muddied picture of how GHB acts in the brain, and researchers cannot yet agree on its mechanism(s) of action,[127] and GHB is a compound that may well have multiple targets. A further challenge is that when the drug is given, it can be readily metabolized to GABA (Figure 47.1). The generation of this additional GABA complicates interpretation of in vivo results because $GABA_A$ and

$GABA_B$ receptors may well be activated by this additional GABA. It remains important to understand GHB's action, as this is a drug widely relied upon to reduce daytime sleepiness and cataplexy in narcolepsy.[128]

HERITABLE AND ACQUIRED CONDITIONS THAT MODULATE SYSTEMIC GABA OR GHB AVAILABILITY IN HUMANS INFLUENCE SLEEP

Several heritable and acquired conditions that modulate systemic GABA or GHB availability and $GABA_A$ receptor signaling in humans reinforce GABA's central role in maintaining normal states of consciousness, including sleep. This function is highly conserved in nature, as evidenced by validating findings in species spanning the spectrum from fruit flies (*Drosophila*) to humans. The most common clinical disorder affecting GABA metabolism is SSADH deficiency, which exhibits autosomal recessive inheritance and chronic elevations of endogenous GABA and GHB (Figure 47.1).[129,130] Associated polysomnographic/multiple sleep latency testing reveals sleep that is highly efficient with a slightly greater proportion of slow-wave sleep and a marked suppression of the onset and total amount of REM sleep, along with daytime hypersomnolence.[131,132] A hyper-GABAergic state resulting from GABA excess also results from inherited deficiency of GABA-T (Figure 47.1). This condition is extremely rare in humans, possibly because it is lethal,[129] and has been investigated by pharmacologic inhibition of GABA-T and genetic manipulation in *Drosophila* to reveal the impact of GABA-T deficiency on sleep.[133] The mechanism of action of the antiepileptic drug vigabatrin is via GABA-T inhibition, and limited data in people with epilepsy suggest that it increases NREM sleep while suppressing REM sleep,[134] an effect mimicked in a rat model of epilepsy.[135] In *Drosophila*, the loss of GABA-T increases sleep, which can be rescued by restoring it in neurons, and particularly in glia.[133,136]

Tiagabine is an antiepileptic that increases synaptic GABA by an alternative means, via selective inhibition of GABA reuptake, and it dose-dependently increases sleep maintenance and NREM sleep in humans.[137] Conversely, human conditions associated with antibodies directed against GAD, the synthetic enzyme for GABA, have been anecdotally associated with recurrent insomnia.[138] Insomnia has also been associated with heritable missense mutations in the β_3 subunit of the $GABA_A$ receptor that produce a more rapid deactivation of GABA-induced inhibitory currents.[139]

CLINICAL PEARL

A recurrent hypersomnia that emerges in concert with the menstrual cycle has been codified in older clinical taxonomies as "menstrual linked hypersomnia" and is thought to reflect actions of naturally occurring, spontaneous fluctuations in neurosteroids upon neural circuits influencing sleep.[140] A potential causal role for progesterone or allopregnanolone, derived in part from 5α-reductase activity, is suggested. This clinical experience reinforces that neurosteroids are among the most potent $GABA_A$ receptor PAMs identified to date, rivaling the actions of BZDs and barbiturates (Figure 47.2). Further elucidation of the molecular, cellular, and network effects of neurosteroids that act on the $GABA_A$ receptor holds promise in advancing treatments for disorders of sleep and hypersomnolence.

CLINICAL PEARL

A substantial scientific and an emerging clinical literature supports new approaches to treating hypersomnolence by antagonizing GABAergic signaling. There is a diversity of potential mechanisms and targets in the $GABA_A$ receptor family through which this might be realized: neurosteroids, endozepine-like substances, and additional domains within the receptor complex (e.g., the chloride channel pore). Additional controlled clinical trials will be critical to establish that such approaches are efficacious and safe. Challenges include defining the most appropriate patient populations, possibly informed by further biomarker development for endogenous $GABA_A$ receptor PAMs.

SUMMARY

GABA agonists and modulators (e.g., Z drugs) that allosterically enhance $GABA_A$ receptors induce sleep, whereas antagonists and NAMs (e.g., clarithromycin) can promote wakefulness (Table 47.1). Natural/endogenous and synthetic/exogenous compounds that modulate GABA's availability and $GABA_A$ receptors are legion and, to the observant clinician, a reminder that GABA modulates a multitude and diversity of human behaviors. Leveraging this clinical experience and expanding knowledge of GABA's biology will point the way to novel treatments for disorders of the wake-sleep continuum. Indeed, GABA and its receptors continue to provide a rich harvest for drugs that influence wake and sleep. Meanwhile, Z drugs remain highly popular sleeping medications. We still lack a complete picture of where and how GABA-mediated inhibition in the brain modulates sleep and wakefulness. Most GABA pathways promote NREM sleep, but a minority, through disinhibition, promote wakefulness. It may turn out that we only need to inhibit key nodes of neural circuitry to induce sleep. Here could lie the future of sleep medicine pharmacology.

ACKNOWLEDGEMENTS

Funded by the U.S. Department of Health and Human Services/National Institutes of Health (NIH) award NS089719 (DBR); and the Wellcome Trust 107841/Z/15/Z (WW) and UK Dementia Research Institute at Imperial College (WW). DBR has received consultancy fees from Eisai Pharmaceuticals, Expansion Therapeutics, Harmony Biosciences, Jazz Pharmaceuticals, and Takeda Pharmaceuticals and royalty fees from Balance Therapeutics for intellectual property surrounding the use of flumazenil and other $GABA_A$ receptor antagonists for the treatment of hypersomnolence (U.S. Patent No. 10,376,524 B2). WW declares no conflict of interest.

SELECTED READINGS

Belelli D, Hogenkamp D, Gee KW, et al. Realising the therapeutic potential of neuroactive steroid modulators of the $GABA_A$ receptor. *Neurobiol Stress*. 2020;12:100207.

Falup-Pecurariu C, Diaconu Ş, Ţînţ D, Falup-Pecurariu O. Neurobiology of sleep (Review). *Exp Ther Med*. 2021;21(3):272.

Farzampour Z, Reimer RJ, Huguenard J. *Endozepines. Adv Pharmacol.* 2015;72:147–164.

Franks NP. General anaesthesia: from molecular targets to neuronal pathways of sleep and arousal. *Nat Rev Neurosci*. 2008;9(5):370–386.

Korpi ER, Grunder G, Luddens H. Drug interactions at GABA(A) receptors. *Prog Neurobiol*. 2002;67(2):113–159.

Masiulis S, Desai R, Uchanski T, et al. GABAA receptor signalling mechanisms revealed by structural pharmacology. *Nature.* 2019;565(7740):454–459.
Nutt DJ, Stahl SM. Searching for perfect sleep: the continuing evolution of $GABA_A$ receptor modulators as hypnotics. *J Psychopharmacol.* 2010;24(11):1601–1612.
Olsen RW, Li GD. In: Brady S, Siegel G, Albers RW, Price D, eds. *Chapter 18: GABA. Basic Neurochemistry.* 8th ed. Academic Press; 2011.
Rye DB, Bliwise DL, Parker K, et al. Modulation of vigilance in the primary hypersomnias by endogenous enhancement of $GABA_A$ receptors. *Sci Transl Med.* 2012;4(161):161ra151.
Smart TG, Stephenson FA. A half century of gamma-aminobutyric acid. *Brain Neurosci Adv.* 2019;3.
Wisden W, Yu X, Franks NP. GABA Receptors and the Pharmacology of Sleep. *Handb Exp Pharmacol.* 2019;253:279–304.

A complete reference list can be found online at ExpertConsult.com.

Chapter 48

Histamine

Patrick M. Fuller; Yves Dauvilliers

Chapter Highlights

- Histamine is a small monoamine signaling molecule that plays a role in many peripheral and central physiologic processes, including the regulation of wakefulness.
- Within the brain, histamine is produced exclusively by neurons of the hypothalamic tuberomammillary nucleus.
- Histamine H3 receptor (H3R) antagonists and inverse agonists have a role in the treatment of some sleep disorders associated with excessive daytime sleepiness. This chapter discusses the basic neurobiology and pharmacology of central histamine and how drugs targeting histamine receptors are used clinically to treat sleep disorders.

CENTRAL HISTAMINE

Histamine is a small monoamine signaling molecule whose role in peripheral vascular and gut smooth muscle activity was first demonstrated more than a century ago. Subsequent studies demonstrated a physiologic role for histamine in many additional peripheral processes. For example, as familiar to most clinicians, histamine functions in the periphery to regulate immune responses and itch when released by mast cells and basophils and regulates acid secretion by enterochromaffin-like cells of the stomach. Perhaps less well appreciated is the fact histamine is also produced in the brain, where it appears to function as a wake-promoting neurotransmitter. Indeed, one need only experience the strongly sedating effect of antihistamines to appreciate the profound effects that histamine can have on the waking state. Central histamine signaling has also been implicated in the regulation of both non–rapid eye movement (NREM) and rapid eye movement (REM) sleep. Although not the focus of this chapter, it should be acknowledged that central histamine can also modulate a wide range of other physiologic and behavioral systems, including thermoregulation, stress, endocrine function, and feeding (for a review, see Hass and colleagues[1]).

Source and Synthesis of Central Histamine

The sole source of neuronal histamine in adult vertebrates is the tuberomamillary nucleus (TMN).[2,3] From a phylogenetic perspective, the TMN is a remarkably conserved structure, both morphologically and anatomically. In mammals, the TMN is located at the level of the posterior hypothalamus and contains approximately 75 to 120,000 neurons that are mostly located around the mammillary body, close to the ventral surface of the brain.[4] Additional "subpopulations" of histaminergic TMN neurons exist in the dorsally-situated medial supramammillary and caudal paramammillary regions. TMN neurons provide widespread innervation of the brain and spinal cord via both ascending and descending projections. The ascending pathways (ventral and dorsal) provide moderate to dense innervation of the hypothalamus, septal nuclei, thalamus, hippocampus, amygdala, basal ganglia, and cortex, whereas the descending pathway provides moderate innervation of the pontine central gray, locus coeruleus, raphe nuclei, trigeminal nucleus, and the spinal cord.[5]

Histamine itself is synthesized from the amino acid histidine through oxidative decarboxylation by histidine decarboxylase (HDC). Once synthesized, histamine is packaged into synaptic vesicles within both the somata and axon varicosities.[6] Upon depolarization of the nerve terminal, histamine is released into the synaptic cleft, where it binds to histamine receptors located on both the presynaptic and postsynaptic membranes (Figure 48.1). Unlike other monoaminergic neurotransmitters, such as serotonin and dopamine, histamine does not appear to have a high-affinity reuptake system but, rather, only the low-affinity organic cation transporter 3 expressed by astrocytes.[7] Instead, histamine is largely inactivated or "cleared" from the extracellular space via its methylation to inactive tele-methylhistamine (tmHA) by the cytosolic-based histamine *N*-methyltransferase (HNMT).

HDC exhibits a fairly high-amplitude diurnal rhythm, with highest expression of *hdc* messenger RNA (mRNA) at the end of the light period (rest phase) and highest HDC protein levels in the dark period (active phase) in mice.[8] Postmortem analysis of brain tissue has revealed a similar diurnal rhythm in *hdc* mRNA in humans, with highest *hdc* mRNA levels during the day.[9] Selective disruption of the core circadian clock gene *Bmal1* in histaminergic TMN neurons severely blunts the amplitude of the 24-hour *hdc* mRNA and HDC protein rhythms, and this loss of circadian variation has been linked to sleep fragmentation.[10]

TMN histamine neurons also express both isoforms of the gamma-aminobutyric acid (GABA) synthetic enzyme glutamate decarboxylase (GAD65 and GAD67), suggesting the possibility that GABA may play an important role in TMN function as a histamine cotransmitter.[11–13] This hypothesis was tested and essentially negated in a recent study in which the effects of selective, albeit incomplete, genetic excision of GAD67 from TMN histamine neurons (i.e., *GAD67*$^{fl/fl}$*::HDCcre* mice) was found to be without

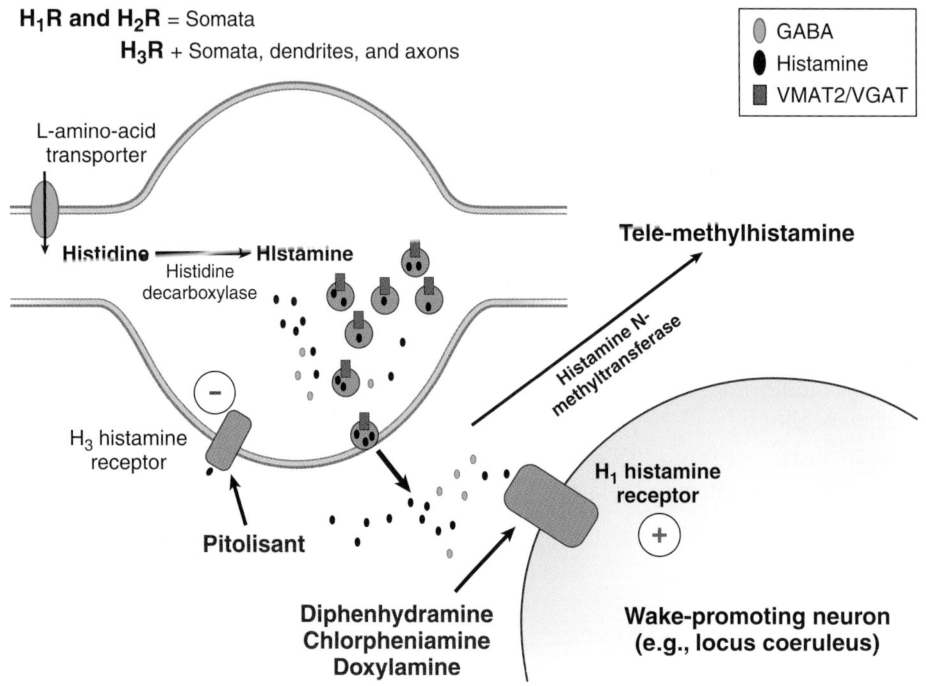

Figure 48.1 Histamine synthesis, metabolism, receptors, and pharmacology. Histamine is produced, largely within varicosities, through the oxidative decarboxylation of histidine by histamine decarboxylase (HDC). Histamine is then packaged into vesicles by the vesicular monoamine transporter (VMAT2) and then released into the extracellular space. Gamma-aminobutyric acid (GABA) is also likely released by histamine neurons, although whether it is packaged into vesicles via VMAT2 or the vesicular GABA transporter (VGAT) remains unresolved. Within the extracellular space, histamine acts on postsynaptic histamine-1 receptors (H_1Rs) or H_2Rs or presynaptic H_3Rs and is inactivated via its methylation to inactive tele-methylhistamine by histamine *N*-methyltransferase. Sleep-promoting antihistaminergics largely act via antagonizing the H_1R on the postsynaptic membrane, whereas wake-promoting inverse agonists act via the H_3R on the presynaptic membrane.

effect on arousal levels.[14] Notwithstanding these findings, it remains unclear whether or not TMN histamine neurons can release synaptic GABA, but if they can, the mechanism for release also remains unclear[14] because TMN neurons do not appear to express the vesicular GABA transporter that is thought to be necessary for synaptic release of GABA, as discussed later. In addition to GABA, TMN histamine neurons may also differentially express other peptides, such as galanin, thyrotropin-releasing hormone (TRH), substance P, and enkephalins in a species-specific manner. The role(s) of these peptides in TMN regulation of arousal remains unknown.

Regulation of Tuberomamillary Nucleus Histamine Neurons

The activity of TMN histamine neurons is under considerable regulation by a wide range of presynaptic inputs, many of which are reciprocal in nature, that is, the inputs arise from cell groups that themselves are postsynaptic targets of TMN histamine neurons. Although a detailed discussion of the channel mechanisms mediating the effects of these inputs is beyond the scope of this chapter, inputs to TMN histamine neurons arise from many of the canonical arousal-related nuclei, including the noradrenergic locus coeruleus, serotoninergic raphe, brainstem cholinergic nuclei, GABAergic preoptic cell groups, glutamatergic hypothalamic and cortical cell groups, and lateral hypothalamic hypocretin/orexin cells.[15] Additional "afferent" input to TMN histamine neurons includes paracrine and humoral factors.[16]

Histamine Receptor Pharmacology

Four distinct metabotropic G protein–coupled histamine receptors (H_1 to H_4) have been identified. The H_1, H_2, and H_3 receptors (H_1Rs, H_2Rs, and H_3Rs) are all expressed in brain, whereas expression of the H_4R appears to be restricted to the periphery.[1] The H_1R modulates postsynaptic excitability and plasticity; is abundantly expressed within the hypothalamus, thalamus, brainstem, hippocampus and cortex; and is necessary for the wake-promoting effects of histamine. Many over-the-counter sleep aids contain antihistamines, such as diphenhydramine or doxylamine that function as H_1R inverse agonists (often incorrectly called "antagonists") to produce sedation. H_1 receptors are also a target of several antipsychotics and antidepressants.

Similar to the H_1R, the H_2R also modulates postsynaptic excitability and plasticity, and it is densely expressed in the cortex, amygdala, basal ganglia, and hippocampus. The H_2R also exhibits constitutive activity, and H_2R deficiency is implicated in learning and memory impairments, as well as increased aggressive behaviors.[17]

The H_3 receptor modulates presynaptic excitability and plasticity; is expressed in particular abundance in the cortex, cerebellum, striatum, posterior hypothalamus, and brainstem; acts as an inhibitory autoreceptor; and is implicated in a wide range of neurobiologic and physiologic processes. The pharmacologic properties of the H_3R are particularly unique insofar as it exhibits robust constitutive activity in vivo and functions as an autoreceptor on the somata, dendrites, and axons of TMN neurons, to inhibit histamine synthesis and release from varicosities. For example, when extracellular histamine tone is high, histamine binds the H_3R on TMN soma, dendrites, and axons and thereby hyperpolarizes the neurons. As such, histamine itself represents another presynaptic regulatory mechanism. Another unique property of the H_3R is that it is expressed as a presynaptic heteroreceptor on a variety of neurons, including cells that make dopamine, serotonin, norepinephrine, acetylcholine, GABA, and glutamate. Hence the H_3R plays an important role in regulating the release of many of the brain's primary peptide and fast transmitters. The unique properties of the H_3R are illustrated by drugs that interfere with, that is, reduce constitutive activity of, H_3 signaling, such as pitolisant, which not only increases brain levels of histamine but also—acting as inhibitory presynaptic heteroreceptors—the levels of serotonin, norepinephrine, dopamine, and possibly other neurotransmitters.[18]

Histamine and Sleep-Wake Behavior

Considerable preclinical research suggests that histamine, likely acting via H_1Rs and H_3Rs, is essential for normal sleep-wake behavior. More specifically, an arousal-promoting role for TMN histaminergic neurons, and histamine itself, has long been posited. In support of this hypothesis, antihistaminergics are often used as over-the-counter treatments for insomnia.[19] whereas the H_3R inverse agonist pitolisant has shown promising efficacy in reducing hypersomnolence and cataplexy in patients with narcolepsy.[20–22] In addition, intracerebral histamine levels are highest during the active period,[23] and TMN histamine neurons themselves exhibit their fastest firing profile during wake, especially active wake. In contrast, TMN neurons fire little during NREM sleep and are essentially silent in REM sleep.[24] TMN histamine neurons are also reciprocally connected with the sleep-promoting ventrolateral preoptic (VLPO) nucleus,[25–30] and it has been shown that histamine release from TMN axon terminals can inhibit the VLPO[31] and hence trigger arousal. TMN histamine neurons similarly innervate, and histamine dose-dependently activates, wake-promoting nuclei, such as the noradrenergic locus coeruleus, suggesting that histamine-induced arousal could also involve, in addition to inhibition of sleep-promoting neurons, activation of wake-promoting neurons.[32] A recent study using chemogenetic activation of TMN histamine neurons reported increased locomotor activity in an open-field challenge,[33] consistent with an arousal-promoting effect of activation. However, another study using a similar approach reported that, although activation of TMN neurons indeed enhanced wakefulness during a behavioral challenge, there was almost no effect upon baseline arousal levels.[14] Acute optogenetic inhibition of ventral TMN histamine neurons has been reported to produce a rapid wake to slow wave sleep transition,[34] although this finding was not reproduced by another group.[14]

Consistent with the absence of a strong arousal-promoting response after selective activation of TMN histamine neurons,[14] it has also been reported that lesions of TMN cells produce limited alterations in sleep or wake in rats.[35–37] In addition, HDC knockout mice exhibit only modest changes in baseline wakefulness,[38,39] although they show less wakefulness after a behavioral challenge, such as a cage change.[38] HDC knockout mice also appear to be drowsier at the start of the active period ("lights off") compared with littermate controls. Similarly, transgenic mice bearing a $GABA_A$ receptor loss-of-function mutation on HDC neurons, which results in increased HDC neuron excitability, exhibit higher arousal after a cage change.[40] Taken together, these findings suggest that other arousal systems can partially compensate for a chronic absence of histamine signaling but also argue that histamine is necessary to produce a high level of arousal under certain conditions, such as a novel environment.

The synthetic enzymes GAD65 and GAD67, for the fast inhibitory transmitter GABA, are also expressed in TMN histamine neurons, suggesting the possibility that TMN histamine neurons may not only produce, but also corelease, GABA and histamine to produce their postsynaptic effects. It has been proposed that synaptic corelease of GABA may counterregulate the wake-promoting effects of histamine. A recent study reported that small interfering RNA–mediated knockdown of the vesicular GABA transporter (VGAT), which is required for packaging GABA into synaptic vesicles for release, selectively in histamine neurons, produces sustained wakefulness and hyperactivity in mice.[33] A more recent study, however, found that very few TMN histamine neurons contain VGAT,[14] suggesting that TMN neurons may package and release GABA by a different mechanism. One possibility is that TMN neurons may instead package and release GABA via the vesicular monoamine transporter VMAT2, which is expressed in TMN neurons and is the mechanism by which dopaminergic neurons of the midbrain release GABA.[41] Hence, although GABA may be released from histaminergic neurons to constrain arousal, it remains to be clarified (1) how targeted knockdown of VGAT, given its apparent absence, in TMN neurons would produce potent arousal effects; and (2) why VMAT2 in TMN neurons appears to colocalize with histamine, not GABA.

GABAergic inhibition of TMN histamine neurons may be an important mechanism by which some drugs promote sleep. For example, zolpidem (Ambien), a $GABA_A$ receptor-positive allosteric modulator and one of the most commonly prescribed insomnia medications, fails to produce sedation in mice with a mutated $GABA_A$ receptor.[42] However, when $GABA_A$ receptor function is selectively restored on histamine neurons, NREM sleep latency is significantly reduced and total NREM sleep time is increased after administration of zolpidem. This finding would suggest that enhanced GABAergic drive onto histamine neurons is sufficient to induce NREM sleep. Thus, for example, increased GABAergic drive from sleep-promoting VLPO neurons may induce natural sleep in part by inhibiting TMN histamine neurons, as has been proposed in the "flip-flop" model of sleep-wake regulation.[43]

For reasons that are incompletely understood, histaminergic TMN neurons appear to possess considerable plasticity. For example, two independent postmortem studies showed that the number of HDC-immunoreactive neurons is increased 64% to 95% in the brains of people with narcolepsy type 1 (NT1), a disease characterized by a severe loss of orexin neurons.[44] Under normal conditions, orexin neurons strongly excite TMN neurons, and their absence appears to produce compensatory changes in TMN neurons. A parsimonious explanation for this finding is that TMN histamine neurons in individuals with NT1 simply express more HDC, making TMN neurons easier to detect by immunostaining. A second explanation for the reported increase in HDC neurons in NT1 may be related to the supposed autoimmune process that kills the orexin neurons in humans. Given strong support for the hypothesis that NT1 is an immune-mediated disease, the increased central nervous system histamine may link to the immune process that produces inflammation and loss of hypocretin neurons in humans.[45] On the other hand, a compensatory increase in TMN histamine neurons numbers was not found in either orexin knockout or orexin/ataxin-3 transgenic mice.[45]

Histamine: Narcolepsy and Other Central Hypersomnolence Disorders

A role for histamine and its main metabolite tmHA in central hypersomnolence disorders has been explored, although the results remain controversial. For example, early studies reported low cerebrospinal fluid (CSF) histamine levels in narcolepsy (both type 1 and type 2) and idiopathic hypersomnia.[46,47] A subsequent and larger study, however, failed to replicate this finding of reduced CSF histamine or tmHA in centrally mediated hypersomnias.[48] As this subsequent study included a well-defined population of patients with narcolepsy and other hypersomnolence disorders and used a far more sensitive assay (liquid chromatographic-electrospray/tandem mass spectrometric assay developed for the simultaneous analysis of histamine and its major metabolite tmHA), these findings suggest that measurements of CSF histamine and tmHA are insufficient to differentiate etiologies of central hypersomnia or to assess the severity of centrally mediated hypersomnia. Moreover, it has been reported that CSF histamine levels do not correlate with subjective (Epworth Sleepiness Scale [ESS]) and objective (Multiple Sleep Latency Test) measures of sleepiness or, for that matter, with CSF orexin-A levels. Repeat CSF sampling in few narcoleptic individuals have also revealed the absence of a significant change in histamine and tmHA levels despite disease progression.[49] In contrast, CSF hypocretin levels measured in the same study decreased from normal/intermediate to undetectable levels in three of the four patients with definite cataplexy and remained stable in the two others with atypical cataplexy. Hence it appears that extracellular histamine levels are likely normal in patients with type 1 narcolepsy, notwithstanding the increase in HDC-immunopositive neurons, bringing into question the utility of CSF histamine or tmHA as useful biomarkers for narcolepsy or other hypersomnolence disorders. It is also worth noting that histamine is a labile molecule and is present only at very low (pM) concentrations in lumbar CSF. In consequence, future efforts to ascertain central histamine levels may require the sampling of extracellular fluids closer to the site(s) of histamine release.

Clinical Use of Histaminergic Drugs for Treating Sleep Disorders

Acute pharmacologic manipulations of TMN histaminergic neurons can produce strong wake-promoting effects, as well as smaller NREM-promoting and REM sleep-suppressing effects. As previously indicated, drugs that block the H_1R are among the most commonly used medications for insomnia. The importance of the H_1R in mediating the sedating properties of many antihistamine is illustrated by the fact that the sedating effect of triprolidine is absent in mice lacking H_1R.[50] First-generation H_1R antagonists, such as diphenhydramine, chlorpheniramine, and doxylamine, all possess high lipophilicity, which facilitates their ability to cross the blood brain barrier. These drugs are also potent in their ability to produce sedation. By contrast, second-generation H_1Rr antagonists, such as fexofenadine and loratadine, are less lipophilic and, predictably, far less sedating. Of note, some antidepressants and antipsychotics, such as doxepin, amitriptyline, and olanzapine, also function as H_1R antagonists and have proven beneficial in treating insomnia.

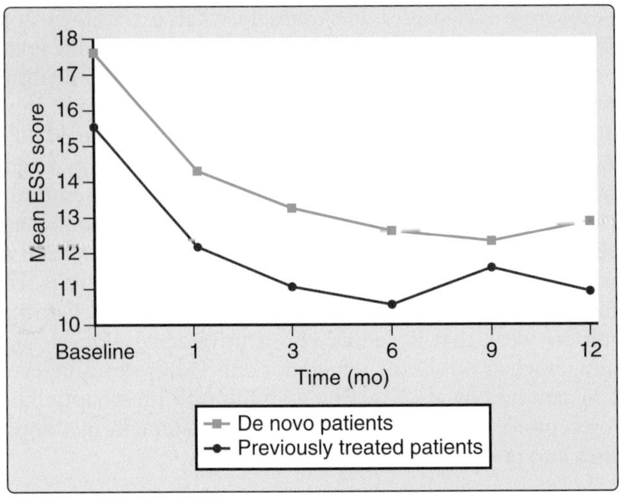

Figure 48.2 Epworth Sleepiness Scale (ESS) scores over time using pitolisant. Improvement in ESS scores was observed at 1 month and continued through 12 months in the two subgroups of de novo patients and those previously exposed to pitolisant.

In contrast to H_1R antagonists, drugs that interfere with H_3 signaling (e.g., ciproxifan, pitolisant) promote wakefulness in mice, likely through an increase in extracellular levels of histamine and other wake-promoting neurotransmitters. The H_3R has become a recent drug target for the treatment of excessive daytime sleepiness in narcolepsy and other hypersomnolence disorders. Pitolisant, for example, is a H_3R inverse agonist that increases brain levels of histamine and potentially other wake-promoting neurotransmitters. In mice lacking orexin, pitolisant increased wakefulness, decreased NREM sleep, and reduced direct transitions into REM sleep (the murine equivalent of cataplexy).[20] In a medium size, class 1 study of patients with narcolepsy (type 1 and type 2), pitolisant at doses ranging from 10 to 40 mg/day (mostly at 40 mg/day) reduced the ESS about 6 points, a reduction similar to modafinil 100 to 400 mg/day.[21] Another study found that pitolisant 10 to 0 mg/day (mostly at 40 mg/day in this flexible-dosing study design) reduced the weekly cataplexy rate by about 75%.[22] The mechanism by which pitolisant reduces cataplexy remains unclear, but it may link to a decrease in total REM sleep. Pitolisant is generally well tolerated, with only few adverse events that include headache, irritability, nausea, and insomnia.[21,22] A recent 2-year open-label, single-arm, pragmatic study using pitolisant confirmed the safety profile and efficacy on excessive daytime sleepiness, cataplexy, hallucinations, and sleep paralysis in narcolepsy[51] (Figure 48.2). Pitolisant has since been approved by the European Medicines Agency and US Food and Drug Administration to treat adults with narcolepsy. Of interest, although most research on H_3 antagonists has focused on their use in narcolepsy, these antagonists also produce improvements in sleepiness in obstructive sleep apnea (OSA) syndrome. A recent study showed that pitolisant significantly reduced self-reported daytime sleepiness and fatigue and improved patient-reported outcomes in sleepy patients with OSA refusing or nonadherent to continuous positive airway pressure.[52] The H_3Rs may thus form the basis of new therapeutic targets to manage daytime sleepiness associated with other neurologic disorders, such as idiopathic hypersomnia, myotonic dystrophy, and Parkinson disease.

ACKNOWLEDGMENT

Regarding conflicts of interest, Yves Dauvilliers is a consultant for and has participated in advisory boards for Jazz Pharmaceuticals, UCB Pharma, Flamel Technologies, Idorsia, Theranexus, and Bioprojet. Patrick M. Fuller has no conflicts to report.

CLINICAL PEARLS

- Drugs that block the histamine-1 receptor (H_1R) are among the most commonly used medications for insomnia.
- The H_3R inverse agonist pitolisant at 10 to 40 mg/day reduces sleepiness and, to a lesser extent, cataplexy in narcolepsy.
- H_3Rs may represent new therapeutic targets to manage daytime sleepiness associated with several other disorders, such as obstructive sleep apnea syndrome and idiopathic hypersomnia.

SUMMARY

The central histaminergic system is thought to play a fundamental, if incompletely understood, role in arousal control. To this end, drugs that selectively target histamine receptors can modulate, profoundly in some cases, the waking and sleeping states. For instance, many H_1R antagonists (e.g., antihistamines such as diphenhydramine, chlorpheniramine, and doxylamine) are potently sedating, whereas drugs that interfere with H_3 signaling (e.g., ciproxifan, pitolisant) promote wakefulness. Notwithstanding the demonstrated clinical efficacy and promise of many drugs that modulate central histamine levels to treat debilitating insomnia and hypersomnolence, preclinical studies support the concept that TMN histamine neurons, and by extension histamine itself, are required for vigilance maintenance under certain environmental and/or behavioral contexts but are neither necessary nor sufficient to promote electrographic or behavioral wake at baseline.

SELECTED READINGS

Dauvilliers Y, et al. Pitolisant for daytime sleepiness in patients with obstructive sleep apnea who refuse continuous positive airway pressure treatment. A randomized trial. *Am J Respir Crit Care Med.* 2020;201(9):1135–1145.

Haas HL, Sergeeva OA, Selbach O. Histamine in the nervous system. *Physiol Rev.* 2008;88(3):1183–1241.

Shan L, Dauvilliers Y, Siegel J. Interactions of the histamine and hypocretin systems in CNS disorders. *Nat Rev Neurol.* 2015;11(7):401–413.

Venner A, Mochizuki T, De Luca R, et al. Reassessing the role of histaminergic tuberomammillary neurons in arousal control. *J Neurosci.* 2019;39(45):8929–8939.

Williams RH, Chee MJS, Kroeger D, et al. Optogenetic-mediated release of histamine reveals distal and autoregulatory mechanisms for controlling arousal. *J. Neurosci.* 2014;34:6023–6029.

Yu X, Ye Z, Houston Catriona M, et al. Wakefulness is governed by GABA and histamine cotransmission. *Neuron.* 2015;87:164–178.

A complete reference list can be found online at ExpertConsult.com.

Chapter 49

Orexin/Hypocretin

Natalie Nevárez; W. Joseph Herring; Luis de Lecea

Chapter Highlights

- The orexins/hypocretins are two alternatively spliced peptides known to regulate sleep and wakefulness through their actions within a highly distributed "arousal network."
- The orexin/hypocretin receptor antagonists suvorexant and lemborexant are approved for the treatment of insomnia, and a number of other orexin/hypocretin receptor antagonists are currently in clinical development for treating arousal-associated disorders. Orexin/hypocretin receptor agonists are being investigated for the treatment of excessive daytime sleepiness.
- This chapter explores the basic anatomy and neurotransmission of the orexin/hypocretin arousal circuit and emphasizes the clinical value of orexin/hypocretin-targeting treatments in sleep disorders and their potential use for other disorders that have associated arousal disturbances such as Alzheimer disease and depression.

INTRODUCTION

Sleep is a physiologically restorative state that is ubiquitous across phylogeny. Understanding the circuits regulating sleep is an area of intense research. One neural population that has received substantial attention is a restricted group of cells within the tuberal hypothalamus defined largely by their shared expression of two peptides: hypocretin (hcrt)-1 and -2 (also known as orexin-A and -B; for a detailed history of their discovery see Selected Readings). These neurons regulate sleep and wakefulness through their extensive and often reciprocal connections within a distributed "arousal network" spanning virtually the entire brain. The development of advanced tools to manipulate and characterize this circuit has revealed a role for these neurons in regulating arousal stability. This is highlighted by narcolepsy, a sleep disorder in which patients aberrantly transition between wakefulness and sleep and in other disorders in which sleep timing, quality, or stability is jeopardized. The fundamental aspect of sleep makes understanding this circuit of high importance for its therapeutic potential. Indeed, two orexin/hcrt receptor antagonists are approved for the treatment of insomnia, and other agents targeting the orexin/hcrt system are in clinical trial testing with promising results for the treatment of sleep disorders and beyond. In this chapter, we discuss the essential "nodes" in this arousal network and the emerging orexin/hcrt-targeting drugs that are revolutionizing the treatment of sleep disorders.

CHARACTERISTICS OF OREXIN/HYPOCRETIN NEURONS

Orexin/hcrt neurons are glutamatergic and their somata are restricted to the tuberal hypothalamus.[1,2] Orexin/hcrt expression varies within this region, with the highest expression in the perifornical area.[3] Orexin/hcrt axons project broadly to create a dispersed "arousal network,"[4] with dense projections observed in the locus coeruleus (LC) and paraventricular thalamus, among other regions. Orexin/hcrt neurons interact with many neurotransmitter systems and coexpress many other signaling molecules including neurotensin, galanin, Narp, dynorphin, and proenkephalin, among others.[5-8] These neurons integrate relevant information (through as yet unknown mechanisms) to influence the probability of sleep-wake transitions.

A Key Role in Wakefulness

Observed patterns of orexin/hcrt neuron activity suggest that these cells play a role in promoting arousal. Orexin/hcrt neurons become active shortly before waking, are phasically active during wakefulness, reduce activity during quiet wakefulness, and have little to no activity during sleep.[9] Similarly, cerebrospinal fluid (CSF) orexin-A concentrations and extracellular orexin-A concentrations are elevated during an animal's active phase.[10] Intracerebroventricular administration of orexin-A to mice and dogs promotes wakefulness and reduces sleep,[11,12] while local infusions into the tuberomammillary nucleus (TMN), pons, basal forebrain (BF), and LC of mice also promote wakefulness.[13-15]

More finely tuned techniques such as optogenetics have provided further evidence for the role of this neural population in regulating wakefulness. Optogenetic stimulation of orexin/hcrt neurons at frequencies above 5 Hz induces wakefulness in mice whereas inhibition of this population promotes non–rapid eye movement (NREM) sleep.[16] This effect is orexin/hcrt dependent, as these manipulations, when conducted in orexin/hcrt-deficient animals, fail to increase wake probability.[16] Furthermore, optogenetic inhibition of orexin/hcrt neurons increases sleep during the active and inactive phase of the daily cycle.[17,18] Similarly, chemogenetic manipulations of orexin/hcrt activity via DREADDs (designer receptors exclusively activated by designer drugs) show that activation of the excitatory (Gq) DREADD promotes wakefulness, whereas activation of the inhibitory (Gi) DREADDs has the opposite effect and causes an increase in NREM sleep.[19]

Altered in Sleep Disorders

Narcolepsy was first described in 1880 by Jean Baptise Edouard Gélineau.[20] However, the earliest data suggesting a role for orexin/hcrt in sleep and narcolepsy occurred over a century later when two studies found that mice and dogs with orexin/hcrt neuron loss showed disrupted sleep-wake cycles and aberrant loss of muscle tone (i.e., cataplexy).[21,22] Further, mice deficient in the *Hcrt* gene have fragmented sleep-wake behavior and behavioral phenotypes similar to human narcolepsy, whereas dogs with mutations in the orexin/hcrt 2 receptor (OX2R; gene name: *HcrtR2*) develop a heritable form of narcolepsy.[23]

Follow-up work in humans found that patients with narcolepsy showed reduced orexin-A in CSF. Subsequent studies of postmortem human narcoleptic brains documented a greater than 85% reduction in the number of orexin/hcrt neurons.[24] The association between reduced CSF orexin-A levels and narcolepsy is so strong that it is a diagnostic metric for the disease.

OVERVIEW OF THE OREXIN/HYPOCRETIN AROUSAL CIRCUIT

As discussed previously in this chapter, the orexin/hcrt network is widely distributed and effects its actions via its connections with many other neurotransmitter systems. Namely, orexin/hcrt neurons send excitatory projections onto noradrenergic cells of the LC, serotonergic dorsal raphe nucleus (DRN), cholinergic nuclei in the BF, and dopaminergic neurons within the ventral tegmental area (VTA). Additionally, orexin/hcrt neurons receive inputs from neuropeptide Y-positive projections from the dorsomedial hypothalamus (DMH) and GABAergic neurons of the ventrolateral preoptic area (vlPOA) and basal forebrain (BF) and glutamatergic inputs from the BF. In the text that follows, we briefly describe some of these connections (organized by neurotransmitter and summarized in Figure 49.1) and the data supporting their activity in relation to arousal (for in-depth discussion of the circuit please see Selected Readings). Importantly, as we will discuss in the clinical portion of this chapter, previous treatments for arousal-related disorders have focused on increasing GABAergic tone; however, current research efforts are shifting to orexin/hcrt, a key orchestrator of sleep and wakefulness, with promising results.

Locus Coeruleus Norepinephrine

The LC receives the densest projections from orexin/hcrt neurons and expresses almost exclusively orexin/hcrt 1 receptor (OX1R).[4] The activity of LC noradrenergic neurons mimics patterns of wakefulness and arousal; these neurons fire tonically during wakefulness, show low activity during NREM sleep and no activity during rapid eye movement (REM) sleep while inhibition of these neurons predictably increases sleep.[25,26] Administration of the Hcrt-1 peptide to

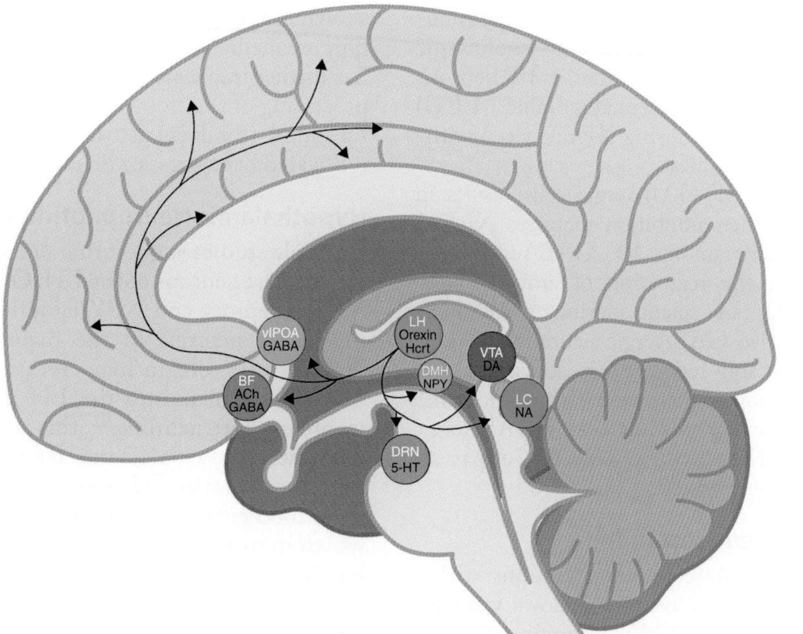

Figure 49.1 Summary of major orexin/hypocretin (hcrt) projections in the human brain. Orexin/hcrt neurons send excitatory projections onto noradrenergic (NA) cells of the locus coeruleus (LC), serotonergic dorsal raphe nucleus (DRN), cholinergic nuclei in the basal forebrain (BF), and dopaminergic (DA) neurons within the ventral tegmental area (VTA). Additionally, orexin/hcrt neurons receive inputs from neuropeptide Y (NPY)–positive projections from the dorsomedial hypothalamus (DMH), gamma-aminobutyric acid (GABA) ergic neurons of the ventrolateral preoptic area (vlPOA), and BF.

the LC increases firing rates and wakefulness and reduces sleep.[26,27] Indeed, the LC is the putative relay in the mechanism that underlies orexin/hcrt-mediated sleep-to-wake transitions.

Zebrafish have provided an additional avenue for the study of the neurotransmitters involved in sleep in vertebrates. NE signaling is necessary for orexin/hcrt-mediated arousal in zebrafish, suggesting that this mechanism is conserved between fish, rodents, and humans. Knocking out NE blocks the excess wakefulness induced by genetic overexpression of Hcrt and by optogenetic activation of orexin/hcrt neurons.[28,29] Limiting NE synthesis in zebrafish increases sleep while reducing arousal thresholds.[28]

In vitro data suggest that the LC can inhibit orexin/hcrt neurons directly or indirectly via the DMH.[30] The DMH relays circadian information from the suprachiasmatic nucleus (SCN) to the LC, especially as it relates to food-entrainable circadian activity. Local administration of orexin/hcrt to the DMH increases c-Fos expression in the DMH and increases feeding in rats.[31,32] Fasting results in dramatic increases in orexin/hcrt c-Fos expression in rodents and nonhuman primates.[33] Reciprocal connections onto the LH provide negative feedback, as suggested by observations that adrenergic agonists induce hyperpolarization in orexin/hcrt neurons in vitro.[34]

Basal Forebrain Acetylcholine and GABA

The BF is a heterogeneous region with reciprocal connections to orexin/hcrt neurons and plays a central role in sustaining arousal states. The individual cell types in the region (cholinergic, GABAergic, and glutamatergic) may sustain individual aspects of arousal. Specifically, cholinergic, GABAergic, and glutamatergic cells from the BF synapse onto orexin/hcrt neurons whereas orexin/hcrt neurons synapse onto cholinergic BF cells.[35,36] DREADD activation of cholinergic BF neurons results in desynchronized electroencephalographic (EEG) activity and decreased delta power during NREM sleep without producing behavioral wakefulness.[37]

In contrast, activation of BF GABAergic cells results in sustained wakefulness and their inhibition increases NREM sleep. There is heterogeneity among BF GABAergic cells regarding their activity in the regulation of arousal states. Somatostatin-positive cells are silent during wakefulness whereas parvalbumin-positive GABAergic neurons are most active during wakefulness and reduce their activity during sleep.[38,39] Targeted stimulation of these neural populations has shown that optogenetic activation of somatostatin GABAergic neurons promotes NREM sleep whereas activation of parvalbumin GABA neurons induces wakefulness.[39]

Tuberomammillary Nucleus Histamine

Orexin/hcrt activates histamine-containing neurons within the TMN. The activity of TMN neurons follows wakefulness and sleep patterns such that TMN histaminergic neurons are active during the onset of wakefulness and silent during sleep.[40] Optogenetic inhibition of TMN histaminergic neurons induces sleep and inhibits wakefulness.[41] However, although this circuit is sufficient to induce wakefulness, it is not required, as histamine-deficient zebrafish show normal sleep-to-wake transitions upon orexin/hcrt neuron stimulation, and mice that lack the enzyme to produce histamine (histamine decarboxylase) still show normal sleep-to-wake transitions.[17,42]

Dorsal Raphe Nucleus Serotonin

Serotonergic neurons of the DRN receive excitatory input from the hypothalamus and send reciprocal inhibitory inputs back onto orexin/hcrt neurons. DRN neurons play a role in promoting wakefulness and in sustaining arousal-related motor activity (i.e., preventing cataplexy).[43] Optogenetic stimulation of DRN serotonergic neurons results in wakefulness.[44] In vitro work suggests that Hcrt increases the firing rate of DRN neurons.[45] Application of orexin/hcrt to the DRN results in wakefulness-like EEG activity.[46]

HcrtR2-knockout mice show cataplectic arrests and the restoration of HcrtR2 into serotonergic DRN cells suppresses these attacks without affecting sleep. Although restoration of orexin/hcrt receptors reduces cataplexy-like attacks, this effect can be blocked by optogenetic inhibition of serotonergic DRN terminals in the amygdala. Indeed, photostimulation of DRN terminals onto amygdala neurons also suppresses these attacks in orexin/hcrt-deficient mice, and orexin/hcrt gene transfer into the amygdala reduces spontaneous and emotion-induced cataplexy.[47,48] Together, these data suggest a multisynaptic circuit among orexin/hcrt neurons, DRN serotonergic cells, and amygdala neurons to drive cataplexy independent of sleep.

Ventral Tegmental Area Dopamine

The VTA has demonstrated roles in motivated behavior and orexin/hcrt may be able to mediate its activity via its dense projections to the region. Infusion of orexin/hcrt into the VTA increases DA release in VTA targets.[49] VTA DA neurons are activated by orexin/hcrt in vitro.[50] In vivo studies have shown that orexin/hcrt-induced hyperlocomotion and stereotypy are mediated by VTA DAergic activity. More recent work has further implicated orexin/hcrt and DA interactions in the processing of cues for food and drug rewards, as well as stressful stimuli (for detailed discussion on the role of orexin/hcrt in motivated behaviors see Selected Readings).[51]

Hypothalamic Neuropeptide Y

Multiple studies suggest that neuropeptide Y (NPY) excites orexin/hcrt neurons of the LH. Orexin/hcrt neurons express NPY receptors and NPY/agouti-related peptide (AgRP)-producing neurons in the hypothalamic arcuate nucleus project onto orexin/hypocretin neurons. Administration of NPY agonists into the LH increases c-Fos expression in orexin/hcrt neurons.[52] This is of important physiologic relevance for arousal and feeding due to NPYs role in ingestive behavior.[53] Indeed, NPY likely relays information from food entrainable oscillators onto orexin/hcrt neurons, which in turn relay to the LC to underlie feeding-mediated regulation of arousal.

Ventrolateral Preoptic Area GABA

GABAergic neurons from the vlPOA project to orexin/hcrt neurons within the LH. These neurons are active during NREM and REM sleep, suggesting that they play a role in inhibiting orexin/hcrt-mediated excitability.[54] Indeed, activation of vlPOA neurons results in NREM sleep, whereas activation of POA GABAergic neurons in slice preparations inhibits orexin/hcrt neurons.[55] Data suggest that this connection is necessary for the maintenance of sleep states in particular, as deletion of GABA-B receptors from orexin/hcrt neurons in the LH results in fragmented sleep episodes.[56]

Integrative Physiology

LH orexin/hcrt neurons engage in complex integrations of central and peripheral signals to modulate arousal. These include hormonal and metabolite messengers that can signal energy balance and stress in the context of health and disease.

Energy Balance

Ghrelin is a gut hormone that is upregulated in response to extended fasting and promotes feeding behavior.[57] Orexin/hcrt neurons express ghrelin receptors (GHS-R) and administration of ghrelin induces c-Fos expression in orexin/hcrt neurons.[58,59] Inhibition of orexin/hcrt signaling blocks ghrelin-induced feeding.[60] Thus orexin/hcrt neurons may be sensitive to ghrelin signaling so as to promote arousal and food seeking under conditions of extended fasting (i.e., metabolic allostasis).

Conversely, leptin is an adipokine-derived hormone that signals satiety.[61] Leptin can directly and indirectly (through neurons that express long-form leptin receptor; LepRB neurons) inhibit LH orexin/hcrt neurons.[5,62] Administration of leptin blocks c-Fos expression in optogenetically stimulated orexin/hcrt neurons.[62] Fasting, on the other hand, increases the activity of orexin/hypocretin neurons.[33,63]

Stress

Stress often triggers increased attention (i.e., hyperarousal) to the environment to protect from impending danger. It is hypothesized that orexin/hcrt integrates stressful stimuli via its interactions with corticotropin releasing factor (CRF) and subsequent activation of the hypothalamic-pituitary-adrenal (HPA) axis.[64] Indeed, activation of orexin/hcrt neurons results in elevation in circulating glucocorticoids that subsequently promotes increased arousal to coordinate an adaptive response to danger.[62,65]

OREXIN/HYPOCRETIN AND THE CLINIC

As we have briefly surveyed, orexin/hcrt network activity is central to the regulation of arousal states. Advanced techniques have allowed for the fine manipulation of "nodes" within this circuit to delineate specific roles for these centers in sleep and wake onset and stability. Importantly, orexin/hcrt is also implicated in integrating physiologic and motivational signals to promote adaptive behavioral responses such as those relating to energy balance and stress. As we continue to expand our knowledge of orexin/hcrt-mediated activity, we will be able to expand the therapeutic potential of this target. In the remainder of this chapter, we will focus on orexin/hcrt-targeting agents for the treatment of insomnia and potential treatment of other arousal-associated disorders.

OREXIN/HYPOCRETIN RECEPTOR ANTAGONISM FOR INSOMNIA

The discovery of the orexins/hcrts and the subsequent determination that the orexin/hcrt signaling system plays a key role in maintaining wakefulness raised the possibility that antagonism of orexin/hcrt receptors could provide a new way to treat insomnia by blocking orexin/hcrt-mediated wake drive. The selective targeting of a neurotransmitter system involved in regulating wakefulness is a distinct approach from the standard treatment of insomnia using Z drugs and off-label use of classical benzodiazepines that promote sleep by enhancing GABA inhibitory effects, with the accompanying generalized depressant effects throughout the central nervous system.[66] Proof-of-concept for the efficacy of orexin/hcrt receptor antagonism in treating insomnia in humans was initially provided by the orexin/hcrt receptor antagonist almorexant.[67,68] Almorexant was discontinued from clinical development because of molecule-specific liver toxicity problems unrelated to the orexin/hcrt mechanism.[69] In 2014 suvorexant became the first orexin/hcrt receptor antagonist to be approved by the US Food and Drug Administration (FDA) for clinical use as a treatment for insomnia, followed by lemborexant in 2019.[70] A number of other orexin/hcrt receptor antagonists are in clinical development including seltorexant[71] and daridorexant.[72] The remainder of this chapter focuses mainly on suvorexant, for which the most extensive published data exists.

OVERVIEW OF SUVOREXANT

Suvorexant (BELSOMRA) is an antagonist for both the OX1R and OX2R receptor subtypes.[73,74] At therapeutic doses, peak concentrations occur at approximately 1.5 to 2 hours, and the mean terminal plasma half-life is approximately 12 hours.[75] Suvorexant's systemic pharmacokinetics are linear, with an accumulation of approximately onefold to twofold with once-daily dosing. Steady state is achieved by 3 days. The mean absolute bioavailability of suvorexant is approximately 80%, and it is mainly eliminated by metabolism, primarily by CYP3A.[76]

In the United States, the current recommended starting dose of suvorexant is 10 mg, which can be increased to a maximum of 20 mg if the lower dose is well tolerated but not satisfactorily effective. This dosing recommendation was based on the FDA view that the lowest effective dose of any insomnia treatment should be used.[77] In some other countries, such as Japan and Australia, regulatory opinion favored a more direct-to-most-effective-dose approach with approval of 15 mg for elderly and 20 mg for nonelderly without titration from a lower dose. The differing doses for elderly and nonelderly in countries such as Japan and Australia reflect the dose regime studied in the Phase 3 trials in which an elderly dose adjustment was made based on available pharmacokinetic data at the time the trials were initiated. It was subsequently determined that age was unlikely to have a significant effect on suvorexant pharmacokinetics; hence, the lack of age-adjusted dosing in the United States. Because CYP3A inhibitors increase suvorexant plasma levels by approximately twofold, in the United States the recommended starting dose for those taking moderate CYP3A inhibitors is 5 mg.

Evidence of Efficacy

The sleep-promoting effects of suvorexant was initially established in animals[74] and healthy people.[75] The efficacy of suvorexant for treating insomnia was evaluated in four randomized placebo-controlled trials comprising an initial dose-ranging trial, two pivotal 3-month Phase 3 trials, and a 1-year safety trial.[78,79] In the initial dose-ranging trial, suvorexant doses of 10, 20, 40, and 80 mg were evaluated in nonelderly insomnia patients and suvorexant efficacy on both objective polysomnography (PSG) and patient self-reported subjective sleep measures was found to be dose related across the range studied.[79] Although the higher doses were more consistently effective across end points than the 10-mg dose, FDA review concluded that the 10 mg data were sufficiently compelling to declare it to be the recommended starting dose in the United States.

Based on results of the dose-ranging trial, doses of 40 mg and 20 mg were selected for evaluation in the two pivotal Phase 3 trials in which both elderly (≥65 years) and nonelderly (<65 years) individuals were assessed.[80] As noted previously in this chapter, in the elderly, doses of 30 mg (instead of 40 mg) and 15 mg (instead of 20 mg) were evaluated to adjust for anticipated differences in exposure based on the data available at the time the Phase 3 studies were initiated. The Phase 3 trials confirmed that suvorexant was effective on both PSG and patient self-reported subjective sleep measures versus placebo both acutely from the earliest time point assessed (night 1 for PSG measures and week 1 for subjective measures), and chronically, with efficacy generally sustained over 3 months (and for up 12 months in the 1-year trial, which only evaluated the 40/30 mg dose). For the approved 20/15 mg dose, at month 3, patients reported an increase from baseline in subjective total sleep time (sTST) of 55 minutes versus 39 minutes for placebo and reported a decrease from baseline in subjective time to sleep onset (sTSO) of −25 minutes versus −19 minutes for placebo.[81] For the PSG end points at the approved 20/15 mg dose at month 3, a reduction from baseline in wake after persistent sleep onset (WASO) of −48 minutes versus −25 minutes for placebo was observed (with a corresponding increase in total sleep time (TST) of 78 minutes versus 51 minutes for placebo). There was a reduction in PSG latency to persistent sleep (LPS) of −28 minutes versus −17 minutes for placebo at night 1, with a smaller difference versus placebo at month 3 (−32 minutes versus −28 minutes for placebo).[81]

Additional analyses of WASO during each hour of an 8-hour PSG recording night showed that the reduction in WASO by suvorexant was apparent from 2 hours and then maintained over the course of the night.[81] While suvorexant reduced WASO, it did not appear to alter the overall number of awakenings during the night as assessed by PSG.[79] An analysis of the microdynamics of suvorexant effects on WASO and awakenings found that, relative to placebo, suvorexant decreased the total number and total time spent in "long" awakenings (>2 minutes) while slightly increasing the total number and total time spent in "short" awakenings (≤2 minutes).[82] On average, a patient returned to sleep from their longest awakening more than twice as fast on suvorexant than on placebo. Furthermore, the reduction in long awakenings increased the odds of patient-reported good/excellent sleep quality twofold while the increase in short awakenings had no effect on sleep quality, supporting the expectation that long awakenings have a greater effect for insomnia patients than short awakenings.[83] The global benefits of the improvements in sleep measures over 3 months were reflected in patient and clinician global assessments of insomnia severity and improvement, and in "responder" analyses.[80,81] For example, the percentage of responders on the patient-rated Insomnia Severity Index,[84] classified as those showing a 6-point or greater improvement[85] at 3 months, was 56% for suvorexant 20/15 mg versus 42% for placebo with an odds ratio of 1.8, indicating that patients taking suvorexant were approximately twice as likely to be a responder than patients taking placebo.[86]

Although many patients use medications to treat insomnia chronically, most randomized controlled drug trials have been less than 3 months in duration. The suvorexant development program addressed this limitation by including a 1-year randomized controlled trial that was primarily designed to assess safety but also evaluated the long-term efficacy of suvorexant 40/30 mg on patient-reported outcomes.[78] Suvorexant effects on sleep onset and sleep maintenance were maintained consistently over 12 months, without evidence of tolerance to long-term nightly treatment. The approved 20/15 mg dose was not included but, based on the pattern of findings with 40/30 mg (and sustained efficacy of the 20/15 mg dose observed in the Phase 3 pivotal trials), it is reasonable to assume that the benefits of 20/15 mg in the 3-month trials would be maintained over longer periods. This is supported by data from a postmarketing survey study of suvorexant in Japan in which median sTSO decreased from 60 minutes at the start of treatment to 30 minutes at month 1, and this improvement was maintained up to month 6. Median sTST increased 60 minutes, from 300 minutes at the start of treatment to 360 minutes at week 1, and this improvement was maintained up to month 6.[87]

Profile of Adverse Effects

In the pooled analysis of the two pivotal Phase 3 trials, most patients completed the planned 3 months of treatment and relatively few discontinued treatment due to adverse events (3.0% for 20/15 mg versus 5.2% for placebo).[81] The most common adverse event associated with suvorexant was somnolence (6.7% for 20/15 mg versus 3.3% for placebo), which occurred mostly early during treatment (within 1–2 weeks), was generally mild to moderate in severity, and rarely resulted in discontinuation. Suvorexant 20/15 mg was also associated with reports of sleep-related hallucinations and sleep paralysis in a small number of patients (<0.5%). Sleep-related hallucinations and sleep paralysis occur spontaneously in the general population and hallucinations have been reported with other sleep-promoting medications (e.g., zolpidem), so it is unknown whether the observed events are specifically related to antagonism of orexin/hcrt receptors.[88,89] There were no reports of somnambulism or other complex sleep behaviors (e.g., sleep eating) for suvorexant 20/15 mg,[81] although there were two reports (0.2% of the Phase 3 population) for the 40/30 mg dose[80]; these appeared qualitatively similar to those reported for other sleep treatments.[90] Data from the Japanese postmarketing survey study support the safety profile of suvorexant: 9.7% of the survey population reported adverse events, and the most common adverse event was somnolence (3.6%).[87]

Use of suvorexant is contraindicated in individuals with narcolepsy given its mechanism of action and the loss of orexin/hcrt neurons associated with this disorder. Individuals known to have narcolepsy were excluded from the Phase

3 trials, so there is no information on the safety profile of suvorexant in this population. Because, in theory, antagonism of orexin/hcrt receptors could mimic signs or symptoms of narcolepsy/cataplexy in nonnarcoleptic individuals, careful monitoring of adverse events potentially related to narcolepsy/cataplexy was performed in the Phase 3 trials. No events, including falls, were confirmed by adjudication (using an independent expert adjudication committee) to be consistent with cataplexy.

With regard to other potential safety issues, there was little evidence that suvorexant caused respiratory depression in patients with mild to moderate chronic obstructive pulmonary disorder[91] or obstructive sleep apnea[92]; however, the effects in patients with severe respiratory disorder have not been evaluated. Animal and human studies suggest that the abuse potential of suvorexant is relatively low[93,94] although suvorexant was placed into Schedule IV in the FDA risk assessment, the same category as most other sleep medications.

Effects of Treatment Cessation

Each of the Phase 3 trials included a randomized discontinuation phase in which, at the conclusion of the primary treatment phase (3–12 months depending on the trial), half of those individuals previously on suvorexant were switched to placebo while the other half remained on suvorexant. Those previously on placebo remained on placebo. The main aim was to assess possible rebound insomnia and withdrawal symptoms. In the two 3-month Phase 3 trials, the randomized discontinuation period lasted for 1 week.[80,81] The effects of discontinuation were most comprehensively examined in the 1-year Phase 3 trial in patients with chronic insomnia which only evaluated the 40/30 mg dose, and where the randomized discontinuation phase lasted for 2 months.[78] Treatment gains during the preceding 12 months were at least partially lost in those previously on suvorexant who were switched to placebo. However, although insomnia symptoms returned upon discontinuation of long-term nightly suvorexant treatment, mean scores in this group did not return to the pretreatment baseline levels and were generally about half of those observed at baseline for both sleep onset and sleep maintenance.

The percentage of patients with rebound insomnia, defined as a return of sleep disturbance greater to any degree than that present at baseline, was also analyzed. The analysis looked at the first 3 nights of the discontinuation phase, where any rebound would be expected to be most apparent. In the discontinuation phase after the 1-year trial, there were no statistically significant differences with regard to worsening of sTST or sTSO for each night or for any of the 3 nights for the prespecified comparison of the group previously on suvorexant who were switched to placebo versus the group previously on placebo who remained on placebo.[78] However, the proportions with rebound insomnia were numerically greater in the group on suvorexant switched to placebo compared with the placebo group. A similar pattern of findings was apparent in the discontinuation phases of the two 3-month treatment trials when looking at rebound insomnia for the 20/15 mg dose, as well as the 40/30 mg.[80,81] Although these findings suggest that rebound insomnia is not an issue for the majority, mild disturbance of sleep may occur in some individuals for 1 or 2 nights after discontinuation of suvorexant.

The Phase 3 trials also investigated the potential for withdrawal symptoms during the discontinuation phase. The proportion of patients with newly emergent or worsening of three or more symptoms on a withdrawal symptom questionnaire for each of the first 3 nights of the discontinuation phase and across the first 3 nights was calculated. The primary comparison of interest was between the group of patients previously on suvorexant who remained on suvorexant versus those previously on suvorexant who switched to placebo. No significant differences were seen in either the discontinuation phase after 1 year of nightly treatment for the 40/30 mg dose, or in the discontinuation phase following 20/15 mg in the 3-month studies.[78,80,81]

Taken together, these findings suggest that patients with chronic insomnia who abruptly discontinue suvorexant in the absence of any other interventions, such as cognitive behavior therapy, are likely to experience a return of insomnia symptoms. However, symptoms of rebound (worsening of insomnia relative to baseline) or withdrawal after long-term use of suvorexant appear to be negligible for most patients.

Use in the Elderly

The elderly constitute a large proportion of those with insomnia and have been shown to have particular problems with sleep maintenance (disrupted sleep), and to shift to a pattern of earlier retiring and early morning awakenings with increased napping during the day.[95,96] The generally poorer sleep of the elderly may reflect degeneration of wake- and sleep-promoting neurons,[97] as well as a phase-advance of the sleep wake system, which could potentially affect the efficacy of sleep treatments. Risk that the elderly may be more prone to nighttime and next-day residual effects, particularly falls, is a concern with some existing sleep treatments.[98,99] In the two 3-month Phase 3 trials of suvorexant, approximately 40% of patients were elderly (≥65 years). In a pooled elderly subgroup analysis, suvorexant doses of 15 mg and 30 mg were found to be effective over 3 months on subjective and objective measures of sleep maintenance and sleep onset.[80] The safety profile in the elderly was similar to that seen in the overall population. Somnolence was the most common adverse event, with no evidence for an increase in falls with suvorexant versus placebo (1.5% for 15 mg, 0.6% for 30 mg, 1.5% for placebo).

Use in Patients with Alzheimer Disease

Sleep disturbance and insomnia are found in up to 40% of patients with Alzheimer disease.[100] Patients and caregivers report symptoms attributable to nighttime sleep fragmentation and nighttime awakenings, early morning awakenings, increased time to fall asleep, decreased deep sleep, and increased daytime napping due to insufficient nighttime sleep. There are concerns about using existing hypnotics, including Z drugs, in these patients because of their potential to increase falls and cause confusion, as well as a lack of data to show that they are effective in this population.[101] Some findings suggest a role for neurodegenerative loss of hypothalamic orexin/hcrt neurons, contributing to disturbed sleep-wake patterns.[102] Progression of Alzheimer disease itself may also cause dysregulation of the orexin/hcrt system, leading to increased orexin/hcrt-ergic output and promotion of inappropriate nighttime wakefulness in patients with Alzheimer disease.[103] A trial evaluated suvorexant for treating insomnia in patients with mild-to-moderate probable Alzheimer disease dementia.[104] It was found that suvorexant was effective in increasing PSG measures of TST and WASO along with evidence for improvement in subjective ratings as performed by the patient's caregiver and their clinician. As well as suggesting a new option for treating insomnia in patients with Alzheimer disease, these findings demonstrate that orexin/hcrt signaling is reasonably functional in patients at the earlier stages of Alzheimer disease dementia, because suvorexant was able to competitively antagonize the action of endogenous orexin/hcrt neuropeptides at orexin/hcrt receptors to improve sleep. Whether this is the case in patients with more advanced disease is unknown.

Neurophysiologic Effects

The neurophysiologic effects of sleep medications have been studied with regard to the amount of time spent in traditional sleep stages consisting of REM and NREM stages N1, N2, and N3/slow wave sleep as assessed by PSG. In pooled analyses of the Phase 3 data, the increase in TST produced by suvorexant was found to be due to increased time spent in all sleep stages compared with placebo.[105] When comparing suvorexant to placebo in terms of changes in percentage of TST spent in each stage, during night 1, there were small decreases of approximately 1% to 2% for N1, N2, and N3 on average, respectively, and an average increase of approximately 4% in REM. The largest differences from placebo were observed at night 1 and generally diminished over time (e.g., REM percent difference dropped to 2% at month 3). Suvorexant reduced REM latency by about 35 minutes during night 1 compared with placebo and by about 16 minutes at month 3.

The neurophysiologic effects of sleep medications have also been evaluated using qEEG spectral analyses of the power in the standard frequency bands (delta, theta, alpha, sigma, beta, gamma). Analyses of pooled Phase 3 data showed suvorexant minimally effected power spectral density during NREM and REM sleep relative to placebo across qEEG frequencies.[105]

Overall, these findings suggest that antagonism of the orexin/hcrt pathway can improve sleep onset and duration without major changes in the patient's neurophysiology as assessed by EEG/PSG. The most notable effects of suvorexant on sleep architecture are minimal mean increases in REM percentage (normalized for the increase in TST). The clinical significance of the effects on REM is unknown. Some data suggest that patients with insomnia may have a deficit in the amount of REM relative to normal sleeper controls,[106] and therefore increasing REM in insomnia patients may have a "normalizing" effect on sleep architecture (making it more closely resemble that of normal sleepers). In the suvorexant Phase 3 PSG population, mean baseline REM latency was approximately 120 minutes, whereas REM latency in normal sleepers is typically close to approximately 90 minutes. Consequently, the observed 35-minute REM latency reduction to a mean of approximately 90 minutes suggests the possibility of a suvorexant-mediated REM latency normalization for these relatively REM-deprived patients.

LEMBOREXANT

Lemborexant (DAYVIGO) was approved by the FDA in 2019 for the treatment of insomnia (unless indicated otherwise, the source for the data in this section is the FDA prescribing information).[107] Like suvorexant, lemborexant is an antagonist for both the OX1R and OX2R receptor subtypes.[108] At therapeutic doses, peak concentrations of lemborexant occur at approximately 1 to 3 hours and the mean terminal plasma half-life is approximately 17 to 19 hours. Lemborexant's systemic pharmacokinetics are approximately linear, with an accumulation of 1.5-fold to 3-fold with once-daily dosing. It is mainly eliminated by metabolism, primarily by CYP3A. In the United States, the recommended starting dose is 5 mg, which can be increased to a maximum of 10 mg based on clinical response and tolerability. Because CYP3A inhibitors increase lemborexant plasma levels, the recommended maximum dose for those taking weak CYP3A inhibitors is 5 mg, whereas concomitant use of lemborexant with moderate or strong CYP3A inhibitors should be avoided. The clinical efficacy and safety profile of lemborexant in Phase 3 clinical trials appeared broadly similar to that described for suvorexant in the preceding sections, although the two drugs have not been directly compared in clinical trials. Lemborexant improved objective (PSG) and subjective measures of sleep onset and sleep maintenance compared with placebo, and the most common adverse event was next-day somnolence. There was no evidence of significant rebound insomnia or withdrawal effects after treatment discontinuation.

Potential Differentiation from GABAergic Drugs

There are no direct head-to-head data regarding the comparative efficacy of suvorexant versus GABAergic drugs such as zolpidem in insomnia patients. However, data exists for the discontinued orexin/hcrt receptor antagonist almorexant and lemborexant.

Zolpidem 10 mg was included as a positive control in a 2-week placebo-controlled RESTORA trial of almorexant 100 mg and 200 mg in nonelderly (<65 years) individuals.[109] Although there was no direct statistical comparison of almorexant versus zolpidem, almorexant appeared to have a larger effect than zolpidem on objective PSG WASO (difference from placebo in change from baseline at week 2 = −14 to −20 minutes for almorexant versus an increase of 4 minutes for zolpidem), but not on patient-reported sWASO (difference from placebo in change from baseline at week 2 = −7 to −10 minutes for almorexant and −13 minutes for zolpidem). With regard to sleep onset, zolpidem appeared to have a larger effect than almorexant on objective PSG LPS (difference from placebo in change from baseline at week 2 = −11 minutes for zolpidem and −4 to −6 minutes for almorexant) but not on patient-reported sTSO (difference from placebo in change from baseline at week 2 = −6 minutes for zolpidem and −4 to −7 minutes for almorexant). These data suggest that orexin/hcrt receptor antagonists maintain sleep over the course of a night more effectively than a GABAergic drug. This advantage was confirmed in the SUNRISE-1 trial where lemborexant was superior to zolpidem extended release 6.25 mg in improving sleep maintenance as assessed by PSG sleep efficiency (TST/time in bed) over the whole night and PSG WASO in the second half of the night in older individuals with insomnia.[110] The extended release formulation of zolpidem used for comparison is marketed for sleep maintenance and may have a weaker sleep onset effect compared with immediate release formulations.[111] Lemborexant showed improved sleep onset versus the zolpidem extended release formulation in the SUNRISE-1 trial.[110]

As noted previously in this chapter, suvorexant has minimal effects on sleep architecture compared with placebo in patients with insomnia when the amount of time spent in each sleep stage is expressed as a percentage of the TST, apart from a small increase in the percentage of REM (and corresponding decrease in the percentage of NREM) and a shortening of latency to REM. Similar findings were observed for almorexant in the RESTORA trial.[109] By contrast, zolpidem was found to reduce the time spent in REM in that trial, with a corresponding increase in the time spent in N2, and to increase the latency to REM consistent with previous findings for zolpidem.[112] Based on preliminary reports, lemborexant was also found to reduce the latency to REM compared with zolpidem in the SUNRISE-1 trial.[113] A direct head-to-head comparison of the effects of suvorexant 20 mg versus zolpidem 10 mg on EEG power spectra during sleep in healthy subjects found that zolpidem reduced EEG spectral density across theta and alpha frequency whereas suvorexant had no significant effects on spectral density.[114] The clinical implications of these sleep architecture/EEG power findings are unknown but could be interpreted as suggesting that orexin/hcrt receptor antagonists produce a more physiologically normal sleep compared with GABAergic drugs.

Animal data suggest that orexin/hcrt receptor antagonists might have a reduced impact on motor coordination, memory, and cognition compared with GABAergic drugs.[115-119] A study in normal healthy subjects found that those taking almorexant performed better on a neurocognitive test battery than those taking zolpidem 10 mg when treatment and testing were administered in the afternoon,[120] but the relevance of these findings for next-day performance after night-time dosing in insomnia patients is not clear. In the RESTORA trial, almorexant and zolpidem 10 mg showed similar incidences of somnolence,[109] while in the SUNRISE-1 trial of older individuals, lemborexant was associated with a small increase in somnolence and falls compared with zolpidem extended release 6.25 mg.[110] Overall, these results suggest that orexin/hcrt receptor antagonists are more effectively able to maintain sleep over the course of a night than Z drugs, without a marked increase in next-day residual effects.

Arousability is a critical element in the definition of sleep, and arousals are typically necessary for normal physiologic responses during sleep. Preclinical studies showing that sleeping dogs and nonhuman primates monkeys given an orexin/hcrt receptor antagonist retain the capacity to awaken to emotionally salient acoustic stimuli while still preserving uninterrupted sleep in response to irrelevant stimuli.[121,122] In contrast, the GABA-A receptor modulators eszopiclone and diazepam impaired the animals' ability to wake to salient stimuli. This suggests that orexin/hcrt receptor antagonists preserve a "normal" arousal threshold whereas the threshold to arouse is higher with drugs that enhance GABA signaling.[122] A study in individuals with insomnia confirmed that suvorexant preserved the ability to respond to nocturnal auditory stimuli, but a GABAergic control drug was not included.[123]

FUTURE DIRECTIONS

The growing realization of the bidirectional nature between sleep and other disorders such as Alzheimer disease and depression has increased awareness of the possibility that orexin/hcrt receptor antagonists could not only improve sleep in patients with these conditions, but may also have beneficial effects on the underlying disorder (i.e., slowing the pathophysiologic changes underlying dementia progression in those with Alzheimer disease, reducing depression in those with major depressive disorder).[124,125] Potential also exists for utility of orexin/hcrt receptor antagonists in settings such as substance abuse disorders, where there is a need for sleep agent alternatives that reduce risk for insomnia-related relapse without the abuse liability profile and respiratory depressant effects of the GABAergic class of drugs.[126] With increasing understanding of the role of sleep in a variety of disorders and the specific role orexin/hcrts play in regulating sleep and wakefulness, important opportunities arise for the potential use of orexin/hcrt receptor antagonists to treat disorders beyond insomnia.[127] Furthermore, research is underway to evaluate the potential therapeutic utility of orexin/hcrt agonists for improving wakefulness in patients with excessive daytime sleepiness and other disorders characterized by impaired arousal[128]; at least one orexin/hcrt agonist has progressed to evaluation in humans.[129]

CLINICAL PEARL

Suvorexant and lemborexant, the first medicines approved by regulatory agencies for targeting the orexin/hcrt signaling system, are orexin/hcrt receptor antagonists that promote sleep by blocking orexin-mediated wake drive. Orexin/hcrt receptor agonists are currently being evaluated as potential treatments for disorders characterized by excessive daytime sleepiness.

SUMMARY

The fundamental biologic nature of sleep makes understanding of the orexin/hcrt circuit of high importance for its therapeutic potential. The development of advanced tools to manipulate and characterize the orexin/hcrt arousal circuit in animal models has allowed for dissection of the circuit with direct implications for translational medicine. Indeed, two orexin/hcrt antagonists have been approved for treating insomnia, and an orexin/hcrt agonist is being evaluated for the treatment of excessive daytime sleepiness. Further research suggests orexin/hcrt antagonists may be effective beyond treatment of sleep-centric disorders with implications for conditions such as Alzheimer disease, depression, and substance abuse.

ACKNOWLEDGMENTS

Christopher Lines from Merck, Sharp & Dohme Corp., a subsidiary of Merck & Co., Inc. (Kenilworth, NJ) contributed to the drafting of the clinical sections of the chapter.

SELECTED READINGS

Berteotti C, Liguori C, Pace M. Dysregulation of the orexin/hypocretin system is not limited to narcolepsy but has far-reaching implications for neurological disorders. Eur J Neurosci. 2021;53(4):1136-1154.

Chen Q, de Lecea L, Hu Z, Gao D. The hypocretin/orexin system: an increasingly important role in neuropsychiatry. *Med Res Rev*. 2015; 35:152–197.

Eban-Rothschild A, Giardino WJ, de Lecea L. To sleep or not to sleep: neuronal and ecological insights. *Curr Opin Neurobiol*. 2017;44:132–138.

Herring WJ, Connor KM, Snyder E, et al. Suvorexant in patients with insomnia: pooled analyses of three-month data from Phase-3 randomized controlled clinical trials. *J Clin Sleep Med*. 2016;12:1215–1225.

Mahler SV, Moorman DE, Smith RJ, et al. Motivational activation: a unifying hypothesis of orexin/hypocretin function. *Nat Neurosci.* 2014;17:1298–1303.

Michelson D, Snyder E, Paradis E, et al. Safety and efficacy of suvorexant during 1-year treatment of insomnia with subsequent abrupt treatment discontinuation: a phase 3 randomised, double-blind, placebo-controlled trial. *Lancet Neurol.* 2014;13:461–471.

Peyron C, Tighe DK, van den Pol AN, et al. Neurons containing hypocretin (orexin) project to multiple neuronal systems. *J Neurosci.* 1998;18:9996–10015.

Sakurai T. The neural circuit of orexin (hypocretin): maintaining sleep and wakefulness. *Nat Rev Neurosci.* 2007;8:171–181.

Takenoshita S, Sakai N, Chiba Y, et al. An overview of hypocretin based therapy in narcolepsy. *Expert Opin Investig Drugs.* 2018;4:389–406.

Tyree SM, Borniger JC, de Lecea L. Hypocretin as a hub for arousal and motivation. *Front Neurol.* 2018;9:413.

Wang C, Holtzman DM. Bidirectional relationship between sleep and Alzheimer's disease: role of amyloid, tau, and other factors. *Neuropsychopharmacol.* 2020;45:104–120.

Wang Q, Cao F, Wu Y. Orexinergic System in Neurodegenerative Diseases. *Front Aging Neurosci.* 2021;13:713201. Published 2021 Aug 17.

Yardley J, Kärppä M, Inoue Y, et al. Long-term effectiveness and safety of lemborexant in adults with insomnia disorder: results from a phase 3 randomized clinical trial. *Sleep Med.* 2021;80:333-342.

A complete reference list can be found online at ExpertConsult.com.

Chapter 50

Serotonin and Sleep

Véronique Fabre; Andrew D. Krystal; Patricia Bonnavion

Chapter Highlights

- Serotonin or 5-hydroxytryptamine (5-HT) neurons have a wake-promoting role, as revealed by pharmacologic studies in humans and animals.
- 5-HT_{1A} receptors primarily mediate suppression of rapid eye movement sleep, while 5-HT_{2A} receptors primarily mediate suppression of non–rapid eye movement sleep.
- 5-HT neurons of the raphe nuclei are highly diverse and organized in functionally distinct subsystems that may underlie a dual role of 5-HT in promoting sleep and wakefulness.
- Conditional gene knockout and genetic neuron silencing/activating experiments reveal a key role for a subgroup of medullary 5-HT neurons in mediating arousal from sleep during hypercapnia, suggesting their potential contribution to sleep-related breathing disorders.

ORGANIZATION OF THE SEROTONIN SYSTEM

In the central nervous system (CNS), 5-hydroxytryptamine (5-HT) neurons are clustered in the raphe nuclei of the brainstem into two major groups.[1] The caudal group includes the nucleus raphe pallidus (RPa; B1/B4), the nucleus raphe obscurus (ROb; B2), and the nucleus raphe magnus (RMg; B3), whereas the rostral group includes the dorsal raphe (DR) nucleus (B6 and B7), the median raphe (MR) nucleus, the caudal linear nucleus, and the pontine raphe nucleus, corresponding to the B5/B8 clusters and the supralemniscal nucleus (B9). Although they show a degree of heterogeneity, 5-HT neurons share the ability to synthetize, store, release, and reuptake 5-HT. These processes require the expression of a core set of genes that define the 5-HT phenotype. In the CNS, differentiation and maintenance of 5-HT neurons is driven by a transcriptional regulatory network in which the transcription factor Pet1 (plasmacytoma expressed transcription factor 1) plays a key role.[1]

5-HT biosynthesis (Figure 50.1) is a two-step process starting by the conversion of the essential amino acid L-tryptophan into 5-hydroxytryptophan (5-HTP) by the brain rate limiting enzyme tryptophan hydroxylase 2 (TPH2). The aromatic L-amino-acid decarboxylase in turn converts 5-HTP to 5-HT, which is accumulated into synaptic vesicles by the vesicular monoamine transporter 2 (VMAT2). Once released in the extracellular space, 5-HT acts on 14 distinct receptor subtypes, divided into seven families ($5\text{-HT}_{1\text{-}7}$)[2]. With the exception of the 5-HT_3 receptor, which belongs to the ligand-gated ion channel superfamily, 5-HT receptors are G protein–coupled receptors. Receptors of the $5\text{-HT}_{1/5}$ families are coupled to $G\alpha_{i/o}$ proteins and negatively modulate cyclic adenosine monophosphate (cAMP) formation by inhibiting adenylate cyclase (AC) activity. In contrast, those of the $5\text{-HT}_{4/6/7}$ families are positively coupled to AC via $G\alpha_s$ proteins and stimulate cAMP accumulation. Receptors of the 5-HT_2 family are coupled preferentially to $G\alpha_{q/11}$ proteins, which activate phospholipases C and A2 and increase cytosolic calcium concentration.

Neurotransmission by 5-HT is tightly regulated by feedback mechanisms that involve 5-HT receptors expressed by 5-HT neurons (autoreceptors) and inactivation through 5-HT reuptake (Figure 50.1). Inhibitory feedback mechanisms include the activation of 5-HT_{1A} and 5-HT_{1B} autoreceptors leading to inhibition of 5-HT neuron firing rate and 5-HT release, respectively. Recent studies[3] also report positive feedback regulation of 5-HT neurons by 5-HT_{2B} autoreceptors: activation of the 5-HT_{2B} receptor increased the firing rate of a subset of DR 5-HT neurons, and mice conditionally lacking 5-HT_{2B} receptors in 5-HT neurons display a hyposerotonergic phenotype. Additionally, single-neuron transcriptome profiles revealed that a subset of 5-HT neurons in the RMg expresses the excitatory 5-HT_{2A} receptors,[4] but experimental data are lacking to evaluate its role as an autoreceptor. Inactivation of the released 5-HT includes its transport back into presynaptic terminals by the high-affinity serotonin transporter (SERT) and its recycling into synaptic vesicles by VMAT2. Alternatively, 5-HT can be cleared from the extracellular space by organic cation transporters, a low-affinity/high-capacity uptake system present in postsynaptic neurons (OCT2 and OCT3).[5] Once transported into cells, 5-HT is ultimately degraded by monoamine oxidase A and B, two mitochondrial isoenzymes that catalyze monoamine degradation.

Detection of the expression of several genes unrelated to 5-HT signaling in raphe neurons has indicated that 5-HT neurons may release a second transmitter.[1] In particular, there is now compelling evidence that a subset of 5-HT neurons, mainly those located in the ventral DR, expresses the vesicular glutamate transporter 3 (VGLUT3), conferring to 5-HT neurons the ability to store and release glutamate. Accordingly, optogenetic stimulation of 5-HT terminals produces

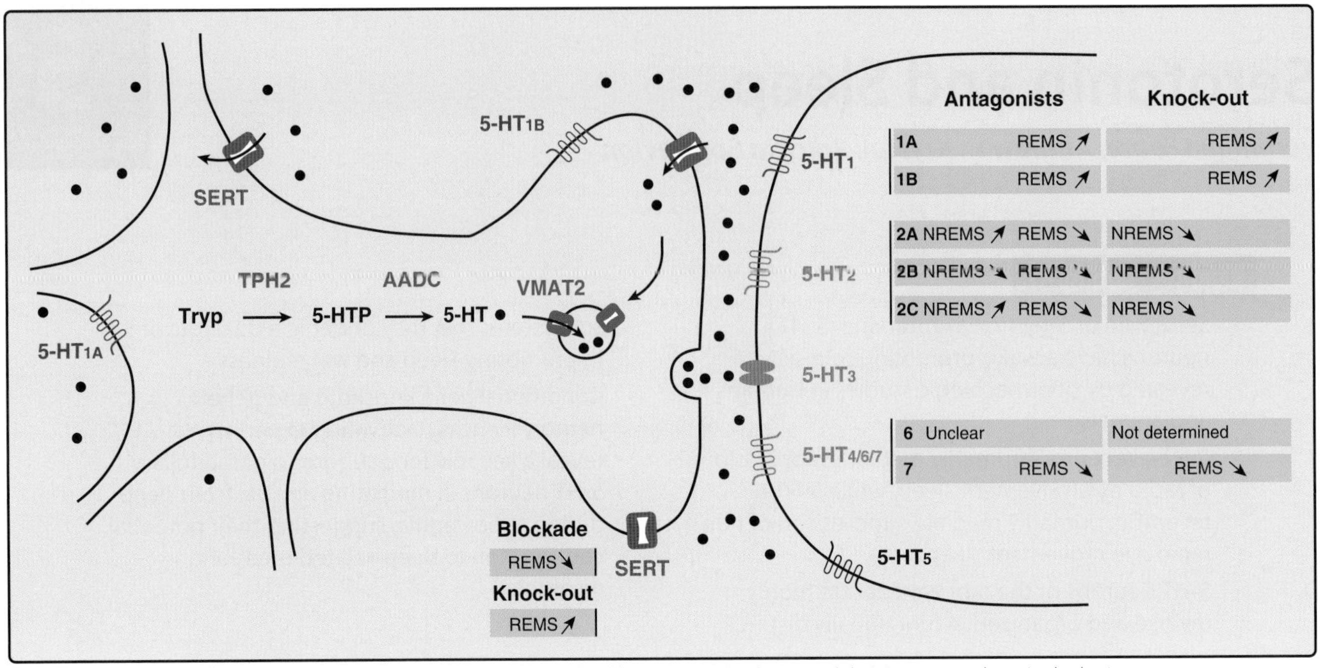

Figure 50.1 The brain 5-hydroxytryptamine (5-HT) system: main players and their impact on sleep. In the brain, 5-HT neurons express a set of genes ensuring 5-HT biosynthesis (*Tph2, Aadc*), storage into synaptic vesicles (*Vmat2*), and reuptake (*Sert*). Once released in the extracellular space, 5-HT can bind to 14 different receptors of the G protein–coupled receptor (subtypes 1, 2, 4, 5, 6, and 7) and ligand-gated ion channel (subtype 3) families. 5-HT$_{1A}$ and 5-HT$_{1B}$ are also expressed by 5-HT neurons exerting an inhibitory control on 5-HT neurotransmission. Pharmacologic studies using 5-HT receptor selective antagonists (except for the 5-HT$_{2B}$ and 5-HT$_{7}$ subtypes) or blocking the SERT support a wake-promoting/REMS suppressing role for 5-HT. Pharmacologic findings were compared with those obtained using gene deletion in constitutive knockout mice. AADC, L-amino-acid decarboxylase; NREMS, NREM sleep; REMS, REM sleep; Tryp, L-tryptophan sleep.

fast glutamate excitatory currents in the hippocampus, ventral tegmental area, and amygdala.[1]

Molecular heterogeneity of 5-HT neurons in mice has been further assessed with the recent development of single-cell transcriptomics.[6] These studies have notably found that a subset of 5-HT neurons in the MR, DR, and RMg expresses mRNA encoding enzymes responsible for gamma-aminobutyric acid (GABA) synthesis and may thus co-release GABA. Similarly, studies using in situ hybridization or immunofluorescence approaches in mice have suggested that some 5-HT neurons of the rostral groups and, more frequently those of the caudal groups, may synthetize GABA.[7] However, functional evidence for GABA release by 5-HT neurons is lacking. Transcriptomic profiling studies also reported expression of mRNAs encoding various neuropeptides including thyrotropin-releasing hormone (TRH), substance P, corticotropin-releasing hormone (CRH), and galanin (Gal) in 5-HT neurons in the mouse brain.[8] Intriguingly, histochemical approaches yielded no evidence of the coexistence of neuropeptides and 5-HT in the mouse DR.[7] This discrepancy may arise from technical limitations. Immunolabeling may lack sensitivity, while single-cell transcriptomes may bias mRNA detection when used in conjunction with cell type-specific driver genes. In some cases, these discrepancies may reflect poor translation of the detected mRNA. In the rat, subpopulations of DR neurons were found to contain both 5-HT and Gal or CRH, revealing robust species differences. Other studies have shown that the coexistence of neuropeptides and 5-HT varies within raphe nuclei, with a higher degree of colocalization in caudal raphe nuclei.[9] For example, *Tac1*, the gene encoding substance P, is predominantly expressed by 5-HT neurons of the ROb and RPa in the mouse.[4] Further investigations are needed to clarify neuropeptide expression in 5-HT neurons across raphe nuclei and across species.

Despite their small number (approximately 26,000 neurons in the mouse brain and approximately 450,000 neurons in humans) and restricted distribution, 5-HT neurons innervate most of the brain and medulla.[1] Broadly, the caudal group innervates the medulla and spinal cord, while the rostral group targets the forebrain and midbrain. In the rostral group, mapping studies also revealed complementary and mostly non-overlapping projection patterns between the DR and MR. Thus 5-HT fibers arising from the DR target the amygdala, cerebral cortex, striatum, substantia nigra, and locus coeruleus, while those from the MR predominantly target subcortical areas, including the hippocampus, septum, caudal hypothalamus, mammillary bodies, interpeduncular nucleus, and mesopontine tegmental nuclei. This organization of the 5-HT system is preserved in many mammalian species, including humans.[10] Recently, whole-brain tracing methods in mice using viral and genetic tools have further highlighted that subsets of 5-HT neurons (defined by their molecular profiles) display specific connectivity, providing further evidence of the diversity of the 5-HT system.[11] A striking example is the 5-HT neurons expressing VGLUT3, mainly found in the ventral DR, that preferentially target cortical structures, while those expressing TRH, mostly observed in the dorsal DR, predominantly innervate subcortical regions such as the thalamus and hypothalamus.[6]

Overall, these molecular and anatomic studies have revealed that 5-HT neurons are highly diverse and organized in distinct anatomic subsystems. This heterogeneity is also supported by functional studies measuring the neuronal activity of raphe neurons across the sleep-wake cycle.

THE ROLE OF SEROTONIN IN SLEEP-WAKE FUNCTION

5-HT Neuronal Activity and Release Across the Sleep-Wake Cycle

Early studies suggested that 5-HT may promote sleep, as electrolytic lesions of the raphe nuclei or inhibition of the 5-HT synthesis using the tryptophan hydroxylase inhibitor para-chlorophenylalanine (PCPA) produced long-lasting insomnia in cats. These data constituted the origin of the monoaminergic theory of sleep in which Jouvet and colleagues proposed that 5-HT promotes sleep.[12] Single-unit recordings were used to further evaluate the role of 5-HT. Initial electrophysiologic studies in anesthetized animals provided evidence that 5-HT neurons have a specific signature characterized by long-duration action potentials following a slow rhythmic firing pattern.[13] These electrophysiologic properties were then used in nonanesthetized animals to identify presumptive 5-HT neurons. Single-unit recordings in freely moving cats provided the first correlative evidence that the vast majority of presumptive 5-HT neurons in the DR are wake-active neurons that exhibit their highest firing frequencies during wake, decreased activity as non–rapid eye movement (NREM) sleep occurs, and almost complete cessation of firing during rapid eye movement (REM) sleep.[14,15] This activity pattern of DR neurons across the sleep-wake cycle has been repeatedly confirmed[16] and was also seen in other raphe nuclei.[17] Microdialysis studies in behaving animals further reported that extracellular 5-HT levels in brain areas targeted by 5-HT neurons consistently vary across the sleep-wake cycle, with higher levels in wake and a progressive decline in NREM and REM sleep.[18] Consequently, 5-HT neurons were thus considered as part of the ascending arousal system that promotes wake, challenging the Jouvet's concept of a sleep-promoting role for 5-HT[12] (however, see the section Manipulating 5-HT Neurons in Adulthood).

This view of 5-HT neurons as a homogenous wake-on population was challenged by subsequent in-depth analysis of larger samples of raphe neurons. Electrophysiologic studies in anaesthetized animals first pointed toward a significant diversity among 5-HT neurons identified using juxtacellular labeling techniques. Thus subsets of 5-HT neurons in the DR were reported to display atypical firing patterns characterized by fast-firing or burst-firing activities in anesthetized rats.[19] Furthermore, the classic criteria used to identify presumptive 5-HT neurons do not allow for unequivocal identification because non–5-HT raphe cells share similar characteristics.[20,21] Importantly, functional diversity is also found in relation to the sleep-wake cycle.[22] Thus a significant proportion of presumptive 5-HT wake-active neurons display atypical behavior as they are tonically active during NREM sleep and some of the latter remain active during REM sleep.[22] More surprisingly, the presence of presumptive 5-HT neurons with highest rate of tonic discharge during sleep was also reported.[22,23]

Although these studies did not assess the chemical identity of the recorded neurons, it is now accepted that DR 5-HT neurons can be differentially categorized into a large population of wake-active neurons with stereotyped electrophysiologic behavior and, to a lesser extent, a wake-sleep–active or sleep-active population displaying mixed electrophysiologic characteristics with both typical and atypical firing profiles. This electrophysiologic diversity suggests that distinct subtypes of 5-HT neurons may underlie specific functions. Consistent with this hypothesis, a study in anesthetized rats showed that fast-firing 5-HT neurons identified by juxtacellular labeling fire phase-coupled to the hippocampal theta rhythm, a rhythm associated with exploration that is prominent in REM sleep.[24] This result suggests that a subset of 5-HT neurons, whose activity is more rapid and phase-locked to theta rhythm, could be involved in information processing. Taken together, studies using single-unit recordings agree that a large proportion of 5-HT neurons (as defined by electrophysiologic criteria) are active during wake, decrease their firing rate during NREM sleep and are nearly silent during REM sleep, but there appears to be greater diversity of firing patterns across the sleep-wake cycle than is generally acknowledged.

PHARMACOLOGIC MANIPULATIONS AFFECTING SEROTONIN SIGNALING AND EFFECTS ON SLEEP

The 5-HT signaling pathways have attracted significant attention as potential drug targets for the treatment of mood and anxiety disorders that are frequently accompanied by sleep complaints, and 5-HT drugs may have beneficial or adverse effects on sleep. This section describes the effects of selective ligands targeting the 5-HT system on sleep in preclinical models (Figure 50.1). Most of these studies have investigated the role of 5-HT_{1A}, 5-HT_2, and 5-HT_7 receptors; less attention has been given to 5-HT_{1B} and 5-HT_6 receptors.

Targeting the 5-HT Transporter: Antidepressants

The SERT is the target of the selective serotonin reuptake inhibitors (SSRIs), which have antidepressant and anxiolytic effects. SSRIs bind selectively to the SERT to block 5-HT reuptake, thereby increasing extracellular 5-HT concentration. In rodents, the acute systemic administration of SSRIs has been consistently reported to inhibit REM sleep and, occasionally, to promote wake. A secondary increase in NREM sleep amounts has also been observed in some cases. In rats and mice, increased REM sleep latency and reduced REM sleep amounts were observed after administration of a single dose of fluoxetine,[25] paroxetine,[26] citalopram,[27] or escitalopram[28] during the lights-on period. Some studies also addressed the impact of chronic SSRI administration. Although reduction of REM sleep amounts persisted after repeated SSRI administration, some tolerance was found.[28] On withdrawal, a REM sleep rebound was not observed after a 3-week treatment with paroxetine.[29]

Targeting 5-HT Receptors

5-HT signaling is remarkably complex because of the diversity of 5-HT receptors. In the 1980s and 1990s, the development of compounds with 5-HT receptor subtype selectivity provided the first framework for understanding the function of individual 5-HT receptors in modulating vigilance states.

Among all 5-HT receptors, the 5-HT_{1A} subtype has been the most extensively studied because of the early identification of the selective agonist 8-OH-DPAT[2] (which is now known to be active at the 5-HT_7 receptor as well) and the synthesis of ligands with anxiolytic properties, the azapirones such as buspirone and ipsapirone.[30] The development of selective silent antagonists such as WAY-100635 further contributed to understanding the role of 5-HT$_{1A}$ receptors in sleep-wake regulation. In rodents, acute administration of 5-HT$_{1A}$ receptor agonists (e.g., buspirone[31]) was consistently shown to markedly enhance wake and strongly reduce REM sleep. Conversely, systemic injection of the 5-HT$_{1A}$ receptor antagonist WAY-100635 tends to increase REM sleep amounts in mice.[32] Importantly, 5-HT$_{1A}$ receptors drive a large portion of the suppressive effects of SSRIs on REM sleep. Indeed, 5-HT$_{1A}$ receptor pharmacologic blockade or genetic inactivation antagonizes the REM sleep reduction induced by citalopram administration in mice.[27]

The mechanisms underlying the effects of 5-HT$_{1A}$ receptor activation on sleep remain unclear. Mapping studies have identified 5-HT$_{1A}$ receptors in most 5-HT neurons of the anterior raphe nuclei (autoreceptors) and on target neurons receiving 5-HT projections (postsynaptic receptors). Target neurons have been implicated in the regulation of sleep by 5-HT$_{1A}$ receptors. Notably, the effects of ipsapirone on sleep persisted after the selective destruction of 5-HT neurons by the neurotoxin 5,7-dihydroxytryptamine.[33] Postsynaptic 5-HT$_{1A}$ receptors are located in a number of brain regions implicated in wake-sleep regulation, including the anterior and lateral hypothalamus, the vertical limb of the diagonal band of Broca, the deep mesencephalic nucleus of the reticular formation/ventrolateral portion of the periaqueductal gray, and pontine reticular nucleus in rodents.[34–36] Notably, 5-HT$_{1A}$ receptors are expressed by sleep-active GABAergic neurons of the VLPO.[37] Although 5-HT$_{1A}$ receptor activation may promote wake by inhibiting sleep-active VLPO neurons, there has been no direct examination of such a mechanism yet. A more recent study has identified a new ponto-hypothalamic pathway through which 5-HT$_{1A}$ receptors can mediate sleep inhibition in mice.[38] This pathway includes GABAergic neurons of the ventral dorsal tegmental (DTg) nucleus of Gudden, which have been shown to strongly express 5-HT$_{1A}$R mRNA.[34] Specifically, local injection of 8-OH-DPAT into the DTg of freely moving mice enhanced wake and reduced REM sleep, mimicking the effects observed after systemic administration. Interestingly, anatomic evidence suggests that DTg neurons make a direct synaptic contact with glutamatergic and histamine neurons in the posterior hypothalamus.[38,39] As the latter are critically involved in wake promotion, 5-HT could promote wake by exerting an inhibitory control on GABAergic neurons of the DTg that project to the posterior hypothalamus through 5-HT$_{1A}$ receptors. Alternatively, REM sleep-active cholinergic neurons of the laterodorsal/pedunculopontine tegmental nuclei have been proposed to trigger REM sleep inhibition induced by 5-HT$_{1A}$ receptors in rats.[40]

Only limited evidence supports the involvement of 5-HT$_{1B}$ receptors in sleep-wake regulation. 5-HT$_{1B}$ receptors are present on axon terminals of 5-HT and non–5-HT neurons and exert an inhibitory control on neurotransmitter release. These receptors are found mainly in the substantia nigra and globus pallidus.[41,42] Acute pharmacologic activation of 5-HT$_{1B}$ receptors reduces REM sleep and increases in wake in mice.[43] Conversely, REM sleep is enhanced after the acute blockade of 5-HT$_{1B}$ receptors in mice.[43] The neural circuits by which 5-HT$_{1B}$ receptors exert their inhibitory control on REM sleep are unknown.

The 5-HT$_2$ receptor family comprises three distinct receptor subtypes: 5-HT$_{2A}$, 5-HT$_{2B}$, and 5-HT$_{2C}$ receptors, with 5-HT$_{2B}$ receptors showing a more restricted expression pattern in the brain than the two other subtypes.[41,42] Interest in the 5-HT$_2$ receptor subtype arose from initial findings showing that the nonselective 5-HT$_{2A/2C}$ antagonist ritanserin had hypnotic properties: acute administration during the light (inactive) period enhanced the duration of NREM sleep and, concomitantly, inhibited REM sleep in rats.[44] Conversely, the nonselective agonist DOI promoted wake in rats.[45] More recently, the respective contribution of each 5-HT$_2$ receptor subtype has been assessed thanks to new drugs with subtype selectivity. In rats, selective 5-HT$_{2A}$ receptor blockade with MDL 100907 enhanced NREM sleep and slow wave activity during NREM sleep when injected during the dark (active) period[46] and inhibited REM sleep in rodents[47] when administered during the light (inactive) period. Selective blockade of the 5-HT$_{2C}$ receptor subtype decreased REM sleep in mice[47] and increased NREM sleep in rats.[48] Together, preclinical studies suggest that 5-HT exerts an inhibitory role on NREM sleep expression by acting on 5-HT$_{2A/2C}$ receptors. Furthermore, they imply that development of pharmacologic agents that antagonize 5-HT$_{2A/2C}$ receptors may lead to novel therapies for insomnia and depression. Blockade of 5-HT$_{2B}$ receptors, unlike that of the 5-HT$_{2A/2C}$ subtypes, resulted in an increase in wake amounts and conversely, their activation increased NREM sleep amounts in mice.[47] These results suggest a peculiar role for the 5-HT$_{2B}$ subtype, in that it is the only 5-HT receptor facilitating NREM sleep upon activation. Interestingly, recent studies have suggested that 5-HT$_{2B}$ receptors are expressed by 5-HT neurons, where they act as a positive modulator of 5-HT tone.[3] Whether the effects of 5-HT$_{2B}$ receptor ligands on sleep can be attributed to postsynaptic or to autoreceptors remains to be addressed.

The 5-HT$_6$ receptor is coupled to the Gs-adenylyl cyclase pathway and is exclusively present in the CNS with its highest expression in the striatum, nucleus accumbens, and hippocampus.[41,42] This receptor has emerged as a target to improve cognition in Alzheimer disease, as 5-HT$_6$ receptor antagonists showed procognitive effects in rodents and humans.[49] 5-HT$_6$ receptor agonists promote wake in rats.[50] However, 5-HT$_6$ receptor antagonists were reported to promote sleep,[46] enhance wake,[51] or have no effect on sleep.[52] More research must be done to identify the role of the 5-HT$_6$ receptor on sleep regulation.

The 5-HT$_7$ receptor is positively coupled to AC through stimulatory G_s/G_{12} proteins; its highest density was detected in hypothalamus, thalamus, hippocampus, cortex, and DR.[41,42] Pharmacologic studies suggest an opposite role for 5-HT$_7$ and 5-HT$_{1A}$ receptors in regulating REM sleep. It has been convincingly reported that blockade of 5-HT$_7$ receptors during the light (inactive) period results in an increase in REM sleep latency and a decrease of time spent in REM sleep.[53,54] One study also found that systemic administration of the selective 5-HT$_7$ receptor agonist LP-211 significantly increases time spent awake.[55] Although surprising at first, these results may be explained by the involvement of 5-HT$_7$ receptor in a local modulatory loop that negatively controls 5-HT neuron activity and release. In this model, locally released 5-HT activates the 5-HT$_7$ receptor located on GABAergic interneurons in the DR, which results in hyperpolarization and reduced firing rate of 5-HT neurons.[56] Accordingly, REM sleep suppression induced by 5-HT$_7$ receptor antagonists may be the result of enhanced 5-HT tone. Interestingly, 5-HT$_7$ receptor antagonists exhibit antidepressant-like properties in preclinical models and potentiate the effects of SSRIs on both REM sleep and behavior.[53,57]

To summarize, reports from pharmacologic manipulations of the 5-HT system in preclinical models are in general agreement (except for the 5-HT_{2B} and 5-HT_7 subtypes) with electrophysiologic and microdialysis findings, which suggests that 5-HT neurons promote wake and inhibit REM sleep.

LESSONS FROM CONSTITUTIVE AND CONDITIONAL MUTANT MICE

Genetic inactivation of different components of 5-HT signaling in constitutive knockout (KO) models leads to sleep-wake deficits that are summarized in Figure 50.1.

The characterization of mice lacking 5-HT receptors first confirmed that 5-HT_{1A} and 5-HT_{1B} receptors exert an inhibitory control on REM sleep expression.[43,58] Thus 5-HT_{1A} and 5-HT_{1B} receptor KO mice display greater REM sleep amounts, as also observed after their pharmacologic blockade. Interestingly, REM sleep homeostasis is also impaired in these mutants. Selective REM sleep deprivation produces changes in the sleep pattern that are mainly characterized by an increase in REM sleep amounts during the recovery period; this REM sleep rebound is abolished in 5-HT_{1A} and 5-HT_{1B} receptor KO mice. Similarly, both mutants exhibited a blunted sleep response to acute stress that is characterized by the absence of a secondary REM sleep increase during the recovery period. Altogether, these data show that 5-HT_{1A} and 5-HT_{1B} receptor subtypes mediate an inhibitory role of 5-HT on REM sleep and are required for REM sleep homeostasis to occur.

In contrast to 5-HT_{1A} and 5-HT_{1B} receptor deficient mice, 5-HT_7 receptor KO mice spend less time in REM sleep.[32,59] This result confirms that 5-HT_7 receptors exert a facilitatory influence on REM sleep expression as previously suggested by pharmacologic studies. Overall, genetic inactivation and pharmacologic tools point toward opposite roles for 5-HT_7 and 5-HT_{1A}/5-HT_{1B} receptors on REM sleep expression.

Further investigations found that 5-HT_{2B} receptor KO mice exhibit reduced amounts of wake.[60] These results are similar to those observed with antagonists at 5-HT_{2B} receptors, providing further evidence that 5-HT_{2B} receptors play an atypical role among 5-HT receptors by contributing to the initiation of sleep.

Divergent results were obtained after constitutive inactivation of certain genes encoding key components of the 5-HT system when compared to their pharmacologic blockade (Figure 50.1). Although SERT blockade with SSRIs suppresses REM sleep, mice with constitutive SERT inactivation have enhanced REM sleep amounts.[61] Similarly, 5-HT_{2A} and 5-HT_{2C} receptor KO mice exhibit increased amounts of wake,[47,62] but antagonists enhance NREM sleep amounts (see previous section). As evidenced for SERT, the sleep-related effects seen in some constitutive KO mice may be causally linked to the influence of 5-HT in brain development. Thus 5-HT brain levels in early development determines, at least in part, brain function during adulthood, particularly during the so-called "critical" developmental stages, ranging from the first to the fourth postnatal weeks in mice and rats.[63] Accordingly, transient changes in 5-HT signaling during this critical period may have striking effects later in life as shown for the regulation of sleep. The best-studied example is SERT KO mice, which have a lifelong increase in brain 5-HT[64] and an increase in REM sleep amounts in adults (see earlier). These sleep alterations in SERT KO mice can be permanently rescued in adulthood by a 2- to 4-week neonatal treatment with an inhibitor of 5-HT synthesis or a selective 5-HT_{1A} receptor antagonist, both of which aim to protect the brain from excessive extracellular 5-HT levels.[65] Conversely, pharmacologic blockade of the SERT during postnatal development by SSRIs induces lifelong alterations of sleep that mimic the SERT KO phenotypes.[66] Future research should address whether the sleep phenotypes of 5-HT_{2A} and 5-HT_{2C} receptor KO mice result from similar modifications of 5-HT signaling during early postnatal life or are a consequence of unrelated mechanisms.

Genetic models lacking brain 5-HT synthesis were generated after the discovery of the gene encoding the tryptophan hydroxylase isoform *Tph2*.[67] TPH2 constitutive KO mice are characterized by a severe and lifelong depletion of 5-HT in the brain.[68] Different laboratories have reported contradictory findings about the sleep phenotype of adult TPH2 KO mice. One study found that mutant mice exhibit more sleep during the light (active) period, supporting the idea that 5-HT promotes wake.[69] However, sleep was defined as periods of immobility lasting at least 5 minutes and was not assessed by polysomnography (PSG). In contrast, PSG studies found that TPH2 KO mice display less REM sleep[70] or more consolidated wake and NREM sleep.[71] Lifelong depletion of 5-HT in the mutants is associated with several dysfunctions early in life, including growth retardation, respiratory deficits, and increased lethality during the first postnatal weeks.[68] It is thus difficult to draw conclusions on the role of brain 5-HT during adulthood by studying constitutive TPH2 KO mice. To overcome these limitations, alternative genetic approaches have been developed. In one study, conditional deletion of the gene encoding *Tph2* was achieved through stereotaxic infusion of Cre recombinase-expressing adeno-associated viruses (AAV) into the rostral raphe nuclei of adult mice carrying a conditional allele of the *Tph2* gene.[72] These mice are characterized by a nearly complete disappearance of TPH2 expression in the rostral raphe nuclei and a marked decrease in 5-HT tissue contents in the forebrain. Indirect evidence from video and motion monitoring suggests that adult 5-HT deficiency affects sleep, but further investigations are needed to properly analyze the sleep pattern of this conditional model.

Another interesting model is the conditional KO Lmx1b (LIM homeobox transcription factor 1 beta) mouse. Lmx1b is a transcription factor that contributes to the differentiation of 5-HT neurons in the CNS. Its inactivation in 5-HT neurons was obtained by crossing mice carrying a conditional allele of the *Lmx1b* gene to Pet1-Cre mice that express Cre recombinase in central 5-HT neurons. As a result, almost all brain 5-HT neurons failed to survive.[73] These mutant mice exhibit severe respiratory dysfunction during the postnatal period with a decrease of ventilation, long-lasting apneas, and a high perinatal mortality.[74] In addition, adult mutant mice housed at an ambient temperature of 23° C display an insomniac-like phenotype characterized by long wake episodes.[75] This phenotype has been proposed to be an indirect consequence of a severe defect in thermoregulation. Indeed, mutant mice lacking 5-HT neurons fail to maintain their body temperature during cold exposure,[75] an effect attributed to medullary 5-HT neurons that regulate thermogenesis.[76] Accordingly, mutant mice display normal sleep-wake patterns when housed at a thermoneutral ambient temperature of 33° C.[75] Interestingly, this insomniac-like profile was also found after pharmacologic inhibition of 5-HT synthesis by PCPA in cats and rats.[12] To investigate whether this phenotype was also caused by thermoregulatory deficits, the sleep-wake patterns of mice treated with PCPA have been analyzed at various ambient temperatures.[77] Similar to mutant mice lacking 5-HT neurons, mice with pharmacologic depletion of 5-HT during adulthood exhibit an insomniac-like phenotype at 23° C but not at 33° C. Altogether, the results obtained after pharmacologic depletion of 5-HT or genetic loss of brain 5-HT neurons suggest that 5-HT does not directly cause sleep but is important for thermogenesis.

A recent study reported the use of a conditional system to perform a selective ablation of central 5-HT neurons in adult mice.[78] Transgenic mice carrying a conditional allele of the diphtheria toxin receptor (DTR) were first crossed with Pet1-Cre mice. Ablation of central 5-HT neurons was then achieved by intracerebroventricular administration of diphtheria toxin in adult Pet1-Cre;DTR mice. The number of 5-HT neurons was decreased by approximately 70% in the DR and by approximately 30% in the other raphe nuclei after administration of the toxin. Accordingly, 5-HT tissue contents were decreased by approximately 50%. Mice with central 5-HT neuron ablation during adulthood exhibited a mild reduction in body temperature during the light (inactive) phase and slightly reduced body weight. They also display less REM sleep and a reduced arousal in response to a novel environment. Although reduced arousal to novelty supports the wake-promoting role of 5-HT neurons, the findings on REM sleep are more surprising and have been proposed to be due to enhanced 5-HT_7 receptor signaling, but this hypothesis remains to be tested.

To summarize, the study of mice with constitutive or conditional gene invalidation has provided new insights into the role of specific components of the 5-HT signaling in sleep regulation and has revealed the importance of 5-HT in brain maturation during early life and its long-lasting impact. However, developmental effects also limit our understanding of the role of 5-HT on sleep in adulthood. Likewise, interpretation of data from constitutive and some conditional KO mutants on sleep is reduced because of the role of medullary raphe 5-HT neurons in breathing and thermoregulation. These latter points underscore the importance of using strategies that enable time- and region-specific gene inactivation.

MANIPULATING SEROTONIN NEURONS IN ADULTHOOD

The development of optogenetics and chemogenetics opens many perspectives to grasp the complex role of the 5-HT system in sleep with specific cell-targeting and temporal control. Only a few studies have used these approaches in adult mice in the context of sleep and arousal. The findings to date suggest that DR 5-HT neurons differentially modulate brain state transitions depending upon their firing discharge mode, circadian period, and arousal context.

Patterned photostimulations were used in optogenetic studies to test the effects of different frequencies and modes of DR 5-HT neurons firing on sleep-wake transitions. Low-frequency tonic (regular) and high-frequency phasic (irregular) photostimulations were shown to differentially modulate brain state toward either sleep or wakefulness, respectively.[79] These opposite effects also seem to depend on the phase of the circadian cycle in which 5-HT system activation was conducted. During the dark (active) phase when the wake state dominates, a slow tonic activation (3 Hz, continuous) of DR 5-HT cells reduces sleep latency by half and extends the duration of sleep episodes.[79] In contrast, during the light (inactive) phase when mice are mostly asleep, high-frequency (20–25 Hz) phasic stimulation of DR 5-HT neurons facilitates wakefulness.[79] Based on these results, optogenetic stimulation of DR 5-HT neurons have bidirectional mode-dependent effects on sleep-wake transitions that vary across the circadian cycle. Interestingly, recent findings using optogenetic functional magnetic resonance imaging with activation of DR 5-HT neurons show that, despite the expression of both excitatory and inhibitory 5-HT receptors in DR projection sites, the net effect of DR 5-HT photostimulation at high frequency (20 Hz) is inhibitory in most brain areas.[80] In addition, such stimulations suppress delta oscillations in the cortex,[80] which could be consistent with cortical activation or changes occurring when animals transition from quiet wakefulness to an active motor behavior. Further investigations are necessary to relate this specific effect to arousal state and its impact on cortical processing.

In future studies, the heterogeneous nature of the 5-HT system involving multiple subsystems among and within each raphe nucleus has to be taken into account.[81] The manner in which optogenetic approaches have been employed to date does not yet allow addressing the functional diversity recruiting a variety of 5-HT subtypes.[80] Future studies using these genetic tools to deconstruct neural circuits could partially address this issue. For instance, it was shown that specific 5-HT DR efferent projections may be specialized to control specific symptoms of narcolepsy in mouse models.[82] A global chemogenetic activation of DR 5-HT neurons was shown to suppress the occurrence of cataplexy-like episodes and decrease REM sleep hypersomnia in narcoleptic mice without affecting wake fragmentation.[83] A follow-up optogenetics study refined 5-HT partners and targets underlying some of these effects.[82] Only activation of DR 5-HT terminals in the amygdala recapitulated anticataplectic effects but did not affect REM sleep amounts. These findings suggest that the control of 5-HT on the excess REM sleep and cataplexy in narcoleptic mice involve distinct 5-HT subpopulations and pathways. Similarly, other optogenetic studies suggest that distinct 5-HT pathways from various DR subdivisions[11] may be differentially engaged in locomotion or anxiety behavior.[84,85]

More efforts should be brought, using these techniques, to better characterize the basal 5-HT operating mode. Recent data suggest that the DR 5-HT nucleus is composed of multiple subsystems with distinct functionalities and inputs that inherently employ different modes of activity that can be selectively recruited upon behavioral context and input signals. In certain contexts, release of 5-HT promotes wake. As discussed earlier, 5-HT is critical to autonomic functions, including thermoregulation and ventilatory responses,[86] and these actions may prime and actually gate 5-HT modulation of sleep-wake states. As also detailed previously, mice genetically engineered to lack 5-HT neurons have impaired thermoregulatory control.[74,75] Their sleep architecture is normal unless mice are exposed to cool ambient temperatures, which leads to increases in the time spent awake.[75] This insomnia is attributable to animals being cold and compensating by increasing motor activity to generate heat and foraging for warmer areas. These mice also exhibit an impaired ventilatory response during sleep, as they do not arouse in response to high levels of CO_2.[75] The importance of 5-HT neuronal activity in generating this lifesaving response was further confirmed with both acute chemogenetic silencing using designer receptors exclusively activated by designer drugs (DREADD) and optogenetic silencing of 5-HT neurons in adults blocking the arousal response to hypercapnic challenges.[87,88] Interestingly, mice lacking 5-HT neurons arouse in response to hypoxic challenges and to auditory and tactile stimuli.[75] These findings indicate that a subset of 5-HT neurons may be specifically involved in inducing arousal in response to hypercapnia.[89,90] In addition, DR 5-HT neurons were found to exhibit phasic firing activity in response to noxious stimuli[91] or aversive cues,[92] which could suggest that hypercapnia-induced arousal may also involve burst firing of 5-HT neurons. Importantly, impairment of this specific response may contribute to sleep-related breathing disorders, such as sudden infant death syndrome or sleep apnea, both of which are consistently associated with 5-HT dysfunction. In summary, these studies highlight the critical influence of 5-HT in homeostatic functions, especially during sleep, and should influence future studies to employ a combination of genetic tools and approaches to tackle this multifaceted role of 5-HT in sleep.

HUMAN STUDIES EVALUATING THE ROLE OF SEROTONIN IN SLEEP-WAKE FUNCTION

Pharmacologic Manipulations Affecting 5-HT Signaling in Humans and Effects on Sleep

A number of studies have been conducted in humans assessing the sleep effects of decreasing 5-HT systemically via consumption of a diet lacking in the 5-HT precursor tryptophan. Because tryptophan is an essential amino acid that must be obtained through dietary intake, the production of 5-HT can be drastically reduced via consumption of a tryptophan-free diet. In a series of double-blind, placebo-controlled, crossover studies, this manipulation was found to result in reduced REM sleep latency in remitted depressed patients receiving SSRIs, depressed patients who had responded to cognitive behavioral therapy for depression, healthy controls, and ecstasy users.[93–96] In addition, in the depressed patients who remitted with SSRIs, rapid tryptophan depletion led to an increase in REM sleep percentage, REM sleep time, REM density, and total sleep time (TST).[93] In healthy controls and ecstasy users, there was also a shortening of sleep-onset latency and increased REM sleep time.[96]

A few small studies evaluated morning rapid tryptophan depletion based on serum tryptophan levels, which has been thought to increase nighttime 5-HT levels. In healthy controls, tryptophan depletion led to decreased stage 2, increase wake percentage, and increased REM density in one study and only an increase in REM sleep latency in another study.[95,97]

Although there is some controversy about whether the rapid tryptophan-depletion paradigm actually decreases neural 5-HT and whether there are confounding side effects, such as nausea and vomiting, as well as some inconsistency of results, these studies broadly suggest that decreasing 5-HT availability reduces REM sleep latency and may also increase the amount and percentage of REM sleep.[97] These findings are generally in agreement with the findings of preclinical models reviewed earlier, which suggest that activation of 5-HT neurons tends to inhibit REM sleep.

Complementing this work are a number of studies that have evaluated the sleep effects of increasing systemic and CNS 5-HT levels with oral L-tryptophan.[98] Double-blind placebo-controlled trials in humans, including groups of healthy controls and individuals with insomnia, suggest that L-tryptophan administration shortens sleep-onset latency.[98-103] However, several studies failed to find therapeutic effects on sleep or found inconsistent effects on sleep-onset latency, including a crossover study in 39 individuals with insomnia, a study of 21 psychiatric patients with insomnia,[104] a study of 90 insomnia patients,[105] and a study of 19 individuals with mild dementia and insomnia.[106] Collectively, these studies suggest that L-tryptophan tends to shorten the latency to sleep onset, but this effect is inconsistent and of limited size and, as a result, do not meaningfully provide insight regarding the role of 5-HT in sleep regulation.

Human Studies of the Sleep-Wake Effects of Drugs with Serotoninergic Effects

A number of different types of medications have serotoninergic effects, several of which have been mentioned previously. Some of these have selective effects that are limited to affecting 5-HT and 5-HT receptors and have been studied in humans, including SSRIs, selective 5-HT_{1A} receptor partial agonists, selective 5-HT_{2A} receptor inverse agonists, selective $5\text{-HT}_{2A/C}$ receptor antagonists, 5-HT_7 receptor antagonists, and L-tryptophan, which, as described previously, is required for synthesis of 5-HT. The sleep effects of these medications are summarized in Table 50.1. There are also a number of medications that have clinically significant pharmacologic effects on 5-HT as well as on at least one other neurotransmitter and/or receptor type, which is not discussed here because the lack of specificity for 5-HT clouds the interpretation of the relationship of clinical effects to 5-HT related mechanisms. These include serotonin/norepinephrine reuptake inhibitors, agomelatine, monoamine oxidase inhibitors, antipsychotic medications, and a number of antidepressant medications with broad pharmacologic effects.[107,108] Examples of antidepressants with such broad effects include tricyclic antidepressants, the chlorophenyl piperazine, trazodone, and the tetracyclic antidepressant mirtazapine.[109,110]

Selective Serotonin Reuptake Inhibitors

As reviewed previously, SSRIs bind selectively to the SERT and block 5-HT reuptake, thereby increasing extracellular 5-HT concentration, which then increases binding to various 5-HT receptors. The findings in studies in humans taking SSRIs mirror the findings reported for studies in animals. The most consistent observation is REM sleep suppression, and the second most consistent finding is a tendency to disturb sleep.[18] Although these findings are relatively consistent across different SSRIs and studies, it is important to note that these agents also have varying degrees of norepinephrine reuptake inhibition, which can also affect sleep-wake function, and results in some heterogeneity of the sleep-wake profiles among this group of agents.[111]

Table 50.1 Effects of Drugs with 5-Hydroxytryptamine Studied in Humans in Placebo-Controlled Trials

Drug Mechanism	Effect on REM Sleep	Effect on NREM Sleep	Associated Sleep Disturbance/ Enhancement
Selective 5-HT reuptake inhibition	Suppression	-	Disturbance
Selective 5-HT partial agonists	Suppression		Disturbance
Selective 5-HT_{2A} inverse agonists	-	Enhancement	Specifically decreases awakenings
Selective $5\text{-HT}_{2A/2C}$ antagonists	-	Enhancement	Specifically decreases awakenings
5-HT_7 antagonists	Suppression	-	-
L-tryptophan (5-HT precursor)	-	-	Inconsistent decrease in sleep-onset latency

There are few placebo-controlled studies that focused on delineating the sleep-wake effects of SSRIs. However, studies employing PSG sleep assessment in both healthy controls and patients with major depressive disorder suggest that these medications tend to increase sleep-onset latency, increase awakenings and wake time after sleep onset (WASO), decrease TST, decrease NREM slow wave sleep, and decrease REM sleep time, REM sleep percentage, and REM sleep latency.[112] These findings tend to be accompanied by self-reported disturbance of sleep in healthy controls but improvement in sleep in depressed patients, which is assumed to reflect therapeutic antidepressant effects.[112]

Additional information regarding the sleep-wake effects of these agents can potentially be gleaned from the side effect profiles seen in clinical trials. Insomnia has been reported in trials of SSRIs in 7% to 22% of patients with depression, which is approximately double the rate of placebo.[113] Notably, daytime somnolence is reported in 4% to 24% of depressed patients, which is also roughly double the placebo rate.[113] However, it is unclear whether this is a direct effect of the SSRIs, a consequence of sleep disturbance, or a consequence of restless legs syndrome or periodic limb movements of sleep causing disruption, which can be triggered by these medications.[114,115]

$5HT_{1A}$ Receptor Agonists/Partial Agonists

A number of selective full or partial agonists at 5-HT_{1A} receptors, including buspirone, have been studied in humans. Consistent with the preclinical data, 5-HT_{1A} receptor agonism tends to enhance wake and suppress REM sleep. Of these, only buspirone is used clinically, having been approved for treatment of generalized anxiety disorder in the United States by the FDA.

Buspirone

Buspirone is a full agonist at presynaptic 5-HT_{1A} receptors and a partial agonist at postsynaptic 5-HT_{1A} receptors.[116,117] Placebo-controlled crossover studies have shown that buspirone was associated with suppression of REM sleep.[117-119] In addition, one study showed that buspirone was associated with fragmentation of sleep.[117] These findings support a role of 5-HT_{1A} receptor agonism in sleep disturbance and REM sleep suppression.

Selective 5-HT_2 Receptor Inverse Agonists and Antagonists

Both 5-HT_2 receptor antagonists and inverse agonists have been studied in humans. These include the selective 5-HT_{2A} receptor inverse agonists APD125 and pimavanserin and the selective $5\text{-HT}_{2A/2C}$ receptor antagonist ritanserin. Only pimavanserin has been approved for clinical use. Consistent with the preclinical work reviewed previously, studies of these agents suggest that 5-HT exerts an inhibitory effect on NREM sleep expression by acting on $5\text{-HT}_{2A/2C}$ receptors.

APD125

APD125, a 5-HT_{2A} receptor inverse agonist, was evaluated in a double-blind, placebo-controlled trial in patients with insomnia and had a notable therapeutic impact on sleep consisting of decreasing the number of PSG-determined awakenings and WASO, and increasing NREM sleep electroencephalographic (EEG) slow wave activity without impacting sleep latency or TST.[120] Also of note, findings on the PSG were much greater than self-reported improvement, which was minimal. These findings suggest that 5-HT_{2A} receptor activation may play a role in maintaining sleep in humans by increasing NREM slow wave sleep. However, $5HT_{2A}$ receptors do not appear to play a role in the aspects of sleep affected by most insomnia therapies: sleep-onset latency and TST. It is unclear why the beneficial effects of 5-HT_{2A} receptor inverse agonism are appreciated only to a modest degree by insomnia patients who take this medication and experience improvement in PSG measures.

Pimavanserin

Like APD125, pimavanserin is a 5-HT_{2A} receptor inverse agonist. The PSG effects of four doses of this medication were compared with placebo in a parallel group study.[121] Similar to APD125, pimavanserin[121] led to a dose-dependent increase in NREM slow wave sleep and decreased the number of awakenings without significantly affecting other sleep parameters.

Ritanserin

Ritanserin is a selective antagonist of 5-HT_{2A} and 5-HT_{2C} receptors. The sleep effects of this medication were evaluated in a number of double-blind placebo-controlled trials carried out in small groups of healthy controls and small groups of individuals with disturbed sleep. These studies consistently indicated that ritanserin significantly increases NREM slow wave sleep time and EEG slow wave amplitude compared with placebo without significantly impacting other sleep parameters.[122,123] The exception to this is that studies evaluating the effects of ritanserin on number of awakenings noted significant improvement in this aspect of sleep.[124] These findings are highly consistent with the effects of 5-HT_{2A} receptor inverse agonists and are consistent with 5-HT_{2A} receptors, mediating a specific effect on disturbing NREM slow wave sleep and enhancing the number of awakenings.

Selective 5-HT_7 Receptor Antagonists

A double-blind, placebo-controlled crossover PSG study of the selective 5-HT_7 antagonist, JNJ-18038683, was conducted in 12 healthy controls.[54] This study indicated that 5-HT_7 receptor antagonism has a REM sleep suppressant effect in terms of a significant increase in REM sleep latency and decrease in REM sleep time compared with placebo.

FUTURE DIRECTION AND CONCLUSION

This chapter summarizes the relationship of 5-HT and sleep. Animal and human studies are strikingly consistent in suggesting a wake-promoting role for the 5-HT system and indicate that activation of 5-HT_{1A} receptors suppresses REM sleep, whereas 5-HT_{2A} receptor activation suppresses NREM sleep.

There is a significant need to carry out research to determine the function of the many 5-HT receptor subtypes for which we currently lack specific ligands in animals and/or humans, including the 5-HT_{2B}, 5-HT_3, 5-HT_{5A}, and 5-HT_6 receptors. Another important area for future research is the clinical significance of specific modulation of REM and NREM sleep. Although it has been the subject of research for more than 30 years, the clinical significance of specifically suppressing REM sleep, enhancing REM sleep, enhancing NREM slow wave sleep, or suppressing NREM slow wave sleep remains unknown. However, in recent years, there has been a significant body of research devoted to the specific roles that REM and NREM slow wave sleep play in maintaining normal health and neuropsychiatric function. Future studies should systematically manipulate these aspects of sleep with 5-HT–related interventions and investigate the impact on key functional and disease outcomes to better delineate the role of the 5-HT system in maintaining health and normal function.

SUMMARY

Serotonin (5-HT) neurons clustered in the raphe nuclei innervate nearly all brain regions to act on a multiplicity of receptors. These neurons are involved in the regulation of a large number of higher functions, including cognition, memory, mood, feeding, and, as detailed in this chapter, the sleep-wake cycle. Evidence from pharmacologic studies in humans and animals supports a role for 5-HT neurons in wake promotion with primary roles for 5-HT_{1A} and 5-HT_{2A} receptors. Curiously, some observations suggest that 5-HT is permissive for sleep. Although 5-HT is intimately linked to the sleep-wake cycle, questions remain regarding its specific role and the mechanisms involved, as well as the implications of this system for sleep medicine and psychiatry. This chapter summarizes key recent findings that, combined with classic data from both animal and human research, refine the role of 5-HT in sleep-wake control.

CLINICAL PEARLS

- 5-HT neurons play a role in wake promotion that is primarily mediated by 5-HT_{1A} and 5-HT_{2A} receptors, which exert inhibitory effects on REM and NREM sleep, respectively.
- Decreasing 5-HT availability enhances REM sleep in terms of shortening of REM sleep latency and perhaps increasing the amount and percentage of REM sleep.
- Increasing 5-HT availability at the synapse results in suppression of REM sleep and a tendency toward sleep disturbance.
- Similar results are observed with selective $5HT_{1A}$ receptor partial agonists, suggesting that the effects of increasing 5-HT may be mediated by $5HT_{1A}$ receptors.
- Studies of selective $5HT_{2A}$ receptor inverse agonism and selective $5HT_{2A/C}$ antagonism suggest that 5-HT exerts an inhibitory effect on NREM sleep expression by acting on 5-HT_{2A} receptors.
- 5-HT_7 receptor antagonism has a REM sleep suppressant effect.
- Human studies largely confirm the findings derived from basic research.

SELECTED READINGS

Buchanan GF, Richerson GB. Central serotonin neurons are required for arousal to CO2. *Proc Natl Acad Sci U S A*. 2010;107:16354–16359.

Maierean AD, Bordea IR, Salagean T, et al. Polymorphism of the serotonin transporter gene and the peripheral 5-hydroxytryptamine in obstructive sleep apnea: what do we know and what are we looking for? A systematic review of the literature. *Nat Sci Sleep*. 2021;13:125–139.

Monaca C, Boutrel B, Hen R, et al. 5-HT1A/1B receptor-mediated effects of the selective serotonin reuptake inhibitor, citalopram, on sleep: studies in 5-HT1A and 5-HT1B knockout mice. *Neuropsychopharmacology*. 2003;28:850–856.

Oikonomou G, Altermatt M, Zhang RW, et al. The serotonergic raphe promote sleep in zebrafish and mice. *Neuron*. 2019;103:686–701.

Popa D, Léna C, Fabre V, et al. Contribution of 5-HT2 receptor subtypes to sleep-wakefulness and respiratory control, and functional adaptations in knock-out mice lacking 5-HT2A receptors. *J Neurosci*. 2005;25: 11231–11238.

Sakai K. Sleep-waking discharge profiles of dorsal raphe nucleus neurons in mice. *Neuroscience*. 2011;197:200–224.

Sakurai T, Saito YC, Yanagisawa M. Interaction between orexin neurons and monoaminergic systems. *Front Neurol Neurosci*. 2021;45:11–21.

Ursin R. Serotonin and sleep. *Sleep Med Rev*. 2002;6:57–69.

A complete reference list can be found online at ExpertConsult.com.

Chapter 51

Melatonin

Helen J. Burgess; Jamie M. Zeitzer

Chapter Highlights

- Melatonin is a hormone produced by the pineal gland and can be found in organisms from single-celled organisms to humans. Melatonin secretion occurs during the biologic night.
- Exogenous melatonin or melatonin agonists are often used as therapeutic agents. Daytime administration of low doses of melatonin can change the timing of the circadian clock, whereas higher doses can help to induce sleep.
- The basic physiology and pharmacology of melatonin as well as the fundamentals of its clinical usage are discussed.

ENDOGENOUS BIOSYNTHESIS AND PHYSIOLOGIC REGULATION

Melatonin is a hormone that is almost exclusively produced by the pineal gland, located above the splenium of the corpus callosum. There is independent, although much smaller, production of melatonin in both the retina[1] and gut.[2] However, these loci are unlikely to contribute to the role that melatonin plays in the regulation of sleep and circadian rhythms. Plasma melatonin concentrations have a stereotypical pattern, with low concentrations throughout the day, a rapid rise 1 to 3 hours before habitual bedtime, elevation throughout the normal sleep period, and a rapid decline approximately 1 hour after wake time (Figure 51.1). The peak nocturnal concentration of melatonin in the plasma and saliva has more than a tenfold variation among healthy adults.[3,4] For clinical and research purposes, melatonin is often assessed from saliva samples. Salivary melatonin concentrations are approximately threefold lower than plasma concentrations and represent the unbound fraction of plasma melatonin.[5] Although the absolute concentrations of melatonin in plasma and saliva are quite different, the relative timing of melatonin concentrations in these two fluids is similar.[6]

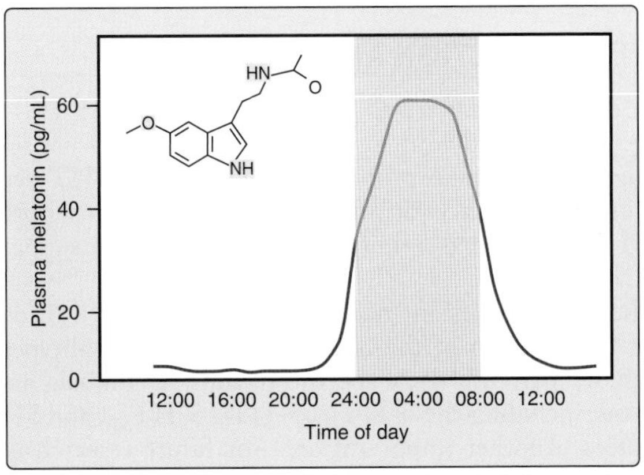

Figure 51.1 The typical pattern of plasma melatonin is for very low concentrations throughout the day, which rise approximately 2 hours prior to habitual bedtime, remain elevated through the sleep period (*gray shaded box*), and decline just after wake time. *Inset,* Molecular structure of melatonin (N-acetyl-5-methoxytryptamine).

PINEAL AFFERENTS

Melatonin production by the pineal gland is controlled predominantly by the suprachiasmatic nucleus (SCN), the site of the central circadian pacemaker.[7,8] Although the pineal gland is located deep within the brain, it is located on the body side of the blood-brain barrier; thus spinal innervation is necessary to connect the SCN with the pineal gland. Efferents from the SCN project to the paraventricular nucleus of the hypothalamus (PVH), which sends axons via the medial forebrain bundle to the intermediolateral column of the spinal cord.[9] These spinal neurons exit the spinal cord in the upper thoracic region (T1-T4) and innervate the superior cervical ganglion (SCG), which, among other targets, innervates the pineal gland. As a sympathetic nerve, the SCG releases noradrenaline that activates both alpha- and beta-adrenergic receptors on pinealocytes, leading to increased intracellular cyclic adenosine monophosphate (cAMP) and calcium that increase the transcription of arylalkylamine-*N*-acetyltransferase, the reported rate-limiting enzyme involved in the synthesis of melatonin.[10] Damage to any of the components of this pathway (i.e., SCN, PVH, spinal cord, SCG, pineal) can lead to abolition of the nocturnal surge in melatonin (see the work by Zeitzer and colleagues[11]). Clinical evidence of damage to this pathway is readily observed by the presence of bilateral oculosympathoparesis (Horner syndrome) as the deficits observed in this syndrome are secondary to dysfunction in the SCG.[12] In addition to the sympathetic innervation of the pineal gland, there is also a parasympathetic innervation from the sphenopalatine ganglion.[13,14] The specific impact of this parasympathetic ganglion on pineal function is unknown, but it has been hypothesized that it inhibits the release of norepinephrine from the SCG via presynaptic muscarinic receptors.[15]

Influence of Light and Chemicals on Melatonin

In addition to circadian control, pineal production of melatonin can be acutely and completely suppressed by light exposure.[16] Light intensity as low as room light can suppress the production of melatonin,[17] with the onset of melatonin being even more sensitive to suppression by light.[18] As such, darkness per se does not stimulate pineal production of melatonin but facilitates its highest levels of production. Medications that interfere with beta-adrenergic receptors (e.g., beta blockers) can also reduce melatonin production.[19] Other chemicals, such as ethanol[20] and nonsteroidal anti-inflammatory medications,[21] may also reduce the amplitude of plasma melatonin. The duration and amplitude of plasma melatonin concentrations can also be influenced by factors that impact the liver, specifically cytochrome P450 (CYP) 1A2,[22] which normally 6-hydroxylates melatonin into 6-hydroxymelatonin, which is conjugated with sulfates and excreted in the urine.[23]

Melatonin as a Circadian Marker

Given the predominance of the circadian clock in the control over the timing of melatonin, under properly controlled conditions (e.g., dim lighting, stable posture), the timing (phase) of the melatonin rhythm has been used as a marker of the timing of the central circadian clock. Various methods have been used to assess the timing of the melatonin rhythm, including the onset of melatonin (dim light melatonin onset) with a fixed or variable threshold, the midpoint of melatonin, the fitted maximum, or a modeled onset.[24] In healthy individuals, most of these techniques give stable assessments of the timing of the central circadian clock.[25]

Molecular Mechanism of Melatonin

Melatonin acts through two high-affinity G protein–coupled receptors, MT_1 and MT_2.[26] MT_1 and MT_2 receptors have a wide distribution in the human brain, including the SCN, cerebellum, thalamus, hippocampus, and cortex.[27] Both MT_1 and MT_2 receptors are expressed by the SCN and appear to have functionally distinct roles. Activation of the MT_1 receptor inhibits SCN firing, especially at the light-dark transition, while activation of the MT_2 receptor, and the MT_1 receptor to a lesser degree, shifts the timing of the SCN.[26] It has been hypothesized that the suppression of SCN firing in the evening may be responsible for a reduction in alertness just before sleep onset.[28]

Activation of the MT_2 receptors in non-SCN areas, such as the reticular nucleus of the thalamus, may also be important for the sleep promotion.[29] There are also melatonin receptors located in many non-brain regions (e.g., gut, heart, pancreas),[30] although these are unlikely to be involved in the sleep-related physiology of melatonin. The importance of endogenous melatonin in normal human sleep is not well understood. In nocturnal mammals, melatonin is still produced at night, when they are maximally active, reinforcing its role as a marker of the night length.[31] Most laboratory strains of mice do not even produce melatonin,[32] with little consequence for sleep.[33] In humans, the chronic loss of melatonin has only a small impact on sleep parameters.[34,35] There are mixed findings on whether the pharmacologic replacement of absent or lower endogenous melatonin levels in humans with clinical conditions can significantly improve sleep.[36-38]

EXOGENOUS PHARMACODYNAMICS

Immediate-Release Formulation

Oral, immediate-release melatonin of varying doses has a similar half-life of approximately 45 minutes and a time to peak blood concentration of approximately 50 minutes.[39] There are a wide variety of doses commercially available, typically from 0.1 mg to more than 10 mg. Daytime oral administration of 0.3 mg of melatonin approximates the normal nocturnal concentrations of melatonin, while doses above 1 mg are supraphysiologic.[40] Given the half-life of melatonin, a single 0.3-mg dose of oral melatonin will produce elevated blood concentrations of melatonin for approximately 5 hours.[40] The higher doses (>10 mg) of oral melatonin produce blood concentrations that are more than 100-fold higher than those normally found in adult humans; these supraphysiologic blood concentrations of melatonin can persist for more than 24 hours[40] and may impact other receptor systems.[41] High doses of melatonin have been used to treated REM sleep behavior disorder (see Chapter 118).

Alternate Routes of Administration

Given its small, highly lipophilic nature, melatonin can readily be administered through alternate routes, including intranasal (spray), transdermal (patch), transmucosal (sublingual), or oral sustained release. The pharmacokinetics of each of these vary considerably based on the exact technology used to introduce melatonin to the bloodstream. In general, intranasal has the shortest (i.e., most rapid acting) time to peak concentration, while transdermal is much slower and has a more sustained profile,[42,43] although there may be considerable between-sex differences in the transfer of melatonin across the skin.[44] Sublingual dosing has a similar pharmacologic profile to oral immediate-release formulations.[45] Oral sustained-release formulations are similar to the transdermal formulations in that they result in an extended time of elevated plasma melatonin concentrations but also have a shorter time to peak concentrations, similar to oral immediate-release formulations.[43] The routes of administration other than through the digestive tract avoid the substantial first-pass metabolism of the exogenous melatonin. Given the very high interindividual variability in endogenous melatonin[3,4] and the high interindividual differences in plasma melatonin concentrations after exogenous administration of melatonin, little research has been conducted to determine whether specific blood concentrations are necessary for the biologic effects of exogenous melatonin.

The Effects of Exogenous Melatonin on Human Sleep

Dose and Timing

Melatonin is well recognized to have soporific effects,[40,46,47] especially when endogenous melatonin levels are low.[37,38] However, there is not a clear dose-response relationship in the soporific effect of melatonin over the range of 0.3 mg to 10 mg, which is the range of melatonin doses most commonly available.[48] The soporific effect is hypothesized to be due to binding to melatonin receptors in the SCN[49] and in the peripheral vasculature,[50] which can induce thermoregulatory changes that promote sleep. Thus, for soporific effects, melatonin is usually taken in the 30 minutes before desired bedtime. Meta-analyses have consistently found that an immediate-release formulation of melatonin can reduce the time taken to fall asleep.[51-53] Exogenous melatonin may also increase sleep duration, although this effect has been less consistently observed and is more likely to occur with a continuous-release formulation.[52] It has been suggested that the soporific effect of supraphysiologic doses of melatonin may be reduced when homeostatic sleep pressure is low (such as after sleep),[44] but this has not been consistently observed.[54]

The Effects of Exogenous Melatonin on Human Circadian Timing

Dose and Timing

Exogenous melatonin administration can shift the circadian pacemaker to both an earlier and later time (phase advance and phase delay, respectively). This was first demonstrated in the rat,[55] with subsequent studies demonstrating this to be true in humans as well.[56,57] In general, exogenous melatonin administration in the late afternoon or early evening leads to phase advances, whereas administration in the late night and early morning leads to phase delays[56,57] (Figure 51.2). There is evidence of a dose-response relationship in circadian phase shifting at lower doses of 0.02 and 0.30 mg.[58] By contrast, when 0.5 mg and 3.0 mg were compared across a range of administration times, maximum phase advance and phase delays were similar.[57] Even higher doses of exogenous melatonin (≥10 mg) may result in *smaller* circadian phase shifts,[59,60] as higher doses increase the duration of melatonin in the circulation, with potential to produce both phase advances and phase delays, resulting in an overall smaller circadian phase shift.[60] For maximal circadian phase shifting, melatonin must be taken during times of usual wakefulness; thus doses of 0.5 mg or lower are recommended to avoid the sleepiness that higher doses of melatonin can produce (see earlier section). People should test their individual soporific response to various melatonin doses before driving or operating heavy machinery.

In an attempt to elicit a circadian phase shift with exogenous melatonin, it is important to also consider the timing of light exposure. Light exposure has stronger phase-shifting properties than exogenous melatonin and can enhance or reduce phase shifts in response to exogenous melatonin. The impact of melatonin on circadian phase can therefore be twofold. First, as described previously, it can directly change circadian phase. Second, because of its hypnotic effects, it can induce a change in sleep timing and, secondarily, light exposure (i.e., mostly dark during sleep). For example, melatonin administration in the evening can elicit phase advances directly (phase-shifting properties) and indirectly by inducing sleep and shielding the pacemaker from exposure to phase-delaying light in the evening. Melatonin administration can also be used adjunctively with light therapy; for example, afternoon administration coupled with morning light administration to promote larger phase advances.[61,62] It is currently unknown whether phase delays obtained with evening light treatment can be increased with morning melatonin. Because of its circadian phase-shifting effects, exogenous melatonin has been recommended to treat circadian rhythm sleep-wake disorders such as jet lag,[63] delayed sleep-wake phase disorder, and non-24-hour sleep-wake disorder.[64]

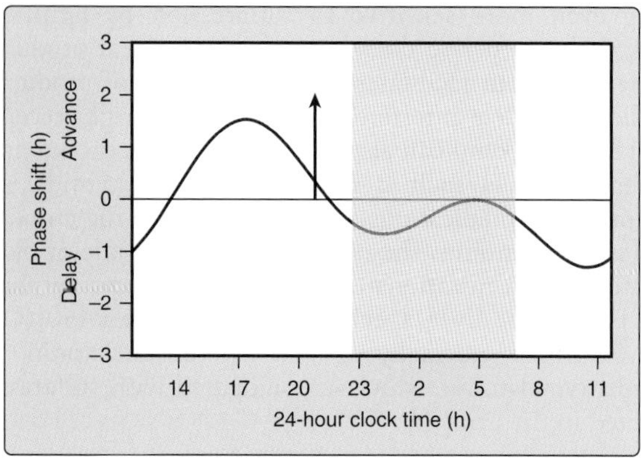

Figure 51.2 A melatonin phase response curve to 0.5 mg of exogenous melatonin applied daily at the same clock time for 3 consecutive days. The *arrow* represents the usual time of the dim light melatonin onset, and the *shaded rectangle* represents the timing of typical nighttime sleep. Late afternoon or early evening administration leads to phase advances, whereas late night and early morning administration leads to phase delay. (Modified from Figure 4 in Burgess HJ, Revell VL, Molina TA, et al. Human phase response curves to three days of daily melatonin: 0.5 mg versus 3.0 mg. *J Clin Endocrinol Metab*. 2010;95:3325–31.[57])

The Effects of Exogenous Melatonin on Human Inflammatory Markers

Melatonin is a potent antioxidant and may have initially evolved as an antioxidant before later evolving into its roles in circadian rhythms and sleep.[65] Large prospective research studies have indicated that lower levels of endogenous melatonin increase the risk for later-developing inflammatory-based diseases such as prostate cancer,[66] breast cancer,[67] and cardiovascular[68] and cardiometabolic disease.[69] In terms of supplemental exogenous melatonin, several placebo-controlled randomized clinical trials have indicated that high doses of exogenous melatonin (6 to 10 mg) taken in the evening can increase total antioxidant capacity[70] and reduce markers of systemic inflammation such as IL-6 and tumor necrosis factor-α[71,72] in individuals with preexisting heightened inflammation.

The Safety of Exogenous Melatonin

Potential Contraindications for Melatonin

Side effects, besides sleepiness, are infrequent with exogenous melatonin, but meta-analyses and in-depth reviews report incidents of increased dizziness, headache, hypertension and hypotension, and gastrointestinal upset.[51,73,74] Individual scientific reports suggest that melatonin may stimulate growth hormone[75] and reduce semen quality.[76] In healthy adult males, a 28-day randomized placebo controlled trial of 10 mg melatonin, a relatively high dose, did not result in any increase in adverse effects relative to placebo, nor any change in a variety of blood and urinary markers.[77] In children, a long-term melatonin administration study (of approximately 3 years) found no effect of melatonin on self-reported markers of pubertal development.[78] However, no study has assessed endocrine markers that could reveal effects of long-term melatonin use.[79] Therefore it is prudent to exercise caution in the administration of melatonin to prepubertal children, particularly in the long term, unless the risk-benefit analysis favors treatment (e.g., in children with significant developmental delay or children with non-24-hour sleep-wake rhythm disorder[64]). It is also advised that pregnant or breastfeeding women, as well as those trying to become pregnant, should not take exogenous melatonin[74] because melatonin is part of the maternal-fetal communication pathway for circadian entrainment.[80]

Generally, it is recommended that people consult with their physicians before taking exogenous melatonin so that any potential contraindications with current medical conditions and/or interactions with other prescribed or over-the-counter (OTC) medications can be considered. Meta-analyses have suggested that exogenous melatonin may interact with oral anticoagulants and should be contraindicated in people with epilepsy.[73] Further, when administered with food, exogenous melatonin (5 mg) may acutely impair glucose tolerance,[81,82] highlighting potential risks for people with prediabetes or diabetes.

Melatonin as an Over-the-Counter Dietary Supplement (in the United States)

Exogenous melatonin has been classified by the U.S. Food and Drug Administration (FDA) as a dietary supplement and, as such, is not subject to the regulation given to pharmaceuticals; the purity and accuracy of dose of exogenous melatonin formulations are not always carefully controlled.[83,84] Choosing an OTC formulation from a manufacturer who participates in the USP Dietary Supplement Verification Program may help with this quality control problem.[85] An important consideration for therapy with melatonin is the low cost (often less than 10 cents per pill).

Other Melatonin Agonists

A variety of prescription-based melatonin receptor agonists and melatonin preparations are also available, all of which are dual MT_1 and MT_2 melatonin receptor agonists. These include ramelteon (approved for the treatment of insomnia), agomelatine (also a serotonin 5-HT_{2c} receptor antagonist approved in Europe and Australia for the treatment of depression), tasimelteon (approved by the FDA for the treatment of non-24-hour sleep-wake rhythm disorder), and circadin (extended-release formulation of 2.0 mg melatonin approved in Europe and Australia for the treatment of primary insomnia). These prescription-based melatonin agonists carry their own potential side effect profiles, including increased risk of liver injury with agomelatine[86,87]; headache, elevated liver enzymes, cardiac conduction changes, upper respiratory and urinary tract infections, and nightmares for tasimelteon[88]; and headache, sleepiness, upper respiratory tract infections, gastrointestinal upset, dizziness, and dysmenorrhea for ramelteon.[89] Circadin is an extended-release formulation of melatonin and has a similar side effect profile to melatonin.[90]

CLINICAL PEARLS

- Low (≤0.5 mg) doses of melatonin or approved doses of melatonin agonists taken in the evening (phase advance) or morning (phase delay) can be an effective chronobiotic.
- Higher doses of melatonin can have a mild hypnotic effect and reduce sleep-onset latency, particularly when taken during the biologic daytime.
- Higher doses of melatonin have been used in REM sleep behavior disorder.
- Pharmacokinetics, cost, and safety of exogenous melatonin and melatonin agonists must be balanced when considering the administration to humans.

SUMMARY

Melatonin is a hormone produced by the pineal gland during the biologic nighttime and is involved in the regulation of sleep and circadian rhythms. Endogenous melatonin, when properly studied, is a robust marker of the timing of the central circadian pacemaker. Endogenous melatonin has a small influence on sleep, but administration of exogenous melatonin during the biologic daytime can be a useful hypnotic or chronobiotic. Dosing and route of administration are critical for the clinical effectiveness of melatonin. Low doses (≤0.5 mg) can advance (evening administration) or delay (morning administration) the timing of the circadian clock. Higher doses are more effective at inducing sleep onset, while sustained-release formulations could be helpful for sleep maintenance. Pharmacokinetics, cost, and safety of exogenous melatonin and melatonin agonists all must be considered when planning the administration to humans.

SELECTED READINGS

Auger RR, Burgess HJ, Emens JS, et al. Clinical Practice Guideline for the Treatment of Intrinsic Circadian Rhythm Sleep-Wake Disorders: Advanced Sleep-Wake Phase Disorder (ASWPD), Delayed Sleep-Wake Phase Disorder (DSWPD), Non-24-Hour Sleep-Wake Rhythm Disorder (N24SWD), and Irregular Sleep-Wake Rhythm Disorder (ISWRD). An Update for 2015: An American Academy of Sleep Medicine Clinical Practice Guideline. *J Clin Sleep Med*. 2015;11:1199–1236.

Axelrod J. The pineal gland: a neurochemical transducer. *Science*. 1974;184:1341–1348.

Burgess HJ, Emens JS. Drugs used in circadian sleep-wake rhythm disturbances. *Sleep Med Clin*. 2020;15(2):301–310.

Burgess HJ, Fogg LF. Individual differences in the amount and timing of salivary melatonin secretion. *PLoS One*. 2008;3:e3055.

Burgess HJ, Revell VL, Molina TA, et al. Human phase response curves to three days of daily melatonin: 0.5 mg versus 3.0 mg. *J Clin Endocrinol Metab*. 2010;95:3325–3331.

Buscemi N, Vandermeer B, Hooton N, et al. The efficacy and safety of exogenous melatonin for primary sleep disorders. A meta-analysis. *J Gen Intern Med*. 2005;20:1151–1158.

Cheng DCY, Ganner JL, Gordon CJ, et al. The efficacy of combined bright light and melatonin therapies on sleep and circadian outcomes: a systematic review. *Sleep Med Rev*. 2021;58:101491.

Emens J, Burgess HJ. Effect of light and melatonin and other melatonin receptor agonists on human circadian physiology. *Sleep Med Clin*. 2015;10:435–453.

Fatemeh G, Sajjad M, Niloufar R, et al. Effect of melatonin supplementation on sleep quality: a systematic review and meta-analysis of randomized controlled trials. *J Neurol*. 2021. https://doi.org/10.1007/s00415-020-10381-w.

Gilat M, Marshall NS, Testelmans D, et al. A critical review of the pharmacological treatment of REM sleep behavior disorder in adults: time for more and larger randomized placebo-controlled trials. *J Neurol*. 2021. https://doi.org/10.1007/s00415-020-10353-0.

Kennaway DJ. Potential safety issues in the use of the hormone melatonin in paediatrics. *J Paediatr Child Health*. 2015;51:548–589.

Lewy AJ, Bauer VK, Ahmed S, et al. The human phase response curve (PRC) to melatonin is about 12 hours out of phase with the PRC to light. *Chronobiol Int*. 1998;15:71–83.

Moroni I, Garcia-Bennett A, Chapman J, et al. Pharmacokinetics of exogenous melatonin in relation to formulation, and effects on sleep: a systematic review. *Sleep Med Rev*. 2021;57:101431.

Reppert SM, Weaver DR, Rivkees SA, et al. Putative melatonin receptors in a human biological clock. *Science*. 1988;242:78–81.

Zeitzer JM, Daniels JE, Duffy JF, et al. Do plasma melatonin concentrations decline with age? *Am J Med*. 1999;107:432–436.

A complete reference list can be found online at ExpertConsult.com.

Chapter 52

Opioid Actions on Sleep and Breathing

Ralph Lydic; David Hillman; Yandong Jiang; Helen A. Baghdoyan; Christopher B. O'Brien

Chapter Highlights

- Ongoing efforts to lessen the morbidity and mortality of opioid use disorder (OUD) have resulted in cross-disciplinary interactions between clinical specialties focused on sleep, anesthesiology, pain, addiction, and pulmonary medicine. The National Institutes of Health is promoting basic research into alternatives to opioids and adjunctive treatments that manage pain using reduced opioid dosing.
- Clinically used and managed morphine and fentanyl effectively decrease pain yet significantly disrupt sleep architecture by increasing wakefulness and decreasing both stage 3 non–rapid eye movement sleep and rapid eye movement sleep. The opioid agonists buprenorphine and methadone, as well as the opioid antagonist naltrexone, are approved by the US Food and Drug Administration to treat OUD. Each of these drugs disrupt sleep, and sleep disruption increases pain, drug craving, and addiction relapse.
- Repeated opioid administration causes tachyphylaxis, requiring higher opioid doses needed to achieve the desired response. This increases the risk of respiratory depression, the prime cause of fatal opioid overdose. This chapter concludes by outlining efforts to develop countermeasures for opioid-induced respiratory depression. These efforts involve cross-cutting collaborations that span cellular and network studies of respiratory neurobiology. Clinical and preclinical data suggest interdependence between opioid effects on sleep, breathing, risk of addiction, pain, and disordered affect. This interdependence calls into question assumptions of independent effects fundamental to inferential statistics.

INTRODUCTION

Opioids are relevant for sleep medicine due to the prevalence of opioid use disorder (OUD) and chronic pain, both of which are comorbid with disordered sleep. Representatives of the World Health Organization and the National Institutes of Health (NIH) concur that OUD is a worldwide epidemic.[1] The goal of lessening OUD must be accomplished while attending to the legitimate need for clinically directed pain management. Chronic pain affects approximately 50 million US adults, and high-impact chronic pain (i.e., pain that interferes with work or life most days or every day) affects 20 million US adults.[2] It has been known for more than 25 years that morphine causes dose-dependent and brain site–dependent disruption of sleep and breathing.[3] In 2019 the American Academy of Sleep Medicine position statement concluded that "chronic opioid use is associated with changes in sleep architecture and an increased risk of respiratory depression during sleep."[4] The concurrence between preclinical and clinical research on opioids and sleep[3,4] is consistent with advocacy for opioid research.[5] The ongoing opioid crisis is dynamic,[6] multifactorial,[7] and characterized by increases in morbidity and mortality caused by extended-release/long-acting opioids.[8] Between 2006 and 2018 the US pharmaceutical industry shipped 76 billion oxycodone and hydrocodone pills.[9] Approximately 2.5 million people in the United States were estimated to have OUD in 2018.[10] This chapter updates clinical and preclinical research on opioid-induced disruption of sleep and breathing.

Opioids disrupt sleep, and comorbidities, including addiction and neuropsychiatric disorders, are not rare in sleep medicine clinics. Opioids have long been known to have the unwanted side effects of sleep disruption[11,12] and exacerbation of sleep-disordered breathing.[13] Insomnia is the most common presenting condition in sleep medicine, and insomnia is comorbid with posttraumatic stress disorder and opioid dependence.[14] With regard to insomnia, data also suggest that prescribed benzodiazepines increase risk for persistent opioid use.[15] Objective, polysomnographic (PSG) studies quantifying how opioids, independent of pain, illness, or addiction, influence the temporal organization of sleep remain rare. This is directly relevant for a scientific approach to sleep disorders because, although self-assessment of sleep quality is clinically valuable,[16] self-assessment of sleep quality can differ significantly from measures provided by objective PSG.[17] Studies also are needed to help understand the paradox that opioid-induced sleep disruption can contribute to increases in the doses of opioids that are needed to achieve pain relief and to the observation that opioids themselves can cause hyperalgesia.[18]

BALANCING THE THERAPEUTIC ROLE OF OPIOIDS AGAINST ADDICTION

A 2010 perspectives paper entitled "A Flood of Opiates, A Rising Tide of Death" pointed out that since the early 1990s opioids have driven a consistent increase in drug overdose deaths.[19] The increase in opioid overdose deaths was paralleled by a 10-fold increase in the medical use of opioids, encouraged by "aggressive marketing of OxyContin, an extended-release form of oxycodone."[19] More recent recommendations aiming to reverse the opioid addiction epidemic are introduced by the view that "the United States is in the midst of the worse drug addiction epidemic in its history."[20] The Centers for Disease Control and Prevention attribute 68% of drug overdose deaths to opioids.[21] This pervasiveness ensures that practitioners of sleep medicine will regularly confront patients who also are on the OUD continuum (Figure 52.1).

Furthermore, some sleep disorders may involve prescribing opioids to opioid-naïve patients. Clinical consensus statements note that, with appropriate cautions, opioids can be used with favorable risk-benefit outcomes to treat restless legs syndrome.[22] The challenge of managing risk-benefit balance involved in opioid prescription is emphasized by the lack of consensus regarding prevalence and incidence of addiction associated with long-term use of opioids.[23,24] A compelling infographic summarizes the current lack of a consistent definition of excessive postoperative opioid use.[25] The present focus on the unwanted, negative side effects of opioids is consistent with evidence that opioid misuse can create medical problems in virtually every organ system,[26] in addition to infections caused by intravenous drug use.[27–29] In 2018 the NIH introduced the Helping to End Addiction Long-term initiative to promote research aiming to enhance pain management and treatment of the more than 2 million people in the United States with opioid OUD.[30]

OPIOID PHARMACOLOGY

In 2016 the US Food and Drug Administration (FDA) asked the National Academies of Sciences, Engineering, and Medicine to create a consensus report addressing why some individuals who use prescribed opioids to alleviate pain go on to develop OUD. The 2017 consensus report addressed the problem of how to mitigate the ongoing opioid crisis while incorporating the legitimate need for pain management.[31] This was followed by a Proceedings Report from a 2019 workshop on how to provide pain management for people with serious illness.[32] Death rates have been analyzed using death certificates with *International Classification of Diseases,* 10th edition codes for subcategories of opioid pharmacology.[21] Subcategories of opioid agonists included morphine and codeine (natural opioids) and oxycodone, hydrocodone, hydromorphone, oxymorphone, and methadone (semisynthetic opioids). Additional semisynthetic opioids include drugs such as buprenorphine, tramadol, and fentanyl. Illicitly manufactured opioids include heroin, fentanyl, and fentanyl analogs.[21] Readers are referred to Yaksh and Wallace[33] for a current update on endogenous opioid peptides (pro-opiomelanocortin, proenkephalin, prodynorphin, and endomorphins), opioid receptors (mu, delta, kappa, and nociceptin/orphanin FQ), and clinical considerations regarding opioid therapy (Figure 52.2).

The mu opioid receptor was named for morphine, and the clinical management of both acute and chronic pain commonly involves administration of mu opioids. Opioid receptors are part of the family of G protein–coupled receptors. This means that opioid receptors are seven membrane-spanning domain receptors that are coupled to G proteins of the Gi/o subtype. Receptor activation closes voltage-gated calcium channels and opens potassium channels, thereby hyperpolarizing neurons and decreasing neuronal excitability.[33] Opioid receptors reside in the central nervous system and also exist in the gastrointestinal system and skin.[34] Multiple opioid

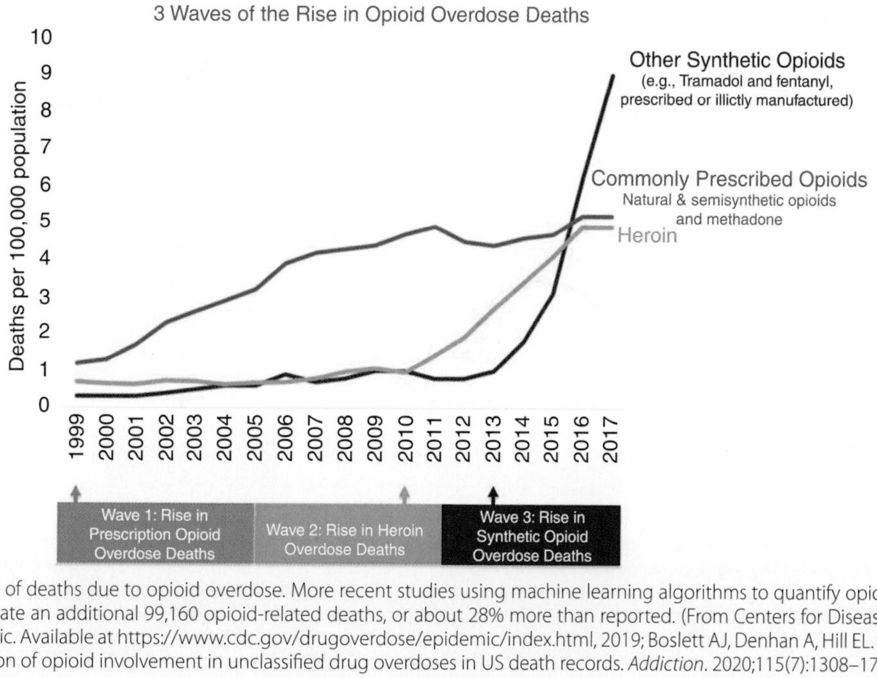

Figure 52.1 Time course of deaths due to opioid overdose. More recent studies using machine learning algorithms to quantify opioid involvement in unclassified drug overdoses indicate an additional 99,160 opioid-related deaths, or about 28% more than reported. (From Centers for Disease Control and Prevention. Understanding the Epidemic. Available at https://www.cdc.gov/drugoverdose/epidemic/index.html, 2019; Boslett AJ, Denhan A, Hill EL. Using contributing causes of death improves prediction of opioid involvement in unclassified drug overdoses in US death records. *Addiction*. 2020;115(7):1308–17.)

receptor subtypes modulate immune function and natural-killer cell activity[35] via their presence on T lymphocytes.[36] Distinctly different opioid receptors can combine to form dimers and/or oligomers that have unique functional roles.[37] Multiple splice variants of mu opioid receptors exist within the brain and spinal cord. Opioids also interact with multiple other receptor systems and, in contrast to opioid inhibition of cell excitability, opioids can also produce neuronal excitation directly or indirectly via disinhibition in different cell types.[38]

Buprenorphine, a mu opioid agonist and kappa opioid antagonist, is one of three drugs currently approved by the FDA for treating OUD.[5] Buprenorphine crosses the blood-brain barrier and is metabolized by cytochrome P450 (CYP450) 3A4 enzymes, which produce the active metabolite norbuprenorphine.[26] An excellent resource on buprenorphine for clinical care providers is entitled "Medications for Opioid Use Disorder: For Healthcare and Addiction Professionals, Policymakers, Patients, and Families" from the US Department of Health and Human Services.[26] This review also cautions that in addition to abuse potential, buprenorphine misuse can cause respiratory depression (see Figure 52.5) and death. When taken by pregnant women, buprenorphine can cause neonatal abstinence syndrome in newborns. In rodents, buprenorphine produces a bell-shaped concentration response curve for analgesia, whereas in primates, buprenorphine causes dose-dependent antinociception and respiratory depression.[39] The respiratory and antinociceptive effects of buprenorphine across a dose range of 0.2 to 0.4 mg/70 kg were compared in 10 healthy human volunteers.[40] While end-tidal partial pressure of carbon dioxide (P_{CO_2}) and partial pressure of oxygen (P_{O_2}) were held constant, breathing frequency was measured, and minute ventilation was calculated. Analgesia was measured as the highest electrical shock to skin covering the shin bone that volunteers would tolerate. Increasing doses of buprenorphine produced increased analgesia but did not produce increased depression of breathing. The results led to the conclusion that across the dose range of buprenorphine tested there was a ceiling in respiratory effect but none in analgesic effect.[40] The use of buprenorphine to treat OUD also must attend to issues of dosing compliance and the potential for drug diversion. These factors have prompted the development of subdermal implants for delivery of long-acting forms of buprenorphine.[41,42]

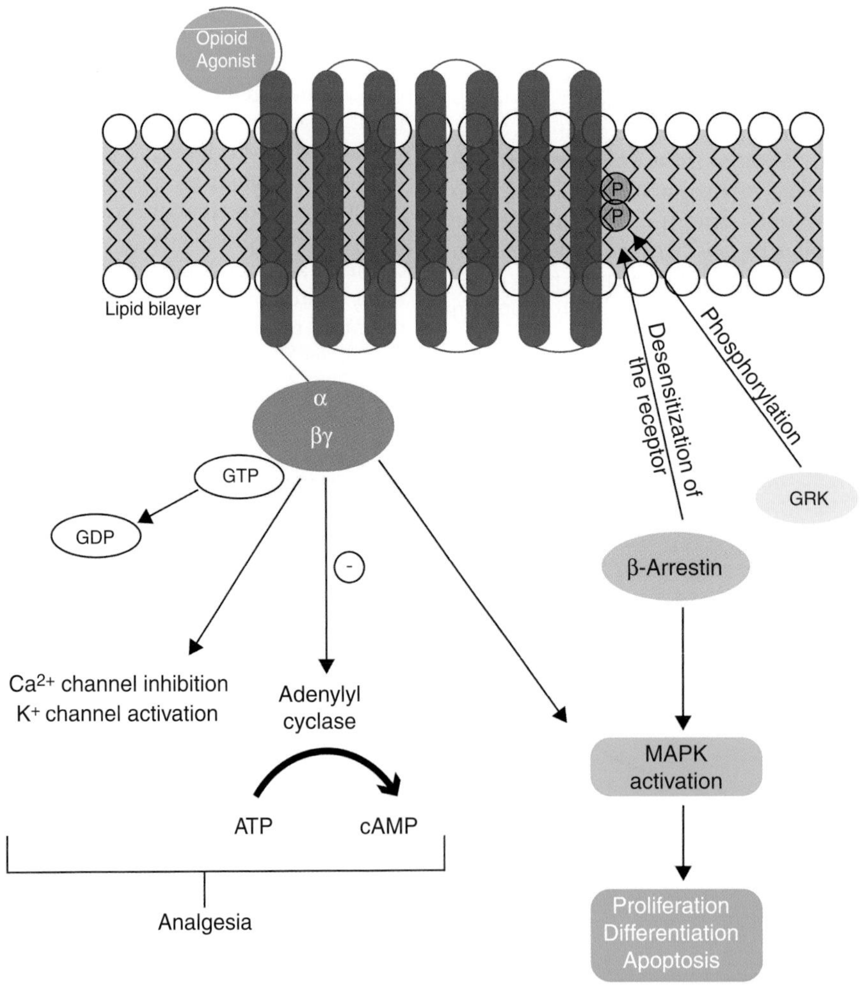

Figure 52.2 Schematic of intracellular signal transduction pathways activated by an opioid agonist binding to an opioid receptor. These pathways (*arrows*) inhibit calcium (Ca^{2+}) channels and activating potassium (K^+) efflux, causing hyperpolarization of the cell. These factors cause both the desired effect (analgesia) and the unwanted side effect of inhibiting neurons that generate sleep and breathing. G proteins inhibit (–) the enzyme adenyl cyclase, which synthesizes cyclic adenosine monophosphate (cAMP) from adenosine triphosphate (ATP). GRK, G protein–coupled receptor kinases; GDP, guanosine diphosphate; G protein—α, β, and γ heterotrimeric subunits; GTP, guanosine triphosphate; MAPK, mitogen-associated protein kinases; P, phosphate. (Modified from Azzam AAH, McDonald J, Lambert DG. Hot topics in opioid pharmacology: mixed and biased opioids. *Br J Anaesth*. 2019;133:e3136–45.)

Sleep disorders medicine and pain management are linked by a shared focus on states of psychophysiology.[43] States of pain are composed of complex psychophysiologic events that include nonnociceptive variables, such as alterations in affect, cognition, and autonomic physiology,[44] each of which varies as a function of sleep and wakefulness. Prevalence data emphasize the relevance of continuing to improve use of opioids for treating cancer-related pain. Data from the American Cancer Society indicate that men and women in the United States have a 1 in 3 lifetime risk of developing cancer.[45] Clinical efforts to manage cancer pain can involve a complex array of pure mu agonists, partial agonists, such as buprenorphine, and opioids with multiple mechanisms of action.[46] Studies characterizing opioid effects on states of sleep and wakefulness using PSG are not presently available for the majority of 20 opioids considered in the context of managing cancer pain.[46]

EFFECTS OF OPIOIDS ON SLEEP STATES AND ELECTROENCEPHALOGRAPHIC TRAITS

J.J. Bonica, the acknowledged founder of pain medicine in the United States, recognized more than 30 years ago that disrupted sleep is a major complaint of patients experiencing pain.[47] A complication for the clinical management of pain is that opioids impair sleep by altering the amount of time spent in states of wakefulness, non–rapid eye movement (NREM) sleep, and rapid eye movement (REM) sleep. Opioid disruption of sleep architecture has been demonstrated in preclinical[48,49] and clinical[50] studies. Opioid-induced sleep disruption can cause hyperalgesia,[51–55] which may increase opioid requirement. Additional data indicate that for patients treated in pain care settings, sleep disturbances are often not systemically evaluated.[56] The paradox of opioids potentially worsening conditions they were deployed to treat also is relevant for addiction. Sleep disorders are 5 to 10 times more common in substances abusers than nonabusers.[57] Poor sleep quality increases drug craving,[58] and increased risk of illicit drug use is associated with insomnia.[59] Sleep disturbance has been described as a "universal risk factor" for addiction relapse.[60] Consistent with the foregoing findings, opioid-assisted treatments for addiction that use methadone or buprenorphine are associated with sleep disruption.[61] One acknowledged limitation is that these associations are based on patient reports rather than objective PSG data.[61] Studies using objective measures of rodent sleep confirm that buprenorphine delays sleep onset, increases wakefulness, and decreases both NREM sleep and REM sleep.[62] The interactions between states of sleep, pain, and addiction derive from the fact that overlapping neuronal networks (Figure 52.3) regulate the physiologic and behavioral traits characterizing these three psychophysiologic states.[63,64]

We are unaware of any PSG data that characterize opioid-induced changes in sleep and wakefulness as a function of age, sex, body habitus, or genotype. This omission is, in part, an

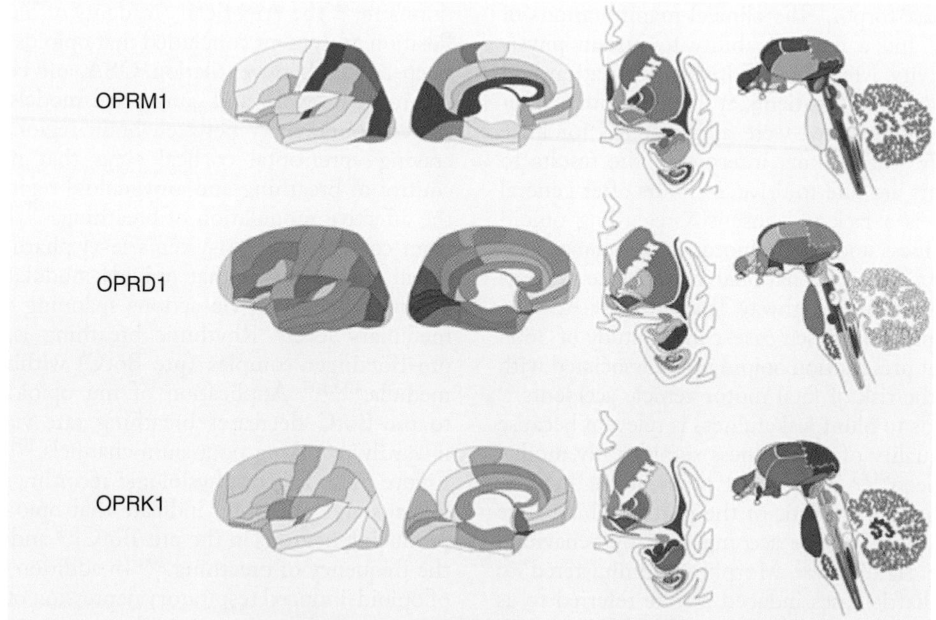

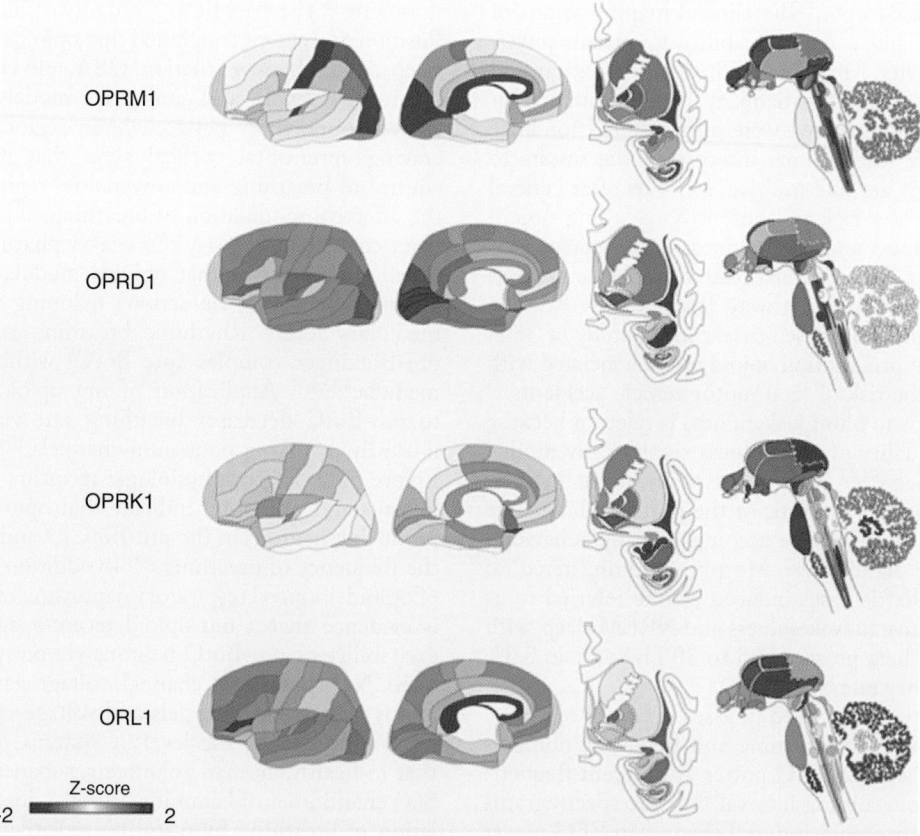

Figure 52.3 Opioid receptor gene expression in human brain shown as normalized Z-scores ranging from 2 (*dark red*) to −2 (*dark blue*). The four columns from left to right show outer cortical surface (*leftmost*), inner cortical surface (*second from left*), subcortical structures in frontal view (*third from left*), and brainstem in sagittal plane (*fourth from left*). Rows illustrate opioid receptors mu (OPRM1), delta (OPRD1), kappa (OPRK1) and the nonopioid receptor, nociceptin (ORL1). This image is from Peciña and colleagues[156] and conveys the wide distribution of opioid receptors throughout the brain. This distribution pattern illustrates that systemically administered opioids exert nonselective influence on neural networks that modulate sleep, pain, and addiction.

extension of the fact that healthy sleep continues to be underappreciated.[65,66] Sleep disorders are associated with an economic loss in the United States of more than $400 billion per year due to disease, lost productivity, and accidents.[67] Furthermore, there are no human PSG data that systematically compare the effects on sleep of different opioids deployed to treat different pain conditions. A recent meta-analysis concerning the relationship between sleep and pain found that only 11% of reviewed studies used objective measures of sleep.[68] Evaluations of the effect of opioid therapy on sleep quality in patients with chronic, nonmalignant pain were unable to conclude that opioid therapy improved sleep through pain reduction.[68] The rare studies using objective PSG measures of sleep (Table 52.1) show that administering clinically relevant doses of opioids to otherwise healthy humans increases light (stage N1) NREM sleep, decreases deeper NREM sleep (stage N3), and inhibits REM sleep.[50,69–73] The data summarized by Table 52.1 distinguish between disruptions in sleep that are caused by opioids and sleep changes that are caused by pain, disease, or addiction. Addressing these gaps in knowledge represents another important opportunity for sleep research.

Electroencephalographic (EEG) recordings remain the standard for objectively measuring the amount of time spent in normal states of sleep and wakefulness and for identifying dissociated states of consciousness produced by disease or drugs.[74] Opioids blunt wakefulness and slow the cortical EEG.[75–79] Systemic delivery of morphine to rats significantly increases low-frequency EEG power.[80,81] Administering opioids to provide pain relief causes an obtunded state of wakefulness referred to as "torpor." The clinical manifestations of torpor are lethargy and a reduced ability to sustain physical and mental activity. Measures of driving simulation and EEG were obtained from 20 patients at 2 and 24 hours after general anesthesia and fentanyl were administered for knee arthroscopic surgery. The authors interpreted the results to indicate that patients are safe to drive 24 hours after general anesthesia.[82] There is a lack of consensus regarding opioid blunting of wakefulness and psychomotor performance. This is illustrated by data from two national surveillance systems maintained by the National Highway Traffic Safety Administration.[83] This population-based case-control study of 3606 cases concluded that prescription opioid use is associated with a 72% increase in the risk of fatal motor vehicle accidents.[83] The action of opioids to blunt wakefulness is relevant because the duration and quality of wakefulness significantly modulates subsequent sleep[84,85] and global brain states.[86] EEG slow wave activity is characteristic of the postmorphine state and, depending on dose, can be accompanied by behavioral torpor and muscle rigidity.[79,81] Morphine administered to 10 postsurgical pediatric cases induced a state referred to as "deep sedation" relative to wakefulness and NREM sleep, with a decrease in EEG beta power (13.5 to 30 Hz) and an 8.3% decrease in respiratory rate.[87]

Multitaper spectrograms, used to asses brain states, transform the EEG waveform into time and frequency domains that quantify and visualize EEG power at different frequencies across an entire recording interval.[88,89] The spectrograms visualize and quantify opioid-induced changes in EEG power and frequency in mouse prefrontal cortex (Figure 52.4).[90] Although morphine and fentanyl are both mu opioid receptor agonists, when administered systemically to mice, these two opioids differentially alter the EEG power spectrum. An important future research opportunity is to systematically characterize opioid-induced alterations in EEG power as a function of drug, dose, route of administration, species, sex, frequency band, and brain region monitored.

OPIOID-INDUCED RESPIRATORY DEPRESSION

The clinical use of opioids must be considered in the context of the ongoing OUD epidemic. Confronting the opioid crisis cuts across clinical specialties. The practice of sleep medicine, addictionology, pain medicine, pulmonology, anesthesiology, and other specialties is impacted by the opioid epidemic. Patients with obstructive sleep apnea (OSA) have increased risks for adverse respiratory and cardiovascular outcomes during and after surgery.[91] The opioid crisis has stimulated three anesthesiology journals to publish special issues focused on opioids.[92–94] The Perioperative Quality Initiative and American Society of Enhanced Recovery have developed consensus guidelines aiming to monitor and minimize use of postoperative opioids.[95] Although there are many nonanalgesic effects of opioids,[26] the most notorious side effect is death due to opioid-induced respiratory depression.[96] In adults with OSA, opioid-induced respiratory depression is an uncontestable issue,[97] and OSA patients require special intraoperative management.[98] Among patients taking opioids for chronic pain, sleep apnea can be predicted by daytime oxyhemoglobin saturation, daily morphine milligram equivalents, and responses to the STOP-BANG (snoring, tiredness, observed apnea, blood pressure, body mass index, age, neck size, gender) questionnaire.[99] The American Academy of Sleep Medicine 2019 Position Statement concluded that opioids are associated with sleep-related hypoventilation, OSA, and central sleep apnea.[4] Neuronal network and conceptual models of addiction note shared connectivity between brain regions involved in drug craving—prefrontal cortical areas that modulate volitional control of breathing and amygdaloid regions contributing to the affective modulation of breathing.[100] These studies range from cellular-level to systems-level pharmacology. An additional complexity is that opioids modulate brainstem regulation of breathing via actions spanning from pontine[101] to medullary levels. Rhythmic breathing is generated by the pre-Bötzinger complex (pre-BötC) within the ventrolateral medulla.[102,103] Application of mu opioid receptor agonists to pre-BötC decreases breathing rate via G protein–gated inwardly rectifying potassium channels,[104] as schematized by Figure 52.2. Electrophysiologic recordings from hypoglossal nucleus and pre-BötC indicate that opioids act on burstlet-producing neurons in the pre-BötC[105] and cause a decrease in the frequency of breathing.[106] In addition to the mechanisms of opioid-induced respiratory depression outlined above, there is evidence that a mu opioid receptor agonist can decrease excitability of pre-BötC neurons via presynaptic modulation of KCNQ (potassium channel, voltage-gated, KQT-like subfamily) potassium channels and voltage-gated calcium channels.[107] Studies at the level of systems pharmacology show that in healthy human volunteers, subanesthetic doses of the S(+) enantiomer of ketamine caused a dose-dependent stimulation of breathing by restoring sensitivity to CO_2 that had been depressed by remifentanil.[108] Common to the foregoing cellular and systems level studies is the goal of decreasing opioid-induced depression of respiration while retaining desired analgesic actions. At present there are no currently

Table 52.1 Polysomnographic Characterization of Opioid-Induced Disruption of Sleep and Wakefulness

Reference	Opiate	Trade Name	n (F/M)	Species, Disposition	Wake Time	Light NREM Sleep Duration	Deep NREM Sleep Duration	REM Sleep Duration	Total Sleep Time	Latency to Onset
69	Morphine	Avinza, Kadian, MS Contin, Roxanol, Roxanol-T	7 (2/5)	Human 24–28 YO, healthy	—	↑	↓	↓	—	—
73	Remifentanil	Ultiva	19 (8/11)	Human 38–62 YO, moderate OSA	—	↑	NS	↓	↓	—
157	Oxycodone	Tylox, Percodan, OxyContin	18 (7/11)	Human 28–32 wk, preterm	NS	↑ (NREM only)	↑ (NREM only)	↓	NS	—
50	Methadone	Methadose, Dolophine	42 (25/17)	Human 18–60 YO, healthy	—	↑	↓	NS	NS	—
62	Buprenorphine	Buprenex, Suboxone, Subutex	26 (0/26)	Sprague Dawley rat, adult, healthy	↑	↓ (NREM only)	↓ (NREM only)	↓	↓	↓
158	Butorphanol	Stadol	6 (0/6)	Horse adult, healthy	↑	↓ (SWS only)	↓ (SWS only)	↓	—	↓

These studies are unique in that they do not include subjects with the potential confounds of surgery, pain, drug addiction, or other comorbid conditions.
F, Female; M, male; NREM, non–rapid eye movement; NS, not significant; OSA, obstructive sleep apnea; REM, rapid eye movement; SWS, slow wave sleep; YO, years old.

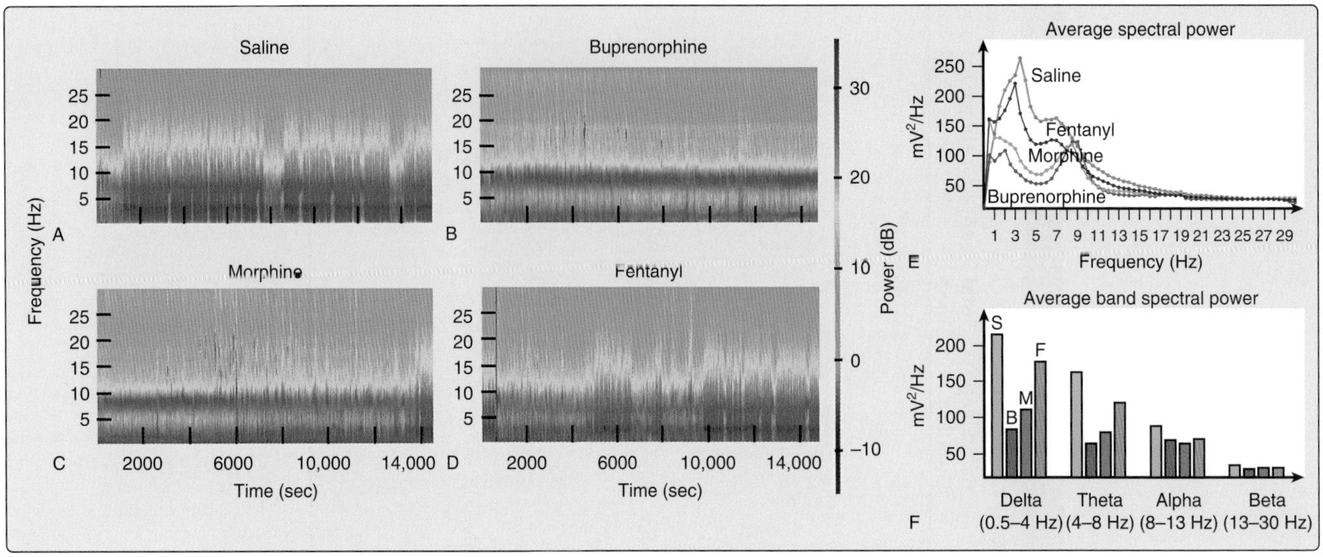

Figure 52.4 Multitaper spectrograms illustrating changes in electroencephalographic (EEG) power and frequency in an adult, male, C57BL/6J mouse that received on different days systemically administered saline **(A)** and antinociceptive doses of buprenorphine **(B)**, morphine **(C)**, and fentanyl **(D)**. Each spectrogram plots EEG frequency in Hertz (Hz, *left ordinate*) and EEG power in decibels (dB, *right ordinate*). Abscissa shows time in seconds for 4 hours after each injection. Data in **E** and **F** show opioid-specific alterations in EEG power, relative to saline. The average EEG spectral power **(E)** on the ordinate is plotted for each half frequency (abscissa) between 0.5 and 29.5 Hz. Data in **(F)** illustrate the average EEG power in four EEG frequency bands (delta, theta, alpha, and beta) after administration of saline (S), buprenorphine (B), morphine (M), and fentanyl (F). (Adapted from O'Brien CB, Baghdoyan HA, Lydic R. Computer-based multitaper spectrogram program for electroencephalographic data. *J Vis Exp*. 2019; e60333.)

available respiratory stimulant drugs that "are adequate for therapeutic use" to lessen or avert respiratory depression caused by opioids.[109]

Obesity functions as a comorbidity for OSA by exacerbating airway obstruction through its effects on airway patency and by predisposing to hypoventilation through excessive mechanical loading of inspiratory muscles. These factors thereby increase the risk of life-threatening respiratory complications induced by the depressant effects of opioids on upper airway muscle activation, ventilation, and protective arousal responses.[110,111] Obese patients need to be closely monitored postoperatively, and therapies such as continuous positive airway pressure, bilevel positive airway pressure, or autotitrating positive airway pressure should be considered.[110] Admonitions for enhanced monitoring of obese patients are consistent with the view that obesity is a disease.[112,113] Data from the National Health and Nutrition Examination Survey and the Behavioral Risk Factor Surveillance System project that approximately 1 in 2 adults in the United States will have obesity by 2030, and the prevalence will be higher than 50% in 29 states.[114]

Paralleling this increase in obesity over the past decade has been an increase in the occurrence of OSA, with as many as 50% of morbidly obese patients experiencing sleep apnea.[115,116] There is also a complex association between sleep-disordered breathing, being overweight or obese, and pain. Sleep-disordered breathing is common in overweight or obese individuals.[117] Obesity itself is associated with increased pain,[118,119] and patients with sleep-disordered breathing have increased reports of pain.[120] When nocturnal hypoxemia was examined independent of sleep fragmentation in OSA patients, it was found that pain reported by the participants upon awakening significantly increased.[120] Use of continuous positive airway pressure to control severe OSA decreased pain experienced by these patients.[121] These findings are consistent with the interpretation that sleep disruption and intermittent hypoxia may amplify pain in OSA patients. Conversely, subsequent work has shown that both adult and pediatric patients with recurrent hypoxia and severe OSA require less opioid administration postoperatively to obtain adequate analgesia.[122,123] The cellular mechanisms mediating the association between sleep-disordered breathing and pain are not understood.[124]

The NIH encourages intensified and better-coordinated research regarding the biologic mechanisms underlying the desired and undesired effects of opioids.[5] Adipocytes secrete leptin, and obese humans have high circulating levels of leptin. Preclinical evidence indicates that leptin modulates nociception in mice possessing a spontaneous mutation that disrupts leptin signaling.[125,126] Nociception in three lines of obese mice with leptin disorders is significantly decreased by the opioid buprenorphine, and leptin status has a greater impact than body weight on nociception.[127] Figure 52.5 illustrates that buprenorphine significantly depresses minute ventilation variability in mice, particularly those with leptin dysfunction.[128] The ability to vary minute ventilation is essential for mounting a successful compensatory response to organismic or environmental challenges to breathing. The extent to which the results from lean and obese, male and female mice also are apparent in humans remains to be determined (see Figure 52.5). Normal mice fed a high-fat diet become obese, and these mice (diet-induced obesity [DIO] mice [Figure 52.5] are homologous to humans who consume more calories than they expend. Mice with DIO also display sleep-disordered breathing.[129] Administering intranasal, but not intraperitoneal, leptin normalized sleep-disordered breathing in mice with DIO.[130] These studies demonstrate how preclinical research can inform and encourage parallel human studies.[131]

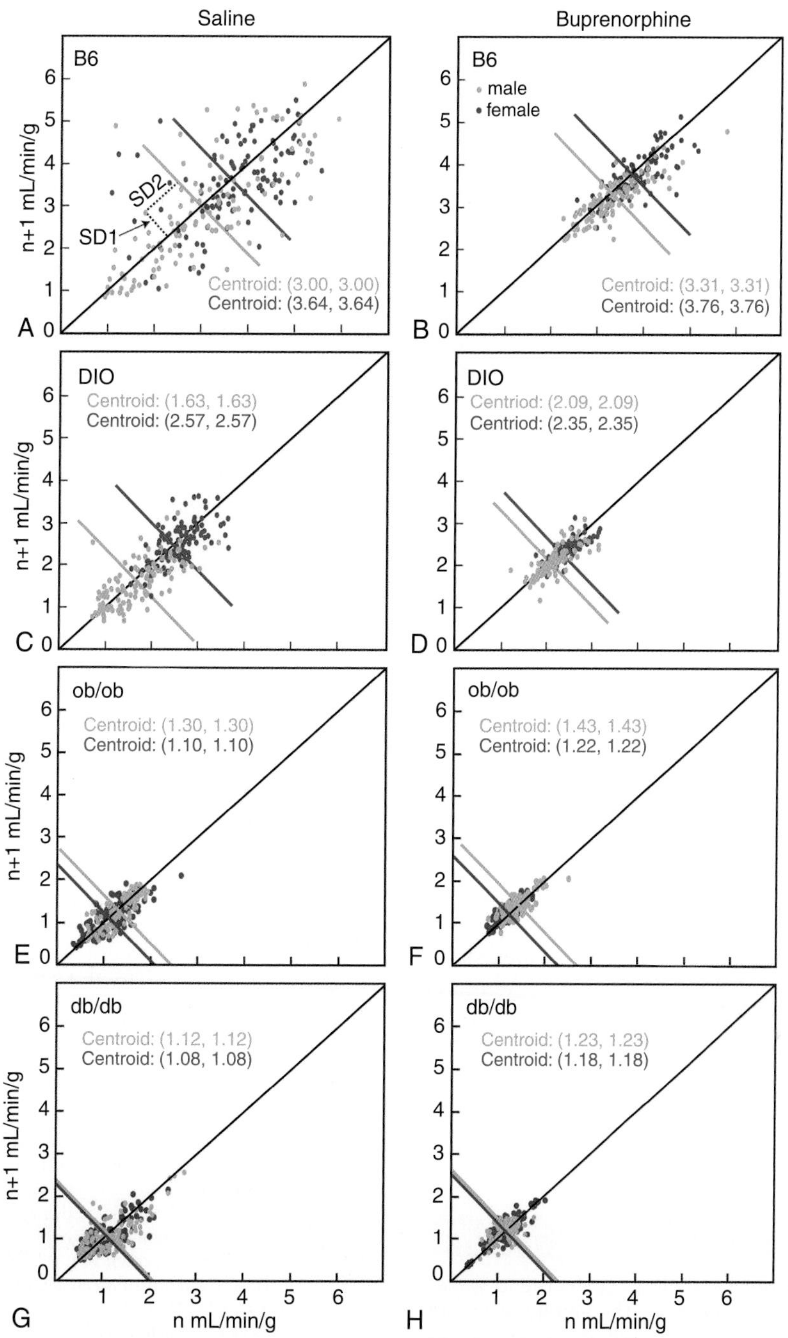

Figure 52.5 Poincaré plots illustrating opioid-induced decrease in minute ventilation in four lines of mice. The *left column* illustrates minute ventilation variability after saline (control) injections. The right column plots the same measure after administration of buprenorphine. From *top* to *bottom,* the rows correspond to four lines of mice (female, *red points;* male, *blue points*). Data are from 80 mice, including C57BL/6J (B6) in rows A and B, B6 mice with diet-induced obesity (DIO) in rows C and D, obese mice (B6.Cg-*Lepr*^{ob}/J [ob/ob]) that fail to produce the satiety hormone leptin (rows E and F), and obese mice (B6.BKS(D)-*Lepr*^{db}/J [db/db]) with dysfunctional leptin receptors (rows G and H). The *x* and *y* portions of each graph are referred to as return plots because minute ventilation during each minute of measurement on the *y*-axis (n+1) is plotted relative to the previous minute of ventilation measurement (n on the *x*-axis). The decrease in minute ventilation variability is apparent in each mouse line by comparing the distribution of points in saline and the buprenorphine conditions. The distributions of points, (x) versus the time delay between breaths (x+1) expresses the standard deviation (SD) of points perpendicular to the line of identity. In **A,** this is illustrated as SD1 and represents breath-to-breath variability. The distribution of points along the line of identity identified as SD2 in **A** represents the long-term variability in minute ventilation over the 1-hour time course of measurement. The center of the line perpendicular to x = y is the centroid and represents the average of all the data points along the line of identity. The *red* and *blue lines* illustrate sex differences in minute ventilation. Considered together, these results show that an antinociceptive dose of buprenorphine significantly decreased breath-to-breath variability (SD1) as a function of mouse line and treatment and significantly altered long-term minute ventilation variability (SD2) as a function of mouse line, sex, and treatment. Thus buprenorphine significantly decreases minute ventilation variability in normal-weight mice (**A** vs. **B**) and causes a greater decrease in obese mice with altered leptin signaling **(C–H).** (From Angel C, Glovak ZT, Alami W, et al. Buprenorphine depresses respiratory variability in obese mice with altered leptin signaling. *Anesthesiology.* 2018;128:984–991.)

Sleep and opioids both impair breathing by reducing respiratory rate and decreasing tonic respiratory drive.[132,133] Decades ago a wakefulness stimulus for respiratory drive was demonstrated by anesthesia research[134] and was subsequently shown to be directly relevant for breathing during sleep.[135] Opioids blunt both the wakefulness stimulus for breathing and chemoreceptive responses to CO_2 and hypoxia, thereby prolonging exhalation time, suppressing tidal volume, and increasing upper airway resistance.[132,133,136,137] Many individuals with OSA remain undiagnosed preoperatively.[110] This is problematic because these people have increased risk of upper airway collapse when asleep or sedated[138] and because accumulating evidence suggests that administration of mu opioid analgesics increases these individuals' risk of respiratory complications in the postoperative period.[122] There is evidence for an increase in endogenous opioids in the cerebrospinal fluid of patients with sleep apnea syndrome, which can increase the sensitivity to opioids in patients with OSA.[139] A dose-dependent relationship exists between chronic opioid use and sleep-disordered breathing regardless of whether or not OSA was a preexisting condition.[132,140–146] Patients with OSA who receive opioids are more likely to develop complex sleep apnea characterized by central and obstructive apneic events.[116,147,148] Central apnea during NREM sleep is the most common effect of chronic opioid use on breathing and sleep.[137,149–151] Seventy percent of patients chronically using opioids developed ataxic breathing and central apneas during NREM sleep compared to an occurrence of 5% in control subjects.[146] In contrast, central sleep apnea was reported to be present in 30% of patients undergoing methadone maintenance therapy.[152] Postoperatively, an increase in the apnea index has been found to be most severe in the first 24 to 48 hours postoperatively.[111,138] During the postoperative period, being elderly and female are risk factors for opioid-induced respiratory depression.[23] Additional risks include OSA, chronic obstructive pulmonary disease, cardiac disease, diabetes mellitus, neurologic disease, renal disease, obesity, two or more comorbidities, opioid dependence, use of patient-controlled analgesia, having multiple prescribers of opioids, and use of two or more opioids.[153]

CLINICAL PEARL

Opioids negatively and significantly impact sleep and wakefulness, as well as control of breathing. The variety of opioid receptors and endogenous opioid neurotransmitters occurring in numerous tissues emphasizes the range of physiologic functions susceptible to modulation by opioids. Opioids also interact with multiple other receptor systems, underscoring the potential synergy of opioids with many compounds. The challenge facing clinicians when prescribing opioids is to achieve an adequate analgesic or other therapeutic effect while minimizing the potential for opioid-induced sleep disruption (which, inter alia, lowers pain thresholds), respiratory depression, tolerance, and risk of addiction.

SUMMARY

Opioids are widely used for the clinical management of acute and chronic pain. Opioids disrupt the temporal organization of sleep by reducing sleep efficiency, increasing time for sleep onset, and reducing NREM (N3) and REM sleep. Such sleep disruption can decrease pain thresholds and promote hyperalgesia counterproductively, even in pain-free individuals. Opioids also blunt wakefulness and can produce dose-dependent states of torpor. Further, they depress the ventilatory responses to hypercarbia and hypoxia, predisposing to hypoventilation, increasing upper airway resistance, and depressing arousal responses. Opioid-induced respiratory depression can be synergistic with comorbid conditions commonly encountered in sleep medicine, such as OSA and sleep-related hypoventilation. Increased vigilance on the part of health care providers is indicated when opioids are part of a treatment plan for obese patients and for patients with preexisting sleep disorders. Furthermore, chronic opioid use is frequently associated with the occurrence of central sleep apnea. In geriatric and pediatric patients, age-specific pharmacokinetics can enhance opioid potency and decrease opioid elimination. The challenge for clinicians when considering prescribing opioids is to achieve adequate analgesia while minimizing respiratory depression, blunting of wakefulness, sleep disruption, drug tolerance, and potential for addiction.

SELECTED READINGS

Angel C, Glovak ZT, Alami W, et al. Buprenorphine depresses respiratory variability in obese mice with altered leptin signaling. *Anesthesiology*. 2018;128:984–991.

Collins FS, Koroshetz WJ, Volkow ND. Helping to end addition over the long-term. The research plan for the NIH HEAL initiative. *J Am Med Assoc*. 2018;320:129–130.

Gupta K, Prasad A, Nagappa M, Wong J, Abrahamyan L, Chung F. Risk factors for opioid-induced respiratory depression and failure to rescue: a review. *Curr Opin Anesthesiol*. 2018;31:110–119.

Ip MSM, Mokhleshi B. Activating leptin receptors in the dentral dervous system using intranasal leptin. A novel therapeutic target for sleep-disordered breathing. *Am J Respir Crit Care Med*. 2018;199:689–691.

Montandon G, Cushing SL, Campbell F, Propst EJ, Horner RL, Narang I. Distinct cortical signatures associated with sedation and respiratory rate depression by morphine in a pediatric population. *Anesthesiology*. 2016;125:889–903.

Overdyk F, Hillman DR. Opioid modeling of central respiratory drive must take upper airway obstruction into account. *Anesthesiology*. 2011;114:219–220.

Rosen IM, Kirsch DB, Carden KA, et al. Chronic opioid therapy and sleep: an American Academy of Sleep Medicine position statement. *J Clin Sleep Med*. 2019;15:1671–1673.

Silber MH, Becker P, Buchfuhrer MJ, et al. The appropriate use of opioids in the treatment of refractory restless legs syndrome. *Mayo Clin Proc*. 2018;93:59–67.

Volkow ND, Collins FS. The role of science in addressing the opioid crisis. *N Engl J Med*. 2017;377:391–394.

Wang D, Yee BJ, Grunstein RR, Chung F. Chronic opioid use and central sleep apnea, where are we now and where to go? A state of the art review. *Anesth Analg*. 2021;132(5):1244-1253.

Wilkerson AK, McRae-Clark AL. A review of sleep disturbance in adults prescribed medications for opioid use disorder: potential treatment targets for a highly prevalent, chronic problem [published online ahead of print, 2021 May 27]. *Sleep Med*. 2021;84:142-153.

A complete reference list can be found online at ExpertConsult.com.

Chapter 53

Clinical Pharmacology of Drugs that Affect Sleep and Wake

Paula K. Schweitzer; Raman K. Malhotra

Chapter Highlights

- Drugs with pharmacologic effects on the neurochemical systems involved in sleep-wake regulation may have therapeutic or impairing effects on sleep-wake behavior. Drugs that inhibit arousal systems may improve sleep but adversely affect wake behavior, whereas drugs that activate arousal systems may improve sleepiness but disrupt sleep. These drugs may also affect duration, timing, and architecture of sleep, in addition to the propensity for abnormalities during sleep such as restless legs, abnormal behaviors, and nightmares.
- The fast neurotransmitters gamma-aminobutyric acid (GABA) and glutamate have key roles in inhibiting and promoting arousal, respectively. Wake-promoting neurotransmitters and neuromodulators include acetylcholine, dopamine, glutamate, histamine, norepinephrine, orexin, and serotonin. Key sleep-promoting mechanisms include enhancement of GABA and inhibition and blocking activation of wake-promoting neuronal systems.
- Pharmacodynamic and pharmacokinetic knowledge is helpful to predict whether a drug will have therapeutic or impairing effects on sleep-wake behavior. Negative effects may be the result of a direct action of a drug (e.g., disturbed sleep from an activating compound or carryover sedation from a long-acting hypnotic) or an indirect action (e.g., inducing or aggravating conditions that disrupt sleep, such as restless legs or nightmares).

Sleep-wake regulation is a highly complex process involving interactions within multiple cell groups resulting in neurochemical changes in (1) the fast neurotransmitters gamma-aminobutyric acid (GABA) and glutamate, which have key roles in inhibiting and promoting arousal, respectively; (2) the wake-promoting neurotransmitters and neuromodulators acetylcholine (ACh), norepinephrine (NE), dopamine (DA), 5-hydroxytryptamine (5-HT; serotonin), histamine (H), orexin/hypocretin, and neuropeptide S; (3) the sleep-promoting neuromodulators adenosine and melanin-concentrating hormone; and (4) the circadian-regulating hormone melatonin.[1-3] Drugs with pharmacologic effects at these neurochemical systems may therefore have effects on sleep-wake behavior. These effects may be therapeutic (e.g., improve sleep or enhance wakefulness) or impairing (e.g., cause sleep disturbance or daytime sedation).

Receptor mechanisms relevant to sleep-wake behavior are listed in Table 53.1.[2,4-8] Drugs can promote sedation or arousal by multiple mechanisms. Inhibition of arousal systems promotes sleep but may adversely affect wake behavior, whereas activation of arousal systems promotes wake but may disrupt sleep. A number of drugs affect both sleep-promoting and wake-promoting mechanisms to varying degrees (e.g., antidepressants, antipsychotics), with the net effect determining the likelihood of sedation or arousal, within the context of circadian phase, drug dose, and drug pharmacokinetics.

Dose, time to peak concentration, and half-life determine the rapidity of onset and the duration of a drug's clinical effect, and the receptor binding profile determines both mechanism of action and adverse events. Potency describes amount of drug required for therapeutic effect and generally correlates with affinity of the drug at specific receptors. However, dose affects receptor occupancy, and as a result, dose can alter the profile of receptors where clinical effects are elicited. For example, doxepin at low doses (3–6 mg) has predominant clinical effects reflecting histamine 1 (H_1) receptor antagonism, whereas at higher doses it exerts clinically significant effects via inhibition of the 5-HT and NE transporters (serotonin transporter [SERT] and norepinephrine transporter [NET], respectively) and also antagonism of adrenergic alpha$_1$(α_1), muscarinic ACh (mACh), and 5-HT$_2$ receptors.[9,10] These properties, in addition to the timing of drug administration, determine whether a drug's action has a desired clinical effect and/or side effects.

In addition to sleep-promoting and wake-promoting effects, drugs may affect duration, timing, or architecture of sleep and the propensity for abnormalities during sleep, such as restless legs syndrome (RLS), periodic limb movements of sleep (PLMS), nightmares, disordered breathing, or abnormal behaviors. This chapter reviews the effects of drugs on sleep-wake behavior with a principal focus on side effects pertinent to sleep and wake. Drugs used to treat insomnia and sleepiness are briefly reviewed. Effects of drugs on sleep architecture are

Table 53.1 Pharmacologic Mechanisms of Drug Effects on Sleep and Wake Behavior

	Mechanism	Promotes Sleep	Promotes Wake	Example Drug(s)
Acetylcholine[a]	Agonism		X	Nicotine, pilocarpine
	Antagonism[b]	X		Oxybutynin, scopolamine, some antidepressants,[c] and antipsychotics[c]
Acetylcholinesterase	Inhibition		X	Donepezil
$Adenosine_{1,2A}$[d]	Agonism	X		Regadenoson
	Antagonism, inverse agonism		X	Caffeine, theobromine, istradefylline
Adrenergic (norepinephrine)	α_1 agonism		X	Phenylephrine
	α_1 antagonism	X		Prazosin
	α_2 agonism	X		Clonidine, guanfacine, methyldopa
	α_2 antagonism		X	Yohimbine, lurasidone
	β antagonism		X	Propranolol
	Reuptake inhibition		X	Stimulants,[c] wake-promoting drugs,[c] antidepressants,[c] antipsychotics[c]
Dopamine	Agonism	X[e]	X	Ropinirole, pramipexole
	Antagonism	X		Most antipsychotics[c]
	Reuptake inhibition		X	Stimulants,[c] wake-promoting drugs,[c] bupropion[c]
$GABA_A$[f]	Positive allosteric modulation	X		Barbiturates,[g] benzodiazepines, nonbenzodiazepine hypnotics (e.g., zolpidem), many antiepileptics[c]
	Negative allosteric modulation		X	Clarithromycin
	Antagonism		X	Ciprofloxacin
Galanin	Agonism	X		
	Antagonism		X	
Glycine	Agonism	X		
	Antagonism		X	Caffeine
Glutamate	Antagonism[h]	X		Esketamine, dextromethorphan, amantadine, memantine, perampanel
$Histamine_1$ (H_1)	Antagonism	X		First-generation antihistamines, low-dose doxepin, many psychotherapeutic drugs[c]
$Histamine_3$ (H_3)	Inverse agonism, antagonism		X	Pitolisant
$Melatonin_{1,2}$	Agonism	X		Ramelteon
Monoamine oxidase	Inhibition[b,i]		X	Phenelzine
Orexin-1,2 (hypocretin-1,2)	Agonism		X	
	Antagonism	X		Lemborexant, suvorexant
Serotonin (5-HT)	$5\text{-}HT_{1A,1B}$ agonism[b]		X	Buspirone, aripiprazole, vortioxetine
	$5\text{-}HT_{2A,2C,3}$ agonism[b]		X	Lorcaserin
	Reuptake inhibition[b]		X	SSRI,[j] SNRI,[k] other antidepressants
	$5\text{-}HT_{1A}$ antagonism	X		Risperidone
	$5\text{-}HT_{2A,2C}$ antagonism,[l] inverse agonism	X		Many antipsychotics,[c] some antidepressants[c]

[a]Acetylcholine binds at muscarinic and nicotinic receptors.
[b]Suppresses rapid eye movement (REM) sleep.
[c]These drugs also have other mechanisms that may promote wake or sleep. Antidepressants and antipsychotics, in particular, have multiple mechanisms that may affect wake or sleep.
[d]$Adenosine_{1,2A}$ receptors regulate the release of a number of neurotransmitters, including dopamine and glutamate. $Adenosine_{2A}$ receptor agonists may induce sleep by inhibiting the histaminergic system through an increase in gamma-aminobutyric acid (GABA).

Table 53.1 Pharmacologic Mechanisms of Drug Effects on Sleep and Wake Behavior—cont'd

[e]Dopamine agonists may promote sleep by variable mechanisms. See text for details.
[f]Drugs act on the gamma-aminobutyric acid A ($GABA_A$) receptor in various ways. Positive allosteric modulators (e.g., benzodiazepines) bind to sites distinct from the GABA binding site on the $GABA_A$ receptor, changing the conformation of the receptor, thereby enhancing the inhibition that occurs when GABA binds to the receptor. Negative allosteric modulators change the conformation of the receptor to decrease GABA inhibition. GABA antagonists inhibit GABA directly.
[g]Barbiturates bind at multiple sites distinct from the benzodiazepine binding site on the $GABA_A$ receptor and also block α-amino-3-hydroxy-5-methyl-4-isoxazolepropionic acid (AMPA) and kainate receptors (subtypes of glutamate receptors).
[h]Glutamate antagonism can occur via N-methyl-D-aspartate (NMDA) receptors (esketamine, dextromethorphan, amantadine, memantine) or AMPA receptors (perampanel).
[i]Inhibition of monoamine oxidase increases dopamine, epinephrine, norepinephrine, and serotonin, thereby promoting wake.
[j]SSRI, selective serotonin reuptake inhibitor.
[k]SNRI, selective serotonin-norepinephrine reuptake inhibitor.
[l]Increases slow wave sleep (SWS).

summarized in Table 53.2. Additional information regarding efficacy, side effects, and other drug properties are included in chapters elsewhere in this volume that discuss clinical management of sleep disorders and sleep in specific diseases.

DRUGS USED TO TREAT INSOMNIA (TABLES 53.3 AND 53.4)

Pharmacotherapy for insomnia includes drugs with US Food and Drug Administration (FDA) indication for insomnia (Table 53.3), drugs used "off-label" (Table 53.4), and over-the-counter and herbal preparations. Effects of these drugs on sleep architecture are summarized in Table 53.2.[11-15]

Drugs with FDA Indication for Insomnia

Mechanisms for sedation of drugs with FDA indication for insomnia (Table 53.3) include enhancement of GABA inhibition via positive allosteric modulation of the $GABA_A$ receptor (benzodiazepines, nonbenzodiazepines [Z drugs]), H_1 antagonism (low-dose doxepin), melatonin agonism (ramelteon), and orexin antagonism (lemborexant, suvorexant).[11] $GABA_A$ positive allosteric modulators differ in their affinities for different $GABA_A$ subunits. Benzodiazepines (estazolam, flurazepam, quazepam, temazepam, triazolam) are nonspecific for the $\alpha_{1,2,3,5}$ subtypes, whereas the nonbenzodiazepines (eszopiclone, zolpidem, zaleplon) have higher affinity for the α_1 subunit, which appears to be more specifically implicated in sleep, and lower but variable affinity for the $\alpha_{2,3}$ subunits.[11] The older benzodiazepines have long elimination half-lives, and some have active metabolites, resulting in a high likelihood for residual sedation and daytime impairment.[16,17]

Doxepin, at the low doses indicated for insomnia (≤6 mg), is a potent H_1 antagonist and lacks clinically significant effects on the noradrenergic and serotonergic systems that are seen with antidepressant doses (≥75 mg).[9] Ramelteon is a potent agonist at both melatonin 1 and 2 (MT_1 and MT_2) receptors but has much higher affinity for the MT_1 receptor, which distinguishes it from both tasimelteon and melatonin. Tasimelteon, which is indicated for the treatment of non-24-hour sleep-wake disorder, has comparable potency to melatonin at the MT_1 receptor but higher affinity for MT_2 compared with MT_1.[18] Suvorexant and lemborexant are dual orexin receptor antagonists with high affinity for both orexin-1 and orexin-2 receptors.[19,20] Despite intermediate to long half-lives, these drugs do not appear to have significant residual effects.[20a,b]

Other drugs with FDA indication for insomnia include the barbiturates, butabarbital and secobarbital. Barbiturates are $GABA_A$ positive allosteric modulators, albeit acting at a binding site other than the benzodiazepine binding site. Barbiturates also inhibit glutamate release by α-amino-3-hydroxy-5-methyl-4-isoxazolepropionic acid (AMPA) and kainate antagonism.[21]

Other Drugs Used to Treat Insomnia

A variety of prescription drugs are increasingly used off-label to treat insomnia (Table 53.4), with trazodone being the most common.[22,23] Amitriptyline, mirtazapine, quetiapine, olanzapine, and gabapentin are also frequently used for insomnia. Most of these drugs promote sleep by antagonism of H_1, α_1, or $5\text{-}HT_{2A,2C}$, but other sleep-promoting mechanisms include dopamine 2 (D_2) antagonism, $5\text{-}HT_{1A}$ partial agonism, postsynaptic α_2 antagonism, alpha2-delta ($\alpha 2\delta$) calcium channel inhibition, and GABA agonism.[11] These drugs affect multiple receptors, however, resulting in variable effects on sleep-wake behavior in addition to side effects not associated with sleep-wake mechanisms. Because most of these drugs have intermediate to long half-lives, they can produce dose-dependent residual sedation. An exception is the antihypertensive agent prazosin, an α_1 antagonist used in the treatment of nightmares and sleep maintenance insomnia in patients with posttraumatic stress disorder (PTSD).[24,25] Receptor mechanisms and sleep architecture effects for these drugs are listed in Table 53.4 and 53.2, respectively, and discussed elsewhere in this chapter in sections that discuss sedation as a side effect. Additional information regarding efficacy, side effects, and use of these drugs in the clinical management of insomnia are discussed elsewhere in this volume.

Common over-the-counter drugs used for insomnia include the hormone melatonin, the H_1 antagonists diphenhydramine and doxylamine, the dietary supplement L-tryptophan (a precursor to serotonin), and the plant extract valerian, which contains multiple constituents. Melatonin is covered more fully elsewhere in this volume. Briefly, melatonin regulates circadian rhythms through its action on MT_1 and MT_2 receptors.[26] Melatonin is considered a dietary supplement in the United States and therefore is not regulated by the FDA. Over-the-counter melatonin is not available in most other countries, but a controlled-release formulation is available by prescription in some countries. In the United States, there is poor quality control of melatonin. In one study, quantification of melatonin content in over 30 commercial supplements revealed wide variation from labeled content, significant lot-to-lot variability, and the presence of serotonin in 26% of the samples.[27] Melatonin has been increasingly used in the treatment of REM behavior disorder (RBD) in doses up to 25 mg.[28] Although sleepiness is typically reported at low incidences with melatonin treatment of insomnia,[29,30] sleepiness was reported in 25% of individuals in a patient-reported outcomes study of RBD, possibly associated with dose.[28]

Clinical trials of diphenhydramine show subjective improvement in some measures of sleep, but most

Table 53.2 Effects of Drugs on Sleep Architecture[a]

Drug Class/Drug	Sleep Latency	Sleep Continuity[b]	SWS	REM[c]
Drugs with FDA Indication for Insomnia				
Benzodiazepines				
Estazolam, flurazepam, quazepam, temazepam, triazolam	↓	↑	↓	↓
Nonbenzodiazepines				
Eszopiclone	↓	↑	↔	↔
Zaleplon	↓	↔	↔	↔
Zolpidem	↓	↑	↔	↓
Other Insomnia Drugs				
Doxepin (≤6 mg)	↓	↑	↔	↔
Ramelteon	↓	↔↑	↔	↔
Lemborexant	↓	↑	↔	↑
Suvorexant	↓	↑	↔	↑
Tasimelteon[d]	↓	↑	↔	↔
Psychotherapeutic Drugs				
Antidepressants				
Tricyclics				
Amitriptyline,[e] clomipramine, doxepin,[e] imipramine, trimipramine	↓	↑	↔	↓[f]
Desipramine, nortriptyline	↔	↔↓		↓
SSRIs				
Citalopram, escitalopram, fluoxetine, fluvoxamine, paroxetine, sertraline	↑	↓	↔↓	↓
SNRIs				
Duloxetine, venlafaxine		↓	↔↓	↓
MAOIs				
Phenelzine, tranylcypromine	↔↑	↓		↓↓
Isocarboxazid, selegiline		↓		↔
Other Antidepressants				
Bupropion	↔	↔	↔	↔↑
Mirtazapine[e]	↔↓	↑	↑	↔
Trazodone[e]	↓	↔↑	↑	↔↓
Vilazodone		↓	↑	↓↓
Antipsychotics				
Chlorpromazine	↓	↑	↑	↓
Clozapine	↔↓	↓	↑	↔↓
Haloperidol	↓	↑	↔	↔↓
Lurasidone[e]	↔	↑	↔	↔
Lumateperone	?	↑	↑	?
Olanzapine[e]	↓	↑	↑	↔↓↑
Paliperidone	↓	↑	↔	↔↑
Quetiapine[e]	↓	↑	↔↓↑	↓
Risperidone[e]	↔↓	↔↑	↔↑	↔
Thiothixene	↓	↑	↑	↔↓
Ziprasidone	↔↓	↑	↑	↓

Table 53.2 Effects of Drugs on Sleep Architecture[a]—cont'd

Drug Class/Drug	Sleep Latency	Sleep Continuity[b]	SWS	REM[c]
Antiepileptics				
Benzodiazepines				
Clonazepam, clorazepate, diazepam, lorazepam, midazolam	↓	↑	↓	↓
Other Antiepileptics				
Phenobarbital	↓	↑	↓	↓
Carbamazepine	?↓	↑	↑	?↓
Ethosuximide		↓	↓	↔↑
Gabapentin[e]	↔	↑	↑	↔↑
Lamotrigine			↔↓	↔↑
Levetiracetam	↔	↑	↑	↓
Phenytoin	↓		↓	↓
Pregabalin[e]	↓	↑	↑	↓
Tiagabine	↔↓	↑	↑	↔
Valproate, valproic acid		?↑	↔	↔
Cardiovascular Drugs				
α_1 Antagonists				
Prazosin		↑		↑
α_2 Agonists				
Clonidine		↔↑	↑	↓
Methyldopa		↑	↓	↑↓
Angiotensin-Converting Enzyme (ACE) Inhibitors				
Enalapril, captopril, lisinopril	↔	↔	↔	↔
Beta Antagonists				
Atenolol, metoprolol, propranolol		↓		↓
Dopamine Agonists				
Pergolide	↓	↑		
Pramipexole			?↑	↓
Ropinirole	↓	↑	↔	↔
Other Drugs				
Alcohol				
Acute ingestion	↓	↑↓[g]	↑	↓
Chronic ingestion	↑	↓	↓	↓
Withdrawal	↑	↓	↓	↑
Antihistamines				
Chlorpheniramine, diphenhydramine, doxylamine, hydroxyzine	↔↓	↔↑	↔↑	↔↓
Pain Medications				
Aspirin, ibuprofen		↓	↓	↔
Opioids, acute	↔↓	↔↑	↓	↓
Opioids, chronic		↓	↓	↓
Stimulants/Wake-Promoting Drugs				
Amphetamine, methamphetamine, methylphenidate	↑	↓	↔↓	↓
Modafinil	↔↓	?	↔	
Caffeine	↑	↓	↓	
Nicotine	↑	↓		↓

Continued

Table 53.2 Effects of Drugs on Sleep Architecture[a]—cont'd

Drug Class/Drug	Sleep Latency	Sleep Continuity[b]	SWS	REM[c]
Other Drugs				
Corticosteroids		↓	↔↓	↓
Melatonin	↓	↔↑	↔	↔↓
Pseudoephedrine	?↑	↓		
Sodium oxybate	↓	↑	↑	↔↓
Theophylline		↓	↓	
Valerian	↔↓	↔↑	↑	↔↑

[a]Information in this table is limited to available polysomnographic data, which may comprise heterogenous samples, including patient groups and healthy individuals. Subjective reports of sleep difficulty may differ.
[b]Sleep continuity refers to the proportion of sleep relative to wakefulness, as reflected by sleep efficiency.
[c]Decreased rapid eye movement (REM) is typically accompanied by increased REM latency and vice versa.
[d]Tasimelteon is indicated for treatment of non-24-hour sleep-wake disorder. Improvement in sleep may be the result of circadian entrainment rather than a direct action of the drug on sleep.
[e]Used off-label to treat insomnia.
[f]Although REM amount decreases, there is an increase in phasic eye movements (REM density).
[g]Alcohol has a biphasic effect on sleep, improving sleep continuity during the first half of the night, but because it is quickly metabolized, disrupting sleep during the second half of the night.
MAOI, Monoamine oxidase inhibitor; REM, rapid eye movement; SNRI, serotonin-norepinephrine reuptake inhibitor; SSRI, selective serotonin reuptake inhibitor; SWS, slow wave sleep; ↑, increase; ↓, decrease; ↔, no change; ?, unclear; blank, unknown.

Table 53.3 Pharmacology of Drugs with FDA Indication for Insomnia

Drug Class/Drug	Indication	Mechanism	Dose (mg)	t_{max} (h)	$t_{1/2}$ (h)[a]	Residual Sedation
Benzodiazepines						
Estazolam (Prosom)	Insomnia	$GABA_A$ PAM	1–2	2.0 (0.5–6)	10–24	++
Flurazepam (Dalmane)	Insomnia	$GABA_A$ PAM	15–30	0.5–4.0	47–120	+++
Quazepam (Doral)	Insomnia	$GABA_A$ PAM	7.5–15	2.0	39–73	+++
Temazepam (Restoril)	Insomnia	$GABA_A$ PAM	7.5–30	1.2–1.6	8–20	+
Triazolam (Halcion)	Insomnia	$GABA_A$ PAM	0.125–0.5	2.0	1.5–5.5	–
Nonbenzodiazepines						
Eszopiclone (Lunesta)	Insomnia	$GABA_A$ PAM	1–3	1.0	6–7	–/+
Zaleplon (Sonata)	Insomnia	$GABA_A$ PAM	5–20	1.0	1.0	–
Zolpidem (Ambien)	Insomnia	$GABA_A$ PAM	5–10	1.6	2.5 (1.4–4.5)	–
Zolpidem ER (Ambien CR)	Insomnia	$GABA_A$ PAM	6.25–12.5	1.5	2.8 (1.6–4.0)	–
Zolpidem sublingual (Intermezzo)	Insomnia	$GABA_A$ PAM	1.75–3.5	0.6–1.25	2.5 (1.4–3.6)	–/+
Zolpidem sublingual (Edluar)	Insomnia	$GABA_A$ PAM	5–10	1.4 (0.5–3.0)	2.7 (1.6–6.7)	–/+
Zolpidem oral spray (Zolpimist)	Insomnia	$GABA_A$ PAM	10	0.9	3.0 (1.7–8.4)	–
H_1 Antagonists						
Doxepin[b] (Silenor)	Insomnia	H_1 antagonism	3–6	3.5	15.3–31	+
Melatonin Agonists						
Ramelteon (Rozerem)	Insomnia	$Melatonin_{1,2}$ agonism	8	0.8 (0.5–1.5)	1.0–5.0	–
Tasimelteon (Hetlioz)	Non-24-hr sleep-wake disorder	$Melatonin_{1,2}$ agonism	20	0.5–3.0	1.3–3.7	–
Orexin Antagonists						
Lemborexant (Dayvigo)	Insomnia	Orexin-1,2 antagonism	5–10	1–3	17–19	+
Suvorexant (Belsomra)	Insomnia	Orexin-1,2 antagonism	10–20	2 (0.5–6)	12	+

Table 53.3 Pharmacology of Drugs with FDA Indication for Insomnia—cont'd

Drug Class/Drug	Indication	Mechanism	Dose (mg)	t_{max} (h)	$t_{1/2}$ (h)[a]	Residual Sedation
Barbiturates						
Butabarbital (Butisol)	Sedative, insomnia	$GABA_A$ PAM[c]	50–100	3–4	100	++++
Secobarbital (Seconal)	Insomnia, preanesthetic	$GABA_A$ PAM[c]	100	2–4	15–40	+++
Drugs in Development						
Daridorexant		Orexin-1,2 antagonism		0.8–1	8.5–9.5	
Seltorexant		Orexin-2 antagonism				

[a]Includes active metabolites when present.
[b]At very low doses (≤6 mg, as used in Silenor), doxepin binds with high specificity and affinity to the H_1 receptor, with negligible binding to 5-HT_{2A}, α_1, NET, and SERT, unlike the higher doses of doxepin used for the treatment of depression and used off-label for insomnia.
[c]Barbiturates also block AMPA and kainate receptors and inhibit glutamate release.
5-HT_{2a}, Serotonin 2A receptor; α_1, alpha adrenergic 1 receptor; AMPA, α-amino-3-hydroxy-5-methyl-4-isoxazolepropionic acid; CR, controlled release; ER, extended release; $GABA_A$, gamma-aminobutyric acid A receptor; H_1, histamine 1 receptor; mACh, muscarinic anticholinergic receptor; NET, norepinephrine transporter; PAM, positive allosteric modulation; SERT, serotonin transporter; $t_{1/2}$, elimination half-life; t_{max} time to peak plasma concentration.

Table 53.4 Pharmacology of Other Drugs Used to Treat Insomnia

Drug Class/Drug	Indication	Receptor Mechanisms: H_1 Antagonism	5-HT_2 Antagonism	α_1 Antagonism	D_2 Antagonism	mACh Antagonism	Other	Usual Dose (mg) for Insomnia[a]	t_{max} (h)	$t_{1/2}$ (h)[b]	Residual Sedation
Antidepressants											
Amitriptyline	Depression	++++	++	+++	+	+++	NET and SERT inhibition	25–150	2–6	5–45	++
Doxepin[c]	Depression, anxiety	++++	++	+++	–	++	NET and SERT inhibition	10–150[c]	2–4	10–30	+++
Mirtazapine	Depression	++++	++	+	–	–	$\alpha_{2A,B,C}$ antagonism, inverse agonism	7.5–30	2–3	20–40	+++
Trazodone[d]	Depression	+	++	++	–	–	α_2 antagonism; SERT inhibition	25–150	1–2	9–14	++
Trimipramine	Depression	+++	++	++	+	++	SERT inhibition	25–150	2–8	15–40	+++
Antipsychotics											
Olanzapine	Schizophrenia, bipolar disorder	+++	+++	++	++	++	D_1 antagonism	2.5–20	4–6	20–54	+++
Quetiapine	Schizophrenia, bipolar disorder	+++	+	++	+	+	D_1 antagonism	25–250	1–2	6	++
Lurasidone	Schizophrenia, bipolar disorder	–	+++	++	+++	–	5-HT_7, D_1 antagonism; 5-HT_{1A} partial agonism	40	1–3	18	++
Risperidone	Schizophrenia, bipolar mania, autistic disorder, irritability	++	++++	+++	+++	+	D_1 antagonism	1–8	1	3–20	++

Continued

Table 53.4 Pharmacology of Other Drugs Used to Treat Insomnia—cont'd

Drug Class/ Drug	Indication	Receptor Mechanisms: H_1	$5\text{-}HT_2$	α_1	D_2	mACh	Other	Usual Dose (mg) for Insomnia[a]	t_{max} (h)	$t_{1/2}$ (h)[b]	Residual Sedation
		Antagonism									
Antiepileptics											
Gabapentin	Neuralgia, seizures	–	–	–	–	–	$\alpha_2\delta$ calcium channel inhibition[e]	300–600	3–4	5–9	+
Pregabalin	Neuropathic pain, fibromyalgia, seizures	–	–	–	–	–		50–300	0.6–1.3	6.3	+
Tiagabine	Seizures	–	–	–	–	–	GAT-1 inhibition	2–12	1–2.5	7–9	+
Benzodiazepines											
Alprazolam	Anxiety	–	–	–	–	–	$GABA_A$ PAM	0.25–1.0	1–2	12–14	+
Alprazolam XR	Anxiety	–	–	–	–	–	$GABA_A$ PAM	0.5–3	1–2	10–16	++
Chlordiazepoxide	Anxiety, alcohol withdrawal	–	–	–	–	–	$GABA_A$ PAM	5–10	1	36–200	+++
Clonazepam	Seizures, panic disorder	–	–	–	–	–	$GABA_A$ PAM	0.25–2.0	1–4	35–40	+++
Diazepam	Anxiety, spasm, seizures	–	–	–	–	–	$GABA_A$ PAM	2–10	0.25–2.5	48–100	+++
Lorazepam	Anxiety	–	–	–	–	–	$GABA_A$ PAM	0.25–2	2	12–18	++
Other Drugs											
Chloral hydrate	Preanesthesia	–	–	–	–	–	Barbiturate-like GABA modulation	500–1000	0.7	8–10	++
Diphenhydramine	Allergy and cold symptoms	++	–	–	–	–	–	25–50	2–3	2.4–9.3	+
Doxylamine	Allergy and cold symptoms	++	–	–	–	–	–	25	1.7	12	++
L-tryptophan	NA	–	–	–	–	–	Tryptophan inhibition	250–15,000	?	?	?
Melatonin	NA	–	–	–	–	–	$MT_{1,2}$ agonism	0.1–75	0.3–1	0.6–1	+?
Prazosin[f]	Hypertension	–	–	++++	–	–	–	1–12	3	2–3	–
Valerian	NA	–	–	–	–	–	Uncertain[g]	400–900	?[f]	?[f]	?

[a]Doses used for insomnia are based on common clinical practice and published studies, not formal dose-ranging studies.
[b]Includes active metabolites when present.
[c]Dose range reported for doxepin reflects use of the antidepressant compound as a hypnotic. Doxepin (Silenor) has US Food and Drug Administration (FDA) indication for insomnia at doses of 3 and 6 mg. At these low doses, doxepin binds with high specificity and affinity to the H_1 receptor, with negligible binding to $5\text{-}HT_{2A}$, α_1, NET, and SERT, unlike the higher doses of doxepin used for the treatment of depression and used off-label for insomnia.
[d]At low doses, trazodone exhibits H_1, α_1, and $5\text{-}HT_{2A}$ antagonism. At moderate to high doses, there is also $5\text{-}HT_{2C}$ and SERT inhibition.
[e]Gabapentin and pregabalin bind to the $\alpha_2\delta$ subunit of voltage-activated calcium channels, attenuating neurotransmitter release of glutamate, noradrenaline, and substance P. See text.
[f]Prazosin is used off-label to treat nightmares and sleep maintenance insomnia in posttraumatic stress disorder.
[g]Mechanism and pharmacokinetics of valerian are uncertain because of multiple constituents; may affect GABA, 5-HT, and adenosine
$5\text{-}HT_{1A}$, $5\text{-}HT_7$, Serotonin receptors 1A, 7; $\alpha_{1,2}$, alpha-adrenergic receptors 1, 2; $\alpha_2\delta$, alpha 2 delta subunit of voltage-dependent calcium channels; D_1, D_2, dopamine receptors 1, 2; GABA, gamma-aminobutyric acid; $GABA_A$, gamma-aminobutyric acid A receptor; GAT-1, GABA transporter; H_1, histamine 1 receptor; mACh, muscarinic anticholinergic receptor; $MT_{1,2}$, melatonin receptors 1 and 2; NET, norepinephrine transporter; PAM, positive allosteric modulation; SERT, serotonin transporter; $t_{1/2}$, elimination half-life; t_{max} time to peak plasma concentration; XR, extended release

polysomnograph (PSG) measures show no difference from placebo.[31,32] Diphenhydramine increases physiologic sleep tendency, as measured by a multiple sleep latency test (MSLT), and decreases performance acutely, but tolerance may develop within 3 to 4 days,[33,34] although driving may continue to be impaired.[35]

Drugs Under Development for Insomnia

Daridorexant, a dual orexin antagonist, has been studied in both younger and older individuals with insomnia.[36,37] Seltorexant, a selective orexin-2 antagonist, is under development for insomnia and major depressive disorder.[38,39] This is of interest because it appears that the orexin-2 receptor is the primary of the two orexin receptors involved in sleep-wake regulation.[40]

DRUGS USED TO PROMOTE WAKEFULNESS (TABLE 53.5)

Stimulants and wake-promoting drugs are used in the treatment of excessive sleepiness in disorders of central hypersomnolence (e.g., narcolepsy, idiopathic hypersomnia), shiftwork sleep disorder, and sleep apnea. Many of these drugs are used in the treatment of attention-deficit/hyperactivity disorder, and some are used for obesity or binge-eating disorder. Guidelines for the treatment of central hypersomnias (Figures 53.1 and 53.2) were updated in 2021.

Stimulants (Sympathomimetics)

Amphetamine and amphetamine-like compounds (dextroamphetamine, lisdexamfetamine, methamphetamine, methylphenidate, amphetamine/dextroamphetamine) promote wakefulness by increasing dopaminergic transmission via direct release of DA and by blocking DA reuptake.[41] These drugs also release NE and block NE reuptake, but the primary mechanism for promoting arousal is presynaptic modulation of DA.[41] There are a number of immediate- and delayed-release stimulants, with half-lives typically 3 to 4 hours for the immediate-release compounds and 8 to 16 hours for the sustained-release formulations, although there are some exceptions. Insomnia may occur with longer-acting drugs, particularly at higher doses.

Wake-Promoting Drugs (Nonsympathomimetics)

Wake-promoting drugs differ from sympathomimetics in that they have no monoamine-releasing properties. The mechanism of action for modafinil and armodafinil is unclear but is at least partially via dopamine transporter (DAT) inhibition.[41,42] Modafinil also appears to modulate noradrenergic, serotonergic, orexinergic, histaminergic, glutamatergic, and GABAergic systems.[43] Solriamfetol inhibits both NET and DAT.[44] Pitolisant is an inverse agonist at the H_3 receptor but also modulates release of DA, NE, and ACh.[45] Insomnia is occasionally reported, generally with higher doses.

Table 53.5 Prescription Drugs Used to Promote Wakefulness

Drug Class/Drug	FDA Indication[a]	Dose (mg)	t_{max} (h)	$t_{1/2}$ (h)	Mechanism
Stimulants					
Amphetamine (Evekeo)	EDS in narcolepsy, ADHD, obesity	5–60	3.5 (2–8)	11.7	Dopamine release and reuptake inhibition; norepinephrine release and reuptake inhibition
Dextroamphetamine (Dexedrine, ProCentra, Zenzedi)	EDS in narcolepsy, ADHD	5–60	8	12	
Amphetamine/dextroamphetamine	EDS in narcolepsy, ADHD				
(Adderall)		5–60	2–3	10 (7–34)	
(Adderall XR)		10–60	7	12	
Lisdexamfetamine (Vyvanse)[a]	ADHD, binge-eating	30–70	4.6	7.9	
Methamphetamine (Desoxyn)[a]	ADHD	5–25	0.5–1	4–5	
	Obesity	15			
Methylphenidate[b]	ADHD				
(Methylin chewable)		10–60	1–2	2.8	
(Methylin oral solution)		10–60	1–2	2.7	
(Ritalin)		10–60	1–3	1.5–3	
(Ritalin LA)		10–60	1.3–4.0	3.5 (6–12)	
Wake-Promoting Drugs					
Armodafinil (Nuvigil)	EDS in narcolepsy, sleep apnea, and shift-work disorder	150–250	2	10–15	DAT inhibition; indirect activation of other wake-promoting neurotransmitters
Modafinil (Provigil)		150–400	2–4	15	
Pitolisant (Wakix)	EDS in narcolepsy; cataplexy	17.8–35.6	3.5	20	H_3 inverse agonism[c]
Solriamfetol (Sunosi)	EDS in narcolepsy and sleep apnea	75–150	2–3	7	NET and DAT inhibition

Continued

Table 53.5 Prescription Drugs Used to Promote Wakefulness—cont'd

Drug Class/Drug	FDA Indication[a]	Dose (mg)	t_{max} (h)	$t_{1/2}$ (h)	Mechanism
Oxybates					
Sodium oxybate (Xyrem)	EDS in narcolepsy; cataplexy	4.5–9 g	0.5–1.25	0.5–1.	$GABA_B$ receptor activity[e]
Low-sodium oxybate (Xywav)[d]	EDS in narcolepsy; cataplexy	4.5–9 g	1.3	0.66	$GABA_B$ receptor activity[e]
Drugs in Development for Hypersomnia Disorders					
AXS-12 (reboxetine)	EDS in narcolepsy; cataplexy		2.4	2.2	NET inhibition
BTD-001 (oral pentetrazol)	idiopathic hypersomnia				$GABA_A$ antagonism
FT218 (controlled-release sodium oxybate)	EDS in narcolepsy; cataplexy		1.5–5		$GABA_B$ receptor activity[e]
Xywav (JZP-258)[e]	Idiopathic hypersomnia;				$GABA_B$ receptor activity[e]
SUVN-G3031	EDS in narcolepsy; cataplexy				H_3 inverse agonism
TAK-925, TAK-994	EDS in narcolepsy				Orexin-2 agonism

[a]Used off-label for EDS in narcolepsy.
[b]The brands of methylphenidate listed are used off-label for EDS in narcolepsy. There are a number of additional formulations of methylphenidate with indication solely for ADHD.
[c]Pitolisant also modulates the release of dopamine, norepinephrine, and acetylcholine.
[d]Xywav is a unique combination of four oxybates (sodium, potassium, calcium, magnesium) with 92% less sodium than that in Xyrem.
[e]The mechanism of action of sodium oxybate is thought to be mediated by $GABA_B$ receptor activity at noradrenergic, dopaminergic, and thalamocortical neurons, and possibly activity at a putative gamma-hydroxybutyric acid (GHBA) receptor.
ADHD, Attention-deficit/hyperactivity disorder; DAT, dopamine transporter; EDS, excessive daytime sleepiness; $GABA_{A, B}$, gamma-aminobutyric acid A, B receptors; H_3, histamine 3 receptor; LA, long acting; NET, norepinephrine transporter; $t_{1/2}$, elimination half-life; t_{max}, time to peak plasma concentration; XR, extended release.

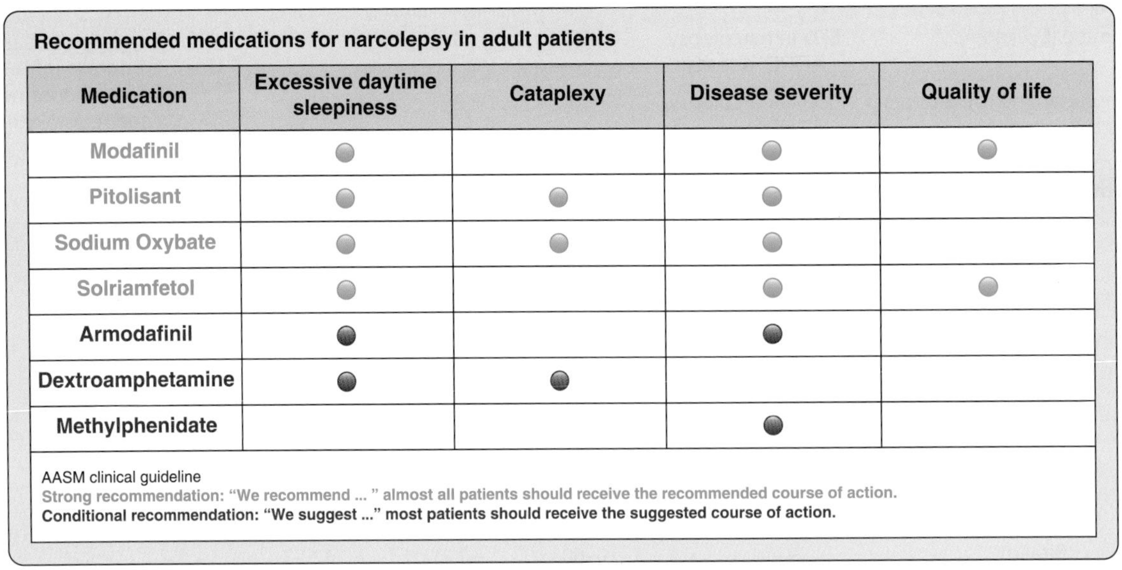

Recommended medications for narcolepsy in adult patients

Medication	Excessive daytime sleepiness	Cataplexy	Disease severity	Quality of life
Modafinil	●		●	●
Pitolisant	●	●	●	
Sodium Oxybate	●	●	●	
Solriamfetol	●		●	●
Armodafinil	●		●	
Dextroamphetamine	●	●		
Methylphenidate			●	

AASM clinical guideline
Strong recommendation: "We recommend ... " almost all patients should receive the recommended course of action.
Conditional recommendation: "We suggest ..." most patients should receive the suggested course of action.

Figure 53.1 Clinical practice guidelines for the pharmacologic treatment of narcolepsy. (Adapted from Maski K, Trotti LM, Kotagal S, et. al. Treatment of central disorders of hypersomnolence: an American Academy of Sleep Medicine clinical practice guideline. *J Clin sleep Med.* Published online April, 2021.)

Oxybates

The mechanism of action of sodium oxybate (Xyrem) for treatment of both sleepiness and cataplexy is not understood, but is thought to be mediated by $GABA_B$ receptor inhibition of noradrenergic, dopaminergic, and thalamocortical neurons, and possibly activity at a putative γ-hydroxybutyrate (GHB) receptor.[46] A low-sodium formulation (Xywav [JZP-258]) is now available and has FDA indications for treatment of idiopathic hypersomnia in adults and for treatment of cataplexy or excessive sleepiness associated with narcolepsy in children and adults.[47,47a] Xywav contains four oxybates (sodium, potassium, calcium, magnesium) and has 92% less sodium (approximately 1000–1500 mg) than that in Xyrem.

Drugs Under Development for Hypersomnia Disorder

FT218, a controlled-release formulation of sodium oxybate that allows for once-nightly dosing, is likely to be approved by FDA in late 2021/early 2022 for treatment of cataplexy or excessive sleepiness in narcolepsy.[48] FT218 is also under study for idiopathic hypersomnia. Additional drugs under development for cataplexy and excessive sleepiness in narcolepsy include two orexin-2 agonists (TAK-925 and TAK-994), AXS-12 (reboxetine), a selective NE reuptake inhibitor approved for treatment of depression in countries outside the US, SUVN-G3031, an H3 inverse agonist, and mazindol, a norepinephrine and dopamine reuptake inhibitor that also exhibits orexin agonism.[49-52] BTD-001, an oral formulation of the GABAA antagonist pentetrazol, is under study for sleepiness in narcolepsy and idiopathic hypersomnia.[53]

DRUGS WITH SEDATING SIDE EFFECTS (TABLE 53.6)

Sedation may be a side effect of drugs that have antagonistic effects at H_1, DA, glutamate, 5-HT, adrenergic α_1, or mACh receptors. Other mechanisms of sedation include enhancement of GABA and activation of opioid μ and κ receptors.

Recommended medications for idiopathic hypersomnia in adult patients

Medication	Excessive daytime sleepiness	Disease severity	Quality of life
Modafinil	●	●	
Clarithromycin	●	●	●
Methylphenidate		●	
Pitolisant	●		
Sodium oxybate	●		

AASM clinical guideline
Strong recommendation: "We recommend ... " almost all patients should receive the recommended course of action.
Conditional recommendation: "We suggest ..." most patients should receive the suggested course of action.

Figure 53.2 Clinical practice guidelines for the pharmacologic treatment of idiopathic hypersomnia. (Adapted from Maski K, Trotti LM, Kotagal S et. al. Treatment of central disorders of hypersomnolence: an American academy of sleep medicine clinical practice guideline. *J Clin sleep Med.* Published on-line April, 2021.)

Table 53.6 Drugs with Sedating Side Effects

Drug Class/Subclass	Drugs	Principal Sedating Mechanism(s)
Antidepressants[a]		
Tricyclics[b]	Amitriptyline, etc.	H_1, mACh antagonism
SSRIs[c]	Citalopram, fluvoxamine	H_1, 5-HT_{2C} antagonism
Atypical drugs	Mirtazapine	H_1, 5-HT_{2A}, 5-HT_{2C} antagonism
	Trazodone	H_1, 5-HT_{2A}, α_1 antagonism
Novel drugs	Brexanolone	$GABA_A$ positive allosteric modulation
	Esketamine	Glutamate antagonism via NMDA receptor
Antipsychotics[d]		
Typical	Chlorpromazine, etc.	H_1, 5-HT_2, α_1, mACh, D_2 antagonism
Atypical	Clozapine, etc.	
Antiepileptics		
Barbiturates	Phenobarbital, primidone	$GABA_A$ agonism, calcium channel inhibition
Benzodiazepines	Clobazam, etc.	$GABA_A$ positive allosteric modulation
Multiple-mechanism drugs	See Table 53.9	See Table 53.9
Other drugs	Cannabidiol (Epidiolex)	GABA enhancement, calcium and adenosine modulation, 5-HT agonism
	Perampanel	Glutamate antagonism via AMPA receptor
	Stiripentol	GABA enhancement
	Tiagabine	GABA reuptake inhibition
Antihistamines[e]		
First generation	Chlorpheniramine, etc.	H_1 antagonism
Second generation	Cetirizine	H_1 antagonism

Continued

Table 53.6 Drugs with Sedating Side Effects—cont'd

Drug Class/Subclass	Drugs	Principal Sedating Mechanism(s)
Antiparkinsonian Drugs		
Anticholinergics	Benztropine	mACh, H_1 antagonism
Dopamine agonists	Pramipexole, ropinirole, rotigotine	See text
Other drugs	Amantadine	Dopamine release and reuptake inhibition, glutamate antagonism
Antiemetics		
Anticholinergics	Scopolamine	mACh antagonism
Antihistamines	Dimenhydrinate, diphenhydramine, meclizine	H_1 antagonism
	Promethazine	H_1, mACh, 5-HT_{2A}, 5-HT_{2C}, α_1 antagonism
Benzodiazepines	Alprazolam, lorazepam, etc	$GABA_A$ positive allosteric modulation
Cannabinoids	Dronabinol, nabilone	Cannabinoid receptor agonism
Benzamides	Metoclopramide	D_2 antagonism
Butyrophenones	Droperidol	D_2, H_1, mACh antagonism, GABA, μ-opioid agonism
Phenothiazines	Prochlorperazine	D_2 antagonism
Cardiovascular Drugs		
α_2 Agonists	Clonidine, guanfacine, methyldopa	α_2 agonism
α_1 Antagonists	Doxazosin, prazosin, terazosin	α_1 antagonism
Pain Medications		
Opioids		
Full agonists	Codeine, fentanyl, hydrocodone, hydromorphone, meperidine, morphine, oxycodone, oxymorphone	μ-opioid and κ-opioid agonism
	Methadone	μ-opioid and κ-opioid agonism, NMDA antagonism
Partial agonists	Tramadol	μ-opioid agonism
Mixed agonist-antagonists[f]	Buprenorphine	μ-opioid agonism
	Butorphanol, nalbuphine, pentazocine	κ-opioid agonism
Muscle relaxants	Baclofen	$GABA_B$ agonism
	Carisoprodol	$GABA_B$ agonism via metabolite meprobamate
	Cyclobenzaprine, orphenadrine	H_1, mACh antagonism
	Dicyclomine	mACh antagonism
	Tizanidine	α_2 agonism
Triptans	Eletriptan, lasmiditan, rizatriptan, zolmitriptan	See text
Antiepileptics	Gabapentin, pregabalin	Inhibition of excitatory neurotransmitters via $\alpha2\delta$ binding
	Felbamate	Glutamate antagonism
	Carbamazepine, lamotrigine	Calcium channel inhibition
	Tiagabine, topiramate	GABA enhancement
Antidepressants	Tricyclics	H_1, mACh antagonism
Other Drugs		
Opioid withdrawal mitigation	Lofexidine	α_2 agonism
Overactive bladder	Oxybutynin	mACh antagonism
Weight loss	Lorcaserin[g]	5-HT_{2C} agonism

[a]See Table 53.7 for a comprehensive list of antidepressants, likelihood of sedation/insomnia, and receptor binding affinity profiles.
[b]Tricyclics with less affinity for H_1 and relatively more norepinephrine reuptake inhibition are less sedating (desipramine, nortriptyline, protriptyline).
[c]Most SSRIs are nonsedating. Citalopram has mild H_1 and 5-HT_{2C} antagonism. Fluvoxamine modulates calcium and sodium release and inhibits melatonin degradation.
[d]See Table 53.8 for a comprehensive list of antipsychotics, likelihood of sedation/insomnia, and receptor binding affinity profiles.
[e]All first-generation antihistamines are sedating. Most second-generation antihistamines are nonsedating; cetirizine is an exception because of central nervous system penetration and moderate affinity for the H_1 receptor.
[f]The activity of mixed agonists-antagonists varies depending on the opioid receptor and dose. See text for details.
[g]Withdrawn from the US market in February 2020 because of cancer risk.
5-HT, Serotonin; 5-$HT_{2,\ 2A,\ 2C}$, 5-HT receptors 2, 2A, 2C; $\alpha_{1,\ 2}$, alpha adrenergic receptors 1, 2; $\alpha_2\delta$, alpha 2 delta subunit of voltage-dependent calcium channels; AMPA, α-amino-3-hydroxy-5-methyl-4-isoxazolepropionic acid; D_2, dopamine 2 receptor; GABA, gamma-aminobutyric acid; $GABA_{A,\ B}$, GABA A, B receptors; H_1, histamine 1 receptor; κ, kappa, mACh, muscarinic cholinergic receptor; μ, mu; NMDA, N-methyl-D-aspartate; SSRI, selective serotonin reuptake inhibitor.

Daytime sedation may also occur indirectly by drugs that interrupt nocturnal sleep. Table 53.6 lists drugs with sedating side effects and the principal mechanisms for sedation.

Antidepressant Drugs with Sedating Side Effects (Tables 53.6 and 53.7)

Drugs classified as antidepressants are used in a variety of disorders, including depression, obsessive-compulsive disorder, anxiety disorders, neuropathic pain, insomnia, smoking cessation, menopausal symptoms, and others. Antidepressant drugs can improve or disturb sleep and can affect waking function. Evaluation of the effects of these drugs on sleep and wakefulness is complicated by the fact that disturbed sleep, daytime fatigue and sleepiness, and decreased cognitive and psychomotor functioning may be associated with the underlying disease for which the drug is taken.[54]

Antidepressants vary considerably in the relative affinity for receptors associated with sleep-wake regulation. Binding affinities (K_i value ranges) of antidepressants for relevant receptors and transporters are noted in Table 53.7. Sedating antidepressants vary in their antagonism of H_1, 5-HT_2, α_1, and mACh receptors. Most antidepressants also exhibit reuptake inhibition of 5-HT and NE, which is the likely mechanism for their therapeutic effect and which may promote wakefulness. Drugs that selectively inhibit reuptake of 5-HT or NE (selective serotonin reuptake inhibitors [SSRIs] and selective serotonin-norepinephrine reuptake inhibitors [SNRIs], respectively) are unlikely to be sedating and may produce insomnia. Sedating antidepressants commonly used off-label for insomnia include amitriptyline, doxepin, trazodone, and quetiapine (Tables 53.2 and 53.4).[14]

Tricyclic antidepressants are among the most sedating antidepressants. These drugs differ from one another in their degree of antagonism of H_1 and mACh receptors and in their relative effects in blocking reuptake of 5-HT versus NE.[55] The more-sedating tricyclics tend to be more antihistaminergic (doxepin, trimipramine) and more anticholinergic (amitriptyline) but also exhibit proportionately greater reuptake inhibition of 5-HT than NE. Tricyclics also exhibit moderate α_1 antagonism. Drugs with less affinity for H_1 receptors (desipramine, nortriptyline, protriptyline) are less sedating and may promote insomnia in some patients. Half-lives generally range from 15 to 30 hours, with active metabolites having slightly longer half-lives.

Generally, tricyclics decrease sleep latency, increase total sleep time (TST), and decrease REM sleep while increasing phasic eye movements during REM, but the more adrenergic drugs (desipramine, nortriptyline) may decrease TST and increase awakenings.[7,11,56-58]

Trazodone has complex effects on the 5-HT system, but the mechanisms for sedation are moderate H_1, α_1, and 5-HT_{2A} antagonism, effects present at low doses. At moderate to high doses, there is also 5-HT_{2C} antagonism and SERT inhibition.[59,60] Trazodone also acts as a partial agonist at 5-HT_{1A}.[59,61] Trazodone (at 25–150 mg) is commonly used off-label as a hypnotic. The half-life is 5 to 9 hours, but the half-life of its active metabolite is 4 to 14 hours; thus residual sedation is likely. Trazodone increases slow wave sleep (SWS), does not affect REM, and may decrease sleep latency, but effects on sleep continuity are equivocal.[62]

Mirtazapine is highly sedating, with potent antagonism of H_1, 5-HT_{2A}, and 5-HT_{2C} receptors. It has no SERT, NET, or DAT reuptake inhibition but does have significant antagonistic/inverse agonist affects at α_{2A}-, α_{2B}-, and α_{2C}-adrenergic receptors, which may promote wakefulness by inhibiting NE release.[63] The decrease in sedation that has been observed with increasing dose may be related to the relative increase in α_2 antagonism at higher doses.[7] Mirtazapine also reduces the release of corticotrophin, resulting in reduced cortisol levels.[60] Mirtazapine is frequently used off-label as a sleep aid. Its potent sedation and long half-life (20–40 hours) make residual sedation a concern. Mirtazapine impairs driving performance, attention, and reaction time.[64]

Brexanolone and esketamine are new antidepressants with novel mechanisms. Both are highly sedating. Brexanolone, approved for the treatment of postpartum depression, is an intravenous formulation of allopregnanolone, a positive allosteric modulator of $GABA_A$ receptors.[65] Esketamine, approved for treatment-resistant depression and delivered intranasally, is a potent antagonist of the glutamate N-methyl-D-aspartate (NMDA) receptor.[66]

Brexanolone is administered intravenously over a 60-hour period. Because of the risk of excessive sedation or sudden loss of consciousness during administration, the drug is available only through a Risk Evaluation and Mitigation Strategy (REMS) program.[65] Esketamine, initially dosed twice weekly and then every 1 to 2 weeks, must also be administered under the direct supervision of a health care provider and must include an observation period of at least 2 hours postadministration. Sleepiness and cognitive performance impairment are significant concerns, and patients are advised not to drive until a day after administration. However, neither cognitive performance nor driving impairment was noted 8 hours after administration.[67,68]

Sedation is unlikely with the majority of SSRIs and SNRIs but occurs more frequently with citalopram, duloxetine, and fluvoxamine. Sedation is likely explained by mild H_1 and 5-HT_{2C} antagonism in citalopram and mild 5-$HT_{2A,2C}$ antagonism in duloxetine. Fluvoxamine is chemically unrelated to other SSRIs and has greater affinity than other SSRIs for the $sigma_1$ (σ_1) receptor, where it acts as an agonist, thereby modulating calcium release and inhibiting sodium channels.[69] Unlike other SSRIs, fluvoxamine also inhibits melatonin degradation.[70]

Lithium, which is used primarily in the treatment of bipolar disorder, is commonly associated with somnolence.[71] Impairment in driving simulator performance has been shown in psychiatric patients taking lithium for periods of time ranging from 2 weeks to longer than 3 months,[72] although it is difficult to determine whether the deficits seen in the patient population are caused by the medication or their psychiatric illness.

Antipsychotic Drugs with Sedating Side Effects (Tables 53.6 and 53.8)

Antipsychotic drugs, particularly the atypical antipsychotics, have complex pharmacologic profiles. Binding affinities (K_i value ranges) for receptors and transporters relevant to sleep-wake mechanisms are noted in Table 53.8. Although their primary indication is use in schizophrenia, many of these drugs are used in the treatment of other disorders, including bipolar disorder, autism, obsessive-compulsive disorder, and major depressive disorder. In addition, these drugs have been used off-label in the treatment of dementia, depression, borderline personality disorder, PTSD, substance abuse, eating disorders, anxiety, and insomnia.[73] Sedation is likely related to

Table 53.7 Antidepressants: Binding Affinities (K_i[a] Range) for Receptors and Transporters Relevant to Sleep-Wake Mechanisms, and Likelihood of Sedation or Insomnia

Class	Drug	Sedation	Insomnia
Tricyclic	Amitriptyline	+++	+
	Amoxapine	+++	+
	Clomipramine	++	-
	Desipramine	+	+
	Doxepin[b]	+++	-
	Imipramine	+++	+
	Maprotiline	++	-
	Nortriptyline	+	+
	Protriptyline	-	+
	Trimipramine	+++	+
MAOI[c]	Phenelzine	+	+++
	Selegiline	-	+
	Tranylcypromine	++	++
SSRI	Citalopram	+	+
	Escitalopram	–	+
	Fluoxetine	+	+++
	Fluvoxamine	++	++
	Paroxetine	–	++
	Sertraline	–	++
SNRI	Desvenlafaxine	–	+++
	Duloxetine	+	++
	Levomilnacipran	–	–
	Milnacipran	–	+
	Venlafaxine[d]	++	++
Atypical	Atomoxetine	+	+
	Bupropion	–	+++
	Mirtazapine	+++	–
	Trazodone	++	–
	Vilazodone[e]	–	++
Novel	Vortioxetine[f]	–	+
	Brexanolone[g]	+++	–
	Esketamine[h]	++++	–

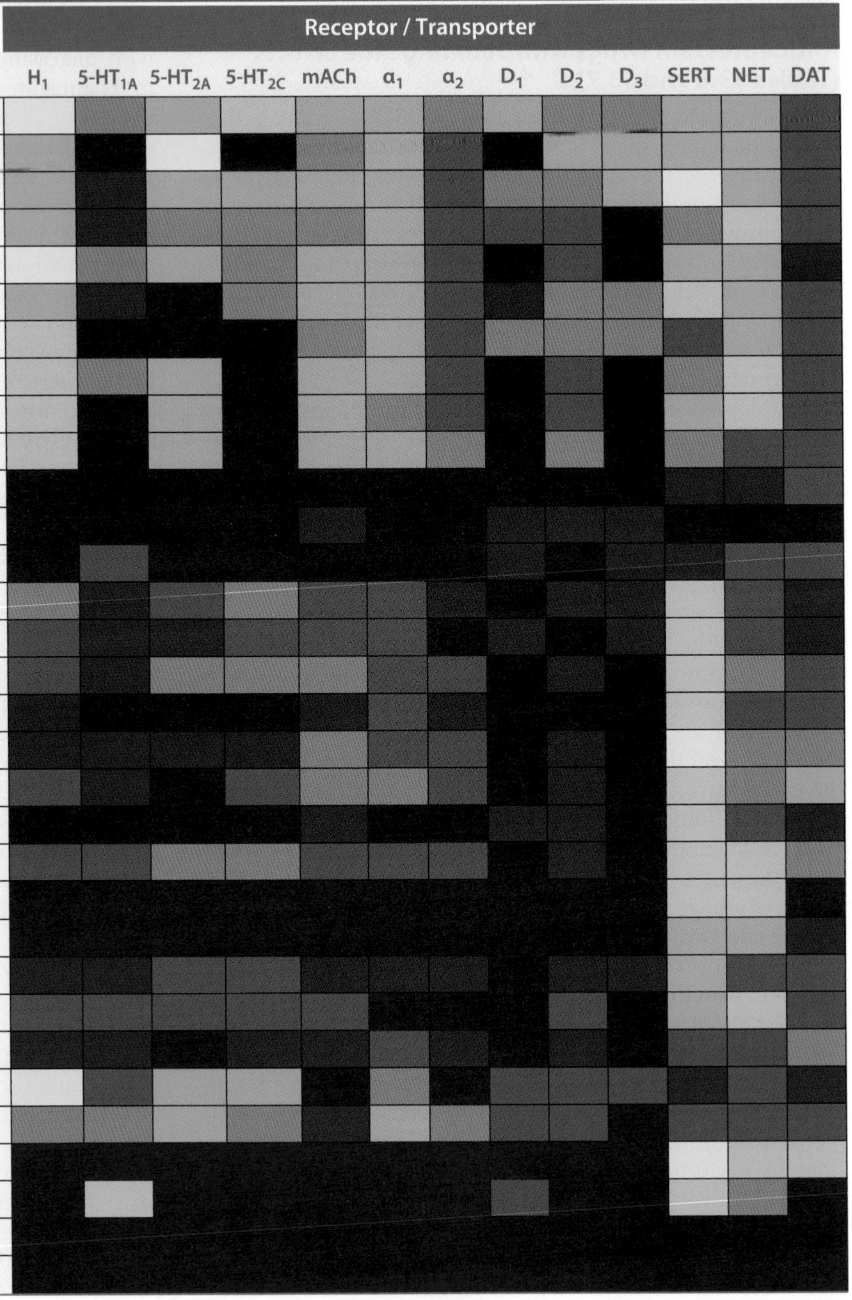

K_i[a] Range (nM)

≤1 | 1–10 | 10–100 | 100–1000 | 1000–10,000 | >10,000 | Not tested

[a]K_i (inhibition constant) values range from ≤1 nM (very high affinity) to >10,000 nM (inactive) and were obtained from the Psychoactive Drug Screening Program (PDSP) K_i database (https://pdsp.unc.edu/databases/kidb.php). Most drugs are antagonists at the indicated receptors; exceptions noted in footnotes and text.
[b]At low doses (≤6 mg), doxepin is primarily an H_1 antagonist.
[c]Inhibition of monoamine oxidase increases dopamine, epinephrine, norepinephrine, and serotonin.
[d]Venlafaxine exhibits greater SERT inhibition at low doses and greater NET inhibition at high doses.
[e]Vilazodone is a partial agonist at $5\text{-}HT_{1A}$.
[f]Vortioxetine is an antagonist at $5\text{-}HT_{1D}$, $5\text{-}HT_3$, and $5\text{-}HT_7$; an agonist at $5\text{-}HT_{1A}$; and partial agonist at $5\text{-}HT_{1B}$.
[g]Brexanolone is a positive allosteric modulator of gamma-aminobutyric acid A ($GABA_A$) receptors.
[h]Esketamine is a potent antagonist of the glutamate NMDA (N-methyl-D-aspartate) receptor.
$5\text{-}HT_{1A, 1B, 1D, 2A, 2C, 3, 7}$, 5-Hydroxytryptamine (serotonin) receptors 1A to 7; $\alpha_{1, 2}$, alpha adrenergic receptors 1, 2; $D_{1, 2, 3}$, dopamine receptors 1 to 3; DAT, dopamine transporter; H_1, histamine 1 receptor; mACh, muscarinic acetylcholine receptor; MAOI, monoamine oxidase inhibitor; NET, norepinephrine transporter; nM, nanomolar; SERT, serotonin transporter; SNRI, serotonin-norepinephrine reuptake inhibitor; SSRI, selective serotonin reuptake inhibitor.

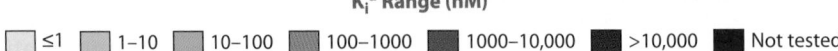

Table 53.8 Antipsychotics: Binding Affinities (K_i[a] Ranges) for Receptors and Transporters Relevant to Sleep-Wake Mechanisms, and Likelihood of Sedation or Insomnia

Class	Drug	Sedation	Insomnia
Typical	Chlorpromazine	++++	–
	Fluphenazine	+	+++
	Haloperidol[b]	++	+++
	Loxapine	++	++
	Molindone	+	–
	Perphenazine	++	+++
	Pimozide	+	+
	Thioridazine	++++	+++
	Thiothixene	+	+
	Trifluoperazine	+	+++
Atypical	Aripiprazole[c]	+	+++
	Asenapine[d]	+++	++
	Brexpiprazole[e]	+	+
	Cariprazine[f]	+	++
	Clozapine[g]	++++	–
	Iloperidone	+	–
	Lumateperone[h]	+++	–
	Lurasidone[i]	++	++
	Olanzapine[j]	+++	++
	Paliperidone[k]	+	–
	Pimavanserin	+	–
	Quetiapine[l]	+++	+
	Risperidone[m]	+++	++
	Ziprasidone[n]	++	+

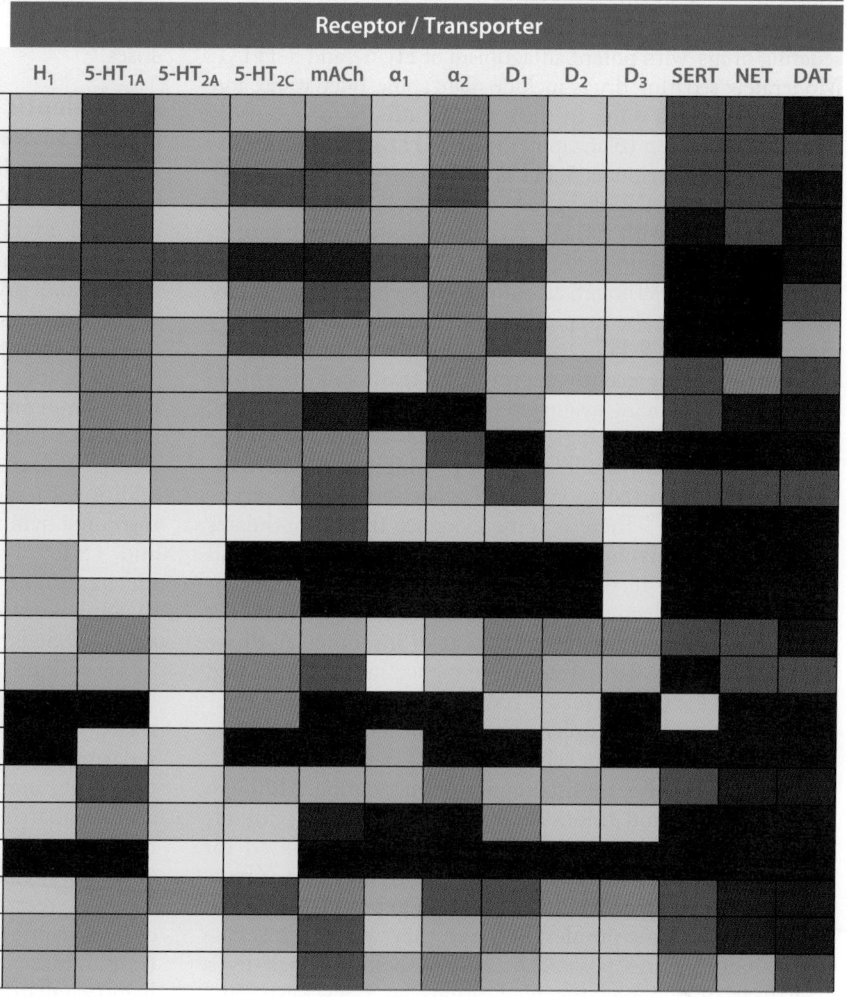

K_i[a] Range (nM)

≤1 | 1–10 | 10–100 | 100–1000 | 1000–10,000 | >10,000 | Not tested

[a]K_i (inhibition constant) values range from ≤1 nM (very high affinity) to >10,000 nM (inactive), values were obtained from the Psychoactive Drug Screening Program (PDSP) K_i database (https://pdsp.unc.edu/databases/kidb.php). Most drugs are antagonists at the indicated receptors; exceptions noted in footnotes and text.
[b]Haloperidol is an inverse agonist at D_2, D_3, and D_4 and an agonist at 5-HT_{1A} and α_2.
[c]Aripiprazole is a partial agonist at 5-HT_{1A}, 5-HT_{2C}, D_2, D_3, and D_4 and an inverse agonist at 5-HT_{2B}.
[d]Asenapine is a partial agonist at 5-HT_{1A}.
[e]Brexpiprazole is a partial agonist at 5-HT_{1A}, 5-HT_{2C}, D_2, and D_3.
[f]Cariprazine is a partial agonist at 5-HT_{1A}, D_2, and D_3 and an inverse agonist at 5-HT_{2C}.
[g]Clozapine interacts with the $GABA_B$ receptor and acts as an agonist at the NMDA receptor.
[h]Lumateperone is a partial agonist at presynaptic D_1 and D_2 receptors and an antagonist at postsynaptic D_1 and D_2 receptors and augments both NMDA and AMPA activity.
[i]Lurasidone is a partial agonist at 5-HT_{1A}.
[j]Olanzapine is an inverse agonist at 5-HT_{2A}, 5-HT_{2B}, 5-HT_{2C}, and H_1.
[k]Paliperidone is the primary active metabolite of risperidone.
[l]Quetiapine is a partial agonist at 5-HT_{1A}.
[m]Risperidone is an inverse agonist at 5-HT_{2A}, 5-HT_{2B}, 5-HT_{2C}, D_3, and H_1.
[n]Ziprasidone is a partial agonist at 5-HT_{1A}, 5-HT_{1B}, 5-HT_{1C}, and 5-HT_{2C}.
5-$HT_{1A, 1B, 1C, 2A, 2B, 2C}$, 5-Hydroxytryptamine (serotonin) receptors 1A-2C; $\alpha_{1, 2}$, alpha adrenergic receptors 1, 2; AMPA, α-amino-3-hydroxy-5-methyl-4-isoxazolepropionic acid; D_1, D_2, D_3, D_4, dopamine receptors 1 to 4; DAT, dopamine transporter; $GABA_B$, gamma-aminobutyric acid B receptor; H_1, histamine 1 receptor; mACh, muscarinic acetylcholine receptor; NET, norepinephrine transporter; nM, nanomolar; NMDA, N-methyl-D-aspartate; SERT, serotonin transporter.

antagonism of DA, H, 5-HT, NE, and ACh, and more likely in drugs that have relatively more potent H_1, ACh, 5-HT_2, and/or α_1 antagonism.[74]

Clozapine, chlorpromazine, and thioridazine are the most sedating drugs, with potent antagonism of H_1, α_1, and 5-HT_{2A}. Moderately sedating drugs include olanzapine, quetiapine, and risperidone, which differ in their relative affinity for receptors promoting sedation (olanzapine: H_1 > 5-HT_{2C} > α_1; quetiapine: α_1 > H_1; risperidone: 5-HT_{1A} > H_1 > mACh, α_1, and α_2). Drugs with less sedation include aripiprazole, lurasidone, and cariprazine, each with variable receptor affinities. For example, lurasidone has no affinity for H_1 and mACh, but potent affinity for 5-HT_{2A}.[74-76] Although all antipsychotics have some affinity for DA receptors, the atypical drugs generally have relatively greater affinity for 5-HT_2 than for D_2 receptors.

Lumateperone, recently approved for treatment of schizophrenia, but also being evaluated for depression and insomnia, has a unique pharmacologic profile.[77] It is a potent 5-HT_{2A} receptor antagonist, moderate SERT inhibitor, a presynaptic D_2 receptor partial agonist, and a postsynaptic D_2 receptor antagonist.[78,79] There is some evidence that it modulates glutamate transmission indirectly via D_1 receptors.[78] D_2 and SERT occupancy increases with dose.[79] Thus at low doses, it functions as a selective 5-HT_{2A} antagonist, which makes it of potential interest for the treatment of insomnia. A Phase 2 trial of patients with sleep maintenance insomnia showed decreased wake and increased SWS without next-day cognitive impairment.[80] Somnolence was the most common adverse effect in clinical trials for schizophrenia.[81,82]

Dose and half-life are also important for sedation. Although chlorpromazine and thioridazine have lower affinity for H_1 than, for example, asenapine, higher doses are required for therapeutic efficacy, increasing the sedating side effect. Ziprasidone and quetiapine would be expected to be sedating, given their pharmacologic profiles; however, they appear less sedating than other drugs, possibly because of their short half-lives.

Effects of antipsychotic medications on PSG sleep variables (Table 53.2) vary somewhat between healthy subjects and patients with schizophrenia, and not all drugs have been evaluated in both populations. Antipsychotic drugs most frequently used off-label for insomnia include quetiapine, olanzapine, and risperidone.[13,14,83] In general, these drugs increase sleep continuity. Olanzapine markedly increases SWS, likely because of 5-HT_2 antagonism. Chlorpromazine, lumateperone, paliperidone, risperidone, and ziprasidone also increase SWS. Olanzapine and paliperidone increase REM in schizophrenia patients but not healthy individuals; most other drugs either decrease or have no effect on REM.[75,84-88] Both clozapine and olanzapine reduce MSLT latencies in schizophrenic patients.[89]

Anxiolytic Drugs with Sedating Side Effects

Drugs with sedating side effects used in the treatment of anxiety include benzodiazepines, antidepressants, antiepileptics, and antipsychotics. Benzodiazepines approved for treatment of anxiety disorders (e.g., alprazolam, clonazepam, diazepam, lorazepam) have similar pharmacologic profiles to benzodiazepines used to treat insomnia and thus similar side effects. Given that these drugs enhance GABA-mediated inhibition at the $GABA_A$ receptor, their most common side effect is sedation.[90] Objective assessment of sleep tendency via MSLT confirms persistence of sleepiness for at least 1 week of daily use of alprazolam and diazepam.[91] Performance impairment, including impairment of actual driving performance, has been demonstrated with daytime administration of benzodiazepines in studies of normal subjects and in patient groups for treatment periods of up to 3 weeks, particularly at higher doses.[92]

Antiepileptic Drugs with Sedating Side Effects (Tables 53.6 and 53.9)

Antiepileptic drugs have diverse pharmacology and chemistry (Table 53.9) but share the common property of reducing neuronal excitability. Although these drugs are used to treat epilepsy, a number of them are used in the treatment of neurologic and psychiatric disease, including neuropathic pain, hyperkinetic movement disorders, migraine, RLS, bipolar disease, and schizophrenia.[93]

Medication-related sleepiness is one of the most common complaints of patients with epilepsy, confirmed by both subjective (Epworth Sleepiness Scale [ESS]) and objective (MSLT) data, and independent of standardized dose, in addition to seizure frequency, age, gender, depression and insomnia symptom severity, apnea-hypopnea index (AHI), and TST.[94] However, sedation is dependent on dose and mechanism of action and is most likely to occur with drugs that enhance GABA, block glutamate, or block calcium channels.[95,96] Sedation is less frequent with drugs acting primarily via sodium channel blockade (carbamazepine, phenytoin). Most drugs have multiple receptor mechanisms (Table 53.9). Based on clinical trials and adverse event reports, the most sedating antiepileptic drugs include the benzodiazepines, the barbiturates, brivaracetam, levetiracetam, stiripentol, and vigabatrin, all drugs that enhance GABA by various mechanisms.

GABA enhancement can occur via direct binding to $GABA_A$ receptors (benzodiazepines, barbiturates); blockade of presynaptic GABA uptake (tiagabine); inhibition of GABA transaminase, the enzyme responsible for GABA metabolism (vigabatrin); or conversion of glutamate into GABA by glutamic acid decarboxylase (gabapentin, valproate).[96] Benzodiazepines used for seizure control include clobazam, clonazepam, clorazepate, diazepam, and lorazepam. Clobazam may also affect voltage-sensitive conductance of calcium ions and the function of sodium channels. Clonazepam may have some action on sodium-channel conductance.

Glutamate blockade can occur via AMPA receptor antagonism (perampanel) or both NMDA and AMPA antagonism (felbamate, topiramate).[96] Felbamate and topiramate also enhance GABA and block both calcium and sodium channels. Felbamate is associated with both sleepiness and insomnia, but the mechanism for insomnia is not clear.[97,98] Levetiracetam and brivaracetam inhibit synaptic vesicle protein 2A (SV2A), which affects calcium channel transmission and GABA release, likely the mechanism for sedation, although the precise function of SV2A is obscure.[99-103]

The mechanism of action of gabapentin and pregabalin is not well understood. However, these drugs appear to inhibit release of excitatory neurotransmitters via binding to the $\alpha_2\delta$ subunits of voltage-activated calcium channels. This action attenuates neurotransmitter release, thereby modulating calcium channel currents and the release of glutamate, noradrenaline, and substance P.[104,105] There is also some evidence that these drugs act on adenosine receptors and voltage-gated potassium currents.[106,107]

Table 53.9 Antiepileptic Drugs: Likelihood of Sedation and Mechanism of Action

Drug	Sedation	GABA Enhancement[a]	Calcium Channel Blockade	Sodium Channel Blockade	SV2A[b] Inhibition	$\alpha_2\delta$[c] Inhibition	Glutamate Blockade[d]	Carbonic Anhydrase Inhibition	Potassium Channel Blockade
Benzodiazepines[e]	++++	Primary							
Brivaracetam	++++			Secondary	Primary				
Cannabidiol[f]	+++	Possible	Possible						
Carbamazepine	+			Primary					
Cenobamate	+++	Primary		Primary					
Eslicarbazepine	+		Secondary	Primary					
Ethosuximide	+		Primary						
Ezogabine	++	Secondary							Primary
Felbamate[g]	++	Possible	Secondary	Primary			Primary		
Fosphenytoin	++			Primary					
Gabapentin	+++	Possible	Secondary			Primary	Secondary		
Lacosamide	++			Primary				Possible	
Lamotrigine	+		Secondary	Primary			Secondary		
Levetiracetam	++++	Secondary	Possible		Primary		Secondary		
Oxcarbazepine	+			Primary					Secondary
Perampanel	+++						Primary		
Phenobarbital	++++	Primary	Secondary	Secondary			Secondary		
Phenytoin	++		Possible	Primary					
Pregabalin	++		Secondary			Primary	Secondary		
Primidone	++++	Primary							
Rufinamide	++			Primary					
Stiripentol	++++	Primary							
Tiagabine	++	Primary							
Topiramate	+++	Primary	Primary	Primary			Primary	Secondary	Primary
Valproate	+	Secondary	Primary	Primary					
Vigabatrin	++++	Primary							
Zonisamide	++		Secondary	Primary				Possible	

Mechanism of Action

(black)	Primary
(dark grey)	Secondary
(light grey)	Possible
(white)	None

[a]Gamma-aminobutyric acid (GABA) enhancement can occur by direct binding to $GABA_A$ receptors (benzodiazepines, phenobarbital), blockade of presynaptic GABA uptake (tiagabine), inhibition of GABA metabolism by GABA transaminase (vigabatrin), and increased synthesis of GABA (gabapentin, valproate).

[b]SV2A, synaptic vesicle glycoprotein 2A. SV2A is a master regulator molecule of neurotransmitter release, present in GABAergic and glutamatergic neurons, and affecting calcium channel transmission and GABA release.

[c]$\alpha 2\gamma$, Alpha 2 delta subunit of voltage-dependent calcium channels. Binding to $\alpha 2\delta$ attenuates neurotransmitter release, thereby modulating calcium channel currents and the release of glutamate, noradrenaline, and substance P.

[d]Glutamate blockade can occur via N-methyl-D-aspartate (NMDA), α-amino-3-hydroxy-5-methyl-4-isoxazolepropionic acid (AMPA), and kainate receptors. Perampanel is a selective AMPA antagonist.

[e]Benzodiazepines include clobazam, clonazepam, clorazepate, diazepam, and lorazepam. Clobazam may also affect voltage-sensitive conductance of calcium ions and the function of sodium channels. Clonazepam may have some action on sodium channel conductance.

[f]Cannabidiol (Epidiolex) is a purified form of cannabidiol. It does not directly bind to or activate cannabinoid receptors at the concentrations used for anticonvulsant effects. Other possible mechanisms include adenosine, glycine, and GABAergic modulation in addition to serotonin agonism.

[g]Felbamate is associated with both sleepiness and insomnia; the mechanism for insomnia is not clear.

Among the newer drugs, stiripentol, indicated for seizures associated with Dravet syndrome in patients taking the benzodiazepine clobazam, is quite sedating, as it enhances GABA and increases the concentration of clobazam via CYP3A4 and CYP2C19. Ezogabine enhances potassium currents and may augment GABA. Epidiolex, a purified formulation of cannabidiol, has multiple mechanisms that promote sedation, including GABA enhancement, calcium and adenosine modulation, and serotonin agonism. Epidiolex does not directly bind to or activate cannabinoid receptors at the concentrations used for anticonvulsant effects.[99,108-110]

PSG studies of antiepileptic drugs show variable effects on sleep in both patients and healthy individuals (Table 53.2).[11,111] Gabapentin, pregabalin, and tiagabine increase SWS.[112-114] Gabapentin, pregabalin, and occasionally tiagabine have been used off-label to treat insomnia.[13,14]

Antihistamines with Sedating Side Effects (Table 53.6)

H_1 Antagonists

The first-generation H_1 antihistamines (e.g., chlorpheniramine, diphenhydramine, hydroxyzine) are lipophilic and easily cross the blood–brain barrier, demonstrating H_1 receptor occupancy of 50% to 80% with standard doses.[115] In addition to H_1 antagonism, these drugs demonstrate mACh antagonism and may also have α-adrenergic and 5-HT effects. They cause decrements in alertness and performance, at least with short-term use.[116,117] Because of the sedating effects, these drugs (in particular, diphenhydramine) are widely used as over-the-counter hypnotics. Subjectively, these drugs decrease sleep latency and increase sleep continuity, but PSG data are mixed. Nighttime dosing may result in next-day performance impairment and sleepiness.[118] Diphenhydramine increases physiologic sleep tendency as measured by MSLT and decreases performance acutely, but tolerance may develop within 3 to 4 days,[119,120] although driving may continue to be impaired.[121]

The second-generation H_1 antihistamines (cetirizine, desloratadine, fexofenadine, levocetirizine, loratadine) are hydrophilic molecules that do not easily penetrate the central nervous system (CNS). Although they are much more selective than the first-generation antihistamines, CNS H_1 receptor occupancy varies from almost negligible (e.g., fexofenadine) to 30% (cetirizine).[121] The majority of studies in normal subjects and atopic individuals generally confirm that these drugs are not sedating and do not impair performance when used in recommended doses.[117] Although MSLT studies indicate that cetirizine is nonsedating,[119] it has been classified as sedating by the FDA, and a number of studies suggest it is more subjectively sedating and more likely to impair performance than other second-generation H_1 antagonists.[122] Meta-analysis of 18 studies concluded that although second-generation antihistamines caused less performance impairment than the first-generation antihistamine diphenhydramine, mild impairment was still present.[123] There is some evidence that fexofenadine and levocetirizine may be less impairing than other second-generation drugs,[115,124] although sedation may emerge with increase in dose.[125]

H_2 Antagonists

H_2 antagonists (e.g., cimetidine, ranitidine, famotidine) are unlikely to impair CNS function because these compounds do not easily cross the blood–brain barrier. However, cimetidine slows the clearance of some benzodiazepine receptor agonists, which may make carryover effects of hypnotics more of a problem.[126] Similarly, cimetidine has been shown to increase levels of theophylline, carbamazepine, and beta blockers with resultant increases in the CNS effects of these drugs.

Antiparkinsonian Drugs with Sedating Side Effects (Table 53.6)

Dopamine Agonists

Sleep disturbances, including daytime sleepiness, insomnia, RLS, PLMS, and RBD, affect over 90% of patients with Parkinson disease (PD).[127-129] A meta-analysis of PSG studies reported decreased TST, REM, and SWS in patients with PD compared with controls, findings that may be associated with disease pathology, PLMS, or the use of antiparkinsonian drugs.[127] Excessive sleepiness, which is reported to affect 15% to 74% of patients, increases with disease progression.[130,131] Etiology of sleepiness may be related to neurodegeneration, disturbed nocturnal sleep, medications, or comorbid disorders. PD is associated with regional brain atrophy, nigrostriatal dopaminergic degeneration, and hypocretin (orexin) cell loss, along with a decrease in hypocretin levels in cerebrospinal fluid, which correlates with objective and subjective measures of sleepiness.[132-135]

DA agonists have been associated with increases in daytime sleepiness, including sudden "sleep attacks" in patients with PD. Meta-analyses suggest a 13% incidence of sleep attacks in patients on dopaminergic medications, most frequently with pramipexole and ropinirole, but it is unclear if these reports indicate a drug-specific etiology.[136,137] MSLT studies of patients with PD are somewhat contradictory and potentially biased by small sample sizes and other methodological issues, but indicate that the frequency of pathologic sleepiness is high in these patients.[138,139] MSLT studies in small samples of healthy individuals in placebo-controlled studies show reduced latencies with pramipexole and ropinirole, suggesting a drug etiology for sleepiness.[140,141]

DA agonists differ somewhat in their selectivity for DA receptor subtypes. There are five subtypes of DA receptors divided into two major classes, D_1-like (D_1 and D_5 subtypes) and D_2-like (D_2, D_3, D_4 subtypes).[142] Rotigotine is a nonselective agonist at D_1, D_2, and D_3, with highest affinity for D_3 (10-fold higher than D_2, 100-fold higher than D_1). However, functional studies indicate similar potencies at D_1, D_2, and D_3.[143] Rotigotine also acts as an antagonist at adrenergic α_{2B} receptors and as a partial agonist at 5-HT_{1A} receptors. Pramipexole and ropinirole act primarily as D_2 and D_3 agonists with no affinity for D_1. Although there have been fewer reports of sleep attacks with rotigotine compared with pramipexole and ropinirole, it is unlikely that the differences in receptor pharmacology account for this finding. Moreover, somnolence is one of the most common adverse effects in long-term studies of rotigotine.[144] The ergot agonist drugs (bromocriptine, pergolide) also have moderately high affinity for D_1; however, these drugs are now rarely used because of association with valvular heart disease. Rotigotine, an extended-release formulation delivered transdermally, was withdrawn from the market in 2008 because of problems with crystallization from the patch, but returned in 2012 when the problem was resolved.

Although DA is considered a wake-promoting substance, the effects of DA agonists on the sleep-wake cycle are complex.[6] Adenylyl cyclase activity is increased by the D_1-like receptors and inhibited by the D_2-like receptors. The D_2 receptor functions as both a neuromodulatory receptor and as an autoreceptor that reduces DA signaling. D_1-like agonists promote wake, whereas D_2-like agonists demonstrate biphasic effects, with low doses reducing wake and increasing SWS and REM (autoreceptor activation) and high doses promoting wake (postsynaptic neuromodulation).[6,145] There is some evidence to suggest that activation of D_3 receptors is sleep-promoting.[6,145] Thus DA agonists may promote sleep by several mechanisms, including activation of D_2 autoreceptors, DA receptor selectivity, dose, and possibly suppression of glutamatergic input to orexin neurons. D_2/D_4 receptor gene polymorphisms may also be relevant.[137]

In an effort to disentangle the contribution of dopaminergic drugs versus disease-related factors in the etiology of sleepiness in PD, researchers have studied patients with RLS treated with DA agonists. In a meta-analysis of 14 randomized controlled short-term trials (1–12 weeks), DA agonists had a relative risk of somnolence of 1.94 in patients with RLS.[146] In a long-term analysis of a group of patients treated with pramipexole for a mean of 8 years and initially followed for 27 months, the percentage reporting sleepiness increased from 5% to 56%, with 10% reporting sleep attacks while driving. However, efficacy in treating RLS decreased with time, dose increase, and additional drug therapy, confounding the interpretation.[147] Although there have been a few case reports of sudden sleep attacks with DA agonists in the treatment of RLS, one study reported a lower incidence of sleep attacks after dopaminergic treatment compared with pretreatment and to controls.[148] However, it is feasible that the decrease in sleep attacks was a function of improved sleep resulting from reduction in RLS symptoms. Nonetheless, the question of sleepiness and sudden sleep attacks among patients with RLS treated with DA agonists is inconclusive.

Antiemetic Drugs with Sedating Side Effects (Table 53.6)

Sleepiness/sedation is a common side effect of medications used for the treatment of nausea/vomiting and motion sickness.[149,150-152] Sedation with these drugs may not always be considered a negative outcome, as for example, with droperidol, which is indicated to reduce the incidence of nausea and vomiting associated with surgical and diagnostic procedures. Mechanisms for sedation include H_1, D_2, and mACh receptor antagonism and $GABA_A$ and cannabinoid receptor agonism.

H_1 antagonists used for nausea include dimenhydrinate, diphenhydramine, meclizine, and promethazine. Promethazine also has moderate mACh receptor antagonism and weak antagonism at $5\text{-}HT_{2A}$, $5\text{-}HT_{2C}$, D_2, and α_1-adrenergic receptors. Scopolamine is a nonselective mACh antagonist; the intranasal formulation appears to be less sedating than the transdermal drug.[153] Dronabinol and nabilone are cannabinoid receptor agonists approved for the treatment of chemotherapy-induced nausea and vomiting. Droperidol, metoclopramide, and prochlorperazine are D_2 antagonists.[151] Droperidol also exhibits H_1, mACh, and nicotinic antagonism; α_2 agonism; dose-dependent GABA agonism/antagonism; sodium channel blockade; and μ-opioid receptor potentiation. Metoclopramide, used in the treatment of gastroesophageal reflux, is also a $5\text{-}HT_3$ antagonist and $5\text{-}HT_4$ agonist at higher doses. Benzodiazepines such as alprazolam, lorazepam, and midazolam and the antipsychotic olanzapine are sometimes used to treat nausea.[154]

Cardiovascular Drugs with Sedating Side Effects (Table 53.6)

Sedation is the most common side effect of clonidine, guanfacine, and methyldopa, centrally acting α_2-adrenergic agonists. Sleepiness usually occurs at treatment initiation and may diminish with time in some individuals.[155] There are also reports of insomnia and nightmares with these drugs. An extended-release formulation of clonidine is approved for treatment of attention-deficit/hyperactivity disorder. Clonidine is used off-label to treat PTSD, opiate detoxification, neuroleptic akathisia, insomnia, menopausal hot flashes, and other disorders.[156]

The α_1 antagonists (doxazosin, prazosin, terazosin) are sometimes associated with transient sedation. Prazosin has been used in the treatment of nightmares and sleep disturbance in PTSD.[24] In placebo-controlled studies, prazosin increased TST, REM, and subjective sleep quality and reduced nightmares.[157,158] Use of α_1 antagonists is associated with a higher risk of sleep apnea in patients with and without hypertension, likely because of decreased genioglossus muscle activity.[159]

Carvedilol and labetalol (beta blockers with vasodilating properties) have been associated with fatigue and somnolence that may be related to the fact that these drugs also block α_1 receptors.[160]

Pain Medications with Sedating Side Effects (Table 53.6)

A variety of medications used in the treatment of pain have sedating side effects. These include opioids, muscle relaxants, triptans, antidepressants, and antiepileptics. Among antidepressants, sedation occurs frequently with tricyclic compounds.[161] Sedating antiepileptic medications frequently used for pain include gabapentin and pregabalin but also carbamazepine, felbamate, lamotrigine, tiagabine, topiramate, and others.[93] Mechanisms for sedation for antidepressant and antiepileptic drugs used for pain[161] are listed in Table 53.6; these drugs are discussed more fully elsewhere in this chapter.

Opioids

Opioid medications exhibit a variety of important clinical effects mediated by one or more opioid receptors, including analgesia (μ, κ, and δ opioid receptors), sedation (μ and κ receptors), and respiratory depression (μ receptors).[162-164] Sedation is one of the principal side effects of opioid agonists, with magnitude affected by dose, duration of use, age, and pain severity. Objective measures of sleepiness indicate persistence of sleepiness 4 to 8 hours postinjection of drugs used for ambulatory surgery.[165] Acute effects of opioids on sleep include decrease in SWS and REM, but effects on sleep latency and TST are inconsistent.[166,167] Chronic use is associated with low sleep efficiency, decreased SWS, possibly decreased REM, and daytime sleepiness.[168-170]

Chronic opioid use is a well-established risk factor for sleep-disordered breathing, especially for central sleep apnea, hypoventilation, hypoxemia, and ataxic breathing.[171] Prevalence of any form of sleep-disordered breathing because of opioid use is unclear but is reported to be in the 30% to 90% range.[171,172] The incidence and severity of sleep disordered breathing from chronic opioid use is affected by increased relaxation of upper airway muscles, changes in hypercapnic and hypoxic ventilatory responses, and blunting of respiratory rhythm.[171] Respiratory depression likely occurs via activation of μ-opioid receptors in the brainstem, with input from other brain areas.[173]

Opioids can be classified as full agonists, partial agonists, mixed agonists-antagonists, and antagonists.[163,174] The majority of opioid medications are full agonists at the μ receptor with some agonist activity at the κ receptor (e.g., codeine, fentanyl, morphine; see Table 53.6). Methadone, used for pain and for the treatment of opioid addiction, is a μ-opioid agonist, NMDA antagonist, and NET and SERT inhibitor.[175,176]

Partial agonists such as tramadol act similarly to full agonists at low doses, but their analgesic effect plateaus as dose increases, with further dose increases augmenting adverse effects. Desmetramadol, the major metabolite of tramadol, is much more potent than the parent drug. Tramadol also exhibits weak NET and SERT inhibition and weak 5-HT_{2C} antagonism.[177]

The activity of mixed agonists/antagonists varies depending on the opioid receptor and dose. Buprenorphine is a partial agonist at the μ receptor and an antagonist at the κ receptor; thus it is indicated to treat pain at all doses and opioid-use disorder at high doses. Buprenorphine monotherapy and in combination with naloxone (a μ-opioid antagonist) is indicated for opioid detoxification treatment. Buprenorphine reportedly promotes analgesia at all doses without an increase in respiratory depression; however, even at standard doses, clinically significant disordered breathing has been noted with both buprenorphine and buprenorphine/naloxone in many patients, predominantly central apneas and ataxic breathing.[178] Butorphanol, on the other hand, is a weak antagonist at the μ receptor and a potent agonist at the κ receptor. The latter activity may potentiate psychotomimetic effects.[179] Because of the weak μ antagonism, respiratory depression may not be significantly increased at higher doses but may be prolonged.[180] Pentazocine, somewhat similar to butorphanol, is a partial agonist at the μ receptor and a full agonist at the κ receptor, leading to analgesic effects at low doses and dysphoria at high doses. Nalbuphine is an antagonist at the μ receptor and an agonist at the κ receptor. At doses above 30 mg, it exhibits a ceiling effect on respiratory depression, and at doses less than or equal to its analgesic doses, may reverse respiratory depression of μ agonists.[181]

Muscle Relaxants

Skeletal muscle relaxants vary in their mechanism of action, but most have CNS activity causing significant sedation.[182] Mechanisms for sedation include GABA potentiation, H and mACh antagonism, and α_2 agonism. Both carisoprodol and its major metabolite, meprobamate, bind to the $GABA_A$ receptor. Cyclobenzaprine and orphenadrine are antagonists at H and mACh receptors. Cyclobenzaprine, similar in structure to tricyclic antidepressants, is also a 5-HT_2 antagonist. Dicyclomine is an mACh receptor antagonist. Tizanidine is an α_2 agonist. Baclofen is a $GABA_B$ agonist that also weakly blocks the $\alpha_2\delta$ subunit containing voltage-gated calcium channels, similar to gabapentin. The sedating effect of baclofen has been demonstrated by improvements in PSG measure of sleep using a transient insomnia model.[183]

Triptans

Most triptans, used in the treatment of acute migraine and cluster headaches, are selective 5-$HT_{1B/1D}$ agonists, with variable affinity for 5-HT_{1D} receptors, but low to no affinity for other types of 5-HT receptors. The exception is lasmiditan, which selectively binds to the 5-HT_{1F} receptor. Sedation with triptans is reported to occur in 4% to 15% of patients and appears to be dose-related.[184,185] However, the mechanism for sedation is unclear. Some data suggest somnolence is the result of unmasking of CNS symptoms associated with the natural resolution of migraine, rather than related to direct pharmacologic effect.[186] On the other hand, drugs with higher lipophilicity and those with active metabolites (eletriptan, zolmitriptan, rizatriptan) appear more likely to be sedating, suggesting there is a central mechanism for sedation.[187]

Other Drugs with Sedating Side Effects

Lofexidine is an α_2 agonist used in the mitigation of opioid withdrawal, with somnolence reported as a side effect in 6% to 42% of patients in clinical trials.[188,189] Oxybutynin, a nonselective mACh antagonist used in the treatment of bladder overactivity, is associated with mild to moderate sleepiness and REM suppression.[190,191] Fatigue is listed as a side effect of lorcaserin, a selective 5-HT_{2C} agonist indicated for weight loss that was withdrawn from the US market in 2020 because of cancer risk.[192,193]

DRUGS WITH INSOMNIA SIDE EFFECTS (TABLE 53.10)

Insomnia may be a side effect of drugs whose mechanisms include agonism of 5-HT, ACh, α_1, DA, or orexin (hypocretin); antagonism of adenosine, GABA, or H_3; and reuptake inhibition of 5-HT, DA, or NE (Table 53.1). Wake-promoting drugs, including caffeine, may cause insomnia if taken too close to bedtime. Drugs that promote or exacerbate RLS symptoms may cause insomnia indirectly. Table 53.10 lists drugs with insomnia side effects and the principal mechanisms for insomnia.

Antidepressant Drugs with Insomnia Side Effects (Tables 53.7 and 53.10)

Most SSRIs and SNRIs are associated with some degree of insomnia.[7,194]Among SSRIs, drugs with more potent NET and/or DAT inhibition (paroxetine, sertraline) are more likely to promote insomnia. Although the primary mechanism of action of SSRIs is potent inhibition of SERT, these drugs are not entirely selective (escitalopram is an exception). Citalopram has mild antihistamine properties; fluoxetine blocks the 5-HT_{2C} receptor, likely enhancing both NE and DA release; paroxetine weakly inhibits NET; sertraline weakly inhibits DAT; and both sertraline and fluvoxamine are active at the σ_1 receptor. These diverse actions may explain why SSRIs are differentially associated with insomnia and/or daytime sedation.[56,195] PSG studies of SSRIs generally indicate disruption of sleep continuity and suppression of REM.[196] Some SSRIs, fluoxetine in particular, have been associated with the presence of prominent slow eye movements during sleep, the so-called "Prozac or SSRI-eyes."[197]

Among SNRIs, those with more potent NET inhibition (desvenlafaxine, duloxetine, venlafaxine) are more likely to promote insomnia.[198] Venlafaxine exhibits greater SERT

Table 53.10 Drugs with Insomnia Side Effects

Drug Class/Subclass	Drugs	Principal Mechanism(s) for Insomnia
Antidepressants[a]		
SSRIs	Fluoxetine, etc.	SERT inhibition
SNRIs	Desvenlafaxine Venlafaxine Duloxetine	NET and SERT inhibition
Tricyclics[b]	Desipramine Nortriptyline Protriptyline	NET inhibition
MAOIs	Phenelzine Selegiline transdermal Tranylcypromine	Increased DA, NE, and 5-HT via MAO-A,B inhibition
Atypical drugs	Bupropion	NET and SERT inhibition
	Vilazodone	SERT, DAT, and NET inhibition
Antipsychotics[c]	Fluphenazine Haloperidol Perphenazine Thioridazine Trifluoperazine Aripiprazole	Unclear, see text; possibly 5-HT_{1A}, 5-HT_{2C} agonism, D_2 antagonism/partial agonism
Antibiotics[d]		
Benzodiazepine antagonists	Flumazenil	$GABA_A$ benzodiazepine binding site antagonism
Beta-lactams	Penicillins Cephalosporins	GABA antagonism
Fluoroquinolones	Ciprofloxacin Levofloxacin	$GABA_A$ antagonism, adenosine antagonism, NMDA agonism
Macrolides	Clarithromycin Erythromycin	$GABA_A$ negative allosteric modulation
Antiparkinsonian Drugs		
MAO type B inhibitors	Selegiline[e] Rasagiline Safinamide	Increased DA via MAO-B inhibition
Adenosine antagonists	Istradefylline	$Adenosine_{2A}$ receptor antagonism
Cardiovascular Drugs		
ACE inhibitors	Captopril Cilazapril	Secondary to cough side effect
Beta antagonists	Propranolol Labetalol Metoprolol	Beta adrenergic receptor, 5-HT antagonism, melatonin suppression; see text
Hypolipidemic drugs	Atorvastatin Lovastatin Simvastatin	Unclear, see text
Nicotine and Drugs for Smoking Cessation		
Nicotine	Tobacco	α7 and α4β2 nicotinic AChR agonism
Nicotine replacement	Nicotine patch Nicotine inhalant Nicotine nasal spray	α7 and α4β2 nicotinic AChR agonism
Non-nicotine drugs	Bupropion sustained release	NET and DAT inhibition
	Varenicline	α4β2 nicotinic AChR agonism
Stimulants and Wake-Promoting Drugs		
Amphetamine-like drugs	Amphetamine Dextroamphetamine Lisdexamfetamine Methamphetamine Methylphenidate[f]	Direct release of DA DAT inhibition

Continued

Table 53.10 Drugs with Insomnia Side Effects—cont'd

Drug Class/Subclass	Drugs	Principal Mechanism(s) for Insomnia
Wake-promoting drugs	Modafinil Armodafinil	Unknown; likely DAT inhibition, indirect activation of other wake-promoting neurotransmitters
	Atomoxetine	NET inhibition
	Solriamfetol	DAI and NET inhibition
	Pitolisant	H_3 inverse agonism
Other drugs	Caffeine Theobromine	Adenosine$_{2A}$ antagonism
Weight Loss Drugs		
Sympathomimetics	Phentermine Diethylpropion Phendimetrazine	NE release or NET inhibition
Combination drugs	Phentermine/topiramate	NE release or NET inhibition
	Naltrexone/bupropion	NET and DAT inhibition
Other Drugs		
Alcohol	Alcohol	Multiple mechanisms, see text
Decongestants	Pseudoephedrine	Adrenergic alpha agonism
Cholinesterase inhibitors	Donepezil Galantamine Rivastigmine	Acetylcholinesterase inhibition
Corticosteroids	Prednisone	Adrenergic agonism, GABA inhibition, possibly glutamate agonism, HPA axis effects
Methylxanthines	Theophylline	Adenosine$_{2A}$ receptor antagonism
NSAIDs	Ibuprofen, etc.	Prostaglandin D_2 inhibition, possibly melatonin suppression
Opioid agonists	Morphine, etc.	Acetylcholine release, adenosine antagonism
Opioid antagonists	Naloxone Naltrexone	μ-opioid receptor antagonism

[a]See Table 53.7 for a comprehensive list of antidepressants, likelihood of sedation or insomnia, and receptor binding affinity profiles.
[b]Most tricyclics are sedating; those with relatively more NET inhibition may promote insomnia.
[c]See Table 53.8 for a comprehensive list of antipsychotics, likelihood of sedation or insomnia, and receptor binding affinity profiles.
[d]Nightmares, hallucinations, and psychiatric symptoms have been noted with fluoroquinolones and macrolides.
[e]In higher doses selegiline inhibits MAO-A, increasing 5-HT and NE. Safinamide inhibits glutamate release and DAT and SERT reuptake.
[f]Methylphenidate also inhibits reuptake of NE.
5-HT, Serotonin; 5-HT$_{1A, 2C}$, serotonin receptors 1A, 2C; ACE, angiotensin-converting enzyme; AChR, acetylcholine receptor; $\alpha 4\beta 2$, alpha 4 beta 2 receptor; $\alpha 7$, alpha 7 receptor; D_2, dopamine 2 receptor; DA, dopamine; DAT, dopamine transporter; GABA, gamma-aminobutyric acid; GABA$_A$, GABA A receptor; H_3, histamine 3 receptor; HPA, hypothalamic-pituitary-adrenal; MAO-A,B, monoamine oxidase receptors A, B; MAOI, monoamine oxidase inhibitor; μ, mu; NE, norepinephrine; NET, norepinephrine transporter; NMDA, N-methyl-D-aspartate; NSAID, nonsteroidal antiinflammatory drug; SERT, serotonin transporter; SNRI, serotonin-norepinephrine reuptake inhibitor; SSRI, selective serotonin reuptake inhibitor.

inhibition at low doses and greater NET inhibition at high doses. In addition to SERT and NET inhibition, duloxetine weakly inhibits DAT and has weak antagonistic activity at 5-HT$_{2A}$, 5-HT$_{2C}$, 5-HT$_6$, and mACh receptors.[198] Insomnia is less frequently reported for levomilnacipran and milnacipran; in the United States, milnacipran is indicated for the treatment of fibromyalgia but not for depression. Duloxetine is also indicated for the treatment of diabetic neuropathy, fibromyalgia, and musculoskeletal pain.

The rate of insomnia for bupropion is similar to that of SSRIs and SNRIs.[7,194] Bupropion is a dual NET and DAT inhibitor with no 5-HT activity, approved for treatment of depression, seasonal affective disorder, and smoking cessation.[199] Bupropion is sometimes used off-label to promote alertness, but there are no controlled studies to support this indication. PSG data show no consistent effects on sleep stage distribution in patients treated for depression.[200,201] Unlike most antidepressants, REM is not suppressed and may be increased in some patients.[202]

Insomnia is also reported with vilazodone, which potently inhibits SERT, weakly inhibits NET and DAT, and binds as a partial agonist with high affinity to 5-HT$_{1A}$, mechanisms involved in wake promotion.[60,203] Vortioxetine, a novel antidepressant that is both a modulator and stimulator of 5-HT, has been associated with a low incidence of insomnia. Mechanisms that may promote sleep include 5-HT$_{1D}$, 5-HT$_3$, and 5-HT$_7$ antagonism, whereas mechanisms that may promote wake include SERT inhibition, 5-HT$_{1A}$ agonism, and 5-HT$_{1B}$ partial agonism.[60] Some data indicate that subjective sleep measures improve independent of depression.[204]

Although most tricyclic antidepressants are sedating, those with relatively more NE reuptake inhibition (desipramine, nortriptyline, protriptyline) may promote insomnia. Protriptyline is not effective in promoting alertness[205] but may be useful in the treatment of cataplexy with minimal sedation.[206]

Monoamine oxidase inhibitors (MAOIs) used in the treatment of depression include isocarboxazid, phenelzine, tranylcypromine, and a transdermal formulation of selegiline. These drugs inhibit both monoamine oxidase type A (MAO-A) and type B (MAO-B), although transdermal selegiline has a greater affinity for MAO-B at low doses. Inhibition of these enzymes increases the concentration of DA, epinephrine, NE, and 5-HT, potentially promoting wake, but melatonin concentration may also be increased. Both insomnia and sedation have been reported, with insomnia more likely at higher doses.[207]

Antipsychotic Drugs with Insomnia Side Effects (Tables 53.8 and 53.10)

Patients with schizophrenia commonly have insomnia and circadian rhythm disturbances, which complicates the assessment of drug-induced insomnia.[208] Objective data of disturbed sleep (via PSG) may differ substantially from patient reports.[84] The incidence of insomnia varies among antipsychotics and cannot reliably be predicted from their pharmacologic-binding profiles (Table 53.8). Possible mechanisms underlying the insomnia include 5-HT and DA agonism/partial agonism, in addition to RLS symptoms secondary to increased availability of 5-HT or dopaminergic blockade.[84,209] Drugs with 5-HT_{1A} and/or 5-HT_{2C} agonism/partial agonism include aripiprazole, asenapine, brexpiprazole, cariprazine, lurasidone, quetiapine, and ziprasidone. Drugs with potent D_2 and/or D_3 antagonism (and potential for RLS) for which insomnia is frequently reported include asenapine, fluphenazine, perphenazine, thioridazine, and thiothixene. Aripiprazole and brexpiprazole are also partial agonists at D_2 and D_3 receptors.[84,210] However, among antipsychotics, insomnia is reported frequently with aripiprazole, fluphenazine, haloperidol, perphenazine, and trifluoperazine; occasionally with asenapine, cariprazine, loxapine, lurasidone, olanzapine, and risperidone; and rarely with other drugs. (See additional information on drugs associated with RLS or PLMS elsewhere in this chapter.)

Antibiotic Drugs with Insomnia Side Effects (Table 53.10)

Insomnia, nightmares, hallucinations, and psychiatric symptoms have been noted with a number of antibiotic drugs, in particular, fluoroquinolones (e.g., ciprofloxacin, levofloxacin), macrolides (clarithromycin, erythromycin), and beta-lactams (e.g., penicillins, cephalosporins). These effects are likely mediated by GABA antagonism or negative allosteric modulation and, for fluoroquinolones, NMDA agonism.[211] The CNS effects appear to be exacerbated by concomitant use of nonsteroidal antiinflammatory drugs (NSAIDs), likely through an interaction that increases the potency of the antimicrobial for the $GABA_A$ receptor.[211]

Flumazenil is a competitive antagonist of the benzodiazepine binding site, by which it antagonizes the sedation, psychomotor impairment, and ventilatory depression produced by benzodiazepines.[212-214] It has no effect on drugs affecting GABAergic neurons by other mechanisms (e.g., ethanol, barbiturates). Flumazenil has been used experimentally to treat hypersomnolence in patients with abnormal cerebrospinal fluid potentiation of $GABA_A$ receptors.[215] The macrolide antibiotic clarithromycin, a negative allosteric modulator of the $GABA_A$ receptor, has also demonstrated improvement in various measures of sleepiness in patients with GABA-related hypersomnia.[216,217] As drugs that decrease the inhibitory effects of GABA, they have the potential to disrupt sleep.

Antiparkinsonian Drugs with Insomnia Side Effects (Table 53.10)

MAO-B inhibitors block the catabolism of DA, resulting in increase in dopaminergic activity in the brain. Selegiline and rasagiline are irreversible MAO-B inhibitors, whereas safinamide is a reversible inhibitor. Selegiline is metabolized to L-methamphetamine, which may result in SERT and NET inhibition.[218] In higher doses, selegiline also inhibits MAO-A, thereby also increasing levels of 5-HT and NE. Safinamide inhibits glutamate release along with DAT and SERT reuptake. Insomnia is reported with these drugs, but the incidence is unclear, particularly with safinamide, for which somnolence has been reported as a side effect.[219,220] There are case reports of confusion, hallucinations, and impulse control disorders with these drugs.

Istradefylline, an adenosine_{2A} receptor antagonist, is used as adjunctive therapy for "wearing-off" symptoms in PD. Low rates of insomnia have been reported in clinical trials.[221] However, daytime sleepiness was reportedly improved in an open-label study.[222]

Cardiovascular Drugs with Insomnia Side Effects (Table 53.10)

Angiotensin-Converting Enzyme Inhibitors

ACE inhibitors (e.g., captopril, cilazapril) reportedly have a low incidence of CNS side effects. However, a dry, irritating cough is a common side effect (apparently induced by increased bradykinin), which may contribute to insomnia.[223] Obstructive sleep apnea has also been reported, and possibly related to rhinopharyngeal inflammation.[224]

Beta Blockers

Insomnia with beta blockers used in the treatment of hypertension is more likely with highly lipophilic compounds that are nonselective for β_1 and β_2 receptors.[225] The more lipophilic compounds have CNS activity in addition to their peripheral effects. Drugs selective for β_1 receptors have lower affinity for 5-HT receptors. However, β_1 blockers suppress melatonin synthesis by blocking sympathetic signaling to the pineal gland, thereby reducing circadian signaling.[226] Sleep quality was improved with melatonin supplementation in hypertensive patients taking beta blockers.[227] Among these drugs, propranolol, which has high lipid solubility and high 5-HT affinity, is most commonly associated with disturbed sleep. Risk for insomnia is also high for metoprolol, moderate for pindolol, and low for other beta-antagonists.

Carvedilol and labetalol also block α_1 receptors, and are thus more likely to be associated with somnolence than insomnia.[165] Other CNS side effects reported with beta antagonists include nightmares and vivid dreams.[228] There have also been case reports of RBD with lipophilic beta antagonists.[229]

Hypolipidemic Drugs

Data mining studies suggest that statins (β-hydroxy β-methylglutaryl-coenzyme A [HMG-CoA] reductase inhibitors), particularly the more lipophilic compounds (atorvastatin, lovastatin, simvastatin), are associated with both insomnia and parasomnias.[230] Observational studies and clinical trials evaluating sleep as a primary outcome indicate mixed results and suggest that further study of statins with higher lipophilicity is needed.[231-234] More recently, a mendelian randomization study based on data from genome-wide association studies showed no association of statin therapy with insomnia, although there was an increased risk of depression.[235] Other studies suggest that neuropsychiatric effects associated with statins are generally rare, typically occurring in susceptible individuals. Mechanisms relating to inhibition of cholesterol biosynthesis have been proposed to explain detrimental effects of statins on the CNS but there is no clear explanation.[236]

Nicotine and Smoking-Cessation Drugs with Insomnia Side Effects (Table 53.10)

Nicotine indirectly alters glutamatergic, dopaminergic, and serotonergic systems in the brain by stimulating the α7 and α4β2 nicotinergic ACh receptors.[237] Sleep disturbances are frequent among smokers and confirmed by PSG studies that show extended sleep latency, decreased TST, delayed REM, and decreased SWS.[238] Nightmares and vivid dreams are also reported. Nicotine withdrawal also leads to insomnia complaints and increased arousals, with severity related to the degree of nicotine dependence.[239]

Nicotine replacement therapy can be provided via gum, inhaler, patch, and nasal and mouth sprays. Side effects are similar to nicotine itself. The nicotine transdermal patch provides continuous nicotine delivery over a 24-hour period. In healthy nonsmokers, it results in dose-dependent reduction in REM followed by REM rebound after cessation.[240] In smokers, transdermal nicotine initially results in prolonged sleep latency and decreased TST along with REM rebound, but over time results in a decrease in arousals and increased SWS despite persistent subjective reports of sleep difficulty.[238] Subjectively, insomnia and vivid dreams are common.[241]

Non-nicotine treatment options include sustained-release bupropion and varenicline. Insomnia and abnormal dreams are reported frequently with both drugs.[241] Bupropion, a NE and DA reuptake inhibitor, is also indicated for depression and discussed elsewhere in this chapter. Varenicline is an α4β2 nicotinic ACh (nACh) receptor partial agonist thought to stimulate the release of sufficient DA to reduce craving and withdrawal while acting as a partial antagonist to block binding of nicotine.

Stimulants and Wake-Promoting Drugs with Insomnia Side Effects (Tables 53.5 and 53.10)

Stimulants (amphetamines and amphetamine-like compounds) and wake-promoting drugs (armodafinil, modafinil, pitolisant, solriamfetol) used to treat sleepiness in narcolepsy, sleep apnea, and shift-work disorder are covered earlier in this chapter (Table 53.5). Insomnia is commonly reported with stimulants, particularly when used at higher doses. The incidence of insomnia with wake-promoting drugs is 5% to 10%, generally occurs with higher doses, and typically diminishes with time.[243-246]

Atomoxetine, used primarily in the treatment of attention-deficit/hyperactivity disorder, is a potent and selective inhibitor of NET but also weakly inhibits SERT and DAT.[247] Insomnia is occasionally reported but may be related to the patient population, as sleep problems are common in both children and adults with this disorder.[248,249]

Caffeine

The alerting effects of caffeine and theobromine are mediated primarily through antagonism of adenosine receptors, which indirectly affects the release of NE, DA, ACh, 5-HT, glutamate, and GABA. Caffeine is metabolized into theobromine, theophylline, and paraxanthine, all of which have CNS-stimulant properties.[250] Theobromine is found in chocolate, tea leaves, and the kola nut. Although the mean half-life of caffeine is 4 to 6 hours, it can range from 1.5 to 9.5 hours because of physiologic and environmental influences such as obesity, pregnancy, altitude, smoking, and medications such as oral contraceptives.[41] Caffeine's most common side effect is disrupted sleep, which is more likely when ingestion occurs within a few hours of bedtime. However, in some individuals, sleep may be disrupted with ingestion of caffeine 6 hours before bedtime.[251]

Weight Loss Drugs with Insomnia Side Effects (Table 53.10)

Weight loss drugs with CNS-stimulating side effects include the adrenergic amines (benzphetamine, diethylpropion, phendimetrazine, phentermine) and the combination drugs phentermine/topiramate and naltrexone/bupropion. The principal mechanism for insomnia with the adrenergic amines is NE release, but 5-HT and DA release may occur to a lesser extent. Common side effects with these drugs include dry mouth, restlessness, dizziness, and insomnia, in addition to tachycardia and elevation of blood pressure.[252] Insomnia is reported with the combination drug phentermine/topiramate, which employs a lower dose of topiramate than the doses used for epilepsy, where sedation is common.[252,253] The mechanism for insomnia reported in clinical trials with naltrexone/bupropion is most likely NE and DA reuptake inhibition via bupropion, but μ-opioid antagonism may play a role.[254]

Other Drugs with Insomnia Side Effects (Table 53.10)

Alcohol

Although the precise mechanism of action of alcohol is unclear, alcohol acts on a variety of mechanisms involved in sleep-wake regulation. Depending on concentration, alcohol acts as a positive allosteric modulator at $GABA_A$, glycine, $5\text{-}HT_3$, and nACh receptors; a negative allosteric modulator of the NMDA, AMPA, and kainate receptors; and a reuptake inhibitor at adenosine and glycine receptors.[255] Secondary to other actions, alcohol also increases DA and endogenous opioids. Alcohol has a biphasic effect on sleep, improving sleep continuity during the first half of the night, but because it is quickly metabolized, disrupting sleep during the second half of the night.[256] Chronic alcohol use is associated with increased insomnia. In individuals with alcohol dependence, abstinence of 2 to 3 weeks produces worsening sleep efficiency, increased REM, and increased frequency of nightmares.[257]

Decongestants

Insomnia is a common adverse reaction with pseudoephedrine, an α- and β-adrenergic agonist.[258,259] High incidences of both insomnia and somnolence have been reported with pseudoephedrine in children.[260]

Cholinesterase Inhibitors

Among cholinesterase inhibitors used in the treatment of Alzheimer disease, insomnia is more common with donepezil and rivastigmine than galantamine (13%–14% versus 4%), and nightmares were more common with donepezil (9%).[261,262] PSG studies of these drugs show an increase in REM duration and density, along with shortened REM latency.[263,264]

Corticosteroids

The daily rhythmicity of plasma glucocorticoids provides synchronizing cues to many physiologic and psychological processes, including arousal, cognition, mood, and sleep.[265] Disruptions in the rhythm of cortisol release that might affect sleep-wake behavior can result from a variety of situations, including misalignment of circadian rhythms because of shift work or jet lag, or suppression of endogenous levels and rhythmicity via synthetic glucocorticoid treatment. Central side effects of glucocorticoid therapy include changes in mood, impairment of memory and cognition, and sleep disturbances.[266] The mechanism by which corticosteroids disrupt sleep appears to be via activation of noradrenergic neurons in the locus coeruleus that subsequently inhibit GABAergic neurons.[267] Insomnia is reported by 30% to 60% of patients on glucocorticoids, with incidence and severity dependent on dose and duration of use.[268] In a cross-sectional survey, insomnia was ranked only behind weight gain as the most important side effect, despite the presence of more serious side effects.[269] Dose and duration of use affect the severity of insomnia.

Theophylline

Disturbed sleep is a common complaint of patients taking theophylline, a respiratory stimulant and bronchodilator chemically related to caffeine and one of the metabolites of caffeine.[270,271] The mechanism underlying this insomnia is likely nonselective adenosine antagonism.[272,273] Peak plasma concentration is usually reached within 2 hours, but the half-life varies by preparation and is typically shorter in children (3.5 hours) and longer in adults (8–9 hours). Absorption is lower at night than in the morning[274] and may be greatly affected by food.[275] Theophylline, administered for up to 3 weeks, has been shown to disturb PSG-recorded sleep in healthy subjects,[276] patients with asthma,[277] children with cystic fibrosis,[278] and patients with sleep apnea[279] or chronic obstructive pulmonary disease.[280] A dose-dependent increase in MSLT latency and performance was noted with short-term administration of theophylline in normals.[281]

Nonsteroidal Antiinflammatory Drugs

NSAIDs may affect sleep because they decrease the synthesis of prostaglandin D2, suppress the normal nocturnal surge in melatonin synthesis, and attenuate the normal nocturnal decrease in body temperature.[282] Prostaglandin D_2 increases proportionally with increased duration of wake and appears to be involved in sleep initiation and maintenance.[283] Limited PSG data are mixed and suggest sleep disturbance with some compounds.[282,284,285]

Opioids

Although sleepiness is a principal side effect of opioid agonists, these drugs can also disrupt sleep. There is increased evidence that opioids act on both sleep- and wake-promoting systems.[286] The mechanisms for sleep disruption may include ACh release and decreased adenosine in brain regions that regulate sleep.[287,288] Chronic use of opioids is associated with low sleep efficiency, decreased SWS, possible decreased REM, and daytime sleepiness.[168-170] Sleep disturbance is highly prevalent in patients on methadone maintenance and does not appear to be limited to methadone, as patients with opioid use disorder treated with methadone, diacetylmorphine, or buprenorphine reported similar sleep disturbance that was significantly higher than in patients with recent opioid detoxification.[289,290]

The opioid antagonists naloxone and naltrexone are indicated for reversal of opioid depression, including respiratory depression. Naltrexone is also indicated for treatment of alcohol and opioid dependence. Disturbed sleep is common with alcohol and opioid dependence; thus it is unclear if insomnia reported with these drugs is specific to the drug.[291-293] However, 9% of patients in a clinical trial of naltrexone for weight loss reported insomnia,[254] and in a small study of healthy individuals, naltrexone decreased REM and SWS and increased wake time.[294]

DRUGS THAT MAY CAUSE VIVID DREAMS OR NIGHTMARES (TABLE 53.11)

Nightmares are clinically reported with numerous drugs.[295,296] However, data are primarily in the form of case reports. In addition, there are very few studies that include drug withdrawal and rechallenge to confirm the relationship. The pharmacologic mechanism explaining how certain medications may trigger nightmares is largely not understood. Nightmares appear to be more common with drugs that have effects on DA, 5-HT, and NE, but drugs affecting GABA and ACh may also produce nightmares. Although withdrawal from REM-suppressing drugs may result in nightmares, the effect of a drug on sleep architecture, particularly REM, does not predict propensity for nightmares.[297] The available literature is even more confusing because some drugs that purportedly cause nightmares have been found to reduce nightmares in clinical trials. Examples include risperidone, clonidine, and tricyclic antidepressants.[298]

Dream recall frequency is often decreased with antidepressants, probably because of the decrease in REM sleep caused by these drugs. However, dream detail may be more vivid, possibly because of effects on cholinergic mechanisms. Nightmares occur more commonly upon withdrawal of these drugs, likely because of REM rebound. Other REM-suppressant drugs with nightmares on withdrawal include alcohol, barbiturates, MAOIs, and benzodiazepines.[299] Bupropion, which does not suppress REM sleep, is the antidepressant most frequently associated with nightmares. Drugs with possible DA-related nightmare mechanisms include DA agonists, levodopa, stimulants, and some antipsychotics.[295]

Certain antimicrobials (e.g., fluroquinolones such as ciprofloxacin, macrolides such as clarithromycin, and beta-lactams such as penicillins and cephalosporins) and antivirals (e.g., amantadine, efavirenz, ganciclovir, mefloquine) have also been associated with increased nightmares, possibly related to modulation of sleep-regulating inflammatory cytokines, although the exact mechanism is unknown.[211] To complicate interpretation, fever itself is associated with increased reports of vivid dreams and hallucinations.[300]

Other drugs associated with nightmares include centrally acting antihypertensive medications such as beta blockers and α_2 agonists. Lipophilic beta blockers such as propranolol and metoprolol are more likely to cause nightmares than hydrophilic drugs such as atenolol.[228] Nightmares have also been reported with cholinesterase inhibitors, particularly donepezil,[262] and some antiepileptic medications.[296]

Table 53.11 Drugs That May Cause Vivid Dreams or Nightmares

Drug/Drug Class	Drug(s)	With Use	On Withdrawal[a]
Alcohol	Alcohol	X	X
Antibiotics, antivirals	Amantadine, ciprofloxacin, clarithromycin, efavirenz, erythromycin, ganciclovir, mefloquine	X	
Antidepressants			
Tricyclics[b]	Amitriptyline, clomipramine, desipramine, doxepin, imipramine, nortriptyline	X	X
SSRIs[c]	Citalopram, escitalopram, fluoxetine, fluvoxamine, paroxetine, sertraline	X	X
SNRIs	Desvenlafaxine, duloxetine, venlafaxine	X	X
MAOIs	Phenelzine, tranylcypromine		X
Other	Bupropion[d], mirtazapine, vilazodone, vortioxetine	X	
Antiepileptics	Ethosuximide, lamotrigine, valproic acid, zonisamide	X	
Antihistamines	Chlorpheniramine	X	
Antiparkinsonian Drugs	Amantadine, cabergoline, levodopa, pergolide, ropinirole, selegiline	X	
Antipsychotics[b]	Clozapine, olanzapine, risperidone	X	
Barbiturates	Phenobarbital		X
Cardiovascular Drugs			
ACE inhibitors	Captopril, enalapril, quinapril	X	
$Alpha_2$ agonists	Clonidine,[b] methyldopa	X	
Angiotensin blockers	Losartan	X	
Beta antagonists	Atenolol, labetalol, propranolol	X	
Calcium antagonists	Verapamil	X	
Other	Amiodarone, digoxin	X	
Cholinesterase Inhibitors	Donepezil, galantamine, rivastigmine, tacrine	X	
Dopaminergic Drugs	Levodopa, pramipexole, ropinirole	X	
NMDA Antagonists	Memantine	X	
Opioids	Buprenorphine, butorphanol, codeine, fentanyl, methadone, morphine, nalbuphine, pentazocine, tramadol	X	X
Sedative Hypnotics			
Benzodiazepines	Temazepam, triazolam, etc.	X	X
Orexin antagonists[e]	Lemborexant, suvorexant	X	
Statins	Atorvastatin, lovastatin, simvastatin	X	
Stimulants	Amphetamine, methylphenidate	X	X

[a]REM rebound occurs on withdrawal with these drugs.
[b]Conflicting data; clinical trials have shown reduction in nightmares with some tricyclic antidepressants, clonidine, olanzapine, and risperidone.
[c]Vivid dreams but decreased recall. Nightmares more common with paroxetine.
[d]Nightmares more frequent with bupropion than with other antidepressants.
[e]Orexin antagonists may be associated with complex behaviors.
ACE, Angiotensin-converting enzyme; MAOI, monoamine oxidase inhibitor; NMDA, N-methyl-D-aspartate; REM, rapid eye movement; SNRI, serotonin-norepinephrine reuptake inhibitor; SSRI, selective serotonin reuptake inhibitor.

DRUGS ASSOCIATED WITH RESTLESS LEGS SYNDROME OR PERIODIC LIMB MOVEMENTS (TABLE 53.12)

Numerous case reports and a few systematic studies suggest that a number of antidepressant, antipsychotic, and antiepileptic drugs are associated with onset or exacerbation of RLS[301-304] and PLMS,[302,305] but the evidence is limited by lack of controlled studies, inadequate use of standardized instruments, heterogeneous populations, and variable study duration. The mechanism by which these drugs may promote RLS or PLMS is not understood but may be associated with increased availability of 5-HT or DA receptor blockade.[7] A review of prospective studies on the influence of antidepressants on RLS and PLMS indicates mirtazapine is associated with high risk, but SSRIs, most SNRIs, and tricyclic

Table 53.12 Drugs that May Be Associated with Restless Legs Syndrome (RLS), Periodic Limb Movements of Sleep (PLMS), REM Sleep without Atonia (RSWA), or REM Behavior Disorder (RBD)

Drug Class	Subclass/Drug	RLS	PLMS	RSWA	RBD
Antidepressants	Tricyclics[a]	Possible	Possible	Definite	Possible
	SNRIs[b]	Probable	Probable	Definite	Probable
	SSRIs[c]	Probable	Definite	Definite	Probable
	MAOIs	Possible	Possible	Definite	Definite
	Mirtazapine	Definite	Definite	Possible	Possible
	Bupropion	None/unlikely	None/unlikely	Possible	Unknown/insufficient data
	Trazodone	Unknown/insufficient data	None/unlikely	Unknown/insufficient data	Unknown/insufficient data
	Other	Unknown/insufficient data	Unknown/insufficient data	Unknown/insufficient data	Unknown/insufficient data
Antipsychotics[d]	Aripiprazole	Possible	Unknown/insufficient data	Unknown/insufficient data	Unknown/insufficient data
	Haloperidol	Possible	Unknown/insufficient data	Unknown/insufficient data	Unknown/insufficient data
	Olanzapine	Probable	Possible	Possible	Possible
	Quetiapine	Probable	Possible	Possible	Possible
	Risperidone	Possible	Possible	Unknown/insufficient data	Unknown/insufficient data
	Thioridazine	Possible	Unknown/insufficient data	Unknown/insufficient data	Unknown/insufficient data
	Other	Unknown/insufficient data	Unknown/insufficient data	Unknown/insufficient data	Unknown/insufficient data
Antiepileptics	Topiramate	Possible	Unknown/insufficient data	Unknown/insufficient data	Unknown/insufficient data
	Zonisamide	Possible	Unknown/insufficient data	Unknown/insufficient data	Unknown/insufficient data
Dopamine agonists[e]	Levodopa	Definite	Unknown/insufficient data	None/unlikely	None/unlikely
	Pramipexole	Definite	Unknown/insufficient data	None/unlikely	None/unlikely
	Ropinirole	Definite	Unknown/insufficient data	None/unlikely	None/unlikely
	Rotigotine	Probable	Unknown/insufficient data	None/unlikely	None/unlikely
	Other	Probable	Unknown/insufficient data	None/unlikely	None/unlikely
Other	Alcohol	Possible	Unknown/insufficient data	Unknown/insufficient data	Possible
	Caffeine	Unknown/insufficient data	Possible	Unknown/insufficient data	Unknown/insufficient data
	Tramadol	Possible	Unknown/insufficient data	Unknown/insufficient data	Unknown/insufficient data

Risk: Definite; Probable; Possible; None/unlikely; Unknown/insufficient data

[a]RLS and PLMS possibly more likely with amitriptyline.
[b]RLS, PLMS, RSWA, and RBD probably more likely with venlafaxine and duloxetine.
[c]RLS and PLMS possibly more likely with fluoxetine and sertraline.
[d]Olanzapine and quetiapine are most frequently reported to be associated with RLS, PLMS, RSWA, and RBD.
[e]For dopamine agonists, increased risk of RLS is in the form of augmentation.
MAOI, Monoamine oxidase inhibitor; REM, rapid eye movement; SNRI, serotonin-norepinephrine reuptake inhibitor; SSRI, selective serotonin reuptake inhibitor.

antidepressants only slightly increase risk.[306] A small study in normal individuals and a prospective study in patients with depression suggest that risk is high with the SNRI venlafaxine.[307] A large (n = 18,980) cross-sectional study reported SSRIs were associated with increased risk for RLS, with overall RLS prevalence in the general population of 5.5%.[308] Bupropion is an exception among antidepressants; it does not exacerbate RLS or PLMS and may improve RLS symptoms, likely because of DAT inhibition.[309]

Among antipsychotics, olanzapine and quetiapine are most commonly associated with RLS, but there are also reports for aripiprazole, asenapine, clozapine, risperidone, haloperidol, loxapine, lurasidone, perphenazine, and thior idazine.[301,302,310-312] Although most of the data consist of case reports, the data are strengthened by the fact that symptoms resolved upon drug discontinuation. PLMS has been reported with olanzapine and quetiapine, but the data are of poor quality.

Among antiepileptic drugs, there are a handful of case reports associating topiramate and zonisamide with RLS.[301,302] There are no studies of PLMS with these drugs.

An estimated 76% of patients with RLS treated with DA agonists require a dose increase and/or show evidence of augmentation with a yearly incidence rate of approximately 8%.[313] Augmentation rates are less than 10% for short-term use, approximately 30% for use duration of 2 to 3 years, and up to 68% at 10 years.[314] Although there are no direct comparative studies, the incidence rate appears to be highest with levodopa and may be higher for shorter-acting (e.g., pramipexole) than longer-acting (e.g., rotigotine) drugs, at least with short-term use.[315] There are case reports of RLS augmentation with tramadol, which, in addition to μ opioid antagonism, shows SERT and NET reuptake inhibition, but no confirmatory data in clinical trials.[316] The use of proton pump inhibitors (e.g., omeprazole) or histamine$_2$ receptor antagonists (e.g., ranitidine) have been associated with the presence of RLS in two large, independent population cohorts of blood donors.[316a] These associations were not mediated by serum ferritin despite the fact that both types of medications are linked to reduced iron.[316b]

Caffeine and alcohol have been reported to exacerbate RLS and PLMS, but most of the data are of poor quality and the results are inconsistent. One epidemiologic study reported that drinking at least three servings of alcohol per day was associated with RLS, whereas drinking one to two glasses was protective for PLMS; in contrast, drinking three cups of coffee per day was associated with PLMS but protective for RLS.[308]

DRUGS ASSOCIATED WITH REM SLEEP WITHOUT ATONIA OR REM BEHAVIOR DISORDER (TABLE 53.12)

Antidepressants are associated with an increased prevalence of REM sleep without atonia (RSWA) and RBD.[302,317-320] This increased prevalence is also seen in patients who take antidepressants for treatment of cataplexy.[321] Among antidepressants, SSRIs and SNRIs (particularly venlafaxine and duloxetine) are most commonly associated with RSWA and, to a lesser extent, with RBD. However, both RSWA and RBD have been reported with mirtazapine, MAOIs, and tricyclics. Trazodone and bupropion have been linked with RSWA but not RBD.

There is also some evidence that antipsychotics (particularly olanzapine and quetiapine) are associated with an increase in RSWA and RBD.[302,320] Two population studies show an association of moderate to heavy alcohol consumption with risk of RBD.[322,323]

Because SSRIs are frequently associated with RSWA/RBD, a serotoninergic mechanism has been proposed via serotonin modulation either at the level of the pons or the spinal cord.[324] However, the diversity of the pharmacologic mechanisms of the drugs associated with RSWA/RBD suggests alternative mechanisms such as DA, glycine, and GABA modulation.[325]

It is unclear if these medications induce RSWA/RBD or merely unmask subclinical RBD. A number of studies have reported prodromal symptoms of synucleinopathy in some individuals who demonstrated medication-triggered RBD.[320,326] Some data suggest that patients in whom RBD symptoms developed after ingestion of antidepressants appear to be less likely to develop neurodegenerative disease than patients with idiopathic RBD.[321,325] This conclusion is supported by the observation that patients with idiopathic RBD, with or without antidepressant use, have higher RSWA than patients without RBD on antidepressants and show a different pattern of tonic and phasic muscle activity.[325]

CLINICAL PEARL

Many drugs have pharmacologic effects on the neurochemical systems involved in sleep-wake regulation. Knowledge of a drug's receptor mechanisms and pharmacokinetics can help predict the effect of the drug on sleep and wake behavior and the likelihood that that effect will be therapeutic or impairing. Drugs that enhance GABA or inhibit arousal systems containing glutamate, H, orexin, NE, 5-HT, ACh, or DA promote sleep but may adversely affect wake behavior. Drugs that activate arousal systems promote wake but may disrupt sleep.

SUMMARY

Drugs with pharmacologic effects on the neurochemical systems involved in sleep-wake regulation may have therapeutic or impairing effects on sleep-wake behavior. Effects on sleep may include changes in sleep duration, timing, or architecture, in addition to abnormalities such as nightmares, restless legs, or abnormal behaviors. Effects on waking function may include changes in alertness, performance, and cognition. The principal neurotransmitters and neuromodulators that affect sleep and wake include GABA, glutamate, ACh, adenosine, DA, H, melatonin, NE, orexin, and 5-HT. Dose, time to peak concentration, and half-life determine the rapidity of onset and the duration of a drug's clinical effect, and the receptor binding profile determines both mechanism of action and adverse events.

The current drugs with FDA indication for insomnia facilitate sleep by enhancement of GABA, antagonism of H or orexin, or melatonin agonism. Most drugs used "off-label" to treat insomnia promote sleep by antagonism of H_1, α_1, or 5-$HT_{2A,2C}$ receptors. These drugs typically affect multiple receptors, resulting in variable effects on sleep-wake behavior in addition to side effects not associated with sleep-wake mechanisms. With the possible exception of orexin antagonists, drugs with intermediate to long half-lives are likely to produce residual sedation.

The principal mechanism for wake promotion among stimulants and wake-promoting drugs is inhibition of DA reuptake and transport and, for sympathomimetics, direct DA release. Other wake-promoting mechanisms include NE release, NET inhibition, and H_3 inverse agonism. Mechanisms among drugs in development include orexin agonism and $GABA_A$ antagonism.

Psychotherapeutic drugs have diverse pharmacologic profiles. Among antidepressants, sedation is more likely with drugs that have more potent antagonism at H_1 or mACh receptors, whereas insomnia is more likely with drugs that have more potent inhibition of NET or DAT, but also occurs with SERT inhibition. Sedation may occur via $GABA_A$ positive allosteric modulation or glutamate antagonism in the novel antidepressants brexanolone and esketamine, respectively. Among antipsychotics, sedation is more common in drugs that have relatively more potent H_1, ACh, 5-HT_2, and/or α_1 antagonism, but may be caused by DA and NE antagonism. Insomnia cannot reliably be predicted from the pharmacologic binding profiles of antipsychotics, but possible mechanisms include 5-HT and DA agonism/partial agonism, along with indirect mechanisms such as RLS symptoms secondary to increased availability of 5-HT or dopaminergic blockade.

In antiepileptic drugs, sedation is most likely to occur with drugs that enhance GABA, block glutamate, or block calcium channels, but may be caused by glutamate antagonism. Gabapentin and pregabalin inhibit release of glutamate, NE, and substance P and may also affect adenosine.

Other drugs with sedating effects include opioids (principally via μ opioid and κ opioid agonism), muscle relaxants ($GABA_B$ agonism, H_1, mACh antagonism), antiemetics (mechanism dependent on drug class), first-generation antihistamines (H_1 antagonism), some antihypertensive drugs ($alpha_2$ agonists and $alpha_1$ antagonists), and some antiparkinsonian drugs. The mechanism for sedation with DA agonists is unclear but may involve activation of D_2 autoreceptors, DA receptor selectivity, and possibly suppression of glutamatergic input to orexin neurons.

Insomnia may occur via GABA antagonism or negative allosteric modulation in some antibiotics, 5-HT antagonism and melatonin suppression in antihypertensive beta blockers, NE release and NET or DAT inhibition in some weight loss drugs, ACh release and adenosine antagonism in opioids, and stimulation of α7 and α4β2 nACh receptors in nicotine.

The pharmacologic mechanism explaining how certain medications may trigger nightmares is largely not understood. Nightmares appear to be more common with drugs that have effects on DA, 5-HT, and NE, but drugs affecting GABA and ACh may also produce nightmares.

The mechanism by which drugs may promote RLS or PLMS is not understood but may be associated with increased availability of 5-HT or DA receptor blockade. A serotonergic mechanism has been postulated for drug-related development of RSWA or RBD. However, the diversity of pharmacologic mechanisms in drugs associated with RSWA or RBD suggests alternative mechanisms such as DA, glycine, and GABA modulation.

Current knowledge of the neurochemical basis of sleep-wake regulation provides a foundation for understanding the effects of medications on sleep and wake behavior. Future research will expand this understanding and lead to the development of targeted sleep-wake medications.

SELECTED READINGS

Alberti S, Chiesa A, Andrisano C, Serretti A. Insomnia and somnolence associated with second-generation antidepressants during the treatment of major depression: a meta-analysis. *J Clin Psychopharmacol.* 2015;35(3):296–303.

Atkin T, Comai S, Gobbi G. Drugs for insomnia beyond benzodiazepines: Pharmacology, clinical applications, and discovery. *Pharmacol Rev.* 2018;70(2):197–245.

Doghramji K, Jangro WC. Adverse effects of psychotropic medications on sleep. *Sleep Med Clin.* 2016;11(4):503–514.

Fang F, Sun H, Wang Z, Ren M, Calabrese J. Antipsychotic drug-induced somnolence: Incidence, mechanisms, and management. *CNS Drugs.* 2016;30:845–867.

Garcia AN, Salloum IM. Polysomnographic sleep disturbances in nicotine, caffeine, alcohol, cocaine, opioid, and cannabis use: a focused review. *Am J Addict.* 2015;24(7):590–598.

Haba-Rubio J, Frauscher B, Marques-Vidal P, et al. Prevalence and determinants of rapid eye movement sleep behavior disorder in the general population. *Sleep.* 2018;41(2):zsx197.

Herrera-Solis A, Herrera-Morales W, Nunez-Jaramillo L, Arias-Carrion O. Dopaminergic modulation of sleep-wake states. *CNS Neurol Disord - Drug Targets.* 2017;16:380–386.

Hirshkowitz M, Neurotransmitters Bhandari H. Neurochemistry, and the clinical pharmacology of sleep. In: Chokroverty S, ed. *Sleep Disorders Medicine.* New York, NY: Springer; 2017.

Holst SC, Landolt H-P. Sleep-wake neurochemistry. *Sleep Med Clin.* 2018;13:137–146.

Hoque R, Chesson AL. Pharmacologically induced-exacerbated restless legs syndrome, periodic limb movements of sleep, and REM Behavior Disorder/REM sleep without atonia: Literature review, qualitative scoring, and comparative analysis. *J Clin Sleep Med.* 2010;6:79–83.

Kolla BP, Mansukhani MP, Bostwick JM. The influence of antidepressants on restless legs syndrome and periodic limb movements: a systematic review. *Sleep Med Rev.* 2018;38:131–140.

Krystal AD. New developments in insomnia medications of relevance to mental health disorders. *Psychiatr Clin North Am.* 2015;38(4):843–860.

Maski K, Trotti LM, Kotagal S, et al. Treatment of central disorders of hypersomnolence: an American Academy of Sleep Medicine clinical practice guideline. *J Clin Sleep Med.* Published online April 2021.

Pagel JF, Helfter P. Drug induced nightmares – an etiology based review. *Hum Psychopharmacol.* 2003;18:59–67.

Piedad J, Rickards H, Besag FM, Cavanna AE. Beneficial and adverse psychotropic effects of antiepileptic drugs in patients with epilepsy: a summary of prevalence, underlying mechanisms and data limitations. *CNS Drugs.* 2012;26(4):319–335.

Thorpy MJ, Bogan RK. Update on the pharmacologic management of narcolepsy: mechanisms of action and clinical implications. *Sleep Med.* 2020;68:97–109.

Vallejo R, Barkin RL, Wang VC. Pharmacology of opioids in the treatment of chronic pain syndromes. *Pain Physician.* 2011;14(4). E343–E360.

Yeung Cavanna AE. Beneficial and adverse psychotropic effects of antiepileptic drugs in patients with epilepsy: a summary of prevalence, underlying mechanisms and data limitations. *CNS Drugs.* 2012;26(4):319–335.

A complete reference list can be found online at ExpertConsult.com.

Section 7

Psychobiology and Dreaming

Chapter 54

Introduction

Robert Stickgold

The COVID pandemic has brought new attention to dreams. People are reporting increased dream recall, many related to the pandemic and its sequelae, more bizarreness in their dreams, and more nightmares.[1] This only brings more attention to our continued poor understanding of the mechanisms and functions of dreaming. Indeed, the study of dreams and dreaming has made remarkably slow progress over the past century. In defense of this slow progress, it is worth noting that it shares with the study of consciousness several unenviable features: (1) it is only poorly defined, and there is no consensus on its definition; (2) it has no clear physiologic correlates, and hence its biologic basis is largely unknown; (3) it has no behavioral correlates and hence has no known function; and (4) its existence in species other than humans is a matter of conjecture. In short, we do not know the cause, nature, or consequence of dreaming. What is, absolutely clear, however, is that dreaming is a highly robust human occurrence experienced nightly by most humans.

DEFINITION

Given our ignorance of underlying biologic mechanisms and functions, it is perhaps not surprising that a clear, agreed-on definition of dreaming has evaded us. Most definitions in science refer either to physical objects or to processes that are defined by their underlying mechanisms or measurable consequences. We have none of these for dreaming. Indeed, a discussion group of the Association of Professional Sleep Societies and the Association for the Study of Dreams concluded that a "single definition for dreaming is most likely impossible given…the diversity in currently applied definitions."[1a] What all discussants did agree on is that its definition must be phenomenologic; that is, dreaming refers to a state of mind and not a state of the brain. Although most discussants argued that dreaming should be restricted to mentation occurring during sleep, some argued that daydreaming should be included. Some insisted that any definition should require the presence of hallucinatory perceptions, thoughts, and emotions that are altered from normal. Still others would require one but not another of these. Some would include any reported mental activity during sleep, even something as simple as a report of "I was wondering when you were going to wake me up."

As a consequence of the agreement to disagree, some authors have eschewed the use of the term altogether, talking instead about *sleep mentation*. Unlike the term *dreaming*, this phrase can be simply defined. Sleep mentation is defined as (1) all mental experiences—perceptions, thoughts, and emotions—occurring during sleep or (2) the process of experiencing perceptions, thoughts, and emotions during sleep. Thus it combines the sense of the words *dream* and *dreaming*. It is this concept, sleep mentation, that is more properly the subject of this section on dreaming.

METHODOLOGY

It is important to understand that researchers do not study dreams directly. Rather, they study dream reports, written, dictated, or, on rare occasions, drawn or acted out after the subject has awakened from sleep, along with their physiologic and psychological correlates. In one or two instances, the acting out of dreams *during sleep* by patients with rapid eye movement (REM) behavior disorder has been studied, although these are usable only when confirmed after awakening.

In one sense, this is not as big a problem as it is often considered. All scientific measurements are derivative. We measure blood pressure with the aid of a pressure cuff applied externally, listening with a stethoscope for the sounds produced by the movement of blood through the brachial artery, depending on our conscious perception of the moment at which the intensity of these sounds drops below our threshold of perception. Yet no one questions the legitimacy of the technique. It certainly is not accurate to more than 5 mm Hg at best, but it is good enough.

The difference between dream reports and blood pressure measurements is in the concept of "good enough." Researchers have confirmed the validity of using pressure cuffs by monitoring blood pressure with indwelling catheters in parallel with pressure cuff measurements and confirming the reliability of the pressure cuff technique. In contrast, there is no way to tell whether a given dream report, or dream reports in general, are good enough, and, despite encouraging functional magnetic resonance imaging studies hinting at dream content,[2] it is not clear that it will ever be possible to record dreams (or any other conscious experiences) with the same level of confidence and reliability that exists for most other measurements in the biologic sciences.

If we make the presumption that dream reports are a good enough representation of the mental experience during the prior period of sleep, the next question is how our data collection procedures affect the data. Table 54.1 outlines some of the parameters of dream collection that vary from one study to the next.

For each of these parameters, changes in the methodology of report collection are known to affect report content, with differences most notable in report frequency, length, bizarreness, and emotional content. But arguments continue in most cases over whether these differences reflect differences in dreaming or just in the accuracy and completeness of the dream reports. Even in the case of laboratory awakenings from REM and non–rapid eye movement (NREM) sleep, arguments continue over how much of the difference seen in reports from the two sleep stages reflects diminished dreaming, as opposed to diminished recall, in NREM. Because a given pair of studies can conceivably differ on all nine of these parameters (allowing more than 3,000 distinct protocols), it is not surprising that disputes over report frequencies, lengths, and features are as common as they are.

Table 54.1 Parameters of Dream Collection

Parameter	Common Values
Location	Home (monitored or unmonitored) Laboratory (monitored)
Awakening	Spontaneous Evoked
Timing	Morning Nocturnal
Sleep stage	REM N1 N2 N3
Time in stage	Constant Random Spontaneous Later in stage (esp. REM) later in the night
Time of night	Constant Variable
Nights	One Several (consecutive, fixed schedule, or ad libitum)
Report style	Written Audio recording
Probes	None Fixed Semistructured

REM, Rapid eye movement.

DESCRIPTION

A proper description of dreaming (defined now as sleep mentation) should describe the nature of the perceptions, thoughts, and emotions experienced by the dreamer and how these change with condition. Several chapters in this section focus on this question. Unfortunately, dreaming remains incompletely characterized even at the descriptive level. Most studies of dreaming focus on dream perceptions—the highly visual, narratively complex, and delusional hallucinations that we all think of when we think of dreaming. A smaller body of research has looked at the emotions of dreams, and a much smaller body has looked at the thoughts in dreams.

Even in the area of dream perceptions, what is studied varies dramatically: from word counts to counts of characters and objects; to classification of characters, objects, and actions as familiar or novel; to identification of bizarreness (on any of a number of ad hoc scales); to measures of "latent content." Thus it is not uncommon for two studies of "dream content" to lack a single outcome measure in common.

Individual and group differences also are poorly understood. Aside from clinical populations and very limited case studies (often from a psychoanalytic perspective), the best comparative data relate to dreaming in children and to the question of whether some individuals dream at all.

Probably the greatest amount of investigation of variability in dreaming relates to the question of REM versus NREM dreaming, and even here, huge disagreements exist. At this time, all that can be safely stated is that the two extreme positions, namely that dreaming occurs only during REM or, conversely, that there is no difference between REM and NREM dreaming, no longer appear to have any champions. But between these two extremes, almost every imaginable theory has been argued.

MECHANISMS

Efforts to explain the mechanisms that produce dreams date back to antiquity, when gods and indigestion were major contenders for the origins of dreams. Over the past 150 years, efforts at finding a brain or mind basis for dreaming have progressed slowly. At the moment, one can discern several schools of thought, which generally fall into the fields of neurophysiology, psychology, psychoanalysis, and, more recently, cognitive neuroscience. At their best, each of these takes an inclusive view, acknowledging the contributions of the other fields but focusing on their own. At their worst, they reject the usefulness of each other, with the usefulness of at least neurophysiology and psychoanalysis explicitly rejected by some groups. All of these, except psychoanalysis, are represented in the chapters that follow.

FUNCTIONS

Theories of the function of dreaming often are unclear as to what is actually being discussed, whether it is the phenomenologic experience of dreaming or the biologic processes that underlie it. This is only important because some researchers state their belief that dreaming per se has no function but that the biologic processes that underlie it have very important functions. For example, they would argue that the activation of neural networks within association cortex during REM might lead to important, long-term changes in network connectivity and also may fleetingly create a dream, but the dream and the process of dreaming itself are irrelevant to the production of these cortical modifications. Other researchers believe that the phenomenologic dream experience (with or without subsequent waking recall) is the critical element in the functionality of the dream and that the underlying biology is important only insofar as it is necessary to create the dream experience. Still others find the distinction unimportant or even meaningless.

This should not be surprising. It exactly parallels discussions of the functionality of consciousness. Philosophers and neurobiologists alike struggle to understand how to even think and talk about such functionality. Some reject any such functionality, others take it as a given, and others believe the distinction reflects a poorly formed question, that consciousness cannot be separated from its underlying brain basis. For the purpose of this section, we will collapse the two questions, talking about the function of dreaming and its underlying brain mechanisms as if they were interchangeable. While not claiming that they actually are interchangeable, it appears safe to say that we do not know how to measure their effects independently.

Theories of the function of dreaming (or lack thereof) go hand in hand with the approaches taken to studying the mechanisms underlying dreaming. Thus physiologic models tend to see little function in dreaming, whereas psychoanalytic models ascribe highly complex functions to dreaming. Psychological and cognitive neuroscience models tend to lie somewhere in between, ascribing various levels of complexity to dream function. But where function is ascribed to dreaming, it invariably involves the offline processing of emotions and memories, a function that has already been well substantiated for sleep more generally.

SUMMARY

In the end, we are left with a field that is a work in progress. There is no more than a hint of an even close-to-complete brain-based model for dream construction, and there is limited experimental evidence of a functional role for dreaming. With that being said, the past 10 years have shown a resurgence of interest and research on dreaming, and brain imaging studies during sleep have fueled the development of new models of dream construction and function. This section provides a snapshot of the state of the field at this time, a warning regarding the questions unanswered, and a guide to how dream research will progress over the next decade.

A complete reference list can be found online at ExpertConsult.com.

Chapter 55

Why We Dream

Robert Stickgold; Erin J. Wamsley

Chapter Highlights

- More than 60 years after the discovery of rapid eye movement sleep launched the field of sleep research, we still have surprisingly little insight into the most fundamental question about the sleeping mind: why do we dream?
- We suggest that dreaming at least partially reflects the activity of brain mechanisms performing off-line memory consolidation during sleep.
- We describe studies suggesting that a multiplicity of memory functions are reflected in the formal properties and content of conscious experience across stages of sleep and wakefulness. Together, these findings suggest both a mechanism and a function for dreaming.
- We present the NEXTUP model of dream mechanism and function, which argues that the conscious experience of dreams serves and evolutionary function.

The search for an understanding of dreaming is thousands of years old. During the past 125 years, three publications have formed the core of most of the scientific discussion of this question: Freud's *Interpretation of Dreams,* published at the end of the 19th century[1]; the report of a correlation between dreaming and the newly discovered rapid eye movement (REM) sleep in the 1950s[2]; and the proposal of the activation-synthesis model of dreams in the 1970s,[3] which argued that dreaming is initiated by random neural activity in the brainstem during REM sleep. Yet now, in the 21st century, there is little on which dream researchers agree.

One relatively new approach, and the focus of this chapter, is to consider dreaming within a larger neurocognitive framework of off-line memory consolidation during sleep. The rationale is that dreaming reflects the activity of the brain and that this activity necessarily includes the reactivation of memories and emotions from earlier experiences. Because neural activity in the brain is well known to induce plasticity, even during sleep,[4,5] neural activity associated with dreaming is likely to modify networks storing memories and emotions. Dreaming then becomes the conscious experiencing of these activated networks in the process of being modified.

BRAIN ACTIVITY DURING SLEEP

To understand how dreams might be produced and the functions they may serve, it is important to understand how brain activity in REM and non–rapid eye movement (NREM) sleep differs from that in wakefulness.[6] In the 1990s positron emission tomography (PET) studies initially demonstrated that, whereas regional cerebral blood flow is generally decreased during slow wave sleep relative to wakefulness, entry into REM sleep is associated with reactivation of some regions along with further deactivation of others.[7,8] This pattern suggested a shift in global brain function in REM sleep away from conscious executive control (decrease in dorsolateral prefrontal cortex activity) and toward hallucinatory (increased activity in sensory association cortices) and emotional (increased amygdala, anterior cingulate, and medial orbitofrontal cortex activity) processing, which might relate to the features of REM dreaming.[9,10]

Yet dreams are also commonly recalled from NREM sleep. Given this, the fundamental neural substrate for dream generation must be active in all stages of sleep. Subsequent imaging studies have been consistent with this notion, stressing that even NREM sleep is not a simple state of "inactivity": in fact, local activation during NREM sleep remains relatively high when controlling for the global decrease in signal, including within several memory-related areas.[11,12] Relative hippocampal activation, for example, has been reported to peak during slow wave sleep, exceeding even that seen during wakefulness.[12] Meanwhile, functional magnetic resonance imaging studies (with vastly superior temporal resolution compared with PET) confirm that brief, transient increases in local brain activation accompany sleep spindles and slow waves. For example, NREM sleep spindles have been associated with transient cortical activation increases in regions of the frontal lobe, as well as in the hippocampus,[13,14] and with increased functional connectivity between the hippocampus and neocortex.[15]

Memory-related brain activity can also be observed on the single-cell level in rats, as patterns of brain activity observed during waking appear to be "replayed" during NREM sleep (for the most part; one study has reported a similar effect during REM sleep[16]). Recordings of single-unit activity demonstrate that sequences of neuronal firing seen as rats explore an environment are later statistically reiterated during sleep.[17,18] First observed in the hippocampus, this effect also occurs in cortical regions.[19]

Similarly, in humans, increasing evidence suggests that patterns of brain activation during the learning of a task are selectively replayed during subsequent sleep, both in REM and NREM sleep.[12,20,21] This reactivation of patterned activity in the sleeping brain is thought to support the consolidation of memory during sleep. Indeed, reactivation has been reported to promote the formation of dendritic spines,[22] and disrupting hippocampal activity during reactivation impairs learning.[23] The discovery that brain networks involved in prior waking experience are reactivated during later sleep has been paralleled by strong evidence from the human behavioral literature that memory consolidation is facilitated by sleep.

MEMORY CONSOLIDATION DURING SLEEP

One interpretation of neural changes during sleep is that they reflect a *homeostatic* process working to restore the brain to its state at the start of the previous day. These "rest" or "restorative" models of sleep argue that sleep serves primarily to reverse deleterious changes that inevitably accrue across the day. A current example of such theories is the synaptic homeostasis model of sleep function.[24] In contrast, a *progressive* model interprets the activation of neural networks during sleep as reflecting *off-line processing* of information obtained during the prior day—consolidating, integrating, and sometimes even selectively reversing changes that occurred during waking.[25] Dreaming, as well, may serve either a *homeostatic* or *progressive* function. Freud, for example, proposed a restorative model of dreaming, specifically considering but then rejecting any progressive model.[1] In contrast, others have questioned[26] or rejected[27] the notion of any sort of evolutionary function for dreams at all.

Although the question of the function of dreaming remains unresolved, there is a growing consensus that sleep serves a function of off-line memory consolidation (see the reviews by Diekelmann and Born[28] and by Stickgold and Walker[25]). As with dreaming, memory consolidation appears to vary across sleep stages. In humans, hippocampus-dependent memory has most strongly been associated with slow wave sleep.[29-31] In contrast, other forms of memory have variously been associated with REM sleep (e.g., emotional memory[32,33] and creative problem solving[34]) or stage 2 sleep (e.g., motor learning[35,36]). The particular model of dream function presented here, then, proposes that dreaming relates to this memory function of sleep, participating in, or at least reflecting, the processing of memories for recent daytime experiences.

SLEEP STAGES AND DREAM CONTENT

If memory processing is differentially activated across sleep stages, and dreaming at least parallels and possibly contributes to these memory processes, one would expect to see changes in the content of dream reports collected from different sleep states. In its simplest form, this is exactly what is seen. Reports are more frequent after awakenings from REM sleep,[37-39] although both REM and NREM sleep reports are more common when awakenings occur later in the night.[39] Reports obtained from REM tend to be longer, more vivid, more story-like, and more bizarre than NREM reports.[26,39] Whereas it has been suggested that some of these differences merely reflect poorer recall after NREM sleep awakenings, little objective evidence supports such a claim, and other REM and NREM sleep differences are not amenable to such an explanation. For example, hallucinations are more prevalent in reports from REM sleep, whereas directed thinking is more common in NREM sleep, a pattern that cannot be explained simply by poorer recall from one stage or another.[40]

Even at this level of analysis, there is the suggestion of homology between dream content and memory function in sleep. In REM sleep, dreams are hallucinatory, emotional, and narrative, with frequent fictive movements (for review, see Hobson and colleagues[26]). Congruently, REM sleep is thought to facilitate consolidation of visual-perceptual and emotional memories.[41,42] In contrast, NREM sleep (particularly slow wave sleep) has been associated with sleep-dependent improvement on a range of hippocampus-dependent tasks, including the memorization of declarative information[29,43] and navigation through spatial environments.[44] Paralleling this mnemonic function, dream reports from NREM sleep tend to be more "realistic" and draw more on material from recent episodic memory.[45] There are exceptions (e.g., improvement on a commonly used motor task is associated with stage 2 sleep,[36,46] but REM sleep dreams are more motoric), but the argument can be made that differences in memory functions across sleep stages are generally reflected in differences in dream content.

DREAMS AND MEMORY SYSTEMS

Most models of dreaming implicitly assume that dreams are constructed from our memories, but they also recognize that this construction need not involve the transparent, direct incorporation of specific memories into the dream scenario. Freud, for example, emphasized that actual memories, events, and their associated emotions underwent "condensation" and "displacement" before appearing in dreams. Whereas he elaborated a complex theory of "dream work" to explain these alterations, modern cognitive neuroscience allows the formation of much simpler, evidence-based explanations. Specifically, dream construction does not include the veridical replay of complete "episodic" memories, whose recall is normally mediated by the hippocampus in waking life. Instead, dreams appear to be constructed from unbound *fragments* of various recent episodes,[47] intermixed with remote memories, semantic memories (facts and general information), and representational memories (sensorimotor images), all stored in and directly accessible in the neocortex.

Within dream content, the distribution of these various types of memory sources appears to differ by sleep stage. Subjects identify episodic memory sources for dream elements more frequently after awakenings from NREM sleep (including sleep onset) than after REM sleep awakenings.[45] This differential rate parallels the decline in directed thinking reported as subjects move from sleep onset to stage 2 NREM sleep and then into REM sleep.[40] At the same time, the frequency of "generic semantic memory sources" is greatest in REM sleep.[45]

Episodic memories are clearly a *source* for the construction of dreams in both REM and NREM sleep, but these episodes are not "replayed" during dreaming in their original form. In one study, subjects identified waking antecedents for 364 dream elements in 299 dream reports. When the extent of congruence between these dreams and their purported waking sources were analyzed, only 3% of dream elements were judged to have the same location, characters, and actions as the identified waking memory source.[47] For this small percentage of reports, dream content may reflect the same hippocampus-mediated process of episodic recall that characterizes waking recall, allowing identification of particular episodes as the source of their dream elements. What, then, is the basis of this association in the remaining 97% of dream elements? The features that showed highest congruence between dream element and putative waking source were theme, emotion, and characters.[47] Whereas the last of these is consistent with the reiteration of a specific episode, the first two are decidedly not. Thematic congruence might instead reflect the activity of nonhippocampal semantic memory systems. As discussed later, evidence from the dreams of amnesiac patients also suggests that the hippocampus is not required for the brain to generate dreams related to recent experience. Yet at the same time, there is increasingly strong evidence that the hippocampal memory system is active during sleep[12,15,17] and may contribute to dreaming in healthy individuals.[48] Next we turn our attention to the activity of hippocampus-dependent declarative memory systems in sleep.

DREAMING AND DECLARATIVE MEMORY CONSOLIDATION DURING SLEEP

A mounting body of evidence suggests that sleep is critically involved in a wide range of types of memory consolidation, ranging from the consolidation of simple visual and motor skills to the consolidation, integration, and extraction of complex, hippocampus-dependent declarative memories.[25]

Several studies have employed the "paired associate" learning paradigm to assess the contribution of sleep to declarative memory performance. In this task, subjects are presented with a series of word pairs, and after the entire list has been presented, they are shown the first word of each pair and asked to recall the second. An early study by Plihal and Born[29] suggested that the deeper, slow wave sleep of NREM sleep early in the night is particularly beneficial for the consolidation of such word pair memory compared with the benefits of wake or late-night, REM-rich sleep. Subsequent studies have consistently confirmed that a period of sleep, relative to wakefulness, benefits the retention of this type of memory and that experimental enhancement of slow wave activity enhances word pair recall.[49,50]

Although most of the literature on sleep and declarative memory focuses on the memorization of verbal or visual stimuli, other research highlights the role of sleep in *reorganization and transformation* of declarative memories across time. For example, numerous studies have now reported that sleep aids in the extraction of generalizations, integration of information, and arrival at creative insights.[25]

In sum, a rapidly accumulating body of research demonstrates that complex, hippocampus-dependent learning is processed during human sleep. Might this reactivation and transformation of declarative memory be expressed within the content of dreams? In partial answer to this question, we discuss evidence that intensive, engaging learning experiences are reliably expressed in the content of dreams during post-training sleep.

INCORPORATION OF WAKING EVENTS INTO DREAMS

Although many studies have described the spontaneous incorporation of everyday waking events into dreams, fewer have successfully influenced dream content by experimentally manipulating waking experience (for review, see Wamsley and Stickgold[51]). Those that have succeeded in doing so have most commonly involved the manipulation of hypnagogic dreams, which occur at sleep onset.[52-55] In one early study,[52] subjects played the video game *Tetris* for several hours across 2 or 3 days. Three groups of subjects were studied: 12 subjects with no prior *Tetris* experience, 10 with extensive *Tetris* experience (experts), and 5 with dense amnesia with extensive medial temporal lobe damage resulting from anoxia or encephalitis. The game involves rotating geometric blocks as they "fall" from the top of the computer screen, with the goal of fitting the pieces together like a puzzle. On each day of game play, subjects were awakened repeatedly during the first hour of their regular overnight sleep and asked to report any thoughts, feelings, or images from the prior sleep period. The majority of participants (64%) reported instances of game imagery during the hypnagogic period, with game images reported in 7.2% of their reports.

Subjects reported remarkably similar imagery, seeing *Tetris* pieces falling in front of their eyes, occasionally rotating and fitting them into empty spaces. Among the 27 reports of imagery, there were no reports of seeing the larger picture surrounding the play window, the scoreboard, or the keyboard or of typing on the keyboard. There were only two reports of seeing a computer screen and none of seeing the desk or room. Thus the imagery was limited to those aspects of the experience that were most salient and to which subjects presumably paid the most attention. Again we see that dreams are not exact "replays" of waking experience but rather are composed of *fragments* of recent episodic material, often intermingled with other content.

Remarkably, three of five patients with amnesia also reported hypnagogic *Tetris* images, despite being unable to recall playing the game before or after the night's sleep. This observation clearly indicates that the hippocampal memory system, which supports the encoding and recall of episodic memories during wakefulness, is *not* necessary for the construction of sleep-onset imagery related to recent experience. Although unable to recall having played the game (or even to recognize the experimenter from session to session), patients nonetheless reported, for example, "little squares coming down on a screen."

An additional point is that two of the five *Tetris* experts reported *Tetris* images explicitly described as being from earlier versions of the game, which they had not played in the last year. One subject reported imagery from a game version that she had not played since high school, 5 years earlier. Thus sleep-onset dream imagery need not be determined only by recent sensory input but additionally can incorporate older, strongly associated memories. Here again, we see that rather than an exact reiteration of waking experience, dreams incorporate salient elements related to recent experience into a novel scenario.

This fact is driven home even more forcefully by a study in which subjects were taught three nonsense sentences across a night, one immediately before going to sleep and two more after awakening from REM sleep.[56] The nonsense sentences (translated from the original Italian) are as follows:

- In the bathroom the raven is painting a fish on a radio and spinning a bust on the custard.
- In the embers a poster is fining a parcel along the bridge and betting a tooth in the game.
- In a liter a cock is tricking a ruble from a palm and nursing a ball in a tub.

Subjects were instructed to memorize the sentences and repeat them back as accurately as possible. When dream reports were collected after the subjects were awakened from the next REM period, dream content was frequently judged as related to the previously memorized sentence. For example, after hearing the first sentence, with its reference to "painting a fish," one subject reported "walking with a friend on the seashore."

Of course, such apparent associations can be spurious. Indeed, when judges scored dream reports from a control night, before subjects had heard any of the sentences, apparent associations were again found. However, the experimental design allowed use of these rates of "pseudo-incorporation," obtained from the control night, to correct for such spurious associations. When this was done, more than one-third of all REM sleep reports collected on the experimental night contained actual incorporations of elements from the learned sentence (72% of reports on the experimental night versus 39% on the control night).

Once again, we see here that dream incorporations are never in the form of an exact replay of the waking episode, in this case, a report of memorizing a sentence. Instead, the brain seems to simply extract specific elements of the memorized sentence (single words or phrases) and to incorporate them into an unrelated scenario.

In another study, after training intensively on the downhill skiing arcade game *Alpine Racer II,* 65% of subjects reported images from the game in their subsequent hypnagogic dreams.[54] These sleep-onset dream reports sometimes included places where they frequently crashed or a particularly steep slope, but the game images were again devoid of their original context, always being reported without the arcade game itself being seen or themselves playing it.[54] In agreement with the findings of the *Tetris* study, subjects with prior downhill skiing experience also reported seeing images related not to the arcade game but to actual skiing experiences from their past.

In the case of *Alpine Racer II,* the nature of game-related sleep-onset imagery also became more abstracted from the original experience across the course of the night. A subset of participants were allowed 2 hours of uninterrupted sleep at the start of each night before being awakened and then, as they fell back asleep, reporting hypnagogic imagery at this later time. In this "delayed awakening" protocol, subjects reported dramatically fewer skiing images. Instead, they reported imagery more indirectly related to the game, for example, of "falling down a hill" or of "moving through some kind of forest" with their "entire upper body incredibly straight."[54] Thus imagery related to recent experience appears to become more abstracted from the original memory source later in the night, a phenomenon also suggested in the transformation of "fish" into "seashore" in the study described previously.[56]

Finally, there is evidence that the incorporation of recent experiences into dream content reflects the process of memory consolidation. When newly learned information is incorporated into dream content, even in abstracted form, this is associated with enhanced memory for that information. De Koninck and colleagues, for example, examined dreams of verbal learning, exploring dream content as a corollary of language learning in an academic setting.[57] Among students enrolled in a French immersion class, those with the strongest language acquisition across the 6-week course incorporated French into dream content more often than students who were less successful in the class. Similarly, our own laboratory has demonstrated that dreaming of a virtual maze navigation task is associated with enhanced consolidation of spatial memory both across a nap[44] and across a full night of sleep.[58]

EMOTION IN THE SLEEPING BRAIN

Dreaming during REM sleep is commonly associated with the experience of intense emotion.[26,39] As such, literature suggesting that sleep supports the reactivation and transformation of *emotional* memories, in particular, may be relevant to our understanding of the dreaming process. In one study, the recall of emotionally charged stories was selectively enhanced after REM sleep. In this protocol, subjects learned both neutral and emotional texts before sleep. Relative to wakefulness, periods of posttraining sleep rich in rapid eye movements were particularly beneficial for these memories.[33] Furthermore, only memory for the *emotional* texts benefited from this REM-rich sleep , but not the neutral material. Remarkably, when the same research participants were again tested 4 years later, the beneficial influence of REM sleep versus wakefulness on memory for the original emotional (but not neutral) texts was maintained.[59] Similarly, research from Payne and colleagues has demonstrated that sleep selectively enhances memory for emotional objects in the foreground of visual scenes, suggesting that sleep selects the information most relevant to an individual for further processing while allowing memory for less salient aspects of an experience to decay.[60,61] These observations are also in line with other literature suggesting that sleep modulates emotional responsiveness more generally.[62]

The most well-known example of emotional processing during sleep is perhaps also the least well understood. This is the phenomenon of "sleeping on a problem," involving situations in which a difficult decision must be made. Anecdotally, people report going to bed at night with such a problem on their mind and waking up the next morning with a clear solution in their mind. There are several features of this phenomenon that are worth noting. First, it is a remarkably robust effect, with most people casually surveyed believing that, as often as not, it successfully yields results over a single night. Second, the decision normally becomes apparent without an explicit rationale. People report knowing at a "gut level" that they have come to the correct decision but without a clear and rational justification for it. Third, there is usually considerable confidence that the decision reached is the correct one and little sense that further deliberation would be of any added benefit. At the same time, the process does not appear to be useful for the recall of forgotten information, such as a phone number or address. Rather, it serves to analyze available information to come to a decision on the basis of some unknown algorithm that appropriately weights the relevant information. Whereas these features of the process are clear from anecdotal observations, few objective studies of the phenomenon have been made. Still, several studies do suggest that laboratory-induced problems are solved more easily following a period of sleep compared with a period of waking incubation.[34,63,64]

A NEUROCOGNITIVE MODEL OF DREAM CONSTRUCTION AND FUNCTION

When memory networks are activated in the brain, they are inevitably altered. This is one of the most striking findings of cognitive neuroscience in the past decade. Indeed, it might be true that no neural circuits are ever activated without being at least subtly altered. This would be true whether the activity of a particular circuit is perceived by the conscious mind or not. Thus every time a young child hears a sentence spoken, neural circuits are activated that over time will extract rules of grammar that will allow her to speak with nearly perfect grammar without explicitly knowing those rules or even that they exist. This is a hallmark of the brain's construction—that it extracts similarities and rules without conscious knowledge that they exist. In addition, studies of mathematical insight[65] and transitive inference[66] have shown that sleep dramatically facilitates this process.

Of course, the activation of memory networks also can be accompanied by conscious experience, as is what is happening as you read and consider the arguments presented here. As there are distinct memory systems in the brain, some accessible to consciousness and some not, so also are there distinct mechanisms for activating and manipulating these memories, some of which are accessible to consciousness and some of which are not. So it should come as no surprise when we suggest, first, that dreaming must inevitably alter the memories accessed in the process of dream construction and, perhaps more important, that dreaming may be a byproduct of mechanisms that evolved to facilitate sleep-dependent memory consolidation and integration.

As in wake, these mechanisms often activate systems that remain outside of our awareness. This perhaps is the case when simple perceptual or motor skills are consolidated during sleep. At other times, the sleep-dependent reactivation of memory networks might occur in a manner that brings the patterns of activation in these networks into conscious awareness. Thus, after training on a hippocampus-dependent virtual maze navigation task, participants dream of the maze, observing the flow of images, thoughts, and feelings that occur during this memory reactivation process, which ultimately correlates with improved memory performance following sleep.[58,67] Critically, we do not necessarily *see* the changes in the memory systems that result from this process, and thus we see the content of dreams but neither their underlying purpose nor their ultimate effects. In short, the content of recalled dreams may not in itself reveal any obvious function; as we saw earlier, dreams typically do not appear to be a rehearsal of things that are important to remember.

The question of the function of dreaming may be reducible to a question of the function of the sleep-dependent memory processes that result in the conscious experience of dreaming. Accumulating evidence suggests that sleep has, as one of its most critical functions, the incremental modification of cortical networks. Such a model has been put forward in some detail elsewhere.[5,25,28] Because sleep has been shown to enhance (1) the experientially controlled modification of visual circuitry during early development[68]; (2) visual,[42] auditory,[69] and motor skill learning[35]; (3) emotional memories[41]; (4) declarative and hippocampus-dependent memories[43,70]; and (5) creative insight,[34] it is clear that sleep's role in memory consolidation spans an impressively wide range of brain circuits and functions. The question of dream function now becomes two questions: (1) For which of these circuits and functions does activity during sleep enter our conscious awareness? (2) Does this conscious awareness in turn have an effect on these brain circuits? As described earlier, there is evidence that the consolidation of memory in the sleeping brain does, in some cases, directly affect dream content. However, there are still no ways to address the question of whether actual conscious experience can ever alter brain activity, either in waking or in sleep.

NEXTUP: A NEW MODEL OF DREAM CONSTRUCTION AND FUNCTION

More recently, a new model of dream construction and function has been proposed, which argues that the conscious experiencing of dreams is necessary for dreaming to serve its evolutionary function. The model, called Network Exploration To Understand Possibilities (NEXTUP),[71] is built on the ideas presented in the previous section.

NEXTUP proposes that dreaming serves as an extension of the sleep-dependent memory processing described previously, an extension that shifts from mechanisms similar to convergent thinking to those of divergent thinking. It differs from previously described forms of sleep-dependent processing, which served to strengthen existing memories or find convergent descriptors of previously learned material in the form of gist, generalizations, or rule discovery. Instead, NEXTUP argues that the function of dreaming is to identify associated memories that are of potential use for interpreting previous waking events and understanding how such events can most effectively be used in guiding future behavior.

Previous work has suggested that the unique neurochemical and neurophysiological state of REM sleep, including the cessation of norepinephrine release[72] and consequent increase in signal-to-noise ratios in cortical neurons,[73] facilitates the discovery of normally weak associations.[74] According to NEXTUP, during sleep, such weak associates of current concerns are identified and then incorporated into dream content in order to permit testing of their potential usefulness. When associations pass this test, their links to current concerns are strengthened.

The core of NEXTUP is this "testing mechanism" and its dependency on the conscious experiencing of dreams. Antonio Damasio[75] has argued that waking consciousness offers two key capabilities to otherwise nonconscious organisms—the ability to construct narratives and to feel emotions. Damasio proposes that without the ability to construct narratives, humans would not be able to imagine the future and therefore couldn't plan ahead. Furthermore, he argues that narratives cannot be constructed outside of consciousness and that consciousness is critical for such planning. Consciously feeling our emotional responses as these narratives play out in our mind then becomes the basis for evaluating these imagined scenarios and determining whether or not such future actions would be to our advantage.

NEXTUP incorporates Damasio's arguments in its description of dreaming. Planning and evaluation during sleep, the model argues, similarly involves narrative construction and emotional evaluation to determine the possible usefulness of discovered associations between older memories with current concerns. Since these processes can only be performed within consciousness, the construction and evaluation of narratives during sleep requires that the brain dream.

Dreaming differs from planning during wake in several ways, especially during REM. The first way, as described previously, is the bias toward incorporating relatively weak associations into the dream narrative. But this is driven further toward unexpected and potentially creative narratives by (1) the lack of incorporation of the related waking concern into the narrative, perhaps due to the inhibition of hippocampal outflow to the cortex during REM[76]; (2) the inhibition of dorsolateral prefrontal cortex (DLPFC) during REM,[77] which would impair normal rational thinking, executive decision-making, and impulse control, perhaps allowing the development of more fanciful and bizarre narratives; and (3) increased limbic activation,[77] which would presumably enhance the emotional response to the ongoing dream narrative. Importantly, the evaluation of any potential value of a discovered association does not proceed to a final decision as to its value, perhaps because of the shutdown of DLPFC and norepinephrine release, the latter of which normally increases prior to any decision-making. Instead, strong emotional response to the narrative, positive or negative, is taken as evidence of the potential usefulness of the association and leads to a strengthening of connections between the waking concern and the newly discovered associate, making it available for later waking consideration.

NEXTUP proposes distinct functions for dreams in different sleep stages (see the section Sleep Stages and Dream Content). N2 and N3 dreams, which are known to have their waking sources in more recent and more episodic memories than REM dreams,[45] are thought to identify more recent and strongly associated memories, ones perhaps more likely to be of use, but at the same time, less likely to offer creative and groundbreaking solutions. In contrast, N1 "dreams," which often lack both narrative development and the embodiment of the dreamer and are often transparently related to events of the previous day, are thought to act by identifying current waking concerns that would profit from later processing by NREM and REM dreams. This view of dream function across sleep stages is consonant with the alternation of sleep stages across the night and with their slow shift from NREM toward stronger and longer REM periods, allowing the brain to consider more and more weakly and potentially creative associations.

Taken as a whole, NEXTUP offers an explanation of the evolutionary function, as well as neurochemical, neurophysiological and cognitive neuroscience mechanisms, of dreaming. It concludes that dreaming is not merely an epiphenomenal correlate of memory processing during sleep, but a unique form of processing that requires conscious awareness of the narrative progression to achieve its evolutionary function. Only time will tell us whether NEXTUP is an accurate representation of what dreams actually are, or whether, in the end, it's just another dream.

CLINICAL PEARL

Emerging data suggest that dream experiences reflect the off-line consolidation, integration, and analysis of recent memories during sleep. As such, studying dreaming may facilitate a greater understanding of the sleep-related processes underlying long-term memory formation, as well as the dysfunction of these processes seen in pathologic conditions such as post-traumatic stress disorder.

SUMMARY

We propose that dreaming is simply the conscious perception of the stream of images, thoughts, and feelings evoked in the brain by one or more of the many forms of off-line learning and memory processing that occur during sleep. At the same time, it reflects one of the most sophisticated forms of processing that the brain performs: the analysis and interpretation of the events of our lives in a manner that provides meaning to these events and can guide our future behavior.

ACKNOWLEDGMENTS

Preparation of this chapter was supported by NSF grant BCS-1849026, BIAL Foundation Bursaries Award 211/16, and NIMH grant MH48832.

SELECTED READINGS

Baylor GW, Cavallero C. Memory sources associated with REM and NREM dream reports throughout the night: a new look at the data. *Sleep*. 2001;24(2):165–170.

Blagrove M, Fouquet NC, Henley-Einion JA, et al. Assessing the dream-lag effect for REM and NREM stage 2 dreams. *PLoS ONE*. 2011;6(10):e26708.

Eichenlaub J-B, Cash SS, Blagrove M. Daily life experiences in dreams and sleep-dependent memory consolidation. In *Cognitive Neuroscience of Memory Consolidation*. Springer; 2017:161–172.

Fosse MJ, Fosse R, Hobson JA, Stickgold RJ. Dreaming and episodic memory: a functional dissociation? *J Cogn Neurosci*. 2003;15(1):1–9.

Graveline YM, Wamsley EJ. Dreaming and waking cognition. *Trans Issues Psychol Sci*. 2015;1:97.

Hobson JA, McCarley RW. The brain as a dream state generator: an activation-synthesis hypothesis of the dream process. *Am J Psychiatry*. 1977;134(12):1335–1348.

Lewis PA, Knoblich G, Poe G. How memory replay in sleep boosts creative problem-solving. *Trends Cogn Sci*. 2018;22(6):491–503. https://doi.org/10.1016/j.tics.2018.03.009.

Malinowski JE, Horton CL. Dreams reflect nocturnal cognitive processes: Early-night dreams are more continuous with waking life, and late-night dreams are more emotional and hyperassociative. *Conscious Cogn*. 2021;88:103071.

Nielsen TA, Stenstrom P. What are the memory sources of dreaming? *Nature*. 2005;437(7063):1286–1289. https://doi.org/10.1038/nature04288.

Nir Y, Tononi G. Dreaming and the brain: from phenomenology to neurophysiology. *Trends Cogn Sci*. 2010;14(2):88–100.

Payne JD, Nadel L. Sleep, dreams, and memory consolidation: the role of the stress hormone cortisol. *Learn Mem*. 2004;11(6):671–678.

Payne JD, Kensinger EA. Stress, sleep, and the selective consolidation of emotional memories. *Curr Opin Behav Sci*. 2018;19:36–43.

Stickgold R, Malia A, Maguire D, Roddenberry D, O'Connor M. Replaying the game: hypnagogic images in normals and amnesics. *Science*. 2000;290(5490):350–353.

Wamsley EJ. Dreaming and offline memory consolidation. *Curr Neurol Neurosci Rep*. 2014;14(3). https://doi.org/10.1007/s11910-013-0433-5.

Wamsley EJ, Tucker M, Payne JD, et al. Dreaming of a learning task is associated with enhanced sleep-dependent memory consolidation. *Curr Biol*. 2010;20(9):850–855.

Wang J, Zemmelman SE, Hong D Feng X, Shen H, Does COVID-19 impact the frequency of threatening events in dreams? An exploration of pandemic dreaming in light of contemporary dream theories. *Conscious Cogn*. 2021;87:103051.

Zadra A, Stickgold R. *When Brains Dream*. New York: W.W. Norton; 2021.

A complete reference list can be found online at ExpertConsult.com.

Chapter 56

Dream Content: Quantitative Findings

Antonio Zadra; G. William Domhoff

Chapter Highlights

- Researchers and clinicians have long been fascinated by the content of dreams, and considerable progress has been made in the systematic study of dream content. The most frequently used methods for collecting dream reports, laboratory awakenings, home dream logs, questionnaires, and most recent dreams collected in group settings all have their uses and inherent advantages and disadvantages. In addition, reliable, comprehensive, and validated instruments for the actual analysis of dream content reports have been developed, and complementary tools are now available to all researchers on the internet.
- Quantitative data on dream content from laboratory and nonlaboratory settings together generally depict a reliable picture about the nature of dream content in the general adult population. Both data sets indicate that, for the most part, dreams are a reasonable simulation of waking life characters, social interactions, activities, and settings and that dreams show systematic relationships to various dimensions of the dreamer's waking life but not to day-to-day events.
- Results from a variety of studies show that developmental changes occur in dream content until the ages of 14 to 15 years, when dream content becomes generally stable and consistent throughout adulthood and old age. In addition, clinically oriented investigations suggest that affect and social interactions are two key dream content variables that are most strongly related to measures of psychological well-being.
- The findings presented in this chapter have several implications for theories of dreaming and provide convincing evidence that dreams are a unique and meaningful product of the mind.

INTRODUCTION

Researchers and clinicians have long been fascinated by the content of dreams. Many contemporary dream researchers suggest that dreaming is functionally significant and may subserve a biologically important function. However, some argue that dreams are a byproduct of neurophysiologic activity during rapid eye movement (REM) sleep and have no value in and of themselves, even though evidence suggests they have psychological meaning. More recently, a neurocognitive perspective on dreams, which argues that dreaming is based in activated portions of the default network during sleep onset and sleep, claims that dreaming is a psychologically meaningful byproduct of the natural selection for waking imagination that is based in the default network.

There is no consensus on what distinguishes "dreaming" from other cognitive processes, such as thinking or daydreaming, nor on what constitutes "dream content." Interdisciplinary groups from the International Association for the Study of Dreams and the American Academy of Sleep Medicine concluded that "a single definition for dreaming is most likely impossible given the wide spectrum of fields engaged in the study of dreaming, and the diversity in currently applied definitions."[1] However, others now argue that dreaming is a form of embodied simulation in which an experiential sense augments the simulations that often occur during waking mind-wandering.[2] Thus, depending on one's perspective, *dreaming* can be synonymous with the term *sleep mentation*, which refers to the experience of *any mental activity* (e.g., perceptions, bodily feelings, thoughts) during sleep, or can be restricted to more elaborate, vivid, and story-like experiences recalled upon awakening. Using a broadly inclusive versus more restrictive definition of dreaming has a direct and significant impact on the nature and sense of empirical data and theoretical modeling in the field.[3]

In this chapter, the term *dream* is conceptualized as having four interrelated meanings. First, a dream is a form of thinking during sleep that occurs when there is a certain, as yet undetermined, minimal level of brain activation in a context in which external stimuli are typically occluded and the cognitive system that keeps us aware of our surroundings is shut down. Second, and as just mentioned, a dream is something people experience as a series of actual events (e.g., a sequence of perceptions, thoughts, and emotions) because the thought patterns simulate waking reality in a manner called *embodied simulation*. Third, a dream is what people remember on awakening, so it is a memory of the dreaming experience. Finally, a dream is the spoken or written report provided to investigators based on the memory of the dreaming experience. The empirical studies discussed in this chapter reveal that the events of a dream always include the dreamer as an observer or participant and that they almost always include at least one other character besides the dreamer (either a person or an animal). In addition, the dreamer or the other characters in the dreams are invariably engaged in one activity or another (e.g., looking, walking, running) or a social interaction. Thus the sense of participation in an event, along with characters, activities, and social interactions, is what distinguishes dreams from the more fleeting, fragmented, and thought-like forms of sleep mentation.

METHODS FOR COLLECTING DREAM REPORTS

Researchers never study dream experiences directly. Instead, they collect and have access to descriptions of the experience, the dream report. The nature and content of the verbal or written report obtained can be influenced by a number of factors. These include the setting (e.g., home, laboratory, classroom, psychotherapy), method of awakening (e.g., spontaneous, induced), time of awakening (e.g., early, middle, or late in the sleep period), sleep stage before awakening (e.g., REM, non–rapid eye movement [NREM] sleep), type of collection instrument (e.g., questionnaire, dream journal), reporting method (e.g., written by the subject, written by the experimenter, audio recording), instructions provided (e.g., report anything that was going through your mind before your awakening, report any dreams you remember having before your awakening), probes on reported content (none, fixed, or semistructured questions), interpersonal situation (e.g., none, reporting directly to an experimenter, clinician), time delay between when the dream was experienced and when it is reported, study duration, and subject characteristics (e.g., sex, personality, habitual level of dream recall).

The degree to which the content of dream reports is influenced by these various factors either individually or in combination varies as a function of the collection method used. The principal sources of dream reports are the sleep laboratory, home dream journals, questionnaires, and classroom or other group settings where a most recent dream report can be collected from everyone willing to participate.

Sleep Laboratory

Sleep laboratories are an excellent source of dream reports because they provide the opportunity for collecting a representative sample of a subject's dream life, both within and across nights, under controlled conditions. Awakening subjects from several REM or NREM periods results in the collection of dream reports that otherwise may have been forgotten by the participants on normal awakening in the morning. On the other hand, frequent awakenings can be difficult for participants, and factors such as sleep inertia and one's desire to return to sleep may interfere with the quality of the dream reports. However, a complementary cued morning report of dreams recalled during the night can yield new and reliable information as to the dreams' original contents.[4]

The main problem with the laboratory collection of dream reports is that it is a very costly and time-consuming process. Furthermore, some types of dreams, including nightmares and sexual dreams, rarely occur in the sleep laboratory. In addition, up to 20% of laboratory REM dream reports reflect direct incorporations of the laboratory environment, even when collected over several consecutive nights. For our purposes, the most important outcome of detailed laboratory studies is that they provide a baseline for assessing the quality of dream reports collected by other methods.

Dream Logs

Prospective daily logs are used by a large number of dream researchers, even though they require a greater investment of time and resources than do questionnaires. In fields such as nightmare research, home journals are considered the gold standard for the measurement of nightmare frequency.[5] Prospective logs can take two different forms. The first is the checklist format in which participants indicate if there was dream recall and, if so, the number and type of dreams recalled (e.g., nightmare). The second is the narrative log, in which participants are requested to provide a complete written transcript of each dream recalled. Findings from one comparison[6] of these two methods of data collection suggest that narrative-log participants, having a more time-consuming task, do not take the required time to provide a narrative of all of their recalled dreams. Instead, they may choose to focus on their more memorable, exciting, or salient dreams. By comparison, people completing checklist logs would be more likely to record all of their dreams (including relatively banal or poorly recalled ones) because each entry is just as quickly completed regardless of dream type.

Although writing down one's dreams remains the most frequently used method to collect dream content, participants may also use dicta phones or cell phones to dictate their reports. This approach may be particularly useful with children and younger adolescents. It also proved very useful in a study of blind participants.[7]

Questionnaires

In questionnaire studies, participants' retrospective self-reported information concerning their dream experiences is viewed as a modest but acceptable way of assessing different aspects of the dream experiences themselves. However, research suggests they are of limited value in assessing the frequency or content of dreams.

Three types of information are generally collected. First, subjects can be queried about the frequency with which they experience certain kinds of dreams (e.g., everyday dreams, nightmares) over a determined period of time. There is increasing evidence, however, that data obtained with retrospective estimates differ considerably from daily prospective home logs and that correlates of retrospective measures of dream recall should not be assumed to be correlates of log measures of dream recall.[8-10]

A second kind of information sometimes elicited by questionnaires focuses on specific dimensions of people's dreams or their beliefs about their general dream life. This approach assumes that there exists a valid relationship between self-reported information on the content of one's everyday dreams and the dream experiences themselves. However, comparisons of self-report measures and log-based data indicate that this assumption may be unwarranted.[11,12]

Third, questionnaires are used to investigate whether participants ever experienced a specific type of dream and, if so, to report the most recent occurrence as best recalled. This approach allows for the investigation of certain types of dreams that, because of their infrequency, are difficult to capture in laboratory settings or with home dream logs (e.g., recurrent dreams, flying dreams) or dreams that stand out in the person's past (e.g., earliest dream recalled, most terrifying nightmare). Although useful in some research settings, the resulting dream content findings must be treated cautiously because of possible memory distortions and biases.

In sum, although some dream questionnaires have good internal consistency and test-retest reliability,[13] studies of their relationship to dream content and frequency obtained from dream journals reveal important discrepancies and raise questions as to their validity.

Classroom and Other Group Settings

Settings such as classrooms provide an objective and structured context for the efficient and inexpensive collection of dream reports. Anonymous participants are instructed to write down the most recent dream that they can recall on a standardized form while revealing only basic background information such as age and sex. The most recent dream method has been used with children as young as ages 10 to 11 years in different countries with surprisingly similar cross-national results.[14] The main drawback with this method is that there is not usually time to collect any personality or cognitive measures about the people providing the reports.

ANALYZING DREAM CONTENT: INSTRUMENTS AND ISSUES

Most past dream research used either rating scales at the ordinal level of measurement ("more" or "less" of a characteristic) or discrete categories at the nominal level of measurement (an element is "present" or "absent"). Rating scales are most useful for those characteristics of dream reports that have degrees of intensity in waking life. Cohen[15] reports that four dimensions of dream salience can be rated by participants in dream studies: emotionality, bizarreness, activity, and vividness. A factor analysis of the ratings of 100 REM dream reports suggests that rating scales boil down to five basic dimensions: (1) degree of vividness and distortion, (2) degree of hostility and anxiety, (3) degree of initiative and striving, (4) level of activity, and (5) amount of sexuality.[16] However, it is often difficult to establish reliability with some scales, and much of the specific information in dream reports is lost or unused with general rating scales.

Of the nearly 150 dream rating and content analysis scales reviewed by Winget and Kramer,[17] the Hall and Van de Castle (HVDC) coding system[18] is the best validated and remains the most widely used system for analyzing dream content. The HVDC system, which was used in many of the findings presented in the rest of this chapter, rests on the nominal level of measurement and uses percentages and ratios as content indicators that can correct for the varying length of dream reports from sample to sample. The dream reports used in the original normative sample, as well as the codings for them, are available to researchers through http://www.dreambank.net.[19] The normative findings reveal a pattern of sex differences that must be taken into account when doing studies of individuals. The coding system employs nonparametric statistics for determining *P* values and effect sizes, which can be obtained instantly after entering codings into the DreamSAT spreadsheet available to all researchers at https://sleepanddreamdatabase.org.[20] The general HVDC norms can be used with confidence for a variety of purposes because they have been replicated in several studies.[2,21] The coding system and the norms also have been found to be useful in studies of college students in several different countries.[22]

As documented by Winget and Kramer,[17] numerous other coding systems exist, and many new ones have been created since their comprehensive review. However, unlike the HVDC system, many of these instruments have only been used by the original investigators (limiting potential for comparisons across laboratories), some use weighting systems of questionable validity, and few are based on clearly defined and objective scoring criteria that yield good interrater reliability. Moreover, as detailed elsewhere,[21] many of these scoring systems can be duplicated by combining two or more elements of the HVDC system.

Finally, because of the time-consuming nature of traditional coding systems, computer programs for word and phrase searches in written dream reports have been created to study specific characters (e.g., "my mother") or activities (e.g., "making love"), and lengthy word strings have been developed for coding concepts characterized by a relatively circumscribed set of terms (e.g., specific situations or emotions). For example, the program for single words, phrases, and word strings available at http://www.dreambank.net calculates frequencies, percentages, *P* values, and effect sizes when two sets of dream reports are compared.[19] A comprehensive set of 40-word strings covers classes of characters, types of activities, natural settings, and much else.[23,24] These 40-word strings have normative findings based on the same dream reports used to create the HVDC norms, and they provide results comparable to the HVDC findings for several categories.

Problems in Studying Emotions and Bizarreness in Dreams

Although both rating scales and the HVDC nominal coding categories have proved useful for most dimensions and elements of dream content, there are methodological problems relating to the study of both emotions and bizarreness in dreaming. Several different studies using external coders find that negative emotions outnumber positive ones.[18,25] Further, a laboratory study that compared ratings of emotions by independent judges with similar ratings by participants immediately after each awakening showed no differences.[26] However, different results emerge when the participants themselves make a global rating of each of their dream reports on a pleasant-unpleasant dimension. Such studies regularly find that the dreamers rate the emotions in their dreams as at least equally pleasant and unpleasant and sometimes as more pleasant.[27,28] Furthermore, some studies[29] show that a greater proportion of laboratory as well as home dream reports are rated as containing emotions when these are scored by the dreamer as compared with external raters. One study[30] of emotional experiences in REM dream reports found that self-ratings of emotions provided by the dreamer on awakening differed from ratings given by external judges using the same rating scales, with self-ratings resulting in greater estimates of emotional dreams, positively toned dreams, and positive and negative emotions per dream.

Generally speaking, dreamers also tend to attribute many more emotions to their home dreams than do blind judges when they are later asked to recall the emotions that accompanied reports they wrote down at an earlier time. In one laboratory study, however, which involved 17 participants who were studied on 2 nonconsecutive nights and questioned after each awakening as to the presence of emotions and the appropriateness of the emotion to the content, there were no differences in their ratings and those of independent judges.[31] Also noteworthy is that the participants in this study reported there was an absence of emotion in 17% of their dream reports in which there would have been emotions in the same context in waking life.

Moreover, dreamers often say their dreams are more pleasant than might be expected based on judges' ratings and attribute more emotions to their home dream reports than judges do when scoring the written dream narratives, which may imply that that a dream's general mood should be differentiated from its specific emotions.[32] Or it may be that these differences result from two extrinsic factors: (1) the demand characteristics of such a rating task and (2) the waking-life assumption that certain emotions would logically be present in many of the situations experienced in the dreams. It is also likely that the use of different rating scales and instructions for the scoring of emotions in dreams (e.g., a dream's overall emotional tone versus number of emotions reported per dream narrative, frequency versus intensity of emotions, number of discrete positive and negative emotions to be rated, scoring of inferred versus explicitly reported emotions) affects the ratings obtained, whether they are self-reported by the dreamer or scored by external judges.

There is also lack of agreement on how to assess unusual or bizarre elements in dreams, which leads to widely varying prevalence and frequency estimates. Using a rating scale based on the degree to which any dimension of the dream differs from waking experience and behavior, researchers found that 75% of 500 REM reports from adult men and women had at least one bizarre aspect, as compared with just 7% to 8% that were bizarre in three or more ways.[33] In studies that focus on clearly impossible events, the figure is 10% or below for large samples of both REM and home dreams.[34,35] When sudden scene changes, uncertainties, and small distortions are included, the figure rises to between 30% and 60%.[36,37] On the other hand, a study in which participants were left alone for up to an hour to think out loud led to the finding that there were as many scene shifts and changes in topics in drifting waking thought as there are in REM dream reports.[38] This study also showed that improbable combinations, such as unusual juxtapositions of objects, were equal in frequency in REM and waking reports, and that identity confusions concerning characters, including the rare occurrences of metamorphoses, appeared more often in the REM reports than the waking reports.[38] These results suggest that, depending on how bizarreness is defined, wandering thoughts can be just as bizarre as dream reports. These findings also highlight the importance of taking into account what the bizarreness is being measured relative to (e.g., waking events and perceptions versus waking mind wandering).

The Importance of Adequate Sample Sizes and Minimum Report Lengths

One important variable that is all too often overlooked when investigating dream content is the sample size required to detect changes in various content variables. The use of an approximate randomization algorithm provides evidence that it takes 100 to 125 dream reports to detect significant content differences between individuals or groups for many of the HVDC content indicators because some dream elements appear in half or less of dream reports; in addition, effect sizes are often modest.[39] It should also be noted that it is unlikely that repeatable and scientifically useful results can be obtained with dream reports much shorter than 50 words, especially when using HVDC content categories.

Finally, although coefficients of internal consistency for dream diaries indicate that everyday dream recall is relatively stable over time,[6,40] several dream content variables appear infrequently in dream reports and show large intraindividual fluctuations. For this reason, it is suggested that correlational studies involving relatively rare or unstable dream content variables be based on at least 20 dream reports from any given participant.[13]

Quantitative Findings on Dream Content

Dream Reports from Laboratory Awakenings

The best starting point for the systematic study of dream content remains the classic studies completed by dream researchers during the heyday of laboratory dream research in the 1960s and early 1970s. They show that dream content simulates everyday life to a far greater degree than had been anticipated based on previous clinical cases.[41] They characterize a prototypical REM dream report as a "clear, coherent, and detailed account of a realistic situation involving the dreamer and other people caught up in very ordinary activities and preoccupations, and usually talking about them."[41]

For example, of all the dream settings that were described, only 5% were "exotic," in the sense of highly unusual or out of the ordinary, and less than 1% were "fantastic," in the sense of unrealistic.[41] Using a conservative standard to guard against imputing any emotions to the dreamers, researchers judged specific emotions to be present in only 30% to 35% of the reports, with unpleasant emotions outnumbering pleasant ones by 2 to 1. Anxiety and anger were the most frequent types of emotions; erotic feelings were reported in only 8 of the 635 reports (1.3%).[41] The dreams were rated as having a low degree of bizarreness. In the longest reports (more frequently rated as bizarre), 50% were rated as having no bizarreness, 30% as having a low degree of bizarreness, 8% as having a medium degree, and 2% as having a high degree.[41]

The issue of emotions in REM dream reports was first investigated in great depth in the sleep laboratory, where participants were quizzed in detail after each awakening as to the presence of emotions and the appropriateness of the emotion to the content. Drawing on ratings by both participants and naïve judges, it was concluded that about 70% of the dream reports had at least some affect.[31] A study in a Swiss sleep laboratory came to very similar conclusions about the frequency and intensity of emotions in dreams.[33]

Several early laboratory studies probed for any changes that might occur in dream content from REM period to REM period, uncovering very few replicable differences. Employing categories for settings, characters, activities, social interactions, and emotions, both quantitative and qualitative analyses find few or no differences from REM period to REM period, but only when corrections are made for the length of report.[27] In the most comprehensive study of this issue, there were two minor differences among 26 analyses employing HVDC categories for the first four REM periods, whether they were nights with single or multiple awakenings, and there were no differences with spontaneously recalled dreams that came from night or morning REM sleep self-awakenings.[42]

However, there may be some degree of thematic continuity from REM period to REM period on a few nights.[33]

REM and NREM Dream Reports

Although there were indications in early laboratory studies that dreaming occurs almost exclusively in REM sleep and that there were differences in the content of REM and NREM reports, many later studies suggest that the differences in recall are not clearly delineated, especially late in the sleep period, and that some of the content differences disappear when there is a control for word length.[43,44] Still, most studies conclude that dreams are more frequent and longer during REM periods and that many NREM reports seem to be "thoughts," not dreams. In fact, NREM reports are more often a continuation of waking thoughts and memories, whereas there are few episodic memory sources in REM or home dream reports.[45,46]

The differences in content relate to a greater character density in REM reports, which in turn leads to the possibility of social interactions.[34,43] Also there is evidence that NREM reports late in the sleep period are more similar to REM reports than are NREM reports from the first few hours of sleep.[47] In the most recent studies of this issue, the thought-like nature of NREM decreased by 56%, and the hallucinatory nature increased by 62% over the course of the night, leading to the conclusion that "as the night progresses, NREM approaches the neurocognitive characteristics of REM."[48] In two separate studies it was found that the major difference between late-night REM and NREM dreams is in aggressive interactions.[49]

Laboratory and Home Dream Comparisons

Several careful investigations reveal relatively few differences between home and laboratory dream reports, even when the dreams are obtained by tape recorders in the sleep laboratory and by written reports at home.[33,34] Furthermore, most of these differences disappear when the proper controls are introduced.[50,51] The one exception to this generalization seems to be hostile and aggressive dream elements, which occur more frequently in the home dream reports of young adults in three different studies.[34,51]

These findings on the relatively small differences between home and laboratory dreams may be explainable in terms of the results from laboratory studies that compare what is reported from REM sleep awakenings with what is still remembered in the morning.[52,53] Such studies reveal that recency and length of report are the primary factors in delayed recall. However, some of these studies also show that intensity can be a tertiary factor in morning recall, which suggests there is some selection bias toward the everyday recall of more emotionally salient content.

Normative Dream Content in Home Dreams

As may be expected from the results of the laboratory-home comparisons, studies of large samples of dream content collected from young college-educated adults outside the laboratory show many similarities with the laboratory results when the same or comparable content categories are employed. Dreams mostly occur in commonplace settings, contain a large number of familiar characters, and revolve around family concerns, love interests, and activities engaged in during waking life.[54] In a study based on a normative nonlab sample containing 991 dream reports from young women and men, 86.9% of the dream reports included a social interaction or shared social activity, 6.7% included the dreamer seeing, hearing, or thinking about another dream character, 2.2% included only the dreamer and at least one animal, and 4.3% included only the dreamer engaging in an activity.[55]

Given the longstanding clinical and popular interest in dreams with erotic or sexual content, this dream content category has received surprisingly little attention. Questionnaire studies indicate that approximately 80% of adults answer positively to the question, "Have you ever dreamed of sexual experiences?"[56] with men reporting sexual dreams more often than women. The normative data from HVDC indicates that 12% of men's dreams and 4% of women's dreams contained sexual content, including having or attempting intercourse, petting, kissing, sexual overtures, and fantasies. However, one study[57] of more than 3500 dream reports found no sex differences, with approximately 8% of dream reports from both men and women containing sexually related activity. The differences with the HVDC data may be partially due to sample composition (college students versus student and nonstudent adults). Alternatively, it is also possible that women actually experience more sexual dreams now than they did 40 years ago or that they now feel more comfortable reporting such dreams because of changing social roles and attitudes, or both.

Age Differences

There appear to be major changes in dream content from the preschool to teen years, but few changes from the late teens to old age. Dream content thus seems to parallel cognitive and emotional development during childhood as well as the stability of adult personality. Much of what is known in a systematic way about children's dreams comes from a classic longitudinal laboratory study of children between the ages of 3 and 15, supplemented by a cross-sectional laboratory replication a few years later with children ages 5 to 8 years.[58] More recently, a 5-year longitudinal laboratory study of Swiss children ages 9 to 15 years has provided additional supporting information.[59,60] Detailed summaries of the methods, samples, and findings can be found elsewhere.[20]

The most unexpected findings in the first study were the low amount of recall from REM periods in 3- to 5-year-olds children (only 27% of the REM sleep awakenings yielded any recall that could reasonably be called a dream) and the static, bland, and underdeveloped content of the few reports that were obtained. The reports became more "dream-like" (in terms of characters, themes, and actions) in the 5- to 7-year-olds children, but it was not until the children were 11 to 13 years old that their dreams began to resemble those of adult laboratory participants in frequency, length, emotions, and overall structure or to show any relationship to personality.[61] A cross-sectional replication of these results[58] with children ages 5 to 8 years supported all of the main original findings.

The results from the longitudinal study of Swiss children ages 9 to 15 years old were generally similar to those for preadolescents and adolescents in the earlier longitudinal study, and there were only relatively small changes in most categories over the 6-year period. The largest change was a decline in bizarreness for both boys and girls, as defined by degrees of deviation from waking experience and social norms; just over 60% of the dream reports had at least some degree of bizarreness at ages 9 to 11 and 11 to 13, but the figure fell to 41% at ages 13 to 15.[59]

In contrast to the changes in dream content from childhood to adolescence, dream content is extremely stable in terms of characters, social interactions, and most other dream elements after age 18, according to cross-sectional studies in the United States, Canada, and Switzerland that are summarized in Domhoff.[21] The elderly recalled fewer dreams in one large longitudinal study,[62] but separate studies suggest their dream content remained generally the same—except perhaps for aggression, in which studies suggest a decline.[63,64]

Dream Content and Well-Being

Considerable research efforts have been expended, trying to establish dream content correlates of standardized personality variables, measures of psychological well-being in nonclinical samples, and indices of psychopathology in clinical populations. Taken as a whole, there is mixed evidence that psychometrically defined personality traits (e.g., neuroticism, extraversion) are related to everyday dream content.[65] Robust relations, however, have been demonstrated between waking levels of well-being and specific types of dreams such as nightmares[5] and recurrent dreams,[66] as well as between dream content and various dimensions of waking life, including people's general waking concerns.[2,39,67] Several studies[68,69] have shown that dream content is reactive to the experience of naturalistic and experimental stressors, but whether dreams play a role in people's actual adaptation to stress remains an open question. In a series of longitudinal studies of REM dream reports from depressed and nondepressed adults undergoing marital separation or divorce, Cartwright and colleagues[67,70] provide suggestive evidence that dream content variables centered around affect and the representation of the ex-spouse are associated with how well people adapt to their situation over time. Similarly, one longitudinal study[71] of normal adults found that participants' dream content from home logs was moderately to strongly correlated to their scores on measures of psychological well-being both at fixed points in time and over a 6- to 10-year period, with content variables of dream affect and social interactions showing the strongest relations. Dream content in severe psychopathologic conditions such as schizophrenia has been reviewed elsewhere,[72,73] and with few exceptions, few consistent findings have emerged from this literature. Furthermore, many studies in this field have methodologic problems, including unclear diagnoses, inadequate controls, unknown effects of medications, few dream reports per patient, and the use of untested coding systems. However, the HVDC system has been shown to be useful in studies of Parkinson disease and those with REM sleep behavior disorder[74,75] as well as women who have had mastectomies.[76]

In addition, unique features of dream content have also been better documented in relation to conditions typically accompanied by distinct waking thoughts and concerns, such as pregnancy,[77] bereavement,[78] and exposure to trauma.[79] A better understanding is also emerging regarding the frequency and contents of specific kinds of dreams, including typical dreams[56,80] (i.e., dreams experienced at least once by a significant proportion of the general population) as well as bad dreams and nightmares.[81]

Studies of Individual Dream Journals

Within the context of the many well-established group findings, studies of individual dream journals can be of great value for both research and possible clinical applications. The dream journals on which such studies are based have value as nonreactive measures that have not been influenced by the purposes of the investigators who later analyze them. The conclusions drawn from nonreactive archival data are considered most reliable and useful when they are based on a diversity of archives likely to have different sources of potential biases.[21]

Studies based on more than a dozen different dream journals first proved their usefulness for scientific purposes by revealing an unexpected consistency in dream content when several hundred dream reports were studied.[21] This consistency begins in the late teens and continues to old age.[82] Two studies of discontinuous dream series show that the consistency revealed in continuous dream journals is not the result of practice effects.[21,83]

Individual dream journals also provided the basis for the most rigorous work to date on the lawfulness of dreams and their relationship to waking conceptual processes. This work[84] shows that the social networks in dreams—that is, the pattern of direct and indirect relationships among the characters—have the same properties as waking social networks in that the paths between characters are short and the clustering of characters is high. Moreover, the frequency distribution of the characters is consistent with Zipf's law, a power law for describing frequency distributions in which the top few entities occur very frequently and most other entities appear very rarely. In a recent extension of this work,[85] the dream and waking-life social networks of a middle-aged woman were compared using 4254 dream reports and information from the dreamer concerning her relationships with her dream characters in waking life. Results showed that people important in one network tended to be important in the other, but that people with different relationships to the dreamer (e.g., family, friends, and coworkers) are mixed together much more in the dream than the waking network. Similar results on the lawfulness of character networks were then reported in a study of five other dream series.[86]

Blind analyses of dream journals[21,87] also have led, through the formulation of inferences that can be accepted or rejected by the dreamer and other respondents, to the conclusion that some dream content is continuous with the dreamers' waking conceptions, concerns, and interests. The most direct continuities involve the main people in a dreamer's life and the nature of the social interactions with them. There also is good continuity for many of the dreamer's main interests and activities. However, these findings on continuity have to be qualified in two ways. First, the continuity is with general concerns, not day-to-day events, as shown by three studies (two based on REM sleep awakenings, one based on morning recall at home) in which judges could not match detailed waking reports of daily concerns with dream reports.[88] This finding is consistent with studies showing low levels of episodic memory in dreams.[45,89] Second, the continuity usually is with both thought and behavior, but sometimes it is only with waking thought. For example, people who have highly aggressive dreams are not always aggressive people in waking life, but they usually admit to many aggressive thoughts and fantasies during the day.[21]

Sensory Experiences and Dreams of Blind Subjects

Although the overwhelming majority of dream reports contain visual and, to a lesser extent, kinesthetic elements, the presence of other sensory modalities has also been noted in both laboratory and home dream reports.[41,90] More than 50% of dream reports contain auditory experiences, whereas explicit references to olfactory, gustatory, and pain sensations occur in less than 1% of all dream reports. One study[90] found that women's dream reports were more likely to contain olfactory or gustatory sensations, whereas references to auditory and pain experiences occurred in a higher percentage of men's dreams. That the more infrequent modalities of smell, taste, and pain occur at all in dreams is an important demonstration of the representational capacities of dreaming.

Perhaps because of the highly visual nature of dreaming, many people have long wondered if blind people dream. Some of the earliest systematic interview studies on dreams dealt with this topic, showing that people who are born blind or become blind before age 4 or 5 years do dream, even though they do not see images in their dreams,[91] a finding that was then supported by laboratory studies.[92] Nor is there much if any difference in dream content, except that there may be less aggression in their dreams.[7,91] There is also much greater mention of touch, taste, and smell in blind people's dreams.[7] It is noteworthy that people who become blind after age 5 or 6 often have visual imagery in their dreams, which suggests that there is a window for the development of the capacity to have visual dreams that parallels what was found in longitudinal studies of children ages 3 to 7 years.[93]

IMPLICATIONS FOR THEORIES OF DREAMING

The array of systematic results presented here suggests that a considerable amount of psychological information can be extracted from dream reports. This conclusion provides support for the core idea of all 20th century dream theories, but it must be stressed that much dream content is not yet understood. The findings also suggest that most dreams focus on a handful of personal concerns revolving around social interactions with family, friends, and coworkers. The greatest variability in dream content seems to concern the appearance of aggression, especially physical aggression.

Despite the originality and creativity that is displayed in the cognitive production of dreams, and even given the aspects of dream content that are not understood, most dreams are more realistic and based on everyday life than is suggested by most traditional dream theories. In addition, much dream content seems more transparent than might be expected by older clinical theories that emphasize disguise or symbolism in understanding dreams. Finally, a significant minority of dreams may not be as emotionally based as theories imply, especially before the adolescent years.[94]

As a starting point, perhaps dreams are best understood as embodied simulations that enact the person's main conceptions and personal concerns, including emotionally salient interpersonal preoccupations. This type of conceptualization is at the heart of the continuity that is found between drifting waking thought and dream content, which suggests there is an important relationship between everyday dream content and personal waking concerns. Although most of the research findings reviewed here are consistent with the continuity concept, much work remains to be done to clarify which specific dimensions of waking life (e.g., particular learning tasks, daily mood, major life events, ingrained behaviors, sustained fantasies, cognitive styles) are most robustly associated to what kind of dream content and the nature of these relationships over time.[45] In the end, dreaming may or may not have a function, but data convincingly show that dream content is a unique and meaningful psychological product of the human brain, and, as such, dreams will continue to interest and challenge clinicians and researchers.

CLINICAL PEARLS

- Examining a series of dreams often yields more meaningful information about a patient's psychological state than focusing solely on one particularly salient dream.
- Affect and social interactions are two key dream content variables that are most strongly related to measures of psychological well-being.

SUMMARY

This chapter reviews methodologic issues in dream research and systematic findings on the content of people's dreams, and it presents the implications of key findings on normative dream content. Quantitative data on the content of laboratory and home dream reports combined depict a reliable picture about the nature of dream content in the general adult population as well as its development in children. At the most general level, these findings indicate that dreams show systematic relationships to various dimensions of the dreamer's waking life and suggest that many dreams are the embodiment of thoughts through dramatizations of life concerns and interests. That a wide range of psychological information can be extracted from dream reports has implications for clinical, theoretical, and empirical approaches to the study of dreams.

SELECTED READINGS

Bulkeley K. Digital dream analysis: a revised method. *Conscious Cogn.* 2014;29:159–170.

Dale A, Lortie-Lussier M, De Koninck J. Ontogenetic patterns in the dreams of women across the lifespan. *Conscious Cogn.* 2015;37:214–224.

Domhoff GW. *The Emergence of Dreaming: Mind-Wandering, Embodied Simulation, and the Default network.* New York: Oxford University Press; 2018.

Domhoff GW, Schneider A. Similarities and differences in dream content at the cross-cultural, gender, and individual levels. *Conscious Cogn.* 2008;17:1257–1265.

Gauchat A, Séguin JR, McSween-Cadieux E, Zadra A. The content of recurrent dreams in young adolescents. *Conscious Cogn.* 2015;37:103–111.

Han HJ, Schweickert R, Xi Z, Viau-Quesnel C. The cognitive social network in dreams: transitivity, assortativity, and giant component proportion are monotonic. *Cogn Sci.* 2015:1–26.

Malinowski JE, Horton CL. Memory sources of dreams: the incorporation of autobiographical rather than episodic experiences. *J Sleep Res.* 2014;23:441–447.

Robert G, Zadra A. Thematic and content analysis of idiopathic nightmares and bad dreams. *Sleep.* 2014;37:409–417.

Sándor P, Szakadát S, Kertész K, Bódizs R. Content analysis of 4 to 8 year-old children's dream reports. *Front Psychol.* 2015;6:534.

Schredl M. Questionnaires and diaries as research instruments in dream research: methodological issues. *Dreaming.* 2002;12:17–26.

Sikka P, Valli K, Virta T, Revonsuo A. I know how you felt last night, or do I? Self- and external ratings of emotions in REM sleep dreams. *Conscious Cogn.* 2014;25:51–66.

Stickgold R, Zadra A. Sleep: Opening a portal to the dreaming brain. *Curr Biol.* 2021;31(7):R352-R353.

Wang J, Zemmelman SE, Hong D, Feng X, Shen H. Does COVID-19 impact the frequency of threatening events in dreams? An exploration of pandemic dreaming in light of contemporary dream theories. *Conscious Cogn.* 2021;87:103051.

A complete reference list can be found online at ExpertConsult.com.

Chapter 57

Neural Correlates of Dreaming

Francesca Siclari; Giulio Tononi

Chapter Highlights

- Dream experiences can occur in every sleep stage.
- Electroencephalographic slow waves and underlying neuronal off periods interfere with the generation of dream experiences in both non–rapid eye movement (NREM) and rapid eye movement (REM) sleep, especially when they occur in posterior cortical regions (posterior hot zone).
- The recall of dream content in NREM sleep is favored by high-frequency power increases in medial and lateral prefrontal regions, likely reflecting increased activity in arousal-related systems.
- Broad perceptual categories (thinking, perceiving, faces, speech, spatial setting, and movement) share similar anatomic substrates across sleep and wakefulness.

The origin and meaning of dreams have intrigued humankind since ancient times. It is therefore not surprising that the advent of electroencephalography (EEG), which allowed researchers to "measure" sleep, also spurred attempts to find objective correlates of dreaming. In 1953, when Aserinsky and Kleitman first described rapid eye movement (REM) sleep in humans, this task seemed accomplished as researchers declared that they had "furnished the means of determining the incidence and duration of periods of dreaming."[1] After all, the electrophysiologic hallmarks of this behavioral state seemed to be highly compatible with dreaming: saccadic eye movements, as if the sleeper were observing an animated scene; low-amplitude, high-frequency EEG activity reminiscent of wakefulness; and muscular atonia, which appeared well suited to prevent dream enactment. More important, when the researchers woke subjects in this sleep stage and asked them whether they had just dreamed, 75% replied in the affirmative, whereas such an answer was given after only 17% of awakenings in other sleep stages.

BETWEEN STATES COMPARISONS: RAPID EYE MOVEMENT SLEEP AS A PROXY FOR DREAMING

In the following decades, dreaming was often equated with REM sleep, and most studies trying to relate changes in brain activity to dreaming were based on comparisons between wakefulness, REM sleep (as a proxy for dreaming), and slow wave sleep (SWS, as a proxy for unconsciousness). With the development of neuroimaging techniques, including functional magnetic resonance imaging (fMRI) and positron emission tomography (PET), it became possible to image local changes in blood flow and metabolism and to create regional maps of brain activity for different behavioral states. Such studies revealed that, compared with SWS, REM sleep was characterized by increased blood flow in a wide variety of brain regions (pons, midbrain, basal ganglia, thalamus, basal forebrain, anterior cingulate, medial prefrontal cortex, anterior insula, parahippocampal cortex, and unimodal sensory areas), while no differences were found for heteromodal association cortices.[2] Compared with wakefulness, REM sleep showed increased blood flow and metabolism in associative visual areas and limbic circuits, consistent with the highly visual and emotional content of dreams, and decreased activity in frontoparietal associative areas, potentially accounting for the lack of insight and reduced reflective consciousness that characterizes dreams.[3] Although these studies allowed researchers to relate dream features to local changes in brain activity, such between-state contrasts also had several limitations. Moreover, it became clear that REM sleep and dreaming can become dissociated in a variety of conditions. Specific forebrain lesions, for instance, induced a cessation of dreaming without affecting REM sleep,[4] whereas pharmacologic suppression of REM sleep did not result in a reduction of dreaming.[5] In addition, studies employing serial awakening paradigms showed that by changing the question from "Tell me whether you had a dream" to more open-ended ones such as "Tell me what was going through your mind," reports of conscious experiences could be obtained in non–rapid eye movement sleep (NREM) sleep in up to 70% of cases.[6,7] Compared with REM sleep dreams, NREM sleep experiences were often shorter, less dreamlike, less vivid, more conceptual, less bizarre, less emotional, under greater volitional control, and more related to current concerns.[8-11] However, in the early morning hours, a substantial proportion of NREM awakenings could yield dream reports that were in every respect indistinguishable from REM reports.[8,11] Finally, in a consistent minority of cases, subjects woken from REM sleep did not report no experience at all.[12] The fact that both dreaming and unconsciousness could occur in two behavioral states with very different EEG patterns challenged researchers and led to many potential explanations, including that dreaming does not occur during sleep but instead is akin to a confabulation produced upon awakening,[13] that there is no relation between conscious experiences in sleep and cortical activation,[14] or that dreaming in NREM sleep results from covert REM intrusions into this stage.[15]

RECENT ADVANCES WITH IMPLICATIONS FOR DREAM RESEARCH

Initial attempts at relating EEG spectral power changes to dreaming resulted in variable findings. For NREM sleep, an increase in the beta band,[16] a decrease in spindle and delta power,[17] and a decrease in right temporal alpha oscillatory activity[18] were reported to precede reports of dreaming. In REM sleep, dream reports were found to be associated with lower frontal and higher occipital alpha power, increased occipital beta power,[17] as well as higher frontal theta activity.[18] This variability in findings likely resulted from the low sampling, as only a limited number of awakenings were performed per subject, but perhaps more importantly from the low spatial resolution of conventional polysomnographic recordings that were used in these studies.

Among many recent conceptual and methodological advances in sleep research, two may be especially important for characterizing the neural correlates of dreaming. First, research in the most recent decades has shown that various neuronal signatures of sleep can occur and be regulated locally. In a number of physiologic and pathologic conditions, sleep and wake-like patterns can coexist in different brain regions (reviewed by Siclari and Tononi[19]). Slow waves, the major hallmarks of NREM sleep, display a characteristic anterior-posterior amplitude gradient in human adults and can vary regionally as a function of prior experience.[20] At the neuronal level, slow waves occur when thalamocortical neurons become bistable and alternate between short periods of hyperpolarization (down states) associated with neuronal silence (off periods), and periods of depolarization (up states), during which neurons fire (on periods).[21,22] In conditions of sleep deprivation, slow waves with associated off periods can also be observed during behavioral wakefulness in humans and rodents, leading to cognitive lapses.[23,24] In addition, slow waves have been recently documented during REM sleep in superficial layers of primary sensory areas in mice[25] and in human scalp recordings.[26,27]

Second, recent work has provided some clues about the neural mechanisms underlying the presence or absence of conscious experiences during sleep. Specifically, there is evidence that the neuronal off period underlying slow waves may interfere with the occurrence of conscious experiences during sleep. Transcranial magnetic stimulation (TMS) applied during SWS, when the absence of dream reports is most likely to occur, induces a slow wave–like response, associated with a breakdown of cortical effective connectivity among specialized thalamocortical regions.[28] Such an altered TMS response has also been observed in other conditions associated with unconsciousness, including general anesthesia and coma.[29,30] Similar responses can be induced during SWS by directly stimulating the cortex in patients with epilepsy implanted with intracranial electrodes as part of a presurgical workup. Importantly, these intracranial studies revealed that neuronal off periods associated with the slow wave break the causal links between brain activity evoked by electrical stimulation and brain activity that resumes after the off period.[31] From a theoretical perspective, this breakdown of causal interactions impairs information integration, an important prerequisite for consciousness.[32] Taken together, these observations suggest that the occurrence, amplitude, and regional distribution of slow waves may account for the presence or absence of dreaming within different behavioral states. To evaluate this possibility, however, it is essential to employ techniques with increased spatial resolution, capable of capturing localized changes in slow waves. Moreover, to account for the variety of conscious states that can occur during sleep, it is important to employ serial awakening paradigms, which permit the sampling of many experiences per subject as well as within-state comparisons.

FROM BETWEEN-STATE TO WITHIN-STATE COMPARISONS

With these considerations in mind, we designed a study in which subjects underwent a serial awakening paradigm[12] coupled with high-density EEG (hd-EEG), a technique that combines the excellent temporal resolution of EEG with a greater spatial resolution, roughly comparable with PET imaging if source modeling is used. Two initial experiments were performed, one with 32 subjects and few awakenings per subject (performed in N2 and REM sleep) and one with seven highly trained subjects who underwent more than 100 awakenings.[33] After each awakening, participants were asked to describe the "last thing going through their mind" before the alarm sounded.

Dreaming versus No Experience

Both experiments yielded highly consistent results: in line with the hypothesis that slow waves interfere with the generation of dreams as conscious experiences, reports of dream experiences (DE) were preceded by lower slow wave activity (SWA, power in the 1 to 4 Hz range) compared with reports of no experiences (NE). Topographically, these differences were restricted to bilateral parieto-occipital regions, encompassing the medial and lateral occipital lobe, and extending superiorly to the precuneus and posterior cingulate gyrus (grouped under the term "posterior hot zone" [PHZ], Figure 57.1, *A*). Similar differences in SWA, localized to the PHZ, were also observed when DE were compared with instances in which subjects reported that they experienced a dream but could not recall the content of their dream (DE without recall of content, DEWR), suggesting that the reduction in SWA in the PHZ accounts for differences in dreaming and not in the ability to recall the dream. Intriguingly, SWA differences in the PHZ were also found when comparing DE and NE in REM sleep, a stage characterized by a highly desynchronized EEG but, as mentioned previously, not devoid of slow waves. Compared with NE, reports of DE were also preceded by increases in gamma activity, putatively reflecting neuronal firing, which extended beyond the PHZ in both NREM and REM sleep.

In a follow-up study we explored how slow wave parameters, including their number, amplitude, slope, and number

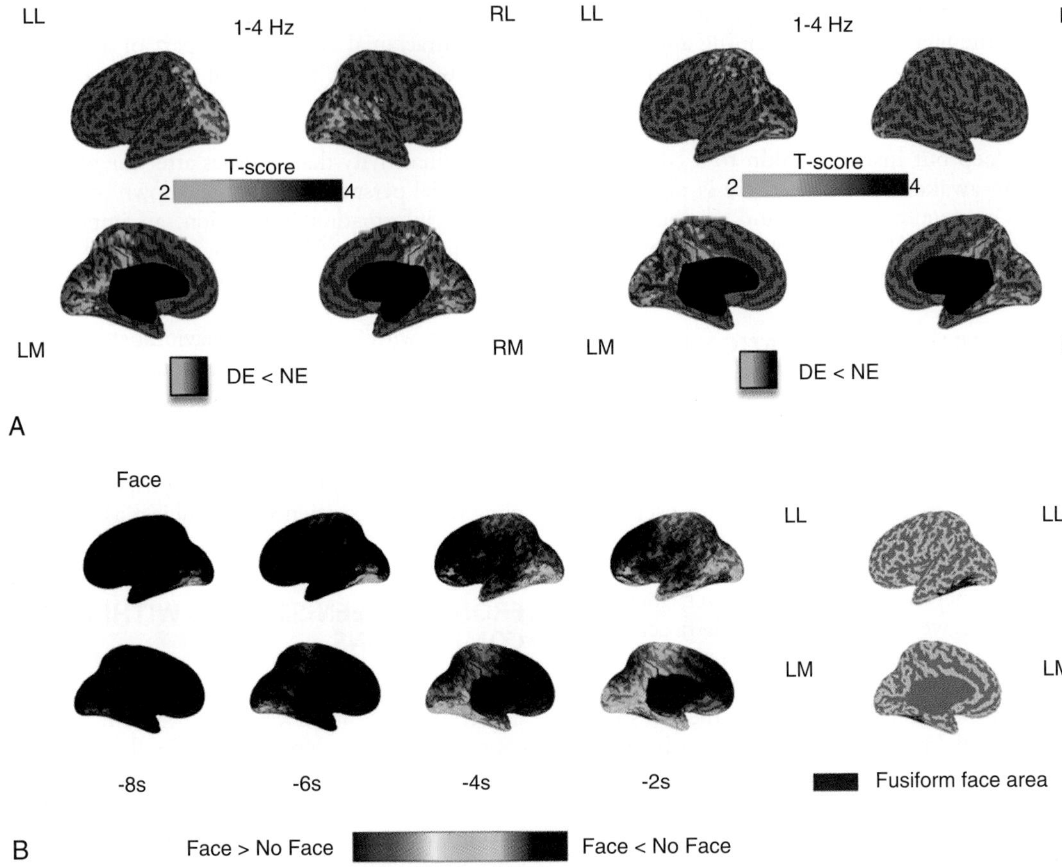

Figure 57.1 The EEG correlates of dream experiences (DEs). **A,** DE versus no experience (NE) in NREM (*left*) and REM sleep (*right*). Reports of DEs obtained after NREM awakenings are preceded by lower low-frequency spectral power (1–4 Hz, *blue-green area, left image*) in a parieto-occipital "hot zone" compared with reports of NE. Spectral power was averaged over the last 20 seconds before awakening the subjects to obtain a report. Only significant differences at the $p < 0.05$ level, obtained after correction for multiple comparisons are shown. **B,** Differences in high-frequency spectral power (25–50 Hz) between dreams with and without a face for different timeframes before the awakening out of REM sleep, highlighting the fusiform face area ($p = 0.023$; one-tailed paired t-test, $n = 7$ subjects, $t6 = 2.52$). The fusiform area is specialized in face recognition in wakefulness. LL, Left lateral; LM, left medial; RL, right lateral; RM, right medial view. (Modified from Siclari F, Baird B, Perogamvros L, et al. The neural correlates of dreaming. *Nat Neurosci*. 2017;20[6]:872–78. doi:10.1038/nn.4545)

of negative peaks, relate to dreaming.[34] We found that reports of dreaming were most likely to occur when the bulk of EEG slow waves (type II slow waves, see the work by Siclari and colleagues[35] and Bernardi and colleagues[36]) were sparse, small, and shallow and had many intra-wave negative peaks, whereas reports of unconsciousness were preceded by numerous steep, high-amplitude slow waves that had few intra-wave negative peaks. Like in our previous study documenting significant SWA differences in posterior cortical regions, these differences in slow wave parameters were most consistent in central and posterior cortical areas. Simulation studies and animal and human experiments have advanced our understanding of how EEG slow wave parameters relate to neurophysiologic processes.[37-39] Slow wave density (number per unit of time) reflects the degree of bistability in thalamocortical neurons, whereas slow wave amplitude reflects the number of thalamocortical neurons that enter the down state at the same time. The descending (surface positive to surface negative) and ascending slopes (surface negative to surface positive) of the slow wave reflect how quickly neurons enter the down state and up state, respectively. Finally, the number of negative peaks within the slow wave reflects the degree of synchronization of the down state across distant neuronal populations, with multipeak waves indicating low synchronization. The fact that reports of unconsciousness were preceded by many steep, high-amplitude slow waves in central and posterior cortical regions suggests that the capacity to generate conscious experiences is reduced when, in a state of high bistability, many neuronal populations within the PHZ enter the down state simultaneously and rapidly. The posterior cingulate gyrus, a central component of the PHZ, is a major cerebral "hub" in the connectivity among many different areas.[40] The occurrence of off periods in the PHZ may thus lead to the fading of consciousness by disrupting the interactions among many brain areas. These results are in line with a TMS study demonstrating that within NREM sleep, reports of dreaming are associated with a larger negative evoked response and shorter phase-locking compared with reports of unconsciousness.[41] A role of posterior brain regions in dreaming is also suggested by studies reporting cessation of dreaming after lesions of the inferior parietal and occipital cortex.[4,42-44] Also, in the course of development, the appearance of dreaming is correlated with the progressive anteriorization of the SWA maximum[45] and the maturation of visuospatial skills, which depend on posterior (parietal) cortical areas.[46]

In the same study, we also evaluated how spindle parameters relate to dreaming. Irrespective of the ability to recall the dream, dream reports were more likely in the presence of fast spindles in a central and posterior brain region, whereas reports of no experience were more likely in the presence of slow spindles in the same area. Spindles that occur during the negative to positive deflection of the slow wave, reflecting the transition to the depolarized up state, are typically faster than spindles occurring during the positive to negative deflection, representing the transition to the down state.[47,35] Thus the association of fast spindles with dreaming may be explained by their tendency to occur in central and posterior regions when slow waves are sparse, shallow, and associated with longer up states.

In summary, these experiments showed that irrespective of behavioral state (REM versus NREM sleep), dreaming is most likely to occur when SWA is reduced locally over posterior cortical regions. A decrease in posterior SWA is more likely during lighter NREM sleep, especially in the morning hours, as well as during REM sleep, when slow waves are small and highly localized. On the other hand, during slow wave sleep early in the night, SWA is highly synchronized across many cortical regions, including the PHZ. Hence, dreams are less likely to occur, and when they do, they are rather fragmentary and lack detail.

RECALLING VERSUS FORGETTING THE DREAM

One of the major difficulties in dream research is disentangling the correlates of the DE from the correlates of the memory of the dream. Conceptually, the absence of a dream report either could mean that the subject did not experience anything or could result from an inability to recall the DE. In our experiments[33] we began to address this question by asking whether so-called white dreams, in which subjects felt that they had dreamed but could not recall any dream content (DEWR), would result in different EEG signatures from dreams whose content subjects could recall (DE). As already described, both DEWR and DE showed reduced of SWA in the PHZ compared with NE, suggesting that reduced SWA is linked to the DE itself, rather than to the ability to recall or report its content. However, comparing high-frequency EEG activity in NREM sleep in DE versus DEWR showed that experiences with recall of content were preceded by increased gamma power in medial and lateral frontoparietal areas, areas known to be involved in working memory. These results suggest that, although dreaming may require low SWA in posterior regions, remembering and subsequently reporting the dream may require the recruitment of frontoparietal areas. An alternative possibility is that DEWR could represent dreams with minimal content, close to the threshold of reportability.[48]

In a subsequent study we showed that, in NREM sleep, dreams that could be recalled were often preceded by the occurrence of isolated, very high amplitude slow waves in frontocentral regions (type I slow waves[35]), especially if these slow waves were followed by local high-frequency increases (microarousals).[34] Indeed, the occurrence of type I slow waves may be triggered by the activation of arousal systems. K-complexes, which share many properties with type I slow waves, are can be induced by sensory stimuli of various modalities. Also, type I slow waves originate preferentially in sensorimotor areas and the posteromedial parietal cortex, the cortical regions with the highest noradrenergic innervation in humans and monkeys,[49-51] and involve predominantly frontomedial areas.[52,53] Consistent with this interpretation, an intermittent activation of arousal systems may favor dream recall, as indicated by the observation that intrasleep awakenings are higher in frequent dream recallers compared with infrequent dream recallers.[54] Importantly, the arousal-promoting neuromodulator noradrenaline favors memory encoding and consolidation both in sleep[55] and wakefulness.[56]

The EEG Correlates of Dream Contents

In another set of analyses, we employed hd-EEG recordings to evaluate the neural correlates of broad perceptual categories that are experienced during dreams, with a focus on REM sleep because of the vividness of dream contents.[33] We first investigated the thinking-perceiving dimension of the most recent DE by asking participants to rate on a scale how perceptual (related to sensory content) or thought-like (unrelated to sensory content) it was. The thought-like aspect was positively correlated with gamma power in mid-cingulate regions (25 to 50 Hz), whereas the perceptual dimension displayed a correlation with gamma power in posterior brain regions, comprising sensory cortices.

A follow-up study directly assessed the neural correlates of thoughts in different behavioral states and found a corresponding activation of mid-cingulate cortex across wakefulness, NREM sleep, and REM sleep.[57] Similar correspondences between sleep and wakefulness[33] were found for dreams containing speech, which were associated with localized high-frequency power increases in Wernicke area (subserving speech perception). Dreams containing a spatial setting displayed gamma power increases in the right posterior parietal cortex, a brain region that is crucial for visuospatial attention. Dreams containing faces show increased gamma power in the fusiform face area, specialized in the perception of faces (Figure 57.1, *B*). Interestingly, dreams in which the dreamer performed body movements were associated with activation of the posterior part of the right superior temporal sulcus. This brain area is not involved in movement preparation or execution as such, but it is active when one views biologic movements. This result suggests that the majority of REM sleep dreams involving movement elicit activation in brain regions involved in the perception of movement rather than in their execution, in line with the motor disconnection that characterizes this state. Note that voluntary movements performed in lucid dreams appear instead to be associated with the activation of sensorimotor cortex.[58] Finally, dreams containing fear activate the midcingulate gyrus and the insula,[59] similarly to wakefulness.

Taken together, these studies suggest that dream and waking experiences engage similar neural substrates and provide a good argument against theories stating that dreams are a form of confabulation produced upon awakening. In addition, for most perceptual categories, relative increases in high-frequency activity were most consistent in the 2 seconds before awakening[33] and decreased when longer time periods before the alarm sound were considered, suggesting that dream reports not only reflect truly experienced dream contents but do so with a surprisingly high temporal accuracy.

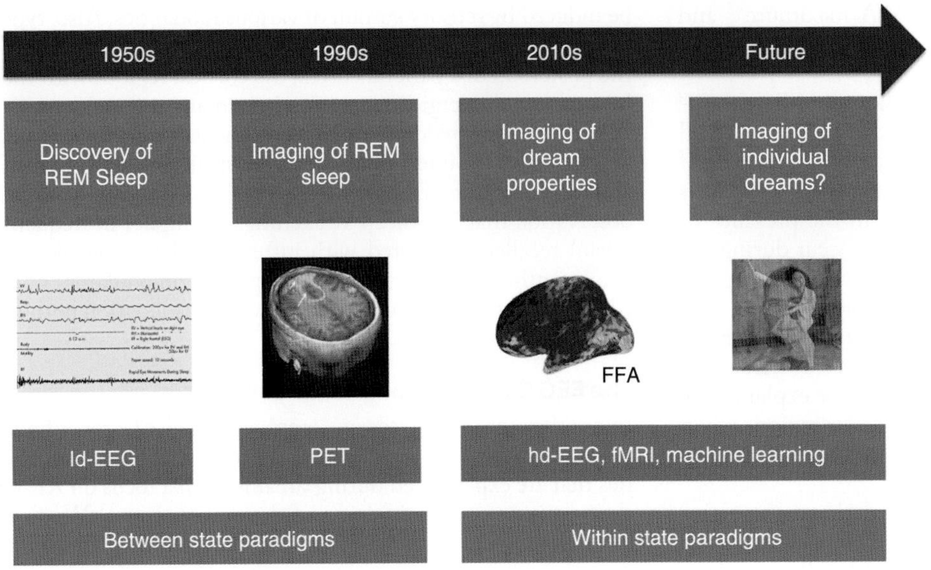

Figure 57.2 Developments in research on the neural correlates of dreaming. *FFA,* Fusiform face area; fMRI, Functional magnetic resonance imaging; hd-EEG, high-density electroencephalography; ld-EEG, low density EEG; PET, positron emission tomography; *REM,* rapid eye movement sleep.

PREDICTING THE OCCURRENCE AND CONTENT OF DREAMING

The findings of reliable EEG correlates of dreaming in serial awakening paradigms opened the possibility that it may be possible to predict dream activity in real time, while subjects were sleeping, based on EEG activation in posterior brain regions. To do so, we evaluated seven subjects who first slept in the sleep laboratory for one undisturbed night. Spectral power distribution in NREM sleep during this baseline night was used to determine individualized thresholds for high and low (above and below the 15th percentile, respectively) delta (0.5–4.5 Hz) and beta power (18–25 Hz). During the next night, spectral power over a posterior set of electrodes was computed in real time, and subjects were awakened whenever the threshold exceeded the predefined cutoffs of cortical activation (dream prediction) and cortical deactivation (unconsciousness prediction). Using this method, we obtained an accuracy for dream prediction in NREM sleep of 91.6%, whereas for unconsciousness prediction it was 80.7%. In another study, Horikawa and colleagues trained a pattern classifier on fMRI data while subjects perceived natural images during wakefulness[60] and succeeded in decoding specific content categories in real time, while subjects were transitioning to sleep.

CLINICAL PEARL

Recent research has outlined major EEG parameters that are associated with dreaming. As a consequence, alterations in sleep microstructure that occur in sleep disorders or as a result of medication, especially changes in SWA or microarousals, have the potential to influence the occurrence and recall of DE.

SUMMARY AND FUTURE DIRECTIONS

Dream research, and, in particular the quest for the neural correlates of dreaming, has recently undergone a transition from between-state contrasts, comparing brain activity between REM sleep as a proxy for dreaming and SWS as a proxy for unconsciousness, to within-subject studies assessing differences in brain activity between dreaming and unconsciousness within both REM and NREM sleep. In addition, motivated by the recent demonstration that sleep-related phenomena occur and are regulated locally, techniques with a low spatial resolution (standard EEG) are progressively being replaced by high-resolution brain imaging techniques including hd-EEG and fMRI. Studies combining these techniques and within-state paradigms have shown that dreaming is associated with a *regional* reduction of SWA in posterior cortical regions in both REM and NREM sleep, two states with a radically different *global* EEG signature. Recalling and reporting the content of the dream are facilitated by the intermittent activation of central and anterior cortical regions, likely promoted by arousal systems. Broad perceptual categories, including faces, spatial setting, movement, speech, and fear, as well as thoughts, have similar neural correlates across sleep and wakefulness. Finally, first attempts to predict the presence and absence of dreaming (in NREM sleep) as well as dream content categories (in the falling asleep period) have yielded promising results. It is therefore conceivable that in the future, it will be possible to predict not only whether someone is dreaming but also individual dream contents during full-fledged sleep (Figure 57.2).

SELECTED READINGS

Horikawa T, Tamaki M, Miyawaki Y, Kamitani Y. Neural decoding of visual imagery during sleep. *Science (80-).* 2013. https://doi.org/10.1126/science.1234330.

Nieminen JO, Gosseries O, Massimini M, et al. Consciousness and cortical responsiveness: a within-state study during non-rapid eye movement sleep. *Sci Rep.* 2016;6(April):1–10. https://doi.org/10.1038/srep30932.

Scarpelli S, Bartolacci C, D'Atri A, et al. Electrophysiological correlates of dream recall during REM sleep: evidence from multiple awakenings and within-subjects design. *Nat Sci Sleep.* 2020;12:1043-1052.

Siclari F, Baird B, Perogamvros L, et al. The neural correlates of dreaming. *Nat Neurosci.* 2017;20(6):872–878. https://doi.org/10.1038/nn.4545.

Siclari F, Bernardi G, Cataldi J, Tononi G. Dreaming in NREM sleep: a high-density EEG study of slow waves and spindles. *J Neurosci.* 2018;38(43):9175–9185. https://doi.org/10.1523/JNEUROSCI.0855-18.2018.

A complete reference list can be found online at ExpertConsult.com.

Chapter
58

The Neurobiology of Dreaming

Dante Picchioni; Shervin Abdollahi; Veda Elisabeth Cost; Hannah Gura; Edward F. Pace-Schott

Chapter Highlights

- The sleep stage, electrophysiologic, and regional brain activity correlates of dreaming are reviewed, including how rapid eye movement (REM) sleep differs from non–rapid eye movement (NREM) sleep in ways that suggest bases for prototypical dreaming.
- Functional connectivity methods and the relationship between dreaming and internally cued cognition during wakefulness are important because information integration across a large number of brain regions has become a central tenet in theories of consciousness. Alterations in this integration resulting from the absence of core nodes or increased randomness may explain the alterations in consciousness that accompany sleep and dreaming.
- Levels of cholinergic and aminergic modulators diminish from waking to NREM, whereas the levels of acetylcholine alone return to waking levels during REM. Observation of these changes contributed to the first neurobiologic theory of dreaming, activation synthesis, in which an elevated cholinergic-to-aminergic ratio accounts in part for differences between dreaming and waking cognition. Other dream theories focus on dopaminergic systems, activation of reward networks, generalized cortical activation, or increased activity in posterior multimodal regions. These latter theories often attempt to explain the neurobiology of dreaming in both REM and NREM.
- Dreaming shares phenomenology with abnormal waking states such as spontaneous confabulation, in which imagined scenarios are accepted as veridical memories, and complex hallucinosis, in which fully formed fictive visual images are perceived. Examinations of underlying neuroanatomy and neurochemistry of these conditions reveal overlap with those of REM sleep.
- Observations from neuroimaging of sleep, cognitive neuroscience, and clinical neuropsychology allow us to construct a putative model of neurobiologic processes that generate dream phenomena, including restored conscious awareness, altered emotion and memory, fictive movement, complex visual hallucinations, fictive space, and impaired executive function.

INTRODUCTION

Dreaming is a universal human experience occurring during sleep. In dreams fictive events follow one another in an organized, story-like manner with interwoven hallucinatory, primarily visual, images that are largely congruent with an ongoing confabulated plot. Most often, during this wholly imaginary experience, it is uncritically accepted in the same manner as are veridical waking percepts and events.

THE ASSOCIATION OF DREAMING WITH BEHAVIORAL STATE

Early speculation that rapid eye movement (REM) sleep was the exclusive physiologic substrate of dreaming[1] was soon followed by awakening studies showing substantial recall of mental experiences from non–rapid eye movement (NREM) sleep.[2] Nonetheless, REM sleep reports are more frequent, longer, more bizarre, more visual, more motoric, and more emotional than are NREM sleep reports.[3] In an extensive review, Nielsen estimates an NREM sleep mental experience recall rate of 42.5%, contrasting with 81.8% from REM sleep, and suggests that brain activation processes occurring outside polysomnographically scored REM sleep ("covert REM") may account for NREM-sleep dreaming.[4]

ELECTROPHYSIOLOGIC ACTIVITY AND CONNECTIVITY DURING SLEEP

REM sleep shows much more gamma frequency (30 to 80 Hz) fast brain waves ("oscillations" or "rhythms") than does NREM.[5,6] In waking, these fast oscillations are associated with attention to stimuli and other forms of active or effortful cognition.[7] During REM-sleep dreaming, fast oscillations

Table 58.1 Summary of Methods Associated with Studying the Preawakening Window

Study	EEG Window Length	Instructions to Subjects	State during Awakening
1986, Williamson[165]	32 s	"During each awakening, subjects were asked to recall their pre-awakening thoughts." (p. 718)	NREM
1987, Wollman[166]	1–5 min	"Please tell me everything that was going through your mind before I called you," and "Was there anything else or can you give me any more details about what you have told me?" (p. 337)	REM
2004, Esposito[167]	3 min	"The experimenter asked the participant what was going on in his/her mind *just* [emphasis added] before the awakening." (p. 290)	REM, NREM
2004, Wittman[168]	32 s	"Subjects were asked what was going through their mind before they heard their names." (p. 44)	NREM
2011, Chellappa[169]	15 min	"How much did you dream? (1: greatly, 2: fairly, 3: relatively little, 4: not at all)" (p. 252)	REM, NREM
2015, Scarpelli[170]	5 min	"After awakening, subjects filled out a sleep and dream diary." (p. 2)	REM
2016, Nieminen[171]	30 s	"Tell me everything that was going through your mind before the alarm sound/you woke up." (p. 2)	NREM
2017, Perogamvros[172]	20 s	"The *last* [emphasis added] thing going through your mind before the alarm sound." (p. 1767)	REM, NREM
2017, Scarpelli[173]	5 min	"Participants were asked to describe everything that was going through their mind during the sleep period." (p. 631)	NREM
2017, Siclari[34]	20–120 s	"The *last* [emphasis added] thing going through your mind before the alarm sound." (p. 872)	Random
2018, Eichenlaub[21]	3 min	"What was going through your mind *immediately before* [emphasis added] you were woken up?" and "Can you remember anything else?" (p. 639)	REM, NREM
2019, D'Atri[174]	15–35 min	"Asked to report if they had or had not a dream experience before awakening." (p. 446)	REM, NREM
2019, Sikka[175]	2 min	"They were first asked to report the *last* [emphasis added] image they had in mind *just before* [emphasis added] awakening, followed by a detailed report of the whole dream." (p. 4777)	REM
2019, Zhang[176]	30–120 s	"Everything that was going through your mind just before I called." (p. 3)	REM, NREM
2020, Sterpenich[20]	20 s	"The *last* [emphasis added] thing going through your mind prior to the alarm sound." (p. 5)	REM, NREM

have been hypothetically associated with cognitive and perceptual processing,[8] memory processing,[9] and the temporal binding of dream imagery.[10] Gamma oscillations in REM sleep become desynchronized between anterior and posterior regions of the brain, a disconnection that may contribute to the hypofrontal and bizarre features of REM-sleep dreaming.[5]

NREM sleep is associated with slower oscillations produced by recurrent interactions between the thalamus and cortex, such as sleep spindles as well as delta (0.5–4 Hz) and cortical slow (<1 Hz) oscillations.[11,12] The latter reflects periods of neuronal quiescence (hyperpolarized or "down" states) that alternate with shorter periods of rapid neuronal firing (depolarized or "up" states).[13] Although human slow wave sleep (SWS) shows less sustained gamma activity compared with REM sleep and waking, intracranial electroencephalography (EEG) has shown that gamma oscillations appear during the transient "up" state of the slow oscillation.[14,15]

STUDIES OF THE PREAWAKENING WINDOW

After waking the dreamer and collecting a dream report, the investigator must choose a length for the window in which to search for a neural correlate. It is difficult to match the timescales of a dream to the corresponding window of brain activity, especially when studying dreaming during NREM sleep, which has a less well-delineated onset compared with the shift to REM sleep. Some suggest moving "beyond the REM-NREM sleep dichotomy and beyond traditional sleep staging"[16] to using randomly distributed awakenings throughout the night.[17] However, this suggestion is subject to the same problem of aligning the dream timeline to the measured brain activity.

Several potential solutions to this problem are available. See Table 58.1 for a selected methodological summary of techniques in this field. Some investigators discard the majority of the dream report and only ask subjects about their most-recent conscious experience (i.e., their mental activity "just" before awakening). This experience is then correlated with a short neural window, such as 2 minutes. Others have emphasized to subjects the importance of reporting the dream in chronologic order and then asked them to divide the report into segments of content. The corresponding EEG segments are then analyzed.[18] Subjects can be asked to estimate the length of the dream. Given the very strong correlation between the length of the REM period and the dream report and between dreamed time and objective time,[19] this approach could allow studying the entire dream report.

Using source localization with 256-channel, high-density EEG, experiencing fear during dreaming has been associated with decreased delta power in the right insula in both NREM sleep stage 2 and REM sleep.[20] The neural correlates of specific content in dreams have also been investigated by measuring the incorporation of recent waking-life experiences[21]: subject-rated incorporation of waking content was positively correlated with REM sleep frontal theta activity. Perhaps the most consistent finding from the studies referenced in Table 58.1 is that slow intrinsic oscillations interfere with ongoing mental activity and lead to a lower frequency of dreams in both REM and NREM sleep.[3] For a more detailed review of EEG studies of dreaming, see Chapter 57.

Very few positron emission tomography (PET) or functional magnetic resonance imaging (fMRI) studies on dreaming during the preawakening window exist. This is a gap in the literature given the inherently high spatial resolution of PET and fMRI compared with EEG. The fMRI scanning of lucidity in REM shows that dreamed hand clenching activates the corresponding sensorimotor cortex[22] and shows greater activation of the prefrontal cortex (PFC) compared with nonlucid REM.[23] Using PET, investigators have also demonstrated that activation of the frontal cortex during sleep in the preawakening window was increased when dreams were coded as having high levels of control.[24] This coding could be interpreted as lying in the same dimension as lucidity. One fMRI study attempted to decode hypnagogic hallucinations by training a machine-learning classifier with data collected during visual stimulus presentation during wakefulness, and the classification was 60% accurate in predicting dream content.[25] Finally, subjects sleeping during PET have been asked about their dreams after awakening and were confirmed to have been dreaming,[26] but dreaming was not investigated as a variable in this study.

NEURAL CORRELATES OF LOW VERSUS HIGH DREAM RECALL AS A TRAIT

The study of neural correlates can extend into studying dream recall as a stable trait.[27] This includes the study of dreaming in patients with brain damage. In 112 patients who reported that they completely stopped dreaming after their injury, it was reported that the supramarginal gyrus (Brodmann area [BA] 40), which is typically referred to as the *temporal-parietal junction*, and medial-prefrontal white matter, typically called the *medial forebrain bundle*, may be necessary for dreaming.[28] Similar neuropsychological investigations implicated the amygdala in the emotions that arise during dreaming.[29] The limitations of these studies are (1) these are clinical populations, (2) baseline levels of dreaming are unknown, and (3) the patients were not awakened from sleep, so dreaming was not directly measured. This research has been extended into healthy controls who are low versus high dream recallers, and the results have some overlap with the neuropsychological data. Medial forebrain bundle density was greater in high versus low recallers,[30] and microstructural integrity in the amygdala was positively correlated with the emotional intensity of the subjects' dreams.[31] An analysis of individual differences in the strength of waking fMRI connectivity revealed that as trait dream recall increases, connectivity in voxels within the visual network decreases, but this was found only during an evening scan and did not replicate during a morning scan.[32] In a hypothesis-based PET neuroimaging study,[33] investigators found that regional cerebral blood flow was greater in high recallers in the temporal-parietal junction and medial PFC/BA 10 during REM sleep, extending neuropsychological and recent EEG[34] data on the importance of these regions for dreaming. Frequent lucid dreaming has been associated with higher functional connectivity during wakefulness between the PFC and inferior parietal lobule as well as lower functional connectivity between the PFC and insula.[35]

Individuals who are high recallers showed less EEG alpha at Pz at 1000 to 1200 ms after hearing their name during wakefulness.[36] When the same stimuli are delivered during NREM sleep stage 2 at 50 dB above waking hearing threshold, several electrodes showed a larger negative potential in the same time window.[37] One interpretation is that high recallers have shallower sleep, which would lead to greater memory encoding of the dream upon awakening.[38] If true, these results would have fewer implications for the neurobiology of dreaming itself.

DREAMING AND PHASIC ACTIVITY IN SLEEP

In cats, a close temporal association exists between REM-sleep rapid eye movements (REM-sleep saccades) and ascending potentials that originate in the brainstem and are termed *ponto-geniculo-occipital* (PGO) *waves*.[3] In the activation-synthesis hypothesis of dreaming,[39] Hobson and McCarley suggest that the brainstem's activation of the forebrain in REM sleep allows the forebrain to synthesize dream scenarios based on currently available information. They suggest that the PGO wave, originating in the pons and arriving at the primary visual cortex by the dedicated visual pathway through the thalamic lateral geniculate nucleus, may be interpreted by the brain as visual information, thereby leading to the visual hallucinosis of dreams.

Early evidence of human PGO waves was derived from scalp EEG recordings temporally locked to REM-sleep saccades.[3,40] Subsequently, PET[41] and fMRI[42] studies also correlated REM-sleep saccades with activation of structures corresponding to the feline PGO wave. Compelling evidence for human PGO waves has recently emerged. First, using magnetoencephalography (MEG), Ioannides and colleagues[43] showed that correlated phasic activity in the pons and frontal eye fields begins before a REM-sleep saccade and intensifies with increasing temporal proximity to saccade onset. Second, using depth electrodes in a patient with Parkinson disease, Lim and colleagues[44] described phasic signals, with waveform and temporal characteristics very similar to the feline PGO, originating in the pedunculopontine nucleus—a structure at the pons-midbrain (mesopontine) junction crucial for generating the feline PGO.[3] Third, using fMRI, Miyauchi and colleagues[45] demonstrated that activity in the pontine tegmentum, ventroposterior thalamus, and visual cortex takes place in the few seconds before REM-sleep saccades. Activation in these regions, relative to the REM-sleep saccade, corresponded to both the neural pathway and time course of the feline PGO wave, that is, pontine tegmentum (–4.7 seconds), ventroposterior thalamus (–3.8 seconds), and primary visual cortex (–2.8 seconds).

The scanning hypothesis, which posits a correlation between REM-sleep saccades and the direction of hallucinated gaze in dreams,[46] continues to generate interesting but conflicting findings. For example, in an event-related potentials study, REM-sleep saccades occurred without the readiness potential that preceded waking saccades, whereas a wake-like potential reflecting visual engagement persisted, suggesting that REM-sleep saccades may trigger rather than follow visual experiences.[47] Nonetheless, Miyauchi and colleagues[45] observed primary visual cortex activation *before* REM-sleep saccades that therefore could not have been triggered by efferent copies from neural activity in the frontal eye fields associated with the saccade, as an alternate explanation may suggest, but rather that REM saccades may have been in response to PGO-initiated dreamed visual imagery.

Convergent evidence does, however, suggest activation of limbic structures in concert with REM-sleep saccades. For example, using low-resolution brain electromagnetic tomography, Abe and colleagues[48] observed a pre–REM-sleep saccade potential with current sources estimated to lie in anterior limbic regions. Using MEG, Ioannides and colleagues[43] also described REM-sleep–saccade-onset–linked current sources estimated to lie in the amygdala and orbitofrontal and parahippocampal cortices. Both groups suggest that this post-saccade limbic activity reflects phasically enhanced emotion processing.[43,48]

RAPID EYE MOVEMENT SLEEP AND NEUROIMAGING MEASURES OF BRAIN ACTIVITY

Deactivation of frontal cortices is one of the first signs of human sleep and can be observed using EEG, MEG, and functional neuroimaging.[40,49] PET studies of NREM sleep show declines in brain activity relative to waking both globally[49] and in many specific regions of the subcortex and cortex,[50,51] findings now replicated using fMRI.[52] Global and regional cerebral activity further decline with the deepening of NREM sleep.[49,51-53] Following sleep onset, EEG studies show greater slow wave spectral power in frontal versus posterior sites.[54] Synchronization of slow waves then spreads progressively to posterior regions,[55] a trajectory also traveled by the slow (<1 Hz) oscillation.[56]

Compared with these deactivated NREM sleep conditions, REM sleep has prominent increases of neural activity in subcortical brain regions, including the pons and midbrain,[26,50] thalamus,[26,50] basal ganglia,[50] and limbic subcortex comprising the amygdala,[26] hypothalamus, and ventral striatum.[50] Increases are also seen in limbic-related cortices anteriorly in the rostral and subcallosal anterior cingulate,[26,50] anterior insula, more posterior orbitofrontal and paracingulate BA 32 cortices, BA 10 in PFC,[50] and more posteriorly in the parahippocampal gyrus and temporal pole.[50] Certain visual association cortices (regions that process higher-order aspects of vision) are also active.[50,57] However, multiple neuroimaging modalities show that lateral prefrontal cortices remain deactivated after the transition from NREM to REM sleep.[26,50,57,58]

When REM sleep is directly compared with waking, there is a relative deactivation of the lateral PFC.[26,50,58] Maquet and colleagues[58] showed that regions most consistently hypoactive in REM sleep compared with waking include middle and inferior frontal gyri as well as inferior parietal and temporal-parietal junction association cortices. However, compared with waking, in REM sleep there is *greater* activation of limbic and paralimbic regions.[26,50,59,60] Nofzinger and colleagues[60,61] termed this region the "anterior paralimbic REM activation area" and described it as a "bilateral confluent paramedian zone which extends from the septal area into ventral striatum, infralimbic, prelimbic, orbitofrontal, and anterior cingulate cortex" (p. 192).[60] It includes the hypothalamus, ventral pallidum, hippocampus, and uncus as well as supplementary motor, pregenual and subgenual anterior cingulate, and insular cortices.[61]

RAPID EYE MOVEMENT SLEEP AND NEUROIMAGING MEASURES OF BRAIN FUNCTIONAL CONNECTIVITY

Connectivity in the context of functional neuroimaging studies is simply correlating the activity of two brain regions. fMRI is ideal for this, but obtaining REM sleep during fMRI is difficult. The acoustic noise could have an effect, but the effect of noise exposure on REM sleep is not agreed upon,[62] whereas converging evidence exists for the decrease in REM sleep during the first night of sleeping in a laboratory environment. Therefore the difficulty in obtaining REM sleep during fMRI may be largely to the result of the first-night effect.[63] There are only four fMRI studies of functional connectivity during REM sleep, and they all have small sample sizes (n = 2–12).[64-67] The results from these studies indicate that connectivity during REM-sleep dreaming exists but may differ from the connectivity observed during waking cognition.

DEFAULT-MODE NETWORK

During rest, a set of brain regions termed the *default-mode network* demonstrates an increase in activation relative to external task performance.[68] This network includes posteromedial parietal (posterior cingulate, precuneus, and retrosplenial cortices), lateral-inferior-parietal/superior-temporal regions, hippocampal formation (hippocampus and parahippocampal cortex), and medial PFC regions.[68,69] Rather than simply labeling them as resting-state networks, this and other such networks can be conceived as *intrinsic connectivity networks* because they are associated with internally cued cognition.[69] Dreaming is another type of internally cued cognition, so it naturally shares many features with waking internally cued cognition.

Default-Mode Network (Simulation Subsystem)

The default-mode network includes two subsystems: one centered on the hippocampal formation (the medial temporal lobe subsystem, henceforth referred to as the *simulation subsystem*) and one centered on the dorsal medial PFC (the dorsal medial PFC subsystem, henceforth referred to as the *self-referential subsystem*). Activity in both correlate strongly with a core network (anterior-medial PFC and posterior cingulate cortex) but weakly with each other.[70,71] The simulation subsystem is active during both retrospective simulation (remembering the past) and prospective simulation (imagining the future),[72] whereas the self-referential subsystem is active during self-relevant tasks and social cognition, including imagining what others are thinking and feeling (i.e., theory of mind).[73]

During SWS, core default-mode network regions are disconnected (e.g., see the work by Fox and colleagues[74]).

During REM sleep, these regions become reconnected,[65,67] and simulation subsystem regions show higher connectivity compared with SWS.[66] The overall similarity in default-mode network connectivity during wakefulness and REM sleep was confirmed using meta-analytic techniques,[75] so the default-mode network simulation subsystem is a primary candidate to explain the dreaming that predominates in REM sleep (e.g., see the work by Pace-Schott[40]).

Default-Mode Network (Self-Referential Subsystem)

Although internally cued cognitions in dreaming and waking share many features, they have notable dissimilarities. Koike and colleagues[66] discovered incomplete reconnectivity in the self-referential subsystem during REM sleep as evidenced by a lack of anterior-posterior connectivity with the dorsal medial PFC. This difference in connectivity in the self-referential network may underlie the high delusional acceptance of dreaming compared with internally cued cognition during waking. Combining data from this study with newer data, Watanabe and colleagues[76] discovered that overall default-mode network connectivity progressively decreases within a single bout of REM sleep, and this reaffirms the heterogeneous and dynamic nature of connectivity during REM sleep.

During dreaming, alterations in default-mode network connectivity may cause the simulation to be perceived as occurring in the present.[40] Without a perception of the self, the dreamer may also confabulate the simulations into a story-like theme as an attempt to interpret them.[77,78] This idea is consistent with the importance of the temporal-parietal junction (BA 40) in dreaming. This region is another node in the self-referential subsystem.[70] Similarly to how Damasio describes alterations in the dream self,[79] perhaps the lack of the integration of the self into cognition is the reason that we cannot properly perceive events experienced during dreaming as a simulation.

LARGE-SCALE NETWORKS

A regular network has many nodes with short-distance connections (similar to a local train). This is inefficient because the average number of jumps needed to travel between all possible pairs of nodes in the network is very high. A random network has more nodes with long-distance connections (similar to an express train), and in such a network, the probability that two nodes are connected is unrelated to distance. This is inefficient because it results in more total wiring, and information may need to travel a long distance to traverse two nodes despite the fact that they are close to each other. During wakefulness, the brain resembles an ideal "small-world" network,[80] which is a compromise between a regular and random network. The importance of information integration across a large number of brain regions has become a central tenet in theories of consciousness,[81-83] and alterations in this integration resulting from the absence of core nodes or increased randomness may explain the alterations in consciousness that accompany sleep and dreaming.[84,85]

During NREM sleep stages 1 and 2, brain connectivity resembles more of a random network compared with wakefulness, and during SWS, the brain resembles more of a regular network compared with wakefulness,[86] although changes to a more regular network have also been observed in NREM sleep stage 2.[87] The shift to a more random network during sleep onset may be correlated with hypnagogic hallucinations.

Although portions of the thalamus are sometimes included in the default-mode network, it may be more appropriate to consider them part of a larger network because many thalamic nuclei project diffusely throughout the brain. Thalamocortical connectivity is weaker in NREM sleep stage 2 and SWS compared with wakefulness[88] and stronger in REM sleep compared with wakefulness and SWS.[67] Heightened thalamocortical connectivity during REM sleep may orchestrate dissociated heteromodal cortical regions and, correspondingly, the forced, confabulatory narrative in dreams.[67] Phasic REM-sleep episodes arising from a tonic REM sleep background showed characteristic changes in forebrain activity, including increased functional connectivity between the thalamus and a broad cortical-limbic-striatal network.[64] Wehrle and colleagues[64] suggest that these changes represent activation, during phasic REM sleep, of networks important to memory and emotion processing. Therefore, like the EEG and MEG studies detailed previously, functional connectivity indicates that phasic REM sleep is associated with brain activity that may reflect intensified dream imagery, attention, and emotion but in the context of a network connectivity that differs from wakefulness.

THE NEUROCHEMISTRY OF DREAMING

Three major neurochemical hypotheses have been advanced to explain differences between dreaming and waking consciousness. First, the activation-synthesis and activation-input-modulation models of Hobson and colleagues suggest that the massive increase in cholinergic (relative to noradrenergic and serotonergic) activation from the ascending reticular activating system (ARAS) during REM sleep contributes strongly to the unique nature of dream consciousness.[3,39] Second, Solms[28] has suggested that stimulation of limbic and prefrontal reward networks by dopaminergic projections from the midbrain ventral tegmental area (VTA) generates motivational impulses that initiate dreaming, a hypothesis recently expanded in the reward activation model of Perogamvros and colleagues.[89,90] Third, Gottesmann suggests that dopaminergic stimulation of the cortex during REM sleep, in the absence of waking's inhibitory serotonergic and noradrenergic modulation, allows emergence of psychotomimetic (psychosis-like) aspects of dream consciousness.[91]

Acetylcholine

The activation-synthesis[39] and activation-input-modulation[3] models suggest that forebrain activation in REM-sleep dreaming originates in ascending activation of the thalamus by mesopontine cholinergic nuclei. Much evidence exists for cholinergic enhancement of both REM sleep and dreaming. Higher mesopontine- and brainstem-derived acetylcholine concentrations during wake and REM versus NREM sleep are seen in the thalamus, including the lateral geniculate nucleus.[92] Cholinergic stimulation potentiates REM sleep when microinjected into the animal brainstem or when systemically administered to humans.[3] Cholinesterase inhibitors can induce REM sleep with dreaming,[93] increase nightmares,[94] and increase hypnagogic hallucinations.[95] Transdermal nicotine[96] and the nicotinic receptor partial agonist varenicline[97] intensify dreams. Compelling evidence for a cholinergic role in dreaming comes from recent studies using the acetylcholinesterase inhibitor galantamine to induce lucid dreaming.

Galantamine, in addition to increasing the frequency of lucid dreams, enhanced ratings of recall, vividness, bizarreness, and complexity.[98] Notably, galantamine also shortens REM latency and increases the percentage of REM sleep.[99]

Dopamine

A key role is assigned to dopamine in psychosis-like[91] and reward-based[28] theories of dreaming. The latter was recently expanded in the reward activation model, which posits that high-saliency memories are selectively processed during dreaming following their replay and prioritization by hippocampal-ventral striatal circuits in NREM sleep.[89,90] Support for this model comes from selective consolidation of salient memories during sleep[100,101] and the fact that administration of a dopamine agonist eliminates this selectivity.[102] In addition, L-dopa and certain other dopaminergic agents can enhance dreaming in patients with Parkinson disease.[28,103,104] However, psychostimulants are not associated with dream enhancement, neuroleptics do not prevent dreaming, some dopamine agonists reduce dreaming, and some dopamine antagonists enhance dreaming.[104] Thus dopamine's dream effects may depend on dosage as well as receptor type and location. This is a particularly important consideration because when dreams were directly measured in patients with Parkinson disease using awakenings from sleep, dopamine agonist dosage was negatively correlated with dreaming.[105]

Roles for dopamine in REM sleep have also emerged from animal studies. For example, enhancing REM sleep intensity increases c-Fos expression in the VTA,[106] and dopamine concentrations in the medial PFC and nucleus accumbens are greater during REM sleep than during NREM sleep.[107] In addition, increased burst firing in the VTA has been observed during REM sleep[108] and may result from increased cholinergic excitation of the VTA by the pedunculopontine nucleus.[109]

Serotonin

Selective serotonin (5-HT) reuptake inhibitors and other serotonergic drugs can intensify dreaming.[110] Animal studies of serotonergic hallucinogens by Aghajanian and colleagues suggest that low or fluctuating cortical 5-HT levels may be conducive to hallucinosis by inducing prolonged excitatory postsynaptic potentials hypothesized to underlie the cognitive-perceptual effects of the hallucinogens.[111] Naturally occurring fluctuations of 5-HT occur during the decline of its release to minimal levels in REM,[3] and this may promote the natural occurrence of hallucinosis.

NEUROPSYCHIATRIC SYNDROMES THAT INFORM THE STUDY OF DREAMING

Confabulation Shares Neural Substrate with REM-Sleep Dreaming

Like the dreamer, patients with spontaneous behavioral confabulation believe they have experienced false events and act on false beliefs, believing them with unshakable conviction.[112-114] Confabulation results from lesions of the ventral medial PFC (vmPFC), the orbitofrontal cortex, and their connections with the basal forebrain, amygdala, thalamic mediodorsal nucleus, and hypothalamus.[113-115] These regions broadly overlap with the anterior paralimbic REM sleep activation region.[61]

One theory on the cognitive deficit resulting in confabulation suggests that vmPFC lesions disrupt a reality-monitoring function that preconsciously suppresses spontaneously activated memories not pertaining to present circumstances.[115] Memories of past experiences are thus perceived as related to the present.[115] An alternative theory posits temporal deficits to be a subset of a more general deficit in strategic retrieval and verification of memories.[114]

In both confabulation[113] and dreaming, altered function of the vmPFC and the orbitofrontal cortex may release from normal inhibitory, reality-monitoring, and executive constraints, innate human tendencies to represent both imagined and experienced events within a narrative structure.[77] Notably, medial PFC regions have also been associated with the production of narrative during wakefulness.[116]

Visual Hallucinosis in Waking and Dreaming

Anatomic regions associated with dreaming and hallucinosis also overlap. Manford and Andermann[117] suggest that hallucinations result when inferior occipital and temporal visual association cortices that identify objects and scenes (the "ventral processing stream") are released from normal restraints under three conditions: (1) loss of exogenous visual input, (2) ARAS damage that alters serotonergic and cholinergic modulation of the cortex, or (3) abnormally excitatory input.[117] Conditions corresponding to each mechanism may contribute to REM-sleep hallucinosis:

1. In Charles Bonnet syndrome, waking hallucinosis results when perceptual input to the visual association cortex is lost because of lesions of the primary visual pathway.[117] In REM sleep there is no retinal input and visual cortices are deactivated,[57] a phenomenon that perhaps decreases their regulatory input on downstream association cortices.
2. As noted previously, the aminergic/cholinergic balance changes with REM/NREM transitions.[3]
3. Abnormal excitation of visual association cortices (the regions active during hallucinations in Charles Bonnet syndrome[118]) can produce epileptic hallucinosis.[117]

Ventral-processing-stream visual association cortices are more active in REM sleep than in either NREM sleep or post-sleep waking[50,57] and are a hypothesized source of dream imagery.[3,28] During REM sleep, PGO waves originating in the mesopontine brainstem[3,44] excite many cortical regions, including visual association regions.[119]

Collerton and colleagues[120] suggest that hallucinations result from combined sensory impairment, attentional deficit, and relatively intact scene perception that allow poorly formed "proto-objects" to resolve into erroneous percepts. In REM-sleep dreaming, ascending activation of visual association cortices may evoke hallucinatory proto-objects that, under the attentionally unstable conditions of REM sleep, resolve into hallucinatory percepts congruent with the ongoing dream plot. Internal consistency of dream plots may then arise because the evolving dream context itself biases resolution of ambiguous percepts into plot-congruent images. Dreams may thus evolve by a "boot-strapping" process, whereby current images provide the context that, in turn, determines succeeding dream imagery.[121] In the absence of working memory capacities that provide continuity to waking experience, the evolving dream plot can be strongly influenced by immediately prior dream experiences.

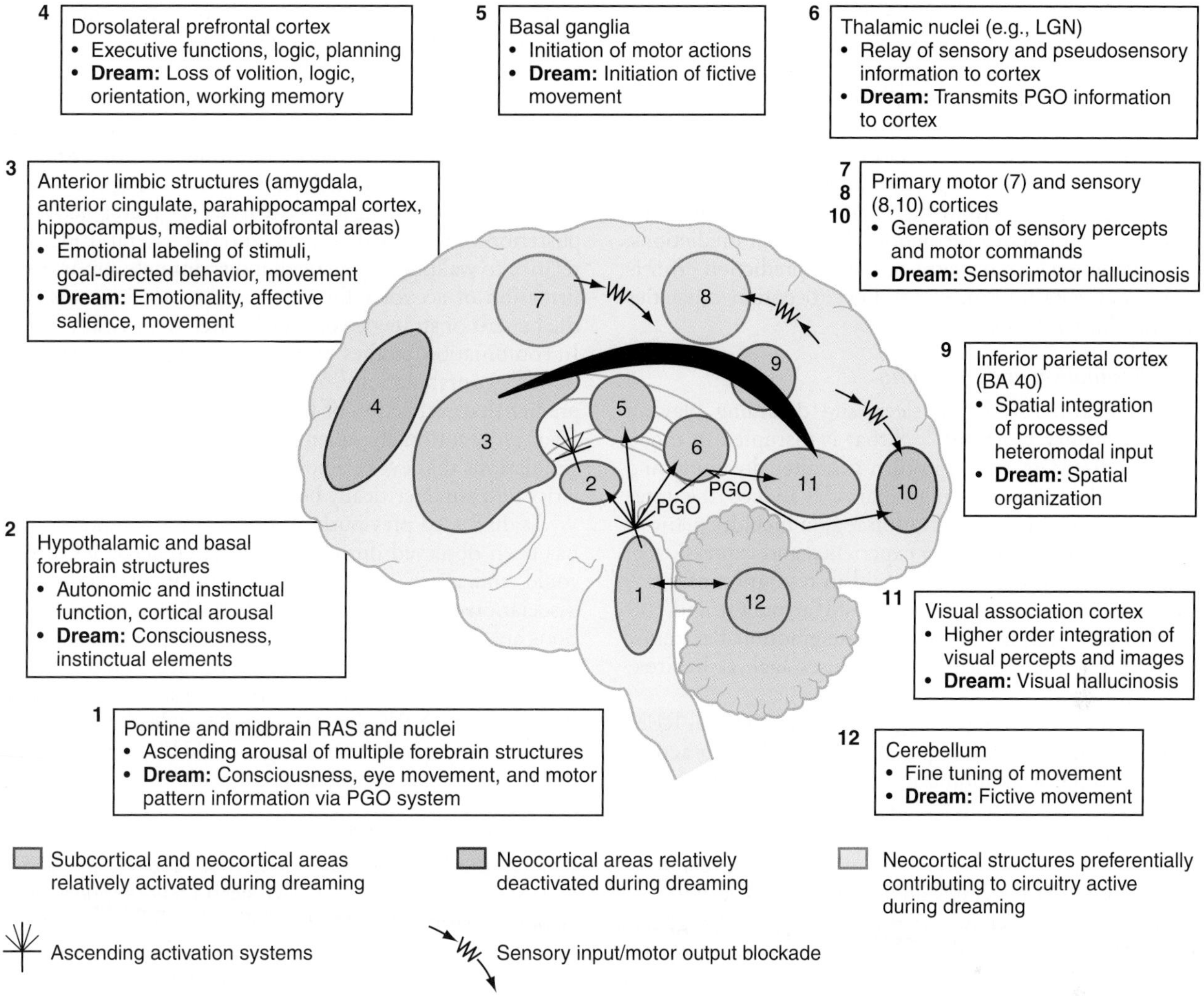
4 Dorsolateral prefrontal cortex
• Executive functions, logic, planning
• Dream: Loss of volition, logic, orientation, working memory
5 Basal ganglia
• Initiation of motor actions
• Dream: Initiation of fictive movement
6 Thalamic nuclei (e.g., LGN)
• Relay of sensory and pseudosensory information to cortex
• Dream: Transmits PGO information to cortex
3 Anterior limbic structures (amygdala, anterior cingulate, parahippocampal cortex, hippocampus, medial orbitofrontal areas)
• Emotional labeling of stimuli, goal-directed behavior, movement
• Dream: Emotionality, affective salience, movement
7 8 10 Primary motor (7) and sensory (8,10) cortices
• Generation of sensory percepts and motor commands
• Dream: Sensorimotor hallucinosis
9 Inferior parietal cortex (BA 40)
• Spatial integration of processed heteromodal input
• Dream: Spatial organization
2 Hypothalamic and basal forebrain structures
• Autonomic and instinctual function, cortical arousal
• Dream: Consciousness, instinctual elements
11 Visual association cortex
• Higher order integration of visual percepts and images
• Dream: Visual hallucinosis
1 Pontine and midbrain RAS and nuclei
• Ascending arousal of multiple forebrain structures
• Dream: Consciousness, eye movement, and motor pattern information via PGO system
12 Cerebellum
• Fine tuning of movement
• Dream: Fictive movement
PGO
PGO
Subcortical and neocortical areas relatively activated during dreaming
Neocortical areas relatively deactivated during dreaming
Neocortical structures preferentially contributing to circuitry active during dreaming
Ascending activation systems
Sensory input/motor output blockade

Figure 58.1 Forebrain processes in normal dreaming—an integration of neurophysiologic, neuropsychological, and neuroimaging data. Regions 1 and 2, ascending arousal systems; region 3, subcortical and cortical limbic and paralimbic structures; region 4, dorsal lateral prefrontal executive association cortex; region 5, motor initiation and control centers; region 6, thalamocortical relay centers and thalamic subcortical circuitry; region 7, primary motor cortex; region 8, primary sensory cortex; region 9, inferior parietal lobe; region 10, primary visual cortex; region 11, visual association cortex; region 12, cerebellum. BA 40, Brodmann area 40, the temporal-parietal junction; LGN, lateral geniculate nucleus; PGO, ponto-geniculo-occipital waves; RAS, reticular activating system. (From Hobson JA, Pace-Schott EF, Stickgold R. Dreaming and the brain: toward a cognitive neuroscience of conscious states. *Behavioral and Brain Sciences* 2000;23:793–842; discussion 904–1121.)

A DESCRIPTIVE NEURAL MODEL OF DREAM PHENOMENOLOGY AND FUNCTION

The following working model of neurobiologic structures and networks subserving REM-sleep-dream phenomenology refers to brain regions depicted in Figure 58.1.[3]

Ascending Arousal Systems

Activation of the forebrain in REM sleep, as in waking, occurs through the ascending arousal systems of the brainstem,[12] basal forebrain,[122] and hypothalamus[123] (regions 1 and 2 in Figure 58.1). However, unlike in waking, ascending activation in REM sleep is primarily facilitated by cholinergic systems, whereas aminergic neuromodulation is attenuated.[3] In NREM sleep, phasic increases in ARAS activity, resulting from endogenous or exogenous stimulation, may transiently stimulate the same forebrain networks activated in REM, potentially creating the subjective experience of NREM-sleep dreaming.

Thalamocortical Relay Centers and Thalamic Subcortical Circuitry

During REM sleep, thalamocortical signaling (region 6 in Figure 58.1) may be interpreted as incoming sensory information by primary and secondary association sensory cortices[39] (region 11) and evoke local activation of stored cognitive representations (hallucinosis of known entities) or novel representations (as in dream bizarreness). The PGO wave may be only one of many pathways for ARAS phasic activation of the cortex by thalamic or basal forebrain intermediaries during REM sleep. For example, in the rat, the pontine p-wave in REM sleep impinges directly on limbic structures such as the amygdala, hippocampus, and entorhinal cortex as well as the visual cortex.[124]

Subcortical and Cortical Limbic and Paralimbic Structures

In REM sleep, selective activation of limbic and paralimbic cortex and subcortex (region 3 in Figure 58.1) suggested to

PET researchers a role for REM sleep in the processing of emotionally influenced memories,[58,125] integration of neocortical functions with basal forebrain and hypothalamic motivational and reward mechanisms,[60] or internal information processing between visual association and limbic regions.[57] Such processes may underlie the emotional and social nature of dreaming.[40,126] Interestingly, the anterior paralimbic cortices have been proposed to be regions that can generate emotional states by active prediction.[127,128] Such predictions, during wakefulness, can be corrected when prediction error is identified on the basis of insight and exteroception-capacities unavailable during dreaming.

Emotion Regulation and Dreaming

It is often hypothesized that sleep and dreaming play an emotion-regulatory function[129,130] that is disrupted in mood and anxiety disorders, which in turn can alter dreaming and result in experiences such as nightmares.[131] Indeed, the anterior paralimbic REM sleep activation region includes many of the structures implicated in the experience and expression of emotion.[132] Although dreams may aid in resolution of intrapersonal conflict (e.g., see the work by Cartwright and colleagues[129]), dreaming may also moderate emotional extremes by universal mammalian learning processes such as habituation and extinction.[131]

Nielsen and Levin[131] have suggested that, in normal REM sleep, activity in the anterior paralimbic REM-sleep activation region regulates emotion through formation of extinction memories when emotionally salient memories appear in safer contexts during dreaming. Human[133] as well as nonhuman-animal[134] studies link formation, retention, and expression of extinction learning to circuitry linking the amygdala, vmPFC, and hippocampus. Notably, a night's sleep promotes generalization of extinction learning.[135,136] Whereas such circuitry may be recruited by cognitive processes subserved by dorsal lateral PFC (dlPFC) in waking,[137] it may function autonomously during REM-sleep dreaming.[131]

Reward systems are also activated in REM sleep, during which positive and negative emotions may be modulated. VTA sources of mesolimbic and mesocortical dopamine are recruited by ascending cholinergic activation[109] and, like their ventral striatal and medial PFC targets, lie well within the anterior paralimbic REM-sleep activation region.[61] In dreaming, hypothalamic-brainstem circuits may initiate instinctively salient behavior[138] that may, in turn, recruit additional forebrain regions to enact appetitive[28] or other adaptive behaviors.[138]

Altered Memory Processing in Dreams

A cholinergically mediated informational barrier between cortex and hippocampus in REM sleep has been proposed to underlie the paucity of episodic memories in dreams.[139] However, despite the inaccessibility of episodic memory, another aspect of declarative memory, "familiarity" or "recognition,"[140] is ubiquitous in dreams. For example, 40% of dream characters may be identified on the basis of "just knowing."[126] Schwartz and Maquet[141] suggest such phenomena result from the sleep-related disconnection of temporal lobe face recognition from prefrontal reality monitoring regions. Alternatively, frequent experiences of familiarity in the absence of accurate replay of episodic memories in dreams may reflect activity of recognition memory mechanisms in anterior perirhinal cortices (BA 35, BA 36) dissociated from hippocampally mediated recall.[140]

During dreaming, frontal contributions to memory retrieval may also be altered. Ventral lateral and dlPFC regions that are deactivated in REM sleep[58] subserve cue-specification and search strategies, respectively.[142] In contrast, posterior vmPFC is active in REM sleep[50] and subserves "feeling-of-rightness"[142] and "feeling-of-knowing,"[143] for which more anterior PFC regions only later provide cognitive verification.[142] Therefore, during REM sleep, greater activation of posterior-ventral-medial than anterior-lateral PFC regions relative to waking may favor an indiscriminate, emotional confirmation of accuracy for any item in consciousness without the benefit of strategic volitional search or critical verification. In combination, studies of mental simulation,[72] active prediction,[128] confabulation,[114,115] and memory verification[142,143] predict that restriction of frontal activation to vmPFC would favor an emotionally salient state prone to producing mental simulations that evoke a powerful sense of veracity and familiarity and are uncritically believed.

As discussed previously, a shift to a more random network has been observed during NREM sleep stage 1.[86] This shift could underlie the discontinuous and incongruous memory associations of dreaming in this stage. Hypnagogic hallucinations are typically short, so it would be difficult to measure the correlation between these bizarre associations and small-world network changes. No similar studies exist for REM sleep, but the data from NREM sleep stage 1 may lead one to predict a similar change, and these changes could be correlated with the bizarreness of the corresponding dream.

Dreaming as a Simulation

Default-mode network simulation subsystem activation and connectivity during REM sleep could support both the elaborate, story-like structure of many REM dreams[77] and the memory function of sleep.[144,145] Although entire memories are often not incorporated into REM-sleep mentation, memory elements may be incorporated depending on their emotional salience and/or cued reward value for subsequent memory consolidation,[140] as discussed previously. In addition to consolidating memories, activity in the default-mode network during dreaming would support the idea that dreams simulate potential future events to prepare for them.[146,147] Imagining future events increases goal-directed actions when the corresponding opportunity later presents itself,[148] so simulation subsystem connectivity and the associated dreaming may increase adaptive behavior, similar to proposals on the functions of internally cued cognition during wakefulness.[70] The sensorially vivid and entirely novel narratives that characterize some dreams[77] speak to the capacity of the brain to involuntarily create fictive experiences, resulting perhaps from both the activation and disinhibition of the predictive capacities of the brain.[149,150]

Social Cognition and Dreams

Brain regions most consistently activated in neuroimaging studies of social cognition include regions that compose the default-mode network self-referential subsystem.[151] Incomplete reconnectivity of this subsystem during REM sleep[66] may underlie the high degree of delusional acceptance of dreams compared with waking cognition, and this may depend on an altered integration of the self into cognition. However, theory of mind, a complex aspect of social cognition,[151] is preserved in dreaming despite notable degradation of reasoning about the physical world.[152,153] This may seem like a contradiction, but social cognition has two components: an ability to perceive ourselves as social agents and an ability to perceive the intentions of others.[154] Subtle disconnections in the self-referential subsystem may disrupt the former and lead to delusional acceptance of dreams, whereas residual connectivity in the self-referential subsystem may preserve the latter and produce the ubiquity of interpersonal interactions and emotions in dreams.[40,58,77,152,155]

Motor Initiation and Control Centers

Strong activation of the basal ganglia[50] (region 5 in Figure. 58.1) may mediate the ubiquitous fictive motion of dreams.[156] The basal ganglia are extensively connected not only with motor cortex but also with mesopontine (e.g., pedunculopontine) nuclei[157] that contain gait circuitry and other motor pattern generators as well as REM-sleep regulatory regions.[3] Activation of brainstem vestibular nuclei and the associated cerebellar vermis[50] during REM sleep may additionally contribute to vestibular sensations interpreted in ways such as flying or falling.

Visual Association Cortex

Medial occipitotemporal cortices (region 11 in Figure. 58.1) are activated in REM sleep.[50,57] These and other visual association regions may generate the visual imagery of dreams.[3,28] As in waking, specific regions of the visual association cortex may process specific visual characteristics of dreaming. For example, the fusiform gyrus both mediates waking face recognition and is activated in REM sleep.[50,57,60] Braun and colleagues[57] suggest that REM sleep constitutes a unique cortical condition of internal information processing (between visual association and limbic cortices), functionally isolated from input from (through primary visual cortex) or output to (through frontal cortex) the external world. Dream image formation may arise as ascending activation impinges on visual and multimodal association regions in occipital, temporal, and inferior parietal cortices.

Inferior Parietal Lobe

The supramarginal and angular gyri of the inferior parietal lobe (BA 39 and 40; region 9 in Figure. 58.1), especially in the right hemisphere, are essential for visuospatial awareness.[158] These regions may generate the fictive dream space necessary for the organized hallucinatory experience of dreaming.[28] Destruction of these regions is alone sufficient to produce global cessation of reported dreaming.[28] Maquet and colleagues have found the right inferior parietal cortex to be relatively activated during REM sleep in some[26] but not all[59] PET studies. In REM sleep, both the previously described visual association cortex and the vmPFC are simultaneously active.[57] Therefore, in REM sleep, self-centric reality simulation, a putative function of the vmPFC,[72] and hallucinatory imagery may arise in concert. Inferior parietal multimodal association cortices may integrate different unimodal inputs and facilitate their incorporation into the emerging plot in the virtual proscenium where the dream is experienced. A recent publication by Siclari and colleagues[34] reports that high frequency activity in a posterior "hot zone," which includes the inferior parietal lobe, predicts the report of dream experience when awakened from either REM or NREM sleep, whereas low frequency activity in this same region predicts the absence of such. These authors equate this region to a putative posterior zone that constitutes the minimum "neural correlate of consciousness."[83]

Dorsolateral Prefrontal Executive Association Cortex

Lesions of the dlPFC (region 4 in Figure 58.1) do not cause cessation or attenuation of dreaming, an observation that suggests that it is nonessential for the generation of dreaming.[28] Unlike vmPFC regions that reactivate, these dorsal lateral prefrontal regions remain deactivated in REM sleep,[26,50,57,58] and this may explain dream mentation executive deficiencies that include disorientation, illogic, impaired working memory, and amnesia for dreams.[3] Additionally, because the PFC regulates posterior sensory cortices,[159] deactivation of the dlPFC in REM sleep[26,50,58] may promote dreaming by disconnection, release, or disinhibition of sensory association cortices (as also suggested by EEG and MEG[5,160,161]). Similar disinhibition may result from lowered activity in the right inferior frontal cortex, a lateral PFC region also associated with inhibition in multiple domains.[162]

This may also be consistent with the absence of the dorsal medial PFC from the default-mode network self-referential subsystem during REM sleep.[66] In addition to considering the dorsal medial PFC as part of the default-mode network self-referential subsystem, it and the lateral portions of the PFC can be considered as part of executive association cortex that includes the superior parietal gyrus, and the disruption of this network may, again, promote dreaming by disinhibition of sensory association cortices.[163] The incomplete reconnectivity of this node in REM sleep may contribute to the bizarre nature of dreaming compared with waking cognition and is closely related to the reconnectivity of the simulation subsystem in REM sleep. Because this reconnectivity co-occurs with a reduction in sensory input, this may elicit the spontaneous and involuntary cognitions of dreaming.[144]

The PFC maintains an online representation of a goal, the means to achieve it, and the ongoing context relevant to this goal to "bias" the functioning of networks elsewhere in the brain toward this particular outcome.[164] With diminished frontal activation during sleep, goal-directed biases in the regulation of circuits subserving working memory and attention (frontoparietal) and memory encoding and retrieval (frontotemporal) may be impaired during dreaming.[3,40]

CLINICAL PEARL

The physician prescribing selective serotonin reuptake inhibitors, transdermal nicotine, varenicline, beta blockers, dopaminergic agents, or a variety of other medications should be alert for possible dream intensification or nightmare induction. Other choices within the same class or a different class of medications may have to be considered if such side effects are intolerable to the patient.

SUMMARY

ARAS, thalamocortical, and basal forebrain-cortical arousal systems activate the forebrain regions involved in dream construction in a manner that is chemically and anatomically different from waking. In REM sleep, such activation may be more frequent and sustained and, perhaps, may proceed through different or more diverse pathways than in NREM sleep. Cortical circuits activated in REM-sleep dreaming are medial circuits that link visual association and paralimbic regions (central crescent in Figure 58.1) but not the primary sensory and lateral frontal executive cortical regions that are active in waking.[57] Therefore dreaming is both positively and negatively emotionally salient (amygdala, ventral striatum, vmPFC), often conflictual (anterior cingulate), and social (vmPFC) while also displaying profoundly deficient working memory, orientation, and logic (lateral prefrontal and parietal deactivation). Subcortical circuits involving the limbic structures, striatum, diencephalon, and brainstem regions are selectively activated in REM sleep. They may contribute to dreaming's emotional (limbic subcortex), motoric (striatum, brainstem, cerebellum), instinctual (hypothalamus), and motivational (midbrain-ventral striatum) properties. Preserved connectivity in default-mode network simulation subsystem during REM sleep may be the neural substrate of dream simulations, whereas altered connectivity in default-mode network self-referential subsystem may underlie the high degree of delusional acceptance of dreams when compared with waking cognition.

ACKNOWLEDGMENTS

Work on which this chapter is based was supported [in part] by the NIH/NIMH R21MH101567 and the Intramural Research Program of the National Institute of Neurological Disorders and Stroke. Dr. Pace-Schott is supported by MH109638, MH115279.

SELECTED READINGS

Baird B, Mota-Rolim SA, Dresler M. The cognitive neuroscience of lucid dreaming. *Neurosci Biobehav Rev.* 2019;100:305–323. https://doi.org/10.1016/j.neubiorev.2019.03.008.

Dresler M, et al. Neural correlates of insight in dreaming and psychosis. *Sleep Med Rev.* 2015;20:92–99. https://doi.org/10.1016/j.smrv.2014.06.004.

Fox KC, Nijeboer S, Solomonova E, Domhoff GW, Christoff K. Dreaming as mind wandering: evidence from functional neuroimaging and first-person content reports. *Front Hum Neurosci.* 2013;7:412. https://doi.org/10.3389/fnhum.2013.00412.

Hobson JA, Hong CC, Friston KJ. Virtual reality and consciousness inference in dreaming. *Front Psychol.* 2014;5:1133. https://doi.org/10.3389/fpsyg.2014.01133.

Hobson JA, Pace-Schott EF, Stickgold R. Dreaming and the brain: toward a cognitive neuroscience of conscious states. *Behav Brain Sci.* 2000;23:793–842; discussion 904 1121. https://doi.org/10.1017/s0140525x00003976.

Manger PR, Siegel JM. Do all mammals dream? *J Comp Neurol.* 2020;528(17):3198–3204.

Maquet P, et al. Human cognition during REM sleep and the activity profile within frontal and parietal cortices: a reappraisal of functional neuroimaging data. *Prog Brain Res.* 2005;150:219–227. https://doi.org/10.1016/S0079-6123(05)50016-5.

Nielsen T, Levin R. Nightmares: a new neurocognitive model. *Sleep Med Rev.* 2007;11:295–310. https://doi.org/10.1016/j.smrv.2007.03.004.

Pace-Schott EF. Dreaming as a story-telling instinct. *Front Psychol.* 2013;4:159. https://doi.org/10.3389/fpsyg.2013.00159.

Perogamvros L, Dang-Vu TT, Desseilles M, Schwartz S. Sleep and dreaming are for important matters. *Front Psychol.* 2013;4:474. https://doi.org/10.3389/fpsyg.2013.00474.

Picchioni D, Duyn JH, Horovitz SG. Sleep and the functional connectome. *Neuroimage.* 2013;80:387–396. https://doi.org/10.1016/j.neuroimage.2013.05.067.

Rechtschaffen A. The single-mindedness and isolation of dreams. *Sleep.* 1978;1:97–109. https://doi.org/10.1093/sleep/1.1.97.

Sterpenich V, Perogamvros L, Tononi G, et al. Fear in dreams and in wakefulness: Evidence for day/night affective homeostasis. *Hum Brain Mapp.* 2020;41(3):840–850.

Wamsley EJ. Dreaming, waking conscious experience, and the resting brain: report of subjective experience as a tool in the cognitive neurosciences. *Front Psychol.* 2013;4:637. https://doi.org/10.3389/fpsyg.2013.00637.

A complete reference list can be found online at ExpertConsult.com.

Chapter 59

Lucid Dreaming

Martin Dresler; Benjamin Baird; Daniel Erlacher; Michael Czisch; Victor I. Spoormaker; Stephen LaBerge

Chapter Highlights

- During lucid dreaming, one is aware of the fact that one is dreaming while continuing to dream. This metacognitive insight often leads to access to waking episodic memory and increased volitional control in the dream.
- Lucid dreaming occurs in physiologically defined rapid eye movement (REM) sleep and can be objectively verified with eye signaling methods with concurrent polysomnography. Lucid dreaming is associated with physiologic activation and autonomic arousal, which reaches its peak during phasic REM sleep.
- Electroencephalographic studies of lucid dreaming have found mixed results, whereas preliminary neuroimaging data indicate that lucid dreaming is associated with prefrontal and parietal cortical regions.
- Lucid dreaming spontaneously occurs infrequently; however, several strategies exist to increase its frequency, including mnemonic techniques, stimulus cues, and pharmacology.
- Lucid dreaming has several potential clinical applications, most notably in the therapeutic treatment of chronic idiopathic nightmares. Other potential applications include treatment of metacognitive deficits in psychosis and development of brain activity markers for patients with disorders of consciousness.

INTRODUCTION

Conscious experience varies strikingly across the sleep-wake cycle. During wakefulness, humans are mostly alert; aware of external and internal stimuli; able to metacognitively reflect on their perceptions, emotions, and thoughts; and capable of a variety of adaptive goal-directed action, both habitual and volitional. Most of these properties of waking consciousness fade during the process of falling asleep but partly or completely reappear during sleep mentation. Conscious experience during sleep is manifold: If not absent as in dreamless sleep, it can include abstract thought fragments, intense emotions, and sensory imagery, up to fully immersive visuomotor hallucinations with a complex interactive dream plot.[1]

The phenomenon of lucid dreaming, which is characterized by many "wake-like" cognitive capabilities, illustrates the upper reaches of cognitive function possible in the dreaming brain. Minimally defined by the criterion that the sleeper is aware of the current dream state as such,[2] lucid dreaming involves insight into the illusory nature of the dream environment, access to short- and long-term memory, and sometimes volitional control within the dream.[3] Despite this increase in wake-like cognitive capability, lucid rapid eye movement (REM) sleep possesses all the defining markers of REM sleep.[2] Of importance, lucid dreaming is not an all-or-nothing phenomenon but can occur in different degrees.[4–6] Questionnaires such as the Metacognitive, Affective, Cognitive Experience (MACE) questionnaire[7] or the Lucidity and Consciousness in Dreams (LuCiD)scale[8] aim to assess different aspects of consciousness in dreams (see Baird and colleagues[9] for extended discussion and criticism of existing questionnaire measures). Because also in nonlucid dream reports some reflective thoughts have been reported and because also during daydreaming and other phases of wakefulness active reflections are frequently absent, it has been argued that metacognitive activity differs only quantitatively and not qualitatively between dreaming and waking consciousness.[10] However, this absence is only a "local," not global feature of such phases: It is hardly imaginable, at least for nonpathologic cases, that the daydreaming subject misinterprets the daydream for reality once paying attention to and reflecting the current state. For the dreaming state, in contrast, this is completely normal—unless the dreamer eventually becomes lucid by such "prelucid" reflections.[4]

Lucid dreaming initially faced skepticism in mainstream sleep research. However, in the late 1970s, the first systematic validation of lucid dreaming as an objective phenomenon occurring during physiologically defined REM sleep was achieved. Based on data showing that rotations of the physical eyes can correlate with subjective gaze direction in dreams, lucid dreamers were asked to indicate the moment they realized they were dreaming by means of a specific preagreed upon dream action (e.g., looking left-right-left-right rapidly in the dream) that was expected to produce observable signs on the polysomnogram.[11] Through this technique, which has become the gold standard in lucid dream research, lucid dream reports could be objectively verified by eye movement patterns as recorded in the electrooculogram (Figure 59.1). By providing objective temporal markers of dream content, this method has allowed for investigations into neural correlates of dreamed behaviors[12–15] and comparisons of temporal intervals

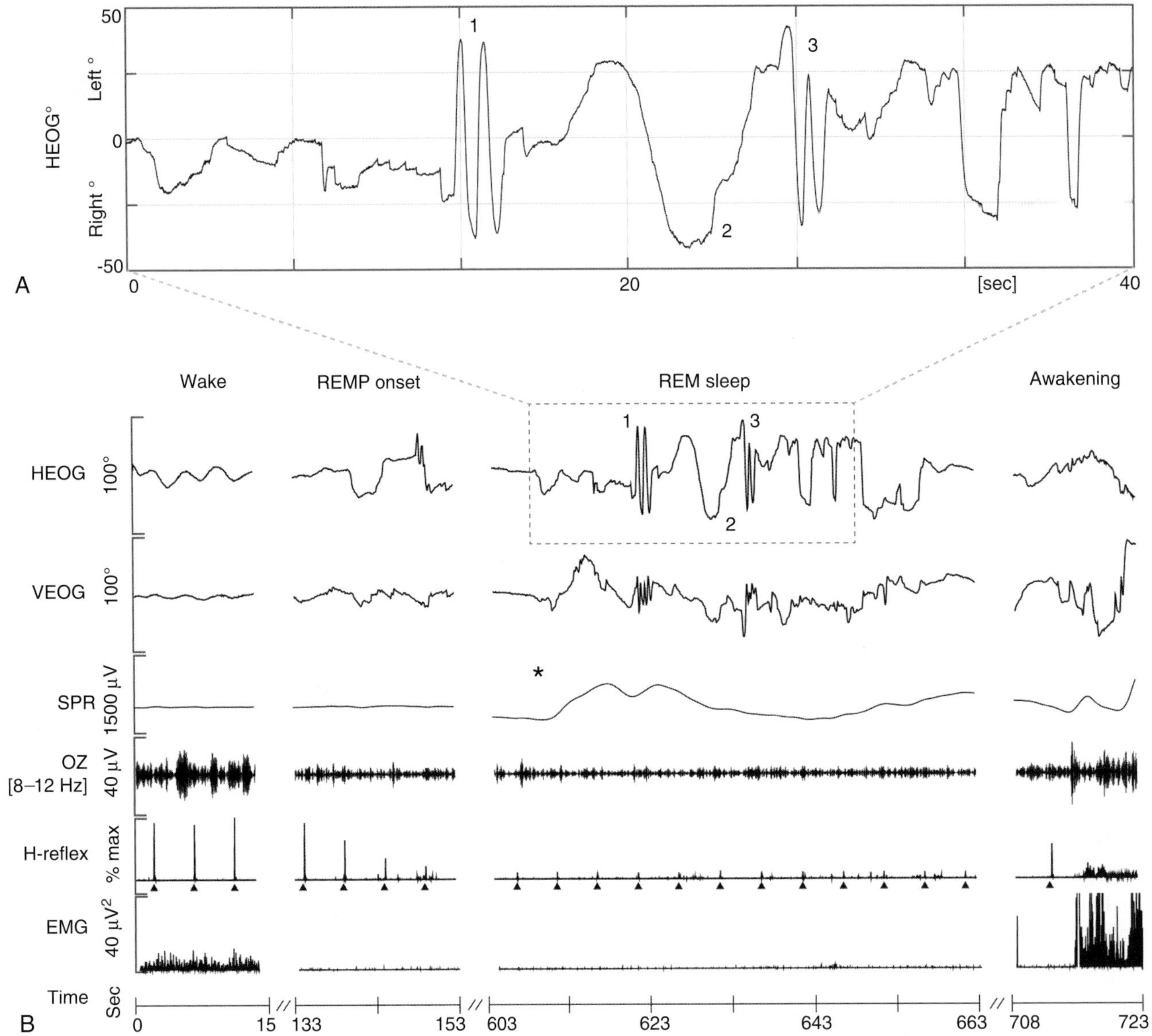

Figure 59.1 Lucid REM sleep–eye movement signaling methodology and line tracking during lucid REM–sleep dreaming. **(A)** Enlarged section showing left-right-left-right (LRLR) eye-movement signals and smooth tracking task as recorded in the horizontal electrooculogram (HEOG). Upon awakening, the subject reported becoming lucid in the dream, making an LRLR signal (1), fully extending his right thumb, and tracking his thumb nail as he slowly swung his arm horizontally from center to approximately 30 degrees left, back through center to 30 degrees right, and finally leftward back to center. While tracking to the right, he noticed moving his head slightly in the direction of tracking both rightward and leftward as he reversed motion back to the center (2). He marked the end of the smooth tracking task (estimated 10 sec) with a second LRLR signal (3). Having completed the task, he spent the remainder of his lucid dream exploring the dream environment, waking approximately 60 seconds later. **(B)** Six channels of physiologic data (HEOG, vertical EOG (VEOG), skin potential response (SPR), occipital electromyogram (EMG) bandpass filtered for alpha (8–12 Hz), H-reflex amplitude (a measure of spinal reflex excitability) (*upward black triangles* mark H-reflex stimulation), and EMG are shown during an initial period of wakefulness, REM-period onset (REMP onset), transition to lucid REM sleep and awakening. Suppression of EMG and H-reflex amplitude along with reduced alpha in EEG confirm that the participant remained in uninterrupted REM sleep during lucid dreaming, including LRLR signals and during completion of the slow tracking task. Lucid dream onset is localized by the autonomic nervous system surprise response (scalp skin potential response [SPR, *black asterisk*]) before the LRLR signal. µV, Amplitude in microvolts.

by counting or subjective estimations experienced during dreaming with objective measurements in the real world.[16–17] However, many of the studies conducted to date have had small sample sizes, in part due to the infrequency with which most subjects have lucid dreams, and thus many experimental results remain preliminary.

PREVALENCE AND INDUCTION METHODS

Lucid dreaming spontaneously occurs infrequently in the general population: Only approximately 50% of the population have had a lucid dream at least once in their lifetime, about 10% to 20% have lucid dreams on a monthly basis, and only a minority of about 1% have lucid dreams several times a week or more.[18–19] Some differences across different populations and cultures seem to exist.[20] Changes in lucid dreaming prevalence across the life span have been reported in some,[21–22] but not other studies,[23] and may be due to confounds such as dream recall. Lucid dreams may spontaneously emerge from nightmares, recognizing recurrent dreams, or reasoning through some peculiarities within the dream. However, lucid dreams can also be intentionally induced by applying various induction and deliberate training strategies,[24–25] including cognitive-behavioral strategies, external stimulation/mnemonic cuing, sleep interruption, pharmacology, and noninvasive brain stimulation.[26]

A number of different cognitive-behavioral strategies have been suggested, including methods where lucidity is initiated from within a dream, that is, a person becomes lucid during a dream (dream-initiated lucid dreams, DILD) and methods where lucidity is initiated from wakefulness, that is, a person retains conscious awareness when falling asleep, for example, after a brief awakening with subsequent sleep-onset REM periods (wake-initiated lucid dreams, WILD). LaBerge[24] developed a reliable cognitive technique for lucid dream induction, referred to as the mnemonic induction of lucid dreams (MILD), which uses a prospective memory technique (see La Berge and colleaugues[27] for more details). Of importance, although cognitive techniques can be used on their own with some success, they also form the foundation for the additional techniques of induction. For example, sleep interruption late in the sleep cycle for 30 to 60 minutes, combined with the MILD technique, significantly increases the number of lucid dreams in the ensuing sleep period.[28] The strategy to intentionally interrupt sleep to induce lucid dreaming is also known as the wake-back-to-bed (WBTB) technique.[29–31] Beyond such purely cognitive-behavioral strategies, technical aids can increase dream lucidity: An external stimulus presented to a sleeping person can be incorporated into their dream and serve as a cue reminding them about the dream state. For such a technique to be effective, an individual must already be sleeping with the goal of becoming lucid and recognizing the cue. One influential cuing device is a sleep mask that flashes light stimuli over a sleeper's closed eyes, and these flashing lights are often incorporated into the sleeper's dream, serving as a memory cue to prompt lucidity.[32,33] Similarly, tactile stimulation[34] or combinations of visual and acoustic stimuli have been used successfully as cues for the induction of dream lucidity.[35]

Several studies have tested whether it is possible to induce lucid dreams through noninvasive brain stimulation methods. Stumbrys and colleagues[36] reported that transcranial direct current stimulation (tDCS) applied to the frontal cortex resulted in a small increase in self-ratings of the unreality of dream objects as assessed by a questionnaire measure. However, it did not significantly increase the number of lucid dreams as rated by judges or the number of lucid dreams confirmed through the eye signaling method. Similarly, Voss and colleagues[37] observed that transcranial alternating current stimulation (tACS) in the low gamma range (25 Hz to 40 Hz) applied to frontolateral cortex increased insight reported in a dream questionnaire after awakening. However, dream lucidity was assessed neither by explicit self-report nor eye signaling, and a recent replication attempt, including these two crucial measures, did not find any advantage of tACS over sham stimulation.[38] Overall, the results of these studies indicate that prefrontal brain stimulation with tDCS or tACS can induce increases in some measures of dream content but currently does not appear viable as a lucid dream induction method (for a more in-depth discussion, see Baird and colleagues[9] and Laberge and colleagues[39]).

Finally, several pharmacologic strategies to increase lucid dreaming have been proposed[40–41]; however, only few have been tested systematically. Based on the role of acetylcholine (ACh) in REM sleep regulation, cholinergically acting substances have been studied. After a proof-of-principle study using the ACh esterase inhibitor (AChEI) donepezil (Aricept),[42] a double-blind, placebo-controlled study found that the AChEI galantamine significantly and in a dose-dependent manner increased lucid dreaming in 121 participants who also practiced the MILD technique.[39] Similar results were reported in a second study using galantamine[43] but not in a study testing the ACh precursor L-alpha glycerylphosphorylcholine.[44]

NEUROBIOLOGY

Dream-like mental activity can be observed during all sleep stages; however, REM sleep dreams are particularly vivid and intense. The specific phenomenal characteristics of dreaming have frequently been associated with neural activation patterns observed during REM sleep. For example, higher visual areas show strong metabolic activity during REM sleep,[45] which is in line with visuospatial hallucinations as the hallmark of typical dreaming.[1] Also the amygdala, medial prefrontal cortex, and anterior cingulate cortex show increased activity during REM sleep.[46,47] All these brain areas have been implicated in emotional processing, mirroring the intense emotions experienced in many dreams. In contrast, the dorsolateral prefrontal cortex and parietal areas, including the supramarginal cortex and precuneus show low metabolic rates during normal REM sleep.[46,47] In particular, prefrontal deactivations have been postulated to underlie cognitive deficiencies that can occur during ordinary dreaming, such as impaired critical thinking, lack of insight that one is dreaming, and restricted volitional control.[48]

Although lucid REM sleep dreaming is characterized by all the defining electroencephalographic (EEG) features of REM sleep, according to the classical Rechtschaffen and Kales[49] or new American Association of Sleep Medicine (AASM)[50] sleep stage scoring, it does show some subtle physiologic changes compared to nonlucid REM sleep, such as higher REM sleep density and increases in respiration, heart rate, and skin potential.[51] Several studies have also reported changes in EEG activity during lucid REM sleep compared to nonlucid REM sleep. Early EEG studies observed higher central alpha activity[4,52] and increased beta-1 activity (13 to 19 Hz) over parietal regions during lucid dreaming.[53] A more recent 19-channel EEG study reported that lucid dreaming is associated with higher activity in the gamma band—the between-states-difference peaking around 40 Hz—and overall EEG coherence compared to nonlucid REM sleep.[54] However, a study with a slightly larger group of narcolepsy patients could not confirm increases in the gamma band during lucid dreaming.[55] In general, scalp EEG measurements in the gamma band can be compromised by electromyogenic artifacts,[56,57] and frontolateral 40-Hz power increases during lucid REM sleep may well be an electomyogenic artifact of

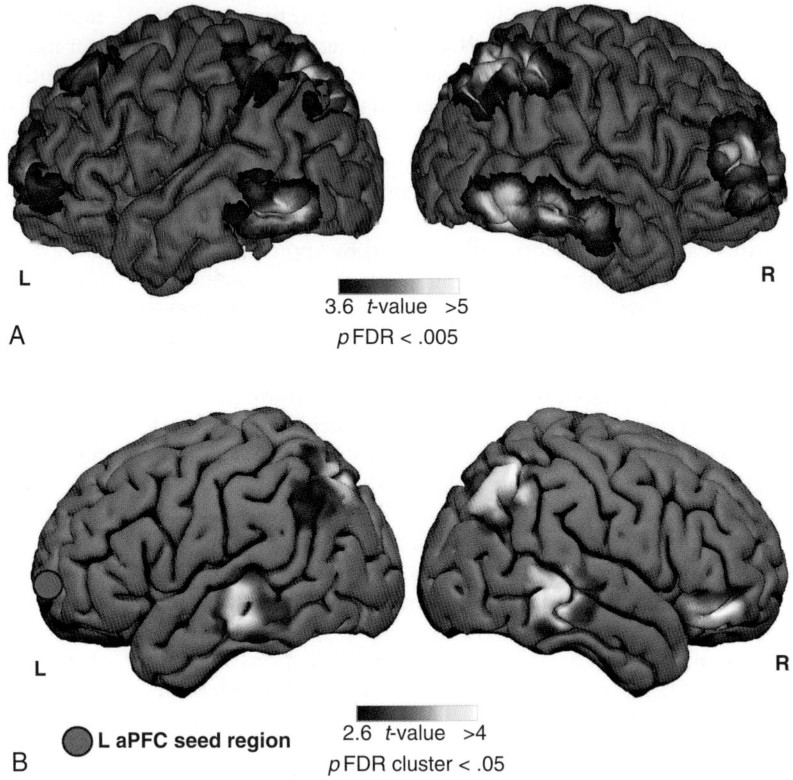

Figure 59.2 Functional magnetic resonance imaging (fMRI) data of lucid dreaming. **(A)** Blood-oxygen-level–dependent (BOLD) activation in fMRI case study of lucid dreaming (Dresler and colleagues, 2012[59]). Clusters show regions with significantly increased BOLD signal during lucid REM sleep (probability false detection rate [pFDR] < .005) in the left lateral hemisphere view (*left*) and right lateral hemisphere view (*right*). Increased activity was observed in anterior prefrontal cortex (aPFC), medial and lateral parietal cortex, including the supramarginal and angular gyrus and inferior/middle temporal gyrus during lucid REM sleep contrasted with nonlucid REM sleep. **(B)** Seed-based resting-state functional connectivity differences between frequent lucid dreamers and controls (Baird and colleagues, 2018a[66]). To estimate connectivity, spherical regions of interest were defined in aPFC based on the peak voxel reported in Dresler and colleagues[59] (*red circle*). Frequent lucid dreamers had increased resting-state functional connectivity between left aPFC and bilateral angular gyrus and bilateral middle temporal gyrus and right inferior frontal gyrus. All clusters are significant at $P < .05$, corrected for multiple comparisons at the cluster level.

(micro-)saccadic spike potentials as a corollary of higher eye movement density.[9] Overall, EEG studies of lucid dreaming have found mixed results, and studies with higher statistical power, better assessment of phenomenologic content, higher spatial resolution EEG montages, and more sophisticated analysis of the EEG signal will be needed to clarify the EEG correlates of lucid dreaming.

In a combined functional magnetic resonance imaging (fMRI)/EEG approach, activations in a network of neocortical regions, including the dorsolateral/frontopolar prefrontal cortex and the parietal cortex, were observed during lucid dreaming compared with nonlucid REM sleep background[59] (Figure 59.2). The frontopolar cortex has been related to the processing of internal states, for instance, the evaluation of one's own thoughts and feelings,[60] metacognitive ability,[61] and supervisory modes,[62] which are impaired in normal dreaming but reinstated in lucid dreaming. Strong activation increases during lucid dreaming were also observed in parietal regions, including the precuneus, inferior parietal lobules, and supramarginal gyrus.[59] Prefrontal-parietal interactions are involved in many higher cognitive processes, such as intelligence or working memory,[63] whereas the medial parietal cortex has been implicated in self-referential processing, such as first-person perspective taking and experience of agency.[64] A limitation of this study is that the participant was performing a task (repeated hand clenching) during the lucid REM sleep segment, and it is therefore possible that some of these activations could reflect task execution rather than lucidity. Systematic group-level fMRI studies of lucid REM sleep before firm conclusions can be drawn regarding fMRI correlates.

Beyond increased activation during lucid dreaming, similar brain regions have also been associated with more trait-like aspects of lucid dreaming propensity: Individuals with high, compared to low or no self-reported, dream lucidity exhibit larger grey matter volume in the frontopolar cortex[65] and increased resting-state functional connectivity between the left frontopolar cortex and the bilateral angular gyrus, bilateral middle temporal gyrus, and right inferior frontal gyrus[66] (Figure 59.2). Baird and colleagues[66] additionally evaluated the association between frequent lucid dreaming and connectivity within established large-scale brain networks, including the frontoparietal control network. Frequent lucid dreamers had increased functional connectivity between the anterior prefrontal cortex (aPFC) and a network of regions that showed the greatest overlap with a frontoparietal control subnetwork.[67] However, overall connectivity within the frontoparietal control network, defined through meta-analysis or parcellation, showed no significant differences between the lucid dream group and the control group. Nevertheless, these results provide preliminary converging support to the proposal that lucid dreaming is linked to large-scale networks that regulate executive control processes, in particular the frontoparietal control network.[3,68]

CLINICAL APPLICATIONS: NIGHTMARES

Lucid dreaming has been suggested as a therapeutic approach for several clinical conditions, including nightmares, posttraumatic stress disorder (PTSD), and schizophrenia. Lucid dreaming frequency is moderately correlated with nightmare frequency,[69] and people with frequent lucid dreams have incidentally reported that their nightmares have triggered lucidity. Theoretically, dream lucidity seems a logical solution to the main problem of nightmares, which encompasses a real emotional response to a nonexisting threat.[70] Once a person realizes the threat is not real, the threat should disappear and thus the emotional response. Neurocognitive models of disturbed dreaming emphasize a hyperresponsivity of the amygdala in nightmare generation, coupled with a failure of medial prefrontal regions to dampen this activation.[71] Lateral prefrontal regions have been shown capable to influence amygdala function through connections to the medial prefrontal cortex.[72] The neurobiology of lucid dreaming with increased lateral prefrontal activation therefore fits well with potential therapeutic effects of lucid dreaming on nightmares.[59]

So far the theory—but does this work as easy in practice? Patients with narcolepsy who frequently suffer from nightmares report that dream lucidity indeed provides relief during nightmares,[73] and a few case studies[74] and one small controlled pilot study[75] have indicated that lucid dreaming therapy was effective in reducing nightmare frequency. In the controlled pilot study, lucid dreaming therapy was superior to a waiting-list regarding nightmare frequency but did not have an effect on secondary anxiety and sleep measures; its efficacy was much higher in an individual than group therapy setting, suggesting confounding therapist effects.[75] A larger online self-help study did not find any additional effect of lucid dreaming therapy as an add-on to other effective cognitive-behavioral techniques, such as imagery rehearsal therapy,[76] although low power and high dropout rates (>50%) limited the scope of the conclusions.

Although lucid dreaming therapy has been included in the recommended therapy options in a recent position paper of the AASM,[77] it should be emphasized that empirical evidence for its efficacy is still sparse.[78] Moreover, it is worth noting that lucid dreaming and nightmares are not mutually exclusive, as the case of lucid nightmares illustrates.[79] In accordance, lucid dreaming therapy can have unexpected issues, such that nightmare sufferers may become lucid but then find themselves unable to change the nightmare,[74] presumably because the expectations about the story line may be too strongly engrained into the brain.[80] Moreover, realizing that one is dreaming does not automatically erase the threat and accompanying (intense) emotions, which also, after complete threat removal, would take some time. As in all lucid dreams, lucidity in nightmares is not exactly an all-or-none phenomenon but rather a staged process, and a prelucid or half-lucid stage may not suffice to fully tackle a seemingly real threat. Moreover, many subjects with frequent nightmares reported a spontaneous change in their nightmares even without obtaining lucidity.[75] This suggests that control over the nightmare, not lucidity, may be the therapeutic factor of successful nightmare treatment. Last, but not least, even in case the promising initial findings that are only partly corroborated in controlled pilot studies are sustained, the effects of lucid dreaming therapy tend to focus more on nightmare aspects (frequency, intensity) than on general sleep quality or mental health characteristics. By contrast, the effects of imagery rehearsal have been much broader in scope.[76]

However, one disadvantage of the nightmare treatments that are currently best supported by experimental evidence, such as imagery rehearsal,[82] exposure therapy,[83] and mixtures of both,[84] also require a repetitive nightmare or theme to work with. If nightmares are too different from night to night, there are no story lines to rescript, as in imagery rehearsal, or no repetitive images to systematically desensitize, as in exposure. Here lucid dreaming therapy has the advantage that, although having a repetitive nightmare or theme is beneficial (to recognize the dream state in a future nightmare), it is not a sine qua non, as people can train to become lucid without having nightmares.[70] Moreover, people can train themselves to link lucidity with feeling anxiety and fear in therapy and thereby preparing themselves for the next time they feel threatened, as it is likely going to occur during a future nightmare. In this manner, lucid dreaming therapy can be useful for people with idiopathic nightmares with very different contents. Naturally, the question arises whether such wildly varying nightmares or bad dreams might be a consequence of more generic negative thinking patterns (such as catastrophic thinking or excessive worrying), which can be addressed directly by standard cognitive-behavioral therapy. One caveat that should be mentioned is that lucid dreaming therapy may not be optimal for posttraumatic nightmares, besides being less evidence based than imagery rehearsal. Because many posttraumatic nightmares may comprise a replication of an original event or parts of an original event,[85] changing the nightmare online during its occurrence may be much harder to achieve than changing it offline in mentation, and even this typically raises questions concerning guilt and "undoing the past." As a consequence, lucidity may have the adverse consequence that patients with PTSD relive their original traumatic event with full consciousness but without the possibility to change a thing.[74] Such an occurrence would rather be retraumatizing than empowering, and although solutions to this inability to change the nightmares have been proposed (e.g., start with changing small background objects in color, and take it from there in small steps), it appears better to avoid experimenting with such inflammable material and to first try the treatments that may work for the majority.

CLINICAL APPLICATIONS BEYOND NIGHTMARES

Lucid dreaming has also been suggested as a therapeutic strategy in the treatment of schizophrenia.[37,86] The idea that normal dreaming can serve as a model for psychosis has a long tradition; however, it is notoriously speculative. One of the most interesting aspects of the dreaming-psychosis model is the issue of insight: Between 50% and 80% of the patients diagnosed with schizophrenia have poor insight into the presence of their disorder,[87] probably due to ineffective self-reflection processes.[88] Because such deficits are thought to lead to more relapses and rehospitalizations and poorer therapy success in general,[89] the concept of insight is becoming an increasingly important area of investigation in schizophrenia research.[90] On the dreaming side of the model, lack of insight into the current state characterizes almost any dream experience, with the obvious exception of lucid dreaming. This suggests that dream lucidity may be a good model for insight in the dreaming-psychosis model. Of interest, historical approaches to psychosis used the term *lucidity* to denote the awareness of the patient into his illness.[91] Although the specific composition the multiple facets of insight in psychosis is still under discussion,[92–93] two crucial dimensions are classically considered to be the recognition that one has a mental illness and the ability to recognize unusual mental events (delusions and hallucinations) as pathologic.[94] Hence, in the dreaming-psychosis model, lucidity during dreaming represents what patients during psychosis lack: full insight into the delusional nature of the current state of consciousness during that state.

Neurobiologically, in particular, prefrontal, medial parietal, and inferior temporal cortical regions that are linked to insight problems in psychosis show striking overlap with brain regions associated with dream lucidity.[86] It has been demonstrated that prefrontal cortex function in schizophrenia patients can be improved through cognitive training.[95] Metacognitive training approaches are of particular interest, because also skilled lucid dreamers typically gained their frequent insight into the dreaming state by metacognitive training, in particular by developing autosuggestions and the habit of frequently contemplating about their state of consciousness.[25,26] By teaching schizophrenia patients such training regimens, enhancing insight-related prefrontal and medial parietal functions might well lead to enhanced insight capabilities during acute psychosis. Of note, psychotic patients have been reported to experience more control in lucid dreams than healthy subjects.[96] However, given the cross-sectional nature of the study, it cannot be decided if lucid dreaming is helpful or detrimental to the patients' condition: It might already be a compensating reaction to psychosis or a training effect due to frequent episodes of dream-like experiences during wakefulness.

Training in lucid dreaming might also be used as an adjunct therapy for parasomnias, such as REM sleep behavior disorder (RBD), for which some patients report that learning to recognize that they are dreaming can keep them from reacting to the dream and thus executing violent or dangerous behaviors during sleep.[97] At the current time, the evidence for a potential therapeutic role of lucid dreaming in RBD remains anecdotal, and experimental studies will be needed to test its efficacy. One last potential clinical application of research on lucid dreaming worth noting is in the development of neuroimaging-based diagnostic markers of (self-) awareness. Such measures have the potential to improve the diagnosis and monitoring of patients who are unresponsive due to traumatic injury, aphasia, motor impairment, or other physical limitations, such as tracheotomy. Research on lucid dreaming could play an important role in this field because, in addition to assessing a patient's capacity for primary consciousness (i.e., if a patient can see, hear, or experience pain), an important clinical goal is to assess whether patients, who may nevertheless be unresponsive via behavioral assessment, are aware of themselves and their state.[98] In accordance, identifying reliable brain activity markers of both primary consciousness and higher-order consciousness has the potential to improve diagnostic accuracy and provide additional means of monitoring rehabilitation for such patients.

NONCLINICAL APPLICATIONS

Lucid dreaming is used also for several nonclinical purposes. Among the most popular intended dream behaviors are flying, communication with dream characters, and sexual encounters during dreaming, with lucid dreaming frequency appearing to predict how successful such intentions are recalled and executed in lucid dreams.[22] Besides such purely recreational applications within dreams, many lucid dreamers also indicate to use lucid dreaming to influence their waking lives.[99] Two examples for which at least some scientific data is available are creative problem solving and practicing motor skills.

Anecdotal reports on scientific discovery, inventive originality, and artistic productivity suggest that creativity can be triggered or enhanced by sleeping and dreaming. Also, theoretical considerations and experimental studies suggest that dreams can improve waking-life creativity. Sleep generally has been suggested to provide an ideal state for creative incubation: The internally generated dream narrative in absence of external sensory data leads to a much more radical renunciation from unsuccessful problem-solving attempts, leading to coactivations of cognitive data that are highly remote in waking life, and both dreaming and creativity have been characterized with primary process thinking, flat associative hierarchies, and defocused attention.[100] In contrast to the more random flow of nonlucid dream narratives, dream lucidity allows a more goal-oriented use of these creativity-related dream characteristics. It has been shown that frequent lucid dreamers are more successful in an insight-based problem-solving task.[101] Surveys among lucid dreamers and experimental studies demonstrate that lucid dreaming can indeed be used to improve creative thinking and problem solving.[99,102]

Motor practice during lucid dreaming is a novel type of mental rehearsal in which a person is using the dream state to consciously practice specific tasks without waking up.[103] It can be compared to mental practice, which is well established in sport theory and sport practice.[104] For both mental and dream rehearsal, movements are simulated with an imagined body on a purely cognitive level, whereas the physical body remains still. One advantage that lucid dreaming has over both mental practice and modern virtual reality simulators is that lucid dreaming offers the potential for practice with all kinesthetic sensations of the dream body in an environment that is experienced with as much vividness and realism as would be encountered in waking experience. In addition, the lucid dreamer, being limited only by his or her imagination and attentional stability, has far greater potential for control over his or her own body, actions, and environment than in mental rehearsal, virtual reality environments, or waking life. In contrast to the vast amount of research on mental practice, however, empirical data on practice in lucid dreams are rather sparse.

In several anecdotal reports, amateur and professional athletes indicated using lucid dreams to improve their waking performance, for instance, in long-distance running, tennis, skating, alpine skiing, or martial arts.[70,105] In a more systematic questionnaire study, 840 German athletes from a variety of sports were surveyed about their experiences with lucid dreams.[106] Although lucid dreaming in athletes had a similar prevalence as in the general population,[19] the percentage of lucid dreams compared to all recalled dreams was found to be increased nearly twofold in athletes. About every tenth athlete who had lucid dreams (5% of the total sample) used lucid dreams to practice sports skills, with most of them having the impression that their performance improved thereby.

Few studies tested possible effects of practice in lucid dreams experimentally. In a qualitative study, subjects were instructed to perform different complex sports skills familiar to them in waking life, such as skiing or gymnastics, in their lucid dreams.[107] Participants reported that they had no difficulties performing these sports skills in their lucid dreams and that their movements improved both in the dream and the waking state. In a quasiexperimental pre-/postdesign study, participants were asked to practice a coin-tossing task in their lucid dreams.[108] Results showed a significant increase in hitting the target from pretest to posttest for the group, which practiced the coin-tossing task in their lucid dreams, but no increase was found for the control group. These results could be replicated with a different motor task (sequential finger tapping). Improvements after lucid dream practice seem to be similar or slightly lower compared to actual physical practice and similar or slightly better to mental practice in wakefulness.[109] More recently, in a sleep laboratory study it was shown that improvement of darts performance after lucid dream practice depends on the number of distractions while rehearsing within the dream.[110] Furthermore, an interview study with athletes revealed that many different sports and movements can be practiced in lucid dreams and that the experiences of lucid dream practice were very realistic, including kinesthetic perception.[111] Lucid dream practice could also be applied in other areas that involve motor learning, such as rehabilitation, surgery, or music.[112]

RISKS

Although the academic and public view on lucid dreaming for many years oscillated somewhere between skepticism, curiosity, and enthusiasm, more recently, concerns about potential risks have been expressed. Besides empirically motivated arguments, for instance, pointing toward an increase in dissociation and schizotypy symptoms longitudinally across periods of deliberate lucid dreaming induction efforts,[113] in particular, practical side effects of lucid dreaming induction strategies and theoretical implications of cultivating a brain state that might not fulfill the evolved functions of sleep have been emphasized.[114–115] These latter possibilities should be seen in perspective though: Any targeted brain interventions with pharmacologic or electric means will come with side effects, which, however, are not intrinsic to the aim of achieving dream lucidity. Interrupting one's night sleep in the early morning to increase lucid dreaming probability will also interrupt the functions early morning sleep serves—just as similarly timed activities such as star gazing or bird watching will do. In case nonlucid dreaming serves biologic functions, as has been proposed,[116] it might be suggested that these would not be served during lucid dreaming. However, determining whether this is the case awaits future experimental study. More research on the neurobiology of lucid REM sleep is needed to understand precisely how it differs from nonlucid REM sleep and whether such differences could influence proposed functions. In this context it is also important to note that lucid dreams commonly last only a few minutes, so such nonlucidity-requiring functions will hardly be affected most of the time. Of note, a recent dream diary study indicates that sleepers feel more rather than less refreshed after a night with a lucid dream.[117] Nevertheless, more empirical research seems warranted, in particular on the reported effects of long-term training of lucid dreaming.

CLINICAL PEARL

Lucid dreaming has been proposed as a natural therapy for nightmares, and there is some clinical support for this indication. It might be particularly suited for idiopathic nightmares but less so for posttraumatic nightmares. As lucid insight into dreaming and insight into psychosis may have overlapping neural correlates, lucid dreaming might also be of value in schizophrenia therapy or in the development of novel antipsychotics. Finally, research on the neurobiology of lucid dreaming may be useful for developing neuroimaging-based diagnostic markers of consciousness.

SUMMARY

In contrast to the lack of insight into one's state during normal dream mentation, lucid dreaming is characterized by awareness of the current state of mind, often leading to considerable volitional control of the dream narrative. Lucid dreaming can be learned and trained by a variety of induction strategies, including prospective memory, external mnemonic cuing, and pharmacology. Although lucid dreaming as a research topic initially faced skepticism within sleep science, the topic is experiencing increasing momentum in recent years. Preliminary findings indicate that lucid dreaming is associated with specific changes in neural activity when compared to nonlucid dreaming, with lateral prefrontal, frontopolar, and medial parietal activations as proposed neural correlates of the increased metacognitive capacity that defines dream lucidity. Lucid dreaming has clinical and nonclinical applications, from nightmare therapy to mental motor skill training and creative problem solving. Reliable induction methods are strongly needed to further explore the potential of lucid dreaming and its scientific study.

SELECTED READINGS

Aviram L, Soffer-Dudek N. Lucid dreaming: intensity, but not frequency, is inversely related to psychopathology. *Front Psychol.* 2018;9:384.

Baird B, Mota-Rolim SA, Dresler M. The cognitive neuroscience of lucid dreaming. *Neurosci Biobehav Rev.* 2019;100:305–323.

de Macêdo TCF, Ferreira GH, de Almondes KM, Kirov R, Mota-Rolim SA. My dream, my rules: can lucid dreaming treat nightmares? *Front Psychol.* 2019;10:2618.

Dresler M, Wehrle R, Spoormaker VI, et al. Neural correlates of dream lucidity obtained from contrasting lucid versus non-lucid REM sleep: a combined EEG/fMRI case study. *Sleep.* 2012;35:1017–1020.

Dresler M, Wehrle R, Spoormaker VI, et al. Neural correlates of insight in dreaming and psychosis. *Sleep Med Rev.* 2015;22:92–99.

Konkoly KR, Appel K, Chabani E, et al. Real-time dialogue between experimenters and dreamers during REM sleep. *Curr Biol.* 2021;31(7):1417-1427.e6.

LaBerge S, LaMarca K, Baird B. Pre-sleep treatment with galantamine stimulates lucid dreaming: a double-blind, placebo-controlled, crossover study. *PLoS One.* 2018;13:e0201246.

LaBerge S, Rheingold H. *Exploring the World of Lucid Dreaming.* New York: Ballantine; 1990.

LaBerge SP, Nagel LE, Dement WC, Zarcone VP. Lucid dreaming verified by volitional communication during REM sleep. *Percept Mot Skills.* 1981;52:727–732.

Mota-Rolim SA, de Almondes KM, Kirov R. Editorial: "Is this a dream?" - Evolutionary, neurobiological and psychopathological perspectives on lucid dreaming. *Front Psychol.* 2021;12:635183. Published 2021 Feb 9.

Purcell S, Mullington J, Moffitt A, et al. Dream self-reflectiveness as a learned cognitive skill. *Sleep.* 1986;9:423–437.

Stickgold R, Zadra A. Sleep: Opening a portal to the dreaming brain. *Curr Biol.* 2021;31(7):R352-R353.

Stumbrys T, Erlacher D, Schädlich M, Schredl M. Induction of lucid dreams: a systematic review of evidence. *Conscious Cogn.* 2012;21:1456–1475.

A complete reference list can be found online at ExpertConsult.com.

Chapter 60

What Is the Function of Nightmares?

Michelle Carr; Tore Nielsen

Chapter Highlights

- The definition of nightmare disorder as a clinical entity by the *Diagnostic and Statistical Manual of Mental Disorders,* fifth edition, and *International Classification of Sleep Disorders*, third edition, suggests that nightmares are symptomatic but not functional.
- The nearly ubiquitous nature of nightmares and dysphoric dreaming in the general population is consistent with the claim that they serve a function related to cognitive-emotional regulation or emotional memory consolidation.
- Theories of nightmare function vary in their emphasis on mechanisms for dealing with emotional regulation and include stress mastery, affect desomatization, fear memory extinction, emotional contextualization, and others.

WHAT IS THE FUNCTION OF NIGHTMARES?

Why do we have nightmares? Are they symptomatic of a clinical condition, or do they serve some homeostatic or affect-regulation function? Or might nightmares be both symptomatic of disease and functional at the same time? The functional characterization of nightmares remains a major unresolved issue of modern sleep medicine with important ramifications for our understanding of mental health and cognitive development. The present review addresses this issue of nightmare function and the available research relevant to the problem.

We consider the term *nightmare* to refer to dreaming during which intense negative emotion is in play, whether or not waking state dysfunction stems from such experiences. The reason for adopting such a broad definition is to include both clinical- and research-based definitions, to encompass dreams with a variety of dysphoric emotions, and to consider dreams that do not immediately awaken the dreamer. This definition, although not shared by all writers, nonetheless corresponds with current clinical definitions (Table 60.1), as well as with earlier *Diagnostic and Statistical Manual of Mental Disorders*, third edition and third edition-revised, definitions of dream anxiety attacks and anxiety dreams and is employed so that a wide swath of nightmare theories may be included in the discussion.

NIGHTMARES ARE A RECOGNIZED CLINICAL ENTITY

Nightmares have been viewed for centuries as pathologic events, and clues to their possible functionality may be found in how they are described clinically. According to the most authoritative sources, the *Diagnostic and Statistical Manual of Mental Disorders*, fifth edition (DSM-5),[1] and *International Classification of Sleep Disorders*, third edition (ICSD-3),[2] nightmares are intensely dysphoric dreams that occur during late-night rapid eye movement (REM) sleep and that are clearly recalled upon awakening (Table 60.1). Basic fear expression seems central to nightmare production in that fear is expressed in 65% to 85% of nightmares, whereas other dysphoric emotions such as anger and sadness prevail in the remainder.[3,4] This clear predominance of fear may mean that nightmares are akin to the symptoms of other fear-dysfunction disorders, such as phobias, generalized anxiety, or social anxiety, but it may also point to a deeper involvement of fear memory, fear extinction, and fear regulation systems that underlie the normal functions of emotional learning and emotional memory consolidation (see reviews in Walker,[5] Levin and Nielsen,[6] and Nielsen and Levin[7]). These are not mutually exclusive possibilities, of course.

The pathologic context of nightmares is striking and has been reviewed in detail elsewhere.[6,8] Pathologic conditions that are comorbid with nightmares range from the mild to the severe, but causality between nightmares and other pathologies has not yet been clearly established. Nightmares are more frequent among those suffering from depressive and anxiety symptoms and neuroticism[6,8] and posttraumatic stress disorder (PTSD)[9] than they are among healthy individuals. Nightmares are also reliably associated with suicidal ideation,[10] suicide attempts,[11] and death by suicide[12]—independent of other psychopathologies.[10,13,14]

Altogether, the description of nightmare disorder as a primarily fear-based disorder and accumulating evidence linking nightmares to various comorbid affective conditions support the position that frequent nightmares reflect a pathologic breakdown in the normal functioning of processes governing fear expression, fear memory, or fear regulation. Nonetheless, despite the distress and suffering caused by nightmares, it remains possible that they also signify—at least up to a certain degree of severity—innate adaptive responses over the long term.

NIGHTMARES MAY BE AN EXPRESSION OF PERCEPTUAL SENSITIVITY

The view of nightmares as a clinical problem has led to a skewed focus on the pathology and comorbid symptoms as described in

Table 60.1 Diagnostic Criteria for Nightmare Disorder from the *Diagnostic and Statistical Manual*, 5th Edition (DSM-5), and *International Classification of Sleep Disorders*, 3rd Edition (ICSD-3)

	DSM-5	ICSD-3
Nature of recalled dream	Repeated occurrence of extremely dysphoric, well-remembered dreams, usually involving threat and occurring in the second half of sleep	Repeated occurrence of extremely dysphoric, well-remembered dreams, usually involving threat and occurring in the second half of sleep
Nature of awakening	Becomes alert and oriented on awakening	Becomes alert and oriented on awakening
Nature of distress	Causes clinically significant distress or impairment	Causes clinically significant distress or impairment in one of the following areas: mood, sleep, cognition, family, behavior, daytime sleepiness, fatigue, occupation, social
Differential diagnosis	Not substance derived	N/A
Differential diagnosis	Not the result of other mental or medical disorders	N/A
Duration	Acute: <1 month	N/A
	Subacute: <6 months	
	Persistent: >6 months	Note: ND only diagnosed in children in cases of persistent distress
Severity	Mild: <1 per week	
	Moderate: 1–6 per week	
	Severe: ≥7 per week	

ICSD-3 criteria have changed only slightly from the ICSD-2. DSM-5 criteria have changed from DSM-4-TR in several respects: (1) DSM-5 introduces categorization of subtypes according to duration and severity (used in ICSD-2), whereas ICSD-3 drops them; (2) terrifying hypnagogic hallucinations in DSM-IV-TR are subsumed in DSM-5 as a sleep onset subtype of nightmares; (3) in DSM-5, nightmare disorder may be diagnosed in cases of RBD, PTSD, and acute stress disorder if nightmares preceded the condition and their frequency or severity necessitates independent clinical attention. Both manuals now include any dysphoric emotional tone and recognize the frequent depiction of threat-related content.
N/A, Not applicable; ND, nightmare disorder.

the previous section. However, growing evidence is consistent with a view that nightmares may reflect a more general personality trait—sensory-processing sensitivity—characterized by heightened emotional reactivity and amplified perceptual and cognitive processing of the environment. Sensory-processing sensitivity is measured using the 27-item Highly Sensitive Person Scale developed by Aron and colleagues,[15] which includes items that assess general emotional reactivity, perceptual sensitivity, and depth of cognitive processing. On the one hand, this trait can be adaptive, enhancing awareness of the environment and augmenting positive outcomes in response to supportive contexts. However, highly sensitive individuals are more easily overwhelmed and distressed when in a stimulating environment. We recently proposed that nightmare-prone individuals may be highly sensitive[16] and have shown in one sample that nightmare distress is correlated with being more highly sensitive.[17] Nightmare sufferers have likewise been described as having "thinner boundaries"—a trait of increased sensitivity across emotional, perceptual, and cognitive domains.[18] Several recent findings support the claim that nightmare-prone individuals may be more sensitive to both negative and positive stimuli. For instance, nightmare sufferers report increased novelty and reward-seeking behaviors,[19] exhibit increased depth of processing of negative and positive semantic stimuli,[20] and report increased responsiveness to social-emotional cues.[21]

The emotional reactivity and sensory sensitivity that characterize the waking experience of highly sensitive individuals would likewise be expressed in the form of intensified dreams, including nightmares, in response to stress. However, more generally, nightmare-prone individuals have an increased dream recall frequency and more vivid and affective non-nightmare dreams.[22] We also found that nightmare sufferers report increased kinesthetic sensations of both negative and positive valences in dreams during a daytime nap.[23] Finally, Perogamvros and colleagues[24] found that patients with nightmare disorder have higher heart-rate–evoked potential, an index of interoceptive awareness, during rapid eye movement (REM) sleep compared with healthy subjects. In our recent study,[17] subjects with higher nightmare distress were more likely to incorporate external stimuli and low-level auditory and visual cues into their dream content. These findings support the notion that heightened sensory processing during sleep is a correlate of nightmare distress. Overall, the model suggests that nightmare-prone individuals experience elevated emotional and perceptual sensitivity that persists during sleep and dreaming. As a wider conceptualization of the nightmare-prone personality, this new view challenges the long-standing view that nightmares are nothing but a symptom of clinical pathology.

NIGHTMARES ARE UBIQUITOUS

Large population studies indicate that not only are nightmares a prevalent clinical problem, but also dysphoric dreaming is much more ubiquitous than is generally appreciated. Nightmare prevalence at a clinically significant frequency, that is, about once per week or more,[1] varies from 0.9% to 6.8% of individuals (see the review by Sandman and colleagues[25]). The two largest cohort studies (i.e., 69,813 participants from the general Finnish population[25] and 87,408 seventh to twelfth graders from Japan)[26] provide consistent estimates. The former study found 4.2% reported "frequent" nightmares in the last 30 days; the latter that 6% reported nightmares "always" or "often" in the same time period. But this is not the complete picture. Nightmares occur at lower frequencies among many more people, for example, 40% of the Finnish cohort reported "occasional" nightmares the last 30 days. A full 85% of adults report at least one nightmare per year.[6] Occasional nightmares are not generally considered pathologic; they may well be evidence of nightmares sustaining a normal, adaptive response. The widespread occurrence of nightmares is also supported by the finding that prospective measures, such as home dream logs, estimate them to be 3 to 10 times more frequent than do retrospective measures, such as questionnaires.[27-29] In addition, there is a much wider spectrum of disturbed and dysphoric dreams,[6,30] including disturbed dreams during bereavement,[31] pregnancy,[32] after trauma or brain surgery,[33] after consuming or withdrawing from various drugs, or in tandem with many mental, physical, and sleep disorders (see reviews by Nielsen[30] and Robert and Zadra[34]). Bad dreams have been distinguished from nightmares in that they do not lead to awakenings and are less emotionally intense.[34] Bad dreams occur up to four times more frequently than do nightmares[29,34] and, combined with nightmares, occur at a rate of about 40 per year among healthy university students[29]; they constitute 13.7% of all dreams reported by 572 subjects (n = 9796 dreams[34]). That bad dreams are thematically similar to nightmares (e.g., physical aggression) yet more likely to resolve positively (38%) than nightmares (22%)[34] suggests that they may be more functional in regulating emotions than are nightmares. Beyond bad dreams, negative emotions constitute from 66% to 80% of all dream emotions in home dreams.[35,36]

In sum, although nightmares are clearly recognized as a clinical entity, the ubiquity of nightmares as part of a wider spectrum of disturbed and dysphoric dreams supports the possibility that they may play a role in emotional regulation or processing of emotional memories; a role that may diminish as nightmares become more severe and disruptive.

Sleep Polysomnographic Findings for Nightmare Sufferers Are Inconclusive

Polysomnography (PSG) has revealed several sleep-dependent memory functions linked to both the proportions of sleep stages and microstructural sleep features such as spindles and rapid eye movement density.[37] REM sleep, in particular, has been linked to the processing of emotional stimuli, such as consolidation of fear and safety memories[38] or of the negative component of complex pictures,[39] and to modulation of emotional reactivity.[37] In light of such findings, the PSG features characterizing nightmare sufferers—and in particular their REM sleep features—may provide clues to nightmare functionality. Two studies of nightmare episodes[40,41] revealed signs of REM sleep activation (e.g., heart rate increase) that could be attributed to increased autonomic arousal accompanying nightmares. However, 60% of cases in the latter study[41] did not exhibit increased autonomic arousal. Other studies have found more eye movements per minute and shorter breath times for dreams that are high versus those that are low in anxiety.[42] For the habitual sleep of nightmare sufferers, studies of PSG abnormalities are inconsistent. Some find REM-specific abnormalities, such as increased skipping of early REM periods, increased REM latency and cycle length, more REM periods,[43] lower REM efficiency,[20] and increased spectral power in the high alpha range (10 to 14.5 Hz)[44] and the "slow theta" range (2 to 5 Hz).[45] Others report changes in non–rapid eye movement (NREM) sleep such as low alpha power,[44] reduced CAP A1 but increased CAP A2 and A3 subtypes,[44] higher density and frequency fast spindles,[46] reduced slow wave sleep,[47] and reduced delta with increased beta and gamma power.[48] Blaskovich and colleagues[48] also find that nightmare sufferers have increased arousals in the 10 minutes preceding, but not following, REM sleep periods compared with control subjects. Other studies report global changes such as more frequent periodic leg movements,[49] more fragmented sleep,[41,50] longer sleep latency, more nocturnal awakenings,[47] and increases in the normalized low-frequency component of the heart rate during recovery sleep after REM sleep deprivation.[51]

These findings are discrepant but could be considered to reflect an increase in arousal during the sleep of nightmare sufferers, be it expressed as leg movements, nocturnal awakenings, or high-frequency oscillations. This notion fits with the subjective experience of increased emotional and physical arousal during nightmares. However, increased arousal in sleep is not a highly specific correlate of known sleep-related functions and does not account for why sometimes nightmares are triggered and sometimes not. Overall, the reviewed studies do not yet allow reliable links to be made between nightmares and known memory or emotion-regulation functions of sleep.

There Is a Spectrum of Nightmare Functionality Theories

In the present work we use the term *functional* to refer to a biologic, adaptive advantage attributed to nightmares (see the review by Revonsuo[52]). The question of whether nightmares are functional has remained contentious since at least the time of Freud[53] and continues to divide opinion today. Although it may be tempting to view existing theories of nightmare functionality as dichotomous, that is, that nightmares either are or are not functional, a closer consideration of the literature and of the dynamic phenomenology of nightmares shows a number of gradations of functionality can be described. As Figure 60.1 illustrates for the case of a simple threat-nightmare, at least five phenomenological steps with five accompanying emotional reactions unfold during a nightmare experience. These include a phase of normal dreaming, a period of building dysphoric emotion, an arbitrary threshold at which the dream passes over into a realm of distress, an awakening, and postawakening reactions.

Theories may attribute functionality or a lack of it to any one or combination of these steps. The lower panel of Figure 60.1 classifies theories according to steps of functionality. Several emotion-regulation theories consider emotional and dysphoric dreams to be functional up to a certain point, but that awakenings triggered by overwhelming distress reflect a failure in function (see row 2 in Figure 60.1). In contrast, threat simulation theory[52] considers threatening dreams and nightmares to be functional, regardless of awakening or postawakening reactions (see row 3 in Figure 60.1). Finally, theories attributing function to postawakening adaptation rely on awakenings to bring nightmare content into the conscious mind for further processing (see row 4 in Figure 60.1). Note that not all possible theories for this five-step functional sequence are shown, and the content of dreaming does not figure into this hypothetical sequence but may nonetheless be decisive. For instance, if a dream replicates a prior trauma, a given step may be hypothesized to be nonfunctional. Thus the

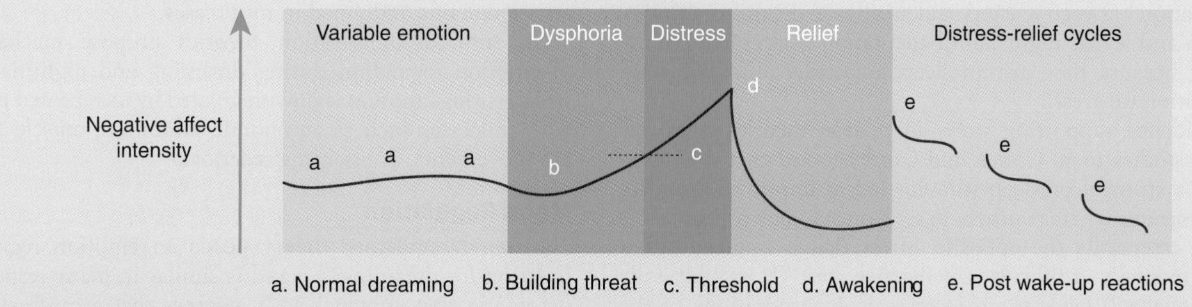

Function step(s)	a	b	c	d	e
1. All nonfunctional	×	×	×	×	×
2. Emotion regulation	✓	✓	×	×	×
3. Threat simulation	×	✓	✓	×	×
4. Postawakening adaptation	×	×	×	✓	✓
5. All functional	✓	✓	✓	✓	✓

×=nonfunctional; ✓=functional

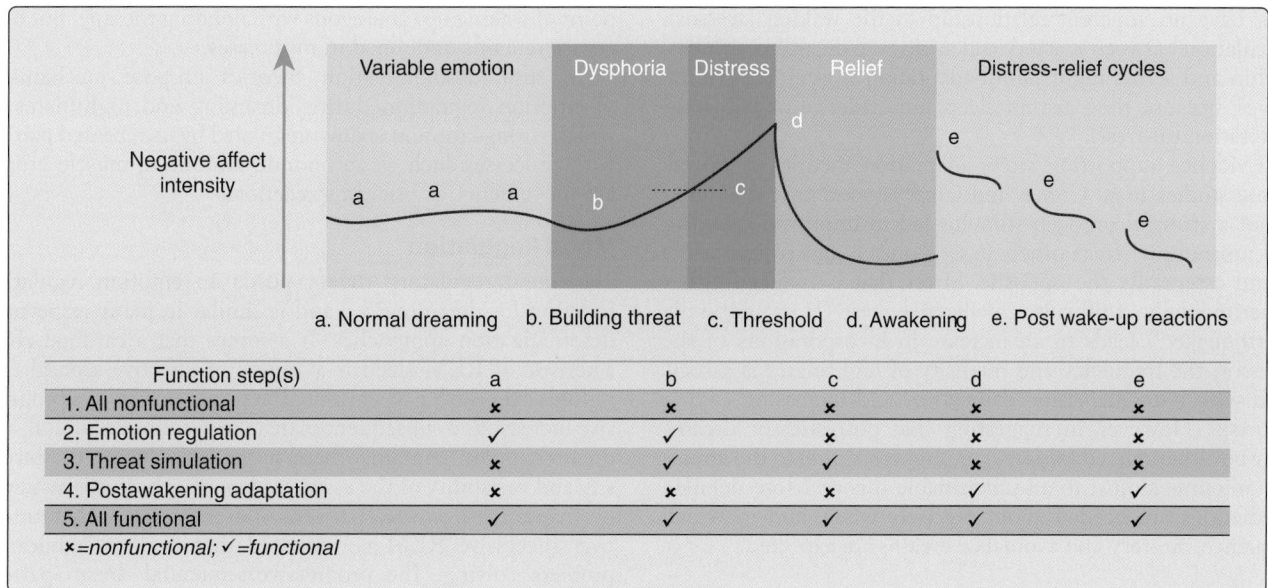

Figure 60.1 Nightmares.

many types of nightmares and other disturbed dreams may or may not all serve the same function.

In the following section, we discuss how several nightmare theories pertain to the question of function. With the growing emphasis on the medicalization of nightmares (DSM-5),[1] as well as evidence linking nightmares to psychopathological conditions, beliefs that nightmares are dysfunctional are widespread. Two theories[54,55] identify nightmare awakenings as evidence that dreaming's function has failed. A third[7] considers failures to regulate fear extinction during dreaming as responsible for dysfunction. On the other hand, several theories share a general assumption that nightmares are implicated in adaptive modification of emotional responses over time. We present these theories separately to highlight the more specific mechanisms of emotion regulation that they bring forward and to summarize the available empirical findings that support or refute each.

Emotion-Defense Regulation

One neo-psychoanalytic theory[56] considered the nightmare awakening a failure in dream function, specifically a failure to contain the overactivation of specific types of emotions. Nightmare awakenings are purportedly triggered by eight basic emotion types: joy, acceptance, surprise, expectation, anger, disgust, sorrow, or fear,[57] each of which produces a distinctive nightmare theme and, frequently, characteristic behaviors upon awakening. For example, fear could lead to a terror nightmare with overt locomotion or speech on awakening; anger could lead to a rage nightmare with fist-clenching; sorrow could lead to a grief nightmare with copious crying; and joy—paradoxically perhaps—could lead to a "pleasure" nightmare with nocturnal orgasm. The failure to contain emotion arousal to an appropriate level triggers awakening, thus interfering with dream function. This eightfold structure of nightmare themes was extended to more general attributes of personality structure, cognitive orientation, psychosomatic organ systems, and so on.[56] An intriguing component of this theory is that every nightmare is thought to contain an element of fear to the extent that there is resistance to fully express a predominant emotion while dreaming, which finally results in awakening (e.g., a fear of letting anger amplify to overt rage or of letting joy/pleasure amplify to the point of orgasm).

Despite its clarity and accessibility, this theory has not been tested empirically and has fostered little research. The theory is, however, generally consistent with current definitions of nightmares as including emotions other than fear as well as studies showing that awakenings from nightmares and other dysphoric dreams are often accompanied by dream-enacting behaviors in both parasomnias such as REM sleep behavior disorder[58] and among the general population.[59]

Adaptation to Stress

Although early theories of dream function emphasized roles for REM sleep and dreaming in facilitating adaptation to stress, most of these dealt only marginally with nightmares. Evidence that presleep stressors are incorporated into dream content or increase dysphoric dream emotions[60-63] was thus generally interpreted to indicate how normal dreaming was able to "master"[60] or "assimilate"[64] daytime stress rather than to explain how stress may trigger nightmares. One exception to this trend was a focus on the possible role of nightmares in "war neurosis,"[65] now known as PTSD, which considered dream function to be mastery of stress and nightmares to reflect continuing attempts to master a trauma.

The disruption-avoidance-adaptation theory[66,67] hypothesized that dreaming enables stress adaptation by its oscillation between two distinct functions: mastery and avoidance. Dreams about unresolved disturbing events are considered *mastery dreams* and have the potential to disrupt sleep—as in the case of awakenings from nightmares. Mastery is hypothesized to occur by a type of creative emotional problem solving that draws on memories of similar, yet successfully resolved, past situations. Emotional mastery is favored by the free-flow of ideas, thoughts, and emotions unique to dreaming. If dreams are too disruptive, however, awakenings and other sleep disturbances may result. *Avoidance dreams* thus complement mastery and prevent sleep disruption by various processes (e.g., presenting dream emotions or specific contents that have no apparent relationship to the waking stressor). Oscillation between mastery and avoidance dreams continues, within and across nights, until adaptation is attained. Nightmares, because they disrupt sleep, are evidence of failure in adaptation to stress.

Evidence supporting stress adaptation theories is mixed. Some studies (e.g., Cohen and Cox[68]) found that dreaming about a stressful presleep stimulus led to improved mood in the morning whereas others (e.g., Koulack and colleagues[69]) found essentially the opposite. Stress that is induced either experimentally (difficult intelligence test[69]) or naturally (earthquake[70]) leads to an increase in incorporations of the stressor; the frequency and intensity of nightmares is associated with both increasing daily stress and increasing coping efforts.[71] However, in suggesting that post-stressor dreams may be either related (*mastery*) or not (*avoidance*) to the stressors amounts almost to an unfalsifiable theory. More detailed predictions are needed about precisely when, and in which sequence, mastery and avoidance dreams are expected.

Desomatization

Fisher and colleagues[41] found that some REM sleep nightmares were not accompanied by the autonomic activation that would be expected for the negative emotions reported. In 60% (12 of 20) of their recorded nightmares, emotion-related autonomic activation, as measured by heart rate, respiratory rate, and eye movement activity, was not seen. In other nightmares, such activity occurred only in the last few minutes of the REM episode. Similar findings were reported in a more recent study.[40] This apparent separation of seemingly fearful dream imagery from its expected autonomic correlates prompted the notion of REM dreaming as a mechanism for "tempering and modulating anxiety, for desomatizing the physiological response to it. . .[for] abolishing or diminishing the physiological concomitants."[41] This desomatization mechanism was thought to help protect REM sleep, to assuage anxiety during dreaming, and to decrease the degree of disruption that occurs in instances of awakening. This serves to prevent the self-perpetuation of anxiety and assist in the mastery of traumatic memories—even after awakening.[41] Nevertheless, a breakdown of the mechanism is suggested by intense autonomic activity while dreaming, as occurred in 40% of their recorded nightmares.

Similar desomatization notions have occurred sporadically in the literature, and slightly different desomatizing mechanisms proposed. Authors of an empirical study on an anxiety-extinction function of nightmares[72] suggested that nightmares facilitate extinction through repeated exposure to fear-inducing stimuli (like implosive therapy), but their own findings did not support the hypothesis.[72] Others have pointed to specific physiologic mechanisms of REM sleep that may be responsible for desomatization. These include REM sleep eye movements desensitizing affect by a mechanism similar to that of eye movement desensitization and reprocessing[73,74]; REM sleep atonia desensitizing the somatic component of negative affect by repeatedly blocking kinesthetic feedback during negative dream imagery[75,76]; and, in a related theory, the repeated pairing of dysphoric dream imagery and REM sleep atonia desensitizing anxiety in a manner analogous to systematic desensitization therapy.[77] In all such models, negative affect is considered to be implicated in desensitization up to a certain threshold; this threshold is clear when it is the point of waking up (analogous with flooding therapy) but otherwise remains undefined in most cases.

In sum, desomatization theories propose mechanisms of emotion regulation during dreaming and nightmares by which strong emotion is downregulated by its repeated pairing with processes such as autonomic inhibition, muscle atonia, eye movements, or orienting reactions.

Mood Regulation

The mood regulatory theory posits an emotion regulation function for dreaming[54,78] and is similar in many respects to desomatization approaches. It assumes that a cardinal characteristic of REM sleep is a "surge" of affective arousal that unfolds over the REM episode. The surge consists of a progressive increase and subsequent plateau in autonomic arousal, and dream content "contains" these surges by reducing the intensity and variability of the associated emotions. This is achieved by *progressive-sequential* patterns of dream content that unfold over successive REM periods and that facilitate emotional problem solving. The progressive-sequential dream pattern is distinguished from a *repetitive-traumatic* pattern, during which an emotional conflict is simply stated and restated without evidence of adaptive change. Nightmares contribute to problem solving up to a point at which the capacity for assimilation of emotional surges is exceeded. Similar mood regulation theories that consider nightmares to function in adaptation to stress have been proposed by others.[71,79]

Apart from REM sleep's recurrent phasic-tonic structure, the physiologic assumption that REM sleep is surge-like remains to be demonstrated empirically. However, dreams are influenced by presleep thoughts and emotions[80] and are related to the next day's mood.[81] Moreover, overnight reductions in negative mood (e.g., unhappiness) correlate with intervening dream content, especially with the number of characters in a dream.[78] Consistent findings were also reported[82,83] by which high presleep depression scores were associated with more dysphoric dreams from the first REM period—but not with sleep physiology variables. Other supporting evidence from this group[84,85] shows that subjects in a marital breakup who report a predominance of early-night negative dreams are more likely to be in remission a year later than are those with more late-night negative dreams. Negative dreams occurring early in sleep may thus reflect a within-sleep mood regulation process similar to the progressive-sequential pattern that is triggered by a major emotional conflict; a predominance of negative dreams late in sleep may reflect a failure of this regulation function.

In sum, mood regulation models posit mechanisms for downregulating intense emotions via the nature and structure of dream content; this may require the regular coupling of emotional surges with a problem-solving dream structure unfolding over time or the timing of negative dream emotion early in the night.

Fear Extinction

A recent theory[6,7] ascribes a fear memory extinction function to dreaming and explains nightmares as a perturbation of this function. Fear extinction during dreaming entails the activation of fear memory elements that are isolated and removed from their episodic contexts, and recombined into novel dream scenarios that support the expression of alternate emotional reactions; this sequence ultimately results in the production of *fear extinction memories*. Fear extinction memories provide a sense of "safety" and thus compete with and, if consolidated, supersede the original fear memories. Fear extinction memories are realized during dysphoric dreams, by coupling fear memory elements with realistic nonaversive contexts. Nightmares occur as a result of disruption of this mechanism. For example, if an entrenched fear memory resists recombining with new contexts, as may be the case for nightmares with recurrent themes, new extinction memories may not be formed.

At the neural level, fear extinction is supported by a network of at least four regions that control the representation and expression of emotions in both sleeping and waking states: the amygdala (Amyg), the medial prefrontal cortex (mPFC), the hippocampal (Hip) complex, and the anterior cingulate cortex (ACC). In the fear extinction model, the recombination of fragmentary memory elements into a dream context is relayed by the Hip, with affective qualities added by the Amyg, and inhibitory afferents from the mPFC and ACC to downregulate excessive emotional activation. This process fails during nightmares, the Amyg may be hyperresponsive to fear-related memory elements portrayed in the dream, while processes in the mPFC or the ACC that normally downregulate Amyg activity may be disrupted, resulting in intense fear activation and inability to extinguish fear. This situation parallels empirically supported models of PTSD pathology.[86]

One test of the theory[87] used neuropsychological tests to assess frontal inhibitory function. Nightmare sufferers showed general slowing on the Emotional Stroop, longer reaction times on the Emotional Go/NoGo, and higher perseveration on Verbal Fluency. We replicated the finding of elevated Verbal Fluency perseveration[88] in frequent nightmare sufferers compared with a control group and showed a positive correlation between perseveration and nightmare severity. Neural support for the model includes recent findings that mPFC[89] activation is lower in frequent nightmare sufferers than in controls, that mPFC and ACC activations during an emotional picture-viewing task are negatively correlated with the severity of dysphoric dreaming,[90] and that ACC regional homogeneity is negatively correlated with severity of the physical consequences of nightmares.[91] Thus there is general support for the cognitive and neural predictions that nightmares are related to a frontal deficit in emotional regulation. Nevertheless, the more precise mechanisms of fear extinction during dysphoric dreaming remain to be tested.

Cognitive Avoidance and the Limits of Fear Extinction: Recurrent Nightmares

Spoormaker[92] proposed a variation of the preceding theory to explain fear extinction failures in the subclass of nightmares with recurrent themes. The recurring storylines are stipulated to be "scripts" in memory that are easily activated by ongoing, neutrally toned dreaming and whose specific contents vary as a function of this prior dreaming. Nightmare scripts may be based upon real traumatic memories or may develop over time with repeated emotional stress, particularly if stressors are habitually responded to in a way that develops and reinforces the underlying script. Cognitive avoidance is the key mechanism by which occasional distressful nightmares may become recurrent. That avoidance of distressing thoughts may encourage dysphoric dreams is supported by research on the "dream rebound" effect; for instance, suppressing unpleasant thoughts is associated with increased dysphoric dreams related to the unpleasant thoughts.[93-96] In the case of nightmares, avoidance strategies (e.g., trying not to think about or remember the nightmare) lead to a failure of fear extinction as well as a reduced likelihood that the nightmare script will be integrated into autobiographic memory or that alternative responses to the nightmare script will be discovered. In detailing the limits of fear extinction processes, this model clarifies the pathologic aspect of nightmare experience.

The theory's emphasis on recurrent themes fits well with the fact that the plot lines of many nightmares are, indeed, recurrent. An unpublished study found that of all nightmares reported by 188 college students, including those that were only occasional, 60% contained a recurrent storyline.[92] Among participants with a clinical nightmare problem (at least once per week), 91% claimed that their nightmares possessed recurrent storylines. The inherent dysfunctionality of recurrent nightmares also fits well with the finding that recurrent dreaming more generally is associated with poorer well-being.[97]

Image Contextualization

The image contextualization theory developed by Hartmann[98,99] highlights the role of emotion in dream formation and considers nightmares—as it does dreaming more generally—to play a role in adaptation to emotional experiences. Hartmann considered dream images to be driven by the emotions associated with current concerns; the more powerful an emotion, the more powerful and salient the central image of the dream. Recurrent and posttraumatic nightmares are among the clearest examples, but dreams of intense emotions of any type are also exemplary. The basic role of dreaming is to *contextualize* the imagery metaphorically within a "safe" context (i.e., during REM sleep when muscular inhibition prevents acting out of the dream). An example of a central, contextualizing dream image is the "tidal wave" dream, in which a powerful wave contextualizes feelings of overwhelming fear or helplessness stemming from a waking concern with similarly intense feelings. Contextualizing depends upon a hyperassociativity of neural networks during dreaming, i.e., increased cross-connectivity among elements of the emotional concern and past similar experiences. As mnemonic connections increase, emotions become less intense and the concern is progressively integrated. The dream's adaptive function is likened to psychotherapy after trauma in that the therapist provides a safe context within which intense emotions may be expressed and linked constructively to other memories.[100]

Supporting evidence includes findings that central images are more frequent following trauma or abuse,[101] that REM sleep participates in the forming of hippocampal dependent memories,[102] and that the hippocampus is central to the consolidation of memory for context.[103]

Threat Simulation

This evolutionary theory developed by Revonsuo[52] suggests that the purpose of dreaming—including nightmares—is to provide a realistic (virtual) environment for confronting threatening situations and practicing threat perception and threat-avoidance skills. Revonsuo claims that repeated threat simulation over time increases the probability of successfully coping with real threats in wakefulness and confers a survival advantage to our species. The threat simulation mechanism is fully activated and thus produces more dreams with threats, when the individual is exposed to heightened levels of daytime threat (e.g., living in a war zone). The high prevalence of dysphoric dreams and nightmares supports the theory as these commonly portray threats. Thus, nightmares of being attacked or chased are considered functional to the extent that these provide opportunities to identify threatening situations that may be met in real life and to practice adaptive reactions to them. Research supporting the theory includes dream content analyses showing that college students report frequent threatening dreams that are both severe and realistic (e.g., aggression, misfortune themes), and during which appropriate responses are enacted by the dreamer.[104] Further, children subjected to high levels of threat (trauma), in fact, do dream more often and more intensely of threatening events.[105] Arguments against threat simulation theory claim that the threats created in dreams are too often unrealistic[106] and that the dreamer is too often unable to react successfully to the threat.[107] Realistic threats appear in less than 15% of recurrent dreams[3] and in only 8% of undergraduates' home dreams.[106] The experiencing of threat dreams also does not correlate with actual adaption to threatening events, as in the case of PTSD, where re-experiencing nightmares are often debilitating. Further, the occurrence of nightmares before or after trauma exposure is often a risk factor for developing PTSD.[108]

Postawakening Adaptations

A number of approaches consider nightmares to be functional to the extent that reactions after waking up may play a homeostatic or adaptive role. One type of theory suggests that a postawakening function can be automatic. The *information-processing* or *memory cycle* theory[109,110] is a neopsychoanalytic approach based on the notion that dreaming's function is incorporation of important new experiences into long-term memory, that is, the affective integration of new with old memories. Anxiety dreams that produce awakenings have a particular functionality in that they signal a failure of normal affective integration but allow waking state processes to modify memory sources of the original anxiety dream. This leads to a modified, *correction,* dream the following night. Associating an anxiety dream with other thoughts, feelings, and memories essentially integrates the latter new sources of information with the original sources and provides new, more adaptive, memory sources for the correction dream. This postawakening integrative function may be automatic and preconscious, resulting simply from "having the dream in mind" during the day, or it may be deliberate, either by intentional reflection on the dream during waking, or by the aid of a therapist. In either case, the corrective feedback leads to a permanent, adaptive reorganization of emotional memory structures. Recurrent anxiety dreams are thought to reflect a failure of affective integration and a failure of the correction dream to correct it. The theory has been subject to very little empirical investigation and is supported only generally by evidence that REM sleep is linked to emotional regulation.

A second type of postawakening theory also considers that using dreams in a self-reflection or therapeutic context leads to biologic adaptations, but the mechanisms for such adaptations are not typically specified. One general goal of some such approaches is to alleviate the suffering associated with the nightmares using pharmacologic or behavioral approaches,[111] but another common goal is to use the nightmares as a source for uncovering focal emotional conflicts, which can then be addressed therapeutically. In this case, nightmare-focused therapies have been documented for a diversity of emotional conditions such as bereavement,[4] drug dependencies,[112] and general psychotherapy.[113] In the general population, nightmares are often reported to be a source of personal insight[114]; more than half the participants in a survey study report that reflecting on the meaning of nightmares can lead to personal realizations.

CONCLUSIONS

Science still remains divided in many ways on whether the darker side of dream experience serves a purpose. Nightmares and other disturbing dreams have been clearly delineated as pathologic conditions that are comorbid with many other illnesses, which is broadly consistent with the notion that nightmares are either nonfunctional or dysfunctional symptoms. However, their association with perceptual sensitivity, their nearly ubiquitous existence in the general population, and evidence for a much wider spectrum of disturbed and dysphoric dreams (e.g., bad dreams), all point to the likelihood that nightmares may, in fact, be a component of cognitive-emotional regulation or emotional memory–processing functions.

Theories of nightmare function fall along a spectrum on which many different parts of a nightmare's progression could be considered as functional. Most functional theories consider nightmares to enable some type of emotion regulation function. Although these are often lumped together under a single category, the mechanisms vary from stress mastery, desomatization of affect, fear memory extinction, emotional contextualization, and others. Postawakening theories of function also share the notion of emotion regulation in which waking reactions to the nightmare have adaptive outcomes. The evolutionary theory of nightmares is distinct in claiming that nightmares enable rehearsal of threat coping skills. Some of the theories are applicable only to certain types of nightmare experience, such as recurrent nightmares,[33,92] fear nightmares,[6,7] or threat nightmares,[52] whereas others[56] deal with such a wide swath of emotions that, paradoxically, even intensely positive dreams are included. Despite this variety, many nightmare theories remain relatively vague as to the key functional mechanism, and predictions as a result are not clear. For those theories that have proposed more detailed explanations, supportive evidence is either still controversial or lacking altogether. All of the theories could benefit greatly from an increase in empirical and comparative investigation.

CLINICAL PEARL

That nightmares are comorbid with many pathologic conditions (e.g., anxiety, neuroticism, and PTSD) indicates that nightmares are symptomatic, but their ubiquity in the general population suggests that they may serve some functional purpose. If nightmares do facilitate emotional regulation or emotional memory consolidation as suggested by some theorists, they may have to be treated only when they are frequent, severe, and disruptive of daily functioning.

SUMMARY

Opinion is divided on whether nightmares have a function. Although the clinical definition of nightmares as pathologic suggests that they do not, epidemiologic evidence of the widespread occurrence of nightmares and other dysphoric dreams in the general population suggests that they do. Theories of nightmare function stipulate many different emotion regulation mechanisms, attributing functionality to several of the phenomenological steps of typical nightmares (e.g., preawakening versus postawakening). Such theories account for emotion regulation by stress mastery, desomatization of affect, fear memory extinction, or emotional contextualization. However, supportive evidence is either controversial or absent.

SELECTED READINGS

Andrews S, Hanna P. Investigating the psychological mechanisms underlying the relationship between nightmares, suicide and self-harm. *Sleep Med Rev.* 2020;54:101352.

Brown RJ, Donderi DC. Dream content and self-reported well-being among recurrent dreamers, past-recurrent dreamers, and nonrecurrent dreamers. *J Personal Soc Psychol.* 1986;50:612–623.

Carr M, Nielsen T. A novel differential susceptibility framework for the study of nightmares: evidence for trait sensory processing sensitivity. *Clin Psychol Rev.* 2017;58:86–96.

Cartwright R. Dreaming as a mood regulation system. In: Kryger MH, Roth T, Dement WC, eds. *Principles and Practice of Sleep Medicine.* Philadelphia: Elsevier Saunders; 2005:565–572.

Hartmann E. Nightmare after trauma as paradigm for all dreams: a new approach to the nature and functions of dreaming. *Psychiatry.* 1998;61:223–238.

Hartmann E, et al. Contextualizing images in dreams and daydreams. *Dreaming.* 2001;11(2):97–104.

Hoel E. The overfitted brain: Dreams evolved to assist generalization. *Patterns (NY).* 2021;2(5):100244. Published 2021 May 14.

Nielsen T, Levin R. Nightmares: a new neurocognitive model. *Sleep Med Rev.* 2007;11(4):295–310.

Sandman N, et al. Nightmares: risk factors among the Finnish general adult population. *Sleep.* 2014.

Siclari F, Valli K, Arnulf I. Dreams and nightmares in healthy adults and in patients with sleep and neurological disorders. *Lancet Neurol.* 2020;19(10):849-859.

Spoormaker VI. A cognitive model of recurrent nightmares. *Int J Dream Res.* 2008;1(1):15–22.

Walker MP. The role of sleep in cognition and emotion. *Annal N York Acad Sci.* 2009;1156(1):168–197.

Zadra A, Desjardins S, Marcotte E. Evolutionary function of dreams: a test of the threat simulation theory in recurrent dreams. *Conscious Cognition.* 2006;15(2):450–463.

A complete reference list can be found online at ExpertConsult.com.

Chapter 61

Dreams and Nightmares in Posttraumatic Stress Disorder

Wilfred R. Pigeon; Michelle Carr

Chapter Highlights

- Trauma-related nightmares appear to be specific to posttraumatic stress disorder (PTSD) and can be a persisting and distressing symptom, although not all dream content reported by persons with PTSD is a direct representation of trauma memories.
- Dreams that more specifically replicate a trauma memory during the early aftermath of exposure are associated with PTSD development. Experimental and naturalistic study findings suggest that dreams can positively influence adaptation to stress and trauma, also suggesting that persisting trauma-related nightmares represent a failure of adaptive mechanisms.
- Among individuals with PTSD, nightmares mostly arise from rapid eye movement (REM) sleep, although they can also be accompanied by non–rapid eye movement (NREM) sleep. PTSD patients also have more fragmented REM sleep than healthy sleepers, which may be predictive of PTSD in the acute aftermath of trauma.
- In contrast to normal dreams, dreams in persons with PTSD often incorporate episodic memories of frightening experiences. These features have implications for understanding dreams' neurocognitive substrates and the development of integrative PTSD pathophysiology models.
- Evidence supports the use of exposure to, and/or cognitive restructuring of, nightmares as a psychological treatment for PTSD-related nightmares. The pharmacologic antagonism of noradrenergic receptors also ameliorates nightmares in PTSD.

REPLICATIVE-TRAUMA NIGHTMARES: HALLMARK OF A DISORDER?

Posttraumatic stress disorder (PTSD) is a psychiatric condition that develops in approximately 5% to 10% of persons who experience severely threatening traumatic experiences.[1] During the 2020-2021 COVID-19 pandemic, there was an increase in PTSD in the general population (prevalence 15% to 20%),[1a] in health care workers (prevalence 10% to 35%),[1b] and in patients who had recovered from infection (prevalence about 10% 3 months after recovery)[1c] (see also Chapter 213). The diagnosis is based on a set of four persisting symptom clusters, which include intrusive symptoms such as reexperiencing the trauma with intrusive images, flashbacks, or nightmares; avoidance of trauma-related stimuli; negative alterations in mood or cognition; and heightened arousal and reactivity. Although the course of PTSD can be self-limited, epidemiologic work suggests a mean duration of 73 months with considerable variance related to the type of trauma exposure leading to the disorder.[2] The fifth edition of the *Diagnostic and Statistical Manual of Mental Disorders* specifically delineates "recurrent distressing dreams in which the content and/or affect are related to the traumatic event" among the intrusive symptoms.[3] In an influential review and theoretical paper, Ross and colleagues emphasized the occurrence of "repetitive replicas" of trauma scenes as a feature of dreams virtually specific to PTSD, further referring to rapid eye movement (REM) sleep disturbance and trauma nightmares as a "hallmark of the disorder."[4] A more recent review of this hypothesis maintains that nightmares constitute a signature feature of PTSD.[5]

Whereas the overall rate of frequent nightmares (one or more per week) is 2% to 6% in the general adult population,[6-9] approximately half of all patients with PTSD have frequent trauma-replicating nightmares, and another 20% to 25% experience nightmares that are thematically or symbolically related to their traumatic event.[10-13] Among children, rates of nightmares range widely from 7% to 20% in the general population and 20% to 81% in trauma-exposed samples, with the highest rates among those with diagnosed PTSD and extreme living situations such as war zones.[14-16] In addition, even compared to patients with idiopathic nightmares, patients with PTSD have an elevated frequency of nightmares.[10,11,17] Moreover, the presence of nightmares at a baseline interview predicted higher PTSD severity 6 months later in 80 recent combat veterans[18] as well as the presence of PTSD 6 months postdeployment in 453 soldiers deployed to combat.[19] Frequent nightmares were found in about 25% of frontline medical workers during the COVID-19 pandemic.[19a] Posttraumatic nightmares seem to be an extreme case of recurrent dreams, which typically feature negative dream content and are associated with high self-reported distress and low self-reported well-being[20-24]; posttraumatic nightmares are even more distressing and more replicative of traumatic experiences than recurrent dreams.

Several studies support the specificity of the relationship between trauma-related nightmares and PTSD.[25-27] In more recent work, PTSD symptoms were associated with nightmare distress, nightmare frequency, and nightmare replicativeness among 62 hospitalized German soldiers.[28] Interestingly, only replicativeness predicted PTSD diagnosis; there were no associations between nightmare variables and depression diagnosis. Trauma-replicating nightmares can persist for decades.[29] The relationship between replicative nightmares and higher PTSD severity has even been observed in patients 40 years after a traumatic event.[30]

Thus there is consistent support for the theory that continuing representation of trauma memories in dreams is a feature of PTSD but not necessarily of trauma exposure absent the diagnosis. Many studies have relied on retrospective and global, categorical assessments of dreams. Esposito and colleagues[31] performed content analysis of dreams elicited from morning diaries in a group of combat veterans receiving treatment for PTSD. About half of subjects' dreams contained direct references to combat experiences, and almost all of the dreams featured threat. Similarly, it was reported that among a group of combat veterans experiencing PTSD symptomotology, about half of the dreams elicited after awakenings in the laboratory setting referred to military experiences.[32] These studies all focused on veterans years after their combat experiences.

Some studies have examined the influence of trauma on dream content during an acute phase after a traumatic event. In one study, hurricane survivors (compared to a large sample surveyed pre-hurricane) reported more with general stressors, with especially stressful life experiences and with content specific to the hurricane.[33] Similarly, evacuees of an urban fire were more likely to have dream content related to death, disasters, and fires than were controls.[34] Among children and adolescents, a similar pattern of trauma event incorporation into early posttrauma dreams has been observed in samples spanning a variety of traumas[35–37] with higher rates of trauma dreams as a function of proximity to the threat or direct versus indirect association with the trauma,[37,38] although findings among children can be more mixed.[14,39] Finally, the relationship of dream content to PTSD status is not commonly assessed. Among adolescent asylum seekers in the UK, nightmare frequency was correlated with PTSD symptoms, although dream content was not assessed.[40] Mellman and colleagues elicited dream content from study participants during the acute aftermath of traumatic injury.[41] A subgroup of the sample described dreams that were distressing and "highly similar" to the traumatic experience (17% of the sample; 56% of those who reported dreams). This group had more severe concurrent PTSD symptom ratings than other dream recallers and higher subsequent PTSD severity than nonrecallers.[41] Wittman and colleagues observed a similar pattern in children acutely after motor vehicle accidents; acute replicative nightmares predicted PTSD symptoms 2 and 6 months later.[42]

Thus trauma-exposed populations tend to report dreams with trauma-related or thematically related content in the acute aftermath of traumas. Dreams that are similar to the memory of the traumatic event are associated with the development of PTSD. Chronic PTSD is associated with recurring dreams that replicate or represent specific memories of a traumatic experience. Nonetheless, the more comprehensive evaluations of dreams during chronic phases of PTSD document that salient dream content is not limited to representations of traumatic memories.

DREAM CONTENT WITH STRESS AND TRAUMA: BEYOND REPLICATION

Although the issue of trauma replication has received considerable attention, there are descriptions of other aspects of content in the literature on dreaming, nightmares, and PTSD. The boundaries of traumatic stress are not always clear, and the topic seems embedded in broader questions of stress and dreaming, including observations of the impact of stressful experiences on dreams, the influence of dreams on adaptation to stressful experiences, and content themes related to trauma exposure and PTSD beyond replication of trauma.

Stress and Dream Content

It has been consistently observed that dream narratives incorporate elements of current concerns, including daily stressors, as distressing dream content.[43] For example, health-related stressors have been evidenced in the home dream content of patients awaiting surgery[44] in hospitalized burn patients,[45] pregnant women,[46,47] and women during the peak hormonal phase of the menstrual cycle.[48] Academic, occupational, and daily life stress have been associated with dream content. This includes increased dream recall in college students a week before exams compared with a control week,[49] increased nightmare frequency in the general population in tandem with increases in daily stress,[50] and dreams of being chased or falling[51] correlated with graduate students' financial stress[52] and stockbrokers' stress levels during market downturns.[53]

Being exposed to adversity is also consistently associated with idiopathic nightmares[54-56]; one recent study found that lifetime adversity in nightmare sufferers was almost twice as high as controls without frequent nightmares as assessed by the Traumatic Antecedents Questionnaire.[56] Living in threatening environments is correlated with increased threatening dreams in traumatized Kurdish children.[57] However, dream reports of South African people living in areas of high crime did not differ in the frequency of threatening content from that of a control Welsh sample.[58] Interestingly, several dream-reporting studies undertaken around the time of the September 11, 2011, terrorist attacks in the United States each concluded, despite varied methodologies, that the attacks were associated with increased intensity of dreams compared to pre–9/11 dreams.[59-62] Only two of the studies, however, found that post–9/11 dream narratives contained explicit references to the terror attacks.[61,62]

Recurring dreams, which have more negative content than nonrecurring dreams, tend to be activated by stressful life experiences.[20,63,64] In a community sample, subjects with active recurring dreams reported greater life stress in the prior 6 months and had more negative dream content than both former recurrent dreamers and dreamers with no recurrent dreams.[65] This was replicated in two college student samples.[49,66] In addition to naturalistic observations, studies using experimental induction of stress (disturbing movies,[67,68] sham intelligence exams,[69,70] and experimentally induced pain[71]) found incorporation of the stressor into dreams on the same night. Overall, experimental stressors are associated with subsequent dreams that are characterized by a negative tone. Unlike in the case of replicative posttraumatic nightmares, it is difficult to distinguish incorporations directly related to stressors as they typically do not appear episodically.[72]

Like relatively innocuous daytime events and concerns that can be incorporated into dreams,[73] the studies reviewed so far demonstrate that stressful waking experiences are also incorporated into dreams and have an impact on the emotional content of those dreams. The relationship of dream incorporation to emotional saliency has led several dream theorists to invoke an emotional information processing function for dreaming.[74-76] The threat simulation theory of dreaming further posits an evolutionary function of dreaming: to simulate realistic threats to rehearse and prepare for future threats in waking life.[77] Although it has been difficult to confirm that threat rehearsal occurs in dreams, several lines of evidence support a relationship between dreams and adaptations to emotional stress.

Dreams and Adaptation to Stress

In one experiment that used viewing a disturbing film as a probe, subjects experimentally deprived of REM sleep were subsequently more distressed by the film than either a non–rapid eye movement (NREM) sleep interruption group or an uninterrupted sleep group.[68] Naturalistic studies suggesting that dream incorporation can aid adaptive processing include several in which dream references to drugs and alcohol were a positive predictor of abstinence.[78-81] Cartwright[74] elicited dream reports after laboratory awakenings from REM sleep in men and women going through divorce. Those who incorporated the ex-spouse into their dreams at the time of the breakup were less depressed and better adjusted at 12-month follow-up than those who did not.

Other research shows that suppressing unpleasant thoughts in waking life is associated with increased distressing dream content[82] that may be specifically related to the unpleasant thought,[83] termed the "dream rebound" effect.[84] This has been proposed as a possible mechanism for nightmare production, in that avoidance of nightmare-related thoughts in waking life may lead to increased expression of nightmares during sleep.[85] Indeed, avoidance of trauma-related stimuli is symptomatic of PTSD[3] and may thus encourage dream rebound in posttraumatic nightmares. Nevertheless, recent evidence has shown that dream rebound may be adaptive; in one study, dreaming of unpleasant thoughts that had been suppressed before sleep was subsequently associated with more pleasant emotional response to the thought, suggesting an emotional processing function of dream rebound.[86]

Observations that dream emotional content serves a functional role in adaptation to stress may initially seem to contradict the observations reviewed earlier of an association between trauma-replicating dreams and the outcome of PTSD. The observations just reviewed, however, refer to incorporation of a reference to or representation of a stressful situation and not necessarily the replication of events. For dreaming to influence emotional adaptation to stress, the neurocognitive activity of sleep must have an enduring influence on memory representations. Support does exist for sleep's role in the consolidation and reprocessing of memory (i.e., learning) that is thoroughly reviewed by Wamsley and Stickgold[87] (see Chapter 55).

Trauma, Posttraumatic Stress Disorder, and Content Themes

Several laboratory-based REM-awakening studies highlight the relationship of dream content to the presence, severity, or course of PTSD. Threatening content was observed in the majority of dreams (83%) in a sample of combat veterans with PTSD.[31] Dreams of combat veterans with PTSD had more anxiety than those of veterans without PTSD,[88] subjects with combat-related PTSD had more frequent aggression in their dreams than healthy controls,[89] and Holocaust survivors symptomatic for PTSD had more anxiety, aggression, and interpersonal conflicts in their dreams than asymptomatic survivors.[90]

In nonlaboratory studies there have been similar associations. For instance, anger ratings in dreams of a PTSD sample were positively correlated with traumatic themes, repetitiveness, and PTSD severity.[91] In two separate studies, the dreams of children exposed to ongoing civil or military violence contained more themes of aggression, persecution, and negative emotions[92] and threat/aggression[57] than the dreams of control subjects in each study, although PTSD status was not assessed. Finally, among patients with recent traumatic injuries, dreams of those who eventually developed PTSD had more content related to general and physical misfortune, as well as more negative emotions, than those who did not develop PTSD.[93]

Thus, compared to other dreams, dreams after trauma have more general negative emotions, anxiety, threat, and aggression. This appears to be most pronounced with PTSD. Beyond emotional content, posttraumatic nightmares contain heightened levels of sensory vividness compared to normal dreams, such as increased olfactory experience,[29] which is typically rare in dreams.[94] The intensified, negative, and trauma-related content of dreams in PTSD led Campbell and Germain[95] to suggest that "dreams themselves could be traumatic for the dreamer."

POLYSOMNOGRAPHIC CORRELATES OF NIGHTMARES IN POSTTRAUMATIC STRESS DISORDER

There is an association, albeit not an absolute one, between dreams—particularly those with content that is more elaborate, visual, emotional, and bizarre—and the REM sleep stage.[96] Other sleep phenomena, such as night terrors and related parasomnias, arise from NREM sleep stages, particularly slow wave sleep.[97] It has been suggested that nightmares in PTSD may also be more associated with NREM than REM sleep. Two small studies support this contention.[25,98]

In contrast, the one spontaneous nightmare awakening that occurred during polysomnography (PSG) recordings in a study by Ross and colleagues[4] and three recorded by Mellman and colleagues were preceded by REM sleep.[99] Hefez and colleagues[100] described a pattern of REM interruption insomnia in a group of subjects with PTSD who experienced nightmares. The largest sample of PSG-recorded spontaneous nightmares (n = 17) for patients with PTSD was reported in an abstract by Woodward and colleagues, who found the probability of REM sleep occurring in the 10 minutes preceding nightmare awakenings was double the probability of nightmares occurring during NREM sleep.[101] In an ambulatory PSG study, 24 of 35 patients with PTSD instructed to press a button at the occurrence of nightmares endorsed nightmares in this manner.[102] Ten of the nightmares occurred in REM sleep, and the remaining 14 arose in NREM stages 1 and 2. Thus overall it seems that nightmares in PTSD may be preceded by REM sleep, but they often emerge from other sleep stages.

In a prospective study of patients hospitalized for traumatic injuries, PSG recordings were obtained close to the time of medical and surgical stabilization. Those who developed PTSD did not differ from those who did not develop PTSD with respect to general measures of sleep maintenance, amount of REM sleep, and increased eye movement density (compared with uninjured controls). The group developing PTSD, however, spent significantly less uninterrupted time in

REM sleep before shifting to waking or other electroencephalography sleep stages,[99,103,104] which was also observed among a community sample with PTSD.[104] A recent meta-analysis reviewed the available PSG studies of PTSD and concluded that PTSD is associated with poorer sleep continuity, less sleep depth, and REM sleep disturbances.[105]

Disrupted sleep characteristics reported during REM sleep of subjects with PTSD are hypothesized to be indices of the heightened arousal that is symptomatic of PTSD and include higher sympathetic heart rate variability indices,[106,107] more periodic leg movements,[108] higher beta frequency power,[103] and lower theta frequency power.[19,109] Similarly, nightmares in REM sleep are associated with acute physiologic arousal, including increased respiration rate, heart rate, and sweating.[110-112] In addition resting pulse rate correlates with nightmare severity.[91] These findings suggest that hyperarousal may characterize individuals with PTSD during both wake and sleep. Finally the most consistent PSG finding in patients with PTSD appears to be one of increased REM fragmentation.[113] It has been hypothesized that this observed fragmentation of REM sleep may compromise REM sleep's potentially adaptive memory-processing functions.[99]

THEORETICAL IMPLICATIONS

Overall, the findings reviewed solidify the representation of traumatic experience memories in dreams as a distinguishing feature of PTSD. Traumatic and stressful experiences appear to influence dream content whether or not people are successfully adapting emotionally. Findings also suggest that nightmares that are replicative of the episodic memory of the trauma experience are associated with the development of PTSD. When PTSD enters a chronic phase, trauma memories continue to be represented in recurring nightmares.

Dream content of patients with established PTSD is not limited to trauma memories and may reflect the negative and restricted emotional state of the dreamer. The literature on stress and dreaming suggests that dream content reflects the dreamer's emotional processing and that dreaming supports emotional adaptation. In contrast, recurring nightmares in patients with PTSD appear to reinforce trauma memories and contribute to distress. The distinguishing feature of replicating or representing the memory of the trauma over time may provide important clues to the overall emotional memory processing of people with PTSD.

Fosse and colleagues[114] have found that dreams recalled by healthy college students do often contain references to recent events, but that events are rarely represented in dreams in their entirety. More recently, Malinowski and Horton[72] also found that dreams do not typically contain episodic memories. As has been discussed, the dreams that characterize PTSD are not necessarily unaltered replays of the traumatic event. However, dreams occurring with PTSD tend to contain more representations of events that include or are closer to unaltered memories (of traumatic events) than normal dreams do. Noncorrespondence to coherent whole-memory representations may be consequent to the selective activation of neural structures during REM sleep. In the generally accepted model of sleep state regulation, neural activation during REM sleep is mediated by firing of cholinergic brainstem nuclei and is further facilitated by inhibition of noradrenergic firing.[115] Experimental evidence indicates that declarative memory for emotionally arousing stimuli is likewise mediated by noradrenergic mechanisms.[116] Therefore impaired inhibition of noradrenergic tone during sleep, consistent with evidence of hyperarousal in sleep of PTSD patients, could be a mechanism underlying the presence of episodic-like, fear-enhanced memories in dreams. Direct support for this hypothesis comes from evidence that pharmacologic blockade of noradrenergic stimulation with prazosin, an alpha$_1$-adrenergic antagonist, ameliorates nightmares in PTSD.[117]

There is a further consideration regarding an adaptive memory-processing function for REM sleep and REM dreaming that may be impaired with PTSD. Normal dream mentation has a hyperassociative quality: characters, places, and sequences that are not typically linked in waking conscious thought tend to be juxtaposed in dreams.[115] Foa[118] has suggested that one of the mechanisms of successful emotional processing during exposure therapy is the development of a new network of associations to the traumatic memories. Such a process may be facilitated by the normal neurocognitive characteristics of REM sleep and impaired by a more selective activation of trauma memories. Nielsen and Levin's neurocognitive model of nightmare production explains how extinction of fear memories can occur through dysphoric dreams.[110,119] The neurocircuitry relies on medial prefrontal cortex regulation of the amygdala during REM sleep, extinguishing fear memories through association with novel, neutral dream elements.

Neurocircuitry models of PTSD posit that the ventromedial prefrontal cortex fails to inhibit the amygdala, leading to attentional bias toward threat, increased fear responses, impaired extinction of traumatic memories, and deficits in emotion regulation.[120,121] If similar activation characterizes sleep in PTSD, it would interfere with neurocognitive functions of REM sleep in extinguishing fear. Germain and colleagues propose that REM sleep amplifies activity of the amygdala and the medial prefrontal cortex, which is permissive of nightmares.[122] Finally, maladaptive REM sleep after trauma may actively consolidate fear; recent work with animal trauma models found that experimental sleep deprivation during the first rest phase after a trauma exposure was associated with reductions in PTSD-like symptoms.[123] Conceptual models that integrate neurobiologic findings from both the sleep and PTSD fields as well as their respective clinical research findings continue to be needed to guide empirical inquiry into the role of recurrent traumatic dreams in PTSD pathophysiology. At the same time, the response of trauma-related nightmares to various treatment strategies can inform models of central PTSD mechanisms. See Chapter 60 for a more detailed coverage of dream nightmare theories as well as Germain and colleagues' recent review of brain-based and intervention research informing conceptual models of PTSD-related sleep disturbances.[124]

TREATMENT OF POSTTRAUMATIC NIGHTMARES

There are five recent clinical practice guidelines (CPGs) for the treatment of PTSD,[125] which give stronger recommendations for nonpharmacologic, trauma-focused interventions compared with pharmacotherapy and/or recommend prioritizing trauma-focused therapies before considering pharmacotherapy. Other than considering sleep intervention when sleep disturbance persists after trauma-focused interventions,

Table 61.1 2018 American Academy of Sleep Medicine Recommendations for the Treatment of PTSD-Associated Nightmares

Recommendation	Pharmacologic Treatments	Psychological Treatments
Recommended[a]	None	Imagery rehearsal therapy (IRT)
May be used[a]	Atypical antipsychotics (olanzapine, risperidone, and aripiprazole); clonidine; cyproheptadine; fluvoxamine; gabapentin; nabilone; phenelzine; prazosin; topiramate; trazodone; tricyclic antidepressants	Cognitive behavioral therapy; cognitive behavioral therapy for insomnia; eye movement desensitization and reprocessing; exposure, relaxation, and rescripting therapy (EERT)
Not recommended[a]	Clonazepam; venlafaxine	None

[a]"Recommended" and "not recommended" indicate a treatment option is determined to be clearly useful (or ineffective/harmful) for most patients; the "may be used" designation is for treatments for which the evidence or expert consensus is less clear, either in favor of or against the use of, a treatment option.
PTSD, Posttraumatic stress disorder.
Modified from Morgenthaler TI, Auerbach S, Casey KR, et al. Position paper for the treatment of nightmare disorder in adults: an American Academy of Sleep Medicine position paper. *J Clin Sleep Med*. 2018;14(6):1041–55.

the guidelines have little to recommend specifically for PTSD-related nightmares. A notable exception is found in the U.S. Department of Veterans Affairs/Department of Defense CPG, which (1) recommends an independent assessment of co-occurring sleep disturbances in patients with PTSD; (2) recommends cognitive behavioral therapy for insomnia in patients with PTSD; but (3) found the evidence for nightmare treatments in PTSD patients to be inconclusive.[126]

There are, nonetheless, four reasons to consider more strongly the use of targeted treatments for PTSD-related nightmares rather than rely on their natural resolution or their amelioration after PTSD treatments. First, although insomnia tends to be more stubbornly persistent than nightmares in the absence of direct intervention, neither do nightmares typically resolve spontaneously.[18] Second, although clinical experience and literature on the treatment of residual sleep symptoms suggest that nightmares do tend to decrease in frequency and intensity as PTSD improves, the relatively limited data available have historically suggested that nightmares are inadequately responsive to first-line interventions for PTSD[127] with more recent work upholding this impression.[128] Third, nightmares clearly have a negative impact on the severity and trajectory of PTSD symptoms,[18,129] exacerbate psychological distress even after controlling for PTSD symptoms,[10] and contribute to suicidal thoughts and behaviors.[8,130] For example, among trauma-exposed participants with PTSD symptoms, suicidal behaviors were endorsed by 62% of those with nightmares compared to 20% of those without nightmares.[131] Finally, treatments for PTSD nightmares are available, grounded in theory, and supported by clinical research evidence.

For instance, a therapeutic effect of postsynaptic blockade of noradrenergic neurotransmission is consistent with the role for noradrenergic activity in mediating traumatic nightmares that was postulated in the previous section. As thoroughly reviewed in a 2018 position paper, the efficacy of prazosin for PTSD nightmares has been demonstrated in both uncontrolled and randomized trials.[132] In this paper,[132] however, the recommendation for prazosin was downgraded from "recommend" to "may be used" because of the negative results of a large clinical trial of veterans with chronic PTSD and current frequent nightmares.[133] Thus there are no clearly recommended pharmacologic treatments for PTSD nightmares. Prazosin remains the first choice for pharmacologic intervention among numerous other medications with a "may be used" designation (Table 61.1). Notably, clonazepam and venlafaxine were not recommended (not clearly useful or ineffective/harmful) for the treatment of PTSD nightmares.[132] An interesting case series from an electronic chart review study underscores the broad clinical landscape in the pharmacologic management of PTSD-related nightmares. Twenty-one individual and 13 different medication combinations were assessed across 480 individual trials, in which only 10% had a full response (no nightmare recall) and 47% had a partial response (some decrease in nightmare frequency or intensity).[134] Alpha$_1$-adrenergic agonists other than prazosin (e.g., doxazosin, terazosin) are being evaluated for nightmare treatment, but the current evidence base for them is too small to properly assess and exists in the larger context of a need for more potent medications for PTSD.[135]

Turning to nonpharmacologic approaches, the idea that dreams are related to emotional processing suggests that recurrent nightmares related to trauma may respond to psychotherapeutic interventions. In fact, several clinical trials have demonstrated good efficacy for nightmare interventions that are based on psychological principles of exposure therapy or cognitive restructuring. Among them, imagery rehearsal therapy (IRT) has the largest evidence base to date.[136] In this technique, patients write out or describe the content of a distressing dream, rescript the content any way they wish, and then rehearse the images of the altered dream scenario. Successful variations of this approach include combining repeated exposure to a disturbing dream, relaxation training with rescripting of the dream (exposure, relaxation, and rescripting therapy),[137] relaxation and exposure without rescripting,[138] and an approach that uses lucid dreaming techniques, in which patients learn to change dream content as the dream actually occurs.[139] Overall, this set of interventions results in significant reductions in nightmare severity and frequency, with more modest improvements in insomnia and PTSD severity. An early meta-analysis found that psychological nightmare interventions were effective as a group with a moderate effect size comparable to that of pharmacologic interventions, but that less involved approaches such as relaxation alone were ineffective.[140] Prior reviews and meta-analyses support IRT as a nightmare treatment.[136,140-144] Here again, the American Academy of Sleep Medicine position paper on nightmare treatments is informative.[132]

Specifically, based on nine randomized trials, it deems IRT to be the only recommended first-line treatment for nightmares (both PTSD nightmares and idiopathic nightmares). Among these a large comparative effectiveness trial (n = 399) compared IRT to exposure therapy, to a self-help audio recording, and to no treatment.[145] IRT and exposure were found to be equally effective in reducing weekly nightmare frequency at posttreatment and an 11-week follow-up, with IRT being superior to self-help. In another randomized trial among 90 individuals with a heterogeneity of mental health diagnoses, IRT was superior to outpatient treatment as usual in reducing nightmare frequency as well as PTSD symptom severity.[146] Interestingly, like the recent negative prazosin trial, one IRT trial in veterans also reported negative results for IRT compared to a standard sleep and nightmare management group.[147] Nonetheless, the weight of the evidence supported a full recommendation for IRT in the treatment of PTSD nightmares.

Psychotherapeutic nightmare interventions such as IRT are consistent with principles from the established cognitive behavior treatments of PTSD that apply exposure or cognitive restructuring, or both, to trauma memories.[148] That such techniques can be effectively applied directly to nightmare content (which in PTSD often features trauma memories) has important implications. One is that clinicians can be realistically hopeful about the potential for alleviating distressing nightmare symptoms. We have previously referred to the apparent paradox that stress-related references in dreams are associated with positive outcome, whereas trauma-replicating nightmares are associated with PTSD. This paradox may be reconciled if the former dreams represent an adaptive emotional processing, possibly related to modification of associative networks, and the latter represent a failure of such a process. Studies of imagery rehearsal suggest that conscious exposure to the content of recurring distressing dreams, along with instruction to modify the dream scenario, facilitates movement toward the more adaptive response.

Benefits of nightmare treatments generalize to other symptom domains; this supports the idea of continuity between waking emotional life and dreaming. Dreams may offer clinicians a unique window into patients' emotional adaptation to trauma and stress along with the status of their processing of traumatic memories. The apparently robust association between PTSD and replays or representations of trauma memories in dreams further provides an important clue to understanding abnormalities of emotional memory processing that differentiate those who suffer with PTSD and those who are more resilient to adverse psychobiologic consequences of trauma. In sum, the literature indicates that treatment of nightmares not only ameliorates sleep disturbances but also can reduce overall symptoms of PTSD, although not to the point of remission. This strongly suggests that nightmare treatments may be combined or sequenced with PTSD treatments for maximal therapeutic effect (see Chapter 100).

One final point regarding the treatment of PTSD nightmares that bears noting is that nightmares often co-occur with insomnia and obstructive sleep apnea. Evidence now suggests that cognitive behavioral therapy for insomnia alone and positive airway pressure alone can each reduce PTSD-related nightmares.[149,150] Accordingly, a potentially productive line of inquiry would be to determine what REM and/or NREM sleep processes may mediate (or what individual variables moderate) the effect on nightmares when the amelioration of disturbed sleep among individuals with PTSD is achieved via insomnia treatment or sleep apnea treatment.

CLINICAL PEARL

The phenomenon of trauma replication in dreams is a distinguishing feature of PTSD. Recurrent trauma nightmares contribute to considerable distress in patients with PTSD. Evidence supports the use of IRT as a psychological treatment for PTSD-related nightmares. Despite some mixed evidence for its use, prazosin remains the most successful pharmacologic treatment for such nightmares. Strong consideration should be given to including targeted nightmare treatments in the course of PTSD treatment.

SUMMARY

Trauma-related nightmares warrant their designation as a hallmark of PTSD. The preponderance of evidence indicates that stressors of increasing strength are incorporated into dream narratives, with severe traumas and PTSD nightmares occupying the extreme end of the continuum. Evidence suggests that dreams indirectly incorporating elements of life stressors or traumatic experiences may be emotionally adaptive in acute posttrauma periods but that persistent and trauma-replicating dreams are maladaptive. Findings from sleep neurobiology, PTSD neurobiology, and PSG studies support that REM sleep is fragmented in PTSD and that increased arousal in PTSD may interfere with a REM sleep function of extinguishing fear. At the same time, the efficacy of some pharmacologic and nonpharmacologic nightmare treatments has been established, which is consistent with the contention that incorporation of actual trauma memories and their affective components into dreams is indicative of neurocognitive substrates.

SELECTED READINGS

Cartwright RD. Dreams that work: the relation of dream incorporation to adaptation to stressful events. *Dreaming*. 1991;1:3–9.

Germain A, McKeon AB, Campbell RL. Sleep in PTSD: conceptual model and novel directions in brain-based research and interventions. *Current Opinion in Psychology*. 2017;14:84–89.

Kobayashi I, Boarts JM, Delahanty DL. Polysomnographically measured sleep abnormalities in PTSD: a meta-analytic review. *Psychophysiology*. 2007;44:660–669.

Lin YQ, Lin ZX, Wu YX, et al. Reduced sleep duration and sleep efficiency were independently associated with frequent nightmares in Chinese frontline medical workers during the Coronavirus disease 2019 outbreak. *Front Neurosci.* 2021;14:631025. Published 2021 Jan 20.

Malinowski JE, Horton CL. Metaphor and hyperassociativity: the imagination mechanisms behind emotion assimilation in sleep and dreaming. *Frontiers in Psychology*. 2015;6:1132.

Mellman TA, Pigeon WR, Nowell PD, Nolan B. Relationships between REM sleep findings and PTSD symptoms during the early aftermath of trauma. *J Trauma Stress*. 2007;20:893–901.

Morgenthaler TI, et al. Position paper for the treatment of nightmare disorder in adults: an American Academy of Sleep Medicine position paper. *J Clin Sleep Med*. 2018;14:1041–1055.

Paul F, Alpers GW, Reinhard I, Schredl M. Nightmares do result in psychophysiological arousal: a multimeasure ambulatory assessment study. *Psychophysiology*. 2019:e13366.

Phelps AJ, et al. An ambulatory polysomnography study of the post-traumatic nightmares of post-traumatic stress disorder. *Sleep*. 2018;41:zsx188. https://doi.org/10.1093/sleep/zsx188.

Ulmer CS, Hall MH, Dennis PA, et al. Posttraumatic stress disorder diagnosis is associated with reduced parasympathetic activity during sleep in US veterans and military service members of the Iraq and Afghanistan wars. *Sleep*. 2018;41:zsy174.

A complete reference list can be found online at ExpertConsult.com.

Chapter 62

Incorporation of Waking Experiences into Dreams

Michael Schredl

Chapter Highlights

- Research on the continuity between waking and dreaming has clearly identified factors that affect the probability that waking-life experiences will be incorporated into subsequent dreams, such as emotional intensity, time interval between waking event and dreaming, and type of daytime activity.
- Because direct empirical tests of possible functions of dreaming are difficult to carry out, research on the continuity hypothesis provides clues about the possible function(s) of dreaming.
- It is still unclear whether dreaming is involved in sleep-dependent memory consolidation.
- The finding that social interactions seem to be integral ingredients of dreams that are closely associated with the waking-life social environment may point to the importance of dreaming in regulating and maintaining social relationships, which have been essential for survival in hunter-gatherer societies over the history of humankind.
- The question of why we dream about things we have never experienced in waking life is yet unresolved.

INTRODUCTION

The questions of how dream content is linked to waking life and why we dream, that is, whether dreaming has a specific function, have fascinated humankind for centuries. The bizarre nature of some dreams has led to various hypotheses, such as (1) dreams are stimulated by a more or less random generator in the brainstem and the mind is constructing meaning out of this mess[1] or (2) dreams reflect those contents the brain should forget, that is, dreams do not serve any function.[2] However, to answer the question regarding a specific dream function, it is necessary to study the relationship between the waking life of dreamers and their dreams in a systematic way; this is the main topic of this chapter.

Regarding function, the question is whether dreaming defined as subjective experiences that occur during sleep[3] has an additional function to the well-established functions of sleep itself (e.g., memory consolidation).[4] Despite the large number of hypotheses regarding dream function, providing conclusive empirical data is difficult. To elicit reports of dream content, study participants are asked to report their dreams upon awakening. However, if the dream is reported in the waking state, how is it possible to differentiate between the original dream and the effects of narrating the dream (e.g., thinking it over)?[5] The aim of this chapter is to address the question of whether we can learn something about the function of dreaming by studying recalled dream content and its relationship to waking life.

DEFINITION OF CONTINUITY AND DISCONTINUITY

Despite the bizarreness of dreams, the occurrence of waking-life experiences in dreams was recognized long ago and termed "day-residues" by Freud.[6] A more specific theory regarding the relationship between waking and dreaming—the so-called continuity hypothesis—was introduced by Hall and Bell[7] and Hall and Nordby.[8] The following quotation[8] illustrates the basic idea:

> This [continuity] hypothesis states that dreams are continuous with waking life; the world of dreaming and the world of waking are one…The continuity may be between dreams and covert behavior (thoughts, feelings, and fantasies) or it may be between dreams and overt behavior ("acting out"). (p. 104)

Whereas the definition of dreams as a recollection of subjective experiences that occur while sleeping is widely accepted,[3] over the years a controversy has emerged about what aspects of waking life (Box 62.1) are continuous to dreaming.[9-14] Empirical findings[3] showed that all of these aspects (e.g., experiences, fantasies, media consumption) can show up in dreams; therefore it may be difficult to falsify the continuity hypothesis. For example, the continuity hypothesis would be disproven if persons who often engage in sports dream less often about sports than persons who are scarcely active. Another challenge for the continuity hypothesis of dreaming[3] is dream elements that are clearly discontinuous with waking

BOX 62.1 DIFFERENT ASPECTS OF WAKING LIFE IN RELATION TO THE CONTINUITY HYPOTHESIS

- Concerns
- Conceptions
- Thoughts
- Emotions
- Experiences
- Preoccupations
- Fantasies
- Actions
- Interests
- Unfinished business
- Psychological issues
- Media consumption
- Personal significant events
- Meta-awareness

Table 62.1 Mathematical Model for the Continuity between Waking Life and Dreaming

Incorporation rate = a (EI, TYPE, PERS) × $e^{-b(TN) \times t}$ + Constant

a (EI, TYPE, PERS)	Multiplying factor, which is a function of emotional involvement (EI), type of the waking-life experience (TYPE), and the interaction between experience and personality traits (PERS)
b (TN)	Slope of the exponential function, which is itself a function of the time interval between sleep onset and dream onset (TN)
t	Time interval between waking-life experience and occurrence of the dream incorporation

life, for example, flying dreams[15] or walking dreams in people with congenital paraplegia.[16]

However, the specific definition of discontinuity is still open to discussion. Hobson, for example, defines discontinuity as misrepresentations of times, places, persons, and actions within the dream and the synthesis of completely original dream features[17] (e.g., dreaming of the workplace but with persons totally unrelated to work). As most dreams do not exactly replay waking-life experiences,[18,19] this broad definition of discontinuity would include almost every dream. Horton[20] suggested that this fragmentation of experiences (i.e., the process of decontextualization of single aspects of the waking-life experience) may serve a function because of the constructive nature of autobiographic memory. A more strict definition of discontinuity was proposed by Michael Schredl in his discussion with Allan Hobson,[17] stating that only dream experiences that cannot be experienced in waking life, such as flying, should be termed discontinuous.

The interesting question of why we dream about topics that we never have experienced in waking life is still unanswered. If the continuity included fantasy, daydreams, and media consumption, some of these bizarre dreams might still be within the range of the continuity hypothesis (e.g., people with congenital paraplegia fantasizing about walking).[16] Interestingly, research in people with limb loss[21,22] indicated that some aspects of dreams (e.g., the own body image) may reflect innate body images that are not based on experience. Another explanation may be provided by the so-called mirror neurons, that is, observing pain experiences by others can result in pain-related brain activation in the observer. So it was not surprising that dreamers could experience pain in their dreams that they have never experienced in waking life (e.g., being shot in the stomach).[23] Given these ideas, the percentage of truly discontinuous dreams, that is, dreams including experiences the dreamer never had in waking life, is still unknown.

STUDYING THE CONTINUITY BETWEEN WAKING AND DREAMING

Model of Continuity

As pointed out previously, the continuity hypothesis in its original form is very broadly defined and therefore difficult to falsify.[9] Schredl[24] formulated a mathematical model (Table 62.1) to specify and investigate factors empirically that may modulate the continuity between waking and dreaming. A very plausible factor is the time interval between waking-life experience and occurrence of the dream: the more distant the waking-life experience or thought is, the less likely it would be incorporated into a dream. Other factors that may modulate continuity have been studied, such as emotional intensity, type of waking-life experience (cognitive activities vs. social activities), or time of the night the dream occurred (see later). The intention of formulating such a formalized model was not to complicate matters but to encourage researchers to look systematically for factors that affect the continuity between waking and dreaming.

BOX 62.2 RESEARCH PARADIGMS FOR STUDYING THE RELATIONSHIP BETWEEN WAKING AND DREAMING

- Assessing temporal references of dream elements
- Diary studies
    - Within-subject approach
    - Between-subject approach
- Experimental manipulation of daytime experiences

Methodological Issues

Over the years, different approaches have been applied for studying empirically the continuity between waking and dreaming (Box 62.2). The major problem with the approach of asking the dreamer to link dream elements with waking life is limited memory capacity. Who can remember every thought, emotion, or experience of the previous day, let alone the previous week or month? To solve this issue, researchers studied the effects of experimental manipulations of waking-life experiences on dreams.[3] For example, De Koninck and Brunette[25] exposed phobic participants to a snake (in a terrarium) and read them different stories before sleep onset. Interestingly, the emotional tone of the story affected the participants' dream emotions but not the dream content. Overall, this line of research showed that experimental manipulation (with the exception of highly immersive video games) did not exert a strong effect on dream content as did real-life stressors such as awaiting major surgery or an intensive group therapy session.[26]

Field studies asking the participants to keep a diary in which they fill in daytime events in the evening and their dreams in the morning were more promising for testing the continuity between waking and dreaming,[27-30] showing the relationship between waking-life emotions and dream emotions or activities such as driving a car and car dreams.

Continuity between Waking and Dreaming: Time Factor

Freud[6] summarized his own experiences and the literature by stating, "Dreams show a clear preference for the impression of the immediately preceding days" (p. 247), the so-called day-residue effect. Subsequent studies[31-33] confirmed that events from the previous day are more often incorporated into dreams compared with events from past days, weeks, or years. Even though a diary study[34] confirmed this decreasing level of incorporation with increasing time intervals between waking-life event and dream, the previously mentioned studies, similar to Freud's observations and the literature he reviewed, applied the approach of assessing the temporal references of the dream elements after the dream was reported. As mentioned previously, this approach, whether including open and/or covert behavior, is limited by the memory capacity of the dreamer: that is, the decrease of more remote references may simply be explained by lack of recalling the corresponding waking experiences.

Several diary studies[28,35-39] have found a day-residue effect (i.e., the highest incorporation rates were for events of the previous day but there was also a so-called "dream lag" effect): the incorporation rate of events that happened 5 to 7 days before the dreams were higher when compared with the period of 2 or 4 days or time intervals longer than 8 days. This has been interpreted as reflection of adaptive processes, especially in regard to social stressors and processes of memory consolidation.[39]

However, diary studies should be viewed with caution because they most likely elicit only rapid eye movement (REM) dreams before awakening in the morning and thus are not representative of all dreams. There is evidence that the first REM dreams of the night are more often affected by experimental manipulations applied before sleep[40,41] when compared with REM dreams later in the same night. Dream elements of late-night REM dreams have more remote references to waking life than dream elements of early REM dreams.[42,43] In addition, early night dreams were more affected by media, whereas late-night dreams were more affected by waking-life activities.[44] This may parallel the findings that different sleep stages play a different role in consolidating different types of memory. For example, slow wave sleep (prominent in the first part of the night) is related to declarative memory, whereas REM sleep (prominent in the second part of the night) is possibly involved in procedural memory and emotional memory consolidation.[4]

Studying the dream lag in laboratory dreams has shown that the dream lag effect was not present in non–rapid eye movement (NREM) dreams but only in REM dreams. The mean time between sleep onset and these REM dreams was 6.16 hours: that is, on average these were dreams of the latter part of the night. To follow up this line of thinking, it would be necessary to collect larger samples of REM dreams stemming from the first part of the night.

To summarize, there is evidence that the time course of incorporating daytime events may not follow a simple exponential function (lower incorporation rates of more remote waking-life experience), but that processes related to memory consolidation or adaption to stressful social events mediate the incorporation of waking-life experiences into dreams.

Continuity between Waking and Dreaming: Effect of Emotional Intensity

In experimental studies[40,45-49] researchers presented different films to subjects before the subjects slept in the lab at night and were awakened during REM sleep to collect dream reports. Interestingly, these studies indicate that direct incorporations of the film topics into dreams occurred very rarely. Even when exposing participants (with fears of snakes) to a real snake (in a terrarium) and telling them a compelling story about meeting the snake in the dark afterward or exposing them to a squirrel and related story (the control condition), De Koninck and Brunette[25] did not receive reports of snake dreams or squirrel dreams. However, the emotional tone of the story (i.e., a positive-tone version included a nice walk in the park by daylight and seeing the animal from a distance versus a negative-tone version with suddenly stumbling over the animal in the dark) had an effect on the emotional tone of the dreams,[25] indicating that it may be more difficult to affect the thematic content of dreams than the emotional tone (see the section Thematic Continuity versus Continuity of Emotions). Formal characteristics of dreams such as colors have also been successfully manipulated by wearing red goggles during the day.[41]

Using the technique of dream incubation (dating back to ancient Greek traditions), the topics the dreamers wanted to dream about before sleep onset did not show up in their dreams.[50,51] If, however, the participants were instructed to think about a current personal problem, the probability of dreaming about this problem increased from 20% to 40%.[31] Similarly, focusing on discrepancies between ideal self and current personality traits before sleep onset increased the probability of dreaming about this trait.[52]

In contrast to the findings regarding dream incubation, a carefully designed study[53] indicated that the instruction to not think about the target person yielded more occurrences in subsequent dreams than thinking about the person, supporting the ironic-process theory.[54] Subsequent studies[55-57] using idiosyncratic intrusive thoughts as targets that should be suppressed (not thought about) replicated the findings of the first study. In a sleep lab study,[58] the same effect was found for sleep-onset dreams, this time using an image of three white bears and the presleep instruction not to think about them.

To summarize, the small effect of experimental manipulation of the presleep situation on dream content may be explained by low salience: that is, even if the film or story is emotionally intense, it is not related to the current personal issues of the dreamer. Paradigms including topics relevant for the dreamer showed a stronger effect, indicating that the subjectively experienced emotions may modulate the continuity between waking and dreaming.

The picture is different for field studies targeting the relationship between waking life and dreaming. Student athletes dream more often about sports,[30,59] music students more often about music,[60] and political science students more about politics[61] compared to students in other fields of study, indicating that relevant waking-life topics clearly showed up in dreams. In one study, about 50% to 70% of the participants stated that TV consumption or reading books has affected their dreams.[62] In children and adolescents, media figures have been found in nightmares frequently.[63,64] There is a direct relationship between time spent with consumption of media with the percentage of media dreams.[65] Computer games such as Tetris or Alpine Racer have shown an effect on subsequent dreams,[66-68] with dream incorporations into up to 47% of reports and by up to 65% of subjects across several awakenings.[69]

Spending time in everyday activities such as reading or driving a car is related to the frequency of these activity in dreams.[29,30] Similarly, spending time with male and female persons during the day is reflected in the ratio of male and female dream characters.[70,71] One's romantic partner not only plays a major role in waking life but also dreams—up to 20% of the dreams include a romantic partner.[72-74] Major life events such as pregnancy[75-79] or divorce[80,81] affect the dreams of the persons involved, again indicating that salient waking-life experiences show up in dreams.

Another area showing continuity between waking and dreaming is dreams in patients with mental disorders, as these dreams clearly reflect specific waking-life psychopathology.[82-86] For example, the severity of depressive symptoms correlated with the intensity of negative dream emotions,[87] and dream bizarreness was related to the severity of psychotic symptoms in schizophrenic patients.[88] Patients with anorexia nervosa dreamed more about rejecting food, and patients with bulimia dreamed more about food in general.[89]

Recurrent nightmares of experienced traumatic events are a hallmark symptom of posttraumatic stress disorder.[90] The effects of waking-life experiences related to the 9/11 terror attacks,[91] sexual assault,[92] childhood sexual abuse,[93] kidnappings,[94,95] accidents,[96,97] and war[98-100] can be detected in dreams even decades after the occurrence of these experiences in waking life.

Overall, trauma studies indicate that emotional intensity may be one of the factors affecting continuity between waking and dreaming, that is, emotionally more intense waking-life experiences are more likely to be incorporated into subsequent dreams than less intense experiences. Interestingly, this plausible hypothesis has rarely been studied directly. From a methodological viewpoint, it seems to be important to use a design in which the emotional intensity of the waking-life event will be rated before the dream occurs. That is, the approach of retrospectively rating the emotionality of events that resurfaced in the dream may be biased by hindsight: I dreamed about this, therefore it must be important.

In a diary study[34] this problem was solved by instructing the participants to keep a diary over a 2-week period to record the five most important events of the day and rate their emotional intensity and valence. The participants also recorded their dreams and checked whether one of the recorded events of the previous days showed up in the dream. The emotional intensity and valence of the incorporated event was compared with the other recorded events of the same day. The findings indicated that emotional intensity was higher for incorporated events, but emotional valence was similar to the events not incorporated.[34] That is, there was no bias toward incorporating more negatively toned waking-life events. The study of Malinowski and Horton[101] replicated this finding: emotional intensity but not stressfulness was crucial for the incorporation into subsequent dreams.

To summarize, the experimental and field studies indicate that the emotional intensity and/or salience of the waking-life experience is affecting the probability that this experience is showing up in subsequent dreams.

Continuity between Waking and Dreaming: Type of Waking-Life Experience

As early as 1909 Meumann[102] observed that reading and writing occurred very rarely in his dreams, although he was engaged in these activities up to 6 hours per day. Hartmann[103] compared the frequencies of reading, writing, and typing with other waking activities such as walking, talking with friends, and sexuality and found that the three Rs (reading, writing, and arithmetic) are less likely to be found in dreams compared to other activities. Based on his findings that emotional intensity of the waking-life activity may not explain these differences (e.g., comparing walking with reading), Hartmann[103] hypothesized that during cholinergically driven REM sleep, focused thinking processes are not that easy for the brain to handle compared with the waking state. Interestingly, thinking in general (e.g., about what other people think or what to do next) is common in dreams.[104]

The findings of Hartmann[103] were confirmed by several studies.[29,30,105] In a diary study[29] so-called cognitive activities (reading, writing, calculating, working with a computer) accounted for 41.6% of the elicited waking-life activities (including talking with friends, driving a car, watching TV, using the phone, and being in nature), whereas only 18.6% of the dream activities fell into this cognitive area. The hypothesis of Schredl[105] that dreams more likely reflect "archaic" themes such as social interactions or being in nature was not supported by Schredl and Hofmann[29]; driving a car, for example, was significantly overrepresented in dreams. The additional finding that talking with friends is also very common in dreams is in line with the findings that persons/characters and emotions showed shorter lag times to be incorporated into dreams[31,106] and may point to a preference of dreams for social topics. Interestingly, daytime emotions related to encounters with friends had the strongest correlations with dream emotions—compared to academic studies or personal issues,[27] indicating again that social interactions during the day have a considerable impact on nighttime dreaming.

Continuity between Waking and Dreaming: Other Factors

As mentioned previously, it was not assumed that the model presented in Table 62.1 encompasses all possible factors affecting the continuity between waking and dreaming. One factor of the model, personality traits, has been not studied in a systematic way, although there is some evidence that the "thin boundary dimension" (being creative, empathic, having unusual experiences, having intense but conflict-laden relationships), which also plays a role in nightmare etiology,[107] can affect continuity, with thin boundary persons more likely to dream about current waking-life problems than thick boundary persons.[108] Interestingly, participants with high trait-thought suppression report more dreams representing their waking-life emotions compared with low trait- thought suppressors.[109] Because of this small number of studies, the modulating effect of personality traits is still unclear. Other trait variables such as attitude toward dreams[110] or beliefs about dream function[111] may also have an effect on the continuity between waking and dreaming as persons with a positive attitude and/or belief in a positive function of dreaming may see more incorporations of waking-life experiences in their dreams.

THEMATIC CONTINUITY VERSUS CONTINUITY OF EMOTIONS

The model shown in Table 62.1 was designed to address the probability of thematic dream content resulting from waking-life experiences and factors affecting this probability. As already indicated by the earlier-cited study of De Koninck and Brunette,[25] there may be different mechanisms at work explaining the topics of the dream compared with the emotional tone of the dream. The findings indicating that current stressors increase nightmare frequency (see Chapter 60) also support the idea that dream emotions may be more continuous with waking life than actual dream content. Most of the nightmare topics, such as being chased, falling, death of close persons, and being paralyzed,[112-114] are not continuous with waking life, but the emotions (e.g., fear, worries) are.

Several studies[27,115,116] showed a very close connection between waking-life emotions and dream emotions. In the study of Sikka, Pesonen, and Revonsuo,[117] peace of mind during waking correlated with positive dream emotions, whereas negative dream emotions correlated with depression and anxiety, again showing the direct effect of waking-life emotions on dreaming. These findings stimulated the idea that one function of dreaming may be to regulate emotions.[118] In terms of research, these findings clearly indicate that the continuity model[24] should be expanded.

CONTINUITY BETWEEN WAKING AND DREAMING IN SLEEP DISORDERS

The most obvious relationship between dreaming and sleep disorders is present in the REM parasomnias, such as nightmare disorder and REM sleep behavior disorder (RBD). In nightmare etiology, current waking-life stressors play a major role[119] and thus indicate a direct effect of waking life on dreaming. The dreams in patients with RBD are typically described as action filled, vivid, and aggressive, but whether this is due to the disorder itself or to daytime stressors related to the disorder is less clear.[120] In some patients with NREM parasomnia, Oudiette and colleagues[121] showed that they enact behavior they practiced in the evening, also indicating a continuity between waking and dreaming, in this case NREM dreaming. In my clinical practice, an adult patient reported that his sleep terror attacks resemble very closely the incident of choking he experienced in adolescence (fear of suffocating). That is, patients with parasomnias may offer a new window to study the relationship between waking life and dreaming.

Although symptom severity (operationalized by the apnea-hypopnea index and/or oxygen saturation nadir) does not correlate with nightmare frequency in patients with sleep-related breathing disorders,[122,123] some studies indicate that successful treatment of the sleep-related breathing disorder with continuous positive airway pressure (CPAP) is accompanied by more positive dreaming.[124] This may indicate that reduction of the stress associated with an untreated sleep apnea syndrome may result in more positive dreams, indicating also continuity between waking and dreaming.

In patients with insomnia, the occurrence of waking-life problems was correlated with the number of problems within the dream.[125] In addition, patients with insomnia showed an elevated nightmare frequency.[126] As current stressors play a role in the etiology of insomnia (see Chapter 91), including questions about dreams and nightmares in the clinical interview may be helpful.

Last, patients with narcolepsy also show altered dreaming with heightened dream recall, more nightmares, more bizarre dreaming, and more lucid dreams.[127-130] However, it has not been studied whether the negative dream experiences reported by this patient group are due to the pathophysiology of narcolepsy with an overactive REM sleep system (see Chapter 111) or—at least partially—due to the daytime distress associated with narcolepsy.

IMPLICATIONS FOR POSSIBLE FUNCTIONS OF DREAMING

Based on the well-documented findings that sleep contributes to memory consolidation,[4] the first question that comes to mind is whether dreaming is somehow associated with the processes involved in sleep-dependent memory consolidation. In a nap study and an overnight study using a maze-learning paradigm, performance gains were higher if task-related dreams were reported.[131,132] For a procedural learning task (mirror tracing), an overnight study[133] did not show any relation between task-related dreams and next-day performance gain in the participants. With use of a paradigm more closely related to autobiographic memory (i.e., remembering a film sequence of 5 minutes), there is some evidence for a relationship between dreaming about the film and memory performance.[134]

Memory consolidation involves processes on the cellular level (long-term potentiation) or network level; therefore the question is whether dreaming (as subjective experience while sleeping that can be recalled upon awaking) is connected or can reflect these processes, similar to waking life when the brain is doing a lot more things than conscious thinking and experiencing. Interestingly, training on a specific task during a lucid dream can enhance performance in the morning,[135-137] although these findings should be viewed with caution as we do not know whether the beneficial effect can be attributed to the dreamed training or the recall of the successful dream training boosting self-confidence and thereby improving performance. To pursue this question, two strategies are warranted. First, it should be demonstrated on a neurophysiologic level using imaging techniques that there is a replay of waking-life experiences in some way during sleep as it has been shown in animals[138]; initial studies in humans yielded promising results.[139,140] To link these replays to dream content, studies investigating the relationship among dream content, respective dream characteristics, and brain activation are necessary. In this area one study using functional magnetic resonance imaging techniques[141] was able to predict images in sleep onset dreaming, and Siclari and colleagues[142] were able to demonstrate links between dreamed faces or speech with activation of the respective brain areas using high-density electroencephalography. Although these first studies seem promising, the question of whether dreaming is associated with or reflects processes crucial to sleep-dependent memory consolidation is not yet answered.

The research regarding the temporal references of dream elements (see the section Continuity between Waking and Dreaming: Time Factor) indicates that new information is integrated with experiences from the distant past in dreams. Second, research indicated that salient events emotionally relevant to the dreamer[34,101] are more likely to show up in dreams. These findings would fit with a function of dreaming in autobiographic memory.[143] Further support for this theory was provided by Schredl and Reinhard,[27] showing that dreams that processed some topics of the previous day are more likely to affect the next day, that is, the same topics may be processed by day (waking consciousness) and night (dreaming).

However, dreams not only consist of previous daytime experiences but also are creative (i.e., they form new associations not yet thought of and feature experiences that never occurred in waking life).[17,144] This parallels processes typically involved in problem solving: first, compare the new incident with already successfully handled experiences, and second, if no strategy is already available, try something new (brainstorming). In view of this analogy, proposing problem solving and adaption as a possible dream function[145] seems plausible.

The balanced ratio of positive and negative dream emotions[146,147] renders dream theories that are solely focused on negative dream emotions, such as the threat simulation theory,[148] unlikely, even though it does not exclude that learning about places that may be dangerous may not be one of the functions of dreaming.

Last, several findings indicate a strong continuity between the social environment of the dreamer in the waking state and social interactions in dreams. Closely related persons often play an important part in dreams,[72,74] emotions related to close persons have strong effects on dreams,[27] the social network is well represented in dreams,[149] and social interactions are overrepresented compared to academic activities.[29] This may point to another evolutionary aspect of dreaming—the importance of the social network for survival in hunter-gatherer societies. That is, it is essential to get along with the other group members and not to be ostracized by the group,[150] and one function of dreams may be to train social skills.[151,152]

To summarize, the findings regarding the continuity between waking and dreaming provide a considerable number of clues to what the function(s) of dreaming may be, even though all these ideas about dream function are, up to now, of course, highly speculative.

FUTURE DIRECTIONS

The review of the research presented in this chapter clearly shows that studying factors that affect the continuity between waking and dreaming, such as emotional intensity, time, or personality traits, still has a long way to go. The model presented in Table 62.1 can guide future research. Methodological problems concerning how to measure waking-life experiences (e.g., type, frequency, intensity) and how to relate these measures to dream content are not yet solved and need more empirical testing. From a neurophysiologic viewpoint, it is very interesting that several researchers[153-155] have suggested that during REM sleep (associated with intense dreaming) the default mode network is active; this network is also active during mind-wandering, daydreaming, and thinking about the past and/or the future in waking life.[156,157] Investigating this parallel on the brain level may help to elucidate the continuity between waking and dreaming on the experiential level.

Last, studying dreams that are clearly not continuous with waking life (e.g., flying dreams) would be most beneficial, because it is completely unknown at this point how we can dream about things (e.g., pain or people with congenital paraplegia dreaming about walking[158]) that we never experienced in our waking life.[23]

CLINICAL PEARL

In clinical practice, a patient may tell you a dream and ask you, a sleep specialist, about its meaning. Based on the findings of thematic continuity, and especially continuity of emotions, the simplest way to relate the dream to the personal life of the dreamer is to identify the basic pattern of the dream. What is the dreamer experiencing in the dream, and what is he or she doing? For example, if the dream is a about being chased by a monster, the basic pattern is fear/panic and avoidance behavior. Thus the patient could be asked if he or she avoids something or someone in his or her waking life, keeping in mind that dream emotions may be an exaggerated version of the corresponding waking-life emotion.

SUMMARY

Research on the continuity between waking and dreaming has clearly identified factors that affect the chances of waking-life experiences to be incorporated into subsequent dreams. Because direct empirical tests of possible functions of dreaming are difficult to carry out, the question arises as to whether the research on continuity may provide hints about the functions of dreaming. At this stage it is still unclear whether dreaming is involved in sleep-dependent memory consolidation. The finding that emotionally salient experiences and social interactions seem to be integral ingredients of dreams that are closely associated with the waking-life social environment may point to the importance of dreaming in regulating and maintaining social relationships, which have been essential for survival in hunter-gatherer societies over the history of humankind. An interesting yet unresolved issue is the question as to why we dream about things we have never experienced in waking life (discontinuity).

SELECTED READINGS

Fosse MJ, Fosse R, Hobson JA, Stickgold RJ. Dreaming and episodic memory: a functional dissociation? *J Cogn Neurosci*. 2003;15:1–9.

Guerrero-Gomez A, Nöthen-Garunja I, Schredl M, et al. Dreaming in adolescents during the COVID-19 health crisis: survey among a sample of European school students. *Front Psychol*. 2021;12:652627. Published 2021 Apr 20.

Hall CS, Nordby VJ. *The Individual and his Dreams*. New York: New American Library; 1972.

Hartmann E. *The Nature and Functions of Dreaming*. New York: Oxford University Press; 2011.

Klepel F, Schredl M. Correlation of task-related dream content with memory performance of a film task – A pilot study. *Int J Dream Res*. 2019;12(1):112–118.

Malinowski J, Horton CL. Evidence for the preferential incorporation of emotional waking-life experiences into dreams. *Dreaming*. 2014;24(1):18–31.

Moverley M, Schredl M, Göritz AS. Media dreaming and media consumption – An online study. *Int J Dream Res*. 2018;11(2):127–134.

Schredl M. *Researching Dreams: The Fundamentals*. Cham: Palgrave Macmillan; 2018.

Schredl M, Reinhard I. The continuity between waking mood and dream emotions: Direct and second-order effects. *Imagin Cogn Pers*. 2009;29:271–282. 2010.

Sikka P, Pesonen H, Revonsuo A. Peace of mind and anxiety in the waking state are related to the affective content of dreams. *Scientific Reports*. 2018;8(1):12762. 2018/08/24.

Skancke J, Holsen I, Schredl M. Continuity between waking life and dreams of psychiatric patients: a review and discussion of the implications for dream research. *Int J Dream Res*. 2014;7:39–53.

Strauch I, Meier B. *In Search of Dreams: Results of Experimental Dream Research*. Albany: State University of New York Press; 1996.

Valli K, Hoss RJ, eds. *Dreams: Understanding Biology, Psychology, and Culture (2 Volumes)*. Santa Barbara: Greenwood; 2019.

Wamsley EJ, Stickgold R. Dreaming of a learning task is associated with enhanced memory consolidation: replication in an overnight sleep study. *J Sleep Res*. 2019;28(1):1–8.

A complete reference list can be found online at ExpertConsult.com.

Chapter 63

Emotion, Motivation, and Reward in Relation to Dreaming

Sophie Schwartz; Lampros Perogamvros

Chapter Highlights

- Emotional and reward brain networks are activated during non–rapid eye movement and rapid eye movement sleep.
- Specific patterns of brain activity during sleep probably determine key features of dream content. Conversely, dream characteristics such as intense emotional experiences offer valuable insights into information processing during sleep.
- The activation of emotional and reward brain circuits during sleep seems to promote the reprocessing of affectively relevant memories, as well as the experience of emotions and the expression of approach and avoidance behaviors in dreams.
- Emotional and reward processing during dreaming may explain its contribution to waking cognitive and emotional processes, including emotion regulation, extinction learning, and performance improvement. This hypothesis is supported by recent experimental evidence.

Recent neuroimaging, neurophysiologic, and clinical studies converge to suggest that emotional and reward networks are activated during sleep. Because these networks are active primarily while the organism interacts with its external environment, of critical relevance is how and why such systems are also activated during sleep. A main hypothesis is that their recruitment during sleep relates to the affective and motivational components of the dreaming experience and has measurable consequences on waking behavior and emotional well-being. This chapter examines how the activation of emotional and reward circuits during sleep may determine the affective and motivational attributes and functions of dreaming.

DREAMING AND EMOTIONAL PROCESSING

More than 50 years ago, the French neurophysiologist Michel Jouvet observed that, when muscle atonia was abolished during REM sleep, cats expressed aggression- or fear-related behaviors.[1] Similarly, patients with rapid eye movement (REM) sleep behavior disorder, who act out their dreams, frequently display aggressive behaviors.[2,3] Consistent with these observations, dream content analyses report generally higher emotional intensity in REM than in non–rapid eye movement (NREM) dreams.[4–7] Although a general intensification of emotions and predominance of negative emotions seems to take place in REM compared with NREM dreams, negative and positive emotions are experienced in both sleep stages.[7] Neuroimaging data also confirm that limbic/emotional and mesolimbic/motivational systems are active during both REM and NREM, presumably promoting affective and memory processing during sleep and dreams.

Specifically, functional magnetic resonance imaging (fMRI) studies of human NREM sleep reported that activity in the insula, anterior cingulate cortex, and superior temporal gyrus was higher during sleep spindles (electroencephalographic [EEG] waves oscillating at a frequency of 11 to 16 Hz),[8] whereas activity in the precuneus, parahippocampal gyrus, and posterior cingulate cortex coincided with slow waves (oscillations of high amplitude, low frequency ≤ 4 Hz).[9] Bilateral increases in regional glucose metabolism from waking to NREM have also been found in the ventral striatum, anterior cingulate cortex, amygdala, and hippocampus.[10] Recently, we provided direct evidence that experiencing fear (vs. no fear) in NREM dreams was associated with the activation of the insula.[6] During wakefulness, the insula participates in the emotional response to distressing cognitive or interoceptive signals.[11] Insular activation during dreaming could thus correspond to the feeling of danger due to integration of sensory and bodily information related to dreamed fearful stimuli.

REM sleep is characterized by the activation of brain regions involved in sensory-motor, memory, and emotion processing, including associative visual areas, motor cortex, medial temporal regions, amygdala, insula, cingulate cortex, and medial prefrontal cortex (mPFC).[12–15] However, until recently, only very few studies investigated the association between these activations and specific emotional experiences in dreams. A brain structural study in humans demonstrated that decreased microstructural integrity in the left amygdala was associated with shorter and less emotional dream reports.[16] During wakefulness, the amygdala is involved in the detection of emotional stimuli and also contributes to emotional learning and extinction, in close interaction with the medial prefrontal cortex.[17] The particular recruitment of the amygdala during REM sleep could thus provide a favorable condition for the reprocessing and regulation of emotionally relevant information during sleep and may elicit intense emotions in dreams.[18–22] More recently, we have demonstrated that experiencing fear (vs. no fear) in REM dreams was associated with the activation of the insula and midcingulate cortex.[6] During wakefulness, the midcingulate cortex is a region known to be critically involved in behavioral/motor responses to dangers.[23] Therefore activation of the midcingulate cortex during REM dreaming could reflect the associated emotional and motor reactions of the dreamer to content containing threatening situations.

Dream content analyses and neuroimaging data thus confirm that emotional processes are active during both REM and NREM sleep stages. Combined EEG/fMRI and phenomenologic studies are needed to further elucidate the exact contribution of subcortical structures, such as the amygdala, in both NREM and REM dreaming.[13,16,24,25] The possible implications related to the processing of emotions during sleep are considered further in the section Implications for Emotion Regulation and Learning.

DREAMING AND REWARD PROCESSING

It has been suggested that an elevated dopamine level in the mesolimbic dopaminergic (ML-DA) system during sleep plays an important role in the generation of dreams.[26,27] The mesolimbic circuit connects dopaminergic neurons of the ventral tegmental area of the midbrain (VTA; source of dopamine activity) with the nucleus accumbens (NAcc), amygdala, hippocampus, anterior cingulate cortex, and frontal cortex (insular and medial orbitofrontal cortex, medial frontal cortex, ventromedial prefrontal cortex). It was proposed that the ML-DA circuit promotes approach-like behaviors and emotional anticipation during both wakefulness and in dreams.[27]

Recent experimental evidence provides support for this proposal. First, during REM sleep, key structures of the ML-DA reward system are activated, including the VTA and the NAcc. In rodents, VTA bursting activity is elevated during REM sleep,[28,29] up to levels observed during reward or punisher anticipation at waking.[30] This activity is significantly higher in REM sleep than in the awake state or in NREM sleep; it is comparable in intensity and duration to activations during waking behaviors, such as feeding, punishment, or sex.[28] Most recently, it was showed that such an activation takes place during NREM sleep of rodents too.[30a] Importantly, a recent paper demonstrated how dreaming per se in humans is related to activation of the midbrain,[30b] supporting the idea that VTA activation during sleep reflects dreaming processes. Moreover, extracellular levels of dopamine are increased in the NAcc during REM sleep in rats.[31] In both animal and human studies, other reward-related regions, including the ventromedial prefrontal cortex and the anterior cingulate cortex, are activated during REM sleep.[13,14,31] Finally, the orexin neurons in the lateral hypothalamus, which are involved in the regulation of sleep-wake states and in reward-seeking behaviors,[32–34] display bursts of activity during REM sleep.[35,36] Further support for an activation of reward-related circuits during REM sleep comes from the observation that, in both animals and humans, the hippocampus exhibits a theta rhythm,[37,38] which is associated with novelty-seeking, exploratory, and instinctual behaviors during wakefulness.[39]

De Gennaro and colleagues[40] studied dreaming in patients with Parkinson disease, which is a well-established model of altered dopaminergic transmission. The authors assumed that the higher the dosages of dopamine agonists administered to these patients, the higher the hypodopaminergic state. They found that dopamine agonist dosage correlated positively with impoverished dream reports, that is, low total word count, emotional load, and bizarreness in dreams. Moreover, visual vividness of dream reports correlated positively with the volumes of bilateral amygdala and with thickness of the left mPFC, whereas emotional load correlated positively with hippocampal volume. These findings, along with previous volumetric measures of the hippocampus-amygdala complex and specific qualitative features of dreaming from the same group,[16] suggest that subcortical mesolimbic nuclei contribute to the dreaming experience and dream recall, and provide an empirical support to the hypothesis that the ML-DA system plays a key role in dream generation. More recent papers confirmed how key structures of the reward system, such as the midcingulate cortex and the insula, are implicated in specific dream content, such as spontaneous thoughts[7] and fear.[6]

Pharmacologic studies offer further evidence that dreaming relates to the activation of the ML-DA system by showing that the administration of dopaminergic (D_2) antagonists is associated with a reduction in dreaming[41] and in nightmares,[42–44] whereas the administration of dopaminergic agents (e.g., pramipexole) causes vivid dreams.[45–47] Furthermore, total or partial sleep deprivation leads to disturbed reward brain functions.[48–50]

How does the activation of reward-seeking mechanisms during sleep influence the content of dreams? Recent research has shown that approach behaviors (e.g., behaviors of exploration, curiosity, or engagement) may be as frequent as "avoidance" behaviors (e.g., avoiding a threat through fleeing, freezing, or hiding) both in dreams[51] and as overtly expressed in parasomnias.[3,52,53] Moreover, dream reports are biased toward content with strong motivational value (e.g., socializing, fighting, sexual content) and less oriented toward content with no such particular value (e.g., typing, washing dishes, buying food at the supermarket).[54] Of importance, frequent approach behaviors are not incompatible with the high prevalence of negative affect in dreams[55] because both the ML-DA system and the amygdala-limbic system are activated during sleep.[56] Combined EEG/fMRI and phenomenologic studies are needed to further elucidate the exact contribution of subcortical mesolimbic structures, such as the VTA and NAcc, in dreaming.

IMPLICATIONS FOR EMOTION REGULATION AND LEARNING

The links between dreaming and emotional or motivational processes, as previously expounded, offer new insights into the possible functions of dreaming. NREM and REM dreams appear to encompass specific emotional/motivational states; NREM dreaming predominantly simulates friendly interactions, self-related information, and actual waking life events, whereas REM dreams contain comparatively more aggressive social interactions.[57] It has been proposed that the variety of emotions that the dreamer experiences may contribute to emotion regulation processes. Evidence in favor of this claim comes from the demonstration that different REM dream characteristics relate to specific daytime affective functions. More specifically, Cartwright and colleagues[58] showed that divorcing participants who were incorporating their ex-spouse into their dreams were psychologically more adapted and less depressed than those who did not dream about their divorce. Moreover, depressed participants whose negative dreams decreased from the beginning to the end of the night were more likely to be in remission 1 year later, compared to those showing the reverse pattern.[59] Cartwright thus suggested that negative emotions in REM dreams have to be integrated with other autobiographic memories for dreaming to have a beneficial emotion regulation function.[60,61] A failure of such integration may explain why a high rate of nightmares and other REM sleep abnormalities (increased REM sleep percentage, shorter REM sleep latency) have been associated with more severe depressive symptoms and suicidality.[62–64]

Being exposed to diverse emotional stimuli (objects, situations, thoughts, memories, and physical sensations) during dreaming, including feared ones, in a safe context that the dream state represents, resembles and may act like desensitization therapy.[65] This assumption is indirectly supported by studies demonstrating that sleep, in general, promotes the retention and generalization of extinction learning.[66–69] Along the same lines, the Finnish psychologist and philosopher Antti Revonsuo proposed the threat simulation theory (TST), according to which dreaming promotes the development and threat-avoidance skills during wakefulness by simulating threatening events during sleep.[21,55] This mechanism would rely on the activation of limbic regions, in particular the amygdala, during REM sleep. Consistent with this hypothesis, persons suffering from posttraumatic stress disorder simulate threatening events in their dreams more often than control subjects.[70] In a recent paper,[6] it was demonstrated that participants with a high propensity to experience fear in dreams had increased activation of the mPFC when facing aversive stimuli while awake. Conversely, and as predicted by TST, the same analysis yielded negative correlations with activity in the right amygdala, right insula, and midcingulate cortex.[6] This finding is consistent with the proposal that dreaming may serve an emotion regulation function through emotional reprocessing, yielding extinction learning, and generalization, which would result in adapted emotional responses to dangerous real-life events during wakefulness.[55,56,60,71]

According to this prediction,[6] nightmares, which represent dysphoric dreams with intensified negative emotions, should also contribute to such an emotional function. As of today, however, it remains unclear whether nightmares, compared to normal dreaming, can offer such an adaptive function. It seems that the more nightmares become severe in frequency and intensity, the less they fulfill such a role. Indeed, it has been shown that nightmare patients show decreased activity in regions associated with extinction learning (e.g., mPFC) at wakefulness[72] and impaired frontal inhibitory functions.[73,74] These findings support that overnight extinction learning fails when fear is exaggerated, as in nightmares.

It has been proposed that nightmare disorder reflects the dysfunction of a network that includes limbic and paralimbic regions (e.g., amygdala, mPFC, hippocampus, anterior cingulate cortex, insula).[71] A recent study reported that the amplitude of the heartbeat-evoked potential (HEP; cortical response to heartbeats), which is typically modulated by interoceptive processing and emotional arousal, was higher in nightmare patients compared to healthy controls over a cluster of frontal regions during REM sleep.[75] These findings suggest that patients with frequent nightmares present elevated emotional arousal during REM sleep, and that the amplitude of HEP may be used as a biomarker of increased emotional processing in these patients.

A second major contribution of dreaming, apart from emotion regulation, seems to pertain to memory processes. Dreaming is a particular state of consciousness during which some memory representations are reexperienced and then potentially reorganized. Evidence for the role of dreaming in the consolidation of memory was recently demonstrated by several studies.[76–79] Improvements in a word–picture association learning task,[77] a spatial navigation task[76,78] or a visuo-olfactory task,[79] have been associated with task-related dreams. Such off-line processes of memory reactivation and reorganization would also explain why sleep may favor creative insights.[80] Using a semantic priming task, Stickgold and colleagues[81] demonstrated that participants awakened from REM sleep showed greater priming by weak primes (than by both unrelated primes and strong primes), consistent with a hyperassociative state of the sleeping mind, reminiscent of the unusual associations of features or events in REM dreams.[82] In a similar experiment, Walker and coworkers[83] demonstrated that subjects awakened from REM sleep exhibited a 32% advantage on an anagram-solving task, compared with the number of correct responses after NREM awakenings. In line with these observations, compared with quiet rest and NREM sleep, REM sleep (but not necessarily dreaming) enhances the integration of initially unassociated information, resulting in more creative problem solving.[84] More experimental studies are needed to better delineate how dreaming per se influences memory consolidation, creativity, and insight.

Taken together, these findings demonstrate that distinct sleep stages contribute to the remodeling of memory stores and that memory reprocessing may be enhanced in the dream state, with important implications for waking performance. On the basis of robust neurophysiologic evidence of emotional and reward circuits activation during sleep, it has been suggested that dreams relate not only to known past events but also to an unexpected, novel, or probabilistic future.[27,85] Dream content analysis provides support for this idea by showing that although past and current waking concerns are common in dreams,[60,86] dreams rarely provide exact replicates of past events; instead they most often represent novel combinations of memory elements.[87,88] Dreaming would thus offer an off-line cognitive and emotional preparation of the dreamer for future significant waking life events. By suggesting that subjective experiences in dreams fulfill important biologic and psychologic functions, as supported by recent neuroimaging evidence in humans,[6] this theoretical proposal also has clinical implications because dream characteristics may represent biomarkers of important brain functions, such as emotion regulation processes.[18]

METHODOLOGIC ISSUES

Recent studies using EEG and fMRI techniques have considerably contributed to a better understanding of the neural correlates and functions of dreaming.[6,7,89] Although it is tempting to relate some aspects of dreaming to motivational and emotional functions, as in work summarized in this chapter and elsewhere (threat simulation theory,[55] protoconsciousness theory,[90] default-mode activation theory[91]), more studies specifically addressing such functional relationship are needed.[6,60,64,76] Moreover, distinct sleep stages and dream states may differ in their contribution to off-line reprocessing of emotional and reward information. NREM sleep and associated dreams would be more specialized in linking memory traces with motivational values,[92,93] whereas REM sleep and related dreams benefit emotional memory consolidation and extinction learning.[69,94] Nevertheless, studies combining dream content analysis, sleep recordings, and an assessment of emotion and/or memory functions are still very scarce.[6,76,95]

CLINICAL PEARL

The demonstration that dreaming affects emotion regulation processes may be useful to promote measures preventing sleep (and dream) restriction. This is particularly important for the most vulnerable populations, such as psychiatric patients or children, whose brains may highly benefit from the reprocessing and simulation of emotions occurring during dreaming. Conversely, dream characteristics constitute biomarkers of important brain functions, such as emotion-regulating processes.

SUMMARY

This chapter summarizes existing evidence for the activation of emotional-limbic and reward-related circuits during sleep. Dreaming seems to be closely related to these specific patterns of neural and behavioral activations, a link that may explain its contribution to important functions such as emotion regulation, associative learning, and social cognition. By simulating defense and approach behaviors, subserved by limbic regions and the mesolimbic dopaminergic reward system, dreaming provides a virtual and safe environment in which the dreamer can be exposed to an important load of aversive or rewarding stimuli. This mechanism provides the person with enhanced learning capacities, which can be potentially used in the waking life. Additional empirical studies are needed to better characterize these proposed roles of dreaming.

ACKNOWLEDGMENTS

Work on which this chapter is based was supported by grants from the Swiss National Science Foundation, the Swiss Center for Affective Sciences, the Boninchi Foundation, and the BIAL Foundation.

SELECTED READINGS

Cartwright R, Agargun MY, Kirkby J, Friedman JK. Relation of dreams to waking concerns. *Psychiatry Res.* 2006;141(3):261–270.

De Gennaro L, Lanteri O, Piras F, et al. Dopaminergic system and dream recall: an MRI study in Parkinson's disease patients. *Hum Brain Mapp.* 2016;37(3):1136–1147.

Diekelmann S, Born J. The memory function of sleep. *Nat Rev Neurosci.* 2010;11:114–126.

Harricharan S, McKinnon MC, Lanius RA. How processing of sensory information from the internal and external worlds shape the perception and engagement with the world in the aftermath of trauma: implications for PTSD. *Front Neurosci.* 2021;15:625490.

Horikawa T, Tamaki M, Miyawaki Y, Kamitani Y. Neural decoding of visual imagery during sleep. *Science.* 2013;340:639–642.

Perogamvros L, Schwartz S. The roles of the reward system in sleep and dreaming. *Neurosci Biobehav Rev.* 2012;36:1934–1951.

Perogamvros L, Baird B, Seibold M, Riedner B, Boly M, Tononi G. The phenomenal contents and neural correlates of spontaneous thoughts across wakefulness, NREM Sleep, and REM Sleep. *J Cogn Neurosci.* 2017;29(10):1766–1777.

Solms M. *The Neuropsychology of Dreams: A Clinico-anatomical Study.* Hillsdale (N.J.): Lawrence Erlbaum Associates; 1997.

Sterpenich V, Perogamvros L, Tononi G, Schwartz S. Fear in dreams and in wakefulness: Evidence for day/night affective homeostasis. *Hum Brain Mapp.* 2020;41(3):840–850.

Valli K, Revonsuo A. The threat simulation theory in light of recent empirical evidence: a review. *Am J Psychol.* 2009;122:17–38.

Wamsley EJ, Tucker M, Payne JD, et al. Dreaming of a learning task is associated with enhanced sleep-dependent memory consolidation. *Curr Biol.* 2010;20:850–855.

***A complete reference list can be found online at** ExpertConsult.com.*

Chapter 64

Dreaming during Pregnancy

Tore Nielsen; Jessica Lara-Carrasco

Chapter Highlights

- Dreaming during pregnancy reflects changing mental representations of the unborn baby and of the woman as a mother.
- Psychological challenges of pregnancy are reflected in more frequent morbid dream contents in late pregnancy.
- Dreaming may facilitate the regulation of negative emotions and the mother's new maternal identity during pregnancy, although it remains unknown whether such adaptations predict real mother-infant interactions after birth.
- Studies on postpartum dreams are few but indicate that mothers dream frequently about their newborns in situations of peril.

INTRODUCTION

Even though dreaming has been studied scientifically for over 65 years, its definition, neurophysiologic substrates, and functions have not been clearly established.[1,2] Nonetheless, in accordance with the hypothesis that dreaming is continuous with daytime thinking,[3,4] some consider that dreaming may function to assimilate daytime worries and emotional concerns to facilitate psychological adaptation to changing life situations.[5-7] The process by which dreaming achieves such adaptions is speculative, but it has been suggested that dream functions may be more evident during periods in which individuals endure major life transitions, particularly transitions implicating the self in relation to significant others.

Pregnancy, which engenders profound and rapid transformations in a woman's life and family, thus affords excellent opportunities to study questions related to the functional roles of dreaming. From a psychological point of view, the transition to motherhood is a major developmental phase that involves important mental reorganizations leading to new relational and identity configurations.[8-10] Being pregnant with a baby whose characteristics are almost completely unknown leads the woman to construct within her mental representational world a constellation of images of herself in relationship with her baby, images that help her to assimilate her maternal identity. It has been suggested that the psychological changes undergone by the mother-to-be must be sustained by different conscious and unconscious cognitive mechanisms, such as dreams.[8,11] However, empirical support for such views is elusive.

This chapter reviews research that assesses changes in dream production and dream content during pregnancy and the postpartum period and the capacity of pregnant women's dreams to predict their psychological adjustment to pregnancy and motherhood. Findings are discussed in relation to how dreams depict emotionally important waking life concerns and to how they may have an adaptive function in maintaining psychological equilibrium during such a major life transition.

CHANGES IN DREAM PRODUCTION AND DREAM CONTENT DURING PREGNANCY

Dream Recall and Disturbed Dream Recall during Pregnancy

The numerous physical, social, and psychological upheavals of pregnancy frequently lead to disturbances in sleep. Because of hormonal and physiologic changes, pregnancy heightens the risk of developing insomnia, restless legs syndrome, and sleep-disordered breathing symptoms.[12,13] Even though not all women will develop such clinical disorders, the majority report alterations in their sleep (e.g., poorer sleep quality, shorter sleep duration, and more frequently interrupted sleep), which will worsen with advancing gestational age—particularly among first-time mothers.[14]

The question of whether cognitive features of sleep, such as dream experiences, are also altered during pregnancy is more controversial. Converging clinical evidence has led to the suggestion that dreams are more easily recalled during pregnancy and that dream imagery is more vivid, frightening, and impactful than during any other period of life.[15,16] To illustrate, a qualitative study showed that 80% of new mothers reported that their dreams were particularly vivid, bizarre, and detailed during pregnancy, and that some of these dreams were disturbing enough to incite them to change their daytime behaviors.[17] However, surprisingly few systematic studies have investigated whether dream production is heightened or more disturbed during pregnancy. To our knowledge, only two studies—both from our research group—have compared pregnant to nonpregnant women for their recall of nondisturbed dreams (Figure 64.1 and Table 64.1). In the first study, similar proportions of pregnant (86%) and nonpregnant (91%) women could recall a recent dream.[18] In another, prospective, study, pregnant and nonpregnant women were equivalent in the number, clarity, and impact of dreams they reported across 14 days.[19] However, retrospective estimates of dream recall were somewhat higher among pregnant women. This subjective impression of heightened dream production

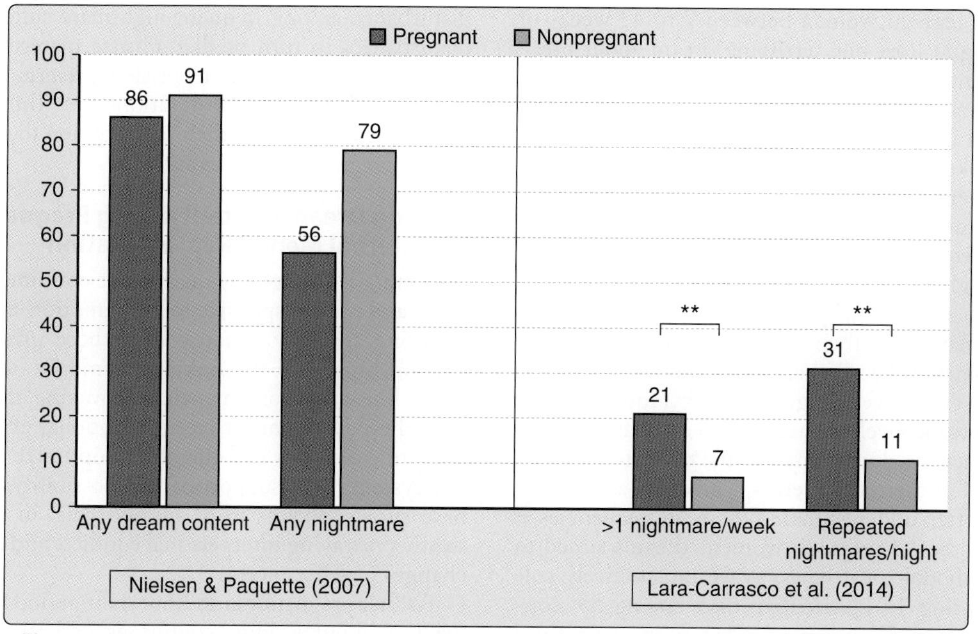

Figure 64.1 Study comparing pregnant to nonpregnant women for their recall of nondisturbed dreams. Prevalence of women in the pregnant (*deep pink columns*) and nonpregnant (*teal columns*) groups who were able to recall any dream and any nightmare contents during the retrospective interview of the study and who prospectively recalled at least one nightmare per week and repeated nightmares per night during a 14-day study. $^{**}P \leq .01$. (Studies by Nielsen & Paquette[18] and Lara-Carrasco and colleagues.[19])

Table 64.1 Group Differences on Dream Measures after Controlling for Potential Confounders[a]

	Pregnant ($n = 57$)	Nonpregnant ($n = 59$)	F	*P*-value[b]	Partial η^2
Prospective Dream Measures[c]					
Dream recall[d]	15.87 ± 0.99	14.68 ± 0.97	0.53	0.47	0.005
Clarity of dream recall[e]	4.26 ± 0.19	4.25 ± 0.19	0.001	0.98	<0.001
Dream impact[e]	3.69 ± 0.22	3.37 ± 0.21	0.77	0.38	0.007
Bad dream recall[d]	2.51 ± 0.31	1.00 ± 0.30	10.24	0.004	0.08
Nightmare recall[d]	1.25 ± 0.21	0.68 ± 0.20	2.78	0.10	0.03
Retrospective Dream Measures[f]					
Retrospective dream recall	3.40 ± 0.17	2.72 ± 0.16	6.24	0.01	0.06
Retrospective bad dream recall	2.49 ± 0.12	2.62 ± 0.12	0.46	0.50	0.004
Retrospective nightmare recall	2.29 ± 0.11	2.45 ± 0.11	1.45	0.23	0.01

[a](Adjusted Mean ± Standard Error). Groups compared using MANCOVA controlling for age, relationship status, employment status, family income, education, and state-anxiety.
[b]Error = Adjusted $P \leq .006$.
[c]Assessed across the 14-day home log
[d]Number of dreams recalled over 14 days
[e]1 = not at all to 9 = very much
[f]1 = never to 5 = always
Modified from Lara-Carrasco et al.[19]

during pregnancy parallels clinical observations that pregnant women become more introspective and conscious of their dreams as a consequence of an increase in the permeability of their boundaries between conscious and unconscious processes.[15] One possible explanation of these observations is that the content of pregnancy dreams piques the future mother's interest, leading to dream recall overestimation. In fact, results from a meta-analysis indicate that interest in dreams is associated with subjective overestimation of dream recall without being related to dream recall frequency per se.[20]

Studies have also reported a wide range of estimates of disturbing dreams (DD) during pregnancy. Nightmares (DD that trigger an awakening[21]) and bad dreams (DD that do not awaken the dreamer[22]) are among the most prevalent DD in the general population: about 85% of adults report at least one nightmare per year, and the frequency of bad dreams is up to four times that of nightmares (see reviews[21,23]). Among pregnant women, one early descriptive study suggests that dreams are commonly disturbed during pregnancy and that they reflect a woman's concerns about the childbearing process, with 25% of 88 pregnant women between 7 to 42 weeks of gestation recalling at least one terrifying dream about pregnancy or the infant.[24] In contrast, four controlled self-report studies suggest that nightmares are not so common during pregnancy. Over a 1-month period, pregnant women of all trimesters were awakened by frightening dreams or nightmares as frequently as were postpartum women.[25] Two other studies found that pregnant women in their third trimester reported bad dreams as frequently as did nonpregnant women[26] and reported fewer nightmares than they did earlier during pregnancy or prepregnancy.[27] Finally, new mothers were less likely to recall a nightmare from their entire pregnancy than were nonpregnant women to recall them from the last 3 months (56% versus 79%, respectively; Figure 64.1).[18] However, none of these studies prospectively measured and compared clearly defined DD frequencies during any specific trimester of pregnancy. Further, all of them used retrospective self-assessment methods, which often underestimate DD recall frequencies.[22]

One of our studies of pregnant women's dreams aimed to correct these methodological flaws, as we prospectively collected dreams during 14 consecutive days among 59 nonpregnant women and 57 pregnant women in their third trimester.[19] Our findings indicate that late pregnancy is a period of markedly increased dysphoric dream imagery, during which nightmares attain a pathologic incidence for a high percentage of women, and that the accumulation of DD over time may deleteriously affect how well women feel they sleep in general (Figure 64.1 and Table 64.1). Indeed, with controls for psychological and demographic characteristics, bad dream recall was 2.5 times higher for pregnant than for nonpregnant women. Further, pregnant women were almost three times more likely than were nonpregnant women to have repeated DD during the same night (31% versus 11%), and among pregnant women average sleep quality for the 14 days of our study was worse when bad dreams and nightmares were frequent. But even more importantly, the prevalence of nightmare recall exceeding once per week—what the *Diagnostic and Statistical Manual of Mental Disorders*, fifth edition (DSM-5)[28] considers to be moderately severe pathology—was three times greater among pregnant (21%) than among nonpregnant (7%) women. These indicators all point to a substantial problem with DD for pregnant women. These findings parallel the qualitative study by Kennedy and colleagues,[17] in which almost all new mothers interviewed reported that their patterns of dreaming had changed; that is, that they had vivid and weird dreams during pregnancy. They also found parallel relationships between DD and sleep disorders such as insomnia in the general population.[29] The increase in DD during pregnancy may be due to hormonal and physiologic changes, or they may be triggered by concomitant psychological changes, such as enhanced introspection and growing concerns about the childbearing process and motherhood. This latter possibility is concordant with the view that a precipitous increase in emotional concerns or "affect load" during pregnancy results in an increase in DD at this time.[21,23] To our knowledge, our study is the first to report such specific frequencies and prevalence rates for prospectively collected DD during pregnancy in comparison with estimates gathered from a normative nonpregnant sample.

The question of DD during pregnancy is of major concern for women's health. DD constitute a substantial sleep disturbance among frequent nightmare sufferers,[30] and sleep disturbances in turn predict adverse maternal and fetal outcomes, such as maternal depression, preterm birth, lower birth weight, and longer labor durations.[31-33] Thus more thorough evaluations of DD and their contribution to sleep impairment during pregnancy are warranted.

Viewing Dream Content during Pregnancy as a Type of Maternal Mental Representation

Dreaming is thought by many to be continuous with daytime life[3,4] and to be responsive to new emotion-evoking situations requiring adaptation, particularly those involving significant relationships.[5,6,34] By linking memories and emotions in a less linear fashion than during waking thought,[35] dreams are believed to connect recent emotional experiences to self-relevant memories and thereby to optimize coherence of the self-system.[5,6] In support of this possibility, content analyses have shown dreams to be highly social in nature, predominantly portraying interpersonal conflicts and concerns[36,37] and changes in self-concept.[38]

As first pregnancy is an important period of mental reorganization about feelings, cognitions, and relationships relating to the self and the unborn baby, pregnant women may well be expected to express these feelings, cognitions, and relationships in their dreams. More specifically, pregnancy is an important transitional phase during which a mental reorganization leads to development of a woman's future maternal identity and competencies.[8,11] Through the activation of a caregiving system reciprocal to attachment,[39] this mental reorganization is thought to involve the elaboration and integration of a constellation of maternal mental representations (MMR) of the unborn baby, of the woman as a mother, of nonmaternal self-features (e.g., the woman as a spouse, a daughter, a friend, a worker), and of other significant relationships (e.g., with the partner, parents, friends, colleagues).[8,11]

Research indicates that the nature and qualities of MMR, including their richness, specificity, and emotional tone, are mostly rooted in the woman's internalized representations of herself and others.[40] They are also likely influenced by contextual factors such as relationships with partner and family, psychological state, and perceived fetal movements.[41,42] Independent of such context, studies also show that the quality of MMR is subject to time-dependent variations. As women progress through their pregnancies, they develop more distinct, differentiated, and emotionally invested MMR,[43] with a substantial presence of fearful imagery about the child when reaching the third trimester.[44] MMR also display peak levels of richness and specificity by the seventh month, with a subsequent decline up until childbirth.[10,45] Since the pregnant woman lacks information about her baby, it has been hypothesized that the development of MMR results from her projections, hopes, attributions, conscious and unconscious fantasies, and dreams.[8-11] However, studies have mainly investigated the more conscious aspects of MMR and given surprisingly little attention to whether more unconscious processes, such as dreaming, also contribute to their organization.

The small number of systematic studies that have assessed dreaming during pregnancy nevertheless indicate that the vast majority of women (67% to 88%) during their pregnancies report having at least one dream relating to a baby, pregnancy, or childbirth.[18,24,46] Some others report that 30% to 62% of pregnant women's dreams refer to at least one of these maternal elements[47-50] and that such dreams increase in frequency with advancing gestational age.[24] Although such pregnancy dreams typically refer to the mother's physical well-being and to the sex of the unborn baby,[47] they also often contain elements of misfortune; injury or threat toward the baby, the mother, or the father[24,46]; and marital and familial issues (e.g., fear of losing the partner, past relational issues with their own mother).[49] Other common themes relate to postpartum parental responsibilities and competencies, including the fear of being an inadequate parent.[46,49] The few available comparative studies indicate that, relative to nonpregnant controls, pregnant women recall more dreams with pregnancy-related themes (e.g., fetus, pregnancy, childbirth, one's own body) and more elements of danger toward the fetus and the self.[18,49-51] The dreams of pregnant women are also more negative[18,50] and contain more masochistic elements (i.e., misfortune, harm, environmental threats) but not more aggressive acts.[50] In sum, although limited in number, studies provide consistent evidence that MMR are expressed during dreaming and that these images are frequently very emotional in nature. However, none of these studies assessed dream content related specifically to MMR.

In one comparative study, we therefore examined whether dreamed MMR, like waking MMR, change from the seventh month of pregnancy to birth, and whether pregnancy-related themes and nonpregnancy characteristics are also transformed.[52] In this study, 60 nonpregnant and 59 pregnant women (37 early and 22 late third trimester) completed demographic and psychological questionnaires and 14-day home dream logs. Dream reports were blindly rated and analyzed according to four dream categories:

1. Dreamed MMR (i.e., *MMR characters* and *social roles of the dreamer*)
2. Quality of baby or child representations (i.e., *intensity of the dreamer's interaction with the baby* and the *specificity and individuality of the baby's personality*)
3. Pregnancy-related themes (i.e., content relating to *pregnancy, childbirth, a fetus, and/or the human body*)
4. Nonpregnancy characteristics, i.e., *development of the dream narrative* using the Dream-Like Fantasy Scale[53]; *dream masochism* using the Masochism Scale for Dreams (see Winget and Kramer's book[54] for an in-depth description of the scale); *aggressive and cooperative movements* and *morbid dream content* derived from the special scores categories of the Exner scoring system for the Rorschach inkblot test. Morbid content refers to an object that is dead, destroyed, injured, or damaged in some way or is characterized by a dysphoric tone (e.g., a sad house[55]) (Table 64.2).

Results show that, controlling for psychological and demographic characteristics, pregnant women reported significantly more dreams depicting themselves as mothers or interacting with babies than did nonpregnant women (Figure 64.2), thus replicating earlier findings.[18,24,46-51] However, there was no evidence that pregnant women dreamed more about themselves in the roles of spouse, daughter, or member of her own family, as expected from an early study reporting that dreams frequently depict marital and familial issues during pregnancy.[49] There were also no differences in the frequencies of dreamers' representations of themselves in the roles of friend, worker, or student. A small cohort study yielded results similar to these in showing that pregnant women in their third trimester dreamed more about babies, but not about the family or the partner, than did nonpregnant women.[51] Therefore, in being focused exclusively on the maternal role during pregnancy, dreams appear to reflect the ongoing daytime processes of remodeling MMR of the self as a mother and of the fetus as a future baby.[8,11]

Another important finding of our study is that baby representations in dreams were less specific in the late third than in the early third trimester and than in the dreams of nonpregnant women. These results concur with MMR studies showing that women in their third trimester of pregnancy report specific and rich images about the unborn baby[43] and that the quality of these representations drops up until childbirth.[10,45] Stern[10] has suggested that this decline may reflect the need for a woman to "undo" her representations to prevent disappointment when faced with the real child after birth. Another explanation is that by the 30th week of gestation, the number of spontaneous fetal movements[56] and nighttime microarousals evoked by fetal movements[57] decreases until birth. In line with the continuity hypothesis of dreaming,[3,4] the lower quality of dreamed representations about babies and children in the late third trimester may parallel this decrease in perceived fetal movements.

Contrary to expectations, however, specific representations of babies were not more negative during pregnancy, thereby failing to support earlier studies showing that babies are commonly depicted as being in danger in pregnant women's dreams (see the work by Nielsen and Paquette,[18] Blake and Reimann,[24] and Van and colleagues[46]). Instead, pregnant groups had more pregnancy, childbirth, and fetus themes, and childbirth content was higher in dreams in the late than in the early third trimester. The latter finding supports previous studies showing that pregnant women's dreams depict greater pregnancy and childbirth themes,[18,51] but they add to this the notion that mental reorganization in the very last stage of pregnancy becomes more focused on preparations for delivery. This shift in focus may parallel the mother's reality of enduring more frequent medical appointments and of undergoing an upsurge of intense ambivalent feelings about the coming event.[15]

Finally, our study[52] shows that the only measure not specific to pregnancy that differentiated the groups was a surplus of morbid dream elements (i.e., dysphoric feelings and negative characteristics attributed to any dream element) in both pregnancy groups as compared to the nonpregnant group (Figure 64.3). This suggests that general dream processes *not* directly related to pregnancy remain relatively stable during pregnancy and that the psychological challenges of pregnancy may be reflected indirectly in a more dysphoric emotional tone in dream content.

In sum, our study, the first to have specifically assessed MMR in dreams, indicates that dreaming during pregnancy reflects daytime processes of remodeling MMR of the woman as a mother and MMR of her unborn baby and parallels a more general decline in the quality of waking-state baby representations in the last trimester of pregnancy. On the other hand, more frequent morbid contents in late pregnancy suggest that the psychological challenges of pregnancy are reflected in a generally more dysphoric emotional tone in dream content. Future studies may assess more directly, using validated scales or objective measures, whether physical, psychological, and social experiences of pregnancy (e.g., obstetrical conditions,

Table 64.2 Description of Dream Measures Assessed in Pregnant Women

Dream Measures	Description
Dream Content Specific to Pregnancy	
Dreamed Maternal Mental Representations	
As daughter-parents	Dreamer as daughter of her parents and dreamer's mother and father representations
As spouse-partner	Dreamer as spouse and dreamer's partner representations
As mother-baby/child	Dreamer as mother and representations of babies and children
As part of own family	Dreamer as part of her own family and representations of dreamer's family
As friend	Dreamer as friend
As professional worker/student	Dreamer as worker or student
Quality of Baby or Child Representations	
Specificity of representations	Intensity of the dreamer's interaction with the baby/child, specificity, and individuality of the personality of the baby/child
Endangered and negative representations	Endangered and negative baby/child representations
Pregnancy-Related Themes	
Pregnancy	Whether or not the content made reference to the dreamer herself or to another dream character (number of occurrences/dream)
Childbirth	Ibid
Fetus	Ibid
Other Dream Characteristics Not Specific to Pregnancy	
Dream development[a]	1 = no recall, 2 = a thought, 3 = a single image, 4 = a dream (two or more images with some connection between them), 5 = a well-developed dream (more than two images with a well-developed plot)
Dream masochism[b]	An unpleasant dream in which the dreamer has negative characteristics and/or the dream's outcome is negative (number of occurrences/dream)
Aggressive movements[c]	Dream action is clearly aggressive, such as fighting, breaking, arguing, being angry, etc. (number of movements/dream)
Cooperative movements[c]	Interactions between two or more dream characters are clearly benevolent, cooperative, or mutually supportive (number of movements/dream)
Morbid contents[c]	Descriptions of dead, destroyed, damaged, polluted, degraded, or broken dream elements or a dysphoric feeling or character attributed to a dream element (number of elements/dream)

[a]Categories derived from the Dream-like Fantasy Scale (see Cartwright et al.[53] for details).
[b]Masochism Scale for dreams (see Winget & Kramer,[54] for an in-depth description of the scale)
[c]Categories derived from the Special scores categories of the Exner scoring system for the Rorschach inkblot test (Exner[55]).
Modified from Lara-Carrasco et al.[52]

frequency of medical appointments, preoccupations relating pregnancy and motherhood, daytime MMR) are associated with such specific themes in the dreams of each trimester of pregnancy.

Can Pregnancy Dreams Predict Maternal and Fetal Outcomes?

Research on dreams during pregnancy is consistent with the notion that a pregnant woman's mental reorganization is focused principally on the construction of her new maternal identity and of representations of her unborn baby. According to some clinicians, this reorganization is likely to be achieved through activation of the caregiving system, a motivational mechanism that guides maternal behaviors and that derives from cognitive and affective representations shaped by the mother's own first relationship experiences.[8,11,39] This transitional process of change in self-concept during pregnancy may require the activation of specific representations of the mother-infant relationship during dreaming, possibly by virtue of dreaming facilitating the integration of recent and remote memories.[5,6]

Some clinical studies go further to support a regulatory function for dreaming in showing, for example, that clinically depressed divorcées who dream emotionally about their ex-spouses at intake are more likely to be psychologically well adjusted several months later than are divorcées who do not report these types of dreams.[53,58] Other studies with healthy subjects find that sadness dissipates across the night, a change that is positively associated with the number of dream characters appearing in the dreams of that night (see the review by

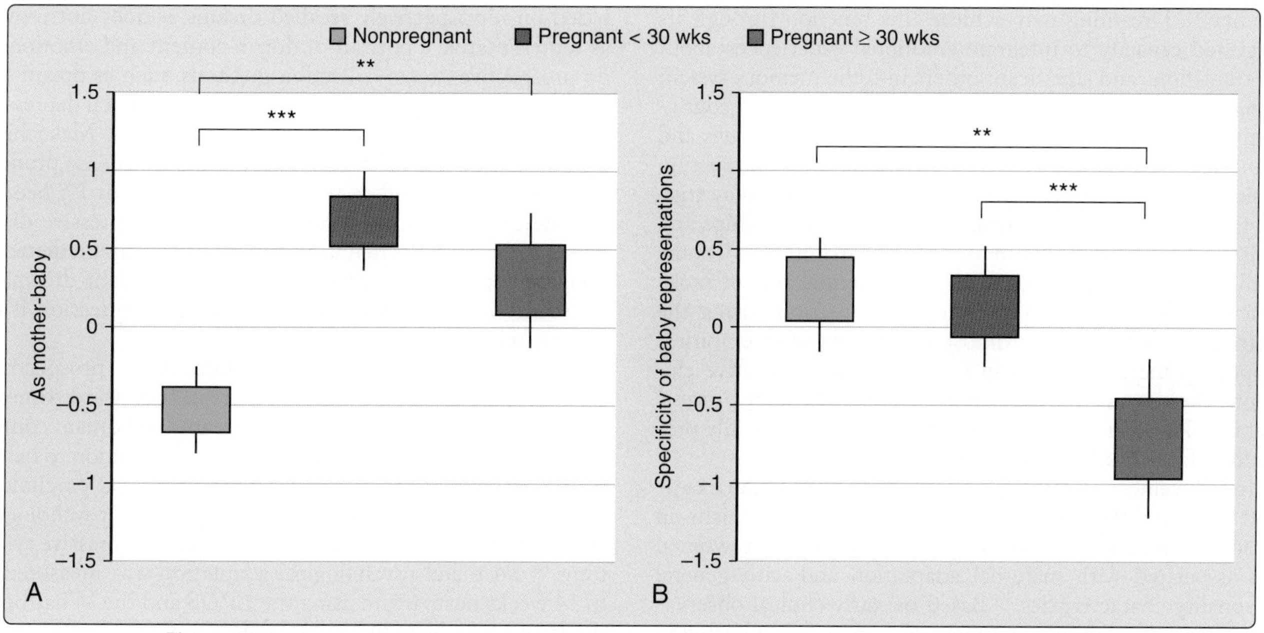

Figure 64.2 Chart showing pregnant women who reported significantly more dreams depicting themselves as a mother or interacting with babies than did nonpregnant women. Pregnant and nonpregnant women differences (mean ± standard error) on "As mother-baby/child" and "Specificity of baby/child representations" dream factor scores. Pregnant women in the early and late third trimester had more representations in their dreams of themselves as mothers and of babies and children (*left panel*) than did nonpregnant women; pregnant women in their late third trimester of pregnancy (≥30 weeks of gestation) had less specific baby and children representations in their dreams than did those in the early third trimester (<30 weeks of gestation) and nonpregnant women (*right panel*). $^{**}P < .01$, $^{***}P < .001$. (From Lara-Carrasco et al.[52])

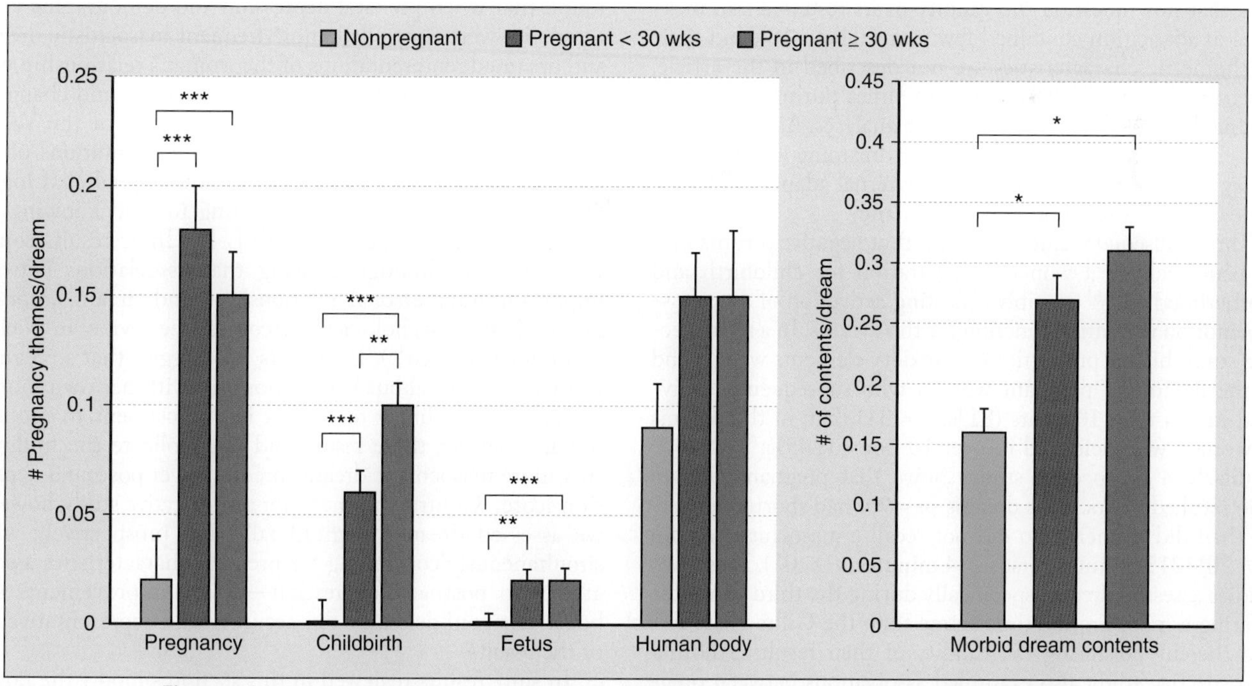

Figure 64.3 Differences between pregnant and nonpregnant women (mean ± standard error) on pregnancy-related themes and on morbid dream contents. Pregnant women in the early and late third trimester had more pregnancy, childbirth, and fetus dream themes than did nonpregnant women, and those in the late third trimester (≥30 weeks of gestation) had more childbirth dream themes (*left panel*) than did those in the early third trimester (<30 weeks of gestation). Morbid dream contents (dysphoric feelings and negative characteristics attributed to any dream element) were more frequent in both pregnant groups than in the nonpregnant group (*right panel*). $^{*}P < .05$, $^{**}P < .01$, $^{***}P < .001$. (From Lara-Carrasco et al.[52])

Kramer[59]). Dreaming may achieve this function through its suggested capacity to integrate emotional experiences about life transitions and significant others into the memory system that defines the self-concept. As dream research has consistently found that dreams are sensitive to relational issues and changes,[36,37] transitional periods implicating the construction of significant new relationships, such as pregnancy, may trigger the activation during dreaming of these relationships and their associated emotions in an adaptive manner.[5,6,31] Some studies have attempted to clarify the potential role of pregnancy dreams in promoting maternal adaptation during the perinatal period.[48,50,60,61] Almost all of them offer empirical support to the notion that in containing more negative elements, dreams may be part of a "working-through process" that enables pregnant women to be more psychologically prepared to face childbirth and to adapt to motherhood.

In this vein, an initial exploratory study by Gillman examined whether the presence of hostility or masochism in dreams collected retrospectively from 44 pregnant women was associated with maternal adaptation and with general personality characteristics.[50] Based on early clinical observations suggesting that new mothers who are poorly adjusted to childbirth are also characterized by depression, hostility, and sado-masochistic fantasies, Gillman tested whether the presence of hostility and masochism in dreams was also associated with maternal adjustment. Positive correlations were found between the absence of masochistic dreams and general measures of psychological adequacy, ability, and strength, but there were no relationships between dream content and specific measures of maternal adaptation. This study, still innovative for the time, nevertheless contains important methodological gaps that now question the validity of its results. First, measures of adaptation contained few items (about 10), and their psychometric characteristics are not described in the article. Also, dreams were collected at four times during pregnancy, mixing dreams of all trimesters in the analyses. As dream content changes throughout pregnancy,[16] dreaming in early pregnancy may not be associated with maternal adaptation to the same extent as dreaming in late pregnancy.

Three subsequent studies suggest that negative dreams may be beneficial for a woman's preparation for childbirth and motherhood,[48,60,61] possibly reflecting activation of a successful emotion regulation function for the dreams. In a retrospective study, higher proportions of anxiety elements were found in the dreams of pregnant women who subsequently delivered in less than 10 hours (81%; $n = 31$) than in the dreams of women who delivered in over 10 hours (≤45%; $n = 16$).[48] Similarly, a prospective study shows that pregnant women who recalled masochistic dreams ($n = 90$) had shorter deliveries than did women who did not recall a masochistic dream ($n = 70$) (215 minutes versus 294 minutes; $P < .01$). These two studies assessed dreams specifically during the third trimester, offering a more limited time frame than the Gillman study[50] and thereby bolstering the validity of their results. Another retrospective study also examined associations between pregnancy dreams and postpartum depression[60] and found that dreams containing masochistic elements and apprehension during pregnancy were more frequent among women who had higher postnatal depression scores (measured 6 to 10 weeks postpartum using the Edinburgh Postnatal Depression Scale [EPDS][62]) than among women who had lower postnatal depression scores. However, because the latter study was based on retrospectively recalled dreams, it does not provide as representative a portrait of dream content and emotions as do prospective dream collection methods, such as dream diaries.[63] Also, the authors did not control for prenatal depression for any socioeconomic factor in their analyses. Masochistic dreams characterize the sleep of individuals who are prone to depression and correlate with depression severity[64]; because pregnancy is a period of increased risk for depressive disorders and because postnatal depression is mostly predicted by prenatal depression,[65] the reporting of masochistic dreams by pregnant women may be confounded with depression if the latter is not appropriately controlled.

Accordingly, in a study (unpublished), we prospectively assessed, among 55 first-time mothers in their third trimester of pregnancy, whether masochistic dreams and dream content about specific maternal representations (i.e., relation to babies, relation to own mother) predict better postnatal psychological adaptation when controlling for prenatal psychological and demographic characteristics—including depressive symptoms.[66] Postnatal psychological adaptation was measured 10 to 14 weeks postpartum using the EPDS and the What Being the Parent of a New Baby is Like–Revised (WPL-R), a questionnaire designed to evaluate maternal adaptation.[67] Relations to babies and to own mother in dreams were used as predictors because clinical research suggests that the reworking of the internalized object and self-representations that sustain both relationships may be among the most important tasks for the woman to achieve her new maternal identity. Dream masochism was also used as a predictor because its presence during pregnancy has been associated with better obstetric and psychological prognoses, as reviewed earlier. We found that when prenatal depression and demographic characteristics were controlled, more frequent masochistic dreams and dreamed representations of the woman's relationship with her own mother predicted less perceived stress and change in her personal and relational life (change scale of the WPL-R). Similarly, more frequent dreamed representations of the woman's relationship with her own mother predicted higher satisfaction from parenting and caring for and knowing her baby (satisfaction scale of the WPL-R). These results concur with previous findings showing that associations between important interpersonal relationships and dream emotions predict better psychological outcomes (see review in Nielsen and Lara-Carrasco[34]). The results also suggest that a pregnant woman's dreams about her relationship with her own mother are particularly likely to predict her adjustment to motherhood. However, these results did not replicate the finding[60] that more masochistic dreams predict lower postnatal depression scores. Contrary to the latter retrospective study, however, we assessed dreams longitudinally and prospectively while simultaneously controlling for prenatal characteristics associated with postnatal depression—design improvements that boost our confidence in the accuracy and representativeness of the results.

In sum, results reviewed in this section support the notion that dreaming facilitates adaptation to emotional life transitions during pregnancy through the regulation of negative emotions. Results also specify that, in being principally centered on the mother-daughter relationship, dreams may help pregnant women assimilate their new maternal identities and adapt to the emotional surge resulting from the achievement of having a baby. Whether the processing of these representations and emotions in dreams are predictive of real mother-infant interactions after birth (beyond subjective psychological adaptation), as was found in studies assessing prenatal waking thoughts, expectations, and representations,[68,69] must be assessed further in longitudinal studies.

Postpartum Dream Changes

A meager literature describes dream changes in the postpartum period; only four studies could be identified for the present review. An initial study[27] of 325 women who were questioned about a range of parasomnias 3 months prepregnancy, throughout pregnancy (in each trimester), and 3 months postpartum revealed that all parasomnias except sleep paralysis decreased in frequency in either the first or second trimesters; sleep paralysis decreased only in the postpartum period. Nightmares in particular decreased from prepregnancy (55.7%) to the first trimester 47.7%, $P < .01$) and remainded low in the second (49.5%) and third (41.2%) trimesters and postpartum (40.3%).

These results were not entirely consistent with those of a second, cross-sectional, study[18] that examined dream content specific to pregnancy and the postpartum period. The dreams of 50 pregnant (28 primiparous; 22 multiparous), 202 postpartum (97 primiparous; 107 multiparous), and 21 nulligravida women were compared for content featuring babies and infants as well as for occurrences of dream-enacting behaviors (motor, verbal, or emotional). Women in the pregnancy and postpartum groups recalled infant dreams and nightmares with equal prevalence, but more postpartum women reported that their dreams contained anxiety (75%) than did those of pregnant women (59%; $P < .05$) and that their dreams depicted the infant in peril (73% versus 42%, $P < .0001$). Motor dream enactments were reported to be present by twice as many postpartum (57%) as pregnant (24%) or nulligravida (25%) women (all $P < .0001$), but emotional dream enactments were less prevalent among postpartum (27%) than among nulligravida (56%) women ($P < .05$) and were not different from pregnant women (37%). Dream enactments were associated with nightmares, dream anxiety, and, among postpartum women, postawakening confusion (51%), anxiety (41%), and an urge to check on their infant (60%). The prevalence of infant dreams and associated behaviors and anxieties may reflect the influence of several factors: the pervasiveness of maternal concerns, altered hormone levels, and severe sleep disruption—rapid eye movement sleep deprivation in particular.

In a third longitudinal study, Coo and colleagues[70] found that dreams from the postpartum period were more likely than those from the third trimester to contain positive dream contents, that is, more likely to reference the newborn baby (23% versus 5%), family members (56% versus 33%), familiar characters (78% versus 57%), and familiar settings (62% versus 55%). Further comparisons of both groups with normative values for nonpregnant women revealed positive themes common to both groups, that is, more references to babies and to family members (fewer friends, however), fewer aggressive actions, more friendly actions, fewer bodily misfortunes, and more successes (but also less sexuality). This study differed from others in suggesting that the postpartum period is not only associated with negative elements in dreams.

Finally, in a cross-sectional study[71] 143 pregnant women completed dream logs during three distinct periods (second trimester, third trimester, postpartum), while 125 nonpregnant controls completed logs on one occasion. Dream contents related to pregnancy and motherhood characteristics and to negative and positive elements were rated by independent judges. Pregnant women were found to experience more direct pregnancy and motherhood contents than were control women, but the groups did not differ on emotional elements. Postpartum women, when compared with women in their third trimester of pregnancy, dreamed more about their babies, of taking care of their babies, and of being a mother and less about fetuses, being pregnant, and childbirth (all $P < .05$). Postpartum women did not have more negative elements in their dreams than either pregnant women or nonpregnant controls.

In sum, only a few studies on dreaming in the postpartum period have been conducted, but these indicate that women continue to dream about their current concerns (e.g., motherhood, care of the infant). This includes dreaming about the infant in peril. However, study results are inconsistent in indicating whether postpartum dream emotions are more or less negative than are those recalled during pregnancy.

CLINICAL PEARLS

- Dysphoric dreams increase markedly in late pregnancy, possibly contributing to impaired sleep at this time.
- Clinically guided management of dysphoric dreaming during pregnancy could improve sleep complaints and pregnancy outcomes.
- More frequent masochistic dreams predict shorter deliveries and less postnatal depression and stress and thus may reflect an emotion regulation function of dreaming.
- Clinical studies could assess whether intentional dream recall during pregnancy enhances a mother's understanding of her parental concerns, relational changes, and shifts in self-concept.

SUMMARY

Most women develop sleep impairments during pregnancy, but dream alterations are seldom studied. However, a marked increase in dysphoric dreams in late pregnancy may contribute substantially to impaired sleep. Because disturbed sleep during pregnancy is related to poor maternal and fetal outcomes, clinically guided management of DD could improve sleep complaints and, ultimately, pregnancy outcomes.

Pregnancy dreams not only express the concerns of pregnant women but also depict representations of a woman's relationship with her unborn child. Such dreams may reflect a regulatory function (e.g., more frequent masochistic dreams predict shorter deliveries, lower postnatal depression, and less postnatal stress). Such findings support the view that life transitions requiring reorganization of the self-concept trigger socially structured dreaming in which memories about relationships and associated emotions facilitate adaptation to a new social context.

Finally, because current investigational designs are mainly correlational, future clinically oriented studies could assess whether intentional dream recall during pregnancy may enhance a mother's understanding of her own parental concerns, relational changes, and self-concept changes, a hypothetical effect of dreaming that otherwise may be achieved only through psychotherapy.

SELECTED READINGS

Blake Jr RL, Reimann J. The pregnancy-related dreams of pregnant women. *J Am Acad Child Psy*. 1993;6:117–122.

Coo S, Milgrom J, Trinder J. Pregnancy and postnatal dreams reflect changes inherent to the transition to motherhood. *Dreaming*. 2014;24(2):125–137.

Dagan Y, Lapidot A, Eisenstein M. Women's dreams reported during first pregnancy. *Psych Clinic Neurosci*. 2001;55:13–20.

Gillman RD. The dreams of pregnant women and maternal adaptation. *Am J Orthopsych*. 1968;38:688–692.

Hedman C, Pohjasvaara T, Tolonen U, Salmivaara A, Myllyla VV. Parasomnias decline during pregnancy. *Acta Neurol Scand*. 2002;105:209–214.

Horton CL, Moulin CJ, Conway MA. The self and dreams during a period of transition. *Consciousn Cogn*. 2009;18(3):710–717.

Korukcu O, Ozkaya M, Boran OF, Bakacak M. Factors associated with antenatal depression during the COVID-19 (SARS-CoV2) pandemic: a cross-sectional study in a cohort of Turkish pregnant women [published online ahead of print, 2021 Mar 26]. *Perspect Psychiatr Care*. 2021. https://doi.org/10.1111/ppc.12778.

Kron T, Brosh A. Can dreams during pregnancy predict postpartum depression? *Dreaming*. 2003;13:67–81.

Lara-Carrasco J, Simard V, Saint-Onge K, Lamoureux-Tremblay V, Nielsen T. Maternal representations in the dreams of pregnant women: a prospective comparative study. *Front Psychol*. 2013;4:551.

Lara-Carrasco J, Simard V, Saint-Onge K, Lamoureux-Tremblay V, Nielsen T. Disturbed dreaming during the third trimester of pregnancy. *Sleep Med*. 2014;15(6):694–700.

Mancuso A, De Vivo AFanara G, Settineri S, Giacobbe A, Pizzo A. Emotional state and dreams in pregnant women. *Psychiat Res*. 2008;160(3):380–386.

Nielsen T, Paquette T. Dream-associated behaviors affecting pregnant and postpartum women. *Sleep*. 2007;30:1162–1169.

Nielsen TA, Lara-Carrasco J. Nightmares, dreaming and emotion regulation: a review. In: Barrett D, McNamara P, eds. *The new science of dreams*. Westport: Praeger Greenwood; 2007:253–284.

Sabourin C, Robidoux R, Pérusse AD, De Koninck J. Dream content in pregnancy and postpartum: refined exploration of continuity between waking and dreaming. *Dreaming*. 2018;28(2):122–139.

van de Castle RL, Kinder P. Dream content during pregnancy. *Psychophysiology*. 1968;4. 375–375.

A complete reference list can be found online at ExpertConsult.com.

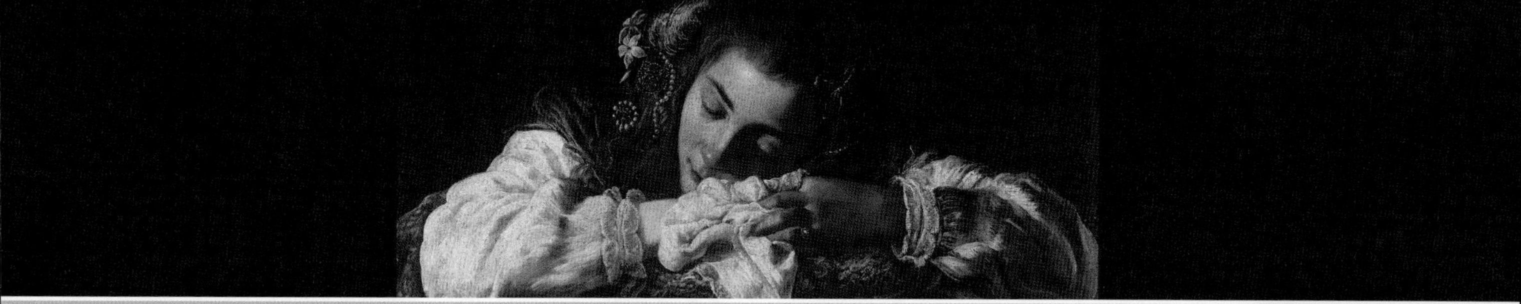

PART II

Practice of Sleep Medicine

Section

8 Impact, Presentation, and Diagnosis

Chapter

65 Approach to the Patient with Disordered Sleep

Beth A. Malow

Chapter Highlights

- This chapter emphasizes the clinical approach to the patient with disordered sleep, focusing on specific aspects of the history and physical examination.
- Patients who complain of disturbed sleep usually describe one or more of three types of problems: insomnia; abnormal movements, behaviors, or sensations during sleep or during nocturnal awakenings; or excessive daytime sleepiness.
- Taking a systematic history that includes medication use, family history, social history, and review of systems can provide important clues regarding the diagnosis.

Patients who complain of disturbed sleep usually describe one or more of three types of problems: insomnia; abnormal movements, behaviors, or sensations during sleep or during nocturnal awakenings; or excessive daytime sleepiness. These sleep complaints are not mutually exclusive, and a sleep disorder may be associated with more than one type. For example, patients with sleep apnea may complain of insomnia, excessive daytime sleepiness, choking or gasping during the night, or all three. Those with narcolepsy may complain of sleep paralysis and hallucinations at sleep onset or on awakening, disrupted sleep, and daytime sleepiness.

CHIEF COMPLAINT AND HISTORY

Evaluation begins with the chief complaint, which provides a focus for delineating the patient's concerns and eliciting the history. It is often useful to ask why the patient is seeking help at the present time, particularly if the problem has been long-standing. If the chief complaint is from the spouse or bed partner, it is important to determine whether the patient recognizes the problem, is unaware of it, or denies its existence. Many clinicians also obtain a brief patient profile during the interview, which includes the patient's age, sex, occupational or academic status, marital status, and living arrangements. The profile often includes valuable information about how the sleep concern is affecting the patient's daily functioning (e.g., difficulty performing job responsibilities or participating in leisure activities with family). After the chief complaint is delineated, details concerning the sleep problem are sought, including its duration, the circumstances at its onset, the factors that lead to exacerbation or improvement, and any associated symptoms.

The patient's daily schedule is reviewed, including the usual bedtime and estimated time to sleep onset, the number and timing of awakenings, and the time of final awakening. Morning symptoms should be elicited, such as increased nasal congestion, dry mouth, or morning headaches. These symptoms may support a diagnosis of obstructive sleep apnea. Daytime symptoms, including during passive or repetitious activities (e.g., watching television or riding in a car), should be investigated to characterize the severity of sleepiness. A comprehensive sleep history also includes questions about the frequency and duration of daytime naps and the presence or absence of cataplexy, hypnic hallucinations, sleep paralysis, and automatic behavior.

Insomnia

Patients with insomnia usually complain that their nocturnal sleep is inadequate in some way. They may describe difficulty falling asleep, frequent awakening, or early morning awakening with inability to return to sleep. It is important to distinguish among these patterns of insomnia because they may have different causes. For example, awakenings from sleep because of obstructive sleep apnea may result in sleep maintenance insomnia but would not result in a patient's complaining of lying awake for hours not being able to fall asleep. The description of insomnia and its course may help determine cause, as outlined in Chapter 93.

Excessive Sleepiness

Patients with daytime sleepiness typically complain of drowsiness that interferes with daytime activities, unavoidable napping, or both. Falling asleep while driving or at other particularly inappropriate or dangerous times is often the impetus that brings the patient to the clinician. Some of these patients complain that they need more sleep at night or that daytime drowsiness occurs regardless of how much sleep is obtained at night. Patients may also complain of difficulty with concentration or memory or increased irritability. Children may exhibit hyperactivity rather than sleepiness.

The differential diagnosis of excessive daytime sleepiness ranges from insufficient sleep to sufficient sleep that is disrupted by pathologic events, such as apneas, or neurologic disorders, such as narcolepsy. Inquiring about sleep routines and bedtimes and wake times is essential in excluding insufficient sleep as a cause of sleepiness. Asking patients who complain of sleepiness about other associated symptoms provides essential information. Loud snoring, gasping, snorting, and episodes of apnea suggest the diagnosis of obstructive sleep apnea syndrome (see Chapter 131). A history of episodic muscle weakness with buckling of the knees, laxity of the neck or jaw muscles, or complete loss of muscle tone associated with laughter, anger, or hearing or telling a joke suggests cataplexy and a diagnosis of narcolepsy (see Chapter 112). Questions assessing mood are needed to identify patients with sleep disorders associated with depression (see Chapter 164). Circadian rhythm sleep disorders should be considered in patients with complaints of nocturnal insomnia and daytime sleepiness (see Chapter 43).

Nocturnal Movements, Behaviors, and Sensations

Information from collateral sources is needed for evaluation of episodic movements and behaviors during sleep. The bed partner should be asked to describe behaviors and vocalizations during the episodes, to relate episodes to sleep onset and time of night, and to note the degree of the patient's responsiveness during the episode. The patient's ability to recall the events is also significant. Episodes of inconsolable screaming and amnesia during the first third of the night suggest sleep terrors (see Chapter 116); episodes of dream-enactment behavior associated with dream recall that occur toward the end of the sleep cycle indicate rapid eye movement sleep behavior disorder (see Chapter 118). Epileptic seizures may occur at any time of the night and should be strongly considered if a history of stereotyped behavior or dystonic posturing is elicited (see Chapter 106).

Medication Use and Medical History

Assessment of medication use, including nonprescription medications, herbal supplements, and illicit drugs, is critical because of the wide variety of medications that alter sleep, wakefulness, and sleep disorders (see Chapter 53).

The history of current or past medical, surgical, and psychiatric illnesses is a source of important information. Seizure disorders, parkinsonism and dementia, arthritic conditions, asthma, ischemic heart disease, migraine or cluster headache, compressive neuropathies, and almost any painful illness can cause significant sleep disturbance. Anemia, renal disease, and pregnancy may cause or exacerbate restless legs syndrome or periodic limb movement disorder. Anxiety disorders, including panic disorder, and mood disorders are psychiatric disturbances that are often accompanied by insomnia, and some patients with depression complain of excessive daytime sleepiness.

Family History

A history of disordered sleep in family members is important information. Specific inquiry should be made about the existence in family members of previously diagnosed sleep disorders or symptoms suggestive of narcolepsy, obstructive sleep apnea, periodic limb movements, enuresis, sleep terrors or sleepwalking, or insomnia. There is a strong genetic contribution to the development of narcolepsy (see Chapter 112), and genetic and familial influences sometimes have a role in the development and expression of obstructive sleep apnea (see Chapter 128) and some of the parasomnias.

Social History

Assessment of psychosocial, occupational, and academic functioning as well as of satisfaction with personal relationships can yield valuable information about the impact of disordered sleep on the patient's life. It is important to identify health disparity problems with financial and geographic access to care, racial discrimination, remote settings, and poor access to telemedicine services (internet, computers). Alcohol, caffeine, nicotine, and illicit drug use should be determined. Alcohol use or abuse may intensify snoring and obstructive sleep apnea, may be a contributor to insomnia, or may produce long-lasting changes in sleep patterns. Caffeine use produces significant sleep disturbance in susceptible persons, and nicotine dependency may lead to nocturnal awakenings.

Use of screens associated with electronic devices (e.g., computers, tablets, cellular phones, televisions) should also be avoided given the combination of stimulating light, especially in the blue light spectrums, and the often stimulating content.

Review of Systems

The review of systems may uncover symptoms of medical illnesses that can cause or contribute to sleep disorders (Box 65.1). Previous infection with SARS-CoV-2 may implicate sleep disorders found in "long COVID" patients (see Chapter 213). Recent weight gain or increase in collar size increases the likelihood of obstructive sleep apnea. Particular attention should be paid to the cardiovascular and pulmonary systems because of their relation to breathing and oxygenation during sleep. Angina, orthopnea, paroxysmal nocturnal dyspnea, and wheezing may indicate that sleep disturbance is

BOX 65.1 SAMPLE SLEEP REVIEW OF SYSTEMS

Sleep Habits
Bedtime on weekdays
Bedtime on weekends
Wake time on weekdays
Wake time on weekends
Time it takes to fall asleep
Awakenings during the night
Time it takes to fall back asleep

Morning Symptoms
Dry mouth
Refreshed
Morning headaches
Nasal congestion

Daytime Functioning
Sleepiness (specific situations when patient has fallen asleep)
Falling asleep while driving
Any accidents caused by sleepiness
Memory problems
Difficulty concentrating
Fatigue
Irritability
Naps (how many, how long, dreams?)

Bed Partner's Observations or What Patient Has Been Told
Loudness of snoring (mild, moderate, severe)
Witnessed apneas
Choking or gasping
Arousals

Sleep-Related Movements
Periodic leg movements
Leg cramps
Restless legs symptoms

Narcoleptic Symptoms
Cataplexy
Hallucinations
Sleep paralysis
Automatic behaviors
Disrupted sleep

Genitourinary System
Nocturia
Impaired sexual functioning

Other
Weight gain in recent years
Sleepwalking
Dream-enactment behavior

due to cardiac or pulmonary disease. Heartburn and reflux of gastric contents into the throat when the patient is recumbent may cause nocturnal choking episodes. Leg cramps and neuropathic pain may be accompanied by sleep disruption. Nocturia is a common cause of disturbed sleep, particularly in older men. Depression or anxiety can contribute to insomnia.

PHYSICAL EXAMINATION

Examination of the head and neck is particularly important in patients with suspected obstructive sleep apnea. Auscultation of the chest may reveal expiratory wheezes in patients with nocturnal asthma attacks. Thoracic abnormalities such as kyphoscoliosis may compromise ventilatory capacity, leading to hypoventilation and nocturnal breathing difficulties. Auscultation may reveal a prominent fourth heart sound originating from the enlarged right ventricle and murmurs related to pulmonary or tricuspid valve insufficiency. On abdominal examination, hepatomegaly may suggest that alcohol abuse is contributing to sleep disturbance or, in conjunction with other findings, that congestive heart failure is a factor. Examination of the extremities may reveal joint swelling or deformity, decreased range of motion across affected joints, and thickening of synovial tissue in patients with disordered sleep resulting from arthritis.

Findings on mental status testing and neurologic examination may indicate the presence of a psychiatric or neurologic disease that causes or contributes to disturbed sleep. Impairment of short-term memory, judgment, language functions, and abstract reasoning suggests the presence of a dementing illness that may cause insomnia or nocturnal confusion. Assessment of mood may suggest the presence of mania or depression, either of which may be associated with insomnia. Delusional thoughts and agitation may indicate that acute psychosis is the cause of insomnia. Reduced alertness with slurred speech and nystagmus may be signs of hypnotic or sedative abuse. Impaired sensation and reduced or absent tendon reflexes may indicate peripheral neuropathy, sometimes accompanied by nocturnal paresthesias or burning pain. Elements of the physical examination relevant to the sleep patient are covered in greater detail in Chapter 67.

CLINICAL PEARL

A complete sleep and medical history often yields a specific cause of the patient's sleep complaint. For example, in patients complaining of excessive daytime sleepiness, the cause can often be pinpointed by close attention to the patient's (and bed partner's) account of nighttime symptoms, bedtime and wake time schedules, medications, and coexisting medical disorders.

SUMMARY

The evaluation of a patient with disordered sleep begins with the chief complaint, which can be classified as insomnia, daytime sleepiness, episodic nocturnal movements or behaviors, or a combination of these concerns. A thorough characterization of these concerns, coupled with a comprehensive sleep history that includes the daily schedule, bedtime routine, and morning and daytime symptoms, forms the foundation for diagnosis. As in other fields of medicine, it is essential to consider other medical and psychiatric conditions, medication use, family history, social history including the psychosocial situation, review of systems, and physical examination before formulating a differential diagnosis and performing diagnostic studies. This systematic approach allows accurate diagnosis and specific interventions for many treatable sleep disorders.

Chapter 66

Cardinal Manifestations of Sleep Disorders

Bradley V. Vaughn; O'Neill F. D'Cruz

Chapter Highlights

- Sleep disorders include a wide range of conditions that impair health and quality of life. To optimize patients' health and quality of life, clinicians must recognize the fundamental symptoms (insomnia, hypersomnia, and unusual sleep-related behaviors) and the more subtle signs to efficiently identify individuals with sleep disorders and direct effective treatment of these conditions.
- Insomnia is a common symptom and diagnosis that can be related to many contributing factors. Features that predispose to, precipitate, and perpetuate the insomnia can be identified in individuals who suffer from chronic insomnias. Insomnia can have an intricate relationship to other medical and psychiatric disorders.
- Hypersomnia is often a presenting feature of other sleep disorders or lifestyle choices. One difficulty is distinguishing sleepiness from fatigue and then determining the underlying contributing features. The pattern of sleepiness, characteristics of sleep length, and response to sleep periods give clues to the etiology. Other symptoms, such as snoring, witnessed apnea, unrefreshing sleep, and morning headache, may indicate potential sleep-related breathing disorders or cataplexy, prompting an evaluation for narcolepsy.
- Unusual nocturnal sensations or events can provide windows into sleep issues. Features of restless legs syndrome, periodic limb movements in sleep, and parasomnias, such as sleepwalking, sleep terrors, and dream enactment, require detailed description of the sleep-related behaviors to help differentiate potential causes. These events may indicate other underlying sleep disorders and brain disease.
- Sleep and circadian rhythm issues can be an early warning feature for other disorders, such as neurodegenerative processes, neurodevelopmental disorders, mood disorders, or other organ system issues. Features of disrupted sleep or changes in circadian rhythm may precede other symptoms or findings by years. Findings of hypertension, unexplained weight gain, or mood or cognitive issues may be important flags to inquire about underlying sleep issues.

Sleep is essential to health, restoring properties that promote wakefulness and a sense of well-being. Sleep disturbance, however, frequently disrupts this sense of well-being and can result in a wide range of systemic and neuropsychological symptoms. Sleep disruption due to intrusion of components of the sleep state into periods of wakefulness may manifest as hypersomnia. Similarly, intrusion of components of wakefulness into the sleep period may manifest as insomnia. Beyond the medical manifestations, sleep disruption frequently decreases this sense of well-being and has societal effects by impairing work performance and psychosocial interactions. As we realize the connection of sleep to good health, we also recognize that sleep disruption may exacerbate symptoms of other diseases. These manifestations may present as worsening of a preexisting disorder or impairment of the patient's ability to cope with their symptoms. The challenge for physicians is to recognize these manifestations and appropriately delineate them as related to dysfunction of sleep.

Most patients referred to sleep centers present with one or a combination of three classic complaints: excessive sleepiness, difficulty attaining or sustaining sleep, or unusual events associated with sleep. These symptoms can be easily recognized as related to sleep and are not mutually exclusive. Patients may note more than one problem, such as difficulty sleeping at night and excessive sleepiness during the day. Others may complain of unusual events at night, daytime sleepiness, or inability to sleep. Each of these symptoms conveys clues to the underlying pathologic process (Figures 66.1 to 66.3). In this chapter we review the cardinal manifestations of sleep disorders and address some of the key features that guide the clinician to pursue further diagnostic evaluations.

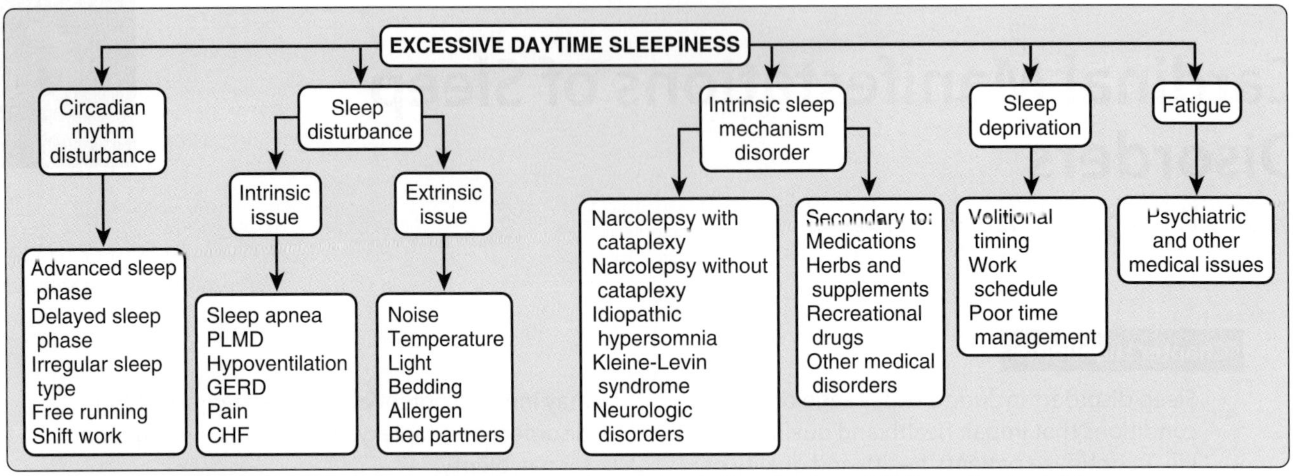

Figure 66.1 Diagnostic flow chart to approach excessive daytime sleepiness. CHF, Congestive heart failure; GERD, gastroesophageal reflux disease; PLMD, periodic limb movement disorder.

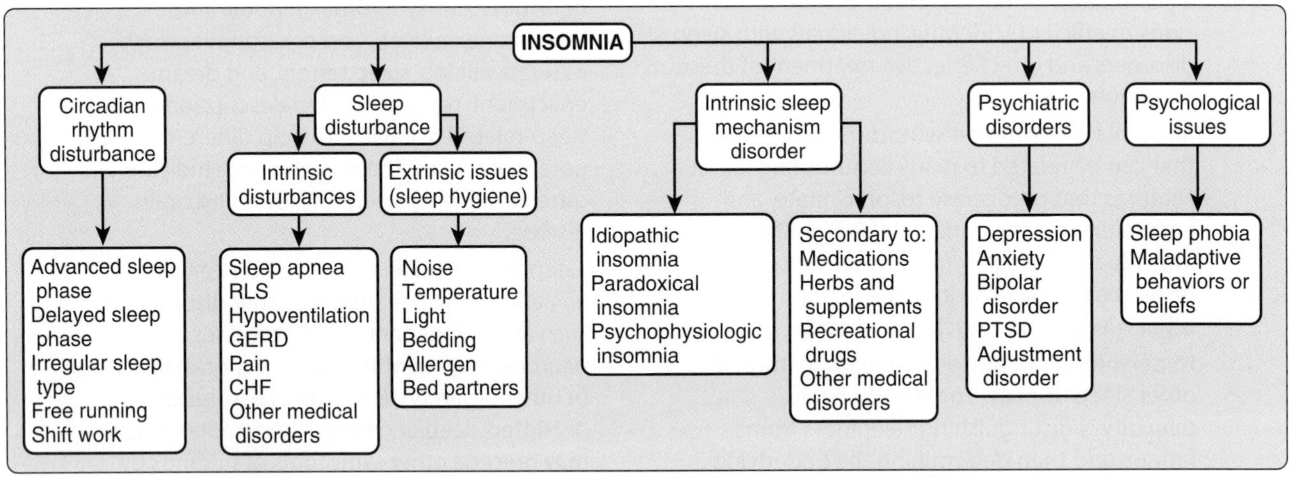

Figure 66.2 Diagnostic flow chart to approach insomnia. CHF, Congestive heart failure; GERD, gastroesophageal reflux disease; PTSD, posttraumatic stress disorder; RLS, restless legs syndrome.

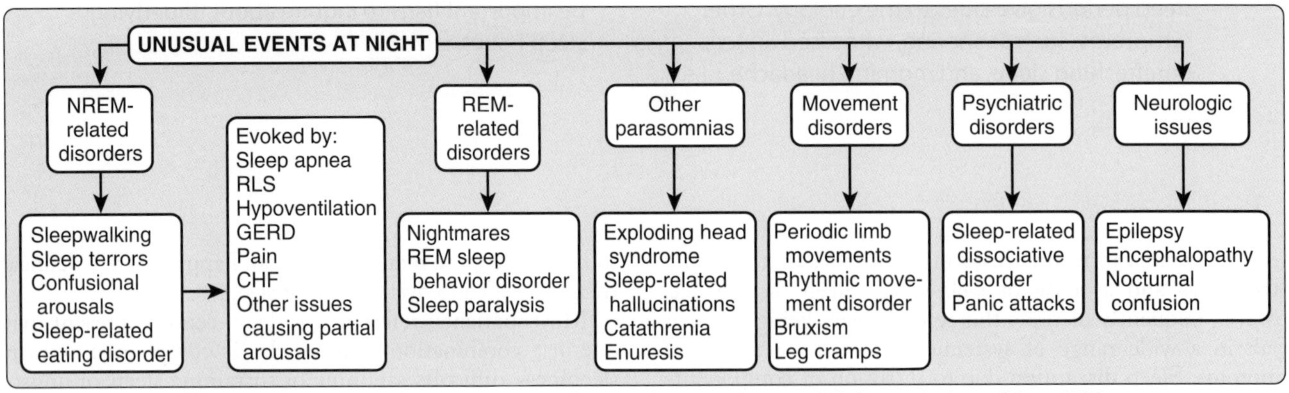

Figure 66.3 Diagnostic flow chart to approach unusual nocturnal events. CHF, Congestive heart failure; GERD, gastroesophageal reflux disease; NREM, non–rapid eye movement; REM, rapid eye movement; RLS, restless legs syndrome.

INSOMNIA

The diagnosis of insomnia is dependent upon the complaint of difficulty initiating or maintaining sleep combined with daytime sequelae. This combination of poor nighttime sleep with an adverse effect on daytime activities is important to establishing the complaint as insomnia. The daytime manifestations of insomnia may take the form of excessive fatigue, impairment of performance, or emotional change. Individual sleep need may vary significantly. Some people may feel fine and note no impairment of performance with 5 hours of sleep per night, whereas others may need more than 9 hours to preserve daytime functioning. Thus the requirement of daytime sequelae differentiates individual sleep need from the complaint of insomnia.

Most people have an occasional night fraught with difficulty falling asleep or trouble maintaining sleep. These occasional nights might be closely linked to the surrounding events of the day, psychological challenges, or sudden changes in environment or medical condition. Surveys have shown that approximately one-third of individuals complain that their sleep is disrupted and that a smaller group, of approximately 1 in 10, have a more persistent insomnia.[1] For these patients, lack of "good-quality" sleep produces a greater disruption of life and may lead to more significant medical or psychological symptoms.

As a symptom, insomnia is directly related to the patient's perception of poor sleep. Patients with insomnia believe that the sleep disruption produces their excessive sleepiness, fatigue, lack of concentration, muscle aches, and depression, and a good night of sleep would reverse these symptoms. Patients with insomnia frequently will describe themselves as tense, anxious, nervous, tired, irritable, unable to relax, obsessively worried, and depressed. Many of these traits may predate the onset of the insomnia, but others may occur after the onset of the poor sleep. Patients with insomnia frequently give historical clues directed toward the mechanisms behind their insomnia. The symptom complex may indicate an underlying disorder related to primary failure of the sleep mechanics or one in which sleep disruption is the byproduct of another disorder. As sleep is an active process, neuronal networks involved with sleep induction must be engaged, and networks involved in wakefulness must be diminished for sleep. Rarely do patients have just one factor responsible for their chronic insomnia (defined as lasting more than 3 months). Most patients have factors that put them at risk for developing and maintaining insomnia. The presence of predisposing, precipitating, and perpetuating factors emphasizes the nature of insomnia as an ongoing process, and clinicians need to search for these contributing factors to outline an effective treatment course (see Chapters 89 to 100).

Epidemiologically, insomnia appears to be more common in women, older individuals, and those with psychiatric or chronic medical illness. Insomnia is also more common in those with lower socioeconomic status and poor education. Behavioral traits, such as obsessive-compulsive nature, frequent rumination, poor coping strategies, and "hyperalert" individuals, are correlated with greater risk for insomnia. "Hyperarousal" documented in multiple modalities, including neuroimaging, electroencephalogram recording, neuroendocrine, and autonomic and metabolic studies, appears to explain the neurophysiologic basis of several of these associated factors predisposing to chronic insomnia.[1]

Insomnia may be initiated by sudden changes in environment or challenges to the body or mind. These challenges may come in the form of acute medical illness, psychological or psychiatric events, shift in schedule, or changes in medications or supplements. Although these events provide good clues to preventing further recurrence of insomnia, initiating events may play little role in the patient's current ongoing process.

Many patients, attempting to improve their sleep, will adopt behaviors that actually perpetuate the insomnia. Patients may employ rituals and endorse "remedies" that convert the short-term insomnia into a chronic form. During this evolution, the patient may take on changes in sleep schedule, depend on certain somnogenic substances, or develop secondary medical or psychological issues. Many of these behaviors conflict with typical sleep hygiene practices, producing an environment detrimental to sleep. Such maladaptive habits may occur during the day or night and include issues such as heavy caffeine or alcohol use, watching television or playing video games while in bed, and even eating or exercising during the usual sleep period. Some patients will describe that television or radio distracts them from intrusive thoughts. Others may develop sleep associations to counterbalance negative experiences. A subgroup of patients actually fear going to bed or have performance anxiety over the oncoming sleep period. This expectation of poor sleep promotes the apprehension toward sleep and may perpetuate counterproductive sleep rituals. These maladaptive behaviors become the predominant feature of psychophysiologic insomnia. Many individuals with these types of negative associations temporarily improve once placed in a new environment.

Timing of the insomnia during the sleep period may also be helpful. Circadian rhythm sleep-wake disorders can masquerade as complaints of insomnia or excessive sleepiness, and patients with insomnia may develop dysfunction of their circadian rhythm. Difficulty with the onset of sleep suggests an underlying delayed sleep phase or occasionally depression in younger adults. Insomnia with early morning arousal raises the possibility of underlying depression or advanced sleep phase. Schedule changes, such as from jet lag or shift work, are important clues, and sleep diaries of bedtime and wake time can be useful in determining potential links to schedule or circadian rhythm issues. Timing may also correlate with other issues, such as restless legs syndrome (RLS), medication, or caffeine intake. Specific questions should explore a daily routine, including the timing of activities that may be stimulating, such as exercise or work or gaming on a computer.

Perception of good sleep is an important factor in evaluating the complaint of insomnia. Some patients exaggerate their symptoms, whereas other patients may not perceive that they are asleep. Paradoxical insomnia is one subtype of chronic insomnia in which individuals do not recognize that they have slept despite the recording of normal physiologic parameters of sleep. Other patients may endorse unrealistic expectations or unobtainable goals, such as 8 hours of uninterrupted sleep every night. These beliefs can be easily addressed with education of the patient.

For some individuals the insomnia may start in childhood and be lifelong. The subtype of chronic insomnia known as idiopathic insomnia is not associated with clear inciting factors. These individuals have insomnia despite change in environment and may have significant family history. These primary insomnias are discussed further in Chapters 91 to 93.

Insomnia can be linked to other illnesses. Insomnia can be an early sign of medical or neurologic issues, and medical or neurologic disorders may precipitate and perpetuate insomnia. Derangement of almost any system in the body can disrupt sleep. Patients with heart, liver, or renal failure or disturbances of the gastrointestinal system or pulmonary disease commonly complain of insomnia. Patients with fulminant rash or significant burns frequently note disturbed sleep, and urologic issues, such as nocturia, may provoke frequent arousals. Neurologic disorders also promote sleep disruption. Patients with neuromuscular disorders may have discomfort or inadequate ventilation at night that provokes insomnia. Some patients with stroke will note insomnia or sleep disruption after their vascular event. Paralysis from central or peripheral nervous system disorders can result in nighttime discomfort from inability to move.

Patients with Parkinson disease may have akinesis, tremor, or medication effect, and patients with dementia may have circadian abnormalities that promote awakenings at night.

Pain can disturb sleep and promote insomnia. Musculoskeletal discomfort may become worse with periods of rest. Arthritis and other rheumatologic disorders frequently can disrupt sleep by increasing nighttime pain and stiffness. Pain from headaches, such as cluster headache, and even pain related to increased intracranial pressure or brain mass lesions can become more intense during sleep, and entrapment neuropathies, such as carpal tunnel syndrome, are typically worse at night. RLS produces a classic urge to move that is worse in the evening.

Nearly all of the psychiatric illnesses have some link to poor sleep. Patients with depression or anxiety disorders may have insomnia years before the presentation of the affective component. Although the cause and effect are still in debate, the association is clear. Insomnia may herald the onset of psychosis or mania, and sleep frequently is a good predictor of mood in bipolar disorders.[2]

The clinician may uncover few physical findings in patients with insomnia. Anxious or hyperalert individuals may demonstrate mild tachycardia, rapid respiratory rate, or cold hands. These individuals may easily startle or be distracted during the interview. The clinician should look carefully for signs of obstructive sleep apnea, narrow airway, and obesity because these too can be manifested as insomnia. Signs of Cushing syndrome (round face and buffalo hump) or hyperthyroidism (tachycardia and excessive sweating) are important clues to an endocrine disorder. Each patient with insomnia should have a complete neurologic examination to look for potential neurologic lesions impairing sleep. This examination should include an assessment of cognition, mood, and affect. Insomnia or interrupted sleep can occur in many forms of neurologic disease states, including several forms of dementia. The Mini-Mental State Examination is one tool that helps assess cognitive abilities and can be followed over time.[3] Clinicians can also use the Minnesota Multiphasic Personality Inventory to identify personality and affect issues, and the Hamilton Anxiety and Depression Scales may be helpful tools in following these individuals.

EXCESSIVE DAYTIME SLEEPINESS

Sleepiness is a common symptom noted by 5% to 20% of individuals.[4,5] Most individuals can relate some instances of falling asleep when they intended to be awake. Sleepiness is a normal feeling as one approaches a typical sleep period or after prolonged wakefulness. Excessive sleepiness may manifest as sleep at an inappropriate setting or episodes of unintentional sleep. Excessive sleepiness can occur in various degrees of severity. In mild sleepiness, one might fall asleep while reading a book or while sitting quietly. This degree of sleepiness may produce only limited impairment in the person's perceived quality of life. Greater degrees of sleepiness may be associated with bouts of irresistible sleep or sleep attacks intruding on such activities as driving, during a conversation, or eating meals. This degree of sleepiness may place the patient at significant risk for accidents and have a major impact on the person's health and sense of well-being.

As with other subjective symptoms, an individual's perception of sleepiness influences the complaint. Some patients may overreport the degree of sleepiness and note sleepiness even during periods of normal wakefulness. Other individuals may underreport and not recognize periods of sleepiness. For some of these individuals, sleepiness may be described as periods of lapse of attention or diminished cognitive abilities, such as missing an exit on the highway or brief delay in performing a task. Perception of sleepiness is also reduced with continued sleep deprivation. Individuals who are chronically sleep deprived become accustomed to their impairment and are less likely to recognize their degree of sleepiness.

Clinicians should always question their hypersomnic patients for clues of potential sleep debt; dyssomnia; medical or psychiatric causes; or use of medications, herbs, or supplements. Sleep deprivation is common in our society, and patients should be queried about their schedule during the week and weekends. Information about sleep habits and environment may disclose important factors contributing to the sleepiness.

Excessive sleepiness may result from a wide range of medical disorders and medication. Patients with heart, kidney, or liver failure and rheumatologic or endocrinologic disorders, such as hypothyroidism and diabetes mellitus, may note sleepiness and fatigue. Similarly, a wide range of medications may cause daytime sleepiness even when taken at night. Neurologic disorders, such as strokes, tumors, demyelinating diseases, and head trauma, can evoke excessive sleepiness. Sleepiness is frequently the cardinal symptom of many sleep disorders. Patients with sleep apnea, narcolepsy, idiopathic hypersomnia, or even parasomnias may note excessive daytime sleepiness as their main complaint. Historical features of snoring, observed apneas, morning headaches, cataplexy, sleep paralysis, hypnagogic hallucinations, and confusion on arousals suggest contributions of a specific sleep disorder. Individuals with idiopathic hypersomnolence have unrelenting daytime sleepiness despite prolonged periods of sleep, which differentiates this disorder from sleep deprivation. Many adults with idiopathic hypersomnia find naps are not refreshing, whereas patients with narcolepsy (type 1 and type 2) note brief naps actually improve their daytime sleepiness.

Physical findings are few in patients with sleepiness. Frequent pauses, slowed responses, drooping eyelids, and repetitive yawning support the complaint of sleepiness. Patients may be asleep when the clinician enters the examination room, and some patients may show signs of chronic sleepiness, such as dark circles under the eyes. The patient's neurologic examination may show findings of inattentiveness or even brief "microsleeps."

Sleepiness can be quantified subjectively by questionnaires or by objective assessments, such as the Multiple Sleep Latency Test (MSLT). The Epworth Sleepiness Scale is one example of a quantifiable subjective measure of sleepiness and has been translated into several languages (Table 66.1).[6] For this scale, the individual is asked to rate on a scale of 0 to 3 (0, no chance; 3, high likelihood) the chance of dozing in a series of eight situations. This score has a modest correlation with physiologic measures of sleep but has a better correlation with the respiratory disturbance index in patients with obstructive sleep apnea (Table 66.2).

Two quantitative tests exist to measure ability to fall asleep and to stay awake: MSLT and Maintenance of Wakefulness Test (MWT). The MSLT quantifies objective sleepiness on the basis of the time to onset of physiologic changes associated with sleep across five trials separated by 2 hours each across

Table 66.1 The Epworth Sleepiness Scale

Name: ________________________________

Today's date: ________________________________
______ Your age (years): ________________________________

Your sex (male = M; female = F): ________________________________

How likely are you to doze off or fall asleep in the following situations in contrast to feeling just tired? This refers to your usual way of life in recent times. Even if you have not done some of these things recently, try to work out how they would have affected you. Use the following scale to choose the most appropriate number for each situation:
0 = would never doze
1 = slight chance of dozing
2 = moderate chance of dozing
3 = high chance of dozing

Situation[a]	Chance of Dozing
Sitting and reading	________
Watching television	________
Sitting, inactive in a public place (e.g., a theater or a meeting)	________
As a passenger in a car for an hour without a break	________
Lying down to rest in the afternoon when circumstances permit	________
Sitting and talking to someone	________
Sitting quietly after a lunch without alcohol	________
In a car while stopped for a few minutes in traffic	________

Thank you for your cooperation.

[a]The numbers for the eight situations are added together to give a global score between 0 and 24.
From Johns MW. A new method for measuring daytime sleepiness: the Epworth Sleepiness Scale. *Sleep*. 1991;14:540–45.

the typical wake period. Sleep is determined by the loss of the posterior dominant rhythm (PDR) in the electroencephalogram or, in the absence of PDR, slow eye movements, vertex sharp waves, and slowing of the background electroencephalographic activity. The MSLT uses these physiologic markers to quantify the time to sleep. Unfortunately, the MSLT is not well correlated with daytime function, and there is significant overlap between individuals deemed "normal" and those deemed to have sleep disruption. Although the MSLT can "quantify" the degree of sleepiness on a particular day, the test is only validated for the diagnosis of narcolepsy (type 1 and type 2). The MWT quantifies the propensity to stay awake across four attempts in a dimly lit room. This test has not been extensively tested in relationship to daytime function. These tests are covered in greater detail in Chapter 207.

FATIGUE

The complaint of fatigue is a complex symptom typically related to the perception of lack of energy. Many patients with excessive daytime sleepiness note fatigue or decreased energy. Patients may be aware of the lack of energy and not perceive the degree of sleepiness or confuse the symptom of fatigue with excessive sleepiness. Although frequently noted in combination, fatigue is distinct from excessive sleepiness. Patients with just fatigue may not have an increased ability to fall asleep but believe that a good night of sleep would improve their lack of energy. Distinguishing sleepiness from fatigue can be difficult even for the most astute clinicians. Detailed questioning regarding ability to fall asleep can be helpful. Sometimes using the Fatigue Severity Scale in combination with the Epworth Sleepiness Scale can help differentiate the two symptoms.[7] Patients with insomnia also frequently complain of fatigue related to disrupted sleep, as well as patients with immunologic, endocrinologic, or organ failure. Similarly, patients with depression frequently have associated fatigue without sleepiness.

SNORING

Snoring is the sound created by turbulent airflow vibrating upper airway soft tissue. Usually more prominent during inspiration, snoring occurs in approximately one-third of adults

Table 66.2 Scores for Various Conditions: Ages and Epworth Sleepiness Scale Scores of Experimental Subjects

Subjects/Diagnoses	Total Number of Subjects (M/F)	Age in Years (Mean ± SD)	Epworth Sleepiness Scale Scores (Mean ± SD)	Range
Healthy control subjects	30 (14/16)	36.4 ± 9.9	5.9 ± 2.2	2–10
Primary snoring	32 (29/3)	45.7 ± 10.7	6.5 ± 3.0	0–11
Obstructive sleep apnea syndrome	55 (53/2)	48.4 ± 10.7	11.7 ± 4.6	4–23
Narcolepsy	13 (8/5)	46.6 ± 12.0	17.5 ± 3.5	13–23
Idiopathic hypersomnia	14 (8/6)	41.4 ± 14.0	17.9 ± 3.1	12–24
Insomnia	16 (6/12)	40.3 ± 14.6	2.2 ± 2.0	0–6
Periodic limb movement disorder	18 (16/2)	52.5 ± 10.3	9.2 ± 4.0	2–16

M/F, Male/female; SD, standard deviation.
From Johns MW. A new method for measuring daytime sleepiness: the Epworth Sleepiness Scale. *Sleep*. 1991;14:540–45.

and in greater than 7% of children.[8,9] Many adults have little knowledge or recognition of their snoring habits, and accounts from bed partners may be more helpful for the clinician.

Snoring is usually worse in the supine position after sleep deprivation or alcohol ingestion. Loud snoring may not disturb sound sleepers, but some patients may report complaints from family members and even neighbors. Snoring may continue for decades. Persistent loud snoring is a classic symptom of obstructive sleep apnea syndrome, but the absence of snoring does not exclude the diagnosis of apnea. Some patients have airway dynamics that are not conducive to snoring. This is especially true in patients who have had upper airway surgical procedures that eliminated flaccid tissue. Other individuals, such as those with neuromuscular disorders, may not generate enough force to produce turbulent airflow.

Snoring, for many people, produces little disruption in their lives, but snoring may have implications on overall health. Individuals who snore have a greater risk of vascular disease. Witnesses may be able to account for snoring occurring in bursts or associated with snorts, gasps, choking, body jerks, and movements. Patients may recall being awoken by their own gasps and relay symptoms of gastroesophageal reflux. These associated symptoms raise the suspicion of obstructive sleep apnea.

SLEEP APNEA

Apnea is the absence of ventilation. In the sleep laboratory, apneas are defined by the cessation of breathing for more than 10 seconds and are usually associated with oxygen desaturation and arousal.[10] Although snoring is very common, witnessed apneas, nocturnal gasping or choking are the most reliable subjective indicators of sleep apnea.[11] Some patients may have hundreds of events in a single night and are unable to obtain quality sleep because of the frequent arousals. These individuals are typically unaware of the arousals, but some may report being aware of the occasional awakening with the gasp or snort. Sleep apnea is classified in two major forms: obstructive and central.

Obstructive apnea is the most common form of sleep apnea. These apneas are due to obstruction in the upper airway and more commonly noted during stage N1, N2, or R (rapid eye movement [REM] sleep). Snoring is a frequent associated complaint, but a wide variety of symptoms may be present. Some questionnaires, such as the sleep apnea section of the Sleep Disorder Questionnaire, STOP-BANG, or Berlin Questionnaire, a combination of items regarding snoring, witnessed apneas, body habitus, and associated disorders such as hypertension (Table 66.3),[12,13] provide a summary score that correlates with presence of obstructive sleep apnea, but the questionnaires have been tested only in selected populations. Thus the questionnaires themselves are rough guides and do not confirm the diagnosis of sleep apnea. Astute clinicians should not exclude patients on the basis of a low score on a questionnaire. The physical examination may show structural evidence for airway obstruction. Many patients are obese and have a large neck or crowded upper airway, yet some have a normal body habitus. Common structural abnormalities, such as narrow nasal passage, long soft palate, large tonsils, or retroflexed mandible leading to a small airway, contribute to airway obstruction. Sleep apnea is associated with significant health risks and lowers the quality of life of both the patient and bed partner. Mounting evidence from multiple studies, such as the Sleep Heart Health Study, indicates that hypopneas with oxygen desaturation correlate with greater risk of vascular disease.[14] These are discussed in greater detail in Chapters 135,136, and 146 to 150.

Central apnea is the absence of ventilation due to an absence of contraction of the lower respiratory musculature. These patients have pauses in respiration also associated with oxygen

Table 66.3 Key Features of the Berlin Questionnaire

Height ________	Age ________
Weight ________	Gender ________
Has your weight changed in the last 5 years?	Increase Decreased No change
Do you snore?	Yes No Do not know
Your snoring is	Slightly louder than breathing As loud as talking Louder than talking Very loud
How often do you snore?	Nearly every day 3 to 4 times per week 1 to 2 times per week 1 to 2 times per month Never or almost never
Has your snoring bothered other people?	Yes No
Has anyone noticed that you quit breathing during your sleep?	Almost every day 3 to 4 times per week 1 to 2 times per week 1 to 2 times per month Never or almost never
Are you tired or fatigued after your sleep?	Nearly every day 3 to 4 times per week 1 to 2 times per week 1 to 2 times per month Never or almost never
During your wake time, do you feel tired, fatigued, or not up to par?	Nearly every day 3 to 4 times per week 1 to 2 times per week 1 to 2 times per month Never or almost never
Have you ever fallen asleep while driving?	Yes No If so, how often does it occur? Nearly every day 3 to 4 times per week 1 to 2 times per week 1 to 2 times per month Never or almost never
Do you have high blood pressure?	Yes No Do not know

Modified from the Berlin Questionnaire; from the editors of *Sleep Breath.* 2000;4:187–92, with the permission of Kingman P. Strohl.

desaturation and arousals. Central apneas can be caused by narcotics or a neurologic abnormality in the brainstem or other areas involved in regulation of respiration. Cheyne-Stokes breathing can have features of both central and obstructive apnea. The classic pattern of crescendo-decrescendo breathing with a central apnea can be seen in individuals with heart failure, neurologic lesions, and metabolic or toxic encephalopathies. This pattern may be present only in sleep and signal underlying disease. Apneas may follow other neurologic events, such as nocturnal seizures, and are more prevalent after acute strokes and seizures. Central apnea is reviewed in Chapters 124 and 125.

CATAPLEXY

Cataplexy is the abrupt loss of muscle tone triggered by strong emotional stimuli or physical exercise.[15] Patients are aware of their surroundings and have clear memory for the complete events. Events can be triggered by a joke, surprise, anger, fear, or athletic endeavors. Individual experiences vary from a mild feeling of weakness to severe falls. Cataplectic attacks start during several seconds and may start with brief waves of loss of tone that may appear like jerks initially. Most symptoms start in the face and neck with features of ptosis, mouth opening, tongue protrusion, and brief head drops, then progress to the rest of the body.[15] Intermixing with brief jerks is common. Patients may describe more subtle events, such as a feeling of slowness to respond or slurring or speech. The events are generally brief, lasting seconds to less than a few minutes. Patients then regain muscle control and have no postictal confusion or memory deficits. Longer events may be ended with the patient's entering sleep and then awakening. Examination of the patient during the cataplectic attack will demonstrate paralysis with diffuse hypotonia, absence of deep tendon reflexes, diminished corneal reflexes, preserved pupillary responses, and many times phasic muscle twitching. Phasic muscle twitching can occur as single jerks or repetitive muscle twitching and is most frequently seen in the face, sometimes being confused with seizure activity.

The combination of excessive daytime sleepiness and cataplexy is nearly always related to narcolepsy type 1. Cataplexy can rarely be seen as an isolated symptom suggestive of an underlying neurologic lesion in the brainstem. Maintenance of consciousness and memory helps differentiate these events from most seizures and syncope. The historical feature of clear emotional triggers differentiates cataplexy from vertebral basilar insufficiency and the group of neuromuscular disorders known to produce periodic paralysis. Cataplexy also is differentiated from myasthenia gravis by the abrupt onset and absence of muscle fatigue with repetitive stimulation that is typical of myasthenia gravis.

SLEEP PARALYSIS

Sleep paralysis is an inability to move during the transition into or out of sleep. The association with intentional sleep distinguishes these events from cataplexy. Patients may describe complete awareness of their surroundings or feeling partially asleep with awareness but be unable to move even their fingers or to speak. Patients may try to scream but produce only a whisper. Some individuals will describe a feeling of suffocation and be able to resume breathing only when the event has passed. Patients frequently describe a strong feeling of impending doom, being chased, or having to escape imminent danger. On occasion, patients may note the feeling that someone else is in the bedroom. Auditory and tactile hallucinations may accompany the events, and patients may recount dramatic stories. These events can be emotionally profound and leave a lasting memory that patients vividly recall years later. Most sleep paralysis episodes last a few minutes and usually end after the patient is touched or is alerted. If the event is allowed to persist, the patient usually reenters sleep and awakens later. These acute events are experienced by many individuals after severe sleep deprivation, schedule disruption, or ingestion of alcohol and more recurrent forms may be more frequently seen in patients with narcolepsy or individuals with posttraumatic stress disorder.[16]

HYPNAGOGIC AND HYPNOPOMPIC HALLUCINATIONS

Hallucinations can occur with sleep onset (hypnagogic) or at the end of sleep (hypnopompic).[17] These hallucinations may include visual, auditory, or tactile components and may last seconds to minutes. The events occur at the transition between wake and sleep and incorporate some dream-like features. They can be relatively pleasant or very terrifying and difficult to distinguish from reality. Patients may note a feeling of weightlessness, falling, flying, or out-of-body experiences and may sometimes terminate with a sudden jerk (hypnic jerk). Visual hallucinations may be described as poorly formed colors and shapes or well-formed images of people and animals. The events are terminated once the patient awakens.

Exploding head syndrome is a loud, painless sound of explosion that occurs near sleep onset. This parasomnia is benign and may be associated with a hallucinatory flash of light or feeling that something occurred inside the patient's head.

In the face of excessive daytime sleepiness, patients with hypnagogic hallucinations should be evaluated for narcolepsy. These events may be repetitive but are not usually stereotypic. This lack of stereotypic feature distinguishes these events from seizures. Individuals may experience these events after sleep deprivation or change in sleep schedule. Alcohol ingestion or withdrawal of REM suppressants may also evoke these events. The relationship of sleep to these hallucinations distinguishes them from hallucinations of psychosis and dementia. Hypnagogic hallucinations are shorter in duration than peduncular hallucinations. Some individuals with dementia have hallucinations at night. These types of hallucinations are associated with cognitive impairment during the day and most commonly are seen in individuals with Lewy body dementia but can occur in other forms of dementia. Small people or animals predominant these hallucinations, and many patients have these events while awake.

AUTOMATIC BEHAVIOR

Automatic behavior is purposeful but inappropriate activities that occur with the patient partially asleep. Patients relay stories of putting milk containers in the microwave oven, cereal bowls in the dryer, or even missing an exit on the highway. Sleep-deprived soldiers have been reported to continue marching in the wrong direction. Patients appear drowsy or groggy during the event and are usually partially or totally amnestic for the actual happenings. Events may last minutes to an hour. Automatic behavior and "sleep inertia," the persistence of profound sleepiness into awake, are more common in individuals with idiopathic hypersomnolence but are also common in patients with a delayed sleep phase.[4]

These events are distinguished from seizures by the lack of stereotypic behavior. Automatisms associated with seizures are usually stereotyped and repetitive, such as picking, rubbing, or lip smacking. Patients with sleep-related automatic behavior appear sleepy but can be alerted and answer questions appropriately, in contrast to postictal confusion and metabolic or toxic encephalopathy. The quick return of orientation with a lack of bewilderment and anxiety also differentiates this from transient global amnesia.

EXCESSIVE MOVEMENT IN SLEEP OR PARASOMNIA

Individuals and bed partners may complain of frequent movement during the sleep period. In part, this complaint may be more concerning to the bed partner than to the patient. This is also a common complaint among patients who complain of insomnia and individuals with sleep apnea. Some individuals will complain of being active sleepers and imply that they are mentally active or have inability to turn off their mind. These individuals need an evaluation focusing on features of insomnia. Those who are physically active need evaluation for the movements or parasomnia.

Parasomnia refers to undesirable physical or behavioral phenomena that occur predominantly during sleep. They include disorders of arousals, such as sleepwalking and night terrors; sleep-wake transition disorders, such as bruxism or rhythmic movement disorder (e.g., head banging); and REM parasomnias, such as REM sleep behavior disorder (RBD). These behavioral events may mimic epileptic seizures or other psychiatric events, and a clear description from a keen observer is very helpful in leading to a diagnosis. The parasomnias are covered in greater detail in Chapters 115 to 120.

Key features of age at onset, time of night of the events, memory for the events, and family history are important in historically distinguishing the etiology of parasomnias. Stereotypic behavior, recurrence of the same behavior with each event, can also help in categorizing the events. Events such as periodic limb movements, rhythmic movement disorder, and epileptic seizures are associated with stereotypic behavior, whereas sleeptalking, sleepwalking, night terrors, and dream enactment incur different behavior with each event. Although historical features can be useful in distinguishing these disorders, most patients require polysomnographic recording to delineate the cause.

Sleeptalking

Sleeptalking is a relatively frequent event of utterances to coherent conversation during sleep. This usually occurs in the lighter stages of non–rapid eye movement (NREM) sleep but can occur in REM (stage R) sleep. The patients have no memory of the events and may convey information that may have little resemblance to the truth. Many people talk in their sleep, and this is considered a normal variant. In the absence of other sleep disturbances, sleeptalking is of little medical concern.

Sleepwalking

Sleepwalking events are usually part of the disorders of arousal indicating incomplete arousal typically from slow-wave sleep (stage N3) occurring during the first half of the sleep period. The events can be minor behaviors and movement or elaborate behaviors, including dressing, unlocking locks, minor tasks, and even driving. Patients usually have little or no memory for the event. Patients can recall various feelings or impressions from the events, and some imagery is more common in adults. The patients do not exhibit significant tachycardia, sweating, or expression of fear. The lack of screaming and autonomic features differentiates sleepwalking from sleep terrors. Both children and adults with a history of recent sleepwalking should be questioned for signs of other sleep disorders. Any disorder evoking arousals may increase the likelihood of these events, and so patients should be carefully questioned for symptoms of other sleep disorders. Patients typically have normal neurologic examination findings during wakefulness.

Sleep Terrors

Sleep terrors are a more intense form of disorder of arousal with a predominance of autonomic expression. Witnesses rarely forget the patient's sudden arousal accompanied by a piercing scream or cry, autonomic output, and behavioral manifestation of intense fear, but the patient has little to no memory for the event. The onset of the events is abrupt, and patients have tachycardia, tachypnea, flushing, diaphoresis, and mydriasis. The patients are confused and disoriented, and attempts to intercede may result in prolongation of the event and potential harm to the person trying to wake the patient. Patients can become violent, resulting in injury to the patient and bed partners. Less than 1% of adults may have these events.[18] They typically occur in the first third of the night, and the events are nonstereotypic. Patients typically have a normal diurnal neurologic examination, and as with sleepwalking, patients should be questioned for the presence of other sleep disorders.

Confusional Arousals

Confusional arousals can occur during any arousal from NREM sleep. These events are characterized by disorientation, slow speech and mentation, or inappropriate behavior. The patients have memory impairment for the event, and the events can be induced with forced arousal. The course of these events usually becomes less frequent with age but may remain stable in adulthood.

Patients may have other complex sleep-related behaviors. One group of individuals may have eating as a sleep-related event, as seen in a patient with a sleep-related eating disorder.[18] These patients will eat high-calorie, sometimes bizarre foods and have no or little memory. They have morning anorexia and unexplained weight gain. Another group may report episodes of sexual intercourse during sleep. Again, these individuals relate no memory for their events.

Sleep-Related Groaning (Catathrenia)

Rarely, patients or families may present because of repetitive nocturnal groaning. Bed partners usually express concern because the patients have long expiratory groans that sound mournful. Patients usually have no recollection of the sound or feeling distressed but may have morning hoarseness. No other detectable abnormalities are found on physical examination.

These groaning events have been compared with central apneas, and the disorder is now classified under sleep-related breathing disorders.[19]

Dream Enactment

REM sleep (stage R) is characterized by diffuse muscle atonia. Normally, only brief phasic muscle activity is noted during REM sleep, but pathologic dream enactment behavior can include punching, kicking, leaping, running, talking, yelling, and any behavior that could occur during a dream.[20] Bed partners are frequently injured, and patients may go to great lengths to protect themselves and bed partners. This dream enactment is commonly seen as part of RBD. Patients usually have a vivid recall of the actual dreams that correlates with the witnessed behavior, and many dreams involve fleeing or defending themes. Dream recall is not uniformly noted, and patients may not be willing to talk about the dream that led them to seek medical attention. These events occur more commonly in the latter half of the night but can occur any time that the patient enters REM sleep. Patients may have multiple events during a single night. Most cases begin in late adulthood, but children with symptoms of RBD have been described. RBD can be induced by medication, and cases have been reported of tricyclic antidepressants, monoamine oxidase inhibitors, and serotonin reuptake inhibitors causing RBD-like behavior. Acute forms of RBD can also occur during alcohol withdrawal and potentially benzodiazepine withdrawal. The more chronic form of RBD may have behaviors occurring for years before presentation for medical evaluation. RBD has been linked to α-synucleinopathies.[21] This group of disorders includes Parkinson disease, multiple system atrophy, and Lewy body dementia. Patients need a complete neurologic evaluation to look for signs of degenerative disorders. Other identifiable neurologic disorders, such as strokes, posterior fossa tumors, and demyelination, have been reported.[21]

Nightmares

Nightmares or recurrent disturbing dream mentation can be a presenting symptom of sleep disturbance. The hallmark of nightmares is emotionally intense dreaming associated with fear, anxiety, anger, sadness, or other negative emotions. Individuals awaken from stage R or light NREM sleep to full alertness and usually recall the event immediately. Nightmares are most commonly associated with a psychologically disturbing event or trauma but may also be a result of medications, such as antihypertensives, antidepressants, or dopamine agonists. Nightmares can occur in patients with narcolepsy and in patients with sleep apnea.

Sleep-Related Rhythmic Movement Disorder

Rhythmic movement disorder can be manifested as a variety of distracting behaviors that occur before sleep onset. The movements are stereotypic, usually involving large muscles, and are sustained into light sleep. Movements may include head banging, body rocking, leg rolling, humming, and chanting and are frequently more concerning to the bed partner and family than to the patient. Many patients are relatively unaware of the movement, and others will describe the movement as a calming effect or as a compulsion before sleep. This behavior is frequently seen in infants and young children, and the prevalence diminishes with age. It is more commonly seen in individuals with mental challenges or autism and is more prevalent in males. Emotional stress may provoke it. Patients can be easily alerted during the events, which helps differentiate these events from seizures (see Chapter 122).

Sleep-Related Bruxism

Sleep bruxism can also occur as a rhythmic or repetitive movement during sleep.[22] Grinding or clenching of the teeth during sleep may produce bizarre sounds, and patients can even rarely vocalize with the episodes. Patients may have abnormal wear of the teeth, jaw pain, headache, facial pain, or tooth pain. They may have hundreds of events per night, and the events increase with emotional stress. Some studies suggest that as much as 85% of the population grinds their teeth to some degree during the day or night. These events often occur in children, and persistence of symptoms is occasionally associated with a familial tendency.

RESTLESS LEGS SYNDROME AND PERIODIC MOVEMENTS OF SLEEP

Patients may complain of an unpleasant crawling, deep aching, or need-to-move sensation in the legs or arms that is improved by motion of the extremities. Diagnostic criteria focus on four main symptoms: the sensation or urge to move the limbs that is worse with rest, improves with movement, and is more frequent in the evening.[23] In addition, the patient must note a symptom of concern, distress, sleep disturbance, or some impairment related to the sensations. Patients with RLS may relay that the discomfort can be debilitating at times, and some individuals are even driven to pursue extreme measures to decrease the symptoms. Most patients experience the symptoms while sitting or lying down and may complain of the need to walk or to have continuous movement of their legs. These symptoms can lead to individuals walking until the early morning hours or trying to sleep with continuous motion in their legs. Other individuals will use a combination of medication and alcohol to reduce the symptoms. Some patients note that their legs will move or dance on their own, indicating periodic limb movements in wakefulness. Some medications used to treat RLS actually make the symptoms worse through a process called augmentation, where the symptoms present earlier in the day and are more intense.

RLS usually occurs along with periodic movements of sleep. Periodic movements of sleep are repetitive stereotyped movements, typically of the lower extremities, that occur during sleep; they consist of the extension of the great toe with dorsiflexion of the ankle and flexion of the knee and hip. Patients or a bed partner may complain of kicking or arm movements at night and rarely can involve the trunk. These movements may occur as periodic events or appear random. The individual movements are relatively brief, lasting 0.5 to 10.0 seconds and occur at 5- to 90-second intervals.[10] Although a majority of individuals with restless legs have periodic limb movements of sleep, only a minority of patients with periodic movements of sleep will have complaints of restless legs, excessive daytime sleepiness, or insomnia. Many patients are unaware of the movements, but bed partners usually are cognizant of the movements. Similar factors that provoke RLS increase the likelihood of periodic limb movements. Periodic movements of sleep have been associated with uremia, anemia, arthritis, peripheral neuropathy, spinal cord lesions, antidepressants, antiemetics, and caffeine use. Further discussion is in Chapter 121.

SLEEP-RELATED HEADACHE

Headaches occurring in the morning or during sleep are a common symptom.[24] Almost three-fourths of the population has occasional headache; this symptom is relatively nonspecific. Morning or waking headache is more specifically linked to sleep dysfunction but may also indicate elevated blood pressure at night or evidence of hypoventilation. Headaches also can occur through the night and may be associated with specific types of headaches, such as hypnic headache, migraine, or cluster headache. Characteristics of the headache, such as location, quality and nature of pain, time of the headache, and potential associations, can aid in determining the etiology. Approximately half of patients with obstructive sleep apnea and hypoventilation note morning headache that is usually dull and generalized and usually clears within an hour of waking. Patients with chronic obstructive pulmonary disease and obstructive sleep apnea may develop morning headache from the increase in carbon dioxide, low oxygen saturation, or vascular changes. Patients with sinus disorders, muscle contraction headache, postalcohol intake, and withdrawal from medication (rebound headaches) may have distinct patterns. Cluster headaches are noted to occur in REM sleep. Hypnic headaches, or alarm clock headache due to their regularity, are throbbing or sharp pains lasting 15 to 60 minutes and awaken the patient typically between 1 a.m. to 3 a.m. Headaches that routinely awaken patients from sleep should be further evaluated, potentially including head imaging. Patients with brain tumors frequently note worsening of headache at night. Headaches in sleep are discussed in greater detail in Chapter 107.

SYSTEMIC FEATURES

The connection of good sleep to good health continues to expand our understanding of the importance of sleep. Sleep plays a role in endocrine regulation, weight, and metabolism and has been hypothesized to improve neuronal network proficiency and function. Therefore sleep disorders may influence both regulatory processes and compensatory mechanisms.

Sleep disorders may influence systemic disorders by three general mechanisms: directly cause the primary physiologic changes that result in systemic disease, exacerbate a preexisting disorder by altering a normal compensatory mechanism, or be the hallmark symptom of the systemic disease, sharing a common pathophysiologic mechanism. Sleep disorders may result in systemic manifestations, as noted in sleep-related breathing disorders. Sleep-related disordered breathing can result in a variety of vascular and autonomic changes that increase the likelihood of hypertension and other vascular disorders.

Physicians must question patients with high-risk disorders, including those with hypertension, vascular disease, heart disease, diabetes mellitus, and obesity, as well as those with cognitive complaints for symptoms of sleep dysfunction that may indicate sleep disorders acting as a cofactor. Sleep disorders, for example, obstructive sleep apnea or hypoventilation, may exacerbate underlying conditions, such as hypertension, diabetes mellitus, congestive heart failure, epilepsy, and depression. Thus the clinician must pay attention to aggravation of symptoms of medical, neurologic, or psychiatric dysfunction as a clue to disordered sleep. The interplay of sleep and brain function makes symptoms of neurologic and psychiatric disease a natural manifestation of sleep dysfunction. This has been documented in individuals with epilepsy and mood disorders and appears to extend to those with other neurologic and psychiatric dysfunction. Patients may not be aware of the connection of sleep to their other medical problems or may not place emphasis on their sleep symptoms. Therefore the clinician needs to consider the potential of sleep disturbance as an aggravating factor and to recognize the relationship of systemic findings to sleep disruption. Patients may also display a systemic illness that may share a common pathophysiologic mechanism with a sleep disorder. In individuals with anemia and restless legs, iron deficiency may be the common link, and thus appropriate treatment of the underlying cause may improve the symptoms of both. Last, the sleep symptom may be the hallmark of another process, as observed with RBD preceding the development of other neurologic disorders, such as Parkinson disease. Although these symptoms may not be considered the typical cardinal manifestations of sleep disorders, they do represent an important aspect and entry point for patients into the medical system. Recognition of the systemic manifestations of sleep disorders is an important step in understanding the full relationship of sleep to the body.

PEDIATRIC CARDINAL MANIFESTATIONS

Symptoms of sleep disorders in children can be strikingly different from those in adults and are likely to be overlooked or misinterpreted.[25] Moreover, disruption of family dynamics, psychosocial factors that influence the family unit, and temperamental differences between parent-child pairs maybe reported as childhood sleep disorders. Sleep-onset associations, cultural norms, and parental expectations can influence the perception of sleep problems in infants and toddlers. Children can present with a range of physical and behavioral manifestations. In young children, sleep disturbances may present as poor growth, learning difficulties, persistent fussiness, inconsolability, or increased oppositional behavior. School-aged children may exhibit suboptimal academic performance, inattention or hyperactivity, or daydreaming behavior in sedentary settings. Adolescents fall asleep in class and may present with affective symptoms that need to be differentiated from primary psychiatric disorders. In children with symptoms of RLS (often reported as "growing pains"), a strong family history is often present, suggesting a hereditary predisposition with age-dependent expression. In all ages, unrefreshing nocturnal sleep is often a clue to sleep disturbance. Although many of these symptoms are nonspecific, the clinician must be aware of the role of sleep dysfunction in the genesis of the symptoms.

CLINICAL PEARL

Patients may present to the clinician with initial complaints that may seem unrelated to sleep, such as morning headache, fogginess during the day, or elevated blood pressure. The patient may not initially be concerned about sleep or even be aware of sleep symptoms. Clarifying functional questions, for instance, describing how they feel during certain activities, such as the process of getting up in the morning or after lunch, may give additional clues. Also, family members may be aware of sleep issues before the patient and thus lend insight into the impact of sleep on the patient's clinical picture.

SUMMARY

Sleep provides the benchmark for many aspects of our lives. The restorative powers of sleep improve our wakefulness and ability to attain higher levels of functioning, whereas poor sleep has a negative impact on health, sense of well-being, and performance. Obvious manifestations of poor sleep, such as daytime sleepiness, insomnia, and sleep-related events, are the hallmark signs for further investigation. Our understanding of the intricate relationship of sleep and health must go beyond the most apparent manifestations of sleepiness. As astute clinicians, we must pay attention to the obvious and discrete signs; predominance of negative over positive memories, trouble with creative solutions, obesity, or poor healing may suggest sleep disruption. We must search for more clues that delineate the connection of sleep to health. Through the insight of the connection between sleep and the body, we will expand our recognition of these cardinal manifestations of sleep disorders. Identification of individuals who need further evaluation and application of appropriate therapies as described in the following chapters will aid both patients and society.

SELECTED READINGS

American Academy of Sleep Medicine. *International Classification of Sleep Disorders: Diagnostic and Coding Manual.* 3rd ed. Westchester, Ill: American Academy of Sleep Medicine; 2014.

Baumann CR, Mignot E, Lammers GJ, et al. Challenges in diagnosing narcolepsy without cataplexy: a consensus statement. *Sleep.* 2014;37:1035–1042.

Boeve BF, Silber MH, Ferman TJ, Lin SC, et al. Clinicopathologic correlations in 172 cases of rapid eye movement sleep behavior disorder with or without a coexisting neurologic disorder. *Sleep Med.* 2013;14:754–762.

Drager LF, McEvoy RD, Barbe F, Lorenzi-Filho G, Redline S. INCOSACT Initiative (International Collaboration of Sleep Apnea Cardiovascular Trialists). Sleep apnea and cardiovascular disease: lessons from recent trials and need for team science. *Circulation.* 2017;136:1840–1850.

Irfan M, Schenck CH, Howell MJ. Non–rapid eye movement sleep and overlap parasomnias. *Continuum (Minneap Minn).* 2017;23(4, Sleep Neurology):1035–1050.

Javaheri S, Barbe F, Campos-Rodriguez F, et al. Sleep apnea: types, mechanisms, and clinical cardiovascular consequences. *J Am Coll Cardiol.* 2017;69:841–858.

Kim TW, Jeong JH, Hong SC. The impact of sleep and circadian disturbance on hormones and metabolism. *Int J Endocrinol.* 2015;2015:591–729.

Morin CM, Drake CL, Harvey AG, et al. Insomnia disorder. *Nat Rev Dis Primers.* 2015;1:15026.

Ophoff D, Slaats MA, Boudewyns A, Glazemakers I, Van Hoorenbeeck K, Verhulst SL. Sleep disorders during childhood: a practical review. *Eur J Pediatr.* 2018;177:641–648.

Stefani A, Högl B. Diagnostic criteria, differential diagnosis, and treatment of minor motor activity and less well-known movement disorders of sleep. *Curr Treat Options Neurol.* 2019;21:1.

Trotti LM. Restless legs syndrome and sleep-related movement disorders. *Continuum (Minneap Minn).* 2017;23(4, Sleep Neurology):1005–1016.

Zeitzer JM. Control of sleep and wakefulness in health and disease. *Prog Mol Biol Transl Sci.* 2013;119:137–154.

A complete reference list can be found online at ExpertConsult.com.

Chapter 67

Physical Examination in Sleep Medicine

Alon Y. Avidan; Meir Kryger

Chapter Highlights

- The physical examination of patients presenting with sleep complaints remains a fundamental requirement based on the presenting symptoms, with appropriate alignment to the patients' age, gender, genetic predisposition, underlying comorbidities, and whether the patient participates in person or virtually.
- Patients should have their vital signs recorded (temperature, heart rate, blood pressure, pulse rate) along with height and weight to calculate the body mass index (BMI).
- Head and neck physical examination is critical for evaluation of people with any sleep complaints but particularly in the setting of evaluation for sleep-disordered breathing (SDB). Examination should include direct visualization of anatomic factors that could hinder airflow at the level of the upper airways using previously validated classification schemes, such as the Mallampati classification.
- In addition to high BMI, other factors that predispose people to SDB include increased neck circumference, macroglossia, retrognathia, tonsillar adenoid hypertrophy, overjet, nasal obstruction, and decreased cricomental space. The chapter reviews specific metrics and anatomic landmarks that serve as predisposing factors in contributing to disordered breathing during sleep.
- Specific phenotypes that contribute to SDB include metabolic storage diseases, such as systemic amyloidosis and mucopolysaccharidosis, which lead to abnormal upper airway tissue infiltration and airway restriction.
- Craniofacial anomalies play a key role in conferring a risk for SDB by reducing upper airway size, particularly in combination with genetic abnormalities in the setting of Down syndrome, Pierre Robin sequence, Treacher-Collins syndrome, and primary mandibular deficiency.
- Facial and body habitus phenotype in specific endocrinopathies, such as acromegaly, Graves disease, Cushing disease, and polycystic ovary syndrome, can predispose people to insomnia and should prompt clinicians to review these complaints in sufficient detail.
- Patients with neurologic disorders have significant sleep comorbidities. Those with neuromuscular disorders and motor neuron disease are especially vulnerable to SDB and nocturnal hypoventilation. Specific neurologic signs, such as bulbar weakness, the Gower maneuver from sitting to standing, and hypophonia, are critical and should prompt the clinician to inquire about breathing patterns at night, excessive sleepiness, and nighttime sleep disruption.
- Patients with abnormal behaviors and movements at night may present with unexplained bruises, ecchymosis, and nonspecific injuries the next day. Those with amnestic sleep-related eating may experience unexplained weight gain and dental disease.
- Symptoms of rapid eye movement sleep behavior disorder (RBD) often precede the onset of α-synucleinopathies, such as Parkinson disease. This is one example why all sleep clinicians should familiarize themselves with the key components of the neurologic examination and be able to identify people with anosmia, autonomic changes, bradykinesia, cogwheel rigidity, masked facies, and resting tremor in the setting of RBD.
- Patients with bruxism occasionally demonstrate dental consequences, including teeth fractures; masseter muscle hypertrophy; tenderness in the masseter, temporal muscle regions, and joints; and inner buccal mucosa ridging.
- Patients with narcolepsy type 1 (NT1) may present with increased BMI, autonomic dysfunction, and cataplexy. Cataplexy is difficult to validate on physical examination, but cataplectic facies manifests in children and consists of tongue protrusion, ptosis, and facial grimacing and is unique to NT1 even in the absence of a stimulus.

The physical examination of the patient presenting with sleep complaints represents a critical opportunity to corroborate the historical narrative and clinical suspicion in support of a presumptive diagnosis of a sleep disorder. Historically, the physical contact through examination provides patients a nonverbal sense of comfort and helps fortify relationships between clinicians and patients. The physical examination legitimizes human connection, particularly in forging a therapeutic alliance between clinicians and their patients.[1] Although touch has diagnostic value for the physician, it also has therapeutic value for the patient because physical touch can implicitly confer comfort and reassurance.[2] The 2020 SAR-CoV-19 (COVID-19) pandemic and the necessary physical distancing has accelerated the transition to a new model of remote sleep medicine care that embraces the capacity to use technologies to deliver and bridge care. Although telemedicine (telesleep) is a solution to address the COVID-19 crisis, it is antithetical to the quintessence of medicine based on human touch—the capacity for intimacy via the physical examination to promote compassion and empathy.[3]

This chapter will review the key attribute of the physical examination as applied to major sleep disorders by using specific illustrations. These include findings observed in sleep-disordered breathing (SDB); hypoventilation syndromes; narcolepsy; parasomnias; movement disorders of sleep, including restless legs syndrome (RLS) and bruxism; and psychiatric conditions. After the narrative medical history, the sleep care provider performs the physical examination, a key and necessary element in evaluating patients with sleep disorders. The examination may provide important clues that lead to elucidation of the etiology and pathophysiology of the sleep disorder. These will help guide the clinician in determining what diagnostic tests will be ordered, what comorbidities require management, and ultimately what therapy will be used. The sleep physical examination is a critical component for monitoring outcome to treatment of many sleep disorders. See also Chapter 169, which is specific to oropharyngeal growth and skeletal malformations.

SLEEP APNEA

Obstructive sleep apnea (OSA) is associated with multiple anatomic and physical risk factors. Some of these require elaborate measurements of nasopharyngeal anatomy, such as cephalometric radiographic techniques, whereas others measure phenotypic attributes that undergo dynamic changes in response to maneuvers. The most commonly used signs are static, anthropometric measurements from simple examination of oropharyngeal and craniofacial structure.[4] However, at the time of the initial evaluation of the patient with suspected SDB, the main physical evaluation relates to obesity, as reflected by elevated body mass index (BMI), and increased neck circumference (NC).[5]

Figure 67.1 summarizes the key anatomic changes that result from increasing age and BMI: The airways become

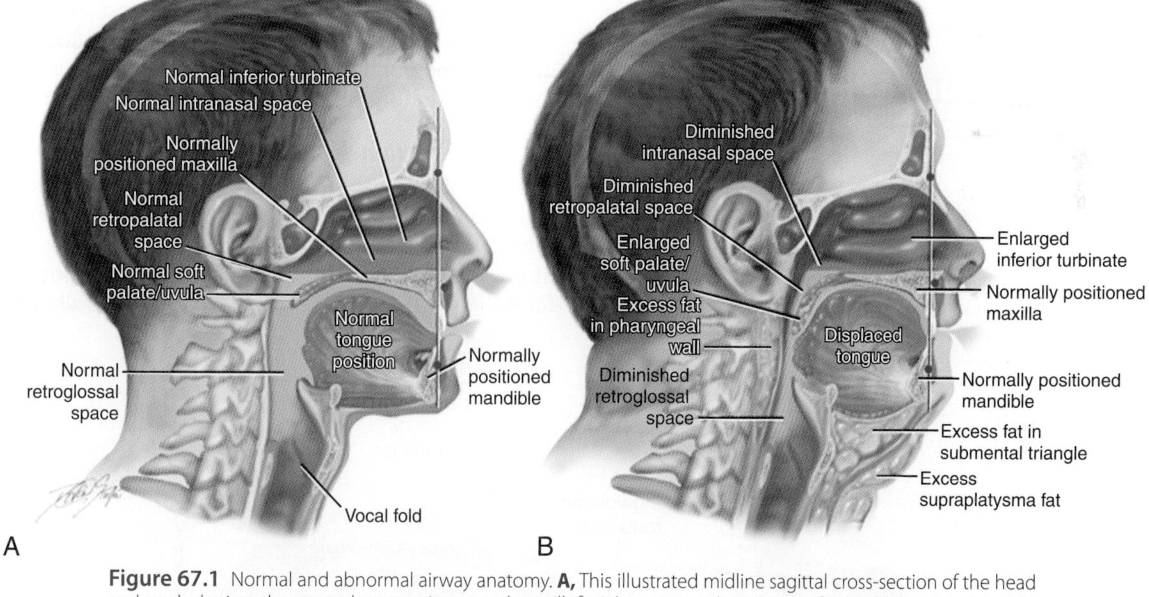

Figure 67.1 Normal and abnormal airway anatomy. **A,** This illustrated midline sagittal cross-section of the head and neck depicts the normal upper airway and maxillofacial spaces and anatomy of a healthy, normal-weight 20-year-old man. The patient has a normal upper and lower facial skeleton and normal soft tissue indicators (soft palate, tongue, tonsils, and adenoids), without any compromise of the intranasal cavity. **B,** With increasing age and weight gain, the same individual, 3 decades later, has an elevated body mass index. Although the anatomy of the upper and lower facial skeleton remains fixed without any changes, fatty tissue consisting of adipose cells has expanded and infiltrated the crevices and space in the upper airway. Particularly compromised are the retropharyngeal and the lateral pharyngeal tissues, the soft palate, and the floor of the mouth, culminating in restricted airflow. At age 20 years, the patient had normal upper airway space; the intranasal, retropalatal, and the retroglossal sites were all well visualized and with appropriate space for air flow to proceed smoothly and unimpeded. At age 50 years, he has developed obstructive sleep apnea: The normal airspace (*green*) is severely compromised because of restriction of the upper airway, intranasal space, and the retropalatal and retroglossal spaces. A perfect storm indeed. (From Posnick JC, ed. Obstructive sleep apnea: evaluation and treatment. In: Posnick JC, ed. *Orthognathic Surgery: Principles and Practice.* Elsevier; 2014:992–1058.)

restricted; the soft palate, which becomes longer and thicker, is now closer to the posterior and lateral pharyngeal walls, restricting the retropalatal space even further.[5] Increased adipose volume in the floor of the mouth displaces the tongue superiorly and posteriorly, thus decreasing the retroglossal airway space. Chronic allergic rhinitis expands the turbinate tissue, leading to diminished intranasal airway space. The spread of adipose volume in the submental triangle and the supraplatysmal regions produces the so-called "double chin" appearance with a full neck phenotype, as seen in two brothers in Figure 67.2.[5]

Anthropometric Measurements in Patients with Suspected Sleep Apnea

Obesity, as measurement of BMI, is strongly associated with obstructive sleep apnea (OSA). However, recent data adds that general body adiposity or regional adiposity are also important risk factors in the evolution of OSA. Besides BMI, other anthropometric obesity indexes, such as waist circumference (WC) and neck circumference (NC), are determined as significant risk factors for the evolution of OSA.[6]

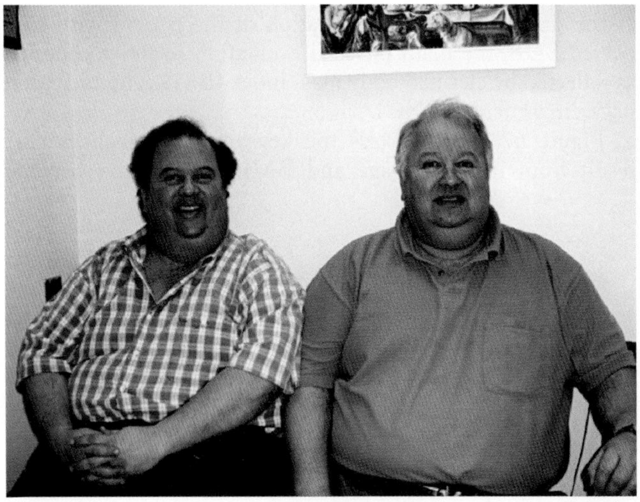

Figure 67.2 Obesity is strongly associated by body mass index (BMI). The example depicts two brothers with sleep apnea with elevated BMI in the morbidly obese range. (From Kryger MH, Avidan A, Berry R. *Atlas of Clinical Sleep Medicine*. 2nd ed. Saunders; 2014: Figures 13.1–3, *A*.)

The following BMI criteria are used to quantitate weight phenotype.

Patients with a BMI below 18.5 are considered underweight, between 18.5 and 24.9 are classified as "normal weight," between 25.0 and 29.9 are classified as "overweight," whereas greater than 30.0 are "obese." Visceral fat accumulation, as depicted in Figures 67.3 and 67.4, is an important risk indicator for sleep apnea, particularly in male patients.[4,5,7] Expansion of regional fat deposition is believed to compromise airway space, whereas visceral/abdominal obesity reduces lung volume and therefore caudal traction on the pharynx.[8]

NC at the superior border of the cricothyroid membrane can be measured to evaluate excessive adiposity in the upper body. This measurement is performed with the patient in the upright position (Figure 67.5). Recent data suggest that in adults with metabolic syndrome, measurement of NC is associated with OSA and should be considered in the definition of metabolic syndrome.[9] In pediatric and adolescent patients, the NC percentile, particularly an NC greater than the 95th percentile for age and sex, may be an additional screening tool for OSA in this cohort.[10] In adults, having a large NC in the context of OSA can predict difficult intubations in the anesthesia setting[11] and has been documented in several metabolic derangements, as in the patients presented in Figure 67.6, *A* and 67.6, *B*.[12]

However, not all patients with OSA are obese but may exhibit reduced oropharyngeal airspace, retrognathia, or micrognathia, which puts patients at risk for OSA (Figure 67.7). In contrast, central sleep apnea usually presents with abnormalities reflective of impaired respiratory effort, including the manifestations of heart failure, central nervous system (CNS) disease, or neuromuscular disease. Hypoventilation may be secondary to obesity but may also reflect pulmonary disease or neuromuscular and chest wall disorders. We review the manifestations of sleep apnea on the basis of anatomic site.

Overall Inspection

As noted in the previous section, sleep apnea often presents in association with obesity, which increases the prevalence 10-fold (20% to 40%).[13] Obesity and, in particular, the central type of obesity (Figures 67.1 and 67.2) are significant risk factors for OSA.[14] They impose increased pharyngeal collapsibility

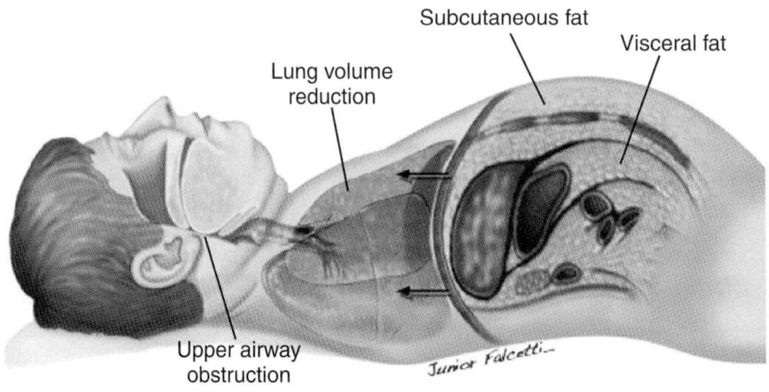

Figure 67.3 The contribution of obesity to obstructive sleep apnea. The illustration depicts the principle anatomic factors that place obese patients at significant risk for obstructive sleep apnea. (From Drager L, Togeiro SM, Polotsky VY, Lorenzi-Filho G. Obstructive sleep apnea: a cardiometabolic risk in obesity and the metabolic syndrome. *J Am Coll Cardiol*. 2013;62[7]:569–76.)

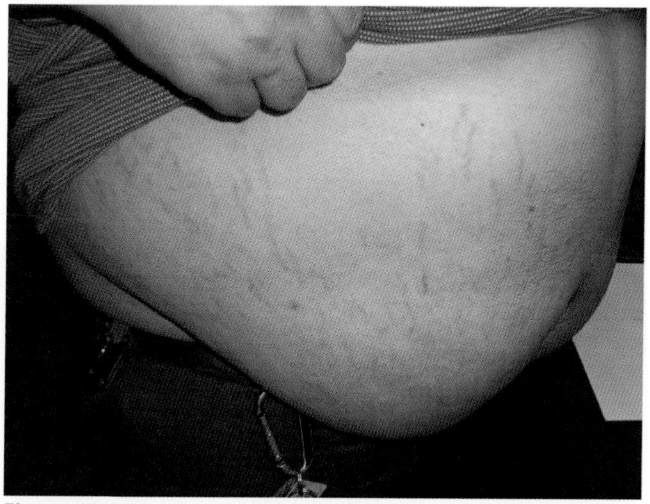

Figure 67.4 Central obesity in obstructive sleep apnea. (From Kryger MH, Avidan A, Berry R. *Atlas of Clinical Sleep Medicine.* 2nd ed. Saunders; 2014: Figures 13.1–42.)

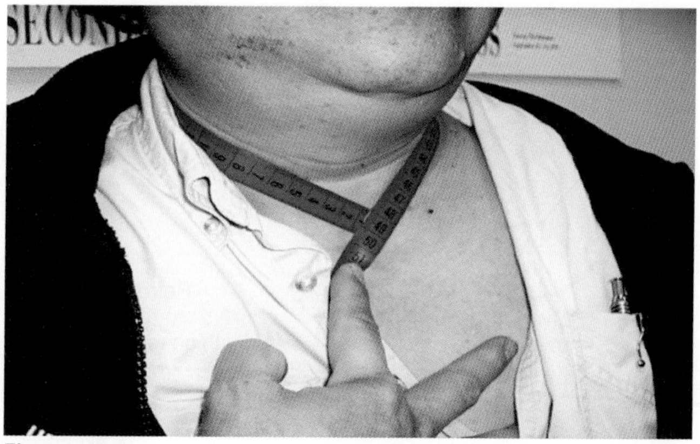

Figure 67.5 Measuring neck collar size. Neck circumference values of 17 inches or greater in men and 16 inches or greater in women are strongly correlated with the risk for obstructive sleep apnea. (From Kryger MH. *Atlas of Clinical Sleep Medicine.* 2nd ed. Saunders; 2014: Figures 13.1–40.)

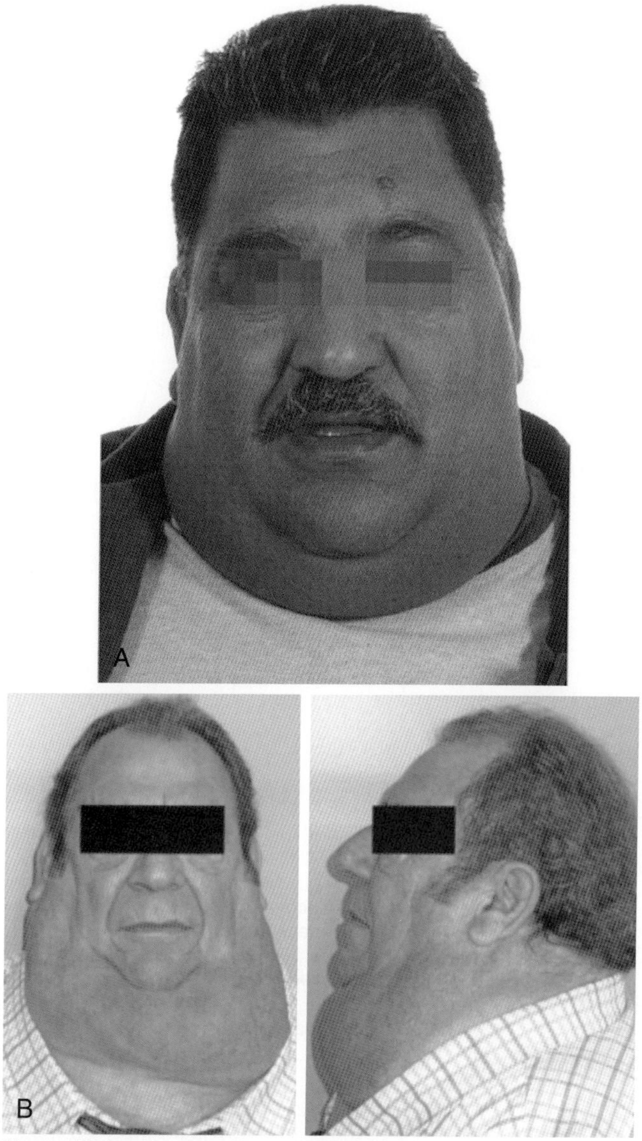

Figure 67.6 **A,** The typical facial features of a patient with obstructive sleep apnea. Notice the width of the neck. **B,** Significantly large neck size due to symmetric accumulation of adipose tissue in a patient with multiple symmetric lipomatosis, a condition characterized by a diffuse, symmetric accumulation of adipose tissue, primarily around the neck. (**A** From Venn PJH. Obstructive sleep apnoea and anaesthesia. *Anaesth Intens Care Med.* 2014;12:313–8; **B** from Esteban Júlvez L, Peréllo Aragónes S, Aguilar Bargalló X. Sleep apnea-hypopnea syndrome and multiple symmetrical lipomatosis. *Arch Bronconeumol.* 2013;49(2):86–7.)

through mechanical compression of the pharyngeal soft tissues and decreased lung volume through CNS-acting signaling proteins (adipokines) that may alter airway neuromuscular control.[14,15] OSA may independently predispose individuals to worsening obesity as a result of sleep deprivation, hypersomnia, and disrupted metabolism.[16]

Sleep apnea is also associated with endocrinopathies, such as hypothyroidism[17,18] and acromegaly.[19] Hypothyroidism is a known cause of secondary OSA; oropharyngeal airway myopathy, edema, and obesity predispose patients to upper airway collapse and obstruction. Acromegaly, as depicted in Figure 67.8, results from excessive growth hormone, resulting in enlarged growth of the craniofacial bones, enlargement of the tongue, referred to as macroglossia (Figure 67.9), and thickening and enlargement of the laryngeal region; all of these factors can contribute to upper airway obstruction.[20] Goiter, which is associated with acromegaly and hypothyroidism and a euthyroid state,[21] can contribute to OSA (Figure 67.10). Patients with Down syndrome (DS) (Figure 67.11) regularly experience snoring and obstructive apneas, two common manifestations of upper airway obstruction in this condition that independently predict neurocognitive impairment.[22] Recent data show significant prevalence of OSA in DS, conferred through several factors, including craniofacial anatomy, high BMI, adenotonsillar hypertrophy, midface hypoplasia, and muscle hypotonia, as summarized in Figure 67.12.[23,24] Metabolic derangement, such as deposition disorders, including mucopolysaccharidosis (MPS) (Figure 67.13), and amyloidosis (Figure 67.14)[25] are strongly correlated to OSA. In fact, in patients with MPS the prevalence of obstructive sleep apnea syndrome can be as high as 70%.[26]

Specific endocrinopathies, in particular polycystic ovary syndrome (PCOS), are extremely common among women of reproductive age but often go undiagnosed.[27] PCOS is associated with metabolic syndrome and carries a greatly increased

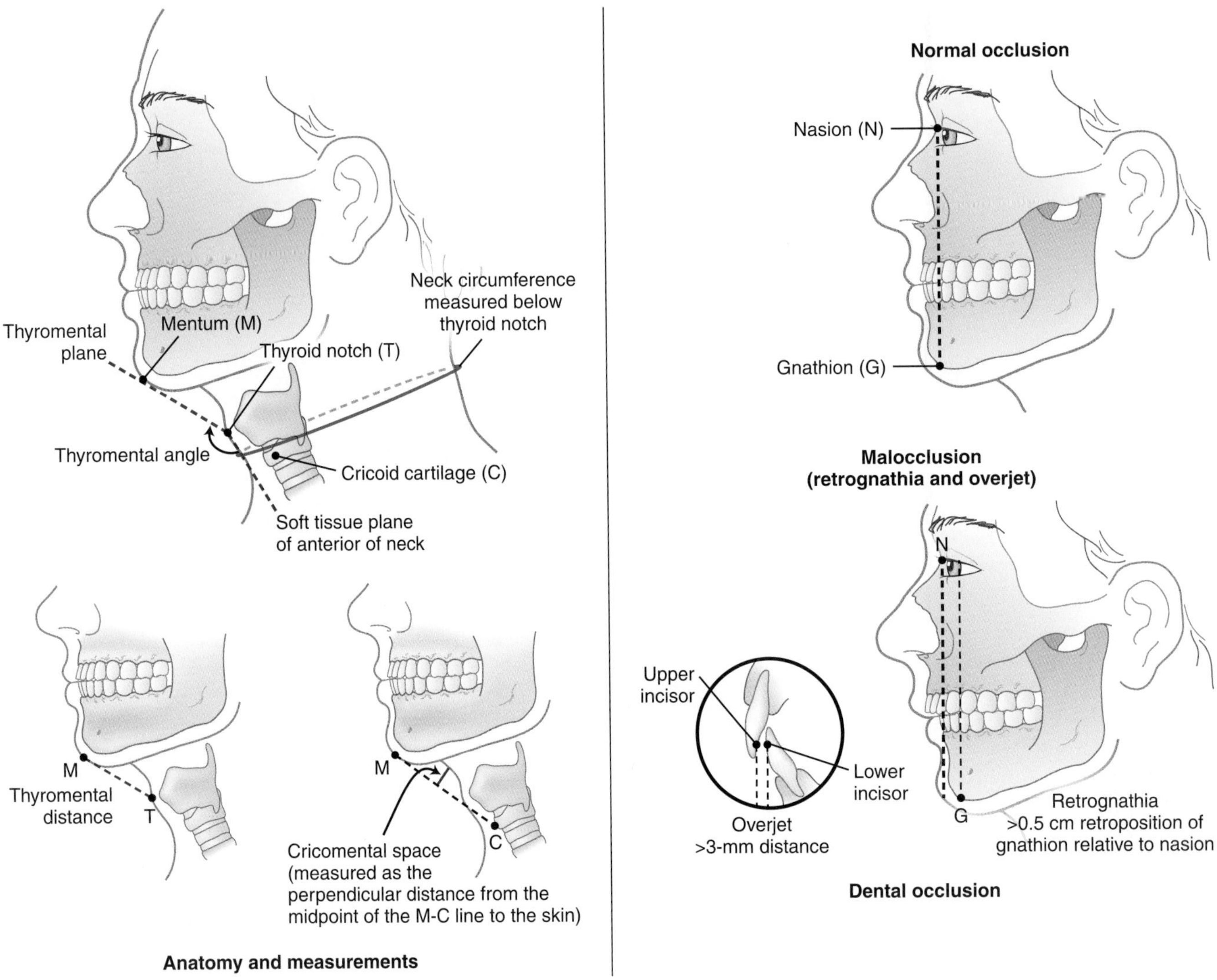

Figure 67.7 Craniofacial landmarks in sleep-disordered beathing. Anatomy and surface measurements in the assessment of a patient with suspected obstructive sleep apnea (OSA). Retrognathia, overjet, and reduced cricomental space are key craniofacial properties that are predictive of OSA. (From Myers KA, Mrkobrada M, Simel DL. Does this patient have obstructive sleep apnea? The rational clinical examination systematic review. *JAMA*. 2013;310:731–41.)

risk for obesity with metabolic syndrome, OSA, impaired glucose tolerance and type 2 diabetes mellitus, and cardiovascular risk.[27] Facial features consist of hirsutism and acne reflective of androgen excess (Figure 67.15).

Craniofacial Factors

As summarized in Figure 67.7, cephalometric measurements reveal that subjects with OSA have significant changes in the size and position of the soft palate and uvula, volume and position of the tongue, hyoid position, and mandibulomaxillary protrusion compared with control subjects. Mandibular retrognathia (Figure 67.16, *A*), micrognathia (Figure 67.16, *B*), and severe micrognathia in the Pierre Robin sequence (Figure 67.16, *C*). The latter presents as symptomatic microretrognathia that leads to glossoptosis (tongue falling posteriorly), resulting in airway blockade.[28] Highlighted in Figure 67.16, *B* is the cricomentalis (CM) space, a unique feature, measured by calculating the distance between the neck and the bisection of a line from the chin to the cricoid membrane, when the head is in a neutral position, which is extremely limited.[29] OSA is unlikely if the CM space is greater than 1.5 cm. However, if the CM distance is less than 1.5 cm, then a diagnosis of OSA is more likely, particularly in the setting of elevated BMI, increased neck size, and older age.[30]

A scalloped tongue (Figure 67.17) may accompany micrognathia.[31] Men with retrognathia or micrognathia may grow a beard to compensate for this anatomic variant. Crowded teeth (Figure 67.18) and overjet (Figure 67.19), with the mandibular teeth (T_2) excessively posterior (>3 mm) when compared to the maxillary teeth (T_1), often accompany retrognathia or micrognathia.

Torus mandibularis, as shown in Figure 67.20, is a bony outgrowth occasionally encountered in the lingual side of the mandible, medial to the canine or premolar region, and typically occurs in pairs as bilateral tori. Although most are asymptomatic, particularly large tori may predispose people to sleep apnea and might impact adherence with positive airway pressure (PAP) therapy.[32] Figure 67.21 depicts the global consequences of primary mandibular insufficiency on the patency

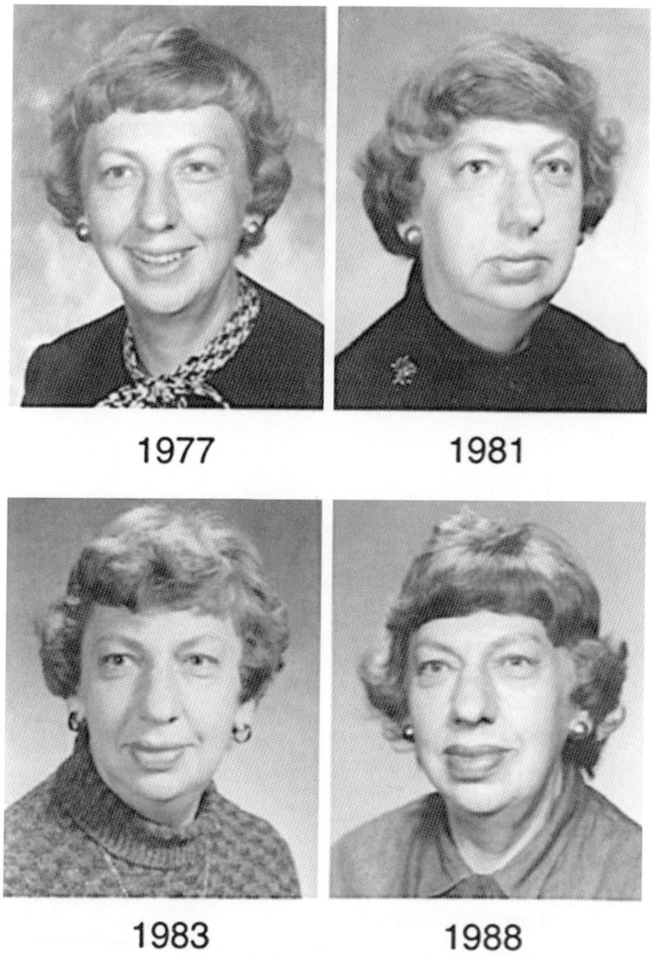

Figure 67.8 Acromegaly as a risk factor for sleep apnea progressive change in facial features in a patient with acromegaly. The onset of physical changes is sometime insidious, and patients may not directly present with specific complaints relating directly to these distinguishing signs of acromegaly. However, patients may be more likely to present with symptoms referred to other conditions, such as diabetes mellitus, hypertension, and obstructive sleep apnea. At the advanced stages of the condition, patients exhibit more dramatic physical characteristics, such as enlarged hands, feet, lips and tongue; prominent supraorbital ridges; and lower jaw protrusion. (From Molitch ME. Clinical manifestations of acromegaly. *Endocrinol Metab Clin North Am.* 1992;21[3]:597–614.)

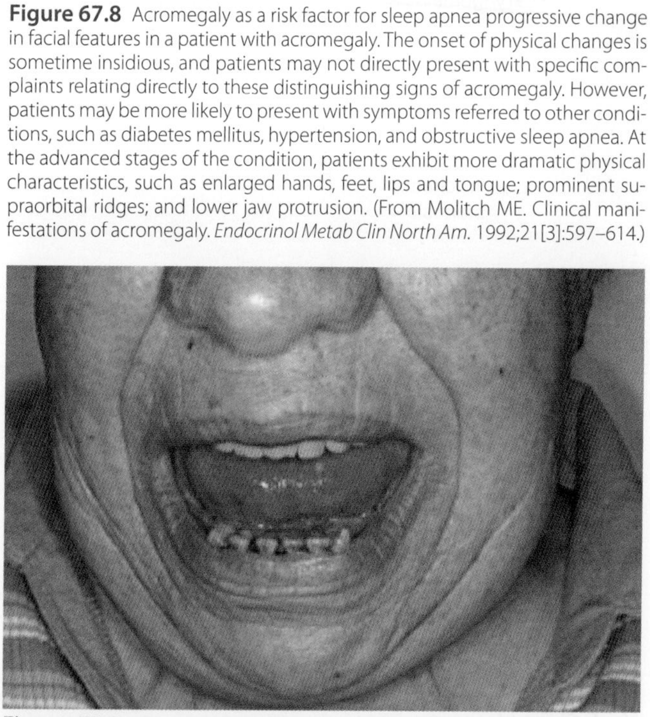

Figure 67.9 Macroglossia patient with acromegaly showing the coarse facial features, macroglossia, and interdental separation typically seen in this condition, which lead to airway restriction and contribute to the development of obstructive sleep apnea. (From Burke G. Endocrine disease. In: Sprout C, Burke G, McGurk M, eds. *Essential Human Disease for Dentists.* Churchill Livingstone; 2006:99–119.)

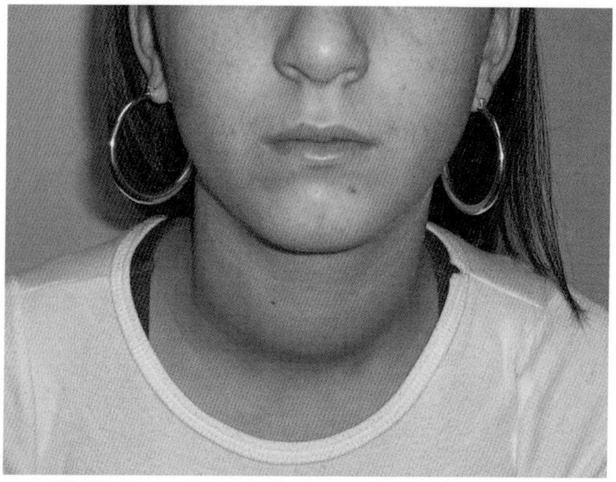

Figure 67.10 Goiter. (From Kryger MH, Avidan A, Berry R. *Atlas of Clinical Sleep Medicine.* 2nd ed. Saunders; 2014: Figures 15.1–8, *B*.)

of the upper airways patency, leading to compromised retronasal, retropalatal, and retroglossal spaces.[5]

Commonly encountered craniofacial features predisposing to sleep apnea consist of mandibular deficiency syndrome, an inferiorly placed hyoid bone relative to the mandibular plane, narrowing of the posterior air space, and elongation of the soft palate.[33] In addition, marfanoid habitus, including the long face phenotype (Figure 67.22, *A*), leads to upper airway restriction, thereby predisposing to OSA.[34] Additional features include notable body proportions consisting of long arm span, abnormally long and slender limbs, fingers and toes (arachnodactyly), and a positive Steinberg sign, with the thumb extending beyond the ulnar border when completely opposed in the clenched hand. Other features include subluxated lenses, everted sternum, and cardiovascular abnormalities, including aortic aneurysms in the aorta or other arteries (Figure 67.22, *B*).

Indeed, when the well-established role of obesity in the development of OSA is taken into account, a model of OSA emerges in which the degree of craniofacial abnormalities determines the extent of obesity required to produce OSA in a given individual. Racial differences in cephalometric properties probably play a major role in conferring risk for OSA in the absence of obesity. For example, in Chinese patients with OSA, a more retropositioned mandible was associated with more severe OSA after controlling for obesity.[35] In Japanese patients with OSA, micrognathia was a major risk factor.[36] Patients with OSA have an increased pharyngeal-narrowing ratio, which is defined as a ratio between the airway cross-section at the hard palate level and the narrowest cross-section from the hard palate to the epiglottis.[37]

Facial type has been classified as follows: (1) The mesocephalic facial type is characterized by equal vertical facial thirds. (2) The brachycephalic facial type appears square with a diminished lower third. (3) The dolichocephalic facial type appears ovoid with an increased lower third (Figure 67.23, *A* to *C*).[38] Recent data illustrate that White patients with sleep apnea were increasingly prone to have the brachiocephalic features, whereas Blacks with sleep apnea were more likely to have a dolichocephalic phenotype. The brachiocephalic cranial shape resulted in small anteroposterior dimensions of the skull base and reduced anteroposterior dimensions of the upper airway.[39]

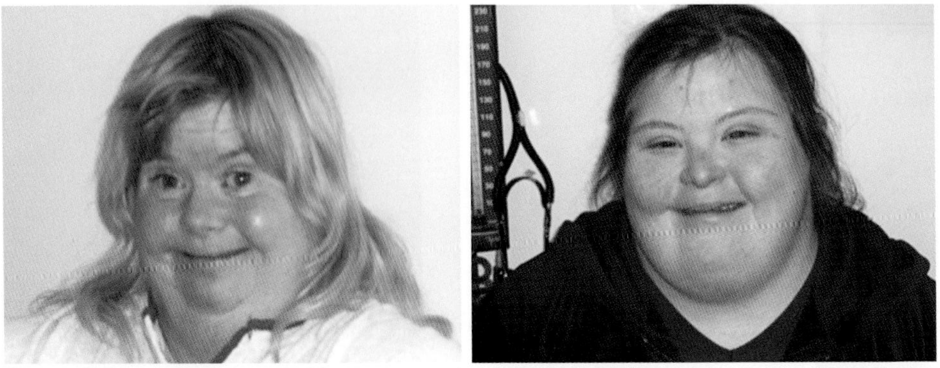

Figure 67.11 Down syndrome (DS). Two patients with the characteristic phenotype of DS. Contributing factors to obstructive sleep apnea in DS include alteration in craniofacial anatomy, adenotonsillar hypertrophy, and muscle hypotonia. (Courtesy Dr. Meir H. Kryger.)

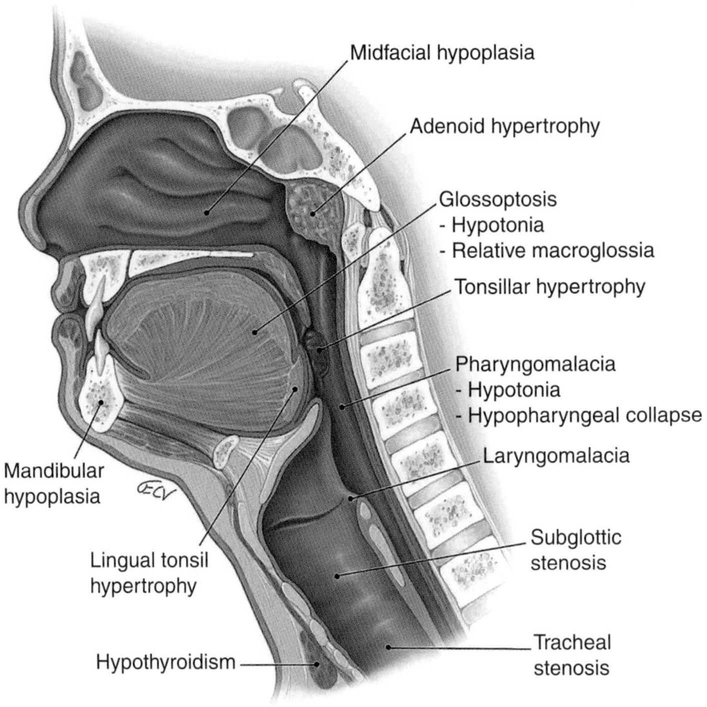

Figure 67.12 Potential sites of airway occlusion in Down syndrome (DS). Midface and maxillary hypoplasia culminate in reduction of the bony dimensions of the airway. Macroglossia emerges due to the reduced bony framework of the small maxilla and mandible. Enlargement of the lingual tonsillars is common in DS and compromise oropharyngeal level. Hypotonia contributes to obstruction at the supraglottic level. Laryngomalacia, defined as collapse of supraglottic structures during inspiration, occurs in as much as 50% of children with DS, whereas subglottic and tracheal stenosis are additional factors that reduced airflow below the hypopharynx. (From Lal C, White DR, Joseph JE, et al. Sleep-disordered breathing in Down syndrome. *Chest.* 2015;147(2):570–9.)

Nasal Factors

The nose represents the initial and preferred port of air entry into the lungs and accounts for 50% of the total upper airway resistance. It is region of strategic importance for normal airflow, which can become obstructed due to anatomic anomalies, such as septal deviation, nasal polyps, turbinate hypertrophy, and rhinitis and contribute to OSA. It is also the port of entry for PAP therapy to prevent airway collapse in OSA.[40]

Examination of the nasal airway should focus on anatomic abnormalities that may contribute to nasal obstruction. These may be congenital, traumatic, infectious, or neoplastic in etiology (Figure 67.24, *A* to *D*). Nasal polyps (Figure 67.25) represent benign pedunculated tumors originating from edematous, chronically inflamed nasal mucosa, and can partially or completely obstruct the nasal airway and may compromise effective continuous positive airway pressure therapy in the setting of OSA.

Neck Circumference

Increased NC (Figures 67.5 and 67.6, *A* and *B*) is an important risk factor for OSA. Patients with an NC greater than 48 cm (19.2 in) have a 20-fold increased risk of having OSA.[41]

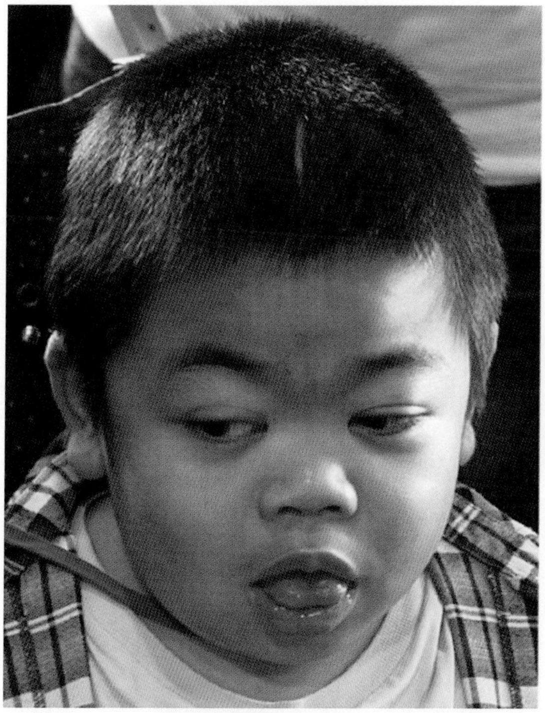

Figure 67.13 Hunter syndrome (mucopolysaccharidosis type II) depicting significant macroglossia, a risk factor for obstructive sleep apnea. In this 8-year-old boy with Hunter syndrome, infiltration of the macroglossia can be seen. Other features include macrocephaly, coarse hair, abnormally short neck, hairy face, puffy eyelids, depressed nasal bridge, upturned nose, full lips, and thick skin texture. (From Chou W-C, Weng C-Y, Lin S-P, Chu S-Y. Postenzyme replacement therapy era for type 2 mucopolysaccharidosis. *Tzu Chi Med J*. 2013;25:128–9.)

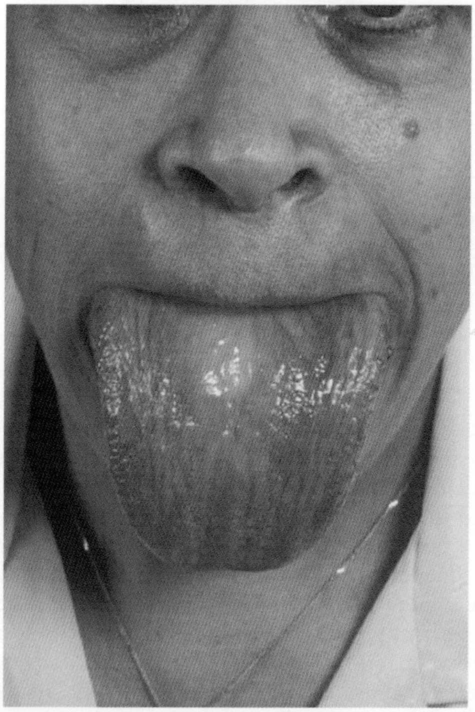

Figure 67.14 Profound enlargement of the tongue (macroglossia) as a result of amyloid infiltration. The patient had severe obstructive sleep apnea. The tongue fills the oral cavity completely, contributing to profound hypopharyngeal and oropharyngeal airway blockade. (From Hoffman R, Benz EJ, Silberstein LE, et al. *Hematology: Diagnosis and Treatment*. Elsevier Health Sciences; 2013:1352, Figure 87.3.)

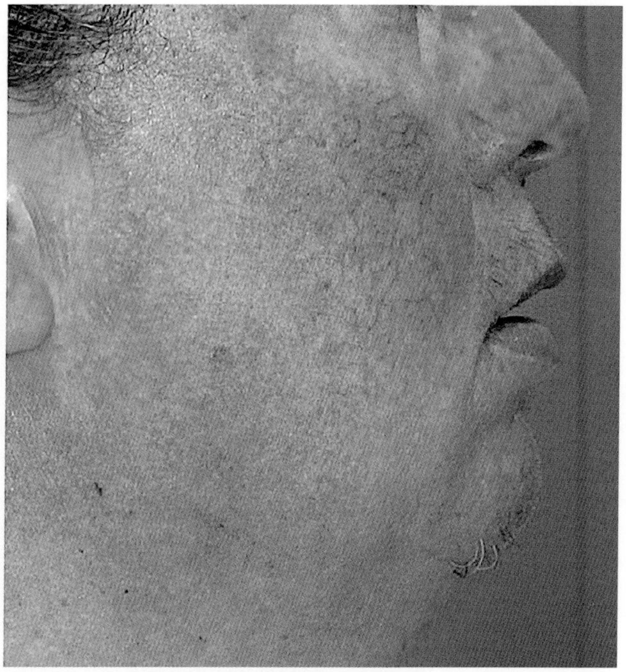

Figure 67.15 A woman with polycystic ovary syndrome (PCOS). The classic facial features include hirsutism, acne, alopecia, and acanthosis nigricans, characteristic of androgen excess. Other features include, type 2 diabetes mellitus, amenorrhea, coronary artery disease, dyslipidemia, hypertension, depression, and anxiety. (From Kryger MH, Avidan A, Berry R. *Atlas of Clinical Sleep Medicine*. 2nd ed. Saunders; 2014: Figure 1.4)

Examination of the Pharynx

There are two well-established classifications to determine the relation of the tongue to the pharynx. The classic "Mallampati classification (MP)" was first hypothesized and described by the anesthesiologist Seshagiri Rao Mallampati. He is best known for proposing the eponymous Mallampati score in 1985 as a method for anesthesiologists to predict difficult tracheal intubation (Figure 67.26).[42] Although the original MP classification comprised three classes, a 4-point scale was subsequently developed by adding class IV in which the soft palate was not visible.

Mallampati Classification. *Instructions:* Examine the oropharynx with the mouth open, without phonating (or saying "ah"), with the tongue protruded.

Class I: Visualization of the soft palate, fauces, uvula and pillars (Figure 67.27).
Class II: Visualization of the soft palate, fauces, uvula (Figure 67.28).
Class III: Visualization of the soft palate and base of the uvula (Figure 67.29).
Class IV: Soft palate is not visible (Figure 67.30).

Modified Mallampati Classification. The modified Mallampati classification (MMP) is also referred to as the Friedman tongue position grading system.

Instructions: Examine the oropharynx with the mouth open, without phonating (or saying "ah") and without protruding the tongue. The combination of a high MMP score, tonsil size, and BMI are reliable predictors of OSA and

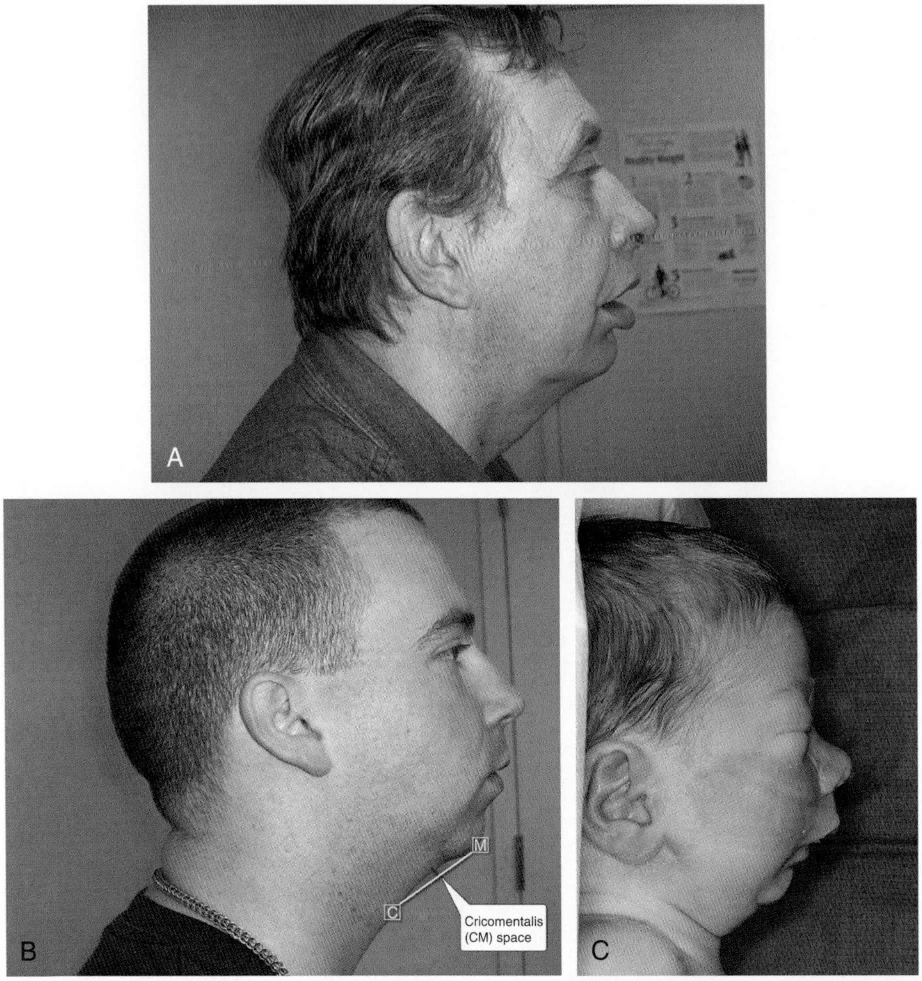

Figure 67.16 **A,** Mandibular retrognathia contributing to obstructive sleep apnea. **B,** An adult with significant mandibular micrognathia contributing to obstructive sleep apnea. The cricomentalis (CM) space (as delineated by the *red line*) is the distance between the neck and the bisection of a line from the chin to the cricoid membrane when the head is in a neutral position and is severely reduced in the adult with mandibular micrognathia. A CM space less than 1.5 cm, increases the likelihood that sleep apnea is present, particularly when associated with age older than 50 years, Mallampati class III and IV, neck circumference greater than 35 cm, the presence of overbite, and body mass index greater than 27 kg/m^2.[30] **C,** Mandibular micrognathia illustrated in this example is in a severely affected newborn who initially presented with difficulties feeding. The patient was noted to have severe micrognathia and a cleft palate at birth. Oxygen desaturations down to the 80s were noted when supine and specifically during feeding, at which time the patient coughed, and saturations dropped to the 60s. The patient was eventually diagnosed with Pierre Robin sequence. (**A** From Kryger MH, Avidan A, Berry R. *Atlas of Clinical Sleep Medicine.* 2nd ed. Saunders; 2014: Figures 13.1–16; **B** from Kryger MH, Avidan A, Berry R. *Atlas of Clinical Sleep Medicine.* 2nd ed. Saunders; 2014; **C** from Resnick CM, LeVine J, Calabrese CE, et al. Early management of infants with robin sequence: an international survey and algorithm. *J Oral Maxillofac Surg.* 2019;77(1):136–56.)

can be coupled with palate position and tonsillar size to serve as good prognostic indicators for successful surgery for SDB.[43]

The MMP classification consists of four grades as follows:

Grade 1: The entire uvula and tonsils of pillars can be visualized.
Grade 2: The uvula can be visualized but not the tonsils.
Grade 3: The soft palate can be visualized but not the uvula.
Grade 4: Only the hard palate can be visualized.

The Friedman tongue position grading system is illustrated in Figure 67.31.

Examination of the Tonsils

Enlarged tonsils and adenoids are a major cause of airway obstruction and sleep apnea in children, but a minority of adults may also have enlargement of these structures, contributing to airway obstruction.[44] Although the adenoids cannot be visualized in a routine physical examination, the examination of tonsils may require use of a tongue blade. Tonsillar size is graded on a scale of 1 to 4 (Figure 67.32). Children with marked adenotonsillar hypertrophy and nasal obstruction have been noted to have a peculiar "dull expression" (i.e., "adenoid facies"), as shown in Figure 67.33, *A* and *B*. Due to the adenoid hypertrophy, the patient becomes an obligate mouth breathers and must keep his mouth open to breathe. Children with chronic sinus allergies may present with an "allergic salute" sign (Figure 67.34).

Craniofacial Abnormalities

Craniofacial abnormalities represent a heterogenous group of conditions, either as part of syndrome or they may occur in

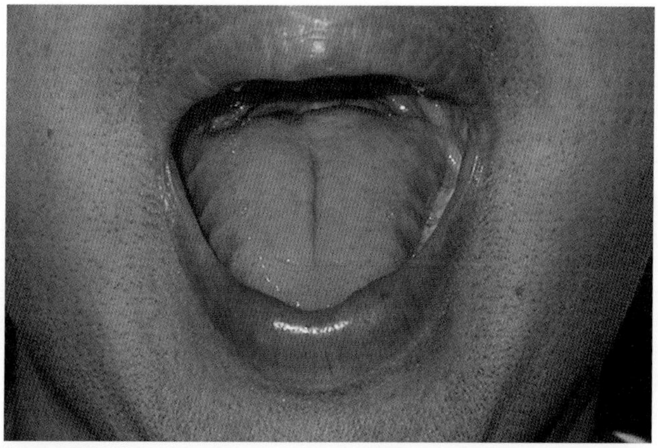

Figure 67.17 Scalloped tongue. The scalloping and furrow result from the tongue's pressing against teeth. This finding may highlight the possibility of sleep apnea, particularly in the presence of other attributes highlighted in Figure 67.16, *B*. (From Moeller JL, Paskay LC, Gelb ML. Myofunctional therapy: a novel treatment of pediatric sleep-disordered breathing. *Sleep Med Clin*. 2014;9(2):235–43.)

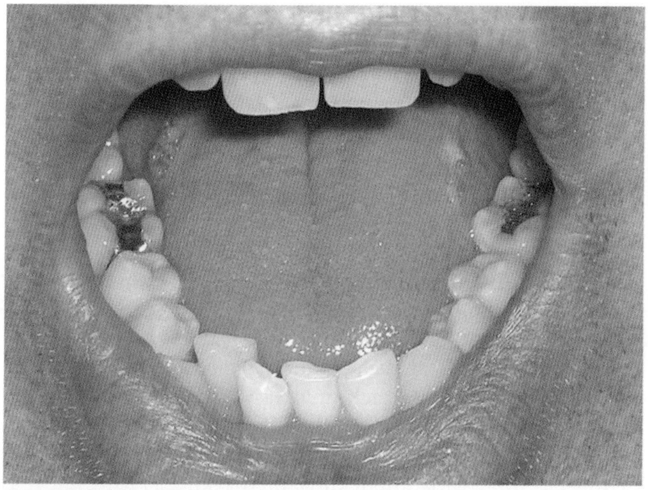

Figure 67.18 Crowded teeth. Crowded teeth indicate a small mandible, contributing to obstructive sleep apnea. (From Kryger MH, Avidan A, Berry R. *Atlas of Clinical Sleep Medicine*. 2nd ed. Saunders; 2014: Figures 13.1–12.)

isolation or as part of a syndrome. Craniofacial clefts consist of cleft lip, cleft palate, or both cleft lip and palate.[45] Sleep apnea is thought to develop from morphologic changes that result in a small midface and mandibular retrognathia. Conditions that present with micrognathia result in OSA due to obstruction at the base of the tongue from glossoptosis (posterior displacement of the tongue toward the pharynx) and reduced oropharyngeal airway size.[46] The Pierre Robin sequence consists of mandibular hypoplasia, glossoptosis, and a U-shaped cleft palate, and it is the most common cause of syndromic micrognathia.[45] Craniosynostoses are congenital conditions that include premature fusion of one or more of the cranial sutures, resulting in abnormal growth of the skull in the direction parallel to the fused suture. OSA can result because of midface hypoplasia, but other factors, such as adenotonsillar hypertrophy and choanal atresia, may lead to OSA. Representative conditions include Apert and Crouzon syndromes.[46] Another key example is Treacher-Collins syndrome, a mandibulofacial craniosynostosis, and it is characterized by hypoplasia of the facial bones, cleft

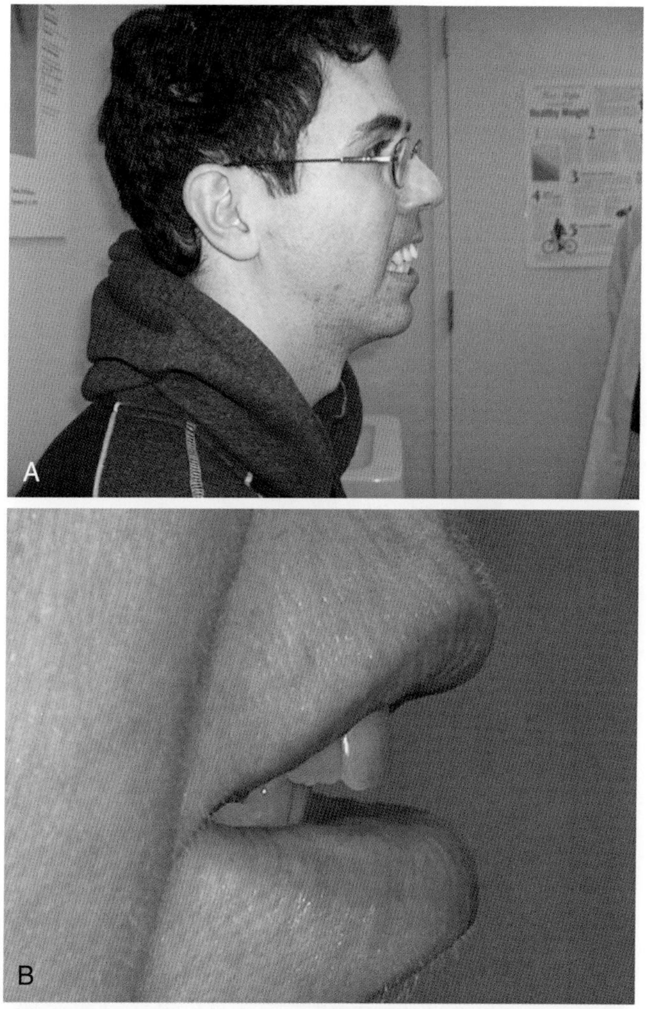

Figure 67.19 Overjet. Overjet is seen as the maxilla protrudes forward relative to the mandible. Overjet is defined as the horizontal overlap of the maxillary incisors (T_1) over the mandibular incisors (T_2) in excess of 3 mm as measured using disposable paper ruler or more sophisticated devices, such as the George gauge, which measures protrusive capacity. (From Kryger MH, Avidan A, Berry R. *Atlas of Clinical Sleep Medicine*. 2nd ed. Saunders; 2014: Figures 13.1–14.)

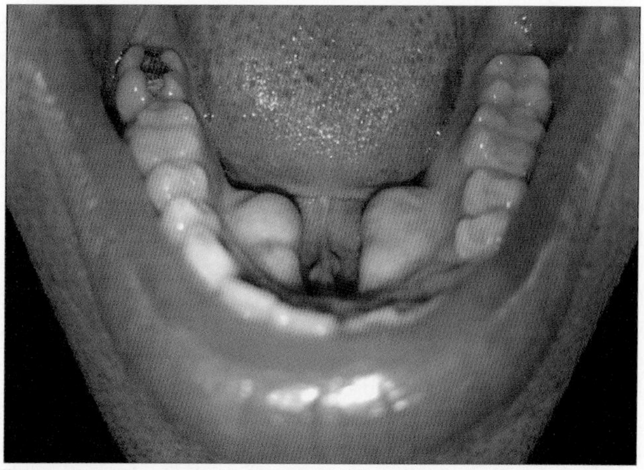

Figure 67.20 Torus mandibularis. Mandibular tori (MT) are outgrowths of bony formation typically found on the lingual surface of the mandible. MT are typically bilateral and symmetric. When prominent, surgical removal might improve the functional space for the tongue and subsequently could improve upper airway size. Their presence may also impact the treatment of sleep apnea, particularly impacting the fitting of mandibular advancement devices.[78] (From Mermod M, Hoarau R. Mandibular tori. *CMAJ*. 2015;187(11):826.)

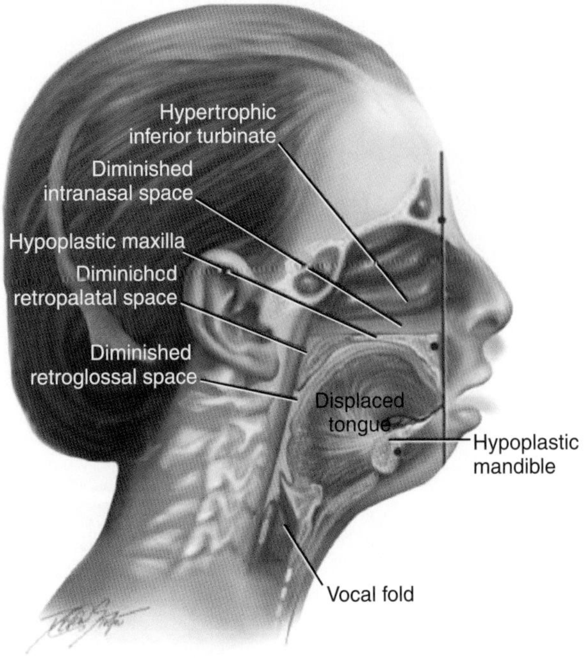

Figure 67.21 Primary mandibular insufficiency: an illustration of a sagittal cross-sectional head and neck view from a 16-year-old patient with primary mandibular deficiency and overjet malocclusion predisposing to obstructive sleep apnea. (From Posnick JC. Obstructive sleep apnea: evaluation and treatment. In: Posnick JC, ed. *Orthognathic Surgery Principles and Practice.* Elsevier Saunders; 2014:992–1058.)

palate, downward-slanting palpebral fissures, colobomas of the lower eyelids, and pharyngeal hypoplasia.[46] Figure 67.35, A to *H* highlights key craniofacial disorders with unique phenotypes representing increased venerability to sleep apnea. Children and adults with DS (Figure 67.36,*A* to *C*) frequently have sleep apnea, most likely related to a combination of craniofacial abnormalities, consisting of mandibular hypoplasia causing narrowing of the hypopharynx and which together with their relative macroglossia, lingual tonsillar hypertrophy, obesity, and reduced muscle tone result in dynamic upper airway collapse.[45]

Neurologic Examination

The neurologic examination may hold important clues to the presence of OSA or central sleep apnea and hypoventilation syndromes. Features of neuromuscular disease evident on physical examination may indicate these syndromes. For example, progressive muscle atrophy and fasciculations of the hand (Figure 67.37, *A* to *D*) or tongue may indicate amyotrophic lateral sclerosis (ALS). In ALS phrenic nerve dysfunction is common and results in diaphragmatic paralysis, with prominent hypoventilation during rapid eye movement (REM) sleep. In addition, coexisting OSA may occur in ALS with bulbar involvement. Weakness of thoracoabdominal or respiratory accessory muscles, often with accompanying kyphoscoliosis, may be observed in poliomyelitis. Post-polio syndrome, muscular dystrophies, myasthenia gravis, and metabolic myopathies may also be manifested with weakness of the chest wall musculature[47] and diaphragm weakness. Myasthenia gravis (Figure 67.38) may also involve facial structures, resulting in OSA. Craniofacial abnormalities may occur in myotonic dystrophy (Figure 67.39) or muscular dystrophy; macroglossia may also occur (e.g., Duchenne muscular dystrophy).[48]

Figure 67.40 depicts a patient with facial weakness in the setting of progressive muscular dystrophy. Figure 67.41 shows a patient with myotonic dystrophy with tightness of muscles (called myotonia), leading to difficulties relaxing certain muscles after using them, such as being able to release grip in a handshake, from a doorknob, or as in the example provided. Figure 67.42, *A* to *E* depicts the classic Gower maneuver in Becker muscular dystrophy. Defects in upper airway neuromuscular control in many of the patients with dystrophinopathies play a critical role in sleep apnea pathogenesis, and the sleep provider must maintain a vigil eye on sleep disturbances in this group of patients.[49] Finally, obesity (e.g., from steroid use, as in Figure 67.43, or inactivity) may also contribute to sleep apnea in neuromuscular disease.

Cardiopulmonary Examination

The presence of congestive heart failure (see Chapter 149) indicates a high likelihood of central sleep apnea. Peripheral edema (Figure 67.44) is a common finding in patients with obesity hypoventilation syndrome, as a manifestation of cor pulmonale, and in some patients with obstructive apnea who also have left ventricular cardiac failure. Resolution of peripheral edema with treatment correlates with clinical improvement. Chronic obstructive pulmonary disease and asthma (see Chapter 137) are also seen in association with OSA. In patients with cardiopulmonary insufficiency, clubbing of digits and nails may be a cardinal sign (Figure 67.45).

CENTRAL NERVOUS SYSTEM HYPERSOMNIA

Narcolepsy

Physical findings in patients with narcolepsy are nonspecific and may be subtle, infrequent, and absent during the clinic visit. During cataplectic spells, patients present with muscle atonia, absence of deep tendon reflexes, and loss of the H-reflex.[50] Cataplexy attacks may range from partial episodes characterized by sagging of the jaw and mild dropping of the head and shoulders, to generalized spells leading to loss of muscle tone with unbuckling of the knee. However, it is very rare to encounter cataplexy during the actual clinic visit/physical examination, which makes it difficult to describe it during routine clinic visits. In general, patients with narcolepsy tend to be obese, with increased predilection to non–insulin-dependent diabetes mellitus, and have a lower basal metabolism compared with control subjects.[51,52] Children with obesity and precocious puberty should be screened for narcolepsy and cataplexy.[53]

Narcolepsy related to medical conditions (symptomatic narcolepsy) is seen in disorders such as CNS tumors, head trauma, multiple sclerosis, neurosarcoidosis, acute disseminated encephalomyelitis, CNS vascular disorders, encephalitis, and neurodegeneration.[54] An abnormal neurologic examination can be an important sign that hypersomnia may be due to a CNS etiology. In lesions of the diencephalon due to inflammatory changes, such as neurosarcoidosis, one finds additional physical findings associated with panhypopituitarism, such as orthostatic hypotension, temperature fluctuations, and other findings of autonomic dysregulation. Patients with narcolepsy type 1 who experience cataplexy are sometimes observed to have a state of peculiar semipermanent ptosis and jaw weakness, during which partial and complete cataplectic attacks were superimposed "cataplectic facies"[55,56] as depicted in Figure 67.46.

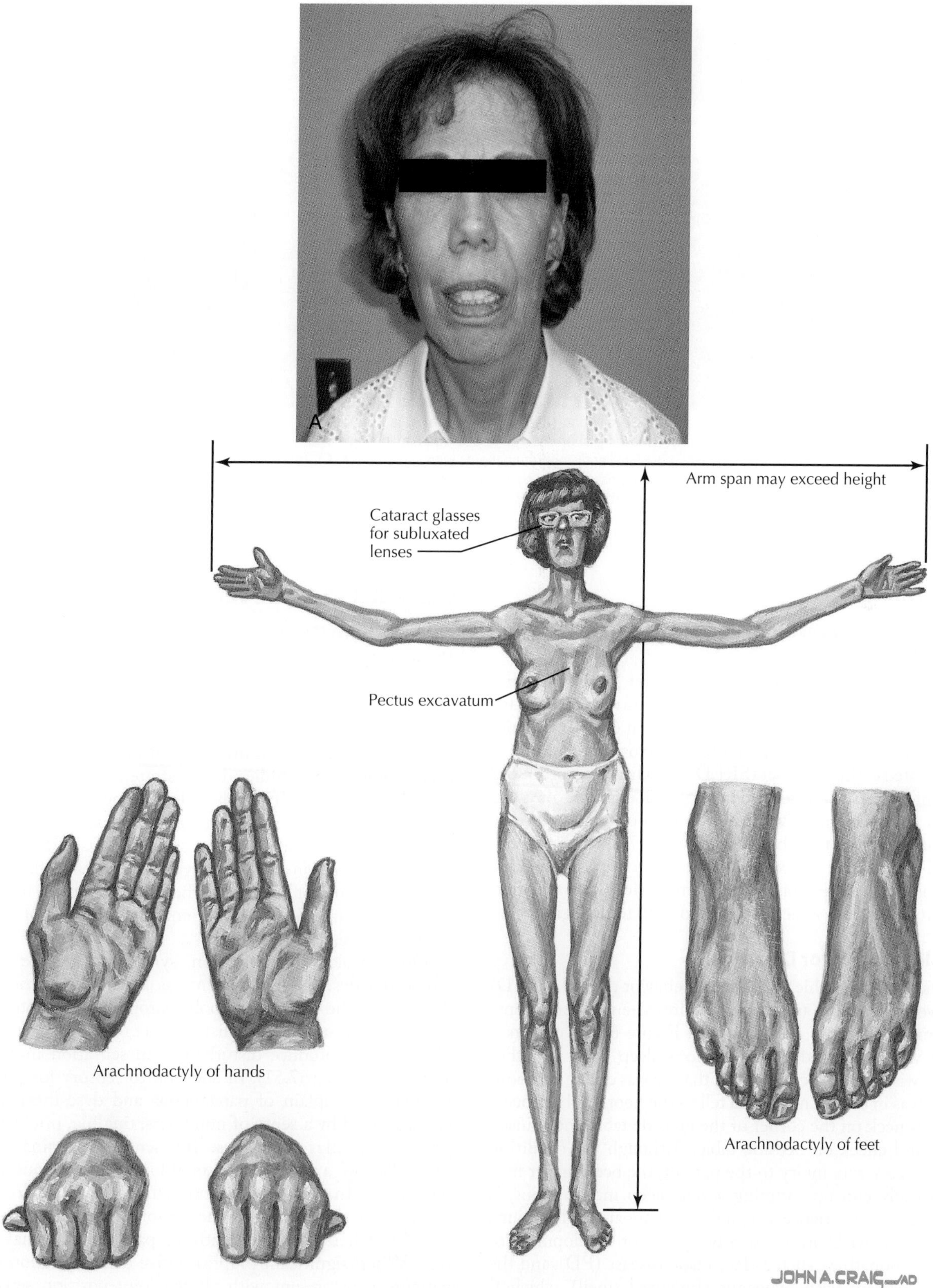

Figure 67.22 **A,** Marfanoid habitus. A patient with the long face syndrome, a well-established risk for obstructive sleep apnea (OSA), that is conferred through an increase of anterior facial height generally associated with retrognathia. **B,** Marfanoid syndrome. Marfan syndrome comprises multiple malformation syndrome involving the connective tissue. Phenotypic features include increased height, disproportionately long limbs and digits, anterior chest wall deformity, joint laxity, and vertebral column deformity. The prevalence of OSA in patients with Marfan syndrome is high and is of importance to the sleep clinicians, particularly in light of a potential association between OSA and aortic dissection, the main cause of morbidity and mortality in this cohort. (From Cochard LR. *Netter's Atlas of Human Embryology.* Updated ed. Elsevier; 2012: Figure 1.17, [Marfan syndrome]. Copyright © 2012. Courtesy Dr. Meir H. Kryger.)

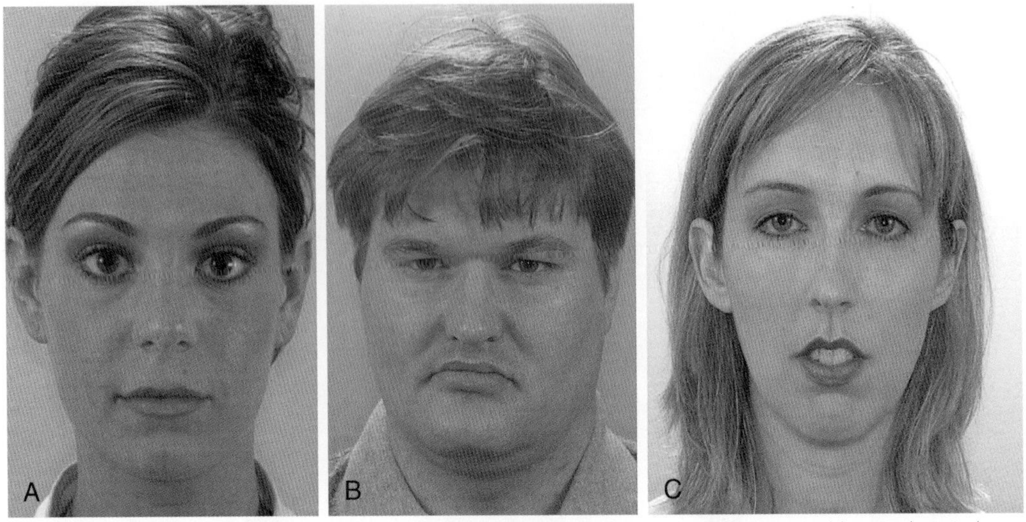

Figure 67.23 Macroaesthetic evaluation **(A)**. The mesocephalic facial type is characterized by equal vertical facial thirds. **B,** The brachycephalic facial phenotype appears square in shape with a diminished lower third. It is likely to be encountered more frequently in White patients with sleep apnea **(C).** The dolichocephalic facial type manifests in an ovoid with an increased lower third and is likely to be encountered more frequently in African Americans with obstructive sleep apnea. (From Sarver D, Jacobson RS. The aesthetic dentofacial analysis. *Clin Plast Surg.* 2007;34(3):369–94.)

PARASOMNIAS

Nocturnal Eating Disorder and Sleep-Related Eating Disorder

In nocturnal eating disorder, patients often manifest compulsive food-searching behaviors and a return to sleep after food ingestion. BMI was abnormally high in 6 of 10 patients after careful exclusion of both anorexia nervosa and bulimia.[57] Sleep-related eating disorder (SRED), which also occurs in the setting of RLS, is characterized by recurrent episodes of eating after an arousal from nighttime sleep with or without amnesia,[58] may also result in obesity. Figure 67.47 illustrates a very unusual and fascinating example of amnestic autocannibalism occurring out of non–rapid eye movement sleep in association with untreated sleep apnea in a person with tetraplegia.[59]

REM Sleep Behavior Disorder

Patients with idiopathic REM sleep behavior disorder (RBD) can develop dramatic and aggressive dream-enactment events sometimes leading to serious injury. Figure 67.48 depicts a patient who presented at the author's sleep clinic together with his wife and who complained that he was dreaming about golfing, was in an argument, and fell to the floor. In the process he hit his neck on the corner of the bedside table and bruised his ear and cheek on bedside table. Although the condition can produce severe injury to the patient, the bed partner may paradoxically end up suffering severe sleep interruptions, is more likely to experience sleepiness, and are at risk for injury. Patients with RBD are frequently at risk for development of α-synucleinopathies, such as Parkinson disease (PD), and the majority present with hyposmia (impaired smell), which is a potential preclinical nonmotor sign of the disease.[60] Odor identification was found impaired in Japanese patients with both idiopathic RBD and PD.[61] Cardinal features in PD are shown in Figure 67.49. Patients with multiple system atrophy may present with inspiratory stridor, which along with RBD may serve as a clue to the disease in a patient with autonomic failure.[62]

SLEEP-RELATED MOVEMENT DISORDERS

Willis-Ekbom Disease

The prevalence of Willis-Ekbom disease (WED), also known as RLS, in type 2 diabetes mellitus is 17.7%,[63] and the prevalence may be higher in patients with hereditary neuropathy.[64] WED occurs in about one-third of patients with polyneuropathy,[65] with preferential involvement of small sensory fibers. Electrophysiologic studies demonstrate that axonal neuropathy is common in WED, which further necessitates comprehensive peripheral nerve evaluations in these patients.[66]

Reduced iron stores can also cause WED. With iron deficiency, examination of the pharynx may reveal inflammation (redness) or loss or atrophy of the lingual mucosa, indicating glossitis (Figure 67.50). The patient may complain of a sore or tender tongue.

On neurologic examination, symptoms include sensory loss, often described by patients as a sense of numbness or tingling. In the generalized polyneuropathies, symptoms frequently begin in the most distal aspect of the longest sensory fibers, which produce disturbances in sensation in the toes and feet (Figure 67.51). In addition to sensory loss, patients frequently complain of paresthesias and dysesthesias, often characterized by a sense of numbness, tingling, prickling, and pins-and-needles sensations. The sensory examination will often disclose a distal to proximal loss of the various sensory modalities. In certain polyneuropathies, pain predominates in the clinical picture, and the sensory examination tends to disclose deficits predominantly of pain and thermal sensation. When significant proprioceptive deafferentation occurs, patients may present with altered joint-position sense that may be manifested as an ataxia or tremor of the affected limbs and an imbalance of gait and station.

Pain may be a significant symptom for many patients with WED in which the etiology is related to a polyneuropathy. It may be described as a dull aching sensation, an intense burning sensation, or, on occasion, intermittent lancinating pulses of pain. On occasion, patients notice that their skin is hypersensitive to tactile stimulation, such as from the touch of bedsheets or clothing or standing on their feet. Some patients note an exaggerated painful sensation resulting from any stimulus to the affected area, a form of pain termed *allodynia*. Various limb deformities and trophic changes may be observed in chronic polyneuropathies. Pes cavus, characterized by high arches and hammertoes, and the clawfoot deformity are typical foot deformities in hereditary polyneuropathies with childhood onset. These deformities are due to progressive weakness and atrophy of intrinsic foot muscles. A similar claw-like deformity may be observed in the hand. Autonomic involvement of a limb may cause the affected area to appear warm, red, and swollen at times and pale and cold at other times owing to dysregulation of small vessels due to autonomic denervation. Various trophic changes, including a tight, shiny skin, may occur. In patients who have had severe sensory loss in the limbs, the affected areas may be subject to incidental traumas, including burns, pressure sores, and other injuries that are not perceived by the patient, in whom repeated injuries and traumas may result in chronic infections and when severe lead to osteomyelitis. A clinical evaluation of peripheral neuropathy is provided by Kelly.[67,68]

Bruxism

Bruxism (see Chapter 170) represents a stereotyped movement disorder clinically characterized by grinding or clenching of the teeth during sleep. The sounds made by friction of the teeth are usually perceived by a bed partner as very unpleasant.[69] The condition is typically brought to the attention of the medical or dental practitioner in efforts to eliminate the disturbing sounds. Bruxism can lead to abnormal

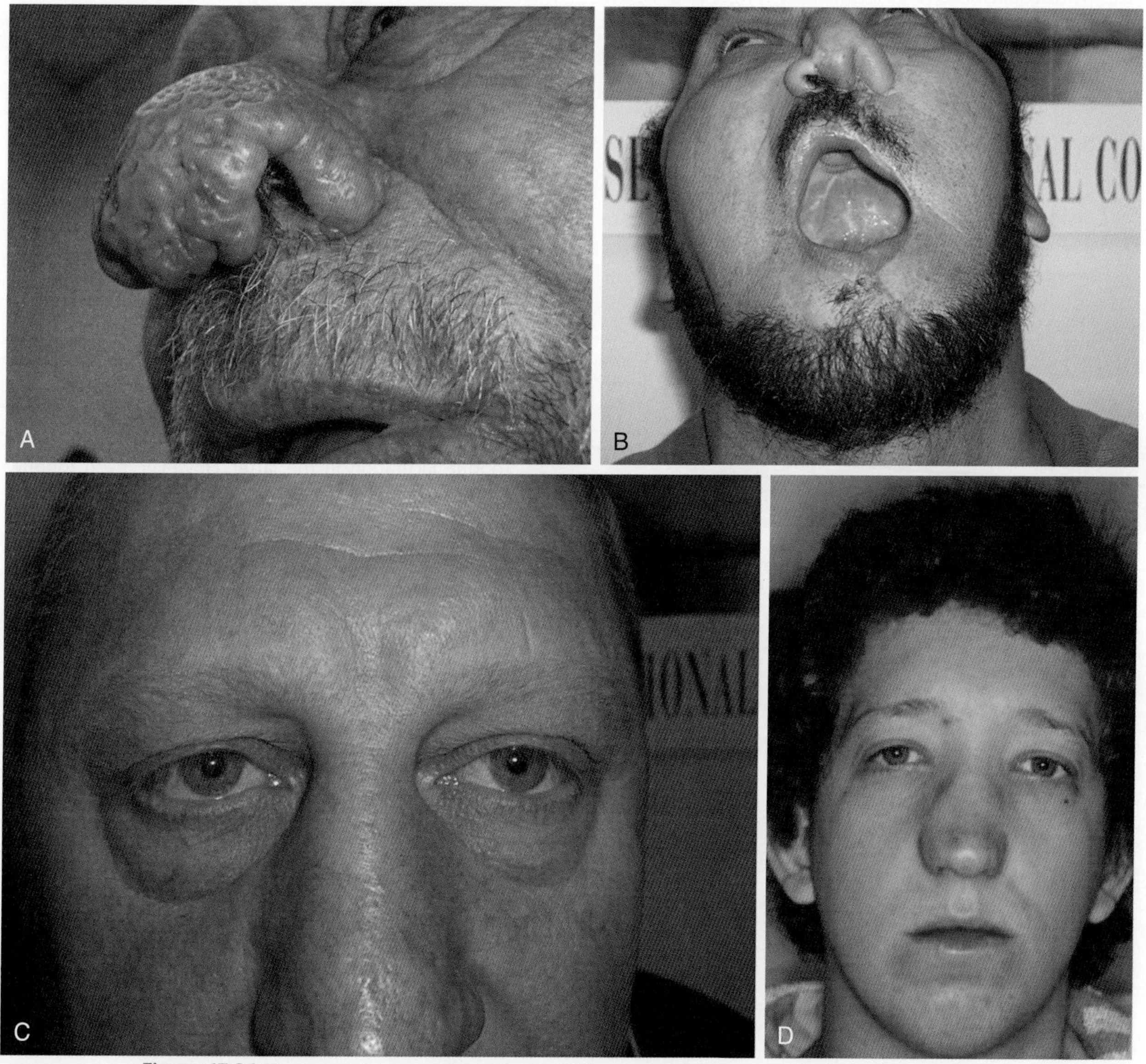

Figure 67.24 The nose and a sleep apnea deformity of the nose can be a very important contributor to sleep-disordered breathing. **A,** Rhinophyma ("bulbous nose" or "phymatous rosacea") is a nodular hypertrophy characterized by progressive thickening of the nose and leading to compromise of the nasal orifice airflow. **B,** Gunshot wound leading to significant facial injury and nasal collapse, requiring maxillomandibular reconstruction and plastic surgery. **C,** Nasal deviations due to remote foot injury. **D,** Nasal deformity due to the presence of nasal polyps. (**A, B,** and **D** Courtesy Dr. Meir H. Kryger; **C** from McGurk M. ENT disorders. In: Sprout C, Burke G, McGurk M, eds. *Essential Human Disease for Dentists.* Churchill Livingstone; 2006;195–204.)

wear of the teeth (Figure-67.52, *A* and *B*), periodontal tissue damage, or jaw pain. Other symptoms include facial muscle, headaches, and tooth pain and damage with abnormal wear to the teeth and damage to the structures surrounding the teeth. Chronically, over time and when untreated, this leads to recession and inflammation of the gums, alveolar bone resorption, muscles of mastication hypertrophy (Figure 67.53), and temporomandibular joint disorders, often associated with facial pain. Additional physical findings include tenderness of the muscles of mastication (masseter, temporalis, pterygoid, sternocleidal), temporomandibular disorders, tongue indentation, subjective appreciation of a tense personality, and hypervigilant patient.[70]

Case reports in patients with bruxism demonstrate bilateral enlargement in the region of the mandibular angle corresponding with the masseter hypertrophy (Figure 67.53).[71] Children with bruxism have a significantly longer and higher palate in the sagittal plane and bigger dental arches compared with normal children.[72] Psychiatric patients have a higher prevalence of bruxism and signs of temporomandibular disorders, possibly related to neuroleptic-induced phenomenon.[73]

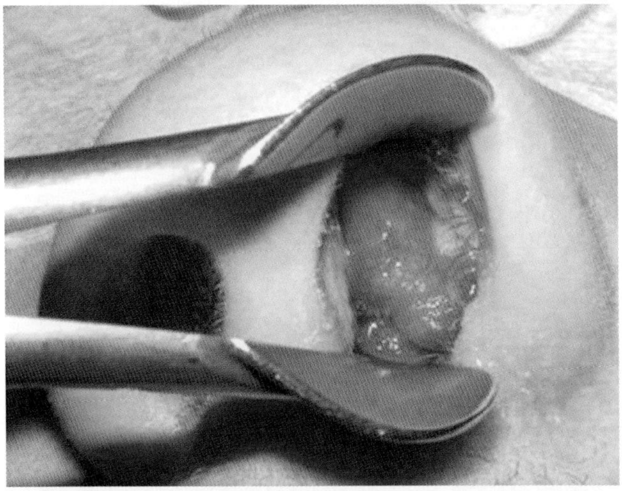

Figure 67.25 Nasal polyps. Nasal polyps are generally painless, soft, and benign, assuming grape-/cyst-like growths from the nasal wall and are generally secondary to chronic inflammation, reactive airway disease, environmental allergies, medication hypersensitivity, and immunologic disorders. (From Manning SC. *Cummings Otolaryngology Head and Neck Surgery*. ed 5. Mosby Elsevier; 2010.)

Ophthalmologic Signs

Patients with Graves disease, an autoimmune disorder and a common cause of hyperthyroidism, is characterized by the presence of exophthalmic eye signs (Figure 67.54), heat intolerance, involuntary weight loss, thyromegaly, tremor, and hyperactivity manifesting as restless sleep and insomnia.[74] Finally, floppy eyelid syndrome (Figure 67.55) is sometimes confused with a patient who may look tired, have a thyroid disorder, or have a neuromuscular disorder and is characterized by flaccid and easily everted upper lids, occurring spontaneously or with minimal manipulation.[75] It is seen in middle-aged males who are overweight, and it has been associated with OSA.[76]

CLINICAL PEARLS

- Overall inspection of the patient, coupled with observation of craniofacial, nasal, and pharyngeal factors, allows detection of key risk factors for sleep apnea.
- Examination of patients with insomnia should focus on the potential associated comorbidities, including hypothyroidism and rheumatologic disorders.
- Patients with motor disorders of sleep and parasomnias also have clinical findings conferred by the underlying medical, neurologic, and associated psychiatric comorbidities. For example, anosmia, orthostatic fluctuations in the setting of dream-enactment behavior and loss of electromyographic tone of polysomnography (PSG) may be predictive of an evolving α-synucleinopathy.
- Clues to the presence of abnormal nocturnal events, such as parasomnias or nocturnal seizures, may include unexplained bruising, lacerations in the former, and tongue laceration in the latter. However, even tongue biting, which is believed to be a clinical sign favoring epilepsy, can also occur in syncope and nonepileptic seizures. These difficulties highlight the importance of a well-tailored approach where the clinical history of coupled with the physical examination and supportive laboratory and PSG data to arrive at the most plausible clinical diagnosis.

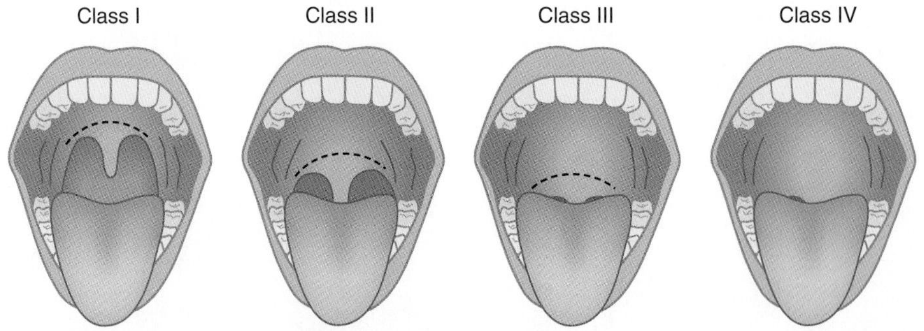

Figure 67.26 The Mallampati classification system. The Mallampati classification system is visualized with the tongue protruded but without the patient phonating. A modified form of the Mallampati system is measured with the tongue remaining on the floor of the mouth. The system was initially developed to predict ease of intubation but was later adopted by sleep medicine to help forecast the severity of obstructive sleep apnea in the ambulatory setting. It can also be used to help predict the appropriateness of upper airway surgery in certain patients by delineating the relationship of the various upper airway structures and noting the tongue size in relation to the uvula, tonsils, soft palate, and oropharyngeal wall. The standard for tongue size measurement involved the patient holding his or her head in a neutral position, opening the mouth as wide as possible, and sticking out the tongue. Class I is characterized by direct visualization of the soft palate, uvula, palatine tonsils, and pillars. However, as these structures become obscured, so does the Mallampati class, until only the hard palate is visible (class IV). (From Townsend CM Jr, Beauchamp RD, Evers BM, et al. *Sabiston Textbook of Surgery.* 19th ed. Elsevier; 2012.)

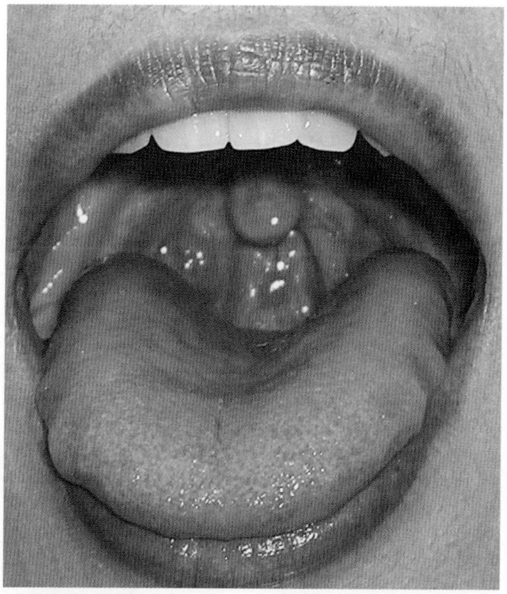

Figure 67.27 Mallampati class I. (From Kryger MH, Avidan A, Berry R. *Atlas of Clinical Sleep Medicine.* 2nd ed. Saunders; 2014: Figures 13.1–28.)

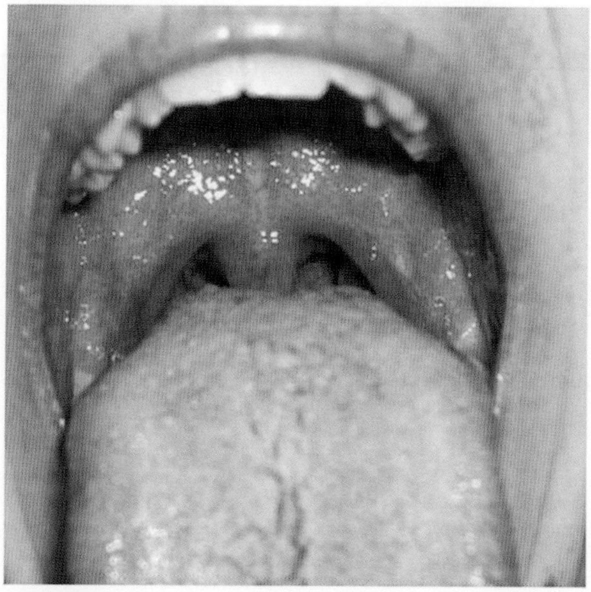

Figure 67.28 Mallampati class II. (From Kryger MH, Avidan A, Berry R. *Atlas of Clinical Sleep Medicine.* 2nd ed. Saunders; 2014: Figures 13.1–29, *A*.)

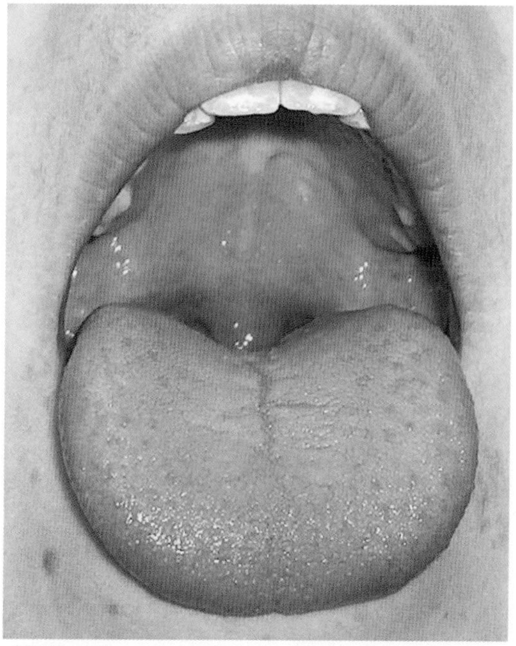

Figure 67.29 Mallampati class III. (From Kryger MH, Avidan A, Berry R. *Atlas of Clinical Sleep Medicine.* 2nd ed. Saunders; 2014: Figures 13.1–30, *A*.)

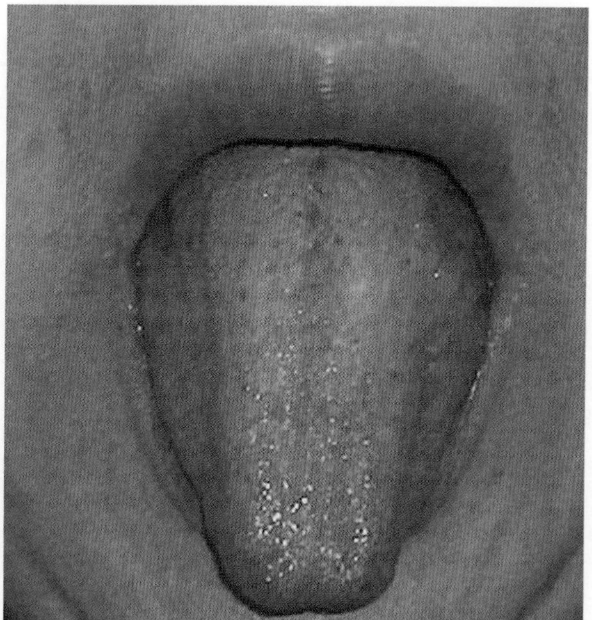

Figure 67.30 Mallampati class IV. (From Kryger MH, Avidan A, Berry R. *Atlas of Clinical Sleep Medicine.* 2nd ed. Saunders; 2014: Figures 13.1–31.)

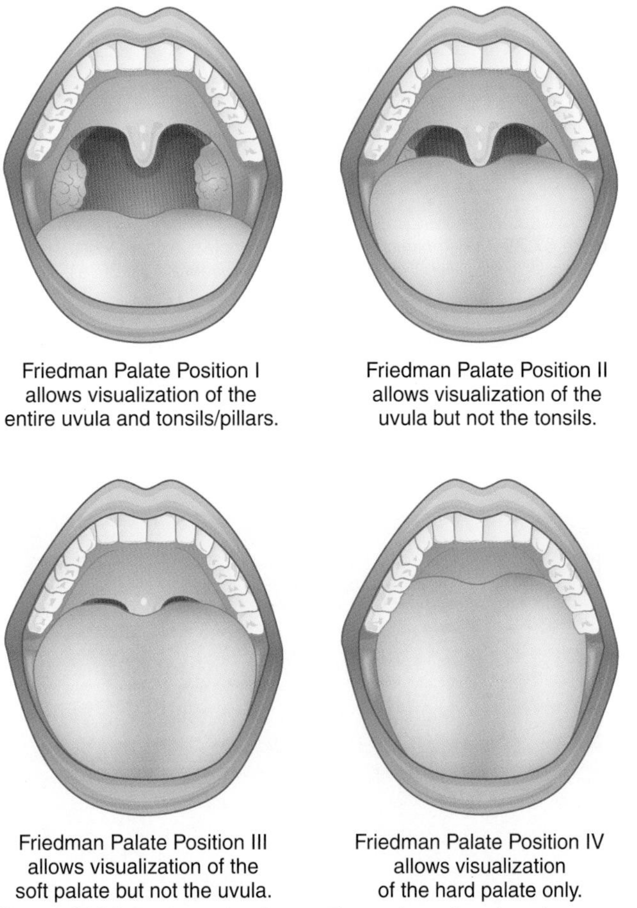
Friedman Palate Position I allows visualization of the entire uvula and tonsils/pillars.
Friedman Palate Position II allows visualization of the uvula but not the tonsils.
Friedman Palate Position III allows visualization of the soft palate but not the uvula.
Friedman Palate Position IV allows visualization of the hard palate only.

Figure 67.31 Friedman classification. This grading is based on the tongue in a natural position inside the mouth. Palate grade I allows the observer to visualize the entire uvula and tonsils or pillars. Palate grade II allows visualization of the uvula but not the tonsils. Palate grade III allows visualization of the soft palate but not the uvula. Palate grade IV allows visualization of the hard palate only. (From Friedman M, Ibrahim H, Bass L. Clinical staging for sleep disordered breathing. *Otolaryngol Head Neck Surg.* 2002;127:13–21.)

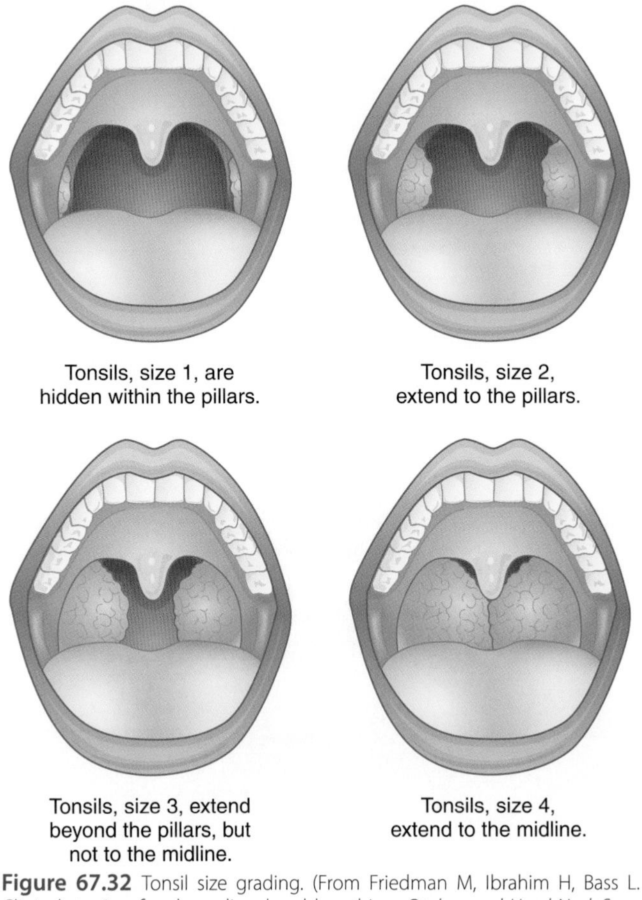
Tonsils, size 1, are hidden within the pillars.
Tonsils, size 2, extend to the pillars.
Tonsils, size 3, extend beyond the pillars, but not to the midline.
Tonsils, size 4, extend to the midline.

Figure 67.32 Tonsil size grading. (From Friedman M, Ibrahim H, Bass L. Clinical staging for sleep-disordered breathing. *Otolaryngol Head Neck Surg.* 2002;127:13–21.)

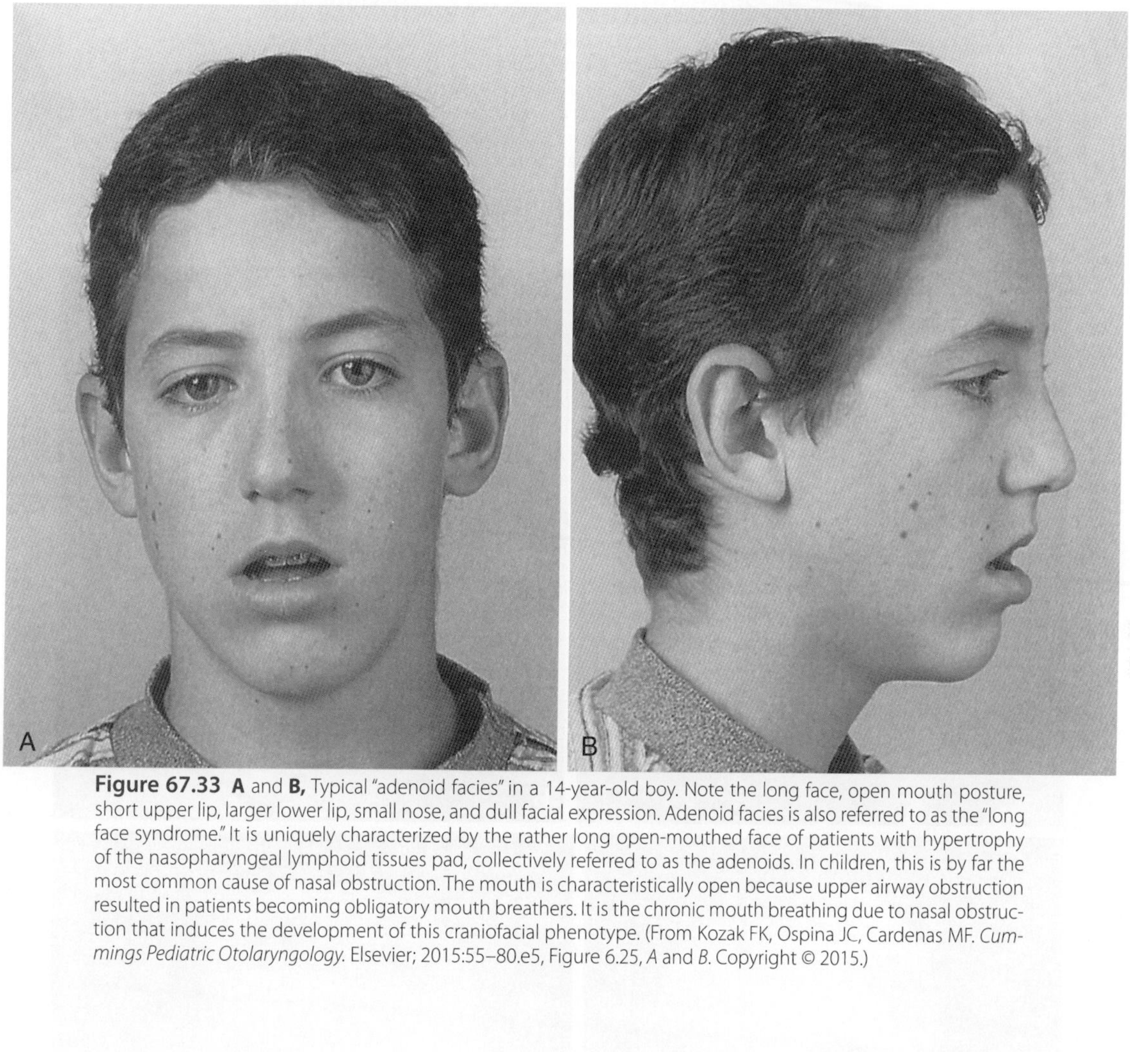

Figure 67.33 **A** and **B,** Typical "adenoid facies" in a 14-year-old boy. Note the long face, open mouth posture, short upper lip, larger lower lip, small nose, and dull facial expression. Adenoid facies is also referred to as the "long face syndrome." It is uniquely characterized by the rather long open-mouthed face of patients with hypertrophy of the nasopharyngeal lymphoid tissues pad, collectively referred to as the adenoids. In children, this is by far the most common cause of nasal obstruction. The mouth is characteristically open because upper airway obstruction resulted in patients becoming obligatory mouth breathers. It is the chronic mouth breathing due to nasal obstruction that induces the development of this craniofacial phenotype. (From Kozak FK, Ospina JC, Cardenas MF. *Cummings Pediatric Otolaryngology.* Elsevier; 2015:55–80.e5, Figure 6.25, *A* and *B*. Copyright © 2015.)

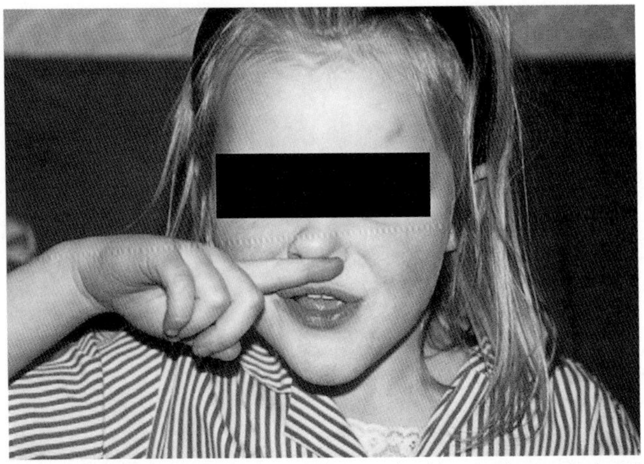

Figure 67.34 Allergic salute sign. "Allergic salute" in a patient with chronic allergic rhinitis. Other associated features include allergic shiners," referred to as infraorbital dark circles, related to venous plexus engorgement, "allergic gape" or continuous open-mouth breathing appearance secondary to nasal blockage, "transversal nasal crease" secondary to vigorous and continuous upward rubbing of the nose, as well as dental malocclusion and overbite resulting from long-standing upper airway problems. (From Scadding GK, Church MK, Borish L. Allergic rhinitis and rhinosinusitis. *Allergy.* 2012;203–26.)

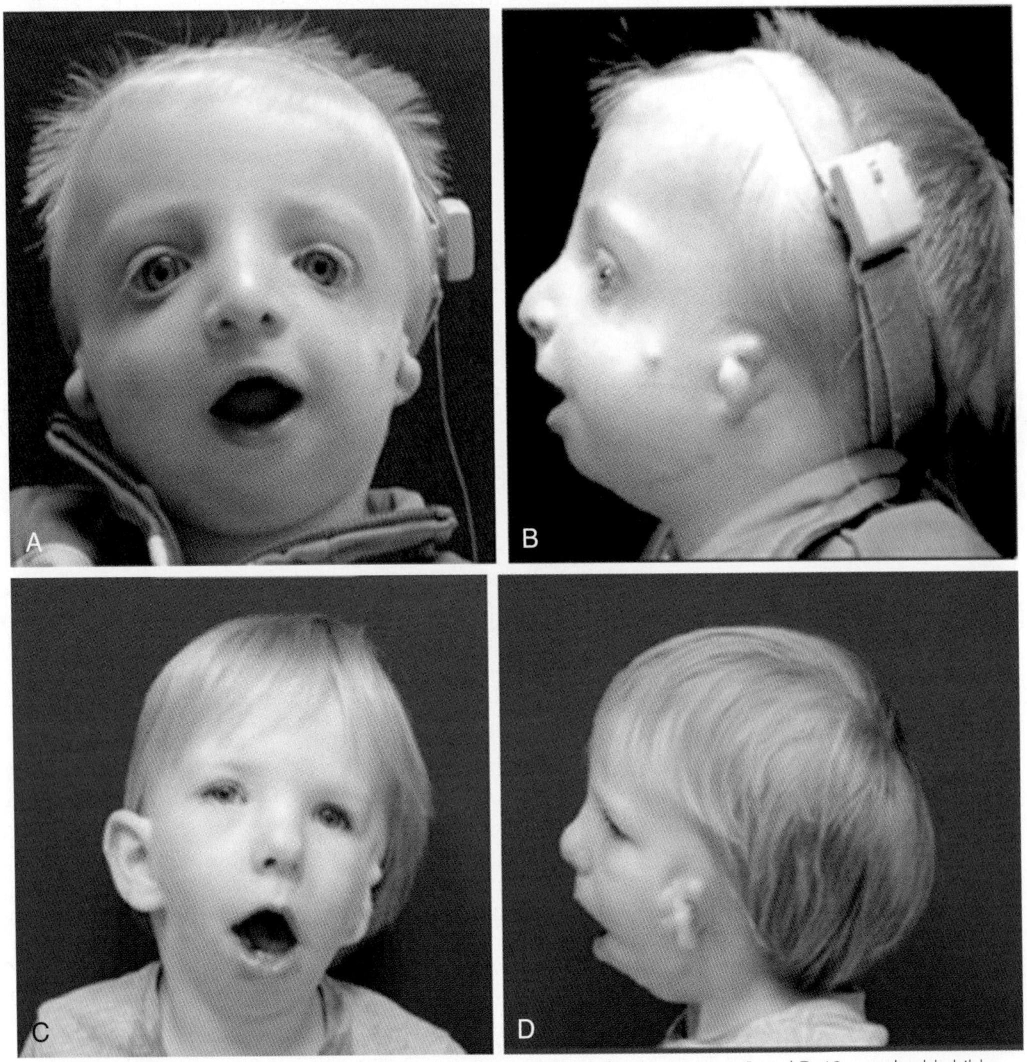

Figure 67.35 Four children with craniofacial syndrome with risk for sleep apnea. **A** and **B,** 13-month-old child with Treacher-Collins syndrome, characterized by down-slanting palpebral fissures, bilateral microtia, and mandibular hypoplasia. **C** and **D,** 22-month-old child with hemifacial microsomia, highlighting mandibular hypoplasia and unilateral microtia.

Continued

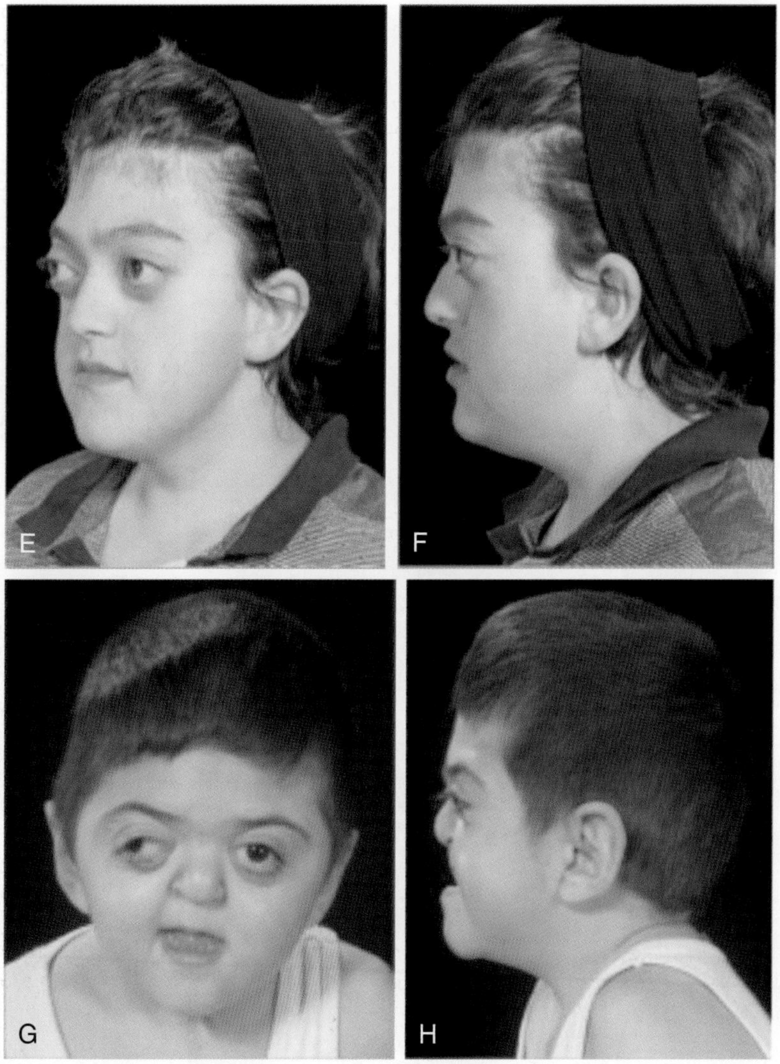

Figure 67.35—cont'd **E** and **F,** 11-year-old child with Crouzon syndrome, highlighting the typical clinical features of brachycephaly, exophthalmos, and maxillary hypoplasia with mandibular prognathism. **G** to **H,** 4-year-old child with Apert syndrome characterized by brachycephaly, strabismus, low set ears, and midface hypoplasia with mandibular prognathism. (**A** to **D** From Cielo CM. Obstructive sleep apnoea in children with craniofacial syndromes, *Paediatr Respir Rev.* 2015;16(3):189–96; **E** to **H** from Tan H-L, Kheirandish-Gozal L, Abel F, Gozal D. Craniofacial syndromes and sleep-related breathing disorders. *Sleep Med Rev.* 2016;27:74–88. Copyright © 2015 Elsevier.)

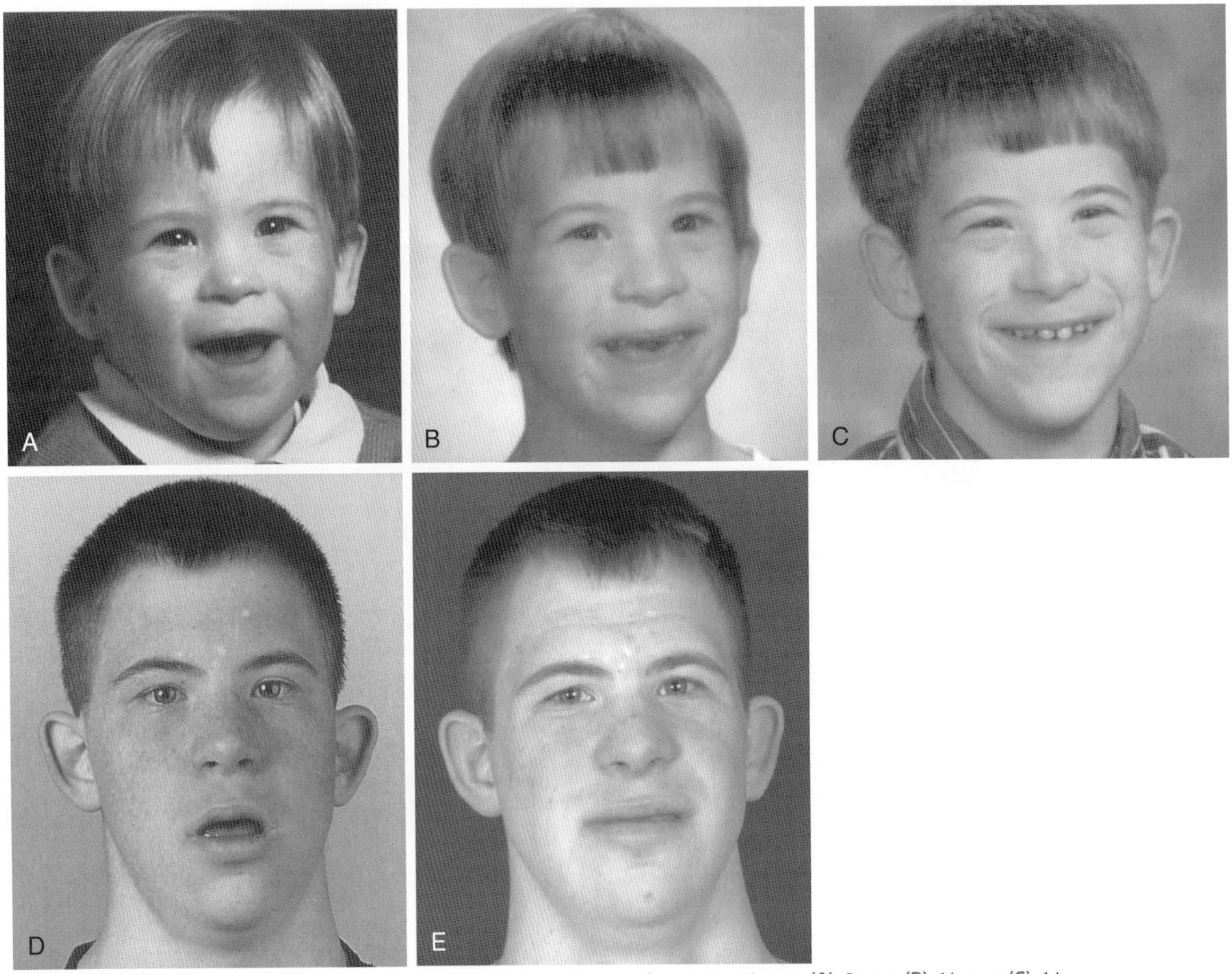

Figure 67.36 Down syndrome (DS) or trisomy 21 in a male patient at 2 years **(A),** 5 years **(B),** 11 years **(C),** 14 years **(D),** and 20 years **(E).** DS is defined by an extra copy of chromosome 21 and is the commonest genetic disorder. As mentioned earlier, risk factors for obstructive sleep apnea (OSA) in children with DS include midface hypoplasia, mandibular hypoplasia, adenotonsillar hypertrophy, and glossoptosis. Contributing factors for OSA in adults with DS are most often due to overlap between the DS phenotype and OSA risk factors. (From Kozak FK, Ospina JC, Cardenas MF. *Cummings Pediatric Otolaryngology.* Elsevier; 2015:55–80.e5, Figure 6.25, *A* and *B*. Copyright © 2015.)

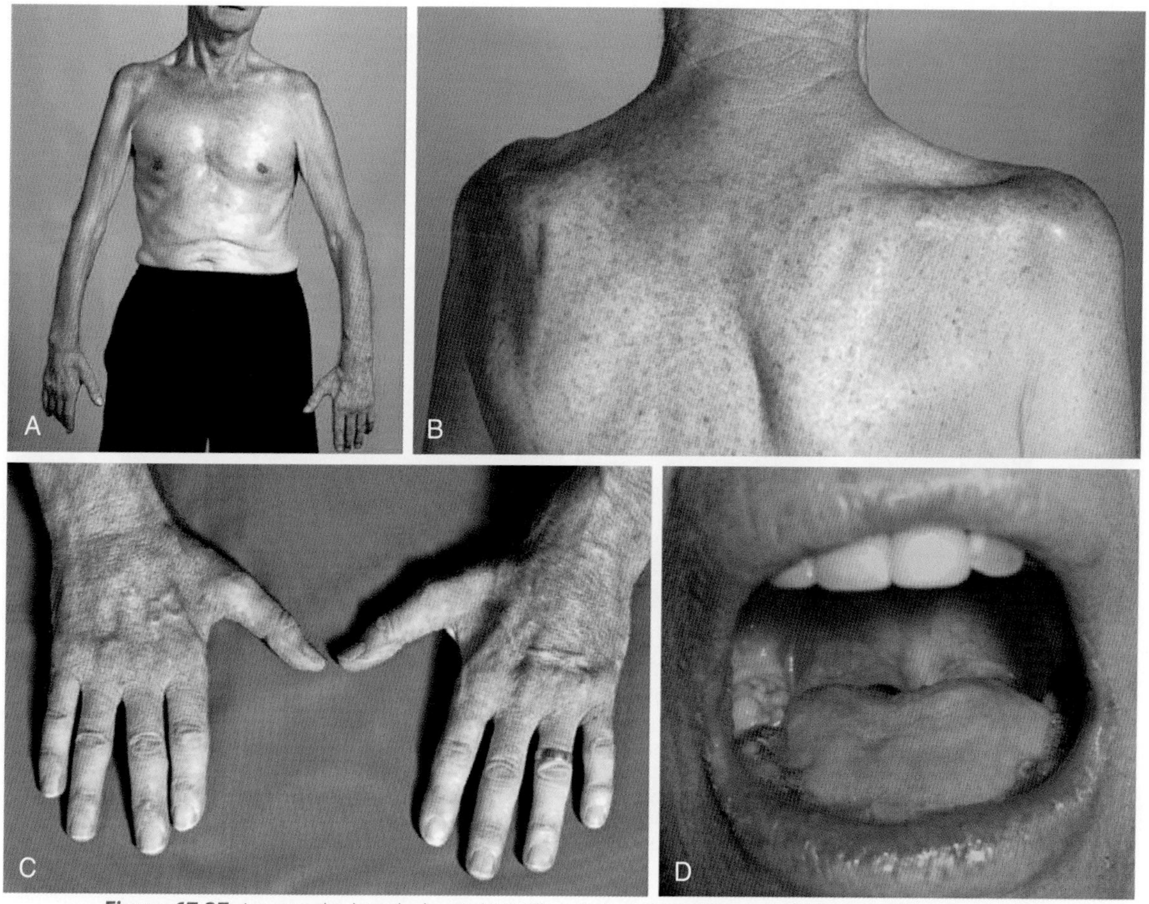

Figure 67.37 Amyotrophic lateral sclerosis (ALS). Clinical phenotypical features of ALS consist of symmetric and proximal upper extremity wasting **(A)** muscle recessions above and below the scapular spine **(B),** indicative of wasting of the supraspinatus and infraspinatus muscles, prominence of the glenohumeral joint making it prone to subluxation. **C,** Wasting of the thenar muscles in a disproportionate manner resulting in the so-called "split-hand." **D,** Substantial wasting of the tongue muscles in bulbar-onset ALS, which is especially critical in sleep-disordered breathing. There is absence of palatal elevation during phonation. (From Kiernan MC, Vucic S, Cheah BC, et al. Amyotrophic lateral sclerosis. *Lancet.* 2011;377(9769):942–55.)

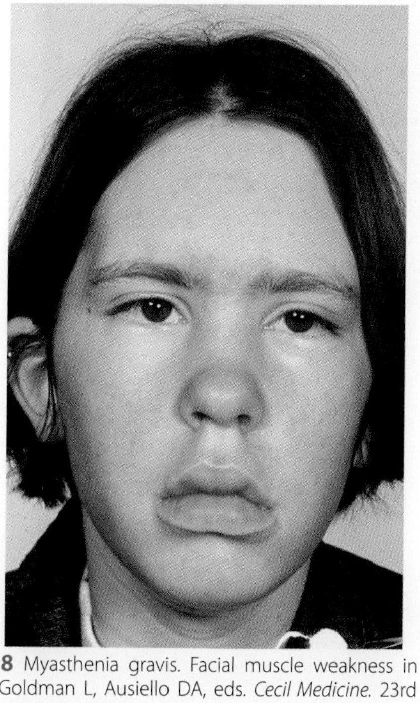

Figure 67.38 Myasthenia gravis. Facial muscle weakness in myasthenia gravis. (From Goldman L, Ausiello DA, eds. *Cecil Medicine.* 23rd ed. Elsevier; 2008.)

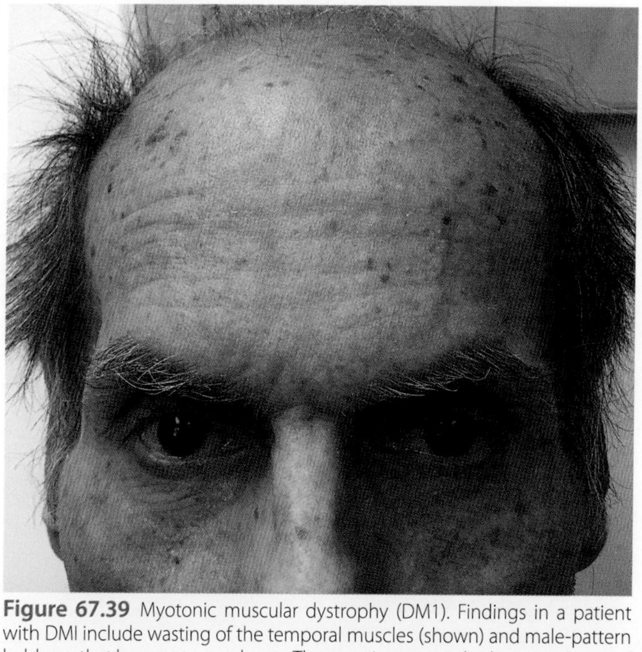

Figure 67.39 Myotonic muscular dystrophy (DM1). Findings in a patient with DMI include wasting of the temporal muscles (shown) and male-pattern baldness that began at an early age. These patients may also have weakness of other facial muscles and micrognathia. (Courtesy Dr. Meir H. Kryger.)

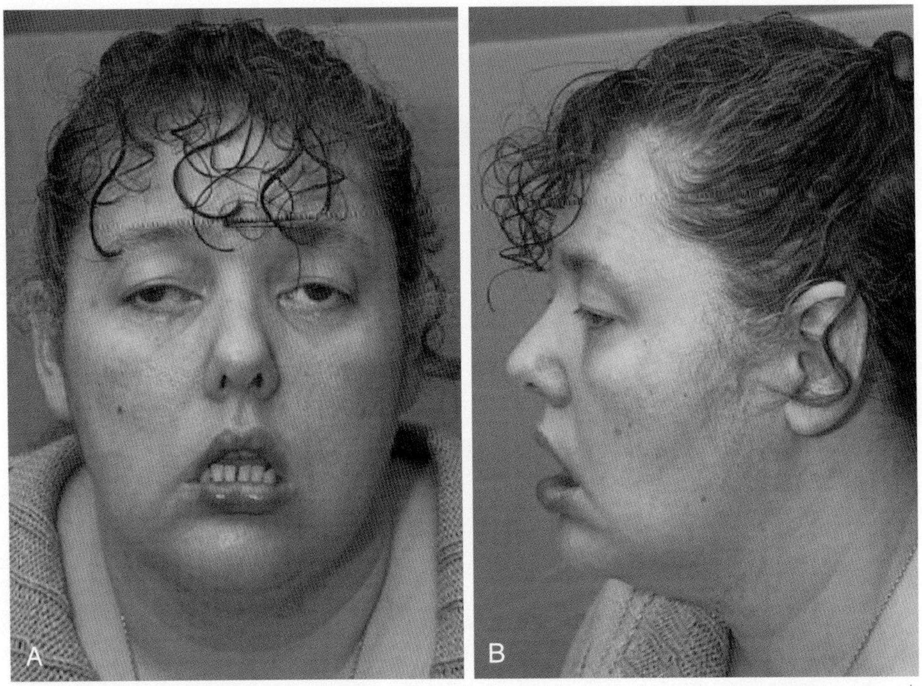

Figure 67.40 Progressive muscular dystrophy. **A** and **B,** Bilateral facial weakness due to progressive muscular dystrophy. The patient exhibits the classic signs, including bilateral ptosis. Facial weakness involves the orbicularis oculi, orbicularis oris, and zygomaticus muscle, producing the characteristic myopathic facial. Weakness of muscles of the thoracic region often leads to respiratory insufficiency, and many patients also present with bulbar symptoms (dysarthria, dysphagia). (From Laina V, Orlando A. Bilateral facial palsy and oral incompetence due to muscular dystrophy treated with a palmaris longus tendon graft. *J Plast Reconstr Aesthet Surg.* 2009;62[11]:e479–81.)

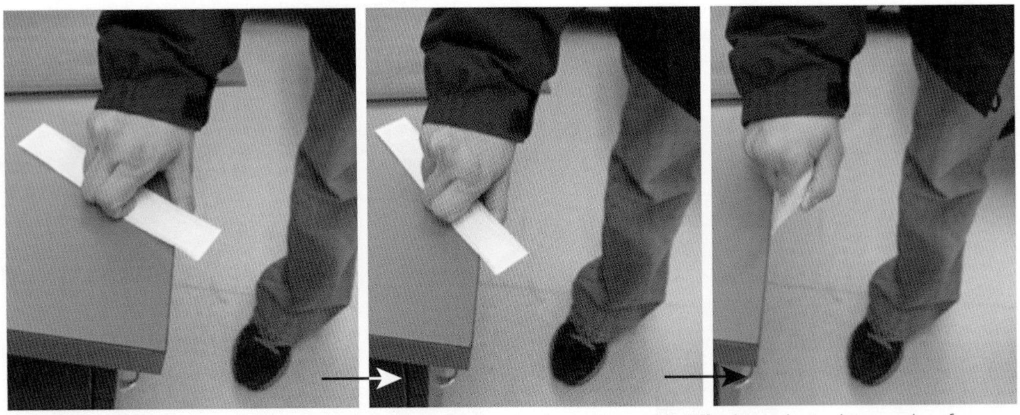

Figure 67.41 Muscular dystrophy. An attempt at grasp by the patient, with difficulties relaxing his muscles after the grasp. (Courtesy Dr. Meir H. Kryger.)

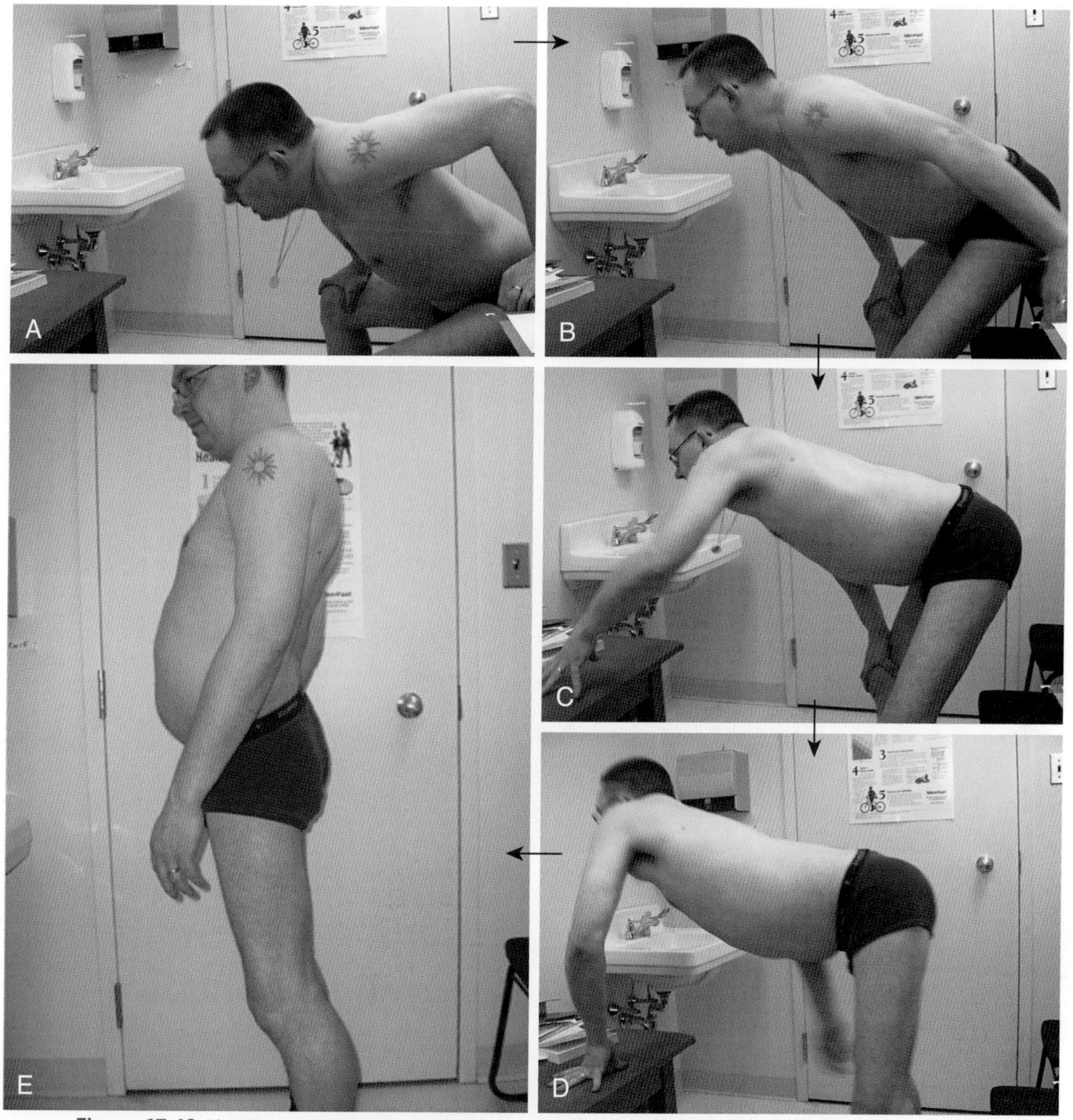

Figure 67.42 The Gower maneuver in a patient with Becker muscular dystrophy caused by an in-frame deletion of exons 45 to 47 in the dystrophin gene. The patient is using the Gower maneuver to rise from a sitting to standing position. While sitting **(A),** he uses the force of his hands to stand (**B, C,** and **D**). In **E,** using his thighs, he pushed himself upright, leading to the characteristic hyperlordosis posture. (Courtesy Dr. Meir H. Kryger.)

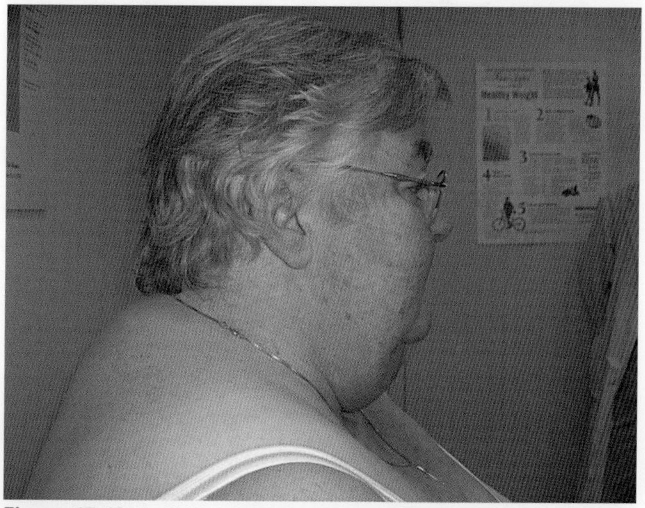

Figure 67.43 "Buffalo hump" in a patient with chronic steroid use. (Courtesy Dr. Meir H. Kryger.)

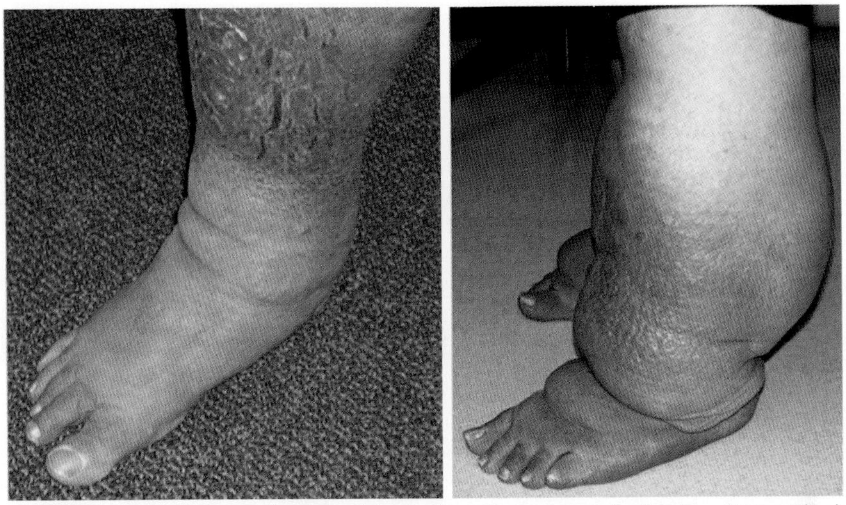

Figure 67.44 Peripheral edema. Chronic peripheral edema is a common finding in patients with obesity-hypoventilation syndrome. (Courtesy Dr. Meir H. Kryger.)

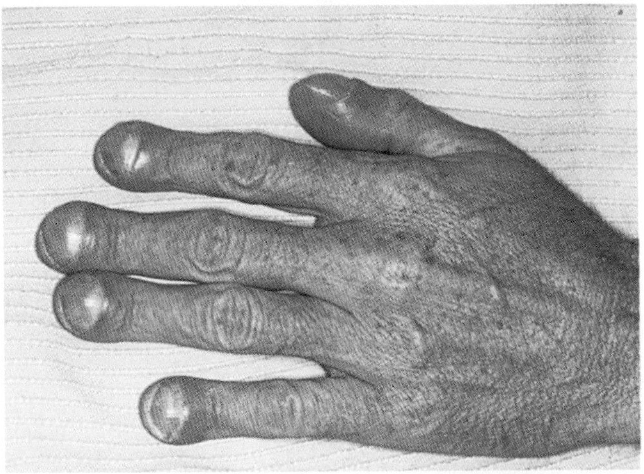

Figure 67.45 Chronic peripheral edema is a common finding in patients with obesity-hypoventilation syndrome. (Courtesy Dr. Meir H. Kryger.)

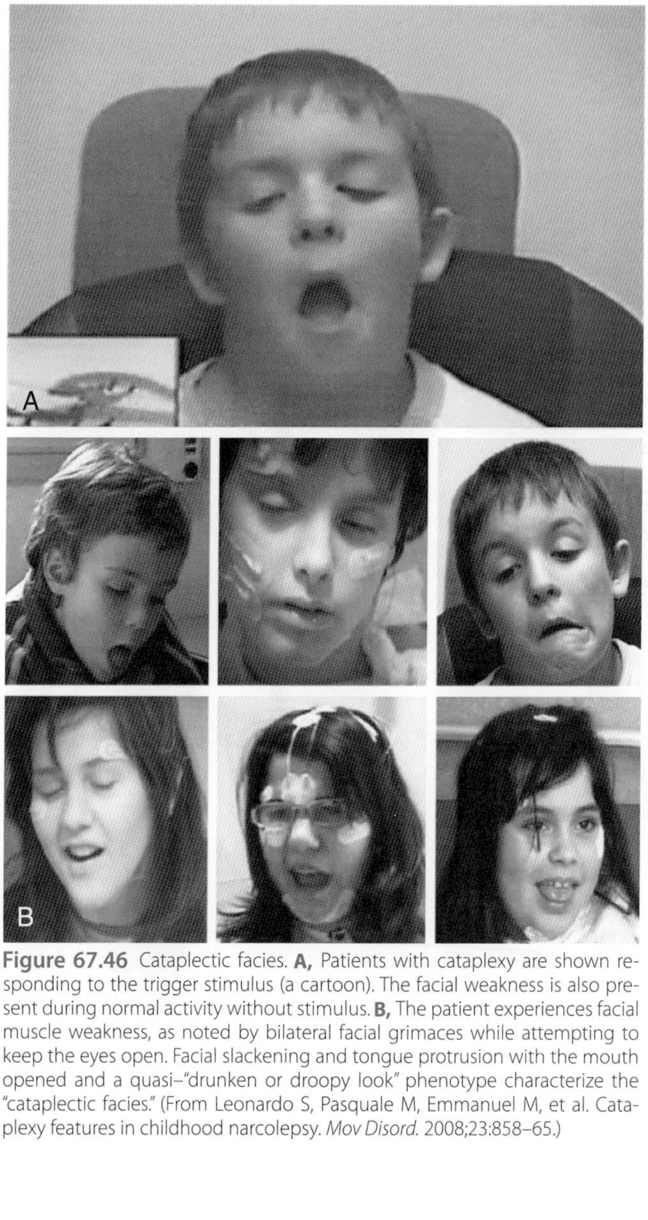

Figure 67.46 Cataplectic facies. **A,** Patients with cataplexy are shown responding to the trigger stimulus (a cartoon). The facial weakness is also present during normal activity without stimulus. **B,** The patient experiences facial muscle weakness, as noted by bilateral facial grimaces while attempting to keep the eyes open. Facial slackening and tongue protrusion with the mouth opened and a quasi–"drunken or droopy look" phenotype characterize the "cataplectic facies." (From Leonardo S, Pasquale M, Emmanuel M, et al. Cataplexy features in childhood narcolepsy. *Mov Disord.* 2008;23:858–65.)

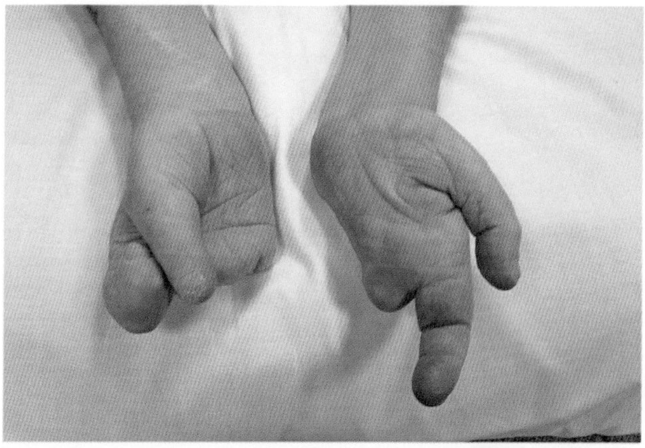

Figure 67.47 Amnestic autocannibalism. A photograph illustrating the damage to the fingers in the setting of a secondary parasomnia induced by untreated obstructive sleep apnea. Amnestic autocannibalism resulted, whereas the perception of pain during the episodes may have been abnormal in the setting of tetraplegia in this male patient. (From Basyuni S, Quinnell T. Autocannibalism induced by obstructive sleep apnea. *Sleep Med.* 2017;37:72–3. (http://www.sciencedirect.com/science/article/pii/S1389945717300801.

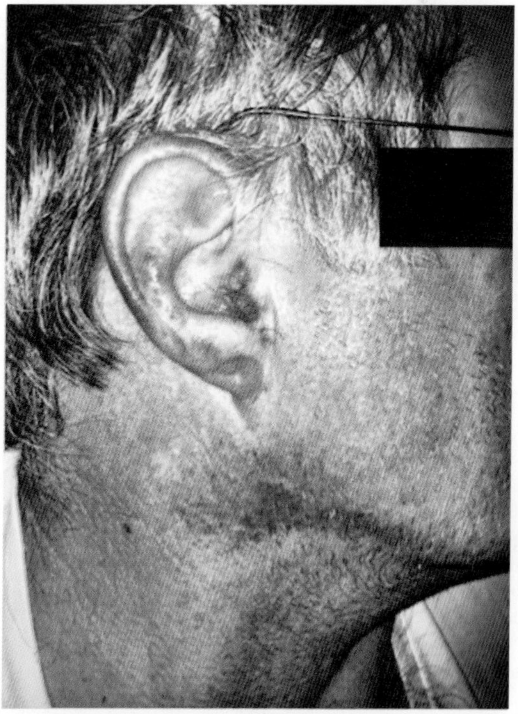

Figure 67.48 Injury in the setting of dream-enactment behavior. A patient with rapid eye movement sleep behavior disorder presented with aggressive dream-enactment behavior, resulting in severe injury during one of his nocturnal episodes. (Copyright Alon Y. Avidan, MD, MPH.)

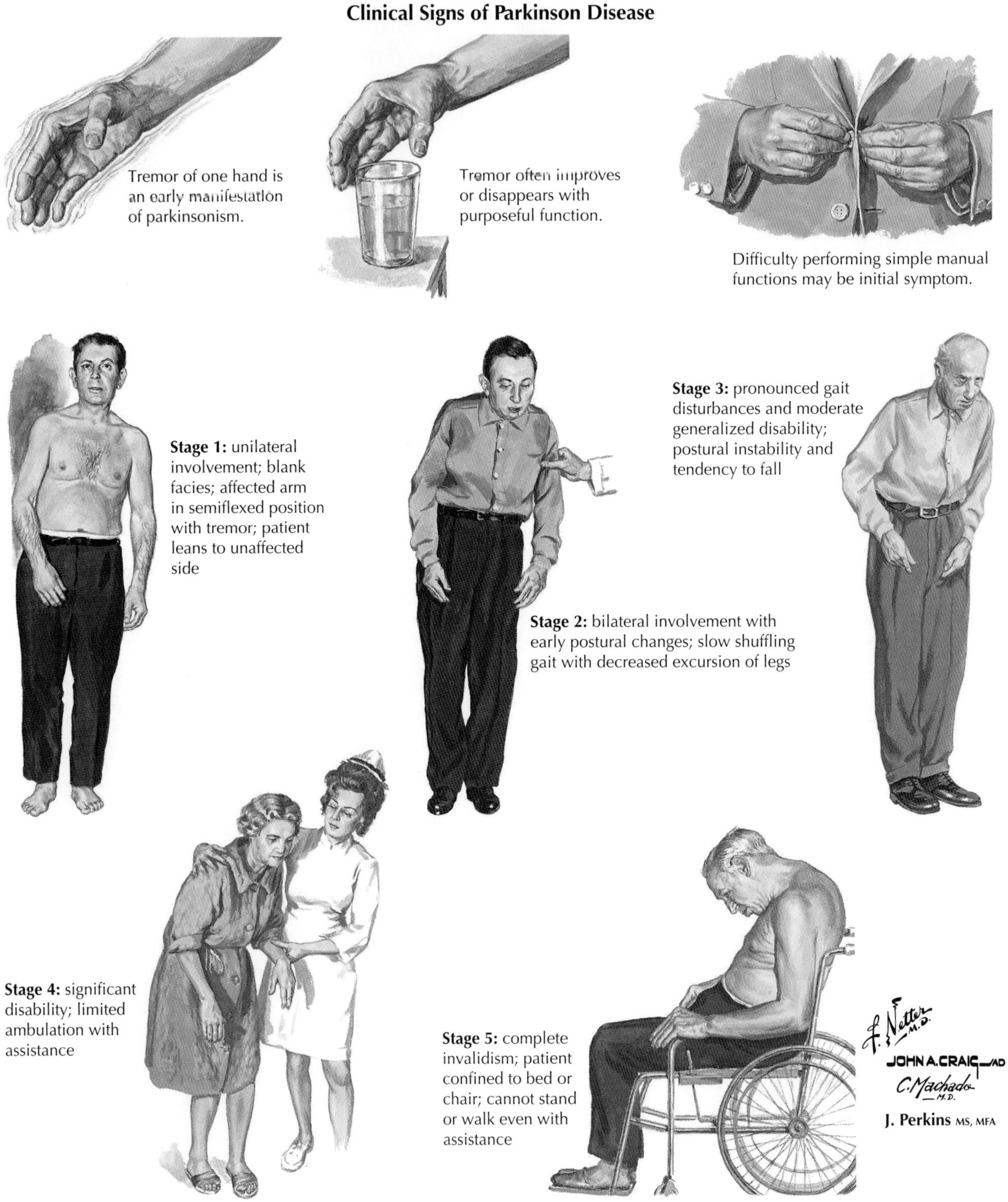
Clinical Signs of Parkinson Disease
Tremor of one hand is an early manifestation of parkinsonism.
Tremor often improves or disappears with purposeful function.
Difficulty performing simple manual functions may be initial symptom.
Stage 1: unilateral involvement; blank facies; affected arm in semiflexed position with tremor; patient leans to unaffected side
Stage 2: bilateral involvement with early postural changes; slow shuffling gait with decreased excursion of legs
Stage 3: pronounced gait disturbances and moderate generalized disability; postural instability and tendency to fall
Stage 4: significant disability; limited ambulation with assistance
Stage 5: complete invalidism; patient confined to bed or chair; cannot stand or walk even with assistance
F. Netter M.D.
JOHN A.CRAIG AD
C.Machado M.D.
J. Perkins MS, MFA

Figure 67.49 The four primary signs of Parkinson disease (PD) include bradykinesia, tremor, rigidity, and gait disturbance. Bradykinesia is a defined as impairment in the ability to initiate movement. This impairs fine motor tasks, such as handwriting, which becomes micrographic. Some patients may present with an expressionless masked facies and reduced blink. The gait becomes shuffling with decreased arm swing, stooped posture, and en bloc turning. Rigidity is characterized by resistance to passive movement. The classic cogwheel quality (stop-and-go effect) results from a tremor overlapping on altered muscle tone. Resting tremor affects up to two-thirds of patients at a frequency of 3 to 7 Hz. Gait impairment and postural instability manifest at later stages of PD, characterized by a change in the center of gravity typified by falling forward (propulsion) or backward (retropulsion) and a festinating (shuffling, slowly propulsive) petit pas (small steps) gait. (From Apetauerova D. Parkinson disease. In: Srinivasan J, Chaves C, Scott B, Small JE, eds. *Netter's Neurology (Netter Clinical Science)*. Elsevier; 2020:346–59, Figure 28.8. Copyright © 2020.)

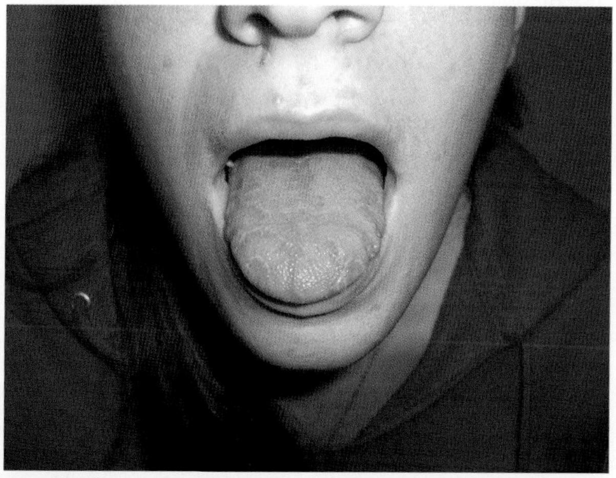

Figure 67.50 Tongue glossitis in iron deficiency. (Courtesy Dr. Meir H. Kryger.)

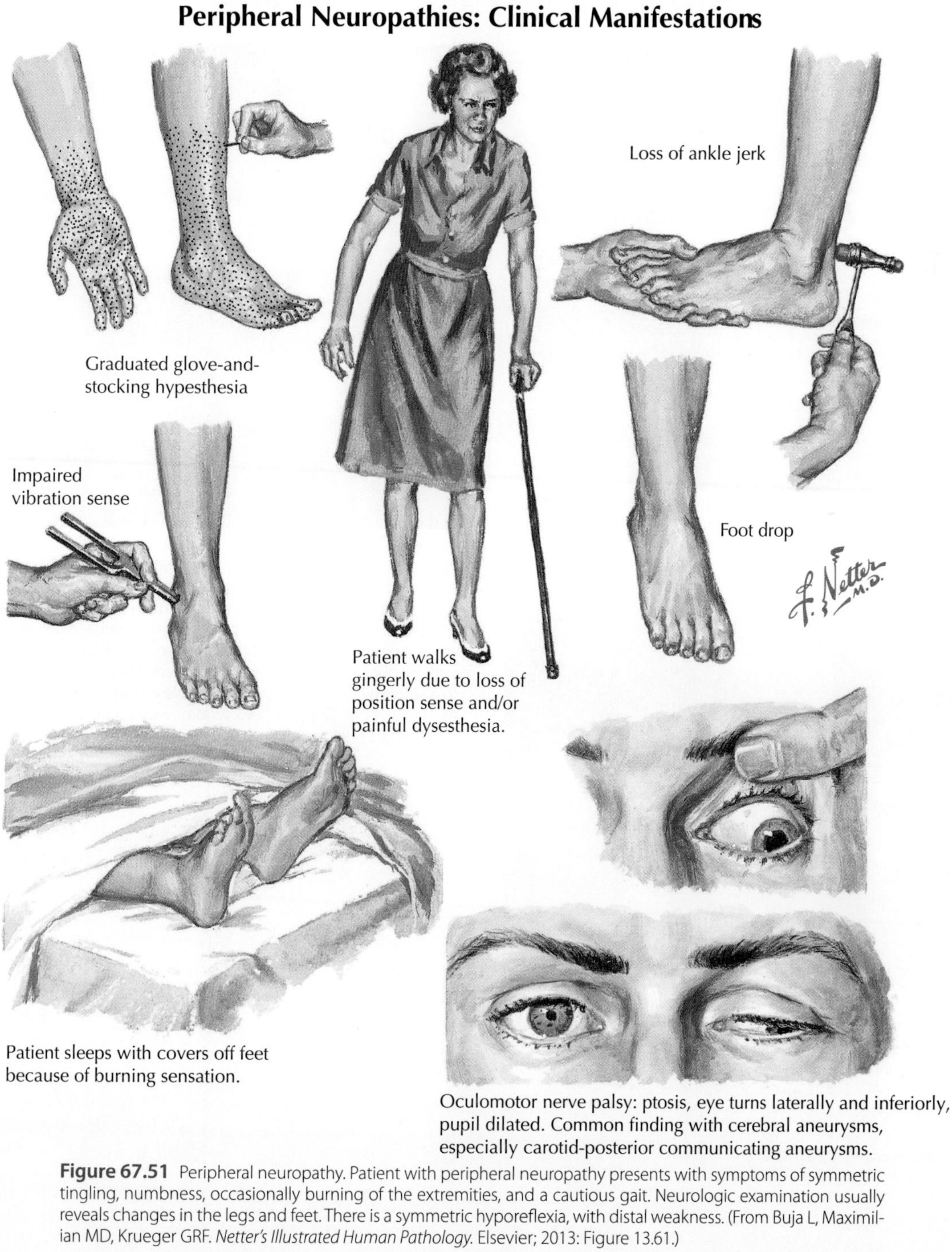
Peripheral Neuropathies: Clinical Manifestations
Graduated glove-and-stocking hypesthesia
Loss of ankle jerk
Impaired vibration sense
Patient walks gingerly due to loss of position sense and/or painful dysesthesia.
Foot drop
F. Netter M.D.
Patient sleeps with covers off feet because of burning sensation.
Oculomotor nerve palsy: ptosis, eye turns laterally and inferiorly, pupil dilated. Common finding with cerebral aneurysms, especially carotid-posterior communicating aneurysms.

Figure 67.51 Peripheral neuropathy. Patient with peripheral neuropathy presents with symptoms of symmetric tingling, numbness, occasionally burning of the extremities, and a cautious gait. Neurologic examination usually reveals changes in the legs and feet. There is a symmetric hyporeflexia, with distal weakness. (From Buja L, Maximilian MD, Krueger GRF. *Netter's Illustrated Human Pathology*. Elsevier; 2013: Figure 13.61.)

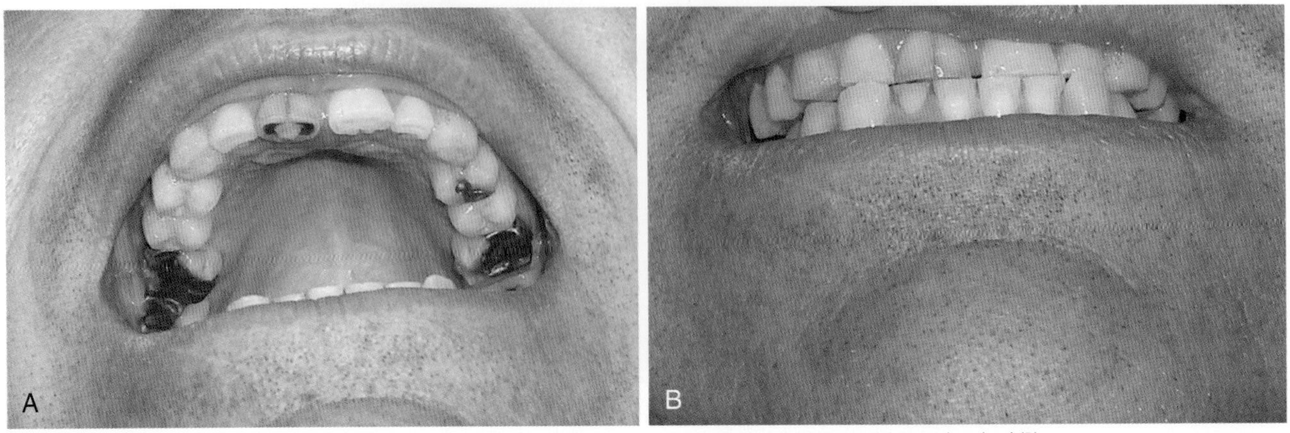

Figure 67.52 Bruxism with abnormal wear of the teeth with mouth open (A), jaw clenched (B).

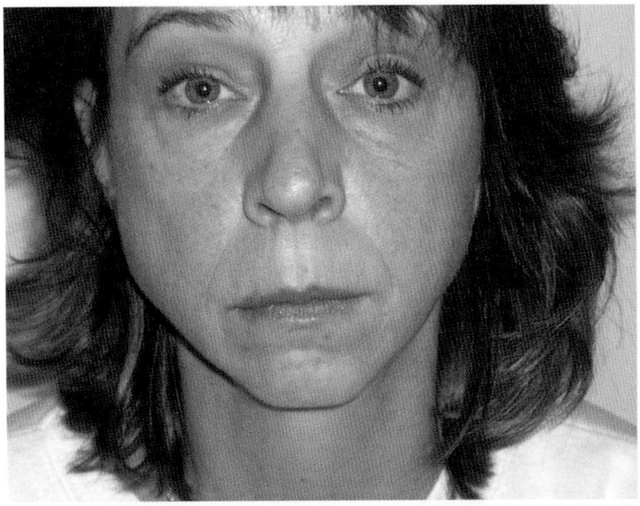

Figure 67.53 Hypertrophic masseter in bruxism. The masseter muscle bulk is markedly increased over the mandibular angle region. (Courtesy Dr. Meir H. Kryger.)

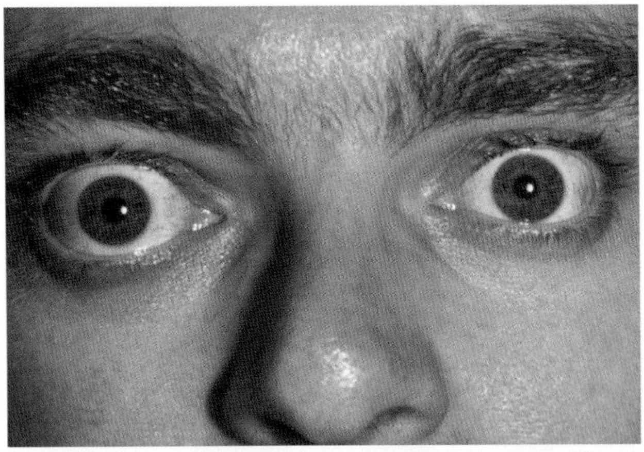

Figure 67.54 Exophthalmic eye signs in the setting of hyperthyroidism. Patient noted increasingly staring eyes. Clinically, he had proptosis and lid lag. (From Quick CRG, Biers SM, Arulampalam Tan HA. *Disorders of the Thyroid, Parathyroid and Adrenal Glands Essential Surgery: Problems, Diagnosis and Management*. Elsevier; 2019:621–35, Figure 49.4. Copyright © 2020.)

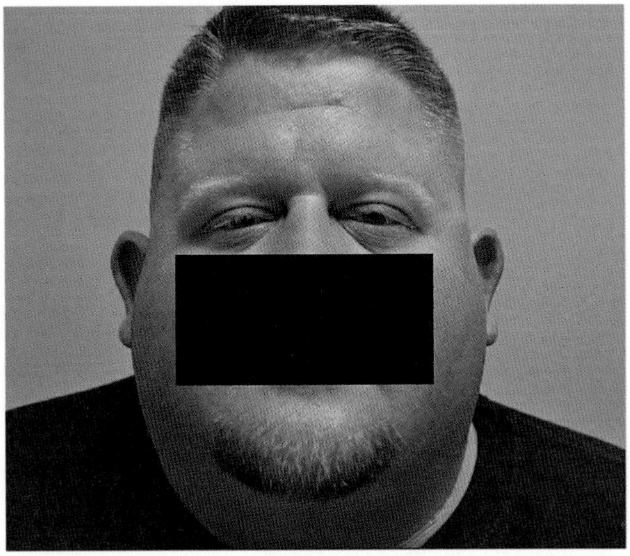

Figure 67.55 Floppy eyelid syndrome is an uncommon unilateral or bilateral condition typically impacting obese, middle-aged, and older men who sleep with one or both eyelids against the pillow, leading to the lid pulling away from the globe. Consequent nocturnal exposure and poor contact with the globe, often exacerbated by other ocular surface disease, such as dry eye and blepharitis, result in chronic keratoconjunctivitis. It may be associated with blepharoptosis (ptosis) and dermatochalasis (eyelid skin redundancy and loss of elasticity), which are also visible in this patient. (From Salinas R, Puig M, Fry CL, et al. Floppy eyelid syndrome: a comprehensive review. *Ocul Surf.* 2020;18(1):31–9.)

SUMMARY

The physical examination of any patient with sleep disorders is the cornerstone for making critical decisions about the possible clinical diagnosis, for determining the need for formal PSG, and for ensuring that treatment is successful. Given that medical trainees often do not receive formalized sleep medicine education in medical school, appreciating the fundamental phenotypical patterns responsible for SDB are critical. A basic appreciation of the abnormal neurologic examination is important for nonneurologists who may encounter patients with parasomnias and motor and movement disorders of sleep. Finally, no clinical examination of the sleepy patient should conclude without a comprehensive review of the background medical endocrine, metabolic, and genetic factors that may contribute to disrupted sleep.

SELECTED READINGS

Myers KA, Mrkobrada M, Simel DL. Does this patient have obstructive sleep apnea? The Rational Clinical Examination systematic review. *JAMA.* 2013;310(7):731–741. https://doi.org/10.1001/jama.2013.276185.

Posnick JC, ed. *Principles and Practice of Orthognathic Surgery*. Elsevier Health Sciences; 2013.

Wilhelm CP, deShazo RD, Tamanna S, et al. The nose, upper airway, and obstructive sleep apnea. *Ann Allergy Asthma Immunol.* 2015;115(2):96–102. https://doi.org/10.1016/j.anai.2015.06.011. PMID: 26250769.

A complete reference list can be found online at ExpertConsult.com.

Chapter 68

Clinical Tools and Tests in Sleep Medicine

Cathy A. Goldstein; Ronald D. Chervin

Chapter Highlights

- A clinician confronted with a complaint about sleep or alertness combines symptoms, signs, and test results to make a diagnostic assessment.
- Information about test performance characteristics, such as sensitivity, specificity, and predictive value, can be weighed with patient preference to select optimal approaches.
- In addition to the history and physical examination, tools and tests used in the evaluation of a patient with sleep-related symptoms may include questionnaires, sleep diaries or logs, actigraphy, nocturnal polysomnography, a home sleep test, or a Multiple Sleep Latency Test.
- The era of big data has ushered in advances in artificial intelligence, which, along with the rapid evolution of sensor technology, have the potential to augment current assessment methods in sleep medicine.

This chapter highlights the clinical reasoning process by which a clinician challenged with a sleep complaint can combine information from different sources, appropriately weigh available evidence, and arrive at sound diagnostic and treatment plans. Here we review the value of tests in evaluations of suspected sleep-disordered breathing, hypersomnolence, insomnia, suspected circadian rhythm sleep-wake disorders, restless legs syndrome (RLS), and suspected parasomnias. A selection of clinical practice guidelines (previously designated as practice parameters), position statements, and their companion review articles are produced by the American Academy of Sleep Medicine (AASM) and can be accessed at https://aasm.org/clinical-resources/practice-standards/practice-guidelines/ (Table 68.1) to supplement the overviews presented in this chapter.

EVALUATION FOR SLEEP-RELATED BREATHING DISORDERS

History

Sleep-related breathing disorders are by far the most common disorders diagnosed at sleep centers, with obstructive sleep apnea (OSA) accounting for nearly 70% of all patients evaluated.[1] Subjective clinical impressions of OSA tend to have inadequate sensitivity (probability of a positive test result or assessment given that the disorder is present) and specificity (probability of a negative test result given that the disorder is absent).[2]

Specific symptoms, such as snoring and excessive daytime sleepiness (EDS), have limited value if taken in isolation.[3,4] For example, snoring has high sensitivity (80% to 90%) but low specificity (20%–50%) for OSA diagnosis; a history of hypertension may be a better predictor.[5] Nocturnal choking or gasping is less sensitive (52%) but more specific (84%) than snoring and, considering a population prevalence of 14%, yields a positive predictive value (PPV) for OSA of 35%, which is greater than the PPV for morning headache, reported apnea, EDS, or snoring.[2]

Combinations of some signs and symptoms can have sensitivity greater than 90%, but because specificity is usually poor, individuals with symptoms suggestive of OSA must undergo objective testing to confirm the diagnosis.

Physical Examination

For detailed information on the physical examination in patients with suspected sleep disorders, see Chapter 67. Neck circumference and body mass index (BMI) correlate well with the presence and severity of OSA,[6] but their predictive value is not large except in extreme ranges.[4,7,8] Patients with OSA who are not obese often have pharyngeal crowding, obstructed nasal passages, or other craniofacial abnormalities associated with narrowing of the upper airway.[9] The predictive value of such findings may differ somewhat between men and women.[10] The Mallampati score, which reflects oropharyngeal crowding on a 4-point scale, is helpful in the assessment of risk for OSA.[11] Each 1-point increase in the score was associated with a 2.5 increase in the odds of OSA and a 5-point higher apnea-hypopnea index (AHI). High blood pressure increases the chance that OSA will be present, especially among the less obese.[12] Signs of congestive heart failure, stigmata of polycystic ovary disease, evidence of prior stroke, or underlying neuropathy or neuromuscular disease are just a few examples of physical findings that may increase the likelihood of OSA.[13]

Table 68.1 Clinical Practice Guidelines, Practice Parameters, and Position Statements Related to the Use of Tools and Tests in Sleep Medicine from the American Academy of Sleep Medicine

Year	Category	Title
2007	Circadian rhythm sleep-wake disorders	Practice Parameters for the Clinical Evaluation and Treatment of Circadian Rhythm Sleep Disorders
2017	Diagnostics	Clinical Practice Guideline for Diagnostic Testing for Adult Obstructive Sleep Apnea: An American Academy of Sleep Medicine Clinical Practice Guideline
2018	Diagnostics	Use of Actigraphy for the Evaluation of Sleep Disorders and Circadian Rhythm Sleep-Wake Disorders: An American Academy of Sleep Medicine Clinical Practice Guideline
2005	Diagnostics	Practice Parameters for Clinical Use of the Multiple Sleep Latency Test and the Maintenance of Wakefulness Test
2008	Insomnia	Clinical Guideline for the Evaluation and Management of Chronic Insomnia in Adults
2010	Pediatrics	Practice Parameters for the Respiratory Indications for Polysomnography in Children
2012	Pediatrics	Practice Parameters for the Non-respiratory Indications for Polysomnography and Multiple Sleep Latency Testing for Children
2017	Pediatrics	American Academy of Sleep Medicine Position Paper for the Use of a Home Sleep Apnea Test for the Diagnosis of OSA in Children
2009	Sleep-related breathing disorders	Clinical Guideline for the Evaluation, Management and Long-term Care of Obstructive Sleep Apnea in Adults
2015	Telemedicine	American Academy of Sleep Medicine (AASM) Position Paper for the Use of Telemedicine for the Diagnosis and Treatment of Sleep Disorders

Physical findings can also be combined into predictive quantitative models to aid in the diagnosis of OSA. Models based on measures that can be obtained during the physical examination, such as BMI, neck circumference, craniofacial measurements, pharyngeal scores, and tonsil size, demonstrate excellent PPV (90% to 100%) but less strong negative predictive value (NPV) (49%–89%).[14–16]

Risk Assessment Tools

Instruments that use a combination of symptoms, comorbidities, and physical findings to assess risk for OSA include the Berlin Questionnaire, STOP, STOP-BANG, and Multivariable Apnea Prediction Questionnaire. The Berlin Questionnaire is a 10-item instrument that identifies high or low risk for OSA by questions related to snoring, apneas, daytime sleepiness, hypertension, and BMI. The STOP instrument assesses snoring, tiredness, observed apneas, and presence of high blood pressure, and the STOP-BANG (Figure 68.1) also incorporates BMI, age, neck circumference, and gender. The Multivariable Apnea Prediction Questionnaire combines three questions regarding the frequency of OSA symptoms with BMI, age, and gender. The pooled sensitivity, specificity, and likelihood ratios from meta-analysis of validation studies that compare these tools to polysomnography (PSG) are summarized in Table 68.2.

More recently, machine learning–derived models that combine medical history with objective patient characteristics were found to outperform models that used self-report symptoms.[17] This finding highlights the inability of subjective symptoms alone to distinguish—with sufficient reliability in clinical practice—between patients with and without OSA. However, as symptoms are relevant in an assessment of risk and whether a patient with sleep-disordered breathing should undergo treatment, the history of present illness remains a vital element in the evaluation of patients with suspected OSA. Clinical prediction tools alone cannot act as a surrogate

SNORING? Do you **snore loudly** (louder than talking or loud enough to be heard through closed doors)?	Yes	No
TIRED? Do you often feel **tired, fatigued, or sleepy** during the daytime?	Yes	No
OBSERVED? Has anyone **observed** you **stop breathing** during your sleep?	Yes	No
PRESSURE? Do you have or are you being treated for **high blood pressure?**	Yes	No
BODY MASS INDEX more than 35 kg/m^2?	Yes	No
AGE older than 50 years?	Yes	No
NECK circumference? Neck circumference greater than 40 cm?	Yes	No
Gender = male?	Yes	No

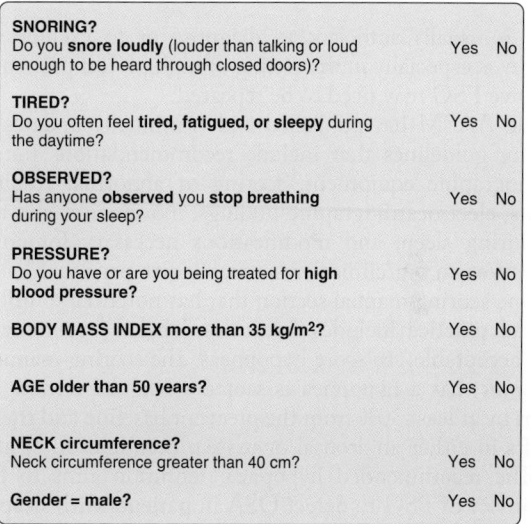

Figure 68.1 The STOP-BANG questionnaire. Low risk for OSA: yes to zero to two questions. High risk for OSA: yes to three or more questions. (From Chung F, Yegneswaran B, Liao P, et al. STOP questionnaire: a tool to screen patients for obstructive sleep apnea. *Anesthesiology.* 2008;108[5]:812–21, with permission.)

for objective testing.[18] However, outside of the sleep disorders center, use of clinical prediction tools may assist with risk stratification.

Nocturnal Polysomnography

Objective testing is required by standard guidelines to diagnose OSA.[19] A nocturnal, laboratory-based PSG (see Chapter 201) is considered the gold standard for OSA diagnosis, assessment of severity, and identification of other sleep disorders that can accompany OSA. The PSG allows direct monitoring and quantification of respiratory events and physiologic consequences, such as hypoxemia, arousals, and awakenings, that are suspected to cause daytime symptoms. A single-night

Table 68.2 Value of Specific Questionnaire Instruments that Combine Symptoms and Physical Findings to Diagnose Obstructive Sleep Apnea

Instrument	PSG AHI Cut-off	Pooled Sensitivity[a]	Pooled Specificity[a]	+LR[a]	−LR[a]
Berlin Questionnaire	≥5	0.76 [0.72, 0.80]	0.45 [0.34, 0.56]	1.38 [1.15, 1.66]	0.53 [0.42, 0.65]
	≥15	0.75 [0.64, 0.83]	0.42 [0.32, 0.52]	1.29 [1.12, 1.48]	0.60 [0.44, 0.81]
	≥30	0.84 [0.77, 0.89]	0.35 [0.26, 0.44]	1.28 [1.17, 1.41]	0.47 [0.30, 0.58]
STOP	≥5	0.88 [0.77, 0.94]	0.33 [0.18, 0.52]	1.31 [1.10, 1.57]	0.36 [0.27, 0.47]
	≥15	0.62–0.98	0.10–0.63	—	—
	≥30	0.91–0.97	0.11–0.36	—	—
STOP-BANG	≥5	0.93 [0.90, 0.95]	0.36 [0.29, 0.44]	1.46 [1.32, 1.62]	0.19 [0.16, 0.23]
	≥15	0.95 [0.94, 0.97]	0.27 [0.20, 0.36]	1.31 [1.18, 1.45]	0.17 [0.12, 0.23]
	≥30	0.94 [0.90, 0.97]	0.30 [0.17, 0.46]	1.34 [1.12, 1.61]	0.18 [0.14, 0.24]
Multivariable Apnea Prediction questionnaire	≥5	0.68–0.85	0.56–0.92	—	—
	≥30	0.80–0.90	0.44–0.72	—	—

AHI, Apnea-hypopnea index; BMI, body mass index; −LR, negative likelihood ratio; +LR, positive likelihood ratio; OSA, obstructive sleep apnea; PSG, polysomnogram.
[a]For instruments with less than five validation studies, a range of sensitivity and specificity is displayed as opposed to pooled values, and therefore likelihood ratios were not reported.
Pooled sensitivity, specificity, and likelihood ratios from meta-analysis of validation studies that compare the Berlin questionnaire, STOP, STOP-BANG, and Multivariable Apnea Prediction Questionnaire to PSG. +LR is the true-positive rate/false-positive rate. −LR is the false-negative rate/true-negative rate.
Modified from Kapur VK, Auckley DH, Chowdhuri S, et al. Clinical practice guideline for diagnostic testing for adult obstructive sleep apnea: an American Academy of Sleep Medicine clinical practice guideline. *J Clin Sleep Med*. 2017;13(3):479–504.

PSG is usually sufficient to diagnose or to exclude OSA. However, especially in the setting of high pretest probability, a negative PSG may need to be repeated.

The AASM has published and continually updates sleep scoring guidelines that include recommendations for polysomnographic equipment; scoring of abnormal respiratory events, electrocardiographic findings, movements, and arousals during sleep; and modifications necessary for children (https://aasm.org/clinical-resources/scoring-manual/).[20]

One scoring manual section that has potential to influence clinical practice includes two rules, labeled "recommended" and "acceptable," to score hypopneas. The scoring manual *recommends* that a hypopnea is scored when the airflow signal drops by at least 30% from the preevent baseline and the event results in either an arousal or oxygen desaturation of at least 3%.The recommended hypopnea definition aims to ensure sensitivity of PSG to detect OSA in patients with sleep fragmentation and daytime impairment but without significant oxygen desaturations.[20] The scoring manual also presents the *acceptable* rule as an alternative method to score hypopneas; this requires an oxygen desaturation of 4% and does not recognize hypopneas that terminate only in arousal.[20]

The distinction between the recommended and acceptable rules for scoring hypopneas is important. In one study, use of a hypopnea definition that required a 4% oxygen desaturation misclassified 40% of symptomatic patients as negative for OSA.[21] Therefore discrepancies in hypopnea definition could result in failure to identify OSA or in underestimation of the severity of sleep-disordered breathing in certain individuals, particularly those who are younger and lean.[21,22] As OSA produces symptoms attributable to sleep fragmentation independent of hypoxemia, laboratories are encouraged to incorporate arousal-based scoring of apneic events.[23]

Most laboratories report an AHI that represents the sum total of apneas and hypopneas per hour of sleep. In addition, the respiratory disturbance index (RDI) calculates the sum total of apneas, hypopneas, and respiratory effort-related arousals (RERAs) per hour of sleep. The *International Classification of Sleep Disorders*, ed. 3 (ICSD-3), uses the RDI to quantify PSG evidence of sleep-disordered breathing and therefore includes RERAs in the diagnosis of OSA.[19] An obstructive RDI of 5 or more per hour of sleep in the context of symptoms attributable to OSA (or 15 or more, regardless of symptoms) is required to meet ICSD-3 diagnostic criteria for OSA.[19] Esophageal pressure monitoring to assess respiratory effort quantitatively or, more commonly, nasal pressure monitoring to assess qualitatively for subtle flow limitation facilitates the scoring of RERAs.

Variability in biologic severity, laboratory equipment, or human scoring performance can also decrease diagnostic precision. Night-to-night variability may be particularly high in subjects with low but clinically significant rates of apneas and hypopneas during sleep. A repeat PSG may confirm OSA in 20% to 50% of individuals who have symptoms suggestive of OSA but initial PSG negative for OSA.[24,25]

The patient's clinical presentation must be considered when interpreting the PSG to help mitigate underdiagnosis and overdiagnosis. Although many clinicians believe that an AHI greater than 5 indicates OSA, the PSG finding of an AHI greater than 5 may not be associated with symptoms. For example, a large population-based epidemiologic study found that only 22.6% of women and 15.5% of men who met this polysomnographic criterion clearly complained of daytime hypersomnolence.[6] Conversely, some patients with an AHI less than 5 may still have OSA that merits treatment to improve symptoms and morbidity.[26,27]

Further research is needed to define and improve the ability of PSGs to measure those aspects of sleep-disordered breathing that most affect health and daytime sleepiness. Massive amounts of electrophysiologic signal are recorded during PSG but are depleted of complexity and meaning by summary metrics such as the AHI. The AHI and minimum oxygen saturation do not correlate strongly with daytime sleepiness, although the AHI may correlate better with cardiovascular morbidity.[28] Other polysomnographic measures that may (or may not) prove to enhance the ability of PSGs to predict outcomes of sleep-disordered breathing include duration of apneas and hypopneas,[29] magnitude and duration of hypoxemia,[30] end-tidal or transcutaneous carbon dioxide readings,[31] pulse transit time,[32] sympathetic activity assessment with peripheral arterial tonometry,[33] scoring of arousals,[34,35] and analysis of respiratory cycle–related electroencephalographic changes.[35,36]

Artificial intelligence (AI), which refers to the capability of computer systems to perform tasks conventionally considered to require human intelligence, is used increasingly to derive meaning from vast data sources. Polysomnographic time-series data may be well suited for analysis with AI, which has already demonstrated the ability to identify distinct phenotypes and predict cardiovascular outcomes among patients with OSA.[37] Continued development of AI approaches could reveal additional phenotypes, capture physiologic heterogeneity, predict treatment response, and forecast health consequences, thus advancing the diagnosis and management of sleep-disordered breathing.[38]

Modified Forms of the Polysomnogram

In comparison to the standard PSG, daytime and split-night studies may reduce costs and expedite evaluation. Studies of daytime PSGs have sometimes found a high NPV with lower PPV, but inconsistent results and the lack of sufficient data explain why daytime PSGs have not generally been recommended.[39]

The split-night PSG protocol refers to the introduction and titration of continuous positive nasal airway pressure (CPAP) after a diagnostic recording for at least 2 hours that demonstrates moderate to severe OSA. A successful split-night study may save a patient from a second night in the sleep laboratory and therefore may be preferred by both patients and insurers. Studies of diagnostic accuracy and treatment outcomes show reasonable results.[40] Concordance is high between AHI measured in the first 2 hours of PSG recording and AHI measured in a full-night PSG (concordance correlation coefficient = 0.93),[41] and with use of an AHI cut-off of 30 events per hour, the first 2 hours of PSG recording has good sensitivity (90%) and specificity (92%)[42]; therefore the split-night protocol may be particularly well suited to individuals suspected to have severe OSA. CPAP efficacy[43] and patient adherence[44] to therapy after a split-night study does not appear inferior to that after traditional, diagnostic PSG coupled with a separate, full-night titration study. Split-night PSGs are not appropriate for all patients who present for evaluation of sleep-disordered breathing, especially those with insomnia, claustrophobia, or individuals hesitant to use CPAP. Diagnostic and management dilemmas may arise if CPAP is introduced during a split-night PSG when OSA is mild, positional, or sleep-stage dependent.[18]

Home Sleep Tests

As the medical community became aware of the prevalence and consequences of OSA and its consequences, the need for a convenient, less resource-intensive, and more widely available diagnostic test was apparent.[45] Portable monitoring tools to diagnose OSA were developed and are now widely used.[46] Studies have demonstrated similar treatment outcomes regardless of whether the diagnosis of OSA was confirmed by a home sleep apnea test (HSAT) or PSG.[47–50]

Different types of HSATs (see Chapter 205) incorporate various physiologic signals. HSAT devices are categorized by type based on the number of sensors used (type II-IV) or by the parameters assessed, which may include sleep, cardiovascular, oximetry, position, effort, and respiratory (SCOPER) measures.[51] At minimum, the AASM recommends that an HSAT include monitoring of nasal pressure, chest and abdominal effort, and oximetry.[18] A peripheral arterial tonometry (PAT) device that also monitors oximetry and actigraphy can be used at home.[18] HSATs are a reliable alternative to confirm OSA in patients who are at high risk for OSA, in whom the accuracy of HSATs (compared to attended PSG) in detecting an AHI greater than or equal to 5 is typically in the 80% to 90% range.[18]

However, the limited variables monitored during HSATs do not typically allow identification of sleep stage or muscle activity and therefore cannot be used for the objective confirmation of sleep disorders other than OSA.

Moreover, without electroencephalogram (EEG), electrooculogram (EOG), and electromyogram (EMG) sensors that are required to distinguish sleep from wake, hypopneas cannot be scored when they terminate in cortical arousal but do not result in oxygen desaturation. In addition, without direct sleep monitoring or estimation of sleep and wake by integrated actigraphy, the number of apneas and hypopneas is often quantified per hour of total recording time as opposed to total sleep time. This produces a respiratory event index (REI) that may be less than an in-laboratory–determined AHI, especially in the setting of significant insomnia. Collectively, these limitations make the HSAT, in comparison to PSG, a less sensitive diagnostic test for OSA, which raises a risk for false-negative results and underestimation of the severity for sleep-disordered breathing.

Based on the potential benefits and limitations posed by HSATs for OSA, the AASM recommends that they be used only in adults with an increased risk of moderate to severe OSA. This level of risk is defined by the presence of EDS and at least two of the following: habitual loud snoring, witnessed apneas or gasping or choking, or hypertension.[18] Further, HSATs should not be used in individuals who take opioids habitually or have significant cardiopulmonary disease, prior stroke, or neuromuscular disease that predisposes to respiratory muscle weakness because these conditions may increase the risk of nonobstructive sleep-disordered breathing (central sleep apnea, sleep-related hypoxemia, or hypoventilation). HSATs are not appropriate in the context of comorbid sleep disorders that may reduce accuracy, such as insomnia, or in patients with personal or environmental barriers that may prevent proper data acquisition.[18]

The use of HSATs to objectively confirm OSA should occur under the guidance of a board-certified or eligible sleep physician, at an accredited sleep disorders center, and in conjunction with a comprehensive clinical evaluation (as seen in Figure 68.2).[18,52] Interpretation of HSATs must include physician review of the raw signal acquired by the portable device.[52] When an HSAT does not confirm the diagnosis of OSA, a PSG rather than a repeat HSAT should be conducted for more definitive evaluation of sleep-disordered breathing.[18]

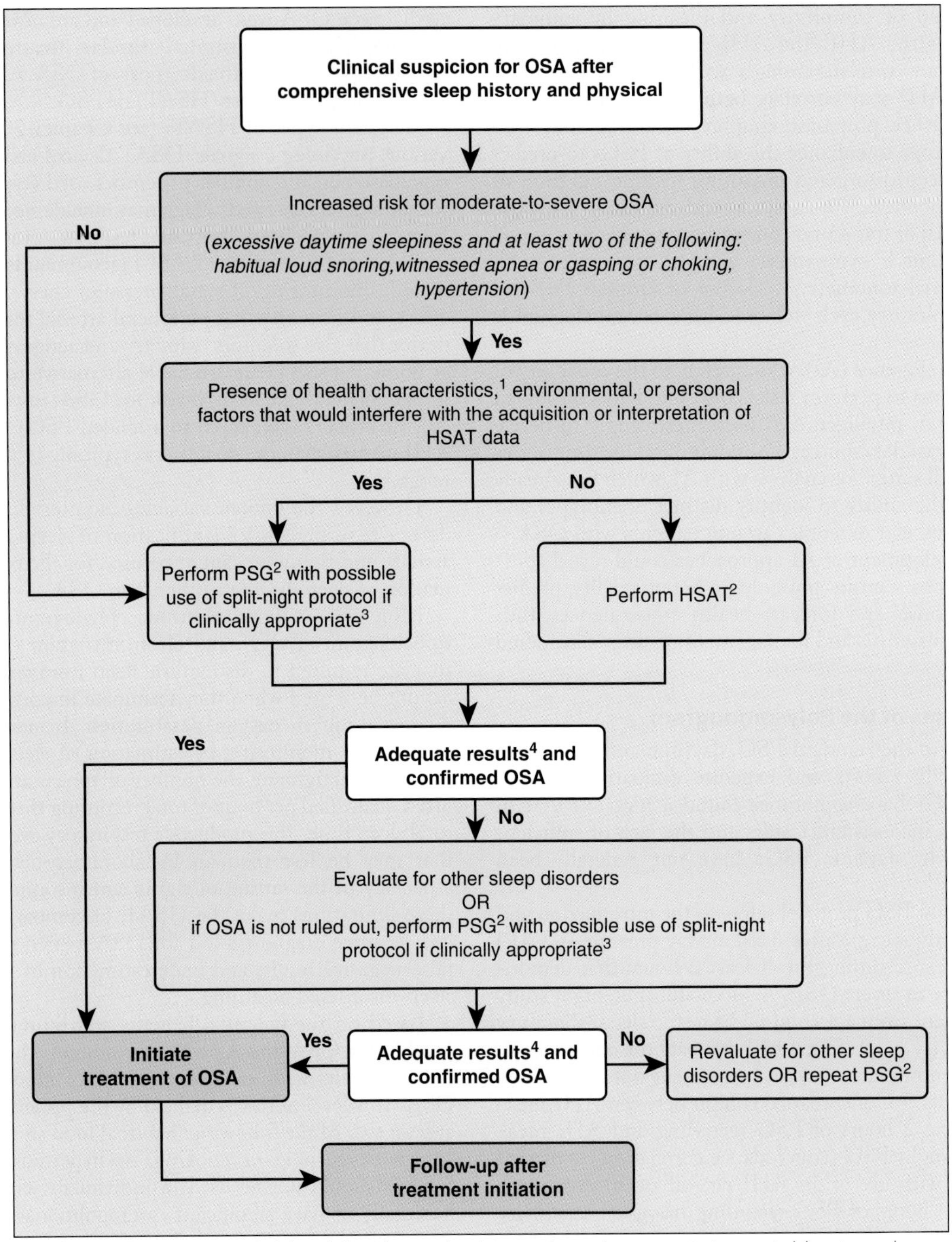

Figure 68.2 Recommended clinical algorithm to select between home sleep apnea test versus in-laboratory polysomnogram. *(1)* Significant cardiopulmonary disease, potential respiratory muscle weakness due to a neuromuscular condition, hypoventilation during wakefulness or high risk of sleep-related hypoventilation, history of stroke, chronic opioid medication use, severe insomnia, symptoms that suggest another significant sleep disorder. *(2)* PSG/HSAT should be administered by an accredited sleep center under the supervision of a board-certified sleep physician. *(3)* Baseline recording of at least 2 hours that demonstrates OSA and a minimum of 3 hours remaining to titrate CPAP. Use of the split-night protocol should be reserved for carefully selected individuals who are free of characteristics that would interfere in the ability to diagnose OSA and titrate CPAP in a single night. *(4)* At least 4 hours of technically adequate oximetry and airflow signal during a time window that overlaps with the usual sleep period are the recommended minimal requirements for HSAT recording. CPAP, Continuous positive nasal airway pressure; HSAT, home sleep apnea test; OSA, obstructive sleep apnea; PSG, polysomnography. (Modified from Kapur VK, Auckley DH, Chowdhuri S, et al. Clinical practice guideline for diagnostic testing for adult obstructive sleep apnea: an American Academy of Sleep Medicine clinical practice guideline. *J Clin Sleep Med.* 2017;13[3]:479–504, with permission.)

Use of HSATs in appropriately selected patients under the care of a sleep specialist generally produces outcomes similar to that observed in individuals evaluated with PSG.[47–50] However, some insurer policies sometimes mandate HSATs, even when they are not the medically indicated test. This can result in false-negative results; patient inconvenience from retesting; or, even more problematic, individuals who fail to return for necessary follow-up testing.[53] Collectively, incorrect use of HSATs has the potential to misclassify individuals with OSA as free of disease and could leave patients untreated and vulnerable to health consequences of sleep-disordered breathing. Conversely, given the ubiquity and ease of use, widespread deployment of HSATs as a screening tool independent of a specialist history could result in false-positive results and unnecessary treatment.

Although HSATs that are low cost and have reasonable sensitivity and specificity for the diagnosis of OSA are often assumed to provide an economic advantage over PSG, cost-effectiveness analyses thus far suggest that full-night PSG is superior to an HSAT.[54,55] Further, economic implications of HSATs must be considered from both payer and provider perspectives,[56] and pretest probability, cost of untreated OSA, and time horizon may all be relevant to models of cost-effectiveness.[57]

Studies of Airway Morphology

Although used in research, imaging of the upper airway is not routinely performed in diagnostic evaluations of patients because they cannot diagnose OSA nor determine its severity. However, visualization of upper airway anatomy may be useful in preoperative identification of sites of obstruction and guide the selection of alternative therapies to positive airway pressure. The primary modalities to visualize the upper airway include cephalometric radiography, computed tomography (CT), magnetic resonance imaging (MRI), nasopharyngoscopy, and drug-induced sleep endoscopy (DISE).

Cephalometric analyses use a lateral radiograph of the head and neck to visualize the airway and boney structures that affect it. The diagnostic value of cephalometrics may be limited in part because only sagittal plane dimensions are provided, whereas coronal plane dimensions or volume may be more pertinent to OSA.[58] In addition, cephalometric images are taken in the upright position, during wakefulness, which does not fully capture the dynamics of the airway most relevant in OSA. Alternatively, CT images are acquired in the supine position and allow cross-sectional assessment and three-dimensional reconstructions to quantify the area and volume of the upper airway and visualize soft tissue and bony anatomy with high resolution. Although use is limited by radiation exposure, CT may provide a more detailed upper airway assessment before surgical interventions, such as maxillomandibular advancement. MRI provides images in sagittal, coronal, and axial planes and, similar to CT, allows the assessment of upper airway area and volume and can provide a three-dimensional reconstruction.[59] Soft tissue can be viewed with high resolution by MRI, and sophisticated algorithms have been used to evaluate fat distribution in the tongue.[60,61] Dynamic sleep MRI protocols may characterize upper airway obstruction better than images acquired during wakefulness.[62–64] MRI does not result in radiation exposure and therefore may be preferred over CT, although patient-specific characteristics that may prevent use include claustrophobia or the presence of certain implantable devices. At this time, the value of MRI in the clinical setting is not well defined.

Nasopharyngoscopy allows the three-dimensional anatomic characterization of the upper airway lumen and can be used with the Müller maneuver to simulate obstruction or during spontaneous or DISE. In addition to determining the site of obstruction, nasopharyngoscopy has been used to assess the response to various OSA treatments, such as oral appliance therapy, hypoglossal nerve stimulation, and uvulopalatopharyngoplasty.[65–67] DISE may reveal the site of airway obstruction better than awake nasopharyngoscopy with the Müller maneuver[68,69] and is used before initiation of hypoglossal nerve stimulation to rule out concentric collapse.

EVALUATION OF HYPERSOMNOLENCE

History and Questionnaires

The history provides important clues to the severity of hypersomnolence. Direct inquiry about sleepiness can be supplemented by questions about sleepiness in sedentary situations, such as driving, desk work, reading, or watching television. However, patients may report little of the EDS suggested by family members, clinical signs, or objective tests. Words other than *sleepiness* are often used by patients with sleep disorders to describe the chief complaint. Terms used by patients include *lack of energy* (40%), *tiredness* (20%), *fatigue* (18%), and *sleepiness* (22%).[70] Furthermore, each of these symptoms tends to resolve after use of CPAP. Patients' opinions about their own sleepiness sometimes show no significant association with results of the Multiple Sleep Latency Test (MSLT).[71]

Questionnaires such as the Epworth Sleepiness Scale[72] and the Stanford Sleepiness Scale[73] (see Chapter 207) provide a more formal and perhaps reliable measure of EDS. The impact of sleepiness on activities of daily living can be assessed with the Functional Outcomes of Sleep Questionnaire.[74] Epworth results correlate reasonably well with patients' self-ratings for overall sleepiness but not well with MSLT results.[75] However, although the Epworth Sleepiness Scale and the Stanford Sleepiness Scale can have clinical utility, for example, in monitoring response to treatment, they do not substitute for well-validated objective measures of sleepiness and may demonstrate some level of variability on sequential testing.[76] Subjective tests of sleepiness should be used in combination with additional clinical information, rather than in isolation, to help assess risk of sleep disorders, prompt changes in management, or predict functional outcomes.

In addition to the severity of EDS, it is critical to assess other symptoms associated with hypersomnolence to determine its etiology. For example, cataplexy is the essential clinical feature that distinguishes narcolepsy type 1 from narcolepsy type 2 and other disorders of sleepiness.[19] Cataplexy must be derived from patient report because it is rarely observed during the clinical evaluation for hypersomnolence. Sleep paralysis and hypnagogic and hypnopompic hallucinations are reported in about 50% of patients with narcolepsy; however, these symptoms are often present in individuals without the disease and thus are not specific.[77] Inquiry about nap duration and quality is also useful because patients with narcolepsy, in contrast to other sleep disorders, may experience a greater (although transient) alerting affect from short naps.[78] In contrast, more than two-thirds of patients with idiopathic hypersomnia report that naps are nonrestorative.[79–81]

Physical Examination

Although the alerting effect of an examination obscures physical signs of sleepiness in most patients, overt signs of sleepiness, such as the inability to stay awake or to keep eyes open in the examination room, have high PPV. The examination may also help distinguish severe sleepiness from stupor due to neurologic impairment or drugs.

Sleep Logs and Actigraphy

The evaluation of hypersomnolence includes assessment of sleep duration and timing to rule out insufficient sleep syndrome or circadian rhythm sleep-wake disorders. The clinician should ask about sleep schedules at the time of clinical evaluation. Unfortunately, singular point estimates of sleep duration and timing demonstrate poor agreement with longitudinal measures.[82–84] Therefore tools such as sleep logs and actigraphy are valuable to track sleep patterns longitudinally over days to weeks.

An actigraph (see Chapter 211) uses an accelerometer to measure movement objectively and, for the purpose of sleep estimation, is typically worn on the wrist.[85] Motion data acquired by the device are then analyzed by an algorithm to estimate sleep and wake. Actigraphy is highly sensitive, but not specific, for EEG-defined sleep and may overestimate true sleep; however, agreement between actigraphy and PSG in the detection of sleep can be high (≈90% in patients without sleep disorders such as chronic insomnia), and this device is accepted as a valid method to evaluate sleep patterns.[85,86]

Data that support the use of actigraphy in individuals with hypersomnolence are derived from the few studies that tracked sleep-wake activity patterns in the days that immediately preceded laboratory testing with PSG and MSLT.[82] There may be a discrepancy between the findings from a sleep log versus actigraphy, with the former suggesting more sleep time than the latter.[82,87] In addition, in contrast to sleep logs, sleep information acquired from actigraphy is objective, passively obtained, and more likely to be complete over the assessment period. Therefore actigraphy is the preferred method to estimate sleep duration and timing in individuals who undergo evaluation for hypersomnolence.[85] The ICSD-3 recommends documentation of sleep-wake patterns with actigraphy, whenever possible, for at least 7 days before an MSLT to provide context for the interpretation of MSLT results.[19] If actigraphy is not feasible, sleep logs may be used as the sole method to estimate sleep-wake patterns before the MSLT.

Actigraphy may also be a useful evaluation tool to estimate sleep in patients who present with hypersomnolence that is likely secondary to insufficient sleep syndrome. In the case of suspected insufficient sleep syndrome, actigraphy is recommended for 2 to 3 weeks to confirm chronically reduced sleep.[85]

Sleep wearable devices (e.g., smart watches) are not currently recommended as a substitute for medical-grade actigraphy to estimate sleep patterns for clinical purposes, including in the assessment of patients with hypersomnolence. Smartphone applications without an associated wearable device may also claim the ability to distinguish sleep from wake and determine sleep stages. There is a lack of validation data against PSG and therefore unclear accuracy to estimate sleep and wakefulness.[88]

Nocturnal Polysomnography

Many patients referred to sleep centers for EDS have sleep disorders, and PSG usually confirms such disorders. The polysomnographic variable that best reflects sleepiness, as measured by the mean sleep latency on the MSLT, is nocturnal sleep latency.[89] The typical summary polysomnographic measures of sleep pathology, such as the AHI and minimum oxygen saturation, show only low magnitudes of correlation with MSLT results.[90] Digital analyses of polysomnographic data, such as respiratory event–linked EEG changes (RCREC),[36,91] may better predict sleepiness. In addition, the use of AI methods, such as deep learning, have already revealed characteristics of nocturnal sleep in patients with type 1 narcolepsy that are not evident with traditional sleep staging and demonstrate the ability to confirm a diagnosis of type 1 narcolepsy from overnight PSG with a specificity of 96% and sensitivity of 91%.[92] However, the use of AI and other computer-augmented sleep scoring methods, although promising, have yet to be adopted in clinical practice.

Multiple Sleep Latency Test

The MSLT is described in detail in Chapter 207. The mean sleep latency on the MSLT is the most commonly used objective measure to assess daytime sleepiness.[93] The MSLT may contribute to diagnosis but is usually not sufficient, alone, to establish a diagnosis. The mean sleep latency is most useful when it is clearly abnormally low. The MSLT can help determine the clinical significance of a sleep disorder or assess response to treatment.

As a general guideline, mean sleep latencies of 8 minutes or less on MSLT are considered abnormal,[93] and latencies less than 5 minutes often indicate severe EDS. However, proper interpretation of MSLT results requires integration of other factors. Results may be misleading if they are affected by age,[94] noise, anxiety, or atypical sleep on the previous night. Medications that are stimulating or sedating, if not properly weaned, may reduce mean sleep latency in the absence of a central disorder of hypersomnolence or result in falsely negative MSLT results. Urine toxicology is recommended before MSLT and may reveal the use of substances relevant to alertness that are not reported by the patient.[95] Sleep apnea and other sleep disorders can make sleep onset more difficult and interfere with the test. In addition, because sleep propensity is dependent on circadian phase, extreme chronotype or the presence of a shift work schedule may produce abnormal mean sleep latency on the MSLT.[96]

In general, the NPV of a long mean sleep latency is less than the PPV of a particularly short mean sleep latency. Therefore, when an MSLT is normal, clinicians must carefully consider other possible explanations before telling a subjectively sleepy patient that there is no objective evidence of EDS. Conversely, community-based samples of adults show mean sleep latencies of 8 minutes or less in well more than 20% of subjects.[96,97] High test-retest reliability among normal subjects[98] does not necessarily generalize to patients. In fact, 40% of central hypersomnia patients had mean sleep latencies that crossed to the other side of the 8-minute threshold when MSLTs conducted about 4 years apart were compared.[99] Interrater reliability can be excellent but adds another source of potential variation in test results.[100]

Nocturnal Polysomnography and Multiple Sleep Latency Test in the Diagnosis of Narcolepsy

The objective sleep laboratory confirmation of narcolepsy requires both reduced mean sleep latency on MSLT and two or more sleep-onset REM periods. Among patients referred to a sleep laboratory, REM sleep-onset latency less than 15 minutes on nocturnal PSG had poor sensitivity (≈40%) but excellent specificity (99.6%) for type 1 narcolepsy.[101] The ICSD-3 allows a sleep-onset REM period on overnight PSG to account for one of the two REM periods necessary to diagnose narcolepsy with an MSLT.[19] The diagnostic criteria for narcolepsy—two or more sleep-onset REM periods (SOREMPs) and short mean sleep latency—were once thought to have high sensitivity and specificity. Original case series suggested that all narcoleptic subjects and virtually no normal control subjects had two or more SOREMPs[102]; the PPV of two or more SOREMPs for the diagnosis of narcolepsy was 98%, and the NPV was 89%.[103] However, two or more SOREMPs were found in 25% of patients with sleep apnea[104] and 17% of normal subjects.[105] Among 2083 patients evaluated with MSLTs at one sleep center, the PPV of two or more SOREMPs was 57%, and the NPV was 98%.[106] Thus the presence of SOREMPs must be interpreted in conjunction with other clinical and polysomnographic findings. The criterion of two or more SOREMPs cannot be used to diagnose narcolepsy when the patient has untreated OSA or participates in shift work, which can increase the odds of a positive MSLT almost eightfold.[96] Antidepressants often suppress REM sleep, and therefore continuation or recent cessation can complicate interpretation of an MSLT.[94] In addition, although the MSLT demonstrates high test-retest reliability in narcolepsy type 1 (narcolepsy with cataplexy),[107] this is not the case when idiopathic hypersomnia or narcolepsy type 2 (narcolepsy without cataplexy) is the underlying cause of sleepiness.[99,107] As an alternative to the MSLT, cerebrospinal fluid hypocretin-1 levels can be used to confirm type 1 narcolepsy, although this approach is not generally used in clinical practice. These levels are low (≤110 pg/mL or ≤one-third of the mean for control subjects) in more than 90% of affected patients but almost never among patients without this diagnosis.[19]

Variations of the Multiple Sleep Latency Test and Other Physiologic Tests

Results of the Maintenance of Wakefulness Test (MWT) can differ markedly from those of the MSLT,[108] but whether the MWT results are more predictive of adverse effects of sleepiness in daily life remains unknown. Results of both the MWT and MSLT can be influenced by the patient's motivation.[109] The MWT results correlate with measures of sleep apnea severity to about the same extent as MSLT results do[110] but may better reflect improvement with treatment.[108] Shorter sleep latencies on MWTs (<20 minutes) are associated with increased errors on driving simulation tests.[111,112] However, until MWT and MSLT results are shown to differ in a clinically meaningful way, the MSLT continues to offer advantages of more published experience, familiarity among clinicians, and relevance to the diagnosis of narcolepsy. The Federal Aviation Administration and other agencies may at times request or require an MWT, but given the dearth of proven real-life predictive value, the role of this test or the MSLT in predicting workplace safety remains controversial.[113,114]

Another available method to assess hypersomnia is the 24-hour PSG. About 40% of patients with idiopathic hypersomnia demonstrate mean sleep latencies greater than 8 minutes on the MSLT despite severe subjective sleepiness.[80,115,116] This finding is more common in patients with long nocturnal sleep durations. In these individuals, prolonged PSG reveals a total sleep duration near 700 minutes over 24 hours.[115] Therefore a 24-hour PSG that documents total sleep time of at least 660 minutes can be used to diagnose idiopathic hypersomnia in patients with symptoms consistent with the disorder but mean sleep latency greater than 8 minutes.[19] The ICSD-3 also allows actigraphy for this purpose[19]; however, few studies have evaluated the validity of actigraphy for this application.[117]

EVALUATION OF INSOMNIA

History and Questionnaires

Like EDS, the complaint of inadequate, insufficient, or nonrestorative sleep can have many different causes. However, causes of insomnia are often diagnosed by history alone.[118] In part because the gold standard is not a physiologic test, few data are available with which to assess the relative value of individual symptoms. Predictive values for some symptoms are likely to be high because symptoms define the disorder.

The Insomnia Severity Index is a seven-item self-report instrument that is typically used in insomnia research.[119] However, this tool may also be beneficial in the clinical setting. A score of 10 or higher on the Insomnia Severity Index identified insomnia with a sensitivity of 86% and a specificity of 88% in a community sample.[120]

Sleep Logs and Actigraphy

Sleep logs are an important tool in the evaluation of insomnia. Patients record sleep-onset latency (SOL) and wake after sleep onset (WASO) on sleep logs, and investigators have tested the ability of different cut-offs of these quantitative parameters to predict insomnia. In one study, SOL or WASO of 31 minutes or longer identified insomnia with a sensitivity of 64% and specificity of 77% in subjects with insomnia at least three times per week for 6 months.[121] A subsequent investigation that also used sleep logs found that SOL or WASO of 20 minutes or more alone identified insomnia with a sensitivity of 94% and a specificity of 80%.[122] Sleep logs are not necessary to establish the presence of insomnia but can help define severity and facilitate identification of causes such as inadequate sleep hygiene or circadian rhythm sleep-wake disorders.

The diagnosis of insomnia does not require objective confirmation. However, actigraphy can be beneficial to estimate certain aspects of sleep in patients with insomnia. Actigraphy should be used with caution in individuals with insomnia due to the tendency for algorithms applied to actigraphic data to score nonmoving wakefulness as sleep. A meta-analysis of investigations in insomnia patients that compared PSG to actigraphy revealed that mean differences in total sleep time and sleep-onset latency were small enough that actigraphy can provide reliable, objective estimates of these variables but not sleep efficiency or WASO.[85] In addition, actigraphic estimates of total sleep time, sleep onset latency, and sleep efficiency were significantly different from sleep logs.[85] Collectively, these findings suggest that actigraphy provides worthwhile, distinct information beyond sleep logs and therefore is recommended by the AASM to estimate sleep variables in patients with insomnia, particularly when ancillary information is required to differentiate insomnia from other diagnoses or to guide treatment.[85] As noted previously, consumer-marketed wearable sleep trackers cannot be used as a replacement for actigraphy, in part due to questionable accuracy that may introduce uncertainty to clinical decision making.

Nocturnal Polysomnography

PSG is not indicated for routine evaluation of insomnia, although when a patient's history and physical examination suggest that insomnia may be due to sleep-disordered breathing, periodic limb movement disorder, paradoxical insomnia, or uncertain causes, a sleep study can be an important aid to diagnosis.[123] In addition, PSG may be indicated if insomnia fails to respond to treatment or in patients who have precipitous arousals with violent or injurious behavior.[118] Of note, injudicious use of PSG can sometimes enhance patient's conviction that insomnia is due to physical rather than behavioral causes or lead to diagnoses that eventually prove irrelevant to the main complaint.

EVALUATION OF SUSPECTED CIRCADIAN RHYTHM SLEEP-WAKE DISORDERS

History and Questionnaires

Discrepancies between the desired time for sleep and wake and the circadian propensity for sleep and wake may present as insomnia or hypersomnolence. Approximately 7% to 16% of patients who present to sleep disorders clinics with symptoms of insomnia are ultimately diagnosed with delayed sleep-wake phase disorder.[124,125] To distinguish circadian rhythm sleep-wake disorders (CRSWDs) from other causes of insomnia and hypersomnolence, examples of useful questions may include, "What time of day do you feel most alert?" and "When do you perform the best?" Comparison of regular sleep schedules to schedules on days free from work or school can reveal discrepancies that help to identify a circadian rhythm disorder.

Questionnaires such as the Horne-Östberg Morningness-Eveningness Questionnaire (MEQ) and the Munich Chronotype Questionnaire (MCTQ) evaluate circadian preference, also known as chronotype.[126,127] The MEQ is the most widely used instrument to assess chronotype and contains 19 self-assessment items to evaluate personal preference for the timing of sleep and other behaviors.[126] The MCTQ is also self-completed but assesses the actual (as opposed to preferred) timing of sleep on work or school days versus free days.[127] The midpoint of sleep on free days and self-rated chronotype derived from the MCTQ both correlate highly with chronotype based on MEQ score.[127,128] In addition to correlating with each other, the MEQ and MCTQ correlate with objective markers of circadian phase.[129–131] The MEQ has also been validated against core body temperature and cortisol secretion.[126,132,133]

Sleep Logs and Actigraphy

Actigraphy is recommended in suspected CRSWD,[85] although sleep logs may be used when actigraphy is not available or feasible.[19] Actigraphy has been validated in patients with CRSWD.[85] Inclusion of ad libitum sleep-wake times (e.g., days off from school or work) will provide a more accurate estimate of true, endogenous circadian phase, and therefore sleep should be tracked with actigraphy or sleep logs for at least 7, and preferably 14, days to guide the diagnosis of a CRSWD.[129,134,135] Vacation times may be particularly revealing; in fact sleep-wake times of individuals on an unrestricted sleep-wake schedule demonstrate higher correlation with dim-light melatonin onset (DLMO) than sleep-wake times of those on a fixed schedule[134]

Whereas actigraphy is typically used to identify sleep and wake periods in suspected CRSWD such that the abnormal pattern of sleep-wake timing can be visualized, mathematical modeling of 24-hour motion signal for days to weeks may be useful to quantify circadian properties of the rest-activity rhythm. Traditionally, cosinor analysis has been applied to actigraphy to estimate acrophase, mesor, period, and amplitude of the rest-activity rhythm; however, this analysis is poorly suited to patterns that change over time, and a growing field of research that uses nonparametric, data-driven methods is likely to reveal more accurate techniques to capture circadian rhythmicity.[136,137] However, these techniques have not yet been incorporated into routine clinical use.

As noted earlier, consumer-marketed wearable sleep trackers are not a reliable substitute to estimate sleep parameters in any suspected sleep disorder; however, given the ability to assess longitudinal biologic patterns beyond movement (skin temperature and heart rate, for example), future research may find a role for such devices to assist in the evaluation of CRSWD.[138]

Nocturnal Polysomnography

PSG is not necessary to diagnose circadian rhythm sleep-wake disorders. A PSG conducted at conventional times may demonstrate a delay of sleep onset or early morning awakening in patients with delayed or advanced sleep-wake phase disorders, respectively.

Multiple Sleep Latency Test

The MSLT is not used to diagnose CRSWDs. However, if obtained, mean sleep latency may be reduced in CRSWD in the setting of sleep loss. Given the circadian regulation of stage R sleep, SOREMPs may also be affected. Of note, in a large epidemiologic study, shift workers (night or rotating) were several times more likely than other subjects to have a mean sleep latency of less than 8 minutes combined with at least two SOREMPs on MSLT.[96] In addition, adolescents with a delay in circadian phase can demonstrate SOREMPs during the MSLT (particularly during the first nap) when they wake according to their school schedule.[139]

Objective Markers of Circadian Phase

The ICSD-3 notes that endogenous markers of circadian phase can confirm the diagnosis of certain circadian rhythm sleep-wake disorders.[19] Salivary (DLMO) or urinary (6-sulfatoxymelatonin, aMT6s) melatonin assays are the most commonly used objective markers of circadian phase. These measures objectively document a stable advance, stable delay, or progressive delay of circadian phase in advanced sleep-wake phase disorder, delayed sleep-wake phase disorder, and non–24-hour sleep-wake rhythm disorder, respectively.[19] Although melatonin assays are infrequently used in clinical practice, at-home DLMO assays correlate well with in-laboratory DLMO assessments.[140] Salivary melatonin assays can capture the onset of melatonin secretion but are not practical to determine the secretion profile overnight. Alternatively, urinary aMT6s can be collected at 8-hour intervals; therefore the first morning void allows for calculation of overnight aMT6s secretion in the home setting.[141] A promising method that leverages the circadian oscillation of gene transcription in the periphery is the analysis of the peripheral blood cell transcriptome.[142] However, further investigation is required to determine whether measurement of circadian phase from a single blood sample is reliable and practical in the clinical setting.

EVALUATION OF RESTLESS LEGS SYNDROME

History and Questionnaires

The diagnosis of RLS is made by a clinical history of an urge to move the limbs that is worse at rest, improved with movement, and worse in the evening or night.[19] These four criteria have a PPV of 76% when expert interview is used as a gold standard.[143] Differentiating RLS carefully from leg cramps or positional discomfort improves the specificity of the four criteria from 84% to 94%.[19,143]

Several instruments exist to assist in the evaluation of RLS or its severity, including the International Restless Legs Syndrome Severity Scale (IRLS), RLS-6, and Johns Hopkins Severity Scale. The IRLS scale is a 10-item questionnaire that assesses the severity of RLS symptoms.[144] This scale has good internal consistency, interexaminer reliability, and test-retest reliability,[144] and a 6-point decrease is considered to be a clinically relevant improvement.[145] Although these scales are used mostly in research, they may be beneficial in the clinic setting to quantify symptom severity; determine the impact of RLS symptoms on patient quality of life, mood, and sleep; measure the progression of RLS symptoms; and evaluate therapeutic response.[146] In addition, a self-administered version of the IRLS (sIRLS) was validated.[147] Therefore the scale can now be completed before or after the patient office visit and independent of the provider, which allows a form of the IRLS to be incorporated into the clinical evaluation with greater ease and flexibility.[147]

Physical Examination

A full neurologic examination is indicated to evaluate for RLS because this condition may arise in the context of other neurologic diseases, such as neuropathy, multiple sclerosis, or Parkinson disease. Assessment of affect and mood to help identify psychiatric disorders is important because mental health morbidity (or the use of medications) frequently coexists with RLS.

Laboratory Tests

Evaluation of a patient with RLS should include serum iron and ferritin levels. More than one-third of individuals with RLS have low serum iron levels, and greater than two-thirds have ferritin values of 50 μg/L or less. Ferritin levels are inversely related to RLS severity,[148,149] and individuals with ferritin levels less than 75 μg/L should be treated with iron supplementation. Iron supplementation may reduce symptoms in RLS, although findings are inconsistent.[150] Therefore evaluation of serum iron and ferritin is an integral part of the evaluation of RLS for both diagnosis and treatment.

Nocturnal Polysomnography

PSG is not routinely indicated in the evaluation of RLS and should be performed only if the clinician suspects a comorbid sleep disorder, such as OSA. Periodic limb movements during sleep are found in up to 90% of patients with RLS. However, periodic limb movements during sleep are nonspecific because they also occur in approximately 25% of individuals without RLS.[151,152]

EVALUATION FOR SUSPECTED PARASOMNIAS

History and Questionnaires

With the notable exception of REM sleep behavior disorder (RBD), parasomnias often can be diagnosed by history alone.[19] Information obtained from a bed partner may contribute more than that obtained from the patient.

Physical Examination

The physical examination of patients evaluated for parasomnias can be useful, but its value is not well quantified. Some signs may suggest sleep apnea as an underlying trigger for confusional arousals, sleepwalking, sleep terrors, RBD, or nocturnal enuresis. A neurologic examination may suggest that the parasomnia arises secondary to another condition, such as a neurodegenerative disorder.

Nocturnal Polysomnography

Few studies have examined the predictive value of PSG for parasomnia diagnoses. When the behavior in question occurs during the PSG, the diagnostic value of the test is likely to be high, especially if appropriate additional recording devices, such as extra EEG leads, extra surface electromyogram (EMG) leads, or video monitoring, are used.[153] Additional EEG leads used during PSG, combined with clinical history, may effectively differentiate sleep-related epilepsy from parasomnias.

However, EEG does not reliably diagnose nocturnal frontal lobe epilepsy (NFLE) because more than 60% of patients with NFLE fail to demonstrate a definite ictal rhythm.[154] Therefore eliciting a detailed description of the appearance of the events is the key to diagnosis. A rigorous decision tree algorithm using video PSG has been developed to distinguish NREM disorders of arousal from NFLE.[154] The following characteristics are suggestive of NFLE as opposed to parasomnia: complete arousal after the ictus, discrete offset of the behavior, presence of head turning to one side or posturing, and persistence of recumbent posture. This decision-tree algorithm classified 94% of events correctly. Unfortunately, PSG often fails to document the behavior—especially in cases of suspected RBD, sleepwalking, night terrors, and epilepsy—either because the behavior does not occur on most nights or perhaps because the sleep laboratory is not an environment familiar to the patient. For evaluation of parasomnias, the NPV of a completely normal study is less clear than the PPV of an abnormal study. In one series of patients with suspected parasomnias, 1 or 2 nights of PSG with video monitoring contributed useful diagnostic information in more than 50% of cases.[153]

Even in the absence of abnormal behaviors on the night of the PSG, other findings can be valuable. Interictal spike and wave complexes may represent an interictal expression of epilepsy. Stage R sleep without atonia (RWA) is the PSG hallmark of RBD and is required to confirm the diagnosis.[19] RWA may be detected manually by the eye or by automated computer programs. When scored manually, RWA is defined by the AASM manual as either tonic, phasic, or any chin EMG amplitude more than double the observed stage R atonia level.[20] Tonic or excessive sustained muscle activity can be designated when more than half of a 30-second epoch of stage R sleep demonstrates EMG tone greater than twice the stage R atonia level. Phasic or excessive transient muscle activity is scored when at least 5 of 10 3-second mini-epochs of stage R sleep contain 0.1- to 5.0-second bursts of muscle activity that are at least twice the stage R atonia level. If stage R atonia is not observed at any point, then the lowest amplitude EMG tone in NREM sleep may be used. The *recommended* rule to designate an epoch as RWA is the presence of either excessive sustained muscle activity in the chin lead or excessive transient muscle activity in the chin or limb leads. In addition, the *acceptable* rule allows an epoch to be designated as RWA if 50% of 3-second mini-epochs contain either any chin EMG amplitude more than double the observed stage R atonia level or phasic limb activity. In addition to these revisions of the definition of RWA, the AASM provides the option to document the RWA index or percentage of stage R epochs with RWA.

A growing number of computer algorithms to automatically detect and quantify RWA are available, including the REM atonia index, the computerized analysis method of the Sleep Innsbruck Barcelona (SINBAR) montage, short/long muscle activity indices, the Frandsen Index, the Kempfner Index, and the supra-threshold REM EMG activity metric.[155–157]

The qualitative visual assessment by the interpreting physician remains the clinical standard to detect RWA, and the AASM scoring manual does not specify a minimum number or proportion of epochs over the course of the night that must contain RWA to meet the PSG criteria to confirm suspected RBD.[20] However, from a research standpoint, different cut points have been investigated. When using the submentalis muscle alone, the presence of RWA (phasic) in 15% of 2-second REM mini-epochs will correctly classify 84% of patients.[158] The SINBAR montage records EMG in both the submentalis muscle and the bilateral flexor digitorum superficialis muscles to score RWA.[159] Use of this montage with specificity set at 100% (no false-positive RBD diagnoses permitted) yields a cut point of 32% of 3-second stage R mini-epochs to diagnose RBD (area under the receiving operator characteristic curve = 0.998).[159] Upper limb as opposed to lower limb EMG more reliably distinguishes patients with RBD from those without RBD.[156] The detection and quantification of RWA remains an area of rapid development, and novel, automated, and data-driven techniques show promise to improve detection of RBD.[160]

DECISION AND COST-EFFECTIVENESS ANALYSES AND THE PROMISE OF EMERGING TECHNOLOGIES

Data on sensitivity, specificity, pretest probability, and utility of outcomes can be used to construct a decision analysis. A clinical decision analysis typically models a choice between diagnostic and therapeutic alternatives. Logical rules are used to weigh information and to make the best decision for an individual patient.[161]

Economic and quality-of-life analyses[162] require quantitative information on costs and outcomes, data that are not often available for sleep disorders. Despite uncertainty of some important data points, cost-utility models have focused on the decision of whether to diagnose OSA with the aid of a full-night PSG, split-night PSG, portable cardiorespiratory monitoring, or no ancillary test.[54,55] The full-night PSG costs less and results in more quality-adjusted life-years than split-night PSG or unattended portable monitoring over the course of an individual's lifetime.[55] Despite the increased upfront cost of full-night PSG, these results reflect the high utility of an accurate OSA diagnosis and the expense of diagnostic mistakes.

The advent of an increasing array of digital analytic approaches now allow derivation of greater meaning from the signals acquired in the sleep laboratory and may reveal distinct clinical phenotypes (see Chapters 128 and 129) and identify physiologic endotypes underlying sleep disorders.[38] When combined with demographic, clinical, genomic, and other -omic information, the field of sleep medicine can leverage AI to move toward precision diagnosis and subsequently personalized treatment. Further, technologic advances have yielded miniaturized sensors for multiple physiologic parameters and therefore allow long-term sleep monitoring in the home. Inexpensive, ambulatory data acquisition may soon provide the possibility for diagnostic testing to take place outside of the sleep laboratory and before provider contact. In addition, prolonged data collection is expected to augment diagnostic accuracy beyond cross-sectional or short-term monitoring.

CLINICAL PEARL

Evaluation of common sleep complaints is based on symptoms, signs, and test results, combined with an understanding of the diagnostic value that each type of data contributes.

SUMMARY

Clinical tools and tests must be used carefully in the evaluation of suspected sleep disorders. All patients with sleep-related complaints should undergo a history and physical examination. Evaluations for obstructive sleep-disordered breathing start with a history and physical examination, which generate valuable information. Symptom-based questionnaires alone usually show inadequate specificity. Laboratory-based nocturnal PSG is a gold standard but not infallible. Final diagnostic decisions should be based on integration of multiple clinical and objective data points rather than on any specific cut-off for one specific variable, such as the AHI or REI. Evaluation for hypersomnolence also relies on historical symptoms collected during an interview or by use of a questionnaire. Objective testing with an MSLT is particularly useful when a shortened mean sleep latency confirms EDS or a shortened latency in addition to sleep-onset REM periods confirm narcolepsy. Results must be interpreted carefully, especially when they are normal, because of potential confounds. Evaluation for insomnia often relies mainly on historical information. Sleep logs and actigraphy can be helpful, but PSG is indicated only when other occult sleep disorders may underlie the insomnia. Questionnaires to determine chronotype and actigraphy are valuable tools when symptoms suggest a CRSWD. RLS is a diagnosis based on clinical history, but serum iron studies provide valuable information with repercussions for treatment. Evaluation for a parasomnia starts with a thorough history, obtained whenever possible from a bed partner in addition to the patient. PSG may confirm a diagnosis or distinguish between several possibilities.

SELECTED READINGS

Andlauer O, Moore H, Jouhier L, et al. Nocturnal rapid eye movement sleep latency for identifying patients with narcolepsy/hypocretin deficiency. *JAMA Neurol.* 2013;70(7):891–902.

Berry RB, Quan SF, Abreu AR, et al. *For the American Academy of Sleep Medicine. The AASM Manual for the Scoring of Sleep and Associated Events: Rules, Terminology and Technical Specifications. Version 2.6.* Darien, IL: American Academy of Sleep Medicine; 2020.

Cesari M, Christensen JA, Kempfner L, et al. Comparison of computerized methods for rapid eye movement sleep without atonia detection. *Sleep*. 2018;41(10):zsy133.

Frauscher B, Ehrann L, Högl B. Defining muscle activities for assessment of rapid eye movement sleep behavior disorder: from a qualitative to a quantitative diagnostic level. *Sleep Med*. 2013;14(8):729–733.

Goldbart A, Peppard P, Finn L, et al. Narcolepsy and predictors of positive MSLTs in the Wisconsin Sleep Cohort. *Sleep*. 2014;37(6):1043–1051.

Kapur VK, Auckley DH, Chowdhuri S, et al. Clinical practice guideline for diagnostic testing for adult obstructive sleep apnea: an American Academy of Sleep Medicine clinical practice guideline. *J Clin Sleep Med*. 2017;13(3):479–504.

Littner MR, Kushida C, Wise M, et al. Practice parameters for clinical use of the multiple sleep latency test and the maintenance of wakefulness test. *Sleep*. 2005;28:113–121.

Malhotra RK, Kirsch DB, Kristo DA, et al. American academy of sleep medicine board of directors. Polysomnography for obstructive sleep apnea should include arousal-based scoring: an American Academy of Sleep Medicine position statement. *J Clin Sleep Med*. 2018;14(7):1245–1247.

Pietzsch JB, Garner A, Cipriano LE, Linehan JH. An integrated health-economic analysis of diagnostic and therapeutic strategies in the treatment of moderate-to-severe obstructive sleep apnea. *Sleep*. 2011;34(6):695–709.

Rosen IM, Kirsch DB, Chervin RD, et al. Clinical use of a home sleep apnea test: an american academy of sleep medicine position statement. *J Clin Sleep Med*. 2017;13(10):1205–1207.

Ruoff C, Pizza F, Trotti LM, et al. The MSLT is repeatable in narcolepsy type 1 but not narcolepsy type 2: a retrospective patient study. *J Clin Sleep Med*. 2018;14(01):65–74.

Smith MT, McCrae CS, Cheung J, et al. Use of actigraphy for the evaluation of sleep disorders and circadian rhythm sleep-wake disorders: an American Academy of Sleep Medicine clinical practice guideline. *J Clin Sleep Med*. 2018;14(7):1231–1237.

A complete reference list can be found online at ExpertConsult.com.

Chapter 69

Classification of Sleep Disorders

Michael J. Sateia; Michael J. Thorpy

Chapter Highlights

- The classification of sleep disorders is necessary to discriminate among disorders and to facilitate an understanding of symptoms, etiology, pathophysiology, and treatment.
- The *International Classification of Sleep Disorders*, third edition (ICSD-3),[1] published in 2014, combines a symptomatic presentation (e.g., insomnia) with one organized in part on pathophysiology (e.g., circadian rhythms) and in part on organ systems (e.g., breathing disorders).
- Major sections of the ICSD-3 include insomnia, sleep-related breathing disorders, central disorders of hypersomnolence, circadian rhythm sleep-wake disorders, parasomnias, and sleep-related movement disorders.
- The ICSD-3 is not only a listing of sleep disorders but also a compendium of major diagnostic features, associated conditions, courses, prognoses, developmental features, epidemiology, and pathophysiology.

The classification of sleep disorders has been of particular interest to clinicians since sleep disorders were first recognized. The first major classification, the *Diagnostic Classification of Sleep and Arousal Disorders,*[2] published in 1979, organized the sleep disorders into categories that formed the basis of the current classification systems. The initial *International Classification of Sleep Disorders* (ICSD) was produced in 1990 and revised in 1997. In 2005 the ICSD, second edition, (ICSD-2) was published and included a significant reorganization of the nosology, an approach that is maintained in the most recent manual (ICSD-3), released in 2014. The *International Classification of Sleep Disorders* is published by the American Academy of Sleep Medicine (AASM) with consultation and review by panels of international experts and sleep societies worldwide. The ICSD system, developed primarily for clinical diagnostic, epidemiologic, and research purposes, has been widely used by clinicians and has allowed better international communication in sleep disorder research.

The ICSD-3 classification (Table 69.1) lists 59 sleep disorders, each presented in detail and with a descriptive diagnostic text that includes specific diagnostic criteria and coding recommendations.[3] The ICSD-3 has seven major sections: (1) insomnia, (2) sleep-related breathing disorders, (3) central disorders of hypersomnolence, (4) circadian rhythm sleep-wake disorders, (5) parasomnias, (6) sleep-related movement disorders, and (7) other sleep disorders.

Two additional sleep disorders classification systems are also in current use. The *Diagnostic and Statistical Manual of Mental Disorders*, fifth edition, (DSM-5)[4] of the American Psychiatric Association includes a sleep disorders section that was designed for mental health and general medical clinicians who are not experts in sleep medicine. Efforts to achieve consistency between DSM-5 and ICSD-3 have been largely successful during the parallel development of these two approaches, although some discrepancies in diagnostic criteria do exist. Notably, the ICSD system is significantly more detailed, as expected in light of the different target audiences. The text revision of DSM-5 (DSM-5 TR) will further reconcile differences between DSM and ICSD. The US clinical modification (CM) of the *International Classification of Diseases,* 10th revision (ICD-10-CM),[5] which was substantially revised with the publication of ICSD-2, includes a classification and coding for sleep disorders, primarily for statistical and epidemiologic purposes. Nevertheless, the crosswalk between ICSD and the ICD system is currently complex in light of the significant differences that exist between these systems. The World Health Organization (WHO) has published the 11th edition of the International Classification of Diseases (ICD-11) to supplant ICD-10. This was approved May 25, 2019, for adoption by member countries and be in effect on January 1, 2022. Implementation of ICD-11 and integration into existing health systems may take years. Table 69.2 is the current classification of sleep disorders in ICD-11. The main sleep wake disorder categories are identical to those in ICSD-3, although the sequence in the table is not.

INSOMNIA

Historically, insomnia has been characterized as either primary or secondary (comorbid).[6] The latter was intended to describe insomnia resulting from a medical or psychiatric illness, another sleep disorder, or substance use. However, current conceptualization of chronic insomnia has resulted in elimination of this dichotomy. ICSD-3 employs a diagnosis of *chronic insomnia disorder,*[7,8] which includes all insomnias of at least 3 months' duration, regardless of presumed etiology. Insomnia of less than 3 months' duration is classified as *short-term insomnia.* A diagnosis of *other insomnia* may be employed when a patient presents with insomnia complaints but does not meet full criteria for either chronic or short-term insomnia.

In ICSD-3 *chronic insomnia disorder* is defined as persistent sleep difficulty despite adequate opportunity and circumstances

Table 69.1 Sleep Disorder Diagnoses and Codes

ICSD-3 Diagnoses	2021 ICD-10-CM Diagnosis and Codes
Insomnia Disorders	
Chronic insomnia disorder	F51.01 (Other insomnia not due to physiologic or substance)
Short-term insomnia disorder	F51.02
Sleep-Related Breathing Disorders	
Obstructive Sleep Apnea	
Obstructive sleep apnea (adult and pediatric)	G47.33
Central Sleep Apnea	
Central sleep apnea with Cheyne-Stokes breathing	R06.3
Central sleep apnea due to a medical disorder without Cheyne-Stokes breathing	G47.37
Central sleep apnea due to high-altitude periodic breathing	G47.32
Central sleep apnea due to drug or substance	G47.39
Primary central sleep apnea	G47.31
Primary central sleep apnea of infancy	P28.3
Primary central sleep apnea of prematurity	P28.4
Treatment emergent central sleep apnea	G47.39
Hypoventilation/Hypoxemia	
Obesity hypoventilation syndrome	E66.2
Congenital central alveolar hypoventilation syndrome	G47.35
Late-onset central hypoventilation with hypothalamic abnormalities	G47.36
Idiopathic central alveolar hypoventilation	G47.34
Sleep-related hypoventilation due to drug or substance	G47.36
Sleep related hypoventilation due to medical or neurologic condition	G47.36
Sleep-related hypoxemia	G47.36
Hypersomnolence Disorders	
Narcolepsy—type 1 (with cataplexy and/or hypocretin deficiency)	G47.411
Narcolepsy—type 2 (without cataplexy or hypocretin deficiency)	G47.419
Idiopathic hypersomnia	G47.11
Kleine-Levin syndrome (recurrent hypersomnia)	G47.13
Hypersomnia due to drug or substance	F10–19
Hypersomnia due to medical condition	G47.14
Hypersomnia associated with psychiatric disorder	F51.13 (Hypersomnia due to mental disorder)
Insufficient sleep syndrome	F51.12
Circadian Rhythm Sleep-Wake Disorders	
Delayed sleep-wake phase disorder	G47.21
Advanced sleep-wake phase disorder	G47.22
Irregular sleep-wake rhythm disorder	G47.23
Non-24-hour sleep-wake rhythm disorder	G47.24
Shift work disorder	G47.26
Jet lag disorder	G47.25
Circadian rhythm sleep-wake disorder, not otherwise specified	G47.20 (Circadian rhythm sleep-wake disorder, not otherwise specified, unspecified)
Parasomnias	
Confusional arousals	G47.51
Sleepwalking	F51.3
Sleep terrors	F51.4
Sleep-related eating disorder	G47.59

Continued

Table 69.1 Sleep Disorder Diagnoses and Codes—cont'd

ICSD-3 Diagnoses	2021 ICD-10-CM Diagnosis and Codes
REM sleep behavior disorder	G47.52
Recurrent isolated sleep paralysis	G47.53
Nightmare disorder	F51.5
Exploding head syndrome	G47.59
Sleep-related hallucinations	H53.16
Sleep enuresis	N39.44
Parasomnia due to a medical disorder	G47.54
Parasomnia not otherwise specified	G47.50
Sleep-Related Movement Disorders	
Restless legs syndrome	G25.81
Periodic limb movement disorder	G47.61
Sleep-related bruxism	G47.63
Sleep-related leg cramps	G47.62
Rhythmic movement disorder	G47.69
Benign sleep myoclonus of infancy	G47.69
Propriospinal myoclonus at sleep onset	G47.69
Sleep-related movement disorder due to drug or substance	G47.69
Sleep-related movement disorder due to medical condition	G47.69
Sleep-related movement disorder not otherwise specified	G47.69

American Academy of Sleep Medicine. *International classification of sleep disorders*, 3rd ed. Darien, IL: American Academy of Sleep Medicine, 2014.

Table 69.2 ICD-11 Classification of Sleep-Wake Disorders

Insomnia Disorders	
7A00	Chronic insomnia
7A01	Short-term insomnia
7A0Z	Insomnia disorders, unspecified
Hypersomnolence Disorders	
7A20	Narcolepsy
7A20.0	Narcolepsy, type 1
7A20.1	Narcolepsy, type 2
7A20.Z	Narcolepsy, unspecified
7A21	Idiopathic hypersomnia
7A22	Kleine-Levin syndrome
7A23	Hypersomnia associated with a mental disorder
7A26	Insufficient sleep syndrome
7A2Y	Other specified hypersomnolence disorders
7A2Z	Hypersomnolence disorders, unspecified
Sleep-Related Breathing Disorders	
7A40	Central sleep apneas
7A40.0	Primary central sleep apnea
7A40.1	Primary central sleep apnea of infancy
7A40.2	Primary central sleep apnea of prematurity

Table 69.2 ICD-11 Classification of Sleep-Wake Disorders—cont'd

Sleep-Related Breathing Disorders	
7A40.3	Central sleep apnea due to medical condition with Cheyne-Stokes breathing
7A40.4	Central sleep apnea due to a medical condition without Cheyne-Stokes breathing
7A40.5	Central sleep apnea due to high-altitude periodic breathing
7A40.6	Central sleep apnea due to a medication or substance
7A40.7	Treatment-emergent central sleep apnea
7A40Y	Other specified central sleep apneas
7A40.Z	Central sleep apneas, unspecified
7A41	Obstructive sleep apneas
7A42	Sleep-related hypoventilation or hypoxemia disorders
7A42.0	Obesity hypoventilation syndrome
7A42.1	Congenital central alveolar sleep-related hypoventilation
7A42.2	Non-congenital central hypoventilation with hypothalamic abnormalities
7A42.3	Idiopathic central alveolar hypoventilation
7A42.4	Sleep-related hypoventilation due to a medication or substance
7A42.5	Sleep-related hypoventilation due to a medical condition
7A42.6	Sleep-related hypoxemia due to a medical condition
7A42Y	Other specified sleep-related hypoventilation or hypoxemia disorders
7A42.Z	Sleep-related hypoventilation or hypoxemia disorders, unspecified
MD11.4	Sleep-related Cheyne-Stokes respiration
7A4Y	Other specified sleep-related breathing disorders
7A4Z	Sleep-related breathing disorders, unspecified
Circadian Rhythm Sleep Wake Disorders	
7A60	Delayed sleep wake phase disorder
7A61	Advanced sleep wake phase disorder
7A62	Irregular sleep wake rhythm disorder
7A63	Non 24 hour sleep wake rhythm disorder
7A64	Circadian rhythm sleep wake disorder, shift work type
7A65	Circadian rhythm sleep wake disorder, jet lag type
7A6Z	Circadian rhythm sleep wake disorders, unspecified
Sleep-Related Movement Disorders	
7A80	Restless legs syndrome
7A81	Periodic limb movement disorder
7A82	Sleep-related leg cramps
7A83	Sleep-related bruxism
7A84	Sleep-related rhythmic movement disorder
7A85	Benign sleep myoclonus of infancy
7A86	Propriospinal myoclonus at sleep onset
7A87	Sleep-related movement disorder due to a medical condition
7A88	Sleep-related movement disorder due to a medication or substance
7B01.0	REM sleep behavior disorder
7A8Y	Other specified sleep-related movement disorders
7A8Z	Sleep-related movement disorders, unspecified

Continued

Table 69.2 ICD-11 Classification of Sleep-Wake Disorders—cont'd

Parasomnia Disorders	
7B00	Disorders of arousal from non-REM sleep
7B00.0	Confusional arousal
7B00.1	Sleepwalking disorder
7B00.2	Sleep terrors
7B00.3	Sleep-related eating disorder
7B00.Y	Other specified disorders of arousal from non-REM sleep
7B00.Z	Disorders of arousal from non-REM sleep, unspecified
7B01	Parasomnias related to REM sleep
7B01.0	REM sleep behavior disorder
7B01.1	Recurrent isolated sleep paralysis
7B01.2	Nightmare disorder
7B01.Y	Other specified parasomnias related to REM sleep
7B01.Z	Parasomnias related to REM sleep, unspecified
7B02	Other parasomnias
7B02.0	Hypnagogic exploding head syndrome
7B02.1	Sleep-related hallucinations
7B02.2	Parasomnia disorder due to a medical condition
7B02.3	Parasomnia disorder due to a medication or substance
6C00.0	Nocturnal enuresis
7B0Y	Other specified parasomnia disorders
7B0Z	Parasomnia disorders, unspecified

for sleep, which is accompanied by daytime consequences that are attributable to the sleep disturbance. Complaints may include difficulty with sleep initiation, sleep maintenance, or early awakening. In addition, resistance to going to bed on an appropriate schedule or difficulty sleeping without the intervention of a parent or caregiver constitutes an insomnia complaint (see Chapters 89 to 93). The disturbance may be reported by the patient or by the patient's parent or caregiver. Although any one of these complaints meets the first criterion for an insomnia diagnosis, it is not uncommon for patients to present with two or more of these symptoms (e.g., difficulty initiating and maintaining sleep). In the case of children or cognitively impaired adults, it is often the parent or caregiver who reports the problem. Symptoms of bedtime resistance or requirement of parent or caregiver intervention applies primarily to these groups. An ICSD-3 insomnia diagnosis also requires associated daytime consequences (e.g., fatigue, impaired concentration, mood disturbance, or other occupational, social, or academic impairment) and adequate opportunity and environmental circumstances for sleep. A duration of at least 3 months and the presence of symptoms at least three times per week are necessary to establish a diagnosis of chronic insomnia. Insomnia symptoms occur frequently in conjunction with many medical and psychiatric disorders. A diagnosis of chronic insomnia disorder should be invoked only when the insomnia component is the focus of independent clinical assessment and treatment.

ICSD-3 discusses previously identified subtypes within the context of chronic insomnia disorder. Although these clinical subtypes are no longer considered independent diagnoses, there may be characteristics of these subtypes that are clinically relevant. Major subtypes of what was previously termed *primary insomnia* include (1) *psychophysiologic insomnia*, characterized by a heightened level of arousal with learned sleep-preventing associations and an excessive concern with the inability to sleep; (2) *paradoxical insomnia* (formerly known as *sleep state misperception*), which is a complaint of severe insomnia that occurs without evidence of objective sleep disturbance and without daytime impairment to the extent that would be suggested by the amount of sleep disturbance reported; (3) *idiopathic insomnia*, a long-standing form of insomnia that appears to date from childhood and has an insidious onset; and (4) *behavioral insomnia of childhood*,[9] including limit-setting sleep disorder and sleep-onset association disorder. The former is a resistance or refusal to go to sleep, which is the result of insufficient limit-setting on the part of care providers. Sleep-onset association disorder occurs when there is reliance on inappropriate sleep associations, such as rocking, watching television, holding a bottle or other object, or specific environmental conditions such as a lighted room or an alternative place to sleep. Previously identified secondary, or comorbid, insomnias include (1) *insomnia due to medical condition*, which has been applied when a medical or neurologic disorder is believed to give rise to the insomnia; (2) *insomnia due to drug or substance*, when excessive use, dependence on, or withdrawal from a substance such as alcohol, a recreational drug, or caffeine is causative; and (3) *insomnia due to mental disorder*, which is employed when an underlying mental disorder is the major etiologic factor.

Patients often present with multiple comorbidities that may contribute to an insomnia complaint. It is often difficult to ascertain the cause-and-effect relationship between comorbidities and the insomnia. When an ICSD-3 diagnosis of chronic insomnia is employed, clinicians are encouraged to list all pertinent comorbidities along with the diagnosis.

Short sleep and *excessive time in bed* are listed as normal variants within the insomnia section. A short sleeper is a person with a routine pattern of obtaining 6 hours or less of sleep in a 24-hour day without sleep complaints or identifiable daytime consequences. In children, this sleep length can be 3 or more hours less than the norm for the age group.

SLEEP-RELATED BREATHING DISORDERS

The disorders in this group are characterized by disordered respiration during sleep (see Chapters 123 to 142). ICSD-3 includes four major categories of sleep-related breathing disorders: (1) *obstructive sleep apnea (OSA)*, (2) *central sleep apnea (CSA) syndromes*, (3) *sleep-related hypoventilation disorders*, and (4) *sleep-related hypoxemia disorder*.

OSA is a disorder in which complete or partial obstruction of the airway during sleep results in absent or reduced airflow despite adequate respiratory effort. Adult OSA[10,11] is characterized by repetitive episodes of cessation of breathing (apneas), reduced breathing (hypopneas), or arousal associated with increased airway resistance and respiratory effort (respiratory effort–related arousal). The term *upper airway resistance syndrome* is no longer employed because the underlying pathophysiology and potential consequences are essentially those of OSA. Heavy snoring is reported in most of these patients. Apneic and hypopneic events are often associated with reduced blood oxygen saturation. Diagnosis requires the presence of five or more obstructive events (apneas, hypopneas, or respiratory effort–related arousals [RERAs]) per hour coupled with at least one sign or symptom (e.g., snoring, observed pauses, excessive sleepiness, insomnia) or medical or psychiatric complications. A predominantly obstructive event frequency of greater than 15 per hour meets diagnostic criteria regardless of the presence or absence of symptoms.

Pediatric OSA[12] is characterized by features similar to those seen in the adult, but cortical arousals may not occur, possibly because of a higher arousal threshold in children. The absence of cortical arousals may give rise to a more sustained pattern of obstructive hypoventilation, which may require CO_2 monitoring for detection. Signs or symptoms are required for a diagnosis of pediatric OSA. These must be coupled with at least one obstructive event per hour of sleep or a pattern of obstructive hypoventilation, as evidenced by $Paco_2$ greater than 50 mm Hg for more than 25% of sleep time.

CSA syndromes[13,14] include those in which airflow is diminished or absent in an intermittent or cyclic fashion as a result of reduced or absent respiratory effort. ICSD-3 includes nine CSA syndromes. All of the adult forms of these disorders, with the exception of high-altitude periodic breathing, require polysomnographic demonstration of a central apnea/hypopnea index (events per hour of sleep) greater than 5. Adult presentations also require associated signs or symptoms (e.g., sleepiness, sleep disturbance, awakening short of breath, snoring, or witnessed apnea), although presence of a medical condition such as congestive heart failure, atrial fibrillation/flutter, or neurologic disorder precludes this requirement in CSA with Cheyne-Stokes breathing. *CSA with Cheyne Stokes breathing*[15-17] is characterized by recurrent central apneas or hypopneas alternating with a respiratory phase in which tidal volume waxes and wanes in a crescendo-decrescendo pattern. This pattern is characteristically seen in non-rapid eye movement (NREM) sleep. *CSA due to a medical condition without Cheyne-Stokes breathing* is generally a result of brainstem lesions of varying etiologies. *CSA due to high-altitude periodic breathing*[18] is seen following recent ascent to altitude, typically greater than 2500 meters, although some individuals may experience the symptoms at lower altitudes. The condition may be diagnosed on the basis of ascent to altitude and symptoms alone, although polysomnography (PSG), if performed, shows a central index greater than 5 per hour. *CSA due to drug or substance*[19,20] is most commonly associated with long-term opioid use. The substance causes a respiratory depression by acting on the μ receptors of the ventral medulla. *Primary CSA* is a disorder of unknown cause characterized by recurrent episodes of cessation of breathing during sleep without associated ventilatory effort. Most of these patients have low normal arterial pCO_2 (<40 mm Hg) during wakefulness. A complaint of excessive daytime sleepiness, insomnia, or difficulty breathing during sleep is reported. The patient must not be hypercapneic (pCO_2 >45 mm Hg).

Primary sleep apnea of infancy (if conceptional age of the child is 37 weeks or greater) or *prematurity* (when conceptional age is less than 37 weeks) is a disorder of respiratory control caused by developmental issues (immaturity of brainstem respiratory centers) or other medical disorders. Diagnosis requires observation of an episode of apnea or cyanosis or detection of apnea or desaturations by monitoring. Recurrent, prolonged (>20 seconds) central apnea or periodic breathing for more than 5% of total sleep time must be demonstrated.

ICSD-3 includes a new CSA diagnosis: *treatment emergent central sleep apnea*.[21] This disorder, which has been referred to in the literature as *complex sleep apnea*, is characterized by predominantly obstructive apnea on baseline PSG, with resolution of obstruction and emergence or persistence of predominantly central apnea during administration of positive airway pressure without backup rate. The term *complex sleep apnea* has also been used to describe emergence of CSA with Cheyne-Stokes breathing or due to drug or substance in the context of treated OSA. However, a diagnosis of treatment emergent CSA should not be applied when another etiology for the CSA is established. In such cases, clinicians should diagnose both OSA and CSA due to Cheyne-Stokes breathing or substance.

Sleep-related hypoventilation disorders[22] comprise six disorders associated with hypoventilation during sleep. Hypoventilation must be established by demonstration of elevated Pco_2 (as defined in the most recent version of the AASM scoring manual) by blood gas or, more commonly, by proxy measures such as end-tidal or transcutaneous CO_2.

Obesity hypoventilation syndrome[23,24] requires demonstration of daytime hypercapnia, whereas other sleep-related hypoventilation disorders require only sleep-related hypoventilation and may or not be associated with daytime hypercapnia. Body mass index is greater than 30 kg/m^2 or above the 95th percentile for age and sex in children. *Congenital central alveolar hypoventilation syndrome*[25] is a failure of automatic central control of breathing associated with mutation of the *PHOX2B* gene. The hypoventilation begins in infancy and worsens during sleep. *Idiopathic central alveolar hypoventilation* refers to sleep-related hypoventilation that is not attributable to another disorder. *Late-onset central hypoventilation with hypothalamic dysfunction*[26] is characterized by onset of symptoms after the first several years of life. In addition to hypoventilation, symptoms may include obesity, endocrine abnormalities of hypothalamic origin, emotional and behavioral disturbances, and neural tumors. *Sleep-related hypoventilation due to a medical condition*[27-29] may result from pulmonary airway or parenchymal disease, extrinsic factors such as chest wall disorder, or neuromuscular disease. Sleep-related hypoventilation may also be caused by substances such as opioid or other respiratory depressants.

Sustained declines in Po_2 (Sao_2 <88% [90% for children] for ≥5 minutes), in the absence of demonstrated elevation of Pco_2, are diagnosed as *sleep-related hypoxemia disorder.*

Snoring is an isolated symptom included in this section and is identified when a respiratory sound, typically associated with inspiration, is disturbing to the patient, a bed partner, or others. This term applies when the snoring occurs without evidence of upper airway obstructive events or sleep-wake complaint such as insomnia or excessive sleepiness. Not only can snoring lead to impaired health, but it may also be a cause of social embarrassment and can disturb the sleep of a bed partner.

CENTRAL DISORDERS OF HYPERSOMNOLENCE

Central disorders of hypersomnolence are characterized by a primary complaint of daytime sleepiness that is not attributable to another sleep disorder (see Chapter 110). Most of these conditions are caused by central nervous system abnormalities or the effects of substances or other disorders on the central nervous system. One exception to this is *insufficient sleep syndrome*, which results from behaviorally induced sleep deprivation. Daytime sleepiness is defined as the inability to stay alert and awake during the major waking episodes of the day, typically resulting in unintended lapses into sleep. Other sleep disorders may be present, and they must first be effectively treated to establish a diagnosis of a hypersomnolence disorder. The disorders previously named *narcolepsy with cataplexy* and *narcolepsy without cataplexy* are now termed *narcolepsy type 1* and *type 2.*[30-32] *Narcolepsy type 1 (NT1)* is diagnosed on the basis of complaint of excessive sleepiness and the presence of definite cataplexy plus Multiple Sleep Latency Test (MSLT) findings (mean sleep latency ≤8 minutes and evidence of two or more sleep-onset rapid eye movement periods [SOREMPs]). Evidence suggests that a SOREMP on PSG before the MSLT is highly specific for NT1.[33] Therefore a nocturnal PSG SOREMP (within 15 minutes of sleep onset) may substitute for one of the MSLT SOREMPs in making the diagnosis. Alternatively, NT1 can be diagnosed when subjective sleepiness and hypocretin deficiency (either <110 pg/mL or <⅓ of mean values obtained in normal subjects with the same assay) are present, even in the absence of cataplexy. Rarely, some patients with hypocretin deficiency may not manifest cataplexy, at least at the time of initial diagnosis. It is for this reason that the term *narcolepsy with cataplexy* has been rendered obsolete. *Narcolepsy type 2 (NT2)* criteria include subjective sleepiness and the MSLT findings described previously for NT1. Cataplexy is absent, and hypocretin levels, if obtained, must not meet type 1 criteria.

Idiopathic hypersomnia[34,35] is the diagnosis given to those with subjective sleepiness complaints that are not explained by other sleep disorders, medical illness, or psychiatric illness. An MSLT latency of 8 minutes or less with fewer than two SOREMPs (including a SOREMP on the preceding night's PSG, if present) or a total 24-hour sleep time of more than 660 minutes is required for diagnosis. It is recognized that some patients with legitimate sleepiness problems may not demonstrate mean latencies of 8 minutes or less. Clinical judgment is required in such cases. Particular care must be exercised to exclude insufficient sleep as a cause or contributing factor before a diagnosis of idiopathic hypersomnia is established.

Kleine-Levin syndrome[36] is a form of recurrent hypersomnia that persists for days to several weeks and is associated with one or more of the following: eating disorder (most commonly hyperphagia), cognitive dysfunction, perceptual disturbance, or uninhibited behavior, often sexual. In some women, recurrent hypersomnia may manifest as a menses-related phenomenon and is now termed *menstrual-related Kleine-Levin syndrome.*

Insufficient sleep syndrome occurs in patients who maintain a habitually short sleep episode relative to age-appropriate norms.[37] These patients typically sleep significantly longer when schedules allow (i.e., weekends or vacation). Extended sleep resolves the sleepiness. Consideration must be given to the possibility of long sleep requirement in patients presenting with otherwise unexplained sleepiness and ostensibly normal sleep times.

Hypersomnia due to medical condition is excessive sleepiness that is caused by a medical or neurologic disorder.[38,39] Cataplexy or other diagnostic features of narcolepsy are not present. Parkinson disease, traumatic brain injury, and certain localized neurologic lesions are among the most common etiologies of this disorder. Residual hypersomnia associated with treated OSA is also classified here. *Hypersomnia due to drug or substance* is diagnosed when the complaint is believed to be secondary to current or past use of drugs.[40] Sedative-hypnotic, opioid, antipsychotic, or antihistamine use are common causes, as well as withdrawal from stimulant medications or substances. *Hypersomnia associated with a psychiatric disorder* is excessive sleepiness that is temporally associated with a psychiatric diagnosis, most commonly atypical, seasonal, or bipolar depression, although, as the name implies, cause-and-effect relationships between true hypersomnolence and psychiatric disorders are not well established and MSLT findings do not typically demonstrate pathologic objective sleepiness.[41]

Long sleeper, a normal variant within the hypersomnolence conditions, applies when a person sleeps more in the 24-hour day than the typical person. Sleep is normal in architecture and quality. Usually, sleep lengths of 10 hours or greater qualify for this diagnosis. Symptoms of excessive sleepiness occur if the person does not get that amount of sleep.

CIRCADIAN RHYTHM SLEEP-WAKE DISORDERS

The *circadian rhythm sleep-wake disorders*[42-44] share a common underlying chronophysiologic basis. The major feature of these disorders is an alteration of the circadian clock or a persistent or recurrent misalignment between the patient's sleep pattern and the pattern that is desired or required by societal demands or the environment (see Chapter 43). Because of the misalignment between circadian sleep-wake propensity and behavioral schedules, these individuals often experience symptoms of both insomnia and excessive sleepiness.

Delayed sleep-wake phase disorder,[45,46] which is seen more commonly in adolescents and young adults, is characterized by a delay in the phase of the major sleep period in relation to the desired sleep time and wake time. By contrast, *advanced sleep-wake phase disorder*, which is seen more commonly in older adults, is characterized by an advance in the phase of the major sleep period in relation to the desired sleep time and wake-up time. In both of these disorders, sleep, when allowed to occur with the circadian sleep propensity, is normal in quality and duration, but at a later (delayed sleep phase) or earlier (advanced sleep phase) time of day than desired. Although chronobiologic factors are clearly of significance in the etiology of these disorders, behavioral/motivational components (e.g., school avoidance) are often a critical component of delayed sleep phase as well. The *irregular sleep-wake rhythm disorder*, a disorder that involves the lack of a clearly defined circadian rhythm of sleep and wakefulness, is most often seen in institutionalized older adults or chronically mentally ill patients and is associated with a lack of synchronizing agents such as light, physical activity, and social schedules.[47] The *non-24-hour sleep-wake rhythm disorder* or *free-running sleep-wake rhythm* is a result of lack of entrainment to the 24-hour light-dark cycle.[48,49] The most common cause of this condition is total blindness, although in a small minority of individuals an unusually long circadian period (which lies outside the range of entertainment) or an abnormal response to light may be causative. These patients generally exhibit cycles of poor sleep alternating with better sleep as their clock moves in and out of phase with the light-dark cycle and conventional sleep-wake times.

Jet lag disorder[50] is related to an abrupt desynchronization between circadian sleep-wake propensity and the environmental day-night cycle as a result of transmeridian travel across two or more time zones. The severity of the disorder is influenced by the number of time zones crossed and the direction of travel, with eastward travel usually being more disruptive. *Shift work disorder*[51] is characterized by complaints of insomnia or excessive sleepiness that occur as a result of work hours that overlap the usual sleep period.

In addition to the subjective reports of insomnia or sleepiness that are attributable to the circadian disturbance, sleep logs that demonstrate the sleep-wake schedule alteration are required for most of these disorders. Although objective measures are not strictly required, increasing emphasis is placed on the use of actigraphy and biomarkers such as dim light melatonin onset (DLMO) to provide more accurate diagnosis and treatment guidance. Other sleep disorders (e.g., chronic insomnia disorder) may mimic or overlap with circadian rhythm sleep-wake disorders and must be identified and addressed as part of the overall therapeutic approach.

PARASOMNIAS

The parasomnias are undesirable behaviors or experiences that accompany sleep (see Chapters 115 to 122). The motor activity of parasomnias is typically more complex than that observed with the sleep-related movement disorders. Experiences may be cognitive-emotional (as in nightmares or sleep terrors) or sensory (e.g., sleep-related hallucinations or exploding head syndrome). The parasomnias can arise during NREM sleep, rapid eye movement (REM) sleep, or sleep-wake transitions. Many parasomnias represent a sleep-wake state disassociation between either NREM and wake (disorders of arousal from NREM) or REM and wake (REM sleep behavior disorder [RBD] and recurrent sleep paralysis). The parasomnias often occur in conjunction with other sleep disorders such as OSA. It is not uncommon for several parasomnias to occur in one patient. NREM parasomnias[52,53] include the disorders of arousal from slow wave NREM sleep (confusional arousal, sleepwalking, and sleep terrors), seen most commonly during childhood, and the closely related sleep-related eating disorder. Confusional arousals are characterized by mental confusion or confusional behavior that occurs during or after arousal from sleep. These arousals are common in children and can occur not only from nocturnal sleep but also from daytime naps. *Sleepwalking* is a series of complex behaviors that arise from sudden arousals from slow wave sleep and result in locomotion during a state of impaired consciousness. *Sleep terrors* also occur from slow wave sleep and are associated with a cry or piercing scream accompanied by intense autonomic system activation and behavioral manifestation of extreme fear. Individuals may be difficult to arouse from the episode and when aroused can be confused and are subsequently amnestic for the episode. These two disorders, sleepwalking and sleep terrors, often coexist and may result in a potentially dangerous state of terror and walking or running. *Sleep-related eating disorder*[54] involves recurrent eating or drinking episodes during partial arousals from sleep. The eating behavior is uncontrollable, typically involves ingestion of unusual or inedible substances, and may be associated with potential injury (e.g., from cooking) or other adverse health consequences, including weight gain. Often the patient has limited or no awareness during the episode and impaired recall of the behavior.

Several parasomnias are typically associated with REM sleep. Pathophysiologic mechanisms related to REM sleep may underlie these disorders. RBD[55-57] involves dream enactment behaviors that occur in REM sleep and may result in injury or sleep disruption. The behaviors are often violent with dream enactment that is action filled. The disorder can occur in narcolepsy and in many patients with Parkinson disease or other synucleinopathies. The delayed emergence of neurodegenerative disorders, primarily synucleinopathies, occurs in a high percentage of patients with idiopathic RBD, especially in men older than 50 years. Recurrent isolated sleep paralysis[58] can occur at sleep onset or on awakening and is characterized by a frightening inability to perform voluntary movements. Ventilation is usually unaffected. Hallucinatory experiences may accompany the paralysis. Nightmare disorder[59] is characterized by recurrent anxiety-laden, often terrifying dreams that occur most commonly in REM sleep and result in an awakening with intense anxiety, fear, or other negative feelings. The disorder is most commonly encountered in the clinical setting in conjunction with posttraumatic stress disorder. The diagnosis should be invoked in this context only when the nightmare component is the focus of independent clinical assessment and treatment.

Sleep enuresis[60] is recurrent involuntary voiding that occurs during sleep. Enuresis is considered primary in a child who has never been dry for 6 months or longer; otherwise, it is considered secondary. Exploding head syndrome is characterized by a loud imagined noise or sense of a violent explosion that occurs in the head as the patient is falling asleep or during waking in the night.

Sleep-related hallucinations are hallucinatory experiences that occur at sleep onset or on awakening. They may be difficult to distinguish from vivid dreams or nightmares but usually are complex images that occur when the patient is clearly awake. Sleep talking, an isolated symptom, may arise during NREM or REM sleep and can be idiopathic or associated with other disorders such as RBD or sleep-related eating disorder.

SLEEP-RELATED MOVEMENT DISORDERS

The sleep-related movement disorders are characterized by relatively simple, usually stereotyped movements that disturb sleep (see Chapter 122). Disorders such as periodic limb movement disorder and restless legs syndrome (RLS) are classified in this section.

RLS[61-64] consists of a complaint of a strong, nearly irresistible urge to move the legs often accompanied by uncomfortable or painful symptoms. The sensations are worse at rest and occur more frequently in the evening or during the night. Walking or moving the legs relieves the sensation temporarily. The disorder is commonly associated with repetitive limb movements during sleep, but a separate diagnosis of periodic limb movement disorder is not used when the movement occurs in the context of RLS, narcolepsy, untreated OSA, or RBD.

Periodic limb movement disorder[63,65] is an independent disorder of repetitive, highly stereotyped limb movements that occur during sleep. The movements must give rise to sleep disturbance or daytime sleepiness to meet criteria. Sleep-related leg cramps[66,67] are painful sensations associated with sudden intense muscle contractions, usually of the calves or small muscles of the feet, which occur during the sleep period and can lead to disrupted sleep. Relief is usually obtained by stretching the affected muscle.

Sleep-related bruxism[68,69] is characterized by clenching of the teeth during any stage of sleep and can result in arousals. Often the activity is severe or frequent enough to result in symptoms of temporomandibular joint pain or damage to dentition. Sleep-related rhythmic movement disorder[70,71] is a stereotyped, repetitive rhythmic motor behavior that occurs during drowsiness or light sleep and results in large movements of the head, body, or limbs. Although typically seen in children, the disorder can also be seen in adults. Head and limb injuries can result from violent movements. Rhythmic movement disorder can also occur during full wakefulness and alertness, particularly in individuals who have intellectual disabilities. Benign sleep myoclonus of infancy[72] is a disorder of myoclonic jerks that occur during sleep in infants. It typically occurs from birth to age 6 months, is not associated with known adverse consequences, and resolves spontaneously. Propriospinal myoclonus at sleep onset[73] is a disorder of recurrent sudden muscular jerks in the transition from wakefulness to sleep. The disorder may be associated with severe sleep-onset insomnia.

Isolated symptoms and normal variants within this section include sleep starts, excessive fragmentary myoclonus, and hypnagogic foot tremor and alternating leg muscle activation.[71,73] Sleep starts (hypnic jerks) are sudden brief contractions of the body that occur at sleep onset. These movements are often associated with a sensation of falling, a sensory flash, or a sleep-onset dream. Hypnagogic foot tremor and alternating leg muscle activation occur at the transition between wake and sleep or during light NREM sleep. These conditions are listed together because they may represent somewhat different manifestations of a single disturbance. Hypnagogic foot tremor consists of rhythmic movement of the feet or toes, whereas alternating leg muscle activation consists of a PSG pattern of repetitive, transient activation of one anterior tibialis muscle group, alternating with activation of the contralateral tibialis. Excessive fragmentary myoclonus is manifest as small muscle twitches in the fingers, toes, or the corner of the mouth that do not cause actual movements across a joint. The myoclonus is often a finding during PSG that may be asymptomatic or associated with daytime sleepiness or fatigue.

OTHER SLEEP DISORDERS

The diagnosis of other sleep disorders is employed when a sleep disorder cannot be classified elsewhere. Disorders that demonstrate clear features of other, more specific categories (e.g., circadian, parasomnia, or movement disorder) but do not meet criteria for a specific diagnosis should be classified within those respective categories as "unspecified."

Sleep disturbance that is purely a function of *environmental disturbance* such as a physical stimulus (e.g., noise or light) or environmental danger does not technically meet criteria for insomnia and should be classified here.

SLEEP-RELATED MEDICAL AND NEUROLOGIC DISORDERS

The ICSD-3 lists six disorders that, although not sleep disorders, per se, are commonly encountered in association with sleep or may have unique presentations during sleep.

Fatal familial insomnia[74] is a progressive disorder characterized by difficulty in falling asleep and maintaining sleep that develops into enacted dreams or stupor. Autonomic hyperactivity with pyrexia, excessive salivation, and hyperhidrosis leads to cardiac and respiratory failure. The disease is caused by a missense mutation of the prion protein gene (*PRNP*), and it leads eventually to death, generally within 12 to 72 months. Sleep-related epilepsy[75] is the diagnosis employed when epilepsy occurs during sleep. Several epilepsy types are associated with sleep, including nocturnal frontal lobe epilepsy, benign epilepsy of childhood with centrotemporal spikes, benign epilepsy with occipital paroxysms, and juvenile myoclonic epilepsy. Sleep-related headaches[76] are cephalgias that occur during sleep or on awakening from sleep. Some are uniquely associated with sleep. Migraine headaches, chronic paroxysmal hemicrania, hypnic headaches, and cluster headaches can all occur during sleep. Sleep-related laryngospasm is a disorder in which patients report choking and difficulty breathing at night typically associated with pronounced fear or panic. Its etiology is not well established, although it is encountered in multisystem atrophy and may be associated with OSA or gastroesophageal reflux. Sleep-related gastroesophageal reflux[77] is characterized by regurgitation of stomach contents into the esophagus during sleep. Shortness of breath or heartburn can result, but occasionally the disorder is asymptomatic. Sleep-related myocardial ischemia is due to reduction of blood flow to the myocardium during the sleep period.

CURRENT AND FUTURE CLASSIFICATION CONSIDERATIONS

Insomnia

From the outset of modern-day sleep disorder classification systems, insomnia has been compartmentalized into primary insomnia and insomnia due to a medical disorder, mental illness, or substance use, with several additional subtypes of primary insomnia identified. The consolidation of insomnia diagnoses in ICSD-3 is not intended to suggest that there may not be important differences among certain subtypes of insomnia. However, from a clinical perspective, differentiation among a number of these subtypes has proved rather unreliable,[78,79] and after treatment of comorbidities is accounted for, therapeutic approaches do not differ significantly among the various subtypes. Nevertheless, there have been some ongoing efforts to identify meaningful subtypes of insomnia.[80-82] The identification of insomnia with objective short sleep duration[83,84] is one notable example of subtyping with important clinical implications, particularly with respect to cardiovascular and metabolic health. Additional research is necessary to determine whether other significant, identifiable differences among insomnias do exist and to what extent these differences may alter therapeutic approaches.

Previous classification systems such as ICSD-2 included a complaint of "nonrestorative sleep"[85,86] in the list of possible insomnia symptoms. However, the nature of this complaint is ambiguous. Although many insomnia patients describe their sleep as "nonrestorative," the majority of these patients have a presenting complaint of sleep initiation or maintenance resulting in extended periods of nocturnal wakefulness. Although a small percentage of patients have an isolated complaint of nonrestorative sleep, it is not clear that this complaint should be categorized as insomnia. Many other disturbances of sleep (e.g., sleep apnea) result in sleep that can fairly be categorized as "nonrestorative." The limited studies of isolated nonrestorative sleep suggest that, although sufferers share many symptoms in common with insomnia patients, they differ in certain respects. Therefore the evaluation and classification of patients with this complaint are left to the judgment of the clinician.

Sleep-Related Breathing Disorders

The pathophysiology (and hence the classification) of central respiratory disorders, including apnea/hypopnea and hypoventilation, is complex. The polysomnographic characteristics of central respiratory disturbances are varied and may be associated with diverse clinical presentations.[87] Moreover, individuals can manifest multiple factors that may contribute to a central respiratory disorder. Although ICSD-3 classification of central breathing disturbance is based on our best current understanding of clinical syndromes, it may not adequately represent the clinical complexity and diversity of these disturbances and, in so doing, unnecessarily confine therapeutic interventions. A more nuanced understanding of the pathophysiology, prognostic significance, and treatment implications of central breathing disturbances will allow for more robust classification of these disorders.

Treatment emergent central sleep apnea first appeared as a diagnosis in ICSD-3. Some controversy has existed regarding the conditions under which it should be applied. The diagnosis is established on the basis of PSG performed during positive airway pressure titration for OSA. However, it has been recognized that a significant degree of CSA that is observed during positive airway pressure titration may resolve spontaneously with continued positive airway pressure[21] or is attributable to another disorder (e.g., opioids, heart failure, or neurologic conditions). Thus potential for overuse of this diagnosis exists and may result in unnecessary application of more complex and expensive treatment modalities such as adaptive servo ventilation (ASV). Further long-term follow-up is necessary to address these issues.

The criteria for pediatric OSA have remain unchanged. However, limited information exists about the appropriate thresholds for treatment intervention in this population.

Central Disorders of Hypersomnolence

Destruction of hypocretin neurons, likely on an autoimmune basis, is the presumptive etiology of NT1.[88] However, 5% to 10% of patients with narcolepsy and cataplexy (type 1) have normal hypocretin levels, suggesting either a downstream problem with hypocretin (e.g., at the receptor level) or an alternative pathophysiologic mechanism. It is unclear whether NT2 shares some common pathophysiologic aspects with NT1 or is a disorder based on an entirely different pathophysiology. The test-retest reliability for MSLT findings in NT2 appears to be no better than 50%, suggesting a significant number of false-positive diagnoses.[89,90] It seems likely that at least a significant percentage of these false positives is due to inadequate pretest attention to factors such as insufficient sleep, inadequately treated sleep-related breathing disorders, circadian phase factors, and medications/substances. Likewise, idiopathic hypersomnia (IH) is still poorly understood because there is no clear pathophysiologic mechanism identified. Diagnosis rests almost entirely on a subjective report of excessive sleepiness accompanied by MSLT latency of less than 8 minutes or a long total sleep time. However, test-retest reliability for the MSLT in idiopathic hypersomnia is reported to be even poorer than that of NT2. There are some patients with NT2 or IH whose diagnostic features change with time, such that a patient diagnosed with NT2 may later fulfill criteria for NT1 and, likewise, a patient diagnosed with IH may later meet criteria for NT2, suggesting that some patients may have a similar underlying pathophysiology that constitutes part of a narcolepsy spectrum disorder. Further research and greater attention to MSLT preparation (e.g., pretest actigraphy) is needed to understand and improve the diagnostic accuracy of these disorders.

Circadian Rhythm Sleep-Wake Disorders

Current research suggests that the role of circadian misalignment in circadian rhythm sleep-wake disorders is variable. For example, a substantial number of individuals with delayed sleep-wake phase disorder (DSWPD) do not demonstrate significant delay of dim-light melatonin onset and, hence, their disorder is considered to be primarily "behavioral" or "motivational" DSWPD.[91] Important treatment implications arise from these observations. Therefore increased application of circadian biologic markers will enhance diagnostic precision and, likely, improve treatment outcome. In particular, salivary dim-light melatonin assays are now readily available and increasingly used for determination of circadian phase. ICSD-3 encourages greater use of these markers for diagnosis in the hope that they will become a diagnostic standard and more widely available.

Parasomnia

Substantial numbers of patients exhibit dream enactment behaviors in the context of OSA or antidepressant use. It remains unclear whether these patients carry the same unfavorable prognosis with respect to development of synucleinopathies as those with idiopathic RBD. This is an especially difficult problem in the decision of whether to inform patients with dream enactment behavior about the risk for development of serious neurologic disease.

CLINICAL PEARLS

- ICSD-3 incorporates all chronic insomnia within a single diagnosis of chronic insomnia disorder. In addition, clinicians should identify all potentially contributing comorbidities.
- MSLT findings in type 2 narcolepsy are not consistently reproducible, possibly because of inadequate attention to pretest total sleep time and attention to circadian misalignment issues. Clinicians should, whenever possible, conduct actigraphy for 1 to 2 weeks before MSLT and, when indicated, assess circadian phase.
- Diagnosis of CSA syndromes is complex. Clinicians should carefully consider the specific polysomnographic patterns of central apnea, accompanying symptoms, accompanying comorbidities, and long-term prognosis before formulating a management strategy.
- Treatment emergent CSA excludes central apneas of known etiology, such as substance-induced central apnea and Cheyne-Stokes breathing.
- Increased utilization of circadian phase markers (e.g., DLMO) will increase diagnostic accuracy and result in more effective management strategies in patients with circadian rhythm sleep-wake disorders.

SUMMARY

The classification of sleep disorders allows accurate diagnosis, improved communication among physicians, and the standardization of data for research purposes. The ICSD-3 identifies six major groups of disorders, including insomnia, sleep-related breathing disorders, hypersomnolence disorders, circadian rhythm sleep-wake disorders, parasomnias, and sleep-related movement disorders. New sleep disorders have been recognized and previous sleep disorders have been clarified with a better understanding of their diagnostic and epidemiologic features. The ICSD-3 increases the refinement of sleep disorder diagnoses because of advances in sleep research. Referral to the ICSD-3 will help clinicians establish a rational differential diagnosis when evaluating patients.

SELECTED READINGS

American Academy of Sleep Medicine. *International Classification of Sleep Disorders*. 3rd ed. Darien, IL: American Academy of Sleep Medicine; 2014.

Berry BR, Quan SF, Abreu AR, et al. For the American Academy of Sleep Medicine. *AASM Manual for the Scoring of Sleep and Associated Events: Rules, Terminology and Technical Specifications*. Darien, IL: American Academy of Sleep Medicine; 2020. version 2.6.

Billiard M, Sonka K. Idiopathic hypersomnia. *Sleep Med Rev*. 2016;29:23–33.

Dauvilliers Y, Schenck CH, Postuma RB, et al. REM sleep behaviour disorder. *Nat Rev Dis Primers*. 2018;4(1):19.

Erickson J, Vaughn BV. Non-REM parasomnia: the promise of precision medicine. *Sleep Med Clin*. 2019;14(3):363–370.

Herkenrath SD, Randerath WJ. More than heart failure: central sleep apnea and sleep-related hypoventilation. *Respiration*. 2019;98(2):95–110.

Scammell TE. Narcolepsy. *N Engl J Med*. 2015;373(27):2654–2662.

Trotti LM. Restless legs syndrome and sleep-related movement disorders. *Continuum (Minneap Minn)*. 2017;(4, Sleep Neurology):1005–1016.

Veasey SC, Rosen IM. Obstructive sleep apnea in adults. *N Engl J Med*. 2019;380(15):1442–1449.

Winkelman JW. Clinical practice. insomnia disorder. *N Engl J Med*. 2015;373(15):1437–1444.

Zee PC, Attarian H, Videnovic A. Circadian rhythm abnormalities. *Continuum (NY)*. 2013;19(1 Sleep Disorders):132–147.

A complete reference list can be found online at ExpertConsult.com.

Chapter 70

Epidemiology of Sleep Medicine

Krisztina Harsanyi; Kavita Ratarasarn; Amy W. Amara; Mary Halsey Maddox

Chapter Highlights

- Sleep medicine is a young field of medicine with evolving classifications of disorders. In addition, most epidemiologic studies in this field rely on subjective data. Current data only scratch the surface, and there is still much to be learned about the epidemiology of sleep disorders.
- Despite significant variability of methods applied in sleep-related epidemiologic studies, they uniformly demonstrate that sleep disorders are extremely common. Insomnia, hypersomnia, and sleep-disordered breathing are the most common disorders reported, and each has proven adverse outcomes for individuals and society.

INTRODUCTION

Defining the epidemiology of sleep medicine proves challenging because of the evolution of diagnostic criteria over time and differences in study methodologies. This chapter highlights the larger epidemiologic studies and attempts to summarize the data available, recognizing that there are gaps in knowledge, particularly in the areas of impact and economic burden. The sections (Sleep-Disordered Breathing [SDB], Hypersomnia, Circadian Rhythm Sleep-Wake Disorders [CRSWD], Insomnia, etc.) in this chapter follow diagnostic criteria based on the *International Classification of Sleep Disorders*, third edition (ICSD-3).

SLEEP-DISORDERED BREATHING

SDB includes a wide spectrum of disorders, from snoring to apnea to hypoventilation disorders. Although disruptions of breathing in sleep had been reported previously (and attributed to hypercapnia), airway obstruction was first recognized as the cause of sleep apnea between 1964 and 1965.[1,2] In the 1970s recognition of obstructive sleep apnea (OSA) expanded with enhancement of polysomnography (PSG) techniques and development of diagnostic parameters.[3] Before the 1980s tracheostomy and weight loss were the only treatments for OSA. In the early 1980s continuous positive airway pressure was introduced and revolutionized the treatment of OSA.

Snoring

Habitual snoring in adults is defined as snoring for 3 or more nights per week with prevalence ranging widely from 14% to 84%, depending on the population studied. Most reports of snoring prevalence do not distinguish between snorers with and without apnea. Snoring is more common in men than women as consistently demonstrated in large cohorts, such as the National Health and Nutrition Examination Survey (37% in men, 22% in women) and the Sleep Heart Health Study (32% to 52% in men, 19% to 29% in women).[4] Of note, in a Swedish population, snoring was perceived as problematic in 17.9% of men and 7.4% of women.[5]

Snoring prevalence is also influenced by body mass index (BMI), age, smoking status, the presence or absence of a bed partner, and ethnicity. For example, Hispanic ethnicity (odds ratio [OR] = 2.25) and Black race (OR = 1.55) were associated with increased snoring risk in women; however, this association held only in Hispanic men, whereas men in other ethnic groups and races had similar prevalence.[6] Evidence also suggests that snoring progresses with age but then tapers beyond the seventh decade of life.

Snoring is associated with adverse clinical outcomes independent of OSA, with investigations that demonstrate twofold increases in bilateral carotid artery stenosis.[7] Furthermore, the severity of snoring may be a relevant factor, as evidenced by carotid atherosclerosis prevalence of 20% in mild snorers and 64% in heavy snorers, despite adjustment for nocturnal hypoxemia or OSA severity.[8]

Obstructive Sleep Apnea

OSA is defined by 5 or more predominantly obstructive respiratory events (apneas, hypopneas, or respiratory event–related arousals) per hour of sleep as measured by PSG or out-of-center sleep testing (OCST) plus a relevant comorbid medical condition, sleep-related complaint (sleepiness, insomnia, nonrestorative sleep), or the presence of nocturnal respiratory disturbances experienced by the patient or observed by the bed partner. Alternatively, OSA is diagnosed when 15 or more predominantly obstructive respiratory events per hour are recorded by PSG or OCST in the absence of other symptoms or comorbid conditions. This definition has not been applied to many of the epidemiologic studies, making interpretation of prevalence challenging, which is further complicated by an evolving hypopnea scoring criteria. However, large population-based studies provide useful information about OSA epidemiology. The Wisconsin Sleep Cohort Study estimated OSA (apnea hypopnea index [AHI] ≥5 in combination with excessive daytime sleepiness [EDS]) affected 2% of women and 4% of men, whereas SDB (AHI ≥5 with or without EDS) was estimated to be 9% in women and 24% in men.[9] The Sleep Heart Health Study reported an AHI greater than or equal to 15 in 18% (25% of men, 11% of women) and an AHI of 5 to 14 in 29% (33% of men, 26% of women).[10] In a Spanish population, 35% had habitual snoring (46% of men, 25% of women), and PSG found an AHI greater than or equal to 10 in 19% of men and 14.9% of women.[11] However, a study from the United States found 7.2% of men and 2.2% of women had an AHI greater than or equal to 10, and 3.9% of men and 1.2% of women had an AHI greater than or equal to 10 plus daytime symptoms.[12]

In summary, mild OSA (AHI >five events/hour) likely affects 1 in 5 adults, with moderate to severe OSA affecting at least 1 in 15 adults.[13–15] These approximations may be underestimated because most of the noted studies evaluated only those with symptoms, and many groups, including those with diabetes, heart failure, Parkinson disease (PD), and others, less frequently present with typical snoring and daytime sleepiness. Male sex appears to be a risk factor for OSA; whereas women, who have fewer typical symptoms, likely are underrepresented in prevalence estimates.[16] Risk factors associated with OSA are summarized in the Table 70.1.

Central Sleep Apnea

A diagnosis of central sleep apnea (CSA) requires at least five central apneas or hypopneas per hour of sleep observed on PSG in the context of symptoms. However, as in the case of OSA, definitions may vary among epidemiologic studies. The Sleep Heart Health Study demonstrated the prevalence of CSA on PSG as 0.9% and that males are more at risk. Heart failure increased CSA prevalence to 4.8%. Compared to those with OSA, patients with CSA are older, less likely to report excessive daytime sleepiness, and have a lower BMI.[17,18] Prevalence of SDB (CSA + OSA; AHI ≥5) in symptomatic heart failure patients was 76% (40% CSA, 36% OSA), with moderate to severe CSA (AHI ≥15) in 21% to 40%.[19] Other medical conditions increase the likelihood of CSA, including atrial fibrillation, stroke, cervical spinal cord injury, and kidney failure.[20–24] CSA occurs in people with Chiari I and II malformation[25] and patients on opioids. Healthy persons commonly develop CSA due to high altitude. CSA in the form of Cheyne-Stokes respirations primarily presents in male individuals older than 60 years and is often associated with heart failure, atrial fibrillation, or stroke.[26,27] Men have been shown to be more at risk for hypocapnic central apnea than women. The differential effects of sex hormones on apneic threshold appears to feed the differences in predilection for CSA between men and women.[28,29]

Sleep-Related Hypoxemia and Hypoventilation

The ICSD-3 recognizes six disorders of hypoventilation, the most common of which are obesity hypoventilation syndrome, chronic hypoventilation due to medical disorders, and hypoventilation due to medication or substance.[27,30,31,32] Because hypoventilation may be the consequence of heterogeneous underlying conditions, the prevalence of hypoventilation cannot be defined uniformly, but rather, it is dictated by the characteristics and severity of the underlying disorder. For example, the prevalence of obesity hypoventilation is 10% among obese people with BMI of 30 to 40 kg/m^2 but 24% among obese people with BMI greater than 40 kg/m.[2,33,34] Other conditions that lead to hypoventilation disorders include neuromuscular disorders (e.g., amyotrophic lateral sclerosis, spinal cord injury, diaphragmatic paralysis, myasthenia gravis, myopathies); chest wall abnormalities, such as kyphoscoliosis, ankylosing spondylitis, and so forth; and severe pleuropulmonary diseases.[32] Primary hypoventilation disorders are rare.[27] Diagnosis of congenital central alveolar hypoventilation syndrome requires confirmation of presence of *PHOX2B* mutation. However, other primary disorders of hypoventilation do not have known genetic disorders and are diagnosed based on clinical features associated with these syndromes.[27]

Health and Economic Impact of Sleep-Disordered Breathing

Among adults, SDB results in increased health care use and increased economic burden. Veterans with OSA have higher odds of having heart failure, hypertension, lung disease, obesity, stroke, depression, diabetes, and other health problems.[35] Patients with OSA use 23% to 50% more health care resources in the 5 years before diagnosis compared to age-matched control subjects, and OSA patients are more at risk to develop heart disease, lung disease, and depression. These lead to decreased work performance and increased risk for work- and leisure-related injuries.[36] In 2000 the estimated cost of sleep apnea–related motor vehicle collisions was $15.9 billion and 1400 lives[37]; however, treatment may reduce these numbers. Treatment of sleep apnea results in significant cost savings compared with untreated sleep apnea. The effects of SDB on other health conditions, such as hypertension, cardiovascular disease, cognitive dysfunction, lung disease, obesity, neurologic disorders, and so forth, are explored in more extensive detail in other chapters in this book.

Pediatric Sleep-Disordered Breathing

Pediatric Obstructive Sleep Apnea and Primary Snoring

Most epidemiologic data for SDB in children report a prevalence of 4% to 11%, with prevalence of OSA ranging from 1.2% to 5.7%.[38–40] Many studies used questionnaires, but some used more objective evaluation with PSG in combination with questionnaires. A study using questionnaires followed by PSG in Chinese school-age children showed prevalence of symptomatic OSA (defined as AHI ≥5) was 5.7% in boys and 3.8% in girls; the prevalence of asymptomatic OSA (AHI ≥5) was 9.1% and 5.7% in boys and girls, respectively.[41] In the United States a study with healthy school-age children showed a prevalence of 1.2% for AHI greater than or equal to 5, 25% for AHI 1 to 5, and 15.5% for primary snoring.[39] A meta-analysis of pediatric SDB reported a prevalence of 4% to 11%. Primary snoring makes up the higher end of the former percentages, ranging from 2.5% in Turkey to 6.2% in Sweden for those who snore "always" (habitual snoring).[40,42–44] For those who snore "often," the prevalence is 3.2% in Iceland, 14.8% in Spain, and 34.5% in Italy.[40,45–47] OSA makes up the lower end of the spectrum, but prevalence depends on the criteria used for diagnosis. Overall, the prevalence of OSA based on PSG ranges from 1% in Hong Kong for AHI greater than 1% to 13% in Italy for an oxygen desaturation index of greater than or equal to 5 per hour.[40,47,48] Parent-reported apnea ranges from 0.2% to 18.6%.[40,47] Based on available studies, the prevalence of pediatric primary snoring appears to range from 1.5% to 27.6%, and the range for OSA is 1% to 5%.[49]

Pediatric Sleep-Disordered Breathing, Age, and Risk Factors

The prevalence of primary snoring in the pediatric population varies by age; specifically, 10% for children 2 to 8 years

Table 70.1 Risk Factors Associated with Sleep-Disordered Breathing

	Categories	Evidence	Reference
Age	Men >65 years of age	26.4% with RDI ≥15	Mehra et al. (2007)[267]
	Men and women 30 to 70 years of age	Each 10-year increase in age leads to 2.2× higher odds of having AHI ≥5	Duran et al. (2001)[11]
	Men and women	Prevalence increases until 60 years of age, then decreases	Bixler et al. (1998 and 2001)[12,18]
	Men and women	OR for increased AHI per 10-year age increase: 2.41 women, 1.15 in men; reduced effect of gender and BMI with increasing age	Tishler et al. (2003)[268]
Race/ethnicity	Hispanics	25.8% prevalence of OSA for AHI ≥5, 9.8% for AHI ≥15, 3.9% for AHI ≥30	Redline et al. (2014)[269]
	Hispanics	3.6× higher odds of frequent snoring	Ramos et al. (2011)[270]
	African Americans	Higher AHI (32.7) compared to Whites (22.4)	Pranathiageswaran et al. (2013)[271]
	African Americans <25 years of age	1.88× higher odds of SDB compared to Whites	Redline et al. (1997)[54]
	African Americans	Stronger association between OSA and cardiovascular disease	Geovanni et al. (2018)[273]
	African Americans	Increased likelihood of more severe OSA (RDI ≥30)	Ancoli-Israel et al. (1995)[274]
	South Asians	Obese South Asians have higher OSA prevalence (85%) compared to obese White Europeans (66%)	Leong at al. (2013)[274]
	Far-East Asian men	Risk of OSA related to craniofacial features in Asian men vs. obesity in White men	Li et al. (2000)[275]
	Chinese	BMI and waist circumference correlated with AHI more prominently in Chinese compared to other racial/ethnic groups	Chen et al. (2016)[276]
Obesity	All ages	Obesity is a clear risk factor for OSA	Peppard et al. (2013)[277]
	Population-based prospective cohort	10% increase in weight →6× higher risk of moderate to severe OSA	Peppard et al. (2000)[278]
	Adolescents	Obesity, male sex, and history of adenotonsillectomy increased likelihood of OSA	Spilsbury et al. (2015)[279]
	Adolescents	OSA prevalence (AHI >1.5) was 45% in moderately to severely obese adolescents	Hannon et al. (2012)[280]
	Pregnant women	OSA prevalence has increasing trend in pregnancy, likely due to increase in maternal obesity	Dominguez et al. (2018)[281]
Comorbidity	Asthma	27% of asthma patients had new-onset OSA at 4-year follow-up	Teodorescu et al. (2015)[282]
	COPD	OSA prevalence 65.9% in patients with moderate to severe COPD	Soler et al. (2015)[283]
	Diabetes	Strong association between OSA and type 2 diabetes	Reutrakul et al. (2017)[284]
	Stroke	AHI ≥ 10 in 62.5% of patients with TIA or stroke	Bassetti et al. (1999)[22]
	Stroke	OSA is an independent risk factor for stroke	Redline et al. (2010)[285]; Campos-Rodriguez et al. (2014)[286]
	Alcohol/benzodiazepine/opioid use	More severe OSA	Issa et al. (1982)[287]; Rosen et al. (2019)[31]

AHI, apnea hypopnea index; BMI, body mass index; COPD, chronic obstructive pulmonary disease; OR, odds ratio; OSA, obstructive sleep apnea; RDI, respiratory disturbance index; SDB, sleep-disordered breathing; TIA, transient ischemic attack.

of age, followed by a decreasing prevalence starting age 9 years.[50] Adenotonsillar hypertrophy is the primary, but not only, contributing factor in younger children. Additional airway anatomic differences, craniofacial features, genetic, and/or neuromuscular factors affecting airway collapsibility, gastroesophageal reflux, infection, and inflammation (chronic rhinitis), and so forth, also contribute.

Obesity has increased in children over the past 30 years and has contributed to a bimodal age distribution of OSA in the pediatric population. Pediatric patients 12 years and older have a 3.5-fold increase in AHI relative to increase in BMI Z-score.[51] The Childhood Adenotonsillectomy Study found that children younger than 9 years with OSA had better resolution of symptoms if they were not overweight or obese regardless of treatment group (adenotonsillectomy or watchful waiting).[52] Follow-up analysis showed less central adiposity, lower AHI, better oxygen saturation, smaller neck circumference, and non-Black race were predictors of spontaneous resolution of OSA.[53] In younger children the strongest risk factors for OSA included living in a disadvantaged neighborhood, African American race, and history of prematurity, whereas during adolescence the risk factors were obesity, male sex, and prior adenotonsillectomy. Further, increased severity of SDB was associated with African American ethnicity, prematurity, and low socioeconomic status.[54–57]

Other risk factors for pediatric OSA include adenotonsillar hypertrophy and neurologic and medical conditions affecting the upper airway anatomy and its neural control, including cerebral palsy, genetic syndromes (e.g., Down syndrome, Prader-Willi, achondroplasia), craniofacial abnormalities (e.g., retrognathia, micrognathia, high arched palate, midface hypoplasia), low birth weight, and history of prematurity, cerebral palsy, muscular dystrophy, and other neuromuscular disorders. Additional contributions to SDB risk include environmental smoke exposure,[58] asthma, allergic rhinitis, and hypothyroidism.

Health and Economic Burden of Pediatric Sleep-Disordered Breathing

Pediatric SDB results in physical health problems. Historically, when SDB was underrecognized, toddlers failed to thrive, developed hypertension, and presented with cor pulmonale. With earlier recognition of pediatric SDB, these outcomes are rarely seen now, but mounting evidence exists for cardiac, inflammatory, and endocrine effects of SDB. The prevalence of such complications is not yet known, but cardiovascular complications include right and left ventricular changes, blood pressure changes, changes in brain natriuretic peptide, changes in cerebral blood flow, and autonomic dysregulation.[49] Although changes in C-reactive protein and insulin levels may be associated with pediatric SDB,[49] more longitudinal studies are needed to further characterize and delineate the prevalence and long-term consequences of these metabolic, cardiovascular, and inflammatory complications of SDB in children. SDB has been linked with poorer academic performance,[59] and an increased lifetime risk for behavioral impairment was observed in children.[60] A dose-dependent association between higher AHI and impaired cognitive performance has been reported in snoring and nonsnoring children[61]; however, general behavioral and cognitive performance may be predicted by snoring severity rather than AHI.[62] Most studies suggest treatment of SDB improves neurocognitive performance,[49] secondary behavioral scores, and quality of life, whereas neurocognitive problems may "catch-up" to control subjects after 1 year.[63] However, treatment of SDB may not result in improvement in executive function and attention scores on neuropsychological testing.[52]

Children with SDB use health care resources 215% more than healthy matched control subjects.[64] Other studies have documented the increased cost in pediatric patients with sleep problems or specific cohorts with other medical problems, such as sickle cell disease, but increased cost has not been delineated for SDB.[65,66] More research is needed, but it stands to reason that children with decreased neurocognitive capabilities and increased medical problems will use more health care and social resources and may not achieve their full potential, a cost that cannot be measured.

Other Sleep-Disordered Breathing in Pediatrics

Other SDB in children includes apnea of infancy, congenital central hypoventilation syndrome, central apnea related to obesity, SDB related to neuromuscular disease, and CSA related to Chiari malformation (both I and II). Regarding prevalence, 81% of children with spina bifida and Chiari II malformation were found to have SDB (moderate to severe in 31%) in a retrospective study at a multidisciplinary spina bifida clinic in patients with sleep complaints.[67] A prospective study of neonates with spina bifida (s/p fetal repair or postnatal repair) and Chiari II demonstrated that SDB in this population is ubiquitous, AHI is higher (34% vs. 19% in control subjects),[68] and this raises awareness that early evaluation for SDB should be considered. The estimated prevalence in pediatric patients with Chiari I is 24% to 70%.[25,69]

HYPERSOMNIA

Excessive daytime sleepiness occurring at least 3 days per week has a reported prevalence between 4% and 21%.[70] Central disorders of hypersomnolence are less common than secondary causes of daytime sleepiness but are more likely to be evaluated and managed within a comprehensive sleep center.

Narcolepsy

The prevalence of narcolepsy has been reported from 0.025% to 0.05%, with two ethnic outliers: (1) People from Japan have the reported the highest prevalence at 0.16%, and (2) strikingly low prevalence was reported in people from Israel (0.0002%).[71] A study combining databases in six European nations and comparing the incidence of narcolepsy with or without cataplexy before, during, and after the H1N1 influenza pandemic reported pooled incidence of about 1 per 100,000 person-years.[72] These results suggested a higher incidence than the 0.6 per 100,000 reported by a study in the US-based study on multistage screening of patients.[73] Similar findings were reported in a study from Minnesota: an incidence of 1.37 per 100,000 person-years for narcolepsy with or without cataplexy and 0.74 per 100,000 person-years for narcolepsy with cataplexy.[74] A review of a US health care claims database in 2019, using the ICSD-3 definitions of narcolepsy type 1 and type 2, found greater prevalence and incidence of narcolepsy than most previous studies: Narcolepsy prevalence overall was 79.4 per100,000 (0.079%), without cataplexy was 65.4 per 100,000 (0.065%), and with cataplexy it was 14.0 per100,000 (0.014%).[75] Although prevalence was highest among the 21- to 30-year age group, incidence was greatest in individuals in their early 20s and late teens. Both prevalent and incident cases were 50% greater for females compared to males across most age groups. North Central United States had the highest prevalence and incidence, whereas the West was the lowest.[75]

After the 2009 H1N1 influenza pandemic in China and the introduction of the ASO3 adjuvant H1N1 vaccine (Pandemrix) in Europe, narcolepsy with cataplexy appeared to have an escalating incidence in certain European countries, especially Sweden, Finland, and in parts of China in which H1N1 influenza was epidemic.[76–78] In Sweden the incidence of narcolepsy with cataplexy in those who received the Pandemrix vaccine was increased threefold in those younger than 20 years, twofold in those 21 to 30 years, and unchanged in those older than 40 years.[79] A systematic review and meta-analysis showed that the Pandemrix-attributable risk of narcolepsy in children and adolescents was small, at 1 per 18,400 vaccine doses, and that benefits of immunization outweigh the risk of vaccination-associated narcolepsy, which remains a rare disease.[80]

Studies show conflicting results regarding whether narcolepsy preferentially affects men or women. There are clear increases in the incidence of narcolepsy in people 10 to 30 years of age compared with other age groups. Age of onset for narcolepsy shown in a study of two large populations of patients in France and Quebec indicated a bimodal presentation, with the first peak occurring around 15 years and a second peak occurring at 35 years of age.[81] The known genetic association with human leukocyte antigen (HLA) DQB1*0602, as well as an increased relative risk in first-degree relatives, suggests an autoimmune mechanism underlying the disorder.[82]

A study reviewing cases of narcolepsy (type 1 and 2 combined) found that African Americans with narcolepsy had a higher mean BMI, an earlier symptom onset, a higher Epworth Sleepiness Scale score, and were more frequently hypocretin deficient compared to other groups. Furthermore, African Americans with low central nervous system hypocretin-1 were 4.5 times more likely to present without cataplexy (28.3%) compared with Whites (8.1%).[83]

The burden of narcolepsy is significant in terms of morbidity, health care costs, and societal costs. A higher rate of motor vehicle crashes is reported in narcolepsy, and drowsy driving is a known risk factor for increased collisions. Furthermore, narcoleptic patients have two to three times the health care use and costs compared with age-matched control subjects, higher rates of short-term disability, and more missed work days, suggesting implications for long-term productivity.[84] A recent population-based study indicated that narcolepsy has negative impact on mental health, health-related quality of life, and leads to economic burdens.[85] Comorbidities associated with narcolepsy include mental illness (31.1%), followed by diseases of the digestive system (21.4%) and diseases of the nervous system/sense organs (excluding narcolepsy; 20.7%).[86] Children and adolescents with narcolepsy type 1 are more likely to have internalizing behaviors and attention-deficit/hyperactivity disorder (ADHD)-like symptoms.[87] Narcolepsy is associated with increased morbidity from endocrine and other sleep-related, neurologic, musculoskeletal, ophthalmic, and respiratory disorders.[88] A mortality rate increase of 1.5 was reported in narcoleptic patients across age groups.[89]

Idiopathic Hypersomnia

The prevalence of idiopathic hypersomnia is not known, although it is estimated to be less than that of narcolepsy based on referrals to sleep centers.[27,70] A recent review estimates the prevalence of idiopathic hypersomnia between 0.02% and 0.010%, with mean age of onset of 21.8 years, and it is associated with several somatic symptoms.[90] Further research is needed in this area to determine true prevalence.

Kleine-Levin Syndrome

Prevalence of Kleine-Levin syndrome, a rare recurrent encephalopathy presenting with hypersomnia and cognitive, psychiatric, and behavioral disturbances, is unknown. Most commonly it presents in the second decade, although there are outliers, and it is far more common in males.[91,92] Prevalence is estimated at 1 to 2 per million based on retrospective studies. In addition, there may be increased risk within families with an affected member.[27,91]

Other Hypersomnia

Hypersomnia due to a medication or substance and its prevalence depend on the substance used and whether the patient is intoxicated or withdrawing. Hypersomnia from stimulant withdrawal occurs most frequently in teens and young adults.[27] Similarly, hypersomnia associated with a psychiatric disorder also depends on the disorder itself and medications used. It is known to occur in more than 50% of people with seasonal affective disorder.[27] More studies are warranted to investigate the epidemiology of various disorders of hypersomnia. Symptoms often present in the second and third decades, therefore frequently making hypersomnia a lifelong disease. Health-related quality of life and adaptive behaviors are often diminished in hypersomnia patients. Family members may suffer stress-related effects of a household member's hypersomnia disorder.

CIRCADIAN RHYTHM SLEEP-WAKE DISORDERS

CRSWDs encompass several disorders as defined by the ICSD-3, including delayed sleep-wake phase disorder (DSWPD), advanced sleep-wake phase disorder (ASWPD), irregular sleep-wake rhythm disorder, non-24-hour sleep-wake rhythm disorder, shift-work disorder, and jet lag. Epidemiologic data are divided according to each disorder; however, true prevalence is not known for most disorders or for CRSWD as a whole.

Delayed Sleep-Wake Phase Disorder

DSWPD prevalence varies depending on the population studied. Overall prevalence is estimated between 0.1% and 10%.[93–95] In sleep clinics, 5% to 10% of patients with insomnia complaints evaluated have DSWPD. It is the most commonly diagnosed circadian rhythm disorder, frequently presenting in adolescence and young adulthood.[96] In adolescents prevalence ranges from 7% to 16%.[27] Prevalence of DSWPD is less than 1% in adults 40 to 64 years of age.[94] Males and females appear equally affected. No studies have examined racial and ethnic differences. DSWPD has a familial pattern in up to 40% of patients, and there is some evidence that it is associated with human *hPer3,* arylalkylamine *N*-acetyltransferase, HLA, and *CLOCK* gene polymorphisms, although it has not been validated in all studies.[27,97] Mutation of the human circadian clock gene *CRY1* can lead to familial delayed sleep phase disorder.[98] DSWPD is associated with hypersomnolence, especially in the morning hours, and it primarily affects teens and young adults. DSWPD can negatively affect academic performance and can lead to higher rates of smoking, alcohol and substance use, anxiety, and depression.[99,100] Hypersomnolence in teens with DSWPD is often worsened by early school start times, thus exacerbating the consequences for affected teens.[100]

Advanced Sleep-Wake Phase Disorder

ASWPD is rare, with an estimated prevalence of less than 1% of the population, although this may be an underestimation because patients may not be sufficiently distressed to seek help.

Older age and neurodevelopmental disorders predispose people to ASWPD.[27] In general, no sex predilection is reported, although one study found a higher prevalence in men.[101] At least two studies indicate a preference for later sleep-onset times in men compared to women, which could cause greater distress in women who experience advanced sleep phase.[102,103] A North American sleep center reported ASWPD prevalence at 0.04%, with a familial history for most cases of young-onset advanced sleep phase.[104]

Irregular Sleep-Wake Rhythm Disorder

Irregular sleep-wake rhythm disorder is infrequent in the general population, and there are fairly limited data regarding its epidemiology.[105,106] It is more common in the elderly, especially with neurodegenerative disorders (e.g., Alzheimer disease, PD, Huntington disease[27]), children with neurodevelopmental disabilities, individuals with traumatic brain injury,[107] and in patients with psychiatric disorders, such as schizophrenia or bipolar disorder.[108,109] There are no clear sex or ethnic differences in prevalence.

Non-24-Hour Sleep-Wake Rhythm Disorder

Non-24-hour sleep-wake rhythm disorder can affect both blind and sighted persons. It is found in up to 63% of completely blind individuals[110] and 5% to 15% of people with other types of blindness.[27,110,111] In blind individuals symptom onset can occur at any age, and there is no sex difference. In sighted individuals this disorder is rare and associated with psychiatric disorders, traumatic brain injury, and male sex.[27,110,112] In a case series of sighted 57 patients with non-24-hour sleep-wake rhythm disorder, 72% were male, 63% had sleep symptom onset in adolescence, psychiatric symptoms preceded the onset of sleep disorder in 28%, and 34% developed major depression after the onset.[112]

Shift-Work Disorder

Shift workers comprise approximately 20% of the workforce in industrialized countries.[113] The prevalence of shift-work sleep disorder is estimated between 1% and 4% in the general population and 10% to 33% in shift workers.[27,114,115] Shift-work disorder results in accidents, including, but not limited to, those related to impaired driving, decreased alertness, decreased quality of life, and increased morbidity and mortality.[116,117] Traffic accidents are of particular concern for night- and early-morning shift workers as they commute during times of extreme sleepiness.[118] Medical interns on night shift have higher risk of accidental needlestick injuries compared with day-shift interns.[119] Rotating shift workers have twice as many work-related accidents compared with day shift workers.[120] In the medical system, increased diagnostic errors, prescription errors, and patient mortality are associated with shift work.[121] In addition to work-related risks, personal adverse health outcomes associated with shift work include development of insulin resistance syndrome and diabetes,[122] gastrointestinal symptoms and peptic ulcer disease,[123] myocardial infarction, ischemic stroke,[124] obesity,[125] breast cancer,[126] and depression and anxiety.[127]

Jet Lag Disorder

The prevalence of jet lag is unknown, although travel via aircraft across multiple time zones is increasingly common. Severity of jet lag symptoms depends on the direction of travel (east is worse) and the number of time zones crossed by the traveler. The relationship between age and propensity for jet lag is unclear as some studies indicate increased predisposition to jet lag with increasing age, but other clinical studies show decreased predisposition.[128,129] The impact of age and sex on the likelihood of developing jet lag has not been clearly defined, although older adults may be less likely to experience symptoms.[130,131]

INSOMNIA

The ICSD-3 has reclassified insomnia, abandoning previous insomnia categories of primary and secondary insomnia for new classifications: (1) chronic insomnia disorder, (2) short-term insomnia disorder, and (3) other insomnia disorder.[27] The criteria for diagnosis of insomnia disorders include a difficulty initiating or maintaining sleep or undesired early awakening despite adequate opportunity for sleep that results in daytime, functional, or social impairment or distress.[27] Many studies on insomnia prevalence were performed before this change in diagnostic criteria, so prevalence estimates of insomnia vary based on the diagnostic criteria used, as evident by the change in prevalence 3.9% to 22.1% when insomnia diagnoses were made based on the *International Classification of Diseases,* 10th revision (ICD-10) criteria versus the *Diagnostic and Statistical Manual of Mental Disorders,* fourth edition (DSM-IV) criteria.[132]

The prevalence range also varies depending on whether patients are evaluated for dissatisfaction with their sleep, any symptoms of insomnia, or actually qualifying for an insomnia diagnosis. For example, in two separate Canadian cohorts evaluated by telephone survey, 19.8% to 25.3% reported sleep dissatisfaction, 29.9% to 40.2% reported at least one insomnia symptom, and 9.5% to 13.4% met criteria for insomnia based on a combination of DSM-IV and ICD-10 diagnostic criteria.[133,134] Another study reported at least one sleep problem more than three times weekly in 29% of subjects, but a prevalence of 19% for those with daytime consequences of the sleep complaint.[135] A study using PSG and a questionnaire showed a prevalence of sleep difficulty in 22.4% and chronic insomnia (symptoms longer than 1 year) in 7.5%.[136] The prevalence range of insomnia diagnosis is likely 4% to 22%, with symptoms of insomnia affecting 20% to 45% of adults.[132,137–139] In individuals without insomnia at baseline, the incidence of chronic insomnia was 9.3% (12.9% in women and 6.2% in men) at 7.5 years.[140] When restricting the diagnosis of insomnia to short-term insomnia, prevalence was reported as 9.5% in the United States and 7.9% in the United Kingdom. The annual incidence of acute insomnia was 31.2% and 36.6%.[141]

Insomnia is more prevalent in women than men.[136,137] A meta-analysis found a risk ratio of 1.4 for men versus women. The higher prevalence among female adults is present at all age groups and increases with age, with a 1.28 higher risk in women ages 15 to 30 years and a 1.73 risk ratio among those older than 65 years.[142] Aging is often identified as a risk factor for insomnia,[143] but some studies show higher rates of incident and persistent insomnia in middle age or in younger age groups.[137,144–146] Insomnia in older adults may be associated with more nocturnal awakenings and early-morning awakening than in younger adults.[147] The association of age with insomnia varies based on the population studied and may depend on the presence of associated health conditions, which could increase with aging, and the increased use of technology among younger age groups.[146] Race, ethnicity, education, marital status, and socioeconomic status may also influence the prevalence of insomnia.[137,147] In addition, the prevalence of insomnia may be underestimated in certain populations because many do not seek help from a physician.[133,148]

Psychological and psychiatric disorders are often associated with insomnia, with up to 40% of insomnia complaint cases presenting with comorbid mental disorders (e.g., depression and anxiety). Additional breakdown of etiology of insomnia cases includes 15% restless legs syndrome (RLS)/periodic limb movement disorder (PLMD), 10% poor sleep hygiene/environmental factors, 5% to 9% SDB, 4% to 11 % medical/neurologic conditions, 3% to 7% psychoactive substance effect, and 12% to 16% with no identifiable cause.[149] Multiple etiologies may coexist in up to 30% of individuals with insomnia.[150] Of importance, insomnia may increase the risk of certain health conditions, for example, chronic insomnia with objective short sleep time may be a cardiovascular disease risk factor.[151]

Over time, an increase has been observed in both the prevalence of insomnia diagnoses (3.1% in 1993 to 5.8% in 2007)[152] and insomnia symptoms (from 16.8% to 23.8% from 2007 to 2015).[153] Use of prescription medications for insomnia has also increased, from 2% in 1999 to 2000, then to 3.5% in 2009 to 2010.[154] One key point is that insomnia results in a societal cost secondary to all the associated medical and psychological consequences of sleep deprivation.

Pediatric Insomnia

Similar to adults, insomnia prevalence rates among adolescents vary based on study design and definitions of insomnia. The ICSD-3 defines insomnia in children under the diagnostic category of Chronic Insomnia Disorder, similar to adults.[27] Previous versions of the ICSD describe several subcategories of pediatric insomnia, and they remain useful considerations in clinical practice[155]: behavioral insomnia of childhood, sleep-onset association, and limit-setting subtypes. Prevalence of pediatric insomnia varies depending on the definition of symptoms and/or categories. If only insomnia symptoms are reported, prevalence ranges approximately from 25% to 35%, whereas the prevalence rates are lower when defined by insomnia diagnostic criteria (DSM-IV or ICSD-2), ranging from 4% to 14%.[156–160]

Insomnia has been reported in up to 41% of those ages 2 to 14 years, with most reports identifying pediatric insomnia prevalence at 10% to 20%. An evaluation of 5- to 12-year-olds found a prevalence of insomnia symptoms in 19.3%, with the highest prevalence among preteen girls.[161] Similar prevalence was found in Australia: 19.8% had mild sleep problems, and 13.8% had moderate to severe sleep problems.[162] Polling of parents revealed sleep problems reported among 6.3% of infants, 10.5% of toddlers, 10.2% of preschoolers, and 10.8% of school-age children. Those with reported sleep problems were more likely to have a later bedtime and to have a parent present at sleep onset.[163] There is considerable impact of parental perception of sleep problems based on cultural and ethnic differences.[164,165]

When restricting the pediatric population to adolescents, the prevalence of insomnia was 23.8% based on DSM-IV criteria, 18.5% based on DSM-5 criteria, and 13.6% based on the quantitative criteria for insomnia, which requires a 6-month duration of symptoms.[166] The presence of insomnia among adolescents can have significant influence on safety, cognition, and mood and may predict future sleep habits.[161,167,168] Studies consistently show a higher prevalence of insomnia among adolescent girls than boys but only after onset of menses.[156,166,167]

During infancy the prevalence of sleep problems is approximately 10%, and most concerns are related to nocturnal awakenings and short sleep duration.[169] Sleep difficulty at this age appears to predict sleep problems during the early childhood years. Infants who do not self-soothe are more likely to have difficulty with sleep onset at age 2 years. Other studies also show that sleep problems at 6 to 12 months of age predict sleep trouble at 3 to 4 years of age.[169–171] These changes may not persist beyond 6 years of age.[172] Insomnia in infants and preschool children is associated with significant parental stress, especially impacting the mother. It has been shown that behavioral infant sleep intervention results in decreased maternal report of depression symptoms.[173]

Difficulties initiating and maintaining sleep and reduced sleep duration are extremely common in children with neurodevelopmental disabilities.[174] Underlying causes in that population are likely multifactorial (e.g., genetic underlying causes influencing initiation and maintenance of sleep, gastroesophageal reflux, spasticity, epilepsy, SDB, altered circadian rhythm, etc.).[175] Similar to the adult population, anxiety and posttraumatic stress disorder in children is often associated with insomnia.[176]

RESTLESS LEGS SYNDROME AND PERIODIC LIMB MOVEMENT DISORDER

Estimates of RLS prevalence in the medical literature vary depending on the methodology or criteria used.[177] In a study in Western Europe, prevalence of RLS symptoms using a screening questionnaire was 7.6%, whereas prevalence decreased to 3.5% when patients underwent physician interview for diagnosis.[178] Similarly, in the United States, prevalence based on the four diagnostic criteria of RLS by questionnaire screening was 7.3%.[179] Using International Restless Legs Syndrome Study Group criteria, prevalence rates are reported between 5% and 15%.[177,180–183] The prevalence of distressing symptoms occurring at least twice weekly is lower, approximately 1% to 10%.[177–179,184]

Regardless of which criteria are used to establish prevalence, RLS is common, likely underdiagnosed, and higher with increasing age. Primary RLS tends to have younger onset of symptoms, whereas secondary RLS usually develops at an older age. Family history can be found in up to 60% of patients, especially with primary RLS. A family study of French-Canadian subjects suggested RLS aggregates in families with variable phenotypic expression.[185] Studies have found possible association of RLS with several genetic variants.[186–189]

Many predisposing conditions have been identified as causes of secondary RLS. Iron deficiency with or without anemia is strongly associated with RLS, especially in absence of family history.[190–192] Likely due to iron deficiency, dialysis patients have a higher likelihood (up to 73%) of RLS, and increased mortality has been reported in these patients.[193–195] Kidney transplant substantially improves symptoms of RLS in dialysis patients. Spinal cord lesions may also trigger RLS/PLMD. Prevalence of RLS between 12% and 57% was reported in a meta-analysis of individuals with multiple sclerosis compared to 2.5% to 18% in general population.[196] Neuropathy can increase prevalence of RLS.[197] Certain medications, such as antihistamines, antidepressants, antipsychotic medications, and many antinausea medications, may precipitate or exacerbate RLS because of their antidopaminergic effect in central nervous system.[198,199] A meta-analysis reviewed possible associations between RLS and movement disorders, including PD, other parkinsonian syndromes, essential tremor, dystonic syndromes, Tourette syndrome, and hereditary ataxias. Possible genetic links have been reported between RLS and PD and between RLS and Tourette syndrome; however, small sample size may affect the strength of association.[200] RLS is consistently reported to be approximately twice as high in women as in men.[177,183] Pregnant women are more likely to be affected by RLS than the general population. Prevalence of RLS increases as the pregnancy progresses, reaching 22% by the third trimester, improving to 4% after delivery.[201] Regarding ethnicity, the prevalence of RLS has been reported to be lower in Asian populations and rare in African populations, although some studies in Asian populations show comparable prevalence rates.[177,202–204]

Adverse health effects associated with RLS include insomnia, daytime sleepiness, increased health care costs, and increased indirect cost related to lost productivity. RLS has been associated in some studies with hypertension,[205] cardiovascular disease,[206,207] gastrointestinal disease, mood disorders,[184,208] stroke,[209,210] chronic kidney disease, and increased mortality in men.[207,211]

PLMD is thought to be uncommon in the general population, but the exact prevalence is not known. In contrast, periodic limb movement of sleep (PLMS) is a common finding on PSG. Prevalence increases with age, affecting up to 57% of older adults even in absence of neurologic comorbid diseases.[212] RLS has a clear relationship with PLMS, disorders present in 85% to 95% of patients with RLS.[213]

Pediatric Restless Legs Syndrome/Periodic Limb Movement Disorder

RLS prevalence in school-age children is estimated to be 2% to 4%.[214] RLS can also be present in young children and infants, although prevalence in these age groups is not known.[215] Prevalence of RLS in adolescents ranges from 1% to 2.8%.[216] Family history of RLS is reported in greater than 70% of affected children.[217] As with adults, iron deficiency is frequently a cause of secondary RLS in the pediatric population.[214,215] History of prematurity is associated with higher prevalence of RLS and elevated periodic limb movement index on PSG, and iron deficiency is a likely contributing factor. Further studies are needed to investigate whether prematurity is an independent risk factor for RLS/PLMD.[218] There is no sex difference in younger children with RLS/PLMD, but female predominance similar to adults is observed after adolescence.[214–216,219] "Growing pains" are more common with RLS compared to control subjects (80.6% vs. 63.2%), whereas sleep disturbance with RLS versus control subjects was 69.4% versus 39.6.[217] Other studies report an association with ADHD, anxiety, depression, insomnia, and daytime sleepiness.[215,219,220] A negative effect on mood was endorsed in 49.5% of children with RLS.[217]

PARASOMNIAS

Epidemiologic studies of parasomnias must be acknowledged, in large part, as rough estimates because most studies are population based, involve varying methodologies, and may involve recall bias because many of the non–rapid eye movement (NREM) parasomnias are more prevalent in childhood. Furthermore, parasomnias may be underestimated in cases in which there is no bed partner or self-report is required. Overall prevalence of parasomnias has been reported as high as 88% in preschoolers and 73% in children ages 3 to 13 years, with lifetime prevalence ranging from 4% to 67% in adults.[221,222]

NREM Parasomnias

NREM parasomnias include confusional arousals, somnambulism (sleepwalking), sleep terrors, and sleep-related eating disorder.[27] Confusional arousals, somnambulism, and sleep terrors tend to initially present in childhood and adolescence; however, somnambulism and confusional arousals may present at any age. All three disorders may persist throughout life with decreasing incidence.[223] NREM parasomnia, irrespective of the type, is associated with HLA DQB1*05:01 genotype.[224] There are no sex differences in prevalence observed in confusional arousals, sleep terrors, or sleepwalking.[223] These arousal disorders can be triggered by other sleep disorders (e.g., OSA, RLS) or environmental stimuli, whereas sleep deprivation and stress are known primers for the occurrence of arousal parasomnias.[27]

Confusional Arousals

There are few epidemiologic studies of confusional arousals. A study involving subjects older than 15 years found a prevalence of 2.9%, with 1.9% of subjects having confusional arousals at least once a month.[225] A telephone study of adults in Norway found a lifetime prevalence of 18.5%, current prevalence (at least once in the last 3 months) of 6.9%, and current prevalence (occurring at least once a week) of 1.8%.[222] No sex difference has been reported. Confusional arousals have been reported more by night and shift workers.[225,226] In pediatric patients, confusional arousals are sometimes misreported as somniloquy by the parents, with prevalence data not well documented.

Sleep Terrors

The prevalence of sleep terrors varies by age, ranging from 2.2% to 2.7% in adults, with a lifetime prevalence of 10% and a much higher prevalence in pediatric populations.[27,222,223] The childhood prevalence of sleep terrors ranges from 1% to 14.7% in 3 to 13 years of age and older to 36.9% in 18-month-olds.[27,227] In a recent study, a similar finding of sleep terror peak prevalence (34%) was shown at 18 months of age, then declining, although it can persist in 40% of children past 5 years of age. One-third of children with night terrors in early childhood had sleepwalking in later childhood. Parental history of sleepwalking was associated with higher rate (32% with parental history present vs. 17% without parental history) of persistent sleep terrors (i.e., beyond 5 years of age) in children,[228] supporting the idea of a common pathophysiology of these parasomnias. Night terrors occur in less than 1% of subjects older than 65 years.[27]

Sleepwalking

Lifetime prevalence based on a telephone survey was 22.4%, current if in the last 3 months was 1.7%, and current if at least once a week was 0.6%.[222] In a European population, reported prevalence of somnambulism (occurs frequently and perceived as problematic by the patient) was 2%.[223] Prevalence of 2.5% was reported in the United States in the late 1970s.[229] Lifetime prevalence of nocturnal wandering was reported as almost 30%.[230] Compiling larger studies of somnambulism reveals a lifetime prevalence of 25% to 30% of sleepwalking or nocturnal wandering and a current prevalence of 0.6% to 3.9%, depending on the definition of "current." Increased prevalence (8.5%) was reported in psychiatric conditions.[231] In pediatrics prevalence rates are higher, at 3.5% to 22.5%.[221,231,235] Sleepwalking is a highly heritable disorder, and one genetic locus associated with sleepwalking was described on chromosome 20.[233] The prevalence of sleepwalking in children was 22.5% if there was no parental history of sleepwalking, 47.4% if one parent had history of sleepwalking, and 61.5% if both parents had history of sleepwalking.[228] Similar factors that can precipitate and prime for confusional arousals can do the same for somnambulism. SDB or RLS/PLMD may trigger sleepwalking, as suggested by improvement or resolution of parasomnias after treatment of those conditions.[234] In addition, "Z-drugs" (nonbenzodiazepine hypnotics) may also precipitate events.[27,235]

Sleep-Related Eating Disorder

Although few epidemiologic studies are available, one telephone survey reported a lifetime prevalence of 4.5%, current prevalence if in the last 3 months was 2.2%, and current prevalence if at least once per week was 0.4%.[222] In a self-reported questionnaire, prevalence in college students was 4.6%, 8.7% in outpatients with an eating disorder, 9.9% in those with psychiatric conditions,[231] and 16.7% in inpatients with an eating disorder.[236] It generally presents in the third decade, tends to be more common in women, and can be associated with sedative-hypnotic use.[27]

REM Parasomnias

REM Sleep Behavior Disorder

REM sleep behavior disorder (RBD) prevalence in the general population is estimated to be 0.38% to 2.1%.[237,238] The prevalence of subclinical RBD (loss of normal REM atonia without history of dream enactment behavior) was reported as 4.95%. A male predominance of RBD has been observed, but this could be due to underreporting in females. RBD is more common in older individuals, typically with an onset older than 50 years.[239–241] A recent study suggests a prevalence of 1.06% in a middle-to-older age population-based sample but with no difference between men and women.[238] Recognition of RBD is important because it can be associated with injury to the patient or bed partner.[239,240] Patients with RBD tend to have increased muscle twitches and periodic limb movements as well.[239]

There is a significant association between RBD and neurodegenerative diseases, such as PD, dementia with Lewy bodies, multiple systems atrophy, and mild cognitive impairment.[240,242–245] Up to 81% to 90% of those with RBD ultimately develop neurodegenerative disease, with risk increasing over time: 33.1% at 5 years, 75.7% at 10 years, and 90.9% at 14 years.[244,246] These strong associations call into question whether idiopathic RBD truly exists. In addition, in those who have a synucleinopathy (e.g., PD, dementia with Lewy bodies, multiple system atrophy), there is an increased prevalence of RBD compared with the general population and those with other neurodegenerative diseases, such as tauopathies (e.g., Alzheimer disease, progressive supranuclear palsy, corticobasal degeneration).[243] A recent meta-analysis of the prevalence of RBD in PD estimated prevalence at 23.6% in PD compared to 3.4% of control subjects[247]; however, only one of the studies in the meta-analysis included diagnosis by PSG.

In multiple-system atrophy, the prevalence of RBD is particularly high, affecting 88% to 100% of patients.[248,249] In younger patients with onset of RBD symptoms before age 50 years, RBD can be associated with narcolepsy, and about one-third of patients with narcolepsy with cataplexy have RBD.[250–252] There may be a genetic predisposition to RBD, as increased odds of having dream enactment behavior were found in family members of patients with confirmed idiopathic RBD.[253] In addition to chronic RBD, there can also be acute episodes that are related to medications, such as selective serotonin reuptake inhibitors, antipsychotic medications, alcohol withdrawal, or drug abuse.[27]

RBD has been described in the pediatric population as well, with one study reporting RBD in 32.3% of narcoleptic patients younger than 19 years.[252] In addition, a chart review on 15 children found that RBD and REM without atonia in children can be associated with neurodevelopmental disabilities, narcolepsy, or medication use.[254]

Nightmare Disorder

Prevalence studies of nightmares are difficult to compare because some studies query "bad dreams" rather than establishing a diagnosis of nightmare disorder. Frequent nightmares that cause distress have been reported to affect 2% to 8% of the general population, although lifetime prevalence is higher.[27,222,255,256] A cross-sectional study of adults reported the lifetime prevalence of nightmares as 66.2% (72% in women and 61% in men), and the prevalence of nightmares in the preceding 3 months as 19.4%. In addition, 2.8% of subjects reported current nightmares occurring at least once per week.[222] Most epidemiologic studies of nightmares in adults show a higher prevalence among women than men, although this sex difference does not seem apparent in children and older adults.[222,256] Nightmare disorder is more common among patients with psychiatric diagnoses and those who have undergone traumatic events.[256,257] A study showed that 29.9% of subjects undergoing outpatient psychiatric treatment reported nightmares at least once per week that resulted in distress. Nightmares can also be associated with insomnia, with a prevalence of approximately 18%.[255,258] In young children a longitudinal study (with parental report at 29, 41, and 50 months of age and at 5 and 6 years of age) showed a 65% to 69% prevalence of nightmares "sometimes," whereas there was only a 1.3% to 3.9% prevalence of nightmares "often."[259] Other studies have reported prevalence up to 80.5% in children between the ages of 4 and 12 years.[260] Frequent nightmares in children can be associated with insomnia, hyperactivity, poor academic performance, and mood disturbances. At the opposite end of the age spectrum, nightmares seem to decrease in frequency and prevalence with aging.

Recurrent Isolated Sleep Paralysis

Recurrent isolated sleep paralysis (RISP) has been described by many names within many cultural contexts, making a true epidemiologic study difficult. Most studies have evaluated small, specific populations, reporting varying prevalence estimates of 4.7% to 41%.[261] Several studies have documented the association of RISP with anxiety and panic disorder, and the association of sleep paralysis with narcolepsy is also well documented.[27,261] An increase in the prevalence of RISP was reported in an African American population compared with reports of the population as a whole.[262] Experience of fear or distress and insomnia has been reported in individuals reporting RISP.[263] RISP usually presents in the second decade and is thought to affect men and women equally.[27]

Sleep-Related Hallucinations

A study using a telephone survey reported an overall prevalence of any type of sleep-related hallucination at 38.7%, but when divided into subgroups, prevalence was 18% for hypnagogic and 4.9% for hypnopompic hallucinations.[264] Hallucinations were more commonly reported in women and in the younger age groups. In a smaller study of medical students, sleep-related hallucinations occurred with greater frequency in those with insomnia.[147] There is, of course, well-documented higher prevalence of sleep-related hallucinations in narcolepsy.[27]

Sleep Enuresis

Sleep enuresis (nocturnal bedwetting) has not been extensively studied in adults, but data suggest a prevalence between 2% and 3%; however, it has been reported to be as high as 6% in the United Kingdom.[265] It occurs with much higher frequency in pediatric patients, with prevalence estimates of 15% to 25% in 5-year-olds and decreasing with age until adulthood.[221] Enuresis has a strong familial component and is associated with SDB in adults and children. In addition, allergic diseases, such as allergic rhinitis, atopic dermatitis, and allergic conjunctivitis, have been shown to increase the chance of sleep enuresis.[266] This disorder can result in significant psychosocial ramifications and expense.[27]

CLINICAL PEARLS

- The epidemiology of sleep medicine depends on the population studied and methodologies used.
- Sleep disorders have significant health, economic, and safety implications.
- Most people have at least one sleep disorder over their lifetime.

SUMMARY

The epidemiology of sleep medicine is a complex topic, and although many excellent studies have been published, more work is needed to define the true prevalence and incidence of each of the sleep disorders, as well as their health and societal implications. The epidemiologic outcomes differ depending on the population studied, the research methodologies used, and the diagnostic criteria used. As the definitions of sleep disorders evolve, we hope that study methodology will be standardized and the burdens of the diseases of sleep medicine will be better identified, allowing for targeted treatments. This chapter summarizes the available data on this broad topic.

SELECTED READINGS

Bertisch SM, Herzig SJ, Winkelman JW, Buettner C. National use of prescription medications for insomnia: NHANES 1999–2010. *Sleep.* 2014;37(2):343–349.

Bixler EO, Vgontzas AN, Lin HM, et al. Sleep disordered breathing in children in a general population sample: prevalence and risk factors. *Sleep.* 2009;32(6):731–736.

Bjorvatn B, Gronli J, Pallesen S. Prevalence of different parasomnias in the general population. *Sleep Med.* 2010;11(10):1031–1034.

Black J, Reaven NL, Funk SE, et al. The Burden of Narcolepsy Disease (BOND) study: health-care utilization and cost findings. *Sleep Med.* 2014;15(5):522–529.

Grandner MA. Sleep, health, and society. *Sleep Med Clin.* 2020;15(2): 319–340.

Iranzo A, Fernandez-Arcos A, Tolosa E, et al. Neurodegenerative disorder risk in idiopathic REM sleep behavior disorder: study in 174 patients. *PLoS One.* 2014;9(2):e89741.

Lumeng JC, Chervin RD. Epidemiology of pediatric obstructive sleep apnea. *Proc Am Thorac Soc.* 2008;5(2):242–252.

O'Connor GT, Lind BK, Lee ET, et al. Variation in symptoms of sleep-disordered breathing with race and ethnicity: the sleep heart health study. *Sleep.* 2003;26(1):74–79.

Ohayon MM, Guilleminault C, Chokroverty S. Sleep epidemiology 30 years later: where are we? *Sleep Med.* 2010;11(10):961–962.

Parthasarathy S, Vasquez MM, Halonen M, et al. Persistent insomnia is associated with mortality risk. *Am J Med.* 2015;128:268–275.

Petit D, Pennestri MH, Paquet J, et al. Childhood sleepwalking and sleep terrors: a longitudinal study of prevalence and familial aggregation. *JAMA Pediatr.* 2015;169:653–658.

Roth T, Coulouvrat C, Hajak G, et al. Prevalence and perceived health associated with insomnia based on DSM-IV-TR; international statistical classification of diseases and related health problems, tenth revision; and research diagnostic criteria/international classification of sleep disorders, second edition criteria: results from the America Insomnia survey. *Biol Psychiatry.* 2011;69(6):592–600.

Schenck CH, Boeve BF, Mahowald MW. Delayed emergence of a parkinsonian disorder or dementia in 81% of older men initially diagnosed with idiopathic rapid eye movement sleep behavior disorder: a 16-year update on a previously reported series. *Sleep Med.* 2013;14(8):744–748.

Wijnans L, Lecomte C, de Vries C, et al. The incidence of narcolepsy in Europe: before, during, and after the influenza A(H1N1)pdm09 pandemic and vaccination campaigns. *Vaccine.* 2013;31(8):1246–1254.

Young T, Peppard PE, Gottlieb DJ. Epidemiology of obstructive sleep apnea: a population health perspective. *Am J Respir Crit Care Med.* 2002;165(9):1217–1239.

Zhang B, Wing YK. Sex differences in insomnia: a meta-analysis. *Sleep.* 2006;29(1):85–93.

A complete reference list can be found online at ExpertConsult.com.

Chapter 71

Sleep Medicine, Public Policy, and Public Health

Raghu Pishka Upender

Chapter Highlights

- The growing interface between sleep medicine and public health is highlighted by surveying the various dimensions of sleep known to affect health outcomes, including sleep duration, sleep timing, sleep efficiency, sleep quality, alertness, and performance.
- The evolving knowledge of sleep physiology and sleep disorders is shaping public policy in various safety-sensitive occupations, such as the transportation and the health care industries. Brief historical backgrounds behind many of the regulations are also discussed.
- The sleep medicine community can shape public policy and improve sleep health and safety by partnering with governmental regulatory agencies and industry stakeholders.

SLEEP MEDICINE AND PUBLIC HEALTH

Sleep is an essential biologic function that is thought to have evolved to help organisms cope with light and dark cycles that occur naturally on Earth. The physiologic importance of sleep is underscored by the fact that humans spend nearly one-third of their lives sleeping. Although the function of sleep remains to be fully elucidated, current evidence suggests key roles in development, neurocognitive performance, mood regulation, and metabolic homeostasis.[1] Accumulating evidence suggests that even partial sleep deprivation has far-reaching consequences on health and well-being.[2] *Sleep health*, a term often encountered in the media, is an apt term emphasizing the strong connection between sleep and health.

Public health interest in sleep has been steadily increasing over the past two decades. This interest is driven not only by the growing knowledge of the physiologic importance of sleep but also by the increasing recognition that sleep deprivation and sleep disorders are pervasive among the general population. The Centers for Disease Control and Prevention (CDC) has been tracking health conditions and risk behaviors in the United States since 1984 through the Behavioral Risk Factor Surveillance System (BRFSS), the largest ongoing telephone health survey system in the world. In the 2014 survey, approximately 35.2% of US adults reported sleeping less than 7 hours per night. The prevalence of those sleeping less than 7 hours per night is even higher among minority groups such as Blacks and Native Americans.[3]

The American Institute of Medicine estimates that 50 to 70 million people have chronic sleep and wakefulness disorders.[4]

Poor sleep in its various manifestations is associated with adverse health outcomes and a huge economic burden at both the individual and societal levels. The costs of sleep loss and sleep disorders are estimated to be billions of dollars. For example, the cost burden of untreated obstructive sleep apnea (OSA) among US adults alone has been estimated at $149.6 billion in both direct and indirect costs related to comorbid medical conditions, hospitalization, accidents, and productivity loss.[5]

Initiatives to increase public awareness of sleep health are underway in many countries. In the United States, for example, the government-sponsored public health initiative *Healthy People 2020* now includes a dedicated section on sleep health to promote public awareness of the ill effects of sleep loss and sleep disorders.[6] The U.S. Army has adopted a program called *Performance Triad* that includes sleep as one of the three pillars of health and performance alongside nutrition and physical activity.[7] Through efforts such as these, sleep health literacy is improving, but the chasm between knowledge and positive changes in health behavior remains formidable. To fully realize the benefits of sleep, public health initiatives must spotlight the various dimensions of sleep—sleep duration, sleep timing, sleep efficiency, subjective sleep satisfaction, and daytime alertness—that have been associated with health outcomes.[8]

Sleep Duration

The amount of sleep required for optimal physiologic function varies across age and individuals. For example, newborns spend 16 hours or more sleeping, much of it in rapid eye movement (REM) sleep. By age 2 years, sleep duration declines to about 11 to 12 hours. School-aged children sleep about 10 hours, whereas adolescents sleep 9 to 10 hours each night.[9] Adults sleep about 8 hours per night when unfettered by lifestyle demands. Total sleep time declines with age at a rate of 10 minutes per decade, and sleep efficiency declines at a rate of 3% per decade. Components of sleep such as slow wave and REM sleep also decrease, but at different rates.[10]

Modern lifestyles with long commutes and long working days are increasingly encroaching on traditional sleep time and creating a society that is chronically sleep deprived. By some reports, average sleep duration in America has declined by 20% over the past century.[11] The advent of the electric light bulb and cheap artificial light has had dramatic effects on the 24-hour sleep-wake patterns of humans. Light exposure activates brainstem arousal systems and attenuates sleep signals by suppressing melatonin. As a result, the peak circadian wake signal that normally occurs at the end of the day is delayed and allows individuals to remain awake well into the night.[12] On the other hand, early start times at school and work prevent compensatory sleep in the morning. Thus the sleep period is squeezed at both ends. A 2010 National Health Survey found that 30% of all employed US adults (40.6 million workers) reported averaging less than 6 hours sleep per night.[13] Even more alarming is the declining sleep duration of school-aged children, adolescents, and young adults. In a 2015 CDC health survey, 72.7% of high school students grades 9 through 12 reported less than 8 hours of sleep per night.[14] The 2006 Sleep in America Poll by the National Sleep Foundation found that sleep duration declined from 8.4 to 6.9 hours per night among 6th and 12th graders, even though physiologic sleep need does not decline significantly across this age span.[15] The problem is global as indicated by a systematic review, which found that sleep duration declined by 1 hour per night over the study period of 1905 to 2008.[16]

Not all studies have shown declining sleep duration. For example, a 2003 face-to-face interview of nearly 2000 British subjects aged 16 to 93 years found that self-reported sleep duration was not significantly different compared with sleep surveys conducted in 1969.[17,18] Another study using time-use diaries from eight surveys across a 31-year period from 1975 to 2006 indicated that the odds of short sleep had not changed for part-time workers, retired workers, homemakers, or the unemployed and that the odds actually decreased for students, who represented less than 5% of the participants. Full-time workers were the only group that showed an increase in the odds ratio of short sleep of 1.19 (95% confidence interval, 1.00, 1.42; $P = .05$) over 31 years. Long work hours were much more common in those sleeping less than 6 hours, suggesting a possible cause-and-effect relationship.[19] Another study examining data from 15 countries over a period spanning between the 1960s and 2000s found that the average sleep duration of adults actually increased in seven countries: Bulgaria, Poland, Canada, France, Britain, Korea, and the Netherlands (range, 0.1 to 1.7 minutes per night each year) and had decreased in six countries: Japan, Russia, Finland, Germany, Belgium, and Austria (range, 0.1 to 0.6 minute per night each year). The findings were inconsistent in the United States and Sweden.[20,21] Some of the conflicting findings noted in these studies could be related to methodological factors. It is important to note that most epidemiologic studies evaluating sleep duration employ subjective measures and are susceptible to recall and response bias. Subjects may confuse sleep time with time in bed. Therefore future public health surveillance of sleep practices should include more objective measures of sleep duration. Low-cost activity monitors and social networking platforms may enable collection of more objective measurement of sleep duration.

A large body of literature has linked sleep duration with health outcomes. One of the earliest associations between sleep duration and mortality risk was found in a prospective study of more than 1 million subjects who were followed for more than 2 years. Those who reported sleeping 7 hours per night had a lower death rate than those who reported sleeping either more or less sleep than this.[22] These findings were corroborated in a study of 7000 subjects in Alameda County, California, who were followed for 9 years.[23] The analysis indicated that those sleeping less than 6 hours or more than 9 hours per night had 1.6 times the total age-adjusted death rate of those sleeping 7 to 8 hours per night. This U-shaped relationship between mortality rates and sleep duration has also been found in a number of studies around the world and holds true across the adult life span.[24] Studies have suggested that short sleep can lead to higher mortality rates even after controlling for comorbidities.[25] Sleep loss is likely to cause higher mortality rates through various adverse effects on physiology. Studies have found higher likelihood of hypertension,[26,27] atherosclerosis,[28] coronary artery disease,[29] ischemic stroke,[30] dyslipidemia,[31] and diabetes[32] in short sleepers. A number of studies in both adult and pediatric populations have shown strong associations between obesity and sleep duration, potentially mediated through alterations in hormones regulating appetite.[33] The rising rates of childhood obesity and diabetes are considered to be partly related to chronic partial sleep loss.

Sleep Timing

Traditional sleep-wake schedules are changing to meet the needs of the 24/7 modern global economy. About 20 million US workers (17.7% of the workforce) are estimated to work in shifts that at least partly fall outside the traditional 6 a.m. to 6 p.m. schedule.[34] As many as 4.3% of workers work primarily during the night. This trend has increased over the past 50 years with globalization of the economy. The rates of nontraditional work hours vary across industry and are the highest among protective services, food service, transportation and health care industry. Nontraditional schedules can have significant effects on intrinsic biologic rhythms known as circadian rhythms, which evolved over millennia to optimize human physiology and behavior during both the light and dark phases of the environment. The circadian system in humans provides alerting signals during the light phase and promotes sleep during the dark phase, coinciding with the period of melatonin secretion. Sleep occurring during the light phase is often fragmented and shorter in duration because of the antagonistic effect of the circadian alerting signal. Studies have shown that night-shift workers average about 30 to 60 minutes less sleep on average then daytime workers.[35] Conversely, maintenance of alertness during the dark phase is extremely difficult for most people, especially in early morning hours when the circadian alerting signal reaches its nadir.

The adverse effects of altered sleep timing are readily apparent to most people who have experienced jet lag from travel across multiple time zones. Rapid travel across multiple time zones leaves circadian rhythms out of sync with the destination's light-dark cycles because circadian rhythms are slower to adapt and can only do so at an average rate of 1 hour per day. Consequently, circadian signals conflict with environmental and social cues in the new location and lead to unpleasant symptoms that include daytime fatigue, irritability, poor concentration, digestive problems, excessive sleepiness, and nocturnal insomnia. Similar but less intense symptoms may be experienced by people who delay bedtime and wake-up time by 1 to 2 hours on weekends. The "Monday morning blues" may partially be due to this "social jet lag."

Circadian misalignment is a perpetual problem for shift workers because it is practically impossible for people to maintain consistent sleep-wake schedules that are out of phase with environmental light-dark cycles. Even small amounts of ambient light can drive circadian phase to shift toward the light or active phase of the rhythm. Sociologic factors force most shift workers to revert to a more traditional sleep-wake schedule on days off to spend time with family and friends and to attend to business affairs. As a result, shift workers are forced to work and sleep during discordant circadian phases. The ability to cope with the physiologic challenges created by circadian misalignment varies across individuals and may be inheritable. Approximately 20% to 30% of shift workers experience what has come to be known as shift-work sleep disorder, persistent symptoms not dissimilar to jet lag that include fatigue, insomnia, impaired concentration, low mood, and memory.[36] Workers with shift-work sleep disorder have higher rates of depression and anxiety and are more prone to accidents.[37] Higher prevalence of gastric ulcers, heart disease, ischemic stroke, obesity, and metabolic syndrome has been noted in the literature.[38] There has been recent interest in the connection between shift work and increased risk for cancers, especially breast cancer.[39] Melatonin is thought to play a role in tumor surveillance, and its suppression by nocturnal light exposure has been hypothesized as a potential mechanism of tumorigenesis in shift workers. Some recent studies have questioned whether this increased risk for cancer is real.[40,41]

Sleep Efficiency and Sleep Quality

Sleep efficiency is defined as total sleep time divided by time spent in bed trying to sleep, a measure that tends to decline with age, partly because of loss of gamma-aminobutyric acid producing neurons in the ventral preoptic area and partly because of medical, psychological, and sociologic factors associated with advancing age. *Sleep quality* is less well defined and more difficult to measure because the subjective experience of it does not always correlate with currently available objective measures. However, there is general consensus that high-quality sleep means falling asleep quickly, sleeping without arousal, and awakening fully rested. Many people believe that quality sleep is a precondition to optimal daytime performance and positive mood. As with sleep efficiency, sleep quality declines with age because of changes in human sleep physiology and concurrent medical, psychologic, and sleep disorders—the latter being important to recognize because of the availability of effective treatments.

One of the most prevalent sleep disorders is insomnia, a condition characterized by difficulty with sleep onset and sleep maintenance. Chronic insomnia affects approximately 30 million Americans and causes much distress to its sufferers.[42] A number of studies have indicated a striking association between insomnia and depression. Some postulate that insomnia may be an early marker for the onset of depression. Although the pathophysiologic relationship remains to be clarified, there may be overlap of neural pathways for anxiety, arousal, and circadian disturbance.[43] The close association of insomnia and depression also raises the tantalizing possibility that treating insomnia may prevent some cases of depression, but limited data are available.[44]

Sleep apnea is another common sleep disorder that is associated with poor sleep efficiency and sleep quality. The prevalence of OSA, as defined by an apnea-hypopnea index greater than 5 and excessive sleepiness, is 9% in women and 24% in men in the adult population.[45] The prevalence of OSA is rising owing to the obesity epidemic and aging demographics. Multiple factors are likely to be responsible for the increasing prevalence of OSA in older individuals. These include age-related weight gain, reduced pharyngeal muscle tone, and declining sensorimotor responsiveness to hypoxia, hypercapnia, and respiratory load.[46] The cessation of apneic and hypopneic events is often contingent on somatic and/or cortical arousal, and therefore sleep fragmentation is intrinsic to the pathophysiology of OSA. Sleep fragmentation is very responsive to continuous positive airway pressure (CPAP) therapy, which provides an opportunity to markedly improve sleep efficiency and quality.

Sleep efficiency is also reduced in patients suffering from restless legs syndrome, a neurologic condition that affects approximately 5% of the general population. Restless legs syndrome is characterized by an irresistible urge to move the legs and is often accompanied by nocturnal periodic limb movements.[47]

A number of studies have shown an association between sleep efficiency, subjective sleep quality, and various health outcomes. For example, a Japanese population-based cohort study of self-reported sleep parameters found that women who reported poor awakening state experienced a higher mortality rate (relative risk, 1.97) compared with those who awakened normally.[48]

Alertness and Performance

The value of sleep for most individuals is its ability to restore alertness and improve performance during the waking period. When sleep is suboptimal, people feel unrested and experience a number of neurocognitive deficits that include poor memory, decreased concentration, slowed reaction times, and impaired judgment. Elegant studies using psychomotor vigilance tests have shown a dose-dependent slowing of response times with increasing sleep restriction.[49] Mean number of lapses on psychomotor vigilance tests increased with increasing sleep restriction. Performance precipitously dropped with sleep durations of less than 5 hours per night. Several nights of recovery sleep were required for performance to be restored to baseline levels.

Beyond their effects on daytime performance, decreased levels of alertness during the day have been linked to poor health. In a study of 5888 individuals, daytime sleepiness was the only sleep disturbance symptom that was associated with mortality, cardiovascular disease, and congestive heart failure.[50] These associations persisted in women after adjustment for age and other factors. In another study of community-dwelling older adults (>65 years old), mortality rate was accelerated by 1.73 times in those who napped most of the time and made two or more errors on cognitive tests.[51]

The importance of alertness and performance is nowhere more relevant than it is in occupational safety. The next section describes the interconnectedness between alertness, fatigue, and performance and how the evolving public policies are aiming to mitigate fatigue-related safety risk in several industries.

SLEEP MEDICINE AND PUBLIC POLICY

Work-related fatigue has long been recognized as a factor contributing to accidents, especially in industries that operate 24/7.

With globalization of the economy in the past century, the number of industries and workers operating around the clock has increased. Commensurately, fatigue-related accidents have become more common and have created a greater threat to the environment and public safety. For example, the Three Mile Island nuclear reactor disaster of 1979 resulted from coalescence of human error and mechanical factors that allowed a large amount of nuclear reactor coolant to escape into the environment. Fatigue was implicated in the accident, not surprisingly because the accident occurred at 4 a.m.[52] Another fatigue-related accident occurred in 1989 when the oil tanker Exxon Valdez struck a reef off the coast of Alaska and spilled 11 to 32 million gallons of crude oil. It was at the time the largest and most devastating human-caused environmental disaster.[53] Although multiple factors played a role in the accident, crew fatigue was identified as a major factor. Investigators found the crew to be understaffed and overworked. Fatigue has also been implicated in the Chernobyl nuclear and space shuttle *Challenger* disasters.[54]

Other examples of preventable fatigue-related accidents abound in the transportation and health care industries. In response to these accidents and to promote public safety, a variety of governmental regulations have been established. Brief histories of these regulations in the transportation and health care industries are discussed next.

Transportation Industry

Railroad

At the end of 19th century after a period of dramatic expansion of railroads in America, it became apparent that train accidents, many related to worker fatigue, were resulting in unacceptable loss of life and economic damages. It was not uncommon for railroad workers to be required to work extremely long hours, especially during harvest time. There was a public outcry for more regulatory oversight, which led to the first public policy attempting to address fatigue-related accidents, the Hours of Service Act of 1907 (45 USC Sect. 61; 1907). The law as originally adopted prevented workers from working more than 16 consecutive hours in a 24-hour period. The act also established a minimum of 10 consecutive hours of rest after a 16-hour shift, and a minimum of 8 hours of rest after an aggregate of 16 hours of work in a 24-hour period. Although it was difficult to assess the direct impact of the law, owing to poor reporting standards, the available data indicated reductions in injuries and fatalities during the 10 years following the enactment of the law despite a rise in passenger and freight traffic.[55] The law was subsequently changed to allow only 14 hours of work in 1969, and 12 hours in 1971. In response to several fatal rail accidents in 2002 and 2008, Congress passed the Rail Safety Improvement Act of 2008 (49 USC 21101; 2008), which enabled the Federal Railroad Administration (FRA), a member of the U.S. Department of Transportation (USDOT), to promulgate new safety regulations governing different aspects of railroad safety, including HOS requirements. This law provided statutory limits on the total on-duty and deadhead time (time spent traveling to duty assignment) to 276 hours per month for rail and signal employees; limited total allowable shift time for employees to 12 consecutive hours; increased uninterrupted off-duty hours from 8 to 10 hours in a 24-hour period; required 2 consecutive days off after 6 consecutive days of work and 3 consecutive days off after 7 consecutive days of work; reduced allowable deadhead time to 30 hours per month; and required electronic HOS recordkeeping.[56] It is important to note that of all transport modes regulated by USDOT, railroad hours-of-service (HOS) standards are the only ones locked into statute (i.e., mandated by law) rather than being adjustable by administrative regulations.

Aviation

Pilot fatigue has long been recognized as a contributing factor to pilot error, which in turn can magnify the dangers inherent to flying an aircraft. In 1931 the U.S. Commerce Department set a monthly flight-time limit of 110 hours as a compromise between the 140 hours wanted by airline operators and the 85 hours advocated by the Airline Pilot Association. In 1938 the Civil Aeronautics Board issued domestic flight-time rules, limiting flight time to 8 hours in a 24-hour period.[57] These flight-time and duty hour regulations evolved over the years, driven by public safety concerns, widely publicized airplane crashes, and better understanding of human fatigue in the operational environment. The Federal Aviation Administration (FAA), the US regulatory body overseeing aviation safety, completed a major overhaul of regulations in 2011.

Key components of the 2011 rules include varying flight and duty time requirements based on the time of day of pilot's first flight, the number of scheduled flight segments, and the number of time zones crossed. Flight duty period is limited to 9 to 14 hours, while flight time is limited to 8 to 9 hours. Pilots are required to have a 10-hour minimum rest period that includes 8 hours of uninterrupted sleep opportunity before the flight duty period, an increase of 2 hours of rest over the previous rules. To address cumulative fatigue, the 2011 rule includes weekly, monthly, and annual limits of flight and duty hours. For example, pilots are required to have 30 consecutive hours off every week. Pilots and airlines are expected to take joint responsibility when considering a pilot's fitness for duty, including fatigue resulting from pre-duty activities such as commuting. Pilots are required to affirmatively state their fitness for duty, and the airlines are required to remove pilots from duty when they are fatigued or unfit to fly.[58] Airlines are also required to implement a comprehensive fatigue risk management plan. The 2011 rules apply only to passenger pilots and exclude pilots who fly only cargo, even though they fly the same types of aircrafts on the same routes and are susceptible to the same levels of fatigue. At the time of this writing, the FAA is considering a plan to amend duty period limits for flight attendants to ensure that they are given at least 10 consecutive hours of scheduled rest period.[59]

Trucking

As in other transportation modalities, concerns about unsafe scheduling practices of commercial drivers in the United States led to the establishment of the Interstate Commerce Commission (ICC), which then had regulatory authority over motor carriers, to promulgate the first governmental regulation in 1938. The original ICC required drivers to be on duty for no more than 15 hours and work no more than 12 hours in a 24-hour period. The rules allowed at least 9 hours off duty (8 for sleep) and 3 hours of duty time for meals and rest breaks. The ICC also set a weekly on-duty limit of 60 hours in any 7 consecutive days or 70 hours in 8 consecutive days, which remains in effect to this day. Shortly after the release of the original rules and under the pressure of competing interests of labor and motor carrier operators, the ICC settled on 8-hour of continuous off-duty rest period and 10-hour driving limit restrictions. Additionally, the industry associations argued for and received a 2-hour extension to these limits for unfavorable weather conditions, which also remains in effect.[60]

The HOS regulations from the late 1930s remained fundamentally unchanged through the end of 20th century, despite accumulating evidence linking driver fatigue and crash risk. In 1989 the USDOT sponsored a field study, the Driver Fatigue and Alertness Study, to determine the relationships among HOS regulations, driver fatigue, and frequency of serious accidents involving commercial motor vehicles. The study was completed in 1996 and found that time of day was the strongest and most consistent factor influencing driver fatigue and alertness. Video recording of drivers' faces showed markedly increased rates of drowsiness during nighttime driving than during daytime driving. Time of day was a much better predictor of decreased driving performance than hours of driving or the cumulative number of trips made. The study also found that drivers spent an average of 5.2 hours in bed, which is about 2 hours less time than their reported "ideal" daily amount of sleep. Drivers with night start time spent the least amount of time in bed, about 4.4 hours. Not surprisingly, there was a negative correlation between sleep duration and the amount of drowsiness during the next driving trip; in other words, less sleep was associated with more drowsiness, as would be expected. Drivers reported being more alert than the performance tests indicated.[61] In a 2004 study analyzing the crash data from three national-scale operators, the crash risk was statistically similar for the first 6 hours of driving and then increased nonlinearly after 6 hours. The 11th hour had a crash risk more than three times the first hour. Multiday driving schedules are also associated with statistically significant increases in crash risk, comparable in magnitude to driving time.[62] Drowsiness was a contributing factor in about 22% to 24% of accidents, according to a 2006 report that analyzed the data from the 100-Car Naturalistic Driving Study.[63]

These and other similar studies prompted the Federal Motor Carrier Safety Administration (FMCSA), which replaced the ICC, to update the regulation in 2003 and then again in 2011. The 2003 rule increased the off-duty period from 8 to 10 hours and reduced the total driving window to 14 hours in an attempt to increase sleep opportunity and move the drivers toward a 24-hour daily clock. Driving time was increased from 10 to 11 hours, and drivers were allowed to restart their duty time calculation whenever they had at least 34 hours of off-duty time. This unfortunately created an opportunity for drivers to drive 14 hours continuously without a break and work 80 hours or more per week. The 2011 rule tried to remedy this safety risk by requiring a minimum of a 30-minute off-duty break after 8 hours of continuous driving, limited the use of the restart provision to once every 168 hours, and reduced the maximum workweek to 70 hours. In consideration of human circadian physiology, the 2011 rule also required that the 34 off-duty time include two periods between 1 a.m. and 5 a.m.[64] This provision gives drivers who routinely work nights and put in very long workweeks an opportunity to sleep during the circadian trough and overcome the chronic fatigue that can build up when working nights.

Regulations continue to evolve, but as of this writing, the following rules are in effect for drivers of passenger and property carrying vehicles.[65]

Property Carrying Drivers:

1. 11-hour driving limit: May drive a maximum of 11 hours after 10 consecutive hours off duty.
2. 14-hour limit: May not drive beyond the 14th consecutive hour after coming on duty, following 10 consecutive hours off duty. Off-duty time does not extend the 14-hour period.
3. 30-minute driving break: Drivers must take a 30-minute break when they have driven for a period of 8 cumulative hours without at least a 30-minute interruption. The break may be satisfied by any non-driving period of 30 consecutive minutes (i.e., on-duty not driving, off-duty, sleeper berth, or any combination of these taken consecutively).
4. May not drive after 60–70 hours on duty in 7–8 consecutive days. A driver may restart a 7–8 consecutive day period after taking 34 or more consecutive hours off duty.

Passenger Carrying Drivers:

1. 10-hour driving limit: May drive a maximum of 10 hours after 8 consecutive hours off duty.
2. 15-hour limit: May not drive after having been on duty for 15 hours, following 8 consecutive hours off duty. Off-duty time is not included in the 15-hour period.
3. 60–70-hour limit: May not drive after 60–70 hours on duty in 7–8 consecutive days.

Additionally, there are provision for sleeper berths and exemptions for bad weather and emergencies.

Marine

Fatigue is also major concern in the marine transport industry, and its operational challenges are unlike those found in other modes of transportation. Crewmembers work away from home, often for 3 to 6 months at a time, and in environments that can often be unpredictable and at times dangerous. Threat to safety is ever present, and maintaining a high level of vigilance at all times is critical to avoiding injury, property damage, and environmental catastrophe. Getting adequate restorative sleep consistently is a luxury that is rarely afforded to mariners, who must work and sleep in shifts around the clock on a noisy moving vessel. The absence of clear separation between work and recreation contributes to increased levels of stress, especially when working with shipmates from different countries speaking different languages. Cramped quarters, environmental noise, vibration, heat, and bad weather compromise sleep quality.[66] Twenty-four–hour operations constrain sleep duration and require some crew members to sleep during the adverse phase of their circadian rhythm. These factors contribute to levels of fatigue that are much greater than those seen in other industries.[67] A study relating fatigue to marine casualties found that 33% of personnel injuries and 16% of critical vessel casualties had crew fatigue as a causal or contributing factor.[68]

The first set of international standards for minimum competence and safety for seafarers was drafted in 1978 by the International Marine Organization, an agency of the United Nations. The resulting Standards of Training, Certification, and Watchkeeping for Seafarers (STCW) included a weekly rest hour minimum that was subsequently increased to the current 77 hours of rest per week. In the United States, the Coast Guard regulates the inland ("brown water") and coastal ("blue water") waterway operations and sets minimum hours of rest regulations based on STCW. Currently, a minimum of 10 hours per 24-hour period and 77 hours per 7-day period of rest is required. Rest hours can be divided into no more than two periods in any 24-hour period, and one of the periods must be at least 6 hours in length.[69]

The inland waterway towboat industry has long adopted the square watch consisting of a 6-hour watch period alternating with 6-hour rest period (6:6:6:6) such that each crew member observes two watch and two rest periods per 24 hours. Although this arrangement limits shift length and thus mitigates time-on-task–related fatigue risk, it does not afford crewmembers the opportunity to sleep continuously for at least 7 hours. Additionally, it necessitates some crewmembers to work and sleep in the adverse circadian phases. For example, crews working the second watch typically work from midnight to 6 a.m. and then again from noon to 6 p.m. Both of these work periods include circadian temperature minimums that can be associated with increased sleepiness, especially in sedentary work environments such as the wheelhouse.

Attempts to introduce HOS regulation by the U.S. Coast Guard (USCG) have been strongly opposed by the industry. For example, the USCG issued a notice in 2011 that it was considering regulations that would require a minimum of a 7- or 8-hour rest period per day. Citing a number of scientific studies, USCG argued that the 6-hour rest periods provided insufficient uninterrupted sleep opportunity and resulted in higher levels of fatigue than an 8-hour rest period.[49,70-75] Industry leaders representing barge operators strongly opposed any changes to the scheduling practices, citing incomplete treatment of the science behind sleep and watchkeeping. A study funded by the American Waterways Organization and barge operators found that both front and back watch wheelhouse crew reported similar time in bed and sleep duration. One of the sleep periods was longer and was described as anchor sleep, whereas the second shorter sleep period was described as a nap. When the sleep periods were combined, the total sleep duration was the same on the boat as at home. Pilots slept on average 6.6 hours, even though they were in bed for about 8.1 hours (sleep efficiency, 81.4%). Sleep quality, on the other hand, was worse for back watch crew, possibly because their sleep periods (6 a.m. to noon and 6 p.m. to midnight) occurred during adverse circadian phases.[76] Whether USCG will pursue future regulations on HOS remains to be seen.

Health Care

The care of the sick necessitates around-the-clock operations, during which continuity of care is paramount. Work shifts tend to be long and thus increase the risk for fatigue-related accidents. This problem is in no place more acute than in the training of physicians and surgeons. In the early years of modern medicine, physician education included brief periods of intense training during which "resident" physicians cared for patients 24 hours a day, 7 days a week. By the latter half of 20th century, "residencies" became multiyear experiences that incorporated new learning modalities.[77] Duty hours remained long and were accepted as being critical to physician training. By the 1970s, congruent with accumulating evidence on the effects of sleep deprivation, it became apparent that postcall residents made more errors.[78] As early as the 1980s some internal medicine and pediatric training programs attempted to balance service and educational needs with personal needs of the residents. The 1984 medication error by residents working 36 hours under insufficient supervision caused the death of Libby Zion in New York and sparked a national debate that continues to this day. It took nearly 20 years for the Accreditation Council for Graduate Medical Education (ACGME) to implement its first common duty hour requirement. The 2003 policy established an 80-hour maximum workweek and reduced shift lengths to no longer than 30 consecutive hours.[79] The standards were further modified in 2011 because of continued concerns over patient safety and resident well-being.[80] The new rules eliminated overnight call responsibilities for the first-year residents by limiting the maximal duty period to 16 hours per 24-hour period and stipulated 1 off-duty day per 7 days.[81]

A number of studies have looked at error rates before and after the implementation of duty hour restrictions. A 2004 study compared the traditional resident work schedules (>24-hour shifts and long workweeks) with newer schedules (shorter, <24-hour shifts and fewer weekly work hours). Interns made 35.9% more serious medical errors during the traditional schedule than during the modified schedule (136.0 versus 100.1 per 1000 patient-days; $P < .001$), including 56.6% more nonintercepted serious errors ($P < .001$). Interns also made 5.6 times more serious diagnostic errors during the traditional schedule as during the intervention schedule (18.6 versus 3.3 per 1000 patient-days; $P < .001$).[82]

Although extant literature suggests that duty hour limits improve resident well-being and sleep duration, they also have had unintended consequences. Some studies have argued that the increased number of handoffs necessitated by duty hour limits disrupts the continuity of care and leads to delayed diagnoses, lengthier hospital stays, and increased number of preventable complications.[83] A study comparing the 2003 and 2011 duty hour regulations found that programs complying with 2011 rules had increased handoffs, decreased resident availability for teaching conferences, and reduced intern presence during daytime work hours.[84]

Faculty of training programs are also concerned that trainees are not gaining adequate exposure to case mix and leaving the already protracted years of postgraduate training with insufficient experience. These concerns lead the ACGME to relax the 2011 rules.[85] The current standards, which went into effect in 2017, offer more flexible scheduling options and include the following rules:

- Maximum 80 hours per week averaged over a 4-week period
- 8 hours off between scheduled clinical work and education periods
- 14 hours free of clinical work and education after 24 hours of in-house call
- Minimum of 1 day off for every 7 when averaged over 4 weeks
- Work periods should not exceed 24 hours of continuous scheduled clinical assignments. Up to 4 hours of additional time may be used for activities related to patient safety, such as providing effective transitions of care, and/or resident education
- In-house call frequency should be no more than every third night when averaged over a 4-week period

A cluster-randomized noninferiority trial comparing the patient safety outcomes in the flexible and standard resident duty hour rules found no significant differences among 30-day mortality, 7-day readmission rates, and other patient safety indicators.[86,87] The study also found no more chronic sleep loss or sleepiness across trial days among interns in flexible programs than among those in standard programs.[87,88]

Hazardous Workplace

In addition to the industries discussed earlier, there are a large number of occupations that operate around the clock and have the potential to affect public safety and health. Workers in these occupations include firefighters, paramedics, police, disaster recovery workers, military personnel, utilities operators, and operators of plants producing hazardous or toxic chemicals. Examples of fatigue-related accidents leading to loss of life, environmental disaster, and economic damages are abundant. The 1986 space shuttle *Challenger* disaster occurred partly because of a sequence of ill-fated decisions made by sleep-deprived individuals.[89] The legacy of the environmental damage caused by the grounding of Exxon Valdez in 1989 by overworked and understaffed crew can still be felt today in Prince William Sound, Alaska.[53]

ROLE OF SLEEP MEDICINE COMMUNITY

Progress in recognizing fatigue as an important factor for health and safety is evident in a number of industries, as described previously. However, much work remains to be done. Sleep clinicians, scientists, and advocates play an important role in socializing the evolving fund of knowledge in sleep medicine and science. In addition to raising awareness and educating the public about sleep's role in health and safety, sleep professionals need to play an active role in developing and promoting industry-specific regulations and best practices that mitigate fatigue-related accidents. While promoting health and safety, these fatigue countermeasures have to be practical and must address operational and economic needs of the stakeholders. Before advocating for a potentially disruptive policy, sleep professionals must gain a reasonable understanding of the operational constraints of a given industry. For example, an evidence-based policy requiring a longer rest period for mariners will fail if it does not account for the economic forces that shaped the unique 6:6:6:6 square watch. This schedule allows two pilots to operate a towboat around the clock with neither of them having to endure fatigue-inducing 12-hour shifts. The downside to this schedule is that it limits sleep opportunities to short intervals and requires some crew members to sleep during the adverse phase of the circadian rhythm. Based on what is currently known about human sleep physiology, this type of work and rest schedule is expected to cause chronic sleep deprivation, performance deficits, and greater risk for accidents. However, without compelling evidence linking the current work-rest schedule with operational safety risk, the industry stakeholders will strongly resist and ultimately prevail against any regulation attempting to change work-scheduling practices. Profit margins in the transportation industry are often thin, and employing an additional pilot to expand the rest periods can render the barge industry unable to compete with other modes of transportation. Additionally, well-intended policies can have unintended consequences as described previously for resident duty hour limits.

Sleep professionals are more likely to be successful in bringing about meaningful changes within an industry when they partner with industry advocates. Policies that aim to improve sleep efficiency and sleep quality are more likely to be accepted by the marine industry than policies that mandate changes to long-observed scheduling practices. For example, the Crews Endurance Management Systems (CEMS), developed by the U.S. Coast Guard, provides a set of industry-specific tools and practices that help maritime operators improve productivity and safety in their work environment.[90] CEMS outlines a number of strategies to mitigate fatigue risk, including the use of artificial light to shift the circadian temperature trough into the off-duty period to improve sleep. Also included are recommendations for sleep quarter improvements (noise and light abatement), sleep hygiene, exercise, nutrition, and stress management.

The historical approach of addressing fatigue by regulating HOS is no longer sufficient. This narrow approach addresses only one of a number of factors contributing to fatigue. Most federal agencies now endorse more comprehensive industry-specific fatigue risk management systems (FRMS). Some of these programs employ mathematical models that attempt to predict the risk for fatigue-related accidents based on factors known to influence alertness and performance.[49] These factors include homeostatic sleep drive, circadian variations in alertness, wake inertia, task type, and time on task. These models are being applied in a number of industries to identify risk of fatigue in nontraditional, rotating work schedules. Although these novel approaches are based on human sleep-wake physiology, caution must be exercised when implementing them in the operational environment. For fatigue models to be applicable, the fatigue scores derived from such modeling must have sufficient positive and negative predictive values for a given operational setting. In other words, the fatigue score must be accurate enough to help management decide which individual should or should not work. Low-accuracy models that falsely indicate high fatigue have the potential to disrupt operations and infringe on labor's income and are unlikely to be implemented successfully. Furthermore, many of the available models do not yet incorporate individual differences in sleep physiology and fatigue susceptibility.

Sleep advocates can also help shape policies that affect public health and workplace safety by engaging governmental regulatory agencies. Familiarity with these agencies and the industries they administer is required to effectively navigate the complex regulatory ecosystem with its various stakeholders vying to promote their own interests. In the United States, the National Transport Safety Board (NTSB) is responsible for investigating major accidents in all modes of transportation and making safety recommendations; however, it lacks the authority to enforce them. The USDOT and its member agencies (i.e., the FAA, FRA, FMCSA, and Pipeline and Hazardous Materials Safety Administration) are responsible for creating and enforcing regulations that govern their respective industries.

The regulatory agencies must consider economic impact, cost-benefit analysis, and industry input when formulating new regulations or policy changes. They are often subject to political pressures. To give an example, in late 2013, the FAA decided to modify rules governing untreated OSA, a disqualifying condition for airmen and traffic controllers when untreated. The proposed modification further mandated that all airmen with a body mass index (BMI) greater than 40 be evaluated by a board-certified sleep specialist and treated for OSA to be medically certified. The policy modification also indicated that the BMI threshold will be gradually lowered until every airman with OSA is treated.[91] Reaction from industry was swift. In a letter to the FAA, the Aircraft Owners and Pilots Association argued that the "policy inappropriately bypasses the rulemaking process; overlooks potentially more effective and efficient solutions; provides no clear safety benefit; and imposes unjustified costs on the user community.... In 2011 the FAA identified 124,973 airmen who are considered obese, making them potential candidates for testing under an expanded policy ... the potential cost to pilots is between $99 million and $374 million for testing alone."[92] As a result of effective lobbying efforts, Congress took action within a matter of days and released legislation that would require the FAA to go through a formal rule-making process before making any policy changes on sleep apnea. The rulemaking process allows the industry and the public to influence policy making in a public forum. The revised guidelines require that "an integrated assessment of history, symptoms, and physical/clinical findings" be used to determine the risk of OSA and "no disqualification of airmen should be based on BMI alone."[93]

This example is typical of how a well-intended policy that promotes sleep health and safety is difficult to implement because of socioeconomic factors. The policies are perceived as an undue burden on individuals, impinging on their right to earn their livelihood, especially in an industry such as aviation, for which the safety record has been strong.

Sleep advocates can help empower industry stakeholders to implement sleep science–based fatigue risk management programs. Even profit-motivated corporations will embrace health- and safety-promoting measures when those measures make economic sense. Berger and colleagues, with the support of Schneider National Incorporated (SNI), created a sleep apnea diagnosis and treatment program that eliminated or lowered many of the barriers to treating sleep apnea. Education about sleep apnea was provided through multiple channels to increase awareness and reduce driver anxiety and misconceptions about the condition. Occupational health professionals, safety officers, and training engineers were trained to monitor for symptoms of sleep apnea. Drivers referred to the program incurred no out-of-pocket expenses, thus eliminating one of the major financial obstacles. Evaluations were performed at locations near major SNI operating centers and allowed for a 2-day turnaround from diagnosis to treatment of apnea, thus minimizing scheduling constraints and time away from work. SNI also explicitly identified what documentation is required of their contracted USDOT physicians to ensure uniform high-standard reporting. Among 348 drivers diagnosed with sleep-disordered breathing and who were treated, medical costs and accident rates declined by 57.8% and 73%, respectively. The driver retention rate of continuous positive airway pressure (CPAP)–treated individuals was 2.29 times greater than the total company driver population.[94]

Success of the SNI sleep apnea program has encouraged other transportation companies to pursue similar programs. To realize the full health and safety benefits, however, programs must go beyond screening and treating sleep apnea to ensure long-term patient engagement and CPAP adherence. A major challenge to the development of such comprehensive sleep apnea monitoring programs is providing care to a geographically distributed workforce. A small study involving towboat wheelhouse crew members showed that centralized care coordination, remote adherence monitoring, and telemedicine tools can provide sleep apnea care that is acceptable to patients and achieves high CPAP adherence rates.[95]

The most important aspect of any fatigue management program is the presence of a corporate safety culture that puts the safety of the employee and the public ahead of corporate profits. Sleep professionals can play an important role in promoting such culture by engaging and educating industry leaders, governmental agencies, and the public at large. They can draw inspiration from past successful public health campaigns that brought about meaningful behavioral changes and societal benefits. Efforts of Ignaz Semmelweis and those who followed helped establish handwashing practices that have saved countless number of lives and much suffering over the past 150 years.[96] The many lives saved by reductions in cigarette smoking and widespread use of seatbelts would not have occurred were it not for the efforts of pulmonologists and emergency medicine physicians. Similarly, sleep medicine has an immense potential to improve public health and safety, especially because sleepiness and sleep disorders have far-reaching influences on health and safety.

CLINICAL PEARL

Sleep medicine has the potential to have an immense positive influence on the public because of the many ways in which sleep and sleep loss affect public health and safety. The promise of sleep medicine will be realized only when there is greater awareness of the importance of sleep. Sleep professionals are in a unique position to increase this awareness through education and advocacy. These professionals have many opportunities to help transform sleep science knowledge to practical solutions that improve public health and safety through partnership with industry and governmental agencies.

SUMMARY

Sleep is an essential biologic function whose physiologic importance has become clear only in the past several decades. Despite this growing knowledge and awareness of sleep's role in health, insufficient sleep is all too common in the modern world. The American Institute of Medicine estimates that 50 to 70 million people suffer from chronic sleep loss. Many factors are driving this worrisome trend toward short sleep. Long work hours, long commute times, ever-expanding 24/7 operations, easy-access on-demand digital entertainment, and pervasive use of social media are creating a culture that champions "work hard and play hard" and leaves too little time for sleep. The availability of inexpensive artificial light has had a dramatic effect on the natural 24-hour sleep-wake patterns in humans. Light exposure interferes with circadian rhythms by delaying the evening peak alertness signal and allows people to extend wake activities well into the night at the expense of sleep. On the other hand, early start times at school and at many workplaces necessitate early arousal. Thus the sleep period is squeezed at both ends. It is estimated that 30% of all employed US adults (40.6 million workers) average less than 6 hours of sleep per night. The sleep deficiency is not unique to employed adults. Sleep trends in school-aged children and adolescents indicate a decrease in sleep time of more than 1 hour over the past 100 years. Insufficient sleep has been associated with a number of chronic medical conditions, such as hypertension, diabetes, and cardiovascular disease, as well as all-cause mortality. When sleep disorders are weighed in, the resulting sleep loss is probably the single most important public health issue of our time. This chapter describes current trends in sleep practices across the age spectrum; their potential effect on health, performance, and public safety; and the role sleep professionals can play in promoting sleep health and public safety.

SELECTED READINGS

Berneking M, Rosen IM, Kirsch DB, American Academy of Sleep Medicine Board of Directors, et al. The risk of fatigue and sleepiness in the ridesharing industry: an American Academy of Sleep Medicine position statement. *J Clin Sleep Med.* 2018;14(4):683–685.

Flynn-Evans EE, Ahmed O, Berneking M, et al. Industrial regulation of fatigue: lessons learned from aviation. *J Clin Sleep Med.* 2019;15(4):537–538.

Gurubhagavatula I, Barger LK, Barnes CM, et al. Guiding principles for determining work shift duration and addressing the effects of work shift duration on performance, safety, and health: guidance from the American Academy of Sleep Medicine and the Sleep Research Society [published online ahead of print, 2021 Jul 8]. *J Clin Sleep Med.* 2021. https://doi.org/10.5664/jcsm.9512.

Gurubhagavatula I, Sullivan SS. Screening for sleepiness and sleep disorders in commercial drivers. *Sleep Med Clin.* 2019;14(4):453–462.

Gurubhagavatula I, Sullivan S, Meoli A, et al. Management of obstructive sleep apnea in commercial motor vehicle operators: recommendations of the AASM Sleep and Transportation Safety Awareness Task Force. *J Clin Sleep Med.* 2017;13(5):745–758.

Gurubhagavatula I, Tan M, Jobanputra AM. OSA in professional transport operations: safety, regulatory, and economic impact. *Chest.* 2020;158(5):2172–2183.

Howard S, Gaba DM, Rosekind MR, Zarcone VP. The risk and implications of excessive daytime sleepiness in resident physicians. *Acad Med.* 2002;77:1019–1025.

Institute of Medicine. *Sleep Disorders and Sleep Deprivation: An Unmet Public Health Problem.* Washington, DC: The National Academies Press; 2006. https://www.nap.edu/catalog/11617/sleep-disorders-and-sleep-deprivation-an-unmet-public-health-problem; [Accessed December 19,2019].

Institute of Medicine. *Resident Duty Hours Enhancing Sleep, Supervision, and Safety.* Washington, DC: The National Academies Press; 2009. https://www.nap.edu/catalog/12508/resident-duty-hours-enhancing-sleep-supervision-and-safety; [Accessed December 19,2019].

Jena AB, Farid M, Blumenthal D, Bhattacharya J. Association of residency work hour reform with long term quality and costs of care of US physicians: observational study. *BMJ.* 2019;366:l4134.

Kancherla BS, Upender R, Collen JF, et al. Sleep, fatigue and burnout among physicians: an American Academy of Sleep Medicine position statement. *J Clin Sleep Med.* 2020;16(5):803–805.

Kancherla BS, Upender R, Collen JF, et al. What is the role of sleep in physician burnout? *J Clin Sleep Med.* 2020;16(5):807–810.

A complete reference list can be found online at ExpertConsult.com.

Section 9

Legal Aspects of Sleep Medicine

Chapter 72

Introduction

Daniel B. Brown

Although the field of sleep medicine is fairly new (see Chapter 1), the legal implications have been present for centuries. Legal systems have tried to deal with the interactions of the mind and actions since the Code of Hammurabi almost 4000 years ago. In Ancient Rome a defendant could be not guilty because of *non compos mentis*, without mastery of mind.[1] When an adverse event or crime occurred, was the perpetrator "guilty" or legally culpable? Was the person's mental status, the *mens rea* (guilty mind), responsible? In the past 4 decades as the field of sleep medicine evolved, so did the legal implications.[2]

In Chapter 73 the forensic implications are discussed. Is someone with a sleep disorder who commits a horrendous action responsible in a legal sense? What are the legal implications of a sleepwalker who kills?[3] Until disorders of arousal were described by Broughton, there was not a strong scientific understanding of what could be responsible for such abnormal behaviors.[4] Now that there is a scientific basis, what is the role of the scientist acting as an expert in a legal case?

Chapter 74 discusses the very many legal implications of disorders that cause daytime sleepiness and impaired performance that could lead to adverse outcomes such as vehicle crashes. What are the responsibilities of the clinician, the patient, and the employer of the patient? What legal protections exist for such patients? Most cases involving sleepiness and crashes involve patients with sleep breathing disorders.

Sleepiness and impaired performance are important issues in fatigue- and safety-sensitive professions such as medicine and aviation.[5] See the section on Occupational Sleep Medicine for a detailed review. The legal implications are discussed in this section in Chapter 76.

Since sleep medicine has become an established field, standards have evolved. Chapters 76 and 77 review the regulations concerning clinical practice and compliance in the United States and Europe.

Clinicians managing patients must be aware of not only the medical aspects of sleep medicine but also the legal aspects.

A complete reference list can be found online at ExpertConsult.com.

Chapter 73

Sleep Forensics: Criminal Culpability for Sleep-Related Violence

Michel A. Cramer Bornemann; Mark W. Mahowald†

Chapter Highlights

- Sleep forensics is the application of neuroscience to somnology and sleep medicine to investigate unusual, irrational, or bizarre human sleep-related behavior associated with alleged criminal activity. This investigation is typically used to form the basis of an expert opinion for use in a criminal trial regarding a defendant's state of mind.
- Consciousness is not an all-or-none state but occurs on a spectrum. In addition, sleep and wakefulness are not mutually exclusive states of consciousness. Wakefulness, non–rapid eye movement sleep, and rapid eye movement sleep may occur simultaneously or oscillate rapidly. This phenomenon is key to understanding the forensic implications of violent parasomnias.
- Consciousness can be dissociated from behavior. Neurophysiologic mechanisms can account for violent or other asocial behaviors associated with sleep.
- In a criminal proceeding, the offer of a clinical diagnosis alone is often insufficient to secure a conviction. Sleep medicine specialists have a role in legal proceedings to describe and address aspects of a defendant's consciousness and culpability.

To blame a person is to express moral criticism, and if the person's action does not deserve criticism, blaming him is a kind of falsehood, and is, to the extent the person is injured by being blamed, unjust to him.

Sanford Kadish, 2000[1]

Philosophers from time immemorial have grappled with the mind-body dilemma. Recent advances in neuroscience put us now on the verge of solving how our brains affect our minds and behavior.

THE DEVELOPMENT OF SLEEP FORENSICS

Sleep forensics is formally defined as the application of the principles and tools of neuroscience as applied to somnology and sleep medicine. These principles and tools have been widely accepted under international peer review as means for investigating unusual, irrational, or bizarre sleep-related behavior associated with alleged criminal activity. The investigation undergoes further examination in a courtroom according to rules of criminal law.

The best application of sleep forensics involves an adaptable conceptual approach. An adaptable approach applies current neuroscientific concepts of consciousness and sleep-wake state dissociation to sleep medicine. This dynamic method is preferred to the approach outlined in the U.S. Model Penal Code (MPC), which uses static definitions and clinical disorder markers from which criminal behavior might be extrapolated.

Therefore a medical expert called on to investigate criminal allegations will need to do more than just evaluate for a possible sleep disorder. Ultimately the expert's determination of the defendant's state of consciousness will prove pivotal. This requires an understanding of the neuroscience of consciousness, an awareness of relevant neuroscientific models for types of potential behaviors that may arise from sleep and a determination concerning the appropriate application of consensus-driven clinical guidelines to assist in determining purported acts of violence arising from sleep.

The medical expert should also recognize the sleep specialist's primary role when interfacing with lawyers, judges, and law enforcement. The sleep specialist can help facilitate the discourse concerning advances in cognitive neuroscience and help develop the framework for further research, particularly in parasomnias.

EVOLUTION OF LEGAL THOUGHT ON CRIMINAL MENTAL STATES

General

Influenced by Sir Edward Coke, Chief Justice of the King's Bench (1613), Anglo-American law defines criminal offenses whereby a person must be in a certain mental state, called the *mens rea* (guilty mind), necessary to have committed a crime. Persons possessed of *mens rea* cannot be convicted absent a corresponding criminal act, called the *actus reus* (guilty act). Traditionally, intention is found within *mens rea,* and the physical part of the offense resides within *actus reus*. Proof of both is essential to secure a conviction.

†Deceased.

Recognition that an impaired mental state might mitigate criminal punishment appears to date back to at least 1772 BCE as recorded in the Code of Hammurabi. The Roman Empire also appeared to recognize a person's altered mental status to find defendants not guilty due to *non–compos mentis*, meaning without mastery of mind.[2]

In 1843 Sir Nicolas Tindal established what has become known as the *M'Naghten Rule*. These rules still provide the conceptual legal framework for excusing a person's criminal act committed while the defendant was suffering from a defect of reason or disease of the mind. For the defense to operate, the actor must be shown to be in a state of mind such that he did "not to know the nature and quality of the act he was doing; or, if he did know it, that he did not know he was doing what was wrong."[3,4]

From a neuroscientific perspective, the criminal act, or *actus reus* component of the crime, is of less interest than the essential *mens rea* element. Implementation of the M'Naghten Rule thereby becomes a watershed moment concerning the influence of neuroscience on criminal law because it is the state of the mind—or perhaps, more accurately, the brain—to which inquiry is focused.

Sleep

With respect to criminal culpability, the inquiry surrounding sleep is whether a person in a sleep state possesses sufficient *mens rea* to support a conviction for the actor's behavior. The first appearance of the "sleepwalking defense" in an American court of law came in *Massachusetts v. Tirrell*[5] in 1846. In this landmark case, Rufus Choate, a skilled orator and US senator, successfully used the "insanity of sleep" defense in the murder trial of Albert Tirrell. The evidence in that case proved that Tirrell brutally killed the victim with a razor, almost severing her head from her body, set the horrifically bloody crime scene ablaze, and then attempted to flee the country.[6] Choate, an innovative legal tactician influenced by the advent of the M'Naghten Rule in the United Kingdom, argued in part that Tirrell, a sleepwalker, murdered the victim in an unconscious sleepwalking state.

Later, in the mid to late 1800s, there were no plausible medical explanations to account for sleepwalking, let alone account for complex violent actions that apparently arose during sleep. Still, courts were willing to adopt and apply defenses to deadly crimes committed by persons in a sleep state by pleas of a temporary "defect of reason" or "disease of mind." See, for example, *HMS Advocate v. Fraser* (1878)[7] and *Fain v. Commonwealth* (1879).[8]

Until physiologic aspects of sleep could be objectively measured and verified using validated neuroscientific instruments, defending criminal behavior arising from sleep often meant associating such behavior with other, better-understood medical or psychiatric conditions, such as insanity or automatism. For example, courts apply the insanity defense to excuse criminal actions resulting from a diseased mind incapable of knowing right from wrong. Where indicated, courts might also withhold criminal punishment for acts caused by a defendant's involuntary bodily movements exhibited even while in a conscious or sane state. Thus a defense of automatism may be appropriate for acts arising from epileptic seizures, fugue states, and limbic psychotic trigger reactions, whereas an insanity plea would be appropriate if the defendant acted in the throes of fulminant delusional paranoid schizophrenia.

The legal community's perspective toward sleep began to shift in 1968 with Roger Broughton's seminal publication characterizing the relationship among somnambulism, nightmares, confusional states of arousal, and rapid eye movement (REM) sleep.[9] By creating a clear demarcation between sleep disorders and other medical or psychiatric conditions, this appears to be the first scientific sleep-related publication with direct legal implications, as demonstrated by the 1992 Canadian criminal case of *Regina v. Parks* (1992),[10] in which Broughton served as an expert witness on behalf of the defense.

The defendant in the *Parks* case claimed that while sleepwalking in the early morning hours he drove to the house of his wife's parents and, provoked to attack by his in-laws' physical contact, killed his mother-in-law with a kitchen knife and left his father-in-law seriously injured.[11] The defendant defended his actions on the basis of automatistic sleepwalking rather than insanity. Expert witnesses for the defense testified that sleepwalking is not a neurologic, psychiatric, or other illness but rather is a sleep disorder very common in children and also found in adults.

The jury acquitted the defendant on the basis of automatism, which is a complete acquittal, as opposed to finding the defendant not guilty by reason of insanity, which typically leads to some institutional incarceration. The Canadian Supreme Court took up the case to decide the single legal issue of whether sleepwalking should be classified as noninsane automatism or insane automatism arising from a "disease of the mind," giving rise to a special verdict of not guilty by reason of insanity. Based on the unchallenged expert testimony that sleepwalking is a sleep disorder rather than a mental defect, the court rejected the characterization of sleepwalking as a mental health disorder.

EVOLUTION OF CONSCIOUSNESS THOUGHT

Criminal law presumes that most human behavior is voluntary and that individuals are consciously aware of their acts. All criminal liability is based on a voluntary act, or an omission to engage in a voluntary act that the defendant would otherwise have been capable of performing. Voluntariness is the first step in establishing *mens rea.* If the state proves *mens rea*, then the state will assess liability according to four levels of culpability: purpose, knowledge, recklessness, and negligence. In criminal law, the level of culpability determines the category of homicide (murder, manslaughter, or negligent homicide), and the category directly influences the severity of punishment.

Because voluntariness is absolutely fundamental to *mens rea,* it is surprising that the MPC offers examples of involuntary acts instead of explicitly defining the term *voluntary acts.* One example of an involuntary act is bodily movement during unconsciousness or sleep. Thus the MPC equates sleep with unconsciousness and deems bodily movements performed in a sleep state to be involuntary and presumably excused from criminal punishment. The other three examples of involuntary acts in the MPC include reflex convulsion; bodily movement that is not otherwise a product of the effort or determination of the actor, either conscious or habitual; and conduct during hypnosis or hypnotic suggestion.[12,13]

Waking Consciousness

A comprehensive review of the neuroscience of consciousness is well beyond the scope of this chapter. However, consciousness involves awareness of our environment, awareness of our bodies, and introspection (self-awareness), and it can only fully occur when we are awake.

To neuroscientists, *consciousness* is a term that has varied meanings, although its definition in the legal realm has held steadfast. In science, for example, consciousness may be used to indicate whether an individual is in a conscious state, as in whether it has been altered, reduced, or even lost. On the other hand, consciousness may be a trait or an attribute of a psychological process, as in the ability to think, see, and feel consciously. With trait consciousness, further distinctions may be made between conscious representations, which are usually phenomenal, and required conscious access.

Unfortunately, a direct objective marker for the neural basis of state and trait consciousness that is independent of a person's external expressions or behavior has yet to be determined. Nevertheless, it is believed that the neuronal processes that mediate access to consciousness take place in a network of fronto-parietal cortical regions of the brain. These networks play an important role in attentional and behavioral selection of incoming and stored information. Because the frontoparietal cortical regions govern behavioral selection, it is not surprising that this region becomes active when patients in a vegetative state recover or becomes further activated when healthy subjects perform demanding perceptual tasks.

Sleep is regularly and actively induced by a shift in neuronal activity and neurotransmitter balance in brainstem nuclei. Functional neuroimaging studies performed on sleeping subjects reveal that during both REM and non–rapid eye movement (NREM) sleep the prefrontal and parietal cortical regions become deactivated in comparison to the resting wakeful state.[14–16] The most active regions during the resting wakeful state include the left dorsolateral and medial prefrontal areas, the inferior parietal cortex, and the posterior cingulate and precuneus.[15] In REM sleep, despite overall increases in cerebral blood flow and energy demands, relatively low regional cerebral blood flow persists in the prefrontal and parietal cortex.[17] Because consciousness can only fully occur when we are awake, the frontal cortex would appear to be indispensable to consciousness.

Another important region is the dorsal thalamus, the "gateway to the cortex," and its accompanying "guardian of the gateway," the reticular complex (part of which is often called the *perigeniculate nucleus*).[18–21] Francis Crick believed that the input and output gating of the reticular complex were topographically arranged to approximate a map of the entire cortex. In his searchlight hypothesis, the reticular complex thereby was able to heat the warmer parts of the thalamus and cool down the cooler parts so that "attention" would remain focused on the most active thalamocortical regions.[22] Although the function of the thalamic reticular complex remains incompletely understood, it is essential for consciousness, whereas cerebellar circuits, in contrast, are not.

Consciousness as a Continuum

The modern concept of consciousness was perhaps first established by influential American scientific psychologist and pragmatist William James (1842 to 1910). Consciousness has been subdivided into nine distinct components (Table 73.1), all of which are seamlessly integrated into our own personal conscious experience.

From the notion that consciousness is graded and not dichotomous, J. Alan Hobson developed the AIM concept.

Table 73.1 The Nine Components of Consciousness

Component	Function
Perception	Representation of input data
Attention	Selection of input data
Memory	Retrieval of stored representations
Orientation	Representation of time, place, and person
Thought	Reflection on representations
Narrative	Linguistic symbolization of representations
Instinct	Innate propensities to act
Intention	Representation of goals
Volition	Decisions to act

This concept creates a four-dimensional "mind space" in time that is transformed by three variables: activation (A), input-output gating (I), and neuromodulation ratio (M) (as measured by the aminergic-to-cholinergic ratio). All of these determine changes in the state of consciousness, which in turn govern the oscillation from wake to sleep.

These variables account for the physiologic properties within each state.[23] The interaction of these variables can cause temporary nonhomeostatic conditions that in turn might trigger or cause undesirable behavior without consciousness or memory. Such behaviors might include violent outbursts related to REM sleep behavior disorder (RBD).[24]

The recurrent pattern of state-determining parameters is amazingly consistent. However, there are numerous clinical and experimental examples of dissociation of state components. Such dissociation can be explained as simultaneous mixtures of clinical and neurophysiologic elements of the three states of being: wake, NREM sleep, and REM sleep. These fall into three categories, as reviewed by Mahowald and Schenck,[25] and include neuroanatomic lesions or stimulation, pharmacologic mechanisms, and sleep deprivation. Neuroanatomic lesions or stimulation include hypothalamic, thalamic, and brainstem manipulation or stimulation inducing state dissociation. Pharmacologic mechanisms include manipulation of the cholinergic or glutamate neurotransmitter systems resulting in a variety of state dissociations. A consequence of general anesthesia is "cognitive unbinding," which further explains state dissociation.[26] As for sleep deprivation, recent studies by Montplaisir and colleagues[27,28] suggest that sleepwalking results from a dysfunction of the mechanism responsible for sustaining stable slow-wave sleep and that sleepwalkers are particularly at risk when exposed to increased homeostatic sleep pressure.

State dissociations are the consequence of timing or switching errors in the normal process of the dynamic reorganization of the central nervous system as it moves from one state (or mode) to another. Elements of one state persist or are recruited erroneously into another state, often with fascinating and dramatic consequences.

Objective support for state dissociation is provided by depth electrode electroencephalographic studies demonstrating areas of wakefulness and sleep occurring simultaneously in humans.[29–32] This concept helps to explain such phenomena

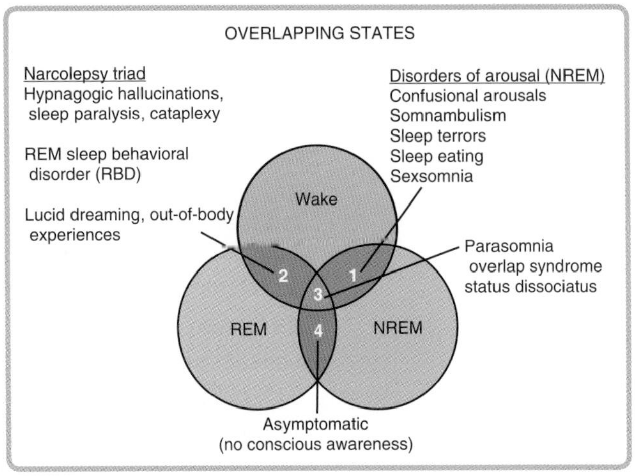

Figure 73.1 Areas of overlap among states of being. NREM, Non–rapid eye movement; REM, rapid eye movement. (Modified from Mahowald MW, Schenck CH. Dissociated states of wakefulness and sleep. *Neurology.* 1992;42:44–52).

as sleep inertia, waking hallucinations, narcolepsy, RBD, lucid dreaming, out-of-body experiences, near-death experiences, repressed or recovered memories of childhood sexual abuse, alien abductions, and disorders of arousal (Figure 73.1).[33–39] The concept of state dissociation supports the notion that consciousness occurs on a continuum.

Fixed Action Patterns and Central Pattern Generators: A Neuroethologic Approach to Behavior

Ethology is the study of whole patterns of animal behavior under natural conditions in a manner that highlights the functions and the evolutionary process of those patterns. With an ever-increasing physiologic approach through the application of refined and elegant laboratory research techniques to animal behavior, neurobiology and ethology have coalesced to develop neuroethology.[40]

An important behavior type in ethology is the fixed action pattern (FAP). This is an instinctive indivisible behavioral sequence that when initiated will run to full completion. FAPs are invariant and are produced by a neural network known as the *innate releasing mechanism* in response to an external stimulus known as a *sign stimulus.*

FAPs are ubiquitous in the animal kingdom and are seen from invertebrates to higher primates. Movements resulting in FAPs may be initiated by central pattern generators (CPGs): "Movements are generated by dedicated network of nerve cells that contain the information that is necessary to activate the different motor neurons in the appropriate sequence and intensity to generate motor patterns. Such networks are referred to as *Central Pattern Generators*."[41]

Tassinari and coworkers[42] recognized that motor events related to certain epileptic seizures and parasomnias share very similar features. This suggests a stereotyped inborn FAP, perhaps initiated by CPGs. Tassinari recognized CPGs as genetically determined neuronal aggregates in the mesencephalon, pons, and spinal cord that, from an evolutionary perspective, were linked with innate primal behavior essential for survival (e.g., feeding, locomotion, reproduction).

In higher primates CPGs are inhibited by the influence of neocortical control. Many of the CPGs are located in the brainstem and in close proximity to processes that govern the wake, NREM sleep, and REM sleep transitions. Despite diurnal neocortical inhibition, Tassinari provides a neuroethologic model whereby both epilepsy and sleep can lead to a temporary loss of control of the neomammalian cortex that is provided a pathway through a common arousal platform initiated by CPGs, which in turn triggers these FAPs (Figure 73.2), resulting in the abrupt onset of bizarre motor or emotional expressions that are uncharacteristic of awake neocortical-mediated diurnal behavior.

Tassinari's concept of the role of CPGs and FAPs provides a physiologic explanation for parasomnias. This concept is particularly useful in sleep forensics because parasomnias and epileptic seizures tend to have patterned stereotyped actions without conscious awareness. When addressing criminal allegations and their potential association with sleep-related conditions, the sleep medicine specialist can use behavior pattern recognition, applying neuroethologic concepts that indicate process fractionation, and neurobehavioral investigative techniques. Such an approach could be particularly beneficial and would be consistent with the direction of current mainstream neuroscience.

Dreaming Consciousness

It is obvious with sleep onset that sensory input is largely lost, and our ability to interact with the external environment is curtailed. The conscious state paradigm outlined by J. Alan Hobson recognizes that all nine components of consciousness change to varying degrees as the brain changes state and does so in a repetitive and stereotyped manner over the sleep-wake cycle. Furthermore, consciousness is graded, and the state changes appear to be of such dramatic magnitude that strong inferences can be made about the major physiologic underpinnings of consciousness.[23] Sleep physicians appreciate, by interpreting polysomnographic studies, the state-determined uniformity of physiologic events that are consistent from patient to patient. To analyze the transitions in process, from wake to sleep or from NREM to REM, and isolate its individual components to deduce its underlying state, including its associated degree of consciousness, is a method called *process fractionation* (Figure 73.3). The application of the conscious state paradigm has led Hobson to declare three important principles.

First, consciousness rides on the crest of the brain activation process. Therefore even a small perturbation in activation level leads to lapses in waking vigilance. Second, the brain remains highly active and capable of processing information even though consciousness may be largely deactivated. Functional imaging studies reveal that the brain remains about 80% active even when consciousness has largely subsided. Last, most brain activity is *not* associated with consciousness. In relation to its evanescence, consciousness "is a very poor judge of its own causation and of information processing by the brain."[23]

There have been seismic shifts in cognitive neuroscience that the legal system has yet to appreciate and incorporate into the legal arena. Rather confusing, the terms *conscious* and *unconscious* are still used in the lexicon of neuroscience, but the ideas and principles behind these terms have been substantially altered and continue to be refined, with one such example being Tononi's information integration theory of consciousness.[43,44]

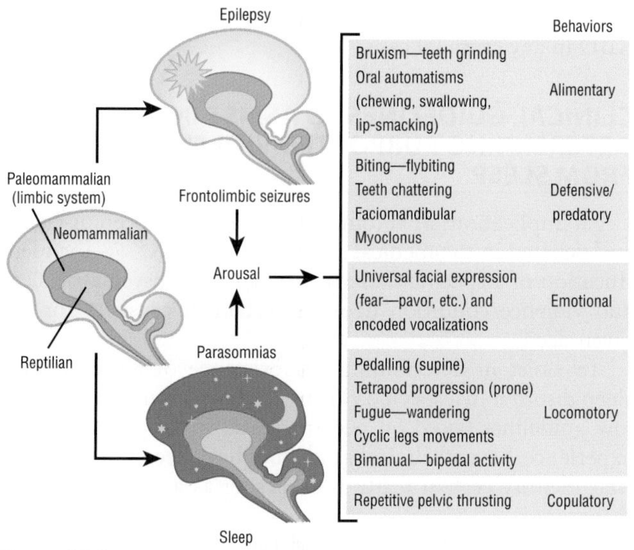

Figure 73.2 The emergence of innate primal behavior facilitated through central pattern generators from the arousal platform. (Modified from Tassinari CA, Rubboli G, Gardella E, et al. Central pattern generators for a common semiology in fronto-limbic seizures and in parasomnias: a neuroethologic approach. *Neurol Sci.* 2005;26:S225–32).

Advances in neuroscience since the 1980s support the existence of a continuum of conscious and unconscious processes, and neuroscience has largely dispensed with Freudian-influenced psychoanalytic concepts and theories. The boundaries between conscious and unconscious, as between wake and sleep, are permeable, dynamic, and interactive. As such, there is no valid scientific support for the sharp dichotomy between consciousness and unconsciousness currently held by the MPC and the legal community. It is this model of state dissociation that assists in the explanation of unusual, irrational, or bizarre human behavior in sleep forensics.

COMPLEX BEHAVIOR ARISING FROM SLEEP

Increasingly, experts in sleep medicine are being called on by attorneys to assist in reviewing legal cases, most of which involve allegations of criminal behavior. The conventional path is to evaluate for parasomnias to explain a wide variety of sleep-related violent behavior. The typical defense strategy is to clothe the behavior as a parasomnia symptom and thus completely exonerate the perpetrator's actions. Case requests to review bizarre nocturnal activities as mere rage reactions

	Wake	NREM	REM	Causal Hypothesis
Sensation & Perception	Vivid, externally generated	Dull or absent	Vivid, internally generated	Presynaptic inhibition, blockade of sensory input
Thought	Logical and progressive	Logical and perseverative	Nonlogical and bizarre	Loss of attention memory and volition leads to failure of sequencing and rule inconstancy; analogy replaces analysis
Attention	Intact, vigilant	Lost	Lost	Decreased aminergic modulation causes a decrease in signal to noise ratio
Orientation	Intact	Unstable	Unstable	Internally inconsistent orienting signals are generated by cholinergic system
Emotion	Inhibited	Weak	Episodically strong	Cholinergic hyperstimulation of amygdala and related temporal lobe structures
Instinct	Inhibited	Weak	Episodically strong	Cholinergic hyperstimulation of hypothalamus and limbic forebrain triggers CPG/FAP axis
Aminergic Inhibition (−)	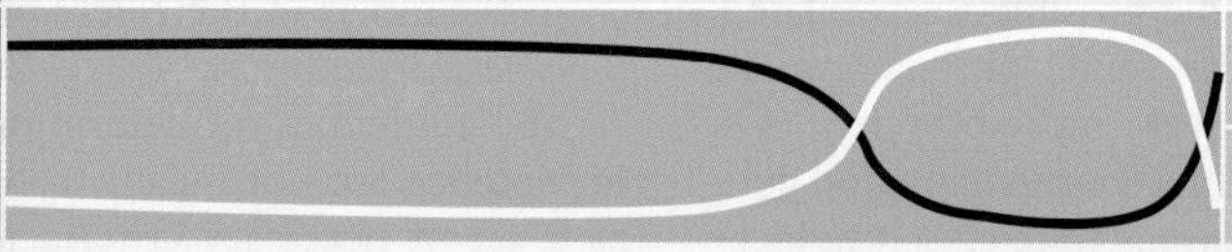			Aminergic Inhibition (−)
Cholinergic Excitation (+)				Cholinergic Excitation (+)

Figure 73.3 Process fractionation: contrasts in components of consciousness between states. CPG, Central pattern generator; FAP, fixed action pattern; NREM, Non–rapid eye movement; REM, rapid eye movement. (Modified from Hobson JA. States of consciousness: normal and abnormal variation. In: Zelazo PD, Moscovitch M, Thompson V, eds. *The Cambridge Handbook of Consciousness*. Cambridge University Press; 2007:69.)

BOX 73.1 CONDITIONS ASSOCIATED WITH AUTOMATIC BEHAVIOR ARISING FROM THE SLEEP PERIOD

Primary Sleep Disorders (Neurologic Conditions)

Disorders of arousal
- Confusional arousal
- Sleep-related abnormal sexual behavior (sexsomnia)
- Sleep terror
- Somnambulism

REM sleep behavior disorder
Nocturnal seizures
Compelling hypnagogic hallucinations
Somniloquy

Psychiatric Conditions

Dissociative states (may arise exclusively from sleep)
Posttraumatic stress disorder
Malingering
Munchausen syndrome by proxy
Psychopathy

REM, rapid eye movement.

attributed to pharmaceutical agents, such as benzodiazepines, and particularly nonbenzodiazepine drugs, are not uncommon.

Incidents of violent sleep-related behavior have been reviewed in the context of automatic behavior in general, with many well-documented cases resulting from a wide variety of disorders. Conditions associated with violence during the sleep period fall into two major categories: neurologic and psychiatric (Box 73.1). Those actions arising from a primary neurologic condition can be explained by applying conceptual approaches based on models of evanescent consciousness, the overlapping physiology of clinical disorders, and the platform of CPGs supported by semiotic neuroethology.

SPECTRUM OF CRIMINAL AND CIVIL ALLEGATIONS ASSOCIATED WITH SLEEP FORENSICS REFERRALS

Referrals to sleep medicine from the judicial system to consider involvement in criminal cases as a medical expert witness are occurring with ever-increasing regularity. There is now overwhelming evidence that very complex behaviors potentially resulting in criminal acts may arise from the foundation of sleep—without memory and conscious awareness. Cramer-Bornemann and colleagues[45] recently provided the first report on the spectrum of legal complaints that were referred by the legal community to a single academic sleep medicine center. From 2006 to 2017, this report documents 351 consecutive legal cases involving 23 categories of criminal and civil complaints, of which murder, manslaughter, assault/battery, and sexual assault were most prevalent (Fig. 73.4). By far the most common criminal complaint was sexual assault, accounting for approximately 41% of all cases. Of the possible sleep-related conditions implicated, parasomnias and pharmaceutical effects, chiefly involving zolpidem, were most prevalent. Of interest, regarding parasomnias, Cramer-Bornemann and colleagues[45] found that forensic implications were closely associated with confusional arousals as opposed to RBD, although the latter is well established as a frequent presenting clinical complaint. Of the 351 cases, although RBD may have been suspected in a few cases, the final analysis did not support RBD in any criminal case.

CLINICAL GUIDELINES TO ASSIST IN DETERMINING PURPORTED VIOLENCE ARISING FROM SLEEP

Legal implications of automatic behavior have been discussed and debated in the medical and legal literature.[46–50] The identification of a specific underlying organic or psychiatric sleep and violence condition does not establish causality for any given deed.

To assist in determining the existence of an underlying sleep disorder in a specific violent act, practitioners should follow guidelines based on peer-reviewed international clinical experience. Several clinical guidelines have been proposed[51–54] that identify certain features occurring as a result of a sleep disorder:

- There should be reason by history to suspect a *bona fides* sleep disorder. Similar episodes, with benign or morbid outcome, should have occurred previously.
- There has to be some degree of interaction with the environment. This behavior cannot be entirely passive in nature.
- The duration of the action is usually brief (seconds), although action of longer duration (minutes) does not necessarily exclude a sleep disorder or a sleep-related behavior. The action is usually abrupt, immediate, impulsive, and senseless—without apparent motivation. Although ostensibly purposeful, it is completely inappropriate to the total situation, out of (waking) character for the individual, and without evidence of premeditation.
- The victim is someone who merely happened to be present, usually in close proximity, and who may have been the stimulus for the arousal. Sleepwalkers rarely, if ever, seek out victims.[54–55]
- Immediately after return of consciousness, there is perplexity or horror, and there is no attempt to escape, conceal, or cover up the action. There is evidence of lack of awareness on the part of the sleepwalker during the event. There is usually some degree of amnesia for the event, but this amnesia need not be complete.
- In the case of sleep terrors, sleepwalking, or sleep inertia, the act may occur on awakening (rarely immediately on falling asleep) and usually at least 1 hour after sleep onset. It occurs on attempts to awaken the subject. The action has been potentiated by sedative-hypnotics or by prior sleep deprivation.
- Last, the violent behavior cannot be better explained by another mental disorder, medical condition, medication, or substance use. Ultimately, to attribute a violent behavior with criminal implications to parasomnia is a diagnosis of exclusion with the explicit understanding that other conditions are often more statistically likely. Note that this final guideline is also in accord with the diagnostic criteria for parasomnias in the *International Classification of Sleep Disorders*, 3rd edition.

The guidelines for determining the role of a sleep disorder in violence are not meant to be perceived as a rigid rule nor as a set of necessary criteria. They merely provide direction to gauge whether an argument in favor of a sleep disorder could be sustained in the formulation of a possible criminal defense. The strength of the argument should consider current

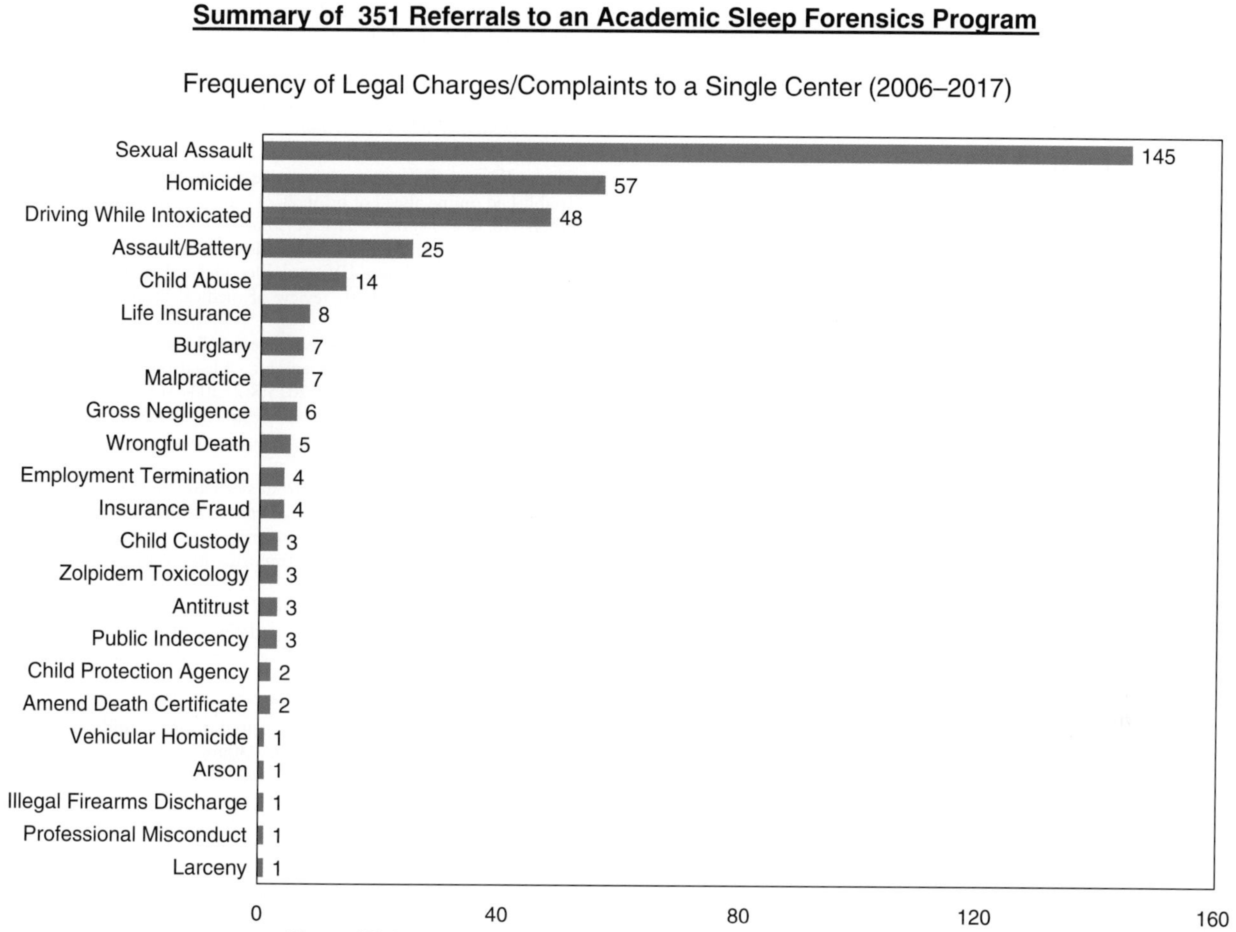

Figure 73.4 Summary of 351 referrals to an academic sleep forensics program.

neuroscientific models of consciousness and behavior as supported by the medical expert's specialized clinical experience.

To address the problem of junk science in the courtroom, some professional societies have developed guidelines for expert witness qualifications and testimony. The American Academy of Sleep Medicine's stance on expert witness testimony is to accept opinions held by the American Medical Association in its 2004 Report of the Council on Ethical and Judicial Affairs.[56]

Expert testimony must remain impartial. The ultimate test for accuracy and impartiality is a willingness to prepare testimony that could be presented unchanged for use by either the plaintiff or the defendant. The practitioner should be willing to submit such testimony for peer review. To establish consistency, the expert witness should make records from his or her previous expert witness testimony available to the attorneys and expert witnesses of both parties.

It is not the role of the medical expert to win the case for a client, although it is not uncommon to use irrelevant disingenuous technicalities in an attempt to deceive and/or to attain an advantage to secure the decision. Instead, the salient ethical decision for those who assume this mantle of medical expert witness is to recognize and value the privileged position given within our society as an educator inside the legal system by promoting current published peer-reviewed science and minimizing bias while rendering an opinion. The goal of the expert witness is not to simply ascertain or promote an argument addressing "reasonable doubt" in any given case because this is best deferred to legal parlance, most often provided during counsel's closing statements. Instead, the role of the expert witness is therefore to attempt to succinctly and clearly communicate scientifically valid information without bias within the context of the case to the jury, who in turn determines culpability based on this information. The weight of the decisions of either guilt or innocence should never rest in the hands of medical experts, whose task is to contribute to the due process of an efficient and functional legal system by ensuring that the jury is educated and well informed.[57]

CLINICAL PEARLS

The Role of Alcohol

In the past alcohol appeared on lists of potential triggers for NREM parasomnias. It was never accompanied by scientific citations that relied on empirical research. More recently, both the *Diagnostic and Statistical Manual of Mental Disorders*, 5th edition (DSM-5) and the *International Classification of Sleep Disorders*, 3rd edition (ISCD-3) have removed alcohol from lists of potential triggers due to the lack of empirical research support.[58,59,60] The ICSD-3 now states: *"Disorders of Arousal should not be diagnosed in the presence of alcohol intoxication."*

There are no empirical studies on the effects of alcohol on clinically diagnosed patients with sleepwalking. On the other hand, there are hundreds of scientific studies of the effects of alcohol on brain and behavior that can account for all behaviors attributed incorrectly to alcohol-induced sleepwalking. In addition, there are millions of cases of alcohol-related violence and sexual assault reported each year.

SUMMARY

Advances in neuroscience are increasing our understanding of how the brain enables action, including everything from simple movement, to thought, to the diurnal and nocturnal variability of sleep-wake processing.

The societal and cultural implications of these scientific advances have yet to be understood or even conceived.[61] However, the legal community is aware of the implications of this new neuroscience because science directly challenges the law's currently held constructs of consciousness as defined by *mens rea* and the voluntary act requirements. To study these problems, the John D. and Catherine T. MacArthur Foundation established the Law and Neuroscience Project in 2007 (www.lawneuro.org), comprising 40 neuroscientists, legal specialists, and philosophers.62 Two important concepts to be incorporated into the legal community are that consciousness is not all-or-none but occurs on a spectrum and that consciousness can be dissociated from behavior.

Sleep forensics does more than provide medical expert testimony in individual legal cases. The growth of cognitive neuroscience will continue to change our understanding of what it means to be human, and as a result, the law will have to change in conformity with it.

The conceptual approach to sleep forensics encourages further research to define and characterize mixed states of wake and sleep and the parasomnias. Understanding all of these is beneficial in understanding the spectrum of complex human behavior. Close collaboration among basic neuroscientists, sleep medicine clinicians, and the legal community will facilitate the development of a commonly shared concept of consciousness and culpability.

SELECTED READINGS

Casartelli L, Chiamulera C. Opportunities, threats and limitations of neuroscience data in forensic psychiatric evaluation. *Curr Opin Psychiatry.* 2013;26(5):468–473.

Cramer-Bornemann MA, Schenck CH, Mahowald MW. A review of sleep-related violence: the demographics of sleep forensics referrals to a single center. *Chest.* 2019;155(5):1059–1066.

Cramer-Bornemann MA. Sexsomnia: a medico-legal case-based approach in analyzing potential sleep-related abnormal sexual behaviors. In: Kothare SV, Ivanenko A, eds. *Parasomnias.* New York: Springer Science+Business Media; 2013:431–461.

Fernandez JD, Soca R. Sexsomnia in active duty military: a series of four cases [published online ahead of print, 2021 Apr 3] Mil Med. 2021;usab126.

Goldrich MS. *Report of the Council on Ethical and Judicial Affairs. CEJA Report 12-A-04.* American Medical Association; 2004.

Ingravallo F, Poli F, Gilmore EV, et al. Sleep related violence and sexual behavior in sleep: a systematic review of medical-legal case reports. *J Clin Sleep Med.* 2014;10:927–935.

Popat S, Winslade W. While you were sleepwalking: science and neurobiology of sleep disorders and the enigma of legal responsibility of violence during parasomnia. *Neuroethics.* 2015;8(2):203–214.

Pressman MR. *Sleepwalking, Criminal Behavior, and Reliable Scientific Evidence: A Guide for Expert Witnesses.* Washington, D.C.: American Psychological Association; 2018.

Pressman MR. Disorders of arousal from sleep and violent behavior: the role of physical contact and proximity. *Sleep.* 2007;30(8):1039–1047.

Pressman MR. Factors that predispose, prime, and precipitate NREM parasomnias in adults: clinical and forensics implications. *Sleep Med Rev.* 2007;11:5–30.

Pressman MR, Mahowald MW, Schenck CH, et al. Alcohol-induced sleepwalking or confusional arousal as a defense to criminal behavior: a review of scientific evidence, methods and forensic implications. *J Sleep Res.* 2007;16:198–212.

Schenck CH, Arnulf I, Mahowald MW. Sleep and sex: what can go wrong? A review of the literature on sleep related disorders and abnormal sexual behaviors and experiences. *Sleep.* 2007;30:683–702.

Tassinari CA, Rubboli G, Gardella E, et al. Central pattern generators for a common semiology in fronto-limbic seizures and in parasomnias: a neuroethologic approach. *Neurol Sci.* 2005;26:s225–s232.

Tononi G. Consciousness as integrated information: a provisional manifesto. *Biol Bull.* 2008;215:216–242.

Zadra A, Desautels A, Petit D, et al. Somnambulism: clinical aspects and pathophysiological hypotheses. *Lancet Neurol.* 2013;12:285–294.

A complete reference list can be found online at ExpertConsult.com.

Chapter

74

Legal Obligations of Persons Who Have Sleep Disorders or Who Treat or Hire Them

Daniel B. Brown

Chapter Highlights

- Patients have a right to refuse treatment for sleep disorders, but they may be liable if the foreseeable results of their sleep-disordered actions cause injury to others.
- Drivers who experience a "sudden blackout" while behind the wheel are excused from liability for damages arising from crashes caused as a result of their unexpected unconsciousness or seizure. However, this legal defense fails if the driver knew that his or her "blackout" or sleep episode was imminent or otherwise foreseeable.
- At least two states, New Jersey and Arkansas, factor fatigue into a criminal finding of reckless driving by drowsy drivers.
- Employers will be found liable for the negligence of their employees if the accident causing the injury occurred during the course of the employee's employment. Thus a trucking company will likely be found liable for injuries caused by an employee truck driver who falls asleep at the wheel while on the job.
- Employers are not likely to be found liable for injuries caused by their employees' sleep-induced actions that occur outside the scope of the employee's employment, even if the employee's fatigue is caused directly by the employer's overscheduling the employee's work hours.
- After passage of the Americans with Disabilities Act Amendments Act (ADAAA) of 2008, a sleep disorder is more likely to qualify as a "disability" for purposes of the ADA.

Sleep disorders such as obstructive sleep apnea (OSA) have been shown to fragment sleep and deprive the sufferer from restful and regenerative slumber.[1] In addition to comorbidities such as cardiopulmonary diseases, untreated OSA can lead to daytime hypersomnolence, which, in turn can directly and adversely affect an OSA sufferer's overall daytime performance on the job or on the road.[2] Sleep deprivation and sleep disorders, such as narcolepsy and idiopathic hypersomnia, can also impair daytime performance.

Legal systems examine a person's adherence to reasonable or statutorily defined standards of conduct and whether variance from such standards causes injury to others. Civil legal remedies generally award monetary penalties to injured parties as compensation for their damages incurred at the hands of a negligent party.[3] Criminal law metes out fines, imprisonment, or other punishments for conduct determined by state or federal statute to be injurious against the public at large.[3]

Legal proceedings under civil law focus on whether the wrongdoer had a duty of care to the injured party and whether the actor's breach of that duty caused the injured party's damages.[3] Criminal court actions focus on whether the actor's conduct violated each element of an activity that a particular statute considers to be criminal.[4]

Because there exists a causal connection between a person's sleep-disordered fatigue and such person's impaired daytime activity, the law will examine whether the sleep-disordered patient or those treating or employing the patient owe any special duty of care. That duty might arise to protect the patient or those with whom the patient may come into contact. This chapter briefly discusses the legal duties owed by sleep-disordered patients, the health care professionals who diagnose and treat them, and those persons or entities who employ potentially fatigue-prone persons under current US law. Most of the legal literature about sleep concern cases of sleep breathing disorders or sleep deprivation. Clinicians should consider that severe sleepiness from any cause may result in impaired performance and thus might have legal consequences.

SURVEY OF SLEEP APNEA IN THE LAW

What ultimately was called *sleep apnea* was described by several European groups in the 1960s, and the first description in a major journal appeared in 1973[5] (see Chapter 1). It was not until the 1980 Social Security benefits case of *Parks v. Harris* that the disorder was first seen in a reported decision in the

United States.[6] Parks, who had recently been diagnosed with sleep apnea, sued to overturn his benefits denial, based on a vocational expert's testimony that Parks suffered from uncontrolled somnolence due to a sleep disorder.[6] This early case did not consider disease treatment as a factor to defeat the disability claim because continuous positive airway pressure (CPAP) treatment for OSA was not available until 1981, or a year after the *Parks* decision.[7]

Legal notice of OSA was slow to develop after *Parks*. For example, in the 9 years after the *Parks* case, references to sleep apnea in all reported US appellate decisions appeared in only 17 cases. However, recognition of OSA in US jurisprudence grew quickly after 1980 and fairly exploded after 2005. References to OSA in reported US cases grew more than 4000% in the 25 years from 1980 to 2005, with 772 cases making some reference to OSA during this period. The references to OSA in US case law grew an astounding 5196 additional cases in the 8-year period between January 1, 2006 and July 1, 2014, with an additional 5581 cases in the following 5.5 years through January 1, 2020. To be clear, most of the 11,566 cases since *Parks* contain only passing references to OSA. For example, OSA often appears only as one of many conditions that make up a defendant's general health profile and has no bearing on the outcome of the case. Only a tiny fraction of these cases addresses a practitioner's liability for failure to diagnose or treat OSA.

Legal Obligations of Persons with Obstructive Sleep Apnea

A long-established general rule states that patients may choose to ignore their medical conditions and refuse treatment without facing legal consequences.[8] That right of refusal does not give those patients the right to ignore the risks to public safety caused by their decisions.[8] In California, for example, there is a statute requiring those with certain infectious diseases to take precautions to avoid the willful spread of their diseases through public contact.[9] Similarly, although an OSA patient may choose not to treat his or her condition with CPAP, oral therapy, or surgery, there can still be legal consequences to driving on the road while fatigued or performing other safety-sensitive activities.

A 1925 Connecticut Supreme Court case addressed the then novel question of a driver's legal duty when possessed by a sleep or other unconscious episode. In *Bushnell v. Bushnell*,[10] Mr. and Mrs. Bushnell drove from Connecticut to Rhode Island to drop their son off at college. On the return trip, Mr. Bushnell dozed off at the wheel and crashed into a tree in a single-car accident. Mrs. Bushnell, who had been sleeping while Mr. Bushnell drove, was injured in the accident.

Mrs. Bushnell sued her husband in negligence for failing to operate the car in a reasonable manner. Mr. Bushnell demurred, arguing in essence that he was to be excused from his duty to maintain control of the car while asleep because sleep, like any other unforeseeable blackout condition, comes about without warning. In essence, Mr. Bushnell argued that he had no duty to adjust his driving conduct that day because the instant of sleep onset cannot be determined in advance.

The Court challenged Mr. Bushnell's assertion that he had no warning of sleep onset. The court received medical evidence indicating that unlike a sudden blackout, sleep displays routine and recognizable precursor conditions. Based on early 20th century medical knowledge, these conditions include sensations of well-being, fatigue, and dulling of the senses. On the basis of this medical evidence the Court ruled that Mr. Bushnell knew, or should have known, that sleep was overtaking his driving and that he should have pulled off the road. Because his sleep episode was foreseeable, the Court found Mr. Bushnell liable for the cost of his wife's injuries. This ruling sets out the rule that an unforeseeable loss of consciousness, such as a suddenly unexpected seizure or blackout, would excuse the driver's duty to exercise due care in driving.

The "sudden blackout" rule is an important legal protection for drivers who suffer from a sudden and unforeseen onset of sleep or seizure disorder. This awareness may exist as a result of disease or past experience of a tendency to either fall asleep or lose consciousness while driving. If a patient knew that he or she suffered from frequent seizures or narcoleptic episodes several times a day, it would be negligent for that individual to get behind the wheel of a car even if the seizure events were unexpected.

An example of the endurance of the sudden blackout rule is seen in a 2006 Vermont case, *State v. Valyou*.[11] In *Valyou*, the defendant dozed off multiple times on the way to work yet continued his drive, eventually colliding with another vehicle after falling asleep.[11] The Vermont Supreme Court recited the Bushnell rule that falling asleep at the wheel does not, in and of itself, constitute gross negligence.[11] "On the other hand, when a driver is on sufficient notice as to the danger of falling asleep but nevertheless continues to drive, the driver's subsequent failure to stay awake may be grossly negligent."[11] The Vermont Supreme Court held the defendant liable because he remained at the wheel despite his knowledge that he was at high risk for falling asleep and injuring others. A Minnesota appeals court cited the Bushnell foreseeability doctrine in its discussion of sleep onset behind the wheel in the 2012 case of *Kellogg v. Finnegan*.[12]

CRIMINAL LIABILITY FOR DROWSY DRIVING

Some states have reviewed their negligent homicide or reckless driving laws and amended these to recognize erratic driving behavior caused by sleep deprivation. The first state to do so was New Jersey through enactment of Maggie's Law in 2003.[13] This law arose after the death of college student Margaret "Maggie" McConnell. McConnell was struck by a driver who had not slept for 30 hours leading up to the crash and had smoked crack cocaine hours before the accident.[14] Unlike drunkenness, no New Jersey statute required the State to consider drowsy driving as a condition or factor in the driver's reckless operation of the car. The judge refused to admit evidence of the driver's sleep deprivation to establish reckless behavior, and the driver received only a $200 penalty for causing the accident.[14]

Maggie's Law is an evidentiary rule establishing that proof of driving after 24 hours of sleeplessness "*shall* give rise to an inference that the defendant was driving recklessly" in order to convict a defendant for vehicular homicide[13] (*emphasis added*). The law also establishes that falling asleep while driving may infer recklessness without regard to sleeplessness.[13]

As finally adopted, Maggie's Law does not criminalize drowsy driving. Fatigued driving provides only inferential evidence that a defendant was driving recklessly. This is to be contrasted with intoxication, the presence of which under Maggie's Law "shall give rise to an inference that the defendant was driving recklessly."[13] Thus, unlike proof of intoxication, evidence of drowsy driving in New Jersey will not, by itself, automatically lead to a conviction of reckless driving.

Unlike inebriation, proof of reckless fatigue under Maggie's Law is itself difficult under the law's definition of sleeplessness. Conviction under Maggie's Law requires proof that the defendant was driving "after having been without sleep for a period in excess of 24 consecutive hours." Under this language, evidence that the driver took a 10-minute nap during the relevant 24-hour period can defeat a prosecutor's offer of the inference of reckless driving due to sleeplessness. Despite its shortcomings, Maggie's Law does open a path for states to consider drowsy driving as a factor in proving reckless driving in vehicular homicide cases.

In 2013 Arkansas became the second state to expand its negligent homicide statute to recognize fatigue as a factor in proving criminal vehicular homicide. The Arkansas law provides that a defendant shall be guilty of a class B felony for negligently causing the death of another person as a result of operating a vehicle, aircraft, or watercraft in a state of intoxication; while passing a stopped school bus; or while fatigued.[15] Fatigue is defined as "having been without sleep for a period of twenty-four consecutive hours," or "having been without sleep for a period of twenty-four consecutive hours and in the state of being asleep."[15] Unlike New Jersey's statute, Arkansas creates no distinction between driving fatigued and driving while intoxicated for purposes of proving negligent homicide.

Over the past 10 years several other states have proposed expanding their reckless driving laws to include drowsy driving.[16] All attempts have failed despite high-profile events, such as the sleep-deprived Wal-Mart truck driver who crashed into comedian Tracy Morgan's limousine in 2014. It appears that the inertia to address drowsy driving aggressively via legislation has abated from the early years of this century.

DUTIES OF PHYSICIANS TO SLEEP DISORDERED PATIENTS

On establishment of the physician-patient relationship, the physician owes the patient the duty of reasonable care present in the community when treating the patient.[17] Very few reported cases can be found that specifically hold a health care provider liable for malpractice surrounding diagnosis or treatment of sleep disorders. A rare example is the 1993 Louisiana case of *Cornett v. State, W.O. Moss Hospital*,[18] which stands for the principle that a physician owes the duty of reasonable care to treat the patient's conditions and warn the patient of potentially fatal risks that may be associated with untreated sleep disorders such as OSA.

In the Cornett case, the hospital treating Mr. Cornett was found liable for his death after he suffered from cardiopulmonary arrest. Mr. Cornett had complained to the hospital's physicians of sleep apnea symptoms, including his falling asleep at the wheel on three separate occasions. Nonetheless, the hospital physicians focused for months on Mr. Cornett's other medical conditions, ordering endocrinology tests for diabetes and acromegaly.

Although the hospital physicians knew that OSA is a potentially fatal condition, Mr. Cornett was never tested or treated for OSA or warned of the risks posed by untreated sleep apnea. At trial, expert witnesses testified that Mr. Cornett's death was likely caused by his untreated sleep apnea. The hospital's own medical expert testified that OSA is an emergency condition. On these facts, the hospital and its physicians were unable to avoid liability for malpractice after the patient's death.[18]

Within the duty of care that a physician owes to patients is the duty to obtain all pertinent information that may be relevant to a patient's health care. In *Feitzinger v. Simon*,[19] the patient, Mr. Feitzinger, was brought in for a routine hernia operation. The anesthesiologist neglected to inquire about Mr. Feitzinger's sleep apnea, and he did not learn about his history of OSA and his current use of CPAP. As a result, CPAP was not recommended for use during the surgery or during recuperation.

Mr. Feitzinger developed pneumonia and died of cardiac arrest 3 days after the hernia operation. His estate sued for malpractice, claiming that if the anesthesiologist had taken Mr. Feitzinger's complete medical history, the anesthesiologist would have known of the patient's OSA and would have recommended CPAP as part of the patient's procedure and recovery. According to expert testimony, CPAP use could have prevented the patient's pneumonia and eventual death. The court determined that the anesthesiologist's failure to check for a sleep-related breathing disorder established sufficient cause to take the trial to a jury.[19]

The principle of informed consent requires a physician who orders surgical treatment for OSA to inform the patient of surgical risks and treatment alternatives such as CPAP.[20] Thus, in *Russell v. Brown*,[20] the plaintiff visited an otolaryngologist complaining of snoring and recurrent tonsillitis. The physician recommended a tonsillectomy for the tonsillitis and the surgical uvulopharyngoplasty procedure for snoring after diagnosing the patient with mild sleep apnea.

The patient suffered complications from the surgery and brought suit against the physician, claiming that the physician never informed the patient of the risks of surgery or the availability of nonsurgical alternatives to his sleep apnea, such as CPAP or laser surgery. The jury nonetheless found in favor of the physician.[20] Medical experts testified at trial that the physician's actions reasonably fell within the accepted standard of care. In addition, the patient had signed a broad consent form that undercut his claim of invalid consent. Although the testimony supported the jury verdict in this case, the judge noted the established rule in informed consent cases that patients must be informed of alternative methods of treatment and the risks and benefits of such treatment.[20]

PHYSICIAN'S DUTIES WITH REGARD TO THIRD PARTIES

In the usual case, a physician is not liable for damages to third parties caused by the negligent or criminal acts of his or her patient.[21] In legal terms, it is atypical for a physician to owe a legal duty to unknown third parties.[21] Whether liability for the acts of a physician's sleep-disordered patient redounds to the sleep physician depends on the facts of the case and the physician's documented warning to patients of the potential adverse effects of failure to adhere to disease treatment.

Under a seminal California case, if a physician knew or should have known that his or her patient was likely to cause serious bodily harm to others, such as a psychiatric patient who tells his psychologist of his plans to kill a woman he was stalking, then a duty arises for the physician to take reasonable steps to prevent the patient causing injury to others.[22] However, this duty rarely attaches in circumstances in which the physician merely dispenses medication or diagnoses a potentially debilitating condition.[23] Although some contrary law exists,[24] courts usually reason that it is beyond a physician's control whether a patient takes the medication prescribed for the patient's condition[25] or, in the case of sleep apnea, whether the patient complies or fails to comply with the patient's CPAP therapy.

If a physician prescribes treatment whose use or nonuse could cause an impaired condition, then the physician has a duty to warn the patient of the risks stemming from use or misuse of the treatment.[26] In *Gooden v. Tips*,[27] a physician prescribed Quaalude tablets for his patient but neglected to warn her of the dangers of driving under the influence of the medication. After taking the pills, the patient injured third parties while driving. The injured third parties sued the physician for damages.

The court ruled that the physician was liable to the injured third parties not because the physician had a duty to prevent his patient from driving but because the physician had the duty to warn the patient not to drive, which he failed to do.[27] A physician treating a patient for OSA or another sleep disorder would have a similar duty to warn the patient about the risks of driving while drowsy or under the influence of medication that impairs performance.

The duty to warn applies only when the physician knows or should have known of the patient's condition that could give rise to injuries. In the case of *Calwell v. Hassan*,[28] the defendant physician examined his patient, Sharon Rylant, who complained of disordered sleep and fatigue. The physician ruled out narcolepsy and prescribed Elavil for Ms. Rylant's excessive daytime sleepiness. Ms. Rylant visited the physician for the next 3 years, but she never complained of drowsy driving during the years after her first visit. Ms. Rylant fell asleep while driving sometime later and ran into Calwell, who was bicycling along the street. Calwell sued the physician for failing to warn Rylant not to drive.

The court determined that the physician was not liable for Calwell's injuries.[28] The court focused on the years-long gap period during which Rylant continued to visit the defendant physician but during which she never complained of hypersomnolence. On these facts, the court determined that the defendant did not breach a duty of care by neglecting to warn Rylant of the dangers that hypersomnolence posed to her driving.[28]

A physician may discharge his or her duty to warn by complying with state public safety disclosure laws. These laws, which are discussed in more detail in Chapter 67, either require or recommend physicians to inform governmental public health or motor vehicle officials of the identity of patients who present a danger to the public by continuing to drive.

EMPLOYER'S DUTIES WITH REGARD TO EMPLOYEES WITH SLEEP DISORDER

In the United States the legal doctrine of *respondeat superior* provides that an employer may be held vicariously liable for the acts of an employee that are performed as part of the employee's duties.[29] Because many employers, such as trucking companies, retailers such as Wal-Mart, or mail delivery services, employ drivers, those employers will be vicariously liable if the driver falls asleep at the wheel and injures a third party in a crash while performing his or her job.[30]

If the accident occurs within the scope of employment, then the trucking company will often try to defend by denying that their driver acted negligently. Thus, when Norman Munnal fell asleep at the wheel of a tractor-trailer and killed a woman when he drifted into oncoming traffic, his employer invoked Ohio's version of the "sudden blackout" doctrine by blaming the accident on Munnal's "sudden unconsciousness."[31]

As discussed, the sudden blackout defense fails if the defendant knew that loss of consciousness was likely to occur and thus was foreseeable.[32] In the Munnal case, Munnal testified that he had a propensity to fall asleep at unpredictable times and that he had fallen asleep at the wheel at least once before.[31] Munnal's fiancé testified that he slept poorly and only slept an average of 3 hours a night despite Munnal's testimony that he slept 8 hours. Munnal was also diagnosed with severe OSA after a sleep test ordered after the accident.[31]

Although there was no evidence that Munnal was aware he had sleep apnea before the test, or that his fiancé had shared her concerns about the quality of his sleep, the court found sufficient evidence that Munnal was aware of his excessive sleepiness. As a result of this knowledge and an expert's testimony that Munnal probably fell asleep rather than suffering from a sudden blackout, the court found Munnal negligent for failing to operate the truck in a safe manner. Munnal's employer was held vicariously liable because Munnal had been operating the rig within the scope of his employment.

EMPLOYER'S OVERSCHEDULING LIABILITY

Some employees who fall asleep at the wheel after the end of an overly long workday have sought to hold their employers liable for scheduling excessive work time. Courts generally refuse to hold employers liable for the postwork actions of their employees, even if the employer contributed to the employee's alleged fatigue.[32]

The case of *Black v. William Insulation Co.*[33] is representative. In that case, Black fell asleep while driving and crossed over into oncoming traffic. The resulting collision killed Black. Black's widow sued her husband's employer, alleging that the trucking company negligently required Black to commute long distances and work long hours and that the employer had failed to provide proper training or safeguards to prevent such an accident from occurring.[33]

The court determined that the employer owed no duty to Black and that it was Black's personal responsibility to ensure that he was capable of safely driving to work.[33] Some of Black's personal decisions, such as working a second job and completing long commutes, were considered more significant contributions to his sleepiness than his working conditions.[33]

In *Barclay v. Briscoe*,[34] Sgt. Barclay suffered catastrophic injuries after a head-on collision with Richardson, who had fallen asleep on his way home after a 22-hour work shift. Barclay sued Richardson's estate and his employer. The court stated that it was the employee's responsibility to get to or from work and that absent special circumstances an employer was not liable for the actions of employees traveling to and from work.[34] The court did not determine the 22-hour shift to be a special circumstance, especially because Richardson elected to complete such a long shift rather than having it forced on him by the company.[34]

As a general rule, businesses providing services through independent contractors instead of full or part-time employees do not assume liability for the acts or omissions of their contracted workforce.[35] Gig workers, such as Uber and Lyft drivers, present novel liability questions for the web-based platforms that set drivers' rates, prohibit anonymous rides, and limit the number of consecutive hours that a driver may work.[36] A recent federal appeals court ruled that sufficient facts exist in arrangements between UberBlack and its drivers to justify further litigation to determine if drivers attain "employee" status for purposes of the Fair Labor Standards Act and analogous Pennsylvania law.[36] A finding of employee status would likely shift liability for accidents caused by hypersomnolent Uber drivers while on the job from the driver to Uber.

EMPLOYER'S DUTY TO ACCOMMODATE AN EMPLOYEE'S SLEEP DISORDER UNDER THE AMERICAN WITH DISABILITIES ACT

The federal Americans with Disabilities Act (ADA) works in conjunction with various state job protection statutes to protect employees with disabilities from discrimination by their employer.[37] The ADA prohibits employers from firing, failing to promote, or failing to provide "reasonable accommodations" to employees who suffer from a protected disability.[37]

A protected disability is one that limits one or more "major life activities" as defined by the court system.[38] The court seldom adds new major life activities, but it has long held that sleeping and breathing are major life activities.[39] As discussed later, few cases of OSA or other sleep disorders rose to the level of a qualified disability under the law before adoption of the ADA amendments in 2008.

To establish an ADA violation, an employee must show that (1) he or she is disabled, (2) he or she is otherwise qualified to perform the essential functions of the job with or without reasonable accommodation, and (3) the employer took an adverse job action against the employee because of the disability or failed to make a reasonable accommodation.[40]

Before passage of the American with Disabilities Act Amendments Act (ADAAA) in 2008,[41] few courts found that a diagnosis of OSA affected either sleep or breathing sufficiently to trigger ADA protections. Upon adoption of the ADAAA, Congress lowered the plaintiff's burden so that he or she needs only to show a "degree of functional limitation," which is a lower standard than the "substantially limits" standard applied before the ADAAA. The ADAAA applies to fact patterns occurring on or after January 1, 2009.

Before the ADAAA, allegations of OSA or sleeping difficulties without proof of an impairment to a major life activity were found insufficient to establish a substantial limitation in the major life activity of sleeping.[42] One court concluded that an individual's inability to get to sleep did not adversely affect the activity of sleep because difficulty sleeping was deemed extremely widespread and because the plaintiff in question did not provide evidence that his difficulties were any worse than difficulties suffered by a large number of other adults.[42] Successful use of oral appliances or positive airway pressure therapy to treat symptoms would also remove OSA as a disability for ADA purposes altogether because the courts found that successful treatment negated disability symptoms.[43]

There were rare circumstances when a court would find OSA severe enough to trigger pre-ADAAA protections,[44] particularly in situations in which therapy such as CPAP failed to relieve fatigue caused by severe sleep apnea.[45] The 2009 Pennsylvania case, *Peter v. Lincoln Technical Institute, Inc.*, is illustrative.[45] There, the plaintiff testified to waking up five to six times a night and falling asleep during the day, even while working and driving to work. The patient's disorder was unresponsive to a variety of therapies, including CPAP, tonsil surgery, oral medication, and pure oxygen therapy. The extreme and untreatable aspects of this particular patient's sleep apnea led to a disability determination.

The ADAAA was designed to refocus ADA cases on determining whether employers are discriminating against their employees, rather than extensively analyzing whether the patient is truly disabled under the legal definition. The plaintiff still possesses a burden of proof to show that he or she is disabled compared with the general population, yet the burden may be met by merely providing physician testimony of a sleeping disorder that interferes with sleep and leads to falling asleep on the job. In addition, successful CPAP treatment no longer acts as a mitigating measure to prevent OSA suffers from claiming a disability under the ADA.

The 2013 case of *Orne v. Christie*[46] showcases several of the changes seen in ADA decisions since the ADAAA was passed. While working as Primary Counsel to the Virginia State Corporation Commission's Bureau of Financial Institutions, Orne was informed he had been sleeping on the job, which he attributed to having difficulty sleeping at night. Orne went to a sleep disorders specialist, was diagnosed with OSA, and was prescribed CPAP. This treatment proved effective in treating Orne's symptoms.

Orne made his employer aware of the diagnosis and treatment plan, yet, after a few months, he was told that he would have to accept a demotion with a pay cut or face termination. The court found that Orne's sleep apnea and the corresponding sleepiness he experienced during the day was sufficient to qualify him as disabled under the new ADAAA standards. In addition, the successful CPAP treatment had no impact on the presence of a disability.[46]

SUMMARY

OSA and other types of sleep disorders or deprivation may result in drowsiness during the day and can impair one's ability to work or drive. Although patients have a right to refuse treatment for sleep disorders, they may be liable if that decision harms others. For instance, new criminal negligence laws in certain states address impaired driving due to fatigue.

Physicians have obligations when treating a patient with a sleep disorder. Physicians who have created a physician-patient relationship must inform patients of the risks of driving while suffering from a sleep disorder that may result in severe sleepiness. Employers will be liable for the negligence of their employees but do not owe any duty to employees for actions after they leave work, even if the employer scheduled the employee to work extremely long hours.

Finally, a 2008 update to the ADA has loosened the definition of a disability for purposes of ADA protections. As a result, sleep-related breathing disorders and other sleep disorders are more likely to qualify as a disability under the ADAAA language.

CLINICAL PEARLS

Clinicians must inform patients they are managing of the risks of operating a motor vehicle or heavy machinery while suffering from a disorder that may result in severe sleepiness.

Clinicians must be familiar with the regulations concerning sleepiness and operating a motor vehicle in their jurisdiction.

SELECTED READINGS

Colvin LJ, Collop NA. Commercial motor vehicle driver obstructive sleep apnea screening and treatment in the United States: an update and recommendation overview. *J Clin Sleep Med*. 2016;12(1):113–125.

Fouladpour N, Jesudoss R, Bolden N, et al. Perioperative complications in obstructive sleep apnea patients undergoing surgery: a review of the legal literature. *Anesth Analg*. 2016;122(1):145–151.

Idzikowski C, Rumbold J. Sleep in a legal context: the role of the expert witness. *Med Sci Law*. 2015;55(3):176–182.

Masullo A, Feola A, Marino V, et al. Sleep disorders and driving licence: the current Italian legislation and medico-legal issues. *Clin Ter*. 2014;165(5):e368–e372.

Rumbold J. Automatism and driving offences. *J Forensic Leg Med*. 2013;20(7):825–829.

Svider PF, Pashkova AA, Folbe AJ, et al. Obstructive sleep apnea: strategies for minimizing liability and enhancing patient safety. *Otolaryngol Head Neck Surg*. 2013;149(6):947–953.

Venkateshiah SB, Hoque R, Collop N. Legal aspects of sleep medicine in the 21st century. *Chest*. 2018;154(3):691–698.

Watling CN, Mahmudul Hasan M, Larue GS. Sensitivity and specificity of the driver sleepiness detection methods using physiological signals: a systematic review. *Accid Anal Prev*. 2021;150:105900.

A complete reference list can be found online at ExpertConsult.com.

Chapter 75

Legal Aspects of Fatigue- and Safety-Sensitive Professions

Daniel B. Brown

Chapter Highlights

- Lack of sleep can cause mistakes in the workplace. These mistakes can have tragic consequences.
- Various industries, including maritime, aerospace, medical, military, nuclear, and shipping, have implemented regulations concerning fatigue and sleep to reduce workplace accidents.
- Drowsy driving regulations have been implemented in many states, potentially resulting in legal liability for those driving without adequate sleep.

Lack of sleep can inhibit performance and cause mistakes in the workplace. Over the past few decades, high-profile incidents resulting from a lack of sleep have created a public awareness of the dangers of sleep deprivation. In response, the US Congress and some governments around the world, as well as many administrative agencies and professional groups, have weighed the harmful risks of lack of sleep and have crafted safety regulations to protect their members in the workplace and the community as a whole.

HISTORY

Lack of sleep can cause mistakes in the workplace that have tragic repercussions. Historically, many accidents have been attributed to lack of sleep. A partial list follows:

- In 1979 a nuclear reactor located on Three Mile Island in Pennsylvania experienced a partial meltdown resulting from human error.[1] Shift workers were suffering from lack of sleep and did not notice that a stuck valve was causing the reactor to lose coolant.[2] Eventually, the core overheated and was damaged.[3]
- In January 1986 the space shuttle *Challenger* exploded moments after launch and resulted in the deaths of all astronauts on board.[4] This incident has been partially attributed to lack of sleep because key managers had had only 2 hours of sleep and had been on duty since 1 a.m., which resulted in poor decision making.[5]
- In April 1986 the Chernobyl nuclear plant experienced a serious meltdown.[6] This disaster was a result of human error in conditions in which employees were fatigued after working more than 13 hours.[7] The aftermath of this event resulted in the most horrific nuclear accident in human history.[8]
- In 1989 the Exxon *Valdez* ran aground and spilled 10.8 million gallons of crude oil into the ocean.[9] This disaster occurred after the third mate stayed awake for more than 18 hours and, being greatly fatigued, did not properly account for the ship's position.[10] This oil spill dealt a great deal of damage to the surrounding wildlife, and the area's environment has still not fully recovered.[11]
- In 1999 American Airlines Flight 1420 crashed during a severe thunderstorm.[12] Although the main cause was the weather, both pilots for the aircraft were near the end of their 14-hour duty shift and displayed poor judgment by trying to land in an area with such dangerous conditions.[13]
- In 2013 an engineer operating a Metro-North train in the Bronx in New York City fell asleep at the controls, which resulted in the train derailing from the track.[14] Although the engineer had no previous record of a sleep disorder, later investigation found that he had sleep apnea.[15]
- In 2020 because of the many sleep-related transportation disasters, two of the ten items of the 2020 MOST WANTED LIST of the National Transportation Safety Board are related to sleep: Reduce Fatigue-Related Accidents and Require Medical Fitness—Screen For and Treat Obstructive Sleep Apnea.

LEGAL OBLIGATIONS REGARDING FATIGUE IN NON–SAFETY-SENSITIVE INDUSTRIES

Businesses engaging in retail, entertainment, lodging, and other activities not generally considered to be safety sensitive typically operate without regulatory limits on employees' hours of service. Employers in these fields are free to schedule their employees for as many hours of service as their employee desires and as the employer is willing to pay. An employer's legal risk in these industries for their employees' impaired job performance as a result of fatigue is far more limited than the risk faced by employers in safety-sensitive industries such as transportation.

For example, courts routinely find employers who overschedule their employees to be free from liability for injuries caused by fatigued employees at the end of their lengthy shift. The case of *Barclay v. Briscoe*, 47 A.3d 560, 427 Md. 270 (Md.,

2012), is instructive. In *Barclay*, a longshoreman fell asleep at the wheel while traveling home after working a 22-hour shift at his job site located at the Port of Baltimore. The longshoreman crashed head-on into a morning commuter, causing catastrophic injuries to the commuter and the longshoreman's own death. The commuter brought suit against the longshoreman's employer for primary negligence in failing to protect the motoring public from an employee driving after an unreasonably long shift.

Following rules laid down by most American state courts, the Maryland Court of Appeals denied the injured commuter's request for damages. The Court found that the employer did no more than establish the work schedule for the job. It did nothing to affirmatively control whether Richardson drove home in a fatigued state. As such, the Court held that an employer has no duty to a third party who may be injured by a commuting employee based solely on the fact that an employee's fatigue was a foreseeable consequence of the employment.[16] In that regard the Court flatly refused "to fashion some type of judicially-imposed maximum working hours standard across all industries."

INDUSTRY REGULATIONS

Unlike employers in non–safety-sensitive industries, employers whose workers' tasks have the direct ability to affect public safety are subject to legal obligations for the fatigue-impaired actions of their employees. These legal obligations arise in the form of government and industry regulation addressing hours of service and fatigue management. The remainder of this chapter discusses a variety of these regulatory schemes.

Maritime

US maritime law, codified in 46 U.S.C. § 8104, has set rules to reduce accidents resulting from fatigue. These rules set limits on how many hours an individual may work per day, while leaving an exception for emergencies.

As stated in § 8104, for vessels leaving port, an officer in charge of deck watch must have been off duty for at least 6 hours of the previous 12 hours.[17] When serving on certain kinds of vessels under 100 gross tons, mariners may not work for more than 9 of 24 hours when in port and more than 12 of 24 hours when at sea.[18] An exception waives these requirements during an emergency.[19] On certain larger vessels over 100 gross tons, mariners on the boat must be split into at least three separate watches, where each watch rotates duty shifts.[20] This allows those not on duty to rest and recuperate. Those on deck or in the engine department may not be required to work for more than 8 hours a day.[21] Again, exceptions can apply in case of an emergency.[22]

Specific rules may apply to certain kinds of vessels. For instance, on towing vessels, mariners may not work for more than 12 hours per day, except in an emergency.[23] Furthermore, on a tanker, a mariner may work up to 15 hours of every 24-hour period or up to 36 hours of a 72-hour period, except for emergencies.[24]

National Aeronautics and Space Administration

The National Aeronautics and Space Administration (NASA) recognizes that circadian disruption caused by shift work or by extended work hours can result in impaired judgment, slowed reaction times, and visual/cognitive fixation.[25] These factors can lead to potential mission critical errors and mishaps. NASA's Procedural Requirements recognize that "[s]afe work practices that minimize human error factors, especially fatigue, require safe work-rest cycles and shift scheduling."[26]

According to NASA's Procedural Requirements (NPR) for noncritical positions, employees may not work more than the following maximum work times: (1) 12 consecutive hours (16 consecutive hours in emergency situations with approval); (2) 60 hours during a 7-day workweek; (3) 7 consecutive days without at least 1 full day off; (4) 240 hours during a 4-week period; and (5) 2500 hours during a rolling 12-month period.[27] The NPR further provides that employees must be given at least 8 hours off duty between shifts.[28] A minimum of 10 hours off duty is preferred, and 12 hours or more is optimal to accommodate employee commute time and domestic and sleep needs.[29]

Medical Residents

New York was the first state to implement residency work duration limits.[30] Support for these regulations grew as a result of the death of a patient resulting from improper medical care, believed to have been a result of overworked physicians and residents.[31] New York's work duration limits on medical residents, codified in 10 CRR-NY § 405.4, states that work hours for medical residents with inpatient care responsibilities must not exceed 80 hours per week over a 4-week period.[32] In addition, residents must not be scheduled to work for more than 24 consecutive hours.[33] On-call duties for surgical residents are exempt from these requirements if (1) such shifts have infrequent interruptions limited to patients that the resident has a continuing responsibility, (2) this responsibility occurs no more than every third night, (3) a continuous assignment that includes a night shift on-call is followed by a nonworking period of at least 16 hours, and (4) additional policies are implemented by the hospital to relieve residents after an unusually active on-call period.[34]

In 2003, after New York implemented these work-hour restrictions, the Accreditation Council for Graduate Medical Education (ACGME) created a new accreditation requirement, mirroring New York's law, which applies to medical residents in all accredited institutions.[35] In 2011 ACGME issued a revised rule, which was further revised in 2017.[36] Currently, ACGME requires that fellowship and residency programs limit clinical and educational duty hours to no more than 24 hours of continuous hours for all residents up to 80 hours per week, averaged over a 4-week period, inclusive of all in-house call activities and moonlighting.[37] A review committee may grant programs a limited exception, up to a maximum of 88 hours per week.[38] Residents must be scheduled for a minimum of 1 free day a week, averaged over 4 weeks.[39] At-home calling cannot be assigned on these free days.[40] Rest facilities are also necessary, even when overnight call is not required, to accommodate the fatigued resident.[41]

United States Military

Unlike many other regulations that mandate compliance, regulations issued by the U.S. Army tend to act more as a guidance; however, that is to be expected given the uncertain day-to-day conditions in the field. The Army's training regulations recommend that each trainee receive 7 hours of sleep per night.[42] The Army's *Combat and Operational Stress Control Manual for Leaders and Soldiers in the Field* describes the factors considered by military personnel when scheduling time for sleep.[43] The Army recommends the best time for sleep as between 11 p.m. and 7 a.m. because of the body's natural circadian rhythms.[44] It also recommends 7 to 8 hours of sleep per 24-hour period and cautions that any reduction in this amount will degrade performance.[45] Although continuous sleep is preferred, sleep may be divided between two or more shorter periods to obtain the full 7 to 8 hours of sleep.[46] The manual also prioritizes the need to sleep based on the task being performed.[47] Leaders making critical decisions have a top priority for sleep.[48] Soldiers on guard duty, performing tedious tasks, or analyzing information have second priority for sleep.[49] Finally, soldiers performing duties that require only physical labor have third priority for sleep.[50]

Nuclear Power Plants

In light of several high-profile nuclear incidents that were at least partially caused by operator fatigue, the U.S. Nuclear Regulatory Commission has mandated limits on the work hours of nuclear power plant operators. As codified in 10 C.F.R. § 26.205, employees may work up to 16 hours per 24-hour period, 26 hours per 48-hour period, and 72 hours per 7-day period.[51] Exceptions may be granted in limited circumstances.[52] Employees must also be provided rest breaks after each work period.[53] These rest break lengths vary depending on how long the employee had been working.[54] For instance, employees must receive at least a 10-hour break after working for at least 10 hours.[55]

In addition, employees must receive a minimum number of days off, depending on their work schedule.[56] For example, employees working 10-hour shifts must have, on average, at least 2 days off of work per week.[57] In the event of an unscheduled preparedness drill, the duration of an employee's unscheduled participation in this drill is not calculated into the hours worked that day.[58]

Railroads

With passage of the Rail Safety Improvement Act of 2008, Congress directed certain railroads to develop and implement a railroad safety risk reduction program.[59] By statute, the program must include a fatigue management plan designed to reduce fatigue experienced by railroad employees and to reduce the likelihood of accidents, incidents, injuries, and fatalities caused by fatigue.[60] This fatigue management plan must consider physiologic and human factors that affect fatigue and promote appropriate fatigue countermeasures to address safety concerns, such as scheduling practices, napping policies, and avoidance of abrupt changes in rest cycles for employees.[61]

Existing regulations address hours of service limitations for railroad employees as follows. These regulations, codified in 49 U.S.C. § 21103, provide that employees may spend up to 276 hours per month working for their carrier.[62] In addition, employees are limited to no more than 12 consecutive hours of work.[63] Each employee must receive at least 10 consecutive hours of off-duty time per 24 hours.[64] Employees must not work more than 6 or 7 consecutive days, depending on how much time the employee had off before that work duration.[65] Exceptions may apply in case of emergency; however, even then, employees are limited to 4 additional hours per 24-hour period.[66]

Trucking

Drowsiness among truck drivers is a highly prevalent risk in the trucking industry. For instance, a study sponsored by the Federal Motor Carrier Safety Administration (FMCSA) found that 45% of US truck drivers sometimes or often had difficulty staying awake while driving.[67] In addition, a number of high-profile accidents have involved truck drivers who fell asleep at the wheel,[68] and a 5-day study found that truck drivers tended to average 4.78 hours of sleep per day with only 5.18 hours in bed per day.[69] As a result, regulations limit the number of hours a truck driver may be on the road.

Trucking regulations cover commercial motor vehicles (CMVs). A CMV vehicle is one that (1) weighs 10,001 pounds or more; (2) is transporting hazardous materials such that it requires a placard; (3) is designed or used to transport 16 or more passengers, including the driver, not for compensation; or (4) is designed or used to transport 9 or more passengers, including the driver, for compensation.[70]

Solo truck drivers that transport property may drive for a maximum of 11 hours after 10 consecutive hours off duty.[71] At the same time, a driver cannot be on duty for more than 14 consecutive hours.[72] Drivers may not drive more than 60 hours per 7-day period or 70 hours per 8-day period.[73] However, truck drivers who reach this hour limit may rest for 34 consecutive hours that include two nights from 1 a.m. to 5 a.m., and then they may resume driving.[74] During the national health emergency for COVID-19, this 1 a.m. to 5 a.m. carve-out is suspended. The "restart" may be used up to once per 168-hour period.[75] Truck drivers are also required to take a 30-minute break during the first 8 hours of a shift.[76]

In light of the COVID-19 emergency, the FMCSA revised these hours of service regulations to provide greater flexibility.[77] In part, the new rules relaxed the 30-minute break requirement to reflect 8 hours of actual driving rather than the 8 hours of duty time, which may not include actual driving.[78] A short-haul exception to the hours of service requirement was expensed to 150 air miles and deems 14-hour work shifts as short-haul trips for purposes of the exception.[79]

The U.S. Department of Transportation (USDOT) is also working toward requiring drivers to undergo sleep apnea testing. Although the USDOT gained the congressional authority to require this testing in October 2013, a lengthy, formal rule-making proceeding must first be completed before this requirement may take effect.[80] A formal rule-making proceeding is a process whereby the administrative agency researches the costs and benefits of a new rule and allows for public comment from the industry.[81] Some applauded this decision, arguing that testing and treatment of obstructive sleep apnea could cost the industry more than $1 billion; the government should take its time to ensure that proper analysis is completed and that suitable regulation language is chosen.[82] Others see the rule-making process as an unnecessary delay in a much-needed rule.[83] These groups worry that the rule-making process will take several years and that new sleep testing requirements may never be implemented.[84]

Airlines

Airline pilots are restricted from working excessive hours by the Federal Aviation Administration (FAA). Pilots of a one- or two-pilot crew may fly for up to 500 hours per calendar quarter, 800 hours per two consecutive calendar quarters, and 1400 hours per calendar year.[85] For a 24-hour period, work duration limits vary depending on whether it is a one- or two-pilot crew.[86] For a one-pilot crew, the total flight time cannot exceed 8 hours.[87] For a two-pilot crew, the total flight time cannot exceed 10 hours.[88] After a duty period, a varying amount of rest is required depending on whether the destination crosses time zones and whether the flight was extended because of unforeseen factors, such as bad weather.[89] For instance, a multiple–time zone flight that had no unforeseen extensions of flight time would require that the pilot rest for at least 14 hours.[90]

Currently, the FAA requires that all pilots diagnosed with obstructive sleep apnea have a generally disqualifying medical condition that must be treated to avoid issuance of a special medical certificate.[91] In November 2013 the FAA's Air Surgeon concluded that OSA is nearly universal in obese people who have a body mass index (BMI) over 40. The surgeon proposed guidance that would have required all pilots with a BMI of 40 or more to be evaluated for OSA and treated for OSA if needed to obtain medical clearance to fly.[92] Reacting to industry and congressional concern, the FAA discarded the objective 40 BMI standard in favor of a more flexible standard.[93] The newer rule sets out guidance for medical examiners to screen for sleep disorders as part of the fitness-to-fly examination.[94] Pilots exhibiting indicia of sleep apnea are issued medical certificates and are expected to undergo a sleep evaluation within 90 days. The evaluation need not be performed by a sleep specialist.[95] Pilots who are diagnosed with sleep apnea must document their initiation, use, and effectiveness of treatment for continued clearance to fly.[95] The FAA has published a flowchart describing the process for screening apnea in pilots consistent with current guidance.[96]

DROWSY DRIVING

Drowsy driving can greatly increase the risk for a collision. For instance, a study found that the risk for a car crash nearly tripled when drivers had less than 5 hours of sleep in a 24-hour period.[97] Drowsiness has also been compared with alcohol consumption. In one study, individuals who had been awake for 24 hours performed like individuals with a blood alcohol concentration of 0.10%.[98] For comparison, the legal blood alcohol concentration limit in the United States is 0.08%.[99]

In addition to regulating professionals' sleep, some states have amended laws to factor sleep deprivation into their definition of criminally reckless driving. The first state to do so was New Jersey, which enacted legislation referred to as "Maggie's Law" as part of the state's criminal code in 1997, following the death of college student Margaret "Maggie" McConnell.[100] A driver, who had not slept for 30 hours before the crash and had smoked crack cocaine hours before the accident, hit McConnell.[101] During litigation, the judge refused to admit evidence of the driver's sleep deprivation to establish reckless behavior, and the driver received only a $200 penalty for causing the accident.[102]

Maggie's Law is an evidentiary rule establishing that proof of driving after 24 hours of sleeplessness "*may* give rise to an inference that the defendant was driving recklessly" (*emphasis added*).[103] The law also establishes that falling asleep while driving may infer recklessness without regard to sleeplessness.[104] Although it may prove difficult to establish that a driver was asleep at the wheel at the time of the collision, or had been awake for the entirety of the 24-hour statutory period, Maggie's Law establishes that drowsy driving, if proven, can uphold a criminal conviction in the state of New Jersey.

In 2013 Arkansas became the second state to pass a drowsy driving amendment to its negligent homicide statute, making it a class B felony to negligently cause the death of another person as a result of operating a vehicle, aircraft, or watercraft while fatigued.[105] "Fatigued" is defined as "having been without sleep for a period of twenty-four (24) consecutive hours," or "having been without sleep for a period of twenty-four (24) consecutive hours and in the state of being asleep."[106]

Several states, including Massachusetts, Tennessee, New York, and Oregon, have attempted to pass statutes similar to those found in New Jersey and Arkansas that would criminalize drowsy driving.[107] Although these attempts have proved unsuccessful thus far, high-profile events, such as the sleep-deprived Walmart truck driver who crashed into comedian Tracy Morgan's limousine in 2014,[108] frequently raise public awareness of the issue and draw significant attention of lawmakers.

CLINICAL PEARLS

- Generally, in situations after work hours, employers do not have a legal duty to protect the motoring public from the drowsy driving of employees whose fatigue may have been caused by the employer overscheduling the employee's work shifts.
- On the other hand, employers are liable under law for the negligent acts of their employees, such as vehicular accidents caused by impaired driving because of fatigue, if the accident occurred during the employee's course of employment.
- To protect the public, the US government imposes hours of service regulations on many safety-sensitive industries, such as commercial trucking, nuclear power, and commercial airlines.

SUMMARY

Lack of sleep can cause mistakes in the workplace and while driving, leading to tragic consequences. Historically, many high-profile accidents have been at least partially attributed to lack of sleep. Various industries, including maritime, aerospace, medical, military, nuclear, and shipping, have implemented regulations concerning fatigue and sleep to reduce workplace accidents. For instance, the ACGME requires that medical residents limit their duty hours for a medical institution to maintain its accreditation. Some states have also implemented drowsy driving regulations, which result in criminal liability for a driver who causes a collision after remaining conscious for at least 24 hours.

SELECTED READINGS

Erin E, Flynn-E, Omer A, et al. Industrial regulation of fatigue: lessons learned from aviation. *J Clin Sleep Med.* 2019;15(4):537–538.

Han SH, Lee GY, Hyun W, Kim Y, Jang JS. Obstructive sleep apnea in airline pilots during daytime sleep following overnight flights [published online ahead of print, 2021 Apr 28]. *J Sleep Res.* 2021:e13375.

Mansfield D, Kryger M. Regulating danger on the highways: hours of service regulations. *Sleep Health.* 2015;1(4):311–313.

National Sleep Foundation. Available at: www.DrowsyDriving.org.

National Transportation Safety Board. 2019-2020 Most Wanted List: https://www.ntsb.gov/safety/mwl/Pages/default.aspx.

Rasleara TG, Gertlerb J, DiFioreb A. Work schedules, sleep, fatigue, and accidents in the US railroad industry. *Fatigue Biomed Health Behav.* 2013;1(1-2):99–115.

Simonelli G, Bellone G, Golombek D, et al. Hours of service regulations for professional drivers in continental Latin America. *Sleep Health.* 2018;4(5):472–475. https://doi.org/10.1016/j.sleh.2018.07.009.

Williamson A, Friswell R. Fatigue in the workplace: causes and countermeasures. *Fatigue Biomed Health Behav.* 2013;1(1–2):81–98.

A complete reference list can be found online at ExpertConsult.com.

Chapter 76

Sleep Medicine Clinical Practice and Compliance—United States

Daniel B. Brown

Chapter Highlights

- The delivery of sleep medicine and the treatment of sleep disorders in the United States are highly fragmented. Government and most commercial insurance payers cover sleep medicine, sleep testing, and sleep therapy under separate reimbursement categories with separate requirements for licensure, accreditation, personnel certification, and coverage conditions. Legal restrictions on patient self-referrals can limit, in certain cases, the ability of treating physicians to dispense continuous positive airway pressure (CPAP), mandibular advancement oral appliance therapy, or other items of durable medical equipment to treat their own patients' sleep disease.
- In-laboratory and home sleep testing (HST) for obstructive sleep apnea performed by physicians and stand-alone sleep centers are reimbursed by Medicare, Medicaid, TRICARE, and most commercial insurance payers. Polysomnography and HST for many other sleep disorders, such as insomnia, restless legs syndrome, and narcolepsy, are not typically covered by government or private insurance.
- Sleep medicine is especially well suited for remote practice via telemedicine. Electronic data from sleep tests and CPAP machines are routinely collected and transmitted via web-based applications for interpretation and monitoring by remote sleep physicians. State legislation has normalized commercial insurance coverage for many telemedicine services across the United States, but Health Insurance Portability and Accountability Act (HIPAA) privacy rules and Medicare coverage conditions severely limit most in-home telemedicine encounters. Emergency rules adopted in response to the COVID-19 pandemic pre-empted most of these impediments on a temporary basis. Relaxation of some of the pre–COVID-19 roadblocks are expected to continue after the emergency ends.
- The government views polysomnography, HST, and CPAP treatment as an activity ripe for fraud and abuse. Accordingly, government health care programs condition reimbursement for sleep medicine services to a wide array of technical requirements, including, but not limited to, a face-to-face examination by a treating physician whose notes must include certain specified notations, testing by laboratories whose programs are accredited by select agencies and who use only certified sleep technicians, test interpretations by physicians who hold certain board certifications, and CPAP dispensing only by durable medical equipment suppliers who, in the case of home sleep tests, are not affiliated with the provider of the home sleep test.

Detection and treatment of obstructive sleep apnea (OSA) and other sleep disorders, like many chronic conditions, trigger a complex range of clinical activity. Patient care plans for sleep-disordered patients include medical examinations, overnight testing, and ongoing respiratory or dental appliance treatment with durable medical equipment (DME), monitoring, and follow-up. This collection of care services touches a wide variety of legal, regulatory, and reimbursement rules, few of which operate in concert to promote seamless delivery of clinical sleep medicine.

This chapter addresses some of the legal, regulatory, and reimbursement roadblocks sleep practitioners in the United States face in offering their services to their sleep-disordered patients.

STATE LICENSING OF SLEEP SERVICES

State Licensing for Sleep Laboratories

Many states allocate health care resources within their borders through the Certificate of Need (CON) process.[1] Obtaining a CON for the operation of a health care facility is a lengthy, expensive, and often adversarial process. Fortunately, sleep laboratories typically fall below the threshold for CON review and escape review requirements in CON states.[2]

Separate from CON review are state laws requiring health care facilities to obtain licensure before operation. Although diagnostic testing performed as part of a hospital or physician practice is almost always exempt from state health care facility licensure, freestanding sleep laboratories may fall within a state's regulatory jurisdiction as a "health care clinic" or other health care facility.[3] Freestanding sleep labs are operated separately from a physician practice or hospital.

At least three states now require freestanding sleep laboratories to obtain health facility licensure before operating: Florida,[4] New Jersey,[5] and Alabama.[6] Licensure requires completing an application and disclosing the laboratory's ownership structure, medical supervision, and affiliations with other health care facilities.[7] Interestingly, these states require facility licensure even if the entity performs only home or portable sleep tests in the absence of any physical health care structure visited by patients. Other states may join in regulating the licensing of freestanding sleep laboratories.

Sleep Physician Certification

Despite its relative newness, sleep medicine is now fully recognized as a medical practice subspecialty in the United States. The American Board of Sleep Medicine (ABSM) began issuing diplomate status in sleep medicine to physicians and PhDs in the late 1970s. The American Board of Medical Specialties (ABMS) began issuing subspecialty board certification to physicians in sleep medicine in 2007 as part of the boards of internal medicine, family medicine, anesthesiology, otolaryngology, pediatrics, and psychiatry and neurology.[8]

As discussed later, government and commercial payers often require that the physicians who interpret polysomnograms or home sleep tests hold ABSM, ABMS, or certain other credentials as a condition for reimbursement. However, one state—Oklahoma—has adopted legislation that prohibits non–board-certified physicians from interpreting sleep tests without regard to the source of payment for the test.

Believing that public safety requires specific regulation of sleep disorders testing, the Oklahoma legislature in 2009 adopted the Oklahoma Sleep Diagnostic Testing Regulation Act.[9] The act establishes minimum medical standards of care in the field of sleep medicine. It declares that it is illegal in Oklahoma for a licensed physician to interpret a sleep test unless the physician is board certified in sleep medicine by the ABSM or ABMS. Alternatively, the interpreting physician must have completed a 1-year sleep medicine fellowship accredited by the Accreditation Council for Graduate Medical Education or received a Certification of Special Qualifications or a Certification of Added Qualifications in Sleep Medicine issued by the American Osteopathic Association. Otherwise, it is illegal for a medical doctor in Oklahoma to interpret the results of a diagnostic sleep test performed in Oklahoma.[9]

Oklahoma also establishes minimum requirements for sleep-testing facilities and their employees.[9] Under the act, (1) sleep diagnostic testing facilities in Oklahoma must be fully or provisionally certified or accredited as a sleep laboratory by the American Academy of Sleep Medicine (AASM), the Accreditation Commission for Health Care (ACHC), or The Joint Commission; (2) Oklahoma sleep laboratories must be supervised by board-certified sleep physicians; and (3) home sleep testing (HST) must be performed by technicians who are supervised by board-certified sleep physicians.[9] In this regard, the Oklahoma law is the most intrusive in the nation.

State Licensing for Nonphysician Polysomnography Technicians

Nonphysician persons who perform and score sleep tests have specialized skills and training. These individuals have enhanced their professional skills and standing by earning certification through organizations such as the Board of Registered Polysomnographic Technologists,[10] the American Association of Sleep Technologists,[11] and the American Board of Sleep Medicine Registered Sleep Technologist program.[12] These credentialing entities generally recognize three levels of sleep technician expertise: trainee, technician, and technologist.[13]

Sleep laboratories are encouraged to use technicians holding a recognized sleep technologist credential. Some payers require the participation of certified technicians as a condition for payment. For example, Medicare will not consider a sleep test performed by a physician practice or by an independent diagnostic testing facility to be medically necessary, unless the technologist attending the overnight test or handling the home sleep test is properly credentialed by a specified professional board and state-licensed to perform the task, if state licensure exists.[14]

Apart from private industry bodies that credential sleep technicians are states that impose state licensure requirements on sleep technicians in their state. For example, the states of Georgia,[15] Louisiana,[16] New Mexico,[17] North Carolina,[18] Maryland,[19] Virginia,[20] District of Columbia,[21] Idaho,[22] Tennessee,[23] New York,[24] and California,[25] among several others, have recognized the allied health profession of polysomnography (PSG) and adopted mandatory licensure or registration requirements for these nonphysician sleep test personnel.

In New York, for example, licensure of PSG technologists requires applicants to be at least 18 years old, complete educational requirements that provide knowledge of PSG technology, pass an examination, and prove "good moral character."[26] Sleep laboratories that fail to use licensed sleep technicians, when required, face potential state law criminal or civil penalties.[27]

State Licensing for Dispensing Continuous Positive Airway Pressure

Continuous positive airway pressure (CPAP) is considered a prescriptive medical device by the U.S. Food and Drug Administration[28] and state law pharmacy and medical equipment regulations. CPAP is also an item of DME for purposes of state law[29] and for insurance reimbursement purposes.[30]

Roughly half of states, including Florida,[31] Tennessee,[32] and Ohio,[33] require persons or entities that dispense DME, like CPAP, to obtain a state license before delivery of DME items to the ultimate consumer. Almost all states that license DME suppliers exempt physicians or other licensed health care practitioners, who dispense devices from their practices to their patients, from licensure.

In addition to state licensure of the supplier, many, but not all, states consider CPAP titration and education to be the practice of respiratory therapy, to be performed only by persons holding respiratory therapy licenses or PSG technology licenses issued by the applicable state.[34] However, persons who hold a state law PSG tech certificate or license are exempt from licensure as respiratory therapists.[35]

REIMBURSEMENT FOR SLEEP MEDICINE SERVICES

Reimbursement drives the delivery of health care services in the United States. The provision of sleep medicine and the types of testing and treatment depend, in large part, on the coverage conditions that health insurance plans impose on the providers of sleep disorders services.

Medicare Coverage for Sleep Testing

The Medicare Part B Program covers in-laboratory and HST performed by physicians or stand-alone independent diagnostic testing facilities as "other diagnostic tests" payable under the under Medicare's Physician Fee Schedule.[36] Medicare reimburses hospitals for the technical components of many outpatient services under the Hospital Outpatient Prospective Payment System.[37] Medicare classifies certain outpatient services into groups called ambulatory payment classifications (APCs), with payment rates established for all activities assigned to each classification group.[38] For example, the technical component of attended, in-lab PSG performed in the outpatient hospital setting is payable under Level 4 APC diagnostic test group 5724,[39] and unattended home sleep tests are in the Level 1 APC diagnostic test group 5721.[40]

Medicare coverage for all diagnostic tests requires a physician's order and proper physician supervision.[41] The Centers for Medicare and Medicaid Services (CMS) has delegated to Medicare administrative contractors (MACs) the authority to specify special medical necessity coverage conditions for activities in the MAC's jurisdiction.

By 2020 Medicare contracted with 6 different contractors to administer the Medicare Part B program in each of 12 different geographic regions known as Part B jurisdictions. Each MAC has adopted a local coverage determination (LCD) or a billing article (Article) addressing the medical necessity requirements for Medicare coverage of in-lab PSG or ambulatory home sleep tests. Each of the current LCDs and Articles mandates a variety of coverage conditions, including the following credentialing requirements: (1) the laboratory must be accredited by the AASM, ACHC, or The Joint Commission; (2) the physician performing the test must be board certified in sleep medicine or a specified related field; and (3) the technicians performing or scoring the test, even a home sleep test, must hold certifications by the Board of Registered Polysomnographic Technologists or evidence of training.[42] These Medicare conditions of medical necessity apply both to physician practice labs and to commercially owned stand-alone sleep centers.[42]

The sleep test LCD issued by First Coast Service Options (Florida) requires that the face-to-face visit notes prepared by the treating physician contain a sleep history and physical examination, the results of the Epworth Sleepiness Scale, as well as notations of the patient's body mass index and neck circumference, and a focused cardiopulmonary and upper airway evaluation.[43] First Coast takes the position that Medicare sleep tests performed without these specific notations are not medically necessary and are ineligible for Medicare coverage, even if all other indications for OSA are present and made clear in the examination notes.[43]

Medicare Coverage for Continuous Positive Airway Pressure Therapy

CPAP therapy is the gold standard treatment for OSA.[44] CPAP machines and supplies are items of DME. As items of DME, CPAP machines and suppliers are part of the home medical equipment supply industry. This means that CPAP delivery, setup, and reimbursement are governed by their own conditions of medical necessity and Medicare fee schedule separate from the rules governing the performance of the diagnostic sleep test.[45]

For example, CPAP suppliers who enroll in the Medicare system must adhere to a complex set of 30 or so supplier standards, including minimum space, insurance coverage, and hours of operation requirements; possession of accreditation from selected accrediting bodies; and the posting of a $50,000 surety bond to offset losses resulting from improper practices.[46] Medicare enrollment and payments are governed by regional DME Medicare Administrative Contractors, each of which adheres to an LCD indicating the conditions of coverage for CPAP reimbursement in the contractor's jurisdiction.[47] According to this LCD, Medicare will reimburse a DME supplier for CPAP to treat OSA only in the following circumstances:

1. The beneficiary has an in-person clinical evaluation by the treating physician before the sleep test to assess the beneficiary for OSA.
2. The beneficiary has a sleep test showing minimum criteria for OSA.
3. The sleep test is performed by a test provider who meets Medicare coverage for sleep testing.
4. The sleep test is interpreted by a board-certified sleep physician or a physician on staff of a sleep center accredited by the AASM, ACHC, or The Joint Commission.
5. The beneficiary shows continued use of the device and that he or she benefits from the device within 90 days of initiation by subjective and objective evidence.[47]

CMS has long believed that the provider of a sleep test may have an inappropriate self-interest in the test result test if the provider, or its affiliate, also supplies the CPAP device. To CMS, affiliations between the test provider and the CPAP supplier incent orders for or more tests than medically necessary and skew positive test interpretations, presumably to drive CPAP sales.[48]

In an effort to curtail these perceived abuses, CMS adopted a special payment rule that prohibits Medicare from paying a DME supplier for CPAP if the CPAP supplier is directly or indirectly affiliated with the provider of the sleep test from which a diagnosis of OSA is obtained.[49] *Affiliation* means a relationship among parties by compensation arrangement or ownership.[50] This special payment prohibition applies only if the underlying sleep test is a home sleep test. In other words, Medicare will reimburse a DME supplier for CPAP even if the DME supplier is affiliated with the provider of the sleep test, as long as the sleep test used to diagnose the patient's OSA was full, in-lab, overnight PSG.[49]

Sleep Dentistry: Medicare Coverage for Oral Appliance Therapy

One alternative to CPAP therapy is an oral appliance worn overnight to advance the jaw and open the patient's airway during sleep.[51] The AASM recommends sleep physicians to prescribe oral appliances to adult patients with OSA who are intolerant of CPAP therapy or prefer alternate therapy in lieu of no therapy at all.[52]

Medicare covers customized oral appliances for the treatment of OSA as an item of DME payable under the Medicare Durable Medical Equipment, Prosthetics, Orthotics and Supplies (DMEPOS) Fee Schedule.[45] Unlike CPAP, which is dispensed and billed by DME suppliers, oral appliances must be dispensed and billed by dentists in their capacity as DME suppliers.[53] In other words, for purposes of Medicare reimbursement, patients seeking oral appliance therapy must visit a licensed, practicing dentist who has enrolled in the Medicare program as a DME supplier.

The diagnosis of OSA and an order of an oral appliance for treatment of the disease state of OSA constitute the practice of medicine that is beyond the scope of a dentist's license.[54] Thus dentists who provide oral appliance therapy may fabricate and fit the devices only on the order of the patient's treating physician.[52]

This also means that dentists should not order nor perform sleep tests, including home sleep tests, for purposes of diagnosing the patient's OSA.[55] Concluding that sleep testing is outside the scope of a dentist's license, the dental licensing boards of a handful of states have outlawed a dentist's use of HST for any purpose.[56]

Dentists who provide oral appliance therapy to Medicare beneficiaries on a physician's order must hew to most of the conditions of participation applicable to Medicare suppliers of DME. The reimbursement paid by Medicare is a lump-sum payment that includes all time, labor, materials, professional services, radiology, and laboratory costs incurred in fabricating and fitting the device, as well as adjustment and professional services required during the 90 days after the initial placement.[57]

Medicaid Coverage

Medicaid is a state-run health care program subsidized with federal funds but operated under terms and conditions adopted by individual states for their citizens. A comprehensive 50-state survey of Medicaid coverage for sleep testing is beyond the scope of this chapter. However, the coverage conditions for Medicaid sleep tests under the State of Minnesota's Medical Assistance program are illustrative.

Minnesota's Health Care Programs, which includes Minnesota Medicaid, will reimburse participating providers for sleep tests only if the study is a full, in-lab test attended by a trained sleep specialist following a careful medical examination.[58] Unattended home sleep tests are not covered by the Minnesota Health Care Programs at this time.[58] However, in-home sleep tests are covered if they are attended in the home by the sleep specialist and if the patient is either nonambulatory or suffering from severe and persistent mental illness.[58]

Commercial Insurance Coverage of Sleep Testing

Almost all commercial health insurance plans cover testing for OSA. The conditions for coverage vary widely according to the terms of the individual plan. Most plans will cover in-lab PSG sessions only if the patient is ineligible for the less expensive home sleep test because of health reasons or if the results of the home test are inconclusive to make a diagnosis of OSA.[59]

FRAUD AND ABUSE LAWS

Health care fraud and abuse laws can be separated into two separate conceptual categories. One category addresses prohibited self-referrals. These laws prohibit physicians from referring their patients to entities in which the physicians or their families have an ownership or other financial interest. On the federal level, the principal regulation in this area is the Stark Law.[60]

The other broad category involves prohibitions on kickbacks, bribes, or other payments to steer patients to a particular health care provider. Anti-kickback laws prohibit any person (not just doctors) from paying or receiving money or other items of value for the referral of a health care service. The federal anti-kickback law extends beyond payments for referrals to include payments, gifts, or other remuneration to anyone who merely recommends or even arranges health care services reimbursed by Medicare, Medicaid, or any other federal health care program.[61]

The Stark Self-Referral Law

Absent an exception, the federal Stark Law prohibits a physician (or an immediate family member of such physician) from making a referral for a designated health service to an entity in which the physician has a direct or indirect ownership or compensation arrangement—if the service is reimbursed by Medicare or Medicaid.[62]

Penalties for violating the Stark Law include denial of payment, refunds of amounts collected in violation of the statute, and a civil money penalty of up to $15,000 for each bill or claim for a service a person knows or should know is for a service for which payment may not be made.[63] If the physician or the entity engages in a circumvention arrangement that the physician or entity knows, or should know, has a principal purpose of indirectly evading the Stark Law, the civil money penalty jumps to $100,000 for each such arrangement or scheme.[64]

Only referrals for designated health services are prohibited. Overnight PSG and HST do not fall within any of the categories of designated health services.[65] Consequently, a physician's referral of a Medicare or Medicaid sleep test falls *outside* the Stark Law prohibition, unless the sleep test is performed in a hospital setting. Inpatient and outpatient hospital services are designated health services, and a physician's referral of a Medicare or Medicaid sleep test performed as an inpatient or outpatient hospital service would be considered a referral of a designated health service. However, a violation would occur only if the referring physician had an ownership or compensation arrangement with the hospital that did not meet a Stark Law exception.

Self-Referrals for Durable Medical Equipment

Unlike referrals for nonhospital sleep tests, referrals for DME *are* referrals for designated health services under the Stark Law.[66] Because CPAP and oral appliances are items of DME, the entirety of the Stark Law applies to these OSA therapies. This means that, absent an exception, a physician may not refer a patient to a DME supplier in which the physician or a member of the physician's family has an investment or compensation interest, if the DME supplier requests payment of the item from a government health care program.

The Stark Law exempts referrals of certain items of DHS that are ancillary to the physician's in-office procedures, such as imaging or prescription drug services. This in-office ancillary services exception permits physicians to refer items of DHS to be furnished by the physician's own practice if certain conditions are met.[67]

Unfortunately, items of DME such as CPAP or oral appliances are not included in the in-office ancillary services exception.[67] This means that physicians may not furnish CPAP to their own OSA patients from the physicians' office if the patients are Medicare or Medicaid beneficiaries, unless another Stark Law exception exists, such as the rural provider or personally performed exceptions.

The AASM petitioned CMS in 2018 to consider a specific Stark Law exception to allow accredited sleep centers and board-certified sleep medicine physicians to dispense Medicare CPAP as part of responsible continuity of care.[68] In 2019 CMS proposed certain Stark Law exceptions to facilitate value-based, coordinated care through otherwise prohibited referred services.[69] The proposal announced by CMS does not address any specific exception for sleep medicine. Instead, CMS continued its suspicion of financial relationships between DME (i.e., CPAP) suppliers and referring physicians. The proposal considers excluding DME suppliers from the value-based Stark Law exceptions being floated under the proposed rule.[70]

State Self-Referral Laws

Many states have their own laws restricting self-referrals. Some states, such as Michigan, adopt language very close to the federal Stark Law.[71] Therefore an exception under the federal law is likely an automatic exception under the state law.[71] Other states, such as Georgia, use their own definitions and exceptions.[72]

Importantly, these states punish self-referrals regardless of the reimbursement of the item or service by a federal or state health care program.[72] Referrals of even private-pay patients to entities owned by the physician or in which the physician has a compensation arrangement not covered by an exception may be unlawful under these laws.

Federal Anti-Kickback Statute

The federal Anti-Kickback Statute makes it unlawful for anyone to knowingly and willfully solicit or receive any payment in return for referring an individual to another person or entity for the furnishing, or arranging for the furnishing, of any item or service that may be paid in whole or in part by any federally funded health care program.[73]

Violations of the law require the solicitation, offer, payment, or acceptance of illegal remuneration.[73] Remuneration includes the transfer of anything of value in cash or in kind, whether made directly or indirectly, and whether made overtly or covertly.[73,74]

The statute is a two-way street. Soliciting for and accepting payments in return for referrals is as bad as paying the kickback itself. A violation of the Anti-Kickback Statute constitutes a felony punishable by a maximum fine of $25,000, imprisonment for up to 5 years, or both.[73] Conviction will also lead to automatic exclusion from Medicare, Medicaid, and other federally funded health care programs.[75]

Civil monetary penalties may be applied to violations of the Anti-Kickback Statute in the amount of $50,000 for each act that violates the statute, plus three times the amount of remuneration unlawfully transferred.[76] Significantly, the imposition of civil monetary penalties requires proof by only a preponderance of the evidence, not proof beyond a reasonable doubt, which is required for criminal penalties.[77] Consequently, it is easier for the government to establish violations in a civil proceeding than in a criminal proceeding. The addition of civil monetary penalties increases the risk associated with practices that implicate the statute but are not protected by statutory exceptions or regulatory safe harbors, discussed later.

Anti-Kickback Exceptions and Safe Harbors

The Anti-Kickback Statute has the breadth to capture almost every health care transaction in the United States. At risk are not only bribes of cash but also a wide array of negotiated business practices—sales commissions, below-market rent, distributions arising from joint ventures with suppliers, expensive gifts, medical director fees, and certain equipment rental arrangements. It is these arrangements that the government or its contractors may review as part of an audit of sleep test services.[78]

Responding to industry concerns, Congress has included several exceptions in the law and approved the promulgation of specific "safe harbor" payment practices.[79] Examples of safe harbor arrangements common in sleep medicine include joint ventures among referring physicians and sleep test providers, medical director and other personal services agreements, and space lease arrangements. Compliance with all aspects of the applicable safe harbor protects the actor from prosecution under the Anti-Kickback Statute. However, failure to meet each of the elements of the applicable safe harbor does not automatically mean that the activity is illegal. The activity may be acceptable in the eyes of the government, depending on a variety of factors.

State Anti-Kickback Laws

Many states have enacted their own anti-kickback laws. Almost all state physician-licensing boards prohibit paying or sharing fees for referrals. Some, like California and Florida, criminalize payments or in-kind exchanges to refer patients notwithstanding the source of the service reimbursement.[80,81]

The Florida Patient Brokering Act makes it illegal for any person, including any health care provider or health care facility, to (1) offer or pay any commission, bonus, rebate, kickback, or bribe, directly or indirectly, in cash or in kind, or engage in any split-fee arrangement, in any form whatsoever, to induce the referral of patients or patronage from a health care provider or health care facility; (2) solicit or receive any commission, bonus, rebate, kickback, or bribe, directly or indirectly, in cash or in kind, or engage in any split-fee arrangement, in any form whatsoever, in return for referring patients or patronage to a health care provider or health care facility; or (3) aid, abet, advise, or otherwise participate in such conduct.[81] The act specifically covers the actions of attorneys and other advisors and participants who counsel persons in the participation of such arrangements.[81]

Federal False Claims Act

Presenting a claim to CMS for payment for an item or service performed in violation of the Stark Law or Anti-Kickback Statute may constitute a false claim under the federal False Claims Act. Enacted during the Civil War to deter war profiteers, the False Claims Act permits private "whistleblowers" to bring actions against health care companies for filing fraudulent claims with the government.[82] Penalties include repayment of the fraudulent claim and a mandatory civil penalty as of June 2020 of at least $11,665 and no more than $23,331 per claim, which amounts can be tripled.[83,84] The whistleblower gets to keep a percentage of the damages and penalties, which could be as much as 30% in some circumstances.[83] Because the penalties could reach in excess of $60,000 per sleep study performed, potential recoveries under the law add up quickly.

The risk to sleep laboratory operators under false claims whistleblower statutes has increased in recent years. A wave of states have adopted state False Claims Acts that mirror the federal False Claims Act in many respects.[85]

Sleep laboratories and sleep physicians participating in government reimbursement programs are well advised to adopt compliance plans, or take other audit and monitoring actions, to ensure compliance with fraud and abuse laws.

TELEMEDICINE AND SLEEP MEDICINE

Sleep medicine is especially well suited for remote electronic practice via telehealth. Real-time internet encounters allow practitioners to conduct interactive histories and treatment and to perform physical and diagnostic testing with peripheral electronic devices, including home sleep tests.

The coronavirus pandemic has accelerated the adoption of telemedicine by easing certain legal impediments and reimbursement prohibitions. For example, before emergency rules adopted in response to the pandemic, Medicare would not cover physician visits that originate in the patient's home. Absent the emergency measure, Medicare would cover telehealth encounters only if the patient was located in a rural area and was physically located in certain health care settings, such as a physician's office, hospital, skilled nursing center, or other designated facility.[86]

COVID-19 measures have also relaxed health care privacy protection laws affecting telehealth. Before the pandemic, HIPAA required that telehealth software platforms include extensive electronic data and security requirements. Many web-based audiovisual software programs commonly available to consumers are unsuitable for health care encounters because of noncompliance with HIPAA standards.

Early in the pandemic, the Office of Civil Rights of the United States Department of Health and Human Services announced that it would waive penalties for HIPAA violations against health care providers who communicate with patients via telecommunications technologies during the pandemic.[87]

Health care industry commentators expect that telemedicine's expansion during the public health emergency will extend long after the emergency ends.[88] During the emergency and afterward, practitioners of sleep telemedicine will face some basic legal conditions, including state licensure, the establishment of professional relationships and consent to treat.

Physician Licensure

Physicians practicing telemedicine must adhere to two cardinal rules applicable in all cases: (1) the practitioner performing the service must be licensed in the state where the patient is situated[89] and (2) the telemedicine practitioner must engage in the encounter in a manner consistent with a valid physician-patient relationship.[90] Some states have granted (at least temporarily) waivers to allow doctors licensed in one state to complete a telemedicine encounter with a patient in another state.

To ease physician licensure in states where the doctor's activity is limited to telemedicine from outside the state, a majority of the states have now relaxed their gatekeeper function by joining the Federation of State Medical Board's Interstate Medical License Compact (the FSMB Compact).[91] Members states of the FSMB Compact look to an interstate commission to operate an expedited licensure process for physicians in good standing in one member state to obtain a license to practice in another member state. Certain other states issue special telehealth licenses or certificates to permit practitioners not licensed in the issuing state to perform telemedicine services in the issuing state.

Whether providing telehealth services under a full license or a limited-use certificate, all physicians who perform telehealth services must establish a valid physician relationship with the remote physician. Failure to establish the relationship may give rise to disciplinary actions.

Depending on state law, indicia of a valid physician-patient relationship in telemedicine encounters typically require real-time audio/video communications, the taking of the patient's history, the ability of the physician to examine the patient using technology or peripherals that are equal to or superior to a personal examination, documenting the encounter and maintaining patient records according to state medical records law, recommendations for follow-up care as needed, and disclosure of the practitioner's contact information for the patient's use.[92]

Consent to Telemedicine Session

According to the Center of Connected Health Policy, a majority of the states and the District of Columbia require telehealth practitioners to obtain a telemedicine consent from the patient before the electronic session.[93] Although not exactly a "consent-to-treat" document, the telemedicine consent provides evidence in the physician's note that the patient agreed to be seen and treated by a distant physician via telemedicine. Draft language for such consents may be available at state medical boards or state Medicaid portals.

Telemedicine Software and Equipment

Persons engaging in telehealth must ensure that the software and equipment used to perform the telemedicine encounter comply with HIPAA and applicable state patient privacy laws. Not all interactive telehealth software platforms satisfy these requirements.

For example, Georgia's Medicaid telemedicine handbook makes clear that services rendered via webcam or internet-based technologies (e.g., Skype, Tango) are inappropriate technologies unless they are used as part of a secured network or specially configured for secure transmission and storage of electronic protected health information.[94] HIPAA guidelines require that software that transmits protected personal health information use end-to-end encryption.[95] Data transmitted and held in or on such platforms must also have functional auditing, archival, and backup capabilities.

SUMMARY

Although sleep testing and CPAP devices may be reimbursed under Medicare, Medicaid, and private payers, many wide-reaching prohibitions on reimbursement fraud and abuse have been established. On the federal level, the Anti-Kickback Statute prohibits medical practices from offering or receiving any direct or indirect remuneration to encourage the referral of patients. In addition, the Stark Law prohibits physicians from referring designated health services to an entity owned by themselves, an immediate family member, or someone with whom the physician has a financial relationship, unless an exception applies. Furthermore, the False Claims Act prohibits medical providers from fraudulently billing for medical services from government payers. States may also have their own fraud and abuse legislation. To provide these services, some states require licensing for technologists performing sleep testing. Oklahoma has even more stringent rules that require physicians to possess specialized credentials to interpret sleep tests.

SELECTED READINGS

Centers for Medicare and Medicaid Services. *Medicare fraud and abuse: prevention, detection, and reporting*. August 2014. http://www.cms.gov/Outreach-and-Education/Medicare-Learning-Network-MLN/MLNProducts/downloads/Fraud_and_Abuse.pdf. Accessed June 1, 2021.

Hunt TL 2nd, Hooten WM. The effects of COVID-19 on telemedicine could outlive the virus. *Mayo Clin Proc Innov Qual Outcomes*. 2020;4(5):583–585.

Office of Inspector General. *A roadmap for new physicians: fraud and abuse laws*. http://oig.hhs.gov/compliance/physician-education/01laws.asp. Accessed June 1, 2021.

Staman J. *Health care fraud and abuse laws affecting Medicare and Medicaid: an overview*. (Congressional. Report No. RS22743). Washington DC: Library of Congressional Research Service, September 8, 2014. https://www.fas.org/sgp/crs/misc/RS22743.pdf. Accessed June 1, 2021.

A complete reference list can be found online at ExpertConsult.com.

Chapter 77

Sleep Medicine Clinical Practice and Compliance—Europe

Thomas Penzel

Chapter Highlights

- European sleep medicine is coordinated through the European Sleep Research Society (ESRS). The ESRS is composed, in part, of the Assembly of National Sleep Societies with delegates from all European sleep societies. The levels of sleep medicine and sleep medicine delivery differ in European countries according to their respective health care systems.
- The ESRS has published European guidelines for certification of sleep physicians, psychologists, scientists, and sleep technologists. Examinations for European somnologists started in 2012. An ESRS textbook on sleep medicine provides the ground for the exam, published in 2014 and updated in 2020.
- European sleep center certification guidelines have been published, and a network of research centers has been created. Harmonized guidelines for sleep medicine center accreditation in Europe are being considered by various European national sleep societies with support from the ESRS.

Sleep medicine research in Europe has a long tradition with a strong focus on basic science. A variety of medical and educational institutions across Europe long engaged in sleep research resulted in pioneering insights in the past century. In 1972 a small group of individual sleep researchers and clinicians sought a forum to exchange and advance scientific ideas relating to sleep research and founded the European Sleep Research Society (ESRS) in Switzerland.[1] Since then the ESRS has become the preeminent aggregator and distributor of sleep research in Europe. Its goals are to promote sleep research in Europe, to improve care for patients with sleep disorders, and to disseminate information regarding sleep research. The ESRS is a founding member of the World Federation of Sleep Research Societies. In 1992 the ESRS founded the *Journal of Sleep Research* and holds biannual conferences in cities all over Europe.

The development and delivery of sleep medicine, unlike sleep research, for European patients suffering from sleep disorders have evolved independently along national lines. This is because the health care systems in Europe differ among the countries. In the beginning, European sleep medicine was closely related to clinical research, which the ESRS exchanged among pioneering sleep medicine groups in various European countries.

Today there are large national sleep societies with a few thousand members in those European countries that have large populations. Many of these national sleep societies outnumber the membership of the ESRS. However, many European countries with smaller populations do not have reasonably sized national sleep societies and do not have the infrastructure to run professional societies. For these countries, the ESRS is of utmost importance to provide support for national sleep medicine needs and services.

In 1994 the ESRS set up a clinical committee to exchange national experiences regarding sleep medicine services in Europe. The committee also sought to coordinate activities among the different insurance and reimbursement schemes across Europe. Additional goals of the committee included the development of standard practice papers and support for the educational exchange of sleep medicine clinicians across Europe.

The Assembly of National Sleep Societies (ANSS) grew out of this committee's work. The ANSS is a membership organization comprising approximately 30 national European sleep societies. The association is devoted to the clinical needs of sleep physicians and is made up of national delegates who exchange ideas and concepts to serve patients with sleep disorders and promote sleep medicine in Europe. The ANSS exists under the auspices of the ESRS and holds annual meetings of delegates and national presidents.

In 2004 the ESRS board met with the national society presidents as representatives of the ANSS for the first time. The ANSS agreed that a number of unifying policies and procedures addressing the delivery of sleep medicine in Europe would be desirable. Acting through task forces, the ANSS and ESRS developed uniform standards for European sleep center accreditation in 2006,[2] certification of sleep professionals in 2009,[3] clinical procedures for adults in accredited sleep centers,[4] and clinical education standards in 2014.[5] Each of these standards and procedures has been published in the *Journal of Sleep Research.*

To address the patchwork standards of European countries that did not adopt ESRS protocols, the ESRS established the Sleep Medicine Committee (SMC) of the ESRS in 2010. The SMC is charged with adopting and promoting (1) standards of practice papers and guidelines for clinical service, (2) certification of sleep medicine professionals (physicians, psychologists, and other scientists, technicians), and (3) accreditation of sleep medicine centers.

The SMC provides certification and accreditation to sleep professionals and sleep centers in countries that do not have access to national certification and accreditation or that desire to supplement national accreditation with the ESRS emblem. Working with national delegates at the ANSS, the SMC works on educational courses and summer schools together with other groups of the ESRS to provide educational opportunities. The SMC acts as an educational clearinghouse to help standardize sleep medicine education throughout Europe.

STANDARDS

Sleep Technicians and Technologists

As elsewhere, performance of overnight polysomnography (PSG) in Europe contemplates the participation by nonphysician technicians and technologists to set up and attend the overnight test. The involvement of trained sleep technicians is part of the ESRS sleep center accreditation standards. Several European countries recognize the separate allied health profession of PSG technician or technologist. Several European countries have established their own sleep technician societies, and the independent European Society of Sleep Technologists (ESST) was formed in 1996. The ESST meets regularly with the biannual ESRS conferences and works closely with the ESRS in terms of education and certification.

Sleep Center Accreditation

The ESRS is also working toward an accreditation of European sleep centers. In 2006 the Steering Committee of the ESRS published European Guidelines for the Accreditation of Sleep Medicine Centres in the *Journal of Sleep Research*. Implementation of an accreditation of European sleep centers is still in progress.

The establishment of institutional sleep medicine programs in Europe is less prevalent than in the United States.[6] This is because many sleep centers in Europe are linked to individuals active in the field who, as yet, have not sold to or otherwise had their centers incorporated into institutional health care systems or facilities. Some scholars view this as a loss because the implementation of academic sleep centers is needed to cover the increasing challenges brought up by the importance of sleep medicine as part of medical health care.[7,8]

CERTIFICATION OF SLEEP MEDICINE PROFESSIONALS

The ESRS inaugurated a sleep medicine committee to serve the needs of the various European national sleep societies and to coordinate sleep medicine standards in Europe. The larger national sleep societies have established national certifications for sleep medicine for sleep professionals in their respective countries. Depending on the national medical education system, these examinations are implemented by the national sleep society or by a chamber of physicians, a university, or some other educational institute.

National recognition of these certifications varies largely across Europe. At this time Germany, France, Spain, and Hungary recognize a national subspecialty in sleep medicine. The German Chamber of Physicians has established the subspecialty in sleep medicine under the primary specialties of pneumology (pulmonology), neurology, psychiatry, pediatrics, and ear-nose-throat medicine.

The lack of universal certification for sleep medicine across Europe has led to a European initiative for all countries to harmonize certifications under the authority of the ESRS. A European certification of sleep professionals started in 2012 based on guidelines for certification requirements published by an ESRS task force in 2009.[3] In general it is recognized that certification of sleep physicians improves health care in patients with sleep disorders.[9]

The task force guidelines specify four different certifications: one for physicians, one for psychologists, one for scientists, and one for sleep technologists, depending on the previous education of the applicant. All certifications are called *European somnologist* with mention of the specific type as an attribute.

The basic requirement for certification includes a full-time clinical training period in a sleep center for 12 months. During this time the applicant should have evaluated at least 100 patients, with cases of sleep-disordered breathing, insomnia, hypersomnia, movement disorder, and circadian disorder. Certification requires experience in clinical interviewing; use of diagnostic criteria and classification systems; use of sleep diaries, questionnaires, and rating scales; psychometric evaluation; and physiologic monitoring. Assessment with actigraphy is required.

PSG experience must include hook-up, nighttime surveillance, scoring, interpretation, and reporting. Experience with the Multiple Sleep Latency Test and the Maintenance of Wakefulness Test as well as other tests must be proved. In relation to treatment, applicants need to show skills in patient education, treatment delivery, and experience with treatment of patients related to their original professional discipline.

The certification programs require proven experience in a variety of sleep disorder treatments, such as pharmacotherapy, continuous positive airway pressure (CPAP), cognitive behavioral therapy, and health behavior. Some of these experiences may be obtained at approved sleep medicine courses.

All certifications require applicants to sit for a written examination. The first examinations in 2012 and 2013 were held according to a grandparenting rule. The regular examinations for physicians, psychologists, and scientists began in 2014 and continue annually. The number of SMC questions increased to 100 for taking the exam. A "practical part" was added, which requires the examinees to score a number of PSG pages and evaluate cases. Sleep technologists had their grandparenting examination in 2014 and 2015. Since 2016 there are also regular technologist examinations annually, in parallel with the examinations for physicians, psychologists, and scientists.

Somewhat parallel to the ESRS push for commonly recognized European sleep specialty certifications is the contemporaneous effort of the European Respiratory Society (ERS) to create European certifications for respiratory sleep physicians.[10] Although the ESRS focuses on the needs of the national sleep societies to have their sleep expert members show proof of qualifications, the ERS approach has been to create a curriculum, then courses, and then certificates to practitioners who successfully completed a final examination after the courses.

The ERS approach is part of a larger framework of certifications for Europeans in respiratory medicine launched in 2009.[11] The framework is a mission to harmonize education in respiratory medicine for European specialists (HERMES) because medical education in Europe is primarily a national duty. European medical associations have been slow to harmonize medical education. The ESRS and the ERS are working together to align their parallel activities in terms of educational content and recognition of educational and examination modules.

ACCREDITATION OF SLEEP MEDICINE CENTERS

Like physician certification, accreditation of sleep centers in Europe is currently a patchwork of rules. The larger national sleep societies in Europe, such as those in Great Britain and Germany, have established an accreditation procedure for their sleep centers. Depending on the national health care system of these particular European countries, the accreditations are recognized by health insurance, by health care officials, or for quality of care. However, sleep center accreditation standards have not been adopted by most European countries.

Although the ESRS has initiated a European somnologist certification, it is not expected that the ESRS will implement a common European sleep center accreditation. In 2009 the *Journal of Sleep Research* published European guidelines for the accreditation of sleep medicine centers.[2] Currently it is envisaged to check national accreditations that are in place in some countries against the published recommendations and endorse these national accreditations if applicable. For countries in which there are no national accreditations, the ESRS will help the national sleep societies to create a national accreditation system or will organize site visits with sleep center accreditation as preferred by the host country.

It is expected that the current accreditation recommendations[2] will be updated to reflect changes in recording and scoring sleep. In addition to the technical update the revisions will include a reflection on sleep medicine services with varying degrees of specialization ranging from the family physician level through sleep medicine services in university-level facilities.[12] Discussions reflect different levels of sleep centers. The top level would be centers offering several sleep medicine services, including outpatient service and daytime and nighttime testing in the sleep center. It would also include training and education in sleep medicine and clinical research programs in sleep medicine. The second level would be similar but without clinical research programs and limited training programs in sleep medicine. The third level would include most kinds of sleep medicine service and most testing options for daytime and nighttime assessment to cover regional clinical needs. Whether specialized sleep centers (e.g., respiratory or neurologic) would fall in this category or another lower category is not yet decided.

MANAGEMENT OF PATIENTS

The management of patients with sleep disorders differs greatly among European countries. This depends much on the health care systems in place and the activity of the local sleep societies. The management of sleep-related breathing disorders had been investigated across Europe.[13] Home sleep testing is prevalent in several European countries for managing patients with sleep-disordered breathing. Some countries require level III home sleep testing, whereas other countries accept level IV home sleep testing as sufficient to diagnose sleep breathing disease and to initiate treatment. Still other countries require cardiorespiratory PSG for the diagnosis of obstructive sleep apnea and the prescription of CPAP therapy.

EDUCATION

The ESRS supports education for researchers and physicians and specialized education for sleep physicians and sleep scientists. In addition to accreditation and certification, the ESRS sleep medicine committee supports the development of educational material for future somnologists in Europe.

A first step will be establishment of a base set of knowledge and skills. A handful of European universities have implemented master classes in sleep science or sleep medicine for a number of selected students. The University of Oxford successfully runs such a program.

In 2014 the *Journal of Sleep Research* published the *Catalogue of Knowledge and Skills for Sleep Medicine*.[5] The catalogue is intended to describe a standardized curriculum for sleep medicine education across Europe. The ESRS Board and its SMC compiled the catalogue based on textbooks, standard of practice publications, systematic reviews, and professional experience. The compilation was later validated by an online survey completed by 110 delegates specializing in sleep medicine from different European countries.

The catalogue is intended to be a basis for sleep medicine education, for sleep medicine courses, and for sleep medicine examinations, serving not only physicians with a medical specialty degree but also PhD and MSc health professionals such as clinical psychologists and scientists, technologists, and nurses, all of whom may be involved professionally in sleep medicine. The treatise comprises 10 chapters covering sleep physiology, pathology, diagnostic and treatment procedures, as well as selected societal and organizational aspects of European sleep medicine. A European textbook on sleep medicine was published following this outline of chapters.[14] Required levels of knowledge and skills are defined, as is a proposed workload of 60 points according to the European Credit Transfer System. Currently, the catalogue is revised to reflect changes in the field of sleep medicine. In parallel with this, the ESRS textbook on sleep medicine was revised, updated, and published in 2020.

COMPLIANCE WITH REGULATIONS AND REIMBURSEMENT

Government regulations for the delivery and reimbursement of sleep medicine in Europe differ as much as the health care systems in European countries differ. Although many countries recognize the need to diagnose, treat, and follow patients with sleep disorders as a matter of good medicine and—with regard to hypersomnolent drivers—public safety, there is little movement to align the disparate regulatory schemes at this time.

A 2007 study indicates that most European countries recognize the public safety risks presented by drivers with excessive daytime sleepiness caused, in part, by sleep-disordered breathing.[15] However, a review of the licensure requirements of 25 different European countries as part of the study showed that less than half of the countries referenced obstructive sleep apnea in their licensure regulations. On July 1, 2014, an update of the European directive on driving was published, which mentions obstructive sleep apnea diagnosed with an apnea-hypopnea index above 15 events per hour and daytime sleepiness specifically.[16] Group one drivers (noncommercial drivers) with sleep apnea must show appropriate treatment and improvement in sleepiness to receive or renew a driving license. A periodical medical review is required every 3 years. Group two drivers (commercial drivers) are required to have a periodical medical review every year. The directive does not specify the qualification of the physician and does not specify how sleepiness is assessed. The directive was adopted by national laws in Europe by December 15, 2015. However, the implementation of these rules is lagging behind, because it has not been clarified which authority has to control the implementation.[17,18]

COVID-19 AND EUROPEAN SLEEP CENTERS

The 2020 pandemic of COVID-19 posed a major challenge to European health care systems. Depending on national health care resources in terms of trained physicians, nurses, hospitals, equipment (e.g., ventilators, oxygen concentrators), countries managed the challenges with some difficulty. Since most sleep centers in Europe are hospital based (estimated 80%), many were closed as part of the pandemic lockdown. Hospital-based sleep centers with predominantly respiratory patients (estimated 20% to 50%) were used to take care of infected patients because expertise with ventilation and oxygen delivery was in place. Patient advice followed AASM recommendations regarding the use of PAP devices.

HEALTH INSURANCE COVERAGE FOR SLEEP MEDICINE: THE GERMAN EXPERIENCE

The insurance and regulatory aspects of covering and delivering sleep medicine in Germany provide one example of the European experience. Almost everyone in Germany has health insurance and expects that all medical care is covered by the insurance. In Germany there are about 100 insurances available to citizens. Very few patients are not insured.

There are two types of insurances: a general basic insurance for more than 85% of the population that is open to anybody and a so-called private insurance for 11% of the population. Although the medical care is the same under each insurance program, small differences exist. Patients with private insurance have a wider choice of physicians and better chances to obtain single-bed rooms if admitted to a hospital. Physician reimbursement is higher for private patients than for general plan patients for the same service.

German citizens with private insurance pay monthly premiums that vary according to age and risk. Thus premiums are relatively low for younger insured persons and higher for older persons. Therefore a person must earn a high salary to be eligible for private health insurance. The cost of health insurance under the general insurance plan is simply a percentage of the insured person's income.

In general, health insurance in Germany covers all costs for a diagnosis of sleep apnea and the treatment of sleep apnea and all replacement and service items. Patients with complaints of irregular snoring or observed apneas go to the family physician to get guidance for their problems. The patient cannot go to a sleep center directly. Sleep centers are only allowed to admit referred and diagnosed patients.

If the patient's family physician suspects sleep apnea, the physician will send the patient to a pneumologist who has a license for home sleep testing. To receive reimbursement for home sleep testing from the health insurance, the pneumologist has to get a license, which requires attending a 5-day course about basics of sleep medicine with an emphasis on sleep-disordered breathing and passing a 60-minute examination at the end of the course.

If the home sleep test is positive in terms of sleep apnea, the pneumologist will refer the patient to a sleep center for CPAP titration with attended PSG. The sleep center has to be accredited by either the German Sleep Society or by another institution to obtain health insurance reimbursement. The patient then returns after 3 to 6 months of treatment to the pneumologist for another home sleep test as a treatment follow-up. Thereafter are no planned follow-ups unless the patient experiences new complaints.

If the health insurance company determines that a diagnosis was wrong or a referral at any step was not justified, the insurance company can ask a control body to review the patient's medical records. These review bodies, called medical service of insurances, typically consist of special physicians employed by the control body. They will check the case and will see whether all diagnostic steps were performed according to guidelines. They will review the pneumologist for credentials and licensure as well as the sleep test data to determine the quality of the recording signals and whether the diagnostic and therapeutic decisions are justified.

The criteria used by the reviewing physicians derive from evidence-based literature and are compiled in a reviewers' guide for sleep-disordered breathing for the medical insurance services. If the reviewing body denies reimbursement for the claim, the pneumologist cannot appeal to the patient nor to the insurance company, but only to the independent control body. The physician is not prohibited from asking the patient to pay privately for the services provided, but as a cultural matter, German patients do not expect to have to pay privately for health care services. Accordingly, providers almost never ask for patients to cover services from their own pockets. If the prescription was found to be erroneous or a procedure was found to be not necessary, then the physician, not the hospital or institution, is liable and will be charged for the prescription. To cover this, German physicians have a professional insurance. Hospitals may cover this claim, if agreed on in the contract with the employed physician.

CLINICAL PEARLS

- Sleep medicine education in Europe is in the process of being developed by creating curricula that are based on evidence and worldwide knowledge on sleep physiology, sleep disorders, and treatment.
- Certification of sleep professionals and accreditation of sleep centers is advancing in all countries, and large efforts are taken to achieve the same consensus on patient service and quality of care independent of the health care system and more dependent on the underlying pathologies.
- Management of sleep disorders is developed through academic institutions that are in the process of installing sleep medicine programs and aligning these programs to achieve comparable goals to finally optimize patient care.

SUMMARY

Europe has a long tradition of sleep research. Sleep medicine evolved in parallel with other countries worldwide. The ESRS covers both sleep science and sleep medicine. Sleep medicine is more a national issue because health care systems are very different across the European countries. Some countries have large national sleep societies with sleep center accreditation and sleep expert certification. Other countries rely heavily on the ESRS. The ESRS tries to set consensus rules for sleep expert certification and sleep center accreditation and provides education for sleep experts and technologists. Publications on these issues are compiled and published in the *Journal of Sleep Research*. The implementation of these steps is coordinated among the European countries and recently is coordinated with similar activities initiated by the ERS. The management of patients with sleep disorders differs among European countries and is strongly linked to reimbursement schemes.

SELECTED READINGS

Bassetti C, Dogas Z, Peigneux P. *Sleep Medicine Textbook*. Regensburg: European Sleep Research Society; 2020.
Garbarino S. Excessive daytime sleepiness in obstructive sleep apnea: implications for driving licenses. *Sleep Breath*. 2020;24(1):37–47.
Grote L, Svedmyr S, Hedner J. Certification of fitness to drive in sleep apnea patients: Are we doing the right thing? *J Sleep Res*. 2018;27(6):e12719.

A complete reference list can be found online at ExpertConsult.com.

Section 10

Occupational Sleep Medicine

Chapter 78

Introduction

Samantha Riedy; Nancy Wesensten; Gregory Belenky

Occupational sleep medicine draws on clinical, experimental, and field research to sustain human performance. It is developing as a subset of sleep medicine with ties to occupational medicine and industrial and organizational psychology. The goal of occupational sleep medicine is to develop tactics, techniques, and procedures for sustaining performance and attendant productivity, safety, health, and well-being in the workplace and in other operational environments.

An operational environment is a workplace in which human performance is critical to system output; if the human fails, the system fails. Occupational sleep medicine applies to all operational environments involving human performance and 24/7 operations. Examples of operational environments include military operations, maritime operations, medicine, land transportation, aviation, security work, energy generation, resource extraction, financial markets, industrial production, the information media, and intelligence-gathering operations.

Sleep loss (time awake), adverse circadian rhythm phase (time of day), and workload (time on task/task difficulty) interact to degrade performance and increase self-reported fatigue and sleepiness. With increasing fatigue, performance degrades, productivity decreases, and the risk of error, incident, and accident increases. Occupational sleep medicine aims to mitigate these adverse effects and provides a basis for enterprise-wide systems of fatigue risk management.

What follows in this introduction are brief overviews of the chapters making up the occupational sleep medicine section.

CHAPTER 79: PERFORMANCE DEFICITS DURING SLEEP LOSS AND THEIR OPERATIONAL CONSEQUENCES

The pattern of sleep-loss–induced neurobehavioral deficits seen during laboratory studies tells us how workplace performance is likely to be affected by insufficient sleep. Under controlled laboratory conditions, performance impairment on neurobehavioral tasks often increases as sleep loss accumulates—an effect that is modulated by circadian phase and thereby exacerbated during the circadian trough. As the ability to sustain attention degrades, time on task becomes more salient, and breaks (time off task) restore performance (Video 78.1).

As discussed in Chapter 79, examples of operationally relevant phenomena associated with the impact of sleep loss include sleep loss–induced performance instability, interaction of sleepiness with time on task, impairment in dynamic decision-making, and sleepiness-induced alternation of regional brain activity. For example, under operational conditions, accidents can occur with exposure to critical events and lapses in sustained attention and/or problems with dynamic attentional control, which themselves are a function of sleep-wake and circadian factors.

CHAPTER 80: SLEEP AND SLEEP DISORDERS IN OPERATIONAL SETTINGS

Sleep disorders commonly observed in the workplace include sleep apnea, insomnia, and shift-work disorder and less frequently narcolepsy, idiopathic hypersomnia, and other sleep disorders. Sleep disorders can cause excessive daytime sleepiness and impaired performance through sleep loss and poor sleep quality. In operational settings, workplace performance degradation, workplace safety risks, and problems with absenteeism, productivity, health, and well-being can be exacerbated by untreated or inadequately treated sleep disorders.

As discussed in Chapter 80, managing sleep disorders in the workplace consists of a tiered approach that starts with screening. Screening may consist of screening for risk factors, using self-report tools aimed at identifying daytime sleepiness and related symptoms, and using functional performance tests for detecting impairment. Workers exceeding cut-offs may be referred to a sleep disorders medicine specialist for diagnosis, treatment, and compliance monitoring. In practical terms, managing sleep disorders in the workplace generally refers to managing obstructive sleep apnea but could be extended to include other common sleep disorders (e.g., insomnia and shift-work disorder).

CHAPTER 81: SHIFT WORK, SHIFT-WORK DISORDER, AND JET LAG DISORDER

In industrial economies, shift work and travel across time zones are common. Both displace sleep and wake from their usual temporal alignments with the 24-hour biologic rhythm. Workers' circadian rhythms will eventually (over days) resynchronize to a new time zone, but in most shift workers, their circadian rhythms do not resynchronize to night-shift work, in part because of light exposure and reverting back to nighttime sleep schedules on off days.

As discussed in Chapter 81, this misalignment can result in insomnia during the daytime period and excessive sleepiness during the nighttime work period, which, when sufficiently severe, are diagnosed as shift-work disorder (SWD). In lieu of organization-level adjustments in shift timing and duration, treatments to mitigate SWD include environmental manipulations, such as nocturnal bright light and daytime sleep in darkness, and pharmacologic interventions, such as stimulants to maintain alertness while on shift at night and sleep-inducing medications to maintain and extend sleep off-shift during the day.

Jet lag is characterized by excessive daytime sleepiness and nocturnal insomnia at the new local time. In contrast to SWD, jet lag is self-limited because the circadian rhythm gradually resynchronizes to new local time as a function of consistent daylight exposure. Thus bright light exposure can facilitate resynchronization if timed appropriately. Naps and caffeine are safe and effective countermeasures that can be implemented to reduce excessive daytime sleepiness.

CHAPTER 82: FATIGUE COUNTERMEASURES

Fatigue countermeasures serve to sustain operational performance and workplace safety in the face of sleep loss, poor sleep quality, sleep inertia, or adverse circadian phase. As such, fatigue countermeasures constitute a means of mitigating performance deficits without necessarily increasing quantity or quality of sleep. As discussed in Chapter 82, fatigue countermeasures can be stratified into four broad categories, including behavioral, environmental, technological, and pharmacologic. Examples of such fatigue countermeasures, respectively, include taking naps and rest breaks, increasing light exposure, using fatigue detection technologies, and using stimulants such as caffeine. Mathematical sleep, sleepiness, and performance prediction modeling can be used to help inform when fatigue countermeasures may be needed in an operation.

CHAPTER 83: SLEEP, SLEEPINESS, AND PERFORMANCE PREDICTION MODELING

Extant mathematical sleep, sleepiness, and performance prediction models are based on the two-process model of sleep regulation. Accordingly, sleep, sleepiness, and performance are governed by two neurobiologic processes: a homeostatic process that is determined by prior sleep-wake and a circadian process with a near 24-hour biologic rhythm. These models can be used to quantify the effect of an actual or predicted sleep-wake schedule on sleepiness and performance.

As discussed in Chapter 83, predictive models traditionally were one-step models that predicted sleepiness or performance directly from sleep-wake data. In recent years, two-step models have been developed to predict sleep-wake behaviors from work-rest schedules, and sleepiness or performance from predicted sleep-wake data. This development has allowed workplaces to use predictive models to proactively assess the likelihood of fatigue during a work-rest schedule and to determine the extent to which fatigue mitigation may be necessary. Application of predictive models as a component of fatigue risk management systems is gaining momentum in operational settings, particularly in transportation.

CHAPTER 84: FATIGUE RISK MANAGEMENT SYSTEMS

Fatigue risk management is an emerging applied arm of occupational sleep medicine. As discussed in Chapter 84, four core components of a fatigue risk management system (FRMS) are policy and documentation, fatigue risk management processes, safety assurance processes, and promotion processes. As indicated by its name, fatigue risk management involves actively managing risk (which in turn implies acceptance of some amount of risk). In contrast, prescriptive hours-of-service (HOS) rules specify shift duration, between-shift intervals, and within-shift breaks, thus imposing a priori boundaries that are designed to eliminate risk. However, because such HOS rules are not based in the physiology that drives performance (i.e., the human circadian rhythm and homeostatic drive for sleep), they are overly restrictive in some aspects (e.g., restricting consecutive hours worked) and potentially unsafe in other aspects (e.g., allowing for 23-hour days and other schedules that are incompatible with circadian physiology).

As discussed in Chapter 84, an FRMS based on sleep-wake and circadian principles affords an alternative to prescriptive HOS rules. An FRMS is adapted to the operational environment and is iteratively reviewed and revised to meet operational demands. Unlike prescriptive HOS rules, in which operators are incentivized to work to HOS limits, an FRMS may incentivize operators to sleep (e.g., in-flight napping) to extend duty hours (e.g., ultra-long–range flights). This unexpected consequence of FRMS implementation results from shifting the locus of responsibility for safety away from the regulator and toward employers and employees.

CHAPTER 85: SAFETY CASES AND ASSESSING ALTERNATIVE MEANS OF REGULATORY COMPLIANCE IN FATIGUE RISK MANAGEMENT

To operate outside of prescriptive HOS rules, an organization may be required to present a safety case and demonstrate that fatigue-related safety risks can be adequately mitigated and managed in the alternative approach. In commercial aviation, for example, airlines may develop an alternative means of compliance to the standard safety operations. As discussed in Chapter 85, to do so, the safety case must detail the proposed exemptions; a risk assessment; risk mitigation measures; and continued monitoring to ensure the continued efficacy of the alternative approach. Developing a robust safety case requires input and expertise from multiple parties, including the workers themselves, unions, management, regulators, and researchers.

CHAPTER 86: FATIGUE PROOFING

Fatigue-proofing strategies are risk-reduction strategies used by individuals and teams that allow workers to work safely even when fatigued. As discussed in Chapter 86, fatigue proofing can also be applied to the system of work; this includes redesigning the system (e.g., fatigue detection technologies) such that there is an additional defense against fatigue that reduces the likelihood of fatigue translating into workplace errors, incidents, or accidents. This shift in perspective away from HOS rules recognizes that fatigue cannot be simply eliminated from shift-work operations and, as such, that fatigue must be both mitigated and managed. As detailed in Chapter 86, important questions going forward will be how these often-informal strategies can be incorporated within a safety culture of an organization, how the efficacy of fatigue-proofing strategies will be assessed, and how they compare relative to other defenses against fatigue.

CHAPTER 87: SLEEP HEALTH IN ATHLETE POPULATIONS: UNIQUE CHALLENGES AND PRACTICAL SOLUTIONS

Obtaining sufficient sleep and reducing circadian misalignment in athlete populations are important for facilitating recovery, sustaining performance, and reducing injury risk. As discussed in Chapter 87, overscheduling, travel schedules, early morning practice times, sleep disorders, and other factors have repeatedly been linked to sleep loss, poor sleep quality, jet lag, and/or circadian desynchrony in athlete populations. However, research on the effects of these factors on athletic performance is limited, particularly in comparison to the well-characterized effects on cognitive performance. Furthermore, the efficacy of treatment for sleep disorders and fatigue countermeasures (e.g., light therapy) for improving athletic performance is not well characterized.

CHAPTER 88: ASSESSMENT OF THE OCCUPATIONAL SLEEP MEDICINE FIELD

Sleep medicine focuses mainly on diagnosis and treatment of specific sleep disorders (e.g., sleep apnea) in the individual patient. Complementing the clinical practice of sleep medicine, occupational sleep medicine is implemented at the group level not only to sustain workplace productivity and safety but also to maintain overall worker health across a career.

As discussed in Chapter 88, occupational sleep medicine is advancing on multiple fronts, including fatigue risk management, development of shift-work policies reflecting the short-term consequences of fatigue on operational performance and safety and long-term consequences on health and well-being, prevention of drowsy driving, mitigation of SWD, behavioral and pharmacologic interventions in special populations (e.g., first responders), and even genetics.

SELECTED READINGS

Borbély AA. A two-process model of sleep regulation. *Human Neurobiology*. 1982;1(3):195–204.

Belenky G, Balkin TJ, Redmond DP, Sing HC, Thomas ML, Thorne DR, Wesensten NJ. Sustaining performance during continuous operations: The U.S. Army's Sleep Management System. *1996 Proceedings of the Army Science Conference*; 1996:1–5.

Belenky G, Wesensten NJ, Thorne DR, et al. Patterns of performance degradation and restoration during sleep restriction and subsequent recovery: A sleep dose-response study. *Journal of Sleep Research*. 2003;12(1):1–12.

Cheng P, Drake C. Occupational sleep medicine. *Sleep Med Clin*. 2016;11(1):65–79.

Jang TW. Work-fitness evaluation for shift work disorder. Int *J Environ Res Public Health*. 2021;18(3):1294.

Van Dongen HPA, Maislin G, Mullington JM, Dinges DF. The cumulative cost of additional wakefulness: Dose-response effects of neurobehavioral functions and sleep physiology from chronic sleep restriction and total sleep deprivation. *Sleep*. 2003;26(2):117–126.

Chapter

79

Performance Deficits During Sleep Loss and Their Operational Consequences

Hans P.A. Van Dongen; Thomas J. Balkin; Steven R. Hursh; Jillian Dorrian

Chapter Highlights

- Sleep loss induces sleepiness and exerts profound negative effects on cognitive performance, increasing the risk of errors and accidents.
- Four operationally relevant phenomena associated with the impact of sleep loss on performance are presented, including sleep-loss–induced performance instability, interaction of sleepiness with time on task, impairments in dynamic decision making, and sleepiness-induced alteration of regional brain activity.
- Current knowledge regarding the impact of sleep loss on performance is summarized, and issues pertaining to the real-world application of this knowledge in operational environments are discussed.

INTRODUCTION

Sleep insufficiency is experienced at least occasionally by everyone and is experienced chronically by a considerable proportion of the adult population. Based on data from the 2014 Behavioral Risk Factor Surveillance System telephone survey,[1] 35% of adults in the United States on average obtain less than the 7 hours of sleep per 24 hours currently recommended.[2] If those with sleep disorders (sleep apnea, insomnia, etc.) are considered along with those who are chronically sleep restricted for other reasons (e.g., shift work, lifestyle), it is estimated that as many as 70 million Americans experience chronic sleep loss[3] and are therefore likely to experience sleepiness and impaired performance on a daily basis. Similar statistics are found across the world; for example, studies in Australia suggest that as many as 40% of adults experience some form of inadequate sleep, and 20% experience excessive daytime sleepiness leading to performance impairment.[4] It is estimated that sleep-loss–induced performance deficits cost the world economy hundreds of billions of dollars per year in accidents, direct health care costs, and lost operational efficiency and productivity.[5,6]

In this chapter, current knowledge regarding the impact of sleep loss on performance is summarized, and issues pertaining to the application of this knowledge to real-world, operational environments are discussed.

THE NATURE OF SLEEP-LOSS–INDUCED PERFORMANCE DEFICITS

Changes in the level of sleepiness, as determined by duration of prior sleep, time since awakening, and circadian timing (see Chapter 39), drive changes in performance on a variety of tasks in a predictable manner. For example, performance on a psychomotor vigilance test (PVT) declines in a dose-dependent fashion, with decreasing amounts of nighttime sleep across multiple days of sleep restriction.[7,8] Even so, identifying and addressing sleep-loss–induced performance deficits in operational settings is challenging because cognitive performance during sleep loss is not solely a reflection of a person's sleepiness level (drive to sleep).[9] In particular, sleepiness-induced declines in performance are not the result of a wholesale shift (general slowing) in the entire distribution of reaction times (RTs), but rather reflect increased trial-to-trial variability in RTs,[10,11] with an increasing proportion of relatively long RTs intermixed with "normal" RTs (i.e., RTs within the range typical of the well-rested state).[11,12]

It has been posited that the increased performance variability that characterizes sleep loss is most likely a manifestation of a reduced level of stability in the physiologic processes by which wakefulness is maintained—specifically, that it is caused by intermittent intrusion of sleep into wakefulness.[11,13] An implication of this hypothesis is that performance deficits due to sleep loss should be generic; that is, sleep loss should impact all facets of cognitive performance. However, evidence from cognitive/behavioral and neuroimaging studies does not uniformly support this hypothesis.[14,15] For example, aspects of working memory, executive mental functioning, and decision making have displayed remarkably little change during sleep deprivation in a variety of studies.[14] Recent evidence regarding the organization of sleep-wake processes suggests that sleepiness has the greatest effect on neural pathways that are used most intensively during performance of a given task. The deleterious effects of sleepiness appear to be most salient for the specific cognitive processes mediated by these neural pathways, in a use-dependent manner.[16,17]

Unfortunately, the relative extent to which different cognitive processes (e.g., information encoding, working memory) are differentially impacted by sleep loss cannot be readily specified, much less quantified. This is because (1) multiple cognitive processes are involved in any given performance task, with each distinct (and typically unobservable) cognitive process being affected by sleep loss to an unknown extent,[18] and (2) there is no scale against which different cognitive processes can be commonly measured and thus compared. Certain cognitive task designs allow for the effects of sleep loss on a specific cognitive process to be assessed by contrasting different task conditions (e.g., performance on a working memory task with two, three, or four items to be held in memory),[19] but these require the assumption that the effects of sleep loss on all other relevant cognitive processes remain invariant under each tested condition.

Although research in this area is gaining traction,[14,18] the experimental and logical challenges to determining the differential effects of sleep loss on various cognitive processes remain considerable. In part, this is because a test's sensitivity to sleep loss varies not only as a function of the sensitivity to sleep loss of the admixture of cognitive processes involved in the task performance, but also as a function of the parameters of the test itself. For example, manipulation of task duration, time pressure, amount of feedback provided during testing, and so forth, can impact the sensitivity of a performance measure to sleep loss[20,21] (see Chapter 38).

Likewise, statistics such as effect size are useful for comparing the sensitivity of specific tests administered with a specific set of test parameters, under specific sleep-loss conditions,[22,23] but they cannot be used as a basis for comparing the extent to which sleep loss generally impacts one cognitive ability versus another. To complicate matters further, large, trait-like individual differences in vulnerability to sleep loss exist.[24–26] These uncertainties also exist in workplace settings, where a job typically involves a wide range of tasks with several individuals performing a given job.

These challenges complicate researchers' efforts to understand the cognitive and neural underpinnings of performance deficits due to sleep loss. However, from a practical standpoint, application of the known principles by which circadian and homeostatic processes mediate alertness and performance can nevertheless be usefully applied in operational environments. That is, although the precise degree to which performance on a particular task will be degraded is not currently predictable for a specific individual, the general trends (both timing and extent) of sleep-loss–induced performance deficits *can* be predicted and usefully applied in operational settings.[27]

In this chapter we discuss four phenomena that characterize sleepiness in operational settings. The first is concerned with the translation of performance instability into errors and accidents in operational settings. The second is the interaction of sleep loss with time-on-task effects. The third is the role of attentional control deficits under rapidly changing circumstances. And the fourth is sleepiness-induced change in the brain activation patterns associated with degraded cognitive performance.

PERFORMANCE INSTABILITY: IMPACT ON ERRORS AND ACCIDENTS

In large-scale correlational studies, work schedules that interfere with adequate daily sleep, including extended work hours and shift work, have been linked to increased risk of human error and accidents,[28–30] resulting in reduced safety and productivity.[31–33] Yet, sleepy people do not make errors or cause accidents simply because they are sleep deprived, just as being fully alert does not guarantee error-free performance. In accident investigations the unequivocal establishment of sleepiness as a causal factor is often impossible, even when the presence of sleepiness is itself undisputed, unless there is convincing evidence that the accident was directly caused by frank sleep onset.[34,35]

There are two reasons for this. First, sleepiness is rarely the sole reason that accidents occur; multiple, diverse factors ranging from personnel shortages to equipment failures and safety-check overrides typically combine with human error to result in adverse outcomes. Second, as previously mentioned, human error due to sleepiness occurs against a backdrop of increased performance *variability*[11] and is therefore at least partly stochastic. In other words, although the likelihood/frequency of decremented performance increases with sleep loss, and is exacerbated during the descending phases of the circadian rhythm of alertness, actual task performance of a sleepy individual can vary from "impaired" to "normal" on a moment-to-moment basis.

Sleep-wake history and circadian rhythmicity interact to determine sleepiness/alertness and performance capability (see Chapter 39). Sleepiness varies as a function of time awake, with longer wakefulness inducing progressively increasing sleep drive. Sleepiness also varies as a function of time of day, with the biological clock's alertness output declining during "nighttime," resulting in elevated drive to sleep (sleepiness). As a consequence, alertness level and performance capability are reduced when working extended hours involving sleep loss and when working at night or in the early morning.[36,37] Moreover, chronic sleep loss leads to cumulative degradation of performance across days and weeks,[7,8] and perhaps longer; definitive longer-term studies have not yet been performed.

Not surprising, it has been determined that the circadian (i.e., time of day) variation in alertness and performance is associated with a circadian rhythm of accident rate and injuries.[28,38] There is less evidence for a relationship between accidents/injuries and changes in performance related specifically to duration of time awake. However, a relationship between duration of time awake and accident risk can be inferred from statistics on road crashes that were attributed to the driver having fallen asleep.[39,40] Although definitive evidence is lacking (and it should be noted that there is a possibility that crash investigators are biased—more likely to attribute accidents to sleepiness when the accident occurred at certain times of the night), it is reasonable to presume that the same interaction between sleep-wake history and circadian rhythm that increases sleepiness and decreases performance capability also increases the probability of driving errors and resulting traffic accidents.[35,41,42]

Many occupationally relevant tasks, ranging from systems monitoring and threat detection to driving, are likely vulnerable to sleep loss, at least in part because these tasks require sustained attention.[43,44] In modern operational settings characterized by extensive automation, such tasks are common. Automation and other technologic innovations have broadly improved safety, but by shifting performance demands to sustained-attention tasks, they may have simultaneously increased the likelihood of human error.[45,46] This is because the ability to sustain attention is negatively impacted by sleep loss and time of day (and time on task, discussed later). The paradoxical result is that although serious accidents are increasingly rare, when they do occur, such accidents can be especially devastating and costly.[47,48]

Because such catastrophic accidents are rare, and because their occurrence also typically depends on the chance convergence of random factors or events, it remains difficult to predict the risk of sleep-loss–induced accidents. Even when considering

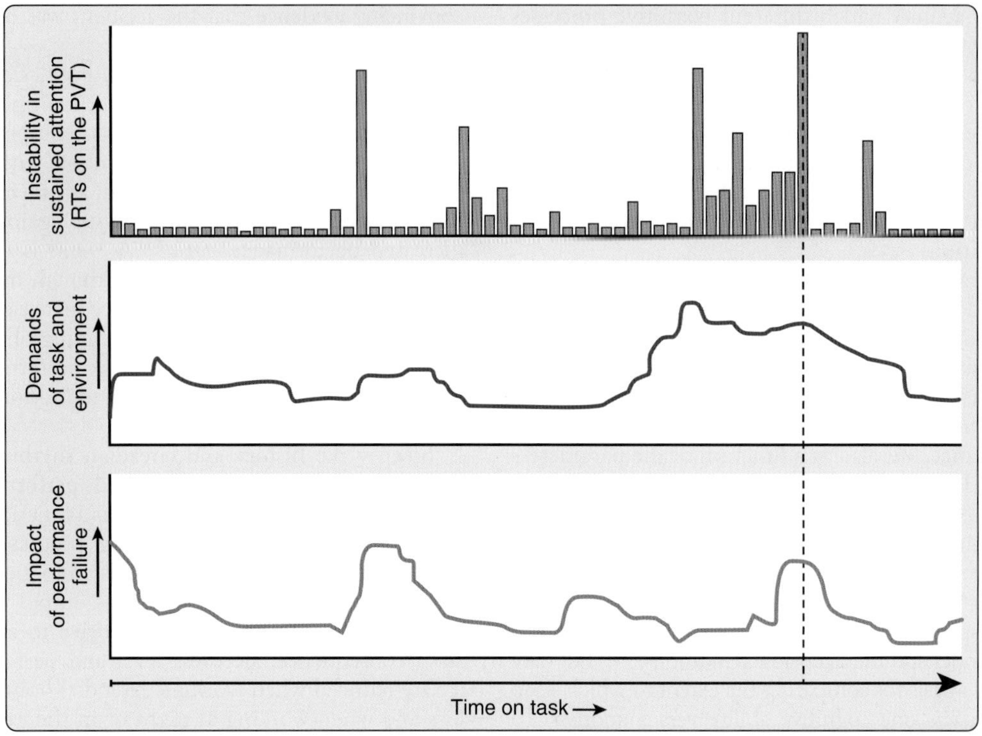

Figure 79.1 Schematic of a proposed mechanism by which sleep loss may contribute to accidents. The *top panel* depicts reaction times (RTs) across a 10-minute span of task performance on a psychomotor vigilance test (PVT) for an individual who continuously maintained wakefulness for 60 hours, as observed during an experiment published by Doran and colleagues[11] (panel reproduced with permission). This illustrates stochastic instability in sustained attention over a 10-minute interval; *longer bars* represent slowed responses indicative of lapses of attention. The *middle panel* shows a hypothetical pattern of changing demands of the task at hand and the environment in which it is performed (upward corresponds to greater demands). The *bottom panel* displays a hypothetical level of impact that human error would have over the course of the task. In this view of how sleepiness contributes to accident causation, intervals of inattention, when cognitive processing demands are high, lead to human error, which in turn, if the impact of error is considerable, results in an accident.[118] Thus, for sleep loss to actually lead to an accident, there must be temporal alignment (illustrated by the *dotted gray line*) of attentional lapses, substantial cognitive processing demands, and high impact of human error.[119] (From Doran SM, Van Dongen HPA, Dinges DF. Sustained attention performance during sleep deprivation: evidence of state instability. *Arch Ital Biol*. 2001;139:253–67.)

incidents more broadly by including near-accidents ("near-misses"[49]) and other performance errors, a relationship between sleepiness and accident rate remains difficult to discern. Consideration of the stochastic nature of performance impairment due to sleep loss may shed some light on this issue.

Figure 79.1 illustrates how sleep-loss–induced instability in performance impairment may lead to an accident. The PVT is a validated assay of sustained attention that is particularly sensitive to sleep loss.[22,50] As such, the series of RTs recorded in a PVT session can be considered a record of task inattentiveness. Assuming for the purpose of illustration that the same admixture of cognitive functions is required for a given task in an operational setting, then long RTs on the PVT would reflect intervals of inattentiveness (lapses of attention) during the task at hand. When the demands for cognitive processing are high during such intervals of inattentiveness, the likelihood of human error increases. And if the negative impact of human error at that specific time is also high, then an accident could result.

For example, if the task is driving a car, and an interval of inattentiveness coincides with the approach to an intersection with a stop sign, then detection and processing of the stop sign might fail and the intersection would be crossed without braking—that is, human error. If at the same time another car enters the intersection, a collision could ensue. Yet, if no other car enters the intersection, or there had been no intersection, and/or if the interval of inattentiveness had occurred a little earlier or later, then the accident would not have occurred.

From this perspective, it is necessary for a period of inattentiveness and significant impact of error to temporally align in a manner that results in an accident. It follows that accident risk is proportional to both total time of inattentiveness (cumulative lapse time) and density of critical task events (i.e., prior risk or exposure[51]). Given information about the latter, it may be possible to predict accident risk by predicting cumulative lapse time. There is a strong positive correlation between the number of lapses of attention and their duration,[50] and so a mathematical model that predicts PVT lapse counts could potentially serve this purpose (see Chapter 83).

THE TIME-ON-TASK EFFECT AND ITS INTERACTION WITH SLEEP LOSS

Hours-of-service regulations intended to mitigate the effects of sleepiness on performance and risk in operational settings are typically focused exclusively on "time on duty" and fail to account for sleep-wake history and circadian rhythm. There are both historical and practical reasons for this.[52] Dealing effectively with sleep-wake and circadian factors would require regulation of the timing and duration of workers' sleep, which would be nearly impossible to enforce. In addition, even when individuals are well rested, performance tends to deteriorate as a function of continuous time working[53] and is improved by rest breaks.[54] However, with the passing of work hours, time awake accrues and circadian time also passes. Depending on

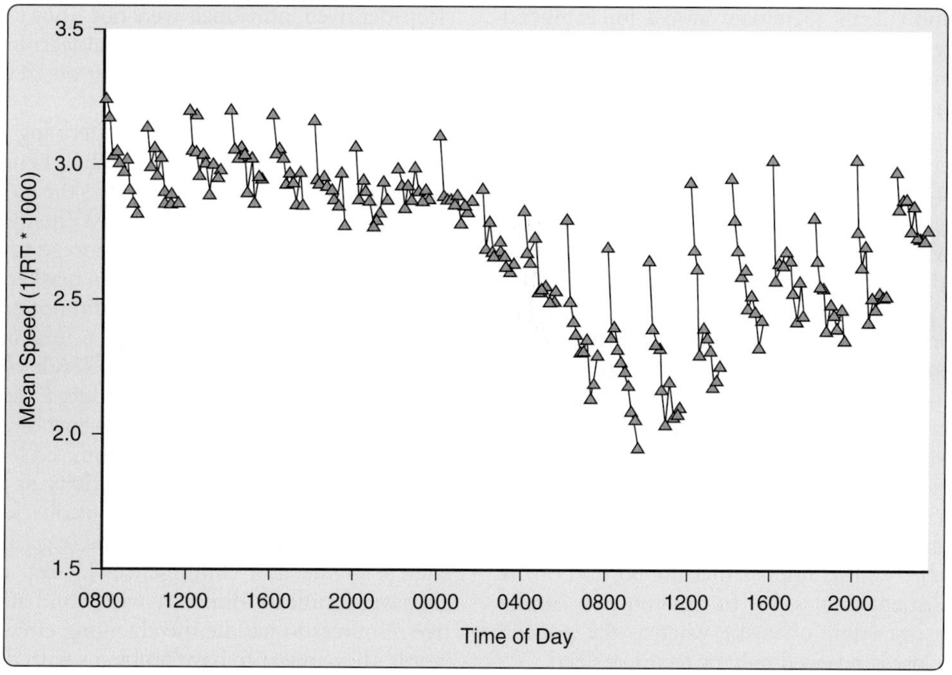

Figure 79.2 Time-on-task effect across a 10-minute psychomotor vigilance test (PVT) during 40 hours of total sleep deprivation. Each set of data points shows average speed (inverse of reaction time [RT]) in consecutive 1-minute bins (not drawn to scale on the time axis) during the 10-minute task duration. Note the changes in overall performance across the 40 hours of sleep deprivation due to the interaction of the effects of time awake and time of day. The time-on-task effect is the steady decline of performance across the 10 1-minute bins in each PVT bout, where the magnitude of the decline is linked to the interaction of the effects of time awake and time of day. Note also the restorative effect of rest breaks, resulting in improvement from minute 10 of one PVT bout to minute 1 of the next PVT bout, 2 hours later, despite the absence of intervening sleep. (Reproduced from Wesensten NJ, Belenky G, Thorne DR, et al. Modafinil vs. caffeine: effects on fatigue during sleep deprivation. *Aviat Space Environ Med.* 2004;75:520–25, with permission.)

whether the circadian rhythm of alertness happens to be in an ascending or descending phase, it will offset or amplify the performance-impairing effects of increasing work time and accumulating time awake. Therefore prescriptive hours-of-service regulations that do not take all of these factors into account will never be more than partially effective.[52,55]

Performance degradation caused by continuous performance on a particular task over time is a phenomenon commonly referred to as the time-on-task effect. This effect is especially pronounced for tasks that require sustained attention, such as the PVT,[56,57] which are also especially sensitive to sleep loss.[20,22,57] The time-on-task effect has been conceptualized as arising from cognitive-effort–related depletion of brain resources over time, resources that, unlike those mediating sleepiness, require only rest (time off task) to effect recuperation.[57] One possibility is that rest-mediated recovery may be the result of sleep-like states in the local neuronal pathways subserving the cognitive processes involved in performance of the task at hand.[16]

The time-on-task effect interacts with time awake and time of day. That is, as homeostatic sleep drive accrues with time awake, performance degrades faster during continuous task performance, and this interaction is mediated by the circadian rhythm of alertness. This is illustrated in Figure 79.2, which depicts minute-by-minute mean response speed on a 10-minute PVT administered every 2 hours across 40 hours of continuous wakefulness.[58] Time-on-task effects were evident before significant sleep loss, that is, from 8 AM to about midnight on the first day. Sleep deprivation exacerbated the time-on-task effect, especially during the night and early morning hours. For example, comparison of the performance change across the 10-minute test at 8 AM on day 1 versus 8 AM on day 2 reveals differences in overall performance *and* in the rate at which performance declined across the 10 minutes.

Of particular interest in Figure 79.2 is the extent to which performance on the PVT recovered from minute 10 on one test to minute 1 on the next test, although there was no intervening sleep. This was evident even when overall performance was degraded most significantly (at around 6 AM to 10 AM on the second day). Mean speed on the PVT at minute 1 on the 8 AM test was greater than mean speed at minute 10 on the 6 AM test, although average 10-minute performance declined across this time interval. In other words, the time-on-task effect is reversed by rest breaks (time off task), even during sleep deprivation.

One reasonable hypothesis is that time-on-task effects are at least partly motivational,[59,60] that is, that the decrements across each 10-minute PVT bout represent a within-bout decline in motivation and that the recovery from the end of one PVT bout to the beginning of the next merely reflects some temporary restoration of motivation. However, it has been found that performance impairment from time on task may carry over to performance of another task performed immediately afterward,[61,62] suggesting that declining motivation does not account for all time-on-task variance. That said, the time-on-task effect does not *necessarily* carry over between tasks performed back to back; in certain cases, performing a different task restores performance similarly to a rest break. It has been hypothesized that time-on-task carryover effects reflect use of common cognitive processes and neuronal pathways, thus preventing rest-mediated recovery in these pathways and resulting in further degradation of performance (as discussed above).[57]

From a practical standpoint, the extent to which sleepiness from time awake and time of day interacts with time on task to produce performance deficits is an important issue. Sleep loss often occurs because of externally imposed (e.g., occupational) requirements for individuals to remain awake for extended periods, performing goal-directed tasks. Thus studies in which the effects of sleep loss are measured on tasks performed nearly continuously may best replicate real-world operational conditions. In one such study, subjects performed cognitively demanding work on a nearly continuous basis across 54 hours of sustained wakefulness, with occasional administration of subjective rating scales (including mood, fatigue, and sleepiness scales) and with short breaks for meals and personal hygiene.[63] The study did not include a comparison condition in which work was performed at a slower pace (i.e., with more frequent and/or longer breaks). Comparison with previously published sleep-deprivation studies using similar tasks but for shorter periods of time, however, suggests that sustained cognitive work accelerates the rate at which performance declines during sleep deprivation.

Thus, the rate and extent to which performance is impaired varies as a function of both time on task and sleepiness (a joint function of the homeostatic sleep pressure and the circadian rhythm of alertness).[58,64] This implies that the portion of the performance impairment that is due to time on task can be reversed by simple rest (time off task), whereas the portion that is due to sleep loss is reversed only by recovery sleep.

IMPAIRMENTS IN DYNAMIC DECISION MAKING DUE TO SLEEP LOSS

The effects of sleep loss on tasks requiring sustained attention have consistently been shown to be substantial. Counterintuitively, the effects of sleep loss on more complex tasks, such as decision making, have been found to be comparatively small and inconsistent.[22,23,65,66] However, evidence is accumulating that when circumstances are fast paced, unfolding over time, and with uncertain outcomes, sleep loss produces substantial deficits in the ability to dynamically adapt decision making to changing conditions.[67,68] In particular, sleep loss causes profound impairments in the ability to use feedback regarding prior decisions to inform and adjust subsequent decision making, a phenomenon that has been called "feedback blunting."[69]

In the study that revealed this phenomenon, participants performed a "go/no go reversal learning task" while under time pressure, and they had to rely on feedback regarding the outcome of choices they made to be able to perform this task. First, the participants used the feedback to learn which four of eight numeric stimuli required a response ("go") and which four required that a response be withheld ("no go"). At an unpredictable time approximately halfway through the task, the "go" and "no go" stimuli were reversed without warning. Participants had to detect and adapt to the reversal, again using the feedback they received on the outcome of their choices. During a baseline day, well-rested participants readily learned which of the stimuli were "go" versus "no go," and they also adapted quickly to the unexpected reversal. But when the same participants were then sleep deprived and asked to perform the task a second time, they showed markedly impaired performance both before and after the reversal, with postreversal responses never rising above chance-level performance. By contrast, the second time the task was administered to participants in a non–sleep-deprived control condition, performance on the task improved both before and after the reversal. Thus, whereas well-rested individuals were able to effectively use choice outcome feedback to guide their decision making, sleep-deprived individuals were not. They exhibited significant impairments during the prereversal learning phase and especially during the more challenging postreversal phase of the task.[69]

Although the mechanisms underlying feedback blunting have yet to be fully elucidated,[68] the phenomenon cannot be fully explained by a failure to process the feedback information due to sustained attention deficits. When well-rested individuals performed a version of the go/no go reversal learning task in which some of the feedback was masked (i.e., obscured) to simulate lapses of attention, they did not experience the same pattern or severity of performance impairment as was seen in the sleep-deprivation study.[69] Results from other experiments suggest that sleep-loss–induced feedback blunting is not the result of degraded stimulus encoding,[70] reduced working memory resources,[19,71] compromised learning due to sleep deprivation,[72] nor enhanced sensitivity to interference.[19,73,74] Rather, it appears that when the feedback received indicates an unanticipated decision outcome (e.g., after an unexpected change in the task contingencies), sleep-deprived individuals have significant difficulty with rapid adaptation of cognitive resources to handle the changing circumstances. In other words, they appear to have problems with dynamic attentional control.[75–78]

When under time pressure, dynamic attentional control problems make it difficult to overcome prior expectations, resulting in reduced cognitive flexibility; failures to update situational awareness; and perseveration,[68,72] a long-recognized, but until recently poorly understood, effect of sleep loss.[79,80] Clearly, these dynamic attentional control problems due to sleep loss can have disastrous consequences in high-risk, high-tempo operational settings, such as military operations, emergency medical scenarios, and disaster response.[72] Prominent accidents that involved poor decision making that were potentially due to sleep-loss–induced problems with dynamic attentional control while under time pressure include the American International Airways flight 808 crash at Guantanamo Bay and the Three Mile Island nuclear catastrophe.

INSIGHTS FROM FUNCTIONAL BRAIN IMAGING STUDIES

Functional brain imaging studies have revealed reduced regional brain activity during sleep deprivation, with greatest reductions manifest in prefrontal cortex, inferior parietal/superior temporal cortex, and thalamus.[81] Based on such findings, specific sleep-loss–induced deficits in various aspects of performance have been predicted. For example, noting that sleep deprivation results in reduced metabolic activity in regions of the prefrontal cortex known to mediate specific aspects of cognitive performance and perception, it has been predicted and confirmed that sleep deprivation causes deficits in certain executive mental functions, such as risky or dynamic decision making[82–86] and moral reasoning and humor appreciation,[87,88] and that it results in reduced ability to differentiate odors.[89]

Although such results suggest a relationship between the level of activity in specific brain regions and cognitive performance, the relationship between regional brain activation and performance is not straightforward.[90] For example, data from functional magnetic resonance imaging (fMRI) studies have revealed not only that sleepiness-related performance deficits

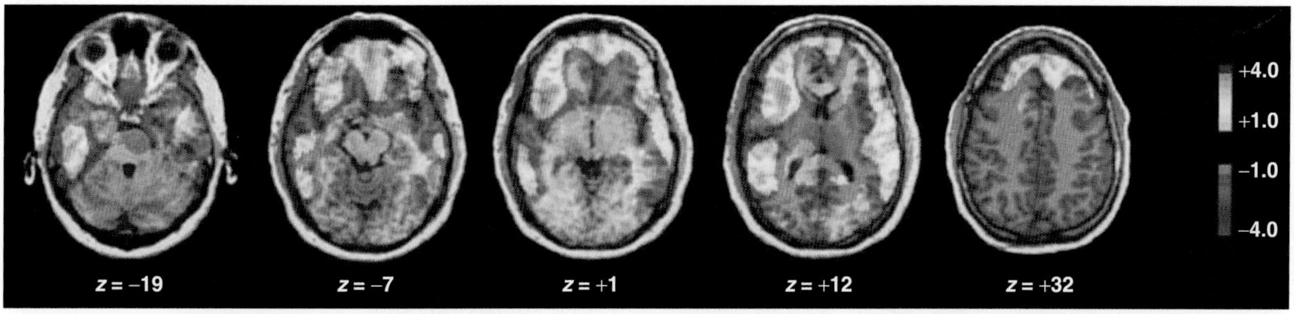

Figure 79.3 Brain map depicting changes in regional cerebral blood flow during the sleep inertia period between 5 and 20 minutes after awakening from stage 2 sleep. Color-coded values are Z-scores representing the significance level of changes in proportionally normalized regional cerebral blood flow in each voxel between scans acquired at 20 versus 5 minutes after awakening. The range Z-scores is coded in the color strip, with *red* designating Z-scores greater than +4.0 and *purple* designating Z-scores less than −4.0. Positive scores reflect relative increases in blood flow from 5 to 20 minutes after awakening; negative scores reflect concomitant, relative decreases during this period. (Reproduced from Balkin TJ, Braun AR, Wesensten NJ, et al. The process of awakening: a PET study of regional brain activity patterns mediating the reestablishment of alertness and consciousness. *Brain*. 2002;125:2308–19, with permission.)

are associated with cortical region-specific reductions in activation (relative to the rest of the brain), but also that the ability to maintain performance near baseline levels on specific tasks during sleep deprivation is associated with relative activation of (usually adjacent) cortical regions that were not comparatively activated during performance of the same task in the well-rested state.[91,92] Individuals whose fMRI images revealed such "new" regional relative activations during sleep deprivation were better able to maintain task performance than those whose fMRI images did not reveal such regional shifts in relative activation. These findings suggest that individual differences in the utilization of resources from other brain regions may underlie some of the task-specific individual differences in resilience to sleep loss.

However, subsequent fMRI studies have painted a more complex picture.[93,94] Results indicate that individuals possess varying degrees of redundant functional neuronal circuitry to process information, in a given task context in the well-rested state,[15] and that sleep deprivation reduces the number of functional neuronal circuits available.[15,94] These findings suggest an alternative explanation for task-specific individual differences in resilience during sleep loss. Namely, individuals with the greatest baseline redundancy in functional neuronal circuits for the task at hand may be the ones who can tolerate the greatest reduction in available circuits during sleep deprivation and are therefore likely to be the most resilient to performance impairment due to sleep loss on that task.[15]

The relationship between sleepiness and performance may also be investigated during the first several minutes after awakening. Paradoxically, this immediate post-awakening period is characterized by profound sleepiness and performance deficits, which rapidly dissipate within about 30 minutes of wakefulness.[95,96] This phenomenon is referred to as "sleep inertia." Studies of sleep inertia characterize a sleepy, yet sleep-satiated, brain that is ascending toward alertness.[97]

It is informative to compare regional cerebral blood flow patterns, as measured with positron emission tomography (PET), which provides information on absolute levels of activity during sleep deprivation, non–rapid eye movement (non-REM) sleep, and sleep inertia. Compared to well-rested wakefulness, sleep-deprived wakefulness is characterized by global reductions in absolute levels of brain activity, with the greatest reductions evident in heteromodal (primarily prefrontal) association cortices and thalamus.[81] A similar pattern is evident when comparing non-REM sleep to well-rested wakefulness: global deactivation (albeit of a greater magnitude than during sleep-deprived wakefulness), with the greatest deactivations evident in anterior (prefrontal) cortical regions and centrencephalic regions, including the thalamus.[98] In contrast, the immediate post-awakening, sleep inertia period is characterized by bidirectional changes in regional cerebral blood flow, with waxing activity in anterior cortical regions and waning activity in centrencephalic regions across the first 5 to 20 minutes of wakefulness[99] (Figure 79.3).

Because deactivated anterior/prefrontal cortex is the only common finding among these three states (sleep-deprived wakefulness, non-REM sleep, and sleep inertia), it has been surmised that activity in the prefrontal cortices is a critical determinant of sleepiness and its attendant performance deficits. Taken together, findings from neuroimaging studies suggest that performance impairment on tasks affected by fluctuations in sleepiness vary as a function of regional brain activity and interregional connectivity patterns,[100] concerning especially those functional connections involving prefrontal cortices.

PERFORMANCE DEFICITS IN THE OPERATIONAL CONTEXT

Sleepiness contributes to hundreds of thousands of road accidents each year[101] and has been cited as a contributing factor in industrial disasters such as the meltdown of the Chernobyl nuclear reactor, the grounding of the Exxon Valdez oil tanker, and the decision to launch the ill-fated Challenger space shuttle. The present chapter provides an overview of current thinking regarding the combined effects of sleep loss, circadian rhythm of alertness, and time-on-task factors on performance.

Figure 79.4 depicts these factors in a larger operational context, where neurobiologic drivers of performance interact with features of the operational setting to determine performance outcomes and the risk of errors, incidents, and accidents. Present-day hours-of-service regulations do not adequately account for this complexity, which limits their utility for promoting safety and productivity in operational environments.[52] Recent developments that integrate mathematical models

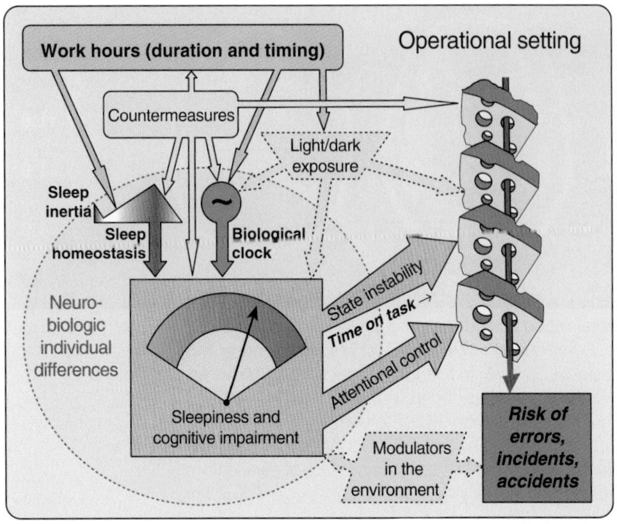

Figure 79.4 Schematic of the interplay of multiple factors shaping the consequences of performance deficits during sleep loss in an operational setting. The timing and duration of work hours determines the timing and (minimal) duration of required wakefulness and thereby the buildup (during wakefulness) and dissipation (during sleep opportunities) of homeostatic sleep pressure. Further, the strength of the alertness drive from the biological clock varies as a function of the timing of the work hours, which in interaction with the homeostatic sleep drive determines the level of sleepiness and the attendant cognitive impairment (see Chapter 38). This manifests as performance instability, which is amplified by the time-on-task effect and deficits in dynamic attentional control. These effects exacerbate the risk of errors, incidents, and accidents. The timing and duration of work hours (and thus wakefulness) also affects exposure to ambient light, which, depending on the timing, duration, and intensity of the light exposure, may (1) influence the rhythm of the biological clock, (2) reduce sleepiness and improve cognitive impairment directly (albeit transiently), and (3) affect risk of errors, incidents, and accidents by impacting vision and visibility.[120] Various factors in the environment, such as the amount of automation,[46] weather conditions, or distractions (see Chapter 38), may modulate the operational risk either directly or by altering sleepiness and cognitive impairment. According to Reason's "Swiss cheese" model of accident causation,[119] accidents occur when risk factors align in space and time (i.e., when the "holes" in the "Swiss cheese" line up so that problems can propagate and turn into accidents). A wide range of countermeasures and mitigations (e.g., rest breaks, nap opportunities, melatonin administration, caffeine intake, safety equipment, and increased staffing) may be used to improve risk outcomes.[113,121] The neurobiologic components in this schematic (in the *purple circle*) exhibit large individual differences, but their dynamics over time are well understood and predictable by mathematical models (see Chapter 83).

predicting cognitive impairment into regulatory frameworks for hours of service can be used to address this issue to some extent (see Chapter 83).

Other indirect effects of sleep loss on performance should be noted. Sleepiness tends to promote impulsivity and risk taking[84,102] and impairs self-monitoring of performance,[70,103] self-regulation of behavior and emotions,[104] and social monitoring and interaction.[104–107] The extent to which these aspects of impaired functioning contribute to errors and accidents is unknown, although risk taking and sleep loss have been noted to be a potentially deadly combination in young male drivers.[108,109] There is also some evidence that sleep loss impacts negatively on communication and team cohesion, with adverse operational consequences.[110]

In the workplace, to the extent possible, the separate and combined effects of all relevant factors should be considered when evaluating the risk of errors, incidents, and accidents (Figure 79.4). The potential costs and consequences of such risk should determine the need for risk management strategies.[52,111–114] Best practice involves doing so in the context of a fatigue risk management system (see Chapter 84).

In the clinic, the consequences of sleep loss and sleepiness and the need to intervene remain difficult to gauge. A clinician seeing objectively or subjectively sleepy patients should discuss with them the risk of errors and accidents. The clinician may also try to estimate risk level by asking questions about the following:

- Type of job
- Nature of job (safety-sensitive/mission-critical)
- Level of risk exposure
- History of accidents and incidents or "near misses"
- Safety measures that could be put in place (e.g., rest breaks, ergonomic tools)
- Habitual sleep-wake/-work schedules
- Duties, tasks, hobbies, and circumstances that intrude on time for sleep
- Potential evidence of the existence of a sleep disorder (e.g., see Chapter 80)
- Length of commute to and from work
- Possible consequences of adverse events

In addition, it is important to consider any legal and ethical requirements that may vary by jurisdiction and by clinical role (e.g., general practitioner, psychologist, occupational medicine specialist). For example, there may be a legal and/or ethical duty of care to report excessive sleepiness to an employer in cases where work safety may be impacted.

Clinical decisions regarding work readiness in this context are frequently complex, and access to legal, ethical, and professional resources is critical to aid clinical decision making.[115] It is often helpful to talk with clients about the potential limitations of their own subjective evaluation of sleep-loss–related impairment, highlighting that people have a tendency to overestimate their own capabilities.[8,9] Furthermore, because of the stochastic nature of human error (Figure 79.1), past performance or safety does not guarantee future performance or safety. Bringing these issues to the attention of clients may assist the clinician to support them in making behavioral or other changes and thereby reducing their risk of sleep-loss–related errors and accidents.

CLINICAL PEARL

Interactions among multiple factors, such as recent and long-term sleep-wake history, circadian rhythm, time-on-task effect, and individual differences in vulnerability to sleep loss, lead to sleepiness-related performance deficits and contribute to errors and accidents. Such factors should be taken into consideration when devising operational work-rest schedules, implementing risk management strategies, and assessing patients who report sleepiness or cognitive performance deficits.

SUMMARY

Inadequate sleep is virtually ubiquitous in operational environments and exacts an inestimable toll on society via generally reduced efficiency and productivity, overestimation of one's performance capabilities, decreased cognitive flexibility and increased errors, and (sometimes catastrophic) industrial accidents. These phenomena manifest as a function of the combined effects of the homeostatic pressure to initiate sleep and the circadian rhythm of alertness, with some evidence for an interaction with task demands.[116,117] In addition, there are considerable trait-like individual differences in the ability to maintain performance under sleepiness-inducing conditions. Future progress will be realized with an improved understanding and appreciation of the interactions between sleep loss and task-related variables, an improved ability to measure these effects, and implementation of alertness/performance management strategies that, unlike most current hours-of-service regulations, effectively address these effects.

ACKNOWLEDGMENTS

This research was supported in part by an appointment to the Research Participation Program at the Walter Reed Army Institute of Research administered by the Oak Ridge Institute for Science and Education through an interagency agreement between the U.S. Department of Energy and U.S. Army Medical Research and Development Command. The views expressed in this article are those of the authors and do not reflect the official policy or position of the Department of the Army, the Department of Defense, the U.S. Government, or any of the institutes with which the authors are affiliated.

SELECTED READINGS

Balkin TJ, Braun AR, Wesensten NJ, et al. The process of awakening: a PET study of regional brain activity patterns mediating the reestablishment of alertness and consciousness. *Brain.* 2002;125:2308–2319.

Belenky G, Wesensten NJ, Thorne DR, et al. Patterns of performance degradation and restoration during sleep restriction and subsequent recovery: a sleep dose-response study. *J Sleep Res.* 2003;12:1–12.

Chee MWL, Asplund CL. Neuroimaging of attention and alteration of processing capacity in sleep-deprived persons. In: Nofzinger E, Maquet P, Thorpy MJ, eds. *Neuroimaging of Sleep and Sleep Disorders.* Cambridge, UK: Cambridge University Press; 2013:137–144.

Dinges DF, Kribbs NB. Performing while sleepy: effects of experimentally-induced sleepiness. In: Monk TH, ed. *Sleep, Sleepiness and Performance.* Chichester, UK: John Wiley & Sons; 1991:97–128.

Drummond SPA, Brown GG, Gillin JC, et al. Altered brain response to verbal learning following sleep deprivation. *Nature.* 2000;403:655–657.

Durmer JS, Dinges DF. Neurocognitive consequences of sleep deprivation. *Semin Neurol.* 2005;25:117–129.

Hudson AN, Van Dongen HPA, Honn KA. Sleep deprivation, vigilant attention, and brain function: a review. *Neuropsychopharmacol Rev.* 2020;45:21–30.

Mantua J, Brager AJ, Alger SE, et al. Self-reported sleep need, subjective resilience, and cognitive performance following sleep loss and recovery sleep. *Psychol Rep.* 2021;124(1):210–226.

Oonk M, Tucker AM, Belenky G, Van Dongen HPA. Excessive sleepiness: determinants, outcomes, and context. *Int J Sleep Wakefulness.* 2008;1:141–147.

Van Dongen HPA, Maislin G, Mullington JM, Dinges DF. The cumulative cost of additional wakefulness: dose-response effects on neurobehavioral functions and sleep physiology from chronic sleep restriction and total sleep deprivation. *Sleep.* 2003;26:117–126.

Wesensten NJ, Belenky G, Thorne DR, et al. Modafinil vs. caffeine: effects on fatigue during sleep deprivation. *Aviat Space Environ Med.* 2004;75:520–525.

Whitney P, Hinson JM, Jackson ML, Van Dongen HPA. Feedback blunting: total sleep deprivation impairs decision making that requires updating based on feedback. *Sleep.* 2015;38:745–754.

Wilkinson RT. Interaction of lack of sleep with knowledge of results, repeated testing, and individual differences. *J Exp Psychol.* 1961;62:263–271.

A complete reference list can be found online at ExpertConsult.com.

Chapter 80

Sleep and Sleep Disorders in Operational Settings

Andrew Vakulin; Shantha Rajaratnam; Ronald Grunstein

Chapter Highlights

- Sleep disorders, including insomnia, obstructive sleep apnea, and disorders of hypersomnolence, are common in operational settings. If left untreated, these conditions contribute to excessive daytime sleepiness and elevated risk of errors and accidents.
- Symptoms of excessive daytime sleepiness and functional performance impairment are highly variable across individual patients/employees, making it essential that a comprehensive fitness-for-duty assessment is conducted on an individual basis.
- When a sleep disorder is identified in an employee, relying on history and self-report is often inappropriate, especially in operational settings, where biased reporting is more likely.
- Sleep specialists and occupational clinicians should consider adopting a formal assessment strategy, including screening and diagnosis of the sleep disorder as well as objective functional alertness/performance testing before finalizing fitness-for-duty recommendations.

INTRODUCTION

The effect of sleep disorders in degrading daytime function is well recognized.[1,2] Patients with sleep disorders in the workplace often have problems such as absenteeism, presenteeism, and increased risk of errors, incidents, and accidents. For some operations, there are regulatory requirements with regard to the presence or absence of sleep disorders. This chapter describes the occupational health issues observed in patients with common sleep disorders, including primary hypersomnia, insomnia, and obstructive sleep apnea (OSA).

PREVALENCE AND IMPACT OF SLEEP DISORDERS IN OPERATIONAL SETTINGS

Narcolepsy and Other Central Disorders of Hypersomnolence

Disorders of hypersomnolence are characterized by excessive daytime sleepiness and pathologically elevated sleep drive that is not caused by nocturnal sleep disruption or circadian misalignment. The disorders collectively fit under an umbrella term, central disorders of hypersomnolence, and include the primary hypersomnia disorders such as narcolepsy and idiopathic hypersomnia,[3,4] which are chronic conditions characterized by excessive daytime sleepiness. These conditions can be associated with decreased quality of life, increased disability, and degraded performance that can affect occupational health and safety. Studies have found that impaired mood, greater psychopathology, and relationship and work problems are more prevalent among patients with narcolepsy relative to that of healthy controls or the general population.[5] Furthermore, increased unemployment, early retirement, welfare enrollment, absenteeism, presenteeism, and lower wages are all seen in patients with hypersomnia.[6-12]

Most of the data on occupational health–related aspects of central disorders of hypersomnolence tend to be from studies of patient populations who are diagnosed with narcolepsy rather than other types of central hypersomnias, such as idiopathic hypersomnolence.[12a] From a practical and regulatory point of view, it is sensible to consider these disorders as part of the same spectrum and to consider the severity of the condition as contributing to the risk to safety and productivity. A possible exception is the motor impairment of cataplexy specific to type 1 narcolepsy, which in addition to hypersomnolence, is characterized by brief episodes of sudden loss of muscle tone, while still awake/conscious. Consequently, cataplexy could lead to additional adverse outcomes ranging from minor injury in a fall to a vehicle crash resulting in injury or death to the patient and others; however, there is limited research supporting these relationships.[13,14] This may be because patients with cataplexy can anticipate the occurrence of a cataplectic attack and adapt their behavior to reduce risk of an incident or accident.[14]

In addition to the effect of the underlying condition, occupational risks can arise from the medications used to treat hypersomnolence. For example, amphetamines and other stimulants have been associated with increased crash risk,[15] and gamma-hydroxybutyrate can impair psychomotor vigilance and driving performance.[16] The reasons for increased accident risk are thought to be multifactorial and include higher risk-taking behavior, poorer compliance with traffic rules, and the after-effects of the medication, including hypersomnolence and fatigue.

Narcolepsy and Other Central Disorders of Hypersomnolence in the Workplace

Narcolepsy, idiopathic hypersomnolence, and other central disorders of hypersomnolence present a major challenge not only for patients but also for clinicians, who are often involved in decisions regarding job suitability, work conditions, and occupational safety.

In a recent analysis of the online-based US National Health and Wellness Survey,[11] 437 individuals reporting a diagnosis of narcolepsy were matched 1 : 2 with 837 controls based on age, sex, race/ethnicity, marital status, education, household income, body mass index, smoking status, alcohol use, exercise, and physical comorbidity. The narcolepsy group had greater comorbidities and substantially higher rates of mental illness. Long-term disability was 70% higher in the narcolepsy group relative to matched controls. Those in the narcolepsy group were less likely to be working and had greater absenteeism and presenteeism. The US BOND study[17] performed a subanalysis of productivity outcomes between 600 subjects with narcolepsy and 2279 matched controls and found that patients with narcolepsy had a higher prevalence of absenteeism, accidents, and disability days related to short-term disability compared with controls. Interestingly, there were no significant differences between the groups in workers' compensation claims. These data highlight the enormous disease burden facing patients with hypersomnias and the complexities of managing the problem. Profound sleepiness can severely limit educational opportunities in narcolepsy, including basic skills needed for employment.[10] Diagnosis and appropriate use of medications will help; however, there is often residual symptomology even with optimum treatment, stigma, and loss of self-esteem that will cause or exacerbate mental illness. The integral role of poor mental health[18] in the disabilities surrounding narcolepsy is critical to acknowledge in understanding the occupational health implications. It has been reported that 30% to 50% of patients with narcolepsy have been dismissed from employment.[9,19]

Narcolepsy and Other Central Disorders of Hypersomnolence in Road Safety

Impaired vigilance is a salient symptom of narcolepsy and other central hypersomnias. Impaired vigilance and other cognitive limitations interact to degrade driving and performance on other critical tasks.[20-22] As a general comment, these studies have relatively few subjects and analyses to determine individuals most at risk are underpowered. Given these relationships, however, it is not surprising that vehicle crashes occur at a higher rate in patients with narcolepsy.[23] A recent study from Taiwan compared narcolepsy cases (n = 329) with matched controls (n = 987) and showed a 6.7-fold higher rate of hospitalization following a MVA in patients with narcolepsy compared to controls.[24] Risk of car accidents is modulated by narcolepsy treatment and has been shown to return risk to control levels after 5 years of sustained treatment.[24,25]

Insomnia

Insomnia is characterized by "difficulty initiating sleep, difficulty maintaining sleep, waking up earlier than desired, resistance to going to bed on appropriate schedule, or difficulty sleeping without parent or caregiver intervention," accompanied by patient reports of functional impairments, occurring at least 3 times per week over at least 3 months, and the symptoms are not better explained by another sleep disorder or by inadequate sleep opportunity (see Chapter 69).[25a] These symptoms may also be indicative of another sleep disorder such as shift-work sleep disorder (see Chapter 81).[25a] There are some inconsistencies in the literature as to which types of neurocognitive impairments are associated with insomnia.[26] These discrepancies could be due to the heterogeneity of the disorder as well as methodological differences between studies. That said, insomnia patients commonly report significant distress and daytime impairments.[27]

Insomnia in Employed Individuals in the General Population

Prevalence of insomnia in working populations has been assessed in national surveys. In a representative sample of US workers from the National Health and Nutrition Examination Survey, insomnia (defined as poor sleep quality) was reported in 19.2% of the full sample, and 30.7% of shift workers.[28] An analysis of the 2008 National Sleep Foundation's Sleep in America telephone poll used available sleep questionnaire items to classify patients into sleep disorder risk categories using diagnostic criteria.[29] The demographic and employment characteristics of the poll sample were close to national labor statistics. The authors found that 26% reported difficulty falling asleep a few nights per week or more, 42% reported frequent awakenings at night a few nights per week or more, and 49% reported experiencing nonrefreshing sleep a few nights per week or more. Those with insomnia symptoms also had increased odds of negative work outcomes, including difficulty with cognitive tasks at work, mood-related problems, and presenteeism and absenteeism. They also had higher odds of experiencing an occupational accident in the previous year. Associations between insomnia symptoms and workplace accidents, errors, and injuries were examined in the America Insomnia Survey, a national survey of subscribers to a large US health plan.[30,31] Prevalence of insomnia in employed individuals, assessed using the Brief Insomnia Questionnaire,[32] was found to be 23% when the duration of symptoms lasted at least 30 days, and 20% when the duration of symptoms lasted at least 12 months.[30] Insomnia was associated with workplace injuries (odds ratio [OR] = 1.9, 95% confidence interval [CI]: 1.4 to 2.6), including after adjusting for sociodemographic confounders (OR = 2.0, 95% CI: 1.4 to 2.8), but not after adjusting for comorbidities (OR = 1.4, 95% CI: 0.9 to 2.0). The estimated proportion of total injuries that was attributed to insomnia was 4.6% after controlling for comorbidities. Insomnia was also significantly associated with costly workplace accidents and/or errors, defined as causing damage or work disruption of $500 or more, with OR of 1.4 after controlling for comorbidities.[31] Compared with the average cost of accidents and errors not related to insomnia, the average costs of insomnia-related accidents and errors was significantly higher. Finally, insomnia was estimated to be associated with 7.2% of all costly workplace accidents and errors and 23.7% of the costs of these events (higher than any other chronic condition identified), which, when projected across the entire US population, would have a combined value of $31.1 billion.[31]

Middle-aged and older employed adults (i.e., age 50 to 70 years) who reported a higher number of insomnia symptoms (i.e., three to four symptoms) showed twice the odds of leaving paid employment as a result of poor health at follow-up.[33] These findings demonstrate that elevated insomnia symptoms are a predictor for leaving paid employment in this age group.

Insomnia in Occupational Settings

The prevalence of insomnia symptoms in occupational settings varies between studies, in part because of differences in population and/or in study methodology. With the Athens Insomnia Scale,[34] large occupational screening studies have found that 6.5% of North American police officers[35] and 6% of US firefighters[36] have symptoms that put them at moderate to severe risk for insomnia. With use of the Insomnia Severity Index, 15.2% of commercial motor vehicle drivers screened as high risk for insomnia,[37] compared with 4.1% of age- and gender-matched controls from the general population.[38] In a sample of emergency medical technicians, 50.3% were found to have delayed sleep onset, and 13.1% were found to have difficulty maintaining sleep using two questions from a broad sleep questionnaire.[39] With use of the National Health Insurance Research Database in Taiwan, the adjusted OR for being treated for insomnia in hospital physicians compared to matched controls was found to be 2.0 (95% CI: 1.9 to 2.1), indicating greater likelihood of being treated for insomnia.[40] Similarly, with the same database, the adjusted hazard ratio for nurses compared with matched controls was 1.4 (95% CI: 1.4 to 1.5).[41] In a sample of workers from a US-based global manufacturing company, 34.5% reported difficulties falling asleep, 60.4% reported difficulty staying asleep, and 35.1% reported waking too early on a short-form version of the Sleep Condition Indicator measuring insomnia symptoms.[42,43] This study also found that insomnia symptoms were associated with impaired workplace productivity.[42] More studies with rigorous sampling methods using validated screening instruments are required.

Impact of Insomnia on Occupational Outcomes

Between 1983 and 2010 a review identified 30 studies that assessed occupational outcomes associated with insomnia, insomnia symptoms, or poor sleep quality.[44] The overall conclusion from this review was that insomnia symptoms are independently associated with reduced workplace safety and productivity, increased sickness-related absenteeism, impeded career progression, and reduced job satisfaction.

There is growing evidence that insomnia and insomnia symptoms are related to occupational accidents and other safety-related events. Results from the 2005 Taiwan Social Development Trend Survey showed that insomnia symptoms, in particular early morning awakenings and nonrestorative sleep, are associated with increased odds of minor accidents during work and leisure time among Taiwanese adults.[45] Similarly, another study found that persistent insomnia symptoms (present at baseline and at a 10-year follow-up) were associated with a higher risk of self-reported occupational accidents among a sample of adults in Sweden, although the results did not show a significantly increased risk of register-reported occupational accidents or sick leave.[46] In a sample of truck drivers, those with insomnia reported more MVA in the 3 years before the study and near-miss accidents in the previous 6 months compared with other drivers, even after controlling for confounders, including OSA.[47]

Few studies have examined the specific impacts of insomnia symptoms on workplace safety behaviors that may ultimately contribute to an adverse safety event. Safety behaviors are defined as those practices and procedures mandated by the workplace to meet and maintain minimal safety requirements, as well as additional voluntary behaviors that further promote safety in the workplace. A recent study in construction workers showed that difficulty falling asleep and maintaining sleep during the past month are associated with fewer reported voluntary safety behaviors.[48] Furthermore, these effects were mediated by workplace "cognitive failure," which is measured by the frequency in which the individual reports engaging in specific behaviors reflecting impaired cognition while at work. Others have also proposed that the relationship between insomnia and increased injury risk may be explained by the influence of insomnia on safety behaviors.[49]

Although the studies described previously focus on the potential impact of insomnia and insomnia symptoms on occupational outcomes, the impact of occupational factors on developing insomnia has received relatively little attention, with the exception of shift work. One study showed in older workers, 18.8% of whom reported insomnia symptoms, that occupational risk factors for insomnia included unemployment, shift work, lack of control and lack of support at work, job insecurity, and job dissatisfaction.[50]

Interactions between Insomnia, Job Stress, and Burnout

Reciprocal relationships between insomnia, job stress, and burnout have been previously described. One prospective study examined insomnia in Norwegian shift-working nurses using the Bergen Insomnia Scale[51] as well as questionnaires assessing personality traits, lifestyle factors, mental health, sleepiness, and work-related stressors both initially and then after approximately 2 years.[52] The authors found that inability to overcome drowsiness, exposure to bullying behavior, and negative spillover between work and family life predicted increased symptoms of insomnia after 2 years. Insomnia and anxiety showed a bidirectional relationship. On the other hand, depression was a predictor of insomnia, but insomnia was not a predictor of depression.

A recent meta-analysis that included 17 studies examined the relationships between job stress variables and insomnia.[53] High levels of job stress, effort-reward imbalance, higher demand, and work-family conflict were found to be associated with greater risk of insomnia. Supporting these findings, a recent prospective study in newly graduated nurses showed that occupational stress was associated with increased severity of insomnia across time points during their first year as nurses.[54]

Reciprocal relationships between insomnia and job stress (including work demands, decision authority, and workplace social support) were shown in a recent prospective study of a large sample of the Swedish working population.[55] In a study of Japanese daytime local government employees, role conflict as well as anxious temperament were associated with insomnia symptoms, highlighting the role of individual characteristics as well as job-related factors in this relationship.[56]

One model that has been applied to explain the reciprocal work stress–insomnia relationship is the work effort–recovery model, in which sleep is regarded as a prototypical recovery activity.[57] The work effort–recovery model states that repeated chronic exposure to a stressful work environment, combined with insufficient recovery and coping possibilities, over time leads to maladaptive reactions to the stressors and starts to negatively impact health.[58] For example, in one study anticipation of increased work stress the following day degraded sleep quality, manifesting as a reduction in slow wave sleep.[59] Strong relationships have been found between sleep quality and occupational stress, rumination, fatigue, and well-being, providing support for the effort-recovery theory.[57]

Burnout is a syndrome resulting from inadequately managed and chronic work-related stress. A systematic review of 36 prospective studies examining physical, psychological, and occupational consequences of burnout found that insomnia was a consequence of burnout in some but not all studies.[60] In North American firefighters, those screening positive for insomnia had higher risk of burnout (adjusted OR 3.60), and two of the dimensions of burnout, high emotional exhaustion (adjusted OR 3.78) and low personal achievement (adjusted OR 2.16).[61] This study also found that sleep during overnight work mediated the impact of having a sleep disorder on burnout risk, suggesting a protective role of sleep and conversely a deleterious role of excessive sleepiness.

Obstructive Sleep Apnea

OSA is a common sleep-related breathing disorder characterized by repeated obstruction of the upper airway, leading to frequent arousals from sleep and oxygen desaturations during sleep.[62] The prevalence of OSA has been rising over the past two decades in parallel with increasing obesity; recent studies report that up to 25% of middle-aged individuals have moderate to severe OSA.[63,64] OSA also tends to be more prevalent among older individuals, males, Asian and Black populations, and postmenopausal women.[62,65-67] OSA is associated with excessive daytime sleepiness, neurobehavioral dysfunction,[1] cardiovascular disease,[68] negative mental health outcomes,[69] reduced quality of life,[70] and premature death.[71,72]

The direct and indirect annual economic cost of OSA has been estimated to range between $65 million and $165 million in the United States[73] and $21 million in Australia.[74] In many operational safety–critical settings such as the transportation industry, OSA may be more prevalent compared with the general population, with repeated reports of over 50% of employees having or being at risk for sleep-related breathing disorders.[38,75,76] This is problematic in occupational settings since OSA has been linked with at least a 2.5-fold increased risk of motor vehicle accidents (MVA),[77] and OSA symptoms have been linked with a twofold increased risk in workplace accidents.[78] Accidents in operational settings can have catastrophic consequences in terms of economic and safety impacts from damage, injury, and loss of life.

Excessive daytime sleepiness is a key symptom of OSA and likely an important driver of fatigue-related workplace accidents. A recent consensus statement indicated that fatigue is a preventable cause of accidents and that up to 20% of accidents in transport operations are fatigue related, surpassing the prevalence of accidents related to alcohol or drug use.[79] OSA has been implicated as a key factor contributing to some major transportation accidents such as the Metro-North train in 2014; Hoboken, NJ, transit in 2016; and Long Island Rail Road in 2016. To mitigate the negative effects of OSA on safety, there is a continued need for systematic screening, diagnosis, and management of OSA in safety-critical occupations.[80]

One significant challenge when screening for OSA in the context of whether one is fit to work/drive is the substantial heterogeneity in daytime sleepiness and alertness performance outcomes between individual patients, which do not strongly relate to work and road errors and accidents. For example, in a case control study of 530 Australian truck drivers who recently had a crash versus 517 Australian truck drivers who had not, 31% and 30%, respectively, had moderate to severe OSA, but this was not associated with crash risk.[81] In laboratory driving simulator studies, it has been found that approximately 35% of OSA patients exhibited significant performance impairment, and the remaining 65% of OSA patients were unimpaired relative to age-matched controls, even if further provoked by sleep restriction or alcohol.[82] Importantly, there was no relationship between driving performance and routine clinical metrics of OSA severity (i.e., apnea-hypopnea index [AHI] or hypoxemia) or excessive daytime sleepiness. The heterogeneity in OSA-related daytime symptoms, functional outcomes, and accident risk highlights the importance of using robust objective functional screening of employees with OSA in operational settings and not relying purely on a diagnosis and confirmation of the condition.

SLEEP DISORDERS SCREENING AND FUNCTIONAL IMPAIRMENT ASSESSMENTS

Screening for sleep disorders from an occupational medicine perspective involves identification of risk factors and recognition of symptoms that trigger referral for diagnostic testing and appropriate therapy if required. Functional performance screening to identify fatigue-related performance impairment is used in some cases when workers are diagnosed with a sleep disorder, and continued follow-up with treatment efficacy and compliance monitoring may be required. Depending on the occupational setting, validated screening questionnaires may be sufficient to identify high-risk employees, although in safety-critical settings further objective diagnosis and testing are usually necessary. Although objective testing is clearly advisable in determining fitness to drive/work, there are no standard criteria or assessment and individual clinician views are often divergent.[83]

In regard to safety-critical occupations, assessment of accident risk is an important part of general clinical assessment of sleep disorders, particularly among professional drivers. The clinical assessment requires a detailed medical history and driving history. Objective testing in professional drivers is a more reliable measure of driving performance than self-report instruments such as the Epworth Sleepiness Scale (ESS),[84] a primary clinical questionnaire used to assess excessive daytime sleepiness related to sleep disorders or lifestyle factors.[85] The major challenge with the use of the ESS in occupational settings such as the transport industry is the significant underreporting or denial of symptoms by the employees.[86] For example, in patients with narcolepsy or other central disorders of hypersomnolence, the ESS does not correlate with driving performance in actual or simulated driving.[22] Similarly in OSA, previous studies using the ESS found that only 4.5% of truck drivers report excessive daytime sleepiness relative to 12% to 33% of individuals in the general population.[87-90]

This is in contrast with anonymized studies with truck drivers, in which 20% reported falling asleep incidents[91] and 15% reported sleepiness-related near-miss events in the previous 5 years.[92] The underreporting by the employees may be out of fear for negative consequence regarding employment or licensing/work restrictions.

The hallmarks of insomnia include difficulty initiating and/or maintaining sleep and/or early morning awakenings, with symptoms accompanied by reported functional impairment occurring at least three times a week for at least 3 months. The Insomnia Severity Index and the Sleep Condition Indicator are commonly used questionnaires that assess the main symptoms and daytime consequences of insomnia. It can be used as an initial screen, and, if necessary, a referral to a sleep specialist may be warranted. Objective measures of fatigue-related functional impairment in operational settings are needed given the relatively inconsistent reports of impact of insomnia on daytime performance and cognitive function.[2]

Validated OSA screening tools include questionnaires such as the STOP-BANG,[93] the OSA50,[94] and the SomniSage questionnaires.[95] These questionnaires gauge risk factors for OSA, including physical and anthropometric characteristics (e.g., obesity, age, and gender) and various symptoms and behaviors (e.g., snoring, breathing pauses, and hypertension).

Objective measurements of OSA symptoms may provide a better assessment of OSA risk. In particular, measurements of obesity or neck/waist circumference are by far the strongest predictors of OSA and are often used to screen for OSA in occupational settings. That said, depending on what screening questionnaires are used and what body mass index (BMI) or obesity cut-offs and metrics are chosen, the prevalence of OSA symptoms and the sensitivity of these measures can vary considerably. For example, with a BMI cut-off of at least 30 kg/m^2 (i.e., the threshold for BMI-defined obesity), a study found that 50% of commercial drivers were identified as high risk for OSA, and 19% of the entire sample were confirmed to have OSA (i.e., an AHI > 10 events/hour).[87,96] In contrast, with a BMI cut-off of 35 kg/m^2 (i.e., the threshold for BMI-defined severe obesity), 12% to 13% of commercial drivers were identified as high risk, and 10% to 12% were confirmed to have OSA.[87,96] Finally, with a higher BMI cut-off of 40 kg/m^2 (i.e., the threshold for BMI-defined morbid obesity), only 6% to 7% of commercial drivers were identified as high risk for OSA, and almost all of these drivers were confirmed to have OSA.[87,95] Therefore it is important to understand the implications of using a given threshold. A BMI of 30 kg/m^2 may be too inclusive and lead to a heavy resource burden with a greater need for objective testing and a higher false-positive rate. A BMI of 40 kg/m^2 will have a higher positive predictive value for OSA, but this threshold will likely miss a lot of true cases of OSA. It is noteworthy that the Federal Motor Carrier Safety Administration and other transport authorities internationally lack a mandate on the use or cut-off of obesity metrics to screen for OSA. In practice, many occupational medicine professionals see a BMI of 35 kg/m^2 as a reasonable middle ground.

Subjective screening tests, objective screening tests, and objective daytime sleepiness assessments that can be used to identify employees at high risk for a sleep disorder are summarized in Table 80.1. Additional objective screening measures of functional impairment and alertness failure risk that are mostly used in research but should be considered when screening for sleep disorders are also summarized in Table 80.1.

Excessive Sleepiness and Functional Impairment Screening (see also Chapter 207)

The Multiple Sleep Latency Test

The Multiple Sleep Latency Test (MSLT) is a clinical diagnostic tool that measures the patient's physiologic tendency to fall asleep during multiple 20-minute nap opportunities during the day in the absence of any alerting factors.[98,113] Sleep latency and rapid eye movement latency are the key parameters measured. The MSLT is used in the diagnosis of narcolepsy and idiopathic hypersomnia and is sometimes used to assess excessive daytime sleepiness in other sleep disorders such as OSA and periodic limb movement disorder. The evidence of the MSLT appropriately assessing the risk of fatigue-related driving impairment and accident risk among private and commercial drivers is inconsistent in studies.[98] For example, one early study reported no difference between the sleep latencies in drivers who have had MVA between 1988 and 1993 compared with those who have not.[114] However, weak correlations have been observed between the MSLT sleep latencies and driving simulator performance in patients with OSA.[115] The MSLT sleep latencies and driving simulator performance have also been shown to improve after continuous positive airway pressure (CPAP) treatment.[116] The inconsistent and often weak relationship between MSLT sleep latency with driving performance and accident risk may be due to a fundamental difference in the cognitive processes assessed by the different tests as well as the context in which the sleepiness is being assessed (i.e., in a laboratory versus in a simulator or on the road). The MSLT may have limited ecological validity because the target is the tendency to fall asleep, whereas vigilance during driving relies on the ability to stay awake. Potential ceiling and floor effects as well as the effects of motivation have also been suggested as potential limitations of the test in differentiating the very alert and very sleepy patients.[113,117] Consequently, the MSLT is not usually used or recommended clinically when screening OSA patients from safety-critical occupations.

The Maintenance of Wakefulness Test

The Maintenance of Wakefulness Test (MWT) assesses the ability to stay awake in a soporific environment during the day using multiple 40-minute daytime tests in which the patient is asked to resist sleep and remain awake, which arguably has higher ecological validity than the MSLT to staying awake while driving. Previous studies assessing the MWT as a predictor of driving performance found a significant inverse relationship between MWT sleep latency and simulator steering deviation,[101] crashes,[100] and inappropriate lane crossings during real on-road driving.[99] One recent study from Finland included experienced driving instructors specializing in performing real-life driving ability assessments to establish whether the patient is safe or unsafe to drive and to hold a group 2 vehicle license.[118] The authors found that the MWT latency scores were useful in differentiating those drivers who qualified via the driving ability assessment versus those who were disqualified.[118] Recent studies suggest that alternative metrics derived from the MWT test, such as microsleeps, may further improve the ability of the test to differentiate between alert and sleepy patients, particularly in patients with sleep latency scores on the borderline of normal clinical thresholds.[119] Despite the link with driving performance, studies

Table 80.1 Subjective Screening Tools and Objective Functional Screening Tools for Sleep Disorders

Screening Tool	Description	Outcomes or Cut-Offs, and Pros and Cons	Deployment Setting
Epworth Sleepiness Scale (ESS)[85]	8-item self-report questionnaire assessing sleepiness by the likelihood of dozing off or falling asleep in 8 situations	• Total score >10 indicates excessive daytime sleepiness • Inconsistent relationships with workplace/ driving accident risk • Potential for significant bias in employee with sleep disorder[89]	The ESS in conjunction with other measures is used to detect excessive daytime sleepiness. Frequently used in clinical and research settings in patients with OSA and central hypersomnia.
Insomnia Severity Index (ISI)[37]	7 item self-report questionnaire assessing the nature, severity, and impact of insomnia	• Total score between 0 to 7 indicates normal sleep, 8 to 14 indicates sub-threshold insomnia, 15 to 21 indicates moderate clinical insomnia, and 22 to 28 indicates severe clinical insomnia • Increasing evidence for an association between insomnia symptoms and workplace safety and productivity outcomes[53,60]	The ISI is used extensively in clinical and research settings in the assessment of insomnia. It is best used in conjunction with functional impairment screening. To date, it is not formally used in employment screening.
Sleep Condition Indicator (SCI)[43]	8-item questionnaire assessing key symptoms and daytime outcomes of insomnia	• A score <16 is suggestive of insomnia • Increasing evidence for an association between insomnia symptoms and workplace safety and productivity outcomes[42,53,60]	The SCI is increasingly used in clinical and research settings. It is best used in conjunction with functional impairment screening. To date, it is not formally used in employment screening.
OSA50 questionnaire[94]	4-item questionnaire that assesses risk of OSA	• Score >5 indicates high risk of moderate to severe OSA • Partially based on objective obesity and age measures • Sensitive to rule in OSA[97] but may be subject to bias in operational settings	The OSA50 is validated for use among clinical populations and is suitable for workplace screening for those at high risk for OSA. It is best used in conjunction with objective diagnosis and functional impairment screening.
STOP-BANG questionnaire[93]	8-item questionnaire that assesses risk of OSA	• Answering "yes" to 0 to 2 questions indicates low risk, 3 to 4 questions indicates intermediate risk, and 5 to 8 questions indicates high risk • Partially based on objective obesity and age measures • Sensitive to rule in OSA but may be subject to bias in operational settings	The STOP-BANG is validated in clinical and general populations and is suitable for workplace screening for those at high risk for OSA. It is best used in conjunction with objective diagnosis and functional impairment screening.
Body mass index (BMI)[86]	A measure of general obesity defined as weight in kilograms divided by height in meters	• Various cut-offs used to screen for high risk OSA including >30, >35 and >40 kg/m^2 • BMI is positively associated with OSA severity • Higher BMI cut-offs have greater sensitivity but lower specificity for objectively confirmed OSA • No mandate or regulations for appropriate BMI cut-off in operational environment	BMI has been used as an index in operational settings to screen for high risk of OSA. It is best used in conjunction with objective diagnosis and functional impairment screening.
Excessive Sleepiness and Functional Impairment Screening			
Multiple Sleep Latency Test (MSLT)[98]	A measure of pathologic daytime sleepiness. It measures propensity to fall asleep during 4–5 20-minute daytime nap opportunities	• Sleep-onset latency ≤ 8 minutes is indicative of excessive sleepiness • Two consecutive ≥ 2 sleep-onset REM periods are indicative of narcolepsy • Indicated for diagnosis of narcolepsy and confirmation of excessive sleepiness in idiopathic hypersomnolence and OSA • Requires controlled sleep laboratory with specialized equipment and staff	The MSLT is used in research settings and clinical settings for diagnosis of narcolepsy and assessment of excessive sleepiness in other sleep disorders such as idiopathic hypersomnolence and OSA. It is also frequently used to assess responses to treatment.

Continued

Table 80.1 Subjective Screening Tools and Objective Functional Screening Tools for Sleep Disorders—cont'd

Screening Tool	Description	Outcomes or Cut-Offs, and Pros and Cons	Deployment Setting
Maintenance of Wakefulness Test (MWT)[98]	A measure of the propensity to stay awake during 4 40-minute daytime tests	• EEG-measured sleep-onset latency is the primary outcome • Sometimes used to assess treatment response in narcolepsy or idiopathic hypersomnia • Some evidence for an association between sleep latencies from MWT and real-world driving and accidents[22,99-101] • Requires controlled sleep laboratory with specialized equipment and staff	The MWT is frequently used in research and clinical settings that measures the ability to stay awake and alert. It has been used to screen employees with OSA in safety-critical occupations.
The Oxford Sleep Resistance (OSLER) test[102]	A behavioral measure of the propensity to stay awake during a 40-minute daytime test, in which where subjects respond to dim light flashes in 3-second intervals	• Absence of response to 7 consecutive stimuli indicates sleep onset • 1 or 2 testing sessions may be informative • Does not rely on EEG or specialized equipment • Can be used to assess treatment response • Some evidence for an association with driving and accidents[102,103] • Modified shorter versions may be suitable for workplace testing of employees with sleep disorders	The OSLER has primarily been used in research settings but has been used in clinical trials.
Psychomotor vigilance test (PVT)	A sensitive assay of sleep loss and consequent alertness failure that measures simple reaction times during a 3-, 5-, or 10-minute test	• Simple reaction time (RT), in which attentional lapses are defined as RTs > 500 ms • >10 lapses considered to be significant vigilance impairment • Some evidence for associations with driving, vigilance performance, and microsleep occurrence[104-107] • Ability to identify phenotypic longer-term future driving impairment and accident risk is uncertain	The PVT has been used in research and clinical settings and may be suitable as a fitness-for-duty, state alertness measure. It may also help to identify employees with sleep disorders who are at increased risk of state alertness failure and fitness for duty before beginning work.
Driving simulators	Variable simulators and driving scenarios used, depending on the context and disorder examined	• Outcome measures include steering deviation, speed deviation, braking parameters, response time, and crash events • Simulator performance is associated with real driving but often exaggerates performance impairment[108,109] • Requires standardization and validation • Further standardization of driving simulator assessment is necessary before wider adoption and use in occupational settings	Driving simulations are increasingly used in research settings, as well as in occupational therapy to assess fitness to drive in a variety of disorders, including elderly drivers, poststroke, Alzheimer's disease, traumatic brain injury, and posttraumatic stress disorder.[109] This has not yet translated into fitness-to-drive assessments in sleep disorders in operational settings.
Ocular measures	Measures eyelid and pupil movements parameters	• Outcome measures include eye blink duration, eyelid closure velocity, percent of time with eyes closed, and saccades • Ocular metrics show promising associations with driving simulator and on-road driving performance, microsleeps, and errors[110,111] • Ability to identify phenotypic longer-term future driving impairment and accident risk is uncertain	Ocular measures are used in research and clinical settings. As technology evolves, it may have potential for occupational functional screening of employees with sleep disorders. Furthermore, it may help identify employees with sleep disorders who are at increased risk of state alertness failure and fitness for duty.
Quantitative sleep EEG	A power spectral analysis of the EEG record. It quantifies EEG power frequencies between 0.4 to 35 Hz	• Outcomes may include predefined frequency ranges (i.e., delta, theta, alpha, sigma and beta), a slowing ratio, power densities, and a delta/alpha ratio • qEEG metrics differ in OSA and insomnia relative to healthy sleepers • Limited evidence of an association between qEEG metrics and vigilance performance including driving[112] • Requires specialized equipment	Quantitative sleep EEG is used in research settings and some clinical settings. Simplified EEG acquisition hardware and analysis may allow workplace functional screening of employees with OSA.

that directly link the occurrence of fatigue-related accidents over the road or in the workplace are currently lacking.

Although the MWT is considered the gold standard test of daytime alertness with an apparent relationship with driving performance and has some utility as a functional screening test, it must be used in combination with careful screening and history. The major limitations of the MWT are that the test is time consuming and costly, and the strength of associations with driving impairment is likely inadequate for routine screening of all employees with OSA in occupational settings. The American Academy of Sleep Medicine recommends that the MWT is used only in patients with overt daytime sleepiness and when the clinician is worried about their driving and workplace safety.[113] Consequently, it is not routinely used in most sleep clinics. MWT findings in relation to driving are also inconsistent, possibly because of ceiling and motivation effects,[117,120] particularly if licensing/work restrictions are at stake when screening employees.[121]

The Oxford Sleep Resistance Test

The Oxford Sleep Resistance (OSLER) test measures maintenance of wakefulness more actively than the MWT by asking the individual to focus on and respond to repeated light stimuli.[102] Unlike the MWT, it does not require an electroencephalogram (EEG). During the OSLER test, a subject remains awake and responds to dim light flashes at 3-second intervals during a 40-minute period. Sleep onset is set if the subject fails to respond to seven consecutive flashes. In comparison with the MWT, the sleep latencies derived from the OSLER test correlate very closely with EEG-measured sleep latencies during the MWT.[122] Furthermore, performance on the test has been shown to significantly improve with and be sensitive to CPAP therapy.[123] These factors, as well as additional performance data that can be derived from the test, such as reaction time to stimuli responses and errors, plus its low technical requirements and lower cost are thought to make the OSLER test useful for large trials. The test may also be better suited to assessing daytime sleepiness in relationship to fatigued driving and fatigue-related accident risk because of the active nature of the test. In this test the patient needs to actively engage and perform a monotonous repetitive task, which may better reflect the act of maintaining vigilance during long haul driving, for example. One study examined sustained attention and used a modified version of the OSLER test in patients with OSA who have had a traffic accident registry–confirmed MVA versus those who have not between 2001 and 2012. The researchers found that the performance metrics from the OSLER test were degraded (i.e., longer reaction times and more lapses in attention) in patients with MVA versus those who had no MVA.[103] In another study, the authors have compared daytime sleepiness in OSA patients and control participants using the OSLER test and found that even a single test is sensitive in identifying patients with excessive daytime sleepiness when using the performance metrics such as reaction times and errors.[124] The OSLER test could be considered as a test of excessive daytime sleepiness to help confirm functional impairment in OSA patients as part of occupational screening in operational environments because of the simpler protocol, lower cost, and potentially the shorter testing time required.

Psychomotor Vigilance Test

The psychomotor vigilance test (PVT) has been used in sleep research for over 30 years and is considered to be a sensitive assay for detecting vigilance impairment resulting from sleep loss or sleep disorders.[125-128] The PVT has been shown to be useful in identifying those individuals in healthy young populations who are vulnerable to sleep loss[106,107,129] and is sensitive to impairment associated with OSA.[126] In a study with commercial drivers and emergency responders, the PVT was found to be useful in identifying employees at risk for severe microsleeps.[105] In a recent study in airline pilots, the PVT was proposed as a feasible way of monitoring alertness in complex operational environments.[104] Another study showed that the PVT was useful in identifying employees from refining/petrochemical plants who were unfit for duty.[130] Although this evidence suggests that the PVT may have utility in identifying employees who have reduced alertness and are more impaired, more research is needed to determine if the PVT is useful in predicting future accident risk in employees with OSA.

Driving Simulator Assessment

Driving simulators are increasingly used by occupational therapists to screen drivers for fitness to drive and offer the advantage of assessing driving performance in a safe and controlled environment.[109] This is important in the context of sleep loss and sleep disorders because the impact of the resultant fatigue can be unpredictable (e.g., lapses in attention) and potentially severe (e.g., falling asleep crashes), making on-road driving assessments less feasible. Driving simulators measure the main aspects of actual driving, including visual tracking and coordination, attention, reaction and vigilance,[108,131] yield reproducible results in studies with patients with different sleep disorders and experimental conditions, and are sensitive to the effects of therapies. Studies have shown that, although simulator studies tend to overestimate some driving abnormalities, the results correlate well with on-road driving performance.[108,132] There are some limitations in using driving simulators to assess fitness to drive; these include motion sickness, motivational factors, varying types of simulators and their validity against real driving, and lack of standardized simulator type and driving scenarios. Despite these limitations, the use of driving simulators has been supported by occupational therapists[109] and increasingly by sleep experts.[108,133] Studies reveal it to be a valid assessment tool in evaluating fitness to drive in a variety of disorders such as poststroke, dementia, and sleep disorders.

Novel Electrophysiologic Objective Markers of Alertness Failure and Driving Risk

There has been a growing interest to identify in healthy subjects biomarkers that quantify sleepiness and explain the wide interindividual variability in susceptibility to sleep loss.[134,135] Several biomarkers have been identified in healthy subjects that appear to explain at least some of the interindividual variability in neurobehavioral response to sleep deprivation including genetic polymorphisms *(PER3, ADORA2A, COMT)*, gene expression, proteomics, inflammatory markers (IL-1, IL-6, TNF-α, CRP), behavioral measures (psychomotor vigilance and posturography), functional brain imaging/spectroscopy, and electrophysiologic measures (electroencephalography, event-related potentials, heart rate variability, and oculography).[135] Some of these novel markers of alertness may have application in occupational screening of employees with OSA; however, a lot more research and validation is likely needed to demonstrate the association with accident risk and its reduction with effective therapy, before adoption in occupational settings and sleep clinics, but it is a step in the right direction.

Sleep Electroencephalography

If an employee with suspected OSA requires a formal diagnosis, there will likely be a need for an overnight polysomnogram (PSG). This involves collecting a substantial amount of electrophysiologic data. Although sufficient for classifying the various sleep stages, cortical arousals, and wake periods, and informing the diagnosis of a sleep disorder, this approach fails to take into account a lot of rich phenotypic information that may relate to patient's daytime function and may help with clinical decisions regarding fitness to drive/work. For example, using power spectra analysis through quantitative EEG (qEEG), it is possible to quantify the sleep microstructure. qEEG techniques have been increasingly used in OSA research studies,[136] showing that patients with OSA demonstrate widespread EEG slowing, both during sleep and wake EEG recordings, compared with healthy control participants. Furthermore, only a few studies with patients with OSA have examined the associations between the EEG activity and daytime outcomes including sleepiness and neurobehavioral function.[136] For example, one study with 10 patients found that, before treatment, those with less slow wave activity in their first non–rapid eye movement period had shorter sleep latencies on an MSLT the next day, suggesting that the sleepiness was associated with reduced slow wave activity.[137] In a more recent study with 76 patients with OSA, quantitative EEG power was a significant independent predictor of steering deviation in a driving simulator, while the routine measures of OSA severity and daytime sleepiness (e.g., apnea and arousal indices) were not related to driving performance.[112] There is also evidence that qEEG is sensitive to CPAP therapy: sleep quality improves on treatment, further supporting the potential utility of EEG as a phenotypic marker. Given that EEG is already collected in routine diagnostic sleep studies makes adopting qEEG metrics to inform clinical decision cost effective and efficient. However, before this happens, larger trials must validate the utility of EEG in phenotyping at-risk OSA patients and importantly link this to on-road/work performance and accident risk.

Ocular Measures of Alertness and Fatigue

Ocular measures of the eye and eyelids have been used to quantify the physiologic alertness state in healthy subjects under various sleep restriction paradigms and have been shown to be sensitive to drowsiness and consequent functional impairment.[110,111,138,139] One study using driving simulation and PVT assessed vigilance performance at baseline and after 24 hours of sleep deprivation with concurrently measured ocular eye blink parameters.[110] The authors found that the proportion of time with eyelids closed and the velocity of eyelid closure significantly correlated with driving simulator crash events and PVT lapses. In another study using actual on-road driving in an instrumented vehicle on a closed track, the ocular measures of blink rate, duration, and amplitude were higher after conditions of sleep deprivation and were associated with higher odds of lane departure events.[139] In a test of the utility of ocular measures in a shift-work population, ocular metrics improved prediction of poor driving performance.[111] Interestingly, one very recent study suggests that ocular measures assessed before driving can predict the impairment that subsequently occurs during the drive, suggesting potential utility of ocular measures as a fitness for duty test. However, the evidence of using ocular metrics in OSA populations is currently lacking, and further validation of the capacity of ocular measures from rested baseline to predict future risk of alertness failure in various population is still necessary.

MANAGEMENT OF SLEEP DISORDERS IN OPERATIONAL SETTINGS

The clinician is often involved in assisting patients, and employers find common ground in ensuring the workplace is safe and supportive. There are very different workplace legislative systems in operations around the world, and not all legislative systems would consider patients with sleep disorders as having a disability. Patients with sleep disorders such as narcolepsy and OSA face issues during interviews, with both health care provider and/or employer, including whether to reveal their diagnosis. Their diagnosis can lead to increased scrutiny for job performance, restriction, and even dismissal or loss of promotion opportunities.

Patient occupational assessment requires detailed knowledge of patient symptomatology, quality of life, functional impairment, and demands of the workplace. Often documents required for workplace disability assessment are structured in a way suitable to physical disabilities or common psychiatric diagnoses but not sleep disorders. Central disorders of hypersomnolence pose a dilemma, even for experienced sleep medicine physicians, in part because of the imprecision of the MSLT, which is required for objective confirmation, and heterogeneity in the presentation of these disorders. There is a need for more systematic assessment tools to help standardize occupational assessments in sleep disorders. For example, a disease severity scale for type 1 narcolepsy (but not other hypersomnias) has recently been published that may be useful for occupational health purposes.[140] In Australia a patient with narcolepsy is not allowed to hold an unconditional driver's license, but a conditional license is permitted with a report from a sleep physician to the road authorities. Professional drivers cannot have a history of cataplexy, must be asymptomatic for 6 months on treatment, and must have a normal sleep latency on the MWT. The nature of the driving (e.g., long distance or local) is considered by the driving authority as well as the frequency of the medical review and restrictions such as maximum journey length. A combination of a 40-minute driving test and a 2-hour simulated driving test has been suggested as a way to assess fitness to drive in patients with narcolepsy or hypersomnia and also to monitor the efficacy of treatment.[22] This suggestion may be impractical for many countries, and an on-road driving test under supervision may not be feasible. Surrogate markers to select those most at risk and then detailed testing in a subset may have greater utility. Disclosure to an employer is a complex issue. Once aware, employers can make accommodation for their employees, such as work hour flexibility and naps. In workplaces, where there is mandatory drug testing, failure to disclose can cause problems for the patient. The role of the clinician can be very important in supporting this process by education of the employer and suggestions that can assist without placing the employer in a situation of financial hardship.

The efficacy of pharmacologic treatment of narcolepsy in improving driving performance has been examined. One study showed that methamphetamine (40 to 60 mg) increased sleep latency during MSLT and reduced error rate on a simple computer driving task returning performance to control levels.[141] In another study, modafinil (400 mg) or placebo was given to 27 patients with central hypersomnia (13 narcolepsy, 14 idiopathic hypersomnolence) and a healthy control group using a crossover design.[142] All participants performed a driving test on a public highway in normal traffic. Relative to placebo, modafinil improved driving performance with a trend to reducing standard deviation of lane position and the number of accidental line crossings. However, patients receiving modafinil still had more accidental line crossing than healthy control participants.[142] Administration of gamma-hydroxybutyrate (50 mg/kg) impairs driving performance and causes off-road accidents on a driving simulator among healthy controls, but no impairment was noted 3 to 6 hours after dosing due to short half of the drug, suggesting safe driving can result after 3 hours.[143] Unfortunately, no data are available in actual patients with narcolepsy despite it being a medication for narcolepsy.

In regard to insomnia management, cognitive behavioral therapy for insomnia (CBT-I) has been implemented and tested in occupational settings, often through an online platform. A systematic review and meta-analysis of randomized controlled trials (RCTs) that examined the efficacy of occupational e-mental health interventions addressing insomnia and mental well-being found a significant moderate effect on insomnia.[144] An RCT comparing an online self-help recovery training program based on CBT-I principles found that six 1-week modules improved insomnia severity scores in the general working population relative to a waitlist control group.[145] These effects persisted even at a 6-month follow-up. The study also showed that work-related rumination and worry mediated the effect of the intervention on sleep.

Results from studies examining the effectiveness of CBT-I for the treatment of shift-work sleep disorder are often inconsistent. One study examined the effectiveness of a 4-week online CBT-I intervention versus a face-to-face outpatient CBT-I intervention and found that both interventions improved sleep efficiency, well-being, and insomnia and depression symptoms.[146] In a small nonrandomized study design that included shift workers with chronic insomnia, CBT-I improved self-reported and actigraphy-measured sleep latency, self-reported sleep quality, and measures of daytime functioning and psychiatric symptoms.[147] These effects persisted over the 6-month follow-up period. A similar study that included a larger group of day-shift workers and shift workers with chronic insomnia found that CBT-I delivered by trained occupational health service nurses resulted in moderate improvement in insomnia severity in 62% of participants who completed a 24-month follow-up.[148] In contrast, an RCT that included shift workers with insomnia found that insomnia symptoms and total sleep time improved with both CBT-I and a sleep hygiene control intervention, but there were no significant differences between the interventions.[149]

Outside of CBT-I and other psychological approaches, such as brief behavioral therapy and digital behavioral therapies, studies evaluating interventions for insomnia in occupational settings are limited. A placebo-controlled crossover study examined the efficacy of melatonin therapy (3 mg taken 30 minutes before bedtime) in improving sleep in shift workers having difficulty falling asleep.[150] The intervention improved sleep latency and sleep efficiency. Despite the growing evidence of the negative impact of insomnia and insomnia symptoms on workplace safety and productivity outcomes, the evidence showing that insomnia treatment improves workplace safety and productivity outcomes beyond sleep benefits is limited. Given the high cost and adverse impacts associated with insomnia, further studies evaluating the effectiveness of interventions are warranted. There are currently no specific guidelines or legislation around the clinical screening and management of insomnia in the operational environment. This may be due to limited evidence of impaired alertness in insomnia and impact on operational performance such as driving and fatigue-related workplace accidents. Historically clinicians have not necessarily viewed insomnia as a sleep disorder representing a significant operational safety risk, but given the growing evidence of a widespread negative impact of insomnia on physical and mental health including safety and productivity, this view is changing and should drive policy.

Regarding management of OSA in operational settings, this ideally should (1) include screening for high-risk cases, including detailed history on OSA symptoms, excessive sleepiness, and accident history by an experienced sleep specialist and diagnostic testing to confirm the presence of OSA and (2) be supported by robust objective evidence of functional fatigue/sleepiness-related impairment risk.[151] This type of management of OSA does not always occur because of lack of accurate and easily deployable objective performance tests. Once the presence of OSA and preferably functional impairment is confirmed, any occupational implications or restrictions must be implemented based on local fitness to work/drive guidelines and, importantly, appropriate OSA therapy initiated. It is then critical to monitor treatment adherence through regular follow-up and functional assessments. In the United States, there is currently no standard regulation or mandate for comprehensive OSA risk assessment in operational settings such as commercial vehicle drivers.[152] Despite many years of evidence gathering and expert consensus and multiple recommendations, there are still significant barriers to translation into legislation in the way OSA is to be screened and managed in operational settings. In Australia there are specific fitness-to-drive recommendations for medical professionals regarding the assessment of drivers with OSA, but the legislation regarding mandatory reporting of high-risk patients differs across states. From the employer perspective there is no systematic, standardized legislation for screening drivers for OSA.

The major clinical challenge with OSA screening and management in operational settings is the focus on confirming the disorder is present and initiating treatment. This simplistic one-size-fits-all approach where the presence of moderate to severe OSA implies high accident risk is likely inappropriate. This occurs often without any confirmation of functional performance impairment, which may not be appropriate. There are large interindividual differences in symptoms and daytime alertness and functioning among OSA patients, perhaps driven by phenotypic differences in individual susceptibility to sleepiness or OSA, neurobehavioral dysfunction, and fatigue-related accident risk.[81,82,153] Consequently, some patients with severe OSA report no daytime sleepiness and have never experienced an accident, whereas others with milder disease experience significant impairment. This is reflected in the current clinical metrics of OSA severity and self-reported daytime sleepiness measures being unreliable and inadequate when it comes to differentiating between OSA patients at high versus low risk of alertness-related work errors and poor driving performance and accident risk.[81,82,112] This is particularly problematic in transportation settings, where most employees report being alert.[89]

In this context, although OSA is a medical condition presenting the greatest risk factor for MVA,[154] this risk relates to only a subset of the OSA population.[81,82,155] The current lack of uniform guidelines and legislation internationally represents a recognition of the lack of best objective metrics and approaches for screening and identifying employees with OSA, who actually represent increased risk and not just the disorder.

CLINICAL PEARL

Sleep disorders are common in operational settings and contribute to negative health, safety, and productivity outcomes. Sleep disorder screening and functional impairment assessments are challenging in the operational settings because of substantial heterogeneity in daytime symptoms, variable impact in functional impairment, and self-report bias of symptoms, making it difficult to rely on history and symptoms alone. Relying on history and screening questionnaires alone is likely insufficient for clinical decision making and objective diagnosis, and functional performance testing should be conducted where possible and appropriate. However, there is a lack of standardized assessment of fitness for work/driving at this stage, and consequently there is no agreed standard or legislation in place to facilitate this. Clinicians should use their clinical judgment and available evidence and variety of tools to assess patients with sleep disorders in operational settings.

SUMMARY

Sleep disorders in operational settings are common and are associated with adverse health, safety, and productivity outcomes. Identifying and managing sleep disorders in operational settings, including the central disorders of hypersomnolence, insomnia, and OSA, are critical to combat the sleep-associated fatigue, absenteeism, functional impairment, and safety risk. The holistic assessment of employees by occupational and sleep physicians, including the approach to screening, diagnosis, and management, and the tools used, must be appropriate to the setting and be guided by a fatigue risk management framework. Given the growing understanding and recognition of the large heterogeneity in daytime outcomes and accident risk among individuals, it is likely that a simple, one-size-fits-all approach to screening and diagnosis, without including risk assessment, is not appropriate. With further research and advances in objective testing and behavioral phenotyping, it should be possible to better link the diagnosis of a sleep disorder with functional impairment and increase in alertness failure risk in operational environments.

SELECTED READINGS

Alakuijala A, Maasilta P, Bachour A. The Oxford Sleep Resistance test (OSLER) and the Multiple Unprepared Reaction Time Test (MURT) detect vigilance modifications in sleep apnea patients. *J Clin Sleep Med.* 2014;10:1075–1082.

Baiardi S, La Morgia C, Sciamanna L, Gerosa A, Cirignotta F, Mondini S. Is the Epworth Sleepiness Scale a useful tool for screening excessive daytime sleepiness in commercial drivers? *Accid Anal Prev.* 2018;110:187–189.

Colvin LJ, Collop NA. Commercial motor vehicle driver obstructive sleep apnea screening and treatment in the united states: an update and recommendation overview. *J Clin Sleep Med.* 2016;12:113–125.

Fortier-Brochu E, Beaulieu-Bonneau S, Ivers H, Morin CM. Insomnia and daytime cognitive performance: a meta-analysis. *Sleep Med Rev.* 2012;16:83–94.

Jennum P, Ibsen R, Petersen ER, Knudsen S, Kjellberg J. Health, social, and economic consequences of narcolepsy: a controlled national study evaluating the societal effect on patients and their partners. *Sleep Med.* 2012;13:1086–1093.

Mulhall MD, Cori J, Sletten TL, et al. A pre-drive ocular assessment predicts alertness and driving impairment: a naturalistic driving study in shift workers. *Accid Anal Prev.* 2020;135:105386.

Sagaspe P, Micoulaud-Franchi JA, Coste O, et al. Maintenance of Wakefulness Test, real and simulated driving in patients with narcolepsy/hypersomnia. *Sleep Med.* 2019;55:1–5.

Stranks EK, Crowe SF. The cognitive effects of obstructive sleep apnea: an updated meta-analysis. *Arch Clin Neuropsychol.* 2016;31:186–193.

Swanson LM, Arnedt JT, Rosekind MR, Belenky G, Balkin TJ, Drake C. Sleep disorders and work performance: findings from the 2008 National Sleep Foundation Sleep in America poll. *J Sleep Res.* 2011;20:487–494.

Virtanen I, Jarvinen J, Anttalainen U. Can real-life driving ability be predicted by the Maintenance of Wakefulness Test? *Traffic Inj Prev.* 2019;20:601–606.

A complete reference list can be found online at ExpertConsult.com.

Chapter 81

Shift Work, Shift-Work Disorder, Jet Lag, and Jet Lag Disorder

Christopher L. Drake; Kenneth P. Wright, Jr.; Philip Cheng

Chapter Highlights

- Shift work that occurs at times normally reserved for sleep has a negative impact on work safety, productivity, and the ability to obtain adequate sleep.
- Workers with long-term exposure to night shifts are at greater risk for a variety of medical disorders, including from the cardiovascular and gastrointestinal systems and cancer.
- Jet lag can also have detrimental effects on sleep and performance, albeit usually of a shorter duration than shift work.
- Individual differences in genes and behavior degrade adaptation to shift work and time zone travel.
- Using circadian principles to inform both behavioral and pharmacologic treatment strategies can be helpful for shift workers and those experiencing jet lag.

Our 24/7 society exposes the workforce to sleep-wake schedules that oppose internal circadian physiology. This misalignment can severely disrupt sleep-wake and other physiologic processes and increase morbidity and mortality. This chapter bridges basic science and laboratory studies of shift work and jet lag and describes the impact of these schedules on underlying physiology and health. Results from occupational health studies that inform the clinician and patient about clinical issues critical to treatment of shift-work disorder (SWD) and travel across time zones (jet lag) are presented and recommendations provided.

CIRCADIAN MISALIGNMENT AND EFFECTS OF LIGHT EXPOSURE RELATED TO SHIFT WORK AND JET LAG

The internal circadian clock regulates physiologic processes across the 24-hour period. Our internal circadian clock differentiates between biologic day and night, in part so that it can promote sleep during the night and wakefulness and related functions during the biologic day.[1] For most individuals, the biologic day and night are aligned with the environmental day and night (i.e., sunlight), and the human circadian clock resets on a daily basis to remain entrained to the 24-hour day.[2] Light is the dominant environmental time cue for circadian entrainment,[3] and the timing of light exposure governs the phase (i.e., timing) of the internal clock. Of importance, the impact of light on the internal clock differs depending on timing of exposure; sometimes, light can phase-delay the internal clock (e.g., push sleep and wake times to be later), which would aid in adaptation to westward travel where time zones move later. At other times, light can phase-advance the internal clock (e.g., pull sleep and wake times to be earlier), which would aid adaptation to eastward travel where time zones move earlier[4] (Figure 81.1). Shift work and transmeridian travel cause misalignment of the normal temporal relationship between the internal circadian clock and the work- or travel-induced schedule of sleep and wakefulness. That is, both shift work and time zone travel frequently require wakefulness during the biologic night and sleep during the biologic day. Altered patterns of light exposure and sleep-wake schedules in shift workers and frequent transmeridian flyers can result in circadian disruption with morbidity in the form of disturbed sleep, impaired alertness, health-related consequences, and severely impacted quality of life.

SHIFT WORK

Prevalence

The working population of the United States is more than 130 million.[5] Estimates regarding prevalence of shift work vary depending on the definition used and region, but US-based estimates in 2015 indicate that 26.6% of employed adults are shift workers.[6] The proportion is higher if estimates included workers engaged in early morning shifts and infrequent or irregular shifts. In the United States, 17.7% to 25.9% of the total workforce start their shifts between 2 p.m. and 6:30 a.m.[7] These data suggest up to 34 million US adults engage in shift work on a regular or rotating basis. Data from other countries also indicate that a high prevalence of the population is engaged in shift work: In Slovenia, the estimated prevalence is 32%, in the United Kingdom, 22%, in Australia, 16%, in Greece, 25%, and in Finland, 25%, and in Japan 22%.[8,9] These estimates include multiple forms of shift-work schedules, which may produce different degrees of circadian misalignment and, by extension, risk for morbidity.

Night-Shift Workers

Night-shift workers with regular start times between 6 p.m. and 4 a.m.[10] make up an estimated 4.3% of the total US

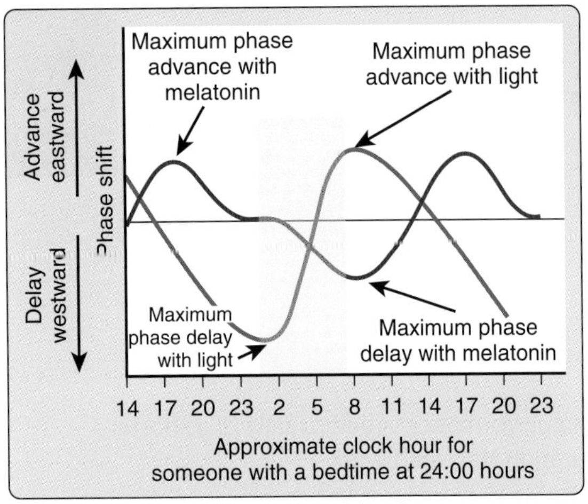

Figure 81.1 Schematic representation of the phase response curves to 1 day of light exposure (6.7 hours) (*blue line*) and 3 days of 3 to 5 mg of exogenous melatonin administration (*red line*) when the circadian system is entrained to local environmental time. The circadian phase resetting response to light and melatonin depends on the internal biologic time of exposure. Generally, bright light exposure before habitual bedtime and several hours thereafter will induce the largest westward phase delays, whereas bright light exposure just before the habitual time of awakening and several hours thereafter will induce the largest eastward phase advances. The time at which phase delays cross over to phase advances is, on average, approximately 2.5 hours before the habitual time of awakening in young adults and 2 hours in older adults. Therefore, bright light exposure close to the crossover point may shift the circadian phase in a direction opposite to what is desired. Opposite to the effects of light, ingestion of exogenous melatonin in the late afternoon will induce the largest eastward phase advances, whereas melatonin ingestion shortly after the habitual time of awakening and several hours thereafter will induce the largest westward phase delays. The time at which melatonin-induced phase delays change to phase advances is, on average, in the early afternoon.

workforce, thus an estimated 5.59 million in 2019. This is a conservative estimate, however, because it does not include workers on variable shift schedules, which often includes night shifts. Although some have speculated that permanent night work may have benefits in terms of circadian adjustment compared to rotating schedules, the extant literature does not support this contention.[11] Rather, results from both objective and subjective metrics generally show that regular night shifts result in greater loss of total sleep time than evening and slow rotating shift schedules.[12–14] Sleep loss accumulates over successive night shifts, resulting in a buildup of homeostatic sleep debt. This sleep debt combines with the sleep and wakefulness disrupting effects of circadian misalignment to negatively impact work performance and safety in shift workers. Comparative studies have shown even modest amounts of sleep loss can impair alertness and performance to levels similar to the legal limit of alcohol intoxication.[15,16] Not surprisingly, the night shift produces the greatest degree of sleepiness relative to daytime work, evening shifts, and even rotating shifts, with sleepiness highest during the early morning hours.[17]

Rotating Shift Workers

Rotating shifts refers to variable work schedules that include some combination of day, early morning, evening, and night shifts. These rotations can be rapid (e.g., multiple changes in work hours during a week) or slow (e.g., 3 weeks per shift schedule). The US population is estimated to include more than 4 million rotating shift workers (2.7% of the total workforce).[7] Owing to the constant flux of rotating shifts, work-related sleep-wake schedules often conflict with internal circadian rhythms. Indeed, nearly all rotating shift workers revert to daytime wakefulness and nocturnal sleep on days off. Thus it is unsurprising that rotating shift workers, like night workers, obtain much less sleep than day workers.[14]

Rotating shift workers face unique challenges related to the speed and direction of shift rotations. Of note, there is much debate regarding the effect of rotation speed on sleep-wake function. Although some data suggest that rapid rotations can produce more *sleep loss* than slow rotations,[14] other more recent studies suggests rapid rotations may have some advantages with respect to sleep quality, sleepiness, and psychosocial impact.[18,19] Due to the relatively slow response of the human circadian pacemaker, rapid rotations may be less likely to cause shifts away from entrainment to daylight, whereas slow rotations (e.g., a week or more per rotation) are more likely to induce shifts in circadian timing. Due to the lower number of consecutive night shifts, fast rotations may provide more time for social and family activities, improved sleep and alertness, and are generally preferred relative to a slow rotating schedule.[18,20] Nonetheless, there remains a lack of consensus regarding the advantages of slow versus rapid shift schedules, a debate which is likely to continue given the myriad of schedules, worker preferences, and prioritization of outcomes (i.e., sleep, performance, health, quality of life).

In terms of direction of shift rotation, both clockwise (i.e., delaying) and counterclockwise (i.e., advancing) rotations can reduce sleep duration compared to day work.[21] These effects are thought to be less severe for clockwise rotations because of the natural tendency of the circadian clock to delay to a later time.[21,22] Although productivity, work satisfaction, and work-life balance can improve when clockwise rotations are used, the effects of shift direction on sleep, alertness, and performance may also be moderated by age and speed of rotation.[20]

Early Morning Shift Workers

The *International Classification of Sleep Disorders* (ICSD-3) classifies early morning shifts as those starting between 4 a.m. and 7 a.m.[10] This is the most common alternate work shift in the United States, with at least 18.1 million workers (12.4% of the US workforce) falling into this category.[23] Given these start times, many early morning shift workers typically awaken before 5 a.m. Thus many early morning workers may be rising before or during their circadian trough, which may contribute to the high rate of excessive sleepiness in this population.[24] In addition, workers on the early morning shift report sleep disturbances almost as severe as night-shift workers,[25] and workers on this shift accrue significantly less sleep than day workers.[24] These factors, coupled with severe sleep inertia in the early morning,[26] suggest that these workers are often on the road when they are sleep deprived and near the low point in circadian alertness, which may pose serious risk for motor vehicle accidents during morning commutes.

Evening/Afternoon Shift Workers

Evening shift workers with regular start times between 2 p.m. and 6 p.m. make up 4.3% of all US workers.[23] Workers in this category are at risk for social isolation and, consequentially, reduced quality of life.[27] Unlike workers on early morning shifts (who obtain less total sleep time), the average evening shift worker sleeps 7.6 hours/night,[14] which is more than most day workers obtain (6.8 to 7.0 hours/night).[28] Because the internal circadian clock has an intrinsic period that is on average slightly longer than 24 hours,[22] the resulting tendency to delay internal rhythms, combined with schedules that allow later morning wakeup times, may account for the increased total sleep time observed in evening shift workers. However, some evening shift workers may have shortened sleep times owing to family obligations that require earlier wakeup times on days off; such reduced sleep time could result in significant impairment over time. Thus not all shift-work schedules are created equal with respect to the risk for morbidity, with evening workers typically no more impacted than what would be expected for an average day-shift schedule. However, as shift work is extended beyond typical 10- to 12-hour shifts significant impairment in occupational performance is likely to occur.[29]

Morbidity Associated with Shift Work

Insufficient Sleep

Consensus statements from the American Academy of Sleep Medicine, the Sleep Research Society, and the National Sleep Foundation agree that sleeping less than 7 hours per night represents an insufficient amount of sleep.[30,31] Findings from a representative nationwide survey (National Health and Nutrition Examination Survey [NHANES]) conducted by the Centers for Disease Control and Prevention (CDC) of more than 6000 adults showed that the prevalence of insufficient sleep (<7 hours/night) in night-shift workers is 61.8%, significantly higher than the 35.9% of daytime workers.[32] Similar findings are observed when sleep is measured objectively using actigraphy, showing that irregular and night-shift workers spend less time in bed than their day-shift counterparts.[33]

Excessive Sleepiness

Given that shift workers experience reduced opportunity for sleep, sleep fragmentation, and lack of circadian alerting signal at night, it is unsurprising that excessive sleepiness is one of the most common and debilitating consequences of shift work.[34,35] After a single night shift, objectively measured levels of sleepiness can be similar to those observed in patients with narcolepsy and sleep-related breathing disorders.[36] Many shift workers have severely fragmented sleep, which can exacerbate their sleepiness. Further, attending to domestic activities during the day (when they should be sleeping) can severely limit opportunities for sleep. The resulting impairment in alertness from these multifaceted contributing factors increases over successive shifts[37,38] and can produce a dangerous accumulation of sleep debt that may warrant a diagnosis of SWD and necessitate clinical attention (see "Shift-Work Disorder" section later).

Sleep Disturbance

An additional and related hazard for the shift-work population is that workers are regularly attempting to sleep during daytime hours when the circadian clock is actively promoting wakefulness,[34,35] leading to difficulties initiating and maintaining sleep. In addition, sleep during the day can be disrupted by other day-active members of the household, traffic noise, and additional external perturbations. The slow rate at which the circadian clock shifts to abrupt changes in sleep wake schedules (requiring days or even weeks), combined with erratic exposure to light,[39] can prevent adaptation of biologic rhythms to shift-work schedules, leading to SWD (see "Shift-Work Disorder" section).[40] Thus, in many shift workers, both sleep disturbance and sleepiness continue even after months or years of shift work or even after discontinuation of long-term shift work.[41]

Fatigue and Sleepiness-Related Accidents

A high proportion of shift workers are involved in safety-sensitive operations, such as first response, emergency health care, security, and transportation. Converging evidence from controlled laboratory settings, large epidemiologic studies, and clinical samples has established an incontrovertible link between shift work and accidents.[42,43]

Motor Vehicle Accidents. In a study of a large sample of nurses, 79.5% of those working the night shift reported at least one drowsy driving incident, equal to an increased odds of 3.96 (95% confidence interval, 3.24 to 4.84) relative to day shift.[44] Other studies have shown that risk increases nearly 10% for every extended shift worked in a month.[45] Driving home from the night shift is a time of particularly high risk, consistent with its proximity to the circadian nadir in alertness.[17,46–48] First-responder occupations, such as active duty police officers, have been studied, and driving simulator performance and alertness are significantly impaired after a standard 10-hour night shift, indicating significant risk for accidents in this safety sensitive population.

Work-Place Accidents. Among medical personnel, an increased number of percutaneous injuries,[49] medical and diagnostic errors,[50] and patient death rates have been documented in those working extended and unconventional shift schedules.[51] The higher rates of medical errors in physician shift workers is not surprising given findings that medical residents on heavy call rotations show levels of impairment similar to those on light call rotations with a blood alcohol concentration of 0.05%.[52] In industrial settings, accidents and injuries increase on the night shift, accumulate over successive shifts, and increase with time awake.[43]

Catastrophes, including Three Mile Island, the American Airlines flight 1420 crash,[53] and the Chernobyl disaster, occurred during the night shift, drawing increased attention to both the risks and costs associated with shift-work schedules.[54] Cost of sleepiness-related accidents in the United States is estimated at up to $40 billion per year, representing 24% of the total cost of traffic accidents in the United States.[55] These data suggest that the economic savings associated with shift work for specific industries should be carefully weighed against the overall cost to society, including increased mortality risk and overall costs of sleep-related accidents.[56]

Work Productivity

The negative impact of shift work is not limited to major adverse events and catastrophes but extends to daily productivity. An association has been demonstrated between shift work and reduced cognitive flexibility,[57] impaired threat detection,[58] and lower work productivity.[59] Thus worker performance is significantly reduced at night in a broad range of occupational settings. Additional evidence shows increased absenteeism in night workers compared with day workers, particularly among those experiencing insomnia and/or excessive sleepiness.[28] The mechanism of these negative impacts on cognition are likely multifaceted, but a well-controlled laboratory study in chronic shift workers provides strong evidence for circadian misalignment as a major contributing factor.[60]

Health Effects of Shift Work

A wealth of information documents the negative health effects associated with shift work.[61] Notable are results from large prospective studies showing a 36% to 60% increased risk of breast cancer[62,63] and, in those exposed to more than 15 years of rotating night work, a 60% increased risk of rectal cancer.[64] The latter effect is particularly evident with increasing years of night-shift exposure suggesting a dose-response relationship. Additional findings associated with shift work include a fourfold increased risk of duodenal ulcers (verified by endoscopy)[65] and increased risk for cardiovascular morbidity and mortality,[66–68] including atherosclerosis and myocardial infarction.[67] Two large prospective cohort studies in women also found an increased risk for coronary heart disease with increasing years of rotating shift work.[69] Overall, shift work increases the risk of type 2 diabetes.[70] However, there is also data suggesting an interaction such that in early chronotypes, the risk for type 2 diabetes increases with increasing duration of shift work exposure whereas that pattern is not observed for evening/late chronotypes.[71] Poor eating habits[72] and other adverse health behaviors among shift workers may account for some of the increased morbidity.[73] Nonetheless, circadian and sleep-wake modulation of the endocrine system[74,75] and experimental evidence for the negative effects of circadian misalignment on insulin resistance suggest that misalignment between endogenous rhythms and the sleep-wake schedule is a major contributing factor to the increased risk for diabetes in shift workers.[75,76]

Effects of Shift Work on Mental Health and Quality of Life

Work factors, including reduced job control, lack of managerial support, high work demands, and an increased prevalence of workplace violence, often contribute to the increased psychosocial stress experienced by shift workers.[77] Night-shift work has consistently been shown to increase the risk for depression[78,79] and anxiety.[76] The development of these conditions in this population is largely mediated by SWD (see section Shift-Work Disorder).[80] Shift work also negatively affects the worker's family and the worker's quality of life, as evidenced by higher divorce rates, reduced job satisfaction, and limitations on family and social interaction.[18,28] After controlling for a number of demographic variables, findings from a 5-year longitudinal study demonstrated a relationship between parental shift work and poor school performance and behavioral problems in children 5 to 12 years of age.[81]

Good Occupational Practice

Globalization and a 24/7 society demand an around-the-clock workforce in first responding, emergent health care, transportation, food service, and myriad other areas. Models of fatigue-risk have provided a useful framework for management of risk and include optimizing the design of shift schedules, implementation of worker education programs, and applying critical fatigue/sleepiness/error detection approaches.[82] The extant literature clearly indicates that no specific shift-work schedule is optimal for all people or for all potential outcomes regarding sleep, alertness, and work performance. These valuable risk-management strategies can be supplemented with personalized medicine approaches to optimize shift-worker sleep, performance, health, and quality of life. Personalized approaches recognize the complexity with regard to worker preferences, physiologic and behavioral vulnerabilities, and family/social activities when deciding on appropriate shift schedules, and or interventions to enhance adjustment to shift work.[40]

Good occupational practice has immense potential to lessen shift-work–related morbidities for the overall population of shift workers. Interventions implemented as part of an overall fatigue-risk management strategy, such as work schedule adjustments, banking sleep before the work shift,[83] specific strategies for caffeine use, and mobile apps that identify circadian phase may be helpful in some shift-work settings.[84,85] Even so, despite best efforts, some shift workers will struggle with their work-enforced sleep-wake schedules. Indeed, people on the same shift schedule differ dramatically with regard to their vulnerability to circadian misalignment, excessive sleepiness, and sleep disruption.[40]

Shift-Work Tolerance

Some workers can tolerate the effects of shift-work schedules and may remain symptom free.[40] In other workers the timing of the internal circadian rhythm (as indexed by endogenous melatonin onset) does not adapt to the work-imposed sleep-wake schedule and is thus chronically misaligned.[86–88] Circadian misaligned workers show reduced daytime sleep relative to that in persons whose melatonin profiles showed adaptation in response to night work. Individual differences in the circadian system itself (e.g., circadian period, circadian amplitude, and the system's response to light) may contribute to maladjustment to shift work. Research suggests that a contributing factor to the individual differences includes physiologically based diurnal preference (i.e., morningness vs. eveningness),[89] which has been linked to polymorphisms of the clock gene, *PERIOD3*.[90,91] Much of the research on diurnal preference and the *PERIOD3* gene focuses on the degree to which sleep loss impairs wake functioning.[91,92] Indeed, night-shift workers who are carriers of the five-repeat allele of the *PERIOD3* gene have higher levels of objective sleepiness on the multiple sleep latency test (MSLT) compared to *PERIOD3* homozygotes.[72]

Previous research has also demonstrated that a subset of individuals are particularly sensitive to sleep disruption from circadian misalignment and other challenges to the sleep system.[93] This trait of sleep disturbance in response to situational challenges or "sleep reactivity" is a heritable predisposition to sleep disturbance and insomnia that manifests in a sleep system that is sensitive or "reactive" to stressful challenges.[94] Prospective data indicate that highly reactive sleepers, even without a history of sleep disorders or mental illness, are highly intolerant to shift work and are at risk for significant morbidity.[80] Together, these data highlight that not only do shift workers vary substantially in shift-work tolerance, but also that a wide variety of factors influence one's ability to tolerate shift work. Unfortunately, a significant proportion of workers struggle to adapt to shift work and ultimately develop SWD.[86]

SHIFT-WORK DISORDER

Disruptions in sleep and wakefulness can reflect normative responses to shift-work exposure. In many individuals these symptoms become chronic and severe, leading to a diagnosis

Table 81.1 Diagnostic Criteria for Shift Work Disorder

***International Classification of Sleep Disorders* (ICSD-3) Criteria: General Criteria for Any Circadian Rhythm Sleep-Wake Disorder**

A. A chronic or recurrent pattern of sleep-wake rhythm disruption due primarily to alteration of the endogenous circadian timing system or misalignment between the endogenous circadian rhythm and the sleep-wake schedule desired or required by the person's physical environment or social/work schedules.
B. The circadian rhythm disruption leads to insomnia symptoms, excessive sleepiness, or both.
C. The sleep and wake disturbances cause clinically significant distress or impairment in mental, physical, social, occupational, educational, or other important areas of functioning.

Specific Criteria for Circadian Rhythm Sleep-Wake Disorder, Shift-Work Disorder (ICD-10-CM code: G47.26)

A. There is a report of insomnia and/or excessive sleepiness, accompanied by a reduction of total sleep time, which is associated with a recurring work schedule that overlaps the usual time for sleep.
B. The symptoms have been present and associated with the shift-work schedule for at least 3 months.
C. Sleep log and actigraphy monitoring (whenever possible and preferably with concurrent light exposure measurement) for at least 14 days (work and free days) demonstrate a disturbed sleep and wake pattern.
D. The sleep and/or wake disturbance are not better explained by another current sleep disorder, medical or neurologic disorder, mental disorder, medication use, poor sleep hygiene, or substance use disorder.

***Diagnostic and Statistical Manual of Mental Disorders, Fifth Edition: DSM-5:* Diagnostic Criteria for Circadian Rhythm Sleep Disorder (307.45)**

A. A persistent or recurrent pattern of sleep disruption that is due primarily to an alteration of the circadian system or to a misalignment between the endogenous circadian rhythm and the sleep-wake schedule required by the person's physical environment or social or professional schedule.
B. The sleep disruption leads to excessive sleepiness or insomnia, or both.
C. The sleep disturbance causes clinically significant distress or impairment in social, occupational, and other important areas of functioning.

Specify Type:

Shift-work type: insomnia during the major sleep period and/or excessive sleepiness (including inadvertent sleep) during the major awake period associated with a shift-work schedule (i.e., recurring unconventional work hours).

of SWD.[10] SWD is a sleep-wake disorder that involves complaints of insomnia during the sleep period and/or excessive sleepiness during the wake period that is directly linked to shift-work exposure (see Table 81.1 for ICSD-3 diagnostic criteria).[10] People who are unable to tolerate the effects of a shift-work schedule present with symptoms of insomnia and/or excessive sleepiness despite adequate time in bed (i.e., 7–9 hours) and an absence of other untreated or inadequately treated sleep disorders. Studies have shown sleep onset and maintenance disturbances using both self-report[95] and polysomnographic (PSG) measures in SWD.[96] Sleep disruption can present in both diurnal and nocturnal sleep periods.[96] Individuals with SWD have difficulty remaining awake during the early morning work and commute hours. These deficits can adversely affect job performance, driving safety, quality of life, work satisfaction, and health. A major challenge for future studies is to determine which specific forms of morbidity in SWD are linked to insomnia, excessive sleepiness, or circadian misalignment, or some combination of these three factors.

Prevalence

Clinical evaluation of insomnia and excessive sleepiness in shift workers is necessary to determine the actual prevalence of SWD. In one representative shift-work sample, the prevalence of the disorder was estimated at 14% to 32% among night-shift workers and 8% to 26% among rotating shift workers depending on the operationalized definition of SWD.[28] Findings from other studies provide similar estimates, with approximately 23% of a sample of oil rig workers in the North Sea,[97] 24% of Japanese nurses working rotating shifts,[98] 38% of general night-working nurses[99] and approximately 32% of night workers from a random population sample.[100] A study using ICSD-3 clinical diagnostic criteria and objective verification of work hours in a Finnish health worker sample found much lower estimates of 3% to 6%, likely due to stringent diagnostic criteria.[101]

Mental Illness in Shift-Work Disorder

Numerous studies have demonstrated that SWD patients have higher levels of depression and anxiety than healthy shift workers and day workers.[80,102] Of importance, SWD incidence mediates the relationship between shift-work exposure and new-onset depression and anxiety.[80]

Medical Morbidity of Shift-Work Disorder

In addition to sleep-wake disturbances, persons with SWD show significant impairments in neurophysiologic measures of attention and memory compared with night-shift workers without SWD.[103] In comparisons of shift workers with and without SWD, those with SWD also show a higher prevalence of ulcers and gastrointestinal disorders,[104,105] absenteeism, difficulties with family and social activities, and higher rates of major depression and mood problems.[28,106,107] Not surprisingly, persons with SWD report higher rates of sleepiness-related accidents[108] than shift workers without

SWD or day workers. Although increased rates of heart disease have been found in shift workers, it is not clear whether this morbidity is directly related to the symptomatology of SWD.[28] In one study, SWD was associated with worse urinary tract symptoms compared to those without SWD.[109] In a study of male workers, testosterone levels were found to be an average of 100.4 ng/dL lower in individuals with SWD compared to night workers without SWD.[110] Additional studies with patients meeting SWD diagnostic criteria are needed before definitive conclusions regarding unique morbidity in SWD, as opposed to shift-work tolerance per se,[40] can be determined.

Clinical Evaluation

The ICSD-3 edition provides diagnostic criteria for SWD (Table 81.1).[10] The diagnosis is made by a thorough sleep history, and PSG is not required per the diagnostic criteria for confirmation of the disorder. However, PSG may be indicated if another sleep disorder (e.g., obstructive sleep apnea) is suspected.[111] The clinical evaluation for SWD is similar to that for other sleep disorders, particularly the other circadian rhythm sleep-wake disorders covered in Chapter 43. Evaluation of the shift worker, however, also requires careful attention to effects of the work-sleep schedule on cognitive, social, and health-related functioning. Ability to maintain wakefulness, particularly during safety-sensitive activities (e.g., commute, dangerous occupational tasks, etc.), should be carefully assessed because patients with SWD still have a twofold increase in sleepiness-related accidents compared with shift workers who do not meet diagnostic criteria.[28] It can be challenging to determine adequate sleep opportunity (i.e., 7 to 9 hours) during the 24-hour day to rule out insufficient sleep (a common occurrence in shift workers), but it should nonetheless be a diagnostic rule-out and considered as part of a comprehensive evaluation.

Clinical evaluation of SWD should include assessing the severity of sleepiness and insomnia symptoms in the patient. The Epworth Sleepiness Scale (ESS) is particularly useful in assessing sleepiness and can be easily administered in the clinical setting. An ESS score greater than 10 is considered to be clinically significant. With excessive sleepiness defined by the ESS threshold of 10, prevalence rates up to 44% have been reported in shift workers,[28] whereas prevalence rates of 24% to 33% have been reported in representative samples of daytime workers using this criteria.[28,112,113]

Standardized and normative assessment tools, such as the Insomnia Severity Index (ISI), the Pittsburgh Sleep Quality Index (PSQI), and the PROMIS sleep disturbance scale, are important for determining the extent and relative impact of sleep disturbance.[28,112–114] Furthermore, such instruments are even more critical when determining the effectiveness of treatment. Extensive clinical guidelines for the general evaluation of insomnia, including its relation to functioning, have been published and should be considered when evaluating a shift worker.[115] Whether the patient reports difficulty initiating sleep, maintaining sleep, or both is important to ascertain for differential diagnosis before considering appropriate treatment strategies. A thorough history of the patient's recent work schedule is essential to diagnosis because many types of shift schedules (particularly rapidly backward-rotating schedules) can cause significant sleep disturbances and excessive sleepiness.[116] If an evening shift worker presents with excessive sleepiness or insomnia, other possible causes of the symptoms should be considered because evening shifts are less likely to trigger SWD; however, SWD might occur in evening workers with a strong morning circadian-phase preference or high social or domestic demands. Sleep-wake information should be collected for workdays and days off as recent studies have determined that patients with SWD are less likely to engage in compensatory sleep on days off, and this may be a valuable clinical indicator.[95]

The clinician also must be aware of potential mental health (e.g., depression, anxiety), gastrointestinal, cardiovascular, cancer, and other health risks associated with shift work. Workers should be encouraged to undergo regular physical examinations to rule out these conditions and take appropriate preventative measures. In addition, health risks related to the use or abuse of substances to relieve insomnia (e.g., illicit drugs and alcohol), poor diet, and nicotine use, which are common in shift workers, also should be thoroughly assessed during the clinical evaluation. Finally, educating the shift worker on appropriate sleep behaviors (i.e., sleep hygiene), with an emphasis on adequate sleep opportunity on days off, is critical.

Although challenging, the use of actigraphy monitoring for at least 7 days is critical for estimating circadian phase in every shift-work patient.[117] Without an accurate measure of circadian phase, the use of circadian interventions (e.g., phase-shifting using bright light/chronobiotics) is severely limited and can even exacerbate symptoms in some patients due to inappropriate timing of treatment. Mathematical circadian models are readily available and have been validated as predictors of circadian phase using actigraphy in night-shift workers.[118] Other valid approaches to determining circadian misalignment, such as sleep-logs/diaries, have been successful and can be another viable alternative approach to verifying the need for circadian adjustment in a patient.[119] Given model availability and ease of use, the ability to accurately predict circadian phase in shift workers and the efficacy of circadian behavioral interventions has the potential to transform the clinical approach from symptomatic management using sleep and wake-promoting medications toward realignment of the underlying circadian rhythm to match the work-imposed sleep-wake schedule.[117]

Treatment

A cardinal feature of SWD is that symptoms are directly linked to the shift-work schedule and thus often remit after returning to daywork.[10] Symptom improvement after returning to a daytime work schedule is indicative of circadian misalignment as the underlying pathophysiologic mechanism. Short of going off the night shift, occupational adjustments, such as moving to an evening shift, changing from backward to forward shift rotation, and incorporating increased worker control by allowing "self-scheduling" of shifts, may be of some benefit.[120] Matching chronotype to work schedules can also be beneficial. Studies have shown that relative to other chronotypes, early chronotypes (i.e., early birds/morningness) have poor sleep adaptation to nocturnal shifts,[121] and both sleep duration and sleep quality can be greatly improved by excluding extreme early chronotypes from night work and excluding extreme late chronotypes from early morning shifts.[122] In most cases, however, clinical intervention is needed because occupational and/or personal and social constraints may prevent major work-schedule adjustments. In accordance, treatment is necessarily targeted at the two symptoms of SWD:

reducing excessive sleepiness and/or improving sleep as achieved through use of medications,[123] behavioral interventions (e.g., cognitive behavioral therapy for insomnia [CBT-I], anchor sleep with naps),[124,125] and circadian interventions (e.g., timed artificial bright light exposure).[82]

Even before the diagnosis of SWD is made, the clinician must first address all potential safety concerns, and the threshold for immediate treatment intervention should be lower in a shift worker presenting with excessive sleepiness while driving and for occupations in which performance is critical for individual or public safety.[10] Shift workers typically have a chaotic sleep-wake schedule and may drastically curtail their time in bed in an attempt to meet their social, occupational, and daily obligations. Potential contributing factors include a short shift transition (i.e., quick returns), long overtime hours to keep up with work demands, a second job, or staying awake to engage in typical family and social activities during the day. All of these factors can make it difficult for the shift worker to get enough sleep opportunity. The clinician needs to address these issues with each patient so that sleep is a health imperative.

Circadian Interventions

Personalized Medicine in Shift-Work Disorder. Although sleep-wake benefits of circadian interventions have been demonstrated in shift workers,[126] the timing of treatment relative to each individual's circadian phase is a critical element to consider. Using a personalized medicine approach, including identification of an individual's circadian phase and chronotype before treatment, is important for matching sleep/work-schedule adjustments to the patient (e.g., morningness vs. eveningness) and for determining the appropriate timing of light and pharmacologic interventions.[122] Without information regarding an individual's endogenous rhythm, light, scheduling, or chronobiotic treatments may inadvertently be applied at the wrong circadian phase, leading to an exacerbation of circadian and sleep-wake disturbances in this population.

Timed Bright Light Exposure. Appropriately timed artificial light (5000 to 10,000 lux) with the aim of shifting endogenous rhythms has been studied in shift workers. For dayworkers, exposure to bright light in the evening near habitual bedtime and for several hours thereafter will induce a phase delay of internal biologic time, whereas exposure to bright light in the morning from approximately 2 hours before habitual wake time and thereafter will induce a phase advance (Figure 81.1). In practice, every hour of properly timed exposure to bright light, can typically induce a 0.5-hour shift in the endogenous biologic clock.

Using these principles, interventions aimed at producing phase delays of the circadian pacemaker (i.e., bright light during the first half of the night shift followed by daytime darkness) have been shown to improve daytime sleep and nocturnal functioning.[127–129] Czeisler and colleagues[129] treated circadian misalignment due to shift work with exposure to 7.5 hours of bright light (7000 to 12,000 lux) on 4 consecutive nights in the laboratory and scheduled sleep in darkness between 9 a.m. and 5 p.m. at home. In comparison with a control group exposed to room light (150 lux) and unscheduled sleep, the treatment group exhibited a 9.6-hour delay (i.e., to a later hour) of their circadian rhythms (i.e., temperature, cortisol, alertness). They also averaged 2 hours more sleep during the day and showed improved nocturnal alertness and cognitive performance.

Compromise Circadian Phase. Despite the ability to achieve large phase shifts in controlled laboratory environments,[127] less robust effects are typically obtained in field studies[130] as this requires near-complete control over the timing of exposure to light and darkness, which is not practical in most work settings. Thus brief intermittent light exposure (15 minutes per hour) to induce a "compromise" circadian phase (i.e., moderate but stable delay of ≈6 hours) has been tested in simulated shift work and shown to improve sleep duration and psychomotor performance.[131] Although this approach is compatible with permanent night work and common day schedules on days off, additional randomized controlled trials of bright light treatment of SWD patients are critically needed as the timing of circadian phase is an order of magnitude more variable in the actual shift-worker population and combined with practical limitations of the work environment may limit effectiveness.

Chronobiotics. Some limited evidence suggests compounds with phase-shifting properties (e.g., chronobiotics) may also be beneficial for shift workers.[123] Exogenous melatonin is perhaps the strongest nonphotic chronobiotic agent in humans. Normally, endogenous melatonin levels rise approximately 2 hours before habitual bedtime,[132] remain high across the night, and decline again near the habitual time of awakening. Use of exogenous melatonin to shift circadian rhythms generally follows the reciprocal of the phase-response curve for light (Figure 81.1). Thus melatonin ingested during the biologic day can be used to phase advance or phase delay the circadian clock.[133,134] In studies of shift work, melatonin (0.5 to 3 mg) improved circadian adaptation through phase delays or advances, depending on the time of administration.[128,135] Properly timed combinations of melatonin and bright light also can be used to induce larger phase shifts than either alone.[136] Of importance, for melatonin to be an effective phase-resetting agent, control over light exposure is critical because inappropriately timed environmental light will easily counter any phase shifts produced by melatonin. Melatonin has been shown to cause performance impairment at doses as low as 5 mg, suggesting caution if wakefulness is intended to be maintained for more than 30 minutes after administration.[128,135] Melatonin preparations certified for purity and dosage level should be used whenever possible.

Improving Diurnal (and Nocturnal) Sleep

Patients with SWD should be encouraged to attempt sleep immediately after the night shift and to maintain a sleep-conducive environment during their sleep time by using light-blocking shades, earplugs, and a comfortable eye mask. Making sleep a priority is particularly important to emphasize in the SWD population as these patients tend to forgo compensating for sleep loss on days off.[95] If sufficient circadian alignment to the night shift is achieved, improvements in daytime sleep occur.[122,127,129] However, the practical limitations of circadian interventions often prevent complete alignment (e.g., diurnal light exposure), thus necessitating interventions directly targeting sleep improvement. This lack of circadian adjustment in shift workers manifests as sleep disturbance during the latter half of daytime sleep.[127]

Anchor Sleep

Use of two sleep periods: (1) an "anchor" sleep period of approximately 4 to 5 hours that represents a time of day (e.g., 8 a.m. to noon when the shift worker is instructed to "always sleep" regardless of its being a workday or day off) and (2) another 3- to 4-hour period of sleep taken at irregular times, depending on the work schedule, may help to stabilize circadian rhythms and increase sleep duration for a given 24-hour period. Results from two studies show that splitting sleep into two phases may provide some advantages including longer duration of daytime sleep[137] and reduced wake after sleep onset.[138]

When used as a nonchronobiotic sleep-inducing agent, melatonin (and melatonin agonists), administered during the biologic day when endogenous melatonin levels are low, can increase total sleep time at doses as low as 0.3 mg.[139–142] In shift workers, some improvements in sleep have been shown with melatonin doses between 5 and 10 mg.[143,144] By contrast, lower doses (1.8 mg) have not produced robust effects.[145]

Hypnotics

Sleep-promoting medications are often used by individuals working night shifts. For example, recent data suggests that 20% of police officers use a sleep-promoting medication.[146] Although hypnotic medications can improve daytime sleep, these effects do not translate into substantially improved alertness during the night shift.[147,148] In contrast with medium-acting compounds (half-life of 5 to 12 hours), short-acting hypnotics (i.e., half-life of 1.5 hours) may be of little benefit in shift workers with isolated sleep maintenance problems (i.e., difficulty staying asleep with no problems falling asleep). Risk for residual sedation is critical in this population and should be considered carefully as shift workers often have safety-sensitive occupations (e.g., fire, police, health care, transportation) and typically have significantly less than a consecutive 7- to 8-hour sleep period.

As in day workers, the use of alcohol for sleep in patients with SWD should be strongly discouraged due to abuse potential and because shift workers may be particularly vulnerable to the sleep disruptive effects of alcohol during the second half of the night.[149] Napping during the day before the night shift and for brief episodes during the night has been effective for improving alertness and performance.[150–152] The combination of an evening nap and caffeine (250 to 350 mg) 30 minutes before the night shift was particularly beneficial for improving alertness and performance for up to 3 nights in one study.[153] Findings from a study of professional drivers demonstrated that a clinically feasible combination of brief naps (two at 20 minutes each) and a short light exposure period (10 minutes at 5000 lux) reduced polysomnographically measured episodes of falling asleep while driving.[152] Finally, a meta-analysis on the effects of napping suggest a moderate benefit of naps to reduce sleepiness during the night shift.[154]

Pharmacologically Enhancing Alertness

Many people who experience sleepiness use caffeine to combat the problem. Caffeine can be used to improve wakefulness and performance during the biologic night.[153,155] Although pre-nap caffeine may be beneficial in reducing the performance-impairing effects of sleep inertia,[156] this approach has yet to be tested in patients with SWD. In a study by Wyatt and colleagues,[157] low-dose caffeine (0.3 mg/kg/hour) administered over periods of extended wakefulness (29 hours) and circadian misalignment helped subjects remain awake and improved memory and psychomotor performance. Overall, evidence supports a role for the use of caffeine to enhance alertness in shift workers.[158] Wake-promoting medication is also used in many occupations involving shift work such as policing.[146] Although other alerting agents have been used, Schedule II stimulant medications, such as amphetamines and methylphenidate, have several disadvantages, including high abuse potential, that offset their ability to enhance alertness in the context of shift work.[159,160]

Medications with US Food and Drug Administration (FDA) indications for enhancing alertness in SWD have been used to promote nocturnal wakefulness in patients. A study on the use of modafinil for treatment of SWD provides evidence for its therapeutic benefit in occupationally related outcomes, including sleepiness while driving. In that study, 204 patients who met the criteria for SWD were given either 200 mg of modafinil or a placebo every night for 3 months during the clinical field trial.[161] The group taking modafinil showed significant improvement over those taking the placebo in psychomotor vigilance and drowsy driving on the commute home, among other end points. Patients also exhibited significant reductions in objectively defined sleepiness on the MSLT during the night shift, although alertness levels did not normalize to those seen during typical daytime assessments. Of importance, modafinil did not have detrimental effects on subsequent daytime sleep when taken at the beginning of the night.[161] Armodafinil, the longer-lasting isomer of modafinil, also has been shown to be effective for the treatment of excessive sleepiness in SWD and has reduced the level of sleepiness during the commute home.[162] In a placebo-controlled driving simulator study in patients with SWD, armodafinil improved driving performance, including reduced standard deviation of lateral position and reduced off-road deviations during the night shift up to 9 a.m.[163] It has been FDA approved for use in SWD and has been shown to significantly reduce excessive sleepiness and to improve overall clinical condition and performance in this patient population.[162] Several investigations have examined the efficacy of combined treatments for promoting wakefulness during the biologic night in normal, healthy volunteers. Combined treatments studied include caffeine and bright light,[155] caffeine and naps,[153] and naps and modafinil.[164] Such wakefulness-promoting treatment combinations have been reported to be of greater benefit than the use of either treatment alone.

Multicomponent Behavioral Treatment

Given that there are multiple contributors to symptoms of SWD, interest in multicomponent approaches to behavioral treatment of SWD has been on the rise. Although not widely tested, a few preliminary studies have showed positive effects on self-reported insomnia symptoms and sleep quality, along with both diary- and/or actigraphy-derived sleep, including sleep-onset latency and sleep efficiency.[125,165,166] These approaches often include typical components of behavioral treatment for insomnia, such as sleep hygiene education, stimulus control, a modified version of sleep restriction (to prevent exacerbation of safety risks due to excessive sleepiness), and stress management strategies (e.g., relaxation techniques, cognitive restructuring). Some have also incorporated strategic use of artificial and natural light as a treatment component.[125,165,167] Of note, only one study used randomized control trial methodology and found no differences between the multicomponent approach and a sleep education control[167]; however, the results showed that shift workers without SWD show more improvements on secondary outcomes (e.g., quality of life, dysfunctional beliefs about sleep, total sleep time on actigraphy), suggesting that interventions may need to be further tailored or intensified for those with SWD.[167] Finally, the interest in multicomponent behavioral treatment has also included use of digital health interventions, with preliminary data showing comparable effects with face-to-face treatment.[125]

Management Guidelines for Shift-Work Disorder

In light of the paucity of clinical tools for assessing and treating SWD, we have proposed a brief set of clinical guidelines (Table 81.2). These guidelines are based on established circadian principles, fatigue-risk management recommendations,[168] and clinical trials in SWD.[162,163,169–171] To the extent possible,

Table 81.2 Clinical Guidelines for Assessment and Management of Shift-Work Disorder

Assessment

- I. Determine circadian misalignment (sleep diaries and actigraphy with concurrent light exposure).
- II. Assess sleep disturbance.
  - A. Determine difficulty falling asleep, staying asleep, or having nonrestorative sleep (both during daytime and nighttime sleeps).
  - B. Measure degree of alertness.
  - C. Assess falling asleep during inappropriate circumstances or times (using Epworth Sleepiness Scale [ESS]), with special attention to drowsy driving.
  - D. Determine important job-related factors: duration of commute after shift, number of consecutive shifts, type of shift, time between shifts.
- III. Determine impact on social and domestic responsibilities.

Management

- I. Shift workers should have regular physical examinations with attention to psychological (e.g., depression), gastrointestinal, cardiovascular, and potential cancer risks associated with shift work.
  - A. Sleep-related comorbidity: Determine risk of sleep-disordered breathing, restless legs syndrome, or other potential sleep disorder.
  - B. Other comorbidity: Identify medical or psychiatric disorders that may contribute to the symptoms of insomnia or excessive sleepiness.
- II. Determine if removal from shift work is appropriate or practically feasible. If patient meets criteria for a diagnosis of shift-work disorder, cessation of the shift-work schedule should be the first option discussed with the patient.
- III. Determine patient-specific therapeutic approach.
  - A. Circadian adaptation
    1. Consider individual difference factors (e.g., age, phase preference).
    2. Consider compromise phase position (e.g., partial phase delay using bright light during first half of night and increased darkness during daytime).
    3. *Night workers*: On days off, adopt a late sleep schedule (i.e., bedtime of 3–4 a.m.).
  - B. Symptom management
    1. Insomnia
       - a. Good sleep behaviors
         - i. Target inappropriate sleep behaviors and encourage use of eye mask, earplugs, and light-blocking shades during daytime sleep.
       - b. Sleep maintenance a primary concern
         - i. Consider intermediate-acting hypnotic (half-life of 5–8 hours).
         - ii. Consider melatonin treatment for daytime sleep (≈3 mg).
       - c. Sleep initiation problems
         - i. Consider short-acting hypnotic.
       - d. Sleep problems on days off
         - i. Consider fixed sleep-wake schedule and consider anchor sleep.
    2. Excessive sleepiness (i.e., ESS score <10)
       - a. Address sleep disturbance if present.
       - b. Consider wake-enhancing medication before shift (e.g., modafinil, armodafinil) or off-label stimulants (e.g., amphetamine, methylphenidate).
       - c. Prophylactic nap before work shift is recommended.
       - d. Judicious use of brief to moderate-length naps (30 to 60 minutes), with recognition of risk of sleep inertia (consider prenap caffeine to reduce sleep inertia).
       - e. Consider combined treatment strategies during the work shift (alerting medications, bright light, anchor sleep and naps).
- IV. Address additional work, social, and domestic factors.
  - A. Social/family/psychological: Improve balance between family/social, work, and sleep time and treat psychosocial stress, depression, or marital discord if present; educate patient's family regarding shift workers need of protected time for sleep.
  - B. Health and safety: Promote improved healthy eating habits with respect to regularity and timing relative to the major sleep period (not within 2 to 4 hours of bedtime), reduce inappropriate substance use, increase exercise at appropriate times (not within 2–4 hours of bedtime), educate on risks of drowsy driving and critical times of performance vulnerability.
  - C. Work-related: Reduce number of consecutive shifts (<4), reduce shift duration (<12 hours), use clockwise rotation, ensure adequate time between shifts (>11 hours), move heavy workload outside circadian nadir (4 to 7 a.m.), address commute time (longer = greater accident risk), move to day or evening shift, consider incorporation of a shift work awareness program.

all clinical approaches to SWD should integrate work-related issues that arise in the context of treatment. Nonetheless, such issues should be approached with the recognition that the Americans with Disabilities Act (ADA) lacks explicit protection for those with SWD as it is not considered a disability. Furthermore, courts have generally not supported the idea that inability to complete shift work should be accommodated under the ADA as change to an evening or night shift is considered a trivial event.[172,173] Although this state of affairs may be addressed in future court cases involving SWD, one novel approach to addressing and preventing the problem of SWD is to provide workers the opportunity and resources to align their circadian system with the shift-work schedule before beginning a specific employer-imposed work shift.

Prevention

Although these described interventions in individuals who are currently symptomatic while performing night work remains a viable approach, preventing the onset of symptoms by shifting circadian rhythms immediately before engaging in a night-shift work schedule may have significant advantages.[174] Shift-work simulation studies using bright light to align circadian rhythms with a shift-work schedule have been successfully conducted and have demonstrated improved sleep, alertness, and performance. However, limitations, including the artificially controlled nature of the laboratory environment and the time typically required to achieve a compromise phase position, will need to be overcome if prevention of SWD is to be translated from circadian science to a viable clinical intervention.[174] In terms of prevention, a fast-forward rotating shift schedule may prevent sleep debt from accumulating during the course of shift work.[175] Markers of risk for SWD, such as sleep reactivity,[80] *PERIOD3* genotyping,[176] and other patient characteristics, including chronotyping, may be important in identifying at-risk individuals and can be used in prospective randomized controlled trials that test the effectiveness of preventative interventions.[176]

JET LAG AND JET LAG DISORDER

Many millions of people travel by airplane each year. Jet lag results from a mismatch between internal biologic time and environmental time caused by rapid eastward or westward travel across multiple time zones. Disturbed sleep and/or shortened sleep duration before and during travel also may contribute to jet lag symptoms.

Severity and duration of symptoms (i.e., tolerance to travel) are dependent on (1) the direction and number of time zones traveled, (2) the ability to obtain sufficient sleep while traveling, and (3) exposure to environmental circadian time cues during travel and in the new time zone. Symptoms include daytime fatigue, sleepiness, and insomnia in the new time zone. Gastrointestinal disturbance is common and may be related to intake of food at a biologic time when the body is not prepared to undertake this function.[177,178] Although the circadian principles used in the management of jet lag are similar to those of shift work, environmental cues (e.g., daytime light exposure) often support adaptation after travel to a different time zone. Thus jet lag symptoms typically subside in a few days, although in some cases symptoms can last for weeks.

Symptoms of jet lag occur because immediately after eastward travel, the traveler attempts sleep in the new time zone before his or her internal biologic night. Sleep in the new time zone is thus disturbed, and such sleep disruption contributes to subsequent daytime sleepiness and reports of fatigue. Daytime sleepiness and fatigue also occur because the traveler must stay awake during his or her internal biologic night. Individual differences in the ability to sleep during the biologic day (vulnerability to insomnia) and to maintain alert wakefulness during the biologic night also may contribute to jet lag symptoms. The cognitive impairments associated with jet lag can have serious consequences, resulting in drowsy driving or aircraft accidents, impaired decision making for the business traveler, and impaired athletic performance. In other cases, jet lag can be an inconvenience leading to difficulty staying awake during sightseeing, attending social events, or having a meal. Sleepiness and fatigue also increase the performance-impairing effects of alcohol.[179–181] Jet lag often is reported to be worse after eastward than westward travel. Westward travel may be easier because the average period of the circadian clock in humans is longer than 24 hours, so the biologic tendency is to go to bed late and sleep in. From 20% to 25% of people, however, have a shorter than 24-hour clock,[182] and such persons may find it easier to adapt to eastward travel.

Treatment

Successful treatment requires a detailed history and knowledge of circadian physiology and of effective countermeasures to improve sleep, wakefulness, and circadian adaptation. Most evidence for jet lag treatments comes from laboratory studies as field trials are limited.[183] Currently, no medications are approved by the FDA for the treatment of jet lag disorder.

Promoting Sleep during Flight and in the New Time Zone

The traveler should be educated on environmental factors that can be controlled to promote sleep.[184] Most flights eastward from the United States to Europe are scheduled at night. Eyeshades and earplugs or noise-canceling headphones may help promote sleep during the flight. Alcohol consumption should be avoided or minimized during the flight. Although alcohol shortens sleep latency, it disrupts sleep continuity.[149] Direct overnight flights provide more opportunity to sleep during travel than do itineraries with multiple stops. On arrival it often is recommended to immediately adapt to the new bedtime and awakening times of the new time zone. Exogenous melatonin can shorten sleep latency and increase sleep duration in a dose-dependent manner when taken during the biologic daytime.[141,142,185] Thus, if sleep is attempted during the biologic daytime while in flight and/or in the new time zone, melatonin may be used to improve sleep quality and duration. Melatonin should be tried in the home time zone before use during travel to determine the response to the chosen dose. Prescription melatonin receptor agonists, such as ramelteon[139] and tasimelteon,[140] are reported to improve sleep during the biologic daytime, so they may be useful in the treatment of jet lag. In a clinical trial, ramelteon (1 mg) was reported to shorten the latency to sleep compared with placebo after eastward air travel across five time zones (from Hawaii to the East Coast of the United States). In addition, 4 mg of ramelteon decreased some daytime symptoms of jet lag.[186] Neither ramelteon nor tasimelteon has been FDA approved for treatment of jet lag. Melatonin and melatonin agonists take about 1 hour or so to initiate physiologic changes to promote sleep, and thus taking melatonin 1 to 2 hours before the preferred bedtime is recommended.

Over-the-counter sleep aids have not been tested to determine their effectiveness in treating jet lag. Several prescription benzodiazepine receptor agonists approved for insomnia have been tested in simulated and actual jet lag trials. Findings from these studies indicate that sleep is improved during jet travel,[187,188] but there is little evidence that subsequent wakefulness is improved by these or other sleep medications. In addition, the side effects of both over-the-counter and prescription sleep-inducing agents must be considered (e.g., cognitive and balance impairments).

Promoting Wakefulness during Flight and in the New Time Zone

Most flights westward from Europe to the United States are scheduled during the daytime. Staying awake until bedtime in the new time zone should promote sleep. Naps when in flight during westward travel and in the new time zone after eastward or westward travel are likely to be effective in promoting subsequent wakefulness.[189,190] Caffeine is perhaps the most commonly used self-selected countermeasure to promote wakefulness during jet travel. As indicated by sleep deprivation and simulated jet travel studies, caffeine can help to promote wakefulness during the biologic night.[155,157,158]

Modafinil has been shown to improve several, but not all, aspects of cognitive function during sleep deprivation combined with circadian misalignment,[191] which are factors common to jet travel. In a clinical trial of patients with jet lag disorder, armodafinil (150 mg) was reported to increase sleep latency on the MSLT and reduce patient ratings of jet lag severity compared with placebo after eastward air travel across six time zones (from the East Coast of the United States to France).[192] However, wakefulness after sleep onset also was higher during the sleep episode in the armodafinil versus placebo condition, and several subjects reported insomnia as a side effect. Thus patients should be monitored for sleep disturbance if armodafinil is used to combat jet lag disorder; alternatively, the shorter-acting compound modafinil may be preferable. Other side effects of armodafinil included headaches, nausea, and heart palpitations.

Circadian Adaptation

Adjustment of the circadian system to a new time zone often takes days. It has been estimated that complete circadian adjustment may require a day or more for each time zone crossed. Proper timing of bright light exposure and dim light or darkness can quicken adaptation of the internal circadian clock to the new time zone (Figure 81.1). Exogenous melatonin also may help to shift the circadian clock during travel. The timing of melatonin administration to induce phase shifts is opposite to that of light (Figure 81.1). For example, if a westward phase delay is desired, exposure to dim light–darkness and melatonin in the morning, coupled with exposure to bright light at night is likely to facilitate a delay (Figures 81.2 and 81.3). Inappropriate timing of light and darkness during and immediately after travel can shift the circadian clock in the wrong direction, thereby increasing the duration of jet lag symptoms from days to more than a week.

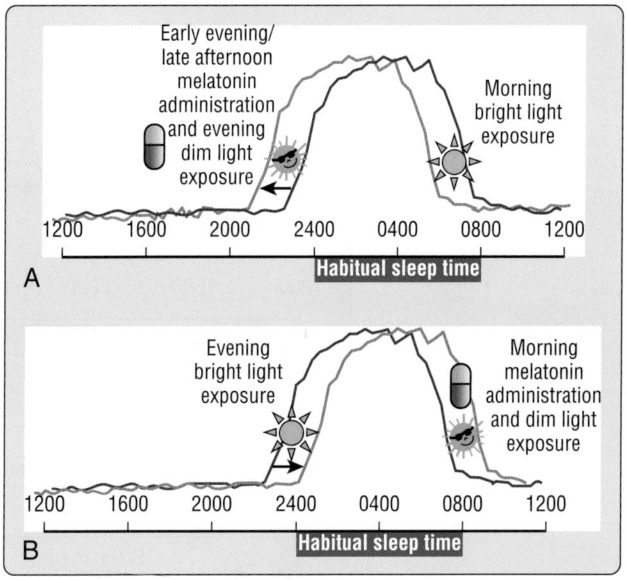

Figure 81.2 Using light and melatonin to phase shift the internal biologic time. **A,** When the traveler is entrained to local time, light exposure during the morning and melatonin ingestion in the afternoon will induce an eastward phase advance shift of the internal circadian clock. *Red line* shows initial melatonin rhythm and *green line* shows advanced melatonin rhythm after treatment. **B,** Light exposure during the evening and melatonin administration in the morning will induce a westward phase delay shift of the internal circadian clock. *Red line* shows initial melatonin rhythm and *green line* shows delayed melatonin rhythm after treatment. Adjustment to eastward travel should include exposure to dim light or darkness in the evening. This can be achieved by wearing sunglasses if the sun has not set and by turning down the lights in the house. Adjustment to westward travel should include exposure to dim light or darkness in the morning. Administration of melatonin when the jet traveler is required to be awake (e.g., for work or driving) should be avoided because melatonin has been reported to impair performance.

Partial Preflight Circadian Adaptation

Partial preadaptation of the traveler's circadian clock before travel[193,194] may shorten the duration of jet lag symptoms. Partial preadaptation involves going to bed and waking up earlier for 1 to 3 days before eastward flight or going to bed and waking up later before westward flight, combined with properly timed exposure to light (Figure 81.3). Earlier awakening before eastward flight should be combined with exposure to bright light (e.g., a sunrise walk or turning up the lights in the house) and exposure to dim light at night. Later bedtimes and wake times before westward flight should be combined with exposure to bright light in the evening and exposure to dim light in the morning. For a full case presentation of successful assessment and treatment using this approach, the reader is referred to the description by Wright[195]; clinical management recommendations have been summarized by Sack.[196]

CONCLUSIONS

Shift work can have debilitating consequences including chronic sleep disruption, social isolation, and circadian misalignment.[197] The negative effects of shift work may involve the gastrointestinal, cardiovascular, and other physiologic systems.[198] Although the direct relation between disruptions of the sleep and circadian systems and corresponding morbidity needs further study, circadian and sleep adaptation to shift work can be improved using interventions that target these systems. Impaired alertness may require management strategies beyond circadian and sleep-related interventions. In people with SWD, treatment should be directed at circadian adjustment to the shift-work schedule and, if necessary, treatment of excessive sleepiness and/or sleep disruption

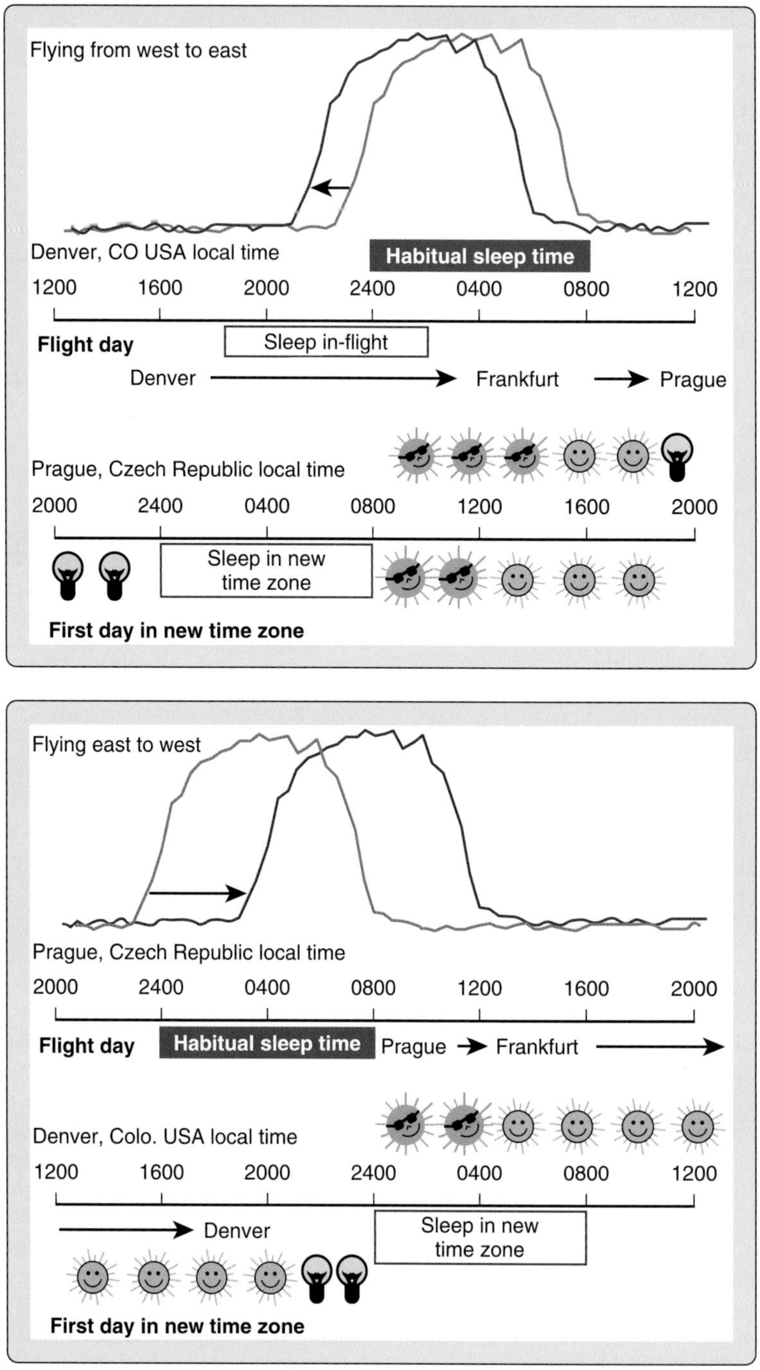

Figure 81.3 Circadian adaptation during jet travel. *Top:* When traveling eastward, the jet traveler needs to advance the timing of his or her sleep schedule and the phase of the internal circadian clock so that both occur earlier. In the current example of a trip from Denver, Colorado, to Prague, Czech Republic, the primary plane flight to Frankfurt (*long black arrows*) occurs during the beginning of the biologic night, when endogenous melatonin levels are high (*green line; top panel*). The traveler should sleep as much as possible on the plane flight to reduce the negative impact of sleep deprivation during jet travel. Exogenous melatonin taken shortly after boarding the plane may help the traveler fall asleep earlier than normal when endogenous melatonin levels are low. In this example the traveler spends several hours in Frankfurt before the flight connection to Prague. Light exposure during most of the biologic night will induce a westward phase delay, opposite to what is needed for an eastward shift; in accordance, the traveler should avoid exposure to bright light (*sun with sunglasses*) and wear an eye mask or sunglasses until after the habitual time of awakening in the home time zone. Subsequent exposure to bright light (*sun without sunglasses and light bulb*) will facilitate the eastward phase advance of the traveler's circadian clock (*red line; top panel*). Sleep timing should be consistent with the local time zone in Prague, and melatonin may again help phase shift the clock and promote sleep onset if taken when endogenous melatonin levels are low. The next day the traveler should at first continue to avoid exposure to bright light. Each day the time of exposure to bright light can be moved earlier by 1 to 2 hours per day. *Bottom:* When traveling westward, the jet traveler needs to delay the timing of his or her sleep schedule and the phase of the internal circadian clock (*green line; bottom panel*) so that both occur later. In the example of a trip from Prague to Denver, plane flights occur across the biologic day when endogenous melatonin levels are low, and the traveler should remain awake for much of the trip, assuming that sleep was adequate before travel. Caffeine and/or a nap can help to support subsequent wakefulness. Exposure to bright light should occur across the entire plane flight and until just before bedtime in the new time zone, to facilitate a westward phase delay (*red line; bottom panel*).

symptoms. Although data on patients diagnosed with SWD are limited, successful treatment approaches have included wake-promoting medications, prophylactic naps, appropriately timed exposure to bright light exposure and darkness, and combined countermeasures (when appropriate). Sleep disturbance, short sleep duration, and circadian misalignment can have a negative impact on productivity, performance, and safety during and immediately after jet travel. Sleep and circadian science principles indicate that appropriately timed exposure to light and darkness before and during the flight and on arrival can hasten adjustment to the new time zone, whereas inappropriately timed exposure to light and darkness during and immediately after jet travel can shift the circadian clock in the wrong direction, thereby increasing the duration of jet lag symptoms.

CLINICAL PEARLS

Shift Work

Shift work disrupts sleep and circadian rhythms and is associated with increased risk for cardiometabolic disease, gastrointestinal disorders, and cancer. Careful application of circadian principles (appropriate timed bright light-darkness exposure and melatonin) can improve adjustment to shift work. Melatonin and prescription hypnotic medications may provide additional benefit in some people. Treatment with FDA-approved alerting medication often is useful in patients with SWD.

Jet Lag

Rapid eastward or westward travel across multiple time zones induces circadian misalignment, which produces insomnia and daytime sleepiness with impaired driving performance and cognition. Circadian adaptation to the new time zone requires appropriately timed exposure to light and darkness. Inappropriately timed exposure to light can shift the circadian clock in the wrong direction, prolonging jet lag symptoms. Wakefulness- and sleep-promoting countermeasures can be used to address symptoms of daytime sleepiness and sleep disruption, respectively, during travel and in the new time zone.

SUMMARY

Shift work and travel across time zones are commonplace. These factors pose circadian challenges because they require abrupt and often large shifts in the timing of sleep-wake schedules. Individual differences exist in the ability to adapt to this mismatch between circadian physiology and sleep-wake behavior that in turn impact sleep-wake, cardiometabolic, and gastrointestinal system functioning. Insomnia and excessive sleepiness, which contribute to other morbidities (e.g., accidents), are the defining symptoms of SWD. Effective treatments for symptoms of SWD include use of nocturnal bright light and daytime darkness, maintenance of anchor sleep with naps to increase 24-hour sleep time, and sleep- and wake-enhancing medications. Jet lag symptoms include gastrointestinal disturbance, daytime fatigue, sleepiness, and insomnia. Cognitive impairments can have serious consequences, including impaired driving and impaired decision making. Interventions such as appropriately timed bright light and darkness can improve circadian adaptation to time zone changes; sleep-promoting agents and melatonin and its agonists (during the biologic daytime) may promote sleep but may not improve wakefulness in the new time zone. Preadaptation of the circadian clock and use of caffeine and brief naps in the new time zone are useful countermeasures to promote wakefulness.

ACKNOWLEDGMENTS

We would like to thank the Division of Sleep Medicine and the staff at the Thomas Roth Sleep Disorders and Research Center at the Henry Ford Health System and the University of Colorado Boulder for their continued support.

SELECTED READINGS

Barger LK, Cade BE, Ayas NT, et al. Extended work shifts and the risk of motor vehicle crashes among interns. *N Engl J Med*. 2005;352:125–134.

Burgess HJ, Sharkey KM, Eastman CI. Bright light, dark and melatonin can promote circadian adaptation in night shift workers. *Sleep Med Rev*. 2002;6:407–420.

Crowley SJ, Eastman CI. Phase advancing human circadian rhythms with morning bright light, afternoon melatonin, and gradually shifted sleep: can we reduce morning bright-light duration? *Sleep Med*. 2015;16(2): 288–297.

Czeisler CA, Johnson MP, Duffy JF, et al. Exposure to bright light and darkness to treat physiologic maladaptation to night work. *N Engl J Med*. 1990;322:1253–1259.

Drake C, Belcher L, Howard R. Length polymorphism in the period 3 gene is associated with sleepiness and maladaptive circadian phase in night-shift workers. *J Sleep Res*. 2015;24:254–261.

Drake CL, Roehrs T, Richardson G, et al. Shift work sleep disorder: prevalence and consequences beyond that of symptomatic day workers. *Sleep*. 2004;27:1453–1462.

Eastman CI, Burgess HJ. How to travel the world without jet lag. *Sleep Med Clin*. 2009;4:241–255.

Gumenyuk V, Roth T, Drake CL. Circadian phase, sleepiness, and light exposure assessment in night workers with and without shift work disorder. *Chronobiol Int*. 2012;29:928–936.

Jang TW. Work-fitness evaluation for shift work disorder. *Int J Environ Res Public Health*. 2021;18(3):1294. Published 2021 Feb 1.

Juda M, Vetter C, Roenneberg T. Chronotype modulates sleep duration, sleep quality, and social jet lag in shift-workers. *J Biol Rhythms*. 2013;28: 141–151.

Monk TH, Buysse DJ, Billy BD, et al. Polysomnographic sleep and circadian temperature rhythms as a function of prior shift work exposure in retired seniors. *Healthy Aging Clin Care Elder*. 2013;5:9–19.

Sack RL, Auckley D, Auger RR, et al. Circadian rhythm sleep disorders: part I, basic principles, shift work and jet lag disorders. An American Academy of Sleep Medicine review. *Sleep*. 2007;30:1460–1483.

Vanttola P, Puttonen S, Karhula K, Oksanen T, HÄrmÄ M. Employees with shift work disorder experience excessive sleepiness also on non-work days: a cross-sectional survey linked to working hours register in Finnish hospitals. *Ind Health*. 2020;58(4):366–374.

Vetter C, Fischer D, Matera JL, Roenneberg T. Aligning work and circadian time in shift workers improves sleep and reduces circadian disruption. *Curr Biol*. 2015;25:907–911.

Wright Jr KP, Bogan RK, Wyatt JK. Shift work and the assessment and management of shift work disorder (SWD). *Sleep Med Rev*. 2013;17:41–54.

A complete reference list can be found online at ExpertConsult.com.

Chapter

82

Fatigue Countermeasures

J. Lynn Caldwell; John A. Caldwell; Anna Anund

Chapter Highlights

- Fatigue is primarily a function of acute or chronic sleep restriction, length of work periods, and attendant body clock disruptions and/or misalignments of the body's circadian rhythms.
- Fatigue degrades health, safety, and well-being.
- Sleep loss has cumulative adverse effects on cognitive performance, including reduced vigilance, increased lapses of attention, degradation in short-term memory, impaired logical reasoning, poor impulse control, and uncontrollable lapses into sleep.
- The effects of fatigue can be mitigated by the implementation of evidence-based fatigue-risk countermeasures.

INTRODUCTION

Fatigue is widespread in the industrialized world because of the high prevalence of around-the-clock operations, irregular work schedules, short and variable off-duty periods, lengthy commutes, and poor sleep environments. Around-the-clock operations and irregular work schedules can result in a misalignment between circadian rhythms and sleep-wake behaviors, which can have consequences for sleep quality and sleep quantity. Short and variable off-duty periods, lengthy commutes, and poor sleep environments further degrade sleep quality and sleep quantity.[1,2]

Increased homeostatic drives for sleep and reduced circadian drives for wakefulness increase fatigue.[3] Although there are individual differences in vulnerability and resilience to sleep loss and fatigue,[4] most fatigued individuals show impairments in alertness, information processing, reaction time, decision making, situational awareness, and memory. They often are not fully aware of the extent to which fatigue is degrading their performance. Despite beliefs to the contrary, individuals do not adapt to sleep loss even with repeated exposure.[5] Furthermore, recovery from fatigue attributable to chronic sleep restriction often takes longer than one would expect given the rapid recovery seen with total sleep deprivation—in many instances up to a week after return to a normal sleep schedule.[6,7]

MITIGATING AND MANAGING FATIGUE

A variety of strategies can help mitigate and manage fatigue. It is important to carefully consider the factors driving fatigue and the context in which fatigue occurs before choosing a mitigation strategy. In this chapter, we concentrate on fatigue resulting from sleep deprivation, sleep restriction, sleep fragmentation, and circadian misalignment. We emphasize fatigue countermeasures and strategies that are suitable for mitigating fatigue-related risks. These strategies fall into four broad categories: behavioral, environmental, technological, and pharmacologic. Within and among these categories, some of the countermeasures are designed to *prevent fatigue from occurring in the first place* (i.e., preventive fatigue countermeasures), while others are designed to *manage fatigue and mitigate the impact of fatigue that already exists* in operational settings (i.e., operational fatigue countermeasures). Preventive fatigue countermeasures include educating personnel about the importance of sleep and teaching personnel how to improve the recuperative value of sleep and ensuring that sleep disorders are properly diagnosed and treated, that sleep-enhancing medications are used properly, that the design and implementation of optimal work/rest scheduling is in place, and to safeguard against mistimed light exposure to minimize circadian and sleep disruptions. Operational fatigue countermeasures include workplace napping, establishment of adequate rest breaks, use of alertness-enhancing medications, optimal work environments (e.g., lighting, ergonomics), and use of technology to identify and/or avoid on-duty fatigue-related performance impairment.

Behavioral Strategies

Behavioral fatigue countermeasures are those that can be implemented by individuals or organizations to mitigate or manage fatigue. Preventive behavioral fatigue countermeasures focus on interventions designed to improve the quantity and quality of sleep, as well as the performance of fatigued individuals.

Education to Improve Sleep and Mitigate Fatigue

Educating workers about the relationships among sleep, circadian rhythms, and fatigue is a first step in optimizing on-the-job performance. Workers should be given an appreciation of the importance of sufficient off-duty sleep for fatigue mitigation, the dangers associated with insufficient sleep, and the strategies that will provide them with the right quantity and quality of sleep needed for complete restoration from waking activity. In addition, it is imperative that both individuals and organizations be given an understanding of the negative effects of undiagnosed sleep disorders so as to promote the recognition and treatment of these alertness-impairing medical conditions. Details on handling these concerns are presented in Chapters 81 and 84.

Napping to Promote Wakefulness

Napping is a strategy that, depending on its application, can be considered either a preventive or an operational workplace fatigue countermeasure. Napping is preventive if the *naps are taken before the duty period* to ensure that the preduty sleep quota has been met and is operational (or strategic) if the *naps are implemented within the work context* to compensate for ongoing job-related sleep loss (such as when excessively lengthy duty periods prohibit adequate sleep). Napping is an effective fatigue countermeasure in situations in which the primary sleep period is inadequate to maintain alertness and performance.[8] Studies on shift workers have shown that napping during the night shift can improve alertness and performance.[9,10] Additionally, napping before the night shift or before a period of extended wakefulness—a strategy often referred to as "banking sleep"—can reduce accumulated sleep debt and improve workplace safety by mitigating acute fatigue.[10-12] Several factors are important to consider before implementing a napping regime.

Nap Timing. Taking naps at optimal times, both with regard to the amount of sleep loss as well as the circadian phase, will influence the effectiveness of a nap. Nap timing should take into account the ease of falling asleep and the probable quality of sleep as a function of the body's internal clock. In addition, nap planning should balance the possible short-term negative effects of napping resulting from sleep inertia (the grogginess that can occur immediately upon awakening) versus the known longer-term positive effects of napping on performance after sleep inertia has dissipated.

Nap Duration. Generally, any length of nap will improve performance and alertness during an otherwise long work/wakefulness session. Bonnet[13] found a dose-response relationship between nap length and performance, concluding that the nap, particularly before an all-night shift, should be as long as possible to produce maximum performance benefits. He also concluded that prophylactic naps, those taken before significant sleep loss, were better than naps that replace sleep that is already lost because of long hours of continuous wakefulness. Brooks and Lack[14] found 20- and 30-minute naps improved overall cognitive performance for as long as 155 minutes compared to the 10-minute nap, which showed cognitive performance effects for only 95 minutes. Driskell and Mullen[15] concluded that naps led to performance benefits equal to, and sometimes greater than, baseline performance levels, with the length of performance benefit directly proportional to the length of the nap (e.g., a 15-minute nap led to 2 hours of benefit while a 4-hour nap led to 10 hours of benefit). However, regardless of nap length, the performance benefit decreased as postnap wakefulness increased (i.e., the benefits of a 4-hour nap were greater shortly after awakening than 10 hours afterward, although performance at the later time still met or exceeded baseline performance).

Sleep Inertia. Whenever napping is proposed as a countermeasure, the effects of sleep inertia, the mental grogginess that occurs immediately after awakening, must be considered. Sleep inertia temporarily impairs performance and reduces alertness after awakening. The duration of sleep inertia depends on many factors, such as the duration of the nap/sleep period, prior time awake, and time of day; however, sleep inertia typically dissipates 1 to 35 minutes after awakening.[16] A common recommendation designed to avoid sleep inertia is to keep naps relatively short in an effort to prevent onset of (and subsequent awakening from) deep sleep. However, this tactic only works in fairly well-rested individuals since sleep inertia has been found to occur with naps as short as 10 minutes when it is taken after an extended period of wakefulness.[17] Sleep inertia is a problematic short-term disadvantage of napping, particularly when returning to work soon after a nap or in cases when performance is critical immediately upon awakening; however, the short-term negative consequences of sleep inertia must be balanced against the known longer-term positive effects of napping on alertness and performance that will persist into the later part of the duty period.

Nap Barriers. In some settings (e.g., the technology sector), napping has gained popularity. However, in other settings (e.g., health care), concerns over adequate personnel coverage, suitable napping facilities, sleep inertia among on-call/emergency personnel, and even unfavorable public opinion over "sleeping on the job" has hindered the implementation of workplace napping strategies.[18]

Rest Breaks to Temporarily Boost Alertness

Rest breaks are a strategy that can be implemented both before and after sleep loss has occurred and are a countermeasure that can be incorporated into most work environments. When the work is monotonous, tedious, or highly automated, short breaks can temporarily increase alertness. Allowing personnel to stand up and move about enhances the benefit of the break,[19] as do social interactions that occur during the break.[20] But regardless of these factors, taking any type of break from the task at hand will briefly improve alertness and performance.[21]

Other Behavioral Strategies to Boost Alertness

A few other strategies have been shown to have minor effects on alertness in individuals who are engaged in extended periods of wakefulness, but these appear to be far less effective than the other techniques noted in this section. A survey of over 3000 drivers found that turning on the radio and opening a window were popular behaviors to counteract sleepiness,[22] despite the lack of evidence that these countermeasures are effective. Reyner and Horne[23] found that "in-car" countermeasures such as turning on the radio or blowing cold air to the face had either no effect on subjective sleepiness or short-term effects lasting about 30 minutes. Schwarz and colleagues[24] supported these findings, concluding that opening the car window and listening to music are not recommended as countermeasures for driver sleepiness.

Another common strategy to improve alertness is exercise. However, there is little evidence that this strategy is beneficial. As with music and cold air, any benefit from exercise is generally short lived[25,26] or does not help higher cognitive functions.[27] If the exercise is lengthy and intense, it can actually increase fatigue and sleepiness over that which would have occurred without the exercise.[25] However, if the exercise is short and implemented frequently, it may benefit night-shift workers.[28]

Environmental Strategies

Environmental strategies can be implemented on the job once sleep loss has occurred but can also be used to boost alertness before significant fatigue becomes an issue. Some types of environmental changes have proven ineffective as fatigue countermeasures. On the one hand, sound and temperature manipulations have been shown to exert little effect on alertness in fatigued workers.[29] On the other hand, manipulation of light exposure has proven quite valuable.

Light Exposure

The correct amount of the right type and correctly timed exposure to light has been proven to benefit both alertness and circadian adjustment.[30] Although the design and implementation of a light-centered strategy is complex, generally speaking, light can be used as a preventive fatigue countermeasure (such as when it helps to ameliorate circadian misalignments and improve preduty sleep quality) or as an on-the-job fatigue countermeasure (such as when it serves to acutely enhance on-the-job alertness and performance).

Increasing Light Exposure. From the standpoint of using light as an effective operational (on-the-job) fatigue countermeasure, most research indicates that light in the blue/green spectrum exerts acute positive effects on alertness and performance, regardless of whether the exposure occurs at night when individuals have not obtained adequate rest or during the day when sleep loss may not be a problem.[31] Exposure to light at the correct times also positively influences the circadian system, allowing faster adjustment to either night shift or a new time zone.[32] Sunlight is an obvious natural light source, but there also are many types of artificial light sources that can provide extra lighting when needed. Determining the best times to maximize light for circadian adjustment (as opposed to acutely enhancing alertness) is, as alluded to earlier, a complicated issue, so a detailed reference should be consulted before relying on lighting modifications to help overcome either jet lag or shift lag.[33]

Avoiding Unwanted Light Exposure. Although light can acutely enhance both alertness and performance, incorrectly timed light exposure can produce undesired effects in terms of adapting to a new time zone or work schedule because ill-timed light can offset desirable circadian adjustment.[30] Travelers should consult an online planning tool (e.g., http://www.jetlagrooster.com) to plan when to avoid (and when to experience) light exposure before flying to distant eastward or westward locations to maximize benefits. Night workers attempting to sleep during the day should avoid light exposure on the drive home by using blue light–blocking glasses. Strategic use of blue light–blocking glasses reduces sleep disruption and improves performance of rotating shift workers.[34] Even in day workers, wearing these glasses in the evening (before bedtime) can significantly improve self-reported sleep quality at night,[35] while wearing them in the morning delays the circadian phase, allowing better daytime sleep following a night shift.[36] These glasses also appear to prevent problems associated with the pre-bedtime use of e-readers, computers, or smartphones.[37] Alternatively, because using electronic devices that emit blue light at the "wrong" times can negatively affect sleep and circadian rhythms,[38] blue light–blocking smartphone and tablet applications should be applied when using these devices in the evening. Better sleep quality, whether at night or during the day, leads to better performance and reduced sleepiness during work hours.

Technological Aids

A category of fatigue countermeasures that is somewhat different to those previously discussed is one that involves technological applications or tools designed to detect fatigue in operational contexts as well as those designed to minimize the impact of fatigue in the workplace. In addition, there are technology-based strategies designed to help develop work/rest schedules that are less fatiguing than those based on prescriptive rules.

Fatigue Detection Strategies

Fatigue detection strategies aim to identify personnel who are showing signs of fatigue-related impairments so that they can be made more self-aware of their potentially problematic fatigue levels, offered an alertness-enhancing countermeasure to the fatigue they are experiencing, and/or removed from the work setting altogether.

On-Duty Ocular Monitoring. The online measurement of eye movements for fatigue assessment appears to hold the most promise of the strategies available. Various strategies have been shown to be useful in research settings, but they have not easily transferred to the real world. The eye movements of alert and sleepy individuals often overlap, creating false positives or false negatives.[39] Measures of pupillary instability have proven reasonably sensitive and specific in terms of estimating time awake and have provided similar temporal profiles as other measures of sleepiness, such as lapses on the Psychomotor Vigilance Task (PVT), electroencephalography (EEG) microsleeps, slow eye movements, and eye closures,[40] but these measurements are not feasible for use in an ordinary workplace. Problematically, ocular measures of fatigue can be confounded by light conditions and other contextual factors.

On-Duty Physiologic Monitoring. Measures such as EEG, event-related brain potentials (ERPs), and heart-rate variability (HRV) have been investigated over the years as potential alertness-tracking/fatigue-detection technologies; however, as with other technologies that are successful at identifying fatigue in the laboratory, these measures are not easily feasible for real-world operation. They tend to be intrusive, uncomfortable, and susceptible to environmental interference and require extensive data processing.[41,42]

On-Duty Head-Position Monitoring. Because sleepy individuals tend to experience head nods or sudden head "snap backs" resulting from a loss of muscle tone in the neck, online identification of such movements has been proposed as an indicator of a serious alertness deficit. However, loss of neck-muscle tone does not occur until someone has already fallen asleep, and at that point, performance has already been seriously compromised. Multiaxis head coordinate monitoring may be a better alternative, but the complex sensor systems required for integrated assessment of x/y/z-axis (forward/rearward, side-to-side, and upward/downward) movements are generally not feasible for operational contexts.

On-Duty Task Performance Monitoring. Embedded measures of performance are desirable for fatigue detection from the standpoints of being "ecologically valid" and nondistracting, but identifying candidates appropriate for every type of operational setting has been difficult. However, one setting in which such systems have shown great promise is vehicle driving. Systems such as lane tracking systems aim to detect or predict unwanted excursions from the desired course of travel, and the use of these systems has increased substantially over the past few years. Such systems provide detection or prediction of driver fatigue as well as driver feedback and warnings designed to prevent serious performance failures. The effectiveness of these techniques is difficult to evaluate,[43] but there is evidence that auditory and/or visual warning systems can reduce involuntary lane departures during relatively short drives.[44] For example, although not generated by vehicle-mounted systems, the noise and vibration created by veering into in-ground rumble strips along roadways have proven successful for cuing drivers to incorrect lane departures.[45]

Automation. Although not a "fatigue monitoring" or "fitness for duty" strategy, automation is often proposed as a helpful technological way to mitigate errors made by fatigued drivers or operators, but since research shows that increased automation actually decreases alertness in drivers[46] and in other settings,[47] it would appear that full automation in which operator input is completely removed is the only true automation-centered fatigue solution. Unfortunately, this level of technology-implementation is not expected within the near future, and in the meantime, partial automation in which the operator is relegated to performing only a relatively inactive supervisory role may lead to more rather than less fatigue-related safety concerns.[48] In the future, a combination of some of the fatigue-detection systems mentioned earlier and the use of automation that takes the user "out of the loop" may be promising.

Technology-Based Schedule Design Strategies

Computer-assisted scheduling tools based on validated biomathematical models aim to improve the ease with which complex science-based scheduling principles can be used to create safer work/rest schedules (see Chapter 83). Biomathematical models predict the temporal profiles of alertness, fatigue, and/or performance using sleep-wake history and time-of-day as model inputs. These tools can be used in a preventive fashion to help develop work/rest schedules that mitigate fatigue. They also can be used to compare the estimated fatigue impact of several potentially viable shift-work schedules so that the best alternative can be selected. If fatiguing schedules must be worked, these tools can identify periods in the work schedules in which fatigue countermeasures may be needed. Finally, modeling tools can assist with determining the optimal timing of an array of counter-fatigue interventions, the conduct of post-hoc accident investigations, and the planning of fatigue mitigation targets for proactive investment.

Pharmacologic Aids

When scheduling, environmental, or work factors prevent proper rest, medications may be an option. Under these conditions, a hypnotic may be used to promote off-duty sleep (when opportunities for sleep are available) or an alertness aid to increase wakefulness when sleep deprivation is unavoidable.

Medications to Improve Sleep

When sleep is difficult, sleep aids are helpful for preventing the sleep deprivation or sleep restriction/disruption that logically can be expected to lead to performance declines. Generally, sleep aids are intended for short-term use when other options are not adequate. For example, when "exogenous" circadian factors (e.g., those encountered with shift lag or jet lag) or unavoidable "sleep disrupters" (e.g., uncomfortable light, noise, and temperature levels in the sleep environment) threaten adequate rest and recuperation, sleep aids may be used to improve sleep.

Medication Options. Numerous prescription options are available to promote sleep, and the decision regarding which one to use should be based on the characteristics of the hypnotic and the situation. A long-acting hypnotic such as temazepam, which has a half-life of 3.5 to 18 hours is useful for maintaining sleep for relatively long periods during the night and/or for optimizing the daytime sleep of night-working personnel who have a sufficiently lengthy sleep opportunity (i.e., 8 to 10 hours).[49,50] A more intermediate-acting medication such as extended-release zolpidem, which has a half-life of 3 to 6 hours may be suitable for shorter sleep opportunities or in situations in which hangover effects are of concern.[51] Another intermediate alternative would be eszopiclone, which has a half-life of 5 to 6 hours. Eszopiclone has been shown to have minimal residual drug effects after as little as 10 hours postdose.[52] For short sleep periods or for sleep initiation—as opposed to sleep maintenance—of major sleep periods occurring earlier than the usual habitual bedtime, zolpidem (mean half-life 2.5 hours) or zaleplon (mean half-life 1 hour) would be preferable to longer-acting hypnotics because their shorter half-lives will significantly reduce the possibility of postsleep sedation.[53,54] Ramelteon (a drug that acts via melatonin pathways) also may be appropriate when a short-acting compound is needed. However, although ramelteon is efficacious for inducing sleep, like extremely short-half-life benzodiazepines or other GABA agonists, it is not optimal for maintaining it.[55] Suvorexant (a medication with a mean half-life of approximately 9 hours) acts differently than both the GABA agonists and the melatonin antagonist. Suvorexant blocks the orexin, which promotes wakefulness, thus inducing sleep, reducing arousals, and improving sleep consolidation.[56] This medication may prove to be another option as an intermediate-acting sleep medication,[57] but its efficacy for daytime sleep and/or jet lag has yet to be tested. Over-the-counter medications and herbs are also available for help with sleep. Most nonprescription sleep aids contain the antihistamines diphenhydramine or doxylamine, and generally these compounds at least offer some improvement in self-reported sleep, despite the fact that they often fail to substantially impact objective measures of sleep. Herbs, such as valerian, and melatonin show little efficacy as well.[58] Although valerian root has been used for centuries as a sleep aid, the research supporting its efficacy is mixed. Generally, there may be some mild benefits, but the evidence does not support the use of valerian root as a general treatment for insomnia.[59] Melatonin possesses weak hypnotic or "soporific" properties that theoretically should facilitate out-of-phase sleep.[60] Substantial evidence indicates that appropriate administration of melatonin can improve circadian adaptation to new time schedules.[61] However, there is little evidence that melatonin improves sleep when taken as a traditional sleep aid by those experiencing insomnia not related to circadian rhythm disturbances.[62] Clinical guidelines for the treatment of primary insomnia do not recommend either diphenhydramine or melatonin as a treatment for sleep onset nor sleep maintenance insomnia.[63]

Choosing the Correct Sleep-Enhancing Medication. The choice of compound depends on the timing of the sleep opportunity, the expected length of the sleep period, and whether there is a high probability of unexpected sleep truncation. It is important to balance the need to optimize sleep with the need to avoid residual effects, but in general, hypnotics can minimize the sleep disruptions associated with shift work and rapid transmeridian travel. With proper planning,[64,65] they can be used without undue concern about postsleep hangover effects. Studies have consistently demonstrated that hypnotics increase the length of daytime sleep in shift workers and out-of-phase sleep in jet-lagged travelers, although the sleep enhancements do not consistently facilitate better performance in night workers or daytime jet lag symptom alleviation in travelers.[66] Nevertheless, the American Academy of Sleep Medicine's Practice Parameters for the Clinical Evaluation and Treatment of Circadian Rhythm Sleep Disorders suggests that hypnotic medications may be used to help deal with shift lag and jet lag, provided that the possibility of adverse effects is kept in mind.[67]

Medications to Improve Alertness

In situations during which alertness is required despite inadequate or ill-timed sleep opportunities and/or poor sleep environments, temporary use of prescription or nonprescription pharmacologic alertness aids should be considered. Generally, prescription aids are recommended to attenuate daytime sleepiness associated with sleep disorders, but they can also help improve alertness resulting from inadequate sleep. Over-the-counter caffeine formulations are freely available (at least in the United States), and these are widely used to overcome the effects of fatigue from insufficient sleep.

Older Prescription Medication Options. Amphetamines such as methylphenidate, dextroamphetamine, and methamphetamine have long been considered the most effective compounds for improving performance during periods of sleep deprivation, and some of these compounds have been found to be particularly useful in military contexts. However, the risk of side effects such as increased anxiety and confusion, elevated blood pressure and heart rate, and increased body temperature, as well as their abuse potential argues against regular recourse to these medication in work or jet lag situations.[67] In fact, none of the amphetamine compounds are FDA approved for the treatment of shiftwork sleepiness disorder or jet lag disorder.

Newer Prescription Alertness-Enhancing Medication Options. Modafinil and armodafinil are newer options that are indicated for the treatment of excessive daytime sleepiness associated with shift-work sleep disorder as well as for sleepiness associated with conditions such as narcolepsy.[68] Both medications are highly effective for alertness maintenance when sleep and circadian factors degrade performance. In a review by Liira and colleagues,[69] modafinil and armodafinil were reported to improve subjective sleepiness and performance on the psychomotor vigilance test in shift workers, so both would presumably improve "real-world" operational performance as well. Modafinil and armodafinil are classified as Schedule IV drugs because of their low abuse potential, thus making them more desirable than Schedule II medications, such as dextroamphetamine.

An Over-the-Counter Alertness-Enhancing Alternative. Caffeine has long been a popular nonprescription means to enhance mental or cognitive functions. Caffeine doses between 200 and 600 mg provide multiple positive performance, mood, and alertness benefits in sleep-deprived individuals, and doses up to 300 mg are beneficial in rested personnel engaged in monotonous activities such as military sentry duty or lengthy periods of highway driving.[70-72] Caffeine is freely and widely available, and it is one of the safest interventions to reduce mental fatigue.

Choosing the Correct Alternative. The choice of whether to use armodafinil, modafinil, or caffeine depends on the availability of these compounds as well as the required duration of action.[73] Both armodafinil and modafinil are longer-acting substances that are only available by prescription, whereas caffeine is a relatively short-acting compound that is widely available in numerous forms such as drinks, candies, gums, and tablets. All three options provide temporary relief from the performance effects of sleep deprivation. The American Academy of Sleep Medicine's Practice Parameters for the Clinical Evaluation and Treatment of Circadian Rhythm Sleep Disorders suggests that both modafinil and caffeine are indicated for alertness enhancement in shift workers, and caffeine is indicated as a good way to counteract jet lag–induced sleepiness.[67] However, in both situations, care should be taken to avoid disrupting any available sleep opportunities.

CLINICAL PEARL

Fatigue from long work hours, insufficient sleep, and circadian disruption and misalignment poses significant performance, health, and safety risks. These risks can be effectively mitigated by a comprehensive set of pharmacologic, empirically based behavioral, and technology-based countermeasures.

SUMMARY

Fatigue resulting from sleep restriction, intense/lengthy work schedules, rotating shifts, jet lag, and other factors poses a substantial risk to safety, performance, health, and general well-being. However, there are empirically validated counter-fatigue strategies that promote more recuperative sleep, optimize circadian adjustment, and mitigate the impact of fatigue in real-world settings. Education regarding the physiologic underpinnings of fatigue and the true seriousness of the problem is an important first step. Once workers are convinced of the importance of proper fatigue management, they can be provided with essential information on regulatory approaches and evidence-based mitigation strategies including (1) behavioral strategies such as the implementation of good sleep hygiene, strategic napping, and appropriately timed rest breaks; (2) environmental tactics such as optimal lighting; (3) technological interventions to include performance monitoring and fitness-for-duty assessments; and (4) pharmacologic interventions such as the use of both alertness enhancers and hypnotics. In addition to these, an emphasis should be placed on the use of biomathematical models to aid in the design of optimal shift-work scheduling and the inclusion of fatigue risk management systems within organizations' overall safety management programs. A fully integrated, scientifically based, multifaceted approach to fatigue management will significantly improve worker health and well-being while bolstering operational safety in today's fast-paced environments.

SELECTED READINGS

Anund A, Fors C, Kecklund G, van Leeuwen W, Åkerstedt T. *Countermeasures for Fatigue in Transportation – A Review of Existing Methods for Drivers on Road, Rail, Sea and in Aviation.* Swedish National Road and Transport Research Institute, VTI report 852A; 2015.

Caldwell JA, Caldwell JL, Thompson LA, Lieberman HR. Fatigue and its management in the workplace. *Neurosci Biobehav Rev.* 2019;96:272–289.

Ehlert AM, Wilson PB. Stimulant use as a fatigue countermeasure in aviation. *Aerosp Med Hum Perform.* 2021;92(3):190–200.

Goel N. Neurobehavioral effects and biomarkers of sleep loss in healthy adults. *Curr Neurol Neurosci Rep.* 2017;17(11):89.

Honn KA, Van Dongen HPA, Dawson D. Working Time Society consensus statements: prescriptive rule sets and risk management-based approaches for the management of fatigue-related risk in working time arrangements. *Ind Health.* 2019;57(2):264–280.

Lowden A, Öztürk G, Reynolds A, Bjorvatn B. Working Time Society consensus statements: evidence based interventions using light to improve circadian adaptation to working hours. *Industr Health.* 2019;57:213–227.

Redeker NS, Carus CC, Hashmi SD, et al. Workplace interventions to promote sleep health and an alert, healthy workforce. *J Clin Sleep Med.* 2019;15(4):649–657.

Sadeghniiat-Haghighi K, Yazdi Z. Fatigue management in the workplace. *Ind Psychiatry J.* 2015;24(1):12–17.

A complete reference list can be found online at ExpertConsult.com.

Chapter 83

Sleep, Sleepiness, and Performance Prediction Modeling

Samantha Riedy; Steven R. Hursh; Drew Dawson; Thomas J. Balkin; Hans P.A. Van Dongen

Chapter Highlights

- Sleep loss and circadian misalignment cause changes in sleepiness and neurobehavioral performance. Biomathematical models have been developed to predict the magnitude and temporal profiles of these changes.
- Most extant biomathematical models predict sleepiness or neurobehavioral performance based on the interplay of two biologic processes: circadian rhythmicity and homeostatic sleep-wake regulation. Sleep inertia may be incorporated as a third process.
- Recent advances among biomathematical models include accounting for the cumulative effects of chronic sleep restriction, individualizing model predictions, improving sleep estimators that predict sleep timing and duration from work-rest schedules, and incorporating dynamic circadian shifting and synchronization.
- Biomathematical models are gaining acceptance in operational settings as tools to help estimate and reduce fatigue-related risk and as components of fatigue risk management systems.

Alertness and neurobehavioral performance vary over time as a function of time of day, time awake, and a variety of person-specific and situational factors. Alertness and performance are degraded during periods of insufficient sleep and/or nighttime wakefulness (see Chapter 39). Equations capturing key neurobiologic processes involved in this degradation have been incorporated in "biomathematical models of fatigue." Such models make quantitative predictions of changes in alertness and performance over time and can be used to describe and predict sleepiness and performance given a wake-sleep or work-rest schedule; inform decisions regarding the application of fatigue countermeasures; help improve work schedules, productivity, and safety; and facilitate fatigue-related accident investigations.

Most extant biomathematical models predict sleepiness or performance based on the quantification of two primary neurobiologic processes: the circadian process and the homeostatic process[1–7] (see Chapter 39). The circadian process is characterized by cyclic variations in physiologic activation reflected in the 24-hour rhythms of nearly all aspects of human physiology and behavior. In the context of modeling sleepiness and performance, the state of the circadian process is determined by time of day, providing a sleepiness-countering drive for alertness and performance that peaks in the evening hours and reaches a trough in the early morning. The timing of the circadian process can be altered by exposure to (bright) light[3] (see Chapter 37). The homeostatic process is characterized by a physiologic pressure for sleep, which builds across time awake and dissipates across time asleep. The state of the homeostatic process is thus determined by current time awake, the number of hours of sleep recently obtained, and prior sleep-wake history. Sleepiness is increased and performance is degraded when homeostatic sleep pressure is high. The homeostatic process interacts with the circadian process to drive changes in sleepiness and performance over time.[8]

In addition to the circadian and homeostatic processes, a third process called sleep inertia is relevant in the context of temporal changes in sleepiness and performance. Sleep inertia refers to the temporary degradation of alertness and performance that occurs immediately after awakening.[9] The magnitude of this effect depends on sleep stage and depth of sleep at the time of awakening, circadian phase, and sleep-wake history.[10] Sleep inertia dissipates rapidly with time awake,[11,12] and the effect of this process is typically negligible within 20 minutes of awakening.

Recent advances among biomathematical models include refinement of the mathematical representations of the circadian, homeostatic, and sleep inertia processes, including added interaction terms to capture nonadditive effects among these processes.[6,13,14] New additions to some models also include components that account for the effects of stimulant use,[15] synchronization of the circadian process by non–light-based time cues,[16] and/or other external factors known to mediate sleepiness and performance.

COMPONENTS OF BIOMATHEMATICAL MODELS

Circadian Process

Performance while awake and the drive to sleep are both controlled, in part, by a circadian process.[3,17,18] For individuals entrained to a nighttime sleep schedule, performance and alertness reach a peak in the early evening and fall to a minimum in the early morning. There is a secondary peak of alertness and performance in the midmorning and a secondary less pronounced nadir in the early afternoon. Negatively correlated with this pattern is the propensity for sleep, which reaches a peak at about the same time performance and alertness reach a trough.

Some models incorporate these major and minor peaks and troughs in performance and alertness using two linked harmonic oscillations (cosine functions), one with a period of 24 hours and the other with a period of 12 hours. This results in a combined function of the form shown in Figure 83.1. More dynamic models of the circadian process use a limit cycle oscillator that yields a function of similar form.[19] There is some evidence that the amplitude of the circadian process (i.e., the magnitude of the difference between the major peak and trough) depends on the state of the homeostatic process (i.e., the level of sleep debt). Implementations of this "nonlinear interaction" between the circadian and homeostatic processes vary across models.[6,20] Some models also account for the effects of individual factors such as chronotype and environmental factors, most notably the timing of sunlight, on the phase (i.e., timing) of the circadian process.[21]

Sleep-Wake Homeostatic Process

The physiologic pressure for sleep and its influence on alertness and cognitive performance is usually modeled as a homeostatic process.[18,22,23] The homeostatic process involves a pressure for sleep that builds during wakefulness and dissipates during sleep. Alertness and performance decrease as the pressure for sleep builds and subsequently increase as the pressure for sleep dissipates. Accordingly, total sleep deprivation produces rapid and significant reductions in alertness and performance, and subsequent recovery sleep results in rapid improvements in alertness and performance.[8]

Laboratory studies have revealed that chronic sleep restriction (anything less than approximately 8 hours per 24 hours) leads to cumulative alertness and performance deficits.[24,25] For sleep durations of more than approximately 4 hours per night, performance declines across days but eventually appears to reach an equilibrium level at which no further sleep debt is accumulated unless daily sleep duration is further reduced.[26,27] This suggests a feedback-modulated control system.[28] The sleep-wake homeostatic process is not infinitely elastic, however, and there is a limit to the extent to which sleep restriction can be tolerated in terms of the ability to maintain a steady, albeit increased, sleep pressure. For sleep durations of less than approximately 4 hours per night, a state of equilibrium is not

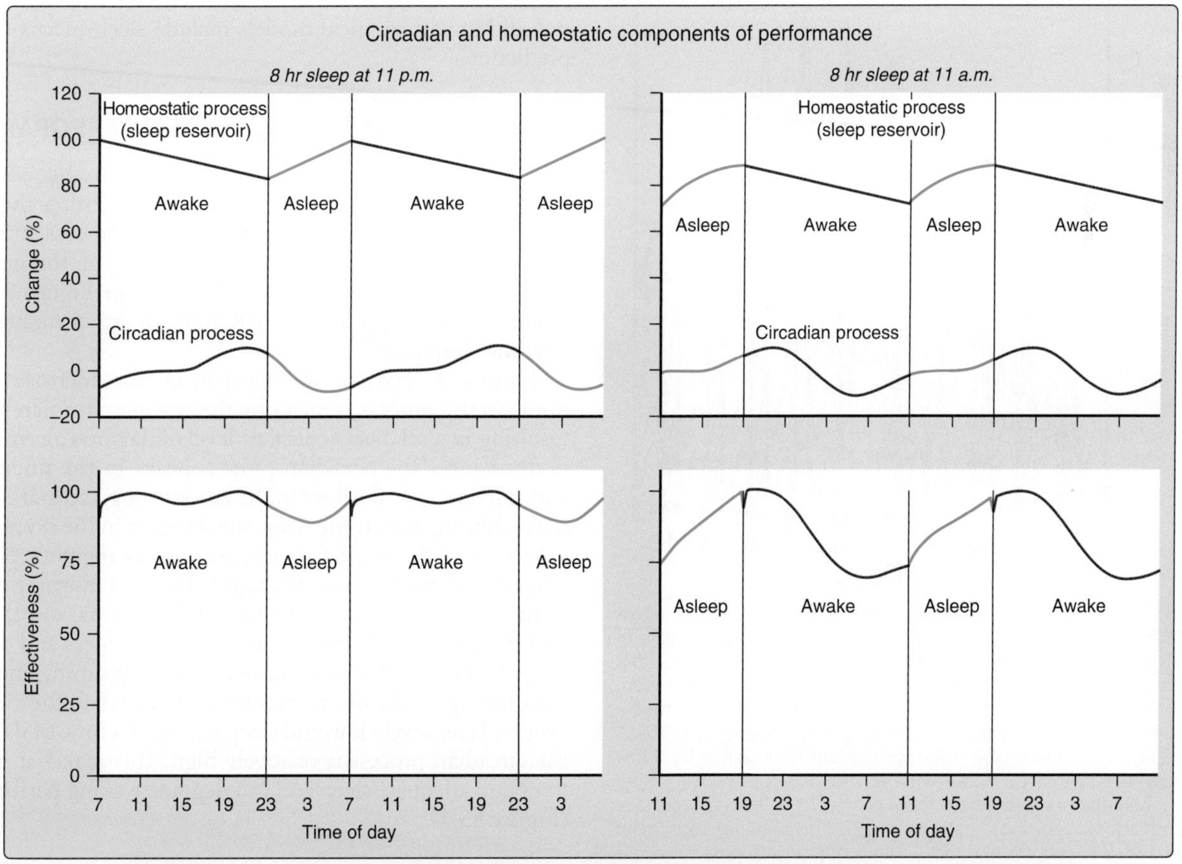

Figure 83.1 The sleep-wake homeostatic process (*top graphs, top curve*) and the circadian process (*top graphs, bottom curve*) and their predicted effects on performance (*bottom graphs*). Graphs are based on a biomathematical model's simulations[5] of cognitive effectiveness during a 16-hour wake/8-hour sleep schedule, with sleep starting at either 11 p.m. (nighttime sleep, *left panels*) or 11 a.m. (daytime sleep, *right panels*). The small dips in predicted effectiveness immediately after awakening reflect sleep inertia. Performance predictions during sleep are estimated because they cannot actually be observed during sleep.

achieved, and alertness and performance continue to decline across days.[26,27] As such, 4 hours of sleep per night can be seen as a threshold below which the buildup of the homeostatic sleep pressure during wakefulness exceeds the dissipation of the homeostatic sleep pressure during sleep. Biomathematical model simulations illustrate this bifurcation (i.e., qualitative change in behavior) for the homeostatic process when sleep is reduced below approximately 4 hours per night[28] (Figure 83.2).

The long-lasting effects of chronic sleep restriction on performance and reduced ability to recuperate suggest that some aspect of the sleep-wake homeostasis process undergoes a gradual change that is slow to recover relative to recovery following total sleep deprivation.[26,27,29] This phenomenon has prompted modelers to revise the sleep-wake homeostatic process by adding a long-term process.[5,28,30] Laboratory research findings also suggest that extending sleep to more than 8 hours per day for an extended period of time provides some resilience to the effects of subsequent sleep loss and reduces recovery time,[31,32] as has also been predicted mathematically.[28] Likewise, recent field research has demonstrated that sleep extension improves cognitive performance, even after

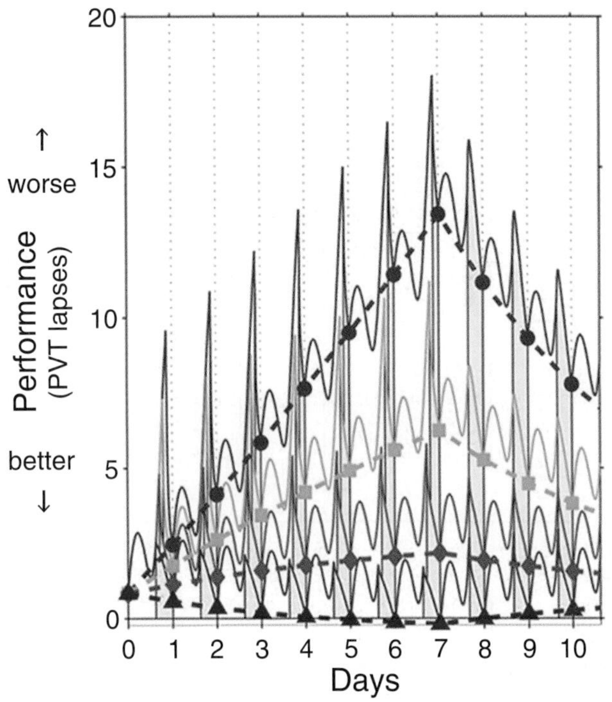

Figure 83.2 Bifurcating (i.e., qualitatively different) dynamic changes in performance impairment on a Psychomotor Vigilance Test (PVT) across days of chronic sleep restriction to less than or more than approximately 4 hours per night. Biomathematical model predictions are shown for a laboratory experiment in which subjects were exposed to baseline days with 8 hours time-in-bed (TIB) (here showing only the last one, as day 0); 7 days of 3, 5, 7, or 9 hours TIB (days 1 to 7); and recovery days with 8 hours TIB (days 8 to 10).[26] *Thin curves* show biomathematical model predictions in the 3-hour (*purple*), 5-hour (*orange*), 7-hour (*brown*), and 9-hour (*blue*) conditions.[28] *Thick dashed curves* show trends across days, exposing the escalation of performance impairment across days of sleep restriction in the 3-hour condition juxtaposed with the gradual dampening of impairment buildup in the 5-hour and 7-hour conditions. Note the gradual performance improvement in the 9-hour condition. *Light gray areas* represent nighttime sleep periods. (Reprinted with permission from McCauley P, Kalachev LV, Smith AD, et al. A new mathematical model for the homeostatic effect of sleep loss on neurobehavioral performance. *J Theor Biol*. 2009;256:227–239.)

resumption of the habitual sleep-wake schedule.[33] Conversely, sleep restriction exacerbates the negative effects of subsequent total sleep deprivation.[34]

Sleep fragmentation, like sleep restriction, negatively affects recuperation and consequently impairs alertness and performance. It is unclear to what extent this is due to a reduction in total sleep time versus a direct effect of sleep fragmentation itself.[35] Regardless of the mechanism, biomathematical models parameterized with time-in-bed data rather than total sleep-time data do not directly account for the effects of sleep fragmentation on subsequent alertness and performance. However, such effects could be approximated by adjusting the rate of recovery in the homeostatic process during sleep. Biomathematical models accounting for sleep fragmentation and the approximate time required to return to restorative sleep after a brief arousal have added a penalty during recuperation, such as a fixed delay from sleep onset until alertness and performance begin to improve.[5]

Sleep Inertia

A third process pertinent to biomathematical models is the transient performance impairment that often occurs immediately after awakening, called sleep inertia.[2] It is typically modeled as an exponentially decreasing performance deficit.[5,36,37] Because of the relatively short duration of sleep inertia, it is relevant mainly in operational contexts in which individuals may be required to perform immediately upon awakening (e.g., first responders and on-call health care providers), and not all biomathematical models include sleep inertia in their predictions.

COMBINED EFFECTS: PREDICTED PERFORMANCE

Alertness and performance are modeled as the combined effect of the mathematical functions representing the circadian process, the sleep-wake homeostatic process, and sleep inertia (if included). The combined effects of the circadian and homeostatic processes are illustrated in Figure 83.1 for a schedule with approximately 8 hours of either nighttime or daytime sleep daily.

During a daytime waking period, the increase in the homeostatic process is offset by the waxing circadian process, resulting in a relatively constant level of daytime alertness and performance. The circadian process peaks in the midevening and subsequently declines in the late evening, facilitating sleep onset. During nighttime sleep, the decrease in the homeostatic process and the waning circadian process together promote sleep maintenance across the night. The next morning the circadian process begins to rise, awakening occurs, and the cycle repeats itself.[1,8,38] During nighttime wakefulness and daytime sleep, there is a misalignment between sleep timing and circadian timing. Wake occurs at a time of day when the circadian process is relatively low, and sleep occurs at a time of day when the circadian process is relatively high. This makes it difficult to obtain adequate sleep and can degrade waking performance (Figure 83.1).

SLEEP PREDICTION

The accuracy of biomathematical model predictions is, to some extent, dependent on accurate measurement or prediction of sleep times and durations. If actual sleep measurements are

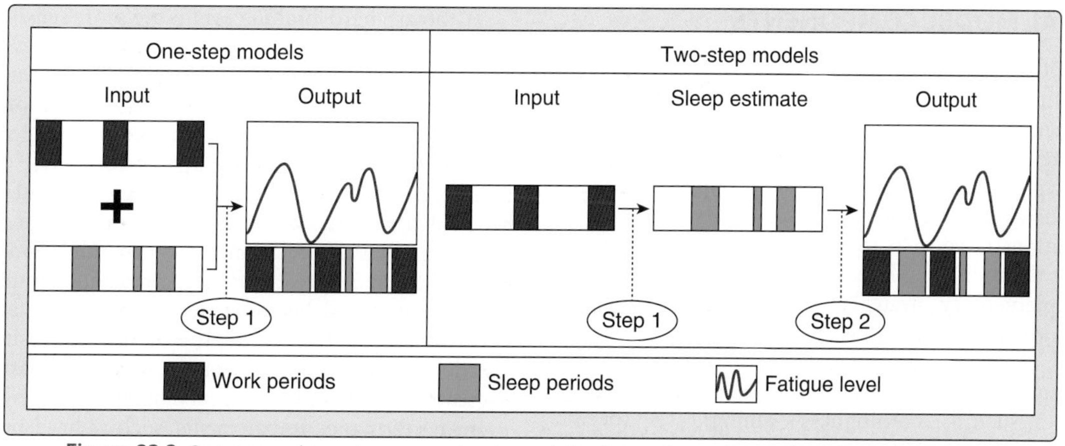

Figure 83.3 One-step and two-step approaches to modeling fatigue for work-rest schedules. In the one-step approach, sleepiness or performance is predicted directly from actual sleep measurements. In the two-step approach, sleep-wake behavior is predicted from work-rest schedules, and sleepiness or performance is then predicted from the predicted sleep-wake behavior. (Reprinted from Kandelaars KJ, Dorrian J, Fletcher A, Roach GD, Dawson D. A review of bio-mathematical fatigue models: where to from here? *Sixth Conference on Fatigue Management in Transportation.* 2005;1–19.)

available, sleepiness and performance can be predicted directly from the actual sleep-wake data ("one-step approach"). If actual sleep measurements are not available, then sleep timing and duration must first be predicted. This can be done mathematically using the two-process model of sleep regulation[39] or mutual inhibition neuronal models.[40–43] Sleepiness and performance can subsequently be predicted using the predicted sleep-wake data ("two-step approach") (Figure 83.3).

One way to develop sleep prediction algorithms is to use the observed likelihood of sleep using sleep-wake and work data collected in field studies.[44–47] The sleep predictions will generally be informed by scheduled work hours and any other constraints on sleep (e.g., commute times), and the predictions will depend on time of day (circadian phase) and homeostatic sleep propensity. Sleep prediction algorithms typically predict sleep at the group level; thus all workers with the same work-rest schedule will have the same predicted sleep-wake behaviors and, as a consequence, the same sleepiness and performance predictions.

Most available sleep prediction algorithms do not account for idiosyncratic social or other factors that drive individuals' sleep-wake behaviors, although first attempts have been made to incorporate such factors.[48–50] Algorithms that account for diversity in sleep behaviors among different individuals regardless of the sources of variability have also been proposed,[51] but they have not yet been made available for use in operational settings.

In recent studies of sleep patterns, it has been observed that the variability in the strategies and practices used by individuals to manage and organize their sleep can vary by operation.[52] For example, in cargo operations that mostly occur at night, a large proportion of sleep occurs during the day, and individuals vary greatly in how they manage daytime sleep.[53] A sleep prediction algorithm that predicts sleep-wake behaviors without accounting for operation-specific constraints may be less accurate for individuals engaged in these operations.[52]

An alternative approach to sleep estimation algorithms is to predict sleepiness or performance directly from the work-rest schedule without predicting sleep in an intermediate step. This has been adopted by a biomathematical model in which work-rest schedules are considered a square wave function that oscillates between work and nonwork periods, each of which are associated with varying fatigue and recovery values.[54]

CIRCADIAN PHASE SHIFTING

After traveling to another time zone or engaging in shift work, the internal circadian oscillator gradually shifts to the new schedule. After traveling to another time zone, the phase of the circadian rhythm may be adjusted to coincide with the new activity pattern.[3,5,56,57] In shift-work operations, however, full circadian adaptation is generally not achieved, in part due to morning light exposure or reverting back to a nighttime sleep schedule on days off.[58,59] Thus biomathematical models often do not include processes to account for any circadian adjustment among shift workers, or the circadian adaptation is predicted to occur at a slower rate.[5]

The factors that are presumed to mediate circadian phase shifts vary across models. A major driver of circadian phase is exposure to sunlight or bright light,[60] especially the blue part of the spectrum[61] (see Chapter 37). In some models, direct measurements of light exposure are required as input to the model and used to predict circadian phase shifts.[3] Other models use a surrogate for sunlight[5] so that light is not required as input to the model. However, this also means that there is no mechanism to account for light exposure when used as a fatigue countermeasure[62–64] (see Chapter 82).

The timing of the sleep period may in and of itself also contribute to circadian adjustment.[65,66] This has been incorporated into biomathematical models through various different mechanisms, including a process that gradually adjusts the phase of the circadian rhythm to coincide with the prevailing sleep-wake pattern without using light as an additional model input[5] and incorporation of a sleep-wake drive and a light drive that act on the circadian pacemaker through circadian sensitivity modulators.[16]

ADDITIONAL MODEL COMPONENTS

Individual differences in responses to sleep loss and adverse circadian timing (e.g., in shift work) represent a substantial source of variance in sleepiness and performance predictions.[8] This constitutes a challenge for most biomathematical models, which were typically developed to predict group-average performance. Individual differences in vulnerability to sleep loss have been demonstrated to be trait-like[67] and thus potentially predictable at the individual level.[68]

Two complementary strategies have been implemented to achieve biomathematical model predictions at the level of individuals.[69] The first is to incorporate predictors of individual differences in specific aspects of the underlying biologic processes, such as morningness-eveningness,[21] specific genetic polymorphisms,[70] or sex,[71] into the model equations. The second strategy is to tailor the parameters of the model to the individual based on real-time or retrospective use of performance measurements. Algorithms for this have been developed.[69,72–75]

SELECTION OF OUTCOME METRICS FOR OPERATIONAL USE

A criticism that has been leveled against biomathematical models is that because they have largely been parameterized and validated using laboratory data, their relevance for actual operational performance is suspect.[76] Of specific concern are questions regarding both their construct validity and ecologic validity, that is, whether the model predictions are relevant to performance in real-world operations and whether predictions from models developed using laboratory data generalize to real-world operational settings.

These concerns could potentially be obviated by constructing models that predict outcomes of operational interest, such as risk of fatigue-related accidents.[77,78] Developing outcomes of operational interest may prove difficult if the outcome measure occurs infrequently and thus requires years of data collection to construct a valid model or if the outcome primarily occurs at severe levels of sleepiness without providing evidence of impairment at lower levels of sleepiness. If the outcome is not sensitive to mild to moderate sleepiness, it also makes it difficult to use a biomathematical model based on the outcome to effectively introduce interventions (e.g., naps, caffeine) *before* severe sleepiness and performance impairment are reached and negative outcomes occur.

Therefore what is needed is an outcome measure more sensitive to varying levels of sleepiness and performance impairment. Hard-braking events in road transportation, for example, constitute a promising outcome metric.[79] Hard-braking events have the virtue of high construct validity and ecologic validity. Hard braking constitutes an evasive action, and most instances that are not associated with an actual accident can reasonably be considered near-miss events. These events also occur at a higher rate than traffic accidents, making this a more utilitarian and feasible outcome measure that can occur with moderate levels of sleepiness, thus facilitating the ability to introduce interventions (e.g., taking a break at a rest stop) to help avoid more severe levels of sleepiness and accidents.

Although hard-braking events are more sensitive to fatigue than traffic accidents, using an outcome metric even more sensitive to fatigue than an actual measure of operational performance, such as performance on the Psychomotor Vigilance Test (PVT),[80,81] can potentially be used to anticipate increased risk. Although the relationship between PVT performance and other measures of fatigue on the one hand, and the risk of accidents on the other hand, is complex,[82] it is reasonable to assume that this relationship is generally monotonic in the moment, that is, greater PVT performance impairment at a given time would be associated with greater fatigue-related accident risk at that time. Thus, using a sensitive outcome metric, such as PVT performance, to measure fatigue provides a greater opportunity to intervene before operationally relevant performance impairments, such as hard-braking events or traffic accidents emerge.

Furthermore, selection of an extremely sensitive outcome measure regardless of direct operational applicability obviates dilemmas associated with selection of outcome metrics for specific operations. There are usually many important outcomes in an operation, each of which is differentially sensitive to the effects of fatigue. A model based on a sensitive measure such as the PVT can be used to identify deteriorating levels of alertness and performance capacity before they reach levels at which operational performance is impacted, thereby facilitating application of optimally timed and effective interventions.

MODELING APPLIED TO OPERATIONAL SETTINGS

Regulations for work and rest times are gradually moving away from predominantly rule-based, prescriptive approaches and toward more performance-based frameworks for managing safety in operational settings.[83] As such, organizations are increasingly required to identify and quantify fatigue-related risks and ensure that appropriate controls or mitigations are in place to ensure safe operations. Biomathematical models provide a convenient methodology to help organizations determine, quantitatively, the expected level of fatigue-related risk associated with any working time arrangement and the extent to which mitigation would be required to continue working safely. That is, biomathematical models provided a clear and simple way in which to quantify the likelihood of fatigue as part of a risk assessment and mitigation process. This has been facilitated, in part, by the development of sleep prediction algorithms (as described earlier), which enable such quantification in the absence of sleep-wake data.

The application of biomathematical models in this context has led to the use of fatigue thresholds, where predictions of fatigue below the threshold would allow work to proceed, whereas predictions of fatigue exceeding the threshold would be considered unacceptable to continue working. However, given inherent uncertainty in the model predictions (e.g., because of the use of predicted sleep-wake behaviors and group-average predictions), potentially imprecise assumptions (e.g., with respect to prior sleep-wake history or initial conditions for the modeling), and the influence of risk factors other than those associated with fatigue, the relationship between a fatigue threshold and operational safety is not robust.

Model-based approaches to fatigue risk management have therefore recommended to move away from the use of fixed fatigue thresholds,[84] favoring instead an approach based on relative comparisons of predicted fatigue[85] or cumulative time of exposure to fatigue[51] between possible work schedules to identify the schedule with the lesser fatigue risk. This comparative approach can also be used to identify possible sources of fatigue risk (e.g., cumulative sleep debt or circadian misalignment) and guide the implementation of mitigations to reduce fatigue risk. When used that way and integrated within a fatigue risk management or overall risk and safety management framework (see Chapter 84), biomathematical models can be an effective tool to help control fatigue-related risk and manage operational safety, in a more flexible way than is possible based on prescriptive work-hour regulations with duty time and rest break thresholds.

Biomathematical models differ in the relative weight they give to the impact of circadian rhythmicity versus homeostatic sleep-wake regulation on fatigue, the way they deal with the estimation of sleep in the absence of actual sleep-wake data, whether and how they take into account the expected quality (or recuperative value) of sleep, and the inclusion of other factors potentially relevant to fatigue, such as geographic location and time of year or the sleep opportunity time lost to eating, personal hygiene, and commuting.[86] They have in common that certain circumstances and effects are simply not predictable; thus no matter which model is used or how sophisticated its implementation, predictions should not be counted on to be always right. Operational validation is important to ensure that a model produces predictions that are meaningful in a given operational setting. Furthermore, it is recommended that the use of a biomathematical model be embedded into a fatigue risk management framework to provide needed checks and balances (see Chapter 84).

A challenge for the use of biomathematical models in operational settings is that people frequently report that their predicted fatigue levels are not consistent with their subjective experience of the fatigue associated with specific working time arrangements, which in practice is often viewed as a failure of the biomathematical models. While this may be the case in some settings,[52] and while subjective and objective fatigue are known to diverge across days with insufficient sleep[27] and between individuals,[87] it also reflects a failure to be clear eyed about what biomathematical models can and cannot be expected to accomplish. In particular, biomathematical models are operationally useful to determine if work schedules provide adequate opportunity for sleep so that fatigue is controlled sufficiently to support a safe work environment. If the actual sleep obtained is substantially less than the opportunity provided, there is likely to be more fatigue than a model would predict, and safety may be compromised.

In addition to their use in model-based fatigue risk management, biomathematical models may also be useful in operational settings as an educational tool to help explain the basic principles of sleep, circadian rhythms, and fatigue. Biomathematical models may also serve as forensic tools in investigations of adverse events, accidents, and injuries, to examine the likelihood that fatigue was involved.[88] However, model predictions by themselves can neither prove nor rule out the involvement of fatigue; additional assessments are needed to increase the confidence in such a determination.[89] Although biomathematical models are no panacea, and in some operational settings, such as emergency medical services, the evidence in support of their use still falls short,[90] they have been widely implemented in commercial aviation[91,92] and railroad transportation,[73,93] and they appear to have significant potential in other operational settings.

LIMITATIONS OF BIOMATHEMATICAL MODELS

Biomathematical models are based on a rapidly evolving science. Accordingly, there are limitations that should be considered when evaluating these models, including (1) the accuracy of model predictions relative to observations obtained from laboratory versus field studies; (2) the generalizability of the model, that is, the extent to which the model is applicable to sleep-wake–work scenarios not used in its development and across different settings and contexts; and (3) the balance between model sensitivity and specificity, that is, the extent to which predictions are liberal or conservative with regard to identifying periods with meaningfully increased or decreased sleepiness and performance within a specific operational environment. These and other modeling issues were discussed at the 2002 Fatigue and Performance Modeling Workshop in Seattle, Washington and documented in the published meeting proceedings.[94] Since then, biomathematical models have undergone further development, rendering some of the information in those proceedings outdated. Nevertheless, the volume continues to provide valuable documentation of biomathematical modeling as a developing science.

The accuracy of model outputs depends on the accuracy of major model inputs. Sleep-wake patterns represent a key input, but often this information is not available in operational settings and must therefore be estimated or assumed, as discussed earlier. Similarly, measures of circadian rhythm are rarely available in the operational environment, and thus estimates of circadian phase and amplitude must be generated from the timing of sleep, light exposure, or other environmental drivers of biological rhythms. Such estimates may suffice for large groups but are likely to be less useful for predicting the performance of individuals who may, for example, be extreme morning or evening types.[95] In such cases, additional information (e.g., recent sleep-wake history) can be applied to reduce this source of error. Adding to the uncertainty is recent evidence that some measures of performance may adapt to time zone changes more quickly than some physiologic systems, such as hormone rhythms and core body temperature.[96] Some models calibrate the rate of adaptation to prior studies of physiologic systems and may therefore underestimate the rate of performance adaptation. More research is needed to address this putative limitation.

Another factor that affects sleepiness and performance and likely represents a residual source of variance in model predictions is the workload borne by personnel on the job. Workload is a very general term that can refer to the length of the duty day, time on task, task load, the complexity of tasks performed, unexpected challenges during the duty day that add additional burdens, and even the lack of experience among coworkers that can increase the effort required of more experienced personnel. Some of these factors are predictable and may be incorporated in biomathematical models.[97] In flight operations, examples include the number of flight segments in a flight duty period, the difficulty of the landing patterns into the airports, the usual congestion at a particular airport, and language difficulties in some regions of the world. Many other potential workload factors cannot be predicted, such as bad weather, equipment failures, and personnel issues. Given this complexity and uncertainty, it is difficult for fatigue models to accurately (1) predict workload, (2) combine these factors into a single metric by which their joint impact can be quantified, and (3) estimate the impact of workload factors on performance and safety.

Another major input to biomathematical models is "initial state." This refers to prior sleep-wake history, circadian phase, and, depending on the specific model, other relevant variables that provide the starting point from which predictions are made. If the initial states are unknown, assumptions regarding the likely sleep-wake history and circadian phase need to be made. The accuracy of these assumptions initially determines the accuracy of the model predictions. However, the influence of the initial state estimates diminishes over time,[98] and the accuracy of the model improves as actual daily sleep measures (e.g., actigraphic sleep measurements) or work schedule–based sleep estimates accrue and are used as model input.

CONCLUSION

Biomathematical models predict physiology-based sleepiness or performance as a function of sleep-wake history, circadian rhythm, and sleep inertia. These model predictions are generally at the group level, although individual-level sleepiness or performance predictions are possible if individual traits are incorporated or individual-level sleepiness or performance data have previously been collected. To obtain accurate group-level or individual-level sleepiness or performance predictions, obtaining accurate actual or estimated sleep-wake data is critical. Furthermore, other factors in addition to sleep-wake patterns, circadian rhythm, and sleep inertia affect sleepiness and performance. Factors such as stimulant use and light exposure have been introduced into some biomathematical models; however, workload, presence of sleep disorders, and other physiologic and nonphysiologic factors remain residual sources of potential error variance in performance and sleepiness predictions. In operational settings, biomathematical models provide a useful tool for assessing the likelihood of sleepiness or performance impairment during a work-rest schedule, and they are increasingly being incorporated into fatigue risk management systems. Unlike prescriptive hours-of-service regulations, these models provide physiology-based, flexible, and quantifiable ways to optimize safety and performance in operational settings.

CLINICAL PEARL

Sleep loss and circadian misalignment produce deficits in neurobehavioral performance. Biomathematical models that predict performance based on these factors are valuable tools that are increasingly being applied in a variety of settings. For personal use, these models can be applied to determine the effects of sleep-wake duration and timing on alertness and performance and thus serve to guide clinical, professional, and personal decision making regarding sleep habits and use of countermeasures. For employers, regulatory agencies, and practitioners in occupational medicine, these models are useful to guide the design of better work schedules, reduce performance errors and accidents, aid in potentially fatigue-related accident investigations, improve the health and well-being of employees, and advance public safety.

SUMMARY

Because insufficient sleep leads to lapses of attention, slowed reaction time, and impaired reasoning and decision making, it is a major proximate cause of errors and accidents in both industrial and military operational settings. Biomathematical models have been developed to predict sleep- and alertness-mediated performance in laboratory and field environments. Such models are being incorporated into scheduling tools to anticipate and avoid performance impairment in operational settings. Most extant models predict performance based on three basic components: circadian variation in alertness and sleep propensity, homeostatic sleep-wake regulation, and sleep inertia. These processes vary over time as a function of sleep-wake patterns and combine to produce changes in alertness and neurobehavioral performance. For a wide range of variations in sleep opportunities or work schedules, current models provide sufficiently accurate predictions of group-average performance. Efforts are underway to further refine these biomathematical models to enhance accuracy of prediction for individuals and incorporate additional factors that determine performance outcomes.

ACKNOWLEDGMENTS

This research was supported in part by an appointment to the Research Participation Program at the Walter Reed Army Institute of Research administered by the Oak Ridge Institute for Science and Education through an interagency agreement between the US Department of Energy and US Army Medical Research and Development Command. The views expressed in this article are those of the authors and do not reflect the official policy or position of the Department of the Army, the Department of Defense, the US Government, or any of the government institutions with which the authors are affiliated.

SELECTED READINGS

Borbély AA, Achermann P. Concepts and models of sleep regulation: an overview. *J Sleep Res*. 1992;1:63–79.

Darwent D, Dawson D, Roach GD. Prediction of probabilistic sleep distributions following travel across multiple time zones. *Sleep*. 2010;33:185–195.

Folkard S, Åkerstedt T. Trends in the risk of accidents and injuries and their implications for models of fatigue and performance. *Aviat Space Environ Med*. 2004;75:A161–A167.

Hursh SR, Redmond DP, Johnson ML, et al. Fatigue models for applied research in warfighting. *Aviat Space Environ Med*. 2004;75:A44–A53.

Åkerstedt T, Ingre M, Kecklund G, et al. Accounting for partial sleep deprivation and cumulative sleepiness in the three-process model of alertness regulation. *Chronobiol Int*. 2008;25:309–319.

Daan S, Beersma DGM, Borbély AA. Timing of human sleep: recovery process gated by a circadian pacemaker. *Am J Physiol*. 1984;246:R161–R178.

Skeldon AC, Phillips AJK, Dijk DJ. The effects of self-selected light-dark cycles and social constraints on human sleep and circadian timing: a modeling approach. *Sci Rep*. 2017;7:45158.

McCauley P, Kalachev LV, Mollicone DJ, et al. Dynamic circadian modulation in a biomathematical model for the effects of sleep and sleep loss on waking neurobehavioral performance. *Sleep*. 2013;36:1987–1997.

Raslear TG, Hursh SR, Van Dongen HPA. Predicting cognitive impairment and accident risk. *Prog Brain Res*. 2011;190:155–167.

Van Dongen HPA, Belenky G. Model-based fatigue risk management. In: Matthew G, Desmond PA, Neubauer C, Hancock PA, eds. *The Handbook of Operator Fatigue*. Farnham: Ashgate; 2012:487–506.

Dawson D, Darwent D, Roach GD. How should a bio-mathematical model be used within a fatigue risk management system to determine whether or not a working time arrangement is safe? *Accid Anal Prev.* 2017;99(Pt B):469–473.

Postnova S, Lockley SW, Robinson PA. Prediction of cognitive performance and subjective sleepiness using a model of arousal dynamics. *J Biol Rhythms.* 2018;33:203–218.

Vital-Lopez FG, Balkin TJ, Reifman J. Models for Predicting Sleep Latency and Sleep Duration [published online ahead of print, 2020 Nov 29]. *Sleep.* 2020;zsaa263.

A complete reference list can be found online at ExpertConsult.com.

Chapter 84

Fatigue Risk Management Systems

T. Leigh Signal; Margo van den Berg; Philippa H. Gander; R. Curtis Graeber

Chapter Highlights

- Fatigue risk management systems (FRMSs) are an example of the application of sleep and circadian science to resolve real-world occupational safety issues. This is achieved as a collaboration between sleep and circadian scientists and stakeholders within the organization, and it requires developing a shared knowledge base and constructive engagement.
- FRMSs are used in a broad range of industries, including aviation, commercial road transport, the offshore oil industry, rail, and health care. The application of FRMS to smaller organizations is an area of increasing focus, as is the integration of FRMSs with other occupational health and safety systems designed to manage risks other than fatigue.
- Each industry has specific fatigue-related challenges and will have unique terminology, but the core FRMS principles and components remain the same. The complexity of an FRMS within an organization needs to be sufficient to manage the associated risks in the work environment.
- The four core components of an FRMS are policy and documentation, FRMS processes, safety assurance processes, and promotion processes. The FRMS processes and the safety assurance processes are two closed-loop systems that use shared data to manage fatigue risk and enable continuous improvement of the FRMS. These are guided and informed by policy. The promotion activities, which include education and communication, promote and support the FRMS within the organization.

This chapter outlines the scientific principles and practical processes that support an effective fatigue risk management system (FRMS). An FRMS is a set of processes that an organization uses to help mitigate and manage the risk that fatigue poses in a particular workplace setting. It is an example of the application of sleep and circadian science to real-world problems.

Globally, work that impacts sleep is increasingly common,[1] with 19% of the European workforce reporting working at night in the last month and 17% reporting doing shift work.[2] Similar proportions are reported in the United States,[3] Norway,[4] Australia,[5] and New Zealand.[6] Shift work can be broadly defined as any work that affects the timing, duration, or quality of sleep. It takes many forms and may involve working early starts, late finishes, night work, on-call work, and patterns of work that are rotating or irregular.[7] The terms nonstandard hours or irregular work are sometimes also used to describe such work, but for simplicity and consistency the term *shift work* will be used throughout this chapter, with the important feature being the impact of work on sleep.

Part-time work[2,3] and independent contracting[8] are prevalent in shift work, and this often results in unstable or inconsistent work schedules.[9,10] In recent years there has been a trend for younger individuals,[5] those who are paid the least,[5] and ethnic minority groups[11] to undertake shift work. The growing prevalence of shift work is driven by many demands, including societal expectations for around-the-clock services, dual-earner households, technology that enables people to work from different locations at different times, globalization, and deregulation of markets.[7]

THE CHALLENGES POSED BY SHIFT WORK

Shift work can pose significant fatigue-related challenges as individuals are required to work at times in the circadian cycle when the pressure for sleep is high and they are less functional. IAs a consequence, sleep may be displaced to a less-than-ideal time in the circadian cycle,[12] which may result in circadian disruption and difficulties with obtaining sufficient good quality sleep.[13] Irregular or changing work hours also make planning adequate sleep opportunities difficult, in conjunction with the other demands of life outside of work.[12]

Fatigue caused through the arrangement of work is of major concern because of the workplace safety consequences. Experimental evidence, largely from laboratory studies, has shown consistent relationships between decrements in multiple aspects of performance and increasing sleep loss,[14,15] prolonged periods of wakefulness,[16,17] and performing at an adverse circadian phase.[18] Shift work is associated with an increased risk of workplace injury,[6,19] reports of accidents and errors,[20,21] and an increased incidence of falling asleep while driving home from work.[22] Fatigue has also been implicated in a number of catastrophic workplace events, for instance,[23–25] demonstrating that the risks posed by unmitigated fatigue in a workplace can be substantial.

In addition to the performance and workplace safety consequences, there is now compelling evidence that shift work that includes night work is an independent risk factor for developing a range of adverse health outcomes.[13] Some of the strongest evidence comes from longitudinal studies comparing the health of large groups of nurses who work night shifts to those who do not. The US Nurses' Health Studies are among the largest prospective investigations into the risk factors for major chronic diseases in women, with more than 275,000 participants since 1976. Robust associations have been found between women working rotating night shifts (defined as at least 3 nights/month) and increased all-cause and cardiovascular disease mortality (after 5 years), and increased lung cancer mortality (after 15 years).[26] Furthermore, other research has shown that night work is associated with increased risk of ischemic stroke,[27] type 2 diabetes,[28] colorectal cancer,[29] and breast cancer.[30] The Danish Nurses Cohort Study reported that nurses working night and evening shifts had an increased risk of developing diabetes,[31] as well as having a higher risk of all-cause mortality and cause-specific mortality (cardiovascular, diabetes, Alzheimer disease, and dementia)[32] when compared to nurses working day shifts only.

Habitual short sleep has also been identified as an independent risk factor for developing some of these conditions.[33] Of interest, among 815 non–shift workers in a New Zealand–based longitudinal cohort study, higher social jet lag scores (difference in timing of midsleep on scheduled days vs. free days) were associated with higher body mass index, greater fat mass, and increased likelihood of being obese and meeting the criteria for metabolic syndrome, after controlling for sleep duration, sex, and chronotype.[34] More research is needed to clarify whether circadian desynchrony and sleep restriction interact and/or independently increase disease risk for shift workers.

In 2019, in response to burgeoning research, the International Agency for Research on Cancer convened a working group to reevaluate the evidence for the carcinogenicity of shift work.[35] The working group confirmed the classification of nightshift work as "probably carcinogenic to humans," based on limited evidence of cancer in humans, sufficient evidence from experimental studies in animals, and strong mechanistic evidence in animal studies. From a scientific perspective, a number of occupational, individual, lifestyle, and environmental factors might mediate, confound, or moderate potential cancer risk in nightshift workers.

DEFINING FATIGUE

The use of the term *fatigue* can create confusion due to the multitude of symptoms it produces and the variability in symptoms expressed by individuals.[36,37] Different regulatory authorities and government agencies have made efforts to define fatigue, for instance,[38–40] with most considering both its causes and consequences. The International Civil Aviation Organization's (ICAO) definition is both comprehensive and useful for application in a work environment. It states that fatigue is

> "A physiological state of reduced mental or physical performance capability resulting from sleep loss, extended wakefulness, circadian phase, and/or workload (mental and/or physical activity) that can impair a person's alertness and ability to perform safety-related operational duties."[41]

This definition clearly indicates there are biological causes of fatigue, it is a physiological state and not a lack of motivation or unwillingness to perform, and it affects both mental and physical performance capability. However, it should be noted that fatigue from health conditions, the environment (e.g., extreme temperature, altitude, or noise), and stress is not covered by this definition, even though these causes of fatigue are relevant in many workplaces.[42,43] Furthermore, fatigue is influenced by activities that occur outside of work. As such, effectively managing fatigue in the workplace requires a shared responsibility between employees and the employer, as well as relevant regulatory agencies.

LEGISLATION AND REGULATIONS FOR THE MANAGEMENT OF FATIGUE

Fatigue is a unique workplace hazard because it can negatively affect many aspects of cognitive and physical functioning relevant to workplace performance. Mitigating and managing fatigue is therefore critical to sustaining safety in around-the-clock operations. Also underpinning the need to manage workplace fatigue are the basic human rights to "just and favourable conditions of work," and "rest and leisure, including reasonable limitation of working hours,"[44] as well as the right to "enjoyment of the highest attainable standard of health."[45]

Depending on the industry and organizational context, there may be different external requirements for the management of fatigue. Organizations often must comply with national working time laws (e.g., the European Working Time Directive[46] and Health and Safety legislation in Australia, New Zealand, and the United Kingdom), abide by labor agreements that stipulate requirements for the management of fatigue, and/or follow prescriptive limits specified by a regulatory agency.

In many safety critical industries (e.g., transportation), a regulatory agency prescribes maximum working hours for a single work period, cumulative working hours (e.g., over a week, month, or year), and minimum rest opportunities within and between work periods. This traditional approach to limiting maximum work hours and specifying minimum rest opportunities is a relatively simplistic, one-size-fits-all model for the management of fatigue that often does not take into account current knowledge in sleep, chronobiology and safety science, and operational knowledge in different industries.[47,48]

Some regulators provide an option for an organization to seek regulatory approval of work-hour limits that are outside the prescriptive approach.[49] This has occurred in conjunction with a general shift to performance-based legislation, which specifies the safety standards that must be met but does not prescribe how this is done.[47] Moving outside the prescriptive limits normally requires an organization to make a safety case to the regulator (see Chapter 85) to demonstrate how they will identify and manage fatigue-related hazards using their proposed alternative approach.

FRMSs have also developed and evolved in conjunction with safety management system (SMS) science. SMSs are focused on the identification and control of all workplace hazards to prevent unwanted events or harm.[50] By extension, FRM involves the modification and application of more general risk management processes to specifically manage fatigue-related hazards.

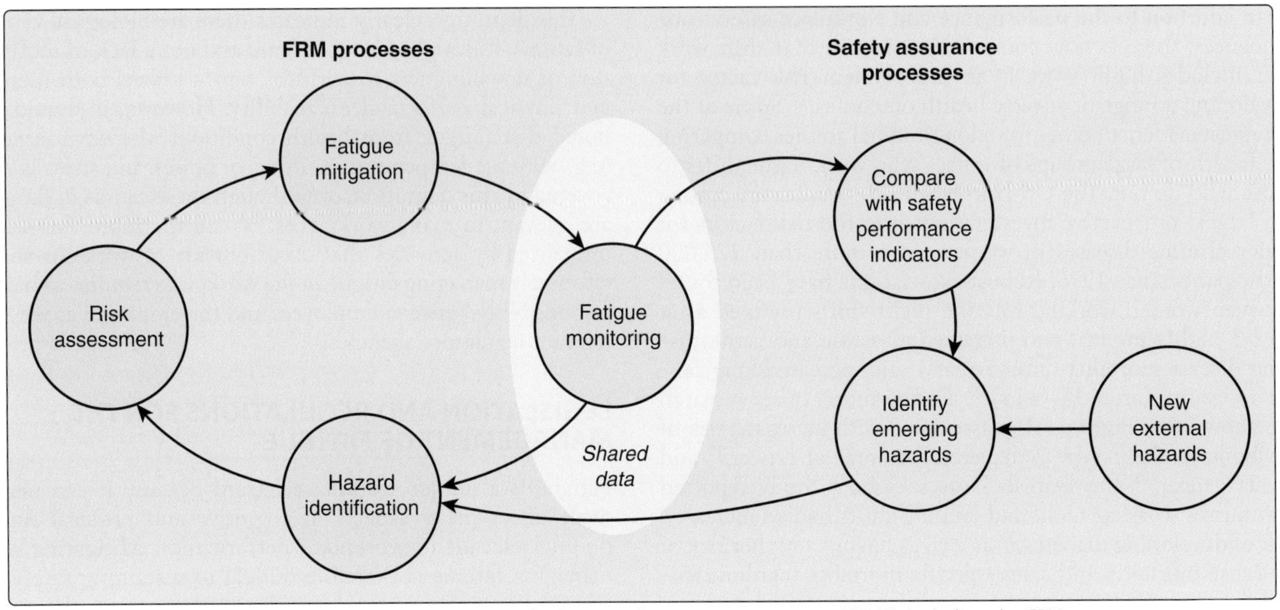

Figure 84.1 Operational components of a fatigue risk management system (FRMS), including the FRM processes and safety assurance processes.

A useful definition provided by ICAO states that an FRMS is

> "A data-driven means of continuously monitoring and managing fatigue-related safety risks, based upon scientific principles, knowledge and operational experience that aims to ensure relevant personnel are performing at adequate levels of alertness."[41]

This highlights a number of important features of an FRMS, including that data are central to the functioning of an FRMS, it is not a static system, and that it requires input from a range of stakeholders. Individuals with expertise in sleep and circadian science can make a significant contribution to the development and ongoing functioning of an FRMS, but this must be done in collaboration with personnel within an organization that have knowledge about its operation and about the risks that a fatigue-impaired person represents in their workplace(s).

THE CORE COMPONENTS OF FATIGUE RISK MANAGEMENT SYSTEMS

The four primary components of an FRMS that also map directly to the ICAO SMS framework are policy and documentation, FRM processes, safety assurance processes, and promotion processes. The FRM processes and safety assurance processes are two closed-loop systems that use shared data to manage fatigue-related risk and together enable continuous improvement of the FRMS (Figure 84.1). The closed loop system describing the FRM processes (on the left of Figure 84.1) follows the basic steps of a typical safety management cycle[50] and details the everyday processes used for collecting data about possible fatigue hazards, determining their potential risk, deciding how to manage and mitigate those risks, and determining if current mitigations are effective. The safety assurance process loop (on the right of Figure 84.1) is focused on ensuring the FRMS is working as intended and includes tracking changes in fatigue metrics over time, comparing the FRMS's performance to its safety objectives, and identifying fatigue-related risks as they emerge. The FRMS promotion activities, which include education and communication, promote and support the FRMS within the organization. The FRMS is guided and informed by policy, and all processes must be documented. These four primary components are discussed in further detail later.

Policy and Documentation

Like any policy, an FRMS policy is an organization's statement of intent but specifically addresses the management of fatigue-related risks. Its purpose is to provide clear guidance to all parts of the organization for decision making around managing fatigue-related risk. As such, it should stipulate what the FRMS aims to achieve (i.e., its safety objectives); the organizational and management commitment to supporting, resourcing, and improving the FRMS; which organizational processes are incorporated into the FRMS; and how they integrate with and relate to other safety processes. Shared responsibility for fatigue management between employers and employees should be clearly outlined in the FRMS policy, and the policy should be signed by an accountable executive. Alongside and including the FRMS policy is the FRMS documentation, which is the record of FRMS activities and changes. Documentation is essential for auditing and oversight of the FRMS.

Fatigue Risk Management Processes

Fatigue Monitoring and Hazard Identification

As clearly indicated in the ICAO definition of an FRMS, the system depends on data from a range of sources to identify potential fatigue-related hazards and to monitor the effectiveness of fatigue mitigations. Data sources must be in a format that is relatively easy to use and interpret in an ongoing manner and need to be periodically reassessed to determine if they provide sufficient, useful information.

Fatigue-related hazard identification can be predictive (i.e., identifying fatigue-related hazards before they have occurred), proactive (i.e., real-time monitoring to identify fatigue-related hazards), and/or reactive (i.e., identifying fatigue-related hazards after an event).

Operational experience, biomathematical modeling tools and existing research evidence can be used to predictively identify fatigue-related hazards. Biomathematical models use sleep and circadian science to predict fatigue levels associated with a pattern of work. However, it is important to note that these models generally predict the fatigue, alertness, or performance of an average individual. The models do not predict the safety risk that a given individual poses in a specific workplace context. See Chapter 83 for additional details on these models.

Proactive data collection involves collecting information on fatigue-related hazards in real time. Fatigue reporting is probably the most widely used proactive tool. Effective fatigue reporting depends on the reporting system being accessible and easy to use, relevant information being collected, and the reports being assessed quickly by individuals with sufficient knowledge to evaluate the fatigue-related risk in the reported scenario. Underpinning the physical processes, an organization must have established an effective safety reporting culture. This is normally supported by "just culture" principles, which accept that humans are fallible, particularly when fatigued, and make mistakes that can be learned from but that intentional actions resulting in reduced safety are not tolerated.[51] Another immediate source of fatigue-related information available to organizations is actual hours worked, which can be important when actual work hours frequently differ from scheduled work hours. Comprehensive proactive data collection, using multiple measures of sleep, fatigue, and performance, is sometimes necessary to better understand a specific fatigue-related hazard and the risk it poses. An example of this is an ultra–long-range (ULR) flight route that is discussed in more detail later.

Data collected after an event allows for reactive identification of fatigue-related hazards. Safety investigations are a common source of reactive data. It is vital that relevant fatigue-related information is sought (e.g., prior sleep history and time of day) and that this information and the nature of the performance decrements that contributed to the event are considered in the safety investigation.[41]

Risk Assessment

The fundamental role of an FRMS is to mitigate and manage the risk that fatigue poses. Individuals can be equally fatigued but pose very different safety-related risks depending on the task they are performing and the context in which they are working (e.g., completing administrative tasks in the office vs. operating safety-critical machinery). The purpose of FRM is to assess the risk posed by a particular fatigue-related hazard in an identified work context so that effective mitigations can be identified, if needed.

The most common approach for assessing the risk posed by a fatigue-related hazard is to use a standard likelihood by severity matrix and apply it to different tasks. However, the usefulness of this approach for quantifying fatigue-related risk is questionable because existing mitigations are not normally taken into account and classifying the severity of a risk usually involves considering the worst possible outcome.[52] It is reasonable to assume that a severely fatigue-impaired individual completing a safety-critical task could produce a catastrophic outcome.

Other options have been proposed, whereby the severity classification is modified to reflect a predicted level of fatigue and the likelihood classification is modified to reflect the frequency with which an individual might be exposed to a fatigue-inducing situation.[41] The predicted level of fatigue of an average individual can be informed by biomathematical models.

Alternatively, the potential causes of fatigue associated with a work pattern can be identified, such as whether the duty may produce sleep loss, extended periods of wakefulness, circadian disruption, or is associated with factors that alter workload. These are considered simultaneously with possible mitigations.[52] The causes of fatigue that cannot be fully mitigated are then summed and categorized to determine acceptability of the remaining fatigue-related risk. Although this approach has merit, it has not yet been validated.

All current fatigue-related risk assessment processes have limitations, and there is no universally agreed upon approach. This highlights the importance of personnel tasked with fatigue-related risk assessment having appropriate FRM training and operational expertise, or access to people who have the necessary expertise.

Mitigations

The mitigations required in a workplace are dependent on the result of the risk assessment processes. If the fatigue-related risks are considered acceptable, mitigations (or further mitigations) may not be required. Otherwise, the fatigue-related risks should be mitigated to as low as is reasonably practicable, and the choice of mitigations should be based on scientific and operational knowledge. Individuals within an organization who have responsibility for managing the FRMS processes should make recommendations about suitable mitigations, but because mitigations often have financial and resourcing costs, final decisions may be made by others with a broader overview of the risks and resources across an organization.

In any safety-conscious industry, there is unlikely to be a single layer of mitigations,[48,53] with limits around periods of work and rest (or the roster design) being only one defensive layer. Mitigations will also range from those employed proactively (e.g., scientifically based rostering practices, workforce education, and appropriate numbers of personnel) to those employed strategically (e.g., workplace napping and the use of light, movement, conversation, and caffeine). These strategic mitigations are addressed in more detail in Chapter 82. In an FRMS, mitigations that are implemented must be recorded and conveyed to all relevant personnel.[54]

Safety Assurance Processes

Safety assurance processes are designed to check that the FRMS is working as intended and look broadly at the activities of the FRMS. The FRM processes and safety assurance processes share common data sources, as is shown in Figure 84.1. Safety performance indicators (SPIs, described in further detail later), are drawn from this shared data and are measures that can be used to track fatigue trends over time and for evaluating the FRMS's performance in relation to its safety objectives as outlined in the FRMS policy.[49] The safety assurance processes also involve looking for changes within the organization and the environment it operates in, to identify emerging fatigue risks and to preempt any adverse consequences by altering the FRMS in advance of the change.[41] Continuous improvement through review and regular audits of the FRMS is also a function of the safety assurance loop. Individuals within the organization that have responsibility for the FRMS may contribute expertise and data as requested to the safety assurance processes, but overall responsibility should rest with individuals who have a broader safety role within the organization.

Safety Performance Indicators

In addition to being monitored over time by the safety assurance processes, SPIs are used to determine whether the FRM processes are adequately managing the day-to-day fatigue-related risks. To determine whether fatigue is adequately managed, SPIs are compared to previously agreed thresholds for acceptable levels of risk. There should be a range of SPIs obtained from data collected as part of the FRMS processes, some of which are operationally focused and others that map to proactive and reactive data. Examples of operational SPIs include work periods not exceeding a certain duration or time off between periods of work not being reduced below a minimum duration. SPIs that relate to proactive and reactive data include the percentage of fatigue reports made, rates of absenteeism and sick leave, and the occurrence of fatigue-related incidents. When data are collected proactively to address a particular fatigue risk, such as the ULR operations described later, then SPIs are used to make decisions about the acceptability of the risk and the effectiveness of the mitigations that have been put in place.[55]

Fatigue Risk Management System Promotion Processes: Training and Communication

Training and communication are key aspects of an FRMS that support the development and maintenance of an effective safety reporting culture and understanding of the need for shared responsibility between the employer and employee in fatigue management.

To support the implementation and sustainability of an FRMS, all individuals who have a role in the FRMS, including senior managers, rostering staff, safety staff, and operational personnel, must have a sufficient understanding of sleep and circadian science, as well as FRMS processes and responsibilities relevant to their role, particularly the need to identify and report fatigue hazards. This should be achieved through competency-based training and training records kept as part of the FRMS documentation.

Regular communication via a range of media (newsletters, bulletin boards, websites, as part of operational meetings and email) should be used to share "lessons learned," successes of the FRMS, and changes in policy and processes and other actions associated with the FRMS.

Responsibilities for the Fatigue Risk Management System

There must be an individual or group of individuals responsible for FRMS activities within an organization. This group is sometimes called a fatigue safety action group (FSAG) and should include representatives from across the organization. It is responsible for the establishment and day-to-day running of the FRMS and for its integration with other parts of the organization.

Fatigue Risk Management System in Aviation

Aviation was one of the first industries to adopt FRMSs. In the early 1990s, one South Pacific airline convened a small group of scientists, pilot representatives, and aeromedical experts to develop a science-based methodology that could be applied to existing long-haul trip patterns. Although all these patterns were within existing contractual and regulatory limits, crew fatigue had periodically been reported as a problem, especially in long-haul operations. Proactive data collection was undertaken on certain routes, and findings were reviewed by an independent panel of sleep and circadian scientists, together with airline management, union representatives, and rostering managers, to assess fatigue-related hazards, the risk they may pose, and determine what, if any, mitigations were required. The Civil Aviation Authority, which had approved the process as alternative means of compliance to the prescriptive limits, also participated in the review. The process became known as the fatigue risk management system (FRMS).

The experience and knowledge gained as a result of this pioneering effort proved invaluable in 2001 when the Flight Safety Foundation (FSF) sought to develop operational and regulatory guidelines for ULR operations. ULR operations refer to flights between a specific city pair and were initially defined as exceeding the traditional flight time limit of 16 hours.[41] ULR flights usually have four pilots who take turns to sleep in bunks in onboard crew rest facilities separated from the passenger cabin. The FRMS developed by this airline became the basis for a consensus agreement among 90 participants (pilots, scientists, manufacturers, airline management, and regulators) from 14 nations.[56] The agreement continues to be implemented successfully to this day as ULR operations have become commonplace worldwide. The same FRMS framework also became the basis for the development of the ICAO's FRMS guidelines adopted for worldwide implementation in 2011.[57]

Although aviation operators may have an FRMS in place for some or all parts of their operation, the application of FRMS in ULR operations are used as an example here.

Hazard Identification

Fatigue hazards associated with ULR operations have previously been identified based on scientific principles and operational experience.[56,58] The long flight and duty times can lead to sleep loss, extended wakefulness, time-on-task fatigue, and also likely require crew to work during adverse times in the circadian cycle. Circadian disruption resulting from rapid time zone changes and some adaptation to the layover time zone will also influence crew members' functioning and ability to sleep on the inbound flight, as well as their rate of recovery posttrip. The extent of sleep loss and circadian disruption experienced by a crew member will, to a large extent, be determined by the timing of flights and layovers relative to a crew member's circadian body clock time.[41]

These fatigue hazards are expected to be the same for flight crew and cabin crew, although recent research with cabin crew has highlighted the importance of considering workload, the cumulative effects of fatigue across the entire ULR trip, and the context of the ULR trip in the entire roster worked.[59–61]

Mitigating and Managing Crew Fatigue Associated with Ultra-Long-Range Flights

Fatigue mitigations that are typically put in place for managing fatigue risk on ULR operations are also primarily based on existing flight crew data and ULR scheduling practices for flight crew.[56,58,62] These include (1) scheduled in-flight rest periods in crew rest facilities, (2) a minimum 2-day layover allowing for at least two major sleep opportunities before the inbound flight, and (3) protected time off duty before and after the ULR trip to assist with preparation for the trip and subsequent recovery. The scheduling of free days before and after the ULR trip is also intended to facilitate reacclimatization to domicile time before starting the next duty period.[58]

The effectiveness of in-flight rest breaks as a mitigation for fatigue depends on the amount and the quality of sleep that crew members are able to obtain in-flight.[63] This is, in turn, dependent on operational factors, such as the flight's local departure time, flight duration, and timing of in-flight rest breaks,[64–66] as well as environmental factors, such as turbulence, noise, and comfort.[59,67,68]

The in-flight sleep of flight and cabin crew members is generally affected by the same factors. However, due to the requirement for all cabin crew to be awake for meal services, they have less time available for in-flight rest than flight crew. In addition, in many countries the regulatory requirements for on-board rest facilities are less rigorous for cabin crew than for flight crew.[69] The high workload of cabin crew can potentially also affect the recuperative value of their in-flight sleep. Compared to flight crew, cabin crews' workload is physically more demanding.[70–75] The stress associated with high work demands and passenger interactions is expected to increase the time needed to unwind, which in turn can impact on subsequent sleep.[76]

Sources of Data for Monitoring Crew Fatigue

Proactive monitoring of crew members' sleep, fatigue, and performance is recommended when fatigue risk is likely to be high or difficult to estimate, such as in a new operation. The choice of measures used for proactive monitoring needs to reflect the anticipated levels of fatigue and safety risk because this type of data collection is relatively time consuming and resource intensive in comparison to other, routinely collected operational data.[41,55,77]

To illustrate this, during the validation of the very first ULR operation, polysomnography (PSG) was used to monitor flight crews' sleep during scheduled in-flight rest breaks, and actigraphy and sleep diaries were used to monitor flight crews' sleep during the 3 days pretrip, throughout the trip, and the 3 days posttrip.[78] In addition, a 10-minute psychomotor vigilance task (PVT)[79] was used to monitor changes in performance across each flight sector. Together these measures enabled a thorough evaluation of flight crew fatigue and the effectiveness of the fatigue mitigations implemented on this first ULR operation.[78]

Subsequent proactive monitoring studies on newly introduced ULR routes (at least those that have been published) have relied on actigraphy and sleep diaries for monitoring the sleep of flight crews[80–83] and used a shorter 5-minute version of the PVT[84,85] to reduce disruption to crew members' workflow. Measures recommended for proactively monitoring flight crew fatigue (actigraphy, sleep/duty diaries, and PVT) are also feasible for use with cabin crew,[61] although differences between these two occupational groups need to be considered.[59–61]

Multiple factors can influence the motivation of crew members to participate in proactive data collection. For example, compared to flight crew monitored on a ULR trip,[80] the response rate and completion rate with cabin crew flying the same route were lower, thus requiring a larger number of cabin crew to be approached to volunteer to obtain sufficient data.[61] Perceived company support may play a role in this.[59,86,87] Nevertheless, recurrent fatigue management training can strengthen crew members' understanding of their role and that of the company in the FRMS, and the training may increase their willingness to participate in proactive data collection.[41]

The usefulness of the PVT for assessing cabin crews' fatigue-related performance changes on ULR flights also needs careful consideration. Distractions in the testing environment and completion of the PVT in a busy cabin are likely to have contributed to the slower preflight performance and large variability observed in subsequent tests reported by van den Berg and colleagues (2015)[61] when compared to flight crew flying the same ULR route.[80] Psychomotor vigilance is only one of many aspects of performance affected by sleep loss, and how an individual crew member's PVT performance relates to team performance is not well understood.[77,88]

Workload has been identified as an important factor contributing to cabin crew fatigue,[60,71,89–92] and the ongoing monitoring of workload is therefore warranted. This can be achieved by including an appropriate workload question in fatigue reports, which form an essential component of FRMS, and by ensuring that in proactive monitoring studies conducted with cabin crew, measures of workload are included.

Compared to quantitative data, which are essential for generating SPIs, qualitative data can provide richer and more in-depth contextual information and identify issues and concerns not readily identified using quantitative methods in an FRMS. Focus groups are a particularly useful method in this context because they enable crew members to share their views and experiences (negative as well as positive), raise any concerns they may have, and offer ideas for possible solutions.[59] They also communicate to the crew members that their feedback is valued. Aviation organizations could include occasional focus groups as part of their FRMS,[93] for example, as part of an evaluation of the fatigue risk mitigations on a newly introduced route. Such efforts can play a key role in building employee confidence in the FRMS and enabling future cooperation.

Fatigue Risk Management System in Health Care

Unlike the transport sector, health care workforces (medical staff, nurses, allied health professionals, etc.) are generally not covered by specific regulatory limits on the length of duty periods and rest breaks, although in some cases professional bodies provide recommended limits, particularly during professional training. An exception is the controversial effort to apply the European Working Time Directive, which limits junior doctors, senior doctors, and nurses to a maximum of 48 hours per week and limits all shift work to a maximum of 13 hours of continuous duty.[94–96]

On the other hand, health care workers are covered by general workplace health and safety legislation. Although specific reference to managing fatigue and shift work is uncommon in such legislation, the legislation can provide a framework for defining responsibilities for FRM. For example, the New Zealand Health and Safety at Work Act[96a] identifies fatigue as one cause of workplace hazards. Hazards and their associated health and safety risks must be managed "so far as is reasonably practicable." The act does not specifically mention shift work, but guidance from the regulatory body that administers the act, WorkSafe New Zealand, identifies shift work as a cause of fatigue. This has provided a regulatory framework to support a new code of practice for managing fatigue and shift work for nurses in New Zealand public hospitals, which has been endorsed by WorkSafe New Zealand and the Council of Trade Unions.[97] The code is based on the approach in commercial aviation[41,98] and was developed by Massey University College of Health researchers in collaboration with the New Zealand Nurses Organization (the main union representing nurses), supported by an advisory group representing all stakeholders. The purpose of this code of practice is to describe the principles that underpin a fatigue and shift work management system and how to build one.

FRM in hospitals in New Zealand and many other countries currently relies heavily on working time limits defined in collective employment agreements. Many different work patterns can be compliant with these requirements, but this does not mean that they are equally safe.[99] Rostering and shift-work–related data management are typically devolved down to the level of individual nursing units, with a widespread expectation among nurses of having choice about the shifts that they work. This results in major variability in work patterns between practice areas, both within and between hospitals. Implementation of the New Zealand Code of Practice is just beginning, and coordinating these units into a system that manages risk across a hospital represents a challenge. Another challenge is that, although more critical incidents must be reported to regulatory authorities and may be investigated, the health care sector in general does not have the emphasis on having an effective safety reporting culture, which, in contrast, is strongly promoted in aviation safety.[100] Fatigue-related issues are difficult to detect if people are unwilling or unable to report them.

This example illustrates that FRMS is not a simple one-size-fits-all solution. It is based on pooling stakeholder knowledge and expertise to come up with better solutions. This requires developing a shared knowledge base and constructive engagement among stakeholders. The complexity of a fatigue and shift work management system needs to be sufficient to manage the associated risk in the work environment(s) where it applies. How it is integrated with existing safety management activities may also differ between organizations and workforce groups.

Fatigue Risk Management Systems in Other Industries

Many other industries also use FRMSs, such as commercial road transport, rail, oil and gas, and the nuclear power industries. It is beyond the scope of this chapter to discuss the application of FRMS in these different sectors, but the principles of FRMS are the same regardless of the industry. The terminology may be different, and each industry has its own unique fatigue-related challenges, but there are many excellent examples of FRMS guidance materials, for instance, in the rail,[40] commercial road transport,[101] and offshore oil and gas industries.[102]

Scaling Fatigue Risk Management Systems for Smaller Organizations

As noted earlier, the scale and complexity of an FRMS should be relative to the fatigue-related risk being managed. For this reason, and because of the resources required to establish and manage an FRMS, they have so far been used mostly by larger organizations. Scaling FRMSs to work effectively in smaller organizations is an important next step in the evolution of FRM. Many smaller organizations want to be proactive in the management of fatigue and experience the safety benefits. In environments where maximum work periods and minimum rest opportunities are prescribed by a regulator, smaller organizations may also wish to avail themselves of the greater operational flexibility that FRMSs allow.

Regardless of the size of the organization, the key elements of an FRMS must still be in place, although the number of personnel involved in managing those processes will be fewer. Consideration needs to be given to the workload placed on these individuals and to ensuring that between them they have the required knowledge and skills. A single person may represent more than one stakeholder group in the FSAG. It may be possible for the responsibilities of the FSAG to be incorporated into other safety-related groups within the organization, such as an existing operational safety committee or a health and safety committee, with fatigue being a standing agenda item each time the committee meets.

The amount of fatigue-related data that can be collected and monitored in an FRMS within a smaller organization will necessarily be reduced. It may be more difficult to see patterns or trends, and smaller numbers of employees may reduce the statistical power for analyzing data and increase the difficulty of maintaining data confidentiality, particularly for those who make fatigue reports. Even in large organizations, anonymity of fatigue reports can be very difficult to achieve; therefore confidentiality of information is often a more realistic expectation.

Groups of smaller organizations working in the same sector of an industry should consider working together to share resources, particularly scientific expertise, training materials and opportunities, communication processes, and, if appropriate, also data so that organizations can learn from each other.

Although there are likely to be additional challenges in managing an FRMS within a smaller organization, there will also be some advantages. Processes do not need to be complex, communication within the organization is likely to be simpler and faster, and change may occur more easily. Across the board, there is still much to be learned about the application of FRMSs in different contexts, and incentives need to be developed so that fatigue management processes become embedded in a broader range of industries and organizations.

Integrating Fatigue Risk Management System and Other Occupational Health and Safety Processes

Most FRMSs focus solely on improving safety, but in the context of SMSs, fatigue can be viewed as a compound hazard, in that it simultaneously affects both safety and health.[100] Ideally, both the immediate and long-term consequences of shift work on health and well-being should be considered as part of an organization's risk management approach. However, in many industries, different legislative and regulatory frameworks are often used to manage safety versus health risks. In several countries, including New Zealand, Australia, and the United

Kingdom, the occupational health and safety (OHS) legislation also describes a four-step process for managing risks, which maps to the FRMS approach[103–105] and requires policy and documentation, risk management training for all relevant personnel, and quality assurance. The New Zealand and Australian OHS legislation also specifically identify fatigue as a cause of hazards.

Because the effects of fatigue are wide ranging from operational safety to health-related problems, FRM may be optimized if the two systems managing these were linked. Rather than FRMS and OHS operating in parallel, some of their components could overlap to ensure effective collaboration and communication. For example, a representative from a health and safety committee could also serve as a member in the FSAG and vice versa.

In addition, fatigue management training and education should be extended to cover the adverse health consequences of chronic sleep restriction and recurrent circadian disruption, further educating employees about the importance of obtaining sufficient sleep as often as possible. It is also important that the company's managers and medical staff understand these negative health consequences, in relation to absenteeism, productivity, and costs, to ensure that the best possible mitigations are implemented.[106]

Although ICAO suggests in their SMS guidance that a compound hazard such as fatigue may be managed more effectively through an integrated risk mitigation system,[100] their FRMS guidance currently focuses solely on operational safety.

Methods and processes for effectively linking FRMS and OHS systems are expected to vary among organizations, but sharing experience should enable principles and guidance to be developed.

CLINICAL PEARL

Fatigue risk management systems (FRMSs) involve the application of sleep, chronobiology, and safety science in conjunction with operational knowledge, to reduce fatigue-related risk in occupational settings. An FRMS includes four key components. The *FRM processes* and the *safety assurance processes* are two closed-loop systems that use shared data to manage fatigue risk and together enable continuous improvement of the FRMS. These are guided and informed by *policy*. The *promotion activities*, which include education and communication, promote and support the FRMS within the organization.

SUMMARY

Any work that disrupts the duration, quality, or timing of sleep can pose a significant fatigue-related challenge. FRMSs are a set of processes that combine scientific knowledge with operational experience. They can be used to improve management of fatigue-related risk in operations with or without prescriptive hours of work limits, or to operate outside the prescriptive regulations. An FRMS comprises two connected closed-loop systems. The first loop comprises FRMS processes, including the ongoing monitoring of a range of data sources to identify fatigue-related hazards, the assessment of risk the hazard poses, the implementation of controls and mitigations to manage the fatigue-related risk, and the monitoring of the effectiveness of the mitigations. The second loop comprises the safety assurance processes and focuses on the overall effectiveness and continual improvement of the FRMS. All FRMS processes are detailed in an organization's FRMS policy and documentation and are supported by training and promotion activities, which are overseen by a group of individuals within an organization with responsibility for the FRMS.

SELECTED READINGS

Canadian Centre for Occupational Health and Safety. *OSH Answers Fact Sheets: Fatigue*; 2017. Available at https://ccohs.ca/oshanswers/psychosocial/fatigue.html.

Dawson D, McCulloch K. Managing fatigue: it's about sleep. *Sleep Med Rev*. 2005;9(5):365–380.

Gander PH. Evolving regulatory approaches for managing fatigue risk in transport operations. *Rev Hum Factors Ergon*. 2015;10(1):253–271. Available at https://doi.org/10.1177/1557234x15576510.

Gander PH, Mangie J, van den Berg MJ, Smith AAT, Mulrine HM, Signal TL. Crew fatigue safety performance indicators for fatigue risk management systems. *Aviat Space Environ Med*. 2014;85(2):139–147. Available at https://doi.org/10.3357/ASEM.3748.2014.

International Civil Aviation Organization. *Manual for the Oversight of Fatigue Management Approaches*. Montréal, Canada: International Civil Aviation Organization; 2016. Available at https://www.icao.int/safety/fatigue-management/FRMS%20Tools/Doc%209966.FRMS.2016%20Edition.en.pdf.

Kecklund G, Axelsson J. Health consequences of shift work and insufficient sleep. *BMJ*. 2016;355:i5210.

Li WC, Kearney P, Zhang J, Hsu YL, Braithwaite G. The analysis of occurrences associated with air traffic volume and air traffic controllers' alertness for fatigue risk management [published online ahead of print, 2020 Sep 13]. *Risk Anal*. 2020. https://doi.org/10.1111/risa.13594.

Maurino D. Why SMS: An introduction and overview of safety management systems (SMS). International Transport Forum Discussion Papers 2017/16, OECD Publishing, 1-61. Available at https://doi.org/10.1787/31ebb8a3-en.

Office of Rail Regulation. *Managing Rail Staff Fatigue*. United Kingdom: Office of Rail Regulation; 2012.

Reason J. Human error: models and management. *BMJ*. 2000;320(7237):768–770.

Safer Nursing 24/7. *National Code of Practice for Managing Nurses' Fatigue and Shift Work in District Health Board Hospitals*. Wellington, New Zealand: Sleep/Wake Research Centre; 2019.

Safe Work Australia. *How to manage work health and safety risks Code of Practice*; 2018. Available at https://www.safeworkaustralia.gov.au/doc/model-code-practice-how-manage-work-health-and-safety-risks.

A complete reference list can be found online at ExpertConsult.com.

Chapter 85

Safety Cases and Assessing Alternative Means of Regulatory Compliance in Fatigue Risk Management

Philippa H. Gander; Amanda Lamp; Thomas Nesthus; Jim Mangie; Don Wykoff; Lora Wu; Lauren Waggoner; Gregory Belenky

Chapter Highlights

- New regulations for managing fatigue-related risks in the workplace are being driven by a growing understanding of the role of sleep restriction, extended time awake, circadian desynchrony, and workload in increasing the likelihood of fatigue-related impairment.
- An alternative regulatory approach allows organizations to develop their own evidence-based fatigue risk management systems (FRMSs) that incorporate scientific principles. To use this approach, an organization is required to present a safety case to assure the regulator that they can adequately predict and manage fatigue-related risks in the operations covered by the FRMS.
- Four successful safety cases are presented in this chapter, which have each enabled an airline to operate outside new prescriptive FRM regulations introduced by the U.S. Federal Aviation Administration (FAA) in 2014. Two of the safety cases allowed an airline to conduct ultra–long-range flights that exceeded the prescribed flight and duty time limits. The other two safety cases allowed airlines to continue flying trips that became noncompliant under the new 2014 regulations.
- Safety cases require the integration of regulatory, operational, and scientific expertise to develop safe and acceptable solutions. To illustrate this process, the chapter presents the perspectives of a regulator, an airline operator, a pilot representative, and a scientist, who each were directly involved in at least one of the safety cases presented.

INTRODUCTION

Transport operators are often required to prepare a safety case if they want to work outside the prescriptive hours of work limits and any other prescriptive fatigue management regulations that govern their operations.[1,2] In a safety case the operator must demonstrate to the regulator that they can adequately predict and manage the fatigue-related safety risks in the operations that they wish to include in their alternative approach. This process requires both operators and regulators to have a sound understanding of (1) the causes of fatigue, (2) the risks associated with a fatigued person working in the relevant operations, and (3) the mitigations that will be effective and workable in those operations. This chapter describes four successful safety cases from commercial aviation, together with perspectives from a regulator, an airline operator, a pilot representative, and a scientist, who each were involved in at least one of the safety cases.

Safety cases and the new regulatory approaches are based on scientific evidence that the diverse signs and symptoms of fatigue reflect a physiologically based state of performance impairment resulting from acute or chronic sleep loss, extended time awake, working and sleeping at suboptimal times in the circadian clock cycle, or physical and mental workload.[2]

Traditional approaches for managing fatigue risk focus primarily on reducing the likelihood of people being fatigued in the workplace by prescribing maximum work hours and minimum breaks.[3] This approach has inherent weaknesses. First, as a stand-alone strategy, it does not adequately address the mentioned causes of fatigue.[4] Second, it cannot eliminate fatigue in 24/7 operations because optimal human functioning requires unrestricted sleep at night. Additional strategies are needed to mitigate and manage residual fatigue-related risk(s). Third, the safety risk associated with a fatigue-impaired person depends not only on that individual's level of fatigue (the focus of hours of work limitations) but also on the nature of the task(s) and the other hazards and safety defenses present in their work environment. The safety risks of an unintended 30-second microsleep are very different for a solo truck driver at night versus an airline pilot on the flight deck with a copilot and the aircraft on autopilot during the cruise portion of flight.

A robust safety case to enable an operator to work outside the prescriptive regulations needs to draw on a range of types of expertise. Scientists and researchers can provide advice about the causes of fatigue, different types of impairment, and the likely effectiveness of different mitigations to reduce fatigue-related risk. People with experience working in the operations covered by the safety case have vital knowledge about the specific safety risk(s) associated with a fatigued individual in that context, as well as about workable mitigations. Managers have essential knowledge about organizational requirements, expectations, and constraints around managing fatigue-related risks. Regulators are responsible for defining a level of risk that is acceptable in the context of their mandate to protect public safety.

REGULATORY CHANGES AND REQUIREMENTS IN COMMERCIAL AVIATION

The safety cases presented here were developed for managing pilot fatigue in commercial aviation in a regulatory environment that is evolving rapidly in response to two key factors: (1) growing understanding that prescriptive flight and duty time limitations do not adequately address all the causes of crew fatigue and (2) advances in technology enabling increasingly longer flights. In 2003 flights longer than 16 hours exceeded the regulatory limits on maximum flight duty periods in most countries and so were not permitted. The Flight Safety Foundation therefore convened a steering committee and held a series of international meetings with regulators, airlines, labor representatives, and scientists, to produce the first recommendations for managing crew fatigue on flights longer than 16 hours (known as ultra-long range [ULR] flights).[5] Based on these recommendations, in 2004 the first ULR commercial passenger flights were approved by the Civil Aviation Authority of Singapore and flown by Singapore Airlines, with an initial period of intensive monitoring by independent scientific organizations.[6]

In 2011 the International Civil Aviation Organization (ICAO) released new international Standards and Recommended Practices (SARPs) for managing the fatigue of airline pilots and cabin crew. They continued to require countries to have prescriptive limits on flight and duty times but also allowed them to introduce a new regulatory option in which airlines could propose their own alternative, evidence-based fatigue risk management system (FRMS) for managing crew-member fatigue on specified operations.[2,7,8] Airlines wishing to operate outside the prescriptive limits, described by ICAO as operating under a "variation," should be required to present a safety case describing how they will manage the expected fatigue risk.[2,7]

Consistent with the 2011 ICAO changes, in 2014 the United States Federal Aviation Administration (FAA) implemented a new regulatory framework that includes both updated prescriptive regulations and the new FRMS regulatory option. To obtain approval to fly specific operations outside the prescriptive regulations, an airline must present a safety case to the FAA describing how it will manage the fatigue-related risk to a level of safety that is at least equivalent to that achieved in operations that comply with the prescriptive regulations.[9] The airline is given an interim approval to fly the operation(s) as proposed in the safety case, so they can collect data to demonstrate that at least an equivalent level of safety can be achieved.

ELEMENTS OF A SAFETY CASE

Demonstrating that an FRMS can deliver at least an equivalent level of safety to operating within the prescriptive requirements is a deceptively simple statement. It has significant implications for regulators, airlines, and their scientific advisors, and it requires agreement on a scientifically defensible approach for measuring the level of safety achieved. Key issues include what to measure, when to collect data, and agreeing on standards for different measures that indicate acceptable levels of fatigue risk (fatigue safety performance indicators).[7]

In commercial aviation, there are four essential elements of a safety case[2,7]:

1. The nature, scope and impact of the proposed exemption(s) from the prescriptive requirements
2. A risk assessment
3. Risk mitigation measures
4. Continued monitoring of the operation to track the effectiveness of FRM

Although these four elements must be addressed, more complex safety cases will be required where the expected fatigue risk is higher and/or where there is more uncertainty about the expected level of fatigue risk. The four safety cases presented in this chapter are complex because commercial aviation is a safety-critical industry, and the safety cases were among the first approved by the FAA after the introduction of ULR flights and its new regulatory framework for managing pilot fatigue[9,10]

SAFETY CASE 1: MANAGING PILOT FATIGUE ON ULTRA-LONG-RANGE FLIGHTS

Regulatory Context

Safety case 1 was developed before the 2011 ICAO regulatory framework and the 2014 FAA regulatory revisions.[9,10] It followed the 2003 Flight Safety Foundation recommendations[5] and was originally approved by the FAA in 2008, with an updated version approved in 2014. As part of this new approval, the airline participated in a three-airline study, requested and overseen by the FAA and designed to compare pilots' sleep and fatigue on ULR flights versus long-range flights that operated within the prescriptive regulatory requirements.[11]

Element 1: Scope of Safety Case 1

The 2003 Flight Safety Foundation recommendations included that ULR operations be flown as a single set of out-and-back flights between two cities, rather than as part of longer sequences of international flights. Each city pair should be considered separately because of the operational differences in flight timing, direction, duration, traffic patterns, seasonal effects, and so forth. The first version of safety case 1 focused on Boeing 777 (B777) flights between Atlanta (ATL) and Mumbai (BOM), India. Both the outbound and inbound flights were scheduled to be longer than 16 hours, which exceeded the prescriptive limits at the time.

Element 2: Risk Assessment

Data for estimating fatigue-related risk on the proposed ATL-BOM-ATL operation were available from studies on the first commercial ULR flights between Singapore (SIN) and Los Angeles (LAX), which followed the Flight Safety Foundation recommendations and were approved by the Civil Aviation Authority of Singapore.

The SIN-LAX-SIN and ATL-BOM-ATL trips were well-matched on key operational features, including flight direction (eastward outbound), duration, number of time zones crossed, and layover duration (48 hours for all BOM layovers and most LAX layovers). The ATL-BOM-ATL flights departed 2.8 to 4.5 hours later, depending on flight direction and season. Both trips had four-pilot crews (two captains and two first officers). One crew flew the take-off on the outbound flight and landing on the inbound flight, and the other crew took the opposite roles. Landing crews were allocated the second and fourth (of four) in-flight rest breaks. The SIN-LAX-SIN ULR operation had flown safely daily for 4 years at the time of preparing safety case 1.

The next step in the risk assessment was to select a biomathematical model to predict the likely levels of pilot fatigue on the ATL-BOM-ATL trip. The predictions of two commercially available biomathematical models were tested against pilots' sleep and fatigue monitored on the SIN-LAX-SIN flights. One model was rejected because it predicted a much greater decline in performance across flights than was observed in pilots' measured psychomotor vigilance task (PVT) performance.[12–15] It also predicted no recovery value of the layover sleep in LAX, which was not consistent with pilots' fatigue and sleepiness ratings or PVT performance. In contrast, the predictions of the second model[16] were within the range of interindividual variability for in-flight sleep measured by polysomnography on the SIN-LAX-SIN trip. This model predicted that ATL-BOM-ATL flights would have higher minimum levels of alertness than many existing two-pilot and three-pilot long-range operations.

Element 3: Fatigue Mitigations

The safety case detailed the following mitigations:

- Although the flight and duty times would sometimes exceed the prescriptive limits, the limits on posttrip rest requirements, cumulative flight times, and duty times would be met.
- A route-specific guidance manual was developed for the pilots by the company and approved by the regulator. This included explanations of the science and principles used to develop the ATL-BOM-ATL trip and recommendations for improving sleep across the trip.
- Mitigations to optimize pilots' in-flight sleep included use of an aircraft with a state-of-the-art rest facility, increasing sleep opportunities during rest breaks by providing meals on the flight deck, and including two captains in the four-pilot crew so that one captain was not responsible for the entire flight (this surpasses the regulatory requirement).
- Mitigations to optimize pilots' sleep during the 48-hour layover in BOM included careful vetting of the layover hotel in accordance with the airline's labor agreement and a procedure whereby the airline's operations control center could notify the hotel of flight delays without disturbing pilots' sleep. Crews were also instructed to try to remain on ATL time (i.e., home base time) during the layover.
- The safety case also detailed planning for managing delays and diversions, which included biomathematical model predictions of fatigue levels in the planning scenarios.

Element 4: Fatigue Monitoring

Pilots could report fatigue issues using established processes for both urgent and nonurgent situations. Designated managers were available in the operations control center around-the-clock to deal with urgent situations. Nonurgent reports were reviewed daily and acted on by flight operations. As an additional safeguard during the first 90 days of the operation, a dedicated duty pilot was in the operations control center to monitor the operation and review and act on any concerns that arose during the first 7 hours and last 4 to 6 hours of each ATL-BOM flight, and during the first 12 hours and last 3 hours of each BOM-ATL flight (potential times of greater operational risk).

This first version of safety case 1 was approved in 2008 under a new FAA regulation (OpSpec A332). However, the airlines strongly challenged OpSpec A332, and it was subsequently withdrawn. The airline independently decided not to introduce the ATL-BOM-ATL trip but developed a similar ULR trip between ATL and Johannesburg (JNB).

Validation Study

With the evolving thinking about regulatory approaches to ULR operations, in 2008 the FAA proposed and oversaw a three-airline study to compare pilots' sleep and fatigue on ULR trips (including the ATL-JNB-ATL trip) versus long-range trips. This study served as an operational validation of the approach to FRM for ULR operations that was proposed in safety case 1.

The study took place in 2009–10 and involved 70 pilots who were monitored before, during, and after the ATL-JNB-ATL ULR trip and a long-range trip between Atlanta and either Dubai, Tel Aviv, or Lagos. The study concluded that there were minimal differences between ULR and long-range trips in sleep patterns (measured by actigraphy), sleepiness ratings (Karolinska Sleepiness Scale[17–19]), fatigue ratings (Samn-Perelli crew status check[20–22]), or PVT performance.[12–15] Where there were differences, fatigue measures were lower at the end of the longer ULR flights, probably due to pilots obtaining more sleep during longer flights.[11]

Conclusions of Safety Case 1

Given that the SIN-LAX-SIN ULR operation had already flown safely daily for 4 years, it was argued that the comparable ATL-BOM-ATL ULR operation, with similar fatigue mitigations, would have a level of safety at least equivalent to that achieved in long-range operations that comply with the prescriptive regulations. The biomathematical model simulations also predicted that ATL-BOM-ATL flights would have higher minimum levels of alertness than many existing two-pilot and three-pilot long-range operations.

In addition, the validation study demonstrated that the level of fatigue-related risk was at least as low on ULR flights managed according to safety case 1 as it was on long-range flights that remained within the FAA daily flight and duty limits. With the validation study, safety case 1 was approved for B777 operations under the new FAA regulatory framework in 2014.

SAFETY CASE 2: EXTENDING SAFETY CASE 1 TO PERMIT FLIGHTS TO BE COMPLETED WHEN UNFORESEEN CIRCUMSTANCES WILL CAUSE THE FAA DAILY FLIGHT AND DUTY TIME LIMITS TO BE EXCEEDED

Regulatory Context

The 2014 FAA flight and duty time regulations for four-pilot crews permit a maximum of 17 flight hours and a maximum

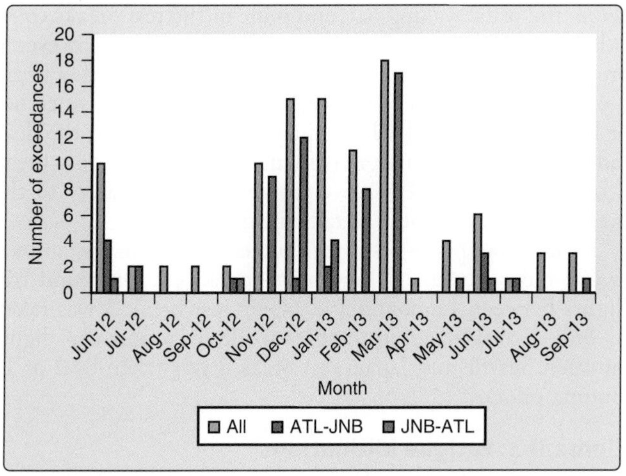

Figure 85.1 Number of Boeing 777 exceedances of flight time limits (17 hours) and/or duty time limits (19 hours) over a 16-month period. ATL, Atlanta; JNB, Johannesberg.

daily duty period of 19 hours.[10] However, unanticipated winds, weather diverts, medical diverts, or other unforeseen circumstances sometimes result in flights and duty periods exceeding these limits.

Element 1: Scope of Safety Case 2

In 2013 a retrospective analysis by the airline of its B777 operations covered by safety case 1 found 22 diversions and 79 delays between June 1, 2012 and September 30, 2013 that had resulted in flights and/or duty periods that exceeded the daily regulatory limits. Of these, 69 (68%) were on the ATL-JNB-ATL ULR trip, mostly on the longer JNB-ATL return sector. Figure 85.1 highlights that exceedances have a marked seasonal pattern. The airline therefore sought an extension of its FRMS based on safety case 1, to be able to complete any B777 flights when unforeseen delays or diversions would result in exceedances of the daily flight and duty time limits. The extension, however, did not allow the airline to schedule beyond those limits.

Element 2: Risk Assessment

Two existing datasets with recommended fatigue safety performance indicators[7] were used to estimate the fatigue risk associated with the exceedances in Figure 85.1: a ULR trip approved by the Singapore Civil Aviation Authority between Changi, Singapore (SIN) and Newark New Jersey (EWR),[23] and a large database combining data from four studies by four airlines that monitored four-pilot crews on long-range and ULR trips, including the B777 validation study in safety case 1.

On the SIN-EWR-SIN ULR trip, average flight durations were 19.1 hours on SIN-EWR flights and 18.5 hours on EWR-SIN flights. By comparison, 98% of exceedances of the FAA 17-hour limit in Figure 85.1 were between 17 hours and 18.5 hours. Average duty durations on the SIN-EWR-SIN ULR trip were 20.7 hours on SIN-EWR flights and 20.4 hours on EWR-SIN flights. By comparison, 89% of exceedances of the FAA 19-hour limit in Figure 85.1 were between 19 hours and 20.5 hours. The SIN-EWR-SIN operational validation study concluded that the alertness levels of pilots on this trip were no lower than on the shorter SIN-LAX-SIN ULR trip and no lower than on other long-range trips that had been studied up to that time.[23]

The combined four airline data set included actigraphic sleep, sleepiness and fatigue ratings, and PVT data from 237 pilots monitored on 13 long-range and ULR city pairs flown by airlines from three continents and governed by three different national regulatory frameworks.[24] This included data for 46 of 729 flights (6.3%) longer than 17 hours and 75 of 730 duty periods (10.3%) longer than 19 hours. Given the range of flights included, the analyses (mixed model analysis of variance) controlled for flight direction, arrival time, and crew position, as well as variability within and between pilots. Fatigue at top of descent (leading into the high workload and safety-critical phase of approach and landing) was lower on longer flights. For every additional hour of flight time, it was estimated that pilots slept 10 minutes longer, and their PVT response speed at top of descent was faster by 0.03 responses per second.

Element 3: Fatigue Mitigations

Safety case 2 was an application to extend the use of the FRMS based on safety case 1, so the mitigations in safety case 1 also applied for managing fatigue on B777 flights that exceeded the daily flight and duty time limits.

Conclusions of Safety Case 2

Applicable data from five monitoring studies were available to estimate the likely fatigue levels on B777 flights that exceeded the daily flight and duty time limits due to unforeseen circumstances. All analyses concluded that pilots' sleepiness and fatigue levels on flights as long as those seen on B777 delays and diversions were no higher than the sleepiness and fatigue levels measured on approved ULR flights and long-range flights that remained within the FAA daily limits.[23,25] Safety case 2 was approved by the FAA in 2017.

SAFETY CASE 3: ALLOCATION OF REST BREAKS ON THREE-PILOT FLIGHTS

Regulatory Context

Longer flights with larger aircraft are permitted when there are more than two pilots on board (the minimum required to fly the aircraft), because with these augmented crews all pilots can have in-flight rest breaks and sleep opportunities. The maximum daily flight and duty times depend on the number of pilots (three or four), the time of day that the duty period starts, and the type of rest facilities available for pilots on the aircraft. The daily limits are longer for four-pilot crews, who each have approximately half of the total available break time, than for three-pilot crews, who each have approximately a third of the available break time.

The 2014 FAA regulatory framework added a new requirement that the pilot flying the landing in an augmented crew (while the other pilot on the flight deck is monitoring) must have a rest break of at least 2 hours in the second half of the flight duty period, to reduce time awake and fatigue levels at top of descent.[1,24] This works for four-pilot crews but has the unintended consequence of forcing the landing pilot to take the third rest break on shorter three-pilot flights.

Element 1: Scope of Safety Case 3

Safety case 3 sought a variation for the airline to allow landing pilots in three-pilot crews to choose break 2 or 3. To ensure they had an adequate sleep opportunity, they would be given at least a third of the total available rest time and no less than 1 hour 45 minutes, with the break beginning up to an hour earlier than the last half of the flight duty period. This request was based on several considerations.

Break 3 does not necessarily provide the best sleep opportunity, which varies depending on when a break occurs in the circadian master clock cycle. Anecdotally, it was also reported that landing pilots preferred break 2, which is between meal services when less activity occurs in the passenger cabin. This is advantageous because on most aircraft used in three-pilot operations pilots take their break in a seat in the passenger cabin, which allows a flat or near-flat sleeping position with privacy curtains.

Three additional factors affect the allocation of rest break time among three-pilot crews. The 2014 regulatory framework requires the pilot monitoring the landing to have 90 consecutive minutes of sleep opportunity. The airline also has a mitigation whereby the third (relief) pilot reduces the workload of the landing and monitoring pilots by taking on all the ancillary and administrative duties from top of descent. Thus the relief pilot also needs to be adequately rested at top of descent. Finally, regulations and established practice give the captain the flexibility to alter break allocations on the day, depending on the fatigue levels of each pilot.

To describe the scope of the operations potentially covered by safety case 3, details were provided on 4151 scheduled flights in 1 month that had three-pilot crews and flight duty periods less than 14 hours (data on departure and arrival cities, number of flights per month, aircraft fleets servicing the flights, scheduled departure times, and maximum flight duty periods).

Element 2: Risk Assessment

The risk assessment for safety case 3 included (1) a literature review, (2) estimation of the sleep opportunities provided by break 2 versus break 3 on the sample of 4151 flights covered by the safety case, and (3) previous studies by the airline that documented pilots' break preferences.

The literature review found that most field studies had focused on four-pilot crew members sleeping in horizontal bunks. By comparison, sleep taken by three-pilot crew members in a seat in the passenger cabin is expected to be more disturbed. Studies with four-pilot crews have demonstrated that in-flight sleep is typically lighter and more fragmented than sleep on the ground.[26] Total sleep varies with the length of breaks and when in the circadian master clock cycle those breaks occur. Less total sleep and longer time awake are associated with greater fatigue and sleepiness at top of descent.[24]

Among the 4151 sample flights, the longest scheduled flight was 11 hours 59 minutes. Assuming three equal breaks and wakeup 20 minutes before the end of the break, at top of descent the pilot flying the landing would have been awake for 4 hours 9 minutes after break 2 and 50 minutes after break 3, that is, not extended periods of wake. For 2063 of the 4151 sample flights, it was reasonable to assume that pilots were adapted to their domicile time zone, so domicile arrival and departure times could be used as a surrogate measure of circadian phase. For each flight, the sleep opportunity offered by break 2 versus break 3 was evaluated relative to the (estimated) time in the circadian cycle that the breaks occurred.[1] For example, the flights departed after the window of circadian low (02:00 to 06:00) and landed before midnight occurred across the usual waking day, and none of the rest breaks coincided with the optimal circadian time for sleep. However, a break that overlaps the afternoon nap window (whether break 2 or 3) will provide a better sleep opportunity than an earlier or later break. Overall, these analyses indicated that the flexibility offered by letting pilots flying the landing choose break 2 or 3 provides at least an equivalent level of safety to the prescriptive requirement to take break 3.[1]

In addition, pilots' rest break preferences were reexamined in two older studies of three-pilot operations. On round-trip flights between Honolulu and Japan, rest break 3 was taken by only 1 of 42 landing pilots,[27] while on round-trip flights between Seattle and Japan, rest break 3 was taken by 2 of 12 landing pilots.[28]

Element 3: Fatigue Mitigations

All pilots involved in three-pilot operations at the airline undertake fatigue management training that meets FAA requirements.[29] Schedulers and others involved in the management of the three-pilot operations are also required to take a 45-minute fatigue management training session that outlines why pilot fatigue is a safety concern, explains the physiology behind fatigue-related symptoms, discusses the role of scheduling in pilot fatigue, and reviews the purpose and processes of the airline's FRM approaches.

Additional FRM strategies implemented by the airline include having a third pilot on some flights that can legally be flown with two pilots, thereby enabling pilots to take breaks and obtain sleep in-flight, and reducing the workload of the landing pilots by allocating ancillary and administrative duties from top of descent to the relief pilot.

Element 4: Fatigue Monitoring

All pilots on flights covered by safety case 3 receive specific training on fatigue reporting mechanisms. They are advised that if they encounter a situation that they consider a fatigue concern, they are responsible for alerting management and, if appropriate, removing themselves from duty or refusing an assignment to duty. Different report forms are required if fatigue represents a flight safety concern versus when it does not. There are also clear processes if a pilot chooses to declare themselves too fatigued for duty.

If flight operations personnel encounter a situation that they consider may cause fatigue-related risk, they must notify the appropriate supervisor or manager. All fatigue reports are acknowledged, evaluated, and acted on (where appropriate) by the pilot fatigue program director and the fatigue safety action team, and regular feedback to pilots is provided.

Validation Study

The FAA requested a validation study to demonstrate that, using the approach described in safety case 3, break 3 does not consistently provide a better sleep opportunity than break 2 during three-pilot augmented operations.[30] Pilots completed a one-page survey on outbound and inbound flights crossing 1 to 7 time zones between 53 city pairs with 1-day layovers (586 surveys). The flights had domicile arrival time in three 4-hour bins (22:00 to 01:59, 02:00 to 05:59, 06:00 to 09:59), with approximately equal numbers of pilot taking break 2 and 3 in each time bin.

On 92% of flights, landing pilots chose break 2. Comparing breaks 2 and 3 across all crew positions, there were no differences in break duration, the likelihood of obtaining sleep (91% in both breaks), total in-flight sleep, subjective sleep quality ratings, or fatigue and sleepiness ratings at the top of descent, after controlling for flight duration. As an additional benchmarking for flights landing 02:00 to 09:59, fatigue and sleepiness ratings at top of descent were compared between these three-pilot flights and four-pilot flights compliant with the FAA requirements. There were no significant differences.

Conclusions of Safety Case 3

The validation study found no supporting evidence to indicate that break 3 consistently provided a better sleep opportunity than break 2 in these three-pilot operations. Overall, it was argued that the flexibility offered by allowing the landing pilot in a three-pilot operation to choose break 2 or 3 provides at least an equivalent level of safety to requiring the landing pilot to take break 3.[1] Safety case 3 received FAA approval in 2015.

SAFETY CASE 4: MANAGING PILOT FATIGUE ON MULTISECTOR DUTY DAYS WITH TOTAL FLIGHT TIMES LONGER THAN 16 HOURS AND DUTY PERIODS LONGER THAN 18 HOURS

Regulatory Context

The 2014 FAA regulations for three-pilot operations with a class 3 rest facility limit the maximum duty day to 15 hours.[10] From a fatigue perspective, the concern is that having a long duty day plus multiple flights adds to pilots' workload and cumulative fatigue.

Element 1: Scope of Safety Case 4

A three-pilot operation flown by an airline for more than 30 years without incident was no longer compliant with these new limits. This operation, often referred to as the "island hopper," provides the primary and sometimes only service for supplies, mail, and transportation to islands in Micronesia and the Marshall Islands. The outbound duty day originates in Guam, makes two to three stops in Micronesia (in Chuuk, Pohnpei, and on some days, Kosrae), two stops in the Marshall Islands (in Kwajalein and Majuro), and ends in Honolulu. After arriving in Honolulu, pilots have a 2- to 3-day layover. The inbound duty day returns from Honolulu to Guam via the same route in reverse. These duty days with five to six flights have duty periods of 15 to 16 hours. Safety case 4 supported an application for an FRMS to manage pilot fatigue on the island hopper trip.

Element 2: Risk Assessment

Before implementation of the 2014 regulations, the airline recognized that the island hopper trip would be noncompliant, and there were no studies on comparable operations to inform risk assessment. A study was therefore conducted that compared sleep and fatigue measures on the island hopper trip (mostly daytime flying) with the much shorter "triangle" trip (mostly night flying), which flew from Guam to Manila to Koror and back to Guam in one duty day and complied with the new regulations. Both trips used B737 aircraft with a crew of one captain and two first officers who flew both the outbound and inbound duty days. Pilots took rest breaks in the passenger cabin, in a reclining seat with a footrest. It was argued that the sleep loss and performance impairment associated with working through the window of low circadian alertness (02:00 to 06:00) increased the likelihood of fatigue-related impairment on the compliant triangle trip, which would at least partially counterbalance the fatigue associated with the extra flight segments and longer duty days on the island hopper trip. Participants were monitored on both trips, and expected times of lowest and highest fatigue were compared between trips, using accepted safety performance indicators (total in-flight sleep, sleep in the 24 hours before the final top of descent, fatigue and sleepiness ratings, and PVT speed). Overall, the evidence indicated a level of safety at least equivalent to the triangle trip.

Even though the initial safety case was favorable, due to the unique nature of the operation, the FAA, their scientific advisors, the operator, and the operator's scientific consultants agreed that an optimal mitigation for operating under the FRMS exemption would be splitting both duty days between two crews (four pilots) as follows. On the outbound day, crew A flies the four to five segments from Guam to Majuro, and crew B flies the final segment from Majuro to Honolulu (a longer flight of about 5 hours). On the inbound day, crew A flies the initial segment from Honolulu to Majuro, and crew B flies the four to five segments from Majuro to Guam.

The FAA requested a validation study comparing this revised island hopper trip with the triangle trip. Participants were again monitored on both trips, and expected times of lowest and highest fatigue were compared between trips. Noninferiority testing was used to identify equivalence and/or superiority.[31] In addition, a commercially available biomathematical model was used to compare "predicted effectiveness" at top of descent on both trips.

Element 3: Fatigue Mitigations

Safety case 4 detailed the following fatigue mitigations for the island hopper trip:

- The trip is flown with two full crews.
- The maximum scheduled duty day is 17.5 hours, which includes a buffer for unforeseen circumstances, and there are daily flight time limits.
- The business or first-class seats used by nonoperating pilots were upgraded to meet the new standards for a class 3 rest facility in the 2014 regulatory framework.
- If the operating crew at any time determines they are no longer fit for duty, the nonoperating crew can seek approval from dispatch to take over as the operating crew for any remaining portion of the trip, so long as they are fit for duty.
- The minimum scheduled layover duration is 48 hours.
- The departure time out of Honolulu at the start of the inbound duty day was delayed allowing an extended sleep opportunity during local night at the end of the layover.
- Crews are recommended to stay on Guam time throughout the entire trip (Guam is 20 hours ahead of Honolulu).

Element 4: Fatigue Monitoring

Pilots can report fatigue issues via established processes for both urgent and nonurgent situations, with designated managers available in the operations control center 24/7 to deal with urgent situations. Nonurgent reports are reviewed daily and acted on by flight operations. Pilots also receive specific information and recommendations about managing fatigue on this unusual trip.

Conclusions of Safety Case 4

The validation study of the island hopper trip flown with two crews, and following the approach in safety case 4, concluded that the evidence supported at least an equivalent level of safety for duty days on the island hopper trip versus the triangle trip. Safety case 4 was approved in 2014.

DISCUSSION

The complexity of these safety cases reflects the safety-critical nature of commercial flight operations and the fact that they were presented when experience with FRMSs was relatively limited. They highlight the need for pooling expertise and sharing data to build a robust safety case. The following sections offer perspectives from four of the authors who worked together on some of the safety cases described earlier. They are offered to provide insight into the different roles of stakeholders in the development of safety cases.

An Operator's Perspective

For operators, the development of a safety case involves many tasks. Once an operation that does not comply with the prescriptive regulatory requirements is defined, areas of possible increased fatigue risk need to be identified. The focus is on how this operation differs from others with which the operator has knowledge and experience. Next, a gaps analysis is undertaken to see if/where additional operational and human performance data are needed. Then the operator is ready to develop the safety case.

The operator is now ready to ask themself "What is needed to run this operation at an acceptable level of safety?" This is the point where scientists, safety professionals, crew members, and regulators should be brought into the discussion. Scientists are needed to guide the effort on how to validate the safety of the operation, including identifying what scientific data are needed and how much data will be sufficient to support the hypotheses. The safety professionals help perform safety risk assessments and identify whether the additional risk fits within tolerable levels defined by the organization. Crew members should be consulted throughout this phase to make sure they understand what the operator is proposing and to provide input as decisions are made. The regulator needs to be fully informed throughout this phase, so they have full confidence in the efforts of the operator and in the information produced and the processes being executed by all stakeholders. All stakeholders should continuously suggest mitigations throughout these discussions.

A Crew-Member's Perspective

The crew member's role can be much more than being a source of data in the data collection process. Motivated and educated representatives of the crew-member workforce can provide vital knowledge about the specific safety risk(s) associated with the operation being considered and about workable mitigations. The need for this operational experience is recognized in the International Civil Aviation Organization's definition of a FRMS. Crew members should also be asking themselves "What is needed to run this operation at an acceptable level of safety?"

Having a full understanding of the proposed operation and the key fatigue safety performance indicators can increase the value and quantity of data collected from crew members. In addition, this deeper understanding and participation in developing the plan has the potential to enhance the crew-member workforce's desire and ability to comply with the plan to mitigate fatigue in the operations covered by the safety case.

The value of an engaged crew-member workforce goes beyond being a component in the development of the type of operation desired. After the plan is developed, approved, and implemented, this same active and engaged workforce can be the "eyes and ears" of the operation to best evaluate the effectiveness of the planned mitigations and provide input for further refinement, thus enhancing safety of the entire flight operation.

A Regulator's Perspective

As long nonstop city-pair operations that exceed prescriptive flight and duty limits increase, safety case development using relevant operational data becomes critical in assuring the regulatory authority that new routes are, indeed, safe for the pilots and the flying public. Designing lucrative city-pair routes using aircraft capable of extended flight operations does not automatically ensure that pilots are not reaching the limits of human endurance. It is therefore of paramount importance that the regulatory authority trusts the air carrier (operator) and their scientific representatives in development of safety cases.

The safety case data not only provide supporting evidence of acceptable performance but also that excessive fatigue is managed with mitigation strategies related to the entire operation, beginning with pretrip preparations, on-board rest procedures, layover sleep, and posttrip recovery before beginning another flight duty period. Without confidence in the safety of the proposed flight operation, the regulatory risk of approving such flight exemptions would be unknown and unacceptable.

From both a regulatory and scientific perspective, publishing data acquired as part of safety cases is strongly recommended. This improves our understanding of the outcomes of extending flight duty periods and other unique operations, as conducted under the conditions and limitations of each safety case. Sharing of data in this manner and providing examples of best practices among air carriers can only improve the safety of flight operations across the globe.

A Scientist's Perspective

The role of scientists in the development of a robust safety case is to provide expertise, being clear about any limitations in the available scientific evidence and taking personal responsibility for their advice. Throughout the development and approval of a safety case, scientists need to remain neutral and trusted by all stakeholders.

This requires a range of skills and tasks that begin with critical evaluation of any relevant previous research. Methodological limitations and knowledge gaps need to be described clearly to all stakeholders for a robust discussion about the adequacy of the available data and findings for estimating operational risk. Scientists usually also have a role in identifying and evaluating proposed mitigations to reduce the expected fatigue-related risk. They must maintain professional integrity by frankly discussing any reservations they may have about the risk estimation and proposed mitigations.

The next key task is designing the data collection study to verify the level of safety achieved when the operations are flown under the provisions of the safety case. This includes the choice of measures, analytical approach, and the number of participants needed to be able to reliably test the agreed hypotheses. The study needs to be designed in collaboration with the operator, who typically pays for the data collection and knows the logistical requirements and constraints in the operations being studied. The regulator needs to approve the study design, which is often an iterative process. It is critical to have sufficient statistical power to reach reliable conclusions based on the data. The regulatory requirement is to demonstrate at least an equivalent level of safety to that achieved by staying within the prescriptive regulations. Some recent studies have met this requirement by using equivalence or noninferiority testing.[31,32]

Gaining independent ethical approval, data collection, analyses, and report writing typically involve people with different roles. In our experience, having a team of scientists with an identified project leader provides a robust process. As well as being the scientific leader, the project leader is the point of contact for the regulator, airline, and labor partners.

From a scientific perspective, publishing studies in the peer-reviewed literature whenever possible is important for building the body of scientific knowledge and for career progression. However, safety cases are confidential documents between an airline and a regulator, and aspects of the work may carry competitive advantage for the airline. It is therefore recommended that, at the planning stage of any data collection project, there is discussion with all stakeholders about which aspects of a project are likely to be appropriate for publication, as well as about authorship and power of veto for any proposed publications.

CLINICAL PEARL

New approaches to fatigue risk management (FRM) are based on scientific evidence that fatigue signs and symptoms reflect a state of performance impairment resulting from acute or chronic sleep loss, extended time awake, working and sleeping at suboptimal times in the circadian clock cycle, or physical and mental workload. Prescriptive regulations that specify limits on duty times and rest breaks aim to reduce workplace fatigue. However, they are increasingly being challenged because they (1) do not adequately address work-related sleep restriction and circadian disruption and (2) are not tailored to the specific risks that a fatigue-impaired person represents in different work settings. When permitted, safety cases offer an alternative approach in which a company, labor groups, and scientists pool their expertise to develop a data-driven FRM system to manage the risks in specified work contexts. In commercial aviation, a safety case must demonstrate to the regulator that the approach it proposes can predict and manage fatigue-related risk at least as well as staying within the prescriptive regulations. Safety cases also highlight gaps in scientific knowledge and can generate new lines of research.

SUMMARY

Safety cases require the pooling of regulatory, operational (management and workforce), and scientific expertise to develop safe and acceptable solutions for operating outside prescriptive FRM regulations, which define the level of risk that a regulator accepts on behalf of the public.

The complexity of the safety cases presented here reflects the diverse and safety-critical nature of commercial aviation. However, the same principles apply at all levels of complexity. The nature, scope, and impact of the proposed exemption(s) need to be defined, the associated safety risk(s) estimated, appropriate mitigation strategies implemented, and their effectiveness evaluated by ongoing monitoring of agreed safety performance indicators. Some regulators also require a validation study during a trial of the approach proposed in the safety case before a full exemption to operate outside the prescriptive requirements is granted.

Safety cases can also make an important contribution to advancing scientific knowledge and to highlighting gaps where more research is needed. Like all transdisciplinary projects, they typically pass through multiple stages of frustration and exhilaration but are ultimately rewarding when they come up with safe, flexible solutions.

SELECTED READINGS

Gander PH, Hartley L, Powell D, et al. Fatigue risk management: organizational factors at the regulatory and industry/company level. *Accid Anal Prev.* 2011;43(2):573–590.

Gander PH, Mangie J, Wu L, et al. Preparing safety cases for operating outside prescriptive fatigue risk management regulations. *Aerosp Med Hum Perform.* 2017;88(7):688–696.

Gander PH, Mulrine HM, van den Berg MJ, et al. Effects of sleep/wake history and circadian phase on proposed pilot fatigue safety performance indicators. *J Sleep Res.* 2015;24(1):110–119.

Gregory KB, Soriano-Smith RN, Lamp ACM, et al. Flight crew alertness and sleep relative to timing of in-flight rest periods in long-haul flights. *Aerosp Med Hum Perform.* 2021;92(2):83–91.

Lamp A, Chen JMC, McCullough, et al. Equal to or better than: the application of statistical non-inferiority to fatigue risk management. *Accid Anal Prev.* 2019;126:184–190.

Wu L, Gander PH, van den Berg M, et al. Equivalence testing as a tool for fatigue risk management in aviation. *Aerosp Med Hum Perform.* 2018;89(4):383–388.

A complete reference list can be found online at ExpertConsult.com.

Chapter

86

Fatigue Proofing

Matthew J.W. Thomas; Drew Dawson

Chapter Highlights

- Fatigue and performance impairment have traditionally been viewed within a "deficit" model of safety and the term *fatigue* described in terms of performance impairment that has significant implications for safety and productivity.
- In the traditional deficit model of safety, fatigue risk management is primarily concerned with eliminating fatigue. In accordance, occupational settings often specify duty time limitations and minimum break requirements. Although this may reduce fatigue, it does not eliminate fatigue in the workplace.
- In occupational settings, skilled workers are able to put in place risk-reduction strategies that allow for safe operation even while fatigued. We call these adaptive and protective-risk reduction strategies "fatigue proofing" strategies.
- The concept of fatigue proofing emphasizes that fatigue is also associated with positive behavioral modification strategies to protect actual job performance and system safety from degradation.

INTRODUCTION

Since World War II we have seen an increasing focus on fatigue as a source of error and a threat to operational safety in a variety of industries, including transport, emergency services, health care, and others. There is a significant extant literature documenting both the causes and effects of fatigue. In brief, prior sleep-wake behavior, time-of-day, and workload are key factors determining the level of fatigue experienced by the individual worker. Slowed cognitive processing and impaired attentional and emotional control all combine to increase the likelihood of task-related errors and thereby compromise judgement, decision making, and ultimately workplace safety.

To reduce the likelihood of fatigue-related error, organizations, often in response to regulatory oversight, have sought to reduce the likelihood of fatigue-related errors by controlling the hours that an individual is able to work. Throughout the developed world we have seen regulatory limits imposed on many workplaces in an attempt to reduce fatigue-related risk and improve safety. In the period 1920 to 1980, we saw significant limits to working hours introduced as part of a general trend toward improved safety and social outcomes.

This trend has been at least partially reversed over the last 40 years as neoliberal governments across the Western World struggle with contradictory community expectations for (1) increased availability of services and (2) reduced taxation and reduced government expenditure on essential services. This has been especially true in fields typically funded by government (e.g., health care and emergency services). As a consequence, working time arrangements have typically expanded with fewer employees working longer hours, more overtime (especially unpaid), and with increased amounts of "on-call" work. See Chapter 84 for further discussion on hours-of-service regulations and fatigue risk management.

For regulators and organizations, it is increasingly difficult to manage fatigue by restricting working time arrangements. The short-term impacts on operational effectiveness, income, and profit make it extremely difficult to restrict working time arrangements. It is also the case that restrictions to shift durations and weekly totals do little to control fatigue due to time-of-day factors. In the past there was a common, albeit mistaken, belief that compliance with working time arrangements was an effective control for mitigating fatigue-related risk. Although fatigue due to sleep loss can be controlled by providing an adequate sleep opportunity, circadian variations in fatigue are not well controlled by such measures. Moreover, there is an increasing awareness that the relative risk associated with fatigue-related errors is often less than the increased risk associated with the withdrawal of services associated with reduced working hours. As we have suggested (controversially) elsewhere "sometimes a tired doctor is better than no doctor at all."[1]

Based on the fatigue science, it is probably fair to say that

- Fatigue cannot be eliminated in any industry that requires people to work overnight.
- Working time arrangements do not ensure that an employee has had sufficient sleep to return to work fit-for-duty (FFD).

The consequences of this realization are profound. That is, regulating working hours cannot never provide an effective control for reducing the likelihood of fatigue-related error because many people have to work at night, where the circadian causes of fatigue are unavoidable, and even if we provide a working time arrangement that provides an adequate opportunity to return FFD, people live complicated lives with many competing family and social obligations that may displace sleep or reduce sleep opportunity and result in uncontrolled fatigue-related risk in the workplace.

We would be better to work on the assumption that a certain amount of fatigue-related risk is inevitable and can never be controlled by regulating the working time arrangement. It is also the case that the risk associated with removing someone from the workplace when fatigued might, paradoxically, increase risk, through a reduction in service availability. We need a new additional paradigm through which to manage fatigue-related risk that cannot be controlled through the regulation of working time. That is, we need ways in which we can ensure that people can work safely while fatigued.

PART ONE: FATIGUE PROOFING THE INDIVIDUAL AND TEAM

At the close of last century, Professor James Reason so eloquently stated, "*human fallibility can be moderated, but it cannot be eliminated.*"[2] Most traditional approaches to safety management have focused on attempts at eliminating human error through strategies such as the prescription of standard operating procedures or through engineering and design.

When catastrophes occur in any high-risk industry, the actions of individuals and teams are often highlighted as primary causal factors. The mantra of *human error* being responsible for the majority of industrial catastrophes is now long entrenched in our constructions of safety management.

Deficit Models of Fatigue

Fatigue has traditionally been seen within a predominantly *deficit* model of safety. Indeed, most definitions of fatigue construct the phenomenon in terms of performance *impairment*.[3] Today, a considerable body of research highlights the ways in which fatigue is associated with degraded performance, from analogues with alcohol intoxication[4] and impaired cognitive performance in the laboratory[5] to impacts on decision making[6] and increased error rates during real-world work performance.[7] In a similar fashion, fatigue has been defined as an archetypal "error-producing condition" that in turn gives rise to suboptimal operator performance and has a direct negative consequence on safety.[8–10]

In recent years, these *deficit* models have received considerable criticism from within the safety science community. Although the construction of the human as the weakest and most variable and unpredictable component of an engineered system has become commonplace, it is a position that does not really reflect the ways in which human operators are able to adapt their performance to mitigate the impacts of factors such as fatigue. In short, the traditional approach fails to celebrate the unique abilities brought to any system of work by the human components.

At this point in time there remains only one intelligent component of any system, the *human* element. We are truly remarkable in our abilities, in our anticipation of change from only the most subtle of cues, our management of complex dynamic scenarios, and in our decision making under the influence of a wide range of stressors.

Ultimately, fatigue proofing rejects the simplistic notion that fatigue should be seen solely in terms of performance impairment. Rather, although fatigue does result in decreased performance on some measures, it is also associated with positive behavioral modification strategies to protect actual job performance and system safety from degradation. As Sidney Dekker asks, "*is the human a problem to control, or a solution to harness*"?[11]

In contrast to the human as deficit model of safety, a new paradigm has been proposed, which has been termed "Safety-II." Within the Safety-II paradigm, safety is defined as an ability "*to make dynamic trade-offs and to adjust performance in order to meet changing demands and to deal with disturbances and surprises,*"[12] Safety is therefore seen as a product of human performance, which may be subject to limitations, but ultimately fundamental in achieving safe operations.

Through the lens of the Safety-II model, fatigue must be seen as something other than simply another error-producing condition. Fatigue must be reconstructed as a natural form of performance variability that in turn must be actively managed in day-to-day operations to mitigate fatigue-related risk and ensure safe operations are maintained. Within this context, the notion of *fatigue proofing* celebrates the solutions humans bring to effectively manage a ubiquitous phenomenon and maintain safe and efficient performance even in the face of fatigue.

Fatigue Countermeasures

The first line of defense proposed against the negative impacts of fatigue on performance has traditionally been the deployment of a range of fatigue countermeasures (see Chapter 82). Indeed, the scientific literature supports the effectiveness of many forms of fatigue countermeasure in the workplace setting.

For instance, the role of rest breaks in maintaining safe operational performance is well known, as is the relationship between inadequate rest breaks and injury and accident risk.[13] Similarly, the effectiveness of short naps on maintaining performance is widely accepted and well supported in the literature.[14–17] Then, the use of caffeine and other stimulants, such as modafinil, have been subject to significant evaluation as fatigue countermeasures and are now widely used in high-intensity sustained operations, especially in the military context.[18–22]

Although these traditional forms of fatigue countermeasures have been found to be effective, they only represent a small component of the ways in which fatigue is effectively mitigated in real-world work environments. To understand the full gamut of fatigue proofing strategies, we need to look beyond this medicant-oriented approach and explore the range of behavioral strategies used by expert operators to mitigate fatigue-related risk.

Control and Compensatory Effort

At an individual level, the simplistic notion that fatigue is automatically and directly associated with performance degradation has been subject to challenge for some decades. In a seminal piece of work in this area, Hockey[23] describes the need to include in our understanding of the relationship between fatigue and performance the operation of a compensatory control mechanism that allocates resources dynamically.

This so called "cognitive-energetical framework" suggests that energy expenditure, or mental and physical effort, is able to be consciously increased or decreased in response to work demands.[23] In situations where fatigue is present, operators are able to conserve resources in times of low work demands and, conversely, increase effort when situations arise that require increased performance. Therefore the negative impacts of fatigue on performance can be overcome through this dynamic allocation of effort in response to varying work demands.

This framework highlights the self-regulatory aspects of human performance and our unique ability to dynamically reallocate resources when required. Although not suggesting this capacity is limitless, the notion of compensatory effort is an important construct in understanding how performance is protected against the negative aspects of fatigue, particularly in high-risk work environments.

Nontechnical Skills and Teamwork

Beyond the confines of compensatory effort at an individual level, further insights into fatigue proofing came from the observation of experts in high-risk industries actively engaging in behaviors that ensured the performance impairment associated with fatigue did not result in any degradation to operational performance.

The first study to suggest the importance of nontechnical skills and teamwork as a fatigue countermeasure was a simulator study conducted at the National Aeronautics and Space Administration Ames Research Center in the mid-1980s.[24] In this study, commercial short-haul airline crews performed a simulated line operation in either a fatigued or rested condition. The findings of the study unexpectedly found that crew who were well rested performed significantly *less effectively* than the fatigued crew. As the findings of the study state:

> "Recent operating experience appears to be a strong influence on crew performance and may have served as a countermeasure to the levels of fatigue present in Post-Duty crewmembers."[24]

In more recent follow-up studies, this finding has been reinforced. For instance, in one study examining the relationship between the sleep-wake history of flight crew and their operational performance, it was observed that although moderate amounts of restricted sleep were associated with significant increases in pilot error, flight crew were able to put in place strategies that increased the effective detection and management of error. In accordance, even in the context of increased error rates associated with fatigue, there was no detrimental impact on operational safety.[7]

Many of these fatigue-proofing behaviors observed can be described in terms of nontechnical skills and especially those relating to communication and teamwork. Long-standing foci of training in high-risk industries, nontechnical skills training programs became the focus of safety enhancement in the 1980s in the form of Cockpit Resource Management (CRM) training.[25–28] In more recent times, CRM training programs have evolved far beyond the commercial aviation flight deck into industries such as healthcare, mining, rail, and many others.[29] Given the recent research into effective error management at the front line of operations, there is little doubt that nontechnical skills training programs are a critical component of fatigue-proofing day-to-day operations.

Harvesting and Formalizing Fatigue-Proofing Strategies

Fatigue-proofing strategies used by individuals and teams are often informal and idiosyncratic in nature.[30] From individual mnemonics and checklists, double and triple checking, and commencing tasks earlier than usual to "buy time," fatigue-proofing strategies are often made up of tacit forms of knowledge that come with expertise. From an organizational perspective, one of the most important considerations is how these informal strategies are "harvested" and formalized through knowledge sharing, training, and in some instances proceduralizing fatigue-proofing strategies.

Observation of expert performance and other knowledge elicitation strategies form an important element of harvesting fatigue-proofing strategies. Techniques such as the Critical Decision Method[31] and variants are especially useful in unpacking tacit knowledge and understanding fatigue-proofing strategies in practice.

The process of harvesting and formalizing fatigue-proofing strategies is, however, constrained to some degree by the underpinning organizational culture and the organization's approach to safety management. In the current milieu, safety is often constructed as a product of work specification through the provision of well-developed standard operating procedures and procedural discipline in execution. This compliance-driven approach to safety fails to capture the dynamic nature of true expertise. Fatigue proofing therefore needs to strike a balance between procedural specification and compliance with the development and deployment of nontechnical skills and error management strategies.

PART TWO: FATIGUE PROOFING THE SYSTEM

Another approach to mitigating fatigue-related risk in day-to-day operations involves fatigue proofing the system of work. Moving beyond behavioral fatigue-proofing strategies put in place by individuals and teams, fatigue proofing the system of work involves the use of technologic additions or system redesign to ensure fatigue does not lead to negative outcomes for productivity or safety.

This approach again is built on the assumption that on occasion, fatigue will be unavoidable, and individuals and teams will be operating at heightened levels of fatigue-related risk. In this situation, additional forms of risk mitigation involve strategies that anticipate performance degradation and put in place mechanisms to prevent fatigue-related impairment leading to negative outcomes.

Fatigue Detection Technologies

In a range of industries, engineered systems have been put in place to detect when an operator might be suffering from reduced alertness or have fallen asleep, and the operator should be alerted or an action initiated to render the system safe.

In the context of rail operations, driver vigilance devices have been used for many decades to prevent incidents or accidents being caused by fatigue-related impairment or incapacitation. Two types of vigilance systems are commonly used in rail. The first, a "dead man's system" is designed such that that the driver must constantly keep a button, pedal, or horizontal bar depressed. The second vigilance system monitors driver input on train controls and in the absence of input requires a button to be pushed. Whenever the constraints of such devises are not met, an auditory and visual alarm prompts a response. If no response is then made within a predetermined period, the train brakes are automatically applied.[32] Derivatives of such vigilance systems are now found in a range of industries and form a reasonable defense against the impacts of drowsiness and microsleeps on performance. However, they may also inadvertently contribute to the monotony of certain driving tasks and thus have an unanticipated deleterious effect.[33]

In recent years, more sophisticated approaches to the monitoring of operator alertness and impairment have been developed. Two main types of systems are currently in operation in the road transport industry. First, driver-facing systems monitor for a range of behavioral symptoms of fatigue, such as eye closure, blink-rate, or head position. Second, forward-facing systems monitor embedded performance measures, such as lane deviation and other vehicle dynamics. Although such technologies have the potential to contribute to fatigue management in contexts such as the transport industry, there is currently a lack of high-quality, independent studies providing converging evidence that support the validity and reliability of these systems in implementation.[34]

Resilience Engineering and Error-Tolerant Design

The final component of fatigue proofing involves adopting an overall system design strategy that anticipates the occurrence of fatigue, understands the risks associated with fatigue in terms of performance variability of individuals and teams and builds barriers that prevent fatigue-related errors resulting in compromised productivity and safety. In complex systems, the total elimination of human error is a futile pursuit, and therefore systems need to be designed to ensure inevitable error does not lead to unacceptable outcomes.[35]

In recent years, this approach has been termed *resilience engineering* and involves the design of systems that are not "brittle" in the face of human performance variability and error. In this sense, a brittle system is one that is vulnerable to the effects of natural perturbations and disturbances in conditions, such as created through human error. In many respects, our traditional approach to safety management has created overly brittle systems. Highly constrained and prescriptive approaches to the specification of work are a classic example. Safety is maintained so long as everything occurs in accordance with the procedure. However, all contingencies seen in real-world operations are not easily captured by a single set of standard operating procedures. When things do not go exactly as planned, brittle systems break.

The allied pursuits of error-tolerant design and resilience engineering provide individuals and teams the freedom to excel. They focus on supporting expert operators effectively managing the complex, dirty, and often unpredictable nature of real-world operations.[11]

Like much of human factors, this approach to fatigue proofing a system celebrates our strengths as experts in the workplace, while being sympathetic to our limitations as brought about by factors such as fatigue.

CONCLUSIONS

Fatigue proofing refers to a wide range of strategies that individuals and teams use to adapt their behavior to ensure that safety and productivity can be maintained even in the face of fatigue. In our opinion, there is little doubt that much of this happens already, albeit informally and in a way that is not documented within the formal safety management system. There is little doubt in our minds that such approaches hold considerable promise and could be easily identified and adopted by organizations. But here lies the challenge. Culturally, we have a century of traditional fatigue risk management characterized only by strategies for controlling the working time arrangement. Although demonstrably ineffective at managing fatigue-related risk with a high degree of specificity and sensitivity, it is administratively straightforward. Regulation of working time arrangements provides simple compliance measures with low levels of ambiguity. A shift is either less than 12 hours or it is not. An employee worked less than 40 hours, or they did not. In many cases, the ease and simplicity of demonstrating compliance has become a proxy for demonstrating a safe system of work. This is understandable. Relative to many hazards, fatigue science is complex. It requires a subtle grasp of the degree to which contributing factors can, or cannot, be controlled. Fatigue proofing requires a detailed understanding of human factors and nontechnical skills acquisition.

Our failure to adopt the rather obvious aspects of fatigue proofing probably reflect the historical and disciplinary origins of how fatigue was initially managed. In most developed countries, hours of work have been negotiated primarily as a financial aspect of work and under the aegis of labour-industrial relations. The primary importance of hours of work has been related to its short-term financial consequences rather than its safety outcomes (i.e., wages cost, employee income, operational effectiveness corporate profitability, etc.). In most of the developed world, managing fatigue through the safety system is a relatively new phenomena that only started in the first decade of this century in some English-speaking countries. In many other parts of the world, it remains either unregulated or managed primarily through compliance and prescription.

Here lies the challenge. Our industrial-labour relations systems and many of our safety regulators are not well equipped for the use of mitigations such as we have outlined earlier. Although likely effective, how does an organization identify, trial, and adopt such measures in the absence of a strong human factors culture? How do regulators determine the appropriateness and effectiveness of fatigue-proofing strategies? Compared with measuring hours of work, it is complicated. What works for one group of workers may not work for others. Even for a similar group of workers, what works in one cultural context (e.g., self-identification of impairment) may be anathema in another. This probably explains why so many of the fatigue-proofing strategies identified in recent years remain as elements of the "informal" safety management system.

The challenge for the next decade is how to reengineer the safety culture of organizations and regulators so that they can help themselves and each other identify, implement, and evaluate effective fatigue-proofing strategies. How do we empower employees to share with their managers how they manage to work safely even when fatigued? How do we support organizational safety professionals to identify, describe, formalize, evaluate, and share potential fatigue-proofing techniques with the rest of their organizations or peers? How do we support regulators to develop the frameworks to support the effective use and dissemination of potential fatigue-proofing strategies? How do we support the training of inspectorates to evaluate whether the organization is effectively implementing such strategies or merely disguising de facto deregulation by being disingenuous?

CLINICAL PEARL

Fatigue proofing refers to the wide range of strategies that individuals and teams use to protect their performance. Fatigue should not be seen solely in terms of degraded performance that poses a threat to safety in high-risk work environments. Rather, fatigue can be seen to generate a range of behaviors that can effectively mitigate risk and ensure that both safety and productivity can be maintained.

SUMMARY

In this chapter we have outlined novel ways in which organizations can approach the task of reducing fatigue-related risk, often while continuing to work. In our view the chapter outlined a whole new class of ways in which organizations can reduce fatigue-related risk without the need to remove the employee from the workplace. Such mitigations can be extremely useful in workplace settings where the removal of the employee carries significant additional risk associated with the nonprovision of a service. That is, where the risk of not providing the service, outweighs the risk of providing it by a fatigued employee.

Based on the Safety II approach, we have identified ways in which employees are simultaneously the problem and the solution. Based on many workplace discussions we have identified ways in which people can control risk and reduce the risk of a fatigue-related error without requiring them to restrict their working time arrangement. These are all the clever ways we adapt (through state-dependent learning) to working while fatigued and increasing the likelihood that we detect or prevent an error before it leads to an adverse outcome.

SELECTED READINGS

Dawson D, Chapman J, Thomas MJW. Fatigue proofing: a new approach to reducing fatigue-related risk using the principles of error management. *Sleep Med. Rev.* 2012;16(2):167–175.

Dawson D, Cleggett C, Thompson K, Thomas MJW. Fatigue proofing: the role of protective behaviours in mediating fatigue-related risk in a defence aviation environment. *Accid Anal Prev.* 2017;99(B):465–468.

Dawson D, Mayger K, Thompson K, Thomas MJW. Fatigue risk management by volunteer fire-fighters: use of informal strategies to augment formal policy. *Accid Anal Prev.* 2015;84:92–98.

Dawson D, McCulloch K. Managing fatigue: it's about sleep. *Sleep Med Rev.* 2005;9:365–380.

Dawson D, Thomas MJW. Fatigue management in healthcare: it's a risky business. *Anaesthesia.* 2019;74(12):1493–1496.

Dawson D, Thomas MJW. Fatigue management in practice—it's just good teamwork. *Sleep Med Rev.* 2019;48:101221.

Thomas MJ, Paterson JL, Jay SM, Matthews RW, Ferguson SA. More than hours of work: fatigue management during high-intensity maritime operations. *Chronobiol Int.* 2019;36(1):143–149.

Australian Long Haul Fatigue Study. In: Thomas MJW, Petrilli RM, Lamond N, Dawson D, Roach GD, eds. *International Aviation Safety Seminar*. Paris, France: Flight Safety Foundation; 2006.

Thomas MJW, Petrilli RM. Error detection during normal flight operations: resilient systems in practice. In: de Voogt A, D'Oliveira T, eds. *Mechanisms in the Chain of Safety*. Aldershot, UK: Ashgate; 2012:107–115.

Thomas MJW. Predictors of threat and error management: identification of core non-technical skills and implications for training systems design. *Int J Aviat Psychol.* 2004;14(2):207–231.

A complete reference list can be found online at ExpertConsult.com

Chapter 87

Sleep Health in Athlete Populations: Unique Challenges and Practical Solutions

Scott Kutscher; Amy Bender; Charles Samuels

Chapter Highlights

- Competitive athletes are generally healthy individuals subject to substantial, repeated physical, psychological, and metabolic demands.
- Training, competition, and travel schedules often require long work hours, high workload, early-morning awakenings, and competing at an adverse circadian phase.
- Sleep loss and circadian desynchrony are prevalent among athletes. Obtaining sufficient sleep and minimizing circadian desynchrony are important health considerations in athlete populations.
- This chapter describes a comprehensive clinical approach that is based on three core principles: (1) ensuring adequate sleep, (2) screening for sleep disturbances and sleep disorders, and (3) managing circadian desynchrony and improving sleep routines.

INTRODUCTION

Athletes are often faced with having to balance training, travel, work, school, and family life, which puts substantial demands on athletes and reduces time for recovery, rest, and sleep. It is well established that sleep is important for mental and physical health, performance, and overall well-being. The sport science community believes that sleep is critical for recovery, sustaining performance, and reducing risk of injury.[1] Although the systematic evidence for this belief is limited, managing sleep and circadian misalignment in athlete populations has become an important part of managing athletes' health at all levels. Sleep clinicians should be aware of the research and evidence currently available and where the evidence is headed in this unique population of potential patients. Improving sleep quantity and sleep quality, detecting and treating sleep disorders, and mitigating the effects of circadian misalignment provide ways for improving athletes' recovery, resiliency, and potentially their athletic performance.

SLEEP LOSS, SLEEP DISTURBANCES, AND SLEEP DISORDERS

Sleep Loss among Athletes

Research studies including surveys of collegiate level athletes have found that insufficient sleep, poor sleep quality, and excessive daytime sleepiness are prevalent among athletes. For example, Mah and colleagues[2] (2018) and Knufinke and colleagues[3] (2018) found that more than one-third of student athletes report sleeping less than 7 hours per night, greater than 40% of student athletes have poor sleep quality as assessed by the Pittsburgh Sleep Quality Index (PSQI), and less than 50% of student athletes experience excessive daytime sleepiness as assessed by the Epworth Sleepiness Scale (ESS; ESS scores > 10).

Overscheduling, improper scheduling, and travel are frequent culprits of sleep loss among athletes. Research has repeatedly demonstrated that athletes obtain less sleep before intense training and competition schedules than before rest days, and this effect is mediated by the time of day.[4] For example, a study involving elite swimmers found that these athletes obtained 5.4 hours of sleep the night before a training day, and sleep was reduced, in part, due to early-morning start times. In contrast, the elite swimmers obtained 7.1 hours of sleep the night before a rest day.[5] In a study involving elite football players, these athletes obtained less sleep before a night match than before a day match or before a regular training day.[6]

Sleep quality and sleep quantity will also depend on a number of other factors, such as an athlete's sleep environment, training load, and travel schedules. These factors can result in displaced, truncated, unpredictable, and/or fragmented sleep opportunities. Further, acute or chronic medical conditions, such as pain, mood disorders, and/or sleep disorders, can reduce sleep quality and sleep quantity. Figure 87.1 outlines the interplay of various individual and environmental factors that can affect sleep opportunity.

Sleep Disturbances and Sleep Disorders among Athletes

There is much for sleep clinicians to consider in the screening, assessment, diagnosis, and treatment of sleep disorders among athletes, such as the context of the training and competitive

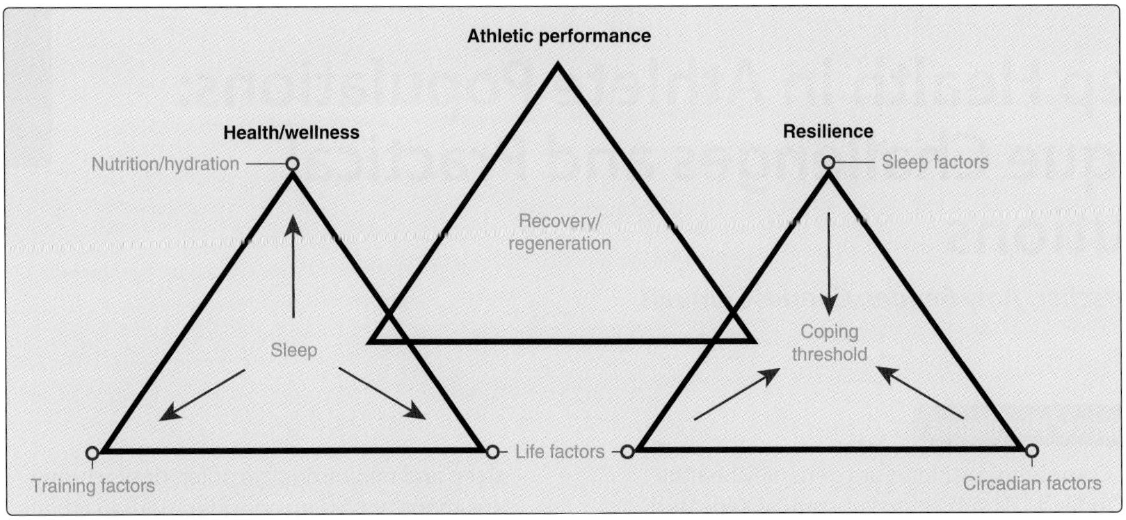

Figure 87.1 Relationship between the sleep state, recovery, and human performance in special populations, such as athletes and occupational athletes. The sleep state serves as the foundation of recovery and a critical physiologic state that stabilizes *human health and wellness,* whereas sleep and circadian factors must be managed to optimize *resilience* and prevent the negative consequences of chronic sleep restriction and circadian disruption due to travel and shift work. Optimal sustained performance is a function of the athlete's health, wellness, and resilience. (Reprinted with permission from Vila B, Samuels C, Wesensten NJ. Sleep problems in first responders and in deployed military personnel. Figure 76.6 in Kryger M, Roth T, Dement WC, eds. *Principles and Practice of Sleep Medicine*, 6th ed. p. 731.)

season. Sleep disorders reduce sleep quality and sleep quantity, which impairs recovery and degrades athletes' health, wellness, and, in some cases, their athletic performance. It is our impression that athletes often tend not to consider sleep and sleep health as important factors in managing their health. Sleep clinicians can have an important role in promoting athletes' sleep health and in educating coaches and support staff on the importance of sleep health and obtaining adequate quality sleep. Effective treatment may be complicated by demands of training, competition, and travel schedules. Use of sleep medications and/or stimulants must be carefully considered. The use of medication and the choice of the medication is complicated by the fact that it needs to comply with the World Anti-Doping Agency banned substance policies.

Across sports, insomnia and obstructive sleep apnea (OSA) are among the most common sleep disorders. Insomnia is the most common sleep disorder among athletes.[7] OSA is not common across all sports. OSA is most frequently observed in power sports, where athletes often have larger neck circumferences and a lower pressure differential keeping the airway open while sleeping. Movement disorders, such as restless legs syndrome and periodic limb movement disorder, are less common, but they are sometimes observed among athletes.[8,9] Our discussion here focuses on insomnia, OSA, and circadian rhythm disruptions. See Chapter 80 for further discussion of sleep disorders in operational settings.

Obstructive Sleep Apnea among Power Athletes

Athletes involved in sports where increased body mass is a performance advantage (e.g., football, rugby, and weightlifting) may be at a higher risk for OSA. As noted earlier, this is in part a result of increased neck circumference and a lower pressure differential making it difficult to maintain airway patency during sleep. In a study with professional football players, George and colleagues[10] (2003) found that 26.9% of the football players screened positive for OSA. Offensive and defensive linemen and players with a large neck circumference or a body mass index greater than 40 were at greater risk of OSA.[11] Treatment of OSA has tremendous potential to improve sleep, health, and possibly athletic performance.

Insomnia

Insomnia symptoms, such as difficulty initiating and maintaining sleep, are common complaints among athletes. The National College Health Assessment—a survey of 8683 United States collegiate athletes—found that 22% of the athletes had insomnia.[12] Similarly, a survey of French athletes found that 22% of the athletes had insomnia,[13] and a survey study of 107 ice hockey players found that 12% of the players had insomnia.[14] In contrast to these findings, a study with Italian Olympic athletes found that only 4% had insomnia.[15] The severity of the symptoms can differ across an athletic season. For example, a survey study of elite athletes found that 64% of the elite athletes reported poorer sleep quality the night before a competition.[16] The treatment of insomnia will depend, in part, on the sleep complaints, but in general, it is recommended that sleep clinicians avoid prescribing long-term use of sedatives and hypnotics. The cornerstone of management should be behavioral therapy for insomnia, and medication should be used only where indicated and as an adjunct to behavioral management strategies.

Circadian Rhythm Desynchrony among Athletes

Training, competition, and travel schedules can result in a misalignment between circadian time and local time. This is important among athletes because even small disruptions to the circadian system can have a large impact on sleep and potentially on their performance.[17,18] Thus identifying and addressing circadian misalignments and circadian rhythm disorders is essential. Of interest, preliminary research suggests that athletes tend to participate in sports that better align with their chronotype (i.e., their circadian preference).[19] For

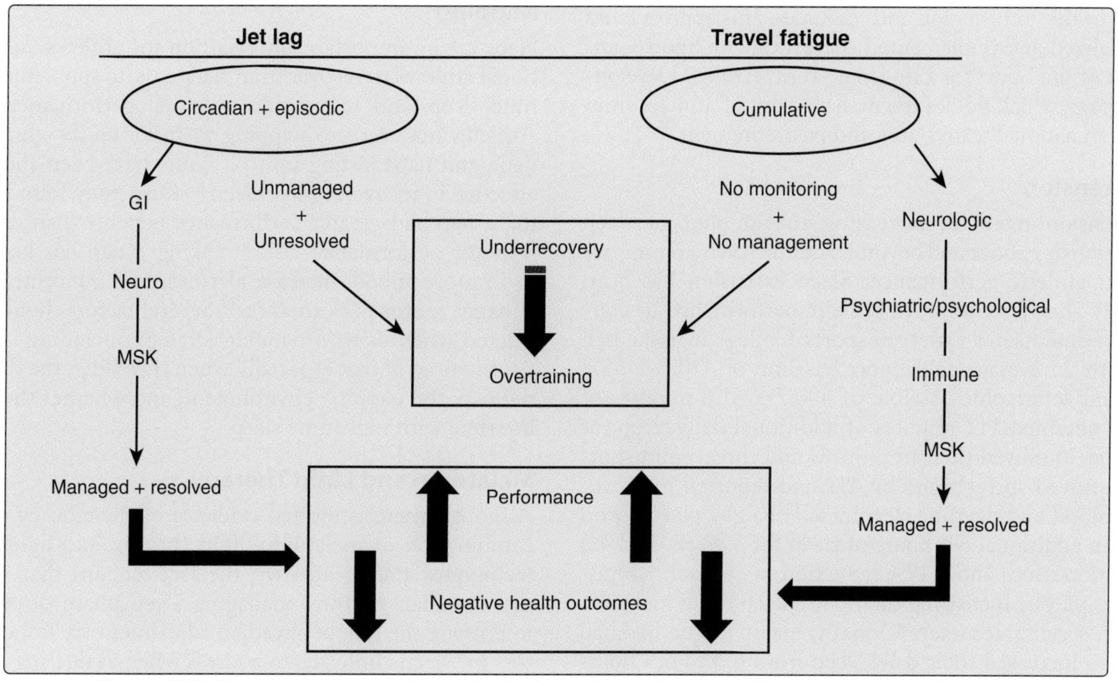

Figure 87.2 The conceptual goal of managing jet lag and travel fatigue in athletes is to preserve the recovery process to prevent underrecovery and overtraining syndrome. Jet lag occurs as an episodic phenomenon, whereas travel fatigue is cumulative. Athletes traveling at high frequency but minimal distance are more at risk for the consequences of travel fatigue and need to have a monitoring system in place. Those athletes who travel long distances with low frequency need to have the jet lag managed. Sleep clinicians must understand the nature of the stress of travel to manage the athlete effectively and proactively. GI, gastrointestinal; MSK, musculoskeletal; Neuro, neurologic. (From Samuels CH. Jet lag and travel fatigue: a comprehensive management plan for sport medicine physicians and high-performance support teams. *Clin J Sport Med.* 2012;22(3):268–73.)

example, sports that require early-morning awakenings, such as swimming, tend to attract athletes who are morning types. Chronotype research in athlete populations reveals there is a high prevalence of morning types in various sports.[18–20] Silvia and colleagues found that evening-type athletes tend to have a higher prevalence of sleep disturbances.[21] Samuels and colleagues[18a] and others have found that there is a high prevalence of morning types in various sports,[20–22] and evening-type athletes tend to have a higher prevalence of sleep disturbances.[23]

Jet lag and travel fatigue are two important factors to consider for traveling athletes.[24] Jet lag is characterized by misalignment between circadian time and local time, and it is associated with short-term sleep disturbances, gastrointestinal symptoms, and physical discomfort. Jet lag is particularly evident after traveling east for three-plus time zones or traveling west for four-plus time zones.[25,26] Travel fatigue is a constellation of physical and cognitive symptoms caused by travel but independent of the misalignment between circadian time and local time.[27] Figure 87.2 describes the relationships between jet lag and travel fatigue and how these factors can impair recovery and contribute to overtraining. Melatonin, light therapy, light-blocking techniques, conservative use of sedatives, and other approaches can help mitigate and manage circadian disruptions associated with travel. See Chapter 81 for further discussion of jet lag.

Screening for a Sleep Disorder

Standardized sleep screening questionnaires can be a starting point to quickly identify athletes with potential sleep disorders. The most widely used sleep questionnaire to date has been the PSQI[26]; however, there have been questions regarding whether the PSQI is valid measure among athletes.[27] The Athlete Sleep Screening Questionnaire (ASSQ) is a newer sleep questionnaire that was developed to detect clinically significant sleep disturbances specifically among athletes.[28] The ASSQ determines whether athletes have no sleep problems, mild sleep problems, moderate sleep problems, or severe sleep problems, and then provides recommendations based on the severity for further intervention. Finally, the Athlete Sleep Behavior Questionnaire (ASBQ) assesses maladaptive sleep behaviors and promotes sleep optimization; however, it has not been validated and requires further study for formal clinical validation.[29]

Daily sleep diaries are used more frequently in sport than sleep screening questionnaires. They are an inexpensive, efficient way to collect daily sleep data without substantial recall bias. Wearable technology is increasingly being used to collect sleep data, and the devices tend to be more accurate than sleep screening questionnaires. Ibáñez and colleagues[29] (2018) conducted a review of the literature and found that wearable devices have sensitivities between 88% to 98% and specificities between 20% and 52%.[30] Accurately collecting sleep data with daily monitoring and wearable technology provides invaluable information on athletes' sleep routines, and these data can be used to advise athletes on how they can improve their sleep routines or implement napping strategies. However, and of importance, wearable technology does not screen for or detect clinically significant sleep disturbance that could indicate that there is a sleep disorder.

Selected Interventions

The basic principles of sleep health management are increasing total sleep time, screening for and treating sleep disorders, managing circadian disruption, and providing athletes and the teams with sleep health information and resources. This approach has been formalized and implemented successfully by Sport Canada as part of the Sport for Life Long-Term Athlete Development program, which guides the management of athletes from childhood to national team status and postretirement.[31]

Sleep Extension

Sleep extension refers to increasing the amount of sleep obtained each day above and beyond baseline levels, to improve subsequent athletic performance. Sleep extension has been consistently shown to improve athletic performance in controlled experiments in a variety of sports. Collegiate basketball players with an average self-report baseline of 470.0 ± 65.9 minutes and actigraphic baseline of 400.7 ± 61.8 minutes of sleep who obtained 111 minutes of additional daily sleep for 5 to 7 weeks improved their free-throw and three-point shots by 9%, improved sprint times by 4%, and reported improvements in mood and daytime sleepiness.[32] Rugby players who obtained an additional 6% hours of sleep for 3 weeks had 4% faster reaction times and a 19% reduction in cortisol.[33] Similarly, tennis players increasing their daily sleep times had a 6% increase in serving accuracy.[34] Finally, major league baseball players who increased their daily sleep from 6.3 to 6.9 hours for 5 nights had improvements in visuospatial search response times.[35] In addition to sleep extension, sleep banking can be used to address anticipated sleep restriction that may arise due to travel, life factors such as family commitments or stressful life events, and training/competition schedules that may affect sleep opportunity. However, sleep banking has not been studied in athlete populations specifically.[36]

Napping

Naps are an important intervention for athletes and occupational athletes to recover from sleep loss, to supplement nighttime sleep, and to provide potential performance benefits. Athletes may turn to napping to make up for chronic sleep debt, and naps lasting up to 2 hours have been shown to be effective in recovering lost sleep.[37] One study found that taking a nap had greater performance benefits than caffeine on a motor performance task.[38] Taking a nap has been shown to improve mood, increase alertness and concentration, and enhance motor performance.[39] Several factors should be considered when using a napping strategy, including sleep inertia; the time of day, especially when travelling; the duration of the nap; the napping environment; and whether the nap may interfere with nighttime sleep.

Melatonin and Light Therapy

Although there is limited evidence of the efficacy of using a combination of melatonin, light therapy, and light-blocking techniques among athletes, the fact remains that stabilizing the circadian rhythm, managing sleep phase disorders, and improving the rate of circadian adjustment are important factors for sleep clinicians to address when evaluating and treating athletes who travel.

Behavioral Sleep Medicine

Behavioral sleep medicine interventions should focus on techniques for reducing arousal, managing sleep routine, increasing total sleep time, napping strategies, and mitigating the negative effects of technology on sleep health.[40–42]

CLINICAL PEARL

It is important for sleep clinicians and researchers who encounter athletes in their work to have a focused approach that considers the fundamental differences in the lifestyle, stressors, and limitations athletes face that have a direct effect on sleep health. Most important, clinicians and researchers must understand the importance of sleep as a key method of recovery in this special population. Recovery is critical for functional resilience and maintenance of health and wellness in an otherwise healthy population that is expected to perform at exceptional levels. Screening for sleep disturbance and sleep disorders is the first step in a focused, systematic approach, followed by appropriate investigations and then interventions that are tailored to the lifestyle and demands of the athlete. Applying standard approaches used in medical and psychiatric populations for sleep and circadian rhythm disturbance rarely are feasible and often fail in athlete populations (Fig. 87.3).

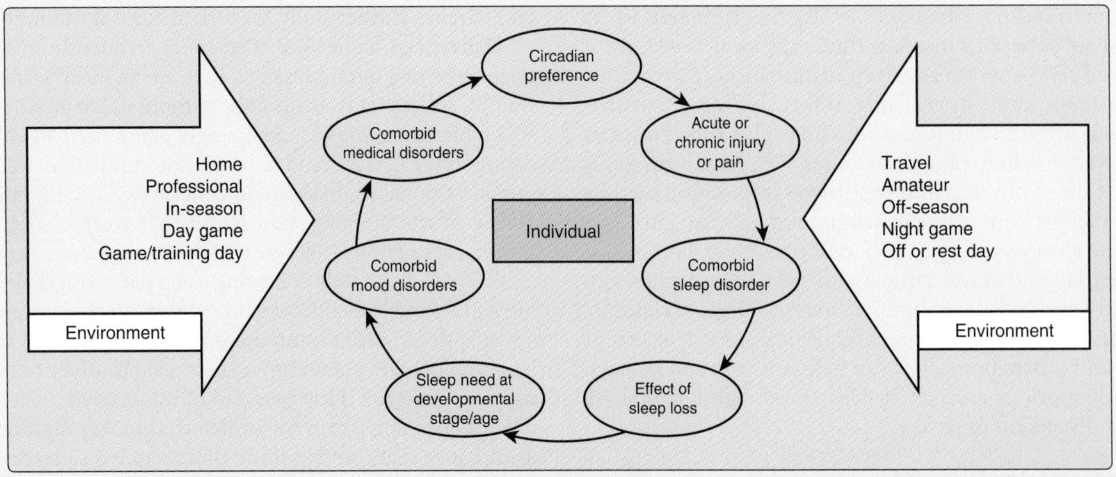

Figure 87.3 Interplay of major factors that influence sleep need to be considered by sleep clinicians when dealing with this special population. An individual athlete's sleep may be challenged by several static or dynamic situations, such as mood, injury, or sleep disorders, which need to be identified and properly addressed. There is also external pressure on sleep from the environment of athletics, often beyond an individual athlete's control, which poses unique circumstances that can further promote or degrade sleep. (Reproduced with permission from Kutscher, SJ. Sleep & elite athletic performance. *Pract Neurol.* 2019;18(3):41, 47–48, 52.)

SUMMARY

Athletes are generally a healthy population that undertake and live a life that puts substantial demands on human physiology, psychology, and metabolic health. Whether the clinician encounters an elite Olympic/professional athlete, a university student athlete, or a high school athlete, the fact is that for the most part these are healthy people in demanding situations that seriously impact sleep health from both a sleep and circadian perspective. Understanding the unique demands of these special populations and learning the unique methods of assessment and intervention will provide the sleep medicine clinician with a more confident, effective, and successful approach and relationship with this special population of sleep medicine patients/clients.

SELECTED READINGS

Gupta L, Morgan K, Gilchrest S. Does elite sport degrade sleep quality? A systematic review. *Sports Med.* 2017;47(7):1317–1333.

Kellmann M, Bertollo M, Bosquet L, et al. Recovery and performance in sport: consensus statement. *Int J Sports Physiol Perform.* 2018;13(2):240–245.

Raikes AC, Athey A, Alfonso-Miller P, et al. Insomnia and daytime sleepiness: risk factors for sports-related concussion. *Sleep Med.* 2019;58:66–74.

Souabni M, Hammouda O, Romdhani M, et. al. Benefits of daytime napping opportunity on physical and cognitive performances in physically active participants: a systematic review [published online ahead of print, 2021 May 27]. *Sports Med.* 2021;10.1007/s40279-021-01482-1.

Vitale KC, Owens R, Hopkins SR, et al. Sleep hygiene for optimizing recovery in athletes: review and recommendations. *Int J Sports Med.* 2019;40(8):535–543.

A complete reference list can be found online at ExpertConsult.com.

Chapter 88

Assessment of the Occupational Sleep Medicine Field

Thomas J. Balkin

Chapter Highlights

- Occupational sleep medicine is a new field that is growing in importance and relevance as the number of shift workers expands to meet the needs of our global, 24-hour society and economy.
- Fatigue risk management systems (FRMSs) offer several advantages over traditional "hours-of-service" regulations, including policies and procedures that enable identification of potentially dangerous decrements in alertness and performance in individual operators in real time, and they facilitate the timely application of appropriate interventions.
- As a component of FRMSs, mathematical performance prediction models (MPPMs) facilitate interpretation of sleep-wake data and the relationships between sleep-wake histories, circadian rhythmicity, and fatigue and performance. There are several impediments slowing the rate at which MPPMs are adopted in operational settings, including a lack of standards for model validation and their failure to account for the many factors that affect fatigue and performance in operational settings.
- Epidemiologic studies have revealed associations between shift work and a variety of pathologies. Animal studies suggest substantial relationships between sleep loss and pathophysiologic changes involving neuroinflammatory processes, beta-amyloid and tau deposition, and oxidative damage, possibly mediated by reduced glymphatic flow.
- As scientific findings continue to accrue, it is anticipated that governments and industries will increasingly adopt policies that reflect not only the short-term effects of shift work on safety and performance but also the long-term effects of shift work on health.

ASSESSMENT OF THE OCCUPATIONAL SLEEP MEDICINE FIELD

The field of "occupational medicine" is the assessment and treatment of work-related injuries and illnesses. It has its beginnings in antiquity, with an early description of the negative effects of work on health dating back to approximately 1700 BCE.[1] The term *occupational sleep medicine* was first coined by Belenky and colleagues in 2011,[2] and as its name implies, this nascent field integrates occupational medicine and sleep medicine. Chief among the reasons that this field was conceived was the recognition that knowledge about sleep and its effects on performance could be usefully applied to enhance both safety and productivity in operational environments. This is a goal that continues to grow in relevance and importance as shift work expands to meet the needs of our global, 24-hour society and economy.

Sleep loss and circadian desynchrony are potential problems for workers in all operational settings but are most prevalent in occupations that require shift work, transmeridian travel, and/or on-call work. As explicated in the other chapters of the Occupational Sleep Medicine section, sleep loss and circadian desynchrony can result in alertness and performance deficits[3,4] and increased risk of accidents.[5] As such, there has long been a general appreciation for the importance of workers obtaining adequate sleep, particularly in operations such as aviation, where lapses in attention, reduced situational awareness, impaired judgment, slow reaction times, and other sleep-loss–induced deficits constitute clear safety risks to both the workers themselves, their coworkers, and the public.[6,7]

Given the clear safety risks, any conditions that result in acute or chronic sleep loss, circadian desynchrony, and/or poor sleep quality (i.e., sleep of diminished recuperative value) that could potentially degrade the alertness and performance of individuals or groups in operational settings fits within the field of occupational sleep medicine.

SLEEP DISORDERS

An important question that occupational sleep medicine researchers and practitioners have begun to grapple with is how to deal with sleep disorders that degrade alertness and performance in operational settings.[8] This is a problem that has increasingly captured public attention over the past several years, likely as a function of growing media attention. For example, after two serious commuter train crashes in 2016 and 2017 in the New York City area, one resulting in a fatality and each resulting in injuries to more than 100 people, it was reported that safety board officials concluded that both train engineers suffered from obstructive sleep apnea, and this was presumed to be a proximate cause of both accidents (https://www.nytimes.com/2018/02/06/nyregion/train-crash-sleep-apnea.html). Such tragedies raise important, difficult questions such as: How should these sleep disorders be detected in operational settings as opposed to clinical settings? If detected, how should the workers be treated, and should treatment be monitored given the potential risks of having a sleep disorder in a safety-sensitive operation? These are only some of the practical and ethical conundrums currently facing safety experts, clinicians, insurance companies, lawyers, researchers, and regulators concerned with mitigating the effects of sleep disorders in operational settings.

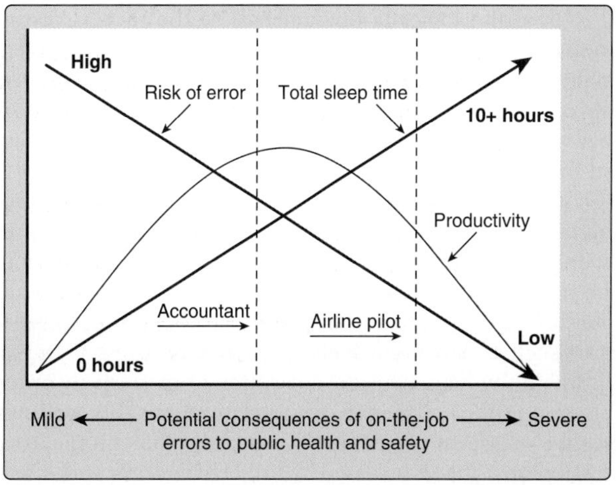

Figure 88.1 A depiction of the interaction of factors that are at least implicitly considered when determining the extent to which timing and duration of work shifts are regulated. As shown here, the risk of making an error on the job is reduced as the number of hours of sleep per night is increased. Productivity initially increases as a function of hours of sleep but levels off at approximately 7 to 8 hours total sleep time for most adults and declines with increasing hours of sleep (i.e., as diminishing returns in terms of productivity are realized as extended sleep time begins to cut into available work time). For airline pilots, the potential consequences of errors are so dire that it makes sense to sacrifice productivity for reduced risk of errors. In occupations for which the consequences of error are less dire (e.g., with respect to public health), it makes more sense to accept a greater risk of error so that productivity is maximized.

THE GENERAL POPULATION OF WORKERS

Of course, the problem of sleepiness- and circadian desynchrony–related performance deficits and risk in operational settings is not limited to workers suffering from sleep disorders. It has been recognized for centuries that working excessively long and continuous shifts can exact a considerable toll on otherwise healthy, normal individuals.[9] This is, in part, why policies have been created that specify duty time limitations and minimum rest break requirements. The recent trend, however, has been toward the development and implementation of evidence-based rules and regulations for managing work hours that aim to improve the safety of workers, as well as those put at risk by fatigued workers. With the development and implementation of rules and regulations that incorporate sleep and circadian science, the overall trend continues to move in a positive direction.

Although the negative effects of sleep loss and circadian desynchrony are not limited to alertness and cognitive performance deficits,[10] it is thought that occupations that primarily entail physical labor are less impacted by sleep loss than occupations that primarily entail mental effort.[11] And, of course, the potential seriousness of job-related errors vary widely as a function of the nature of the occupation. As an obvious example, the potential consequences of errors by nuclear power plant operators (e.g., death and injury on a large scale and environmental devastation) are more dire than the potential consequences of errors by workers at package sorting facilities (e.g., lost or damaged packages, injuries associated with lifting and handling of packages). As notionally depicted in Figure 88.1, the potential for catastrophic errors varies by occupation and largely determines the risk/productivity trade-off that society or government regulations deem acceptable for that occupation.

HOURS-OF-SERVICE RULES

It is notable that for most of the past approximately 200 years the primary (and often only) "tools in the toolbox" to address workplace alertness and performance deficits and their attendant risks have been manipulations of work-rest schedules, also known as hours-of-service (HOS) rules and regulations that limit the duration of allowable work hours for various occupations. Without a doubt, when introduced, HOS regulations provided a way to improve the health, safety, and quality of life of workers. That said, there are obvious limitations to their effectiveness: (1) Although work schedules that allow for adequate sleep opportunities are clearly a minimum requirement, such work schedules do not guarantee that workers will actually obtain adequate sleep on any given night (e.g., due to child care requirements, family emergencies, transient insomnia associated with anxiety-inducing events, chronic sleep disorders, etc.), and (2) HOS regulations fail to account for individual differences in both sleep needs and sensitivity to the effects of sleep loss. Thus one-size-fits-all HOS regulations might provide dangerously inadequate protection for some individuals, for instance, for the rare individual who obtains 7 hours of sleep per night but needs 9-plus hours of nightly sleep to maintain normal daytime alertness and functioning, or for those who are especially sensitive to the alertness- and performance-decrementing effects of sleep loss.

FATIGUE RISK MANAGEMENT SYSTEMS

To a significant extent, some of the inadequacies of HOS rules have been addressed by the addition of fatigue risk management systems (FRMSs) in a number of operational settings, often on top of existing HOS rules. Although the particulars vary from one industry and occupation to another, and from one FRMS to another, comprehensive FRMSs generally include several components: fatigue management policies that comply with industry regulations; relevant education and training programs; processes for reporting subjective fatigue by operators; procedures for investigating, reporting, and recording possible fatigue-related events; and the ability to subsequently implement and assess the efficacy of interventions designed to reduce fatigue-related risk.[12] Also included in FRMSs, and logically fundamental to the success of such systems, is the ability to actually monitor and measure operationally relevant levels of fatigue. This is because, as succinctly summarized by Dr. Greg Belenky (personal communication), "That which cannot be measured in the field, cannot be managed in the field."

Of course, in most operational environments, the most straightforward way to assess sleepiness and fatigue is to simply rely on the operators' self assessments. Such self-assessments largely reflect the duration and timing of work shifts, which can affect sleep timing and duration, but they can also reflect factors such as perceived levels of job-related stress.[13] In general, for individuals who do not suffer from sleep disorders, subjective ratings of sleepiness correlate reasonably well with objective measures of sleepiness, especially the chronic, trait-like sleepiness that is assessed by subjective rating scales, such as the Epworth Sleepiness Scale.[14] However, for more acute fluctuations in sleepiness, such as those that may occur across an 8-hour work shift, the relationship between subjective and objective measures is more tenuous (e.g., see Saletin and colleagues[15] and Tremaine and colleagues[16]), and objective measures are often more sensitive to the effects of acute sleep loss than subjective self-assessments.[17] This is especially true for individuals suffering from sleep disorders, such as obstructive sleep apnea[18] and narcolepsy,[19] who may experience some subjective habituation to reduced alertness over time. In addition, subjective measures are more likely to be skewed by non-fatigue-related factors in real-world operational settings, where operators may be hesitant to report excessive fatigue for a variety of non-fatigue-related reasons, including fears about job security, overconfidence in personal abilities, and reluctance to burden coworkers with extra work, to name but a few. Accordingly it is reasonable to expect that the use of objective fatigue and performance measures will generally enhance safety and productivity to a greater extent than exclusive reliance on subjective self-assessments. However, of course, self-assessments of excessive fatigue should always be taken seriously, regardless of what is indicated by objective measures.

Efforts to objectively identify workers who become debilitated while performing safety-critical jobs, and efforts to mitigate the consequences of these events, have a long history. One early example is the "driver safety device" (DSD, also known as "dead man switch") that was first installed in streetcars in the 1890s. This device required the driver to maintain pressure on a lever while the streetcar was in motion. If the driver fell asleep or lost consciousness for any reason, the resultant removal of pressure on the lever would automatically activate the brakes. Therefore this device helped protect passengers from a driver who suddenly became totally incapacitated. However, it did not protect passengers from a driver who was only partially impaired (e.g., sleepy or intoxicated to a potentially dangerous extent), as long as that driver maintained consciousness and enough self-awareness to sustain pressure on the DSD lever.

More recent efforts have appropriately been focused on development of methods to identify more sensitive indicators of impairment that potentially reflect deficits in operationally relevant mental capabilities, such as judgment, situation awareness, and problem solving, and/or methods that indicate that an operator's fatigue and performance is trending in a negative direction. These have included behavioral measures (e.g., head nodding[20]), measures of physiologic state (e.g., via psychophysiologic measures reflecting reduced alertness, such as frequency and duration of eyelid closures,[21] increased theta activity in the electroencephalogram,[20] etc.), and/or detection of actual performance decrements with embedded measures that suggest reduced operator alertness (e.g., lane deviations by those operating a motor vehical[22]). Such measures can be used to trigger an alarm when a meaningful threshold has been crossed, alerting the affected operator, and possibly those up the chain of command, that an intervention may be warranted.

Relative to HOS regulations alone, the advantages conferred by an FRMS that uses fatigue monitoring are clear: Potentially dangerous decrements in alertness and performance can be identified in real time, facilitating the ability to intervene in an optimally timely manner. In addition, FRMSs also introduce the prospect of increased flexibility in work scheduling because work hours can be more fluidly determined based on operator performance capacity, both extant and anticipated (see next section on mathematical modeling), instead of being based solely on rigid HOS regulations. However, although FRMSs constitute a significant leap forward toward the goal of improved workplace safety and performance, they, like the HOS rules that preceded them, are not without problems. For example, the relationship between measures of drowsiness and meaningful risk to performance can be difficult to assess.[21] Accordingly it can also be challenging to determine the correct threshold for triggering alarms based on operator monitoring, a difficulty that has considerable implications for the ultimate utility of an FRMS: If the threshold is set too low (e.g., if an alarm is triggered in response to normal fluctuations of daytime alertness that, in reality, do not appreciably alter the risk of error or accident), then those alarms could eventually lose their informational value and be ignored. However, if the threshold is set too high, then potentially dangerous decrements in alertness and performance will be missed, obviating the utility of monitoring operator fatigue.

MATHEMATICAL PERFORMANCE PREDICTION MODELS

Mathematical performance prediction models (MPPMs) are increasingly being used in occupational settings. MPPMs predict sleepiness, fatigue, and/or performance based on recent sleep history and circadian rhythm (see Chapter 83 by Riedy and colleagues for a review). These MPPMs incorporate our scientific understanding of sleep and circadian rhythms and their relationships with alertness, sleepiness, fatigue, and/or performance. Although presently used most often as a tool to inform construction of work-rest schedules (e.g., trip schedules in aviation), their greater utility will be realized as they are increasingly incorporated into FRMSs. Indeed, their utility is already expanding from construction of work-rest schedules to the examination of fatigue likelihood in postaccident investigations and the development of safety cases. In the future, MPPM predictions could also be used effectively in occupational settings to (1) suggest prophylactic interventions before significant alertness/performance decrements are manifest and/or (2) continuously and automatically update operator's predicted level of impairment when partnered with continuous monitoring of the operator's sleep-wake behaviors.

IMPEDIMENTS TO IMPLEMENTATION OF MATHEMATICAL PERFORMANCE PREDICTION MODELS

Mathematical Performance Prediction Models Are Based on Group Data

MPPMs are developed based on group data. Consequently, their predictions reflect the alertness and performance of the "average person," and their utility for predicting an individual's performance depends on the extent to which that person's "need for sleep" and "sensitivity to sleep loss" approximate the group averages. This drawback is currently being addressed via development of at least one individualized MPPM (i.e., the Unified Model of Performance, instantiated in the "2B-Alert" app) that "learns" how individuals respond to sleep loss.[23] One drawback to this approach is that it requires the individual to occasionally perform a Psychomotor Vigilance Test (PVT). Importantly, the more often PVTs are performed, and the greater the variability in nightly sleep durations that precede these PVTs, the more accurate the individualization process.

Mathematical Performance Prediction Models are Based on Psychomotor Vigilance Test Data

Another criticism of MPPMs is that they are based (largely) on PVT data, a measure for which the real-world operational relevance is largely unknown. Another way to frame this problem is that MPPMs lack a meaningful, widely understood performance decrement scale. There are currently three potential, non–mutually exclusive solutions to this problem. (1) The effects of sleep loss on more operationally meaningful performance measures could be tested, providing the data necessary to construct occupation-specific MPPMs. *Note:* Creating an occupation-specific MPPM would be a costly process that would be logistically and practically difficult or even impractical for many occupations. (2) MPPM predictions can be reported in terms of an already widely accepted impairment scale (i.e., blood alcohol concentration [BAC]).[24] However, despite the fact that there is overlap in the types of deficits resulting from sleep loss and alcohol intoxication, the overlap is not perfect (e.g., alcohol has a greater effect on hand-eye coordination). (3) A third possibility is that a new, PVT-based scale could eventually acquire meaningfulness and acceptance with its continued use,[25] in much the same way that BAC—a measure that was probably mostly devoid of meaning for a majority of the populace when it was first introduced as a scale of sobriety—has now become a standard measure and a well-understood term within the lexicons of most modern nations.

Failure to Account for Interventions

Another criticism of MPPMs is that they do not currently or adequately account for all factors that putatively degrade operational performance (e.g., time on task and cognitive load) or improve operational performance (e.g., rest breaks, stimulants, and other fatigue mitigation strategies). In addition, experienced operators may develop and use their own risk-mitigation strategies to ensure adequate performance and safety when fatigued (see Chapter 86). As such, the MPPM predictions may not necessarily reflect the true risk of error or an accident.

Especially conspicuous is the fact that most models do not account for the alertness and performance sustaining effects of even common interventions such as caffeine, which is probably the most widely available and used intervention to combat alertness and performance deficits in the world. An exception is the MPPM currently under development by U.S. Army scientists (i.e., the Unified Model of Performance), which provides evidence-based predictions of the performance effects of caffeine under conditions of sleep loss[26] and guidance regarding optimal timing and dosing regimens of caffeine during sleep loss.[27] It is anticipated that as MPPMs continue to be developed they will account for increasing numbers of factors that contribute to work performance variance and as such will be increasingly incorporated into FRMS in a variety of occupational settings.

Lack of Validation Standards

Last, the fact that there are no agreed-upon standards for the validation of MPPMs, which are often proprietary, constitutes a potential impediment to their widespread adoption, or at least slows the rate at which they are likely to be adopted widely. Because there are no standards, it is always possible to argue that more data and research is needed before a model can be appropriately implemented in a particular operational setting. Nevertheless, even in the absence of such standards, MPPMs are increasingly being used by governments and industry. This may be, at least in part, because model-based alertness/performance predictions are not only based on scientific evidence, but they are also generally consistent with logic and human experience. What the models add is objectivity and specificity by quantifying the level of predicted performance and/or risk produced by the confluence of relevant factors such as the phase of the "circadian rhythm of alertness," "recent sleep history," and perhaps at some future point, "time on task" and/or "cognitive load," presuming these latter two factors are found to account for a meaningful portion of the variance in performance and risk.

CHALLENGES TO ORTHODOXY

Although the sleep duration-mediated trade-off between productivity and risk depicted in Figure 88.1 is straightforward, it has been argued that this relationship does not necessarily reflect the relationship between impairment and risk for all occupations. For example, and very notably, it has been argued that the relationship does not apply to US medical residents because of the well-documented risks associated with medical handoffs (i.e., transferring responsibility and information about patients' extant health status from one medical professional to another). It is reasoned that because handoffs are risky to patient health, patient safety is enhanced by keeping the number of handoffs to a minimum, which is accomplished by subjecting medical residents to shift durations of up to 28 continuous hours. This, of course, is a level of acute sleep loss that produces significant reductions in prefrontal cortical activity and reduced cognitive performance,[28] including decrements in the performance of medical personnel,[29] which logic dictates should constitute an obvious threat to patient safety. In fact, based on the relationship depicted in Figure 88.1, it can be surmised that the riskiness of medical handoffs is most likely exacerbated if those on either the giving and/or receiving end of this information transfer are sleep deprived. Nevertheless, there is some evidence that patient safety is not appreciably reduced by these long shifts,[30,31] possibly (although this is conjecture) because of fail-safe procedures

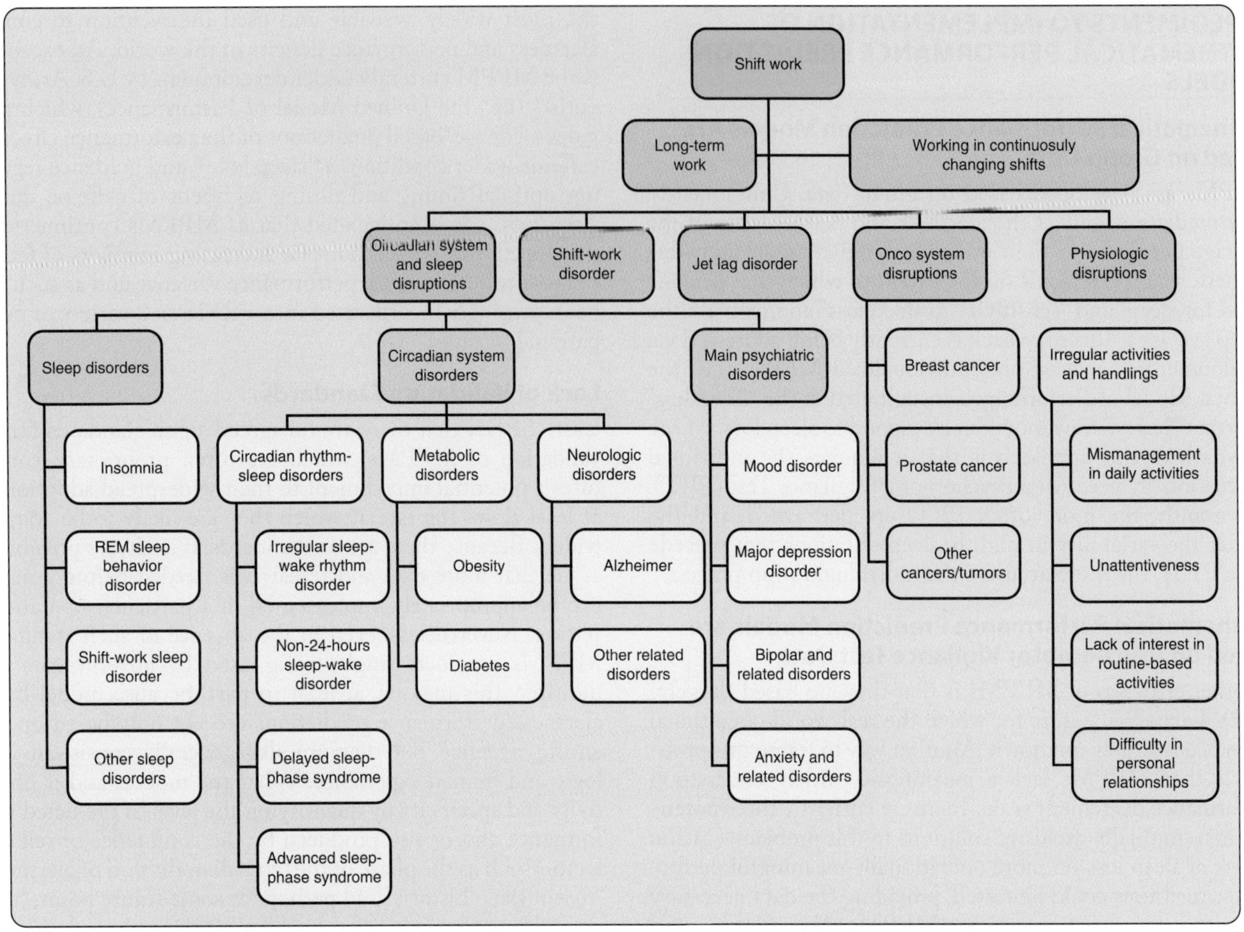

Figure 88.2 A list of disorders categorized according to putative shift-work–related pathophysiologic mechanisms. (Reprinted from Khan S, Duan P, Yao L, Hou H. Shiftwork-mediated disruptions of circadian rhythms and sleep homeostasis cause serious health problems. *Int J Genomics.* 2018;2018:8576890. https://doi.org/10.1155/2018/8576890)

and shared responsibility for patient care and safety that tend to reduce the consequences of errors by fatigued medical residents.

It is beyond the scope of this chapter to review all the literature related to this topic or to render an opinion regarding the relative merits and risks of continuously working medical residents on shifts of up to 28 hours' duration. But it can be predicted that the shift-work schedules of medical residents will at some not-too-distant point be brought more into line with those working in other occupations. This is not because it is likely that questions regarding the relative risks to patient safety will have been settled, but because it will be determined that patient safety is not the sole factor that should be considered when determining shift parameters: Increasingly taken into consideration will be the health and well-being of the medical residents working these shifts.

EFFECTS OF SHIFT WORK ON HEALTH

As indicated at the beginning of the present chapter, the birth of occupational medicine can be traced to approximately 1700 BCE, when a description of the negative effects of work on health were first recorded. In contrast, the relatively nascent field of occupational sleep medicine has, up to this point, been concerned primarily with facilitating short-term alertness and performance of workers in the operational environment, so as to enhance productivity and prophylactically reduce the risk of accidents and injuries. But based on a growing body of scientific evidence, the field of occupational sleep medicine is currently expanding its scope, with an increasing emphasis on the potential effects of shift work and sleep loss on the health and well-being of workers, thus harkening back to the ancient roots of the occupational medicine field.

The evidence that shift work has long-term, negative effects on the health of workers is swelling.[32,33] It is often unclear whether the negative effects of shift work are due directly to circadian desynchrony, the sleep disturbances and sleep loss that invariably accompany circadian desynchrony, or the combined effects of both.[34] It is also possible that some negative health outcomes are due to, or exacerbated by, secondary effects of shift work, including dietary choices[35] and artificial light exposure at night, which has been associated with increased risk of breast cancer in night-shift workers.[36] As depicted in Figure 88.2, there are currently a wide variety of disorders putatively associated with shift work,[37] although it should be noted that the quantity and quality of scientific evidence linking shift work to these various disorders varies considerably.

Not surprising, much of the evidence showing significant associations between shift work and long-term health outcomes is from epidemiologic studies and is therefore correlational. However, there is an expanding body of experimental evidence from animal studies that not only confirms that sleep loss, which is a virtually unavoidable consequence of shift work, has long-term effects on health but also suggests possible physiologic mechanisms that may underlie a cause and effect relationship. Animal studies to determine the neurochemical, neurophysiologic, and neurostructural consequences of sleep restriction currently point to three possible pathophysiologic processes.

Neuroinflammation

Sleep disruption has been shown to upregulate proinflammatory cytokines in the brain,[38] most likely the result of microglial activation.[39] And neuroinflammatory activation of both microglia and astrocytes after sleep loss have been shown to result in phagocytosis of cortical synaptic elements.[40] Additional studies have similarly revealed dystrophic changes in cortical and subcortical neurons and synapses during sleep deprivation.[41]

Oxidative Damage

Likewise, several studies suggest that sleep deprivation is associated with oxidative stress in animals.[42] And in mice it has been found that sleep restriction is associated with the generation of reactive oxygen species and depletion of antioxidant enzymes in the locus coeruleus and orexinergic/hypocretinergic neurons in the lateral hypothalamus, potentially resulting in neuronal death and attendant loss of efferent cortical projections from these nuclei.[43]

Tau and Beta-Amyloid Deposition

In addition, beta-amyloid[44] and tau protein,[45] both of which are implicated in the pathophysiology of Alzheimer disease, are increased in central nervous system interstitial fluid in rodents after acute sleep deprivation. It has been hypothesized that this is a consequence of sleep loss–mediated reduction in glymphatic flow.[46]

Although the extent to which neuroinflammation and oxidative damage mediate glymphatic flow (which may, in turn, mediate tau and beta-amyloid deposition in the brain) is unclear, the accrued evidence in this area points to the strong possibility that these processes either singly or interactively underlie at least some of the disorders associated with sleep restriction that are listed in Figure 88.2.

IMPLICATIONS FOR POLICY

Consistent with Australia's well-deserved reputation for leading-edge research on, and implementation of, fatigue management practices, the Parliament of Australia in 2019 became the first government entity to formally acknowledge the emergent scientific evidence broadly linking shift work to health. The first recommendation in their official report on "Sleep Health Awareness" is "Committee recommends that the Australian Government prioritize sleep health as a national priority and recognize its importance to health and well-being alongside fitness and nutrition." In addition, the 11th recommendation in this report included the suggestion that the government fund research focused on "The impact of long-term shift work on sleep health and potential measures to minimize the associated health risks…" (https://www.aph.gov.au/Parliamentary_Business/Committees/House/Health_Aged_Care_and_Sport/SleepHealthAwareness/Report/section?id=committees%2Freportrep%2F024220%2F26554).

Given the growing public awareness and appreciation of the effects of inadequate sleep on safety and performance in operational settings, as well as the accrual of scientific evidence suggesting a causal relationship between shift work and long-term negative health outcomes, it seems likely that the governments of other industrialized nations will soon take notice and follow suit.

CLINICAL PEARL

Relative to hours-of-service regulations alone, evidence-based fatigue risk management systems (FRMSs) can enhance both safety and productivity in operational environments. Accordingly it is anticipated that further development and adoption of FRMSs in commercial and government operations will continue to proliferate. However, because scientific evidence that shift work contributes to negative health outcomes is rapidly accruing, it is likely that these long-term health effects will increasingly be reflected in the next generation of shift-work policies and regulations and in the FRMSs that will be used to implement them.

SUMMARY

Occupational sleep medicine encompasses all operationally relevant issues pertaining to sleep, sleep loss, circadian desynchrony, and sleep disorders. FRMSs constitute a significant advancement in the management of operational safety and performance. FRMSs include several components, but their utility ultimately derives from technology: the ability to sensitively measure and accurately monitor operationally relevant levels of fatigue and performance and to use these data streams to predict future operational performance and associated risk (e.g., as output from a MPPM). In addition, because scientific evidence that shift work produces long-term negative effects on health is rapidly accruing, it is anticipated that government and industry policies will be adopted that increasingly reflect not only the short-term effects of shift work on safety and performance but also the long-term effects of shift work on health.

ACKNOWLEDGMENTS

This research was supported in part by an appointment to the Research Participation Program at the Walter Reed Army Institute of Research, administered by the Oak Ridge Institute for Science and Education through an interagency agreement between the U.S. Department of Energy and U.S. Army Medical Research and Development Command. The views expressed in this article are those of the author and do not reflect the official policy or position of the Department of the Army, the Department of Defense, the U.S. Government, or any of the government institutions with which the author is affiliated.

SELECTED READINGS

Abushov BM. Morphofunctional analysis of the effects of total sleep deprivation on the CNS in rats. *Neurosci Behav Physiol.* 2010;40(4):403–409.

Belenky G, Wu LJ, Jackson ML. Occupational sleep medicine: practice and promise. *Prog Brain Res.* 2011;190:189–203.

Bellesi M, de Vivo L, Chini M, et al. Sleep loss promotes astrocytic phagocytosis and microglial activation in mouse cerebral cortex. *J Neurosci. 2017.* 2017;37(21):5263–5273.

Capaldi VF, Balkin TJ, Mysliwiec V. Optimizing sleep in the military: Challenges and Opportunities. *Chest.* 2019;155(1):215–226.

Dawson D, Ferguson SA, Vincent GE. Safety implications of fatigue and sleep inertia for emergency services personnel. *Sleep Med Rev.* 2021;55:101386.
Gander P, Hartley H, Powell D, et al. Fatigue risk management: Organizational factors at the regulatory and industry/company level. *Accid Anal Prev.* 2011;43:573–590.
Holth JK, Fritschi SK, Wang C, et al. The sleep-wake cycle regulates brain interstitial fluid tau in mice and CSF tau in humans. *Science.* 2019;363(6429):880–884.
Liu J, Ramakrishnan S, Laxminarayan S, et al. Real-time individualization of the unified model of performance. *J Sleep Res.* 2017;26(6):820–831.
Mehra R, Wang L, Andrews N, et al. Dissociation of objective and subjective daytime sleepiness and biomarkers of systemic inflammation in sleep disordered breathing and systolic heart failure. *J Clin Sleep Med.* 2017;13(12):1411–1422.
RamakrisKhnan S, Wesensten NJ, Kamimori, et al. A unified model of performance for predicting the effects of sleep and caffeine. *Sleep.* 2016;39(10):1827–1841.
Villafuerte G, Miguel-Puga A, Rodriguez EM, et al. Sleep deprivation and oxidative stress in animals: a systematic review. *Oxid Med Cell Longev.* 2015;2015:234952. https://doi.org/10.1155/2015/234952. [Epub Apr 6, 2015].
Xie L, Kang H, Xu Q, et al. Sleep drives metabolite clearance from the adult brain. *Science.* 2013;342(6156):373–377.
Zhu Y, Fenik P, Zhan G, et al. Intermittent short sleep results in lasting sleep wake disturbances and degeneration of locus coeruleus and orexinergic neurons. *Sleep.* 2016;39(8):1601–1611.

A complete reference list can be found online at ExpertConsult.com.

Insomnia

Section 11

Chapter 89

Advances in Insomnia Pathophysiology and Treatment: An Introduction

Christopher L. Drake; Julio Fernandez-Mendoza

"One thing about insomnia is the longer it lasts, the weirder it gets."

William C. Dement

Everyone is familiar with sleeplessness in some way, and many curse its grip on our lives. Insomnia is an uninvited houseguest, both coda to the day's harshness and a prelude to tomorrow's worries. At times this houseguest visits just for the night, gone by the morning; other times, insomnia overstays so long we cannot remember what brought its arrival. Yet, we hope that if we lie in bed for just a little longer, it will take the hint and leave. Instead, insomnia makes itself comfortable, humming unsleepable nocturnes with its feet up on the bed.

This seventh edition of *Principles and Practices of Sleep Medicine* (PPSM) is the most comprehensive and timely literature review covering the vast area of insomnia. This edition comprises diverse perspectives from epidemiologists, psychologists, psychiatrists, pediatricians, and basic scientists, among many other experts across disciplines. These viewpoints indicate that difficulties with sleep initiation and maintenance do not adequately capture insomnia; instead, these thought leaders emphasize the underlying complexities of insomnia etiology, evaluation, and treatment throughout the life span. Readers will learn the most up-to-date estimates of insomnia prevalence, persistence and incidence rates in the population, differences across ethnicities and cultures, what we know (and still do not know) about the underlying pathophysiology of insomnia disorder, and the adverse consequences of untreated or undertreated insomnia, including the well-established risk for the development of psychopathology.

Research on behavioral treatments of insomnia has demonstrated robust effectiveness in providing long-term relief of insomnia symptoms, improving quality of life, and reducing risk for mental health comorbidity. As a result, this edition of PPSM has expanded its coverage of behavioral insomnia treatments, including newer evidence-based therapies, such as novel sleep restriction paradigms or mindfulness-based therapy. In addition, increased access to behavioral treatments, including support for telemedicine and digital therapeutics, is as timely as ever during this global COVID-19 pandemic. In response to the inadequate treatment effects of insomnia therapy on cognitive and physiologic hyperarousal and barriers to real-world implementation of cognitive behavioral therapy for insomnia (CBT-I), expanded treatment coverage also allows us to consider the shortcomings of current treatments and delivery methods.

This edition of PPSM includes several new topics worth highlighting, including a detailed review by McCrae and colleagues (see Chapter 90) on insomnia disparities across racial, ethnic, and cultural groups, which are more complex than previously posited and deserve greater and urgent attention. In addition, this edition includes a long-overdue chapter on pediatric insomnia by Barclay and colleagues (see Chapter 92) that describes its developmental trajectories and genetic and environmental determinants. This edition gives a fresh look at the polygenetic nature of insomnia. Readers are kept abreast of the current state-of-the-science on wearable technology in assessing insomnia, as well as issues regarding insomnia diagnosis and subtyping in Chapter 93 by Ong and colleagues. This edition also features a compelling chapter by Hall and colleagues (see Chapter 94) on the role of multidimensional, multimethod frameworks, including the role of objective sleep measures as phenotypic markers of severe sequelae in insomnia and multidimensional sleep health as a critical public health need. Readers are guided through the exciting area of insomnia with short sleep duration, which has gained recognition as a more biologically severe phenotype of insomnia, potentially requiring specific treatment approaches. This growing area of insomnia research has called into question current practices of relying solely on patient reports of symptoms and urges sleep scientists to reconsider how best to use objective sleep measurements to better conceptualize insomnia as a multidimensional sleep disorder. This edition devotes a new chapter by Vedaa and colleagues (see Chapter 97) to digital and telemedicine therapeutics' efficacy in treating insomnia, including logistic barriers to successful implementation. Many chapters in the section challenge widely held views on the hyperarousal concept of insomnia, insomnia being purely symptom based, and CBT-I being highly efficacious across all patient populations, thus moving the insomnia field forward into the future.

INSOMNIA NATION

Difficulty falling asleep. Trouble staying asleep. Waking up too early and unable to resume sleep. Sleep continuity disturbance. Poor sleep. Sleeplessness. All these descriptors characterize the phenomenology of insomnia as the most common sleep affliction in adults. At any given time, approximately 1 in 3 adults struggles with symptoms of insomnia, whereas 1 in 10 adults meets the diagnostic criteria for insomnia disorder. Insomnia is generally considered nocturnal in terms of sleep initiation and maintenance. For patients, sleeplessness can feel both unsafe and unpredictable. When considering these experiences and the potential impact insomnia has on daytime functioning (fatigue, depression, anxiety, poor concentration), we see a common, if not universal, occurrence that has a corrosive effect on our patients' quality of life. The impairments can be debilitating, thus warranting further research and clinical attention.

Burgeoning literature emphasizes that untreated insomnia deteriorates quality of life, social interactions and well-being, and increases the risk of mental disorders. It is no wonder that insomnia is a heavy burden on the nation's health care resources, as insomnia patients make more visits to the emergency department, take more prescription drugs, and use outpatient clinics far more than good sleepers. The economic burden can be suffocating to those who have insomnia. They spend billions on prescription and over-the-counter sleep aids, turn to alcohol and drugs to aid sleep, are absent from work more frequently, and when they go to work, become less effective than their well-rested coworkers. In the United States it is estimated that 367 million workdays are lost annually, amounting to $92 billion per year. Estimates from other developed countries around the world echo these figures. In addition, undertreated insomnia is a risk factor for future work disability at a magnitude similar to that of depression. Insomnia also appears to be a strong risk factor for disability among young adults in the workforce. Indeed, contemporary evidence elucidates insomnia as an independent clinical entity rather than a byproduct of other so-called primary disorders (e.g., depression). This paradigm shift now emphasizes that insomnia is a critical intervention target on its own that merits increased public health attention.

COUNTING ON A WILD SHEEP CHASE

For decades we conceptualized the etiology of insomnia behaviorally via the 3-P model (predisposing, precipitating, and perpetuating factors). However, over the past 30 years, our understanding of vulnerabilities and mechanisms facilitating insomnia development has grown tremendously. Although traditional behavioral and cognitive frameworks have endured the test of time, more recent perspectives from human models incorporate findings from neurobiologic, physiologic, and genetic studies. Several chapters review laboratory experiments, epidemiologic studies, and long-term prospective studies on insomnia trajectories, which cover the most cutting-edge discoveries in the development and maintenance of insomnia. With excitement, nonhuman models have become increasingly relevant and strongly influence our understanding of human insomnia's etiology. Perlis and colleagues (see Chapter 91) cover recent evidence from rodent and *Drosophila* studies that may inform us about how insomnia develops in humans and reveals the mechanisms by which our interventions may deliver their benefits.

Icelos on the Shore

Although the term *insomnia* may carry myriad definitions and conceptualizations, insomnia disorder is clearly defined in the *International Classification of Sleep Disorders,* third edition (ICSD-3) and the *Diagnostic and Statistical Manual of Mental Disorders,* fifth edition (DSM-5). Ong and colleagues (see Chapter 93) emphasize the essential overlap between diagnostic systems and highlight the minor differences between DSM-5 and ICSD-3 criteria. Of note, the assessment chapter has been updated to reflect the current nosological conceptualizations of insomnia disorder's relationship with other comorbid conditions. The chapter reflects the prevailing zeitgeist that insomnia disorder should not be considered secondary and requires independent treatment even in the context of comorbid conditions. Furthermore, the authors evaluate currently available diagnostic tools, ranging from clinical interviews to self-report surveys and the emerging wearable technology, and how each contributes to diagnostic decision making, case conceptualization, and insomnia phenotyping.

Sleeping Like a Child

For the first time, this edition of PPSM includes a chapter by Barclay and colleagues (see Chapter 92) on insomnia's developmental trajectories, starting in infancy and extending into adulthood. Sleep homeostasis and the circadian clock take months to develop after birth, and frequent nighttime awakenings are normal in the approximately the first 6 months of life. However, children whose sleep patterns do not normalize or become disrupted after a period of normal sleep may suffer from childhood insomnia. Although behavioral insomnia of childhood shares overlapping features with insomnia in adolescents and adults, it is uniquely characterized by bedtime resistance to a developmentally appropriate schedule and/or an inability to sleep independently without parent or caregiver intervention. This exciting new chapter covers pediatric insomnia and answers questions about genetics, risk factors, treatment options for different developmental stages, and the relationship to parental sleep, stress, and mental health. This chapter also delves into more conceptual matters: Is pediatric insomnia an early manifestation of adult insomnia? If so, in whom? Or are they distinct conditions? To this end, readers will explore the current science of insomnia over the human life span, including evaluations of how symptoms and etiologic factors of insomnia evolve.

Hear the Wind Sing

In the era of precision medicine, optimal treatment of insomnia requires clinicians to think beyond the nocturnal symptoms. Several chapters discuss these additional considerations, including the understanding of how predisposing factors may play a role, how insomnia interacts with specific comorbidities (e.g., sleep apnea, pain) and populations (e.g., shift workers and pregnant women), the role of psychosocial support or lack thereof, and finally, how insomnia, hyperarousal, and the daytime impact can produce a vicious cycle over time that contributes to nocturnal and daytime effects with growing risk for both physical and mental health disorders. These and other issues discussed throughout this Insomnia section of PPSM emphasize the need for our treatments to evolve beyond a focus on sleep self-reports to address a range of contextual, dimensional, and patient-centered factors.

New to the seventh edition of PPSM, coverage of behavioral treatment has been expanded and split into three chapters from Drs. Carney, Manber, and Vedaa. The authors explore evidence for tried and true behavioral sleep strategies, including sleep restriction, stimulus control, and cognitive therapy, which are often packaged together into CBT-I. CBT-I and brief behavioral therapies are not only effective in treating insomnia but also in alleviating symptoms of common comorbid mental health conditions. Readers will learn about patient populations for whom behavioral insomnia therapy is successful and people for whom behavioral sleep strategies should be appropriately modified to maximize outcomes (e.g., pregnant women, the elderly with fall risk). Despite the efficacy of CBT-I, implementation and patient access issues (i.e., effectiveness) have hindered its promise. The authors discuss how to improve its integration into health care systems and increase its dissemination across different patient populations that currently have inadequate access to insomnia therapies.

Telemedicine and digital health care approaches have exploded in recent years and accelerated even further since the COVID-19 pandemic hit. In this new edition of PPSM, the chapter by Vedaa and colleagues (see Chapter 97) has compiled the quickly accruing data on the efficacy of CBT-I delivered via telemedicine and digital methods. Not only are readers presented with the current state of the science supporting these novel delivery systems for insomnia therapies, they are also offered data on different levels of digital delivery: fully automated digital therapy, supportive digital therapy, and therapist-guided digital therapy. Despite the immense potential of telemedicine and digital therapeutics, only a few studies directly compare these new delivery methods with the efficacy of face-to-face treatment, making it challenging to gauge the relative effectiveness of digital therapies and telemedicine approaches. An important area of digital insomnia therapy is identifying ways to maximize patient engagement through strategies such as adaptive approaches and stepped-care models. Innovative strategies are needed to reach the "digital threshold" and address the challenges of scale and efficacy before CBT-I can be realized as "the standard of care in insomnia" and an alternative to hypnotic medications as first-line treatment in routine clinical care.

THE CONTEXT OF THE COVID-19 PANDEMIC

Work on the seventh edition of PPSM started long before the COVID-19 pandemic began. Even so, our discussion would be incomplete without acknowledging how the pandemic has informed not only our approach to treatment but also our perspective on the field overall. In mid-2021, the course of the pandemic around the globe remained uncertain and in flux. COVID-19 abruptly became the third leading cause of death in the United States and other parts of the world. It is still too early for the research community to understand how long the risk of SARS-CoV-2 infection will disrupt daily life and to what extent the development of COVID-19 will determine the natural course of insomnia and new treatment needs among the population at large. Nevertheless, early signs point to the COVID-19 pandemic changing many aspects of health care. Although the impact on sleep researchers, clinicians, and technologists has varied immensely across the globe, the shift toward more technology-based ambulatory assessment and treatment approaches is likely to continue. Multiple surveys were conducted during the peak of the COVID-19 pandemic and indicate a rise in insomnia symptoms and insufficient sleep in many, and changes in sleep duration and circadian timing in others. An entire world of frontline health care workers—an already sleep-deprived population—has been in overdrive with no respite in sight; the overwhelming evidence shows that their sleep quality and duration are suffering significantly in a disproportionate manner. During this time, the burgeoning research areas of telemedicine and digital insomnia therapeutics have become more essential than ever. Nearly all sleep-focused journals have produced or are in the planning stages of special issues on sleep in relation to the pandemic. Only time will tell how COVID-19 will shape the world, the field of sleep medicine, and how health care services are delivered (see Chapter 213).

Meeting Future Challenges in Insomnia

Finding solutions for untreated or disengaged patients, particularly those who have limited access to care, remains a formidable challenge to the field—specifically, studies using evidence-based approaches to address the most severe treatment-refractory individuals with insomnia. Current progress includes elegant studies combining pharmacologic and behavioral interventions, as reviewed by Edinger and colleagues (see Chapter 100) in their excellent contribution to this section, investigating treatment outcomes in specific populations (e.g., people with insomnia and comorbid depression) and assessing the benefits of CBT-I for non–sleep-related outcomes (e.g., pain, depression, anxiety). These strategies and other treatment advances, including Sequential Multiple Assignment Randomized (SMART) trials, adaptive interventions, and matching patients to the most effective pharmacologic agents, will help carry on the mission begun by those we have lost over the last decade: Art Spielman, Dick Bootzin, Peter Hauri, and the father of sleep medicine, the beloved William (Bill) Dement.

Although these expanding options are gaining popularity with the public, providers face significant limitations and challenges to our approaches, despite their convenience, accessibility, and efficacy. These include scalability, access at the cost of reduced effectiveness, personalization in the case of digital CBT-I, and the unknown utility of matching insomnia phenotypes to behavioral therapies or specific medications in pharmacologic management. Concomitantly, telehealth approaches are being increasingly used, although the impact remains in question.

Treatment in the context of specific patient characteristics (e.g., pain, depression) has yielded much success. However, personalized/tailored treatment that enhances patient engagement and adherence, improving insomnia remission beyond the current 50% to 60%, remains limited. Progress in these areas will depend upon the willingness of the field and its stakeholders to recognize several of the critical shortcomings we must face as stewards of this scientific discipline, namely, that our most highly recommended behavioral treatments are in short supply. Other challenges remain, including optimally combining, matching or tailoring behavioral and pharmacologic approaches, and translating scientific knowledge regarding safety and efficacy of hypnotics, as reviewed by Bertisch and Buysse (see Chapter 98) and Krystal (see Chapter 99), into the clinic, where patients can benefit from these advances.

NIGHT SKY WITH EXIT WOUNDS

The field has largely dismissed the utility of objective sleep measures in insomnia assessment, phenotyping, and management, and CBT-I has been heralded as the "Swiss Army Knife" of behavioral sleep medicine. Today, we know that insomnia is an independent condition with unique detriments on mental and physical health, objective sleep disturbance in insomnia heralds a more severe phenotype, and insomnia therapy needs to be enhanced to better treat specific populations and phenotypes and better alleviate physiologic and cognitive hyperarousal.

As the section editors, we are excited and incredibly proud to present the seventh edition of PPSM's Insomnia section. As previous editions of this volume have contributed to the rise of sleep medicine, we hope that this section continues to pave the way for the future of insomnia treatment as previously led by Drs. Allison Harvey and Daniel Buysse in the previous sixth edition of PPSM. Our goal is to present the clinical foundation for understanding the current state-of-the-science on the assessment, pathophysiology, and consequences of insomnia and its myriad treatments. Just as earnestly, we believe it is important to travel beyond the boundaries of scientific evidence in many cases where the insomnia field has established a robust and longstanding evidence base and enter into the ones where new findings rekindle our inherent thirst for exploration. The field of insomnia will require further innovations, including approaches to prevention, discovering additional etiologic mechanisms, and developing new pharmacologic strategies. More important, these innovations need to be translated into the clinical setting so that more of our patients can be treated to remission safely. These innovations must not only be evidence based but will need to be accessible and used by the largest number of patients possible to truly impact all of those suffering from insomnia.

Chapter 90

Insomnia: Epidemiology, Risk Factors, and Health Disparities

Christina S. McCrae; Daniel J. Taylor; Megan E. Petrov; Michael A. Grandner; Ashley F. Curtis

Chapter Highlights

- Insomnia prevalence estimates vary widely, depending on how insomnia is defined, with approximately 30% of the general population reporting insomnia symptoms, 10% to 20% reporting frequent symptoms (3 or more nights per week), and 10% reporting insomnia disorder.
- Yearly incidence reports also vary, with 31% to 50% reporting symptoms and 2% to 15% reporting insomnia disorder.
- Of importance, although more than three-quarters of cases reporting insomnia symptoms remit within 3 months, residual subclinical symptoms are common, and those that do not remit are unlikely to do so without intervention.
- Evidence generally shows minimal racial/ethnic group differences in insomnia prevalence. However, differences in how insomnia is perceived may result in underestimation of clinically significant insomnia in non-White racial ethnic groups, particularly in Blacks.
- Advancing age, female sex, and low socioeconomic status are strong insomnia correlates, and they may moderate racial/ethnic differences and other risk relationships.
- Cognitive, physiologic, and neural arousal, often referred to as hyperarousal, have long been considered risk factors for insomnia, but empirical support is limited. Emerging research suggests hyperarousal-related factors, such as environmental awareness related to cortical arousal, and the responsiveness of sleep to stress may emerge as insomnia risk factors.
- Insomnia serves as a risk factor for psychiatric comorbidities (e.g., depression, substance abuse, posttraumatic stress disorder) and vice versa. However, mechanisms, causal paths, and mediators/moderators of these relationships are poorly understood. It may also be a risk factor for medical comorbidities (e.g., hypertension, chronic pain), but more evidence is needed.
- Recurrent bouts of acute insomnia and genetic factors are becoming recognized as important risk factors for insomnia disorder.
- Future priorities include increased use of standardized diagnostic criteria for insomnia and more research involving longitudinal studies; expanded examination of medical comorbidities, genetic variables, and sleep health disparities; and increased understanding of perceptions of insomnia in non-White racial ethnic groups, hyperarousal, and related factors; as well as other mechanisms, causal paths, and mediators/moderators of insomnia risk relationships.

Insomnia is the most common sleep disorder and is among the most prevalent of all mental health disorders. Evaluating the epidemiology of insomnia is challenging because insomnia is an umbrella term used to describe a wide range of sleep behavior—from a single, acute complaint to insomnia disorder (chronic, clinically significant insomnia)—that not surprisingly results in a wide range of prevalence estimates. Interpretation of any given prevalence rate requires understanding how insomnia is defined and assessed.

A robust literature supports insomnia as a risk factor for psychiatric disorders, whereas a smaller but growing literature indicates it can also be a risk factor for medical disorders. The reverse is also true, with psychiatric and medical disorders predicting insomnia risk. Evidence of minimal racial/ethnic differences may underestimate clinically significant insomnia in non-White groups. The mechanisms, causal paths, and mediators/moderators of these risk relationships are not currently well understood. Age, sex, and genetics are static risk factors that may moderate other insomnia risk relationships, including racial/ethnic differences.

Hyperarousal, a component of most, if not all, insomnia models, is a traditional insomnia pathophysiologic mechanism. Hyperarousal is a complex term and, when used in the context of insomnia, typically refers to cognitive, physiologic, and/or neural arousal that interferes with the initiation and/or maintenance of sleep. However, limited, largely cross-sectional support combined with emerging support for hyperarousal-related factors raises new questions regarding hyperarousal's role in insomnia. This chapter reviews the current literature on the epidemiology of insomnia and risk factors for insomnia, describes its weaknesses, and suggests areas for research prioritization and methodological improvement.

EPIDEMIOLOGY

Definition of Insomnia

Defining insomnia is a complex task for several reasons. First, insomnia can occur as symptom(s) (e.g., difficulty initiating and/or maintaining sleep, early-morning awakening), syndrome (e.g., difficulties occurring at least 3 nights per week along with associated daytime impairment/distress), or disorder (e.g., clinician-verified diagnosis). Second, insomnia that begins as a symptom of another disorder or stressful life event often evolves over time into an independent chronic syndrome or disorder. Third, as a disorder, insomnia is heterogeneous, with varying types and etiologies. Fourth, insomnia severity often fluctuates over time.

The literature contains numerous insomnia definitions, ranging from broad and inclusive to narrow and exclusive. Epidemiologic studies of insomnia are often secondary analyses of population-based studies in which sleep or insomnia was assessed with as few as one question. Some epidemiologic studies rely on respondents to provide their own definitions by simply asking whether or not they have trouble sleeping,[1] whereas other studies define insomnia more narrowly, using quantitative severity threshold criteria (e.g., >30 minutes of sleep-onset latency or wake time after sleep onset).[2] Varied definitions of insomnia provide different population prevalence rates that range from 4% to 48%, with rates decreasing as the definition narrows from symptom(s) (highest) to syndrome to disorder (lowest).[3,4] Efforts to standardize diagnostic criteria for insomnia have narrowed this range.[5] Recent revisions of the *International Classifications of Sleep Disorders*, third edition (ICSD-3)[6] and the *Diagnostic and Statistical Manual of Mental Disorders*, fifth edition (DSM-5)[7] specify sleep complaints at least three times per week for at least 3 months with associated daytime impairment to diagnose chronic insomnia disorder.

Evaluation

Epidemiologic studies and clinical practice settings traditionally rely on self-report data from a few items. Large-scale objective assessment (polysomnography [PSG] or actigraphy) can be expensive and cumbersome, and diagnostic criteria for insomnia does not require objective assessment, unless needed to rule out other sleep disorders (e.g., sleep-disordered breathing [SDB]). Further, self-report instruments better capture sleep perception and associated distress than objective methods, which may be important targets for treatment and treatment adherence.[5]

Epidemiologic surveys rely heavily on self-reported, retrospective sleep assessments, which are prone to inaccuracies and unreliability and may overestimate insomnia symptoms because they use time periods that are either unspecified (e.g., participants report how they "usually" or "generally" sleep) or require averaging across multiple nights (increasing risk for recall errors and recency bias [responding based on prior night's sleep]),[2] that are vulnerable to temporary situational influences and emotional states (e.g., work-related stress, depressed mood), and often lack information on sleep environment adequacy and other context-specific circumstances that might explain reported sleep disturbance.

Prospective assessments of insomnia symptoms and insomnia disorder through nightly sleep diaries improve upon retrospective biases but do not provide sufficient information on their own to identify individuals with insomnia symptoms or disorder (e.g., duration, daytime impairment, rule out other sleep disorders) and are more time and resource intensive, which can affect feasibility for epidemiologic research. Therefore examining retrospective insomnia-related items in publicly available datasets has merit and highlights the need for greater clinical and research focus on insomnia, but such data should be interpreted with knowledge of their limitations. Alternatives to sleep diaries and insomnia-related items are validated, short retrospective instruments that can differentiate normal sleepers from people with probable insomnia[8] and those meeting DSM-5 criteria for insomnia disorder.[9,10]

Prevalence

Most population-level estimates suggest approximately 30% of the US population reports insomnia symptoms.[11] This estimate, frequently reported in the literature, largely derives from classic insomnia epidemiologic studies[12] and consensus statements.[13] Ohayon[3] reviewed the literature in 2002 and found the population prevalence of insomnia symptoms was similarly approximately 33%. When the definition of insomnia is restricted to those reporting frequent or moderate to severe symptoms, population prevalence estimates drop to approximately 10% to 28%.[3] When the definition is further restricted to include daytime consequences, this estimate is reduced to approximately 10% (Table 90.1).[3]

Nationally representative, weighted estimates from the 2007 to 2008 National Health and Nutrition Examination

Table 90.1 Insomnia Prevalence Rates by Four Main Definitional Categories and Three Symptom Categories

Category	Prevalence (%)
Definitional Category (No. of Studies)	
DSM-IV insomnia diagnosis (*n* = 5)	4–6
Dissatisfaction with sleep quantity or quality (*n* = 11)	8–18
Insomnia symptoms plus daytime consequences (*n* = 8)	9–15
Insomnia symptoms[a] (*n* = 21)	10–48
Symptom Category	
Insomnia symptoms only	30–48
Insomnia symptoms plus frequency criteria (≥3 nights/week or often/always)	16–21
Insomnia symptoms plus severity criteria (moderately to extremely)	10–28

[a]Insomnia symptoms included difficulty initiating or maintaining sleep. Some studies also included nonrestorative sleep as a symptom.

DSM-IV, *Diagnostic and Statistical Manual of Mental Disorders*, 4th edition, text revision.

Modified from Ohayon MM. Epidemiology of insomnia: what we know and what we still need to learn. *Sleep Med Rev.* 2002;6:97–111.

Survey (NHANES) suggest 18.8% of the US population reports a sleep latency of more than 30 minutes.[4] This study also reports the relative frequency of insomnia symptoms (difficulty initiating and/or maintaining sleep, early-morning awakenings) and nonrestorative sleep, which is related to insomnia (Figure 90.1). Rates of individuals reporting difficulty initiating or maintaining sleep or early-morning awakenings at least five times per month are 19.4%, 20.9%, and 16.5%, respectively. Future research will determine whether the COVID pandemic will have changed prevalence data.

Incidence, Persistence, and Remission

A longitudinal study of the natural history of insomnia in US and UK samples[14] found approximately 4.4% of the general population develops acute insomnia symptoms per month (61.1% of which are a first-onset problem). This reflects an annual incidence of acute insomnia symptoms estimated at 36.6%. This was attenuated to 31.2% when the criteria are restricted to individuals with likely insomnia disorder—those who met DSM-V diagnostic criteria and also reported sleep latency and/or wake after sleep onset of at least 30 minutes and reduced quality of life. Similarly, a national US-based study documented annual incidence at 27.0% for acute insomnia.[15] A provincial Canadian study described an incidence of "insomnia syndrome" (defined as insomnia symptoms at least 3 nights per week for at least 1 month, in the presence of daytime dysfunction) to be 3.8% at 1 year, 9.3% at 3 years, and 13.9% at 5 years, among those who did not report insomnia symptoms at baseline.[16] A subset of 100 individuals randomly selected from this larger study completed 12 monthly assessments and demonstrated that among those who were good sleepers at baseline, 48.6% experienced some insomnia symptoms during the year, and 14.5% reported an "insomnia syndrome."[17] Another US-based prospective study[18] found that 18.4% of the general population developed insomnia symptoms, and 9.3% developed chronic insomnia after 7 years of follow-up.[19]

In the US/UK study, 78.6% with insomnia symptoms remitted by the third month after symptom onset; this was 67.0% for those who met criteria for an acute insomnia disorder. These findings suggest many new cases with insomnia symptoms emerge each month, and although most remit, a portion become chronic (7.8% of the population for insomnia symptoms and 10.3% for insomnia disorder). In the US-based study, similarly, 72.4% remitted.[15] In the other US-based study from the Penn State Sleep Cohort, 44% of those with insomnia symptoms fully remitted, whereas only 25% of those with chronic insomnia did after 7.5 years of follow-up; of those who did not remit, 58% maintained their insomnia; and 62% partially remitted, still experiencing insomnia symptoms.[18,20] These findings supported earlier natural history studies,[21,22] which suggest once insomnia becomes chronic (i.e., 3 months), it is unlikely to remit on its own. This was supported by the Canadian study, which observed that a 3-month window was reliable for defining chronic insomnia.[17] Persistence of insomnia symptoms has been shown to be predicted by both physical health conditions and mental health disturbances,[18,23,24] as well as being female.[23] Of note, even among those who remit, residual symptoms are common, including fatigue (24.7%), mood disturbance (23.0%), and cognitive disturbances (22.6%).[23]

Some hypothesize that recurrent episodes of acute insomnia *kindle*[26] the development of chronic insomnia. Over time, acute episodes become progressively more independent from precipitating stress-related triggers and deteriorate the body's adaptive stress response system. These episodes can become more dependent on perpetuating factors (e.g., worry about

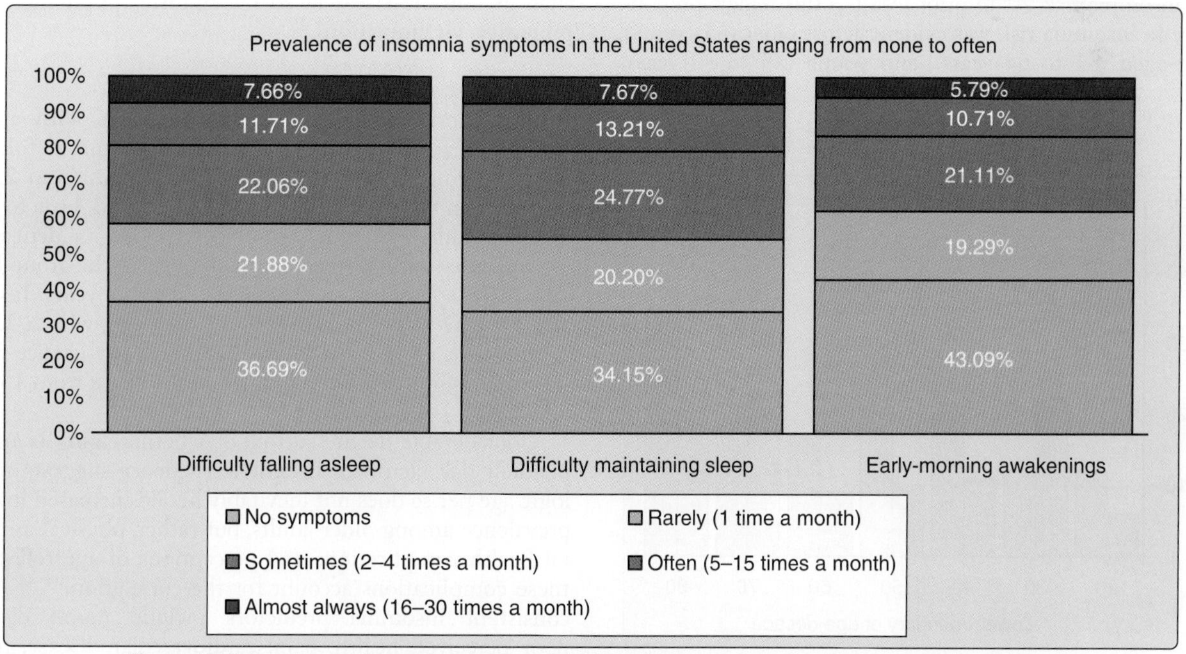

Figure 90.1 Prevalence of insomnia symptoms in the United States. Relative frequency of a number of symptoms of insomnia (difficulty initiating sleep, difficulty maintaining sleep, early-morning awakenings) in the US general population. Frequencies are based on nationally representative weighted estimates from the Centers for Disease Control and Prevention's 2007 to 2008 National Health and Nutrition Examination Survey (NHANES).

sleep ability, daytime consequences of sleep loss[27]) or maladaptive sleep-related behavior (e.g., increased time in bed, activities conducted in the bedroom).

Demographic Factors and Health Disparities

Sex and Gender

Insomnia is more common in women than men. Lichstein and colleagues[2] reviewed 42 epidemiologic studies (33 reporting sex comparisons). Overall, women were more likely to report insomnia symptoms (18.2%) than men (12.4%). Results from the associated prospective study further support greater overall prevalence of insomnia in women (Figure 90.2). There was no reliable difference in quantitative sleep parameters (e.g., sleep-onset latency, total sleep time) of men and women with insomnia. A decade-by-decade breakdown shows women exhibited greater insomnia prevalence than men across the life span, with the exception of before puberty onset[28] and the decade of ages 30 to 39 years. Specifically, insomnia prevalence for women ranged from 12% (ages 20 to 29 and 30 to 39 years) to 41% (ages 80+ years). For men, rates ranged from 6% (ages 20 to 29 years) to 23% (ages 70 to 79 and 80+ years). Although prevalence rates are generally higher for women, insomnia may be particularly problematic for men because in men (not women), mortality risk is associated with insomnia and short sleep duration (<6 hours).[29]

A meta-analysis[30] of 29 epidemiologic studies (n = 1,265,015; 718,828 females/546,187 males) found women exhibited a higher risk ratio (RR) of 1.4. That risk varied depending on sample size and strength of study methodology, with women exhibiting higher insomnia risk ratios in larger, more rigorous studies (RR, 1.64) than in smaller, less rigorous studies (RR, 1.32). Similarly, a review of 21 population-based prospective studies in adults ages 50+ years found the most consistent independent risk factor for insomnia was female sex.[31] Across reviewed studies, females experienced elevated odds ratios (OR) of 1.44 to 2.44 relative to men (0.52) for future insomnia risk. As in prior results,[2] this female preponderance in insomnia risk was evident across older (65+ years), middle-aged (31 to 64 years), and young (15 to 30 years) adults.

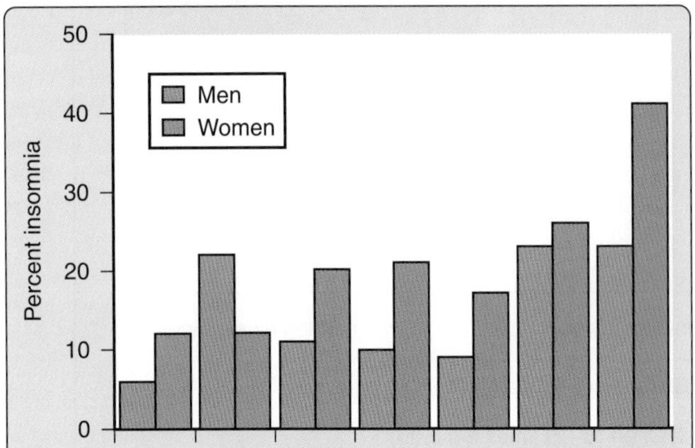

Figure 90.2 Insomnia prevalence by sex and age. Each value on the abscissa represents the beginning of an age decade as in 20 (to 29) and 30 (to 39). (Data from Lichstein KL, Durrence HH, Riedel BW, et al. *Epidemiology of Sleep: Age, Gender, and Ethnicity.* Erlbaum; 2004.)

This risk may begin as young as prepubescence; a study[32] of children (n = 700; ages 5 to 12 years) found insomnia symptom prevalence (controlling for anxiety, depressive symptoms) was 10% to 14% higher in girls ages 11 to 12 years compared with boys and younger girls. Another study suggests late puberty may exacerbate sex differences. A large school-based study[33] (n = 7507, ages 6 to 17 years) found that there were fewer sex differences in the prevalence of insomnia symptoms in early puberty stages and larger sex differences showing higher prevalence of insomnia symptoms emerge only during late puberty and beyond. Associated behavioral and emotional symptoms also differed between females and males throughout puberty, potentially representing gender role–specific differences, as females with insomnia are more likely to exhibit emotional and relationship problems, whereas males are more likely to exhibit maladaptive behavior (e.g., smoking/drinking).[33] More work is needed to delineate sex (biologic disposition) versus gender role differences in insomnia symptoms and associated daytime functioning.

There is emerging evidence suggesting higher rates of insomnia disorder in sexual and gender minority (lesbian, gay, bisexual, and transgender [LGBT]) populations. A national survey[34] in the United States (n = 9396) found that individuals who identified as a sexual minority reported greater insomnia symptoms than individuals who identified as heterosexual. In addition, women were more likely than men to report both insomnia symptoms. A systematic review[25] of 31 articles evaluating insomnia symptoms in heterosexual versus sexual minority groups found that the majority of findings show that adolescent and adult LGBT populations are at increased risk of greater self-reported insomnia symptoms, even after controlling for age, sex, socioeconomic status (SES), race/ethnicity, substance use, and physical/mental health problems. Overall, more research is needed to evaluate objective sleep parameters in LGBT populations and identify potential underlying factors of sleep disparities, such as chronic stress faced by minority populations (e.g., prejudice, victimization).[25]

Aging

Insomnia prevalence and severity increases with age.[2,3,35] Average yearly incidence of chronic insomnia at follow-up times ranging from 1 to 4 years then ranges from 2.4% to 4.2%[36–38] in young to middle-aged adults and 3.6% to 15.2% in older adults.[39–42] One study[40] determined incident insomnia increases with age and nearly doubles in the group having 75+ years, compared to those ages 65 to 74 years. Insomnia also appears to be more persistent with age, with a 1.1-fold greater odds each decade of life.[43] Annual persistence rates of insomnia symptoms among older adults range from 13.3% to 22.7%.[39,41]

Considerable debate surrounds whether aging is an independent risk factor for insomnia. Evidence suggests chronologic age per se does not inevitably herald increased insomnia prevalence among older adults, but rather, physical and mental health complications and perceptions of age reflected by these complications account for the correlation.[44–46] Indeed, consistent insomnia predictors include mood disorders, poor perceived health, pain, cardiovascular disease, respiratory symptoms, stressful life events, somatic complaints, and memory problems.[39,41] Incident, persistent, and even remitted insomnia during older adulthood may increase the risk of physical and/or emotional impairments,[42] potentially through accelerating cellular aging.[47]

Race and Ethnicity

In the last few decades, interest in race/ethnicity as an important explanatory factor has grown, given data indicating sleep health disparities by racial/ethnic group. Most epidemiologic data on race/ethnicity and insomnia compares non-Hispanic Whites and non-Hispanic Blacks. A meta-analysis of 13 studies found racial differences in the reported insomnia symptoms: Whites were more likely to report difficulty maintaining sleep and early-morning awakenings but not difficulty initiating sleep, compared to Blacks.[48] Age and gender were noteworthy moderators in Black versus White differences, with advancing age attenuating differences. Among women the difference in difficulty maintaining sleep was smaller, whereas the difference in early-morning awakenings was larger. Socioeconomic indicators as moderators could not be computed in this meta-analysis. After this meta-analysis, results from community- and population-based studies on insomnia symptoms have been mixed.[49,50] Further, studies examining actual prevalence of Black versus White differences in insomnia disorder remain scant. Of the limited data available, Black adults are more likely to have current or remitted insomnia disorder with short sleep duration,[51] an insomnia phenotype most associated with negative physical and mental health outcomes.[52–54]

These discrepant findings may be partly accounted for by study design and differences in insomnia criteria used. The interpretation of questions about insomnia may also vary by race/ethnicity. A national survey found Blacks less likely to report insomnia symptoms than Whites, yet they were more likely to report sleep-onset latencies of more than 30 minutes.[4] This result indicates Blacks may underreport clinically meaningful insomnia symptoms. Moreover, underexplored moderation by age, gender, and historical and current SES indicators may also be a factor.[30,32,55–58] In a population-based, multiethnic sample of middle-aged to older adults, insomnia severity increased with age across all racial/ethnic groups but was most pronounced among Hispanics compared to non-Hispanic Whites.[59] In contrast, no racial/ethnic differences were found among studies of multiethnic adolescents and young adults.[60,61] Also, insomnia prevalence was lower among Whites with greater educational attainment but higher among Hispanic adults with greater educational attainment, compared to Whites.[57]

Available data on differences in insomnia prevalence among other racial/ethnic groups remain minimal. A large, national survey found Blacks, Mexican Americans, and other Hispanic/Latino groups less likely to report insomnia symptoms than Whites,[4] although other studies suggest the Hispanic/Latino-White difference is inconsistent.[62] Studies are mixed regarding differences in symptom reporting between Asian groups and Whites.[4,55,63] Overall, racial/ethnic minority groups appear less likely to report insomnia symptoms than Whites. This does not necessarily mean these groups are not at increased risk for insomnia, particularly among Blacks.

Education and Socioeconomic Status

Epidemiologic studies consistently show low SES is associated with poor sleep.[3] In general, studies examining SES and insomnia are more complex than simply measuring education because many variables contribute to SES (e.g., immigration status, occupation, income, health care access, food insecurity).[64] A study[55] of US adults (n = 159,856, ages 18+ years) found higher odds (twofold to sevenfold) of insomnia symptoms (trouble falling asleep, staying asleep) for unemployed versus employed individuals. Among the unemployed, men had a higher likelihood of these insomnia symptoms than women. Sex also affected the relationship as the association between greater insomnia symptoms and lower education was stronger in men who did not finish high school.[3] Thus social and economic health determinants may be potential factors underlying the sex differences described earlier. Another study[65] found persons with lower individual and household education were more likely to experience insomnia disorder and report greater insomnia-related impairment. Of importance, education level was related to insomnia disorder even after controlling for race, sex, and age.

PREDISPOSING AND PRECIPITATING RISK FACTORS

It is believed that certain predispositions make people more susceptible to developing insomnia after exposure to a precipitant, similar to a *diathesis-stress model*.[66] Conversely, insomnia might aggravate or serve as a precipitant for developing a comorbid disease (e.g., depression).[67] Longitudinal research designs are the primary means of determining risk by assessing presence of a predisposition (e.g., genetics or precipitant [e.g., stress]) before insomnia onset.

To follow, we review studies (primarily prospective) investigating risk factors for insomnia and insomnia as a risk factor for other disorders. More static risk factors (e.g., gender, race/ethnicity) were previously reviewed.

Personality

Cross-sectional studies indicate neuroticism, agreeableness, internalization, less openness, and perfectionism are personality traits associated with insomnia, with neuroticism demonstrating the strongest and most consistent association across studies.[68–70] Unfortunately, little longitudinal data exist.[70] Those available find neuroticism, arousability, anxious-ruminative traits, depressive traits, social introversion, and low ego strength predict incident insomnia symptoms or chronic insomnia.[18,19,71,72] However, examining personality without considering the roles of genetic predisposition, coping styles, and stress reactivity makes longitudinal data difficult to interpret.[73]

Arousability

All insomnia models (i.e., physiologic, behavioral, cognitive, neurocognitive) assume some degree of heightened arousability predisposes to the onset of insomnia. Unfortunately, virtually all evidence for this relationship is cross-sectional and involves comparing people with and without insomnia on current levels of arousal.[74,75] The evidence is also quite mixed and of low effect, raising concern that (1) the relationship either does not exist, (2) is of such small and unreliable effects that it is not meaningful, or (3) that the presence of physiologic hyperarousal in people with insomnia is heterogeneous and is present only in specific phenotypes. Newer neurocognitive studies investigating spectral electroencephalography[76] and neuroimaging[77] suggest physiologic hyperarousal thought to cause insomnia may be cortical arousal resulting in increased environmental awareness. The absence of longitudinal evidence of these associations makes it impossible to delineate causal paths. Although individuals with hyperarousal may be predisposed to developing insomnia, hyperarousal may also be a downstream effect of insomnia.

Genetics

Familial aggregation analysis determines whether a disorder (i.e., insomnia) occurs more commonly in family members than in nonrelated persons. Existing insomnia familial aggregation studies used a variety of different methodologies (e.g., adults with insomnia, children with insomnia, no-insomnia control subjects), insomnia definitions (e.g., severity scales, DSM-III, DSM-IV), and confounding factors (e.g., age, sex, work schedules, comorbidities).[78,79] Therefore results have varied greatly, indicating genetic risk from 20% to 73%.[80–86]

Twin studies, which are methodologically more rigorous than aggregation studies, report heritability of a composite insomnia syndrome of 28% to 58%,[87–93] which appear to hold longitudinally in adolescents,[94] young adults,[95] and adults.[91] Regarding insomnia symptoms, adult studies report heritability rates of 28% to 32% for difficulties falling asleep and 33% to 45% for difficulties maintaining sleep.[89,92] One study of children was more variable depending on the parent (79%) or child (17%) reporting, both of which are somewhat questionable, given the young age of the children (8 years) and potential parental reporting biases.[96] A longitudinal study in children and adolescent twins, ages 8 to 18 years, observed moderate heritability for insomnia (based on DSM-III–defined "clinically significant insomnia") at all four waves of measured ages—8, 10, 14, and 15 years (mode ages), showing 33%, 38%, 14%, and 24% genetic heritability, respectively.[94] Lower heritability values in adolescents relative to children highlight the importance of nonshared environment, as adolescents often experience additional environmental and social changes, which may play a larger role than heritability in sleep interference.[94] Of interest, another longitudinal twin study of 7500 adults from the Virginia Adult Twin Studies of Psychiatric and Substance Use Disorders[91] found sex differences in heritability of a latent insomnia factor, with women showing higher heritability (58%) than men (38%).

Several research groups attempted identification of specific genetic mechanisms or polymorphisms underlying insomnia risk or serving as a perpetuating mechanism. The most commonly studied genes are the period circadian clock gene (i.e., *PER, CLOCK*), serotonin transporter genes (i.e., *5-HTTLPR*[78]), and dopaminergic system genes (e.g., APOE). More recent studies identify as many as 57 different single-nucleotide polymorphisms associated with insomnia that replicated in multiple large biobanks.[97]

Stress and Life Events

Adverse life events can produce physiologic changes to the hypothalamic-pituitary-adrenal and sympathetic-adrenal-medullary systems, which can prompt long-term changes in how individuals experience and manage stress.[98] Studies show activation of the stress system is associated with insomnia,[99–101] which may explain why individuals experience worse sleep after stressful life events,[102,103] especially traumatic ones.[104,105] Stress, particularly its role in arousal, is widely hypothesized to be a key factor in developing insomnia.[74,75] Yet, the relationship between insomnia and stress is complicated. Prospective evidence suggests stress reactivity is a risk factor for insomnia.[71] As some individuals with insomnia may not present with increased stress reactivity,[106] perhaps the relevant issue is the degree to which an individual's sleep responds to that stress exposure. There is relatively extensive work showing that individuals whose sleep reacts to life stress are at increased risk for insomnia.[74,87,107–109] A longitudinal study shows those who experience stressful events are 13% more likely to develop insomnia at 1 year, and those who experience stress-induced cognitive intrusions are 61% more likely, with intrusions mediating stressful-event impact and sleep reactivity accounting for this effect.[110]

Comorbidities

Insomnia is frequently comorbid with other conditions. The conceptualization, though, of comorbid insomnia has changed in recent years. Rather than considering insomnia as either a primary disorder or secondary to another condition, current nosologies consider insomnia disorder as either present or absent, irrespective of whether another condition is present.[6] This is because it is established that evidence does not support the concept of "secondary insomnia." Further, insomnia treatments are generally effective whether or not comorbidities are present.[111,112] When other conditions co-occur with persistent and frequent insomnia, they are considered comorbid, and the insomnia is treated as a separate disorder.

Psychiatric Disorders

Examining the risk relationship between insomnia and psychiatric disorders is complicated.[113] Insomnia is a symptom of many psychiatric disorders, raising the possibility these disorders cause sleep disturbance, but the balance of prospective research shows insomnia is a risk factor for these disorders. Nevertheless, reciprocal exacerbation likely exists between insomnia and psychopathology.[113] A recent meta-analysis demonstrated that insomnia symptoms at baseline in nondepressed individuals are associated with increased likelihood of incident of depression (OR, 2.83), anxiety disorders (OR, 3.23), alcohol abuse (OR, 1.35), and psychosis (OR, 1.28).[114]

Depression

Research suggests depression is the most common insomnia comorbidity.[115] As much as 84% of patients with major depressive disorder report insomnia symptoms versus 10% to 30% of the general population.[12,116,117] Depression or depressive symptoms increase the risk (OR, 1.1 to 8.6)[43,118–121] of developing insomnia across age groups and populations. Of interest, only 23% to 29% of patients report insomnia symptoms developing after depression, whereas 41% to 69% report insomnia symptoms developing before depression, and 8% to 29% report both started at the same time.[122,123] Prospective research has definitively established insomnia as a risk factor for depression.[124]

One recent meta-analysis[125] found insomnia symptoms resulted in nearly two times greater risk (RR, 1.89 to 2.71) of depression. Two studies show that persistence of chronic insomnia[126] or transitioning from acute to chronic insomnia[126,127] portends a first-onset major depressive episode, and this risk may be moderated by short sleep.[126]

Suicide

Considerable evidence supports insomnia as a risk factor for suicide. A recent meta-analysis found that insomnia symptoms were significantly associated with suicidal ideation (2.8-fold), suicide attempts (3.5-fold), and completed suicide (2.4-fold),[128] a finding confirmed in Japanese adults[129] and Chinese psychiatric outpatients.[130] A recent study replicated these results, cross-sectionally *and prospectively*, in active duty military (n = 380) but found the relationships were fully mediated by depression severity.[131] A similar, larger (n = 1896) civilian study found "thwarted belongingness" (i.e., not feeling accepted by others), but not anxiety or depression, mediated the relationship between insomnia and suicide.[132] Insomnia is an extremely important "modifiable" risk factor for suicide because patients, military or not, may be more willing to disclose sleep-related problems than mood disturbances. This hypothesis was validated in a larger sample showing insomnia severity, and not suicidal symptoms, was the best predictor of US Army recruits attending mental health visits and the only predictor of later major depressive episodes.[133]

The only study that examined suicidal ideation and attempts as risk factors for insomnia found that baseline suicidal ideation did not predict insomnia symptoms at follow-up after controlling for baseline insomnia symptoms and other relevant predictors, including hopelessness, depression, posttraumatic stress disorder (PTSD), anxiety, and substance use/abuse.[134]

Anxiety

Insomnia is also closely associated with anxiety disorders, with as much as 64% of patients with generalized anxiety disorder reporting insomnia symptoms (for a more thorough review see Chapter 165).[135] Similar to depression, until recently, insomnia was considered a symptom of anxiety. In contrast to depression, 44% to 73% of patients report insomnia symptoms developing after an anxiety disorder, whereas only 16% to 18% reported insomnia symptoms developing before an anxiety disorder, and 11% to 39% report they started at the same time.[122,123] Anxiety disorders are a risk factor for insomnia symptoms in adults (RR, 1.39 to 4.24) and adolescents (RR, 2.3 to 5.5) in multiple cultures.[43,120,121]

Several studies establish insomnia is a risk factor for developing anxiety disorders. One literature review found people with insomnia were 1.97 to 6.3 times more likely to develop an anxiety disorder than those without insomnia.[124] More recently, research[43] found that having insomnia at baseline increased the risk of developing incident anxiety disorders by 1.43 to 3.64 times, after controlling for age, sex, SES, and baseline depression and pain. Similar results (OR, 2.44 to 5.86) were found in a Korean older-adult sample, after controlling for demographics, socioeconomic factors, and comorbid anxiety and medical illnesses.[136]

Posttraumatic Stress Disorder

Approximately 41% to 51% of people with PTSD report insomnia symptoms,[137,138] and in the US Army, as much as 56% of soldiers reporting insomnia also report comorbid PTSD.[138] Few longitudinal studies examine the relationship between insomnia and PTSD. Even fewer found evidence or even investigated PTSD as risk factor for insomnia. However, several found insomnia and other sleep disturbances are risk factors for PTSD.

One study of Palestinian adults living amid ongoing violent political turmoil found baseline PTSD was not associated with increased "difficulty sleeping" at 6-month follow-up, but baseline "difficulty sleeping" was associated with increased PTSD, depression, and intrapersonal resource loss after controlling for baseline sleep problems.[139] A similar study of US soldiers also found PTSD symptoms at 4 months of postdeployment did not predict change in insomnia at 12 months of postdeployment, again controlling for baseline insomnia.[140] Conversely, in both studies, baseline insomnia predicted PTSD symptoms at follow-up, even after controlling for baseline PTSD. However, in a study of Dutch service members assessed before and after military deployment, insomnia symptom severity at baseline did not predict PTSD symptoms at 6 months (0.86 to 1.16), after controlling for multiple factors.[141] A more recent study investigating bidirectional associations between daily PTSD symptoms and sleep quality in World Trade Center responders (n = 202) found increased PTSD symptoms on a given day were prospectively associated with worse sleep quality, but not vice versa.[142]

Substance Use and Abuse

One early systematic review found people with insomnia symptoms at baseline were 2.35 times more likely to develop alcohol abuse or dependence disorders and 7.18 times more likely to develop drug abuse or dependence disorders than people without insomnia symptoms.[124] These results were not replicated in a study examining whether insomnia presence in adolescence predicted young adult substance use, after controlling for higher report of substance use in adolescents with versus without insomnia (OR, 1.26 to 2.85).[143] However, recent interest and evidence in this topic has increased substantially, with multiple studies in the past decade demonstrating baseline insomnia symptoms predict increased alcohol and drug use, abuse, and problems in adolescents.[144–150] One study found 25% of college students report using alcohol or marijuana as a sleep aid, and those who reported doing so at baseline were much more likely to have increased alcohol use, abuse, and problems at follow-up (average of 68 days later).[151] Not surprising, one review found difficulty falling asleep consistently predicted relapse among persons recovering from alcohol addiction, which the authors theorized may generalize to other psychoactive substances (i.e., nicotine, cocaine, amphetamines, opioids, sedative-hypnotics).[152] A more recent study only partially supports this hypothesis, showing pretreatment insomnia levels predicted 12-month cocaine relapse (OR, 1.04 to 1.62), but not heroin or alcohol relapse.[149]

Table 90.2 Prevalence of Medical Problems in People with or without Insomnia

Medical Problem	Prevalence of Medical Problem (%)[a] PWI	PNI	Adjusted Odds Ratio[b] (95% CI)
Heart disease	21.9	9.5	2.27 (1.13–4.56)[c]
Cancer	8.8	4.2	2.58 (0.98–6.82)
Hypertension	43.1	18.7	3.18 (1.90–5.32)[d]
Neurologic disease	7.3	1.2	4.64 (1.37–15.67)[c]
Breathing problems	24.8	5.7	3.78 (1.73–8.27)[e]
Urinary problems	19.7	9.5	3.28 (1.67–6.43)[e]
Diabetes mellitus	13.1	5.0	1.80 (0.78–4.16)
Chronic pain	50.4	18.2	3.19 (1.92–5.29)[d]
Gastrointestinal problems	33.6	9.2	3.33 (1.83–6.05)[d]
Any medical problem	86.1	48.4	5.17 (2.93–9.12)[d]

[a]Percentage of people with or without insomnia who report that particular disease.
[b]Adjusted for depression, anxiety, and sleep disorder symptoms.
[c]$P < .05$
[d]$P < .001$
[e]$P < .01$
CI, Confidence interval; PNI, people not having insomnia; PWI, people with insomnia.
Modified from Taylor DJ, Mallory LJ, Lichstein KL, et al. Comorbidity of chronic insomnia with medical problems. *Sleep.* 2007;30:213–8.

Table 90.3 Prevalence of Insomnia in People with or without Medical Disorders

Medical Problem	Insomnia Prevalence (%)[a] PHM	PNM	Adjusted Odds Ratio[b] (95% CI)
Heart disease	44.1	22.8	2.11 (1.07–4.15)[c]
Cancer	41.4	24.6	2.50 (1.01–6.21)[c]
Hypertension	44.0	19.3	3.19 (1.87–5.43)[d]
Neurologic disease	66.7	24.3	5.21 (1.22–22.21)[c]
Breathing problems	59.6	21.4	2.79 (1.27–6.14)[c]
Urinary problems	41.5	23.3	3.51 (1.82–6.79)[d]
Diabetes mellitus	47.4	23.8	2.03 (0.86–4.79)
Chronic pain	48.6	17.2	3.16 (1.90–5.27)[d]
Gastrointestinal problems	55.4	20.0	3.00 (1.66–5.43)[d]
Any medical problem	37.8	8.4	5.26 (2.82–9.80)[c]

[a]Percentage of people with or without that particular disease who report insomnia.
[b]Adjusted for depression, anxiety, and sleep disorder symptoms.
[c]$P < .05$
[d]$P < .001$
CI, Confidence interval; PHM, people who reported having the medical problem; PNM, people who did not report having the medical problem.
Modified from Taylor DJ, Mallory LJ, Lichstein KL, et al. Comorbidity of chronic insomnia with medical problems. *Sleep.* 2007;30:213–8.

MEDICAL DISORDERS

Medical disorders are ubiquitous in insomnia (Table 90.2). One could argue that even though this is based mostly on cross-sectional data, when insomnia prevalence runs two to five times the population prevalence (Table 90.3), as is the case in many severe medical conditions,[138,153,154] these conditions are likely a risk factor for insomnia. The few longitudinal studies examining medical status find general health status or having greater than one medical disorder are insomnia risk factors (OR, 1.3 to 3.8).[18,19,71,118,119] One study found baseline kidney/bladder problems and migraines, and, to a lesser extent, allergy/asthma and anemia, were risk factors for incident chronic insomnia, but these significant results were lost after controlling for baseline mental health problems.[19] A similar study of the same sample found both medical (e.g., obesity, sleep apnea, and ulcer) and mental (e.g., depression) health conditions and behavioral factors (e.g., smoking and alcohol consumption), when considered simultaneously (i.e., controlling for all factors) increased incident insomnia symptoms (i.e., poor sleep).[18]

Even fewer studies investigated insomnia as a risk factor for medical disorders, which is surprising considering people with severe insomnia report more medical problems, more physician office visits, being hospitalized twice as often, and more medication use than good sleepers.[155] A recent Norwegian large, prospective, population-based study found insomnia was a significant risk factor for *incidence* of many medical problems: fibromyalgia (OR, 1.51 to 2.79), rheumatoid arthritis (OR, 1.29 to 2.52), arthrosis (OR, 1.43 to 1.98), osteoporosis (OR, 1.14 to 2.01), headache (OR, 1.16 to 1.95), asthma (OR, 1.16 to 1.86), and myocardial infarction (OR, 1.06 to 2.00), even after controlling for confounding factors.[156] Chapter 94 addresses these issues in more detail.

Cardiovascular Disease and Hypertension

Cardiovascular disease is a risk factor for insomnia, but of great interest is insomnia as a risk factor for hypertension and cardiovascular diseases. Most studies reporting on insomnia as a risk factor for incident hypertension consistently suggest a positive relationship. A meta-analysis of prospective studies finds insomnia is associated with a 5% to 20% increased risk for hypertension.[157] However, this meta-analysis, along with several other studies, did not adequately account for PSG-confirmed SDB, and oftentimes hypertension was self-reported or based on single time-point blood pressure assessments.[158] Also, the literature is somewhat unclear regarding whether these risks apply to insomnia symptoms or insomnia disorder or both. Longitudinal studies accounting for some of these weaknesses indicate insomnia symptoms and chronic insomnia remain as risk factors for hypertension, but only in the presence of objectively measured short sleep duration.[24,159] A recent systematic review concluded insomnia of greater frequency, chronicity, and/or associated with objective short sleep duration or physiologic hyperarousal is associated with increased hypertension risk.[160]

Prospective studies also demonstrate heightened risk for incident cardiovascular disease events among persons with insomnia compared to normal sleepers. Prior meta-analyses find insomnia symptoms increase risk (28% to 45%) for several cardiovascular outcomes (e.g., myocardial infarction, stroke).[161,162] However, consistency in insomnia definitions and assessment is lacking. Similar to the studies on hypertension, the insomnia with objective short sleep duration phenotype appears to be associated with 29% increased risk for incident cardiovascular disease.

WORK

Compared to people working full-time, insomnia symptoms are more common among those unemployed or unable to work[55] and those with insecure employment.[163] Several studies show insomnia impacts an individual's ability to work. Compared to good sleepers, employees with insomnia report lower self-esteem at work, less work satisfaction, and decreased work efficiency.[164] Workers with insomnia demonstrate approximately 6.1% productivity loss, whereas good sleepers report approximately 2.5% productivity loss (3.6% absolute difference).[165] These results are similar to another study showing that, compared to good sleepers, workers with frequent trouble sleeping report an absolute difference of 3.6% in ratings of their own work performance and 2.4% difference in the discrepancy between their own performance and perceived performance of a typical person in that job, controlling for age, sex race/ethnicity, education, income, and overall health.[166] This study further shows work performance decreased by 1.1% for every 1-point increase on a 5-point scale.[167] This study also shows that persistent trouble sleeping is associated with absenteeism and increased health care costs, and over a 1-year period, if sleep worsened, these outcomes also worsened. These results are consistent with findings by others that show that insomnia is associated with absenteeism,[168–172] occupational injuries/accidents,[169,170,173,174] and likelihood of disability payments.[167,175–177]

CONTROVERSIES

Drawing conclusions based on epidemiologic studies is challenging because methodological approaches (i.e., different insomnia definitions, inadequate control for alternative explanations) vary considerably. Some studies examined sleep "problems" or "disturbances" rather than insomnia symptoms, syndrome, or diagnosis but may assess insomnia components, which further contributes to even greater methodological variation. Careful consideration of these methodological differences is important when interpreting epidemiologic findings. In addition, insomnia is often comorbid with other undiagnosed sleep disorders (e.g., obstructive sleep apnea),[178,179] but the prevalence of sleep comorbidities is unclear.

SUMMARY

The prevalence of chronic insomnia is 10%, but insomnia symptoms occur in a much larger portion of the population. Differences in how insomnia is perceived may produce underestimates of clinically significant insomnia among racial/ethnic minority adults. Advancing age, female sex, and low SES are strong insomnia risk factors. Empirical support for hyperarousal as an insomnia predisposing risk factor is limited, but emerging evidence suggests that hyperarousal-related factors (e.g., cortical arousal/environmental awareness, responsiveness of sleep to stress) warrant additional study. Recurrent acute insomnia and genetics are emerging risk factors. Insomnia also serves as a risk factor for psychiatric and possibly medical conditions, but the mechanisms and important mediators/moderators underlying that risk remain poorly understood. Research priorities include increased use of standardized insomnia criteria; longitudinal studies; expanded examination of medical comorbidities, genetics, and sleep health disparities; and increased understanding of perceptions of insomnia in non-White racial ethnic groups, hyperarousal, and related factors, as well as other mechanisms, causal paths, and mediators/moderators of insomnia risk.

CLINICAL PEARLS

- Although 30% of individuals report occasional insomnia symptoms, chronic insomnia impacts 10% of the general population.
- Most newly reported insomnia symptoms remit within 3 months. Those that do not typically require intervention.
- Advancing age, female gender, and low socioeconomic status are the strongest risk factors of insomnia.
- Insomnia is a risk factor for psychiatric (e.g., depression, substance abuse, posttraumatic stress disorder), and possibly medical comorbidities (e.g., hypertension, chronic pain, asthma), but more evidence is needed. In addition, mechanisms, causal paths, and mediators/moderators of these risk relationships are poorly understood.
- Differences in the perception of insomnia may contribute to fewer insomnia complaints and result in underestimation of clinically significant insomnia among racial/ethnic minority adults.

SELECTED READINGS

Chen X, Wang R, Zee P, et al. Racial/ethnic differences in sleep disturbances: the Multi-Ethnic Study of Atherosclerosis (MESA). *Sleep*. 2015. https://doi.org/10.5665/sleep.4732.

Fernandez-Mendoza J, Vgontzas AN, Bixler EO, et al. Clinical and polysomnographic predictors of the natural history of poor sleep in the general population. *Sleep*. 2012;35(5):689–697.

Grandner MA, Ruiter Petrov ME, Rattanaumpawan P, Jackson N, Platt A, Patel NP. Sleep symptoms, race/ethnicity, and socioeconomic position. *J Clin Sleep Med*. 2013. https://doi.org/10.5664/jcsm.2990.

Hertenstein E, Feige B, Gmeiner T, et al. Insomnia as a predictor of mental disorders: a systematic review and meta-analysis. *Sleep Med Rev*. 2019. https://doi.org/10.1016/j.smrv.2018.10.006.

Jansson-Fröjmark M, Linton SJ. The course of insomnia over one year: a longitudinal study in the general population in Sweden. *Sleep*. 2008;31:881–886. https://doi.org/10.1093/sleep/31.6.881.

Kalmbach DA, Pillai V, Arnedt JT, Anderson JR, Drake CL. Sleep system sensitization: evidence for changing roles of etiological factors in insomnia. *Sleep Med*. 2016. https://doi.org/10.1016/j.sleep.2016.02.005.

Kaufmann CN, Mojtabai R, Hock RS, et al. Racial/ethnic differences in insomnia trajectories among US older adults. *Am J Geriatr Psychiatry*. 2016;24(7):575–584.

Khachatryan SG. Insomnia burden and future perspectives. *Sleep Med Clin*. 2021;16(3):513–521.

Liu T, Wu D, Yan W, et al. Twelve-month systemic consequences of COVID-19 in patients discharged from hospital: a prospective cohort study in Wuhan, China [published online ahead of print, 2021 Aug 14]. *Clin Infect Dis*. 2021:ciab703.

Mai QD, Hill TD, Vila-Henninger L, Grandner MA. Employment insecurity and sleep disturbance: evidence from 31 European countries. *J Sleep Res*. 2019. https://doi.org/10.1111/jsr.12763.
Meira E, Cruz M, Kryger MH, et al. Comorbid insomnia and sleep apnea: mechanisms and implications of an underrecognized and misinterpreted sleep disorder. *Sleep Med*. 2021;84:283–288.
Morin CM, Jarrin DC, Ivers H, Merette C, LeBlanc M, Savard J. Incidence, persistence, and remission rates of insomnia over 5 years. *JAMA Netw Open*. 2020. https://doi.org/10.1001/jamanetworkopen.2020.18782.
Ohayon MM. Epidemiology of insomnia: what we know and what we still need to learn. *Sleep Med Rev*. 2002. https://doi.org/10.1053/smrv.2002.0186.
Petrov ME, Lichstein KL. Differences in sleep between black and white adults: an update and future directions. *Sleep Med*. 2016. https://doi.org/10.1016/j.sleep.2015.01.011.
Taylor DJ, Mallory LJ, Lichstein KL, et al. Comorbidity of chronic insomnia with medical problems. *Sleep*. 2007;30:213–218.

A complete reference list can be found online at ExpertConsult.com.

Chapter 91

Etiology and Pathophysiology of Insomnia

Michael L. Perlis; Jason G. Ellis; Kai Spiegelhalder; Dieter Riemann

Chapter Highlights

- Up until the late 1990s, there were only two models regarding the etiology and pathophysiology of insomnia; namely, the Stimulus Control and 3P models.
- Since the 1990s, there has been a proliferation of theoretical perspectives on the etiology and pathophysiology of insomnia that includes both human and animal models.
- The newer models of insomnia integrate the concepts gained from research in humans, experimental mammals, and insects *Drosophila*.
- The human models of insomnia include classical stimulus control, the three-factor (3-P) model, the neurocognitive model, the psychobiological inhibition model, and the neurobiological model.
- The models based on non-human findings include the Cano-Saper rodent model, the Shaw *Drosophila* model, and the Kayser-Belfer *Drosophila* model.
- The models have implications that affect current and future therapeutics.

INTRODUCTION

Until the late 1990s there were only two models regarding the etiology and pathophysiology of insomnia—namely, the stimulus control and three-factor (3P) models. The relative lack of theoretical perspectives was due to at least three factors. First, the long-time characterization of insomnia as a symptom carried with it the clear implication that insomnia was not itself worth modeling as a disorder or disease state. Second, the widespread conceptualization of insomnia as owing directly to hyperarousal (levels of physiologic or central nervous system [CNS] arousal that are sufficiently high as to directly prohibit sleep) may have made it appear that further explanation was not necessary. Third, for those inclined toward theory, the acceptance of the behavioral models (i.e., the stimulus control model[1] and the three-factor model[2]), and the treatments that were derived from them, might have had the untoward effect of discouraging the development of alternative or elaborative models.

Since the 1990s there has been a proliferation of theoretical perspectives on the etiology and pathophysiology of insomnia that includes both human and animal models. In the prior edition of this volume, nine of the human models were described and critiqued. The models presented spanned from the classical behavioral perspectives, to the traditionally cognitively focused frameworks, to the more modern cognitive information-processing perspectives, to an interaction paradigm that takes into account basal arousal and sleep requirement, to the neurocognitive and neurobiologic models that essentially frame insomnia, from a functional and neurophysiologic point of view, as a hybrid state. In the present chapter, five human and three animal models are reviewed: the classical stimulus control[1] and three-factor models,[2] the neurocognitive model,[3] the psychobiological inhibition (PI) model,[4] the neurobiologic model,[5] the Cano-Saper rodent model,[6] the Shaw *Drosophila* model,[7] and the Belfer-Kayser *Drosophila* model.[8] Each of these models are reviewed here based on their theoretical importance and the extent to which they have been impactful (have endured over time and are frequently cited). A more comprehensive coverage of the existing models is provided in the sixth edition of this volume (see Table 91.1).

DEFINITION OF INSOMNIA

The *Diagnostic and Statistical Manual of Mental Disorders,* fifth edition (DSM-5)[9] and *International Classification of Sleep Disorders,* third edition (ICSD-3)[10] define *Insomnia Disorder* as difficulty initiating or maintaining sleep on 3 or more nights per week for at least 3 months. This definition further stipulates that the diagnosis of insomnia must take into account sleep opportunity, level of daytime impairment and distress, whether symptom presentation (in the case of children and elders) varies with caregiver presence, and the possibility that the insomnia is not better explained by (or does not occur exclusively during the course of) other sleep disorders or medical or psychiatric illnesses. For further consideration of how this definition differs from prior formulations and for commentary regarding the implications of the changes, please see Chapter 93 in this volume.

Table 91.1 Central Concepts of Insomnia Models in Order of Date of Description

Human Models	Animal Models
Stimulus dyscontrol promotes wakefulness	Psychosocial stress induces sleeplessness
Sleep-related stimuli may become conditioned stimuli for wakefulness	Induced sleeplessness is associated with abnormal activity within the anterior hypothalamus (VLPO)
Stress induces sleeplessness	Induced sleeplessness is associated with cortical activation
All individuals may be at risk for insomnia (acute insomnia)	Insomnia-like sleep patterns are heritable (and subject to genetic/laboratory selection)
Insomnia may be a part of the flight-or-fight response	Selectively bred short sleep (low sleep ability) is associated with sleep continuity disturbance
Insomnia may occur as an override to the normal homeostatic and circadian imperatives for sleep	Sleep continuity disturbance and short sleep are associated with daytime deficits in *Drosophila*
Sleep extension (the mismatch between sleep opportunity and ability) serves to perpetuate sleeplessness	Experimentally mismatching sleep opportunity and ability in wild type flies is "insomnogenic"
Altered sensory and information processing are features of chronic insomnia	Mutant short sleeping flies exhibit a mismatch sleep opportunity and ability
Chronic insomnia entails an attenuation of the normal mesograde amnesia of sleep	The mismatch in sleep opportunity and ability can be rectified by changing the light: dark period
The "inhibition of sleep-related de-arousal" (as opposed to hyperarousal) gives rise to enduring sleep continuity disturbance.	
Problematic perceptions and the engagement of behaviors that perpetuate insomnia occur due to a shift in attention, intention, and effort from stressor to sleeplessness (A-I-E Pathway)	
Chronic insomnia may occur as a hybrid state (part NREM sleep and part wake)	
Chronic insomnia may occur as a hybrid state with local neuronal wakefulness during NREM sleep	

HUMAN MODELS

Stimulus Control Model

Basic Description

Stimulus control, as originally described by Bootzin in 1972,[1,11] is based on the behavioral principle that one stimulus may elicit a variety of responses, depending on the conditioning history (Figure 91.1). A simple conditioning history, wherein a stimulus is always paired with a single behavior, yields a high probability that the stimulus will yield only one response. A complex conditioning history, wherein a stimulus is paired with a variety of behaviors, yields a low probability that the stimulus will yield only one response. In individuals with insomnia, the normal cues associated with sleep (e.g., bed, bedroom, bedtime, etc.) are frequently paired with behaviors other than sleep. For instance, to cope with insomnia, the individual may spend a large amount of time in the bed and bedroom awake and engaging in behaviors other than sleep. These coping behaviors appear to the individual to be both reasonable (i.e., staying in bed is at least permissive of "rest") and reasonably successful (i.e., engaging in alternative behaviors in the bedroom appears to sometimes result in improved sleep). These practices, however, set the stage for stimulus dyscontrol, that is, reduced probability that sleep-related stimuli will elicit the desired response of sleepiness and sleep. Figure 91.1 provides a schematic representation of stimulus control and stimulus dyscontrol.

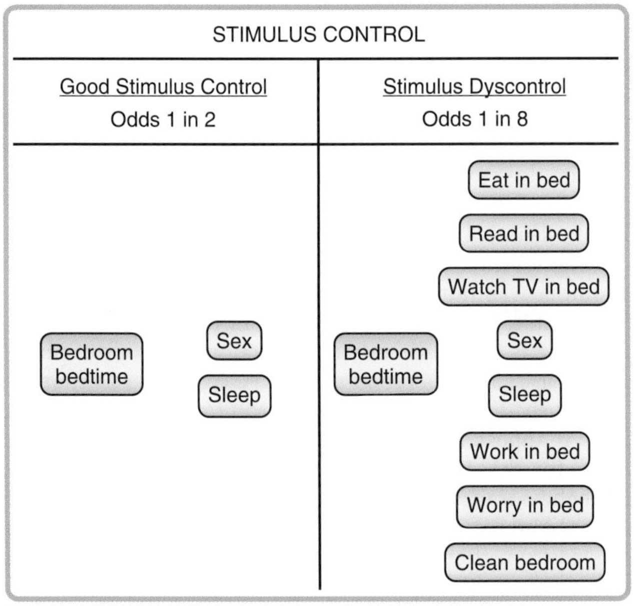

Figure 91.1 The schematic represents the instrumental conditioning perspective on stimulus control. In the *left frame* (good stimulus control) the bedroom is tightly coupled with sleep and sex where, given the orthogonality and equal probability of events, the probability of association of bedroom to sleep is 1 in 2. In the *right frame* (stimulus dyscontrol) the bedroom is no longer a strong associate of sleep and sex where, given the orthogonality and equal probability of events, the probability of association of bedroom to sleep is 1 in 8. The treatment implication of stimulus dyscontrol is the voluntary elimination (hence instrumental conditioning) of the nonsleep associates, except that sex should make it more likely that sleep will occur in the bedroom.

Strengths and Limitations

The treatment derived from stimulus control theory is one of the most widely used behavioral treatments, and its efficacy has been well established.[12–16] The success of the therapy, however, is not sufficient evidence to say that stimulus dyscontrol is responsible for the etiology or pathophysiology of insomnia. In fact, one investigation found that the reverse of stimulus control instructions also improved sleep continuity.[17] Another limitation of the stimulus control perspective is that it focuses on instrumental conditioning. That is, there are behaviors that reduce or enhance the probability of the occurrence of sleep. The original model does not explicitly delineate how classical or pavlovian conditioning may also be an operational factor. Specifically, the regular pairing of the physiology of wakefulness with sleep-related stimuli may lead to sleep-related stimuli becoming conditioned stimuli for wakefulness. This latter possibility, although not part of the classical stimulus control perspective, is clearly consistent with it.[11]

Implications for Current and Future Research and Therapeutics

Given the efficacy of stimulus control therapy, as a monotherapy and as a component of cognitive behavior therapy for insomnia (CBT-I), it would be useful to determine how much of treatment outcome may be related to this treatment modality (compared to sleep restriction, sleep hygiene, and cognitive therapy). More than this, it would be informative to conduct a dismantling study for stimulus control itself, given that the treatment contains not only the instruction to "limit activities in the bedroom to sleep and sex" but also instructions to go to bed only when sleepy, leave the bedroom when awake, get up at the same time every morning irrespective of how much sleep is obtained, and not nap during the day. Any of these components, alone or in combination, may account for the efficacy of stimulus control and may do so through addressing pathogenic factors other than stimulus dyscontrol, such as sleep-wake scheduling irregularity, conditioned wakefulness (pavlovian conditioning), and sleep homeostasis dysregulation. By way of one example, the prescription to get up at the same time every morning, irrespective of how much sleep is obtained, prevents the deleterious effects of excessive time in bed (see Spielman's three-factor model [later]) and may ensure that sleep loss will prime for better sleep on subsequent nights.[18] In a related vein, the instruction to leave the bedroom when awake may serve as a means of ensuring that patients are fully awake (vs. microsleeping) and thus may also improve sleep through sleep homeostatic processes (vs. simple stimulus control). More than this, it may be that being fully awake at night may allow for a greater-than-normal "homeostatic prime" and in doing so account for, in part, the efficacy of stimulus control.[19]

Three-Factor Model

Basic Description

This model, alternatively referred to as the Spielman model, 3P model, or behavioral model, delineates how sleep continuity disturbance occurs acutely and how this becomes both chronic and self-perpetuating[2] (Figures 91.2 and 91.3), leading to insomnia disorder. The model is based on the interaction of three factors. The first two factors (predisposing and precipitating factors) represent a stress-diathesis conceptualization of how insomnia comes to be expressed. The third factor (perpetuating factor) represents how behavioral considerations modulate chronicity.

Predisposing factors extend across the entire biopsychosocial spectrum. Biologic factors include, for example, the genetic predisposition for insomnia or related etiologic factors, increased basal metabolic rate, hyperreactivity, sleep reactivity, and fundamental alterations to the neurotransmitter systems associated with sleep and wakefulness. Psychological factors include worry or the tendency to be excessively ruminative. Social factors, although rarely a focus at the theoretical level, include factors such as the bed partner keeping an incompatible sleep schedule and social pressures to sleep according to a nonpreferred sleep schedule (e.g., child rearing).

Precipitating factors are acute occurrences that trigger sleep continuity disturbance. The primary "triggers" are thought related to life stress events (real or perceived threat), including medical and psychiatric illness.[20–22] It should be noted that acute sleep continuity disturbance is remarkably common (27% to 36% incident rates per annum) with only a fractional percentage of affected individuals (15% to 20%) going on to develop insomnia disorder.

Perpetuating factors refer to the behaviors adopted by the individual that are intended to compensate for (or cope with) sleeplessness, but that actually reinforce the sleep problem. Perpetuating factors include the practice of nonsleep behaviors in the bedroom, staying in bed while awake, and spending excessive amounts of time in bed. Stimulus control speaks to the first two of these (as reviewed earlier). The classic version of the three-factor model focuses primarily on the last of these. Excessive time in bed (or sleep extension) may involve going to bed early, getting out of bed late, and/or napping as ways of coping with insomnia. Such compensatory behaviors are enacted to increase the opportunity to get more sleep and are likely to be highly self-reinforcing because they allow lost sleep to be "recovered" and the daytime effects of lost sleep to be ameliorated. Extension of sleep opportunity can lead to a mismatch between sleep opportunity and sleep ability.[2,23] The greater the mismatch, the more likely the individual will spend prolonged periods of time awake during the given sleep period, regardless of what factors predisposed or precipitated the insomnia.

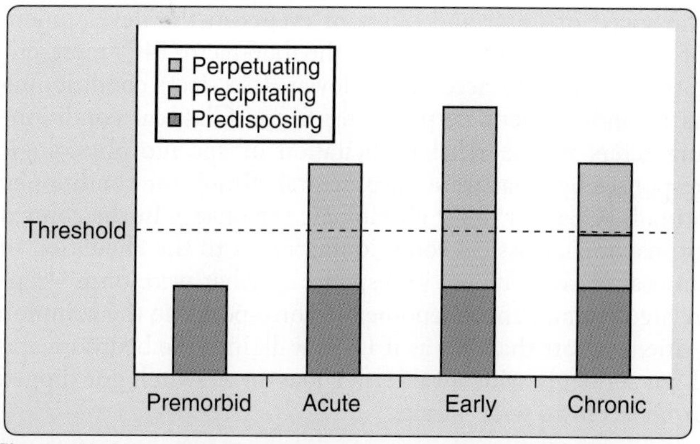

Figure 91.2 The diagram represents the classic 1987 rendition of the three-factor model. There are two more recent representations in Figure 91.3. The reader is encouraged to compare the three versions of the model.

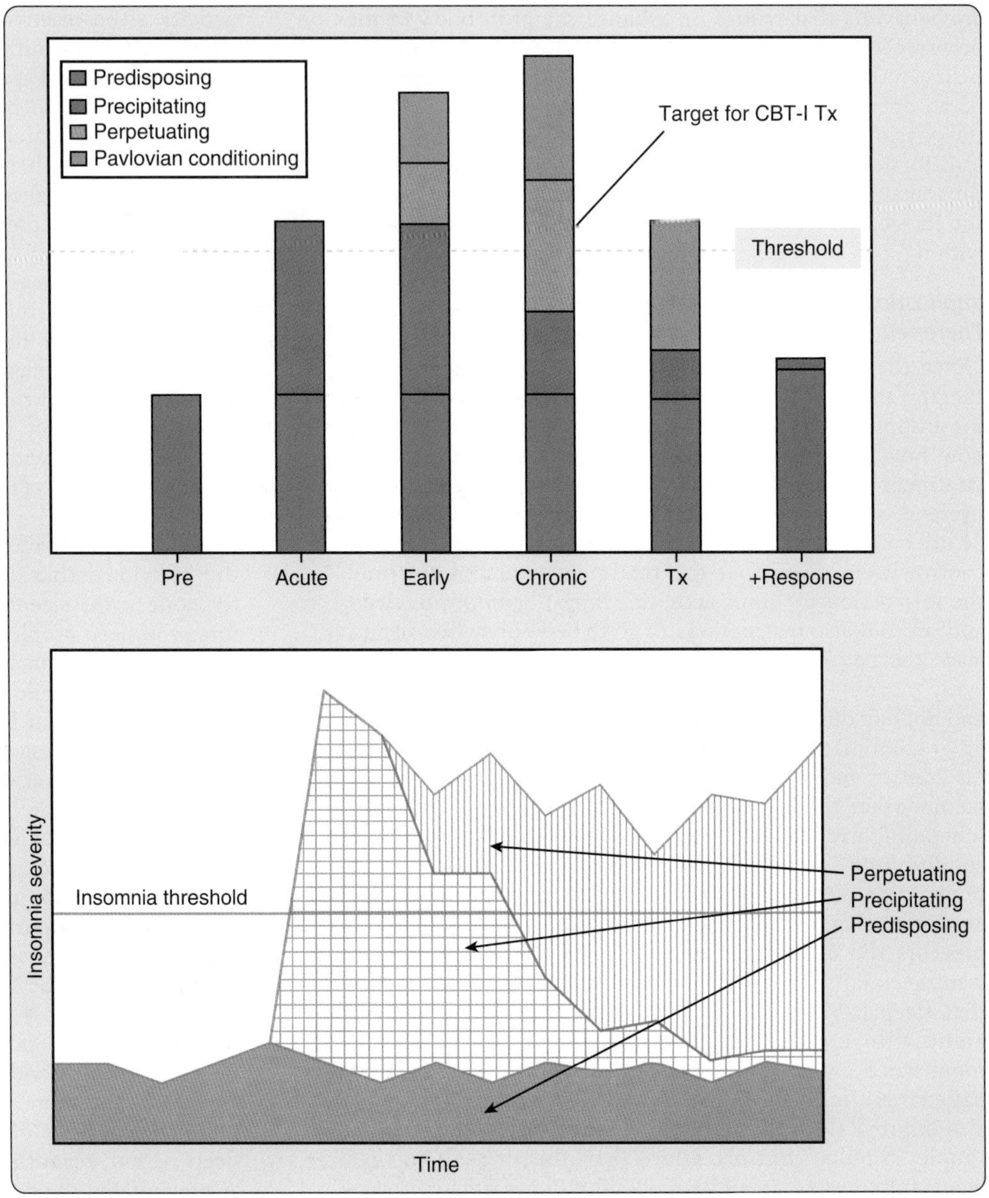

Figure 91.3 The dynamic version of the three-factor model (Figure 91.2) has the added value, compared with the original model, of illustrating the temporal course of each of the factors. The four-factor model has the added value of (1) explicitly incorporating pavlovian conditioning and how this factor affects the clinical course of insomnia and (2) depicting response to cognitive behavior therapy for insomnia (CBT-I) at the end of treatment and 6 to 12 months after treatment discontinuation. Tx, Therapy.

The three-factor model and its graphic representations have been periodically updated.[24] Two examples are provided in Figure 91.3. One version, proffered by Spielman, represents the speed of onset and offset of events in the development of insomnia. The other version, the four-factor (4P) representation, takes into account pavlovian (classical) conditioning as an independent perpetuating factor. Classical conditioning refers to the reliable elicitation of specific physiologic responses by what were once neutral stimuli (or conditioned stimuli [CSs] for other physiologic responses). In the context of insomnia, classical conditioning refers to the elicitation of arousal or wakefulness in response to what were once sleep-related stimuli. This phenomenon corresponds to the common patient report that "it's as if I just walk into the bedroom and I am suddenly wide awake…it's like some switch got flipped from sleepy to wide-awake."

Strengths and Limitations

The three-factor model is conceptually appealing and comports well with both clinical experience and with the two-process model of sleep-wake regulation.[25] The model has good face validity for both patients and clinicians, and the therapy derived from the model (sleep restriction) is efficacious. This said, there have been few studies evaluating sleep restriction therapy as a monotherapy[26] and no studies evaluating the relative efficacy of sleep restriction therapy as a component of CBT-I (i.e., no dismantling studies). It is therefore difficult to assess the extent to which treatment efficacy supports the model. Further, even if studies could show that sleep restriction therapy accounted for most clinical gains with CBT-I, formal validation of the model would still require a natural history study showing that the transition from acute to chronic insomnia is largely mediated by sleep extension.

Another limitation of the original model is the implication that the predisposition for insomnia varies across individuals but is a trait factor within the individual. With respect to between-subjects variability, this means that some individuals are less prone to insomnia disorder, some are marginally at risk, and still others are at high risk. Although it stands to reason that the vulnerability for insomnia exists on a continuum, it is also plausible that *all individuals* are at risk for insomnia (acute insomnia) and that this may be so to the extent that insomnia represents an adaptive response to stress; that is, a real or perceived threat (as part of the flight-fight response) triggers a systemic response that overrides the normal homeostatic and circadian imperatives for sleep (see also, the Cano-Saper model [later]).[27,28] This said, although some predispositions may indeed be "hard wired," some predispositions may vary over the life span (e.g., new sleep environments or partners, pregnancy or child rearing, altered hormonal status, aging effects, prior insomnia experience). Of interest, the newer rendition of the Spielman model (Figure 91.3) portrays predisposing factors varying with time.[24]

Implications for Current and Future Research and Therapeutics

Several avenues for research are possible. Predisposition to insomnia could be, and has recently been, evaluated using genetic data.[29,30] As a complement to this approach, medical anthropologic studies could be used to assess vulnerability to insomnia at the cultural level (industrial vs. nonindustrial societies and the effects of artificial light and other factors associated with urbanization[31]), and natural history studies could be used to assess vulnerability to insomnia at the individual level (the biopsychosocial factors that mediate the transition from good sleep to acute insomnia).[22]

As for the tenets of the three-factor model, the model has served as the conceptual basis for one treatment modality in particular: sleep restriction. This therapy, although believed by many to be the single most potent component of CBT-I, was developed to target one particular perpetuating factor, *sleep extension*. In multicomponent CBT-I, other treatment components address other perpetuating factors. For instance, stimulus control addresses the engagement of nonsleep behaviors in the bedroom and the tendency to remain in bed when awake; cognitive therapy addresses the problem of catastrophic or dysfunctional thinking about insomnia; and sleep hygiene addresses, for instance, the misuse of counterfatigue measures. The relative efficacy of each of these treatment components needs to be further assessed, perhaps with dismantling studies that target *single factors,* as opposed to particular therapies. An example of such a study was recently conducted by Maurer and colleagues,[32] where they showed that sleep restriction produced superior outcomes compared to simple sleep schedule regularization.

This said, it should be noted that there have been at least two studies evaluating the relative efficacy of treatment modalities (e.g., cognitive vs. behavioral therapy for insomnia[33,34]), and these represent an equally worthy effort to determine which components of CBT-I are essential and/or account for the most "therapeutic bang for the buck." The first of the two studies suggested that stimulus control and sleep restriction produce comparable outcomes. The second study suggested that behavioral and cognitive treatments produce comparable outcomes, although behavioral therapy showed a more rapid "onset of action" (more treatment responders at the end of therapy [vs. follow-up assessments]).

Finally, the three-factor model may also help to identify alternative treatment targets for insomnia. For instance, the model could be used to guide the development or adaptation of existing therapies to target predisposing (as opposed to perpetuating) factors. Such treatments could be used to increase treatment response, to diminish the risk for recurrence, or (prophylactically) to prevent first episodes of insomnia.

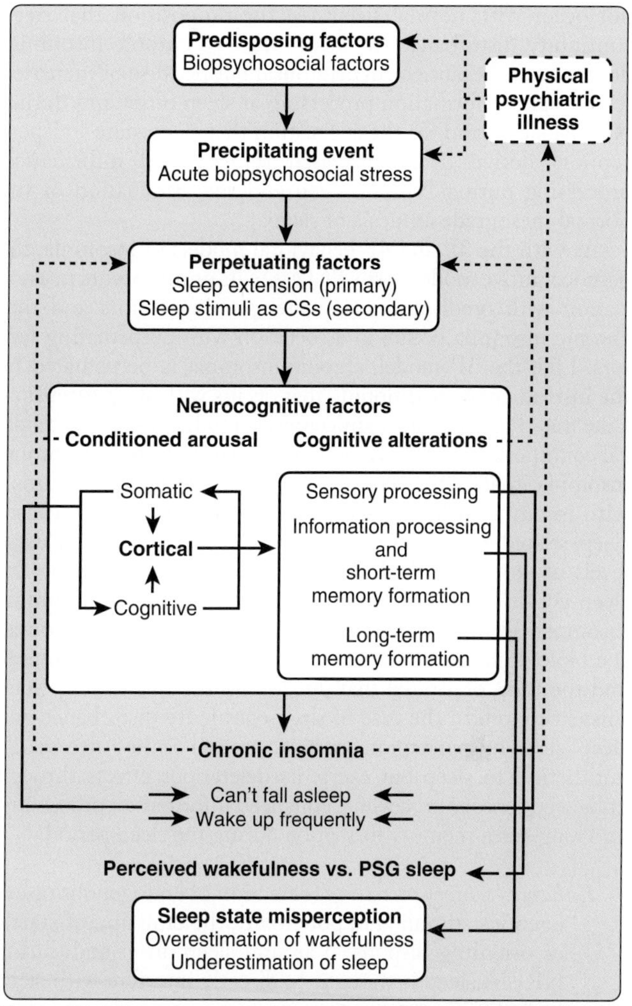

Figure 91.4 The schematic is different from prior publications of the neurocognitive model in several ways: (1) *Dotted lines* are provided to highlight feedback loops (*solid lines* represent feed-forward loops); (2) The examples provided for perpetuating factors have been changed. The primary factor is designated as "sleep extension" (previously denoted as increased time in bed and staying awake in bed). The secondary factor is designated as "sleep stimuli as CSs." This is meant to represent when "sleep stimuli" become CSs for wakefulness (arousal); The section of the diagram denoted "neurocognitive factors" may well correspond to the "persistence of wakefulness" (when such events occur before sleep onset proper) and the "failure to inhibit wakefulness" (when such events occur during non–rapid eye movement sleep). The latter may correspond to what is characterized by Cano and Saper[6] as "hybrid state" (not entirely sleep or wakefulness) and may be accounted for by "local neuronal wakefulness" as posited by Buysse and colleagues.[5] CSs, Conditioned stimuli; PSG, polysomnography.

Neurocognitive Model

Basic Description

The neurocognitive model is based on, and is an extension of, the 3P and 4P models[3] (Figure 91.4). The central tenets of the neurocognitive model include (1) a pluralistic perspective of hyperarousal (cortical, cognitive, and somatic arousal); (2) the specification that cortical arousal (as opposed to cognitive or somatic arousal) is central to the etiology and pathophysiology of insomnia; (3) the proposition that cortical arousal, in the context of chronic insomnia, occurs as a result of classical conditioning and is permissive of cognitive processes that do not occur with normal sleep; (4) the proposition that sleep continuity disturbance (in the context of chronic insomnia) do not occur because of hyperarousal but because of increased sensory and information processing at sleep onset and during NREM sleep; and (5) the suggestion that sleep state "misperception" derives from increased sensory and information processing during NREM sleep and the attenuation of the normal mesograde amnesia of sleep.

As with the 3P and 4P behavioral models of insomnia, the neurocognitive model posits that acute insomnia occurs in association with predisposing and precipitating factors and that chronic insomnia occurs in association with perpetuating factors. Like the 3P model, chronic insomnia is perpetuated by the instrumental conditioning that occurs with sleep extension. Like the 4P model, the neurocognitive model posits that classical conditioning also serves as a perpetuating factor for chronic insomnia; that is, the repeated pairing of sleep-related stimuli with insomnia-related wakefulness (arousal) ultimately causes sleep-related stimuli to elicit (or maintain) higher than usual levels of cortical arousal at around sleep onset or during the sleep period. This form of arousal is, in the context of chronic insomnia, is thought to be independent of somatic arousal; the biologic substrate for, and precipitant of, cognitive arousal; and the form of arousal that directly contributes to sleep state misperception. In the case of sleep continuity disturbance and sleep state misperception, cortical arousal is not necessarily antithetical to sleep but exerts its deleterious effects through enhanced sensory processing, enhanced information processing, and long-term memory formation during the sleep period.

Enhanced sensory processing (detection of endogenous or exogenous stimuli and, potentially, the emission of startle or orienting responses) around sleep onset and during NREM sleep is thought to directly interfere with sleep initiation or maintenance.

Enhanced information processing (detection of, and discrimination between, stimuli and the formation of a short-term memory of the stimulating events) during NREM sleep is thought to blur the perceptual distinction between sleep and wakefulness and thus contribute to sleep state misperception.

Enhanced long-term memory (the recollection of stimulating events hours after their occurrence) around sleep onset and during NREM sleep is thought to interfere with the subjective experience of sleep initiation and duration and thus contribute to the discrepancies between subjectively and objectively assessed sleep continuity.

Finally, conditioned cortical arousal is hypothesized to be self-reinforcing and thus like sleep extension, serves to perpetuate insomnia in the absence of the original precipitants. That is, each time sleep-related stimuli (i.e., the specifics of the sleep environment) elicit cortical arousal, this reinforces the potential of sleep-related stimuli to serve as conditioned stimuli for enhanced sensory and information processing or long-term memory formation.

Strengths and Limitations

In general, the major strengths of the neurocognitive model are that it allows a pluralistic perspective on the concept of arousal, does not require that hyperarousal be so intense as to directly interfere with sleep initiation and maintenance, delineates a mechanism beyond that of instrumental conditioning (i.e., classical conditioning as a perpetuating factor), allows a distinction between the type and intensity of arousal responsible for acute insomnia and that which is responsible for chronic insomnia, specifies how chronic insomnia "takes on a life of its own" (i.e., is self-reinforcing); and is based on hypotheses that are falsifiable.

To date the evidence for the model derives from observations about individuals with insomnia compared with good sleepers exhibiting increased cortical or CNS arousal using such measures as quantitative electroencephalography[35–42] and positron emission tomography,[43,44] increased sensory or information processing using such measures as evoked response potentials,[45,46] an attenuation of the normal mesograde amnesia of sleep using such measures as implicit and explicit memory tests for semantic stimuli presented during sleep,[47] and an association between sleep state misperception and objective measures of cortical arousal or evoked response potential abnormalities.[48–50]

The primary limitations of the neurocognitive model are that it does not adequately account for the transition from acute insomnia to good sleep (recovery), the importance of circadian and homeostatic influences on sleep in which brain regions or circuits are abnormally activated around sleep onset and during NREM sleep, the likely possibility that abnormal activation may also occur in subcortical regions, and the neurobiologic mechanisms by which insomnia may occur as a hybrid state (as a *status dissociates* disorder of wake and NREM sleep, as presaged by Mahowald and Schenck in 1991[51]). Some speculations regarding the functional anatomic substrate of the neurocognitive model have been published since the model was first introduced.[52,53]

Implications for Current and Future Research and Therapeutics

Many of the model's central tenets require further empirical validation. For instance, laboratory studies are needed to demonstrate that neurocognitive processes (sensory and information processing and long-term memory formation) are reliably altered in patients with insomnia disorder, that the alterations occur with the onset of chronic insomnia, and the magnitude of the alterations are strongly correlated with insomnia severity. Further, it must be shown that there is *a conditioned aspect* to the "insomnia response" (i.e., neurocognitive processing is conditionable) and that altered neurocognitive processing has clear (1) *neurobiologic substrates* (e.g., altered activity in specific brain regions or the occurrence of local neuronal wakefulness) and (2) *functional consequences* (sleep continuity disturbance and sleep state misperception). In short, novel experimental paradigms need to be developed to test the model's core hypotheses.

The neurocognitive model may provide some insight into the potential mechanisms of action of existing therapies and also some guidance regarding potential targets for new treatments. In the case of existing therapies, pharmacotherapy might be effective to the extent that the various compounds block sensory and information processing or promote amnesia for episodic memories formed during the sleep period. This idea, first espoused by Mendelson,[54–59] seems probable given the effects of benzodiazepines and benzodiazepine receptor agonists on arousal thresholds and memory formation. Sleep restriction therapy might also work through these mechanisms to the extent that this treatment modality serves to deepen sleep, which may augment the endogenous form of sleep-related mesograde amnesia.[60,61] Potential avenues for new medical treatments include the assessment of compounds that have greater-than-normal amnestic potential for their efficacy as hypnotics, provided that such effects can be limited to the desired sleep period. Given that this is not possible, potent amnestics may be used experimentally to determine the extent to which amnesia for events occurring during the sleep period influences morning recall about sleep continuity and sleep quality. Alternatively, it may be possible to use stimulants during the day (e.g., modafinil) to promote wake extension and thereby decrease nocturnal cortical arousal through increased sleep pressure. Potential avenues for behavioral treatment include protocols that use more intensive forms of sleep restriction to promote counterconditioning, such as intensive sleep retraining therapy.[62]

Psychobiologic Inhibition Model

Basic Description

The PI model posits that good sleep is ensured by automaticity and plasticity (Figure 91.5).[4,63] Automaticity refers to the involuntary nature of sleep initiation and maintenance, governed by processes such as homeostatic and circadian regulation.[25] Plasticity refers to the ability of the system to accommodate real-world circumstances. Under normal circumstances, sleep occurs passively (without attention, intention, or effort). Within the context of normal sleep, stressful life events precipitate both physiologic and psychological arousal, which can result in inhibition of sleep-related dearousal and the occurrence of selective attending to the life stressors. In acute insomnia, physiologic and psychological arousal interfere with the normal homeostatic and circadian regulation of sleep. Acute insomnia may, in turn, resolve or be perpetuated based on whether the stressor resolves or the individual attends to the insomnia symptoms that occur with the acute insomnia. The shift of attention from the life stressor, implicitly or explicitly, to the insomnia symptoms is posited to be the first of three critical events that transition acute sleep continuity disturbance to self-perpetuating insomnia disorder. Collectively, the three events (attention, intention, and effort) are referred to as the A-I-E pathway. When individuals are unable to sleep, their attention is drawn to an otherwise automatic process. The very process of attending, in turn, prevents perceptual disengagement and behavioral unresponsiveness (sleep). Because a primary function of attention is to promote action in response to perceived need, an intentional process (purposeful attempt to sleep) is initiated that acts to further inhibit the normal downregulation of arousal. Finally, the intention to fall asleep triggers sleep effort, and this effort, like enhanced attention and intention, serves only to further inhibit sleep-related dearousal. Ultimately, the inhibition of sleep-related dearousal reflects ongoing or elicited sleep-related attention, intention, and effort in chronic insomnia.

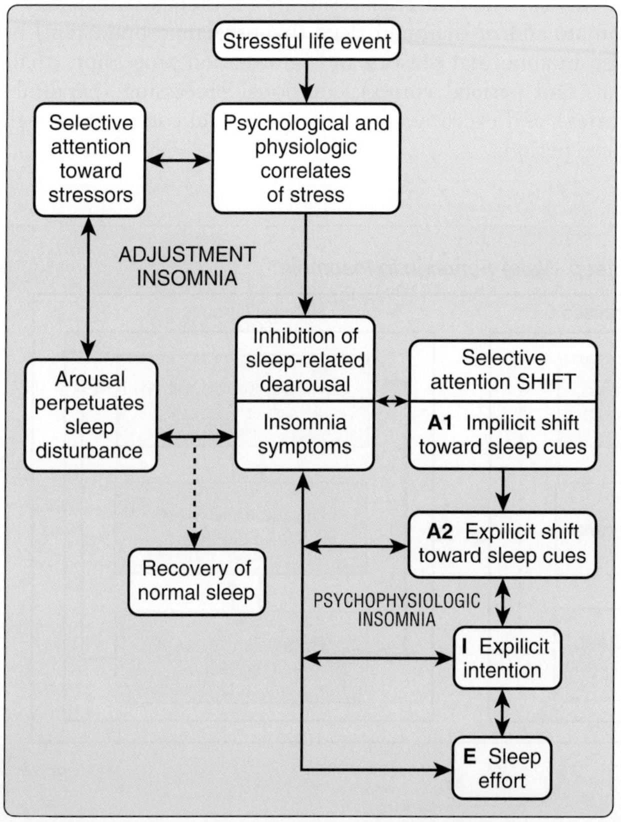

Figure 91.5 The psychobiologic inhibition model focuses on how insomnia may be perpetuated by (1) the inhibition of sleep-related dearousal and (2) increased sleep-related attention, intention, and effort.

Strengths and Limitations

A major strength of the PI model is that it differentiates between acute sleep continuity disturbance and insomnia disorder and delineates the mechanisms that are thought to mediate the transition between these conditions. This differentiation is particularly important because it allows for the possibility that acute sleep continuity disturbance (followed by recovery of normal sleep) is a normative, if not an adaptive, phenomenon[28] (see also, the Cano-Saper model [later]). The delineation of mediational variables is not only conceptually clear and compelling, but there is substantial support for attention bias or selective attention as operational in insomnia,[64–77] although experimental manipulation of selective attention in insomnia has produced mixed results for sleep-related outcomes.[78,79]

Another strength of the PI model is that it allows objective measurement of cognitive processes in insomnia. Individuals with insomnia commonly complain of cognitive events interfering with sleep, such as intrusive thoughts, racing thoughts, worry, and inability to disengage from environmental "noise" or bodily sensations. The identification of such cognitive events relies on self-report. The constructs of the model can be operationally defined and tested with objective measures, such as the computerized emotional Stroop task, the induced-change blindness task, and the dot probe task.[64–79]

Finally, and perhaps most important, is that the PI model proposes that the inhibition of sleep-related dearousal (rather than hyperarousal) may be responsible for both acute and chronic insomnia. In acute insomnia the inhibition of dearousal is engaged by the psychologic and physiologic correlates of stress. In insomnia disorder the engagement of sleep-related attention, intention, and effort serve to chronically inhibit dearousal. This reconceptualization represents a potential paradigm shift regarding the pathophysiology of chronic insomnia. This is not only true from a psychological and behavioral vantage point but also from a neurobiologic perspective, as it is possible that hyperarousal and the inhibition of dearousal have different neurobiologic substrates. For example, hyperarousal may be associated with hypercortisolemia[80–82] and increased sympathetic tone,[83–89] whereas the inhibition of dearousal may be associated with reduced gamma-aminobutyric acid–ergic (GABAergic) tone[90,91] and/or hyperactivation of the orexin system.[92]

The primary limitations of the PI model are that it does not adequately address the importance of circadian and homeostatic influences on sleep or take into account behavioral mediators or moderators, such as sleep extension and stimulus dyscontrol. These factors could be considered forms of sleep effort and thus be accounted for implicitly within the model. This said, explicit inclusion of sleep extension and stimulus dyscontrol would allow the PI model to be more comprehensive and integrative. Other limitations include the conceptualization of attentional bias (AB) as only a perpetuating factor for insomnia (it is possible that AB may also serve as a predisposing factor for acute or recurrent insomnia[93]); a lack of conceptual detail regarding the transition from acute sleep continuity disturbance back to good sleep (although it is featured in the model); and a lack of detail regarding how the inhibition of dearousal is similar to, and different from, the more traditional concept of hyperarousal.[94] Finally, as with all of the prior models, there is only limited empirical evaluation of model components, including the intention[95] and effort aspects of the A-I-E pathway[96] and the "tonic inhibition of dearousal."

Implications for Current and Future Therapeutics and Research

The PI model may help to explain the efficacy of many existing elements of CBT-I. Any behavioral or cognitive intervention that potentiates sleep-related dearousal or promotes the disengagement of attention, intention, and effort should help to restore normal sleep. For example, sleep restriction may help to reinstate sleep automaticity by increasing homeostatic pressure and overcoming the effects of increased attention, intention, or effort. Similarly, stimulus control may strengthen adaptive and automatic bed-sleep dearousal associations. Finally, relaxation, distraction, and imagery methods may reduce worry about sleep, and paradoxical intention methods may entirely refocus the A-I-E pathway away from sleep preoccupation. With respect to the development of new approaches, the PI model supports the rationale for sensory gating training and mindfulness therapies (e.g., mindfulness-based therapy for insomnia [MBT-I][97,98]).

Neurobiologic Model

Basic Description

The neurobiologic model of insomnia focuses on the changes in brain activity and function that may account for chronic insomnia (Figure 91.6; see also Riemann colleagues[99] for a review on neurobiologic findings in insomnia). Specifically, Buysse and colleagues[5] posit that insomnia is "a disorder of sleep-wake regulation characterized by persistent wake-like activity in neural structures during NREM sleep, resulting in simultaneous and regionally specific waking and sleeping neuronal activity patterns" (p. 133 of source). Wake-like levels of activity during cortically defined NREM sleep are specified as occurring in the prefrontal and parietal cortices, the paralimbic cortex, the thalamus, and the hypothalamic-brainstem arousal centers. Localized activation within these regions (local wakefulness) during what is otherwise more globally sleep can be expected to be associated with "persistent awareness of the environment" (p. 133 of source).[5] Put differently, coactivation of this sort may directly result in an attenuated capacity to initiate and/or maintain sleep (hypothalamic-brainstem) but also in abnormal sensory and information processing (thalamus and parietal cortex), emotional processing (paralimbic cortex), and executive function (prefrontal cortex) during the sleep period.

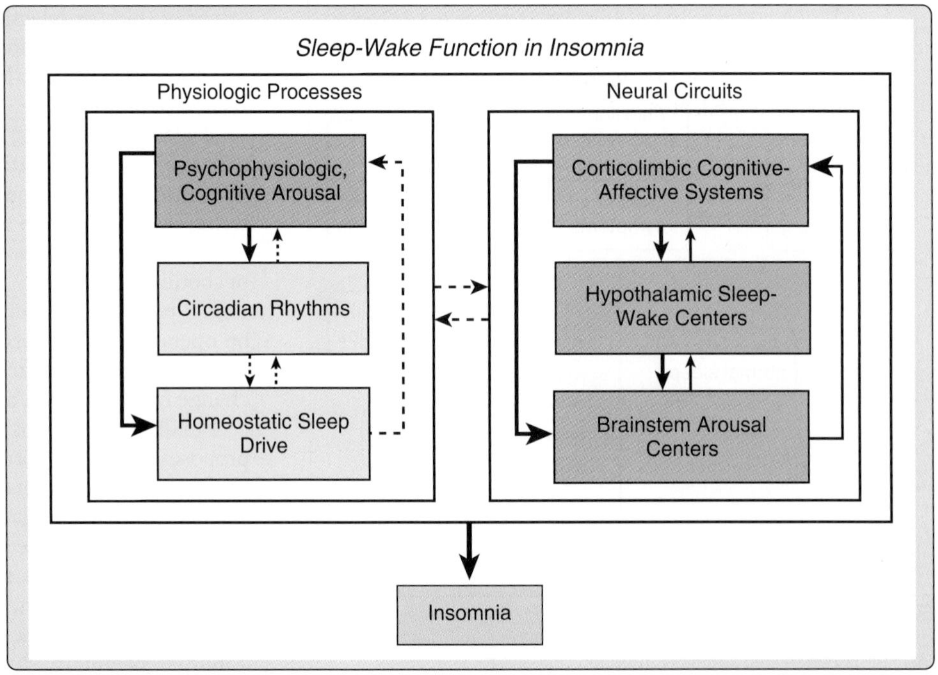

Figure 91.6 The neurobiologic model is primarily a state model that focuses on how insomnia may be a hybrid state that has as its neurobiologic substrate "local neuronal wakefulness" during non–rapid eye movement sleep.

Strengths and Limitations

The neurobiologic model is an integrative model that proposes a more specific mechanism for insomnia than provided by the general concept of hyperarousal or the inhibition of "sleep-on" systems. This model defines insomnia as a hybrid state (part sleep and part wakefulness) that occurs with local neuronal variations in sleep depth and may help to explain clinical features of insomnia. The model is informed by the neurocognitive model,[3] the neuronal transition probability model,[100] the two-process model of normal sleep-wake regulation,[25] and recent findings within neuroscience regarding both the sleep switch[101] and the phenomenon of local neuronal sleep.[102] Further, the neurobiologic model echoes the concept of *status dissociates* disorders as propounded by Mahowald and Schenck,[51] which suggests that hybrid states of consciousness (coactivations of wake, NREM, and REM sleep) may occur in a variety of the sleep disorders, including narcolepsy, REM sleep behavior disorder, and confusional arousals. Of interest, Mahowald and Schenck[51] did not propose that insomnia might be yet another example of *status dissociates* disorder.

The proposal that insomnia represents an aberrant state of persistent awareness that occurs as a result of local neuronal wakefulness adds to the existing literature in two ways. First, the model is explicit about what other models only imply: Insomnia is, in part, a disorder of persistent wakefulness that may occur globally (objective insomnia/with short sleep duration) or more locally (subjective insomnia/with normal sleep duration [i.e., sleep state misperception]). Second, the application of the concept of local sleep provides a mechanistic explanation for the proposition that insomnia entails aberrant levels of sensory and information processing or memory formation during the sleep onset period or during sleep. The model also provides a framework for understanding the phenomena of shallow sleep or sleep state misperception and the paradox that small or no objective treatment gains are regularly paralleled by larger subjective effects.[103] With respect to paradoxical treatment gains, small treatment-related changes in the polysomnogram may be associated with larger subjective improvements, given reduced local waking neural activity in critical regions or circuits, such as the default mode network or the thalamocortical system.

The first limitation of the neurobiologic model is that it is not an etiologic model. It does not focus on how good sleep transitions to insomnia nor on how acute sleep continuity disturbance transitions to insomnia disorder. Future elaborations of this model could address how local wakefulness develops and how the functional and physiologic abnormalities that occur with this phenomenon map onto the symptoms of insomnia (difficulties initiating and maintaining sleep). A second limitation is that, like the neurocognitive model, it focuses primarily on aberrant brain activity during NREM sleep that does not take into account recent findings on the role of fragmented REM sleep for insomnia.[104,105]

Implications for Current and Future Research and Therapeutics

Future investigations of the neurobiologic model are likely to rely heavily on neuroimaging (and potentially also dense-array electroencephalogram [EEG] studies) before and during sleep to document regional and circuit-level brain dysregulation in individuals with insomnia. Extending such paradigms cross-sectionally and longitudinally could address the transition between acute sleep continuity disturbance and insomnia disorder.

The therapeutic implications of the model are varied and include the exploration of whether present medical and cognitive-behavioral approaches minimize or eliminate neuronal local wakefulness. CBT-I may accomplish this by increasing homeostatic pressure for sleep, and medical treatment with benzodiazepines and benzodiazepine receptor agonists may do this through modulation of central nervous system GABA activity. Neuromodulation techniques to increase regional brain activity during wakefulness or to decrease such activity during sleep may also warrant further study.

ANIMAL MODELS

Cano-Saper Rodent Model

Basic Description

A rat model of acute stress-induced insomnia was developed using a species-specific psychosocial stressor. In the cage exchange paradigm, stress is induced by manipulation of the social context.[6] This is accomplished by transferring a male rat from his home cage, at the peak of the sleep period, to a soiled cage previously occupied by another male rat. Because rats are very territorial, exposure to the olfactory and visual cues of a competitor, even in its absence, induces a stress "fight-or-flight" response, including autonomic and hypothalamic-pituitary-adrenal axis activation. Several hours later, when the physiologic indicators of acute stress are attenuated, this manipulation continues to elicit disturbed sleep (i.e., the manipulation produces both sleep-onset and maintenance insomnia).

The brain circuitry activated during the late sleep-disturbed period was assessed by examining the expression of Fos, a transcription factor widely used as a marker of neuronal activity. Increased activation was observed in the cerebral cortex, limbic system, some arousal-related brain areas (locus coeruleus and tuberomamillary nucleus), and part of the autonomic system. Surprisingly, there was also simultaneous activation of the sleep-promoting areas (ventrolateral preoptic area [VLPO] and median preoptic nucleus). This coactivation results in a unique pattern of brain activity that differs from those observed during wake or normal sleep as the sleep circuitry appears to be like that in a sleeping rat, whereas the arousal system and the cortex show a level of activation similar to wakefulness. The high level of cortical activation was also associated with high-frequency EEG activity (distinctive of wakefulness) during NREM sleep and is consistent with elevated beta EEG activity found in individuals with insomnia.[3,35,36,42,106–109] Subsequent experiments revealed that inactivation of discrete limbic or arousal regions, via cell-specific lesions or pharmacologic inhibition, allowed for the recovery of specific sleep parameters and changed the pattern of brain activity in the cage exchange paradigm.[6] This suggests that stress-induced insomnia requires the occurrence of a cascade of neuronal events along with the normal propensity for sleep. This cascade likely includes sensory inputs (i.e., olfactory and visual cues of a competitor) that activate limbic areas, which in turn activate part of the arousal system that subsequently activates the cerebral cortex. This latter event (cortical activation) may be measured as high-frequency EEG activity during NREM sleep, and it is eliminated after inactivating parts of the arousal system.

The proposition that this particular stress paradigm may induce a novel intermediate state needs to be considered within the context of normal sleep-wake control.[110,111] As proposed by Saper and colleagues,[111] in normal animals there is a reciprocal inhibitory innervation between the main sleep-promoting neuronal group (VLPO), whose neurons are active during sleep, and the neuronal groups that comprise the arousal system (the histaminergic tuberomammillary nucleus, the serotonergic dorsal raphe, and the noradrenergic locus coeruleus), whose neurons are active during wakefulness. This reciprocal inhibition provides for a control system that is analogous to an electrical flip-flop switch. In this case, when one side is strongly activated, it inhibits and deactivates the other side, which decreases the inhibitory input to itself (disinhibition) and reinforces its own activity. In the absence of other factors, this configuration renders a "bistable" circuit (stable in one or the other state) with rapid and complete transitions between states and no occurrence of intermediate states (coactivation).

In the present context, the simultaneous activation of the VLPO and the arousal system in the cage exchange paradigm is surprising. A possible explanation is that during stress-induced insomnia the VLPO is fully activated due to both the homeostatic and circadian drives, but it is unable to turn off the arousal system because this is being excited intensely by inputs from the cortical and limbic systems. At the same time, the arousal system cannot turn off the VLPO because it is highly active due to the stronger homeostatic pressure caused because the stressed rats are partially sleep deprived. This results in the simultaneous activation of opposing systems that normally are not activated in tandem, and the bistable circuit becomes inherently unstable (i.e., the switch is forced into an intermediate position). This scenario is represented in Figure 91.7.

Strengths and Limitations

The rat model's cage exchange paradigm has several strengths. One is the conceptualization of acute sleep continuity disturbance as part of, or precipitated by, the flight-or-fight response. It uses a psychosocial stressor (perceived territorial threat) to induce sleep continuity disturbance, and it successfully produces a form of acute insomnia that includes both initial and late subtypes. It identifies specific neuronal effects within regions implicated in the regulation of sleep and wakefulness and produces quantitative EEG findings that are consistent with those found in human insomnia. Its overall findings are consistent with the conceptualization of insomnia as a disorder of hyperarousal, and its neuronal findings suggest that acute insomnia is a hybrid state resulting from the coactivation of systems that normally function in a bistable fashion.

The explicit characterization of acute insomnia as part of, or as a consequence of, the flight-or-fight response is particularly useful. This suggests that insomnia may be, as a transitory phenomenon, an adaptive response to real or perceived threat and is consistent with Richardson's proposal in 2007 that "insomnia reflects the overactivity of systems extrinsic to the sleep-wake circuitry that can temporally override normal sleep-wake control to facilitate a more imperative function, the stress response."[27] It should be noted that this concept was presaged by Spielman and Glovinsky in 1991, when they stated

> "*The fact that arousal should take precedence over sleep makes sense from an evolutionary perspective. No matter how important sleep may be, it was adaptively deferred when the mountain lion entered the cave*" (p. 3 of source).[112]

Finally, the suggestion that insomnia may exist as a hybrid state is an important refinement of the hyperarousal concept and is consistent with several of the human models and one that is not covered in the present chapter—the neuronal transition probability model put forward by Merica and colleagues.[100]

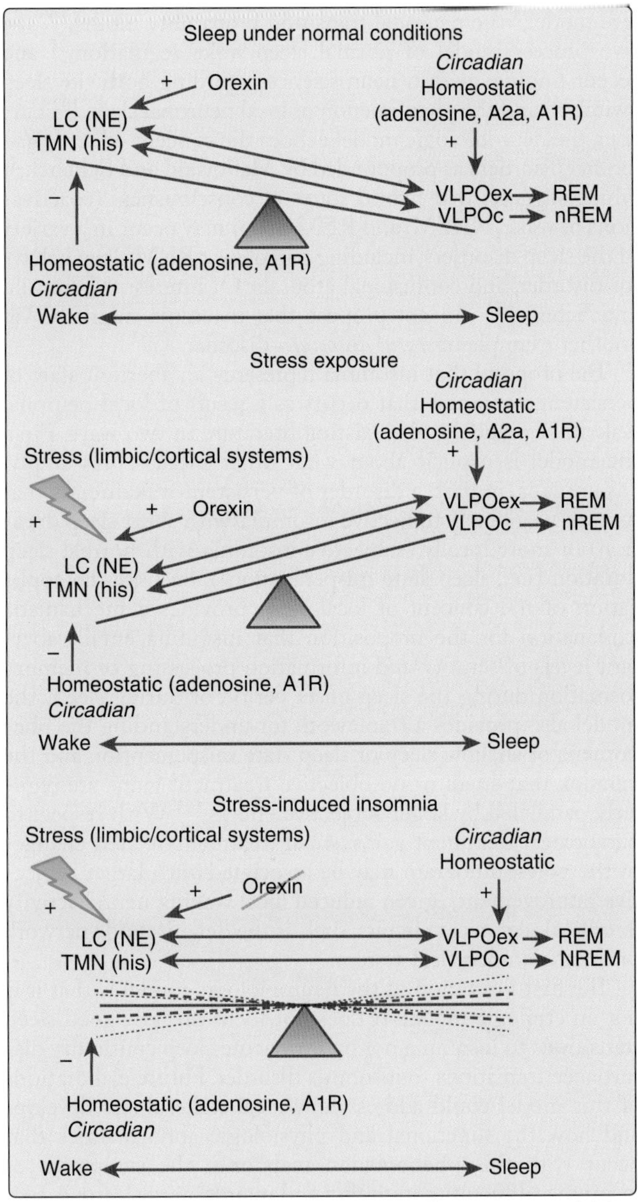

Figure 91.7 This illustration is a representation of Cano-Saper model. During normal sleep, the circadian and homeostatic drives enhance the activity of the sleep-promoting areas and simultaneously inhibit the arousal system, favoring the sleep state (the homeostatic effect is mediated in part by adenosine acting on A1 and A2a receptors). Stress activates part of the arousal system via cortical and limbic inputs, and this activation opposes the direction of the circadian and homeostatic drives. In stress-induced insomnia, the cortical, limbic, and arousal activation persists, but the homeostatic pressure is stronger than usual because the rats are partially sleep deprived; the circadian drive still favors the sleep state. Because these two forces are opposing and strong, the sleep-wake switch is forced into an unstable position, allowing the emergence of an intermediate state in which both sleep and wake circuitries are activated simultaneously, but each state is unable to sufficiently inhibit the other to prevent it from firing. A1R, A1 receptor; his, histamine; LC, locus coeruleus; NE, norepinephrine; NREM, non–rapid eye movement; REM, rapid eye movement; TMN, tuberomammillary nucleus; VLPOc, ventrolateral preoptic nucleus core; VLPOex, ventrolateral preoptic nucleus extended.

The rat model of acute insomnia has some limitations. As with all animal models, it is unable to establish the subjective complaint of insomnia, and as an analogue of acute insomnia, it might not be relevant for assessing chronic insomnia, which most would argue is the more clinically relevant condition. Although there is no question that modeling chronic insomnia (e.g., using a conditioning paradigm) would be useful, the acute model might nevertheless serve as a guide for what to expect in or how to move toward a chronic insomnia model. For example, the model clearly identifies brain regions of interest and clearly delineates one kind of brain activation pattern that may be characteristic of both acute and chronic insomnia, namely, the coactivation of both sides of the flip-flop switch. Another limitation of the model may be its reliance on the Fos measure. Not all neuronal groups express Fos in association with action potential activity. Thus this might limit the resolution of the neurobiologic effects of the cage exchange paradigm to regions that express Fos.

Implications for Current and Future Therapeutics and Research

Observations from the rat model might help identify putative targets for pharmacologic manipulation that can guide the development of new therapies. One essential finding is that the sleep-promoting neuronal groups are fully active in the rat model, and the problem seems to be the anomalous residual activation of the arousal and limbic systems at a time they should be completely off. This suggests that shutting down the residual activity of these systems might be a better approach to treat stress-induced insomnia (and perhaps chronic insomnia) rather than potentiation of the sleep system. Further, identifying the phenotype of these neurobiologic abnormalities may be helpful in the search for more specific pharmacologic treatments, which may in turn yield fewer unwanted side effects.

Shaw *Drosophila* Model

Basic Description

The conceptual basis for the Shaw *Drosophila* model is that insomnia occurs, in part, in relation to genetic predisposing factors[29,30] and that a portion of the variance in the incidence of insomnia is related to factors that are heritable. Given the complexity and number of traits observed for insomnia, it seems unlikely that single-gene mutations will result in an animal model that adequately captures the human condition. An alternative approach is to identify natural variants in a population that simultaneously exhibit several behavioral characteristics of insomnia. The phenotypic variation in these individuals is likely to be the result of minor changes in many genes and, as a consequence, is more likely to reflect the diversity of the human disorder.[113] This natural polygenic variation was thus amplified over successive generations using laboratory selection and identified using whole-genome arrays.[114] This is the approach that undergirds the Shaw *Drosophila* model.

Evaluation of a normative dataset of wild-type *Canton-S (Cs) Drosophila* indicated that they display a sufficient range of sleep times and activity levels to make them suitable for laboratory selection (Figure 91.8).[7] *Drosophila* that demonstrated reduced sleep time in combination with increased sleep latency, reduced sleep bout duration, and elevated levels of waking activity (*insomnia-like*, referred to as *ins-l* flies) were selected and bred over successive generations. As seen in Figure 91.8, total sleep time (TST) was progressively reduced during selection. At generation 65, more than 50% of *ins-l* flies obtained less than 60 minutes of sleep in a day. As with human insomnia, *ins-l* flies showed increased latency from lights off to the first sleep bout of the night, suggesting that they have difficulty initiating sleep.[115] The *ins-l* flies also exhibited difficulties maintaining sleep as evidenced by an inability to consolidate sleep into long bouts.

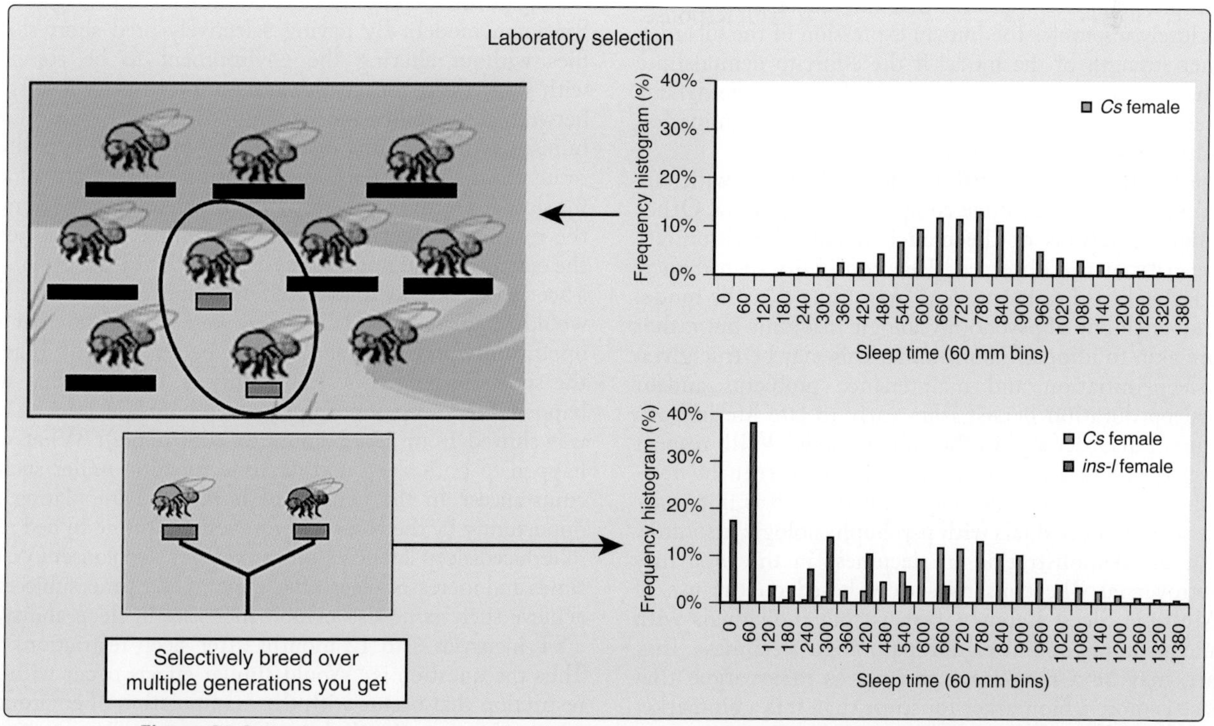

Figure 91.8 The figure above represents the laboratory selection process responsible for the creation of short-sleeping insomnia flies (*ins-l*) in the Shaw model.

To assess the extent to which the sleep patterns of the selectively bred *Drosophila* represent a reasonable analogue of human chronic insomnia, the sleep of the *ins-l Drosophila* was evaluated for chronicity (i.e., stability of the abnormal sleep pattern over the life span), and the wake state of the *ins-l Drosophila* was evaluated for typical daytime consequences (i.e., fatigue, sleepiness, impaired concentration or memory) or health outcomes (increased mortality) of insomnia. With respect to chronicity, it was found that the sleep profile remained stable in *ins-l Drosophila* over time. With respect to daytime consequences, *ins-l* flies showed elevated levels of amylase (a putative biomarker for sleepiness) relative to *Cs* flies during their primary wake period. Learning, as assessed using aversive phototaxic suppression,[116] was significantly impaired in the shortest sleeping *ins-l* flies compared to *Cs* flies. Motor and/or coordination difficulties were observed in *ins-l* flies by assessing the number of spontaneous falls during walking in an obstacle-free environment. Finally, and perhaps most dramatically, *ins-l* flies were shown to have a reduced life span compared to *Cs* flies, paralleling such findings in epidemiologic studies of insomnia and/or short sleep duration.[117–119]

In summary, the selection procedure approach was effective in producing animals with reduced TST, increased sleep latency, and shortened sleeping-bout duration. These sleep effects were found to be persistent and were associated with a variety of daytime function sequelae. These findings suggest that the *Drosophila* model might be a reasonable analogue of human chronic insomnia.

Strengths and Limitations

A major strength of the *Drosophila* model is its approach: A naturally occurring set of sleep parameters, parameters that are commonly found in human insomnia, were operationally defined for use in the fly and amplified over successive generations using laboratory selection. In particular, the use of multiple parameters ensures that the analogue condition more closely resembles the human expression of the disorder. Another strength of the model is the effort to demonstrate that the aggregate phenotype also exhibited daytime deficits with respect to sleepiness, learning impairment, coordination difficulties, and reduced life span.

One limitation is the inability to establish, as with any animal model, the subjective complaint of insomnia. Other potential limitations of the model include the chronicity and severity of the observed sleep continuity disturbance. With respect to chronicity, some may argue that the model is not an analogue of psychophysiologic insomnia but rather is more akin to idiopathic insomnia. This may be true given that sleep-initiation and maintenance problems and/or short sleep duration persist from early to late life in both the human disorder and in the animal model. With respect to severity, TSTs are a fraction of the TST seen in *non–ins-l* flies (1 to 2 hours per day), and this too is not commonly seen in individuals with psychophysiologic insomnia. Finally, the demonstration of sleepiness in the *ins-l* flies is controversial. The consensus view, based on the use of the Multiple Sleep Latency Test, is that individuals with chronic insomnia do not exhibit pathologic sleepiness. This, in part, may be a measurement issue as many argue that amylase is more a biomarker for stress than it is a biomarker for sleepiness.[120]

Implications for Current and Future Therapeutics and Research

There are a variety of possible directions for future research. Given the complexity of insomnia, it is likely that independent selections would potentially yield alternative outcomes. That is, the genes identified in the *ins-l* flies may only represent one potential pathway to insomnia. Thus a greater understanding of insomnia may be advanced with additional selected lines and determining if any identified genetic mutations are present in the human condition. Further, the use of molecular-genetic and genomic strategies may be useful for the identification of the genes that are associated with the various aggregate phenotypes. Given this latter strategy, it is important to acknowledge that gene profiling in *Drosophila* obtained by laboratory selection is likely to reveal two classes of genes: those that are causative for a given behavior and those that are a consequence of the behavioral change.[121] Most studies have focused on identifying genes that are causative for a given behavior. However, given that extended waking results in substantial physiologic impairment,[122,123] including death,[124,125] the latter set of genes may also be particularly important in the context of insomnia.

The Shaw *Drosophila* model might be more relevant to the human condition than has been appreciated. The manipulation may have, in fact, not only produced low "sleep ability," but the assessment paradigm itself may have produced a direct analogue of (had the same consequences as) sleep extension in humans—the enactment of a "sleep opportunity" that is greater than sleep ability.

Belfer-Kayser *Drosophila* Model

Basic Description

The primary point of departure for the Belfer-Kayser *Drosophila* model was the possibility that Shaw and colleagues'[7] work not only served as an exploration of the genetic predisposition to insomnia but was also relevant for issues pertaining to the perpetuation of insomnia (as presaged by the Spielman model). By having selectively bred short-sleeping flies without altering the environment to be compatible with short sleep, the investigators put into place a mismatch between sleep ability and sleep opportunity (Figure 91.9). In humans with insomnia disorder, this mismatch is posited to result from sleep extension (expansion of the time allocated for sleep, to recover lost sleep). In the Shaw *Drosophila* model, the mismatch occurred because the animal could not escape the environmental imperative for sleep (12:12 LD cycle). Such a scenario naturally lends itself an empirical question: What would happen if the LD cycles were altered so that sleep opportunity and sleep ability were better aligned? That is, if the short-sleeping fly's sleep ability is 4 hours, what would happen if the sleep opportunity was 4 hours (i.e., the LD cycle was shifted from 12:12 hours to 20:4 hours)? What would happen to both sleep and daytime function under such circumstances? In the context of humans, manipulating sleep opportunity by the voluntary restriction of time in bed results in reduced sleep latencies and wake after sleep onset (WASO) times and increased sleep efficiency.[23] Over time, subjects that achieve such gains also exhibit increases in sleep ability (i.e., TST increases 6 to 12 months after sleep restriction).[127,128] Thus the question is "Would similar effects occur with sleep restriction that occurs with the manipulation of environmental cues for sleep (i.e., light and temperature)"?

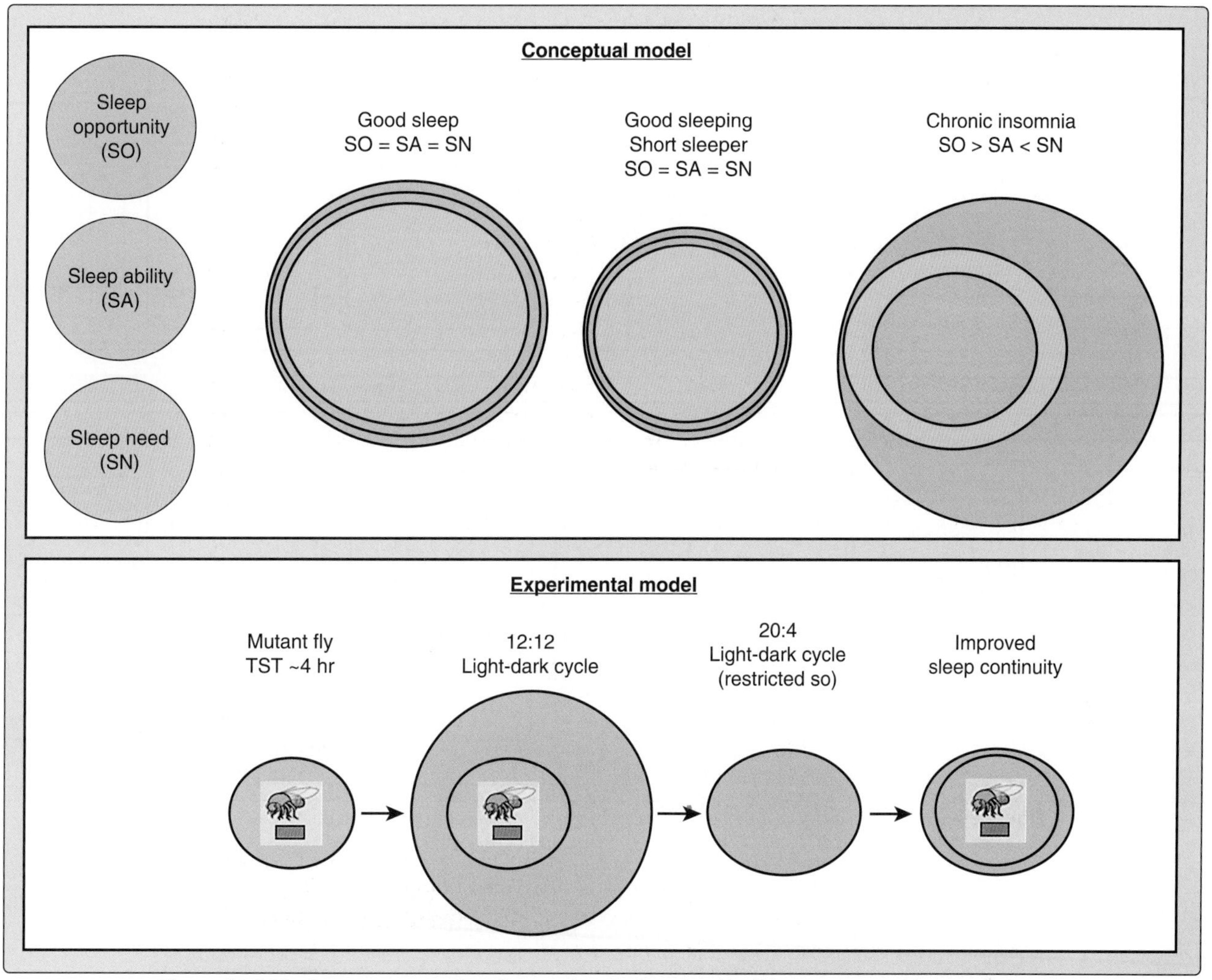

Figure 91.9 The figure represents three factors related to "good and bad" sleep continuity (sleep need, sleep ability, and sleep opportunity) and presents a schematic representation of good sleep, good/short sleep, and the insomnia that necessarily occurs when sleep ability and sleep opportunity are mismatched. TST, total sleep time.

In 2019 Belfer, Kayser, and colleagues[8] presented data on the systematic evaluation of the association between sleep opportunity and ability. Over the course of a series of studies, wild-type and short-sleeping mutant flies were subjected to altered LD cycles as a means to manipulate sleep opportunity; as in humans, darkness is sleep promoting in flies. Using a paradigm in which the dark period was either extended (10:14 LD or 8:16 LD) or restricted (20:4 LD or 18:6 LD), the investigators demonstrated that (1) dark-period extension (expansion of sleep opportunity) in wild-type flies decreased sleep efficiency and resulted in longer sleep latencies and increased WASO times; (2) dark-period restriction (compression of sleep opportunity) through manipulation of environmental cues increased sleep efficiency and resulted in decreased sleep latency and reduced WASO times in multiple short-sleeping *Drosophila* mutants; and (3) the alignment of sleep ability and opportunity was associated with extended life span in a fly model of Alzheimer disease that normally exhibits sleep deficits. These effects were dependent on ongoing environmental inputs (maintenance of the experimental conditions) but independent of circadian considerations.

Strengths and Limitations

The Belfer-Kayser model provides for a unique approach to the investigation of the neurobiologic basis of the Spielman model and the effects of sleep restriction and provides a platform that can be exploited toward unravelling the mechanistic basis of behavioral therapy and the development of novel treatment targets for insomnia. Moreover, the findings attest to potential universality of the Spielman model (i.e., insomnia occurs partly as a mismatch between sleep opportunity and ability) and the therapeutic effects of sleep restriction therapy (i.e., sleep restriction can reverse sleep initiation and maintenance problems and that this can have significant positive effects on function). At a more macro level, the successful application of the model suggests that it is possible to reverse genetically mediated sleep abnormalities with behavioral manipulations. A limitation of the model, partly owing to the shortness of the *Drosophila* life span (≈30 days) and the difficulties of extended observation, is that it is difficult to model the titration process that also is a component of sleep restriction (i.e., the systematic extension of sleep opportunity over time [usually 15-minute increments over 7-day periods, initiated based on a criterion sleep efficiency of 85% or 90%]).

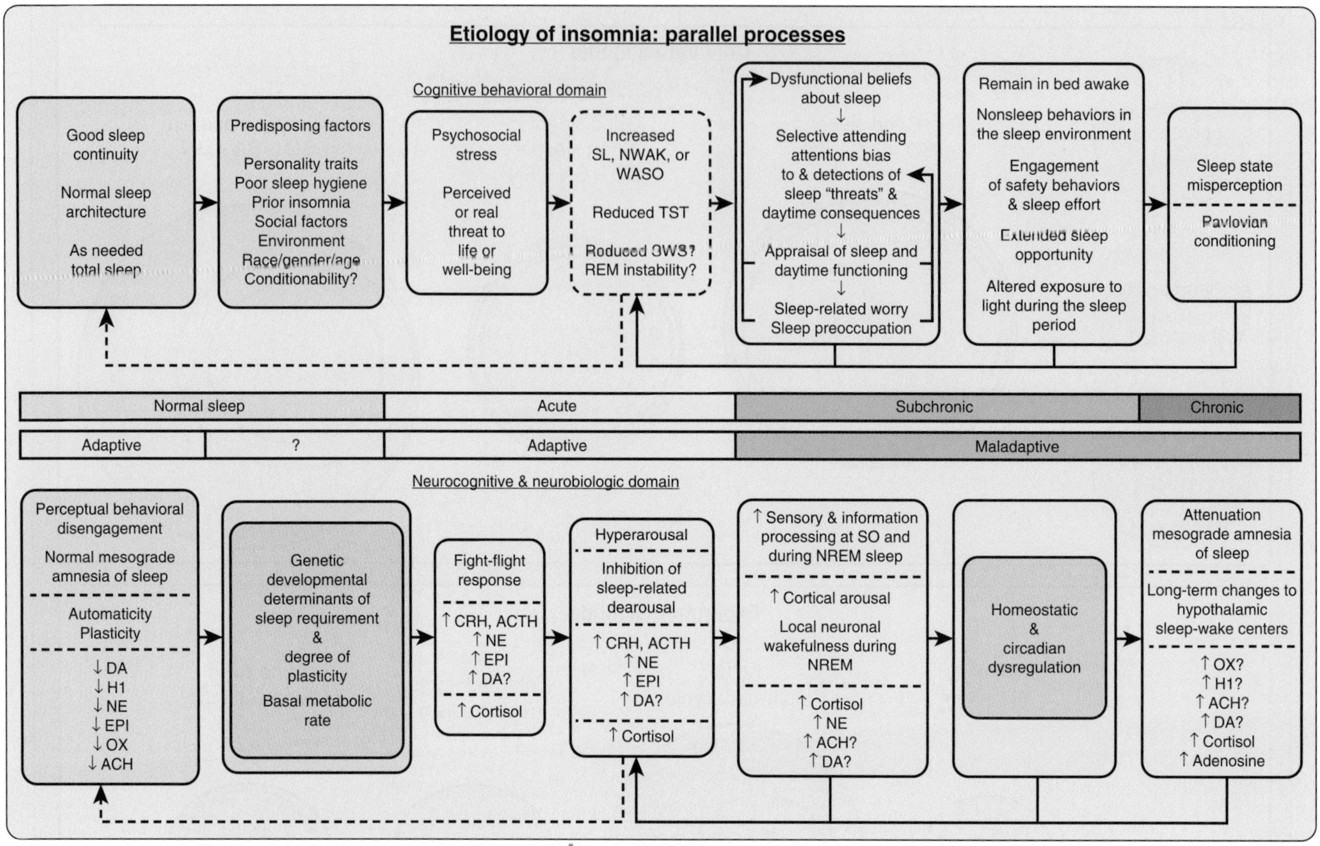

Figure 91.10 The parallel process model. The parallel process model is provided to illustrate how (1) all the identified factors may be contributory and (2) the cognitive and behavioral domains may be viewed as parallel processes to the neurocognitive and neurobiologic domains. ACH, Acetylcholine; ACTH, adrenocorticotropic hormone; CRH, corticotrophin-releasing hormone; DA, dopamine; EPI, epinephrine; H1, histamine-1 receptor antagonist; NE; norepinephrine; NWAK, number of awakenings; OX, orexin; SL, sleep latency; SO, sleep onset; TST, total sleep time; WASO, wake after sleep onset. (From Perlis ML, Ellis JG, Kloss JD, et al. Chapter 82—etiology and pathophysiology of insomnia. In: Kryger MH, Roth T, Dement WC, eds. *The Principles and Practice of Sleep Medicine*. St. Louis: Saunders Elsevier; 2017:769–784.)

In the current version of the Belfer-Kayser protocol, titration was accomplished using a fixed rule: 2-hour increases in sleep opportunity every other day, regardless of sleep efficiency. Under these conditions, it is not surprising that therapeutic gains were not achieved with respect to TST. This said, even with standard CBT-I titration schedules, TST gains during acute treatment are minimal (±20 minutes), with appreciable gains only evident in the 6 to 12 months after treatment response.[127–129] In future studies, it may be informative to develop a titration process that more closely approximates how this is conducted in humans.

CONCLUDING REMARKS

The Spielman, neurocognitive, PI, neurobiologic, and the Cano-Saper models share at least two central tenets: (1) Stress (threat or perceived threat) is a major precipitant of acute insomnia and (2) chronic insomnia involves a "hybrid state" where there is simultaneously higher-than-normal levels of CNS activation and a failure to inhibit processes normally associated with wakefulness.

The neurocognitive model and the PI model differ with respect to the role of cognitive processes as they occur in chronic insomnia. The PI model allows for cognitive processes to assume a central role in the perpetuation of insomnia (i.e., one is awake *because he/she is worrying and/or is attending to not sleeping*). The neurocognitive model takes into account cognitive processes but does not ascribe a primary role to such phenomena (i.e., one is worrying and/or is attending to not sleeping *because he/she is awake*). Thus cognitive phenomena may serve as "the flame" for the PI model and "wind to the flame" for the neurocognitive model.

The Cano-Saper model differs from the human models at the conceptual level because of its mechanistic emphasis on the "sleep switch" (as opposed to functional or environmental factors) and dysregulation of the "sleep switch" as it occurs acutely with homeostatic and circadian dysregulation. This difference is, however, not as profound as one might think. The question is "What happens over time?". Is it possible that rodents may develop chronic insomnia, and if so, does this occur in a fashion that is analogous to, or relevant for, the human condition? In the absence of data, it stands to reason that the conditioning factors that appear to be operative with human insomnia are also likely to be operational in the rodent. If true, an animal model of chronic insomnia is possible and may be used to explore the effects of conditioned arousal and/or conditioned wakefulness on persistent sleep continuity disturbance, brain function, physiology, and anatomy.

In the final analysis, the differences between the models may not be a matter of which is correct but, rather, at what point the various models are more or less relevant. Although the assessment of such a proposition awaits empirical evaluation, it stands to reason that most, if not all, the factors—stress response (in terms of reactivity, intensity, and recovery), attention bias, sleep extension (i.e., the mismatch between sleep opportunity and ability), sleep effort, conditioning, and altered neurobiology (cortical activation, alterations to the "flip-flop" circuit, and local wakefulness during NREM sleep)—all play a role in the etiology and/or pathophysiology of insomnia disorder. In recognition of this, we provide in an integrative perspective, parallel process model (Figure 91.10). This model is intended to represent each of the core components from the eight models within one framework, the perspective that the cognitive-behavioral and the neurocognitive and neurobiologic domains represent two sides of the same phenomena, and the possibility that acute insomnia is adaptive. In framing the various factors in this manner, we hope to stimulate new ideas for both research and possible interventions.

CLINICAL PEARL

Although many consider theory to be largely an academic enterprise, the models presented in this chapter provide a framework for understanding how insomnia becomes chronic, why the disorder presents as it does, and how and/or why different treatments may work. Such frameworks, although inevitably imperfect and incomplete, help in the conceptualization of both individual cases and the directions for future research.

SUMMARY

Since the 1990s there has been a proliferation of theoretical perspectives on the etiology of insomnia that includes five human and three animal models. Each is summarized in this chapter, reviewed for its strengths and limitations, and evaluated for its potential to generate new therapeutics and research. After the summaries, overall limitations of existing models are considered, and an integrative perspective is provided.

SELECTED READINGS

Belfer SJ, Bashaw AG, Perlis ML, et al. A *Drosophila* model of sleep restriction therapy for insomnia. *Mol Psychiatry*. 2021;26(2):492–507.

Bootzin RR. Stimulus control treatment for insomnia. In: *Proceedings of the 80th Annual Convention of American Psychological Association*; 1972:395–396.

Buysse D, Germain A, Hall M, et al. Neurobiological model of insomnia. *Drug Disc Today Dis Mod*. 2011;8:129–137.

Cano G, Mochizuki T, Saper CB. Neural circuitry of stress-induced insomnia in rats. *J Neurosci*. 2008;28:10167–10184.

Ellis JG, Gehrman P, Espie CA, et al. Acute insomnia: current conceptualizations and future directions. *Sleep Med Rev*. 2012;16:5–14.

Espie CA. Insomnia: conceptual issues in the development, persistence, and treatment of sleep disorder in adults. *Annu Rev Psychol*. 2002;53:215–243.

Perlis ML, Giles DE, Mendelson WB, et al. Psychophysiological insomnia: the behavioural model and a neurocognitive perspective. *J Sleep Res*. 1997;6:179–188.

Riemann D, Nissen C, Palagini, et al. The neurobiology, investigation, and treatment of chronic insomnia. *Lancet Neurol*. 2015;14:547–558.

Seugnet L, Suzuki Y, Thimgan M, et al. Identifying sleep regulatory genes using a *Drosophila* model of insomnia. *J Neurosci*. 2009;29:7148–7157.

Spielman A, Caruso L, Glovinsky P. A behavioral perspective on insomnia treatment. *Psychiatr Clin North Am*. 1987;10:541–553.

A complete reference list can be found online at ExpertConsult.com.

Chapter 92

Pediatric Insomnia and Its Developmental Trajectories

Nicola L. Barclay; Mari Hysing; Børge Sivertsen; Alice M. Gregory

Chapter Highlights

- Nocturnal awakenings in newborn infants are considered *normal* and to be *expected,* yet the persistence of difficulties initiating sleep and frequent nocturnal awakenings beyond the first 6 months of life may in certain cases be problematic. For some, these difficulties may develop into insomnia disorder.
- In this chapter we outline how behavioral insomnia of childhood may, to some extent, be distinct from insomnia that presents in adolescence or adulthood in terms of symptomology and etiology.
- This chapter outlines longitudinal research that examines the trajectories of insomnia from infancy to adulthood, proposing a combination of genetic, neurophysiologic, environmental, cognitive, and behavioral factors in its genesis and maintenance. We highlight factors that may contribute to the stability of insomnia over time and those that may contribute to change.
- Knowledge of the etiology of insomnia across the life span has the potential to inform clinicians as to the best treatment approach. There is a paucity of studies on the efficacy and effectiveness of behavioral and pharmacologic interventions in pediatric insomnia.
- Behavioral approaches are the recommended first-line treatment for pediatric insomnia, whereas pharmacologic treatments have a limited evidence base.

INTRODUCTION

During infancy, changes in sleep are dramatic. An irregular sleep pattern and frequent awakenings at night are considered normative during the first months of life. Newborns have an underdeveloped sleep homeostat, and rhythmic circadian melatonin secretion is first established around 2 to 3 months of age.[1,2] Night feeds are also common during these first months and for most a necessity. The consolidation of sleep during the first 6 months must thus be seen as a normal process and a key developmental task. Yet when difficulties getting to sleep and frequent nocturnal awakenings persist beyond 6 months of age and impact on daily life, additional consideration may be warranted.

Sleep difficulties in infancy carry high family burden and are associated with maternal depression, fatigue, and stress, as well as mood and behavioral difficulties in the child/adolescent.[3–5] Disrupted sleep in early life is also associated with a plethora of mental health problems concurrently and longitudinally.[6] Although persistence of insomnia from infancy through childhood, adolescence, and adulthood is sometimes found, insomnia is transient in certain people. There are also changes in the manifestation of insomnia at different stages of life. Indeed, behavioral insomnia of childhood is in many ways distinct from the difficulties with sleep onset that occur in adolescence and adulthood.

This chapter outlines evidence from longitudinal studies of the developmental trajectories of insomnia and summarizes evidence from quantitative genetic studies that have contributed to our understanding of the relative importance of genetic and environmental factors in insomnia across the life span. This research has highlighted that the persistence of insomnia appears to be due to a combination of genetic, neurophysiologic, environmental, cognitive, and behavioral factors. This chapter also provides evidence-based guidelines on the treatment of pediatric insomnia from a synthesis of the relatively few studies that exist in these populations. Finally, the chapter discusses future directions for research and clinical practice to enhance our understanding of the factors contributing to insomnia across the life span, with the goal of developing tailored treatment approaches to optimize patient care and family well-being.

Developmental Trajectories of Insomnia Across Infancy, Childhood, and Adolescence

Sleep undergoes major changes throughout infancy and early childhood, and both the prevalence and presentation of symptoms of insomnia during childhood shows a developmental pattern. In an international study of almost 30,000 parents, babies were reported to wake about twice a night during their first couple of months.[7] At 6 months of age, nocturnal awakenings remain frequent, with studies showing that the majority of infants (69%) still wake up every night[8] but with high individual variability. A pattern of sleep consolidation and a reduction in awakenings occur during the first 2 years of life,[9] a pattern that has been shown across assessment methods.[10] Despite this general reduction of nocturnal awakenings, 44% of infants awakening three or more times every night at 6 months of age still awaken at least once every night at 18 months.[8] Overall however, there are improvements over time, and a Swedish general population study of 10,000 children concluded that with increasing age the number of nocturnal awakenings reduced and the quality of sleep improved across the preschool years.[11] A pattern of improved sleep and a reduction in awakenings over time has also been shown in a longitudinal study of early adolescence from 10 to 13 years of age.[12] This was also confirmed in a longitudinal study of sleep problems, based on sleep-related items of the Child Behavior Checklist (CBCL), among 492 children, with a 50% decline in sleep problems from 4 to 15 years of age.[13] Similarly, another longitudinal study using latent growth curve analyses and the CBCL found that parent-reported sleep problems gradually declined during preschool and remained relatively stable across the childhood years.[14]

Although some studies have found a general decline in broadly defined sleep problems from childhood to early adolescence,[13] others have reported a sharp *increase* in difficulties, specifically focused on initiating and/or maintaining sleep from early childhood to late adolescence,[15] and that such difficulties occurring in preschool years are likely to persist into the school-age years.[16,17] In adolescents, one study demonstrated that 52% of those exhibiting insomnia symptoms at baseline continued to experience insomnia symptoms 4 years later.[18] Finally, multiple studies have documented that those who woke frequently early in life are at increased risk of awakenings several years later.[8,11,19]

Defining Pediatric Insomnia

Pediatric studies of sleep problems focus on a range of measures and definitions, so their relevance to insomnia is not always clear. In this section, we consider the definition of pediatric insomnia.

Diagnostic Criteria

In the *Diagnostic and Statistical Manual of Mental Disorders,* fifth edition (DSM-5),[20] insomnia disorder is listed as 1 of 10 sleep-wake disorders and features difficulties falling asleep, awakening during the night, or awakening early in the morning.[20] Although pediatric and adult cases are considered within a single category, the two types can present differently, and information is provided that can help diagnose childhood cases. For example, the need for caregiver intervention may be the key in certain cases of childhood insomnia, which may show the child's "difficulty initiating sleep without caregiver intervention" or "difficulty returning to sleep without caregiver intervention." As with adults, diagnoses are only given when the sleep difficulty causes clinically significant impairment and occurs at least three times a week for a duration of 3 months or more. Co-occurring mental, physical, withdrawal, and sleep disorders also need to be considered before a diagnosis can be made.[20]

The *International Classification of Sleep Disorders,* third edition (ICSD-3),[21] also categorizes child and adult insomnia together. "Behavioral insomnia of childhood" is categorized within the general category of "chronic insomnia disorder." As with DSM-5, ICSD-3 criteria focus on difficulties initiating and maintaining sleep and awakening earlier than desired. The ICSD-3 also includes criteria that are particularly relevant to children. These include "resistance to going to bed on appropriate schedule" and "difficulty sleeping without parent or caregiver intervention." Some of these behaviors may be a result of anxiety, such as separation anxiety from the caregiver, nightmares, or "fear of the dark" in young children. The ICSD-3 diagnostic criteria for chronic insomnia disorder also stipulate that difficulties must occur despite adequate opportunity for sleep, must result in daytime impairment, occur three or more times a week, and last for at least 3 months. The presentation should not be explained by an alternative sleep disorder. The family context of childhood insomnia is highlighted, and it is noted that caregivers may miss out on their own sleep because of their child's sleep difficulty and as a result struggle during the day. Disagreement concerning management of child sleep can result in caregiver arguments, and there may be negative feelings toward sleepless children.

Interpreting the Diagnostic Criteria

Information is provided in the ICSD-3[21] to facilitate the interpretation of criteria. For example, "difficulty initiating sleep" has the potential to be interpreted in different ways. It is suggested that sleep-onset latency or nocturnal awakenings that are greater than 20 minutes may be noteworthy (shorter periods may occur outside the context of insomnia). Furthermore, the time a child goes to sleep should be considered when deciding whether a specific early-morning awakening is problematic. Waking can be particularly early in prepubescent children, and data suggest that children go to bed and wake early when they are young, with timing becoming progressively later around adolescence, until the second decade of life[22] or perhaps even later.[23] Age is important when considering nocturnal awakenings too, and given that children younger than 6 months regularly wake at night, an insomnia diagnosis in younger children should only be considered in severe cases. In accordance with the *Diagnostic Classification of Mental Health and Developmental Disorders of Infancy and Early Childhood* (DC:0-5),[24] the child must be at least 6 months of age to consider a sleep-onset disorder, or 8 months of age for a night waking disorder, which are the equivalent of behavioral insomnia.[24] Thus one should avoid using the term *behavioral insomnia* until the child reaches 6 months of age.

Other aspects of development, including when a child transitions to a bed and develops certain cognitive skills are all likely to be important when considering a child's sleep. Familial, cultural, and historical differences in sleep must also be considered.[25] Families choosing to co-sleep may be less likely to report difficulties sleeping without caregiver intervention, for example, and there are extensive individual differences between families in terms of expectations about behavior that is considered acceptable and that which is considered problematic. These may also include considerations such as parents' unrealistic sleep expectations, neurodevelopmental comorbidities, abuse or attachment difficulties, parents' boundary issues, parents' overinvolvement or psychopathology, social determinants, and environmental factors such as a cramped living space.[26]

Subtypes of Insomnia

Despite the DSM-5 and ICSD-3 abandoning the subtyping of insomnia, there is considerable heterogeneity within the disorder, and certain subtypes may be particularly relevant to children. For example, the term *idiopathic insomnia* was used in ICSD-2 to refer to adult insomnia with a reported childhood onset and without a known cause. Similarly, within "behavioral insomnia of childhood" three types had been suggested.[21] First, the "sleep-onset association type," which could involve a child needing a particular object or setting to fall asleep. This subtype is often reported in young infants. Second, the "limit-setting type" might be the result of caregivers failing to set consistent and appropriate boundaries. This subtype is often reported in older infants who are able to challenge caregiver authority. Finally, the "mixed type" arises from a combination of the aforementioned processes.[21]

Other subtypes have also been highlighted. For example, it has been proposed that youth with reported insomnia symptoms (i.e., difficulties falling asleep and/or nocturnal awakenings) may also differ in their objective sleep duration, as measured by polysomnography (PSG).[27] Insomnia symptoms coupled with objective short sleep duration is considered to be a more severe and biologically driven subtype, whereas insomnia symptoms and objective normal sleep duration is attributed to the behavioral processes mentioned earlier. A study focusing on 700 children ages 5 to 12 years and 421 adolescents ages 12 to 23 years found that hypothalamic-pituitary-adrenal (HPA) axis activity (i.e., morning and nighttime cortisol levels) differed from control subjects in children with parent-reported insomnia symptoms and who had objective short sleep duration, but not for those obtaining normal sleep duration.[28] In line with work focusing on adults, this might suggest a different etiology in insomnia with objective short sleep duration subtype (i.e., physiologic hyperarousal). Furthermore, the insomnia with objective short sleep duration subtype has been associated with internalizing symptoms, whereas the insomnia with the normal objective sleep duration subtype has been associated with difficulties with limit setting, rule breaking, and aggression.[29,30]

As in adults, pediatric insomnia has also been subtyped based on symptom presentation, including specific developmental nuances (restless sleep). Three clinically distinct groups were identified after the assessment of 338 children ages 6 to 48 months presenting with "insomnia."[31] These groups were characterized by (1) difficulties falling asleep and nocturnal awakenings (with restless sleep), (2) early awakening, and (3) difficulties falling asleep and nocturnal awakenings (without restless sleep). Comorbid restless legs syndrome (RLS) was associated with group 1, whereas allergies were associated with group 3, suggesting that there might be distinct etiologies for these three subtypes.

The information from these different studies using multimethod approaches is potentially valuable, although further research is required to corroborate these subtypes. It is possible that distinct etiologies account for age-specific presentations of insomnia, given that sleep and circadian rhythms change across the life span.

Predictors of Stability and Change of Insomnia Across the Life Span

There might be a complex developmental shift in insomnia trajectories from childhood to adolescence, in which the individual stability may be higher *within* individual time periods of childhood or adolescence compared to *between* these periods.[32] This may be understood in a framework with different factors that influence sleep across these time periods. For example, the relative contribution of genetic and environmental influences on sleep may change at different stages of the life course.[32–34] The nature of behavioral insomnia may also change. Although frequent nocturnal awakenings are a key characteristic of infancy and childhood, and are in line with parental perceptions of sleep problems,[11] difficulties initiating sleep and the related long sleep-onset latency are the key components of adolescent insomnia.[35,36] This may account for the discontinuity of insomnia before and after puberty.

The developmental shifts in behavioral insomnia may in many ways reflect normative changes in sleep and sleep problems. For the affected child and family, as well as health care providers, individual stability of sleep across time is another important dimension to consider. As discussed earlier, although there is a general reduction of sleep problems across age, for some children, symptoms may persist.

It is clear that for some individuals manifestations of insomnia occurring in childhood contribute to the development of insomnia throughout adolescence and beyond. The following section describes the etiologic underpinnings of insomnia, with particular focus on risk factors for childhood insomnia and outlines evidence for predictors of stability of insomnia throughout adolescence and adulthood, as well as predictors of change.

Predictors of Stability

Genetics

The quantitative genetic literature provides robust evidence to suggest that genetic factors are involved in insomnia symptoms at different stages of life (see Barclay and Gregory[37] for a review). The heritability of insomnia symptoms has been estimated at 17% to 79% in children at age 8 years,[32,38] 37% in older childhood, age 12 years[39]; 41% in adolescents, age 16 years[40]; and 35% in young adults, age 20 years.[41] Although the variability in heritability estimates could be related to the use of different insomnia definitions across studies, they may also indicate that different genetic and environmental influences may be important at distinct stages of life. A longitudinal twin study of children ages 8 to 15 years showed that, although there was overlap in genes conferring risk for insomnia symptoms across that age period, different genes came into play at age 10 years.[32] Genes involved in the transition from childhood to adolescence, such as those relating to puberty, could be plausible candidates. Thus genetic factors may contribute to both the stability and change of insomnia across time.

Environment

Not all factors predisposing to insomnia are biologically based and could also include environmental adversity. In one study of infants age 3 months, neighborhood deprivation—conceptualized as poverty, the necessity of receiving food stamps, low parental education, and lack of a male adult in the household—was associated with increased nocturnal awakenings measured by actigraphy.[42] Similar findings were observed in a study of children age 11 years, where neighborhood economic deprivation was associated with shorter sleep and poorer sleep efficiency, measured using actigraphy.[43] Different environmental influences may act as triggers for an episode of insomnia in those at risk. Precipitating factors that may be relevant in youth include trauma, death of a close relative, moving home or school, abuse (particularly sexual abuse, which may lead to negative bedroom associations), and bullying.[44–48]

Childhood trauma and abuse have consistently been shown to have long-term consequences for disturbed sleep through to adulthood.[47]

Environmental factors may also impact on insomnia via epigenetic mechanisms (i.e., modification of gene expression), principally across developmental time points. In particular, early-life stress has been hypothesized to be etiologically important in the development of insomnia. It is likely that the stress of the mother in the child's prenatal period may lead to heightened vulnerability, for example, via HPA axis activity.[49] For example, a study showed that women experiencing preconceptional psychological distress predicted greater likelihood of infant night waking at 6 and 12 months of age, independent of whether the mother experienced postnatal depression.[50] Another study showed that increased nocturnal awakenings in infants at 12 months was predicted by a greater number of stressful life events experienced by the mother during early pregnancy,[51] and this is echoed by others that have highlighted the importance of maternal psychological health as predictors of disturbed sleep in infancy.[52] However, overall, there is a dearth of research on the epigenetics of insomnia, highlighting an avenue for further exploration into its complex etiology.

Behavior

Internalizing and externalizing behaviors, or emotional disorders, are likely to account for stability of insomnia. Data from an Australian cohort study demonstrated bidirectional relationships between sleep problems (akin to insomnia) and externalizing difficulties from data collected at five time points through the ages of 4 to 12 years, particularly during the elementary school transition period. Internalizing symptoms were predicted by sleep problems longitudinally, but the reverse association was not borne out.[53] That said, a study examining persistence of sleep problems across a 4-year period in children who were between 1 and 6 years of age at the study inception, demonstrated that prolonged sleep problems were predicted by anxiety and depression, as well as aggression, social, and attention problems.[54] One could also hypothesize that separation anxiety or externalizing behaviors might interfere with parent's attempts at limit setting.

Furthermore, behavioral factors, such as excessive time in bed, may also play a role in the perpetuation of insomnia in children. For children, parents often set bedtimes and rise times, and these may not always correspond with the child's biologically-driven sleep drive or circadian clock. Thus some children may be spending excessive time in bed, and this could conceivably allow negative, sleep-incompatible cognitions about the bedroom environment to take hold. These behaviors could then persist into adulthood. In addition, difficulty sleeping at night time may increase daytime naps, which has shown to be common in adolescents[55] and may drive daytime inactivity due to tiredness, all of which may further perpetuate nighttime sleep difficulties.

Predictors of Change

Despite the presence of multiple contributors to the stability of pediatric insomnia, some of these and other factors also help to explain change in symptoms from childhood, adolescence, and adulthood. Such factors may help to explain those adolescents or adults whose insomnia is not preceded by insomnia in childhood and in those whose pediatric insomnia remits. Quantitative research has shown that environmental influences on insomnia across childhood and adolescence are largely time specific and may account for change in insomnia over time.[32]

Longitudinal studies have shown that environmental factors occurring *early in life* may predict the *later* development of insomnia. In a longitudinal study that examined the incidence of insomnia in children ages 9 to 14 years, Zhang and colleagues[56] showed that lower paternal education was associated with new incidence of insomnia at follow-up. Gregory and colleagues[57] showed that exposure to family conflict in childhood, at ages 7 to 15 years, was associated with increased likelihood of developing insomnia at age 18 years even after controlling for sleep problems at 9 years. Similarly, childhood adversity has been shown to be associated with greater incidence of poor sleep quality in adulthood,[58] an association that was mediated by neuroticism.[59] Thus identification of early and time-specific environmental triggers, as well as personality type perpetuators, is important as strategies to modify the environmental risk can then be implemented.

Changes in cognitive abilities also likely account for differences in sleep from childhood onward. Infants and toddlers commonly experience separation anxiety, including anxiety sleeping alone or difficulty settling to sleep without their caregiver by their side. The necessity of the presence of the caregiver to settle to sleep is a psychological comforter and consistent with "sleep-onset association"–type insomnia.[21] Around the age of 6 years, nightmares may increase in frequency[60] and may contribute to fear of going to bed, heightened arousal, and the development of cognitions/behaviors consistent with insomnia. Nightmares tend to decline by around the age of 10 years.[60]

Cognitive development could also account for differences in insomnia from childhood and adolescence as maladaptive cognitions may be more relevant as we get older. Dysfunctional beliefs about sleep and presleep cognitive arousal have been shown to be associated with insomnia-related items on a self-report measure in children ages 8 to 10 years,[61,62] and catastrophic worry has been shown to be associated with Pittsburgh Sleep Quality Index–derived sleep quality in a sample of early adolescent girls from the general population.[63]

Besides early-life stress and changes in cognitive abilities, we are likely to see distinct changes in sleep during adolescence. Adolescents go through a host of changes—hormonally, physiologically and psychologically—that combine to impair sleep. It is during the teenage years that we may see sex differentiation in insomnia-related symptoms.[64] Although there are few gender differences in early childhood, females are more likely to experience poorer quality and more disrupted sleep from adolescence and beyond,[64] and the sex differences observed in insomnia prevalence during adolescence may be explained by the onset of puberty.[64,65] Thus there may be something etiologically distinct around puberty that predicts insomnia in girls but not boys. Plausible candidates may be hormonal changes and differences in stress reactivity between boys and girls during adolesence.[64,66] An alternative explanation is related to the circadian rhythm. Males and females differ in chronotype: Females typically go to bed and rise from bed earlier than males.[67,68] One study examining sleep-time preferences across the life span (from ages 10 to 87 years) found that girls exhibited a much greater phase advance (that is, the circadian rhythm exhibits earlier timing) than boys, but only during the adolescent years, implicating the sex hormones in this phase difference.[69] The phase advance rhythm could explain the increased prevalence of apparent insomnia symptoms. Females appear to be sleeping at an earlier time than males, and thus earlier sleep offset may be perceived as a symptom of insomnia (early-morning awakenings).[64]

Regardless of the apparent sex differences in insomnia and circadian phase during adolescence, we see a marked shift in the circadian system in both sexes.[22,70] Physiologically, adolescents exhibit a phase delay, that is, their circadian rhythm becomes shifted later such that they find it difficult to initiate sleep until a much later clock-time, often in the early hours of the morning. It is common to interpret difficulty initiating sleep, such as that seen in delayed sleep-wake phase disorder, as insomnia, given the frustration that may be apparent when attempting sleep at a time that is out of sync with the body's physiologic propensity for sleep, which is common in teenagers. However, growing awareness of the normalcy of late sleep and rise times has led to the shift in interpretation of teenagers as being "lazy" in the mornings, with a growing appreciation of their delayed timing as *normal* and *expected*.

Other research has focused on neurophysiologic correlates of insomnia, with one study showing that children exhibiting high-frequency electroencephalogram activity, specifically beta activity during non–rapid eye movement sleep, were more likely to report new insomnia symptoms 7.5 years later during adolescence, compared to normal-sleeping children.[71] Thus cortical hyperarousal appears to be a premorbid factor for the later development of adolescent insomnia.

Taken together, this body of cross-sectional and longitudinal research demonstrates the multifaceted etiology in pediatric insomnia and that a combination of genetic, neurophysiologic, environmental, cognitive, and behavioral factors may contribute to its stability and change across time.

Clinical Approach to Pediatric Insomnia

Insomnia symptoms in children and adolescents exhibit vast heterogeneity in presentation and etiology. As such, treatment approaches vary from child to child. Although there are a range of evidence-based behavioral and pharmacologic tools that are used to treat insomnia in adults, these approaches require modification to be applied to pediatric populations. Akin to the treatment of insomnia in adult patients, behavioral approaches are superior and are the recommended first-line treatment.[72] However, access to therapy in primary care is limited due to the lack of trained providers globally. On the other hand, pharmacologic treatments for insomnia in children and adolescents lack a clear evidence base.[73] Although prescription medications are frequently provided by general practitioners (off-label in many cases, particularly in the context of attention deficit hyperactivity disorder [ADHD][74]), the small evidence base is rife with inconsistencies concerning their efficacy, lack of knowledge of potential long-term side effects, and no clear dosing guidelines. This section provides practice-based guidelines for the evaluation of pediatric insomnia and discusses the empirical literature to date on the efficacy, effectiveness, and application of behavioral and pharmacologic treatments.

Initial Evaluation

Chapter 93 provides a thorough description of diagnosis and assessment of insomnia more generally. In this section we provide information on the specific nuances of diagnosis and assessment in pediatric populations. The first step toward developing a treatment pathway for pediatric insomnia is to consider age-specific recommendations for healthy sleep length, such as those outlined by the American Academy of Sleep Medicine,[75] and to identify the nature of the sleep problem. The second step is to consider the potential cause of the sleeplessness and to rule out other sleep or medical disorders that may account for the difficulties with sleep initiation or maintenance, such as obstructive sleep apnea (OSA), RLS, circadian rhythm disorders, or neurodevelopmental disorders, that often exhibit disturbed sleep as a comorbid condition requiring attention (e.g., autism spectrum disorder [ASD], or ADHD). In addition, children with chronic pain, type 1 diabetes mellitus, gastroesophageal reflux, colic, anxiety or depression, and those that have experienced traumatic brain injury or those using certain medications are also likely to experience disturbed sleep, and so identifying potential comorbidities is essential. Behavioral treatments for insomnia should be tailored in the context of comorbidities, and some studies are now addressing the acceptability and feasibility of such approaches in children with insomnia, for instance, sleep difficulties associated with traumatic brain injury.[76,77]

Third, the clinician should evaluate sleep hygiene by gaining a picture of the bedroom environment (e.g., evaluate temperature, light, noise), bedtime routine, bed(room)-sharing, sleep-wake scheduling, and the environmental conditions surrounding bedtime, such as light exposure, social interactions, and media use. A comprehensive checklist for assessing sleep hygiene and appropriate parental advice is provided by Mindell and Owens.[78] Sleep hygiene advice and sleep education directed at parents and children may be sufficient in cases where sleep disruption occurs as a result of unhealthy sleep practices.

If other causes of the sleep disturbance have been ruled out, the next step, for younger children at least, is to determine whether the insomnia symptoms may be the result of poor limit-setting associated with behavioral resistance or learned sleep-onset associations. Identification of the specific type of insomnia occurring can direct the clinician to the most appropriate behavioral treatment approach. Yet, before implementing any behavioral strategy, it is important first to establish good daytime and nighttime routines. For example, it is important to get up at a consistent time each morning, ensure that daytime naps are timed and of age-appropriate duration according to the sleep need of the child, and make sure that the hours leading up to bedtime are calm and consistent. These are the starting point for any further treatment.

Behavioral Treatments for Pediatric Insomnia

A small number of studies consistently demonstrate the efficacy and effectiveness of behavioral interventions for pediatric insomnia.[79] Determining which behavioral strategy to use depends on the child's age, their temperament, and preferences of the caregivers.[26,79a] Young children may benefit from short behavioral techniques that are implemented by the parent/caregiver, whereas older children and adolescents may benefit from more comprehensive cognitive behavioral therapy (CBT-I) for insomnia. Evidence-based behavioral techniques for younger children (typically from infancy to 4 years of age) include behavioral extinction and its variants (including modified variants, such as "camping out"), parental education of positive routines, bedtime fading, and scheduled awakenings.[80]

Behavioral extinction techniques are based on psychological learning principles. The goal of behavioral extinction is for the child to develop positive, independent methods of falling asleep alone and to reduce the necessity of the caregiver being present. Graduated extinction, of which there are a vast number of variants, involves putting the child to bed at a consistent time each night, the caregiver leaving the room, and returning after a predefined period of time has elapsed (e.g., 1 minute). Each time, the duration of time before returning to the bedroom is increased until the child is asleep, although some variants suggest returning after a fixed amount of time (e.g., 5 or 10 minutes). The amount of time decided upon depends on the child's age and temperament, as well as parental tolerance to crying.[80] The procedure is repeated if the child wakes in the middle of the night. Children eventually learn to go to sleep without caregiver intervention, and sleep-onset associations are reduced. Graduated extinction has been shown to reduce sleep-onset latency, wake-after-sleep onset, and number of awakenings in infants ages 6 to 16 months.[81] An alternative type of graduated extinction, known as "camping out," involves the caregiver remaining in the room with the child but gradually moving further away from the child at set intervals, eventually leaving the bedroom altogether.

There is concern among some parents about the potential long-term harm of extinction-based approaches and whether young children should be expected to "self-soothe." Although there is some evidence that such approaches have no short-term harm in terms of emotional and behavioral development, as well as parent-child attachment,[81] we acknowledge the sensitivity of this topic and appreciate that family preferences must be considered centrally in any recommendations.

Contrary to extinction-based techniques, bedtime fading involves stimulus control techniques to develop positive associations around sleep onset. Bedtime fading involves removing the child from the bed if they do not fall asleep. Bedtime is then delayed for a set period of time, after which the child is returned to bed. The child is repeatedly removed from bed if they do not fall asleep quickly. This method maintains positive parent-child interactions and allows the child's homeostatic sleep pressure to build so that they eventually fall asleep rapidly. No maladaptive sleep-onset associations are generated, and gradually the child will learn to fall asleep independently, bringing forward bedtime by 15 minutes over a few nights until a desired, age-appropriate bedtime is achieved. Bedtime fading has been shown to reduce sleep-onset latency, wake-after-sleep onset, and bedtime tantrums in children ages 1 to 4 years, with improvements in sleep sustained for at least 2 years.[82]

For some children, nocturnal awakenings occur at a predictable time after sleep onset. Scheduled awakenings by caregivers can then be timed around 15 minutes before the expected awakening. The caregiver may gently tap the child on the shoulder to induce an arousal, and the child is then permitted to go back to sleep. This method appears to reduce the number of spontaneous awakenings after several weeks, and the frequency of scheduled awakenings can eventually be faded out.[80] Although empirical research is limited, a review of the evidence concluded that there is some support for bedtime fading and scheduled awakenings in improving pediatric insomnia.[80]

Although many families have benefitted from behavioral interventions for insomnia in young children, certain families do not. There are parental and child factors that predict response to behavioral interventions. Such factors may include marital discord,[83] maternal depression[84] child anxiety,[85] and parental cry tolerance.[86] The presence of such factors should be considered when deciding whether to recommend a specific intervention. For example, one study demonstrated greater improvements in parent-reported sleep problems, using the Brief Infant Sleep Questionnaire, and reported night wakings after graduated extinction or camping-out for families with higher parental cry tolerance.[86] Another study found greater treatment success, in particular a reduction in wake-after-sleep onset, for the camping-out method compared to graduated extinction in children with high separation anxiety.[85] It is further suggested that bedtime fading, which involves little distress for the child, may be even better suited to children with separation anxiety, yet no studies have addressed this.

For older children and adolescents, CBT-I may be more age appropriate, given that the nature of the sleep disturbance may be more akin to adult insomnia. CBT-I is a multicomponent therapy that encompasses sleep hygiene advice, stimulus control, challenging maladaptive sleep-related cognitions, sleep restriction, and relaxation training. The small number of randomized controlled trials (RCTs) in children and adolescents suggest that CBT-I is effective in these populations,[87–89] although there are far fewer studies in these populations compared to those in the adult literature, warranting further pediatric research.[79]

Pharmacologic Treatments for Pediatric Insomnia

In cases that do not respond to behavioral treatments, pharmacologic treatments can be used as an adjunct therapy.[26,89a] Yet, there are no approved medications for insomnia in the pediatric population, and most medications are used off-label. This is surprising given that one study demonstrated that around 81% of visits to the general practitioner for pediatric insomnia resulted in the prescription of a medication to tackle the sleep disturbance.[90] Although these prescriptions may include sedative antidepressants, nonbenzodiazepine sedative hypnotics, melatonin, or antihistamines, there is concern about potential risks; there is no standard guidance on dosing and very little data on their efficacy and/or side effects. Our review of the literature concludes that the few RCTs of pharmacologic treatments for pediatric insomnia are largely limited to melatonin in the context of neurodevelopmental disorders,[91] with very little good-quality evidence for other medications and populations. A summary of the current evidence for these lines of therapy is presented later.

Antidepressant medications, such as selective-serotonin-reuptake inhibitors (SSRIs) are not indicated for infants and children. Serotonin precursors, such as L-5-hydroxytryptophan, have shown some evidence of positive effects on sleep, including reduced sleep-onset latency and increased slow-wave sleep,[92] although in children, this has only been examined in the context of reducing sleep terrors.[93]

Benzodiazepines and Z-drugs, such as clonazepam, zolpidem, and zopiclone, have often been used to treat insomnia in adults. However, these drugs have a very limited evidence base in children regarding their efficacy and potential side effects[26] and so are not recommended until further data are available. Two RCTs, one each of zolpidem and eszopiclone in children with ADHD, showed no improvement in sleep latency or ADHD symptoms.[94,95]

First-generation H_1 antihistamines are frequently used to treat sleep difficulties in children and are well accepted by caregivers despite the fact that studies on their efficacy are limited. Positive effects have been observed for some histamine H_1-receptor antagonists, including niazeprine, which in one study improved various indices of poor sleep in children ages 6 months to 6 years with no apparent adverse side effects.[96] A handful of studies evaluating trimeprazine and diphenhydramine, however, have provided mixed results in their treatment of pediatric sleep disturbances, particularly night waking.[97–101] Although adverse side effects have not been consistently documented, children frequently consuming sedative antihistamines may exhibit lethargy, daytime sleepiness, and consequent difficulties in learning and attention, as well as hyperactivity, tachycardia, and dry mouth.[102] Due to the lack of evidence in pediatric populations on the efficacy of first-generation antihistamines and lack of knowledge on adverse side effects, they are only recommended in children with particular problems (limited to urticaria, dermatitis, and anaphylaxis) for whom sedation might be a benefit for the primary condition.[103] Furthermore, rapid tolerance to their sedating effects precludes their use to treat chronic cases of insomnia.[104]

Exogenous melatonin is available in numerous countries as an over-the-counter sleep aid, and thus the use of melatonin as a "hypnotic" appears to be on the rise. Given its potential to advance sleep onset,[105] one may reason that it may aid with difficulties initiating sleep. However, the evidence for its efficacy in typically developing children is limited. Children with ADHD and ASD exhibit variations in the amplitude of melatonin secretion across the 24-hour period, which may account for difficulties with sleep onset and circadian rhythm disruption observed in these populations. These children may benefit from melatonin, but there is little evidence in other populations. A systematic review of pharmacologic treatments for sleep disorders in children identified 18 placebo-controlled trials focusing on melatonin.[91] All but 5 of these studies evaluated insomnia in the context of ADHD, ASD, or another neurodevelopmental disorder. Only one of these studies was considered good-quality evidence (the remainder deemed "fair"), and this study evaluated controlled-release melatonin singly and in combination with CBT-I for insomnia in children with ASD.[106] Melatonin was most effective at reducing insomnia symptoms and increasing sleep duration, particularly when combined with CBT-I, in the short term.[106] However, the results across all melatonin trials included in the review were mixed regarding changes in sleep-onset latency, awakenings, and sleep duration.[91] It is important to note that all of the studies on melatonin were short term (≤4 weeks), and there is little information regarding their longer-term potential for adverse reactions. Because melatonin is a hormone, concerns have been raised that long-term use may adversely affect pubertal development and fertility.[107,108] Furthermore, there are no specific guidelines on how to use melatonin in children with and without neurodevelopmental disorders,[109] highlighting a clear need for further research to develop optimal dosing regimens.

In summary, there is some evidence that melatonin treatment in conjunction with CBT-I improves sleep-onset latency and duration, particularly in children with ASD, ADHD, or neurodevelopmental disorder, but evidence is lacking on the efficacy both in the short and long term and in potential adverse effects of medications used for pediatric insomnia.

FUTURE DIRECTIONS

Further research should acknowledge the following considerations. First, many different definitions of pediatric insomnia are used across the field. Some studies broadly define "sleep problems" or "sleep disturbances," and other studies use clinical or research diagnostic criteria. Standardizing the approach to assessment will enable greater consistency between studies and in translating the empirical research to clinical contexts. On the other hand, exploring these potentially distinct constructs more explicitly will enable a better appreciation of the complex manifestations of insomnia and disturbed sleep more generally.

Second, much of the research to date uses different methods to assess insomnia. Questionnaires, clinical interviews, parent-report, self-report, sleep diaries, polysomnography, and actigraphy have all been used in research to contribute to the assessment of insomnia. Different results are often obtained depending on the method of assessment used, and it is possible that each of these methods is measuring a different construct that stems from distinct etiology. As such, future research should use consistent measurements to assess insomnia, aligned to diagnostic criteria.

Third, it is necessary to embed theories of insomnia in a developmental context. For example, the distinction between insomnia with and without objective short sleep duration suggests different etiologic underpinnings. It is also possible that these different subtypes represent distinct developmental trajectories, yet very little research explores etiologic differences in those with and without objective short sleep duration in pediatric populations. There is also the question of whether childhood-onset insomnia is harder to treat than adult-onset cases. Some evidence demonstrates poorer insomnia treatment response in childhood-onset cases of insomnia comorbid with depression, compared to adult-onset cases for both disorders.[110] Further research is needed to understand whether different treatment approaches are warranted based on these distinctions.

Fourth, there are a dearth of studies assessing the efficacy of behavioral treatments during adolescence. Transdiagnostic behavioral interventions that target both circadian rhythm disturbances and insomnia may be particularly useful when considering co-occurring mental health problems.[111] In all contexts, it is also necessary to determine whether treatment has concomitant effects on secondary outcomes, such as general and mental health, mood, academic performance, and behavior, as has been found previously.[112,113] Long-term follow-up studies of behavioral and/or pharmacologic treatments are also required to determine how long positive treatment outcomes are maintained, as well as their long-term potential side effects on mood, behavior, and development.[80] In particular, research should focus on establishing the potential long-term side effects of melatonin on pubertal development before this treatment can be routinely endorsed.

Finally, further research should examine potential predictors of treatment response. Identification of factors beyond parental cry tolerance or child anxiety that can predict who is likely to benefit from which behavioral and/or pharmacologic treatment will pave the way toward personalized medicine, maximizing treatment outcomes and enhancing clinical efficiency.

From a clinical standpoint, our synthesis of the literature has highlighted considerations that should be addressed in routine practice. Perhaps most important, pediatric clinicians should be educated in the identification, diagnosis, and management of sleep disorders in the primary care setting. This may be challenging, given that current rates of screening for sleep disorders in this context are low.[114] There are very few trained providers of CBT-I worldwide, particularly in pediatric care, despite the growing rise of "sleep coaches," who are often not appropriately trained and for whom there is no formal credentialling.[115] The focus now should be on educating health care providers on the behavioral treatment of insomnia and its application in numerous populations. That said, digital therapies for insomnia (see Chapter 97) have the potential to increase access to clinical care and should be tested in pediatric populations.

In addition, there should be a development of evidence-based parental education materials, focusing on the management of normal sleep difficulties using sleep hygiene and behavioral techniques. Given that the family context is so influential for sleep, particularly in younger populations, the focus should be on both preventative and management solutions to hinder the development of long-term sleep problems. There are excellent guidelines and resources available, such as Meltzer and McLaughlin Crabtree[116] and Mindell and Owens,[78] and a growth of expert-led websites providing free access to evidence-based, age-specific advice and techniques to tackle childhood sleep problems, such as www.babysleep.com and accessible popular science books (e.g., by Gregory[117]).

CLINICAL PEARL

Pediatric insomnia is etiologically complex, with the likelihood of many genetic, neurophysiologic, environmental, cognitive, and behavioral factors involved. The relative importance of these factors varies across development, and the exact nature of these influences is time specific. Treatment of insomnia at any stage of life should acknowledge the environmental circumstances that may have contributed to its genesis. Behavioral treatments for pediatric insomnia are effective and have the potential not only to improve sleep but also to contribute positive effects to mood, cognition, behavior, and general health.

SUMMARY

Epidemiologic, quantitative genetic, and molecular genetic research has highlighted the multifactorial etiology of insomnia. A combination of genetic, neurophysiologic, environmental, cognitive, and behavioral factors work in concert to influence pediatric insomnia, and a distinct set of influences contribute to its persistence. Research has uncovered some of the environmental factors that are particularly potent disruptors of sleep, including early-life stress, which predicts both current and future insomnia, and suboptimal socioeconomic circumstances and certain parenting practices that make the conditions for sleep challenging. Treatment of pediatric insomnia should be tailored according to the child's age, the nature of their insomnia (i.e., sleep-onset association type or limit-setting type), consideration of potential comorbidities, and environmental circumstances. Increasing access to behavioral treatments, be it through training of sleep practitioners in primary care or through parental education programs, is of utmost importance to decrease the burden of insomnia and to limit its enduring trajectory from infancy to adulthood.

SELECTED READINGS

Barclay NL, Gregory AM. Quantitative genetic research on sleep: a review of normal sleep, sleep disturbances and associated emotional, behavioural, and health-related difficulties. *Sleep Med Rev*. 2013;17:29–40.

Bruni O, Angriman M. Pediatric insomnia: new insights in clinical assessment and treatment options. *Arch Ital Biol*. 2015;153:144–156.

Ekambaram V, Owens J. Medications used for pediatric Insomnia. *Child Adolesc Psychiatr Clin N Am*. 2021;30(1):85–99.

Gregory AM. *Nodding Off: The Science of Sleep*. London: Bloomsbury Sigma; 2020.

Hysing M, Harvey AG, Torgersen L, Ystrom E, Reichborn-Kjennerud T, Sivertsen B. Trajectories and predictors of nocturnal awakenings and sleep duration in infants. *J Dev Behav Pediatr*. 2014;35:309–316.

Meltzer LJ, Mindell JA. Systematic review and meta-analysis of behavioral interventions for pediatric insomnia. *J Pediatr Psychol*. 2014;39:932–948.

Meltzer LJ, Wainer A, Engstrom E, Pepa L, Mindell JA. Seeing the whole elephant: a scoping review of behavioral treatments for pediatric insomnia. *Sleep Med Rev*. 2021;56:101410.

Mindell JA, Owens JA. *A Clinical Guide to Pediatric Sleep: Diagnosis and Management of Sleep Problems*. Lippincott Williams & Wilkins; 2015.

Sivertsen B, Harvey AG, Pallesen S, Hysing M. Trajectories of sleep problems from childhood to adolescence: a population-based longitudinal study from Norway. *J Sleep Res*. 2017;26:55–63.

A complete reference list can be found online at ExpertConsult.com.

Chapter 93

Insomnia Diagnosis, Assessment, and Evaluation

Jason C. Ong; J. Todd Arnedt; David A. Kalmbach; Michael T. Smith

Chapter Highlights

- This chapter provides an overview of the state-of-the-science for the clinical assessment of insomnia disorders.
- The tools for conducting a clinical assessment of insomnia are described. The essential tools include the clinical interview, sleep diaries, and self-report measures. Objective measures, including polysomnography and actigraphy, are not routinely used but can be useful with certain populations or to rule out other sleep disorders.
- Considerations for case formulation, assessing treatment progress, and variations in clinical setting are discussed.
- Consumer devices for monitoring sleep are not yet validated for clinical settings but could provide opportunities for enhancing the assessment of insomnia in the future.

INTRODUCTION

This chapter provides an overview of the state-of-the-science for the clinical assessment of insomnia. The first section reviews diagnostic criteria of current classification systems. The second section describes components of clinical assessment of insomnia with expanded discussion on the role of consumer devices. The third section provides considerations for insomnia assessment based on clinical context, patient population, and quality metrics. The chapter concludes with a discussion on the renewed interest in objective measures and the rising interest in emerging consumer technologies.

THE DIAGNOSIS OF INSOMNIA

Insomnia is characterized by difficulty falling/staying asleep or awakening earlier than desired. These sleep disturbances are considered insomnia symptoms, which, by themselves, lack specificity and do not sufficiently capture the complexities of the sleep problem or the impact on daytime function (see Chapter 89). In some cases these symptoms are isolated or transient and do not require clinical attention. In other cases the symptoms are persistent and cause significant distress or impairment, prompting patients to seek clinical attention.

The main classification systems to diagnose insomnia include the *Diagnostic and Statistical Manual of Mental Disorders* (DSM-5)[1] and the *International Classification of Sleep Disorders* (ICSD-3).[2] Essential elements for an insomnia disorder include these patient-reported criteria:

A. A predominant complaint of dissatisfaction with sleep quantity or quality, associated with difficulty initiating sleep, maintaining sleep, or early-morning awakenings
B. Distress or impairment that is caused by the insomnia symptoms
C. Frequency at least 3 nights per week
D. Duration at least 3 months
E. Adequate opportunity for sleep
F. The insomnia is not better explained by the course of another sleep-wake disorder
G. The insomnia is not attributable to the effect of a substance
H. Coexisting mental disorders or medical conditions do not adequately explain the insomnia

To properly diagnose insomnia, the sleep disturbance (criterion A) must be related to daytime distress or impairment, such as fatigue or concerns about daytime functioning (criterion B). There are requirements for frequency (criterion C), duration (criterion D) of sleep problems, and adequate opportunity for sleep (criterion E). The remaining criteria (F to H) involve discerning other potential explanations, attributions, or comorbid conditions that could account for the insomnia symptoms. In contrast to previous versions, DSM-5 and ICSD-3 do not distinguish between primary and secondary insomnia and do not include insomnia subtypes (e.g., psychophysiological). Evidence did not support the value of DSM-IV-TR primary versus secondary categories nor ICSD-2 insomnia subtypes regarding treatment or prognosis, and these distinctions failed to demonstrate adequate validity and reliability.[3]

At present, the DSM-5 uses a single diagnosis of Insomnia Disorder.[1] Specifiers are used to indicate the presence of another comorbid condition (mental, medical, or other sleep disorder) and the natural course of the insomnia symptoms (episodic, persistent, or recurrent). DSM-5 assigns the diagnosis of Other Specified Insomnia Disorder with the specifier Brief Insomnia Disorder when the insomnia symptoms last less than 3 months but fulfill all other diagnostic criteria. In contrast, the ICSD-3 uses two diagnoses based on duration: Chronic Insomnia Disorder (≥3 months, consistent with DSM-5) and Short-term Insomnia Disorder (≥1 month but less than 3 months).[2] Finally, DSM-5 and ICSD-3 insomnia diagnoses can be applied to both adults and children.

ASSESSMENT OF INSOMNIA

The clinical assessment of insomnia should include a clinical interview, self-report measures of global insomnia symptoms, and sleep diaries. Objective measures, such as polysomnography and actigraphy are not necessary but may be required to rule out other sleep disorders when additional signs and symptoms are present and considered if patients fail to respond to standard treatments. Conceptual models for the development and maintenance of insomnia can provide a useful framework for organizing assessment data from multiple sources. The three-factor model[4] guides assessment of predisposing factors (e.g., family history of insomnia), precipitating events associated with the onset of insomnia (e.g., stressful life events), and perpetuating factors that maintain insomnia (e.g., excessive time in bed). Etiologic models of hyperarousal[5] and the role of cognitions (e.g., worry about insomnia and its consequences, unrealistic sleep expectations)[6] can be useful to inform case conceptualizations and treatment planning.

The Clinical Interview

The clinical interview should yield a detailed account of the chief complaint, a comprehensive list of differential *diagnoses,* and a logical treatment plan. Of importance, insomnia patients typically seek treatment because of daytime impairment; thus therapeutic targets should include both nighttime and daytime symptoms. An assessment outline with general category areas and key specific areas of inquiry can be found in Table 93.1. Structured clinical interviews have also been developed for research settings with evidence to support reliability and validity.[7,8]

Interviews often begin by eliciting the primary insomnia symptom, which typically fall along a limited number of dimensions: inability to fall asleep, inability to stay asleep, waking too early, poor-quality sleep, too little sleep, work or lifestyle interfering with sleep, or inability to sleep without medications.[9] Clinicians should assess nightly frequency and duration of symptoms to determine whether nocturnal symptoms meet the frequency and duration criteria for a DSM-5 and ICSD-3 diagnosis and to aid later evaluation of quantitative changes with treatment. Although quantitative criteria for sleep parameters are not required for a diagnosis, sleep-onset latency greater than 30 minutes and wake after sleep onset greater than 30 minutes are often considered clinically significant levels of difficulty falling and staying asleep in adults, respectively.[10] The perceived severity of the nighttime problem and its impact on daytime consequences should also be gauged.

Daytime consequences of nighttime symptoms are necessary for insomnia diagnosis. Patients commonly report that sleep problems lead to and/or exacerbate daytime fatigue, irritability, cognitive-emotional problems, attention and memory deficits, physical illness, and work/school issues.[5,11,12] As daytime issues prompt patients to seek treatment, these symptoms deserve full attention in the assessment of insomnia and in tracking treatment progress. If the patient has a bed partner, assessing the extent to which the patient's sleep is impacted by the bed partner's sleeping habits can reveal important contextual information.

Current sleep patterns under normal life circumstances should be documented in the interview. Information to collect includes bedtime, "lights out time," rise time, sleep latency, number and duration of awakenings during the night, final wake-up time, frequency and duration of daytime naps, total sleep time, perceived sleep quality, and morning restfulness. Clinicians should assess whether sleep patterns differ between weekdays/workdays versus weekends/nonworkdays (e.g., sleeping in on weekends), on and off sleep medication, and on good nights versus bad nights. Many patients report their sleep to be invariable, unpredictable, and resistant to environmental circumstances, but the patient should nevertheless be challenged to consider differences between good and bad nights. In addition, clinicians should assess whether there is adequate opportunity for sleep. For example, individuals working multiple jobs or shift workers who also have family responsibilities might not allocate enough time in their schedule to obtain sufficient sleep.

The clinician should additionally inquire about presleep activity (e.g., use of electronics), perceived causes of difficulty falling asleep or waking in the night (e.g., stress, environmental factors), coping responses when unable to sleep (e.g., remain in bed, watch television, sleep in a different room), and factors that improve or worsen sleep. Understanding the patient's response to sleep disturbances (e.g., distress levels after a bad night of sleep) and daytime consequences (e.g., napping due to fatigue) can inform case formulation and identify treatment targets.

Individuals with insomnia often self-treat with over-the-counter (OTC) sleep aids, herbal remedies, and alcohol.[13] The clinical interview should assess current and past treatments, including prescription and OTC medications, alcohol and other substances, and nonmedication approaches. Inquiring about medications and substances for other conditions that might be used to treat insomnia is also important, as self-treatment might include off-label or inappropriate use of substances not intended to treat insomnia. Treatments should be assessed for type, dosage, frequency of use, time of administration, typical response, and the conditions surrounding deviations from this pattern. The interviewer should establish whether prior treatments were given an adequate trial because past failures can result from suboptimal treatment. Consideration should also be given to the timing of the insomnia disorder relative to the initiation of medications/substances and alterations in sleep as a function of use, extended exposure, and discontinuation.

Sleep-incompatible behaviors (e.g., using the bed and bedroom for activities other than sleep) and thoughts (e.g., daytime consequences of poor sleep) often precipitate and/or perpetuate insomnia and should be assessed in detail.[4,5] These behaviors include poor sleep hygiene practices,[14] but most patients have already attempted to remedy these before seeking treatment. Maladaptive beliefs and attitudes about sleep and sleep-incompatible cognitive reactions to sleep disturbances can serve to maintain the disorder. Ruminating on insomnia and its daytime consequences is especially harmful and may increase risk for comorbid psychiatric disorders. The importance of assessing maladaptive cognitions during the clinical interview is to maximize treatment gains through their modification.[15,16] Assessment of sleep-compensatory behaviors used to increase nighttime sleep (e.g., spending excessive amount of time in bed awake trying to sleep, erratic

Table 93.1 Clinical Interview Assessment Outline

Category	Specifics
Chief complaint	Difficulty falling asleep, staying asleep, waking up too early, poor-quality sleep, too little sleep, work/lifestyle interferes with sleep, inability to sleep without medications Define frequency (weekly, monthly), duration, severity, and course (episodic, seasonal variation)
Circumstances surrounding onset	Age of onset, precipitating event(s), sudden/gradual onset, premorbid sleep pattern/quality, previous insomnia episodes
Daytime consequences	Fatigue vs. sleepiness, napping, cognition, performance, and mood
Current sleep-wake schedule	Bedtime, wake time, rise time, sleep latency, frequency, and duration of nighttime awakenings, estimated total sleep time Define average night and variability (e.g., weekdays vs. weekends, medication vs. nonmedication), identify factors that ameliorate and exacerbate sleep pattern Identify prebedtime activities and environment
Current and past treatments, adequacy of trial, efficacy	Type (prescription, over-the-counter, behavioral), dosage, efficacy, adequacy of trial
Perpetuating factors: Behavioral	Practices intended to improve sleep (e.g., going to bed early, staying in bed late, increasing time in bed, falling asleep with TV/radio, staying in bed during awakenings, delayed rise time on weekends) Practices intended to counter fatigue (e.g., napping vs. dozing vs. resting, increasing caffeine ingestion, decreasing physical activity)
Cognitive	Worry about: (1) consequences of insomnia (fatigue, performance deficits, health, appearance), (2) sleeplessness ("I'll never get to sleep tonight"), (3) self-perception ("I'm not together," "I can't even sleep like a normal person," "My sleep is out of control, just like my life") *False beliefs:* Misconceptions about sleep ("Everybody sleeps 8 hours," "I can't function on less than 7 hours of sleep"), catastrophizing ("Insomnia is ruining my life"), requirements for sleep ("I cannot sleep without sleeping pills," "I must sleep alone")
Other	Alcohol, noise, pets sleeping in the same bed, clock watching during the night, getting home late without enough time to wind down
Work	Stress, work schedule incompatible with sleep schedule or contributing to insomnia
Family/social	Childhood habit of staying up late with a parent Family history of sleep and psychiatric disorders Stressful life events (past stressful events may be precipitants, and present stressful events may be perpetuators) Environmental factors (safety, neighborhood)
Medical factors	Pain and other medical conditions that can interfere with sleep
Pharmacologic considerations	Activating and sedating drugs that interfere with the sleep-wake cycle (consider type, dosage, frequency, and timing), side effects, history of hypnotic use
Psychiatric factors	*Key features of depression:* Sadness, anhedonia, suicidal thoughts/behaviors, hopelessness, worthlessness, negative repetitive thinking, social withdrawal *Key features of anxiety:* Exaggerated worry, tension and irritability; restlessness, headaches, trembling, sweating and sleep disturbance Key features of substance use disorders: Excessive and persistent use of substance(s) with evidence of impaired control, use in risky circumstances, and/or significant social impairment Consider relationship with current insomnia symptom and status of treatment
Other sleep disorders	Sleep-related breathing disorders (see Section 15) Central disorders of hypersomnolence (see Section 13) Circadian rhythm sleep-wake disorders (see Chapter 43) Parasomnias (see Section 14) Sleep-related movement disorders (see Chapters 121-122)
Significant other report	Obtain collateral information from bed partner when possible about sleep pattern and other sleep disorders

sleep schedules) and/or dealing with the daytime consequences of poor sleep (e.g., napping, increased caffeine intake) can uncover targets for behavior modification.

Family history of insomnia and psychiatric disorders can provide insight into predisposing factors to insomnia. Insomnia patients often have first-degree relatives with sleep disturbances, with the mother being the most commonly affected family member.[17–19] Social determinants of health apply to insomnia such that individuals with low income, lower education attainment, who are unemployed, experience racial or gender discrimination, and live in unsafe neighborhoods are more likely to experience insomnia.[20] Assessing these social determinants can provide an important context and may help to identify treatment targets or barriers. Assessing social history, including occupational or school performance, quantity and quality of interpersonal support, and life stressors can also elicit potential therapeutic targets. Finally, assessment of work hours and timing (e.g., multiple jobs, night shifts) and caregiver demands can determine if adequate opportunity to achieve sufficient sleep exists or if the sleep symptoms might be better explained by another sleep-wake disorder.

A significant and critical portion of the interview is devoted to evaluating psychiatric and substance use disorders, medical conditions, and other sleep disorders that co-occur with insomnia (Table 93.2).[21,22] The interviewer should establish the nature of the relationship between insomnia and the comorbid condition, including temporal precedence and possible causality. In some circumstances an unstable psychiatric or medical disorder may require a primary initial focus in the sequence of care and/or influence insomnia treatment planning options, such as the decision to initiate cognitive-behavioral therapy versus pharmacotherapy or combination approaches.

Table 93.2 Medical and Psychiatric Conditions Commonly Comorbid with Insomnia

Medical Conditions	Psychiatric Conditions
Neurologic (e.g., headache, neuropathic pain conditions, stroke, seizure disorders, brain injury, dementia, Parkinson disease)	Mood disorders (e.g., major depressive disorder, persistent depressive disorder, bipolar disorder, seasonal affective disorder)
Cardiovascular (e.g., hypertension, angina, congestive heart failure)	Anxiety disorders (e.g., generalized anxiety disorder, posttraumatic stress disorder)
Pulmonary (e.g., chronic obstructive pulmonary disease, asthma)	Psychotic disorders (e.g., schizophrenia)
Digestive (e.g., irritable bowel syndrome, reflux, peptic ulcer)	Eating disorders: bulimia nervosa, anorexia nervosa
Endocrine (e.g., hyperthyroidism, diabetes mellitus)	Attention deficit and hyperactivity disorder
Musculoskeletal (e.g., rheumatoid arthritis, chronic pain disorders)	Adjustment disorder
Reproductive (e.g., pregnancy, menopause)	Personality disorders (e.g., borderline)
Genitourinary (e.g., incontinence, enuresis, benign prostatic hypertrophy)	
Other sleep disorders (e.g., sleep apnea, restless legs syndrome, periodic limb movement disorder)	

Modified from Schutte-Rodin S, Broch L, Buysse D, Dorsey C, Sateia M. Clinical guideline for the evaluation and management of chronic insomnia in adults. *J Clin Sleep Med.* 2008;4(5):487–504.

Insomnia symptoms are essential features of several psychiatric disorders, with rates of comorbidity for insomnia disorder ranging from 40% to more than 50%.[23] Thus it is important to assess for undiagnosed or inadequately treated psychiatric conditions that may be contributing to, or being exacerbated by, the sleep disturbance. It is also important to note that the comorbid condition should not be the sole focus of treatment[23] because insomnia and/or changes in sleep patterns are often a prodromal, initial symptom manifesting before a major depressive or manic episode and often persist after resolution of comorbid psychiatric illness.[24,25] Cotreatment of insomnia and comorbid psychiatric disorders is the recommended approach and yields higher remission rates for the psychiatric disorder compared to treatment of the psychiatric disorder alone.[26]

Mood disorders are often comorbid with insomnia, with 40% of individuals with depression also meeting criteria for a comorbid insomnia disorder.[27] Patients with bipolar disorder may report intermittent insomnia, which might arise due to heightened arousal/activation during mania. A history of bipolar disorder should be considered in treatment planning, as sleep deprivation from sleep restriction in insomnia treatment may increase risk of a manic episode.[28] Insomnia is also an independent risk factor for suicidal behavior, particularly in patients with major depression and chronic pain.[29,30] Evaluating current suicidal risk and previous suicidal ideation and behavior should be a routine part of the insomnia evaluation. Insomnia is common in patients with anxiety, namely panic disorder and generalized anxiety disorder, and in patients with trauma and stress-related disorders, such as posttraumatic stress disorder (PTSD). In comparison, patients with social phobia, obsessive compulsive disorder, or simple phobias are less likely to have insomnia.[31,32] Although anxiety can occur at night, assessing thought contents and the situational context can aid in determining whether patients with anxiety have comorbid insomnia or if the sleep disturbance is a symptom of the anxiety condition.

One-third to more than three-quarters of patients with a substance use disorder report insomnia symptoms.[33,34] Rates of clinically significant insomnia (occurring more than 3 nights per week for at least 1 month) among treatment-seeking individuals with alcohol use disorder, for example, are as high as 50%,[35] and the presence of insomnia in early abstinence consistently predicts alcohol relapse.[34,36,37] Insomnia patients with alcohol misuse should be evaluated for comorbid substance use disorders and whether alcohol is used as a compensatory behavior in response to sleep disturbance. Similarly, attention should be given to how patients are using prescription medications to treat insomnia. Clinicians should assess for indications of dependence and tolerance, as well as adverse effects (e.g., memory loss) or potential safety issues (e.g., residual daytime grogginess, falls in the middle of the night). Misuse of other substances, such as stimulants (e.g., methylphenidate, cocaine) and depressants (e.g., cannabis, opioids), may be exacerbated by or contribute to insomnia. The use of cannabis for insomnia has increased in recent years, despite inconclusive efficacy.[38,39] Similarly, "use to get sleep" is among the top motivations for nonmedical use of opioids among adolescents.[40]

Medical comorbidity is high in insomnia disorder,[41] and accompanying medical conditions often exacerbate insomnia and interfere with treatment progress (Table 93.2). A review of systems and inquiry of the patient's medical history should be part of the assessment. If available, a review of medical records or self-report questionnaires before the interview can facilitate the medical evaluation. Depending on the setting and training of the clinician, a physical examination and/or further laboratory testing might be warranted if there is suspicion of an undiagnosed medical condition that could contribute to the patient's insomnia symptoms.

If another sleep disorder is suspected, the clinician should determine whether the insomnia is better explained by the other sleep disorder or if the insomnia is comorbid with the other sleep disorder. If an occult sleep disorder is suspected, an in-laboratory polysomnography (PSG) or home sleep apnea test (HSAT) should be considered. Greater than 40% of patients with obstructive sleep apnea (OSA) report insomnia symptoms,[42] and the comorbidity of insomnia and OSA is very common in patients presenting to sleep medicine clinics.[43] Typically, these patients will report frequent nighttime awakenings with difficulty returning to sleep, although some can also report difficulty with sleep onset. Critically, OSA patients with insomnia may be less tolerant to positive airway pressure, the gold-standard treatment of OSA.[44] Given the high rates of comorbidity between patients with insomnia and OSA, clinicians should assess for additional risk factors for sleep apnea, including obesity, excessive daytime sleepiness, endorsement of loud snoring, and neck circumference greater than or equal to 17 inches.[45] Restless legs syndrome (RLS) is characterized by an irresistible urge to move the legs, usually accompanied by abnormal sensations.[46] RLS patients can present with insomnia because the symptoms are worse in the evening/night and can disturb the ability to fall and stay asleep. Most RLS patients have periodic limb movements during sleep,[47] which can increase nighttime waking and contribute to sleep maintenance insomnia.

Insomnia related to misalignment between the patient's endogenous circadian rhythm and the external environment may reflect a circadian rhythm sleep-wake disorder (CRSWD). The distinction between insomnia and a CRSWD can be informed by asking whether sleep problems are resolved when the patient is able to choose a preferred schedule, such as on weekends. Patients with CRSWD-delayed sleep phase type report severe difficulty falling asleep at typical hours and difficulty waking up in the morning. Those with CRSWD-advanced sleep phase type report sleepiness several hours before bedtime but then waking up much earlier than their planned times. If insomnia can be directly attributed to an unconventional work schedule, it may reflect and be better explained by CRSWD–shift-work type.

Self-Report Measures

Self-report measures of insomnia, daytime impairment, co-occurring symptoms, and other relevant factors provide important information to augment interview data. Table 93.3 includes a summary of the most common self-report measures used in clinical and research settings in the assessment of insomnia. These measures can be particularly useful in assessing treatment progress or treatment outcomes during follow-up visits.

Sleep diaries are a prospective form of insomnia assessment wherein patients complete a series of questions each morning about their prior night's sleep. A standard sleep diary is available[48] that assesses bedtime, sleep latency, number of nighttime awakenings, rise time, and other parameters. Diaries are kept for 1 to 2 weeks to capture a representative sample of data. An advantage of sleep diaries is their prospective nature, which is less subject to bias (e.g., primacy, recency effects), compared to information about during a clinical interview. They also yield a series of quantitative values that provide individualized accounts of patient sleep patterns and can be useful in guiding behavioral treatments and tracking treatment-related changes in sleep parameters. In addition, daily monitoring of sleep can offer valuable insights—for

Table 93.3 Summary of Self-Report Measures

Domain	Measure	Utility/Purpose
Sleep/wake patterns	Consensus Sleep Diary	Prospective estimates of sleep parameters, bedtimes, sleep quality ratings, and daytime naps
Global measures of insomnia	Insomnia Severity Index Pittsburgh Sleep Quality Index PROMIS Sleep Disturbance PROMIS Sleep-related Impairment	Assess severity of insomnia symptoms and change in symptoms during follow-up
Other measures	Dysfunctional Beliefs and Attitudes about Sleep Scale Pre-Sleep Arousal Scale Glasgow Sleep Effort Scale Daytime Insomnia Symptom Response Scale Epworth Sleepiness Scale Fatigue Severity Scale Flinders Fatigue Scale Patient Health Questionnaire-9 Generalized Anxiety Disorder-7 Item Scale Morningness-Eveningness Questionnaire Sleep Hygiene Index Ford Insomnia Response to Stress Test Arousal Predisposition Scale	Assess daytime functioning, presence of psychiatric symptoms, sleep behaviors, or etiologic factors (e.g., predisposing or perpetuating factors)

PROMIS, Patient-Reported Outcomes Measurement Information System.

patients and clinicians—into nightly variations in sleep quality and factors (e.g., triggers, behaviors) that improve or impair sleep quality. One disadvantage of sleep diaries is the potential to become hypervigilant about monitoring time when recording sleep patterns, which could lead to heightened anxiety and rumination about sleep.

Global measures of insomnia provide an index of insomnia severity in relation to normative data. In treatment, these measures are often administered at follow-up visits to track patient progress.[49] At present, the most common self-report insomnia measure in clinical practice and research is the Insomnia Severity Index (ISI).[50] The ISI consists of 7 items on nighttime and daytime symptoms and assesses severity over the prior 2 weeks. Scoring is straightforward and yields a total score with validated cut-offs that can be used to identify those with clinically significant insomnia. The ISI is commonly used as a screening tool and as an outcome measure in clinical practice and trials,[51] allowing for the determination of treatment response and remission. Another option is the Pittsburgh Sleep Quality Index (PSQI), which has been translated into more than 50 languages and is one of the most widely used sleep questionnaires in the world.[52] It consists of 18 items that assess multiple facets of sleep over the past month, including sleep duration, latency, efficiency, sleep-interfering behaviors, and daytime impairment. The primary disadvantage of its use as an insomnia measure is that it broadly assesses sleep disturbance; thus not all items on the PSQI assess insomnia (e.g., difficulty sleeping due to breathing problems). Although insomnia patients score high on the PSQI, elevated scores (five points or higher) may be due to other sleep disorders. The Sleep Disturbance Scale and Sleep-Related Impairment Scale from the National Institutes of Health Common Fund's Patient-Reported Outcomes Measurement Information System (PROMIS) initiative assesses nighttime and daytime symptoms of sleep disturbance, respectively.[53] Similar to the PSQI, the PROMIS scales are not specific to insomnia, although many items are relevant to insomnia.[54]

Assessment of sleep-interfering cognitions and arousal can inform case conceptualization and treatment targets. The Dysfunctional Beliefs and Attitudes about Sleep Scale (DBAS)[55] assesses the degree to which patients harbor maladaptive beliefs about sleep. Item-level analysis of the DBAS often reveals important cognitive inaccuracies that can inform target areas for therapy. DBAS scores often decrease with successful insomnia treatment, reflecting a normalization of attitude toward sleep. Key measures of insomnia-related cognitive arousal include the Pre-Sleep Arousal Scale's cognitive factor[56] (nocturnal cognitive arousal), the Glasgow Sleep Effort Scale[57] (effort and pressure to sleep), and the Daytime Insomnia Symptom Response Scale[58] (insomnia-focused rumination). As cognitive arousal is transdiagnostic to psychiatric disorders, non-sleep-specific measures can also provide insight into cognitive phenomena contributing to sleep disturbance, daytime impairment, and/or psychiatric comorbidities (e.g., Perseverative Thinking Questionnaire,[59] Ruminative Response Scale,[60] and Penn State Worry Questionnaire[61]).

Individuals with insomnia typically seek treatment when their daytime functioning becomes impaired because of their sleep problems. Most insomnia patients report fatigue or sleepiness; thus measuring these domains can reveal changes in daytime impairment. The Flinders Fatigue Scale[62] captures insomnia-related fatigue, whereas the Fatigue Severity Scale and Epworth Sleepiness Scale[63] are not specific to insomnia. Psychiatric symptoms may be of interest given the high rates of mental illness in insomnia. Measures of depression (e.g., Patient Health Questionnaire-9) and anxiety (e.g., Generalized Anxiety Disorder 7-Item Scale) can inform the presence of mood disturbances and can be used to monitor improvements in comorbid mental illness as insomnia is alleviated or to identify barriers to improvement when patients do not respond well to treatment. Interpretation of these measures should consider the overlapping items on insomnia symptoms.

Assessing other aspects of the insomnia experience and etiologic/perpetuating factors may be informative. Circadian tendencies or chronotypes (e.g., Morningness-Eveningness Questionnaire[64]) can be useful for differential diagnosis with CRSWD and also provide information to help clinicians tailor recommendations regarding the timing of sleep behaviors. The Sleep Hygiene Index[65] can also provide insights into sleep-incompatible behaviors that can serve as the target of behavioral treatments. Sleep reactivity is a trait-like degree to which stress exposure disrupts sleep and has been found to decrease with treatment for some insomnia patients, and posttreatment sleep reactivity may predict relapse. It can be measured by the Ford Insomnia Response to Stress Test (FIRST).[66] General arousability is a robust predictor of insomnia and may even predict treatment response. The Arousal Predisposition Scale measures trait-like arousability, which includes cognitive-emotional and physiologic aspects of arousal.[67]

Objective Measures

PSG is the gold-standard objective measure of sleep. However, it is not indicated for the routine evaluation of a transient or chronic insomnia disorder, which places primacy on self-reported symptoms for the diagnosis of insomnia.[68] PSG is indicated to rule out the presence of a sleep-related breathing disorder (SRBD) (e.g., OSA), periodic limb movement disorder (PLMD), or when the initial insomnia treatment fails.[68] However, emerging evidence suggests that SRBDs, in particular, may be underrecognized causes of insomnia, even among individuals who deny cardinal SRBD symptoms on initial presentation.[69] Although insomnia patients often report daytime sleepiness, the Multiple Sleep Latency Test (MSLT), the standard assessment tool for objective measurement of daytime sleepiness,[70] is not indicated for the evaluation of sleepiness in insomnia.[71] Patients with insomnia may show longer sleep latencies on the MSLT than normal control subjects, which is attributed to their heightened physiologic arousal.[72] A major limitation of traditional PSG is that 1 to 2 nights of PSG may not adequately capture a representative sleep period for the patient. Thus it is less useful in the context of insomnia, where assessing the pattern of habitual sleep is important. In recent years, in-home PSG has become increasingly feasible as home sleep testing devices initially developed to screen for sleep apnea have become more advanced.

Actigraphy is another well-validated objective measure of sleep-wake patterns, with some clinical-grade devices approved by the U.S. Food and Drug Administration (FDA).[73] Actigraphs are small motion sensor detectors, typically triaxial accelerometers, that measure occurrence and degree of movement over time. The accelerometer is encased in a unit about the size of a wristwatch and can be worn continuously for days to months. Following technical guidelines, sleep can be reliably inferred during times at which low activity occurs.[74,75] Dedicated software using one of several validated algorithms provides summary measures of behavioral sleep-wake activity and circadian rhythm parameters. It should be noted that actigraphy is not considered a replacement for self-report assessment of insomnia but, rather, provides important additional and distinct information.

Current practice guidelines suggest that clinicians use actigraphy in the assessment of adults and pediatric patients with insomnia disorder when there is a need for objective measurement of sleep-wake patterns.[76] It is especially useful in patient populations who have difficulty adhering to diary monitoring or who may be unable to report diary information, such as in infants, young children, or individuals with cognitive deficits. In pediatric populations diagnosed with insomnia, actigraphy was generally consistent with diary estimates but more sensitive in identifying sleep maintenance problems (increased wake after sleep onset time) and reduced sleep duration. Actigraphy may also be useful in evaluating patients who report extremely low habitual sleep duration, to determine potential discrepancy or agreement between the self-reported sleep duration and objectively measured sleep duration.[76] In cases where actigraphy reveals relatively normal amounts of sleep, the findings can be used as part of treatment to provide education and alleviate anxiety regarding insufficient sleep. In cases where actigraphy corroborates low sleep duration, it may provide diagnostic information regarding other medical or psychiatric causes (e.g., mania, endocrine imbalance).

Several limitations should be considered when using actigraphy in the assessment of insomnia. First, the scoring algorithms for sleep and wakefulness can vary across the different devices, manufacturers, and patient populations. Therefore it is important to consider using specific algorithms and sensitivity settings with specific insomnia subpopulations.[77,78] Also, actigraphy is generally less accurate at detecting sleep compared to PSG for several sleep parameters, with the accuracy diminishing with increasing amounts of nighttime wakefulness.[79] Finally, actigraphy does not provide a measure of sleep architecture, which could be an important consideration when assessing insomnia and sleep disturbances in a research context.

Consumer Sleep Monitoring Devices

With the rapid growth in mobile technology, consumer devices for monitoring sleep and daytime activity levels are becoming increasingly popular and could potentially play a role in the assessment of insomnia. These devices use one or more sensors to estimate sleep and include two broad categories: wearable and nonwearable devices. Wearable devices are worn on the wrist or finger and typically use an accelerometer to measure sleep (e.g., Fitbit). Other wearable devices, such as the Oura, are worn as a ring and use multiple sensors to measure sleep (pulse rate, heart rate variability, pulse amplitude, motion, body temperature). Nonwearable devices measure sleep using a mattress pad (Beddit) or using biomotion technology (S+).

Given the rapid uptake of these consumer devices, experts in the field recently developed guidelines and recommendations for the use of wearables in sleep and circadian research.[80] Overall, the available evidence revealed that consumer wearable and nonwearable devices have limitations in reliability and validity that limit their clinical utility. Furthermore, many validation studies suffered from major limitations, including small sample sizes, lack of comparison with gold-standard measures of sleep, and heterogeneity with respect to the sample characteristics (e.g., nonclinical). As a result, the group concluded that consumer devices should not be considered as a replacement for PSG or actigraphy using a clinical grade (FDA approved) device and recommended further independent studies to examine the reliability and validity of these devices. At present, clinical evaluation of self-reported nocturnal and daytime symptoms remains the gold standard for assessment and treatment evaluation in patients presenting with insomnia symptoms.

Despite these limitations, many sleep clinic patients use sleep monitoring devices at home. Thus clinicians should be prepared to discuss the benefits and limitations of this technology with patients. The low cost, accessibility, and convenience of these devices provide an opportunity to gather naturalistic data over long periods of time, which can inform treatment. Conversely, nightly sleep monitoring can fuel sleep anxiety, especially for insomnia patients.

CONSIDERATIONS FOR CONDUCTING THE CLINICAL ASSESSMENT OF INSOMNIA

Several factors should be considered when assessing insomnia, including clinic setting, clinician discipline, patient populations, reports from bed partners, and treatment side effects. The type of clinical setting may influence the length of the assessment and resources available for using sleep diaries or objective sleep measurement. If the assessment occurs in primary care, the assessment will be conducted in a short amount of time and should focus on making a clear diagnosis or the need for further sleep evaluation and PSG referral. Brief self-report measures, such as the ISI, can be particularly helpful to aid in clinical decision making or to track changes in response to treatment. Furthermore, assessment of any medications or substances used for sleep is particularly important because primary care settings are typically where patients first seek help for sleep disturbance, and the initial treatment is often using hypnotic medication.

If the assessment occurs in a sleep clinic, the focus should be on a comprehensive sleep evaluation for insomnia and careful differential diagnosis from other sleep disorders, medical, and psychiatric conditions. The sleep clinician's training background and discipline will play a role in the assessment process. Physicians who conduct physical examinations can further inform the need for a PSG as part of the assessment. Evidence of a crowded upper airway, large tonsils, or enlarged turbinates may suggest the presence of SRBD and the need for PSG. Assessments conducted by psychologists will typically emphasize a functional analysis of the sleep schedule or differential diagnoses between insomnia and psychiatric disorders. Ideally, an interdisciplinary care model that includes a sleep physician and a sleep psychologist can cover the entire biopsychosocial spectrum of causes and contributors to insomnia.

Patient populations are critical contextual factors in sleep assessment. Assessing children or those who might not be able to provide accurate self-reports (e.g., cognitive impairment) might rely more on objective measures than the clinical interview or questionnaires. Further, certain patient populations are at increased risk for insomnia (women, especially pregnant women), short sleep (e.g., Black or African American, pregnant women), and SRDB (e.g., Eastern Asian, Black or African American, older men, pregnant women, obese persons).[20,81]

Whenever available, gathering information from the bed partner is a source of valuable information in the evaluation of the person with insomnia. Bed partners provide collateral information about the nature of the sleep difficulty, including symptom frequency, severity, and duration, as well as the nature and degree of the daytime impairment, and may be helpful when evaluating treatment response. Of note, patient-partner discrepancies in sleep reports can be useful therapeutically, especially as bed partners can provide insight into important differential diagnoses, such as the presence of symptoms of SRDB, PLMD, or parasomnias.

FUTURE DIRECTIONS

As discussed throughout this chapter, insomnia is diagnosed through self-reported measures and clinical interviews. The inability to identify a reliable biomarker of insomnia has been a limitation in both research and clinical settings. Therefore new approaches to phenotyping insomnia using objective measures may lead to further understanding of the etiology of insomnia. In addition, emerging consumer technology for monitoring sleep-wake patterns can provide new opportunities in the assessment of insomnia.

Objective sleep measures had fallen out of favor in insomnia assessment, but the field is reconsidering their utility. Growing evidence suggests that about half of patients with insomnia disorder may have short sleep duration as measured by PSG or actigraphy.[82–85] In biomarker and outcome-based research, the insomnia with objective short sleep phenotype has been consistently associated with stress system activation, more medical comorbidities, distinct psychological profiles, and poorer long-term prognosis relative to those with normal objective sleep.[83,84] Retrospective studies examining treatment response have been equivocal, with some studies reporting that insomnia with objective short sleep is less responsive to cognitive-behavioral therapy than patients with normal objective sleep,[86,87] whereas other studies have shown no difference in treatment response between these phenotypes.[88–90] Research is needed using prospective trial designs to elucidate the diagnostic value of objective short sleep in insomnia and to inform treatment considerations for this phenotype.

Future research is also poised to use multimethod, data-driven approaches combining various sources of data (e.g., self-report, objective measures, biomarkers) to identify insomnia phenotypes.[83] For example, one study using clinical and PSG measures identified three insomnia subtypes: (1) high subjective wakefulness, (2) mild insomnia, and (3) insomnia-related distress.[91] Another study using a large dataset in a general population that included a number of variables, including life events, biomarkers, and treatment response found five insomnia subtypes: (1) highly distressed, (2) moderately distressed but reward sensitive, (3) moderately distressed and reward insensitive, (4) slightly distressed with high reactivity, and (5) slightly distressed with low reactivity.[92] By leveraging large datasets, these bottom-up approaches could provide a pathway toward personalized sleep medicine.

With the rapid growth and proliferation of research-grade and consumer wearable technology, future research should also clarify how these tools can be used and interpreted by clinicians to inform insomnia case conceptualizations and treatment planning. For example, wireless electroencephalogram devices that can be self-applied and worn for multiple nights is rapidly becoming a feasible clinical endeavor and may provide more nuanced data better characterizing insomnia profiles and subtypes to develop tailored treatment approaches and morbidity risk profiles.[93] Technology can also provide more opportunities to intervene, either by notifying clinicians of changes in a patient's sleep patterns or through automated algorithms that can provide feedback to patients about behavioral recommendations. As new technology emerges, collaborations between clinicians, sleep researchers, and industry partners will be particularly important to establish when and how these tools can be used to improve the clinical management of insomnia.

CLINICAL PEARL

Insomnia symptoms are the most commonly reported form of sleep-wake disturbance. A comprehensive clinical assessment using a clinical interview, self-report questionnaires, and sleep diaries should be used to determine a diagnosis of an insomnia disorder and to characterize the nocturnal sleep disturbance, daytime distress or impairment related to the sleep disturbance, the temporal pattern of these symptoms, and etiologic factors related to the disorder.

SUMMARY

The clinical assessment of insomnia includes a comprehensive clinical interview, sleep diaries, and self-report measures. These tools enable the clinician to characterize the nocturnal sleep disturbance, identify daytime distress or impairment related to the sleep disturbance, and determine the course or temporal pattern of these symptoms. In addition, etiologic factors that predispose, precipitate, or perpetuate insomnia should be assessed, including sleep-interfering cognitions and behaviors, circadian preferences, sleep-related arousal, and comorbid medical or psychiatric conditions. Polysomnography and actigraphy are not routinely used in the assessment of insomnia but can be useful in certain populations or to rule out other sleep disorders. The data gathered from these tools should inform case formulation and treatment planning. Ongoing assessment during treatment should be conducted to monitor progress and potential side effects. Consumer devices for monitoring sleep are not yet validated for clinical settings but could provide opportunities in the near future for enhancing the assessment of insomnia with an eye toward personalized sleep medicine.

SELECTED READINGS

Buysse DJ, Ancoli-Israel S, Edinger JD, Lichstein KL, Morin CM. Recommendations for a standard research assessment of insomnia. *Sleep.* 2006;29(9):1155–1173.

Carney CE, Buysse DJ, Ancoli-Israel S, et al. The consensus sleep diary: standardizing prospective sleep self-monitoring. *Sleep.* 2012;35(2):287–302.

Depner CM, Cheng PC, Devine JK, et al. Wearable technologies for developing sleep and circadian biomarkers: a summary of workshop discussions. *Sleep.* 2020;43(2):254. https://doi.org/10.1093/sleep/zsz254.

Galbiati A, Sforza M, Leitner C, et al. The reliability of objective total sleep time in predicting the effectiveness of cognitive-behavioral therapy for insomnia [published online ahead of print, 2021 Mar 25]. *Sleep Med.* 2021;82:43–46.

Schutte-Rodin S, Broch L, Buysse D, Dorsey C, Sateia M. Clinical guideline for the evaluation and management of chronic insomnia in adults. *J Clin Sleep Med.* 2008;4(5):487–504.

Smith MT, McCrae CS, Cheung J, et al. Use of actigraphy for the evaluation of sleep disorders and circadian rhythm sleep-wake disorders: an American Academy of Sleep Medicine clinical practice guideline. *J Clin Sleep Med.* 2018;14(7):1231–1237.

Vgontzas AN, Fernandez-Mendoza J, Liao D, Bixler EO. Insomnia with objective short sleep duration: the most biologically severe phenotype of the disorder. *Sleep Med Rev.* 2013;17(4):241–254.

A complete reference list can be found online at ExpertConsult.com.

Chapter 94

Insomnia with Short Sleep Duration and Multidimensional Sleep Health

Martica H. Hall; Julio Fernandez-Mendoza; Christopher E. Kline; Marissa A. Evans; Alexandros N. Vgontzas

Chapter Highlights

- Sleep is inherently a multidimensional biobehavioral process. Research seeking to understand why and how we sleep is best approached from a multidimensional perspective.
- Examples of multidimensional sleep approaches linked to health and functioning include the insomnia with objective short sleep duration (ISS) phenotype (clinical perspective) and multidimensional sleep health (MSH; public health perspective).
- The ISS phenotype perspective views insomnia as a heterogeneous disorder in terms of degree of objective sleep disturbance, etiology, relative contribution of behavioral versus biologic perpetuating factors, clinical features, natural history, and association with morbidity and mortality—specifically, adverse cardiometabolic and brain health outcomes.
- The MSH perspective views sleep in the general population as inexorably linked to biobehavioral processes, including daytime functioning. Emerging evidence suggests that each is linked to important indices of mental and physical health.
- Moreover, the ISS phenotype and MSH indices may be stronger predictors of adverse health outcomes compared to single indices, such as insomnia symptoms, sleep duration, or sleep quality alone.
- A multidimensional, multimethod approach to understanding sleep disorders (clinical) and sleep health (population) will help us better predict the adverse health outcomes associated with poor sleep, treat it in clinical settings, and prevent it in the general population.

INTRODUCTION

Sleep is, by its very nature, multidimensional. It can be described by the amount of sleep obtained, its continuity, depth, architecture, timing, regularity, and subjective quality, among others. For example, two people may report the same severity of insomnia complaints but differ in the objective amount of time it took them to fall asleep, the amount of time they were awake, or the amount of time they were asleep during their time in bed. Furthermore, two people may have the same duration of sleep but differ in the amount of time it took them to fall asleep or the amount of time they were awake during their time in bed. Similarly, individuals who obtain the same amount of sleep may spend different proportions of the night in slow wave or rapid eye movement sleep and thus display different sleep architecture profiles despite identical sleep durations. These multidimensional aspects of sleep can differ between individuals, within individuals, and across the night or nights.

Despite the wealth of variables that describe sleep, many of which may be measured across self-reported, behavioral, and/or physiologic modalities, research has tended to focus on individual variables (e.g., self-reported sleep duration) or classes of variables (e.g., sleep continuity, architecture, etc.). Yet, none of these approaches account for the multidimensional nature of sleep, nor does the assessment of multiple, individual sleep characteristics account for their potential interactions and overlapping nature. Only in recent years have sleep researchers started to use multidimensional, multimethod approaches to better understand the holistic nature and impact of sleep, a concept known as "sleep health."

This chapter highlights two conceptual approaches developed as a result of advances in sleep and circadian science: the ISS phenotype and MSH concept. The ISS phenotype uses a multidimensional clinical approach to understand the etiology, pathophysiology, clinical features, and natural course of insomnia and its downstream consequences to health and functioning by relying on both self-reported (i.e., insomnia symptoms) and objectively measured (i.e., sleep duration) domains. The concept of MSH uses a public health perspective to characterize and evaluate the importance of sleep and rhythms to health and functioning in the general population by primarily relying on self-reported (i.e., regularity, satisfaction, alertness, timing, efficiency, and duration) domains. The MSH perspective views sleep as inexorably linked to biobehavioral (circadian) rhythms, including daytime functioning, and thus complements the more clinically oriented and objectively characterized ISS phenotype. Each of these approaches has advanced our understanding of sleep and biologic rhythms, including how and why we sleep. Most important, these approaches have improved our understanding of the association of insomnia with adverse health outcomes.

INSOMNIA WITH OBJECTIVE SHORT SLEEP DURATION PHENOTYPE

Insomnia and short sleep duration are each highly prevalent sleep problems that are linked to a variety of adverse mental and physical health outcomes. These sleep problems reflect independent characteristics; whereas insomnia is characterized by sleep dissatisfaction resulting primarily from symptoms of difficulty initiating and/or maintaining sleep, short sleep duration is defined by a restricted and insufficient amount of sleep, which can be either voluntary (behavioral) or due to underlying (biologic) factors. As such, these sleep characteristics have historically been evaluated in isolation.

More recent work has considered the combined, synergistic influence of insomnia and short sleep duration on health. Many of these studies have found that their concurrent presence increases health risk, compared to the presence of insomnia alone or short sleep duration alone, or compared to the absence of either of these sleep problems.[1,2] This clustering of sleep problems, recently termed the *insomnia with objective short sleep duration* (ISS) phenotype, emphasizes the clinical importance of considering the quality *and* duration of sleep, as well as its perceived *and* objective aspects in regard to understanding the pathophysiology, clinical features, and adverse health risk associated with insomnia. In this section we will define the ISS phenotype, discuss how it has been operationalized in research, and summarize the emerging literature on its associations with physical health, mental health, and mortality, and its potential impact on treatment response.

Definition, Measurement, and Clinical Features of the Insomnia with Objective Short Sleep Duration Phenotype

Although not yet called the ISS phenotype, research into this cluster of sleep problems first appeared in the late 1990s. In these studies, well-characterized young adult insomnia samples with objectively verified poor sleep (e.g., polysomnographic [PSG] sleep efficiency < 85%) were found to exhibit greater autonomic dysfunction (e.g., catecholamines) and hyperactivity of the hypothalamic-pituitary-adrenal (HPA) axis (e.g., cortisol) relative to good sleepers or to relate positively to the degree of objective sleep disturbance.[3–5] As shown in Table 94.1, previous efforts had focused on the "subjective" versus "objective" nature of poor sleep but not on assaying for an objective sleep dimension that could predict the health impact of the disorder. Thus

Table 94.1 Studies on the Association of Insomnia Phenotypes Based on Objective Sleep Measures with Hyperarousal Biomarkers

Study (Design)	*N* (Men, Age [years])	Definitions (Self-Report + Objective)	Outcomes
			Alertness
Sugerman et al., 1985[17] (Cross-sectional)	24 (25%, 21–55)	Good sleep	Ref.
		Insomnia + PSG criteria (subjective)[a]	↓ MSLT
		Insomnia + PSG criteria (objective)[a]	← MSLT
Stepanski et al., 1988[18] (Cross-sectional)	115 (59%, 48.1 ± 12.6)	Good sleep	Ref.
		Poor sleep + PSG shorter sleep duration	↑ MSLT
Bonnet et al., 1995[19] (Cross-sectional)	20 (N/A, 18–50)	Good sleep	Ref.
		Insomnia + PSG < 85% sleep efficiency	↑ MSLT
Bonnet et al., 1997[20] (Cross-sectional)	18 (78%, 18–50)	Good sleep	Ref.
		Insomnia + PSG criteria (sleep misperception)[b]	← MSLT
Dorsey et al., 1997[21] (Cross-sectional)	31 (55%, 18–25)	Good sleep	Ref.
		Poor sleep + PSG criteria (subjective)[c]	← MSLT
		Poor sleep + PSG criteria (objective)[c]	↑ MSLT
Roehrs et al., 2011[22] (Cross-sectional)	150 (46%, 22–70)	Good sleep	Ref.
		Insomnia + PSG < 85% sleep efficiency	↑ MSLT
		Insomnia + PSG < 85% + MSLT < 10 min sleep latency	Ref.
			↓ PSG sleep duration
		Insomnia + PSG < 85% + MSLT > 16 min sleep latency	
Li et al., 2015[23] (Cross-sectional)	315 (33%, 40.0 ± 10.2)	Good sleep + MSLT < 14 min sleep onset	Ref.
		Insomnia + MSLT < 14 min sleep onset	← PSG sleep duration
		Insomnia + MSLT > 14 min sleep onset	↓ PSG sleep duration
		Insomnia + MSLT > 17 min sleep onset	↓ PSG sleep duration

Table 94.1 Studies on the Association of Insomnia Phenotypes Based on Objective Sleep Measures with Hyperarousal Biomarkers—cont'd

Study (Design)	*N* (Men, Age [years])	Definitions (Self-Report + Objective)	Outcomes
			Autonomic
Bonnet et al., 1995[19] (Cross-sectional)	20 (N/A, 18–50)	Good sleep Insomnia + PSG < 85% sleep efficiency	Ref. ↑ metabolic rate
Bonnet et al., 1997[20] (Cross-sectional)	18 (78%, 18–50)	Good sleep Insomnia + PSG criteria (sleep misperception)[b]	Ref. ↑ metabolic rate
Bonnet et al., 1998[5] (Cross-sectional)	24 (N/A, 18–50)	Good sleep Insomnia + PSG < 85% sleep efficiency	Ref. ↓ HRV
Spiegelhalder et al., 2011[24] (Cross-sectional)	104 (38%, 39.5 ± 11.8)	Good sleep Insomnia + PSG > 85% sleep efficiency Insomnia + PSG < 85% sleep efficiency	Ref. ← HRV ↓ HRV
Bonnet et al., 2014[25] (Cross-sectional)	19 (N/A, 18–50)	Insomnia + PSG criteria (sleep misperception)[b] Insomnia + PSG < 85% sleep efficiency	Ref. ↑ metabolic rate
Miller et al., 2016[26] (Cross-sectional)	96 (36%, 23–75)	Good sleep Insomnia+ PSG cluster I (INS)[d] Insomnia + PSG cluster II (ISS)[d]	Ref. ← HRV ↓ HRV
Castro-Diehl et al., 2016[27] (Cross-sectional)	527 (46%, 68.3 ± 8.8)	Good sleep + ACT > 7 h sleep duration Poor sleep + ACT > 7 h sleep duration Poor sleep + ACT < 7 h sleep duration	Ref. ← HRV ↓ HRV
Huang et al., 2018[28] (Cross-sectional)	1047 (39%, 43.0 median)	Poor sleep + PSG > 5.5 h sleep duration Poor sleep + PSG < 5.5 h sleep duration	Ref. ↑ HR
Jarrin et al., 2018[14] (Cross-sectional)	180 (37%, 49.9 ± 11.3)	Insomnia + PSG > 6 h sleep duration Insomnia + PSG < 6 h sleep duration	Ref. ↓ HRV
			Neuroendocrine
Vgontzas et al., 2001[4] (Cross-sectional)	24 (62%, 29.4 ± 6.8)	Good sleep Insomnia + PSG > 70% sleep efficiency Insomnia + PSG < 70% sleep efficiency	Ref. ← 24-h cortisol ↑ 24-h cortisol
Fernandez-Mendoza et al., 2014[29] (Cross-sectional)	327 (46%, 5–12)	Good sleep + PSG > 7.7 h sleep duration Poor sleep + PSG > 7.7 h sleep duration Poor sleep + PSG < 7.7 h sleep duration	Ref. ← a.m./p.m. cortisol ↑ a.m./p.m. cortisol
D'Aurea et al., 2015[30] (Cross-sectional)	30 (17%, 30–55)	Insomnia + PSG > 5 h sleep duration Insomnia + PSG < 5 h sleep duration	Ref. ↑ a.m. cortisol
Castro-Diehl et al., 2015[31] (Cross-sectional)	600 (47%, 69.1 ± 9.0)	Good sleep + ACT > 6 h sleep duration Insomnia + ACT > 6 h sleep duration Insomnia + ACT < 6 h sleep duration	Ref. ← CAR ↓ CAR
Castro-Diehl et al., 2016[27] (Cross-sectional)	527 (46%, 68.3 ± 8.8)	Good sleep + ACT > 7 h sleep duration Poor sleep + ACT > 7 h sleep duration Poor sleep + ACT < 7 h sleep duration	Ref. ← alpha amylase ↑ alpha amylase
Mohammadi et al., 2018[32] (Cross-sectional)	53 (60%, 14 ± 62)	Good sleep Insomnia + PSG criteria (paradoxical)[e] Insomnia + PSG criteria (psychophysiologic)[e]	Ref. ↑ a.m. cortisol[h] ← a.m. cortisol
			Immune
Vgontzas et al., 2002[33] (Cross-sectional)	22 (64%, 29.4 ± 6.6)	Good sleep Insomnia + PSG < 80% sleep efficiency	Ref. ↑ IL-6 shift
Fernandez-Mendoza et al., 2017[34] (Cross-sectional)	378 (54%, 12 ± 23)	Good sleep + PSG > 7 h sleep duration Poor sleep + PSG > 7 h sleep duration Poor sleep + PSG < 7 h sleep duration	Ref. ← CRP ↑ CRP
Tempaku et al., 2018[35] (Cross-sectional)	925 (45%, 48.1 ± 19.8)	Good sleep + PSG > 6 h sleep duration Poor sleep + PSG > 6 h sleep duration Poor sleep + PSG < 6 h sleep duration Insomnia + PSG > 6 h sleep duration Insomnia + PSG < 6 h sleep duration	Ref. ← telomere length ← telomere length ← telomere length ↓ leukocyte telomere length

Continued

Table 94.1 Studies on the Association of Insomnia Phenotypes Based on Objective Sleep Measures with Hyperarousal Biomarkers—cont'd

Study (Design)	*N* (Men, Age [years])	Definitions (Self-Report + Objective)	Outcomes
			Cortical
Krystal et al., 2002[36] (Cross-sectional)	50 (38%, 54.4 ± 10.5)	Good sleep	Ref.
		Insomnia + PSG criteria (subjective)[f]	↓ δ, ↑ σ/β power
		Insomnia + PSG criteria (objective)[f]	↑ σ power
Parrino et al., 2009[37] (Cross-sectional)	40 (20%, 45.0 ± 8.0)	Good sleep	Ref.
		Insomnia + PSG criteria (paradoxical)[g]	↑ CAP/A2 rate
Turcotte et al., 2011[38] (Cross-sectional)	78 (38%, 25–55)	Good sleep	Ref.
		Insomnia + PSG criteria (paradoxical)[e]	↑ N1/P2/attention
		Insomnia + PSG criteria (psychophysiologic)[e]	↓ N1/P2/inhibition
St-Jean et al., 2012[39] (Cross-sectional)	67 (40%, 25–55)	Good sleep	Ref.
		Insomnia + PSG criteria (paradoxical)[e]	↓ L/↑ R frontal activation
		Insomnia + PSG criteria (psychophysiologic)[e]	↑ R parietal activation
Spiegelhalder et al., 2012[40] (Cross-sectional)	54 (37%, 47.1 ± 6.0)	Good sleep	Ref.
		Insomnia + PSG criteria (subjective)[f]	← δ/σ/β power
		Insomnia + PSG criteria (objective)[f]	
Bastien et al., 2013[41] (Cross-sectional)	88 (37%, 25–55)	Good sleep	Ref.
		Insomnia + PSG criteria (paradoxical)[e]	↑ N1/↑ P2 amplitude
		Insomnia + PSG criteria (psychophysiologic)[e]	↑ N1 amplitude
St-Jean et al., 2013[42] (Cross-sectional)	67 (40%, 25–55)	Good sleep	Ref.
		Insomnia + PSG criteria (paradoxical)[e]	↓ δ power
		Insomnia + PSG criteria (psychophysiologic)[e]	
Chouvarda et al., 2013[43] (Cross-sectional)	30 (33%, 37.9 ± N/A)	Good sleep	Ref.
		Insomnia + PSG criteria (paradoxical)[g]	↑ A3-B3/A1-B1 rate
		Insomnia + PSG criteria (psychophysiologic)[g]	↑ A3-B3 rate
Pérusse et al., 2015[44] s(Cross-sectional)	113 (42%, 25–55)	Good sleep	Ref.
		Insomnia + PSG criteria (paradoxical)[e]	↑ wake intrusion REM
		Insomnia + PSG criteria (psychophysiologic)[e]	
Normand et al., 2016[45] (Cross-sectional)	70 (36%, 25–55)	Good sleep	Ref.
		Insomnia + PSG criteria (paradoxical)[e]	↓ spindles length
		Insomnia + PSG criteria (psychophysiologic)[e]	← spindles length
Fernandez-Mendoza et al., 2016[46] (Cross-sectional)	44 (36%, 16.6 ± 2.0)	Good sleep	Ref.
		Poor sleep + PSG > 85% sleep efficiency	↑ β power sleep latency
		Poor sleep + PSG < 85% sleep efficiency	↑ β power sleep latency
			↑ β power NREM

[a]Sugerman et al.[17] identified "subjective" and "objective" subgroups using PSG; "objective insomnia" was defined by the presence of an average latency to stage 2 >30 min or an average sleep efficiency <90%; otherwise, subjects were classified as "subjective insomnia."

[b]Bonnet et al.[20] identified a "sleep state misperception" subgroup using PSG criteria; sleep state misperception was defined by PSG sleep latency <30 min and sleep efficiency >90%, overestimation of sleep latency at 100%, and sleep latency estimates ≥20 min on both PSG nights.

[c]Dorsey et al.[21] identified subjective and objective subgroups using PSG; subjective insomnia was defined by a ratio of self-reported sleep latency/PSG latency to stage 2 >1.5; subjects were classified as having objective insomnia if their subjective latency/PSG latency ratio was <1.5.

[d]Miller et al.[15] identified insomnia subgroups using cluster analysis of PSG total sleep time, sleep onset latency and wake after sleep onset; insomnia clusters were named ISS and INS commensurate with their total sleep time below and above 6 h, respectively.

[e]Mohammadi et al.,[32] Turcotte et al.,[38] St-Jean et al.,[39,42] Bastien et al.,[41] Pérusse et al.,[44] and Normand et al.[45] identified "paradoxical" and/or "psychophysiologic" subgroups using PSG criteria; paradoxical insomnia was defined by PSG total sleep time >6.5 hours and sleep efficiency >85%, a discrepancy of >60 min between subjective and PSG total sleep time or of >15% between subjective and PSG sleep efficiency or sleepless nights on sleep diaries most of the time; otherwise, subjects were classified as having psychophysiologic insomnia.

[f]Krystal et al.[36] and Spiegelhalder et al.[40] identified subjective and objective subgroups using PSG; subjective insomnia was defined by (1) total sleep time ≥6.5 h, (2) age <60 yr: total sleep time 6.0–6.5 h and sleep efficiency >85%, or (3) age ≥60 yr: total sleep time 6.0–6.5 h and sleep efficiency >80%; otherwise, subjects were classified as having objective insomnia.

[g]Parrino et al.[37] and Chouvarda et al.[43] identified paradoxical and/or psychophysiologic insomnia subgroups using PSG criteria; paradoxical insomnia was defined by PSG total sleep time >6.5 h, PSG sleep latency <30 min, underestimation total sleep time (subjective versus PSG) ≥120 min and subjective estimation of sleep latency >20% of PSG sleep latency; otherwise, subjects were classified as having psychophysiologic insomnia.

[h]Mohammadi et al.[32] included adolescents (ages 14–62 yr) and 42% males with insomnia, whereas only adults (ages 26–59 yr) and 81% males with good sleep were included.

ACT, Actigraphy; ACTH, adrenocorticotropic hormone; a.m., morning; CAP, cyclic alternating pattern; CAR, cortisol awakening response; CRP, C-reactive protein; good sleep, absence of poor sleep or insomnia (i.e., good sleeping controls); HR, heart rate; HRV, heart rate variability; IL-6, interleukin-6; INS, insomnia with normal sleep duration; insomnia, diagnostic criteria or a complaint of chronic insomnia (i.e., insomnia disorder); ISS, insomnia with short sleep duration; MR, metabolic rate; MSLT, Multiple Sleep Latency Test; N/A, not available; NREM, non–rapid eye movement sleep; poor sleep, difficulty initiating sleep, difficulty maintaining sleep, early morning awakening, and/or nonrestorative sleep, typically moderate to severe or frequent (>3 times/wk), without chronicity or diagnostic criteria (i.e., insomnia symptoms); p.m., evening; PSG, polysomnography; Ref., reference group for comparison(s); REM, rapid eye movement sleep; SL, sleep latency; TST, total sleep time.

it was not until 2013, when Vgontzas and colleagues[1] published a review on the topic, that the ISS phenotype was first introduced, and it was proposed that objective short sleep duration could serve as an index of the biologic severity of insomnia.[1] They characterized the ISS phenotype as a disorder of physiologic hyperarousal (i.e., enhanced autonomic, neuroendocrine, immune, and central activation) with a chronic and unremitting course and linked to cardiovascular, metabolic, neurocognitive, and psychiatric morbidity.[1] In contrast, the insomnia with objective normal sleep duration (INS) phenotype was characterized as a disorder of cognitive-emotional and concomitant cortical arousal that is more likely to remit and linked to sleep misperception and psychiatric morbidity,[1] a phenotype that would include a larger number of cases previously termed *subjective, sleep state misperception,* or *paradoxical* insomnia.[6] This phenotyping was consistent with Bonnet and Arand's[7] early proposal that the alertness (i.e., Multiple Sleep Latency Test [MSLT]) and autonomic (e.g., heart rate variability [HRV]) findings in insomnia "supported the contention that objectively-measured sleep ability is a combination of sleep drive and level of central nervous system arousal, where arousal has both state and trait components." Although much of the initial research empirically supporting these phenotypes came from the research of Vgontzas and colleagues, using data from the Penn State Adult Cohort (PSAC), other research groups have since supported the clinical significance of this multidimensional, multimethod approach to phenotyping insomnia.

In the PSAC, investigators used a multidimensional approach by which self-reports defined the presence of normal sleep (i.e., absence of sleep complaints), poor sleep (i.e., moderate-to-severe insomnia symptoms), and a chronic (i.e., ≥1 year) insomnia complaint, whereas a single night of laboratory-based PSG with an 8-hour sleep opportunity defined the presence of objective short sleep duration (i.e., <75% sleep efficiency equivalent to <6 hours of sleep).[1] Insomnia has been operationalized in various ways in other studies, ranging from the self-report of poor sleep (i.e., insomnia symptoms), to meeting diagnostic criteria for insomnia disorder (i.e., symptoms along with daytime impairment and sufficient frequency and chronicity); because much of the research on this phenotype has come from large-scale epidemiologic studies, they are often limited in their ability to diagnose individuals with chronic insomnia disorder. The threshold of less than 6 hours has largely been adopted by other research groups in their operationalization of the ISS phenotype. As the gold standard objective measure of sleep, PSG has been recommended as the best way to classify short sleep duration in insomnia cases and, as a result, serve as an assay for the health risk associated with the disorder.[8] However, PSG is expensive, impractical, and often restricted to a single night of assessment. As a substitute for PSG, many studies instead have used actigraphy (ACT) or self-reports due to their scalability and ability to assess sleep over multiple nights in one's habitual environment.

Minimal research has directly addressed measurement issues regarding the ISS phenotype. Rosa and Bonnet,[9] and more recently Castro and colleagues,[10] have demonstrated that self-reported insomnia symptoms or criteria are poor predictors of PSG-defined sleep disturbance, which highlights the orthogonal nature of these two sleep dimensions and the heterogeneity within those with insomnia self-reports. Other evidence suggests that PSG provides a unique characterization of the ISS phenotype. A study in the PSAC showed that both ISS and INS phenotypes report a similar amount of habitual or in-laboratory subjective sleep duration, which does not accurately discriminate between the two phenotypes.[11] Moreover, it was found that "sleep misperception" (i.e., underestimation of PSG sleep duration >1 hour) was significantly more frequent in the INS phenotype than the ISS phenotype, which was relatively accurate or overestimated its sleep time,[11] a finding that replicated early studies on sleep misperception using initial criteria for "subjective" and "objective" insomnia.[6] In a study of adults who met diagnostic criteria for insomnia, Erwin and colleagues[12] observed poor concordance between short sleep (<6 hours) assessed with a single night of PSG and either sleep diary– or ACT-assessed habitual short sleep (<6 hours), suggesting that different thresholds may be needed depending on the measure used. In addition, research using both PSG and self-reports to characterize sleep duration among adults with insomnia has shown less robust health risk identified with self-reports of less than 6 hours, compared to PSG.[13–15] With regard to whether a single night is sufficient for characterization of short sleep, Gaines and colleagues[16] examined the short-term and long-term concordance of short sleep classification from a single night of laboratory-based PSG with an 8-hour sleep opportunity. Among adults who spent 3 consecutive nights in the sleep clinic or who were assessed on two occasions separated by approximately 2.6 years, there was greater than 70% concordance in sleep duration classification from the first night of PSG using the median sleep duration.[16] Together, this small body of literature suggests that self-reported and ACT data may not identify short sleep as precisely as PSG when using the same cut-offs, that a single night of PSG may be acceptable to characterize PSG-assessed short sleep duration in individuals with insomnia, and that validation studies are needed to replace PSG with more ecologic, but similarly reliable, objective sleep measures.

Overall, the ISS phenotype has been examined so far using a variety of approaches. Outside of the original studies using PSG, other studies have examined the combined influence of self-reported poor sleep and short sleep duration (assessed via subjective reports or ACT). Some of these studies have shown that self-reports of poor sleep[1] and of sleep duration[13] show less precision than studies with a stronger operationalization of insomnia and sleep duration assessed by PSG.[2] This latter issue is of particular importance when examining health risk.

Insomnia with Objective Short Sleep Phenotype and Physical Health

A proposed hallmark of the ISS phenotype is physiologic hyperarousal, reflecting 24-hour activation of both limbs of the stress system, which is incompatible with stable sleep ability.[1] As shown in Table 94.1, a large number of observational studies have found greater indices of hyperarousal (e.g., increased MSLT, high cortisol levels, blunted HRV, elevated high-frequency electroencephalographic [EEG] activity) in individuals with insomnia and objective sleep disturbance.[4,5,17–48] Although most of these studies used PSG, similar findings have been reported in three recent studies using ACT.[27,31,48] The cardiac autonomic dysfunction, HPA axis dysregulation, and low-grade inflammation observed in the ISS phenotype are presumed to be mechanisms linking this phenotype to increased cardiovascular and metabolic morbidity.[1]

As presented in Table 94.2, the simultaneous presence of insomnia symptoms and short sleep duration has been consistently associated with increased cardiovascular disease (CVD) risk. In many of these studies, risk is greatly attenuated or no

Table 94.2 Studies on the Association of Insomnia Phenotypes Based on Objective Sleep Measures with Adverse Health Outcomes

Study (Design)	*N* (Men, Age [years])	Definitions (Self-Report + Objective)	Outcomes
			Cardiovascular Health
Vgontzas et al., 2009[50] (Cross-sectional)	1741 (48%, 20–88)	Good sleep + PSG > 6 h sleep duration	Ref.
		Poor sleep + PSG > 6 h sleep duration	OR = 0.79 HTN
		Insomnia + PSG > 6 h sleep duration	OR = 1.31 HTN
		Poor sleep + PSG 5–6 h sleep duration	OR = 1.48 HTN
		Insomnia + PSG 5–6 h sleep duration	OR = 3.53[a] HTN
		Poor sleep + PSG < 5 h sleep duration	OR = 2.43[a] HTN
		Insomnia + PSG < 5 h sleep duration	OR = 5.12[a] HTN
Fernandez-Mendoza et al., 2012[58] (Longitudinal, 7.5-yr follow-up)	786 (49%, 20–84)	Good sleep + PSG > 6 h sleep duration	Ref.
		Poor sleep + PSG > 6 h sleep duration	OR = 0.50[a] HTN
		Insomnia + PSG > 6 h sleep duration	OR = 0.85 HTN
		Poor sleep + PSG < 6 h sleep duration	OR = 1.34 HTN
		Insomnia + PSG < 6 h sleep duration	OR = 3.75[a] HTN
Nakazaki et al., 2012[56] (Cross-sectional)	86 (29%, 73.6 ± 4.9)	Good sleep + ACT > 5 h sleep duration	Ref.
		Insomnia or ACT < 5 h sleep duration	↑ CIMT
		Insomnia + ACT < 5 h sleep duration	↑ CIMT, CPS
Li et al., 2015[23] (Cross-sectional)	315 (33%, 40.0 ± 10.2)	Good sleep + MSLT < 14 min sleep onset	Ref.
		Insomnia + MSLT < 14 min sleep onset	OR = 1.17 HTN
		Insomnia + MSLT > 14 min sleep onset	OR = 3.27[a] HTN
		Insomnia + MSLT > 17 min sleep onset	OR = 4.33[a] HTN
Bathgate et al., 2016[13] (Cross-sectional)	255 (35%, 46.2 ± 13.7)	Insomnia + PSG-1 > 6 h sleep duration	Ref.
		Insomnia + PSG-1 < 6 h sleep duration	OR = 3.33[a] HTN
		Insomnia + PSG > 6 h sleep duration	Ref.
		Insomnia + PSG < 6 h sleep duration	OR = 3.5 [a] HTN
Johann et al., 2017[59] (Cross-sectional)	328 (38%, 44.3 ± 12.2)	Insomnia + PSG-1 > 6 h sleep duration	Ref.
		Insomnia + PSG-1 < 6 h sleep duration	OR = 0.80 HTN
		Insomnia + PSG-2 > 6 h sleep duration	Ref.
		Insomnia + PSG-2 < 6 h sleep duration	OR = 1.82 HTN
Bertisch et al., 2018[15] (Longitudinal, 11.4 year follow-up)	4994 (47%, 64.0 ± 11.1)	Good sleep + PSG > 6 h sleep duration	Ref.
		Poor sleep or insomnia + PSG > 6 h sleep duration	HR = 0.99 CVD
		Poor sleep or insomnia + PSG < 6 h sleep duration	HR = 1.29[a] CVD
Fernandez-Mendoza et al., 2018[70] (Cross-sectional)	1741 (48%, 20–88)	Good sleep + PSG > 6 h sleep duration	Ref.
		Poor sleep or insomnia + PSG > 6 h sleep duration	OR = 1.33 CVD
		Poor sleep or insomnia + PSG < 6 h sleep duration	OR = 1.85[a] CVD
Huang et al., 2018[28] (Cross-sectional)	1047 (39%, 43 median)	Poor sleep + PSG > 5.5 h sleep duration	16.6% HTN
		Poor sleep + PSG < 5.5 h sleep duration	27.5%[a] HTN
Hein et al., 2019[57] (Cross-sectional)	1272 (53%, 44.9 ± 12.3)	Insomnia + PSG < 18 h sleep fragmentation	Ref.
		Insomnia + PSG > 18 h sleep fragmentation	OR = 1.59[a] HTN
		Insomnia + PSG > 85% sleep efficiency	Ref.
		Insomnia + PSG > 65%–85% sleep efficiency	OR = 0.92 HTN
		Insomnia + PSG < 65% sleep efficiency	OR = 1.57[a] HTN
		Insomnia + PSG > 7 h sleep duration	Ref.
		Insomnia + PSG 5–7 h sleep duration	OR = 0.89 HTN
		Insomnia + PSG < 5 h sleep duration	OR = 1.91[a] HTN
Hein et al., 2019[54] (Cross-sectional)	703 (45%, 45.0 ± 12.3)	Insomnia and MDD + PSG > 85% sleep efficiency	Ref.
		Insomnia and MDD + PSG > 70%–85% sleep efficiency	OR = 1.15 HTN
		Insomnia and MDD + PSG < 70% sleep efficiency	OR = 2.19[a] HTN
			Metabolic Health
Vgontzas et al., 2009[61] (Cross-sectional)	1,41 (48%, 20–88)	Good sleep + PSG > 6 h sleep duration	Ref.
		Poor sleep + PSG > 6 h sleep duration	OR = 1.52 T2D
		Insomnia + PSG > 6 h sleep duration	OR = 1.10 T2D
		Poor sleep + PSG 5–6 h sleep duration	OR = 1.55 T2D
		Insomnia + PSG 5–6 h sleep duration	OR = 2.07 T2D
		Poor sleep + PSG < 5 h sleep duration	OR = 1.06 T2D
		Insomnia + PSG < 5 h sleep duration	OR = 2.95[a] T2D

Table 94.2 Studies on the Association of Insomnia Phenotypes Based on Objective Sleep Measures with Adverse Health Outcomes—cont'd

Study (Design)	*N* (Men, Age [years])	Definitions (Self-Report + Objective)	Outcomes
Vasisht et al, 2013[66] (Cross-sectional)	28 (39%, 48.0 ± 9.0)	Insomnia + PSG > 6 h sleep duration Insomnia + PSG < 6 h sleep duration	Ref. ↑ insulin sensitivity
D'Aurea et al., 2015[30] (Cross-sectional)	30 (17%, 30–55)	Insomnia + PSG > 5 h sleep duration Insomnia + PSG < 5 h sleep duration	Ref. ↑ fasting glucose
Johann et al., 2017[59] (Cross-sectional)	328 (38%, 44.3 ± 12.2)	Insomnia + PSG-1 > 6 h sleep duration Insomnia + PSG-1 < 6 h sleep duration Insomnia + PSG-2 > 6 h sleep duration Insomnia + PSG-2 < 6 h sleep duration	Ref. OR = 1.39 T2D Ref. OR = 2.30 T2D
Hein et al., 2018[62] (Cross-sectional)	1311 (53%, 45.1 ± 12.4)	Insomnia + PSG > 8 h sleep duration Insomnia + PSG 6.5–8 h sleep duration Insomnia + PSG < 6.5 h sleep duration	Ref. OR = 1.11 T2D OR = 1.81[a] T2D
Castro-Diehl et al., 2018[67] (Cross-sectional)	2007 (46%, 45–84)	Good sleep + ACT > 6 h sleep duration Poor sleep + ACT > 6 h sleep duration Poor sleep + ACT < 6 h sleep duration	Ref. ← adequate diet ↓ adequate diet
			Brain Health
Bonnet et al., 1995[19] (Cross-sectional)	20 (N/A, 18–50)	Good sleep Insomnia + PSG < 85% sleep efficiency	Ref. ↓ cognition
Bonnet et al., 1997[20] (Cross-sectional)	18 (78%, 18–50)	Good sleep Insomnia + PSG criteria (sleep misperception)[b]	Ref. ← cognition
Fernandez-Mendoza et al., 2010[76] (Cross-sectional)	678 (40%, 50.4 ± 11.5)	Good sleep + PSG > 6 h sleep duration Insomnia + PSG > 6 h sleep duration Insomnia + PSG < 6 h sleep duration	Ref. ← cognition ↓ cognition
Edinger et al., 2013[77] (Cross-sectional)	184 (48%, 20–79)	Good sleep Insomnia + MSLT < 8 min sleep onset Insomnia + MSLT > 8 min sleep onset	Ref. ← cognition ↓ cognition
Miller et al., 2016[26] (Cross-sectional)	96 (36%, 23–75)	Insomnia+ PSG cluster I (INS)[c] Insomnia + PSG cluster II (ISS)[c]	Ref. ↓ cognition
Biddle et al., 2017[78] (Cross-sectional)	74 (100%, 50–75)	Insomnia and MDD + ACT > 80% sleep efficiency Insomnia and MDD + ACT < 80% sleep efficiency	Ref. ↓ cognition
Miller et al., 2017[79] (Cross-sectional)	47 (32%, 23–56)	Good sleep Insomnia+ PSG cluster I (INS)[c] Insomnia + PSG cluster II (ISS)[c]	Ref. ← metabolites ↓ metabolites
Khassawneh et al., 2018[80] (Cross-sectional)	89 (29%, 35.1 ± 12.8)	Good sleep Insomnia + PSG > 6 h sleep duration Insomnia + PSG < 6 h sleep duration	Ref. ← cognition ↓ cognition
Fan et al., 2019[81] (Cross-sectional)	86 (39%, 46.4 ± 8.5)	Good sleep Insomnia + PSG > 6 h sleep duration Insomnia + PSG < 6 h sleep duration	Ref. ← cognition/BDNF ↓ cognition/BDNF
Fernandez-Mendoza et al., 2019[82] (Cross-sectional)	1741 (48%, 20–88)	Good sleep + PSG > 6 h sleep duration Poor sleep + PSG > 6 h sleep duration Insomnia + PSG > 6 h sleep duration Poor sleep + PSG < 6 h sleep duration Insomnia + PSG < 6 h sleep duration	Ref. OR = 0.46 CI OR = 0.66 CI OR = 2.26[a] CI OR = 2.65[a] CI
			Behavioral Health
Bonnet et al., 1995[19] (Cross-sectional)	20 (N/A, 18–50)	Good sleep Insomnia + PSG < 85% sleep efficiency	Ref. ↑ tense/depressive
Bonnet et al., 1997[20] (Cross-sectional)	18 (78%, 18–50)	Good sleep Insomnia + PSG criteria (sleep misperception)[b]	Ref. ↑ anxious/ruminative
Dorsey et al, 1997[21] (Cross-sectional)	31 (55%, 18–25)	Good sleep Poor sleep + PSG criteria (subjective)[d] Poor sleep + PSG criteria (objective)[d]	Ref. ↑ neuroticism ↑ introversion

Continued

Table 94.2 Studies on the Association of Insomnia Phenotypes Based on Objective Sleep Measures with Adverse Health Outcomes—cont'd

Study (Design)	N (Men, Age [years])	Definitions (Self-Report + Objective)	Outcomes
			Cardiovascular Health
Edinger et al., 2000[87] (Cross-sectional)	125 (50%, 40–79)	Good sleep + PSG criteria (subjective) Good sleep + PSG criteria (objective) Insomnia + PSG criteria (subjective)[e] Insomnia + PSG criteria (objective)[e]	↓ anxious, beliefs, ↑ mood Ref. ↑ anxious, beliefs, ↓ mood Ref.
Fernandez-Mendoza et al., 2011[88] (Cross-sectional)	866 (52%, 20–88)	Good sleep + PSG > 6 h sleep duration Insomnia + PSG > 6 h sleep duration Insomnia + PSG < 6 h sleep duration	Ref. ↑ anxious/ruminative ↓ coping skills ↑ depressive/somatic
Fernandez-Mendoza et al., 2015[89] (Longitudinal, 7.5 year follow-up)	1137 (52%, 20–88)	Good sleep + PSG > 6 h sleep duration Poor sleep + PSG > 6 h sleep duration Insomnia + PSG > 6 h sleep duration Poor sleep + PSG < 6 h sleep duration Insomnia + PSG < 6 h sleep duration	Ref. OR = 1.80,[a] 1.33 MDD OR = 1.80,[a] 1.00 MDD OR = 1.82,[a] 1.59 MDD OR = 2.81,[a] 2.20[a] MDD
Fernandez-Mendoza et al., 2016[90] (Cross-sectional)	397 (58%, 12–23)	Good sleep + PSG > 7 h sleep duration Poor sleep + PSG > 7 h sleep duration Poor sleep + PSG < 7 h sleep duration	Ref. ↑ externalizing ↑ internalizing
Calhoun et al., 2017[91] (Cross-sectional)	700 (46%, 5–12)	Good sleep + PSG > 7.7 h sleep duration Poor sleep + PSG > 7.7 h sleep duration Poor sleep + PSG < 7.7 h sleep duration	Ref. ↑ externalizing ↑ internalizing
			Mortality
Vgontzas et al., 2010[95] (Longitudinal, 12-yr follow-up)	1741 (48%, 20–88)	No insomnia + PSG > 6 h sleep duration Insomnia + PSG > 6 h sleep duration Insomnia + PSG < 6 h sleep duration No insomnia + PSG > 6 h sleep duration Insomnia + PSG > 6 h sleep duration Insomnia + PSG < 6 h sleep duration	Ref. OR = 1.10 women OR = 0.36 women Ref. OR = 0.74 men OR = 4.00[a] men
Bertisch et al., 2018[16] (Longitudinal, 11.4-yr follow-up)	4994 (47%, 64.0 ± 11.1)	Good sleep + PSG > 6 h sleep duration Poor sleep + PSG > 6 h sleep duration Poor sleep + PSG < 6 h sleep duration	Ref. HR = 0.99 HR = 1.07

[a] *P* value for point estimate < .05.
[b] Bonnet et al.[20] identified the "sleep state misperception" subgroup using PSG criteria; sleep state misperception was defined by the presence of sleep latency <30 min and sleep efficiency >90%, overestimation of sleep latency by at least 100% and sleep latency estimates of 20 min or more on both PSG nights.
[c] Miller et al.[26,79] identified insomnia subgroups using cluster analysis of PSG total sleep time, sleep onset latency and wake after sleep onset; insomnia clusters were named ISS and INS commensurate with their TST below and above 6 hours, respectively.
[d] Dorsey et al.[20] identified "subjective" and "objective" subgroups using PSG; subjective insomnia was defined by a ratio of self-reported sleep latency to stage 2 sleep latency >1.5; otherwise, subjects were classified as having objective insomnia if their subjective latency/objective latency ratio was <1.5.
[e] Edinger et al.[87] identified subjective and objective subgroups using PSG; subjective insomnia was defined by the presence of (1) TST ≥6.5 h, (2) age <60 yr: TST 6.0–6.5 h and sleep efficiency >85%, or (3) age ≥60 yr: TST 6.0–6.5 h and sleep efficiency >80%; otherwise, subjects were classified as having objective insomnia.
ACT, Actigraphy; BDNF, brain-derived neurotrophic factor; CI, cognitive impairment; CIMT, carotid intima-media thickness; CPS, carotid plaque score; CVD, prevalent or incident cardiovascular diseases in cross-sectional and longitudinal studies, respectively; good sleep, absence of poor sleep or insomnia (i.e., good sleeping controls); HR, hazard ratio; HTN, prevalent or incident hypertension in cross-sectional and longitudinal studies, respectively; insomnia, diagnostic criteria or a complaint of chronic insomnia (i.e., insomnia disorder); MDD, prevalent or incident major depressive disorder in cross-sectional and longitudinal studies, respectively; MSLT, Multiple Sleep Latency Test; OR, odds ratio; poor sleep, difficulty initiating sleep, difficulty maintaining sleep, early morning awakening, and/or nonrestorative sleep, typically moderate to severe or frequent (>3 times/wk), without chronicity or diagnostic criteria (i.e., insomnia symptoms); PSG, polysomnography; PSG-1, polysomnography on first night; PSG-2, polysomnography on second night; Ref., reference group for comparison(s); T2D, prevalent or incident type 2 diabetes in cross-sectional and longitudinal studies, respectively; TST, total sleep time.

longer present in those with insomnia or short sleep duration alone. One of the most consistent findings is an increased risk of hypertension (HTN) in the ISS phenotype,[49] supported by 11 cross-sectional studies.[13,23,28,50–57] In the only longitudinal cohort study published to date, Fernandez-Mendoza and colleagues[58] found that the ISS phenotype was associated with 3.75 times greater likelihood of incident HTN compared to good sleepers over a 7.5-year follow-up. Of note, the INS phenotype (odds ratio [OR], 0.85) and good sleepers with short sleep duration (OR, 0.88) were not associated with a greater likelihood of incident HTN.[58] Only one cross-sectional study using PSG-assessed sleep duration has found contrasting results. In that study, the ISS phenotype was not significantly or consistently (OR, 0.80; OR, 1.82, respectively) associated with a greater likelihood of prevalent HTN (43.5%) when compared to the INS phenotype (28.5%) in a clinical sample.[59]

As shown in Table 94.2, the ISS phenotype has also been linked to metabolic dysfunction in 7 studies, including impaired glucose metabolism[60] and both prevalent[55,61–64] and incident[65] type 2 diabetes (T2D) risk. In addition, 2 small laboratory-based studies found that adults with the ISS phenotype, compared to the INS phenotype, had altered metabolic function, as indicated by increased fasting blood glucose levels in 1 study[30] and increased insulin sensitivity (i.e., lower insulin secretion in the fasting state and in response to an oral glucose challenge) in the other study.[66] One study has also shown that people with the ISS phenyotype are more likely to have a metabolically unhealthy diet.[67] However, 4 of the 10 studies in the extant literature relied on self-reported sleep duration,[55,61,63,64] and 1 additional study that relied on PSG-assessed sleep duration failed to demonstrate a significant association between the ISS phenotype with prevalent T2D in a clinical sample (OR, 2.30).[59]

Another set of evidence linking the ISS phenotype to cardiometabolic morbidity comes from 10 studies that have shown a greater risk of prevalent or incident CVD,[15,56,68–75] including atherosclerosis, myocardial infarction, and coronary heart disease, for the combined effect of insomnia and short sleep duration. However, 8 of these studies relied on self-reported sleep duration, and 2 provided mixed findings.[74,75] The only longitudinal cohort study that has used PSG to identify the ISS phenotype in relation to incident CVD comes from Bertisch and colleagues,[15] who analyzed data from the Sleep Heart Health Study and found that the ISS phenotype, but not the INS phenotype, was associated with a 29% increased risk of incident CVD (Table 94.2).[15] Finally, recent work provides suggestive evidence that the ISS phenotype could increase the risk for age-related diseases through accelerated cellular aging. In a cross-sectional study of 925 adults, those with the ISS phenotype had approximately 4.2 times greater odds of having short leukocyte telomere length compared to good sleepers with normal sleep duration,[35] a finding consistent with the immune changes previously reported in the literature (Table 94.1).

Overall, the majority of existing research suggests that the ISS phenotype is associated with elevated cardiovascular and metabolic risk, particularly with HTN, T2D, and CVD, whereas the INS phenotype is not. However, many large, cohort studies have examined the combined influence of self-reported poor sleep (as a proxy for insomnia) and short sleep duration (assessed via self-report) on health outcomes. Although those studies have reported significant health risk associated with this self-reported sleep clustering, the magnitude of effect is often less robust and shows less precision than studies with a stronger operationalization of insomnia (e.g., chronic complaint or disorder) and objective assessment of sleep duration (e.g., PSG or ACT),* as has already been tested and shown in three studies.[13–15] Furthermore, the lack of objetive measures also does not allow an adequate control for factors (e.g., sleep apnea) that are commonly comorbid with insomnia phenotypes. Thus, although a causal link between the ISS phenotype and cardiovascular and metabolic morbidity is suggested, future prospective and mechanistic research using objective sleep measures should clarify this link.

Brain health has been another traditional area of investigation for insomnia research and its phenotyping. Although cognitive deficits remained elusive in early studies of insomnia, accumulating evidence indicates poorer executive functioning among individuals with insomnia and objective sleep disturbance.[19,20,26,76–82] Specifically, cognitive deficits in processing speed, sustained attention, set-switching attention, or working memory and increased likelihood of prevalent cognitive impairment have been reported for adults with the ISS phenotype, but not for those with the INS phenotype (Table 94.2),[19,20,26,76–82] with one additional study relying on self-reported sleep duration.[83] Furthermore, recent studies that did not replicate previous findings of decreased gamma-aminobutyric acid (GABA) levels or impaired default mode network (DMN) connectivity in individuals with insomnia found that shorter PSG-measured sleep duration was associated with lower GABA levels in the anterior cingulate cortex[84] and that lower PSG-measured sleep efficiency was associated with greater waking connectivity between the retrosplenial cortex/hippocampus and various nodes of the DMN.[85] Two novel studies have suggested that the ISS phenotype may be associated with altered brain-based biomarkers, such as decreased glutamate metabolites and brain-derived neurotrophic factor.[79,81] Together, these data are consistent with the proposed link between the ISS phenotype with altered neurocognitive function and potential increased risk of cognitive impairment.[1] However, few brain health studies have been performed, compared to the number of cardiometabolic health studies, and those completed have been cross-sectional. Thus there is a need for longitudinal studies using objective cognitive and sleep measures that follow individuals with insomia long enough for cognitive changes to be observed.

Insomnia with Objective Short Sleep Phenotype and Mental Health

Insomnia is an established predictor of adverse mental health, including depression and anxiety.[85,86] In their initial characterization, investigators surmised that both insomnia phenotypes (ISS and INS) would demonstrate increased risk for psychiatric disorders.[1] The altered cortical dynamics observed in the ISS and INS phenotypes (Table 94.1)[36–46] were presumed to be one of the shared mechanisms linking both phenotypes to increased psychiatric risk.[1] However, they also hypothesized that the ISS phenotype would predispose to psychopathology through chronic physiologic hyperarousal (e.g., HPA axis hyperactivity), whereas the INS phenotype would be linked to psychopathology through cognitive-emotional factors (e.g., coping resources).[1] Accumulating research[19–21,87–92] now suggests that the ISS phenotype is associated with significantly greater risk of prevalent[55] and incident psychopathology[93,94] compared to the presence of insomnia or short sleep duration alone. The INS phenotype has been shown to present with elevated anxiety, rumination, and maladaptive beliefs and coping resources in adu lts[20,21,87,88] and externalizing behaviors in children and adolescents (Table 94.2).[90,91] However, some recent studies that relied on self-reported short sleep duration reported even higher rates or levels of mental health disorders, such as anxiety or depression.[55,92] Given the known discrepancy between self-reported and objective sleep duration (i.e., sleep misperception) within the ISS and INS phenotypes, there is still a need for longitudinal studies, including objective sleep measures that can help us better understand the degree of association and underlying mechanisms of the impact of ISS and INS phenotypes on mental health.

*References 13, 14, 23, 28, 30, 50, 54, 56–58, 61, 62, 66, 70.

Insomnia with Objective Short Sleep Phenotype and Mortality

In contrast to its impact on physical and mental health, evidence that the ISS phenotype increases mortality risk is mixed (Table 94.2).[16,95] In the PSAC, the ISS phenotype was associated with increased all-cause mortality risk when compared to good sleeping control subjects; however, this effect was only observed in men and was stronger when HTN or T2D was present.[95] In other words, men appeared to be more vulnerable to the impact of ISS, and the increased mortality risk was higher if they had already developed cardiometabolic morbidity. Other studies have also noted increased risk for all-cause[96] or CVD mortality[97] among those with the ISS phenotype. However, the ISS phenotype has not been linked to increased all-cause mortality risk in other cohort studies.[15,74] Overall, the uncertain relationship between the ISS phenotype and mortality risk seems to be similar to the equivocal findings for self-reported insomnia symptoms and mortality.[98]

Insomnia with Objective Short Sleep Phenotype and Treatment

As will be extensively reviewed in the chapters that follow, cognitive-behavioral therapy for insomnia (CBT-I) is the recommended first-line treatment for the disorder, with hypnotic medication suggested when CBT-I is unsuccessful.[99] Vgontzas and colleagues[1] initially proposed that optimal treatment for the ISS phenotype may differ from the INS phenotype. Specifically, treatments that target underlying physiologic hyperarousal (e.g., via medication) may be indicated for the ISS phenotype, whereas the INS phenotype might respond better to CBT-I alone.[1]

Prospective randomized clinical trials (RCTs) to examine the efficacy of targeted therapies for those with the ISS and INS phenotypes have not yet been conducted. However, researchers have examined the adherence and treatment response of adults with insomnia based upon PSG- or ACT-assessed sleep duration at baseline in existing RCTs. As shown in Table 94.3,[100–106] four studies have found that objective short sleep duration at baseline is associated with lower remission rates in patient-reported outcomes after various forms of CBT-I,[100,102,103,106] whereas three other studies have reported identical remission rates after CBT-I, regardless of objective sleep duration at baseline.[101,104,105] Of interest, the pooled remission rate across these seven CBT-I studies that used objective sleep measures is about 20% higher in the INS phenotype (53%, n = 214) than in the ISS phenotype (30%, n = 196). In addition, studies that relied on self-reported short sleep duration have provided mixed findings in terms of adherence (drop-out)[107–109] and treatment response to CBT-I.[110]

No research has been published on whether the ISS phenotype responds more favorably to medication than the INS phenotype. However, recent research has evaluated the impact of insomnia treatment on indices of physiologic hyperarousal. Minimal changes in common indices of physiologic hyperarousal (e.g., cortisol, HRV) have been observed after CBT-I,[111–113] whereas zolpidem use may lead to reduced evening salivary cortisol.[114] Preliminary research has compared trazodone against CBT-I in adults with the ISS phenotype,

Table 94.3 Studies on the Association of Insomnia Phenotypes Based on Objective Sleep Measures with Behavioral Treatment

Study (Design)	N (Men, Age [Years])	Definitions (Self-Report + Objective)	Outcomes: Response[a]	Outcomes: Remission[b]
Troxel et al., 2013[100] (Retrospective)	39 (33%, 72.5 ± 6.6)	Insomnia + PSG > 6 h sleep duration Insomnia + PSG < 6 h sleep duration	N/A N/A	81.3%[c] 18.8%
Lovato et al., 2016[101] (Retrospective)	91 (47%, 63.3 ± 6.4)	Insomnia + PSG > 6 h sleep duration Insomnia + PSG < 6 h sleep duration	N/A N/A	51.9% 55.6%
Bathgate et al., 2017[102] (Retrospective)	60 (48%, 56.2 ± 10.1)	Insomnia + ACT > 6 h sleep duration Insomnia + ACT < 6 h sleep duration	100.0%[c] 48.6.0%	88.0%[c] 2.9%
Miller et al., 2018[103] (Retrospective)	39 (37%, 41.4 ± 11.8)	Insomnia+ PSG cluster I (INS)[d] Insomnia + PSG cluster II (ISS)[d]	70.0%[c] 37.0%	30.0% 32.0%
Rochefort et al., 2019[104] (Retrospective)	159 (39%, 50.3 ± 10.1)	Insomnia + PSG > 6 h sleep duration Insomnia + PSG < 6 h sleep duration	60.0% 58.3%	46.0%[e] 25.0%
Crönlein et al., 2020[105] (Retrospective)	92 (22%, 50.8 ± 11.5)	Insomnia + PSG > 6 h sleep duration Insomnia + PSG < 6 h sleep duration	N/A N/A	54.5% 51.7%
Kalmbach et al., 2020[106] (Retrospective)	113 (0%, 56.4 ± 5.3)	Insomnia + PSG > 85% sleep efficiency Insomnia + PSG < 85% sleep efficiency	N/A N/A	61.8%[c] 37.8%

[a]Clinically significant improvement in insomnia symptoms by post-treatment (decline of at least 8 points in the Insomnia Severity Index in Lovato et al.[100] and Rochefort et al.[103] and decline of at least 6 points in Miller et al.[102]) or by 6-month follow-up (decline in sleep diary–measured total wake time of at least 25% or more in Bathgate et al.[101]).

[b]Absence of clinically significant insomnia symptoms at posttreatment (Insomnia Severity Index < 8 in Lovato et al.,[100] Miller et al.,[102] Rochefort et al.,[103] and Kalmbach et al.[106]; Pittsburgh Sleep Quality Index < 5 in Troxel et al.[99]; and Regensburg Insomnia Scale < 12 in Crönlein et al.[104]) or at 6-mo follow-up (Insomnia Symptoms Questionnaire < 39.5 in Bathgate et al.[101]).

[c]P value for point estimate < .05.

[d]Miller et al.[102] identified insomnia subgroups using cluster analysis of PSG total sleep time, sleep-onset latency and wake after sleep onset; insomnia clusters were named ISS and INS commensurate with their TST below and above 6 h, respectively.

[e]P value for point estimate < .09.

All studies were retrospective analyses of existing randomized clinical trials.

ACT, Actigraphy; insomnia, diagnostic criteria or a complaint of chronic insomnia (i.e., insomnia disorder); N/A, not available; PSG, polysomnography; TST, total sleep time.

suggesting that trazodone, the second most prescribed sleeping aid, with increasing trends over the last decade in the US, may improve markers of physiologic hyperarousal (e.g., cortisol, non–rapid eye movement beta-frequency EEG activity) and lengthen objective sleep duration to a greater extent than CBT-I in this insomnia phenotype.[115,116]

Overall, the evidence is mixed as none of the studies reviewed herein were prospective RCTs designed to test the differential adherence rate and therapeutic response to CBT-I or to medication across the ISS and INS phenotypes.

Future Directions

In the short time since the term was first defined, the ISS phenotype has proved useful for its ability to predict significant adverse health risk, particularly cardiovascular, metabolic, and neurocognitive outcomes. Much remains to be learned about this phenotype, however. First, we need to understand how to best identify this phenotype; in particular, more studies testing whether more practical (i.e., non-PSG) objective measures can reliably and accurately identify this phenotype are needed. Second, we need to better understand the underlying pathways through which the ISS phenotype confers greater risk of physical health, including the magnitude of risk. More longitudinal studies that use objectively assessed sleep duration and account for key confounders (e.g., sleep apnea) are greatly needed. These studies will also help understand the potential cardiometabolic resilience of the INS phenotype, in the face of increased psychiatric risk. Finally, research is needed to identify how to optimally treat these insomnia phenotypes in prospective RCTs; specifically, understanding whether improvement results from decreased physiologic arousal will be critical. Overall, the importance of the ISS phenotype has been demonstrated over the past decade; future refinements to its assessment, identification of health risk, and tailored treatment will further clarify the importance of this insomnia phenotyping for the assessment, diagnosis, and treatment of a highly prevalent disorder.

MULTIDIMENSIONAL SLEEP HEALTH

Multidimensional sleep health (MSH), which captures the 24-hour experience of sleep by considering nighttime sleep, behavioral rhythms, and daytime functioning, is an emerging concept in sleep and circadian science.[117] The focus of MSH is on sleep at the population level and the *presence* of healthy sleep. This movement away from the medical model of disease and toward a state of wellness was succinctly captured in the World Health Organization charter of 1948: "Health is a state of complete physical, mental and social well-being and not merely the absence of disease or infirmity."[118] However, neither sleep epidemiology nor clinical sleep medicine have used this framework in the past 50-plus years. Sleep health provides a positive frame of reference for sleep, can be evaluated in everyone in the population, and specific cut-offs for "optimal" sleep health may provide clear targets for improving sleep, rather than the mitigation of negative symptoms.[117] In this section of the chapter, we will discuss the definition and measurement of sleep health and the emerging literature on the associations between sleep health and physical health, mental health, and mortality.

Definition, Measurement, and Features of Multidimensional Sleep Health

Although the term *sleep health* has been used by others, this chapter will use the multidimensional perspective articulated in 2014 by Buysse[117]: "Sleep health is a multidimensional pattern of sleep-wakefulness, adapted to individual, social, and environmental demands, that promotes physical and mental well-being. Good sleep health is characterized by subjective satisfaction, appropriate timing, adequate duration, high efficiency, and sustained alertness during waking hours." After the publication of Buysse's definition, regularity was included as another component of sleep health and defined as the consistency of sleep timing. These six multidimensional components of sleep health—*r*eg*u*larity, *s*atisfaction, *a*lertness, *t*iming, *e*fficiency, and *d*uration—can be referred to by the mnemonic "RU SATED."

Several studies have used the RU SATED concept to evaluate associations among MSH and important indices of mental and physical health. However, one issue for consideration as this research progresses, and as highlighted by the later inclusion of regularity in the RU SATED concept, is whether the identified components are all necessary (i.e., Are all components needed?) and/or whether these dimensions are sufficient (i.e., Should other characteristics be included?). In the only validation study published to date, Becker[119] reported good convergent validity and reliability for the six RU SATED components. However, confirmatory factor analyses revealed that the MSH items loaded onto a single factor, minus sleep efficiency, suggesting this item may not be necessary.[119] A different study that included three epidemiologic cohorts of older adults tested the relative power of numerous dimensions of sleep health in relation to mortality.[120] Results showed that a composite sleep health measure was a stronger predictor of mortality than any individual sleep dimension, suggesting good sleep health may present developmental (age-related) differences when predicting life expectancy.

Another important measurement issue is how to best combine the individual components of sleep health into a single composite score. To date, most studies, including those summarized in this chapter, have dichotomized individual components, then summed them to create a composite score (see Table 94.4 for the definitions and cut points for sleep health studies).[119–133] Creating cut points for each component has predominantly been based on norms in the literature and statistical methods of observed data distributions.[129] One study obtained empirically derived cut points for six sleep health components by creating receiver operating characteristic (ROC) curves to assess specificity and sensitivity in one sample; these cut points were then used to generate a composite score in a second, related sample.[123] It is important to note that the ROC curves generated by Brindle and colleagues[123] were used to predict cardiometabolic morbidity; these ROC-defined cut points may not be optimal for studies focused on other populations and outcomes. Future work might additionally use alternative, more sophisticated statistical methods for creating composite scores.[134] It is also worth considering how to optimize the composite score for ease of use in clinical settings, similar to cardiovascular risk score calculators.[135] Overall, the goal of improving the measurement and validity of MSH indices will be critical to advancing our understanding of the role of sleep and rhythms in key indicators of health and functioning, including health span and life span measures.

Multidimensional Sleep Health and Physical Health

Eight studies have linked MSH with physical health, particularly cardiometabolic morbidity. Dalmases and colleagues[124]

Table 94.4 Study-Specific Definitions of "Good" Sleep Health Components

Citation	Regularity	Satisfaction	Alertness	Timing	Efficiency	Duration
Becker et al., 2018[119]	Wake up at about the same time daily (within 1 h)	Satisfied with sleep	Awake all day without dozing	Asleep (or trying to sleep) between 2 and 4 a.m.	<30 min of SOL and WASO	6–8 h
Bowman et al., 2020[121]	Standard deviation of sleep midpoint <60 min	Moderately, quite a bit, or extremely rested upon awakening	≤10 on ESS	Sleep midpoint 2–4 a.m.	>85% sleep efficiency	6–8 h
Brindle et al., 2018[122]	Standard deviation of sleep midpoint <29 min for men, <26 min for women	Median split at 66.66 (scale of 0–100)	≤10 on ESS	Sleep midpoint 2:27–3:38 a.m. for men, 2:41–3:54 a.m. for women	≥85% sleep efficiency	7–8 h
Brindle et al., 2019[123]	Standard deviation of sleep midpoint <1 h 5 min	<2.8 (scale of 1–5)	<2.2 (scale of 1–5)	Sleep midpoint 2:24–3:30 a.m.	>83% sleep efficiency	5 h 20 min to 7 h 6 min
Dalmases et al., 2018[124]	Did not include	Satisfied with sleep	Awake all day without dozing	Asleep (or trying to sleep) between 2 and 4 a.m.	<30 min of SOL and WASO	6–8 h
Dalmases et al., 2019[125]	Did not include	Satisfied with sleep	Awake all day without dozing	Asleep (or trying to sleep) between 2 and 4 a.m.	<30 minutes of SOL and WASO	6–8 h
DeSantis et al., 2019[126]	Standard deviation of sleep duration <1 h	>3 (scale of 1–5)	Did not include	Sleep midpoint earlier than 4 a.m.	≥85% sleep efficiency	6–8 h
Dong et al., 2019[127]	Standard deviation of sleep midpoint <1 h	"Very good" or "fairly good" rating of sleep quality per the PSQI	≤7.5 on a 10-item sleepiness scale	Sleep midpoint 2–4 a.m.	≥85%	9–11 h for 10- to 13-year-olds, 8–10 h for 14-to 18-year-olds
Ensrud et al., 2020[128]	Did not include	Sleep duration is greater than or equal to individual's perceived sleep need	≤10 on ESS	2nd–7th octiles of sleep midpoint in the sample	<30 min SOL	7–9 h
Furihata et al., 2017[129]	Did not include	Never, rarely, or sometimes do not get enough sleep	Never, rarely, or sometimes feel excessively sleepy	Sleep midpoint 2–4 a.m.	<30 min SOL	7–9 h
Furihata et al., 2020[130]	Did not include	Very sufficient or sufficient sleep obtainment	Never, seldom, or sometimes feel excessively sleepy	2nd–4th quintiles of sleep midpoint in the sample	Never, seldom, or sometimes DIS, DMS, EMA	≥6 h
Kubala et al., 2020[131]	Wake up at about the same time daily (within 1 h)	Satisfied with sleep	Awake all day without dozing	Asleep (or trying to sleep) between 2 and 4 a.m.	<30 min of SOL and WASO	6–8 h
Wallace et al., 2018[132]	Standard deviation of wake time <45 min, and a measure of rhythmicity—PsF, ≤785.60	"Very good" or "fairly good" rating of sleep quality per the PSQI	≤10 on the ESS	Sleep midpoint 2–4 a.m.	<88 min WASO	5.3–7.5 h
Wallace et al., 2019[120]	Did not include	Sleep quality from the PSQI	ESS and napping	Bedtime, wake-up time	Sleep efficiency and SOL	Total sleep time, time in bed
Wallace et al., 2019[133]	Did not include	Sleep quality from the PSQI	≤10 on the ESS	Sleep midpoint 2–4 a.m.	≥85% sleep efficiency	6–8 h

DIS, Difficulty initiating sleep; DMS, difficulty maintaining sleep; EMA, early-morning awakenings; ESS, Epworth Sleepiness Scale; PsF, actigraphy pseudo-F statistic; PSQI, Pittsburgh Sleep Quality Index; SOL, sleep-onset latency; WASO, wake after sleep onset.

reported that self-reported MSH was a better predictor of self-reported health status than self-reported sleep duration alone and that better self-reported MSH was more strongly associated with better self-reported physical health than were established risk factors, including diet, physical activity, alcohol consumption, and smoking.[125] Only two studies have linked better ACT-assessed MSH with established risk factors for morbidity and mortality, including lower self-reported health limitations[126] and odds of cardiometabolic morbidity, defined as self-report of physician diagnosis or current medication use for HTN, T2D, stroke, or CVD, or hemoglobin A1c values consistent with T2D.[123] In contrast to the studies linking MSH to morbidity and mortality, three studies reported that MSH was not significantly associated with objectively assessed body mass index, including obesity.[121,126,127] Using data from the Study of Osteoporotic Fractures and medical claims data, better MSH was associated with lower total health care costs in the following 3 years, but this association was not significant after adjustment for functional limitations, chronic medical conditions, and depressive symptoms, suggesting that these factors may be important confounders or mediators of the sleep health-medical cost link.[128] Of interest, these studies showed that the link between sleep health and physical health was more robust and consistent for the multidimensional index of sleep health than for each individual sleep dimension alone (Table 94.4). Overall, six of the studies linking MSH with physical health outcomes examined cross-sectional associations (Table 94.5),[121,122,124–127,131] and only two studies have examined longitudinal associations (Table 94.6).[121,128] There is a clear need for longitudinal and experimental studies to evaluate temporal and causal associations between MSH and objectively measured physical health. Also important will be research that evaluates pathways linking MSH to physical health and identification of important effect modifiers, such as age, sex, sociodemographic characteristics, and preexisting conditions.

Multidimensional Sleep Health and Mental Health

MSH has been associated with mental health in three studies of adolescent, midlife, and older adult samples. One study reported that adolescents with better diary-assessed sleep health scores had lower depressive symptoms, lower anxiety symptoms, lower cognitive problems, fewer social problems with friends and family, and fewer somatic symptoms.[127] DeSantis and colleagues[126] reported that midlife adults with five or six indices of good sleep health assessed by ACT had lower levels of psychological distress, including symptoms of anxiety and depression. Among older adult women, there was a dose-response relationship between number of good self-reported sleep health indices and lower odds of prevalent and incident depression at 6-year follow-up.[129]

Table 94.5 Multidimensional Sleep Health: Cross-Sectional Studies

Citation	Sample	MSH Method	Description	Key Finding
Furihata et al., 2017[129]	*N* = 6485 older women from SOF cohort	Five components, self-report	MSH associations with depression symptoms	MSH was associated with depression symptoms in a graded fashion
Dalmases et al, 2018[124]	*N* = 4385 adults from CHS survey	SATED questionnaire and self-report sleep duration	MSH associations with number of chronic disorders	SATED had a higher AUC than sleep duration in ROC analysis
Dalmases et al., 2019[125]	*N* = 4385 adults from CHS survey	SATED questionnaire	SATED vs. other behavioral health risk factors in relation to overall health	MSH was a stronger risk factor than physical activity, diet, tobacco, and alcohol
Brindle et al., 2019[122]	*N* = 432 and 271 from MIDUS cohort	Sleep diary, actigraphy	MSH associations with cardiometabolic outcomes	MSH was associated with lower cardiometabolic morbidity
DeSantis et al., 2019[126]	*N* = 738 low-income Black adults	Actigraphy	MSH associations with psychological distress, BMI, physical function	MSH was associated with lower psychological distress and better physical function scores
Dong et al., 2019[126]	*N* = 176 adolescents at risk for poor health	Sleep diary	MSH vs. composite risk factors in relation to five health domains	MSH was related to emotional, cognitive, and social health risks
Kubala et al., 2020[131]	*N* = 114 mid- and late-life adults	RU SATED questionnaire	MSH associations with pedometer-assessed physical activity	MSH was associated with higher moderate- and vigorous-intensity physical activity
Furihata et al., 2020[130]	*N* = 2482 female hospital nurses	Five components, self-report	MSH associations with depression symptoms	MSH was associated with depression symptoms in a graded fashion
Bowman et al., 2020[121]	*N* = 221 midlife women from SWAN cohort	Actigraphy	MSH associations with body mass index and waist to hip ratio	MSH was not associated with body mass index or waist to hip ratio after adjusting for covariates

AUC, Area-under-the-curve; BMI, body mass index; CHS, Catalan Health Survey; MIDUS, Midlife in the United States; MSH, multidimensional sleep health; ROC, receiver operator characteristics; RU SATED, questionnaire assessing sleep *regularity*, *satisfaction*, daytime *alertness*, *timing*, *efficiency*, and *duration*; SATED, questionnaire assessing sleep *satisfaction*, daytime *alertness*, *timing*, *efficiency*, and *duration*; SOF, Study of Osteoporotic Fractures; SWAN, Study of Women's Health Across the Nation.

Table 94.6 Multidimensional Sleep Health: Longitudinal Studies

Citation	Sample	MSH Method	Description	Key Finding
Furihata et al., 2017[129]	N = 3806 older women from SOF cohort	Five components, self-report	Prospective associations between MSH and depression symptoms	MSH was prospectively associated with depression symptoms in a graded fashion
Wallace et al., 2018[132]	N = 2897 older men from MrOS cohort	Seven components, self-report and actigraphy	MSH as a predictor of mortality risk	MSH was related to mortality risk in a graded fashion
Wallace et al., 2019[120]	N = 8668 older adults from SOF, MrOS, SHHS cohorts	Nine components, self-report	Variable importance of 47 health-related measures and domains (including MSH) for predicting mortality	MSH was a significant predictor of all-cause and cardiovascular mortality and was stronger than the self-reported health and heart failure
Wallace et al., 2019[133]	N = 1722 older adults (sex- and age-equated) from SOF and MrOS cohorts	Five components, self-report	Associations among three MSH phenotypes and all-cause mortality	Heightened sleep propensity phenotype conferred the greatest risk for all-cause mortality compared to average sleep and insomnia with short sleep phenotypes
Ensrud et al., 2020[128]	N = 1459 older women from SOF cohort	Five components, self-report	Prospective associations between MSH and health care costs and utilization	MSH was prospectively associated with total health care costs in a graded fashion
Bowman et al., 2020[121]	N = 221 midlife women from SWAN cohort	Actigraphy	Prospective associations between MSH and body mass index and waist to hip ratio	MSH was not prospectively associated with body mass index or waist to hip ratio after adjusting for adiposity values at the time of the sleep study

MrOS, Outcomes of Sleep Disorders in Older Men; MSH, multidimensional sleep health; SHHS, Sleep, Heart, Health Study; SOF, Study of Osteoporotic Fractures; SWAN, Study of Women's Health Across the Nation.

Adverse life circumstances known to increase psychiatric morbidity have also been linked to poor MSH in two studies. In one study, retrospectively reported childhood trauma was associated with poorer self-reported and ACT-assessed MSH in midlife adults.[122] Another study showed that adverse housing and neighborhood conditions predicted disparities in ACT-assessed sleep duration, sleep efficiency, wake after sleep onset, and self-reported sleep quality.[136] These data suggest that developmental and environmental factors may influence sleep health, which, in turn, may adversely affect mental health.

Similar to the physical health literature, these studies focused on mental health have also suggested that a composite measure of MSH is more strongly associated with adverse outcomes than are each of its individual sleep indices alone. However, most of the existing studies are cross-sectional (Table 94.5),[126,127,129,130] and more longitudinal studies are needed (Table 94.6).[129] As will be reviewed in the following chapters, efforts have been made on understanding how improving insomnia can lead to improved mental health, such as in major depression or anxiety disorders. There is, nevertheless, a need for pragmatic, population-based trials that evaluate strategies to improve MSH as a strategy for preventing psychiatric morbidity and improving the clinical course of mental health disorders.

Multidimensional Sleep Health and Mortality

Emerging evidence suggests that MSH may be a significant predictor of mortality. MSH, assessed in older adults by the six RU SATED measures and an ACT-derived index of daily rhythmicity, was a stronger predictor of time to all-cause mortality than established risk factors, including T2D, HTN, history of stroke, race, or smoking status.[132] Moreover, MSH and mortality risk were associated in a graded fashion.[132] A larger follow-up study of harmonized data from the Sleep Heart Health Study, Study of Osteoporotic Fractures, and Outcomes of Sleep Disorders in Older Men Study cohorts created a self-reported MSH measure consisting of indices of sleep timing, duration, efficiency, daytime napping and sleepiness, subjective sleep quality, symptoms of sleep apnea and insomnia, and use of medications that affect sleep.[120] Variable importance metrics evaluated MSH and established risk factors in relation to all-cause and cardiovascular mortality. MSH was a significant predictor of both all-cause and cardiovascular mortality.[120] Although less predictive than multidimensional indices of sociodemographic, physical health, and medication use, MSH was a stronger predictor of both outcomes than were a number of established risk factors for mortality such as health behaviors, including alcohol and nicotine use and physical activity.[120] However, these studies included individuals with symptoms of other sleep disorders beyond insomnia (e.g., sleep apnea) and medications (e.g., hypnotics) known to be associated with morbidity and mortality in the definition of MSH.

Overall, the extant literature is mostly based on studies of older adults who were, for the most part, White, which limits their generalizability to the general population. There is a need to examine how health disparities may impact the association between MSH and mortality. Moreover, the mechanisms underlying this association have not been evaluated. As with insomnia and its phenotypes, the link of MSH and mortality requires better control for existing disorders (e.g., sleep apnea) and examination of potential sex/gender differences before firm conclusions can be reached.

Future Directions

In summary, the emerging literature is compelling in support of the hypothesis that MSH is associated with physical and mental health and, potentially, mortality. Out of the 12 current studies, few have reported contradictory findings, and the majority of studies suggest that MSH is more strongly associated with adverse health outcomes than its individual sleep dimensions. Although much of the initial evidence on MSH is coming from the research of Buysse and colleagues, using data primarily from two US cohorts, more research is needed in large sleep cohorts from other investigators using a multidimensional, multimethod approach. Many questions remain to be answered, including further psychometric evaluation and development of improved methods, definitions, and standardization. For example, it remains unclear whether the six RU SATED items are the most predictive of physical and mental health or whether additional or alternative sleep dimensions should be considered. It also needs to be examined whether each dimension is equally weighted or whether some are more important than others. In addition, it needs to be tested whether the same dimensions and the same weightings are equally predictive for any and all populations and health outcomes or whether specific dimensions and weights are most relevant to, for example, youth or older adults or when examining morbidity versus mortality. Furthermore, it needs to be tested whether exclusion of individuals with symptoms or diagnoses of sleep disorders known to impact morbidity and mortality modifies the magnitude of risk associated with MSH. Certainly, experimental studies that evaluate mechanisms are critical to evaluating the extent to which MSH is causally related to health and functioning, as they may overlap, or not, with those identified for insomnia phenotypes. Important too is the identification of who and under what circumstances MSH affects mental and physical health and mortality. Finally, development of a scalable measure of MSH will be critical for translating this construct into a tool that can be used in clinical practice. For example, there is a need to optimize a composite MSH score, similar to cardiovascular risk score calculators, that can be readily available for clinical settings, particularly primary care. Such an MSH score needs to be tested in clinical samples to better understand which of its dimensions, or none, require self-reports or objective measures to predict morbidity and mortality in individuals with chronic sleep disorders such as insomnia.

CLINICAL PEARLS

- On the basis of seminal findings in the 1990s, researchers first proposed that objective sleep measures could serve as an index of the biologic severity of insomnia and its phenotypes.
- Studies conducted in the past decade continue to support that the ISS phenotype is associated with physiologic hyperarousal and increased risk of cardiovascular, metabolic, and neurocognitive morbidity, whereas the insomnia with objective normal sleep duration phenotype is not.
- Recent studies also indicate that both insomnia phenotypes are associated with psychiatric morbidity, albeit through potentially different psychobiologic mechanisms.
- Novel studies have included developmental approaches, at-home actigraphy, diagnostic accuracy measures, and retrospective examination of their response to cognitive-behavioral therapy.
- The multidimensional sleep health (MSH) perspective is an important step forward in understating the association of good sleep with health in the general population.
- Optimized MSH indices may help us develop sleep health risk scores similar to those used in cardiovascular disease.
- Simple MSH measures may be used in primary care settings and preventative sleep campaigns and may be of use to sleep clinicians alike.

SUMMARY

Despite the high comorbidity rates observed in individuals with poor sleep, the impact of insomnia on physical health has remained elusive. Sleep is a multidimensional biobehavioral process, and a wealth of variables can describe it and may be measured across self-reported, behavioral, and/or physiologic modalities. Still, most research has tended to focus on individual variables (e.g., self-reported sleep duration) or classes of variables (e.g., sleep architecture) to understand the association of poor sleep with adverse health outcomes. In recent years, sleep researchers have started using multidimensional, multimethod approaches to better understand the nature and impact of sleep health. The clinical perspective has focused on the ISS phenotype, although the public health perspective has begun to focus on MSH. The clinical perspective views insomnia as a heterogeneous disorder in terms of degree of objective sleep disturbance, etiology, role of behavioral versus biologic perpetuating factors, clinical features, natural history, and association with morbidity and mortality—specifically, adverse cardiometabolic and brain health outcomes. MSH phenotypes insomnia by relying on both self-reported (i.e., insomnia symptoms) and objectively measured (i.e., sleep duration) domains. The public health perspective views sleep as inexorably linked to biobehavioral rhythms and integrates their importance by relying on regularity, satisfaction, alertness, timing, efficiency, and duration domains primarily by self-report. Most important, the ISS phenotype and MSH indices may be stronger predictors of adverse health outcomes compared to single indices, such as insomnia symptoms, sleep duration, or sleep quality alone. Such a multidimensional, multimethod approach to understanding sleep disorders (clinical) and sleep health (population) will help us better predict the adverse health outcomes associated with poor sleep, treat it in clinical settings, and prevent it in the general population.

SELECTED READINGS

Insomnia with Objective Short Sleep Duration Readings

Bathgate CJ, Edinger JD, Wyatt JK, Krystal AD. Objective but not subjective short sleep duration associated with increased risk for hypertension in individuals with insomnia. *Sleep*. 2016;39(5):1037–1045.

Bertisch SM, Pollock BD, Mittleman MA, et al. Insomnia with objective short sleep duration and risk of incident cardiovascular disease and all-cause mortality: Sleep Heart Health Study. *Sleep*. 2018;41(6):zsy047.

Fernandez-Mendoza J. The insomnia with short sleep duration phenotype: an update on its importance for health and prevention. *Curr Opin Psychiatry*. 2017;30(1):56–63.

Jarrin DC, Ivers H, Lamy M, Chen IY, Harvey AG, Morin CM. Cardiovascular autonomic dysfunction in insomnia patients with objective short sleep duration. *J Sleep Res*. 2018;27(3):e12663.

Vgontzas AN, Fernandez-Mendoza J, Liao D, Bixler EO. Insomnia with objective short sleep duration: the most biologically severe phenotype of the disorder. *Sleep Med Rev.* 2013;17(4):241–254.

Multidimensional Sleep Health Readings

Brindle RC, Yu L, Buysse DJ, Hall MH. Empirical derivation of cutoff values for the sleep health metric and its relationship to cardiometabolic morbidity: results from the Midlife in the United States (MIDUS) study. *Sleep.* 2019;42(9):zsz116.

Buysse DJ. Sleep health: can we define it? Does it matter? *Sleep.* 2014;37(1):9–17.

DeSantis AS, Dubowitz T, Ghosh-Dastidar B, et al. A preliminary study of a composite sleep health score: associations with psychological distress, body mass index, and physical functioning in a low-income African American community. *Sleep Health.* 2019;5(5):514–520.

Furihata R, Hall MH, Stone KL, et al. An aggregate measure of sleep health is associated with prevalent and incident clinically significant depression symptoms among community-dwelling older women. *Sleep.* 2017;40(3).

Wallace ML, Buysse DJ, Redline S, et al. Multidimensional sleep and mortality in older adults: a machine-learning comparison with other risk factors. *J Gerontol A Biol Sci Med Sci.* 2019;74(12):1903–1909.

A complete reference list can be found online at ExpertConsult.com.

Chapter 95

Behavioral Treatment I: Therapeutic Approaches and Implementation

Colleen E. Carney; Meg Danforth

Chapter Highlights

- Behavioral techniques are highly effective, even as monotherapy techniques, but most commonly as a multicomponent treatment; they are the backbone of a frontline treatment approach to chronic insomnia.
- Key behavioral techniques in a multicomponent cognitive behavioral therapy (CBT) include stimulus control to manage conditioned arousal and sleep restriction therapy to increase the drive for sleep.
- There are several treatment delivery options available to fill gaps in access to providers for cognitive behavioral therapy for insomnia (CBT-I), including digital and bibliotherapy options, or offering group therapy to serve more clients at once.
- It is important to include a self-reported questionnaire to assess clients' perspectives on their symptoms, such as the Insomnia Severity Index, and most essentially, a daily monitoring tool (the Consensus Sleep Diary) to track treatment targets and improvements.

INTRODUCTION

Behavioral approaches are effective for treating chronic insomnia, even in those with comorbid medical or psychiatric conditions. In this chapter we will outline how behavioral approaches are based on research on the factors that cause, perpetuate, or exacerbate sleep difficulties. Based on these factors, behavioral principles guide treatment development, which are then tested and refined until they are shown to be efficacious. We will discuss successful behavioral strategies, such as stimulus control (SC), sleep restriction therapy (SRT), relaxation training, and counterarousal strategies, as well as combinations of these methods into a treatment called cognitive behavioral therapy for insomnia (CBT-I). We will also discuss implementation and delivery issues, the use of these tools in comorbid disorders and other special populations, and a discussion of common treatment tracking tools.

BEHAVIORAL APPROACHES TO INSOMNIA

The tradition of behavioral approaches to conditions such as insomnia involves the identification of precipitating and perpetuating factors for the condition[1] and the application of learning principles to develop and test interventions to address these putative etiologic factors. The assumption is that changing behaviors can positively affect sleep regulatory systems, indirectly challenge beliefs that may be unhelpful for sleep, and alleviate insomnia symptoms. This is not to say that a behavioral failure on the part of the patient is to blame; instead, the assumption is that behavior can exert a powerful influence on biology and provide relief, irrespective of the original cause. A classic example is SC, a behavioral treatment to address the inadvertent pairing of the bed with wakefulness characteristic of most protracted insomnias.[2] When the bed loses its stimulus value for sleep, clients can reestablish an association of the bed with sleep with a set of behavioral rules. Key in behavioral therapy is the idea that the intervention is tested and shown to be efficacious. Some treatments that are integral to multimodal CBT-I have demonstrated efficacy as a monotherapy as well. We describe each approach herein; treatment approaches and their components are summarized in Table 95.1.

Stimulus Control

The conceptual model behind SC[2] is that a stimulus can become associated with a variety of responses. Ideally, the bedroom environment is associated with sleep, and there develops high stimulus value of the bed for the sleeping response. In insomnia the bed loses its stimulus value for sleep because initial nights of sleep disturbance in the bed is paired with wakefulness and thus begins to elicit wakefulness. The goal in treatment is to restrict stimuli at the initiation of sleep to stimuli associated with sleep only and/or to avoid stimuli associated with wakefulness before sleep initiation. At the core of SC is the recognition that in the early stages of sleep disruption, there will be more time awake in bed than previously experienced. Over time, the bed is paired with the experience of wakefulness and can become a conditioned stimulus for the response of wakefulness. This is outside of the awareness of people with insomnia and may be the consequence of having acute sleep disturbance. Once the acute sleep disturbance resolves, the expectation is that normal sleep resumes; however, if conditioned wakefulness/conditioned arousal occurs,

Table 95.1 Behavioral Approaches

Psychological Treatments	Treatment Summary
Stimulus control	Follow five rules to reassociate the bed with sleep only: 1. Do not go to bed until you are sleepy (e.g., actively falling asleep). 2. If you are in a sleep-incompatible state while in bed, leave the bed/bedroom; do not return until you are sleepy. 3. Get out of bed at the same time every morning, irrespective of how you slept. 4. Reserve the bed for sleep only (do not engage in wakeful activities in bed). 5. No naps.
Sleep restriction therapy	Restrict time in bed to the average total sleep time of the last 2 weeks. After implementing the prescription for 2 weeks: 1. If the sleep problem has resolved, continue with the prescription. 2. If there is evidence of excessive sleepiness, extend the time in bed prescription by 15 to 30 minutes for the next 2 weeks, and continue extending at subsequent appointments until sleepiness has resolved. Any reemerging sleep problems are addressed by restricting time in bed back to the previously effective prescription
Relaxation therapy	Collection of relaxation practices that entail daily practice of one or more of the following: 1. Progressive muscle relaxation 2. Imagery/autogenic training 3. Deep/diaphragmatic breathing
Paradoxical intention	Instruction to go to bed at regular time and initiate effort to stay awake while in bed, all night long.
Cognitive therapy	Direct challenge of sleep believes using one or more of the following: 1. Thought records 2. Socratic questioning 3. Behavioral experiments
Counterarousal Strategies	Addressing active mind in the presleep period. Commonly used counterarousal strategies include 1. Buffer zone (wind-down time before bed) 2. Constructive worry or scheduled worry hour 3. Daily mindfulness practice
Sleep hygiene	Set of rules derived from basic sleep research to correct habits that could interfere with sleep: 1. Caffeine: cessation by early afternoon and limit use to no more than (dose and timing instructions tend to vary) 2. Nicotine reduction/elimination 3. Exercise regularly but not within a few hours of bedtime 4. Avoid middle-of-the-night eating 5. Reduce alcohol, marijuana, and other sleep-interfering substances 6. Optimize environment: limit light, noise, and extremes in temperature
Cognitive behavioral therapy for insomnia	Multicomponent, empirically based and empirically supported therapy to modify sleep-interfering behaviors. The most common elements are 1. Stimulus control 2. Sleep restriction 3. Cognitive therapy 4. Counterarousal strategies; some versions have relaxation therapy 5. Sleep hygiene
Mindfulness	Daily practice of directing one's attention to the present moment, nonjudgmentally

this becomes a perpetuating factor and will likely turn the acute problem into a chronic insomnia. The answer then is to address the conditioned arousal by reassociating the bed with sleep by being in bed only when asleep.

To accomplish the reassociation of the bed/bedroom with sleep, clients are instructed to wait for the experience of sleepiness to guide their decision to get into bed. Sleepiness is characterized by behaviors observed at sleep onset (e.g., head falling forward or back because of a loss of muscle tone, eyes rolling back into the head, lapses in attention, falling asleep, etc.). Waiting for sleepiness and associated behaviors, rather than using the clock to determine when to get into bed, increases the likelihood of falling asleep quickly (i.e., because they are already actively falling asleep). If after getting into bed, the client notices that they are no longer sleepy, they are in an arousing or sleep-incompatible state, or 15 minutes has elapsed (i.e., sleepiness is present when sleep onset occurs in less than 15 minutes), they leave the bed/bedroom and return only when sleepiness returns.[3] Most providers resist giving time guidance (i.e., 15 minutes) because it may encourage clock watching; however, case formulation can provide guidance on this issue. If a client is not getting out of bed for long periods of time while awake, the 10-minute/sleepiness guideline may help with adherence to this rule. In contrast, clients who watch the clock are told to turn away the clock from view and to focus on the internal sensation of sleepiness/readiness to sleep. This step is repeated as many times as is needed to reestablish the association of the bed with sleep (breaking the association of the bed with wakefulness). The third rule is to get out of bed at the same time every morning irrespective of the previous night's sleep. This helps to establish a firm time and a place for a sleep opportunity, thereby establishing stimulus value for the bed within a certain window associated exclusively with sleep. There is not a way to establish a set bedtime given that sleepiness must be present to go to bed, but rise times are easily set with an alarm clock. Prohibited are wakeful activities in bed because wakefulness in the bed weakens the association of the bed with sleep. Some couples choose to move sexual activity to a different room (i.e., because it is a wakeful activity), whereas other couples choose to make sex an exception and continue to have sex in their bed/bedroom. Daytime naps are disallowed, to further establish the bed and a particular window of sleep opportunity with sleep. Chapter 96 is dedicated to reviewing its efficacy, but briefly; multiple studies support the use of SC on its own, including studies enrolling those with sleep-onset insomnia,[4–6] older adults,[7,8] and those in group and individual therapy.[5–8] Although SC has support as a monotherapy,[7] it is most commonly combined with SRT in clinical practice.

Sleep Restriction Therapy

SRT[9] is derived from biologic drive studies demonstrating that responses are increased by removing or limiting access to it. For example, remove food and increased food-seeking behaviors occur. Remove the opportunity to sleep and there is a greater propensity to sleep once access is provided. Behaviors such as eating, drinking, and sleeping are homeostatically controlled, and SRT leverages this principle with impressive effects. Clients are asked to spend less time in bed—engage in less sleep effort and build sufficient drive for sleep. This results in greater consolidation of sleep and sleep depth.[10,11]

SRT is an unfortunately named treatment, as the goal is to restrict the time in bed to closely match the current average sleep duration, rather than reducing sleep duration. Many providers refer to this treatment as "time-in-bed restriction."[12] Time-in-bed restriction leverages the homeostatic system by prescribing only the mean total sleep time as a window for time in bed for the 2-week period preceding the appointment. There are some variations in the prescription, wherein some time is added to the window (e.g., 30 minutes to account for normative sleep-onset latency).[3] Typically, there is a minimum prescription (e.g., 5 to 6 hours) to protect against excessive sleepiness; but again, there is some variation in this practice and no empirical studies available to guide this clinical decision. This restriction in time in bed creates greater sleep efficiency and consolidation of sleep. This procedure, in addition to greater efficiency, can result in sleepiness, and hence extension of time in bed is prescribed as therapy progresses.[13,14] An extension in the time-in-bed prescription typically occurs in the context of a complaint of subjective sleepiness, a mean sleep-onset latency less than 10 minutes, and/or a mean sleep efficiency greater than 85% or 90%. When delivered alone, the number of weekly treatment sessions vary from two to six. It is a well-established treatment on its own,[7,15,16] particularly for the gold standard outcomes of Insomnia Severity Index (ISI) and sleep diaries, but is most often used as part of a multicomponent CBT-I.

Relaxation Therapy

Relaxation therapy (RT) refers to a collection of empirically supported relaxation practices to reduce 24-hour basal levels of arousal. The RT strategies tested in insomnia include those involving breathing, imagery, and muscle relaxation techniques. Various relaxation strategies are effective in insomnia, although there are smaller effect sizes with RT relative to CBT-I.[17,18] Lichstein and colleagues[19] suggest that most relaxation therapies used for insomnia should conform to Benson's[20] recommendations for relaxation, that is, practicing in a quiet environment and in a comfortable position, with an object to dwell upon and a passive attitude. Most of the relaxation therapy studies in insomnia were published decades ago, focusing on sleep-onset insomnia, so it is unclear whether it generalizes to sleep maintenance or more mixed insomnia presentations.

Guided imagery is a relaxation technique that uses continuous visualization of a relaxing scene/situation. Instructions are similar to other forms of relaxation in that clients are asked to practice during the day and eventually at night, in a comfortable position and place in which they are less likely to be disturbed. The first visualization is typically in the therapist's office and is often recorded to take home for at-home, between-session practice. The visualization is typically something autobiographically relevant, in the past, and a scenario that was relaxing and relatively easy to contemplate. When clients experience difficulty recalling such a scene, the therapist and client collaboratively discuss possible relaxing scenes until the client settles on one that is personally relevant. For example, the client may picture moments from a beach vacation and visualize the sights, sounds, tastes, touch, and smell of the imagined scene.

Progressive muscle relaxation (PMR) involves tensing and then releasing 16 muscle groups in a gradual paced progression, focusing on the contrasting sensations of tension and release.[21] This practice is typically taught in-session, led by the therapist, and then practiced daily with an audio recording between sessions. The use of audio between sessions is considered an important part of skill acquisition.[22] PMR is a deep relaxation technique used widely for problems such as stress, anxiety, and in chronic conditions, such as headaches or anxiety. There are varying instructions as to when the practice occurs, but in general, the instruction is to practice it during the day to build the skill of releasing tension and lowering basal levels of tension, and then eventually PMR is completed in the presleep period to produce a state of relaxation presleep.[23]

Autogenic training[24] is a relaxation training technique in which clients lay down, or assume a suitably comfortable position, and repeat in their mind suggestions of feeling warmth and heaviness. Sometimes there are repetitions of statements such as "I am at peace." Imagining warmth and heaviness progressing through the body purportedly creates a physiologic state of vasodilation and reduced muscle tone, a state conducive to lowered arousal. Similar to PMR, this technique is taught across multiple sessions with a therapist and through daily practice.[25] The daily practice eventually also includes use of the technique in the pre-sleep period.

Paradoxical Intention

Paradoxical intention has been tested as a treatment for sleep-onset insomnia with a relatively simple instruction to "go to bed and attempt to stay awake all night long in bed." There may be several reasons why this is an effective treatment. First, it is an exposure of sorts to a significant fear in those with insomnia: staying awake all night. In addition, Espie and colleagues[26] have built a body of research supporting that one major issue in insomnia is that people with insomnia exert effort to sleep. Exerting effort to sleep is counter to the state needed to enter sleep; thus the paradoxical suggestion to exert effort to resist sleepiness makes it difficult to do so. Whereas some clients may believe they already stay awake all night in bed, the key difference in this treatment is that they are intentionally avoiding effort to sleep. The length of treatment sessions varies between two sessions,[27] 4 sessions[6,28] and eight sessions.[4] The flexible number of sessions and strong empirical support raises the issue of whether there is any benefit of multicomponent CBT-I over this approach. However, most people with insomnia do not have sleep-onset insomnia exclusively, perhaps limiting the utility of this treatment.

Cognitive Therapy and Counterarousal Strategies

Each of the behavioral interventions described earlier is an individually effective therapy for chronic insomnia.[29] The "C" in CBT-I stands for "cognitive" therapy (CT); at the time of this writing, there are not enough published empirical tests of CT as a monotherapy to establish it as a treatment on its own; however, there is extensive evidence for the effectiveness of CT used in combination with other therapies. Reading descriptions of CT from past CBT trials, there appeared to be some variability in what was labeled CT. Belief change is targeted in many ways, including psychoeducation, direct challenge of beliefs typically via Socratic questioning, thought records, and behavioral experiments. There has been one large scale randomized controlled trial (RCT) in CT, and in this contemporary version, there is the predominant use of behavioral experiments as the tool.[30] Presumably the shift toward behavioral experiments has occurred because of research supporting an advantage for behavioral experiments over verbal challenge (i.e., in thought records).[31] Behavioral strategies are effective on their own, leading some to conclude that CT is unnecessary, but one possibility is that CT may be important because belief change may help sustain long-term benefits of CBT-I over behavioral approaches.[14] Moreover, decreasing the rigidity of sleep beliefs is linked to multiple indices of clinical improvement.[32] Clearly, more studies are needed to understand the role of cognition and methods to modify thinking in resolving chronic insomnia.

Worry in the presleep period is one of the strongest cognitive predictors of delayed sleep-onset latency.[33] For those who tend to worry in bed, the behavioral insomnia therapies are proven strategies: SC eliminates the bed as a conditioned stimulus for worry and wakefulness, whereas SRT may increase the homeostatic drive for sleep to the point that the client ceases to worry because they are asleep. However, there are a variety of processing/problem-solving techniques that have focused more directly on presleep cognitive arousal. One of the original problem-solving cognitive strategies is a writing procedure that takes place in the evening, developed by Espie and Lindsay[34]; this technique is similar to a procedure called constructive worry.[35] The premise is that unresolved problems lead to worry and interfere with sleep onset by increasing arousal. Creating a plan during the day to address the problem decreases the likelihood that such worries will follow the person to bed. With constructive worry, clients are asked to set aside time several hours before bedtime to identify the problems that have the greatest likelihood of keeping them awake at night as well as the next, most immediate steps they can take toward resolving the problem. When combined with the behavioral insomnia therapies, the constructive worry procedure reduced insomnia symptom severity and worry to a greater degree than did behavioral therapy (combined SC and SRT) alone.[36]

Mindfulness

Mindfulness is a treatment that trains clients to observe, describe, and experience the present moment, nonjudgmentally. In therapy sessions a trained facilitator presents key principles of mindfulness (e.g., beginner's mind, nonstriving, letting go, nonjudging, and acceptance) and guides individuals through various formal meditations (e.g., mindful eating, body scan, and walking meditation). Thereafter person/group members are invited to participate in a brief period of inquiry regarding their in-session and at-home practice of mindfulness. Essential to mindfulness therapy are daily, between-session exercises of attentional training. Relative to behavioral strategies in which there is a change in sleep habits only, mindfulness approaches require a greater daily time commitment but may appeal to those who view their arousal as key in maintaining their insomnia. Mindfulness may also be easier to adhere to for those who do not wish to or find it difficult to change their sleep habits; however, there is no evidence that insomnia can be effectively treated without sleep behavior change. Three RCTs have tested mindfulness along with effective behavioral insomnia strategies as a group therapy with promising results.[37–40]

Sleep Hygiene

Sleep hygiene (SH) is the number one disseminated treatment strategy on the internet and the number one cited treatment strategy among providers,[41] but this is unfortunate, as SH is used effectively as a placebo control treatment in clinical trials[42–44] and has not been adequately tested as a stand-alone treatment in insomnia clients with specific abnormal sleep hygiene behaviors. The reason SH is used as a placebo control condition is that it is credible to patients but is generally not an efficacious stand-alone therapy for insomnia disorder.[45,46] Perhaps one of the reasons SH continues to be a component of CBT-I is that it is a low-resource treatment, typically consisting of a handout of recommendations only, and is occasionally clinically relevant for selected patients. It should be noted that SC, an effective treatment, can be delivered as a handout set of instructions. Unlike SC and SRT, or even CT, SH was not tested in those with insomnia except in the context of answering other research questions. The variability in the instructions makes it difficult to say anything definitive about this "treatment." Addressing sleep hygiene factors in treatment may occasionally be necessary, but it is insufficient as an isolated insomnia intervention. In other words, drinking caffeine before bed is ill-advised because the stimulant properties will have a negative effect on sleep, but reducing or even eliminating caffeine is rarely sufficient to address sleep in individuals with insomnia disorder. Thus SH remains in CBT-I for cases in which this might be an issue, but because good and poor sleepers do not reliably differ on SH practices,[47–49] and as it is less tied to those with insomnia,[50] it is often unnecessary. It is also possible that SH actually causes harm. For instance, receiving this advice could delay effective treatment, its lack of efficacy could affect the perception of effective therapies such as CBT-I, and inclusion in CBT-I approaches may unduly burden clients, but this has not been studied empirically.

Multicomponent Cognitive Behavioral Therapy for Insomnia

The most common treatment for insomnia is the combination of SC, SRT, SH, CT, and RT and/or other types of counterarousal techniques, thus receiving the name of multicomponent CBT-I. Multimodal CBT-I is typically defined by the inclusion of at least SRT and SC.[51] Multicomponent therapy is highly effective,[7] and CBT-I is effective and durable even across those with comorbid conditions.[51] See Table 95.2 for an example of a session-by-session outline of CBT-I.

Brief behavioral therapy for insomnia (BBTI) is a multicomponent treatment that combines psychoeducation, SC, and a prescription of SRT based on a pre–session-one sleep diary. It is purportedly brief, although the number of treatments has varied across studies. For example, BBTI was initially delivered in two sessions,[52] but several studies have increased it to two in-person sessions plus two phone or electronic follow-ups,[53] which is the optimal dose of sessions for CBT-I.[54] Another study combined BBTI with imagery rehearsal therapy for nightmares for eight sessions.[55] Given that the session length of BBTI may be as long as CBT-I, and CBT-I is a more established treatment with direct techniques to address unhelpful thinking that may improve adherence, why use BBTI? One reason BBTI is regarded as a useful alternative is that BBTI is a strictly behavioral approach and may appeal to providers with less experience or training in CT.

Table 95.2 Sample Session-by-Session Outline for a Four-Session Model

Week	Therapeutic Activities
Week 1 Week 2	Diagnostic and treatment planning assessment, assign diaries
Week 3	Completion of sleep diaries Begin psychoeducation, stimulus control, sleep restriction therapy, and sleep hygiene instructions
Week 4	At-home implementation of strategies
Week 5	Troubleshoot adherence to homework and determine if changes are necessary to schedule Begin cognitive therapy and time permitting, add counterarousal strategies/relaxation therapy
Week 6	At-home implementation of strategies
Week 7	Troubleshoot adherence and determine if changes are necessary to schedule Continue with cognitive therapy; add counterarousal strategies (if it was not added at session 2) Introduce termination issues
Week 8	At-home implementation of strategies
Week 9	Troubleshoot adherence Determine if changes are necessary to schedule Finish cognitive therapy Termination issues and relapse prevention

From Edinger JD, Carney CE. *Overcoming Insomnia: A Cognitive-Behavioral Therapy Approach, Therapist Guide*. 2nd ed. Oxford University Press; 2015:141.

Also, BBTI combines two behavioral treatments with demonstrated efficacy as monotherapies, does not require in-clinic follow-ups, and is primary care friendly.

IMPLEMENTATION OF COGNITIVE BEHAVIORAL THERAPY FOR INSOMNIA

Individual Treatment Format and Dosing

The most commonly used and most researched method of delivery for CBT-I has been individual therapy consisting of one-on-one outpatient sessions between a clinician and a single patient.[21,54] Most published RCTs using this treatment format have used doctoral-level or graduate student psychologists as therapists, although many have trained other professionals, such as nurses, with similar success rates.[56] Several meta-analyses and systematic reviews suggest that individual CBT-I is an effective short-term and long-term treatment for insomnia disorder.[57] CBT-I is designed to be a brief intervention, with most protocols consisting of four to eight sessions of individual therapy.[58] Edinger and colleagues[54] found that four individual, biweekly sessions represents the optimal dosing of multicomponent CBT-I, with greater short- and longer-term improvement in sleep relative to fewer or more treatment sessions.

Table 95.2 provides a sample four-session outline. Assumed in this four-session model is that a full diagnostic and treatment planning assessment occurred before the start of session one. In this model, once a diagnosis of insomnia disorder is made, and the provider and client agree to proceed with CBT-I, clients are provided with daily sleep diary instructions and assigned 2 weeks of monitoring. Providers query any anticipated barriers in completing the diaries daily and engage in troubleshooting of barriers (e.g., placing the diary in a conspicuous spot, setting a timer reminder for the morning to complete it, challenging catastrophic beliefs that answering questions about habits could worsen, rather than improve, sleep, etc.). Thus treatment session one begins with the sleep diary data necessary for creating a schedule for the time-in-bed prescription.

Other Delivery Methods

Many organizations, including the American College of Physicians,[59] have formally endorsed CBT-I as the first-line treatment for adults with chronic insomnia. When offered a choice, most patients prefer CBT-I to the use of hypnotic medications,[60] as do prescribers.[61] That said, one barrier to the more widespread dissemination of CBT-I has been a lack of trained clinicians to deliver this treatment. In the last decade there have been calls for a stepped-care model for the treatment of insomnia.[62,63] To this end, researchers have established efficacy for alternative methods of delivering CBT-I to patients, including group therapy,[64] self-help books,[65] abridged protocols for primary care settings,[14,56,66,67] telephone- and video-based therapy,[68,69] and digital CBT-I.[70–72] Innovative approaches were implemented during the COVID-19 pandemic (see Chapter 213).[72a]

Use in Older Adults and Those with Co-occurring Mental Health and Medical Conditions

There is ample support for the effectiveness of unaltered CBT-I in older adults and those with co-occurring medical and mental health conditions.[46,51,73] This is not surprising, as older insomnia patients and those with comorbid conditions share the same chronic insomnia perpetuating factors with adults who present only with insomnia: behaviors that prevent adequate "buildup" of homeostatic sleep drive, behaviors that interfere with the circadian timing of sleep, and hyperarousal. For example, there can be decreased activity and increased time in bed in older adults and those with co-occurring conditions; as such, the treatment targets in these comorbid patients are the same.[74]

Although CBT-I is effective in an unaltered state for older adults and those with co-occurring conditions, some have argued for modifications. For example, Smith and colleagues[75] (2005) speculated there may be unique delivery issues among particular populations that require special alterations of, or additions to, CBT-I to optimize insomnia treatment outcomes (e.g., the partial sleep deprivation occurring in SRT may increase risk for panic attacks, psychotic or manic symptoms). In such cases clinicians may opt for countercontrol,[76] which replaces the SC rule of leaving the bedroom with sitting-up and giving up the effort to sleep until sleepiness returns. Thus, during the countercontrol modification of SC, patients remain in bed. Countercontrol is primarily used in those with high fall risk (e.g., frail older adults, those with medication that may make them less steady on their feet at night, physical limitations or housing limitations that prevent going to another room). In addition, there may be a number of situations in which (1) SRT is modified (e.g., setting a prescription limit of no less than 6 hours), (2) SRT is replaced with sleep compression so that time in bed is reduced more gradually (i.e., 30 minutes per week),[77] or (3) SRT is removed altogether[78] to limit potential negative effects (e.g., lowering seizure or panic attack thresholds, or increasing mania or psychotic symptoms).

Although there are some situations in which CBT-I may be adapted, in addition, there have been some notable augmentations to CBT-I. Fatigue is notable problem in cancer populations, so one augmentation to CBT-I has been to add fatigue management.[79] Although not specific to older adults, cognitive and psychoeducation preparation for hypnotic medication taper has been added to CBT-I, as well as post–CBT-I support during a medically supervised taper, for older adults who are hypnotic dependent.[80] Those with posttraumatic stress disorder often receive a nightmare treatment (e.g., imagery rescripting and rehearsal therapy),[81] in which they rehearse alternative dream scenarios to address co-occurring nightmares. In those with serious mental illness, most notably in those with psychotic disorders[78] and bipolar disorders,[82,83] there is often circadian treatment targets of extreme variability and phase delay, which are not explicitly targeted by CBT-I. Thus CBT-I has been augmented in various ways, for instance, targeting sleep inertia with morning strategies to help those with bipolar disorder adhere to morning rise time goals.[83] Such approaches are labeled transdiagnostic, to recognize that some populations may have more sleep problems than insomnia only, and broader behavioral sleep medicine techniques would be most helpful.[84]

ASSESSMENT TOOLS USED IN COGNITIVE BEHAVIORAL THERAPY FOR INSOMNIA

Assessment Tools for Treatment Monitoring in CBT-I

Insomnia disorder is diagnosed based on the person's reported symptoms, which take precedence over any objective findings. As such, self-report measures of symptoms are essential, and the sleep diary represents a critical tool to identify behavioral targets for insomnia intervention, to guide the implementation of behavioral interventions, to identify challenges with treatment adherence, and to measure treatment outcomes.[85] Although there are several versions of sleep diaries available in the literature, the Consensus Sleep Diary (CSD)[86] was developed in consultation with a group of 25 leading experts to provide a standardized diary. The CSD is a prospective tool completed upon awakening that queries the subjective experience of the previous night. Examples of core items include the time the patient got into bed, the estimated amount of time it took to fall asleep, and the time at which they got out of bed. An expanded version includes optional items querying habits, such as naps, medications, alcohol, and so forth. Indices such as naps, alcohol, time in bed, and the variability of bedtimes and rise times, calculated by examining the difference between the earliest and latest times, provide information to generate hypotheses about possible behaviors to target. Ongoing completion of the CSD over the course of treatment allows the clinician to test hypotheses using the patient's own data (e.g., decreasing time in bed by 1 hour should lead to improved sleep indices) and to modify treatment in response. The CSD is especially critical to the implementation of SRT in CBT-I: The initial time-in-bed prescription is derived from the patient's average total sleep time on the CSD, and in subsequent sessions, the clinician uses data from CSD to assess adherence to behavioral targets and to make adjustments to the time-in-bed prescription. The CSD is also used in CT to test beliefs the patient has about their sleep system. For example, data collected using the CSD may challenge the accuracy of a patient's all-or-nothing statement about "not sleeping." The CSD has good treatment sensitivity for the diary in detecting improvement after CBT-I.[87]

Another important self-report measure is the ISI.[88] The ISI is a seven-item measure of perceived insomnia severity assessing initial, middle, and late insomnia; satisfaction with sleep; sleep-related preoccupation; and the impact and noticeability of sleep difficulties. Each item is rated on a five-point scale, and the summation of the items yield a total score ranging from 0 to 28. Cut-off scores of 10 in community samples and 14 in primary care clinics have been recommended to detect insomnia, although a change score of 8 points has been suggested to define an optimal treatment response.[89,90] The ISI has been shown in several studies to be sensitive to therapeutic changes, which is why it may be particularly useful to track treatment progress.[30,91,92] Although there are strong psychometric properties for the ISI, it remains unclear as to what clients "mean" by their ISI score. Construct questions are essential to understand in a patient-centered approach, and more answers are needed.

Actigraph

An actigraph is a device used to monitor cycles of activity and rest, usually worn around the nondominant wrist. Movement and/or light data are recorded on the device over an extended period of time (days to weeks) and are transformed with mathematical algorithms into estimates of sleep parameters (e.g., total sleep time, sleep latency, wake after sleep onset). Actigraphy does not measure sleep directly, nor the subjective experience of sleep as with the CSD, but rather draws inferences about sleep and wake patterns based on movement. As such, those lying awake motionless for hours or those awake but in sedentary jobs all day pose challenges to the assumptions underlying this technology. Actigraphy has acceptable correlations with other estimates of global sleep-wake parameters, such as total sleep time and sleep efficiency, but are much less accurate in estimating discrete or event-to-event sleep-wake parameters, such as sleep onset latency and time awake after sleep onset. Thus, if it is ever used in a clinical setting for insomnia, it would most likely assess 24-hour global patterns, which is most often done to assess sleep-wake patterns in those with atypical circadian rhythms, or adherence to into time-in-bed prescriptions.[93] Its use in clinical settings for insomnia is limited due to questionable validity, cost, and limited coverage by third-party payers. Of note, in recent years, consumer-grade sleep-tracking devices have become increasingly available, affordable, and popular. Clinicians and their patients should be aware that the vast majority of these devices have been developed commercially without supporting evidence for reliability and validity.[94] Although a potentially useful complement to self-report and polysomnography measures, actigraph devices and algorithms are not all equivalent and there may be significant variability in the reliability and validity of nocturnal sleep-wake data,[95] as well as nap data derived from different devices.[96] This equipment does not capture subjective experience—the quintessential feature of this disorder.

There are many other valuable assessment tools, including those for other symptoms, such as fatigue; assessment tools of most relevance to cognitive therapy; and tools that are useful in other sleep disorders, such as polysomnography, but the primary tools used in behavioral insomnia treatment are (1) prospective subjective diaries and (2) retrospective subjective questionnaires, such as the ISI.

SUMMARY

- Behavioral approaches are those grounded in learning theory and empirically tested and supported; the assumption that altering behavior can affect change in physiology and thoughts is common across behavioral approaches.
- The behavioral approaches with the strongest support include SC, SRT/time-in-bed restriction, and a multicomponent treatment that combines these two with other techniques.
- Relaxation therapy and other counterarousal techniques are effective in their own right, albeit with smaller effect sizes than SC and SRT.
- There are many effective delivery methods, including brief individual and group therapy, self-help books, telephone- and video-based therapy, and digital CBT-I; such variability is important to meet the needs of areas with limited access to therapists.

CLINICAL PEARLS

- Sleep hygiene education is not an effective treatment for insomnia; for a primary care–friendly alternative, consider stimulus control (SC), which can be used as a monotherapy. Like the other behavioral therapies, SC will require some follow-up, which can be done by phone.
- It is important to assess clients' perspectives on their symptoms using a self-report questionnaire, such as the Insomnia Severity Index, and to track treatment targets and improvements using the daily Consensus Sleep Diary.
- Sleep diary data are essential for calculating the initial time prescription for sleep restriction therapy and making adjustments to this in subsequent sessions; this cannot be done using clients' retrospective estimates of sleep time.
- Patients who cannot access in-person individual cognitive behavioral therapy for insomnia (CBT-I) should consider alternative delivery mechanisms, including digital CBT-I.

SELECTED READINGS

Bastien CH, Vallières A, Morin CM. Validation of the Insomnia Severity Index as an outcome measure for insomnia research. *Sleep Med.* 2001;2:297–307.

Becker PM. Overview of sleep management during COVID-19 [published online ahead of print, 2021 Apr 24]. *Sleep Med.* 2021;S1389-9457(21)00248-3.

Bootzin RR. Stimulus control treatment for insomnia. *Proc Am Psychol Assoc.* 1972;7:395–396.

Buysse DJ, Ancoli-Israel S, Edinger JD, Lichstein KL, Morin CM. Recommendations for a standard research assessment of insomnia. *Sleep.* 2006;29:1155–1173.

Carney CE, et al. The consensus sleep diary: standardizing prospective sleep self-monitoring. *Sleep.* 2012;35:287–302.

Espie CA, Lindsay WR, Brooks DN, Hood EM, Turvey TA. Controlled comparative investigation of psychological treatments for chronic sleep-onset insomnia. *Behav Res Ther.* 1989;27:79–88.

Geiger-Brown JM, et al. Cognitive behavioral therapy in persons with comorbid insomnia: a meta-analysis. *Sleep Med Rev.* 2015;23:54–67.

Moss TG, Lachowski A, Carney CE. What all treatment providers should know about sleep hygiene recommendations. *Behav Ther.* 2013;36:76–84.

Ong JC, et al. A randomized controlled trial of mindfulness meditation for chronic insomnia. *Sleep.* 2014;37:1553–1563.

Qaseem A, et al. Management of chronic insomnia disorder in adults: a clinical practice guideline from the American College of Physicians. *Ann Intern Med.* 2016;165:125–133.

Siriwardena AN, et al. General practitioners' preferences for managing insomnia and opportunities for reducing hypnotic prescribing. *J Eval Clin Pract.* 2010;16:731–737.

Spielman AJ, Saskin P, Thorpy MJ. Treatment of chronic insomnia by restriction of time in bed. *Sleep.* 1987;10:45–56.

Vincent N, Lionberg C. Treatment preference and patient satisfaction in chronic insomnia. *Sleep.* 2001;24:411–417.

A complete reference list can be found online at ExpertConsult.com.

Chapter 96

Behavioral Treatment II: Efficacy, Effectiveness, and Dissemination

Rachel Manber; Norah Simpson; Lauren Asarnow; Colleen E. Carney

Chapter Highlights

- Over the past 10 years, cognitive behavioral therapy for insomnia (CBT-I) has increasingly been recognized as the "gold-standard" treatment (or standard-of-care treatment) for chronic insomnia by several major medical/health care organizations. These include the American College of Physicians, the American Academy of Sleep Medicine, the British Association for Psychopharmacology, and, more recently, the European Sleep Research Society.
- There is a wealth of empirical evidence for the efficacy of CBT-I in reducing insomnia severity and improving sleep among individuals with insomnia, either alone or comorbid with other disorders. This chapter also discusses evidence for the effects of CBT-I on a range of outcomes beyond sleep. The discussions in each subsection also highlight areas for future research.
- The chapter describes real-world implementation of CBT-I, including known barriers to large-scale implementation of CBT-I and strategies to overcome these barriers.
- There are efforts to increase access to CBT-I through training of additional providers, including evidence of real-world effectiveness, and the use of alternatives to the currently prevailing delivery model that relies on individual psychotherapy in the clinician's office, for example, using group, telehealth, and direct-to-consumer self-help options, including digital programs.
- This chapter discusses how use of these alternative models of delivery can help overcome some of the known barriers to treatment access and engagement, as well as how stepped-care implementation models combine different delivery methods to facilitate the broad dissemination of CBT-I.

EFFICACY

Cognitive behavioral therapy for insomnia (CBT-I) is a brief and effective multicomponent treatment that alters behaviors and thoughts associated with insomnia disorder (see Chapter 95 for a detailed description of treatment components and how to implement them). Many meta-analytic studies and reviews provide robust empirical support for CBT-I as an effective treatment for insomnia disorder across a range of insomnia and sleep outcomes. The discussion that follows focuses primarily on evidence for efficacy of CBT-I relative to a control condition. Among the many outcome measures in efficacy trials, remission of a disease is the most desired outcome and is an index of clinically meaningful outcome. A meta-analysis of five randomized controlled trials (RCTs) of adults with insomnia reports a remission rate of 53%[1]; these studies determined remission based on established cut-off score on the Insomnia Severity Index or the Pittsburgh Sleep Quality Index. Remission rates are lower when insomnia co-occurs with another disorder, as demonstrated by a meta-analysis of 22 RCTs that enrolled participants with both insomnia and another medical or psychiatric conditions. This meta-analysis estimated that slightly more than one-third of patients who received CBT-I experienced remission of their insomnia disorder, which, after controlling for publication bias, yielded an odds ratio of 2.6 relative to control conditions.[2] Regarding change in insomnia symptom severity, although based on a small number of studies, meta-analyses suggest moderate to large effects relative to control conditions.[1,3,4] For subjective estimates of sleep parameters based on sleep diaries, meta-analyses found medium to large effect sizes for sleep onset latency, time awake after sleep onset, sleep efficiency, and subjective sleep quality relative to control conditions.[2,5] For sleep duration, which is an important component of overall sleep health (see Chapter 94)[6] that treatment-seeking patients wish to improve, results are more nuanced. Although the cited meta-analyses did not find an increase in subjective total sleep time with CBT-I relative to control conditions immediately posttreatment, a meta-analysis conducted by Okajima and colleagues[3] (2011) found a statistically significant increase in self-reported sleep duration at follow-up assessments conducted at 3 and 12 months posttreatment, with a small effect size relative to control conditions. In contrast to the robust evidence for improvement in subjective sleep, meta-analyses examining objective sleep parameters yielded mixed results.

Okajima and colleagues'[3] meta-analysis of 14 studies reported moderate effect sizes for wakefulness after sleep onset and sleep efficiency.[3] In contrast, Mitchell and colleagues'[5] meta-analysis of 12 controlled studies reported an absence of significant effects on polysomnography (PSG)-defined sleep, small or no effects on actigraphy-based sleep continuity parameters, and a moderate reduction in total sleep time posttreatment.[5] Thus, whereas the effects of CBT-I on subjective sleep parameters are robust, effects on objective sleep parameters (PSG and actigraphy) are mixed and more modest. It is important for future research to develop a nuanced understanding of the impact of treatment for insomnia disorder on sleep outcomes. However, given that symptoms bring patients with insomnia disorder into contact with health care providers, efficacy of CBT-I in subjective domains remains of primary importance.

The documented positive effects of CBT-I on self-reported outcomes immediately posttreatment are also durable. Two meta-analysis of follow-up data provide evidence for continued efficacy of CBT-I at 3, 6, and 12 months posttreatment relative to control conditions,[3,7] with moderate effect sizes for sleep onset latency, minutes awake after sleep onset, sleep efficiency, and insomnia severity. Although the effects tended to decline over time, they remained clinically meaningful at the 12-month follow-up.[7] Whereas most RCTs of CBT-I include follow-up periods of 1 year or less, several studies have included longer follow-ups. A seminal study by Morin and colleagues[8] demonstrated sustained gains from CBT-I over a 2-year naturalistic follow-up period.[8] A recent study of web-based CBT-I reported a large effect size for insomnia severity over a 3-year posttreatment follow-up period relative to control conditions.[9] Further, an observational clinic-based study reported significant improvements in sleep that were maintained for up to 10 years (mean follow-up, 7.8 years[10]). Given evidence for some decline in effect sizes during follow-up and the potential bias in long-term follow-up, where one may not assume that data are missing at random, there is a critical need in the field to assess the long-term benefits of CBT-I using strategies for minimizing attrition. Knowledge gained from such research could guide the development of strategies for relapse prevention and possibly scheduling additional maintenance sessions.

Evidence for the efficacy of CBT-I is further strengthened by studies of CBT-I that were conducted in populations with medical and psychiatric comorbidities and in different age groups. Meta-analyses have concluded that CBT-I is an effective treatment of insomnia among cancer survivors[11] and adults with pain conditions,[12] as well as in samples with a mix of medical and psychiatric conditions.[2,13,14] There is also evidence from adequately powered randomized controlled trials that CBT-I is effective among postmenopausal[15] and pregnant women[16] and among adults with depression, including those taking antidepressant medications.[17,18] There is strong evidence that CBT-I improves insomnia and sleep among older adults[19] and emerging evidence that it is also effective among adolescents.[20] Although efficacy of CBT-I among those with comorbidities is clear, it is less clear if there is differential efficacy of CBT-I among people with or without comorbidities, although, as noted earlier, remission rates in meta-analyses of CBT-I in samples with comorbidities are somewhat smaller than in analyses when comorbidities were excluded. Meta-analyses that have examined differential efficacy by comorbidity and age have done so as secondary analyses, pooling results from studies designed to answer questions of efficacy relative to control treatment rather than comparative efficacy among subgroups of patients. Knowing how specific patient-level attributes relate to outcomes is important as it could inform further refinement of CBT-I to tailor it to specific patient presentations. One promising approach is to conduct pooled patient level meta-analyses. At the time of this writing, efforts to pool individual patient data to address this important question are underway.[21]

Meta-analyses have concluded that CBT-I is also effective across treatment modalities[22] and for specific modalities.[23–25] Among self-help interventions, internet-delivered treatments are increasing in popularity and are effective.[26,27] A meta-analysis of an internet CBT-I conducted by Zacharie and colleagues[27] identified higher dropout rates as a predictor of smaller effect sizes. This finding highlights the importance of identifying and addressing factors that can increase patient engagement in self-help CBT-I. There is already some evidence that internet-based interventions that offer a higher intensity of support produce larger effect sizes compared to those with low or no support interventions.[23,27–29] Researchers have also compared the efficacy of different delivery methods, with some meta-analyses suggesting that individual treatment is more effective than group or self-help treatments.[13,22] Although efficacy across treatment modalities provides further support for the robust nature of CBT-I, the range of observed effect sizes based on delivery method has led to increased interest in development and testing of stepped-care models of insomnia treatment delivery to most effectively and efficiently deliver treatment resources to help the largest number of patients in need (see Dissemination and Implementation section.)

EFFECTIVENESS: IMPACT ON OTHER SYMPTOMS

Increasingly, studies examining the efficacy of CBT-I also examined it effectiveness, that is, the effects of CBT-I on symptoms beyond insomnia and sleep. Some of these effectiveness studies have specifically selected individuals with comorbidities or with specific symptoms (e.g., those with elevated depression scores but not meeting formal diagnostic criteria for major depression) and examined the impact of CBT-I on the target comorbid disorder or symptom severity. Other effectiveness studies have examined the impact of CBT-I on nonsleep outcomes in general samples of individuals with insomnia. To follow, we review the literature on the effectiveness of CBT-I on the following outcomes: depression, anxiety, pain, fatigue, and quality of life. In addition, because multiple professional and medical organizations, including the American Academy of Sleep Medicine, encourage minimizing the use of hypnotic medications,[30,31] we also discuss the effects of CBT-I on hypnotic medication use.

Depression Symptom Severity

Three meta-analyses have concluded that behavioral and cognitive behavioral interventions for adults with insomnia lead to decreases in depressive symptom severity.[32,33] Whereas pretreatment to posttreatment effect sizes for improvement in depression symptom severity in these meta-analyses are moderate to large,[33] effect sizes relative to a control condition are small to medium.[32,34] When considering treatment type (behavioral vs. cognitive behavioral) and modality (self-help, group, and individual), only individual CBT-I (i.e., individually provided treatment that included cognitive and behavioral treatment for insomnia) was associated with greater improvement in depressive symptoms compared with control conditions.[32] However, studies of self-help CBT-I that were included in this analysis consisted of a mix of digital and other self-help modalities and did not include two very large digital CBT-I studies.[35,36] This is particularly important, given increase in availability of digital CBT-I. These two large studies reported small to moderate effects of digital CBT-I on depression symptom severity.

Many of the analyzed studies in these three meta-analyses excluded participants that met, or were likely to meet, diagnostic criteria for a depressive disorder. As a result, it is possible that the effects of CBT-I alone on depression severity among individuals with meaningful depressive symptoms is smaller than these meta-analyses suggest. Moreover, these three meta-analyses focused on the effects on depression of CBT-I alone, rather than as an adjunct to an antidepressant intervention. Two RCTs of patients with comorbid insomnia and depression diagnoses provided CBT-I (or a control intervention for insomnia) plus a depression intervention. Both studies found that there was no additive effect of CBT-I on depressive symptom severity.[17,18] Nonetheless, in one of these studies, Manber and colleagues[18] found that improvements in insomnia severity over the first 6 weeks of insomnia treatment mediated the remission from depression over the entire 12-week treatment period; in other words, early change in insomnia severity symptoms predicted depression remission in the CBT-I but not in the control treatment arm.

The large heterogeneity in samples and study designs among studies on the effects of CBT-I on depressive symptoms precludes definitive conclusions. The results do, however, point to three directions for further research that could have clinically meaningful implications. The first pertains to the potential utility of CBT-I for the prevention of depression among those at risk for depressive disorder. Two recent prevention studies that used digital CBT-I suggest that this may indeed be a promising approach,[35,37,38] particularly among those with low depression severity at baseline and hence at risk for developing a depressive disorder. The second direction for future research is to identify attributes of patients with dual diagnoses of insomnia and depression who are particularly likely to experience additive benefit from incorporating CBT-I into their depression management. For example, Asarnow and colleagues[39] identified greater eveningness tendencies as one such characteristic.[9] Specifically, they found that individuals with co-occurring depression and insomnia who had a stronger evening tendency had better depression outcomes if assigned to CBT-I plus an antidepressant medication condition compared with the control insomnia intervention plus an antidepressant medication condition. The third clinically meaningful direction for future research is to focus on ways to enhance depression outcomes among patients with dual insomnia-depression diagnoses. For example, findings from a recent study conducted by Kalmbach and colleagues[40] suggest that the cognitive component of CBT-I might be particularly important for reducing depressive symptoms.

Anxiety Symptom Severity

A 2011 meta-analysis identified 50 controlled and uncontrolled studies of CBT-I that included measures of anxiety and anxiety-related constructs (e.g., perceived stress).[41] This analysis found that effect sizes for in-person CBT-I on anxiety and related symptoms were small for comparisons between treatment and control conditions (20 studies) and moderate for pretreatment to posttreatment (within-subject) comparisons (30 studies). Of interest, studies that integrated a hypnotic withdrawal component into the CBT-I protocol had a near-zero effect size for anxiety outcomes. This intriguing finding suggests that additional attention to anxiety might enhance the effectiveness of CBT-I protocols that target hypnotic-dependent patients and include a hypnotic taper component (see Chapter 100 for more detailed discussion). The results of this meta-analysis have limited generalizability for those with comorbid anxiety disorder because only 4 studies in this large meta-analysis had samples with dual diagnoses of insomnia and anxiety disorders.[41] A more recent meta-analysis of 8 RCTs that evaluated change in anxiety symptom severity with CBT-I found a low effect size for comparisons between CBT-I and control conditions[26]; similarly, none of the included studies focused on patients with a comorbid anxiety disorder. In contrast, a 2016 meta-analysis focused exclusively on the effects of psychological treatments for improving sleep among individuals with posttraumatic stress disorder (PTSD) symptoms or syndrome[42] found a moderate effect size on PTSD symptoms. However, it is difficult to tease out the impact of CBT-I alone on PTSD symptoms because only 3 of the 8 studies used CBT-I as a monotherapy; the rest included interventions that targeted nightmares, either alone or in combination with CBT-I. Taken together, there seems to be a small effect size of CBT-I on anxiety symptoms among individuals without comorbid anxiety disorder and paucity of research on the effects of CBT-I on anxiety symptoms among individuals with diagnoses of comorbid insomnia and anxiety disorders

Pain

CBT-I protocols that do not directly address pain have been tested in a variety of pain conditions. In a meta-analysis of six such studies among those with pain-related conditions, Tang and colleagues[12] (2015) found a small effect size on pain. Similarly, in a meta-analysis of four studies on group-delivered CBT-I protocols that did not include a target pain intervention, Koffel and colleagues[24] (2015) found a small effect size for pain improvement among adults with insomnia, although participants were not specifically selected to also have a pain condition. A 2019 review considered the evidence to date about the potential benefits of CBT-I in the management of pain conditions.[43] This review included several studies published after 2015 and have similarly concluded that "the effect sizes for pain reduction after behavioral sleep interventions are modest and variable but comparable or even superior to those of psychological therapies for pain." Three small studies and a more recent larger RCT tested hybrid interventions that simultaneously address sleep and pain among those with pain conditions and suggest that this hybrid approach could be beneficial for the management of chronic pain.[44–46] There is also convergence of evidence that the beneficial effects of CBT-I alone or in combination with behavioral pain interventions on pain outcomes are greater at 3- to 6-months follow-up than at posttreatment.[47,48] Given that insufficient sleep is particularly relevant to the pain experience,[49] it is possible that the lag in benefits is related to the fact that total sleep duration often continues to increase after CBT-I is completed, likely due to patients continued use of cognitive-behavioral components (i.e., maintenance) after the initial treatment phase.[3] It is therefore important that future research on the effects on CBT-I on pain include long-term follow-up and consider and evaluate treatment protocols that include a maintenance treatment phase.

Fatigue

Fatigue is a frequent complaint of individuals with insomnia disorders and therefore an important outcome to assess. Fatigue is not a well-defined construct among both patients and researchers. One of the challenges for synthesizing the literature on the impact of CBT-I on fatigue is that the construct of fatigue is multidimensional and not uniformly defined in research. As a result, different studies likely measure different aspects of fatigue. Regardless, studies that have focused on populations known to have high levels of fatigue, such as cancer patients, generally find improvement in fatigue after CBT-I. A meta-analysis of CBT-I among those with pain-related conditions (cancer and fibromyalgia) found a moderate overall effect size for reduction in fatigue posttreatment (six studies) and at 3- to 12-month follow-up (three studies). Only two of the six studies included in this meta-analysis had a treatment component that specifically addressed fatigue,[12] suggesting that CBT-I alone could help reduce fatigue in these populations. The available RCTs of CBT-I among patients with other medical comorbidities, such as patients on peritoneal dialysis and hemodialysis[50] and with COPD,[51] also found improvements in fatigue levels after CBT-I, as did a recent trial among those with menopausal symptoms.[52] The effects of CBT-I on fatigue in mixed samples of patients with varying levels of fatigue at baseline are less clear. A network meta-analysis, which included samples with and without comorbidities and varying levels of fatigue at baseline, found a moderate effect size for fatigue after individually delivered CBT-I; however, after examining heterogeneity among studies, the meta-analysis concluded that there were no significant effects on fatigue.[32] A few studies published after this meta-analysis reported fatigue improvements after internet-delivered CBT-I[36,53] and therapist-delivered CBT-I.[54] Many studies on the effects of CBT-I on fatigue did not report having a fatigue-specific treatment component; however, because concerns about next-day fatigue are often identified by patients with insomnia as an obstacle to implementing time-in-bed restriction, it is likely that even therapists who implement strictly behavioral protocols end up addressing fatigue. It is possible that adding a component that explicitly addresses fatigue to general CBT-I protocols, as previously done in a study in CBT-I among cancer patients (e.g., Savard and colleagues[55]), could further enhance fatigue outcomes. Explicitly addressing fatigue could also enhance adherence to the behavioral components of CBT-I, which in turn may strengthen efficacy for CBT-I on insomnia symptoms.

Quality of Life

Quality of life is an important outcome in insomnia because chronic insomnia is one of the top contributors to reduced quality of life.[56] It is therefore surprising that quality of life has been understudied as an outcome after CBT-I. One meta-analysis of RCTs of CBT-I suggest it is associated with statistically significant improvements in measures of global quality of life.[57] The improvements in quality of life seen with CBT-I may be more modest among those with comorbid mental health conditions.[14] There also is some evidence for delivery-specific effects; for instance, telephone-delivered CBT-I did not improve quality of life, even though it did improve sleep.[58] In contrast, recent data suggest that digital CBT-I improves sleep-related quality of life, that is, aspects of quality of life that patients believe are impaired by poor sleep.[36] Taken together, although available data are limited, CBT-I appears to improve quality of life, but the size of the effects may be variable depending on domain-specific quality of life, coexisting conditions, and method of CBT-I delivery.

Hypnotic Use

CBT-I protocols that do not directly target hypnotic reduction seem to significantly reduce hypnotic medication use, nonetheless. One of the earliest studies to demonstrate that CBT-I leads to reduction in hypnotic medication use was based on data from a series of 100 patients in a university-based sleep center who received CBT-I.[59] In this study the number of habitual users of sleep medication decreased by 54% posttreatment. Subsequent controlled studies have similarly shown that, without therapists' explicit attention to discontinuing medication, close to half of habitual users decreased their hypnotic medication by half of their baseline use after CBT-I, compared to only 17% of those receiving usual care.[60] Several additional studies have examined the effect of CBT-I protocols that have included a targeted medication taper component (e.g., information about taper and encouragement to include discontinuation or tapering as a treatment goal). A 2019 meta-analysis of eight studies examined the effects of adding CBT-I to a schedule for gradual taper of medication on hypnotic medication use.[61] It concluded that the addition of CBT-I leads to greater reduction in hypnotic use than gradual medication taper alone in the short (<3 months) but not long term (12 months). Studies in this meta-analysis were heterogeneous with respect to the extent to which the CBT-I protocol provided targeted attention to support the taper. The studies were also heterogeneous with respect to representation of frequency and chronicity of hypnotic use in the sample. Not included in this meta-analysis is an RCT of internet-based CBT-I, conducted in a sample in which about half the participants took hypnotic medications at baseline. After treatment and during a 3-year follow-up, roughly a quarter of those assigned to CBT-I were using sleep medications; at the 3-year follow-up, the difference between CBT-I and control conditions was statistically significant and clinically meaningful (29% vs. 47%[9]). In clinical practice, many behavioral medicine specialists integrate into CBT-I strategies to help patients reduce or eliminate hypnotic use, often collaborating with prescribing physicians regarding the specific taper schedule.[62] Given increasing professional guidelines to minimize the use of hypnotic medications,[63] it will be important for future research in this area to identify patient factors that predict spontaneous reduction in hypnotic use after CBT-I alone. It will also be important to formalize and refine strategies to encourage and facilitate successful hypnotic taper among those who are less likely to do so with standard CBT-I alone. Chapter 100 of this book includes additional discussion of hypnotic discontinuation protocols.

DISSEMINATION AND IMPLEMENTATION

Limited access to CBT-I is a major barrier to its wide-scale implementation as a first-line treatment of insomnia and ergo to the successful implementation of the insomnia treatment guidelines made by multiple professional organizations. Efforts to overcome this limitation have included training of providers and the development of new models for delivering CBT-I that promote greater and better access to trained CBT-I providers and use of digital technology. These efforts are discussed as follows.

Dissemination via Provider Training

The traditional paths for training treatment providers to deliver CBT-I has been through graduate programs and/or postdoctoral fellowships within the psychology discipline. These training paths involve courses on general principles of CBT and on sleep science and sleep disorders. Although the majority of psychology graduate programs and psychiatry residencies offer training in CBT for a variety of mental health disorders, few offer specialty training in CBT-I. In response to high demand for CBT-I services, the Veterans Health Administration has developed a CBT-I training program for licensed mental health providers from different professional disciplines. This 4-month training program provides a model for increasing the ranks of licensed clinicians who can effectively provide CBT-I. In the past 10 years it has trained 900 Veterans Affairs (VA) mental health providers nationwide to deliver CBT-I. In addition to a didactic portion, which included learning about sleep architecture, sleep regulation, and common sleep disorders, training involves experiential learning, both through role-plays and ongoing expert consultation and feedback on sampled work throughout the training period. Expert consultation and feedback in this initiative aim to optimize competency and promote continued use of CBT-I. Although the VA training uses a traditional six-session protocol, a case-conceptualization–driven approach guides therapists on how to adapt and tailor the protocol to patients with complex presentations, who often experience insomnia in the context of comorbid medical and mental disorders. Tailoring includes guidelines for selecting which components of CBT-I to emphasize and in what order to present them based on the case-conceptualization framework. Consultants (expert-level providers in CBT-I involved in the training program) also listen to recorded sessions and use a program-developed competency rating form, which, unlike standard fidelity checklists, rates the level of competency in delivering each of the CBT-I treatment components, not merely whether these components are present or absent.

Program evaluation of this VA training program provides evidence on real-world effectiveness of CBT-I, examining patient outcomes, therapists' fidelity, and the extent to which those trained continue to use CBT-I.[64,65] To promote sustainable impact, the VA CBT-I training initiative developed a mechanism for identifying and training outstanding high-utilization graduates to become consultants and trainers themselves. This allows the training program to keep growing in scope and amplifies its impact. As a result, CBT-I is now available to veterans seen in a wide range of practice settings, including general and specialty mental health clinics, primary care, and those in residential and home-based care. To enhance the reach of CBT-I, the program also developed supplemental training to deliver CBT-I in a group format, which is available to those who have already obtained competency and became experienced practitioners of individual CBT-I.

Implementation Models

Currently, the most prevalent model for delivering CBT-I is individual face-to-face therapy by specialty-trained providers, usually mental health professionals. However, there are many barriers for patients to engage in CBT-I within the currently prevailing model. One of these barriers is the need to travel to the provider's office. This is a challenge for patients with limited mobility and for those who live in communities that do not have qualified providers nearby. Telemedicine helps mitigate this barrier to access to therapist-led CBT, allowing therapists to use secure video conferencing technology to deliver CBT-I. Eliminating the need to travel to the therapist's office also minimizes the time off from work and reduces child care burden for patients. Digital CBT-I, such as online- or app-based programs, also addresses these barriers and additionally reduces potential stigma and embarrassment about seeking mental health care, eliminates waiting time for therapy, and offers flexibility in pace of treatment. However, as reviewed earlier and in Chapter 97, although digital CBT-I programs are effective, there is also evidence that they are less effective than therapist-delivered treatment. There are also barriers for use of digital CBT-I, such as patient preferences and proficiency and comfort with digital technology. Some individuals may do better with hybrid models that provide some human guidance and encouragement while they are using a digital program. Indeed, there is evidence from one meta-analysis that a higher degree of support leads to greater efficacy of digital interventions.[27] Examples of low level of support include automated text messages; examples of higher level of support include access to brief phone consultation with a provider. Additional ways to increase support within hybrid models include supplementing digital CBT-I with short visits with a provider (professional or paraprofessional) and use of a chatbot (or virtual coach). Hybrid models can also be used in clinical settings to promote patient engagement and adherence to treatment recommendations offered in the course of digital CBT-I.

Stepped-care implementation models combine digital and therapist delivery but do so sequentially rather than concomitantly. One approach is to provide digital CBT first and then offer therapist-delivered CBT-I to those whose insomnia does not remit. Another approach is to triage patients into digital or therapist-delivered CBT-I at the first step of care, based on their clinical presentations, and then offer therapist-led CBT-I to those who have not sufficiently benefited from digital CBT-I. Testing of this model is currently underway (NCT03532282). Regardless of implementation model, real-life implementations will need to take into account patient preferences. The COVID-19 pandemic of 2020-2021 has accelerated acceptance of newer modes of CBT-I delivery.[66]

As CBT-I becomes more widely disseminated using the variety of delivery modes and implementation strategies, it will be important to understand how to best optimize its effectiveness in real-world settings. Some important unanswered effectiveness questions include the following: What are the best methods to ensure therapists' fidelity to CBT-I treatment in the field? How is patients' engagement best promoted in real-world clinical settings rather than within the context of a research setting? How do financial considerations, such as health insurance coverage for online interventions, factor into the use of CBTI-I in the community? What resources do physicians need to support their patients' engagement in CBT-I? Future large-scale pragmatic trials can answer these and related questions and examine the efficacy of CBT-I in real-world settings.

SUMMARY

The evidence reviewed in this chapter indicates that CBT-I is highly effective treatment in diverse patient populations, including those with comorbid conditions and across the life span. At the end of treatment, patients typically experience improvements in insomnia and sleep outcomes, except for total sleep time. The benefits are durable long after treatment ends, and total sleep duration tends to increase over time. CBT-I also has modest benefits on some outcomes beyond sleep, such as quality of life, mood, pain, and fatigue, as well as reduction in hypnotic medications use. Digital CBT-I has vastly increased access to CBT-I; however, recent data suggests that it may be less effective than therapist-led treatment. Stepped-care models that triage patients to digital or therapist-led CBT-I have the potential for increasing access to CBT-I in a manner that could optimize patient care and available resources.

CLINICAL PEARLS

- After completing cognitive behavioral therapy for insomnia (CBT-I), patients are expected to experience reduction in insomnia severity and meaningful improvements in sleep outcomes, except for total sleep time, for which improvements are expected to gradually increase after treatment ends.
- CBT-I is an effective treatment for patients with insomnia, including those with a range of comorbid conditions, and also might have value in management of some symptoms of the comorbid conditions.
- Individuals receiving CBT-I may also experience modest benefits in some other life domains, such as quality of life, mood, pain, and fatigue.
- Access to CBT-I can be enhanced with telehealth, web-based CBT-I programs, and combinations of technology-assisted therapy options. Stepped-care models that triage people to digital or therapist-led CBT-I might increase access to CBT-I in a manner that could optimize patient care and available resources. These efforts may facilitate integration of behavioral sleep medicine /CBT-I in accredited sleep centers.

SELECTED READINGS

Altena E, Baglioni C, Espie CA, et al. Dealing with sleep problems during home confinement due to the COVID-19 outbreak: practical recommendations from a task force of the European CBT-I academy. *J Sleep Res.* 2020;29(4):e13052.

Ballesio A, Bacaro V, Vacca M, et al. Does cognitive behaviour therapy for insomnia reduce repetitive negative thinking and sleep-related worry beliefs? A systematic review and meta-analysis. *Sleep Med Rev.* 2021;55:101378.

Espie CA, Emsley R, Kyle SD, et al. Effect of digital cognitive behavioral therapy for insomnia on health, psychological well-being, and sleep-related quality of life: a randomized clinical trial. *JAMA Psychiatry.* 2019;76(1):21–30.

Gee B, Orchard F, Clarke E, Joy A, Clarke T, Reynolds S. The effect of non-pharmacological sleep interventions on depression symptoms: a meta-analysis of randomised controlled trials. *Sleep Med Rev.* 2019;43:118–128.

Manber R, Carney C. *Treatment Plans and Interventions for Insomnia: A Case Formulation Approach.* New York: Guilford Press; 2015.

Mitchell LJ, Bisdounis L, Ballesio A, Omlin X, Kyle SD. The impact of cognitive behavioural therapy for insomnia on objective sleep parameters: a meta-analysis and systematic review. *Sleep Med Rev.* 2019;47:90–102.

Okajima I, Komada Y, Inoue Y. A meta-analysis on the treatment effectiveness of cognitive behavioral therapy for primary insomnia. *Sleep Biol Rhythms.* 2011;9(1):24–34.

Parsons CE, Zachariae R, Landberger C, Young KS. How does cognitive behavioural therapy for insomnia work? A systematic review and meta-analysis of mediators of change [published online ahead of print, 2021 Apr 3]. *Clin Psychol Rev.* 2021;86:102027.

Sateia MJ, Buysse DJ, Krystal AD, Neubauer DN, Heald JL. Clinical practice guideline for the pharmacologic treatment of chronic insomnia in adults: an American Academy of Sleep Medicine clinical practice guideline. *J Clin Sleep Med.* 2017;13(2):307–349.

Selvanathan J, Pham C, Nagappa M, et al. Cognitive behavioral therapy for insomnia in patients with chronic pain - A systematic review and meta-analysis of randomized controlled trials [published online ahead of print, 2021 Feb 2]. *Sleep Med Rev.* 2021;60:101460.

Takaesu Y, Utsumi T, Okajima I, et al. Psychosocial intervention for discontinuing benzodiazepine hypnotics in patients with chronic insomnia: a systematic review and meta-analysis. *Sleep Med Rev.* 2019;48:101214.

van Straten A, van der Zweerde T, Kleiboer A, Cuijpers P, Morin CM, Lancee J. Cognitive and behavioral therapies in the treatment of insomnia: a meta-analysis. *Sleep Med Rev.* 2018;38:3–16.

van der Zweerde T, Bisdounis L, Kyle SD, Lancee J, van Straten A. Cognitive behavioral therapy for insomnia: a meta-analysis of long-term effects in controlled studies. *Sleep Med Rev.* 2019;48:101208.

Zachariae R, Lyby MS, Ritterband LM, O'Toole MS. Efficacy of internet-delivered cognitive-behavioral therapy for insomnia: a systematic review and meta-analysis of randomized controlled trials. *Sleep Med Rev.* 2016;30:1–10.

A complete reference list can be found online at ExpertConsult.com.

Chapter 97

Behavioral Treatment III: Digital and Telehealth Approaches

Øystein Vedaa; Katherine E. Miller; Philip R. Gehrman

Chapter Highlights

- Despite the demonstrated efficacy of cognitive behavioral therapy for insomnia, many patients do not have access to face-to-face treatment. There has been a surge of interest in technological means of treatment delivery, including internet, mobile, and telehealth approaches.
- Internet treatment delivery has a strong evidence base demonstrating efficacy when compared to control conditions. Available data on mobile and telehealth delivery indicate that these modalities are associated with clinically important improvements in insomnia severity as well.
- There is a lack of evidence directly comparing technological means to face-to-face delivery, so it is not clear if there is a loss in the magnitude of improvements. There is also a need to determine which modalities are best suited for particular patient populations (e.g., pregnancy). This is likely to be an area of increased growth in coming years.

INTRODUCTION

The costs of offering cognitive behavioral therapy for insomnia (CBT-I) and lack of trained clinicians have so far prevented sufficient dissemination of the treatment to the broad population of people with insomnia. The standard means of delivery of CBT-I is face-to-face, individual therapy with a sleep specialist, but this is also the most resource intensive and limited in availability. Alternative treatment delivery models have therefore been proposed, including brief face-to-face interventions,[1] delivery in a group therapy format,[2] and telephone consultations,[3] among others. These are delivery models that may increase service efficiency and help reach more people with effective treatment for chronic insomnia but still require considerable resources. During the COVID pandemic, when face to face CBTi sessions were not possible, telehealth approaches were often explored (see Chapter 213).

Since the mid-1990s there has been a steady increase in the use of technological means for delivering cognitive behavioral therapy (CBT) for mental health problems and medical conditions (i.e., conditions in which behavior is a component). In particular, many solutions have been developed to deliver CBT through digital platforms or over the internet. The highly structured nature of CBT makes it especially suitable for a manual- and algorithm-based delivery. In the literature, the conceptual apparatus for describing this type of technological innovation in the delivery of CBT has not yet established itself: some refer to internet CBT, electronic CBT, computerized CBT, or digital CBT.[4] The U.S. Food and Drug Administration (FDA) seems to have accepted the term *digital*, in which digital CBT can be categorized as a digital therapeutic, within the subset of digital health.[5]

In recent review studies, a distinction has been made between three levels of delivering digital CBT (Figure 97.1).[4,6] First, in supportive digital CBT, the digital content often has a more simplistic nature and serves a purely supportive function in conjunction with the face-to-face expert therapy. Second, in therapist-guided digital CBT, the therapeutic content is communicated and sequenced primarily through the technological platform that also may incorporate some degree of automation, to which the therapist only has a supportive function. Third, fully automated or self-guided digital CBT typically involves more sophisticated algorithm-based delivery of the therapeutic content, which often uses interactive and tailoring features for better user engagement and experience, but without any support from a clinician. Important differences between these digital CBT delivery levels include the amount of clinician time they require and the level of automatization they provide, which in turn also indicate the expected costs and the scalability of the delivery modes.

The goal of this chapter is to review the burgeoning area of research on technological means of delivering CBT-I. The focus is on internet, mobile, and telehealth approaches to treatment delivery, although other technological solutions have been proposed.

DELIVERY OVER THE INTERNET

The success of internet-based (i.e., digital) interventions for mental health problems has been demonstrated in more than 200 trials over the past two decades. A recent review of new meta-analyses found moderate to large average effect size improvements on panic disorder, social anxiety disorder, general anxiety disorder, posttraumatic stress disorder (PTSD), and major depression, with digital CBT interventions.[7] The

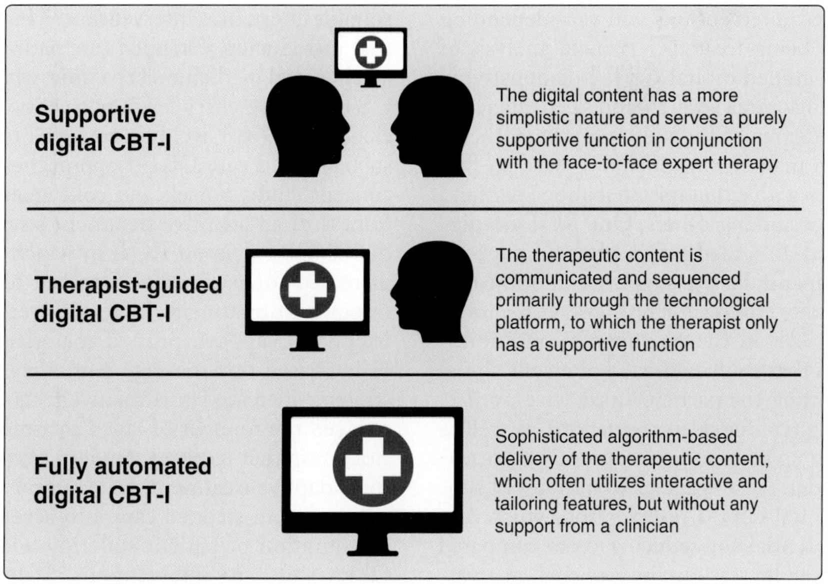

Figure 97.1 Three levels of delivering digital cognitive behavioral therapy.

first randomized controlled trial (RCT) that demonstrated the effects of internet therapy for insomnia was published by Ström and colleagues in 2004, in which written self-help material was made available to participants through a webpage.[8] Since then, online adaptations of CBT-I have become increasingly interactive and personalized, which seems to have enhanced the effect size improvements with such interventions (see the reviews by Ritterband and colleagues[9] and Espie and colleagues[10]).

Digital CBT-I programs are usually designed to mimic face-to-face CBT-I[11] in terms of content and form. Typically, they consist of six weekly sessions that cover the basic topics of CBT-I, including sleep restriction, stimulus control, cognitive restructuring, relaxation strategies, sleep hygiene, and relapse prevention.

In one recent well-conducted RCT, more than 300 adults with insomnia were recruited from the general population and given access to either fully automated digital CBT-I or a webpage containing information about sleep hygiene. The authors found that use of digital CBT-I was associated with reductions in insomnia severity and improvements in sleep-wake patterns (assessed via online sleep diaries).[12] Other large, well-conducted trials have demonstrated the efficacy of fully automated digital CBT-I on reductions in depressive symptoms,[13] improved functional health, psychological well-being, and sleep-related quality of life.[14] Further, in a sample of more than 3000 students, use of digital CBT-I was associated with significantly greater reductions in symptoms of paranoia and hallucinations, compared with usual care.[15] These findings are in line with those of several meta-analyses on the effects of digital CBT-I (including trials on both therapist-guided and self-guided interventions), with the overall conclusion that the interventions lead to significant and sustained improvements on daytime and nighttime symptoms of insomnia, with a magnitude that is comparable to that typically obtained with traditional face-to-face treatment.[16-18] Number needed to treat (NNT) is a measure of how many participants need to receive the intervention for one individual to respond or recover. The most recent meta-analysis of digital CBT-I calculated an average NNT of 2.2 for insomnia severity, based on treatment response or estimates from effect sizes.[17] This is comparable to the NNT reported in studies using in-person CBT-I, which in one RCT was 3.2 for cases of recovery on insomnia severity,[19] and in another RCT was 2.4 for participants who no longer met the criteria for insomnia disorder.[1]

A number of studies have demonstrated a high rate of comorbid medical or mental health conditions with chronic insomnia.[20-22] RCTs have so far found meaningful improvements in insomnia severity among participants with comorbid medical or mental health conditions.[12] Furthermore, in participants with comorbid depressive disorder, it is fairly well documented that digital CBT-I not only reduces complaints of sleep problems but also reduces depressive symptomatology.[13,23] Digital CBT–I has also been demonstrated as a viable intervention for cancer survivors experiencing insomnia,[24,25] for individuals with Parkinson disease and comorbid insomnia,[26] and for individuals with comorbid pain and insomnia.[27] In a recent RCT of digital CBT-I for pregnant women with insomnia, it was found that insomnia severity and sleep quality, as well as symptom severity of depression and anxiety, improved after the intervention period when compared with standard of care.[28]

The question often raised in the discussion of internet delivery of CBT is whether there is value in the addition of therapist support. This is an important question because a digital intervention without therapist support would be preferred over an intervention that requires therapist support, given that they are equally effective, as dissemination of the former would be easier and associated with lower costs. Whether the effects of an intervention changes as a factor of the level of support could also have implications for how digital interventions are implemented, for example, in the context of a stepped care model.[29] There is some evidence to suggest that therapist support is needed to gain the full potential of digital interventions (see, for example, the report by Andersson and Cuijpers[30]). However, few studies have compared digital interventions with and without therapist support in controlled study designs. It is also reasonable to expect that the effects of unguided, fully automated interventions will vary depending on the condition that is being treated.[31] A meta-analysis of both supported and self-guided digital CBT-I demonstrated larger improvements for insomnia severity and sleep efficiency in studies with a higher degree of therapist support.[17] Therapist support can come in many forms; including face-to-face sessions, videoconferences with a therapist, telephone sessions, and email correspondence, among others. One RCT on digital CBT-I demonstrated an added effect of email support, in which 59% of participants in the support condition met the insomnia severity index criteria for response at 6-month follow-up, compared to 32% in the no-support condition.[32] The support condition in that study consisted of emails aimed at reminding and motivating the participants, advice on participants sleep scheduling (confer sleep restriction), as well as support aimed at clearing up common misconceptions' intrinsic to the insomnia disorder. An average of 40 minutes of support was added to the digital CBT-I intervention, which may indicate a significant potential for reducing costs compared to the traditional six to eight sessions in face-to-face treatment. There are also studies that have demonstrated improved adherence to target behaviors in insomnia treatment through support by means of automated reminders.[33] However, there is potential for further development of personalized automated support in digital CBT-I, in the form of tailor-made feedback and encouragement to increase user engagement and adherence to the intervention.

Although meta-analyses indicate that digital CBT-I leads to improved sleep and daytime functioning with effect sizes comparable to those typically obtained with face-to-face treatment,[17,18] there are very few trials that have directly compared automated digital interventions with face-to-face treatment. One trial compared guided digital CBT-I with individual face-to-face CBT-I (n = 30 in each group) and demonstrated superior effects of face-to-face treatment on reduction of insomnia symptoms and improved sleep-wake patterns.[34] In another noninferiority trial, fully automated digital CBT-I was compared with face-to-face treatment ($n \approx 50$ in each group) and demonstrated superior effects of the face-to-face approach in terms of reducing insomnia severity at 9-week follow-up.[35] In particular, 52% of participants in the face-to-face group were in remission at 9-week follow-up, compared to 18% in the digital CBT-I group, which represent a statistically and clinically significant 34% difference in the proportion of participants in remission. However, the difference in insomnia severity between the groups at 6-month follow-up did not differ significantly from the noninferiority margin. In both of the previously mentioned trials, guided and fully automated digital CBT-I were associated with large effect size improvements on insomnia symptoms among participants.[34,35] Although the limited data available suggest some advantage for face-to-face over digital in the short term, additional research is needed to clarify the effect of fully automated digital CBT-I compared to face-to-face CBT-I on sleep and functional health outcomes.

It is reasonable to expect that digital CBT-I will not be suitable for everyone. Self-help solutions such as internet-based or digital programs should be organized in the larger context of a stepped care approach.[20] This would ensure that those who do not benefit from such interventions, or for other reasons are believed to have an unacceptable risk of undesirable effects of fully automated programs, are provided a suitable alternative intervention.[29] Indeed, one study indicated that introducing a stepped care pathway in routine practice at a behavioral medicine sleep clinic, with fully automated digital CBT-I as the entry level intervention, increased service efficiency by 69%.[36] RCTs are needed to evaluate the efficacy of such stepped care CBT-I approaches. Further, in a proof-of-concept study, Forsell and colleagues[37] investigated the usefulness of an adaptive treatment strategy in therapist-guided digital CBT-I in an RCT, in which treatment intensity was increased for participants deemed to be at risk of failing to respond to treatment. Increased treatment intensity entailed telephone support, printed materials via regular mail, and/or increased text message reminders. The adaptive treatment strategy increased treatment effects for at-risk patients and reduced the number of failed treatments, compared to a control group that received standard of care.[37] The authors argued that adaptive treatment strategies may be an important step in moving from stepped care into accelerated care to minimize the duration of patient suffering and time spent in unhelpful low-intensity interventions. Adaptive treatment strategies should be further developed in terms of identifying both the effective outcome prediction algorithms and the appropriate components of added treatment intensity.

MOBILE DELIVERY OF COGNITIVE BEHAVIORAL THERAPY FOR INSOMNIA

With mounting evidence for the efficacy of digitally delivered CBT-I[4,38] and the ubiquity of smartphone use,[39] mobile health applications (*apps*) could serve as another route in the stepped care model to increase access to evidence-based interventions for insomnia.[40,41] As smartphones are typically carried on the person and rarely turned off, apps offer convenient, private access to treatment, allowing patients to take advantage of opportunities to engage with content when they may not otherwise do so (e.g., in public). Although there are some available apps built on evidence-based principles for improving insomnia symptoms, not all available apps, particularly free apps, are created equal. Yu and colleagues[42] conducted a review of freely available smartphone apps for insomnia and found that few of these apps use evidence-based principles to help users practice the behavioral and cognitive skills shown to best manage insomnia. In addition to potential quality control issues with app content, few of the available programs have been formally tested in research studies.[43] This lack of validation and rigorous testing potentially puts users at risk for receiving an app-generated treatment plan that is based on inaccurate or invalid data. Therefore it may be important for providers to review an app before suggesting it to their patients. In this section, we highlight the available apps using evidence-based cognitive-behavioral principles for treating insomnia and the current state of their efficacy.

As described previously, digitally delivered treatments vary based on the level of clinician involvement, level of automatization, costs, and scalability. Similar to internet-delivered treatment options, available apps fall into these categories or as companions to other digital platforms (Table 97.1). The first category includes mobile apps that augment in-person CBT-I, typically as a resource for patients to store sleep diary entries, track treatment progress, review educational materials, and practice relaxation strategies outside of session. Potential advantages of these apps are to increase accessibility of

Table 97.1 Examples of Mobile Apps Delivering Insomnia Treatment by Category

Example Apps	Description	Intended User	Outcome, Feasibility, Usability, or Case Studies
Support Face-to-Face Treatment			
CBT-i Coach	Used in conjunction with face-to-face CBT-I	Individuals with insomnia	Reilly, Robinson[47]; Koffel, Kuhn[46]; Babson, Ramo[44]
Win-Win aSleep [WWaS]	Used in conjunction with face-to-face CBT-I	Older adults with insomnia	Chen, Hung[45]
Guided Programs with Clinical Support			
interactive Resilience Enhancing Sleep Tactics (iREST)	Bidirectional exchange of data to clinician portal for delivery of a just-in-time adaptive intervention based on brief behavioral therapy for insomnia	Patients with sleep disorders under provider care. Focus on military populations	Pulantara, Parmanto[48]; Pulantara, Parmanto[49]
Companion App to Web-Based Program			
Sleepio	Companion app to fully automated subscription-based CBT-I web program	Adults with insomnia symptoms	See studies noted in internet-delivered section
Fully Automated			
SleepRate	A fully automated, subscription-based CBT-I program	Individuals with sleep difficulties	Eyal and Baharav[51] (abstract supplement); Baharav and Niejadlik[55] (abstract supplement)
Night Owl: Sleep Coach	Fully automated delivery of a 56-day CBT-I program	Individuals with insomnia symptoms	Harbison, Cole[52] (abstract supplement)
Sleep Ninja	Fully automated delivery of a 6-week CBT-I informed program	Adolescents with insomnia or sleep disturbance	Werner-Seidler, Wong[56]
SleepCare (commercial version called Lyla Coach)	Fully automated delivery of a 6- to 7-week CBT-I program	Adults with insomnia	Horsch, Lancee[54]; Horsch, Spruit[57]

materials and improve adherence to recommendations. These apps are found to be user friendly and perceived as helpful[44]; however, they may need further tailoring for use by older adults.[45] A small RCT comparing CBT-I alone to CBT-I with the addition of an app (CBT-i Coach) found that app users consistently used the app as intended, and integration of the app into treatment did not compromise the therapy.[46] Although a nonsignificant finding, there also was a large effect for app use being related to better adherence to therapist recommendations. More recently, Reilly and colleagues[47] published outcomes of a pilot trial assessing the use of CBT-I Coach as a self-management tool for insomnia in veterans. Although originally intended to be used in conjunction with provider-delivered CBT-I, this study used the app with a self-management guide that instructed the participant on what materials to review or features to use from the app during each week of the 6-week intervention. Significant improvements in insomnia severity and overall sleep quality and sleep-related functioning were reported by those who completed treatment, suggesting that this app could be used to manage insomnia without the aid of a therapist, thereby reducing clinical resources.

The second category includes mobile apps that interface with a clinician portal from where clinicians can review patient data and send individualized recommendations, such as sleep restriction and stimulus control prescriptions, to the patient's app. This category reduces the need for in-person appointments while simultaneously providing clinician monitoring. An example of this type of system is the interactive Resilience Enhancing Sleep Tactics (iREST) platform.[48,49] A usability study of this platform found that participants rated the platform as easy to use and learn, and participants used the app daily to record their sleep.[49] Results from an open pilot investigation of iREST in a sample of military personnel and veterans with sleep disturbance revealed a significant reduction in self-reported insomnia symptoms from pre- to postintervention along with improvements in depression, anxiety, and PTSD symptoms.[48] Notably, the treatment response and remission rates observed in this study were comparable to those found in other trials of provider-delivered CBT-I.

Along the continuum of accessibility, the third category of mobile interventions includes fully automated models that do not require clinician input. Apps within this category may stand alone (e.g., Sleeprate, Sleep Ninja) or serve as a companion to internet-based CBT-I programs (e.g., Sleepio). Typically, these programs are structured to guide the user through modules and daily tasks and to provide recommendations based on sleep diary entries or other user input. This category of apps has no clinical oversight but has the advantage of reaching diverse individuals who may not otherwise have access to treatment (i.e., individuals living in rural locations, shift workers). These types of apps are viewed favorably in feasibility studies[50] and results from pre- to postintervention show improvements in sleep outcomes (see the reviews by Eyal and Baharav,[51] Harbison and colleagues,[52] and Kang and colleagues[53]). Horsch and colleagues[54] were among the first to conduct an RCT investigating a fully automated app delivering CBT-I (SleepCare, recently transformed to a commercial version called "Lyla Coach"). They found significant interaction effects in favor of the app compared to the waitlist condition for improving the main outcomes of insomnia severity and sleep efficiency in adults with mild insomnia symptoms. Together, the outcomes from these pilot investigations support the applicability of using automated app-delivered insomnia treatment and show promise in benefitting users.

Although the past few years have seen a rise in published studies on app-based programs for sleep disturbances, most research on app-only programs remains in the pilot or feasibility stage. The exception is the evidence for the internet-delivered programs, described in the previous section, that can also be offered through an app (e.g., Sleepio or Shuti, now called Somyrst). Additional trials are needed to ensure the efficacy and safety of fully automated apps in diverse patient populations.

TELEHEALTH DELIVERY OF COGNITIVE BEHAVIORAL THERAPY FOR INSOMNIA

Widespread implementation of CBT-I is limited by the lack of clinicians who are trained in this treatment.[58] Although increasing the number of certified providers is critical, additional strategies to increase access to care, particularly for patients in more rural locations where providers are particularly scarce, is paramount. One means of increasing access to CBT-I is to use telemedicine, defined as "the use of electronic communications and information technology to provide and support health care when distance separates the provider from the patient."[59] Although there are several types of telehealth, CBT-I delivery fits into clinical video telehealth (CVT), in which video technology is used to connect the patient and provider, as opposed to face-to-face treatment. CVT is increasingly used to provide mental health services remotely, known as telemental health. Studies have examined the feasibility of medical management via video teleconferencing (e.g., see the reports by Nieves and colleagues[60] and Himle and colleagues[61]), and several noninferiority studies on telemental health have demonstrated comparable outcomes to that of in-person treatment.[62-64] Because of the consistency of results across mental health conditions and types of treatment, there is now a general consensus that telemental health treatment is not inferior to in-person treatment, resulting in a move away from further head-to-head studies. Although it may be argued that this type of global statement is premature, it represents the thinking of many in the field. Few studies, however, have addressed the telemedicine delivery of an intervention targeted to chronic insomnia.

The first published study of CVT delivery of insomnia treatment was a small, uncontrolled pilot study of CBT for combined insomnia and depression.[65] As such it was not specifically CBT-I. Adults age 50 and above with insomnia and depression were recruited from rural primary care clinics. Treatment was delivered using Skype and consisted of 10, 50-minute weekly sessions. Eighteen patients were enrolled in treatment, but only five completed the study because of several factors. There were improvements in both insomnia and depression posttreatment. The working alliance was also rated as being comparable to face-to-face therapy. A subsequent study[65a] reported on the results of a larger trial of 40 participants randomized to receive combined CBT for insomnia and depression or a usual care condition. CBT treatment led to significant improvements in both insomnia and depression compared to usual care at posttreatment and 3-month follow-up. Similar results were found in an uncontrolled case series of group CBT-I delivered by CVT in a general veteran population.[66] These studies demonstrate the CBT delivered by CVT is associated with significant improvements and highlights the potential of using technology to reach patients in rural settings, where access to health care providers may be limited.

An important next question is how the efficacy of CBT-I delivered by CVT compares to other modalities of treatment delivery. Holmqvist and colleagues conducted a clinical trial in which 73 adults with insomnia were randomized to telehealth or web-based CBT-I.[67] Both treatment groups demonstrated significant improvements in insomnia severity, with some evidence of larger effects in the telehealth treatment group. However, patient preferences were stronger for web-based delivery given the greater convenience of this format. A final study compared group CBT-I delivered by CVT to face-to-face treatment for veterans with PTSD in a randomized, noninferiority trial.[68] This study is the only one thus far to formally test whether telehealth delivery of treatment is inferior to face-to-face treatment. Although only preliminary results of the trial have been reported, they suggest that there is not a loss of treatment efficacy in using CVT to deliver care. This finding is consistent with a growing body of evidence that clinical services can be delivered using video telehealth technology without a loss of effectiveness for patients with insomnia[65,67] and other disorders.[62,64]

In summary, telehealth delivery of CBT-I is a means of increasing access to evidence-based treatment for insomnia by reducing barriers such as a lack of trained providers in many locations. Patients and providers can increasingly feel confident that they can use these technologies without sacrificing clinical improvement. It would be helpful to have more controlled trials comparing telehealth CBT-I to in-person treatment, although as stated previously, the telemental health field as a whole is moving away from these studies. Future studies should also examine whether certain individuals are more suited for this modality than others. For example, patient preferences may be an important determinant success in each approach. Also, there may be ways to use the telehealth technology to modify the delivery and/or content of CBT-I components.

SUMMARY

Given the high prevalence of insomnia, there has been a tremendous growth in the interest of using technology to deliver CBT-I to address the limited availability and scalability of face-to-face treatment. Internet, mobile, and telehealth technologies have received the most attention, although there are other means of using technology to deliver care. Evidence suggests that treatment delivered via these means is efficacious and effective in numerous RCTs. What is less certain is how these modalities stack up against face-to-face treatment, as there have been few direct comparisons. The limited evidence suggests that technological delivery is only slightly less effective, or even not inferior, compared to in-person treatment. The advantages of increased access to care may outweigh any disadvantages in terms of reduced efficacy, particularly in the context of stepped care approaches. However, much more work is to be done. In parallel to determining which technological treatments "work," it is important to determine for whom so that individuals can be matched to the type of intervention from which they are most likely to benefit. Digital delivery of CBT-I has a bright future ahead and will help to increase the accessibility of proven treatments to match the number of patients in need.

CLINICAL PEARL

The demand for CBT-I outweighs the availability of trained providers. Technology-delivered CBT-I, via internet platforms, mobile devices, or CVT, is a means of increasing access to treatment and may serve as an important tool in the stepped care pathway. Technological means of treatment delivery may also reduce costs of treatment, although this has not been directly tested. There are not yet sufficient data to guide treatment decisions of which patients would most benefit from each approach, so selection of modality should be made in discussion with patients. Although still burgeoning, evidence indicates that treatment delivered via these means is efficacious and effective for improving insomnia severity. If their patients express openness to technology, providers may consider incorporating digitally delivered CBT-I in their treatment plan.

SELECTED READINGS

Espie CA, Emsley R, Kyle SD, et al. Effect of digital cognitive behavioral therapy for insomnia on health, psychological well-being, and sleep-related quality of life: a randomized clinical trial. *JAMA Psychiatry*. 2019;76:21–30.

Gehrman P, Bellamy SL, Medvedeva E, et al. Telehealth delivery of group CBT-I is non-inferior to in-person treatment in veterans with PTSD. *Sleep*. 2018;41(Suppl):A141–A142.

Holmqvist M, Vincent N, Walsh K. Web- vs. telehealth-based delivery of cognitive behavioral therapy for insomnia: a randomized controlled trial. *Sleep Med*. 2014;15(2):187–195.

Horsch CHG, Lancee J, Griffioen-Both F, et al. Mobile Phone-delivered cognitive behavioral therapy for insomnia: a randomized waitlist controlled trial. *J Med Internet Res*. 2017;19(4):e70.

Hsieh C, Rezayat T, Zeidler MR. Telemedicine and the management of insomnia. *Sleep Med Clin*. 2020;15(3):383–390.

Kallestad H, Langsrud K, Vedaa Ø, Stiles T, Vethe D, Lydersen S, et al. 0371 A randomized noninferiority trial comparing cognitive behavior therapy for insomnia (cbt-i) delivered by a therapist or via a fully automated online treatment program. *Sleep*. 2018;41(suppl 1):A142–A.

Koffel E, Bramoweth AD, Ulmer CS. Increasing access to and utilization of cognitive behavioral therapy for insomnia (CBT-I): a narrative review. *J Gen Intern Med*. 2018;33(6):955–962.

Lancee J, van Straten A, Morina N, Kaldo V, Kamphuis JH. Guided online or face-to-face cognitive behavioral treatment for insomnia: a randomized wait-list controlled trial. *Sleep*. 2016;39:183–191.

Luik AI, Kyle SD, Espie CA. Digital Cognitive Behavioral Therapy (dCBT) for insomnia: a state-of-the-science review. *Curr Sleep Med Rep*. 2017;3:48–56.

Luik AI, van der Zweerde T, van Straten A, Lancee J. Digital delivery of cognitive behavioral therapy for insomnia. *Curr Psychiatry Rep*. 2019;21:50.

Ritterband LM, Thorndike FP, Ingersoll KS, et al. Effect of a web-based cognitive behavior therapy for insomnia intervention with 1-year follow-up: a randomized clinical trial. *JAMA Psychiatry*. 2017;74:68–75.

Zhang C, Yang L, Liu S, Xu Y, Zheng H, Zhang B. One-week self-guided internet cognitive behavioral treatments for insomnia in adults with situational insomnia during the COVID-19 outbreak. *Front Neurosci*. 2021;14:622749.

A complete reference list can be found online at ExpertConsult.com.

Chapter 98

Pharmacologic Treatment I: Therapeutic Approaches and Implementation

Suzanne M. Bertisch; Daniel J. Buysse

Chapter Highlights

- Several guidelines support the use of benzodiazepine receptor agonists as one of the first-line agents for chronic insomnia disorder in adults.
- Guidelines also support use of other US Food and Drug Administration (FDA)–approved agents from other medication classes, including melatonin receptor agonists, tricyclic antidepressants (i.e., low-dose doxepin), and dual orexin receptor antagonists for chronic insomnia disorder in adults.
- Over-the-counter agents such as antihistamines and dietary supplements, including melatonin, have little evidence supporting their use in the treatment of chronic insomnia disorder.

A MODEL OF SLEEP-WAKE REGULATION RELEVANT TO SLEEP-PROMOTING DRUGS

Findings from the basic and clinical neuroscience of sleep-wake regulation underlie the pharmacologic targets of hypnotic medications. One sleep-regulation model in Figure 98.1 depicts a simplified circuit diagram describing the control of sleep and wakefulness as the dynamic interaction among several neural systems.[1] The ascending activity of monoaminergic neurons in the rostral brainstem and the caudal hypothalamus and the wake-promoting activity arising from the parabrachial nucleus and cholinergic regions generate wakefulness and arousal states.[2] These wake-promoting regions are excited by orexin-A and orexin-B (hypocretin-1; hypocretin-2) neurons in the perifornical lateral hypothalamus (LHA), which also produce glutamate and dynorphin.[3] At sleep onset, gamma-aminobutyric acid (GABA) and galaninergic neurons in the ventrolateral preoptic (VLPO) area and median preoptic nucleus (MnPO) of the hypothalamus inhibit the wake-promoting areas in the caudal hypothalamus and brainstem. Nuclei in the basal forebrain, parafacial zone, and cortex promote sleep. In addition, the "sleep switch" model proposes that mutual inhibition of the LHA and VLPO/MnPO areas is in dynamic equilibrium to ensure stable sleep-wake states (see Chapter 7).[4,5]

Sleep-promoting medications may affect sleep-wake regulatory systems at several levels. Benzodiazepine receptor agonists (BzRAs) may directly affect the sleep-wake state-switching system and have direct cortical, thalamic, and brainstem effects because of the widespread distribution of gamma-aminobutyric acid type A ($GABA_A$) receptors. Sedating antidepressant and antipsychotic medications, through their activity on monoaminergic systems, affect corticolimbic systems and brainstem-hypothalamic arousal systems. Antihistamines antagonize histamine-1 (H_1) receptors in the hypothalamus and cortex that receive projections from the tuberomammillary nucleus. Melatonin and melatonin receptor agonists, through their effects on melatonin 1 and 2 (MT_1 and MT_2) receptors, influence the "wake signal" from the suprachiasmatic nucleus and circadian timing system. Orexin antagonists[6] inhibit orexin/hypocretin's effect on brainstem/hypothalamic arousal centers, and 5-HT_2 antagonists most likely have corticolimbic and brainstem sites of action. Thus sleep-promoting drugs achieve their effects through very different actions on the sleep-wake regulatory system.[7]

TRENDS IN PRESCRIPTION MEDICATION USED FOR INSOMNIA

Pharmacoepidemiology

Data from the National Health and Nutrition Examination Survey[8] and National Ambulatory Medical Care[9] indicate that zolpidem and trazodone are the two most commonly prescribed medications for insomnia in the United States. Prescriptions for zolpidem increased during the 1990s through the early 2010s, with about 3.5% of US adults reporting prescription medication use for insomnia in the past month.[8] More current data from a large national pharmacy database of individuals with employer-provided insurance in the United States suggest that zolpidem prescriptions have declined from 4.6% in 2011 to 2.5% in 2018, whereas trazodone rates have modestly increased from 1.3% to 1.8% over the same period.[10] As these data indicate, off-label prescribing of medications for

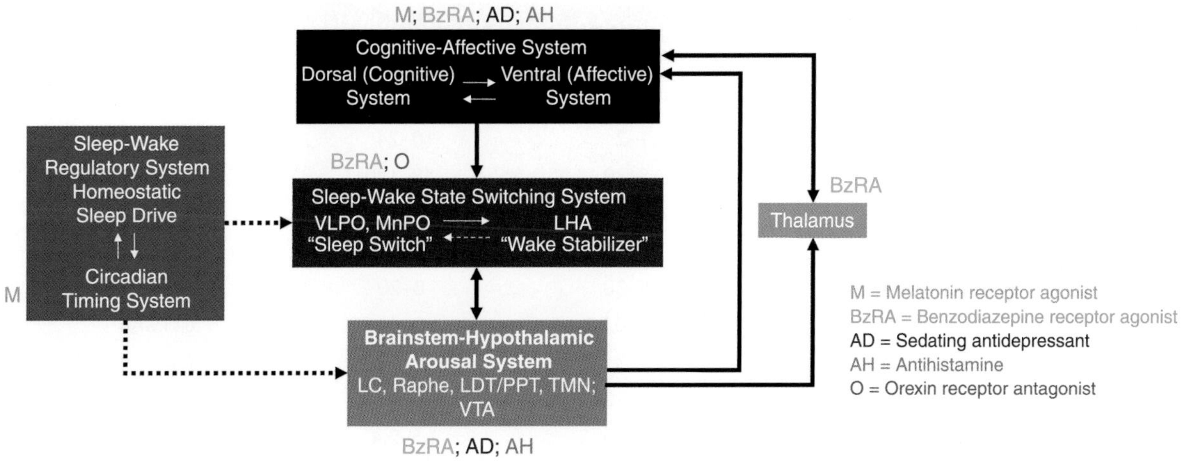

Figure 98.1 *Solid arrows* indicate direct anatomic or physiologic pathways. *Dotted arrows* indicate indirect pathways. LC, Locus coeruleus; LDT, laterodorsal pontine tegmentum; LHA, lateral hypothalamus perifornical area; PPT, pedunculopontine tegmentum; TMN, tuberomammillary nucleus of the posterior hypothalamus; VLPO, ventrolateral preoptic area; VTA, ventral tegmental area. (Adapted from Buysse DJ, Germain A, Hall M, et al. A neurobiological model of insomnia. *Drug Discov Today Dis Models*. 2011;8:129–137.

insomnia is common, with one study in Canada estimating that 83% of trazodone prescriptions, 36% of doxepin prescriptions, 23% of amitriptyline prescriptions, and 3% of mirtazapine prescriptions written by primary care physicians are for insomnia.[11]

Additionally, further evidence suggests that rates of use of over-the-counter (OTC) medications for sleep, such as diphenhydramine, may be as high as 19% in the general adult population[8] in a given month, with rates of melatonin use, particularly among children,[12] increasing over the past several years. Prescription medications for sleep are frequently taken in combination with alcohol,[13] opiates,[14,15] and other drugs, leading to increased toxicity and mortality. Despite the common use of medications to treat insomnia, significant concerns remain regarding their use, including limited data on short- and long-term efficacy and safety. Because many drugs commonly used off-label or available OTC have not been rigorously evaluated for insomnia, vital information regarding appropriate dose, efficacy, and side effects remains sparse (see also Chapter 53).

MEDICATION CLASSES

Benzodiazepine Receptor Agonists

Pharmacodynamics and Receptor Pharmacology. BzRA drugs include benzodiazepines (e.g., temazepam, triazolam) and nonbenzodiazepine benzodiazepine receptor agonists (e.g., eszopiclone, zaleplon, zolpidem). BzRAs bind to specific $GABA_A$ receptors, which produce sedative/hypnotic, anxiolytic, amnestic, myorelaxant, and anticonvulsant effects. The effects of each agent depend on their specificity for the different $GABA_A$ receptor subtypes responsible for these effects.[16] For example, zolpidem is relatively specific for $GABA_A$ receptors containing $\alpha 1$ subunits, which give it relatively greater specificity for sedative/hypnotic versus other effects (e.g., anxiolytic).[17] Although some BzRAs are US Food and Drug Administration (FDA)–approved for insomnia and others for anxiety, they have similar pharmacodynamic properties. Thus clonazepam and lorazepam are sometimes used as hypnotics when anxiolytic properties and a longer duration of action are desired. Concurrent use of BzRA agents for different indications (e.g., lorazepam for anxiety, temazepam for insomnia) can lead to additive effects.[18]

Pharmacokinetics. Clinical differences between the effects of specific BzRAs primarily result from their pharmacokinetic properties, particularly terminal elimination half-life. Most BzRAs used for insomnia have a rapid absorption and onset of action (Table 98.1).[19] More slowly absorbed BzRAs (e.g., oxazepam) are less useful for insomnia. Elimination half-lives of hypnotic BzRAs vary widely, with predictable clinical effects. For example, with a half-life of 1 hour, zaleplon reduces sleep-onset latency (SOL) but has no impact on wake after sleep onset (WASO); flurazepam and its metabolite have half-lives up to 120 hours, resulting in reduced WASO and greater potential for residual daytime sleepiness.

Effects on Insomnia. The efficacy of BzRAs has been established in randomized controlled trials (RCTs) that demonstrate short-term, clinically significant improvements in SOL, WASO, sleep efficiency, total sleep time (TST), and sleep quality, with some heterogeneity by duration of action (Table 98.1).[17,20] Additional double-blind RCTs have demonstrated the efficacy of BzRAs for up to 6 months of nightly[21] or intermittent use[22] and up to 12 months in open-label studies.[20,23]

Side Effects. Relative contraindications to BzRA use include alcohol or sedative abuse/dependence, severe pulmonary failure, hepatic failure, and hypersensitivity to the drug class. BzRAs should be used with caution in patients with depression and in older adults.[24] Adverse effects of BzRAs include morning sedation, anterograde amnesia, and impaired balance, in addition to a higher risk of falls[25] and hip fractures,[26] though data have been inconsistent.[27,28] BzRAs are also associated with sleep-related behaviors such

Table 98.1 Characteristics of Benzodiazepine Receptor Agonists Commonly Used for Insomnia

Generic Name	Receptor Binding Specificity	Dose Range (mg)	Elimination Half-Life (hr)	Metabolism
Estazolam	Nonspecific	1–2	10–24	CYP3A
Flurazepam	Nonspecific	15–30	48–120[a]	CYP3A4
Lorazepam[b]	Nonspecific	0.5–2	8–12	CYP3A4
Quazepam	Nonspecific	7.5–15	39–73[a]	Not available
Temazepam	Nonspecific	15–30	8–20	None
Triazolam	Nonspecific	0.125–0.25	2–6	CYP3A4
Eszopiclone	$GABA_A$, α1,2,3	1–3	6	CYP3A4, CYP2E1
Zaleplon	$GABA_A$, α1	5–20	1	Minor: CYP3A4
Zolpidem	$GABA_A$, α1	5–10	1.5–2.4	CYP3A4, CYP2C9
Zolpidem extended-release	$GABA_A$, α1	6.25–12.5	1.6–4.5	CYP3A4, CYP2C9
Zolpidem sublingual tablet	$GABA_A$, α1	5–10	1.5–2.4	CYP3A4, CYP2C9
Zolpidem oral spray	$GABA_A$, α1	5–10	1.5–2.4	CYP3A4, CYP2C9
Zolpidem sublingual lozenge	$GABA_A$, α1	1.75–3.5	1.5–2.4	CYP3A4, CYP2C9

Adapted from 6th edition, Chapter 87.
[a]Refers to elimination half-life of active metabolite.
[b]This medication is not approved by the US Food and Drug Administration (FDA) for the treatment of insomnia.
CYP, Cytochrome P-450 (letters and numbers refer to specific CYP enzymes); $GABA_A$, gamma-aminobutyric acid, type A receptor complex.

as sleepwalking, sleep eating, driving, and sexual behavior[19] and have resulted in injuries from falls, car accidents, and accidental overdoses, which led to an FDA-issued black box warning for the sleep medications eszopiclone, zaleplon, and zolpidem.[29] Additional concerns regarding BzRAs include rebound insomnia, withdrawal, and dependence. Abuse can occur with benzodiazepines and nonbenzodiazepine benzodiazepine receptor agonists, particularly in individuals with a history of alcohol or other sedative abuse.[30,31] Increased risk of cognitive impairment, dementia,[32] and mortality have been associated with use of BzRAs at therapeutic doses in some studies,[33] though confounding by indication and the effects of comorbidities likely influence these findings.[34,35] See Chapter 99 for a further discussion of side effects.

Sedating Antidepressants

Over two dozen drugs are FDA-approved as antidepressants in the United States, and several of these are commonly used for the treatment of insomnia. These include the tricyclic antidepressants (TCAs) doxepin, trimipramine, and amitriptyline and the heterocyclic drugs trazodone and mirtazapine. Only low-dose doxepin is FDA-approved for insomnia. Sedating antidepressants affect receptors for multiple neurotransmitters in the ascending arousal system (histamine, acetylcholine, serotonin, and norepinephrine). Detailed pharmacokinetic properties of these drugs are summarized in Table 98.2. These medications are used off-label for insomnia at doses lower than those indicated for antidepressant or anxiolytic effects. Most data regarding the effects of antidepressant drugs on human sleep come from studies in patients with depression. Formal dose-ranging studies have not been conducted to determine the optimal doses in insomnia, with the exception of doxepin.

Trazodone

Pharmacodynamics and Receptor Pharmacology. Trazodone is a relatively weak but specific inhibitor of the serotonin reuptake transporter with minimal affinity for norepinephrine or dopamine reuptake. Trazodone also inhibits 5-hydroxytryptamine (serotonin; $5\text{-HT})_{1A}$, 5-HT_{1c}, and 5-HT_2 receptors. It has practically no affinity for M_1 receptors, but it does have moderate H_1 receptor antagonism. Finally, trazodone is a relatively weak antagonist of α_2 adrenergic receptors and a somewhat more potent antagonist of α_1 receptors.[36,37]

Pharmacokinetics. Trazodone is rapidly absorbed, with peak plasma concentrations occurring 1 to 2 hours after oral doses. Like TCAs, it is highly (85%–95%) protein-bound. Trazodone's half-life is approximately 5 to 9 hours.

Effects on Sleep and Insomnia. Studies of trazodone effects on human sleep have been limited by small sample sizes, particularly in polysomnographic (PSG) studies, and by study designs that have typically included sleep only as a secondary endpoint. Given limited data from clinical trials evaluating the efficacy of trazodone for insomnia and measurable apparent risk of harms, recent guidelines recommend that clinicians not use trazodone to treat sleep-onset or sleep-maintenance insomnia (versus no treatment) in adults without significant comorbidity.[38] A meta-analysis that included seven RCTs of trazodone and included patients with comorbidities (e.g., major depressive disorder, Alzheimer disease), demonstrated improvements in perceived sleep quality and modest reductions in nighttime awakenings, but no other clinically meaningful changes in objective sleep measures.[39]

Table 98.2 Pharmacokinetic Properties of Sedating Antidepressant Drugs

Generic Name	Drug Class	Dose Range, Hypnotic (mg)[a]	Elimination Half-Life, hr (range)	Metabolism, CYP Enzymes
Trazodone[b]	Phenylpiperazine	25–150	9 (3–14)	3A4, 2D6
Mirtazapine[b]	Noradrenergic and specific serotonergic antidepressant	15–30	25 (13–40)	3A4, 2D6, 1A2
Doxepin	Tricyclic	3, 6	20 (10–30)	Major: 2D6, 2C19; Minor: 1A2, 3A4
Amitriptyline[b]	Tricyclic	25–150	30 (5–45)	Major: 2D6, 2C19; Minor: 1A2, 3A4

Adapted from 6th edition, Chapter 42.
[a]Except doxepin, hypnotic doses are based on published studies and common clinical practice without formal dose-ranging studies for this indication.
[b]This medication is not approved by the US Food and Drug Administration (FDA) for the treatment of insomnia.
CYP, Cytochrome P-450 (letters and numbers refer to specific CYP enzymes).

Side Effects. Trazodone can produce side effects, including orthostatic hypotension, lightheadedness, and weakness.[37] Unlike TCAs, trazodone does not have anticholinergic side effects,[40] but it can have antihistiminergic effects such as weight gain. A potentially rare, but serious effect of trazodone is priapism—sustained painful erections in men. The risk appears to be higher in men over 40 (1.5 versus 2.9 per 100,000 person-years)[41] and earlier in the course of treatment. Meta-chlorophenylpiperazine, the metabolite of trazodone, can contribute to serotonin syndrome. Concerns regarding abuse potential are minimal.[42] Trazodone does not worsen sleep-disordered breathing.[43] Although no information has been published regarding its long-term effects on sleep, rebound insomnia has been observed after several weeks of use.[44]

Mirtazapine

Pharmacodynamics and Receptor Pharmacology. Mirtazapine is a very weak inhibitor of noradrenergic reuptake and has no effect on serotonin reuptake.[45] However, similar to TCAs, it increases serotonergic and noradrenergic neurotransmission through blockade of α_2 autoreceptors and heteroreceptors.[46] It also has prominent antagonist activity at 5-HT_2, 5-HT_3, H_1, and α_1 adrenergic receptors,[47] which may contribute to its hypnotic effects.

Pharmacokinetics. Mirtazapine is rapidly absorbed, undergoes extensive first-pass metabolism, and is about 85% protein-bound, yielding bioavailability of about 50%. Mirtazapine has an elimination half-life of approximately 20 to 40 hours.[48]

Effects on Sleep and Insomnia. Mirtazapine is reported to be subjectively sedating in clinical studies of depression.[49] In PSG studies in healthy adults and adults with depression, mirtazapine decreased SOL, continuity, and TST.[50,51] Although potentially promising, mirtazapine has not yet been adequately evaluated as a hypnotic. The S(+) enantiomer of mirtazapine, esmirtazapine, was investigated in an RCT of 419 patients with insomnia. The groups randomized to 3.0 and 4.5 mg of esmirtazapine had significantly reduced WASO and number of awakenings, increased TST, and improved insomnia severity at 6 weeks compared with placebo.[52]

Side Effects. In addition to commonly causing sedation, mirtazapine is associated with dry mouth, increased appetite, weight gain (acutely and over the long term), and elevated serum cholesterol. Clinical observations suggest that mirtazapine may be less sedating at doses >30 mg per day than at lower doses. This is hypothesized to be related to greater noradrenergic effects relative to antihistiminergic and serotonergic effects at lower doses.[53] Mirtazapine has not been associated with serious toxicity or death in overdose.

Tricyclic Antidepressant Drugs

TCAs share a cyclic core structure and are classified according to their different side-chain structures as tertiary or secondary amines. Tertiary TCAs are generally more sedating than secondary TCAs.

Pharmacodynamics and Receptor Pharmacology. TCAs interact with receptors of a variety of neurotransmitters, including serotonin, norepinephrine, acetylcholine, and histamine. Amitriptyline is the most anticholinergic of all antidepressants, and doxepin is a more potent antihistamine than many drugs marketed as antihistamines, including diphenhydramine. Doxepin at low doses is also highly selective for this effect, with more than seven times greater affinity for the H_1 receptor relative to any other receptor type.[54,55] As a result, low doses of doxepin (3 and 6 mg) can achieve selective H_1 blockade, with no serotonergic, adrenergic, and cholinergic effects.[56-59] Like other tricyclic drugs, doxepin is not scheduled by the Drug Enforcement Administration (DEA).

Pharmacokinetics. Doxepin is rapidly absorbed (fasting T-max 3.5 hours), undergoes extensive first-pass metabolism, and is about 80% protein-bound. Doxepin has an elimination half-life of approximately 15 hours.[60,61] Doxepin is highly lipophilic, ensuring high distribution and concentration in the brain. Ingestion with a high-fat meal increases the bioavailability and delays the peak plasma concentration by ≈3 hours.

Effects on Insomnia and Sleep. Doxepin is FDA-approved for insomnia at doses of 3 to 6 mg and for depression at doses more than 10-fold higher (i.e., 100 to 200 mg). Guidelines recommend doxepin for treating sleep maintenance insomnia based on objective improvements in TST, WASO, and small-to-moderate improvements in sleep quality compared with placebo.[38] Studies using low doses of doxepin (1, 3, and 6 mg) also demonstrated improved sleep efficiency,[56-59] particularly the last quarter of the night, without demonstrable effect on next-day alertness psychomotor performance. The PSG effects of TCAs in depression have been studied extensively and indicate reduced SOL and WASO and increased sleep efficiency from amitriptyline[62-64] and trimipramine.[65,66] In contrast, secondary TCAs (e.g., desipramine) have little or no effect on sleep onset or continuity in depressed patients.[62,63]

Side Effects. Anticholinergic side effects of high/moderate doses of doxepin and amitriptyline include dry mouth, constipation, and urinary retention. More serious effects include precipitation of ocular crises in patients with narrow-angle glaucoma, seizures, and anticholinergic delirium, which are dose-related.[67] Side effects related to antihistaminergic properties include sedation and weight gain. Studies of very low-dose doxepin (1–6 mg) show a low incidence of side effects, with somnolence and headache being the most common.[56–59] Side effects related to α_1 antagonism include orthostatic hypotension with attendant risks of lightheadedness, syncope, and falls. TCAs can cause prolongation of the QRS duration and PR and QT intervals and heart block, although these QT interval effects have not been observed with low-dose doxepin (up to 50 mg) in younger, healthy individuals.[68] TCA overdose causing cardiovascular lethality is largely the result of their α_1 adrenergic receptor antagonism,[69] which can occur at doses as low as 5 to 10 times the therapeutic antidepressant daily dose.[70]

Orexin Antagonists

Orexin (hypocretin) is a peptide neurotransmitter localized to the perifornical neurons of the lateral hypothalamus. Orexinergic neurons have widespread excitatory projections to the brainstem and posterior hypothalamic arousal centers, which are key neuropeptides responsible for generating and maintaining wakefulness.[71-73] Two receptors respond to orexin signaling: orexin 1 receptor (OX_1R) and orexin 2 receptor (OX_2R), and both have partially overlapping nervous system distributions. Dual orexin antagonists (DORAs) are the newest class of medications to be FDA-approved for insomnia disorder.

Pharmacodynamics and Receptor Pharmacology. Suvorexant and lemborexant are potent and selective antagonists of OX_1R and OX_2R.[2] Similar to suvorexant, lemborexant exhibits reversible competitive antagonism to receptors OX_1R and OX_2R but displays higher affinity for OX_2R and faster receptor on/off kinetics.[74]

Pharmacokinetics. Suvorexant's peak concentrations occur at a median T_{max} of 2 hours (30 minutes–6 hours) under fasting conditions. The mean absolute bioavailability of 10 mg is 82%. It is extensively bound (>99%) to plasma proteins and has a terminal half-life of 9 to 12 hours.[6] Lemborexant's peak concentrations occur at 1 to 3 hours, with a terminal half-life of 17 to 19 hours (5- and 10-mg doses, respectively). Lemborexant is primarily metabolized via CYP3A4,[75] and no significant differences in pharmacokinetics have been observed by age, sex, race/ethnicity, or body mass index.[76]

Effects on Insomnia. Guidelines recommend suvorexant at the currently approved FDA doses (10–20 mg) for sleep maintenance insomnia only.[38] This recommendation was based on clinical trial data demonstrating objective improvements in WASO and sleep efficiency and lack of clinically meaningful improvement in subjective or objective SOL. More recent studies of suvorexant have evaluated its efficacy in targeted populations, including older adults with mild-to-moderate Alzheimer disease, for which it is FDA-approved.[77] Two Phase 3 clinical trials have examined the efficacy of lemborexant in chronic insomnia. In a 6-month study, participants randomized to either 5 or 10 mg of lemborexant on average reported a shorter SOL, lower WASO, and greater sleep efficiency.[78] In a 1-month study in women aged 55 years and older and men aged 65 years and older, lemborexant improved SOL, sleep efficiency, and WASO assessed via PSG.[79]

Side Effects. The most common adverse events are somnolence, fatigue, dry mouth, and headache. Other safety concerns for DORAs include potential for residual sedation, rapid onset of somnolence if administered during the daytime, motor impairment, middle-of-the-night balance impairment, driving impairment, and hypnogogic hallucinations.[80,81] The risk of parasomnias is low and unpredictable. Patients should be monitored for cataplexy; reduced orexinergic neurotransmission contributes to this symptom in narcolepsy. Given the stricter FDA policy for hypnotics to use the lowest effective dose to minimize safety risk (e.g., next-day somnolence), 10- and 20-mg strengths of suvorexant have been approved,[80] as opposed to the 30- and 40-mg doses tested in Phase 3 trials.[82] Because of DORA's mechanism of action, drug-drug interactions are of lesser concern relative to other classes of hypnotics, though concurrent use of moderate-to-strong CYP3A inhibitors (e.g., fluconazole) and inducers (e.g., rifampin) should be avoided. Concerns regarding cognitive impairment and addiction potential remain low. Of note, unlike suvorexant, lemborexant has not been studied in patients with moderate-to-severe obstructive sleep apnea or chronic pulmonary obstructive disease.

Melatonin and Melatonin Receptor Agonists

Melatonin (N-acetyl-5-methoxytryptamine) is a hormone endogenously synthesized from tryptophan and produced in the pineal gland, retina, and intestinal tract. Pineal melatonin is normally secreted in a circadian fashion during the dark phase of the circadian cycle. Two synthetic melatonin receptor agonists, ramelteon and tasimelteon, have been tested in clinical studies. Tasimelteon, which has a similar mechanism of action and effects to ramelteon, is FDA-approved for the treatment of non-24-hour sleep-wake disorder[83] and is discussed elsewhere in this volume.

Pharmacodynamics and Receptor Effects. Three subtypes of melatonin receptors have been identified, with MT_1 and MT_2 subtypes being most prevalent in the SCN and retina. MT_1 and MT_2 receptors mediate the phase-shifting effects of melatonin.

Pharmacokinetics. Exogenous oral melatonin is rapidly absorbed, with peak levels occurring in about 30 to 60 minutes.[84,85] It has a 40- to 60-minute elimination half-life. Bioavailability is low, with substantial interindividual variability,[86] with approximately 85% of an oral dose removed by hepatic first-pass metabolism. Ramelteon is also rapidly absorbed, with time to maximal concentration of 0.75 to 1 hour and elimination half-life of 0.8 to 2.5 hours.[87]

Effects on Insomnia. In humans, melatonin has been studied both as a chronobiotic and as a hypnotic. Clinical trials evaluating melatonin have used a wide range of doses, from less than 1 to more than 80 mg. A clear dose-response effect has not been demonstrated. Clinical guidelines suggest against the use of melatonin for adults with sleep-onset or sleep-maintenance insomnia.[38] This recommendation was based on weak evidence deriving from trials of 2-mg doses that demonstrated equivocal data for sleep onset, a paucity of data for sleep-maintenance insomnia, and little evidence about harms. However, the task force noted that among elderly adults, the possible improvement in SOL was equal to potential harms.

Guidelines recommend using 8 mg ramelteon as a treatment for sleep-onset insomnia based on a meta-analysis of PSG evidence from short-term clinical trials demonstrating ramelteon reduces PSG SOL on average by about 9 minutes compared with placebo. This review also reported ramelteon marginally increases TST and does not produce consistent changes in WASO or other sleep continuity measures, with similar results for self-reported data.[38] In a 6-month RCT, compared with placebo, ramelteon modestly improved objective and self-report SOL, but TST and sleep continuity were similar between groups.[88]

Side Effects. Exogenous melatonin has a wide therapeutic index in humans and is typically well tolerated at doses from 0.1 mg to 10 mg.[89] Despite the widespread use of melatonin at low doses, no apparent public health risk has yet emerged. Nonetheless, the longer-term risks remain unknown. The most common side effect of melatonin is headache. Melatonin should not be used during the daytime because of sedation. Caution should be used in patients taking anticoagulants.[38] Melatonin does not lead to dependence or produce withdrawal symptoms.

Melatonin is classified as a dietary supplement in the United States, where its production is regulated differently than foods and medications, which raises safety concerns. As highlighted in a review of 31 available melatonin products, inconsistent standardization of doses (range 83%–478% of the labeled dose; more than 70% varied by at least 10%) and contamination (26% of products contained unlabeled serotonin) are common.[90] Thus consumers should only use melatonin products that are third-party verified (e.g., US Pharmacopeia Convention).

Ramelteon is generally well-tolerated, with the most common side effects including headache, dizziness, somnolence, fatigue, and nausea. Rebound insomnia has not been observed, and there is no evidence for abuse potential. Caution in women of reproductive age should be exercised because of potential hormonal effects and limited long-term studies. Ramelteon has no effect on sleep-disordered breathing in patients with sleep apnea.[91,92]

OTHER PRESCRIPTION AGENTS

Gabapentin

Gabapentin, an alpha-2-delta voltage-gated calcium channel ligand, was initially developed as an anticonvulsant, but investigators subsequently found widespread use in treating neuropathic and fibromyalgia pain, restless legs syndrome, bipolar mood disorder, and insomnia. Gabapentin and its analog pregabalin are consistently associated with improvement in self-reported sleep measures in patients with various pain conditions (e.g., fibromyalgia, neuropathic pain, postherpetic neuralgia, postsurgical pain).[93,94] Although gabapentin is sometimes used clinically for insomnia disorders, including insomnia with pain conditions, and restless legs syndrome or patients who have a contraindication to BzRAs (e.g., history of substance abuse), it has not been systematically evaluated for the treatment of chronic insomnia. The side effects of gabapentin and pregabalin include sedation and fatigue, dizziness, headache, ataxia, peripheral edema, weight gain, and, less commonly, a risk of leukopenia. The FDA has mandated a black box warning for gabapentin for causing respiratory depression, particularly among patients with concurrent use of other central nervous system (CNS) depressants, including opioids, anxiolytics, antidepressants, and antihistamines.

Quetiapine

The second-generation antipsychotic drugs have high rates of somnolence in clinical trials.[95] This effect may be clinically useful in treating insomnia, particularly among patients with severe depression, bipolar disorder, and psychotic disorders. Quetiapine is one of the drugs most commonly used in nonpsychotic and nonbipolar patients for this purpose. Quetiapine is an antagonist of serotonin 5-HT_{2A}, H_1, α_1, and dopamine D_2 receptors. Quetiapine is rapidly absorbed and reaches peak concentration in about 1.5 hours and has a terminal elimination half-life of approximately 6 hours. Quetiapine has a lower incidence of extrapyramidal side effects than traditional antipsychotics. However, it can cause hypotension. In addition, quetiapine has been associated with weight gain and glucose intolerance and neurocognitive impairment at higher doses. Quetiapine has also been associated with QT_c prolongation. One double-blind RCT evaluating the efficacy of quetiapine 25 mg in primary insomnia showed no significant improvement of self-reported TST and SOL.[96] Given antipsychotics' potentially significant neurologic and metabolic side effects, they are best reserved for the treatment of individuals who have insomnia comorbid with major psychiatric disorders, particularly psychotic and bipolar disorders.

OVER-THE-COUNTER AGENTS

Antihistamines

Antihistamine drugs used in the treatment of insomnia are reversible antagonists of H_1 receptors. First-generation agents include doxepin (discussed earlier), diphenhydramine, doxylamine, chlorpheniramine, hydroxyzine, meclizine, promethazine, and cyproheptadine. Essentially all of the over-the-counter antihistamine drugs marketed as sleep aids include diphenhydramine, the prototype of this class, or doxylamine. The second-generation nonsedating antihistamine drugs are used primarily to treat allergies and allergic responses, rather than insomnia.

Pharmacodynamics and Receptor Pharmacology

Histamine is widely present throughout the CNS and the body. Three types of histamine receptors have been described, labeled H_1, H_2, and H_3. The neurons of tuberomammillary nucleus, the source of CNS histamine, fire actively during wakefulness, reinforced by excitatory input from the lateral hypothalamus's orexin neurons. Histamine also suppresses the ventrolateral preoptic area, which in addition to the median preoptic nucleus, contains neurons that promote non–rapid eye movement (NREM) sleep.[2] Paradoxically, a minority of patients respond with CNS activation, including restlessness, anxiety, and increased alertness. H_1 antihistamines also have minor effects on antagonizing respiratory smooth muscle, relaxing bronchospasm, and promoting vasodilation.[97] Many of the early sedating antihistamines, including diphenhydramine, have muscarinic anticholinergic effects similar to atropine. In addition, diphenhydramine increases serotonergic neurotransmission and antagonizes adrenergic receptors. Unlike first-generation antihistamines that readily penetrate the blood–brain barrier, second-generation H_1 antagonists minimally penetrate the blood–brain barrier and thus are nonsedating.[98]

Pharmacokinetics

Antihistamines are well absorbed from the gastrointestinal tract and widely distributed throughout the body. Most first-generation antihistamines, including diphenhydramine and doxylamine, achieve peak plasma concentrations in 2 to 4 hours, and effects usually last 4 to 6 hours. Diphenhydramine has an elimination half-life of 4 to 8 hours.[99]

Effects on Sleep and Insomnia

First-generation antihistamines are associated with subjective drowsiness and sleepiness, leading to widespread use as OTC hypnotic agents. However, their efficacy has not been well studied. The largest published trial compared a diphenhydramine and valerian-hops combination with placebo in a total of 184 adults.[100] Diphenhydramine was associated with greater improvement in self-reported sleep efficiency, but not in SOL or TST, relative to placebo. A global measure of self-report outcome, the Insomnia Severity Index, showed significantly greater reductions in the diphenhydramine than placebo groups that were modest at 2 weeks. No significant differences were observed at 4 weeks. PSG-measured SOL, sleep efficiency, and TST showed no significant group differences. Guidelines recommend against the use of diphenhydramine for insomnia, given the absence of clear benefits and the potential for side effects and tolerance to its sleep-enhancing effects.[38]

Side Effects

Impairment of psychomotor performance with diphenhydramine has been well documented.[101] Epidemiologic studies have also suggested diphenhydramine is associated with cognitive impairment in the elderly[102] and incident dementia.[103] Other side effects related to CNS activity include dizziness, fatigue, and tinnitus. Peripheral side effects can include decreased appetite, nausea, tachycardia, urinary retention, constipation, and weight gain.

Dietary Supplements

Valerian

Pharmacodynamics and Receptor Pharmacology. The exact mechanism of action of *Valerian officinalis* preparations is unknown. The GABA-like activity of valerian extracts is suggested by their sedative, anxiolytic, myorelaxant, and possible anticonvulsant effects.[104] Valerian extracts contain a small amount of GABA, but GABA is not transported across the blood–brain barrier.

Pharmacokinetics. Valerian preparations are mainly derived from the roots of *V. officinalis.* These extracts contain a number of chemicals with CNS activity, including sesquiterpenes, valepotriates, valerenic acid, and various other alkaloids, in unknown proportions.[105] The constituents of a specific valerian preparation also depend on the valerian species used and the extraction process. Because of the multiple constituents found in valerian preparations, their pharmacokinetics have not been well described.

Effects on Sleep and Insomnia. The effects of valerian on sleep in humans have been investigated in healthy young adults and middle-aged and older adults with insomnia, generally with insomnia symptoms and not insomnia disorder. Although RCTs suggest valerian improves sleep in healthy adults, the data demonstrate minimal benefit for patients with insomnia disorder. A meta-analysis examining valerian for insomnia disorder (14 RCTs, $n = 1602$) found no short-term (≤6 weeks) differences between the valerian and placebo arms. It is important to note that a wide range of preparations and doses were studied, and given limited information on preparation methodology, the risk of bias could not be assessed.[106] Guidelines also recommend against its use for insomnia.[38]

Side Effects. Side effects associated with valerian have been reported to be few and mild and include headache and weakness.

Other Dietary Supplements

Beyond melatonin and valerian, few clinical trials have evaluated other dietary supplements for insomnia. German chamomile (*Matricaria recutita*) has been used as a medicinal herb for thousands of years.[107] Common preparations include tea or tinctures (1–4 mL/day). Preclinical studies suggest chamomile's mechanism of action is the result of the flavone, apigenin, which modulates GABA receptors.[108] Chamomile has been studied in a small number of short-term trials. The most rigorous RCT examined high-grade chamomile extract (270 mg, twice a day) versus placebo among 34 patients with primary insomnia and found minimal differences between groups, though a small sample size limits conclusions.[109] Chamomile is in the same flower family as ragweed and should be used with caution in patients with a history of hay fever, as allergic reactions, including rare cases of anaphylaxis, have been reported.[107]

Exogenous consumption of the amino acid l-tryptophan has also been purported to induce sleep, although data are limited. Based on limited evidence for efficacy, the American Academy of Sleep Medicine recommends against the use of l-tryptophan for chronic insomnia.[73] In the 1990s, l-tryptophan was recalled from the market because of safety concerns, as it was linked to more than 1500 reports of eosinophilia-myalgia syndrome.

Lavender, specifically English lavender (*Lavandula angustifolia*), usually in the form of oil or tea, has been used to promote sleep. Several small, very short-term (<1 week) studies suggest that lavender oil may improve sleep quality in healthy adults.[110] Lavender is generally well tolerated in adults,[111] although prepubertal gynecomastia has been linked to lavender oils.[112]

Cannabinoids

Drugs cultivated from the flowering plant genus *Cannabis* are among the most commonly used worldwide.[113] Cannabis plants produce over 100 terpenophenolics, with delta-9-tetrahydrocannabinol (THC), the most psychoactive cannabinoid; cannabidiol (CBD); and cannabinolic acid as the predominant compounds.[114] Cannabinoids interact with the endogenous cannabinoid (endocannabinoid) system, a widespread network that modulates various physiologic processes, including pain, mood, memory, inflammation, and metabolism. The endocannabinoid system includes two G protein–coupled cannabinoid receptors, CB1 and CB2,[115,116] and endogenous ligands, including, 2-arachidonoyl-glycerol (2-AG) and arachidonoyl ethanolamide (AEA or anandamide). THC, the main phytocannabinoid in cannabis-derived drugs such as marijuana and hashish, is a partial agonist of the CB1 and CB2 receptors[117] and may exert sleep-promoting effects via direct CB1 receptor activity.[118] CBD has a weak affinity for the CB1 receptor, preferentially binding to the CB2 receptor.[119] The effects of other cannabinoids, such as terpenes, on the endocannabinoid system is uncertain.

The hypnotic effects of cannabis have long been reported,[120] and insomnia is among the most common reasons for "medical marijuana" use.[121] In contrast to the widespread use of cannabis in the community, scientific understanding of the role of the endocannabinoid system and the effects of cannabinoids' (phyto- and synthetic) on sleep is nascent. In PSG studies, healthy adults acutely exposed to THC had reduced SOL, WASO, and REM sleep and more slow-wave sleep compared with control nights.[122-125] Several recent reviews have summarized the data to date on cannabinoids for sleep, but although potentially promising, cannabinoids have not yet been adequately evaluated for chronic insomnia disorder.[117,126-128] Most trials focused on symptomatic treatment of other chronic conditions and assessed sleep as a secondary outcome.[126] One review that did not require a clinician diagnosis of insomnia identified two RCTs: one PSG study of nine patients with mild insomnia evaluated the impact of THC on SOL,[129] and one crossover trial (n = 31) compared 2 weeks of nabilone (0.5–1.0 mg), a synthetic cannabinoid, to 2 weeks of amitriptyline (10–20 mg), for chronic insomnia in patients with fibromyalgia.[130] In these studies, sleep parameters and insomnia severity improved. Given these limited data, no conclusions on the efficacy of cannabinoids can be drawn at this time. However, several RCTs are actively evaluating various cannabinoids for chronic insomnia that will provide evidence on their efficacy and safety. Short-term side effects reported in clinical trials of cannabinoids for medical use include balance problems, confusion, dizziness, disorientation, diarrhea, euphoria, dry mouth, hallucination, nausea, and vomiting.[131] Long-term use of THC has been associated with altered brain development with initial use in adolescence, an increased risk of temporary hallucinations, paranoia and worsening symptoms in patients with schizophrenia, and cannabinoid hyperemesis syndrome.[132] The legality of cannabinoid use for medical purposes varies widely among individual states in the United States, and practitioners should be familiar with regulations in their area.

CONSIDERATIONS FOR PHARMACOTHERAPY

As many patients may present with insomnia symptoms rather than insomnia disorder, it is critical to ensure the proper diagnosis before initiating pharmacologic therapy. Several professional societies have published guidelines on the pharmacologic management of insomnia for adults in the outpatient setting, including the American Academy of Sleep Medicine (2017),[38] American College of Physicians (2016),[133] British Association of Psychopharmacology (2019),[134] European Sleep Research Society (2017),[135] Mexican Institute of Social Security (2014),[136] and the Veterans Affairs/Department of Defense (VAV/DOD, US, 2020).[137] Of note, several guidelines recommend limited use of sedative-hypnotics, particularly in older adults (Choosing Wisely Canada, US, and Australia; Canadian Family Physicians). See Chapter 100 for an in-depth discussion of sequential treatment and hypnotic discontinuation. Most international guidelines recommend cognitive-behavioral therapy for insomnia as first-line treatment before pharmacotherapy is initiated. These guidelines recommend that practitioners and patients should jointly consider the risks and benefits of pharmacotherapy, especially in circumstances such as unavailability or failure to respond to behavioral therapy, or the presence of comorbidities that would preclude engagement in behavioral treatments.[137] Careful assessment of the risk of dependence or abuse is critical when considering BzRA hypnotics; evidence-based alternatives with no/low abuse liability, such as doxepin, ramelteon, and suvorexant, are available.

Given limited comparative effectiveness data, existing guidelines provide few recommendations on sequencing medications. Despite concerns regarding dependence, tolerance, and safety, several guidelines include BzRAs as first-line agents, given their proven short-term efficacy,[133-137] for patients with sleep-onset or maintenance difficulties. Patients who report morning sedation may benefit from a BzRA with a shorter half-life; patients with sleep-maintenance difficulties may benefit from a drug with a longer half-life. In patients with coexisting anxiety disorders, benzodiazepines can be used advantageously to reduce anxiety at bedtime or during waking hours. Long-acting benzodiazepines should be avoided in the absence of daytime anxiety, as should the concurrent use of more than one BZRA, given additive effects.[138,139]

Several guidelines also recommend other non-BzRA agents as treatment options: ramelteon for sleep-onset insomnia[38] or insomnia in older adults[134] and suvorexant[38,133] and doxepin for sleep-maintenance insomnia.[38,106] Among guidelines that make specific recommendations for first-line agents, in addition to use of nonbenzodiazepine BzRAs, the British Association of Psychopharmacology recommends prolonged-release melatonin for adults older than 55 years of age, the European Sleep Research Society recommends sedating antidepressants, and the VA/DOD recommends doxepin as first-line treatment for chronic insomnia.

Given limited data on comparative effectiveness, algorithms on sequencing of insomnia therapies are sparse (see Chapter 100 for a discussion of sequencing).[140] As such, medications should be selected based on patient characteristics (the type of insomnia, comorbidities, previous and current use of sleep medications), pharmacologic properties (timing of onset, duration of action), efficacy, safety, and cost. Given the specific pharmacokinetics and receptor pharmacology of these agents, clinicians should educate patients about the dose, timing, and duration of their use in addition to other routine prescribing instructions (e.g., avoidance of alcohol and opiates). For example, shorter-acting medications (e.g., ramelteon, triazolam, zaleplon, zolpidem) are reasonable first-line agents for sleep-onset insomnia, whereas for sleep-maintenance insomnia, longer-acting agents could be considered. Clinicians must educate patients about the prescribed hypnotics' side effects and provide ongoing care to assess effectiveness, side effects, and discontinuation. It is also essential to set realistic expectations for patients, including how sleep medications work with the brain's control of sleep. To minimize the impact of sedation/drowsing and associated risks, we support an initial trial of a shorter-acting BzRA agent, low-dose doxepin, or DORA at the lowest effective dose and consideration of intermittent use if long-term therapy is warranted. If desired outcomes are not achieved, reevaluation of adherence to current medication, dose, and patient use should be reviewed. If the patient is adhering to instructions, considering different dosages, medications within the class (e.g., change from zolpidem to eszopiclone), or another class of drugs (e.g., BzRA agonist to orexin antagonist, low-dose doxepin) should be considered. Cost and formulary availability may also influence the choice of medications. Given limited data on efficacy, lack of regulation, and evidence indicating inconsistent dosing and contamination, we do not recommend using dietary supplements, such as melatonin, valerian, and tryptophan for insomnia disorder or cannabinoids. We also advocate for behavioral therapy use in conjunction with sleep medications or assist with the deprescribing of sleep medications.

Additional Considerations

Despite limited data, some medications could be considered for patients with specific comorbidities, such as headache disorders (e.g., amitriptyline). Similarly, the alpha-2-delta ligand agents gabapentin and pregabalin may be considered to treat insomnia when comorbid with neuropathic pain conditions, fibromyalgia, hot flash–associated insomnia, or restless legs syndrome. As noted, special consideration should be given to patients with a history of substance abuse disorders, given that several recommended medications have abuse potential. For such patients, low-dose doxepin, ramelteon, DORAs, and gabapentin may be considered. Additionally, given the increased risk of cognitive impairment, delirium, falls,[25] fractures,[26] and motor vehicle crashes in adults aged 65 years and older, the 2019 American Geriatrics Society Beers Criteria for potentially inappropriate medication use in older adults strongly recommends against BzRAs and TCAs (except low-dose doxepin) in older adults.[24] However, confounding by sleep symptoms has remained a concern, and it is plausible that both insomnia and sleep medication use are independent risk factors for falls.[27,28] Therefore potential risks must be discussed with patients and the implementation of fall-reduction strategies, including evaluating physical limitations (e.g., vision, bone density) and environmental assessments (e.g., removal of loose mats, carpeting of slippery floors). See Chapter 99 for a comprehensive discussion of adverse effects.

Given the documented sex differences in pharmacokinetics, the FDA has revised the recommendations for starting a dose of selective BzRAs for women. Additionally, there is limited evidence for the use of pharmacologic medications for insomnia during pregnancy and lactation. Although there are some conflicting data, the use of BzRAs during pregnancy is not associated with congenital malformations or low birth weight. However, some studies suggest their use is associated with preterm birth and spontaneous abortion.[141] Additionally, a few small studies in perimenopausal women with insomnia have benefited from zolpidem,[142] eszopiclone,[143] ramelteon,[144] and suvorexant.[145]

CLINICAL PEARL

The first step to pharmacologic management of insomnia is ensuring the proper diagnosis and performing a comprehensive clinical assessment. Although recent guidelines recommend cognitive-behavioral therapy for insomnia as first-line treatment, medications are recommended through a shared decision-making process with the patient. The selection of a pharmacologic agent to treat insomnia should consider patient characteristics (the type of insomnia, comorbidities, previous and current use of sleep medications), pharmacologic properties (timing of onset, duration of action), efficacy, safety, and cost. The use of OTC medications is generally not supported by current guidelines. Given the known side effects of all medication classes, educating patients on proper use and close clinical follow-up are warranted to maximize effectiveness and minimize harm.

SUMMARY

Numerous OTC and prescription medications are available to treat insomnia. The most commonly used prescription medication is the BzRA zolpidem. However, guidelines support the use of other medication classes, including melatonin receptor agonists, TCAs (i.e., low-dose doxepin), and the recently developed DORAs. Other commonly used classes of medications, such as heterocyclic antidepressants (trazodone, mirtazapine), antipsychotics (quetiapine), TCAs (high-dose doxepin, amitriptyline), and gabapentin, can be considered in certain patients, although evidence supporting their efficacy for insomnia disorder is limited. OTC agents such as antihistamines and dietary supplements, including melatonin, have little role in the treatment of insomnia disorder.

ACKNOWLEDGMENT

The authors wish to acknowledge the contributions of Drs. Shachi Tyagi, James Walsh, Thomas Roth, and Andrew D. Krystal to Chapters 42, 87, and 88 in *Principles and Practice of Sleep Medicine,* 6th ed., 2017, from which this chapter was adapted.

SELECTED READINGS

Bertisch SM, Herzig SJ, Winkelman JW, Buettner C, et al. National use of prescription medications for insomnia: NHANES 1999-2010. *Sleep.* 2014;37(2):343–349.

Kesner AJ, Lovinger DM. Cannabinoids, endocannabinoids and sleep. *Front Mol Neurosci.* 2020;13:125.

Morin CM, Inoue Y, Kushida C, et al. Endorsement of European guideline for the diagnosis and treatment of insomnia by the World Sleep Society. *Sleep Med.* 2021;81:124–126.

Qaseem A, Kansagara D, Forciea MA, Cooke M, Denberg TD, et al. Management of chronic insomnia disorder in adults: a clinical practice guideline from the American College of Physicians. *Ann Intern Med.* 2016;165(2):125–133.

Riemann D, Baglioni C, Bassetti C, et al. European guideline for the diagnosis and treatment of insomnia. *J Sleep Res.* 2017;26(6):675–700.

Sateia MJ, Buysse DJ, Krystal AD, Neubauer DN, Heald JL, et al. Clinical practice guideline for the pharmacologic treatment of chronic insomnia in adults: an American Academy of Sleep Medicine clinical practice guideline. *J Clin Sleep Med.* 2017;13(2):307–349.

Wilt TJ, MacDonald R, Brasure M, et al. Pharmacologic treatment of insomnia disorder: an evidence report for a clinical practice guideline by the American College of Physicians. *Ann Intern Med.* 2016;165(2):103–112.

Wong J, Horwitz MM, Bertisch SM, Herzig SJ, Buysse DJ, Toh S, et al. Trends in dispensing of zolpidem and low-dose trazodone among commercially insured adults in the United States, 2011-2018. *JAMA.* 2020;324(21):2211–2213.

Zhou ES, Gardiner P, Bertisch SM. Integrative medicine for insomnia. *Med Clin.* 2017;101(5):865–879.

A complete reference list can be found online at ExpertConsult.com.

Chapter 99

Pharmacologic Treatment II: Efficacy, Effectiveness, and Contraindications

Andrew D. Krystal

Chapter Highlights

- Efficacy research is a determination of how a treatment performs under ideal circumstances that are designed to provide the most sensitive assay for detection of a therapeutic effect, if one exists.
- Effectiveness research seeks to determine how treatments actually perform in clinical practice.
- There are a set of meta-analyses of insomnia medications that have been carried out that summarize the efficacy research supporting the use of existing medications for specific types of sleep problems.
- Together with information on relative contraindications to the use of particular agents, these data provide a framework for optimization of insomnia pharmacotherapy by choosing the medication(s) for each individual that has the strongest empirical support for efficacy for the specific type of sleep problem and with the least associated risks.
- A personalized medicine paradigm for insomnia pharmacotherapy is presented.

INTRODUCTION

A number of medications are used for the treatment of insomnia. This chapter focuses on reviewing the evidence indicating whether these medications are helpful. It employs a traditional framework for carrying out such a review: evaluation of the evidence of efficacy and effectiveness. Studies assessing efficacy evaluate how well a medication functions under ideal circumstances for determining therapeutic effects, which typically includes careful selection of a subset of subjects from among the patient population of interest, use of randomization (typically including a placebo), and administration under ideal circumstances (e.g., absence of concomitant medications, comorbidities, in a sleep laboratory).[1] As a result, efficacy trials function as a standardized assay to determine if therapeutic effects are present but do not reflect how therapies perform when prescribed to patients encountered in clinical practice. That is the aim of effectiveness trials (also known as pragmatic trials), which seek to determine the overall risk-to-benefit ratio of treatment as delivered in usual health care practice.[1] Although the distinction between these two types of studies seems straightforward, there is a great deal of confusion surrounding efficacy and effectiveness, which motivates further consideration. Given that one's goal in determining whether a potential treatment is therapeutic for a given condition is to ultimately assess whether treatments are beneficial when administered in clinical practice, it is reasonable to ask whether there is any need to consider efficacy trials at all when evaluating therapeutic value. However, effectiveness trials carry with them significant risks of providing false-positive and false-negative indications of therapeutic benefit.[2] They may fail to indicate beneficial effects when they exist because of patient nonadherence to therapy, clinicians choices about whom they prescribe the treatment to, lack of availability of the treatment, or patients' nonacceptance of the therapy.[2] Effectiveness trials may also falsely suggest beneficial effects when they do not exist because of their being tested: in disorders with high placebo response rates; in disorders with which there is a significant rate of spontaneous remission; or where there is clinician or patient bias toward the treatment being therapeutic.[3] As a result, regulatory agencies primarily require trials to have key components of efficacy trials when assessing whether there is evidence for therapeutic benefit.[3] For example, beginning in 1962 the U.S. Food and Drug Administration (FDA) added the requirement of "substantial evidence of effectiveness" to the existing requirements of safety to the Federal Food, Drug, and Cosmetic Act. This referred to the more generic concept of overall therapeutic benefit and was defined as "evidence consisting of adequate and well controlled investigations" deemed necessary to distinguish drug effects "from other influences, such as spontaneous change in the course of the disease, placebo effect, or biased observation."[4] It was intended to address the growing problem of "misleading and unsupported claims." Requirements have evolved such that current requirements include double-blinding, randomization, placebo/sham controls, end points that minimize bias, and appropriate patient selection as standards of rigor and reproducibility.[3] However, the FDA indicates that other designs can provide evidence of effectiveness depending on the nature of the condition under study and study specifics. As one example, studies without placebo are acceptable in conditions in which it is well established that there is no placebo response.

Based on the previously mentioned considerations, our review of the therapeutic effects of insomnia pharmacotherapeutic agents will consider evidence from *efficacy studies* as an indicator of therapeutic effect that takes into account the placebo response and spontaneous remission and is relatively less affected by bias. This chapter also considers data from *effectiveness studies* to provide an indication of real-world, clinical practice risk-to-benefit ratio. This body of work forms the research evidence that supports the use of pharmacologic treatments and provides the foundation for the cutting edge of insomnia pharmacologic therapeutics: moving toward a personalized medicine paradigm for insomnia pharmacotherapy. This chapter also considers this paradigm as well as future directions for insomnia pharmacotherapy.

THE SCIENTIFIC BASIS FOR ASSESSING THE EFFICACY OF INSOMNIA MEDICATIONS AND CONTRASTING EFFICACY AND EFFECTIVENESS RESEARCH

Optimizing the design of efficacy studies for insomnia requires including trial design features that maximize the ability to detect a treatment effect if one actually exists.[2] The goal is to use the most sensitive possible assay for determining the existence of a true therapeutic effect. This requires use of an appropriately selected control, method of patient assignment to treatment (e.g., randomization), minimizing bias (e.g., blinding), patient selection, method of treatment administration, and valid and reliable outcome assessments.[2,3] In contrast, optimizing the design of effectiveness trials requires including all features that maximize the ability to determine how well a treatment performs in *real-world* clinical practice.[2] However, many effectiveness studies employ some features that deviate from clinical practice based on practical considerations. This section reviews factors related to optimizing these components for efficacy studies of insomnia pharmacotherapy, contrasting them with the typical features of effectiveness studies.

Control Therapy

For efficacy trials of insomnia, pharmacotherapy placebo pills are used because there is a robust, highly reproducible placebo response that has been universally evident in insomnia efficacy studies and accounts for 69% of the effect size of insomnia therapies.[5] In contrast, in effectiveness studies placebos are generally not included because they are not administered in clinical care. However, comparison to another intervention that is administered clinically is common.

Method of Patient Assignment to Treatment

The standard for assigning patients to treatments for efficacy trials is randomization of subjects to the drug being studied versus placebo.[2] Essentially all efficacy studies of insomnia pharmacotherapies have employed randomization, usually involving assignment of equal numbers of patients to the active drug and placebo. However, to maximize drug exposure some studies have randomized a greater number of patients to active therapy than placebo such as an esmirtazapine trial employing a 3:1 drug-to-placebo randomization.[6] Alternative ratios are also sometimes employed in studies evaluating multiple doses of a drug or including an active comparator such as a 5:5:5:4 randomization for a study of 2 doses of lemborexant, zolpidem CR, and placebo.[7] Designs employing adaptive randomization are being increasingly used, particularly for Phase 2a studies in which multiple doses are employed. The goal of such studies is typically to select the best subset of dosages from a set of dosages of interest. This is achieved by varying randomization over the course of the trial based on interim analyses and increasing the randomization to more efficacious dosages based on prespecified criteria. For example, a recent Phase 2a study of lemborexant used frequent interim analyses to update randomization ratios to 1 of 6 dosing groups by increasing the randomization toward dosages with greater scores on a utility function that combined measures of therapeutic improvement and daytime sleepiness (placebo randomization was kept constant at 1 in 7).[8]

In effectiveness research, treatment assignment is ideally determined by practitioner choice as occurs in clinical practice. However, many studies identified as effectiveness trials employ randomization and/or nonclinician-determined treatment assignment and are actually hybrids, including a mix of efficacy and effectiveness components.

Minimizing Bias

Employing double-blinding and randomization involving a placebo control is the best way to minimize the likelihood that subject and clinician expectation bias will affect the outcome of efficacy trials of insomnia pharmacotherapies.[2] Randomization ensures that clinician treatment choices do not affect the assessment of efficacy, and it decreases the impact of patient acceptance of the treatment on study outcome.

Patient Selection

Selection of a subset of the patients is typically employed in efficacy research to identify a subgroup who are most likely to demonstrate a response to treatment if one exists.[2] This approach is optimal for identifying a therapeutic effect, but generalizability to clinical practice is unknown until effectiveness studies have been performed. For efficacy studies, patient selection is achieved through use of strict inclusion and exclusion criteria, which typically include selecting individuals based on insomnia disorder diagnosis, meeting objective and/or subjective severity thresholds, comorbid medical and/or psychiatric conditions, concomitant medications, and factors related to their ability to participate in the trial (e.g., cognitive status).[2]

Efficacy trials typically establish the diagnosis of the disorder of interest in a standardized way, often using a validated instrument for this purpose based on the major sleep nosologies.[9,10] This ensures that variability in how diagnostic criteria are understood, interpreted, and applied by clinicians does not affect the ability of the study to detect an effect. Including individuals without the condition of interest adds noise to study results, as they can be false nonresponders. Excluding individuals who actually have insomnia because of systematic biases in the application of diagnostic criteria introduces the risk of not treating some important subgroups of the insomnia population, which could affect study outcomes and generalizability (e.g., the most treatment-responsive subgroup may be eliminated).

The use of a severity threshold to select subjects addresses the problem that individuals without symptoms on a measure at baseline cannot improve on that measure with treatment. As a result, efficacy trials typically require participants to have at least a moderate degree of elevation on the key outcome measures at baseline. Experimental evidence supporting this practice is a post hoc analysis from an eszopiclone study (n = 788), indicating that greater baseline wake time after sleep onset (WASO) predicted a greater drug versus placebo effect size on WASO with treatment.[11]

Those with comorbid medical and psychiatric conditions are frequently excluded from efficacy studies because of their limited ability to complete study procedures and to reduce noise in outcome assessment because of fluctuations in their comorbid condition.

Because this makes studies less representative of populations seen in clinical practice, this practice is limited or absent in effectiveness research. However, effectiveness trials often exclude subjects who are at elevated risk if they participate. This is sometimes justified on the grounds that such individuals ought not to receive the intervention in clinical practice.[2,12]

The issue of the inclusion of individuals with comorbidities is complicated by the fact that insomnia disorder includes individuals with sleep problems occurring concomitantly with medical and psychiatric conditions.[10] This represents a change that was introduced with the DSM-5. Before that change, insomnia efficacy trials nearly always included "primary insomnia" (insomnia without a co-occurring condition) for the reasons noted previously. The design of an insomnia efficacy trial must balance (1) the introduction of noise associated with comorbidities with (2) the desire to identify a generalizable therapeutic effect. As a result, there is an increasing inclusion of patients with comorbidities in efficacy trials of insomnia agents.

Another factor adding noise to insomnia study outcomes is concomitant medications that are often needed for treating the comorbid condition. The noise arises because of the potential for interactions with the study drug, the potential for adverse effects to occur that have to be considered as possible study drug side effects and could increase insomnia or affect outcome ratings, and the potential for improvements occurring in associated conditions occurring in the middle of the trial. For this reason, concomitant medications are typically not allowed in pure efficacy studies. When they are allowed, they are generally required to remain at stable dosages throughout the study. However, excluding concomitant medications undermines generalizability to clinical practice. Thus this type of exclusion is minimized or absent in effectiveness studies.

One final factor typically employed in efficacy studies is the exclusion of individuals unlikely to be adherent to study procedures. This is necessary because such individuals undermine the ability of studies to be sensitive assays for the detection of the benefits of effective treatments.

Treatment Administration

In efficacy research all those participating in the study are provided treatment.[2] This addresses the problem faced in effectiveness research of limitations to treatment access because of variations in insurance coverage, patient financial resources, transportation, mobility, or other factors.

Assessment of Outcome

The goal of outcome assessment selection for insomnia efficacy trials is to identify the measure that provides the most sensitive assay of treatment therapeutic insomnia effect, if one exists. In effectiveness trials the goal is to select outcome measures that best reflect how outcome is assessed in clinical care. The choice of outcome measures that are appropriate for efficacy trials of insomnia treatments depends on how insomnia is defined.

The current definition of insomnia defines the universe of features of the condition that one should seek to measure in assessing outcome. Based on the DSM-5 definition this consists of a self-report of: (1) difficulty initiating sleep; (2) difficulty maintaining sleep, characterized by frequent awakenings or problems returning to sleep after awakenings; (3) early-morning awakening with inability to return to sleep; and (4) clinically significant distress or impairments in social, occupational, educational, academic, behavioral, or other important areas of functioning.[10]

To be able to include an assessment in an efficacy trial intended to reflect one or more of these components of insomnia requires that there be a measure of that aspect of insomnia that has been established to have suitable measurement properties. This ensures that the assessment will measure what it is intended to measure and do so with minimum associated measurement error so as to maximize study assay sensitivity. The set of measurement properties typically considered includes test-retest reliability (stability of scores over time when no change is expected), inter-rater reliability (for clinician-rated measures; degree of agreement among raters), internal consistency (degree to which items within a scale are correlated/measure the same thing), content validity (the extent to which the instrument reflects the concept of interest in terms of the components being "appropriate and comprehensive relative to its intended measurement concept, population, and use"), construct validity (the degree to which the "relationship among items, domains, and concepts conform to a priori hypotheses concerning logical relationships that should exist with measures of related concepts or scores produced in similar or diverse patient group"), and ability to detect change (the extent to which the instrument reflects changes over time occurring in the construct of interest in the patient group of interest).[3.] Outcomes for assessing effectiveness are intended to mirror clinical practice and typically involve a clinician carrying out a rating such as a Clinical Global Impression (CGI) scale, in which they codify their impression of the patient's experience.[13]

In consideration of efficacy outcome measures it is important to note that the major insomnia diagnostic criteria all consist only of self-reported features. As a result, it is critical to include self-report when assessing outcome. This is necessary for ensuring content validity. A type of high content validity self-report measure that has been employed in a very large number of efficacy trials, including many reviewed by regulatory agencies leading to treatment approval, is the sleep diary. The sleep diary represents a family of scales that vary in terms of the specific questions they ask and the format of those questions. Typical outcome measures derived from these scales include sleep parameters such as average sleep-onset latency (SOL), average WASO, or average total sleep time (TST). A number of versions have content validity, construct validity, and established ability to detect change. The "consensus sleep diary" is the only one in which development was systematically based on expert consensus input and patient focus group feedback.[14-16] Syndromal measures that assess overall insomnia disorder severity are also commonly employed in efficacy research. They are retrospective measures with the advantage that they can be obtained in a short period of time. The Insomnia Severity Index (ISI)[17,18] and the Pittsburgh Sleep Quality Index[19] have content and construct validity, internal consistency, test-retest reliability, and the ability to detect change.

Many efficacy studies, including pivotal trials of treatments approved by major regulatory agencies include polysomnographic (PSG) outcome measures. This may seem to limit generalizability given that insomnia is a diagnosis based on patient report and PSG is not generally obtained in clinical practice. However, PSG studies serve very valuable functions for insomnia efficacy studies. They represent the most standardized assay for objectively determining the effects of an insomnia drug, and they provide a means to ensure that self-reported effects do not just reflect global effects of an agent on subjective state that may impact all types of ratings but do, in fact, reflect effects on physiologic sleep. As a standardized assay, undergoing a study in the laboratory eliminates noise (i.e., measurement error) because of uncontrolled factors at home that, while more generalizable, undermine assay sensitivity. This laboratory approach does not reflect habitual sleep and introduces effects including a new sleeping environment and the burden of recording equipment. As a result, this procedure is not useful for effectiveness research but is critical for efficacy research where detection of effects through tight controls and minimization of variability in extraneous variables is a primary concern.

Last, it is important to consider which among the many measures generated by PSG and sleep diaries to include as outcome measures for a particular insomnia medication efficacy study. For purposes of specificity, regulatory agencies generally require use of SOL to demonstrate beneficial effects on ability to fall asleep and either WASO or number of awakenings as an indicator of effects on ability to stay asleep. A benefit of this approach for regulatory purposes is that it allows a determination of the specific type of sleep problem improved, which can allow the designation of a specific indication or indications for the use of the drug. This is not possible with measures such as TST or sleep efficiency (SE%), because they include contributions of a component of sleep-onset effect and sleep maintenance effect, which is not possible to disentangle from TST without considering other measures.

Also, to improve the specificity of delineation of therapeutic effects, some efficacy studies have incorporated measures obtainable with PSG, indicating the nature of therapeutic effects with greater specificity than can be achieved with self-report measures. This includes hour-by-hour wake time, which reflects the particular part of the night where therapeutic effects occur. This methodology has allowed the demonstration that doxepin 3 to 6 mg and hypocretin/orexin antagonists suvorexant and lemborexant are uniquely therapeutic in the last third of the night, including specifically in the last hour of an 8-hour night in the laboratory.[7,20-22] As medications with other types of very specific effects may emerge, it will be important to identify the types of measures that best reflect their unique effects.

RESEARCH EVIDENCE THAT SUPPORTS THE USE OF INSOMNIA MEDICATIONS

The research evidence base that supports the use of medications for treating insomnia consists of a sizable body of efficacy studies as well as a small number of studies oriented more toward assessing effectiveness. Here we review this literature to provide a high-level view of the evidence supporting the use of these agents.

Efficacy

To summarize the findings of efficacy studies I rely primarily on recent meta-analyses that have used systematic methods to characterize the therapeutic effects of individual agents as well as broader groupings of insomnia medications. Because the methodologies and goals of these efforts differ and all provide some unique contribution to understanding the effects of insomnia medications, this summary incorporates the findings of the set of meta-analyses carried out in the last 5 years (Table 99.1).[23-26] It is important to note that the set of medications covered in this review are those included in at least one of those meta-analyses. These include nearly all of the medications approved by the major regulatory agencies around the world for the treatment of insomnia plus the agents most commonly used off-label to treat insomnia. It does not, however, include the FDA–approved hypocretin/orexin antagonist lemborexant, which was not included in any of these meta-analyses because of the very recent publication of results from trials for this medication.[7,27]

Other medications not included in this review are those in which too little research has been carried out to support meta-analysis. This includes some very commonly used insomnia treatments, including the antihistamine doxylamine, various tricyclic antidepressants such as amitriptyline, various atypical antipsychotic agents including quetiapine, and anticonvulsants such as gabapentin. Importantly, clinical approaches to the use of these agents are reviewed in Chapter 98. The results of the meta-analyses are compiled in Table 99.1 in the form of the means and 95% confidence limits for the therapeutic effect versus placebo of each medication for which there was a statistically significant therapeutic effect versus placebo on key sleep parameters (global outcomes [CGI, ISI, sleep quality ratings], sleep-onset effects [SOL for self-report and SOL or latency to persistent sleep for PSG], sleep maintenance effects in terms of WASO, and effects on TST for both self-report and PSG).

The first of the meta-analysis considered, that of Wilt and colleagues, was carried out for a clinical practice guideline by the American College of Physicians and included 35 double-blind randomized, placebo-controlled trials of at least 4 weeks' duration evaluating pharmacotherapies approved by the FDA for the treatment of insomnia.[23] This meta-analysis was limited to consideration of self-reported outcomes only and did not include benzodiazepines. The second meta-analysis by Sateia and colleagues was undertaken as part of the development of clinical practice guidelines for the pharmacologic treatment of chronic insomnia in adults by the American Academy of Sleep Medicine.[24] Forty-six studies were included, which had an initial sample size of at least 20, and were carried out in adults with insomnia without significant comorbidities. Another meta-analysis by Samara and colleagues restricted its attention to studies of at least 5 days' duration carried out in individuals over 65 years of age.[25] The last meta-analysis considered, that of Zheng and colleagues, included randomized, double-blind, placebo-controlled trials of insomnia medications carried out in adults with insomnia disorder based on the DSM and who had no comorbidities nor concomitant medication use.[26] The sleep medications studied were those approved by the FDA for the treatment

Table 99.1 Meta-analysis Evidence Supporting the Use of Insomnia Medications

Insomnia Medication	Wilt et al., Size of Drug-Placebo Differences Favoring Drug: Mean [95% CI]	Sateia et al., Size of Drug-Placebo Differences Favoring Drug: Mean [95% CI]	Samara et al., Size of Drug-Placebo Differences Favoring Drug in Older Adults: Mean [95% CI]	Zheng et al., Model Estimated Size of Drug-Placebo Differences Favoring Drug: Mean [95% CI]	Summary
Triazolam 0.125–0.5 mg Benzodiazepine GABA-A Positive Allosteric Modulator					
Global Outcome					
SOL				Mix 16.0 [5.4 26.6]	**
WASO					
TST				Mix 20.7 [4.6 45.3]	**
Flurazepam 15–30 mg Benzodiazepine GABA-A Positive Allosteric Modulator					
Global Outcome					
SOL				Mix 9.2 [2.3 16.0]	**
WASO				Mix 12.6 [3.2 22.0]	**
TST				Mix 26.1 [9.5 42.8]	**
Temazepam 7.5–15 mg Benzodiazepine GABA-A Positive Allosteric Modulator					
Global Outcome		SQ NS	SQ 0.5 [0.1 0.9]		
SOL		SR 20.1 [1.1 39.1] PSG 37.1 [21.3 52.8]	SR 11.4 [6.5 16.3]	Mix 16.0 [5.4 26.6]	***
WASO				Mix NS	
TST		SR 64.4 [8.1 121] PSG 99.1 [63.4 135]	SR NS	Mix 19.1 [3.1 35.1]	*
Zolpidem 5–10 mg Non-Benzodiazepine GABA-A Positive Allosteric Modulator					
Global Outcome		SQ 0.6 [0.03 1.3]	SQ NS		*
SOL	SR 15.0 [7.8 22.1]	SR 19.6 [14.2 24.9] PSG 11.7 [4.2 19.2]	SR NS	Mix 13.6 [10.0 17.2]	*
WASO	SR NS	SR 13.6 [7.3 19.8] PSG 25.5 [17.9 33.0]	SR 14.9 [0.3 29.4]	Mix 19.7 [12.8 26.6]	*
TST	SR 23 [2.0-43.9]	SR 30.0 [15.1 45.0] PSG 28.9 [10.9 47.0]	SR NS	Mix 25.8 [18.9 32.7]	*
Zolpidem Extended Release 6.25 mg Non-Benzodiazepine GABA-A Positive Allosteric Modulator					
Global Outcome	CGI 1.8 [1.6-2.0]				**
SOL	SR 9 [CI NR]	SR NS		Mix 10.1 [2.6 17.6]	*
WASO	SR 16 [CI NR]	SR 13.0 [3.6 22.5]		Mix 19.9 [12.1 27.6]	***
TST	SR 25 [CI NR]			Mix 32.1 [18.1 46.0]	***
Transoral Zolpidem 3.5 mg Non-Benzodiazepine GABA-A Positive Allosteric Modulator					
Global Outcome					
SOL	SR MOTN 18 [CI NR]				**
WASO					
TST	SR 9 [CI NR]				**
Zaleplon 10 mg Non-Benzodiazepine GABA-A Positive Allosteric Modulator					
Global Outcome		NS	SQ NS		
SOL		SR 11.4 [4.6 27.4] PSG 9.6 [0.2 18.8]		Mix 12.9 [9.4 16.4]	***
WASO		NS PSG		Mix NS	
TST		NS SR		Mix 12.6 [6.3 18.9]	*
Eszopiclone 2–3 mg Non-Benzodiazepine GABA-A Positive Allosteric Modulator					
Global Outcome	ISI: 4.6 [3.9 5.3]	SQ 1.5 [0.8 2.1]	SQ 0.4 [0.3 0.5]		***

Continued

Table 99.1 Meta-analysis Evidence Supporting the Use of Insomnia Medications—cont'd

Insomnia Medication	Wilt et al., Size of Drug-Placebo Differences Favoring Drug: Mean [95% CI]	Sateia et al., Size of Drug-Placebo Differences Favoring Drug: Mean [95% CI]	Samara et al., Size of Drug-Placebo Differences Favoring Drug in Older Adults: Mean [95% CI]	Zheng et al., Model Estimated Size of Drug-Placebo Differences Favoring Drug: Mean [95% CI]	Summary
SOL	SR 19.1 [14.1 24.1]	SR 25.0 [13.9 36.1] PSG 13.6 [3.7 23.4]	SR 12.5 [5.5 19.4]	Mix 16.4 [12.2 20.6]	***
WASO	SR 21.6 [13.6 29.6]	SR 15.1 [8.2 22.1] PSG 14.7 [11.7 17.7]	SR 12.5 [4.5 20.4]	Mix 18.0 [12.4 23.6]	***
TST	SR 44.8 [35.4 54.2]	SR 57.1 [37.5 76.8]	SR 23.9 [3.3 44.6] PSG 25.5 [13.5 37.5]	Mix 34.6 [25.4 43.7]	***
Melatonin Various Dosages Melatonin Receptor Agonist					
Global Outcome		SQ NS	SQ 0.7 [0.2 1.3]		*
SOL	SR 6.0 [2.1 10.0]	PSG 8.9 [2.4 15.5]	SR NS		*
WASO	SR NS	PSG NS	SR 24.0 [11.1 36.9]		*
TST	SR NS		SR NS		
Ramelteon 8 mg Melatonin Receptor Agonist					
Global Outcome		NS			
SOL	SR NS	SR 11.4 [3.3 19.6] PSG 9.6 [6.4 12.8]	SR 10.0 [4.1 15.9]	Mix 10.3 [5.2 15.3]	*
WASO	SR NS	SR NS PSG 3.5 [2.8 4.2]		Mix NS	*
TST	SR NS	SR NS PSG 6.6 [1.4 11.8]	SR NS	Mix NS	*
Doxepin 3–6 mg Selective H1 Histamine Antagonist					
Global Outcome		SQ 0.3 [0.1 0.5]	SQ 0.4 [0.2 0.7]		***
SOL		SR NS PSG NS	SR 16.8 [7.2 26.3]	Mix 5.5 [0.1 10.9	*
WASO		SR 14.4 [3.9 24.9] PSG 23.4 [16.5 30.3]	SR 17.8 [7.3 28.0]	Mix 20.6 [14.9 26.2]	***
TST		SR 43.6 [5.2 82.0] PSG 32.3 [24.2 40.3]	SR 31.2 [5.1 57.2] PSG 23.6 [6.9 40.3]	Mix 25.4 [16.2 34.7]	***
Suvorexant 10–20 mg Selective Dual Hypocretin/Orexin Receptor Antagonist					
Global Outcome	ISI 1.2 [0.6 1.8]				**
SOL	SR 6.0 [1.9 10.0]	SR 5.2 [0.3 10.1] PSG 8.1 [2.4 13.9]	SR 7.3 [1.8 12.9]		***
WASO	SR 16.0 [4.7 27.2]	PSG 16.6 [8.3 24.9]	SR 24.3 [14.1 34.4]		***
TST	SR 4.7 [0.5 8.9]	SR 10.6 [1.8 19.4]			***
Trazodone 50 mg					
Global Outcome		SQ NS			
SOL		SR 10.2 [9.0 11.4]			**
WASO		SR 7.7 [6.5 8.9]			**
TST		SR 21.8 [20.1 23.5]			**
Diphenhydramine 25–50 mg					
Global Outcome		SQ NS	SQ 0.1 [0.03 0.2]		*
SOL		SR NS PSG NS	SR NS		
WASO					
TST		SR NS PSG NS	SR NS		

*Indicates mixed evidence for efficacy across the meta-analyses.
**Indicates evidence of efficacy for the one meta-analysis reporting results for this end point.
***Indicates consistent evidence of efficacy across the meta-analyses.
Absence of information in the table indicates that the drug or outcome was not considered in the meta-analysis.
CGI, Clinical Global Impression Scale; CI, confidence interval; ISI, Insomnia Severity Index; Mix, mixture composed of whatever self-reported and PSG data were available were included in the estimate; MOTN, after middle of the night awakening; NR, not reported; NS, no statistically significant advantage for drug versus placebo; PSG, polysomnographic outcome; SOL, sleep-onset latency; SQ, sleep quality rating; SR, self-reported outcome; TST, total sleep time; WASO, wake after sleep onset.

of insomnia, including flurazepam, temazepam, triazolam, eszopiclone, zaleplon, zolpidem, suvorexant, ramelteon, and doxepin. The authors evaluated SOL, WASO, and TST as end points and relied on any type of measure that was available (self-reported, PSG, or both) and combined them into a single outcome for each of these. To address the problem of data being available for different time points and missing data, they employed a regression-based modeling approach to estimate treatment versus placebo effects and the associated 95% confidence intervals.[26] A total of 44 studies met their a priori criteria and were included in the analysis.

Taken together, these studies provide an overall indication of the extent to which the available research studies provide evidence for the efficacy of each medication for the end points considered (Table 99.1). There is no standard methodology for achieving this goal. However, useful information can be gained by identifying medications as demonstrating relatively convincing evidence of efficacy for an end point when a significant effect versus placebo was found in more than one of the meta-analyses without any of the studies failing to find such an effect. In addition, it is of interest to identify those studies in which a medication was found to have evidence of efficacy when it was the only study where results were reported for a given variable. Last, agents are noted as having some but less convincing evidence of efficacy when there were mixed results across studies. From this point of view, the meta-analyses as a whole provided relatively convincing evidence of efficacy for the following: temazepam for sleep onset; zolpidem ER for WASO and TST; zaleplon for sleep onset; eszopiclone for global outcome, sleep onset, WASO, and TST; doxepin for global outcome, WASO, and TST; and suvorexant for SOL, WASO, and TST. There is evidence of efficacy for the one meta-analysis reporting results for the following: triazolam for sleep onset and TST; flurazepam for sleep onset, WASO, and TST; zolpidem ER for global outcome; transoral zolpidem for returning to sleep in the middle of the night and TST; suvorexant for onset, WASO, and TST; and trazodone for sleep onset, WASO, and TST. The meta-analyses provided mixed evidence of efficacy for the following: temazepam for TST; zolpidem for global outcome, onset, WASO, and TST; zolpidem ER for sleep onset; zaleplon for TST; melatonin for global outcome, onset, and WASO; ramelteon for onset, WASO, and TST; doxepin for sleep onset; and diphenhydramine for global outcome. These findings represent the base of efficacy research that supports the use of insomnia pharmacotherapies. It is important to note that for a number of the medications considered here and a number not considered, the absence of a relatively positive indicator of evidence is more of a reflection of limitations of the research studies that have been performed with those agents and what was reported in papers reporting studies (many papers do not report the results in a format that allows the results to be included in meta-analyses) than evidence that the medications lacked efficacy. Of the medications considered, triazolam, flurazepam, and trazodone are particularly notable in this regard, each being included in only one of the four meta-analyses.

Effectiveness

One recent study that primarily incorporated effectiveness study features is considered here. It is one of very few studies that provide an indication of likely performance of two of the most commonly prescribed medications for insomnia in the United States, zolpidem and trazodone, in clinical practice settings.[28] This study was a sequential multiple-assignment trial, in which 211 patients meeting insomnia disorder diagnostic criteria were assigned in a single-blind manner to behavioral therapy (BT) versus zolpidem 5 to 10 mg and those who did not remit entered a second stage, where zolpidem nonremitters were randomized to trazodone 50 to 150 mg or behavioral therapy and BT nonremitters were randomized to zolpidem 5 to 10 mg or cognitive therapy. Both zolpidem and trazodone doses were titrated based on side effects and degree of improvement, mirroring clinical practice. Because this chapter focuses on pharmacotherapy, we consider only the findings with zolpidem and trazodone (see Chapter 100 for other findings). In stage 1, zolpidem was associated with a response rate of 49.7% (odds ratio [OR] of response 1.18, 95% confidence interval [CI] 0.60 to 2.33) and remission rate of 30.3% (OR 1.41 95% CI 0.75 to 2.65). For patients who had failed to remit to BT in stage 1, the addition of zolpidem led to a significant 62.7% response rate (OR 2.46, 95% CI 1.14 to 5.30) and 55.9% remission rate (OR 2.06, 95% CI 1.04 to 4.11). For those who failed to remit to treatment with zolpidem in stage 1, switching to trazodone did not significantly increase the response rate but did increase the remission rate from 31.4% to 49.4% (OR 2.13, 95% CI 0.91 to 5.0). It was also noted that response and remission rates were sustained for up to a year in these groups. This study suggests that zolpidem is likely to be helpful for patients as initial therapy in clinical practice as well as for those who fail to remit to BT. Furthermore, a significant number of patients who fail to remit with zolpidem in clinical practice are likely to do so if switched to trazodone therapy.

CONTRAINDICATIONS TO INSOMNIA PHARMACOTHERAPY

There are no absolute contraindications to pharmacotherapy for patients with insomnia. There are, however, relative contraindications that increase the risks of therapy. For each patient it is necessary to weigh the risks of treatment against both the expected benefit and the risks of not treating the patient for insomnia. For example, an individual with a substance use disorder (e.g., alcoholism) has increased risks when treated with a benzodiazepine for insomnia resulting from significantly heightened abuse liability. However, a risk-benefit analysis may favor treatment with a benzodiazepine in patients facing serious medical complications if they resume drinking, but the only way they can avoid resuming drinking is through institution of effective therapy for their severe sleep-onset insomnia, and the only treatment that is effective for this is a benzodiazepine. In this case, the risk of abuse-related problems, which would normally preclude prescribing such an individual a benzodiazepine/non-benzodiazepine, is outweighed by the medical benefit of preventing resumption of alcohol consumption. In this context, this section considers some of the most important relative contraindications as a basis for such risk-benefit analysis, including liver failure, severe obstructive sleep apnea (OSA)/chronic obstructive pulmonary disease, pregnancy, suicidality, abuse liability, and interactions with other medications (Table 99.2). However, it is important to be aware that there are some relative contraindications that are stronger than others. Among the strongest are a history of an anaphylactic or other serious reaction to prior use of a medication and

Table 99.2 Some Important Relative Contraindications for Use of Insomnia Medications

Insomnia Medication	Liver Failure Toxicity Risk	Pregnancy Category[a]	Excreted in Breast Milk	0–100 Rating of Abuse Liability[35,b]	DEA Abuse Liability Category	Drugs Increasing Risks
Triazolam	High	X	Yes	42	IV[c]	Strong CYP3A4 inhibitors; erythromycin, cimetidine, ranitidine
Flurazepam	High	X	Unknown	38	IV	
Temazepam	Moderate	X	Yes	50	IV	
Zolpidem	High	C	Yes	33	IV	Strong CYP3A4 inhibitors
Zolpidem ER	High	C	Yes	33	IV	Strong CYP3A4 inhibitors
Transoral Zolpidem	High	C	Yes	33	IV	Strong CYP3A4 inhibitors
Zaleplon	High	C	Yes	50	IV	Cimetidine
Eszopiclone	High	C	Unknown	50	IV	Strong CYP3A4 inhibitors
Ramelteon	High	C	Unknown	0	No	Strong CYP3A4, CYP1A2, and CYP2C9 inhibitors
Doxepin	High	C	Yes	NR	No	Monoamine oxidase inhibitors; cimetidine
Suvorexant	High			NR	IV	Strong CYP3A4 inhibitors
Trazodone	High	C	Yes	0	No	Strong CYP3A4 inhibitors; monoamine oxidase inhibitors
Diphenhydramine	High	B	Yes	25	No	

[a]Pregnancy categories: X, Studies have demonstrated fetal abnormalities and/or that there is positive evidence of human fetal risk based on adverse reaction data from investigational or marketing experience, and the risks involved in use of the drug in pregnant women clearly outweigh potential benefits; C, Animal reproduction studies have shown an adverse effect on the fetus and there are no adequate and well-controlled studies in humans, but potential benefits may warrant use of the drug in pregnant women despite potential risks; B, Animal reproduction studies have failed to demonstrate a risk to the fetus and there are no adequate and well-controlled studies in pregnant women OR Animal studies have shown an adverse effect, but adequate and well-controlled studies in pregnant women have failed to demonstrate a risk to the fetus in any trimester.

[b]100 is the greatest possible abuse liability and 0 is no abuse liability.

[c]DEA Category IV indicates a low potential for abuse and low risk of dependence. Drugs that are strong inhibitors of the liver enzyme cytochrome P450 3A4 include ketoconazole, itraconazole, posaconazole, clarithromycin, nefazodone, ritonavir, saquinavir, nelfinavir, indinavir, boceprevir, telaprevir, telithromycin, and conivaptan. Drugs that are strong inhibitors of the liver enzyme cytochrome P450 1A2 include fluvoxamine. Drugs that are strong inhibitors of the liver enzyme cytochrome P450 2C9 include fluconazole.

DEA, Drug Enforcement Agency; NR, not rated.

the use of some of the medications considered in pregnancy. A subset of the agents considered have been identified as associated with a relatively high risk of significant adverse outcomes when used in pregnancy, particularly early in pregnancy; this has been viewed as a contraindication to the use of those agents.

Another key consideration related to the risk-benefit ratio is age. In general, prevalence of adverse drug reactions in those over 65 is double than that of those under 65.[29] Key contributors to this are greater sensitivity and vulnerability to side effects (worse consequences from falls, heightened sensitivity to cognitive impairment, higher rate of medical conditions such as coronary artery disease and hypertension), higher blood levels of drugs (resulting from changes in drug absorption, distribution, metabolism and excretion, and changes in volume of distribution), and greater likelihood of drug-drug interactions as a result of being more likely to be taking concomitant medications. It is important to take such considerations into account when considering insomnia pharmacotherapy in older adults.

Liver Failure

The risk of treating patients with liver failure with insomnia medications occurs because all of these medications are broken down by liver enzymes. In patients with significant liver dysfunction these medications are not as effectively deactivated and, as a result, there is a substantial risk that blood levels will be substantially higher than usual, increasing the risk of toxicity. As a result, all medications used to treat insomnia should be used with caution in individuals with substantial liver dysfunction. However, the specific pathway by which each of the medications is metabolized has an impact on the degree to which liver failure increases the toxicity risk. Those metabolized by the liver cytochrome p450 microenzymes are relatively more affected than those metabolized by glucuronide conjugation, which are associated with somewhat lower toxicity risk. Of the medications considered here, only temazepam is metabolized by glucuronide conjugation and, as a result, may be associated with a lower, although still significant, risk of toxicity.[30]

Pregnancy

Nonmedication therapies are preferable, when possible, for treatment of insomnia in pregnant women to minimize treatment risks. The medications used for insomnia differ in their risk levels when used in pregnancy. There is some evidence that the use of benzodiazepines during pregnancy, especially early in pregnancy, may be associated with fetal damage. As a result, triazolam, flurazepam, and temazepam have been assigned pregnancy category X, which is assigned when the FDA believes that "the risks involved in use of the drug in pregnant women clearly outweigh potential benefits." Otherwise, all of the other medications considered have been assigned category C, which is an indication that "animal reproduction studies have shown an adverse effect on the fetus and there are no adequate and well-controlled studies in humans, but potential benefits may warrant use of the drug in pregnant women despite potential risks." The exceptions to this are melatonin, which is not assigned a pregnancy category by the FDA because, as a supplement, it does not oversee this medication, and diphenhydramine, which was assigned category B, indicating that "animal reproduction studies have failed to demonstrate a risk to the fetus and there are no adequate and well-controlled studies in pregnant women OR animal studies have shown an adverse effect, but adequate and well-controlled studies in pregnant women have failed to demonstrate a risk to the fetus in any trimester."

Suicidality

Population-based research suggests that the use of insomnia medications is associated with elevated risks for suicide.[31] Whether this association is causal remains unclear as the studies did not control for conditions such as major depression that occur frequently in individuals who are prescribed these medications. Review of the available literature suggests that there may be two factors that could be responsible for such an association: the lethality of insomnia medications when taken in overdose and the possibility that parasomnias induced by the medications could lead to self-harm or suicidal behavior in individuals not known to have suicidal thoughts.[31] The latter appears to be rare and is somewhat speculative. As a result, the focus here is on the fact that prescribing a medication to suicidal individuals brings with it the possibility that the individuals may take an overdose of the medication in an attempt to end their life. Death from single-drug overdose with insomnia medications considered here occurs rarely, despite the fact that some of the agents have been taken in overdose many times.[32] All of the agents have been associated with lethal single-agent overdose in at least one case, with the exception of ramelteon and suvorexant. However, this reflects, at least to a degree, that relatively fewer individuals have been prescribed these two agents compared with all of the other medications considered.[31-34] All of the prescription medications considered here except for suvorexant were ranked on lethality in overdose in a recent analysis, taking into account available data: they were all given essentially the same risk rating, except for ramelteon, which was assigned a lower level of risk.[34] More common than single-agent overdose deaths are deaths in overdose when taken in combination with other CNS depressants such as alcohol and opioids. Whether these agents contribute significantly to the lethality in those circumstances is difficult to determine. Given the potential for lethality, care must be exercised when considering prescribing all of these medications to individuals at risk for suicide. In individuals at high suicide risk with sleep-onset insomnia, ramelteon may be an option to consider.

Abuse Liability

The available evidence suggests that drugs prescribed for the treatment of insomnia that have abuse liability based on animal and human studies are used for recreational purposes only in a small, predisposed subset of individuals.[35] The U.S. Drug Enforcement Agency assigns a liability class to all medications approved for use by the FDA based on animal data and on abuse liability studies in which the drug is given to known poly-substance abusers. As a result, these categories can provide an indication of the risks of prescribing an agent to an abuse-prone individual. These categories appear in Table 99.2. The majority of agents are assigned category IV, which indicates that, although abuse liability exists, there is "a low potential for abuse and low risk of dependence." The exceptions are doxepin, melatonin, ramelteon, trazodone, and diphenhydramine (as well as other OTCs), which are not scheduled because they are not identified as having abuse liability. A ranking of abuse liability of all of the medications considered here except for suvorexant was recently carried out in an analysis that took into account all available human and animal studies.[36] The medications were assigned a risk score from 0 to 100, with 100 being the greatest risk (Table 99.2).

Drug Interactions

All agents that promote sleep have additive effects with other drugs that have sedative effects, including alcohol. As a result, drugs used to treat insomnia should be used with caution when taken with other agents that promote sleep. Special concerns have been raised about the use of medications for the treatment of insomnia with opioids because of observational studies suggesting an increase in mortality compared with use of opioids alone. This is presumed to be due to enhanced respiratory depression and profound sedation that has been observed with combinations of opioids and benzodiazepines. However, there are no data to provide reassurance with any of the other medications except for diphenhydramine, for which there has been some experience with concomitant use with opioids.[37] As a result, caution should be exercised when considering combining any of these medications with opioid medications.

Risks are also increased when combining these agents with agents that impede that the metabolic action of the pathway or pathways responsible for their breakdown. The resulting elevation in blood levels increases the risk for toxicity. A number of insomnia medications can be affected by specific inhibitors of liver cytochrome P450 microenzymes. Increased toxicity risks exist when using triazolam, zolpidem, eszopiclone, ramelteon, suvorexant, and trazodone along with strong inhibitors of the P450 CYP3A4 microenzymes, which include ketoconazole, itraconazole, posaconazole, clarithromycin, nefazodone, ritonavir, saquinavir, nelfinavir, indinavir, boceprevir, telaprevir, telithromycin, conivaptan, and cimetidine (Table 99.2). Increased toxicity risks exist when using ramelteon with drugs that strongly inhibit P450 CYP1A2, including fluvoxamine and that strongly inhibit P450 CYP2C9, such as fluconazole. Cimetidine blocks several liver microenzymes involved in metabolism of these drugs and increases risks with triazolam, zaleplon, and doxepin. The use of drugs that block the enzyme monoamine oxidase, which is responsible for the breakdown of a number of monoamines as well as tyramine, increases the risks of serotonin syndrome or hypertensive reactions occurring with doxepin and trazodone. However, these risks are believed to be associated with their antidepressant dosages, which are higher than dosages typically used to treat insomnia, particularly for doxepin.

Severe Obstructive Sleep Apnea/Chronic Obstructive Pulmonary Disease

Because of blunting of arousal and the capacity to depress respiratory drive, precautions should be taken when treating patients with severe OSA and chronic obstructive pulmonary disease (COPD) with these medications. For a number of these medications, studies have been carried out with individuals with mild to moderate OSA and COPD demonstrating safety, but no studies have been carried out in individuals with severe disease.

DEFINING THE CUTTING EDGE OF INSOMNIA PHARMACOTHERAPY

I reviewed the evidence for efficacy, effectiveness, and relative contraindications of the major medications used to treat insomnia. Different types of medications have therapeutic effects on different types of sleep problems among the set of problems experienced by patients with insomnia. These medications differ in their risk profiles among groups of patients with insomnia. As a result, optimizing treatment requires personalization of therapy by selecting a medication for individuals that best addresses the specific type of sleep problem they are experiencing while accompanied by the least possible side effects and risks. This has only been possible to a limited degree in the past because of the availability of medications with only a limited set of mechanisms of action and the lack of medications with highly specific pharmacologic effects.

Although we have had some medications with highly specific pharmacologic effects such as benzodiazepines, which generally have as their only pharmacologic effect binding to a specific site on the GABA-A receptor complex, these medications exert broad clinical effects because of the wide distribution of GABA-A receptors in the brain. The result is that they can affect all of the major sleep problems experienced by people with insomnia, along with symptoms of some common comorbid conditions (anxiety and pain) and other conditions (seizures), but the trade-off that comes along with this can include unwanted effects, such as impairment in cognition, impairment in psychomotor function, and abuse liability.

We have also long had medications available that exerted clinically significant effects via mechanisms other than those of the benzodiazepines. For example, histamine H1 receptor antagonism, which occurs with the antidepressant amitriptyline or the antipsychotic medication thioridazine; however, these medications exert clinically significant effects at other types of receptors that result in both broader impact on sleep problems but also a significant number of unwanted adverse effects. It is only relatively recently that studies have been carried out with treatments that had H1 antagonism as their *only* clinically significant effects.[38] Another example of such specific drugs relatively recently studied include hypocretin/orexin receptor antagonists.

The personalization approach is only viable when there are medications with high pharmacologic specificity, because such medications have effects on subsets of the possible set of sleep problems experienced by patients with insomnia, and because they affect a single pharmacologic system, their potential side effect profile is relatively more circumscribed. The result of using such a medication with highly specific effects matched to the needs of an individual is a better risk-to-benefit ratio than is possible to achieve with medications that exert more global/generalized nonspecific effects.

This review of efficacy/effectiveness and contraindications of insomnia medications suggests that such personalization is possible to a degree that is likely to impact clinical care quality. Here these opportunities are summarized: the type of sleep problems experienced by patients with insomnia, their associated medical conditions and concomitant medications, and the interventions best suited for treatment of individuals with those problems in a personalized medicine insomnia treatment framework (Table 99.3). For this purpose it is assumed that agents with the strongest available evidence for a therapeutic effect for the type(s) of sleep problem that an individual has (indicated by *** in Table 99.1) should be considered first, followed by those agents with supportive evidence in the one meta-analysis reporting results for the outcome of interest (indicated by ** in Table 99.1), followed by those agents with mixed supportive evidence from the meta-analyses (indicated by * in Table 99.1). Relative contraindications are taken into account by choosing the medication with the strongest evidence for efficacy for the patients' specific type of sleep problem that does not have a significant relative contraindication weighing against its use (Table 99.2).

One efficacy-related issue that was not considered in the meta-analyses reviewed here that is relevant to personalization is the need to take a more specific approach to sleep maintenance therapy. It is possible to have difficulties staying asleep that affect the entire night or are restricted to a portion of the night. Because there is clear evidence that the medications with demonstrated sleep maintenance effects differ in the time of night when they exert these effects, there is an opportunity to optimize sleep maintenance therapy by matching the time of night of the patient's sleep problem to the time of night of drug therapeutic effects. Zolpidem ER demonstrated therapeutic effects only in the first 6 hours of the night, whereas doxepin 3 to 6 mg and suvorexant have been found to be unique in having therapeutic effects in the last third of the night.[20,22,39] As a result, taking into account the time of night of sleep maintenance effects is incorporated into this personalized medicine framework for insomnia medications. Further, flurazepam is not considered because its excessively long half-life has led its use to be minimal in recent years. The resulting personalized medicine framework is presented in Table 99.3.

FUTURE DIRECTIONS

The preceding review of the existing evidence base for pharmacologic therapies suggests some important gaps in the available treatments that provide opportunities for future treatment development. These include medications that are effective and can be taken by pregnant women without increasing risks; agents without abuse liability risk that are highly effective for helping individuals with sleep onset problems and the combination of onset and maintenance problems; and medications that are effective for onset and maintenance problems without increased risk in those with hepatic failure. Opportunities for developing new agents include mechanisms that have been established to affect sleep-wake function but have not

Table 99.3 Personalized Medicine Paradigm for Insomnia Pharmacotherapy

Type of Sleep Problem										
Sleep Onset	Sleep Maintenance	Early Morning Waking	No Meds or Medical Conditions	Liver Failure	Pregnancy	High Substance Abuse Risk	Taking CYP3A4 Inhibitor	Taking CYP1A2 or CYP2C9 Inhibitor	Taking Cimetidine	Taking MAO Inhibitor
X			1-TE ZA ES S 2-TI TR 3-Z ZE M R D	1-TE	None; Cat C- ZA ES S	2-TR 3-M R D	1-TE ZA 3-M D	1-TE ZA ES S 2-TI TR 3-Z ZE M D	1-TE ES S 2-TR 3-Z ZE M R	1-TE ZA ES S 2-TI 3-Z ZE M R
	X		1-ZE ES D S 2-TZ TR 3-Z M R	None	None; Cat C- ZE ES D S	1-D 2-TR 3-M R	1-D 3-M	1-ZE ES D S 2-TZ TR 3-Z M R	1-ZE ES S 2-TZ TR 3-Z M R	1-ZE ES S 2-TZ 3-Z M R
		X	1- D S	None	None: Cat C- D S	1-D	1-D	1-D S	1-S	1-S
X	X		1-ES S 2-TR 3-Z M R D	None	None: Cat C-ES S	2-TR 3-D M R	3-D M	1-ES S 2-TR 3-Z ZE M R D	1-ES S 2-TR 3-ZE Z M R	1-ES S 3-Z M R
X	X	X	1-S	None	None: Cat C-S	None	None	1-S	1-S	1-S

1, Treatments with best supported efficacy based on the meta-analyses. 2, Treatments with only one meta-analysis reporting results but that suggested efficacy. 3, Treatments with mixed evidence for efficacy in the meta-analyses.
Cat C, Pregnancy Category C; D, doxepin; E, eszopiclone; M, melatonin; R, ramelteon; S, suvorexant; TI, triazolam; TE, temazepam; TR, trazodone; TZ, transoral zolpidem; Z, zolpidem; ZA, zaleplon; ZE, zolpidem ER.

been capitalized upon for insomnia medication development. These include those targeting adenosine, galanin, dopamine, and a number of neuropeptides. Last, there is a need for more effectiveness studies and more studies comparing existing treatments that would allow us to better understand how to personalize and optimize therapy with the available options.

CLINICAL PEARL

Clinical management of patients with insomnia has long been a one-size-fits-all endeavor. Clinicians tend to identify a treatment that they use in most if not all of their patients with insomnia. However, over time a body of evidence has accumulated, indicating that medications have effects on specific types of sleep problems and differ in their relative contraindications to use based on the clinical circumstances of the patient. This body of evidence represents a guide for optimizing care by selecting the medication for each patient that is most likely to improve the type of sleep problem they are experiencing with the least associated risks.

SUMMARY

There are a number of medications available for the treatment of insomnia. There is a body of efficacy research summarized in meta-analyses that documents which treatments are effective for the specific types of sleep problems experienced by patients with insomnia. This includes (1) sleep onset difficulties for which the evidence base most strongly supports temazepam, zaleplon, eszopiclone, and suvorexant; (2) sleep maintenance problems without early-morning awakening for which the evidence base most strongly supports the use of zolpidem ER, eszopiclone, doxepin, and suvorexant; and (3) sleep maintenance problems with early-morning awakening, for which the existing research most strongly supports the use of doxepin and suvorexant. In addition, a number of relative contraindications to the use of specific agents exist. Such contraindications include use in those with liver failure, during pregnancy, in those at high risk for substance abuse, and those taking concomitant medications with interactions. Together the efficacy and contraindications data provide a framework for selecting the insomnia medication(s) that are most likely to have the best risk-benefit ratio for each individual patient and form the basis for a personalized medicine approach to insomnia pharmacotherapy.

SELECTED READINGS

Lou BX, Oks M. Insomnia: pharmacologic treatment. *Clin Geriatr Med.* 2021;37(3):401–415.

Samara MT, Huhn M, Chiocchia V, et al. Efficacy, acceptability, and tolerability of all available treatments for insomnia in the elderly: a systematic review and network meta-analysis. *Acta Psychiatr Scand.* 2020;142(1):6–17.

Sateia MJ, Buysse DJ, Krystal AD, Neubauer DN, Heald JL. Clinical practice guideline for the pharmacologic treatment of chronic insomnia in adults: an American Academy of Sleep Medicine Clinical Practice Guideline. *J Clin Sleep Med.* 2017;13(2):307–349.

Singal AG, Higgins PD, Waljee AK. A primer on effectiveness and efficacy trials. *Clin Transl Gastroenterol.* 2014;5(1):e45.

U.S. Department of Health and Human Services Food and Drug Administration (USFDA), Center for Biologics Evaluation and Research (CBER), Center for Drug Evaluation and Research (CDER). Demonstrating Substantial Evidence of Effectiveness for Human Drug and Biological Products Guidance for Industry. 2019.

Wilt TJ, MacDonald R, Brasure M, et al. Pharmacologic treatment of insomnia disorder: an evidence report for a clinical practice guideline by the American College of Physicians. *Ann Intern Med.* 2016;165(2):103–112.

Zheng X, He Y, Yin F, et al. Pharmacological interventions for the treatment of insomnia: quantitative comparison of drug efficacy [published online ahead of print, 2020 Apr 1]. *Sleep Med.* 2020;72:41–49. https://doi.org/10.1016/j.sleep.2020.03.022.

A complete reference list can be found online at ExpertConsult.com.

Chapter 100

Pharmacologic Treatment III: Sequenced and Combined Psychologic and Pharmacologic Treatments for Insomnia

Jack D. Edinger; Charles M. Morin; Wilfred R. Pigeon

Chapter Highlights

- Psychological/behavioral insomnia therapies as well as various forms of pharmacotherapy have been widely used for insomnia treatment. The psychological/behavioral treatments produce gradual treatment benefits but have durable effects over time, whereas pharmacotherapies produce more rapid symptomatic relief but may not have durable benefits with sustained use. Yet neither form of treatment is universally effective, and there may be times when combining or switching treatment modality produces the best outcomes.
- Although limited, past and recent research has examined such questions as: (1) Does past exposure to pharmacotherapy dampen response to the psychological/behavioral insomnia therapies?; (2) What are the best approaches for combining or sequencing these two forms of therapy?; (3) Is there value added to switching treatment modality (i.e., psychological/behavioral therapy to pharmacotherapy and vice versa) when the initial treatment modality fails to produce optimal improvement?; (4) Can the psychological/behavioral insomnia therapies be effectively combined with other forms of psychological treatments to address sleep problems and concurrent comorbidities?; (5) What approaches are most effective to help patients discontinue hypnotics?
- This chapter reviews outcomes of combined and sequenced insomnia therapies and highlights treatment combinations and sequences that show promise for improving care of persons with insomnia.

INTRODUCTION

Chronic insomnia is widely prevalent and associated with impaired daytime functioning, increased risks for psychiatric and medical illnesses, and enhanced health care costs for millions worldwide.[1-9] Currently the most viable and best-supported treatments for insomnia include various forms of pharmacotherapies (e.g., benzodiazepine-receptor agonists, melatonin-receptor agonists, orexin antagonists, sedative antidepressants, and over-the-counter antihistamines) and the psychological/behavioral therapies, particularly cognitive behavioral therapy for insomnia (CBT-I). Medications produce rapid symptomatic improvements, are widely available, and are consequently the first treatment most insomnia patients receive. Such medications are generally well tolerated, but there are concerns about potential adverse effects (e.g., daytime sedation) and risk of tolerance and dependence with longer-term use.[10,11] Furthermore, there are limited data documenting sustained benefits of the available pharmacologic agents with prolonged usage or after their discontinuation.[12,13] In contrast, CBT-I has shown both short-term and durable sleep improvements, is well tolerated and preferred by many patients, and has a generally favorable side effect profile vis-à-vis medication.[14-17] As a consequence, CBT-I has become the recommended first-line insomnia therapy for all adults who suffer from insomnia disorders.[18,19]

Yet it should be recognized that no single therapy, whether CBT-I or some form of pharmacotherapy, is effective or beneficial for all patients. If we consider the CBT-I literature, for example, 35% to 40% of all patients receiving such treatment fail to show a "clinically significant" improvement in symptoms, whereas less than 50% receiving such treatment achieve insomnia remission.[3,14] Hence a substantial portion of insomnia patients who receive CBT-I alone do not achieve desired treatment outcomes. This observation raises a number of questions about the available insomnia therapies. Since many insomnia patients are exposed to a pharmacotherapy before CBT-I, does such prior treatment exposure dampen their response to this subsequent treatment? Second, it seems possible that some patients may require an adjunctive pharmacotherapy to optimize their treatment outcome. So, the question then is how best to combine pharmacologic and CBT-I approaches to optimize treatment outcomes. Also, are there certain treatment sequences such as pharmacotherapy to CBT-I or CBT-I to pharmacotherapy that show better outcomes than providing CBT-I alone? Finally, it is important to note that most patients with insomnia do not experience this condition in isolation but rather have concurrent sleep-disruptive comorbid conditions (e.g., major depressive disorder, chronic pain). Then, the question is whether treatments for the comorbid conditions should be combined with the insomnia therapy to optimize insomnia treatment outcomes.

In this chapter we address these various questions. In the first section we examine the literature to determine if those having prior exposure to pharmacotherapy for insomnia show a blunted response to CBT-I as compared with medication-naïve patients. Second, we review the results of studies testing various CBT-I medication treatment combinations to determine if there is an optimal model for such a combined treatment approach. Third, we review the limited literature on CBT-I–pharmacotherapy treatment sequences to ascertain the value of such treatment used as first- and second-stage interventions. Fourth, we provide a review of studies that tested combined psychological therapies with CBT-I to concurrently address insomnia and associated comorbid conditions. Finally, we consider strategies for helping persons who are hypnotic dependent achieve hypnotic abstinence. The chapter concludes with a general summary of our findings and suggestions for much-needed future research.

PRIOR HYPNOTIC EXPOSURE AND SUBSEQUENT OUTCOMES WITH PSYCHOLOGICAL TREATMENTS

Those who have conducted clinical trials to test psychological/behavioral therapies for insomnia are well aware that a majority of patients entering such trials have a long history of insomnia before their first exposure to such treatments. In fact, it is not uncommon for these trial participants to have suffered from insomnia for 10 or more years before their first exposure to the sort of nonpharmacologic interventions offered in these trials. Of course, during the time period leading up to their first exposure to a psychological/behavioral therapy, many patients seek other insomnia remedies and a substantial subset come to rely on a prescription hypnotic for insomnia management. As a result, many insomnia patients are chronic hypnotic users at the time they seek their first exposure to psychological/behavioral insomnia treatment either through research study participation or via clinical referral.

It is important to note that management of insomnia via pharmacotherapy and psychological/behavioral therapies involve distinctive behavioral and cognitive "sets" on the part of the patient. From the patient's viewpoint, pharmacotherapy involves the production of sleep "on demand" via use of a sedative hypnotic. Patients who find their pharmacologic agent effective may be able to exercise somewhat flexible sleep schedules, within reason, and may not have to change their sleep habits significantly to be able to sleep better. In contrast, many of the psychological/behavioral insomnia therapies, including CBT-I specifically, mandate following a fairly rigid sleep-wake schedule and altering a number of current sleep habits to improve sleep. Rather than expecting to be able to produce sleep *on demand*, they must accept the belief that they can make their sleep more reliable by making significant alterations in their sleep habits and cognitive stance toward the sleep process. Whereas adopting the behavioral and cognitive changes required by these therapies may be relatively less difficult for the hypnotic-naïve patient, the paradigm shift required by the psychological/behavioral insomnia therapies may be more challenging for the chronic hypnotic user to effect. Thus it seems reasonable to speculate that their prior hypnotic exposure could make patients less responsive to psychological/behavioral interventions.

A review of the published literature, however, generally suggests that patients who use hypnotics are no less responsive to the psychological/behavioral interventions for insomnia than are hypnotic-naïve patients. Table 100.1, for example, provides a list of studies and their observed outcomes for hypnotic users and medication-free patients with insomnia across a variety of sleep measures used to assess sleep improvements. All but one of these trials showed that hypnotic users achieved comparable sleep improvements across the outcome measures assessed as did the medication-free patients. The one trial showing better treatment response of medication-free patients was a small trial of only 20 participants. Moreover, many of the remaining trials showed comparable sleep improvements by the hypnotic users and medication-free patients, and they showed many of the hypnotic users reduced or discontinued their hypnotic use once provided a psychological/behavioral therapy, even in studies without formal medication-tapering instructions.

More recent data supporting the findings shown in Table 100.1 come from a trial[20] testing an online version of CBT-I. In this large trial, patients with insomnia were randomized to treatment with the online CBT-I or a waitlist control. Results of this trial in general showed significantly better sleep and insomnia symptom improvements in the treatment group as compared with control. However, unpublished data extracted from this trial showed that those who were using hypnotics at the time of their trial entry did as well with the online CBT-I intervention as did those who were medication free at the time of trial entry (Figure 100.1). Along with these findings, an earlier study[21] with the same online CBT-I intervention showed hypnotic users who received this treatment were significantly more likely to discontinue their hypnotics than were hypnotic users who were assigned to a waitlist control. This literature suggests that the incidental pairing of hypnotic use with psychological/behavioral insomnia therapies by virtue of a patient being on hypnotics at the time of treatment initiation should not reduce expectations for a positive insomnia treatment outcome.

TREATMENT OUTCOMES OF CONCURRENT COGNITIVE BEHAVIORAL THERAPY FOR INSOMNIA AND HYPNOTIC COMBINATIONS

Despite the extensive literature documenting the effects of CBT-I and various classes of medications for the management of insomnia,[22,23] there are surprisingly very few studies

Table 100.1 Response of Hypnotic Users and Nonusers to Psychological/Behavioral Insomnia Therapies[74-83]

Study Citation	Active Treatments	*n* (Sample Size / % Females)	Findings
Backhaus et al., 2001	CBT-I + relaxation	20/65%	5 of 12 discontinued hypnotic use; unmedicated showed greater improvement than hypnotic users
Baillargeon et. al, 1998	Stimulus control	15/67%	SOL declined and hypnotic use decreased by 84%
Dashevsky et al., 1998	Stimulus control + sleep restriction + sleep hygiene + relaxation	48/75%	SOL, WASO, SE%, and TST all improved 53% of sample reduced hypnotic use by at least 50%
Espie et al., 2001	CBT-I + relaxation	138/68.8%	SOL & WASO improved 50 of 74 hypnotic users were hypnotic free at 1-year follow-up
Lichstein et al., 1999	Medication withdrawal and/or relaxation	40/57.5%	Medicated patients had decreased hypnotic use by 78% by the 3-month follow-up
Morgan et al., 2004	CBT-I + medication withdrawal	209/67.5%	PSQI improved; 39% of those receiving CBT-I reduced hypnotics by >50% of their baseline levels by the 6-month follow-up
Reidel et al., 1998	Stimulus control and/or medication withdrawal	41/54%	Medicated and unmedicated showed similar improvements
Semeit et al., 2004	CBT-I and progressive relaxation or autogenic training	229/75.1%	Sleep improvement occurred and medication use decreased among those receiving CBT-I
Strom et al., 2004	Internet CBT-I	109[a]/65.1%	Greater reduction in unhelpful beliefs and hypnotic use among CBT-I group relative to controls
Verbeek et al., 1999	CBT-I + relaxation + medication withdrawal	86/65.1%	Hypnotic users achieved sleep improvements that were comparable to the medication-free patients

[a]Sample size listed included 28 treatment dropouts.
The table shows the response of hypnotic users and non-users to various types of psychological and behavioral insomnia therapies. All except the first study listed showed that hypnotic users and nonusers responded comparably to the treatment listed. CBT-I, Cognitive behavioral therapy for insomnia; PSQI, Pittsburgh Sleep Quality Index; SE%, sleep efficiency; SOL, sleep-onset latency; TST, total sleep time; WASO, wake after sleep onset.

(less than a dozen) that have directly compared the benefits of these two treatment modalities (Table 100.2). The evidence available is rather convincing that when used as monotherapies, both CBT-I and medication produce significant improvements on several sleep-wake parameters (sleep-onset latency, wake after sleep onset, total sleep time) and other patient-reported outcomes, such as perceived insomnia severity symptoms, mood symptoms, and daytime fatigue. Effect sizes derived from meta-analyses indicate that CBT-I may have an advantage for reducing sleep continuity parameters such as sleep-onset latency and time awake after sleep onset, whereas medication is more effective for increasing total sleep time.[15,22-24] What is also clear is that there is no single treatment, whether psychological or pharmacologic, that is effective or acceptable to all patients with insomnia. Each treatment modality has its own advantages and limitations. As we previously noted, medication produces quick symptomatic relief. However, with some exceptions, these benefits are lost upon drug discontinuation. Conversely, CBT-I may take longer to improve sleep, yet those improvements are well sustained over time. Based on these observations, there seems to be a good rationale for combining CBT-I and medication to capitalize on the quicker benefits derived from medication and the longer-lasting effects of CBT-I.

The first few studies investigating the effect of combined therapies compared triazolam against various combinations of relaxation and stimulus control therapy[25,26] or a hybrid sleep hygiene intervention mixed with relaxation.[27] Those early investigations were conducted with relatively small samples and showed that medication produced improvements on sleep latency and total sleep time, sometimes in the very first week of therapy, whereas behavioral therapy showed slightly delayed benefits during the course of treatment. In a study comparing estazolam plus muscle relaxation or guided imagery against estazolam plus sleep education,[28] significant improvements were obtained on measures of wake after sleep onset, sleep efficiency, and total sleep time in the two groups combining medication with behavioral treatment, but only on total sleep time for those receiving estazolam with sleep education. Collectively, these early uncontrolled studies also showed that patients treated with behavioral interventions, with or without concurrent medication, maintained their sleep improvements more consistently than those receiving medication alone at 1-, 6-, and 10-month follow-ups.

Three randomized controlled trials (RCTs) have examined the impact of CBT-I, medication, and combined therapy against a drug placebo control condition. The first such placebo-controlled trial[29] compared CBT-I and temazepam, singly and combined, with drug placebo in 78 older adults. All three treatments were more effective than placebo on the primary end point of wake after sleep onset, with the combined approach yielding slightly superior benefits over CBT-I or temazepam alone. Medication was discontinued at the end of the 8-week treatment period and naturalistic follow-ups were conducted 3, 12, and 24 months later. Patients treated with medication lost their initial benefits over time and those

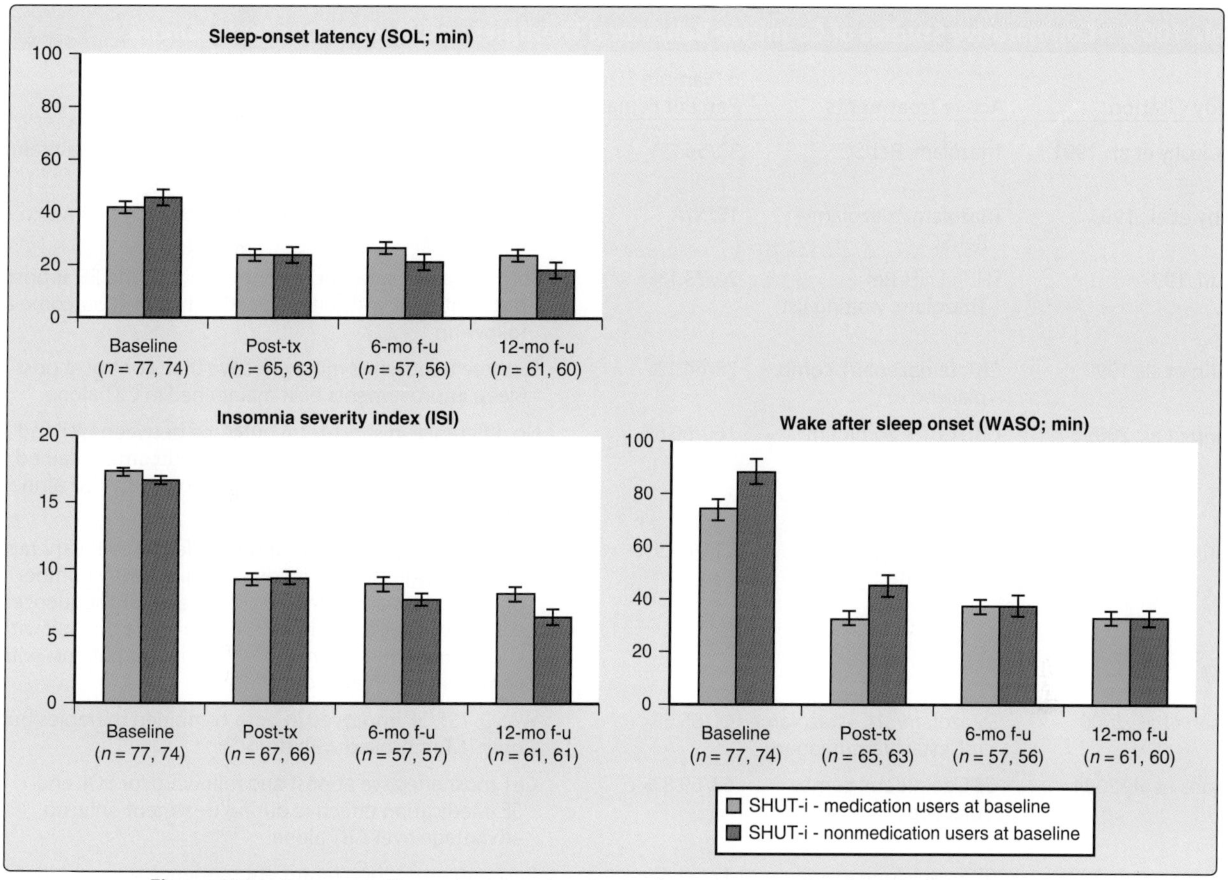

Figure 100.1 Responses of hypnotic users and medication-free patients to online CBT-I. The figure shows that SHUT-i was equally effective for improving sleep measures in medication users and nonusers. The SHUT-i group was subdivided into users and nonusers of medication at baseline. Medication use was defined as having taken any medication for sleep based on sleep diaries at baseline. Samples sizes for each are displayed as *n* = medication users, nonusers. For all measures the group × time interaction was nonsignificant. (Data from Ritterband LM, Thorndike FP, Ingersoll KS, et al. Effect of a web-based cognitive behavior therapy for insomnia intervention with 1-year follow-up: A randomized clinical trial. *JAMA Psychiatry.* 2017;74[1]:68–75.)

treated with CBT-I retained their sleep improvements best over time. Long-term outcomes were variable among patients treated with combined therapy, with some patients retaining their benefits and others not. Overall, long-term treatment effects were weaker for the combined condition relative to CBT-I alone. Of additional interest in this study was the use of polysomnography (PSG) at baseline and at the end of treatment. In general, the magnitude of improvements was smaller on PSG measures compared to patients' reported outcomes, but the PSG findings were clearly in the same direction of improvements reported by patients in the three treatment conditions.

Similar findings were reported in two other placebo-controlled trials using temazepam[30] or zolpidem[31] as comparators. In a study of 71 adults, Wu and colleagues[30] reported that their three active treatments were more effective than placebo and that patients treated with medication improved more on sleep-onset latency, sleep efficiency, and total sleep time than CBT-I patients at the end of the 8-week treatment period. However, at 3- and 8-month follow-ups, CBT-I patients maintained their sleep improvements best and reported additional benefits on self-report measures of nighttime pre-sleep arousal, daytime functioning, and dysfunctional sleep beliefs, whereas medicated patients gradually lost their initial benefits; the combined group showed variable long-term effects. In another similar trial conducted with 63 young and middle-aged adults with chronic sleep-onset insomnia,[31] CBT-I produced the largest effects on sleep latency and sleep efficiency, as well as the highest proportion of patients in remission after treatment. Combined treatment provided no advantage over CBT-I alone, whereas pharmacotherapy (zolpidem) produced moderate improvements during treatment but returned toward baseline insomnia severity after medication discontinuation. In yet another study comparing CBT-I to zopiclone and a drug placebo in 46 older adults,[32] CBT-I produced the best outcomes on three of four measures, whereas zopiclone did not differ from placebo. At 6-month follow-up, total sleep time was similar in all three groups, but patients using CBT-I had better sleep efficiency than those taking zopiclone or placebo.

Collectively, these controlled studies yielded similar findings, showing that psychological and pharmacologic interventions produce significant short-term benefits and, in some cases, faster relief for medication. Studies examining long-term outcomes have shown that sleep improvements are well maintained with CBT-I but not with hypnotic medication

Table 100.2 Comparative Studies of Cognitive Behavioral Therapies and Medications for Insomnia

Study Citation	Active Treatments	*n* (Sample Size/ Percent Females)	Findings
McClusky et al., 1991	Triazolam, Rel/SC	30/56.7%	Both treatments decreased SOL but gains only maintained in Rel/SC
Milby et al., 1993	Triazolam, triazolam + Rel/SC	15/N/A	Greater changes in TST in combined therapy relative to drug alone
Hauri, 1997	SH/Rel, SH/Rel + Triazolam, waiting list	26/73.1%	Both therapies superior to control on SOL and SE at post, but treatment without medication had best outcome at follow-up
Morin et al., 1999	CBT, temazepam, comb, placebo	78/64.1%	All three treatments more effective than control at post. Sleep improvements best maintained in CBT alone
Morin et al., 2009	CBT, CBT + zolpidem	160/60.6%	No difference in short-term outcome between CBT and combined therapy. Best long-term outcome obtained with combined therapy initially followed by CBT alone (medication discontinued)
Morin et al., 2016	BT, zolpidem, CT, trazodone	211/62.5%	No difference between BT and zolpidem as initial therapy. Second-stage therapy increased significantly number of responders and remitters. Best treatment sequences were those starting with BT. Second-stage therapy with CT and trazodone were more effective for patients with comorbid psychiatric disorders
Rosen et al., 2000	Estazolam/SH, estazolam/rel, estazolam/imagery	41/65.6%	WASO, TST, SE improved in both combined therapies but only TST improved with drug/SH
Jacobs et al., 2004	CBT, zolpidem, comb, placebo	63/69.8%	CBT most effective at post and follow-up for SOL and SE. Medication effective during treatment only; no advantage over CBT alone.
Vallières et al., 2005	CBT, zopiclone, comb	17/58.8%	Best outcome when treatment sequence started with CBT
Sivertsen et al., 2006	CBT, zopiclone, placebo	46/47.8%	Best short and long-term outcomes for CBT compared to medication on 3 of 4 variables
Wu et al., 2006	CBT, temazepam, comb, placebo	71/N/A	Three treatments more effective than control at post. SOL, TST, SE were more improved in medication relative to CBT at post, but all variables more improved in CBT relative to medication or combined therapy at follow-up.

BT, Behavior therapy; CBT, cognitive behavioral therapy; comb, combined; CT, cognitive therapy; N/A, not applicable; post, posttreatment; rel, relaxation; SC, stimulus control; SE, sleep efficiency; SH, sleep hygiene; SOL, sleep-onset latency; TST, total sleep time; WASO, wake after sleep onset.

alone, and mixed outcomes have been reported for combined therapy. The outcomes for combined therapy have been replicated at short (1 month), intermediate (6 months), and long-term follow-ups (12 and 24 months). In all studies that included a combined behavioral and drug therapy condition, these two therapies were initiated and discontinued concurrently, which may explain the more variable long-term outcomes. Indeed, it is plausible that patients who are prescribed a sleep medication, whether it is combined with CBT-I or not, may be less inclined to invest their time and efforts in changing maladaptive sleep behaviors and cognitions known to perpetuate insomnia. As such, the sole availability of a drug may undermine the patient's efforts and motivation for behavioral changes. Furthermore, if patients attribute their initial sleep improvements to the hypnotic drug alone, without integration of self-management skills, they may remain at greater risk for relapse once the medication is discontinued. As sleep-incompatible behaviors and unhelpful sleep-related cognitions often contribute to perpetuating insomnia, behavioral and attitudinal changes are essential to producing sustained sleep improvements. Thus, instead of discontinuing both medication and CBT-I at the same time, a more effective strategy may be to taper medication (under supervision) while patients are still engaged in CBT-I to ensure they fully integrate the newly learned behavioral and cognitive skills.

DOES MAINTENANCE THERAPY ENHANCE OUTCOMES?

Recent studies have addressed the issue of how best to sequence medication and CBT-I and examined whether the addition of maintenance therapies enhanced long-term outcomes. In a small investigation using single-case design methodology to test different treatment sequences with 15 patients, the best outcome was obtained when CBT-I was introduced first in the sequence, regardless of whether it was used alone or combined with medication.[33] The issue of maintenance therapy and treatment sequencing was further addressed in a larger study comparing CBT-I against CBT-I plus zolpidem in a two-stage, sequential multiple-assignment RCT (SMART design), testing four different treatment sequences with 160 patients with chronic insomnia disorder.[34] After an initial 6-week course of CBT-I or combined CBT-I and zolpidem, patients treated with CBT-I alone were randomized to an extended 6-month CBT-I that involved monthly booster sessions or no additional therapy. Patients treated with combined therapy initially were randomized to a 6-month extended CBT-I treatment alone (i.e., medication was discontinued) or to an extended CBT-I plus medication condition in which the drug was used on an as-needed basis (i.e., no more than two to three times per week) as opposed to an every-night regimen as in first-stage therapy. Following the initial 6-week treatment phase, similar rates of success were obtained when CBT-I was used alone (60% of patients achieved a treatment response and 39% were in remission) or in combination with zolpidem (61% responders and 44% remitters). After the 6-month extended treatment, there was a higher remission rate for those who were initially treated with combined therapy (56%) than those who used CBT-I alone (43%), and this higher remission rate was sustained throughout the 24-month follow-up.[35] Among patients who received combined CBT-I plus zolpidem as their initial treatment, those who continued with maintenance CBT-I but discontinued medication during extended therapy achieved better long-term outcomes than those who continued using medication intermittently (2 to 3 nights per week). Taken together, these findings suggest that, although medication may provide an added value during the initial course of treatment, the most effective long-term strategy is to discontinue medication after the initial course of therapy but while patients are still engaged in CBT-I.

SPEED OF RECOVERY AND TRAJECTORY OF CHANGES

In addition to documenting short- and long-term treatment outcomes, it is important to examine the speed of recovery during the course of therapy, as delayed therapeutic benefits may lead some patients to early or premature treatment discontinuation. In a secondary analysis of the same data set presented previously with 160 patients treated with CBT-I alone or combined with medication, the speed and trajectory of changes of insomnia symptoms/sleep-wake parameters were tracked on a week-by-week basis during the first 6-week course of treatment.[36] Patients treated with combined CBT-I plus medication exhibited faster improvements on most sleep parameters (sleep-onset latency, wake after sleep onset, total sleep time, sleep quality) (Figure 100.2). These improvements emerged during the first week of treatment for the

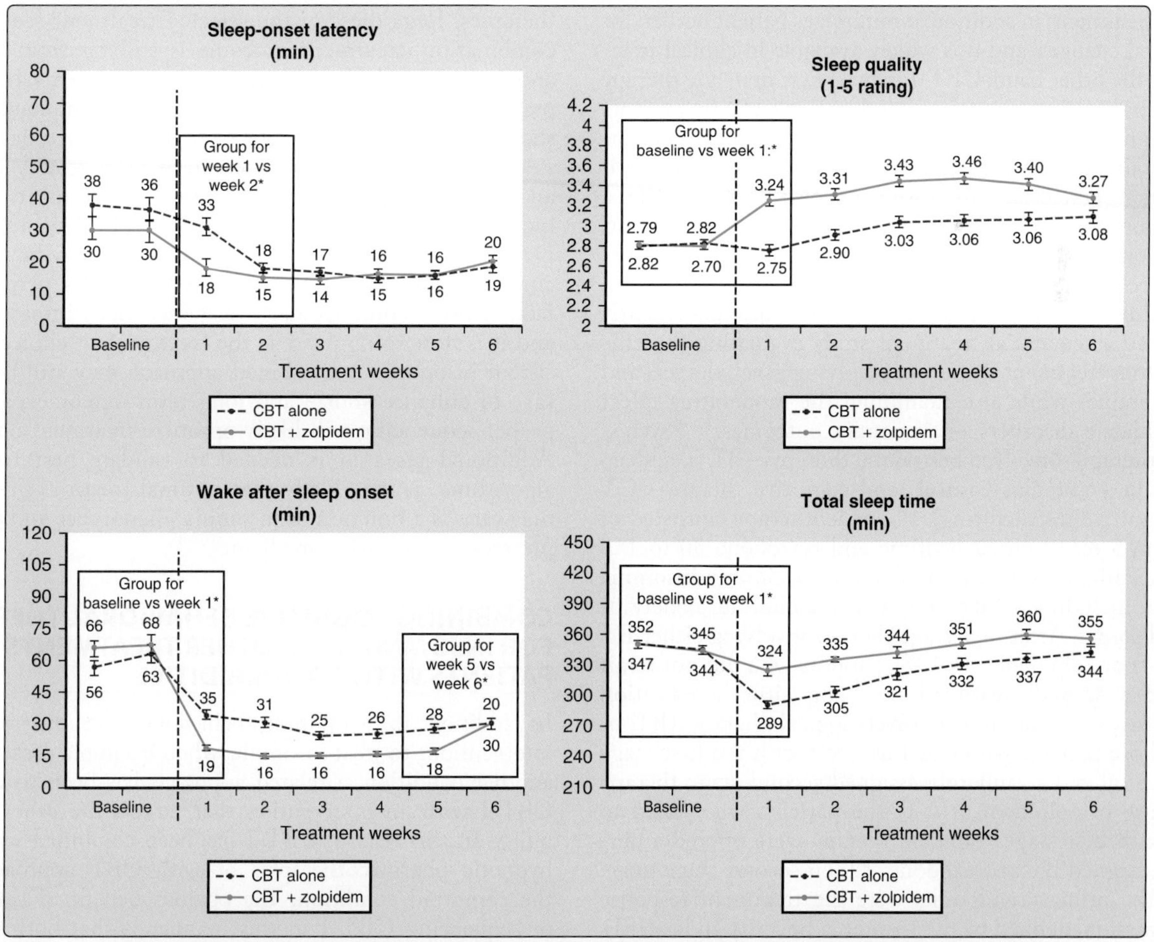

Figure 100.2 Speed and trajectory of change in CBT-I treatment. Data shown are changes in measures taken from sleep diaries during the course of treatment. CBT-I, Cognitive behavioral therapy for insomnia; min, minutes. (Data from Morin CM, Beaulieu-Bonneau S, Ivers H, et al. Speed and trajectory of changes of insomnia symptoms during acute treatment with cognitive-behavioral therapy, singly and combined with medication. *Sleep Med.* 2014;15[6]:701–707.)

combined approach compared with 2 to 3 weeks for CBT-I alone. Despite this initial advantage for combined therapy, sleep improvements were no longer different during the last 2 weeks of treatment. Furthermore, early treatment response did not reliably predict posttreatment recovery status. One potential advantage of combined therapies early in treatment is that medication often contributes to increased total sleep time, which may be an important factor to enhance compliance with behavioral interventions, particularly with sleep restriction therapy.

WHAT SHOULD BE OUR FIRST TREATMENT AND HOW SHOULD WE PROCEED WITH THOSE WHO FAIL INITIAL THERAPY?

An important question when sequencing therapies is whether our first treatment should involve pharmacotherapy or psychological/behavioral therapy. Often the selected treatment is a direct function of the provider's clinical training, such that a physician will most likely prescribe medication, whereas a psychologist will rely on CBT-I. From a purely empirical basis, there is little information to guide the decision about what should be our first treatment and how best to proceed when initial treatment fails. Medication may be preferred as initial therapy because it produces rapid therapeutic effects and may short-circuit the vicious cycle of sleep anticipatory anxiety early in treatment; in addition, it minimizes patient burden for behavioral changes, and it is widely available in clinical practice. On the other hand, CBT-I may be best first-line therapy because it directly targets the underlying perpetuating factors of insomnia (sleep-incompatible behaviors and misconceptions about sleep), it minimizes risk of adverse events, and it produces sustained sleep improvements over time even after a short-course of CBT-I. The downside is that it requires time, motivation, and a good dose of effort before sleep improvements become noticeable.

To address these questions, Morin and colleagues recently completed a sequential treatment study evaluating the efficacy of four treatment sequences involving psychological and drug therapies while also examining the moderating effect of psychiatric disorders on insomnia outcomes.[37] Psychological therapies involved behavioral therapy—BT (i.e., sleep restriction + stimulus control) and cognitive therapy—CT (i.e., cognitive restructuring). Pharmacotherapy consisted of zolpidem 5 to 10 mg at bedtime and trazodone 50 to 150 mg h.s. Patients were 211 adults with a chronic insomnia disorder, including 74 patients with a comorbid anxiety or mood disorder. After first-stage therapy involving either BT (n = 104) or zolpidem (n = 107), patients who did not remit received a second treatment involving either medication (zolpidem or trazodone) or psychological therapy (BT or CT). Those patients who failed to remit with the first-stage BT were offered a randomly assigned second-stage therapy consisting of zolpidem or CT. The patients who failed to remit with first-stage zolpidem therapy were offered a randomly assigned BT or trazodone as their second-stage treatment. The primary endpoints were the treatment response and remission, defined by the Insomnia Severity Index (ISI). First-stage therapy with BT or zolpidem produced equivalent rates of responders (BT = 45.5%, zolpidem = 49.7%) and remitters (BT = 38.0%, zolpidem = 30.3%). For nonremitters, second-stage therapy produced significant increases in response rate for the two conditions starting with BT (BT followed by zolpidem = from 40.6% to 62.7%; BT followed by CT = from 50.1% to 68.2%), but no significant change for the second-stage treatments after zolpidem treatment. A significant increase in the percentage of remitters was also observed with two second-stage therapy sequences (BT followed by zolpidem = from 38.1% to 55.9%, zolpidem followed by trazodone = from 31.4% to 49.4%). Although response/remission rates were lower among patients with psychiatric comorbidity, treatment sequences that involved either BT followed by CT, or zolpidem followed by trazodone, yielded better outcomes for the patients with comorbid insomnia. Overall, sequential therapy was an effective strategy to optimize insomnia management. Adding a second-stage treatment produced an added value for those who failed to remit with initial therapies. Patients with comorbid insomnia and psychiatric disorders benefited most from therapies that targeted mood in addition to sleep (CT, trazodone).

In summary, although there is a solid conceptual rationale for combining psychological and pharmacologic therapies, the evidence is still equivocal as to whether outcome is superior with combined therapies. Although it is clear that combined therapy is superior to medication alone, it is unclear whether there is an advantage to adding medication to CBT-I. Furthermore, there are still many unanswered questions as to how best to proceed when using combined or sequential therapies. Regardless of the selected treatment sequence or combination, treatment outcome is still far from optimal, and there is much room for further improvements. In clinical practice, selection of a treatment or a treatment combination should be based on both practical and evidence-based considerations. Medication is likely to be more readily available and produces rapid relief of insomnia symptoms; its primary indication remains for the management of acute insomnia, although an intermittent-use regimen may be useful in chronic insomnia. CBT-I is likely to address perpetuating factors and to produce more sustained sleep improvements, and it is now recognized as the treatment of choice in persistent insomnia. A combined approach may still be necessary to enhance short- and long-term outcomes, although proper sequencing will likely optimize treatment outcomes. Additional research is needed to validate best treatment algorithms, as it is likely that optimal treatment responses may vary as a function of insomnia phenotypes and patients' preferences (precision medicine[38,39]).

COMBINING COGNITIVE BEHAVIORAL THERAPY FOR INSOMNIA WITH OTHER TREATMENTS IN PATIENTS WITH COMORBIDITIES

In addition to combining behavioral and pharmacologic interventions to treat insomnia, when insomnia presents with another condition, a related approach has been to combine CBT-I with an intervention that targets the other comorbidity. In this regard, CBT-I has been combined with nonhypnotic pharmacotherapies or with CBT approaches for the comorbid condition. The obvious benefit of combining or sequencing CBT-I in this manner is that both presenting conditions (e.g., insomnia and depression) are addressed by a condition-specific treatment. Additional benefits can include delivering both interventions in the same setting (often by the same interventionist), creating opportunities to cross-reinforce treatment strategies from each intervention, and (if both interventions are nonpharmacologic) avoiding medication side effects.

Insomnia and Nightmares and Posttraumatic Stress Disorder

One of the first patient populations for which CBT-I principles were combined or sequenced with another behavioral and/or cognitive intervention was individuals with insomnia and nightmares. As detailed elsewhere in this volume, imagery rehearsal therapy (IRT) is an effective form of psychological/behavioral therapy for patients with posttraumatic nightmares.[40] It generally consists of nightmare psychoeducation, selection of a target nightmare to rescript, and imaginal rehearsal of the rescripted dream both in session and between sessions. Several uncontrolled, open-label trials and case series have been published, demonstrating both the feasibility of combining CBT-I+IRT and the effects of doing so on both insomnia and nightmare symptoms.[41-45] In each of these studies the interventions were delivered as one combined treatment as opposed to sequencing the interventions. The results suggested that combined IRT+ CBT-I could be delivered across a variety of sample populations (survivors of natural disasters, victims of violent crimes, and combat veterans with posttraumatic stress disorder [PTSD]), delivery formats (group and individual), and number of sessions. Within-group effect sizes for insomnia and for nightmares ranged considerably from small to large but certainly supported the need for RCTs to assess how the combined intervention performed compared with control conditions.

One pilot RCT study (n = 22) compared six individual, biweekly sessions (three CBT-I followed by three IRT sessions) to a treatment-as-usual condition among veterans with PTSD, current nightmares, and at least moderate insomnia severity (ISI score > 14).[46] Compared to controls, the sequential CBT-I+IRT condition showed statistically significant reductions in insomnia severity and nightmare frequency, more insomnia remitters (11% versus 0), more insomnia responders (44% versus 0), and a PTSD remission rate of 50% compared to none of the controls. Germain and colleagues conducted a three-arm trial comparing prazosin, placebo pill, and combined brief behavioral treatment of insomnia (BBTI)+IRT and delivered over 8 weeks in at least five individual face-to-face sessions and up to three phone sessions.[47] The randomized sample of 50 veterans were experiencing nightmares and moderate-to-severe insomnia. At posttreatment, both active intervention arms had significantly greater reduction in insomnia severity and nightmare frequency than did the placebo arm. Among completers, a higher sleep-specific treatment response rate was observed in those randomized to BBTI+IRT or to prazosin (79% in each condition) than in those receiving placebo (39%). At a 4-month follow-up assessment, nightmare frequency was not assessed, but improvements in insomnia severity were greater in the BBTI+IRT group compared to the prazosin group. In contrast, a very recent dismantling trial randomized 108 veterans with chronic, combat-related PTSD and frequent nightmares to receive six weekly, individual sessions of either CBT-I alone or combined CBT-I+IRT delivered together over the same six-session period.[48] Both conditions led to significant improvements on nightmare frequency and distress, but there was no advantage of combined CBT-I+IRT over CBT-I alone at either posttreatment or at 3- and 6-month follow-ups. The effects on insomnia severity were not reported.

Thus no large RCT comparing combined CBT-I+IRT to a control condition exists to more reliably assess the effects of this combined approach on insomnia, nightmares, and important clinical outcomes such as PTSD severity. Taking into account both controlled and uncontrolled studies, combining cognitive-behavioral treatment of insomnia and nightmares in populations exposed to serious trauma is clearly feasible. Second, data on the effect of the combined intervention on reducing the severity of insomnia and nightmare symptoms are mixed. Third, the extent to which gains in sleep improvements were associated with clinically meaningful attenuation of PTSD symptoms also differed across studies, but reductions in PTSD severity were evident. Given that there does appear to be some reduction in PTSD severity in some samples, this raises the possibility that CBT-I and/or IRT may also be combined with or sequenced with standard PTSD treatments for maximal effect in trauma populations. One RCT tested a sequencing approach[49] but has only reported results in abstract form.[50] This trial randomized 110 participants with insomnia, major depression, and PTSD related to interpersonal violence to receive either 4 individual CBT-I sessions followed by 12 individual sessions of cognitive processing therapy (CPT) or attention control followed by CPT over the same time course. As currently reported, compared with the sequenced control+CPT group, the sequenced CBT-I+CPT was associated with large, statistically significant improvements in insomnia, depression, and PTSD severity. As with trauma-related nightmares, the limited available data with respect to PTSD suggest that CBT-I and CBT-I+CBT-P can be sequenced with evidence-based psychological treatments for PTSD with some clinical benefit in trauma populations with sleep disturbances.

Insomnia and Depression

Combination or sequencing strategies with CBT-I have also been tested in patients with comorbid insomnia and depression. The first of these was a small, uncontrolled pilot study (n = 5) using a combination approach.[51] Lichstein and colleagues delivered 10 sessions of combined CBT-I and CBT for depression (CBT-D) in weekly individual sessions over real-time audio and video telehealth to older adults with insomnia and depression. The first five sessions were mixed CBT-I and CBT-D; the last five sessions focused primarily on CBT-D. Pre-post effects of the combined CBT-I+CBT-D were large and significant. Although not reported in terms of remission rates, the mean ISI, which was in the moderate range at baseline, was in the normal/remitted range (ISI <8) after treatment; the same was true with respect to depression. The second study was a small trial (n = 41) in youth ranging from 12 to 20 years in age who were randomized to receive either 10 weekly individual sessions of CBT-D+CBT-I or of CBT-D+sleep hygiene.[52] Each combined treatment commenced with either three to four sessions CBT-I or of sleep hygiene followed by four to six sessions of CBT-D. Although no group differences were observed between conditions on either insomnia severity or depression severity, insomnia remission rates were higher in the CBT-D+CBT-I condition (60% at 12 weeks and 68% at 26 weeks) compared to CBT-D+sleep hygiene (43% at 12 weeks and 43% at 26 weeks). Two RCTs have been conducted to test the effects of combining CBT-I with antidepressant

(AD) pharmacotherapy in patients with insomnia and major depressive disorder. Manber and colleagues[53] randomized 150 participants to receive seven sessions of either a credible insomnia control treatment (sleep education with sleep anxiety desensitization) or to CBT-I plus a standardized AD algorithm. Depression remission did not differ significantly between conditions (44% in CBT-I+AD; 36% in control), but the CBT-I+AD condition was associated with greater reduction in insomnia severity. It was also determined that greater improvements in insomnia at week 6 mediated depression remission. Given the design of this study, a comparison of the combined CBT-I+AD to either intervention alone was not possible. Such a comparison was possible in a trial of 107 participants conducted by Carney and colleagues.[54] In this three-arm study, participants were randomized to either four sessions of CBT-I+AD (escitalopram), CBT-I+placebo pill, or AD+4-session sleep hygiene control. There were large and significant pre-post reductions in both the ISI and the depression severity scale in each condition, but no differences between groups. Similarly, insomnia remission was higher in both CBT-I+AD and CBT-I+placebo (22% each) compared with control (6%), but this was not a significant difference. Both conditions with CBT-I (either with AD or with placebo) had PSG-measured improvements in total wake time, whereas the AD+sleep hygiene condition worsened; a similar pattern was observed for sleep efficiency. Finally, depression remission of approximately 40% was observed in all three conditions, even the CBT-I+placebo condition that received no depression treatment. Overall, there is a modest advantage to combining CBT-I with a depression treatment (as opposed to depression treatment alone or depression treatment plus a control condition) for patients presenting with comorbid insomnia and depression (Table 100.3).

Insomnia and Chronic Pain

Three RCTs have assessed the combination CBT-I with CBT for pain (CBT-P) to address comorbid insomnia and chronic pain. The first of these was a small effectiveness pilot study ($n = 21$) comparing waitlist control to 10 individual sessions of CBT-I alone, CBT-P alone, and combined CBT-I+CBT-P.[55]

Table 100.3 Randomized Controlled Trials of Combined Interventions for Comorbid Insomnia

Study Citation	Comorbid Condition	Active Treatments	*n* (Sample Size/ % Females)	Remission Rates by Treatment Condition	ES[a] (Other Findings)
Ulmer et al., 2011	PTSD & nightmares	CBT-I+IRT TAU	22/33%	Insomnia: 11%; PTSD: 50% Insomnia: 0%; PTSD: 0%	ISI: 2.15 NM: 0.60 PTSD: 1.76
Germain et al., 2012	Trauma & nightmares	BBT-I+IRT Prazosin Placebo	50/12%	Overall Sleep & NM: 62% Overall Sleep & NM: 62% Overall Sleep & NM: 25%	-
Harb et al, 2019	PTSD & nightmares	CBT-I CBT-I+IRT	108/14%	-	No group differences
Pigeon et al., 2017	PTSD	CBT-I+CPT Attention+CPT	110/97%	PTSD: 70% PTSD: 43%	PTSD: 0.53
Clarke et al., 2015	Adolescent depression	CBT-I+CBT-D SH+CBT-D	41/63%	Insomnia: 68%; depression: 84% Insomnia: 43%; depression: 67%	No group differences
Manber et al., 2016	Major depression	CBT-I+AD Sleep Educ+AD	150/73%	Depression: 44% Depression: 36%	
Carney et al., 2017	Major depression	CBT-I+placebo CBT-I+AD SH+AD	107/68%	Insomnia: 22%; depression: 39% Insomnia: 22%; depression: 39% Insomnia: 6%; depression: 41%	Large ES for each group; no group differences
Pigeon et al., 2012	Chronic pain/neck, back, and shoulder	CBT-I CBT-P CBT-I+CBT-P Waitlist	21/67%	-	ES for ISI (vs Waitlist): CBT-I: 1.64 CBT-P: 0.07 CBT-I/P: 2.99
Vitiello et al., 2013	Chronic pain/ osteoarthritis	CBT-I+CBT-P CBT-P Educ Control	367/78%	Insomnia (response): 52% Insomnia (response): 52% Insomnia (response): 28%	ISI: 0.48 No differences in pain outcomes
Lami et al., 2018	Chronic pain/ fibromyalgia	CBT-I+CBT-P CBT-P Medical TAU	126/100%	-	CBT-I/P superior sleep quality improvement and 'better' overall results

[a]Effect size of CBT-I Combined Condition Compared to Control Condition(s) reported as Cohen's d

AD, Antidepressant medication; BBTI, brief behavioral treatment of insomnia; CBT-D, cognitive behavioral therapy for depression; CBT-I, cognitive behavioral therapy for insomnia; CBT-P, cognitive behavioral therapy for pain; CPT, cognitive processing therapy; ES, Cohen's *d* effect size; ISI, Insomnia Severity Index; IRT, imagery rehearsal therapy; NM, nightmare; PE, prolonged exposure; PTSD, posttraumatic stress disorder; SH, sleep hygiene; TAU, treatment as usual.

Despite the small sample size both the CBT-I and combined CBT-I+CBT-P were associated with significantly greater reductions in insomnia severity and depression severity than the control condition (with large effect sizes). No intervention had a significant effect on pain outcomes compared to control, and the combined intervention did not appear to be more or less effective than CBT-I alone.

The Lifestyles Trial[56] was a large (n = 367) RCT comparing three, 6-week group interventions for comorbid osteoarthritic pain and insomnia in older adults, including combined CBT-I+CBT-P, CBT-P alone, and an education-only control. Participants in the CBT-I+CBT-P group experienced greater reductions in insomnia severity than either the education-only control or CBT-P alone groups at posttreatment and at 9-month follow-up, whereas changes in pain severity did not differ between the three arms. The same pattern of outcomes was observed with respect to achieving a clinically significant reduction (30% from baseline) in insomnia severity (52% in the CBT-I+CBT-P condition compared to 28% in CBT-P alone; OR = 2.2); however, there were no differences between treatment groups in terms of pain severity.

The most recent of the three RCTs was also a three-arm study.[57] It compared CBT-I+CBT-P and CBT-P alone to treatment as usual (pain medical care). The interventions were delivered in nine weekly 90-minute group sessions, and the sample consisted of 126 women with fibromyalgia (n = 126). Significant time (pre-post) by group interactions were observed for sleep quality favoring the CBT-I+CBT-P condition, which was the only study arm to show a significant pre-post improvement in sleep quality. No group differences were observed on pain or mood outcomes. As the authors concluded, the best clinical response pattern overall was experienced by those receiving CBT-I+CBT-P, which is a fair summary of the three studies assessing combined CBT for insomnia and pain. In fact, the data reviewed in this entire section on comorbid conditions are perhaps best summarized in a similar manner (Table 100.3). Combining or sequencing CBT-I with another psychological/behavioral therapy to address a comorbid condition both is feasible to achieve and continues to hold high face validity across the conditions where data are available. From the relatively limited set of RCTs conducted, a combined or sequenced approach is certainly superior to control conditions and generally appears to produce better overall clinical outcomes than a stand-alone intervention for the comorbid condition. Less clear is whether a combined or sequenced approach is superior to CBT-I alone as data to assess this question are limited and mixed.

USE OF PSYCHOLOGICAL/BEHAVIORAL INSOMNIA THERAPIES TO ASSIST HYPNOTIC DISCONTINUATION

Most people with insomnia seek treatment at primary care practices, where *the first and usually only insomnia treatment* is a hypnotic prescription.[58,59] In fact, available data suggest prescription hypnotic treatment is highly common: it has been estimated that people with insomnia spent well over $285 million in 1995 alone for prescription sleeping pills.[60] In 2010, 5% to 10% of US adults were prescribed a total of more than 15 million daily doses of hypnotic medication for relief of their sleep difficulties,[61] making hypnotics some of the most widely prescribed treatments in adult medicine. Among older adult populations, hypnotic usage rates appear to be even higher: community studies suggest as many as 14% of older adults are hypnotic users.[62] Although hypnotic use is short term or episodic for many patients, a sizeable proportion fall in a more frequent and chronically using group. For example, one recent study showed that about one-third of the 10,000 hypnotic users identified in an electronic health record dataset used more than 90% of the hypnotics prescribed for the entire patient group. Moreover, epidemiologic studies show that at least 65% continue their hypnotic use for at least 1 year, and at least 30% use such medications for at least 5 years.[62,63]

Whereas many chronic hypnotic users express interest in discontinuing their hypnotic medications, they commonly also express doubts about their abilities to do so. It appears such doubts are warranted: current evidence suggests that reducing or discontinuing hypnotic medications after extended use is challenging for many patients. Successful self-initiated attempts to decrease or abstain from hypnotics are, in fact, relatively rare.[64] Perhaps the best estimate of self-initiated discontinuation rates comes from studies of "minimal interventions," such as a personalized letter from one's health care provider advising long-term users to gradually quit. One recent study using this sort of minimal intervention found that only 14% (285) of 2004 chronic benzodiazepine users reported quitting their benzodiazepine use within 3 months after receiving such a letter.[65] Thus it is clear that the majority of chronic hypnotic users are unlikely to achieve hypnotic abstinence without some sort of formal assistance.

To assist such patients, it is important to understand what factor(s) may sustain hypnotic dependence. In this regard, clinical and research observations suggest that psychological factors play a central role in chronic hypnotic use and the difficulties achieving hypnotic abstinence. Observational research, for example, shows hypnotic users believe themselves to be more out of control of their sleep, and they have much stronger beliefs in their need for sleep medication than other groups of insomnia sufferers who are not hypnotic users.[66] For such individuals, the challenge of *knowingly* trying to sleep with less or no medication is anxiety provoking, particularly during the designated sleep period. For many, such anxiety is sufficient to elicit sleep disruptive arousal that leads to either a return of insomnia or a worsening of existing insomnia symptoms. Rather than attributing their enhanced sleep disturbance to their anxiety, such individuals most typically assign blame to their medication reduction/elimination and thus resume their hypnotic use. The resumption of the medication, of course, reduces sleep-disruptive performance anxiety, which, in turn, leads to sleep improvement. The belief that medication is necessary is reinforced, and the vicious cycle is perpetuated.[67] Given such considerations, effective management of patients' anxiety-provoking, sleep-related beliefs during the medication-tapering process seems central to the success of interventions designed to achieve hypnotic abstinence.

Given such observations, it seems reasonable to expect that CBT-I should play a useful role in assisting hypnotic users achieve hypnotic discontinuation. Specifically, its cognitive components would seemingly be useful for addressing the previously mentioned unhelpful sleep-related beliefs that support medication dependence, whereas the behavioral components would seemingly be useful in helping patients establish more effective sleep-promoting behaviors. Moreover, the CBT-I package ultimately can serve as a substitute or replacement insomnia therapy once hypnotic medication is discontinued, thus moving the patient from medication dependence to a self-management approach toward sleep. Indeed, providing an effective replacement treatment such as CBT-I to hypnotic-dependent patients would be expected to produce more successful outcomes than medication tapering alone.

To date, there have been surprisingly few studies examining the usefulness of CBT-I for assisting hypnotic-dependent patients to achieve hypnotic abstinence, but the evidence available suggests this therapy can be a useful intervention in this regard. Morin and colleagues[68] conducted an RCT with 76 benzodiazepine hypnotic users who all wished to discontinue their hypnotic use. Patients in this trial were assigned to a 10-week intervention comprising CBT-I alone, a physician-supervised medication tapering (SMT) intervention alone, or the combination of the two interventions. The CBT-I intervention included standard components including stimulus control therapy and sleep restriction to help patients develop sleep-promoting habits, and cognitive therapy to address patients' unhelpful sleep-related beliefs. The SMT provided physician guidance and support during tapering and followed a series of steps as shown in Box 100.1. All three interventions produced significant reductions in both the quantity (90% reduction) and frequency (80% reduction) of benzodiazepine use with the largest improvements shown by the group receiving the combined CBT-I+SMT intervention. Figure 100.3 shows the proportion of each intervention group who achieved hypnotic abstinence by the end of the 10-week intervention. As can be seen, the majority (85%) of those assigned to the combined CBT-I+SMT intervention achieved hypnotic abstinence by the end of treatment, whereas only 54% of the CBT-I group and 48% of the SMT group were medication free by the end of the treatment phase. The patients in the two groups that received CBT-I perceived greater subjective sleep improvements than those who received medication taper alone. PSG data showed an increase in the percent of time spent in sleep stages N3 and rapid eye movement (REM) sleep and a decrease in stage N2% and total sleep time across all three conditions from baseline to posttreatment. The decrease in PSG total sleep time at the posttreatment time point is not atypical of CBT-I given its inclusion of sleep restriction instructions. Initial benzodiazepine reductions were well maintained up to the 12-month follow-up, and sleep improvements became more noticeable over this period.

Whereas the results of this study show the use of CBT-I greatly enhances outcomes with regard to hypnotic discontinuation, data from two additional studies have provided somewhat less impressive results. In one of these studies O'Connor and colleagues[69] enrolled 86 hypnotic-dependent patients wishing to discontinue their hypnotic medications into a trial that evaluated an SMT and psychological interventions for insomnia. An initial cohort of 41 patients were provided solely the SMT intervention comprising *treatment as usual* (taper only) plus physician counseling in the same clinic. A second cohort of 45 patients were then randomly assigned to group CBT-I+SMT or group support (GS)+SMT. At a 3-month follow-up results obtained for the CBT-I and GS conditions were equivalent, although an intent-to-treat analysis showed slight advantages for the CBT-I condition. In a second study, Belleville and colleagues[70] randomly assigned 53 hypnotic-dependent patients to an 8-week SMT used alone or combined with a self-help CBT-I (weekly mailed booklets with therapy instructions). The treatment instructions contained the common CBT components included in in-person CBT-I, but patients in this study received no CBT-I therapist contact. Results of this study did not show greater reductions in hypnotic use by those who received SMT+self-help CBT-I versus those who received SMT alone. For both groups, weekly hypnotic use decreased from nearly nightly use at baseline to less than once per week at posttreatment. Nightly medication dosage (in lorazepam dose equivalents) decreased from 1.67 mg to 0.12 mg. However, those receiving SMT+self-help CBT-I did show greater sleep improvements than did those receiving SMT alone. SMT+self-help CBT-I recipients improved their sleep efficiency by 8%, whereas those receiving only the SMT remained stable. Furthermore, total wake time per night decreased by 52 minutes among SMT+self-help CBT-I recipients but increased by 13 minutes among those receiving solely the SMT. A follow-up secondary analysis by Belleville and Morin[71] showed that lower insomnia severity at the end of the trial predicted increased likelihood of remaining medication free through a 6-month follow-up period. Thus it appears that the greater sleep improvements shown by the CBT-I group translated into better long-term hypnotic abstinence rates.

To date, only one study[72] has compared the short- and longer-term outcomes of various hypnotic tapering interventions. This report was a follow-up study of the earlier-cited study by Morin and colleagues[68] and provided follow-up data at 3, 12, and 24 months posttreatment solely for those (n = 47) original study participants who achieved hypnotic abstinence by the end of the initial 10-week intervention. Figure 100.4 shows the percentages of these participants in each treatment group who had

BOX 100.1 COMPONENTS OF THE SUPERVISED MEDICATION TAPERING PROTOCOL

- Change from multiple hypnotics to one hypnotic
- Each week set a goal for medication use
- Reduce dose of hypnotic 25% every 2 weeks
- Progressively introduce drug-free nights
- Plan drug-free nights in advance

Morin CM, Bastien C, Guay B, Radouco-Thomas M, Leblanc J, Vallieres A. Randomized clinical trial of supervised tapering and cognitive behavior therapy to facilitate benzodiazepine discontinuation in older adults with chronic insomnia. *Am J Psychiatry.* 2004;161(2):332-342.

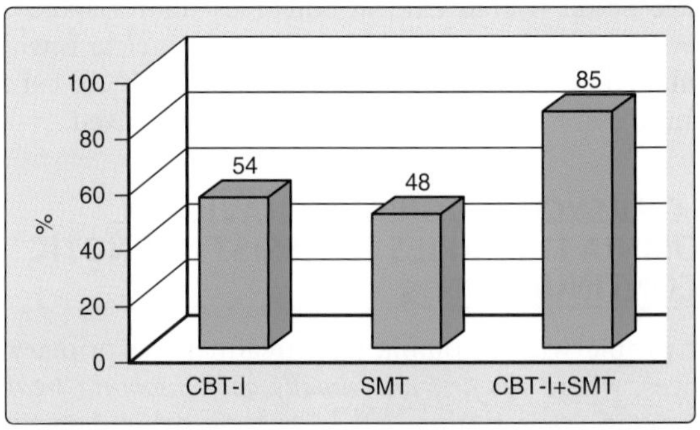

Figure 100.3 Percentage of each intervention group who discontinued hypnotics by the end of treatment. Values shown are the percentage of hypnotic users in each group who discontinued hypnotic use by the end of treatment time point. CBT-I, Cognitive behavioral therapy for insomnia; CBT-I+SMT, the combined treatment; SMT, supervised medication taper. (Data reported by Morin CM, Bastien C, Guay B, Radouco-Thomas M, Leblanc J, Vallieres A. Randomized clinical trial of supervised tapering and cognitive behavior therapy to facilitate benzodiazepine discontinuation in older adults with chronic insomnia. *Am J Psychiatry.* 2004;161[2]:332–42.)

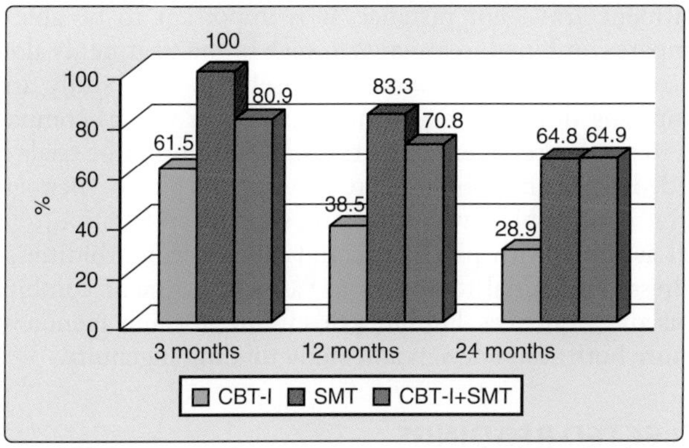

Figure 100.4 Hypnotic abstinence rates over time for those who discontinued hypnotics by the end of treatment. The sustained abstinent rates across time for the subgroups of hypnotic users in each treatment condition that discontinued hypnotic use by the end of the treatment phase. CBT-I, Cognitive behavioral therapy for insomnia; CBT-I+SMT, the combined treatment; SMT, supervised medication taper. (Data shown in figure were reported in Morin CM, Belanger L, Bastien C, Vallieres A. Long-term outcome after discontinuation of benzodiazepines for insomnia: A survival analysis of relapse. *Behav Res Ther.* 2005;43[1]:1–14.)

discontinued hypnotic use by the end of their respective treatment and remained abstinent at the various time points mentioned. Figure 100.4 indicates that the SMT and SMT+CBT-I interventions show better sustained hypnotic abstinence than does CBT-I used in isolation, yet the combined intervention produces the best long-term outcomes for its recipients. Nonetheless, it is also noteworthy that even this treatment results in long-term hypnotic abstinence in only slightly more than half of the patients who receive it. Moreover, the hypnotic resumption rates are sizeable across all three treatment conditions. Hence, although the combination of an SMT and CBT-I produces the best overall short- and longer-term results, a substantial proportion of those patients who receive even this "optimal" treatment do not seem able to abstain from hypnotic use.

Beyond posttreatment insomnia severity, it is not clear what other factor(s) may contribute to the relatively high hypnotic resumption rate among hypnotic users who enroll in clinical trials desiring to discontinue their sleep medications. However, one possible explanation concerns the type of tapering approach used in the previous trials. Although gradual tapering has been the general approach, previous trials have exclusively employed an "open-label" approach, wherein patients are aware of their nightly medication dosage as well as when reductions in that dosage occur throughout the tapering process. In this regard Roehers and colleagues[13] have shown that individuals taking hypnotics on a nightly basis for insomnia management generally do not show a worsening of their sleep when they are blindly switched to a placebo for periods of 7 consecutive nights. Thus, *knowing* versus *not knowing* what one's hypnotic dosage on a particular night may be a factor influencing hypnotic discontinuation.

Based on this rationale, Edinger and colleagues[73] recently completed an RCT with 78 hypnotic-dependent patients who all reported a desire to quit their hypnotic usage. In this RCT, enrollees first completed baseline measures and then underwent four sessions of individual CBT-I. Subsequently they were randomized to one of three 20-week, double-blinded tapering protocols, wherein their medication dosage either remained unchanged (control) or was reduced by 25% or 10% every 2 weeks. During tapering, all enrollees were given biweekly contact with the study physician, who provided support and guidance while monitoring medication withdrawal effects. At the end of the 20-week period the study blind was eliminated, and those who completed one of the two blinded tapering protocols entered a 3-month follow-up period, whereas participants in the control group were offered an open-label taper before completing the follow-up.

Preliminary analyses showed no differences in outcomes for the two blinded tapering groups, so their data were combined and compared with data from the control group who received open-label tapering. At the end of the 20-week tapering period 92.9% of those completing the blinded taper discontinued their hypnotics, whereas 77.3% of those receiving the open-label taper were medication free at this time point. At the 3-month follow-up, 72.1% of those who underwent blinded tapering remained hypnotic free, whereas only 52% of those who underwent open-label tapering were abstinent from hypnotics. Additional comparisons at the 3-month follow-up indicated those who received blinded tapering were using hypnotics significantly less frequently ($P = .042$; effect size = .62) and at significantly lower doses (diazepam dose equivalents; $P = .041$; effect size = .53) than were those in the control group who were provided open-label tapering. Although the nature of this study design precludes definitive conclusions about blinded tapering, results suggest further direct comparisons of blinded and open-label hypnotic tapering are warranted.

Overall, there has been relatively little research testing the usefulness of CBT-I alone and combined with SMT for hypnotic discontinuation, a perplexing fact given the plethora of studies conducted to test sleep interventions among patients with and without significant sleep disruptive comorbidities. Admittedly, much more research is needed in this area. Given that factors such as higher initial medication dosage, more severe insomnia symptoms, greater anxiety and distress, and lower self-efficacy have been shown to be negative prognosticators in hypnotic discontinuation trials,[69,71,72] studies testing more intensive interventions to target these factors would seem useful. Also, it remains unclear as to whether the sequencing of the treatments provided affects outcomes. For example, CBT-I and tapering interventions were provided to patients simultaneously, except in the study by Edinger and colleagues,[73] which provided the treatments sequentially with patients completing CBT-I before beginning their hypnotic tapering. It seems possible that the contrasting treatment sequences could have some influence on eventual hypnotic discontinuation outcomes. Of course, much future research will be needed to address these and other questions that arise as we learn more about hypnotic discontinuation interventions.

CLINICAL PEARL

Psychological/behavioral insomnia therapies, particularly CBT-I, can be effective for patients who have had prior hypnotic drug exposure. Moreover, there are emerging data exploring the optimal sequencing of CBT-I and hypnotics to achieve the best treatment results. Since neither psychological/behavioral insomnia therapies nor pharmacotherapies are universally effective, there may be value added to switching treatment modalities when the initial modality does not produce satisfactory results.

SUMMARY

Psychological/behavioral insomnia therapies and particularly CBT-I are widely recommended as first-line treatments for insomnia disorder, but pharmacotherapy is by far the more commonly used approach. Neither approach alone produces clinically meaningful treatment outcomes in more than 50% to 60% of patients. In addition, chronic insomnia more frequently presents with a sleep-disruptive comorbid condition, which requires its own treatment. Given these realities, the optimal approach to manage chronic insomnia for many patients may be to combine or sequentially deliver more than one intervention.

Available clinical trial data suggest that CBT-I can be initiated in patients who are using a hypnotic medication. Contrary to some clinical expectations, the data suggest that hypnotic exposure does not reduce responsiveness to CBT-I and related behavioral insomnia therapies. Furthermore, some hypnotic users are able to discontinue hypnotics once exposed to CBT-I, even if they are provided no formal hypnotic-tapering instructions. However, efforts to combine psychological/behavioral treatment with hypnotic medication to improve outcomes have provided mixed results. Seemingly the best results have been obtained when the hypnotic medication is used in the beginning stages of treatment and then withdrawn while the psychological/behavioral intervention is continued. Nonetheless, one recent trial has suggested that switching behavioral therapy to medication or from medication to behavioral therapy may benefit some patients who do not achieve optimal results with the initial treatment provided. For the many patients who present with insomnia and a co-occurring condition, there is good evidence that CBT-I can be combined or sequenced with a psychological therapy targeting the comorbid condition. Such supporting data are not overwhelmingly present or strong but do exist for the benefits of CBT-I *combined* with IRT for nightmares, CBT-I *sequenced* with psychological treatments that target PTSD symptoms, and CBT-I *combined* with psychological treatment that targets pain disorders. The evidence for *combining* CBT-I with CBT-D is surprisingly sparse and inconclusive in terms of its added benefit. Finally, when hypnotic discontinuation is desired, CBT-I may prove helpful, especially when combined with (or followed by) a supervised hypnotic-tapering plan.

Over the past decade the literature on combining and sequencing the use of psychological/behavioral insomnia therapies has expanded. The field is now in a place to consider several future directions to serve the purpose of a personalized medicine approach to insomnia care. In almost all instances, whether addressing CBT-I and hypnotics, CBT-I and another psychological treatment or CBT-I and tapering strategies, what is needed are large RCTs that can accommodate multiple treatment arms. For instance, it is important to be able to compare combined treatments to each of the treatments alone. In sequencing trials, it would be useful to have study arms comparing differing treatment sequences as well as comparison to single-treatment conditions. In addition, large trials are needed that can accommodate a variety of phenotypes, such as those with objective normal and short sleep duration,[8,38] as well as those with psychiatric and medical comorbidities, to address differential responses to various treatment combinations and sequences. Fulfilling this future research agenda will require both study design and study funding ingenuity.

SELECTED READINGS

Carney CE, Edinger JD, Kuchibhatla M, et al. Cognitive Behavioral Insomnia Therapy for those with insomnia and depression: a randomized controlled clinical trial. *Sleep*. 2017;40(4).

Edinger JD, Arnedt JT, Bertisch SM, et al. Behavioral and psychological treatments for chronic insomnia disorder in adults: an American Academy of Sleep Medicine systematic review, meta-analysis, and GRADE assessment. *J Clin Sleep Med*. 2021;17(2):263–298.

Krakow BJ, Melendrez DC, Johnston LG, et al. Sleep Dynamic Therapy for Cerro Grande Fire evacuees with posttraumatic stress symptoms: a preliminary report. *J Clin Psychiatry*. 2002;63(8):673–684.

Morin CM, Bastien C, Guay B, Radouco-Thomas M, Leblanc J, Vallieres A. Randomized clinical trial of supervised tapering and cognitive behavior therapy to facilitate benzodiazepine discontinuation in older adults with chronic insomnia. *Am J Psychiatry*. 2004;161(2):332–342.

Morin CM, Belanger L, Bastien C, Vallieres A. Long-term outcome after discontinuation of benzodiazepines for insomnia: a survival analysis of relapse. *Behav Res Ther*. 2005;43(1):1–14.

Morin CM, Colecchi C, Stone J, Sood R, Brink D. Behavioral and pharmacological therapies for late-life insomnia: a randomized controlled trial. *J Am Med Assoc*. 1999;281(11):991–999.

Morin CM, Edinger JD, Krystal AD, Buysse DJ, Beaulieu-Bonneau S, Ivers H. Sequential psychological and pharmacological therapies for comorbid and primary insomnia: study protocol for a randomized controlled trial. *Trials*. 2016;17(1):118.

Morin CM, Edinger JD, Beaulieu-Bonneau S, et al. Effectiveness of sequential psychological and medication therapies for insomnia disorder: a randomized clinical trial. *JAMA Psychiatry*. 2020;77(11):1107–1115.

Pigeon WR, Moynihan J, Matteson-Rusby S, et al. Comparative effectiveness of CBT interventions for co-morbid chronic pain & insomnia: a pilot study. *Behav Res Ther*. 2012;50(11):685–689.

Ritterband LM, Thorndike FP, Ingersoll KS, et al. Effect of a web-based cognitive behavior therapy for insomnia intervention with 1-year follow-up: a randomized clinical trial. *JAMA Psychiatry*. 2017;74(1):68–75.

Roehrs TA, Randall S, Harris E, Maan R, Roth T. Twelve months of nightly zolpidem does not lead to rebound insomnia or withdrawal symptoms: a prospective placebo-controlled study. *J Psychopharmacol*. 2012;26(8):1088–1095.

Vitiello MV, McCurry SM, Shortreed SM, et al. Cognitive-behavioral treatment for comorbid insomnia and osteoarthritis pain in primary care: the lifestyles randomized controlled trial. *J Am Geriatr Soc*. 2013;61(6):947–956.

A complete reference list can be found online at ExpertConsult.com.

Index

Page numbers followed by "*f*" indicate figures, "*b*" indicate boxes, and "*t*" indicate tables.

B

F

G

I

J

K

Q

R

U

V

W

X

Y

Z

Principles and Practice of
SLEEP MEDICINE

Meir Kryger MD, FRCPC
Professor
Department of Pulmonary Critical Care and Sleep Medicine
Yale University
New Haven, Connecticut

Thomas Roth PhD
Director
Sleep Disorders Center
Henry Ford Hospital
Detroit, Michigan

Cathy A. Goldstein MD
Associate Professor
Department of Neurology
University of Michigan
Ann Arbor, Michigan

William C. Dement MD
Lowell W. and Josephine Q. Berry Professor of Psychiatry and Behavioral Sciences
Stanford University School of Medicine
Department of Sleep Sciences & Medicine
Palo Alto, California

Principles and Practice of SLEEP MEDICINE

Seventh Edition

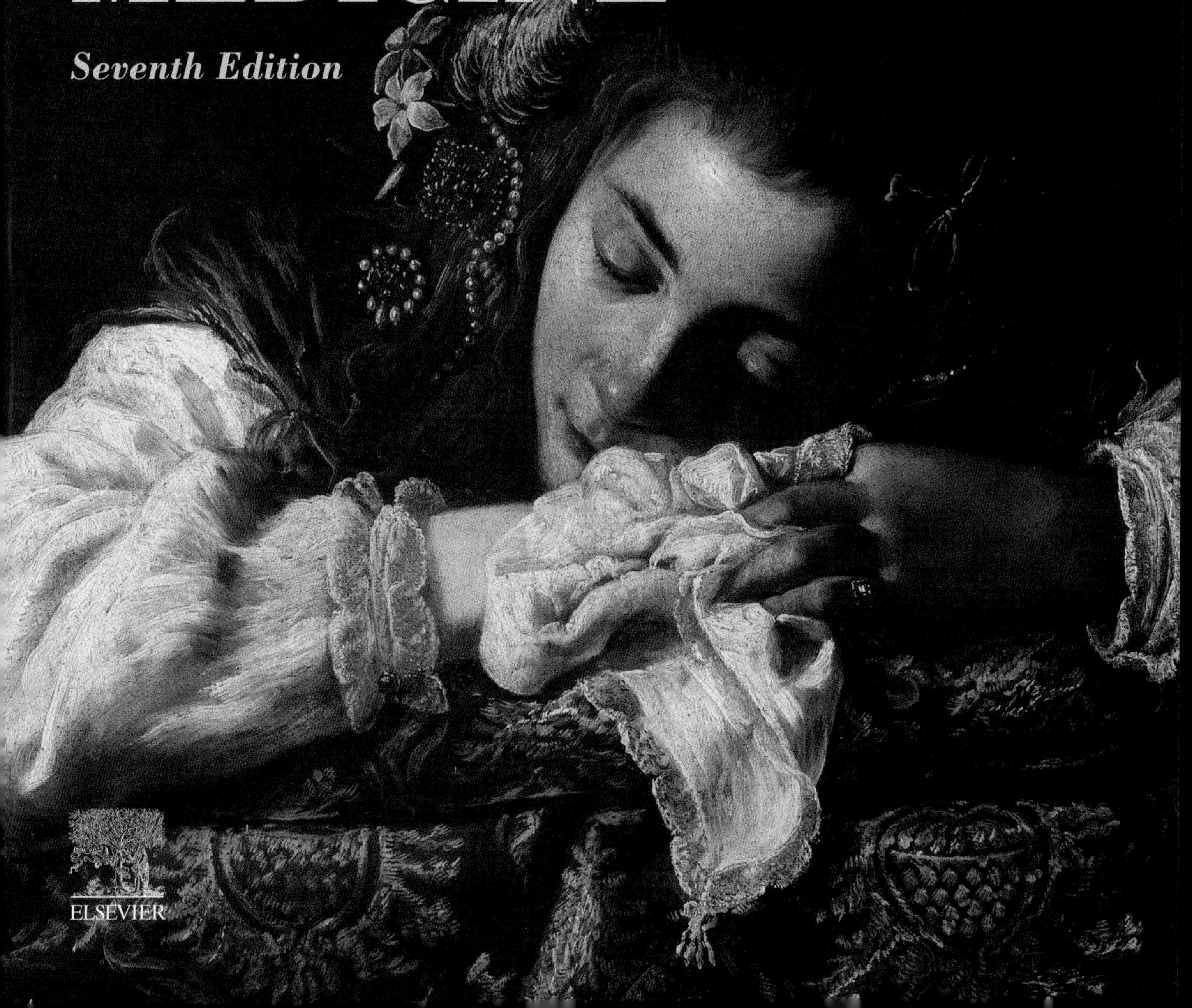

ELSEVIER

ELSEVIER
1600 John F. Kennedy Blvd.
Ste 1600
Philadelphia, PA 19103-2899

PRINCIPLES AND PRACTICE OF SLEEP MEDICINE
ISBN: 978-0-323-66189-8
VOLUME 1 ISBN: 978-0-323-88220-0
VOLUME 2 ISBN: 978-0-323-88221-7

The cover illustration: "Sleeping Girl or Young Woman Sleeping is an oil on canvas painting by an unknown 17th century artist active in Rome, sometimes dated to c.1620 and previously attributed to Theodoor van Loon or Domenico Fetti." Wikipedia.org: https://en.wikipedia.org/wiki/Sleeping_Girl_(17th_century_painting)

Previous editions copyrighted 2017, 2011, 2005, 2000, 1994, and 1989.

ISBN: 978-0-323-66189-8

Senior Acquisitions Editor: Melanie Tucker
Senior Content Development Strategist: Lisa Barnes
Publishing Services Manager: Catherine Jackson
Senior Project Manager: Kate Mannix
Design Direction: Amy Buxton

Printed in India

Last digit is the print number: 9 8 7 6 5 4 3

We dedicate this volume to

Barbara Kryger, Jay and Shelley Gold, Emily and Michael Kryger, Steven Kryger and Barr Even

Toni Roth, Daniel and Jeanne Roth, Adam and Carol Roth, Jonathan and Cheyna Roth, Andrea and Justin Leibow

Tadd, Evan, and Cole Hiatt, Larry and Tamara Goldstein, and Carolyn Hiatt

In Memoriam

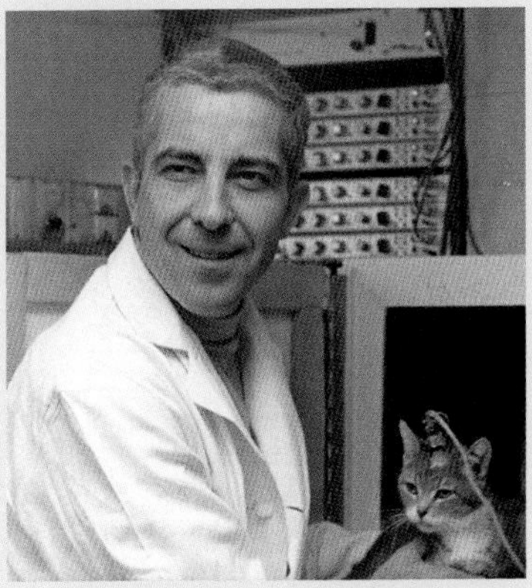

William C. Dement
1928–2020

William C. Dement, the father of sleep medicine, was the inspiration for *Principles and Practice of Sleep Medicine* and was a chief editor starting with the first edition in 1989.

Bill was a brilliant scientist, mentor, teacher, and leader. He did some of the ground-breaking research on rapid eye movement sleep; mentored many of the most productive scientists doing sleep research; taught the most popular course ever at Stanford University, *Sleep and Dreams*; and played a key role in advocating for the importance of sleep to science, governments, and the public. He has affected millions of lives!

I (TR) met Bill for the first time in 1972 when he came to Cincinnati for a CME course on sleep medicine. He invited me to give two lectures and we spent most of the day together. During that day I learned about his intellect, passion for educating the public about sleep medicine, and importantly, his generosity. Over the next 40 years we had many interactions; in every instance they reinforced those initial impressions. It is important recognize that without Bill Dement, the book you are holding would not exist.

I (MK) met Bill for the first time in 1978 at a sleep meeting being held in Stanford. After I gave my presentation (I think I was the only pulmonary trained person in the room) Bill came over to me and said, "My God, you're just a kid." I guess I was. That was the beginning of a beautiful friendship.

In about 1985, we had been discussing and thinking about whether a sleep medicine textbook was needed. We were hesitant to proceed and were actually discouraged by some colleagues who told us there wasn't enough science to warrant a textbook. When presented with the question, Bill said, "You can't have a field without a textbook!" The rest is history. The first edition came out in 1989; it had 730 pages. The sixth edition (2017) was exactly 1000 pages longer. Bill was instrumental in creating the field of sleep medicine. His contributions will never be forgotten. We will miss him.

Meir Kryger Tom Roth Cathy Goldstein

From the Performing Arts

Every Tuesday, Queen Elizabeth II of the United Kingdom (played by Dame Helen Mirren) had a private audience with her Prime Minister in the Private Audience Room on the first floor of Buckingham Palace. This is dramatized in Peter Morgan's play The Audience. *In this scene, Elizabeth is meeting with Prime Minister Gordon Brown.*

Elizabeth: So, back to your weekend, and all this industriousness. Were you up very early?
Brown: Four thirty.
Elizabeth: Oh, dear.
Brown: It's all right. I never sleep much.
Elizabeth: Since when?
Brown: Since always.
Elizabeth: Harold Wilson always used to say, "The main requirement of a Prime Minister is a good night's sleep … and a sense of history." Mrs. Thatcher taught herself to need very little towards the end. But I'm not sure how reassured I am by that. I like the idea of any person with the power to start nuclear war being rested. (*A beat.*) Besides, lack of sleep can have a knock-on effect in other areas.
Brown: Such as?
Elizabeth: One's general sense of health.
A silence.
And happiness.
A silence.
And equilibrium.
Brown looks up. A silence.
I gather there's been some concern …
Brown: About what?
Elizabeth: Your happiness. Don't worry. You wouldn't be the first in your position to feel overwhelmed. Despondent.
She searches for the right word.
Depressed.

From Morgan, Peter. THE AUDIENCE, Faber and Faber, 2013.
Used with permission of Mr. Peter Morgan.

But the tigers come at night
With their voices soft as thunder
As they tear your hope apart
As they turn your dream to shame.

From I Dreamed a Dream, LES MISÉRABLES, with permission, Cameron Mackintosh, producer © 1985 Alain Boublil Music Ltd. Used with permission 1991, CMI.

From Literature

Blessings on him who first invented sleep.—It covers a man all over, thoughts and all, like a cloak.—It is meat for the hungry, drink for the thirsty, heat for the cold, and cold for the hot.—It makes the shepherd equal to the monarch, and the fool to the wise.—There is but one evil in it, and that is that it resembles death, since between a dead man and a sleeping man there is but little difference.

From DON QUIXOTE
By Saavedra M. de Cervantes

"To sleep! To forget!" he said to himself with the serene confidence of a healthy man that if he is tired and sleepy, he will go to sleep at once. And the same instant his head did begin to feel drowsy and he began to drop off into forgetfulness. The waves of the sea of unconsciousness had begun to meet over his head, when all at once—it was as though a violent shock of electricity had passed over him. He started so that he leapt up on the springs of the sofa, and leaning on his arms got in a panic on to his knees. His eyes were wide open as though he had never been asleep. The heaviness in his head and the weariness in his limbs that he had felt a minute before had suddenly gone.

From ANNA KARENINA, Part IV, Chapter XVIII
By Leo Tolstoy

The Body Electric

Every cell in our bodies contains a pore
like a door, which says when to let in
the flood of salt-ions bearing their charge,
but the power in us moves much slower
than the current that rushes into wires
to ignite the lamp by which I undress,
am told to undress by sparks that cross
the gap of a synapse to pass along
the message, *It's time for sleep.* As I pull
back the sheets, ease into bed, I think
if I could only look beneath my skin,
I'd see my body as alive as Hong Kong,
veins of night traffic crawling along
the freeways as tiny faces inside taxis
look up from the glow of their phones,
sensing that someone is watching.

James Crews, Dec. 3, 2020. *New York Times Magazine.* Used with permission of the poet.

Contributors

Ghizlane Aarab, MD
Associate Professor
Department of Oral Kinesiology
The Academic Center for Dentistry
Amsterdam, The Netherlands

Sabra Abbott, MD, PhD
Assistant Professor
Department of Neurology
Center for Circadian and Sleep Medicine
Northwestern University Feinberg School of Medicine
Chicago, Illinois

Shervin Abdollahi, BS
Research Analyst (Contractor)
National Institute of Neurological Disorders and Stroke
Bethesda, Maryland

Philip N. Ainslie, PhD
Professor
Department of Health and Exercise Sciences
The University of British Columbia
Kelowna, British Columbia, Canada

Cathy Alessi, MD
Director
Geriatric Research, Education and Clinical Center
VA Greater Los Angeles Healthcare System;
Professor
Department of Medicine
David Geffen School of Medicine
University of California, Los Angeles
Los Angeles, California

Richard P. Allen, PhD
Professor
Department of Neurology
Johns Hopkins University
Baltimore, Maryland

Fernanda R. Almeida, DDS, MSc, PhD
Associate Professor
Oral Health Sciences
University of British Columbia
Vancouver, British Columbia, Canada

Aurelio Alonso, DDS, MS, PhD
Department of Anesthesiology
Orofacial Pain–Duke Innovative Pain Therapies
Center for Translational Pain Medicine
Duke University
Durham, North Carolina

Neesha Anand, MD
Critical Care Fellow
University of Pittsburgh
Pittsburgh, Pennsylvania

Amy W. Amara, MD
Associate Professor
Department of Neurology
University of Alabama at Birmingham
Birmingham, Alabama

Sonia Ancoli-Israel, PhD
Professor Emeritus
Professor of Research
Department of Psychiatry
University of California, San Diego
La Jolla, California

Anna Anund, PhD
Reserach Director
Department of Human Factors
Swedish National Road and Transport Research Institute;
Associate Professor
Rehabilitation Medicine
Linköping University
Linkoping, Sweden

Taro Arima, DDS, PhD
Lecturer
Division of International Affairs
Graduate School of Dental Medicine
Hokkaido University
Sapporo, Japan

J. Todd Arnedt, PhD
Departments of Psychiatry and Neurology
University of Michigan Medical School
Ann Arbor, Michigan

Isabelle Arnulf, MD, PhD
Sleep Disorders Unit
Pitie-Salpetriere University Hospital
Sorbonne University
Paris, France

Vivian Asare, MD
Assistant Professor
Department of Medicine (Pulmonary, Critical Care, and Sleep Medicine)
Yale University School of Medicine
New Haven, Connecticuit

Lauren Asarnow, PhD
Assistant Professor
Psychiatry
School of Medicine
University of California–San Francisco
San Francisco, California

Hrayr Attarian, MD
Professor
Department of Neurology
Northwestern University
Chicago, Illinois

Alon Y. Avidan, MD, MPH
Director
University of California, Los Angeles Sleep Disorders Center;
Professor
Department of Neurology
University of California, Los Angeles,
Los Angeles, California

Nicoletta Azzi, MD
Sleep Disorders Center
Department of Medicine and Surgery
University of Parma
Parma, Italy

M. Safwan Badr, MD,MBA
Professor
Department of Internal Medicine
The Liborio Tranchida MD Endowed Chair
Wayne State University
Detroit, Michigan

Helen A. Baghdoyan, PhD
Beaman Professor
University of Tennessee
Knoxville, Tennessee;
Joint Faculty, Biosciences Division
Oak Ridge National Laboratory
Oak Ridge, Tennessee

Sébastien Baillieul, MD, PhD
Pneumology-Physiology Department
Grenoble Alpes University Hospital;
INSERM U1300, HP2 Laboratory
Grenoble Alpes University
Grenoble, France

Benjamin Baird, PhD
Wisconsin Institute for Sleep and Consciousness
Department of Psychiatry
University of Wisconsin–Madison
Madison, Wisconsin

Fiona C. Baker, PhD
Director, Center for Health Sciences
SRI International;
Honorary Senior Research Fellow
Brain Function Research Group
School of Physiology
University of the Witwatersrand
Johannesburg, Gauteng, South Africa

Thomas J. Balkin, PhD
Senior Scientist
Behavioral Biology Branch
Walter Reed Army Institute of Research
Silver Spring, Maryland

Siobhan Banks, PhD
Professor
UniSA Justice and Society
University of South Australia
Magill, South Australia

Nicola L. Barclay, BA(Hons), MSc, PhD
Sleep and Circadian Neuroscience Institute (SCNi)
Nuffield Department of Clinical Neurosciences
University of Oxford
Oxford, Great Britain

Steven R. Barczi, MD
Professor of Medicine
Department of Medicine
University of Wisconsin School of Medicine & Public Health;
Director of Clinical Programs
Madison VA Geriatric Research, Education, and Clinical Center
Wm. S. Middleton Veterans Affairs Hospital
Madison, Wisconsin

Mathias Basner, MD, PhD, MSc
Professor of Sleep and Chronobiology in Psychiatry
Unit for Experimental Psychiatry
Division of Sleep and Chronobiology
Department of Psychiatry
Perelman School of Medicine
University of Pennsylvania
Philadelphia, Pennsylvania

Claudio L.A. Bassetti, MD
Professor
Chairman and Head
Neurology Department
Inselspital University Hospital
Bern, Switzerland

Celyne Bastien, PhD
School of Psychology
Laval University
Quebec City, Quebec, Canada

Christian R. Baumann, MD
Department of Neurology
University Hospital Zurich
Zurich, Switzerland

Louise Beattie, PhD
Institute of Health and Wellbeing
University of Glasgow
Glasgow, Great Britain

Bei Bei, DPsych(Clinical), PhD
NHMRC Health Professional Research Fellow
Clinical Psychologist
School of Psychological Sciences
Monash University
Clayton, Victoria, Australia

Gregory Belenky, MD
Research Professor
Sleep and Performance Research Center
Washington State University
Spokane, Washington

Amy Bender, MS, PhD
Adjunct Assistant Professor
Department of Kinesiology
University of Calgary;
Senior Research Scientist
Calgary Counselling Centre
Calgary, Canada

Suzanne M. Bertisch, MD, MPH
Division of Sleep and Circadian Disorders
Brigham and Women's Hospital
Harvard Medical School
Boston, Massachusetts

Carlos Blanco-Centurion, PhD
Department of Psychiatry and Behavioral Sciences
Medical University of South Carolina
Charleston, South Carolina

Benjamin T. Bliska, DDS
Faculty of Dentistry
University of British Columbia
Vancouver, British Columbia, Canada

Konrad E. Bloch, MD
Professor
Respiratory Medicine, Sleep Disorders Center
University Hospital Zurich
Zurich, Switzerland

Bradley F. Boeve, MD
Professor of Neurology
Department of Neurology
Mayo Clinic
Rochester, Minnesota

Patricia Bonnavion, MD
Lab of Neurophysiology
ULB Neuroscience Institute
Université Libre Bruxelles
Brussels, Belgium

Scott B. Boyd, DDS, PhD
Professor of Oral and Maxillofacial Surgery, Retired Faculty
Department of Oral and Maxillofacial Surgery
Vanderbilt University School of Medicine
Nashville, Tennesee

Alessandro Bracci, DDS
Adjunct Professor
Department of Neuroscience
School of Dentistry,
University of Padova
Padova, Italy

Tiffany Braley, MD
Associate Professor of Neurology
Department of Neurology
Multiple Sclerosis and Sleep Disorders Centers
University of Michigan
Ann Arbor, Michigan

Josiane L. Broussard, MD
Assistant Professor
Department of Health and Exercise Science
Colorado State University
Fort Collins, Colorado

Daniel B. Brown, JD
Partner, Taylor English Duma, LLP
Atlanta, Georgia

Luis F. Buenaver, PhD
Assistant Professor of Psychiatry and Neurology
Director, Johns Hopkins Behavioral Sleep Medicine Program
Johns Hopkins University School of Medicine
Baltimore, Maryland

Helen J. Burgess, PhD
Professor
Department of Psychiatry
University of Michigan
Ann Arbor, Michigan

Keith R. Burgess, MBBS, MSc, PhD, FRACP, FRCPC
Clinical Associate Professor
Department of Medicine
University of Sydney
Sydney, Australia

Orfeu M. Buxton, PhD
Professor
Department of Biobehavioral Health
Pennsylvania State University
University Park, Pennsylvania

Daniel J. Buysse, MD
UPMC Professor of Sleep Medicine
Professor of Psychiatry and Clinical and Translational Science
University of Pittsburgh School of Medicine
Pittsburgh, Pennsylvania

Sean W. Cain, PhD
Associate Professor
School of Psychological Sciences
Turner Institute for Brain and Mental Health
Monash University
Clayton, Victioria, Australia

J. Lynn Caldwell, BS, MA, PhD
Senior Research Psychologist
Naval Medical Research Unit Dayton
Wright-Patterson Air Force Base, Ohio

John A. Caldwell, BS, MA, PHD
Senior Scientist
Fatigue and Sleep Management
Coastal Performance Consulting
Yellow Springs, Ohio

Michael W. Calik, PhD
Assistant Professor
Department of Biobehavioral Nursing Science

Assistant Professor
Center for Sleep and Health Research
University of Illinois Chicago College of Nursing
Chicago, Illinois

Francisco Campos-Rodriguez, MD
Respiratory Department
Hospital Valme
Seville, Andalucía

Craig Canapari, MD
Associate Professor
Department of Pediatrics
Yale University
New Haven, Connecticuit

Michela Canepari, PhD
Department of Humanities, Social and Cultural Enterprises
University of Parma
Parma, Italy

Michelle T. Cao, DO
Clinical Associate Professor
Department of Neurology
Stanford University School of Medicine
Palo Alto, California;
Clinical Associate Professor
Psychiatry and Behavioral Sciences
Stanford University School of Medicine
Redwood City, California

Colleen E. Carney, PhD
Professor
Department of Psychology
Ryerson University
Toronto, Ontario, Canada

Michelle Carr, PhD
Department of Psychiatry
University of Rochester Medical Center
Rochester, New York

Santiago Carrizo, MD
Servicio de Neumología
Hospital Universitario Miguel Servet
Zaragoza, Spain

Mary A. Carskadon, PhD
Professor, Psychiatry and Human Behavior
Alpert Medical School of Brown University;
Director, Chronobiology and Sleep Research
EP Bradley Hospital
Providence, Rhode Island

Diego Z. Carvalho, MD
Assistant Professor
Center for Sleep Medicine
Department of Medicine
Mayo Clinic College of Medicine and Science
Rochester, Minnesota

Anna Castelnovo, MD
Faculty of Biomedical Sciences
Università della Svizzera Italiana
Lugano, Switzerland

Eduardo E. Castrillon, DDS, MSc, PhD
Associate Professor
Section for Orofacial Pain and Jaw Function
Department of Dentistry and Oral Health
Aarhus University
Aarhus, Denmark

Lana M. Chahine, MD
Assistant Professor
Department of Neurology
University of Pittsburgh
Pittsburgh, Pennsylvania

Etienne Challet, PhD
Institute of Cellular and Integrative Neurosciences
Strasbourg, France

Philip Cheng, PhD
Assistant Scientist
Division of Sleep Medicine
Thomas Roth Sleep Disorders and Research Center
Henry Ford Health System
Detroit, Michigan;
Research Assistant Professor
Department of Psychiatry
University of Michigan School of Medicine
Ann Arbor, Michigan

Ronald D. Chervin, MD, MS
Professor of Neurology
Michael S. Aldrich Collegiate Professor of Sleep Medicine
Director, Sleep Disorders Center
University of Michigan Health System
Ann Arbor, Michigan

Soo-Hee Choi, MD, PhD
Associate Professor
Department of Psychiatry
Seoul National University College of Medicine;
Associate Professor
Department of Psychiatry
Seoul National University Hospital
Seoul, Korea

Ian M. Colrain, PhD
President
SRI Biosciences
SRI International
Menlo Park, California;
Professorial Fellow
Melbourne School of Pscyhological Sciences
The University of Melbourne
Parkville, Victoria, Australia

Veda Elisabeth Cost, BA
Research Fellow
National Institute of Neurological Disorders and Stroke
Bethesda, Maryland

Anita P. Courcoulas, MD
Professor of Surgery
Division of Minimally Invasive Bariatric and General Surgery
University of Pittsburgh Medical Center
Pittsburgh, Pennsylvania

Michel A. Cramer Bornemann, MD, DABSM, FAASM
Lead Investigator
Sleep Forensics Associates;
Visiting Professor, Sleep Medicine
Fellowship, Minnesota Regional Sleep Disorders Center
Hennepin County Medical Center
Minneapolis, Minnesota;
Co-Director of Sleep Medicine Services
CentraCare
Saint Cloud, Minnesota

Ashley F. Curtis, PhD
Assistant Professor
Psychiatry
Psychological Sciences
University of Missouri
Columbia, Missouri

Charles A. Czeisler, PhD, MD
Frank Baldino, Jr., Ph.D. Professor of Sleep Medicine
Department of Medicine
Director
Division of Sleep Medicine
Harvard Medical School;
Chief, Division of Sleep and Circadian Disorders
Department Medicine
Brigham and Women's Hospital
Boston, Massachusetts

Michael Czisch, MD
Max Planck Institute of Psychiatry
Munich, Germany

Armando D'Agostino, MD, PhD
Department of Health Sciences
Università degli Studi di Milano
Milan, Italy

O'Neill F. D'Cruz, MD
OD Consulting and Neurological Services, PLLC
Chapel Hill, NC

Steve M. D'Souza, MD
Resident
Eastern Virginia University Medical School
Norfolk, Virginia

Meg Danforth, PhD
Clinical Psychology
Duke University Faculty Practice in Psychology
Durham, North Carolina

Yves Dauvilliers, MD, PhD
Professor
Sleep Unit, Department of Neurology
Gui de Chauliac Hospital
Montpellier, France

Drew Dawson, PhD
Professor
Appleton Institute
Central Queensland University
Wayville, Australia

David de Ángel Solá, MD
Staff Physician
Department of Pediatrics
Yale School of Medicine
New Haven, Connecticut;
Faculty Physician
Department of Neurology
VA Caribbean Healthcare Systems;
Faculty Physician
Department of Pediatrics
San Juan City Hospital
San Juan, Puerto Rico

Luis de Lecea, PhD
Department of Psychiatry and Behavioral Sciences
Stanford University
Palo Alto, California

Massimiliano de Zambotti, PhD
Principle Scientist, Human Sleep Research
Center for Health Sciences
SRI International
Menlo Park, California

Tom Deboer, PhD
Associate Professor
Cell and Chemical Biology
Leiden University Medical Center
Leiden, The Netherlands

Lourdes DelRosso, MD
Associate Professor
Department of Pediatrics
Seattle Children's Hospital
University of Washington
Seattle, Washington

William C. Dement, MD†
Lowell W. and Josephine Q. Berry Professor of Psychiatry and Behavioral Sciences
Stanford University School of Medicine
Department of Sleep Sciences & Medicine
Palo Alto, California

Jerome A. Dempsey, PhD
Professor Emeritus
Population Health Sciences;
Director
John Rankin Laboratory of Pulmonary Medicine
University of Wisconsin–Madison
Madison, Wisconsin

Massimiliano DiGiosia, DDS
Orofacial Pain Clinic
Division of Diagnostic Sciences
Adams School of Dentistry
University of North Carolina at Chapel Hill
Chapel Hill, North Carolina

†Deceased.

Derk-Jan Dijk, PhD
Professor
Surrey Sleep Research Centre
Department of Clinical and Experimental Medicine
Faculty of Health and Medical Sciences
University of Surrey;
Investigator
Dementia Research Institute Care Research and Technology Centre
Imperial College London
University of Surrey
Guildford, Great Britain

David F. Dinges, MS, MA(H), PhD
Professor and Director, Unit for Experimental Psychiatry
Chief, Division of Sleep and Chronobiology
Department of Psychiatry
Pereleman School of Medicine
University of Pennsylvania
Philadelphia, Pennsylvania

G. William Domhoff, PhD
Distinguished Professor Emeritus and Research Professor in Psychology
Department of Psychology
University of California
Santa Cruz, California

Jillian Dorrian, PhD, MBiostat
Professor and Dean of Research
Behavior-Brain-Body Research Centre
University of South Australia
Adelaide, South Australia

Anthony G. Doufas, MD, PhD
Professor
Department of Anesthesiology, Perioperative and Pain Medicine
Stanford University School of Medicine
Palo Alto, California

Luciano F. Drager, MD, PhD
Associate Professor of Medicine
Department of Internal Medicine
University of Sao Paulo
Sso Paulo, Brazil

Christopher L. Drake, PhD, FAASM, DBSM
Director of Sleep Research
Division of Sleep Medicine
Henry Ford Health System;
Professor
Department of Psychiatry and Behavioral Neuroscience
Wayne State University School of Medicine
Detroit, Michigan

Martin Dresler, PhD
Radboud University Medical Center
Department of Cognitive Neuroscience
Donders Institute for Brain, Cognition, and Behavior
Nijmegen, The Netherlands

Jeanne F. Duffy, MBA, PhD
Division of Sleep and Circadian Disorders
Departments of Medicine and Neurology
Brigham and Women's Hospital;
Division of Sleep Medicine
Harvard Medical School
Boston, Massachusetts

Peter R. Eastwood, PhD
Director, Flinders Health and Medical Research Institute
Dean of Research and Matthew Flinders Fellow
College of Medicine and Public Health
Flinders University
Adelaide, South Australia

Danny J. Eckert, PhD
Professor and Director
Adelaide Institute for Sleep Health
Flinders Health and Medical Research Institute
Flinders University
Bedford Park, South Australia

Jack D. Edinger, PhD
Professor
Department of Medicine
National Jewish Health
Denver, Colorado;
Adjunct Professor
Psychiatry and Behavioral Sciences
Duke University Medical Center
Durham, North Carolina

Bradley A. Edwards, PhD
Department of Physiology
School of Biomedical Sciences and Biomedical Discovery Institute
Monash University
Melbourne, Victoria, Australia

Jason G. Ellis, MD
Northumbria Sleep Research
Faculty of Health and Life Sciences
Northumbria University
Newcastle, United Kingdom

Daniel Erlacher, PhD, MD
Institute of Sport Science
University of Bern
Bern, Switzerland

Gregory Essick, DDS, PhD
Professor
Division of Comprehensive Oral Health
Adams School of Dentistry
University of North Carolina at Chapel Hill
Chapel Hill, North Carolina

Marissa A. Evans, MS
Department of Psychiatry
University of Pittsburgh
Pittsburgh, Pennsylvania

Véronique Fabre, PhD
Neuroscience Paris Seine
INSERM
Sorbonne Université Paris
Paris, France

Francesca Facco, MD
Associate Professor of Medicine
Department of Obstetrics, Gynecology, and Reproductive Sciences
University of Pittsburgh School of Medicine
Pittsburgh, Pennsylvania

Ronnie Fass, MD
Director, Division of Gastroenterology and Hepatology
Department of Medicine
MetroHealth Medical Center;
Professor of Medicine
Case Western Reserve University
Cleveland, Ohio

Luigi Ferini-Strambi, MD
Professor of Neurology
Department of Clinical Neuroscience
Università Vita-Salute San Raffaele
Milano, Italy

Julio Fernandez-Mendoza, PhD, CBSM, DBSM
Associate Professor
Director, Behavioral Sleep Medicine Program
Sleep Research & Treatment Center
Department of Psychiatry and Behavioral Health
Penn State University College of Medicine
Penn State Health Milton S. Hershey Medical Center
Hershey, Pennsylvania

Fabio Ferrarelli, MD, PhD
Associate Professor of Psychiatry
Department of Psychiatry
University of Pittsburgh
Pittsburgh, Pennsylvania

Raffaele Ferri, MD
Sleep Research Centre
Department of Neurology I.C.
Oasi Research Institute - IRCCS
Troina, Italy

Stuart Fogel, PhD
Associate Professor
School of Psychology
University of Ottawa
Ottawa, Ontario, Canada

Jimmy J. Fraigne, PhD
Senior Research Associate
Department of Cell & Systems Biology
University of Toronto
Toronto, Canada

Paul Franken, PhD
Associate Professor
Center for Integrative Genomics
University of Lausanne
Lausanne, Switzerland

Karl A. Franklin, MD, PhD
Assistant Professor
Department of Surgery
Surgical and Preoperative Sciences
Umeå University
Umeå, Sweden

Neil Freedman, MD, FCCP
Head, Division of Pulmonary and Critical Care
Department of Medicine
NorthShore University Healthsystem;
Clinical Professor of Medicine
University of Chicago Pritzker School of Medicine
Chicago, Illinois

Liam Fry, MD, CMD, FACP
Division Chief of Geriatrics and Palliative Medicine
Department of Internal Medicine
University of Texas Dell Medical School;
President
Austin Geriatric Specialists
Austin, Texas

Patrick M. Fuller, MS, PhD
Professor of Neurological Surgery
Vice Chair of Research
University of California, Davis School of Medicine
Sacramento, California

Constance H. Fung, MD, MSHS
Geriatric Research, Education and Clinical Center
VA Greater Los Angeles Healthcare System;
Associate Professor
Department of Medicine
David Geffen School of Medicine
University of California, Los Angeles
Los Angeles, California

Carles Gaig, MD, PhD
Multidisciplinary Sleep Unit
Neurology Department
Hospital Clinic Barcelona
Barcelona, Spain

Philippa H. Gander, PhD, FRSNZ, ONZM
Professor Emeritus
Sleep/Wake Research Centre
Massey University
Wellington, New Zealand

Sheila N. Garland, PhD
Associate Professor
Department of Psychology, Faculty of Science
Discipline of Oncology, Faculty of Medicine
Memorial University
St. John's, Newfoundland, Canada

Philip R. Gehrman, PhD
Associate Professor
Department of Psychiatry
University of Pennsylvania Perelman School of Medicine
Philadelphia, Pennsylvania

Martha U. Gillette, PhD
Alumni Professor
Cell and Developmental Biology
Professor
Beckman Institute for Advanced Science & Technology
Molecular and Integrative Physiology
Director
Neuroscience Program
University of Illinois at Urbana-Champaign
Urbana, Illinois

Kevin S. Gipson, MD, MS
Assistant in Pediatrics
Department of Pediatrics
Massachusetts General Hospital;
Instructor
Harvard Medical School
Boston, Massachusetts

Peter J. Goadsby, MD, PhD, DSc
Department of Neurology
University of California, Los Angeles
Los Angeles, California;
National Institute for Health Research–Wellcome Trust King's Clinical Research Facility
King's College London
London, United Kingdom

Avram R. Gold, MD
Associate Professor of Clinical Medicine
Pulmonary, Critical Care, and Sleep Medicine
Stony Brook University School of Medicine
Stony Brook, New York

Cathy A. Goldstein, MD
Associate Professor of Neurology
Sleep Disorders Center
University of Michigan Health System
Ann Arbor, Michigan

Joshua J. Gooley, PhD
Associate Professor
Program in Neuroscience and Behavioral Disorders
Duke-NUS Medical School
Singapore

Nadia Gosselin, PhD
Associate Professor
Department of Psychology
Université de Montréal;
Researcher
Center for Advanced Research in Sleep Medicine
Hôpital du Sacré-Coeur de Montréal
Montreal, Quebec, Canada

Daniel J. Gottlieb, MD, MPH
Medical Service
VA Boston Healthcare System;
Division of Sleep and Circadian Disorders
Departments of Medicine and Neurology
Brigham and Women's Hospital;
Division of Sleep Medicine
Harvard Medical School
Boston, Massachusetts

R. Curtis Graeber, BA, MA, PhD
Honorary Fellow
Sleep/Wake Research Centre
Massey University
Wellington, New Zealand

Michael A. Grandner, PhD, MTR
Assistant Professor
Department of Psychiatry
University of Arizona
Tucson, Arizona

Harly Greenberg, MD
Professor of Medicine
Northwell Sleep Disorders Center;
Chief, Division of Pulmonary, Critical Care, and Sleep Medicine
Professor of Medicine
Donald and Barbara Zucker School of Medicine at Hofstra-Northwell
New Hyde Park, New York

Alice M. Gregory, BSc, PhD
Professor
Department of Psychology
Goldsmiths
University of London
London, Great Britain

Edith Grosbellet, PhD
Institute of Cellular and Integrative Neurosciences
Strasbourg, France

Ludger Grote, MD, PhD
Professor
Sleep Disorders Center
Department of Respiratory Medicine
Sahlgrenska University Hospital
Gothenburg, Sweden

Ronald Grunstein, MBBS, MD, PhD, FRACP
Professor
Sleep and Circadian Research Group
Woolcock Institute of Medical Research
Sydney, Australia

Christian Guilleminault, MD, BioL†
Professor
Department of Psychiatry and Behavioral Sciences
Sleep Medicine Division
Stanford University School of Medicine
Redwood City, California

Andrew Gumley, MD
Institute of Health and Wellbeing
University of Glasgow
Glasgow, United Kingdom

Hannah Gura, BS
Research Fellow
National Institute of Mental Health
Bethesda, Maryland

†Deceased.

Monika Haack, MD
Associate Professor of Neurology
Department of Neurology
Beth Israel Deaconess Medical Center
Boston Massachusetts

Martica H. Hall, PhD
Professor
Department of Psychiatry
Clinical and Translational Science
University of Pittsburgh
Pittsburgh, Pennsylvania

Erin C. Hanlon, PhD
Research Associate Professor
Department of Medicine
Section of Pediatric and Adult Endocrinology, Diabetes, and Metabolism
University of Chicago
Chicago, Illinois

Ronald M. Harper, PhD
Distinguished Professor
Department of Neurobiology
David Geffen School of Medicine
Distinguished Professor
Brain Research Institute
University of California at Los Angeles
Los Angeles, California

Krisztina Harsanyi, MD
Assistant Professor
Department of Pediatrics
University of Alabama at Birmingham
Birmingham, Alabama

Eric Heckman, MD
Instructor in Medicine
Division of Pulmonary, Critical Care, and Sleep Medicine
Department of Medicine
Beth Israel Deaconess Medical Center
Harvard Medical School
Boston, Massachusetts

Jan Hedner, MD, PhD
Professor
Sleep and Vigilance Disorders
Department of Internal Medicine
Sahlgrenska University Hospital
Gothenburg, Sweden

Brent E. Heideman, MD
Clinical Felow
Department of Medicine
Division of Allergy, Pulmonary, and Critical Care Medicine
Vanderbilt University Medical Center
Nashville, Tennessee

Raphael Heinzer, MD, MPH
Director
Center for Investigation and Research in Sleep (CIRS)
University Hospital of Lausanne;
Associate Professor
University of Lausanne
Lausanne, Switzerland

Luke A. Henderson, BSc, PhD
Professor
Department of Anatomy and Histology
Brain and Mind Centre
University of Sydney
Sydney, Australia

Rebecca C. Hendrickson, MD, PhD
Northwest Network Mental Illness Research Education and Clinical Center (MIRECC)
Department of Psychiatry and Behavioral Sciences
University of Washington
Seattle, Washington

Alberto Herrero Babiloni, DDS, MS
PhD Candidate
Department of Experimental Medicine
McGill University
CUISS NIM
Montreal, Quebec, Canada

W. Joseph Herring, MD, PhD
Associate Vice President
Clinical Neuroscience
Merck & Co., Inc.
Kenilworth, New Jersey

Elisabeth Hertenstein, MD
University Hospital of Psychiatry and Psychotherapy
University of Bern
Bern, Switzerland

David Hillman, MBBS, FANZCA
Emeritus Physician
Sir Charles Gairdner Hospital;
Clinical Professor
Medical School, Surgery and School of Human Sciences
University of Western Australia
Perth, Australia

Max Hirshkowitz, PhD
Professor (Emeritus)
Department of Medicine
Baylor College of Medicine
Houston, Texas

Aarnoud Hoekema, MD, DMD, PhD
Oral and Maxillofacial Surgery
Tjongerschans Hospital
Heerenveen, The Netherlands;
Department of Oral Kinesiology
Academic Centre for Dentistry Amsterdam
Amsterdam, The Netherlands

Birgit Högl, MD
Head of the Sleep Disorders Clinic
Department of Neurology
Innsbruck Medical University
Innsbruck, Austria

Richard L. Horner, PhD
Professor
Department of Medicine and Department of Physiology
University of Toronto;
Canada Research Chair in Sleep and Respiratory Neurobiology
Toronto, Ontario, Canada

Amanda N. Hudson, BS, MA
Graduate Research Assistant
Sleep and Performance Research Center
Elson S. Floyd College of Medicine
Washington State University
Spokane, Washington

Steven R. Hursh, PhD
President
Institutes for Behavior Resources, Inc.;
Adjunct Professor
Department of Psychiatry and Behavioral Biology
Johns Hopkins University School of Medicine
Baltimore, Maryland

Nelly Huynh, DDS
Faculty of Dental Medicine
Université de Montréal
Montréal, Quebec, Canada

Mari Hysing, MD
Department of Psychosocial Science
University of Bergen
Bergen, Norway

Octavian C. Ioachimescu, MD, PhD, MBA
Section Chief and Medical Director
Sleep Medicine Center
Atlanta VA Clinic
Decatur, Georgia;
Professor of Medicine
Department of Medicine
Division of Pulmonary, Critical Care, and Sleep Medicine
Emory University School of Medicine
Atlanta, Georgia

Mary Ip, MD
Chair and Professor
Department of Medicine
The University of Hong Kong
Hong Kong, China

Alex Iranzo, MD, PhD
Neurologist
Neurology Service
Hospital Clinic de Barcelona
Institut d'Investigació Biomèdiques;
Associate Professor
University of Barcelona
Barcelona, Spain

Bilgay Izci Balserak, PhD
Associate Professor
Department of Biobehavioral Health Science
Center for Sleep and Health Research
University of Illinois College of Nursing
Chicago, Illinois

Chandra L. Jackson, MD
Epidemiology Branch
National Institute of Environmental Health Sciences
National Institutes of Health
Department of Health and Human Services
Research Triangle Park, North Carolina;
Division of Intramural Research
National Institute on Minority Health and Health Disparities
National Institutes of Health
Department of Health and Human Services
Bethesda, Maryland

Shahrokh Javaheri, MD
Professor Emeritus
Department of Pulmonary Critical Care and Sleep
University of Cincinnati
Cincinnati, Ohio;
Adjunct Professor
Department of Cardiology
The Ohio State University
Columbus, Ohio

Sogol Javaheri, MD, MPH, MA
Physician
Department of Sleep Medicine
Brigham and Women's Hospital
Boston, Massachusetts

Peng Jiang, PhD
Research Assistant Professor
Center for Sleep and Circadian Biology
Northwestern University
Evanston, Illinois

Yandong Jiang, MD, PhD
Professor
Department of Anesthesiology
University of Texas, Houston
Health Science Center
Houston, Texas

Hadine Joffe, MD, MSc
Paula A. Johnson Professor of Psychiatry in the Field of Women's Heath
Executive Director of Mary Horrigan Connors Center for Women's Health and Gender Biology
Executive Vice Chair for Academic and Faulty Affairs
Department of Psychiatry
Brigham and Women's Hospital
Harvard Medical School
Boston, Massachusetts

David A. Johnson, MD, MACG, FASGE, MACP
Professor of Medicine and Chief
Department of Internal Medicine
Division of Gastroenterology and Hepatology
Eastern Virginia Medical School
Norfolk, Virginia

Karin Johnson, MD, FAASM, FAAN
Associate Professor
UMMS - Baystate Regional Campus
Neurology at UMMS-Baystate;
Medical Director
Baystate Health Regional Sleep Program
Springfield, Massachusetts

Anne E. Justice, MA, PhD
Assistant Professor of Population Health Sciences
Geisinger Health System
Danville, Pennsylvania

Marc Kaizi-Lutu, BA
Unit for Experimental Psychiatry
Division of Sleep and Chronobiology
Department of Psychiatry
Perelman School of Medicine
University of Pennsylvania
Philadelphia, Pennsylvania

David A. Kalmbach, PhD
Thomas Roth Sleep Disorders & Research Center
Division of Sleep Medicine
Henry Ford Health System
Detroit, Michigan

Elissaios Karageorgiou, MD, PhD
Division Chief
Sleep & Memory Center
Scientific Director
Neurological Institute of Athens
Athens, Greece

Eliot S. Katz, MD
Assistant Professor of Pediatrics
Harvard Medical School;
Division of Pulmonology
Boston Children's Hospital
Boston, Massachusetts

Brendan T. Keenan, MS
Co-Director, Biostatistics Core
Division of Sleep Medicine
Department of Medicine
University of Pennsylvania Perelman School of Medicine
Philadelphia, Pennsylvania

Sharon Keenan, PhD
Director
Department of Sleep Medicine
The School of Sleep Medicine, Inc.
Palo Alto, California

Thomas Kilduff, PhD
Center Director, Center for Neuroscience
Biosciences Division
SRI International
Menlo Park, California

Douglas Kirsch, MD
Medical Director
Department of Sleep Medicine
Professor
Department of Medicine and Neurology
Atrium Health
Charlotte, North Carolina;
Professor
Department of Medicine
University of North Carolina School of Medicine
Chapel Hill, North Carolina

Christopher E. Kline, PhD
Assistant Professor of Health and Physical Activity
Department of Health and Human Development
University of Pittsburgh
Department of Health and Physical Activity
Pittsburgh, Pennsylvania

Melissa P. Knauert, MD, PhD
Assistant Professor
Section of Pulmonary, Critical Care and Sleep Medicine
Department of Internal Medicine
Yale University School of Medicine
New Haven, Connecticuit

Kristen L. Knutson, PhD
Associate Professor
Department of Neurology
Northwestern University
Chicago, Illinois

Abigail L. Koch, MD, MHS
Assistant Chief
Division of Pulmonary Medicine
Miami VA Healthcare System
Miami, Florida

George F. Koob, MD
National Institute on Alcohol Abuse and Alcoholism
National Institutes of Health
Bethesda, Maryland

Sanjeev V. Kothare, MD, FAAN, FAASM
Director, Division of Pediatric Neurology
Department of Pediatrics
Cohen Children's Medical center
New Hyde Park, New York;
Director, Pediatric Neurology Service Line for Northwell Health
Professor of Pediatrics and Neurology
Zucker School of Medicine at Hofstra Northwell
Lake Success, New York

Kyoshi Koyano, DDS, PhD
Professor
Department of Implant and Rehabilitative Dentistry
Faculty of Dental Science
Kyushu University
Fukuoka, Japan

James M. Krueger, PhD, MDHC
Regents Professor
Integrative Physiology and Neuroscience
Washington State University
Spokane, Washington

Meir Kryger, MD, FRCPC
Professor
Pulmonary, Critical Care, and Sleep Medicine
Yale University School of Medicine
New Haven, Connecticuit

Andrew D. Krystal, MD, MS
Ray and Dagmar Dolby Distinguished Professor
Department of Psychiatry
University of California, San Francisco
San Francisco, California

Samuel T. Kuna, MD
Professor of Medicine
Department of Medicine
Perelman School of Medicine at the University of Pennsylvania;
Chief
Sleep Medicine Section
Department of Medicine
Corporal Michael J. Crescenz Veterans Affairs Medical Center
Philadelphia, Pennsylvania

Scott Kutscher, MD
Associate Professor
Department of Sleep Medicine
Stanford University
Redwood City, California

Stephen LaBerge, PhD
Research Associate
Department of Psychology
Stanford University
Palo Alto, California

Annie C. Lajoie, MD
Respirology Fellow
Department of Respirology
Institut Universitaire de Cardiologie et de Pneumologie de Québec
Quebec City, Quebec, Canada

Amanda Lamp, BS, MS, PhD
Research Assistant Professor
Sleep and Performance Research Center
Washington State University
Spokane, Washington

Hans-Peter Landolt, PhD
Human Sleep Psychopharmacology Laboratory
Institute of Pharmacology and Toxicology
Sleep and Health Zürich
University Center of Competence
University of Zürich
Zürich, Switzerland

Jessica Lara-Carrasco, PhD
Clinical Psychologist
Hôpital Maisonneuve-Rosemont
CIUSSS del'Est-de-l'île-de-Montéal
Montreal, Quebec, Canada

Gilles Lavigne, DMD, FRCDI, PhD
Professor
Faculty of Dental Medicine
Université de Montréal
CIUSS NIM and CHUM-Stomatology
Montréal, Quebec, Canada

Michael Lazarus, PhD
International Institute for Integrative Sleep Medicine
University of Tsukuba
Tsukuba, Japan

Han-Hee Lee, MD
Department of Cell and Systems Biology
University of Toronto
Toronto, Ontario, Canada

Guy Leschziner, MBBS, MA, PhD, FRCP
Consultant Neurologist
Sleep Disorders Centre
Guy's and St Thomas' NHS Trust;
Professor of Neurology and Sleep Medicine
Institute of Psychiatry, Psychology, and Neuroscience
King's College London
London, Great Britain

John A. Lesku, PhD
Associate Professor
School of Life Sciences
La Trobe University
Melbourne, Australia

Christopher J. Lettieri, MD
Professor of Medicine
Department of Pulmonary, Critical Care, and Sleep Medicine
Uniformed Services University of the Health Sciences
Bethesda, Maryland

Vicki Li
Project Assistant
Research Institute
California Pacific Medical Center
San Francisco, California

Paul-Antione Libourel, PhD
Neurosciences Reseach Center of Lyon (CRNL)
Team SLEEP
Lyon, France

Melissa C. Lipford, MD
Center for Sleep Medicine
Department of Neurology
Division of Pulmonary and Critical Care Medicine
Mayo Clinic
Rochester, Minnesota

Frank Lobbezoo, DDS, PhD
Professor and Chair
Department of Orofacial Pain and Dysfunction
Academic Centre for Dentistry Amsterdam (ACTA)
Amsterdam, The Netherlands

Geraldo Lorenzi-Filho, MD, PhD
Associate Professor
Department of Cardio-Pulmonology
University of Sao Paulo
Sao Paulo, Brazil

Judette Louis, MD, MPH
James M. Ingram Professor and Chair
Department of Obstetrics and Gynecology
Morsani College of Medicine
University of South Florida
Tampa, Florida

Brendan P. Lucey, MD, MSCI
Associate Professor of Neurology
Sleep Medicine Section Head
Washington University School of Medicine
Saint Louis, Missouri

Ralph Lydic, PhD
Professor
Department of Psychology
University of Tennessee
Knoxville, Tennessee;
Joint Faculty
Biosciences Division
Oak Ridge National Laboratory
Oak Ridge, Tennessee

Madalina Macrea, MD, PhD, MPH
Department of Pulmonary and Sleep Medicine
Salem Veterans Affairs Medical Center
Salem, Virginia;
Associate Professor
University of Virginia
Charlottesville, Virginia

Mary Halsey Maddox, MD
Associate Professor
Department of Pediatrics
University of Alabama at Birmingham
Birmingham, Alabama

Mark W. Mahowald, MD†
Professor of Neurology
University of Minnesota Medical School;
Visiting Professor
Minnesota Regional Sleep Disorders Center
Hennepin County Medical Center
Minneapolis, Minnesota

Atul Malhotra, MD
Professor of Medicine
Peter C. Farrell Presidential Chair in Respiratory Medicine
Department of Pulmonary, Critical Care, and Sleep Medicine
University of Southern California, San Diego;
Research Chief of Pulmonary, Critical Care, and Sleep Medicine
University of California, San Diego School of Medicine
La Jolla, California

Raman K. Malhotra, MD
Associate Professor of Neurology
Washington University School of Medicine
Saint Louis, Missouri

Beth A. Malow, MD, MS
Professor
Department of Neurology and Pediatrics
Director
Sleep Disorders Division
Department of Neurology and Pediatrics
Vanderbilt University Medical Center
Nashville, Tennessee

Rachel Manber, PhD
Professor
Psychiatry and Behavioral Sciences
Stanford University
Palo Alto, California

Daniele Manfredini, DDS, MSc, PhD
Professor
School of Dentistry
University of Siena
Siena, Italy

Jim Mangie, BS
Aeronautical Studies Program Director
Pilot Fatigue Flight Operations Delta Air Lines
Atlanta, Georgia

Edward Manning, MD, PhD
Intensivist, Pulmonologist
Veterans Affairs Connecticut Healthcare System;
Instructor
Pulmonary and Critical Care Medicine
Yale School of Medicine
New Haven, Connecticut

Pierre Maquet, MD, PhD
Sleep and Chronobiology Laboratory
GIGA-Cyclontron Research Center/In Vivo Imaging
University of Liège;
Professor
Department of Neurology
Liège University Hospital
Liège, Belgium

†Deceased.

Jose M. Marin, MD
Head
Respiratory Sleep Disorders Unit
Hospital Universitario Miguel Servet;
Professor of Respiratory Medicine
Department of Medicine
University of Zaragoza
Zaragoza, Spain

Marta Marin-Oto, MD
Respiratory Department
Clinica Universidad de Navarra
Pamplona, Spain

Jennifer L. Martin, PhD
Associate Director for Clinical and Health Services Research
Geriatric Research, Education and Clinical Center
VA Greater Los Angeles Healthcare System;
Professor
Department of Medicine
David Geffen School of Medicine
University of California, Los Angeles
Los Angeles, California

Miguel A. Martínez-Garcia, MD, PhD
Servicio de Neumologia
Hospital Universitario y Politécnico La Fe
Valencia, Spain;
Centro de Investigación Biomédica en Red de Enfermedades Respiratorias (CIBERES)
Madrid, Spain

Kiran Maski, MD, MPH
Associate Professor
Department of Neurology
Boston Children's Hospital
Boston, Massachusetts

Ivy C. Mason, PhD
Postdoctoral Research Fellow
Medical Chronobiology Program
Division of Sleep and Circadian Disorders
Departments of Medicine and Neurology
Brigham and Women's Hospital;
Research Fellow
Division of Sleep Medicine
Department of Medicine
Harvard Medical School
Boston, Massachusetts

Christopher R. McCartney, MD
Professor of Medicine
Department of Medicine
Division of Endocrinology and Metabolism
University of Virginia School of Medicine
Charlottesville, Virginia

Colleen McClung, PhD
Professor
Departments of Psychiatry and Clinical and Translational Science
University of Pittsburgh School of Medicine
Pittsburgh, Pennsylvania

Christina S. McCrae, PHD
Professorr
Department of Psychiatry
University of Missouri-Columbia
Columbia, Missouri

Dennis McGinty, PhD
Adjunct Professor
Department of Psychology
University of California
Research Service
VA Medical Center, GLAHS
Los Angeles, California

Andrew W. McHill, PhD
Research Assistant Professor
Oregon Institute of Occupational Health Sciences
Oregon Health & Science University
Portland, Oregon

Reena Mehra, MD, MS
Professor of Medicine
Sleep Disorders Center, Neurologic Institute
Cleveland Clinic Lerner College of Medicine of Case Western Reserve University;
Respiratory Institute
Department of Molecular Cardiology
Lerner Research Institute
Heart and Vascular Institute
Cleveland, Ohio

Emmanuel Mignot, MD, PhD
Director
Center For Sleep Sciences and Medicine
Stanford University
Palo Alto, California

Katherine E. Miller, PhD
Cpl. Michael J Crescenz VA Medical Center
Philadelphia, Pennsylvania

Brienne Miner, MD, MHS
Assistant Professor
Department of Internal Medicine
Section of Geriatrics
Yale University
New Haven, Connecticut

Jennifer W. Mitchell, PhD
Department of Cell & Developmental Biology
Neuroscience Program
University of Illinois at Urbana-Champaign
Urbana, Illinois

Murray Mittleman, MD, DrPH
Associate Professor
Department of Medicine
Harvard Medical School;
Associate Professor
Department of Epidemiology
Harvard School of Public Health
Boston, Massachusetts

Vahid Mohsenin, MD
Professor (Emeritus)
Department of Medicine
Yale University
New Haven, Connecticuit

Babak Mokhlesi, MD, MSc
J. Bailey Carter Professor of Medicine
Chief, Division of Pulmonary, Critical Care and Sleep Medicine
Co-Director, Rush Lung Center
Department of Internal Medicine
Rush University Medical Center
Chicago, Illinois

Jacques Montplaisir, PhD
Professor
Department of Psychiatry
Université de Montréal;
Center for Advanced Research on Sleep Medicine
CIUSSS du Nord-de-l'Île-de-Montréal
Hôpital du Sacré-Coeur de Montréal
Montreal, Quebec, Canada

Charles M. Morin, PhD
Professor
Department of Psychology
Director
Center for the Study of Sleep Disorders
Canada Research Chair in Sleeping Disorders
Laval University
Quebec City, Quebec, Canada

Mary J. Morrell, PhD
Professor of Sleep and Respiratory Physiology
National Heart and Lung Institute
Imperial College
London, Great Britain

Tanvi H. Mukundan, MD
Program Director, Sleep
Veterans Administration
Portland, Oregon

Erik Musiek, MD, PhD
Associate Professor
Department of Neurology
Washington University School of Medicine
Saint Louis, Missouri

Carlotta Mutti, MD
Sleep Disorders Center
Department of Medicine and Surgery
University of Parma
Parma, Italy

Alexander D. Nesbitt, BM BCh, PhD, FRCP
Consultant Neurologist and Sleep Physician
Sleep Disorders Centre and Department of Neurology
Guy's and St Thomas' NHS Foundation Trust
London, Great Britain

Thomas Nesthus, PhD, FRAeS, FasMA
Engineering Research Psychologist
Aerospace Human Factors Research Division
FAA, Civil Aerospace Medical Institute
Oklahoma City, Oklahoma

Natalie Nevárez, MD
Department of Psychiatry and Behavioral Sciences
Stanford University
Palo Alto, California

Tore Nielsen, PhD
Professor
Department of Psychiatry and Addictology
Université de Montréal;
Director, Dream & Nightmare Laboratory
Center for Advanced Research in Sleep Medicine
CIUSSS du Nord-de-l'Île-de-Montréal (Hôpital du Sacré-Coeur)
Montreal, Quebec, Canada

Christoph Nissen, MD
University Hospital of Psychiatry and Psychotherapy
University of Bern
Bern, Switzerland

Eric A. Nofzinger, MD
Adjunct Professor
Department of Psychiatry
University of Pittsburgh
Pittsburgh, Pennsylvania

Christopher B. O'Brien, BS
Department of Psychology
University of Tennessee
Knoxville, Tennessee

Louise M. O'Brien, PhD, MS
Associate Professor
Division of Sleep Medicine
Associate Professor
Department of Obstetrics & Gynecology
Associate Research Scientist
Oral & Maxillofacial Surgery
University of Michigan
Ann Arbor, Michigan

Bruce O'Hara, PhD
Professor
Department of Biology
University of Kentucky
Lexington, Kentucky

Yo Oishi, PhD
International Institute for Integrative Sleep Medicine
University of Tsukuba
Tsukuba, Japan

Eric J. Olson, MD
Division of Pulmonary and Critical Care Medicine
Center for Sleep Medicine
Mayo Clinic
Rochester, Minnesota

Jason C. Ong, PhD
Associate Professor
Department of Neurology
Center for Circadian and Sleep Medicine
Northwestern University Feinberg School of Medicine
Chicago, Illinois

Mark R. Opp, PhD
Professor and Chair
Integrative Physiology
University of Colorado Boulder
Boulder, Colorado

Edward F. Pace-Schott, PhD
Assistant Professor of Psychiatry
Harvard Medical School
Boston, Massachusetts;
Massachusetts General Hospital
Charlestown, Massachusetts

Allan I. Pack, MB, ChB, PhD, FRCP
John Miclot Professor of Medicine
Division of Sleep Medicine
Department of Medicine
University of Pennsylvania Perelman School of Medicine
Philadelphia, Pennsylvania

John Park, MD
Associate Professor of Medicine
Division of Pulmonary and Critical Care Medicine
Mayo Clinic
Rochester, Minnesota

Liborio Parrino, MD
Professor
Department of Medicine and Surgery
University of Parma
Parma, Italy

Sara Pasha, MBBS
Assistant Professor
Pulmonary, Critical Care, and Sleep Medicine
University of Kentucky
Lexington, Kentucky

Michael Paskow, MPH
Associate Director
Epidemiology, Global Real-World Evidence Generation
Washington, DC

Susheel P. Patil, MD, PhD, ATSF
System Director, UH Sleep Medicine
Section Chief, Sleep Medicine
Division of Pulmonary, Critical Care, and Sleep Medicine
Clinical Associate Professor of Medicine
Case Western Reserve University School of Medicine
Cleveland, Ohio

Alexander Patrician, MSc
Department of Health and Exercise Sciences
The University of British Columbia
Kelowna, British Columbia, Canada

Milena K. Pavlova, MD, FAASM
Medical Director, Faulkner Sleep Testing Center
Department of Neurology
Brigham and Women's Hospital;
Associate Professor of Neurology
Department of Neurology
Harvard Medical School
Boston, Massachusetts

John H. Peever, PhD
Professor
Department of Cell and Systems Biology
University of Toronto
Toronto, Ontario, Canada

Philippe Peigneux, PhD
Full Professor
Neuropsychology and Functional Neuroimaging at Centre for Research in Cognition and Neurosciences
Universite Libre de Bruxelles
Bruxelles, Belgium

Yüksel Peker, MD, PhD
Professor
Department of Pulmonary Medicine
Head of Sleep Medicine Unit
Koç University School of Medicine
Istanbul, Turkey

Rafael Pelayo, MD
Clinical Professor
Sleep Medicine Division
Stanford Univeristy School of Medicine
Stanford, California

Thomas Penzel, MD
Research Director of Sleep Center
Interdisciplinary Sleep Medicine Center
Charité–Universitätsmedizin Berlin
Berlin, Germany

Jean-Louis Pépin, MD, PhD
Pneumology-Physiology Department
Grenoble Alpes University Hospital;
INSERM U1300, HP2 Laboratory
Grenoble Alpes University
Grenoble, France

Michael L. Perlis, PhD
Department of Psychiatry
University of Pennsylvania
Philadelphia, Pennsylvania

Lampros Perogamvros, MD
Department of Medicine
University Hospitals of Geneva
University of Geneva
Geneva, Switzerland

Dominique Petit, PhD
Research Associate
Center for Advanced Research in Sleep Medicine
CIUSSS du Nord-de-l'Île-de-Montréal – Hôpital du Sacré-Coeur de Montréal
Montreal, Quebec, Canada

Megan E. Petrov, PhD
Assistant Professor
College of Nursing and Health Innovation
Arizona State University
Phoenix, Arizona

Dante Picchioni, PhD
Scientist (contractor)
National Institute of Neurological Disorders and Stroke
Bethesda, Maryland

Grace W. Pien, MD, MSCE
Assistant Professor of Medicine
Department of Medicine
Johns Hopkins University School of Medicine
Baltimore, Maryland

Wilfred R. Pigeon, PhD
Professor
Psychiatry & Public Health Sciences
University of Rochester Medical Center
Rochester, New York;
Executive Director
Center of Excellence for Suicide Prevention
U.S. Department of Veterans Affairs
Canandaigua, New York

Margaret A. Pisani, MD, MPH
Associate Professor
Internal Medicine–Pulmonary, Critical Care, and Sleep
Yale University
New Haven, Connecticuit

Melanie Pogach, MD, MMSc
Assistant Professor of Medicine
Tufts University School of Medicine
SEMC/SMG Pulmonary, Critical Care, and Sleep Medicine
Director, Chronic Respiratory Failure Program
St. Elizabeth's Medical Center
Brighton, Massachusetts

Donn Posner, PhD
Department of Psychiatry and Behavioral Science
Stanford University
Palo Alto, California

Ronald Postuma, MD, MSc
Professor
Department of Neurology
McGill University
Montreal, Quebec, Canada

Naresh Punjabi, MD, PhD
Division of Pulmonary and Critical Care Medicine
Department of Medicine
Johns Hopkins University
Baltimore, Maryland

Stacey Dagmar Quo, DDS, MS
School of Dentistry
University of California San Francisco
San Francisco, California

Shadab Rahman, PhD
Instructor in Medicine
Division of Sleep Medicine
Harvard Medical School;
Associate Neuroscientist
Division of Sleep and Circadian Disorders
Departments of Medicine and Neurology
Brigham and Women's Hospital
Boston, Massachusetts

David Raizen, MD, PhD
Associate Professor of Neurology
Perelman School of Medicine
University of Pennsylvania
Philadelphia, Pennsylvania

Preethi Rajan, MD
Division of Pulmonary, Critical Care, and Sleep Medicine
Department of Medicine
Northwell Heath;
Donald and Barbara Zucker School of Medicine at Hofstra-Northwell
New Hyde Park, New York

Shantha Rajaratnam, MD
School of Psychological Sciences
Turner Institute for Brain and Mental Health
Monash University
Melbourne, Victoria, Australia

Kannan Ramar, MD
Center for Sleep Medicine
Division of Pulmonary and Critical Care Medicine
Mayo Clinic
Rochester, Minnesota

Winfried J. Randerath, MD
Department of Clinic of Pneumology
Bethanien Hospital
Institute of Pneumology at the University of Cologne
Solingen, Germany

Karen Raphael, PhD
Professor
Department of Psychiatry and Behavioral Sciences
University of Washington;
Behavioral Sciences Director
Mental Illness Research, Education and Clinical Center
VA Puget Sound Health Care System
Seattle, Washington

Murray Raskind, MD
Professor
Department of Psychiatry and Behavioral Sciences
University of Washington;
Behavioral Sciences Director
Mental Illness Research, Education and Clinical Center
VA Puget Sound Health Care System
Seattle, Washington

Kavita Ratarasarn, MBBS
Associate Professor
Department of Medicine
Medical College of Wisconsin
Milwaukee, Wisconsin

Niels C. Rattenborg, PhD
Group Leader
Avian Sleep
Max Planck Institute for Ornithology
Seewiesen, Germany

Susan Redline, MD, MPH
Peter C. Farrell Professor of Medicine
Department of Medicine
Brigham and Women's Hospital
Beth Israel Deaconess Medical Center;
Department of Medicine
Harvard Medical School
Boston, Massachusetts

Kathryn J. Reid, PhD
Research Professor
Ken and Ruth Davee Department of Neurology
Center for Circadian and Sleep Medicine
Northwestern University Feinberg School of Medicine
Chicago, Illinois

Kathy Richards, PhD, RN, FAAN, FAASM
Research Professor
School of Nursing
University of Texas at Austin
Austin, Texas

Samantha Riedy, PhD, RPSGT
Senior Statistician
Behavioral Biology Branch
Walter Reed Army Institute of Research
Silver Spring, Maryland

Dieter Riemann, PhD
Department of Psychiatry and Psychotherapy
Medical Center–University of Freiburg;
Faculty of Medicine
University of Freiburg
Freiburg, Germany

Timothy Roehrs, PhD
Senior Bioscientist
Division of Sleep Medicine
Thomas Roth Sleep Disorders and Research Center
Henry Ford Health System;
Professor
Department of Psychiatry & Behavioral Neuroscience
Wayne State University
Detroit, Michigan

Thomas Roth, PhD
Director
Division of Sleep Medicine
Thomas Roth Sleep Disorders and Research Center
Henry Ford Hospital
Detroit, Michigan

James A. Rowley, MD
Professor of Medicine
Chief, Pulmonary, Critical Care & Sleep Medicine
Wayne State University School of Medicine
Detroit, Michigan

David B. Rye, MD
Sleep Center
Department of University
Emory University
Atlanta, Georgia

Ashima S. Sahni, MD
Assistant Professor of Clinical Medicine
Division of Pulmonary, Critical Care, Sleep and Allergy
University of Illinois Hospital and Health Science System
Chicago, Illinois

Charles Samuels, MD, CCFP, DABSM
Clinical Assistant Professor
Family Medicine
Adjunct Professor
Faculty of Kinesiology
University of Calgary;
CANMedical Director
Centre for Sleep and Human Performance
Calgary, Alberta, Canada

Anne E. Sanders, MS, PhD, MS
Assistant Professor
Divison of Pediatric and Public Health
Adams School of Dentistry
University of North Carolina at Chapel Hill
Chapel Hill, North Carolina

Clifford B. Saper, MD, PhD
James Jackson Putnam Professor of Neurology and Neuroscience
Harvard Medical School;
Department of Neurology
Beth Israel Deaconess Medical Center
Boston, Massachusetts

Michael J. Sateia, MD, FAASM
Professor of Psychiatry (Sleep Medicine), Emeritus
Geisel School of Medicine at Dartmouth
Hanover, New Hampshire

Josée Savard, PhD
Professor
School of Psychology
Université Laval
CHU de Québec-Université Laval Research Center
Quebec City, Quebec, Canada

Marie-Hélène Savard, PhD
Research Associate
CHU de Québec Cancer Research Center
Québec City, Québec, Canada

Thomas E. Scammell, MD
Professor
Department of Neurology
Beth Israel Deaconess Medical Center;
Professor
Department of Neurology
Boston Children's Hospital;
Professor
Harvard Medical School
Boston, Massachusetts

Matthew T. Scharf, MD, PhD
Assistant Professor
Medical Director, Robert Wood Johnson Sleep Laboratory
Comprehensive Sleep Center
Division of Pulmonary and Critical Care Medicine
Robert Wood University Medical School
Rutgers University
New Brunswick, New Jersey

Steven M. Scharf, MD, PhD
Director
University of Maryland Sleep Disorders Center;
Professor of Medicine
University of Maryland School of Medicine
Baltimore, Maryland

Frank A.J.L. Scheer, PhD, MSc
Professor of Medicine
Department of Medicine
Harvard Medical School;
Director, Medical Chronobiology Program
Department of Medicine and Neurology
Brigham and Women's Hospital
Boston, Massachusetts

Logan Schneider, MD
Staff Neurologist
Stanford/VA Alzhemier's Center
MIRECC Investigator
Department of Psychiatry and Behavioral Sciences
Palo Alto Veteran's Affairs Healthcare System
Palo Alto, California

Michael Schredl, PhD
Head of Research
Sleep Laboratory
Central Institute of Mental Health;
Medical Faculty
Mannheim/Heidelberg University
Mannheim, Germany

Sophie Schwartz, PhD
Professor of Neuroscience
Department of Neurosciences
University of Geneva
Geneva, Switzerland

Paula K. Schweitzer, PhD
Director of Research
Sleep Medicine and Research Center
St. Luke's Hospital
Chesterfield, Missouri

Bernardo Selim, MD
Assistant Professor of Medicine
Section of Pulmonary and Critical Care
Department of Medicine, Sleep Medicine
Mayo Clinic
Rochester, Minnesota

Frédéric Sériès, MD
Centre de pneumologie
Department of Medicine
Institut Universitaire de Cardiologie et de Pneumologie de Québec
Quebec City, Quebec, Canada

Barry J. Sessle, PhD
Professor
Department of Physiology
Neuroscience Platform
University of Toronto
Toronto, Ontario, Canada

Amir Sharafkhaneh, MD, PhD
Professor of Medicine
Department of Medicine
Baylor College of Medicine
Sleep Disorders & Research Center
Medical Care Line
Michael E. DeBaky VA Medical Center
Houston, Texas

Katherine M. Sharkey, MD, PhD
Associate Professor
Department of Medicine
Associate Professor
Psychiatry & Human Behavior
The Warren Alpert Medical School of Brown University
Providence, Rhode Island

Paul J. Shaw, PhD
Professor
Department of Neuroscience
Washington University in St. Louis
St. Louis, Missouri

Ari Shechter, PhD
Assistant Professor of Medical Science
Department of Medicine
Columbia University Medical Center
New York, New York

Stephen H. Sheldon, DO
Professor of Pediatrics and Neurology
Northwestern University Feinberg School of Medicine
Sleep Medicine Center
Division of Pulmonary and Sleep Medicine
Ann & Robert H. Lurie Children's Hospital of Chicago
Chicago, Illinois

Fahmi Shibli, MD
Research Fellow
MetroHealth Medical Center;
Visiting Scholar
Case Western Reserve University
Cleveland, Ohio

Priyattam J. Shiromani, PhD
Professor
Department of Psychiatry
Medical University of South Carolina
Charleston, South Carolina

Tamar Shochat, DSc
Full Professor
Department of Nursing
University of Haifa
Haifa, Israel

Francesca Siclari, MD
Center for Investigation and Research on Sleep
University Hospital Lausanne
Lausanne, Switzerland

Jerome M. Siegel, PhD
Professor of Psychiatry and Biobehavioral Sciences
David Geffen School of Medicine
University of California, Los Angeles;
Chief Neurobiology Research
Veterans Affairs Greater Los Angeles Healthcare System
Los Angeles, California

T. Leigh Signal, Bav, MA (hons), PhD
Lecturer
Sleep/Wake Research Centre
School of Health Sciences
Massey University
Wellington, The Netherlands

Michael H. Silber, MBChB
Professor of Neurology
Center for Sleep Medicine
Department of Neurology
Mayo Clinic College of Medicine
Rochester, Minnesota

Norah Simpson, PhD
Clinical Associate Professor
Psychiatry and Behavioral Sciences
Stanford University School of Medicine
Palo Alto, California

Mini Singh, MBBS
Assistant Professor
Department of Neurology
Medical University of South Carolina
Charleston, South Carolina

Børge Sivertsen, MD
Department of Health Promotion
Norwegian Institute of Public Health
Bergen, Norway

Lillian Skeiky, BS
Graduate Research Assistant
Sleep and Performance Research Center
Elson S. Floyd College of Medicine
Washington State University
Spokane, Washington

Anne C. Skeldon, PhD
Department of Mathematics
Faculty of Engineering and Physcial Sciences
University of Surrey;
UK Dementia Research Institute Care Research and Technology Center
Imperial College London
University of Surrey
Guildford, United Kingdom

Carlyle Smith, MD
Psychology Department
Trent University
Peterborough, Ontario, Canada;
Neuroscience Department
Queens University,
Kingston, Ontario, Canada

Michael T. Smith, PhD
Professor of Psychiatry, Neurology and Nursing
Director, Division of Behavioral Medicine
Johns Hopkins School of Medicine
Baltimore, Maryland

Virend K. Somers, MD, PhD
Alice Sheets Marriot Professor of Medicine
Department of Cardiovascular Medicine
Mayo Clinic
Rochester, Minnesota

Kai Spiegelhalder, MD PhD
Department of Psychiatry and Psychotherapy
Medical Center–University of Freiburg
Faculty of Medicine
University of Freiburg
Freiburg, Germany

Arthur J. Spielman, PhD, FAASM†
Cognitive Neuroscience Doctoral Program
The City College of the City University of New York
Center for Sleep Medicine
Weill Cornell Medical College
New York, New York

Victor I. Spoormaker, PhD, MD
Max Planck Institute of Psychiatry
Munich, Germany

Erik K. St. Louis, MD, MS
Associate Professor
Center for Sleep Medicine
Departments of Neurology and Medicine
Mayo Clinic College of Medicine
Rochester, Minnesota

Robert Stansbury, MD
Associate Professor and Director
WYU Sleep Evaluation Center
Section of Pulmonary, Critical Care, and Sleep Medicine
Department of Medicine
West Virginia University School of Medicine
Morgantown, West Virginia

†Deceased.

Murray B. Stein, MD, MPH
Distinguished Professor
Psychiatry and Public Health
University of California, San Diego
La Jolla, California;
Staff Psychiatrist
Psychiatry Service
Veterans Administration San Diego Healthcare System
San Diego, California

Robert Stickgold, PhD
Professor
Department of Psychiatry
Beth Israel Deaconess Medical Center;
Professor
Department of Psychiatry
Harvard Medical School
Boston, Massachussetts

Katie L. Stone, MA, PhD
Senior Scientist
Research Institute
California Pacific Medical Center
San Francisco, California

Riccardo Stoohs, MD
Director
Sleep Disorders Clinic
Somnolab
Dortmund, Germany

Robyn Stremler, RN, PhD, FAAN
Associate Professor
Lawrence S. Bloomberg Faculty of Nursing
University of Toronto;
Adjunct Scientist
The Hospital for Sick Children
Toronto, Ontario, Canada

Patrick J. Strollo Jr., MD, FACP, FCCP, FAASM
Professor of Medicine and Clinical and Translational Science
Pulmonary, Allergy, and Critical Care Medicine
Vice Chair for Veterans Affairs
Department of Medicine
Vice President, Medical Service Line
VA Pittsburgh Health System
Pittsburgh, Pennsylvania

Shannon S. Sullivan, MD
Clinical Professor
Division of Pediatric Pulmonary, Asthma, and Sleep
Department of Pediatrics
Division of Sleep Medicine
Department of Psychiatry
Stanford University
Palo Alto, California

Peter Svensson, DDS, PhD, Dr.Odont
Professor and Head
Section for Orofacial Pain and Jaw Function
Department of Dentistry and Oral Health
Aarhus University
Aarhus, Denmark

Steven T. Szabo, MD, PhD
Assistant Professor
Psychiatry and Behavioral Sciences
Duke University Medical Center;
Attending Psychiatrist
Mental Health Service Line
Durham Veterans Administration Medical Center
Durham, North Carolina

Ronald Szymusiak, PhD
Adjunct Professor
Department of Medicine
David Geffen School of Medicine
University of California, Los Angeles;
Research Scientist
Research Service
VA Greater Los Angeles Healthcare System
Los Angeles, California

Mehdi Tafti, PhD
Department of Biomedical Sciences
University of Lausanne
Lausanne, Switzerland

Renaud Tamisier, MD, PhD, MBA
Professor of Medicine
Section of Pulmonary and Physiology Medicine
Departmetn of Thorax and Vessel Medicine
Director, Sleep Disorders CCenter
Université Grenoble Alpes
Grenoble, France

Esra Tasali, MD
Associate Professor
Department of Medicine
Section of Pulmonary/Critical Care
University of Chicago
Chicago, Illinois

Daniel J. Taylor, MD, PhD
Professor
Department of Psychology
University of Arizona
Tucson, Arizona

Mihai C. Teodorescu, MD
Associate Professor
Department of Medicine
University of Wisconsin
Madison, Wisconsin

Matthew J.W. Thomas, PhD
Associate Professor
School of Health, Medical, and Applied Sciences
Appleton Institute
Central Queensland University, Australia

Robert Joseph Thomas, MD, MMSc
Associate Professor of Medicine
Division of Pulmonary, Critical Care, and Sleep Medicine
Department of Medicine
Beth Israel Deaconess Medical Center
Harvard Medical School
Boston, Massachusetts

Michael J. Thorpy, MD
Professor of Neurology
The Saul R. Korey Department of Neurology
Albert Einstein College of Medicine at Yeshiva University;
Director
Sleep-Wake Disorders Center
Montefiore Medical Center
Bronx, New York

Lauren A. Tobias, MD
Assistant Professor
Pulmonary, Critical Care, and Sleep Medicine
Yale University School of Medicine
New Haven, Connecticuit

Giulio Tononi, MD, PhD
Professor
Department of Psychiatry
University of Wisconsin
Madison, Wisconsin

Irina Trosman, MD
Attending Physician, Sleep Medicine
Health System Clinician of Pediatrics (Pulmonary Medicine)
Northwestern University Feinberg School of Medicine
Chicago, Illinois

Fred W. Turek, PhD
Charles E.& Emma H. Morrison Professor of Biology
Departments of Neurobiology and Physiology
Director, Center for Sleep and Circadian Biology
Northwestern University
Evanston, Illinois

Raghu Pishka Upender, MD, MBA
Medical Director, Associate Professor
Department of Neurology
Vanderbilt University Medical Center
Nashville, Tennessee

Andrew Vakulin, PhD
FHMRI Sleep Health
Flinders Heath and Medical Research Institute
College of Medicine and Public Health
Flinders University
Adelaide, Austria

Philipp O. Valko, MD
Neurology
University Hospital Zurich
Zurich, Switzerland

Eve Van Cauter, PhD
Frederick H. Rawson Professor
Department of Medicine
Section of Pediatric and Adult Endocrinology, Diabetes, and Metabolism
University of Chicago
Chicago, Illinois

Margo van den Berg, PhD
Lecturer
Sleep/Wake Research Centre
School of Health Sciences
Massey University
Wellington, New Zealand

Hans P.A. Van Dongen, MS, PhD
Professor and Director
Sleep and Performance Research Center
Elson S. Floyd College of Medicine
Washington State University
Spokane, Washington

Eus Van Someren, MD
Netherlands Institute for Neuroscience
Amsterdam, The Netherlands

Olivier M. Vanderveken, MD, PhD
Department of Ear, Nose and Throat, Head and Neck Surgery
Antwerp University Hospital;
Professor
Faculty of Medicine and Health Sciences
University of Antwerp
Antwerp, Belgium

Gilles Vandewalle, PhD
Sleep and Chronobiology Laboratory
GIGA-Cyclontron Research Center/In Vivo Imaging
University of Liège
Liège, Belgium

Andrew W. Varga, MD, PhD
Assistant Professor
Department of Medicine
Icahn School of Medicine at Mount Sinai
New York, New York

Ivan Vargas, PhD
Department of Psychological Science
University of Arkansas
Fayetteville, Arkansas

Bradley V. Vaughn, MD
Professor of Neurology
Department of Neurology
University of North Carolina
Chapel Hill, North Carolina

Øystein Vedaa, PhD
Department Director
Department of Health Promotion
Norwegian Institute of Public Health
Bergen, Norway;
Researcher
Department of Mental Health
Norwegian University of Science and Technology
Trondheim, Norway

Richard L. Verrier, PhD
Associate Professor
Department of Medicine
Harvard Medical School
Beth Israel Deaconess Medical Center
Boston, Massachussetts

Alexandros N. Vgontzas, MD
Professor of Psychiatry
Department of Psychiatry and Behavioral Health
Director, Sleep Research and Treatment Center
Penn State University College of Medicine
Penn State Health Milton S. Hershey Medical Center
Hershey, Pennsylvania

Aurelio Vidal-Ortiz, MD
Laboratory of Sleep Neuroscience
Ralph H. Johnson VA Medical Center
Charleston, South Carolina

Aleksandar Videnovic, MD, MSc
Associate Professor
Department of Neurology
Harvard Medical School/MGH
Boston, Massachusetts

Martha Hotz Vitaterna, PhD
Research Professor
Department of Neurobiology
Deputy Director
Center for Sleep and Circadian Biology
Northwestern University
Evanston, Illinois

Lauren Waggoner, BS, MA, PhD
Fatigue Scientist
Flight Safety, CSSC
Delta Air Lines, Incorporated
Atlanta, Georgia

Arthur S. Walters, MD
Professor of Neurology
Department of Neurology
Vanderbilt University School of Medicine
Nashville, Tennessee

Erin J. Wamsley, PhD
Associate Professor
Department of Psychology
Furman University
Greenville, South Carolina

Paula L. Watson, MD
Assistant Professor
Pulmonary, Critical Care, and Sleep Medicine
Vanderbilt University Medical Center
Nashville, Tennessee

Terri E. Weaver, PhD, RN
Dean and Professor
Biobehavioral Nursing Science
Professor
Division of Pulmonary, Critical Care, Sleep, and Allergy
University of Illinois Chicago College of Medicine
Chicago, Illinois

Gerald L. Weinhouse, MD
Associate Physician
Brigham and Women's Hospital;
Assistant Professor of Medicine
Harvard Medical School
Boston, Massachusetts

Pnina Weiss, MD
Vice Chair of Education
Department of Pediatrics
Yale University School of Medicine
New Haven, Connecticut

Nancy Wesensten, PhD
Air Traffic Organization Safety and Technical Training Safety Services (AJI-15)
Federal Aviation Administration
Washington, DC

Sophie West, MD
Lead
Newcastle Regional Sleep Centre
Newcastle upon Tyne Hospitals National Health Service Trust
Newcastle upon Tyne, United Kingdom

Ephraim Winocur, DMD
Clinical Assistant Professor in Orofacial Pain (ret.)
Section of Function, Dysfunction & Pain in the Stomatognathic System,
Department of Oral Rehabilitation
The Maurice and Gabriela Goldschleger School of Dental Medicine
Tel Aviv University
Tel Aviv, Israel

William Wisden, MA, PhD
Professor
Department of Life Sciences
UK Dementia Research Institute
Imperial College London
London, Great Britain

Lisa F. Wolfe, MD
Associate Professor of Medicine
Division of Pulmonary, Critical Care, and Sleep Medicine
Northwestern University Feinberg School of Medicine
Chicago, Illinois

Christine Won, MD, MS
Associate Professor
Department of Medicine (Pulmonary, Critical Care, and Sleep Medicine)
Yale University School of Medicine;
Medical Director
Yale Centers for Sleep Medicine
New Haven, Connecticuit

Jean Wong, MD, FRCPC
Staff Anesthesiologist
Anesthesia and Pain Management
Toronto Western Hospital;
Staff Anesthesiologist
Department of Anesthesia and Pain Management
Women's College Hospital;
Associate Professor
Department of Anesthesia
University of Toronto
Toronto, Ontario, Canada

Kenneth P. Wright, Jr., PhD
College Professor of Distinction
Department of Integrative Physiology
University of Colorado Boulder
Boulder, Colorado

Lora Wu, PhD
Senior Research Officer
Sleep/Wake Research Centre
Massey University
Wellington, New Zealand

Mark Wu, MD, PhD
Professor
Departments of Neurology, Medicine, and Neuroscience
Johns Hopkins University
Baltimore, Maryland

Don Wykoff, BBA, FRAeS
President Emeritus, Fatigue Working Group
Chair, Flight Time Duty Time Committee
International Federation of Airline Pilots' Associations
Montreal, Quebec, Canada

Lichuan Ye, PhD, RN
Associate Professor
School of Nursing
Bouvé College of Health Sciences
Northeastern University
Boston, University

Magdy Younes, MD, FRCPC, PhD
Distinguished Professor Emeritus
Department of Internal Medicine
University of Manitoba
Winnipeg, Manitoba, Canada

Antonio Zadra, PhD
Professor
Department of Psychology
Université de Montréal;
Researcher
Center for Advanced Research in Sleep Medicine
Hôpital du Sacré-Coeur de Montréal
Montreal, Quebec, Canada

Phyllis C. Zee, MD, PhD
Professor
Department of Neurology
Director, Center for Circadian and Sleep Medicine
Northwestern University Feinberg School of Medicine
Chicago, Illinois

Jamie M. Zeitzer, PhD
Associate Professor
Stanford Center for Sleep Sciences
Stanford University;
Health Science Specialist
Mental Illness Research, Education, and Clinical Center
VA Palo Alto Health Care System
Palo Alto, California

Eric Zhou, PhD
Faculty
Division of Sleep Medicine
Harvard Medical School;
Staff Psychologist
Perini Family Survivors' Center
Dana-Farber Cancer Institute;
Staff Psychology
Department of Neurology
Boston Children's Hospital
Boston, Massachusetts

Andrey V. Zinchuk, MD, MHS
Assistant Professor of Medicine
Section of Pulmonary, Critical Care, and Sleep Medicine
Yale University School of Medicine
New Haven, Connecticut

Ding Zou, MD, PhD
Center for Sleep and Vigilance Disorders
Institute of Medicine
Sahlgrenska Academy
University of Gothenburg
Gothenburg, Sweden

Foreword

Celebrating *PPSM*: Connected, Collaborative, Global

From birth of the first edition in 1989 to the seventh edition in 2021, *Principles and Practice of Sleep Medicine (PPSM)* has been the gold standard of knowledge for this fast-changing discipline. Today, sleep medicine is a well-established medical discipline that stands on a strong foundation of scientific and clinical knowledge, but just a little over 30 years ago (which for some of us, seems like only yesterday), the landscape was quite different. A search of PubMed revealed only about 300 publications matching the term "sleep medicine," compared to nearly 12,000 publications in 2020. The exponential growth in knowledge has fueled the rapid increase in the number of clinical sleep medicine centers and doctoral and postdoctoral training programs in the US and all over the world. Advances in basic and clinical sleep and circadian science continue to open up exciting, innovative approaches to diagnose and treat sleep and circadian disorders, and for defining the role of sleep as a fundamental requirement for the maintenance of health and well-being of people at all stages of life and within the context of health disparities.

It was indeed a "dream come true" when in 2017 the Nobel Prize in Physiology or Medicine was awarded for the discovery of the genetic mechanisms of circadian rhythms. The burgeoning evidence that circadian clocks regulate metabolic, immune, cardiovascular, and neural activity in central and peripheral tissues is gaining attention. Circadian medicine is now an emerging clinical specialty. In the past, there was an artificial separation of circadian and sleep science, but it is increasingly clear that the alignment of these two systems at the molecular, cellular, and system levels is critical for health. The potential of integrating the time domain in medicine has many implications for the future of sleep medicine, and medicine as a whole.

Since the previous edition of *PPSM*, sleep medicine has become even more connected, collaborative, and global. The World Sleep Society, founded in 2016, represents individual members and more than 40 sleep societies in the world. International conferences, courses, and events, such as World Sleep Congress and World Sleep Day, help promote sleep and circadian health, develop training programs for sleep professionals, and foster the development of sleep medicine worldwide. The COVID-19 pandemic highlights that our well-being is deeply interconnected and reinforces the importance of global collaboration to translate scientific discoveries into the clinic and share new perspectives in sleep and circadian medicine. This edition of *PPSM* celebrates the vision and contributions of the pioneers and giants of our field and delivers the most comprehensive state of knowledge of this exciting interdisciplinary field.

Phyllis C. Zee, MD, PhD
Director, Center for Circadian and Sleep Medicine
Northwestern University Feinberg School of Medicine
President-Elect World Sleep Society

Sleep Is Essential to Health

On behalf of the American Academy of Sleep Medicine (AASM) and its more than 11,000 members and accredited sleep centers, we congratulate the editors for completing a new edition of this landmark textbook in this most challenging and difficult time marked by a worldwide pandemic. Each edition of *Principles and Practice of Sleep Medicine* serves as a celebration of how far the field of sleep medicine has come in a relatively short period of time. This latest edition showcases an even greater understanding of the role of sleep and the circadian system in other medical disorders and overall health. As scientists have tirelessly worked to better comprehend sleep and wake physiology, this edition contains sections dedicated to new and exciting pharmacotherapeutics that target novel receptors in the central nervous system to help treat sleep disorders. Although much has changed in content as you turn the pages of this latest edition, which describes the latest findings in areas such as genetics, chronobiology, and consumer sleep monitoring, one constant remains: this textbook serves as the standard reference and guiding light for the field of sleep medicine. Even as the AASM develops innovative training models for sleep medicine physicians, obtaining and reading *Principles and Practice of Sleep Medicine* continues to serve as initiation for our trainees and students as they enter our exciting field, and the textbook remains a reliable companion for the seasoned clinician to reference while taking care of patients with sleep disorders.

At the AASM, we strive to continue the spirit and determination of our founder, and one of the founding editors of this book, Dr. William Dement. Although sleep medicine professionals around the world mourn losing him in 2020, his passion to spread the significance of sleep health has not only emboldened sleep clinicians and scientists to carry on this mission, but it also fostered significant progress in educating our public policy makers and society about the importance of sleep. Recently we have seen the creation of the first ever Sleep Health Caucus in the United States Congress, as well as ongoing progress in legislation to delay school start times, ensuring that our adolescents are better able to achieve sleep health. This textbook plays a central role in supporting the AASM vision that sleep is recognized as essential to health. The AASM and its members look to this textbook to properly care for patients, train our clinicians and scientists, and also allow other specialists to learn about how sleep is essential for the health of their patients.

The textbook represents what we have accomplished as a field thanks to sleep clinicians and scientists, past and present, and perhaps more importantly, it also provides a roadmap for researchers, whose findings will undoubtedly appear in future editions. Completed during a worldwide pandemic, this textbook highlights the resiliency of our many colleagues to continue to explore sleep and circadian science through research, and it is a testimony to the many sleep specialists and clinicians who continue to provide evidence-based, up-to-date clinical care for their patients with sleep disorders while enduring the pandemic. As with many devastating events, growth and progress emerge out of necessity, exemplified in our field through advances such as embracing telemedicine, utilizing home diagnostic testing and monitoring of sleep disorders, and recognizing the prevalence of sleep health disparities. Undoubtedly, adaptation and innovation within sleep medicine will allow us to rise up to future challenges and disruption within the field. The AASM and its members applaud the editors and all of the authors for completing this influential tome amid such obstacles. We thank them for their efforts, which will further the AASM's mission of advancing sleep care and enhancing sleep health to improve lives.

Raman K. Malhotra, MD, FAASM
President, American Academy of Sleep Medicine (2021-2022)
Associate Professor of Neurology, Sleep Medicine Center
Washington University in St. Louis School of Medicine

Acknowledgments

We have been working on *Principles and Practice of Sleep Medicine* for about a third of a century. Thousands of people have been involved in the production of the seven editions. This has been a challenge to produce a volume during a pandemic. Contributors and Elsevier staff worked in the context of lockdowns, isolation, evacuations, while some were caring for hospitalized patients, while others caring for outpatients. As much as we would like to personally thank each person, there is no way that we can thank them all. Some have retired, some have died, and some have made important contributions in the production of the various editions but are unknown to us. This group includes secretaries, copyeditors, artists, designers, people who dealt with the page proofs, internet programmers, and those who physically produced the books.

We would like to acknowledge all the extraordinary Elsevier editors who gave birth to each previous edition of the book. These include Bill Lamsback, Judy Fletcher, Richard Zorab, Cathy Carroll, Todd Hummell, and Dolores Meloni. They fueled the dream that helped establish a new field of medicine.

Many people helped in the preparation of the content of this volume, the seventh edition, including those listed below.

The staff members at Elsevier who helped this book in its seventh journey were Nancy Duffy, Laura Kuehl-Schmidt, Lisa Barnes, Kate Mannix, Melanie Tucker, Amy Buxton, and many others involved in production and design for both the printed volume and the online content.

We also must acknowledge the family members of all the people involved in the book because they indirectly helped produce a work that we believe may have had important positive impact on the lives of thousands, perhaps millions, of people.

Finally, we wish to thank the many hundreds of authors and the magnificent work of the section editors and their deputy editors. All their contributions were so great that they cannot be measured.

Section and Deputy Editors

1E 1989

Mary Carskadon
Michael Chase
Richard Ferber
Christian Guilleminault
Ernest Hartmann
Meir Kryger
Timothy Monk
Anthony Nicholson
Allan Rechtschaffen
Gerald Vogel
Frank Zorick

2E 1994

Michael Aldrich
Mary Carskadon
Michael Chase
J. Christian Gillin
Christian Guilleminault
Ernest Hartmann
Meir Kryger
Anthony Nicholson
Allan Rechtschaffen
Gary Richardson
Thomas Roth
Frank Zorick

3E 2000

Michael Aldrich
Michael Chase
J. Christian Gillin
Christian Guilleminault
Max Hirshkowitz
Mark W. Mahowald
Wallace B. Mendelson
R.T. Pivik
Leon Rosenthal
Mark Sanders
Fred Turek
Frank Zorick

4E 2005

Michael Aldrich
Ruth Benca
J. Christian Gillin
Max Hirshkowitz
Shahrokh Javaheri
Meir Kryger
Mark W. Mahowald
Wallace B. Mendelson
Jacques Montplaiser
John Orem
Timothy Roehrs
Mark Sanders
Robert Stickgold
Fred Turek

5E 2011

Sonia Ancoli-Israel
Gregory Belenky
Ruth Benca
Daniel Buysse
Michael Cramer-Bornemann
Charles George
Max Hirshkowitz
Meir Kryger
Gilles Lavigne
Kathryn Aldrich Lee
Beth A. Malow
Mark W. Mahowald
Wallace B. Mendelson
Jacques Montplaisir
Tore Nielsen
Mark Sanders
Jerome Siegel
Fred Turek

6E 2017

Sonia Ancoli-Israel
Robert Basner
Gregory Belenky
Dan Brown
Daniel Buysse
Jennifer DeWolfe
Max Hirshkowitz
Shahrokh Javaheri
Andrew Krystal
Gilles Lavigne
Kathryn Aldrich Lee
Beth A. Malow
Timothy Roehrs
Thomas Roth
Thomas Scammell
Jerome Siegel
Robert Stickgold
Katie L. Stone
Fred Turek
Bradley V. Vaughn
Erin J. Wamsley
Christine Won

7E 2021

Sabra Abbott
Cathy Alessi
Fiona C. Baker
Bei Bei
Gregory Belenky
Daniel B. Brown
Jennifer Laurel DeWolfe
Christopher L. Drake
Julio Fernandez-Mendoza

Section and Deputy Editors—cont'd		
Constance H. Fung	Eric A. Nofzinger	Renaud Tamisier
Max Hirshkowitz	John Park	Robert Joseph Thomas
Shahrokh Javaheri	Rafael Pelayo	Bradley V. Vaughn
Thomas Kilduff	Samantha Riedy	Erin J. Wamsley
Andrew D. Krystal	Thomas Scammell	Nancy Wesensten
Hans-Peter Landolt	Paul J. Shaw	Lisa F. Wolfe
Gilles Lavigne	Stephen H. Sheldon	Christine Won
Guy Leschziner	Jerome M. Siegel	Kenneth P. Wright, Jr.
Beth A. Malow	Robert Stickgold	Phyllis C. Zee
Jennifer Martin	Erik K. St. Louis	Andrey V. Zinchuk
Kiran Maski	Shannon Sullivan	

Preface

This edition of *PPSM* had a very difficult gestation. It was during the pandemic that washed over our unprotected planet in brutal waves. All our lives were upended and changed. Our beloved friend and co-editor, Bill Dement, died. Most of us knew people infected with COVID or who had died of COVID. We were all deeply concerned that our families and friends might be affected. That was the context of the gestation of the book.

Before the pandemic, Cathy Goldstein had joined the senior editorial team of the book. Section editors and authors had agreed to contribute. Then, in early 2020, contributors in Europe were impacted, followed by contributors from other continents. Some contributors, when contacted, told us they were in the hospital with COVID or had family members with COVID. Many contributors were conscripted to take care of hospitalized patients. Some contributors were banished from their offices with work from home orders and did not have access to the things they needed to complete their chapters. Even the forest fires in California impacted the book, trapping some authors, while others had to evacuate their homes. And at the end of the day, all the contributors produced magnificent chapters.

The book has 22 sections, including a new section on "Transition from Childhood." About 75% of the sections have new editors. The book retains its philosophical underpinnings with content from the diverse disciplines (basic and clinical) with contributors from 4 continents.

While the book was being produced, several contributors from this and previous editions died: Richard Allen, Rosalind Cartwright, Bill Dement, Christian Guilleminault, Mark Mahowald, Art Spielman, and Mario Terzano. Their contributions to medicine will impact the field for generations to come. May their memories be a blessing and an inspiration.

Just as some of the greatest wines come from grapes that survive in the most difficult terrains, we believe that this edition, having weathered a difficult gestation, has produced a volume worthy of the field of sleep medicine and continues the vision outlined over 30 years ago.

Meir Kryger
Cathy Goldstein
Tom Roth

FIRST EDITION PREFACE

Medical disorders related to sleep are obviously not new. Yet the discipline of sleep disorders medicine is in its infancy. There is a large body of knowledge on which to base the discipline of sleep disorder medicine. We hope that this textbook will play a role in the evolution of this field.

Douglas Hofstadter reviewed how ideas and concepts evolve and are transmitted.[1] In 1965, Roger Sperry[2] wrote the following: "Ideas cause ideas and help evolve new ideas. They interact with each other and with other mental forces in the same brain, in neighboring brains, and thanks to global communication, in far distant, foreign brains. And they also interact with the external surroundings to produce *in toto* a burstwise advance in evolution that is far beyond anything to hit the evolutionary scene yet, including the emergence of the living cell." Jacques Monod[3] wrote the following in *Chance and Necessity:* "For a biologist it is tempting to draw a parallel between the evolution of ideas and that of the biosphere. For while the abstract kingdom stands at a yet greater distance above the biosphere than the latter does above the non-living universe, ideas have retained some of the properties of organisms. Like them they tend to perpetuate their structure and to breed; they too can fuse, recombine, segregate their content; indeed they too can evolve, and in this evolution selection must surely play an important role." Hofstadter has called this universe of ideas the ideosphere analogous to the biosphere. The ideosphere's counterpart to the biosphere gene has been called meme by Richard Dawkins.[4] He wrote "just as genes propagate themselves in a gene pool by leaping from body to body via sperm or eggs, so memes propagate themselves in the meme pool by leaping from brain to brain. … If a scientist hears or reads about a good idea, he passes it on to his colleagues and students. He mentions it in his articles and his lectures. If the idea catches on it can be said to propagate itself spreading from brain to brain … memes should be regarded as living structures, not just metaphorically but technically."

Thus, this textbook represents an attempt to summarize the body of science and ideas that up to now has been transmitted verbally, in articles, and in a few more specialized books. The memes in this volume are drawn from a variety of disciplines, including psychology, psychiatry, neurology, pharmacology, internal medicine, pediatrics, and basic biological sciences. That a field evolves from multidisciplinary roots certainly has precedents in medicine. The field of infectious diseases has its in microbiology, and its practitioners are expected to know relevant aspects of internal medicine, surgery, gynecology, and pediatrics. Similarly, oncology has its roots in surgery, hematology, and internal medicine, and its practitioners today must also know virology and molecular biology. Patients with sleep problems have in the past 'fallen through the cracks.' It is not uncommon to see a patient with classic narcolepsy who has seen five to ten specialists before a diagnosis is finally made. There is a clinical need for physicians to know about sleep and its disorders.

[1]Hofstadter DR. Chapter 3. In: *Metamagical Themas: Questing for the Essence of Mind and Pattern*. Toronto: Bantam Books; 1986.
[2]Sperry R. Mind, brain, and humanist values. In: Platt JR, editor. *New Views of the Nature of Man*. Chicago: The university of Chicago Press; 1965.
[3]Monod J. *Chance and Necessity.* New York: Vintage Books; 1972.
[4]Dawkins R. *The Selfish Gene.* Oxford: Oxford University Press; 1976. p. 206.

Contents

Video Contents

Neurologic Disorders

Section 12

Introduction

Chapter 101

Guy Leschziner

Despite it long being recognized that "sleep is of the brain, by the brain and for the brain,"[1] it has always been somewhat surprising that, until recently, the wider neurologic community seemed broadly disinterested in sleep. Physicians specializing in disorders of the brain appeared disinclined to address a central neurologic function or dysfunction. Perhaps this was as a result of sleep being seen as not neurologically "pure," but rather a confluence of the neurobiologic, the psychological, the environmental, and the behavioral.

If my own neurologic training—not so far in the dim and distant past—is anything to go by, most neurologists were mindful of the association between sleep disturbance and conditions such as migraine and epilepsy, but largely limited themselves to purer neurologic sleep disorders, conditions such as narcolepsy, restless legs syndrome, and sleep-related hypermotor epilepsy. Insomnia was poorly understood, poorly assessed, and poorly treated. Circadian rhythm disorders went largely unspoken of. Sleep apnea was simply a mechanical issue of the airway, left to pulmonologists.

How times have changed. The last decade or two has seen an explosion of interest. Neurologists in the fields of inflammation, dementia, stroke, neurorehabilitation, epilepsy, and movement disorders all now appreciate the fundamental importance of sleep and its disorders in their patients. And it is not purely a function of quality of life, or that patients with particular neurologic disorders may be at increased risk of certain sleep disorders. We now know that untreated, these sleep disorders may influence the natural history of these conditions, may affect recovery, or may complicate symptoms and signs; that some of these sleep disorders may actually have a role in the pathophysiology of the conditions we see in our clinics, such as stroke or dementia; that some sleep disorders may be a useful clinical tool, to clarify or narrow the differential diagnosis of the underlying neurologic disorder; or even that some sleep disorders may herald broader neurologic disorders by decades or permit prognostication about the path that a particular patient follows.

The chapters that follow are a superb summary of the huge amount of progress that has been made in recent years, the wealth of understanding of the relationship between sleep and neurologic disorders acquired through the efforts of clinicians and scientists from around the world.

In Chapter 102, Isabelle Arnulf and Ron Postuma illustrate the impact of sleep disorders on Parkinson disease, but also the impact of Parkinson disease on sleep. We learn how the identification and treatment of sleep disorders may have positive effects for both the patient and their partner, provide prognostic information, and in rare cases save lives.

Claudio Bassetti (Chapter 103) discusses the role of sleep apnea and sleep disturbance, in general, in the pathophysiology of stroke and how sleep disorders may hinder recovery.

Sleep disturbances and sleep-disordered breathing are highly relevant components in the multidisciplinary evaluation and management of patients with neuromuscular disease and are detailed by Michelle Cao, Kevin Gipson, and the late Christian Guilleminault in Chapter 104.

Dominique Petit and colleagues (Chapter 105) describe the bidirectional relationship between sleep and neurodegeneration—an area of particular research focus at present in an effort to identify modifiable risk factors for dementia—and demonstrate the characteristics of sleep disturbances in individuals with dementias and how they should be treated.

In the sphere of epilepsy, Milena Pavlova and Sanjeev Kothare (Chapter 106) guide us through the relationship between the circadian rhythm, sleep disturbance, and epilepsy, and the complex nature of that relationship. We learn of the effects of sleep on epilepsy, the effects of epilepsy on sleep, and the subtleties of epilepsy management and its impact on sleep quality.

"Alex Nesbitt and Peter Goadsby" (Chapter 107) highlight those primary headache disorders most clearly sleep associated and some of the mechanistic and treatment considerations in this patient group.

The rapidly expanding literature surrounding traumatic brain injury and sleep is beautifully summarized by Christian Baumann and Philip Valko in Chapter 108. They stress the hefty burden and prevalence of sleep disorders in patients with traumatic brain injury and the particular difficulties of clinical evaluation of sleep in this patient group, where subjective experience of sleep and objective measures often correlate extremely poorly. In this group of patients in particular, the timely diagnosis and treatment of sleep disorders compromise not only quality of life but also rehabilitation.

Tiffany Braley, Carles Gaig, and Mini Singh explore the autoimmune neurologic disorders (Chapter 109). We learn of the nature of sleep disorders in multiple sclerosis and how they contribute to the fatigue and mood disturbances that impact quality of life. And they also discuss the exciting area of autoimmune encephalitides and how we are beginning to better understand the nature of sleep disturbances of many forms in these disorders. Finally, infection with SARS-CoV-2 can have both acute and chronic effects on the nervous system, which can impact sleep. This topic is covered in Chapter 213.

The reality is that there is a significant selection bias for those neurologists or other physicians who seek out the pages of this book. They will already be aware of the importance of sleep and its disorders in the management of patients in the neurology clinic. For those clinicians, these chapters will serve as a useful reminder and a guide for the finer details of the management of these conditions. They illustrate how much our knowledge of this area of medicine has moved forward in the last few years and also highlight how much more we have to learn. But for those yet to understand the complex nature between sleep and neurologic disorders, these pages will be a fantastic educational and training resource, when they are pointed toward them.

A complete reference list can be found online at ExpertConsult.com.

Chapter 102

Parkinsonism

Ronald Postuma; Isabelle Arnulf

Chapter Highlights

- Sleep problems are extremely common in patients with Parkinson disease (PD) and are major causes of disability. Neurodegeneration in sleep regulatory structures and motor impairment are primary sources of sleep-related issues in patients with PD.
- Although obstructive sleep apnea (OSA) is not clearly increased in PD, treatment of severe OSA may improve somnolence in some patients. Inspiratory nighttime stridor can be associated with sudden respiratory death and mandates continuous positive airway pressure treatment in most cases.
- Insomnia is generally characterized by sleep maintenance problems and can be treated by optimizing therapy for nighttime motor symptoms, rigorous exercise, cognitive behavioral therapy for insomnia, and pharmacotherapy (eszopiclone, doxepin, trazodone, and possibly atypical neuroleptics).
- Restless legs syndrome (RLS) is commonly associated with PD. Differential diagnosis is often made difficult, as motor fluctuations and other related symptoms can mimic RLS. Patients with PD may be particularly prone to augmentation, given their requirement for constant dopaminergic therapy.
- Somnolence is more common in advanced PD and may result from degeneration of arousal systems, although medications for PD may also contribute. Potential mitigation strategies include medication reduction, bright light therapy, modafinil, caffeine, methylphenidate, and possibly sodium oxybate.
- Rapid eye movement sleep behavior disorder occurs in up to 60% of patients who have PD, and often starts years before motor manifestations. Primary treatments include bed safety measures, clonazepam, and melatonin.

Parkinsonism is a frequent and disabling condition that affects approximately 2% of adults older than 65 years. During the last decades, there have been major advances in the treatment of motor symptoms, at least in idiopathic Parkinson disease (PD). Therefore nonmotor and treatment-resistant symptoms (falls, dementia, etc.) are now the major determinants of prognosis. In the past, abnormal sleep in parkinsonian patients was mostly considered "collateral damage" of the disease, until key observations documenting the centrality of sleep disorders were made over the last decade. The increasing interest in nonmotor PD overall has led to the first treatment trials for sleep disorders in PD.

DEFINITION

Parkinsonism: A General Introduction

Parkinsonism describes a syndrome characterized by bradykinesia plus either rigidity or a 4- to 6-Hz rest tremor, of which PD is the most common cause. Motor PD is generally characterized by asymmetry, a slow progressive worsening, and sustained response of symptoms to levodopa.[1] Onset and disease progression have been increasingly characterized and linked to specific patterns of neurodegeneration, with a final common clinical picture of end-stage motor and cognitive symptoms.[2] PD is caused by diffuse synuclein-mediated neurodegeneration, often first involving olfactory and lower brainstem areas (e.g., nucleus of the vagus nerve) before spreading to the substantia nigra and eventually the cortex. PD is primarily a disease of aging. Its prevalence increases with age from about 0.5% among persons age 60 to 69 years, to 2% to 3% among persons older than 80 years, with a 1.5-fold male preponderance.[3] Very few develop parkinsonism before age 45 years, and young-onset patients are more likely to have genetic causes. The most important genetic causes include mutations in leucine-rich repeat kinase 2, glucocerebrosidase, and the α-synuclein gene, as well as *parkin* and PINK-1 for young-onset cases; however, many causative genes and genome-wide association study linkages are discovered each year.[4]

The primary motor treatment of PD is levodopa (L-DOPA), which can be supplemented by other dopaminergic agents (e.g., dopamine agonists, monoamine oxidase inhibitors, etc.). Often, after several years of symptomatic control on dopaminergic treatment, patients develop motor complications, including dyskinesias (abnormal involuntary movements) at the peak dose, and off periods, with generalized slowing and pain when the effect of L-DOPA wears off. Patients then use dopaminergic treatment on daily schedules that become stricter and more frequent as the disease progresses. Many with a 10-year disease duration may take 20 tablets per day, including frequent doses of levodopa, dopamine agonists, monoamine oxidase-inhibitors, and medications to avoid the side effects of dopamine treatment (nausea, orthostatic hypotension, hallucinations) and to treat nonmotor symptoms. Functional neurosurgery or continuous dopaminergic infusion therapy is used for those experiencing severe motor fluctuations and dyskinesia.

Recently, there has been increasing recognition that PD is much more than a motor disease. Pathologic staging systems of PD have documented structures involved in control of autonomic regulation, olfaction, mood, and sleep degeneration early in PD, whereas cognition is impaired especially in those with advanced age.[5,6] These symptoms are generally not levodopa-responsive and often occur years before the first motor symptoms, although many are treatable by other means. Once PD has commenced, further levodopa-resistant motor symptoms, such as falls, freezing, dysarthria, drooling, and swallowing dysfunction, often occur. Because motor symptoms are involved relatively late in the pathologic process of PD, prodromal PD can be defined by a diverse array of nonmotor symptoms, including constipation, urinary dysfunction, erectile dysfunction, orthostatic hypotension, depression, anxiety, cognitive loss, olfactory loss, and cognitive and behavioral changes.[7] Sleep disorders, including rapid eye movement sleep behavior disorder (RBD), restless legs syndrome (RLS), and somnolence, can also be features of prodromal PD.

Dementia with Lewy bodies (DLB) is the second most frequent cause of dementia after Alzheimer disease. Like PD, DLB is a synuclein-related Lewy body disorder and is not a mutually exclusive diagnosis from PD (patients can legitimately carry both diagnoses if they meet criteria for both).[8] DLB patients develop cognitive impairment mostly affecting attention/vigilance, visuospatial performance, and impaired memory retrieval. Clinical hallmarks include visual hallucinations, parkinsonism (frequently levodopa-sensitive), and fluctuations of alertness and vigilance over days or weeks. RBD is rare in Alzheimer disease and other non–Lewy body dementias so that the existence of RBD in a dementia syndrome is a strong diagnostic marker for DLB.[9] In fact, in the current DLB criteria, polysomnography (PSG)-proven RBD in a dementia patient is sufficient by itself to meet criteria for DLB diagnosis.[10]

Atypical Parkinsonism

It is important to differentiate PD from atypical parkinsonism, as treatment and prognosis are different. Indeed, greater than 10% of patients have atypical parkinsonism characterized by different neuropathologies, primarily other synucleinopathies (multiple system atrophy [MSA]), tauopathies, or drug-induced parkinsonims.[11] The tauopathies comprise progressive supranuclear palsy with parkinsonism, saccade slowing, vertical gaze impairment, swallowing problems, dysarthria, frontal cognitive impairment, and early falls or corticobasal syndrome. In general, the prognosis of atypical parkinsonism is worse, with reduced or absent dopaminergic response. Sleep problems are particularly frequent and severe in MSA (e.g., stridor, see later). This disorder is characterized by progressive, non–DOPA-sensitive parkinsonism, cerebellar syndrome and pyramidal impairment, and autonomic failure in various combinations. Stridor, in association with parasomnia and sleep apnea, has also been recently described in a rare tauopathy associated with immunoglobulin-like cell adhesion molecule-5 (IgLON-5) antibodies.[12] "Vascular parkinsonism," which can occur in isolation or as a comorbidity of PD, results from multiple infarcts in the frontal white matter and basal ganglia and is characterized by prominent gait dysfunction, symmetric akinetic-rigid symptoms, and an absence of most nonmotor features. Other rare parkinsonian diseases are Guadeloupean parkinsonism[13] and Parkinson-hypoventilation syndrome. Mild parkinsonian symptoms can also be observed in patients with Huntington disease and spinocerebellar ataxia. The aforementioned neurodegenerative disorders are classified according to whether the mechanism of neuronal loss is associated with deposition of α-synuclein in Lewy bodies, *tau* protein, or is secondary to a genetic polyglutamine disease (Table 102.1). Although the major emphasis in this chapter is on PD, much of the discussion also applies to the other degenerative disorders associated with parkinsonism.

Table 102.1 Prevalence of Rapid Eye Movement Sleep Behavior Disorder in Neurodegenerative Diseases

Disease	Prevalence (%)
Synucleinopathies	
Parkinson disease[60,61,122]	15–60
Multiple system atrophy[68]	88–90
Dementia with Lewy bodies[59,123]	76–86
Tauopathies	
Progressive supranuclear palsy[54,55]	10–11
Alzheimer disease[124]	4.5–7
Corticobasal degeneration[59]	Case reports
Frontotemporal dementia[59]	0
Pallidopontonigral degeneration[125]	0
Guadeloupean parkinsonism[126]	78
Genetic Diseases	
Huntington disease[127]	8
Spinocerebellar ataxia type 3[128]	56
Parkin mutation[129,130]	9–60

PATHOGENESIS

The disruption of normal sleep and wakefulness in patients with parkinsonism may be caused by (1) neurodegenerative damage in brain areas responsible for sleep and arousal regulation; (2) behavioral, respiratory, and motor system phenomena accompanying the disease; and (3) deleterious effects of medications that may induce nightmares, nocturnal movements, insomnia, or sleepiness.

These three elements contribute to various degrees to the clinical symptoms; for example, there is stronger evidence for neuronal loss as the primary cause of RBD than there is for insomnia.

Insomnia and Sleep Fragmentation

Insomnia is a nonspecific symptom that does not necessarily result from a selective lesion in any sleep system. General factors, such as aging, anxiety, and depression may account for some nocturnal sleep disruption in PD. Poor sleep quality correlates with depression and anxiety scores and, as in the general population, mood disorders may contribute to early-morning awakening specifically.

Of all the causes of impaired sleep, motor phenomena and disability at night are perhaps the most important. The frequency of insomnia increases with advanced motor stages of PD and a need for higher daily dose of dopaminergic therapy.[14] Slow movements, nocturnal akinesia with difficulties turning in bed and adjusting blankets, pain, cramps, nocturnal or early morning dystonia (often a claw-like contraction of the toes), and frequent need to urinate are reported by patients with advanced PD as main causes of their insomnia. Older patients with on-off phenomena and those with hallucinations are particularly vulnerable to severe sleep disruption. The role of the dopaminergic system in the pathogenesis of insomnia is illustrated by improvements in wake time and subjective sleep quality after using subthalamic nucleus stimulation at night.[15,16] RLS unrelated to off periods may cause insomnia that is typically sleep-onset in nature. The emergence of RLS and periodic limb movements of sleep (PLMS) during subthalamic stimulation suggests that RLS is not controlled by the basal ganglia.

There is still controversy as to whether the circadian system is affected in PD, especially in patients displaying nighttime insomnia and daytime sleepiness. Some patients may demonstrate a circadian phase advance because even patients with mild PD (i.e., without any motor problems) consistently report early bedtimes and rise times. The nocturnal profile of core body temperature is similar in patients with PD and in control subjects, whereas the nocturnal temperature fall is blunted in patients with MSA.[17] However, studies suggest a blunting of the circadian rhythm of melatonin secretion in PD, which is more pronounced in patients with somnolence.[18]

Finally, deleterious effects of medications may also contribute to poor sleep in PD. These can be direct; for example, selegiline is metabolized to amphetamines, and dopaminergic agents may have alerting properties, although somnolence effects are more common clinically. Attempts to improve the motor state can also paradoxically worsen sleep if underlying hallucinations or psychosis is exacerbated. Dopamine agonists are associated with dopamine dysregulation syndrome and impulse control disorders, with resultant hyperactive behaviors at night, such as computer usage, gambling, compulsive online shopping, binge eating, or hypersexuality, leading to sleep deprivation. These impulse control disorders affect up to 11% patients with PD, and are mostly seen with high doses of dopamine agonists.[19]

REM Sleep Behavior Disorder

RBD in parkinsonism is probably caused by a nondopaminergic lesion of the system controlling atonia during REM sleep.[20–22] The substantia nigra does not seem to be implicated in generating RBD.[23] Lesioning the locus coeruleus peri-alpha (pons) in the cat, an area adjacent to the noradrenergic locus coeruleus, produces an animal model of RBD and complex behaviors during REM sleep, including grooming, leaping, being on watch, and hunting invisible prey, are observed.[24] Muscle atonia is also reduced in rat models after lesioning of an analogous region, the sublaterodorsal nucleus.[25,26]

The equivalent of these nuclei in humans is the subcoeruleus nucleus, a pontine region known to degenerate in both PD and MSA.[27,28] Of note, the magnetic resonance imaging neuromelanin signal in the coeruleus/subcoeruleus complex is decreased in patients who have PD with RBD (and not in patients who have PD without RBD or in control subjects) in proportion to the loss of muscle atonia in REM sleep.[29] Cholinergic neurons located in the pedunculopontine tegmental nucleus have also been hypothesized to contribute to muscle atonia during REM sleep, but they are similarly damaged in patients who have DLB or MSA with and without RBD.[30] Loss of areas in the ventral medulla, which also controls REM atonia, may contribute to RBD.[31]

In addition, RBD can be triggered or exacerbated pharmacologically, especially by the use of antidepressants such as serotonin reuptake inhibitors. This may be due to direct serotonergic activation of motor neurons.[21] As RBD symptoms in PD are associated with relative neocortical, limbic cortical, and thalamic cholinergic denervation but not with differential serotoninergic or nigrostriatal dopaminergic denervation,[32] the presence of RBD symptoms might signal cholinergic system degeneration.

In atypical parkinsonism, the lesions are extensive, complicating clinicopathologic correlations. As shown in Table 102.1, synucleinopathies are more often associated with RBD than the tauopathies and polyglutamine diseases, suggesting that the neurons responsible for muscle atonia in REM sleep are more vulnerable to α-synuclein–related neurodegeneration than to other mechanisms of damage.

The key regions that cause RBD degenerate early in PD. Lewy bodies containing α-synuclein deposits are detected in the brains of 10% to 15% of clinically normal people older than 60 years; when not associated with PD, this is termed *incidental Lewy body disease.* The subcoeruleus/coeruleus complex is frequently affected in incidental Lewy body disease.[33] Moreover, recent staging systems of PD have proposed that α-synucleinopathy initially affects the olfactory areas and medulla oblongata and progresses to more rostral brain areas in a hierarchical sequence.[33,34] In this model the subcoeruleus nucleus, which is located in the pons, should be affected earlier than the substantia nigra, located in the mesencephalon.[35] This provides a pathologic basis for the fact that RBD anticipates PD. However, only one-third of patients with PD develop RBD before parkinsonism onset, and RBD prevalence is not 100%, even in patients with advanced PD; therefore this staging model is not always observed clinically.

Excessive Daytime Sleepiness

The mechanisms of sleepiness and sleep attacks in PD may include complex drug-disease interactions. Most arousal systems (Table 102.2) are affected by neuronal loss and Lewy bodies in the brains of those who have PD, including the noradrenaline neurons in the locus coeruleus,[36] the serotonin neurons in the raphe,[36] the hypocretin neurons in the hypothalamus,[37,38] and the cholinergic neurons in the pedunculopontine tegmental nucleus and basal forebrain.[36] Of note, deep brain stimulation of the pedunculopontine nucleus area in patients with PD can cause immediate sleepiness when the nucleus is blocked by high-frequency current and alertness when it is stimulated by low-frequency current.[39,40] In contrast, the wake-active dopamine neurons in the ventral periaqueductal gray matter and the histamine neurons in the hypothalamus are intact in the brains of those who have PD.[41] In MSA there is also a marked decrease of hypocretin neurons.[42] As much as 28% of patients with MSA complain of daytime sleepiness,[43] whereas 36% of show a narcolepsy-like phenotype.[44]

Table 102.2 Neuronal Loss in Arousal Systems in Patients with Parkinson Disease

Nucleus	Main Neurotransmitter	Neuronal Loss in Parkinson Disease Brain (%)
Locus coeruleus[36]	Noradrenaline	40–50
Median raphe[36]	Serotonin	20–40
Ventral periaqueductal gray matter	Dopamine	9
Pedunculopontine tegmental nucleus	Acetylcholine	50
Tuberomammillary nucleus	Histamine	Unchanged enzymatic activity
Lateral hypothalamus[37,38]	Hypocretin	23–62
Basal forebrain[36]	Acetylcholine	32–93

In PD sleepiness is more frequent in patients with advanced disease.[45] Sleep deprivation due to insomnia is often considered a potential cause of somnolence, but in PD daytime sleepiness is actually associated with longer sleep time at night, suggesting overall increased sleep drive.[46,47] Similarly, sleep apnea (observed in 20% to 30% of PD patients), PLMS. and sleep fragmentation do not correlate with daytime sleepiness[46,47] in PD; however, his does not imply that treatment will not be beneficial in individual cases. As discussed later, dopamine medications increase the risk of sleep attacks,[48] and some patients may sleep half an hour after levodopa intake. It remains unknown how drugs that stimulate the alerting system (particularly at bedtime) are also sedating. This effect cannot be explained, at these high doses, by the biphasic effect (presynaptic sedative effect at low dose, postsynaptic alerting effect at high dose) of dopamine agonists that has been described in animals. Rather, a different selectivity for D1 or D2 receptors may be important; D1 agonists and small doses of dopamine increase the firing of hypocretin neurons in rat hypothalamus, whereas high concentrations of dopamine and D2 agonists decrease or even block this firing.[49] If one applies this concept to PD, patients with a partial hypocretin deficiency would be sedated by D2-D3 agonists or high doses of levodopa.

CLINICAL FEATURES AND EVALUATION OF SLEEP DISORDERS IN PARKINSONISM

In clinical practice, parkinsonian patients are usually referred to sleep centers for three main complaints: insomnia, abnormal movements when asleep, or daytime sleepiness. These symptoms may arise alone or in association. A detailed interview, sometimes followed by a video polysomnogram, is essential to understand and adequately treat these patients. The sleep history in parkinsonism should include the same features obtained from any patient with a sleep complaint. In addition, the physician should query disease-specific questions on nocturnal akinesia, daytime fatigue in relation to medication intake, and psychiatric symptoms. A careful description from the bed partner is essential to determine the presence, timing, and frequency of movements during sleep, arousals and awakenings, and periods of daytime sleepiness. Although general population sleep questionnaires are often very useful, there are also two PD-specific scales, the PD Sleep Scale and the SCOPA-Sleep, which can be helpful for research purposes on sleep quality in PD.[50,51] A checklist of useful questions when investigating a sleep complaint in a PD patient is displayed in Table 102.3.

Insomnia and Sleep Fragmentation

Sleep problems, and especially insomnia, are common in all forms of parkinsonism. A community-based survey determined that 60% of patients with PD had sleep problems, significantly more than in patients with diabetes mellitus (45%) or in aged control subjects (33%).[52] These percentages increase up to 76% in patients with PD who report "broken sleep" in hospital samples. As many as 53% of patients with MSA complain of sleep fragmentation, compared to 39% of patients with PD.[53] Insomnia can be very severe in patients with progressive supranuclear palsy.[54,55]

In general, patients with PD have more problems with sleep maintenance than with sleep onset.[52] Many patients report two to five long awakenings during the night (twice more than control subjects), lasting 30% to 40% of the night.[56] In patients with moderate to severe PD, special attention should be paid to anxiety, depression, hallucinations, and sensory/motor symptoms during the night. Sensory discomfort during the night is common in PD and may manifest as motor restlessness and painful dystonia. Early-morning dystonia consists of long-lasting, sometimes painful contractions of the toes in flexion or extension (sometimes with internal rotation of the ankle) that occur during both the end of the night and upon awakening. Severe dystonia or rigidity of the leg, neck, and back muscles may occur only at night, when dopamine levels are low. Patients also commonly experience nighttime bradykinesia, with difficulty turning in bed, readjusting the blankets or pillow, sitting up, and walking to the toilet. Difficulty moving during the night can further increase anxiety levels. Collectively, these symptoms may curtail sleep by one-third, if not more, by prolonging awakenings.

Restless Legs Syndrome

Restless legs syndrome (RLS), a frequent cause of insomnia in the general population, has a 15% to 20.8% prevalence in PD.[57,58] However, estimates of prevalence are uncertain, as RLS can be difficult to distinguish from other symptoms of parkinsonism, including leg pain, general increased pain threshold in off periods, off-dystonia, and so forth.[57] Patients who have PD with RLS have lower ferritin levels than those without, suggesting that RLS itself is responsible for some symptoms.[57] Prevalence of RLS clearly increases with disease duration. One important cause may be augmentation: Those who may have had subclinical RLS express full RLS because the frequent use of levodopa has triggered augmentation.

Table 102.3 Sleep and Night Problems in Parkinson Disease and Suggested Management

Problem	Potential Diagnosis	Proposed Management
Frequent Nocturia (± Two Episodes/Night)		
Normal volumes	Sleep apnea syndrome	Check for sleep apnea and treat appropriately
Small volumes, poor stream	Prostatism	Refer to urologist
Small volumes, good stream	Parkinsonism: associated nocturia	Intranasal desmopressin, oral amitriptyline, or transdermal rotigotine patch; if detrusor instability: oxybutynin, tolterodine, myrbetriq
		Decrease evening fluid intake; empty bladder before bed; avoid evening dosing with diuretics, antihypertensives, or vasodilators; have a urinal at the bedside table
Difficulty Initiating Sleep		
Early in the evening	Too early lights-off	Switch off lights later
	Anxiety or behavioral insomnia	Sleep hygiene; treat anxiety Evening melatonin, eszopiclone, doxepin
With restlessness	Restless legs syndrome	Check for low ferritin; remove antidepressant drugs; if the diagnosis is uncertain, consider polysomnography with leg monitoring; try gabapentin, pregabalin or opiates, such as tramadol, if not confused
Late in the night	Altered circadian cycle	Sleep hygiene; decrease levodopa/dopamine agonists in the evening Melatonin 1–2 hours before the desired bedtime
Late in night, hypomanic	Assess for impulse control disorder	Decrease dopamine agonists; keep on levodopa monotherapy; close neuropsychological follow-up
Difficulty Resuming Sleep		
With cramps, muscle pain, slowness	Nocturnal bradykinesia	Immediate-release levodopa with a glass of water during awakenings Continuous drug delivery (ropinirole transdermal patch; pramipexole or extended-release ropinirole; apomorphine infusion; intrajejunal levodopa-carbidopa infusion)
		Satin bed sheets to aid movement in bed
With restlessness	Restless legs syndrome	Similar to nocturnal bradykinesia treatment
With anxiety	Anxious disorder	Evening antidepressants (mirtazapine, doxepin, paroxetine)
With low mood	Depressive disorder	Treat the depression
Nightmares, Agitation		
Confused at night when awake	Hallucinations, psychosis, confusion	Remove or reduce the evening dose of dopamine agonist or antidepressant; assess for sleep apnea; Antipsychotics (quetiapine, clozapine)
Kicks, shouts, slaps	REM sleep behavior disorders	Secure the bed environment; discontinue antidepressant; assess likelihood of sleep apnea (video-PSG before treating) Melatonin, 3–9 mg in the evening, clonazepam, 0.5–2 mg in the evening
Daytime Sleepiness		
Falls asleep unexpectedly	Sleep attack	Check for possible sedating drugs (e.g., dopamine agonists) and remove or change them; warn patient not to drive
Falls asleep more often than before		Consider the Epworth Sleepiness Score; ask about associated hallucinations; consider PSG and MSLT
		Treat sleep apnea if severe
		Decrease/stop the dopamine agonist during daytime, and other sedative drugs
		Caffeine, modafinil, methylphenidate

MSLT, Multiple Sleep Latency Test; PSG, polysomnography; REM, rapid eye movement.

RLS can be seen early in disease and may precede the clinical diagnosis of PD. One study found that diagnosis of recent RLS in men was associated with an approximately 1.5-fold risk of being diagnosed with PD in the following 4 years.[58] However, there is no evidence that RLS symptoms early in life predispose to the subsequent development of PD.

REM Sleep Behavior Disorder and Other Parasomnias

Abnormal movements during sleep typically represent either a parasomnia or PLMS. Stereotypic and periodic movements suggest PLMS, whereas nonstereotypic movements suggest a parasomnia, usually RBD. Other potential sleep movements include myoclonus, rest tremor, dystonia, and bruxism, which are absent in sleep but can emerge during arousals.

RBD is covered in detail in Chapter 118. RBD affects 30% to 90% of patients with synucleinopathies but is uncommon in other neurodegenerative disorders.[59] The prevalence of RBD in the various diseases with parkinsonism is shown in Table 102.1. Cross-sectional studies generally find that one-third of patients with PD report at least one RBD episode per week.[60] Studies using PSG, which can detect asymptomatic RBD or asymptomatic loss of REM atonia, generally find RBD in 40% to 60%.[60,61] Note that RBD often waxes and wanes throughout the course of disease, so the lifetime prevalence of RBD in PD is likely higher. Most,[62,63] but not all,[60,61] series of RBD patients with parkinsonism demonstrate a male predominance, which is less consistent in idiopathic RBD.[64] Of note, RBD is very common in all synucleinopathies, occurring in approximately 75% of patients with MSA and DLB.

Clinically, RBD consists of dream-enactment behavior, such as laughing, talking, crying, kicking, fighting invisible enemies during sleep, and so forth.[65] RBD can be violent enough to disrupt sleep and induce self- or bed-partner injury, although this is relatively uncommon in PD (Video 102.1). Compared to patients with idiopathic RBD, who were usually selectively referred for violent behaviors, RBD in PD is less frequent and violent.[63] Indeed, quiet behaviors, including eating/drinking, singing, or giving a lecture, are often mentioned incidentally by the bed partner.[66] In addition to fully expressed complex behaviors, patients can also have abrupt movements and jerks, such as simple, "aborted," proximal or distal movements of the limbs. Patients with RBD generally have normal sleep patterns except for higher numbers of PLMS than those without. RBD does not generally cause daytime sleepiness or insomnia. Some patients with PD are disturbed by nightmares and awakenings due to vocalizations or by violent movements, including falling from bed.

Non–rapid eye movement (NREM) parasomnia can often mimic RBD. In general, RBD and NREM parasomnia can be distinguished by history. One should note, however, that patients who have PD with both sleepwalking and RBD have been reported (i.e., parasomnia overlap).[67]

A unique finding is the disappearance of parkinsonism during an RBD episode. In a large series, spouses of patients with PD reported that the patient had unusually strong and rapid movements during RBD, as if they were transiently "cured" from PD.[60] This clinical improvement has been confirmed on sleep and video monitoring, performed after a 12-hour withdrawal of dopaminergic drugs (Video 102.2). Similar findings have been reported in MSA and progressive supranuclear palsy.[68] Understanding the cause of this spontaneous improvement could lead to development of novel treatments (e.g., novel surgical targets) and help to elucidate mechanisms of motor control during sleep. Basal ganglia motor loops may be bypassed during REM sleep, and therefore the deleterious influence on movements in PD is released. This theory is strengthened by the type of movements,[60] lack of coupling between the subthalamic and motor cortex activities,[69] and absence of activity in the basal ganglia observed with functional imaging during RBD movements in patients with PD, despite the fact that the motor cortex is at work.[70]

Whereas RBD is experienced by 30% to 60% of patients with PD, there is increasing evidence that RBD marks a subtype of PD. Patients with RBD have less tremor, more falls and freezing, more cardiovascular autonomic dysfunction (especially orthostatic hypotension), and manifest more cognitive dysfunction on detailed neuropsychological testing in an early population. As such, RBD may be a marker of a "diffuse malignant" subtype of PD.[71] Of special significance is a strong link between RBD and dementia in PD; the presence of baseline RBD increases relative risk of dementia fivefold or more in most studies.[72,73]

Arguably, the most important implication of isolated RBD in general is that it can predict development of PD and other synucleinopathies. In a 5-year follow-up of their original idiopathic RBD cohort, Schenck and colleagues[74] found that 38% eventually developed PD, and on continued follow-up, 81% developed a neurodegenerative disease. This finding has now been confirmed in many independent cohort studies.[75–78] Recently, the RBD study group reported a 23-center study of neurodegenerative outcome in 1280 patients and found an overall phenoconversion rate of 6% to 7% per year.[79] If other neurodegenerative signs are present (e.g., olfactory loss, subtle motor dysfunction), annual conversion rates can increase to 10% to 20%. Patients are at approximately equal risk for either primary parkinsonism (PD and MSA) or primary dementia (DLB); eventually most patients will develop both parkinsonism and dementia. This very high risk has critical implications for neuroprotective therapy against PD because idiopathic RBD patients are ideal candidates for neuroprotective trials and future candidates for definitive neuroprotective therapy once it becomes available.

Daytime Sleepiness

On average, excessive daytime sleepiness affects one-third of patients with PD. Case-control studies performed in various countries consistently find higher sleepiness scores and higher percentages of subjects with abnormal somnolence in patients with PD (from 16% to 74%) than in age- and sex-matched control subjects.[44,45,56] Sleepiness is infrequent at PD onset in the absence of medications.[80] Sleepiness may, however, precede the onset of PD because sleepy adults in a large Asian longitudinal study developed PD later in life 3.3 times more often than nonsleepy adults.[81] Sleepiness in PD develops with time, with an incidence of 6% per year in a prospective series.[82] Those with dementia very commonly have somnolence, perhaps underlying some of the fluctuations in attention/concentration that are a hallmark of the disease.

Somnolence is a common side effect of all dopaminergic medications, including levodopa. Levodopa-induced somnolence commonly occurs at peak doses; many patients note the need to sleep 30 to 60 minutes after any large levodopa dose. Dopamine agonists particularly cause sleepiness during uptitration of doses. Some experience sleep attacks (or sudden onset of sleep), often falling asleep during stimulating life conditions, such as eating a meal (the head drooping in the plate), walking, attending work, and in the most dangerous situation, while driving a car.[83] Due to the high risk of accidents in sleepy drivers, the level of daytime sleepiness must be regularly checked in PD patients, especially when dopaminergic treatment is changed. The percentage of PD patients having experienced sleep attacks or "sudden onset of sleep without a prodrome" varies from 1% to 14%, whereas 1% to 4% PD patients report having experienced sleep attacks while driving.[84,85] Fortunately, most patients have some warning beforehand.

The Epworth Sleepiness Score is the most commonly used and well-validated scale for somnolence in PD,[86] with an abnormal threshold above 10, but it is poorly predictive of sleep attacks.[84] Some authors have added specific questions on the ability to fall asleep when driving, eating, working, or having a home routine activity[84] that better predict the risk of driving accidents. Questioning patients with daytime sleepiness about hallucinations, and vice-versa, is useful because these two symptoms are often associated and are underreported because many patients are afraid of being considered mentally ill. Although self-report can be useful, the key to a reliable somnolence history is the presence of a caregiver because some patients are remarkably unaware of their sleepiness.

Sleep Apnea and Stridor

The role of sleep apnea in parkinsonism is controversial. A large majority of studies have not identified an increased incidence of obstructive sleep apnea (OSA) among patients with PD when compared to the general population, which may be related to certain features that protect patients with PD against OSA, such as lower body weight and preserved tone in REM sleep. Moreover, most clinical studies fail to detect measurable differences between patients who have PD with or without OSA; even somnolence has not been consistently linked to OSA in PD.[87,88] Studies that assess the effectiveness of OSA treatment are limited and show modest and inconsistent effects. One randomized trial demonstrated improvement in somnolence measures but without cognitive benefits.[89] However, further studies on the potential benefit of OSA treatment are ongoing.

Stridor is caused by partial obstruction of the larynx, resulting in a harsh, high-pitched inspiratory noise (Video 102.3). Unlike OSA, which does not expose patients to immediate risk, stridor is a life-threatening condition. The larynx obstruction usually begins during the night and is observed in 42% of unselected patients with MSA.[90] It can be recognized quite easily by mimicking it to the caregiver or by an audio recording during the night but is not detected on usual apnea monitoring devices. Of interest, nighttime stridor is alleviated by the application of nasal continuous positive airway pressure (CPAP), which can avoid tracheotomy and provides a long-term benefit on quality of sleep and median survival time.[90,91] The choice of ventilation depends on whether stridor is isolated (fixed CPAP), or associated with obstructive (autoadjusting CPAP) or central (adaptive servoventilation) sleep apnea.[92]

Sleep Benefit

In PD, a specific, positive restoration of fluent mobility is observed on awakening from sleep, before drug intake, and is named "sleep benefit." Based on questionnaires, prevalence of this phenomenon among PD patients is variable and estimated between 10% and 55%. The restored mobility lasts a mean of 84 minutes, and patients may be able to skip their first dose of levodopa. However, when examining patients with sleep benefit on awakening, the motor benefit may be objectively absent or minor[93] and appears unrelated to the sleep structure, levodopa serum levels, or chronotype.[94]

POLYSOMNOGRAPHY IN PARKINSON DISEASE

As with other diseases, the clinical interview is crucial for diagnosing the causes of sleep complaints in patients with parkinsonism (Table 102.3). However, in parkinsonism, the information brought by video PSG is important and useful, provided that all aspects of the disease (motor aspects, both during sleep and wake) and sleep are carefully analyzed. The recording of a patient with parkinsonism in a sleep unit can be difficult when the team is not used to monitoring disabled, anxious patients, who awaken frequently with nocturia, require drug dosing every few hours, need assistance regularly during the night, require massage when they have violent cramps or dystonia, and must be reassured when they are confused or subject to hallucinations.

Video PSG should include the usual sleep montage (electroencephalography [EEG], electrooculography, chin electromyography [EMG]), electrocardiography, nasal pressure, thorax and abdomen efforts, oxygen saturation, leg EMG, but also audio monitoring, as stridor may be mistaken for snoring. If RBD is suspected, a synchronized infrared video and upper limb EMG electrodes (hand rather than shoulder/arm muscles) increase sensitivity to detect RBD.[95] Video monitoring also allows recognition of other frequent night-related motor problems in PD, including cramps, dystonia, tremor, and restless legs behavior. Sleep staging may be particularly difficult and time consuming in patients with parkinsonism because stages are often unstable, with multiple awakenings. Therefore video monitoring can also assist with sleep staging because altered EEG features interfere with the ability to distinguish episodes of RBD from wakeful behaviors. Video is also essential in accurately diagnosing stridor. Specific pitfalls in EEG interpretation should be considered. For example, the number of sleep spindles during NREM is reduced in PD, and EEG alpha activity may occur in all sleep stages in PD, giving the false picture of complete wakefulness throughout the night. By contrast, in patients suffering DLB or progressive supranuclear palsy, the alpha background rhythm during wakefulness may turn to a slow, regular rhythm closer to 5 to 7.5 Hz, with a further shift of all NREM sleep frequencies toward slow wave activity, so that an awake patient with open eyes may have a concomitant EEG consistent with N3 sleep.[96] In addition, sequences of slow or REMs may be observed during NREM sleep.[97]

In contrast to the quiescence of sleep in normal persons, increased muscle tone and abnormal simple and complex movements are common and also complicate the scoring of PSGs in patients with PD. Tremor may produce a 4- to 6-Hz regular artifact at the level of the chin or the legs during wakefulness (Figure 102.1); although this disappears with

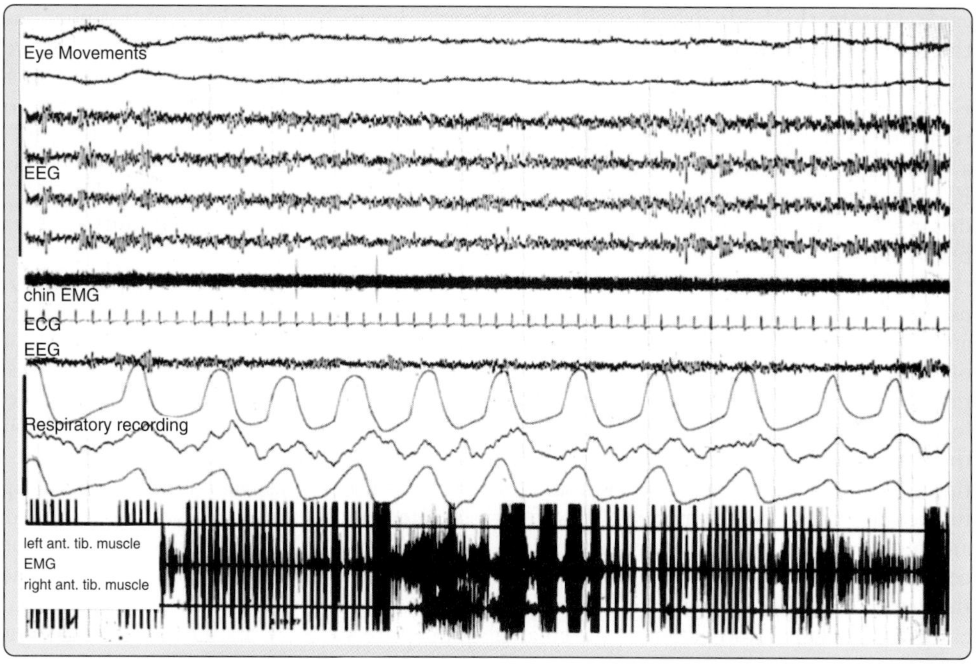

Figure 102.1 Polysomnogram in a patient with Parkinson disease and nocturnal rest tremor of the right leg occurring between wakefulness and stage 1 sleep. The regular unilateral rest tremor is interrupted by bilateral motor activity. Channels from top to bottom: 1 to 2: eye movements; 3 to 6: EEG; 7: chin EMG; 8: ECG; 9: additional EEG; 10 to 12: respiratory recording with thoracic and abdominal belts; 13: no recording; 14: EMG of left anterior tibialis muscle; 15: EMG of right anterior tibialis muscle. ECG, Electrocardiogram; EEG, electroencephalogram; EMG, electromyogram.

the onset of N1 sleep, tremor may persist as an isolated PSG finding during awakenings, arousals, and body movements from N1 sleep. Other atypical patterns of simple motor activity during sleep include repeated blinking at sleep onset, REMs during NREM sleep, blepharospasm at REM sleep onset, and prolonged tonic muscle activity of limb extensor or flexor muscles during NREM sleep. Chin muscle tone may be enhanced during REM sleep, a feature frequently associated with clinical RBD (Figure 102.2). Of note, not only the time spent with enhanced muscle tone is increased during REM sleep in patients with PD but also the amplitude of tonic muscle tone, suggesting that both PD-related hypertonia and RBD-related enhanced muscle tone coexist during REM sleep.[98] An example of sleep recordings during an RBD episode is shown in Figure 102.2.

EEG and video analysis of PSG in PD generally results in a hypnogram that shows severely fragmented sleep. In addition to usual reporting, PSG reports may benefit from a more detailed description of the EEG, for example, the frequency of the alpha background rhythm, as slow (e.g., 6.5 to 7.8 Hz) rhythms have been associated with RBD and possibly cortical degeneration. The presence of abnormal sleep stages, including REMs during NREM sleep, and REM sleep without atonia should also be specified. As much as 51% of patients with de novo PD (vs. 15% of controls) exhibit minor behavioral events during REM sleep that do not qualify for RBD but may precede its onset. Patients with this pattern are more likely to eventually develop full RBD.[99]

Sleep architecture has been studied in large, case-control series. At PD onset, there is no change in sleep structure compared to control subjects, except for longer REM sleep latency.[100] Patients with treated or more advanced PD have shorter total sleep time, lower sleep efficiency, longer REM latency, higher N1 percentage, and lower REM sleep percentage than control subjects.[101] Examples of hypnograms obtained in patients with PD are shown in Figure 102.3. When daytime sleep was assessed in a series of 54 patients with PD by nap opportunities during the Multiple Sleep Latency Test (MSLT), more than half of sleepy patients fell asleep within 5 minutes, an objective indication of pathologic sleepiness.[46] Moreover, 41% of sleepy patients had at least two sleep-onset REM periods (SOREMPs).[46] This "narcolepsy-like" pattern of short sleep means sleep latency with SOREMPs on MSLT is observed in 15% of unselected patients with PD, in some cases of MSA, and in dementia with Lewy bodies, but not in progressive supranuclear palsy.[44] In patients who have PD with severe hallucinations, the hallucinations are temporally associated with REM sleep during the night and with sleep onset in REM periods during the daytime, as in narcolepsy.[97] In other patients with PD, hallucinations occur after REM sleep during the night, and during wakefulness or N1 sleep during the daytime. Sleep attacks may also consist of rapid transitions into N2 sleep.[102]

TREATMENT

The management of sleep disorders in parkinsonism depends on the causes identified by the history and sleep laboratory tests. A list of common problems and corresponding, experience-based management is given in Table 102.3.

Insomnia

Despite the fact that insomnia is frequent in PD, research on its treatment remains limited. The treatment of insomnia in patients with PD is therefore more experience based than evidence based.[103]

The comfort of the parkinsonian patient during the night can be improved by using sheets that enable easy movement, silk pajamas without buttons, levodopa tablets and

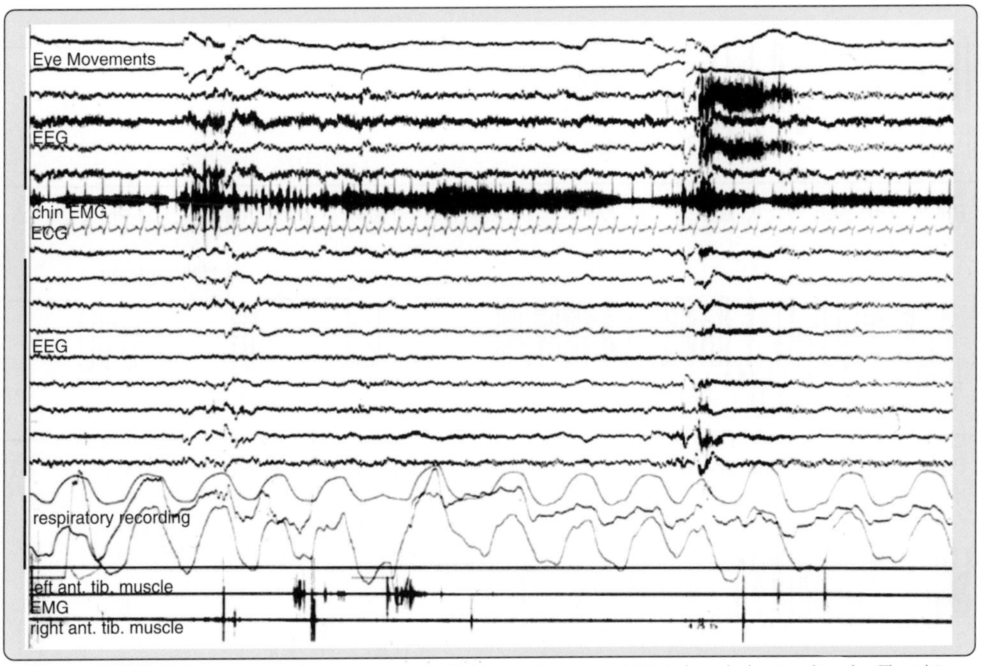

Figure 102.2 Polysomnogram in a patient with Parkinson disease and REM sleep behavior disorder. The chin EMG shows a highly elevated muscle tone, and motor activity occurs in the recording, with typical muscle twitches in the EMG channels of both legs. Channels from top to bottom: 1 to 2: eye movements showing a typical REM sleep pattern; 3 to 6: EEG; 7: chin EMG with increased muscle tone; 8: ECG; 9 to 17: further EEG channels showing muscle artifacts of eye movements; 18 to 20: respiratory recording with thoracic and abdominal belts; 21: no recording; 22 to 23: EMG of left and right anterior tibialis muscle. ECG, Electrocardiogram; EEG, electroencephalogram; EMG, electromyogram.

a bottle of water on the bed table, and transitory blockade of nighttime polyuria with an evening intranasal dose of desmopressin. In advanced stages of the disease, the patient's spouse might be inclined to sleep in a different bed or room, but unfortunately these patients are often in need of a nocturnal caregiver to assist with getting out of bed, using the bathroom, and administering nocturnal L-DOPA. Inadequate rest for the spouse or other caregiver may make the patient's sleep disturbance intolerable and lead to institutionalization.

In patients with motor fluctuations, reestablishing continuous dopaminergic stimulation during day and night may be the first-line strategy to improve nighttime motor disability. A careful record of the time of the symptoms, in correlation with time of drug intake, can help identify a nighttime gap in dopaminergic stimulation. However, the benefit of dopaminergic agents in the evening and night must be weighed against potential alerting effects.[104] The use of levodopa in the evening or at bedtime improves subjective sleep quality and decreases nighttime movements. Sustained-release forms of levodopa in the evening have not been compared systematically to normal-release forms of levodopa. In small unblinded trials, sustained-release preparations do not improve subjective aspects of sleep (general quality, sleep-onset latency, total sleep time, number of awakenings), but they have a mild benefit on nocturnal akinesia. We have had good experience with rapid-release forms of levodopa soluble in water or crushed regular levodopa tablets taken upon awakening in the middle of the night. Transdermal rotigotine during the day and night improved most aspects of sleep quality and symptom control, including early-morning akinesia.[105] When comparing rotigotine to oral pramipexole three times a day for motor symptoms, similar results were obtained in advanced PD.[106] Subthalamic nucleus stimulation consistently improves sleep duration, reduces nocturnal awakenings, and reduces early-morning dystonia in patients with advanced PD[15,16,107] but can worsen restless legs symptoms (probably due to decrease of dopamine agonists).

Beyond dopaminergic optimization, a small randomized controlled trial of cognitive behavioral therapy demonstrated benefits on subjective sleep measures.[108] A study of a sleep hygiene intervention showed improvements in subjective sleep, without benefits on PSG sleep measures.[109] More notable, this same study demonstrated dramatic benefits of an exercise program on PSG but not subjective sleep efficiency. A small randomized study suggested benefits of low doses (10 mg) of doxepin, a sedating antidepressant.[108] This is analogous to findings in Alzheimer disease, in which a randomized controlled trial of 50 mg trazodone demonstrated clear benefits.[110] Theoretical concerns about cognitive side effects of trazodone and doxepin due to anticholinergic effects have generally not been borne out in these studies because anticholinergic properties are not seen at these low doses. Another randomized trial showed equivocal benefit of eszopiclone; although the primary outcome (total sleep time) was negative, there was benefit on some subjective measures.[111] Pimavaserin, a serotonin 5-hydroxytryptamine 2A (5-HT2A) inverse agonist had beneficial effects on sleep disturbances in patients who have PD with psychosis.[112] Similarly, small open-label studies have suggested that quetiapine reduces insomnia (somnolence is a very common side effect).[113] These medications, including

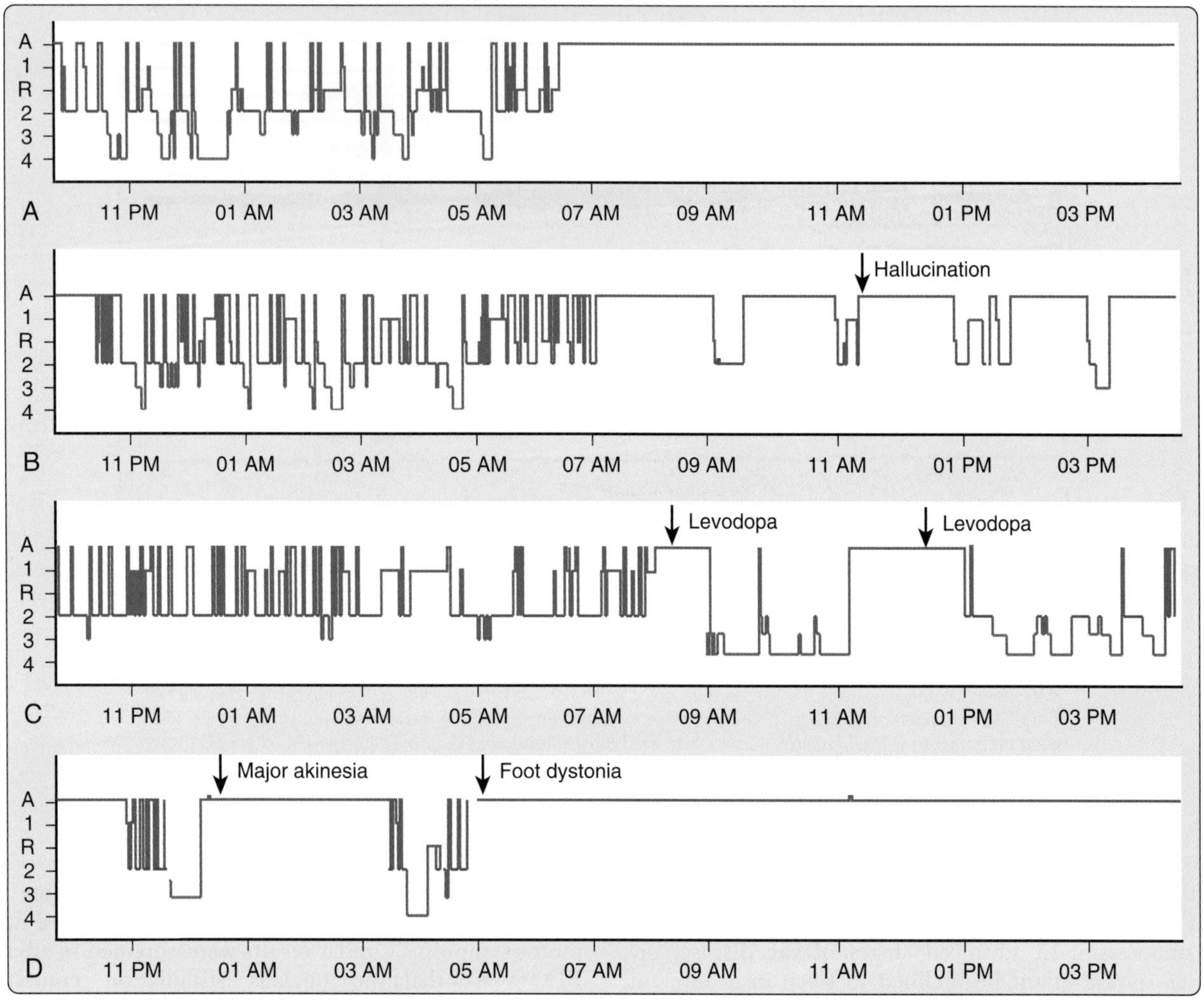

Figure 102.3 Four 24-hour hypnograms. **(A)** A healthy 60-year-old woman with normal sleep. **(B)** A 54-year-old woman with Parkinson disease (PD) treated with levodopa 300 mg/day and bromocriptine 30 mg/day, reporting frequent nighttime awakenings, daytime sleepiness, and hallucinations (indicated by the *arrow:* saw a stranger in the room, here synchronous with abnormal daytime REM sleep onsets [narcolepsy-like phenotype]). **(C)** An 80-year-old man with mild PD complaining of falling asleep 2 to 3 hours after each levodopa intake (*arrow*), who displayed severe hypersomnia. **(D)** A 72-year-old man with advanced PD and on-off motor fluctuations. After a midnight awakening (*arrow*), he developed severe bradykinesia with an axial, painful dystonia that prevented him from resuming sleep. Later, at 4:30 a.m., he had foot dystonia (early-morning dystonia). All these motor phenomena lengthened his time awake. The *x* axis displays the time of night and day (clock hours), and the *y* axis displays the stages of sleep and wakefulness: with awakening (A), non-REM sleep stage 1 (1), stage 2 (2), stage 3 (3), stage 4 (4), and REM sleep (R).

clozapine with an appropriate monitoring of leukocyte count, can be particularly useful if disturbing hallucinations or other psychotic symptoms are present. Other hypnotics are frequently used in clinical practice; surveillance is required for worsening of preexisting RLS, RBD, hallucinations, or daytime sleepiness.

Apart from iron supplementation when indicated, the treatment of nocturnal RLS in PD may be complex. Because RLS may be due to a deficit of dopamine stimulation at night, an evening additional dose of dopamine agonist may be beneficial. However, this is complicated by the possibility of increased augmentation from chronic dopaminergic treatment of otherwise subclinical RLS. In patients without PD who experience augmentation, a reduction in the daily dose of dopamine is usually beneficial; however, this is not a practical strategy in PD, given the potential to worsen motor disability. Therefore it is unclear to what degree dopaminergic manipulation is warranted. Evening gabapentin/pregabalin and, more rarely, opiates (in nondemented patients without hallucinations) may be carefully used; however, minimal guidance to embark on these alternatives is available in the literature.

REM Sleep Behavior Disorder

For patients with potentially dangerous manifestations of RBD, safety of the sleeping environment is crucial. When pharmacotherapy is required, clonazepam (0.5 to 2 mg at bedtime) treatment provides moderate or greater improvement in 78% of patients.[114] Although generally well tolerated, in patients with PD clonazepam can cause daytime somnolence, worsen sleep apnea, exacerbate cognitive impairment, and increase the risk of falls. Therefore careful monitoring for these side effects is required, and in mild cases without injury, clonazepam may not be warranted. Observational non-randomized studies have suggested that melatonin (3 to 9 mg at bedtime) provides at least moderate improvement in 48% of patients (lower than clonazepam) but with a mean reduction in RBD visual analogue scale ratings similar to clonazepam.[114] Melatonin may have less cognitive or gait side effects than clonazepam.[114] Dopaminergic therapy may be helpful for RBD, although findings are mixed. We personally have experienced variable effects of dopaminergic therapy on RBD, including both reduction and, less commonly, exacerbation of dream enactment. Often, idiopathic patients with RBD who phenoconvert to parkinsonism note at least a transient reduction in RBD symptoms with initiation of levodopa. Other potential treatments, which have been documented only in case studies or small series, include donepezil and zopiclone.[115]

Excessive Daytime Sleepiness

Finding and treating the cause of daytime sleepiness in patients with PD requires a careful interview on nocturnal disturbances, hallucinations, recent changes in dopaminergic and psychotropic treatment, and sometimes a nighttime PSG to identify a treatable cause such as OSA. The short-term benefit of CPAP on sleepiness (measured with the MSLT but not with the Epworth Sleepiness Scale) was recently demonstrated in patients who have PD with sleepiness and a moderately increased apnea-hypopnea index.[89] In addition, efforts should be made to reduce any sedative drugs (clonazepam, other benzodiazepines, dopamine agonists, sedative antidepressants, opioids, atypical neuroleptics). In a randomized controlled trial, bright light therapy resulted in a 2.8-point improvement in Epworth Sleepiness Scores compared to the dim red light placebo condition.[116] Subjective and actigraphy sleep parameters were also improved. Given its safety and low cost, bright light therapy can be considered a first-line treatment option, particularly for patients who have low light exposure at baseline (e.g., during winter in high latitudes, institutionalized patients, etc.). Chronotherapies in general, including morning bright light, evening melatonin, and daytime exercise, might be low-cost interventions for improving both daytime sleepiness and nighttime insomnia in patients with PD.[117]

Several medication options are available if required. Caffeine may provide a modest improvement in sleepiness scales but is temporary[118] and therefore well suited for the short term, as-needed use, in situations in which one wishes to remain alert (e.g., episodic social engagements). Modafinil is well tolerated in patients with PD and has had positive benefit demonstrated in two of three randomized trials.[119] However, alerting effect is limited, with less than one-third of patients responding.[119] Methylphenidate is another option and decreased excessive daytime sleepiness by 3 points on the Epworth Sleepiness Scale without worsening sleep quality in a recent controlled trial aimed at alleviating gait freezing.[120] Caution is required in using stimulants in cognitively impaired patients because confusion and violent behaviors may occur. A recent randomized trial of sodium oxybate, taken at bedtime and then again in the middle of the night, improved Epworth scores by 4.2 points compared to placebo and reduced sleep latency on MSLT by 2.9 minutes.[121] Considerable caution is required, given its strong sedative properties, and its cost may be prohibitive in many contexts.

CLINICAL PEARLS

- In patients with parkinsonism, clinicians should inquire about nighttime bradykinesia, off-period dystonia, early-morning akinesia, tremor, restless legs syndrome, respiratory disturbances, insomnia, rapid eye movement behavior disorder, or psychosis from medication-associated factors and their contribution to the sleep problem.
- Specific interventions may then improve quality of sleep and reduce daytime sleepiness, thus enhancing quality of life in PD.
- Nocturnal stridor is a life-threatening symptom in multiple system atrophy that can benefit from continuous positive airway pressure.

SUMMARY

As much as 60% patients with PD suffer from insomnia, 30% to 60% from RBD, and 30% from excessive daytime sleepiness. These frequencies can be higher in atypical parkinsonism. The disruption of sleep and wakefulness in parkinsonism is caused by a combination of neurodegenerative damage in brain areas responsible for sleep; arousal and clock control; side effects of medications; and behavioral, respiratory, and motor phenomena accompanying the disease. Sleep maintenance insomnia may be intrinsic to PD but is also promoted by motor disability, painful dystonia, RLS, dysuria, anxiety, and depression. Improving motor control during the night with therapy; treating nocturia, anxiety, and depression; and recommending rigorous exercise, benzodiazepine receptor agonists, doxepin, trazodone, pimavanserin, and quetiapine can help. RBD is often violent, enacted dreaming that can cause nighttime injuries and is generally caused by neurodegeneration in the REM sleep atonia system. RBD often precedes parkinsonism (or dementia with Lewy bodies), with up to 90% of idiopathic RBD patients eventually developing a synucleinopathy. In accordance, idiopathic patients with RBD often have other signs of neurodegeneration, including olfactory, cognitive, and autonomic disturbances; decreased dopaminergic transmission; and slowed electroencephalographic rhythms. Parkinsonism can be temporarily reversed during RBD episodes in some patients with PD. RBD is treated primarily with melatonin and clonazepam, although efficacy remains to be established. Daytime sleepiness and a narcolepsy-like profile are also seen in PD, and somnolence is a common side effect of medications. Bright light therapy, medication adjustment, and psychostimulants may mitigate excessive daytime sleepiness. Patients with MSA also can develop a life-threatening stridor during sleep that should be rapidly treated with positive airway pressure.

SELECTED READINGS

Cristini J, Weiss M, De Las Heras B, et al. The effects of exercise on sleep quality in persons with Parkinson's disease: A systematic review with meta-analysis. *Sleep Med Rev*. 2021;55:101384.

Fernandez-Arcos A, Morenas-Rodriguez E, Santamaria J, et al. Clinical and video-polysomnographic analysis of rapid eye movement sleep behavior disorder and other sleep disturbances in dementia with Lewy bodies. *Sleep*. 2019;42(7):zsz086.

Knudsen K, Fedorova TD, Hansen AK, et al. In-vivo staging of pathology in REM sleep behaviour disorder: a multimodality imaging case-control study. *Lancet Neurol*. 2018;17:618–628.
Mollenhauer B, Trautmann E, Sixel-Doring F, et al. Nonmotor and diagnostic findings in subjects with de novo Parkinson disease of the DeNoPa cohort. *Neurology*. 2013;81:1226–1234.
Postuma RB, Iranzo A, Hu M, et al. Risk and predictors of dementia and parkinsonism in idiopathic REM sleep behaviour disorder: a multicentre study. *Brain*. 2019;142:744–759.

A complete reference list can be found online at ExpertConsult.com.

Chapter 103

Sleep-Wake Disturbances and Stroke

Claudio L.A. Bassetti

Chapter Highlights

- Sleep-wake disturbances (SWDs) and stroke are common and intertwined neurologic problems; each may cause the other, and they can arise from similar predisposing factors.
- Clinicians who treat patients with SWD or stroke should be aware of this potential comorbidity and its clinical implications.
- In patients with stroke, SWDs are frequent (20%–50% of patients), and their treatment may improve outcome and reduce the risk of stroke recurrence.

HISTORY

A link between sleep and stroke was observed already in the 19th and early 20th centuries. Sleep-disordered breathing (SDB) after stroke was reported by Cheyne (1819) and Broadbent (1887).[1,2] Charcot (1884) and Wildbrand (1887) described a loss of dreaming with occipital stroke, and Freund (1913) and Lhermitte (1922) observed hypersomnia after thalamic and midbrain stroke.[3,4]

In the last 30 years a complex bidirectional relationship between sleep and stroke was recognized, including the following elements: (1) SDB and other nonapneic sleep-wake disturbances (SWDs) represent independent risk factors for stroke; (2) SDB and SWD are frequent in stroke patients and may have negative impacts on outcomes; (3) sleep interventions in animal experiments and humans can positively influence stroke evolution and outcome; and (4) sleep electroencephalogram (EEG) changes ipsilesionally and contralesionally may offer a unique window to understand the neuroplasticity processes that take place after stroke.

STROKE

Stroke is a focal neurologic deficit of acute onset and vascular origin; about 65% of patients have ischemic stroke, 15% intracerebral hemorrhage, and 20% transient ischemic attacks (TIAs) in which neurologic deficits resolve within 1 hour.

Stroke has an estimated lifetime risk for those aged 25 years or older of 25% and represents the second most common cause of mortality and disability-adjusted life years (DALY[5]) worldwide. Despite a declining stroke incidence related to improvement in prevention and treatment measures, the number of strokes is anticipated to increase in the next few decades because of the population aging.[6]

Risk factors for stroke include atrial fibrillation, arterial hypertension, dyslipidemia, disorders of glucose metabolism, overweight body habitus (specifically, abnormal waist-to hip ratio), excessive alcohol consumption, cigarette smoking, and physical inactivity. Patients with heart disease, asymptomatic carotid stenosis, history of TIA, depression, psychosocial stress, and age older than 65 years are also at higher risk for stroke.[7] Primary prevention of stroke includes treatment of risk factors, physical exercise, reduction of body mass index, anticoagulation for atrial fibrillation, and endarterectomy.

Emergency treatment includes the systemic use of fibrinolytic agents and endovascular treatment (thrombectomy). Management of acute stroke includes placement of patients in a stroke unit, early recognition of medical complications, and prescription of agents that inhibit platelet aggregation. Surgery may be considered in patients with accessible (e.g., cerebellar) hemorrhages and malignant middle cerebral artery strokes.

After stroke, treatments include neurorehabilitation and the prevention of recurrent events with platelet antiaggregants, blood pressure–lowering medications, statins, management of other risk factors, and in selected patients anticoagulation and endarterectomy.

SLEEP-WAKE DISTURBANCES BEFORE STROKE: INDEPENDENT RISK FACTORS FOR STROKE

There is increasing evidence that not only SDB (see Chapter 150) but also nonapneic SWDs may independently increase the risk of stroke.[8-13] Table 103.1 summarizes the current knowledge on the role of different SWDs on stroke risk.

SLEEP DURATION

In a systematic review and meta-analysis published in 2019, eight studies were reported in which sleep duration and stroke risk were assessed.[9] Most studies included cerebrovascular risk factors (but only two depression/depressive symptoms) as covariates. The majority of the studies were considered of good quality. Seven of eight studies reported a significant association between long sleep duration, or more than 8 hours of sleep, and ischemic stroke death or incidence. The relative increase in risk (RR) ranged from 0.24 to 3.90. Only one study reported and increased risk in ischemic stroke for short sleep duration (<7.5 hours versus >7.5 hours of sleep). A major limitation of large studies published is the absence of objective measures of sleep duration.

Table 103.1 Sleep-Wake Disturbances as Risk Factors for Stroke[a]

	Studies	Impact
Sleep-disordered breathing (SDB)	37 studies	OSA doubles the risk (RR 2.02–2.24)
Treatment of SDB	13 studies	CPAP may reduce the risk in patients using >4 hr/day
Sleep duration	8 studies	Long sleep duration increases the risk (RR 1.24–3.90)
Intervention	None	
Insomnia	6 studies	Effect uncertain
Treatment of insomnia	3 studies	Benzodiazepines may increase the risk
Excessive daytime sleepiness (EDS)	17 studies	EDS increases the risk (RR 1.09–1.98)
Intervention	None	
Restless legs syndrome (RLS)/PLMS	34 studies (26 RLS/8 PLMS)	RLS does not, whereas PLMS may increase the risk
Treatment of RLS/PLMS	None	
Circadian disturbances	50 studies	Shift work/long work hours modestly increase the risk
Intervention	None	

[a]The results of the most recent systematic reviews (SRs)/meta-analyses (MAs)[1-5] are summarized.
CPAP, Continuous positive airway pressure; OSA, obstructive sleep apnea; PLMS, periodic limb movements of sleep; RR, relative risk.
1. Gottlieb E, Landau E, Baxter H. The bidirectional impact of sleep and circadian rhythm dysfunction in human ischaemic stroke: A systematic review. *Sleep Med Rev*. 2019;45:54-69. 2. Rivera AS, Akanbi M, Dwyer LC, et al. Shift work and long work hours and their association with chronic health conditions: A systematic review of systematic reviews with meta-analyses. *PLOS One*. 2020;15/4):e0231037. 3. Wang BH, Liu W, Heizhhati, et al. Association between excessive daytime sleepiness and risk of cardiovascular disease and all-cause mortality: A systematic review and meta-analysis of longitudinal cohort studies. *J Am Med Dir Assoc*. 2020;S1525:https://doi.org/10.1016/j.jamda.2020.1005.1023. 4. Lin HJ, Yeh JH, Hsieh MT, et al. Continuous positive airway pressure with good adherence can reduce risk of stroke in patients with moderate to severe obstructive sleep apnea: An updated systematic review and meta-analysis. *Sleep Med Rev*. 2020;54:101354. doi: 101310.101016/j.smrv.102020.101354. 5. Bassetti CLA, Randerath W, Vignatelli L, et al. EAN/ERS/ESO/ESRS statement on the impact of sleep disorders on risk and outcome of stroke. *Eur J Neurol*. 2020;55:1117-1134.

The increase in stroke risk may be related to the association of long sleep with such cardiovascular risk factors as high C-reactive protein (CRP) levels, white matter disease, and atrial fibrillation.[9,14-16] However, sleep duration could represent only a marker of poor health with increased sleep needs.

No study assessed the effect of a change in sleep duration on stroke risk.

Insomnia

In a systematic review and meta-analysis published in 2020, six studies were found in which insomnia and stroke risk were assessed.[13] Most studies were considered of good quality. Contrary to previous publications,[9,17] this analysis concluded that, although insomnia slightly increases the risk for cardiovascular events (CVEs), the effect on stroke is uncertain.[13]

A subsequently published 10-year cohort study from China including data from 487,200 adults (ages 30–79) reported an association not only between insomnia symptoms (difficulties initiating or maintaining sleep, early morning awakening, and/or daytime dysfunction for at least 3 days a week) and risk of ischemic heart disease but also ischemic and hemorrhagic stroke.[18]

Limitations in most studies published include the inconsistent definitions of insomnia and the lack of objective measures of sleep quality/insomnia. Insomnia with objective short sleep duration appears in fact to be associated with cardiovascular risk factors such as hypertension and diabetes.[19]

The effect of treatment/reduction of insomnia on stroke risk is poorly studied, but benzodiazepines may increase the risk of stroke, particularly in the presence of high dosages and chronic consumption.[13,20]

Several mechanisms were suggested to explain the link between insomnia and CVE, including sympathetic activation, impaired glucose tolerance, and elevated levels of inflammatory cytokines.[15,21]

Experimental studies have shown that sleep deprivation and fragmentation during the first days after stroke have long-term detrimental effects on functional recovery and structural/molecular markers of neuroplasticity.[22-24] Conversely, slow-wave sleep-enhancing drugs (gamma-hydroxybutyrate baclofen) were shown in both rats and mice to promote functional recovery and poststroke neuroplasticity.[25,26]

Noteworthy, sleep deprivation (as a form of ischemic preconditioning) immediately preceding stroke was shown experimentally to be neuroprotective.[27,28] The favorable change in the signaling response to ischemia was linked to an increase of rapid eye movement (REM) sleep and orexin/melanin-concentrating hormone transmission.[27]

Excessive Daytime Sleepiness

In a systematic review and meta-analysis published in 2020, 17 studies were found in which excessive daytime sleepiness (EDS) and stroke risk were assessed.[10] EDS was found to represent a modest but statistically significant predictor for CVE, coronary heart disease, stroke, and all-cause mortality. The pooled relative increase in risk was 0.47 (range 0.9–1.98).

The link between EDS and stroke can be explained by the fact that EDS is a marker of disease burden resulting often from overlapping causes or comorbid multicontributors.

No study assessed the effect of treatment/reduction of EDS on stroke risk.

Restless Legs Syndrome/Periodic Limb Movements of Sleep

In a systematic review and meta-analysis published in 2020, stroke risk in restless legs syndrome (RLS) (26 studies) and periodic limb movements of sleep (PLMS) (8 studies) were reported.[13] Most studies were considered of moderate to low quality. Confirming some, but not all, previous analyses, this most study concluded that whereas PLMS may increase the risk factor of stroke, RLS does not.[13,29,30] Several mechanisms were suggested to explain the link between PLMS and stroke, including sympathetic activation and elevated levels of inflammatory cytokines.[31,32] No study assessed the effect of treatment of RLS/PLMS on stroke risk.

Circadian Disturbances

Ischemic stroke, like myocardial infarction and sudden death, occurs most frequently in the morning hours, particularly after awakening. A meta-analysis of 31 publications reporting the circadian timing of 11,816 strokes found a 49% increase in stroke of all types (ischemic stroke, hemorrhagic stroke, TIA) between 6 A.M. and noon.[33] Possible explanations for this pattern are circadian or postural changes in platelet aggregation, thrombolysis, blood pressure, heart rate, and catecholamine levels that occur with awakening and resumption of physical and mental activities.[34,35] In addition, the most prolonged REM sleep period, during which autonomic system instability is known to occur, occurs close to awakening.[36] Treatment with aspirin does not modify the circadian pattern of stroke onset.[37]

In a systematic review and meta-analysis published in 2020, 50 studies were found in which shift work or long work hours and risk of CVE (including stroke) were assessed.[12] Most studies were considered of moderate to low quality. A modest increase of stroke risk was found with shift work (RR: 1.13, 1.08–1.20) and long work hours (RR: 1.33, 1.11–1.61). Two studies reported an increased risk of stroke in subjects with a late chronotype.[38,39] Circadian misalignment, which mimics shift work, is associated with a negative effect on cardiovascular system/risk profile.[40] No studies assessed the effect of treatment/improvement of circadian disturbances (CDs) on stroke risk.

Others and Combinations

One study reported an increased stroke risk in patients with probable REM sleep behavior disorder, as assessed by a validated questionnaire.[41] In a study of 385,292 participants initially free of cardiovascular disease (CVD) from the UK Biobank, patients with sleep disturbances had over a follow-up period of 8.5 years a 34% (25%–42%) higher risk of stroke compared with those without sleep disturbances. In this study, five sleep characteristics defined the referent group as follows: early chronotype, sleep 7 to 8 hours per day, never/rarely insomnia, no snoring, and no frequent EDS.

SLEEP-WAKE DISTURBANCES AFTER STROKE: PREVALENCE AND IMPACT ON OUTCOME AND STROKE RECURRENCE

There is increasing evidence that SDB (see Chapter 150) and nonapneic SWDs are frequent in stroke and negatively affect its evolution and outcome.[8,9,13] A prospective study of 438 patients also suggests that the presence of multiple SWDs may significantly increase the risk of subsequent cardio/cerebrovascular events.[42] These negative effects may be linked to inflammatory processes, sympathetic activation, and decreased synaptic plasticity. Table 103.2 summarizes the current knowledge on the frequency of different SWDs in stroke patients and their impact on stroke outcome.

Several experimental studies and few clinical observations suggest that, on the other hand, treatment of SWD (e.g., continuous positive airway pressure [CPAP] for obstructive sleep apnea [OSA]) and sleep enhancement (e.g., pharmacologically, optogenetically) may be neuroprotective and have a favorable effect on neuroplasticity and functional outcome.[25,26,43]

Finally, few experimental and first clinical observations suggest that neuroplasticity processes taking place after stroke may be reflected by wake and sleep EEG changes taking place perilesionally and contralesionally.[44-48] The study of sleep offers, in other words, a unique window to monitor and understand the plasticity changes that accompany and promote stroke recovery.[49-54]

Table 103.2 Sleep-Wake Disturbances after Stroke: Frequency and Impact on Outcome[a]

	Studies	Frequency	Impact
Sleep-disordered breathing (SDB)	132 studies, 13 RCT	AHI >30 in 30%	OSA increases the recurrence risk/may worsen outcome
Treatment of SDB			CPAP may improve outcome
Insomnia	28 studies	20%–30% (2%–59%)	Associated with worse outcome
Treatment of insomnia	None		
Fatigue	24 studies	50%	
Treatment of fatigue	None		
Excessive daytime sleepiness (EDS)/hypersomnia	27 studies	10%–20% (9%–72%)	
Treatment of EDS/hypersomnia	None		
Restless legs syndrome (RLS)/periodic limb movements of sleep (PLMS)	15/10 studies	5%–15%	Associated with worse outcome
Treatment of RLS/PLMS	None		
Circadian disturbances	8 studies	In most cases	Associated with worse outcome
Intervention	None		

[a]The results of the most recent studies and systematic reviews (SRs)/meta-analyses (MAs) are summarized. (Gottlieb et al.[9]; Bassetti et al.[13]; Hasan F, et al. Dynamic prevalence of sleep disorders following stroke or transient ischemic attack. Systematic review and meta-analysis. *Stroke.* 2021;52.; Cumming, et al. The prevalence of fatigue after stroke. *Int J Stroke.* 2016;11:968-977.; Lin HJ, et al. Continuous positive airway pressure with good adherence. *Sleep Med Rev.* 2020;54.)
AHI, Apnea-hypopnea index; CPAP, continuous positive airway pressure; OSA, obstructive sleep apnea; RCT, randomized controlled trial.

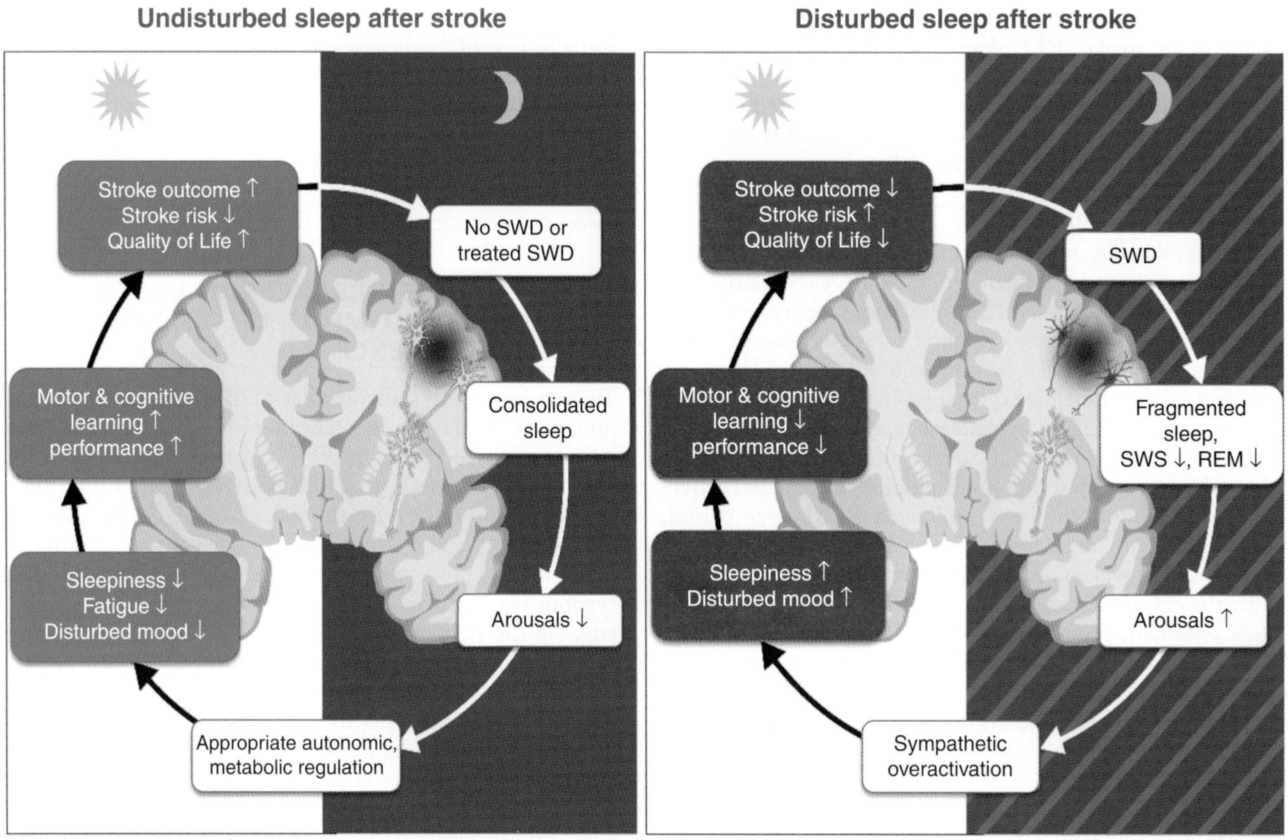

Figure 103.1 Sleep neuroplasticity and outcome after stroke. The two circles illustrate the impact of undisturbed sleep (and treatment of sleep-wake disturbances [SWDs]) and disturbed sleep (sleep deprivation, SWD) on stroke evolution and outcome. (Modified from Duss et al. *Curr Neurol Neuorsci Rep*. 2018.)

The effects of undisturbed sleep/treated SWD and disturbed sleep/SWD are schematically shown in Figure 103.1 (modified after[55]).

Sleep Duration

Sleep duration after stroke has rarely been studied. Few series suggest an increase sleep duration in patients with paramedian thalamic strokes and in patients with severe strokes and the possibility to document it by actigraphy.[56,57] The pathophysiology and clinical significance of this change are unclear.

Insomnia

Epidemiology and Impact

In a systematic review and meta-analysis published in 2020, eight studies were found in which the frequency and impact of insomnia poststroke were assessed.[13] Most studies were considered of moderate to low quality. The frequency of poststroke insomnia was estimated to be around 30%. The different methods used to assess insomnia and intervals after stroke in which patients were studied explain the high variability in results found in the literature (from 2.3% up to 59.5%).[58,59]

The evolution of poststroke insomnia is poorly known. Some data suggest the possibility of a persistence over years.

Associations and Pathophysiology

Poststroke insomnia is associated with female gender, depression, anxiety, and poorer functional outcome.[9,13] On rare occasions, strokes can cause insomnia "de novo" through disruption of sleep mechanisms. Examples include patients with

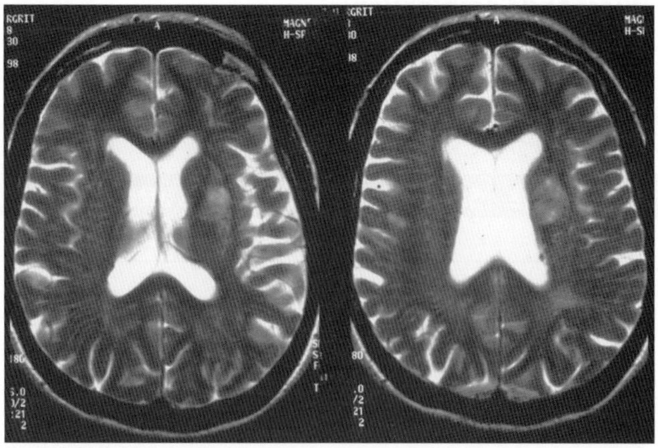

Figure 103.2 Insomnia after subcortical stroke. A 68-year-old female patient with left subcortical hemispheric stroke (corona radiata). Clinically mild right hemisyndrome, National Institute of Health (NIH) Stroke Score = 6. In the first poststroke week, almost complete insomnia and excessive daytime sleepiness (EDS). Two weeks later, recovery of EDS and improvement of insomnia (2–3 hours sleep/night). Normalization of sleep-wake functions after 4 weeks.

pontine strokes, with almost complete insomnia persisting for 1 to 2 months.[60-62] Patients with caudate or subcortical (Figure 103.2), thalamic, thalamomesencephalic, and tegmental pontine stroke can present with insomnia accompanied by an inversion of the sleep-wake cycle, with insomnia and agitation during the night and EDS/hypersomnia during the day.[61,63,64] Poststroke insomnia may be also be the result of a

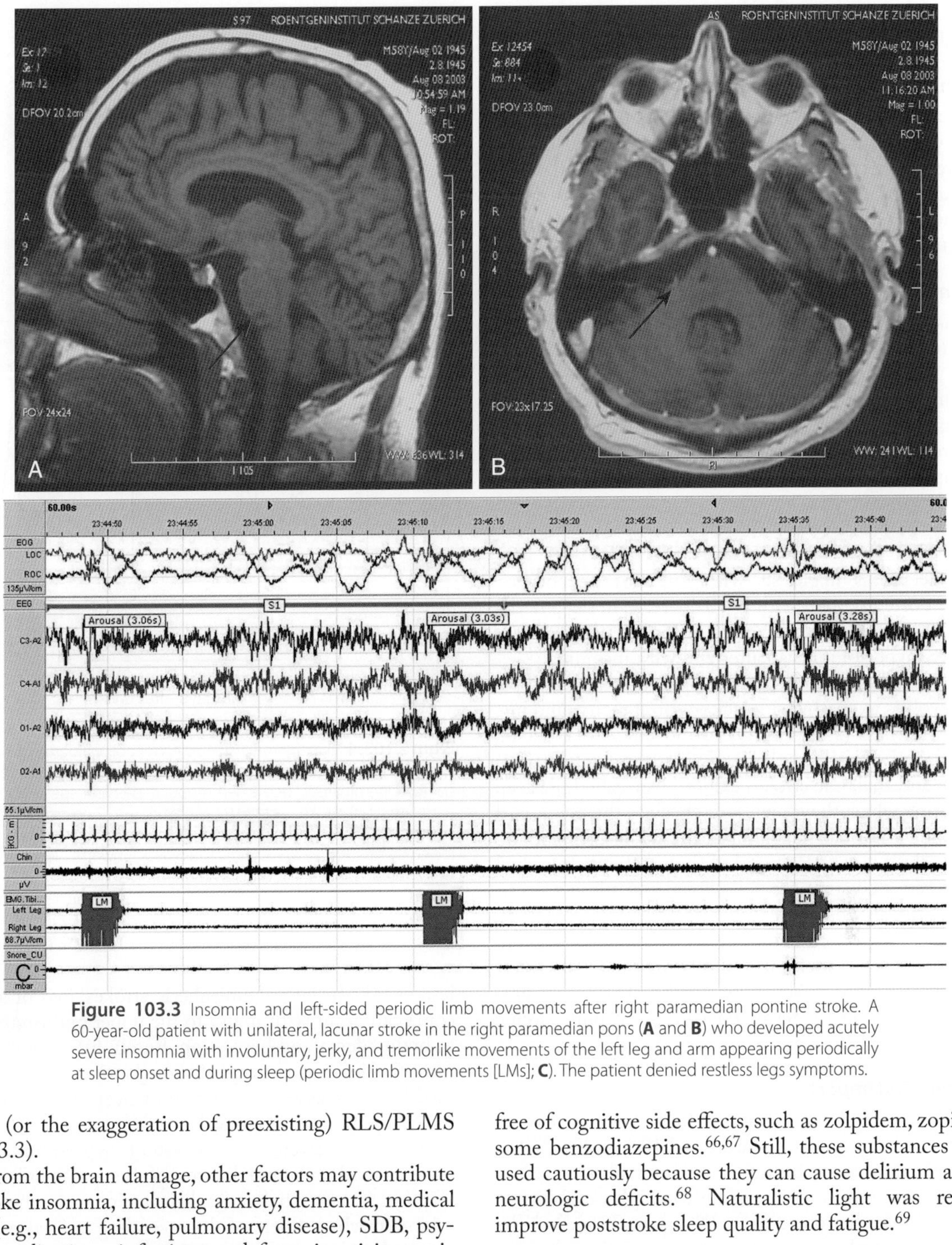

Figure 103.3 Insomnia and left-sided periodic limb movements after right paramedian pontine stroke. A 60-year-old patient with unilateral, lacunar stroke in the right paramedian pons (**A** and **B**) who developed acutely severe insomnia with involuntary, jerky, and tremorlike movements of the left leg and arm appearing periodically at sleep onset and during sleep (periodic limb movements [LMs]; **C**). The patient denied restless legs symptoms.

new onset (or the exaggeration of preexisting) RLS/PLMS (Figure 103.3).

Aside from the brain damage, other factors may contribute to poststroke insomnia, including anxiety, dementia, medical disorders (e.g., heart failure, pulmonary disease), SDB, psychotropic medications, infections and fever, inactivity, environmental disturbances, stress, and depression.[65]

Diagnosis and Treatment

Diagnosis is made on clinical grounds. Questionnaires (e.g., Insomnia Severity Index) and actigraphy can be useful for the recognition of poststroke insomnia.[58] Polysomnography should be used only for unclear, severe, or persisting poststroke insomnia.

Treatment of poststroke insomnia should focus on behavioral measures such as placing patients in private rooms at night, protection from nocturnal noise and light, and mobilization with exposure to light during the day. If necessary, one could consider temporary use of hypnotics that are relatively free of cognitive side effects, such as zolpidem, zopiclone, and some benzodiazepines.[66,67] Still, these substances should be used cautiously because they can cause delirium and worsen neurologic deficits.[68] Naturalistic light was reported to improve poststroke sleep quality and fatigue.[69]

Fatigue

Fatigue is defined as a feeling of physical tiredness and exhaustion with lack of energy accompanied by a strong desire for sleep with usually normal (or paradoxically decreased) sleep propensity.

Epidemiology and Impact

In a series of 235 patients assessed 0.3 to 2 years after stroke, 46% reported abnormal fatigue (Fatigue Severity Scale [FSS] ≥4.0); no correlation was found between fatigue and interval poststroke.[70] Using the same cutoff, a systematic review and meta-analysis of 24 studies published in 2016 found a similar frequency of poststroke fatigue of 50%.[71] Poststroke fatigue not infrequently persists over time.[72] In such cases it predicts institutionalization and mortality.[73]

Associations and Pathophysiology

In a systematic review and meta-analysis published in 2020, 14 studies were found in which risk factors for poststroke fatigue were assessed.[74] Female gender, depression, thalamic stroke, leukoaraiosis, depression, sleep disturbances, diabetes mellitus, and anxiety were found to be associated with poststroke fatigue.

Diagnosis and Treatment

Diagnosis is made on clinical grounds. Questionnaires (e.g., FSS) are often used for the recognition of poststroke fatigue.[70] Activating antidepressants amantadine, tirilazad mesylate, and modafinil can improve poststroke fatigue.[72,75] Naturalistic light was also reported to improve poststroke fatigue.[69] A systematic review and meta-analysis reported on the effects of several nonpharmacologic interventions, including cognitive behavioral therapy.[75]

Excessive Daytime Sleepiness and Hypersomnia

Poststroke sleepiness manifests with different phenotypes. Patients most often present with EDS, increase in sleep needs (hypersomnia), or a combination of both (Figure 103.4). Occasionally, EDS/hypersomnia can alternate with insomnia.[76]

Hypersomnia is often preceded by sopor or coma and typically often evolves to apathy with lack of spontaneity (and initiative) and slowness (and poverty) of movements (so-called *akinetic mutism*). Rarely, patients with deep (subcortical) hemispheric and thalamic strokes exhibit a so-called presleep behavior, during which they yawn, stretch, close their eyes, curl up, and assume a normal sleeping posture while complaining of a constant sleep urge.[77] Removal of these patients from bed can result in repeated attempts to lie down and adopt a sleeping posture. During what appear to be daytime sleep periods, relatively quick responses to questions or requests suggest, however, a preserved wakefulness. For this peculiar dissociation between lack of auto-activation in the presence of preserved heteroactivation, the term *athymormia*, or "pure psychic akinesia," was coined.[78]

Epidemiology and Impact

Based on 27 studies in the literature, the frequency of poststroke EDS can be estimated to be around 10% to 30%.[79] The different methods to assess insomnia and intervals after stroke in which patients were studied explain the high variability in results found in the literature (from 9% up to 72%).[58,79] The frequency of poststroke hypersomnia is essentially unknown. The evolution of poststroke EDS is poorly known. Some data suggest the possibility of a persistence over years.

Poststroke hypersomnia usually improves, but in severe cases (e.g., after paramedian thalamic stroke) it can persist over years[80] (Figure 103.5).

Associations and Pathophysiology

Reduced arousal because of lesions involving the ascending arousal pathways is the most common cause of poststroke hypersomnia, whereas SDB is rarely the underlying main cause.[81] Mental arousal seems to be affected more severely by medial lesions, whereas motor arousal (including spontaneous motor activities) is impaired more strongly by lateral

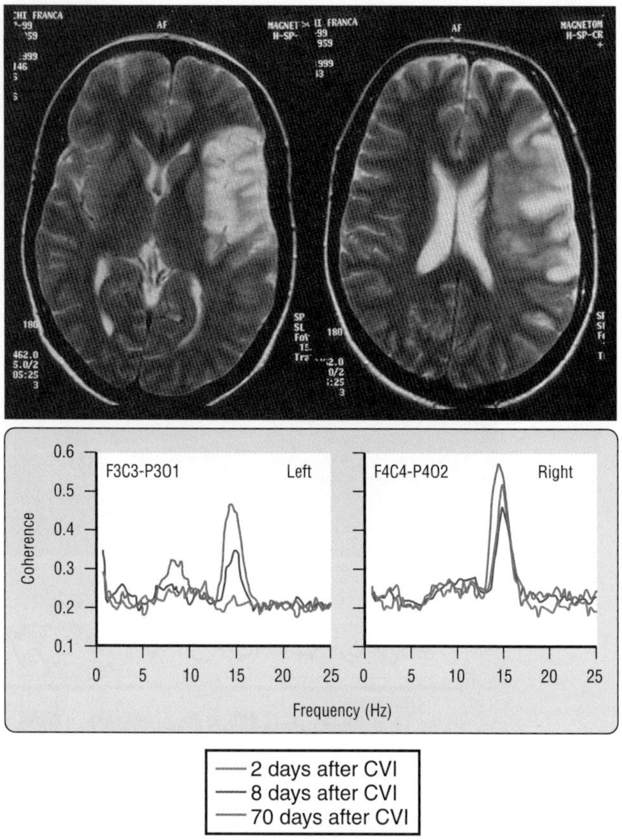

Figure 103.4 Hypersomnia/sleep electroencephalogram (EEG) changes after left middle cerebral artery stroke. A 39-year-old female patient with aphasia, right hemiparesis, depressed mood, and crying spells. National Institute of Health (NIH) Stroke Score = 16. In the first 1 to 2 poststroke weeks, increase in sleep needs (12 hours/day compared with 7 hours/day before stroke), followed by mild excessive daytime sleepiness (Epworth Sleepiness Score = 12). At 12 months, patient reports a decrease in sleep needs (10/24 hours). Repeated polysomnographic recordings (day 2, 8, and 70 days after stroke) demonstrate a progressive recovery of spindling activity (coherent activity around 12 Hz) over both the affected *(left)* and the nonaffected *(right)* hemispheres.

lesions.[82,83] In large hemispheric strokes, loss of arousal and coma can occur with injury to the upper brainstem secondary to brain edema and herniation. Rarely, hypersomnia resulting from thalamic, mesencephalic, or pontine stroke is accompanied by an excessive production of sleep, which can be documented polysomnographically.[56,80,84,85]

The most severe and persistent hypersomnia occurs in patients with bilateral lesions of the paramedian thalamus (Figure 103.5), thalamo-subthalamic area, and tegmental midbrain where fibers of the ascending arousal pathways are bundled and can be severely injured even by relatively small lesions. Hypersomnia after hemispheric stroke (Figure 103.4) usually occurs with large lesions, on the left more than on the right, and anteriorly more than posteriorly.[86-88] Upper tegmental pontine and paramedian pontomedullary lesions can also be accompanied by EDS/hypersomnia (Figure 103.6).[84,89]

Aside from the brain damage, other factors may contribute to poststroke EDS/hypersomnia, including medical disorders (e.g., heart failure, pulmonary disease, infections), SDB, psychotropic medications, and depression.[79]

Diagnosis and Treatment

Diagnosis is made on clinical grounds. Questionnaires (e.g., Epworth Sleepiness Scales) and actigraphy can be useful for

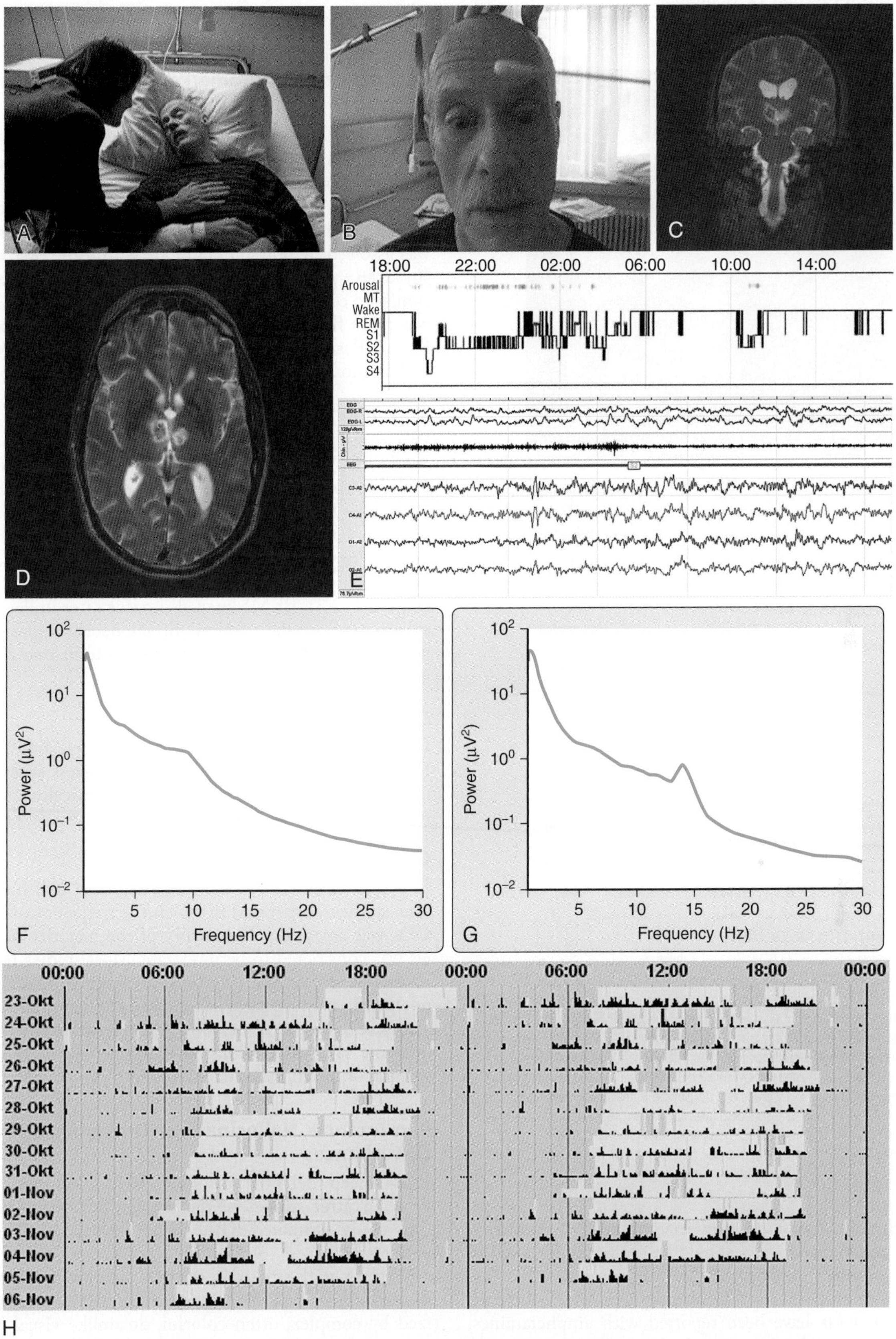

Figure 103.5 Hypersomnia after bilateral paramedian thalamic stroke. A 65-year-old male patient with initial coma, followed by severe hypersomnia **(A),** vertical gaze palsy **(B),** amnesia, and disturbed time perception ("Zeitgefühl"). Brain magnetic resonance imaging (MRI) shows a bilateral paramedian thalamic stroke (**C, D**). Polysomnography performed 12 days after stroke onset demonstrates **(E)** a drastic reduction of sleep spindles **(F)** and loss of spindle peak (12–14 Hz activity) on spectral analysis (compared with normal control **[G]**). A severe central apnea (apnea-hypopnea index of 54/hr) was observed in the acute phase (in the absence of any signs of cardiac dysfunction) but not on follow-up a few months later. Actigraphy performed within the first month after stroke shows time "asleep" (rest or sleep) during 61% of the recording time (2 weeks) **(H).** One year after stroke, the patient still reports increased sleep needs (15 hours per day), apathy (athymormia), and attentional/memory deficits. Modafinil at a dose of 200 mg per day improved his hypersomnia. (Modified from Bassetti, Sleep and stroke. In: Handbook of Clinical Neurology. Sleep disorders, 2011.)

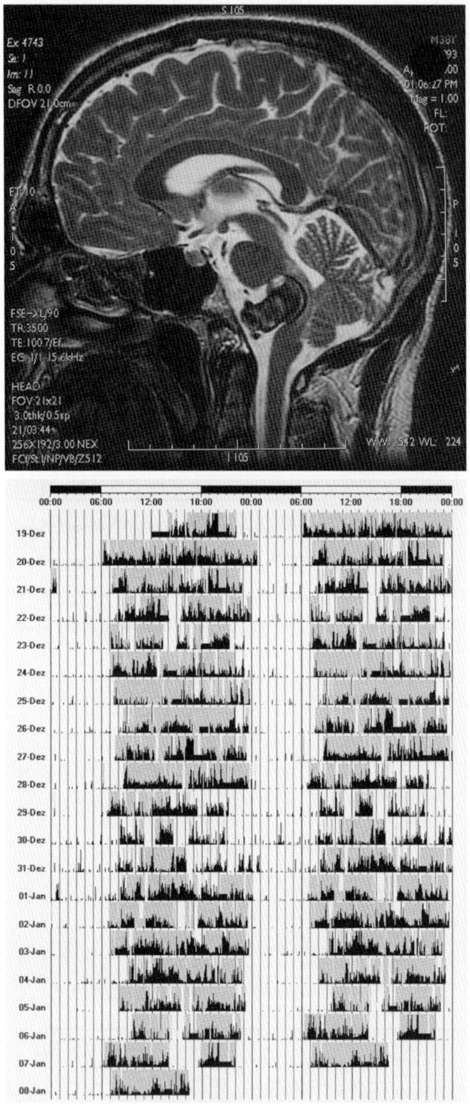

A

B

Figure 103.6 Hypersomnia/excessive daytime sleepiness (EDS) after ponto-medullary stroke in a 39-year-old male patient with ponto-medullary ischemia after subarachnoid hemorrhage and embolization of a giant aneurysm of the basilar artery (A). Clinically brainstem syndrome with singultus; left IX, X, and XII palsy; dysarthria; gait ataxia; and mild left hemiparesis. Postintervention severe EDS (Epworth Sleepiness Score: 23/24) and increased sleep needs (12–14 hr/day). Polysomnography (not shown): sleep efficiency 97%, slow wave sleep 8% (of total sleep time), no sleep apnea, no periodic limb movements of sleep. Multiple sleep latency test: mean sleep latency 1 minute, no sleep-onset REM periods. Actigraphy (B): time "asleep" (rest or sleep) during 43% of the recording time (2 weeks). Normal cerebrospinal fluid levels of hypocretin-1. Patient declined treatment for his EDS/hypersomnia.

the recognition of poststroke hypersomnia.[58,80,81] Polysomnography and vigilance tests should be used only for unclear, severe, or persisting poststroke EDS/hypersomnia.

Treatment of poststroke hypersomnia is often difficult, but improvements have been reported with amphetamines, modafinil, methylphenidate, and dopaminergic agents.[81] Bromocriptine may improve apathy and presleep behavior.[78] Treatment of an associated depression with stimulating antidepressants may also help. It is noteworthy that a favorable influence on early poststroke rehabilitation was reported for both methylphenidate (5 to 30 mg/day) and levodopa (100 mg/day), an effect that may be partially related to improved arousal.[90,91]

Restless Legs Syndrome/Periodic Limb Movements of Sleep

Epidemiology and Impact

The frequency of poststroke RLS can be estimated, based on eight studies in the available literature, to be around 5% to 15%.[13,58,92-94] In one study RLS was more frequent in stroke patients then in controls.[93] In the SAS-CARE study PLMS was assessed by polysomnography within the first week after stroke (n = 169) and 3 months later (n = 191) and found to be similar to controls.[95] In a more recent study, poststroke PLMS was more frequent in patients with RLS than those without RLS.[94] Poststroke RLS predicts a worse stroke outcome at 3 and 12 months and a lower quality of life.[96,97]

Associations and Pathophysiology

Poststroke RLS was reported to be associated with female gender, depression, and low serum ferritin levels.[94] Poststroke RLS can appear "de novo" or represent a preexisting condition. Poststroke RLS appears to be more frequent with subcortical (e.g., caudate), thalamic, and pontine stroke.[92,98-101] It can be bilateral or involve the paralyzed side.[99] After stroke, PLMS can worsen (and even appear de novo) and lead to insomnia (Figure 103.3). PLMS may also occur after unilateral hemispheric and spinal strokes. Spontaneous improvement of poststroke RLS was noted in one study in one out of four patients.[92]

Diagnosis and Treatment

Diagnosis is made on clinical grounds. Questionnaires (e.g., RLS Severity Score) are often used to assess severity. Treatment of poststroke RLS was not systematically studied. Few reports suggest a good response to dopaminergic drugs.[92]

Circadian Disturbances

In a systematic review and meta-analysis published in 2019, nine studies were found in which the frequency of poststroke CDs was assessed.[9] The quality of the majority of the studies was considered to be moderate. Most studies reported an alteration of circadian rhythms (as assessed by actigraphy or nocturnal serum melatonin) but also self-reported chronotype after stroke and an association with a less favorable functional outcome.[9] An association was found between CD and stroke severity or functional outcome.[9]

Parasomnias, Hallucinations/Dreaming, and Other Disturbances

REM sleep behavior disorder (RBD) has been reported to occur after strokes in the tegmentum of the pons.[102,103] One study estimated RBD to be present in 11% of stroke patients.[104]

Patients with strokes in the pons, midbrain, or paramedian thalamus may experience peduncular hallucinosis, characterized by complex, often colorful, dreamlike visual hallucinations, particularly in the evening and at sleep onset (Figure 103.7).[4,105,106] Peduncular hallucinosis may represent a release of REM sleep mentation and can be associated with insomnia.

Cessation or reduction of dreaming occurs in the Charcot-Wilbrand syndrome and can be limited to an alteration of the visual component of dreams.[107,108] This syndrome can occur with parieto-occipital, occipital, or deep frontal strokes, which are often bilateral.[109-111] Patients frequently also exhibit

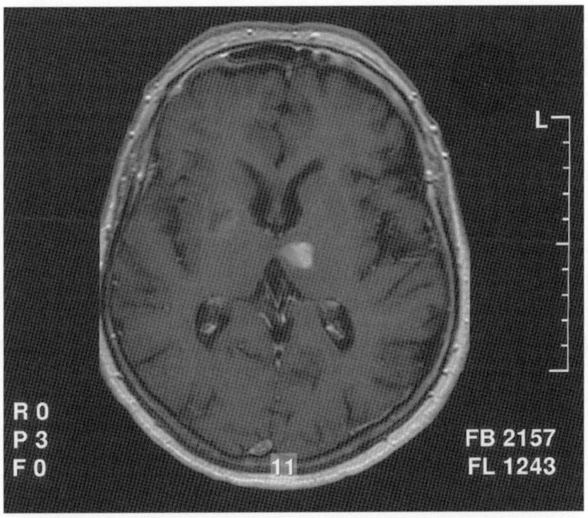

Figure 103.7 Dreamlike hallucinations after unilateral paramedian thalamic stroke in a 62-year-old patient (PV) with left paramedian thalamic stroke who presented clinically with confusional state, abulia, anomia, and moderate-severe amnesia in the absence of major sleep-wake disturbances. In the first few days after hospital admission, recurrent episodes of visual and acoustic hallucinations in the form of human figures (mostly relatives, partial insight), seen on the right side of the visual field, which the patient describes as dreamlike. At 7 months after stroke, the patient had persistent memory problems and reported almost daily episodes of psychic hallucinations ("sensed presence") and a disturbed time perception ("Zeitgefühl").

deficient revisualization, topographic amnesia, and prosopagnosia. REM sleep may be preserved.[110] Loss of dreaming with insomnia was reported also after lateral medullary stroke.[64] An increased frequency or vividness of dreaming may occur after stroke, particularly with thalamic, parietal, and occipital strokes.[111]

Focal (temporal) seizures secondary to stroke can lead to the syndrome of dream-reality confusion or to recurrent nightmares, which may be more frequent with right-sided lesions.[112]

A few patients with severe motor deficits may report the persistence of seemingly normal motor function within their dreams for up to several years after stroke. Waking up in the morning is a source of great distress in these patients. In other patients, motor handicap may, conversely, be apparent and incorporated in dreams within a few days of stroke onset.

Other disturbances include an abnormal transition from wakefulness to sleep and vice versa (with a dream-reality confusion) and an altered perception of time (so-called *Zeitgefühl*, Figures 103.5 and 103.7).[113,114]

POSTSTROKE SLEEP EEG/POLYSOMNOGRAPHY

In a systematic review and meta-analysis published in 2016, 44 studies were found in which patients after stroke were assessed by polysomnography/sleep EEG, 15 of which included also a control group.[48] The meta-analysis revealed that patients with stroke have poorer sleep (lower sleep efficiency, shorter total sleep time sleep, less time in stage 2 sleep) than controls. The systematic review revealed a strong bias toward studies in the early phase of stroke.[48]

Changes in sleep EEG after stroke depend on the following factors: (1) preexisting condition (e.g., age, SDB); (2) topography and size of the brain lesion; (3) complications of stroke (e.g., SDB, fever, infections, depression, anxiety); (4) medications; and (5) interval after stroke onset. The influence of noncerebral factors is stressed by the fact that acute myocardial infarction patients also experience sleep EEG changes.[115]

Several studies suggest that acute poststroke sleep EEG changes such as low sleep efficiency, decreased spindles, slow-wave sleep, and REM sleep are associated with a worse functional outcome.[47,53,116,117]

Like the wake EEG, the sleep EEG also undergoes changes in the postacute phase of stroke, reflecting overall recovery but also neuroplasticity processes and possibly even therapeutic interventions.[47,49,51,54,55,118]

Supratentorial Strokes

Reductions in non–rapid eye movement (NREM) sleep, total sleep time, and sleep efficiency can follow acute supratentorial stroke.[117,119-123] Reduced spindling can be observed with thalamic and cortical-subcortical strokes (Figure 103.5).[56,80,124,125] With unilateral thalamic strokes, sleep spindles may be preserved.[56,80,126,127] Spindling and slow-wave sleep can occasionally increase in the acute stage of large middle cerebral artery stroke.[116,120] In some cases, the increase in slow-wave sleep with cortical stroke reflects an increase in lesional delta activity during both sleep and wakefulness.[44,128]

A reduction in REM sleep can be observed in the acute phase of a supratentorial stroke in both experimental animals and humans and be linked with a poorer outcome.[53,116,120,121,129] Sawtooth waves can be decreased bilaterally in large hemispheric strokes, especially in those that involve the right side.[123] Cortical blindness has been associated with a reduction of rapid eye movements.[130]

In hemispheric strokes, sleep EEG changes can recover over time even in patients with large lesions (>50 mL in volume).[123] In paramedian thalamic strokes, clinical recovery can occur despite the persistence of reduction in spindles/NREM sleep (Figure 103.5).[56,80]

Infratentorial Strokes

Mesencephalic (midbrain) strokes can increase REM sleep. Ponto-mesencephalic strokes can decrease NREM sleep without effects on REM sleep.[62] Unilateral pontine strokes can not only alter the sleep EEG ipsilesionally, but also abolish selectively REM or REM sleep.[131-135] Bilateral infarcts in the dorsal pons can reduce both NREM and REM sleep.[84,134,136-139] Isolated REM sleep loss can persist for years without obvious cognitive or behavioral consequences.[137,138]

> **CLINICAL PEARLS**
>
> - Clinicians should consider SWD as a potential risk factor for stroke in addition to modulators of its outcome.
> - The study of poststroke SWD offers a unique opportunity to expand our knowledge about the brain mechanisms involved in sleep-wake regulation.

SUMMARY

SWDs, including OSA, long sleep duration, insomnia, EDS, PLMS (but not RLS), and CDs, are independent risk factors for stroke. In stroke patients, OSA and nonapneic SWD are observed in 20% to 50% of strokes that arise from preexisting factors (e.g., age), brain damage, and stroke complications (e.g., pain, mood changes, immobilization, drugs) and negatively affect stroke evolution and outcome. Poststroke sleep EEG changes reflect the topography and severity of stroke but also neuroplasticity changes and recovery processes involved in functional outcome. Animal and human observations support the hypothesis that sleep and treatment of SWD may positively influence stroke outcome.

SELECTED READINGS

Bassetti CLA, Randerath W, Vignatelli L, et al. EAN/ERS/ESO/ESRS statement on the impact of sleep disorders on risk and outcome of stroke. *Eur J Neurol*. 2020;55:1117–1134.

Facchin L, Schöne C, Mensen A, et al. Slow waves promote sleep-dependent plasticity and functional recovery after stroke. *J Neurosci*. 2020. in press.

Fan M, Sun D, Zhou T, et al. Sleep patterns, genetic susceptibility, and incident cardiovascular disease: a prospective study of 385 292 UK biobank participants. *Eur Heart J*. 2020;41:1182–1189.

Gottlieb E, Landau E, Baxter H. The bidirectional impact of sleep and circadian rhythm dysfunction in human ischaemic stroke: a systematic review. *Sleep Med Rev*. 2019;45:54–69.

Mensen A, Pigorini A, Facchin L, al e. Sleep as a model to understand neuroplasticity and recovery after stroke: observational, perturbational and interventional approaches. *J Neuroscience Methods*. 2019;313:37–43.

A complete reference list can be found online at ExpertConsult.com.

Chapter 104

Sleep and Neuromuscular Diseases

Kevin S. Gipson; Christian Guilleminault†; Michelle T. Cao

Chapter Highlights

- Patients with neuromuscular diseases (NMDs) are at risk for sleep-related problems, including sleep-disordered breathing (SDB), nocturnal hypoventilation, and when most severe, diurnal hypoventilation and respiratory insufficiency.
- Many factors may contribute to poor sleep quality and quantity in NMDs.
- Perhaps the greatest advances in the medical treatment of NMDs have come from increasingly effective management of SDB. The use of noninvasive ventilatory support devices has improved morbidity and mortality in this patient group.

Neuromuscular diseases (NMDs) are disorders of the motor unit comprising the lower motor neuron, nerve root, peripheral nerve, myoneural junction, and muscle.

Patients with neuromuscular syndromes are at increased risk for sleep-related problems. Weakness, rigidity, and spasticity may limit a person's ability to move and reposition themselves during sleep, causing discomfort, pain, and sleep disruption. Difficulty maintaining comfortable positions may lead to cramping, abnormal and uncontrolled movements, and weakness, all of which also contribute to poor sleep. Abnormal sphincter control may induce nocturia, incomplete emptying or incontinence, constipation, or painful defecation.

Sleep-related changes in breathing put the patient with a neuromuscular disorder at risk by impairing ventilation. In most NMDs, chronic respiratory muscle failure typically develops over years. It may initially present with sleep-disordered breathing (SDB), followed by progression to nocturnal hypoventilation, then diurnal hypoventilation, cor pulmonale, and eventual respiratory failure and end-stage disease. The slow progression of ventilatory failure in some disorders may go undetected for some time and, as a consequence, may contribute to increased mortality in this population.

Often, insufficient attention is paid to the impact of sleep-related issues in patients with NMD, particularly because most sleep medicine providers see only a small number of patients with neuromuscular disorders. Even in specialized neuromuscular clinics, a minority of patients are asked about their sleep problems or have undergone a prior sleep evaluation.[1] Moreover, some sleep medicine specialists are uncomfortable managing the common problems in this population, such as spasticity, sphincter dysfunction, pain, abnormal movement, and confusional arousal, which can contribute to sleep fragmentation, insomnia, parasomnias, daytime fatigue, and hypersomnolence. As such, patients with neuromuscular disorders benefit from a multidisciplinary approach to treatment, and this should be considered the standard of care.

†Deceased.

EPIDEMIOLOGY AND GENETICS

Each neuromuscular syndrome has a distinct pathogenesis and unique epidemiologic characteristics. Although robust cumulative data to describe the overall prevalence of NMD remains elusive, one recent Canadian study suggests that the prevalence of NMD is increasing by around 8% to 10% per year across all age groups in the context of declining mortality rates.[2] Many neurologic disorders, such as maltase deficiency, myopathy, myotonic dystrophy (MD), Rett syndrome, and familial dysautonomia, have a clear genetic origin. Other neuromuscular disorders may be secondary to traumatic, infectious, vascular, malignant, or degenerative diseases.

Although much research has addressed abnormal sleep and breathing in patients with NMDs, there are few large studies that characterize the prevalence of SDB in these patients.[3–6] One study from New Mexico attempted to gather information from its entire neuromuscular clinic population.[1] Although complete data were available for only 60 patients (20% of the clinic population), the investigators demonstrated that sleep and breathing abnormalities were present in more than 40% of patients.[1] Such a high prevalence is not surprising, given the vulnerability of such patients to sleep-related reductions in muscle tone and overall ventilation. Patients with spinal cord injury (SCI) have been better studied. Compared with the normal population, individuals with SCI have significantly greater difficulties falling asleep and subjectively poor sleep; they also frequently require prescriptions for sleep aids, sleep more hours, take more frequent and longer naps, and have a greater incidence of snoring.[7]

PATHOPHYSIOLOGY

The diaphragm is the major muscle of respiration during wakefulness and sleep. During non–rapid eye movement (NREM) sleep, there is an overall reduction in ventilation due to altered chemosensation and increased impedance of the respiratory system. However, rib cage activity is maintained (albeit reduced), as is diaphragmatic activity. The importance of the diaphragm is particularly evident during rapid eye movement (REM) sleep. During REM sleep, there is postsynaptic inhibition of somatic motor neurons, causing further reduction or complete loss of tone in the intercostals and other muscles of respiration; however, the diaphragm is relatively unaffected. Any process affecting the diaphragm, whether through a myopathy or a disruption of its innervation, can significantly reduce ventilation and oxygenation during REM sleep. In patients with bilateral diaphragmatic paralysis who are dependent on the accessory respiratory muscles for breathing, marked oxygen desaturations can occur during REM sleep.[8,9] The REM sleep-related inhibition of intercostal and accessory muscles leads to profound hypoventilation during this sleep stage. A "vicious cycle" occurs wherein muscle weakness and chest wall restriction leads to low tidal volumes and thus persistent microatelectasis, worsened lung compliance, and ventilation/perfusion mismatch.[10]

In some genetic neuromuscular disorders, muscle weakness may begin early in development, interfering with normal development of the skull and facial bones. For example, orofacial muscle weakness can affect growth of the maxilla and mandible, resulting in in the "long face" seen in congenital MD.[11] In rhesus monkeys, experimental reduction of nostril size by ligature, with consequent impairment of nasal breathing, leads to abnormal facial muscle contraction and secondary abnormal orofacial bone growth.[12,13] Similarly, in humans impaired nasal breathing leads to abnormal masseter contractions, consequently limiting orofacial growth.[14] Narrowing of dental arches, reduction in maxillary arch length, anterior crossbite, maxillary overjet, and overall narrowing of the facial skeleton are a result of changes in muscle contractions. These facial skeletal changes decrease upper airway diameter, consequently increasing its collapsibility during sleep.

Depending on the type of neuromuscular disorder, sleep-related breathing abnormalities may present as central apneas, obstructive apneas, nasal airflow limitation, or periods of prolonged hypoventilation, or there may be a combination that renders the neuromuscular patient at times difficult to treat. Sleep disruption with frequent cortical arousals may be due to discomfort with certain positions, muscle spasm, difficulty in clearing secretions, sphincter control, or an increase in upper airway resistance related to muscle weakness and secondary craniofacial changes. Hypoventilation is quite prevalent in NMD.[15] Periods of hypoventilation can contribute to arousals, reduced sleep time, and sleep deprivation from ventilatory and arousal responses to changes in oxygen and carbon dioxide (CO_2) levels. Although these changes may protect ventilation in the short term, over time ventilatory responses to changes in oxygen and CO_2 levels become blunted, leading to further worsening of hypoventilation, eventually occurring during both wakefulness and sleep.

CLINICAL FEATURES COMMON TO MOST NEUROMUSCULAR DISORDERS

Nonspecific complaints, such as increased fatigue, daytime hypersomnolence, or disrupted sleep, are the often subtle initial manifestations of a slowly evolving NMD of adult onset.[1] Such nonspecific complaints may also be the sole indication of a progressive neuromuscular disorder. Problems of oropharyngeal airway clearance and gastrointestinal transit can lead to significant drooling, esophageal reflux, or pulmonary infections from aspiration or retained secretions. Impairment of cough mechanisms may further impair the ability to clear secretions.

Autonomic dysfunction may manifest as abnormal sensitivity to temperature or pressure, with discomfort related to the use of sheets and blankets. As in other chronic diseases, patients with neuromuscular disorders may be at increased risk for the development of anxiety, depression, and insomnia. Pharmacologic agents for NMD that are prescribed to be taken in the evening may have alerting effects, whereas others used in the morning may lead to daytime sleepiness. In all, patients with chronic neuromuscular disorders may have many factors disrupting sleep, consequently worsening daytime function and quality of life (QOL).

Neurodegenerative Diseases Involving the Motor Neuron

Amyotrophic lateral sclerosis (ALS) is a degenerative motor neuron disease involving upper and lower motor neurons, leading to muscle weakness and atrophy throughout the body. ALS affects an estimated 0.005% of the population of the United States. Although ALS has not been shown to directly affect the sleep-regulating areas of the brain, it is likely that indirect effects of the disease contribute to sleep disruption.[16–18] SDB is reported in 17% to 76% of patients with ALS.[19] ALS patients with normal respiratory function, normal phrenic motor responses, and preserved motor units on electromyography may still have SDB with periodic oxygen desaturations independent of sleep stage (REM or NREM).[20] However, respiratory-related sleep disruption is generally not significant until phrenic motor neurons are involved and the diaphragm becomes weak. When there is involvement of the diaphragm, severe hypoventilation and hypoxemia occur during REM sleep, and nearly all these patients will need some form of ventilatory support. Periodic limb movements associated with arousals and SDB may cause sleep disruption in ALS patients. Some ALS patients without any respiratory disturbance or periodic limb movements still experience sleep fragmentation, independent of age. This suggests that other factors contribute to disturbed sleep, such as anxiety, depression, pain, coughing or choking, excessive secretions, muscle fasciculation, cramps, and the inability to find a comfortable position or turn oneself freely in bed. Orthopnea, a frequent complaint in ALS, may also contribute to sleep disruption.[17,18]

Spinal Cord Disease

Poliovirus infection targets the nervous system in several ways by injuring cranial motor nuclei and spinal cord anterior horn cells, resulting in acute paresis and impairing normal breathing. Abnormalities in central regulation of breathing in patients with acute and convalescent poliomyelitis were described in 1958 by Plum and Swanson.[21] Subsequently, central, mixed, and obstructive apneas have been noted.[22] Sleep and breathing abnormalities are seen not only in patients who are on respiratory assistance (e.g., rocking beds used to augment ventilation) during sleep but also before ventilatory assistance is initiated.[23] These abnormalities include decreased sleep efficiency, increased arousal frequency, and varying degrees of apnea and hypopnea. After treatment of sleep and breathing abnormalities, many symptoms frequently attributed to the postpolio syndrome (PPS) do improve. Although not all symptoms of the PPS can be explained, excessive daytime sleepiness and fatigue may be explained by poor sleep quality related to abnormal respiration during sleep.[24,25]

Poliomyelitis can alter central and peripheral respiratory function decades after the acute infection, an important element of PPS.[24] Muscle atrophy and immobility can lead to kyphoscoliosis and restricted ventilation. The anatomic deformities resulting from poliomyelitis may cause chronic pain and consequent sleep abnormalities. Bulbar involvement may affect upper airway muscles, contributing to SDB and airway clearance problems. SDB is reported in 31% of patients with PPS.[24] Prolongation of REM sleep latency may result from prolonged recruitment time related to damaged neurons in the pontine tegmentum.[26]

Inherited metabolic diseases, such as subacute necrotizing encephalomyelopathy (Leigh disease), typically appear in childhood and may be associated with respiratory disturbance. Rarely, this disease may appear in adulthood with respiratory failure during sleep.[27] Syringomyelia can be associated with central, mixed, and obstructive apneas when it involves the bulbar and high cervical neurons.[28] Malformations of the skull base or high cervical junction (platybasia, Chiari malformations) may cause both central and obstructive types of sleep apnea.[29]

Traumatic SCI has dramatically increased in frequency over the past 30 years owing to an increase in traffic accidents and military conflicts. Incidence rates are highest in the second to fourth decades of life, and with improvements in long-term supportive care providing longer life expectancy, the prevalence of SCI will likely continue to increase.[30] Overall, morbidity and mortality are higher with cervical and high thoracic spinal cord lesions, especially in ventilator-dependent individuals.[31–33] In an epidemiologic survey from Stockholm, muscle spasm, pain, paresthesias, and voiding problems were reported as the most important causes of sleep disturbance.[7]

In tetraplegic patients, the higher the spinal cord lesion, the more significant the impairment, not only with diaphragm, intercostal, and abdominal muscle weakness but also with impaired cough and other reflexes for laryngeal and lung clearance.[32,33] Gastrointestinal problems related to autonomic dysfunction, including impairment of gastrointestinal motility and worsened reflux, are common.[32,33] In addition, spinal cord injury increases the development of neurogenic obesity.[33a] All these elements together can impair breathing, especially during sleep.[31,33] High cord lesions can interrupt pathways to the superior cervical sympathetic ganglion that regulate melatonin secretion.[34,35]

Pharmacologic agents used by patients with SCI (antispasmodics, analgesics, drugs for dysautonomia, psychoactive substances) can also disrupt sleep and wakefulness. An important feature seen in cervical lesions is progressive ventilatory impairment during sleep noted between the 15th day and the 13th week after the injury, often after the patient has been released from an acute care setting. Such worsening may lead to a higher percentage of deaths during sleep, as reported in a cohort of patients with mid to lower cervical SCI during this time period.[36]

Polyneuropathies

The most common polyneuropathy associated with SDB is Charcot-Marie-Tooth disease (CMT).[37] CMT is characterized by chronic degeneration of peripheral nerves and roots, resulting in distal muscle atrophy that begins at the feet and legs and later involves the hands. SDB may occur in these patients as result of a pharyngeal neuropathy leading to upper airway obstruction (obstructive apnea, upper airway resistance syndrome) or secondary to diaphragmatic dysfunction.[38,39] Secondary autonomic neuropathies, for example that related to uncontrolled type 1 diabetes, may be associated with impaired chemosensitivity to CO_2, although the effects on sleep and breathing are inconsistent.[40]

Neuromuscular Junction Diseases

Myasthenia gravis (MG) is an autoimmune disorder of the neuromuscular junction resulting in weakness and fatigability of skeletal muscles. Sleep breathing abnormalities can occur as a result of diaphragmatic or pharyngeal weakness. Risk factors for the development of sleep-related ventilatory problems in patients with MG include age, restrictive pulmonary syndrome, diaphragmatic weakness, and daytime hypoventilation.[41] Younger patients with a shorter duration of illness are less likely to experience sleep-related hypoventilation or hypoxemia, whereas older patients with increased body mass index, abnormal total lung capacity, and abnormal daytime blood gases are more likely to develop hypopneas or apneas, particularly during REM sleep.[42,43] In one study, sleep apnea was diagnosed in 60% of patients with MG, even when the disease was in a clinically stable stage.[44,45] A prospective study by Nicolle and colleagues[46] found that obstructive sleep apnea (OSA) was the predominant abnormality, occurring in 36% of MG patients, with significant associations with older age, male gender, elevated body mass index, and corticosteroid use.

Other neuromuscular disorders that can disturb sleep include congenital myasthenic syndromes, botulism, hypermagnesemia, and tick paralysis.[47] Taking a careful history is extremely helpful in making the diagnosis in these circumstances. Dyspnea that worsens with activity, morning headache, paroxysmal nocturnal dyspnea, fragmented sleep, and daytime somnolence are among the commonest symptoms that suggest SDB in these syndromes.

Muscle Diseases

Myotonic Dystrophy

MD is an autosomal dominant disorder that causes myotonia, muscle weakness, and daytime sleepiness. In this illness, there is consistent involvement of facial, masseter, levator palpebrae, sternocleidomastoid, forearm, hand, and pretibial muscles; MD is, in a sense, a distal myopathy. However, pharyngeal and laryngeal muscles may also be involved, as well as respiratory muscles, in particular the diaphragm.

Central nervous system abnormalities also occur in MD type 1 and 2 (although more severe in type 1), causing excessive daytime sleepiness by different mechanisms.[11,48,49] For example, neurodegeneration in the dorsomedial nuclei of the thalamus can lead to a medial thalamic syndrome characterized by apathy, memory loss, and mental deterioration. Loss of 5-hydroxytryptamine (serotonin) neurons of the dorsal raphe nucleus and the superior central nucleus, as well as dysfunction of the hypothalamic hypocretin-orexin system, can result in short sleep latencies and sleep-onset REM periods on the Multiple Sleep Latency Test.[48–51] Daytime sleepiness is particularly common in patients with MD, occurring in 33% to 77% of patients, and is associated with lower QOL scores.[52,53]

Involvement of the respiratory muscles may result in SDB, including alveolar hypoventilation predominantly in REM sleep, obstructive apneas, and central apneas.[54–56] However, the development of SDB abnormalities in MD is not solely caused by muscle weakness. When patients with MD were compared with patients with nonmyotonic respiratory muscle weakness, periods of hypoventilation and apneas (central and obstructive) occurred at higher frequencies in those with MD than in nonmyotonic patients who had the same degree of muscle weakness (measured by maximal inspiratory and expiratory pressures).[57] This finding suggests that changes in the central nervous system control of respiration contribute to abnormal breathing in patients with MD.

Similarly, decreased ventilatory responses to hypoxia and hypercapnia and extreme sensitivity to sedative drugs suggest a central origin of the breathing impairments in MD.[58,59] The differential diagnosis requires further testing. A standard technique for assessing control of respiration is to study the increase in ventilation as a response to increased arterial CO_2. However, when respiratory muscles are weak, as in MD, it may be difficult to interpret a reduced ventilatory response. That is, chemoreceptor activity and efferent signaling to respiratory muscles may be intact, but weak or inefficient respiratory muscles may not produce a normal ventilatory response to a hypercapnic or hypoxic stimulus. Another method of assessing impairment of respiratory center output is measurement of mouth pressure developed at the beginning of a transiently occluded breath (occlusion pressure, $P_{0.1}$).[60,61] In patients with MD, $P_{0.1}$ may be as high or higher than that of control subjects at rest and during stimulated breathing, although overall ventilation is lower.[59,62] The finding of a high transdiaphragmatic pressure (P_{di}) despite overall lower ventilation suggests that increased impedance of the respiratory system accounts for incomplete transformation into ventilation of normal or increased respiratory center output.

Magnetic stimulation of the cortex, in conjunction with phrenic nerve recordings, can also be used to test the corticospinal tract to phrenic motor neuron pathways and is a reliable method for diagnosing and monitoring patients with impaired central respiratory drive.[63,64] The use of transcortical and cervical magnetic stimulation demonstrates that greater than 20% of MD patients have impaired central respiratory drive.[64] The finding of neuronal loss in the dorsal central, ventral central, and subtrigeminal medullary nuclei in MD patients with alveolar hypoventilation and the severe neuronal loss and gliosis in the tegmentum of the brainstem also support a central abnormality.[65,66]

Another problem in MD patients is orofacial growth impairment early in life. Craniofacial muscle weakness can negatively affect bone growth during development, particularly on orofacial muscles that are involved with stimulation of growth areas, such as the intermaxillary synchondrosis that usually becomes inactive near 15 years of age. As a consequence of muscular weakness, development of craniofacial structures in patients with MD is impaired. These patients may experience more vertical facial growth than normal subjects and so may have relatively narrowed maxillary arches and narrow palates as measured between the palatal shelves, with deeper depths. These craniofacial changes may contribute to the development of obstructive sleep apnea owing to a smaller maxilla and mandible, consequently restricting the size of the upper airway and leading to upper airway collapse during sleep.

Other Myopathies

Abnormalities in sleep and breathing have been reported in isolated series of patients with various neuromuscular disorders, such as congenital myopathies (nemaline or congenital fiber-type disproportion myopathy) or metabolic myopathies (mitochondrial myopathy such as Kearns-Sayre syndrome and acid maltase deficiency).[67–71] In all these cases there are various alterations in respiratory control and breathing pattern changes, including hypoventilation, obstructive apneas, and central apneas. All genetic myopathies with orofacial weakness have similar risks for impaired bone growth, particularly on the maxilla and mandible, as in MD.[13,14] Severe central sleep apnea and marked hypoxemia, particularly during REM sleep, resulting in hypoxia-induced pulmonary hypertension, excessive daytime sleepiness, heart failure, morning headaches, and rare nocturnal seizures, may be seen in patients with congenital muscular dystrophy.[72] OSA has also been described in Thomsen disease (myotonia congenita).[73]

Myopathies such as Duchenne muscular dystrophy (DMD) can cause restrictive lung disease and chest wall deformities.[74,75] These changes also contribute to ventilatory impairment, fragmented sleep, hypercapnia and hypoxemia (more profound during REM sleep), development of deformities, chronic pain, and discomfort.[76,77] There is a bimodal presentation of SDB in children with DMD, wherein OSA is more common in younger children in the first decade of life.[78,79] In younger children with DMD, OSA can improve with adenotonsillectomy, whereas in older children who have already developed hypoventilation, OSA is better managed with noninvasive ventilation (NIV). Young patients with DMD may be predisposed to central obesity related to chronic glucocorticoid therapy.[80] Overall, DMD patients experience significantly decreased sleep efficiency, an increase in REM sleep latency, decreased total REM, and worsened apnea-hypopnea index (particularly as obstructive apneas).[81]

Acid maltase deficiency myopathy can cause SDB, with rapid and significant diaphragmatic impairment noted long before the weakness of other skeletal muscles.[82] In fact, SDB and the secondary daytime fatigue may be presenting symptoms of the myopathy.[82]

Facioscapulohumeral muscular dystrophy (FSHD) is an autosomal dominant disease and the third most frequent form of muscular dystrophy, after DMD and MD. Della Marca and colleagues[83] evaluated FSHD patients and found that impaired sleep quality was directly correlated to the severity of the disease. Among 46 FSHD patients, 27 had snoring and 12 reported respiratory pauses during sleep.[83]

DIAGNOSTIC EVALUATION

An effective diagnostic strategy will be informed by the type of neurologic disorder, the degree of sensory and motor impairment and resulting disability, the associated autonomic defects, and the impact of the illness on the patient's mood. Understanding the patient's interaction with society and family is a critically important factor for making actionable treatment decisions. A detailed sleep history is required to outline the severity and type of sleep-related problems. Even in those cases where a clinician is mindful of the increased risk of SDB in the NMD population, efforts to screen patients for sleep breathing disorder may be frustrated by the unique nature of SDB in this group. In the earliest manifestations of SDB in NMD, patients are often not sleepy, and so the Epworth score may not be a useful screening tool.[84] General assessment should also determine the degree of pain and discomfort (particularly in the supine position and during sleep), the presence or absence of sphincter problems and urinary or digestive dysfunction during wake and sleep, and any evidence of autonomic dysfunction already present during wakefulness and suspected during sleep. Patient report of orthopnea in particular (e.g., a sense of dyspnea when lying in bed or when reclining in a bath) is a discerning screening finding that may indicate diaphragmatic weakness. Other additional diagnostic tests may supplement the evaluation of sleep in the patient with NMD. These include a disability index scale, a sleep disorder questionnaire, and a sleep log or actigraphy (helpful for the investigation of daily rhythms and sleep-wake disturbances during the 24-hour period).[1] The severe respiratory insufficiency questionnaire, a multidimensional health-related QOL instrument, may be used for patients with neuromuscular disorders on assisted ventilation.[85]

Clinicians should carefully look for craniofacial abnormalities, including high and narrow hard palate, teeth crowding, tongue indentations, and Mallampati and Friedman rating scales for evaluating the size of upper airway.[85,86] Routine measures of pulmonary function (spirometry, maximal inspiratory pressure [MIP], maximal expiratory pressure [MEP]), and gas exchange (arterial partial pressure of oxygen [Pao_2] and arterial partial pressure of carbon dioxide [$Paco_2$]) should be performed in all patients at initial presentation. Static lung volume measurements, both upright and after 15 minutes in supine position, often demonstrate significant changes caused by respiratory muscle weakness, particularly diaphragmatic weakness. A forced vital capacity (FVC) less than 50% of predicted, a $Paco_2$ greater than 45 mm Hg, and a base excess of 4 mmol/L or greater indicates significant ventilatory impairment, and initiation of nocturnal (at minimum) noninvasive ventilatory support should be implemented. An overnight polysomnography should be considered if the patient exhibits signs suggestive of early nocturnal respiratory impairment, particularly if FVC is greater than 50% predicted or other testing of daytime respiratory function (MIP, MEP) is minimally impaired or within normal range. Supine inspiratory vital capacity measurements of less than 70%, 50%, and 25% is expected to result in hypoventilation during REM sleep, full night, and daytime, respectively.[3,75,87] Diaphragmatic strength is best surveilled through a combination of MIP, changes from upright to supine FVC measurement, formal overnight oximetry recordings, and $Paco_2$ measurement.[88] Although MIP is an important surrogate for diaphragmatic strength in patients with NMD, accurate measurement can be adversely impacted by suboptimal patient effort and patient difficulty with the MIP interface due to bulbar and facial weakness.[89] "Sniff" nasal inspiratory pressure (SNIP) may be helpful in these cases, where available. Mean inspiratory and expiratory pressures and cough peak flow can additionally provide insight into a patient's cough strength and their ability to clear their airway of secretions (Table 104.1).

Overnight polysomnography is the key to a definitive evaluation of sleep and breathing in those patients in early stages of their disease (see Chapter 201 for further discussion). Attended in-laboratory evaluation permits important measurements, such as transcutaneous or end-tidal CO_2, allowing continuous tracking of ventilation during sleep and guiding the decision for nocturnal ventilatory assistance.[89a] Of note, as most sleep laboratories no longer routinely include esophageal manometry or diaphragm electromyography, diaphragm weakness in NMD may be misinterpreted as central or obstructive apneas.[90] Level I attended in-laboratory polysomnography remains the standard of care for children with known or suspected NMD.[91] Home sleep testing is not recommended for adults with NMD.

Table 104.1 Diagnostic Testing for Respiratory Insufficiency

Test	Recommended	Considered
Pulmonary Function Test (PFT)	Yes	
Supine PFT	Yes (normal upright PFT)	
Maximal inspiratory pressure and maximal expiratory pressure	Yes	
Peak cough flow	Yes	
Overnight polysomnogram with CO_2 monitoring ($Tcco_2$, $Etco_2$)	Yes (normal PFT)	
Sniff nasal inspiratory pressure		Yes
Arterial blood gas		Yes
Overnight pulse oximetry		Yes
Serum bicarbonate		Yes

CO_2, Carbon dioxide; $Etco_2$, end-tidal carbon dioxide; $Tcco_2$, transcutaneous carbon dioxide.

TREATMENT OF SLEEP ABNORMALITIES AND SEQUELAE IN PATIENTS WITH NEUROMUSCULAR DISEASE

Some of the greatest advances in the medical management of neuromuscular disorders has emerged from the early diagnosis of nocturnal or diurnal ventilatory impairment and the timely implementation of NIV.[92] The goal in these patients is restoration of normal sleep architecture, with subsequent improvement of sleep, daytime function, and QOL. Simple measures, such as bedding, are often overlooked. Specialized beds and mattresses are available to facilitate ease of positional changes fostering avoidance of skin lesions at pressure points and offer segmental inflation or deflation (e.g., air mattresses), thus improving autonomic dysfunction, cramps, spastic contraction, and rigidity. Great efforts should be made to diminish pain and discomfort of any type. Treatment of abnormal behavior and confusional arousals may necessitate use of sedatives, such as benzodiazepines, but such therapy should be considered only after careful evaluation of ventilatory function and risk for worsening the sleep-related abnormal breathing. Treatment of abnormal breathing during sleep should be based on polysomnographic findings and should be adjusted with regular follow-up, considering clinical symptoms and polysomnographic studies. Various therapies may improve nocturnal hypoventilation or offset the attendant oxygen desaturation.

Supplemental oxygen has been used to alleviate the REM sleep–related oxygen desaturation in patients with DMD but does not clearly improve sleep.[93] Repeated nocturnal hypoxia may worsen muscle weakness, which begets further oxygen desaturation, and reversal of the hypoxemia may arrest the muscle weakness. In one patient with acid maltase deficiency treated with nocturnal oxygen, hypoxemia and muscle weakness did not progress over an 8-year period.[94] Because most of the hypoventilation occurs during REM sleep, pharmacologic suppression of REM sleep with a tricyclic antidepressant is a theoretical option. In a small study of patients with DMD, protriptyline markedly improved the nocturnal oxygen saturation profile.[95,96] However, anticholinergic side effects limit the widespread use of such therapy. Inspiratory muscle training has improved waking respiration in one patient with acid maltase deficiency, with major improvement in the nocturnal oxygen saturation.

In children two syndromes have a high prevalence of sleep hypoventilation: DMD and spinal muscular atrophy. Both conditions can cause progressive hypoventilation during sleep and, as the disease progresses, hypoventilation during wakefulness. In this young age group, the appropriate time to begin airway clearance and to introduce noninvasive ventilatory support that can preserve or enhance lung growth and chest wall mobility must be carefully assessed. The presence of an imbalance between mechanical load and the capacity of the respiratory muscles must be evaluated because fatigue may occur, leading to respiratory failure. Inspiratory muscle training can significantly improve respiratory parameters in these patients.[97] Children with impaired orofacial bone development as a consequence of abnormal muscle contractions secondary to the genetically induced generalized muscle dystrophy may benefit from myofunctional reeducation (i.e., orofacial muscle exercises aiming at improving suction, mastication, swallowing, and nasal breathing).[98,99]

Judicious use of wake-promoting drugs, such as modafinil or armodafinil, can improve daytime alertness without nocturnal sleep disruption. Studies of patients with MD, ALS, and multiple sclerosis have shown beneficial effects of modafinil in improving daytime fatigue.[100–102] Baclofen can reduce muscle spasms and help nocturnal sleep but may worsen daytime sleepiness. Treatment of pain with opioids can complicate treatment of SDB by inducing sleep hypoventilation or central sleep apnea.

Noninvasive Positive Airway Pressure

Mechanical ventilation has been a mainstay in supporting ventilation since the days of the poliomyelitis epidemic. Rocking beds, negative-pressure "iron lung" ventilators, positive-pressure ventilation through tracheostomy, and cuirass ventilation have been long-term options in the past.[103] However, all these options are cumbersome, severely limit the mobility of patients, and may have unwanted complications. In response, other forms of assisted ventilation have been developed, including phrenic nerve pacing and noninvasive positive-pressure ventilation (NIPPV) devices.[104,105]

Positive airway pressure (PAP) devices, including bilevel therapy with backup respiratory rate and advanced PAP devices targeting tidal volume and minute ventilation by way of variable inspiratory pressure support have been used to treat hypoventilation in NMD. Treatment of hypoventilation requires adequate delivery of tidal volume and maintenance of minute ventilation to effectively eliminate CO_2, which is why continuous positive airway pressure (CPAP) is of limited utility in treating hypoventilation. As bilevel therapy acts as a noninvasive ventilator and supports ventilation, it also treats CO_2 retention, which is commonly seen in patients with advanced NMD. Low-flow oxygen can be bled into the nasal mask during nocturnal sleep, but it is usually not required and not routinely recommended. CPAP is contraindicated in NMD as it can increase work of breathing.

In the past 2 decades, NIPPV has significantly improved the natural course of NMD, and is now considered the first-line intervention for respiratory impairment. NIPPV has been shown to improve QOL and increase survival in neuromuscular disorders.[106–110] In PPS the median time for prolongation of life expectancy is more than 20 years. In patients with spinal muscular dystrophy types 2 and 3, DMD, and acid maltase deficiency, the median improvement in life expectancy is 10 years. In MD the median improvement in life expectancy is 4 years, and in ALS it is 1 to 2 years.[106,111,112] Compared with ventilation through tracheostomy, NIPPV through nasal interfaces and portable ventilators is now the preferred means of assisting ventilation because it is much simpler to administer, is more comfortable, and reduces costs.

With eradication of poliomyelitis in most of the world, ALS has become the most common neuromuscular disorder for which NIPPV is used. In the only randomized controlled clinical trial that demonstrated the value of noninvasive ventilatory support, ALS patients with orthopnea, maximum inspiratory pressure less than 60% of predicted, or symptomatic daytime hypercapnia, NIPPV significantly improved QOL, sleep-related symptoms, and survival in those without severe bulbar dysfunction.[106] NIPPV is now the standard of care, and implementation is recommended earlier than the study's entry point. Improvements from NIPPV continue to be greater than those achievable with any currently available pharmacotherapy. Therefore, for palliative indications, a trial of NIPPV in ALS patients may be warranted even in those with severe bulbar dysfunction. Recent studies also have demonstrated good tolerance of NIPPV in severe bulbar patients.[113]

Patients may require more ventilatory support during sleep, particularly with progressive muscle and diaphragm weakness. Advanced NIPPV devices are available specifically for treatment of hypoventilation during sleep by targeting tidal volume or minute ventilation (e.g., average volume-assured pressure support [AVAPS] and intelligent volume-assured pressure support [iVAPS]).[114] As the volume-assured devices adjust pressure support based on the patient's respiratory cycle breath by breath, they adapt to changes in severity of disease and therefore are ideal for sleep hypoventilation or progressive respiratory insufficiency (see Chapter 140 for further discussion). VAPS ventilation uses proprietary algorithms to dynamically adjust pressure support to meet a patient's ventilatory need. Newer devices also offer autotitrating expiratory positive airway pressure (EPAP), which has been found to be noninferior to fixed EPAP settings and which offers the promise of better maintaining airway patency throughout the night.[115,116] Study of sequential titration through bilevel ST (spontaneous timed) and AVAPS PAP modalities in patients with NMD demonstrated improved tidal volume, nadir NREM peripheral capillary oxygen saturation, respiratory rate, transcutaneous CO_2, and arousal index with AVAPS.[117] Adaptive servoventilation (ASV), an anticyclic PAP device, has been considered when opioid intake complicates the clinical presentation because of a high number of central apneas, provided that hypoventilation is not significant.[118,119] However, ASV is generally contraindicated in NMD, given its algorithm that targets a lower minute ventilation or peak flow compared to patient's own ventilation, resulting in some degree of hypoventilation during sleep. ASV is also contraindicated in patients with low cardiac ejection fraction in the setting of diffuse myopathies.

The choice of settings when choosing NIPPV can influence sleep architecture and quality in patients with NMD. Tailoring the settings (options available depending on portable ventilator used) to the individual's respiratory effort, rather than the usual or default parameters, is highly recommended and associated with better nighttime gas exchange, percentage of REM sleep, and sleep quality[120] (Table 104.2). The AVAPS mode, for example, requires predetermined tidal volume that is calculated from the patient's ideal body weight (IBW), with a recommended 6 to 8 mL/kg of IBW used instead of actual body weight. However, if rib cage and abdominal muscles are weak, the recommended volume setting for the patient may be too high, and pain may develop during chest expansion; in these cases we recommend decreasing the predetermined tidal volume to 6 to 7 mL/kg IBW.

Another parameter that may directly impact a patient's comfort and compliance is the "rise time" (i.e., the speed at which airflow is delivered from expiration to inspiration in 10ths of a second). It is adjusted based on the severity of thoracic muscle weakness, lung inflation capabilities, and amount of secretion accumulated in the airway. The inspiratory time is another important parameter that, when properly set, prevents premature ending of inspiratory cycle. Neuromuscular patients may be able to spontaneously trigger, but respiratory muscle weakness may prevent the ability to achieve a full inspiratory cycle, and therefore the patient's spontaneous inspiratory cycle may be prematurely cut off. When this occurs, the full tidal volume may not be delivered. We recommend an inspiratory cycle of at least 1.0 to 1.5 seconds in the stable outpatient setting. For certain devices, the inspiratory time is only activated in the pressure control modality, whereas in other devices the clinician is able to program a minimum and maximum inspiratory time, therefore guaranteeing a minimum inspiratory time duration. We highly recommend that the clinician become familiar with a given device's algorithms and technical features as this is important for effective ventilatory management.[121]

NIV mask interface selection is a nuanced and often underappreciated aspect of successful therapy. Treatment-induced upper airway obstruction has been associated with the use of oronasal masks in patients with ALS and other NMDs, and may be related to posterior displacement of the tongue or jaw.[122] In patients with NMD, nasal mask or pillow interfaces may be preferable as they are associated with improved comfort and adherence and do not carry this risk of worsened obstruction. Patients with NMD may habitually mouth-breathe secondary to masseter weakness, and so some degree of leak/oral pressure venting may need to be tolerated.[88]

Many patients benefit from daytime ventilatory support, which may help to both preserve ventilation and maintain lung volume recruitment, as well as preserve cough and swallow strength.[123–125] Mouthpiece ventilation (MPV), otherwise known as sip ventilation, can be a helpful daytime adjunctive respiratory support in patients with NMD, permitting as-needed positive pressure to facilitate breath-stacking and lung-volume recruitment during the day via "sips" of positive pressure from a small mouthpiece.[126] MPV is a noninvasive option only available on specific portable ventilators that can be programmed with two or more distinct modes for use during day and night. Success of MPV is demonstrated in the DMD population, given the relative lack of bulbar impairment. MPV has been shown to prevent hypoventilation, tracheostomy, preserve FVC, cough, speech, and swallowing strength in DMD.[148] For ALS, MPV can be successful for patients without bulbar weakness.[150]

Table 104.2 Suggested Settings for NIPPV for Neuromuscular Respiratory Failure

Setting	Recommendation
Mode	ST, PC, ±VAPS
EPAP	Low
Auto-EPAP	No (use set EPAP)
IPAP/PS	Medium to high
Vt	6–8 mL/kg (ideal body weight)
Rise time	Medium or slow (for bulbar weakness)
Ti	Long
BUR	Yes
AVAPS rate (if available)	Medium
Trigger sensitivity	High
Cycle sensitivity	Low

AVAPS, Average volume-assured pressure support; BUR, backup rate; EPAP, expiratory positive airway pressure; IPAP, inspiratory positive airway pressure; NIPPV, noninvasive positive-pressure ventilation; PC, pressure control; PS, pressure support; S, spontaneous; ST, spontaneous/timed; Ti, inspiratory time; VAPS, volume-assured pressure support; Vt, tidal volume.

Unlike endotracheal intubation or tracheostomy, which bypasses the upper airway, NIV requires a patent upper airway before ventilation can be effective.[121] Therefore we recommend always keeping a low EPAP, between 4 and 6 cm H_2O to maintain upper airway patency. High EPAP can increase work of breathing during exhalation. Besides determination of appropriate inspiratory and expiratory pressures, the need for a backup respiratory rate is recommended to augment ventilation during periods of severe hypoventilation or if a patient is unable to consistently trigger support.[80] The backup rate is commonly set at about 10 to 12 breaths/minute but will need adjustment over time based on the severity and evolution of the syndrome. The use of NIPPV has dramatically improved QOL and mortality for patient with NMDs and has allowed patients to return to work and even travel, something previously impossible when constrained by reliance on a rocking bed or the complications of tracheostomy for nocturnal ventilatory support.

Decision to Assist Nocturnal Ventilation

Nocturnal NIPPV should be started when nocturnal hypoventilation is present. Clinical symptoms and physiologic markers of hypoventilation assess disease severity and assist in the decision to initiate nocturnal NIPPV. Patients usually first develop nocturnal hypoventilation, followed by diurnal hypoventilation with associated clinical symptoms, which can lead to acute respiratory failure. Continuous monitoring of arterial CO_2 by end-tidal CO_2 or transcutaneous CO_2 during an overnight sleep study is necessary to document nocturnal hypoventilation, which may occur exclusively during REM sleep. Arterial blood gas and serum chemistry can document daytime hypoventilation with elevated arterial CO_2 ($Paco_2$), low arterial oxygen (Pao_2), relatively normal pH, and high serum bicarbonate. Many clinicians consider starting NIPPV for an arterial Pco_2 greater than 45 mm Hg and an arterial Po_2 less than 70 mm Hg. An isolated change in nocturnal oxygen saturation alone is insufficient for deciding whether the patient needs ventilatory assistance. However, sustained nocturnal oxygen desaturations may be an indicator of nocturnal hypoventilation.

In summary, there is long-standing consensus on the management of severe progressive neuromuscular disorders, in which respiratory failure plays a significant part of the natural history of the disease.[127,128] The positive impact of noninvasive ventilatory support in NMD patients has become very clear since the introduction of PAP in 1980s and, shortly after, the introduction of NIV. The most effective time to introduce NIPPV is when SDB, including nocturnal hypoventilation, develops. It can be argued that initiating NIV when pulmonary function tests decline (e.g., FVC < 50% predicted) is late and we have missed the opportunity to intervene when early respiratory impairment has begun. Issues such as QOL and family/caregiver support must be considered. When initiating NIV therapy, close follow-up to ensure optimal early experience and to facilitate acclimation is central to fostering adherence, as is patient family/caregiver education.[129] Each patient must be assessed in detail, and the clinician must bear in mind that nocturnal (and later, 24-hour) ventilation will treat only one (albeit important) aspect of the disorder.

Looking ahead, new and emerging medical therapies offer great promise in improving the usual trajectories of pulmonary decline in neuromuscular disorders. Young patients with DMD treated with the exon-skipping drug eteplirsen experienced significantly less decline in respiratory muscle function as measured by FVC (% predicted) compared to control subjects.[130,131] In one study of children with spinal muscular atrophy who were treated with the intrathecal antisense oligonucleotide therapy nusinersen since infancy, at approximately 3 years follow-up all were still alive, and none had required permanent ventilatory support.[132,133] How these remarkable medical therapies and other advancements will ultimately impact the complex interplay of breathing and sleep in patients with NMD remains to be seen, but doubtless this will remain a vibrant field for the sleep medicine specialist in the future.

CLINICAL PEARLS

- Sleep is a vulnerable state for patients with neuromuscular disorders because normal rapid eye movement (REM) sleep–related changes in ventilation are magnified as a result of muscle weakness, resulting in hypoventilation and oxygen desaturation.
- In addition to sleep-disordered breathing, sleep may also be disturbed by spasticity, poor secretion clearance, sphincter dysfunction, inability to turn, pain, and autonomic dysfunction. All of these factors can impair sleep and worsen daytime disability.
- Noninvasive ventilation is the gold standard treatment for neuromuscular disease patients with respiratory involvement by reducing morbidity and improving life expectancy.
- The most effective time to introduce noninvasive ventilatory support is when sleep-disordered breathing develops, including REM and non–rapid eye movement sleep hypoventilation.
- Continuous positive airway pressure is contraindicated in neuromuscular patients with neuromuscular respiratory weakness. Rather, respiratory assist devices with backup respiratory rate or portable ventilators are recommended, depending on the stage of respiratory involvement.
- Newer advanced modes of noninvasive ventilation, such as volume-assured pressure support, are being use frequently (although with limited evidence for superiority over basic bilevel positive airway pressure modes) for ventilatory insufficiency in neuromuscular patients because it targets tidal volume or minute ventilation and therefore treats hypoventilation and carbon dioxide retention.
- The overnight polysomnography remains the gold standard test to diagnose nocturnal respiratory impairment, but it is not a required test to initiate noninvasive ventilatory support, depending on the stage of respiratory impairment.

SUMMARY

Neuromuscular disorders consist of central and peripheral neurologic disorders with impairment of the motor system. The disability of patients with a neuromuscular disorder worsens during sleep, and the abnormal sleep and secondary impairment of daytime function further degrade QOL. Nocturnal sleep disruption can result from pain and discomfort related to weakness, rigidity, or spasticity that limits movement and posture. Sleep disruption may also be caused by autonomic dysfunction, poor sphincter control, problems with clearance of secretions, and abnormal movements and behaviors during sleep. Most important, sleep-related hypoventilation is common with neuromuscular disorders, and overlooking this may lead to death. Daytime evaluation will determine the severity of the disability but may not identify the presence and severity of an associated sleep-related disorder. Nonspecific symptoms of daytime fatigue and sleepiness can indicate poor sleep in these patients. Polysomnography with continuous monitoring of CO_2 is the only test that can objectively identify and evaluate the severity of sleep-related disorders, as well as ventilatory impairment. By recognizing and treating sleep-related problems early, before daytime respiratory impairment ensues, these patients can enjoy improved survival and better QOL.

SELECTED READINGS

Aboussouan LS. Sleep-disordered breathing in neuromuscular disease. *Am J Respir Crit Care. Med.* 2015;191:979–989.

Alves RSC, Resende MBD, Skomro RP, et al. Sleep and neuromuscular disorders in children. *Respir Physiol Neurobiol.* 2009;169:165–170.

Camacho M, Certal V, Abdullatif J, et al. Myofunctional therapy to treat obstructive sleep apnea: a systematic review and meta-analysis. *Sleep.* 2015;38:669–675.

Contal O, Janssens JP, Dury M, et al. Sleep in ventilator failure in restrictive thoracic disorders. Effects of treatment with noninvasive ventilation. *Sleep Med.* 2011;12:373–377.

De Braekeleer K, Toussaint M. Transcutaneous carbon dioxide measurement in adult patients with neuromuscular disorders: a quality level assessment. *J Neuromuscul Dis.* 2021;8(2):305–313.

Devivo MJ. Epidemiology of traumatic spinal cord injury: trends and future implications. *Spinal Cord.* 2012;50:365–372.

Finder JD, Birnkrant D, Carl J, et al. Respiratory care of the patient with Duchenne muscular dystrophy: ATS consensus statement. *Am J Respir Crit Care Med.* 2004;170:456–465.

Gurbani N, Pascoe JE, Katz S, Sawnani H. Sleep disordered breathing: assessment and therapy in the age of emerging neuromuscular therapies. *Pediatr Pulmonol.* 2021;56(4):700–709.

Hukins CA, Hillman DR. Daytime predictors of sleep hypoventilation in Duchenne muscular dystrophy. *Am J Respir Crit Care Med.* 2000;161:166–170.

Kryger MA, Chehata VJ. Relationship between sleep-disordered breathing and neurogenic obesity in adults with spinal cord injury. *Top Spinal Cord Inj Rehabil.* 2021;27(1):84–91.

Selim B, Junna M, Morgenthaler T. Therapy for sleep hypoventilation and central apnea syndromes. *Curr Treat Options Neurol.* 2012;14:427–437.

Seshagiri DV, Huddar A, Nashi S, et al. Altered REM sleep architecture in patients with myotonic dystrophy type 1: is it related to sleep apnea? *Sleep Med.* 2021;79:48–54.

Skatrud J, Iber C, McHugh W, et al. Determinants of hypoventilation during wakefulness and sleep in diaphragmatic paralysis. *Am Rev Respir Dis.* 1980;121:587–593.

Steindor M, Wagner CE, Bock C, et al. Home noninvasive ventilation in pediatric subjects with neuromuscular diseases: one size fits all. *Respir Care.* 2021;66(3):410–415.

Udd B, Krahe R. The myotonic dystrophies: molecular, clinical, and therapeutic challenges. *Lancet Neurol.* 2012;11:891–905.

A complete reference list can be found online at ExpertConsult.com.

Chapter 105

Alzheimer Disease and Other Dementias

Dominique Petit; Erik K. St Louis; Diego Z. Carvalho; Jacques Montplaisir; Bradley F. Boeve

Chapter Highlights

- This chapter gives an overview of sleep disturbances, characteristics of sleep architecture and microstructure in mild and major neurocognitive disorders, including amnestic and nonamnestic mild cognitive impairment (MCI), Alzheimer disease, progressive supranuclear palsy, Parkinson disease, dementia with Lewy bodies, vascular dementia, Huntington disease, Creutzfeldt-Jakob disease, and frontotemporal dementia.
- Recent research that has clarified the bidirectional relationships between the sleep state and neurodegeneration is reviewed, including how the sleep state influences protein biomarker turnover in the central nervous system, which likely influences pathogenesis of neurodegenerative diseases.
- Certain sleep disorders, including rapid eye movement (REM) sleep behavior disorder (RBD) combined with MCI, substantially increase the risk for developing dementia and parkinsonism.
- Treatment of sleep disturbances in patients with dementia should focus on managing specific symptoms, including insomnia or fragmented sleep; excessive daytime sleepiness; alterations in the sleep-wake circadian rhythm; and excessive motor activity during the night, including RBD, periodic leg movements (PLMS) during sleep, and nocturnal agitation or wandering.

With the steady increase in life expectancy, the prevalence of dementia and neurodegenerative diseases is rising at a rapid pace. It is estimated that the prevalence of dementia doubles every 5 years after age 65 years. The *Diagnostic and Statistical Manual of Mental Disorders,* fifth edition, has classified neurodegenerative disorders as mild or major neurocognitive disorders, with the distinction in severity being drawn by preservation or impairment in independent daily functioning. In neurodegenerative disease, myriad comorbid sleep disturbances and disorders may aggravate cognitive deficits, worsen the patient's and caretaker's quality of life, and, in those with dementia, may lead to premature institutionalization. On the other hand, sleep disturbances can sometimes help in making a differential diagnosis or in predicting who may be at greater risk for developing dementia.

ALZHEIMER DISEASE

Alzheimer disease (AD) is a neurodegenerative disorder characterized by a gradual onset and progressive decline in memory and other cognitive domains. AD is the primary cause of irreversible dementia in old age. Diagnostic criteria, first established by the National Institute of Neurological Disorders and Stroke–Alzheimer's Disease and Related Disorders Association Work Group, were revised in 2011[1] in light of the discovery of new markers, brain imaging findings, and analyses of amyloid-β (aβ) and tau proteins in cerebrospinal fluid (CSF). Although aβ and tau proteins are normally present in healthy brains, in AD these proteins aggregate abnormally and accumulate in the brain. Accumulation of phosphorylated tau (p-tau) protein appears to mediate neuronal dysfunction more so than aβ deposition. Classic AD pathologic staging described earliest and most prominent involvement of the entorhinal cortex, followed by limbic structures (hippocampus and amygdala) and basal forebrain (nucleus basalis of Meynert) before eventual diffuse neocortical spreading. However, more recently it has become evident that tau pathologic involvement begins earlier in subcortical nuclei, particularly in the locus coeruleus and in other nuclei with diffuse cortical projects related to the sleep-wake cycle. Neuropathology findings include neurofibrillary tangles, neuritic plaques, and neuronal loss.

Of interest, sleep may play a protective role in preventing toxic protein accumulation, and the brain's "glymphatic" system, the interstitial space surrounding glia and neurons, appears to play a key role in protein homeostasis in the central nervous system because there is substantially higher clearance of aβ during sleep and drug-induced anesthesia compared with wakefulness.[2] Further animal and human research will be necessary to demonstrate whether this "housekeeping" role of the brain's glymphatic system during sleep influences potentially toxic protein accumulation and neurodegeneration. The bidirectional relationships between sleep, neurodegeneration, and protein homeostasis/turnover in the central nervous system are discussed in following sections.

Sleep Problems

Sleep disturbance occurs in up to 25% of patients with mild to moderate AD and in about 50% with moderate to severe AD. Several types of sleep problems with multifactorial causes can be seen, including both excessive daytime sleepiness and insomnia. Difficulties in falling asleep primarily, as well as problems maintaining sleep, may occur due to frequent nocturnal arousals and premature morning awakening.[3] Sleep problems pose additional functional consequences; daytime sleepiness is associated with greater impairments in AD patients independent of cognitive impairment severity,[4] and sleep disturbances are a major cause of early institutionalization.

Perhaps the most burdensome sleep problem of patients with AD is sundowning, a delirium-like state characterized by confusion, agitation, anxiety, and frequent aggression in the evening or night, with potentially injurious nocturnal wandering. This phenomenon can be explained, at least in part, by an alteration in the biologic clock due to impaired functioning of the hypothalamic suprachiasmatic nucleus (SCN).[5] The secretion rhythm of many hormones is affected in elderly people, but it is even more disrupted in AD patients.[6] The timing of the biologic clock is shifted earlier, as evidenced by two common markers: core body temperature and plasma melatonin.[6]

A series of pathophysiologic findings has shed some light on the circadian rhythm disorder of AD patients. Melatonin production and rhythm are disrupted,[7] even in the early preclinical stages of AD.[8] This might be caused by dysfunction in the sympathetic regulation of pineal melatonin secretion by the SCN.[7] The SCN is under the modulatory influence of the nucleus basalis of Meynert,[9] which degenerates early in AD. In addition, sundowning could result from defective nucleus basalis control of arousal signal processing to the neocortex.[9]

Obstructive sleep apnea (OSA) is more frequent in AD patients than in the general population.[10] A relationship between AD and apolipoprotein E (ApoE), a lipoprotein made in the liver and brain and involved in cholesterol transport and deposition, was first noted in the early 1990s.[11] The risk for developing AD is associated with ApoE-ε4 allele homozygosity and heterozygosity. An association has been also found between the ApoE-ε4 allele and OSA.[12] In fact, OSA and AD share many other neuropathologic processes, such as oxidative stress, metabolic disturbances, inflammation, and amyloid and tau pathology; markers of these processes have been reviewed in both OSA and AD.[13]

Finally, rapid eye movement (REM) sleep behavior disorder (RBD) is rarely reported in association with AD; most RBD cases are instead associated with underlying synucleinopathy neurodegenerative pathology.[14]

Polysomnography Findings

Sleep architecture is often abnormal in patients with AD, with most changes representing an acceleration of usual age-related disturbances. AD patients show an increased number and duration of arousals and increased N1 percentage. Compared with elderly control subjects, AD patients also show reduced N3 (slow wave sleep [SWS]) percentage,[15] which is the most consistently reported change in mild to moderate AD. Sleep architecture disturbances tend to worsen with increasing severity of AD.[15]

Altered N2 electroencephalographic (EEG) features in AD include sleep spindles and K-complexes that are poorly formed and of lower amplitude, shorter duration, and lower number than those seen in age-matched control subjects.[16,17] Reduction in fast spindles has been linked to worse immediate recall in AD.[18] With advancing AD severity, distinguishing N2 from N1 becomes more difficult, given loss of characteristic N2 EEG features. The proportion of indeterminate non–rapid eye movement (NREM) sleep increases even further with the disappearance of high voltage (>75 μV) delta waves of SWS.

Conversely, other sleep changes observed in AD are not consistent with acceleration of aging manifestations. Although the percentage of REM sleep remains stable in normal aging, REM sleep is reduced in AD patients compared with control subjects, mostly because of decreased mean REM sleep episode duration.[16] However, REM sleep initiation and other characteristic features, including REM density, number of REM sleep episodes, REM sleep latency, muscle atonia, and phasic electromyographic activity, are usually unchanged in mild AD,[16,19] probably because these aspects of REM are under the control of cholinergic neurons in the mesopontine tegmentum that are relatively spared in mild AD. Lower REM sleep percentage could be due to degeneration of the cholinergic nucleus basalis of Meynert, which normally exerts an inhibitory influence on the thalamic nucleus reticularis.[20] Without strong long-lasting inhibition, the rhythm generator of the thalamus can trigger spindle oscillations, thus curtailing the REM periods (see Chapters 7 and 8).

In AD there are also changes in the waking EEG activity, which is characterized by a slower dominant occipital rhythm than in healthy older people, with increased theta and delta activity compared with age-matched control subjects. Several studies have attempted to correlate quantitative waking EEG with clinical severity of AD, with variable results.

EEG slowing is more apparent during REM sleep than during wakefulness in AD patients,[21,22] with a distinctive topographic pattern of temporoparietal and frontal regional REM sleep EEG slowing in AD patients,[24] which parallels findings from neuroradiologic[23] and neuropathologic[24] studies, a pattern not observed for the waking EEG. The REM sleep EEG power ratio, but not the waking EEG power ratio, was also correlated with the Mini-Mental State Examination and with a measure of interhemispheric asymmetry of regional cerebral blood flow in AD.[25] Possibly, the superiority of REM sleep EEG over wakefulness EEG to identify AD-related neurodegeneration is due to the fact that the basal forebrain cholinergic neurons, among the first to degenerate in AD, are more active during REM sleep than during wakefulness[26] and that cholinergic activity is not as masked by other activating neurotransmitter systems as it is during wakefulness.

Because EEG delta activity is prominent throughout sleep, distinguishing pathologic from normal physiologic delta waves during NREM sleep is particularly challenging. Patients with AD have shown less frequent and lower amplitude elicited K-complexes in response to auditory stimulation than age-matched control subjects,[27] suggesting that AD patients may have an impaired ability to generate normal physiologic high-amplitude slow waves during NREM sleep.

Mild Cognitive Impairment as a Prodrome of Alzheimer Disease

One of the major advances in AD research during the past 20 years is an improved understanding of the prodromal phase known as mild cognitive impairment (MCI). The conversion rate from MCI to AD is about 50% over 3 years.[28] The amnestic MCI subtype is more likely to evolve toward AD, whereas nonamnestic MCI more frequently converts to dementia with Lewy bodies (DLB). Sleep problems are one of the four most common neuropsychiatric symptoms of MCI. A meta-analysis confirmed that 15% to 59% of MCI subjects report sleep disturbances.[29] MCI subjects, especially in ApoE-ε4 carriers, have a higher density of SWS arousals and shorter REM sleep duration than control subjects.[30] As shown for AD, REM sleep measures are more helpful than those taken during wakefulness to discriminate amnestic MCI patients from control subjects.[31,32] Amnestic MCI patients also show fewer sleep spindles and spend less time in SWS.[33] MCI subjects also have greater wake after sleep onset, increased REM sleep latency, and earlier dim-light melatonin onset relative to control subjects (but similar levels of total melatonin secreted).[34] This advanced melatonin onset is associated with poorer memory in MCI patients.[34]

The Sleep State and Neurodegenerative Disease Pathogenesis

Recent research has clarified possible contributions of normal and abnormal sleep toward the pathogenesis of neurodegenerative diseases, suggesting there is a bidirectional relationship between sleep and neurodegeneration, especially in Alzheimer disease.[35] Amyloid-β and other potentially neurotoxic proteins presumed to be involved in neurodegenerative disease pathogenesis may chiefly accumulate for two basic reasons: increased protein production and/or decreased protein clearance. Sleep may contribute toward pathogenic protein accumulation through both of these mechanisms, because extended wakefulness and/or sleep disruption could cause increased protein production, whereas decreased sleep quantity would likely decrease protein clearance. The sleep state has been shown to be intimately related to aβ, tau, and synuclein homeostasis in both animal models and humans. Even a single night of sleep deprivation has been associated with increased levels of aβ and tau in mice brains and human CSF, as well as with selective accumulation of aβ in limbic structures as demonstrated by amyloid positron emission tomography brain imaging studies.[36–40] Sleep extension proportionately decreases these same AD markers. N3 sleep reduction and disruption has also been associated with increased aβ-42 amyloid in the CSF.[41–43] The relationship between aβ pathology and sleep disturbance has also been shown to be bidirectional in cognitively normal community-dwelling adults long before AD onset; measures of sleep fragmentation have been associated with aβ CSF levels.[39,43] Symptoms of excessive daytime sleepiness are associated with accelerated brain aging and longitudinal aβ accumulation.[44–45] What degree and amount of sleep loss is necessary to potentiate amyloid and other pathologic protein increases in CSF remains unclear because one recent study of chronic partial sleep restriction (4 hours per night × 5 nights) showed no impact on CSF amyloid, tau, or other neuronal or glial marker levels, although modest and likely adaptive increases in CSF hypocretin were seen.[46] Self-reported sleep reduction in middle life predicted later life temporal lobe amyloid and tau burden, which was also correlated, respectively, with reduced slow wave amplitude and slow wave spindle coupling.[47] There is also evidence from animal models that amyloid and tau pathology alters hippocampal neuronal excitation and possibly also both local and broadly distributed neuronal network excitability, which in turn may alter sleep slow wave oscillations. Sleep slow waves can be enhanced by externally administered acoustic stimulation or transcranial alternating current stimulation in both younger and older healthy adults, and enhanced sleep slow waves have been correlated with improvements in memory performance.[48–50] Whether sleep slow wave oscillations may be harnessed toward preventing or reversing the progression of neurodegenerative protein accumulation and memory impairments in patients with symptomatic cognitive impairment remains a research frontier.

PROGRESSIVE SUPRANUCLEAR PALSY

Progressive supranuclear palsy (PSP), also called Steele-Richardson-Olszewski syndrome, is a neurodegenerative tauopathy characterized by progressive axial rigidity, postural instability, and supranuclear gaze palsy. Dementia in PSP primarily reflects dysfunction in the frontal subcortical neural networks.[51]

Excessive daytime somnolence is common in PSP. Hypocretin 1 (orexin A) levels were found to be low in PSP, and these levels were inversely correlated with the duration of PSP.[52] Patients with PSP show a longer sleep latency, a reduced sleep efficiency, less SWS, and much less REM sleep than control subjects.[53–55] RLS is frequent in PSP and may contribute to reduced sleep efficiency and duration.[56] RBD and REM sleep without atonia (RSWA) has been reported to occur in 15% to 20% of patients with PSP despite reductions in REM sleep duration;[57] RSWA appears to be markedly less frequent in PSP than in patients with Parkinson disease (PD) or multiple system atrophy (MSA); the presence of RSWA tends to distinguish patients who have an underlying synucleinopathy.[53,58,59] A weaker circadian signal (mesor, amplitude, and robustness) was also reported in PSP and found to be associated with increased disease severity.[60]

Cognitive decline is, in turn, reflected by a slowing of the frontal EEG during wakefulness[55] that is consistent with neuropsychological frontal lobe functional deficits. Absence of EEG slowing during REM sleep[55] suggests that waking EEG slowing is likely not due to a cholinergic deficit, consistent with findings of normal neocortical and hippocampal choline acetyltransferase activity in PSP.[61] However, dopamine levels are severely reduced in the caudate, putamen, and substantia nigra in PSP patients.[61] Frontal deafferentation resulting from striatopallidal complex dopaminergic deficiency may be responsible for PSP impairments because there are extensive fiber connections between these deep nuclei and the prefrontal region.

PARKINSON DISEASE WITH DEMENTIA

PD is a progressive neurologic disorder characterized by rigidity, resting tremor, bradykinesia, and an impairment of postural reflexes and gait that is caused in part by degeneration of dopaminergic neurons in the substantia nigra. Sleep alterations experienced by patients with PD are discussed in Chapter 102; therefore this chapter only focuses on information relevant to dementia associated with PD.

The incidence of overt dementia in PD is relatively high. In a population-based study of dementia in PD, approximately 80% of nondemented PD patients developed dementia within 8 years.[62] Risk factors include advanced age at onset of symptoms, severe motor symptoms (particularly bradykinesia), levodopa-related confusion or hallucinations, speech and axial involvement, depression, and atypical neurologic features, such as modest response to dopaminergic agents or early autonomic dysfunction.[63]

Demented patients with PD often experience hallucinations. One study found that patients with REM sleep anomalies have more hallucinations than patients without such anomalies.[64] Sleep reduction, particularly REM sleep reduction, could trigger hallucinations due to emergence of REM sleep features during wakefulness. Hallucinations are significantly correlated with the presence of RBD and the amount of dopaminergic medication, independent of age, gender, disease duration, or Unified Parkinson's Disease Rating Scale score.[65] There is growing evidence that RBD is an early manifestation of a neurodegenerative disorder, particularly the synucleinopathies (e.g., DLB, PD, and MSA)[66,67] and the strongest risk factor for rapid and severe cognitive decline in PD. The 5′-region variant of *SNCA*, the coding gene for α-synuclein, is associated with PD with dementia, DLB, and idiopathic/isolated RBD.[68] The occurrence of RBD in PD was estimated at 15% with a structured questionnaire[69] but rises to 33% using polysomnographic recordings,[70] with only half of these cases detected during clinical interview. RSWA may lead to difficulties in distinction of REM sleep when sleep staging is performed according to the standard criteria. Challenges in staging accuracy in the setting of RSWA may at least partially explain reported reductions in REM sleep in PD patients because accurate recognition and staging of REM sleep in the context of RSWA requires a high degree of experience and application of alternative scoring criteria.[71]

Approximately one-third of patients with PD have EEG slowing regardless of the presence of dementia,[65] and although focal temporal-occipital and frontal regional EEG slowing occurs even in some nondemented PD patients,[72] only PD-RBD patients have slowing of the dominant occipital EEG frequency.[73] PD-RBD and idiopathic RBD patients have higher theta power during wakefulness in frontal, temporal, parietal, and occipital regions compared to those without RBD and control subjects.[74] Polysomnography (PSG) EEG characteristics have also been found to be altered with PD and dementia, with reduced sleep spindle density shown in most studies,[75–77] except one.[78] Lower-amplitude sleep spindles in the parietal and occipital regions also predict conversion to dementia in PD patients.[79]

Patients with PD-RBD also have significantly worse performance on standardized tests of episodic verbal memory, executive functions, and visuospatial and visuoperceptual processing compared with both patients having PD without RBD and control subjects.[80] Of interest, patients with idiopathic/isolated RBD also have worse performance on tests of executive function and verbal memory compared with control subjects.[81]

The association of RBD with dementia in PD was more directly demonstrated by one study.[82] Of 65 patients with PD, 24 had RBD. The frequency of RBD was significantly higher in a PD with dementia group compared with a PD without dementia group (77% vs. 27%). Patients who had PD without RBD had a lower rate of dementia (7.3%) compared with patients with PD-RBD (42%).

There are compelling reasons to believe that RBD may often represent prodromal PD with dementia or DLB. The topography of EEG slowing observed in PD-RBD is similar to that of DLB-associated functional neuroimaging hypoperfusion and hypometabolism.[83,84] Also, the profile of cognitive impairments noted in PD-RBD resembles that of DLB,[85] and many RBD patients later develop DLB.[86,87] Thus the presence of RBD in patients with PD may be an early sign of an evolution toward dementia. Some evidence suggests that cortical Lewy body–type degeneration is the main source of dementia in PD.[88] Other studies have suggested that α-synuclein–positive cortical (especially frontal) Lewy bodies are associated with cognitive impairment, independent of AD-type pathologic process.[89,90] More studies are necessary to determine the pathologic and neurochemical underpinnings of dementia in PD.

DEMENTIA WITH LEWY BODIES

DLB is the second most common neurodegenerative cause of dementia in old age. The core clinical features of DLB are progressive cognitive decline, spontaneous parkinsonism, recurrent visual hallucinations, fluctuating cognition and vigilance, and RBD.[91] Autonomic dysfunction is also often present.[91] DLB is characterized by the presence of Lewy bodies in limbic and neocortical structures.

A questionnaire study showed that patients with DLB had more overall sleep disturbances, more movement disorders while asleep, and more daytime sleepiness than AD patients.[92] Based on results from the Epworth Sleepiness Scale, 50% of patients with DLB experience excessive daytime sleepiness.[93] However, normal hypocretin-1 levels were found in the CSF of DLB patients with daytime sleepiness, suggesting that sleepiness in DLB is not related primarily to dysfunctional hypocretin neurotransmission.[52,94] Moreover, contrary to popular belief, fluctuating daytime alertness as measured by objective methods was not found to be related to fluctuations in cognition.[95] A polysomnographic study[96] found that 72% of patients with DLB had a sleep efficiency lower than 80%. Sleep efficiency was not, however, correlated with dementia severity. A high proportion of these patients had pathologic respiratory disturbances indices (70.5%) or PLMS during sleep associated with arousal (45%).[96] As in PD, restless legs syndrome (RLS) and PLMS are indeed common in DLB and can play a part in sleep-onset insomnia, nocturnal arousals, and awakenings.[97] However, a significant proportion of DLB patients have high arousal indices not accounted for by PLMS or respiratory disturbances.[96]

A number of studies or review papers have reported that RBD is common in DLB.[86,87] In a large cohort of 78 DLB patients, 96% had a history of recurrent dream-enactment behaviors, and RSWA with or without behavioral manifestations was confirmed in 83% of patients.[96] Inclusion of RBD in the list of core criteria improves sensitivity and specificity of DLB diagnosis,[85,87,98] leading to RBD as being considered as a core feature for the diagnosis of DLB in the fourth report of the DLB consortium.[91] Of interest, the presence or absence of concomitant RBD was found to be associated with distinct clinical and pathologic characteristics of DLB; patients with concomitant RBD had earlier onset of parkinsonism and visual hallucinations, shorter duration of dementia, lower Braak stage, and lower neuritic plaque scores.[99] Quantitative EEG studies have reported EEG slowing during wakefulness in DLB that correlates with fluctuating cognition and the severity of dementia.[100–104]

VASCULAR DEMENTIA

The term *vascular dementia* covers a range of problems of various etiologies and includes the entities known as multiinfarct dementia (MID, now a rather outdated term), subcortical ischemic vascular dementia, and Binswanger disease. The most studied form of vascular dementia in sleep medicine is probably MID, realizing misdiagnoses are not uncommon. An actigraphy study found that patients with MID had a significantly greater disruption of sleep-wake cycles associated with poor sleep quality than AD patients.[105] There was no correlation, however, between the degree of sleep disruption and the severity of intellectual deterioration. OSA was more strongly associated with MID than with AD or other dementias.[106,107] Sleep apnea is considered a risk factor for vascular dementia.[108] Patients with vascular dementia were found to have twice the risk for suffering from insomnia compared with AD patients.[107] A population cohort also demonstrated that, compared with men without sleep disturbances, elderly men with daytime sleepiness at baseline had 4.44 times the risk for developing dementia of vascular origin 10 years later, even after adjustment for possible confounding factors, including cognitive function.[109] Spectral analysis of the waking EEG of patients with vascular dementia have revealed significant slowing, both generalized and in the occipital region, with variable correlation with mental status and neuropsychological functioning, possibly enabling distinction from AD patients.[110–115]

HUNTINGTON DISEASE

Huntington disease (HD) is an autosomal dominant hereditary condition associated with atrophy of basal ganglia structures, especially the caudate nucleus, and characterized by choreic movements and progressive dementia associated with psychotic features. A cytosine-adenosine-guanine (CAG) trinucleotide repeat in the *HTT* gene located on the short arm of chromosome 4 is the cause of this condition.[116]

Patients with HD have a disrupted night-day activity pattern, and similar patterns are seen in animal models. Transgenic mice carrying the HD mutation showed a disruption of night-day activity, which worsened as the degeneration progressed, but also showed a marked reduction in the expression of *mPer2* and disrupted expression of *Bmal1* in the SCN, the motor cortex, and the striatum.[117] Ubiquitin-proteasome dysfunction has been suggested to play a role in the pathogenesis of HD,[118] and such inclusions have also been found in the SCN of HD transgenic mice.[119] In humans a postmortem study found that patients with HD had 85% fewer vasoactive intestinal peptide neurons and 33% fewer arginine-vasopressin neurons in the SCN.[120] Dim-light melatonin onset was delayed by 1½ hours in HD patients, and daytime melatonin levels were correlated with severity of functional impairment.[121] Delayed sleep phase is also associated with depression, higher anxiety, and poorer cognitive performance in HD patients.[122,123] Daily treatment with alprazolam in HD transgenic mice reversed dysregulated expression of *Per2* and *Prok2*, an output factor of the SCN that controls behavioral rhythms, and also markedly improved cognitive performance in a visual discrimination task.[124] The combination of bright-light treatment and restricted periods of voluntary exercise was also shown to improve the behavioral synchronization to the light-dark cycle and to delay the disintegration of the rest-activity rhythm in the transgenic mouse model.[125] Restoring circadian rhythms in HD patients might thus improve cognitive dysfunction, the most devastating feature of HD.

A meta-analysis of polysomnographic findings demonstrated that patients with HD had lower sleep efficiency, lower percentages of SWS and REM sleep, and higher percentage of N1 sleep than age-matched control subjects.[126] Sleep disturbances, including less SWS and more time spent awake, correlate with the degree of caudate atrophy and the severity of clinical symptoms.[127] REM sleep duration was significantly reduced in presymptomatic carriers of abnormal CAG repeat expansion in the *HTT* gene and decreased as disease severity increased. Three out of 25 patients with HD had RBD. Finally, patients with HD did not have more daytime sleepiness but had more PLMS than control subjects. Contrary to patients with other neurodegenerative diseases, HD patients showed a higher density of sleep spindles compared with healthy control subjects.[76,127] However, no correlation was found between CAG repeat length and sleep disturbances.[128] Finally, no difference was found on sleep respiratory variables between patients with HD and control subjects.[128] Waking EEG exhibits gradual slowing and diminished amplitude as HD progresses, with waking quantitative EEG showing slowing compared to control subjects, but similar in degree to patients with AD.[129]

CREUTZFELDT-JAKOB DISEASE

Creutzfeldt-Jakob disease (CJD) is a prion-related transmissible spongiform encephalopathy causing extensive neuronal degeneration and pathologic changes, especially in the cortex, resulting in myoclonic jerks and rapidly evolving dementia and leading to death. CJD typically develops between the fifth and the seventh decades of life. Younger age of onset is associated with an increased likelihood of sleep disturbances and other symptoms.[130] The mean survival duration is 4 to 8 months,[131] although 5% to 10% of patients have a clinical course that spans 2 years or more.

Three large-sample studies[132–134] reported that more than half of CJD patients experienced sleep disturbances and sometimes hypersomnia but mostly severe insomnia. In some patients, sleep disturbances were a prodromal or presenting symptom,[132] and there is a continuum between CJD and fatal familial insomnia (FFI).[135] A mutation of the prion protein at codon 178 is present in both CJD and FFI. A concomitant polymorphism at codon 129 (valine vs. methionine) appears to determine whether CJD or FFI will ensue. However, the 129 polymorphism alone (common in the general population) does not appear to be associated with important changes in PSG variables or insomnia complaints.[136] Predominant thalamic pathology with little cortical involvement is characteristic of FFI, whereas predominant progressive cortical dysfunction is more usual in CJD.[137] Polysomnographic studies of CJD reveal disorganized sleep patterns with sudden transitions between sleep stage, few sleep spindles and K-complexes in N2 (which may be difficult to distinguish from N3), decreased slow waves and SWS, and lower REM sleep percentage and REM density.[134,138–140] Episodes of nocturnal oneiric, sometimes aggressive behavior with dream-reality confusion, have been reported in some patients.[132,139] An indeterminate state (neither clear wakefulness nor clear sleep) has also been observed in these patients[139] and in patients with FFI.[140] The absence or paucity of sleep (with disrupted architecture) along with autonomic hyperactivation and motor overactivity are the defining features of agrypnia excitata, which was initially described in FFI and attributed to thalamic degeneration causing intralimbic disconnection, leading to disinhibition of the hypothalamus and brainstem reticular formation. A similar presentation with thalamolimbic dysfunction was subsequently observed in patients with voltage-gated potassium channel autoimmunity causing limbic encephalopathy and delirium tremens during alcohol withdrawal.[141] Sleep apnea, central or obstructive, are also frequent in CJD.

The hallmark awake EEG feature in patients with CJD is periodic sharp wave complexes within a background of generalized slow but low-voltage EEG, consistent with diffuse cerebral pathology.[131,142] Periodic sharp wave complexes, usually generalized biphasic complexes, are invariably present by the time patients evolve clinically evident myoclonus and typically present by 3 months after symptom onset.[142] Periodic sharp wave complexes are part of the diagnostic criteria for probable CJD[143] because they are present in about two-thirds of patients and show a high specificity, occurring in only 9% of patients with another neurodegenerative disorder.[144] Sleep EEG studies also report the presence of periodic sharp wave complexes as early as 1 to 3 months after the onset of symptoms.[145,146] Cyclic changes with periodic complex phases alternating with semirhythmic theta-delta activities have been described.[145,146]

FRONTOTEMPORAL DEMENTIA

Frontotemporal dementia (FTD) is a neurobehavioral syndrome associated with accumulation of tau (e.g., Pick disease, corticobasal degeneration, progressive supranuclear palsy) or transactivation response (TAR) element DNA-binding protein, molecular weight 43. FTD is a progressive, degenerative condition characterized by loss of executive or language abilities and several other neurobehavioral features, such as loss of insight, overactivity, lack of social awareness, disinhibition, and lack of personal hygiene.[147] Approximately 5% to 15% of patients with dementia have a disorder within the FTD spectrum. FTD is likely underdiagnosed because of its similarities with AD, especially later in the progression of the disease. However, unlike AD, FTD initially manifests with progressive aphasia and/or personality changes, whereas memory tends to remain relatively intact. Structural and functional brain imaging shows atrophy, reduced cerebral blood flow, or diminished glucose metabolism in frontal and anterior temporal areas.[147]

As in AD, FTD is generally accompanied by a disturbance of the alpha rhythm and of the sleep-wake rhythm, which worsens with progression of the disease.[148] Patients with FTD show more nighttime activity,[149] particularly behavioral variant–FTD (85%) compared with the semantic variant of primary progressive aphasia (3%),[150] less morning activity, and lower sleep efficiency compared with control subjects.[149] For a comparable level of cognitive impairment, patients with FTD showed more sleep disruption and a worse sleep macrostructure than patients with AD, regardless of sleep apnea or other primary sleep disorders.[151] Sleep-disordered breathing seems as prevalent in FTD as in AD.[152] REM sleep parameters, however, were found to be more altered in AD than in FTD.[153] EEG slowing during wakefulness is observed in FTD, especially with increased delta and theta power in anterior head regions.[154–156]

TREATMENT OF SLEEP DISORDERS IN PATIENTS WITH DEMENTIA

One useful approach to address sleep disorders in patients with dementia involves considering symptoms within four major categories: insomnia or fragmented sleep, excessive daytime sleepiness, alteration in the sleep-wake circadian rhythm, and excessive motor activity during the night, including RBD, PLMS, and nocturnal agitation or wandering.[157] Sleep disturbances could be due to RLS, OSA, mood or pain disorders, malnutrition, infections, medication effects (often polypharmacy), bladder catheterization, fecal impactions, or disturbing environmental factors. Management frequently requires identification and treatment of underlying medical or psychiatric disorders. For each of these four categories of sleep disorders, we review the appropriate pharmacologic and nonpharmacologic treatment strategies. A summary of selected medications with suggested dosage and titration schedule also appears in Table 105.1.

Insomnia

Insomnia may affect between 40% to 60% of patients with dementia.[152] Insomnia that is comorbid with other sleep disturbances is a common occurrence in patients with dementia (described in a recent review by Dauvilliers[158]). Patients with cognitive impairment are often unable to explain why they are unable to sleep through the night, so caregivers and physicians should carefully investigate possible sources for insomnia. Evaluations of pain, concomitant medical conditions, and medications are essential to treat the patient successfully. For example, both untreated depression and some antidepressant medications (venlafaxine, fluoxetine, and bupropion) can lead to insomnia. Cholinesterase inhibitors, such as donepezil, which can improve cognitive and behavioral symptoms in AD patients, can also cause insomnia. "Activating" antidepressants, cholinesterase inhibitors, and stimulants may cause or aggravate insomnia, especially when given at night before bedtime. This problem usually can be avoided if the medication is administered no later than the evening meal, although in some individuals, these medications must be given in the morning to avoid causing or aggravating insomnia. Melatonin was ineffective in treating insomnia in patients with AD in multicenter, placebo-controlled trials.[159,160]

Behavioral interventions should be tried first, including instituting a regular sleep schedule and routines, limiting caffeine and alcohol intake, and increasing activity and exercise during the daytime with avoidance of prolonged daytime napping. One recent randomized controlled trial of walking, bright-light exposure, or combination therapy in community-dwelling adults with possible or probable AD found that all three active interventions decreased night time spent awake.[161] Before prescribing medication to treat insomnia, the clinician should keep in mind that many hypnotic agents, especially benzodiazepines, can exacerbate cognitive deficits and OSA and aggravate daytime sleepiness because of carryover effects. Use of sedative-hypnotics is associated with longer hospital stays and significantly increased fall risk in the acute care setting.[162] If no cause is found for insomnia, trazodone or chloral hydrate may be considered, although some studies have shown little alteration in actigraphic sleep parameters in institutionalized patients with dementia receiving sedative-hypnotic medications.[159] The hypocretin antagonist suvorexant 10 to 20

Table 105.1 Sleep Disorders and Disturbances in Dementia: Selected Medications with Suggested Dosing Schedules[a]

Initial Medication	Starting Dose	Suggested Titrating Schedule	Typical Therapeutic Range
Insomnia			
Trazodone	25 mg qhs	Increase in 25-mg increments q3–5d	50–200 mg/night
Chloral hydrate	500 mg qhs	Increase in 500-mg increments q5–7d	500–1500 mg/night
Melatonin	3 mg qhs	3–6 mg nightly	3–12 mg/night
Quetiapine	25 mg qhs	Increase in 25-mg increments q3d	25–100 mg/night
Zolpidem	5 mg qhs	Increase to 10 mg qhs if necessary	5–10 mg/night
Suvorexant	10 mg qhs	Increase to 20 mg qhs if necessary	10–20 mg/night
Restless Legs Syndrome, Periodic Limb Movements in Sleep			
Pramipexole	0.125 mg qhs	Increase in 0.125-mg increments q2–3d	0.125–0.50 mg/night
Gabapentin	100 mg qhs	Increase in 100-mg increments q2–3d	300–1800 mg/night
Pregabalin	25–50 mg qhs	Increase in 25- to 50-mg increments q3–7d	100–600 mg/night
Excessive Daytime Somnolence			
Methylphenidate	2.5 mg q a.m.	Increase in 2.5- to 5-mg increments q3–5d in bid dosing (a.m. and noon)	5 mg q a.m. to 30 mg bid
Modafinil	100 mg q a.m.	Increase in 100-mg increments q5–7d in bid dosing (a.m. and noon)	100 mg q a.m. to 400 mg/day (400 mg q a.m. or 200 mg bid)
Armodafinil	50 mg q a.m.	Begin with 50 mg q a.m., increase gradually up to 250 mg q a.m.	50–250 mg q a.m.
Amphetamine/ dextroamphetamine	5 mg q a.m.	Increase in 5-mg increments q7d in qd-bid dosing (a.m. and noon)	5 mg q a.m. to 20 mg bid
Rapid Eye Movement Sleep Behavior Disorder			
Clonazepam	0.25 mg qhs	Increase in 0.25-mg increments q7d	0.25–2.0 mg/night
Melatonin	3 mg	3–6 mg/night	3–12 mg/night
Psychotic Features, Behavior Dyscontrol, Nocturnal Agitation, Nocturnal Wandering			
Donepezil	5 mg q a.m.	Increase to 10 mg q a.m. 4 wk later	5–10 mg q a.m.
Rivastigmine[b]	1.5 mg bid	Increase in 1.5-mg increments q4wk in bid dosing (a.m. and hs)	3–6 mg bid
Galantamine[b]	4 mg bid	Increase in 4-mg increments q4wk in bid dosing (a.m. and hs)	4–12 mg bid
Risperidone	0.5 mg qhs	Increase in 0.5-mg increments q7d in bid dosing (a.m. and hs)	0.5 mg qhs to 1.5 mg bid
Olanzapine	5 mg qhs	Increase in 5-mg increments q7d in bid dosing (a.m. and hs)	5 mg qhs to 10 mg bid
Clozapine[c]	12.5 mg qhs	Increase in 12.5-mg increments q2–3d	12.5–50 mg qhs
Quetiapine	25 mg qhs	Increase in 25-mg increments q3d	25–100 mg qhs
Valproic acid[c]	125 mg qhs	Increase in 125-mg increments q3–7d in bid to tid dosing	250 mg qhs to 500 mg tid
Carbamazepine[c]	100 mg qhs	Increase in 100-mg increments q3–7d in bid to tid dosing	200 mg qhs to 200 mg tid

[a]*Disclaimer:* The choice of which agents to use and which dosing schedules to recommend must be individualized. It is the responsibility of the clinician to consider potential side effects, drug interactions, allergic response, life-threatening reactions (e.g., leukopenia with clozapine), dosing changes due to renal or hepatic dysfunction, etc., before administering any drug to any patient, including those listed above. Drs. Petit, Montplaisir, Carvalho, St. Louis, Boeve, their respective institutions, and Elsevier will not be held responsible for any adverse reactions of any kind to any patient regarding the content of this information.
[b]If insomnia is problematic, the second dose should be given no later than the evening meal.
[c]Requires periodic laboratory monitoring; refer to the manufacturer's instructions for laboratory monitoring.
bid, two times daily; hs, at bedtime; q, every day; qd, every day; qhs, every night at bedtime; tid, three times daily.
Modified from Boeve BF. Update on the diagnosis and management of sleep disturbances in dementia. *Sleep Med Clin.* 2008;3(3):347–60.

mg was also demonstrated to significantly improve objectively measured total sleep time in a recent randomized controlled trial in patients with Alzheimer disease and insomnia.[163]

In some cases insomnia can result from unrecognized or untreated RLS. In two recent studies, RLS occurred in approximately 4% to 5% of patients with dementia and probably is at least as common as in the general population.[152,164] RLS may be difficult to diagnose in patients with cognitive impairment, and in one recent study analyzing probable RLS in 59 patients with dementia, two expert raters found that probable RLS occurred in 24% of patients and that probable RLS was associated with nocturnal agitation behaviors.[165] In another recent study, patients with RLS and early dementia often showed repetitive mannerisms and restlessness, and RLS behaviors were associated with selective serotonin reuptake inhibitor use and a polysomnographic PLMS index greater than 15 per hour.[166] Several medications, especially dopamine agonists, have been efficacious and well tolerated in RLS (for a review, see Chapter 121), although the efficacy and safety of these agents in patients with dementia has not been reported. In some patients dopaminergic agents can be stimulating and cause insomnia, whereas in others sleepiness may be seen, or these drugs can trigger or exacerbate psychosis.

Excessive Daytime Sleepiness

Excessive daytime sleepiness has been reported mainly in PD. Daytime sleepiness may result from poor sleep, dopaminergic therapy, circadian disorders, or comorbid OSA, or it may be due to PD itself.[167] Somnolence not resulting from another primary sleep problem can also affect patients with AD, DLB, and FTD. In such cases methylphenidate (at a low dose), modafinil, or armodafinil can be effective in improving alertness without producing significant adverse effects, although careful monitoring of blood pressure is indicated to ensure hypertension does not evolve during stimulant medication administration.

Hypersomnolence can also result from OSA, a condition often associated with degenerative disorders, especially AD and vascular dementia. The relationship between sleep apnea syndrome and dementia is complex. OSA is associated with cognitive deficits, some of which may be improved with continuous positive airway pressure (CPAP) therapy.[168] There have been cases of patients with OSA whose cognitive impairment improved with CPAP therapy.[169] One study showed that long-term CPAP treatment succeeded in slowing cognitive deterioration and improving sleep and mood in patients with AD and OSA.[170] Although our clinical experience suggests only a minority of patients with dementia significantly improve both functionally and on psychometric testing with CPAP therapy, a significant proportion of patients tolerate CPAP and use it nightly, and spouses enjoy a more consolidated sleep when their bed partners with dementia are on CPAP therapy.[170]

Circadian Rhythm Disorders

Several studies have demonstrated disruption of the sleep-wake rhythm in patients with dementia, especially in AD and FTD. In fact, insomnia and excessive daytime somnolence can be the manifestation of a primary circadian disorder. Degenerative changes in the biologic clock, the hypothalamic SCN, and the pineal gland, accompanied by reduced melatonin production, may be responsible for the disorganization and flattening of the circadian rhythms.[6,8] Melatonin can be helpful for sleep-wake cycle disturbances in patients with dementia, improving sleep, reducing sundowning, and slowing the progression of functional impairment in AD.[171,172] Bright-light therapy administered in the evening may alleviate sleep-wake cycle disturbances in patients with dementia and improve consolidation of their nighttime sleep.[173-175] In some patients, regular daylight exposure is also effective for day-night reversal problems.

Excessive Motor Activity during the Night

RBD and RSWA during PSG are more frequent in, and can aid diagnostic distinction of, the synucleinopathies when compared with AD, FTD, and PSP.[14] Two recent studies of polysomnographic RSWA, comparing patient with clinically probable cognitive (DLB) and motor (PD, MSA) synucleinopathies to Alzheimer disease and other tauopathies (PSP, corticobasal degeneration), found that elevated RSWA well distinguished those with a synucleinopathy.[58,176,177] There is a high interpatient variability in the severity of RBD, but the symptoms generally decrease with disease progression. It is important to differentiate RBD from nocturnal wandering by taking a careful history. When diagnosis is uncertain and the potential for injury is present, PSG with video recording is indicated. The first step in the management of RBD is to ensure the safety of the patient by removing potentially dangerous objects from the bedroom, placing a soft mattress on the floor next to the bed, and removing any firearms from the bedroom. Clonazepam, the traditional treatment of choice for RBD in nondemented persons, can potentially worsen cognition and can aggravate OSA. Before prescribing clonazepam, it is essential to exclude OSA, or to assure that patients with OSA are adherent to CPAP therapy at an effective treatment pressure. Clinical experience suggests that clonazepam is generally well tolerated and produces few cognitive side effects, although melatonin has also been shown to improve RBD symptoms and may be better tolerated in the elderly.[178–180] If depression is also present, treatments other than nefazodone should be considered because this drug increases REM sleep, contrary to most other antidepressants, and can therefore potentiate RBD. Agomelatine, a melatonergic antidepressant, may improve RBD symptoms and may also help treat comorbid depression.[181] The cholinesterase inhibitor rivastigmine also improved RBD symptom frequency in a pilot treatment trial in patients with PD.[182] A higher level of evidence from well-powered, definitive randomized controlled treatment trials is necessary to support specific RBD treatments.[183]

The prevalence of PLMS in dementia has not been clearly estimated. However, PLMS are known to be increased in dementia populations, especially in the synucleinopathies.[184] Without a polysomnographic recording, the severity and clinical significance of PLMS are difficult to assess. If PLMS are bothersome to the patient or cause daytime sleepiness as a result of sleep fragmentation, treatment with dopaminergic agonists can be considered. Dopaminergic agents should be used particularly cautiously in patients with psychotic features.

One of the heavier burdens on families of elderly demented patients and a primary cause of institutionalization is the lack of sleep because of nocturnal agitation or nocturnal wandering. Nocturnal agitation could be the result of discomfort (constipation, full bladder, clothing, heat, cold), pain (pressure sores, infection), or environmental interruptions (staff noise, light); hence verifying potential sources of discomfort and pain is crucial. As for insomnia management, eliminating alcohol and restricting caffeine intake to the morning can improve nocturnal agitation. Behavioral techniques should be tried before resorting to psychotropic or sedative-hypnotic medications. However, if necessary, medication options, including atypical neuroleptics (risperidone, olanzapine, clozapine, quetiapine), antiepileptic drugs (carbamazepine, lamotrigine, valproic acid, gabapentin), benzodiazepines (clonazepam, lorazepam), trazodone, or chloral hydrate, can be effective in treating nocturnal agitation (see Table 105.1 for dosages and titration schedule). Cholinesterase inhibitors can significantly reduce hallucinations for patients who are frightened or significantly bothered by them. In these patients medications with hallucinatory side effects (levodopa, dopamine agonists, anticholinergics, amantadine, selegiline) should be decreased or eliminated.

CONCLUSIONS

Sleep disturbances are frequent in patients with dementia. Although a common pattern of sleep impairment can be observed in dementia, the study of specific sleep variables may be valuable tools in aiding diagnosis and evaluating for behavioral and pharmacologic treatments.

CLINICAL PEARLS

- Patients with dementia often have important and disturbing sleep problems that can lead to premature institutionalization.
- When managing sleep disturbances in patients with dementia, clinicians should carefully look for underlying causes.
- Nonpharmacologic treatments and basic healthy sleep principles should be undertaken before considering psychotropic or sedative-hypnotic medications that could exacerbate cognitive deficits or obstructive sleep apnea, which should also be promptly diagnosed and treated when identified.
- When a pharmacologic treatment is necessary, one useful approach is to directly target the symptoms, which can be grouped in four categories: (1) insomnia or fragmented sleep, (2) excessive daytime sleepiness, (3) alteration in the sleep-wake circadian rhythm, and (4) excessive motor activity during the night, including rapid eye movement sleep behavior disorder, periodic leg movements during sleep, and nocturnal agitation or wandering.

SUMMARY

Sleep disturbances are frequent in patients with dementia. Sleep is usually more fragmented, with more frequent awakenings and a longer duration of time awake; SWS is decreased; sleep spindles and K-complexes are less well formed or less numerous, so sleep stages are more difficult to distinguish; and REM sleep may be reduced. Patients with dementia frequently present with comorbid sleep disorders, including OSA, PLMS, and RBD. As dementia advances, sleep disturbances typically worsen in parallel with progression of neurodegeneration.

ACKNOWLEDGMENTS

Dr. Montplaisir is supported by grants from the Canadian Institutes of Health Research. Dr. Boeve is supported by grants AG045390, AG052943, AG038791, AG056270, AG054256, NS100620, AG050326, AG056639, AG062677, AG063911 from the National Institutes of Health, the Mangurian Foundation, the Little Family Foundation, and the Turner Foundation. Dr. St. Louis is supported by the National Institutes of Health, National Institute on Aging, National Institute of Neurological Disorders and Stroke, and National Heart, Lung, and Blood Institute, the Michael J. Fox Foundation, Sunovion Pharmaceuticals, Inc., and Mayo Clinic Center for Clinical and Translational Science grant 1 UL1 RR024150-01. Dr. Carvalho has no disclosures.

SELECTED READINGS

Arnulf I, Nielsen J, Lohmann E, et al. Rapid eye movement sleep disturbances in Huntington disease. *Arch Neurol.* 2008;65(4):482–488.

Boeve BF. Update on the diagnosis and management of sleep disturbances in dementia. *Sleep Med Clin.* 2008;3(3):347–360.

Boeve BF, Silber MH, Ferman TJ, et al. REM sleep behavior disorder and degenerative dementia: an association likely reflecting Lewy body disease. *Neurology.* 1998;51(2):363–370.

Gagnon JF, Fantini ML, Bedard MA, et al. Association between waking EEG slowing and REM sleep behavior disorder in PD without dementia. *Neurology.* 2004;62(3):401–406.

Hita-Yanez E, Atienza M, Gil-Neciga E, Cantero JL. Disturbed sleep patterns in elders with mild cognitive impairment: the role of memory decline and ApoE epsilon4 genotype. *Curr Alzheimer Res.* 2012;9(3):290–297.

Kundermann B, Thum A, Rocamora R, et al. Comparison of polysomnographic variables and their relationship to cognitive impairment in patients with Alzheimer's disease and frontotemporal dementia. *J Psychiatr Res.* 2011;45(12):1585–1592.

Landolt HP, Glatzel M, Blattler T, et al. Sleep-wake disturbances in sporadic Creutzfeldt-Jakob disease. *Neurology.* 2006;66(9):1418–1424.

McCarter SJ, Tabatabai GM, Jong HY, et al. REM sleep atonia loss distinguishes synucleinopathy in older adults with cognitive impairment. *Neurology.* 2020;94(1):e15–e29.

Montplaisir J, Petit D, Lorrain D, et al. Sleep in Alzheimer's disease: further considerations on the role of brainstem and forebrain cholinergic populations in sleep-wake mechanisms. *Sleep.* 1995;18(3):145–148.

Osorio RS, Gumb T, Pirraglia E. Alzheimer's Disease Neuroimaging Initiative. Sleep-disordered breathing advances cognitive decline in the elderly. *Neurology.* 2015;84(19):1964–1971.

Pao WC, Boeve BF, Ferman TJ, et al. Polysomnographic findings in dementia with Lewy bodies. *Neurologist.* 2013;19(1):1–6.

Peter-Derex L, Yammine P, Bastuji H, Croisile B. Sleep and Alzheimer's disease. *Sleep Med Rev.* 2015;19:25–38.

Wang C, Holtzman DM. Bidirectional relationship between sleep and Alzheimer's disease: role of amyloid, tau, and other factors. *Neuropsychopharmacology.* 2020;45(1):104–120.

A complete reference list can be found online at ExpertConsult.com.

Chapter 106

Epilepsy, Sleep, and Sleep Disorders

Milena K. Pavlova; Sanjeev V. Kothare

Chapter Highlights

- Seizures may disrupt sleep, whereas sleep loss and sleep disorders may worsen epilepsy. This chapter describes the complex and bidirectional interactions of sleep and epilepsy.
- Epilepsy is a chronic disease, and seizures often occur at specific times of day and in certain stages of sleep.
- This chapter describes epilepsy syndromes that present with predominantly nocturnal seizures.
- The differentiation between nocturnal seizures and parasomnias can be challenging, and this chapter provides clinical pearls that help better identify seizures.

INTRODUCTION

Epilepsy and sleep disorders are considered by many to be common bedfellows. Sleep can affect seizure occurrence, threshold, and spread, whereas epilepsy can have a profound effect on the sleep-wake cycle and sleep architecture. Many factors can contribute to sleep disruption in patients with epilepsy, including inadequate sleep hygiene, coexisting sleep disorders, circadian rhythm disturbances, epilepsy per se, seizure frequency, and the effects of antiepileptic medications.

WHAT IS EPILEPSY?

Epilepsy is characterized by the tendency to have repeated, unprovoked seizures. The seizures can occur spontaneously or can be triggered reflexively by flashing lights or other sensory stimuli. The diagnosis of epilepsy[1] requires one of the following:

- At least two unprovoked (or reflex) seizures occurring more than 24 hours apart
- One unprovoked (or reflex) seizure and a probability of further seizures similar to the general recurrence risk (at least 60%) after two unprovoked seizures, occurring over the next 10 years
- A diagnosis of an epilepsy syndrome.

Epilepsy may result from genetic, structural, metabolic, traumatic, infectious, or unknown causes.

An individual seizure is the transient occurrence of signs and/or symptoms due to abnormal, excessive, or synchronous neuronal activity in the brain. A seizure can be focal (or partial) if it originates from a process within one hemisphere or generalized if it arises from both hemispheres. The seizure can be further classified by the type of motor activity observed—hypomotor, hypermotor, or automotor—or may include tonic and or clonic movements, or may be atonic (sudden loss of muscle tone) or myoclonic. When the seizure is focal, a variety of activity can be observed, depending on the brain region that leads to the seizures (epileptogenic zone), such as a stereotypic phrase or movement; stereotypic sensation (e.g., a specific sense of smell or hallucination); versive movement of head, eyes, or extremities; automatisms; or sometimes an abrupt cessation of activity. These abnormalities may be associated with alteration of consciousness.

Electrographically, seizures can be identified by distinct, rhythmic, epileptiform patterns (Figure 106.1) that disrupt the normal electroencephalographic (EEG) background, evolve in amplitude and frequency, often spread to involve other brain regions, and end abruptly, often followed by slowing or suppression of the EEG rhythms of the affected area. In between seizures, patients with epilepsy frequently have EEG abnormalities called "spikes" and "sharp waves," which are sharply contoured waves that stand out from the background and are often followed by a slow wave (Figure 106.2). Spikes are usually 30 to 70 microseconds in duration, whereas sharp waves are 70 to 200 microseconds in duration. Both have similar clinical significance.

Epilepsy Syndromes

Many patients exhibit a constellation of specific clinical and electrographic characteristics that allow identification of a specific epilepsy syndrome. In others the epilepsy is nonsyndromic. More than 50 distinct epilepsy syndromes have been defined, and the next sections review several of the syndromes that have a consistent association with sleep.

Sleep-Related Epilepsy Syndromes

Syndromes in Childhood

Benign Rolandic Epilepsy. Also called benign epilepsy with centrotemporal spikes, benign rolandic epilepsy is the most common partial epilepsy syndrome in children, with an onset between ages 3 and 13 years and remission in adolescence.[2] The typical presentation is a partial seizure with paresthesias and tonic or clonic activity of the lower face associated with drooling and dysarthria. The seizures are mostly nocturnal, with 55% to 59% of patients having seizures exclusively during sleep.[3] The EEG shows characteristic central and

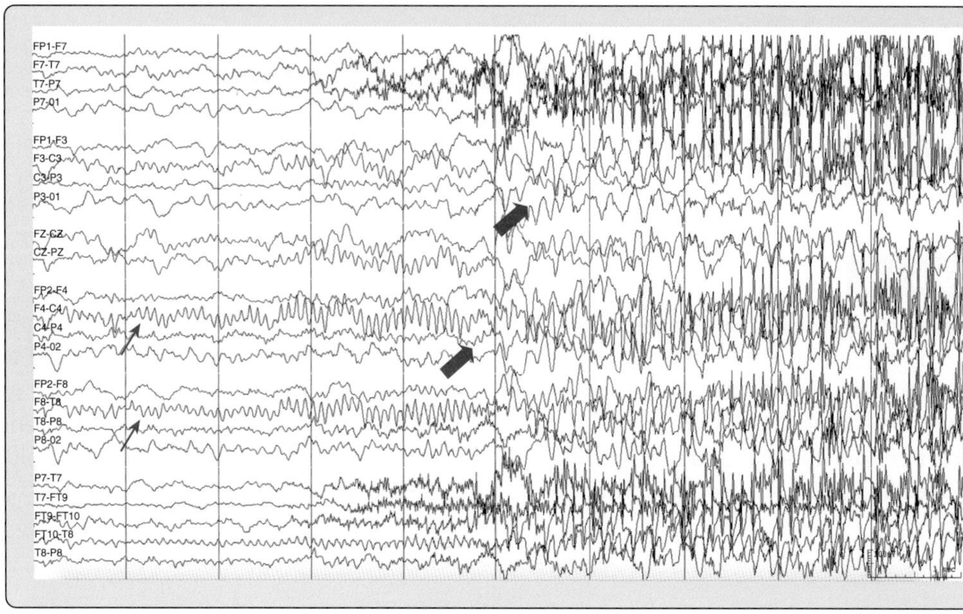

Figure 106.1 Electroencephalogram depicting a focal seizure with secondary generalization. Rhythmic activity starts in the centrotemporal area (F4/C4-F8/T8, *small arrows*), and over the next several seconds, it spreads to both hemispheres (*large arrows*).

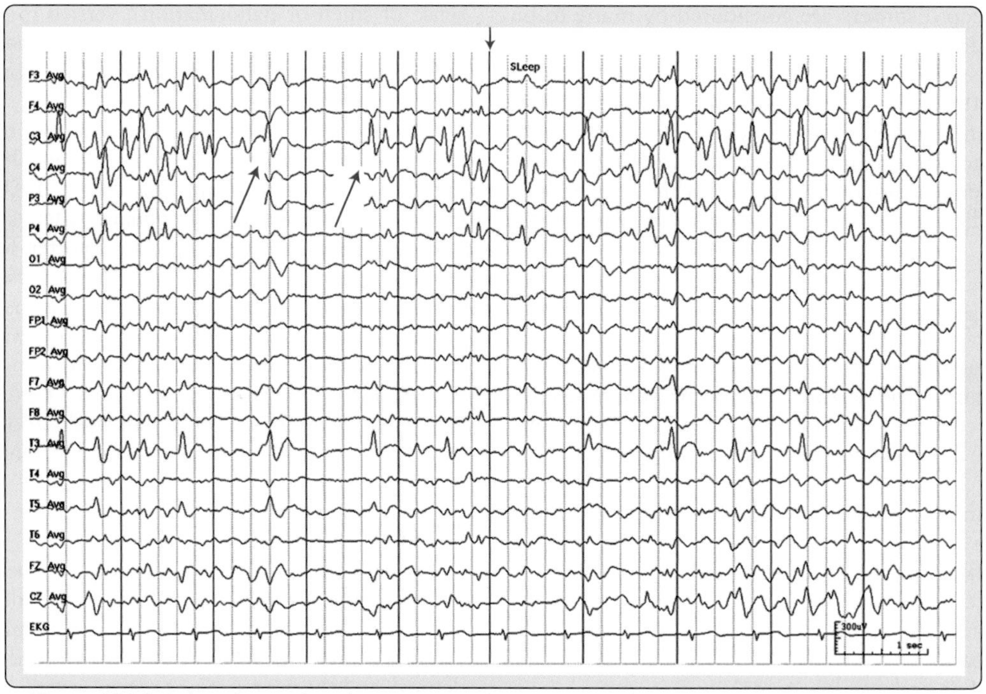

Figure 106.2 Spikes: abnormalities that are commonly seen on EEG of patients with epilepsy. Multiple spikes (*arrows*) are seen in a patient with benign epilepsy with centrotemporal spikes. The spikes are maximal in the centrotemporal areas bilaterally, but they occur independently (channels C3-T3 to C4-T4).

temporal spikes that occur bilaterally but independently and are potentiated during non–rapid eye movement (NREM) sleep (Figure 106.3). The discharge rate is increased during drowsiness and light sleep, compared to the waking record, with no change in spike morphology. Despite the increased frequency of seizures and spikes during sleep, the sleep architecture is unaffected, and sleep is not disrupted. The response to medications is excellent, and the prognosis is universally benign from an epilepsy perspective. However, these children often have deficits in visuospatial short-term memory, attention and cognitive flexibility, picture naming, visuoperceptual skills, and visuomotor coordination. These deficits may be related to nocturnal spiking. Reducing the nocturnal spike index has resulted in improved cognition, albeit at the cost of significant side effects.[4] These spikes are often seen incidentally in patients undergoing sleep studies to rule out obstructive sleep apnea (OSA) and in those who have never had overt seizures.[5]

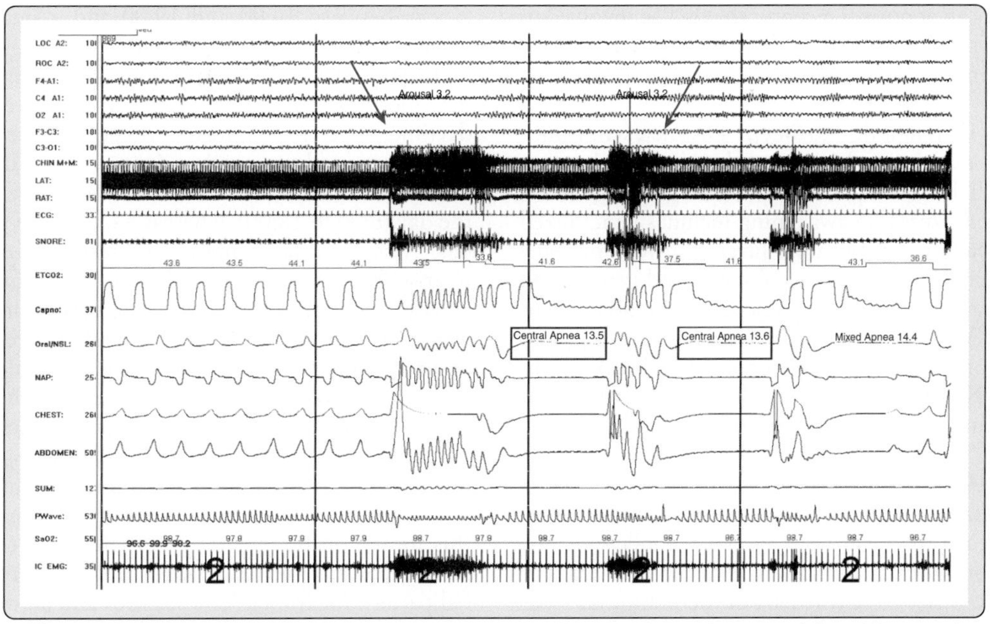

Figure 106.3 Tonic seizures (*arrows*) with tachypnea and tachycardia during the events, followed by central apneas.

Benign Occipital Lobe Epilepsy. This infantile variant of benign epilepsy of childhood with occipital paroxysms (also known as Panyiotopoulos syndrome) is another benign epilepsy syndrome seen in children age 2 to 6 years that is characterized by prolonged periods of eye deviation and autonomic instability (vomiting, temperature, heart rate, respiration, blood pressure) and hemiconvulsive and generalized tonic-clonic seizures in sleep, with vomiting on awakening. Interictal EEGs show occipital spikes, whereas ictal EEGs show electrographic seizures emanating from the occipital region during sleep.[6] Almost always, the epilepsy goes into remission within 2 years of onset.

Electrical Status Epilepticus in Slow Wave Sleep. Electrical status epilepticus in slow wave sleep (ESES) is characterized by spike-wave complexes "continuously" during NREM sleep but not during wake or rapid eye movement (REM) sleep.[7] The term *continuous* is applied only to EEG abnormalities with spikes occurring frequently (≥85% or epochs) during NREM sleep and persisting on three or more recordings over a period of 1 month.

Seizure onset typically occurs at 4 to 5 years of age. These seizures are partial or generalized and occur predominantly during sleep, with staring spells (atypical absence seizures) when awake, along with behavioral and language regression. Cognitive decline and mental retardation are noted in 50% of patients. Aggressive treatments to abolish paroxysmal EEG changes include corticosteroids, intravenous gammaglobulins, and high-dose antiepileptic medications.

Landau-Kleffner Syndrome. Landau–Kleffner syndrome (LKS) is an acquired disorder with epileptic aphasia in which children, usually 3 to 8 years of age, who have developed age-appropriate speech experience language regression with verbal auditory agnosia, epileptiform activity during sleep, behavioral disturbances, and sometimes overt seizures, more often in sleep.[7] Seizures arise out of sleep (generalized tonic-clonic, focal clonic, and/or atypical absences) and are less frequent and less severe than in ESES (absent in 20% to 30%). Behavioral problems are also less severe than in ESES.

There are several similarities between ESES and LKS. Both conditions demonstrate a normal EEG background during wakefulness, with rare focal or generalized spike-wave discharges. In ESES, however, discharges during sleep are generalized, whereas in LKS, spike-wave activity is mainly in the temporal channels. In ESES, epileptiform activity becomes virtually continuous during NREM sleep such that it may be impossible to distinguish sleep stages.

Infantile Spasms. This is a catastrophic epilepsy syndrome characterized by a triad of epileptic flexor/extensor spasms of the body, variable intellectual disability, and chaotic (otherwise termed *hypsarrythmic*) EEG, with onset between ages 3 and 18 months. Of interest, these spasms tend to cluster upon awakening in the morning.[8]

Syndromes Predominantly in Adulthood

Acetylcholine Receptor Mutations. Autosomal dominant nocturnal frontal lobe epilepsy (ADNFLE) is an adult epilepsy syndrome that presents with nocturnal seizures. Typical onset is in young adulthood (in the 20s), but it may also start in childhood and teenage years.[9] The clinical manifestations vary between individuals, although within the same individual, the seizures are stereotypic. These behaviors can include sudden awakenings with dystonic or dyskinetic movements (in 42% of patients from recent literature),[10] complex behaviors (13%), and sleep-related violent behavior (5%). The corresponding EEG findings include ictal epileptiform abnormalities, predominantly over frontal areas in 31% of patients, or rhythmic ictal slow wave activity over larger anterior cortical areas in another 47%. The disorder likely results from a mutation in the genes coding for the alpha4 and beta2 subunits of the nicotinic acetylcholine receptor (CHRNA4 or CHRNB2). At present, this is the only epilepsy syndrome in which the identified cause is an abnormal receptor that is also involved in the regulation of sleep. A third of patients also have associated NREM parasomnias.

Other Epilepsies with Relation to Sleep. Distinct, syndrome-specific patterns of seizures have been described with other syndromes as well. For example, as the name suggests, generalized tonic-clonic seizures on awakening includes generalized seizures that occur in the morning. Juvenile myoclonic epilepsy is characterized by myoclonic, absence, and generalized tonic-clonic seizures, and the myoclonic seizures tend to occur in the morning. A common symptom is myoclonus (a jerk of an extremity) soon after awakening, often before breakfast. In addition to ADNFLE, frontal lobe seizures generally occur at night and during sleep, as described in further detail later.

Patterns of Seizure Frequency

The timing of seizures from any cause (mesial temporal sclerosis, tumor, vascular malformations, etc.) often follows a pattern. It depends on time of day and stage of sleep, and varies by the epileptogenic-onset zone (the part of the brain that leads to the individual seizure).

Effect of Sleep Stage on Seizures

Many studies have examined the frequency of seizures in specific sleep stages and in wakefulness. The most striking and consistent finding is that seizures are extremely rare in REM sleep. A recent review of 42 studies (scalp and intracranial EEG recordings), which included a total of 1458 patients, reported that the lowest number of seizures are seen in REM sleep, compared to all other states.[11] More specifically, compared to REM sleep, in wakefulness there are eight times more focal seizures. The highest proportion of seizures occurs in N1 and N2 stages of NREM sleep, (respectively, 87 and 68 times more than in REM sleep), whereas in N3 sleep, seizures are slightly less frequent (51 times more than in REM sleep).

It is unclear what characteristics of REM sleep physiology are responsible for this unusual phenomenon. Some researchers hypothesize that the EEG desynchronization of REM sleep may reflect a unique pattern of neuronal connectivity that provides some protection against seizures.

Effect of Circadian Rhythms on Seizures

Even within the same state, the frequency of seizures varies with time of day, possibly due to the effects of endogenous circadian rhythms on brain activity. Several studies have described seizures captured in the hospital during continuous EEG monitoring. Early studies have reported a midafternoon peak in the frequency of temporal lobe seizures,[12] with a similar distribution of seizures in adults with temporal lobe epilepsy, as also observed in an animal model[13] and assessed by cosinor analysis (a distribution by fluctuating wave). Seizures originating from different brain locations had different times of occurrence,[13] with 50% of all temporal lobe seizures occurring between 15:00 to 19:00, whereas extratemporal seizures had a different distribution, suggesting that the peak times of seizure frequency varies by epileptogenic region. Further studies in adults using more precise localization techniques (performed with intracranial electrodes) confirmed consistent peaks in the timing of seizures depending on their location: occipital between 16:00 to 19:00; parietal between 4:00 to 7:00; frontal between 4:00 to 7:00; and mesial temporal with a peak between 16:00 and 19:00 and a smaller peak in the morning between 7:00 to 10:00.[14,15]

In children the patterns are slightly different. Clonic, atonic, hypomotor, and myoclonic seizures are more common in the daytime, whereas nighttime predominance was noted for automotor and hypermotor seizures, especially during sleep.[16] Generalized and occipital seizures were more common during the day (6:00 to 18:00), whereas a nighttime pattern (18:00 to 6:00) was noted for temporal and frontal seizures, which tend to arise from wakefulness and sleep, respectfully.

All of the above studies have significant limitations. All were performed within the hospital, where many activities occur at regular intervals (vital signs, scheduled examinations, etc.). Light levels are generally higher, and this may affect circadian rhythms by suppressing melatonin secretion or altering its pattern of secretion. In addition, weaning of antiepileptic medications (often done to facilitate recording of seizures) may also affect the timing of seizures. One study addressed this limitation by including patients with continuous home EEG recording and a diary of symptoms. It revealed a nocturnal pattern for frontal lobe seizures and an evening predominance for temporal lobe seizures.[17]

Much more advanced information has been obtained recently due to a novel method of treatment for epilepsy. The responsive nerve stimulation system is an intracranially implanted device that treats seizures by stimulating the brain region that generates the seizure. To exert this effect, the neurostimulator is connected to two four-contact leads (depth or subdural strip electrodes) implanted at the site of one or two seizures-onset regions. This also allows monitoring of the seizure frequency in long-term recordings with direct intracranial input, thus minimizing the likelihood that a seizure will be obscured by artifact outside the brain and opening the possibility to analyze data over much longer periods of time than can be obtained during outpatient scalp EEG. Using this method, Spencer and colleagues[18] have described circadian and ultradian patterns of epileptiform discharges from 191 adults with epilepsy. They found that brief epileptiform discharges show a strong, nocturnal pattern, which was visible in all tested seizure zones, whereas longer bursts had different patterns based on location. Seizures of neocortical origin had a strong monophasic circadian pattern with an acrophase in the early-morning hours, whereas mesial temporal seizures often had a biphasic pattern. These data support the previous reports that the timing of seizures relative to clock time is strongly dependent on the location of seizure onset.

Dosing Antiepileptic Medications to Reduce Nocturnal Seizures

The knowledge of this pattern of seizure frequency may be used to optimize therapy. A recent study[19] reported treatment of 17 children with nocturnal or early-morning seizures who were switched to a proportionally higher dose of antiepileptic medications in the evening and were retrospectively reviewed for seizure outcome and side effects. This differential dosing improved the patient's health, with seizure freedom in 65% (11/17) of patients and greater than 50% reductions in seizures in 88% (15/17).

Effects of Epilepsy on Sleep

Patients with epilepsy frequently have fragmented sleep and excessive daytime somnolence.[20–22] Causes include primary sleep disorders that disrupt sleep (e.g., sleep apnea, limb movements), nocturnal seizures that cause sleep fragmentation, and effects of medications. Insomnia is reported by 40% to 51% of epilepsy patients.[23,24] Furthermore, epilepsy patients with insomnia also have a higher frequency of depressive symptoms and poorer quality of life.[23]

Sleep fragmentation is a common complaint, and in many patients the cause of sleep disruption may be nocturnal seizures. An early publication included a visual example of individual seizures causing awakenings during a polysomnogram (PSG) of a patient with epilepsy who was not treated with antiepileptic medication.[25] After treatment, the patient's sleep became more continuous.

Sleep architecture may also be altered in patients with epilepsy. A decreased amount of REM sleep has been reported by several researchers.[26,27]

Primary sleep orders are relatively common in patients with epilepsy. A recent report includes the results from a cohort of 40 children with epilepsy[28] who underwent a sleep study because of various sleep complaints. Thirty-three patients (83%) exhibited snoring (42.5%), sleep-disordered breathing (obstructive hypoventilation in 12.5%; OSA in 20%; and upper-airway resistance syndrome in 7.5%), or periodic limb movements of sleep (10%). Children with poor seizure control had significantly lower sleep efficiency, a higher arousal index, and a higher percentage of REM sleep compared with children who were seizure free or exhibited good seizure control. Patients with epilepsy and OSA had significantly higher body mass index (BMI), longer sleep latency, higher arousal index, and lower apnea-hypopnea index, but significantly more severe desaturation compared with patients with uncomplicated OSA. A significant proportion of children with epilepsy referred for PSG with diverse sleep problems manifest sleep-disordered breathing, including OSA, and adults with epilepsy also have a higher prevalence of OSA.[29]

Effects of Sleep on Epilepsy

Effects of Sleep Deprivation on Seizures

Epilepsy patients frequently identify sleep loss as a major factor that provokes seizures. In a recent study,[30] greater than 97% of patients with epilepsy report at least one factor that provokes seizures, and the top three are acute and probably also chronic sleep loss, fatigue, and stress.

Sleep deprivation is often used in epilepsy monitoring units to increase the frequency of seizures. In addition, interictal epileptiform discharges are also more apparent after sleep deprivation.[31]

Effects of Obstructive Sleep Apnea on Epilepsy

When PSGs were performed on patients with medication-resistant epilepsy,[32] one-third of the patients were found to have OSA (apnea-hypopnea index ≥5). Furthermore, older adults with poorly controlled seizures have more frequent OSA.[33] A pilot placebo-controlled trial of the effectiveness of positive airway pressure (PAP) to help seizure control revealed that, among epilepsy patients with OSA, a 50% reduction in seizure frequency was seen more frequently among those who were treated with therapeutic continuous positive airway pressure (CPAP) (32%) than those receiving sham CPAP (15%). Some patients in this study with large reductions in seizure frequency had only mild OSA.[34] Although this study was not powered to detect subtle differences or for stratification by apnea severity or patient characteristics, the study's overall findings support the notion that treatment of the sleep apnea leads to better seizure control.

In a recent study of CPAP compliance in adults with epilepsy and OSA, 28 patients were CPAP compliant and 13 were not CPAP compliant.[35] In the compliant group, CPAP use reduced seizure frequency from 1.8 per month to 1 per month ($P = .01$). In the noncompliant group, no significant difference in seizure frequency was noted between baseline (2.1 per month) and follow-up at 6 months (1.8 per month, $P = .36$). Sixteen of the 28 CPAP-compliant subjects became seizure free, whereas only 3 of 13 non-CPAP–compliant subjects were seizure free (relative risk, 1.54; $P = .05$). Thus good CPAP compliance in patients with epilepsy and OSA can reduce the frequency of seizures.

Similar findings have been seen in children. A recent study followed 27 children with epilepsy and OSA who were treated with adenotonsillectomy.[36] Three months after the surgery, 10 (37%) patients became seizure free, 3 (11%) had greater than 50% seizure reduction, and 6 (22%) had smaller reductions in seizure frequency, whereas 2 (7%) demonstrated unchanged seizure frequency and 6 (22%) manifested a worsening of seizure frequency. The median seizure frequency per month before surgery was 8.5 (interquartile range, 2 to 90), and after surgery it was 3 (interquartile range, 0 to 75), with a 53% median seizure reduction. Multivariate analysis demonstrated a trend toward seizure freedom with each percentile increase in BMI and early age of surgery. Thus adenotonsillectomy for OSA in children may decrease seizure frequency, especially in children with elevated BMI scores and younger age at time of surgery.

Effect of Epilepsy Treatments on Sleep

Antiepileptic treatment may affect sleep.[37–39] Effects vary by type of medication and comorbidities. In general, with improvement of seizure control, the regularity of the sleep cycle improves, and sleep becomes more consolidated. However, some antiepileptic medications have been associated with insomnia and others with excessive daytime sleepiness (Table 106.2).[37]

Vagus nerve stimulation (VNS) is a nonpharmacologic therapy approved for use in patients with refractory epilepsy. An implanted device is programmed to stimulate the vagus nerve with electrical impulses and is typically used when pharmacologic therapy has been unsuccessful or a surgical approach is not indicated or has failed. VNS may also affect sleep, specifically sleep architecture and breathing. Some studies have found improvement of sleepiness and sleep architecture with VNS treatment.[40] However, VNS may also increase the incidence of sleep-related breathing disturbances, leading to OSA.[41] Therefore evaluation and treatment of OSA, if present, may be warranted for patients undergoing VNS therapy. Newer versions of VNS (Sentiva) allow changes in programming differentially in the daytime and in sleep and allows detection of supine and prone sleep, thus allowing positional intervention and monitoring.

Differential Diagnosis of Nocturnal Seizures from Other Events

Clinically, it can be a challenge to distinguish nocturnal epileptic seizures from movement disorders, psychogenic nonepileptic seizures, and parasomnias. Unlike periodic limb

Table 106.1 Differential Diagnosis of Nocturnal Seizures versus Parasomnia

Characteristic	Seizure	Parasomnia
Age of onset	Variable	Usually childhood onset
Course over time	Stable	Typically disappears in adulthood
Stage of sleep	NREM: more frequently N2	Slow wave sleep
Time of night	Any time, often first half	Typically first third of the night
Duration	≈30 sec to 2–3 min	Few minutes, may last as long as ≈30 min
Course of the individual event	Beginning, evolution, and end	Can be waxing-waning
Type of behavior	Stereotypic, nonpurposeful. Versive movements and dystonic posture can be seen	Complex, variable from event to event. Can appear purposeful
End of the event	Abrupt	Gradual emergence of consciousness
Number of events in the same night	Often multiple (>3)	1–2
EEG during the event	When visible, focal rhythmic activity with evaluation in time and space and abrupt end can be seen. Often, muscle artifact may obscure EEG	Normal Often, muscle artifact may obscure EEG
EEG between events	Interictal discharges are highly specific; however, a normal EEG does not rule out epilepsy	Normal

EEG, Electroencephalogram; NREM, non–rapid eye movement.

movement disorder, the rhythmic movements seen during an epileptic convulsion are much faster in frequency and have a distinct beginning, evolution, and end. Psychogenic nonepileptic seizures rarely arise during sleep, although individual patients have been described.[42] Psychogenic events are usually longer, have a waxing-waning pattern, and usually occur when the event can be witnessed by others.

Most critical is distinguishing nocturnal seizures from a NREM parasomnia. As the events occur at night, history is often sparse, and the immediately available tests can be difficult to interpret, which can lead to incorrect diagnosis. For example, several authors report that more than half of the patients with ADNFLE have been incorrectly diagnosed as having parasomnia.[10,42] The distinction is difficult because both disorders occur at night, impair sleep, and can be worsened by stress or sleep fragmentation. In addition, both types of events can be associated with amnesia for the event, and the interictal epileptiform abnormalities, which are so helpful in the positive identification of epilepsy, are uncommon in patients with any form of frontal lobe epilepsy and thus may be absent on a routine 30-minute EEG or even on an overnight recording.

Helpful elements in the presenting history include age of onset, duration, occurrence of multiple events in the same night, event frequency, and any description of the events. Derry and colleagues[43] created a standardized instrument—the frontal lobe epilepsy and parasomnia (FLEP) scale, which systematizes the approach to history. Typically, characteristics that indicate a higher likelihood of nocturnal seizures include a relatively short duration (<2 minutes), stereotypic behaviors, clustering (multiple events in the same night), and prominent dystonic posturing or tonic limb extension (Table 106.1). This scale has been successfully used in clinical practice.[44]

Capturing an event on video and/or EEG is extremely helpful. However, the absence of typical EEG features does not completely rule out seizures. Muscle artifact from movement can obscure the EEG, and a focal seizure may simply not be visible with a standard PSG montage.[45] Using an extended EEG montage better detects focal seizures and interictal discharges.[46]

Table 106.2 Side Effects Associated with Antiepileptic Drugs

Moderate to Severe Somnolence	Insomnia	Anxiety or More Severe Depressive Symptoms
Brivacetam	Lamotrigine	Brivacetam
Carbamazepine	Felbamate	Levetiracetam
Clobazam		Oxcarbazepine
Clonazepam		Perampanel
Diazepam		Tiagabine
Eslicarbazepine		Topiramate
Gabapentin		Valproate
Lacosamide		
Levetiracetam		
Lorazepam		
Oxcarbazepine		
Perampanel		
Phenobarbital		
Phenytoin (Dilantin)		
Pregabalin		
Primidone		
Rufinamide		
Tiagabine		
Topiramate		
Valproate (Depakote)		

Regarding analysis of the video recording, Derry and colleagues[47] proposed a decision tree to distinguish seizures from NREM parasomnias, based on the following characteristics:

1. *Whether there is a clear arousal to full consciousness and how this occurs.* If the patient does arouse, whether this occurs abruptly or gradually and whether the patient remains

supine or prone or engages in more complex behaviors with sitting, for instance, getting up from bed after the event.

2. *Presence of any versive movements or dystonic posturing during the event.* Versive movements or dystonic posture, or an abrupt ending with the patient remaining prone, would suggest a seizure, whereas complex behaviors and getting up from bed would point toward parasomnia.

Capturing the individual events on a single-night PSG is difficult, as these events are relatively rare, and they may not occur on the night of recording. Extending the length of the recording may be helpful in many clinical situations. The most reliable diagnosis is achieved via hospital admission with continuous video-EEG monitoring, with the goal of capturing one or more events. This allows (1) a long recording, which increases the likelihood of capturing interictal abnormalities; (2) examining the EEG for ictal abnormalities; (3) review of the video for any typical ictal phenomena or, if multiple events are captured, for stereotypy. In situations when this is not economically or logistically feasible, an outpatient continuous recording of EEG can be considered. The yield of outpatient testing is limited by lack of video and by the potential for loss of EEG signal from disconnected electrodes. The typical length of ambulatory EEG recordings is 48 to 72 hours. Longer recordings are technically possible, but with the multitude of activities and movements the patients engage in, the EEG signal progressively deteriorates and eventually becomes difficult to interpret.

Seizures that involve the frontal lobes, either because they originate from this area or because they have spread to involve the frontal lobes, often may manifest with vigorous movements, which makes the differential diagnosis between epilepsy and parasomnia particularly complex. To aid with this complexity, a specific disorder, sleep-related hypermotor epilepsy (SHE) was described. The causes of seizures are diverse; however, per statement publication,[48] the established criteria are as follows:

"SHE is characterized by the occurrence of brief (<2 minutes) seizures with stereotyped motor patterns within individuals and abrupt onset and offset. HE consists of "hypermotor" events. Seizures of SHE occur predominantly during sleep; however, seizures during wakefulness may occur."

The criteria include:

"Diagnosis of SHE is primarily based on clinical history. The absence of clear interictal and ictal EEG correlates, both during wakefulness and sleep, does not exclude the diagnosis of SHE."

"Certainty of diagnosis can be categorized into 3 levels: witnessed (possible) SHE, video documented (clinical) SHE, and video-EEG documented (confirmed) SHE."

Consequences of Epilepsy

Cardiorespiratory Abnormalities during Seizures

Epilepsy is associated with increased morbidity and mortality. The most devastating consequence is sudden unexpected death in epilepsy patients (SUDEP), a leading cause of death in young and otherwise healthy patients with epilepsy. Sudden death is at least 20 times more common in epilepsy patients compared to patients without epilepsy. A recent paper found SUDEP to be as common in the pediatric population as seen in adults, at 1 in 1000.[49,50] Most patients with SUDEP are found dead in sleep in the prone position. A significant proportion of patients with epilepsy experience cardiac and respiratory complications during seizures, which may contribute to SUDEP.

Respiratory changes often occur with generalized and focal seizures, especially those arising out of the mesial temporal structures. These include central and obstructive apneas; hypoventilation with hypercapnia and oxygen desaturation; as well as respiratory and metabolic acidosis, bradypnea, and tachypnea.[51] Cardiac abnormalities include tachycardia, bradycardia, hypotension, hypertension, tachyarrhythmias, bradyarhythmias, including asystole, and prolongation of the QTc interval.[52] These depend on multiple factors, including age and severity of epilepsy. A recent study found postictal central apnea to be a reliable predictor of SUDEP in the near future.[53] It appears that sleep stage may also affect physiologic distress from seizures. A recent study performed in mice[54] reported that seizures in REM sleep were universally fatal.

It appears that state of consciousness may directly affect how life-preserving mechanisms get activated or fail to activate during a seizure. For example, seizures from sleep lead to particularly severe respiratory abnormalities: The desaturation is more severe and associated with a longer time to return to preictal levels.[55] A recent epidemiologic study[56,57] examined the national database in Sweden, which compared individuals who had died of SUDEP versus individuals who were alive and had epilepsy in terms of type of seizures and living conditions. They identified 255 cases of SUDEP and compared their risk factors to 1148 sex-matched individuals with epilepsy who were still alive. The main finding was that the risk of SUDEP was 15 times greater in those who had nocturnal convulsions within the previous year. Further risk was associated with intervention: Those who lived alone had a 5 times greater risk of dying, and more than two-thirds of the deaths of those who had lived alone could potentially be prevented. Other risk factors included use of recreational drugs and alcohol.

The risk of SUDEP is by no means specific for SHE or any specific epilepsy. Patients with generalized epilepsy also have a substantial risk of SUDEP.[58] Thus nocturnal seizures, particularly nocturnal convulsions, should serve as an alert to any treating clinician regardless of specialty. Assessing mitigating factors and optimizing treatment to minimize nocturnal seizures, as well as addressing lifestyle and comorbidities, including sleep disorders, may be lifesaving.[58]

CLINICAL PEARLS

- Patients with epilepsy have frequent sleep complaints, and sleep disorders may worsen epilepsy.
- Treatment of sleep disorders may improve control of epilepsy.
- Seizures occur in patterns that depend on sleep stage and circadian factors. Integrating the treatment of seizures with knowledge of the chronobiologic pattern may improve treatment.
- Distinguishing seizures from non–rapid eye movement parasomnias is sometimes difficult. Clustering (multiple events in the same night), stereotypic behaviors, and dystonic posture or versive movements suggest seizures, whereas longer duration and complex behaviors are more common with parasomnias.

SUMMARY

Epilepsy is a chronic disease characterized by recurrent seizures. The frequency of seizures can be influenced by sleep stage and circadian rhythms, depending on the seizure focus. Several epilepsy syndromes present with predominantly or exclusively nocturnal seizures. These include syndromes with benign prognosis in childhood, such as benign epilepsy with centrotemporal spikes and benign occipital epilepsy, some adult epilepsies, such as ADNFLE, and other syndromes with poorer prognosis, such as electrical status epilepticus of sleep. Other seizures, such as those of temporal lobe origin, tend to occur during wakefulness, most often in the mid to late afternoon.

Nocturnal seizures should be differentiated from movement disorders and from parasomnias. Behaviorally, seizures have stereotypic presentation, short duration (30 seconds to 2 minutes), and a tendency for clustering (multiple events in the same night), whereas parasomnias have a more fluctuating course during the night and may include complex, nonstereotypic behaviors. Adequate diagnosis is established by identifying typical EEG patterns (ictal or interictal) and careful analysis of any events captured on video for stereotypic features.

SELECTED READINGS

Buchanan GF, Gluckman BJ, Kalume FK, et al. Proceedings of the sleep and epilepsy workshop: section 3 mortality: sleep, night, and SUDEP [published online ahead of print, 2021 Mar 31]. *Epilepsy Curr.* 2021; 15357597211004556.

Derry CP, Harvey AS, Walker MC, Duncan JS, Berkovic SF. NREM arousal parasomnias and their distinction from nocturnal frontal lobe epilepsy: a video EEG analysis. *Sleep.* 2009;32(12):1637–1644.

Ferlisi M, Shorvon S. Seizure precipitants (triggering factors) in patients with epilepsy. *Epilepsy Behav.* 2014;33:101–105.

Fisher RS, Acevedo C, Arzimanoglou A, et al. ILAE official report: a practical clinical definition of epilepsy. *Epilepsia.* 2014;55(4):475–482.

Hollway JA, Aman MG. Sleep correlates of pervasive developmental disorders: a review of the literature. *Res Dev Disabil.* 2011;32(5):1399-421.

Latreille V, Abdennadher M, Dworetzky BA, et al. Nocturnal seizures are associated with more severe hypoxemia and increased risk of postictal generalized EEG suppression. *Epilepsia.* 2017;58(9):e127–e131.

Latreille V, St Louis EK, Pavlova M. Co-morbid sleep disorders and epilepsy: a narrative review and case examples. *Epilepsy Res.* 2018;145:185–197.

Manni R, Terzaghi M. Comorbidity between epilepsy and sleep disorders. *Epilepsy Res.* 2010;90(3):171-177.

Mayer G, Jennum P, Riemann D, Dauvilliers Y. Insomnia in central neurologic diseases—occurrence and management. *Sleep Med Rev.* 2011;15(6):369–378.

Pavlova MK, Ng M, Allen RM, et al. Proceedings of the sleep and epilepsy workgroup: section 2 comorbidities: sleep related comorbidities of epilepsy [published online ahead of print, 2021 Apr 12]. *Epilepsy Curr.* 2021; 15357597211004549.

Pavlova M, Singh K, Abdennadher M, et al. Comparison of cardiorespiratory and EEG abnormalities with seizures in adults and children. *Epilepsy Behav.* 2013;29(3). 537-41.

Pavlova MK, Woo Lee J, Yilmaz F, Dworetzky BA. Diurnal pattern of seizures outside the hospital: Is there a time of circadian vulnerability? *Neurology.* 2012;78(19):1488–1492.

Quigg M, Bazil CW, Boly M, et al. Proceedings of the sleep and epilepsy workshop: section 1 decreasing seizures-improving sleep and seizures, themes for future research [published online ahead of print, 2021 Mar 31]. *Epilepsy Curr.* 2021;15357597211004566.

Sandhu MRS, Dhaher R, Gruenbaum SE, et al. Circadian-like rhythmicity of extracellular brain glutamate in epilepsy. *Front Neurol.* 2020;11:398. Published 2020 May 15.

A complete reference list can be found online at ExpertConsult.com.

Chapter 107

Sleep and Headache

Alexander D. Nesbitt; Peter J. Goadsby

Chapter Highlights

- Headache is one of the commonest reasons to seek medical attention. There are multiple potential levels of overlaps between sleep, biologic rhythms, and primary headache disorders. These include mechanistic, clinical, and therapeutic interactions.
- Hypnic headache, cluster headache, and migraine are the most closely sleep-associated primary headache disorders, with sleep apnea headache perhaps being the most familiar disorder among sleep physicians. The clinical features of each of these disorders and their associations with sleep and biologic rhythms are outlined.
- The chapter emphasizes how to recognize and differentiate between each of these disorders, as their treatment options, which are also considered herein, differ considerably.

Headache is one of the commonest reasons to seek medical attention. Worldwide, it is estimated that 3 billion people will experience a primary headache disorder, such as migraine, annually. Socioeconomic studies estimate approximately 153 million sufferers in Europe alone, with an economic burden of a magnitude of 43 billion Euros per annum.[1] So high is this burden, largely as a result of reduced productivity associated with the problem, that the World Health Organization lists headache as one of the 20 most significant causes of disability worldwide. Although the potential relationships between sleep, biologic rhythms, and headache have long been postulated, they remain largely speculative and underused therapeutically. These interactions are thought to feature prominently in several headache disorders, namely, hypnic headache (HH), cluster headache (CH), and migraine, in which attacks can arise from, be modulated by, and are associated with sleep, as well as being probabilistically more likely to occur at certain times during the 24-hour period. A more focused and detailed understanding of these relationships is likely to be fruitful for headache sufferers. This chapter reviews what is currently known about these relationships from a mechanistic, clinical, and therapeutic viewpoint.

MECHANISTIC CONSIDERATIONS

The pain of headache is thought to be a consequence of activation or perception of nociceptive signaling pathways within the trigeminovascular system (Figure 107.1).[2,3] This system integrates a network of both ascending somatosensory and descending modulatory neural pathways, which are centered around the trigeminocervical complex (TCC), located in the spinal trigeminal nucleus caudalis and the upper cervical cord (C1 and C2). The ascending pathways comprise sensory afferents of the trigeminal nerve, which innervate the larger blood vessels and dura of the cranium, synapsing in the TCC and then ascending to the thalamus and onward to a diffuse cortical sensory network. A reflex connection from the TCC to the superior salivatory nucleus of the facial nerve also exists, which forms the basis of the trigeminal autonomic reflex, thought to be important in perpetuating the pain and generating some of the specific cranial autonomic features of some headache disorders (Figure 107.1). The trigeminovascular system is under the modulatory control of a number of descending pathways, originating in various different brain regions, including the hypothalamus, brainstem, and limbic system, which differentially convey excitatory or inhibitory influences on it. It is thought that dysfunction of these modulatory pathways is responsible for the generation and maintenance of headache.

Many of the structures and neurotransmitters involved in the trigeminovascular system are also considered to be relevant to arousal, sleep-wake control, and, to a lesser extent, biologic rhythmicity.[4] These particular regions and molecules, and the basic and clinical evidence supporting their roles in headache, are summarized in Tables 107.1 and 107.2, respectively.

HEADACHE DISORDERS ASSOCIATED WITH SLEEP

At outset, a clear distinction must be made between one-off and briefly appearing, recurrent attacks of very severe headache, which may wake a sufferer from sleep, and those occurring more regularly and over a longer period of time. In the former group, subarachnoid hemorrhage can famously arise as an extreme thunderclap headache from sleep, as can consecutive attacks of reversible cerebral vasoconstriction syndrome, typically only occurring a handful of times. Acute-angle glaucoma is also thought more likely to occur in the early hours of the morning, often waking sufferers from sleep, and the pronounced ophthalmic manifestations usually (although not always) help easily distinguish it.

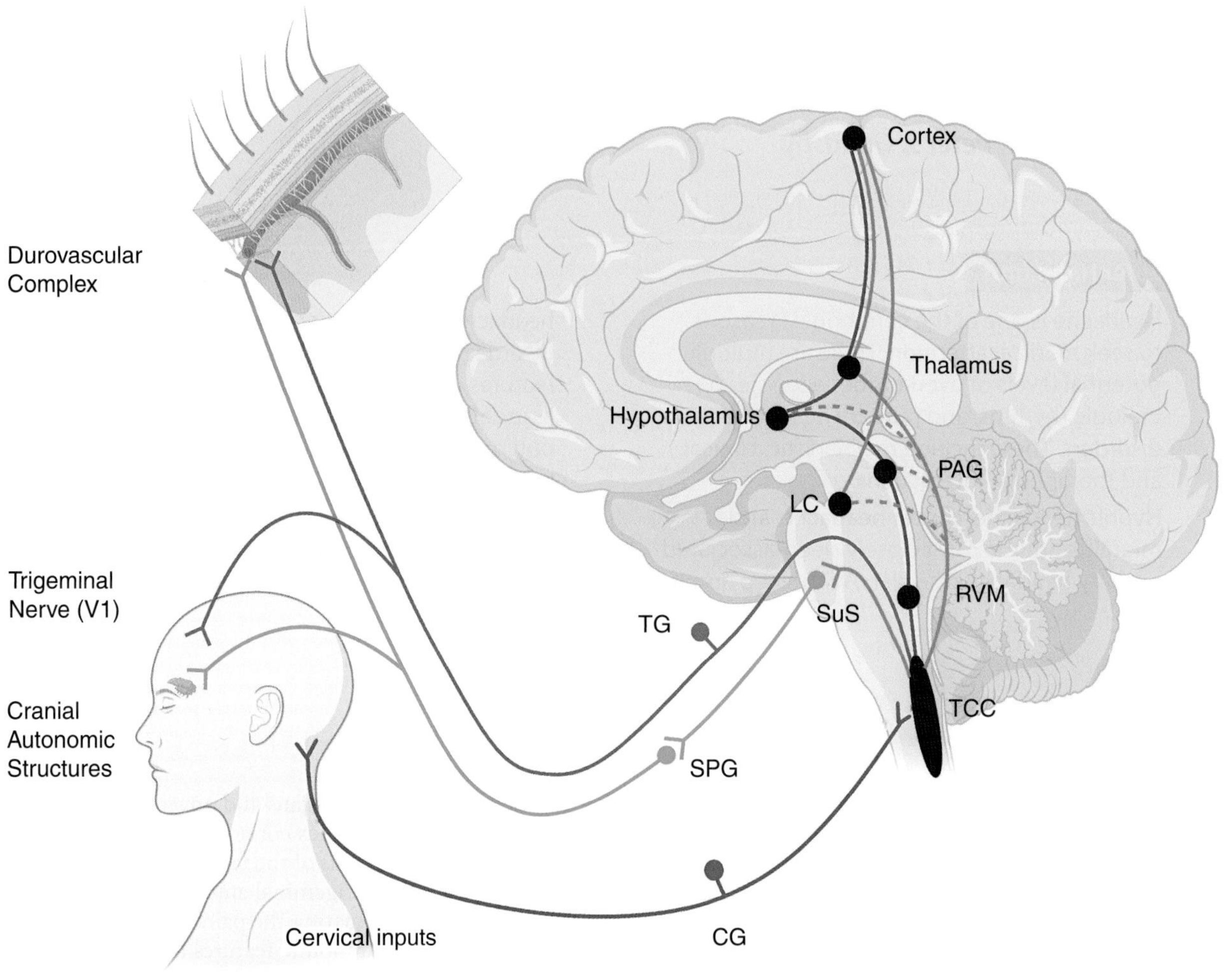

Figure 107.1 The trigeminovascular system. Sensory fibers innervating the head and neck, including the pain-sensing blood vessels and dura of the cranial vault (the durovascular complex), travel as either the trigeminal nerve or greater occipital nerve via the cervical ganglion (CG) to the trigeminocervical complex (TCC), where they synapse with second-order neurons (shown in *pink*). These ascending second-order neurons project to the thalamus via the quintothalamic tract (shown in *blue*) and are also thought to have direct projections to the locus coeruleus (LC), periaqueductal gray (PAG), and hypothalamus (shown in *dashed blue lines*). These structures in turn send ascending signals to the cortex. There is also a reflex connection of second-order neurons in the TCC to the superior salivatory (SuS) nucleus of the facial nerve, which provides parasympathetic outflow to the cranial vasculature within the durovascular complex, as well as to cranial autonomic structures, such as the lacrimal gland, via the sphenopalatine ganglion (SPG) (shown in *green*). This trigeminal autonomic reflex is responsible for the cranial autonomic features seen in response to head pain in several primary headache disorders, such as cluster headache. There are also descending projections from the cortex to the thalamus, hypothalamus, and LC (shown in *red*). Descending modulation of TCC neurons is mediated by the hypothalamus and PAG via its connections with the rostroventral medulla (RVM). TG, Trigeminal ganglion.

Recurrent, stereotypic attacks of headache arising from sleep are more suggestive of primary headaches: headache disorders that are not symptoms of other pathologies, some of which are noted to have stronger associations with sleep than others. These associations range from those disorders, which arise exclusively from sleep, and never from wakefulness, to those which typically arise from wake but can also emerge during sleep, in which a sufferer may awaken with a headache, rather than be awoken by one. In rank order of their associations with sleep, these disorders are discussed later, and the features which distinguish them are summarized in Table 107.3. This section then goes on to discuss secondary headache disorders, those in which headache is a symptom of another condition, and their association with sleep, in particular sleep apnea headache.

Hypnic Headache

Considered to be the archetypal sleep-related primary headache disorder, HH was only first described in the mid-1980s.[5] The attacks are exclusively sleep locked and never arise from wakefulness.[6] A specific feature of the disorder is that sufferers must be woken *by* the headache, rather than awakening *with* a headache. True HH is considered to be very rare, with a recent systematic review of all published cases yielding 348 descriptions.[7,8] These cases form our current clinical understanding of the disorder and define its current diagnostic criteria (Box 107.1),[9] which makes HH harder to distinguish from migraine, even in specialist settings. Unusually for a headache disorder, onset, in at least 90% of cases, seems to occur after the age of 50 years.[8] Despite this, rare cases are reported in pediatric populations.[10–12] There is a slight female preponderance of around 65%.[8]

Table 107.1 Brain Regions Involved in Sleep-Wake Regulation and Headache

Structure	Reported Roles in Headache
Ventrolateral periaqueductal gray	Stimulation inhibits pain-evoked firing in TCC Block of P/Q-type calcium channels facilitates pain-evoked firing in TCC
Rostroventral medulla	ON neurons are pronociceptive OFF neurons are antinociceptive
Locus coeruleus	Region active in functional imaging studies Stimulation causes intracranial vasoconstriction and extracranial vasodilatation Lesioning inhibits pain-evoked firing in TCC Lesioning lowers CSD triggering threshold
Hypothalamus (posterior)	Region active in functional imaging studies of TAC attacks Volumetric changes seen in CH and HH DBS of region therapeutic in TACs Nociceptive dural stimulation causes activation, especially in hypocretinergic neurons
Paraventricular	Modulates trigeminovascular processing, particularly in response to stress
A11	Activation reduces pain-evoked firing in TCC Disruption increases pain-evoked firing in TCC Role in RLS pathophysiology
Suprachiasmatic	*CSNK1D* mutation causes FASPD2 (FASPD plus migraine with aura) *CSNK1D* mutant mice have lowered CSD triggering threshold
VPM of thalamus	Variety of headache drugs act on VPM neurons
Cortex	NREM increased in response to CSD Cortex has been shown to be both hyperexcitable and hypoexcitable in migraine

CH, Cluster headache; CSD, cortical spreading depression; *CSNK1D*, gene coding for casein kinase 1 delta; FASPD2, familial advanced sleep-wake phase disorder type 2; HH, hypnic headache; NREM, non–rapid eye movement; RLS, restless legs syndrome; TAC, trigeminal autonomic cephalalgia; TCC, trigeminocervical complex; VPM, ventral posteromedial nucleus.

Approximately two-thirds of sufferers report a mild to moderate dull headache, with the remainder describing a more intense pain severity, with a possible throbbing sensation.[8] The attacks are typically bilateral and usually frontotemporal or holocranial in location, although occasional unilateral cases have been described.[13,14] Twenty percent of patients will report some nausea, but typically only a much smaller number (7%) report any degree of photophobia or phonophobia during an attack.[8] Cranial autonomic features are typically absent, but mild nasal symptoms have been reported in up to 15% of cases.[15,16] The majority of patients with HH are said to leave the bed with an attack and to perform some other activity,

Table 107.2 Neuropeptides and Neurotransmitters Involved in Sleep-Wake Regulation and Headache

Peptide/ Transmitter	Reported Roles in Headache
Melatonin	Trigeminovascular activation enhanced by pineal ablation and trigeminovascular activation normalized by exogenous melatonin administration Melatonin may inhibit CSD Low melatonin amplitudes seen in CH and chronic migraine Melatonin therapeutic in migraine and CH
Hypocretin	Hypocretin-1 administration into hypothalamus reduces pain-evoked firing in TCC Hypocretin-2 administration into hypothalamus increases pain-evoked firing in TCC
Adenosine	A1 receptor agonists antinociceptive A1 receptor agonists attenuate nociceptive blink reflex Receptor polymorphism described in migraine with aura
PACAP	Hypothalamic administration facilitates trigeminal nociception May have a role in light aversion in migraine
Nitric oxide	Nitric oxide donors can trigger migraine, including premonitory phase (yawning, etc.)
Melanopsin	ipRGCs mediate light aversion response in migraine

A1, Adenosine 1; CH, cluster headache; CSD, cortical spreading depression; ipRGC, intrinsically photosensitive retinal ganglion cell; PACAP, pituitary adenylate cyclase–activating polypeptide; TCC, trigeminocervical complex.

such as watching television or drinking water, in contrast to migraine, in which sufferers typically remain in bed,[16,17] and patients with CH, who often leave the bed with a profound sense of psychomotor agitation. The attacks of HH occur at least on a third of nights a month, with most experiencing them on a mean of 20 nights a month. The attacks are typically said to be short lasting, although two-thirds of patients can have attacks that continue for 2 hours or more, with some series suggesting they may go on longer.[18]

HH secondary to tumors of the posterior fossa[19–21] or pituitary gland[22,23] are reported. In addition, nocturnal hypertension has also been described as a causative factor in a small number of reports.[24–26] Given these associations, magnetic resonance imaging (MRI) and blood pressure recordings during attacks of HH are prudent. Sleep studies are helpful in ruling out obstructive sleep apnea (OSA).

Caffeine is reported to be the most useful acute treatment to use on waking with an attack,[16,17,27–29] followed by aspirin,[6,27,30] although the short attack length leaves open the possibility of natural history resolving individual attacks. Lithium carbonate, caffeine, and indomethacin, taken nightly before sleep, are the most frequently reported preventive treatments.[8] These medications are, however, not without their potential adverse effects, especially when taken long term. Note should

Table 107.3 Differences between the Main Sleep-Related Primary Headache Disorders

	Hypnic Headache	Cluster Headache	Migraine
Attacks arising from sleep	Exclusively	Very often	Occasionally
Woken by or wake with attack	Woken by attack	Woken by attack	Wake with attack
Daytime attacks as well?	Never	Often	Very often
Nocturnal timing	Second third of night	First third of night	Final third of night
Recurrent attacks per night	Very rare	Common	No
Prevalence	Very rare	Rare (≈0.12%)	Very common (≈14.4%)
Usual age of onset	6th decade onward	3rd decade onward	2nd decade onward
Gender	Women > men	Men > women	Women > men
Pain severity	Moderate	Very severe	Moderate to severe
Pain characteristic	Dull, constant	Sharp, stabbing	Throbbing, dull
Pain location	Bilateral	Unilateral	Unilateral or bilateral
Cranial autonomic symptoms	No	Marked, ipsilateral to side of pain	Occasional, mild
Pain duration	<2 h	15 min–3 h	4–72 h
Attack frequency	>15 nights/mo	1/48 h to 8/24 h; occurring in bouts	Variable; chronic ≥15 days/mo
Attack behavior	Get out of bed and do something	Pacing, rocking, hitting head, 90%	Stay still in bed
Associated nausea	Unusual	Possible: up to 50%	Very common
Pain worsened by movement	No	No	Yes
Pain worsened by light and noise	No	Possible: up to 50%; usually limited to same side as the attack	Yes
Acute treatments	Caffeine, aspirin	High-flow oxygen, subcutaneous or nasal sumatriptan, nVNS	NSAIDs, triptans
Preventive treatments	Caffeine, indomethacin, melatonin	Verapamil, topiramate, lithium, melatonin, nVNS, CGRP antibodies in episodic cluster headache	TCAs, propranolol, topiramate, onabotulinum toxin A, CGRP antibodies

CGRP, Calcitonin gene–related peptide; NSAIDs, nonsteroidal antiinflammatory drugs; nVNS, noninvasive vagus nerve stimulation; TCAs, tricyclic antidepressants.

BOX 107.1 *INTERNATIONAL CLASSIFICATION OF HEADACHE DISORDERS,* THIRD EDITION: DIAGNOSTIC CRITERIA FOR HYPNIC HEADACHE

A. Recurrent headache attacks fulfilling criteria B–E
B. Developing only during sleep and causing wakening
C. Occurring on ≥10 days/mo for >3 mo
D. Lasting from 15 min up to 4 h after waking
E. No cranial autonomic symptoms or restlessness[a]
F. Not better accounted for by another ICHD-3 diagnosis

[a]Cranial autonomic symptoms include conjunctival injection, lacrimation, ptosis/miosis, eyelid edema, forehead and facial sweating, aural fullness.
ICHD-3, *International Classification of Headache Disorders*, third edition.

also be made that concurrent indomethacin use can cause lithium toxicity.[31] Indomethacin can worsen OSA, and lithium can worsen restless legs syndrome (RLS) and periodic limb movements.[32] Topiramate, melatonin, and gabapentin have also been reported as potential preventive treatments in individual cases.[8]

Timing of Hypnic Headache

Consistent timing of awakening with an attack of HH is a widely reported phenomenon,[16–18] and has given rise to the moniker "alarm clock headache."[27] Unlike the attacks of CH, which typically happen within the first 2 hours of sleep onset, and may then repeat through the night, HH attacks are said to be more likely to occur between 02:00 to 04:00, suggesting, if we assume population average sleep-wake timings in these patients, that they are occurring later during the nocturnal sleep episode. The attacks usually occur once at night, although some reports of multiple attacks per night do exist.[6,16,18,33,34] Of interest, attacks can also arise from daytime naps[27,35] and at the same time after sleep onset, regardless of local time zone, as described in a case report of a patient flying from Brazil to Portugal.[36] This might be taken as anecdotal evidence to suggest homeostatic sleep-related mechanisms are more important than circadian timing in the onset of these attacks.

Sleep and Hypnic Headache

Despite the apparent rarity of HH, many polysomnographic (PSG) studies exist.[33,34,37–42] However, none of these studies have shown any consistent association with any sleep stage or other qualitative sleep electroencephalographic (EEG) parameters. Some of these studies have demonstrated coexistent OSA,[34,38] although only two patients have been documented to have had contemporaneous improvement in HH attacks with treatment of OSA: one with continuous positive airway pressure (CPAP)[38] and one with a mandibular advancement

BOX 107.2 INTERNATIONAL CLASSIFICATION OF HEADACHE DISORDERS, THIRD EDITION: DIAGNOSTIC CRITERIA FOR CLUSTER HEADACHE

A. At least five attacks fulfilling criteria B–D
B. Severe or very severe unilateral orbital, supraorbital, and/or temporal pain lasting 15–180 min (when untreated)
C. Either or both of the following:
   1. At least one of the following symptoms or signs, ipsilateral to the headache:
      a. Conjunctival injection and/or lacrimation
      b. Nasal congestion and/or rhinorrhea
      c. Eyelid edema
      d. Forehead and facial sweating
      e. Miosis and/or ptosis
   2. A sense of restlessness or agitation
D. Occurring with a frequency between one every other day and eight per day
E. Not better accounted for by another ICHD-3 diagnosis.

ICHD-3, *International Classification of Headache Disorders*, third edition.

device.[43] Periodic limb movements have also been described, possibly reflecting treatment with lithium.[44]

In addition to clinical sleep studies, voxel-based morphometric imaging has demonstrated significant volume reductions in posterior hypothalamic areas, particularly, and somewhat puzzlingly, more so on the left side than right[45] in patients with HH. This is in contrast to two studies in CH, one that demonstrated an increase in volume in the same area,[46] and another that found no difference.[47] An electrophysiologic study found no decrement in facilitation or habituation in response to either the nociceptive blink reflex or trigeminal pain-related evoked potentials in HH,[48] which is in contrast to all other electrophysiologically studied categories of primary headache disorders.[49] Furthermore, individuals with HH appear to have normal melatonin secretion profiles.[50]

Cluster Headache

Few, if any, medical disorders inflict more intense pain than CH.[51] Patients describe the pain of a single attack as being worse than anything else they have ever experienced, including childbirth. The term *cluster headache* originates from the tendency of the attacks to cluster together into bouts ("in-bout") lasting several weeks at a time, with longer periods of remission lasting at least a month between bouts ("out-of-bout"). CH is the most common subtype of a group of primary headache disorders called trigeminal autonomic cephalalgias (TACs), which all share the feature of prominent symptoms such as lacrimation and redness of the eye, nasal congestion, and rhinorrhea, ipsilateral to the side of most often extreme head pain[52] (Figure 107.1).

The diagnostic criteria for CH are outlined in Box 107.2, and the clinical features differentiating CH from other sleep-related headache disorders are summarized in Table 107.3. It must also be emphasized that the treatment of CH differs from that of other headache disorders.[51] For individual attacks, the rapidity of onset necessitates the use of parenteral triptans (subcutaneous or nasal sumatriptan, or nasal zolmitriptan) or high-flow oxygen, both of which will typically abort an attack within 15 minutes of treatment.[51,53] Preventive pharmacotherapy aims to reduce the frequency and intensity of attacks, typically using verapamil, topiramate, or lithium. High doses of melatonin are sometimes used as an adjunct treatment, particularly in chronic CH.[54] More recently, galcanezumab, a monoclonal antibody directed toward calcitonin gene–related peptide (CGRP), has shown efficacy as a preventive treatment for episodic CH.[55] Targeted local anesthetic and corticosteroid block of the greater occipital nerve is often useful while preventive treatments are initiated,[56,57] or oral corticosteroids.[58] Recently, devices purported to stimulate noninvasively the vagus nerve,[59] and minimally invasively stimulate the sphenopalatine ganglion,[60] have demonstrated efficacy in both acute and preventive treatment approaches.

Timing and Cluster Headache

The attacks of CH last between 15 and 180 minutes; however, they may, rarely, last longer. Attack frequency is between one attack every 48 hours, to eight separate attacks in any 24-hour period. A large British cohort study found the mean maximum number of attacks experienced per day to be 4.6, with 37% reporting a predictable time of onset during the day and 72% reporting attacks occurring at predictable times during the night, waking them from sleep.[61] This striking, regular, ultradian periodicity of CH attacks, probably alluded to as early as the 17th century in Western medical literature,[62,63] has been more systematically documented in the 20th century.[64–67] Data from other large retrospective clinical series confirm about 70% of patients reporting predictable timing of attacks,[61,68–76] although this may become less striking the longer the disorder continues. Studies of individual attack timing patterns recorded retrospectively have revealed quite consistent early-morning, midafternoon, and prominent evening peaks in attack likelihood.[77–79] Case reports of individual patients prospectively recording thousands of attacks have also found potential ultradian peaks in attack frequency but did note a high degree of variability.[80,81]

Most people with CH experience one bout of attacks a year, with a unimodal frequency distribution and mean bout duration of 8.6 weeks found in the British series. However, individuals may go for several years without a bout (up to 20 in some cases), and others may suffer more frequent bouts each year.[61] The bouts of attacks are said to occur with greater frequency at particular times of year (typically spring and autumn), and in some patients with chronic CH, the frequency and intensity of attacks may also show a similar seasonal worsening.[61,82–84]

These remarkable clinical observations regarding the temporal characteristics of CH attacks have strengthened a rather nebulous notion that possible dysregulation of circadian timing systems might underpin the disorder's pathophysiology. This idea gained traction from functional imaging studies demonstrating hypothalamic regions at the core of the attacks[85] and subsequent deep brain stimulation of this region proving to be therapeutic in some patients with chronic CH.[86] However, no compelling evidence exists to support dysfunction of biologic timing systems in CH, and what does exist remains circumstantial. For example, application of the Munich Chronotyping Questionnaire in a large patient cohort showed a slightly higher prevalence of later-evening types in episodic CH compared to chronic CH and control subjects,[87] and a recent study also found that women with CH may experience a slightly earlier peak in the timing of their attacks than men.[88] A genetic analysis of *PER3* variable number tandem repeat polymorphisms in patients with CH has not shown any consistent association.[89,90] However, the same cohort was used to demonstrate additional associations with another polymorphism in a *CLOCK* variant gene, which did show some association, albeit not a particularly strong one.[91] Several earlier clinical investigations have found a variety of changes in melatonin secretion in patients with CH, most notably a reduction in amplitude associated with the in-bout state,[92–96] although the significance of this finding is difficult to interpret, especially as the pineal gland receives innervation from the sphenopalatine and superior cervical ganglia, the former being highly activated during CH attacks.[97,98]

Sleep and Cluster Headache

A recent study in a large clinical cohort confirmed poorer sleep quality, as measured by the Pittsburgh Sleep Quality Inventory, in CH versus control subjects, which, given the nocturnal preponderance of attacks, is perhaps not surprising.[87] Although early PSG studies in small numbers of patients reported attacks of CH arising exclusively from rapid eye movement (REM) sleep,[99,100] the current body of evidence suggests that this is not the case, with the most recent studies unable to demonstrate any clear association between the attacks and macroscopic PSG variables.[101,102] However, an interest in REM physiology in CH persists, with a prolonged REM latency in in-bout CH patients being the only finding to date of statistical significance.[103–105] Sleep latency, time in bed, and total sleep time, derived from PSG and actigraphy studies, appear to be increased in patients who are in-bout.[106,107] A small number of PSG and polygraphy studies have suggested a coassociation between CH and OSA,[108–112] whereas more recent series have not necessarily found this to hold true,[105] except for one case-control study that showed a higher incidence of OSA during in-bout episodic CH.[113] OSA is a common disorder, particularly in male smokers,[114] who are perhaps overrepresented in the CH clinical population, which might contribute to this potential, yet inconclusive, association.[115] Furthermore, treatment of OSA with CPAP does not necessarily have any impact on CH,[113] bar a few isolated reports.[116,117] It is reported that chronic insomnia is found be coassociated in 40% of patients.[106,118] Unlike migraine, there appears to be no coassociation with RLS in a small case-control cohort study.[119] One case report of bruxism with OSA in CH exists.[120]

Although much interest has been attributed to the potential role of the hypocretin system in CH, the supportive clinical data are mixed. Two genetic association studies found polymorphisms in the hypocretin receptor gene in patients with CH,[121,122] which was not reproduced in subsequent studies.[123,124] One cerebrospinal fluid study of patients with CH found slightly lower but within accepted normal range hypocretin-1 levels in CH patients versus sleep clinic–based control subjects.[125]

Other Trigeminal Autonomic Cephalalgias and Sleep

In contrast to the striking timing patterns and sleep associations seen in CH, far less is known about these associations in the rarer TACs.[52] Although case series[126,127] and reports[128] of patients with paroxysmal hemicrania suggest that attacks can occur at night, awakening sufferers from sleep, the preponderance of sleep-related nocturnal attacks is not nearly as high as that seen in CH.[126] Only one PSG recording exists, suggesting attacks were REM locked, although this has never been replicated.[129] Similarly, in short-lasting, unilateral, neuralgiform headache attacks with conjunctival injection and tearing (SUNCT) and in short-lasting, unilateral, neuralgiform headache attacks with autonomic symptoms (SUNA), the attacks also do not show a clear nocturnal preponderance, with only 7% of SUNCT patients and no SUNA patients reporting predominantly sleep-associated attacks in a small case series.[130] The association between SUNCT-like attacks and pituitary tumors is quite well-established,[131] and indeed, one patient reporting exclusively nocturnal attacks of SUNCT was found to have a pituitary microadenoma,[132] reiterating that pituitary function testing and imaging is of value in this disorder. In the only sleep study reported, one patient with SUNCT successfully treated by posterior hypothalamic deep brain stimulation showed frequent awakenings from REM sleep, with a pronouncedly increased wake after sleep onset time.[133] In a case series of hemicrania continua, just more than a third reported irregular sleep increasing the likelihood of an exacerbation.[134]

Migraine

Perhaps less associated with sleep and biologic rhythms than the primary headache disorders described earlier, it is clear that migraine can still be profoundly influenced by sleep. Attacks can begin before or during sleep, and sufferers may frequently wake with the headache of a migraine attack, although it is perhaps more unusual to be woken by it. Furthermore, patients report that sleep can be therapeutic once the attack is established. Sleep as a trigger for migraine is also widely feted, although often in a very nonspecific way, both in terms of the description of sleep or sleep disturbances or in the nature of the ensuing headache itself.[135]

Migraine is the most common of the primary headache disorders,[136] and indeed, estimated to be the second most common disorder of humans worldwide, with an estimated population prevalence of 14.7% for episodic migraine[137] and 2% for chronic migraine.[138] It broadly exists in two forms—migraine with and without aura—and may be either episodic or chronic. In addition to characteristic head pain, the migraine attack presents a constellation of symptoms resulting from episodic dysfunction within the central nervous system. These often begin with premonitory symptoms suggestive of hypothalamic dysfunction, including fatigue and food cravings, as well as autonomic symptoms, such as lacrimation, yawning, and increased urination,[139,140] many of which may manifest during the daytime before a migraine attack that arises during sleep. These premonitory features may be followed, in 30% of individuals, by a range of transient and positive neurologic symptoms, such as visual disturbances or paresthesia, typically lasting between 5 and 60 minutes, which represent depolarization and repolarization of cortical neurons, which spreads anteriorly as wave, a process known as cortical spreading depression.[141]

In just more than half of patients the pain will be unilateral and throbbing, and the majority report the pain worsening with exertion. The median duration of attacks is 24 hours (range, 4 hours to 72 hours).[142] Other widely reported symptoms with the attacks include photophobia and phonophobia, as well as allodynia of the scalp. Nausea occurs in just more than half of patients.[143] After cessation of an attack a proportion of suffers will experience postdromal symptoms, which might include various sleep complaints, including hypersomnolence or insomnia.[144]

Treatment is separated into acute therapy, used to terminate individual attacks, the mainstay of which are nonsteroidal antiinflammatory drugs or triptans, and preventive treatment for high-frequency episodic and chronic migraine. Options for preventive treatments include amitriptyline, propranolol, and topiramate, as well as onabotulinum toxin A injections, the latter for chronic migraine, and more recently monoclonal antibody treatments directed at CGRP or its receptor involved in trigeminal nociception.[145,146]

Attack Periodicity in Migraine

The periodicity of migraine attacks has been studied in analyses of retrospective patient diaries. In terms of timing within the 24-hour period, two studies found significantly higher peaks of migraine onset on waking in the morning. The first found a peak, particularly in women, between 04:00 to 09:00,[147] and the second, a peak between 06:00 and 12:00, with a much lower probability of occurrence in prebed evening hours.[148] A study using Twitter found morning peaks in migraine content across a week's sample in the United States.[149] What these studies do not reveal, however, is whether this is a circadian influence or merely sleep related. Two further conflicting studies found patterns in occurrence probability by day of the week, with Sundays being reported the most likely day for an attack to arise in one study[150] but the least likely day in another,[151] which showed an even spread of probability across the days of the week, except Sundays.

January has been reported as being the most likely month for higher frequencies of migraine attacks.[150] Conversely, another study from the Arctic circle suggested a higher frequency of migraine with aura attacks in women in lighter summer months, which the authors suggested might relate to comorbid insomnia seen during this period.[152]

One well-conducted, albeit small, recent study showed that the phase angle (between sleep onset and melatonin peak) was greater in chronic migraineurs reporting higher migraine severity scores, suggesting that circadian misalignment of sleep may be of importance.[153] Similar to CH, lower levels of melatonin have been shown in patients with chronic migraine compared to control subjects.[154]

Sleep in Migraine

In comparison to CH and HH, PSG studies in migraine are relatively scarce. However, studies that have examined sleep EEG in migraine have reported a variety of findings of questionable significance. These have included a trend toward lower arousal rate during REM sleep compared to control subjects in three studies[155–157]; a slightly reduced sleep latency in premonitory phases; a slightly increased arousal index in patients reporting migraine on awakening; higher levels of slow wave activity, suggesting prior sleep deprivation[158,159]; and lower sleep efficiency and lower slow wave.[160] Reduced REM and slow wave sleep have been shown in children, too.[161]

There is a paucity of dynamic or therapeutic sleep studies testing migraine variables. One study that attempted to explore these relationships reported lower trigeminal pain thresholds in migraineurs with higher proportions of N3 sleep. This was taken to imply they were potentially more likely to be chronically sleep deprived.[162]

Sleep Disorders and Migraine

Perhaps the strongest coassociation is migraine and RLS, confirmed to have a pooled odds ratio of 4.19 in case-controlled studies and 1.22 in cohort studies, from a recent meta-analysis, that suggested the association is dependent on study design.[163] This association is of interest, as an anatomic locus potentially linking the two disorders has been located in the dopaminergic A11 nucleus of the hypothalamus.[164,165] There are currently no studies examining the risk of conversion from episodic to chronic migraine with untreated RLS or assessing the impact of RLS treatment on migraine frequency.

Insomnia appears to be the next strongest coassociation, with meta-analyses of large-scale population-based studies showing an odds ratios of between 1.4 and 1.7, rising to 2.0 to 2.6 for severe or chronic headache, including migraine.[166] Again, some of the studies analyzed perhaps lack the specificity to distinguish migraine from other headache disorders and insomnia from other sleep disorders. The association has, however, been lent some support from a theoretically sound biobehavioral model linking the two disorders.[167]

Chronobiologically, one important link between migraine and biologic rhythms does exist. Dominantly inherited mutations in the *CSNK1D* gene, which codes for casein kinase 1 delta, an enzyme that phosphorylates PER2 protein, and is hence involved in the transcriptional translational feedback loop mechanisms of the suprachiasmatic nucleus, not only cause the rare problem of familial advanced sleep-wake phase disorder but also seemingly have linkage to migraine with aura.[168] Although small case series have suggested coassociations between migraine and OSA,[169,170] narcolepsy,[171,172] Kleine-Levin syndrome,[173] parasomnias,[174] and delayed sleep-wake phase disorder,[175] no robust epidemiologic evidence exists to support these associations at present.

Sleep Apnea Headache

Within the *International Classification of Headache Disorders*, third edition, sleep apnea headache is considered a secondary headache attributed to a disorder of homeostasis and subgrouped under headache attributed to hypoxia and/or hypercapnia (Box 107.3). However, this categorization is not supported by any significant mechanistic evidence.

Sleep apnea headache is present on waking in the morning and is essentially bilateral in location, pressure-like in quality, and without any additional features of migraine, such as nausea, photophobia or phonophobia, or cranial autonomic features. It typically fades within 4 hours of waking and would typically be present on half or more of the mornings a month. The *sine qua non* of the disorder are the presence of OSA (defined in the diagnostic criteria as having an apnea-hypopnea index ≥ five events per hour), and clear resolution of headache after adequate treatment of the OSA.[176] Without these conditions, it would be considered to be an undifferentiated headache on waking.

Good extrapolations of prevalence can be made from cross-sectional studies in adults, which found the symptom of morning headache to be present often or very often in 11.6% to 18% of patients with snoring and/or OSA, but only in 4.6% to 7.6% of the nonsnoring and/or non-OSA population.[176] Of interest, there is no discernible difference in headache prevalence in patients with OSA when they are stratified according to OSA severity.[177] Further detailed epidemiologic studies from Norway have also demonstrated no coassociation between either migraine or tension-type headache and OSA.[169,178]

BOX 107.3 *INTERNATIONAL CLASSIFICATION OF HEADACHE DISORDERS*, THIRD EDITION: DIAGNOSTIC CRITERIA FOR SLEEP APNEA HEADACHE

A. Headache present on awakening after sleep and fulfilling criterion C
B. Sleep apnea with apnea-hypopnea index ≥5 has been diagnosed
C. Evidence of causation demonstrated by at least two of the following:
   1. Headache has developed in temporal relation to the onset of sleep apnea
   2. Either or both of the following:
      a. Headache has worsened in parallel with worsening of sleep apnea
      b. Headache has significantly improved or remitted in parallel with improvement in or resolution of sleep apnea
   3. Headache has at least one of the following three characteristics:
      a. Recurring on ≥15 days/mo
      b. All of the following:
         i. Bilateral location
         ii. Pressing quality
         iii. Not accompanied by nausea, photophobia, or phonophobia
      c. Resolving within 4 h
D. Not better accounted for by another ICHD-3 diagnosis.

ICHD-3, *International Classification of Headache Disorders*, third edition.

Although one population-based mechanistic study showed patients with sleep apnea headache understandably spent longer with oxygen saturations of lower than 90% and had lower oxygen nadirs than patients with morning headache without OSA, no other sleep variables differed between the groups.[177] These data suggest that hypoxia is not a pathophysiologic substrate for sleep apnea headache.

It is clear that other types of sleep-disordered breathing can also be associated with headache, although this area is less well studied. Snoring may cause sleep fragmentation, which may contribute to headache experienced by some snorers in the absence of OSA,[179] and at the other end of the spectrum, patients who experience headache on waking with comorbid obesity hypoventilation syndrome may indeed have hypoxia and hypercapnia contributing to their symptoms, perhaps via similar mechanisms operating in high-altitude headache.

Recurrent Headache on Waking

Regularly waking with a headache, usually after the major sleep episode, but sometimes also after a usually prolonged nap, is a recognized complaint, yet it is symptomatically and etiologically poorly defined. In similarity with sleep apnea headache, one might expect waking or morning headache to be bilateral, mild to moderate, and featureless, and expected to dissipate quite quickly after waking or getting up.

In the absence of features diagnostic of migraine, or indeed OSA, this can present a challenge. Anecdotally, however, there are frequently other reasons why their sleep disruption might be culpable, including insomnia; insufficient sleep and chronic sleep restriction; "rebound" sleep extension, often at weekends; marked sleep fragmentation from arousals (spontaneous, autonomic, snore or limb-movement associated, or parasomnia associated); and perhaps, albeit rarely, with misalignment of sleep relative to circadian phase (in shift workers and with jet lag). Bruxism may also be associated with morning headache, independent of temporomandibular joint dysfunction.[180] There may be comorbid medical disorders that contribute to poor sleep continuity or fragmentation, including nocturia (in the absence of OSA), epilepsy with nocturnal seizures, nocturnal hypertension, type 1 diabetes mellitus with morning hypoglycemia, and other endocrine disorders, such as corticosteroid insufficiency and chronic pain disorders. Just as important there may be comorbid psychiatric disorders, such as depression and anxiety, all having at least equally sleep-disrupting effects. Recurring headache on waking can arise as a result of medication side effects and may rarely be a manifestation of surreptitious drinking, or even an environmental hazard, such as carbon monoxide emissions from poorly maintained heating systems.[181]

There is often concern that there might be a postural component to the headache, and it results from raised intracranial pressure, exacerbated when supine. Although this can occur, there are usually other clinical features, such as vomiting, blurred vision, and worsening of the pain with cough, sneeze, Valsalva maneuver, or bending forward. Often other signs of raised intracranial pressure may be present, such as papilledema. Raised intracranial pressure can result from intracranial tumors, particularly of the posterior fossa compartment, and in the disorder idiopathic intracranial hypertension. This disorder is often said to be associated with OSA.[182,183] However, although theoretical associations linking OSA to increased pressure dynamics within the skull are described, clinical evidence linking the two disorders is less apparent.

Recurring headache on waking is likely to be an epiphenomenon of unrefreshing sleep in some individuals and may potentially be more likely to occur in individuals with comorbid primary headache disorders, other markers of primary headache biology, such as a family history of migraine, an antecedent history of travel sickness, or experience of significant hangovers after alcohol consumption. However, this area is largely unexplored, and further work characterising headache on waking phenotypes and associations is needed.

Miscellaneous

Although the disorder exploding head syndrome is often mentioned in reviews of sleep and headache, it is not a headache disorder, but rather a hypnagogic sensory phenomenon.[184–186] However, 4% of sufferers have been reported to experience a very brief, sharp, and usually mild sensation of pain in the head with the contemporaneously occurring loud bang or explosion.[187] However, about a third of sufferers in case-series report a variety of comorbid primary headache disorders, including rarer headache types, such as migraine with brainstem aura, primary stabbing headache, primary exercise headache, and primary headache associated with sexual activity.[187–189] This coassociation has led some to speculate that exploding head syndrome may represent a migraine aura phenomenon in some individuals.[190,191] Indeed, in some more severe cases of the disorder, medications that also have preventive use in chronic migraine have also been reported as being efficacious.[187,192]

Sleep and Headache in Children

Particular attention has been paid to the potential coassociation of childhood headache disorders with sleep disorders,

Table 107.4 Commonly Used Headache Drugs and Their Sleep Effects

Treatments	Uses	Sleep Effects	Cautions
Acute treatments			
NSAIDs			
Ibuprofen, naproxen, diclofenac	Migraine	Little; reduces melatonin	
Aspirin	Migraine, HH	Little; reduces melatonin	
Indomethacin	HH	Reduces melatonin	OSA (precipitates or worsens)
Caffeine	HH	Increases SL; increases SWS in second cycle	Insomnia
Triptans (sumatriptan, zolmitriptan, etc.)	Migraine, CH[a]	Reduces melatonin; somnolence reported but unclear if side effect or treatment-emergent effect of migraine	
Preventive Treatments			
Tricyclics (amitriptyline, nortriptyline, etc.)	Migraine	Increased REM latency; reduced REM; sleep inertia	RLS; sleep inertia
Beta-blockers (propranolol, etc.)	Migraine	Reduces melatonin; REM fragmentation; vivid dreams	Insomnia; nightmares
Verapamil	CH		Potentiates benzodiazepines and Z-drugs
Lithium	CH, HH	Increased SWS; reduced REM; circadian effects?	RLS; toxicity when given with indomethacin
Indomethacin	HC, PH, HH	Reduces melatonin	OSA (precipitates or worsens)

[a]Only parenteral triptans have been shown to be effective in cluster headache.
CH, Cluster headache; HC, hemicrania continua; HH, hypnic headache; NSAIDs, nonsteroidal antiinflammatory drugs; OSA, obstructive sleep apnea; PH, paroxysmal hemicrania; REM, rapid eye movement; RLS, restless legs syndrome; SL, sleep latency; SWS, slow wave sleep.

especially that of migraine.[193] In fact, one clinic-based study of teenagers and younger adults from Italy found that the commonest associated problem in children with migraine was a sleep disorder, followed by anxiety.[194] As other observers have pointed out, there is a causality dilemma as to what extent` sleep disruption contributes to, or is part of, migraine, particularly in children. What is anecdotally apparent is that sleep disruption, namely, shortened or extended sleep, seems to have a clearer contribution to childhood migraine attacks than seen in adulthood, and, similarly, sleep is more deeply therapeutic and can terminate an attack more often in children than it can in adults.

In children there appears to be a stronger coassociation between non–rapid eye movement (NREM) arousal parasomnias and development of migraine, especially chronic migraine in adolescence.[174,195,196] The apparent strength of this association has led some to suggest that NREM arousal parasomnias in childhood could be a migraine precursor disorder, similar to cyclical vomiting syndrome.[196] Nocturnal enuresis in childhood also appears to be associated with later development of migraine.[197] As in adults, RLS appears to be comorbid with migraine in children,[198] with perhaps also a more pronounced relationship with OSA and bruxism also.[199,200] Case reports of headache in teenagers associated with delayed sleep-wake phase disorder exist.[175]

THERAPEUTIC CONSIDERATIONS

Behavioral

In adults, two small randomized controlled trials of cognitive behavioral therapy for insomnia (CBT-I) versus control sham treatments in patients with comorbid chronic migraine and chronic insomnia have shown a trend toward lower frequency of headache in the CBT-I group and improvement in sleep parameters, which were sustained at follow-up.[201,202] A single-treatment arm study of CBT intervention in teenagers with both migraine and insomnia has also demonstrated that this approach could be feasible and acceptable to teenagers.[203]

It certainly makes theoretical sense that improving sleep behavior may help patients with migraine. These approaches may include fixing a morning anchor and ensuring adequate time-in-bed opportunity in those with insufficient sleep, as well as introducing stimulus control in those with insomnia and the avoidance of daytime napping. Migraine is a relative contraindication for the sleep restriction therapy component of CBT-I, and a gentler sleep compression paradigm should be used instead.

Pharmacologic

Generally speaking, the pharmacologic treatment of headache is divided into acute and preventive strategies, many of which may impact sleep.[204] The commonest sleep effects of these medications and the areas in which cautious prescribing should be noted are summarized in Table 107.4.

A small evidence base exists for the use of melatonin as a preventive treatment for certain primary headache disorders. In migraine a small randomized controlled trial suggested superiority and better tolerability of 3 mg immediate-release melatonin over 25 mg amitriptyline as a preventive,[205] with another showing no difference between 2 mg sustained-release melatonin and placebo.[206] In CH, one very small randomized controlled trial suggested superiority of melatonin over placebo.[207] Small case series and case reports also document the use of melatonin in HC,[208] as well as HH[16] and primary stabbing headache.[209]

CLINICAL PEARL

Accurate clinical phenotyping of sleep-related headache, with particular reference to the differences in the diagnostic criteria of hypnic headache (HH), cluster headache, and migraine, is very important, as the management of each disorder differs considerably. Magnetic resonance imaging and blood pressure measurement during an attack is mandatory in HH. Identification and treatment of comorbid insomnia, RLS, and snoring in migraine may prove valuable in terms of reducing the risk of conversion from the episodic form of the disorder to chronic migraine. Sleep apnea headache appears to occur independently of the severity of OSA and is not pathophysiologically associated with oxygen desaturation. Pharmacotherapy of headache produces a range of potential sleep effects, which can potentially prove to adversely affect sleep or enhance it, and attention should be paid to these considerations when sleep is a significant cofactor.

SUMMARY

The influence of sleep, and indeed biologic rhythms, on headache disorders and vice versa has long been noted yet remains relatively underexplored. Numerous levels of potential overlap exist. These include common neuroanatomic loci and physiologic mechanisms generating both head pain and alterations in the vigilance state within the brain, including sleep; clinical observations of the role of sleep and biologic timing in the triggering or modulation of the individual attacks of various primary headache disorders; and the symptom of headache as a result of a range of sleep pathologies. The most striking associations with sleep occur with HH, CH, and migraine; these associations are introduced here with further detailed review of their sleep-related manifestations. Furthermore, the less-well–defined symptoms of headache as it relates to sleep disorders, most notably sleep apnea headache, are outlined. The intensity of overlap between sleep and headache is reported to be more apparent in children than in adults, and some of these observations are discussed. Headache disorders remain some of the most treatable neurologic conditions, and the effects of these treatments on sleep, both complementary and adverse, are outlined.

SELECTED READINGS

Barloese M. Current understanding of the chronobiology of cluster headache and the role of sleep in its management. *Nat Sci Sleep.* 2021;13:153–162.

Bertisch SM, Li W, Buettner C, et al. Nightly sleep duration, fragmentation, and quality and daily risk of migraine. *Neurology.* 2020;94(5):e489–e496.

Dodick DW. Migraine. *Lancet.* 2018;391:1315–1330.

Gelfand AA, Goadsby PJ. The role of melatonin in the treatment of primary headache disorders. *Headache.* 2016;56:1257–1266.

Goadsby PJ, Holland PR. An update: pathophysiology of migraine. *Neurol Clin.* 2019;37(4):651–671.

Holland PR. Headache and sleep: shared pathophysiological mechanisms. *Cephalalgia.* 2014;34:725–744.

Liang JF, Wang SJ. Hypnic headache: a review of clinical features, therapeutic options and outcomes. *Cephalalgia.* 2014;34:795–805.

Nesbitt AD, Goadsby PJ. Cluster headache. *BMJ.* 2012;344:37–42.

Nesbitt AD, Leschziner GD, Peatfield RC. Headache, drugs and sleep. *Cephalalgia.* 2014;34:756–766.

Ong JC, Park M. Chronic headaches and insomnia: working towards a biobehavioural model. *Cephalalgia.* 2012;32:1059–1070.

Russell MB, Kristiansen HA, Kvaerner KJ. Headache in sleep apnea syndrome: epidemiology and pathophysiology. *Cephalalgia.* 2014;34:752–755.

Vgontzas A, Pavlović JM. Sleep disorders and migraine: review of literature and potential pathophysiology mechanisms. *Headache.* 2018;58(7):1030–1039.

A complete reference list can be found online at ExpertConsult.com.

Chapter 108

Sleep Disorders after Traumatic Brain Injury

Philipp O. Valko; Christian R. Baumann

Chapter Highlights

- Traumatic brain injury (TBI) is among the most frequent causes of chronic disability, especially in younger adults, but the high prevalence and burden of posttraumatic sleep-wake disorders have only recently been recognized.
- The most frequent posttraumatic sleep-wake disturbances are conditions with impaired arousal, including excessive daytime sleepiness, hypersomnia, and fatigue. Insomnia is also frequent but probably overdiagnosed, as disturbed nighttime sleep resulting from posttraumatic circadian sleep-wake disorders is often mistaken for posttraumatic insomnia.
- TBI survivors do not correctly perceive their sleep-wake disturbances, and marked underestimation of various sleep-wake disturbances is particularly common after moderate-severe TBI. Since overlooked sleep-wake disturbances may compromise recovery from TBI and impair quality of life, careful examination is mandatory even if TBI patients deny any disturbances.
- Posttraumatic sleep-wake disturbances are the result of multiple coexisting causes, and the approach to such patients is therefore challenging and should be multidisciplinary. Current treatment strategies are limited, but recent insights into the underlying pathophysiology spark potential for the development of novel and tailored therapeutics.

INTRODUCTION

Each year, roughly 10 million people worldwide sustain a traumatic brain injury (TBI),[1] and males are more often victims than women are. TBI represents the leading cause of death and long-term disability among children and young adults.[2,3] Based on a literature review covering the period 1990 to 2005, the annual incidence of TBI was estimated between 108 and 332 cases per 100,000.[4] Because a large proportion of patients with mild TBI never seek medical attention, the true incidence of TBI is likely far greater. According to a recent epidemiologic study from New Zealand, the incidence may be as high as 749 new TBI cases per 100,000 people/year.[5] Motor vehicle accidents are the most frequent cause of TBI among young adults, while the growing proportion of elderly people has led to an increased frequency of TBI resulting from falls.[2] Other common causes of TBI are high-contact sports such as American football and boxing and warfare-related events, including blast injuries, blunt force trauma, and penetrating injuries.[6,7]

From a clinical perspective, the acute phase of TBI is characterized by loss of consciousness, anterograde and retrograde amnesia, and other neurologic symptoms. The severity of TBI is clinically classified using the Glasgow Coma Scale (GCS) as mild (GCS 13–15), moderate (GCS 9–13), or severe (GCS 3–8) TBI (Figure 108.1).[8] The core neurologic deficit in acute TBI is a quantitative and qualitative impairment of vigilance, ranging from coma in severe TBI to drowsiness and inattention in mild TBI.

Recovery from TBI may last many months up to several years. Because of the marked heterogeneity in etiology, mechanical impact, secondary injuries (in particular brain swelling with increased intracranial pressure and subsequent impairment of cerebral perfusion), comorbidities, and individual vulnerability, it is challenging to predict outcome after TBI (Figure 108.2). However, the number of TBI survivors is steadily growing, because the incidence of TBI continues to rise, the identification of patients with mild TBI has improved, and mortality after severe TBI has decreased from approximately 55% to 20% over the last two decades.[9-11] As a consequence, medical and public awareness of the long-term neurologic and neuropsychiatric sequelae has substantially improved over the last years, including better recognition of sleep-wake disturbances.[12-15]

This chapter reviews the current knowledge regarding posttraumatic sleep-wake disturbances from a clinical perspective and outlines the management we have found useful over the years. It does not, however, deal with the pathophysiology and mechanisms underlying such disturbances. These are addressed in Chapter 32, which delves more deeply into translational research in this rapidly growing field. As stated by Sandsmark, Elliott, and Lim, given the heterogeneity of human TBI and sleep-wake sequelae, rigorous translation of animal models to

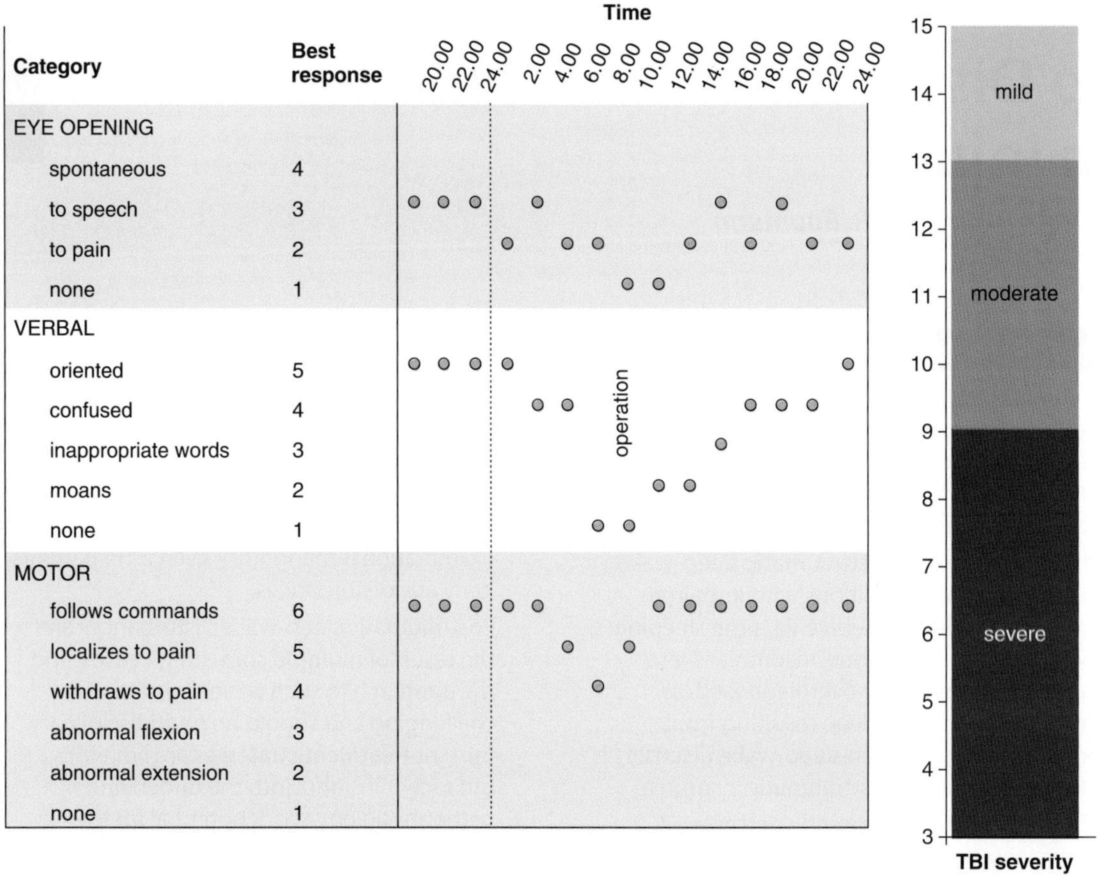

Figure 108.1 The Glasgow Coma Scale is used for initial classification of traumatic brain injury (TBI) severity and for serial assessment.

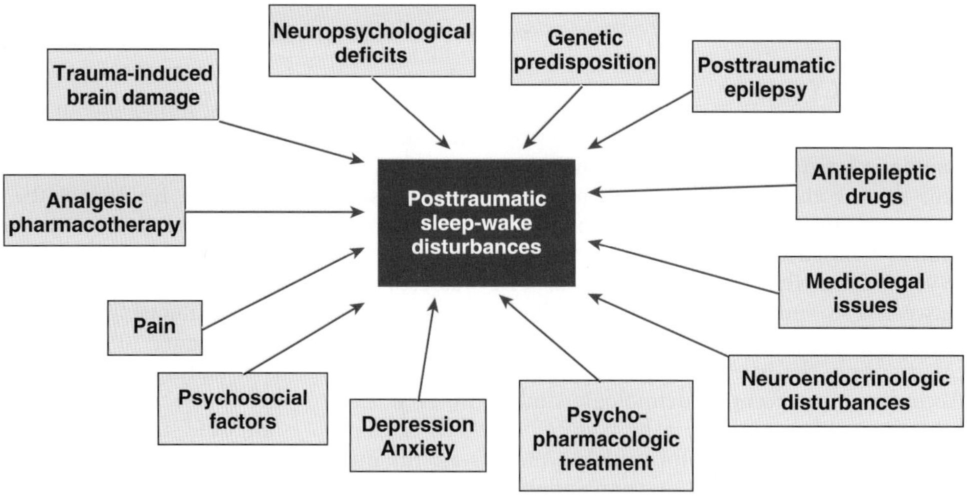

Figure 108.2 Potential contributors to posttraumatic sleep-wake disturbances.

the human condition is critical to our understanding of the mechanisms and of the temporal course of sleep-wake disturbances after injury.[16]

OVERVIEW OF POSTTRAUMATIC SLEEP-WAKE DISTURBANCES

In 1949 the British neurosurgeon Sir Hugh Cairns focused his Victor Horsley memorial lecture on disturbances of consciousness and reported on several patients with acute coma induced by TBI.[17] One patient, a young soldier, had sustained severe TBI with prolonged coma and remained hospitalized for more than 5 months. It took him several weeks to regain full consciousness, and after 5 months he still complained of difficulty "in grasping the meaning of pictures." When observing the gradual recovery of consciousness, Cairns noted, "We have no words to describe these states which lie between coma and full consciousness."[17] This account can be read as an early illustration of the wide range of posttraumatic arousal disturbances. Although Cairns did not use such words as *arousal, sleepiness, increased sleep need*, or *fatigue*, there is nevertheless no doubt that his patient did present all these arousal disturbances at different times. After 5 months, the soldier still had some kind of mental fatigue, but whether he continued to suffer from posttraumatic sleep-wake disturbances is unknown. In the scientific literature, the problem of posttraumatic sleep-wake disturbances remained neglected for a long time. When researchers from Oklahoma some 30 years later observed differences of sleep recordings between controls and patients with TBI 6 to 59 months after injury, they wondered, "Do patients continue to show sleep abnormalities more than 6 months after injury?"[18] Another decade later, a questionnaire-based study from Israel compared frequency and type of subacute and chronic posttraumatic sleep-wake disturbances in 22 inpatients of a rehabilitation center and 77 already-discharged patients.[19] Among the hospitalized patients with TBI (median 3.5 months after injury), 73% had sleep-wake disturbances, whereas in the second group, with a median latency since TBI of 29.5 months, still more than half (52%) suffered from sleep-wake disturbances. The two groups, however, differed with regard to the type of their complaints. During the subacute phase, 81.2% of all patients exhibiting posttraumatic sleep-wake disturbances had insomnia, namely difficulty initiating and maintaining sleep, while excessive daytime sleepiness (EDS) was the predominant symptom in the chronic TBI group, accounting for 72.5% of posttraumatic sleep-wake disturbances.[19] Importantly, the authors also noted a negative impact of posttraumatic sleep-wake disturbances on occupational outcome and emphasized the need to manage posttraumatic sleep-wake disturbances early in the rehabilitation process.

The first systematic and prospective studies in this regard appeared only in 2007.[20,21] We now know that sleep-wake disturbances are highly prevalent 3 to 6 months after TBI and may persist for several years.[20-22] Six months after TBI, 47 of 65 consecutive patients (72%) presented with de novo sleep-wake disturbances, that is, the patients denied having similar complaints before the accident.[20] Arousal disturbances were the most common type, with EDS/fatigue in 55% and posttraumatic hypersomnia (defined as needing at least 2 hours more sleep per 24 hours compared to pre-TBI) in 22% of the patients.[20] Furthermore, 43% of patients had no identifiable etiology of the posttraumatic sleep-wake disturbance (e.g., obstructive sleep apnea syndrome, depression, insufficient sleep syndrome), suggesting a direct causative role of the trauma-induced brain damage (Figure 108.3). In a follow-up study, the authors reevaluated 51 patients 3 years post-TBI, and the prevalences of posttraumatic sleep-wake disturbances

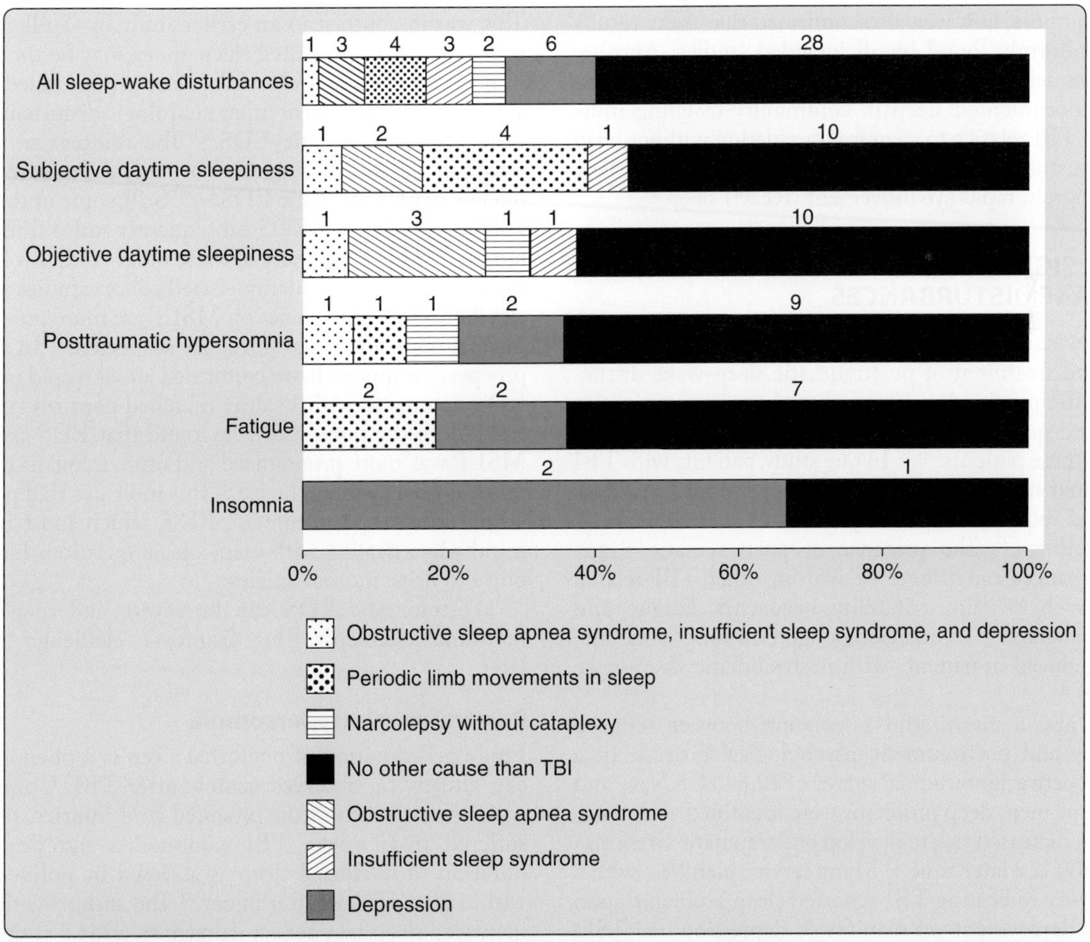

Figure 108.3 Overview of various conditions and comorbidities that could be identified as potential causes of posttraumatic sleep-wake disturbances. In a substantial proportion of patients, the etiology remained unclear despite extensive diagnostic workup. In these patients, trauma-induced brain damage could be primarily responsible for the sleep-wake disturbances. *TBI*, Traumatic brain injury. (Reproduced from Baumann et al 2007,[20] with permission from Oxford University Press.)

were still remarkably high: 67% of patients still had symptoms, including fatigue (35%), posttraumatic hypersomnia (27%), EDS (12%), and insomnia (10%).[22] Another prospective clinical and sleep laboratory study performed at least 3 months after TBI showed similar results with sleep-wake disturbances in 46% of patients and with EDS in 25%.[21]

In a controlled prospective study in 42 patients 6 months after TBI and healthy people who have been matched for age, sex, and sleep satiation, the average sleep need per 24 hours as assessed by actigraphy was markedly increased in TBI patients as compared with controls (8.3 hours versus 7.1 hours), and objective daytime sleepiness was found in 57% of trauma patients compared with 19% of healthy subjects.[23] Patients, but not controls, markedly underestimated both excessive sleep need and EDS when assessed only by subjective means. A follow-up study 18 months after trauma confirmed that sleepiness and posttraumatic hypersomnia—and also the neglect toward these symptoms—persist for a long time.[23]

Several recent reviews and meta-analyses have dealt with posttraumatic sleep-wake disturbances, and each team draws slightly different conclusions, reflecting the heterogeneity of studies in this field. One systematic review and meta-analysis focused on sleep architecture after TBI and concluded that moderate-severe TBI is associated with elevated slow wave sleep and reduced sleep efficiency, whereas mild TBI was not associated with any significant alteration of sleep architecture.[24] The authors, however, also confirmed that these results were not uniformly found by all included studies. Another meta-analysis selected studies if they compared polysomnographically documented sleep in community-dwelling individuals with TBI relative to a control population without head injury.[25] This study did not find an increase in slow wave sleep but a reduction in rapid eye movement (REM) sleep.[25]

CLINICAL SIGNIFICANCE OF POSTTRAUMATIC SLEEP-WAKE DISTURBANCES

Increasing evidence demonstrates the importance of timely diagnosis and treatment of posttraumatic sleep-wake disturbances. Posttraumatic sleep-wake disturbances compromise health-related quality of life, and they impact rehabilitation outcome of these patients.[26,27] In one study, patients with TBI with disrupted nighttime sleep patterns had poorer daytime function and required longer stays in both acute and rehabilitation settings.[28] The presence of posttraumatic sleep-wake disturbances can trigger or worsen other TBI-related symptoms such as pain, irritability, headaches, fatigue, and cognitive deficits.[29,30] In addition, long-term functional outcomes are reduced in patients with posttraumatic sleep-wake disturbances.[31]

There is also a meaningful association between reduced sleep quality and posttraumatic psychological distress. In a recent, prospective, longitudinal survey of 29,640 US Navy and Marine Corps men, sleep problems were identified as an early marker of an increased risk to develop posttraumatic stress disorder (PTSD) at a later time.[32] Many service members with a medical history indicating TBI reported sleep problems upon return from deployment yet manifested depression or PTSD only several months later.[32] A more recent study applied overnight polysomnography and examined brain coherence markers in 76 veterans with and without PTSD.[33] The authors found that sleep electroencephalography (EEG)-based brain coherence markers can be utilized as an objective instrument for determining the presence and severity of PTSD.

Finally, many TBI survivors struggle with medicolegal issues. One study reported that more than 50% of patients with posttraumatic EDS had exhausting discussions with their insurers and other financial problems.[34] Overall, TBI survivors with posttraumatic sleep-wake disturbances may exhibit a poorer occupational outcome.[35]

Posttraumatic Excessive Daytime Sleepiness

Despite major methodological differences, most studies have identified EDS as one of the most prevalent posttraumatic arousal disturbances. EDS can be defined as subjective (Epworth Sleepiness Scale [ESS] score > 10) or objective, that is, based on a short mean sleep latency on the Multiple Sleep Latency Test (MSLT) or the Maintenance of Wakefulness Test (MWT). The correlation between ESS scores and MSLT findings are generally poor.[36,37] In the same line, no correlation existed between ESS scores and mean sleep latency on MSLT in 71 adults examined 38 ± 60 months after TBI.[38] In this study, 47% had a mean MSLT sleep latency of 10 minutes or less, and 18% had latencies 5 minutes or less.[38] Of note, 30% had objective EDS but normal respiratory and periodic limb movement indices in the polysomnography, suggesting the cause of EDS was not disturbed sleep, rather an underlying cause of posttraumatic EDS other than disturbed sleep. This was in contrast to an earlier study by Guilleminault and colleagues, who suggested sleep apnea may be the main cause of posttraumatic EDS,[39] while other groups failed to uncover any major sleep-wake or other neurologic disturbances responsible for posttraumatic EDS.[20] The findings of prospective longitudinal studies suggested a gradual decrease of the frequency of posttraumatic EDS.[22,40] Still, some of these patients who recovered from EDS subsequently suffer from persistent fatigue.[22] However, many of these older studies were not controlled, and large population-based cohort studies suggest that short mean sleep latencies on MSLT are more prevalent in the normal population than formerly suspected.[41] In a controlled prospective approach, we confirmed an increased prevalence of EDS compared with healthy matched controls (unpublished results). In the same study, we found that EDS as assessed by MSLT was more pronounced and more frequent than subjective EDS assessed by the ESS. This indicates that patients may underestimate posttraumatic EDS, which must be borne in mind when dealing with medicolegal questions like the capability to drive motor vehicles.

Posttraumatic EDS can be severe and may sometimes resemble narcolepsy. This diagnostic challenge is discussed later.

Posttraumatic Hypersomnia

Prolonged duration of nocturnal sleep is a phenomenon that can already be observed acutely after TBI. Compared with patients with orthopedic or spinal cord injuries, subjects who suffered from severe TBI exhibited a significantly longer duration of nocturnal sleep as assessed by polysomnography within 20 ± 15 days after injury.[42] The authors concluded that increased sleep may reflect damage to critical sleep-wake regulation brain areas, or the brain's need for consolidated and long sleep to enhance recovery.

In the subacute and chronic stages after injury, increased sleep need is a major problem after TBI and has hitherto been referred to as posttraumatic hypersomnia. However, the definition of hypersomnia is inconsistent and has been used interchangeably for sleepiness.[40,43] Importantly, increased sleep need after TBI is not always accompanied by EDS, yet significantly prolonged sleep times may represent a debilitating symptom even in the absence of EDS. Affected patients may face difficult limitations on their social, family, and work-related activities. Thus it became necessary to find a more appropriate term for this apparently frequent condition in patients with TBI, and we recently proposed the word *pleiosomnia*, originating from the Greek word "pleio" (more, excessive) and the Roman word "somnus" (sleep).[44] We defined pleiosomnia as increased sleep need of 2 hours or more per 24 hours compared with pre-TBI conditions.

In a large, prospective study, we diagnosed pleiosomnia in 22% of our patients with TBI.[20] In a follow-up study to more specifically characterize posttraumatic pleiosomnia, two of three patients with posttraumatic pleiosomnia had no subjective EDS but had longer sleep times per 24 hours and increased slow wave sleep.[44] Likewise, on MSLT, only 42% of the patients had a mean sleep latency of less than 8 minutes, that is, objective EDS (Figure 108.4). One important observation was that several patients with posttraumatic pleiosomnia displayed actigraphy patterns consistent with insufficient sleep syndrome, with compensatory increased sleep on weekends. Thus patients with posttraumatic pleiosomnia may be at risk for secondary development of EDS as a consequence of insufficient sleep syndrome, especially younger patients returning to work and/or those parenting small children. In addition, there is novel evidence based on actigraphy recordings of 56 individuals at 1 month after mild TBI suggesting that increased sleep need may be associated with the presence of pain.[45]

Last, patients with TBI may underestimate their actual amounts of sleep; reports of sleep times per 24 hours on sleep logs by patients with pleiosomnia are significantly shorter than simultaneous actigraphy measures (unpublished results).[20,44]

Posttraumatic Fatigue

Fatigue is usually defined as a subjective feeling of exhaustion, physical and mental tiredness, apathy, and a persistent lack of energy.[46,47] The current literature offers a large variety of self-report questionnaires on fatigue, but there is no objective measure. It is thus not surprising that the rapidly increasing literature on posttraumatic fatigue provides inconsistent and often divergent results. The prevalence of fatigue in TBI survivors ranges from 16% to 80%.[48] Posttraumatic fatigue is one of the most persistent symptoms after TBI and still emerged as the most frequent complaint (together with balance problems) in a longitudinal study at 10 years postinjury.[49-52] A recent study of 22 adults with moderate to severe TBI demonstrated

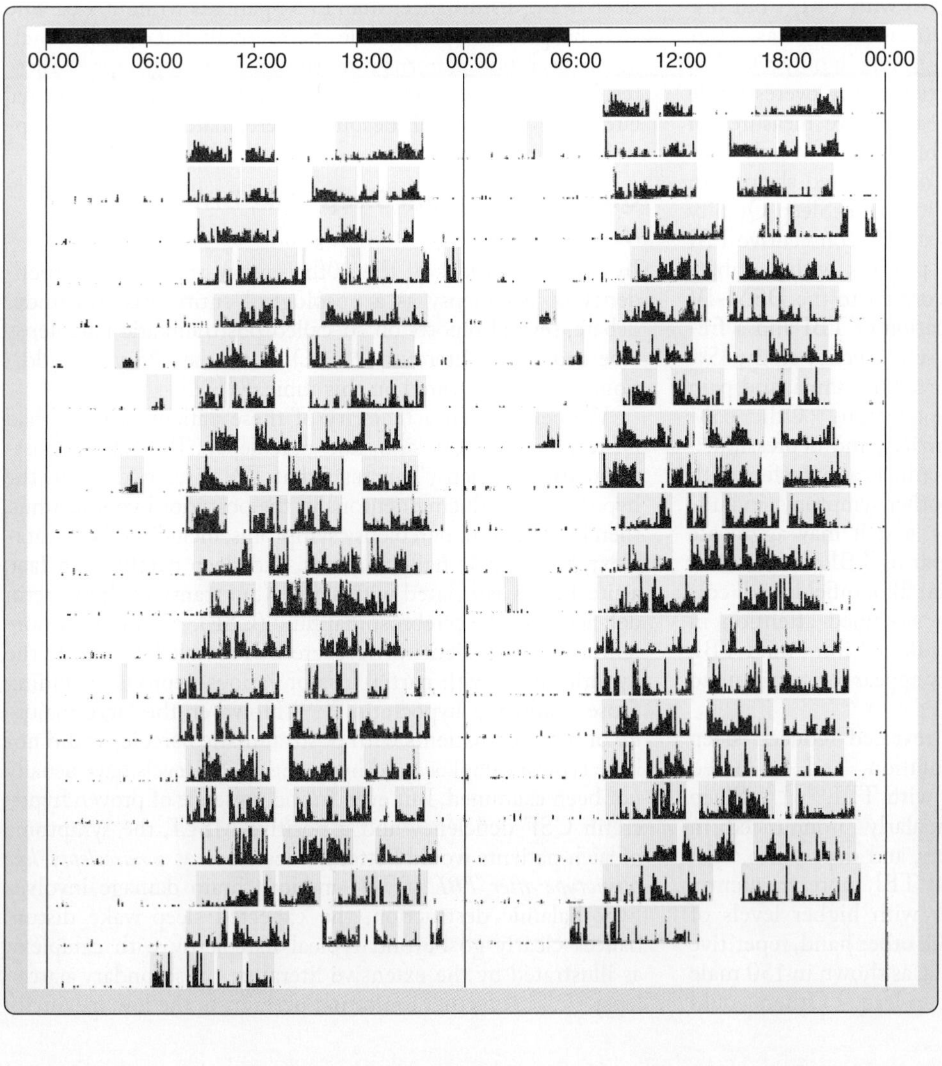

Figure 108.4 Actigraphy in a patient with posttraumatic hypersomnia. The actigraphy was performed 12 months after mild traumatic brain injury and demonstrated increased sleep amount per 24 hours (54%), with prolonged sleep times during the night and multiple rest periods during the day. Mean sleep latencies were 18 minutes on the Multiple Sleep Latency Test and 40 minutes on the Maintenance of Wakefulness Test. This patient demonstrates posttraumatic hypersomnia without accompanying excessive daytime sleepiness.

that 1 to 11 years after injury, fatigue is more prominent than EDS.[53] Posttraumatic fatigue is associated with limited daily functioning.[54] Higher levels of posttraumatic fatigue are associated with reduced quality of life.[55,56] The effect of posttraumatic fatigue on other symptoms is unclear. For instance, several groups reported a correlation between posttraumatic fatigue and worse cognitive performance,[56,57] whereas other studies failed to detect any robust relationship.[58,59] Among many other causes, neuroendocrine abnormalities have been suggested to influence posttraumatic fatigue; in particular, lower basal cortisol levels have been correlated with higher fatigue scores.[60,61] Depression and anxiety are frequent after TBI, and an association with fatigue has been shown repeatedly.[22,48,56] However, a substantial proportion of patients with posttraumatic fatigue do not present mood disturbances, suggesting another cause and thereby illustrating the multifaceted etiology of this condition. More specifically, in the context of TBI, evidence supports two potential causes of posttraumatic cognitive fatigue: first, it may result from increased efforts required for the brain to process information after trauma-induced damage, and second, it may be related to posttraumatic sleep-wake disturbances.[62]

Posttraumatic Insomnia

Estimations of the prevalence of posttraumatic insomnia are varied mainly because of methodological differences and inconsistent definitions. The majority of reports indicate that insomnia affects 30% to 70% of patients with TBI,[26] but one prospective study that used objective measures such as actigraphy and polysomnography found insomnia in only 5%.[20] In fact, others have shown that TBI patients may overestimate insomnia symptoms: compared with subjective measures of insomnia that included a questionnaire, 2 nights of polysomnography revealed lower frequencies of disrupted sleep.[63] In a prospective, questionnaire-based (Pittsburgh Sleep Quality Index) study, insomnia occurred in 30% of 50 consecutive TBI patients.[64] Among 116 consecutive patients with combat-related TBI, 55.2% had insomnia according to the DSM-IV criteria.[65] Pain is a common complication of TBI and a frequent cause of disturbed sleep.[66] In a retrospective study, 45% of 184 somnolent TBI survivors reported insomnia, and pain appeared as the predominant underlying feature.[40] Other contributing factors include dizziness, anxiety, and depression.[67] On the other hand, posttraumatic insomnia can interfere with rehabilitation, as it often exacerbates other symptoms, including headache and emotional distress, and it may aggravate cognitive impairment.[68] Indeed, comparing TBI patients with and without posttraumatic insomnia, Bloomfield and colleagues reported significantly poorer sustained attention in the former group.[69] In workers who suffered from mild TBI, insomnia, pain, depression, and anxiety appear to contribute to higher disability.[70,71]

Studies using polysomnography revealed reduced sleep efficiency, increased sleep fragmentation, and increased sleep-onset latency among patients with TBI.[68,72-74] Sleep fragmentation appears to be particularly pronounced in those patients with mild TBI, anxiety, and depression.[73] In fact, patients with a history of mild TBI more frequently report insomnia symptoms together with higher levels of fatigue, depression, and pain.[68] On the other hand, repetitive TBI increases the severity of insomnia, as shown in 150 male military patients seen in a TBI clinic in Iraq.[75] Others could not find a correlation between injury variables and occurrence of insomnia.[76]

Posttraumatic Circadian Sleep-Wake Disorders

Few studies have reported circadian sleep-wake disorders after TBI, but most lacked temperature and melatonin measurements.[14,20] However, posttraumatic circadian disturbances may be underestimated, since problems such as initiating or maintaining sleep are easily confused with insomnia. In fact, when Ayalon and colleagues systematically studied 42 patients with insomnia complaints after mild TBI by means of actigraphy, saliva melatonin measurements, and body temperature determination, they found circadian rhythm sleep disorders—consisting of both delayed sleep-wake phase disorder and irregular sleep-wake rhythm disorder—in 36% of patients (Figure 108.5).[77] Other groups confirmed a high prevalence of posttraumatic circadian rhythm disorders.[78-82] In addition, evening melatonin production was significantly lower in 23 patients with TBI more than 1 year after injury than in 23 age- and sex-matched healthy controls.[83] In patients with severe TBI, others found attenuated melatonin production overnight and delayed timing of melatonin secretion.[83] These findings indicate that TBI may be associated with persistent circadian sleep-wake disorders and impaired melatonin synthesis.[84]

In the acute phase after TBI, however, the situation is not as clear. In 42 patients with acute (about 1 month after injury) moderate-to-severe TBI, a recent study found more serious sleep-wake disturbances than in 34 patients without TBI who were hospitalized in the same environment, but circadian melatonin secretion patterns were similar in both groups.[85] These results indicate that patients with acute TBI have a normal circadian clock signal, despite a deregulated 24-hour sleep-wake cycle.

Other Posttraumatic Sleep-Wake Disturbances

Narcolepsy

In the first decades of the 20th century, when the independency of narcolepsy as a nosological entity was still under debate, several reports on so-called posttraumatic narcolepsy emerged in the literature.[86-89] Over the last 25 years, additional reports appeared on this topic.[20,34,90-97]

We believe that a majority of these patients actually had posttraumatic EDS and not narcolepsy. The name "posttraumatic narcolepsy" suggests that TBI directly destroys the hypocretin-producing neurons in the posterior hypothalamus, thereby leading to narcolepsy symptoms, including EDS, cataplexy, hypnagogic hallucinations, and sleep paralysis. In fact, acute TBI is associated with severe (but transient) hypocretin deficiency in the cerebrospinal fluid (CSF),[20,98] and postmortem studies of patients with severe TBI revealed damage to the hypothalamus with partial loss of various neurons, including those producing hypocretin.[99,100] However, the large majority of reported patients with posttraumatic narcolepsy did not have typical cataplexy, and hypocretin CSF levels have usually not been examined. But even in the presence of proven hypocretin CSF deficiency and a positive MSLT, the symptoms of such patients would better be described as a *narcolepsy-like phenotype after TBI*. If TBI-induced brain damage involves hypothalamic destruction, the expected sleep-wake disturbances clearly go beyond typical narcolepsy with cataplexy, as illustrated by the extensive literature on secondary narcolepsy.[101,102] A further limitation pertains to the low specificity

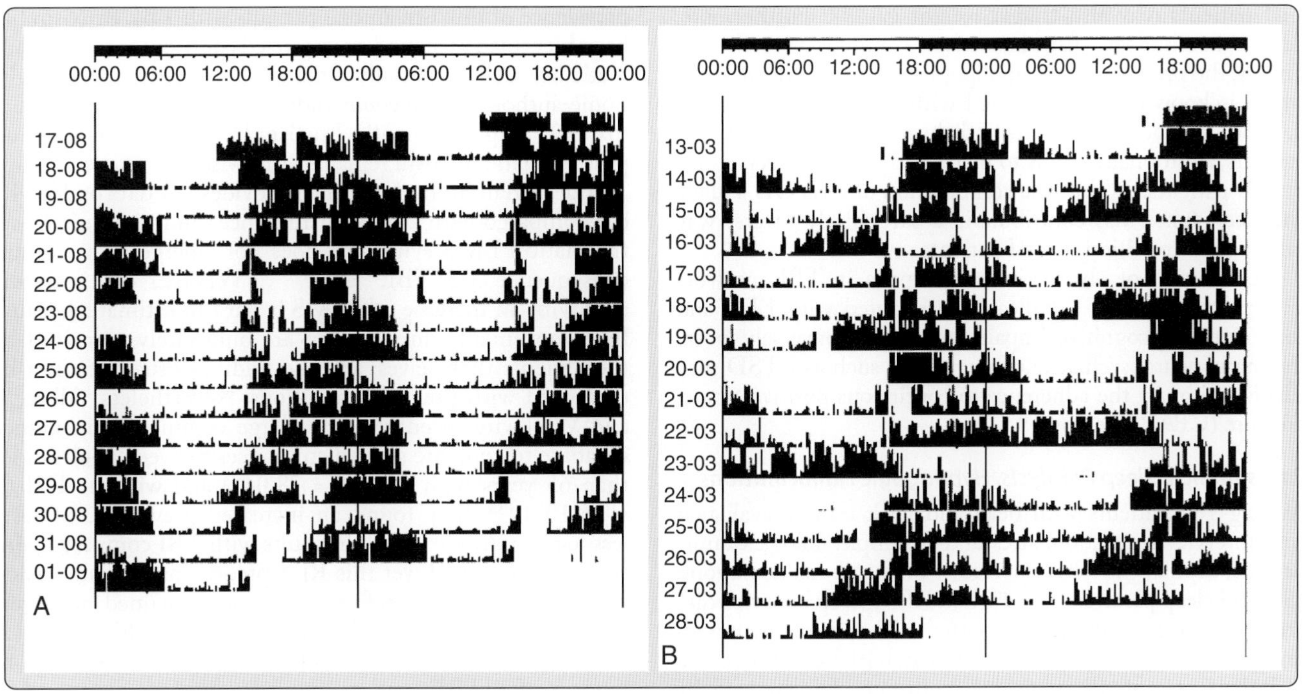

Figure 108.5 Actigraphy in two patients with different posttraumatic circadian sleep-wake disorders. The first patient **(A)** has delayed sleep phase syndrome, and the second patient **(B)** has an irregular sleep-wake pattern. (Reproduced from Ayalon L, Borodkin K, Dishon L, Kanety H, Dagan Y. Circadian rhythm sleep disorders following mild traumatic brain injury. *Neurology*. 2007;68:1136–140 with permission from Lippincott, Williams & Wilkins.)

of the MSLT-based diagnosis of narcolepsy without cataplexy, consisting of mean sleep latency lower than 8 minutes and multiple sleep-onset REM sleep periods (SOREMPs).[103] The recent report on a 27-year-old man presenting narcolepsy-like EDS 6 years after TBI, including multiple SOREMPs and mean sleep latency of 4.5 min on MSLT, may serve as an example.[96]

On the other hand, we found a history of TBI in 7 out of 37 consecutive patients with narcolepsy with clear-cut cataplexy, with proven CSF hypocretin deficiency and positive HLA DQB1*0602 haplotype.[97] The latency between TBI and narcolepsy onset was 2 years or less in all but one patient. This unexpectedly high prevalence of TBI (19%) among narcolepsy patients suggests some kind of causal relationship. It can be speculated that partial loss of hypocretin neurons resulting from TBI may be sufficient to reduce hypocretin signaling in susceptible patients, subsequently giving way to the emergence of overt narcolepsy.[97]

Kleine-Levin Syndrome

Kleine-Levin syndrome is a very rare sleep disorder of presumed hypothalamic origin, characterized by recurrent episodes of extreme hypersomnia and behavioral disturbances such as hypersexuality and hyperphagia.[104] First described almost a century ago, the etiology of this disorder remained a mystery. Several researchers observed a temporal link between onset of Kleine-Levin syndrome and TBI.[105-111] Billiard and Podesta recently reviewed most of these cases and concluded that most patients presented with genuine Kleine-Levin syndrome, while in others the delay between TBI and occurrence of symptoms argued against a causal relationship between the two conditions.[112] The largest review on Kleine-Levin syndrome included 186 cases, and in 9% of them TBI was identified as a precipitating factor, compared with 38% of cases triggered by infections.[105] The exact mechanism of how TBI may contribute to the development of Kleine-Levin syndrome remains uncertain, but hypothalamic dysfunction seems to be involved, as suggested by reversible changes in CSF hypocretin-1 and histamine levels in patients with Kleine-Levin syndrome.[113,114] Traumatic damage to the hypothalamus may thus potentially favor the emergence of hypothalamic dysfunction, and fluctuating CSF hypocretin-1 levels have recently been shown in a Japanese patient with mild brain trauma-induced Kleine-Levin syndrome.[115]

Obstructive Sleep Apnea

In our prospective study on posttraumatic sleep-wake disturbances, only 11% had obstructive sleep apnea,[20] whereas other groups reported higher frequencies ranging from 23% to 36%.[21,34,65,116] One group extensively evaluated pre-TBI behavior, including bed partner interviews, and concluded that obstructive sleep apnea emerged in a large proportion of TBI survivors as a de novo posttraumatic feature.[34] Among 116 patients with combat-related TBI, multivariate analysis identified blunt trauma (as opposed to blast injury) as a significant predictor of obstructive sleep apnea.[65]

The link between TBI and sleep-disordered breathing is unclear. Preexisting EDS resulting from obstructive sleep apnea increases the risk of TBI, especially while driving. Thus sleep apnea may represent a risk factor for TBI in many patients, rather than a posttraumatic consequence. On the other hand, posttraumatic sequelae such as physical disability, depression, pain-related immobility, and pharmacologic treatment for posttraumatic epilepsy or mood disturbances could cause weight gain and thus increase the risk of obstructive sleep apnea.[66] Partial loss of neurons producing hypocretin in

TBI patients may also trigger weight gain.[100] Furthermore, neuroendocrinologic disturbances are common after TBI.[117] Finally, the presence of the apolipoprotein ε (APOE) 4 allele, which is known to be associated with cognitive decline and development of dementia in both healthy subjects and TBI patients, additionally seems to increase the risk of sleep apnea in TBI patients.[118] Thus the combination of ε APOE 4 allele and sleep apnea may contribute in a particularly adverse way to impaired cognition in TBI patients.

Recognition of obstructive sleep apnea in TBI survivors is important, as it is significantly associated with EDS and contributes to cognitive impairment.[39,119] Conversely, posttraumatic neuropsychiatric consequences such as PTSD may adversely impact the adherence to continuous positive airway pressure (CPAP) therapy.[120]

Parasomnias, Sleep Paralysis, Hypnagogic Hallucinations

Among 184 patients with head and neck trauma evaluated with interviews, questionnaires, and electrophysiologic examinations, as many as 53% reported hypnagogic hallucinations, 15% had sleep paralysis, and 9% had REM sleep behavior disorder.[34] Rodrigues and Silva reported a 28-year-old man with severe TBI who slowly recovered after an initial 2-month coma and then presented a transient syndrome characterized by narcolepsy-like EDS, polysomnography-documented REM sleep behavior disorder, and periodic limb movements of sleep (PLMS).[121] In another retrospective study of 60 patients with TBI, a quarter of all patients had various parasomnias, sometimes in combination, including acting out dreams (8.3%), nightmares (6.7%), sleepwalking (8.3%), sleep paralysis (5%), nocturnal enuresis (5%), cataplexy (3.3%), and nocturnal eating (3.3%).[116] Apparently, none of the patients had any sleep complaints before the TBI,[116] suggesting that trauma-induced damage to brain circuits that regulate sleep-wake behavior contribute to posttraumatic parasomnias. In our own study, we found a similarly low incidence of sleep paralysis (5%) and hypnagogic hallucinations (5%), which is even lower than the prevalences of these features in the normal population.[20] On the other hand, TBI survivors with PTSD were more likely to develop REM sleep behavior disorder, independent of whether they had additionally suffered a TBI.[122]

Disturbed Dreaming

Dreaming can be differently altered in TBI patients depending on time point after TBI, presence of other comorbidities, and memories concerning the moments immediately before the TBI. In the acute phase after TBI, dream recall seems decreased and may even be completely lost despite normal REM sleep.[18,123] During recovery, when TBI survivors tend to have longer and more consolidated sleep, dream recall was still found to be reduced, and patients indicated less vivid dreams.[124,125] On the other hand, persistent nightmares are highly prevalent in TBI survivors and may in turn worsen posttraumatic sleep-wake disturbances, in particular by interrupting sleep.[126,127] Guilleminault and others reported nightmares in up to 41% of patients with TBI.[34]

Sleep-Related Movement Disorders

Bruxism is a very common sleep-related movement disorder characterized by teeth grinding or jaw clenching during sleep and subsequent orofacial pain. Risk factors are anxiety and stress, and it seems therefore reasonable to suspect a high prevalence of bruxism among patients with TBI. Bruxism has been identified as an underrecognized contributor to posttraumatic headache, especially if the latter is poorly controlled.[128] Some authors have recommended treatment with botulinum toxin-A in posttraumatic bruxism.[129-131] The literature on posttraumatic bruxism remains otherwise very scarce.

The current literature on TBI provides few data on PLMS, but compared with arousal disturbances and insomnia, posttraumatic PLMS syndrome does not emerge as a relevant consequence after TBI.[20,21,38,116,132] Whether TBI is associated with an increase of PLMS is hard to estimate, because limb movements during sleep are only rarely perceived by the patients themselves, and the findings usually cannot be compared with pre-TBI conditions. Nevertheless, Albrecht and Wickwire recently used a large commercial insurance database to compare sleep disturbances between adults older than 65 years with TBI (n = 78,044) and without TBI (n = 76,107).[133] They found an increased prevalence of restless legs syndrome (RLS) in adults with TBI compared with those without TBI, yet this RLS predominance had existed already 12 months before TBI and remained relatively unchanged 12 months after TBI.[133] Hence, although RLS increases the risk of TBI, RLS prevalence does not seem to increase after TBI.

If TBI is associated with spinal cord injury, the situation is clearly different. Several groups observed the frequent occurrence of PLMS in patients sustaining spinal cord injuries at various levels.[134-137] Moreover, a polysomnography-based study found significantly higher PLMS indices in 24 patients with spinal cord injury compared with 16 control subjects.[138]

Posttraumatic Sleep-Wake Disturbances in Children

Although TBI is the most common cause of long-term disability in children, there is a striking paucity of data regarding posttraumatic sleep-wake disturbances in this age group.[139-141] In light of the growing evidence emphasizing the importance of sleep for learning, memory, and neural plasticity, more studies on this topic are urgently needed.[142-144]

One study assessed 19 adolescents with sleep disturbances 3 years after TBI.[145] Compared with controls, polysomnography and actigraphy revealed significantly lower sleep efficiency with more awakenings and more wake time. Another prospective and longitudinal study confirmed the persistence of sleep disturbances up to 24 months after TBI.[146] The authors identified mild TBI, frequent pain, and psychosocial problems as risk factors for disturbed sleep. Conversely, sleep disturbances predicted poorer functional outcome in children with moderate-to-severe TBI.[146] In a larger study comparing questionnaire and actigraphy outcomes in 50 adolescents with mild TBI and 50 healthy adolescents, subjective and objective sleep disturbances including poorer actigraphic sleep efficiency persisted up to 1 year after injury.[141] Acute TBI was also reported to alter sleep patterns in infants and young children.[140]

The few available studies on posttraumatic sleep-wake disturbances mostly focus on sleep problems and less on impaired daytime vigilance.[147-149] A prospective study compared the frequency of sleep problems between children aged 6 to 12 years with a history of moderate TBI (n = 56) or severe TBI (n = 53) and controls with only orthopedic injuries (n = 80) at 6, 12, and 48 months post-TBI.[148] They found more sleep problems only in the severe TBI group, while children from the moderate TBI and orthopedic group did not differ. In contrast, another study of children of the same age range also considered the parents' perspective and revealed greater parental reports of sleep disturbances 6 months after mild TBI compared with parents of children with only orthopedic injuries.[149] Of note, the affected children with mild TBI did not self-report greater sleep problems, thus indicating the importance of a rigorous search for sleep-wake disturbances in children with TBI. Using actigraphy and questionnaires in 15 moderate-severe children with TBI, Sumpter and colleagues confirmed an increased prevalence of poor sleep with prolonged sleep onset and impaired sleep maintenance but did not find any evidence for circadian rhythm disorders or more frequent daytime napping.[150]

DIAGNOSIS OF POSTTRAUMATIC SLEEP-WAKE DISTURBANCES

Timely evaluation and management of posttraumatic sleep-wake disturbances is paramount. It is fundamental to realize that the optimal approach to patients with TBI should be multidisciplinary. In addition to sleep specialists and neurologists, awareness for posttraumatic sleep-wake disturbances is also mandatory not only among neurosurgeons and physicians working in the intensive care unit and in the rehabilitation centers but also among general practitioners and psychiatrists. Type, frequency, and severity of sleep-wake disturbances may change over time. Particularly in the acute and subacute phase after TBI, the presence of sleep-wake disturbances may be obscured by other more salient clinical symptoms. In addition, apart from intracranial hemorrhage, which is associated with posttraumatic hypersomnia, there are no useful risk factors or biologic markers heralding the development of certain sleep-wake disturbances soon after the TBI.[23] Hence, we should consider the possibility of sleep-wake disturbances in every patient with TBI; ideally this screening should be repeated at several time points. A detailed overview on this topic has been published a few years ago.[151]

Assessment of posttraumatic sleep-wake disturbances includes a structured interview, questionnaires for semi-quantitative measurement and longitudinal monitoring, and sleep laboratory examinations such as whole-night polysomnography, MSLT, MWT, and actigraphy. Many self-report instruments are available to assess sleep-wake disturbances; most of them, however, have not been developed and validated specifically for patients with TBI.[152]

A detailed history and self-report questionnaires are crucial diagnostic aids, but many studies have found a marked discrepancy between subjective estimates and the results of sleep laboratory examinations. The observed discrepancies went in both directions, with underestimation of sleep-wake disturbances being very common in patients with moderate-to-severe TBI and a tendency to overestimation in individuals with mild TBI. Table 108.1 gives an overview of studies reporting discrepant findings between subjective and objective measures of posttraumatic sleep-wake disturbances. Paradoxically, this under- and overestimation of sleep-wake disturbances by patients with TBI is actually one of the most consistent findings throughout most studies on posttraumatic sleep-wake disturbances.[20,38,44,49,68] The underlying mechanisms for this discrepancy are unknown, but potential explanations include distorted perception resulting from neurologic or neuropsychiatric comorbidities, deficits in frontal-executive functioning, and impaired self-awareness.[44,84,152-154] The Patient Competency Rating Scale is a common tool to assess self-awareness in patients with TBI.[155] Comparing 30 patients with TBI with high levels of self-awareness and 32 patients with TBI with impaired self-awareness, Noé and colleagues observed better neuropsychological function and higher functional independence in the group with appropriate perception of symptoms.[153] The deleterious effects of impaired self-awareness after TBI may include poorer treatment outcome, longer hospital and rehabilitation stay, and poor compliance.[154]

In addition, one study determined the validity of different sensitivity settings of actigraphy analysis to optimize its use as a proxy for recording sleep patterns in patients with TBI by comparing actigraphy to standard polysomnographic determination of sleep on a single overnight study.[156] In 227 consecutive, medically stable patients with TBI, the authors found that actigraphy underestimates the level of sleep disruption and has poor concordance with polysomnography-determined sleep. Although another group found a better sensitivity, specificity, and accuracy of actigraphy for nighttime sleep monitoring in 17 hospitalized TBI patients compared with polysomnography,[157] this finding corroborates the important role of polysomnography and other in-lab EEG-based sleep examinations in TBI cohorts and scrutinizes the sole application of activity-rest-based sleep-wake investigations in animal TBI models.

In the diagnostic management of patients with TBI, this peculiarity has to be taken into consideration. As a consequence, a high degree of clinical suspicion is crucial when searching for potential sleep-wake disturbances in patients with TBI. Whenever possible, the clinician should obtain the perspectives and ratings of relatives and caregivers. Finally, the threshold to perform sleep laboratory examinations should be low.

TREATMENT OF POSTTRAUMATIC SLEEP-WAKE DISTURBANCES

Posttraumatic sleep-wake disturbances often have multiple causes, which should be considered by the treating physician. For instance, insomnia will likely persist despite successful treatment of sleep-disordered breathing if concomitant features such as pain and depression are not addressed. This may explain why several treatment studies in TBI patients failed to obtain significant improvements of posttraumatic sleep-wake disturbances.[158,159] On the other hand, successful treatment of posttraumatic sleep-wake disturbances may improve pain, communication, cognition, and mood disturbances, thereby optimizing recovery and outcomes.[160] Currently, the number of inadequately treated patients with TBI appears very high. For instance, Ouellet and colleagues reported that 60% of patients with TBI with chronic and severe insomnia syndromes were not on any treatment.[68]

Treatment of posttraumatic sleep-wake disturbances includes pharmacologic and non-pharmacologic therapy. Good sleep hygiene should be encouraged in all patients with TBI, although this approach failed to produce significant improvements in a recent study.[161] Some promising effects of cognitive-behavioral therapy have been reported in patients suffering from posttraumatic insomnia.[162,163]

Table 108.1 Several Studies Emphasized the Poor Correlation between Subjective Estimation and Objective Sleep Laboratory Findings in Patients with TBI

Type of Sleep-Wake Disturbance	Study	Study Design	Patients (Age)	TBI	Subjective Measurement	Objective Measurement	Outcome
Insomnia	Ouellet et al (2006)[63]	Prospective	14 TBI patients 14 healthy good sleepers	Mild: $n = 4$ Moderate: $n = 5$ Severe: $n = 5$	Insomnia Severity Index TBI: 18.3±3.5 Controls: 1.7±1.6	Sleep latency/ efficiency (PSG) TBI: 23 ± 21 min/87 ± 7% Controls: 20 ± 9 min/91 ± 3	Despite showing similar findings in the polysomnography, patients with TBI had significantly higher subjective insomnia measures.
Hypersomnia	Sommerauer et al (2013)[44]	Retrospective case-control	36 patients with posttraumatic hypersomnia (36 ± 12 years) 36 age-/sex-matched controls	Mild: $n = 13$ Moderate: $n = 7$ Severe: $n = 16$	Sleep logs TBI: 9.4 h (6.8–15.0 h) Controls: 7.5 h (6.1–9.3 h)	Actigraphy TBI: 10.8 h (8.0–15.6 h) Controls: 7.3 h (5.7–9.2 h)	Patients with TBI significantly underestimated their sleep need ($p = 0.02$). Conversely, controls showed good agreement between self-reported and actigraphically measured sleep need.
EDS	Baumann et al (2007)[20]	Prospective	65 patients (39 ± 17 years), 6 months post-TBI	Mild: $n = 26$ Moderate: $n = 15$ Severe: $n = 24$	Epworth Sleepiness Scale 7.5 (range 2–20) ≥10 in 18 patients (28%)	MSLT Mean sleep latency: 9 ± 5 min, ≤5 min in 16 patients (25%)	The combined presence of both subjective and objective EDS was observed in 38%, but only in 9% did subjective and objective EDS concur. Likewise, ESS score and MSLT results did not correlate.
EDS	Masel et al (2001)[38]	Prospective	71 patients (32 ± 11 years) 38 ± 60 months after injury Patients with objective EDS ($n = 33$) are compared to those without ($n = 38$)	Various head injuries (83% with accidental TBI)	Epworth Sleepiness Scale without obj. EDS: 6.0 ± 5.3 with obj. EDS: 6.5 ± 4.3	Mean sleep latency (MSLT) without obj. EDS: 14.3 ± 2.4 min with obj. EDS: 6.4 ± 1.9 min	Patients with objective EDS (mean sleep latency on MSLT ≤ 10 min) estimated their sleepiness similar to patients without EDS, indicating an inability to perceive posttraumatic EDS.
Amelioration of EDS with modafinil	Kaiser et al (2010)[168]	Double-blind, randomized, placebo-controlled	20 patients with EDS or fatigue	GCS: 7–8 2 years after injury	Estimation on vigilance impairment amelioration with 100–200 mg modafinil or placebo	MWT (increase of mean sleep latency) Modafinil: 8.4 ± 9.6 min Placebo: 0.4 ± 6.2 min	Similar subjective estimation of vigilance improvement between modafinil and placebo groups, but significantly improved ability to remain awake at daytime ($p = 0.005$)

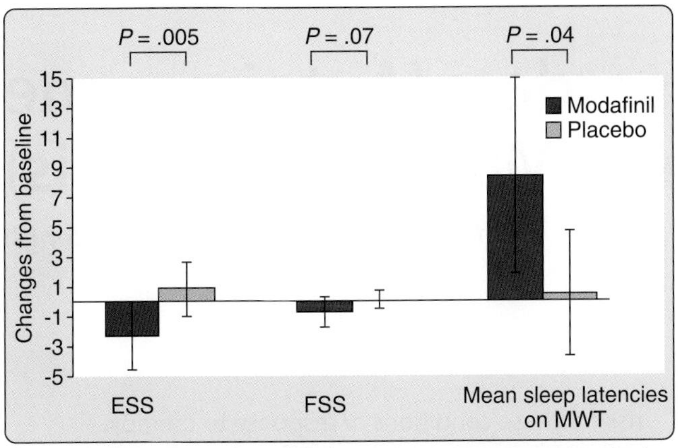

Figure 108.6 Effects of modafinil on posttraumatic excessive daytime sleepiness (EDS) and fatigue. Modafinil (100–200 mg daily) improves subjective and objective posttraumatic EDS but not fatigue. ESS, Epworth Sleepiness Scale; FSS, Fatigue Severity Scale; MWT, Maintenance of Wakefulness Test. (Reproduced from Kaiser PR, Valko PO, Werth E, et al. Modafinil ameliorates excessive daytime sleepiness after traumatic brain injury. *Neurology*. 2010;75:1780–785 with permission from Lippincott, Williams & Wilkins.)

In a comprehensive review, the following key components of cognitive-behavioral treatment were recommended for patients with insomnia after TBI: stimulus control, sleep restriction, cognitive therapy, sleep hygiene education, and management of fatigue.[164]

Using a randomized, placebo-controlled study, Sinclair and colleagues reported positive effects on posttraumatic fatigue and EDS with blue light therapy.[165] Such a positive effect on fatigue after severe TBI was confirmed in a more recent randomized controlled trial.[166] Furthermore, such interventions may directly benefit brain damage recovery and repair: in a randomized, double-blind, placebo-controlled trial of blue wavelength light exposure on sleep and recovery of brain structure, function, and cognition after mild TBI, an elegant behavioral and neuroimaging study found that morning blue light advances sleep timing, reduces daytime sleepiness, and improves executive functioning.[167] In addition, this intervention was associated with increased volume of the posterior thalamus (i.e., pulvinar), greater thalamocortical functional connectivity, and increased axonal integrity of these pathways, altogether corroborating the hypothesis that circadian and sleep systems play an important role in brain repair.[167]

Pharmacologic therapy may play a role in mitigating symptoms from TBI-related sleep-wake rhythm disorders, although few data are available. In a double-blind, randomized, placebo-controlled study, 100 to 200 mg modafinil significantly improved ESS scores and mean sleep latencies on MWT (Figure 108.6).[168] In addition, actigraphy suggested in increase in wakefulness of almost 2 hours per day without, however, reaching statistical significance. Modafinil did not improve fatigue,[168] but fatigue may improve with treatment of associated pain or depression. In a randomized double-blind placebo-controlled crossover study in 33 patients with mild to severe TBI, 2 mg prolonged-release melatonin reduced global Pittsburgh Sleep Quality Index scores relative to placebo, indicating improved sleep quality.[169]

CLINICAL PEARL

Sleep-wake disturbances are common among TBI survivors but are often undiagnosed. Arousal disturbances are the most common type of posttraumatic sleep-wake disturbance, including hypersomnia, EDS, and fatigue. Recognition of these problems requires a high degree of clinical suspicion, as they are often underreported by patients with TBI. Untreated sleep-wake disturbances may negatively influence recovery and functional outcomes.

SUMMARY

This chapter provides an overview on epidemiologic aspects of posttraumatic sleep-wake disturbances, their clinical diversity, as well as diagnostic and therapeutic challenges. The characterization of different types of sleep-wake disturbances, encompassing conditions with impaired vigilance, disturbed sleep consolidation, and disrupted circadian rhythm, is presented. We also outline less frequent sleep-wake disorders, such as posttraumatic narcolepsy, sleep apnea syndrome, and parasomnias, in which the causal link to TBI is often unclear. Pediatric TBI is addressed separately, as the detrimental effects of posttraumatic sleep-wake disturbances on psychosocial function, school performance, and productivity are particularly serious in this age group. The chapter aims to offer a guide for management and treatment of patients with TBI with disturbed sleep and wakefulness.

SELECTED READINGS

Ayalon L, Borodkin K, Dishon L, Kanety H, Dagan Y. Circadian rhythm sleep disorders following mild traumatic brain injury. *Neurology*. 2007;68:1136–1140.

Baumann CR, Werth E, Stocker R, Ludwig S, Bassetti CL. Sleep-wake disturbances 6 months after traumatic brain injury: a prospective study. *Brain*. 2007;130:1873–1883.

Collen J, Orr N, Lettieri CJ, Carter K, Holley AB. Sleep disturbances among soldiers with combat-related traumatic brain injury. *Chest*. 2012;142:622–630.

Guilleminault C, Yuen KM, Gulevich MG, et al. Hypersomnia after head-neck trauma: a medicolegal dilemma. *Neurology*. 2000;54:653–659.

Imbach LL, Büchele F, Valko PO, et al. Sleep-wake disorders persist 18 months after traumatic brain injury but remain underrecognized. *Neurology*. 2016;86(21):1945–1949.

Imbach LL, Valko PO, Li T, et al. Increased sleep need and daytime sleepiness 6 months after traumatic brain injury: a prospective controlled clinical trial. *Brain*. 2015;138(Pt 3):726–735.

Macera CA, Aralis HJ, Rauh MJ, MacGregor AJ. Do sleep problems mediate the relationship between traumatic brain injury and development of mental health symptoms after deployment? *Sleep*. 2013;36:83–90.

Mollayeva T, Kendzerska T, Colantonio A. Self-report instruments for assessing sleep dysfunction in an adult traumatic brain injury population: a systematic review. *Sleep Med Rev*. 2013;17:411–423.

Ouellet MC, Beaulieu-Bonneau S, Morin CM. Sleep-wake disturbances after traumatic brain injury. *Lancet Neurol*. 2015;14:746–757.

Shekleton JA, Parcell DL, Redman JR, et al. Sleep disturbance and melatonin levels following traumatic brain injury. *Neurology*. 2010;74:1732–1738.

Sommerauer M, Valko PO, Werth E, Baumann CR. Excessive sleep need following traumatic brain injury. a case-control study of 36 patients. *J Sleep Res*. 2013;22:634–639.

Werner JK Jr, Baumann CR. TBI and sleep-wake disorders: pathophysiology, clinical management, and moving towards the future. *Semin Neurol*. 2017;37(4):419-432.

A complete reference list can be found online at ExpertConsult.com.

109

Autoimmune Disorders (Autoimmune Encephalitides and Multiple Sclerosis)

Tiffany Braley; Carles Gaig; Mini Singh

Chapter Highlights

- Multiple sclerosis (MS) and autoimmune encephalitis are inflammatory diseases of the central nervous system. Many patients who suffer from these conditions also suffer from sleep disorders and severe, disabling fatigue.
- Sleep disturbances are particularly common in persons with MS. Approximately 50% of individuals with MS report some form of sleep disturbance, including insomnia, central or obstructive sleep apnea, and restless legs syndrome. Recent studies have also shown that sleep disturbances contribute to fatigue and depression, which may diminish functional outcomes and quality of life.
- Sleep disorders may also be prominent in some autoimmune encephalitides and are related to direct involvement by the immunologic attack of neural areas that regulate sleep and wakefulness.
- The most common and noteworthy sleep disorders in MS are reviewed in the context of disease-specific variables that may influence risk for these conditions or response to therapy. This provides a practical and efficient approach to the evaluation and treatment of sleep disorders in MS. Another inflammatory disorder, neuromyelitis optica spectrum disorder, is also discussed briefly.
- Sleep problems in the autoimmune encephalitides (i.e., anti-Ma2 encephalitis, encephalitis associated with leucine-rich glioma inactivated 1 antibodies, CASPR2 encephalitis, anti–*N*-methyl-D-aspartate (NMDA) receptor encephalitis, and anti-IgLON5 disease) are addressed. Sleep problems in these autoimmune encephalitides include excessive daytime sleepiness with narcoleptic-like features, severe insomnia with loss of the circadian sleep-wake rhythm, abnormalities in sleep architecture, rapid eye movement sleep behavior disorder and other parasomnias, and sleep breathing difficulties such as hypoventilation, obstructive apneas, and stridor during sleep.

SLEEP DISORDERS IN MULTIPLE SCLEROSIS

Multiple sclerosis (MS) is a chronic, progressive, autoimmune disease of the central nervous system (CNS) that causes myelin destruction and axonal degeneration. This debilitating neurologic disorder is estimated to affect nearly 1 million Americans and 2.3 million people worldwide.[1] MS is also the leading cause of nontraumatic disability among young adults.[2]

The natural course of MS is highly variable from individual to individual. Approximately 85% to 90% will first present with relapsing remitting multiple sclerosis (RRMS). The RRMS course is characterized by discrete episodes of neurologic dysfunction (relapses or exacerbations) punctuated by periods of clinical quiescence, characterized as remissions.[3]

In most untreated cases, however, the discrete relapses associated with RRMS are eventually replaced by a slow, more insidious progression of symptoms, usually in the form of paraparesis, hemiparesis, or subcortical dementia.[4] Most patients with RRMS transition to secondary progressive disease within 10 to 20 years of initial symptoms. A primary-progressive multiple sclerosis (PPMS) subtype occurs in a smaller percentage of patients, characterized by a slow deterioration in neurologic function from onset, without antecedent relapses. The most common clinical phenotype of PPMS is spastic paraparesis, followed by cerebellar dysfunction and hemiplegia.

In addition to physical disability, persons with MS (PwMS) suffer disproportionately from a variety of "invisible" symptoms that may profoundly impact quality of life, including cognitive impairment, pain, depression, anxiety, and fatigue. Such symptoms are experienced in all MS subtypes.

Cognitive dysfunction is one of the most common and impactful symptoms of MS. Impairments in processing speed, working memory, executive function, visuospatial processing, and language function affect an estimated 40% to 70% of individuals with MS.[4] Cognitive decline often occurs early in the disease. Cognitive impairment is more prevalent in progressive compared to relapsing disease, and the quality of dysfunction may differ between the two.[5]

Fatigue is another common and debilitating symptom reported by patients and is present in more than 80% of patients over the course of the disease.[6] This highly debilitating symptom imposes significant socioeconomic consequences and is a leading cause of diminished quality of life among individuals with MS. Nevertheless, fatigue in MS remains poorly understood, in part, because of its subjectivity and lack of a unified definition as well as a gold standard for measurement. One commonly used definition is "a subjective lack of physical and/or mental energy that is perceived by the individual or caregiver to interfere with usual or desired activity"[7]; however, many patients use other terms to describe this symptom, such as tiredness or exhaustion.

Although the last two decades have seen major advances in the development of immune-based treatments to prevent progression of MS-related disability, interventions to ameliorate existing symptoms such as fatigue or neurologic deficits remain extremely limited. Consequently, an important component of MS care includes the identification of treatable conditions that contribute to existing symptoms, disability, and quality of life. *Among such treatable conditions, sleep disturbances have recently gained recognition for their prevalence and potential consequences in PwMS.* The prevalence of sleep disorders in PwMS has been conventionally underestimated. However, several patient series have estimated the prevalence to be higher in PwMS than in the general population, ranging from 25% to 54%.[8-11] Furthermore, sleep disturbances have been linked to several of the most debilitating symptoms of MS, including fatigue, pain, and depression,[12] implicating sleep as a promising potential therapeutic target to alleviate these symptoms. Bidirectional relationships between sleep disturbances, pain, and depression are also common.[13,14]

The following sections review the most common sleep disorders and their consequences in PwMS. Potential MS-related risk factors that may predispose this population to sleep disorders, and caveats for diagnosis and treatment are also discussed.

Sleep-Related Breathing Disorders

Sleep-related breathing disorders (SRBDs) are respiratory disturbances that occur during sleep. PwMS are at risk for both obstructive sleep apnea (OSA) and central sleep apnea (CSA). Although reasons for this require additional exploration, one potential explanation implicates the disruption of important brainstem pathways that are responsible for maintenance of nocturnal upper airway patency or respiratory drive. Refer to Section 14 for a detailed review of this topic.

Two published studies that assessed the prevalence of OSA in PwMS suggest that 4% to 21% of patients may carry an OSA diagnosis.[15,16] Additionally, both studies also showed that a higher proportion (38% to 56%) of PwMS were at elevated risk for OSA based on a validated screening tool for OSA, the STOP-BANG Questionnaire,[17] suggesting a significant disparity in the recognition of OSA among PwMS.

Aside from general risk factors such as age, body mass index, and male sex, underlying neuroanatomic and immunologic features associated with MS may in part explain this elevated OSA prevalence. Maintenance of upper airway patency during sleep requires an increase in pharyngeal tone, which is mediated primarily by efferent motor output from cranial nerves X and XII to the palatal and genioglossus muscles, respectively. This process is influenced largely by afferent sensory input from pressure receptors in the upper airway, peripheral chemoreceptors in the aortic and carotid bodies, and brainstem respiratory generators.[18,19] Pathophysiologic processes that disrupt these tightly regulated brainstem pathways therefore have the potential to impair nocturnal respiration.[20,21] In a previous study of patients referred to an academic sleep center for overnight polysomnography, PwMS, and particularly those patients with radiographic evidence of brainstem involvement, were found to have more severe OSA than patients without MS also referred to a sleep laboratory.[22] Among PwMS, progressive MS subtypes also predicted apnea severity, suggesting a potential role for global CNS damage as a risk factor for OSA as well. Conversely, disease-modifying therapy use emerged as a strong predictor of *reduced* apnea severity, raising interesting possibilities about the role of local and/or systemic inflammation in OSA.[22]

In contrast to OSA, CSA refers to hypopneas or apneas that occur as a result of complete or partial lack of respiratory effort.[23] The prevalence of CSA in PwMS has been estimated to be between 1% and 4% based on prior studies[24,25]; the highest rate is noted to be 8% in patients with MS without other comorbidities.[26] Although the exact prevalence of CSA in MS is still unknown, several case studies and two recent cross-sectional studies would suggest that PwMS, particularly those with brainstem involvement or patients with more disability, are also at elevated risk for CSA.[27,28] In the aforementioned study by Braley and colleagues, CSA was also found to be more severe in PwMS with brainstem involvement.

Furthermore, central alveolar hypoventilation syndrome, previously described as "Ondine's curse," has been rarely reported to affect PwMS.[29] This condition is marked by normal respiration during wakefulness but hypoventilation and hypercapnia during non–rapid eye movement (NREM) sleep. Although most often referenced in its congenital form, the acquired type is associated with lesions in pontine and medullary respiratory generators along with the solitary nucleus. Autopsy case reports of two patients with MS who died during sleep revealed the presence of plaques within the medullary reticular formation.[30]

Current evidence suggests that the consequences of untreated OSA in MS may be far-reaching. In addition to the serious health consequences reported in the general population, the detrimental effects of OSA in MS are well documented. PwMS with an OSA diagnosis and those at elevated risk for OSA have been shown to have increased fatigue compared with undiagnosed or low-risk patients.[17,24,31,32] OSA is also a predictor of diminished quality of life in MS,[33] and preliminary research suggests that apnea severity may correlate with impaired cognition in MS.[34] The etiology of cognitive dysfunction in OSA is believed to be multifactorial with sleep fragmentation and hypoxemia as key contributors. Nocturnal hypoxia in OSA can cause neuroimaging and neuropathologic abnormalities in regions of the cortex that may be disproportionately affected in MS.[35]

Given the overlap between OSA, chronic MS symptoms, and the potential risk of further increasing disability from complications related to untreated sleep apnea, clinicians should maintain a low threshold for OSA screening and referral to a sleep specialist. All PwMS should be asked about traditional OSA symptoms, including snoring, pauses in breathing witnessed by a bed partner, gasping or choking upon awakening, nonrestorative sleep, excessive daytime hypersomnolence or fatigue, cognitive disturbances, and nighttime awakenings, any of which could arise in part from underlying OSA. Dysarthria or dysphagia, which may reflect signs of brainstem dysfunction, may also signal high risk for OSA or CSA. Non-MS anatomic risk factors for OSA (obesity, increased neck circumference, crowded oropharyngeal inlet, retrognathia, or micrognathia) should, in conjunction with the previously mentioned symptoms, prompt clinicians to consider a sleep clinic referral.

No algorithm for assessment of OSA risk, specific for patients with MS, has been validated; however, one of the most commonly used screening tools for OSA in MS research is the STOP-BANG questionnaire.[36] Although the STOP-BANG has yet to be validated in MS, it may provide a useful means to assess general OSA risk factors among patients with MS. However, because this tool does not include additional questions about MS-specific risk factors (e.g., features of brainstem involvement), a low STOP-BANG score should not supersede clinical judgment when determining the need to pursue diagnostic workup.[37]

In terms of diagnosis, in-laboratory PSG, rather than home sleep apnea testing, is recommended. The latter has not been well studied in patients with neurologic conditions such as MS and may not be as sensitive to concomitant CSA, which may be more common or severe in MS.[38]

The management of PwMS with sleep-disordered breathing requires a multidisciplinary approach and consideration of the patient's primary apnea subtype, apnea severity, comorbidities and behaviors, neurologic symptoms, and MS-related deficits.[38] Positive airway pressure (PAP) therapy improves fatigue as well as sleepiness in patients without MS and is the gold standard treatment for patients with MS with OSA.

Although rigorous demonstration of effectiveness in patients with MS has yet to be published, the general health and symptomatic benefits of PAP therapy are thought to be similarly beneficial among PwMS as compared with the general population and should be discussed with the patient.[39] If PAP therapy is selected, existing neurologic deficits and symptoms should be taken into consideration when selecting a mask interface. For patients with significant dexterity issues or hemiparesis, masks that involve complex fasteners or setup should be avoided. Patients with a history of trigeminal neuralgia may benefit from masks that minimize facial contact. Currently, no studies to evaluate the relative efficacy of alternative treatments such as oral appliances or surgery (such as uvulopalatopharyngoplasty) in MS patients with OSA have been conducted. Although no absolute contraindications to surgery exist, the possible neuroanatomic underpinnings of sleep-disordered breathing, and anticipation of changing neurologic function among patients with MS, generally makes surgery a less attractive option.[37] In addition, careful consideration of postsurgical risks in the setting of MS are also necessary, especially for patients who are on disease-modifying therapies that affect immune system function. These risks should be discussed with the patient if surgery is considered.[39]

Treatment of CSA should be tailored to the underlying etiology and may involve limiting the use of CNS depressant medications such as opiates or antispasmodics, which may also worsen CSA. In patients with CSA and significant brainstem pathology, therapy should be individualized. Several modalities including bilevel ventilation in spontaneous timed mode, tracheostomy with mechanical ventilation, or diaphragm pacing could be used.[40,41]

Sleep-Related Movement Disorders

Sleep-related movement disorders include restless legs syndrome (RLS, also known as Willis-Ekbom disease) and periodic limb movement disorder (PLMD). Although considered separate clinical entities, both conditions have the potential to cause disrupted sleep, share a similar pathogenesis, and have an increased prevalence among PwMS.[42,43]

RLS and PLMD are reviewed in detail in Chapter 121. The prevalence of RLS in MS is estimated to be three to five times higher than general population estimates. Studies published to date have reported prevalence ranges from 13.3% to 65.1%.[44,45]

RLS is thought to be a result of disordered dopaminergic transmission. Low iron stores are also implicated in the pathogenesis of RLS, as iron is a cofactor in the synthesis of dopamine.[46] Dopaminergic neurons located in the A11 region are the source of dopaminergic pathways for the spinal cord. Some investigators have proposed a role for dysfunction of downstream dopaminergic pathways in RLS pathogenesis, namely diencephalospinal and reticulospinal pathways that project to the spinal cord from the A11 region.[47] These pathways are responsible for the suppression of sensory inputs and motor excitability and are susceptible to damage from diseases that affect the spinal cord. This hypothesis may explain the increased prevalence of RLS in certain neurologic conditions, including spinal cord injury and MS. This hypothesis is also supported clinically by work from Manconi and colleagues, who demonstrated associations between RLS and measurements of decreased myelin integrity in the cervical spinal cord.[42,48] Additional clinical evidence from the same group of investigators also demonstrated a link between RLS and primary progressive MS subtype, as well as increased levels of neurologic disability[49] (Figure 109.1).

One study suggests the prevalence of PLMD in patients with MS is 36%, compared to 8% in healthy controls.[24] Interestingly, PwMS and PLMD have been associated with higher magnetic resonance imaging lesion load in infratentorial regions, as compared with PwMS without PLMD.[26] Although not sufficiently studied in PwMS, in non-MS populations, PLMD also occurs frequently in the absence of RLS.[49]

Persons with MS and RLS report greater excessive daytime sleepiness (EDS), reduced sleep quality, worse clinical disability, and reduced quality of life than PwMS who do not have RLS.[50-52]

In contrast to PLMD, which requires polysomnogram confirmation, RLS is a clinical diagnosis, characterized by four essential diagnostic criteria (all must be met): (1) unpleasant sensations in the legs (or less likely the arms); (2) worsening of the symptoms during rest; (3) relief of the symptoms by movement; and (4) exacerbation of the symptoms in the evening or at night. *Additionally, ICSD-3 requires that these symptoms not be explained by another medical or behavioral disorder and cause distress, sleep disturbances, or daytime impairment.*[53] This is particularly important to consider when evaluating PwMS, who may also experience comorbid cramping, clonus, spasticity, or neuropathic pain[54] that may be mistaken for RLS.[54,55] Neuropathic pain is an RLS "mimicker" commonly encountered in PwMS. This symptom may also be more noticeable to patients at night, in the absence of distractions, which may suggest a circadian predilection. In this case, endorsement of relief with movement, even if the relief is only temporary while the movement continues, provides support for RLS. Conversely,

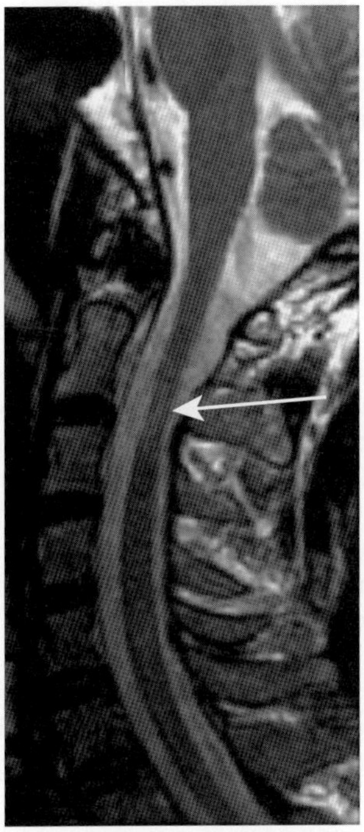

Figure 109.1 Sagittal T2-weighted image from a 54-year-old male with primary progressive multiple sclerosis demonstrates a hyperintense lesion in the cervical spinal cord. The presence of spinal cord lesions is associated with a higher risk of RLS. (From Zivadinov R, Cox JL. Neuroimaging in multiple sclerosis. In: *International Review of Neurobiology*. Academic Press; 2007:449–74.)

persistent pain that is not ameliorated by movement suggests neuropathic pain. Spasticity or clonus may also become more noticeable to the patient at night, and during times of fatigue later in the day. Symptoms of leg tightness relieved by voluntary movement suggest RLS, whereas involuntary spasms, even if a circadian component is endorsed, suggests spasticity. Rhythmic involuntary movements triggered by stretch or certain leg positions suggest clonus. In this regard, the Restless Legs Syndrome Diagnostic Index (RLS-DI) may be a useful tool to rule out false-positive diagnoses.

As in persons without MS, treatment of RLS should first focus on the alleviation of reversible cause, such as iron deficiency or iatrogenic causes that are suspected to cause or worsen RLS or PLMD. Medications that may exacerbate RLS, including dopamine antagonists, lithium, selective serotonin reuptake inhibitors, serotonin–norepinephrine reuptake inhibitors, antihistamines, tricyclic antidepressants, alcohol, tobacco, and caffeine should be minimized if possible. Screening for low iron stores is also recommended. Supplemental iron is recommended if serum ferritin levels are equal to or less than 75 ng/mL.[56-59] If no exacerbating features are found (or if addressing these factors does not provides adequate symptom relief), pharmacologic treatment may be indicated. Dopamine agonists (pramipexole, ropinirole, and rotigotine) and the α-2-δ ligand, gabapentin enacarbil, are the only first-line therapies approved by the US Food and Drug Administration (FDA) for moderate to severe RLS. However, other α-2-δ ligands (gabapentin or pregabalin) can be also helpful for RLS, with concomitant benefit of treating neuropathic pain symptoms.[60] Such agents should be considered as useful alternatives to dopamine agonists in cases in which the side effects of dopaminergic therapy, or augmentation, are a concern. Augmentation—a phenomenon that involves worsening of RLS symptoms earlier in the day with geographic spread to other body regions—is associated with dopaminergic agents in up to 80% of patients.[61]

A recent study has recognized the relationship between physical activity, patterns of sedentary behavior, and RLS severity in MS. Results from the study suggest that light physical activity and the pattern of sedentary behavior may be important targets for prospective behavioral interventions that target the management of RLS in PwMS who have mild RLS severity.[62]

Insomnia

Insomnia is characterized by difficulty initiating or maintaining sleep. Insomnia can exist as a symptom or as a disorder—in which case symptoms of insomnia must be associated with some form of distress about poor sleep or lead to impairments in social, academic, or vocational functioning. This topic is discussed in detail in Section 10. Although population-based estimates are scant, the prevalence of insomnia in the MS population is estimated to be around 30% to 40%.[63]

All PwMS who endorse daytime impairment or express concerns about prolonged sleep latency, fragmented sleep, unrefreshing sleep, or early terminal awakenings should be evaluated for insomnia. A useful screening tool to identify such patients is the Insomnia Severity Index (ISI). The ISI is a seven-item questionnaire designed to assess the nature, severity, and impact of insomnia in adults.[64]

Some of the most common symptoms experienced by patients with MS, including nocturia from neurogenic bladder, pain syndromes, spasticity, and mood disorders (e.g., depression and anxiety), commonly contribute to sleep initiation or sleep maintenance insomnia.[63]

Medications used to alleviate chronic MS symptoms, including over-the-counter medications, also have the potential to interfere with sleep. Selective serotonin reuptake inhibitors, while helpful for depressive symptoms, may worsen insomnia.[63] Stimulants, which are often used for fatigue, may interfere with sleep initiation if taken during the late afternoon or early evening hours. Antihistamines, which are used as sleep aids by up to 25% of patients with MS,[66] may worsen RLS and thereby worsen sleep-onset insomnia.

A systematic approach to the treatment of insomnia is recommended for PwMS. Medications or substances that may contribute to insomnia should be limited or discontinued, if possible. Stimulants should be used cautiously, and if necessary, earlier dose administration is recommended. Overactive bladder symptoms should be treated and referred to urology if indicated. This recommendation is underscored by an ancillary analysis of data provided by the North American Research Committee on MS (NARCOMS) Registry that showed only 43.3% of patients with moderate to severe overactive bladder symptoms were evaluated by urology, of which only 51% were treated with an anticholinergic medication.[67]

Immunomodulatory treatment, particularly interferon therapy, is a frequent but underrecognized contributor to insomnia. Flu-like side effects, fatigue, reduced sleep efficiency, and insomnia are all common side effects of these medications[68] and may be minimized by switching to a morning administration schedule.[69]

Chronic pain, neuropathic or neuromuscular, is another frequent symptom that interferes with both sleep quality and daily life activities. Treatment with tricyclic antidepressants and the α-2-δ ligand pregabalin are useful agents for neuropathic pain in MS and have the potential to cause sleepiness.[70] Similarly, antispasmodic agents such as baclofen or tizanidine may offer secondary benefits of hypersomnolence. Benzodiazepines are effective muscle relaxants and may be used in selected cases; however, these agents may also lead to next-day carryover effects of sedation.[37]

Depression affects approximately 50% of patients with MS at some point during the disease course, and recent studies show that rates of insomnia are higher in patients with MS and depression than in those with MS who do not have depression.[37] Treatment of insomnia should therefore commence beyond the treatment of the underlying comorbid psychological disorder.

If the symptoms of insomnia are persistent despite the treatment of comorbidities and in PwMS who have no significant comorbid symptoms, psychological and behavioral therapies can be considered. Initial steps include emphasizing the importance of sleep hygiene. However, a more structured and formal regimen may be indicated. Cognitive behavioral therapy for insomnia (CBT-I) promotes healthy sleep habits and modifies factors that perpetuate insomnia, including behavioral factors, psychological factors, and physiologic factors.[37] CBT for insomnia is also an effective approach when treating patients with MS with comorbid depression.[71]

Pharmacologic therapies can be considered if more conservative strategies have been exhausted or are not fully effective. Benzodiazepines, benzodiazepine agonists (zolpidem, zolpidem extended release, zaleplon, eszopiclone), and a melatonin receptor agonist (ramelteon) are the most extensively studied pharmacologic hypnotic therapies for chronic insomnia in patients without MS. Orexin receptor antagonists have also gained recognition as novel therapies for insomnia. In August 2014 the FDA approved the first orexin receptor antagonist (suvorexant) for the treatment of chronic insomnia. Although generally well tolerated, potential side effects include increased daytime somnolence or sedation, vivid dreams, worsening depression, and complex nighttime behaviors. Orexin antagonists are contraindicated in patients with concomitant narcolepsy.[37]

Hypersomnolence in Multiple Sclerosis

Hypersomnolence (or EDS) is an underrecognized symptom in MS; it is distinct from fatigue. It is defined as "the inability to stay awake and alert during the day, leading to episodes of irrepressible need for sleep or unintended lapses into drowsiness or sleep." EDS predisposes to impairments in daily functioning.[72] In contrast, fatigue is defined as "a subjective lack of physical and/or mental energy that is perceived by the individual or the caregiver to interfere with usual and desired activities."[6] PwMS are at risk for both symptoms.

EDS can be measured subjectively using the Epworth Sleepiness Scale (ESS) and objectively using the Multiple Sleep Latency Test (MSLT). Using these tools, several studies have found evidence of sleepiness among PwMS with concomitant fatigue. Furthermore, relationships between sleepiness and the Pittsburgh Sleep Quality Index score, sleep efficiency index, sleep continuity index, wake time after sleep onset, total arousal index, and periodic limb movement arousal index were found to be abnormal, which led to the conclusion that MS may cause sleep fragmentation.[73]

Narcolepsy

Narcolepsy is a central disorder of hypersomnolence that affects about 1 in 2000 people.[74] This topic is detailed further in Chapters 111 and 112.

The prevalence of narcolepsy among PwMS is unknown, as no large studies have been conducted. A study on the secondary causes of narcolepsy has revealed that MS is the fourth most common cause after inherited disorders, CNS tumors, and brain injury. In this study, 12% of the cases of secondary narcolepsy were due to MS. It is known that both diseases are related to human leukocyte antigen DQB1*0602, which may suggest that a similar autoimmune process may be important in the development of fatigue and sleepiness.[74] Hypothalamic MS lesions resulting in low cerebrospinal fluid (CSF) hypocretin levels have been described in patients with hypersomnia.

Neuromyelitis optica (NMO) is an autoimmune inflammatory disease of the CNS characterized by severe attacks of optic neuritis (ON) and myelitis. Since the discovery of a specific autoantibody against aquaporin-4 (AQP4), the diagnosis of NMO has evolved from the historical description into a broader spectrum disorder (NMO spectrum disorder [NMOSD]).[75]

In 2006 Pittock and colleagues reported that asymptomatic brain lesions were common in NMO and that NMO brain lesions characteristically occurred in the hypothalamus and periventricular areas, which correspond to brain regions with high levels of AQP4 expression. Furthermore, Nakashima and colleagues detected abnormalities on brain MRI in 71% of NMO-IgG-positive Japanese patients.[76] Hypersomnia or narcolepsy can be the initial presentation or signify a relapse in NMO. Many of these cases have associated hypothalamic lesions identified on neuroimaging (Figure 109.2).

As in patients without MS, if narcolepsy is suspected in PwMS, consultation with a sleep specialist is recommended for narcolepsy evaluation and management. An MSLT is required to establish the diagnosis. In terms of management, scheduled naps may improve alertness and psychomotor performance. Wake-promoting agents or stimulants may be used to increase wakefulness and vigilance, in addition to MS fatigue. Sodium oxybate (an endogenous metabolite of gamma-aminobutyric acid [GABA] is FDA approved for cataplexy and hypersomnia) and may be used in select patients. Rapid eye movement (REM)–suppressing antidepressants may be useful for cataplexy and sleep paralysis. In cases of secondary narcolepsy, if new MS or NMO lesions hypothalamic lesions are identified, a trial of high-dose steroids should be considered. Patients refractory to steroids may warrant plasmapheresis.[37]

REM Sleep Behavior Disorder

REM sleep behavior disorder (RBD) is a parasomnia characterized by a loss of motor inhibition during REM sleep, resulting in excessive and sometimes violent nocturnal vocal or motor activity and dream enactment. Both idiopathic (primary) and secondary forms exist.[37] RBD is discussed in detail in Chapter 118.

Secondary forms of RDB are most commonly associated with conditions that affect pontine REM generators,

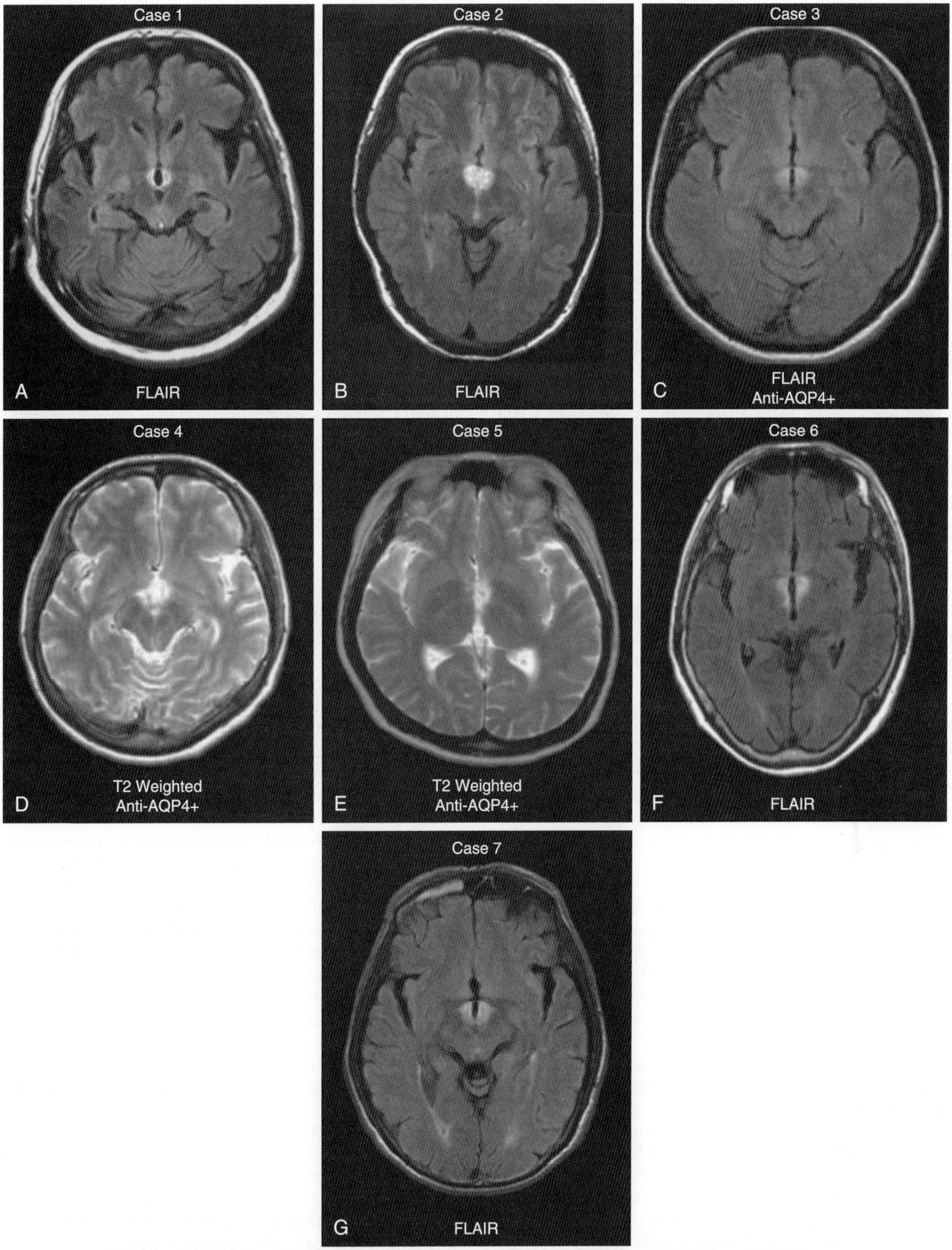

Figure 109.2 Magnetic resonance imaging findings of a series of patients with neuromyelitis optica spectrum disorder. A typical horizontal slice including the hypothalamic periventricular area from each case is presented. AQP4, Aquaporin 4; +, positive. (From Kanbayashi T, Shimohata T, Nakashima I, et al. Symptomatic narcolepsy in patients with neuromyelitis optica and multiple sclerosis: new neurochemical and immunological implications. *Arch Neurol*. 2009;66[12]:1563–66.)

including MS.[77] Case reports have described symptoms of RBD in relation to acute MS attacks and as the initial clinical manifestation of MS.

Overnight PSG is required to confirm loss of REM atonia and rule out other conditions that may exacerbate or mimic RBD, such as sleep apnea, nocturnal seizures, or other parasomnias. Given that RBD is exceptionally rare in otherwise healthy young adults, such individuals who present with symptoms of RBD should undergo a complete neurologic workup with consideration for a MRI of the brain. Patients with known MS with new-onset RBD should also be evaluated for signs of radiographic progression.[37]

As in patients without MS, the first steps toward treatment should focus on the safety of the patient and the bed partner. If symptoms are sufficiently bothersome or potentially hazardous despite safety measures, clonazepam is typically the drug of choice. If RBD is suspected to occur in association with an acute brainstem inflammatory lesion, high doses of methylprednisolone should be considered. Melatonin and zopiclone have also been shown to be effective in patients with RBD. In contrast, antidepressant medications such as tricyclic antidepressant agents and selective serotonin reuptake inhibitors (SSRIs) may trigger or exacerbate RBD.[37]

SLEEP IN AUTOIMMUNE ENCEPHALITIDES

Autoimmune encephalitides are neurologic disorders characterized by an immune-mediated attack directed against different brain areas. These disorders typically are associated with antibodies in serum and CSF that target proteins of the neuronal surface (e.g., ion channels or receptors) or intracellular proteins. Some of these encephalitides can be paraneoplastic as they are associated with specific malignancies.[78] Patients with autoimmune encephalitides can present prominent sleep problems, particularly when there is an involvement of the diencephalic and brainstem structures that regulate the sleep and wake cycle. In this section, autoimmune encephalitides in which sleep disorders are especially common are reviewed (Table 109.1).

Anti-Ma2 Encephalitis

Anti-Ma2 encephalitis is a paraneoplastic neurologic syndrome usually linked to testicular and lung carcinomas that affects limbic, diencephalic, and brainstem structures. Anti-Ma2 antibodies target both intraneuronal and tumoral proteins. This encephalitis has a subacute onset with memory loss, seizures, parkinsonism, gaze palsy, and hypothalamic dysfunction (e.g., hyperthermia, diabetes insipidus, weight gain). Hypersomnia and other sleep problems are present in one-third of the patients and are related to hypothalamic and brainstem involvement.[79] EDS is usually severe and characterized by narcolepsy-like features, including cataplexy, hypnagogic hallucinations, low hypocretin-1 levels in CSF, and multiple sleep-onset REM episodes in the MSLT. Video-polysomnography (video-PSG) may show disrupted sleep architecture with absence of sleep spindles or RBD. The HLA DQB1*0602 typical of narcolepsy is usually absent.[80,81] Brain MRI may show hypothalamic hyperintensities but sometimes can be normal despite of severe hypersomnia. Postmortem examination demonstrates inflammation with cytotoxic $CD8^+$ T lymphocytes in the hypothalamus with loss of the hypocretin producing neurons.[82] The impact of immunotherapy and treatment of the primary cancer on sleep problems is variable, but prognosis of this paraneoplastic encephalitis is often poor.

Limbic Encephalitis Associated with LGI1 Antibodies

This encephalitis affects elderly or middle-aged individuals and is related to antibodies against the leucine-rich glioma inactivated 1 (LGI1) protein that is part of the voltage-gated potassium channel complex located in the neuronal surface. The condition is usually benign as only 10% of the cases are associated with tumors, mainly thymoma and lung cancer. The immunologic insult is directed mainly to the mesial temporal lobe, including the hippocampus and amygdala, leading to a typical clinical picture of limbic encephalitis with subacute cognitive impairment with episodic memory loss and hyponatremia, with faciobrachial dystonic seizures and mesial temporal lobe hyperintensity on brain MRI.[78] Sleep disorders such as insomnia, EDS, and RBD are present in some patients. Video-PSG may show increased electromyographic activity in REM sleep associated with prominent limb jerking typical of RBD. Interestingly, the association of this limbic encephalitis with RBD supports the notion of a pathophysiologic link between this parasomnia and the limbic system and may explain the intense emotions typically occurring in dreams of RBD. Hypocretin-1 levels in the CSF are normal. The clinical syndrome, including RBD and other sleep disturbances, can improve partially or completely with immunotherapy (Figure 109.3).[83,84]

Encephalitis Associated with CASPR2 Antibodies

Other antibodies against the potassium channel complex bind the contactin-associated protein-2 (CASPR2) and result in a subacute neurologic disorder that affects predominantly older males. Tumors such as thymomas or lung cancer are present in only 5% of patients. CASPR2 encephalitis consists in cognitive decline, seizures, peripheral nervous system hyperexcitability (e.g., neuromyotonia, myokymia, cramps, and fasciculations), or cerebellar symptoms. A combination of these symptoms with a prominent sleep-wake disorder with severe insomnia and autonomic dysfunction (e.g., excessive perspiration, tachycardia, and hypertension) is known as Morvan syndrome, and most cases of this syndrome are linked to CASPR2 antibodies.[78,85,86] Insomnia in Morvan syndrome is severe and associated with an altered sleep-wake pattern in which circadian rhythmicity is lost and accompanied with mental confusion, visual hallucinations, and nearly continuous abnormal motor activation throughout the 24 hours with agitation, myoclonic jerks, and dream-enactment behaviors.[85] Video-PSG shows extremely reduced sleep efficiency. During short periods of sleep the background electroencephalography consists of theta activity with brief intrusions of REM sleep (labeled as stage N1-REM or subwakefulness) alternated with sparse epochs of REM sleep without muscle atonia. There is a severe reduction and disappearance of K-complexes, spindles, and slow wave activity, leading to a virtual absence of stages N2 and N3. Behavior at night or during relaxed wakefulness is characterized by frequent episodes of dream-enacting behaviors reminiscent of routine daytime activities such as eating, drinking, dressing, setting up a device, or pointing or handling a nonexistent object. These episodes have been designated as "*oneiric stupor*," can occur with open or closed eyes, are often associated with dream-like mentation or hallucinations (e.g., single oneiric scene), and can emerge from any sleep-wake state

Table 109.1 Sleep Abnormalities in Autoimmune Encephalitides

	General Clinical Features		Sleep Abnormalities				
	Age, Gender, and Associated Tumors	Neurologic Syndrome	Excessive Daytime Sleepiness	Insomnia	NREM Sleep	REM Sleep	Sleep Breathing Disorders
Anti-Ma2encephalitis	Middle age, males > females (2:1), testicular germ-cell tumor or lung cancer(~100%)	Subacute memory loss, seizures, parkinsonism, gaze palsy, hypothalamic dysfunction (diabetes insipidus), hypersomnia	Severe hypersomnia with narcolepsy features (cataplexy, hypocretin deficiency, multiple episodes of REM sleep in the MSLT)	–	NREM sleep architecture can be altered with absence of sleep spindles and K complexes	RBD can be present	–
LGII limbic encephalitis	Elderly or middle age, males > females (2:1), thymomas or small cell lung cancer (~10%)	Subacute limbic encephalitis with memory loss and confusion, faciobrachial seizures	Mild to moderate daytime sleepiness	Mild to moderate insomnia	–	RBD can be present	–
CASPR2 encephalitis	Older males, thymomas or small cell lung cancer (~5%)	Subacute sleep disorder with insomnia, dysautonomia and neuromyotonia (Morvan syndrome), cognitive impairment, seizures, cerebellar symptoms	–	Severe insomnia with loss of the circadian sleep-wake pattern with episodes of dream enactive behaviors (oneiric stupor)	Theta activity with brief intrusions of REM sleep (stage N1-REM or subwakefulness). Absence of K complexes, spindles and slow wave activity (disappearance of stages N2 and N3)	Short periods of REM sleep without atonia	–
Anti-NMDA receptor encephalitis	Children and young women, ovarian teratoma (~50%)	Acute psychosis, amnesia, confusion, seizures, movement disorders, catatonia, autonomic instability, coma	Daytime somnolence after recovery	Severe insomnia in the early phase	–	–	Central hypoventilation
Anti-IGLON5 disease	50–80 years, males = females, no association with tumors	Chronic sleep disorder with NREM and REM parasomnia with sleep breathing disorder, bulbar symptoms (dysarthria, dysphagia), gait instability (falls), chorea, cognitive impairment	Mild to moderate daytime somnolence can occur	Mild to moderate reduction in sleep efficiency, complaints of nonrestorative and poor quality sleep (circadian sleep-wake rhythm preserved)	Abnormalities in NREM sleep initiation with undifferentiated NREM sleep and poorly structured N2 sleep with frequent vocalizations, movements and complex behaviors. Periods of normal NREM sleep (stages N2 and N3)	REM sleep without atonia with frequent limb and body jerks	Stridor (due to vocal cord palsy) and frequent obstructive sleep apnea

MSLT, Multiple Sleep Latency Test; RBD, rapid eye movement behavior disorder.

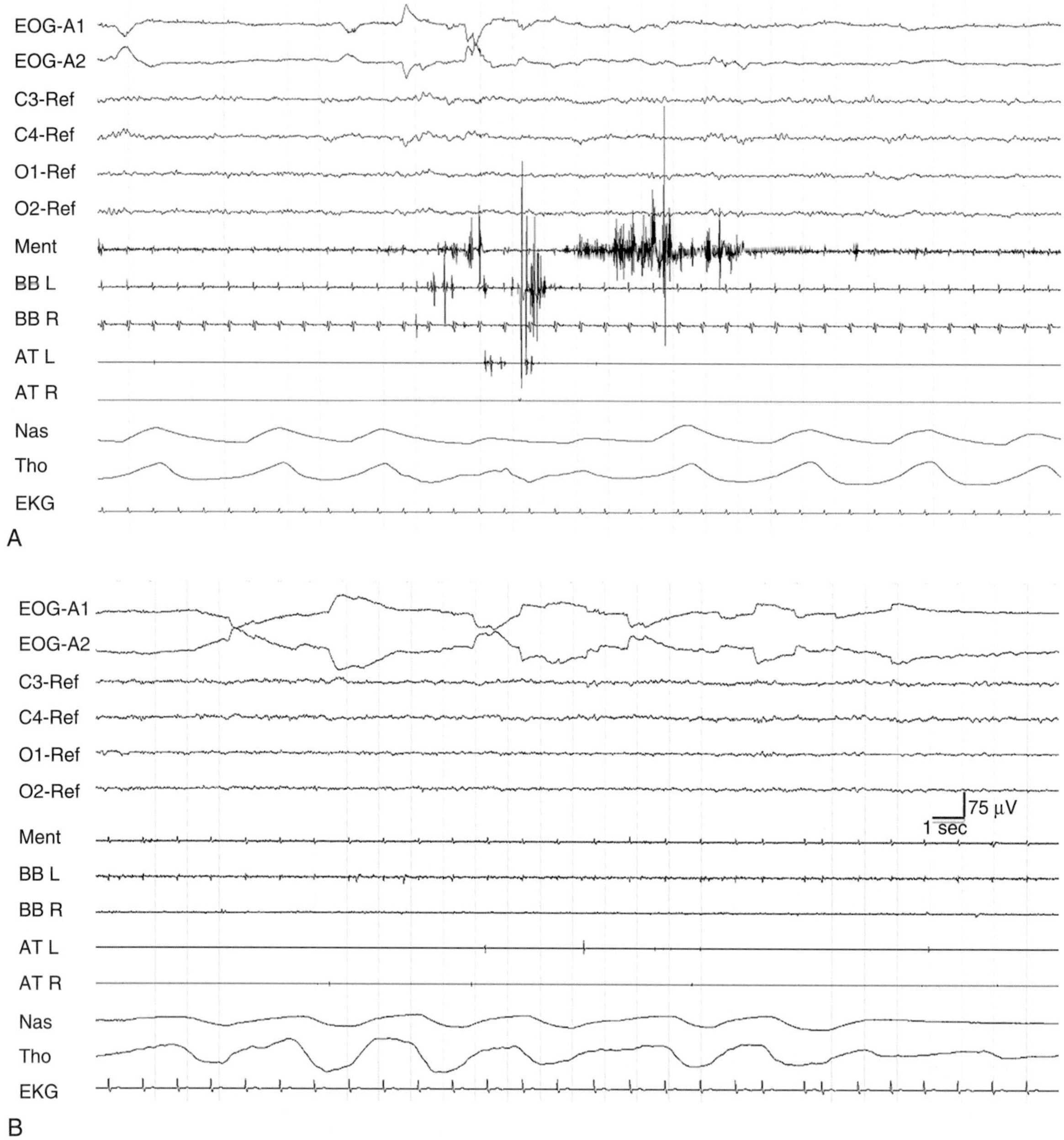

Figure 109.3 REM sleep behavior disorder in encephalitis associated with leucine-rich glioma inactivated 1 (LGI1) antibodies. **A,** REM sleep with excessive tonic and phasic electromyographic (EMG) activity in the mentalis and limb muscles typical of a REM sleep behavior disorder in a 65-year-old male with LGI1 encephalitis. **B,** Three months after immunotherapy (intravenous immunoglobulins and steroids) REM sleep was normalized with preserved muscle atonia. AT, EMG of anterior tibialis left (*L*) and right (*R*); BB, EMG of biceps brachii muscle left (*L*) and right (*R*); EKG, electrocardiogram; EOG, electrooculogram; Ment, electromyography (EMG) of mentalis muscle; Nas, nasal air flow; Tho, thoracic respiratory movement. Note the calibration mark for time/electroencephalogram (EEG) voltage. All figures represent a 30-second epoch. Ref: EEG electrodes were referenced to both ears.

(relaxed wakefulness, stage N1-REM or REM sleep without atonia).[87] *Agrypnia excitata* is a syndrome characterized by this severe sleep-wake disorder accompanied with motor agitation and symptoms of autonomic hyperactivation that, in addition to Morvan syndrome, can also occur in delirium tremens or a prionic disorder such as fatal familial insomnia. The underlying pathophysiology of *agrypnia excitata* and its sleep-wake disorder is related to a severe thalamolimbic dysfunction that in patients with Morvan syndrome and CASPR2 antibodies are considered to be immune mediated.[88] In most cases of CASPR2 encephalitis, Morvan syndrome and sleep symptoms including insomnia, *oneric stupor*, and sleep-wake cycle disorganization respond to immunotherapy.

Anti-NMDA Receptor Encephalitis

This is the most frequent autoimmune encephalitis and is related to pathogenic antibodies against the *N*-methyl-D-aspartate (NMDA) receptor of the surface of the neuron. This disorder can occur at any age but typically affects children or young women in whom ovarian teratomas are often found. Anti-NMDA receptor encephalitis typically starts with changes in behavior (e.g., anxiety, irritability, agitation), delusions, hallucinations, confusion, and short-term memory loss that in days or weeks progress to seizures, movement disorders (orofacial and limb dyskinesias), autonomic instability, coma, and central hypoventilation. Brain MRI is normal in most patients, but mesial temporal lobes, basal ganglia, and brainstem abnormalities can be detected. Patients usually recover after immunotherapy and tumor removal.[78] Sleep problems are common in anti-NMDA receptor encephalitis but have not been studied in detail. The most frequent sleep abnormality is severe insomnia occurring during the early phase in combination with psychosis. Inversion of sleep pattern with mild to moderate insomnia at night and daytime somnolence can be present after recovery, and confusional arousal can occur in some patients.[89-91]

Anti-IgLON5 Disease

This neurologic disorder is associated with antibodies against IgLON5, a cell adhesion protein of unknown function in the neuronal surface. The disease usually starts in ages between the 50s and 70s and is not associated with cancer. Symptoms frequently have an insidious onset and slow progression.[92] Anti-IgLON5 disease presents a prominent sleep disorder associated with symptoms of bulbar dysfunction (e.g., dysarthria, dysphagia, vocal cord palsy, or episodes of respiratory failure), gait instability, and less frequently other neurologic problems, including cognitive decline, chorea, oculomotor abnormalities, mild dysautonomia, and peripheral nervous system hyperexcitability (e.g., stiffness, spasms, cramps or fasciculations). Brain MRI and CSF analysis is usually normal, but the disease is strongly associated with the *HLA DRB1*1001* and *DQB1*0501* alleles present in 60% to 80% of the patients. Some patients can improve after immunotherapy. Mortality, however, occurs in up to 60% of the patients, frequently because of sudden death occurring either during sleep or wakefulness.[93,94] Neuropathologic examination in anti-IgLON5 disease shows features of a novel neuronal tauopathy with neuronal loss and deposits of tau protein in the tegmentum of the brainstem and hypothalamus.[92] The exact pathogenesis of this disorder is at present unclear, but all these features suggest that neurodegeneration and autoimmunity may be involved.

Sleep problems can be present in up to 90% of the patients with anti-IgLON5 disease and are characterized clinically by abnormal sleep-related vocalizations, movements, and behaviors. Patients are unaware of their abnormal sleep behaviors that are only noted by bed partners, who also often report breathing apneas and a "loud" respiratory noise during sleep. Patients usually complain of insomnia with poor quality and nonrestorative sleep and mild to moderate EDS. The circadian sleep-wake rhythm is preserved, and the total nocturnal sleep time is only mildly reduced.[94] Video-PSG shows a complex parasomnia involving both NREM and REM sleep, with frequent OSA and stridor. NREM sleep initiation, either at sleep onset or following an awakening during the night, is abnormal and occurs as undifferentiated NREM sleep (characterized by diffuse irregular theta activity without vertex waves, K-complexes, sleep spindles, or delta slowing) and poorly structured N2 NREM sleep (with sparse but well-defined sleep spindles and K-complexes) (Figure 109.4). Undifferentiated NREM sleep and poorly structured N2 sleep are associated with abnormal motor activation linked to vocalizations (e.g., murmuring, whispering, groaning, or talking) and simple (e.g., raising the arm, finger tapping or grasping) or purposeful-looking movements (e.g., resembling an activity of daily life, such as eating, manipulating wires, or picking up objects). In contrast to the oneiric stupor of Morvan syndrome, behaviors of anti-IgLON5 disease occur in periods of sleep, always with the eyes closed, never invade daytime wakefulness, and are not associated with dream mentation or hallucinations. In patients with anti-IgLON5 disease, if an awakening does not interrupt abnormal NREM sleep, there is a progressive normalization of NREM sleep with periods of normal stage N2 and N3 with frequent sleep spindles, K-complexes, and delta slowing without motor activation. REM sleep is characterized by loss of muscle atonia accompanied with frequent limb and body jerks typical of RBD. Finally, OSA and stridor are particularly frequent and prominent during periods of normal NREM sleep. The sleep disorder of anti-IgLON5 disease usually does not improve with immunotherapy, but OSA and stridor can be eliminated with continuous positive air pressure therapy or tracheotomy.[95]

CLINICAL PEARL

Early recognition and treatment of sleep disorders in MS provide an opportunity to ameliorate chronic symptoms, particularly daytime fatigue experienced by patients with MS. Dedicated screening tools are therefore essential to aid in prompt diagnosis.

A prompt diagnosis of an autoimmune encephalitis is important because an early treatment with immunotherapy (and oncologic treatment when a cancer or tumor is present) can lead to significant improvement and even to a full recovery from neurologic symptoms, including sleep problems. Conversely, identification of a specific sleep disorder (e.g., oneiric stupor, NREM parasomnia and RBD with OSA and stridor, or hypersomnia with narcoleptic features) in a patient with a neurologic condition is important to suspect certain autoimmune conditions (CASPR2 encephalitis, anti-IgLON5 disease, or anti-Ma2 encephalitis, respectively) and prompt antineuronal antibodies testing to confirm the diagnosis.

SUMMARY

Patients with MS are at an increased risk for sleep disturbances, and all clinicians who treat such patients should routinely screen these patients for sleep disorders. Increased efforts are also needed to facilitate early recognition and treatment of sleep disorders among PwMS. Some of the most common and treatable sleep disorders among patients with MS include chronic insomnia, OSA, and RLS. Significant improvements in the symptoms of MS and overall quality of life may be achieved by an increased awareness and appropriate treatment of sleep disorders in this patient population.

Sleep disorders are also frequent in some autoimmune encephalitides prone to involve the brain areas that generate and regulate the sleep and wake cycle. Anti-Ma2 encephalitis affects the hypothalamus and can cause a severe hypersomnia with narcoleptic features secondary to hypocretin deficiency. Anti-IgLON5 disease presents a distinctive parasomnia involving both NREM and REM sleep in addition to

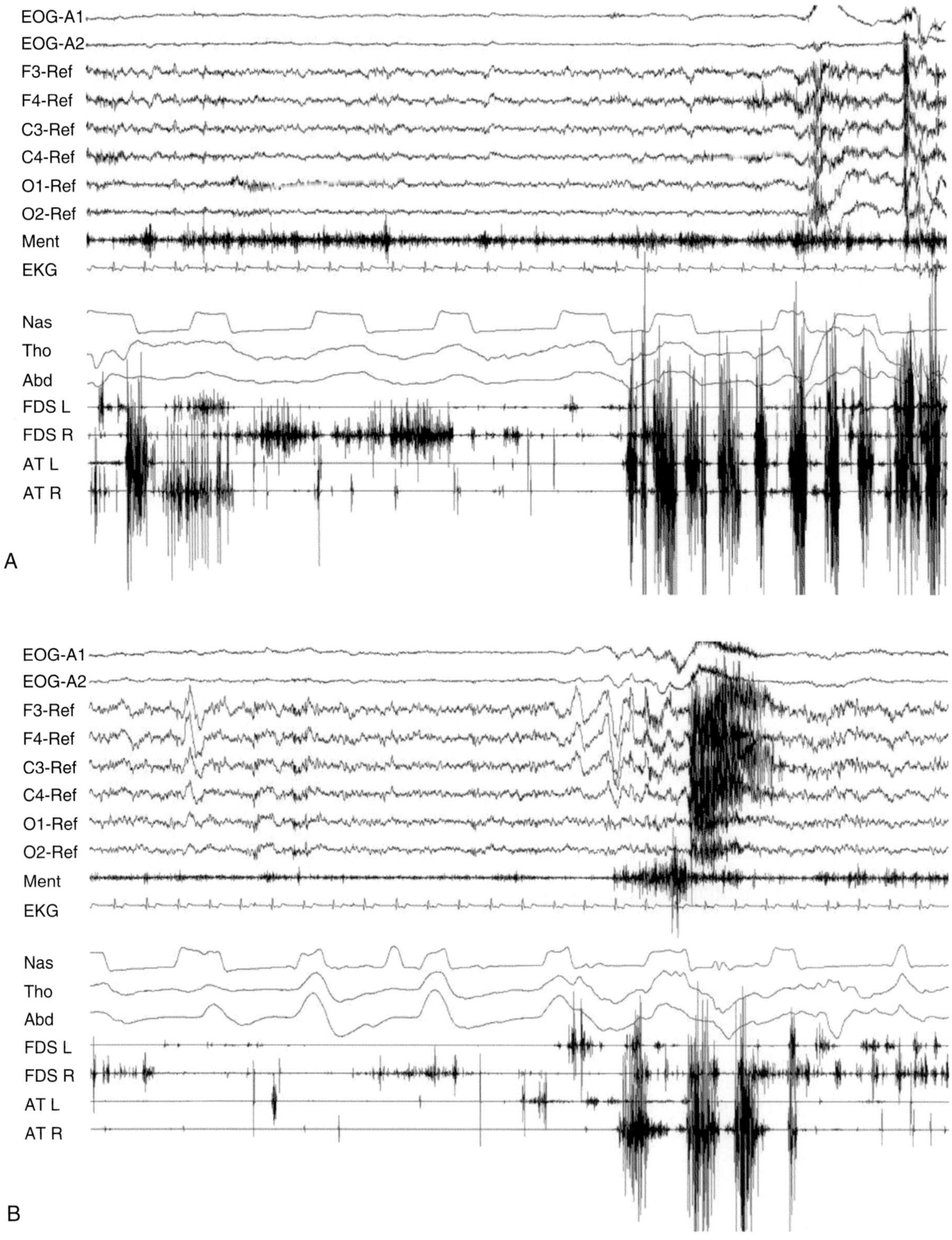

Figure 109.4 NREM parasomnia in anti-IgLON5 disease. **A,** Undifferentiated NREM sleep with diffuse irregular theta activity in a 62-year-old male with IgLON5 antibodies. **B,** Poorly structured N2 NREM sleep with sparse but well-defined K-complexes in the same patient. Undifferentiated NREM sleep and poorly structured N2 NREM sleep are associated with frequent muscle activity in electromyogram (EMG) of the limbs that correlates with vocalizations and simple and quasi-purposeful movements. Abd, Abdominal respiratory movement; AT, EMG of anterior tibialis left (L) and right (R); EKG, electrocardiogram; EOG, electrooculogram; FDS, EMG of flexor digitorum superficialis muscle left (L) and right (R); Ment, electromyography (EMG) of mentalis muscle; Nas, nasal air flow; Tho, thoracic respiratory movement. Note the calibration mark for time/EEG voltage. All figures represent a 30-second epoch. Ref: EEG electrodes were referenced to both ears.

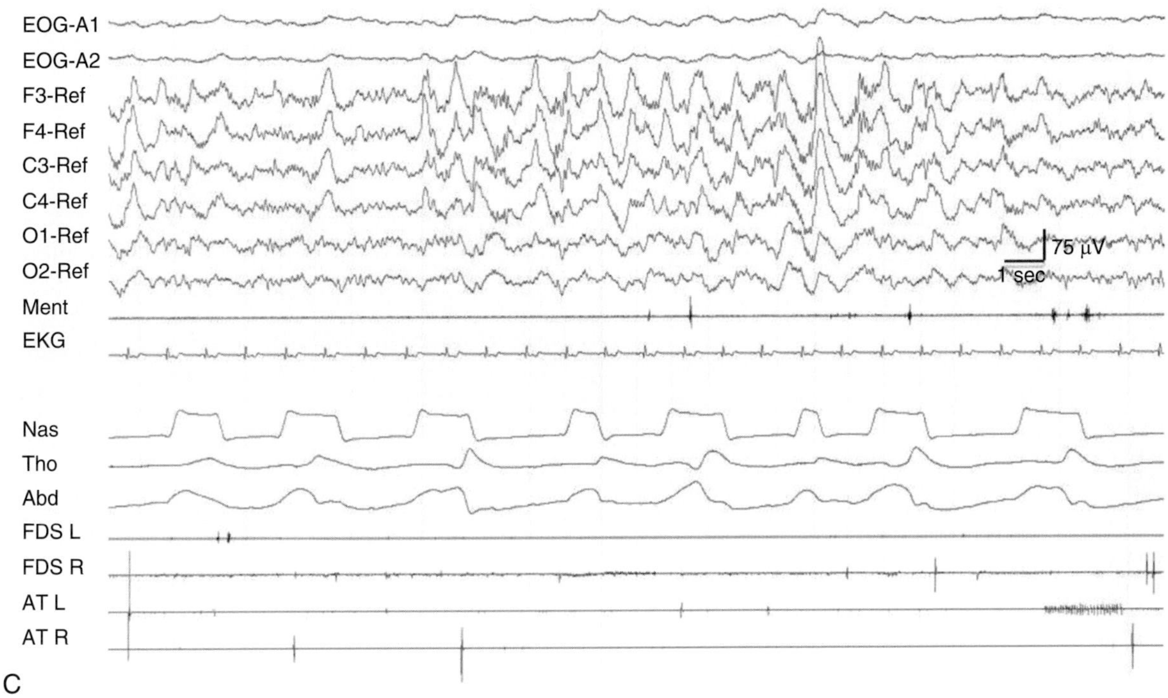

Figure 109.4—cont'd **C,** Period of normal stage N3 in this patient. Abd, Abdominal respiratory movement; AT, EMG of anterior tibialis left (L) and right (R); EKG, electrocardiogram; EOG, electrooculogram; FDS, EMG of flexor digitorum superficialis muscle left (L) and right (R); Ment, electromyography (EMG) of mentalis muscle; Nas, nasal air flow; Tho, thoracic respiratory movement. Note the calibration mark for time/EEG voltage. All figures represent a 30-second epoch. Ref: EEG electrodes were referenced to both ears.

OSA and stridor. These sleep disturbances are explained by the pathologic involvement of the hypothalamus and tegmentum of the brainstem that regulate NREM and REM sleep and control vocal cord motility and respiration during sleep. CASPR2 encephalitis is linked to Morvan syndrome, characterized by severe insomnia and extreme state dissociation with breakdown of the sleep-wake boundaries because of immune-mediated thalamolimbic dysfunction. LGI1 encephalitis is associated with limbic encephalitis, and some patients can present with RBD, while insomnia is prominent in the early phase of anti-NMDA receptor encephalitis.

SELECTED READINGS

Braley TJ, Segal BM, Chervin RD. Sleep-disordered breathing in multiple sclerosis. *Neurology*. 2012;79(9):929–936.

Braley TJ, Segal BM, Chervin RD. Underrecognition of sleep disorders in patients with multiple sclerosis. *J Clin Sleep Med*. 2015;11(1):81.

Braley TJ, et al. sleep and cognitive function in multiple sclerosis. *Sleep*. 2016;39(8):1525–1533.

Foschi M, et al. Sleep-related disorders and their relationship with MRI findings in multiple sclerosis. *Sleep Med*. 2019;56:90–97.

Gaig C, Iranzo A, Cajochen C, et al. Characterization of the sleep disorder of anti-IgLON5 disease. *Sleep*. 2019b:pii: zsz133. https://doi.org/10.1093/sleep/zsz133.

Guaraldi P, Calandra-BuonauraG, Terlizzi, et al. Oneiric stupor: the peculiar behaviour of agrypnia excitata. *Sleep Med*. 2011;12:S64–S67.

Iranzo A, Graus F, Clover L, et al. Rapid eye movement sleep behavior disorder and potassium channel antibody–associated limbic encephalitis. *Ann Neurol*. 2006;59:178–182.

Kaminska M, et al. Sleep disorders and fatigue in multiple sclerosis: Evidence for association and interaction. *J Neurol Scie*. 2011;302(1):7–13.

Lugaresi E, Provini F, Cortelli P. Agrypnia excitata. *Sleep Med*. 2011;12:S3–S10.

Overeem S, Dalmau J, Bataller L, et al. HCRT-1 CSF levels in anti-Ma2 associated encephalitis. *Neurol*. 2004;62:138–140.

Sabater L, Gaig C, Gelpi E, et al. A novel non-rapid-eye movement and rapid-eye-movement parasomnia with sleep breathing disorder associated with antibodies to IgLON5: a case series, characterisation of the antigen, and post-mortem study. *Lancet Neurol*. 2014;13:575–586.

A complete reference list can be found online at ExpertConsult.com.

Section 13

Hypersomnias

Chapter 110

Central Disorders of Hypersomnolence

Kiran Maski; Thomas E. Scammell

INTRODUCTION

The central disorders of hypersomnolence in this section are conditions that cause persistent sleepiness, most likely due to dysfunction of the central nervous system. In the *International Classification of Sleep Disorders,* third edition (ICSD-3),[1] these central disorders of hypersomnolence include narcolepsy type 1 (NT1), narcolepsy type 2 (NT2), idiopathic hypersomnia (IH), and Kleine-Levin syndrome (KLS).

Researchers and clinicians sometimes use the terms *excessive daytime sleepiness* (EDS), *excessive need for sleep, hypersomnolence,* and *hypersomnia* interchangeably, but these terms should be used with more precise meanings. Hypersomnolence is defined as "daily episodes of an irrepressible need to sleep or daytime lapses into sleep" in the ICSD-3, and this term thus encompasses the symptoms of excessive need for sleep and excessive daytime sleepiness (inability to stay awake during the normal wake period of the day). In contrast, hypersomnia is derived from the Greek words "hyper," meaning "over," and "somnus," or "sleep,"[2] and thus should refer to a need or tendency for an increase in the amount of sleep per 24 hours. For example, compared to patients with narcolepsy, patients with IH have longer sleep durations, higher nocturnal sleep efficiency, and fall asleep less quickly in the daytime.[3] Patients with KLS have recurrent periods of hypersomnia with about 18 hours of sleep per 24 hours during an episode. In contrast, patients with NT1 typically sleep about 7.5 to 8 hours per 24 hours, but they have great difficulty sustaining wakefulness and complain of severe daytime sleepiness. NT2 seems to be a more heterogeneous condition that lies in the borderland of NT1 and IH; its cause is unknown, but some patients may have a partial loss of hypocretin neurons, with mildly lower cerebrospinal hypocretin levels.

DIAGNOSTIC CHALLENGES

Disorders of chronic hypersomnolence can be difficult to diagnose because many disorders cause sleepiness, terminology can be confusing as noted earlier, symptoms are reported inconsistently, and the conditions are heterogeneous. The Multiple Sleep Latency Test (MSLT), preceded by an overnight polysomnogram (PSG), is an excellent method to objectively assess EDS and sleep-onset rapid eye movement (REM) periods, and it has high diagnostic validity and reliability in people with NT1.[4] However, in people with IH, routine PSG and MSLT do not measure the high amount of sleep per 24 hours that is a core symptom of IH, possibly contributing to poor validity and reliability. In NT2 the severity of EDS and REM sleep dysregulation may be more variable, contributing to low reliability of the PSG and MSLT. The poor reliability of MSLT may improve with more focus on sleep satiation before the test, correction or consideration of circadian phase, and appropriately stopping medications/substances that affect wake and sleep. At present, most health care providers rely on the PSG and MSLT for diagnosing IH because other objective testing options encouraged by the ICSD-3 (actigraphy and extended 24-hour PSG) are generally not accessible or reimbursed. As new evidence becomes available, diagnostic testing and protocols may change in the coming years.

Thus, to a great degree, the diagnosis of hypersomnolence disorders relies upon taking a careful history from the patient and family and using diagnostic tests with an understanding of their appropriateness and limitations. For example, in patients with IH, the traditional PSG is not helpful, but a 36-hour extended PSG has impressive validity and reliability.[5] IH patients often complain of profound sleep inertia,[6,7] and this may be objectively measured using attention, working memory, and cognitive throughput tasks.[8] KLS can impact behavior and thinking between episodes, and functional brain imaging during asymptomatic periods shows mild hypoperfusion of the parietotemporal junction and of the mesiotemporal lobe, as well as asymmetric perfusion of the thalamus, which may help support the diagnosis.

CURRENT AND FUTURE TREATMENTS

An improved understanding of sleep-wake mechanisms has helped drive the development of better therapies. Most progress has been made in the treatment of NT1 because the symptoms are well defined, it can be diagnosed with confidence, and we know that it is caused by a selective loss of the hypocretin-producing neurons. Just in the last few years, researchers have begun to define the underlying immune pathophysiology of NT1, and in the future, immune-modulating medications could be tested to slow or stop the disease. As hypocretin deficiency likely underlies most symptoms of NT1, there are now substantial efforts underway to develop small-molecule hypocretin agonists expected to help people with NT1 and, perhaps, other disorders with partial reductions in hypocretin tone. Treatments for IH and NT2 have received less attention, in part because of heterogeneous symptoms that may produce more variable treatment responses and difficulty obtaining insurance support for medications, but clinical trials focused on these disorders are now underway. KLS is quite rare, so clinical trials are a challenge. Recent research suggests that intravenous steroids can shorten long KLS bouts[9] and is a step in the right direction.

Central disorders of hypersomnolence impair performance in school and work, impact social interactions and family dynamics, and present real risks with driving. As noted in these chapters, listening to the patient is crucial for correct diagnosis and management. Allowing patients to describe their symptoms in their own words and distinguishing daytime sleepiness, excess sleep needs, and fatigue can point the clinician toward the correct diagnostic testing. Identifying and treating the patient's most burdensome symptoms, providing academic/work accommodations and anticipatory guidance on driving, and routinely screening for medical, cognitive, and psychiatric comorbidities can also improve quality of life immensely.

A complete reference list can be found online at ExpertConsult.com.

Chapter

111

Narcolepsy: Pathophysiology and Genetic Predisposition

Emmanuel Mignot

Chapter Highlights

- Narcolepsy, a term reserved in the past for individuals with cataplexy, is now used for patients with unexplained daytime sleepiness and a positive Multiple Sleep Latency Test (MSLT). As a result, narcolepsy type 1 (with cataplexy; NT1) and narcolepsy type 2 (without cataplexy; NT2) are now differentiated in international classifications. NT1 is a discrete disease entity with a specific cause, hypocretin/orexin deficiency. In contrast, NT2 may be overdiagnosed in the context of false-positive MSLTs that are not repeatable and may not be easily differentiable from idiopathic hypersomnia. We can anticipate changes in the international classification in the future.
- NT1 is a T cell–mediated autoimmune disease targeting the hypocretin/orexin neurons, wake-promoting neurons located in the posterior hypothalamus. Among people with NT1, 97% carry the gene for *DQB1*06:02*, so absence of this human leukocyte antigen (HLA) in a marker almost excludes the diagnosis. Hypocretin deficiency can be demonstrated by measuring hypocretin-1 (orexin A) in cerebrospinal fluid (CSF), a test highly specific and sensitive, providing it is performed in a patient who is not critically ill.
- NT1 results from genetic predisposing factors that increase T-cell responses in particular ways, followed by exposure to very specific pathogens that can trigger an autoimmune attack on the hypocretin neurons. Specific influenza A subtypes such as H1N1 can trigger a strong T-cell reaction that cross-reacts with posttranslationally modified portions of the hypocretin peptides, resulting in hypocretin cell loss. The cell loss is irreversible, thus narcolepsy is lifelong.
- Current therapies, although effective, act mostly through the modulation of monoaminergic (antidepressants and stimulants) and GABAergic systems (sodium oxybate). Our improved understanding of narcolepsy is leading to novel treatments and may improve diagnostic procedures. It may be possible to prevent narcolepsy using modified flu vaccinations that do not contain specific epitopes and would not only protect against the flu but also prevent immune response that could be cross-reactive. If caught early, immune suppressants may stop hypocretin neuron loss before it is too late. Most importantly, hypocretin/orexin receptor 2 agonists are now in development and are showing very promising efficacy in animal models and humans.

INTRODUCTION

Narcolepsy has long been characterized by "excessive daytime sleepiness associated with cataplexy and other rapid eye movement (REM) sleep phenomena such as sleep paralysis and hypnagogic hallucinations."[1] Cataplexy, a sudden occurrence of muscle weakness in association with laughing, joking, or anger, was thus considered necessary for the diagnosis.[2-4] Almost all reported patients had cataplexy, except for a few individuals who would typically develop cataplexy within a few years, although rarely this could take decades. Recently, more patients have been recognized in early childhood or close to disease onset, and in these individuals, cataplexy can be atypical, with global hypotonia without any obvious emotional triggers, or with spontaneous grimaces or jaw-opening episodes with tongue thrusting.[5] Patients with narcolepsy can rapidly transition into REM sleep, and the Multiple Sleep Latency Test (MSLT), a 5 nap test during the daytime initially designed to measure sleepiness, was adjusted to measure sleep-onset REM sleep periods (SOREMPs). Multiple SOREMPs during naps[6] and soon after nocturnal REM sleep onset were found to be highly specific (97%) and sensitive (92%) to diagnose narcolepsy, a practical way to objectively confirm the diagnosis.[7] In testimony to the wisdom of these older clinical descriptions, narcolepsy type 1 (NT1; narcolepsy with cataplexy) is a discrete disease entity with a strong association with HLA-*DQB1*06:02* and a unique autoimmune pathophysiology targeting the hypocretin/orexin neurons, as demonstrated by low CSF hypocretin-1 levels in most patients.[8] Specific polymorphisms modulating antigen presentation by dendritic cells to $CD4^+$ T cells and $CD8^+$ T cell activity have been identified in people with NT1.[9] The autoimmune condition can be triggered by influenza A, notably H1N1, and involves a process in which $CD4^+$ T cells targeting specific flu peptide sequences cross-react with the hypocretin peptides, with subsequent recruitment of $CD8^+$ T cells that kill the hypocretin neurons.[10] Armed with these new findings, we are now witnessing progress likely to lead to immune-modulating therapies and development of hypocretin agonists for NT1. These will supplement current therapies that are modulating symptoms through downstream effects on monoaminergic transmission. These results should also improve our understanding and treatment of narcolepsy type 2 (NT2) and idiopathic hypersomnia, two poorly defined conditions that can be hard to distinguish.

PREVALENCE AND INCIDENCE OF TYPE 1 NARCOLEPSY

Because cataplexy can be identified using questionnaires, many studies have evaluated the prevalence of narcolepsy with cataplexy (NT1) in population-based samples and found it is consistent across most countries, with estimates generally ranging from 0.02% to 0.05%.[11-13] In most studies, patients with cataplexy are verified through interviews, MSLT testing, and human leukocyte antigen (HLA) positivity. Many are unaware of their condition, in line with estimations suggesting that only half of patients with NT1 are diagnosed even in countries where awareness is high. The explanation may be that the disease is not always recognized by the medical profession, and that patients do not report their symptoms, believing these to be part of a normal continuum. Another factor is that symptoms are usually most severe around disease onset and lessen with time, with decreased cataplexy severity over years. Incidence studies have been sparser, and only in Scandinavian countries when medical care is systematic and widespread enough can these be trusted. In Finland, Noheynek[160] reported basal yearly incidence of narcolepsy with cataplexy at 0.31 per 100,000 person-years in children and adolescents, which, considering that the disease is lifelong with approximately half of patients starting disease onset before age 18, is roughly congruent with a prevalence of 0.023% reported in Finland. Other incidence estimates are in similar ranges, 0.5 to 1 of 100,000 individuals per year.[15] Peak onset age of narcolepsy has been well established in multiple populations, with exceptional patients before age 3, rare before age 7, peaking around age 15, with a possible smaller peak of onset around age 30 and rare onsets in late adulthood.[16,17] Onset in childhood is now more often reported, which may reflect a real shift toward earlier onset (possibly related to the appearance of the H1N1 2009 flu, see later), improved recognition resulting from increased awareness, or both.

FAMILIAL ASPECTS OF HUMAN NARCOLEPSY

Westphal[18] was the first to report familial occurrence of narcolepsy-cataplexy in 1877. In all studies, the risk of a first-degree relative to develop narcolepsy-cataplexy has been shown to be 1% (see the work by Mignot[11] and Yan and colleagues[19]). A larger portion of relatives (2%–4%) may have isolated daytime sleepiness, when other causes of daytime sleepiness have been excluded.[11] These figures are important to keep in mind because they are helpful in reassuring patients regarding the risk to their children and relatives. A 1% risk is 10- to 40-fold higher than in the general population but remains manageable. A 2% to 4% risk for daytime sleepiness is not negligible, but similar values have been reported for excessive daytime sleepiness in the general population independent of narcolepsy.[20-23] As mentioned later, a subset of these family members with unexplained sleepiness and no cataplexy may have mild forms of NT1 involving partial hypocretin deficiency.[19]

SPECTRUM DISEASE OF TYPE 1 NARCOLEPSY

In addition to this, some individuals likely have partial autoimmune loss of hypocretin neurons and can thus be considered "milder" NT1 without cataplexy. This is illustrated by one postmortem case in which loss of neurons was 85% as opposed to more than 90% in cases with cataplexy.[24] Although narcolepsy without cataplexy but with hypocretin deficiency is rarely ascertained in sleep clinics (most have normal CSF hypocretin-1), they may represent a larger group in the general population based on several observations. First, patients without cataplexy but with low CSF hypocretin-1, HLA-*DQB1*06:02*, and positive, repeatable MSLTs, although rare in sleep clinics, have been long described (representing perhaps 15% of patients in older series), with about half estimated to develop cataplexy within their lifetime.[25] These individuals generally have more SOREMPs on the MSLT than other subjects.[25] Second, milder presentations of narcolepsy without cataplexy have long been described in family members of patients with NT1,[11] of whom approximately 1% of first-degree relatives have NT1 with cataplexy, and another 1% have positive MSLT, HLA positivity, and in some cases low CSF hypocretin but no cataplexy.[19] Third, although systematic MSLT testing in population samples with exclusion of confounding etiologies and repeated sleep tests has been performed only in a small number of subjects; in one cohort of 1300 subjects, one case with and one case without cataplexy were reliably identified.[26] Finally, a number of studies suggest that cataplexy improves with age; thus it is conceivable some older patients do not experience this symptom anymore. Overall, these studies suggest that perhaps up to 0.1% of the general population may have a hypocretin-deficient NT1 condition, with half to a third with clear cataplexy and only a portion properly diagnosed, most commonly in the presence of cataplexy. These findings are reminiscent of what is found in other autoimmune diseases in which milder forms are common, sometimes characterized only by the presence of autoantibodies. In the future, it may become possible to test this idea if a blood test is developed to detect hypocretin autoimmunity.

TWIN STUDIES IN NARCOLEPSY

Studies of more than 30 monozygotic twins with NT1 show that only 25% to 30% are concordant for the disorder.[11,27-30] This low concordance in genetically similar individuals thus suggests that narcolepsy requires additional stochastic and environmental factors to develop. This is also substantiated by the fact that onset is not at birth but rather in adolescence,[16,17,31-33] suggesting triggering factors in childhood or adolescence. As detailed later, it is likely that a main triggering factor is influenza, and that onset is modulated by prior history of exposure to various infections.

CANINE NARCOLEPSY AND INVOLVEMENT OF HYPOCRETIN/OREXIN

For the last 40 years, narcolepsy research has been facilitated by the existence of a unique animal model, canine narcolepsy. Knecht[34] and Mitler[35] first reported the existence of canine narcolepsy in 1973. Early attempts to establish genetic transmission were unsuccessful, suggesting a nongenetic etiology in most cases. In 1975, two narcoleptic Dobermans were reported in a single litter,[36] and breeding found autosomal recessive transmission with full penetrance, allowing the establishment of a colony at Stanford University. Familial canine narcolepsy was also reported in Labrador retrievers and dachshunds.[36,37] Interestingly, dogs heterozygous for the gene have subclinical abnormalities; for example, drugs that increase cholinergic and reduce monoaminergic transmission (manipulations known to promote REM sleep) can induce cataplexy at specific developmental times in heterozygous animals.[38]

The parallel between human NT1 and canine narcolepsy is striking. In MSLT-like procedures, narcoleptic canines have short latencies to enter non–rapid eye movement (NREM) and REM sleep.[39] Twenty-four–hour recordings show sleep fragmentation and more daytime sleep.[40] Finally, as in humans, muscle weakness akin to cataplexy occurs with strong positive emotions, typically with appetizing food or while at play (Figure 111.1). These episodes last a few seconds and preferentially affect the hind legs, neck, or face and may escalate into complete paralysis with abolition of tendon reflexes. During these episodes, the animal is conscious and most often able to visually track nearby movement (Video 111.1). Polygraphic recordings indicate a desynchronized, wake-like EEG pattern at the onset of cataplexy, followed by increased theta activity and genuine REM sleep in long-lasting episodes.[41]

In 1999 positional cloning studies showed that autosomal recessive canine narcolepsy is due to mutations in the gene coding for hypocretin receptor-2 (also known as orexin 2 receptor).[37,42] Three different mutations causing complete dysfunction of the receptor were identified.[37,42] Sporadic cases of canine narcolepsy were later shown to be associated with low CSF hypocretin and almost absent brain hypocretin peptide content,[43] as found in human narcolepsy.[24,44] In contrast, familial canine narcolepsy cases have normal CSF hypocretin but lack the orexin 2 receptor.[43]

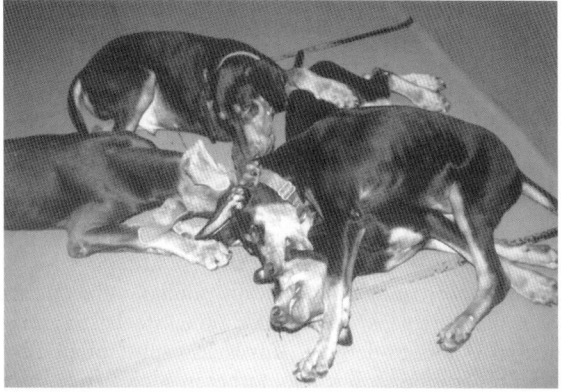

Figure 111.1 Narcoleptic Doberman pinschers during attacks of cataplexy. Note that the eyes are open. Autosomal recessive forms of canine narcolepsy are due to mutations in the hypocretin receptor-2 gene. (Modified from Lin L, et al. The sleep disorder canine narcolepsy is caused by a mutation in the hypocretin [orexin] receptor 2 gene. *Cell.* 1999;98[3]:365–76.)

The effects of more than 200 compounds with various modes of action have been examined in human patients and narcoleptic canines (see the work by Nishino and Mignot[39] for review). In almost all cases, similar effects were found in humans and canines.[39] For example, antidepressants were found to primarily decrease cataplexy through inhibition of adrenergic reuptake,[45,46] while stimulants increased wakefulness through inhibition of dopaminergic reuptake or increased dopaminergic release.[47-50] Almost all the significant effects have been reported for monoaminergic and cholinergic compounds. As cataplexy is easier to study than sleep in canines, most research in narcoleptic dogs has focused on cataplexy. For cataplexy, the findings were generally consistent with pharmacologic studies of REM sleep. As with REM sleep, cataplexy is increased by drugs that enhance cholinergic signaling and reduced by drugs that increase monoaminergic tone.[39] Muscarinic M2 or M3 receptors mediate the cholinergic effects, while monoaminergic effects are mostly modulated by postsynaptic adrenergic alpha-1 receptors and presynaptic D2/D3 autoreceptors.[39]

A number of studies have shown that the wake-promoting effect of these amphetamines and amphetamine-like drugs is mostly due to dopamine (DA) release and reuptake inhibition, although adrenergic release and reuptake inhibition may have additional, independent wake-promoting effects in humans, notably for solriamfetol. Most likely, modafinil selectively inhibits DA uptake. Illustrating this, these compounds have been found to be ineffective in DA transporter knockout mice, suggesting a primary promotion of wake via dopaminergic systems.[48] Interestingly, in dogs, compounds selective for dopaminergic transmission have no effect on cataplexy, whereas amphetamine-like compounds with combined dopaminergic and adrenergic effects have some anti-cataplectic properties at high doses.[45,51] Adrenergic effects of amphetamine-like stimulants also correlate with the respective effects of these compounds on normal REM sleep.[39,51] DA-specific uptake blockers like modafinil have little effect on REM sleep when compared with adrenergic or serotonergic compounds.[39] The most important effects of dopaminergic uptake blockers are to reduce total sleep time and slow wave sleep.[52] An exception to this may be solriamfetol, which, in spite of its dual adrenergic and dopaminergic reuptake inhibition effects, has no effect on cataplexy. The reason for this discrepancy is unclear and illustrates the complexity of translating preclinical pharmacology into clinical practice.

Although the primary cause of NT1 is hypocretin deficiency, studies have shown abnormal cholinergic and monoaminergic receptor density and neurotransmitter levels in human or canine narcolepsy brain and CSF samples.[39,53-57] Local injection studies in selected brain areas of narcoleptic canines have also shown functional relevance for some of these abnormalities.[58-60] As a result, cholinergic hypersensitivity, dopaminergic abnormalities, and abnormal histaminergic tone are likely to be critical downstream mediators of hypocretin deficiency in the expression of the narcolepsy symptomatology.[54,57-60] The cholinergic/monoaminergic imbalances observed in narcolepsy are best illustrated by the finding that in asymptomatic dogs heterozygous for the hypocretin receptor-2 mutation, combining cholinergic agonists with an alpha-1 blocker or a D2/D3 agonist, can trigger cataplexy.[38] Further, the brains of NT1 patients have an increased number of histaminergic neurons,[55,56] and focal expression of the hypocretin receptor 2 in the posterior hypothalamus rescues sleepiness in these mutant mice.[61] An application of these findings is illustrated by the recent development of histaminergic H3 antagonists such as pitolisant, drugs that are known to stimulate histamine release via the H3 receptor, as novel wake-promoting stimulants and anticataplectic agent for the treatment of narcolepsy.[62,63] In 2019 pitolisant was approved by the US Food and Drug Administration for the treatment of sleepiness in narcolepsy in the United States, although it has been available in Europe for this indication for several years.

RODENT HYPOCRETIN/OREXIN MODELS OF NARCOLEPSY

Multiple rodent models of narcolepsy are available. Chemelli and colleagues[64] developed prepro-hypocretin knockout mice, reporting fragmented sleep, rapid transitions from wakefulness into REM sleep, and a reversible state of paralysis akin to cataplexy.[64] In other models, toxic transgenes are driven by the hypocretin promoter, producing various levels of hypocretin-containing cell loss and narcolepsy.[65,66] In these models, more than 90% loss of the hypocretin neurons produces narcolepsy. A rat model with partial hypocretin cell loss[67] and mice lacking either of the two hypocretin receptors, hypocretin receptor-1 and -2, are also available.[61,68-70] In these models, only hypocretin receptor-2 receptor knockouts experience cataplexy, although episodes are few and not as clear as in hypocretin peptide knockout mice.[68] Interestingly, hypocretin receptor-1 knockout animals are almost normal, having only mildly fragmented sleep and REM sleep abnormalities but no cataplexy.[69] Dual hypocretin receptor-1 and -2 knockout mice recapitulate the full phenotype of hypocretin peptide knockout, suggesting that in mice hypocretin receptor-1 increases the severity of the hypocretin receptor-2 phenotype,[68] leading to a full narcolepsy phenotype only when both receptors are inactivated.

LIMITATIONS OF ANIMAL MODELS

The use of these models, together with recent developments that make it possible to increase firing rate selectively in hypocretin cells through optogenic stimulation,[71] is revolutionizing research in this area. However, it is important to keep in mind that humans are more genetically diverse than inbred rodent lines and have distinct ecologic niches, most likely explaining interspecies differences in the regulation and functions of hypocretin.[72] This may explain why hypocretin receptor-2 mutants have clearer cataplexy in dogs versus mice, or why hypocretin receptor-2 mutations causing narcolepsy have not yet been identified in humans (e.g., the phenotype may be too mild in humans to raise concern). Similarly, food deprivation (up to 31 hours) in mice increases wakefulness, most likely because of the acute need to search for food, but this response is severely blunted in mice lacking hypocretin.[73] Yet, metabolically, mice have high metabolic demands and low energy reserves, unlike humans. Further, in contrast to these results, patients with narcolepsy frequently use food restriction to stay awake and have binge-eating abnormalities, especially at night.[74-76] Similarly, we found that the small decrease in food intake found in rodents with hypocretin deficiency could partially be explained by wake fragmentation.[67] Finally, as discussed later, pharmacologic responses vary across species. As an example, the alpha-2 antagonist yohimbine is a strong wake-promoting compound and anticataplectic agent in canines, yet has little effect in humans.[39] Similarly, in dogs, the anti-cataplectic effects of antidepressants is mediated by inhibition of adrenergic reuptake,[45] while clinical experience suggests that in humans, dual inhibition of adrenergic and serotoninergic reuptake (e.g., using venlafaxine), may be more effective than serotonin-only (escitalopram) or adrenergic-only (atomoxetine) medications.[77]

STRONG HUMAN LEUKOCYTE ANTIGEN DQ0602 ASSOCIATION IN NARCOLEPSY

HLA genes, also called major histocompatibility complex genes, are a specialized set of immune-regulatory genes located on human chromosome 6. These genes and their resulting proteins are unusual: they are extremely polymorphic in a small region of the protein that functions as a peptide binding area.

HLA molecules present foreign antigens (e.g., peptide fragments derived from a virus or bacteria) to T cells, major effector cells of the immune system. Because each person has a specific set of HLA genes, these bind slightly different sets of peptide antigens (peptide repertoire), and thus T cells of each individual can only "see" a specific set of antigenic peptides. HLA polymorphisms are thus at the origin of much of the interindividual genetic variation in immune responses. As such, immune responses to infection vary by HLA subtype (and these genes are submitted to strong evolutionary pressure), although as most infections involve thousands of epitopes and multiple genes, the effect at the level of individual genes on infection outcome is modest, and HLA polymorphisms modulate infectious disease severity rather than occurrence. Rather, as is discussed later, most of the diseases that are strongly associated with HLA are autoimmune, likely involving the presentation of a few specific autoantigens by specific HLA subtypes, therefore explaining the strong associations.

The observation that narcolepsy is strongly associated with HLA was first reported in Japan[78,79] with HLA-DR2 and DQ1 (Figure 111.2, *A*). Subsequent studies found that the true culprit is *DQ0602*, encoded by *DQA1*01:02* and *DQB1*06:02*, alleles of *DQA* and *DQB*, two genes located within 20 kb of each other.[80,81] The functional HLA-DQ protein is a heterodimer composed of a DQα chain (encoded by DQA) and a DQβ chain (encoded by DQB). Because these genes are located close together, there is high linkage disequilibrium between these two genes so that specific combinations of DQA1 and DQB1 alleles are found as haplotypes (such as *DQA1*01:02* and *DQB1*06:02*). The presence of these nonrandom combinations of DQA1-DQB1 haplotype has been shaped by evolutionary constraints, as some but not all DQα and DQβ chains can bind together. Indeed, functional studies have shown that the DQα chains of the broad DQ1 subtype (subseparated into DQ5 and DQ6) can heterodimerize together, but not with other subtypes that are very distinct in term of their sequence homology. The sequence homology is reflected by the nomenclature with gene products of the DQ1 family being associated with DQA1*01 and DQB1*05 or DQB1*06 subtypes. As

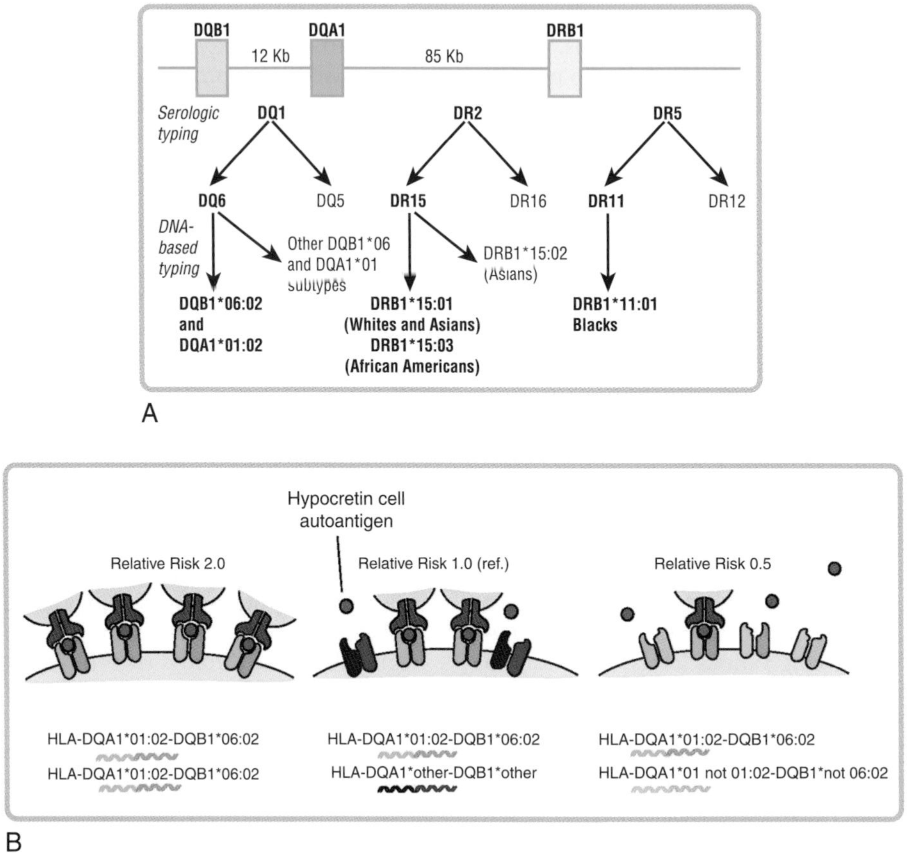

Figure 111.2 Human leukocyte antigens (HLA) DR and HLA DQ alleles typically observed in narcolepsy. **(A)** The DR and DQ genes are located very close to each other on chromosome 6p21 and are part of the HLA class II family of HLA genes. These genes encode heterodimeric HLA proteins composed of an α and a β chain that interact with T-cell receptors (TCRs) located on $CD4^+$ T cells. In the DQ locus, both the DQα and DQβ chains have numerous polymorphic residues and are encoded by two polymorphic genes, *DQA1* and *DQB1*, respectively. Polymorphisms at the DR(αβ) level are mostly encoded by the *DRB1* gene, so only this locus is depicted in this figure. *DQB1*06:02*, a molecular subtype of the serologically defined DQ1 antigen (later split into DQ5 and DQ6), is the most specific marker for narcolepsy across all ethnic groups. It is always associated with the *DQA1* subtype, *DQA1*01:02*, forming the DQ(αβ) heterodimer DQ0602. **(B)** Studies suggest that the allelic dose of DQ0602 influences narcolepsy risk. Because of this, homozygotes are at approximately twice the risk of developing narcolepsy, whereas subjects heterozygous with other DQ1 subtypes are at reduced risk. (Modified from Ollila et al.[86])

a consequence, only very rarely would a DQB1*06 subtype be found adjacent to a non-DQA1*01 DQα chain; in these patients a nonfunctional heterodimer would result and thus would likely be eliminated by evolution.

A number of other DQ haplotypes in the population carry *DQA1*01:02* without *DQB1*06:02* (instead, other DQB1*05 or *06 subtypes that can dimerize with *DQA1*01:02* are present), and those do not predispose to narcolepsy.[82] Conversely, although *DQB1*06:02* subjects are almost always *DQA1*01:02* positive, rare haplotypes with *DQB1*06:02* but without *DQA1*01:02* are observed in the control population but not in narcolepsy subjects.[82] Thus both the *DQA1*01:02* and the *DQB1*06:02* alleles together (also known as the DQ0602 heterodimer) are needed for narcolepsy predisposition,[82] which is logical because polymorphism in both the DQα and DQβ region contributes to peptide binding.

Across multiple ethnic groups, *DQ0602* (the combination of *DQA1*01:02* and *DQB1*06:02*) is nearly required for developing narcolepsy, and individuals homozygous for DQ0602 are at approximately two times greater risk of developing narcolepsy,[83-86] suggesting that the amount of DQ0602 heterodimer increases risk.[87] In addition, DQB1*05:01, DQB1*06:01, DQB1*06:03 and other DQ1 alleles that are non-DQ0602 appear protective.[84-86,88-90] These DQ1 alleles, unlike those of the other broad DQ groups (DQ2, 3, and 4), are "compatible" with each other, meaning that they have sequence similarity and proper folding as selected by invariant chain binding (in contrast, non-DQ1 subtypes such as DQ2 and DQ3 are generally compatible with each other) (Figure 111.2, *B*). Estimating relative risk, we noted that risk of DQ0602/other DQ1 is about one-half of DQ0602/other, suggesting that there is competition of trans-encoded DQ1 alleles that are non-DQ0602, reducing the amount of DQ0602, and thus risk, a phenomenon we call allele competition[85,86] (Figure 111.2, *B*). This model nicely explains why DQ0602/DQ0601, DQ0602/DQ0603, and DQ0602/DQ0501 are relatively protective against narcolepsy.

Intriguingly, *DQB1*06:02*/DQB1*03:01 increases risk versus other combinations,[84-86,88,91] an effect difficult to explain because it occurs in the context of multiple DQα-associated alleles (d, DQA1*03:02, DQA1*05:05, and DQA1*06:01), suggesting it is not mediated via DQα/β heterodimers (further, these DQA1 would not heterodimerize with *DQB1*06:02*. The reason for this additional effect is unclear, but unlike DQ0602 dose, DQB1*03:01 reduces age of onset of narcolepsy so that the association is stronger in early-onset narcolepsy.[92] One possibility may be that the presence of DQB1*03:01 shapes the T-cell receptor (TCR) repertoire in subjects with DQ0602 in a way that increases the risk of carrying pathogenic autoimmune $CD4^+$ T-cell clones.[93]

OTHER HUMAN LEUKOCYTE ANTIGEN LOCI MODULATING NARCOLEPSY RISK

Although HLA-DQ is the primary genetic factor associated with narcolepsy (DQ0602 dose and DQB1*03:01 for early onset), additional effects within the HLA region add further modulation. Ollila and colleagues[94] compared controls and narcolepsy subjects fully matched for HLA-DQ and found protective effects of *DPB1*04:02* (odds ratio [OR] ≈ 0.5) and susceptibility effects of *DPB1*05:01* (OR ≈ 2). Additional matching for HLA-DP (i.e., matching for DR, DQ, and DP) revealed weak but significant residual effects in the HLA class I region (Figure 111.3). Because HLA-Class II interacts with $CD4^+$ T cells (see later), whereas HLA-Class I interacts with $CD8^+$ T and NK cells, these data suggest that multiple immune populations are involved in the pathophysiology of narcolepsy, as discussed later.

ROLE OF HUMAN LEUKOCYTE ANTIGEN TYPING IN CLINICAL PRACTICE

The usefulness of HLA typing in clinical practice is limited by several factors. First, the HLA association is very high (97%) only in patients with NT1, and as seen in clinical practice, most patients with NT1 have cataplexy. Second, a large number of control individuals (approximately 12% in Japan, 25% in Whites and Chinese, 38% in Blacks) have *DQB1*06:02* without having narcolepsy. In a recent study, four of nine subjects lacking *DQB1*06:02* with documented low CSF hypocretin-1 were *DPB1*09:01* positive, a rare subtype (≈3%).[95] Practically, determining if a patient carries *DQB1*06:02* is only helpful to exclude hypocretin deficiency as the cause of the clinical complaint, especially before a lumbar puncture for CSF hypocretin-1 determination. Whether or not having an ultimate biologic basis for symptoms is important is a matter of individual clinician preference. In my opinion, establishing if a patient is hypocretin deficient helps clinicians decide whether to be more aggressive with selected therapies, whereas symptoms without a clear cause must lead to a constant reevaluation of the situation. For this reason, we believe that CSF hypocretin is most useful in HLA-positive borderline patients in whom it is difficult to determine if the patient has true cataplexy or for whom the MSLT results were unexpectedly normal.

GENETIC FACTORS OTHER THAN HUMAN LEUKOCYTE ANTIGEN

As mentioned earlier, genetic factors other than HLA can increase the risk of developing narcolepsy. The increased familial risk in first-degree relatives (10-fold in Japanese, 20- to 40-fold in Whites) cannot be explained solely by the sharing of HLA subtypes, which are estimated to explain a twofold to threefold increased risk.[11] Further, as discussed later, other associations have been established through genome-wide association studies (GWAS). Finally, polymorphisms in the catechol-*O*-methyltransferase gene, a key enzyme in the degradation of catecholamines, may modulate disease severity.[96,97]

Additionally, the existence of rare HLA-negative families (and occasional unexplainable cases with typical symptoms and normal CSF hypocretin) suggests disease heterogeneity and the possible involvement of other genes. Many of these individuals have normal CSF hypocretin but lack mutations in hypocretin receptor genes.[95] In a rare multiplex family with *DQB1*06:02* negativity and low CSF hypocretin levels, a mutation in myelin oligodendrocyte glycoprotein (MOG) was found to be associated with narcolepsy.[98] MOG mutations have not yet been found in any other HLA-negative patients with low CSF hypocretin.[95] A single case of preprohypocretin mutation was found in an individual with cataplexy and HLA negativity of very early onset (6 months of age).[44]

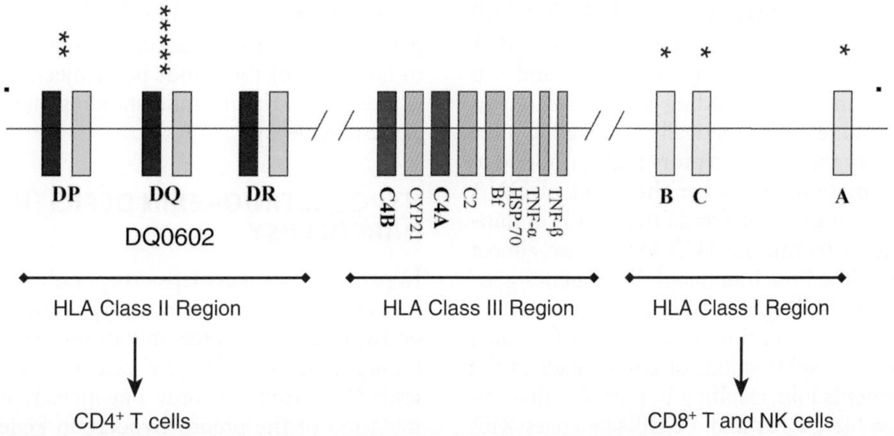

Figure 111.3 Effects of human leukocyte antigen (HLA) loci other than HLA-DQ. HLA loci other than DQ also influence narcolepsy, notably HLA class II genes DPB1*04:02 (protective) and DPB1*05:01 (predisposing). In addition, effects of specific HLA class I gene alleles are also evident. HLA class I genes present peptides to T-cell receptors located on $CD8^+$ cytotoxic T cells or may interact with natural killer (NK) cells, suggesting involvement of these cells in the pathophysiology of narcolepsy. (From Ollila et al.[9])

Since 2000, studies have moved toward systematic genome coverage using GWAS designs.[9,90,92,99-102] In a first study, Miyagawa and colleagues[99] found involvement of rs5770917, a polymorphism located between *CPT1B* and *CHKB*, genes that regulate cholinergic metabolism and beta chain fatty acid oxidation, respectively. A similar effect of rs5770917 (and a significant HLA association) was also observed in patients with "essential hypersomnia syndrome," a milder form of narcolepsy defined by sleepiness, refreshing naps but no cataplexy,[99] suggesting a disease continuum.

Using a larger sample, Hallmayer and colleagues[100] found that narcolepsy is strongly associated not only with HLA but also with a specific polymorphism in the TCRα gene.[100] Although genetic risk was not high (OR ≈2) when compared with effects found with HLA polymorphism, the finding was remarkable: it further demonstrated a role of the immune system in narcolepsy. It is also an unusual finding, as none of the other autoimmune disorders subjected to GWAS analysis have TCR loci as a susceptibility factor.

Further studies in larger samples that also included other ethnic groups, notably Chinese, Japanese, and Blacks, identified other associated genes, most known to be involved in other autoimmune diseases,[9,92,101,102] or in viral immune responses. These include TCRα and β genes; TNFSF4, a costimulatory receptor for T-cell activation; cathepsin H, an enzyme likely involved in antigen processing and associated with type 1 diabetes; ZNF365, a transcription factor associated with inflammatory bowel disease; *IFNAR1*, a gene important for the regulation of the type 1 interferon response involved in viral immunity; langerin, a protein important for flu virus entry into dendritic cells; P2RY11, an ATP receptor, regulating immune cell death and chemotaxis and perforin, a cytolytic molecule involved in the killing of target cells by $CD8^+$ T cells.

T-CELL RECEPTOR POLYMORPHISMS ASSOCIATED WITH NARCOLEPSY SHAPE THE T-CELL RECEPTOR REPERTOIRE

As mentioned previously, a striking finding of these genetic analyses is that in addition to HLA, NT1 is strongly associated with specific TCRA polymorphisms, with weaker effects within the TCRB loci.[9,100] $CD4^+$ and $CD8^+$ cells express TCRs, and TCRs are activated when peptides are presented to these cells in the presence of HLA Class II (DR, DQ, DP) and Class I (A, B, C) molecules, respectively. Like most HLA genes, TCRs are heterodimers constituted of an α and a β chain, although in this instance, encoding of the two chains is on different chromosomes and genetically unlinked. Unlike HLA, sequence diversity for these receptors is also not due to genetically encoded variation, but rather the result of DNA recombination events in individual T cells that result in joining V, D, and J segments within the TCR locus in an almost random fashion, much like how immunoglobulin genes generate antibody diversity. TCR genes have approximately 50 different V and J sequences, multiple D sequences for some loci, and even additions or subtractions of amino acids at the level where these segments join, resulting in a system that can create billions of possible TCRα and TCRβ sequences with the potential to recognize any peptide bound to HLA.

These random, "recombinant" T cells are next filtered in the thymus for functionality (positive selection) and removed if cross-reactive with self-antigens (negative selection), resulting in a repertoire of naïve T cells (and regulatory T cells when recognizing self-antigens with low affinity). When the TCR binds a matching peptide presented by HLA, the corresponding T-cell clone will proliferate and participate to the immune response. Thus TCR sequences in adult identical twins are almost as different as in unrelated subjects because TCR diversity is mostly stochastic; T-cell clones grow, depending on infections or other environmental factors encountered across life.

Based on the previously mentioned material, how could polymorphisms in TCR loci affect narcolepsy predisposition? TCR repertoire differences across individuals are indeed mostly stochastic and dependent on past infection history, but polymorphisms within TCR loci slightly modulate TCR repertoire composition, either when there is a coding polymorphism within a V, D, or J segment, or when regulatory sequences surrounding these segments modify the probability of expression of recombination of specific V, D, or J segments with each other.[93] Finally, preferential usage of various segments is partially determined by HLA types, as some HLA molecules preferentially interact with specific TCR sequences, creating positive selection in the thymus.

In the case of NT1, the two TCR polymorphisms associated with the disease have very specific effects. One, located within the TCRA, changes an amino acid L to F in the J24 sequence in an area where the resulting TCRs are predicted to bind the peptide presented by HLA. Because this polymorphism is also associated with other nearby DNA changes, this NT1-associated polymorphism also decreases the occurrence of J24 positive clones (so that the ratio of J24F/L sequences is only about 40% in heterozygotes) and increases the occurrence (also called "usage") of J28 positive clones, probably by modulating expression.[93] In the case of the TCRB-associated polymorphism, the effect is simpler, and the polymorphism simply increases the usage of VB4-2 segments in the repertoire.[93,100] Based on this result, it is strongly suggested that somewhere in the pathophysiology of narcolepsy, T-cell clones that contain J24F rather than L or having J28 in their TCRα sequences, and a TCRVB4-2 in their TCRVβ chain, must be important in triggering narcolepsy. For example, if a TCRα/β containing these sequences recognized an autoantigen presented by DQ0602, it could result in hypocretin cell loss. Of note, only about 0.7% to 0.8% of TCRs contain either of these segments, thus the finding likely reduces the population of potential narcolepsy-causing receptors from several billions to hundreds of thousands per subject.[100] The J24 phenomena is likely essential in understanding how certain TCR clones cause narcolepsy.

HYPOCRETIN/OREXIN DEFICIENCY IN HUMAN NARCOLEPSY

In people, most narcolepsy is sporadic and not fully genetic as in dogs or mice, so it is not surprising that prepro-hypocretin or hypocretin receptor mutations have not been found in human narcolepsy despite extensive genetic screening studies.[37,44,103] Thus far, only one person with a signal peptide mutation of the prepro-hypocretin gene has been identified. This individual had an extremely early onset (6 months), severe narcolepsy-cataplexy, *DQB1*06:02* negativity, and undetectable hypocretin-1 cerebrospinal fluid (CSF) levels.[104] This important observation indicates that hypocretin system gene mutations can cause narcolepsy in humans as in animals, but they appear to be exceedingly rare.

Following the cloning of the canine narcolepsy gene, we and others found that most patients with sporadic, HLA-*DQB1*06:02* positive narcolepsy with cataplexy have undetectable or low (≤110 pg/mL) hypocretin-1 immunoreactivity in CSF.[105-110] Subsequent neuropathologic studies in 10 patients with narcolepsy also indicated dramatic loss of hypocretin-1, hypocretin-2, and prepro-hypocretin mRNA in the brain and hypothalami of patients with narcolepsy (Figure 111.4).[24,44] As mentioned previously, these subjects have no hypocretin gene mutations and the typical peri- or postpubertal disease onset[32] as opposed to a 6-month onset in the subject with a prepro-hypocretin mutation.[44]

CEREBROSPINAL FLUID HYPOCRETIN-1 AS A DIAGNOSTIC TEST FOR NARCOLEPSY

The observation that CSF hypocretin-1 is decreased in NT1 provides a useful diagnostic method (Table 111.1 and Figure 111.5). Quality receiver operating curve (QROC) analysis has shown that a cut-off value of 110 pg/mL (30% of mean control values) was most predictive in patients with cataplexy.[8]

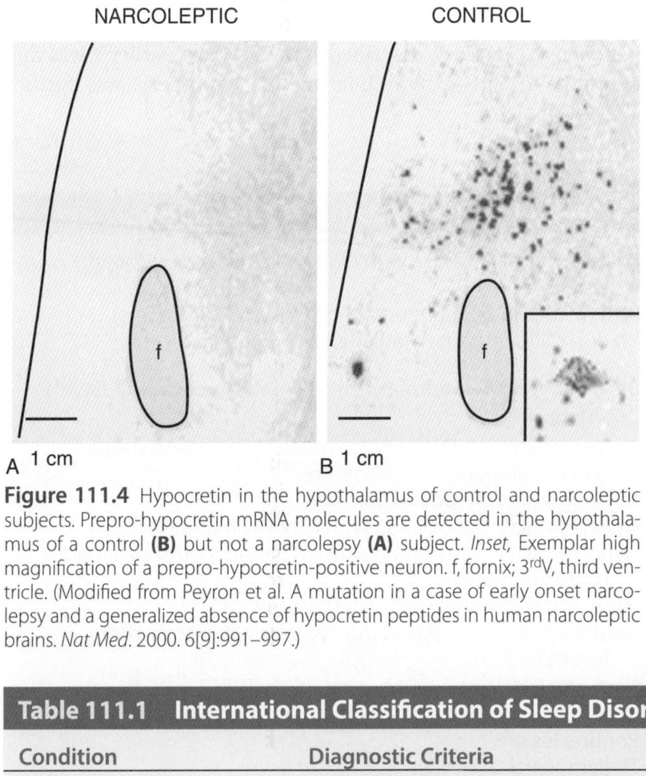

Figure 111.4 Hypocretin in the hypothalamus of control and narcoleptic subjects. Prepro-hypocretin mRNA molecules are detected in the hypothalamus of a control **(B)** but not a narcolepsy **(A)** subject. *Inset,* Exemplar high magnification of a prepro-hypocretin-positive neuron. f, fornix; 3rdV, third ventricle. (Modified from Peyron et al. A mutation in a case of early onset narcolepsy and a generalized absence of hypocretin peptides in human narcoleptic brains. *Nat Med.* 2000. 6[9]:991–997.)

In patients without cataplexy, in QROC analysis a cut-off value of 200 pg/mL is most predictive, highlighting that in a minority of patients with NT2, partial hypocretin deficiency can be present. In addition, some patients with NT2 may later develop cataplexy and even lower hypocretin levels.[25]

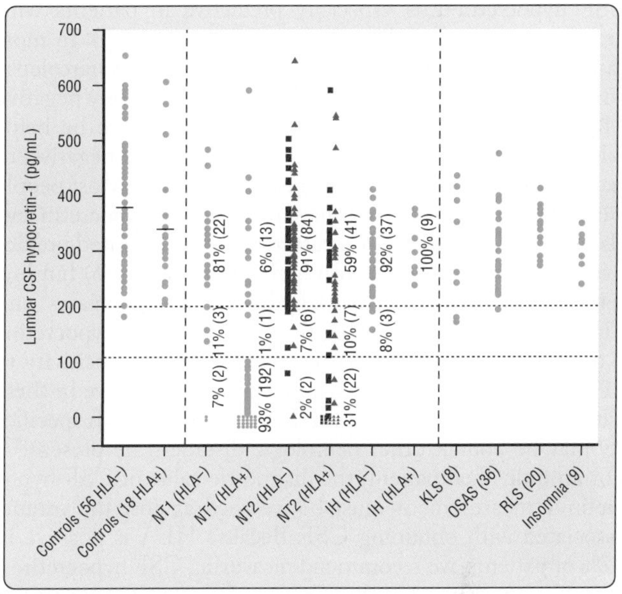

Figure 111.5 Lumbar cerebrospinal fluid (CSF) hypocretin-1 concentrations in controls versus subjects with narcolepsy and other sleep disorders (from the Stanford Center for Narcolepsy Research database). Each point represents the concentration of hypocretin-1 as measured in unextracted lumbar CSF of a single individual. Subjects are differentiated according to HLA DQB1*0602 status and include controls (samples taken during both night and day). Patients are classified as narcolepsy with or without cataplexy, and individuals without cataplexy are subdivided into those with atypical (triangle) and no cataplexy (squares). Clinical subgroups include patients with narcolepsy with cataplexy (NT1) and without cataplexy (NT2), idiopathic hypersomnia (IH), Kleine-Levin syndrome (KLS), obstructive sleep apnea syndrome (OSAS), restless legs syndrome (RLS), and insomnia. Individuals with secondary narcolepsy/hypersomnia are not included. The *dashed lines* indicated hypocretin levels that are low (<110 pg/mL), intermediate (111–200 pg/mL), or normal (>200 pg/mL). Note that these pg/mL values are largely artificial and meant to represent approximately 30% of mean control value as tested in a given center using direct radioimmunoassay and a set of healthy controls.[8] Mean CSF hypocretin-1 concentration was not significantly different between HLA DQB1*0602 positive and negative controls. Low hypocretin levels are noted in 7%, 93%, 2%, and 31% of NT1, HLA-; NT1, HLA+; NT2, HLA-, and NT2, HLA+ patients, respectively. Intermediate hypocretin levels are noted in 11%, 1%, 7%, 10%, and 8% of NT1, HLA-; NT1, HLA+; NT2, HLA-; NT2, HLA+, and IH, HLA- patients, respectively. Normal hypocretin levels are noted in 81%, 6%, 91%, 59%, 92%, and 100% of patients with NT1, HLA-; NT1, HLA+; NT2, HLA-; NT2, HLA+; IH, HLA-, and IH, HLA+ patients, respectively.

Table 111.1 International Classification of Sleep Disorders (ICSD-3): Definitions and Pathophysiology

Condition	Diagnostic Criteria	Pathophysiology
Type 1 narcolepsy	Presence of ≥2 of the following: cataplexy, positive MSLT, and/or low CSF hypocretin-1	Hypocretin deficiency 98% HLA-*DQB1*06:02*
Type 2 narcolepsy	Positive MSLT; most often with no or unclear cataplexy	Unknown, heterogenous ~16% hypocretin deficiency ~40% HLA-DQB1*0602
Secondary narcolepsy	As above, but due to neurologic conditions	With or without hypocretin deficiency; various disorders (Table 111.2)
Idiopathic hypersomnia	No cataplexy, no SOREMPs during the MSLT	Unknown, likely heterogeneous

Positive MSLT: sleep latency ≤8 min and ≥2 SOREMPs, including a nocturnal SOREMP. For details, see International Classification of Sleep Disorders, 2014.[214]
CSF, Cerebrospinal fluid; MSLT, Multiple Sleep Latency Test; SOREMPs, sleep-onset REM sleep periods.

Hypocretin levels are normal in patients with idiopathic hypersomnia, sleep apnea, restless legs syndrome, or insomnia. CSF hypocretin cannot be interpreted in the context of coma or serious neurologic defects (e.g., head trauma), as it can be reversibly low.[111]

With use of the 110 pg/mL cut-off, the measurement of CSF hypocretin-1 is especially predictive in patients with definite cataplexy (100% specificity, 83% sensitivity). In most case series, approximately 8%–12% of patients with narcolepsy with cataplexy or hypocretin deficiency have a falsely negative MSLT. Measuring CSF hypocretin may therefore be helpful in patients with cataplexy when the MSLT is negative, to exclude a possible functional neurologic disorder. Most people with atypical or no cataplexy have normal CSF hypocretin levels, and CSF hypocretin-1 measurements have limited predictive power in this group, with high specificity (99%) but low sensitivity (16%) (see the work by Mignot and associates[8] and Figure 111.5).[8,108,110] Raising the cut-off of CSF hypocretin-1 to 200 pg/mL with HLA positivity increases sensitivity to 41%, suggesting that 200 pg/mL may be informative in these patients in combination with HLA typing, although specificity may be poor if other neurologic disorders are present.[111] For an individual patient, the diagnostic value of CSF hypocretin-1 measurement must be weighed against the trauma associated with obtaining CSF. Because HLA is positive in 97% of patients, we recommend measuring CSF hypocretin-1 only after verifying that the subject is *DQB1*06:02* positive. If the subject is 0602 negative, low hypocretin is very unlikely; only approximately 2% to 3% probability if the subject has cataplexy and probably less if without cataplexy.[95]

Another potential application for CSF hypocretin-1 testing lies in the complex field of narcolepsy and hypersomnia related to neurologic disorders associated with trauma, tumor, infection, degenerative diseases, as well as genetic disorders (Box 111.1). von Economo was the first to suggest that narcolepsy may have its origins in the posterior hypothalamus. In his classic study of encephalitis lethargica, von Economo recognized three categories of patients: a group with hypersomnia and eye movement abnormalities (somnolent-ophthalmoplegic), a group with insomnia and hyperkinetic movement disorder (sometimes with reversal of the sleep cycle), and a group with Parkinsonism ("amyostatic-akinetic," often as a residual form).[112] Neuropathologic studies revealed involvement of the midbrain periaqueductal grey matter and posterior hypothalamus in the hypersomnolent variant (with extension to the oculomotor nuclei, explaining the oculomotor symptoms). Involvement of the anterior hypothalamus with extension into the basal ganglia was observed in the insomnia variant (explaining the frequently co-occurring chorea). This led von Economo to speculate that the anterior hypothalamus contained a sleep-promoting area, while an area spanning from the posterior wall of the third ventricle to the third nerve (encompassing part of the posterior hypothalamus and the periaqueductal midbrain region) was involved in promoting wakefulness. He also speculated that narcolepsy-cataplexy, described some 50 years earlier[18] was due to injury to this general area.[113] This hypothesis was further

BOX 111.1 CLINICAL DISORDERS THAT CAN INCLUDE LOW CEREBROSPINAL FLUID HYPOCRETIN-1[a]

Secondary Hypersomnia with Hypocretin-1 <110 pg/mL

- Acute disseminated encephalomyelitis (ADEM) with sleepiness
- Autosomal dominant cerebellar ataxia, deafness, and narcolepsy (*DNMT1* mutations)
- Large pituitary adenoma with probable hypothalamic involvement
- Late-onset hypoventilation syndrome, probably rapid-onset obesity with hypothalamic dysfunction, hypoventilation, and autonomic dysregulation (ROHHAD)
- Multiple sclerosis patients with bilateral hypothalamic plaques
- Paraneoplastic syndrome (seminoma) with anti Ma2 and sleepiness, cataplexy
- Hypothalamic tumors and surgery postremoval of such tumors
- Prader-Willi syndrome (15q11-q13)
- Steroid-responsive encephalopathy associated with autoimmune thyroiditis
- Whipple disease with central nervous system involvement (with hypersomnia)[b]
- Postdiencephalic stroke with hypothalamic and midbrain lesions
- Post head trauma (but unclear if mediating symptoms)
- Prader-Willi syndrome (15q11-q13)

Secondary Hypersomnia with Intermediate Hypocretin-1 Levels (110–200 pg/mL)

- Autosomal dominant cerebellar ataxia, deafness, and narcolepsy (*DNMT1* mutations)
- Moebius syndrome
- Niemann-Pick type C with cataplexy (*NPC1* mutations)
- Norrie syndrome (deletion of *MAO* genes on the X chromosome)

Secondary Hypersomnia with Normal Hypocretin-1 Levels (>200 pg/mL)

- Acute disseminated encephalomyelitis (ADEM) with sleepiness
- HIV encephalopathy with sleepiness
- Hypersomnia with depression
- Hypersomnia in association with Parkinson disease
- Hypersomnia in association with myotonic dystrophy type 1 (*DM1* mutations)
- Myotonic dystrophy type 1 (*DM1* mutations)
- Neurocysticercosis cysts in the hypothalamus and other locations
- Niemann Pick type C without cataplexy (*NPC1* mutations)
- Narcolepsy-cataplexy posthypothalamic irradiation
- Pontine lesions
- Thalamocortical strokes

Other Pathologies with Intermediate or Low Levels (No Reported but Possible Sleep Symptoms)[c]

- Traumatic brain injury (probably transient)
- Encephalitis of infectious origin
- Guillain-Barré syndrome and other inflammatory neuropathies
- Coma caused by infection or trauma

[a]Patients tested at Stanford University or in centers that used the same standard CSF samples for comparisons are included; measurements in other laboratories cannot be compared.
[b]In another patient with Whipple disease with long-lasting resistant insomnia without hypersomnia, intermediate CSF hypocretin levels were found.
[c]These may reflect nonspecific effects, or be indirectly affecting the hypothalamus, with potentially reversible changes in CSF hypocretin-1.

refined by others who noted that tumors or lesions located close to the third ventricle were also associated with secondary narcolepsy.[114,115] A postulated hypothalamic cause of narcolepsy was widespread until the 1940s but was subsequently ignored during the psychoanalytic boom, to be replaced by a brainstem hypothesis.[116]

Narcolepsy can be caused by a variety of lesions near the third ventricle (hypothalamus and upper midbrain).[113,115,117-119] In addition to encephalitis, narcolepsy-like symptoms have been reported after traumatic brain injury, acute disseminated encephalomyelitis, hypothalamic sarcoidosis or histiocytosis X, and in association with multiple sclerosis (MS) and Parkinson disease (PD).[111,120,121] In some patients, lesions of the hypothalamic region containing the hypocretin neurons have been clearly identified using magnetic resonance imaging (MRI), as in MS or anti-aquaporin-4 lesions in the hypothalamus, and tumors of the third ventricle.[111,120,121] Cataplexy may be present in these individuals, and CSF hypocretin-1 levels may be either in the narcolepsy range (<110 pg/mL) or in the intermediate range[8,111] (Table 111.2). Similarly, postmortem studies have shown a 30% and 50% decrease in hypocretin cell counts in end-stage Huntington disease and PD,[111] respectively, with maintenance of normal CSF hypocretin-1 levels.[8] Such intermediate or normal levels may reflect damage to nearby hypocretin projection sites, with sufficient preservation of cell bodies to maintain detectable levels of hypocretin-1. In addition, injury to other types of wake-promoting neurons in the upper midbrain and hypothalamus may also contribute to the symptomatology, especially sleepiness and increased sleep time, as initially proposed by von Economo.[113]

Autoimmune diseases frequently co-occur. Unfortunately, although rare cases of NT1 co-existing with multiple sclerosis, lupus, or other common autoimmune conditions have been reported, there is no consistent pattern of co-occurring autoimmune conditions in patients or family members. Rather, the possibility that narcolepsy is an autoimmune disease is supported by the rare existence of autoimmune narcolepsy with documented low CSF hypocretin-1 as part of two other autoimmune diseases. The first is a rare paraneoplastic syndrome associated with anti-Ma2 antibodies in the context of seminomas.[122,123] Interestingly, in one case, a $CD8^+$ T-cell infiltration largely restricted to the hypothalamus and with an almost complete loss of hypocretin neurons was observed.[124] Similarly, in one case of late-onset hypoventilation syndrome, a disorder with reported hypothalamic abnormalities,[125] very low CSF hypocretin-1 levels were found in an individual with otherwise unexplained sleepiness and cataplexy-like episodes.[8] More recently, this disorder has been renamed rapid-onset obesity with hypothalamic dysfunction, hypoventilation, and autonomic dysregulation and has been suggested to be autoimmune based on the finding of extensive infiltrates of lymphocytes and histiocytes in the hypothalamus of some patients.[126,127]

Therefore, as illustrated previously, CSF hypocretin-1 levels can be helpful in complex clinical situations in which the history, polysomnogram, and/or MSLT data are difficult to interpret (Table 111.2). However, hypocretin values should be cautiously interpreted, as in a large series of individuals with various neurologic disorders, we found that up to 15% had CSF hypocretin-1 values within the intermediate range; most of these patients had severe brain pathology, most notably head trauma, encephalitis, and subarachnoid hemorrhage.[106,111] Decreased hypocretin-1 levels in these patients may reflect damage to hypocretin neurons, changes

Table 111.2 Cerebrospinal Fluid Hypocretin-1 and Human Leukocyte Antigen Results: Selected Examples in Secondary Narcolepsy and Hypersomnias

Clinical case	CSF Hypocretin-1	Notes
8-year-old boy without cataplexy (onset within 6 months)	88 pg/mL HLA+, MSLT+	Type 1 narcolepsy, treatment with modafinil, later developed cataplexy and treated with venlafaxine
17-year-old boy with rape hallucinations, suspicious and difficult to interview, possible cataplexy	Undetectable (<40 pg/mL) HLA+, refused venlafaxine MSLT	Type 1 narcolepsy, associated with psychosis, positive effect of venlafaxine testing
16-year-old woman with a 5-year history of depression and drug resistant insomnia; cataplexy on interview	Undetectable (<40 pg/mL) HLA+, MSLT not interpretable	Type 1 narcolepsy, now successfully treated with sodium oxybate, modafinil, and atomoxetine
32-year-old man, postresection of hypothalamic craniopharyngioma, very impaired, possible cataplexy	152 pg/mL HLA-, MSLT impossible	Secondary narcolepsy; possibly lesions of other areas; partial effect of stimulants
33-year-old woman successfully treated with D-amphetamine and fluoxetine, no cataplexy	Undetectable (<40 pg/mL) HLA+No MSLT	Type 1 narcolepsy No change in treatment but considering modafinil
15-year-old woman with sleepiness, no cataplexy	310 pg/mL HLA+, MSLT+	Type 2 narcolepsy Treatment with modafinil
A 67-year-old man diagnosed with undetectable narcolepsy without cataplexy at age 50, currently with falls not typically triggered, AHI = 25 events/hour, non-CPAP compliant	Undetectable (<40 pg/mL) HLA+	Type 1 narcolepsy First tried on venlafaxine without effect, then with sodium oxybate with very positive response

HLA+, HLA-*DQB1*06:02* positive; MSLT+, MSL <8 minutes, ≥2 SOREMPs, including a nocturnal SOREMP.

in CSF flow or in protease levels affecting peptide degradation, or binding to CSF proteins, as recently suggested by one study.[127a] Other authors have shown that CSF hypocretin-1 increases with locomotor activity in animals and decreases with serotonin reuptake inhibitors (but never to near-undetectable, narcolepsy-like levels).[128] Finding hypocretin-1 levels in the intermediate range should therefore alert the clinician to the possibility of underlying brain pathology, which may require additional clinical evaluation, laboratory testing, or imaging. Whether genuine hypocretin deficiency explains abnormal sleep in these neurologic disorders requires further investigation.[111]

HYPOCRETIN INVOLVEMENT IN GENERATING NARCOLEPSY SYMPTOMS

Since the discovery of the hypocretins/orexins, much has been learned about how they regulate sleep. Central (intracerebroventricular or local injections) but not peripheral administration of hypocretin-1 stimulates wakefulness and reduces REM sleep. Hypocretin antagonists promote NREM and REM sleep in animals and humans,[129,130] whereas the opposite is true of newly described hypocretin agonists.[131] In rats and monkeys, cisternal CSF hypocretin-1 fluctuates, with maximal levels at the end of the active period (night in rodents) and minimum levels at the end of the inactive period (amplitude is about 40% of the maximum).[132-134] Using in vivo dialysis, a similar profile is observed in the rat brain extracellular fluid.[132] In diurnal, wake-consolidated squirrel monkeys, hypocretin-1 levels in CSF collected from the cisterna magna peak in the late evening, around their bedtime with a diurnal amplitude about 40%.[134] These results suggest that hypocretin may help promote wakefulness in the evening in primates. In this model, hypocretin would oppose the sleep pressure that has accumulated since early morning, allowing a constant level of wakefulness through the day.[134] Additional studies suggest that diurnal fluctuations in hypocretin release are driven both directly by the circadian clock and indirectly by the increased sleep pressure.[72] The circadian role may explain why a polymorphism located within the HCRTR2 region has been associated with morningness-eveningness,[135] and as hypocretin levels remain high during sleep deprivation, a role in resisting sleep pressure is likely, explaining the need to nap every few hours in narcolepsy. However, it is still unclear how hypocretin release/activity fluctuates across the various sleep stages (REM versus NREM sleep), although single cell activity suggests reduced activity during NREM and REM sleep. Of note, CSF is usually collected from the lumbar space in humans, and it shows only a 10% diurnal fluctuation in hypocretin levels with lowest levels in the morning, suggesting a dampening and delay of changes when reaching the lumbar sac.[128] Because measurement of hypocretin in lumbar CSF has such poor temporal resolution, the time of CSF collection has no significant effect for narcolepsy diagnostic purposes.[8,136]

The densest reported hypocretin projections are to the monoaminergic cell groups of the locus coeruleus (which makes norepinephrine), substantia nigra/ventral tegmental area (which makes DA), raphe magnus (which makes serotonin), and tuberomammillary neurons (which make histamine). DA and histamine cell groups have a very high hypocretin receptor-2 density[137] and may be especially important.[37,138-140] An increased DA level in the amygdala is one of the most consistent neurochemical abnormalities reported in canine narcolepsy,[53,57] and GABAergic neurons in this area are likely important for triggering cataplexy.[141] Decreased histamine levels are also observed in the brain of narcoleptic canines,[142] although in humans, increased numbers of histidine decarboxylase–positive cells have been reported,[55,56] with possibly decreased histamine levels in CSF.[143-145] In vivo dialysis studies have indicated a critical role for the DA mesolimbic and mesocortical system in the regulation of alertness and the triggering of cataplexy by emotions. Histaminergic transmission has long been recognized as a critical wake-promoting neurotransmitter.[146] DA and histaminergic projections may thus be centrally involved in controlling both cataplexy and alertness.[61] Similar to REM sleep, cataplexy is probably controlled by pontine cholinergic REM-on cells and aminergic locus coeruleus REM-off cells.[39] Loss of excitatory hypocretin projections to monoamine cell groups could decrease monoaminergic tone and produce a cholinergic-aminergic imbalance, resulting in the sleepiness and abnormal REM sleep of narcolepsy. Hypocretin projections to the basal forebrain area, an area with cholinergic hypersensitivity in narcoleptic animals, are also likely to be involved.[39] It is also likely that hypocretin helps integrate sleep regulation with metabolic status, although the importance of this effect could be species dependent. Recent models of sleep wake regulation integrate the hypocretin/orexin system within a complex network of sleep and wake-promoting neurons,[147-149] although in most likelihood, many additional unknown systems are yet to be discovered.

ROLE OF INFLUENZA AND OTHER UPPER AIRWAY INFECTIONS IN TRIGGERING TYPE 1 NARCOLEPSY

Upper airway infections such as influenza and maybe *Streptococcus pyogenes* may trigger the development of narcolepsy, at least in children. Starting in the 2000s, increased recognition of narcolepsy in younger children led to the realization that the disorder often followed strep throat, and that close to narcolepsy onset, subjects often had elevated titers of antistreptolysin-O, a marker of recent infection with *S. pyogenes*.[150] Epidemiologic studies also indicated a link,[13] but because *S. pyogenes* often coinfects viral upper airway pathology, this could be secondary to the influenza effect. Han and colleagues, studying onset in more than 1000 patients, found strong annual fluctuations of onset of narcolepsy in children, with onsets six times more frequent in spring and summer than in winter (Figure 111.6), suggesting that winter infections trigger a process that, over months, results in hypocretin cell loss.[10]

In the spring of 2010 a number of events converged to indicate that the 2009 H1N1 pandemic influenza triggered narcolepsy in young children (Figure 111.6). To review the background: in the spring of 2009, a new strain of influenza A (H1N1) of likely swine origin appeared in Mexico, spreading rapidly in humans, and affecting young adults with a high reported case fatality rate of 0.4%.[151] This caused alarm, as with such a high mortality rates, millions of deaths were possible worldwide when the new virus hit the world population the following winter. Faced with such a threat, the World Health Organization (WHO) and other organizations encouraged vaccine makers to initiate large-scale production of vaccines targeting the new strain, which had not been included in the 2009–2010 regular trivalent seasonal flu vaccine.[152] To generate these vaccines, almost all manufacturers

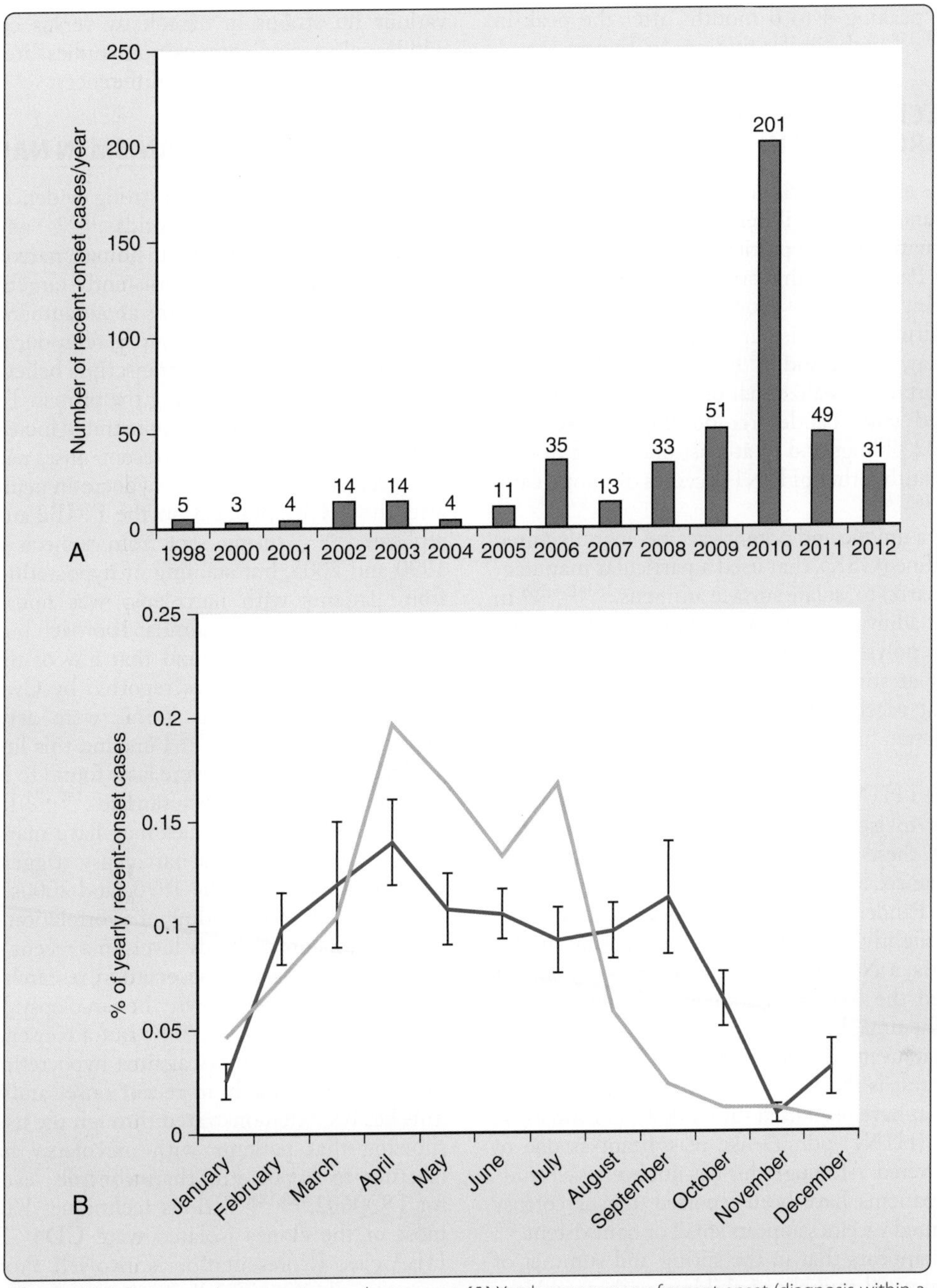

Figure 111.6 Temporal patterns in narcolepsy onset. **(A)** Yearly occurrence of recent onset (diagnosis within a year of onset) showing a dramatic increase in 2010, following the H1N1 pandemic of 2009, with return to baseline condition the following years. **(B)** Seasonal pattern of onset of narcolepsy in Chinese patients showing highly increased risk in spring and summer versus early winter. Data are represented as a yearly fraction of 12 months, that 0.083 (8.3%) would be the expected value of each month if onsets were randomly distributed across the year. The *blue line* represents the mean ±SEM of this yearly fraction for years 2002 to 2009, with very low levels of new onset in late winter. The *red line* represents the numbers for 2010, following the 2009 pH1N1 pandemic, and shows a more pronounced circannual pattern peaking in spring and summer. (**A** modified from Han F et al. Decreased incidence of childhood narcolepsy 2 years after the 2009 H1N1 winter flu pandemic. *Ann Neurol.* 2013;73[4]:560; Han F et al. Narcolepsy onset is seasonal and increased following the 2009 H1N1 pandemic in China. *Ann Neurol.* 2011:70[3]:410–17.)

used a A/California/7/2009 (H1N1)-pdm09–like reassortant virus containing hemagglutinin type 1, neuraminidase type 1 (thus H1N1), and polymerase basic 1 proteins from A/California/7/2009, on a backbone H1N1 virus PR8, derived from an older, A/Puerto Rico/8/1934, H1N1 virus.[153-155]

As predicted, pandemic 2009 H1N1 spread rapidly and became the dominant influenza strain the following winter. Fortunately, mortality was not as high as anticipated, ranging closer to that of a regular seasonal flu.[156] However, in the spring of 2010, we noted that a much higher number of children with recent narcolepsy onset were referred to Stanford when compared with prior years.[157] Further, in China, the number of children with new-onset narcolepsy was increased 3- to 5-fold over prior years in the spring and summer of 2010

(Figure 111.3, *B*), peaking 4 to 6 months after the peak in H1N1 infections,[10,158] with similar findings in Taiwan.[159]

H1N1 2009 VACCINATION WITH PANDEMRIX TRIGGERED NARCOLEPSY IN EUROPE

In parallel with this and most strikingly, in both Finland[160,161] and Sweden,[162] hundreds of children developed NT1 a few months after vaccination with a particular pH1N1 flu vaccine formulation called Pandemrix; this brand of vaccine increased the risk of developing narcolepsy about 10-fold in children.[157] Other studies confirmed that this particular vaccine had similar effects in Norway,[163] England,[164] France,[165] and Ireland,[15] although it is important to realize that only about 1 in 15,000 children vaccinated with Pandemrix developed narcolepsy (including DQ0602 siblings and in at least one case a discordant twin). Importantly, other pH1N1 vaccines did not clearly trigger narcolepsy.[166,167]

Pandemrix was a unique and potent vaccine, manufactured by Glaxo Smith Kline (GSK), that used a particular manufacturing process (Fluarix) to isolate surface antigens.[153-155,168] In addition, a specific adjuvant, AS03A, a mix of squalene, DL-α-tocopherol, and polysorbate 80, was added. This AS03A adjuvant is potent at stimulating CD4+ T-cell responses,[169] and it is clear that vaccine efficacy was high; one injection was sufficient to obtain high coverage as measured by the HA antibody assays.[153-155]

Other adjuvanted H1N1 vaccines were manufactured using different protocols to isolate surface antigens and/or different adjuvants, but these did not clearly increase narcolepsy risk.[166,167,170] Arepanrix, a vaccine also produced by GSK, was almost identical to Pandemrix, except that it was made at a different site using a slightly different process for isolating surface antigens.[154] Focetria, a Novartis vaccine, also relatively similar to Pandemrix, used the MF59 adjuvant containing squalene only, and a purer hemmaglutinin preparation.[153,154,168] In the United States, nonadjuvanted or live attenuated H1N1 vaccines were used. Of interest is the fact all seasonal trivalent split or subunit vaccines that have been used since 2009 still contain A/California/7/2009 (H1N1)-pdm09-like reassortant as one of the three strains covered. Although this has not been well studied and sporadic patients have been reported, the narcolepsy risk for nonadjuvanted vaccines appears small or nonexistent.[171]

In summary, it appears that in the spring and summer of 2010, a larger than usual number of children with narcolepsy were observed in China and probably in other countries (Germany, Taiwan, and the United States) independent of any vaccination.[10,158,159] In addition, narcolepsy in children also occurred in reaction to Pandemrix, although overall risk was small (1 in 16,000 vaccinees). The effects of other pH1N1 vaccines were either milder or nonexistent.[166,167] Antigens common to the wild type virus and Pandemrix may have been involved.[154] Why Pandemrix but not other vaccines triggered narcolepsy is unknown, but it may be related to the way these vaccines were produced,[154] geographic factors (genetics and prior infections), and different flu vaccines.[166] Pandemrix was used in Europe coincident with the pandemic flu infection itself, and this may have increased the risk of developing narcolepsy if subjects were vaccinated while they were infected, especially young children exposed to their first flu (most children get their first flu infections before 7 years of life).[166] Further studies aiming at studying prior immune history to various flu strains in narcolepsy versus controls, as well as additional vaccine composition studies, are needed to pursue our understanding of these differences.

AUTOIMMUNE MECHANISM IN NARCOLEPSY

Researchers have not found strong evidence of autoantibodies targeting the hypocretin peptides,[172-175] and immunostaining of hypothalamic tissue with human narcolepsy sera has not revealed autoantibodies consistently targeting the hypocretin neurons.[176-178] Several claims about autoantibodies have been made, but these have been hard to reproduce. Cvetkovic-Lopes and colleagues[179] isolated transcripts believed to be increased in hypocretin cells, including the protein Tribbles homologue 2 (TRIB2). The authors demonstrated increased Trib2 autoantibodies in individuals with recent-onset narcolepsy, and some cross-reactivity of sera with hypocretin neurons.[176-178] Shortly after the TRIB2 publication, the TRIB2 antibody finding was replicated[180,181] using sera from subjects collected between 1990 and 2005, but staining of hypocretin neurons with sera from patients with narcolepsy was not observed.[176-178,182] Further studies using a similar approach but another mRNA-binding protein also found that few of the genes expressed in hypocretin neurons as reported by Cvetkovic-Lopes and colleagues,[179] including *Trib2*, were actually enriched in hypocretin neurons.[183-185] Pursuing this line of investigation, TRIB2 autoantibodies were later found to be generally absent in more recent narcolepsy samples.[157,175] It is our hypothesis that TRIB2 autoantibodies may have marked a co-infection present together with a narcolepsy trigger in some patients with disease onset in the 1990s and 2000s. This hypothesis is substantiated by the finding of a correlation between A/H1N1 and TRIB2 autoantibody levels in a recent study.[130]

Because of the TCR association, research has moved toward seeking T-cell autoreactivity in narcolepsy. Initial experiments were generally negative,[186,187] but a consensus is now emerging that T-cell reactivity against hypocretin itself is increased in narcolepsy, notably in recent onset and young subjects.[188] This has been demonstrated through the use of cellular assays, showing that patients with narcolepsy have more T cells reacting to hypocretin than controls, even when matched for DQ0602.[188,189] Various techniques have been used, and most of the clones isolated were CD4+ T cells, suggesting HLA class II presentation is involved. Problematically, however, overall CD4+ T-cell reactivity to hypocretin fragments is immune dominated by HLA-DR presentation of hypocretin fragments,[189] not HLA-DQ, and thus does not really explain why NT1 is associated with HLA DQ. In one study, reactivity was found only in children but not in adults.[186]

In light of this limitation, Luo and colleagues[190] and Jiang and colleagues[191] took a different approach, focusing on HLA-DQ0602–restricted T-cell reactivity, a minor portion of overall T-cell reactivity to all hypocretin fragment presented by all HLA alleles. As early as 2005, my colleagues and I noticed that the C terminal portion of hypocretin peptides and pH1N1 $pHA_{275-287}$, sequences that both bind to DQ0602, were homologous, suggesting that molecular mimicry of T cells with these epitopes could explain why NT1 was triggered by H1N1.[190] In 2018 Luo and colleagues screened all potential DQ0602 binders located within key flu proteins abundant in the virus and Pandemrix for T-cell reactivity when presented by DQ0602 in patients and controls after vaccination with Pandemrix and found increased reactivity to $pHA_{275-287}$ in comparison with other H1N1 epitopes.[190] Furthering this observation, we also found increased T-cell reactivity in narcolepsy to the C terminal portion of hypocretin peptides ($HCRT_{56-68}$ and $HCRT_{87-99}$), but only when the carboxy terminal of this antigen was amidated (denoted as $HCRT_{NH2}$ for simplification) as naturally occurs with the secreted hypocretin-1 and -2 peptides.[190]

Further revealing was the fact that some clones recognizing both $HCRT_{NH2}$ and $pHA_{275-287}$ used VB4-2 and that clones recognizing $HCRT_{NH2}$ used TRAJ24 (TCR segments modulated by TCR polymorphisms associated with narcolepsy), suggesting that these T-cell clones may be involved in molecular mimicry and autoimmunity.[190] Slightly different findings were reported by Jiang and colleagues,[191] who found J24 recognition of the same HCRT sequence, although not the deamidated segment. These results suggest that narcolepsy may be the result of excessive reaction to $pHA_{275-287}$, which, when presented by DQ0602, may in some cases cross-react with the $HCRT_{NH2}$ autoantigen. This response may then recruit additional $CD4^+$ T cells recognizing other fragments of HCRT in the context of HLA DR and other HLA class II antigens (epitope spreading),[189] eventually involving $CD8^+$ T cells recognizing other hypocretin cell–containing proteins and leading to HCRT cell loss ($CD8^+$ T cells are known to more frequently target intracellular antigens). In line with this hypothesis, higher numbers of $CD8^+$ T cells reactive to intracellular HCRT cell-enriched transcription factors such as Lhx3 and Rfx4 have been reported in DQ0602-positive patients versus controls.[192] Such a model involving CD4 helper T cells and CD8-mediated T cell killing of hypocretin neurons has been artificially created in an animal model expressing a neoantigen in HCRT cells, showing this mechanism can kill HCRT neurons. CD8 involvement is also suggested by the fact a perforin hypomorph polymorphism is genetically protective of narcolepsy.[9] Figure 111.7 summarizes the likely autoimmune process involved in narcolepsy, with the hypothesis that both $CD4^+$ and $CD8^+$ T cells are involved.

NARCOLEPSY AND NARCOLEPSY-LIKE SYMPTOMS IN GENETIC SYNDROMES

Narcolepsy-like symptoms, including daytime sleepiness, SOREMPs, and/or cataplexy-like symptoms have been

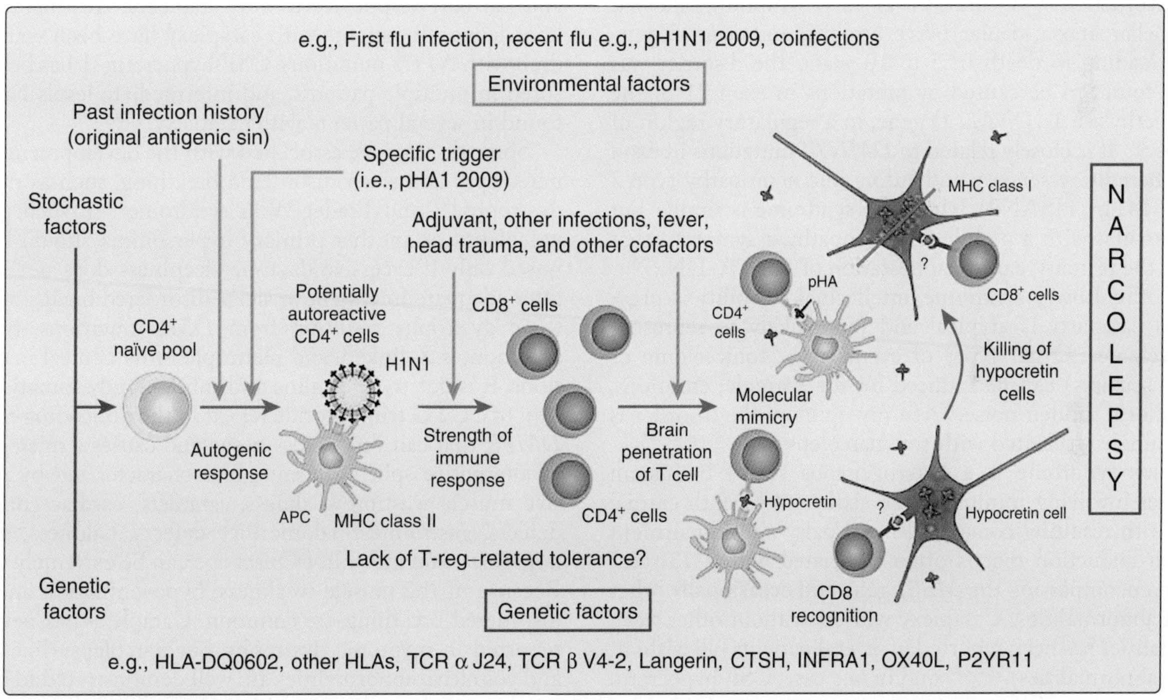

Figure 111.7 Hypothetical pathophysiologic model for autoimmune narcolepsy. Narcolepsy is likely an autoimmune disease involving specific subpopulations of $CD4^+$ and $CD8^+$ T cells and may have little if any B-cell, autoantibody involvement. The development of narcolepsy probably results from many unlikely events. First, DQ0602 must almost always be present, and genetic background at other loci also influences predisposition. $CD4^+$ T cells bearing specific receptors are generated stochastically, although with influence of T-cell receptor loci polymorphisms, and autoreactive cells are removed by the thymus, while others are released as naïve T cells. We hypothesize that only a subset of the population may have naïve T cells with the potential to become pathogenic and narcolepsy-inducing, most likely cells reacting to $HCRT_{NH2}$ when presented by DQ0602. In many patients, these cells may become anergic or will be moved into a regulatory T cell compartment that rather inhibits autoimmunity, although escape from negative selection is favored by the fact the thymus does not typically present posttranslationally modified antigens such as secreted C-amidated HCRT. In some unlucky individuals, an immune reaction to an external infection such as 2009 H1N1 may engage these cross-reactive naïve T cells through cross-reactivity with sequences resembling $HCRT_{NH2}$ such as hemagglutinin $pHA_{275-287}$. This may be more likely to occur in younger individuals with a particular history of infections (or lack of). Indeed, in many subjects, such infection would first stimulate memory $CD4^+$ T cells that recognize shared epitopes and are not pathogenic. Other factors that may participate in tilting the balance toward developing narcolepsy could be the strength of the immune response (co-infection, adjuvant), a leaky blood-brain barrier, and so on. Following engagement of $CD4^+$ T cells, $CD8^+$ T cells are also likely to be involved and may be important in mediating the actual hypocretin cell killing.

reported in a variety of genetic disorders, including autosomal dominant cerebellar ataxia, deafness, and narcolepsy (*ADCA-DN, MIM 604121, DNMT1* mutations), Coffin-Lowry syndrome (*MIM 303600, RSK2* mutations),[193] Moebius syndrome (*MIM 157900,* heterogeneous),[194-196] myotonic dystrophy (*MIM 160900* and *602668, MD1* and *2* mutations),[197] Niemann-Pick Type C1 (*MIM 257219, NPC1*),[8,198-200] Norrie disease (*MIM 310600, Xp11.4-p11.23* deletions encompassing the *NDP* and in patients with cataplexy, the *MAO* genes),[194,201,202] and Prader-Willi syndrome (*MIM 176270,* most often the result of 15q11.2 deletions encompassing the paternal copies of the imprinted *SNRPN* and *NDN* genes).[8,194] DQ0602 is not associated with these disorders. We have explored CSF hypocretin-1 levels in such pathologies and have found that most have normal or intermediate CSF hypocretin-1 levels (>110 pg/mL).[8] These special etiologies are described in the following sections.

Autosomal dominant cerebellar ataxia, deafness, and narcolepsy (ADCA-DN) is a late-onset neurodegenerative disorder (age 30 to 40 years) with ataxia, deafness, and narcolepsy-cataplexy with intermediate to low CSF hypocretin-1.[203] Narcolepsy is an early manifestation, and at this stage, CSF hypocretin-1 may be normal, dropping only in the late stage of the disorder.[203-205] Deafness is an early symptom, followed by cerebellar ataxia, ocular nerve atrophy, and neurodegeneration, leading to death in 5 to 10 years. The disorder was recently found to be caused by mutations in exon 21 of the DNA methylase 1 (*DNMT1*) gene, in a regulatory region of the gene.[205] It is closely related to *DMNT1* mutations in exon 20 and hereditary sensory and autonomic neuropathy type 2 (MIM 614116, HSAN2), where the syndrome is similar but manifests first with a peripheral neuropathy, a symptom that is rarely the primary, early manifestation of ADCA-DN.[204]

In Coffin-Lowry syndrome, intellectual disability is present, and cataplexy is atypical and more likely to represent atonic seizures. Other types of events (e.g., tonic-clonic or absence seizures) can be induced by, for example, emotions, surprise, or a sudden noise.[193] In my opinion, the disorder is not genuinely associated with true narcolepsy.

Mobius syndrome is a heterogeneous set of brainstem anomalies involving minimally the sixth and seventh cranial nerves with resulting congenital facial palsy and impairment of ocular abduction that is often associated with a 13q12.2 deletion encompassing the *MBS1* gene and occasionally other skeletal abnormalities. Cataplexy with or without other sleep abnormalities has been reported in several patients (all without skeletal abnormalities),[194,196] and in one case, CSF hypocretin was intermediate.[195] One case was responsive to antidepressant. In these patients, brainstem impairment affecting REM sleep–regulating centers of the pons is likely causal. The condition can be complicated by the existence of sleep-disordered breathing.

In its typical manifestation, Norrie disease is an X-linked recessive disorder characterized by very early childhood blindness resulting from degenerative and proliferative changes of retinal neurons, and frequently hearing deficits and neuropsychiatric symptoms.[206] Many cases are secondary to an Xp11.3-p11.4 deletion that encompasses the *NRD* gene. As mutations of *NRD* also cause Norrie disease with its ocular manifestations, the syndrome is causal to this gene. Patients with cataplexy have been described in various microdeletion syndromes but not in individuals with isolated *NDP* mutations.[194,201,202] Further, families or cases with deletions encompassing both monoamine oxidase genes and that did not affect the *NDP* gene show severe developmental delay, intermittent hypotonia, and stereotypical hand movements.[207,208] I saw one patient with cataplexy, intellectual disability but without ocular symptoms, and a deletion limited to the *MAO* genes, suggesting these monoaminergic genes are indeed crucial to this manifestation. This observation may be of interest, considering that optogenetic stimulation of the noradrenergic locus coeruleus can produce arousal followed by behavioral arrests,[209] and cataplexy is exacerbated by prazosin.[39]

Niemann-Pick type C is a lysosomal storage disease associated with mutations in *NPC1* and *NPC2* genes and abnormal cholesterol metabolism. Onset is usually before age 10 (with death before age 20), but the disease can manifest at much later age. Niemann-Pick type C has a wide clinical spectrum that may include hepatosplenomegaly and a wide range of neurologic abnormalities (e.g., cerebellar ataxia, tremor, seizures, dysphagia, dysarthria, hypotonia, dystonia, psychosis, dementia, and other psychiatric symptoms). Vertical gaze palsy with involvement of the third cranial nerve is often an early and typical feature. This condition is remarkable as cataplexy can be clear, triggered by typical emotions (laughing),[198] and partially responsive to anticataplectic treatment. To my knowledge, all patients with cataplexy have been young children with *NPC1* mutations. CSF hypocretin-1 has been measured in multiple patients, and intermediate levels have been found in several patients with cataplexy.[8,200]

Some diseases are associated with the development of both narcolepsy and sleep-disordered breathing, such as myotonic dystrophy[197] and Prader-Willi syndrome[8]; in such patients, narcolepsy or another primary hypersomnia should be diagnosed only if excessive daytime sleepiness does not improve after adequate treatment of sleep-disordered breathing. Myotonic dystrophy resulting from *DM1* mutations, the most common, is X-linked, and pleitropic in its clinical manifestations. It is due to a germline and subsequently somatic expansion of a CTG trinucleotide repeat in the noncoding region of *DMPK* that can vary across tissue and causes a misregulation of alternative splicing events. It is characterized by progressive muscle wasting/weakness, cataracts, cardiac conduction defects, gastrointestinal motility defects, baldness, endocrinopathies, and infertility. Onset age can be extremely variable. Because of the muscle weakness, hypoventilation and sleep-disordered breathing are common. Cataplexy has never been reported in myotonic dystrophy, but narcolepsy-like MSLTs and cognitive abnormalities are well demonstrated to be independent of sleep-disordered breathing.[210] CSF hypocretin is generally normal or slightly decreased.[211]

Prader-Willi syndrome is caused by a loss of function of genes in the 15q11.2 region, with likely involvement of the small nuclear ribonucleoprotein polypeptide N (*SNRPN*) and necdin (*NDN*) genes leading to a complex cascade of genetic dysregulations. Most patients (70%) have a deletion of paternal origin (in this case a loss of function occurs when the maternal copy is imprinted), and in most of the other patients, it is due to maternal uniparental disomy (inheritance of two inactivated maternal copies). It is characterized by a typical facial appearance, intellectual disability, hypotonia, hyperphagia, and many other symptoms. Because of obesity and hypotonia, hypoventilation plus sleep-disordered breathing is a complication that can contribute to sleepiness, although

SOREMPs are common on the MSLT, and CNS effects are almost surely involved.[212] Prader-Willi syndrome is interesting because patients rarely can have typical cataplexy triggered by laughing. In one patient with a 15q deletion I saw, obesity was not a striking feature thanks to food restriction, and cataplexy was improved by the adrenergic reuptake inhibitor atomoxetine, although at a higher dose it exacerbated absence seizures also observed in this patient. CSF hypocretin is generally intermediate.[213]

In conclusion, a few genetic disorders are associated with REM sleep abnormalities and cataplexy-like features. It is likely that the study of the downstream mechanisms involved could shed light on REM sleep regulation and type 2 narcolepsy.

NARCOLEPSY TYPE 1 VERSUS TYPE 2 NARCOLEPSY AND IDIOPATHIC HYPERSOMNIA

Confounding the issue of what narcolepsy is has been a broadening of the definition of narcolepsy in clinical practice. Indeed, a new definition of the disease slowly emerged that includes patients with sleepiness and abnormal REM sleep, SOREMPs during the MSLT, sleep paralysis, or hypnagogic hallucinations ("narcolepsy without cataplexy"). These patients were diagnosed with narcolepsy without cataplexy ("type 2"; NT2) (Table 111.1),[214] and they generally have normal CSF hypocretin and only a slightly elevated frequency (40%) of HLA DQB106:02, suggesting a different etiology in most patients. Little has been written on the neuropathology of NT2, but hypocretin neurons were very decreased in one subject[24] with modest, if any, loss in two other patients.[215]

Although initially the number of patients with NT2 were low (representing 10% to 15% of cases in older cohorts), it has now increased to the point that most sleep centers are diagnosing NT2 more frequently than NT1 based on a single MSLT. Problematically, however, considering the prevalence of NT1 (0.02% to 0.1%) and the rate of false positivity of the MSLT (≈3%),[26,216] conducting MSLTs in a large number of subjects complaining of sleepiness (>4% of the population) will result in false-positive diagnoses. Illustrating this, four recent studies found that positive MSLTs in subjects with NT2 are repeatable in only 10% to 40% of patients,[217-220] suggesting that, in many, the diagnosis of NT2 is falsely positive. Positive MSLTs are also more frequent in the context of circadian abnormalities such as shift work, or chronic sleep restriction.[26] As it is hard to clinically distinguish NT2 from idiopathic hypersomnia,[221] a revised nosology is urgently needed.

HYPOCRETIN COMPOUNDS AS IDEAL FUTURE NARCOLEPSY TREATMENTS

Researchers have studied the effects of hypocretin on sleep after nasal, systemic, and central administration (e.g., intracerebroventricular injection and/or local perfusion in selected brain areas). Central administration of hypocretin-1, for example, into the lateral ventricle of wild-type rodents or normal canines, is strongly wake-promoting[222] and reverses cataplexy and sleep abnormalities in narcoleptic mice.[223] The effect is likely to be partially mediated by the hypocretin receptor-2 as intracerebroventricular hypocretin-1 at the same dose (10–30 nmoles) has no effect in hypocretin receptor-2 mutated narcoleptic canines.[222] Interestingly, intracerebroventricular hypocretin-2 administration has few, if any, central effects even in normal animals, perhaps because it is biologically unstable and rapidly degraded. This instability may also explain why hypocretin-2 is undetectable in native CSF.[224]

Experiments conducted after intravenous administration of hypocretin-1 have been performed in hypocretin receptor-2 mutated canines and in two hypocretin-deficient narcoleptic dogs. In spite of a previous report,[225] my colleagues and I were unable to detect any significant effect even at extremely high doses in hypocretin receptor-2 mutated animals. This result was not surprising, considering the lack of effects after central administration of the same dose in these animals lacking hypocretin receptor-2 (see previously).[222] More interestingly, a possible very slight and short-lasting suppression of cataplexy was observed in a single hypocretin–deficient narcoleptic animal at extremely high doses.[222]

The effect of hypocretin-1 intranasal administration in rodents and humans has also been studied,[226-229] with the hope that hypocretin-1 would penetrate into the brain via the cribriform region. Deadwyler and colleagues[228] found a significant reversal of MRI abnormalities induced by sleep deprivation after intranasal administration of hypocretin-1 (1.0 μg/kg) in rhesus monkeys. Weinhold and colleagues[229] found improved attention, decreased wake to REM sleep transitions, and less REM sleep in patients with narcolepsy after intranasal hypocretin-1 (435 nmol), but no effects on daytime tests of maintenance of wakefulness, suggesting limited clinical significance. My colleagues and I also examined the possibility of intrathecal administration (up to the very large dose of 96 μg/kg) by implanting a Medtronic pump with catheterization of the cisterna magna in a single hypocretin-deficient narcoleptic canine.[230] Our hope was that at a high dose, some reverse flow would occur back into deeper brain structures, providing therapeutic relief. A positive result would have had therapeutic application, as these pumps are frequently used in humans for the treatment of pain or spasticity using intrathecal administration. Preliminary results in mice suggested potential.[231] Disappointingly, however, we did not observe any significant effect on cataplexy,[230] probably because the hypocretin did not diffuse into upper ventricular compartments. Additional studies using intraventricular rather than intracisternal injections are needed to verify that hypocretin-deficient narcoleptic canines are responsive to supplementation.[226] In mice, however, intrathecal hypocretin was found to inhibit cataplexy.[231]

The discovery of hypocretin and its involvement in narcolepsy has led some drug companies to develop hypocretin receptor antagonists for insomnia. Two of these compounds, suvorexant and lemborexant, dual hypocretin receptor 1 and 2 antagonists (called DORAs, dual orexin receptor antagonists), have been approved for the treatment of insomnia,[130] and many others are under development. More relevant to narcolepsy, brain-penetrant hypocretin agonists have now been successfully synthesized. These compounds are wake-promoting and successfully reverse all abnormalities in mouse models of narcolepsy lacking orexin.[131] One of these compounds, TAK925, has been studied in human patients with narcolepsy in the context of a proof of concept study, with the caveat that because it had a short half-life and is not well absorbed, it was given intravenously. Nonetheless, at doses that had only modest effects in controls, it dramatically improved the Maintenance of Wakefulness Test (MWT) sleep latencies in patients with NT1 from a baseline to a few minutes to almost constant wakefulness in every 40-minute nap, a strongly promising result.[232] Newer orally available compounds such as TAK-994 are now entering clinical trials. Of note, however, current compounds are mostly agonists of the hypocretin receptor 2 (orexin receptor 2), the main receptor involved in the cause of narcolepsy based on animal studies. It may be that dual hypocretin receptor 1 and 2 agonists will be needed to fully restore function (because patient lack both hypocretin-1 and -2, both receptor 1 and receptor 2 transmission should be deficient), or that single-receptor agonists will find preferential indications in the treatment of various sleep disorders.

CONCLUSION

NT1 is both a common neurologic disorder and a model disorder to further our understanding of REM sleep and sleepiness regulation. Over the last 50 years, research has been greatly facilitated by the existence of a canine narcolepsy model, now replaced by rodent models. Narcolepsy-cataplexy, now reclassified as NT1, is most commonly caused by a loss of hypocretin-producing neurons in the hypothalamus. Low CSF hypocretin-1 can be used to diagnose NT1. The disorder is associated with HLA-*DQB1*06:02*, other HLA genes, and polymorphisms in immune system genes such as TCR polymorphisms, indicating that the cause in most patients is an autoimmune destruction of the hypocretin neurons. Studies in narcoleptic canines have substantiated a tight parallel between the pharmacologic control of cataplexy and that of REM sleep. Using this model, researchers found that the mode of action of stimulant medications is presynaptic stimulation of dopaminergic transmission while anticataplectic compounds exert their therapeutic effects primarily via adrenergic uptake inhibition. The hypocretin system sends strong excitatory projections onto monoaminergic cells, and the loss of hypocretin is likely to create a cholinergic-monoaminergic imbalance in narcolepsy. Abnormally sensitive cholinergic transmission and depressed dopaminergic and histaminergic transmission are believed to underlie abnormal REM sleep and daytime sleepiness in canine narcolepsy. This model explains why monoaminergic compounds such as amphetamines, antidepressants, and H3 antagonists are active on narcolepsy, but not why gamma hydroxybutyrate (GHB) has positive effects when administered at night. However, GHB, a known GABAB agonist,[233-236] is known to modulate dopaminergic transmission[39,233,235] and may increase DA store available for daytime alertness. Although these compounds have great efficacy in treating narcolepsy, an ideal theoretical treatment would be hypocretin agonists, which have been recently successfully produced and in one case pilot tested in patients with NT1 with very promising results.

There is increasing evidence that the autoimmune destruction of hypocretin cells is triggered by upper airway infections, notably the flu. In children, when narcolepsy onset is often more abrupt, a history of strep throat is often reported. The onset of narcolepsy in children is seasonal and peaks in spring and summer, strongly suggesting that winter infections may precipitate narcolepsy a few months later. Most strikingly, increased incidence of childhood narcolepsy was found in early 2010 in China, following the 2009 H1N1 swine flu pandemic, and possibly in the United States as well. Strongly suggesting that H1N1 itself is involved, H1N1 vaccinations in Europe using Pandemrix increased the number of new narcolepsy cases many fold. More mysteriously, however, risk was not increased with other brands of H1N1 vaccines, maybe because the content of the various vaccines varied and AS03 is a particularly strong adjuvant for stimulating $CD4^+$ T cells.

The most recent research now suggests that narcolepsy is primarily a T cell–mediated disease, and that the process is initiated by $CD4^+$ T cell confusing flu peptides with hypocretin itself when presented by DQ0602. This would trigger a cascade of events that leads to $CD8^+$ T cell destruction of hypocretin neurons. It may be possible to use CSF hypocretin-1 testing to evaluate the extent of hypocretin cell loss in early stages of the disease (e.g., in children), thus facilitating the development of treatments that may arrest or at least delay disease progression. Similar strategies using immunosuppression have been used in other autoimmune diseases, such as type I diabetes mellitus. In one case, 2 months after an abrupt onset, my colleagues and I tried high-dose prednisone but did not observe significant effects on symptoms and CSF hypocretin-1 levels[237]; however, in this case, very low hypocretin-1 levels were already observed, suggesting the possibility that irreversible damage to the hypocretin neurons had already occurred. In other patients with recent onset, intravenous immunoglobulin administration was reported to have positive effects in some but not all open-label studies,[238-243] suggesting the need for placebo-controlled studies.[244] More fruitful interventions could involve T-cell suppressants such as compounds blocking CNS entry of T cells. We anticipate that, in time, patients at risk for narcolepsy will be identified through genetic typing, monitored with biomarkers (e.g., measuring T-cell populations bearing specific TCR idiotypes, occurrence of specific infections), therefore allowing early intervention to stop hypocretin cell immune destruction. One of these interventions may involve modification of existing flu vaccine sequences.

CLINICAL PEARL

Narcolepsy remains a clinical diagnosis. If cataplexy is clear and present, the MSLT is done as a confirmation and to exclude the possibility of conversion disorder. In these patients, the cause of sleepiness and of other symptoms is established, and treating narcolepsy should be the priority above all other associated sleep disorders (e.g., sleep apnea) unless these are life threatening. If the patient does not have clear cataplexy the clinician should not lean too heavily on the presence of SOREMPs on the MSLT in making the diagnosis. Other causes of daytime sleepiness, such as medical conditions, sleep apnea, sleep deprivation, and circadian issues, should be excluded carefully, and then symptomatic therapy can proceed using compounds similar to those used for NT1, keeping in mind that cause and evolution of the underlying problem are not established. HLA typing and CSF hypocretin-1 measurements are mostly helpful in patients with suspected conversion disorder or psychiatric comorbidities, or in a patient without cataplexy who has a high probability of having NT1 without cataplexy (e.g., multiple SOREMPs on multiple MSLTs) as a positive result will justify more aggressive therapy.

SUMMARY

Narcolepsy includes two diagnostic entities, NT1 and NT2, subtypes that have been defined clinically and through the diagnostic use of the MSLT. In NT1 the condition is caused by a deficiency in the hypocretin/orexin hypothalamic neuropeptide system, and almost all diagnosed individuals have cataplexy, low CSF hypocretin-1, and HLA DQ0602. NT1 is also associated with multiple genetic polymorphisms in immune-related genes, notably in the T-cell receptor (TCRA and TCRB) loci. Both genetic and environmental factors are implicated in predisposition to NT1, with upper airway infections, notably influenza 2009 pandemic H1N1, playing a role in triggering an autoimmune process that ultimately results in hypocretin cell loss through a T cell–mediated autoimmune reaction targeting hypocretin peptides. In contrast, patients with NT2 have a positive MSLT, generally lack cataplexy, and have normal CSF hypocretin-1. NT2 can be hard to distinguish from idiopathic hypersomnia based on current diagnostic criteria. On rare occasions, narcolepsy and narcolepsy-like conditions can be caused by genetic disorders, brain tumors, traumatic brain injury, or inflammatory disorders, some of which injure the hypothalamus and/or the hypocretin system. Still, decreased CSF hypocretin-1 can also occur nonspecifically in patients with severe brain pathology. Current therapies include behavioral modification, stimulants, antidepressants, and gamma hydroxybutyrate (sodium oxybate). Hypocretin/orexin agonists are under development with very promising early results.

SELECTED READINGS

Chemelli RM, et al. Narcolepsy in orexin knockout mice: molecular genetics of sleep regulation. *Cell.* 1999;98:437–451.

Cogswell AC, et al. Children with Narcolepsy type 1 have increased T-cell responses to orexins. *Ann Clin Transl Neurol.* 2019;6(12):2566–2572.

Daniels LE. Narcolepsy. *Medicine.* 1934;13(1):1–122.

Edwards K, et al. Meeting report narcolepsy and pandemic influenza vaccination: what we know and what we need to know before the next pandemic? A report from the 2nd IABS meeting. *Biologicals.* 2019;60:1–7.

Han F, et al. Narcolepsy onset is seasonal and increased following the 2009 H1N1 pandemic in China. *Ann Neurol.* 2011;70(3):410–417.

Jiang W, et al. In vivo clonal expansion and phenotypes of hypocretin-specific CD4(+) T cells in narcolepsy patients and controls. *Nat Commun.* 2019;10(1):5247.

Latorre D, et al. T cells in patients with narcolepsy target self-antigens of hypocretin neurons. *Nature.* 2018;562(7725):63–68.

Lin L, et al. The sleep disorder canine narcolepsy is caused by a mutation in the hypocretin (orexin) receptor 2 gene. *Cell.* 1999;98(3):365–376.

Luo G, et al. Autoimmunity to hypocretin and molecular mimicry to flu in type 1 narcolepsy. *Proc Natl Acad Sci U S A.* 2018;115(52):E12323–E12332.

Mignot E, et al. The role of cerebrospinal fluid hypocretin measurement in the diagnosis of narcolepsy and other hypersomnias. *Arch Neurol.* 2002;59(10):1553–1562.

Ollila HM, et al. Narcolepsy risk loci are enriched in immune cells and suggest autoimmune modulation of the T cell receptor repertoire. *BioRxiv.* 2018:373555.

Peyron C, et al. A mutation in a case of early onset narcolepsy and a generalized absence of hypocretin peptides in human narcoleptic brains. *Nat Med.* 2000;6(9):991–997.

Trotti LM, Staab BA, Rye DB. Test-retest reliability of the multiple sleep latency test in narcolepsy without cataplexy and idiopathic hypersomnia. *J Clini Sleep Med.* 2013;9(8):789–795.

A complete reference list can be found online at ExpertConsult.com.

Chapter

112

Narcolepsy: Diagnosis and Management

Kiran Maski; Christian Guilleminault†

Chapter Highlights

- Narcolepsy disrupts the maintenance of wake and sleep states, resulting in daytime sleepiness and disrupted nighttime sleep. It also can produce states intermediate between wake and rapid eye movement sleep that manifest as cataplexy, hypnagogic hallucinations, and sleep paralysis.
- Some symptoms, such as cataplexy, are highly specific to narcolepsy, but others, such as daytime sleepiness, hypnagogic hallucinations, and sleep paralysis, can be seen in other sleep disorders and with insufficient sleep.
- Narcolepsy type 1 (NT1; narcolepsy with cataplexy) is caused by loss of the hypocretin/orexin-producing neurons, and diagnosis is usually straightforward. The cause of narcolepsy type 2 (NT2; narcolepsy without cataplexy) is unclear, and its diagnosis is challenging as it requires significant understanding of available diagnostic tests and their limitations.
- As hypocretins/orexins influence many neurologic functions, narcolepsy is associated with multiple comorbidities, and it is important to recognize and to treat these comorbid conditions in addition to treating narcolepsy.
- Although there is no cure for narcolepsy, treatments are often effective and include both behavioral and pharmacologic approaches.

Gélineau[1] first coined the term *narcolepsy* in 1880 to designate a pathologic condition characterized by irresistible and brief episodes of sleep recurring at close intervals. Although Westphal[2] and Fisher[3] previously published reports of patients with excessive daytime sleepiness (EDS) and episodic muscle weakness, Gélineau was the first to characterize narcolepsy as a distinct syndrome. He wrote that falls, or "astasias," sometimes accompanied attacks. Henneberg[4] later referred to these attacks as cataplexy. In the 1920s von Economo[5,6] hypothesized that narcolepsy is caused by injury to neurons in the hypothalamus. In the 1930s Daniels[7] emphasized the association of daytime sleepiness, cataplexy, sleep paralysis, and hypnagogic hallucinations with the syndrome. Referring to these symptoms as the clinical tetrad, Yoss and Daly[8] and Vogel[9] reported nocturnal sleep-onset rapid eye movement (REM) periods in narcolepsy patients, a finding confirmed in the following years.[10–11]

In the last 20 years, our understanding of narcolepsy has vastly improved with the discovery of the hypocretin/orexin neuropeptides (often called orexins),[11,12] the mapping of hypocretin/orexin projections from the lateral hypothalamus to many parts of the brain, including the sleep-wake and autonomic nervous regulatory system,[13] and the discovery that the hypocretin/orexin-producing neurons are destroyed in the brains of people with narcolepsy.[14,15]

Narcolepsy with cataplexy is likely caused by an autoimmune attack on the hypocretin/orexin-producing neurons (see Chapter 111).[16] Honda and Juji[17] were the first to discover that narcolepsy is associated with human leukocyte antigen (HLA) DR2. Further studies have now established across all ethnic groups that this DR2 association is specifically due to the DQB1 allele, DQB1*0602.[18] Recent studies have identified $CD4^+$ T-cells[19] and cytotoxic $CD8^+$ T-cells[20] in people with narcolepsy that target fragments of the hypocretin/orexin peptides. These T cells also cross-react with influenza antigens,[21,22] suggesting that molecular mimicry may underlie the attack on the hypocretin/orexin-producing neurons. Much less common, nonspecific destruction of the hypocretin/orexin neurons or their projections by other pathologic processes (e.g., trauma, tumors, infections)[23] can cause secondary narcolepsy with cataplexy.[24]

The hypocretin/orexin-producing neurons control many functions, and narcolepsy is more than just sleepiness and abnormal REM sleep. Narcolepsy destabilizes wake and sleep stages; people with narcolepsy can produce full wakefulness, non-REM (NREM), and REM sleep but are unable to maintain these states. In addition, people with narcolepsy can have intermixed sleep states, such as cataplexy and sleep paralysis, which likely represent a combination of wakefulness with the paralysis of REM sleep.[25]

CLINICAL FEATURES

The third edition of the *International Classification of Sleep Disorders* divided narcolepsy into narcolepsy type 1 (NT1; narcolepsy with cataplexy) and narcolepsy type 2 (NT2; narcolepsy without cataplexy).[26] The classic pentad of symptoms

† Deceased.

includes EDS plus variable amounts of cataplexy, sleep paralysis, hypnagogic and/or hypnopompic hallucinations, and disrupted nighttime sleep. All people with narcolepsy have EDS, but only about one-quarter of them have all five of these symptoms. Automatic behaviors (stereotyped or repetitive behaviors done without awareness while sleepy) also commonly occur. Symptoms suggestive of narcolepsy can occur in any person who is severely sleep deprived, but *only* cataplexy is unique to narcolepsy. Narcolepsy has a population prevalence of 0.02% to 0.06%[27–30] and affects both sexes equally.

SLEEPINESS

Most people with narcolepsy have unwanted episodes of sleep several times a day, typically during monotonous sedentary activity or after a heavy meal, but on occasion, people will doze off when fully involved in a task. The duration of sleep may vary from a few seconds to hours, depending on the situation and time of day. Many people with narcolepsy intentionally take one or two brief (15 to 30 minutes) naps each day and feel alert for the next 1 to 2 hours. These relatively short and refreshing naps can help differentiate people with narcolepsy from people with idiopathic hypersomnia, who often take long and unrefreshing naps. Despite feeling sleepy during the day, people with narcolepsy generally do not sleep more in 24 hours compared with those without narcolepsy. Apart from quick transitions into sleep (sometimes referred to as "sleep attacks"), people with narcolepsy also report feeling persistently drowsy, resulting in poor performance at school and work, inattention, and memory lapses.

Cataplexy

Cataplexy occurs in 60% to 70% of people with narcolepsy.[26,31] It is episodes of abrupt and transient decreases in muscle tone, most frequently elicited by strong emotions, such as laughter, anger, and surprise. Cataplexy can also be induced by a feeling of elation while listening to music, reading a book, or watching a movie, but a certain intensity of the associated emotion triggered by the abrupt new situation is an important element. Cataplexy can be triggered merely by remembering a happy or funny situation, anticipation, and/or surprise.

Cataplexy may involve certain muscles or most voluntary muscles. At the onset of cataplexy, abrupt muscle inhibition can be interrupted by recurrent bursts of normal muscle tone, resulting in rhythmic weakness that can mimic a tremor. The severity and extent of cataplexy attacks can vary from a state of complete cataplexy, which involves all voluntary muscles, leading to collapse, to partial cataplexy with limited involvement of certain muscle groups or no more than a fleeting sensation of weakness. If it involves the upper limbs, the patient may complain of "clumsiness," reporting activity such as dropping cups or plates or spilling liquids when surprised and laughing. With typical full episodes of cataplexy, the jaw sags, the head falls forward, the arms drop to the side, and the knees buckle. Rarely, in a severe cataplexy attack, there is complete and rapid loss of muscle tone causing a fall and injuries. With most episodes, people with narcolepsy may perceive this growing weakness and simply sit down or stand against a wall to prevent a fall. Awareness is preserved throughout the attack. The skilled physician must be cautious not to overdiagnose normal phenomena, such as the "rubber knees" that precede the anxiety of public speaking or "rolling on the ground laughing."

Partial cataplexy is more common than full cataplexy. In one study, people with NT1 reported 29 episodes of partial cataplexy and 8 episodes of full cataplexy over a month.[32] Partial cataplexy presents with head drops, speech slurring, and/or jaw slackening with/without tongue protrusion. Because mild cataplexy does not resemble the "classic" full-blown attack of cataplexy, it can be overlooked by family and physicians.[33] If the weakness involves only the jaw or speech, the patient may present with wide masticatory movements, dysarthria, or an unusual attack of stuttering speech.

Short attacks are the most common presentation of cataplexy. The duration of each cataplexy attack, whether partial or complete, is variable, lasting from a few seconds to 2 minutes, with rare episodes lasting up to 30 minutes. Status cataplecticus is a rare manifestation of prolonged cataplexy lasting hours. In adults it mainly occurs with sudden withdrawal of cataplexy-suppressing medications or insufficient sleep, but in children it can be a presenting symptom.

In children and rarely in adults, more complex forms of cataplexy can occur without emotional triggers, usually in the first 6 months after symptom onset.[9] One form of this complex cataplexy is characterized by negative motor symptoms—persistent, generalized hypotonia, usually with an unsteady gait and "cataplectic facies" (slack jaw, tongue protrusion, and ptosis).[34,35] Positive motor movements similar to dyskinesias (i.e., tongue thrusting, chewing movements with the mouth) can also occur in children with NT1, particularly those with negative motor symptoms.[34,35] These more complex forms of cataplexy tend to improve months after symptom onset and then evolve into more typical emotionally triggered cataplexy.[36]

Sleep Paralysis

Sleep paralysis occurs on falling asleep or awakening from sleep. The symptoms are likely occurring during REM sleep-wake state transitions and represent a combination of the atonia of REM sleep with the consciousness awareness of wakefulness. People with narcolepsy may feel awake but paralyzed, unable to move the limbs, to speak, or even to breathe deeply. The patient is fully aware of the condition and can recall it completely later. This state can be accompanied by hallucinations. In many episodes of sleep paralysis, but especially the first occurrence, the patient may experience anxiety about the immobility, which can be intensified by the accompanying hallucinations. With time, the patient usually learns that episodes are brief and benign, rarely lasting longer than a few minutes, and sleep paralysis rarely requires treatment with medications. Sleep paralysis can also occur as an isolated and intermittent phenomenon in 7.6% of the general population.[37]

Hallucinations

Vivid and often unpleasant auditory, visual, or tactile hallucinations can occur at sleep onset (hypnagogic) or upon awakening (hypnopompic), during daytime naps, or at night.[38] These sleep-related, transient hallucinations likely reflect a state of wakefulness mixed with the dream-like imagery of REM sleep. The visual hallucinations can consistent of threatening imagery (i.e., scary figure) as well as simple forms (colored circles, parts of objects) that are either constant or changing in size. The image of an animal or a person may present abruptly and often in color. The auditory hallucinations can range from a ringing phone to an elaborate melody. These hallucinations are often perceived as so vividly realistic that the patient finds them frightening. In some cases of unrecognized narcolepsy with daytime hypnagogic/hypnopompic hallucinations, the patient may be mistakenly diagnosed as having a psychosis.[39]

Dreams/Nightmares

People with narcolepsy commonly report nightmares, vivid dreams, and lucid dreams (dreams in which a person is consciously aware of dreaming).[40] Even more uniquely, people with narcolepsy report dream delusions. Dream delusions are described as dreams so vivid and realistic that they produce false memories leading to a false belief that could persist for days or weeks.[12] In one study, 83% of people with narcolepsy reported that they had confused dreams with reality, compared to only 15% of healthy control subjects.[41] For example, one man with narcolepsy asked his wife to turn on the local news because he had dreamt that a young girl had drowned in a nearby lake and had full expectation that the event would be covered in the news.

Sleep Disruption

People with narcolepsy commonly experience disrupted nighttime sleep.[13] Ironically, people with narcolepsy complain of difficulty staying asleep at night, although they may fall asleep repeatedly during the daytime. Based on polysomnographic studies, their sleep is often interrupted by repeated awakenings, and more time is spent in light sleep compared to healthy control subjects.[42] Other narcolepsy sleep-related symptoms include periodic limb movements and REM sleep behavior disorder. Periodic limb movements can be severe, with 10% of people with narcolepsy having a periodic limb movement index of greater than 15 per hour.[43] Perhaps due to dysregulated REM sleep physiology in the setting of hypocretin deficiency, 20% to 60% of adults and children with narcolepsy have REM sleep behavior disorder.[44–46] People with narcolepsy tend to have pantomime- or gesture-like behavior during their dream enactment[45,47] as opposed to the more violent dream enactment described in people with Parkinson disease.

COMORBID ASSOCIATIONS

Overweight and obesity are common, and weight gain can be rapid in younger children at the onset of narcolepsy.[47a,b,c] Precocious puberty occurs in 17% of children with narcolepsy and develops independent of obesity.[48]

Autonomic dysfunction is reported in NT1 during sleep, with a lack of expected blood pressure drop (nondipping pattern)[49] and blunted heart rate with physiologic triggers such as arousals.[50]

Psychiatric comorbidities are frequent, including depression, anxiety, obsessive compulsive disorder, and, more rarely, schizophrenia.[51] Symptoms similar to attention deficit hyperactivity disorder (ADHD) are common in both adult and children with narcolepsy[52] and can affect job and academic performance. Although inattention is likely related to EDS, improving sleepiness with wake-promoting medications alone does not reverse the ADHD-like symptoms,[52] suggesting intrinsic executive dysfunction may be present in people with narcolepsy.

Collectively, narcolepsy symptoms and comorbidities substantially reduce quality of life.[53–56] A large study in the United States involving 55,871 subjects, including 9312 in the narcolepsy group and 46,559 matched control subjects, characterized health care utilization, costs and productivity in a large population of patients diagnosed with narcolepsy; it showed that narcolepsy with its comorbidities was associated with substantial personal and economic burdens, as indicated by significantly higher rates of health care utilization and medical costs.[57] Narcolepsy is also associated with higher rates of accidents, employee absence due to short-term disability, job dismissal, and early retirement.[58] When needed, clinicians should provide work and/or school accommodations that permit scheduled naps, movement breaks, and other supports people with narcolepsy find necessary to function effectively.

ONSET OF CLINICAL SYMPTOMS AND LONGITUDINAL COURSE

The peak age of narcolepsy symptom onset ranges between 10 to 25 years.[49,60] A survey of 157 narcolepsy patients found that about 80% experienced symptoms before the age of 30 years,[61] but a second, small peak of onset has been noted between 35 and 45 years and near menopause in women. In those who developed narcolepsy at age 60 years or later, cataplexy was the most common initial symptom.[61] On the other end of the life span, there is one case report of NT1 developing in a 6-month old baby due to a hypocretin/orexin gene mutation.[62]

In 2009 to 2010, a number of children and adolescents in northern Europe developed NT1 soon after receiving Pandemrix, a specific brand of H1N1 influenza vaccine no longer in use, resulting in an 5- to 14-fold increase in NT1 incidence.[63] In these postvaccination cases, NT1 began at an earlier age and presented with more severe symptoms than in non–vaccine-related cases.[64–66]

EDS is usually the first symptom of narcolepsy and can be most severe close to disease onset.[36] Sleepiness and its impact on daily life may lessen slightly with age but do not resolve completely. Cataplexy can develop years after onset of EDS,[67] resulting in changes in diagnosis from NT2 to NT1. Cataplexy varies in frequency from a few episodes during the patient's entire lifetime to one or several episodes per day and can fluctuate with life events, such as pregnancy and life stresses. More recent longitudinal data suggests that cataplexy attacks are less frequent with age.[68]

DIAGNOSIS OF NARCOLEPSY

The diagnosis of NT1 and NT2 requires a clinical history of EDS (and cataplexy in the case of NT1) and a confirmatory Multiple Sleep Latency Test (MSLT) result, with a mean sleep-onset latency of 8 minutes or less and two or more sleep-onset REM periods (SOREMPs).[26] A nocturnal SOREMP (REM sleep within 15 minutes of sleep onset) can be included in the tally of SOREMP[26] and is a highly specific biomarker of NT1 in adults and children independently.[69,70]

Alternatively, NT1 can be diagnosed if the hypocretin/orexin level is low in cerebrospinal fluid (CSF). Greater than 90% of people with NT1 have a CSF hypocretin-1/orexin A level less than or equal to one-third that of healthy subjects; on the standard radioimmunoassay, this cut-off is 110 pg/mL.[71]

Although NT1 is a distinct phenomenon with strong consensus on diagnostic criteria, researchers debate whether NT2 is a distinct phenomenon or part of a spectrum of narcolepsy and idiopathic hypersomnia. This ambiguity is fueled in large part by the poor reproducibility of MSLT results in NT2 (discussed further in this section) and the lack of additional biomarkers as CSF hypocretin/orexin levels are nearly always normal in NT2. Thus clinical judgement is crucial for differentiating the more typical REM sleep-related symptoms of NT2 from the nonrestorative sleep and long sleep times of idiopathic hypersomnia.[72]

A correct diagnosis of narcolepsy is often delayed more than 10 years, especially if cataplexy is initially absent.[73] This delay is attributed to health care providers' general lack of awareness of narcolepsy symptoms[74] and misdiagnosis of narcolepsy as other conditions, such as epilepsy, mood disorders, and attention deficit disorder.[75]

EVALUATION OF SLEEPINESS

The Epworth Sleepiness Scale is most commonly used as an index of subjective sleepiness in adults (see Chapter 207). The Epworth Sleepiness Scale for Children and Adolescents (ESS-CHAD)[76] and Pediatric Daytime Sleepiness Scale[77] are validated for use in children and teenagers. Typically, people with narcolepsy will report severe EDS (score of 15 or higher) on the Epworth scales. The Stanford Sleepiness Scale,[78] a 7-point scale, was developed to quantify the subjective sleepiness in individuals throughout the day, but it is often difficult for people to accurately rate themselves every 15 to 20 minutes.

Polysomnography

A PSG should always be performed on the night before MSLT as it measures the amount of nocturnal sleep and helps rule out other sleep disorders, such as obstructive sleep apnea (OSA). The first 15 minutes of the PSG should be scrutinized for the presence of REM sleep (nocturnal SOREMP) as REM sleep within 15 minutes of sleep onset is highly specific for NT1 and associated with low CSF hypocretin-1/orexin-A levels.[79] People with narcolepsy may also have PSG findings of REM sleep without atonia, increase in N1 sleep, and frequent transitions from wake or N1 sleep to REM sleep; these electrophysiologic biomarkers support a narcolepsy diagnosis.[44,46,80] Other sleep disorders, including REM behavior disorder and periodic limb movements of sleep, may be detected among people with narcolepsy.[43] OSA can co-occur with narcolepsy. In one study, authors reported that 25% of narcolepsy patients had an apnea hypopnea index greater than 10 per hour,[81] and this finding may delay narcolepsy diagnosis if OSA is interpreted as the primary diagnosis.

Multiple Sleep Latency Test

The MSLT (see Chapter 207) measures physiologic sleep tendencies in the absence of alerting factors.[82] This test consists of five scheduled naps, usually at 10 a.m.; noon; and 2, 4, and 6 p.m., during which the subject is polygraphically monitored in a comfortable, soundproof, dark bedroom while wearing street clothes. After each 20-minute monitoring period, the patient stays awake until the next scheduled nap. Major end points on the MSLT are the latency for each nap (time between lights out and sleep onset), the mean sleep latency across all naps, and the presence of REM sleep during the naps.[83] A mean sleep-onset latency less than 8 minutes is generally considered to be diagnostic of sleepiness; those greater than 10 minutes are considered to be normal. Mean latencies of 8 to 10 minutes represent a gray area.[54] REM sleep that occurs during one of these naps is considered a daytime SOREMP. A positive PSG-MSLT supportive of a narcolepsy diagnosis requires a mean sleep-onset latency of 8 minutes or less plus two SOREMPs (including nocturnal SOREMP).

There is controversy about the reliance on a positive MSLT result in diagnosing narcolepsy. General population investigations have shown that healthy people can have two or more SOREMPs, especially those with short sleep duration and shift work.[85] One study showed that 16% of adolescents with delayed sleep phase disorder can have multiple daytime SOREMPs.[86] Thus it is very important to document prior sleep history, ideally by use of actigraphy, or at least sleep logs 2 weeks before testing, and to correct sleep irregularities to avoid false-positive tests. Furthermore, use of REM sleep–suppressing medications, such as selective serotonin reuptake inhibitors (SSRIs), serotonin-norepinephrine reuptake inhibitors (SNRIs), clonidine, guanfacine, and traditional stimulants, can cause false-negative testing and thus need to be weaned off 2 weeks or more before testing.[87]

Although the MSLT is an objective measurement of sleepiness, it comes with limitations. Prepubertal children appear to be hyperalert compared to postpubertal children,[88] and this can lengthen sleep latencies on MSLT. A recent study showed that the current PSG-MSLT diagnostic values are valid for the diagnosis of NT1 in people 9 to 18 years of age,[89] but there were too few subjects younger than 9 years to assess the influence of very young age. The MSLT also ignores brief microsleeps that can lead, in borderline cases, to daytime impairment not scored by conventional analysis, resulting in underestimation of objective EDS. Another potential drawback of the MSLT is related to methodology. Despite published guidelines from the American Academy of Sleep Medicine on how to conduct the MSLT,[90] sleep laboratories vary widely in methodology, including enforcement of protocols and interscorer reliability in identifying SOREMPs.

Still, the PSG-MSLT with cut-offs of mean sleep latency of 8 minutes or less and two or more SOREMPS is considered valid and reliable for diagnosing NT1, with sensitivity of 80%, specificity of 95%,[71] and reliability of 81% to 87%.[91,92] These PSG-MSLT cut-off values are less reliable for NT2. The diagnostic consistency among people with NT2 assessed with two separate PSG and MSLT tests at different times was only 18% to 47% due to differences in mean sleep latency and sleep-onset REM periods.[91–93] This poor test-retest reliability may be due to unstable NT2 physiology or inconsistencies in patient behavior and PSG and MSLT testing protocols. Currently, it is recommended that the PSG and MSLT be repeated if there is diagnostic uncertainty about the NT2 diagnosis.

Genetic Testing

Genetic factors affect the risk of developing NT1. The concordance rate in monozygotic twins for NT1 is approximately 20% to 30%.[58] Furthermore, only 1% to 2% of first-degree relatives of a person with NT1 are affected by the disease. Although this frequency is small, the relative risk for first-degree family members of people with NT1 is approximately 10- to 40-fold higher than that in the general population.[94]

Genetic testing is sometimes used in the clinical diagnosis of narcolepsy. HLA DQB1*06:02 is the most common genetic marker for narcolepsy across all ethnic groups, and it is found in 85% to 95% of people with NT1.[1] Further, homozygosity for DQB1*06:02 increases the risk of NT1 and NT2 twofold to fourfold.[95] However, in NT2 only 40% of subjects have DQB1*06:02,[16] so HLA testing is generally unhelpful in people without cataplexy. Of importance, this genetic testing alone is insufficient for the diagnosis of narcolepsy as DQB1*06:02 is found in 12% to 25% of the general population.

Other HLA alleles and genes affect the risk of narcolepsy. For example, DQB1*03:01 and DRB1*15:01 increase the risk, whereas DQB1*05:01 and DQB1*06:01 are protective.[96–98] NT1 is also associated with polymorphisms in the genes coding for the T-cell receptor alpha subunit, cathepsin H, and OX40L, which may affect antigen presentation and T-cell function. Overall, these genetic associations highlight the role of the immune system in the development of narcolepsy.

Hypocretin-1/Orexin-A Measurement in Cerebrospinal Fluid

Measurement of hypocretin-1/orexin-A in CSF is the most accurate technique for diagnosing NT1. Hypocretin/orexin neurons are selectively killed in people with narcolepsy with cataplexy,[99] and a very low or nonexistent level of hypocretin/orexin in CSF can confirm the diagnosis of NT1.[100–104] CSF hypocretin-1/orexin-A levels less than 110 ng/L (measured using the radioimmunoassay) have a high positive predictive value (94%) for narcolepsy type 1.[99,105] In contrast, hypocretin-1/orexin-A levels are usually normal in NT2; specifically, only 24% of people with NT2 have low CSF hypocretin-1/orexin-A levels, and this appears more common in African Americans with NT2.[106] In rare cases CSF hypocretin-1/orexin-A levels may be low due to a neurologic condition that injures the hypocretin/orexin neurons, such as brain tumors, encephalitis, vascular diseases, and brain trauma.[99]

Maintenance of Wakefulness Test

The Maintenance of Wakefulness Test (MWT) is not used in standard practice for diagnosis of narcolepsy but can be helpful in assessing treatment efficacy and evaluating the risk of falling asleep associated with specific jobs or activities.[107] The MWT tests the patient's ability to remain awake in a comfortable sitting position in a dark room for different trials given at 2-hour intervals during the daytime. The test is composed of four sessions at 2-hour intervals (9 a.m., 11 a.m., 1 p.m., and 3 p.m.), and the patient is instructed to remain awake for 40 minutes. Falling asleep in an average of less than 8 minutes during the test is considered abnormal. One study showed that a mean sleep latency of less than 12 minutes on the MWT had a sensitivity of 84% and a specificity of 98% for narcolepsy.[108] The MWT has been validated with different performance tests, including driving simulation,[109] and is commonly used in clinical drug trials.

TREATMENT

The goal of all therapeutic approaches is to optimize control of narcolepsy symptoms and to allow the patient to have a full personal and professional life. Treatment goals should focus on improving symptoms most bothersome to people with narcolepsy, which are typically EDS and cataplexy. When selecting medications, clinicians must consider possible side effects because narcolepsy is a lifelong illness, and people will have to receive medication for years. The treatment of narcolepsy must balance the maintenance of an active life with the avoidance of side effects and tolerance to medications.[110]

Behavioral Approaches

Behavioral approaches are an important aspect of treating narcolepsy. Daytime sleepiness often improves for 1 to 2 hours after a 15- to 20-minute daytime nap, and some people with narcolepsy benefit from two naps. When needed, clinicians should work with schools and employers to help implement opportunities for a nap. In addition, other important behavioral treatment targets include maintaining a regular sleep-wake schedule, avoiding frequent time zone changes, and practicing good sleep hygiene (Tables 112.1 and 112.2).

Career counseling is also important because people with narcolepsy and their employers must be educated about jobs that may be challenging to perform with daytime sleepiness, including jobs that require shift work and on-call schedules. People with narcolepsy should be discouraged from work that

Table 112.1 Examples of Initial Treatment Packages for Children[a]

Prepubertal Children	Adolescents
General Measures	
Contact school to alert teachers	Contact school to alert teachers
Emphasize need for regular nocturnal sleep schedule, and at least 9–11 hours of nocturnal sleep	Emphasize need for regular nocturnal sleep schedule, and at least 8–10 hours of nocturnal sleep
Naps <30 minutes 1–3 times per day	Naps <30 minutes 1–3 times per day
Medications for Sleepiness	
Modafinil 50–200 mg/day[b,c]	Modafinil 100–400 mg/day[b]
	Armodafinil 50-250 mg[b]
Sodium oxybate is based on patient weight if under 45 kg[d,e]	Sodium oxybate 6–9 g[d,e]
Methylphenidate IR or ER 0.5–1 mg/kg/day (typical max dose 40 mg/day)	Methylphenidate ER 18–54 mg (typical max dose 60 mg/day)
Dextroamphetamine-amphetamine IR/ER[e] 5–40 mg/day	Adderall IR/ER 5–40 mg/day
Atomoxetine 0.25–1.2 mg/kg/day	Atomoxetine 10–80 mg/day
Medications for Cataplexy[e]	
Sodium oxybate is based on patient weight if under 45 kg[d,e]	Sodium oxybate 6–9 g[c,d]
Venlafaxine XR 37.5 mg–150 mg in a.m.[f]	Venlafaxine XR 37.5–225 mg in a.m.[c]
Fluoxetine 5–20 mg in AM	Fluoxetine 10–40 mg in AM

[a]Doses and safety are not established in children < 18 years of age for all medications except sodium oxybate and traditional stimulants. Medication dosages for children ≥ 6 years of age are based on Lexicomp and Lecendreux M, et al: *Pediatr Drugs* 16:363-372, 2014.
[b]Modafinil and armodafinil are not U.S. Food and Drug Administration (FDA) approved for people <17 years of age.
[c]Dosage based on clinical experience.
[d]Sodium oxybate requires titration.[171] Maximum dosing: 20 to <30 kg is 3 g twice nightly; 30 to 45 kg maximum dos is 3.75 g twice nightly and ≥45 kg is 4.5 g twice nightly.
[e]Has received approval by the FDA for use in pediatric narcolepsy.
[f]Lexicomp specifies 75 mg, but clinically the dosage may be higher.
ER, Extended release; IR, immediate release; XR, extended release.

Table 112.2 Examples of Initial Treatment Packages for Adults

General Measures

Avoid shifts in sleep schedule.
Avoid heavy meals and alcohol intake.
Regular timing of nocturnal sleep: 10:30 p.m. to 7 a.m.
Naps: Strategically timed naps if possible (e.g., 15 minutes at lunchtime, 15 minutes at 5:30 p.m.)

Medications for Sleepiness

The effects of stimulant medications vary widely among people with narcolepsy. The dosing and timing of medications should be individualized to optimize performance. Additional doses, as needed, may be suggested for periods of anticipated sleepiness.
Modafinil[a]: 100–200 mg (taken when waking up in the morning) and 100–200 mg at lunchtime *or*
Armodafinil: 50–250 mg/day
Pitolisant: 17.8–35.6 mg taken once in the morning *or*
Solriamfetol: 75–150 mg taken once in the morning *or*
Sodium oxybate[b] at bedtime: dosage must start low at 2.25 g taken twice while in bed (at bedtime and 2.5–4 hours after bedtime); increase to total dosage by 0.75 g/dose every week to dose of 3.5-4.5 g twice nightly. Do not increase above 9 g because of risk of serious side effects during sleep. It may take more than 2 months for daytime symptoms to improve, and cataplexy may improve faster than excessive daytime sleepiness. If the patient is already taking a daytime stimulant, it may be possible to reduce the stimulant dose or to discontinue it once a therapeutic dosage of sodium oxybate has been reached.
Methylphenidate XR: 18-54 mg in the morning or methylphenidate IR 5–20 mg twice to three times per day. Better action is always obtained if the drug is taken on an empty stomach

If Persistent Difficulties

Modafinil: 200 mg in the morning and 200 mg at lunch (total daily dosage, 400 mg) *or*
Pitolisant: 17.8–35.6 mg taken once in the morning *or*
Solriamfetol 75–150 mg taken once in the morning *or*
Add sodium oxybate (GHB) at bedtime: dosage must start low as indicated above
Methylphenidate (SR): 20 mg in the morning; IR 5 mg afternoon nap; 5 mg at 4 pm *or*
Amphetamine[c] (XR): 10–20 mg in the morning; IR 5 mg afternoon nap; 5 mg at 4 pm *or*
Atomoxetine (possibly; more in teenagers): start at 0.5 mg/kg within 1 week to appropriate dosage of 1 to 1.2 mg/kg taken in the morning

Medications for Cataplexy[c]

Sodium oxybate (see above)
Venlafaxine XR 37.5–225 mg
Fluoxetine 20–60 mg

If No Response

Clomipramine: 10–75 mg, *or*
Protriptyline 2.5–5 mg tid

[a]
[b]Response to sodium oxybate is slow.
[c]Medications may be taken in the evening near bedtime (sodium oxybate, clomipramine, imipramine), only in the morning (fluoxetine), or in the morning and at lunchtime (viloxazine, venlafaxine). The only medications specifically approved for use in narcolepsy by the U.S. Food and Drug Administration are modafinil, amphetamine, and sodium oxybate.
ER, Extended release; IR, immediate release; SR, sustained-release tablet; tid, three times daily.

requires continuous attention for long hours without breaks, particularly under monotonous conditions, such as commercial driving and the transportation industry.

Narcolepsy impacts numerous aspects of life, and many patients benefit from participation in a patient support group. These are sometimes organized by local sleep disorders centers or national organizations, such as Narcolepsy Network, Wake Up Narcolepsy, and similar organizations in other countries. People with narcolepsy can also find helpful information on the websites of the American Academy of Sleep Medicine, Stanford University, and Harvard University.

Pharmacologic Treatments

Pharmacologic treatments are listed in Tables 112.1 to 112.3.

Excessive Daytime Sleepiness

Modafinil. Modafinil is a wake-promoting drug that likely promotes wakefulness by blocking the reuptake of dopamine.[111–114] Mice lacking the dopamine transporter do not show an increase in wake with modafinil.[114] In contrast, amphetamines block the reuptake of dopamine, norepinephrine, and serotonin, and some people with narcolepsy find modafinil less potent in promoting wakefulness than amphetamines.

Modafinil improves EDS in people with narcolepsy with relatively few side effects. Headache is the most common complaint, followed by nervousness, nausea, and dry mouth. These symptoms can be reduced by a slow increase in dosage. Blood pressure should be monitored as the drug may cause elevated pressures. Rarely, modafinil can cause Stevens-Johnson syndrome or other serious rashes. Modafinil has a

Table 112.3 Narcolepsy Drugs Currently Available

Drug	Usual Dosage[a]
Treatment of Sleepiness[b]	
Modafinil	100–400 mg each day
Methylphenidate	10–60 mg/day
Atomoxetine	10–25 mg/day
Dextroamphetamine	5–60 mg/day
Sodium oxybate	6–9 g/night (split between bedtime and 3–4 h later)
Pitolisant	17.8–35.6 mg/day
Solriamfetol	75–150 mg/day
Treatment of Cataplexy	
Sodium oxybate	6–9 g/night (split between bedtime and 3–4 h later)
Venlafaxine XR	37.5–225 mg/day
Fluoxetine	10–60 mg/day
Duloxetine	60 mg/day
Protriptyline	2.5–20 mg/day
Imipramine	25–200 mg/day
Clomipramine	25–200 mg/day
Desipramine	25–200 mg/day

[a]On occasion, depending on clinical response, the dose may be outside the usual dosage range.
[b]Depending on the half-life, some wake-promoting medications should be administered in divided doses, commonly in the morning and at lunchtime.
XR, Extended release.

very low potential for addiction, abuse, or tolerance. Modafinil can be given as a single dose in the morning (200 to 400 mg) as its half-life is 10 to 12 hours, but some people with narcolepsy find it helpful to split the dose between morning and midday. Modafinil can reduce the efficacy of oral contraceptives, and therefore people with narcolepsy should use alternative methods of birth control. Modafinil may be teratogenic, and it should be stopped before conception, pregnancy, and lactation.[115]

Armodafinil. Armodafinil is the active *R*-enantiomer of modafinil and is approved by the US Food and Drug Administration (FDA) for the treatment of EDS in narcolepsy. In a multicenter, randomized, double-blind, placebo-controlled trial of 196 subjects with narcolepsy, armodafinil significantly improved EDS throughout the day.[116,117] It may produce longer improvements in EDS than regular modafinil due to its longer half-life of 12 to 15 hours. Doses range from 50 to 250 mg/day. Side effects are similar to those of modafinil, which include headache, nausea, dizziness, and insomnia.

Amphetamines and Amphetamine-like Central Nervous System Stimulants. Stimulants include amphetamines, such as dextroamphetamine and mixed amphetamine salts, and amphetamine-like drugs, including methylphenidate. Like modafinil, these drugs block the reuptake of dopamine, but they also block the reuptake of norepinephrine and serotonin. At higher doses, amphetamines can cause efflux of these monoamine neurotransmitters from nerve terminals, and this sudden rise in monoamines may contribute to their addictive potential. These neurotransmitters all promote wakefulness and suppress REM sleep, and in consequence, stimulants improve EDS, increase the latency to NREM and REM sleep, and reduce the percentage of REM sleep. Amphetamines IR are usually administered in two or three divided doses, typically 10 to 20 mg in each dose. The slow-release form may provide gradual and delayed responses during the daytime. Methylphenidate and amphetamines at more than 60 mg/day tend to produce side effects, including more nocturnal sleep disruption and a higher frequency of psychosis, paranoia, and psychiatric hospitalizations. Rebound hypersomnia is more frequent with higher dosages of amphetamines. These stimulants have a high potential for abuse and development of tolerance, and therefore should be administered at the lowest effective doses.

Pitolisant. Pitolisant is a histamine H3 receptor inverse agonist approved for use in Europe in 2016 and in the United States in 2019 for the treatment of EDS in people with NT1 and NT2. In the brain, histamine promotes wake and may suppress REM sleep. The H3 receptor is an inhibitory autoreceptor that reduces release of histamine, acetylcholine, and other monoamine neurotransmitters.[118] Pitolisant blocks this effect, resulting in higher levels of histamine and these other neurotransmitters.[119]

Pitolisant is a moderately potent treatment for EDS, superior to placebo and similar to modafinil.[120] In addition, pitolisant modestly reduces cataplexy frequency compared to placebo[121] but is not yet approved in the United States as an anticataplexy agent. Pitolisant is given once daily at 8.9 mg/day, and it may be increased up to 35.6 mg/day. Pitolisant is generally well tolerated, with mild adverse effects; nausea and musculoskeletal pain are most frequent, and it can also cause headache, insomnia, abdominal pain, and prolonged QT interval, but anxiety is uncommon.[120] Limited data are available about the effects on pregnancy and lactation. Pitolisant is not scheduled as a controlled substance because of its low abuse potential.[122] Of note, pitolisant is hepatically metabolized and is contraindicated in people with severe hepatic impairment.

Solriamfetol. Solriamfetol is a selective dopamine and norepinephrine reuptake inhibitor approved in the United States in 2019 for the treatment of adults with EDS due to narcolepsy. In contrast to amphetamines, solriamfetol does not promote the release of monoamines.[123]

In a phase 3 randomized, placebo-controlled study of adults with narcolepsy, people treated with solriamfetol showed large improvements in subjective and objective measures of EDS over placebo.[124] Side effects were mild to moderate and included headaches, nausea, appetite suppression, anxiety, insomnia, and small dose-dependent increases in blood pressure and heart rate. The starting dose of solriamfetol is 75 mg once daily. Doses may be increased every 3 days as needed to 150 mg daily (maximum dose approved in the United States). The mean half-life of the drug is 7.1 hours, and it is excreted predominantly in the urine. Limited data are available about the effects on pregnancy and lactation. Concomitant use of monoamine oxidase inhibitors or use within last 14 days is contraindicated with solriamfetol.

Sodium Oxybate. Sodium oxybate is the sodium salt of gamma-hydroxybutyrate and is approved by the FDA for the treatment of sleepiness and cataplexy in narcolepsy. How sodium oxybate improves the symptoms of narcolepsy is only partially understood. Sodium oxybate promotes deep non-REM sleep, and this acute sedating effect is likely mediated by gamma-aminobutyric acid–B receptors.[125] Over the course of weeks to months, sodium oxybate also improves daytime sleepiness and cataplexy, but how this occurs is unknown.

In large, multicenter studies, sodium oxybate has shown efficacy in improving the EDS and cataplexy of narcolepsy.[126,127] The drug is normally taken at bedtime with the patient already in bed to avoid falls due to acute and sometimes intense sedation. A second dose is taken approximately 2.5 to 4 hours after the first one while the patient is in bed. Its half-life is 90 to 120 minutes. Many people with narcolepsy start with a total nightly dose of 4.5 to 6 g, and the dose is gradually titrated up over 2 to 3 months to 6 to 9 g, based on improvements in EDS and cataplexy. These doses can also reduce sleep fragmentation, sleep paralysis, hypnagogic hallucinations, and nightmares.[128] Deeper nighttime sleep is apparent early in treatment, but it may take more than 3 months to see the full benefits of the medication on EDS and cataplexy. Sodium oxybate can have additive effects on EDS when used in combination with modafinil.[129] Acute withdrawal does not produce intense rebound cataplexy or sleepiness.

If people with narcolepsy wake 1 to 2 hours after dosing, they can have confusion, nausea, and enuresis, especially at higher doses and when first starting the drug. Sodium oxybate can cause respiratory depression (notably when combined with sedating substances) and obstructive and central apnea,[126–138] and it should be used cautiously in narcolepsy patients with sleep-disordered breathing. It is not recommended in pregnancy. Sodium oxybate is contraindicated in combination with sedatives or alcohol and in people with succinic semialdehyde dehydrogenase deficiency. In the United States clinical use of sodium oxybate necessitates close safety monitoring through a federal drug safety program (Risk Evaluation and Mitigation Strategy, or REMS).

Atomoxetine. Atomoxetine, an serotonin-norepinephrine reuptake inhibitor, has been studied for the treatment of narcolepsy in retrospective cohort studies and case reports.[139,140] In one study, improvements in daytime sleepiness, cataplexy, and disrupted sleep were reported among children with NT1, but standardized outcome measures were not used.[139] Side effects include appetite suppression and mood disorder. Currently, evidence of treatment efficacy is quite limited.[141–143]

Cataplexy and REM Sleep-Related Symptoms

Cataplexy is thought to be an intrusion of REM sleep atonia into wakefulness. REM sleep is strongly suppressed by norepinephrine and serotonin, and drugs that increase levels of these neurotransmitters are often effective in suppressing cataplexy. Expert consensus supports the off-label use of antidepressants for cataplexy treatment due to their REM sleep-suppressing capabilities, but there are no randomized controlled trials establishing their efficacy.

Monoamine Nonspecific Reuptake Inhibitors. Tricyclic antidepressants were the first medications used to treat cataplexy. The older tricyclic antidepressants include imipramine, clomipramine, and protryptiline.[144–146] Tricyclic antidepressants inhibit monoamine (serotonin, norepinephrine, dopamine) reuptake and block cholinergic, histaminergic, and alpha-adrenergic transmission and were formerly drugs of choice, particularly protriptyline. However, they have significant anticholinergic side effects, including dry mouth, sweating, constipation, tachycardia, difficulty urinating, and particularly sexual dysfunction that led to impotence in greater than 40% of males with narcolepsy. Tricyclic antidepressants are now used infrequently when a patient desires a potent medication for occasional use during times when cataplexy is likely.

Selective Serotonin Reuptake Inhibitors. SSRIs are considered effective and well tolerated for cataplexy management. Typical fluoxetine starting doses for cataplexy are 10 to 20 mg in the morning, and it can be increased to 60 mg/day. Fluvoxamine at 25 to 200 mg/day has also been shown to be mildly effective for cataplexy. Compared with the classic tricyclic antidepressants, SSRIs have fewer side effects and are quite effective. Adverse effects include insomnia, nausea, and sexual difficulties. Tolerance to this class does not develop.

Serotonin-Norepinephrine Reuptake Inhibitors. SNRIs substantially reduce cataplexy, sleep paralysis, and hypnagogic/hypnopompic hallucinations and are the recommended drugs because they have fewer side effects and greater efficacy. The most commonly used drug of this class is venlafaxine XR, a potent inhibitor of serotonin and noradrenergic reuptake and a weak inhibitor of dopamine reuptake. At a dose of 37.5 to 225 mg, venlafaxine XR has been the most widely used of these compounds both in adults and in children; it has good efficacy and is better tolerated than the tricyclic antidepressants. Duloxetine (60 mg each morning) is another SNRI that reduces cataplexy.[147]

SNRIs and SSRIs are category C drugs (paroxetine is category D) when used during pregnancy. Information about the use of antidepressant medication use in pregnant women comes from mostly observational studies, but data suggest no teratogenic effects.[148] Antidepressants can also produce periodic limb movements during sleep[149,150] and the development of REM sleep behavior disorder,[151] but it is unknown if these symptoms worsen in people with narcolepsy taking SSRI/SNRI medications.

Treatment of Children

Most data regarding drug treatment efficacy and safety in children with narcolepsy are based on observational data. In a study of 13 children (mean age, 11.0 years), modafinil (mean dose, 346 mg/day) increased sleep latencies on MSLT (from 6.6 to 10.2 minutes) and reduced sleep attacks in 90% of subjects, and it appeared to be safe and well tolerated for more than a year.[152] Modafinil 50 to 200 mg seems to work best when it is administered in the morning and at noon. A low dose of immediate-release methylphenidate may be added when the child returns from school, if needed. The drug should not be given too late to avoid inducing sleep-onset insomnia.

Modafinil and armodafinil are not FDA approved for people younger than 17 years due to case reports of Stevens-Johnson syndrome. In a meta-analysis of modafinil use in a pediatric narcolepsy cohort, side effects included irritability, dry mouth, nausea, loss of appetite, and headaches, but no severe adverse reactions were reported.[153] If modafinil cannot be prescribed, methylphenidate is the second best option; it comes in immediate-release, slow-release, and extended-release formulations.[154] In children the recommended dose is based on weight (typically 0.5 to 1 mg/kg/day with a maximum dose <50 to 60 mg/day), and we use long-acting formulations for better adherence and to reduce addiction potential. We prefer methylphenidate over amphetamines as a study of children with ADHD showed a higher risks of psychosis with amphetamines.[155]

In a randomized controlled trial, sodium oxybate improved EDS and cataplexy in children/adolescents with NT1, and the therapeutic response was sustained over the 1-year study period without development of tolerance.[156] Side effects were generally mild and comparable to those seen in adults, including nausea, weight loss, dizziness, and nocturnal enuresis. However, some subjects had depression, suicidal ideation, and obstructive and central sleep apnea.[156] Sodium oxybate can also produce NREM parasomnias (e.g., sleep walking, night terrors), particularly at higher dosages.[157]

Emerging Therapies and Pharmacologic Agents under Investigation

Ideally, one would treat NT1 with hypocretin/orexin peptides, but this approach has several challenges. One limitation is that the peptide has to cross the blood-brain barrier to reach the central nervous system.[158–162] Small studies of intranasal hypocretin-1/orexin-A in people with NT1 showed reductions in REM sleep time and fewer wake-to-REM sleep transitions but no improvements in sleepiness or cataplexy.[163,159] Transplantation of hypocretin/orexin-producing neurons generated from pluripotent stem cell could be considered, although poor survival of grafted hypocretin/orexin-producing neurons and an autoimmune attack on these cells are major concerns.[162]

Emerging treatments for narcolepsy include hypocretin/orexin agonists, immunotherapy, SNRIs, brain-penetrable agonists for trace amine-associated receptor 1 (TAAR1), reformulations of existing drugs, and combinations or variations of currently used therapies and other therapies.[128,129] TAK-925, a hypocretin/orexin 2 receptor agonist, robustly increased wakefulness in murine models of NT1,[164] and clinical trials to evaluate safety, tolerability, and pharmacokinetics of hypocretin/orexin agonists are underway. Another emerging narcolepsy treatment involves trace amines, metabolites of amino acids with structural similarity to classical biogenic amines. Novel, brain-penetrable agonists for TAAR1 act as negative modulators of monoaminergic neurotransmission and show a dose-dependent increase in wakefulness and reductions in REM sleep in mice and rats.[165] Another monoaminergic approach is reboxetine (AXS-12), which specifically blocks norepinephrine reuptake and treats cataplexy better than serotonin reuptake inhibitors in hypocretin/orexin-deficient mice.[166] A clinical trial for reboxetine to treat cataplexy and EDS in people with NT1 is underway.

As NT1 is likely caused by an autoimmune process, investigators are also exploring immunotherapy as a treatment for NT1, including corticosteroids, plasmapheresis, and intravenous immune globulin.[167–170] An open-label intravenous immune globulin study reported limited success and reduction of symptoms, suggesting that if a therapeutic benefit is obtained, it may be limited by timing of treatment (i.e., at onset of disease) and severity of symptoms.[153] Currently, intravenous immune globulin and corticosteroids are not recommended, and further trials are needed to determine the possible role of immunomodulators in the treatment of narcolepsy.[170]

CLINICAL PEARLS

- Narcolepsy is characterized by the clinical pentad of excessive daytime sleepiness (EDS), cataplexy, sleep paralysis, hypnagogic/hypnopompic hallucinations, and disrupted nighttime sleep. All people with narcolepsy have EDS, but other symptoms are present only in some individuals. Cataplexy is unique to narcolepsy, but other symptoms are nonspecific.
- Narcolepsy is associated with multiple comorbid conditions, including obesity, sleep apnea, and mood disorders, including depression.
- The diagnosis of narcolepsy type 1 (NT1) requires a history of EDS and one of the following: (1) low cerebrospinal fluid hypocretin-1/orexin-A level or (2) cataplexy and a positive Multiple Sleep Latency Test (MSLT) result. The diagnosis of narcolepsy type 2 (NT2) requires a history of EDS and a positive MSLT result.
- Genetic testing for human leukocyte antigen (HLA) DQB1*06:02 is positive in 95% of people with NT1 and in 40% of people with NT2, However, as this allele is found in 18% to 35% of the general population, HLA testing is not recommended as a diagnostic tool.
- The MSLT must be preceded by nighttime polysomnography to rule out other sleep disorders and to document adequate sleep. The MSLT can be falsely positive due to shift work, sleep apnea, or sleep deprivation, and it is influenced by age, sex, and puberty.
- Modafinil, armodafinil, pitolisant, and solriamfetol can reduce EDS and have fewer side effects than amphetamines.
- Sodium oxybate can improve cataplexy, EDS, and disrupted nighttime sleep.

SUMMARY

Narcolepsy is a chronic neurologic sleep disorder due to hypocretin/orexin neuron loss, resulting in EDS, disturbed nocturnal sleep, and intrusions of aspects of REM sleep into wakefulness, such as cataplexy, sleep paralysis, and hypnopompic/hypnagogic hallucinations. The syndrome is associated with multiple comorbidities. MSLTs taken after overnight PSG show short sleep latencies (mean sleep-onset latency of 8 minutes or less) and two or more SOREMPs. Narcolepsy with cataplexy is associated with likely autoimmune destruction of the hypocretin/orexin neurons that are located in the lateral hypothalamus, resulting in a severe reduction of CSF hypocretin-1/orexin-A. Medications for narcolepsy have improved over time, with the newer compounds providing good efficacy with fewer side effects compared with amphetamines and tricyclic antidepressants. Modafinil, armodafinil, solriamfetol, and pitolisant improve daytime sleepiness, and sodium oxybate improves multiple narcolepsy symptoms, including cataplexy and daytime sleepiness. Individualized treatment plans are recommended based on patient needs, risks and benefits of medications, cost to patient, and adherence. Behavioral approaches, including school and work accommodations, nap opportunities, sleep hygiene, and psychological supports for coping with this chronic disease, are critical to optimize disease management.

ACKNOWLEDGMENT

Christian Guilleminault wrote the original versions of this chapter, and we are saddened by his passing. We appreciate his excellent work and that of Michelle Cao who contributed to earlier versions of this chapter.

SELECTED READINGS

Andlauer O, Moore H, Jouhier L, et al. Nocturnal REM sleep latency for identifying patients with narcolepsy/hypocretin/orexin deficiency. *JAMA Neurol.* 2013;70:891–902.

Andlauer O, Moore 4th H, Hong SC, et al. Predictors of hypocretin/orexin (orexin) deficiency in narcolepsy without cataplexy. *Sleep.* 2012;35:1247–1255.

Baumann CR, Mignot E, Lammers GJ, et al. Challenges in diagnosing narcolepsy without cataplexy: a consensus statement. *Sleep.* 2014;37:1035–1042.

Black J, Reaven NL, Funk SE, et al. The Burden of Narcolepsy Disease (BOND) study: health-care utilization and cost findings. *Sleep Med.* 2014;15:522–529.

Goldbart A, Peppard P, Finn L, et al. Narcolepsy and predictors of positive MSLTs in the Wisconsin Sleep Cohort. *Sleep.* 2014;37:1043–1051.

Kornum BR, Knudsen S, Ollila HM, et al. Narcolepsy. *Nat Rev Dis Primers.* 2017;3:16100.

Lopez R, Doukkali A, Barateau L, et al. Test-retest reliability of the Multiple Sleep Latency Test in central disorders of hypersomnolence. *Sleep.* 2017;40(12).

Maski K, Pizza F, Liu S, et al. Defining disrupted nighttime sleep and assessing its diagnostic utility for pediatric narcolepsy type 1. *Sleep.* 2020;43(10):zsaa066.

Maski K, Steinhart E, Williams D, et al. Listening to the patient voice in narcolepsy: diagnostic delay, disease burden, and treatment efficacy. *J Clin Sleep Med.* 2017;13(3):419–425.

Maski K, Trotti LM, Kotagal S, et al. Treatment of central disorders of hypersomnolence: an American Academy of Sleep Medicine clinical practice guideline. JCSM. Forthcoming.

Mignot E, Hayduk R, Black J, et al. HLA-DQB1*0602 is associated with narcolepsy in 509 narcoleptic patients. *Sleep.* 1997;20:1012–1020.

Mignot E, Lammers GJ, Ripley B, et al. The role of cerebrospinal fluid hypocretin/orexin measurement in the diagnosis of narcolepsy and other hypersomnias. *Arch Neurol.* 2002;59:1553–1562.

Pizza F, Franceschini C, Peltola H, et al. Clinical and polysomnographic course of childhood narcolepsy with cataplexy. *Brain.* 2013;136(Pt 12):3787–3795.

Sansa G, Iranzo A, Santamaria J. Obstructive sleep apnea in narcolepsy. *Sleep Med.* 2010;11:93–95.

Sasai-Sakuma T, Kinoshita A, Inoue Y. Polysomnographic assessment of sleep comorbidities in drug-naïve narcolepsy-spectrum disorders—a Japanese cross-sectional study. *PLoS One.* 2015;10(8):e0136988.

Scammell TE. *Narcolepsy. N Engl J Med.* 2015;373(27):2654–2662.

Serra L, Montagna P, Mignot E, Lugaresi E, Plazzi G. Cataplexy features in childhood narcolepsy. *Mov Disord.* 2008;23(6):858–865.

A complete reference list can be found online at ExpertConsult.com.

Chapter 113

Idiopathic Hypersomnia

Yves Dauvilliers; Claudio L.A. Bassetti

Chapter Highlights

- Idiopathic hypersomnia (IH) is a rare central nervous system hypersomnolence disorder characterized clinically by excessive daytime sleepiness often associated with long and unrefreshing naps, prolonged and undisturbed nocturnal sleep, and great difficulty waking up and "getting going" (sleep inertia) after sleep.
- Polysomnography often shows normal nighttime sleep with high sleep efficiency without sleep apneas or periodic limb movements. A short mean sleep latency (<8 minutes) on the Multiple Sleep Latency Test is required with one or less sleep-onset rapid eye movement periods. Alternatively, IH can be diagnosed by total sleep time of more than 10 hours on continuous 24-hour monitoring polysomnography or average total sleep time of more than 10 hours across at least 7 days of actigraphy testing.
- The pathophysiology of IH remains unclear. In the absence of a specific biologic marker, IH is a diagnosis of exclusion with a broad differential diagnosis, including atypical forms of depression, narcolepsy type 2 (NT2; narcolepsy without cataplexy), sleep apnea syndrome, and behaviorally induced insufficient sleep syndrome.
- Pharmacologic options for IH are similar to the treatments for narcolepsy, including modafinil, methylphenidate, pitolisant, dextroamphetamine, and sodium oxybate.
- Symptoms of IH may be severe and long lasting, but spontaneous improvement in hypersomnolence occurs in about one-third of patients.

HISTORY

The term idiopathic hypersomnia (IH) was used as early as 1829 ("die idiopathische chronische Schlafsucht") for excessive daytime sleepiness (EDS) of undetermined origin.[1] In the late 1950s, Bedrich Roth was the first to describe a syndrome characterized by EDS, prolonged sleep, and sleep drunkenness and by the absence of "sleep attacks," cataplexy, sleep paralysis, and hallucinations. The terms "independent sleep drunkenness" and "hypersomnia with sleep drunkenness" were initially suggested.[2-5] Overlapping features with narcolepsy were identified from the beginning and led to the use of such labels as essential narcolepsy, independent narcolepsy, and non–rapid eye movement (NREM) sleep narcolepsy.[6,7] Other terms, including idiopathic central nervous system hypersomnolence, functional hypersomnia, hypersomnia with automatic behavior, harmonious hypersomnia, and IH, were also put forward in the 1990 version of the *International Classification of Sleep Disorders* (ICSD). The 2005 version of the ICSD differentiated between IH with long sleep time (>10 hours; polysymptomatic, classic form of IH) and IH without long sleep time (monosymptomatic form). The most recent ICSD (third edition, ICSD-3) now pools both conditions (with and without long sleep time) into one heterogeneous condition because researchers were unable to objectively separate both forms of the disease based on the length of nocturnal sleep; patients above the cut-off of 10 hours of sleep showed no significant differences in daytime sleepiness assessed by the Epworth Sleepiness Scale (ESS), Multiple Sleep Latency Test (MSLT), and no differences in the percentage of subjects with sleep inertia or unrefreshing naps.[8,9] Although recent research provides some intriguing findings, the pathophysiology of IH remains unclear. EDS is a multidimensional complaint and qualitatively different from an increased need for sleep. People with IH present with different expressions of hypersomnolence, typically with a combination of EDS or an increased need for sleep (i.e., hypersomnia when objectively assessed). The absence of a specific biomarker for IH, together with the presence of subtle forms of sleep-disordered breathing and chronic sleep insufficiency that may mimic IH, raises questions about the "true" frequency and clinical picture of IH.

EPIDEMIOLOGY

In the absence of systematic studies, the exact prevalence and incidence of IH remain unknown. A few reports suggest that patients with IH represent only about 1% of patients seen in neurologic sleep centers and are 5 to 10 times less common than people with narcolepsy.[8,10] Hence, the prevalence of IH in the general population may be estimated at approximately 50 per million people, a figure much lower than the 300 to 600 per million people suggested until the early 1980s.[4,5,11] In a large series published, people with IH represented 1% of 6000 patients seen at a single respiratory sleep center. Because IH was twice less frequent than narcolepsy, questions about the diagnostic accuracy arise.[12-14]

The age of onset of symptoms varies, but it is frequently between 10 and 30 years. In contrast to narcolepsy type 1 (NT1; narcolepsy with cataplexy), the age of onset is sometimes difficult to pinpoint because of the insidious onset of the hypersomnia. When established, symptoms are generally stable and long lasting. Spontaneous improvement in EDS may be observed, however, in up to one-third of patients.[10,12,15] A female preponderance was found in some but not all series.[9,10,12,15]

PATHOGENESIS

Genetic and Environmental Factors

IH can present in families in one- to two-thirds of cases, and these individuals are more likely to have long sleep time. On rare occasions, IH and narcolepsy may occur in the same family.[8,10,16] An autosomal dominant mode of inheritance has been discussed, and females may be affected more frequently[9]; however, no well-done studies in the field have been performed. In a few case series, an association with diabetes or obesity was observed.[10,17]

Given the existence of overlapping features between IH and narcolepsy (see later), there has been an interest in potential human leukocyte antigen (HLA) markers for IH. Despite reports of an increase in HLA-DQ1,[10] -DR5, -Cw2,[18] and -DQ3,[19] and of a decrease of HLA-Cw3,[20] no consistent findings have emerged. HLA typing currently does not play a role in the diagnosis of IH.

A recent study investigated the dynamics of the expression of circadian clock genes in dermal fibroblasts of 10 patients with IH compared with healthy controls. The amplitude of the rhythms in *BMAL1, PER1,* and *PER2* mRNA was dampened in cells from IH patients over two circadian periods, and the overall expression of *BMAL1* was significantly reduced.[21]

Hypersomnolence usually starts insidiously. Occasionally, EDS is first experienced after transient insomnia, abrupt changes in sleep-wake habits, overexertion, mood change, general anesthesia, viral illness, or mild head trauma; however, these potential triggers are not specific to IH.[10]

Neurochemistry

Montplaisir and colleagues found a decrease in dopamine and indoleacetic acid in patients with IH and those with narcolepsy.[21] Faull and associates found dysregulation of the dopamine system in narcolepsy and of the norepinephrine system in IH.[22-24] These metabolic data suggest the possibility of a dysfunction of aminergic arousal systems in IH. Additional experimental and human data give some support to this hypothesis. In the cat, both hypersomnia and disturbances of monoamines can be induced by a lesion of ascending noradrenergic pathways.[25] Cerebrospinal fluid (CSF) hypocretin-1 levels are normal in IH.[15,26-28] Several studies have examined CSF levels of histamine in patients with IH and other central hypersomnias with discordant results.[29-31] Based on a highly sensitive and selective ultraperformance liquid chromatography tandem mass spectrometry assay to quantify simultaneously histamine and its major metabolite tele-methylhistamine, Dauvilliers and colleagues found no differences for these two amines between patients with narcolepsy type 1 (NT1), narcolepsy type 2 (NT2), or IH and patients with a complaint of EDS without any objective underlying etiologies.[31] Moreover, no association was found between CSF histamine and tele-methylhistamine, subjective or objective daytime sleepiness, or use of psychostimulants.

Rye and colleagues examined modulators of gamma-aminobutyric acid (GABA) signaling in patients with non–hypocretin-deficient central nervous system hypersomnia, some of whom met criteria for IH. They found that in the presence of GABA, CSF from these patients enhanced $GABA_A$ receptor function in an in vitro electrophysiologic assay (i.e., a whole-cell patch-clamp recording to measure the potentiation of $GABA_A$ receptor currents).[32] In this assay, inhibitory chloride currents were increased when cells were exposed to GABA combined with CSF from patients with hypersomnia compared with controls. Moreover, flumazenil, a drug that antagonizes the sedative-hypnotic actions of benzodiazepines, reversed this enhancement of $GABA_A$ signaling and may have improved vigilance in some hypersomnolent patients. However, no differences were observed between different central disorders of hypersomnolence (CDH), no correlation was found between GABA potentiation and measures of vigilance, and the bioactive CSF component remains unknown. In addition, even still controversial, these results were not confirmed using an in vitro voltage–clamped *Xenopus laevis* oocyte assay in a different population of patients with well-characterized IH compared with patients with NT1 and controls.[33-35] In this study, no potentiation of GABA–A receptor signaling was found in CDH, with no significant differences between hypocretin– and non–hypocretin–deficient patients compared with neurologic controls and control subjects with only subjective reports of sleepiness. Further studies including well-phenotyped patients are required to better understand the pathophysiology and identify specific biomarkers of IH.

Neurophysiology

Researchers have hypothesized that the sleepiness of IH could be caused by homeostatic and circadian disturbances of sleep regulation as well as deficient activity in arousal systems.

Some investigators have reported an abnormally high level of slow wave activity (SWA) because of either an abnormally slow decay of SWA or to a normal decay of an enhanced level of SWA.[36,37] In another study, patients with IH exhibited reduced cyclic alternating pattern rate in slow wave sleep, suggesting more stable slow wave sleep in IH than in normal subjects but no differences in the percentage of slow wave sleep.[38] A more recent meta-analysis of 10 studies on the nocturnal sleep in IH showed that patients with IH had decreased slow wave sleep percentage and increased rapid eye movement (REM) sleep compared with controls.[39] These findings, which partially contrast with previous observations, suggest an alteration of sleep microstructure in IH, with potentially less restorative sleep and daytime sleepiness in IH.

Reports of increased sleep spindles activity at the beginning and at the end of sleep and of a delayed start (and decline) of melatonin and cortisol secretion suggest a primary circadian deficit in IH.[40,41] Unfortunately, core temperature recordings (a more reliable circadian measure) have not yet been reported in IH.

The detection of delayed and smaller P300 potentials after awakening in IH suggests a cortical activation problem possibly related to sleep inertia, but the origin of this phenomena is unknown.[37,42]

CLINICAL FEATURES

Excessive Daytime Sleepiness

Patients with IH describe a constant, daily EDS that only rarely leads to involuntary naps ("sleep attacks"). The Epworth Sleepiness Scale (ESS) score is typically increased (>11/24). As with other forms of EDS, alcohol, exercise, heavy meals, and warm environments can accentuate EDS. Daytime drowsiness leads to naps that are usually prolonged (typically >1 hour), and in contrast to patients with narcolepsy, patients with IH typically describe naps as unrefreshing.[10] The unrefreshing quality of napping and the sleep inertia associated with awakenings lead patients to fight sleepiness and avoid naps as long as they can.

Patients who do not nap are particularly prone to episodes of drowsiness and automatic behavior. During these episodes, patients may stare and have purposeful but inappropriate actions resulting from EDS. Patients have reported finding themselves miles from their homes while driving, sprinkling salt on coffee, putting dirty plates in a clothes dryer and turning on the machine, writing incoherent sentences during classes, having loud and irrelevant bursts of speech, and so on. Amnesia of such occurrences is common, although patients are usually aware that they have had one of their "drowsy" episodes when they are later confronted with the results of their automatic behavior.

Some patients with IH, typically with normal sleep duration, may present with symptoms that overlap with narcolepsy. In these narcolepsy/IH "borderland" cases, people report occasional episodes of irresistible sleep as well as short and refreshing naps.[10]

Nocturnal Sleep

Nocturnal sleep is typically reported as subjectively long and undisturbed, usually with more than 10 hours of sleep. In most people with IH, EDS does not improve with prolonged sleep. With unconstrained sleep, people with IH may report sleep times of 12 to 19 hours per day (weekends and holidays).

Patients are hard to awaken and experience sleep inertia, which is a transitional state between sleep and wake, marked by impaired performance, reduced vigilance, and a desire to return to sleep.[43] Sleep inertia is typically described upon emerging from nocturnal sleep, but it can also occur when patients wake from naps. People with IH report being aggressive and verbally and physically abusive during that twilight state if they are awakened, even at their own request. The patient may be confused and unable to react adequately to external stimuli on awakening. The time it takes to "get going" in the morning may be as long as 2 to 3 hours; when severe, it is sometimes called sleep drunkenness (see the work by Evangelista and colleagues[13]). Sleep drunkenness or confusional arousal (also called *syndrome d'Elpénor* after the youngest of Ulysses' comrades who fell to his death during an episode of incomplete awakening) is reported by 40% to 60% of people with IH[5,10,12,13] but can be seen also in other forms of EDS. Sleep inertia is also common when patients are awakened from naps.

Associated Features

Sleep paralysis and hallucinations are common in narcolepsy but less common in IH.[10,28,44] Notably, depressive symptoms have been reported in 15% to 25% of patients with IH.[5,10,15,45,46] Mood changes not qualifying for the diagnosis of affective disorder may precede or follow the onset of EDS and evolve independently. The presence of primary major depression is incompatible with the diagnosis of IH (discussed further later). Migraine- and tension-type headaches are reported in about 30% of people with IH. Pain complaints of other localizations are occasionally observed. Neurovegetative symptoms such as cold hands or feet, lightheadedness on standing up, orthostatic hypotension, or syncope have been observed.[3,10,14,17,18] The frequency of these symptoms is, however, similar in narcolepsy and IH.[14] In case series, patients with IH were found to have increased body mass index.[10,16]

To assess the clinical burden of IH, a recent study developed and validated the Idiopathic Hypersomnia Severity Scale (IHSS).[49] The IHSS is a brief self-report questionnaire to evaluate symptom frequency, severity, and consequences in people with IH. IHSS scores were higher in patients with IH who were drug free than in controls, and lower in treated than in untreated patients, thus showing treatment sensitivity.

DIAGNOSIS

Definition Criteria

The ICSD-3 redefined the criteria of IH, resulting in a more heterogeneous diagnosis than in the previous edition (ICSD-2), which distinguished two forms with and without long sleep time. ICSD-3 diagnostic criteria include the following:

1. More than 3 months' duration of daily periods of irresistible need to sleep or daytime lapses into sleep
2. Absence of cataplexy
3. Fewer than two sleep-onset rapid eye movement periods (SOREMPs) on MSLT (or fewer than one if nocturnal REM latency was ≤15 minutes)
4. The presence of at least one of the following:
   - MSLT showing a mean sleep latency of 8 minutes or less
   - Total 24-hour sleep time of 660 minutes or longer (typically 12 to 14 hours) on 24-hour polysomnography (PSG) monitoring (performed after the correction of chronic sleep deprivation) *or* by wrist actigraphy in association with a sleep log (averaged over at least 7 days with unrestricted sleep)
5. Insufficient sleep syndrome ruled out (if deemed necessary, by lack of improvement of sleepiness after an adequate trial of increased nocturnal time in bed, preferably confirmed by at least 1 week of wrist actigraphy)
6. EDS or MSLT findings that are not better explained by another sleep disorder, medical or neurologic disorder, mental disorder, medication use, or substance abuse. Drugs known to affect sleep, sleep latency, and daytime alertness must be carefully evaluated and should be withdrawn for a minimum of 2 weeks before objective tests.

Some authors recently suggested more stringent criteria for the diagnosis of IH, including severity criteria, as well as a more active exclusion of potential causes of EDS such as sleep deprivation and shift work.[49]

Polysomnography

While not part of diagnostic criteria, typical PSG findings of IH include a short sleep latency and a high sleep efficiency (typically >90%; Figures 113.1 and 113.2).[3,10,12,50] A recent meta-analysis on nocturnal sleep architecture in IH showed increased total sleep time and REM sleep and decreased

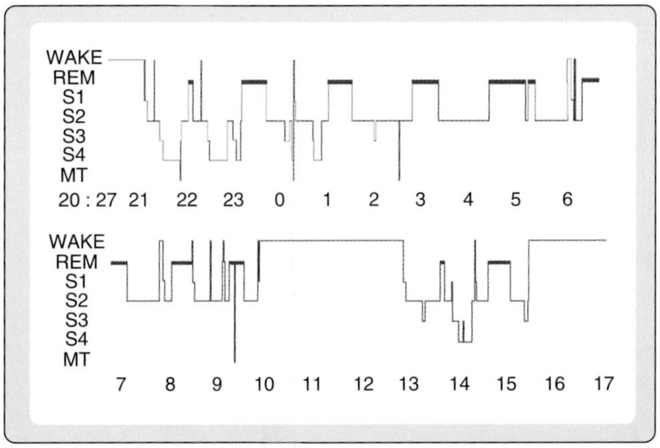

Figure 113.1 A 24-hour continuous hypnogram in idiopathic hypersomnia. A 24-year-old woman presented with excessive daytime sleepiness (EDS), prolonged unrefreshing sleep, and sleep drunkenness. Her Epworth Sleepiness Scale score was 18/24. She had frequent hallucinations while falling asleep or on awakening, but no sleep paralysis or cataplexy. Her body mass index was 24, and she had a positive family history for EDS. The polysomnogram was notable for a sleep efficiency of 98%, sleep latency to NREM 2 sleep of 10 minutes, and slow wave sleep 26% of total sleep time. She had no snoring, apneas, or periodic limb movements. Her Multiple Sleep Latency Test showed a mean sleep latency of 4.8 minutes but no sleep-onset REM period. A 24-hour continuous polysomnogram revealed a total nighttime sleep time of 12 hours, 44 minutes and daytime sleep of 2 hours, 36 minutes (a single long nap). Hypocretin-1 in cerebrospinal fluid was normal. HLA-DQB1*0602 positive. Psychiatric assessment was normal. Her EDS improved slightly with modafinil up to 600 mg/day, but her sleep inertia was unchanged.

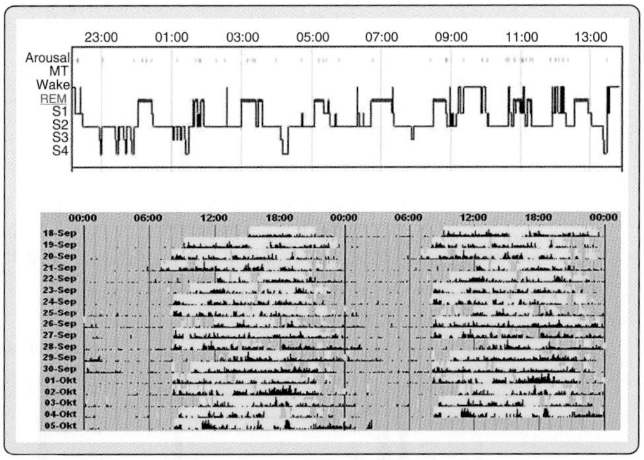

Figure 113.2 Hypnogram and actigraphy in idiopathic hypersomnia. A 32-year-old man presented with excessive daytime sleepiness (EDS), prolonged unrefreshing sleep up to 13 to 18 hours, and sleep drunkenness. His Epworth Sleepiness Scale score was 19/24. He had occasional sleep paralysis and hallucinations. He had migraine headaches, a body mass index of 27, and no family history of EDS. Polysomnography ad libitum over 16 hours showed a sleep efficiency of 92% with a total sleep time of 14.7 hours, latency to NREM 2 sleep of 22 minutes, and slow wave sleep 6% of sleep period time. He had no snoring, apneas, or periodic limb movements. His Multiple Sleep Latency Test showed a mean sleep latency of 4.3 minutes and no sleep-onset REM period (SOREMP). Two weeks of actigraphy revealed a mean sleep time (rest/sleep) over 48% of the recording time. His cerebrospinal fluid hypocretin-1 level was normal, and HLA-DQB1*0602 was negative. Psychiatric assessment was normal. He did not improve with modafinil, methylphenidate, or melatonin.

sleep-onset latency and slow wave sleep percentage relative to healthy persons.[39] These findings are nonspecific and can be seen also in patients with behaviorally induced insufficient sleep syndrome (BIISS; see later). The number of sleep spindles (throughout the sleep period or at the beginning and end of the night) may be elevated in IH[8,40] (Figure 113.3). Sleep-onset REM sleep episodes are rare, and typically the arousal, apnea-hypopnea, and periodic limb movement indexes are low.

Multiple Sleep Latency Test

The MSLT typically shows a mean sleep latency of 8 minutes or less, and a few IH patients have mean sleep latencies of less than 5 minutes.[9,10,12] A SOREMP occurs in 3% to 4% of naps, but never more than once.[10,12]

The MSLT may be of limited diagnostic value in IH patients with long sleep time.[8,9] The first reason is the usual difficulty keeping the patient awake before the test and between sessions of the test. The second reason is the obligation to wake the patient in the morning to perform the MSLT, thus precluding the recording of prolonged nighttime sleep (a typical and diagnostic symptom of IH with long sleep time). Regarding these limits, some patients with IH may have mean sleep latencies longer than 8 or even 10 minutes.[8-10,12] In addition, one study demonstrated poor test-retest reliability of the MSLT in a clinical population of people with non–hypocretin-deficient central nervous system hypersomnias (such as IH) who underwent two diagnostic MSLTs.[51] No correlation was found between the mean sleep latencies on the first and second tests, with a change in diagnosis occurring in 42% of patients because of differences in the mean sleep latencies. Two more recent studies confirmed these findings with the absence of stable PSG-MSLT measures in patients with IH, resulting in frequent diagnostic changes.[52,53]

Other Polysomnography Protocols

Because the typical PSG-MSLT approach has these limitations, a prolonged (up to 24 to 32 hours) continuous PSG on an ad libitum sleep-wake protocol has been proposed as a diagnostic tool for IH.[8] This protocol allows the documentation of a major sleep episode (>10 hours) and of daytime sleep episodes of more than 1 hour duration (see Figures 113.1 and 113.3). Hypersomnia is hence confirmed when there is objective evidence for increased sleep need using actigraphy and PSG. Some researchers have even suggested several 24-hour recordings to ensure that the patient has had sufficient sleep duration.[48,54]

These protocols, however, have several drawbacks. First, standardization and validation are still lacking, especially regarding the level of physical and social activity allowed during the recording. For example, should the patient remain in bed during the full recording or perform some physical activity, and to what degree? Do these prolonged polysomnograms have to be performed in an ambulatory or only in a laboratory setting? Do age and gender modify both night and daytime quantity of sleep obtained in normal controls and in patients with IH? Second, prolonged sleep times are not specific for IH and are seen in patients with hypersomnia related to neurologic disorders and rarely in depressed patients with EDS.[55-58] Third, a standard MSLT would still be required if a diagnosis of NT2 is possible. Fourth, a prolonged PSG recording adds considerable cost to the diagnostic workup.

Based on all these limitations, a recent study quantified the total sleep duration in a 32-hour controlled bed-rest condition protocol preceded by a PSG-modified MSLT procedure in patients with hypersomnolence and controls to better define the sleep duration cut-off for the IH diagnostic criteria.[13] In standardized and controlled stringent conditions, the optimal

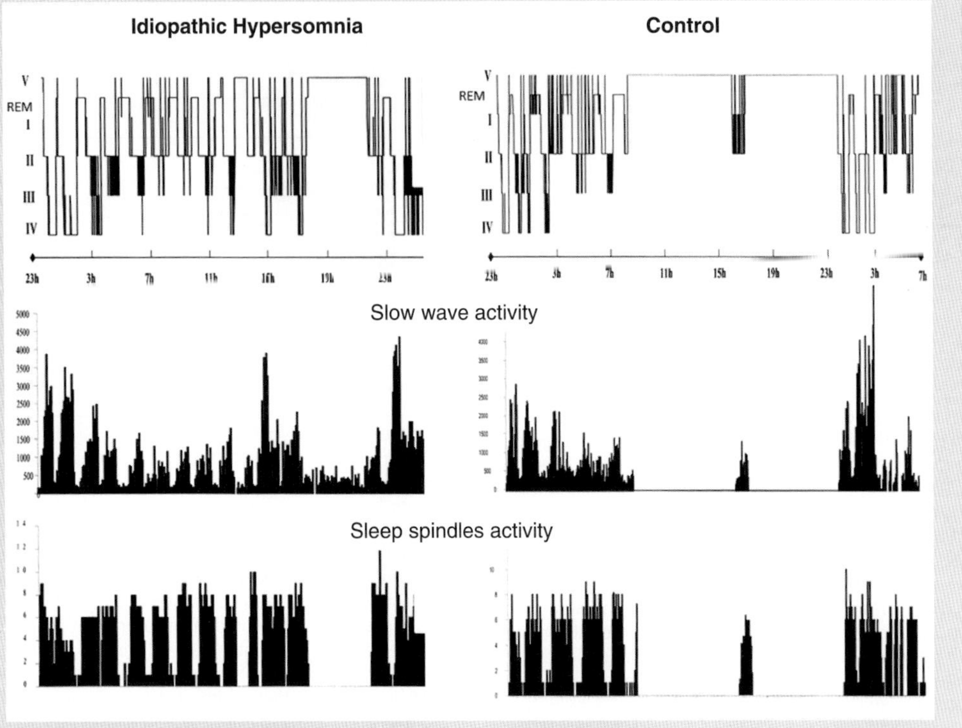

Figure 113.3 Increased sleep, slow waves, and spindles in idiopathic hypersomnia (IH). Prolonged (32 hours) polysomnograms in a 26-year-old woman with IH and long sleep time (*left*) and a 28-year-old control (*right*). The patient with IH has increased total sleep time, persistently high slow wave activity (SWA), and persistent sleep spindles. This patient also has an increase in daytime sleep, including high SWA at about 3 p.m.

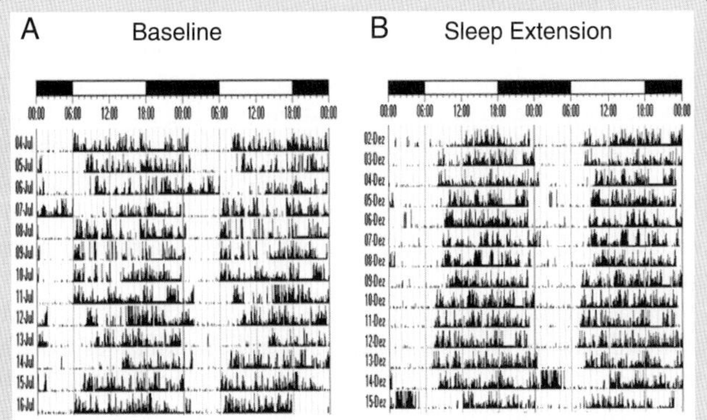

Figure 113.4 Actigraphy in hypersomnia associated with chronic sleep insufficiency. A 22-year-old man presented with excessive daytime sleepiness (EDS) and sleep drunkenness. His initial Epworth Sleepiness Scale (ESS) score was 20/24. He had occasional sleep paralysis on awakening. He had no cataplexy or hallucinations. His body mass index was 24, and there was no family history of EDS. Initially, he denied sleep deficiency. His Multiple Sleep Latency Test showed a mean sleep latency of 6 minutes and 3 sleep-onset REM periods. **A,** Two weeks of actigraphy (during working days) showed irregular sleep-wake rhythms with a mean sleep time (rest/sleep) more than 35% of the recording time. Hypocretin-1 in cerebrospinal fluid was normal. HLA-DQB1*0602 was positive. Psychiatric assessment was normal. **B,** After sleep extension of more than 1 h/day, with a mean sleep time (rest/sleep) more than 41% of the recording time, he had complete resolution of his subjective sleepiness and normalization of the ESS score (4/24).

cut-off best discriminating patients with IH from patients without IH was 19 hours of total sleep over a 32-hour testing period (sensitivity 91.9%, specificity 81.2%). Moreover, patients with shorter sleep latencies on the MSLT also tended to have greater total amounts of sleep.

Actigraphy

Instead of additional 24-hour PSG, ambulatory actigraphy monitoring over several days can demonstrate the prolonged rest episodes characteristic of IH (see Figure 113.2).[16] In addition, actigraphy is helpful to rule out BIISS (see later) and other circadian disorders that may lead to EDS. However, actigraphy protocols have not been standardized or validated in IH, and the differentiation between sleep and rest while awake (clinophilia) is difficult, especially in the context of mild depression.[16] Accordingly, a recent study in a small population of IH showed that actigraphic settings should be carefully considered when estimating sleep duration.[59]

Other Testing

Brain magnetic resonance imaging, HLA typing, and assessment of CSF hypocretin-1 levels are not useful in the diagnosis of IH (see earlier) but may be considered to rule out other causes of EDS.

DIFFERENTIAL DIAGNOSIS

Narcolepsy Type 1 and Type 2

Narcolepsy is a common differential diagnostic consideration, but it is not the most difficult, as demonstrated also by large comparative studies.[8,10,12,14] NT1 is usually easy to diagnose in patients with EDS plus clear-cut (definite) cataplexy, two or more SOREMPs on the MSLT, and low or undetectable CSF hypocretin-1 levels (ICSD-3). Conversely, a diagnosis of IH is supported by long nocturnal sleep times, sleep inertia or drunkenness, high nocturnal sleep efficiency, and only one or no SOREMPs during the PSG-MSLT. As pointed out before, some patients fulfilling the current ICSD-3 criteria for IH report irresistible sleep episodes, as well as short and refreshing naps. On the other hand, patients with NT1 have been reported to present with nonimperative EDS, prolonged naps, and long nocturnal sleep.[10,44,60] People with narcolepsy may initially present as EDS without or with mild or rare cataplexy, and the positive diagnosis may be in doubt for months or even years. Finally, an overlap may exist between IH and NT2 because similar clinical symptoms may be shared in both conditions, and changes in the number of SOREMPs over two consecutive MSLTs occur in patients with central hypersomnolence that may modify the diagnosis. CSF hypocretin-1 level has been found to be normal in most patients with either narcolepsy without cataplexy (80% of patients) or IH (100% of patients).[16,26,27] When low or absent CSF hypocretin-1 levels are found in patients with CDH, even without cataplexy, they are reclassified as having NT1, according to ICSD-3 criteria.

Sleep-Disordered Breathing Syndromes

IH should be distinguished from sleep-disordered breathing syndromes, including upper airway resistance syndrome (UARS).[61] Patients with UARS complain of isolated EDS and snoring. Examinations reveal a triangular face or a steep mandibular plane, a highly arched palate, a class II malocclusion, and, at times, retroposition of the mandible, but patients need not be obese. Cephalometric radiographs have indicated the presence of a small space behind the base of the tongue (posterior airway space), often near the location of the hyoid bone. In one study, a subset of subjects with IH presented with repetitive short ("transient") alpha electroencephalographic arousals lasting 3 to 14 seconds, which regularly interrupted the abnormally high inspiratory efforts that otherwise did meet the definition of hypopneas or apneas.[61] Standard PSG recordings of these subjects evoked the diagnosis of UARS from the presence of these repetitive, transient increases in snoring just before the arousal, and an increase in inspiratory time and a decrease in expiratory time, which were determined with the use of well-calibrated sensors. No significant change in Sao_2 was seen, and the respiratory disturbance index was low (<5/hour).

A nasal pressure cannula and, in rare, doubtful cases, esophageal pressure monitoring must be included in all sleep studies to confirm the diagnosis of UARS. In patients with isolated snoring and IH, a continuous positive airway pressure trial may be warranted. Lack of improvement would support the latter diagnosis.[10,62]

Behaviorally Induced Insufficient Sleep Syndrome, Chronic Sleep Insufficiency, and Long Sleepers

A careful history is needed to differentiate patients with IH from those with BIISS (chronic insufficient nocturnal sleep) who present with EDS.[63,64] The patient should establish a regular sleep-wake schedule and complete sleep diaries (or actigraphy) for at least 2 weeks before PSG. Typically, patients with BIISS sleep 2 to 3 hours longer on weekends than weekdays. PSG and MSLT findings in BIISS may be similar to those in IH (see earlier).

Actigraphy is often necessary to rule out BIIS because the history may be misleading or inconclusive. Particularly difficult is recognizing relative sleep insufficiency in long sleepers. It is possible that besides long sleepers, some individuals may simply be more prone to develop hypersomnolence in association with sleep insufficiency (see Figure 113.4).

Some authors have suggested that IH may represent an extreme phenotype of long sleepers.[8,37] However, patients with insufficient sleep, but rarely those with IH, exhibit a subjective and objective improvement of EDS with prolongation of sleep times or when allowed to sleep ad libitum.

Excessive Daytime Sleepiness/Hypersomnolence Associated with Psychiatric Disorders

Hypersomnia associated with psychiatric disorders (e.g., atypical depression, bipolar depression, dysthymia or neurotic depression, neurotic hypersomnia) can be difficult to differentiate from IH.[65,66] Both conditions can include nonimperative EDS, long unrefreshing naps, long sleep times, sleep inertia, and depressed mood. The term *atypical* or *vegetative depression* has been used for the association of major depression with these symptoms. Particularly difficult is distinguishing between IH and mild depression or dysthymia. PSG findings may be very similar, although patients with hypersomnia associated with psychiatric disorders generally have higher amounts of NREM stage 1, less SWS, and lower sleep efficiency.[67-69] In patients with EDS/hypersomnia associated with psychiatric disorders, the MSLT typically shows normal mean sleep latencies, although up to 25% of these patients may have abnormal MSLT results.[65,70] In addition, these patients may spend a large amount of time in bed and acknowledge much time resting but awake (clinophilia). Patients with hypersomnia associated with psychiatric disorders may exhibit apparent mean sleep times of up to 50% to 60% of the entire actigraphy recording times, but it is uncommon for them to have greater sleep duration on ad libitum PSG compared with healthy controls.[16,71-73] Finally, worse EDS in winter months, obesity, and improved EDS with antidepressants are other typical features of hypersomnia associated with psychiatric disorders, including seasonal affective disorder.

Hypersomnolence associated with psychiatric disorders may also, however, be accompanied by abnormal MSLT findings (in 36% of cases in one series[70]), and conversely, patients with IH may exhibit normal MSLT findings.[11,16,74] In unclear cases, formal psychiatric assessment is needed. Treatment with activating antidepressants (selective serotonin reuptake inhibitors [SSRIs], monoamine oxidase inhibitors [MAOIs], norepinephrine reuptake inhibitors) rather than stimulants may be considered in patients in whom a psychiatric disorder is likely to cause EDS.

Chronic Fatigue Syndrome

Chronic fatigue syndrome (CFS) is characterized by persistent or relapsing fatigue that does not resolve with sleep or rest. One of the clinical difficulties is that CFS is a poorly defined diagnosis, and patients and clinicians may have difficulty differentiating fatigue from a desire for sleep, EDS, and need for sleep. The clinical presentation of CFS is similar to that seen in patients with hypersomnolence associated with psychiatric disorders. In addition to fatigue, patients complain of cognitive difficulties, poor mood, anxiety, fever, and myalgias. In CFS, the PSG may show decreased sleep efficiency and recurrent alpha intrusions, and the MSLT is typically normal. A few patients with CFS may have a specific sleep diagnosis (e.g., sleep apnea, restless legs syndrome [RLS], periodic limb movement disorder [PLMD]).[75]

Restless Legs Syndrome and Sleep-Related Movement Disorders

Sleep-related movement disorders include several conditions such as RLS and PLMD. Patients or bed partners may complain of movements before or during sleep. Nocturnal sleep disturbances and complaints of fatigue and EDS are common.[76]

A clinical interview should address symptoms such as nocturnal restlessness and discomfort of the extremities during periods of inactivity that are relieved with movement. PSG shows periodic and highly stereotyped limb movements during sleep, exceeding more than 15 per hour in adults. PLMD must be interpreted in the context of a patient's related complaint, with an important overlap between symptomatic and asymptomatic patients according to the leg movement index.[113]

Circadian Disorders

EDS during the morning hours in patients with a delayed sleep phase syndrome and EDS during the afternoon hours in patients with advanced sleep phase syndrome may lead to questions regarding the diagnosis. However, an appropriate sleep history, sleep logs covering 15 days, and, if needed, actigraphy indicate a normal total sleep time but abnormal sleep-onset and wake-up times, which differentiates from IH.

Excessive Daytime Sleepiness/Hypersomnolence and Neurologic and Medical Disorders

A medical condition may produce hypersomnolence and mimic IH with EDS, automatic behaviors, prolonged sleep episodes, and sleep drunkenness. EDS usually is associated with other manifestations of the underlying condition. Rarely, hypersomnia, EDS, or fatigue may be the only or main symptom.

Several neurologic disorders may cause hypersomnia and EDS, with large variation in severity and clinical presentation.[77-79] Brain tumors, encephalitis, stroke, and other lesions in thalamus, hypothalamus, or brainstem can cause hypersomnolence that may mimic clinical symptoms of IH but typically also include alteration in sleep continuity and obvious abnormalities on the neurologic exam, including abnormal eye movements, corticospinal weakness, and impaired memory and cognition.[80] Neurodegenerative conditions such as Alzheimer disease, Parkinson disease, or multiple-system atrophy are also associated with EDS and hypersomnia.[81] Although intrinsic hypersomnolence exists in those neurologic disorders, other possible causes of EDS, such as nighttime sleep fragmentation, sleep-disordered breathing, drugs, and periodic limb movements, must be excluded.

Patients with specific genetic disorders (Norrie disease, Niemann-Pick type C, Prader-Willi syndrome, myotonic dystrophy) may present with severe EDS, which can be attributed also to comorbid sleep-related breathing disorders or periodic limb movements.

Hypersomnia and EDS are occasionally observed in diabetes, metabolic encephalopathy (e.g., hepatic, uremic, hypercarbic), hypothyroidism, and acromegaly. The EDS in these conditions may also be attributed to comorbid sleep-related breathing and PLMD. Hypophyseal insufficiency and obesity without sleep-disordered breathing can be associated with apathy, EDS, or hypersomnia.[82,83]

Posttraumatic hypersomnolence is another cause of neurologic hypersomnolence and is discussed in detail in Chapter 32. In a study of patients with traumatic brain injury (TBI) 6 months after injury, 28% of patients reported subjective EDS (ESS score ≥10) and 25% had objective EDS (mean sleep latency on MSLT of <5 minutes).[84] In addition to hypersomnolence, patients post-TBI commonly had nighttime sleep-wake disturbances, impaired memory and concentration, and headaches that were strongly associated with poorer quality of life.

After an acute viral infection (e.g., mononucleosis, pneumonia), patients may develop a (postviral) syndrome of EDS or hypersomnia with features similar to those of chronic fatigue and IH.[85] In some of these patients, an encephalitic process or elevated levels of inflammatory cytokines may play a role.[86,87]

African trypanosomiasis, which is due to the transmission of trypanosomes by tsetse flies, is a frequent cause of severe hypersomnolence in western Africa (*Trypanosoma brucei gambiense*) and eastern Africa (*Trypanosoma brucei rhodesiense*). After an extensive immune reaction during the initial stage, severe sleep and wakefulness impairment follow, and the disorder at this point is referred to as "sleeping sickness." Over the last 20 years, trypanosomiasis has become less common, but it should be considered in travelers and individuals migrating from Africa with EDS.

Periodic Hypersomnias

Periodic and recurrent hypersomnias, including Kleine-Levin syndrome, are usually easy to differentiate from the chronic sleepiness of IH by history alone.[88-92]

Drugs and Substance Use and Abuse

Many medications can cause fatigue, EDS, and hypersomnia, including beta blockers, other antihypertensive agents, dopaminergic agents, antidepressants, and opioids.[93] In doubtful cases, it may be helpful to screen for drugs in urine at the time of MSLT.

TREATMENT

Because the underlying causes of IH are unknown, treatment is symptomatic. Prolongation of sleep times has been suggested[10] but has generally proved to be ineffective for improving daytime function. Still, behavioral approaches and sleep hygiene are always recommended to prevent relative insufficient sleep, with at least 9 hours of sleep per night often recommended in this population. Restriction of time in bed and short duration of planned naps may be advantageous to decrease sleep inertia on awakening but may have little positive impact alone.

The pharmacologic options for IH are similar to the treatments of EDS in narcolepsy. Treatment response, however, is often less frequent and robust than in narcolepsy and especially in patients with prolonged nighttime sleep.[10] Many medications have been tried in IH patients, including the stimulant drugs (i.e., modafinil, methylphenidate, pitolisant, mazindol, and dextroamphetamine) and sodium oxybate, flumazenil, clarithromycin, tricyclic antidepressants, MAOIs, SSRIs, clonidine, levodopa (isolated or in combination), bromocriptine, selegiline, and amantadine. Overall, only about 50% to 70% of patients report significant improvement, most commonly with modafinil or amphetamines.[10,12]

We use modafinil as a first-line treatment for IH. The dose is typically started at 100 mg and gradually increased. The dosage usually prescribed is between 200 and 400 mg/day, taken once or twice a day, with doses up to 600 mg prescribed in some cases, although this is off-label.[94] The most common side effect is headache, and this is less problematic if the dose is increased gradually. A positive effect has also been observed in children with IH.[95] In some series, a good treatment response was found in a more than half of IH patients.[10,12,96,97] Modafinil seems to have good benefit-to-risk ratio in IH, similar to its effect in narcolepsy.[97] Differences between studies are probably due to the more or less strict criteria used by different researchers to exclude other causes of hypersomnia (some of which respond to stimulants). A recent randomized, placebo-controlled study including 33 patients with IH reported that modafinil improved the ESS score but did not improve performance on the Maintenance of Wakefulness Test.[98] Another randomized, crossover, double-blind placebo-controlled trial showed improved driving performance with modafinil in patients with IH in the same way as in narcolepsy.[99]

Other medications that increase monoamine signaling may be effective in IH. Recently, two retrospective studies reported a favorable benefit-to-risk ratio of mazindol (a tricyclic, anorectic, nonamphetamine stimulant) and pitolisant (a wake-enhancing drug that increases the histamine release in the brain by blocking presynaptic histamine-3 reuptake)[100] in drug-resistant patients with hypersomnolence disorders including IH.[101,102] However, sleep inertia often persists in IH despite medication.[8] Treatment with antidepressants (SNRIs, certain SSRIs, and rarely, MAOIs) rather than stimulants may be first considered in patients in whom a psychiatric or depressive disorder cannot be ruled out with certainty. Fantini and Montplaisir reported improvement in half of their 10 patients, in whom melatonin (2 mg of slow-release form at bedtime) was attempted.[62] One retrospective single site study highlighted the potential benefit of sodium oxybate in IH: patients with IH had comparable improvement in EDS to those with NT1, and 71% reported improvement in sleep inertia. However, this study had a high overall dropout rate and patients with IH reported more frequent adverse effects to sodium oxybate than those with NT1.[103] Unpublished (as of the publication of this edition) data from a randomized controlled trial of the lower sodium formulation of sodium oxybate that demonstrated improved Epworth sleepiness scale, Patient Global Impression of Change, and Idiopathic Hypersomnia Severity Scale were submitted to the US Food and Drug Administration (FDA), and the medication was granted approval for the indication of IH in August of 2021. The low sodium formulation of sodium oxybate is the first FDA-approved medication for IH."

Based on the hypothesized abnormal $GABA_A$ receptor activity in IH, researchers have studied the effects of the benzodiazepine antagonist flumazenil. Approximately 63% of 153 patients with central disorders of hypersomnolence reported that flumazenil improved their symptoms in one observational study, but it is unknown how this benefits IH specifically. In addition, adverse side effects included a transient ischemic attack and a lupus vasculopathy (authors note it was unknown if these events were due to flumazenil use).[104] In another study, seven patients with hypersomnia on flumazenil had improved vigilance as assessed by the Psychomotor Vigilance Test and Stanford Sleepiness Scale.[32]

Clarithromycin, an oral agent with potential antagonism of the $GABA_A$ receptor, has also been studied. Clinical experience with clarithromycin has been reported in patients with hypersomnolence refractory to conventional psychostimulants, whose spinal fluid potentiated $GABA_A$ receptor function in vitro.[105] Two-thirds of the patients reported subjective improvement in sleepiness during short-term treatment and 38% with long-term treatment in a single-blinded study, but potential side effects include gastrointestinal problems, antibiotic resistance, and infection. A randomized, placebo-controlled, double-blind, crossover trial of 2 weeks of clarithromycin 500 mg performed in 20 patients with hypersomnolence syndromes (e.g., a mix of IH and NT2, some already treated with wake-promoting medications) showed subjective improvement on the ESS, but no objective improvement on the Psychomotor Vigilance Test.[106]

The recommendations for treating EDS in IH with modafinil or other stimulants is currently based on expert opinion only. Further studies are required to assess both efficacy and safety of these medications in well-designed controlled trials in IH.[107] The FDA approval of sodium oxybate for IH is promising, though greater clinical experience with use of the medication in IH will be revealing. Moreover, employment of validated diagnostic criteria for IH and clinical instruments such as the IHSS that evaluate severity and consequences of major symptoms are required in future clinical trials to more precisely assess responses to treatments.[49]

CLINICAL COURSE AND PREVENTION

The overall psychosocial burden of IH is similar to that of narcolepsy.[108-110,112] At times, the severity of the impairment can place lives in jeopardy; for example, there are reports of patients with IH having automatic behavior episodes resulting in sustained third-degree burns or turning on gas furnaces or stoves without lighting them, leading in one case to a severe explosion.[110] In IH, symptoms may be stable and long lasting, but spontaneous improvement in EDS may occur in up to one-third of patients.[10,12,14,52] No prevention is possible in this disorder.

PITFALLS

Because IH is rare and essentially a diagnosis of exclusion, the main pitfall is failing to make an accurate diagnosis. The terms *EDS, hypersomnolence, hypersomnia, IH,* and *hypersomnia* of unknown origin are not synonymous. Different research groups have historically used different diagnostic criteria, making comparisons across studies difficult. This is particularly true of case series that did not exclude mild forms of sleep-disordered breathing, BIISS, and hypersomnolence associated with psychiatric disorders.

Careful history, sleep questionnaire, actigraphy, full physical examination, overnight PSG, and MSLT are essential for diagnosis and, more important, to rule out other causes of EDS. Demonstration of increased sleep times using prolonged PSG, formal psychiatric testing, CSF hypocretin-1 measurements, and brain magnetic resonance imaging may be necessary in unclear cases to confirm the diagnosis and rule out other causes of EDS.

The main controversies relate to (1) the different procedures between sleep centers to diagnose patients with IH around the world, (2) the clinical and neurophysiologic overlap between IH and hypersomnolence associated with psychiatric disorders, mild sleep apnea, NT2, and BIISS; (3) the potential for spontaneous improvement; (4) change in diagnostic category resulting from the low test-retest consistency of the MSLT in IH; and (5) the currently unknown pathophysiology of IH. Further studies are required to understand the pathophysiology of IH, to determine whether there are distinct clinical subtypes of IH (e.g., forms with and without long sleep time), and to validate current and future biomarkers for better diagnosis and personalized treatment. Finally, prospective studies are needed to obtain objective evidence for the efficacy of medications in treating IH and to clarify whether mood changes in IH are consequent to difficulty adapting to the disease or indicate a primary brain dysfunction.[111]

CLINICAL PEARLS

- Clinicians should consider IH in the differential diagnosis of patients with EDS (mean age at onset, 15 to 25 years), prolonged unrefreshing sleep, and difficulty waking up in the morning or after a nap.
- Before diagnosing IH, clinicians should rule out other causes of EDS, including insufficient sleep syndrome, atypical forms of depression, sleep apnea syndrome, and narcolepsy.
- The symptoms of IH are often severe and long lasting, and treatment requires stimulant drugs as in narcolepsy.
- IH can remit in about 20%–40% of patients, and clinicians should periodically reevaluate the diagnosis and treatment plan.

SUMMARY

IH is a rare disorder characterized clinically by EDS with long and unrefreshing naps, prolonged and undisturbed nocturnal sleep, and great difficulty waking up and "getting going" (sleep inertia) after sleep. Physiologically, the key features of IH are PSG findings of high sleep efficiency and long sleep times and MSLT findings of decreased mean sleep latencies and one or no SOREMPs. The pathophysiology of IH is unknown but may include genetic factors and deficient monoaminergic and abnormal GABAergic signaling. In the absence of a specific biologic marker, IH is a diagnosis of exclusion with a broad differential diagnosis, including NT2, atypical forms of depression, circadian rhythm disorder, and BIISS. The response to stimulants is variable, and remission is possible.

SELECTED READINGS

Anderson KN, Pilsworth S, Sharples LD, et al. Idiopathic hypersomnia: a study of 77 cases. *Sleep*. 2007;30:1274–1281.

Bassetti C, Aldritch MS. Idiopathic hypersomnia. A series of 42 patients. *Brain*. 1997;120:1423–1435.

Cook JD, Eftekari SC, Leavitt LA, Prairie ML, Plante DT. Optimizing actigraphic estimation of sleep duration in suspected idiopathic hypersomnia. *J Clin Sleep Med*. 2019;15(4):597–602.

Dauvilliers Y, Dellallée N, Jausssent I, et al. Normal cerebrospinal fluid histamine and tele-methylhistamine levels in hypersomnia conditions. *Sleep*. 2012;35:1359–1366.

Dauvilliers Y, Evangelista E, Barateau L, et al. Measurement of symptoms in idiopathic hypersomnia: The Idiopathic Hypersomnia Severity Scale. *Neurology*. 2019;92(15):e1754–e1762.

Dauvilliers Y, Evangelista E, Lopez R, et al. Absence of γ-aminobutyric acid-a receptor potentiation in central hypersomnolence disorders. *Ann Neurol*. 2016;80(2):259–268.

Dauvilliers Y, Lopez R, Ohayon M, Bayard S. Hypersomnia and depressive symptoms: methodological and clinical aspects. *BMC Med*. 2013;11:78.

Evangelista E, Lopez R, Barateau L, et al. Alternative diagnostic criteria for idiopathic hypersomnia: A 32-hour protocol. *Ann Neurol*. 2018;83(2):235–247.

Lammers GJ, Bassetti CLA, Dolenc-Groselj L, et al. Diagnosis of central disorders of hypersomnolence: a reappraisal by European experts. *Sleep Med Rev*. 2020:101306.

Lavault S, Dauvilliers Y, Drouot X, et al. Benefit and risk of modafinil in idiopathic hypersomnia vs. narcolepsy with cataplexy. *Sleep Med*. 2011;12:550–556.

Lopez R, Arnulf I, Drouot X, Lecendreux M, Dauvilliers Y. French consensus. Management of patients with hypersomnia: Which strategy? *Rev Neurol (Paris)*. 2017;173(1-2):8–18. https://doi.org/10.1016/j.neurol.2016.09.018.

Maski K, Trotti LM, Kotagal S, et al. Treatment of central disorders of hypersomnolence: an American Academy of Sleep Medicine clinical practice guideline. *J Clin Sleep Med*. Published on-line April, 2021.

Mayer G, Benes H, Young P, et al. Modafinil in the treatment of idiopathic hypersomnia without long sleep time-a randomized, double-blind, placebo-controlled study. *J Sleep Res*. 2015;24(1):74–81.

Plante DT. Sleep propensity in psychiatric hypersomnolence: A systematic review and meta-analysis of multiple sleep latency test findings. *Sleep Med Rev*. 2017;31:48–57.

Plante DT. Nocturnal sleep architecture in idiopathic hypersomnia: a systematic review and meta-analysis. *Sleep Med*. 2018;45:17–24.

Rye DB, Bliwise DL, Parker K. Modulation of vigilance in the primary hypersomnias by endogenous enhancement of GABAA receptors. *Sci Transl Med*. 2012;4. 161ra151.

Šonka K, Šusta M, Billiard M. Narcolepsy with and without cataplexy, idiopathic hypersomnia with and without long sleep time: a cluster analysis. *Sleep Med*. 2015;16:225–231.

Trotti LM. Waking up is the hardest thing I do all day: Sleep inertia and sleep drunkenness. *Sleep Med Rev*. 2017;35:76–84.

Trotti LM, Saini P, Bliwise DL, et al. Clarithromycin in γ-aminobutyric acid-Related hypersomnolence: a randomized, crossover trial. *Ann Neurol*. 2015;78:454–465.

Trotti LM, Staab BA, Rye DB. Test-retest reliability of the multiple sleep latency test in narcolepsy without cataplexy and idiopathic hypersomnia. *J Clin Sleep Med*. 2013;9:789–795.

Vernet C, Arnulf I. Idiopathic hypersomnia with and without long sleep time: a controlled series of 75 patients. *Sleep*. 2009;32:753–759.

Yaman M, Karakaya F, Aydin T, et al. Evaluation of the effect of Modafinil on cognitive functions in patients with idiopathic hypersomnia with P300. *Med Sci Monit*. 2015;21:1850–1855.

A complete reference list can be found online at ExpertConsult.com.

Chapter 114

Kleine-Levin Syndrome

Isabelle Arnulf

Chapter Highlights

- Kleine-Levin syndrome (KLS) is a rare remitting-relapsing disease affecting mostly adolescents. It is characterized by episodes lasting 1 to several weeks with hypersomnia, as well as cognitive, behavioral, and psychiatric disturbances.
- Patients are normal between episodes, but after recurrent episodes, 15% develop some residual mild cognitive impairment, and 20% (mostly girls with psychiatric symptoms during episodes) develop psychiatric anxiety and mood disorders.
- The syndrome mostly affects male (two-thirds) and female (one-third) teenagers, but KLS begins before age 12 in about 10% of patients and after age 20 in about 10%.
- The sudden, severe (more than 18 hours of sleep per day), and recurrent hypersomnia plus the mental slowness help differentiate KLS from other psychiatric mimics.
- Derealization (a striking feeling of being in a dream), confusion, and apathy occur in all patients during episodes, while disinhibited behavior (megaphagia, hypersexuality, or lack of politeness) is less frequent. One-third of patients with KLS have psychotic symptoms during episodes.
- The episodes tend to be less frequent and to disappear with advancing age, with less severe hypersomnia. However, 28% of patients have long (>30 days) episodes, and around 15% have no sign of recovery after more than 20 years of the disease.
- Patients with severe episodes may benefit from lithium therapy for preventing episodes, and IV steroids during long episodes.

Kleine-Levin syndrome (KLS) is a rare disease characterized by recurrent episodes of severe hypersomnia as well as cognitive, behavioral, and psychological disturbances.[1] The typical presentation is a teenager who was completely normal the day before but who suddenly (usually in a context of flu, alcohol use, or sleep deprivation) looks exhausted, needs to sleep 18 to 20 hours a day, becomes mute, answers just "yes" or "no" to questions, and reports feeling "unreal." The patient sleeps in his darkened room for 1 or 2 weeks, comes out only for brief meals and use of the toilet, and then immediately goes back to bed. The teen stops answering the cell phone and stops using social networks and computer games. After a couple of weeks in most cases, the episode ends with 1 or 2 days of insomnia. The teen is then talkative and resumes normal sleep, cognition, and behavior for several weeks or months until a new episode begins.

Because the hypersomnia is prominent, KLS has been classified among the hypersomnias of central origin, but many symptoms are suggestive of a wider brain dysfunction, perhaps involving the association cortex. These symptoms include exhaustion, mental slowness, severe apathy with loss of spontaneous auto-activation, and a striking derealization that is perceived as highly disagreeable. In some but not all patients, the behavioral changes include various forms of disinhibition similar to frontal lobe dysfunction, including rudeness, ravenous intake of certain foods, or inappropriate overt sexual offers. Blunted or sad mood (with a typically unexpressive face) and possibly hallucinations and paranoiac delusions are other, more psychiatric symptoms. Functional brain imaging is now a widely used research tool in KLS, both between and during episodes (which can be challenging). It shows persistent, reduced activity, mostly in the parietotemporal and mesiotemporal associative cortex.[2,3] The cause of KLS is unknown, but genetic factors may contribute because multiplex families represent 2% to 5% of cases. In addition, inflammatory/autoimmune origins are suspected.[4]

HISTORY

Reports suggestive of KLS are found in the 19th century (Box 114.1).[5] In 1925 Kleine reported on nine patients with periodic hypersomnia (two with increased food intake, and one with menstruation-linked hypersomnia).[6] In 1936 Levin emphasized the association of periodic somnolence with morbid hunger in a single patient.[7] In 1942 Critchley coined the eponym Kleine-Levin syndrome (KLS). He claimed that male gender, onset in adolescence, periodic hypersomnia, compulsion to eat, and spontaneous remission were mandatory characteristics of KLS, dismissing as "doubtful" the previously reported female cases and the patients without hyperphagia.[8] His opinion prevailed[9] until a series of women with KLS[10] as well as numerous patients without hyperphagia[11,12] were reported. After 2000, several large case series from all continents better characterized the spectrum of KLS,[3,11,13-28] finding that in addition to

Box 114.1 REPORT OF THE FIRST PROBABLE CASE OF KLEINE-LEVIN SYNDROME IN 1862

Dr. Wilson, a doctor in the Middlesex hospital (United Kingdom), observed a very remarkable case of "double-mind" in a child. This patient was defiant, timid, and modest; he ate with moderation. In his usual state, he showed by his acts that he had an honest and scrupulous nature, but as soon as the disease reoccurred, he lost all these qualities. He slept a lot, was difficult to arouse, and as soon as he was awakened, he extemporaneously sang, recited, and acted with great ardor and aplomb. When he was not asleep, he ate ravenously. As soon as he got out of his bed, he would go close to another patient's bed and overtly seize, without any scruple, all the food he could find. Apart from this intriguing disease, he was intelligent and skillful (author's translation).[5]

Box 114.2 DIAGNOSTIC CRITERIA OF KLEINE-LEVIN SYNDROME (ICSD-3)

A. The patient experiences at least two recurrent episodes of excessive sleepiness of 2 days' to 5 weeks' duration.
B. Episodes recur usually more than once a year and at least once every 18 months.
C. The patient has normal alertness, cognitive function, behavior, and mood between episodes.
D. The patient must demonstrate at least one of the following during episodes: cognitive dysfunction, altered perception, eating disorder (anorexia or hyperphagia), or disinhibited behavior (such as hypersexuality).
E. The hypersomnia and related symptoms are not better explained by other sleep disorders; other medical, neurologic, or psychiatric disorders (especially bipolar disorder); or use of drugs or medications.

hypersomnia, slowed cognition, apathy, and derealization, only one-third to one-half of patients had socially disruptive symptoms such as hypersexuality and hyperphagia, and not with each episode.[11,15,17] Current KLS research focuses on residual symptoms during "asymptomatic periods,"[17,20,24] functional brain imaging,[3,29] genetics,[22,28] possible autoimmunity,[19] and treatment.[18,26]

CLINICAL FEATURES

Episodes

The international criteria for diagnosing KLS are indicated in Box 114.2.[1] The disease is typically relapsing-remitting (Figure 114.1). KLS episodes start abruptly (i.e., within a few hours) in half of the cases and progressively (i.e., within a few days) in the others.[11] When the end of an episode is sudden, patients frequently experience some insomnia and mild elation for 1 to 3 nights, although this is not the case when the end is gradual. Episodes last a median 13 days, occurring every 3 months on average.[11,17] However, the picture is highly variable, including short episodes (e.g., 7 days) occurring every month in young patients as well as prolonged episodes of 6 months or more with mostly apathy and altered cognition. Prolonged (more than 1 month) episodes are observed in one-third of patients.[11,17] In contrast, some patients (mostly when treated) have mini-episodes of exhaustion and derealization lasting 1 day or even a few hours, which disappear after sleeping.[18] In most patients, the episodes are monophasic, with all symptoms always present during the full episode, while some rarer patients have biphasic episodes, consisting of a first phase of excitation, disinhibition, and sometimes insomnia for a few days, followed by a longer period of hypersomnia (in this order or in the reverse order). The frequency and duration of episodes are unpredictable. Patients with long episodes at KLS onset usually continue to have long episodes later and longer disease duration.[17] In a series of 108 cases, patients averaged 19 episodes of 13 days' duration.[11] The mean interval between episodes was 5.7 months, with ranges of 0.5 to 66 months. Over the course of several years, the frequency and duration of episodes often lessen[12,13] but are stable after 5 years.[26]

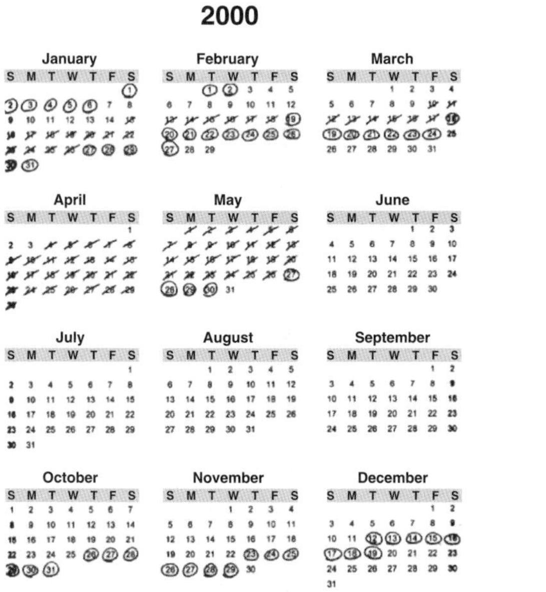

Figure 114.1 Diary of Kleine-Levin syndrome episodes during the first year of disease in a 15-year-old girl as reported by her mother. *Circles* indicate the days with complete hypersomnia, whereas *slashed* days indicate abnormal feelings (derealization, apathy, confusion) but no hypersomnia.

Disease Duration

The episodes tend to be less frequent and then disappear with time. Indeed, most affected teenagers have no more episodes in their 30s.[4,12,13] The accurate disease duration can be only evaluated in patients with long follow-up, especially because patients followed by pediatricians can be lost to follow-up in the transition to adulthood, and because patients may not inform the physician of late relapses (sometimes after 15 years of remission). If one defines the end of the disease as no more episodes after a time that is the double of the longest interval between episodes, the disease duration was evaluated using an actuarial curve as a median of 13.6 ± 4.3 years in a recent series.[11] High episode frequency at the beginning of the disease was associated with a shorter course in a meta-analysis of 168 cases in the literature,[30] but this was not apparent in a recent single-center large study.[17] Male sex, age of onset before 12 or after 20, as well as the presence of hypersexuality during episodes predicted longer disease duration.[4,11] About 15% of patients (including more than half of those with an adult onset) still have recurrent episodes after 25 years of disease.[11,17]

Triggering Events

Eighty-nine percent of patients remembered an event closely associated with disease onset, most often infections (72%; 25% with a cold-like syndrome with fever), alcohol use (23%), sleep deprivation (22%), unusual stress (20%), physical exertion (19%), traveling (10%), head trauma (9%), and marijuana use (6%). In infection-triggered KLS, symptoms of KLS occurred shortly (between 3 and 5 days) after the onset of fever. The agents responsible for the first infection included mostly viruses (e.g., Epstein-Barr, varicella-zoster virus,[11,31] H1N1 and other seasonal influenza,[17,32,33] enterovirus[34]) and *Salmonella typhi*[35] and *Streptococcus*.[36,37] Rare postvaccine onset includes combined typhoid and tetanus vaccine,[36] tuberculosis vaccine,[11] papilloma virus vaccine, and H1N1 vaccine.[17] Factors that trigger relapses are similar, although nothing can be identified in 15% to 20% of recurrences. In a cohort of 30 teenagers in Taiwan with KLS who were carefully followed for at least 2 years, the timing of disease onset and of recurrent episodes correlated significantly (the coefficient of correlation was between 0.45 and 0.55) with community outbreaks of upper respiratory infections such as acute bronchitis, bronchiolitis, pharyngitis, and nasopharyngitis.[15]

SYMPTOMS DURING EPISODES

Some core symptoms are almost always present, at least in the first years of the disease, including hypersomnia, cognitive impairment, derealization, apathy, and psychological changes. The frequency of other symptoms such as hypersexuality, hyperphagia, hallucinations, delusions, and headache varies among patients and between episodes.[15]

Sleep Symptoms

All patients with KLS have hypersomnia, and it is required for diagnosis. One of the major characteristics of hypersomnia during a KLS episode is the extremely prolonged duration of sleep (especially in teenagers) with a median 18 hours of sleep per day. In recent series, sleep was enormously increased during episodes, averaging 18 ± 4 hours per 24 hours.[11,17] Most patients are difficult to awaken and report intense dreaming and frequent hypnagogic hallucinations during episodes. Sleep paralysis is uncommon and cataplexy is absent. However, patients remain arousable, waking up spontaneously to void and eat, but are irritable or aggressive when awakened or prevented from sleeping. Sleep symptoms change from frank hypersomnia during the first episodes to a heavy fatigue accompanied by a feeling "as if in twilight between sleep and waking" during later episodes,[13] especially during long episodes. Most patients have a main, prolonged sleep episode during the night that ends around midday followed by a nonrestorative, long nap in the afternoon. There may be a small window of clarity and wakefulness at around 6 p.m. in the evening.

Cognitive Symptoms

During an episode, the most obvious cognitive sign is bradyphrenia, or slow thinking. Patients look exhausted; they do not initiate conversation and are slow to answer and answer with just "yes" or "no" (examples in Videos 114.1 and 114.2). They are frequently disoriented in time and less often in space. Still, they can write, read, and calculate when asked and can distinguish left from right. What they write or the short messages they send are frequently confused (Figure 114.2). These confused communications can raise concern of alcohol or substance use. Anterograde amnesia is frequent. Some teenagers improperly sent to school during episodes were unable to follow the lessons and complete examinations and had no memory of what they were taught. A mild apraxia is possible: some patients report that they do not remember how to dress with a T-shirt or how to use tools. The patients report that they do not "understand" the world around them: they can watch TV without understanding what happens. Beyond this abnormal mental status, the remainder of the neurologic exam is normal. These findings, together with the frank apathy and derealization, suggest dysfunction of the association cortex during episodes. Altered cognition may persist during a few days or weeks after the end of an episode, especially with episodes that end gradually, so some caution is needed before sending a teenager back to school.

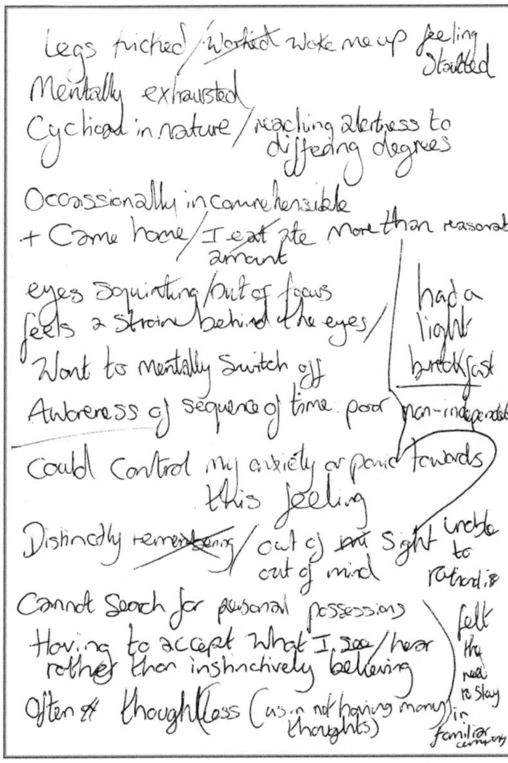

Figure 114.2 Symptom report of an 18-year-old boy with Kleine-Levin syndrome during an episode. Note both the symptoms and the abnormal, sometimes incoherent writing that illustrates his cognitive problems.

Derealization

Almost all (98% to 100%) patients report that the world around them seems unreal, as if they were "in a bubble" or "in a dream,"[38] feeling that their perceptions are unreal or changed, observing the scene from a distant perspective, or as a mind-body disconnect.[3] In contrast, an out-of-body experience is highly unusual. Some young patients have asked their mothers: "Am I dead or alive?"[11] Seeing (like through a glass window, or seeing space in two dimensions and with difficulties discerning contours), hearing (hypersensitivity to noise, voices seeming far), touching, smelling, tasting, feeling cold/hot and pain may feel "wrong," which is unpleasant and leads some patients to test their environment by, for example, spraying fresh water into their faces or counting their fingers to reassure themselves that things are normal. Taking a shower can be disagreeable because patients could see water flowing on their body without feeling it exactly at the same time, in addition to difficulties evaluating its temperature, suggesting difficulties dealing with cross-modal sensory stimulations. Some do not like looking at their face in the mirror, as they can have difficulty recognizing themselves.[3] Patients scored much higher during episodes (70 ± 22) than they did between episodes (13 ± 18) on the Depersonalization/Derealization Inventory.[17]

Apathy

Striking apathy affects almost all patients with KLS.[17] In sharp contrast to their usual teenage habits, patients suddenly stop using their cell phones, playing videogames, watching shows on TV, going on social media, seeing friends, combing their hair, putting on makeup or hair gel, taking showers (unless pushed by their parents), initiating conversation, and/or smoking. Instead, they stay in their rooms lying in bed with window curtains/shutters closed. When observed in the hospital during an episode, they look exhausted, sleeping or keeping their eyes closed, totally unconcerned by the medical interview. Indeed, interviewing the family is much more informative than the patient's interview and examination. The average apathy score on the Starkstein Apathy Scale (range 0 to 40) was 30 ± 8 during symptomatic periods versus 9.5 ± 5 during asymptomatic periods, indicating an almost complete loss of autoactivation.[17] Speaking often seems like it requires an effort. Some patients remain able to mechanically perform their daily routines. A young patient (normally an talented skier) followed his brother during an episode skiing like a robot, without taking any risk or initiative.[4] This complex inability to properly interpret novel environments renders patients unfit to drive during episodes. One of our patients who followed his brother's car while driving during the beginning of an episode inappropriately followed the wrong car more than 600 km, crossed a border, bought gas, and finished in a car crash with complete amnesia of the event. Decreased appetite and decreased sexuality are common (see later).[21]

Disinhibited Behavior

Hyperphagia and hypersexuality are often quoted as characteristic or typical symptoms of KLS,[9,39] yet only 9% to 57% of patients have hyperphagia, and only 18% to 53% have hypersexuality, and these occur only in some but not all episodes.[11,15,17,21,40] Single case reports likely have overreported these symptoms,[9,39] as these were mandatory[41] for KLS diagnosis before the 2005 and 2013 international definitions.[1,42] Hyperphagia is different from bulimia: there is no voluntary vomiting or attempt at controlling weight. Patients are disinhibited toward specific food and good manners, to the point of "stealing candies in their friend's bag," or "eating all available food."[5,43] Some patients report that they eat a large amount of food once a day and immediately resume sleep. Parents may find candies and cakes hidden under the patient's bed. Some patients had obsessive ideas about certain foods (e.g., demanding only orange juice, but 8 L per day). Many patients had some episodes of increased eating, and others had episodes of decreased eating. On the contrary, 34% to 59% of patients actually eat less (as part of the major apathy), sleeping all the time, and when they are called to the family table, they eat mechanically.[17,21,40,44,45]

Hypersexuality affects 18% to 53% of the patients during at least one episode but is unusual in other psychiatric syndromes (which may help recognizing KLS). It is one of the most embarrassing symptoms in public and may lead to forensic problems if not prevented. This mental, physical, and behavioral loss of sexual inhibition affects boys more often than girls (58% versus 35%), with increased masturbations ("to the point of bleeding"), increased demands on their sexual partners, inappropriate sexual behaviors such as exposing or touching oneself, masturbating in the presence of parents and physicians, swearing, asking sexual questions to their teacher, touching a nurse's breast, and making inappropriate proposals.[35,46] As an example, one of our patients mechanically accompanied his family to the beach during an episode. Once in his swimsuit on the beach, he started to overtly masturbate in front of his grandmother, aunt, parents, and little sister. A 13-year-old patient entered the bathroom where his stepmother was taking a shower and proposed sexual relations to her. The plasma levels of sex hormones (testosterone, luteinizing hormone, follicle-stimulating hormone) were normal in 14 patients and mildly decreased in two patients.[30] Importantly, testosterone is not increased during KLS episodes.

Some patients exhibit regressive behaviors such as skipping or playing with one's fingers,[47] speaking with a childish voice (Videos 114.1 and 114.2), using childish words, or asking their mother to sleep nearby them.[11,45] Some parents qualify each episode with a specific (low) mental age. Young patients have tantrums, especially when prevented from rest or sleep, or when brought to medical care.[48-51] Repetitive, compulsive behaviors are also frequent. One-third of patients sing, pace (Videos 114.3 and 114.4), tap, snap fingers, repeatedly listen to the same music, or watch the same video in a continuous loop.[11,15,52,53]

Mood, Anxiety, and Psychotic Symptoms

Flattened affect and sad mood are observed in 50% to 62% of the patients.[11,15,24] Depressive mood tends to be more common among girls than boys.[11,24] Suicidal ideation and thoughts of death are reported by 18% to 22% of patients (mostly in response to the unbearable episode experience, the massive anxiety caused by derealization, or with the idea that the episode would never end), but they rarely led the patients to attempt suicide (1.8%).[24,54,55] The major apathy may have prevented this outcome. When sadness is present, it is associated with rare feelings of guilt or hopelessness, although the cognitions associated with sadness are poor (general cognitive slowness).[24] The abrupt termination of an episode is commonly characterized by a feeling of relief and elation lasting 1 to 3 days, with some logorrhea and a febrile desire to recover the missing time. When an episode ends slowly, the sad mood may persist. Anxiety (52% of patients) can be high during episodes. Patients may fear being left alone at home and can be panicked when left alone in unusual environments such as a hospital, when going outside, or when meeting people.[45] Typically, patients stay in their room, refusing the visits of friends or grandparents. During milder episodes, they are able to stay a few hours in the family room, and in rare cases accept to go out of the house but mostly in non-crowded places. They do not open the door to visitors.

From 33% to 46% of patients report brief, elementary hallucinations (visual: a snake near the bed, a dangerous man with a bear in the hospital lift, auditory: being called by their name, but not any insulting content).[24,45] Delusions, when present, are most often isolated. The predominant delusive ideas are ideas of reference (i.e., the feeling of being scrutinized by others when the patients are outside of their home and a feeling of surrounding hostility). Sometimes patients experience the disagreeable feeling that their uneasiness is perceptible to others. In rare cases, delusive ideas are part of a psychotic-like episode and consisted of interpretations with a theme of persecution (e.g., "There are hidden movie cameras watching me") or with megalomaniacal ideas ("I can drive this plane," "I know where every car is going," and "I am Jesus").[24,56] Psychotic symptoms usually last only a few hours to a few days and stop spontaneously.

Autonomic Symptoms

Headache, photophobia, and painful hyperacousia are frequent. Most patients remain lying in their room in the dark. The face of teenagers during episodes often has an exhausted look, an absence of mimic and an empty gaze. Patients may void less often (e.g., only once a day) and have, in rare cases, urinary retention. Orthostatic hypotension and low 24-hour blood pressure are common, especially if the patient has been spending much time in bed.[21] Other autonomic signs are exceptional. They include abnormally high blood pressure,[44] bradycardia or tachycardia,[57] and ataxic or rapid ventilation.[58,59]

"Asymptomatic" Periods

During asymptomatic periods, patients generally have normal amounts of sleep and no psychiatric or cognitive symptoms (Videos 114.2 and 114.4), normal anxiety, depression, and eating attitude test scores and higher[11] or normal body mass index.[17] One long-term follow-up study reported that 25 patients were in good health several years after the cessation of their KLS episodes, suggesting that complete recovery and a good prognosis are the rule for KLS.[13] However, case reports and recent longitudinal studies partially challenge this rule, indicating that after a mean 5 years of KLS, a subset (15% to 20%) of patients have residual, mild sleep, cognitive, or psychiatric symptoms during "asymptomatic" periods. These recent results should be placed in perspective with abnormal perfusion or metabolism in several brain area in functional imaging during asymptomatic periods.[3]

Residual Sleep Symptoms

In a controlled study, the 120 patients with KLS went to sleep earlier, slept better and longer (half an hour on average), and had higher alertness during the daytime than controls.[17] Whether they spontaneously noticed that sleep deprivation could trigger episodes and consequently had better sleep hygiene than controls, or whether this is a long-term consequence of repeated episodes of hypersomnia is unknown.

Residual Cognitive Symptoms

During asymptomatic periods, cognition is supposedly unaffected.[1] After an episode, teenagers return to school and complete their missed lessons. However, half of them note decreased work or academic performance.[17] Plus, whereas cognitive tests were rarely performed in the 168 cases published between 1925 and 2004,[30] case reports from Sweden have described persistent cognitive impairment, in link with residual hypoperfusion of the temporal lobe between episodes.[16] In a systematic study of cognitive status during asymptomatic periods, the 124 patients with KLS had lower logical reasoning and nonverbal IQ scores, slower processing speeds, reduced attention, and reduced retrieval strategies in episodic verbal memory compared with healthy controls. Specifically, 37% of patients with KLS had altered immediate recall verbal episodic memory, but not delayed recall, indicating difficulties in information retrieval immediately after encoding (pointing to a problem in the frontal-subcortical cognitive network rather than a hippocampal defect). Executive function, visuoconstruction ability, and nonverbal memory were intact. In 44 of these patients, cognitive status was reevaluated 2 years later: processing speed remained reduced and retrieval strategies for verbal episodic memory worsened. Consequently, the 15% of patients with mild cognitive impairment may reduce their workload at school, pause regularly while doing homework, and be given extra time to complete an exam. Cognitive remediation and use of methylphenidate can also be advised on an individual basis.

Residual Psychiatric Symptoms

The question of whether KLS promotes bipolar disease or psychosis in a subsample of patients is recurrent, but the actual information does not support this outcome. Contrasting with the high frequency of siblings affected in patients with bipolar disorders, a familial history of severe depression and bipolar disorder is rare in meta-analysis of cases[30] and similar to controls in two large controlled studies.[11,24] In a cohort of 115 young patients with KLS regularly followed by a psychiatrist, only one patient with KLS developed bipolar I disorder after KLS onset, an expected low percentage, as in the normal population.

However, these regular psychiatric evaluations during follow-up in 115 patients with KLS resulted in new information about comorbid (nonbipolar) psychiatric disorders, which emerged in 21% of patients during asymptomatic periods within an average 5-year period after KLS onset.[24] Mood disorders were particularly prominent (14 of 23), whereas anxiety disorders (7 of 23) and various other disorders (6 of 23, including one with schizoaffective disorder in one, and one with psychotic disorder) were rarer. As anxiety and mood disorders are the most common psychiatric disorders associated with chronic medical illness, this outcome is not surprising. Risk factors for developing psychiatric disorders included female gender, longer KLS course, longer incapacitated time, and more frequent psychiatric symptoms during episodes. Patients with psychiatric disorders were also more often hospitalized in a psychiatric ward, more frequently had minor residual symptoms of anxiety and depression during asymptomatic periods, and had more difficulty adjusting to KLS. The present study suggests paying attention to emerging psychiatric disorders in KLS, especially in patients with female sex, a long disease course, and depression during episodes, to carefully follow them and suggest lithium therapy in this vulnerable subgroup.

CLINICAL SUBTYPES OF THE DISEASE

KLS may be mild, moderate, or severe. In mild forms, teenagers experience 1-week symptomatic periods two to three times a year. In moderate, rapid cycling forms (mostly observed in children and teenagers), patients may experience 7- to 10-day episodes every month.[60,61] Episodes lasting more than 1 month are observed in one-third of the patients, often since disease onset. A recent study suggests that when KLS starts after the age of 20, evolution toward curing may not be absolute, as less than 50% of these patients were cured after 25 years of disease.[11] This last result suggests that in some rare cases, especially adult onset, KLS never fully resolves.

Familial KLS cases are observed in 8% of the cases (corresponding to 4% of multiplex family (see Genetics in Kleine-Levin Syndrome). Their clinical symptoms are similar to those of sporadic cases, although slightly less severe (less frequent episodes, sharper termination of episode, less postepisode insomnia).[22] Siblings do not have the episodes at the same periods of the year.

Menstrual-Related Hypersomnia

When episodes are temporally related with menstruation (just before or at time of), the condition was named "menstrual related hypersomnia"[62] and was reported in only 18 women worldwide.[9] Hypersomnia episodes in these cases are associated with compulsive eating in 65%, sexual disinhibition in 29%, and depressed mood in 35%.[9] Episodes last 3 to 15 days and recur less than three times a year. Of note, a boy with KLS had a sister affected by "menstrual-related hypersomnia."[63] Plus, girls with typical KLS episodes mostly but not exclusively associated with menstruations are reported.[6,33,36] Because these symptoms are similar to those of KLS, menstrual-related hypersomnia is now considered a variant of KLS in ICSD-3. Improvement with contraceptive doses of estrogen and progesterone has been reported in rare cases.[64]

DIFFERENTIAL DIAGNOSIS

As KLS is exceptionally rare, several more common diagnoses should be considered first. When brought to the emergency room during a first episode, most patients undergo a classical workup for acute confusion and sudden behavioral changes in teenagers: checking for alcohol, prescription drug, and illegal substance intake; magnetic resonance imaging (MRI) or other imaging studies to rule out a tumor, trauma, or stroke; or inflammation such as in multiple sclerosis. Tumors within the third ventricle (such as colloid cysts, pedunculated astrocytomas, or, in some cases, craniopharyngiomas) may produce intermittent obstructions of ventricular flow, leading to headaches, vomiting, and a paroxysmal impairment of alertness. An electroencephalogram (EEG) helps to exclude complex partial seizures. A few, nonspecific EEG sharp waves and localized or generalized background of EEG slowing may be observed in up to 70% of KLS cases. Beside basic laboratory tests, checking serum ammonia helps to rule out hyper-ammonemic encephalopathy, carnitine,[65] folate, B_{12}, pyruvate, and lactate levels. Evaluation for possible endocrinopathies and autoimmune diseases, as well as tests for intermittent porphyria and Lyme disease, may be useful. A spinal tap (especially in a context of fever) is usually advised to exclude encephalitis.[66] Severe basilar migraine may mimic KLS but is usually shorter.[17,67]

Differentiating KLS from recurrent psychiatric disorders may be tricky. Recurrent episodes of sleepiness can occur with psychiatric disorders, such as depression, bipolar disorder, seasonal affective disorder, and somatoform disorder.[17,68] Disinhibition may also be prominent in some teenagers with attention-deficit/hyperactivity disorder. Hallucinations and delusions in a previously normal teenager are evocative of brief psychosis episodes. As a consequence, some patients with KLS may be admitted to a psychiatric ward before the correct diagnosis is made. KLS with psychotic symptoms differs from psychotic disorders by the sudden occurrence and disappearance of delusions and hallucinations in KLS, the absence of long-term adherence to the delusional belief, the presence of associated symptoms (mainly hypersomnia, slowness, confusion, and amnesia), and the recurrence of symptoms. The difference between KLS with mood changes and a depressive disorder is how suddenly the symptoms come and go in a previously happy teenager, and the association with cognitive and behavioral symptoms. Sleepiness associated with chronic mood disorders typically alternates with periods of insomnia, while insomnia is very brief (2 to 3 days) in KLS, and only at the onset or offset of episodes. Excessive sleepiness can occur with drug or substance use, obstructive sleep apnea, narcolepsy, idiopathic hypersomnia, or insufficient sleep. In these disorders, however, sleepiness occurs daily and is usually not recurrent; in idiopathic hypersomnia, the level of sleepiness may fluctuate with some "better" periods but sleep still remains prolonged (e.g., 12 to 14 hours/day).[69] "Idiopathic" stupor is a rare and debated entity, occurring usually in middle-age subjects, with stuporous episodes lasting no more than 48 hours, associated with benzodiazepine intoxication.[70]

POLYSOMNOGRAPHY

The polysomnography results depend on whether sleep is monitored only for the night or for 24 hours, at the beginning or the end of episodes, or at onset of the disease or later in its course. Twenty-four–hour polysomnography demonstrates prolonged total sleep time (12 to 14 hours),[12-14] up to 18 hours or more in some reports.[71] In a meta-analysis, the mean total sleep time was 445 ± 122 minutes (N1, 6%; N2, 56%; N3, 19%; rapid eye movement [REM] sleep, 19%) during the night in 40 patients.[30] However, in 15 patients monitored for 24 hours, sleep time was 740 minutes. In a series of 14 patients in Israel, sleep efficiency was decreased, with frequent awakenings and excess stages N1 and N2.[13] Nocturnal sleep time increased from an average 384 minutes during asymptomatic periods to an average of 568 minutes during symptomatic periods.[13] In 17 children with KLS, nighttime slow wave sleep percent was decreased during the first half of episodes, and REM sleep decreased during the second half of episodes.[72] In seven Chinese patients, the nighttime sleep time and structure were normal during KLS episodes.[73]

The results of the Multiple Sleep Latency Test depend on the subject's willingness to cooperate and may either be normal[72] or abnormal with short latencies[73] or multiple sleep-onset REM periods and a narcolepsy-like pattern in up to 21% of patients.[30] With disease development, patients may not sleep continuously but stay in their bed with eyes closed. They report that this attitude is driven by heavy fatigue and reduces the feeling of being unreal.

OTHER TESTS

Spinal fluid studies have shown no abnormalities in cells, protein, or oligoclonal bands. Cerebrospinal levels of hypocretin-1 are mostly within normal range during episodes,[21,43,74,75] although they are one-third lower during symptomatic versus asymptomatic periods,[21] a result that may hardly explain the major hypersomnia during episodes. Dopamine and serotonin metabolism was normal in a cerebrospinal fluid analysis in six patients with

KLS, showing that KLS is not a monoamine biogenic disorder and that apathy may not be related to a hypodopaminergic state.[76] Computed tomography scans and magnetic resonance imaging are normal or contain incidental findings unrelated to the disease. The most interesting tests are brain functional imaging, which are abnormal in most cases (see Pathogenesis).

EPIDEMIOLOGY

The exact prevalence of KLS is unknown, but it is considered as an extremely rare disease, with a prevalence of 3 to 4 per million inhabitants,[11,13,15,17,68] and a yearly incidence of 0.3 new case per million and per year.[17] However, it has been described in all continents and most countries. Whereas cases were initially frequently reported in Israel,[13] KLS seems more common in Jewish populations in the United States,[11] but not in France.[17] The male/female ratio varies from 2 : 1 to 3 : 1.[11,15,17,77] In large series, 80% of the patients had their first episode between 13 and 19 years old, while 10% had it before 13 years old (childhood forms), and 10% (adult forms) started after 20 years old.[11,17,21] The youngest disease onset is 4 years old,[78] while the oldest is 82 years old.[79]

Birth and developmental problems are risk factors for developing the syndrome, with up to one-third of patients in two large series having suffered from delivery or developmental problems.[11,17] In 115 patients (and their family) regularly interviewed by the same psychiatrist, 16.5% of patients had some various psychiatric disorders (anxiety disorders during childhood in 84% of them) preceding the onset of KLS.[24] As this frequency is observed in the general population, there is no indication here that psychiatric disorders in childhood predispose to later development of KLS.

PATHOGENESIS

Mechanism of Symptoms

Many neuropsychiatric KLS symptoms such as derealization, apathy, and disinhibition are suggestive of altered function in association cortex. Possibly, dysfunction of the thalamus, hypothalamus, and basal forebrain contributes to hypersomnia.[2,29] Functional brain imaging during episodes show hypometabolism in the thalamus,[15] hypothalamus, mesialo temporal lobe, and frontal lobe, persisting during asymptomatic periods in half of the patients.[2,3,29] SPECT imaging in 41 patients during asymptomatic periods showed hypoperfusion in the hypothalamus, thalamus (mainly the right posterior area), the caudate nucleus, and cortical association areas (anterior cingulate, orbitofrontal, and right superior temporal cortices) compared with controls (Figure 114.3).[3] Two additional hypoperfused areas emerged during symptomatic periods, located in the right dorsomedial prefrontal cortex (possibly underlying apathy) and the right parietotemporal junction (possibly underlying derealization).[3] Patients with KLS performing a working memory task need to recruit a different network (including increased thalamic activity and decreased cingular activity and adjacent prefrontal cortex, as shown by functional MRI) to achieve similar or lower performances than controls, suggesting a more effortful process and some compensation during asymptomatic periods in patients.[81,82] In 138 untreated patients with KLS studied with FDG-PET/CT during asymptomatic periods, 70% had hypometabolism, mostly affecting the posterior associative cortex and the hippocampus. Hypometabolism was associated with younger age, recent (<3 y) disease course, and a higher number of episodes during the preceding year.[83]

Mechanism of the Disease

The mechanism of KLS is unknown. KLS is probably not a form of epilepsy because epileptiform activity is very rare,[84-86] and the symptoms are not improved by anticonvulsants during episodes. Several mechanisms have been hypothesized to cause KLS, including autoimmune, genetics, and metabolic origin, leading to a localized, recurrent encephalitis.

Brain Examination Suggests a Localized Encephalitis

Neuropathologic examination in four patients with KLS (2 primary and 2 secondary cases) suggests mild localized encephalitis.[58,87-89] Three subjects showed perivascular lymphocytes in the hypothalamus, amygdala, and the grey matter of the temporal lobes, the thalamus, and the diencephalon and

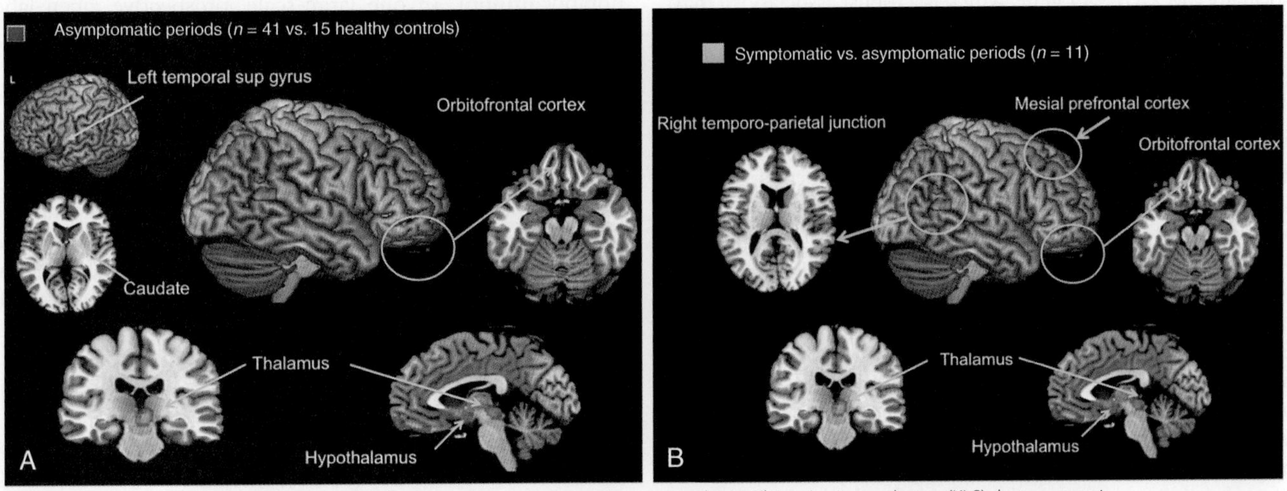

Figure 114.3 Single-photon emission computed tomography in Kleine-Levin syndrome (KLS), between episodes **(A)** and during episodes **(B)**. This group analysis in 41 patients with KLS shows decreased perfusion (*red*) during asymptomatic periods in the hypothalamus, thalamus, caudate nucleus, left temporal superior gyrus, and orbitofrontal cortex, when compared with healthy controls **(A)**. During episodes, the right parietotemporal junction and the right dorsomedial prefrontal cortex show hypoperfusion (*green*) compared with the asymptomatic period **(B)**. The right parietotemporal junction is more hypoactive in patients with more severe derealization.[3]

the midbrain. In the fourth case, a smaller locus coeruleus and decreased pigmentation in the substantia nigra were reported.

Autoimmunity in Kleine-Levin Syndrome

An autoimmune basis for the disorder is suggested clinically by the onset during adolescence, often in conjunction with an infection, a head trauma, and alcohol intake (which increases blood-brain barrier permeability and may promote the passage of antibodies)[90] by the relapsing-remitting aspect, the recurrences and by the partial benefit of IV steroids. To date, no HLA genotype or antibodies are associated with KLS. An association with HLA DQB1*02 in 30 European patients[14] was not replicated in 108 American patients,[11] in 28 children in Taiwan,[15] nor in 120 French patients.[17] Serum cytokine levels are normal during symptomatic and asymptomatic periods in 51 patients with KLS.[19] The recent discoveries of new autoimmune encephalitis with major sleep symptoms (see Chapter 109) should prompt future research into autoantibodies in KLS.

Genetics in Kleine-Levin Syndrome

Although familial risk is low (1% per first-degree relative), 8% of cases have an affected family member, suggesting a 1280- to 6400-fold increased risk in first-degree relatives.[22] Several multiplex KLS families have been reported, including transmission within the same generation (four monozygotic twin pairs,[22,91,92] six siblings,[11,17,43] and vertical transmission (mother-son,[14] fathers-sons,[11] a father and 5 of his 10 children,[93] an uncle and two of his nephews).[17,94,95] Karyotyping is normal in 112 patients from France, except for a patient with sporadic KLS who had a duplication in Xp22.31.[22] Linkage analysis and exome sequencing in a large multiplex KLS Saudian family have identified a low-frequency variant in *LMOD3* (a gene located in chromosome 3, associated with nemaline myopathy).[28] In addition, 7 of 38 European sporadic KLS cases (18.4%) carried an *LMOD3* missense variant and 4 of 51 UK sporadic cases (8.9%) also carry two *LMOD3* variants.[28] Genome-wide association studies of 844 patients found that a gene polymorphism in *TRANK1* (a gene located in chromosome 3 too) is more frequent (OR: 1.48 to 1.54) in affected patients who had birth difficulties than in controls.[28a] All in all, several genes (and especially the *TRANK1* gene, which is a robust association) may increase the risk of KLS without directly causing the disorder.

TREATMENT

General Management

There is no formal established treatment protocol for KLS, although there is class IV evidence of benefit with intravenous steroids for reducing episode duration during prolonged (>30 days) episodes,[26] and with lithium for reducing episode frequency in patients with frequent (>4 per year) episodes.[18] Patients and families benefit from reassurance, simple hygiene rules, and home management. During the episodes, it is recommended to let the patient sleep at home in a familiar environment under family supervision rather than hospitalizing them, given the anxiety related to novelty and the risk of embarrassing public behaviors; therefore this approach promotes patient safety. It is important to explain to the family that attempts to wake up or stimulate the patient are useless and painful. Driving should be firmly forbidden during episodes, as sleepiness, automatic behavior, and altered perception increase the risk of a road accident. The family should regularly check during an episode if the patient drinks and eats enough (in case of reduced eating/drinking) or not too much (in case of hyperphagia), urinates at least once a day (in case of urine retention), and has no suicidal ideas or major aggressiveness (hospitalization will be required in these instances). During asymptomatic periods, patients should keep a regular sleep-wake schedule (as sleep deprivation can trigger episode), avoid alcohol, cannabis, and contact with others who may be infectious.

Medications during Episodes

Once an episode has begun, there is no evidence that medications can stop its development, except for intravenous methylprednisolone 1 g/day for 3 days, which can abort episodes within a median of 7 days in 40% of patients, and, if given within the first 10 days of an episode, more than 60% of patients respond.[26] Because the delay in organizing infusions combined with their delay of action often exceeds 7 days, this agent is not to be recommended for brief (7- to 10-day) episodes, but only for patients who previously had long (>30-day) episodes. Intravenous steroids are well tolerated, with only a few minor side effects (such as insomnia) and no megaphagia or manic switching.[26] In other cases, amantadine (an antiviral and stimulant therapy) could be tried at least once, because it may help abort episodes, as reported by half of patients in a cross-sectional interview.[11]

During episodes, stimulants (modafinil, methylphenidate, amphetamine) may partially improve alertness, but these medications have no effect on apathy, derealization, and confusion, as reported by 20% of patients[11] and by 40% of physicians,[30] so many patients prefer to sleep rather than enduring the derealization. When psychotic symptoms are prolonged and prominent, risperidone seems more helpful than other neuroleptics in retrospective and cross-sectional series.[11,30] In cases in which major anxiety occurs, a benzodiazepine or hydroxyzine can be of some help.

Drugs Preventing New Episodes

When episodes are frequent (e.g., more than 3 to 4 per year), disabling (e.g., with major symptoms such as severe delusion or aggressiveness), or prolonged (e.g., at least one episode longer than 1 month), preventive medications can be suggested, notably lithium. In one large-scale, prospective, open-label controlled study, the benefit–risk ratio of lithium therapy in 71 patients was superior to that of abstention in 49 patients, thereby supporting the idea that lithium has antiinflammatory/neuroprotective effects.[18] When serum lithium levels were kept within 0.8 to 1.2 mmol/L (as measured 12 hours after drug intake), episodes were completely stopped in 35% of patients and were less frequent or less severe in a further 45% of patients, with immediate relapse within 2 days when lithium was discontinued (and only 20% of nonresponders).[18] The potential risks of lithium therapy are thyroid and kidney insufficiency,[96] hence the importance of adequate hydration, and regularly monitoring serum lithium level, thyroid-stimulating hormone, and creatinine.[18] Lithium may be tapered after a few years of complete benefit or after age 30.

Antiepileptic mood stabilizers (e.g., valproate) seem less effective than lithium in our experience.[11,30] In women with menstrual-associated KLS, estrogen-progesterone may be tried,[62] although our team has not seen any obvious benefit (except from preventing undesired pregnancy with severe sexual disinhibition). Antidepressants appear to have no benefit in KLS.[11,30]

CLINICAL PEARLS

- The interview of the patient's family is the most important part of KLS diagnosis as the patient's report is often blurred by amnesia and altered perceptions during KLS episodes. Videos of behavioral changes made by the family during episodes are very helpful. Sleep monitoring during episodes is too inconsistent to aid in diagnosis.
- It is mandatory to document clear-cut episodes (at least two) with altered sleep, cognition, and behavior, as well as clear-cut asymptomatic periods, at least during the first years of the disease. Parents should keep a calendar tracking episodes and good periods.
- The diagnosis is essentially clinical and retrospective, hence the importance of the history, focused on symptoms of apathy (e.g., patient not using their cellphone) and derealization (feeling "in a dream" or "unreal"). Functional brain imaging, which is easily feasible during asymptomatic periods, often shows (70%) mild hypoperfusion of the posterior associative cortex and hippocampus.
- Long (more than 1 month) episodes affect 28% of patients. They can begin with disease onset and are associated with longer disease duration and larger impact on quality of life.
- There is class IV evidence of benefit with intravenous steroids for reducing episode duration during prolonged episodes and with lithium for reducing episode frequency.

SUMMARY

Kleine-Levin syndrome is a rare, remitting-relapsing disease of unknown origin. The disease usually starts during adolescence with a male (66%) predominance, and one-third of patients have a history of birth or developmental problems. It is characterized by recurrent episodes of hypersomnia (>18 hours of sleep/day) lasting 1 to several weeks with cognitive impairment, derealization, apathy, and behavioral changes. Less frequently, episodes include disinhibition with hyperphagia and hypersexuality, or depression, hallucinations, and delusions. Between episodes, patients have normal sleep, mood, cognition, and behavior for 1 to several months, but 15% to 20% of them develop after 5 years of KLS, some emerging mild cognitive impairment or psychiatric disorders. Episodes may be triggered by infection, alcohol intake, or sleep deprivation. Episodes usually become less frequent and less severe by age 30. There is no diagnostic test for KLS, but functional brain imaging is often abnormal, both during and between episodes. Lithium therapy decreases the frequency of the episodes, and IV steroids reduce long episodes' duration.

SELECTED READINGS

Ambati A, Hillary R, Leu-Semenescu S, et al. Kleine-Levin syndrome is associated with birth difficulties and genetic variants in the *TRANK1* gene loci. *Proc Natl Acad Sci U S A*. 2021;118(12). e2005753118.

Arnulf I, Lin L, Gadoth N, et al. Kleine-Levin syndrome: a systematic study of 108 patients. *Ann Neurol*. 2008;63:482–493.Arnulf I, Rico T, Mignot E. Diagnosis, disease course, and management of patients with Kleine-Levin syndrome. *Lancet Neurol*. 2012;11:918–928.

Engstrom M, Latini F, Landtblom AM. Neuroimaging in the Kleine-Levin syndrome. *Curr Neurol Neurosci Rep*. 2018;18(9):58.

Gadoth N, Kesler A, Vainstein G, Peled R, Lavie P. Clinical and polysomnographic characteristics of 34 patients with Kleine-Levin syndrome. *J Sleep Res*. 2001;10:337–341.

Huang Y, Guilleminault C, Lin K, Hwang F, Liu F, Kung Y. Relationship between Kleine-Levin Syndrome and upper respiratory Infection in Taiwan. *Sleep*. 2012;35:123–129.

Huang YS, Guilleminault C, Kao PF, Liu FY. SPECT findings in the Kleine-Levin syndrome. *Sleep*. 2005;28:955–960.

Kas A, Lavault S, Habert MO, Arnulf I. Feeling unreal: a functional imaging study in 41 patients with Kleine-Levin syndrome. *Brain*. 2014;137:2077–2087.

Leu-Semenescu S, Le Corvec T, Groos E, Lavault S, Golmard JL, Arnulf I. Lithium therapy in Kleine-Levin syndrome: an open-label, controlled study in 130 patients. *Neurology*. 2015;85:1655–1662.

Lin C, Chin WC, Huang YS, et al. Different circadian rest-active rhythms in Kleine-Levin syndrome: a prospective and case-control study [published online ahead of print, 2021 Apr 14]. *Sleep*. 2021:zsab096.

Wang JY, Han F, Dong SX, et al. Cerebrospinal fluid orexin A levels and autonomic function in Kleine-Levin syndrome. *Sleep*. 2016;39(4):855–860.

A complete reference list can be found online at ExpertConsult.com.

Section 14

Parasomnias

Chapter 115

Parasomnias and Sleep-Related Movement Disorders: Overview and Approach

Bradley V. Vaughn

Chapter Highlights

- Parasomnias and sleep-related movement disorders are part of a larger group of disorders that produce nocturnal events.
- Parasomnias can be divided into those associated with non–rapid eye movement sleep, those associated with rapid eye movement sleep, and those associated with transitions or no specific sleep stage.
- Sleep-related movement disorders are most commonly present at the transition from wake to sleep or in light sleep.
- The evaluation of parasomnias and sleep-related movements depends on an accurate history and clear description of the events.
- Key features in the history, physical examination, and polysomnography help distinguish the parasomnias and sleep-related movements.
- Parasomnias and sleep-related movements offer an opportunity to diagnose other potential sleep, medical, neurologic, or psychiatric disorders.

Parasomnias and sleep-related movements are part of a larger group of disorders that produce nocturnal events. Most of us envision these nocturnal events as part of entertaining stories from bed partners or roommates. Yet, diligent clinicians understand that these events may result in injuries, sleep disruption, and psychosocial impairment, as well as hold the opportunity to diagnose other underlying sleep or medical disorders provoking the behavior.[1] The larger group of nocturnal events can be typically subdivided into parasomnias, sleep-related movements, or other neurologic, medical, or psychiatric events.

Parasomnias are defined as undesirable physical events or sensory experiences that occur with entry into, during, or arousing from sleep. Many times these events may involve common and usual behaviors, but they also may include bizarre and unusual events, such as seemingly purposeful movements, perceptions, dreaming, and autonomic output.[2] Sleep-related movements are primarily characterized by discrete, usually specific, movements that disturb or fragment sleep.[3]

The *International Classification of Sleep Disorders*, third edition, categorizes parasomnias into three major categories: non–rapid eye movement (NREM) sleep–related parasomnias, rapid eye movement (REM) sleep–related parasomnias, and other parasomnias[4] (Table 115.1). Beyond parasomnias, some patients may have movement disorders that present in the transition period between wake and sleep or during sleep and that can be confused with parasomnias but still represent a risk for harm.[3] Nocturnal events may also include pathophysiology that goes beyond the state of sleep and offers an

Table 115.1 Parasomnia Classification

NREM Sleep–Related Parasomnias
Disorders of arousal (from NREM sleep)
Confusional arousals
Sleepwalking
Sleep terrors
Sleep-related eating disorder
REM Sleep–Related Parasomnias
REM sleep behavior disorder
Recurrent isolated sleep paralysis
Nightmare disorder
Other Parasomnias
Exploding head syndrome
Sleep-related hallucinations
Sleep enuresis
Parasomnia due to a medical disorder
Parasomnia due to a medication or substance
Parasomnia, unspecified

NREM, Non–rapid eye movement; REM, rapid eye movement.

opportunity to diagnose and potentially treat other medical, neurologic, or psychiatric events.[2,3] This section (see Chapters 115 to 122) addresses the classic parasomnias of NREM and REM sleep–related events and reviews the expansion of other parasomnias and movement issues in sleep.

CLASSIFICATION OF PARASOMNIAS

The categorization of nocturnal events has progressed as our understanding of the mechanisms involved with sleep and wake have advanced. Early classification and nomenclature used the nature of the behavior as the prominent distinguishing feature to categorize the events. Some remnants of this convention still exist in terms such as *sleepwalking*, *sleep-related eating*, and *sexsomnia*. However, as we have developed further understanding of the neurologic drivers of sleep-wake states and the components of consciousness, we have grouped events toward the originating sleep-wake state and, to some extent, limited common pathologies.[2,4] The brain's three distinct states allow us to understand that the starting physiologic state provides the substrate for which these parasomnias may exist and form the basis of parasomnias associated with NREM sleep, those associated with REM sleep, and those associated with transitions between wake and sleep.[5] This classification scheme also allows us to move toward a classification structure more aligned with physiology and subsequently underlying pathology.

Some parasomnias may represent a mixture of states.[2,5,6] This model is best exemplified when considering the NREM sleep–related parasomnias or disorders of arousal (see Chapter 116). The disorders of arousal (sleep terrors, sleepwalking, and confusional arousals) are associated with mixture of NREM sleep and wake (Table 115.1). These disorders are most likely not distinct but instead represent a continuum of behaviors that share components of NREM sleep associated with minimal cognitive functioning and amnesia for the events, with features of wake, such as eyes open (Table 115.2). These events are more likely to be triggered by stimuli, occur after sleep deprivation or psychosocial stressors, and involve a variety of nonstereotypic behaviors. Some patients report a memory of vague visual imagery and auditory impressions. Although no clear neuropathology has been uniformly identified, early studies suggest that these individuals may have compromised ability to inhibit or fully permit arousal from sleep.[7,8] Therefore these parasomnias may be an early indicator of other sleep disruption. Similarly, one NREM parasomnia, sleep-related eating disorder, is goal directed toward the behavior of eating. This disorder has some unique characteristics that distinguish it from general sleepwalking and in some patients may also have links to other underlying psychological issues.[8]

Of the REM sleep–associated parasomnias, recurrent isolated sleep paralysis may represent a mixture of wake and REM sleep (Table 115.2; see Chapter 118). Although many times associated with narcolepsy, this disorder in isolation is characterized by the intrusion of REM sleep–related paralysis into wakefulness.[9,10] Other REM sleep parasomnias are confined to the state. Nightmare disorder is typically isolated to REM, but the distressing features carry over into wakefulness (see Chapters 60, 61, and 119).[10,11] REM sleep behavior disorder is an example of neurologic impairment of the circuitry that produces the REM sleep–associated atonia.[10,12] This disorder is characterized by dream enactment, typically violent, and lack of the usual paralysis of REM sleep[12] (Table 115.2). REM sleep behavior disorder has been associated with Parkinson disease, multiple system atrophy, and dementia with Lewy bodies and may predate other symptoms by decades.[12,13] This disorder represents an example of how sleep-dedicated neural circuitry may be uniquely more vulnerable to specific types of degeneration or injury.[14]

Many of the disorders categorized as "other parasomnias" represent events that occur during the transition between wake and sleep (Table 115.1; Chapter 120). Some sensory events, such as exploding head syndrome and sleep-related hallucinations, are events that may occur as the patient enters light sleep but that also may occur on awakening.[4,15,16] Additionally in this group are parasomnias that occur across the spectrum of sleep states or represent a loss of sleep-wake state distinction. Parasomnias can be initiated by medications or other neurologic, psychiatric, or medical disorders.[8,17–21] Some hypnotics with short half-lives have been implicated in initiating parasomnia behavior.[8,17,18] Medical issues that provoke arousals, such as chronic obstructive pulmonary disease or renal disease, have been reported to cause parasomnia behaviors. Parasomnias have been associated with other neurologic degenerative and autoimmune disorders.[19,22] Recent identification of a novel parasomnia disorder associated with antibodies directed toward immunoglobulin-like cell adhesion molecule 5 raise a new pathophysiologic mechanism for nocturnal events.[22,23] Several researchers have postulated the existence of an overlap disorder in which patients lose the neurologic ability to express discrete sleep stages.[24]

Events can also occur during the night that may not be truly part of sleep. Approximately 20% of patients with known epilepsy have seizures occurring predominantly at night, and the behaviors may frequently overlap with those seen in parasomnias.[25,26] The key element is that these events have stereotypic behavior, usually at the beginning of the event. Other neurologic disorders can present with nighttime events, such as confusion in association with delirium or dementia.[27] Psychiatric disorders, such as panic attacks or dissociative events, may be predominantly expressed during the night hours as nocturnal events.[28] Other medical disorders can also evoke arousals with disturbed mentation. Hypoglycemia, from nocturnal insulin administration, can cause arousal with cognitive

Table 115.2 Distinguishing Features of Nocturnal Events

Feature	Disorders of Arousal	Sleep-Related Eating Disorder	REM Behavior Disorder	Recurrent Isolated Sleep Paralysis	Exploding Head Syndrome	Periodic Limb Movements of Sleep	Psychogenic Events	Nocturnal Seizures
Behavior	Confused; semipurposeful movement with eyes open	Eating typically high-calorie foods; eyes open	Sometimes combative with eyes closed	Episodes of inability to move	Painless sensation of explosion inside the head	Typically triple flexion of the leg	Variable	Dependent on the portion of brain involved
Age of onset	Childhood and adolescence	Variable	Older adult	Variable	Adult	Any but more common in adults	Adolescence to adulthood	Variable
Time of occurrence	First third of night	First half of night	During REM	Typically on awakening	Usually near sleep onset but can be variable	More common in the first half of night	Anytime	Anytime
Frequency of events	Less than one per night	Variable	Multiple per night	Variable less than weekly	Rare	Every 10–90 sec	Variable	Frontal seizures: multiple per night
Duration	Minutes	Minutes	Seconds to minute	Seconds to minutes	Seconds	Typically less than 5 sec	Variable minutes or longer	Usually <3 min
Memory of event	Usually none	Usually none or limited	Dream recall	Yes	Yes	Variable	None	Usually none
Stereotypic movements	No	No	No	No	Similar sensation	Yes	No	Yes
Polysomnogram findings	Arousals from slow wave sleep	Arousal from NREM sleep	Excessive electromyogram tone during REM sleep	Arousal from REM sleep	Usually occurs in light sleep	Periodic limb movements	Occur from awake state	Potentially epileptiform activity

NREM, Non–rapid eye movement; REM, rapid eye movement.

impairment typically in the early morning.[21] Similarly, cognitive depressant medications taken before bedtime may also impair cognition in individuals when waking at night.

Sleep-related movements also present a challenge to distinguish. One of the most recognized of these is periodic limb movements in sleep and its contribution to the sensory syndrome of restless legs syndrome (see Chapter 121). This link of restless legs syndrome to periodic limb movements creates a dynamic opportunity to understand the complex world of sensory motor interaction and perception.[29,30] Although most periodic limb movements are relatively subtle, some of these movements can be more dramatic and easily confused with other movement disorders. Other movements in sleep can cause significant sleep disruption or distress (see Chapter 122).[30] These other disorders may be confused with or provide clues to underlying sleep or other neurologic conditions.

APPROACH TO DISTINGUISHING NOCTURNAL EVENTS

The goal of any evaluation of a patient with nocturnal events is to prevent subsequent harm. The initial consultation should focus on the following questions. (1) Is the patient at risk for potential harm or causing harm to someone else? (2) What may be driving the appearance of these events? (3) Are these events indicating another underlying disorder?

In general, one can differentiate parasomnias by looking for key distinguishing features (Table 115.2). The foundation of any evaluation of nocturnal events is a thorough history and physical examination. Although there are no absolutes, the underpinning of the evaluation is based on a clear description of the events from witnesses who can give an accurate testimony of the behaviors. Historical features, such as time of night, duration, frequency of occurrence, behavioral characteristics with each event, eyes open or closed, memory recall, age of onset, and family history of nocturnal events, may help differentiate these disorders.[2,4] The physician should also search for factors that precipitate parasomnias, such as poor sleep environment, improper sleep hygiene, sleep deprivation, circadian rhythm abnormalities, other sleep disorders, medical issues, fever or other illnesses, emotional stress, medication use, and ingestion of alcohol or sedatives before sleep onset.[2,17,18,31] Additional search for other neurologic symptoms, such as decreased sense of smell, constipation, or other autonomic issues, may give clues to REM sleep behavior disorder. Similarly, features suggesting cognitive decline in an adult may provide the opening for further investigation of encephalopathic processes or dementia.

Polysomnography can provide important information in determining the etiology of the nocturnal events, with the goals of capturing the physiology of each sleep state and evaluating the possibility of other contributing sleep disorders.[4] Overnight polysomnography is necessary if the history is atypical, sleepiness is significant, other sleep disorders are suspected, or the patient is at risk for self-harm or harming others (Table 115.3).[32,33] Studies should include complete respiratory monitoring, time-synchronized video monitoring, additional electromyographic recording from all four limbs, a complete set of cephalic electrodes, and ability to extensively review the electroencephalogram.[32–34] Incorporation of a full 10- to 20-electrode array and ability to view the tracing in 10-second windows are necessary in evaluating for seizures and the differentiation of the epileptiform discharges from potential normal variants or artifacts.[34]

Table 115.3 Indications for Polysomnography in Patients with Nocturnal Events

Atypical presentation for a parasomnia (time of night, behavioral description)
Events injurious or with significant potential for injury
Significant disturbance to patient's home life
Unusual age of onset
Events stereotypic or repetitive
Unusual frequency of the events
Patient has excessive daytime sleepiness or complaints of insomnia
Complaints suggestive of sleep apnea, periodic limb movements, or other sleep disorders

CLINICAL PEARL

Disorders of arousal are more common in children but can also present in adults. When patients have a recurrence of somnambulism, sleep terrors, or confusional arousals, the clinician should ask about other features that may be causing arousals. Sleep-related events, such as sleep apnea, limb movements, or even medications, may provoke parasomnias for which the parasomnia is the sentinel symptom hallmarking the other sleep issue.

SUMMARY

Parasomnias as part of a greater group of nocturnal events allow us to examine the interaction of behaviors we associate with wakefulness during sleep. Although we recognize the three normal states of being as wakefulness, NREM, and REM sleep, we understand that these distinct states may not be as distinct as "a flick of a switch" phenomenon. Disruption of the neuronal processes determining a state of being can cause a mixture of these states. Thus behaviors normally accompanying one state may intrude into another. The mechanisms determining the state distinction also may be impaired and allow the mixture of these states, such as in disorders of arousal. This process of state change can be disrupted by disorders causing arousals, such as sleep apnea or poor sleeping environment. Similarly, nocturnal events can be the manifestation of a vulnerability of a neuronal circuit to disease process, such as in REM sleep behavior disorder. In addition, sleep-related movements may be easily misinterpreted as part of a parasomnia, as may other medical, neurologic, or psychiatric disorders. A detailed history and clear description of the events may aid in establishing clues about the underlying etiology. The challenge for the clinician is to recognize the prospect of using these nocturnal events as the trigger to diagnose and treat other underlying issues.

SELECTED READINGS

Dauvilliers Y, Schenck CH, Postuma RB, et al. REM sleep behaviour disorder. *Nat Rev Dis Primers*. 2018;4(1):19.

Erickson J, Vaughn BV. Non-REM parasomnia: the promise of precision medicine. *Sleep Med Clin*. 2019;14(3):363–370.

Foldvary N, Caruso AC, Mascha E, et al. Identifying montages that best detect electrographic seizure activity during polysomnography. *Sleep*. 2000;23:221–229.

Iranzo A. Parasomnias and sleep-related movement disorders in older adults. *Sleep Med Clin*. 2018;13(1):51–61.

Khachiyants N, Trinkle D, Son SJ, Kim KY. Sundown syndrome in persons with dementia: an update. *Psychiatry Investig*. 2011;8:275–287.

Korotun M, Quintero L, Hahn SS. Rapid eye movement behavior disorder and other parasomnias. *Clin Geriatr Med*. 2021;37(3):483–490.

Pedersen MJ, Rittig S, Jennum PJ, Kamperis K. The role of sleep in the pathophysiology of nocturnal enuresis. *Sleep Med Rev*. 2019;49:101228.

Pilon M, Montplaisir J, Zadra A. Precipitating factors of somnambulism: impact of sleep deprivation and forced arousals. *Neurology*. 2008;70:2274–2275.

Proserpio P, Loddo G, Zubler F, et al. Polysomnographic features differentiating disorder of arousals from sleep-related hypermotor epilepsy. *Sleep*. 2019;42(12).

Silber MH, Buchfuhrer MJ, Earley CJ, et al. The management of restless legs syndrome: an updated algorithm. *Mayo Clin Proc*. 2021;96(7):1921–1937.

Stefani A, Högl B. Diagnostic criteria, differential diagnosis, and treatment of minor motor activity and less well-known movement disorders of sleep. *Curr Treat Options Neurol*. 2019;21(1):1.

Zucconi M, Galbiati A, Rinaldi F, Casoni F, Ferini-Strambi L. An update on the treatment of restless legs syndrome/Willis-Ekbom disease: prospects and challenges. *Expert Rev Neurother*. 2018;18(9):705–713. Review.

A complete reference list can be found online at ExpertConsult.com.

Chapter 116

Disorders of Arousal

Alon Y. Avidan

Chapter Highlights

- Non–rapid eye movement (NREM) parasomnias encompass a broad clinical spectrum from mild, nondisruptive episodes, such as mild confusion with sleep talking, to aggressive and potentially injurious motor disturbances such as sleepwalking and sleep terrors. Typically, the episodes last for a few seconds to minutes and are associated with partial or complete amnesia.
- NREM-related parasomnias are thought to take place during an incomplete transition from NREM deep sleep to wakefulness.
- Essential physiologic drives, such as hunger, aggression, and sex, may be manifested by sleep-related eating, violence, or sexual behaviors. Despite their odd and peculiar clinical presentations, NREM parasomnias are readily explainable, diagnosable, and manageable.
- Comorbid sleep disorders, such as sleep apnea, may cause partial arousals that provoke a NREM-related parasomnia event.

DEFINITION

Non–rapid eye movement (NREM)-related parasomnias are defined as undesirable and often abnormal motor or subjective phenomena that arise during arousals from NREM sleep.[1-5] The episodes may include abnormal movements, behaviors, emotions, and autonomic activity, most of which are readily diagnosable and manageable.[2,4,6-9] These parasomnias may occur in response to intrinsic events, such as apneic episodes and fever, or may be triggered by external stimuli.

The third edition of the *International Classification of Sleep Disorders*, third edition (ICSD-3)[10] organizes the NREM parasomnias as follows. Disorders of arousal (DOA) include confusional arousals, sleep terrors, sleepwalking, and sleep-related eating disorder (SRED).[11-13] Sexsomnia is classified as a subtype of confusional arousals but is also associated with sleepwalking. However, some sleep specialists consider it a distinct parasomnia.[14]

CLASSIFICATION OF THE DISORDERS OF AROUSAL

The ICSD-3 diagnostic criteria for the DOA are outlined in Box 116.1.[10] Table 116.1 highlights how unique behavioral manifestation may help differentiate between the various subtypes of DOA. As a rule, all episodes are associated with amnesia. The behavioral episodes commonly begin as partial arousals from stage N3 slow wave sleep and typically are brief but can be protracted, lasting up to 30 minutes.

Universal features of DOA consist of[3,5,15-17]

- Diminished cognition: Impairment or absence of higher cognitive functioning.
- Confused demeanor and stare: During an episode, the eyes are often wide open, with a confused "glassy" stare.
- Absence of or inappropriate response to external stimuli: The patient may be very difficult to awaken, and even when the efforts succeed, the patient does not return to baseline function readily.
- Sudden onset: The patient typically experiences an abrupt to explosive onset associated with a variety of abnormal motor, behavioral, autonomic, or sensory symptoms.

Although patients are typically amnestic, some may report dreamlike mentation or similar altered states of consciousness. Arousals may emerge from any NREM sleep stage but arise primarily from stage N3 sleep and therefore have a propensity to occur during the first third of the night.[18]

DOA are common in children and are typically considered a normal age-related sleep manifestation, generally not requiring specific interventions.[19,20] Predisposing factors include febrile illness, emotional stress, sleep deprivation, alcohol use, a full bladder, and central nervous system (CNS)-acting medications, as illustrated in Figure 116.1.[20-24] In both adults and children, primary sleep disorders such as sleep apnea and disruptive periodic limb movements also may provoke DOA.[25]

PATHOPHYSIOLOGY OF THE DISORDERS OF AROUSAL

Several physiologic mechanisms have been proposed to help explain DOA, but the current prevailing theory is that they occur as a result of an incomplete transition from one sleep state into another.[1,22,26] Sleep stage progression entails the coordination of several neuronal centers for an equivocal declaration of stage. As illustrated in Figure 116.2, vulnerability to incomplete transition is at a maximum between NREM sleep and the awake state. During this period of sleep-stage admixture, the intrusion of one state into another may result in complex behaviors.[17] Some evidence for this admixture rests on studies showing that affected patients may have impaired awakening mechanisms. The partial arousal state may activate discrete central pattern generators in the neuroaxis, producing complex involuntary motor events such as walking, highlighted in Figure 116.3.[27,28]

Box 116.1 ICSD-3 CRITERIA FOR THE DISORDERS OF AROUSAL

All five criteria must be met to establish the diagnosis. The episodes generally emerge during the major sleep episode.[14] The patient generally appears to be disoriented and confused for several minutes or longer after the episode. Because disorders of arousal emerge from stage N3, slow wave sleep, they typically occur during the third or first half of the typical sleep period, or at other periods that deepen slow wave sleep, such as during recovery sleep after sleep deprivation, but very rarely after a daytime nap.

1. Repeated episodes of partial or incomplete awakening from NREM sleep.
2. Patient responds inappropriately, or does not respond to efforts of observers to intervene or redirect him or her during the episode.
3. Little or absent cognition or dream imagery after the event.
4. Fragmented or no recollection of the episode.
5. Absence of other primary sleep disorder, mental disorder, medical condition, medication, or substance use to help explain the disturbance.

Modified from American Academy of Sleep Medicine. *The International Classification of Sleep Disorders, Revised: Diagnostic and Coding Manual.* 3rd edition. Darien, Il: American Academy of Sleep Medicine; 2014.

CLINICAL FEATURES OF DISORDERS OF AROUSAL

The DOA are classified as such based on the following common characteristics: (1) underlying pathophysiology characterized by impaired arousal classically from stage N3 sleep, (2) genetic and familial patterns of inheritance, (3) exacerbation by sleep fragmentation, (4) impaired cognitive functioning during the event, and (5) partial or total amnesia for the event.[3,13,19,26,29,30]

DOA also share unique features based on the following attributes:

Behavior and semiology are usually complex, and clinical features vary. Many times, the patient's eyes are open, and the patient does not seem to interact with his or her environment. Confusional arousals present with abrupt awakening associated with confusion, disorientation, and, at times, utterances of unintelligible speech.[3,19,31] If displacement takes place out of bed, the event is reclassified as sleepwalking and may include a range of behaviors from simple automatic non–goal-oriented behavior, which is common, to more complex, violent, inappropriate, agitated behavior, which tends to be less common.[3,12] The hallmark of sleep terrors is a piercing scream signaling an abnormal arousal associated with increased sympathetic activity and aggression.[32]

Age at onset is often childhood or adolescence with resolution after puberty, but DOA may persist into young adulthood.

Frequency and timing of events is usually a few times per month or week, but rarely with more than one event per night, and the events usually occur in the first half of the night. If they do occur more frequently, the clinician should consider other provocative factors such as sleep apnea contributing to the events.

Duration of events is typically from 20 seconds to minutes and may be protracted, especially when sleep inertia is prolonged.[32]

Table 116.1 Clinical Spectrum of the Behavioral Manifestation of the Disorders of Arousal as a Key for Differentiating among Them Based on the Behavior Observed

Behavioral Semiology	Disorders of Arousal
Arousal progressing to sitting up in bed, verbal confusion, puzzled behavior, and disorientation. If displacement occurs, then categorize as sleepwalking.	Confusional arousal
Arousal followed by confusion, disorientation, automatic behavior, and displacement from the bed. May range from simple automatic non–goal-oriented behavior to more complex, violent, inappropriate, agitated behavior.	Sleepwalking
Eating behavior of edible and nonedible compounds.	Sleep-related eating disorders (subtype of sleepwalking)
Sexually inappropriate behavior, out of character with typical behavior orientated toward bed partner or bystander next to patient.	Sexsomnia (subtype of confusional arousal)
Piercing scream, increased sympathetic response, and aggression. Attempts to interrupt behavior deepen confusion and aggression.	Sleep terror

All episodes are associated with universal amnesia as a rule.
Modified from American Academy of Sleep Medicine. *The International Classification of Sleep Disorders, Revised: Diagnostic and Coding Manual.* 3rd edition. Darien, IL: American Academy of Sleep Medicine; 2014.

Although DOA share these common characteristics, the events are phenomenologically distinguished by their semiology: "a fingerprint" of unique clinical presentations and behaviors. Sleep terrors begin with a sudden explosion of sympathetic activity, distress, and expression of fear, which diminish over time, whereas confusional arousals and sleepwalking rarely begin with distress. Confusional arousals usually consist of normal arousal behaviors, with abnormal duration rarely manifesting in explosive distress or motor behavior.[31-33] Somnambulism consists of normal arousal behaviors at the onset, proceeding to nonagitated motor behavior, including walking with a lack of distress.[34,35] Figure 116.4 extrapolates in a graphic format the spectrum of behavioral manifestations of the arousal disorders, depicting characteristic attributes for each: the duration, the magnitude of displacement or ambulation, and the degree and intensity of distress as a function of time.[30] Occasionally, an admixture of multiple behavior types may wax and wane simultaneously.[30] All events usually emerge out of stage N3 sleep and terminate either in wakefulness or during lighter NREM sleep. The episodes typically are brief (solid lines in Figure 116.4) but may occasionally be

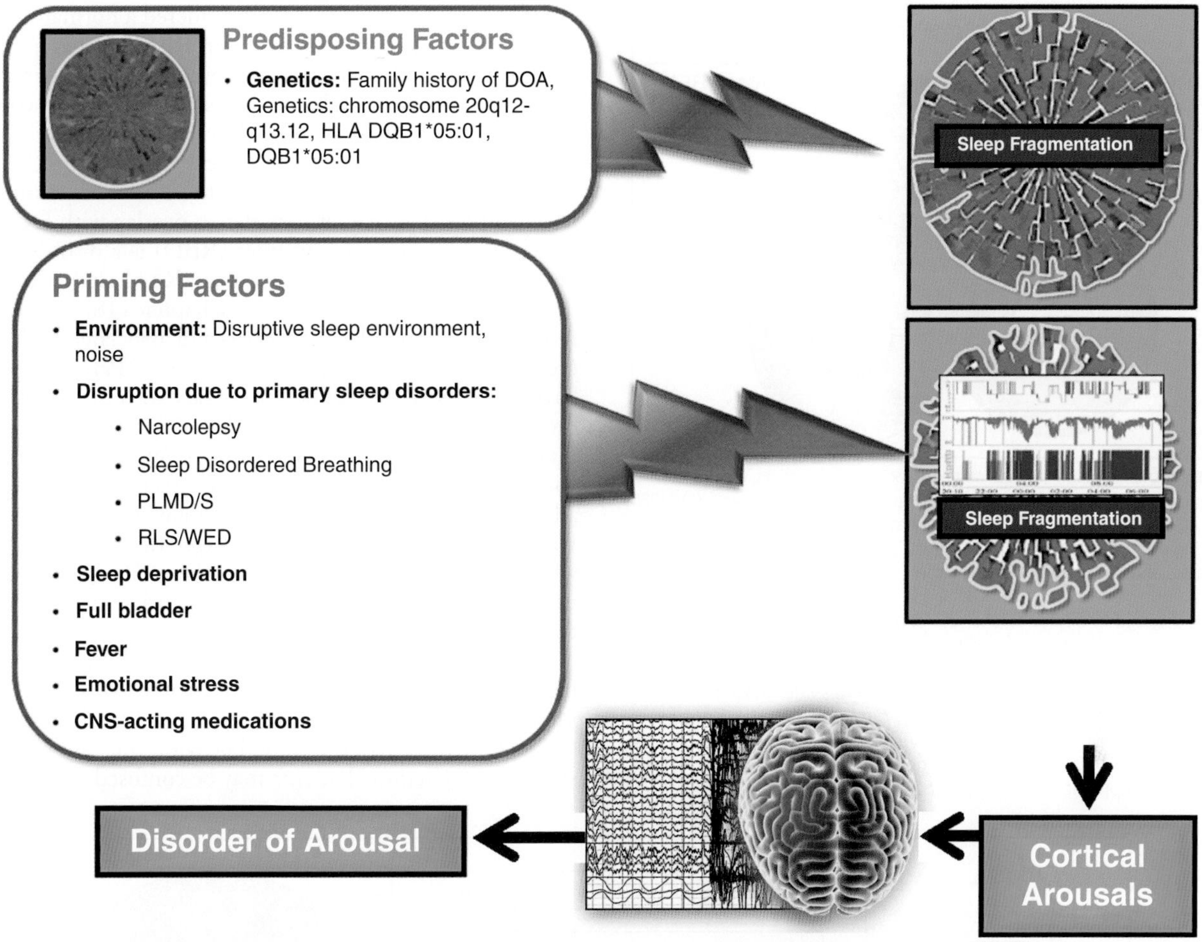

Figure 116.1 Predisposing conditions responsible for the disorders of arousal. Predisposing factors, such as obstructive sleep apnea in this case, lead to fragmentation of sleep architecture as exemplified by the hypnogram highlighting apneic spells (*bottom blue bars*), arousals (*top blue bars*), and oxygen desaturations (*red tracing*). In susceptible individuals (i.e., with a family history of NREM parasomnias), the precipitating factor triggers EEG arousals that lower the threshold for the arousal disorder. CNS, Central nervous system; DOA, disorders of arousal; OSA, obstructive sleep apnea; PLMD/S, period limb movement disorder or syndrome; RLS, restless legs syndrome; WED, Willis-Ekbom disease. (Courtesy of Alon Y. Avidan, MD, MPH.)

prolonged (hatched lines). This may be seen occasionally if an attempt is made by an observer to interrupt the behavior.[30]

CLINICAL EVALUATION OF DISORDERS OF AROUSAL

The evaluation of patients suspected to have DOA should focus on key clinical attributes, ideally with an observer—a family member or bed-partner—to aid in establishing the diagnosis. These key attributes rely heavily on historical features provided by the patient and the observer, as well as a search for other associated features and priming factors.[19,26] In general, patients with NREM parasomnias do not require in-laboratory investigation unless they are at risk of injuring themselves or others or are suspected of having another comorbid sleep or medical disorder, or if the events lead to insomnia, hypersomnia, or impairment in daytime functioning. The key elements of the clinical semiology—the age at onset, frequency, severity, complexity, and duration—are established in the initial evaluation.[1,32] A clear and detailed description of the separate events, from both the patient's and the witness's perspective, is essential to provide focus toward the most likely etiology. Patients may have some type of video recording, usually demonstrating the later portions of an event. Although these recordings can be helpful, important details regarding the start of the events may be missed, as the witness may be asleep. In addition to a detailed history, patients should also undergo a general physical examination and detailed neurologic examination to evaluate for clues of other sleep or neurologic disorders (see Chapter 115). Most of these patients have normal findings, but the presence of physical or neurologic findings may suggest the need for further evaluation. Furthermore, signs of injury should be questioned and considered as to the potential for the patient to have injurious behaviors during events. These findings reinforce the need for polysomnography.[36]

DIFFERENTIAL DIAGNOSIS OF DISORDERS OF AROUSAL

The DOA must be differentiated from other parasomnias and nocturnal events. If the behavior associated with the events is strictly related to eating, then sleep-related eating disorder is considered. Among other NREM events, all of the DOA behaviors may also include a variety of utterances and random dialog; however, talking in sleep in isolation with no

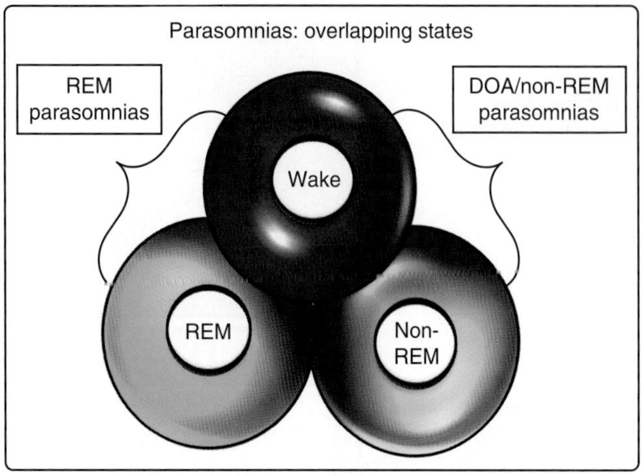

Figure 116.2 Parasomnias as state dissociation disorders. Under various conditions, abnormal admixtures of the three sleep-wake states—(1) NREM sleep, (2) REM sleep, and (3) wakefulness—may occur, with consequent overlap, giving rise to parasomnias. Wakefulness and sleep are not mutually exclusive states, and sleep-to-wake dissociation, incomplete transition, or oscillation from one sleep state to another leads to the parasomnias. Parasomnias are hypothesized to be due to changes in brain organization across multiple sleep-wake states: incursion of wakefulness into NREM sleep leads to the disorders of arousal, and intrusion of wakefulness into REM sleep produces REM sleep parasomnias, of which REM sleep behavior disorder (RBD) is the most dramatic and clinically important. (Modified from Mahowald MW, Schenck CH. Non–rapid eye movement sleep parasomnias. *Neurol Clin*. 2005;23:1077–106, vii; and Avidan AY, Kaplish N. The parasomnias: epidemiology, clinical features, and diagnostic approach. *Clin Chest Med*. 2010;31:353–70.)

other behavior or movement is considered a normal variant.[10] The clinician should also consider REM-related parasomnias, sleep-related epilepsies, and other causes of paroxysmal encephalopathies (see Chapter 115).[30,37,38] The most common two etiologies that need to be differentiated are REM parasomnias and sleep-related epilepsies.[39] Although other nocturnal events can occur, these are the two most common to have features that may, at first glance, overlap with DOA.

REM sleep behavior disorder (RBD) is a disorder of loss of the typical normal atonia of stage REM sleep along with dream enactment behavior (see Chapter 118).[40,41] RBD is more common in older individuals and associated with dream mentation and reasonable recollection.[42] Patients typically have eyes closed, and the behaviors vary with the dream. These events are more common in the latter third of the night and may occur as multiple events throughout the night. Patients with RBD rarely get more than a few feet from the bed, usually instantly waking and realizing their dream enactment.[42] RBD can present in patients younger than 50 years of age, where it coexists with narcolepsy, other NREM parasomnias, use of serotonergic antidepressants, attention-deficit/hyperactivity disorder spectrum, or epilepsy.[43-45]

Sleep-related epilepsies may also occur multiple times during the night or may be only rare events (see Chapter 106). The key finding associated with seizures is that the events usually start with nearly the same behavior, thus are considered stereotypic in nature. Patients may be confused after events or

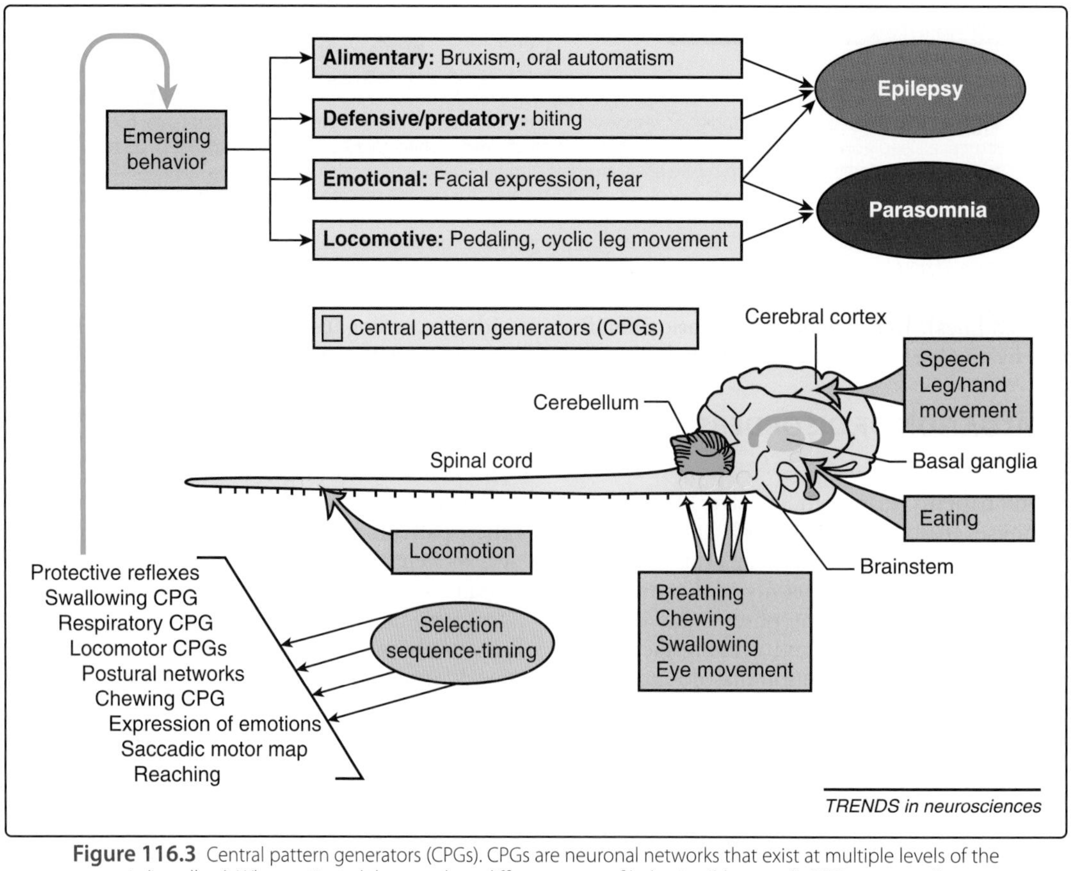

Figure 116.3 Central pattern generators (CPGs). CPGs are neuronal networks that exist at multiple levels of the neuraxis (in yellow). When activated they produce different types of behavior (*blue panel*). CPGs can contribute to monomorphic and stereotyped behaviors in which the pattern is consistent with sleep-related epilepsy or complex (locomotive) polymorphic behavior in which the etiology may attributed to a parasomnia. (Modified from Grillner S. The motor infrastructure: from ion channels to neuronal networks. *Nat Rev Neurosci*. 2003;4:573–586; and Tassinari C, et al. Neuroethological approach to frontolimbic epileptic seizures and parasomnias: the same central pattern generators for the same behaviours. *Rev Neurol (Paris)*. 2009;165:762–8.)

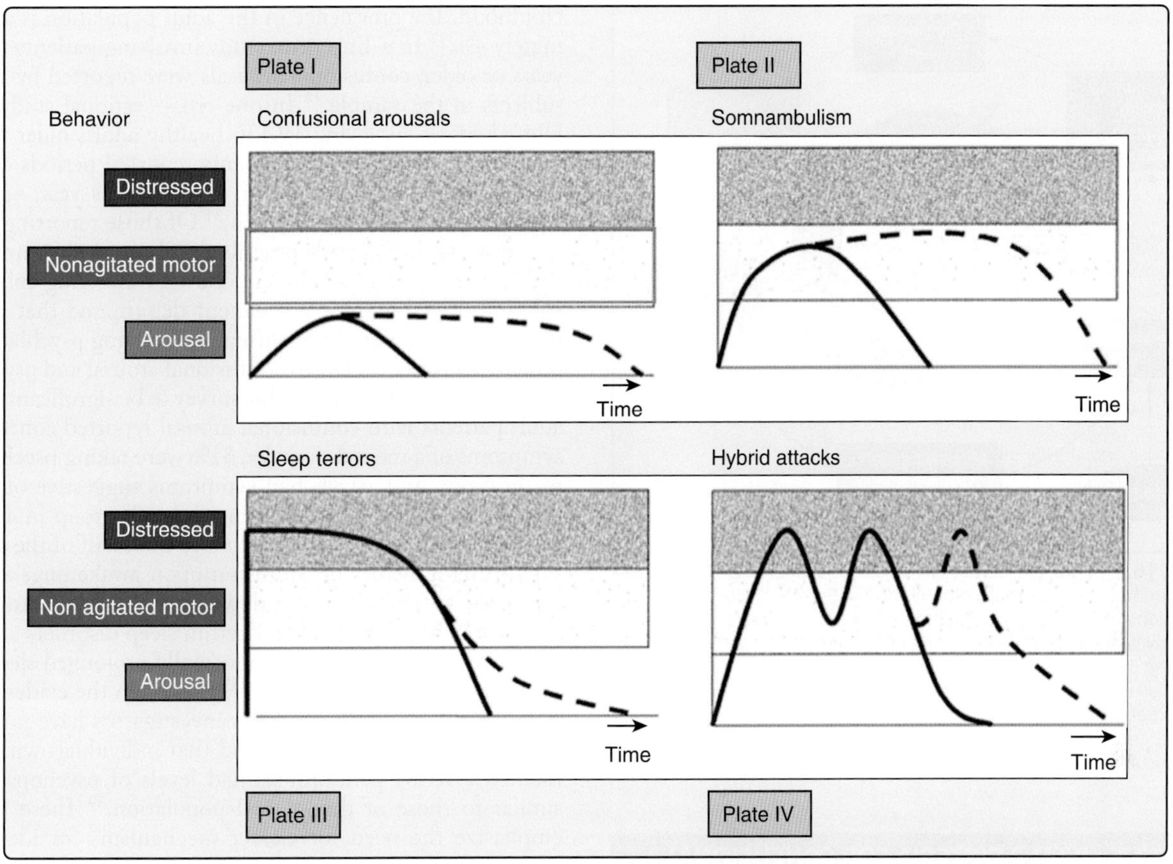

Figure 116.4 Semiology of disorders of arousal as a function of time. Diagrammatic representation of the common behavioral semiologic pattern as a function of time for the key disorders of arousal (NREM parasomnias). Depicted are hierarchical combinations of the three behavior states on the vertical axis (arousal → nonagitated motor → distressed state) as a function of time (1–10 minutes) on the horizontal axis. Plate I represents a typical confusional arousal spell. The parasomnia consists of normal arousal behaviors but of abnormal duration only. Plate II depicts a classic somnambulistic event comprising normal arousal behaviors at onset, proceeding to nonagitated motor behavior. Plate III illustrates a typical episode of sleep terrors, beginning with an intense autonomic discharge, appearance of distress, and experience of predominantly negative emotional behavior typically of sudden onset; motor and normal arousal behaviors usually are also seen during these events, either at onset or thereafter. Plate IV is a mixed type, comprising two different arousal disorders, referred to hybrid attacks or hybrid parasomnias, with waxing and waning of the multiple behavior types. All events usually start in stage N3 NREM sleep and terminate either in wakefulness or in lighter NREM sleep. The episodes typically are brief (*solid lines*) but sometimes can be prolonged (*hatched lines*). Patients who start out with a confusional arousal who experience locomotion and displacement from the bed would be categorized as experiencing somnambulism. (Modified from Derry CP, et al. NREM arousal parasomnias and their distinction from nocturnal frontal lobe epilepsy: a video EEG analysis. *Sleep*. 2009;32:1637–44.)

note complete wakefulness. Memory for the events is highly variable as the seizure must involve both medial temporal lobe structures to cause amnesia.[46] Sleep-related epilepsies typically emerge between the ages of 10 and 20 years but can manifest later in life.[47,48]

In comparison with sleep-related epilepsy, parasomnias are typically less frequent and more complex and polymorphic, as opposed to the stereotypical semiology and higher frequency of events in a given night with sleep-related epilepsy (SRE).[49]

SPECIFIC DISORDERS OF AROUSAL

Confusional Arousals

Essential and Associated Characteristics

Confusional arousals, also referred to as "sleep drunkenness," consist of brief periods of confusion and disorientation after arousal from slow wave sleep.[50,51] To an observer, patients appear confused and disoriented, as they display inappropriate behaviors and slow or poor mentation. The timing of the episodes is most common during the first half of the night, in keeping with the higher propensity for arousal out of stage N3 sleep.[36] Confusional arousals typically last a few minutes and end when the patient falls back asleep (as summarized in Figure 116.5). The episodes are associated with retrograde amnesia (inability to recall past memories after the arousal) and anterograde amnesia (difficulties making new memories after the arousal). Sexsomnias are considered a subtype of confusional arousals and consist of inappropriate amnestic sexual behaviors, sometimes triggered by primary sleep disorders.[52-55] Box 116.2 summarizes diagnostic criteria for confusional arousals as defined by ICSD-3.

The proposed pathophysiology of confusional arousals is an incomplete awakening from slow wave sleep leading to intensification and prolongation of the normal period of sleep

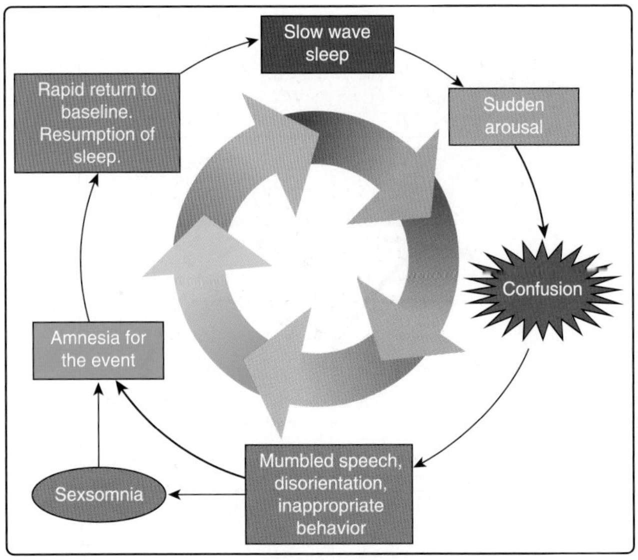

Figure 116.5 Characteristic pattern of confusional arousal. Confusional arousals are sudden and abrupt arousals from deep sleep with demarcated by confusion mentation, inappropriate behavior, and minimal motor or autonomic activity, but typically terminating in rapid return to baseline with amnesia to the preceding event. Sexsomnias are classified by the *International Classification of Sleep Disorders,* third edition (ICSD-3) as a subtype of confusional arousals manifested by inappropriate sexual behaviors typically oriented at the bed partners followed with complete amnesia for the behavior.[14] (Courtesy of Alon Y. Avidan, MD, MPH.)

Box 116.2 ICSD-3 CRITERIA FOR CONFUSIONAL AROUSALS

To establish the diagnosis of confusional arousals, the ICSD-3 requires that the following criteria be met:

1. Repeated episodes of partial or incomplete awakening from NREM sleep.
2. Patient responds inappropriately, or does not respond to efforts of observers to intervene or redirect him or her during the episode.
3. Little or absent cognition or dream imagery after the event.
4. Fragmented or no recollection of the episode.
5. Absence of other primary sleep disorder, mental disorder, medical condition, medication, or substance use to help explain the disturbance.

Modified and revised from American Academy of Sleep Medicine. *The International Classification of Sleep Disorders, Revised: Diagnostic and Coding Manual.* 3rd edition. Darien, IL: American Academy of Sleep Medicine; 2014.[14]

inertia. Predisposing factors may include sleep deprivation and recovery from sleep deprivation, circadian rhythm sleep disorders (especially shift work disorder), fever, sleep-disordered breathing, central nervous system (CNS) depressants (particularly alcohol, sedative-hypnotics, and antihistamines), exposure to stimulants, or any other factor that deepens sleep and increases the arousal threshold.[36,56] Confusional arousals may be experimentally induced by attempts at forced arousal from slow wave sleep and, in adults, during recovery from sleep deprivation.

Demographic Features and Epidemiology

Confusional arousals are almost universal among children younger than 3 years of age and are less common in older childhood. The prevalence in the adult population is approximately 4%.[57] In a European study involving patients aged 15 years or older, confusional arousals were reported by 2.9% of subjects in the sample.[33] In one cross-sectional study in the United States surveying 19,136 healthy adults older than 18 years of age, 15.2% of participants reported periods of mental confusion on awakening in the previous year, occurring equally among men and women.[31] Of those reporting confusion on awakening, 8.6% described full or partial amnesia for the episodes, and 14.8% had nocturnal wandering episodes.[31] In adults, demographic assessment determined that populations at risk include those with an underlying psychiatric disorder. The overlap between confusional arousal and psychiatric comorbidities was found in this survey to be significant: 37% of adult patients with confusional arousal reported concomitant symptoms of a mental disorder, 31% were taking psychotropic medications, and 70.8% had symptoms suggestive of underlying sleep disorders.[31] The same research group in a similar epidemiologic study found that more than half of the subjects supporting a history of confusion upon awakenings also had symptoms of anxiousness or depressive mood.[33,58] Additional risk factors include circadian rhythm sleep disorders and both insufficient sleep, as well as abnormally prolonged sleep, with a duration of 9 hours or longer.[31] Although the evidence does raise important questions, other investigators have not found such a robust link. Labelle found that individuals with documented NREM parasomnias had levels of psychopathology similar to those of the general population.[59] These findings emphasize the need for clearer mechanisms for identifying those with parasomnias.

Objectively Verifiable Indicators

Polysomnographic Features. Confusional arousals represent an admixture of wakefulness into NREM sleep.[36] Patients awaken partially exhibiting marked confusion, slow mentation, disorientation, perceptual impairment, and errors of logic. Polysomnographic recordings during the episodes demonstrate arousals from deep, slow wave associated with brief episodes of delta activity, stage N1 theta patterns, with repeated microsleeps, or a diffuse and poorly reactive alpha rhythm (Figure 116.6).[36] The duration of the episode typically is between 30 seconds and several minutes, and the electroencephalogram (EEG) during the recordings depicts characteristics of stage N3 sleep, with delta-to-theta range activity.[60] Unlike in somnambulism and sleep terrors, motor events in confusional arousals are less complex and typically do not include any form of ambulation or sympathetic activation (as illustrated in Figure 116.7).[60]

Differential Diagnosis

Distinguishing confusional arousals from other paroxysmal disorders, and normal arousals can present a diagnostic challenge (Table 116.2). Confusional arousals are differentiated from other parasomnias, such as somnambulism, by the lack of displacement out of bed or walking. Confusional arousal episodes lack an acute fear component, intense screaming/crying, and increased autonomic hyperarousal, seen with sleep terrors, nor are there the complex dream enactment behaviors of RBD.[17] Unlike in RBD, confusional arousal episodes tend to occur in children during stage N3 sleep and in the first half of the night. Amnesia for the event preceding the arousal is typical in confusional arousals. Complex partial

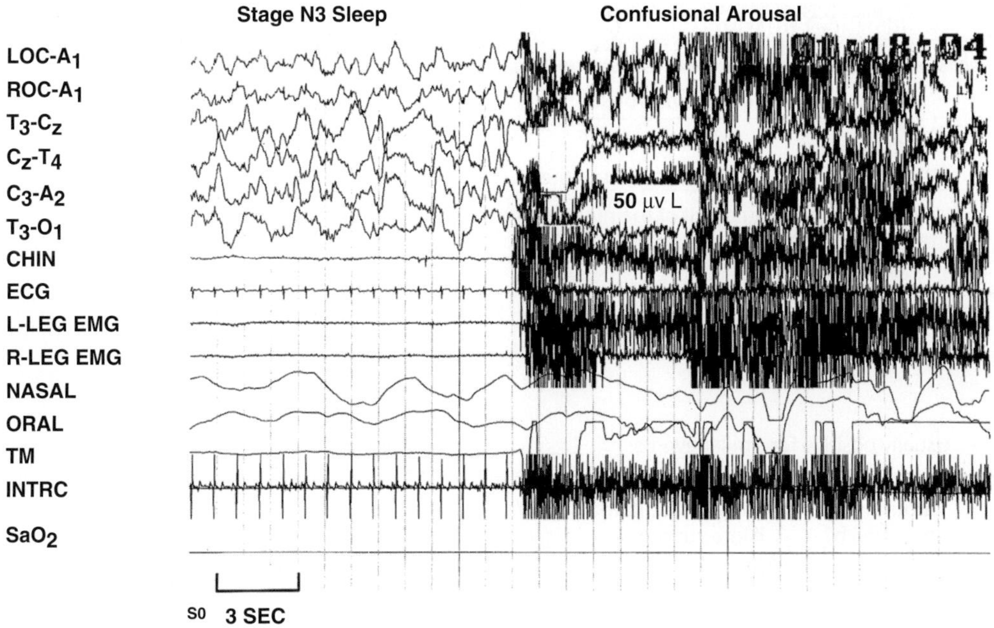

Figure 116.6 A 45-year-old woman with a history of psychosocial stresses presented to clinic with "abrupt awakening from sleep in confusion and panic." A polysomnogram captured her typical spells where she suddenly woke up as she sat up during stage N3 sleep. Her demeanor was frightened and confused, but slowly improved, returning to baseline waking level of cognitive funtioning with vaguely described mental imagery, but without specific recollection of a dream sequence of the specific event.

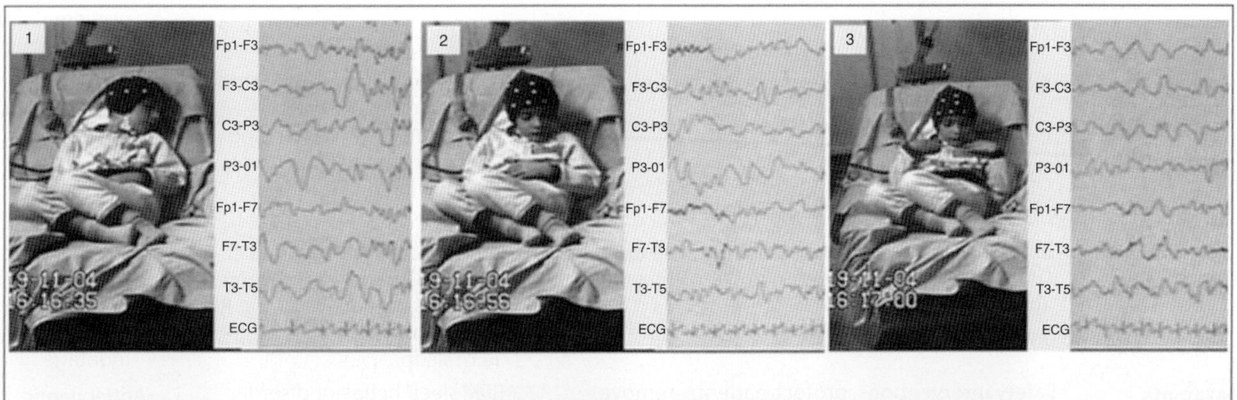

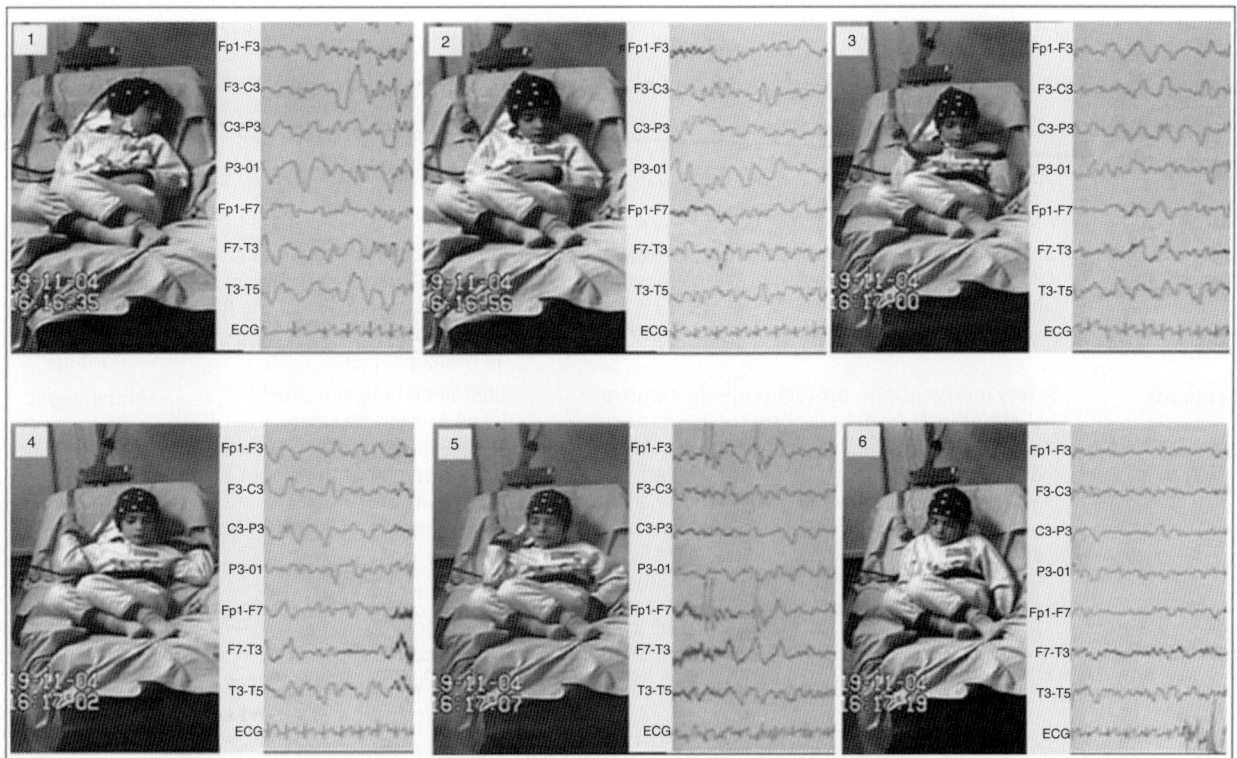

Figure 116.7 A 7-year-old boy with confusional arousals. This parasomnia begins with the patient in stage N3 NREM sleep (1) depicted by delta activity in the right panel of fragment 1. The episode progresses with raising the head (2), placement of the hands on his chest (3), after which he then raises his arms to touch the armchair (4), and repositioning his body on the armchair (5 and 6). The total duration of the episode was longer than 30 seconds, but the EEG remained characteristic of slow wave sleep as exemplified by delta-to-theta range activity in the face of motor behavior. As opposed to patients with sleepwalking and sleep terrors, patients with confusional arousals present with less complex ambulatory events in bed but never with walking or terror behavior. (From Tinuper P, Bisulli F, Provini F. The parasomnias: mechanisms and treatment. *Epilepsia.* 2012;53[Suppl 7]:12–9.)

Table 116.2 Key Similarities and Differentiating Features among the Non–Rapid Eye Movement and Rapid Eye Movement Parasomnias, as well as Nocturnal Seizures

	Disorders of Arousal			REM Parasomnias		
	Confusional Arousals	Sleepwalking	Sleep Terrors	REM Sleep Behavior Disorder	Nightmares	Nocturnal Seizures
Timing at night and sleep-stage specificity	Usually occur in the first half of the night and typically out of stage N3 slow wave sleep.			Occur from REM sleep and typically occur in the last third of the night.		At any time of night, but usually out of NREM sleep. Favoring occurrence when EEG is synchronized.
Family history	Usually positive for similar events			No	May be positive	May be positive.
Behavior semiology	Sudden arousals followed by confusion, disorientation, and amnesia for the event	Abrupt arousal confused/agitated if interrupted. Amnesia at the end	Sudden arousal intense screaming, inconsolable crying, agitation, and heightened autonomic discharge	Purposeful dream enactment behaviors, including yelling, punching, kicking, to fighting a supposed intruder/animal	Paroxysmal awakenings with anxiety and dream recall.	Stereotyped, monomorphic, paroxysmal events often with dystonic limb posturing, vocalizations, and confusions. May encounter partial recall/ amnesia.
Event duration	Few seconds to minutes	Usually 1–10 minutes	Few seconds to minutes	Usually <10 minutes	Few seconds to minutes	Few seconds to few minutes.
Frequency	Few times per month-week, very rarely >1 episode in a single night					Frequent: may occur multiple times in a night.
Postspell behavior	Limited to no recall of the events with confusion			Recall is usually present at times with vivid details. Patients with RBD often describe needing to protect themselves from an attacker (animal/intruder)		Complete/ partial recall to amnesia and confusion.
Polysomnography	Abrupt arousal from slow wave sleep (stage N3) with expression confusion/ambulation/intense fright in CA/SW/ST, followed by return to sleep. Increase cyclic alternating pattern (CAP)			Abnormal increased chin or limb EMG tone (atonia is noted during normal REM sleep).	Dense eye (phasic) movements during REM	Epileptiform activity/muscle artifact/or normal EEG if limited montage
Treatments	Safety interventions, protect patients, remove sharp objects from bedroom, cover windows, barricade furniture, place door alarms. Avoidance of precipitating factors, protecting sleep environment, improving sleep hygiene, avoidance of sleep deprivation. Hypnosis, anticipatory awakenings are helpful. If episodes are frequent, severe, and disruptive to sleep continuity, or result in daytime sleepiness or injury, consider pharmacotherapy			REM sleep behavior disorder Level A: Promote safety Level B: Pharmacotherapy with Melatonin or Clonazepam Nightmares: Reassurance, avoid injury, treat precipitating factors.		Antiepileptic drugs, carbamazepine most frequently used for normal seizures.

Modified after Avidan AY, Kaplish N. The parasomnias: epidemiology, clinical features, and diagnostic approach. *Clin Chest Med*. 2010;31:353–70.

nocturnal seizures of frontal lobe or inferiomesial temporal origin may manifest with confusional amnestic semiology. Unlike confusional arousals, however, SRE with ictal confusion episodes begin with more stereotypical behavior, have a variable frequency, and may be associated with an ictal EEG waveform.[46,61]

Kleine-Levin syndrome (KLS) is classified as a disorder of CNS hypersomnolence and is described as a periodic hypersomnolence disorder. Its association with sleep inertia/drunkenness may lead to diagnostic challenges, as it may be difficult to differentiate from confusional arousals. Unique features of KLS are periods of prolonged sleep with intermingled brief

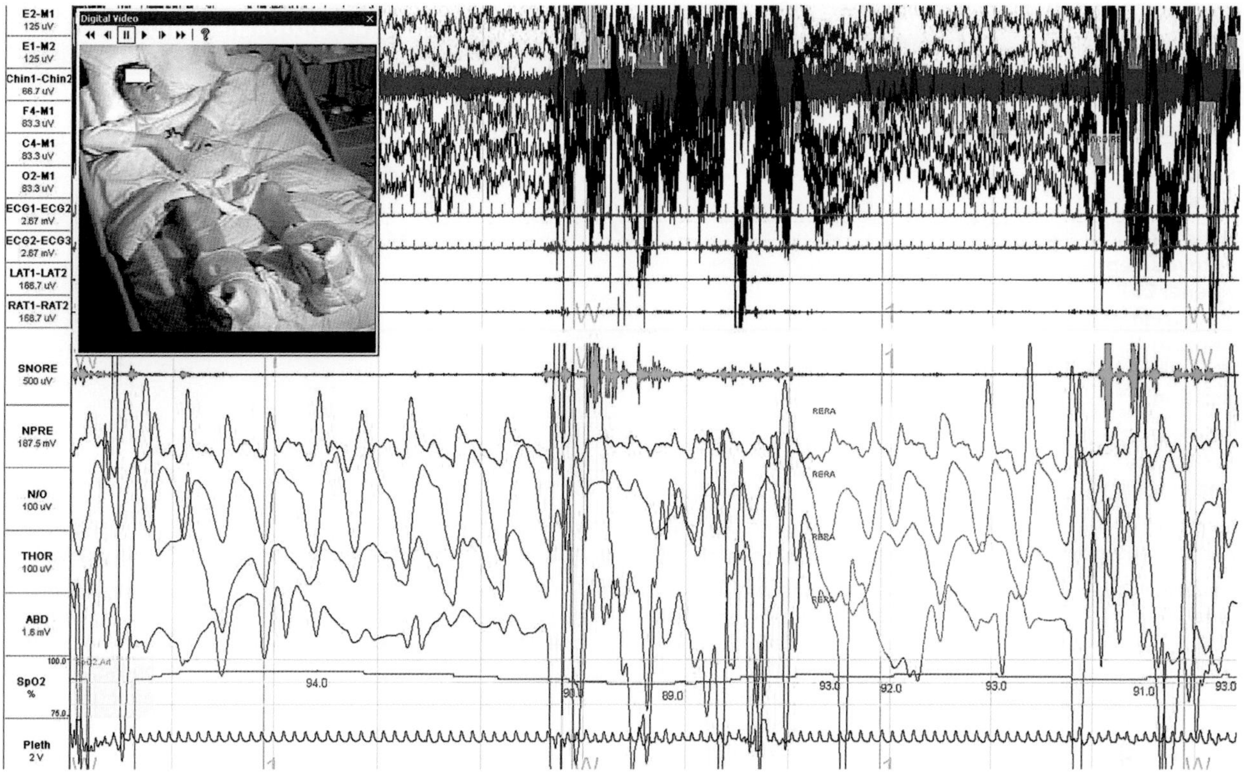

Figure 116.8 Confusional arousal secondary to sleep-disordered breathing. A 120-second epoch of a diagnostic polysomnogram (PSG) conducted to evaluate arousals with confusion and singing behavior in a 54-year-old man. A representative event for the patient is illustrated: an arousal from slow wave sleep, as demarcated by the star, with the patient's arms abducted (in "flapping" his arms; he also was described by the technicians to be "quacking like a duck"). Channels are as follows: electrooculogram (*left*: E1-M2; right: E2-M1), chin EMG (Chin1-Chin2), EEG (*left*: frontal-F3, central-C3, occipital-O1, left mastoid-M1; right: frontal-F4, central-C4, occipital-O2, right mastoid-M2); two ECG, two-limb EMG (LAT, RAT), snore, nasal-oral airflow-N/O, nasal pressure signal-NPRE, respiratory effort (thoracic, abdominal), and oxygen saturation (Sao_2). ECG, Electrocardiogram; EEG, electroencephalogram; EMG, electromyogram; LAT, left anterior tibialis; RAT, right anterior tibialis. (Modified from Avidan AY, Kaplish N. The parasomnias: epidemiology, clinical features, and diagnostic approach. *Clin Chest Med*. 2010;31:353–70.)

periods of wakefulness during which there are mental confusion, incoherent speech, irritability, cognitive impairment, hyperphagia, and hypersexuality,[62,63] KLS also may be associated with episodes of sleep eating and sleep sexual activity, which blurs the clinical distinction, but the other sleep features help distinguish this disorder.[62,64]

Epidemiologic data showed that 13.2% of patients with confusional arousals had obstructive sleep apnea, compared with 2% of those without such arousals.[33] Patients with sleep-related breathing disorders may engage in a variety of peculiar behaviors after an apneic episode. Figure 116.8 demonstrates a diagnostic polysomnogram of a 54-year-old man who presented with a history of disruptive nighttime confusion and singing behaviors. During the recorded event, arousal from slow wave sleep, the patient is seen with the arms abducted; he was then observed to "flap" his arms and was described by the technicians to be "quacking like a duck."[26] In the setting of sleep apnea, confusional arousals may result from the apnea triggering arousal during sleep, and in some cases, the hypoxemia may provoke waking neurobehavioral deficits.[33]

Behavioral and Pharmacologic Treatment Options

As with other parasomnias, treatment should focus on safety measures. The sleep environment should be reviewed for possible safety issues: bed on the floor, windows guarded, no sharp or dangerous articles nearby. In most cases, the disorder remits with age, and episodes can be prevented or limited by avoidance of the facilitating factors (e.g., sleep deprivation, stimulants, other issues causing arousals). Confusional arousals may be managed conservatively by avoiding sleep deprivation, preventing irregular sleep-wake schedule patterns, limiting exposure to CNS depressants, and managing coexisting sleep disorders. If identified, other sleep disorders such as sleep apnea should be treated. Pharmacologic management often is not necessary because the arousal episodes are self-limiting. In refractory cases, some patients respond to tricyclic antidepressants, such as clomipramine (Table 116.3).

Sexsomnias (a Subtype of Confusional Arousals)

One of the more bizarre disorders of arousal is a variant of confusional arousals known as sexsomnia, somnambulistic sexual behavior, or "sleepsex."[14,52] Sexsomnias consist of abrupt nocturnal episodes of often inappropriate sexual behaviors occurring with limited awareness during the act, relative unresponsiveness to the external environment, and amnesia for the event.[55]

Patients with sexsomnia engage in often inappropriate amnestic sexual behavior ranging from masturbation,

Table 116.3 Treatment Options for Disorders of Arousal: Prevention, Behavioral Approaches, and Pharmacotherapy

Component	Confusional Arousal	Sexsomnias	Somnambulism (Sleepwalking)	SRED	Sleep Terrors
Environmental safety	✔	✔	✔	✔	✔
Reassurance, improve sleep hygiene, CBT, MBSR, treat comorbid sleep/medical condition	✔	✔	✔	✔	✔
Scheduled/ anticipatory awakening	✔		✔		✔
"Universal" pharmacotherapy	Clonazepam, melatonin (preferred because of better safety and side effect profile). Melatonin may also have a role in disorders of arousal in the setting of sleep disorders in children with neurodevelopmental disabilities.				
Behavioral management	Reassurance of benign nature. Avoid precipitants: Sleep deprivation, alcohol, CNS depressants	Enhancing sleep hygiene, ensuring optimal sleep duration. Psychotherapy and stress management Comorbid mood disorder or anxiety	Avoid precipitants: Sleep deprivation, nonbenzodiazepine BZRAs	Avoid BZRAs	Reassurance of benign nature Relaxation therapy Hypnosis/autogenic training[b] Psychotherapy
Specific pharmacologic management	**Benzodiazepines:** Clonazepam **Antidepressants:** Imipramine, clomipramine	**Benzodiazepines:** Clonazepam **Antidepressants:** SSRIs, sertraline **AEDs:** Lamotrigine, valproic acid	**Benzodiazepines:** Clonazepam, diazepam, triazolam, flurazepam **Antidepressants:** TCA: Imipramine SSRIs: Paroxetine, sertraline **Antipsychotics:** Quetiapine, temazepam, olanzapine, biperiden **Melatonergic agents:** Melatonin	**Benzodiazepines:** Clonazepam, dopamine agonists **Antidepressants:** SSRIs **AED:** Topiramate[a] **Melatonergic agents:** Agomelatine or melatonin extended release	**Benzodiazepines:** Clonazepam, diazepam (adult patients) **Melatonergic agents:** Melatonin (pediatric patients) **Antidepressants:** SSRIs: Paroxetine TCA: Imipramine, clomipramine, trazodone **Antidepressants:** Hydroxytryptophan

[a]Side effects include weight loss, cognitive impairment, paresthesias, visual symptoms, and less frequently, renal calculi.
[b]Autogenic training is a special relaxation technique similar to meditation.
AED, Antiepileptic drug; BZRA, benzodiazepine receptor agonist; CBT, cognitive-behavioral therapy; CNS, central nervous system; GABAergic, gamma-aminobutyric acidergic; MBSR, mindfulness-based stress reduction, SRED, sleep-related eating disorder; SSRI, selective serotonin reuptake inhibitor; TCA, tricyclic antidepressant.
Sources: Drakatos P, et al. NREM parasomnias: a treatment approach based upon a retrospective case series of 512 patients. *Sleep Med*. 2019;53:181–8. Proserpio P, et al. Drugs used in parasomnia. *Sleep Med Clin*. 2018;13:191–202.

attempting sexual activity with a partner co-sleeping in the same bed, and may include attempted sex with a nonpartner with whom the patient does not share a bed or a room.[14] The consequences of sexsomnia can be serious, leading to marital distress and even forensic repercussions in aggressive, inappropriate cases or those involving minor children.[14] Although the underlying cause of sexsomnia is unknown, factors such as fatigue, stress, alcohol use, and substance abuse, and physical contact with another person in the bed can precipitate the episodes.[65] The prevalence of sexsomnia is unknown, and the disorder probably is underreported. A recent review from Spain, behavioral semiology in the sexsomnias ranges from gentle and affectionate with the bed partners to violent explosive sexual acts, typically out of character for the affected person.[65] As with any behaviors, sexual behaviors can occur in a variety of disorders, including as part of disorders of arousal, RBD, epileptic seizures, and psychiatric events.[65] These events can have significant forensic implications (see Chapter 73). Anecdotal evidence suggests that successful amelioration of sexsomnia events entails the following approach: optimizing safety, enhancing sleep hygiene measures, ensuring optimal sleep duration, and, especially in patients with anxiety,

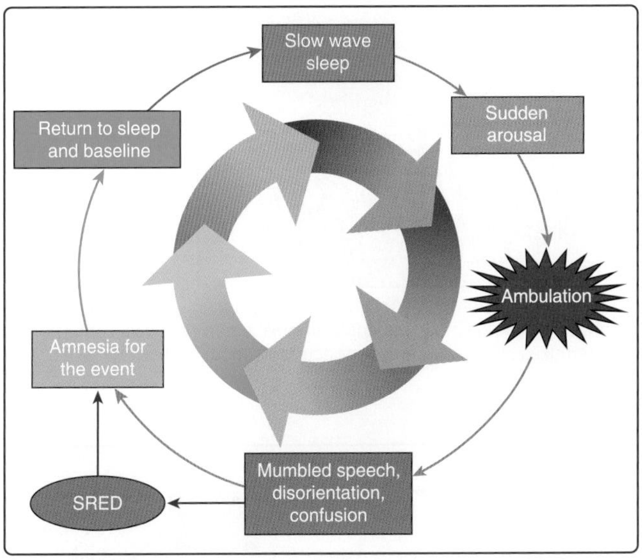

Figure 116.9 Characteristic pattern of sleepwalking. Somnambulism consists of a sudden arousal followed by bizarre motor activity, typically walking, but occasionally with other semipurposeful tasks such as moving objects, expression of unintelligible speech with minimal aggressive, autonomic, or affective involvement. When eating or drinking occurs, then sleep-related eating disorders are diagnosed. (Courtesy of Alon Y. Avidan, MD, MPH.)

Box 116.3 ICSD-3 CRITERIA FOR SLEEP WALKING

Diagnostic Criteria

Requires that both criteria A and B are met.

A. The disorder meets general criteria for NREM disorders of arousal criteria as outlined in Box 116.1.
B. The arousals are associated with walking (ambulation) but could also include other complex behaviors out of bed.

Modified from American Academy of Sleep Medicine. *The International Classification of Sleep Disorders, Revised: Diagnostic and Coding Manual.* 3rd edition. Darien, IL: American Academy of Sleep Medicine; 2014.

psychotherapy, and stress management techniques.[52,54,66] Benzodiazepines, particularly clonazepam, may be considered for first-line pharmacotherapy, with a recommended dosage ranging from 0.25 mg to 2 mg at bedtime (see Table 116.3).[67]

Sleepwalking/Somnambulism

Essential Features and Associated Characteristics

Somnambulism, or sleepwalking, consists of complex behaviors that are initiated during slow wave sleep and result in walking during sleep (Figure 116.9). The episodes generally last from 1 to 5 minutes and may consist of a wide range of activities. Typical spells consist of complex behaviors ranging from simple and calmly sitting up in bed, simple walking to agitated walking, and rarely, in extreme cases, frantic efforts to escape a perceived threatening situation, sometimes accompanied by inappropriate behavior such as urinating.[68] Typical frequency ranges from several times a week to only when precipitating factors are present.[4,69] Somnambulism occasionally may result in falls and injuries incurred during attempts to "escape" or while walking. Box 116.3 summarizes diagnostic criteria for sleepwalking as defined by ICSD-3.

Although most who experience sleepwalking are children, this usually benign and self-limiting condition can be associated with violent behaviors, injury to the sleepwalker or the bed partner, sleep disruption, hypersomnia, anxiety, psychological distress, and altered quality of life.[70,71] Precipitating factors include the use of sedatives, acute sleep deprivation, and specific causes of arousals such as extrinsic stimuli (e.g., noise).[71] In addition, drugs with effects recognized as possible contributing factors include selective serotonin reuptake inhibitors (SSRIs),[72,73] bupropion,[74] mirtazapine,[75] paroxetine,[76] and norepinephrine reuptake inhibitor.[77]

Other medical events and conditions such as fever, untreated sleep apnea, stress, and distended bladder may exacerbate the frequency of sleepwalking episodes. These occurrences demonstrate that sleep fragmentation and deprivation increase sleepwalking episodes and support the hypothesis that impairment of either the sleep homeostatic mechanism or the arousal mechanism is at the root of these events.[49,50]

Demographic Features and Epidemiology

In a recent review of data for a large population of adults, the lifetime prevalence of nocturnal wandering with an abnormal state of consciousness was 29.2%, whereas 3.6% of the sample subjects experienced more than one episode in the previous year. This number is extremely high, and the clinician should remember that nocturnal wandering may have many underlying neurologic or psychiatric etiologies and may include sleepwalking. The prevalence of sleepwalking in the general pediatric population is between 1% and 17% and approaches 4% in adults.[59,78] A large study involving more than 1000 children from Los Angeles reported a prevalence of 2.5% of sleepwalking,[79] whereas a study of Swedish schoolchildren revealed a prevalence of 7%[80] peaking between the ages 4 and 8 years.[81,82] The male-to-female ratio is 1, and familial patterns are common.[2] Recently a specific human leukocyte antigen gene (*DQB1*) was found to increase susceptibility to sleepwalking.[83]

Objective Verifiable Indicators

Polysomnographic Features. The utility of formal polysomnography in the evaluation of somnambulism is mainly in the exclusion of potential mimics such as nocturnal seizures and RBD and of other primary sleep disorders that may potentially contribute to this parasomnia. However, two fundamental difficulties impede the ability to accurately describe them: (1) Somnambulistic behaviors do not occur nightly, and (2) when the episodes do occur, they are often less dramatic or complex than previously described by the patient or family members. Polysomnographic findings in patients with sleepwalking episodes usually show frequent arousals from slow wave sleep, the emergence of hypersynchronous slow wave EEG just before and during arousals, and diminished delta activity. These findings may represent instability of slow wave sleep in the early portion of the sleep period[18,84,85] (Figure 116.10). However, these frequent polysomnographic variables are neither diagnostic nor confirmatory for sleepwalking. The lack of specificity and sensitivity for these biomarkers degrades their usefulness as tools in the clinical or forensic confirmation of parasomnias.[85,86]

Imaging and EEG. A recent EEG and imaging study confirmed that the motor manifestations during sleepwalking events are preceded by arousal-related activation of the cingulate motor area.[23] These data illustrate a fascinating hypothesis

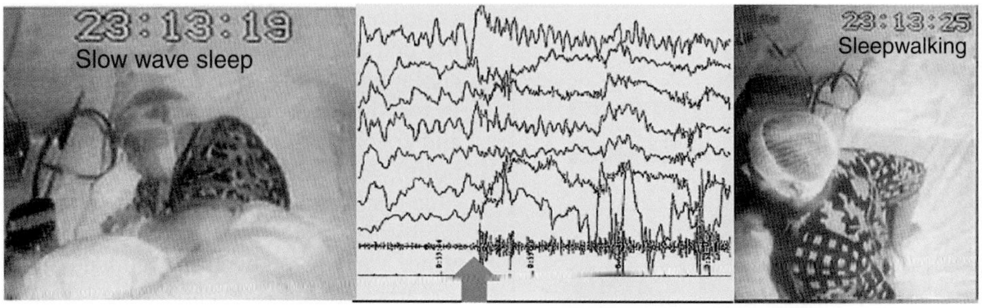

Figure 116.10 Polysomnography in sleepwalking: slow wave sleep instability. Polysomnographic fragment highlights instability during stage N3 during sleepwalking episode (*arrow*), demarcated by sudden onset of a diffuse, high-voltage rhythmic delta activity. The patient is ambulating and appears confused; the electroencephalogram (EEG) recorded concurrently shows a diffuse theta activity with intermixed alpha, beta, and delta activities. (Modified from Bassetti C, et al. SPECT during sleepwalking. *Lancet*. 2000;356:484–5.)

that the event and resulting movement may be related to pathologic blunting of the arousal-related disinhibition of cortical geographies responsible for the control of movement.

Differential Diagnosis

Considerations in the differential diagnosis for sleepwalking include other disorders of arousal, such as sleep terrors and confusional arousals, and RBD. Whereas in RBD, patients are in REM sleep and appear to be acting out a dream sequence, sleep terror and confusion arousals are more abrupt in onset, with the typical association of hypersynchronous and high-amplitude delta activity on polysomnography.[87,88] Similarly, patients with RBD rarely make more than a few steps from the bed without awakening. Early reports of sleep-related partial complex seizures with ambulatory automatisms appeared almost four decades ago, published by Pedley and Guilleminault, who termed these events "episodic nocturnal wanderings," characterized by paroxysmal ambulation and bizarre behavioral manifestations during sleep.[49,67] Episodic nocturnal wandering episodes may represent complex partial seizures but also can be seen as a postictal state, during alcohol intoxication, as a manifestation of dementia, or related to a CNS active drug.[89]

Behavioral and Pharmacologic Treatment Options

Maximizing safety interventions is the best practice approach to the effective management of sleepwalking and the other disorders of arousal. This may be achieved by avoiding the precipitating factors and ensuring a safe living environment by removal of sharp-edged furniture, covering windows, eliminating obstacles that may lead to injury during a sleepwalking episode, locking doors, using door alarms, and providing the safest possible sleeping environment, on the ground floor rather than upstairs, or on the lower rather than an upper bunk bed. Frequent travelers with sleepwalking may want to book hotel rooms on the ground floor, ask for rooms without balconies, or a room without access to a swimming pool. Behavioral intervention using scheduled awakenings can successfully ameliorate sleepwalking episodes but, compared with pharmacologic treatment modalities, has the added advantage of avoidance of CNS-acting medications.[68] The technique calls for the parents to gently wake the patient approximately 15 to 30 minutes before the child typically experiences their typical sleepwalking episode. Once the child responds, parents are instructed to allow the child to fall back asleep. Parents are instructed to continue the scheduled awakenings for up to 4 weeks and to log the frequency of the episodes during this period.[90] Although robust efficacy data are currently lacking, the theory behind the scheduled awakening technique suggests that altering the patient's sleep patterns decreases the disruption in slow wave sleep.[91] Alternatively, the technique may condition the patient for self-arousal just before the arousal event, thereby avoiding it altogether, or may normalize the patient's total sleep time and improve sleep efficiency.[90] In adults with sleepwalking, sleep disorder–focused psychotherapy and hypnosis constitute effective alternatives to pharmacotherapy.[72,92] Definitive pharmacotherapy with tricyclic antidepressants or benzodiazepines is sometimes deemed necessary when the episodes are refractory to behavioral/environmental modifications and when frequent, severe, or associated with injury.[2,87–92] Treatment of sleepwalking is summarized in Table 116.3.

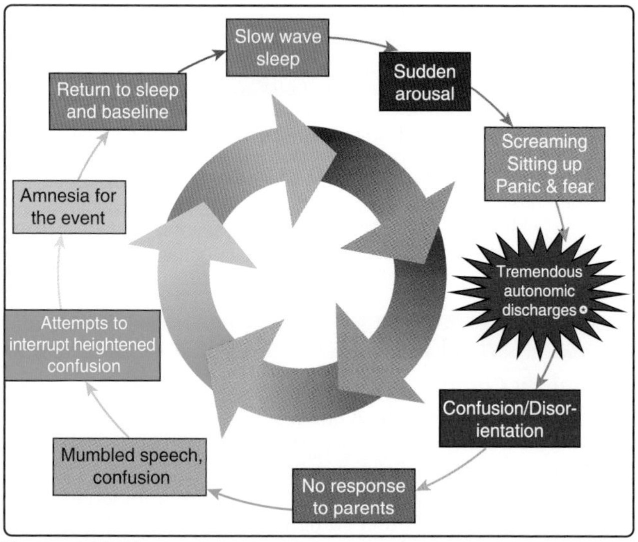

Figure 116.11 Clinical course of sleep terrors. Sleep terrors (pavor nocturnus) are dramatic events characterized by a sudden and abrupt arousal associated with a panicky scream, agitation, intense anxiety, and heighted autonomic activity ✪. The general duration is about a minute, but they can last for up to 10 minutes. Inconsolability is almost universal, and the patient is unresponsive to the efforts of others to console him. The child is incoherent and has an altered perception of the environment, appearing confused. This behavior may potentially be dangerous and could result in injury. (Courtesy of Alon Y. Avidan, MD, MPH.)

Sleep Terrors

Essential Features and Associated Characteristics

Sleep terrors, also known as night terrors (*pavor nocturnus*), consist of sudden arousal from deep sleep manifested by a piercing scream accompanied by heightened autonomic arousal and behavioral manifestations of extreme fear (Figure 116.11). This

Box 116.4 ICSD-3 CRITERIA FOR SLEEP TERRORS

Criteria A–C must be met.

A. The disorder meets general criteria for NREM disorders of arousal.
B. The arousals are characterized by episodes of abrupt terror, typically beginning with an alarming vocalization such as a frightening scream.
C. There is intense fear and signs of autonomic arousal, including mydriasis, tachycardia, tachypnea, and diaphoresis during an episode.

Modified from American Academy of Sleep Medicine. *The International Classification of Sleep Disorders, Revised: Diagnostic and Coding Manual*. 3rd edition. Darien, IL: American Academy of Sleep Medicine; 2014.

is the most dramatic of the DOA and is characterized further by extreme panic and confusion, associated with increased sympathetic activity manifested by tachycardia, tachypnea, reduced galvanic skin resistance reflecting diaphoresis, flushing of the skin, and mydriasis (dilated pupils). Affected patients are in a state of cerebral hyperresponsiveness manifested by extreme agitation, escape behavior, and marked confusion.[3,90] The episodes are typically followed by amnesia and disorientation and occasionally prominent motor activity and displacement resulting in bodily injury.[4,93-95] Sleep terror episodes may become violent, potentially resulting in injury to the patient and bed partner, with evidence from the literature of episodes with forensic implications.[96-98] The duration of the event usually is between 30 seconds and a few minutes. A universal feature is inconsolability, Any attempt by the parent, bed partner, or observer to interrupt the episode or soothe the patient further exacerbates, intensifies, or prolongs the episodes. The patient typically appears to be awake and may sometimes misperceive the nature of the environment or engages in automatic activity such as running for a door or window. Box 116.4 summarizes diagnostic criteria for sleep terrors as defined by ICSD-3.[99]

Demographic Features and Epidemiology

The prevalence or sleep terrors is approximately 1% to 6% among prepubertal children and 1% among adults. Males are more commonly affected than females, with a peak incidence between 5 and 7 years of age.[100,101] Episodes tend to decrease in frequency or cease during early adolescence. Psychopathology is uncommon in affected children but may have a more significant role in adult sufferers.[92] As with sleepwalking, sleep terrors are perhaps more prevalent in adults than has been generally acknowledged.[99]

Objectively Verifiable Indicators

Polysomnographic Features. Although sleep terrors usually are diagnosed on the basis of clinical criteria alone, video-polysomnography, with multiple EEG channels included in the recording montage, may be performed for atypical episodes (i.e., repetitive episodes, occurrence several times per night, or a stereotypical behavior pattern) or in patients with possible underlying sleep disorders or neurologic or psychiatric issues.[36,85,102]

The onset of sleep terror episodes typically is within the first few hours of the night, during stage N3 sleep. Before a sleep terror spell, the EEG typically reveals high-voltage, symmetric, hypersynchronous slow wave activity. The characteristic polysomnogram during the sleep terror episode may reveal sudden and incomplete arousal from slow wave sleep associated with a regular, rhythmic slow wave activity pattern, accompanied by a marked increase in muscle tone and change in respiratory and heart rates, inconsolable crying along with screaming, and sympathetic hyperactivation.[94-96] Although these changes may be difficult to appreciate consistently, the arousal from N3 sleep, as noted by the star in Figure 116.12, may be appreciated on polysomnography.

In children with sleep-disordered breathing, disruptive periodic limb movements in sleep may precipitate sleepwalking or sleep terrors; and treatment of these primary sleep disorders may reduce the parasomnia behaviors.[11,15,16] When patients with DOA undergo formal polysomnography, a detailed examination of the nasal cannula/pressure transducer system and/or esophageal manometry is crucial to identify apneas and hypopneas or more subtle indications of upper airway resistance, in particular, provoking the parasomnia.[15,16]

Differential Diagnosis

The differential diagnosis should include REM sleep nightmares, nocturnal anxiety attacks related to obstructive sleep apnea, nocturnal cardiac ischemia, and SRE. Differentiation from nightmares is most important. Nightmares are distinguishable from sleep terrors in that the former often is associated with a vivid recall of the dream event during REM sleep, the clinical presentation is less dramatic, and many patients do not experience the typical autonomic hyperarousal that characterizes the latter[2,3,35] (Table 116.4). Sleep terrors preferentially occur during stage N3 slow wave sleep[95] and are universally characterized by amnesia, but fragmentary indistinct recollections of threats (spiders, monsters, snakes) from which patients have to defend themselves are sometimes reported. Differentiating between sleep terrors and SRE can sometimes be difficult, and the use of electroencephalography is helpful in patients in whom the episodes are atypical, unusually frequent, or less responsive to management.[49,103] Nocturnal seizures, especially complex partial seizures of temporal and frontal origin, may have a major fear component and manifest with many of the characteristics found in sleep terrors, including screaming, panic, fear, tachycardia, and vague frightening perceptions (Figure 116.13).[49] For this reason, history and clinical semiology alone are not sufficient to conclusively differentiate sleep terrors from seizures. In these challenging cases, video-polysomnographic recording with a full set of EEG electrodes is essential when the spells are frequent, repetitive, or refractory to conventional therapy or have atypical features.[37] Video-polysomnographic recordings capturing multiple events may be helpful in demonstrating stereotypic behaviors suggestive of an epileptic origin, even in the face of no EEG change.[103]

Behavioral and Pharmacologic Treatment Options

Treatment again should focus on the safety of the patient. If the episodes are rare, treatment may be conservative, but more aggressive therapy is essential when events are frequent, intense, disruptive to the patient's sleep, and place the patient at risk or others for harm. An essential first step is to facilitate safety measures because these are paramount in protecting the patient from injury. As with sleepwalking, the security and protection of the patient from harm in the external environment are prudent. Typical measures include (1) ensuring that the patient's sleeping area is on the ground floor, (2) avoiding

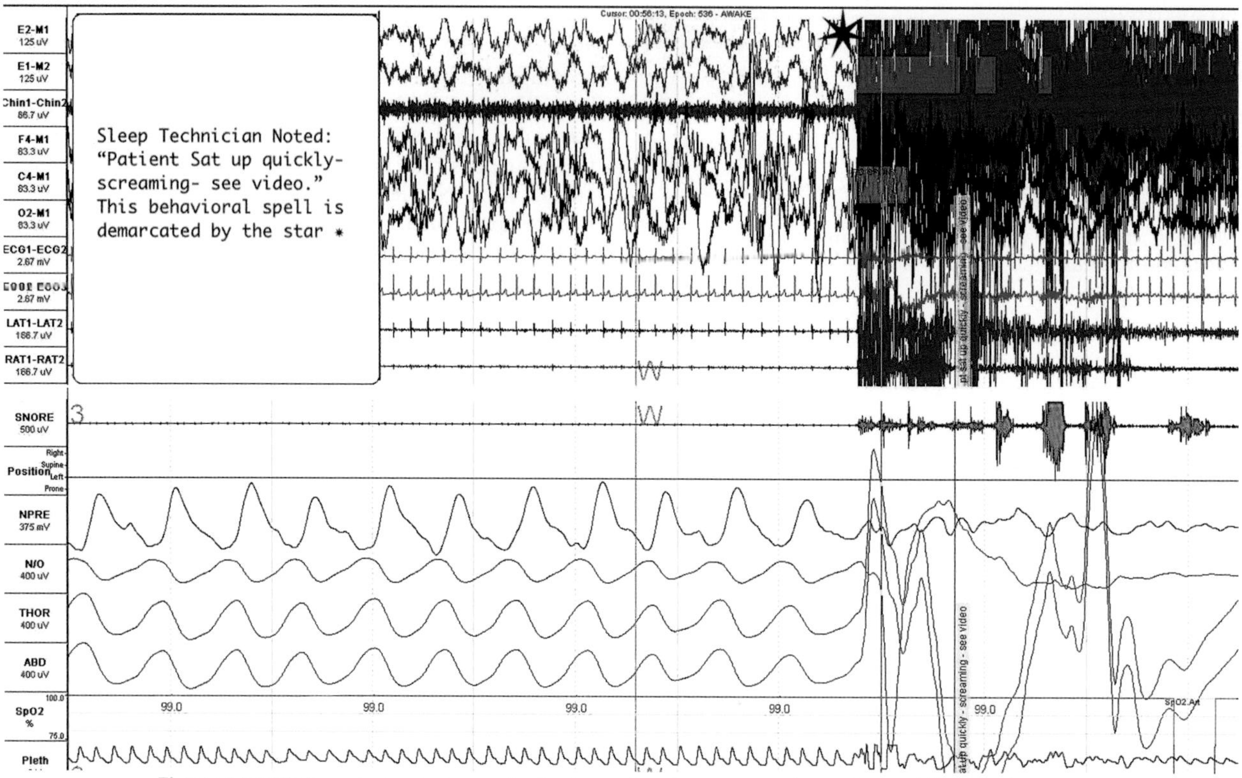

Figure 116.12 Two minute minute epoch of a diagnostic polysomnogram from a 9-year-old boy performed to evaluate for arousals associated with screaming and inconsolable crying. The figure illustrates one of the patient's representative spells, illustrating an arousal with screaming arising out of slow wave sleep with the patient's arms flexed and held close to chest (as if afraid and protecting himself). Channels are as follows: electro-oculogram (left: E1-M2, right: E2-M1), chin electromyogram (Chin1-chin2), electroencephalogram (right: frontal-F4,central-C4, occipital-O2, right mastoid-M2), two ECG channels, 2 limb EMG (LAT, RAT), snore channel, nasal-oral airflow-N/O, nasal pressure signal-NPRE, respiratory effort (thoracic, abdominal), and oxygen saturation (SaO_2). (Polysomnogram slide courtesy Timothy Hoban, MD, Professor of Pediatrics and Neurology, University of Michigan, Ann Arbor, Michigan.)

Table 116.4 Comparisons between Sleep Terrors and Rapid Eye Movement Sleep Nightmares

Characteristic	Sleep Terror	Nightmare
Timing during the night	First third (deep slow wave sleep)	Last third (REM sleep)
EEG characteristics	Stage N3 sleep	Stage REM
Movements	Common	Rare
Anxiety level	High (difficult to control)	Minimum
Severity	Severe	Mild
Vocalizations	Common	Rare
Autonomic discharge	Severe and intense	Mild
Recollection	No (amnestic, occasional fragmentary recall of frightening images)	Yes (good recollection)
State on waking	Vague, confused, disoriented	Function well, vivid and clear
Injuries	Common	Rare
Violence	Common	Rare
Displacement from bed	Common	Very rare

Modified from Avidan AY, Kaplish N. The parasomnias: epidemiology, clinical features, and diagnostic approach. *Clin Chest Med.* 2010;31:353–70.

the upper deck of a bunk bed, (3) removing sharp furniture close to the bed area, (4) blocking windows, (5) providing special bolts for windows and doors, and (6) using door alarms and bells to alert the family members should the child leave the room.[98] The parents and the patient need to be educated and reassured that these episodes are transient and self-limiting and typically will be outgrown with time. Additional measures should focus on maintaining a regular sleep-wake schedule and reducing or entirely eliminating caffeinated beverages. As with the other arousal disorders considered here, it

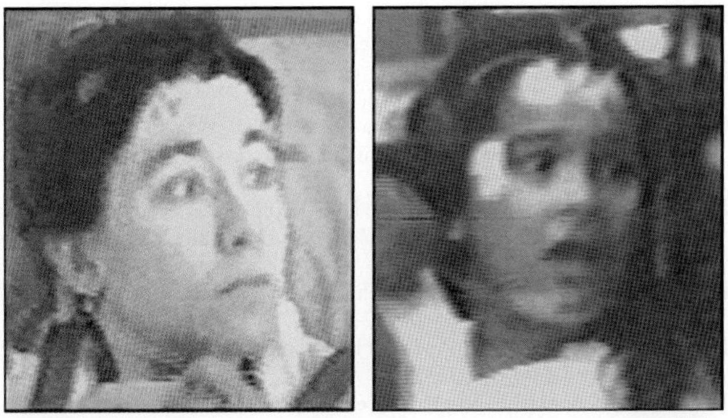

Figure 116.13 Facial emotion expressing surprise during a temporal lobe seizure (*left*) and fear during a nocturnal frontal lobe seizure (*right*). (Modified from Tassinari CA. Relationship of central pattern generators with parasomnias and sleep-related epileptic seizures. *Sleep Med. Clin.* 7:125–34. Copyright © 2012 Elsevier Inc.)

is best not to confront, restrain, or awaken the patient during the episodes because such interventions may prolong, intensify, or worsen the behaviors.[98]

Scheduled or anticipatory awakenings before the time of the regular occurrence of episodes are of significant benefit.[91,104,105] The technique is especially helpful when the episodes occur at a consistent time. The technique of anticipatory or scheduled awakening consists of three distinct phases.[106] The *baseline-phase* consists of data collection specific to the timing of the episodes using a sleep log. This period typically lasts for about 1 to 2 weeks until sufficient data are available to calculate the optimal time for awakenings. The *intervention phase* follows next, in which the parents/observers are instructed to awaken the child lightly between 15 and 30 minutes before the usual time of occurrence of episodes. This period usually occurs 90 to 180 minutes after sleep onset. The parents or observers are instructed to ensure that when the child/patient awakens he or she responds with eyes open. The treatment concludes with the *treatment fading and termination phase,* to evaluate for a reduction in the parasomnia behavior while the sleep diary continues to be monitored. The sequence is repeated if parasomnia behavior recurs. Scheduled awakenings are hypothesized to treat DOA by alteration of the sleep state. The advantage is of comparable efficacy to medications but without the side effects of sedation or daytime somnolence. Potential complications include the effect on the parents' sleep and risk of sleep fragmentation or deprivation.[106]

Hypnosis is another practical, inexpensive, and effective treatment, especially when posthypnotic suggestions are used to help decrease awareness of the unpleasant nocturnal sensory experience.[75,99-102] Adult sufferers with a history of a psychiatric disorder may benefit from psychotherapy and stress reduction, as well as reassurance.[6,104-106] Pharmacotherapy should be reserved for patients with severe, frequent, and refractory sleep terror episodes. Treatment options consist of clonazepam and tricyclic antidepressants. Low-dose benzodiazepines (clonazepam, diazepam) may be effective when administered close to bedtime[107] (see Table 116.3).

Sleep-Related Eating Disorder (See Chapter 117)

Sleep-related eating can be seen as part of a spectrum of behaviors in confusional arousals and sleepwalking. Often the SRED consists of episodes of amnestic nocturnal sleepwalking associated with compulsive eating behavior, occurring with fluctuating levels of impaired consciousness and sometimes associated exposure to psychotropic agents (e.g., zolpidem, olanzapine).[24,107,108] These events of eating occur after partial arousal from sleep, and the patient may consume unusual food items, such as inedible substances (e.g., bar of soap) or unusual or odd food choices or combination (e.g., eating mayonnaise out of a jar, consuming a frozen pizza, or preparing a cat food–dish soap sandwich). The main concerns with SRED are related to the safety and welfare of the patient during the preparation of food (i.e., cutting and cooking) and the potential metabolic consequences (obesity, poor glucose control). The disorder is further described in Chapter 117.

CLINICAL PEARLS

Identification

Disorders of arousal may place patients at high risk for sleep-related injuries and can adversely affect quality of life. Accordingly, clinicians and health care providers need to adequately screen for, correctly classify, and appropriately manage these disorders.[32,36]

Predisposition

As was alluded to earlier, family history and genetics play a significant role in priming patients with an autosomal-dominant pattern of inheritance, whereas sleep fragmentation (e.g., from obstructive sleep apnea) and CNS depression are considered precipitating factors (see Figure 116.1).

Investigation

Evaluation of nocturnal events can be challenging to even the most ardent clinician and requires careful attention to detail. Formal evaluation with nocturnal polysomnography is required in certain scenarios, particularly when seizures are suspected, and prolonged video EEG can assist in the differentiation between parasomnias, other sleep events, sleep-related epilepsies, and other nonepileptic events if full montage EEG is combined with video-polysomnography.[36,103] Polysomnographic fingerprints of DOA include hypersynchronous slow waves but also EEG abnormalities within the K complexes of N2 sleep.[109] Unique genetic markers for DOA include chromosome 20q12-q13.12, HLA DQB1*05:01, and DQB1*05:01.[88,110,111]

Management

Identification and elimination or resolution of factors that provoke parasomnias is a crucial component to treatment; factors to assess and intervene on include environmental issues, medications and other substances, and concomitant sleep disorders.[35] Minimization of stimuli in the bedroom, including extraneous sounds and lights, may limit the occurrence of events. Alcohol remains a known precipitant for some arousal disorders, but its role in provoking somnambulism is controversial.[35,112] Formal evaluation and treatment of other sleep disorders are key to successful management. One of the largest studies to date, of more than 500 patients from Europe of mostly adult patients with DOA over 7.5 years, highlights the value of improving sleep hygiene advice as the first step and proceeding with the management of comorbid sleep disorders and treatment of priming factors such as anxiety, and finally resorting to pharmacotherapy, which has efficacy in up to 60% of patients.[88] Interestingly, the data support conservative nonmedication modalities with efficacy of up to a third of our patients.[110] Clonazepam has demonstrated efficacy in two-thirds of patients and may be considered as first-line therapy in the setting of DOA associated with injury. Melatonin is also effective and may be preferred given its superior safety profile.

SUMMARY

The DOA are a unique group of sleep disorders that share similar characteristics and have a common underlying pathophysiology. Successful treatment is dependent on accurate diagnosis, which includes identification of key distinguishing features. Often reassurance, addressing safety issues, and education are sufficient for less dramatic, nonviolent parasomnias. Safety precautions and good general sleep hygiene measures are vital recommendations because such disorders can be exacerbated by sleep deprivation and various other factors. When the nocturnal episodes are frequent or involve aggressive or dramatic behaviors, pharmacotherapy with a benzodiazepine, particularly clonazepam, at bedtime is an effective approach. Another therapy relies on the use of short-acting benzodiazepines, such as diazepam and alprazolam, or tricyclic antidepressants in the case of sleep terrors. Relaxation training and guided imagery may be helpful strategies for some patients, especially those with DOA.

SELECTED READINGS

Baldini T, Loddo G, Sessagesimi E, et al. Clinical features and pathophysiology of disorders of arousal in adults: a window into the sleeping brain. *Front Neurol.* 2019;10:526.

Castelnovo A, Lopez R, Proserpio P, Nobili L, Dauvilliers Y. NREM sleep parasomnias as disorders of sleep-state dissociation. *Nat Rev Neurol.* 2018;14(8):470–481.

Cochen De Cock V. Sleepwalking. *Curr Treat Options Neurol.* 2016;18(2):6.

Drakatos P, Marples L, Muza R, et al. NREM parasomnias: a treatment approach based upon a retrospective case series of 512 patients. *Sleep Med.* 2019;53:181–188.

Dubessy AL, Leu-Semenescu S, Attali V, Maranci JB, Arnulf I. Sexsomnia: a specialized non-REM parasomnia? *Sleep.* 2017;40(2).

Ekambaram V, Maski K. Non-Rapid eye movement arousal parasomnias in children. *Pediatr Ann.* 2017;46(9):e327–e31.

Erickson J, Vaughn BV. Non-REM parasomnia: the promise of precision medicine. *Sleep Med Clin.* 2019;14(3):363–370.

Grigg-Damberger M, Foldvary-Schaefer N. Eyes wide open minds shut best identify disorders of arousal in adult sleepwalkers. *J Clin Sleep Med.* 2020;16(1):7–8.

Irfan M, Schenck CH, Howell MJ. Non-Rapid eye movement sleep and overlap parasomnias. *Continuum (Minneap Minn).* 2017;23(4, Sleep Neurology):1035–1050.

Kotagal S. Sleep Wake disorders of childhood. *Continuum (Minneap Minn).* 2017;23(4, Sleep Neurology):1132–1150.

Leung AKC, Leung AAM, Wong AHC, Hon KL. Sleep terrors: an updated review. *Curr Pediatr Rev.* 2019.

Loddo G, Sessagesimi E, Mignani F, et al. Specific motor patterns of arousal disorders in adults: a video-polysomnographic analysis of 184 episodes. *Sleep Med.* 2018;41:102–109.

Lopez R, Shen Y, Chenini S, et al. Diagnostic criteria for disorders of arousal: a video-polysomnographic assessment. *Ann Neurol.* 2018;83(2):341–351.

Ntafouli M, Galbiati A, Gazea M, Bassetti CLA, Bargiotas P. Update on nonpharmacological interventions in parasomnias. *Postgrad Med.* 2020;132(1):72–79.

Proserpio P, Terzaghi M, Manni R, Nobili L. Drugs used in parasomnia. *Sleep Med Clin.* 2020;15(2):289–300.

Rodriguez CL, Foldvary-Schaefer N. Clinical neurophysiology of NREM parasomnias. *Handb Clin Neurol.* 2019;161:397–410.

Sarilar AC, Ismailogullari S, Yilmaz R, Erdogan FF, Per H. Electroencephalogram abnormalities in patients with NREM parasomnias. *Sleep Med.* 2019.

Simon SL, Byars KC. Behavioral treatments for non-rapid eye movement parasomnias in children. *Curr Sleep Med Rep.* 2016;2(3):152–157.

A complete reference list can be found online at ExpertConsult.com.

Chapter 117

Sleep-Related Eating Disorder

Lauren A. Tobias

Chapter Highlights

- Sleep-related eating disorder (SRED) is a non–rapid eye movement parasomnia characterized by recurrent episodes of partial arousals from sleep with uncontrollable food consumption with impairment of consciousness and no or partial memory of the event.
- Patients with SRED typically experience symptom onset in early adulthood; it can be associated with comorbid psychiatric disorders, including eating disorders.
- Many patients have episodes on a nightly basis that can vary in frequency up to multiple times per night, with consumption of high-calorie and sometimes bizarre foods or inedible substances.
- Weight gain and obesity are the primary adverse health consequences of SRED. These may be refractory to usual treatment because of the involuntary nature of food consumption.
- The episodes of nighttime eating related to SRED can be distinguished from nocturnal eating syndrome by the impairment of consciousness during events.
- The presence of SRED should prompt a thorough evaluation for potential triggers, including hypnotic medications and sleep-disordered breathing (SDB). For these patients, remission may occur with reduction or cessation of precipitating medications or treatment of underlying SDB.
- For those not provoked by medication or SDB, pharmacologic therapy may help.

INTRODUCTION

Sleep-related eating disorder (SRED) is characterized by recurrent episodes of eating and drinking during partial arousals from nocturnal sleep. This non–rapid eye movement (NREM) sleep parasomnia is considered distinct from the disorders of arousals (DOAs): the predominant behavior is related to the consumption of food. Patients typically describe the events as involuntary or "out of control," and their recall for the event is impaired or absent. Schenck and colleagues initially described SRED in 1991.[1] Since then, our understanding of SRED has continued to evolve, and it is likely that it remains underrecognized.[2]

SRED may contribute to adverse health consequences resulting from weight gain and obesity and can negatively impact quality of life. Patients often perceive that their sleep quality is impaired because of morning lethargy and decreased daytime functioning.

SRED can be provoked by specific medications, particularly hypnotics or other sleep disorders; thus a thorough clinical evaluation of the patient is crucial to determining a therapeutic strategy. SRED may also occur as part of other NREM parasomnias.

DEFINITION

SRED is considered a subtype of the NREM parasomnias, which are undesirable physical events or sensory experiences that occur in association with sleep or with the onset or offset of sleep. This NREM parasomnia is separate from the DOAs, even though some patients with DOAs may exhibit eating behaviors during events. For SRED, the primary parasomnia behavior is related to the consumption of food. Although SRED was once considered a variant of a daytime eating disorder, the current conceptualization is that these represent distinct entities.

The *International Classification of Sleep Disorders*, third edition (ICSD-3), diagnostic criteria for sleep-related eating disorder (ICD-9 327.49, ICD-10 G47.59) are outlined in Box 117.1. Key components of the definition include the recurrent nature of nocturnal feeding episodes arising abruptly from sleep; a lack of conscious awareness during the eating episode; feeding events including consumption of peculiar foods or substances or resulting in a consequence; and exclusion of other contributing sleep disorders or substances.

DEMOGRAPHICS

Parasomnias overall are most common in children and young adults, and SRED specifically tends to begin in the mid to late 20s.[3] Perhaps owing to the potential for social stigma, patients have often been symptomatic long before receiving a diagnosis. In one study following 34 patients over a 5-year period, symptoms preceded the onset of the SRED diagnosis by an average of 8 years, suggesting a chronic course.[3] SRED has a female predominance; women have accounted for 60% to 83%

Box 117.1 SLEEP-RELATED EATING DISORDER DIAGNOSTIC CRITERIA

A. Recurrent episodes of dysfunctional eating that occur after an arousal during the main sleep period
B. The presence of at least one of the following in association with the recurrent episodes of involuntary eating:
  - Consumption of peculiar forms or combinations of food or inedible or toxic substances
  - Sleep-related injurious or potentially injurious behaviors performed while in pursuit of food or while cooking food
  - Adverse health consequences from recurrent nocturnal eating
C. There is partial or complete loss of conscious awareness during the eating episode, with subsequent impaired recall.
D. The disturbance is not better explained by another sleep disorder, mental disorder, medical disorder, medication, or substance use.

Modified from the *International Classification of Sleep Disorders: Diagnostic & Coding Manual*, 3rd ed. ICSD; 2014.

of patients in case series to date.[1,4,5] However, a more recent population study in Japan showed that only 53% of individuals characterized as having SRED events were female.[6] SRED also appears to be much more common in those with underlying eating disorders. One survey of patients with eating disorders across settings found symptoms consistent with SRED in 17% of inpatients and 8% of outpatients.[7] Conversely, another study by the same group found that 40% of those with SRED were also diagnosed with an eating disorder.[8]

It is difficult to estimate the prevalence of SRED in the general population. While a study of college students found that nearly 5% reported symptoms of SRED,[7] another sample of patients referred to a sleep center found that only 0.5% fulfilled criteria for SRED.[2] The Japanese survey estimated 2.2% of the population endorsed SRED-like behavior.[6] A higher prevalence has been reported among those with a psychiatric diagnosis, perhaps owing to medication-related SRED in this group.[9] Symptoms of SRED are probably underreported by adults who live alone, since they may fail to recognize symptoms. This is suggested by a study showing a higher likelihood of reporting sleepwalking in couples than in single individuals.[10]

RISK FACTORS

Although no large-scale population studies have identified risk factors, some case series appear to identify some specific associations (Box 117.2). Most case series of SRED show the events are associated with either a primary sleep disorder or use of a sedative-hypnotic medication. Several investigators have observed a high prevalence of past or current sleepwalking among patients with SRED, and many conceptualize SRED as a specialized form of sleepwalking.[5] It is common for patients to carry a prior sleep diagnosis; one study reported that nearly 80% of patients had another sleep disorder, most often restless legs syndrome (RLS), periodic limb movements of sleep (PLMS), or somnambulism.[8] In one survey of patients with RLS, more than a third reported symptoms consistent with SRED.[11] It is also common for patients to have

Box 117.2 RISK FACTORS FOR SLEEP-RELATED EATING DISORDER

- Young adulthood (mid-20s)
- History of eating disorder
- History of NREM parasomnias
- Hypnotic medication use

comorbid sleep-disordered breathing (SDB), the treatment of which may improve SRED.

The past decade has seen an increase in research examining a potential familial predisposition toward the development of parasomnias, including associations with certain human leukocyte antigen (HLA) genotypes.[12] Although several series suggest a familial relationship in SRED,[2,8,13] no clear genetic pattern of inheritance has been identified.

CLINICAL FEATURES

Episodes of SRED are characterized by repeated episodes of uncontrolled nocturnal eating associated with impaired consciousness. Patients have partial or complete amnesia for eating episodes and may describe themselves as "half-awake, half-asleep." As with other parasomnias such as sleepwalking, it may be difficult to bring patients to a level of full consciousness during events, and their recollection of episodes is typically impaired. Although the events have a central theme of eating, these events vary in their behavior and are not stereotypic. Some events may only last a few minutes, while others may be more elaborate in scope, lasting longer than 10 minutes. Episodes typically occur during the first half of the night, when NREM sleep predominates, and generally begin 2 to 3 hours after sleep onset. A majority of patients describe nightly episodes, although frequency ranges from once a week to up to 10 times in the same night.[1]

For many patients the events of eating may take on strange and bizarre features. Patients may choose foods that are extremely different from their daytime diet.[14] These foods are commonly high-fat or high-sugar foods but may also include unusual items such as raw bacon or frozen pizzas or even nonnutritive or inedible substances such as cigarettes, coffee grounds, egg shells, soap, glue, cologne, or cat food.[15] Patients may engage in behaviors of food preparation, including cooking, which may be potentially dangerous given their impaired level of consciousness. Typically, patients are messy during food preparation and consumption, spilling food on themselves, matting food into their hair, or dropping and scattering food on the floor of their home.[1] Upon awakening, patients may have continued inertia or even feel "hungover" with morning anorexia as a result of overeating during the prior night.

DIFFERENTIAL DIAGNOSIS

As a parasomnia, SRED should be differentiated from other nocturnal events (Box 117.3). Etiologies of nocturnal events include other parasomnias, nocturnal seizures, and other behavioral events. Within the parasomnias, SRED is distinguished by the act of eating as a primary behavior, whereas for other NREM and rapid eye movement (REM) parasomnias, the behaviors will vary and less often include food

Box 117.3 DIFFERENTIAL DIAGNOSIS FOR SLEEP-RELATED EATING DISORDER

- Night eating syndrome (NES)
- Bulimia nervosa with nocturnal eating
- Binge eating disorder
- Hypoglycemic states
- Kleine-Levin syndrome
- Dissociative disorder
- Klüver-Bucy syndrome
- Disorders of arousal
- Medication-induced delirium

consumption. Nocturnal seizures also rarely involve eating behavior, and events should be stereotypic.

Most important, SRED must be distinguished from the other nighttime eating disorder, nocturnal eating syndrome (NES).[16-18] Table 117.1 provides a comparison between SRED and NES.

NES is an *eating disorder* characterized by nocturnal hyperphagia in *fully conscious* patients,[19] in which patients consume at least a quarter of their daily calories after the evening meal. Patients demonstrate evening hyperphagia, insomnia with food ingestion during awakenings, and morning anorexia[20] and typically exhibit episodes of nocturnal ingestion at least twice weekly. NES is thought to be related to a circadian delay in food intake, which may even dissociate from the sleep-wake rhythm.[21] Although the exact prevalence of this disorder is unclear, it is estimated that 1% to 4% of the general population and 6% to 16% of obese patients meet criteria for NES.[22,23] Since NES is not a standalone diagnosis in the *Diagnostic and Statistical Manual of Mental Disorders*,[24] patients are typically given a diagnosis of "eating disorder, other specified feeding and eating disorder."[25]

Clinically, SRED and NES can be distinguished on the basis of whether the patient appears to have impaired consciousness or impaired memory for the episodes. Full memory is typically seen in NES, although some persons may describe eating as "automatic." Patients with NES may describe cravings for specific foods, distress about sleep disruption, a sense of compulsion to eat, or beliefs that they must eat to get to sleep. Comorbid depression and anxiety are common in patients with NES, and episodes may increase during times of stressful life events.

Although some have suggested that SRED and NES may lie upon a continuum, they are currently considered independent disorders with distinct clinical presentations. Speaking broadly, patients with SRED should be thought of as sleepwalkers who happen to eat, whereas those with NES have a binge eating disorder that happens to manifest at night.[26] Unfortunately, the terminology that has evolved to characterize these two disorders has been at turns both divergent and overlapping, resulting in confusion. Part of this lack of clarity may stem from the fact that the prior diagnostic criteria (ICSD-2) allowed for "lumping" both diagnoses together, since there was no definitional requirement for impaired consciousness in SRED. To make matters more confusing, some have reported a high rate of co-existence between these disorders.[4] One potential explanation for the overlap between entities is that SRED may be primed by sedating medications, while patients with NES who take sedating medications may have exhibited a blunted awareness of episodes. Given the shared features of these two disorders, it can be difficult to establish with certainty whether an individual patient's presentation is most consistent with SRED or NES.

Table 117.1 Comparison of Sleep-Related Eating Disorder and Nocturnal Eating Syndrome

	SRED	NES
Consciousness during episodes	Impaired awareness	Fully aware
Memory of event	Amnesia or partial recall	Full recall
Timing of food intake	Awaken from sleep to eat	May eat either before bed or during nighttime awakenings
Consumption of inappropriate or bizarre substances	May be present	Absent
Comorbid sleep disorders	Common	Uncommon
Prevalence	Low	High
Binge eating during nocturnal ingestions	Absent	Present
Evening hyperphagia	Absent	Present
Morning anorexia	Variably present	Present
Induced by hypnotics	Yes	Unknown

NES, Nocturnal eating syndrome; SRED, sleep-related eating disorder.

EVALUATION AND DIAGNOSIS

As a clinical diagnosis, accurately diagnosing SRED relies upon obtaining a thorough sleep history, including a description of the events from witnesses. Some patients may be embarrassed or reluctant to describe their events. Yet clear detailed description of several events is paramount to establishing the diagnosis. Aspects of the individual behaviors, time of night, eyes open or closed, pattern of speech, potential provoking stimuli, and other associated features are helpful information for diagnosis. As with other parasomnias, clinicians should inquire about potential triggers, including insufficient sleep, circadian disruption, other sleep disorders such as SDB, medical issues, fever or other acute illness, medication use, and consumption of alcohol or illicit substances. Patients should be asked about their sleep environment and the nature of their episodes, with particular attention to stimuli that may initiate a parasomnia event as well as assessing both the patient and family to ensure they are safe from potential injury. A family history of parasomnias may also provide clues to predisposing features. Patients should be questioned regarding their relationship to food and diet. SDB is highly prevalent among patients with eating disorders (9% of outpatients and 17% of inpatients in one study),[7] and thus a thorough assessment of eating disorders should accompany evaluation of these patients. In patients with obesity refractory to standard weight loss treatment, both

SRED and night-eating syndrome should be considered. For some patients, events become more prominent with new stress or smoking cessation, so a review of underlying stressors may help identify other triggers.[27]

POLYSOMNOGRAPHIC FINDINGS

Although polysomnography (PSG) is not required to make the diagnosis of SRED, these overnight studies offer the opportunity to capture characteristic episodes and identify other sleep issues that may be provoking events. Typically sleep-related eating events arise from stage N2 or N3 sleep, and rarely from stage R. During typical episodes, PSG may demonstrate mixed features of wakefulness with varying degrees of slowing of the background EEG activity. Patients have eyes open and appear slowed down or confused.

PSG may also demonstrate whether events are provoked by either sleep-related breathing or an underlying movement disorder. Situations in which PSG is recommended include those in which the patient's history is atypical, events place the patient or bed partner at risk of harm (e.g., because of weight gain or toxic ingestion), or there is suspicion for other neurologic events such as seizures; an extended EEG montage is recommended in these cases. For DOAs in general, the chances of capturing an event increase with sleep deprivation, shifting the sleep period to daytime, and the introduction of auditory stimuli during slow wave sleep; the applicability of these interventions to patients with SRED has yet to be determined.[28]

CLINICAL CONSEQUENCES

Patients with SRED commonly describe nonrestorative sleep and a feeling of fullness in the morning. Daytime symptoms include fatigue and sleepiness, possibly resulting from fragmentation of sleep or the underlying disruption from the parasomnia. The other physical consequences may be more pronounced.

One of the more pressing clinical consequences of SRED is weight gain and obesity resulting from the excess calories consumed. Patients often consume calorie-dense foods during episodes, and the involuntary nature of their eating makes weight gain difficult to control. Weight gain can have adverse metabolic consequences, including impaired glucose control or diabetes and hyperlipidemia.[28] Case series have estimated the prevalence of overweight or obesity in SRED to range from 15% to 39%. However, it is worth noting that these studies were conducted 2 decades ago, before the obesity epidemic reached its current proportions, so current rates of overweight/obesity among patients with SRED are likely higher.

Sleep-related injury is also an important concern in those with SRED. Case reports describe individuals consuming noxious or even toxic substances. There is the potential for internal or external burns from consuming or spilling hot foods and liquids, or from using the stove or toaster in a haphazard manner. Patients may also exhibit careless handling of kitchen utensils, and there have been reports of people lacerating digits while cutting food. Finally, there are adverse consequences for one's dentition; falling asleep with an oral bolus of food in the setting of a circadian decline in salivation increases one's risk of dental caries.

Box 117.4 PHARMACOLOGIC AGENTS LINKED TO DRUG-INDUCED SLEEP-RELATED EATING DISORDER[4,37-45]

- Clonazepam
- Bromazepam
- Etizolam
- Flunitrazepam
- Lithium
- Mirtazapine
- Nitrazepam
- Olanzapine
- Risperidone
- Triazolam
- Zaleplon
- Zolpidem
- Zopiclone

RELATIONSHIP BETWEEN SLEEP-RELATED EATING DISORDER AND MEDICATIONS

Sedative hypnotic medications are a notorious contributor to all NREM parasomnias, and their role in SRED has been documented extensively (Box 117.4). In one review of 30 patients with SRED, the authors observed that a third of cases were likely related to a precipitating medication (most often benzodiazepines or benzodiazepine-receptor agonists) as suggested by the temporal relationship with initiation of the drug.[4] Importantly, symptoms of SRED resolved completely after dose reduction or cessation of these medications. In another case series of 28 patients with sleepwalking with or without SRED, quetiapine was the most commonly implicated medication.[29] The authors observed remission from SRED in all cases when antipsychotics were stopped or the dose reduced, or when comorbid sleep apnea was treated with continuous positive airway pressure. Taken together, these findings support the notion that most cases of medication-induced SRED are potentially reversible. As one may expect, the frequency of sleep-associated amnestic behaviors has risen in parallel to the use of sedative-hypnotic medication.[30]

MANAGEMENT

The goal of SRED treatment is to reduce the frequency of nocturnal eating episodes to prevent weight gain and to prevent injury. Regardless of the therapeutic path chosen, close and consistent clinical follow-up is strongly recommended until episodes are well controlled. The purpose of these visits is to reassess symptom severity, evaluate response to treatment, and monitor for any side effects. Similarly, patients should be reevaluated if the frequency of events suddenly increases or if the character of the events change. Patients should be encouraged to keep a calendar with known events and possible triggers so that slow changes can be easily identified.

Patients and families frequently come to clinicians with misunderstanding and confusion regarding their events. Counseling of patients should be founded on three major components: safety for the patient and family; understanding the disorder; and strategizing to avoid aggravating and provocative factors. A key aspect of SRED management is prevention of sleep-related injuries. Patients should be counseled to examine their bedside for furniture or objects that could potentially injure themselves or bed partners. If necessary, the bedroom environment should be modified to prevent sleep-related injury. Patients may attempt to lock doors and kitchen cabinets to prevent consumption of certain food. Patients should also be counseled to avoid triggers and ensure the bedroom is a dark, quiet, and comfortable setting.

Regardless of the therapy chosen for SRED, all patients should be educated regarding appropriate sleep hygiene and avoidance of sleep deprivation, as well as counseling about ensuring a safe sleep environment.[31]

Avoidance or Removal of Triggers

Avoidance of precipitating factors is key to management of SRED. A detailed sleep history should include attention to factors that might contribute to sleep disruption or sleep deprivation (Box 117.5). It is also important to screen for symptoms of SDB or RLS given their strong association with SRED. For example, dysfunctional nocturnal eating can often be controlled by identifying and treating comorbid RLS.[11] As noted previously, certain pharmacologic agents including sedative-hypnotics may be responsible for nighttime eating events. Switching from extended release to immediate release of a sedative-hypnotic agent was helpful in one small study.[32]

Pharmacologic Treatments

The decision to initiate medications for SRED should be dictated by how frequent and troublesome the episodes are to the patient, as well as their impact on weight gain. For example, when excessive caloric intake results in significant excess weight or other metabolic consequences, treatment may be considered.

Although there are no high-quality randomized controlled trials evaluating the efficacy of pharmacologic treatments for SRED, several promising pharmacotherapies are reported in the literature.[31] One small randomized controlled trial of 34 subjects showed that topiramate significantly reduced the frequency of events by more than half.[33] In another descriptive study of SRED patients, in whom 77% were managed with pharmacologic therapy, topiramate was used most commonly. SRED episodes successfully resolved or decreased in 85% of patients. However, 30% of patients discontinued topiramate because of adverse effects, with dizziness reported most often. Topiramate was also found to be effective in a case series of 25 patients with SRED, with 68% classified as responders. Its tolerability was again a barrier, however: nearly half of patients discontinued the medication at 1 year because of adverse effects.[34] Others have proposed that first-line therapy should consist of a selective serotonin reuptake inhibitor (SSRI) and melatonin-related agents.[35,36] Benzodiazepines, such as clonazepam, are frequently prescribed for SRED, although they lack approval for this indication. Their precise mechanism is unclear but probably relates to the suppression of arousals.

The choice of treatment may also be driven by comorbid sleep disorders. Treatment of SDB is well documented to improve parasomnia events. Similarly, dopaminergic agents may improve events in patients with RLS-related SRED. Pramipexole, a dopamine agonist, was shown in a small, double-blind, placebo-controlled trial to reduce nighttime activity as documented with actigraphy.[13]

Box 117.5 POTENTIAL PRECIPITANTS FOR SLEEP-RELATED EATING DISORDER EPISODES

- Sleep deprivation
- Irregular sleep-wake cycles
- Stress
- Alcohol use
- Smoking cessation
- Dieting
- Sedative hypnotic use
- Stimulant medications
- Fever
- Pain
- Sleep-disordered breathing

CLINICAL PEARLS

- SRED is characterized by recurrent amnestic episodes of "out-of-control" nighttime food consumption arising out of arousals from NREM sleep.
- SRED is a clinical diagnosis based on ICSD-3 criteria (Table 117.1). Video polysomnography may be considered in cases in which the history is atypical, where symptoms overlap with those of night eating syndrome, when events put the patient or bed partner at risk of harm, or when there is suspicion for a concurrent neurologic or sleep disorder such as SDB.
- It is likely that SRED is underrecognized, stemming from patients' embarrassment about volunteering symptoms and clinicians' low awareness of the disorder.
- SRED is frequently seen in the setting of psychotropic medication use. A significant proportion of patients will experience marked symptom improvement or even resolution of SRED when hypnotic medications are stopped or their doses are decreased.
- SRED often co-occurs with other sleep disorders, including SDB, RLS, and PLMS; treatment of comorbid sleep disorders may improve SRED.

SUMMARY

SRED represents a unique type of NREM parasomnia characterized by recurrent episodes of compulsive nocturnal eating after partial arousals from sleep. The definition of SRED and its distinction from NES have evolved over time, and they are currently considered to represent separate disorders, with SRED distinguished by the presence of impaired consciousness. Affected patients are most often female, present in young adulthood, and commonly have comorbid eating disorders. Episodes most often occur nightly, and patients may describe consumption of peculiar or inedible substances. Symptoms are often present for nearly a decade before the diagnosis is established. The major clinical consequences of SRED are weight gain and obesity, with resulting metabolic and cardiovascular complications. Initial management should focus on reducing or removing precipitating factors such as psychotropic medications, comorbid sleep-related breathing disorders, and insufficient sleep. Although it is considered a chronic disease, symptoms of SRED may abate or resolve when medication triggers are addressed.

SELECTED READINGS

Allison KC, et al. Proposed diagnostic criteria for night eating syndrome. *Int J Eat Disord.* 2010;43(3):241–247.

Chiaro G, Caletti MT, Provini F. Treatment of sleep-related eating disorder. *Curr Treat Options Neurol.* 2015;17(8):361.

Chopra A, et al. Sleepwalking and sleep-related eating associated with atypical antipsychotic medications: case series and systematic review of literature. *Gen Hosp Psychiatry.* 2020;65:74–81.

Erickson J, Vaughn BV. Non-REM parasomnia: the promise of precision medicine. *Sleep Med Clin.* 2019;14(3):363–370.

Howell MJ. Parasomnias: an updated review. *Neurotherapeutics.* 2012;9(4);753–775.

Morgenthaler TI, Silber MH. Amnestic sleep-related eating disorder associated with zolpidem. *Sleep Med.* 2002;3(4):323–327.

O'Reardon JP, Peshek A, Allison KC. Night eating syndrome : diagnosis, epidemiology and management. *CNS Drugs.* 2005;19(12):997–1008.

Proserpio P, et al. Drugs used in parasomnia. *Sleep Med Clin.* 2020;15(2):289–300.

Santin J, et al. Sleep-related eating disorder: a descriptive study in Chilean patients. *Sleep Med.* 2014;15(2):163–167.

Schenck CH, et al. Additional categories of sleep-related eating disorders and the current status of treatment. *Sleep.* 1993;16(5):457–466.

Winkelman JW. Clinical and polysomnographic features of sleep-related eating disorder. *J Clin Psychiatry.* 1998;59(1):14–19.

Winkelman JW, Johnson EA, Richards LM. Sleep-related eating disorder. *Handb Clin Neurol.* 2011;98:577–585.

A complete reference list can be found online at ExpertConsult.com.

Chapter 118

Rapid Eye Movement Sleep Parasomnias

Michael H. Silber; Erik K. St Louis; Bradley F. Boeve

Chapter Highlights

- Rapid eye movement (REM) sleep behavior disorder (RBD) is a unique parasomnia characterized by loss of REM sleep atonia and dream-enactment behavior. This chapter explores the epidemiology, clinical features, pathophysiology, diagnosis, and management of the condition.
- RBD is commonly seen in patients with a group of neurodegenerative disorders known as the synucleinopathies, including Parkinson disease, dementia with Lewy bodies, and multiple system atrophy. RBD is designated as idiopathic when the disorder takes place without a comorbid neurologic disorder or identifiable cause. Robust evidence confirms that a majority of patients with idiopathic RBD also harbor synucleinopathy pathology. RBD may be associated with antidepressant use, certain rare autoimmune disorders, and narcolepsy.
- RBD is diagnosed through clinical history and polysomnography. Quantitative assessments of muscle activity in REM sleep can result in greater diagnostic accuracy.
- Management includes prognostic counseling and injury prevention by addressing bedroom safety and the use of medications such as melatonin and clonazepam.
- Other REM sleep parasomnias include nightmare disorder, recurrent isolated sleep paralysis, and sleep-related painful erections. The epidemiology, clinical features, and management of the latter two conditions are discussed in this chapter.

RAPID EYE MOVEMENT SLEEP BEHAVIOR DISORDER

Overview

Rapid eye movement (REM) sleep comprises a complex combination of phasic and tonic phenomena, including desynchronized electroencephalographic activity, rapid eye movements, dreaming, and skeletal muscle atonia (Figure 118.1). In disorders such as narcolepsy, these phenomena can dissociate, resulting, for example, in intrusion of muscle paralysis during wakefulness (cataplexy and sleep paralysis). Conversely, muscle atonia can become dysregulated or lost during REM sleep, a finding known as REM sleep without atonia (RSWA) (Figure 118.2). This allows dream-enactment motor activity to occur in the condition known as REM sleep behavior disorder (RBD).

The first description of such a dissociated state was in experimental cats in which introduction of pontine lesions resulted in motor behaviors during REM sleep.[1] Retained muscle tone in REM sleep caused by clomipramine was described in human subjects in 1972.[2] Similar findings were reported in sleep during alcohol withdrawal, a state given the name "stage 1 REM sleep."[3] The definitive descriptions of the disorder, as well as its name, are attributed to Carlos Schenck and Mark Mahowald,[4,5] who published reports of 10 cases in 1986 and 1987, 3 of which were associated with neurodegenerative disorders. Extensive subsequent studies of the clinical features, pathophysiology, etiology, and management have led to a deeper understanding of the complexity and broad implications of this unique parasomnia.

Epidemiology

Several population-based studies of older subjects have attempted to determine RBD prevalence. In a Hong Kong community-based study of 1034 subjects 70 years of age or older, prevalence of RBD was estimated at 0.38%.[6] The age- and sex-adjusted estimate for polysomnography (PSG)-confirmed RBD in a Korean population age 60 years or older was 2.01%, and the idiopathic RBD (iRBD) prevalence estimate was 1.34%.[7] A Spanish study of subjects age 60 years or older, including video PSG, suggested a prevalence of 0.74% for iRBD.[8] A Swiss study of subjects with mean age 59 years that included PSG suggested a prevalence of 1.06% for RBD.[9]

RBD occurs more frequently in men. Pooled data for 717 patients in six series from the United States, Europe, and China indicate a male predominance of 79%.[10–16] This difference is less marked in patients with RBD younger than 50 years (52% to 59% of men).[12,13,17] RBD commences most frequently in middle-aged to older persons; the mean age at

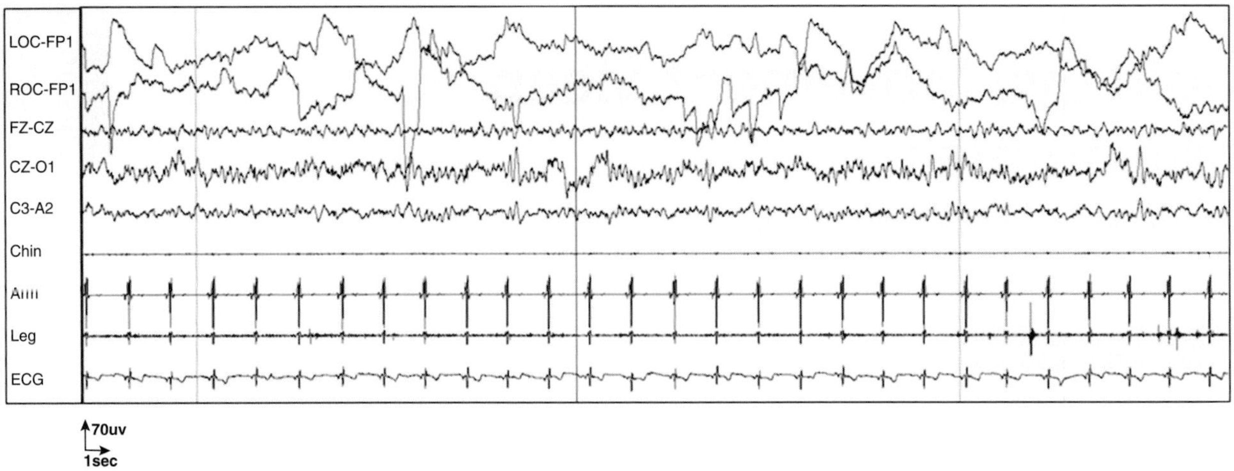

Figure 118.1 Normal REM sleep atonia. A 30-second polysomnogram epoch demonstrates normal REM sleep levels of atonia in submentalis, arm, and anterior tibialis leg leads on the electromyogram.

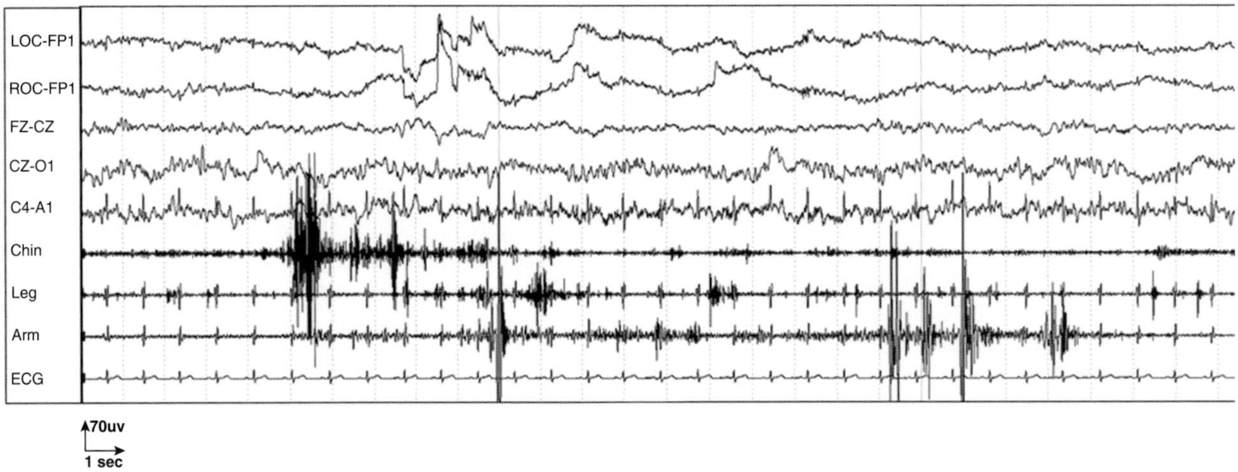

Figure 118.2 Abnormal REM sleep without atonia. Increased phasic/transient muscle activity is shown in the submentalis, anterior tibialis, and arm electromyographic leads in this 30-second polysomnogram epoch. A more sustained lower-grade elevation of muscle tone lasting for longer than one-half of the epoch represents abnormal tonic muscle activity, seen in the submentalis and arm channels of the electromyogram.

onset of symptoms ranged between 45 and 63 years in several large series,[10–13,16] and the mean age at diagnosis, between 52 and 68 years.[10–13,15,16]

In a questionnaire series of 316 patients with iRBD, a proxy-reported family history of presumed RBD was found in 13.8% of cases, compared with 4.8% of control subjects.[18] A community-based study suggested that RBD was significantly associated with lower education levels, coal mining, less physical activity, head injury, and various cardiovascular risk factors.[19] An environmental risk factor study of 347 patients with iRBD found cigarette smoking, previous head injuries, farming occupation, and pesticide exposure to be associated with RBD more frequently than in control subjects.[20] The association with smoking was confirmed in a separate case-control study.[21] Although many of these factors have also been linked to Parkinson disease, smoking, by contrast, is associated with lower risk for Parkinson disease.[22]

Clinical Features

Patients with RBD exhibit abnormal motor behaviors during REM sleep, predominantly while in bed. These behaviors include talking, screaming, swearing, gesturing, arm flailing, punching, kicking, and leaping or falling off the bed.[11,16] Walking or running away from the bed occurs in 11% of patients, in addition to the more typical in-bed activities.[11] Although violent behaviors are most common, nonviolent activities such as laughing, whistling, singing, and masturbation occur at times in 18% of patients.[23] Self-injuries are reported in 32% to 76% of patients,[11,13,16,24] including lacerations, ecchymoses, limb fractures, and subdural hematomas,[11,22] requiring medical attention in approximately 11% of the cases. Injuries occur when patients fall off the bed or strike the limbs against the wall, a headboard, or bedside furniture. Occasional patients have attempted to leap through a window.[11] Sixty-four percent of bed partners report being assaulted, and about 21% have been injured.[11,16,22] Injurious behaviors include punching, slapping, kicking, pulling of hair, and attempted strangulation.[6,11,22] Periorbital hematomas and dental injuries have been reported.[5,11] Not understanding the organic nature of the disorder, patients and their partners often are mortified by the behaviors; some patients have built elaborate barriers in their beds or even slept in restraints to avoid injuring their spouse.[11,25] The frequency and severity of behaviors are highly variable. In some patients with concomitant neurodegenerative disorders, the frequency of events appears to diminish over time, for uncertain reasons.[11,26]

Dream content changes in RBD and becomes more violent in nature in most cases. In a series of 93 cases, dreams involved defense of the sleeper against attack in 80% (65% human assailants and 35% animal), defense of relatives against attack in 7%, adventures in 9%, sporting activities in 2%, but aggression by the dreamer in only 2%.[11] In a study of 98 dreams reported by patients with RBD compared with 69 control dreamers, the RBD dreams featured a higher level of aggression and a higher frequency of animal characters.[27] Despite the aggressive nature of the dreams, daytime aggressiveness questionnaire scales have yielded findings in the normal range[28] or have even shown lower values on the physical aggressiveness subscale than for control data.[27]

Etiology and Associated Disorders

Association with Neurodegenerative Disorders

Synucleinopathies are a group of neurodegenerative disorders in which the protein α-synuclein accumulates abnormally to form inclusions in the cell bodies or axons of neurons or oligodendrocytes. The synucleinopathies include Lewy body disease—manifested as phenotypes of Parkinson disease, dementia with Lewy bodies, or pure autonomic failure—and multiple system atrophy. Associated RBD is very common in these disorders, and increasing evidence suggests that most cases of apparent iRBD are due to otherwise asymptomatic synucleinopathies.

Parkinson disease, characterized clinically by often asymmetric rest tremor, rigidity, and bradykinesia responsive to levodopa, as well as postural instability, is associated on histopathologic examination with α-synuclein–containing intraneuronal Lewy bodies in substantia nigra and other structures, with resultant degeneration of the dopaminergic nigrostriatal pathway.[29] The reported frequency of RBD in Parkinson disease ranges between 15% and 65%.[30–34] Clinical features of Lewy body dementia differ from those of Alzheimer disease and may include impaired attention and visuospatial organization, fluctuating course, visual hallucinations, parkinsonism, delusions, and depression.[35] Lewy bodies are found in cortical, limbic, and substantia nigra neurons. When dementia develops before or concomitant with motor features of parkinsonism, dementia with Lewy bodies is diagnosed, whereas when dementia occurs at least 1 year after onset of motor features, the designation Parkinson disease with dementia is used. Patients with dementia and RBD have clinical and psychometric features much more suggestive of Lewy body dementia than of Alzheimer disease.[36–38] The frequency of RBD in dementia with Lewy bodies is reported to be 68% to 80%.[39]

Multiple system atrophy is a neurodegenerative disorder with dysautonomia and variable combinations of parkinsonism (poorly responsive to levodopa) and dysfunction of the cerebellar and corticospinal systems.[40] Sleep-disordered breathing, including obstructive sleep apnea (OSA), central sleep apnea, and nocturnal stridor, is common. In contrast with Parkinson disease and dementia with Lewy bodies, α-synuclein is found in non–Lewy body inclusions in oligodendrocytes. RBD occurs in 60% to 90% of patients with multiple system atrophy, both the cerebellar and the parkinsonian phenotypes.[41,42]

Many cross-sectional studies have demonstrated that patients with the apparently idiopathic form of RBD have

Table 118.1 Prodromal Features of Fully Expressed Synucleinopathies in Patients with Idiopathic Rapid Eye Movement Sleep Behavior Disorder

Physiologic Abnormalities
Reduced olfaction
Reduced color vision
Autonomic dysfunction (symptoms, cardiovascular tests,[123] I-MIBG myocardial scintigraphy)
Motor dysfunction
Cognitive dysfunction
EEG power abnormalities
Imaging Abnormalities
Midbrain: transcranial sonography
Striatal dopamine transporters: SPECT scans
Putaminal volume: MRI scans
Parkinson disease–related covariance pattern: PET and SPECT scans
Hyperperfusion and hypoperfusion of various brain regions: SPECT scans
Pons and midbrain abnormalities: MRI diffusion tensor imaging
Hippocampal gray matter: voxel-based morphometry
Cerebellum and pontine tegmentum: voxel-based morphometry
Increased cholinergic innervation of brainstem: PET scan
Pathologic Abnormalities
α-Synuclein deposits in:
Skin
Salivary glands
Colonic mucosa

EEG, Electroencephalogram; MIBG, metaiodobenzylguanidine; MRI, magnetic resonance imaging; PET, positron emission tomography; SPECT, single-photon emission computed tomography.

physiologic and imaging abnormalities suggestive of the prodromal phase of a synucleinopathy[43] (Table 118.1). Loss of olfactory function has been noted in 58% to 93% of patients with iRBD, significantly more than in control subjects[44–45] and similar to that in patients with Parkinson disease.[46] Similarly, abnormalities in color vision have been detected both in patients with iRBD and in those with Parkinson disease.[47] The presence of abnormalities of olfaction and color vision in patients with iRBD at baseline increases the risk of phenoconversion to parkinsonism or dementia over 5 years.[48] Autonomic symptoms[49,50] and abnormalities on tests of cardiovascular autonomic function[50–51] are more frequent in patients with iRBD than in control subjects. Pathologic studies have shown the presence of intraneuronal aggregates of phosphorylated α-synuclein in autonomic and somatosensory nerve fibers in the skin in proximal and distal sites,[52,53] in autonomic fibers in the submandibular salivary glands,[54,55] and in the colonic mucosa in patients with RBD.[56] Subtle abnormalities in motor function, including altered gait and decreased hand dexterity, have been detected in patients with iRBD.[49,57] Abnormalities in visuospatial functioning are evident on cognitive testing,[58] and electroencephalogram (EEG) spectral analysis has demonstrated increased theta power during wakefulness, decreased beta power during REM sleep,[59] and increased delta power in non–rapid eye movement (NREM) sleep[58] compared with control data.

A range of advanced imaging studies have shown abnormalities in patients with iRBD, particularly in the nigrostriatal system implicated in parkinsonism (Table 118.1). Transcranial sonography has shown midbrain hyperechogenicity in 36% to 63% of patients with iRBD,[45,60–61] a finding also noted in patients with Parkinson disease. Single-photon emission tomography (SPECT) scans with use of the tracer ^{123}I-fluoropropyl (FP)-CIT (2β-carbomethoxy-3β-[4-iodophenyl]-*N*-[3-fluoropropyl]-nortropane) or ^{123}I-IPT ([*N*]-[3-iodopropene-2-yl]-2β-carbomethoxy-3β-[4-chlorophenyl] tropane) have shown reduction of striatal dopamine transporters in 36% to 40% of patients with iRBD.[45,61,62] Reduced activity has been associated with progression to a fully expressed synucleinopathy.[61,63] In volumetric measurements on 3T magnetic resonance imaging (MRI) scans, putaminal volumes were smaller in patients with iRBD than in control subjects.[64] ^{18}F-fluorodeoxyglucose positron emission tomography (PET) and ethyl cysteinate dimer SPECT scans assessing a brain network known to be abnormal in Parkinson disease (i.e., Parkinson disease–related covariance pattern) showed similar increased activity in patients with iRBD, and those exhibiting such abnormalities had a greater likelihood of subsequent phenoconversion to Parkinson disease or dementia with Lewy bodies.[65,66] A PET study assessing cholinergic activity showed increased cholinergic innervation in brainstem areas associated with REM sleep, presumably representing compensatory upregulation.[67] MRI diffusion tensor imaging has shown abnormalities in the pons and midbrain of patients with iRBD.[68,69]

These data conclusively indicate that many patients with iRBD have abnormalities found in fully expressed synucleinopathies and that the presence of many of these changes predicts phenoconversion to parkinsonism or dementia. The rate of such conversion has been assessed in several prospective studies. In an early study a parkinsonian disorder emerged over a mean of 3.7 years in 38% of 29 men with iRBD diagnosed after the age of 50 years.[70] When the same cohort was reassessed 16 years later, parkinsonism or dementia had developed in 80.8%, with a mean of 14.2 years from iRBD onset to phenoconversion.[71] In a study of 93 patients with iRBD,[72] a survival analysis estimated the risk of phenoconversion to parkinsonism or dementia at 12 years from diagnosis to be 52.4%. In a series of 174 patients with iRBD followed for a mean of 4 years from diagnosis, survival analysis predicted phenoconversion rates of 33.1% at 5 years, 75.7% at 10 years, and 90.9% at 14 years.[73] The largest prospective study of 1280 patients seen in 24 sleep centers in Europe, Asia, and the Americas found a predicted conversion rate at 12 years from diagnosis of 73.5%, with an annualized overall phenoconversion rate of 6.25% per year[74] (Figure 118.3). Increased conversion rate was found in patients with olfactory deficit, color vision impairment, erectile dysfunction, and abnormal dopamine-transporter SPECT. Thus it appears that parkinsonism or dementia will develop in most patients with iRBD if they live long enough. A significant conversion rate has been confirmed in the only community-based study of 44 neurologically normal subjects with iRBD and age 70 to 89 years. After a median of 3.8 years, mild cognitive impairment, generally a precursor of dementia, had developed in 14, and Parkinson disease in 1. Compared with that in control subjects, the risk of phenoconversion estimated by hazard ratio was 2.2 (range, 1.3 to 3.9).[75] The latency between the onset of iRBD and phenoconversion can be extremely prolonged. A retrospective study of 27 patients diagnosed with iRBD at least 15 years before development of a fully-expressed neurodegenerative syndrome found a median interval of 25 years and a maximum interval of 50 years.[76]

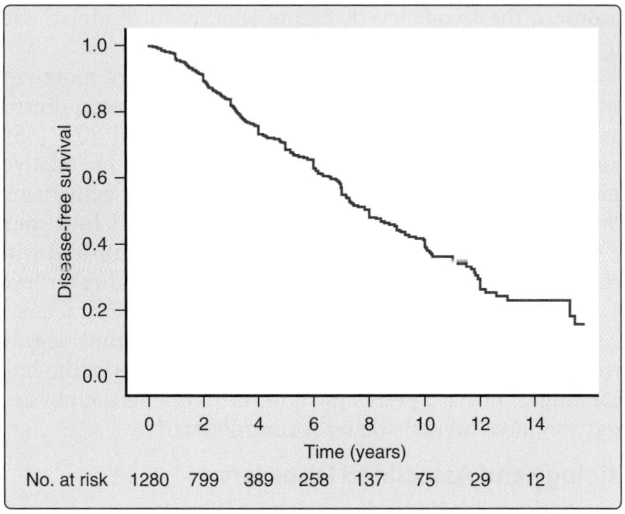

Figure 118.3 Progression from idiopathic REM sleep behavior disorder (iRBD) to fully developed synucleinopathies. Kaplan-Meier curve showing the rate of progression from iRBD to fully developed synucleinopathies. (Modified from Postuma RB, Iranzo A, Hu M, et al. Risk and predictors of dementia and parkinsonism in idiopathic REM sleep behavior disorder: a multicenter study. *Brain*. 2019;142:744–59; with permission.[74])

RBD occasionally has been reported in other neurodegenerative disorders that are not synucleinopathies. In a series of 45 patients with clinically diagnosed progressive supranuclear palsy (PSP), a disorder associated with tau protein inclusions, 13% were reported to have PSG-confirmed RBD, and another 14% had RSWA.[77] By contrast, none of the bed partners of 9 patients with PSP, 1 with the diagnosis subsequently confirmed pathologically, reported the presence of dream-enactment behavior.[78] In a series of 15 patients with clinically diagnosed Alzheimer disease, 1 patient (7%) had PSG-confirmed RBD, and 27% had RSWA.[79] However, the pathologic changes of Lewy body dementia and Alzheimer disease often occur concurrently in patients with suspected Alzheimer disease, and this may not be diagnosable ante mortem. RBD also has been described in association with Huntington disease[80] and with Guadeloupean parkinsonism, another tauopathy.[81]

The association of RBD with synucleinopathies has been confirmed in an international study of 172 patients with RBD, diagnosed either clinically or by PSG, who subsequently underwent autopsy.[82] Synucleinopathies were found in 93% (95% of 82 patients with PSG-confirmed RBD). These included 82% with Lewy body pathology (34% with concomitant Alzheimer-type changes) and 11% with multiple system atrophy. In the group with PSG confirmation, Alzheimer disease alone was found in only 1 patient, and PSP in another. In 1 patient with iRBD who died without the development of another overt neurologic disease, pathologic changes of Lewy body disease were found at autopsy, confirming an earlier reported similar case.[83] Whether a specific neurodegenerative disorder is associated with RBD appears to depend on the propensity for the disorder to involve pontomedullary neurons and not on the chemistry of the accumulating protein. This issue is discussed further in the subsequent Pathophysiology section.

Association with Other Neurologic Disorders

REM sleep motor dyscontrol is a common feature of narcolepsy. PSG studies found RBD in 32.5% of children with narcolepsy type 1[84] and increased REM sleep muscle activity in narcolepsy patients compared to control subjects.[84,85] RBD starts at a younger age in patients with narcolepsy than in patients without narcolepsy[86] and may be present at the start of the illness.[87]

RBD has been described in several rare paraneoplastic and autoimmune encephalopathies. Voltage-gated potassium channel complex (contactin-associated protein 2 [CASPR2] or leucine-rich glioma-inactivated protein 1[LGI1]) antibodies are associated with limbic encephalitis and Morvan syndrome, a disorder characterized by profound insomnia, dysautonomia, and peripheral neuromuscular irritability, sometimes associated with tumors such as malignant thymoma. RBD has been described in patients with both phenotypes.[88,89] Ma1 and Ma2 autoantibody-related encephalopathies are associated with testicular and other cancers. The clinical phenotype may include narcolepsy and RBD.[90,91] Autoantibodies directed against IgLON5, a neuronal cell adhesion molecule, have been associated with a distinctive neurologic syndrome characterized by progressive gait disturbances, bulbar symptoms, stridor, central hypoventilation, dysautonomia, and abnormal ocular movements.[92] All 8 affected patients exhibited abnormal movements during REM and NREM sleep, with RBD being diagnosed in the 4 patients in whom REM sleep was recorded during PSG.[93] These associations are uncommon and highly specific; a controlled study of 318 patients with iRBD did not reveal a higher frequency of autoimmune diseases in the RBD group.[21]

RBD also has been described in patients with a range of other neurologic disorders, including Machado-Joseph disease (spinocerebellar atrophy type 3),[94,95] adult-onset autosomal dominant leukodystrophy,[96] myotonic dystrophy type 2,[97] autism,[98] Tourette syndrome,[99] Möbius syndrome,[100,101] and Smith-Magenis syndrome.[101] Structural brainstem lesions occasionally may cause RBD, including multiple sclerosis,[102] astrocytomas,[101] acoustic neuroma,[103] vascular malformations,[104,105] central nervous system vasculitis,[106] and cerebral infarcts.[107,108]

Association with Antidepressants

RSWA[109,110] and RBD[12,111] have been related to antidepressant use. One study showed quantitatively increased REM sleep muscle activity in patients taking antidepressants even without RBD, compared to untreated patients with depression.[112] In comparison with patients with iRBD not taking antidepressants, RBD commenced earlier in patients in the antidepressant group, which also had a higher percentage of women.[113] In a study of early- versus late-onset RBD, the frequency of psychiatric diagnoses and antidepressant use was higher in the early-onset group.[16] A multicenter, controlled study that included 318 iRBD cases showed a higher percentage of depression and antidepressant use for the RBD group.[94] Various hypotheses have been suggested to explain this apparent association.[16,114] Antidepressants might cause RBD idiosyncratically in a minority of treated patients through a mechanism unrelated to synucleinopathies. Alternatively, antidepressants might unmask RBD in patients with otherwise subclinical synucleinopathies, resulting in an earlier presentation of RBD. Finally, antidepressant use may be a surrogate marker for depression, which is known to be an independent prodromal feature of synucleinopathies.[115] To address these possibilities, 100 patients with iRBD, 27 of whom were taking antidepressants, were followed for a mean of 4.5 years.[114] The groups with and without antidepressants showed the same frequency of abnormalities in olfactory, color vision, autonomic, and motor tests, suggesting that the antidepressant group patients were no less predisposed to development of a fully expressed synucleinopathy. However, the rate of phenoconversion to a diagnosis of a fully expressed synucleinopathy was slower in the antidepressant group, implying that RBD had emerged earlier than it would have if the patients were not taking antidepressants. By contrast, if depression were the initial manifestation of a synucleinopathy, one might have predicted phenoconversion to occur at least at the same rate as for the group not taking antidepressants, and perhaps faster.

Association with Other Drugs

An acute, transient form of RBD induced by withdrawal from barbiturates[116] and ethanol[117] has been described. Beta blockers and caffeine abuse also may possibly induce RBD.

Pathophysiology

The primary generator of REM sleep lies in the lateral pontine tegmentum in a small area ventral and slightly rostral to the locus coeruleus. Depending on researchers and species studied, the region has been termed the subcoeruleus nucleus, perilocus coeruleus alpha, sublateral dorsal tegmental nucleus, or nucleus reticularis pontis oralis.[118,119] Predominantly, glutamatergic neurons in the vicinity of this nucleus are responsible for regulation of REM sleep atonia. These neurons project both directly to inhibitory interneurons in the ventral horn of the spinal cord and also to neurons in the ventromedial medulla, including the gigantocellular and magnocellular neuronal groups.[119,120] The spinal interneurons and ventromedial medullary neurons inhibit anterior horn cells in the ventral horn of the spinal cord by release of the inhibitory neurotransmitters glycine and gamma-aminobutyric acid (GABA), resulting in skeletal muscle atonia.[118,120] Theoretically, then, RBD could arise from interruption of these pathways at pontine, medullary, or spinal cord levels.

Various animal models confirm these hypotheses, illustrated by the following examples.[121] Bilateral pontine tegmental lesions in cats cause loss of REM atonia and dream-enactment behavior, depending on the exact site and extent of the lesions.[122] Loss of REM atonia and complex motor behavior in REM sleep are seen in rats with lesions in the sublateral dorsal nuclei in the pons.[123] Lesions of the medullary gigantocellular nuclei result in loss of REM atonia in cats.[124] Transgenic mice expressing reduced glycine and GABA inhibitory activity exhibit motor behaviors during REM sleep with loss of REM atonia.[125] In humans, rare cases of focal lesions in the pontine tegmentum have been reported to cause RBD.* In Parkinson disease, Lewy bodies are found in neurons in the subcoeruleus nuclei in the pons and magnocellular reticular formation in the medulla.[128] In an MRI study of 24 patients with Parkinson disease, 12 with RBD and 12 without, reduced signal intensity was seen in the locus coeruleus–subcoeruleus complex, more marked in the subgroup with RBD.[129] The degree of signal intensity reduction correlated with the percentage of abnormal muscle activity in REM sleep.

*References 102, 104, 106, 121, 126, 127.

This model fits with the Braak staging scheme for the pathologic features of Parkinson disease.[130] In this scheme, pathologic changes of Lewy body disease develop first in the dorsal nucleus of the vagus in the medulla and the olfactory bulb—stage 1—and subsequently ascend to affect pontomedullary structures, including the magnocellular and subcoeruleus/sublateral dorsal nuclei—stages 2 and 3. Only in stage 4 is substantia nigra involved, resulting in overt parkinsonism, whereas mild cognitive impairment and dementia develop with cortical involvement in stages 5 and 6. This anatomic progression can explain the phenomenon of iRBD being in many cases a prodrome for the later development of Parkinson disease. Experimental evidence suggests that this relatively stereotypic progression of pathology may be explained by a prion-like mechanism, whereby α-synuclein aggregates can be induced transneuronally and serve as templates for further misfolding of the protein and subsequent neurodegeneration.[131]

Although an attractive hypothesis supported by experimental evidence, this model alone does not explain all aspects of the disease. As discussed earlier, patients with iRBD showed subclinical reduced sense of smell, impaired color vision, dysautonomia, and cognitive inefficiencies, suggesting involvement of multiple regions of the central and peripheral nervous system early in the disorder. In addition, iRBD patients have α-synuclein deposits in nerve fibers in the colonic mucosa, skin, and salivary glands.[53–57] Thus a multifocal origin for synucleinopathies remains possible, with certain regions showing increased selective vulnerability for the pathology. In addition, the Braak staging scheme does not fit all cases of Lewy body disease. In some patients with Parkinson disease, RBD develops simultaneously with the onset of parkinsonism or thereafter,[11] whereas in Lewy body dementia, cognitive impairment precedes definite parkinsonism.[128] Further animal and human studies are needed to define more precisely the nature of the origin and progression of RBD-associated neurodegeneration.

Diagnosis

Diagnostic criteria for RBD include the presence of RSWA (Figure 118.2) on PSG, sleep-related injurious or potentially injurious disruptive behaviors by history, and/or abnormal REM sleep behaviors during PSG, absence of epileptiform activity during REM sleep (unless RBD can be clearly distinguished from any concurrent REM sleep-related seizure disorder), and no better alternative explanation for the sleep disturbance.[132] In view of the resource-intensive nature of confirmatory PSG, however, a designation of "probable RBD" can be applied to patients presenting with a clear-cut clinical history of dream-enactment behaviors but lacking PSG evidence for RSWA, either owing to unavailability of the test or absence of recorded REM sleep during PSG. Also, because dream enactment is only rarely captured during in-laboratory PSG, RBD diagnosis usually instead relies on the history of dream-enactment behaviors, together with recording of RSWA.[132,133]

For use in epidemiologic research studies or clinical practices without readily accessible PSG, well-validated questionnaire screening instruments for probable RBD are available.[134–141] The REM Sleep Behavior Disorder Single-Question Screen (RBD1Q) poses a single "yes/no" question about dream enactment, providing 93.8% sensitivity and 87.2% specificity for RBD diagnosis in Parkinson disease in a large, multicenter validation study.[137] The Mayo Sleep Questionnaire (MSQ), a screening questionnaire that can be administered to either the patient or the bed partner, is another well-validated tool, with an Informant (Bedpartner) Version being particularly useful in older patients.[141,142] The MSQ-Informant (Bedpartner) Version is 100% sensitive and 95% specific,[141] and the MSQ-Patient Version is 100% sensitive and 73% specific for RBD diagnosis.[143] The REM Sleep Behavior Disorder Questionnaire–Hong Kong (RBDQ-HK) poses 13 questions about the frequency and severity of dream-enactment behavior, with a cut-off score of 18 of 100 possible points, yielding positive and negative predictive values greater than 80%.[135] The REM Sleep Behavior Disorder Screening Questionnaire (RBDSQ) is a 10-item questionnaire self-rated by the patient, with scores ranging from 0 to 13 points, yielding average scores of 9.5 in patients with RBD and 4.6 in control subjects without RBD.[135] Despite the usefulness of these measures for screening purposes, excluding mimickers of RBD (e.g., OSA with atypical arousals during REM sleep, NREM sleep parasomnias, and nocturnal epilepsy) is difficult and usually requires confirmation of RSWA by PSG.[14,28,132,144–147]

Polysomnographic RSWA manifests in submentalis, anterior tibialis, and arm leads of the electromyogram (EMG), especially flexor digitorum superficialis (FDS) and biceps brachii,[133,148–150] An EMG montage including the FDS has been shown to be most sensitive for identifying RSWA.[149,150] The prevailing gold standard for RSWA determination is the use of visual scoring methods as first proposed in 1992,[151] with subsequent modifications.[133,149,150,152,153] RSWA is classified as either excessive phasic (transient) or tonic muscle activity (Figure 118.2). Phasic RSWA is scored when at least 50% of the 3-second "mini-epochs" (with each 30-second epoch containing 10 mini-epochs) contain phasic (transient) muscle activity bursts exceeding the REM background EMG amplitude by at least two times and lasting for 0.1 to 5.0 seconds.[133,148,151,152] Tonic muscle activity is scored when the REM EMG background exceeds twice the background voltage amplitude and lasts longer than 15 seconds within a 30-second epoch.[133,148,152] The designation "any" muscle activity refers to phasic activity, tonic activity, or both present within a 3-second mini-epoch and is a more inclusive and readily applied metric for clinical use.[151,152] The most recent American Academy of Sleep Medicine scoring manual designated any chin or limb EMG activity as acceptable method to score RSWA, if the activity is greater than twice the amplitude of atonia during stage REM sleep and is present in greater than 50% of 3-second mini-epochs.[133] Percentage muscle activity for phasic, tonic, and "any" muscle activity is then determined by dividing the total number of 3-second mini-epochs (for phasic and "any") EMG activity and the number of 30-second tonic epochs by total REM time (after first accounting for, and deleting from the calculations, any physiologic REM sleep muscle activity that occurs during normal REM sleep arousals, which are not considered to be RSWA).[148,151,152] Many studies have shown clear elevations of phasic and tonic muscle activity in patients with RBD over that in control subjects without RBD, with diagnostic cut-offs determined for both individual and combined muscles.[148,150,152,154,155]

Various phasic, tonic, and "any" muscle activity cut-off values have been established for RBD diagnosis with 100% specificity. The SINBAR ("Sleep Innsbruck Barcelona") group of investigators has proposed a 31.9% "any" muscle activity cut-off for RBD diagnosis using combined submentalis and bilateral FDS EMG derivations.[150] A 43.4% "any" muscle activity diagnostic cut-off has been suggested for the commonly used combined submentalis and anterior tibialis EMG derivations from either split- or full-night PSGs in patients with RBD having comorbid OSA.[152] Measuring the phasic muscle burst duration was found to further help distinguish patients with RBD from control subjects.[152] Submentalis phasic and "any" muscle activity cut-offs have appeared quite similar across several studies from different centers: found to be between 15% to 20% (Montreal 15%, SINBAR 18%, Mayo 21.6%).[148,150,152] However, normative RSWA values in a large sample of adults without dream enactment found considerably lower-cohort 95th percentile amounts, suggesting that case-control study designs may have set the bar too high for RBD diagnosis.[153] In this study of 118 adults age 21 to 88 years without dream-enactment behaviors, 95th percentile muscle activity percentages in the submentalis muscle were phasic 8.6%, "any" 9.1%, and tonic 0.99%, whereas for the anterior tibialis muscle, phasic/"any" were both 17%, and combined submentalis/anterior tibialis muscles were phasic 22.3% and "any" 25.5%.[153]

Isolated elevations in RSWA levels are also a frequent incidental finding during PSG recordings in patients without dream-enactment behavior, seen especially in older adult males and in patients taking antidepressants.[153,156,157] The significance of isolated RSWA for future development of dream enactment or neurodegeneration remains unclear, although anecdotal cases of progression to synucleinopathy have been reported.[136] In addition, a longitudinal pilot study of 14 patients with isolated RSWA found, after a mean of 8.6 ± 0.9 years, that 1 patient developed RBD, 4 patients had substantia nigra hyperechogenicity, and 10 (71%) had presence of at least one neurodegenerative marker, including objective hyposmia, orthostatic hypotension, decreased color vision discrimination, fine motor task slowing, or cognitive impairment similar to "soft signs" of synucleinopathy identified in idiopathic RBD[136,157] Isolated RSWA without clinical dream enactment occurs frequently in Parkinson disease and other synucleinopathies, suggesting that additional lesions in other structures may be required to mediate full RBD.[31]

Several computerized automated methods for RSWA analysis have demonstrated comparable diagnostic yield to labor-intensive visual methods, including the REM Atonia Index,[153–155] an enveloping technique for mentalis short- and long-duration muscle activity measurement,[158] an automated SINBAR method analyzing combined submentalis and FDS muscle activity,[159] and a data driven, machine learning method.[160] These methods await further external validation in large multicenter cohorts to determine their eventual clinical utility and adoption.

REM Sleep Behavior Disorder Variants

RBD has been described in association with three variant syndromes in which dream enactment and RSWA are associated with other parasomnias or disturbances of sleep architecture. Overlap parasomnia disorder is characterized by overlapping clinical features of both NREM disorder of arousal parasomnias, such as sleepwalking, night terrors, confusional arousals, or related events, including sleep eating or sexsomnia behaviors and RBD.[161,162] A recent review of 144 cases suggested that overlap parasomnia disorder is a distinct clinical entity. In 69% of patients with this disorder, the RBD plus parasomnia was idiopathic, with an earlier age at onset than for patients with typical RBD alone. Patients with overlap parasomnia exhibited more prominent NREM than REM parasomnia characteristics, with RBD either being mild or discovered incidentally.[163] The association of overlap parasomnia with synucleinopathies also appears to be less clear than for typical RBD, although overlap parasomnia has been described in Parkinson disease. Further research is necessary to clarify whether overlap parasomnia has a natural history different from that for typical RBD.[164]

Status dissociatus is a rare condition involving completely eroded wake and sleep-state boundaries, with resultant disturbances in vigilance, cognitive functioning, and sleep motor control. Conventional sleep-stage scoring during PSG is almost impossible owing to the characteristic admixture of neurophysiologic features of wake, NREM, and REM sleep states.[165,166] Agrypnia excitata is another rare, closely related condition with the distinctive features of inability to fall asleep, coupled with excessive motor and autonomic hyperactivity. PSG in agrypnia excitata shows absence of N3 sleep, spindles, and K complexes, with persisting N1 architecture and brief periods of REM sleep with loss of normal atonia.[167] Oneiric behaviors (complex motor acts resembling simple daytime activities and gestures, such as chewing, hair combing, or pointing) also are characteristic of agrypnia excitata.[168] Status dissociatus may be seen in certain pontomesencephalic brain lesions and late-stage neurodegenerative disorders, including multiple system atrophy and other synucleinopathies. Agrypnia excitata is thought to arise from thalamic-limbic dysfunction associated with delirium tremens, fatal familial insomnia, and certain autoimmune encephalopathies, including voltage-gated potassium channel (CASPR2 or LGI1) antibody (Morvan) syndrome.[169] Clonazepam has been reported to be effective in the treatment of status dissociatus[165]; treatment approaches for agrypnia excitata beyond supportive care have not been described.

Differential Diagnosis

Mimickers of RBD include nightmares, NREM parasomnias, nocturnal epilepsy, OSA with "pseudo-RBD"–type confusional arousals from REM sleep, the proposed parasomnia trauma-associated sleep disorder, and psychiatric disorders, such as posttraumatic stress disorder (PTSD) or nocturnal panic disorder.[144,170,171] Patients with nightmare disorder may vocalize or move minimally during their dreams, but dream enactment involving complex motor behaviors paralleling dream content usually is lacking. These patients do not exhibit RSWA during PSG. Nocturnal epilepsy, particularly frontal lobe or extratemporal seizures, may very closely mimic RBD in some cases, although nocturnal epilepsy usually is distinguished by relative stereotypy across events and lack of paralleling dream mentation. Video EEG PSG, including a full EEG montage, is necessary in some cases to rule out nocturnal epilepsy with confidence. OSA may manifest with dream-enactment behavior that subsides with successful nasal continuous positive airway pressure therapy, and in patients with OSA alone, without comorbid RBD, RSWA is not observed during PSG.[170]

Trauma-associated sleep disorder, a proposed parasomnia, is characterized by violent nocturnal behaviors associated with dream enactment, specifically related to a previous significant life trauma, and presents in a substantially younger group of patients than would be typical for RBD. Trauma-associated sleep disorder was initially described in four young, male active duty US soldiers (age 22 to 39 years).[171] It remains unclear if trauma-associated sleep disorder is simply RBD or possibly a NREM parasomnia variant because RSWA was not seen in all cases, or whether it is a distinctive parasomnia. Prazosin was reported to be helpful in controlling disturbing nocturnal behaviors associated with trauma-associated sleep disorder. Psychiatric disorders, such as PTSD and panic disorder, are sometimes difficult to distinguish from RBD, and indeed PTSD has also been associated with both RBD and RSWA. Of 394 military veterans (94% men, 54.4 to 15.5 years) who were studied with PSG, symptoms of dream enactment without RSWA were present in 31% of patients, whereas 9% had RBD, and 7% had isolated RSWA. In this cohort, RBD diagnoses were most frequent in those with PTSD (15%) and especially in patients who also had a history of traumatic brain injury (11%).[172] RBD and RSWA are frequently associated with depression and antidepressant use, and some patients with underlying depression, PTSD, or panic disorder may have both conditions. Confident RBD diagnosis requires a thorough clinical history and examination and confirmation of RSWA by the gold standard of PSG.[14,132,144]

Management

The goals of RBD treatment are to reduce dream-enactment behavior frequency and severity and to prevent injury. Bedroom safety principles should be advised for all patients, including removal or padding of bedside furniture with sharp corners, minimizing fall-related injury potential by adding bed rails, lowering the mattress to floor level or placing cushions near the bed, erecting pillow barriers between the patient and the bed partner, and removing firearms from the bedroom.[136,144] A bed alarm system also may be useful to alert the patient or caregiver if the patient leaves the bed.[173]

Melatonin and clonazepam are the two mainstays of RBD pharmacologic treatment[11,174–176] and appear to be similarly effective in reducing dream-enactment behaviors. However, although clonazepam and melatonin both appear to reduce RBD symptoms, these drugs only rarely actually stop the behaviors.[174] In consequence, additional prospective treatment trials and development of other novel agents to treat RBD are needed.[177]

Clonazepam has been the traditional drug of choice for RBD, with a reported median effective dose between 0.25 and 2.0 mg at bedtime. Approximately 90% of subjects in open-label studies reported a partial or complete response to the drug, although no adequately powered controlled trials have been performed. A small pilot, placebo-controlled, randomized trial of clonazepam (0.5 mg) found no difference in Clinician Global Impression scores after 1 month,[11,174,176,178] Clonazepam has several adverse effects that may limit its application in most elderly patients, including worsened OSA; cognitive dysfunction; and dose-related adverse effects of sleepiness, dizziness, unsteadiness, and sexual dysfunction.[144,174] Both melatonin and clonazepam variably decrease PSG motor activity during REM sleep.[151,175,176,179–182]

Several retrospective and small prospective studies support the use of melatonin treatment for RBD.* Melatonin may have a slightly more robust effect in reducing injuries, with fewer adverse effects,[174] although a prospective comparison with clonazepam has not been performed.[177] Melatonin may be more effective and tolerable in elderly patients, especially those with cognitive impairment or parkinsonism.[174] Adverse effects of melatonin include daytime sleepiness and dizziness, with headache and hallucinations occasionally reported.[173,174] Use of melatonin doses between 3 and 15 mg at bedtime (with occasional patients using doses up to 25 mg) has been reportedly effective, with a median dose of 6 mg[174] (Table 118.2). However, a recent small, randomized, placebo-controlled symptomatic treatment trial of melatonin in RBD associated with Parkinson disease has raised doubt concerning the efficacy of this treatment as it showed no statistically significant difference between prolonged-release melatonin (4 mg) and placebo.[175]

Other drugs also have been reported to reduce RBD symptoms, including pramipexole,[186,187] zopiclone,[179] zonisamide,[188] donepezil,[189,190] ramelteon,[191] agomelatine,[192] memantine,[193] cannabidiol,[194] and the herbal supplement Yi-Gan San.[195]

* References 173,174,178,180,181,183–185.

Table 118.2 Principal Treatments for Rapid Eye Movement Sleep Behavior Disorder

Drug	Possible Mechanism of Action	Dose	Adverse Effect(s)
Clonazepam	$GABA_A$ receptor agonist	0.25–2 mg	Sedation, dizziness, sexual dysfunction, worsened sleep-disordered breathing
Melatonin	Unknown	3–15 mg	Sedation

$GABA_A$, Gamma-aminobutyric acid type A (receptor).

OTHER RAPID EYE MOVEMENT SLEEP PARASOMNIAS

Nightmare Disorder

Nightmare disorder is discussed in Chapter 119.

Recurrent Isolated Sleep Paralysis

Sleep paralysis has long been recognized in different cultures, often with postulation of a supernatural explanation.[196] It consists of an inability to move or speak at sleep onset or on awakening from sleep, with at least partial preservation of consciousness. The trunk and all four limbs are affected.[197,198] The paralysis resolves after sensory stimulation, such as with someone touching the patient. At least initially, events usually are associated with severe anxiety.[197] Visual hypnagogic or hypnopompic hallucinations are experienced by 21% to 24% of patients with sleep paralysis,[199,200] but associated kinetic, tactile, and auditory hallucinations may be even more common.[200] Events occur more commonly on awakening than at sleep onset.[199] Insomnia,[200] sleep starts, sleep-related cramps, and sleeptalking[199] are more common in patients with sleep paralysis than in control subjects. PSG studies have suggested that sleep paralysis may occur during dissociated REM sleep, with persistence of consciousness and alpha activity intruding into the otherwise desynchronized REM sleep EEG.[196]

Sleep paralysis is common in narcolepsy but occurs frequently in isolation in the general population. Reported prevalence of sleep paralysis varies widely between studies, with higher rates reported in samples of students, patients with psychiatric illnesses, and patients with panic disorder.[201] The prevalence within a large population-based study of 8085 subjects was 6.2%.[199] Predictive variables for sleep paralysis included bipolar disorder and the use of anxiolytic medications. Sleep paralysis can start at any age, but onset may be most common during young adulthood and middle age.[199] Familial sleep paralysis has been described,[197] with recognition of three- to four-generation families and a possible maternal inheritance pattern.[198]

Sleep paralysis should be considered a disorder only if it is recurrent and results in clinically significant distress, including bedtime anxiety or difficulty initiating sleep.[132] Explanation and reassurance usually are sufficient to address the patient's concerns. Antidepressants occasionally have been tried, presumably to suppress REM sleep phenomena, but no adequately reported studies of pharmacologic interventions are available.

Sleep-Related Painful Erections

Sleep-related painful erections is a rare disorder of uncertain etiology. The mean age at diagnosis is 39.8 years, with symptoms present for a mean of 5.4 years.[202] Painful erections occur during REM sleep, usually nightly and sometimes several times a night.[203] Erections are painless during intercourse or masturbation.[204] Structural abnormalities of the penis are not present. PSG shows reduced sleep efficiency, increased wake time after sleep onset, and decreased percentage REM sleep compared with control data.[203] One study showed reduced vagal activity during sleep and a trend toward heart rate acceleration during spontaneous body movements.[203] Various medications have been reported to be effective for weeks to months in single-patient or short-series reports,[204] including propranolol,[202] clonazepam,[205] baclofen,[205] and various antidepressants (amitriptyline,[205] paroxetine,[202] and venlafaxine[205]), but no controlled or systematic long-term study of management has been performed.

CLINICAL PEARLS

- Rapid eye movement sleep behavior disorder (RBD) occurs predominantly in men (79% of patients), but this difference becomes less marked when the disorder commences before the age of 50 years.
- RBD can result in serious injuries to both patients and their bed partners, including fractures, subdural hematomas, ecchymoses, lacerations, and dental injuries.
- RBD is strongly associated with fully expressed synucleinopathies (Parkinson disease, dementia with Lewy bodies, and multiple system atrophy), and in 74% of patients with idiopathic RBD, a fully expressed synucleinopathy will develop within 12 years of RBD diagnosis.
- In patients with idiopathic RBD, decreased olfaction, changes in color vision, and autonomic findings may indicate a greater risk for an underlying synucleinopathy.
- Although both clonazepam and melatonin are effective in treating RBD, clonazepam has many side effects, especially in elderly and neurologically disabled persons, and melatonin should be the first drug tried in these patients.
- Recurrent isolated sleep paralysis may occur in 6% of the population but should be regarded as a disorder only if it results in significant distress, including bedtime anxiety or difficulty initiating sleep.

SUMMARY

Dissociation of the phenomena characterizing the REM sleep state results in a number of disorders, with broad implications for elucidation of sleep and neurologic disease. Clinical and basic science research over the past 50 years has resulted in an understanding of RBD that exceeds that of any other parasomnia. It is an example of a sleep disorder in which the anatomic, physiologic, and pathologic substrate correlates closely with the clinical and PSG manifestations. Increasingly sophisticated diagnostic tools are becoming available, and effective forms of management have emerged. RBD serves as a biomarker for the development of fully expressed synucleinopathies, and an important goal of future research will be finding therapeutic agents that may delay or prevent phenoconversion to overt neurodegenerative disorders. The contribution of antidepressants to the pathogenesis of RBD remains unsettled, and further studies are needed to determine definitively whether these drugs are primary etiologic agents or merely unmask an evolving synucleinopathy. Other REM parasomnias range from the very common (nightmares and sleep paralysis) to the rare (sleep-related painful erections). Further investigations of their pathophysiology and optimal management are needed.

SELECTED READINGS

Boeve B, Silber MH, Ferman TJ, et al. Clinicopathologic correlations in 172 cases of rapid eye movement sleep behavior disorder with or without a coexisting neurologic disorder. *Sleep Med.* 2013;14:754–762.

Boeve BF, Silber MH, Saper CB, et al. Pathophysiology of REM sleep behavior disorder and relevance to neurodegenerative disease. *Brain.* 2007;130:2770–2780.

Doppler K, Jentschke H, Schulmeyer L, et al. Dermal phospho-alpha-synuclein deposits confirm REM sleep behavior disorder as prodromal Parkinson's disease. *Acta Neuropathol.* 2017;133:535–545.

Feemster JC, Jung Y, Timm PC, et al. Normative and isolated rapid eye movement sleep without atonia in adults without REM sleep behavior disorder. *Sleep.* 2019;42(10):zsz124.

Fernandez-Arcos A, Iranzo A, Serradell M, Gaig C, Santamaria J. The clinical phenotype of idiopathic rapid eye movement sleep behavior disorder at presentation: a study in 203 consecutive patients. *Sleep.* 2016;39:121–132.

Frauscher B, Iranzo A, Högl B, et al. Quantification of electromyographic activity during REM sleep in multiple muscles in REM sleep behavior disorder. *Sleep.* 2008;31:724–731.

Gilat M, Marshall NS, Testelmans D, Buyse B, Lewis SJG. A critical review of the pharmacological treatment of REM sleep behavior disorder in adults: time for more and larger randomized placebo-controlled trials [published online ahead of print, 2021 Jan 7]. *J Neurol.* 2021;10.1007/s00415-020-10353-0.

Haba-Rubio J, Frauscher B, Marques-Vidal P, et al. Prevalence and determinants of REM sleep behavior disorder in the general population. *Sleep.* 2018;41(2):zsx197.

Iranzo A, Borrego S, Vilaseca I, et al. α-Synuclein aggregates in labial salivary glands of idiopathic rapid eye movement sleep behavior disorder. *Sleep.* 2018;41(8). https://doi.org/10.1093/sleep/zsy101.

McCarter SJ, Boswell CL, St Louis EK, et al. Treatment outcomes in REM sleep behavior disorder. *Sleep Med.* 2013;14:237–242.

McCarter SJ, St Louis EK, Duwell E, et al. Diagnostic thresholds for quantitative REM sleep muscle densities, phasic burst duration, and REM atonia index in REM sleep behavior disorder with and without co-morbid obstructive sleep apnea. *Sleep.* 2014;37:1–14.

Olson EJ, Boeve BF, Silber MH. Rapid eye movement sleep behavior disorder: demographic, clinical and laboratory findings in 93 cases. *Brain.* 2000;123:331–339.

Postuma RB, Gagnon JF, Bertrand JA, et al. Parkinson risk in idiopathic REM sleep behavior disorder: preparing for neuroprotective trials. *Neurology.* 2015;84:1104–1113.

Postuma RB, Gagnon JF, Tuineaig M. Antidepressants and REM sleep behavior disorder: isolated side effect or neurodegenerative signal? *Sleep.* 2013;36:1579–1585.

Postuma RB, Iranzo A, Hu M, et al. Risk and predictors of dementia and parkinsonism in idiopathic REM sleep behavior disorder: a multicenter study. *Brain.* 2019;142:744–759. 2012;71:49–56.

A complete reference list can be found online at ExpertConsult.com.

Chapter 119

Nightmares and Dream Disturbances

Isabelle Arnulf

Chapter Highlights

- Nightmares are common and have many causes.
- Nightmare disorder is the condition of distressing dreams that result in clinically significant distress or impairment in social, occupational, or other areas of functioning.
- Distressing dream mentation can occur with other sleep and neurologic disorders.
- Approximately 70% of adults with a disorder of arousal will have one event with memory of dream-like and nightmarish mental content associated and congruent with the motor episodes of sleepwalking or sleep terror.
- Patients with rapid eye movement (REM) sleep behavior disorder are more likely to report dreams containing elements of aggression and animals, with behavior isomorphic to the dream content.
- Patients with narcolepsy have long and intense dreams during sleep onset in REM periods (with pleasurable flying expeditions) with a high number of lucid dreams and nightmares. The multimodal hypnagogic hallucinations in narcolepsy suggest awake dreaming.

Classically, awakening nightmares are defined as frightening or distressing dreams from sleep. However, patients may use the term *nightmare* in various situations, including the classical rapid eye movement (REM) sleep nightmare disorders, posttraumatic stress disorder, distressing dreams linked with psychiatric conditions, disturbed dreaming associated with drugs and substances or with neurologic diseases or conditions, hypnagogic hallucinations, sleep terrors (ST), REM sleep behavior disorder (RBD), *status dissociatus*, and epic dreaming. The sensorial characteristics of their mental experience, its construction, timing, duration, and context, along with associated behaviors, concomitant autonomic signs, the ability to recognize the unreal nature of the experience, and associated disorders, as well as aspects and timing of polysomnography help to determine a diagnosis (Table 119.1). A good example of this complexity is in a 62-year-old patient who experienced recurrent nightmares in which he was obliged to swallow several big, yellow snakes every night. As a consequence, he was scared of going to bed and delayed his bedtime every night. Through a long interview, my colleagues and I realized that this patient did not use any provocative drugs, have posttraumatic stress disorder, nor have experience with snakes. Video polysomnography and Multiple Sleep Latency Tests demonstrated no evidence of ST nor RBD, and my colleagues and I concluded he suffered from hypnagogic hallucinations linked to narcolepsy.

This case illustrates that patients complaining of nightmares or disturbed dreaming may not restrict the use of the word *nightmare*, as a sleep specialist would, to REM sleep–associated nightmares. In terms of mechanisms, recent insights have shown that many of these disturbed mental experiences in neurologic diseases may give us clues to the network involved in the sleep-wake state.

NIGHTMARE DISORDER

Diagnosis

Nightmare disorder is characterized by recurrent episodes of intense dysphoric dreaming (involving feelings of threat, anxiety, fear or terror, anger, rage, embarrassment, and disgust) that arise primarily during REM sleep, often result in awakening with rapid reorientation, and cause clinically significant distress or impairment in social, occupational, or other area of functioning.[1] The episodes tend to occur during the second half of the major sleep episode when the REM pressure is most pronounced. Nightmare content most often focuses on imminent physical danger to the individual but may also involve other distressing themes. Most patients are able to detail the nightmare's contents upon awakening. Nightmares are distinct from anxiety dreams (or "bad dreams"), which are frightening dream experiences remembered only after waking in the morning, usually less emotionally intense than nightmares.[2] Physical aggression is the most frequently reported theme in nightmares, whereas interpersonal conflicts predominate in bad dreams.[2] Nightmare disorder can lead to sleep avoidance and deprivation, and thereby to more intense nightmares, which can produce insomnia or other daytime sequelae. The disorder is distinct from parasomnia-associated nightmares by the absence of dream enactment.

Criteria

Patients with nightmare disorders should meet the following criteria:

1. Repeated occurrences of extended, extremely dysphoric, and well-remembered dreams usually involve threats to survival, security, or physical integrity.
2. On awakening from the dysphoric dreams, the person rapidly becomes oriented and alert.

Table 119.1 Causes and Semiology of the Complaints of "Nightmares" and Disturbed Dreaming in Neurologic Diseases

	Aspects	Associated Disorders
Vivid dreaming	Dreams of flight, nightmares	Narcolepsy
	Fights with animals, aggression	Parkinson disease Dementia with Lewy bodies
	Associated with autonomic dysfunction and *status dissociatus*	Guillain-Barré syndrome
Hypnagogic hallucinations	Multimodal, frightening Often associated with sleep paralysis and RBD	Narcolepsy
	Presence, passage, visual hallucinations of humans and animals	Parkinson disease Dementia with Lewy bodies
	Visual, spatial tilt, auditory Associated with autonomic dysfunction and *status dissociatus*	Guillain-Barré syndrome
NREM parasomnia	Associated with screams, tachycardia, sudden arousal, escaping from the bed Mostly misfortunes (buried alive, collapsing ceiling, life-threatening danger)	Sleep terrors Confusional arousals
REM parasomnia	Enacted dreams with aggression by humans or animals, kicking, boxing, shouting, swearing	REM sleep behavior disorder (idiopathic, Parkinsonism, dementia, narcolepsy)
Status dissociatus	Continuously enacted dreams with visual hallucinations (patients may seem awake)	Guillain-Barré syndrome *Delirium tremens* Fatal familial insomnia Morvan's chorea and neurodegenerative diseases

RBD, REM sleep behavior disorder.

3. The dream experience, or the sleep disturbance produced by awakening from it, causes clinically significant distress or impairment in social, occupational, or other important areas of functioning.[1]

Epidemiology

Occasional nightmares are frequent in children (60% to 75%, beginning as young as 2½ years old and peaking between 6 and 10 years old). Nightmares are repeated more than once a week in only 2% to 8% of the children, but they often persist in adulthood.[3] Girls and boys are equally affected until late adolescence, when girls are more affected than boys. Around 4% of adults suffer from nightmare disorder. The nightmare frequency is higher in psychiatric disorders, including posttraumatic stress disorder, substance abuse, stress and anxiety, borderline personality, and other psychiatric illnesses such as schizophrenia spectrum disorders. Nightmares particularly occur immediately after a traumatic stress. Nightmares beginning within 3 months of a trauma are present in up to 80% of patients with posttraumatic stress disorder. Approximately 50% of posttraumatic stress disorder cases resolve within 3 months, but posttraumatic nightmares may persist throughout life.

Evaluation

Overnight polysomnography is not routinely used to assess nightmare disorder but may be appropriately performed to exclude other parasomnias or sleep-disordered breathing. Sleep recordings during actual nightmares occasionally show abrupt awakenings from REM sleep preceded by accelerated heart and respiratory rates. Of note, posttraumatic nightmares emerge both from REM sleep (sometimes just after less than 1 minute of REM sleep) and non–rapid eye movement (NREM) sleep (including sleep onset). Highly disturbing dream content frequently contrasts strikingly with relatively minor autonomic changes (e.g., no visible tears) and lack of vocalization or motor behavior (no shouting, no attempt to suddenly escape the bed), which constitutes the main differences with ST. One exception to this rule has been described in a few veterans during the acute phase of posttraumatic stress disorder. Some patients may indeed yell, scream, attack their bed partners, or run out of bed when dreaming of replaying the traumatic experience. These occasional enacted nightmares in posttraumatic stress disorder have led some authors to suggest building a new category of parasomnia, named trauma-associated sleep disorder, in the next edition of the *International Classification of Sleep Disorders* (ICSD).[4]

RBD, in contrast, does demonstrate significant movement, typically defending against aggressors, in the absence of previous trauma experience, and takes place exclusively in REM sleep. Hallucinations and sleep paralysis may be described as "nightmares," but they specifically occur at sleep onset and offset, and the paralysis affects the whole body and induces a dyspnea. Nocturnal panic attacks are not associated with detailed mental imagery. Severe sleep apnea may be associated with disagreeable sleep-associated mentation that resolves with the treatment of apnea.

Neurophysiology

Recently, a series of experiments combining serial awakenings with dream recall, high-density electroencephalography

(EEG), and brain functional imaging in normal subjects showed the following:

1. The insula and midcingulate cortex activity increase during dreams containing fear (as they would do when experiencing fear during wakefulness).
2. Subjects reporting a higher incidence of fear in their dreams show reduced emotional arousal and functional magnetic resonance imaging response to fear-eliciting stimuli in the insula, amygdala, and midcingulate cortex while awake.
3. Consistent with better emotion regulation processes, the same participants display increased medial prefrontal cortex activity.[5]

These findings support that emotions in dreams and wakefulness engage similar neural substrates and suggest that experiencing fear in dreams is associated with more adapted responses to threatening signals during wakefulness.

Treatment

The most well-established treatment of idiopathic nightmare disorder is image rehearsal therapy, while systematic desensitization and progressive deep muscle relaxation training is also suggested.[6] During image rehearsal therapy, patients are trained to change nightmares into dreams.[7] After writing down the less distressing of their recurrent nightmares, patients are invited to identify in the report the point when the story takes a negative turn. From this point, they are instructed to imagine some changes in the nightmare storyline (e.g., change a character, change the end of the story toward a more ordinary or happy end) that will result in more positive emotions. It is mandatory that the changes are trained by mental imagery, not just written. Each evening before sleeping, they should rehearse the new dream scenario by mental imagery, until they stop experiencing this particular nightmare. Exercises of mental imagery are performed too. Systematic desensitization is a behavioral therapy that uses the principle of gradually exposing the patients to what they fear.[8] The patients are trained to cope with and manage the stressors gradually before they are actually exposed to the feared object or situation.

There is lower-grade evidence for using lucid dreaming therapy and self-exposure therapy. Among the pharmacologic treatment of posttraumatic stress disorder–associated nightmares, prazosin carries a level-A recommendation, while the benefit of clonidine is less clear. However, a recent randomized trial in military veterans failed to find a benefit of prazosin in posttraumatic nightmares.[9] Treatments with lower-grade evidence include several drugs such as trazodone, atypical antipsychotic medications, topiramate, low-dose cortisol, fluvoxamine, triazolam and nitrazepam, phenelzine, gabapentin, cyproheptadine,[10] and tricyclic antidepressants. Some behavioral therapies such as exposure, relaxation, and re-scripting therapy, sleep dynamic therapy, hypnosis, eye-movement desensitization and reprocessing, and the testimony method also have low-grade or limited evidence of effect.

DRUG-ASSOCIATED NIGHTMARES

Recurrent nightmares may also be a deleterious effect of various drugs that are commonly prescribed (Table 119.2),[11] including antidepressants (more those with serotonin reuptake activity than tricyclics),[10] antihypertensives (beta blockers,[12] alpha agonists, enalapril, losartan, verapamil), dopamine-receptor agonists, cholinesterase blockers (donepezil, rivastigmine, and tacrine),[13,14] varenicline (a nicotinic acetylcholine blocker),[15,16] nicotine patches,[15,16] and ganciclovir. Similarly, the withdrawal of REM sleep suppressive agents (antidepressants, benzodiazepine, barbiturate, ethanol) or the end-of-night REM sleep rebound after using short-acting hypnotics such as zolpidem can promote nightmares.

DREAM-LIKE AND NIGHTMARISH MENTATIONS DURING AROUSAL DISORDERS

General Context

Sleepwalking (SW) and ST consist of a series of abnormal mental experiences and complex behaviors associated with sudden adrenergic discharges occurring during partial awakenings from slow wave sleep (or NREM sleep N3 stage), hence their name "disorders of arousal."[1] Most motor episodes begin with raising the head, opening the eyes, and looking about in a confused manner, sometimes with concomitant verbal utterances.[17] In addition to this common pattern, sleepwalkers will stand up and walk, and patients with ST begin their events with a scream and signs of intense fear (see Chapter 116).[17]

Mentation Associated with Sleepwalking and Sleep Terrors

Contrary to common belief, more than 70% of adults with SW/ST will remember at least one event with dream-like content (which they frequently identify as a dream or a nightmare) associated with their abnormal motor behavior.[19] The dreams are mostly short, visual, and frequently unpleasant, involving a threat to them or a loved one. There is no major difference regarding the frequency and nature of the dream content in SW versus ST. In another series of 73 adults with SW/ST, 53% reported nightmarish mental content combined with the sensation of a vital threat and the need to escape danger during the motor episodes.[20]

The patients with SW/ST describe the presence of a person in the associated dream mentation (39% of patients), either unknown to the dreamer or a relative of the dreamer (33%). Animals (11%) have also been described and are generally frightening.[19] Most (80%) mental contents are negative, associated with aggression (26%) and misfortune (54%), and 84% are apprehensive. The patient is never the primary aggressor. In reports of acts of friendliness (12%), the patient befriends someone and attempts to protect them (generally a relative) from danger.[19] In another series, as much as 70% of dream mentation during SW/ST contained threats, which were more commonly misfortunes and disasters than aggressions. The scenario included their bedroom in nearly half of the sleepwalkers' dreams.[21] The projection of the mental images on the room background suggests a concomitant activation of mental images and real images seen through the eyes of the sleepwalker (Figure 119.1).[22] A few case reports confirmed the mind-body isomorphism using a video of the event, followed by a detailed report of a dream coherent with the previously observed behavior (Videos 119.1 and 119.2).[23]

Mechanisms

There have been several hypotheses regarding the mechanisms of these abnormal dream mentations. The brief scenes may be hypnagogic hallucinations emerging from N3 sleep rather than more classical dreams; alternatively, they could be the

Table 119.2 Influence of Common Drugs Promoting or Reducing Nightmares

Type of Drug	Effect on CNS	Type of Altered Dreaming
Antiallergic and Antiinflammatory Drugs		
Cyproheptadine[10]	Reduces 5-HT	Reduces posttraumatic nightmares
Montelukast (leukotriene receptor antagonist)	Not elucidated	Promotes nightmares
Antidepressants[67]		
Selective serotonin reuptake inhibitors; serotonin and norepinephrine reuptake inhibitors	Increases 5-HT, NA (α2), DA, ACh, reduces H	Promotes nightmares and REM sleep behavior disorder
Antihypertensives		
Beta blockers, especially lipophilic ones passing the blood brain barrier (propranolol, labetalol, metoprolol)[12]	Blocks NA (beta) receptor Reduces melatonin release	Promotes nightmares, disturbing and vivid dreams
Prazosin	Blocks NA (alpha-1) receptors	Reduces posttraumatic nightmares in acute[68] but not in chronic PTSD[9]
Dopaminergic Drugs		
Pramipexole,[69] levodopa[53]	Increases DA	Promotes vivid dreams and nightmares
Antiinfectious Agents		
Efavirenz[70]	Increases 5-HT_2	Promotes unusual and bad dreams
Mefloquine[71]	Reduces 5-HT and GABA Blocks gap junctions	Promotes abnormal dreams
Drugs Used for Smoking Cessation		
Varenicline[15,16]	Increases ACh (agonist of nicotinic receptors)	Promotes abnormal dreams and dream-/sleep-related behaviors
Nicotine patches[16]	Increases ACh (nicotinic) and DA	Promotes abnormal dreams
Hypnotics		
Nonbenzodiazepine receptor agonists (zolpidem, zaleplon, zopiclone)[72]	Increases GABA	Promotes nightmares, dream-like hallucinations, and dream-/sleep-related behaviors (automatism-amnesia syndrome)
Nabilone[73]	Cannabinoid receptors	Reduces posttraumatic nightmares
Memory-Enhancing Drugs		
Cholinesterase inhibitors (galantamine, donepezil)[13,14]	Increases ACh	Promotes nightmares

ACh, Acetylcholine; CNS, central nervous system; DA, dopaminergic transmission; GABA, gamma-aminobutyric acid; 5-HT, serotonergic; H, histaminergic; NA, noradrenergic; PTSD, posttraumatic stress disorder.

terminal part of a longer dream partially forgotten at the time of arousal[19] or a phasic, short mental creation elicited before or just at the time of arousal, by ambient noises or physical contacts.[22,24] Notably, the adrenergic arousal occurs 4 seconds before motor arousal from N3 sleep, suggesting that an alarming event during sleep (possibly a worrying sleep mentation or a local, subcortical arousal) causes the motor arousal.[25] The negative emotions associated with the mentations parallel the activation of the amygdala–temporo-insular areas disengaged from the control of the prefrontal cortex (motor and emotional activation, such as fear and wandering) observed in functional imaging and deep EEG during SW.[26,27] The emotional and motor features of parasomnias could be interpreted as a release of inhibition of the subcortical central pattern generators, which regulate innate behavioral automatisms and survival behaviors.[28] The relatively consistent mental contents during ST across individuals (ceiling collapse, being buried alive, and escaping a life-threatening event) followed by a common flight response support this concept,[21] as predicted by the threat simulation theory of dreams.[29] These mental contents may also be biased toward unpleasant experiences in clinical series because these patients would more frequently seek medical advice.

Distressing mentation and nightmares during ST/SW may suggest abnormal processing of emotion during sleep. Psychological trauma has been reported to influence the content, and recent stressful events may trigger SW/ST episodes.[30] Compared with sleepwalkers, higher levels of anxiety, obsessive-compulsive traits, phobias, and depression have been found in adult patients with ST in one study.[31] However, most studies showed no psychiatric disorders in these patients. Patients with SW/ST score slightly higher than healthy controls on

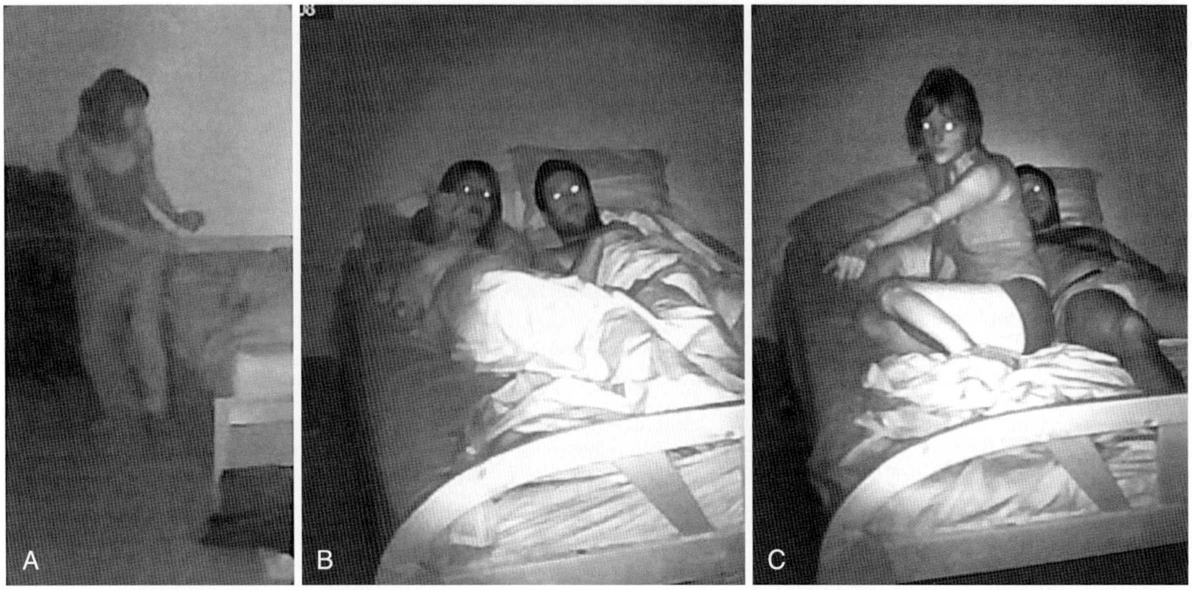

Figure 119.1 A 33-year-old woman with sleepwalking dreamed that her baby was about to fall from her cradle. She suddenly stood up, caught the baby, and brought her cautiously (with slightly folded knees) onto her bed, illustrating the isomorphism between dream content during sleepwalking and real behavior (**A,** From infrared video clip). During several episodes, the patient stared and pointed with her finger toward an invisible person, trying to convince her husband of the apparition, as if she were hallucinating (**B** and **C**), illustrating how the dreamed images are projected on the real bedroom scene.

depression and anxiety scales,[32] but their scores do not differ from those of patients with RBD.[21] In addition, they have normal daytime aggression scores.[21]

Another study of 105 sleepwalkers showed depression and anxiety scores are similar to those of the general adult population, but those with psychopathology had higher frequency of nightmares and with potentially injurious behaviors.[33] The successful treatment of a comorbid depressive disorder in 100 adults with SW/ST had no effects on the course of parasomnias, suggesting that the concurrent psychopathology did not play an essential role or that the improvement in mood is a different mechanism from the parasomnia.[34]

Treatment

SW and ST that cause distressing dreams should be treated with similar standard therapy for disorders of arousals: safety measures (avoiding sleep deprivation and other priming factors such as alcohol, heavy meals, hyperthermia, or daytime stress; quietly guiding the patient back to bed; closing windows and doors), behavioral therapy (relaxation training, hypnosis), or medications (benzodiazepines, antidepressants, carbamazepine, gabapentine). However, none of these therapies has been tested with randomized trials. In the experience of my team, the treatment of patients with SW/ST typically improves the dreams too.

DISTURBED DREAMING IN RAPID EYE MOVEMENT SLEEP BEHAVIOR DISORDER

Dreams and Nightmares in REM Sleep Behavior Disorder

Patients with RBD enact violent dreams during REM sleep in the absence of normal muscle atonia.[1] This disorder is highly frequent in patients with synucleinopathies (60% to 100% of patients, including dementia with Lewy bodies, Parkinson disease, and multiple sleep atrophy and may precede these diseases by several years) and rare in patients with other neurodegenerative disorders (see Chapter 118). RBD constitute a unique window to study the dreaming process from a point of view external to the dreamer and are usually different from those experienced by patients before RBD onset. Most descriptions emphasize the forceful and violent aspect of these motor behaviors, which are usually associated with vivid, unpleasant, and active dreams (Video 119.3).[35,36] Usual, nonaggressive behaviors can be observed in around 20% of patients (Video 119.4).[37] Similar to RBD, dream content of patients with Parkinson disease (whether they have RBD or not) includes heightened aggressiveness and an increased presence of animals compared with normal subjects.[38]

Mechanisms of Abnormal Dreaming in REM Sleep Behavior Disorder

RBDs are strongly linked to brainstem focal or neurodegenerative lesions within the system causing muscle atonia during REM sleep.[39,40] Although the exact origin of the dream content is unclear, in animal models with focal brainstem lesions that cause RBD, the RBD behaviors also contain a majority of violent behaviors (chasing or fighting) and a minority of nonviolent behaviors (licking self or grooming).[41] The aggressive dream content correlates with more severe frontal dysfunction in Parkinson disease, regardless of whether concomitant RBD is present.[38] In this case, disturbed dreaming in RBD may be a consequence of the concomitant frontal dysfunction rather than of a brainstem lesion. In addition, the intense apparent emotions observed in patients with RBD suggest an increased activation of the amygdala, as shown in normal REM sleep. Another mechanism could be related to the general function of dreams, as suggested by the threat simulation theory.[29] This theory suggests that the function of dreaming is to simulate threatening events in a virtual environment and to rehearse threat perception and threat avoidance for the evolutionary purpose of increased survival. If true, this threat simulation would be exacerbated in the dreams of patients with Parkinson disease, possibly linked with the frontal dysfunction. These dreams of fighting wild animals and aggressors are not a consequence of personality changes, as they contrast with the placid personality and absence of aggressiveness during the daytime in patients with RBD.[21,35]

Treatment

Several large series show the benefit of melatonin (3 to 12 mg before sleeping; one study was double blinded and placebo controlled[42]) and clonazepam (0.5 to 2 mg before sleeping)[36] on nightmares and the corresponding behaviors during RBD.[43] A few recent observations suggest that zopiclone and cholinesterase inhibitors (rivastigmine, donepezil) may also help with the nightmares.[44] Whether these drugs attenuate the negative emotions in dreams or just reduce the motor expression of dreams is yet incompletely determined.

DISTURBED DREAMING, NIGHTMARES, AND HALLUCINATIONS IN NARCOLEPSY

Patients with narcolepsy often report frequent and intense dreaming (Figure 119.2). In a controlled series of 53 patients, patients with narcolepsy remembered, on average, 49 dreams per month, versus 15 dreams per month in controls, including more frequent dreams of false awakening.[45] The intense characteristics of dreaming activity are more obvious during sleep onset in REM periods,[46] with reports containing longer and a more complex organization.[47] The emotional tone of dreams is high, including a negative tone that is more frequent in narcoleptics' than in healthy controls' dreams.[48] Patients with narcolepsy also experience more recurrent dreams than controls,[45] or insomniacs.[49] Between 33% and 83% of patients with narcolepsy report nightmares (Figure 119.2),[45,50,51] more frequently[45] or as frequently[51] in narcolepsy with than without cataplexy and more frequently than in controls[45] and in insomniacs.[49]

As many as 85% of people with narcolepsy also experienced "dream delusion," or difficulty distinguishing between dream and reality, and they mistake the memory of a vivid dream for a real experience.[52] One man, after dreaming that a young girl had drowned in a nearby lake, asked his wife to turn on the local news in full expectation that the event would be covered.

Around three-fourths of patients with narcolepsy are frequent lucid dreamers[45,46] and use lucidity to turn recurrent nightmares into agreeable dreams, as illustrated in the following examples[45]:

- "I was chased by an aggressor and had to kill myself by throwing myself onto an electrified fence to avoid the aggressor and wake up."
- "I was chased by soldiers and chose to fly to escape them."
- "I built a panic room in myself where I mentally went during my nightmare to escape dangerous people."
- "I was seeing my family tortured to death and decided that it was not true, because we were rehearsing a play or a movie. I was behind the camera."[45]

Whether the nightmares result from an overactive REM system, sleep onset in REM periods with more perceived sleep paralysis, fragmented REM sleep, abnormal amygdala activation in narcolepsy, overall higher daytime stress, or side effects of antidepressants and stimulants is yet undetermined. Patients with narcolepsy with nightmares had longer wakefulness time and higher percentages of N1 stage sleep, suggesting either that nightmares disrupted sleep or that superficial sleep promoted their onset.[51] A small (11%, 6 of 54 patients) proportion of patients reported that nightmares had been eliminated by narcolepsy medications, mostly anticataplectic drugs.[51]

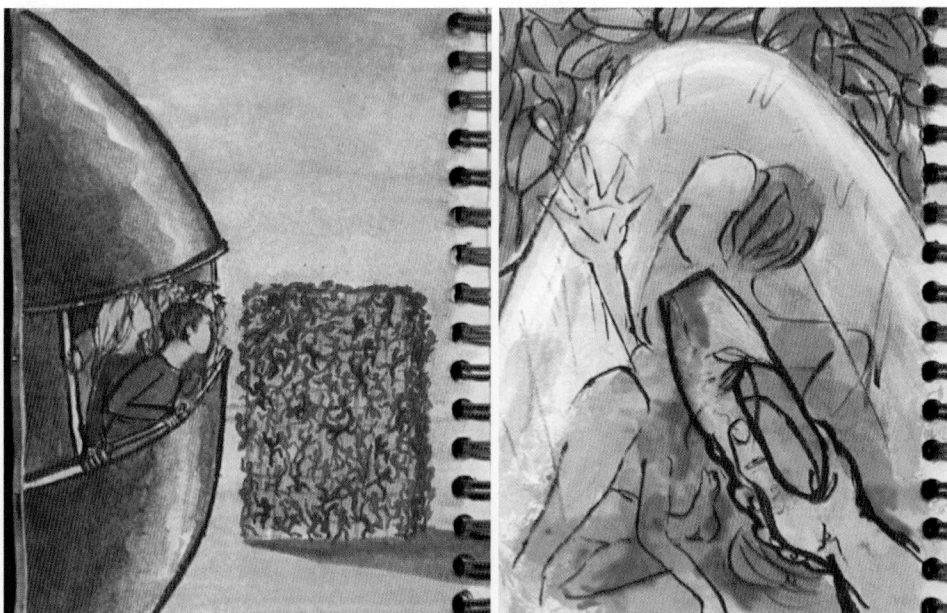

Figure 119.2 Vivid dreams painted by their author, a 19-year-old patient with narcolepsy. "We were on field trip with my class, traveling in a giant ball silently floating over a desert. Suddenly, we saw a large building with a moving surface. As we approached, we discovered that the moving surface was composed of thousands of Spidermen. We leaned with interest" (*left image*). "In this nightmare, I was obliged to kill my whole family in a tube placed in the backyard. I had to kill them with a ballroom shoe, which was a long, tedious, and horrible experience" (*right image*).

DREAM DISTURBANCES IN OTHER NEUROLOGIC DISEASES

Parkinson Disease

One-third of patients with Parkinson disease report "vivid" dreams and a high frequency of nightmares, especially when dopaminergic therapy is introduced.[53] Lower emotional load and bizarreness in patients' dreams (compared with controls) is associated with amygdala and mesial prefrontal cortex thickness,[34] two key structures implicated in current models of dreaming and emotion regulation during sleep. In contrast, Borek and colleagues found a relatively higher frequency of aggressive features in patients with Parkinson disease with versus without RBD, although dreams were less aggressive in women with Parkinson disease than in men.[55] The altered dreaming activity was associated with more frequent awakenings and illusions/hallucinations, but not with specific (levodopa, dopamine agonist) medications.[56] A "kindling" phenomenon, starting from altered dreaming, evolving toward illusions, hallucinations of minor then major severity, and eventually psychosis, was suspected.[57] However, the presence of vivid dreams/nightmares correlated with concurrent hallucinations but did not predict the future development of hallucinations when they occurred in non-hallucinators in a 10-year prospective study.[58] Yet the presence of RBD at entry into cohorts proved to be a major determinant for concurrent and incident hallucinations, as well as later development of psychosis and dementia.[58,59] Of note, 15% to 20% of patients with Parkinson disease (mostly those with excessive daytime sleepiness) have a narcolepsy-like phenotype, with daytime sleep onset in REM periods, which contribute to hallucinations and disturbed dreaming in this population.[60]

The treatment of nightmares and hallucinations in Parkinson's disease and other neurodegenerative diseases usually requires decreasing or stopping the priming drugs (usually dopamine agonists and antidepressants), assessing for RBD (and treat adequately with melatonin or clonazepam), and, if severe, using atypical neuroleptic drugs such as quetiapine or clozapine.

Guillain-Barré Syndrome

Guillain-Barré syndrome is a rare, acute, and severe polyradiculopathy, probably of autoimmune origin. Although it mostly affects the peripheral nervous system, signs of central nervous dysfunction such as RBD,[61] sleepiness, hallucinations, abnormal antidiuretic hormone secretion, and low cerebrospinal fluid levels of hypocretin are noted.[62] In a consecutive series of 139 patients with Guillain-Barré syndrome without any psychotropics and opiates, patients frequently reported vivid dreams (19%), illusions (30%, including an illusory body tilt), hallucinations (60%, mainly visual), and delusions (70%, mostly paranoid).[63] In patients monitored during the hallucinatory period, the polysomnography showed a *status dissociatus* characterized by major insomnia; REM sleep without atonia in all hallucinators; bursts of rapid eye movements during stage N2 sleep; sleep onset in REM periods; and continuous, rapid switching between waking, N1, and REM sleep stages across day and night. In addition, there were signs of dysautonomia. The *status* progressively disappeared when hallucinations subsided. In this case, *status dissociatus* (rather than "isolated" RBD) was concomitant with disturbed dreaming and hallucinations.

Delirium Tremens, Fatal Familial Insomnia, and Morvan's Chorea: Agrypnia Excitata

Notably, some forms of *status dissociatus* include continuous dreaming and hallucinations, motor activity, and a complete loss of wake-sleep boundaries, with patients fluctuating continuously between N1/REM and wakefulness.[64] Such *status dissociatus* is also observed in Parkinson disease, dementia with Lewy bodies, Guillain-Barré syndrome, alcohol withdrawal syndrome (*delirium tremens*), fatal familial insomnia, and Morvan's chorea.[65] This phenomenon has been named *agrypnia excitata* by the Bologna investigators and *oneirism* in French literature, but these names refer to the same observation of severe visual hallucinations and enacted dreams (resembling a continuous RBD, but with open eyes). A specific variants of *status dissociatus* included poorly structured stage N2 sleep with simple movements and finalistic behaviors and RBD in patients with the IgLon-5 autoimmune encephalitis.[66]

CLINICAL PEARL

The clinician should realize that some patients use the words "disturbed dreaming" and "nightmares" not only for indicating the classical REM sleep nightmare disorder; posttraumatic stress disorder; and distressing dreams associated with psychiatric conditions, drugs, and substances, but also for reporting the mental experiences associated with hypnagogic hallucinations, ST, SW, RBD, and *status dissociatus*. The characteristics (type, construction, timing, duration, and context) of their mental experience, along with associated behaviors, concomitant autonomic signs, and associated disorders, as well as aspects on video and timing on polysomnography, are crucial for making a diagnosis.

SUMMARY

Most adult patients with arousal disorders remember a mental content timely associated with SW and ST, mostly a brief visual scene including misfortune, apprehension, and life-threatening, imminent dangers that they must flee. The concomitant observed behaviors and speeches are congruent with the mental content. During RBDs, patients mostly enact violent dreams in which they are aggressed by humans and animals and counter attack, despite their placid personality when awake. However, around 20% of the behaviors and concomitant dreaming are elaborated, nonviolent content, including laughing, performing their job, or speaking with people. In narcolepsy, patients have longer, more intense and lucid dreams than controls, with more frequent nightmares, timely associated with sleep onset in REM periods. Vivid dreams, illusions, hallucinations, and psychosis in several neurologic diseases caused by neurodegeneration (mostly synucleinopathies, including Parkinson disease and dementia with Lewy bodies), autoimmunity (primary narcolepsy, Guillain-Barré syndrome, Morvan's chorea), and alcohol withdrawal (*delirium tremens*) seem linked to abnormal REM sleep and *status dissociatus*.

SELECTED READINGS

Antelmi E, Ferri R, Iranzo A, et al. From state dissociation to status dissociatus. *Sleep Med Rev*. 2015;28:5–17.

Arnulf I, Bonnet AM, Damier P, et al. Hallucinations, REM sleep and Parkinson's disease. *Neurology*. 2000;55:281–288.

Baldelli L, Provini F. Differentiating oneiric stupor in agrypnia excitata from dreaming disorders. *Front Neurol*. 2020;11:565694.

Bugalho P, Paiva T. Dream features in the early stages of Parkinson's disease. *J Neural Transm*. 2011;118:1613–1619.

Castelnovo A, Loddo G, Provini F, Miano S, Manconi M. Mental activity during episodes of sleepwalking, night terrors or confusional arousals: differences between children and adults. *Nat Sci Sleep*. 2021;13:829–840.

Cochen V, Arnulf I, Demeret S, et al. Vivid dreams, hallucinations, psychosis and REM sleep in Guillain-Barre syndrome. *Brain*. 2005;128:2535–2545.

Fénelon G, Mahieux F, Huon R, Ziegler M. Hallucinations in Parkinson's disease: prevalence, phenomenology and risk factors. *Brain*. 2000;123:733–745.

Fortuyn HA, Lappenschaar GA, Nienhuis FJ, et al. Psychotic symptoms in narcolepsy: phenomenology and a comparison with schizophrenia. *Gen Hosp Psychiatry*. 2009;31:146–154.

Konkoly KR, Appel K, Chabani E, et al. Real-time dialogue between experimenters and dreamers during REM sleep. *Curr Biol*. 2021;31(7):1417–1427.e6.

Leclair-Visonneau L, Oudiette D, Gaymard B, Leu-Semenescu S, Arnulf I. Do the eyes scan dream images during rapid eye movement sleep? Evidence from the rapid eye movement sleep behaviour disorder model. *Brain*. 2010;133:1737–1746.

Scarpelli S, Alfonsi V, Gorgoni M, Giannini AM, De Gennaro L. Investigation on neurobiological mechanisms of dreaming in the new decade. *Brain Sci*. 2021;11(2):220.

Siclari F, Valli K, Arnulf I. Dreams and nightmares in healthy adults and in patients with sleep and neurological disorders. *Lancet Neurol*. 2020;19(10):849–859.

Stefani A, Högl B. Nightmare disorder and isolated sleep paralysis. *Neurotherapeutics*. 2021;18(1):100–106.

Uguccioni G, Golmard JL, de Fontreaux A, Leu-Semenescu S, Brion A, Arnulf I. Fight or flight? Dream content during sleepwalking/sleep terrors vs rapid eye movement sleep behavior disorder. *Sleep Medicine*. 2013;14:391–398.

Valli K, Frauscher B, Peltomaa T, Gschliesser V, Revonsuo A, Högl B. Dreaming furiously? A sleep laboratory study on the dream content of people with Parkinson's disease and with or without rapid eye movement sleep behavior disorder. *Sleep Medicine*. 2016;16:419–427.

A complete reference list can be found online at ExpertConsult.com.

Chapter 120

Other Parasomnias

Alex Iranzo

Chapter Highlights

- The heterogeneous group of "other parasomnias" includes sleep-related hallucinations, exploding head syndrome, and sleep enuresis. Sleeptalking, considered an isolated symptom or normal variant, will also be covered here.
- Other parasomnias are very frequent, transient, and usually benign in nature, but some may indicate rare underlying disorders that are progressive and devastating.
- In most cases the physician should provide patients with education and reassurance that these sleep-related experiences are harmless. Therapy is rarely warranted but could be considered when experiences are bothersome, unpleasant, terrifying, or very frequently causing sleep difficulties.
- Although most cases are benign and idiopathic, some are associated with serious conditions. For example, sleep-related hallucinations may manifest as hypnagogic hallucinations in patients with narcolepsy or complex nocturnal visual hallucinations in subjects with brainstem strokes. Sleep enuresis in children may indicate underlying obstructive sleep apnea or recurrent urinary tract infections.

INTRODUCTION

Parasomnias are undesirable physical events or experiences that occur during entry into sleep, within sleep, or during arousal from sleep.[1] *The International Classification of Sleep Disorders*, third edition (ICSD-3) classifies "other parasomnias" to include a miscellaneous group of phenomena not linked to a specific sleep stage. This group includes disorders such as sleep-related hallucinations, exploding head syndrome, sleep enuresis, parasomnias secondary to a medical disorder and to a medication or substance, and the normal variant of sleeptalking.[1] This chapter describes the conditions listed in the "other parasomnias" category and will discuss the possible epidemiology, pathophysiologic consequences, and clinical approach.[1]

SLEEP-RELATED HALLUCINATIONS

Definition, Diagnostic Criteria, and Classification

Hallucinations are sensory experiences that are perceived in the absence of environmental stimuli. Consciousness is preserved, and subjects are able to describe in detail their perceptions with or without insight into their unreality. Hallucinations should be distinguished from illusions that correspond to misperceptions or distorted perceptions of real external stimuli. They also should not be mistaken for dreams, which are experiences that occur when the individual is asleep and are recalled upon awakening.[2] Hallucinations are the result of abnormal neuronal sensory processing in the setting of the wake-sleep transition (e.g., hypnagogic hallucinations [HHs], hypnopompic hallucinations [HPHs]), sensory deprivation (e.g., severe vision loss in the Charles Bonnet syndrome), structural brain lesions (e.g., stroke), neurologic diseases (e.g., Parkinson disease, dementia with Lewy bodies), psychiatric diseases (e.g., schizophrenia), metabolic diseases (e.g., hypoxic encephalopathy), and the use or withdrawal of a medication (e.g., dopaminergic agents).

Although hallucinations can occur during daytime wakefulness, sleep onset, and upon awakening from sleep, daytime hallucinations are more frequent than sleep-related hallucinations.[2,3] According to the ICSD-3, diagnostic criteria of sleep-related hallucinations include (1) a complaint of recurrent hallucinations that are experienced just before sleep or upon awakening during the night or in the morning, (2) the hallucinations are predominantly visual, and (3) the disturbance is not better explained by another sleep disorder (especially narcolepsy), mental disorder, medical disorder, medication, or substance use.[1]

Sleep-related hallucinations may be classified into two different forms according to their time of occurrence, clinical characteristics, and underlying substrate: (1) HHs (those that occur at sleep onset) and HPHs (those that occur upon awakening), which are experiences that are either idiopathic or related to other conditions, particularly narcolepsy, and (2) complex nocturnal visual hallucinations (CNVHs) that occur after sudden awakening during the night, are not simple experiences, and are almost always linked to an underlying pathology, usually neurologic, psychiatric, metabolic, and ophthalmic in nature.[2]

Hypnagogic and Hypnopompic Hallucinations

Clinical Findings. HH and HPH are visual (e.g., feeling someone or something present in the room; simple elementary forms, such as sparks, lines, flashes, confetti, and shadows; complex forms, such as waterfalls, cucumbers, animals, known or unknown people or faces, dwarfs, thieves, firemen, and lifelike scenes); auditory (e.g., footsteps, explosions, shots, a beep from a cell phone, voices of known or unknown people, familiar or unfamiliar songs); tactile (e.g., someone grabbing the subject, bugs crawling on the skin, tingling, pain) gustatory (e.g., metallic taste); olfactory (e.g., perfume, cologne, feces, smoke); and kinetic (e.g., floating, flying, jumping, falling, out of body experiences, levitation). Most of the people who experience HH and HPH know that the perceptions are not real. Despite this, some hallucinations, such as seeing and hearing persons, may be unpleasant, frightening, and so vivid that they are difficult for the person to distinguish from true events.[3,4] Kinetic hallucinations are so bizarre that they may lead to paranormal beliefs or be mistaken for delusional psychosis.

Epidemiology. Epidemiologic studies are scarce and give different estimations of prevalence due to methodological differences in the definition of hallucination and the accuracy of how data was obtained (telephone interviews, questionnaires). HH are more common than HPH. In a community sample of 49,772 people from the United Kingdom, ages 15 to 100 years, and interviewed by telephone, 37% reported HH and 12.5% reported HPH.[5] In an observational study involving 134 healthy medical students from Spain with a mean age of 22 years, 13% reported sleep-related hallucinations.[6]

Associations. There is no known familial or genetic predisposition. The most important precipitant in predisposed individuals is sleep deprivation leading to HH or HPH during daytime naps or during the night. Many drugs and psychoactive substances have been related to HH and HPH, such as hashish, opiates, amphetamines, cocaine, hypnotics, and zopiclone.[4] Simultaneous occurrence of HH or HPH with sleep paralysis is common in narcoleptics and healthy people in the context of sleep deprivation.

In *narcolepsy*, HHs are more frequent than HPHs. In one study, hallucinations occurred in 59% of the patients with cataplexy and in 28% without cataplexy.[7] They were experienced in the context of sleep onset (55%), sleep offset (3%), and onset/offset (42%). Hallucinations were visual in 95% of the patients, auditory in 75%, kinetic in 55%, tactile in 33%, and 10% experienced passage or presence of a real person. Olfactory and gustatory hallucinations were not reported. When narcoleptics experience sleep paralysis, the most common simultaneous hallucinations are tactile (e.g., a frightening pressure on the chest) and visual (e.g., feeling the presence of someone or a shadow). For some, the events are so vivid that some undiagnosed narcoleptics may be convinced that they are experiencing paranormal events.[8] In narcolepsy, HHs and HPHs occur predominantly in the supine position, potentially because of the exacerbation of rapid eye movement (REM)-related obstructive sleep apnea (OSA) in the supine position, which can lead to partial arousals resulting in hallucinatory experiences.[9]

Etiology. HH and HPH are thought to be intrusions of the characteristic dream-like phenomena of REM sleep into wakefulness. Acetylcholine, serotonin, and dopamine dysfunction is involved in the mechanisms underlying hallucinations.[10]

Management. When HH and HPH are idiopathic in normal healthy individuals, patients need to be assured that they are normal phenomenon and not a sign of psychosis, narcolepsy, or a paranormal experience. Patients with narcolepsy should be informed that hallucinations are part of the disease process. When treatment is needed because hallucinations are frequent or bothersome, clomipramine 10 to 75 mg at bedtime may be effective, particularly for those associated with sleep paralysis. Antipsychotics, such as quetiapine, may also be effective at bedtime. Sodium oxybate has an unclear impact on such events in patients with narcolepsy.[11,12]

Complex Nocturnal Visual Hallucinations

Clinical Findings. Complex nocturnal visual hallucinations (CNVHs) usually occur after a sudden awakening. They may be primary or much more frequently secondary to an underlying condition. Despite the variety and large number of conditions that may cause CNVHs, the type of visual hallucinations are very similar among them. CNVHs are complex, vivid, detailed, relatively stereotypic, static or mobile, and colorful images of people, animals, and elaborate scenes resembling a dream. They can be brief, lasting a few seconds, or prolonged, lasting several hours. They usually disappear if the eyes are opened or if the lights of the room are switched on. Sometimes the images are distorted in shape or size, such as those seen in the Alice in Wonderland syndrome. In rare cases, visual hallucinations can be associated with auditory hallucinations (e.g., a song, a crowd of people talking or chanting) or tactile hallucinations (e.g., tingling, pain). Insight regarding the hallucinations is more reduced than in HHs and HPHs, and subjects may believe they are true and leave the bed to investigate if the images are real or not. In other patients, insight is preserved, but hallucinations are perceived as bothersome and distressing. CNVHs may co-occur with HH and HPH. The secondary, but not the primary, form of CNVHs may coexist with hallucinations during wakefulness.[1,13,14]

Associations. Precipitants of CNVHs depend on the nature of the underlying condition and include sleep deprivation, fever, trauma, electrolyte disturbances, changes in medication, poor vision, and low ambient illumination. In contrast to HHs and HPHs, CNVHs are secondary to a large number of conditions of different origin (Box 120.1).[13–29]

In *Parkinson disease,* hallucinations occur in about 25% of the patients.[15] Risk factors are older age, long disease duration, increased motor disability, depression, cognitive impairment, hypersomnia, REM sleep behavior disorder (RBD), and the use of dopaminergic agonists and anticholinergics.[7,15] In Parkinson disease, minor hallucinations often precede the onset of well-structured visual hallucinations.[30] Hallucinations are mostly visual, recurrent, static or mobile, stereotypic, or vivid, involving shadows, silent moving animals and people, and the presence or passage of a quiet known person or pet. They appear mostly in dim surroundings or at night. Tactile, auditory, and kinetic hallucinations are rare. Although the etiology of these hallucinations in Parkinson disease is unclear, the connection to REM sleep intrusions into wakefulness or perceptual disturbance is debated.[7,16–18,31]

Dementia with Lewy bodies is dependent upon visual hallucinations as one of the major diagnostic criteria.[19] In patients with idiopathic RBD, the occurrence of CNVHs may be an indicator of impending cognitive impairment. In one study, a patient with dementia with Lewy bodies experienced an episode of CNVH, and polysomnography (PSG) showed that it

BOX 120.1 CONDITIONS ASSOCIATED WITH SLEEP-RELATED HALLUCINATIONS

Hypnagogic and Hypnopompic Hallucinations
Sleep deprivation[1]
Narcolepsy[7,8]

Complex Nocturnal Visual Hallucinations
Parkinson disease[7,13,15–17]
Dementia with Lewy bodies[19,20]
Peduncullar hallucinosis[13,21,23,24]
Charles Bonnet syndrome[13,25]
Schizophrenia[13]
Metabolic encephalopathy[13]
Posterior cerebral artery infarction[13]
Delirium tremens[13]
Migraine[13]
Focal epilepsy[13]
Guillain-Barré syndrome[28]
Sleepwalking[1,2,29]
Night terrors[1,2]
Idiopathic hypersomnia[14]
Anxiety disorder[14]
Acute alcohol withdrawal[12]
Acute barbiturate withdrawal[14]
Acute benzodiazepine withdrawal[14]
Lipophilic beta blockers[1,2]
Dopaminergic agents[1,2]
Substances with hallucinogenic properties, such as mescaline, LSD, amphetamine, and cocaine[1,2]

LSD, Lysergic acid diethylamide.

resulted from an awakening arising from N2 sleep stage.[20] In another case, video-PSG showed a patient gesturing (picking nonexisting objects from the air) with the eyes closed, and the electroencephalogram (EEG) showed diffuse slow theta/delta activity of moderate amplitude that attenuated with the quasi-purposeful behaviors. This EEG pattern was also seen when the patient was resting quietly, awake with the eyes closed, and lights on.[32] Another patient with a 6-year history of talking for hours during the night was found, on video-PSG, to have complex motor and vocal manifestations with the eyes closed and hand gesturing, kissing-like movements, and speaking for 3 hours about several topics. Simultaneous EEG during the speech episode showed alpha rhythm intermingled with theta activity, theta/delta slowing, and no alpha rhythm during quiet wakefulness with the eyes closed and the lights on.[32] Many patients with dementia with Lewy bodies and other forms of dementia may find it very difficult to distinguish CNVHs from dreams.

Peduncular hallucinosis is characterized by CNVH in the setting of pontine, midbrain, or thalamic damage.[13,21] The most common etiology is vascular, but tumors and inflammatory processes have also been described.[22] These stereotypic events are usually self-limited, starting a few days after a stroke, and are commonly associated with hypersomnia. These events typically occur in the evening, last several minutes or hours, and disappear when the eyes are opened.[13] Patients may lack insight and may interact with the hallucinations by performing pseudopurposeful activities (e.g., using a screwdriver, putting on trousers, or talking). PSG studies have shown that the hallucinations occur during wake-sleep transitions with preserved occipital alpha activity.[23,24]

Charles Bonnet syndrome is characterized by CNVHs in elderly subjects with severe visual loss secondary to bilateral ocular pathology (e.g., macular degeneration, cataracts, glaucoma).[33] The hallucinations are visual and consist of vivid objects that tend to reoccur. The syndrome may be caused by any lesion affecting the visual pathway, including the optic nerve, optic chiasm, and temporal and occipital lobes. For these patients, CNVHs occur in the evening and night when the patient is drowsy but eyes are still open. Patients usually have insight into the nature of their perceptions, and their cognitive and psychiatric assessments are normal.[34] The course and treatment depend upon the underlying pathology. Symptomatic therapy with atypical antipsychotics, such as olanzapine, and anticonvulsants, such as levetiracetam, may be effective.[13,25]

Polysomnography. The very few studies that have described the PSG pattern of CNVHs have shown that CNVHs arise from N2 and N3, and not from REM sleep. During the events, the EEG shows occipital alpha rhythm without epileptic activity, indicating that the subject is awake.[14,26] CNVHs experienced by patients with Parkinson disease may arise from four distinct circumstances: (1) during REM sleep without atonia; (2) upon arousal from non–rapid eye movement (NREM) sleep; (3) in the daytime during drowsiness within the wake-NREM sleep transition; and (4) during the wakeful state.[27] In the setting of dementia with Lewy bodies, CNVHs may arise from wakefulness, and the EEG may show slow activity that is the same as that found during wakefulness.[32]

Etiology. The anatomic substrate of CNHV shares a final common pathway where the occipital visual cortex generates false images from reduced sensory inputs. Input reduction may arise from the occipital cortex itself (e.g., in dementia with Lewy bodies) or its afferents from the thalamus (e.g., peduncullar hallucinosis), the brainstem (e.g., Parkinson disease), and the retina (e.g., Charles Bonnet syndrome).[13]

Management. In most cases reassurance is sufficient. Adequate treatment of the underlying condition may eliminate the CNVHs. Withdrawal of the offensive agent (e.g., beta-adrenergic antagonist, dopaminergic agents, anticholinergics) often results in resolution of CNVHs.[14] In cases for which therapy is warranted, antidopaminergic psychotics (e.g., risperidone, quetiapine, olanzapine, and clozapine), anticholinesterase inhibitors (e.g., rivastigmine), or melatonin may be effective.[35]

EXPLODING HEAD SYNDROME

Definition and Diagnostic Criteria

Exploding head syndrome (EHS) is a sense of a loud explosion in the head that awakens the individual.[36] Diagnostic criteria in the ICSD-3 include (1) a complaint of a sudden noise or sense of explosion in the head, either at the wake-sleep transition or upon awakening in the night; (2) the individual experiences abrupt arousal after the event, often with a sense of fright; and (3) the experience is not associated with significant complaints of pain.[1] Because pain is usually absent, EHS cannot be considered a form of headache.

Clinical Findings

Patients are abruptly woken by an imagined, sudden, violent, and frightening sensation of explosion deep in the center or the back of the head or near them.[36,37] Patients have a clear recollection of the events without any postictal confusion. Episodes last between a split second and a few seconds and disappear completely the moment the subject is awakened.[38] The majority of subjects report episodes of EHS during wake-sleep transitions but during sleep-wake transitions is not uncommon.[39] The noise is perceived over both ears,[40] although a few subjects describe hearing the sound in only one ear.[41,42] In one study, although some subjects perceived EHS sounds as emanating from the right (26%) or the left (19%), the majority (55%) experienced them bilaterally.[39] Patients report noise, not pain, and describe the experience in many ways, such as "a sudden bang in the head,"[37] "thunderclap,"[37] "shouts,"[40] "shotgun,"[43] "loud metallic noise,"[43] "clash of cymbals,"[43] "door slamming,"[43] "the earth moved,"[43] "electric shocks,"[43] "bomb-like explosion,"[43] "electrical current running,"[44] "a beep,"[45] "a buzzing noise,"[46] "screaming sounds,"[47] "dropping an object from a height,"[39] "high-pitched noise,"[39] "someone or something hitting a wall,"[39] "fireworks,"[39] "thud,"[39] "breaking glass,"[39] "car crash,"[39] "door knock,"[39] "ding dong,"[39] "train noise,"[39] "drumming,"[39] "metal pans banging together,"[39] and "things being broken apart."[39] Some patients are so alarmed by its violence that they think that it is a symptom of a stroke or a brain tumor.[40] The explosive noise may occasionally be accompanied by a simultaneous flash of light in front of the eyes,[40,43] hypnic jerks of the whole body[40] or one limb,[46,48] and the sensations of fear,[43] difficult breathing,[39] palpitations,[39] sensations around the stomach and the heart,[39] out-of-body sensations,[39] feeling the body floating,[39] and autoscopy.[39] In one case, EHS was followed by episodes of sleep paralysis.[45] Attacks occur exclusively during sleep; during the transition from wakefulness to sleep; or, less often, on awakening from sleep, particularly during the nighttime. In a few cases the attacks only appear on awakening from nighttime sleep[41,47] or during daytime naps.[47] EHS is likely to occur when sleeping in a supine position.[39]

Epidemiology

There are fewer than 150 cases reported in the medical literature, but it is suspected to be much more common and generally underreported.[36,37] In fact, epidemiologic studies have shown that EHS occurs at least in 10% of the general population. In a study involving 211 undergraduate students with a mean age of 20 years, 18% experienced lifetime EHS, and 16% experienced recurrent EHS.[49] In another study with 199 female undergraduate students (mean age, 20 years), the lifetime prevalence of EHS was 37.19%, with 6.54% experiencing at least one episode a month.[50] In another sample from the same study with 1683 participants (mean age, 34 years, 53.0% female), the lifetime prevalence of EHS was 29.59%, with monthly episodes occurring in 3.89% of participants.[50] Onset is usually after the age of 50 years, but it may start in childhood and adolescence. There is a slight predominance in females.

Natural Course

The frequency and course of episodes is highly variable, ranging from two or three spells in a lifetime up to several per night for several weeks. Some patients have clusters of lasting weeks to few months separated by prolonged periods of remission. The majority of the patients do not seek medical advice as only a minority consider the experience to be clinically significant. The condition improves and resolves spontaneously.[36]

Laboratory Investigations

Neurologic examination, brain magnetic resonance imaging, angiography, EEG, and interictal PSG are normal. Sleep studies reveal that the attacks may either evolve at the transition from wakefulness to N1[40,51] and from N2[42,51] or in the transition from N1 to wakefulness.[46] During PSG the episodes can be induced by intermittent photic stimulation.[52] No epileptic activity, apneic events, or electrocardiographic abnormalities are seen in the episodes.

Associations

Family history of EHS may occur, but it is very uncommon.[46] There are no identifiable precipitants, although a few patients state that attacks tend to occur when they are under stress or very tired. Events are not associated with any type of neurologic, psychiatric, and auditory diseases. It occurs in 37% of the subjects with isolated sleep paralysis.[49] It is also reported in subjects with many types of headaches, such as migraine with or without aura, chronic tension-type headache, primary stabbing headache, and primary headache linked to sexual activity.[53] EHS has been described in one case in association with spontaneous sleep-related orgasms plus hypnic jerks and central sleep apnea.[54] Insomnia is also common in subjects with EHS.[50]

Etiology

The etiology of the EHS is unknown. It is an abnormal sensory phenomena occurring at the transition from wakefulness to sleep. The events may represent an auditory sleep-related hallucination or a sensory variant of hypnic jerks.[2] Some investigators suggest events may be related to abnormalities in the brainstem reticular formation,[48] an acoustic migraine aura,[51] or middle ear eustachian tube dysfunction.[41]

Management

Treatment is generally not required because EHS is a benign disorder that remits with time. Education and reassurance that EHS is a harmless condition can be necessary to reduce fear and anxiety. A medication can be tried when episodes interfere with sleep or cause stress. There are no clinical trials investigating treatment options for EHS. Anecdotal reports suggest benefit with clomipramine,[55] amitriptyline,[53] topiramate,[46] flunarizine,[48] nifedipine,[56] duloxetine,[52] clobazam,[57] or clonazepam.[54]

SLEEP ENURESIS

Definition

Sleep enuresis (SE), also termed *bedwetting* and *nocturnal enuresis,* is defined as involuntary recurrent micturition during sleep in subjects older than 5 years at least twice a week for more than 3 months.[1]

Classification

SE is classified into primary and secondary forms, depending if the patient has been dry during sleep for at least 6 months. Primary sleep enuresis is characterized by the absence of a 6-month period free of enuresis, whereas secondary enuresis is designated when there is a 6-month period free of enuresis. This distinction is made because the primary and secondary forms have different etiology despite the symptomatology being the same. Primary SE is more frequent than secondary SE.[1]

Primary Sleep Enuresis

Diagnostic Criteria. According to the ICSD-3, diagnostic criteria include the following: (1) the patient is older than 5 years; (2) the patient exhibits recurrent involuntary voiding during sleep, occurring at least twice a week; (3) the condition has been present for at least 3 months; and (4) the patient has never been consistently dry during sleep for at least 6 months.[1]

Epidemiology. SE affects approximately 4% to 16% of school children.[58–60] A study on the development of parasomnias from childhood to early adolescence showed that enuresis occurred in 16% of 1353 children and persisted into adolescence in 12% of these cases.[60] The prevalence of SE decreases with time, being present in about 10% of 6-year-olds and 3% of 12-year-olds.[60] Adult enuresis is rare, occurring in about 0.5% to 3% of the population and is usually linked to an underlying condition. In children primary SE is more common in boys than in girls. In adults it is more frequent in women.[1]

Polysomnography. Sleep studies show that the episodes of SE occur from wakefulness to any sleep stage. During sleep, 39% of the episodes occur in N2, 20% in N3, and 9% in REM sleep. Most of the events occur in the first third of the night. PSG studies show an increased number of arousals.[61] OSA occurs in 8% to 47% of children with SE.[62]

Associations. About two-thirds of cases of primary SE are familial and one-third are sporadic. SE occurs in 77% of the children when both parents had SE and in 44% when one of the parents had a history of SE.[63] There is a higher concordance rate for monozygotic twins than for dizygotic twins.[64] Models of heritance can be either autosomal dominant or autosomal recessive.[64] Linkage studies have demonstrated associations with chromosomes 4, 8, 12, 13, and 22.[64] Primary SE is usually not associated with involuntary voiding during wakefulness. SE may cause embarrassment and low self-esteem, causing psychosocial stress for the patient.

Etiology. The etiology of primary SE is unknown, but several mechanisms are implicated in its pathophysiology: (1) polyuria leading to nocturia, (2) reduced bladder functional capacity (the volume at which the bladder empties itself is reduced), (3) increased nocturnal bladder activity, (4) decreased nocturnal secretion of vasopressin (the antidiuretic hormone), and (5) central difficulty of arousing from sleep. The later may be the most important factor in primary SE. Some researchers have hypothesized the enuresis is due to a developmental delay of central nervous system processing, leading to a failure in the arousal system in response to the sensation of a full bladder. Enuretic boys are found to be more difficult to arouse from sleep than age-matched control subjects,[65,66] and a small proportion of children with primary SE have reduced vasopressin levels during sleep, resulting in higher nocturnal urinary volume.[67]

Management. Parent and children involvement, motivation, and cooperation are crucial. To avoid embarrassment and low self-esteem causing the patient psychosocial stress, parents must be supportive of the child and use positive reinforcement for desired behaviors. Fluid restriction in the evenings and scheduled awakenings in the middle of the night for urination are not usually effective. Treatment includes behavioral therapy with daytime bladder control training,[68] alarm systems as a conditioning therapy,[69,70] and drugs, such as imipramine, oxybutynin, and desmopressin.[71]

Secondary Enuresis

Diagnostic Criteria. According to the ICSD-3, diagnostic criteria include the following: (1) the patient is older than 5 years; (2) the patient exhibits recurrent involuntary voiding during sleep, occurring at least twice a week; (3) the condition has been present for at least 3 months; and (4) the patient has been consistently dry during sleep for at least 6 months.[1]

Associations. Secondary SE is the result of an acquired factor, including excessive liquid intake, diabetes mellitus, diabetes insipidus, malformations of the genitourinary tract, recurrent urinary tract infections, chronic constipation and encopresis producing an extrinsic pressure on the bladder, significant psychosocial stress, attention deficit hyperactivity disorder, developmental disorders in children with mental retardation, OSA, congestive sleep heart failure, nocturnal epilepsy, stroke, Parkinson disease, multiple sclerosis, multiple system atrophy, dementia of any type, neurogenic bladder in spinal cord lesions and multiple sclerosis, and the use of diuretics.[1]

Etiology. Etiology depends on the underlying condition. Overall, pathophysiology of secondary SE includes an inability to concentrate urine, increased urinary production, hyperactivity of the bladder, and genitourinary tract malformations. Failure of arousal from sleep when the bladder is full of urine may also occur in a few cases with secondary SE, but this is a factor mostly associated with primary SE.

Management. The underlying cause should be treated first (urinary infection, urinary malformation, sleep apnea, diabetes mellitus, diabetes insipidus) before symptomatic therapy. In children specific therapy for primary SE should be tried in patients with secondary SE.

SLEEPTALKING

Definition and Classification

Sleeptalking (ST), also known as somniloquy, consists of talking while the individual is asleep. This should be distinguished from periods of talking during nocturnal awakenings or during arousals. ST may not be mistaken for other sounds occurring in sleep, such as catathrenia, snoring, stridor, chocking, and coughing. There are two forms of ST: (1) a primary form in which ST is an isolated manifestation and (2) a secondary form where it is one of the clinical features of a different underlying condition, such as a disorder of arousal and RBD (see Chapters 116 and 118).

Isolated Sleeptalking

Clinical Findings. Isolated ST is a normal sleep variant, a benign phenomenon where the individual remains immobile, except for the act of talking, and is usually amnestic for the event the next morning upon awakening. In most of the instances the spells do not cause an awakening and are noticed by the bed partner or household members who report them.[72] In most of the individuals the episodes are sporadic, self-limited, and brief, usually lasting less than 1 minute. Sometimes the events may occur nightly in clusters, particularly when the subject is under emotional stress. Episodes may range from speaking a single word or a sentence to a long elaborated dialogue. Content may be either meaningful or nonsense. Sleeptalkers seem to be either talking to themselves or having a dialogue. The voice can be the same or different as in the waking state. Sometimes ST may be accompanied by other sounds and vocalizations, such as whispering, muttering, humming, moaning, weeping, giggling, and shouting. ST is rarely accompanied by crying, laughing, and singing.[72] In a study performed in the Basque country, a region in northern Spain in which two completely different official languages are spoken (Euskera and Spanish), most children used their dominant (native) language during sleeptalk, but 4% used their nondominant language.[73]

Epidemiology. ST is very common in the general population. About half of the children present somniloquy at least once a year, but less than 10% present it every day.[73,74] Sleeptalking in children decreases with time and is slightly more common in boys (53%) than in girls (47%).[60]

Natural Course. Onset is usually between the ages of 3 and 10 years, but it may start in adolescence and even in early adulthood. The course is variable because it may be present for a few days only, recur in clusters, or may last for several months or many years. In children, ST usually resolves spontaneously during adolescence or adulthood.

Polysomnography. There are few formal studies assessing isolated ST with PSG. These have shown that ST occurs in all sleep stages: 50% to 60% associated with N1 and N2, 20% to 25% with N3, and 20% to 25% in REM sleep.[75] Some subjects only experience ST during NREM sleep, others exclusively in REM sleep, and the majority in both NREM and REM sleep.[75] When a person is experiencing ST and is experimentally awakened, dream recall occurs in 79% of the episodes arising from REM sleep, in 46% of the events arising from N2, and in 20% of the spells arising from N3. ST episodes related to REM sleep are longer and clearer than those occurring in N2 and N3.[58] In REM sleep, episodes of ST are characterized by sustained alpha EEG trains.[76]

Associations. Most cases of ST are not associated with a medical illness or psychopathologic conditions. Predisposing factors include anxiety, sleep deprivation, and fever. Children are more likely to experience recurrent ST if parents had sleepwalking during childhood.[77]

Etiology. The etiology is unknown. Some cases may have a clear familial predisposition, suggesting a genetic background.[78]

Management. Isolated ST is benign and an uncommon reason for consultation in a sleep center. However, ST may become disturbing for both the sleeptalker and the bed partner if frequent and excessively long or loud, and if the content includes obscenities and discusses intimate experiences. Isolated ST has no specific medical treatment, but adequate sleep hygiene and reduction of emotional stress may help.

Secondary Sleeptalking

ST may occur as one of the clinical manifestations of several disorders (Box 120.2)[1,79–91] that are covered in Chapters 116 to 118.

BOX 120.2 CONDITIONS ASSOCIATED WITH SECONDARY SLEEPTALKING

Confusional arousals[79]
Night terrors[79]
Sleepwalking[79]
Sleep related eating syndrome[80]
Sexsomnia[81]
REM sleep behavior disorder[82–85]
Status dissociatus[86]
Parasomnia overlap disorder[87]
Agrypnia excitata[88]
Anti-IgLON5 disease[89]
Sleep-related hypermotor epilepsy[1]
Periodic limb movement disorder[90]
Obstructive sleep apnea[91]
Nocturnal panic attacks[1]
Sleep-related dissociative disorder[1]

IgLON5, Immunoglobulin-like cell adhesion molecule 5; REM, rapid eye movement.

PARASOMNIA DUE TO A MEDICAL DISORDER

Parasomnia due to a medical disorder is diagnosed when the parasomnia is attributable to an underlying neurologic disorder or medical condition.[1] Secondary NREM sleep and REM sleep parasomnias are covered in other chapters.

NREM Sleep Parasomnias

Confusional arousals, night terrors, and sleepwalking are idiopathic disorders of arousal that are not linked to any specific psychiatric, psychological, neurologic, or medical disorder (see Chapter 116). Patients with disorders of arousal do not develop a neurodegenerative disease with time. Although these are not associated with other disorders, episodes of disorders of arousal can be precipitated by sleep deprivation, night shifts, fever, alcohol, noise, touch, psychological stress, and anxiety.[92] Coexistent OSA and periodic leg movements in sleep may provoke partial arousals, resulting in episodes of disorders of arousal and sleepwalking variants (sleep-related eating disorder, sleep driving, and sexsomnia) in predisposed individuals. Sleep-related eating disorder is associated with sleepwalking, sleep smoking, sexsomnia,[81] narcolepsy with cataplexy,[93] restless legs syndrome,[94] nocturnal eating syndrome,[94] and depression (see Chapter 117).[80,95]

Combined NREM and REM Sleep Parasomnias

Parasomnia Overlap Disorder

Parasomnia overlap disorder is the coexistence of a disorder of arousal (NREM parasomnia) and RBD (REM parasomnia) in the same patient (see Chapter 118). This entity mainly affects young subjects in whom NREM sleep clinical and polysomnographic features of the parasomnia predominate over RBD. However, only few of the reported cases have documented these two parasomnias by video-PSG.[96,97] Two-thirds of these patients have an idiopathic form,[86,87,98] and the remaining third is linked to several heterogeneous disorders, such as Möbius syndrome,[86] narcolepsy,[86] multiple sclerosis,[86] removal of a fourth ventricle astrocytoma,[86] head trauma,[86] atrial fibrillation during sleep,[86] posttraumatic stress disorder,[86] ethanol abuse,[86] harlequin syndrome,[99] hyperekplexia due to mutation of the glycine receptor gene,[100] and brainstem structural lesions.[101] On the other hand, the link

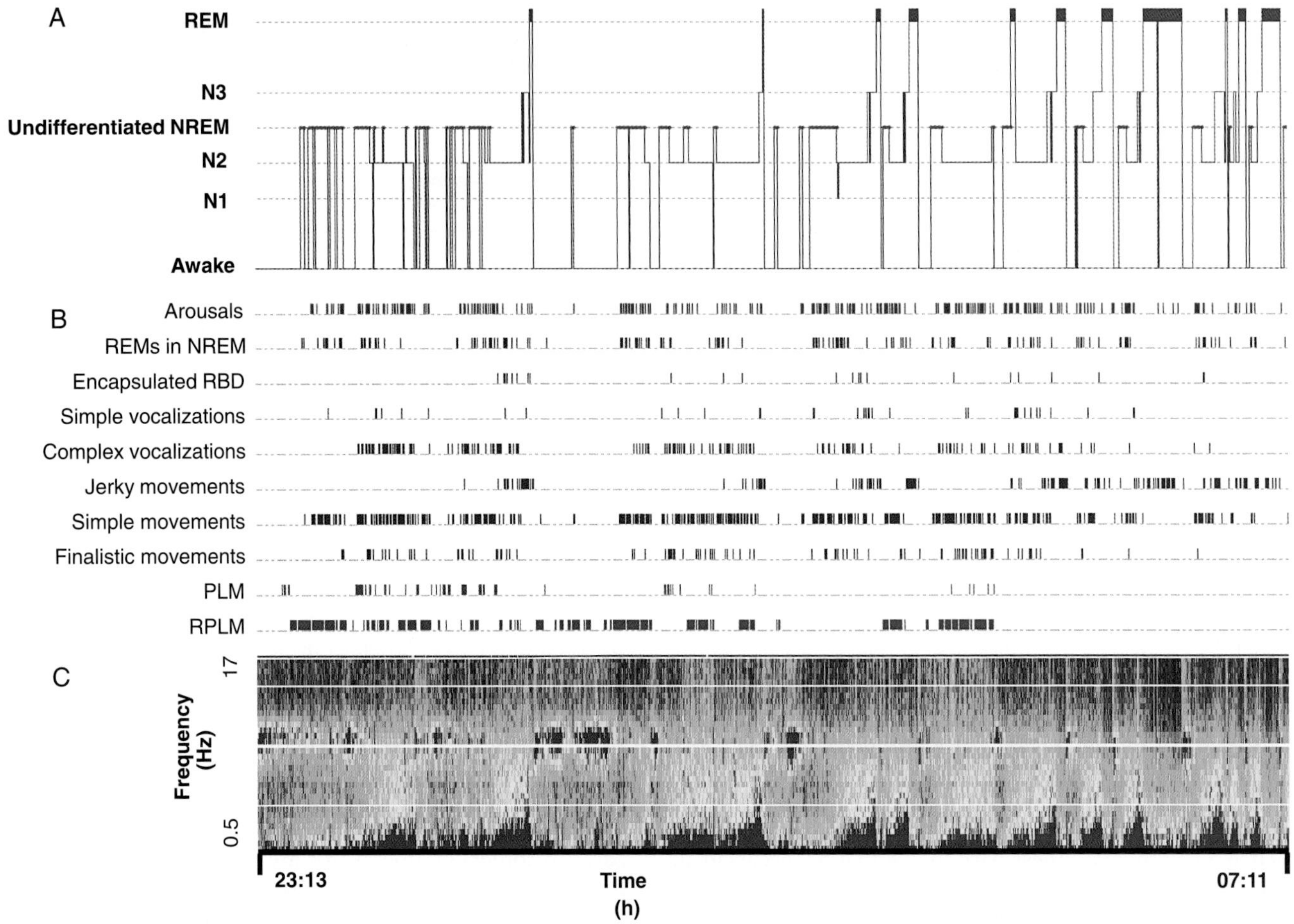

Figure 120.1 Sleep recording with CPAP in a patient with IgLON5 parasomnia. **(A)** Hypnogram. **(B)** Arousals, dissociations, and abnormal movements. **(C)** Density spectral array showing the power spectrum of electroencephalographic frequencies (0–17 Hz) in electrode C3 referenced to electrode O2. Warmer colors indicate more dominant frequencies. CPAP, Continuous positive airway pressure; IgLON5, immunoglobulin-like cell adhesion molecule 5; NREM, non–rapid eye movement; PLM, periodic limb movement; RBD, REM sleep behavior disorder; REMs, rapid eye movements; RPLM, rapid periodic leg movement.

between a NREM sleep parasomnia and RBD can be by chance in an older subject who has had a disorder of arousal since childhood and persists and decades later develops RBD. The NREM parasomnia usually consists in sleep terrors, confusional arousals, and sleepwalking, but sleep-related eating and sexsomnia can also be part of the clinical picture.[96,102] In more severe cases of overlap disorder, patients have degradation of sleep and wake features and behaviors to the point of the being indistinguishable in status dissociatus.

Anti-IgLON5 Disease. The anti-IgLON5 (immunoglobulin-like cell adhesion molecule 5) disease[89] is a novel neurologic disorder clinically characterized by neurologic and sleep symptomatology. Patients presented clinically with witnessed apneic events, stridor, insomnia, excessive daytime sleepiness, abnormal sleep behaviors, and additional waking neurologic symptoms, such as gait instability, dysarthria, dysphagia, chorea, cognitive impairment, and dysautonomia.[103,104] Patients have no previous history of disorders of arousal and are unaware of their sleep behaviors, which are only noted by the bed partner. Video-PSG shows a very complex distinct pattern characterized by (1) normal occipital alpha rhythm during wakefulness; (2) mild to moderate reduction of total sleep time and sleep efficiency; (3) initiation of sleep and reentering of sleep after awakenings characterized by prolonged periods of theta activity with motor activation and rapid repetitive leg movements that do not fit criteria for periodic leg movements in sleep; (4) reduced amount of normal N2 sleep; (5) periods of diffuse delta activity, typical of normal N3 sleep, mixed with spindles; (6) poorly structured stage N2 sleep characterized by clear spindles and K complexes with frequent vocalizations (e.g., talking, laughing, crying) and simple (e.g., raising the arm, punching) and finalistic behaviors (e.g., goal-directed behaviors, such as sucking the thumbs while apparently eating, manipulating wires); (7) sleepwalking, night terrors, and confusional arousals do not occur; (8) RBD characterized by limb and body jerks but no violent or finalistic behaviors; and (9) OSA and inspiratory stridor secondary to vocal cord palsy, particularly intense during normal N3 stage (Figures 120.1 and 120.2). Autoantibodies against IgLON5, a neuronal cell adhesion protein, are identified in all patients. The haplotypes DQB1*0501 and DRB1*1001 are very common. Prognosis seems to be poor, but some patients may experience clinical improvement with immunotherapy. Neuropathology shows a tauopathy, mainly involving the tegmentum of the brainstem and the hypothalamus, making the underlying pathophysiologic process unclear.

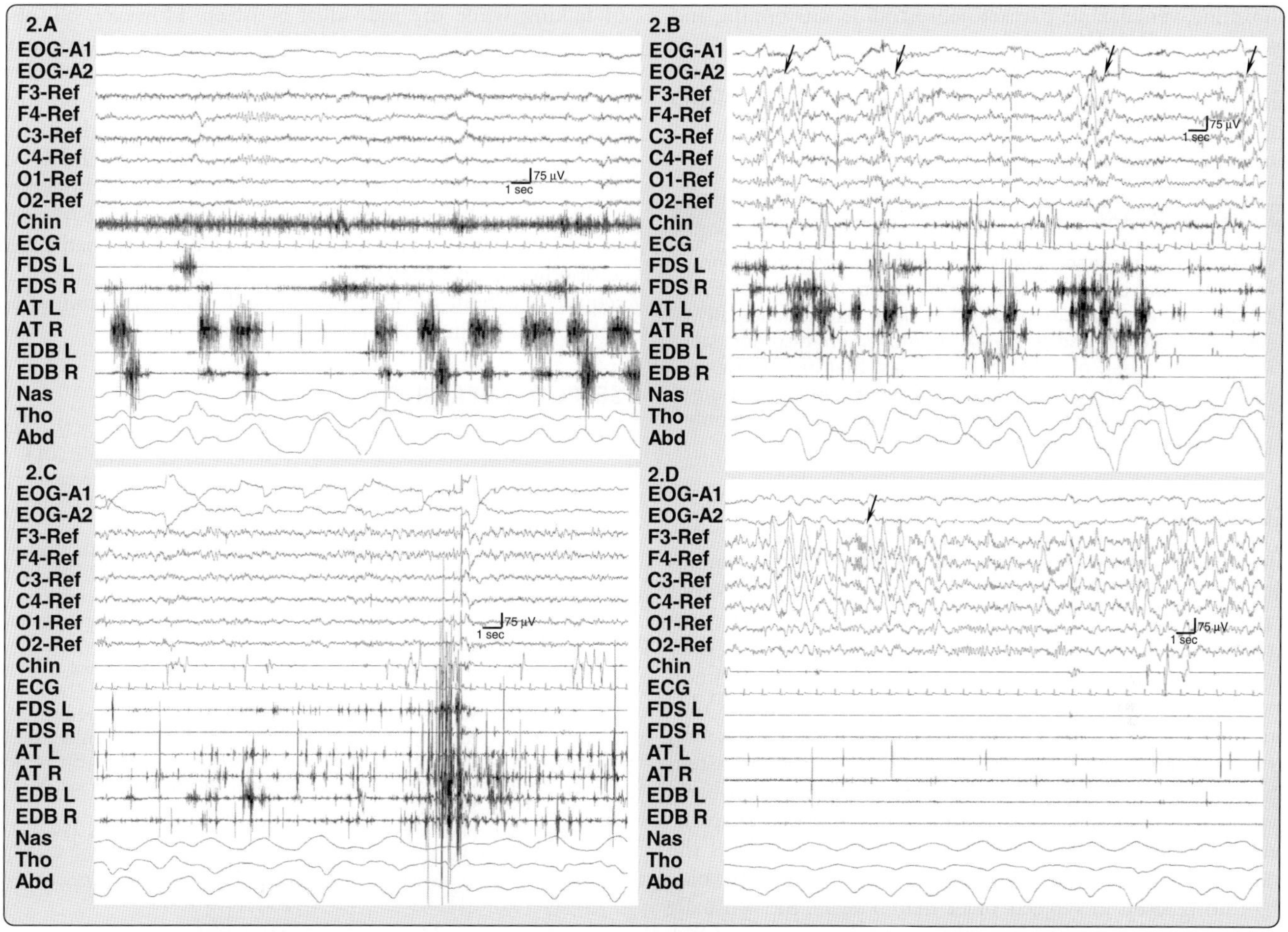

Figure 120.2 Polysomnographic epochs illustrative of each sleep state in a patient with the IgLON5 parasomnia. **(A)** Sleep onset characterized by undifferentiated NREM sleep with diffuse theta activity and rapid periodic leg movements particularly prominent at the right anterior tibialis electromyographic channel. **(B)** N2 sleep with chains of two or three consecutive K complexes (*arrows*) with frequent muscular phasic activity in EMG surface of the limbs that correlate with finalistic movements. **(C)** REM sleep with typical rapid eye movements and EEG features with excessive phasic muscular activity and limb jerks indicative of REM sleep behavior disorder. **(D)** N3 with diffuse delta activity mixed with well-defined sleep spindles at 13 Hz (*arrows*) without vocalizations nor movements. Abd, Abdominal respiratory movement; AT, anterior tibialis left (L) and right (R); Chin, electromyography of mentalis muscle; EDB, extensor digitorum brevis left (L) and right (R); EEG, electroencephalogram, EMG, electromyogram; EOG, electrooculogram; IgLON5, immunoglobulin-like cell adhesion molecule 5; FDS, flexor digitorum superficialis left (L) and right (R); Nas, nasal airflow; NREM, non–rapid eye movement; REM, rapid eye movement; Tho, thorax respiratory movement.

REM Sleep Parasomnias

As pointed out in the ICSD-3, when diagnostic criteria for RBD are met, the more specific diagnosis of RBD should be made, as with the other parasomnias.[1] In some instances, RBD may be an important clinical feature, and in others it is not clinically significant and is overlooked by other symptoms and signs (e.g., dementia, confusion, seizures). RBD is frequent among 25% to 58% of patients with Parkinson disease,[82,105–108] 50% to 80% with dementia with Lewy bodies,[32,82,105,109] and 90% to 100% with multiple system atrophy,[82,105,110] as well as other neurodegenerative diseases, autoimmune diseases such as narcolepsy, and structural brainstem lesions (see Chapter 118).[82]

PARASOMNIA DUE TO A MEDICATION OR SUBSTANCE

The assumption of drug-induced parasomnia is based on the temporal association between the introduction of the drug and the onset of the abnormal sleep behaviors and their cessation after the drug is stopped. The emergent parasomnia can be de novo parasomnia, the aggravation of a chronic intermittent parasomnia, or the reactivation of a previous parasomnia.[1]

NREM Sleep Parasomnias

The most common drugs inducing NREM sleep parasomnias are zolpidem (used at therapeutic doses for insomnia)[111] and sodium oxybate (used at high doses within the normal range for narcolepsy).[112] Both medications can cause sleepwalking, sleep-related eating disorder, sleep driving, and sleep sex.[111,112] There is no strong evidence that alcohol causes sleepwalking or other NREM parasomnias, but alcohol could increase sleep apnea, evoking a parasomnia event.[1]

REM Sleep Parasomnias

Antidepressants, including tricyclics, selective serotonin reuptake inhibitors, and selective noradrenaline reuptake inhibitors, have been described to trigger or aggravate RBD. They include clomipramine, imipramine, nortryptiline, mirtazapine, fluoxetine, venlafaxine, paroxetine, sertraline, citalopram, and escitalopram.[82,113,114]

The introduction of lipophilic beta blockers, such as bisoprolol, can also induce RBD.[115] There are also reports of RBD induced by withdrawal from meprobamate and alcohol.[116] Suvorexant may induce sleep paralysis.[117]

CLINICAL PEARL

When facing a patient who seeks medical advice for abnormal behaviors or experiences during sleep, clinicians should be aware that, in addition to NREM sleep parasomnias, REM sleep parasomnias and sleep-related movement disorders still remain in a group of "other parasomnias" that include sleep-related hallucinations, exploding head syndrome, sleep enuresis, and ST. These disorders require careful history to identify key features for the diagnosis.

SUMMARY

This chapter comprises a miscellaneous group of parasomnias that are included in the ICSD-3 under the category "other parasomnias." Sleep-related hallucinations are experiences perceived in the wake-sleep transition or upon awakening during the night or in the morning. HH and HPH are common in the general population and in narcolepsy, whereas CNVHs are usually linked to an underlying pathologic condition, such as Parkinson disease, dementia with Lewy bodies, brainstem structural lesions, and severe vision loss. EHS is possibly a type of auditory hallucination characterized by a benign, painless sense of a loud explosion in the head that awakens the individual. SE is characterized by recurrent involuntary voiding during sleep in subjects older than 5 years. SE is usually idiopathic and transient, but other conditions such as OSA and genitourinary tract malformations may be associated. Isolated ST is a very common normal sleep variant that consists of talking while the individual is asleep. However, ST also occurs in the setting of the NREM- and REM-related parasomnias, and these parasomnias can hallmark or be evoked by other medical conditions. Similarly, medications can provoke NREM- and REM-related parasomnias, particularly in the case of zolpidem and NREM parasomnias. Anti-IgLON5 disease is characterized by OSA, abnormal sleep architecture, and abnormal behaviors during both NREM and REM sleep in subjects with a brainstem and hypothalamic taupathy and antibodies against the protein IgLON5. All of these disorders require a careful detailed history and physical examination before considering a laboratory evaluation.

SELECTED READINGS

American Academy of Sleep Medicine. *International Classification of Sleep Disorders*. 3rd ed. Darien, IL: American Academy of Sleep Medicine; 2014.

Arkin AM, Toth MF, Baker J, Hastey MS. The frequency of sleep talking in the laboratory among chronic sleep talkers and good dream recallers. *J Nerv Ment Dis*. 1970;151:369–374.

Irfan M, Schenck CH, Howell MJ. NonREM disorders of arousal and related parasomnias: an updated review. *Neurotherapeutics*. 2021;18(1):124–139.

Leu-Semenescu S, De Cock VC, Le Masson VD, et al. Hallucinations in narcolepsy with and without cataplexy: contrasts with Parkinson disease. *Sleep Med*. 2011;12:497–504.

Manford M, Andermann F. Complex visual hallucinations. *Brain*. 1998;121:1819–1840.

Sabater L, Gaig C, Gelpi E, et al. A novel non-rapid-eye movement and rapid-eye-movement parasomnia with sleep breathing disorder associated with antibodies to IgLON5: an observational study: a case series, characterisation of the antigen, and postmortem study. *Lancet Neurol*. 2014;13:575–586.

Sharpless BA. Exploding head syndrome. *Sleep Med Rev*. 2014;18:489–493.

Wen JG, Wang QW, Chen Y, Wen JJ, Liu K. An epidemiological study of primary nocturnal enuresis in Chinese children and adolescents. *Eur Urol*. 2006;49:1107–1113.

A complete reference list can be found online at ExpertConsult.com.

Chapter 121

Restless Legs Syndrome (Willis-Ekbom Disease) and Periodic Limb Movements during Sleep

Richard P. Allen†; Jacques Montplaisir; Arthur S. Walters; Birgit Högl; Luigi Ferini-Strambi

Chapter Highlights

- Restless legs syndrome, also called Willis-Ekbom disease, (WED/RLS) is defined by its clinical symptoms, involving an urge to move the legs, engendered or worse with rest, relieved by movement, and most prominent in the evening and night.
- Periodic limb movements in sleep, relatively common in the general population, are a sensitive but nonspecific motor sign of RLS.
- RLS/WED varies both in severity, from annoying to disabling, and in natural course, from intermittent (remission and reoccurrence) to gradually progressive. More severe disease can significantly impair work productivity, quality of life, and possibly cardiovascular health.
- Iron status has a close relation to RLS/WED. Oral and intravenous iron treatment should always be considered first in treatment planning and for some may improve disease course.
- Dopamine agonists treatment should be used cautiously because they often produce RLS/WED augmentation, altering the disease process to create worse RLS/WED symptoms.
- Alpha-2-delta ligands and opioid medications are as effective and with no risk of augmentation.

DESCRIPTION AND MAJOR CLINICAL CHARACTERISTICS

Primary Sensory Manifestations

Restless legs syndrome/Willis-Ekbom disease (RLS/WED) is defined by its sensory symptoms and three factors that regulate expression of these symptoms (Box 121.1). RLS/WED has been described for centuries, with an early description by Willis in 1672,[1,2] but only in 1945 was it singled out as a distinct clinical entity by the Swedish neurologist Carl Ekbom.[3] Patients with RLS/WED when resting in the evening or night report an urge to move (akathisia) focused on the legs. This focal akathisia is usually, but not always, associated with dysesthesia.[4] Patients with dysesthesias describe them very differently, for instance, as uncomfortable, unpleasant, creepy-crawly, jittery, internal itch, or shock-like feelings; up to 50% of RLS/WED patients describe their sensations as painful. Some, however, describe only an urge to move without any other sensory component. Symptoms are usually felt over large areas of the thighs or calves in either or both legs. These feelings are typically expressed as coming from deep within the legs, rarely limited to the joints, and often do not include the feet.

The term *restless legs* can be somewhat misleading. The RLS leg akathisia is not fidgety—general restlessness like that occurring for many when sitting too long; rather, it is a focused, strange, consciously perceived feeling of an urge or drive for movement limited to the legs. The urge to move must involve the legs but also sometimes expands to a focus on other specific body parts, for instance, the arms.[5]

Three critical features regulate occurrence of the sensory symptoms defining RLS/WED (Box 121.1). *First, the symptoms are engendered or worsened by rest or inactivity.*[4] Typically, patients describe onset or exacerbation of symptoms in soporific situations, for instance, watching television, driving/flying long distances, attending meetings, going to bed. Symptoms worsen with decreasing alertness. *Second, activity relieves the symptoms.*[4] Patients use different motor strategies to relieve the discomfort, for instance, eating, showering, moving their legs vigorously, flexing, stretching, or crossing them one over the other, getting up, and walking. Partial or complete relief usually begins immediately or soon after the activity starts and persists as long as the activity continues. The symptoms, however, may return after movement stops. In severe cases, patients may walk for hours in the evening or night to relieve the discomfort. Some, however, with very severe RLS/WED find limited symptom relief even from strenuous movement. *Third, the symptoms are worse in the evening or during the night.*[4] Differing overall activity levels does not explain the evening predominance. Three studies using modified constant routine protocols demonstrated a circadian rhythm of the symptoms, maximal near midnight and independent of overall general activity effects.[6–8] The symptoms' circadian rhythm correlated with that of subjective vigilance, core body temperature,

† Deceased.

Box 121.1 DIAGNOSTIC CRITERIA ESTABLISHED BY THE INTERNATIONAL RESTLESS LEGS SYNDROME STUDY GROUP

Essential Features (All Five Must Be Met to Make a Diagnosis)

1. An urge to move the legs usually but not always accompanied by or felt to be caused by uncomfortable and unpleasant sensations in the legs.
2. The urge to move the legs and any accompanying unpleasant sensations begin or worsen during periods of rest or inactivity, such as lying down or sitting.
3. The urge to move the legs and any accompanying unpleasant sensations are partially or totally relieved by movement, such as walking or stretching, at least as long as the activity continues.
4. The urge to move the legs and any accompanying unpleasant sensations during rest or inactivity only occur or are worse in the evening or night than during the day.
5. The occurrence of the above features is not solely accounted for as symptoms primary to another medical or a behavioral condition (e.g., myalgia, venous stasis, leg edema, arthritis, leg cramps, positional discomfort, habitual foot tapping).

Specifiers for Clinical Course of RLS/WED

1. Chronic-persistent RLS/WED: symptoms when not treated would occur on average at least twice weekly for the past year.
2. Intermittent RLS/WED: symptoms when not treated would occur on average less than two times per week for the past year, with at least five lifetime events.

Specifier for Clinical Significance of RLS/WED

The symptoms of RLS/WED cause significant distress or impairment in social, occupational, educational, or other important areas of functioning by their impact on sleep, energy/vitality, daily activities, behavior, cognition, or mood.

Nonessential but Common Features

1. PLMs: presence of PLMs in sleep or resting wake at rates or intensity greater than expected for age or medical/medication status
2. Dopaminergic treatment response: reduction in symptoms at least initially with dopaminergic treatment
3. Family history of RLS/WED among first-degree relatives
4. Lack of profound daytime sleepiness

PLMs, Periodic leg movements; RLS/WED, restless legs syndrome/Willis-Ekbom disease.
From Allen RP, Picchietti DL, Garcia-Borreguero D, et al. Restless legs syndrome/Willis-Ekbom disease diagnostic criteria: updated International Restless Legs Syndrome Study Group (IRLSSG) consensus criteria—history, rationale, description, and significance. *Sleep Med*. 2014;15(8):860–73.

and salivary melatonin secretion. Thus the sensory symptoms should come on with rest more quickly and intensely in the evening or night than morning and follow changes in circadian entrainment, for instance, jet lag.

Other Major Clinical Features

RLS/WED has marked symptom variability and frequency. Symptom intensity ranges from mild and annoying to a disabling compulsion to keep moving. Symptom frequency also varies from less than yearly to daily. A large population-based study in Europe and the United States found 37% of all with RLS/WED symptoms had moderate to severe disease (bothersome symptoms two or more times a week).[9]

Disrupted nocturnal sleep occurs with little daytime sleepiness. In a study of 133 patients, 85% reported problems falling asleep, and 86% were frequently woken by symptoms.[10] The sleep problems occurred for moderate to severe RLS patients but not for about two-thirds of mild RLS patients.[11] Sleep laboratory studies confirm moderate to severe RLS/WED patients compared to control subjects and indicate increased wake after sleep onset, decreased sleep time, decreased stage 2 and increased stage 1 sleep with little change in rapid eye movement (REM) or slow wave sleep.[12] Daytime fatigue is commonly reported, but most RLS/WED patients do not report the level of sleepiness expected for their degree of sleep loss.[13,14] Thus RLS/WED appears to occur with some increased arousal process counteracting the sleep-loss effects.

Motor Sign of RLS/WED: Periodic Leg Movements in Sleep

Periodic limb movements in sleep (PLMS) are reasonably sensitive but nonspecific as a motor sign of RLS/WED. These are described in the previous section and shown in Figure 121.1 and Videos 121.1 to 121.5.

Clinical Course

RLS/WED can start at any age from childhood to late adult life. Familial cases of RLS/WED have an earlier age of onset, typically before age 30 years.[15–17] Symptom severity and frequency often fluctuate throughout life and can be dramatically affected by iron status and activity levels. Patients with a dramatic worsening of RLS should be evaluated for change in iron status. Some, however, report remissions, lasting for months or even years, and also relapses, both without any apparent reason.[18] Severely affected patients commonly report a progressive increase in symptom severity with advancing age.[18]

EPIDEMIOLOGY AND BURDEN OF DISEASE

Epidemiology

RLS/WED is one of the most common sleep-related disorders. The prevalence in European and American populations is about 7%[9] for any RLS/WED symptoms during a year and 2.7% for moderate to severe symptoms.[9] Physician-identified, medically significant RLS/WED occurs in 2.7% of patients seen in general medical practices in Europe.[11] The prevalence of moderate to severe RLS/WED symptoms increases with age from about 0.5% for children[19] to 5% for ages older than 70 years.[9] In adults older than 40 years, RLS/WED occurs about twice as often in women than men, but there is no gender difference for children[19] or young adults.[9] The gender difference appears related to pregnancy because nulliparous women have the same rate of RLS/WED as men.[20,21]

Burden of the Illness

Mild or minimal RLS/WED does not appear to have significant social or medical impact.[22] In contrast, moderate to severe RLS/WED significantly and adversely impacts work performance, quality of life, cognition, and health. Work productivity is diminished by 20% for moderate to severe RLS/WED and by 50% for very severe RLS/WED.[22] Quality of life (QOL) is similarly significantly diminished as shown by marked impairment in the Short Form (SF)-36 QOL

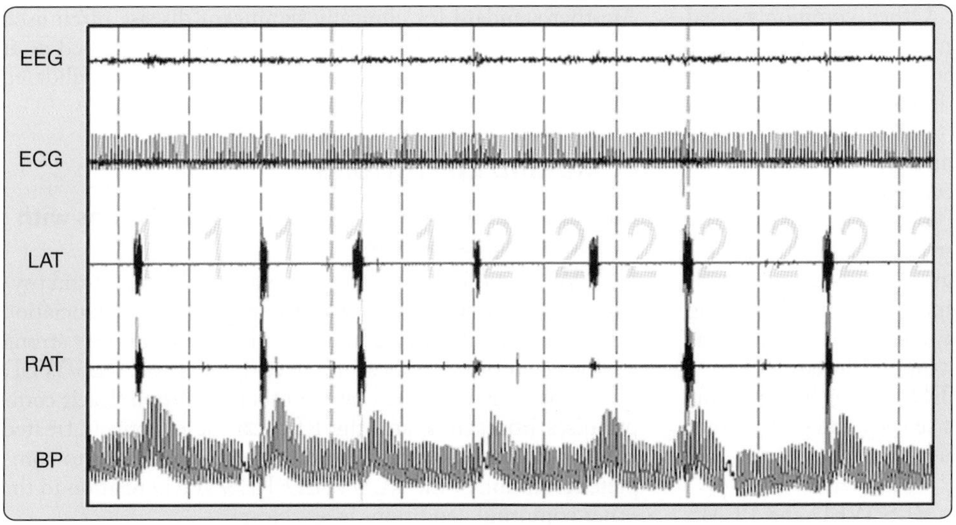

Figure 121.1 Polysomnogram of an RLS/WED patient with periodic limb movements in sleep. The figure shows the periodicity of leg movements and reveals significant increases in blood pressure associated with every periodic limb movement. BP, Blood pressure; ECG, electrocardiogram; EEG, left central electroencephalogram; LAT, left anterior tibialis electromyogram; RAT, right anterior tibialis electromyogram; RLS/WED, restless legs syndrome/Willis-Ekbom disease.

questionnaire dimensions of vitality, role physical, pain, physical functioning, and general health, and somewhat less impairment in social functioning, role emotional, and mental health.[9] This disruption in QOL is at least as great as the disruption caused by other chronic medical conditions, such as diabetes mellitus, depression, osteoarthritis, or hypertension.[9] RLS/WED patients also show impaired cognitive function involving mostly prefrontal cognitive tasks sensitive to sleep loss.[23,24]

Cardiovascular Disease, Cardiovascular Events, and Hypertension

Cross-sectional and longitudinal studies have produced mixed results on RLS associations, with increased risks of cardiovascular disease (CVD), cardiovascular events (CVEs), and hypertension. A 2017 systematic review of 20 cross-sectional general-population studies on RLS association with CVD found 14 supported a relationship, whereas 6 found no relation.[25] This review also found 13 longitudinal studies of at least 1-year duration that evaluated 18 cohorts reporting on possible CVE and all-cause mortality association to populations with primary RLS or PLMS determined by a sleep study. The CVEs included stroke, arrhythmias, congestive heart failure, and incidents related to coronary artery disease. The association between RLS and CVEs was evaluated in 8 cohorts and was significant for only 4 of these. The RLS association with all-cause mortality was evaluated in 8 cohorts and found to be significant in only 3. The only two relevant studies on PLMS reported significant relations between PLMS and both CVEs and mortality. Overall, the evidence supporting RLS predicting CVEs or related mortality is mixed and inconclusive. Significant prediction of CVEs was, however, found for two studies with secondary RLS[26,27] and one with longer-term RLS exposure.[26] Two studies reporting PLMS, without or with arousal, significantly predict CVEs and mortality.[28,29]

The possible relation between RLS/WED and hypertension is based mostly on several cross-sectional studies showing a relationship[30–35] but some not finding a relation particularly when controlling for other risk factors.[36–38] A recent meta-analysis reported an overall significant association of RLS/WED with hypertension, but this was largely attributed to other risk factors, particularly smoking.[39] There is one retrospective cohort study[27] showing a limited predictive relation. A significant nondipping blood pressure pattern was reported for RLS/WED, possibly increasing risk for developing hypertension.[40]

These population studies have several limitations. The diagnostic methods in these studies used mostly questionnaires. This approach produces populations in which 50% do not have RLS.[11] Thus the cross-sectional studies are not adequate and longitudinal studies are few, and many studies failed to control for alternate factors, such as smoking or medication. Furthermore, evidence exploring mechanisms for health impact of RLS/WED is limited. Three exceptions are (1) the relation of PLMS to transient heart rate and blood pressure increases,[41–44] (2) a recent study on nondipping blood pressure,[40] and (3) the attention to frequent, often brief arousals disrupting sleep.[27] A recent study indicated that PLMS associated with arousal may provoke nonsustained ventricular tachycardia.[45]

DIAGNOSIS AND SEVERITY ASSESSMENT

Clinical Diagnosis

No biologic assay is available for diagnosing RLS/WED; thus the diagnosis is based on the clinical evaluation of the patient. In 1995 the International RLS/WED Study Group (IRLSSG) established four essential criteria for the diagnosis of RLS/WED that were further refined at a National Institutes of Health RLS/WED consensus workshop.[46] These sufficed for clinical practice; however, when used in population-based surveys, about half of the participants identified with RLS/WED did not have the disorder but rather an RLS "mimic."[11,47] The revised 2014 IRLSSG official diagnostic criteria therefore include a fifth criterion, requiring differential diagnoses to exclude mimicking conditions.[4] The diagnosis cannot be made by questionnaire but requires a careful clinical evaluation to exclude mimics.[11] The current five essential RLS/WED diagnostic criteria[4] are listed in Box 121.1. These also address "clinical significance" and "clinical course," emphasizing heterogeneity of RLS/WED manifestations and the need to code these important disease dimensions. In addition, diagnostic uncertainty can be reduced by supportive clinical features, such as an RLS/WED family history, a high rate of PLMS, and a therapeutic response to dopaminergic medications.

Medical Evaluation

Iron status should be evaluated in every patient, given its importance for RLS. This must include morning fasting serum values for iron, ferritin, total iron-binding capacity (TIBC), and percent transferrin saturation. Other commonly used blood tests are not sensitive for iron deficiency; for instance, hemoglobin or hematocrit can be normal despite significant iron deficiency. When lower iron levels are found, further medical evaluation is recommended to determine any possible cause, often involving blood loss or an iron-poor diet.[48]

Medication history should be reviewed for any temporal relation to exacerbation or onset of RLS/WED, particularly for medications known to engender or exacerbate RLS, for instance, antidepressants (other than bupropion and trazodone),[49] lithium carbonate, dopamine D_2 receptor–blocking agents, (neuroleptics, dopaminergic antiemetics), antihistamines, alcohol, and doxepin (antihistamine effects).

A significant number of RLS/WED patients have peripheral neuropathy,[50,51] so the history of sensory and motor functions should be reviewed with further evaluation if indicated for neuropathy.

When taking the medical history, RLS/WED and PLMS should be differentiated from other state-dependent sensorimotor disorders, for instance, positional discomfort, hypnic myoclonus, painful legs and moving toes syndrome, nocturnal leg cramps, neuroleptic-induced akathisia, and vascular or neurogenic intermittent claudication. Whenever the diagnosis is doubtful, a polysomnogram (PSG) with measures of PLMS or a multinight leg activity meter[52] can be considered.

Sleep Laboratory Diagnosis with Periodic Leg Movement in Sleep

Although not routinely indicated, a PSG can be used to measure PLMS, the motor sign of RLS/WED. PLMS provides useful objective support for both diagnosis and assessment of RLS disease severity. The diagnosis of RLS is supported by rate of PLMS per hour greater than or equal to 3 for children[53] and 13 for adults,[54] but PLMS also occurs with multiple other conditions and older age (see the sections Periodic Limb Movements in Sleep and Periodic Limb Movement Disorder [PLMD]). PSG also helps identifying other sleep disorders contributing to the patients' sleep complaints.

Suggested Immobilization Test

The suggested immobilization test (SIT) measures both sensory and motor manifestations of RLS/WED in wakefulness.[55] Patients recline in bed at 45-degree angle with their legs outstretched and eyes open for 1 hour, usually just before bedtime. They are told to stay relaxed, awake but not moving (Video 121.6). Mean leg discomfort scores (every 5 minutes) and PLMS per hour during wake provide sensitivity and specificity for RLS diagnosis of about 80% to 85%.[56] The SIT can be repeated a few times during the day, with tests separated by 1 hour to capture variability and circadian pattern of RLS.[57]

Severity Assessments

The 10-question IRLSSG International RLS Severity Scale Group (IRLS) is well validated and the accepted standard for assessment of RLS severity[58,59] (sample copy at IRLSSG.org). This scale has a single total score (range, 0 to 40) and two subscales: symptoms and symptom-impact scales.[58,60] Scores less than 10 indicate minimal symptoms, and scores greater than 24 indicate moderate to severe symptoms.[61] Scores greater than 15 are required for entry into most clinical trials. This scale and the standard clinical global impression (CGI) of change are used in almost all pharmacologic clinical trials. Another standard for clinically significant disease often used in surveys is symptoms at least twice a week described as at least moderately bothersome.[9] The RLS-6 is another validated but less-used RLS severity scale.[62]

COMORBID CONDITIONS

Comorbid Conditions with Strong Associations with Restless Legs Syndrome

RLS/WED has been related to several other medical and psychiatric conditions, but in only a few cases is the association well documented. Three of these conditions have a very strong comorbid relation indicating development of RLS/WED symptoms may be caused by the other condition. Each compromises iron status, and the RLS can be effectively treated with iron. Resolution of these conditions often leads to complete resolution of the RLS/WED. RLS/WED relation to the other comorbid conditions is less clear.[63]

Uremia

RLS/WED occurs with uremia, and 20% to 60% of patients on hemodialysis have RLS/WED.[64–67] Several factors can predispose uremic patients to RLS/WED, particularly anemia and compromised iron regulation. Iron appears to be critical as intravenous (IV) iron reduces RLS/WED symptoms.[68] RLS/WED relates to increased mortality rate in patients with end-stage renal disease.[69] Kidney transplantation leads to complete resolution of RLS/WED, and return of RLS/WED symptoms can be an early indicator of transplant failure.[70]

Anemia

RLS/WED occurs in about 35% of patients with iron deficiency anemia[71,72] and at only a slightly lower rate in patients with iron deficiency without anemia.[73] IV iron treatment resolving the anemia also completely resolves the associated RLS/WED in most patients.[74]

Pregnancy

RLS/WED occurs in about 15% to 30 % of pregnant women, mostly during the last trimester. It may abate shortly before delivery and generally resolves quickly afterward.[75–77] Iron deficiency, common during pregnancy, relates to the co-occurrence of RLS/WED.[78,79] IV iron treatment reduced or resolved the RLS/WED during pregnancy for 2 women with low serum ferritin (≤50 mcg/L)[80] and for 19 women with serum ferritin less than 35 mcg/L or hemoglobin less than 11 g/dL.[81] The excellent treatment response indicates iron compromise during pregnancy is a primary factor driving the development of the associated RLS/WED.

Other Comorbid Medical Conditions Associated with Restless Legs Syndrome

Neuropathy

Neuropathy appears to increase the risk of RLS/WED. The studies, however, are complicated by problems of both differential diagnosis of neuropathy and RLS/WED and also by the limited use of control subjects for detecting possible confounding pain effects. One study using a pain control group and carefully validated diagnostic procedures found RLS/WED occurred in 8% of patients with diabetic neuropathy compared with 3.9% with osteoarthritis.[82] It is, however, unclear if these results would generalize to all neuropathies.

One study showed a high rate (32%) of subclinical small-fiber neuropathy in RLS/WED patients that significantly related to no family history and later age of symptom onset of RLS/WED.[51] Thus it seems there is some as yet unexplained relation between neuropathy and RLS/WED.

Parkinson Disease

Parkinson disease (PD) deserves special mention because RLS/WED occurs commonly in patients with PD, and the major dopaminergic drugs for RLS/WED are also used for PD. RLS/WED in PD often appears after starting dopamine treatment for PD, and the prevalence of RLS/WED is not increased in untreated PD.[83] Thus RLS/WED is not comorbid with PD; rather, treatment of PD with dopaminergic agents will often engender or exacerbate RLS/WED.

Other Medical and Neurologic Disorders

Several other medical conditions have been found to have a significantly high rate of RLS/WED. All conditions associated with iron deficiency appear to show increased risk of RLS/WED, including celiac disease,[84] frequent blood donors,[73] and irritable bowel syndrome.[85] RLS/WED has also been noted to occur with a wide range of medical conditions, for instance, hypothyroidism and hyperthyroidism, chronic lung disease, leukemia, Isaac syndrome, stiff-man syndrome, Huntington chorea, multiple sclerosis, essential tremor, migraine, and amyotrophic lateral sclerosis. Considering the high prevalence and the differential diagnostic uncertainty of RLS/WED for many studies, these associations should be interpreted with caution. However, the rate of occurrence of RLS/WED may increase in patients with multiple comorbid medical conditions,[86] suggesting multiple, complicated interactions increasing the expression of RLS/WED. There is likely a major confounding in all of these studies with inflammatory processes, possibly greater with more medical conditions, compromising iron status and thereby driving the relation to RLS. Overall, unless shown otherwise, iron status should be the presumed relation of any condition to RLS.

Comorbid Psychiatric Conditions

One population-based sample of 1024 participants using excellent diagnostic procedures found the odds ratios (95% confidence range) of psychiatric conditions occurrence in the past year for those with RLS/WED versus not RLS/WED was 2.0 (0.6 to 7.3) for generalized anxiety disorder, 2.7 (1.1 to 6.7) for major depressive disorder, 5.6 (1.4 to 21.9) for obsessive compulsive disorder, and 5.3 (2.0 to 14.0) for panic disorder.[87] RLS/WED appears to increase the risk of having these other disorders rather than the reverse, possibly because of some shared biologic features or a response to the stress of living with RLS/WED.

ETIOLOGY AND PHYSIOPATHOLOGY

Genetics

Substantial evidence suggests a genetic contribution to RLS/WED. Greater than 50% of idiopathic cases report a positive family history of RLS/WED.[3,15,18,88,89] In most pedigrees the disorder follows an autosomal-dominant inheritance pattern, with a penetrance rate greater than 90%.[15] Multiple linkage studies of familial RLS/WED have, however, identified mostly marginal associations over a wide range of chromosomes. Thus far none have identified any specific gene associated with RLS/WED.

In contrast, modestly large, genome-wide association studies have discovered specific common allelic variants strongly associated with increased risk of RLS/WED occurring at loci for specific genomic regions of *MEIS1, BTBD9, PTPRD, MAP2k/SKOR1, TOX3/BC034767,* and at an intergenic region on chromosome 2 (rs6747972). Variants in *MEIS1* appear to carry the largest relative risk for RLS/WED, indicating possible neurodevelopmental factors for RLS/WED consistent with this gene's role in early development.[90,91] The *BTBD9* variant is associated with reduced serum ferritin[92] in RLS/WED, indicating a possible genetic role in the iron relation to RLS/WED. The *BTBD9* variants are also strongly associated with PLMS independent of RLS/WED,[92] and most of the other variants associated with RLS/WED also relate to some degree to PLMS.[93] The known common variants associated with RLS/WED, however, account for only 7% of RLS heritability.[94,95] The missing genetic factors may involve as yet undetected common alleles, rare variants, or epigenetic features. For example, association with RLS has been found both for nine new low-frequency rare variants[96] and also for rare allelic variants of *MEIS1* altering transcription.[95]

Iron

Iron has a major, possibly dominant, role in the physiopathology of RLS. Several clinical aspects of RLS relate to an underlying iron deficiency: Most if not all conditions compromising iron also increase risk of RLS, iron deficiency has a central role for virtually all medical conditions comorbid with RLS, and iron treatments of RLS are very effective.[97,98] This central role of iron was recognized in the middle of the 20th century by Ekbom's and Norlander's pioneering medical studies of RLS.[3,99] The RLS iron pathophysiology has two major features: (1) brain and not peripheral iron deficiency and (2) regional more than total brain iron deficiency, particularly involving the substantia nigra (SN) and thalamus. Two independent studies, one in the United States and the other Japan, showed that despite normal peripheral iron RLS, patients had decreased CSF ferritin, indicating likely brain iron deficiency.[100,101] Brain iron deficiency was found in 23 of the 25 studies of brain iron in RLS patients compared to control subjects. These studies included 8 using magnetic resonance imaging (MRI),[102–109] 3 with cerebrospinal fluid (CSF) analyses,[100,101,110] 5 with autopsy,[111–115] and 7 with midbrain ultrasound imaging.[106,116–121] Two brain regions appear to be most involved in RLS brain iron deficiency. The SN was iron deficient in 5 of the 8 MRI studies, all of the ultrasound studies, and 4 of the autopsy studies. Two studies using different, more recently developed, susceptibility measures found iron deficiency in the thalamus of RLS patients.[103,105] SN and thalamic brain iron deficiency have obvious significance for the sensory-motor symptoms of RLS. Underlying the brain iron deficiency is a complex pattern of abnormal iron metabolism as revealed by autopsy analyses of RLS SN tissue, that is, increased mitochondrial ferritin, decreased cytosolic ferritin,[112] decreased transferrin receptor despite iron deficiency,[115] altered regulation at the blood-brain interface,[122] and association with increased hypoxia-inducible factor despite no actual hypoxia.[123]

Of interest is the role of iron in dopaminergic transmission in the central nervous system (CNS). Experimentally induced brain iron deficiency produces increased extracellular dopamine, decreased dopamine transporter (DAT), and decreased D_2 and D_1 receptors in the striatum of rats similar to the findings in RLS/WED.[124] A forward genetic animal model produced RLS SN brain iron deficiency without low peripheral iron and also produced circadian RLS-like behavior,[125] providing strong support for a putative causal relationship.[126] Thus abnormalities in iron metabolism or environmental factors producing brain iron deficiency may be one primary cause of RLS/WED. In this regard the finding that pregnancy increases the risk of RLS/WED in later life[20,21] raises the interesting concept that environmental factors with significant iron deficiency may produce epigenetic changes, altering susceptibility to developing RLS/WED.

Neural Substrates

The iron deficiency in the brain of RLS would be expected to impair myelination, possibly reducing brain white matter with limited effect on grey matter. Studies generally confirm this. There is no known significant cell loss or degeneration in the peripheral nervous system or CNS in RLS/WED.[115,127] There were, on autopsy, no overall histopathologic abnormalities for RLS/WED brains[115] and, in particular, none for the major RLS/WED dopaminergic areas (SN[115] and A11[127]). MRI studies generally find no morphologic abnormalities nor grey matter loss.[128,129] White matter, however, appears, as expected, to be decreased in RLS/WED,[130] particularly in the corpus callosum, anterior cingulum, and precentral gyrus.[111,131,102] The abnormal myelination loss is consistent with that in iron-deprived animals.[111] These abnormalities involve key somatosensory circuits that may underlie RLS sensory symptoms.

Central Nervous System Functional Abnormalities

Mild abnormalities in CNS functioning appear to be widespread in RLS/WED during the times without symptoms. Changes in cortical[132–134] and spinal[135] excitability have been reported, although the later may result from loss of cortical inhibition.[135] Connectivity in the asymptomatic resting state appears to be altered for the thalamus,[136] the thalamic sensory-motor associated circuits,[137] and in ventral and dorsal attention, cingulate, and brainstem networks.[138] The documented default mode network abnormalities in asymptomatic RLS/WED have both a circadian pattern[139] and a response to dopaminergic treatments.[140] These changes are generally consistent with the abnormalities in neural substrates.

Neurotransmitter Dysfunction

Dopamine

Levodopa and dopamine agonists (DAs) dramatically reduce RLS/WED symptoms and PLMS, indicating possible altered dopamine signaling involvement. Initial brain-imaging studies had somewhat conflicting results, but recent analyses have overall consistent findings. Positron emission tomography (PET) studies showed decreased membrane-bound DAT in RLS/WED,[141] but single-photon emission computed tomography studies showed no change in overall DAT.[142,143] Iron-deprived animals similarly show a decrease mostly in membrane-bound DAT.[144] Raclopride binding for dopamine receptors is decreased in PET studies of more severe RLS/WED patients,[145] and, in an autopsy study, striatal D_2 receptors had a significant decrease, correlated with RLS/WED severity.[146] The decreases in DAT and the D_2 receptors are consistent with increased striatal dopamine.[145] CSF studies showed increased 3-orthymethyldopamine, indicating possible increased dopamine production.[147] Thus, overall, RLS/WED appears to have increased, not decreased, presynaptic dopaminergic activation leading to a possible compensatory decreased postsynaptic response, with circadian inadequacy at the nadir of the dopamine cycle producing the circadian RLS symptoms. A small increase in dopamine at this nadir may suffice to normalize dopamine signaling and reduce the RLS symptoms. Overall, RLS/WED appears best characterized as a striatal hyperdopaminergic condition.[124]

Opioid

The positive pharmacologic response to opioid treatment[148–150] and the reversal of that treatment with opiate receptor blocker naloxone[151–153] indicates possible endogenous opiate system dysfunction in RLS/WED and PLMS.[151] Pharmacologic studies suggest that opioids may benefit RLS by effects on dopamine signaling.[154,155] A PET scan study showed no abnormalities in postsynaptic opiate receptor binding for RLS/WED patients.[156] An autopsy study showed decreased endogenous opioids beta endorphin and met-enkephalin in RLS/WED patients.[157] An in vivo total opiate knockout mouse model of RLS showed significant hyperactivity during the inactive period, but there were no significant changes in D_1 and D_2 receptors or dopamine levels in the striatum.[158]

Other Neurotransmitters

The RLS brain iron deficiency has been associated with producing neurotransmitter changes other than dopamine, that is, glutamate, histamine, and adenosine.[159] Abnormal glutamate in RLS has been reported in one MR spectroscopy study,[160] and alpha-2-delta ($\alpha 2\delta$) ligands reducing glutamatergic activity provide effective treatment for RLS.[161,162] Adenosine A1 receptors in rats are reduced by RLS-like mild iron deficiency with associated hyperactivity,[163] providing another target for new RLS treatments.[164] Dipyridamole increases extracellular adenosine by inhibiting adenosine transporters and in a small open-label trial was effective in reducing RLS symptoms.[165] Striatal histamine abnormalities with increased histamine 3 receptors occur for rats on an iron-deficient diet known to produce SN iron deficiency, and this occurs with development of PLMS that can be reduced by treatment with a histamine 3 receptor antagonist.[166] There have been, however, no reports of clinical evaluation of this potential treatment for RLS.

TREATMENT FOR ADULTS

Nonpharmacologic

It is important that RLS patients maintain good sleep hygiene to prevent developing psychophysiologic insomnia, frequently encountered in RLS/WED. Patients should also refrain from drinking alcohol in the evening because it aggravates symptoms in most individuals. Some patients report benefit from activity during times symptoms tend to occur and delaying sleep times to later when symptoms have abated.[6]

Iron

Iron replacement, unlike the other treatments for RLS, attempts to ameliorate or correct a basic biologic abnormality of the disorder, the brain iron deficiency. It should always be the first choice of treatment because it may reduce any doses needed for other treatments. Morning fasting serum levels of iron, TIBC, transferrin saturation, and ferritin should be routinely obtained for all RLS patients at initial treatment, when continuing iron treatments, and whenever there is a change in RLS symptoms. Iron treatments should not be used for patients with fasting morning transferrin saturation greater than or equal to 45%. Oral versus IV iron choice depends primarily on oral treatment limits, that is, limited and slow iron uptake into the blood and multiple common adverse effects, and it is counterindicated for common medical conditions. Official guidelines for iron treatment[167] with minor updates are summarized here.

Oral Iron

Oral iron treatment is indicated when the patient's ferritin level is less than 75 mcg/L.[168] Ferrous sulfate, 325 mg, or its equivalent, with vitamin C, 100 to 200 mg, can be taken once a day preferably, if tolerated on an empty stomach. Hepcidin regulation blocking iron uptake into blood is increased for several hours after a dose of oral iron, so there is little benefit but increased adverse effects with more than once-a-day treatment.[169] It may take several weeks for oral iron to produce symptom relief, but if little occurs within 3 months, consider using IV iron. The need for continued treatment on oral iron should be determined by a trial off the iron, but treatment may need to be continued indefinitely to maintain adequate iron levels.

Intravenous Iron

IV iron provides effective treatment for adult RLS at doses of 1000 to 1500 mg but not 500 mg.[170] IV iron formulations differ considerably in how rapidly they release iron into blood. Two formulations, iron sucrose (Venofer) and ferric gluconate (Ferrlecit), release iron rapidly, leading to increased free iron not taken up by transferrin. Free iron produces the common adverse effects of flushing, bloating, and nausea. These formulations therefore need to be given in five repeated 200-mg doses spaced 2 to 5 days apart. These are not recommended for IV iron treatment of adults. Iron dissociates slowly into blood over several hours for the other major formulations, that is, low–molecular-weight (LMW) iron dextran (Dexferrum), iron isomaltoside (renamed ferric derisomaltose, Monoferric), ferric carboxymaltose (FCM), and ferumoxytol (Feraheme). These formulations can generally be given in one 1000-mg dose or two doses of 500 to 750 mg separated by 5 days.

There are three blinded placebo-controlled clinical trials for 1000-mg FCM treatment of RLS. Two showed significant efficacy at the planned end point of 4 and 6 weeks,[98,171] and the third showed efficacy at 12 weeks but not at the planned end point at 4 weeks after treatment.[172] These data met criteria for the evidenced-based recommendation that 1000 mg FCM IV is effective for treatment of RLS. The other formulations with slow release of iron have not been adequately studied for evidenced-based recommendations but are assumed likely to be effective for treating RLS. The duration of benefit from IV iron treatment varies considerably, with about 30% of the patients showing long-term efficacy without added RLS treatments for at least 4 to 6 months. Repeated doses when RLS symptoms return have been found to be effective for some but not all patients.[173]

IV FCM and LMW iron dextran treatments of RLS were effective in several studies and well tolerated without significant adverse events[98,170–172,174] as confirmed in one meta-analysis.[175] There is very limited risk of anaphylaxis or severe adverse effects with IV iron treatments aside from that seen with LMW dextran,[176] a formulation no longer available. Standard anaphylaxis treatment options should, nonetheless, be readily available. The LMW dextran (Dexferrum) treatment requires a small test dose followed by an observation period before giving the remaining total dose, but this is not required for the other formulations.

There are three major unusual features of IV iron that should be noted: (1) delayed clinical response, sometimes immediate but usually not until 4 to 6 weeks after treatment. The patient needs to be informed of this delay with appropriate management as needed. (2) About 30% to 40% of patients do not respond, and limited data indicate an added or increased dose may not be helpful with these patients.[98] At this point there is no established way to identify those who would respond. (3) The clinical studies included only a few patients with ferritin values in the 100- to 200-mcg/L range, with about half responding to treatment.[167] The consensus guidelines, however, based on concerns about safety and limited clinical experience, restrict IV iron treatment to patients with serum ferritin less than or equal to 100 mcg/L for initial treatment and less than or equal to 300 mcg/L for repeated treatments.

A puzzle with IV iron is the complete lack of response for 30% to 40% of RLS patients. A preclinical study indicated IV iron normalizes the brain iron deficiency in a murine model of RLS iron status.[177] A small study demonstrated that the IV iron treatment was more effective for patients showing greater SN iron deficiency on sonography before treatment, but all patients except one had substantia nigra iron deficiency on sonography.[178] Lower transferrin saturation before treatment (<30%) may also indicate more likely response to IV iron treatment.[172,179] Patients with more severe iron problems may respond better to IV iron, but there are many other significant factors, such as iron storage, transport, loss, and measurement accuracy. IV iron also does not correct the basis for the RLS brain iron deficiency that may persist, complicating long-term outcomes.

Pharmacologic Treatment for Adults

RLS treatments, other than iron, involve many years of essentially palliative drug treatments. Unfortunately, most of the controlled clinical treatment studies for RLS/WED lasted only 3 to 6 months, but some of the most significant dopaminergic treatment complications arise after the first 6 months of treatment.[180] The following emphasizes medication choices assuming long-term treatment.

Four categories of medications are commonly prescribed to treat RLS/WED: dopaminergic medications, α2δ ligands, opioids, and benzodiazepines.

Dopaminergic Medications

Dopaminergic medications, although dramatically effective, should generally be avoided or, when needed, the dose should be maintained as low as possible. They have been the most commonly prescribed medications for RLS/WED, with typically excellent short-term benefit producing a false impression that these are the most effective long-term medications for RLS/WED. A well-controlled 1-year treatment trial showed an α2δ ligand was, if anything, more effective than a DA.[180]

Dopaminergic medications also have serious adverse effects emerging with long-term treatment.

Long-term complications with dopaminergic treatments present three major problems: (1) Augmentation (worsening of the underlying RLS/WED symptoms) develops in the majority of patients, usually insidiously and with longer duration of treatment.[181] (2) Compulsive behaviors and profound sleepiness develop in a few patients, mostly with higher doses.[182] (3) Strong withdrawal symptoms occur with profound sleep loss,[183] making it difficult to stop the medications.

RLS/WED augmentation is a phenomena in which RLS/WED symptoms become worse than they were before treatment so that they occur earlier in the day, have greater intensity when present, involve more of the body (e.g., more of the legs, arms as well as legs), have increased periodic leg movements, and shorter periods of relief after taking the medication.[46,181,184,185] Augmentation leads to a need for increased dose to control symptoms and doses earlier in the day to block the earlier onset of symptoms. Thus, in clinical practice, the most common symptoms of augmentation are the need for increasing dosing earlier in the day (afternoon, morning) to block the augmentation effects.[181] Augmentation can produce RLS/WED symptoms 24 hours a day even while taking high doses of dopaminergic medications. The extreme distress with severe RLS/WED augmentation is shown in Video 121.7 for sensory/motor symptoms and Video 121.8 for in-bed continuous movement.

The rate of augmentation varies by medications and is generally higher with shorter-acting medications and can develop over at least 10 years.[186] About 75% of the patients in a population study developed augmentation over 1 to 8 years of DA treatment.[181] The risk of augmentation can be reduced by using longer-acting DA, keeping the dose low, and in particular, not exceeding the approved dose levels and not increasing the dose after stable treatment has been established. A clinical need to increase the dose is a warning sign of possible augmentation.

The recommended treatments for augmentation all require discontinuing the current dopaminergic medication.[185] The treatments include switching to a much longer-acting DA or gradually tapering off the dopaminergic drug. Switching to a longer-acting dopaminergic drug seems unlikely to be a satisfactory final solution because even the continually active transdermal DA rotigotine eventually produces a high rate of augmentation.[187,188] Switching to a nondopaminergic drug is preferred. This can be done as a gradual withdrawal from the DA and then, after 5 to 7 days off all treatment, starting a nondopaminergic drug. Alternatively, a new nondopaminergic can be gradually introduced during the taper of DA dose to reduce the marked withdrawal effects. This involves less suffering for the patient but complicates determining minimum effective medication dose after completing DA withdrawal. It may, however, take several weeks to months to fully recover from augmentation.[189]

Once augmentation has occurred with long-term treatment, it may reoccur more rapidly if the dopaminergic agent is restarted after withdrawal,[190] suggesting augmentation may produce long-term changes in sensitivity to dopaminergic stimulation.

Compulsive behavior and sleepiness can occur with long-term use of the higher doses of currently used DAs, presumably related to overstimulation of D_2-like receptors.[182,191] DAs have produced excessive gambling with significant financial loss and also inappropriate sexual behaviors. All patients being treated for RLS/WED with dopaminergics should be cautioned about these problems. The patient, however, will generally not recognize these as abnormal behaviors. Profound sleepiness, sometimes with sudden onset, also occurs but only rarely and at higher dopaminergic doses.[182]

Abrupt or even tapered dose discontinuation of a DA can produce insomnia and increased RLS/WED symptoms for at least the first 2 to 5 days off the medication,[183] which may lead some patients to reinitiate DA. Withdrawal symptoms appear less common for $\alpha 2\delta$ medications.[183]

Commonly used dopaminergic medications include levodopa and the DAs pramipexole, ropinirole, and rotigotine.

Levodopa. Several open-label and placebo-controlled studies have documented the benefits of levodopa, given with a DOPA-decarboxylase inhibitor, either benserazide or carbidopa, in idiopathic RLS/WED[192–196] and RLS/WED associated with uremia.[197–199] Adverse effects included nausea, vomiting, tachycardia, orthostatic hypotension, hallucinations, insomnia, daytime fatigue, and daytime sleepiness. Morning rebound of RLS/WED symptoms can occur, with symptoms presenting in the morning at the end-of-dose efficacy. Augmentation is common (60% to 82%) and may be severe, requiring medication adjustment.[184,200] With levodopa, augmentation can occur within the first 6 months of treatment and even at a low dose (50 mg levodopa).[200] The use of as needed, lower doses (50 to 100 mg daily) at a frequency of once or twice a week appears to have limited risk of augmentation.

Dopamine Agonists. DAs are more effective and produce fewer adverse effects (especially augmentation) than L-DOPA,[201] and therefore they had become one of the first-line treatments for RLS/WED. They are now are used more cautiously as a second choice at lower doses to avoid long-term treatment complications, particularly augmentation. Several agonists have been studied in RLS/WED.

The long-acting ergoline-derivative DA cabergoline, although effective for treatment of RLS,[202,203] can produce retroperitoneal and pleuropulmonary fibrosis[204] and is not recommended for RLS/WED treatment.

Two intermediate-duration non–ergoline-derivative DAs, pramipexole and ropinirole, have been extensively studied for the treatment of RLS/WED. Both are effective and well tolerated. Pramipexole, a full agonist for the D_2 subfamily of receptors with preferential affinity for the D_3-receptor, has sustained efficacy for 3 to 12 months[205–208] and is approved for RLS treatment by the U.S. Food and Drug Administration (FDA) for evening doses of 0.25 to 0.5 mg and by the European Medicines Evaluation Association (EMEA) for doses of 0.25 to 0.75 mg. Ropinirole, a DA pharmacologically similar to pramipexole, but with a somewhat shorter half-life, has sustained efficacy for up to 12 months[209,210] and is approved by the FDA and EMEA for RLS treatment for evening doses up to 4 mg.

Augmentation occurred in about one-third of patients over 3 years of treatment[207,211] and 75% of patients treated for up to 8 years.[181,186]

Rotigotine. Rotigotine, with a 24-hour transdermal delivery, provides continuous dopamine stimulation and effective treatment of RLS/WED[188,212–214] sustained for 5 years.[188] It has high affinities for the D_2 receptor family and also, unlike pramipexole and ropinirole, has significant affinity for D_1, D_5, and alpha$_{2B}$-adrenergic receptors. Rotigotine is approved by the FDA and EMEA for treatment of moderate to severe RLS/WED at doses of 1 to 3 mg per 24 hours. In a prospective 5-year rotigotine treatment trial, 39% continuing on drug were essentially free of all RLS/WED symptoms,[188] but 50% stopped treatment, 30% because of adverse effects and 11% for lack of efficacy. The annual augmentation occurrence rate averaged over 5 years was 7.2% and 2.6% for clinically significant augmentation.[188] Pramipexole and ropinirole longer-acting formulations may also effectively treat RLS with possibly less augmentation,[215] but they have not been adequately studied.

Alpha-2-Delta Ligands

Alpha-2-delta ligand medications act on the $\alpha 2\delta$ subunit of voltage-dependent calcium channels to reduce the influx of calcium ions into the neuron, thereby reducing release of some neurotransmitters, particularly glutamate, norepinephrine, and substance P. Unlike dopaminergics, these drugs do not appear to cause augmentation with long-term treatment.[162] They are therefore the preferred first-line treatment for RLS/WED when their adverse effects are not a problem. The primary adverse effects for these drugs are dizziness, somnolence, peripheral edema, and weight gain. This class of drugs has been marked by the FDA for possible development of suicidal ideation. This has not been documented as a problem in the RLS/WED studies, but caution is advised when prescribing these drugs for patients with major depression and suicidality diagnoses. In general, $\alpha 2\delta$ ligand medications should be started at low doses, with a gradual increase in dose about once a week until therapeutic levels are reached. Unlike the DAs, the response to these drugs may not occur on the first night of treatment; rather, the clinical response may be delayed usually by the need to gradually increase the dose to therapeutic levels. Three $\alpha 2\delta$ agents are currently used to treat RLS/WED.

Gabapentin Encarbil. Gabapentin enacarbil, which is FDA approved for RLS/WED at a dose of 600 mg daily, is an oral prodrug for gabapentin that provides better absorption and allows for a higher continuous blood level of gabapentin. It has been found to be very effective for treatment of RLS/WED over a full 24-hour period, reducing daytime as well as evening and nighttime symptoms.[216–220]

Pregabalin. Pregabalin is commonly used to reduce pain. Pregabalin 100 mg, is as effective as 0.5 mg pramipexole and more effective than 0.25 mg pramipexole over 12 months of treatment.[180] It has no significant augmentation rate compared to placebo over a full year of (1.7% vs. 1% to 2%),[221] significantly less than the 9.0% for pramipexole 0.5 mg.[180] The low reported augmentation rates for placebo and pregabalin reflect nonpharmacologic processes in the natural course of the disease, for instance, symptom fluctuation or gradual progression of the disease rather than augmentation.

Gabapentin. Gabapentin has been widely used to reduce neuropathic pain, and several very small open-label trials[222–226] and one small placebo-controlled, crossover study[227] showed it is also effective for treatment of moderate to severe RLS/WED. Its efficacy is reduced by problems with absorption limiting actual doses that can be achieved, and serum levels can be variable for a given dose.[228] Neither pregabalin nor gabapentin are approved by the FDA or EMEA for treatment of RLS/WED.

Opioids

The therapeutic effects of opioids were noted by Ekbom[3] and confirmed in several open-label and controlled clinical trials.[149,150,229,230] Persisting efficacy of opioids was demonstrated in long-term follow-up studies.[229,230] Opioids are often prescribed for severe cases of RLS/WED, especially in patients unresponsive to other treatments. A prolonged-release oxycodone combined with naloxone (doses of 5 to 40 mg oxycodone/2.5 to 20 mg naloxone, twice daily) was found in a placebo-controlled study to provide significant benefit for RLS/WED patients not responding well to their current, mostly dopaminergic, medications.[150] This medication is approved for use in Europe as a second-line treatment. Methadone has also been used for treatment of severe RLS/WED in patients refractory to other treatments.[230] The total daily dose of methadone for RLS/WED is usually 2.5 to 20 mg per day, lower than that for analgesia. It has the major advantage of less problems with drug dependence, and it does not activate some primary pathways possibly associated with addiction to opiate medications.[155]

Although there is little evidence of tolerance or addiction to opioids in the RLS/WED literature, the data are sparse, and therefore prescription of opioids should be restricted to patients without a previous history of substance abuse. Opioids should also be used cautiously in patients who snore and are at risk for having sleep apnea syndrome.[229,231] Constipation, lethargy, depressed mood, and sleepiness are common adverse effects of opioid treatments of RLS.

Benzodiazepines

The benzodiazepines clonazepam,[232] nitrazepam,[233] and temazepam[44,234] have been found to improve sleep quality and reduce PLMS-related arousals in patients with RLS/WED and PLMS. However, the therapeutic effects of benzodiazepines on subjective ratings of RLS/WED symptoms were either modest or not significant. Curiously, although these medications reduce arousal, they do not consistently reduce the rate of PLMS.[232] Benzodiazepines and other gamma-aminobutyric acid–active hypnotics are mostly used to improve sleep and may suffice as treatment for patients who appear not to be awakened by their RLS symptoms.

Clinical Approach

In summary, oral and IV iron should be a primary initial consideration in treatment of RLS/WED, and the morning fasting serum iron panel is critically important. The $\alpha 2\delta$

ligand medications, when they are tolerated, are considered a good first choice for standard pharmacologic treatment because they provide excellent long-term treatment without RLS augmentation. They are specifically preferred for patients with anxiety, sleep disturbance, and either RLS or neuropathic pain. They should also be considered if the RLS/WED course is intermittent, and future trials off medication are contemplated because unlike DA they appear to have few withdrawal symptoms.[183] Among these medications, only gabapentin enacarbil has been approved by the FDA for RLS/WED treatment. Because of gabapentin absorption problems, some patients who fail to respond to gabapentin may respond to gabapentin enacarbil or pregabalin.

DAs, owing to the risk of augmentation, are now considered a second-line treatment for long-term management of RLS/WED. They are particularly useful for patients with depression and increased risk of falls. They have the major advantage of often producing a rapid therapeutic response with relatively limited immediate adverse effects. Ropinirole, pramipexole, and rotigotine are the only DAs with FDA and EMEA approval. Some patients who respond poorly to the shorter-acting DAs may respond better to a longer-acting medication, such as rotigotine or long-acting formulations of ropinirole and pramipexole.[215] The significant problems with long-term use of DAs can be reduced by keeping the dose low, that is, less than maximum FDA-approved daily doses (0.5 mg pramipexole, 4 mg ropinirole, and 3 mg rotigotine) and, rather than increasing dose, changing to another medication class if symptoms reemerge.

RLS/WED symptoms can spontaneously remit for weeks or even months. Pharmacologic treatments may permit, as needed, use of medications during symptomatic periods. Daily pharmacologic treatment should be considered if patients complain of RLS/WED occurring at least 2 nights per week and find the symptoms distressing and affecting their functioning. An occasional drug holiday can be considered to evaluate the need for continued treatment. All pharmacologic treatments other than iron are palliative and do not reduce the underlying disease process. Iron appears in some patients to possibly alter the disease process, providing long-term treatment benefit that can last for several months without the need for other medications. This possibly occurs by reducing RLS brain iron deficiency, as shown in preclinical studies[177] and one small clinical study using sonography to measure SN iron status.[178] Long-term treatment with dopaminergic medications, in contrast, can make the condition worse. Therefore the clinician should carefully assess the therapeutic benefit of the treatments for long-term care versus the severity of adverse effects. Choice of treatment should also consider cost differences.

A therapeutic flowchart is shown in Table 121.1. Each drug is presented with its commonly used therapeutic dosage, its most common side effects, and the appropriate countermeasures to adopt. Higher doses may be considered with caution for all drugs, particularly for dopaminergic medications where the risk of augmentation increases with dose.[162] Prolonged-release oxycodone/naloxone[150] and methadone[186,230] are considered good second-line treatments. IV iron, the opioids and, particularly, methadone are considered effective for refractory hard-to-treat patients who do not have RLS augmentation.[176,230] Patients with significant RLS augmentation can be treated with $\alpha 2\delta$ agents or opioids, especially methadone, but it is not certain if iron treatments will reduce augmentation.

RESTLESS LEGS SYNDROME IN CHILDHOOD

RLS/WED and PLMS occur in children[235–237] (Video 121.9) with a prevalence of 0.5% to 2%.[19] The pediatric RLS/WED diagnosis[237] requires meeting the adult criteria (Box 121.1). Older children may describe the leg discomfort in their own words. Like adults, RLS/WED children respond to dopaminergic therapy.[238] PLMS, the motor sign of RLS, occurs at low to moderate rates for most RLS children (>2/hour), but rarely for healthy children, unlike common occurrence for healthy older adults.[53,239] Thus, for children, PLMS strongly supports the diagnosis of RLS, provided other childhood conditions with PLMS can be excluded, for instance, narcolepsy,[53] attention-deficit/hyperactivity disorder (ADHD),[240–242] and sleep apnea.[243] Some children with clinically significant restless sleep do not have RLS or PLMS but, rather, may meet criteria for the newly proposed pediatric restless sleep disorder.[244,245] Pediatric RLS/WED has mostly the same comorbid conditions as adult RLS, for instance, migraine headaches[246] and chronic kidney disease,[247] and is associated with common childhood conditions of growing pains,[248] ADHD,[249–251] and anxiety disorders.[251]

Pharmacologic treatment of RLS in children is not well studied. The options that have been evaluated include a few studies on low doses of levodopa[238,252] and, for two patients, the DA pergolide.[252] Oral iron treatments are recommended in children with fasting morning serum transferrin saturation less than 45% and ferritin less than 50 mcg/L, and they can be effective for both RLS and PLMS.[167,253–257] IV iron has also been reported to provide effective treatment for children with RLS,[167,258] especially when oral iron fails, but given limited experience, it should be used very cautiously.

PERIODIC LIMB MOVEMENTS IN SLEEP

Description and Measurement

PLMS occur during sleep as patterned movements, mostly of the legs repeating about every 20 to 40 seconds for periods of a few minutes to a large part of sleep. PLMS classically consist of dorsiflexion at the ankle with extension of the big toe, but more extreme leg movements can occur. Video 121.1 shows classic PLM foot flexion at the ankle with extension of the large toe. Larger and more varied PLMS in Videos 121.2 to 121.5 reflect the large variation of PLM severity.

The World Association of Sleep Medicine (now the World Sleep Society) and the IRLSSG have established the standards for recoding and scoring PLMS.[259] Leg movements are defined as anterior tibialis electromyograph (EMG) signals greater than or equal to 8 μV above baseline, lasting 0.5 to 10 seconds, and separated by at least 0.5 seconds of EMG activity less than 2 μV above baseline. EMG from both legs define a

Table 121.1 Management of RLS/WED for Adults

Agent/Daily Dosage	Side Effects	Countermeasures
Step 1: Oral Iron: First-Line Treatment for RLS with Serum Ferritin ≤75 mcg/L and Transferrin Saturation <45%, Provided Not Counterindicated or Cannot Tolerate		
Step 1A: Ferrous sulfate (325 mg with vitamin C, 100 mg once a day) Evaluate efficacy after 12 wk; if not effective consider IV iron	Constipation, stomach upset, and pain	Reduce dose, discontinue, take with food Switch to IV iron if not tolerated or treatment response is too limited or slow
Step 1B: IV Iron Infusion: First-Line Treatment for RLS with Serum Ferritin ≤100 mcg/L and Transferrin Saturation <45%, Provided Oral Iron Could Not Be Used or Was Ineffective		
Ferric carboxymaltose, 500–750 mg 2×, 5 days apart (1000–1500 mg total) LMW dextran, 1000-mg dose or 500 mg 2×, 5 days apart Other formulations are either not recommended or have not been adequately tested in RLS	Transitory facial flushing, dizziness, nausea, systolic blood pressure increase	Observe, should resolve in 30 min, after injection LMW dextran ONLY requires small test dose, followed by 30-min observation, with remainder of dose given if no significant adverse effects occur
Step 2: α2δ Agents: First-Line Treatment, Particularly if Sleep Disturbance, Pain, or Anxiety Is Present[a]		
FDA APPROVED Gabapentin enacarbil Evening or before bed starting daily dose by age/ClCr[a] <65 yr, 600 mg ≥65 yr or ClCr <30 mL/min, 300 mg Usual effective daily dose 600–1200 mg *NOT APPROVED BY FDA* Pregabalin Evening or before bed Starting daily dose by age/ClCr[a] <65 yr, 75 mg ≥65 yr or ClCr <30 mL/min, 50 mg Usual effective daily dose 150–400 mg Gabapentin Evening/bedtime or divided dose over day Stating daily dose by age or ClCr[a] <65 yr, 300 mg ≥65 yr or ClCr <30 mL/min, 100 mg Usual effective daily dose, 900–2400 mg Divided dosing for higher doses	Depression–suicidal ideation	Mild depression: reduce dose, add alternate medication class or discontinue and switch to alternate medication class Suicidal ideation, moderate depression: discontinue and switch to alternate medication class
	Dizziness	Reduce dose and add alternate medication class as needed If fall risk, then discontinue and change to alternate medication class
	Somnolence, daytime fatigue	Reduce dose and add alternate medication class as needed, If significant, discontinue and change to alternate medication class
	Tolerance	Discontinue, drug holiday with return to medication Switch to alternate medication class
	Weight gain	Reduce dose and add alternate medication class as needed If significant discontinue and change to alternate medication class
Step[3a]: Dopamine Medications: Second-Line Treatment unless Depression Is a Significant Problem for First Trying α2δ Treatment (Limit Increases to Minimize the Risk of Augmentation)		
Step 3A: Dopamine Agonists		
Start at lowest dose and gradually (every 3–7days) increase to efficacy or maximum dose Gradually (every 3–7days) increase to efficacy or maximum dose Pramipexole, 0.125–0.5mg (0.75 mg in Europe)[a,b] Ropinirole, 0.5–4.0 mg[b] Rotigotine, 1–3 mg/24 h	Nauseas and orthostatic hypotension	Decrease dose, then slowly increase dose and/or add domperidone if available (10–30 mg)
	Insomnia	Add/switch to α2δ agent Use a small dose of benzodiazepines in association with DA agonists
	Daytime fatigue and somnolence	Reduce dosage or discontinue DA agonists
	Compulsive or impulsive behavior	Reduce dose and add alternate medication class as needed If significant, discontinue and change to alternate medication class
	Tolerance	Discontinue and switch to longer acting DA agonist or alternate medication class
	Augmentation	Discontinue and switch to alternate medication class or longer-acting DA agonist

Continued

Table 121.1 Management of RLS/WED for Adults—cont'd

Agent/Daily Dosage	Side Effects	Countermeasures
Step 3B: Dopamine Precursors: Useful for Intermittent Treatment (e.g., twice a week)		
Levodopa/benserazide or levodopa/carbidopa (regular or slow release), 100/25 or 200/50 mg[c]	Same as for DA agonists	See countermeasures for DA agonists
	Morning rebound or augmentation of RLS in early evening	Use small extra dose of levodopa during daytime or reduce dosage or combine levodopa with DA agonists or benzodiazepines or discontinue levodopa (if severe and persistent)
	Augmentation	Do not use daily; discontinue and switch to DA agonists or a nondopamine medication
Step 4: Benzodiazepines: Useful for Sleep Promotion		
Clonazepam, 0.5–2.0 mg[d] Temazepam, 15–30 mg[d] Nitrazepam, 5–10 mg[a]	Daytime somnolence	Reduce dosage
	Tolerance	Drug holiday for 2 wk, then return to lower dosage
Step 5: Opioids: Second-Line Treatment		
Oxycodone-naloxone (10/5–40/20 mg/day) Methadone, 2.5–20 mg/day Oxycodone, 5–40 mg	Constipation	Symptomatic treatment
	Dependency	Drug holiday Discontinue and switch to alternate medication

ClCr, Creatinine clearance; DA, dopamine; IV, intravenous; LMW, low-molecular-weight; prn, as needed; RLS/WED, restless legs syndrome/Willis-Ekbom disease.
[a]ClCr, renal clearance: adjust dose for low ClCr.
[b]1 h before onset of symptoms in the evening or 1–2 h before bedtime if symptoms are not present in the evening.
[c]Considered most appropriate for prn dosing ≥3 times a week rather than daily use.
[d]Before bedtime, usually to promote sleep with RLS.

PLMS sequence as four or more consecutive leg movements with onsets separated by 10 to 90 seconds. PLMs vary considerably over nights, requiring 3 to 5 nights for evaluation of a single person.[52] PLMs occur mostly in NREM sleep and cluster into episodes lasting several minutes to hours. The electrographic picture can be a sustained contraction with one to multiple peaks but must have a 0.5-second period of sustained activity with median EMG greater than or equal to 2 μV above threshold. The number of PLMs per hour of sleep are referred to as the PLMS index or PLMI. The less commonly used PLMS periodicity index, defined as the percentage of all leg movements that are PLMS, has less within-subject variability over nights.[260,261]

Leg activity meters provide an alternative for evaluation of PLMS when sleep-disordered breathing is not an issue. They provide data over 3 to 5 nights, correcting for the large internight variability of PLMS.[52]

Relationship of Periodic Leg Movement in Sleep to Restless Legs Syndrome and Other Conditions

PLMS support the diagnosis and indicate severity for RLS. A PLMI greater than or equal to 13 has an 85% sensitivity and 87% specificity for diagnosis of adult RLS when compared to healthy control subjects.[54] This is assumed to hold for Americans and Europeans, but high rates of PLMS occur in only about half of Korean RLS patients.[262] PLMS measure RLS severity[263] and indicate brain iron deficiency, particularly for the thalamus.[103]

PLMS also occur at high rates in other medical conditions,[264] for instance, REM behavior disorder,[265] narcolepsy,[266–268] ADHD,[241,250] and also with healthy older age. The average rate in healthy adults is 5 to 15 per hour for those younger than 60 years but greater than 20 per hour for older healthy adults.[239]

Clinical Significance

About one-third of PLMS in RLS/WED patients is associated with cortical electroencephalographic (EEG) signs of arousal.[269] PLM events are also associated with transient episodes of tachycardia[269] and also increased systolic and diastolic blood pressure (on average, 22 mm Hg and 11 mm Hg, respectively) (Figure 121.1).[42,43] These increases are greater in RLS patients than healthy adults[270] and also when associated with EEG arousals.[42] They may adversely affect cardiovascular health and increase risks of arrythmias.[45,271–273]

Periodic Limb Movement Disorder

PLMD is diagnosed for patients who have a high rate of PLMS, a sleep-related complaint related to poor sleep (e.g., insomnia, sleepiness, fatigue) and no apparent other cause for the PLMS (e.g., medications, other medical or sleep disorder, including RLS). The clinically reported relation between sleep complaints and PLMS may, however, be coincidental, given the high rates of both PLMS and sleep complaints in older adults. Studies generally support this view, failing to find a relation between PLMS and sleep-wake problems in adults.[274–278] One study, however, reported a significant relation between PLMS per hour and subjective sleep quality in middle-aged adults.[279] Given the conflicting data, the diagnosis of PLMD should be used cautiously, particularly for older adults. PLMS in children, however, commonly occur with significant sleep-wake problems, and PLMD is considered a useful pediatric diagnosis.[280–282]

CLINICAL PEARL

Patients with RLS/WED can use a wide variety of terms describing the uncomfortable urge to move or difficulty comfortably staying still while resting. The disorder is common and underdiagnosed despite the more recent rise of therapies. The tetrad of symptoms and careful elimination of mimics are important for the astute clinician to recognize. The disorder has a strong genetic component and correlation to brain iron deficiency. The key to treatment is accurate clinical assessment, assessment of aggravating conditions, and morning fasting evaluation of iron status to include serum ferritin, total iron-binding capacity, transferring saturation, iron, and hemoglobin. After correction of iron status, use of α2δ agents provide effective long-term treatment with less risk of augmentation than with levodopa and dopamine agonists.

SUMMARY

RLS/WED is a neurologic disease defined by its primary clinical features of an urge to move the legs, often with abnormal sensations that occur during resting in the evening and night more than in the morning or day. The diagnosis is based on clinical history and can be supported by PLMS and a family history. Its severity ranges from annoying to disabling. Moderately severe RLS/WED reduces sleep, quality of life, and work productivity. It is associated with possible increased risk of cardiovascular disease. Moderate to severe RLS/WED occurs in about 1% to 3% of adults and 0.5% of children.

RLS/WED occurs with many medical conditions. It commonly involves brain iron abnormalities and is closely related to iron status, as documented by epidemiology, biology, and iron treatments. RLS/WED often occurs in families. Genome-wide association studies have identified common and rare allelic variations that increase the risk of RLS/WED.

Iron status and treatments should be considered first. They often provide long-term benefits and frequently enhance other treatments. α2δ agents provide effective first-line treatment without significant risk of augmentation. Short- to intermediate-acting dopamine medications should be used cautiously because, despite excellent initial treatment, they often produce augmentation (worsening) of the disease with long-term use. Opioids, particularly methadone, are effective for hard-to-treat severe RLS.

SELECTED READINGS

Allen RP, Chen C, Garcia-Borreguero D, et al. Comparison of pregabalin with pramipexole for restless legs syndrome. *N Engl J Med.* 2014;370(7):621–631.

Allen RP, Ondo WG, Ball E, et al. Restless legs syndrome (RLS) augmentation associated with dopamine agonist and levodopa usage in a community sample. *Sleep Med.* 2011;12(5):431–439.

Allen RP, Picchietti DL, Auerbach M, et al. Evidence-based and consensus clinical practice guidelines for the iron treatment of restless legs syndrome/willis-ekbom disease in adults and children: an IRLSSG task force report. *Sleep Med.* 2018;41:27–44.

Allen RP, Picchietti DL, Garcia-Borreguero D, et al. Restless legs syndrome/Willis-Ekbom disease diagnostic criteria: updated International Restless Legs Syndrome Study Group (IRLSSG) consensus criteria—history, rationale, description, and significance. *Sleep Med.* 2014;15(8):860–873.

Allen RP, Walters AS, Montplaisir J, et al. Restless legs syndrome prevalence and impact: REST general population study. *Arch Intern Med.* 2005;165(11):1286–1292.

Bae H, Cho YW, Kim KT, Allen RP, Earley CJ. Randomized, placebo-controlled trial of ferric carboxymaltose in restless legs syndrome patients with iron deficiency anemia. *Sleep Med.* 2021;84:179–186.

DelRosso L, Bruni O. Treatment of pediatric restless legs syndrome. *Adv Pharmacol.* 2019;84:237–253.

Ferré S, Garcia-Borreguero D, Allen RP, Earley CJ. New insights into the neurobiology of restless legs syndrome. *Neuroscientist.* 2019;25(2):113–125.

Fulda S, Allen RP, Earley CJ, et al. We need to do better: a systematic review and meta-analysis of diagnostic test accuracy of restless legs syndrome screening instruments. *Sleep Med Rev.* 2021;58:101461.

Garcia-Borreguero D, Silber MH, Winkelman JW, et al. Guidelines for the first-line treatment of restless legs syndrome/Willis-Ekbom disease, prevention and treatment of dopaminergic augmentation. *Sleep Med.* 2016;21:1–11.

Silber MH, Becker PM, Buchfuhrer MJ, et al. The appropriate use of opioids in the treatment of refractory restless legs syndrome. *Mayo Clin Proc.* 2018;93(1):59–67.

Yang X, Yang B, Ming M, et al. Efficacy and tolerability of intravenous iron for patients with restless legs syndrome: evidence from randomized trials and observational studies. *Sleep Med.* 2019;61:110–117.

A complete reference list can be found online at ExpertConsult.com.

Chapter 122

Sleep-Related Movement Disorders and Their Unique Motor Manifestations

Lana M. Chahine; Aleksandar Videnovic

Chapter Highlights

- The *International Classification of Sleep Disorders*, third edition, recognizes 10 sleep-related movement disorders characterized by relatively simple, stereotypic movements that disrupt sleep initiation, maintenance, or quality. It also recognizes four isolated movement-related symptoms that are considered normal variants.
- A familiarity with all sleep-related movement disorders is required to identify those that are clinically significant and determine when they are a manifestation of neurodegenerative or other neurologic or medical disorders.

A variety of simple and complex movements can occur during sleep. Some are considered normal variants, but several may be clinically relevant. The third edition of the *International Classification of Sleep Disorders* (ICSD-3)[1] includes 10 sleep-related movement disorders (SRMDs) and four isolated sleep-related movements. SRMDs share in common the occurrence of relatively simple, stereotyped movements that disturb sleep or sleep onset.[1] SRMDs are important to recognize and to differentiate from normal physiologic movements during sleep; other nocturnal disorders, such as parasomnias; and mimics of movement disorders, including nocturnal seizures. This chapter provides an overview of the movements commonly observed during sleep (Figure 122.1) and focuses primarily on the sleep-related movements (both physiologic and pathologic) that are not specifically covered in other designated chapters. These movements of sleep are considered in three categories: (1) normal physiologic movements, (2) isolated sleep-related movements and normal variants, and (3) SRMDs. Normal physiologic movements and isolated sleep-related movements are benign, rather than indicators of coexistent pathologic processes. SRMDs include a range of simple and repetitive movements that are associated with clinical symptoms. Several features are useful clues to distinguish normal movements from clinically significant events during sleep, including elements in the history, age at onset, movement semiology, affected body region, time of occurrence, and findings on polysomnography (PSG).

NORMAL PHYSIOLOGIC MOVEMENTS OF SLEEP

An understanding of normal physiologic movements of sleep is needed to ensure consideration of a comprehensive differential diagnosis of movements that occur before and during sleep. These include phasic twitches of rapid eye movement (REM) sleep and major body movements (MBMs).

Phasic Twitches during REM Sleep

Twitches during REM sleep are sudden, brief contractions of skeletal muscle that typically occur during phasic REM sleep. The brief contractions may translate into brief twitches of the face or extremities but do not cause movements across large joints. The contractions can be seen in surface electromyography (EMG) leads and take on a short (usually <0.10 second) repetitive burst pattern that is superimposed on the "atonic" background EMG signal (Figure 122.2).

Major Body Movements

The American Academy of Sleep Medicine (AASM) Scoring Manual recognizes the phenomenon of MBMs as a normal manifestation of body movements due to individuals moving or shifting position during a sleep period.[2] An MBM may be scored when muscle or movement artifacts obscure more than half of the epoch. For a given epoch that contains an MBM, if that epoch contains a posterior dominant rhythm and/or wake precedes that epoch, then the epoch that contains the MBM is scored as a wake state. Otherwise, the epoch with MBM is scored as whatever scoring is applied to the epoch that follows the MBM, as contiguous with the sleep stage that occurred before and after the MBM epoch if the preceding epoch does not demonstrate overwhelming evidence of prolonged arousal or awakening (e.g., slow eye movements). If evidence suggests prolonged arousal or awakening within the epoch after the MBM, the MBM epoch is considered a wake state; if the body movement occurs contiguous with two definitive wake epochs of wakefulness, it is also considered a wake epoch.

ISOLATED SLEEP-RELATED MOVEMENTS AND NORMAL VARIANTS

Four isolated sleep-related movements and normal variants are identified in the ICSD-3.

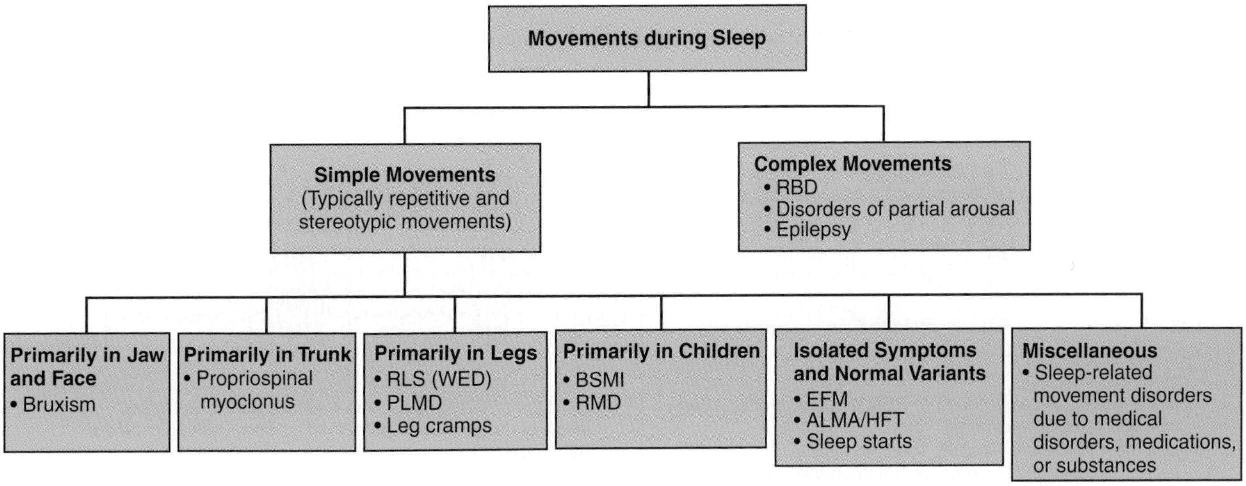

Figure 122.1 Flow chart for the approach to the differential diagnosis of sleep-related movement disorders. ALMA, Alternating leg muscle activation; BSMI, benign sleep myoclonus of infancy; EFM, excessive fragmentary myoclonus; HFT, hypnagogic foot tremor; PLMD, periodic limb movement disorder; RBD, rapid eye movement (REM) sleep behavior disorder; RLS/WED, restless legs syndrome/Willis-Ekbom disease; RMD, rhythmic movement disorder.

Excessive Fragmentary Myoclonus

Excessive fragmentary myoclonus (EFM) is characterized by quick bursts of muscle activity that may produce minor movements around the corners of the mouth, fingers, or toes. EFM is characterized by EMG bursts seen lasting at least 20 minutes during non–rapid eye movement (NREM) sleep with at least 5 bursts per minute, each of a duration of approximately 150 milliseconds (Figure 122.2).[2] EFM is usually not associated with changes in the electroencephalogram (EEG), such as microarousals. However, in the case of relatively high-amplitude EFM bursts, associated K-complexes or shifts to faster EEG frequencies may be observed.[3] EFM predominantly occurs in adult men. EFM is usually seen during NREM sleep and is typically a benign incidental EMG finding. On rare occasions, EFM may result in sleep fragmentation and may be associated with sleep-related breathing disorders, narcolepsy, periodic limb movement disorder (PLMD), and insomnia.[1]

Hypnagogic Foot Tremor

Hypnagogic foot tremor (HFT) is marked phenomenologically by rhythmic muscle contractions and movement of the feet or toes that occurs at the transition between wake and sleep or during light sleep.[4] The movements appear similar to foot tapping and are characterized by at least four EMG bursts, 250 to 1000 milliseconds in duration, and a frequency range of 0.3 to 4.0 Hz, typically lasting a few to 15 seconds (Figure 122.2). HFT appears as trains of recurrent EMG potentials or movements in one or both legs and can be similar to alternating limb movement activity (ALMA; described later). In contrast to HFT, periodic limb movements in sleep (PLMS) have a longer interval between the movements (5 seconds). HFT appears to be a common disorder, at least among patients with sleep disorders. In a single-center study of 375 consecutive patients with sleep disorders, the prevalence of HFT was 7.5%.[4] Although HFT may be comorbid with PLMS and sleep disorders, including restless legs syndrome (RLS [Willis-Ekbom disease]) and obstructive sleep apnea (OSA), it generally is regarded as a benign incidental finding.[4]

Alternating Leg Muscle Activation

ALMA represents alternating EMG bursts in the lower extremities during sleep. Typically lasting over seconds, ALMA consist of at least four movements at a frequency of 0.5 to 3.0 Hz that alternate between the legs, with each single contraction lasting 100 to 500 milliseconds (Figure 122.2). Although the pathophysiologic mechanism of ALMA is unknown, a relation between ALMA and serotoninergic and dopaminergic pathways in the spinal networks has been postulated. These movements are differentiated from PLMS by the much shorter intermovement interval. Although ALMA does not require treatment in most cases, treatment may be considered in select patients who also exhibit sleep disruption. Although there is scant evidence to guide treatment, anecdotal evidence indicates that pramipexole, a dopamine agonist, may reduce the occurrence of ALMA and associated insomnia and daytime sleepiness.[4]

Sleep Starts (Hypnic Jerks)

Sleep starts, also referred to as hypnic jerks, hypnic myoclonus, or hypnagogic startle, usually consist of a single, rapid focal or axial contraction that often affects the body asymmetrically. Sleep starts occur at the wake-sleep transition and are usually not repetitive.[1] These myoclonic jerks may be either spontaneous or induced by tactile or auditory stimuli. PSG recordings show that hypnic jerks generally occur during transitions from wakefulness to sleep, often at the beginning of a sleep episode. Surface EMG recordings of involved muscles show brief (75 to 250 milliseconds) high-amplitude potentials that may be isolated or occur in succession. The motor activity is often associated with sensory phenomena (e.g., a feeling of falling, pain, tingling), auditory (e.g., banging, snapping, or crackling noises), or visual (e.g., flashing lights) hallucinations. A sharp cry may occur simultaneously with the movement. Individuals who manifest hypnic jerks may not recall the movements if they do not result in an awakening. Sleep starts affect all ages and both sexes. Originally reported in individuals with head trauma,[5] sleep starts are also associated neurodegenerative

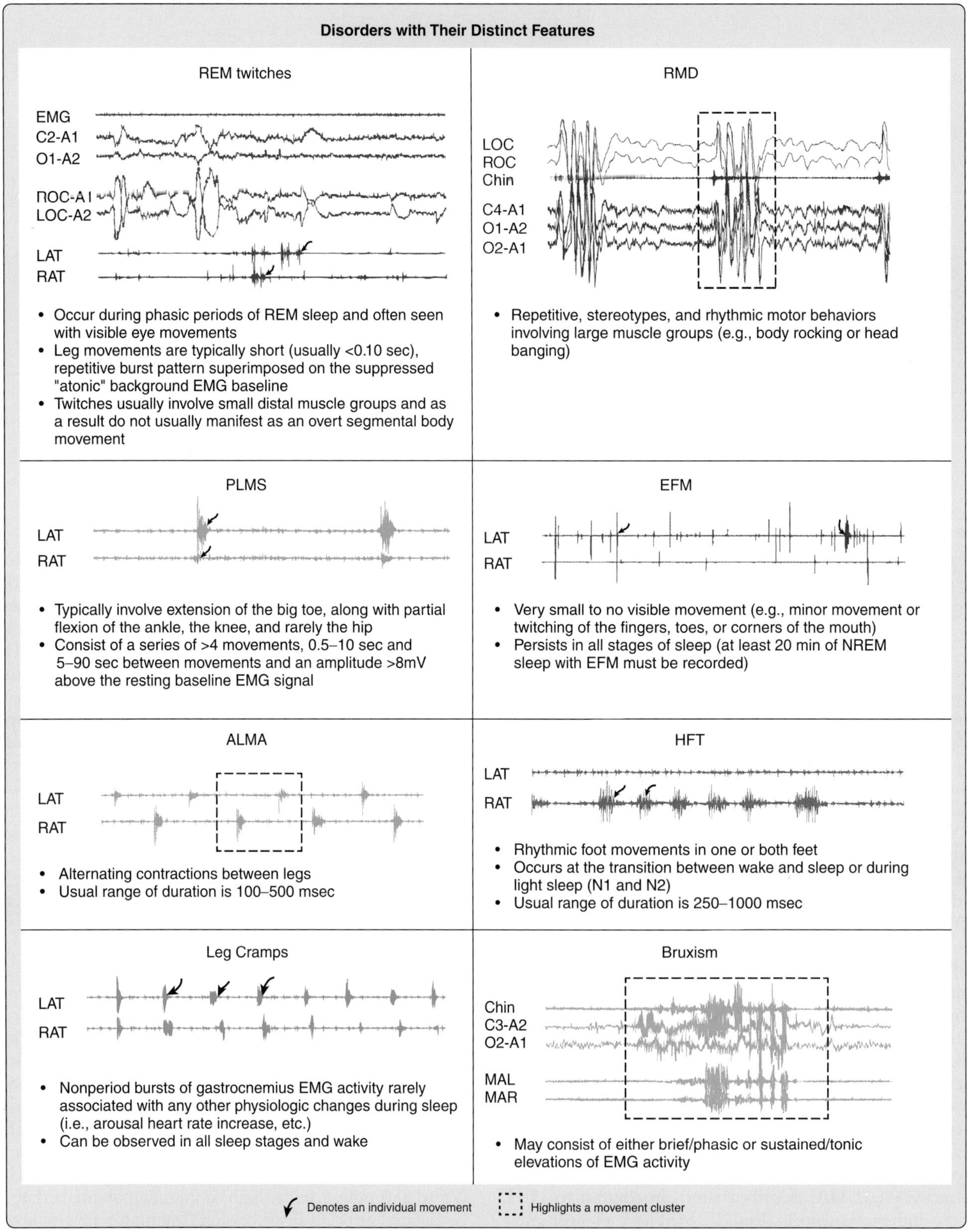

Figure 122.2 Common movements in sleep. Distinct clinical and polysomnographic features of rapid eye movement (REM) twitches, rhythmic movement disorder (RMD), periodic limb movements in sleep (PLMS), excessive fragmentary myoclonus (EFM), alternating leg muscle activation (ALMA), hypnagogic foot tremor (HFT), leg cramps, and bruxism. A, Auricle (as in C4-A1); C, central (as in C4-A1); EMG, electromyography; LAT, left anterior tibialis; LOC, left outer canthus; MAL, masseter muscle left; MAR, masseter muscle right; NREM, non–rapid eye movement; O, occipital (as in O1-A2); RAT, right anterior tibialis; ROC, right outer canthus.

parkinsonian disorders[6] and epilepsy,[7,8] where appropriate evaluation of PSG with extended EEG coverage and time-synchronized video is critical to prevent misdiagnosis as myoclonic seizures. In the general population, sleep starts are very common, affecting more than half of adults[1,9] and most often are benign physiologic myoclonus. Their management therefore largely centers around reassurance and patient education. However, when sleep starts are frequent, intense, or repetitive, they could potentially result in insomnia. Excessive caffeine or other stimulant intake, intense physical work or exercise before bedtime, sleep deprivation, strange sleeping environment, and emotional stress all can increase the frequency and severity of sleep starts. Counseling regarding these triggers and exacerbating factors are important to discuss with patients who have concerns about sleep starts.

Periodic Limb Movements in Sleep

PLMS can be frequently seen in adults and raise suspicion of possible disorder. If the PLMS are benign—sporadic episodes of involuntary leg movements that occur during sleep but do not lead to symptoms or have other clinical consequences or implications—these are considered an isolated sleep-related movement. PLMS are characterized semiologically by extension of the big toe in combination with partial flexion of the ankle, knee, and hip.[1] Although these movements predominantly occur in the legs, the upper extremities may be involved as well. According to the AASM scoring criteria, PLMS consist of a series of four or more consecutive movements, each lasting 0.5 to 10 seconds with an interval of 5 to 90 seconds between movements and an amplitude greater than 8 mV above the resting baseline EMG signal (Figure 122.2). The PLMS index is defined as the number of PLMS divided by the observation time in hours. In general a PLMS index is considered abnormal if there are more than 5 per hour in children and more than 15 per hour in adults.[1] Approximately 5% of adults demonstrate incidental, asymptomatic PLMS on PSG, and in these cases they are considered benign epiphenomena. Figure 122.2 illustrates unique physiologic features that distinguish PLMS from other isolated sleep movements and normal variants that can be mistaken for PLMS on PSG. In PLMS that are associated with symptoms, further clinical evaluation is recommended. The reader is referred to Chapter 121 for discussion of PLMs as they relate to PLMD, RLS, and other sleep disorders.

Sleep-Related Movement Disorders

SRMDs encompass a broad range of simple, stereotypic movements that are variably associated with clinical dysfunction (e.g., poor sleep quality, nonrestorative sleep, fatigue). The motor features seen in SRMDs are helpful clues in distinguishing them from the more complex movements observed in parasomnias. The ICSD-3[1] encompasses the 10 disorders: RLS, PLMD, sleep-related leg cramps, bruxism, sleep-related rhythmic movement disorder, benign sleep myoclonus of infancy, propriospinal myoclonus at sleep onset, SRMD due to medical disorder, SRMD due to medication or substance use, and SRMD unspecified. Etiologies of SRMD due to medical disorder and SRMD due to medication or substance use are shown in Table 122.1. RLS and PLMD are discussed elsewhere in this book (see Chapter 121) and are not considered here.

Sleep-Related Leg Cramps

Clinical Features

Sleep-related leg cramps are sudden and intense involuntary contractions that usually occur in the calf or small muscles of the foot and manifest with tightening and pain.[1] The diagnosis requires that the painful muscle spasm occur during the sleep period and that the pain is relieved by forcefully stretching the affected muscle. Although the sleep-related leg cramps usually have a sudden onset, they may also begin slowly. These cramps can last for several seconds up to several minutes. Individuals with sleep-related leg cramps report, in general, more sleep disturbances, snoring, less adequate sleep, excessive daytime sleepiness, and lower quality of life.[10] Nocturnal leg cramps may be idiopathic but have also been associated with vascular disease, lumbar canal stenosis, cirrhosis, hemodialysis, pregnancy, neuromuscular disorders, and other medical conditions (e.g., metabolic disorders). Moreover, certain medications may also result in sleep-related leg cramps (as described later). Individuals with secondary causes of sleep-related leg cramps may be more likely to have daytime cramps as well,[11] In patients with complaints of sleep-related leg cramps, secondary etiologies should be considered.[12,13] Thorough physical examination is necessary, and laboratory testing and other

Table 122.1 Causes of Sleep-Related Movement Disorders Due to Substance or Medical Condition

Sleep-Related Movement Disorder	Substances that Induce Specified Disorder	Medical Condition Causative of Specified Disorder
Sleep-related leg cramps	Diuretics, β2-agonists, statins	Hypokalemia Neurodegenerative parkinsonian syndromes Renal disease Neuropathy Pregnancy
Bruxism	Selective serotonin reuptake inhibitors Serotonin norepinephrine reuptake inhibitors	
Propriospinal myoclonus	Quinolone Penicillins	Spinal cord lesions Functional (psychogenic) movement disorder

testing, including EMG/nerve conduction studies, may be indicated where appropriate.[11]

Epidemiology

Occasional leg cramps are common, arising at least once in most adults over age 50 years. In 6% of the general population, leg cramps may occur five or more times a month,[14] and may result in insomnia. Although age is a risk factor for nocturnal leg cramps,[12,13] they may occur at any age.[14,15] Sleep-related leg cramps occur in about 7% of children and adolescents, typically not occurring before the age of 8 years. Pregnancy has also been associated with sleep-related leg cramps[11]; about 33% to 50% of pregnant women experience leg cramps that also tend to become worse as pregnancy progresses but tend to go away after delivery. Vigorous exercise, use of certain medications (e.g., naproxen, intravenous iron sucrose, conjugated estrogens, and teriparatide), dehydration, fluid and electrolyte disturbances, and disorders that reduce mobilization in individuals can trigger nocturnal cramps. In addition, individuals with certain medical disorders, such as diabetes, sleep apnea,[16] blood vessel disease, metabolic disorders, and nerve or muscle diseases, may be more likely to have sleep-related cramps.

Differential Diagnosis

Sleep-related leg cramps may be confused with the leg discomfort experienced by individuals with RLS. RLS may manifest with cramping sensations, and thorough clinical history and physical examination are needed to distinguish between these disorders. The critical differentiating sleep-related leg cramps is occurrence of an involuntary, palpable, painful, often visible sustained muscle contraction, which is not seen in RLS. Furthermore, leg cramp events tend to be a more defined period of occurrence compared to the typical symptoms of RLS, occurring across an evening or early night. Focal seizures are also on the differential diagnosis of nocturnal leg cramps. Features that distinguish between the two include the typically much shorter duration and much more focal distribution of leg cramps. Focal dystonia of the feet can be distinguished electrophysiologically from leg cramps by demonstration of ongoing co-contraction of agonist and antagonist muscles. In addition, episodic dystonia is rare, and when it occurs, episodes last longer than the few seconds that leg cramps last.

Polysomnography Scoring Criteria and Motor Features

Sleep-related leg cramps manifest electrophysiologically with nonperiodic bursts of gastrocnemius EMG activity that arise without any specific preceding physiologic changes during sleep.[1] Sleep-related leg cramps may be observed throughout all sleep stages.

Pathophysiology

Sleep-related leg cramps result from sustained recruitment of motor units innervating the involved muscles. They are associated with high-voltage spontaneous firing of anterior horn cells. Possible pathophysiologic mechanisms that have been hypothesized include excitability in the spinal cord,[12] spinal disinhibition, abnormal terminal motor nerve excitability, and enhanced muscle contraction propagation resulting from cross-activation of adjacent neurons.[12,13] Local ischemia or metabolic abnormalities may account for the associated pain. Several medications can be a cause of sleep-related leg cramps as shown in Table 122.1.

Treatment

Treatment of leg cramps includes nonpharmacologic measures, such as frequent stretching or massaging of the affected muscle, application of heat, and movement of the affected limbs.[17] A systemic review focused on pharmacotherapy found that quinine reduces the number of cramps per night, their severity, and nights with cramps.[18] Risks of quinine are serious and include thrombocytopenia and cardiac arrhythmias, although there was a low incidence with short-term use (<60 days). Other treatments that may be tried, although with limited evidence of efficacy, include magnesium, diltiazem, and anticonvulsants, such as gabapentin. Use of continuous positive airway pressure in patients with moderate to severe sleep apnea may improve nocturnal leg cramps.[16]

Sleep-Related Bruxism

Clinical Features

Bruxism (from the Greek word *brugmos,* for "gnashing of teeth") is marked by repetitive jaw muscle activity resulting in clenching or grinding of the teeth and extension of the mandible occurring in both wake and sleep. Bruxism typically involves a constellation of stereotypic somatic complaints, such as dental attrition, tooth pain, temporomandibular joint dysfunction, and headaches. Sleep-related bruxism can be determined when there is a clinical history of frequent tooth grinding sounds during sleep associated with at least one of the following: abnormal tooth wear, morning jaw muscle pain or jaw muscle fatigue, temporal headache, and jaw locking on awakening.[1] The intensity and duration of sleep-related bruxism are variable, but contractions may occur hundreds of times during a sleep period. Temporal headaches, often present on awakening or beginning soon after, are common in individuals with bruxism and may be the presenting feature. Other associated symptoms include tooth pain, limited range of motion of the jaw, pain on jaw movement, temporal tenderness and pain, tooth wear, and, in extreme cases, tooth fracture. Buccal mucosa lesions may result from excessive bruxism.[1,19] Bed partner sleep may be disrupted from bruxism as well.

Epidemiology

Sleep-related bruxism is often familial, with up to half of affected individuals having one or more family members with a history of tooth grinding. The genetic etiology remains to be identified. Bruxism is more common during childhood but may persist into adulthood in more than half of childhood cases. Prevalence is approximately 8% in the general adult population and 3% in older adults (although underdiagnosis may occur in older adults).[1,19] Precipitating factors include stressful life events and anxiety.[1] Nicotine and caffeine exposure in the hours before sleep may contribute to the occurrence of sleep-related bruxism[19] (Table 122.1).

Differential Diagnosis

Sleep-related bruxism needs to be differentiated from other causes of faciomandibular movements occurring during sleep, such as seizures, myoclonus, REM sleep behavior disorder (RBD), and jaw-closure dystonia. The presence of daytime symptoms and examination findings help distinguish sleep bruxism from oromandibular dystonia. Gastrointestinal disorders that are on the differential include abnormal swallowing and gastroesophageal reflux disease.

Polysomnography Scoring Criteria and Motor Features

Although typically a clinical diagnosis, the PSG findings may help in diagnosis. Bruxism can be recorded on surface EMG channels. Although the diagnosis can be made on clinical grounds alone, PSG may be indicated to evaluate for associated respiratory disturbances and/or to distinguish from other etiologies.[1] Audio-video recordings help confirm the nature of the sounds (e.g., grinding, snoring) and the type of movements (e.g., clenching or rhythmic jaw movement). Contractions may be incidentally seen as sustained (tonic) or brief (phasic) elevations of chin EMG activity that is greater than twice the baseline. When a history of bruxism is present and PSG is specifically evaluating for it, surface EMG electrodes should be placed over the masseter and temporalis during PSG,[2] Phasic elevations occur in a regular sequence at least three times with each elevation and about 0.25 to 2 seconds in duration and may be associated with a click sound (Figure 122.2). For tonic elevations, EMG activity must occur for more than 2 seconds to be scored as bruxism. A separate episode of bruxism is scored after a period of at least 3 seconds of stable background chin EMG activity.[20] Associated recording of loud "grinding sounds" on audiovisual recording confirms the diagnosis. Bruxism-related EMG changes must be differentiated from those associated with simple movements, myoclonus, head banging, and other rhythmic oromandibular activities (e.g., sleep chewing automatism). There are no standard criteria for reports of bruxism episodes; usually indices are used to give the total number of episodes per hour of sleep.

Pathophysiology

Sleep-related bruxism can be primary or idiopathic when there is no identified cause or secondary when it is linked with medication, recreational drugs, or a variety of neurologic disorders (e.g., Parkinson disease, RBD, cerebral palsy, and Down syndrome).[1] Sleep-related bruxism may also occur in those with sleep-related breathing disorders and is noted to have a common association with OSA.[1] Catecholamines (e.g., norepinephrine and dopamine) have been proposed as having a role in the pathophysiologic process of bruxism.[21]

Treatment

Due to the association of other sleep disorders accentuating bruxism, the astute sleep specialists should evaluate and treat secondary causes of bruxism, including medications and undiagnosed sleep apnea, epilepsy, tics, or oromandibular dystonia. Dental splints and mouth guards may be helpful in the appropriate patient, as well as behavioral modifications, and interventions to reduce anxiety may also be indicated, and in some instances, pharmacotherapy. Chemodenervation with botulinum toxin injection into the masseter and or temporalis muscle has been shown to be efficacious in randomized controlled trials.[22] Botulinum toxin reduces the intensity of muscle contraction[23] and should be considered, especially in severe cases.

Sleep-Related Rhythmic Movement Disorder

Clinical Features

Sleep-related rhythmic movement disorder (RMD) is characterized by repetitive, stereotypic, and rhythmic motor behaviors that interfere with normal sleep or lead to significant daytime symptoms and/or risk of bodily injury. The diagnosis is based on the patient's history and neurologic examination. Subtypes of RMD include body rocking, head banging, head rolling (side-to-side movements of the head), and a combined type involving two or more of the individual types. Rhythmic humming may be heard along with the movements.[1] Other movements, such as body rolling, leg banging, and leg rolling, may also be reported. A combination of several RMD patterns may sometimes occur in the same individual during the same night.[24] The episodes usually last less than 15 minutes, but the duration may vary from a few minutes to an hour. The repetitive movements occur with a frequency of 0.5 to 2 per second. The movements and the associated sounds may be quite loud. Environmental noise or distractions during the movements may lead to cessation of the event. Sleep-related RMD may occur in states of drowsiness or during any stage of sleep.[1,25] Children with RMD may experience insomnia, parasomnia (e.g., sleepwalking), and daytime sleepiness. Although patients may find these stereotypic movements as self-soothing, the movements may be concerning to their bed partner or other family members. Insomnia and significant daytime sleepiness may also be observed in adults.[26] Aside from consequences on sleep/sleepiness, RMD is associated with risk of injury. In adults RMD is more likely to be reported in association with other primary sleep disorders, such as OSA, narcolepsy, RBD, and attention-deficit hyperactivity disorder. RMD during sleep onset for an individual with RLS may even be used as a strategy to relieve internal dysesthesia symptoms of RLS. Individuals with narcolepsy demonstrate rhythmic movements[27] that may associated with termination of episodes of sleep paralysis.[28]

Epidemiology

Although seen in adults, sleep-related rhythmic movements are primarily observed in children. At 9 months of age, 59% of all infants have been reported to exhibit one or more sleep-related rhythmic movements; the overall prevalence has been reported to decline to 33% by 18 months and to 5% by 5 years.[1] Sleep-related rhythmic movements severe enough to constitute a disorder, that is, RMD, are estimated to occur in 5% of preschool children[29,30] Although RMD often occurs in otherwise healthy children or adults, risk factors for RMD include developmental delay, behavioral disorders, attention-deficit disorder, and anxiety.[31] As mentioned, other sleep disorders, including RLS, sleep apnea, and RBD are also associated with increased risk of RMD.

Differential Diagnosis

The diagnosis of RMD is one of exclusion. Diagnosis of RMD is usually established by clinical history or video recordings provided by the patient. PSG is indicated when the clinical history alone is insufficient to provide diagnostic certainty or when the movements are atypical or violent. Occurrence of bowel or bladder incontinence, tongue biting, foaming at the mouth, or a personal or family history of seizures should raise concern for seizures on the differential diagnosis. In these circumstances a full EEG montage should be considered during PSG. Parasomnias, such as RBD, is in the differential for RMD. RBD episodes tend to be complex and "goal directed," whereas RMD is more monophasic and not goal directed. Other conditions in the differential diagnosis include sleep myoclonus and bruxism. RMD should be distinguished from tremor, which, like RMD, is characterized by rhythmic involuntary movement of any body part but is predominantly a disorder of wakefulness, although it may persist in N2 and N3 sleep. In contrast to RMD, stereotypies are repetitive rhythmic movements often seen in children during wakefulness or in states of quiet/drowsiness that do not disrupt sleep, lead to daytime sleepiness or injury.

Polysomnography Scoring Criteria and Motor Features

The diagnostic criteria for RMD, based on the AASM Scoring Manual, require presence of a minimum of four stereotypic movements occurring in a cluster pattern at a frequency of 0.5 to 2.0 Hz (Figure 122.2). Video-PSG studies have demonstrated that the majority of rhythmic movements occur during wakefulness but are also common during stages N1, N2, and/or REM sleep.[31] Of interest, the rhythmic movements exclusive to REM occur more frequently in adults.

Pathophysiology

The pathophysiology of RMD is not well understood. Because RMDs are common in infants and young children, it has been proposed that that the cause is related to a self-soothing effect generated by vestibular stimulation.[31] Because of their occurrence during drowsiness and/or sleep transitions, fluctuations in arousal mediated by central motor pattern generators in the brainstem have also been implicated.[7]

Treatment

Most patients with minor movements do not require treatment. Treatment should be considered if the RMD causes significant sleep disruption, daytime sleepiness, or risk of bodily injury to the patient or the bed partner. Safety precautions are typically emphasized (i.e., protective head gear). Based on a limited amount of efficacy data, clonazepam[32] and imipramine may be considered, but many times the movements persist despite medication. Other treatments that may be useful based on anecdotal evidence include behavioral interventions, hypnosis, and sleep restriction. Treatment of OSA may improve comorbid RMD.[11]

Benign Sleep Myoclonus of Infancy

Clinical Features

Benign sleep myoclonus of infancy (BSMI) (also referred to benign neonatal sleep myoclonus) is characterized by myoclonic jerking movements in the limbs, trunk, or rarely the face, occurring in neonates and infants (e.g., birth to 6 months of age), and is only considered in the SRMD group because of its easy confusion with epileptic seizures.[1] The movements tend to be bilateral and high amplitude. Symptoms may be present for a few days or may last for several months. These movements occur during sleep and sometimes during transition from sleep to wakefulness, but not when the infant is awake.[33] The majority of affected infants are neurologically normal[33]; diagnosis of BSMI can only be made if symptoms are not better explained by other etiologies, such as medication or another sleep, medical, or neurologic disorder.[1]

Epidemiology

The prevalence of BSMI is unknown, and the incidence has been estimated at 0.8 to 3 per 1000 live births.[34] Males are affected more than females.

Differential Diagnosis

BSMI is considered benign but is often confused with epilepsy, particularly myoclonic seizures and myoclonic encephalopathy.[33] An EEG recording with time-synchronized video during episodes of myoclonus helps make the diagnosis as there will be no epileptiform activity. Neurologic examination is typically normal in infants with BSMI. However, in some patients, nonspecific neurologic signs or expressive language delays have been reported. The evaluation includes EEG with time-synchronized video, a metabolic panel, and screening for toxins. Gentle rocking may induce a BSMI event and may be a useful provocative measure during EEG monitoring to help differentiate BSMI from seizures. Other key features to distinguish BSMI from other neurologic disorders are listed in Table 122.2.

Table 122.2 Common Mimics of Benign Sleep Myoclonus of Infancy

Mimics	Distinguishing Features
Myoclonic seizures	BSMI occurs only during sleep and stops abruptly and consistently when infants are aroused, whereas seizures can occur during wakefulness. Epileptiform activity on electroencephalogram (EEG) is present during epileptic myoclonus but not with BSMI. BSMI is seen typically in neurologically and developmentally normal infants, whereas myoclonic seizures may be associated with perinatal disorders (i.e., hypoxic-ischemic encephalopathy, infection, or metabolic abnormalities).
Infantile spasms (West syndrome)	Often seen after the first month of life Manifested by sudden head flexion with arm extension and lower extremity flexion Epileptiform activity on EEG is present; usually associated with an abnormal EEG pattern known as hypsarrhythmia
Pyridoxine-dependency seizures	Can occur while infants are awake, whereas BSMI will stop abruptly and consistently when infants are aroused EEG slowing is supportive of encephalopathy versus BSMI Responsive to vitamin B_6 (pyridoxine)
Hyperekplexia (startle disease)	Generalized stiffness while awake Exaggerated startle reflex Typical movements occur as an excessive response to stimulation, such as touch or loud noise
Jitteriness	Occurs during wakefulness in response to tactile or auditory stimuli, whereas BSMI occurs during sleep

BSMI, Benign sleep myoclonus of infancy.

Polysomnography Scoring Criteria and Motor Features

On PSG, a BSMI event appears as paroxysmal body jerks that typically occur in clusters of 4 or 5, with a duration of 40 to 300 milliseconds. Once the BSMI episode has ensued, the paroxysmal body jerks can recur in clusters for a few minutes and rarely continue past an hour. Video-PSG during an episode of BSMI shows the events occurring during sleep, and no arousals or awakenings are typically observed. Absence of ictal or interictal epileptiform activity helps differentiate BSMI from seizures.

Pathophysiology

The pathophysiology of BSMI remains unknown. Immaturity of descending supraspinal inhibitory mechanisms, including the underdeveloped state of myelination of the central nervous system in infancy, has been proposed.[1]

Treatment

Parental education and reassurance are critical components of the management of BMSI. This is a self-limited disorder, and it is important to accurately diagnosis it to avoid unnecessary intervention.

Propriospinal Myoclonus at Sleep Onset

Clinical Features

Propriospinal myoclonus at sleep onset is a rare disorder characterized by jerks involving axial musculature of the abdomen and trunk, occurring at the transition from wakefulness to sleep.[1,35] The clinical history is one of sudden jerks, mainly of the trunk, in the neck or abdomen, and during relaxed wakefulness and drowsiness. The jerks disappear with sleep onset and are not observed during sleep. These movements can be quite distressing to patients and their bed partners and lead to insomnia and impaired quality of life. Movements may be precipitated by assuming a supine position.[36]

Epidemiology

Propriospinal myoclonus is a rare condition, and epidemiologic data are sparse. It is likely more common, or at least more often reported, among males.[35]

Differential Diagnosis

Because of the stereotypic and rhythmic pattern of the often "full-body jerking" appearance of propriospinal myoclonus, it may be confused with epileptic myoclonus and other seizure semiologies. However, a normal ictal EEG distinguishes the two. A simple clinical history helps distinguish the involuntary movements of propriospinal myoclonus from voluntary movements triggered by dysesthesias in RLS. Propriospinal myoclonus does not demonstrate the rhythmicity seen in PLMs. Hypnic jerks, or sleep starts, can be confused with propriospinal myoclonus but are usually briefer and electrophysiologically do not propagate in the pattern of propriospinal myoclonus.

Polysomnography Scoring Criteria and Motor Features

PSG shows high-amplitude surface EMG activity occurring during wakefulness or transition to sleep. Discharges arise from cervical or thoracic spinal segments and spread slowly rostrally and caudally but spare cranial segments.[36] Discharges typically last 100 to 300 milliseconds, with both reciprocal and co-contracting agonist-antagonist activity. Jerks may be isolated or may recur at quasi-periodic intervals (every 5 to 40 seconds).

Pathophysiology

Although the pathophysiology of propriospinal myoclonus remains unknown, the spinal cord may serve as the underlying generator for the movements in some cases. Of interest, persistent propriospinal myoclonus occurring during the day has been linked to structural spinal cord disease.[1] In other cases, propriospinal myoclonus is not associated with structural spine lesions but, rather, is due to a psychogenic/functional etiology.[35]

Treatment

As with most SRMDs, education is recommended for treatment after a thorough evaluation to rule out more serious disorders. Some patients may respond to clonazepam or valproic acid.[35]

CLINICAL PEARLS

- Sleep-related movement disorders (SRMDs) are marked by simple or stereotypic movements occurring in drowsiness, in transition to sleep, or during sleep.
- Different SRMDs are more likely to occur in different age groups. Benign myoclonus of infancy occurs only in neonates/the neonatal period. Rhythmic movement disorder and bruxism are more common in childhood but may persist into adulthood. Nocturnal leg cramps occur in all ages, especially in older adults.
- There are several etiologies to nocturnal leg cramps, and through history, examination, and laboratory evaluation are part of the evaluation.
- Propriospinal myoclonus may result from spinal cord pathology but more often is psychogenic.

SUMMARY

The ICSD-3 currently recognizes 10 different SRMDs and four isolated sleep-related movements. They may result in sleep disruption and reduced quality of life. They are relatively common and demonstrate significant overlap with several other disorders. A thorough history and examination are critical in evaluating patients with suspected SRMDs. These, along with electrophysiologic findings, help distinguish them from parasomnias or seizures.

ACKNOWLEDGMENT

The authors wish to acknowledge Mr. Anthony Kwan for his original work on Figure 122.1 and Ms. Seulah Choi for her original work on Figure 122.2.

SELECTED READINGS

Baldelli L, Provini F. Fragmentary hypnic myoclonus and other isolated motor phenomena of sleep. *Sleep Med Clin*. 2021;16(2):349–361.

Bergmann M, Stefani A, Brandauer E, Holzknecht E, Hackner H, Högl B. Hypnagogic foot tremor, alternating leg muscle activation or high frequency leg movements: clinical and phenomenological considerations in two cousins. *Sleep Med*. 2019;54:177–180.

Berry RB, Quan SF, Abreu AR, et al. *The AASM Manual for the Scoring of Sleep and Associated Events: Rules, Terminology and Technical Specifications*. Darien, Illinois: American Academy of Sleep Medicine; 2020. Version 2.6.

Chervin RD, Consens FB, Kutluay E. Alternating leg muscle activation during sleep and arousals: a new sleep-related motor phenomenon? *Mov Disord*. 2003;18(5):551–559.

Delacour C, Chambe J, Lefebvre F, et al. Association between physical activity and Nocturnal Leg Cramps in patients over 60 years old: a case-control study. *Sci Rep*. 2020;10(1):2638.

Frauscher B, Gabelia D, Mitterling T, et al. Motor events during healthy sleep: a quantitative polysomnographic study. *Sleep*. 2014;37(4):763–773B.

Gogo E, van Sluijs RM, Cheung T, Gaskell C, Jones L, Alwan NA, Hill CM. Objectively confirmed prevalence of sleep-related rhythmic movement disorder in pre-school children. *Sleep Med*. 2019;53:16–21.

Grandner MA, Winkelman JW. Nocturnal leg cramps: prevalence and associations with demographics, sleep disturbance symptoms, medical conditions, and cardiometabolic risk factors. *PLoS One*. 2017;12(6):e0178465.

Marx C, Masruha MR, Garzon E, Vilanova LC. Benign neonatal sleep myoclonus. *Epileptic Disord*. 2008;10:177–180.

Rana AQ, Khan F, Mosabbir A, Ondo W. Differentiating nocturnal leg cramps and restless legs syndrome. *Expert Rev Neurother*. 2014;14:813–818.

Stefani A, Högl B. Diagnostic criteria, differential diagnosis, and treatment of minor motor activity and less well-known movement disorders of sleep. *Curr Treat Options Neurol*. 2019;21(1):1.

Trotti LM. Restless legs syndrome and sleep-related movement disorders. *Continuum (Minneap Minn)*. 2017;23(4, Sleep Neurology):1005–1016.

van der Salm SM, Erro R, Cordivari C, et al. Propriospinal myoclonus: clinical reappraisal and review of literature. *Neurology*. 2014;83(20):1862–1870.

A complete reference list can be found online at ExpertConsult.com.

Section 15
Sleep Breathing Disorders

Chapter 123
Introduction

Robert Joseph Thomas; Andrey V. Zinchuk

IN THE BEGINNING

BC/AC: before CPAP (continuous positive airway pressure), after CPAP. Most readers of this book will have no personal experience of what sleep medicine and sleep apnea care was like before CPAP. The simplicity and biologic efficacy of CPAP is one of the unrivaled treatments in medicine. CPAP not only made lives better, it saved lives and took on mythical properties in the 1980s. The past 3 decades have seen developments of new machines, interfaces, and alternative therapies, but this simple tool to support a collapsing upper airway continues to reign supreme, driving the field and industry of sleep medicine.

The chapters in this section take us through a fascinating journey of sleep breathing medicine, from pathophysiology to clinical manifestations to phenotypes to therapy and to current understanding of impact on brain structure and function. An online chapter complements by describing various complementary phenotyping approaches. It is, however, sobering that for the average patient much of this material has yet not born fruit, and, other than ergonomic improvements in machines and interfaces, sleep apnea is treated largely using the same conceptual approaches as 3 decades ago. This needs to change. Armed with the new knowledge described in enclosed chapters, the field is now taking first steps to develop new treatments, to understand who is most susceptible (or resilient) to apnea-related stresses, and to personalize care for our patients.

WHAT IS SLEEP APNEA?

When respiratory tidal volume and rhythm fluctuate beyond certain thresholds, respiratory events are scored. When the frequency of events crosses a threshold, sleep apnea is diagnosed. However, these thresholds may hold meaning for some patients but not others. As a large minority of the population have substantial frequency of events but are asymptomatic both subjectively and even in terms of downstream biologic impact, the importance of differentiating the measurement phenomenon from disease is critical. For example, the impact/biologic associations of respiratory events can range from none to autonomic activation, arousals, sleep fragmentation, perceptions of choking, triggering of arrhythmias, or parasomnias. Biologic recovery from respiratory abnormality at both individual event and cumulative levels over duration of the disease need to be better understood to determine what is and what is not biologically significant and relevant for the individual. Chapters 125 to 129 and 138 provide a description of the conventional and emerging understanding of sleep breathing disorders, and Chapter 141 gives insight into key mechanisms of sleep apnea by challenging humans respiratory system at high altitude.

WHEN DOES SLEEP APNEA START AND HOW DOES IT CHANGE WITH AGING?

At conception? The upper airway, respiratory control and sleep homeostatic systems are regulated by a large number of genes. The familial risks of sleep apnea likely engage all these systems. Craniofacial morphology showing constricted upper airway passages during childhood is a risk factor, though true long-term follow-up data is scant and exceptionally difficult to generate (e.g., serial cephalometry or magnetic resonance imaging over decades starting in childhood). Nevertheless, more precise phenotypes such as cephalometric measures, tongue fat and nonanatomic endotypes (e.g., respiratory event duration and arousal threshold) and large-scale multidimensional datasets have recently elucidated a number of genes that predispose to sleep apnea and contribute to its consequences: inflammation, endothelial function and cognitive impairment. Can early intervention prevent sleep apnea (obesity being controlled)? Can the natural history of obstructive sleep apnea be changed, other than targeting ideal body weight? Chapters 128, 142 and 139 provide insight on these topics.

An apnea-hypopnea index (AHI) of 1 which suddenly transforms into an AHI 5 as thresholds of abnormality based on age leaves much to be desired. Normative data across all ages[1,2] is limited as there are racial differences, night to night variability, and individual differences (e.g., slow wave power, apnea length, arousal intensity) that are minimized by current scoring guidelines.

ARE THE ASYMPTOMATIC PROTECTED OR SHOULD THEY BE TREATED?

Patients at the extreme ends of the measured pathology-clinical impact relationship often provide novel insights into disease pathobiology. For example, severe asymptomatic sleep apnea is a bit of clinical mystery. There is insufficient evidence to know if those who have substantial sleep apnea but are asymptomatic are protected or at risk. Epidemiologic data suggest that those free of sleepiness are not at higher risk of cardiovascular outcomes,[3] however, mechanistic studies of sleep apnea treatment show improvements in endothelial function,[4] a precursor of cardiovascular disease. Perhaps blood biomarkers, endothelial function, ambulatory blood pressure and brain imaging and functional studies can determine who is at risk or at the early stages of tissue injury. Our understanding in these topics is explored in Chapters 131, 136, and 137. Sleep-disordered breathing rarely occurs in isolation, how it interacts with other chronic disorders common to our patients is described in Chapters 137 and 138 and throughout the chapters devoted to diagnostic categories (e.g., obstructive [Chapter 131], central apneas [Chapters 124 and 126], and hypoventilation [Chapter 138]).

PHENOTYPE TALK, NEXT, PHENOTYPE WALK

Several chapters in this edition address phenotypes in sleep apnea (Chapters 128, 129 and 130, and those devoted to diagnostic categories). It is fashionable to talk about pathogenic or clinical presentation phenotypes at conferences, in publications, but far harder to move it into clinical testing and practice. Recent work sheds light on clinical (sleepy vs. insomnia versus minimally symptomatic), polysomnographic (hypoxic vs. arousal predominant), and endotypic (high vs. low loop gain) sleep apnea subtypes that exhibit differences in tolerance of CPAP, cardiovascular outcomes, and response to non-CPAP therapies. This new knowledge has yet to reach the patients. For example, although a third of sleep apnea presents with an insomnia phenotype, the clinical practice guidelines for insomnia management does not include objective sleep testing, especially for sleep apnea. The field is poised to make progress in diagnosis and tailoring therapies to those at highest risk of adverse events and most likely to respond to treatment. Because adjunctive therapies targeting driver phenotypes, such as oxygen, sedatives and acetazolamide are largely generic, a collaboration between the government, academic institutions, and the industry is needed to move the field beyond one-size-fits all approaches.

SINGLE VERSUS MULTIMODAL APNEA THERAPY

If multiple disease (apnea) drivers are present, it is unlikely that targeting only one of them will adequately treat the disease. It is time for evaluation of multimodal therapy, targeting disease drivers, downstream effects, and perhaps even recovery kinetics.

From a business/product development perspective, it is understandable that single therapies are evaluated and US Food and Drug Administration (FDA) approval sought. However, in clinical practice, in virtually every disease where multiple therapies are available, combinations of therapy are routine (e.g., diabetes, asthma, rheumatologic diseases, heart failure). Yet in sleep apnea, typically single therapies are used. Medicare in the United States, for instance, prohibits combined therapy with an oral appliance and positive airway pressure (PAP). We thus have a vast opportunity to evaluate, based on biologic principles, combination therapies. Such combinations could reasonably target driver mechanisms and/or downstream impact, such as hypertension and endothelial dysfunction. Chapters 132 and 140 discuss the core therapy of PAP, advanced technologies in this area and how to tailor PAP to specific disorders (e.g., adaptive servoventilation for periodic breathing in heart failure). Adjunctive therapies (Chapters 133, 134, and 139) can be used to target one pathology (such as obstruction) or coexisting pathologies (such as high loop gain).

DEFINING SUCCESSFUL THERAPY BEYOND "MINIMAL ACCEPTABLE ADHERENCE"

Current metrics of success for the first-line and most common treatment, CPAP, are largely set by insurance. The use of 4 hours per night on 70% of the nights in the first few months of therapy for an essentially lifelong disease does not do it justice. Because data show that symptoms and function improve with every hour of CPAP use, it is time to retire "4 hours 70% of the time" as the metric. Using such a metric as a gold standard limits our understanding of patients and treatment factors that impact benefits of therapy. From letters from CPAP providers sent to patients in the United States:

> *"Congratulations! You have used your CPAP for at least 4 hours for 70% of nights during a 4-week period in the first 3 months." (To a patient with severe residual sleepiness and residual AHI of 17 per hour of sleep.)*

> "You have not used your CPAP for at least 4 hours for 70% of nights during a 4-week period in the first 3 months. *As you have not used this treatment, it is not medically necessary.* You will be contacted for arrangements to return the CPAP." (To a patient with severe obstructive apnea, heart failure and repeated hospitalizations.)

BEYOND APNEA-HYPOPNEA INDEX AND EXCESSIVE DAYTIME SLEEPINESS, BUT CHANGE IS HARD

Efficacy of therapy metrics that integrate total sleep times, residual apnea on therapy, and residual apnea off therapy may be more relevant. Importantly, effectiveness must incorporate subjective, patient-centered outcomes (e.g., symptoms and function).

Several chapters in this edition discuss approaches to sleep-breathing characterization beyond the AHI and excessive daytime sleepiness (Chapters 129 and 130). Machine learning and computational methods can extract novel information from respiratory signals, whereas clinical phenotypes such as sleepy, asymptomatic, and insomnia are readily recognized in the sleep clinic too. The field is working toward addressing whether tailored treatments provide benefits above and beyond CPAP for all approach.

Two additional key sleep phenotypes that can change the base platform of sleep-disordered breathing efficacy are short and long sleep. Short sleep may be natural or a component of insomnia, anxiety, depression, atrial fibrillation, heart failure, traumatic brain injury, neurodegeneration, or bipolar disease (even in remission). Long sleep most commonly occurs with idiopathic hypersomnia but also after traumatic brain injury; depression, especially with seasonal worsening; and natural long sleepers. Clearly, the standard adherence requirements need to be modified to accommodate sleep duration.

PALLIATIVE THERAPY

Treatment of sleep apnea rarely considers palliative therapy, but this could be relevant based on patient preferences, life expectancy, and quality of life considerations. Why not a sedative for insomnia? The role of arousals in non–rapid eye movement (NREM) sleep amplifying apnea is now better understood. Milder non-REM-dominant apnea could be a possible phenotype which may respond well enough to a sedative. A wake-promoting medication for excessive daytime sleepiness? A bedtime dose of antihypertensive for blood pressure nondipping? Oxygen for nocturnal hypoxia or periodic breathing? In many diseases we focus on symptoms reduction and quality of life, why not sleep apnea? This is an area with scant published work and an opportunity for development.

CONSUMER DIAGNOSTICS AND MOBILE TRACKING OF OUTCOMES

Expect that FDA-approved medical grade sleep apnea diagnostics will be available over the counter and all the associated upheaval in the field that will follow. Current and developing technology allows tracking of respiration, sleep, heart rate kinetics, movements, cognition, mood, and quality of life through wearables usually coupled with a Smartphone. Simple feedback about use and efficacy of CPAP to patients on a daily basis improves use.[5,6] Longitudinal, multidomain data gathered by mobile devices, has the potential to provide unparalleled insights into sleep apnea burden and engage our patients in management of their disease.

ACCURACY OF DEVICE DATA TRACKING

Respiratory event detection during therapy uses manufacturer-specific proprietary algorithms with no standardization across vendors or even recommendations from scientific societies. Such rule-based algorithm accuracy varies and does not estimate stable breathing. The adaptive ventilators are even more inaccurate than CPAP and bilevel as the pressure profile of the device is not considered in estimating treatment efficacy. Despite the association with reduced adherence, the implications of residual unstable breathing are largely unknown. It is critical to know if blood pressure, autonomic indices, or residual sleepiness/cognition is impacted by residual respiratory instability, but to do so estimation of breathing instability must be standardized and accurate.

TARGETING DOWNSTREAM PATHOLOGY

The focus on insurance-mandated expectations of device or therapy use has deemphasized clinically significant and measurable downstream effects of sleep apnea. These include mood, attention, inflammation, cardiac hypertrophy, white matter hyperintensities, metabolic and endothelial dysfunction, and blood-based biomarkers of health. Compared to a condition such as diabetes, where multiorgan system effects are tracked and managed, apnea-related multisystem derangements are not yet part of clinical practice. Adjunctive pharmacotherapy for downstream cardiovascular consequences of sleep-disordered breathing, for example, may benefit patients with sleep apnea who lack contemporary clinical indications for their specific prescription.[7] This is an area of immense opportunity for research and translation.

RECOVERY KINETICS IN SLEEP APNEA

There is some understanding of the time course of recovery of excessive daytime sleepiness, but little about other associated features such as impaired mood, inattention, migraine, high blood pressure, endothelial dysfunction, inflammation, cerebral white matter changes among others. We do not know the predictors of a clinical presentation in a given patient (e.g., fatigue vs. sleepiness, high vs. normal C-reactive protein), or factors which enhance recovery. Studies to fill this critical knowledge gap must be done and creation of collaborative registries might be one approach given the inherent expense of such research.

SLEEP AND BRAIN HEALTH

Can sleep apnea cause dementia? Vascular dementia seems more intuitive, with nocturnal hypertension causing white matter injury. There is however accumulating evidence for apnea-linked amyloidogenesis. It is plausible that apnea steepens the slope of loss of cognitive reserve with aging. However, research-based testing of interventions to treat apnea to modify dementia is a daunting long haul. Chapters 135 and 142 address the advances and future directions in this area.

Can treatment of sleep apnea improve depression outcomes, including treatment-resistant forms? Clinical trials support improvement in symptoms of depression even with low (3 hours or so) CPAP use. Perhaps it should not be CPAP versus no CPAP or placebo CPAP but "sleep apnea treatment" (one or more of CPAP, oral appliance, hypoglossal nerve stimulation, maxilla-mandibular advancement, bariatric surgery) versus a control condition.

ATRIAL FIBRILLATION

Although sleep apnea triggering cardiac arrhythmias, including atrial fibrillation, seems well supported, is routine screening for apnea in atrial fibrillation patients justified? There are two specific challenges: the large proportion of patients with substantial apnea who are asymptomatic and the high prevalence of high loop-gain apnea. The time has come to assess the effectiveness of sleep apnea diagnosis and treatment in this population through a clinical trial.

HEART FAILURE

In countries where there is reasonable sleep care, apnea directly causing heart failure is less common now than before. Treatment trials with unimodal therapy (oxygen, PAP) may be an uphill battle when considering the complex pathophysiology of sleep apnea in heart failure with elements of obstruction, high loop gain, and sleep fragmentation freely admixed.

PATIENT ENGAGEMENT (IN RESEARCH AND CARE)

We have been examining "hard outcomes" in trials (mortality, incidence of heart disease, 2-mm Hg decreases in blood pressure with CPAP); however, we need to hear from patients about what is important to them. Metrics such as function and quality of life are critical to assess the effectiveness sleep apnea treatment and studies funded by Patient-Centered Outcomes Research Institute are outstanding examples.

CORONAVIRUS

This is the other BC/AC that has impacted sleep medicine. Undoubtedly the field will move to more ambulatory and disposable sleep apnea diagnostics. Learning how to manage patients of moderate or greater complexity without classic laboratory testing may be necessary. Such management will require careful data tracking and improvements in the quality of remote data monitoring. Time will tell if there will be a lasting change in the practice of sleep breathing medicine.

HOW DO WE END? A NEED TO PERSONALIZE SLEEP APNEA THERAPY

After decades of "standardizing" management of disorders, the movement to "personalize" care is gaining momentum, perhaps best demonstrated in oncology. There is ample opportunity to personalize sleep breathing care,[8–10] including (1) severity; (2) disease driver phenotyping and targeting; (3) symptom phenotypes; (4) natural sleep duration; (5) downstream impact of respiratory abnormality on directly linked (e.g., hypoxia, autonomic activation) and more distal (e.g., endothelial dysfunction) effects; (6) precision requirements (What is "normalization"? How precise should sleep apnea treatment be: elimination of every single respiratory perturbation even to levels not seen in the general public or something less? Glycemic control is rarely normalized in diabetes. Would precision need to be personalized? That is, should the end point for hypoxic apnea be different from minimally hypoxic apnea but substantially increased upper airway resistance? How would the presence of comorbidities influence goals?); (7) pretreatment risk stratification (e.g., heart failure, chronic obstructive lung disease, fatty liver, depression, migraine, cognitive impairment); (8) patient preferences; and (9) palliative and adjunctive strategies targeting specific symptoms, such as daytime sleepiness and insomnia, or specific biologic downstream effects, such as hypertension, inflammation, and dysglycemia.

Welcome to a brave new world of sleep and sleep breathing management.

A complete reference list can be found online at ExpertConsult.com.

Chapter 124

Central Sleep Apnea: Definitions, Pathophysiology, Genetics, and Epidemiology

Madalina Macrea; Eliot S. Katz; Atul Malhotra

Chapter Highlights

- The various clinical entities comprising sleep breathing disorders are the result of pathophysiologic mechanisms that frequently overlap. Defining the types of central sleep apnea (CSA) within the sleep breathing disorder spectrum is essential for a common language among clinicians, educators, and researchers.
- CSA includes several heterogeneous syndromes, many heavily represented in day-to-day medical practice. Recent scientific evidence allows a more comprehensive understanding of CSA epidemiology, genetics, pathophysiology, and associated morbidity and mortality.
- Several mechanisms participate in the control of breathing. Chemical, mechanical, and neural pathophysiology involved in CSA, and their clinical implications, are detailed.
- Considerable progress has been made in our understanding of control of breathing related to CSA, with major implications of these new findings for patient care. Only by further mechanistic research are new therapeutic strategies likely to emerge.

DEFINITION AND CLASSIFICATIONS

Sleep breathing disorders (SBDs) are characterized by repetitive periods of cessation in breathing (i.e., apneas) or reductions in breathing (i.e., hypopneas) that occur during sleep. The various clinical entities belonging to SBDs are the result of pathophysiologic mechanisms that frequently overlap; centrally driven events are primarily due to a temporary loss of output from the pontomedullary pacemaker that generates breathing rhythm, resulting in loss of the respiratory pump muscles (diaphragm, thorax, abdomen). Alternatively, obstructive events are primarily due to inward collapse of the oropharynx when the pharyngeal dilator muscles are relaxed, resulting in loss of airflow because of upper airway narrowing.[1] Both obstructive and central respiratory events converge in their symptoms of frequent nocturnal awakenings and excessive daytime sleepiness.

Defining the end points of SBDs polysomnographically (i.e., central sleep apnea [CSA] and obstructive sleep apnea [OSA]) is often a straightforward process. In CSA, both oronasal flow and thoracoabdominal excursions are absent; that is, there is an absence of respiratory effort during the cessation of airflow, whereas in OSA, there are ongoing respiratory efforts during the absence of oronasal flow. In contrast, differentiating rigorously between events within the SBD spectrum (i.e., "central" and "obstructive" hypopnea) is difficult without quantification of respiratory effort as recorded by esophageal pressure monitoring. Because esophageal manometry is mildly invasive and rarely employed clinically, thoracic and abdominal excursions assessed by respiratory inductance plethysmography are widely used to detect asynchrony of these excursions during hypopnea (consistent with obstruction) or in-phase breathing (consistent with decreased central drive). Thus central hypopnea is characterized by a proportional and synchronous decrease in thoracic and abdominal excursions, whereas obstructive hypopnea is characterized by paradoxical inward rib cage movement or asynchronous decrease in the thoracic and abdominal excursions (Figure 124.1). Nasal pressure recordings are sometimes used as a surrogate for upper airway narrowing because inspiratory flattening has been shown to correspond with inspiratory flow limitation. Additionally, obstructive and central apneas may overlap within the same event: such "mixed" apneas have features of both conditions, when an apnea begins with loss of central drive to breathe ("central" apnea) but then proceeds with increasing effort against an occluded upper airway ("obstructive" apnea).

Definitions

As defined by the *International Classification of Sleep Disorders,* third edition (ICSD-3), CSA includes six heterogeneous adult syndromes (Box 124.1).[2,3] Several of these have in common a waxing and waning ventilatory pattern.

1. *Cheyne-Stokes breathing* (CSB) is an abnormal pattern of breathing characterized by oscillations of tidal volume between apnea or hypopnea at the nadir of ventilation and hyperpnea at the height of ventilation with a spindle-like

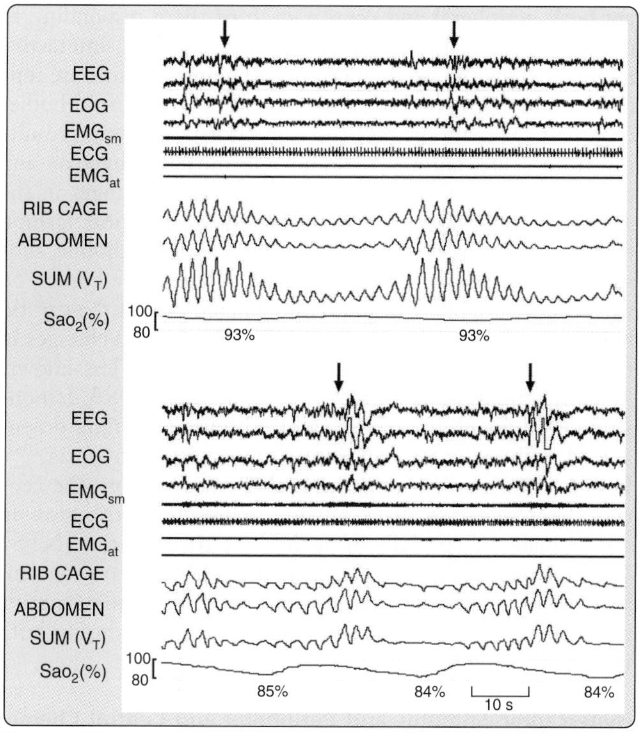

Figure 124.1 Polysomnographic recordings of central and obstructive hypopneas from patients with heart failure with use of respiratory inductance plethysmography. The *upper panel* shows a central hypopnea during stage 2 NREM sleep in a patient who has central sleep apnea with Cheyne-Stokes breathing. Note in-phase gradual waxing and waning of tidal volume (V_T) during hyperpnea and only minimal O_2 desaturation during hypopnea. Arousal occurs several breaths after termination of the hypopnea. The *lower panel* shows an obstructive hypopnea in a patient with obstructive sleep apnea. Note that in contrast to central hypopnea, rib cage and abdominal motion are out of phase and O_2 desaturation is greater during hypopnea, and the rise in ventilation after its termination is more abrupt and hyperpneas are shorter. In addition, arousals occur earlier at hypopnea termination. ECG, Electrocardiogram; EEG, electroencephalogram; EMG_{sm}, submental electromyogram; EMG_{at}, anterior tibial EMG; EOG, electrooculogram. Arrows (↓) indicate arousals. (From *Central sleep apnea and Cheyne-Stokes respiration*, vol 5, issue 2, The Proceedings of the American Thoracic Society.)

BOX 124.1 HETEROGENEOUS ADULT SYNDROMES OF CENTRAL SLEEP APNEA

Central sleep apnea with Cheyne-Stokes breathing
Central sleep apnea due to a medical disorder without Cheyne-Stokes breathing
Central sleep apnea due to high-altitude periodic breathing
Central sleep apnea due to a medication or substance
Primary central sleep apnea
Treatment emergent central sleep apnea

crescendo-decrescendo pattern in the depth of breathing.[4] According to the American Academy of Sleep Medicine (AASM),[5] CSB in adults is scored when both of the following are met: (1) there are episodes of three or more consecutive central apneas or central hypopneas, or both, separated by a crescendo and decrescendo change in breathing amplitude with a cycle length of at least 40 seconds (typically 45 to 90 seconds) and (2) there are five or more central apneas or central hypopneas, or both, per hour associated with the crescendo and decrescendo breathing pattern recorded over a minimum of 2 hours of monitoring. In terms of nocturnal oxygen desaturation, there is generally less desaturation during central apnea and hypopnea than during obstructive events in patients with heart failure.[6]

2. *Primary CSA* resembles CSA-CSB, except that the cycle duration is shorter, arousals occur earlier (at the termination of apnea versus during or near the peak ventilatory effort), and resumption of breathing is more abrupt and not crescendo, typically with a large-volume breath. The diagnostic polysomnography (PSG) shows five or more apneic episodes per hour of sleep, the number of central apneas or central hypopneas more than 50% of the total number of apneas and hypopneas, and absence of CSB. The disorder is not better explained by a medical or neurologic disorder, medication use, or substance use disorder.
3. *High-altitude periodic breathing* is seen in normal persons at elevations greater than 7600 meters and in some at lower altitudes (see Chapter 144). This ventilatory pattern is characterized by periods of alternating hyperpnea and apnea,[7] the cycle length typically being between 12 and 34 seconds. PSG, if performed, demonstrates recurrent central apneas or hypopneas primarily during non–rapid eye movement (NREM) sleep at a frequency of five or more per hour.
4. *CSA due to a medical condition without CSB* is encountered in individuals with cardiac, renal, and neuromuscular disease who have CSA without the CSB.
5. *Central sleep apnea due to a medication or substance* is commonly seen in patients with long-term opioid use that causes respiratory depression by acting on the μ receptors of the ventral medulla. PSG demonstrates lack of CSB and five or more central apneas or central hypopneas, or both,[1] per hour of sleep, with the number of central apneas or central hypopneas, or both, 50% or greater than the total number of apneas and hypopneas.
6. *Treatment emergent central apnea* (or "complex" sleep apnea) is included in the ICSD-3 and refers to CSA not explained by another CSA disorder (e.g., CSA with CSB or CSA resulting from a medication or substance). The diagnostic PSG shows five or more predominantly obstructive respiratory events per hour of sleep. The continuous positive airway pressure (CPAP) titration PSG without a backup rate shows resolution of obstructive events and emergence or persistence of central apnea or central hypopnea with both a central apnea-central hypopnea index of five or more per hour and number of central apneas and central hypopneas 50% or greater than total number of apneas and hypopneas.

PATHOPHYSIOLOGY

As Cherniack[8] noted in the early 1980s, breathing in an awake, healthy person involves a smooth and regularly recurring sequence of inspiration and expiration without pauses. The rate and depth of breathing are regulated by a negative-feedback control system aimed at maintaining arterial partial pressures of carbon dioxide ($Paco_2$) and oxygen (Pao_2) at relatively constant levels. When diseases of the lung or chest wall produce hypoxemia and hypocapnia or hypercapnia, they usually do so without affecting the regularity of breathing. Several mechanisms and their corresponding controls influence the rhythmicity of breathing. A synopsis of the following roadmap we used in the discussion of CSA pathophysiology and its clinical translation is detailed in Tables 124.1 and 124.2.

Table 124.1 Common Noncardiac Conditions Associated with Central Sleep Apnea Events

Medical Condition	Prevalence (%)	Authors
Multiple sclerosis	18	Braley et al[154]
Central nervous system tumor survivors	12.9	Mandrell et al[155]
Cerebrovascular accident	7	Johnson et al[156]
Congenital muscular dystrophies	55	Pinard et al[158a]
End-stage renal disease on hemodialysis	17	Tada et al[157]
Diabetes	3.8	Resnick et al[158]

Table 124.2 Roadmap Used in Discussion of the Central Sleep Apnea Pathophysiology

Mechanism	Control	Clinicopathophysiologic Translation
Chemical	Metabolic	Cheyne-Stokes breathing OHS Sleep transition apnea CCHS
Mechanical	Metabolic Neural	Muscular degenerative Postarousal/postsigh central apnea
Neural	Neural	Stroke CCHS

CCHS, Congenital central hypoventilation syndrome; OHS, obesity hypoventilation syndrome.

Mechanisms

Several types of receptors and their associated afferent and efferent pathways are involved in maintaining the regular normal breathing.

Chemical Aspects of Ventilation

Ventilatory responses vary widely between the awake and asleep state, as well as between rapid eye movement (REM) and NREM sleep. Ventilation during sleep is largely regulated by the same mechanisms that drive breathing while awake,[9] except that behavioral influences[10] become suppressed in transition to, and during, sleep. Therefore central apneic events are rarely present during the awake state[11,12] or REM sleep.[13] During NREM sleep, however, changes in the respiratory pattern are primarily controlled chemically, being the result of a fine balance among a critical $Paco_2$ level, below which there is a central cessation of breathing (i.e., apneic threshold); its triggering factors (mainly hypocapnia); and respondent receptors (i.e., central and peripheral chemoreceptors). Additionally, the level of ventilation in respiratory dysrhythmias is augmented by arousals from sleep, resulting in transient hyperventilation with hypocapnia below the apneic threshold[14] and therefore initiation of central apneic events, primarily during NREM sleep.

Hypoxic Stimulus and Peripheral and Central Chemoreceptors. The chemoreceptors involved in the ventilatory response are both peripheral and central, each of them responding to changes in arterial Po_2 *and* Pco_2 in a complex, interactive manner. In mammals, the peripheral chemoreceptors are represented by the aortic and carotid bodies. The carotid bodies represent the main drive of the ventilatory stimulation resulting from acute, chronic,[15,16] and intermittent[17] hypoxia and contain the glomus cells that respond to the changes in the arterial blood oxygen concentration in a curvilinear fashion through several neurotransmitters, such as acetylcholine, substance P, and adenosine triphosphate.[18] The aortic bodies, on the other hand, likely become upregulated only if the carotid bodies are chronically absent and then respond to changes in the arterial Po_2[19] through mechanisms that are less known. Notably, studies in patients with long-standing OSA demonstrated the possibility of the carotid bodies becoming desensitized with extended exposure to intermittent hypoxia.[20-22] In comparison with the peripheral chemoreceptors, the central chemoreceptors have a wide anatomic distribution in the brainstem (especially in nucleus tractus solitarius [NTS], locus coeruleus, raphe nuclei, and the retrotrapezoid nucleus [RTN]) and respond to central nervous system–specific hypoxia by augmentation of alveolar ventilation during both wakefulness[23] and sleep.[24]

Hypercapnic Stimulus and Peripheral and Central Chemoreceptors. In addition to responding to hypoxia, the carotid bodies also act as a sensitive detector of the adequacy of alveolar ventilation.[25] However, in the absence of concomitant changes in arterial pO_2, the carotid chemoreceptor ventilatory response appears to be slow with more than 10 mm Hg increase in $Paco_2$ above eupneic air-breathing being required before triggering a hyperventilatory response of more than 10 liters per minute.[26] In the absence of an exact biologic definition for the central chemoreceptors, most consideration is given to the possibility that these cells are glial or vascular cells that regulate the activity of surrounding neurons through paracrine mechanisms and respond promptly to the changes of the local neuronal pH.[27,28] Anatomically, the RTN is considered to be the predominant location of integration of the central chemoreceptor drive.[29] In contrast to the highly sensitive vascular reactivity of most of the cerebral vasculature to hypercapnic-induced vasodilation and hypocapnic-induced vasoconstriction, the RTN vasculature seems nonresponsive to local changes in arterial pCO_2; thus its H^+ homeostasis is being sacrificed as an exchange of preserving a hypersensitive RTN chemoresponsiveness.

Apneic Threshold and Implications for Central Sleep Apnea. During NREM sleep, motor output to respiratory muscles is dramatically reduced compared with wakefulness, causing mild to moderate sustained hypoventilation in all healthy subjects (+2 to +8 mm Hg $Paco_2$). If relative hyperpnea occurs and $Paco_2$ falls below a characteristic value for each individual (the apneic threshold), a central apnea occurs (Figure 124.2).[30] The hypocapnia-induced apneic threshold is not a constant value but usually occurs at a level very close to the eupneic $Paco_2$ present during wakefulness after a very small reduction in $Paco_2$, from 2 to 5 mm.

Mechanistically, to reach the apneic threshold, transient ventilatory overshoots are necessary, commonly provided by transient arousals with consequent brief hyperpnea with hypocapnia. Alternatively, to overcome the apneic threshold

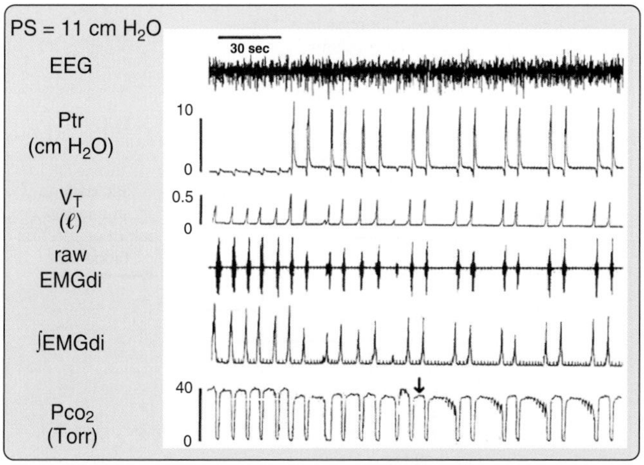

Figure 124.2 Polygraph record of one pressure support (PS) trial (11 cm H_2O) in which ventilatory instability was achieved in dogs. A reduced diaphragmatic electromyelogram (EMGdi) and inspiratory effort on the seventh ventilator cycle was insufficient to trigger a ventilator breath. Clear periodicity developed after the ninth ventilator cycle. The *arrow* marks the petCO_2 considered to be the apneic threshold. EEG, Electroencephalogram; Ptr, tracheal pressure; V_T, tidal volume. (Modified from Nakayama H, Smith CA, Rodman JR, et al. Effect of ventilatory drive on carbon dioxide sensitivity below eupnea during sleep. *Am J Respir Crit Care Med.* 2002;165:1251–61.)

and therefore reinitiate the breathing rhythm, a $Paco_2$ higher by 1 to 4 mm Hg than the apneic threshold is needed; this difference reflects a postapneic control system termed *inertia,* aimed at enhancing the chemoreceptor stimulus after the ventilatory overshoot.

Interactions between the Central and Peripheral Chemoreceptors. Several anatomic and functional connections (e.g., the RTN receives direct input from the NTS and thus the carotid body)[31] serve a dual chemotactic role (peripheral and central), raising the question of interdependence between the two types of chemoreceptors. Failing to demonstrate unequivocally the existence of only one model because of variations in the experimental protocol, the literature describes three possible interactions: additive (the two responses simply sum), hyperadditive (the two responses multiply), or hypoadditive (the sum of each response is less than their mathematical sum). Regardless of the specifics of the final augmentative response, it is postulated that carotid chemoreceptors act as the immediate hypocapnic sensors,[32] given the lack of short-term response of the central chemoreceptors to systemic hypocapnia when normocapnia and normoxia are maintained at the level of the carotid bodies.[33] However, peripheral receptors do not primarily induce hypocapnic apnea by themselves, as demonstrated by experimental models involving isolated carotid body hypocapnia that fails to result in apnea.[34] Therefore it appears that both central and peripheral chemoreceptors must interact and respond to hypocapnia for the ventilatory overshoot to induce central apnea during sleep.

Mechanical Aspects of Ventilation

Dysfunction of upper airway mechanics represents the basis of OSA pathophysiology. Such dysfunction, however, is also observed in CSA because of upper airway collapsibility, resulting in ventilatory instability.

The two primary collapsing forces of the upper airway are intraluminal negative pressure (generated by the diaphragm during inspiration) and extraluminal soft tissues (e.g., generated by fat deposition within bony structures surrounding the airway). These forces are opposed primarily by the pharyngeal dilator muscles, whose activity either varies from breath to breath (phasic respiratory muscles such as genioglossus) or stays similar throughout the respiratory cycle (tonic muscle, such as the tensor palatini). Additionally, activity of these muscles is dependent on mechanoreceptor and chemoreceptive influences. Studies in animals have shown that chemoreceptor activation resulted in an augmented depolarization of the inspiratory and expiratory hypoglossal motoneurons, thus providing evidence for the arterial chemoreceptors' contribution to maintaining upper airway patency throughout the respiratory cycle.[35] Additionally, the activity of the most important pharyngeal dilator muscle, the genioglossus, is accentuated by hypoxia and abolished by hyperoxia.[36] Alternatively, hypercapnia at the level of peripheral and central chemoreceptors leads to increased afferents to hypoglossal motoneurons and decreased threshold of the genioglossus activation. In comparison of the quantitative participation of mechanoreceptors with chemoreceptors as modulators of upper airway activation, it has been suggested that chemoreceptors are stronger, although the two stimuli in combination may interactively augment upper airway muscle activity more than either stimulus alone.[37] Besides the upper airway muscles, the fluctuations in chemical stimuli also affect the diaphragm. Animal studies demonstrate a linear chemoreceptor-driven recruitment of the diaphragm electromyogram.[38] Endoscopy performed during both induced and naturally occurring central apnea demonstrated that upper airway obstruction occurs without evidence of an inspiratory effort in the first 10 seconds of a CSA episode.[39] Consequently, neuromuscular respiratory pathology overlaps in these different types of SBDs, making a clear adjudication between obstructive and central events difficult in many cases.

Neural Aspects of Ventilation

The respiratory neurons are divided into two groups, inspiratory and expiratory. The former belong to the dorsal respiratory group localized in the area of the NTS; the latter belong to the ventral respiratory group localized adjacent to the nucleus ambiguous.[40] Although the hypoxic and hypercapnic afferent responses of the peripheral and central chemoreceptors activate certain populations of respiratory neurons, the details of such intricate processes are still missing; likewise, the relative contribution of each neuronal population to central apnea pathogenesis is also unknown.[41] Studies of several congenital disorders have provided information on the central apnea neuronal ventilatory impairment and helped in understanding better the sudden infant death syndrome. Such rare congenital diseases include Leigh syndrome, a mitochondrial encephalopathy whose manifestations include frequent post-sigh apneic episodes resulting from lung stretch receptors ending their vagal afferents into abnormal NTS,[42] and Fukuyama-type congenital muscular dystrophy, in which sudden death is commonly encountered as a result of migration defects of the brainstem structures involving pathology of the arcuate nucleus that acts as a central chemoreceptor sensitive to hypercapnia.[43]

As Harper and colleagues[44] reviewed recently, however, CSB with or without CSA affects the brain structure and function beyond the rhythmicity of breathing and includes hormonal, autonomic, and behavioral (affect, memory, and cognition) functions. Neural injuries of the ventrolateral and dorsal medullary areas are common in patients with heart failure who demonstrate CSB patterns with or without CSA, affecting the final pathway of sympathetic outflow and sympathetic tone regulation.[45] Congenital central hypoventilation syndrome (CCHS) neuropathology also involves the ventrolateral medulla, with subsequent dysfunction of the respiratory phase switch.[46] Neurotransmitter system injuries have been also recognized in CCHS in the raphe system, locus coeruleus (noradrenergic neurons), ventral midbrain, hypothalamus, and basal ganglia (dopaminergic fibers).[47] The cerebral cortex is not spared in either of these conditions; ischemic damage to the right insula is significantly accentuated in patients with heart failure who also have a high prevalence of OSA and CSB.[48] Essentially, because of hippocampal injury, short-term memory and cognitive impairments are also common in CCHS.

Ventilatory Control in Central Sleep Apnea

Metabolic Control of Ventilation

Normal respiratory rhythmicity during sleep is maintained by a complex feedback mechanism best described by the concept of "loop gain," with CO_2 responsiveness between the eupnea and apneic threshold contributing.[49] *Loop gain* is an engineering term that describes the dynamic feedback of several stabilizing ventilatory mechanisms composed of three elements: (1) the controller gain (chemoresponsiveness, including ventilatory response to Pao_2 and $Paco_2$ above and below eupnea); (2) the plant gain (effectiveness of CO_2 excretion from such ventilatory response); and (3) mixing gain (e.g., from circulation delay between the lungs and the peripheral and central chemoreceptors). Simplistically, the loop gain could be defined as the ratio of the amplitude of the ventilatory response to a ventilatory disturbance. A loop gain of less than 1 accompanies a stable ventilatory system with low respiratory variability because disturbances lead to smaller responses, ensuring a rapid return to a stable pattern. On the contrary, a loop gain of greater than 1 accompanies an unstable ventilatory system with high respiratory variability, in which disturbances lead to disproportionately large responses, resulting in a perpetual waxing and waning pattern. The ventilatory control system is dynamic, with both chemical and nonchemical inputs contributing to the breath-by-breath variability, as detailed by Khoo[50] (Figure 124.3).

Ventilatory variability is due to the feedback instability of the hypoxic and hypercapnic chemosensitivities. For example, a transient episode of hyperpnea leads to an eventual decrease in ventilation, but given the lag in the chemical response resulting from the circulation time, the initial correcting ventilatory response occurs well into the hyperpneic episode. This brief episode of hypopnea or apnea elicits a similarly delayed response, resulting in an ongoing oscillatory pattern of hyperpnea-hypopnea, whose magnitude and duration depends heavily on the *net effects* of the ventilatory control system. Several factors influence each of the gains: (1) the controller gain is affected by the sensitivity of the peripheral chemoreceptors to changes in gas partial pressure, sensitivity of central centers to peripheral chemoreceptors, and the excitability and integrity of the lower motor neurons supplying the respiratory muscle; (2) the plant gain is determined by the respiratory cycle frequency, $Paco_2$, Pao_2, ventilation-perfusion matching, and dead-space ventilation[51]; (3) the mixing gain is dependent on the circulatory delay time, thoracic blood volume, and brain

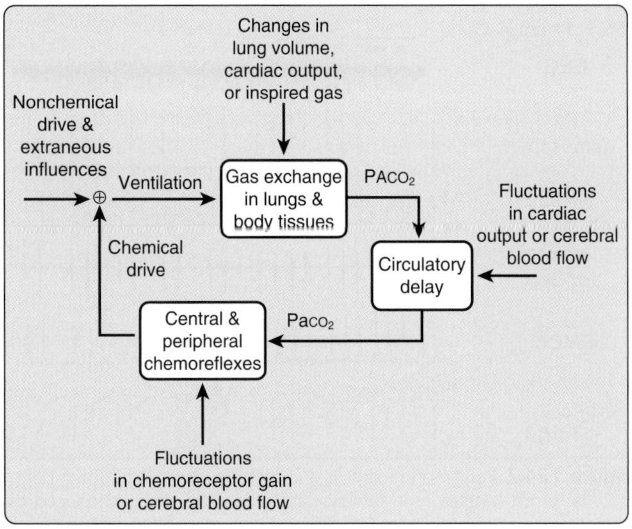

Figure 124.3 Chemical and nonchemical inputs contributing to the breath-by-breath variability.

extracellular fluid volume. In addition to the loop gain, another factor affecting ventilatory stability is the $Paco_2$ reserve, that is, the difference between the eupneic $Paco_2$ and the $Paco_2$ at the apneic threshold. The lower the $Paco_2$ reserve, the smaller the increase in the ventilation required for reaching the apneic threshold and developing central apnea. Conversely, when the apneic threshold for $Paco_2$ is far away from the eucapnic $Paco_2$, large ventilatory changes are necessary to lower the $Paco_2$ below the apneic threshold, decreasing the likelihood of developing central apnea. Several factors are shown to alter the apneic threshold. $Paco_2$ reserve is widened by testosterone suppression with leuprolide acetate in healthy men[52] and by hormone replacement therapy in postmenopausal women.[53] Alternatively, $Paco_2$ reserve is lowered with aging, explaining the increased propensity for central apneas in elderly adults during NREM sleep.[54]

The theoretical applications of the concepts of ventilatory instability and loop gain have been translated clinically by several clinical experiments. Common to all of them is the pathophysiologic relationship between alveolar ventilation (VA) and alveolar Pco_2 described best by several authors[55-57]; a compiled explanation is given by Dempsey and colleagues[49] and depicted in Figure 124.4.

In hypoxic and normoxic acetazolamide-induced metabolic acidosis, the accompanying hyperventilation results in an increase in the VA required to reduce the $Paco_2$ to the apneic threshold, protecting against apnea and respiratory instability. Despite a similar conceptual pathway of *reduced plant gain* for both hypoxic and normoxic hyperventilation, in hypoxia the slope of the ventilatory response increases and therefore the CO_2 reserve below eupnea is decreased, predisposing to ventilatory instability compared with nonhypoxic hyperventilation (Figure 124.5).[58]

Ventilatory instability is also promoted by *increasing plant gain,* such as is seen with $NaHCO_3$-induced metabolic alkalosis that narrows the CO_2 reserve without a change in the slope of the CO_2 response below eupnea.[59] For the controller gain, both increased and decreased controller gain have been demonstrated using pharmacologic manipulations of the peripheral chemoreceptor sensitivity; intravenous administration of dopamine resulted in a fall in ventilation and reduced

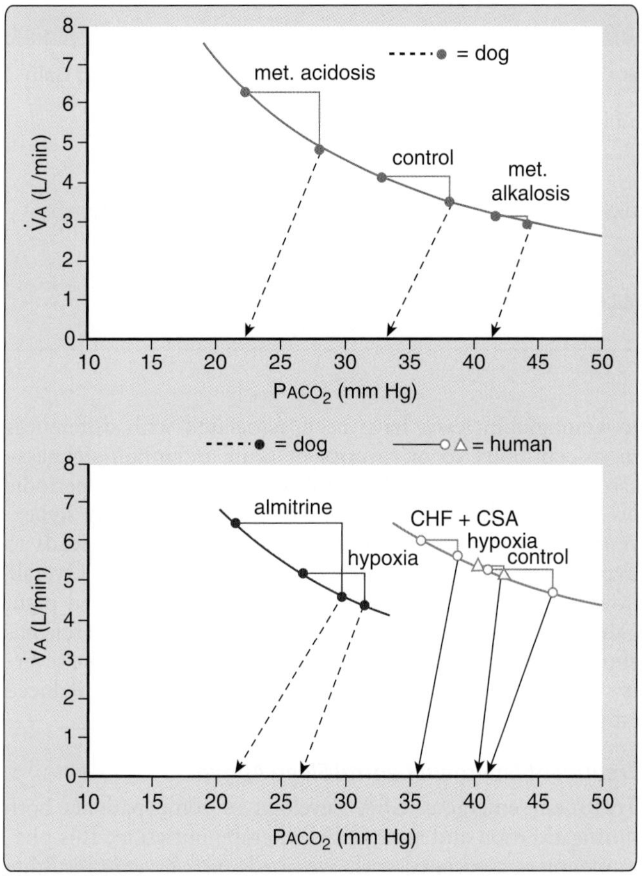

Figure 124.4 The effects of changing background ventilatory drive on the gain of the ventilatory responsiveness to CO_2 below eupnea, on "plant gain," and on the CO_2 reserve (ΔP_{ETCO_2} eupnea − apnea) in sleeping dogs and humans. Data are plotted on separate isometabolic lines for dogs [CO_2 flow ($\dot{V}CO_2$) = 150 mL/min^{-1}] and for humans ($\dot{V}CO_2$ = 250 mL/min^{-1}). The *diagonal dashed* or *continuous lines* join eupneic and apneic points, and their slopes indicate the gain below eupnea of the ventilatory response to hypocapnia in each condition. The height of the *vertical bar* above the isometabolic line indicates the increase in $\dot{V}CO_2$ required to reduce the Pa_{CO_2} to the apneic threshold (i.e., the inverse of plant gain). The CO_2 reserve is the difference in P_{ACO_2} between eupnea and the apneic threshold. CHF, Congestive heart failure; CSA, central sleep apnea.

O_2 sensitivity[60] (i.e., *reduced controller gain*), whereas administration of the dopamine D_2-receptor antagonist domperidone resulted in increased carotid body sensitivity to O_2 (i.e., *increased controller gain*).[61] As detailed in Figure 124.5, the steeper the slope of the V_{ACO_2}–P_{ACO_2} relationship, the smaller the change in Pa_{CO_2} required to reach the apneic threshold, and therefore the higher the controller gain. Numerous clinical entities are associated with one or more abnormalities of loop gain, as summarized in Table 124.3.

Neural Control of Ventilation

Neural mechanisms of ventilatory control in central apnea are likely as important as the metabolic pathways, dictating behavior during wakefulness, affecting airway patency, and controlling respiratory plasticity. The wakefulness stimuli to breathe include tonic excitatory inputs from the so-called reticular formation, brainstem aminergic systems, and hypothalamic orexin neurons.[62] Younes,[63] using correlational analysis, demonstrated that an effective neural control of the upper airway and chest wall respiratory muscles was more important than the inherent passive collapsibility of the airway.

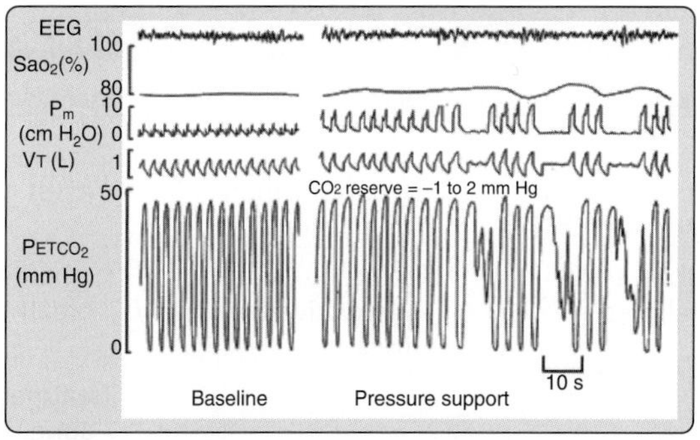

Figure 124.5 Hypoxia reduces the CO_2 reserve. A healthy human is exposed to moderate hypoxia (Pa_{O_2} 80%) for 15 to 20 minutes during NREM sleep, causing mild hyperventilation. When pressure support ventilation is subsequently applied, note that a transient reduction of only 1 or 2 mm Hg in P_{ACO_2} is required to cause apnea and periodic breathing. This effect contrasts with the 3- to 5-mm Hg ΔP_{ACO_2} required in the normoxic control condition. The CO_2 reserve is markedly reduced in hypoxia despite the reduced P_{ACO_2} and plant gain because the slope of the $\Delta \dot{V}_A$–ΔP_{ACO_2} relationship below eupnea is significantly increased. EEG, Electroencephalogram; P_m, mean airway pressure; V_T, tidal volume. (From Braley TJ, Segal BM, Chervin RD. Sleep-disordered breathing in multiple sclerosis. *Neurology.* 2012;28:929–36.)

Respiratory plasticity translates into *long-term facilitation* (LTF), a term used to describe the increase in the respiratory activity that persists after the conclusion of an acute episode of intermittent hypoxia.[64] Mediated through several receptors, including serotonergic and *N*-methyl-D-aspartate, this response in sleeping humans is aimed at stabilizing ventilation through increased minute ventilation (i.e., ventilatory LTF),[65] decreased inspiratory upper airway resistance,[66] and increased genioglossus electromyographic activity (i.e., upper airway LTF).[67] However, concentrating on central apnea pathophysiology, Chowdhuri and colleagues[68] demonstrated that, in healthy participants undergoing nasal noninvasive ventilation for promoting hypocapnic central apnea, the increase in the hypocapnic ventilatory response resulted in a significant decrease in the CO_2 reserve, thus offsetting the protective effect of LTF.

Examples of Pathophysiologic to Clinical Applications

Cheyne-Stokes Breathing with or without Central Sleep Apnea

CSB is characterized by a destabilizing interplay of several gains: specifically, controller and plant, with CSA presenting when this destabilization is most accentuated. A *high controller gain* is due to a hypersensitive ventilatory chemoreflex response to CO_2. Although the exact mechanism for this increase in chemosensitivity is not yet known, both congestive (e.g., pulmonary edema[69] and left atrial stretch[70]) and noncongestive (e.g., reduced carotid arterial blood flow[71]) factors result in vagal afferents that stimulate central respiratory control centers and fail to allow the Pa_{CO_2} to increase at sleep onset.[72] Ventilatory control is also affected in patients with congestive heart failure (CHF) because of an attenuated cerebrovascular reactivity to the changes in Pa_{CO_2} levels.[73] *The mixing gain* is a concept sometimes used to define how a delay in the circulation can be destabilizing for ventilation. The fact that the chemoreceptors are in the carotid bodies and brainstem rather than in the lung is one factor that can contribute to instability because periodic breathing would be unlikely if chemoreceptors were in the lung. Circulatory delay was induced in classic experiments by Guyton and colleagues,[74] who showed

Table 124.3 Loop Gain Abnormalities in Clinical Disorders

Increased Plant Gain	Decreased Plant Gain	Increased Controller Gain	Decreased Controller Gain	Increased Mixing Gain
Obesity-hypoventilation syndrome (OHS)	Congenital central hypoventilation syndrome	Cheyne-Stokes breathing (CSB)	OHS	CSB
Neuromuscular weakness	Hypercapnic chronic obstructive pulmonary disease	High-altitude periodic breathing		Idiopathic pulmonary hypertension
		Treatment emergent central apnea		

that delays of several minutes (beyond what could occur clinically) were sometimes required to induce periodic breathing in animals. Subsequent studies suggested that circulatory delay was similar in patients with CSB with CHF compared with patients without CSB matched for the severity of heart failure. However, some studies have shown that improvements in circulatory delay are associated with improvement in loop gain (and hence improved apnea-hypopnea index [AHI]). Thus, in aggregate, the data suggest that circulatory delay is necessary but not enough to destabilize ventilation in most cases. Therefore the overall response in CSB is that of an increased loop gain manifesting as increased ventilatory instability. During CSB with CSA, arousals mostly occur within the first half of the hyperpneic phase or close to hyperpnea onset.[75] Recent work in patients with CHF suggests that the CSB with CSA is characterized by two patterns: a positive pattern where end-expiratory lung volume remains at or above functional residual capacity and a negative pattern where it falls below functional residual capacity. Patients who had a negative CSB with CSA pattern had evidence of worse cardiac function than those with a positive pattern.[76]

CSB with CSA had been also noted in individuals with cerebrovascular accident (CVA) and chronic renal failure. Among patients with CVA and CSA, the presence of CSB with long hyperpnea and cycle durations and a gradual rise to peak tidal volume during hyperpnea was associated with left ventricular systolic dysfunction but was not related to the location or type of stroke. The authors indicated that the presence of CSA with CSB was more closely associated with left ventricular systolic dysfunction than it was with the stroke itself.[77] Similarly, Yamamoto and Mohri,[78] studying the influence of chronic renal insufficiency on SBDs in patients with symptomatic chronic heart failure, found that most of these patients had unspecified central events, with estimated glomerular filtration rate comparable between non-SBD and SBD groups. The authors suggested that renal dysfunction played a relatively minor role in determining breathing abnormalities in chronic heart failure.

High-Altitude Periodic Breathing

High-altitude periodic breathing is another example of ventilatory instability that occurs during sleep in individuals during ascent to moderate and high altitude (see Chapter 144). Individual susceptibility to high-altitude periodic breathing is driven by multiple genetic factors; polymorphisms in numerous genes, including the hypoxia-responsive transcription factor subunit *EPAS1/HIF2α* and additional genes in the hypoxia-inducible factor (HIF) pathway linked to hemoglobin level, have been associated with differences in susceptibility to or severity of acute mountain sickness–associated conditions.[79,80] In this case, high-altitude periodic breathing is the result of ambient hypoxia inducing hyperventilation (*increased controller gain*), which further leads to hypocapnia and consequently to *decreased plant gain*. Overall, however, the controller gain dominates the decreased plant gain, resulting in periodic breathing.[78] Recent research has shown that increasing cerebral blood flow decreases the severity of high-altitude periodic breathing because of reduced stimulation of the central chemoreceptors.[81]

Treatment Emergent Central Sleep Apnea

Treatment emergent CSA develops in some patients both during titration and after CPAP therapy initiation. This phenomenon is associated with *increased controller gain* resulting from lowering upper airway resistance with perhaps a contribution of the air leak washing out the anatomic dead space.[82] Treatment emergent CSA is associated with a higher baseline OSA or CSA index and a higher residual AHI on the CPAP titration study.[83] A recent study that monitored trajectories of treatment emergent CSA in week 1 and week 13 after CPAP initiation for OSA showed that the CSA was transient in 55.1% of patients and persistent in 25.2%. As in a pilot study, loop gain was higher in patients with treatment emergent CSA in whom central apneas persisted after 1 month of CPAP therapy; loop gain measurement in these patients may enable a priori determination of those who need alternative modes of positive airway pressure.[84]

Obesity-Hypoventilation Syndrome

Obesity-hypoventilation syndrome (OHS) is characterized by a combination of obesity (body mass index > 30 kg/m^2) and arterial hypercapnia during wakefulness ($Paco_2$ > 45 mm Hg) (see Chapter 138). OHS is the result of an interplay between respiratory mechanics and ventilatory drive, with leptin, a circulating protein produced mainly by adipose tissue, playing a role. A deficiency of this adipokine, as seen in the leptin-deficient *ob/ob* mouse mode, results in impaired respiratory mechanics, depressed ventilatory responsiveness, and awake hypercapnia.[85] In mice, leptin administration relieved upper airway obstruction in sleep apnea by activating the forebrain, possibly in the dorsomedial hypothalamus.[86] Thus, as leptin replacement in these mice reverses their OHS, recent work has focused on the potential role of leptin in individuals with OHS. It is presumed that the development of central leptin resistance or relative leptin deficiency in OHS could contribute to the development of awake hypoventilation by altering respiratory drive output as well, affecting the mechanical properties of the lungs and chest wall and attenuating the normal compensatory mechanisms used by individuals to cope with obesity-related respiratory loads.[87] These patients have decreased ventilatory responsiveness to hypoxia and hypercapnia compared with similarly obese non-OHS patients and also respond with large increases in $Paco_2$ to small decreases in ventilation (*increased plant gain*), increasing overall the probability of developing central apneic events.[82]

Congenital Central Hypoventilation Syndrome

CCHS is a rare congenital disease caused by mutation in *PHOX2B* gene leading to lack of central drive and decreased ventilatory response to $Paco_2$ (decreased controller gain) despite normal lungs and respiratory muscle function.[88]

Opioid-Induced Central Sleep Apnea

The exact pathophysiologic mechanism of opioid-induced apnea remains poorly understood but is likely related to opioid-induced suppression of inspiration generated by the pre-Bötzinger complex in the brainstem.[89] Both a periodic, nonwaxing waning breathing pattern and a cluster-type breathing pattern, each with central apneas, have been reported during NREM sleep in individuals receiving chronic opiates.[90] Chronic opioid use is a risk factor for the development of CSA and ataxic breathing,[91] but it is only rarely associated with daytime hypercapnia.[92]

GENETICS

Congenital Central Hypoventilation Syndrome

Most CSA disorders in adults have not been linked to specific genotypes. The one clear exception is CCHS, which is a monogenetic disorder of central respiratory control associated with diffuse autonomic dysregulation,[93] and, at times, Hirschsprung disease and tumors of neural crest origin.[94] CCHS is characterized by a specific facial phenotype, such as boxy facies and an inferior inflection of the lateral segment of vermillion border on the upper lip.[95] CCHS has a familial presentation, and the *PHOX2B* mutation located on chromosome 4p12 has been identified and confirmed as the disease-defining gene.[96-99] CCHS, a lifelong disease, is diagnosed in the absence of other systemic pathology and a positive *PHOX2B* screening test or whole-gene *PHOX2B* sequencing test.[100] Clinically, CCHS is defined by an inability to adapt appropriately to needed ventilatory changes; these patients have altered or absent perception of shortness of breath when awake and profound and life-threatening hypoventilation during sleep.[101] Patients with CCHS develop apnea or severe bradypnea during NREM sleep. However, expression of the disease is highly variable, with some patients presenting as neonates and others presenting in adulthood, largely depending on the genotype. Approximately 90% of mutations involve excessive polyalanine repeats of the *PHOX2B* gene beyond the normal 20/20 pattern observed in the normal population. Polyalanine repeat patterns of 20/25 to 20/33 typically present at birth with hypoventilation. By contrast, people with a 20/24 pattern may present after the neonatal period, including as adults. Approximately 10% of CCHS patients have nonpolyalanine repeat mutations (frameshift, missense, or nonsense), and they are typically affected at birth with hypoventilation during wakefulness and sleep. Therapeutically, CCHS patients require intratracheal or noninvasive positive pressure ventilation during sleep, and about one-third also require additional ventilator support during wakefulness, including positive pressure ventilation or diaphragmatic pacing.[102] Generally, adults present with the 20/24 CCHS genotype, which typically involves only mild hypoventilation that can be managed with noninvasive ventilation during sleep only.

EPIDEMIOLOGY

Risk Factors

Several independent risk factors have been established for CSA-CSB. In patients with CHF and reduced left ventricular ejection fraction, risk factors for CSA-CSB include age older than 60 years, male gender, presence of atrial fibrillation, and hypocapnia.[103-105] For patients with treatment emergent CSA, a high baseline AHI or arousal index, hypertension, opioid use, coronary artery disease, stroke, and CHF all appear to be risk factors.[106]

Prevalence

CSA is estimated to account for 5% to 10% of patients with SBDs that, according to ICSD-3, includes OSA, sleep-related hypoventilation disorders, and sleep-related hypoxemia disorder.[107] Additionally, variations in the hemodynamic profile of CHF patients predispose them to alterations day to day and sometimes within the same night of the predominant type of apnea—from OSA to CSA, and vice versa.[108,109] In patients with left ventricular dysfunction with predominantly CSA, both the frequency and duration of CSA increase during the later segments of NREM sleep.[110]

Cheyne-Stokes Breathing

CSA-CSB is highly prevalent in patients with left ventricular dysfunction regardless of the etiology (ischemic versus idiopathic), type (preserved or low ejection fraction), New York Heart Association (NYHA) class, and acuity of event (acute or chronic heart failure).[111] CSA-CSB can present during wakefulness and sleep when the central apnea burden (number and duration) increases during later hours of sleep.[108] Nocturnal CSA-CSB has been studied mostly in stable compensated heart failure and is present in up to 69% of patients who have heart failure with a reduced ejection fraction (HFREF)[112-113] and in up to 27% of patients who have heart failure with a preserved ejection fraction.[114] CSA-CSB during wakefulness is common, occurring in 57% in patients with systolic heart failure.[115] CSA-CSB has been demonstrated after myocardial infarction and unstable angina; in both situations, it is a common occurrence, being present in more than 60% of these patients.[116]

Primary Central Sleep Apnea

Primary CSA, formerly categorized as "idiopathic" CSA, is uncommon. The general population prevalence of primary CSA is not known. However, within the sleep center population, the prevalence has been reported to be 4% to 7%. A higher prevalence of idiopathic CSA has been reported in older patient populations.[117] These individuals usually complain of excessive daytime sleepiness, insomnia, or difficulty breathing during sleep.[118]

High-Altitude Periodic Breathing

Despite considerable heterogeneity in the susceptibility to altitude illness, periodic breathing in the form of cyclic central apneas and hypopneas occurs in almost all individuals at a sufficiently high altitude.[119]

Treatment Emergent Central Sleep Apnea

When treatment emergent CSA (or "complex" CSA) is simply defined as the emergence of central apneas and hypopnea both during and after the application of PAP therapy in patients with OSA, its estimated aggregate point prevalence in the general sleep center patient population is 8% with the estimated range varying from 5% to 20%. The prevalence tends to be higher for split-night studies compared with full-night titration studies. Risk factors include male gender, higher baseline AHI, and central apnea index at the time of diagnostic study.[120] Treatment emergent CSA was found to be transient in 55.1% and persistent in 25.2% of patients after 13 weeks of CPAP initiation.

Central Sleep Apnea Due to a Medical Disorder

A synopsis of several common noncardiac medical conditions associated with CSA events is described in Table 124.1. In cardiac conditions not related to left heart disease, CSA events were identified by PSG in 10.6% of a cohort of such patients[121] who developed NYHA class II or III disease as a result of a variety of conditions, such as idiopathic pulmonary hypertension, chronic thromboembolic disease with pulmonary hypertension, chronic obstructive pulmonary disease, and interstitial lung disease. PSG and ambulatory cardiorespiratory sleep studies documented concomitant CSA in up to 39% of patients with idiopathic pulmonary hypertension and NYHA class II to IV chronic thromboembolic disease with pulmonary hypertension[122] and in up to 20% of patients with hypertrophic cardiomyopathy.[123]

Central Sleep Apnea Due to a Medication or Substance

Opioid-induced CSA has been recognized[124] only since about 2000, with a reported prevalence, for example, of 30% of patients in a methadone pain program[125] or in cancer patients receiving opioids for pain.[126] Given the progressive increase in opioid use for symptom management in both neoplastic and chronic diseases, it is expected that such CSA will be increasingly identified in clinical sleep practice.

Age

In both general and heart failure populations, CSA-CSB seems to be more commonly encountered in patients of advanced age.[127] In children with CHF, CSA-CSB is quite rare,[128] whereas in a random sample of men aged 20 to 100 years, using sleep laboratory evaluation subsequent to a telephonic survey, Bixler and colleagues[129] noted CSA in 0.4% of those 45 to 64 years old and in 1.1% for those 65 to 100 years old. Others[130] have reported an even higher occurrence of 17% in a population aged 71 years and older.

Gender

Among healthy middle-aged adults, CSA syndromes are overall much more common in men (7.8%) than in women (0.3%).[131] For example, a study including a large proportion of women with stable HF reported unspecified CSA in only 0.05% of those with HF and in none of those with preserved ejection fraction heart failure.[132] CSA is uncommon in premenopausal women, who are less susceptible to hypocapnic CSA than men.[133] Although OSA is increasingly recognized in postmenopausal women, similar consistent data for CSA are lacking.

Race

No data are available on the racial distribution of CSA syndromes to our knowledge.

Morbidity

Central Sleep Apnea and Cardiac Hemodynamics

In CSA-CSB, intermittent surges in blood pressure and heart rate occur in association with oscillations in ventilation. Such surges can be precipitated by cyclic increases in sympathetic nervous system activity targeting the heart and peripheral vasculature.[134,135] Studies concentrating on these hemodynamic responses have confirmed that the frequency and peaks of heart rate and blood pressure oscillations are dependent primarily on periodic oscillations in ventilation.[136] The clinical significance of this finding is not certain, but surges in blood pressure during hyperpnea may be one factor related to the poorer prognosis in patients with heart failure with CSB compared with those without it.[137] More recently, Yumino and colleagues[138] assessed the beat-to-beat stroke volume from before until the end of central respiratory events during sleep in patients with HFREF and demonstrated an increase in stroke volume by a mean of 2.6% ($P < .001$ for the difference).

Central Sleep Apnea and Cardiac-Related Hospital Readmission

The only study to date[139] that prospectively evaluated cardiac readmission associated with SBD in a cohort of hospitalized patients with acutely decompensated HFREF demonstrated CSA-CSB to be a predictor of both 1-month and 6-month readmission (univariable rate ratios of 1.5 and 1.63, respectively). Ongoing studies are evaluating whether treating CSA-CSB prevents such readmission.

Central Sleep Apnea and Cerebrovascular Accident

Using near-infrared spectroscopy in individuals with acute and subacute CVA, Pizza and colleagues documented asymmetric patterns of cerebral hypoxia during unspecified CSA events, with significantly larger changes on the unaffected compared with the affected hemisphere.[140]

Central Sleep Apnea and Atrial Fibrillation

A recent large prospective, multicenter study of community-dwelling older men (older than 65 years) who participated in the MrOS Sleep (Outcomes of Sleep Disorders in Older Men) Study, showed that CSA, including Cheyne-Stokes respiration, were significantly associated with incident atrial fibrillation even after accounting for confounders, including cardiovascular risk and disease.[141] Although the exact pathophysiologic mechanisms by which CSA increases atrial arrhythmogenesis are not yet identified, they include augmented respiratory chemoreflexes and autonomic nervous system dysfunction[142] and cardiac electric instability resulting from hypocapnia.[143]

Mortality

As the oxyhemoglobin desaturations, arousals, increased sympathetic output, and negative intrathoracic pressure (during hyperpnea that follows central apnea in CSA-CSB) contribute to myocardial ischemia, CSA-CSB could contribute to excess mortality in patients with heart failure. Relatively large studies looking specifically at the mortality associated with unspecified CSA and CSA-CSB have provided divergent results, some likely deriving from the lack of a strict definition for CSA or for CSA-CSB. Javaheri and colleagues[144] evaluated survival in HFREF (ejection fraction <45%) over a period of 51 months and demonstrated that patients with unspecified CSA had half the survival time of those without such CSA, 45 and 90 months, respectively ($P = .01$), independent of systolic function, NYHA functional class, heart rate, serum digoxin and sodium concentrations, hemoglobin, and age. In contrast, Andreas and colleagues[145] noted that, in patients with HFREF, nocturnal CSA-CSB had no prognostic impact. Both Andreas and colleagues and Lange and Hecht[146] reported that awake CSA-CSB was associated with a high likelihood of death within 1 to 24 months. Roebuck and colleagues[147] noted that systolic heart failure patients with unspecified CSA had decreased survival at 500 days, but similar long-term survival compared with those without such CSA. Luo and colleagues[148] demonstrated that unspecified CSA had no effect on the prognosis of middle-aged patients with CHF, whereas Bakker and colleagues[149] provided contrasting evidence by demonstrating a significantly lower survival rate in patients with heart failure and unspecified CSA compared with both heart failure and OSA (mean survival time difference, 3.8 years; $P = .005$) and those with heart failure only (mean survival time difference, 4 years; $P = .01$). Additionally, within the group of patients with HFREF and unspecified CSA, mortality is reported to be significantly higher in the "severe" (AHI > 22.5/hour) unspecified CSA group compared with the "mild" unspecified CSA group (AHI < 22.5/hour; 38% versus 16%; unadjusted $P = .002$ and adjusted for the confounders age and NYHA class $P = .035$).[150] Notably, all of these studies have focused on understanding mortality in untreated patients with heart failure and CSA with or without CSB. The randomized controlled multicenter trial, the Canadian Continuous Positive Airway Pressure for Patients with Central Sleep Apnea and Heart Failure Trial (CANPAP)[151] and its post-hoc analysis,[152] showed that death and heart transplantation events did not differ between the control group and the CPAP group. The post-hoc analysis showed improved survival without heart transplantation in the CANPAP group when CPAP therapy was associated with a reduced frequency of CSA-CSB events to fewer than 15 events per hour.

Similar benefits were not noted in a recent large ($n = 1325$) randomized controlled trial examining the impact of adding adaptive servo-ventilation (ASV) to guideline-based medical treatment on survival and cardiovascular outcomes in patients who had heart failure with reduced ejection fraction and predominantly CSA.[153] In this landmark study, Treatment of Sleep-Disordered Breathing with Predominant Central Sleep Apnea by Adaptive Servo Ventilation in Patients with Heart Failure (SERVE-HF), ASV decreased the central apnea-hypopnea index, from 25.2/hour at baseline to less than 4/hour after 48 months of therapy. However, all-cause mortality and cardiovascular mortality were higher in the ASV group than in the control group. The first event of death from any cause, lifesaving cardiovascular intervention (cardiac transplantation, implantation of a ventricular assist device, resuscitation after sudden cardiac arrest, or appropriate lifesaving shock), or unplanned hospitalization for worsening heart failure were similar between the groups. Thus utility of PAP therapy in patients with CSA and heart failure remains uncertain.

CLINICAL PEARLS

- Centrally driven respiratory events are primarily the result of a temporary loss of output from the pontomedullary pacemaker that generates breathing rhythm, resulting in loss of diaphragmatic activity.
- CSA with CSB is a form of periodic breathing, commonly observed in patients with heart failure, in which central apneas alternate with hyperpneas that have a waxing-waning pattern of tidal volume.
- Nocturnal CSB has been studied mostly in stable compensated heart failure and is present in up to 69% of patients with low ejection fraction and in up to 27% of patients with preserved ejection fraction. However, variations in the hemodynamic profile of heart failure patients predispose them to day-to-day and sometimes within-night alterations of the predominant type of apnea—OSA to CSA, and vice versa.
- Ventilatory control in CSA is largely chemically driven, especially during NREM, and is the result of a fine balance between a critical Pa_{CO_2} level, below which there is a central cessation of breathing (i.e., apneic threshold); its ventilatory triggering factors (mainly hypocapnia); and respondent receptors (i.e., central and peripheral chemoreceptors). This complex feedback mechanism is best described by the concept of loop gain.
- CSA-CSB is likely an independent risk for increased mortality or cardiac transplantation in patients with heart failure.
- Definitive outcome data on the effect of PAP therapy on the natural progression of CSA and CSA-CSB in patients with heart failure are still lacking.

SUMMARY

In CSA, both oronasal flow and thoracoabdominal excursions are absent; that is, there is an absence of respiratory effort during the cessation of airflow. CSB and treatment emergent (or "complex") CSA are the most common clinical CSA patterns. CSA with CSB is characterized by oscillations of ventilation between apnea and tachypnea, with a waxing and waning crescendo-decrescendo pattern in the depth of respirations and is highly prevalent in patients with heart failure. Treatment emergent CSA most commonly refers to the development of CSA with the application of CPAP in patients with OSA; in most cases, this breathing pattern resolves spontaneously with ongoing therapy. Nighttime, daytime, and 24-hour moderate-to-severe CSB-CSA is associated with increased cardiac mortality. It remains unclear whether improving the frequency of CSA-CSB in sleep improves clinical outcomes in this setting or, conversely, resolution of the CSA-CSB is simply a marker of a good prognosis.

SELECTED READINGS

Coniglio AC, Mentz RJ. Sleep breathing disorders in heart failure. *Heart Fail Clin.* 2020;16(1):45–51.

Costanzo MR, Khayat R, Ponikowski P, et al. Mechanisms and clinical consequences of untreated central sleep apnea in heart failure. *J Am Coll Cardiol.* 2015;65:72–84.

Dempsey JA. Crossing the apneic threshold: causes and consequences. *Exp Physiol.* 2004;90:13–24.

Eckert DJ, Jordan AS, Merchia P, et al. Central sleep apnea: pathophysiology and treatment. *Chest.* 2007;131:595–607.

Javaheri S, Dempsey JA. Central sleep apnea. *Compr Physiol.* 2013;3:141–163.

Jordan AS, McSharry D, Malhotra A. Adult obstructive sleep apnea. *Lancet.* 2014;383:736–747.

Nishino T, Lahiri S. Effects of dopamine on chemoreflexes in breathing. *J Appl Physiol.* 1981;50:892–897.

Orr JE, Ayappa I, Eckert DJ, et al. Research priorities for patients with heart failure and central sleep apnea. An official American Thoracic Society Research Statement. *Am J Respir Crit Care Med.* 2021;203(6):e11–e24.

A complete reference list can be found online at ExpertConsult.com.

Chapter
125

Central Sleep Apnea: Diagnosis and Management

Andrey V. Zinchuk; Robert Joseph Thomas

Chapter Highlights

- Pathologically enhanced respiratory chemoreflexes result in a spectrum of polysomnographic breathing patterns and disorders, including central sleep apnea (CSA), periodic breathing/Cheyne-Stokes breathing, high-altitude sleep apnea, and treatment-emergent CSA.
- A narrow carbon dioxide (CO_{2+}) reserve (difference between eupneic and apneic partial pressure of carbon dioxide [$Paco_2$]), high loop gain and sleep state, and stage instability are the primary mechanisms of hypocapnic CSA.
- A pathologically decreased chemoreflex can result in hypercapnic CSA.
- Opiate use causes a disintegrative CSA disorder with unique polysomnographic features.
- Identification of central hypopneas and chemoreflex activation is challenging using current visual (individual event rule-based) scoring polysomnographic standards.
- Predominance of events in non–rapid eye movement sleep and persistent or enhanced respiratory instability during treatment with therapy for upper airway obstruction are key features that help in the recognition of respiratory control–mediated sleep-disordered breathing.
- Adaptive servo ventilation is a major advance in noninvasive ventilatory therapy for CSA. However, long-term benefits are not proven, sleep fragmentation may persist despite reduction in central apneas, and there is potential for harm in patients with heart failure. Several other off-label approaches can be considered as primary or adjunctive therapy.
- Volume-assured positive pressure ventilation can improve oxygenation and ventilation in hypercapnic CSA and hypoventilation syndromes but may cause sleep fragmentation if pressure fluctuations are excessive.
- Residual disease during treatment is common in CSA syndromes. The long-term persistence of the residual central apnea depends on etiology and associated disorders.

INTRODUCTION

The term *central sleep apnea (CSA)* describes both the pattern of an individual respiratory event and the clinical syndrome characterized by repeated episodes of apneas during sleep caused by an impaired respiratory drive system.[1,2] This is in contrast to obstructive apneas, where respiratory drive remains active during the apnea, which is associated with upper airway occlusion (Figure 125.1).

Although central apneas are less frequent than obstructive, they present in ways and settings that are diverse. CSA breathing patterns can vary from the rhythmic sequences of apnea and recovery breaths in congestive heart failure (CHF) to the ataxic respiratory patterns in patients with opioid use.[3,4] Most humans exhibit central apneas during transitions into sleep, and they appear in travelers to high altitude. CSA patterns are associated with a range of medical conditions, from end-stage renal disease to multiple system atrophy and from opioid dependence to congenital central hypoventilation syndrome.[5-9] CSA is important to recognize because of complications ranging from frequent nighttime awakenings and excessive sleepiness to adverse cardiovascular outcomes and mortality.[10-12]

Central respiratory events in sleep rarely occur in isolation, and many patients with sleep apnea appear to live on a phenotypic spectrum between the obstructive and central apneas. In heart failure and opioid-induced sleep apnea, central and obstructive apneas often coexist.[8,13] In treatment-emergent CSA (TE-CSA), alleviation of obstructive apneas with positive airway pressure (PAP) amplifies a sensitive chemoreflex with resultant centrally mediated apneas and periodic breathing.[14] Identifying where the patient is on the obstructive-to-central spectrum and focusing on the factors responsible for this physiology are critical for an accurate diagnosis of CSA and its management.

DEFINITIONS

Current definitions for central apnea and hypopnea are based on polygraphic data and are reviewed in Chapter 125

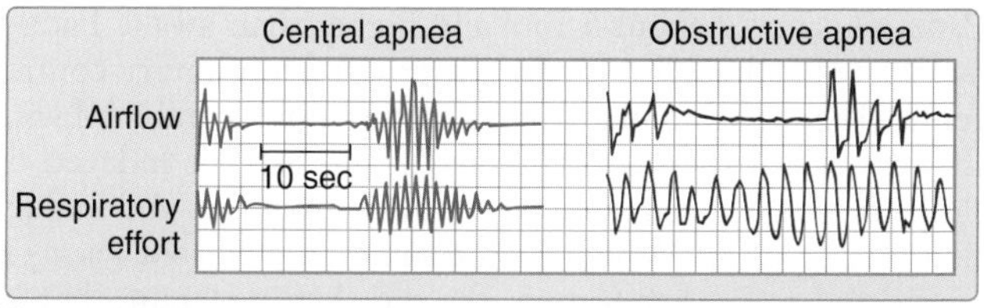

Figure 125.1 Central and obstructive sleep apnea. The relationship between airflow and respiratory effort in central and obstructive apnea. During central apnea, cessation of airflow is shown with and without associated ventilatory effort. Respiratory effort is present during an obstructive apnea.

in addition to the American Academy of Sleep Medicine (AASM) scoring manual.[15,16] A CSA syndrome is defined when five or more central apneas *and/or* central hypopneas are present per hour, that is, a central apnea-hypopnea index (CAHI) of greater than 5, with CAHI comprising more than 50% of all respiratory events.[17] For the various CSA syndromes, additional criteria related to signs and symptoms and specific etiologic entities are required.[16]

Assessment of central respiratory events and the underlying pathophysiological mechanisms is difficult using conventional scoring approaches. Evidence of upper airway obstruction on polysomnography (PSG), including flow limitation, does not rule out central apneas/hypopneas,[18-20] and esophageal manometry is rarely used in practice. Unclassified hypopneas are thus summed into the overall apnea-hypopnea index (AHI), not the specific CAHI, biasing toward obstructive sleep-disordered breathing (SDB).[2,14,21] Integrated analysis of polysomnographic features can improve identification of central hypopneas,[22] including predominance during non–rapid eye movement (NREM) versus rapid eye movement (REM) sleep, arousal after and flow restoration pattern at hypopnea termination, and lack of thoraco-abdominal paradox. Automation of hypopnea phenotyping is possible, but accuracy in comparison with esophageal manometry is limited (69%).[23] Ultimately, automated assessments of pathophysiological traits reflecting SDB mechanisms such as loop gain, derived from routinely collected signals (e.g., nasal pressure), will be required to bring SDB phenotyping into practice.[24]

CLASSIFICATION OF CENTRAL SLEEP APNEA SYNDROMES

The *International Classification of Sleep Disorders,* 3rd ed. (ICSD-3) group provides one framework for classifying CSA syndromes[16] (see Chapter 124). The approach in this chapter (Table 125.1) aims to be complementary and demarcates physiologic and pathologic states in which CSA occurs, linking mechanisms to therapies. Notably, because multiple mechanisms often coexist in a given patient, multimodality therapy may be required to stabilize breathing.

Pathophysiology of Central Sleep Apnea Syndromes that Affect Diagnosis and Treatment

The pathophysiology of CSA is discussed in detail in Chapter 124, including the chemical, mechanical, and neural aspects of respiratory control; the feedback loop between the sensors and the respiratory center; the loop gain (measure of respiratory system stability) and its components (controller, plant, mixing); and other important features. Figure 125.2 summarizes the interplay between ventilatory drive (controller) and the lung's ability to excrete CO_2 (plant) in relation to normal (eupnea) and cessation (apnea) of breathing. In this section we highlight the physiologic concepts important for our approach to diagnosis and treatment and discuss them in the context of specific CSA syndromes.

Table 125.1 Pathophysiologic Classification of Central Sleep Apneas

Physiologic	Pathologic

• Sleep transition
• Phasic REM
	• Nonhypercapnic
	  • Medical condition related:
	    • Congestive heart failure
	    • Post stroke
	    • ESRD
	    • PAH
	    • Atrial fibrillation
	  • High altitude
	  • Idiopathic
	• Hypercapnic
	  • Congenital central hypoventilation syndrome
	  • Primary chronic alveolar hypoventilation syndromes
	  • Other CNS disorders associated with CSA
	    • Encephalitis, tumors, strokes
	    • Anatomic abnormalities
	    • Neurodegenerative disorders
	  • Muscular and PNS disorders associated with CSA (selected examples)
	    • Muscular dystrophies
	    • Acid maltase deficiency
	    • Charcot-Marie-Tooth disease and other neuropathies
	    • Postpolio syndrome
	    • Myasthenia gravis
	• Disintegrative (e.g., brainstem injury, opioid-induced)
	• CSA with OSA or upper airway disorders (including treatment emergent central sleep apnea)

CNS, Central nervous system; CSA, central sleep apnea; ESRD, end-stage renal disease; OSA, obstructive sleep apnea; PAH, pulmonary arterial hypertension; PNS, peripheral nervous system; REM, rapid eye movement.

Pathophysiologic Changes that Lead to Central Sleep Apneas and Periodic Breathing

Interactions of three factors predispose an individual to ventilatory instability and central apneas/hypopneas during sleep[2]: (1) low CO_2 reserve (CO_2 reserve = $Paco_2$ eupneic − $Paco_2$ apneic), (2) abnormally high *or* low loop gain (a product of controller, plant, and mixing gains), and (3) sleep state and stage instability.

CO_2 reserve is affected by changes in plant and controller gains. For example, CO_2 reserve is decreased in metabolic alkalosis (increased plant gain; Figure 125.2), promoting the risk for central apneas and ventilatory instability, whereas it is increased with metabolic acidosis (decreased plant gain),[25] which protects against central apneas (Figure 125.2). Administration of oxygen (which reduces the hypoxic stimulus to breathing) has been shown to decrease ventilation and responsiveness to $Paco_2$ during sleep.[26] This stabilizes breathing

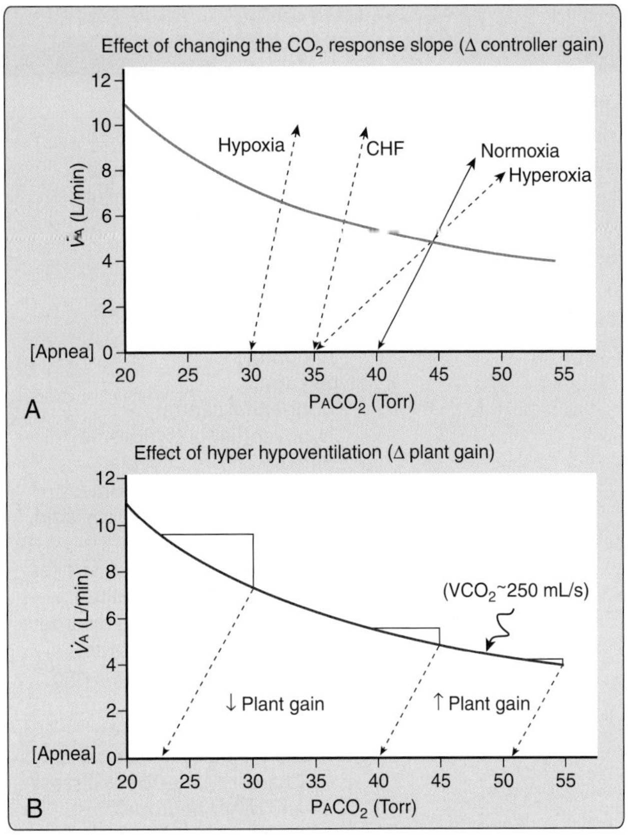

Figure 125.2 Changing plant gain *(top, A)* and controller gain *(bottom, B)* influences on CO_2 reserve. Diagrammatic representation of the steady–state relationship between alveolar ventilation and alveolar P_ACO_2 ($Paco_2$) at a fixed resting CO_2 production of 250 mL/min. The schematic figure shows how changing plant gain (**A**) or controller gain (**B**) will influence the "CO_2 reserve" or $\Delta Paco_2$ between eupnea and apnea. **A,** Changing the background drive to breathe without changing the slope of the ΔV_A versus ΔP_ACO_2 relationship (controller gain) above or below eupnea. For example, background hyperventilation (via metabolic acidosis or specific carotid body stimulation with almitrine) raises V_A and lowers P_ACO_2 along the isometabolic hyperbola (decreased plant gain). This means that a greater transient increase in V_A and reduction in P_ACO_2 is required to reach the apneic threshold than it would be under controlled, normocapnic conditions. The reverse is true for conditions that reduce the background drive to breathe and cause hypoventilation (for example, metabolic alkalosis). **B,** At any given level of background P_ACO_2, changing the slope (or responsiveness) of the relationship below eupnea would alter the CO_2 reserve or the amount of reduction in P_ACO_2 required to cause apnea. Changing the slope of the ventilatory response to CO_2 above eupnea would alter the susceptibility for transient ventilatory overshoots. Often both plant and controller gains may change together—note the reduced plant gains and increased controller gain—with hypoxia or with congestive heart failure (CHF) patients. The increased controller gain dominates, and the net effect is a decreased CO_2 reserve and instability. (Adapted with permission from Javaheri S, Dempsey JA. Central sleep apnea. *Compr Physiol.* 2013;3(1)146–163.

through reduction in controller gain and increase in $Paco_2$ reserve, whereas hypoxia leads to opposite effects (Figure 125.2). In addition, inherent delays in the negative feedback loop controlling ventilation (mixing gain) increase loop gain. This delayed recognition of blood gases by the controller (as in those with systolic CHF) predisposes to unstable and periodic breathing, which can abate with improvement in cardiac output.[27]

During sleep, brief and abrupt transitions to wakefulness, termed "arousals," can result in ventilatory instability, with the level of ventilatory response and arousal threshold playing important roles. With a sudden arousal, the sleep eupneic $Paco_2$ (normally about 5 mm Hg higher than awake $Paco_2$) is detected as hypercapnic by the aroused respiratory control center. This signal to increase ventilatory drive, combined with the removal of the upper airway (UA) resistance induced by sleep, results in increased ventilatory response and reduction in $Paco_2$.[28,29] When sleep resumes, the current $Paco_2$ is considered to be hypocapnic for the sleeping brain, that is, below the apneic threshold, resulting in central apnea. Thus any process that leads to frequent sleep-wake transitions, such as sleep-maintenance insomnia, sleep apnea, maladaptation to continuous positive airway pressure (CPAP), or periodic limb movement disorder, can increase the propensity to ventilatory overshoots, periodic breathing, and CSAs, especially in a setting of high chemosensitivity.[29-32]

Pathophysiologic Changes in Specific Central Sleep Apnea Syndromes

Nonhypercapnic Central Sleep Apnea

Disorders manifesting as nonhypercapnic (eupneic or hypocapnic) CSA have two physiologic phenomena in common: (1) normal or slightly low awake steady-state $Paco_2$ and (2) increased ventilatory responsiveness to $Paco_2$ or hypoxemia (increased loop gain). In the setting of arousals, CSAs are perpetuated because of the so-called "inertial" effect (see Chapter 124).

Central Sleep Apnea and Periodic Breathing of Heart Failure. Heart failure is associated with Cheyne-Stokes breathing (CSB), which occurs at times during wakefulness and frequently during sleep (see Chapter 149). CSB is characterized by a crescendo-decrescendo pattern of tidal volumes, with central apnea or hypopnea occurring at the nadir of the cycle (typically 60–90 seconds; Figure 125.3). It is in part a consequence of increased loop gain resulting from a heightened chemoreflex (sensitive controller)[33,34] and lack of the "normal" increase in $Paco_2$ with sleep onset (decreased CO_2 reserve).[35] These are superimposed on prolonged circulation time from impaired cardiac output (increased mixing gain), resulting in cyclical ventilatory instability.[36] Support for these mechanisms comes from studies showing that acetazolamide and oxygen, which reduce loop gain, and cardiac resynchronization, which augments cardiac output, improve CSA-CSB.[37-40]

Periodic breathing of shorter cycles occurs in other settings and conditions with "hyperactive" chemoreflex (as described later). Although ICSD-3 defines CSB with specific cycle lengths (≥40 seconds) and intervening apneas, we feel CSB represents one end of the chemoreflex activation severity spectrum, whereas at the other end of the clinical spectrum, although poorly recognized in practice, is nonapneic short-cycle (≤30 seconds) periodic breathing.

Central Sleep Apnea Because of High-Altitude Periodic Breathing. In contrast to CSB in heart failure, the cycle time of periodic breathing at high altitude is short (probably because of elimination of the mixing gain defect). The mechanism involves exposure to hypoxemia with resultant chemoreceptor-mediated hyperventilation during sleep. After approximately 10 minutes of hypoxia in a sleeping human, tidal volumes oscillate in a waxing and waning pattern. The oscillations increase in magnitude as hypoxia is maintained, and $Paco_2$ falls to the level of the apneic threshold.[28] At this point, overt periodic breathing occurs with cycle times of 15 to 25 seconds (two to five large tidal-volume breath clusters followed by apneas of 5–15 seconds).[2,41-43] There is wide variation in O_2 during this time. The predominant mechanism is increased loop gain manifested as a reduced $Paco_2$ reserve (1–2 mm Hg) with increased chemosensitivity (Figure 125.2).[26,44] The marked increase in arousals and decrease in slow wave sleep potentiate respiratory instability. Key role of narrowed CO_2 reserve manifested as hypocapnia in this disorder is reflected by improvement with administration of small amounts of CO_2 (increase in $Paco_2$ reserve),[45] increasing dead space (increase in $Paco_2$ reserve),[46] and acetazolamide (reduction in plant gain and increase in $Paco_2$ reserve).[47]

Primary Central Sleep Apnea. Primary (idiopathic) CSA is a rare disorder characterized by repetitive episodes of central apneas in NREM sleep, which are short and irregular (rather than periodic) and terminate with an abrupt, large breath (Figure 125.4), in contrast to CSA-CSB. The most clearly demonstrated pathophysiology is an increased hypercapnic ventilatory response during wakefulness.[26,33] In addition, impairment of switching between expiration and inspiration has been found in these patients.[48] It has been speculated that the long expiratory pause that typically occurs with these CSA events may be attributable to this impairment.

Other Nonhypercapnic Central Sleep Apnea Syndromes and Their Associated Medical Conditions. Common chronic medical conditions such as end-stage renal disease (ESRD),[49] cerebrovascular accident (CVA), and pulmonary hypertension have been associated with nonhypercapnic CSA. In patients with ESRD, the central apnea index (CAI, or frequency of central apneas) inversely correlates with $Paco_2$ and cardiac silhouette enlargement,[50] and ultrafiltration increases $Paco_2$ with an associated decline in the CAHI by 55%.[6]

CSB occurs in 7% to 12% of patients after CVA.[51,52] Although in many cases post-CVA, the CSB is associated with left ventricular dysfunction and hypocapnia,[53] some authors note an increased prevalence of CSB in patients with lacunar strokes (≈20%) and without left ventricular dysfunction.[54] CSA and CSB have been reported in patients with idiopathic pulmonary arterial hypertension (PAH), and CSA is independently associated with pulmonary hypertension in epidemiologic studies.[55] The postulated mechanisms include decreased stroke volume and increased mixing gain,[56] although, as in the case of CVA, no PAH-specific studies have been done.

Hypercapnic Central Sleep Apnea

Hypoventilation resulting from a failed or failing automatic control (and effector) system is the pathophysiologic hallmark of disorders that manifest with hypercapnic CSA. They can be

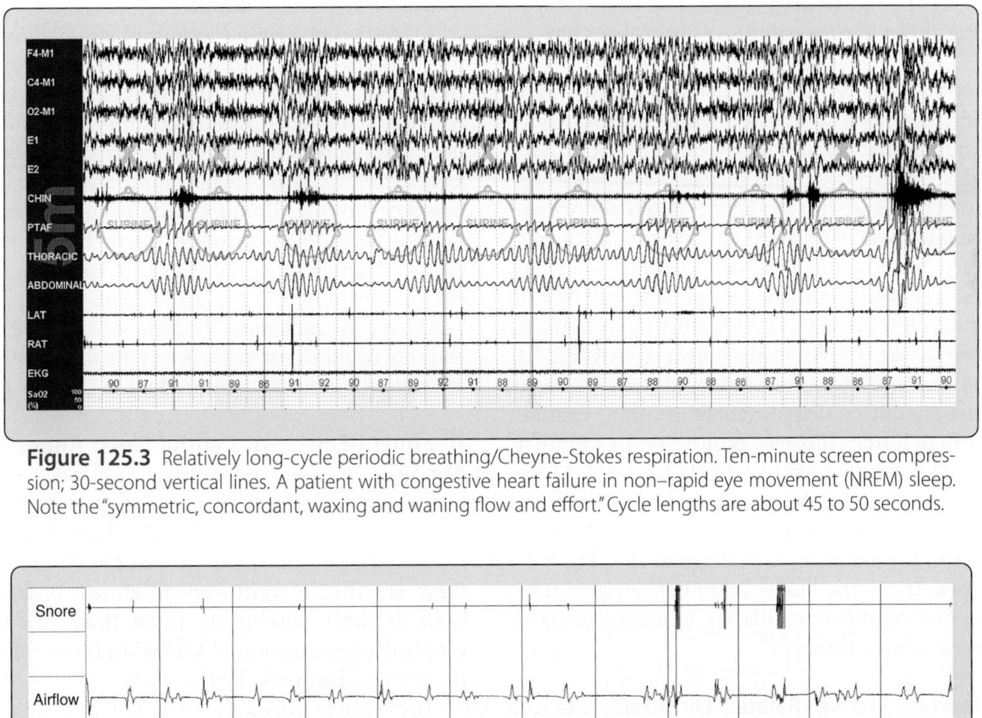

Figure 125.3 Relatively long-cycle periodic breathing/Cheyne-Stokes respiration. Ten-minute screen compression; 30-second vertical lines. A patient with congestive heart failure in non–rapid eye movement (NREM) sleep. Note the "symmetric, concordant, waxing and waning flow and effort." Cycle lengths are about 45 to 50 seconds.

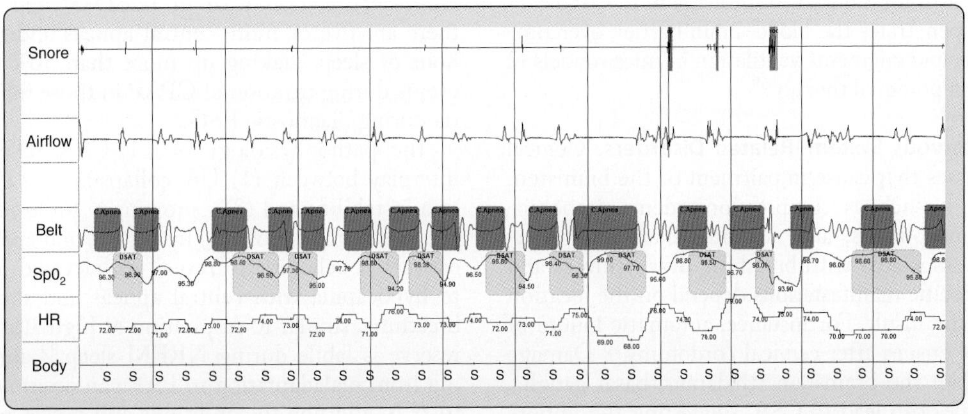

Figure 125.4 Idiopathic sleep apnea. A home sleep study on a medication-free, 27-year-old, nonobese man presenting with mild daytime sleepiness (Epworth Sleepiness Scale 9/24), nocturnal awakenings, and unrefreshing sleep. Note the short cycles (about 20 seconds) of pure central respiratory events.

broadly approached as disorders of impaired central drive ("*won't* breathe") or impaired respiratory muscle control ("*can't* breathe"). In general, the former category is the result of processes involving the brainstem respiratory centers (e.g., congenital central alveolar hypoventilation syndrome), whereas the latter is the result of neuromuscular weakness disorders (e.g., amyotrophic lateral sclerosis). Most of these disorders are associated with pathologically *low* loop gain (either because of controller or plant components) and worsening of hypoventilation and apneas during REM sleep (in contrast to hypocapnic CSA, which is NREM-dominant). The latter occurs primarily because of intercostal muscle atonia during REM. Most of these conditions are classified under the sleep-related hypoventilation disorders in the ICSD-3.

Congenital Central Alveolar Hypoventilation Syndrome and Idiopathic Central Alveolar Hypoventilation. Congenital alveolar central hypoventilation syndrome (CCHS, or Ondine curse) is a rare disorder of respiratory control and autonomic systems first reported by Mellins in the 1970s.[57] Small tidal volumes and monotonous respiratory rates result in hypoventilation, and the wakefulness and behavioral stimuli supply the respiratory drive. With sleep onset, worsened hypoventilation, hypercapnia, and hypoxemia ensue because of the impaired automatic control system. In many cases, if not identified early, this leads to asphyxia and death.[57] Mutations of the *PHOX2B* gene are disease-defining.[58] This gene encodes a transcription factor responsible for the fate of early autonomic nervous system cells, including those in the respiratory control centers.[59]

Obesity Hypoventilation Syndrome ("Pickwickian Syndrome"). A clinical diagnosis of obesity hypoventilation syndrome (OHS) requires that obesity (body mass index [BMI] ≥30 kg/m^2) and daytime hypoventilation ($Paco_2$ >45 mm Hg) be present without other causes for the latter.[58] PSG abnormalities include progressive hypoventilation and hypoxemia during REM sleep and further impairment in NREM sleep.[60] Mechanisms are complex and insufficiently investigated in the face of the obesity epidemic. They include (1) ventilatory abnormalities of obstructive sleep apnea (OSA, nearly universal in OHS[21]), (2) obesity-related changes in the respiratory system (reduced lung volumes, impediment of diaphragmatic motion, ventilation/perfusion mismatch from intrinsic positive end-expiratory pressure),[61,62] and (3) blunted chemosensitivity (decreased loop gain).[63-65] Resistance to leptin, a hormone produced by adipocytes that normally augments ventilatory response to $Paco_2$, is a possible mechanism for reduced controller gain in OHS.[66-68] Intranasal leptin penetrates the blood–brain barrier, overcoming this resistance, and augments ventilation in mice models of OHS, suggesting a potential therapy.[69]

Other Central Nervous System–Related Disorders. Central neurologic processes that cause impairment of the brainstem respiratory centers, such as compression, edema, ischemia, infarct, tumor, encephalitis, and Arnold-Chiari malformations, have been associated with breathing dysrhythmias and CSA.[70-79] The specific manifestations depend on the location and the type of the insult. For instance, automatic failure of breathing control ensues after cervical cordotomy.[80] Damage to areas other than the brainstem (thalamus, basal ganglia, centrum semiovale) can lead to CSA, suggesting the importance of the descending signals for generation of the automatic breathing stimulus.[81]

Peripheral Nerve and Muscle Disorders. Neuromuscular diseases, such as muscular dystrophy, myasthenia gravis, Guillain-Barre syndrome, amyotrophic lateral sclerosis, postpolio syndrome, and Charcot-Marie-Tooth disease, can lead to awake alveolar hypoventilation, with worsening hypoventilation during sleep. This is occasionally associated with central apneas, although sleep-related hypoventilation without outright central apnea is the more prominent feature. Ventilation during sleep in patients with respiratory muscle disease often deteriorates well before awake ventilation is affected.

Disintegrative Central Sleep Apnea and Hypoventilation Associated with Opiates. Although the respiratory depressant effects of opioids are well known, the effects of opiates on sleep are widespread and complex.[55] With chronic use, hypoventilation and obstructive and central apneas can occur in a single patient, fulfilling diagnostic criteria for several disorders under the ICSD-3 classification. Two unique patterns of breathing tend to occur in patients taking chronic opioids: (1) cluster breathing characterized by cycles of deep breaths with relatively stable tidal volumes, with interspersed central apneas of variable duration and (2) Biot breathing (ataxic breathing) with variable tidal volumes and rates.[82] In addition, patients taking chronic opioids with nearly pure OSA on initial PSG evaluation can develop TE-CSA.[2] In chronic opioid use, there is also a high prevalence of obstructive events and nocturnal hypoventilation.

Of the various opioid receptors, stimulation of μ and κ receptors tends to drive respiratory depression,[83] primarily in the pre-Bötzinger complex.[8,84] At low doses, tidal volumes decline,[85] whereas at higher doses, respiratory rate and rhythm generation are suppressed.[86] Morphine given to normal human subjects acutely decreases hypercapnic and hypoxic controller gain[8]; however, chronic administration results in decreased hypercapnic but increased hypoxemic chemosensitivity.[87] Mechanisms of ataxic breathing (Figure 125.5), common among those taking chronic opioids (nearly 70%) and those taking higher doses (>200 mg of morphine[88]), have not been elucidated. Similar features could occur with injury to the carotid bodies, such as after head and neck chemoradiation (Figure 125.6).

Treatment-Emergent Central Sleep Apnea ("Complex Sleep Apnea"). In some patients with OSA, central apneas and periodic breathing "emerge" during initiation of continuous positive airway pressure (CPAP). This phenomenon is termed *treatment-emergent CSA* in ICSD-3[4] and is defined when there are five or more central apneas and/or hypopneas per hour of sleep, making up more than 50% of all respiratory events during titration of CPAP in those fulfilling OSA criteria during diagnostic PSG.

The pathophysiology of TE-CSA reflects a disordered interplay between (1) UA collapsibility, (2) ventilatory system instability, and (3) a propensity for arousals. The relief of UA obstruction provided by CPAP, oral appliance, or tracheostomy is believed to "reveal" an elevated loop gain leading to hypocapnia with central apneas and short-cycle periodic breathing, similar to respiration at high altitude.[16] The $Paco_2$ reserve is labile during NREM sleep,[89] and arousals resulting from maladaptation to PAP can occur and drive instability.[90] In addition to conditions and processes predisposing to CSA in general, OSA severity may play a role in raising loop gain, as prevalence of TE-CSA is higher among patients with

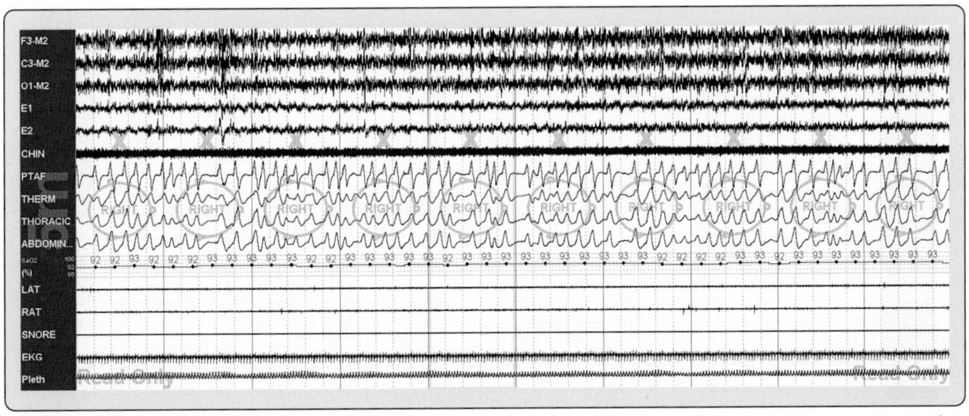

Figure 125.5 Opiate-induced central sleep apnea and ataxic breathing. Ten-minute screen compression; each vertical line is 30 seconds. A methadone-treated 56-year-old woman. The most characteristic feature of opiate-related disease is the variability in expiratory duration, although tidal volumes also vary. These polysomnographic features are readily recognizable and occur in non–rapid eye movement (NREM) sleep.

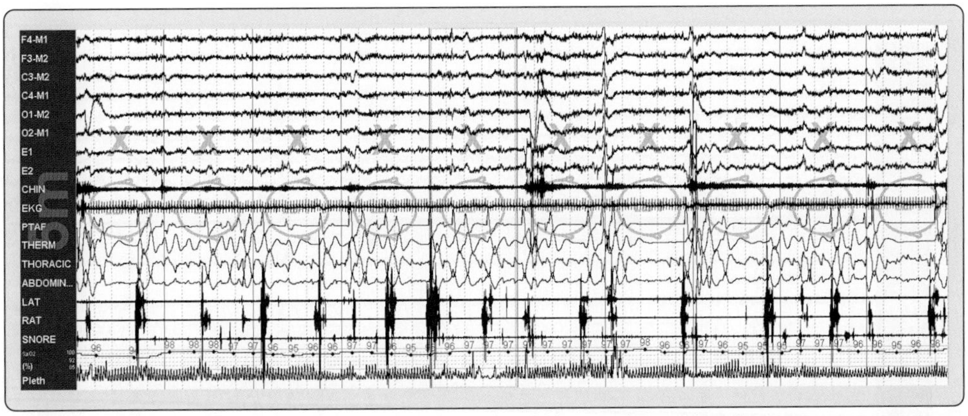

Figure 125.6 Central sleep apnea associated with head-neck chemoradiation. Ten-minute screen compression; each vertical line is 30 seconds. A 71-year-old man treated with radiation and platinum-based chemotherapy for laryngeal cancer. He presented with severe insomnia, multiple nocturnal arousals, and daytime fatigue. Note the variable-duration central apneas, mixed features, and sleep fragmentation.

severe versus mild OSA. Additional proposed contributors include CO_2 washout (i.e., anatomic dead-space reduction) with effective PAP or leak[14] and overactivation of lung stretch receptors with PAP therapy (particularly at higher pressures),[91] although TE-CSA also occurs at low pressures (5–8 cm of water). Evidence showing elevated loop gain and easy arousability (low arousal threshold) are key pathophysiologic traits of OSA[92,93] and support the notion that OSA and CSA exist on a phenotypic spectrum and in some cases of unstable chemoreflex and arousability can drive SDB.

The term "complex sleep apnea" refers to the pathophysiologic coexistence of obstructive and nonobstructive pathophysiologic components, essentially high–loop gain OSA.[94] TE-CSA is an outcome of targeting the UA alone in patients with high–loop gain OSA. A similar pattern may be seen whenever overventilation occurs, such as excessive CPAP or bilevel ventilation. The key feature of complex apnea and TE-CSA is NREM-dominant central hypopneas or periodic breathing with obstruction (Figure 125.7), resolving spontaneously during REM sleep. NREM dominance may be readily seen during positive pressure titration (Figure 125.8). Publications use, and insurance coverage criteria require, conversion of OSA to CSA by stringent conventional criteria.[95] In these patients, short-cycle (≤30 seconds) periodic breathing can occur, with features of admixed obstruction, which is highly reminiscent of high-altitude periodic breathing.[95]

A consistent feature of patients with treatment-emergent or complex sleep apnea is sleep fragmentation, which often persists despite reasonable respiration-targeted therapy. Because arousals amplify hypocapnic instability, inadequate cohesion of the NREM sleep–related network activity seems to be the core pathology in some of these patients. This phenomenon is reminiscent of reports of CHF patients in whom sleep fragmentation persists beyond that attributable to respiratory events.[96]

A pertinent question is whether the findings of the treatment-emergent or complex sleep apnea phenotype persist with continuous use of CPAP. Lack of persistence may imply that it is simply a marker of the severity of OSA and the dynamics of its improvement, or it may reflect an artifact of scoring approaches that ignore or misidentify central hypopneas (see the Definitions section). Some studies report resolution in 78% to 86% of patients[97,98] with 2 to 12 months of CPAP treatment, whereas others note treatment success rates of about 50%.[99] In the largest prospective study (n = 675) by Cassel and colleagues,[100] the prevalence was 12% at 3 months follow-up, when defined as CAI greater than or equal to 5/hour or predominant periodic breathing pattern on effective CPAP (obstructive AHI <5 /hour). Importantly, there are

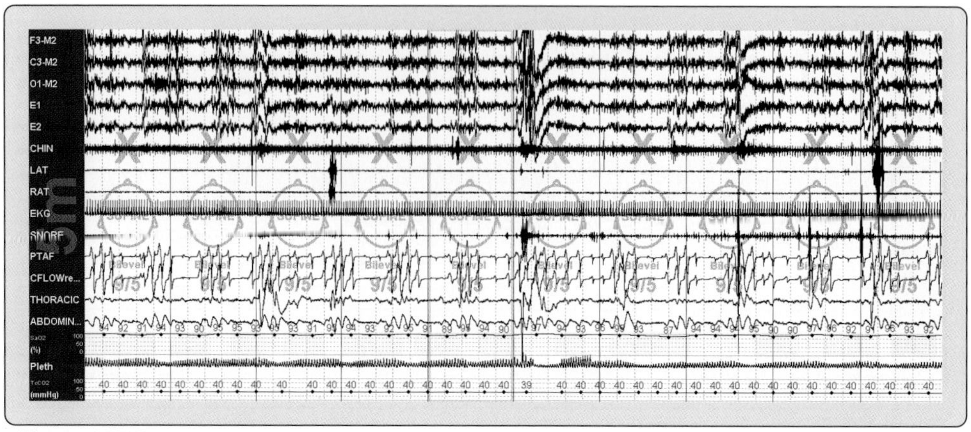

Figure 125.7 Key feature of non–rapid eye movement (NREM)-dominant apnea. Ten-minute screen compression; each vertical line is 30 seconds. Periodic breathing with short cycles (30 seconds or less) with variable degrees of obstruction. Conventional scoring typically identifies these events as "obstructive." Flow limitation is often seen, but the waxing-waning characteristic is usually evident.

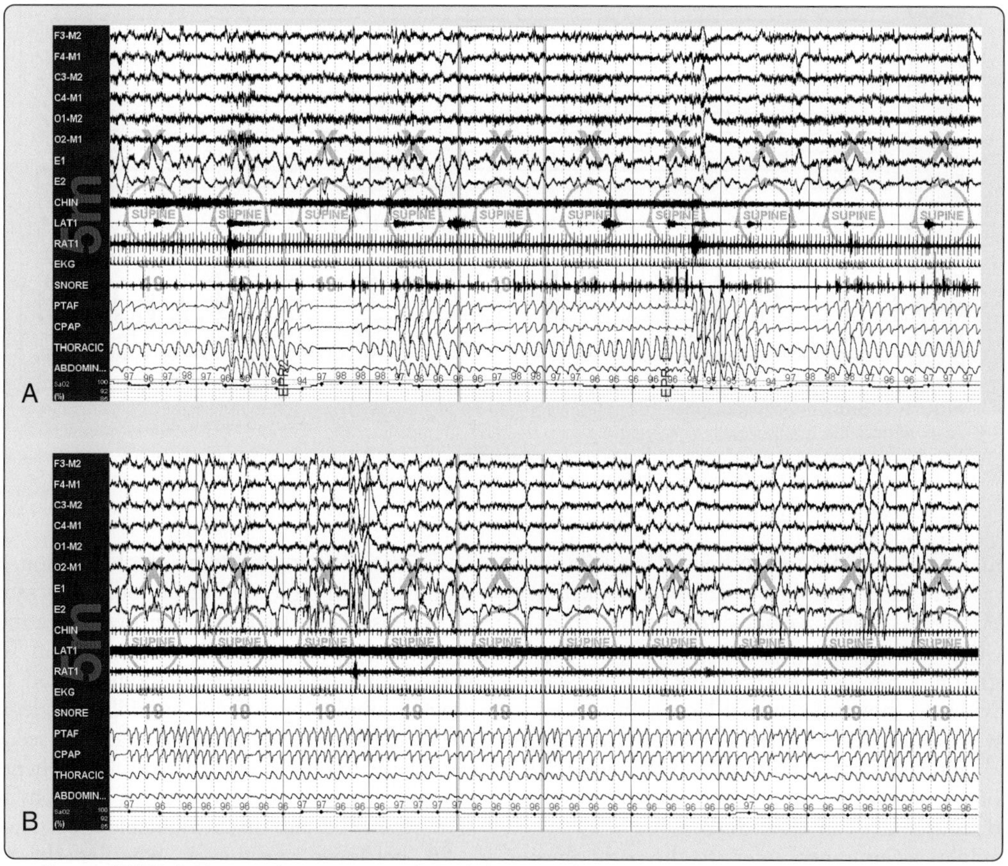

Figure 125.8 **A,** Non-rapid eye movement (NREM)-dominant sleep apnea; continuous positive airway pressure (CPAP) during NREM sleep. Ten-minute screen compression; each vertical line is 30 seconds. Unresolved respiratory events across a range of CPAP pressures (5–19 cm), with long cycle events, some periodic breathing features, and clear obstructive features. **B,** NREM-dominant sleep apnea during rapid eye movement (REM) sleep. Ten-minute screen compression; each vertical line is 30 seconds. The same subject as in **(A),** with spontaneous transition to REM sleep showing resolution of all abnormality. The CPAP pressures were progressively reduced to 10 cm with continued maintenance of stable breathing in REM sleep.

three trajectories of TE-CSA: resolution, persistence, or late emergence.[101] Cassel found that among those who had TE-CSA on initial titration or at 3 months follow-up, it resolved in 57%, persisted in 20%, and emerged during 3 months in 23%.[100] These findings are remarkably similar to a retrospective analysis of U.S. PAP telemonitoring data in 133,000 patients of which 3.5% were found to have CAI greater than or equal to 5/hour at baseline.[102] Resolution occurred in 55%, persistence in 25%, and late emergence in 20%. A key limitation of the latter study is the likely underestimation of overall prevalence resulting from a lack of central hypopnea scoring and reliance on device-generated metrics.

One approach to quantifying the persistence of TE-CSA is to measure residual respiratory events after several months of

Table 125.2 Clinical Characteristics of Patients with Sleep Apnea

Central		Obstructive
Nonhypercapnic	Hypercapnic	
Insomnia	Daytime sleepiness Morning headache	Daytime sleepiness
Mild intermittent snoring	Snoring	Prominent snoring
Awakenings (choking/ dyspnea)	Respiratory failure	Witnessed apneas/ gasping
Normal body habitus	Normal or obese	Commonly obese
	Polycythemia	Upper airway narrowing
	Cor pulmonale	

CPAP use, using the flow data available in current-generation devices. In a study of 217 patients after an average of 6 months of CPAP therapy, the manually scored AHI_{FLOW} of greater than or equal to 10/hour of use was seen in 23%, and the CAI at the baseline sleep study was the only predictor of residual disease.[103]

The predominant role of the CO_2 control instability in pathogenesis of treatment-emergent or complex sleep apnea is supported by resolution with small increases of inhaled CO_2.[104,105] The mechanisms for improvement in chemoreflex events after prolonged use of CPAP include reduction in controller gain and increase in $Paco_2$ reserve.[106] Stabilizing central respiratory motor output via prevention of transient hypocapnia (see Treatment of Central Sleep Apnea) prevents most cases of OSA in selected patients with a high chemosensitivity and a collapsible upper airway, whereas increasing respiratory motor output through moderate hypercapnia eliminates "obstructive" apnea in most patients with a wider range of chemosensitivity and CO_2 reserve.[107] Recent experiments suggest that in those with elevated loop gain and mild UA collapsibility, reducing chemosensitivity through hyperoxia may be effective.[104,108]

Epidemiology of Central Sleep Apnea and Its Subtypes

This topic is discussed in detail in Chapter 124. The epidemiology data for CSA are largely based on standard AASM definitions of respiratory events in sleep[108] and may underestimate the prevalence of CSA. This is largely the result of the inability to effectively distinguish central from obstructive hypopneas without esophageal manometry, leading to classification bias toward obstructive SDB (see Definitions section).

As alternative measures for detecting centrally mediated SDB are developed and automated, CSA prevalence may rise. For example, central apneas, periodic breathing, and CSB are patterns that suggest chemoreflex-mediated respiratory control dysfunction.[109] A biomarker of heightened chemoreflex activity (narrow-band elevated low-frequency coupling [$e\text{-}LFC_{NB}$]) has been described using an electrocardiogram-based analysis of heart rate variability and heart rate/respiratory coupling. This metric quantifies the metronomic self-similar oscillations that characterize nonhypercapnic CSA and periodic breathing.[110] One-third of a large, community-based patient cohort with SDB (the Sleep Heart Health Study) exhibited the $e\text{-}LFC_{NB}$, which is associated with CSA and periodic breathing.[111] This proportion is roughly in keeping with detailed phenotyping experiments performed over the years,[94,112] as detailed in Chapter 129.

Clinical Features and Diagnosis of Central Sleep Apnea and Its Subtypes

Clinical Presentation

The clinical presentation of patients with CSA varies by the etiology and subtype (Table 125.2). Symptoms and signs are not specific to CSA per se and often overlap with those of OSA, in addition to the underlying conditions leading to CSA (e.g., dyspnea on awakening in patients with heart failure[113]).

Polysomnographic Features Important in Central Sleep Apnea

Diagnosis of CSA syndromes generally requires a full night recording of standard PSG, with special attention to inspiratory effort, to differentiate central (no inspiratory effort throughout event) from obstructive apneas. Although this differentiation is simple for apneas, for hypopneas, it requires esophageal manometry.[114,115] Respiratory inductance plethysmography excursions are present in both central and obstructive hypopneas, and determining whether decreases in effort and flow are proportionate can be arbitrary and difficult to operationalize.[116] Finally, cardiopulmonary coupling signal analysis, as described previously, and nasal pressure/electrocardiogram (ECG) signal estimated loop gain analyses[15] may also be used to differentiate central predominant (chemoreflex driven) from obstructive SDB phenotypes,[117] but require clinical validation.

A consistent feature of nonhypercapnic, heightened, chemoreflex-mediated central apnea and hypopnea is the predominance of events during NREM sleep, especially during non-slow wave sleep stages.[27,110,118-122] Flow limitation can occur because of a fluctuating neural drive to the UA, which makes applying conventional scoring criteria challenging. A metronomic self-similar appearance is typical, in contrast to opiate-induced CSA, in which variability of the expiratory phase is characteristic. Additional features of chemoreflex modulation during sleep are noted in Table 125.3. In contrast, in many cases of hypercapnic CSA (and in OSA), the severity of SDB worsens markedly during REM sleep, especially if the motor neurons of the diaphragm are involved.[2,123] Notable exceptions are CCHS and opioid-induced CSA, in which SDB worsens in NREM sleep. Finally, objective measures of hypoventilation are needed, such as arterial, transcutaneous, or end-tidal Pco_2 (P_{ETCO_2}) to confirm hypercapnia in sleep.[119]

Propensity for sleep fragmentation and UA collapsibility can both worsen CSA and have specific treatment implications (see Treatment of Central Sleep Apnea). A sleep fragmentation phenotype on PSG can be suggested by prolonged sleep-wake transitional instability (>10 minutes), low sleep efficiency (<70%), persistently high N1 stage during PAP titration (>15%), and poor evolution of slow wave sleep (< 1 Hz).[16] UA collapsibility can be measured by P_{crit}, derived from relationships between maximal inspiratory airflow and

Table 125.3 Recognition of Strong Chemoreflex Modulation of Sleep Breathing[259]

Polysomnographic Feature	Relatively Pure Obstructive Sleep Apnea	Chemoreflex-Modulated Sleep Apnea
Periodic breathing, Cheyne-Stokes	Rare	Typical (often short cycle, <30 seconds in absence of CHF)
Respiratory event timing	Variable (each event tends to have different durations)	Self-similar/metronomic
Severity during sleep state	Greater severity in REM	Minimal severity in REM
Effort signal morphology	Well maintained during obstructed breath	Complete or partial loss between recovery breaths
Flow-effort relationship	Discordant: flow is reduced disproportionately to reduction in effort	Concordant: flow and effort follow each other in amplitude
Arousal timing	Early part of event termination	Crests event, often in the center of the sequence of recovery breaths
Oxygen desaturation	Irregular, progressive drops, V-shaped contour	Smooth, symmetric, progressive drops rare

CHF, Congestive heart failure; REM, rapid eye movement.

nasal or mask pressure in OSA patients,[94,118] or estimated from clinical titration, with equal to or less than 8.0 cm water therapeutic pressures predicting mild UA collapsibility.[124] Noninvasive methods of estimating a low arousal threshold (sleep apnea trait associated with sleep fragmentation), UA collapsibility, and loop gain from routine clinical PSG have been developed,[125,126] and studies on prediction of treatment responsiveness are ongoing. A detailed description of SDB phenotyping can be found in Chapters 128 and 129.

Because of the challenges in diagnosing CSA without esophageal manometry, we recommend taking into account an array of the PSG features to distinguish between central and obstructive phenotypes, as described previously (and in Table 125.3). Such an approach, combined with complementary measures of chemoreflex hyperactivity (e.g., cardiopulmonary coupling analysis, loop gain estimates [Chapter 129]) and identification of propensity for sleep fragmentation and airway collapsibility (Chapter 129), can augment recognition of and treatment of CSA. Identifying a mildly collapsible airway or high loop gain/low arousal threshold would help identify patients who are more likely to respond to drugs targeting these pathogenic mechanisms.

Unique Features of the Disorders

Nonhypercapnic Central Sleep Apnea

Heart Failure and Central Sleep Apnea. Clinical features, implications, and treatment of central apneas in CHF are discussed in detail in Chapters 140 and 149. In brief, age older than 60 years, male sex, atrial fibrillation, diuretic use, and daytime hypocapnia appear to be risk factors for CSA among those with CHF.[127,128] Patients generally present with CHF symptoms, fatigue, and weakness rather than sleepiness.[114,129-131] Symptoms and apneas improve with position changes, including lateral positioning, and are independent of the postural effects on the upper airway,[132] suggesting that J-receptor activation or oxygen stores play a role in the pathogenesis of CSA-CSB. Arousals occur midcycle at the peak of the recovery.[133]

Central Sleep Apnea at High Altitude. Travelers to high altitudes often experience restlessness, frequent brief arousals, and unrefreshing sleep[134] at least in part because of periodic breathing and CSA (see Chapter 141). Men are twice as likely to be affected as women, and at altitudes above 5000 feet it is nearly universal. PSG features are discussed in the section Pathophysiology of Central Sleep Apnea Syndromes that Affect Diagnosis and Treatment.

Primary Central Sleep Apnea. Patients with primary CSA often present with insomnia or frequent awakenings during the night, rather than daytime sleepiness, as seen in OSA.[42,135] Cycles of central apneas in idiopathic CSA are shorter (20–40 seconds) and not as gradual as in CSA with CSB (CSA-CSB; see Pathophysiology of Central Sleep Apnea Syndromes that Affect Diagnosis and Treatment). Underlying medical conditions must be ruled out before diagnosis.

Other Medical Conditions Associated with Central Sleep Apnea. CSA is also found in patients with ESRD, CVA, PAH, and atrial fibrillation. There are no particular clinical features with high predictive value for CSA among these patients (hypocapnia may be a clue); thus diagnosis requires heightened clinical suspicion and PSG.

Patients with ESRD and CSA (concomitant obstructive and mixed apneas are common) are generally male, older, and more frequently volume overloaded.[136,137] Ultrafiltration improves Pa_{CO_2} and CAHI,[138] suggesting an initial avenue for the management of CSA in ESRD. Higher suspicion for CSA is also warranted in those with larger territory and more severe CVAs.[51,55] Patterns of CSA include CSB with long cycle times in CVA patients with left ventricular dysfunction and periodic breathing with shorter cycle lengths in those without left ventricular dysfunction.[139-141] Although some studies suggest CSA resolution as patients recover from their stroke,[142,143] more recent data suggests persistence[144]; therefore monitoring is prudent. In patients with PAH, older age and sleepiness (Epworth Sleepiness Scale [ESS] score of >10) are predictive of SDB,[145] and CSB is the predominant CSA pattern, with a cycle of about 45 seconds. The presence of atrial fibrillation should raise suspicion for CSA and vice versa.[146-149] In community cohorts, increasing CAI correlates with increasing prevalence, and incidence of atrial fibrillation and presence of CSA-CSB is associated with an odds ratios of 2.0 to 4.5 for new atrial fibrillation, even when controlled for cardiac comorbidities, including CHF.[148,150,151]

Hypercapnic Central Sleep Apnea

Hypercapnic CSA and hypoventilation should be considered if a condition associated with them (Table 125.1) or certain clinical features (Table 125.3) are present. A PSG and an assessment of sleep hypoventilation through nocturnal $Paco_2$ (or surrogate) are recommended. In cases in which hypercapnic CSA and hypoventilation are discovered during a PSG obtained for another indication (e.g., OSA), a careful clinical approach to identify the underlying cause is warranted. Our initial assessment is based on locating the lesion along an anatomic pathway that could result in hypoventilation: corticobulbar tracts, brainstem, bulbospinal tracts to cervical spinal cord, anterior horn cells, lower motor neurons, neuromuscular junction, and diaphragmatic muscles. Lung and chest wall abnormalities are generally apparent on examination, and basic diagnostic studies can help identify the underlying medical disorder (e.g., chronic obstructive pulmonary disease) in those with hypercapnic CSA and hypoventilation. Selected conditions are discussed next.

Congenital Central Alveolar Hypoventilation Syndrome. The classic feature of presentation for CCHS is mild awake and marked sleep-related alveolar hypoventilation with hypercapnia and hypoxemia (Figure 125.9). Although usually diagnosed at birth, some patients can present as late onset in childhood or even in adulthood because of variable penetrance of the *PHOX2B* mutations (polyalanine repeat mutations [PARMs]).[152-156] In these individuals, alveolar hypoventilation can be unmasked by administration of central nervous system (CNS) depressants and anesthetics or recent severe pulmonary infections. CCHS should also be considered in those without another explanation for hypoventilation or parents of those with CCHS.[157,158] Clinical associations that should raise suspicion for CCHS include Hirschsprung disease, tumors of neural crest origin, autonomic dysfunction, facial dysmorphology, and dermatographism.[59,159,160] The ventilatory response and sensation of dyspnea are greatly diminished or absent in children with CCHS.[161] The respiratory pattern during sleep

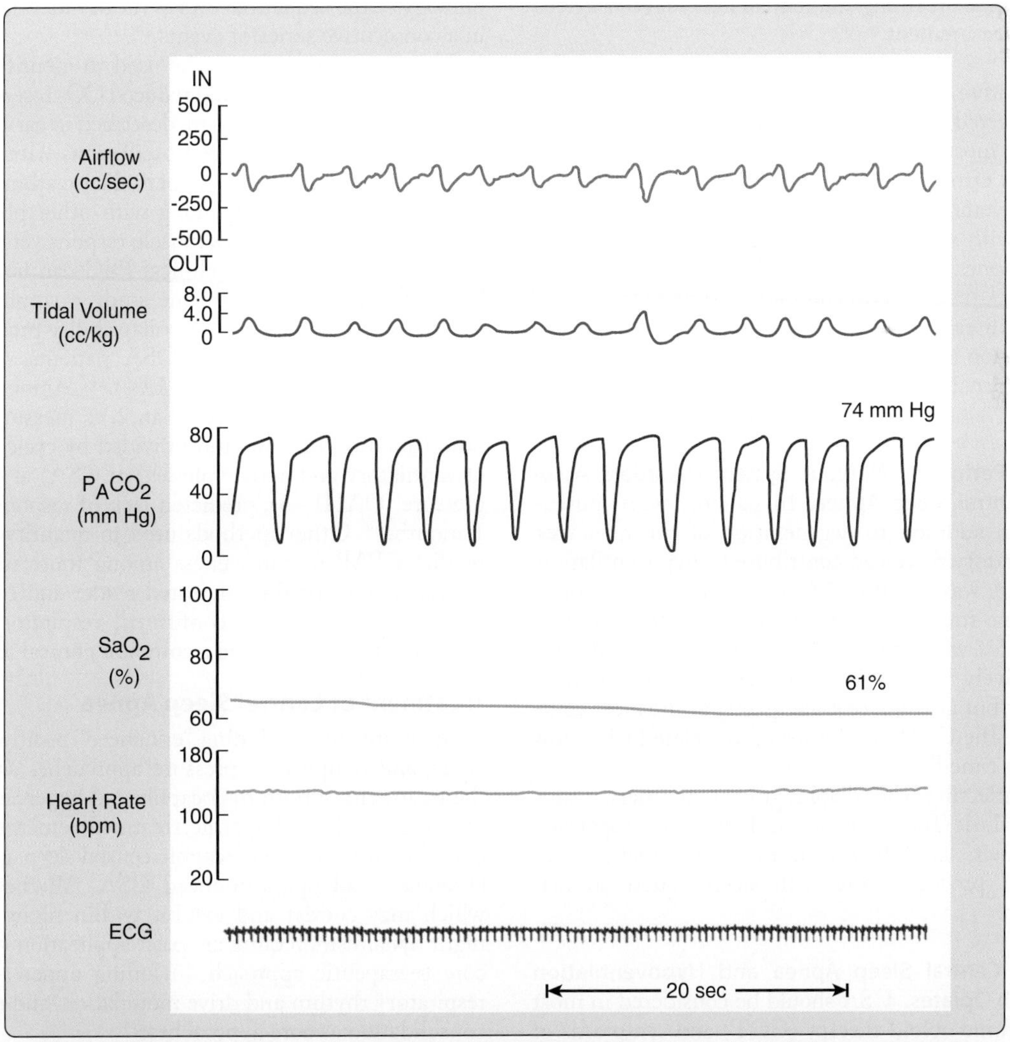

Figure 125.9 Congenital central hypoventilation. Polygraph tracing from 28-month-old girl demonstrating typical breathing pattern during non–rapid eye movement (NREM) sleep in congenital central alveolar hypoventilation syndrome (CCHS). Note inappropriately regular (20 breaths per minute), shallow breathing (tidal volumes averaging 3.5 mL/kg). Progressive hypercapnia and hypoxemia did not stimulate ventilation, arousal, or beat-to-beat heart rate variability. (Adapted with permission from Weese-Mayer et al.[9])

is characterized by markedly diminished tidal volumes and inappropriately constant respiratory rate in the face of hypercapnia and hypoxemia.[9,162] Ventilation is more stable during REM versus NREM sleep. There are variations in clinical phenotype with PARM genotype. For example, individuals with 20/25 (normal alanine repeat genotype being designated as 20/20) rarely require 24-hour ventilatory support, whereas for genotypes 20/27 to 20/33, continuous ventilatory support is needed.[163-165] Care for patients with CCHS should be provided through centers with extensive expertise in the condition, as children diagnosed early and managed effectively can achieve markedly improved quality of life as adults.[12,166]

Obesity Hypoventilation Syndrome. OHS is described in detail in Chapter 138. The diagnosis hinges on increased awake $Paco_2$ (>45 mm Hg) in the absence of other known causes of hypoventilation (e.g., chronic obstructive lung disease, restrictive lung disease) and obesity (BMI of ≥30 kg/m^2). A bicarbonate level of greater than or equal to 27 mEq/L has 92% sensitivity for $Paco_2$ greater than 45 mm Hg (specificity of 50%[167]) among those with OSA and, if present, $Paco_2$ measurement should be performed. Resting O_2 saturation of less than 94% while breathing ambient air also suggests a need for blood gas measurement.[60,168]

Neurodegenerative Disorders. CSA and hypoventilation should be suspected in patients with neurodegenerative disorders. They are most common in multiple sclerosis (MS) and multiple system atrophy (MSA).[7,169] Patients with MS with brainstem involvement manifest with central apneas, in contrast to those with nonbrainstem lesions and controls.[170] In MSA, central apneas, CSB, and apneustic breathing have all been reported.[171-173] CSA is uncommon in Alzheimer disease and Parkinson disease.[7,174-177] In amyotrophic lateral sclerosis, hypoventilation is the most common presenting feature of SDB, with nocturnal symptoms preceding daytime ventilatory failure.

Muscular and Peripheral Nervous System Disorders Associated with Central Sleep Apnea. In patients with muscular disorders, in addition to degeneration of the myocytes, impaired respiratory drive can contribute to hypoventilation. This abnormality was found in 20% of a myotonic dystrophy cohort.[178] In one study of 85 patients with myotonic dystrophy, 11% and 15% were found to have CSAs and mixed sleep apneas, respectively, with 39% having OSA.[179] These patients were not sleepy, but noted poor sleep quality as the most common symptom. The CAHI in this group correlated with slow oral swallowing time.[180]

Disorders affecting the diaphragm or its nerve supply (Charcot-Marie-Tooth disease and other neuropathies, myasthenia gravis, and other neuromuscular junction disorders) present predominantly with sleep-related alveolar hypoventilation.

Disintegrative Central Sleep Apnea and Hypoventilation Associated with Opiates. CSA should be considered in most patients on chronic opioid therapy (COT) and symptoms of disturbed sleep.[181] Pure opioid receptor agonists (e.g., methadone, oxycodone) and combinations of partial agonists and antagonists (i.e., buprenorphine and naloxone) result in significant SDB, both central and obstructive.[182] In those with CSA, case series suggest that there is increased sleep fragmentation, increased stage 2 sleep, and decreased REM and slow wave sleep,[183] consistent with NREM predominance of central events. CSA in COT can present during the initial PSG or emerge after treatment of predominantly obstructive disease (TE-CSA).[184] There is some consistency in published reports that decreased tolerance, efficacy (high residual sleep apnea), and compliance with CPAP are present in this setting of CSA (see Treatment of Central Sleep Apnea). Disintegrative CSA patterns may also be seen in patients with brainstem injury, such as with stroke and MS. Finally, hypoventilation is not unique to the use of opioids and can be seen with anesthetics, sedatives, and muscle relaxants.

Treatment-Emergent Central Sleep Apnea. Any therapy targeting UA obstruction (e.g., oral appliances) can trigger or unmask elevated chemoreflex activation, though it is most commonly described with continuous or nonadaptive bilevel PAP is increased to control airway obstruction in patients diagnosed with OSA.[83] The most useful feature enabling recognition is not the exact morphology of individual events, but rather the NREM sleep dominance and the timing and morphology of the sequential events (nearly identical, self-similar) in a consecutive series of events.[14,118,185]

Various techniques may be used to identify patients with heightened chemoreflex and reduced CO_2 reserve. Time-series analysis of electrocardiogram, described in earlier sections, can provide a map of state sleep oscillations with e-LFC_{NB} as a marker of central apneas and periodic breathing in those with TE-CSA.[108] Loop gain, along with other phenotypic traits in OSA (UA collapsibility, muscle responsiveness, and arousal threshold) assessed from clinical PSG can be helpful in tailoring therapy.[110,126,127] In one study, a combination of elevated loop gain and low UA collapsibility predicted response to supplemental oxygen in OSA patients with equivalent AHIs (Δ AHI of 59% versus 12%).[117] Among patients with TE-CSA, loop gain greater than 2, as measured by the duty ratio (duration of ventilation divided by cycle duration [sum of ventilatory and apneic phases] of CSA) at optimal CPAP pressure (OAHI <5), predicted lack of response to CPAP at 1 month.[186] Other methods used to quantify loop gain and predict CPAP responsiveness among those with CSA-CSB are referenced for the interested reader and can be found in Chapter 129.[187-190] If confirmed, respiratory chemoreflex phenotyping may become a common clinical reality.

Treatment of Central Sleep Apnea

Positive pressure, including "enhanced" positive pressure (see later), and nonpositive pressure approaches are available for the treatment of both hypocapnic and hypercapnic CSA syndromes, including idiopathic, treatment-emergent or complex, periodic breathing, hypercapnic central sleep apnea of various etiologies, and opiate-induced CSA. All these phenotypes, which may coexist and exhibit within night and night-to-night dynamism, require an exact application of a multimode core therapeutic approach, including upper airway support, respiratory rhythm and drive modulation, and enhanced sleep consolidation as core approaches.[34]

Positive Pressure–Based Therapy

AASM recommends CPAP as an initial option for CSA, based on the premise that UA obstruction is relevant for hypercapnic and nonhypercapnic types of CSA.[118] However, there are now enough data that demonstrate CPAP alone is poorly effective and tolerated in nonhypercapnic CSA syndromes, whereas adaptive servo ventilation (ASV) and enhanced CPAP (used with respiratory stabilization approaches that include hypocapnia minimization, sedatives, carbonic anhydrase inhibition, and oxygen) may be superior for suppression of central apneas and periodic breathing patterns on the PSG. Nonadaptive (fixed pressure) bilevel positive pressure ventilation alone is also suboptimal: this tends to exaggerate CSA and periodic breathing.[191] Although using a backup rate with fixed bilevel positive pressure ventilation can reduce central apneas as the machine-delivered mandatory breaths substitute for lack of patient-derived effort, comparative studies with ASV show the latter to achieve superior elimination of central apneas. Because individual adaptive ventilator algorithms are substantially different, specific patient subsets may have differential responses (e.g., short- versus long-cycle periodic breathing). Such individual differences in responses are currently not predictable from diagnostic PSG features.

ASV devices provide expiratory support, inspiratory pressure support, and backup supportive responses guided by measures of ventilation or flow averaged over several minutes. These devices are primarily designed for patients with elevated loop gain and thus nonhypercapnic CSA, but can be beneficial when hypoventilation is not the primary and sole abnormality. Opiate-induced CSA, for example, is difficult to treat with PAP, and ASV is superior, with one study showing a residual CAI of 20/hour and 0/hour on CPAP and ASV, respectively.[192] Although patients with opiate-induced CSA do not have classic periodic breathing and are characterized by ataxic breathing and central apneas of variable lengths, ASV devices can impose a rhythm in these individuals. When used in patients with TE-CSA and heart failure, central apneas are decreased in frequency, and numerous neurohumoral and cardiac function parameters are improved.[193,194] Muscle sympathetic activity is reduced by adaptive ventilation, but not CPAP, in patients with CHF and CSA-CSB.[195] ASV is better tolerated than CPAP by patients with TE-CSA, and switching from CPAP to ASV improves residual respiratory events, adherence, and sleepiness.[193,196,197] Positive effects on sleep architecture are less impressive. The criteria for success and the respiratory event scoring criteria (often 4% desaturation association for hypopneas) can overestimate effectiveness. A randomized prospective trial of CPAP versus ASV in TE-CSA used a success threshold of suppressing central AHI (essentially central apneas) below 10/hour of sleep as a criterion for success.[198] ASV was superior to CPAP in suppressing respiratory events and success was achieved in 90% versus 65% of participants treated with ASV versus CPAP, but sleep quality, sleepiness, and quality of life were not different between the groups. These findings raise the question about the best approach to quantify effectiveness beyond merely apnea suppression. Alternative indices such as variability of minute ventilation (ratio of 95th percentile to median ventilation) and delivered pressure, which correlate with clinical global improvement impressions, may provide useful information.[199] ASVs can also induce patient-ventilator asynchrony and therefore need to be carefully titrated with a focus on patient symptoms and quality of life. Cycle lengths likely influence outcomes, and it is our observation that ASVs are less effective in patients with short-cycle (≤30 seconds) periodic breathing. A subset of patients demonstrate immediate ASV intolerance and desynchrony, and this effect does not resolve with added time. Patients with prolonged sleep-wake transitional instability can have the pathology markedly amplified by an ASV. The normal fluctuations of respiration during REM sleep can inappropriately trigger the adaptive algorithms of ASVs and cause arousals, but this seems rare in clinical practice. Chapter 140 describes ASVs and their function in detail.

Recognition of Efficacy and Scoring of Respiratory Events During Adaptive Servo Ventilation Use

Scoring respiratory events during adaptive ventilation should use the pressure output signal from the ventilator. This is roughly equal and opposite to the patient's respiratory output. The flow and effort signals combine patient and ventilator contributions and give a false sense of success. See Figure 125.10 for excessive "pressure cycling," which is a response of an adaptive ventilator to ongoing periodic breathing. When

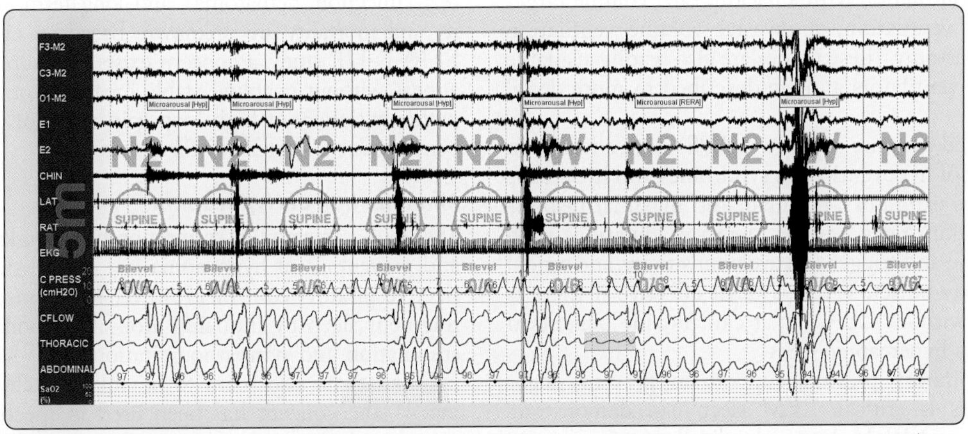

Figure 125.10 Pressure cycling during adaptive ventilation treatment. Ten-minute compression snapshot; 30-second vertical lines. The C-PRESS channel is the pressure output from the adaptive ventilator (Adapt SV). This 56-year-old man had predominantly central apneas, which were eliminated. However, respiratory instability, repetitive arousals, and pressure cycling continued without resolution, despite adjustments of pressure support. Persistent pressure cycling is readily recognized during home use by generating expanded night data using the device software, with attention to tidal volume and pressure traces. The device may not automatically detect respiratory events during such periods.

pressure cycling persists, sleep fragmentation can be severe even if respiration is "improved." This pattern means that periodic breathing pathology is ongoing, necessitating the continued pressure response. When the ventilator enables stable respiration, cycling between the minimal and maximal pressure support zones is minimal. Further details on algorithms and titration strategies may be obtained from comprehensive reviews[200,201] and in Chapter 140. Bench testing of ASV algorithms shows device-specific response characteristics, but stable breathing does not readily occur across a range of simulated central apnea patterns.[202]

ASVs are powerful devices, and if there is patient-ventilatory asynchrony, they can induce hypocapnia, excessive cycling of pressures, arousals, distorted flow patterns, and physical discomfort. Increased mortality through sudden cardiac death and no benefits, including in quality of life, were found in the SERVE-HF clinical trial comparing ASV with medical management in patients with systolic heart failure (ejection fraction ≤45%) and AHI >15/hour with 50% or more central events.[203] Those at highest risk had an ejection fraction of <30% and CSB occurring during >50% of the night.[198] Hypocapnia, metabolic alkalosis, hemodynamic perturbations, and excessive sympathetic driving associated with pressure cycling are speculative mechanisms of adverse outcomes.[204] It also remains unclear if the risk is related to the specific ASV device or ASVs in general.[205] While the results of another large trial on ASV therapy in CHF (ADVENT-HF)[206] are awaited, ASV use in patients with CHF with reduced ejection fraction should be avoided.[207] Caution is recommended in other vulnerable populations such as CHF with preserved ejection fraction and stroke. Tracking of device data such as tidal volume stability, degree of pressure cycling, and surrogate signs of patient-ventilator asynchrony (e.g., wide variations in expiratory durations), regardless of underlying disease state, and not relying on manufacturer-derived AHIs alone are prudent.

Considerations for the Treatment of Hypercapnic Central Sleep Apnea

Management of the sleep-related breathing disorders of the hypoventilation syndromes is a complex process; a few key points are noted here.[208] Respiratory support may be provided by bilevel ventilation with a backup rate, volume target pressure-support ventilation, or invasive volume ventilation through a tracheostomy. These modes are also readily available on several home ventilators and are described in more detail in Chapter 140.

Volume-assured pressure support (VAPS) is an advance in the management of hypoventilation syndromes and hypercapnic CSA. Besides expiratory, minimal, and maximal inspiratory support, backup rates, various breath modulations such as inspiratory time and trigger and cycle sensitivity, and a tidal volume target may be set. VAPS is most effective if there is hypoventilation without CSA, but it can provide benefits if used cautiously in hypercapnic CSA.

Sufficient expiratory pressure support to prevent major obstructive events is critical. REM sleep can demonstrate greater severity than NREM sleep and typically requires greater ventilation than NREM sleep. However, NREM dominance may also be seen, as in opiate-induced CSA. An autoexpiratory pressure function can aid in managing patients with markedly higher REM sleep settings. The backup rate is usually set slightly below the patient's native rate. However, if there is bradypnea (e.g., respiratory rate below 6 breaths/minute) or tachypnea (e.g., rate above 20 breaths/minute), entraining the patient to a different rate may be difficult and result in patient-ventilator desynchrony. Substantial inspiratory support (e.g., 25 cm H_2O) may be required to enable optimal ventilation.

Positive pressure ventilation therapy for hypercapnic CSA poses the specific challenge of inducing relative hypocapnia and respiratory instability and associated sleep fragmentation by overly aggressive ventilation.[209] There is a trade-off between improving ventilation and oxygenation versus sleep quality because excessive volume targets and the associated pressure rises can induce sleep fragmentation. The rate of change in pressure support can be prescribed in these devices, providing one form of "brake" to prevent pressure-related sleep fragmentation. In the absence of PSG titration, when sleep versus wake and NREM versus REM sleep treatment requirements are not estimated, treatment may be less precise than possible. An iterative approach of two or three PSG titrations with transcutaneous CO_2 monitoring, separated by a few months, can result in greater precision of therapy and sleep quality, allowing resetting of the respiratory controller.

Alternative Approaches to Positive Pressure Therapy

Phrenic Nerve Stimulation

Unilateral phrenic nerve stimulation activating the diaphragm during central apneas has been shown to markedly improve CAI and arousals in patients in CSA.[210,211] In a clinical trial of 151 individuals (64% with CHF) who underwent device implantation, stimulation versus no stimulation reduced the CAI by 23/hour and arousals by 15/hour, with improvements in oxygen saturation, sleep efficiency, REM sleep, and sleepiness (ESS increase of 3.4 units). Although a promising modality for relatively "pure CSA," caution in use is warranted for two reasons. First, patients included in the studies had minimal, if any, obstructive disease (OAHI <20/hour) and stimulation did not improve hypopneas or obstructive events (residual OHI 19.9/hour). Because many patients with CSA also exhibit obstructive SDB, and phrenic stimulation can induce upper airway occlusion,[212] careful patient selection or a combination of phrenic stimulation with pharyngeal stabilization (CPAP or mandibular advancement) are warranted. Second, 9% of patients experienced serious adverse events (e.g., infection, hematoma), and long-term effects on morbidity and mortality are unknown. Based on experience with the SERVE-HF study, a concern exists that suppression of central apneas without enabling stable breathing or targeting the core pathophysiology of high loop gain may not provide long-term benefits. See Chapter 149 for details.

Minimization of Hypocapnia

That CO_2 can stabilize respiration has been known for decades, and prevention of hypocapnia is a critical stabilizing factor in sleep respiratory control. However, high concentrations of CO_2 fragment sleep by inducing arousals secondary to respiratory stimulation and sympathoexcitation.[213,214] More modest CO_2 manipulations also seem to be able to stabilize sleep breathing.[214] The concept has been used in mechanical ventilation to reduce hypocapnia for several years and more recently has been successfully used to treat CSA-CSB in heart failure.[108] Combining hypocapnia minimization with positive pressure keeps CO_2 just above the apnea threshold, an approach called *enhanced expiratory rebreathing space (EERS).*[215] EERS consisted of 50 to 150 mL of tubing and a nonvented mask (dead space) added to PAP therapy, which markedly improved AHI and sleep efficiency (Figure 125.11). There is no or minimal increase in inspiratory CO_2 (increase in ET_{CO2} from 38 ± 3 to 39 ± 3 mm Hg) because of the positive pressure–induced washout. CO_2 manipulation can also be done by bleeding CO_2 into the circuit by a more precisely controlled flow-independent method. Successful treatment of mixed OSA and CSA using a proprietary investigational device, the positive airway pressure gas modulator (PAPGAM), has been reported.[105] Dynamic CO_2 manipulation (delivery restricted to a specific phase of the respiratory cycle) may, in future studies, improve the stabilizing effects of CO_2.[106]

Oxygen

Supplementary O_2 can reduce chemosensitivity and has a long history in treating CSA and periodic breathing without CSA.[216,217] Because hypoxic burden is a marker of mortality in patients with CHF and CSA-CSB, some propose that it may be particularly useful in those patients.[218,219] Small clinical trials show improvements in respiratory indices and patient function, but residual sleep apnea and sleep fragmentation are common.[217,220-222] Adding oxygen to CPAP may benefit CSA and TE-CSA by reducing responsiveness of peripheral chemoreceptors and loop gain.[192,223] A study in U.S. Veterans showed a 25% increase in reaching CAI below 5/hour using CPAP and

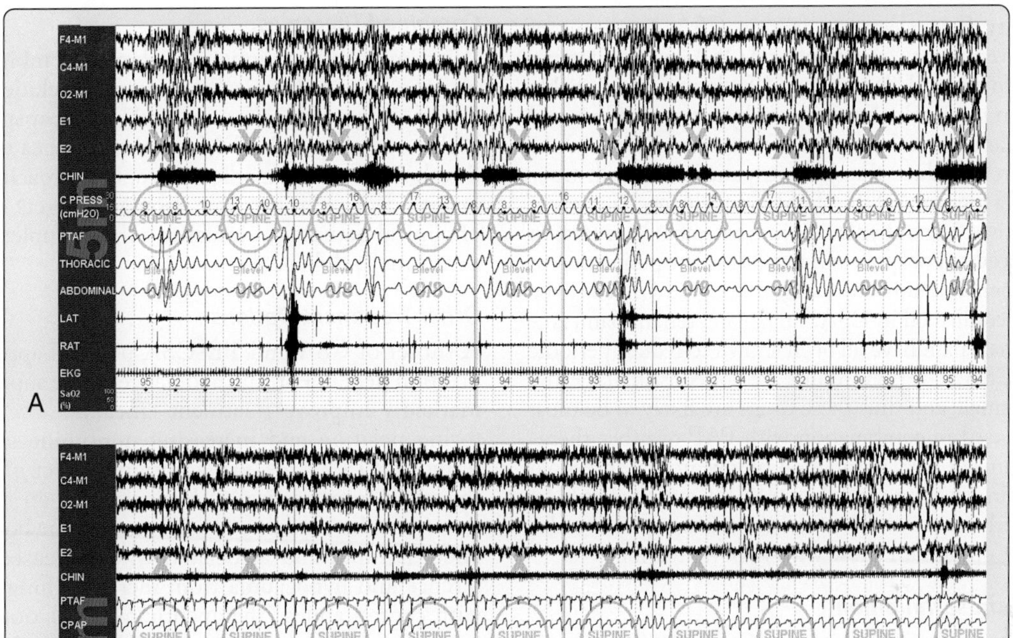

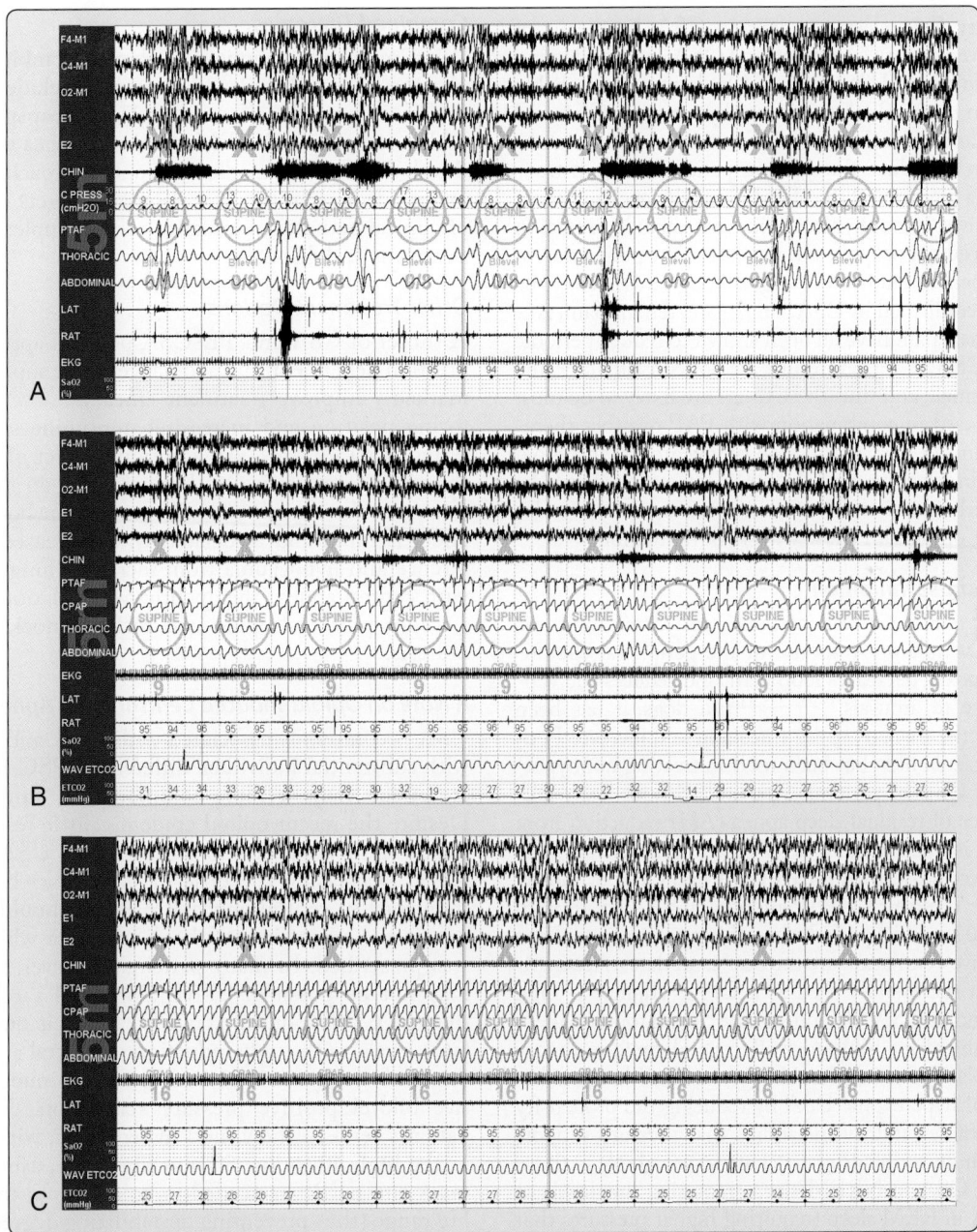

Figure 125.11 A-C, Efficacy of CO_2 manipulation for stabilizing respiration. A 72-year-old with congestive heart failure (same patient as in Figure 125.6). **A,** Adaptive servo-ventilation failure; note excessive cycling of pressure (the C-PRESS channel) and the associated arousals. **B,** After addition of 50 mL enhanced expiratory rebreathing space (EERS); note stabilization of respiratory rhythm but residual flow limitation and mild residual periodic breathing. **C,** With 100 mL EERS; note normalization of sleep and respiration. The end-tidal CO_2 (ET_{CO_2}) signal plateau is slightly blunted and thus the CO_2 measured is falsely low. However, the resting wake ET_{CO_2} of this patient was 30 mm Hg, a level that can be readily seen in patients with congestive heart failure.

oxygen compared with CPAP alone.[224] Respiratory event cycles can lengthen with the use of O_2. Such a change may "reduce" the respiratory event index but not imply a true stabilization of respiration. Use of O_2 also negates use of a desaturation parameter to score hypopneas. Beneficial effects of oxygen for PSG metrics in CSA are not limited to those with oxygen saturations below thresholds used for long-term nasal oxygen therapy (e.g., ≤88%); however, given recent concerns about safety in nonhypoxic patients, we advise against sustained nocturnal saturations greater than 94%.[225] Use of O_2 is currently off-label for CSA, and a long-term trial in patients with CHF and CSA-CSB (LOFT-HF, Clinical trials # CT03745898) is ongoing.

Enhancing Sleep Consolidation

Easy arousability from sleep can worsen CSA, by means of hyperpnea and ventilatory overshoot, and OSA, by not allowing sufficient time to recruit UA muscles.[226] Sedatives can probably be used safely in minimally hypoxic, nonhypercapnic CSA and NREM-dominant apnea in general. For example, eszopiclone has been shown to reduce the AHI in patients with obstructive apnea with a low arousal threshold.[32] Likely mechanisms of benefit of sedatives in nonhypercapnic CSA include reduction of arousal-induced hypocapnia and increasing the proportion of NREM sleep spent in stable breathing, although this needs to be experimentally confirmed in CSA. Triazolam, temazepam, zolpidem, and clonazepam have all been shown to reduce periodic breathing and CSA,[227-231] but results are not consistent.[228] The effect sizes are small, and thus these drugs are likely to be most effective when used in combination with PAP or other therapies, as shown in OSA.[232] Estimation of low arousal threshold may be helpful in selecting candidates.[233,234] Caution should be used in the elderly; those at risk of falls; those using other sedatives, alcohol, or opioids; or those with hypoventilation.

Carbonic Anhydrase Inhibition

Acetazolamide, a diuretic and carbonic anhydrase inhibitor, diminishes the ventilatory response of the peripheral chemoreceptors to hypoxia, decreases loop gain, and reduces the ventilatory response to arousals.[38,227,235,236] In dogs, it has been shown to lower the P_{ETCO_2} apnea threshold and increase P_{CO_2} reserve.[237] Acetazolamide has been used in treating nonhypercapnic CSA or CSB in patients with and without heart failure.[26] The degree of residual sleep apnea (AHI reduction from 57 to 34/hour) is unacceptable as sole long-term therapy. The drug may convert those with mixed OSA and CSA to mostly obstructive (the reverse of CPAP-induced CSA). Those with short-cycle (≤30 seconds) periodic breathing not responding to EERS or adaptive ventilation are the best candidates. Acetazolamide has been successfully used as a CPAP adjunct at high altitude[238,239] and in OSA.[240] Zonisamide[241] and topiramate[242] have carbonic anhydrase inhibitory effects and could in theory be used in the place of acetazolamide. Acetazolamide can aid in the treatment of hypercapnic CSA by reducing the propensity for worsening of respiratory instability that pressure support ventilation can induce. The drug may have a special role in those with coexisting CSA in NREM sleep (requiring low levels of PAP) and OSA in REM sleep (requiring higher pressures that could exacerbate CSA in NREM sleep).

Other Drugs with Possible Benefits in Nonhypercapnic Central Sleep Apnea

Clonidine and[243] the 5-α reductase inhibitor finasteride[244] have been shown to improve breathing stability. Inhibition of H_2S (gaseous signal transmitted in the carotid body) in a rodent model of CHF nearly normalized chemosensitivity and breathing instability[245] and may serve as a new therapeutic target. A case report of unilateral carotid body denervation in a man with systolic heart failure and moderate CSA showed that chemosensitivity and sleep apnea severity were reduced and shifted to an obstructive phenotype at 2 months after treatment, accompanied by an improvement in quality of life.[246] A recently completed trial of carotid body denervation in people with systolic heart failure may provide key risk-benefit information (ClinicalTrials.gov Identifier: NCT01653821) on pharmacologic targeting of carotid body function.

Combined Therapies

With improved phenotyping, a logical combination of therapies can be tested clinically. Examples include PAP + oxygen, PAP + acetazolamide for sea-level high-loop-gain sleep apnea, PAP + sedative for NREM-dominant apnea with low arousal threshold, or even a medication-only approach for CSA (acetazolamide + sedative). This approach targets multiple drivers of clinical pathology, similar to other complex disorders such as asthma and diabetes.

Other Treatment Options

A subset of CSA and TE-CSA patients appear very supine position dependent, and avoidance of the supine position can markedly improve treatment efficacy.[133,247] Devices monitoring position and increasing nonsupine sleep have been tested in OSA.[248,249] An additional effect of body position, this time from vertical to horizontal, is on fluid redistribution from the caudal to cranial parts of the body.[51,250-254] The effect is rapid and associated with increased neck circumference and hypocapnia from increased lung water in those with central apnea. Therapeutic manipulation could include a wedge pillow, sleeping in a recliner, stockings, or careful diuresis.

A Note on Opioid-Induced Central Sleep Apnea

CSA is commonly associated with COT and is dose related with substantial individual differences. PSG features of opiate effects may be more common than clinical symptoms. Despite the recent opioid epidemic, little research has been done on the impact and treatment of CSA on health in COT. Decreasing the dose of COT may help reduce the frequency of central apneas[255,256] and should be attempted within the constraints of the disorder for which medication was prescribed. In many patients, however, stopping COT may not be possible. CPAP alone will rarely be effective therapy. COT-induced ataxic breathing is quite sensitive to CO_2 levels, with ready induction of central apnea and worsening of dysrhythmic breathing on continuous or nonadaptive bilevel positive pressure ventilation. Although these patients tend to show mild hypercapnia, with ET_{CO_2} levels in the high 40 to low 50 mm Hg range, using a nonvented mask and EERS as needed to hold CO_2 in the mid-40 mm Hg range (thus preventing destabilizing degrees of hypocapnia despite supporting the UA) can be helpful regardless of the positive pressure mode used. We have found the use of acetazolamide of benefit as an adjunct to PAP.[257] Adaptive ventilation is a double-edged sword in these patients—being able to both enable stable breathing and markedly destabilize breathing.[193,258,259]

CLINICAL PEARLS

- Sleep apnea caused by a pathologically activated respiratory chemoreflex results in a wide PSG spectrum of disease, with variable features of UA obstruction mixed with more traditionally accepted central patterns.
- Pathophysiology guides treatment. Treatment end points should aim to normalize sleep and sleep-breathing biology, not merely suppression of scored events to an arbitrary threshold.
- Recognizing NREM sleep dominance of disease in nonhypercapnic CSA and minimizing the importance of concomitant UA flow limitation when identifying otherwise typical periodic breathing are applicable in clinical and research assessments. Hypercapnic CSA may be REM dominant, with the exception of opiate-induced CSA, and require ventilatory support for management. Unlike OSA, CSA is relatively difficult to treat and increases the risk for poor compliance, residual symptoms, ongoing sleep fragmentation, and high residual respiratory events despite therapy.
- It is useful to consider CSA as taking hypercapnic and nonhypercapnic forms. Accurate phenotyping of sleep apnea is increasingly important because several on-label and off-label therapies (e.g., acetazolamide, oxygen), singly or in combination, have improved therapeutic options for CSA syndromes.

SUMMARY

CSA caused by pathologic activation of the respiratory chemoreflex includes idiopathic CSA, periodic breathing, high-altitude sleep apnea, and treatment-emergent or complex sleep apnea. A narrow NREM sleep CO_2 reserve and propensity for arousal and sleep fragmentation are key pathophysiologic drivers. A unifying theme for nonhypercapnic CSA is predominance in NREM sleep and a metronomic appearance; cycle times, the duration of the respiratory event from peak to peak or trough to trough, can be short (≤30 seconds). Sleep fragmentation is often severe, but hypoxia is relatively moderate in nonhypercapnic CSA. The prevalence and evolution of residual CSA phenotypes with treatment remain to be accurately estimated because of limitations of current approaches to PSG scoring; new methods need to be validated to outcomes. Noninvasive adaptive ventilation provides pressure support approximately equal and opposite to patient-generated ventilation, with substantial differences in individual device algorithms. Off-label approaches may be considered as adjuncts to improve therapeutic efficacy, including minimization of hypocapnia with dead space adapted to PAP, acetazolamide, and sedatives to reduce the arousal threshold.

Hypercapnic CSA is associated with pathologically reduced activation of the respiratory chemoreflex and may be seen in association with hypoventilation syndromes and neurologic disorders. Disease severity can be maximal in REM sleep, although successful ventilation (and reduction in hypercapnia) may result in respiratory instability in NREM sleep as a result of relative hypocapnia. Noninvasive bilevel ventilation with a backup rate and volume-assured ventilation are primary therapeutic options; acetazolamide may improve respiratory drive and reduce NREM-related instability.

SELECTED READINGS

Chowdhuri S, Javaheri S. Sleep disordered breathing caused by chronic opioid use: diverse manifestations and their management. *Sleep Med Clin.* 2017;12(4):573–586.

Costanzo MR, Ponikowski P, Javaheri S, et al. Transvenous neurostimulation for central sleep apnoea: a randomised controlled trial. *Lancet.* 2016;388(10048):974–982.

Cowie MR, Woehrle H, Wegscheider K, et al. Adaptive servo-ventilation for central sleep apnea in systolic heart failure. *N Engl J Med.* 2015;373(12):1095–1105.

Dempsey JA, Smith CA, Przybylowski T, et al. The ventilatory responsiveness to CO(2) below eupnoea as a determinant of ventilatory stability in sleep. *J Physiol.* 2004;560:1–11.

Dempsey JA, Xie A, Patz DS, Wang D. Physiology in medicine: obstructive sleep apnea pathogenesis and treatment—considerations beyond airway anatomy. *J Appl Physiol.* 2014;116:3–12.

Eckert DJ, White DP, Jordan AS, et al. Defining phenotypic causes of obstructive sleep apnea: identification of novel therapeutic targets. *Am J Respir Crit Care Med.* 2013;188:996–1004.

Gaig C, Iranzo A. Sleep-disordered breathing in neurodegenerative diseases. *Curr Neurol Neurosci Rep.* 2012;12:205–217.

Javaheri S, Dempsey JA. Central sleep apnea. *Compr Physiol.* 2013;3:141–163.

Jordan AS, O'Donoghue FJ, Cori JM, et al. Physiology of arousal in obstructive sleep apnea and potential impacts for sedative treatment. *Am J Respir Crit Care Med.* 2017;196(7):814–821.

Liu D, Armitstead J, Benjafield A, et al. Trajectories of emergent central sleep apnea during cpap therapy. *Chest.* 2017;152(4):751–760.

Masa JF, Mokhlesi B, Benítez I, et al. Long-term clinical effectiveness of continuous positive airway pressure therapy versus non-invasive ventilation therapy in patients with obesity hypoventilation syndrome: a multicentre, open-label, randomized controlled trial. *Lancet.* 2019;393(10182):1721–1732.

Murtaza G, Turagam MK, Akella K, et al. Pacing therapies for sleep apnea and cardiovascular outcomes: a systematic review. *J Interv Card Electrophysiol.* 2021;61(1):11–17.

Oldenburg O, Costanzo MR, Germany R, McKane S, Meyer TE, Fox H. Improving nocturnal hypoxemic burden with transvenous phrenic nerve stimulation for the treatment of central sleep apnea. *J Cardiovasc Transl Res.* 2021;14(2):377–385.

Pavsic K, Herkenrath S, Treml M, et al. Mixed apnea metrics in obstructive sleep apnea predict treatment-emergent central sleep apnea. *Am J Respir Crit Care Med.* 2021;203(6):772–775.

Rao H, Thomas RJ. Complex sleep apnea. *Curr Treat Options Neurol.* 2013;15:677–691.

Thomas RJ. Alternative approaches to treatment of central sleep apnea. *Sleep Med Clin.* 2014;9:87–104.

Voigt J, Emani S, Gupta S, Germany R, Khayat R. Meta-Analysis comparing outcomes of therapies for patients with central sleep apnea and heart failure with reduced ejection fraction [published online ahead of print, 2020 Apr 24]. *Am J Cardiol.* 2020;S0002-9149(20):30379-9. https://doi.org/10.1016/j.amjcard.2020.04.011.

Xie A, Teodorescu M, Pegelow DF, et al. Effects of stabilizing or increasing respirator motor outputs on obstructive sleep apnea. *J Appl Physiol.* 2013;115:22–33.

Zeineddine S, Badr MS. Treatment-emergent central apnea: physiologic mechanisms informing clinical practice. *Chest.* 2021;159(6):2449–2457.

A complete reference list can be found online at ExpertConsult.com.

Chapter 126

Anatomy and Physiology of Upper Airway Obstruction

James A. Rowley; M. Safwan Badr

Chapter Highlights

- Upper airway patency is determined by craniofacial structure, surrounding tissues, intrinsic properties of the upper airway, and the neuromuscular function of the upper airway.
- With sleep, the loss of the wakefulness drive to breathe is associated with decreased neuromuscular activity of the upper airway, and in particular decreased afferent reflexes, and is further modified by such factors as lung volume, hypercapnia, and age. Upper airway caliber decreases with a resultant increase in upper airway resistance and compliance, and upper airway collapsibility.
- Mechanistically, crowding of the oropharynx, within a small rigid bony enclosure, may promote upper airway narrowing. This oropharyngeal crowding can occur either due to increased upper airway soft tissue (e.g., with obesity and/or a small maxilla/mandible size.
- This chapter describes and discusses the factors that influence the determinants of upper airway obstruction in humans. However, further research is needed to understand how these determinants interact to maintain upper airway patency.

INTRODUCTION

Sleep-disordered breathing is a relatively common disorder with substantial adverse health consequences. From the earliest descriptions it has been known that upper airway obstruction plays an important role.[1] The mechanisms underlying increased propensity to sleep-related upper airway obstruction in some, but not all, individuals remain poorly understood. This chapter reviews the anatomy and physiology of the upper airway as it relates to upper airway patency and propensity to obstruct during sleep. See Chapter 168, which reviews the abnormalities of craniofacial structures that contribute to sleep-disordered breathing in some patients. The occurrence of collapse during sleep and not wakefulness implicates the removal of the wakefulness drive to breathe as a key factor underlying sleep-related upper airway obstruction. The determinants of upper airway patency—upper airway neuromuscular activity and nonneuromuscular factors including craniofacial structure, surrounding tissues, and intrinsic properties of the upper airway itself—are discussed.

This chapter additionally reviews the effect of sleep on upper airway properties such as patency, resistance, compliance, and collapsibility. Within each area, the factors that influence these properties, including host factors (e.g., gender and body mass index), disease (e.g., tonsillar hypertrophy, fluid overload), and obstructive sleep apnea (OSA) itself, are examined.

BASELINE DETERMINANTS OF UPPER AIRWAY PATENCY

Upper Airway Function and Structure

The human upper airway is unique in that it serves as a multipurpose passage. It both transmits air to the lungs (via the nose and mouth) and liquids and solids to the esophagus (via the mouth). The upper airway, particularly the nose, also serves as a heat exchanger. Furthermore, the upper airway in humans, particularly the larynx and lips, is important for vocalization. However, because it serves multiple purposes, portions of the upper airway lack rigid support, and hence are prone to collapse.

The upper airway is classically divided into five regions based upon anatomic structures (see Figure 126.1, *A*). Each of these regions is either rigid and resistant to collapse or semirigid and susceptible to collapse. Whether rigid or semirigid, however, each region can become occluded due to other anatomic variants or abnormalities. Although the nose is a rigid section of the upper airway because of its bony components, it can become obstructed due to nasal congestion and polyps, altering upper airway mechanics. The nasopharynx is defined as the area from the posterior aspect of the nasal turbinates to the horizontal plane of the soft palate. Thus the proximal portion of the nasopharynx tends to be rigid but the distal region is semirigid. Nasopharyngeal patency can be compromised by local mass lesions and palatal and uvular hypertrophy or edema. The oropharynx is defined as the area from the soft palate to the base of the tongue and is semirigid. It can be further divided into an area posterior to the soft palate (retropalatal) and tongue (retroglossal). Oropharyngeal patency is generally compromised from tonsil hypertrophy, palatal or uvular enlargement, and/or macroglossia. Because the nasopharynx and oropharynx are semirigid, these two areas are the site of collapse in the majority of patients with OSA. The hypopharynx extends from the base of the tongue to the larynx and is relatively rigid and resistant to collapse. Finally, the larynx, the most distal portion of the upper airway, is rigid, composed of both cartilage and muscle.

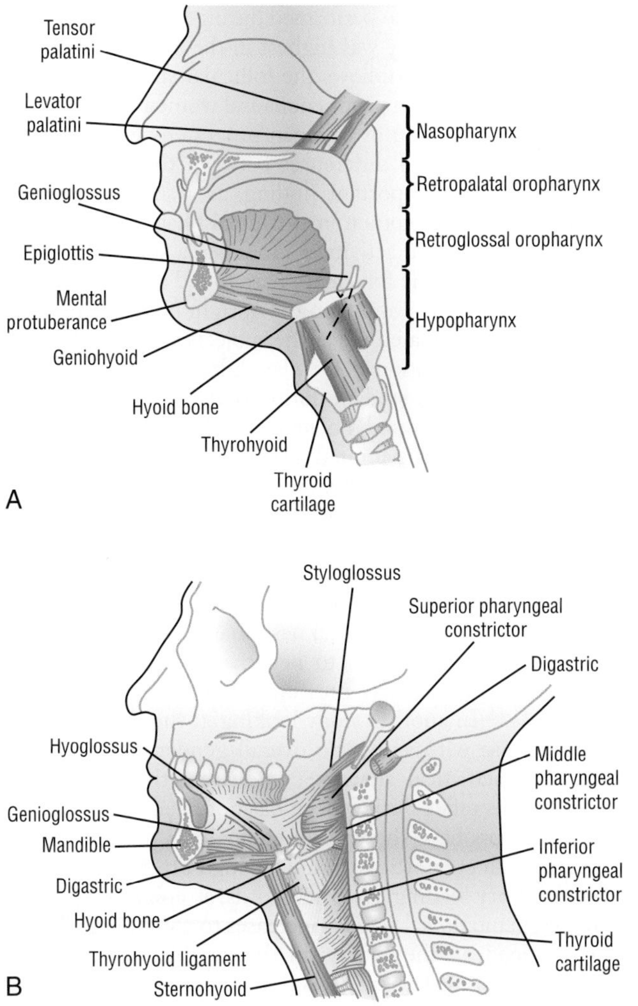

Figure 126.1 **A,** Schematic diagram of upper airway anatomy showing the classic divisions of the pharynx and key upper airway muscles. **B,** Schematic diagram of upper airway muscles and other key landmarks such as the hyoid.

Neuromuscular Function of the Upper Airway

The upper airway musculature consists of 24 pairs of striated skeletal muscles extending from the nares to the larynx (see Figure 126.1, *B* for major anatomic landmarks and muscles).[2,3] These pharyngeal muscles have complex anatomic relationships but can generally be classified into groups that regulate the position of the soft palate, tongue, hyoid bone, and pharyngeal walls. The muscles are generally activated in groups to control the major functions of the upper airway such as phonation and swallowing.

There are two general patterns of electrical discharge from upper airway muscles when these are studied with multiunit electromyograms (EMGs): tonic (constant) activity, independent of phase of respiration, and phasic activity, occurring during one part of the respiratory cycle. There are at least ten upper airway muscles that may be classified as pharyngeal "dilators," innervated by multiple cranial nerves. Some, such as the genioglossus are classified as dilators by virtue of their phasic inspiratory activity. Others, such as the tensor palatini, do not clearly have a dilating effect, but demonstrate activity throughout the respiratory cycle (tonic activity), and are presumed to "stiffen" the upper-airway wall and decrease pharyngeal collapsibility. It is widely accepted that upper airway dilators play a critical role in preserving pharyngeal patency.[4] There is evidence from EMG studies that activity of upper airway dilators begins about 200 milliseconds before onset of thoracic pump activity in normal subjects.[5,6]

Upper airway narrowing and/or obstruction during sleep is associated with a sleep-related decrease in upper airway muscle activity. The effect of non–rapid eye movement (NREM) sleep on upper airway muscle function is complex and difficult to study because of the challenges in isolating the multitude of influences on upper airway muscle activity, such as changes in air flow, magnitude of negative pressure in the pharyngeal airway, and lung volume. Available evidence indicates that NREM sleep is associated with a reduction in tonic and/or phasic EMG activity in numerous upper airway muscles,[3] including the levator palatini,[7] tensor palatini,[8] palatoglossus,[7] and geniohyoid.[9] Studies measuring single motor unit activity of the genioglossus muscle also noted decreased activity of the phasic inspiratory motor units at sleep onset[10] and NREM stage 2 sleep with increased discharge frequencies and duration in NREM stage 3 sleep.[11] The EMG changes are accompanied by upper airway narrowing and increased upper airway resistance.

The effect of rapid eye movement (REM) sleep on upper airway muscle activity is more clearly documented. Activity of antigravity muscles is reduced during REM sleep, and there is strong evidence that activity of phasic upper airway dilating muscles, such as the genioglossus, is greatly attenuated during REM sleep,[12,13] particularly during periods of phasic rapid eye movements.[14,15] Reduced activity has also been shown for the alae nasi[14] and geniohyoid muscles.[9] Similar findings have been found for single motor unit activity of the genioglossus.[16] In summary, the sleep state is associated with decreased upper airway muscle activity.

The response of upper airway muscle to chemical and mechanical perturbations may be more relevant to upper airway narrowing than reduced baseline activity. Negative pressure applied to the upper airway results in a brisk reflex response in upper airway muscle activity. This reflex is attenuated with application of topical lidocaine, indicating mediation through local mechanoreceptors.[17] Large changes in pressure (>10 cm H_2O) still result in activation of upper airway muscles even in the presence of local anesthetic.[18] Studies of reflex activity in the genioglossus, palatoglossus, and tensor palatini muscles show that this negative pressure reflex response is attenuated during NREM[19-21] and REM sleep[22] compared with wakefulness. Similarly, responsiveness of the genioglossus muscle to hypercapnia is attenuated during sleep.[23] These data suggest that upper airway dilator muscles are less able to maintain upper airway patency in the face of chemical or mechanical perturbations. Furthermore, there is evidence that lung volumes alter genioglossus muscle activity during NREM sleep, with decreases in end-expiratory lung volume being associated with increased genioglossus activity above baseline.[24]

There is evidence that activation of the genioglossus (and presumably other upper airway dilators) is important in maintaining upper airway patency. For instance, the critical closing pressure of the upper airway (see section Surrounding Tissues and Pressures for full discussion) correlated to the responsiveness of the genioglossus to negative pressure.[25] In another study, obese participants without OSA had a greater response in genioglossus activation with changes in epiglottic pressure than subjects with sleep apnea.[26] In both animal models and human studies, a variety of neurotransmitters have been found to be associated with reduction in genioglossus activity, such as noradrenaline, histamine, and serotonin.[27] Desipramine, an antidepressant with noradrenergic effects, was found to increase tonic genioglossus activity during NREM sleep while reducing airway collapsibility.[28] Finally, stimulation of the hypoglossal nerve results in decreased collapsibility (i.e., a stiffer airway) and decrease surrounding pressure in animal models.[29,30] Existing studies indicate that supraphysiologic electrical stimulation of the hypoglossal nerve using a surgically implanted upper airway stimulation device in patients with OSA lead to significant improvements in the severity of the sleep-disordered breathing in a select group of patients.[31,32]

However, the large number of upper airway muscles and their complex interactions mandate caution in extrapolating findings from studies focusing on the genioglossus or hypoglossal nerve activity alone, particularly as measurement of electrical activity of the muscle is not always an appropriate surrogate for muscle fiber shortening or for upper airway dilatation. In fact, there is evidence that upper airway muscle activation is not necessarily sufficient to dilate the upper airway under either physiologic or loading conditions, including resistive loading due to airway resistance,[33] or elastic loading due to either increased soft or fat tissue[34-36] or small mandibular enclosure.[37] Nor may such activation be necessary; for example, in sleeping humans, increased end-expiratory lung volume has been found to result in decreased upper airway resistance and increased retropalatal cross-sectional area in association with *reduced* EMG activity of the genioglossus.[38] In patients with OSA, increased lung volume causes a substantial decrease in sleep-disordered breathing during NREM sleep[39] and an inverse correlation between continuous positive airway pressure (CPAP) requirements and lung volume in patients with OSA has been found.[40]

It is also unclear whether complete atonia of the pharyngeal muscles increases upper airway collapsibility. For example, the pharyngeal airway becomes more collapsible in dead infants,[41,42] but not in paralyzed animal preparations.[43,44] In addition, REM sleep, associated with decreased neuromuscular stimulation, is not associated with changes in upper airway compliance or collapsibility in human studies of upper airway physiology.[45,46] Likewise, increased pharyngeal compliance in patients with sleep apnea cannot be attributed to decreased upper airway dilating muscle activity per se, because patients with OSA show increased activity of the genioglossus muscle during wakefulness[47] and sleep,[48] perhaps as a compensation for anatomically reduced caliber. Similarly, when the pharyngeal airway is narrowed during hypocapnic central apnea,[49] more pronounced narrowing (or even closure) occurs in patients with OSA relative to normal control subjects despite complete inhibition of upper airway dilating muscle activity in both groups.

Gender and Upper Airway Neuromuscular Activity

OSA is more prevalent in men than in premenopausal women (approximately 3:1 ratio). Hence, many investigations have been performed to determine whether the gender difference can be explained by upper airway neuromuscular activity. There have been several studies investigating a gender difference in baseline neuromuscular activity. During wakefulness, Popovic and White found that women had both higher peak phasic and expiratory tonic genioglossal EMG activity compared with men.[50] In a subsequent study, Popovic and White compared genioglossus activity between pre- and postmenopausal women and between the luteal and follicular phase in the premenopausal women.[51] This study, also performed during wakefulness, found that genioglossal activity was highest in the luteal phase of the menstrual cycle, which follows the follicular stage. Genioglossal activity was lowest in postmenopausal women and improved with the administration of estrogen/progesterone replacement therapy. The finding of differences between the follicular and luteal phases is an important finding, as a subsequent study comparing men and women in the luteal phase found no difference in genioglossal activity.[52] However, a study comparing men and women in the follicular phase found a higher baseline genioglossal EMG in women in the upright body position; the difference was attenuated when the subjects were compared in the supine body position.[53] Gender differences in genioglossal activity have been studied during both NREM and REM sleep; both studies found no gender differences in baseline activity.[15,54] Hence, the limited available evidence would suggest there is not a gender difference in baseline neuromuscular activity when women in the luteal phase of the menstrual cycle are compared with men.

Regarding the upper airway negative pressure reflex, only a few studies have investigated gender differences. In a study investigating the role of topical nasopharyngeal anesthesia on genioglossal responsiveness to negative pressure, no gender differences in the negative pressure reflex were found during wakefulness.[55] In another study looking at the change in this reflex response with aging, no overall gender difference was noted after statistical analysis.[56] However, the influence of gender on this reflex during sleep has not been studied.

Investigators have shown that genioglossal muscle activity correlates with epiglottic pressure during both tidal breathing and inspiratory loading. In other words, as epiglottic pressure decreases, genioglossal activity increases to compensate for the increased load on the airway; in theory, this reflex helps to maintain upper airway cross-sectional area. This relationship has been shown to be present during both wakefulness and sleep and under a variety of conditions including hyper- and hypocapnia. One study specifically compared this relationship in men and women. Jordan and colleagues studied 24 men and women and found no difference in the relationship between men and women (slope of the change in epiglottic pressure to change in genioglossal activity, men $-0.63 + 0.20$ and in women $-0.69 + 0.33$).[52] In general, gender differences in OSA prevalence do not appear to be due to gender differences in upper airway neuromuscular activity.

Aging and Upper Airway Neuromuscular Activity

As the prevalence of OSA increases with age, there have been investigations into the effect of aging on upper airway neuromuscular activity. There have been few studies on the effect of aging on baseline neuromuscular activity of upper airway muscles. In the Malhotra and colleagues, study of 38 men and women of varying ages, both tonic and phasic genioglossus muscle activity was measured.[56] In this study, there was no difference in either tonic or phasic genioglossus activity with aging (with age as a continuous variable). Fogel and colleagues studied the change in genioglossus activity during sleep onset in a group of younger (18–25 years) versus older (45–65 years) men. Genioglossus activity was higher in the older men during wakefulness, and both groups showed a decrease in genioglossus activity during sleep onset; however, only the older men showed a recruitment of genioglossus activity during the transition to more stable sleep.[57] There are a limited number of studies on the influence of aging on upper airway reflexes that contribute to upper airway collapsibility. Malhotra and colleagues studied the genioglossal reflex to negative pressure in a group of 38 men and women during wakefulness and found that the reflex response decreased with age in the total group.[56] However, this effect of aging was significant only in men, not women. The influence of aging on this reflex has not been studied during sleep. Another group compared the genioglossus EMG response to hypoxia in a group of younger (20–40 years) compared with older (41–60 years) subjects. This group found that the genioglossus response to hypoxia was decreased in the older subjects.[58] Finally, Murtolahti and colleagues studied the perception of inspiratory loading in a group of younger (11–20 years) and older (59–82 years) subjects. The group found that younger subjects detected increased resistance at lower flow rates, suggesting an increased sensitivity to changes in inspiratory loading than older subjects.[59] Collectively, these studies show that upper airway reflexes are decreased in older subjects than younger subjects and could explain, in part, age-related changes in upper airway collapsibility.

Nonneuromuscular Factors Contributing to Upper Airway Patency and Obstruction

Upper Airway Muscle Histology

There is a large body of research examining upper airway muscle histology in patients with OSA, based upon the hypothesis that pathologic changes in upper airway muscle histology may promote upper airway obstruction by increasing propensity to upper airway muscle fatigue and/or delay reopening via impairment of sensorimotor function. Studies have shown a variety of histologic changes including edema and mucosal gland hypertrophy,[60] neurogenic injury,[61] changes in muscle enzyme activity,[62,63] and leukocytic inflammation.[64,65] A consistent finding across studies is an increase in type II fast-twitch fibers in the genioglossus muscle of patients with OSA.[61,66-68] As type II fibers are more likely to fatigue than type I fibers, these studies suggest that upper airway muscles in OSA patients are more susceptible to fatigue than in normal subjects. In contrast, there is no consistent finding for differences in tongue protrusive force[69,70] in patients with OSA compared with normal subjects.

Changes in sensorimotor activity of the upper airway in OSA patients have been studied based upon evidence that upper airway sensory receptors contribute to apnea-terminal arousal, and that topical anesthesia impairs these responses. In patients with OSA, changes in two-point discrimination, vibratory sensation, upper airway muscle reflex response to short air pulses, and sensory perception to varying air flow rates have been observed.[71-73] Increased pain threshold correlated with worsened apnea-hypopnea index (AHI) and hypoxemic indices.[74] These changes may explain the observation that inspiratory load sensation is decreased in patients with OSA.[75,76] Such impairment of upper airway sensorimotor function may contribute to decreased upper airway muscle activity in response to upper airway obstruction, loading, or collapse.

Although the aforementioned studies indicate changes in upper airway neuromuscular histology and sensorimotor function in patients with OSA, there is only minimal evidence linking specific histologic changes or sensorimotor changes to changes in upper airway mechanics or propensity of the upper airway to collapse. In fact, the noted histologic changes, if secondary to recurrent airway collapse, may not be contributing to an increased propensity to collapse. For instance, treatment with nasal CPAP has been associated with improvement in genioglossus muscle force production[67] and vibratory thresholds.[71] Thus, further investigation is necessary to determine to what extent changes in upper airway histology and function seen in patients with OSA are primary or secondary, and whether and how such changes, primary or secondary, contribute to the noted increased propensity to collapse in sleep in patients with OSA.

Craniofacial Structure

Craniofacial structure is an important determinant of upper airway patency. See also Chapter 168. Although obesity is the most common risk factor, in a study in a large sample of men, obesity alone explained only 26% of the variance in the AHI, and obese patients with unfavorable airway dimensions were susceptible to larger increases in OSA severity.[77] The importance of craniofacial structure is most evident in children with craniofacial abnormalities such as Pierre Robin sequence and Treacher Collins syndrome, each of which is associated with an increased prevalence of OSA.[78] Mandibular size was found to be smaller in children with residual sleep apnea after tonsillectomy,[79] indicating the importance of craniofacial structure in contributing to airway patency during sleep in children. In adults, several anatomic abnormalities have been associated with OSA, including retrognathia, micrognathia, overjet, and a high arched palate.[80,81]

Several investigations have used lateral cephalometry to analyze the contribution of craniofacial structure to the development of OSA (Figure 126.2).[77,82-88] These studies vary widely in methodology, sample size, gender ratios, and the presence and degree of obesity. In these studies, common craniofacial abnormalities that have been associated with increased severity of sleep apnea include (1) smaller airway dimensions, particularly those involving the maxilla and mandible; (2) mandibular retrognathia; (3) decreased posterior airspace; (4) an inferiorly placed hyoid bone; and (5) increased soft palate dimensions and length. These abnormalities decrease the dimensions of the naso- and oropharynx, likely increasing the risk of upper airway obstruction. The aforementioned studies primarily compared cephalometrics in subjects with and without OSA and did not attempt to correlate dynamic upper airway collapse. Mittal and colleagues showed that cephalometric parameters, particularly the sella-nasion-A point angle (a common cephalometric angle relating the sella and nasion) and posterior airway space at the level of the mandible, predicted obstruction on sleep induced endoscopy.[89] In addition, Genta and colleagues showed that pharyngeal closing pressure is correlated with hyoid position (in relation to the mandibular plane), as well as pharyngeal length.[90] These latter two studies show that craniofacial structure affects both pharyngeal airway size and function.

Magnetic resonance imaging (MRI) has also been used to compare upper airway craniofacial structure and soft tissue between subjects with and without OSA. Important differences have been found in men and include a wider mandibular divergence, smaller mandibular length, and smaller area at the mandibular plane being associated with OSA.[91,92] Although the hyoid bone was inferiorly placed in these studies in subjects with OSA, it was not a primary determinant of upper airway obstruction. Finally, Chi and colleagues studied craniofacial structure using MRI in a cohort of subjects with and

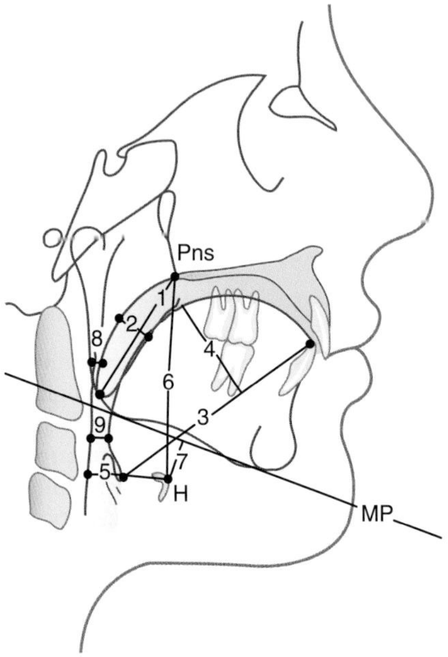

Figure 126.2 Cephalometric landmarks and soft tissue, hyoid position, and airway size variables frequently used in cephalometric studies. Landmarks: Pns, posterior nasal spine; H, hyoid bone; MP, mandibular plane (tangent line from the symphysis to the inferior border of the mandibular angle). Variables: *(1)* SPl: the length of the soft palate; *(2)* Spw: the width of the soft palate; *(3)* Tl: the length of the base of the tongue; *(4)* Tw: the width of the tongue; *(5)* H-Ph: the distance from the hyoid bone to the posterior wall of the pharynx; *(6)* H-Pns: the distance from the hyoid bone to Pns; *(7)* H-MP: the distance from the hyoid bone to the mandibular plane; *(8)* SPAS: the upper posterior pharyngeal space; and *(9)* IPAS: the lower posterior pharyngeal space. In one study, critical closing pressure was predicted by the length of the soft palate *(1)*, distance from hyoid bone to posterior wall of the pharynx *(5)*, and the distance from the hyoid bone for the posterior nasal spine *(6)*. (From Sforza E, Bacon W, Weiss T, Thibault A, Petiau C, Krieger J. Upper airway collapsibility and cephalometric variables in patients with obstructive sleep apnea. *Am J Respir Crit Care Med.* 2000;161(2 Pt 1):347–52.)

without OSA and their siblings (Figure 126.3).[91] After correction for differences in age, sex, ethnicity, height, and weight, several factors were found to demonstrate significant heritability including mandibular width, maxillary width, and size of the oropharyngeal space. The heritability of these structures was similar in normal and OSA subjects.

Craniofacial indices derived from both cephalometric and MRI data have been used to compare OSA susceptibility between races. Redline and colleagues found that bony and soft tissue factors and brachycephaly were associated with OSA in Whites, while only soft tissue factors were similarly associated in African Americans.[86,93] In contrast, Polynesian men with OSA were shown to have more mandibular retrognathia and larger nasal aperture width than White men, whereas neck circumference, tongue, and soft palate dimensions were associated with the respiratory disturbance index in the White subjects.[94] In Japanese patients with OSA, obesity and other upper airway soft tissue indices were less important than craniofacial structures; studies have found smaller mandibular length and area at the mandibular plane and has been observed, as has constriction of the maxillary dental arch in relationship to a mandible positioned rearward relative to the maxilla.[79,92,95] Similar findings of craniofacial restriction have also been observed in Chinese patients OSA[96] that showed that subjects with moderate-severe OSA have greater collapsibility than White subjects with OSA, suggesting a relationship between structure and upper airway function.[97] Taken together, these data indicate that race-specific craniofacial and neck structural factors contribute to the likelihood of having OSA.

Only one study has specifically compared gender differences in craniofacial and structural factors which could contribute to a propensity for OSA. Using MRI, Malhotra and colleagues[98] found that men had increases in airway length, soft palate cross-sectional area, and airway volume, presumably contributing to a diathesis for upper airway obstruction.

It should be noted that in many of these craniofacial studies, obesity remained an important etiologic factor for OSA, with abnormal craniofacial structure most important in nonobese patients with OSA. In addition, several studies have been performed to determine whether craniofacial structure measurements could predict response to non-PAP therapies such as mandibular advancement devices (MAD) or surgery. Several of these studies, though not all, found no correlation between craniofacial structure and treatment response. Hence, although craniofacial structure is clearly an important determinant of airway patency, it is not a primary factor.

Surrounding Tissues and Pressures

A collapsing upper airway transmural pressure can be generated either by a negative intraluminal pressure or a collapsing surrounding pressure. The role of negative intraluminal pressure in the pathogenesis of upper airway obstruction is widely hypothesized,[4] whereby a subatmospheric intraluminal pressure generated by the thoracic pump muscles causes upper airway collapse by "sucking" the hypotonic upper airway. However, there are no data showing that such subatmospheric intraluminal pressure causes upper airway obstruction in sleeping humans. In addition, upper airway narrowing and/or obstruction does not appear to require negative pressure. For example, studies using fiberoptic nasopharyngoscopy have shown that the upper airway narrows during hypocapnia-mediated central inhibition.[49,99] Isono and colleagues compared the mechanics of the pharynx in anesthetized and paralyzed normal subjects and in patients with OSA.[100] The pharynx was patent at atmospheric intraluminal pressure in normal subjects and required negative intraluminal pressure for closure. In contrast, patients with OSA had a positive closing pressure; that is, the pharynx was occluded at atmospheric intraluminal pressure. Similarly, the critical closing pressure in patients with OSA has been generally found to be positive, as opposed to the negative critical closing pressure in normal subjects.[101,102]

The disconnect between the occurrence of upper airway obstruction and of negative intraluminal pressure supports the possibility that upper airway patency is, in part, determined by the extrinsic or surrounding pressure contributed to by properties of soft tissue structures of the upper airway. Using MRI technology, three factors have been found to be most significantly associated with an increased risk of OSA: increased tongue size, increased size of lateral pharyngeal walls, and increased total soft tissue volume (Figure 126.4).[103] The association of increased tongue and lateral pharyngeal wall size with OSA has also been noted in computed tomography (CT) and cephalometric studies of the upper airway,[87,104] as well as in clinical studies.[80] Subsequent work has shown that these same factors show familial aggregation, even after correction for confounding factors such as gender and age.[91,105] Thus, the known familial predisposition to OSA[106] may in part be explained by heritable soft tissue factors.

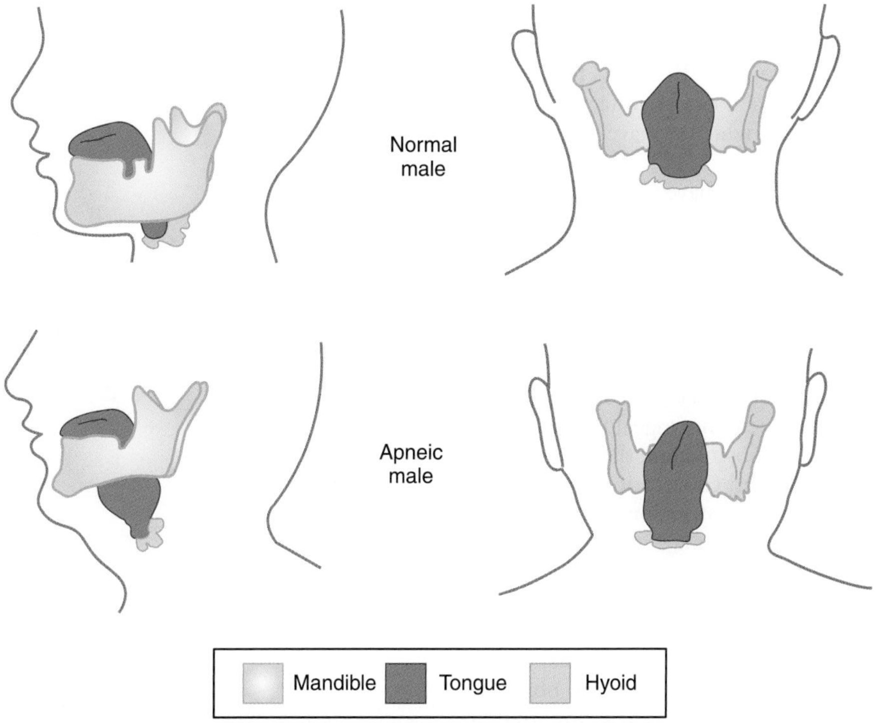

Figure 126.3 Three-dimensional reconstruction of hyoid, tongue, and mandible in a patient with obstructive sleep apnea (*bottom:* male, apnea/hypopnea index [AHI] 86 events/hour; body mass index [BMI] 31 kg/m^2; 49 years of age) and a normal subject (*top:* male, AHI 5 events/hour; BMI 25 kg/m^2; 44 years of age) illustrating the inferior-posterior positioning of hyoid and enlarged tongue volume. Note that the hyoid is more inferior-posteriorly positioned in the apneic subject than in the normal subject; tongue volume is greater in the apneic subject than in the normal subject. (From Chi L, Comyn FL, Mitra N, et al. Identification of craniofacial risk factors for obstructive sleep apnoea using three-dimensional MRI. *Eur Respir J.* 2011;38(2):348–58.)

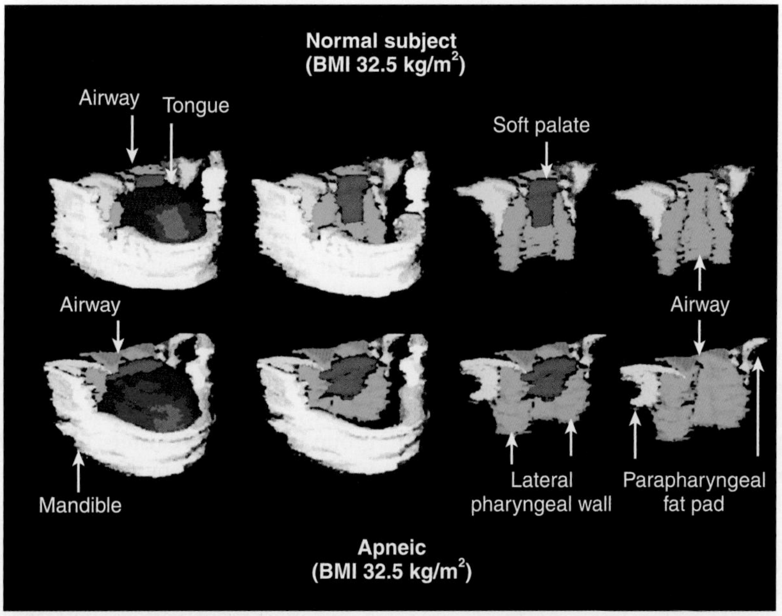

Figure 126.4 Volumetric reconstruction of axial magnetic resonance (MR) images in a normal subject and a patient with sleep apnea both with an elevated body mass index of 32.5 kg/m^2. The mandible is depicted as gray, tongue as orange/rust, soft palate as purple, lateral parapharyngeal fat pads as yellow, and lateral/posterior pharyngeal walls as green. Note that the airway is larger in the normal subject than in the apneic patient. The tongue, soft palate, and lateral pharyngeal walls are larger in the patient with sleep apnea. (From Schwab RJ, Pasirstein M, Pierson R, et al. Identification of upper airway anatomic risk factors for obstructive sleep apnea with volumetric magnetic resonance imaging. *Am J Respir Crit Care Med.* 2003;168(5):522–30.)

Enlarged tonsils have also been shown to be associated with an increased risk of OSA even after correction for body mass index and neck circumference.[80] Enlarged tonsils and adenoids are particularly noted as a causative factor in children, adolescents, and thin adults, who may have resolution of OSA after tonsillectomy.[107,108]

CT and MRI of the upper airway have also demonstrated evidence of increased soft tissue volume and pharyngeal fat at the level of the nasopharynx in males,[109] which could explain, in part, their higher prevalence of OSA. Pharyngeal fat volume was found to correlate with the AHI in one study[36] but not in other studies.[103,104] Jang and colleagues studied the relationship between pharyngeal fat measured by CT scan and objective outcomes of drug-induced endoscopy. Although they found no relationship between pharyngeal fat and apnea hypopnea index or the degree of obstruction, there was a correlation between pharyngeal fat and concentric type obstruction (rather than antero-posterior obstruction).[110] This study suggests that pharyngeal fat volume may contribute to the propensity of collapse, though not the severity of collapse as measured by AHI.

There is an association of soft tissue structures in relationship to the craniofacial structures. The term "oropharyngeal crowding" has been introduced: this refers to the observation that some subjects with OSA have a jaw size that is not sufficiently large relative to tongue size or upper airway soft tissue volume. In particular, Tsuiki and colleagues studied a group of subjects with and without OSA with various craniofacial dimensions.[111] They found that individuals with OSA had larger tongue sizes in relation to mandibular dimensions that subjects without OSA, suggesting that the oropharynx was "crowded." In a subsequent larger study, the same group found that a measure of oropharyngeal crowding, the ratio between tongue size and lower cage face (measured using cephalometry and related to the bony enclosure of the upper airway), correlated with AHI in in both obese and nonobese subjects; in obese subjects, the contribution of the ratio was larger than that of body mass index (BMI).[112] The group hypothesizes that the relationship between soft tissue structures and craniofacial structure is itself an important determinant of airway patency independent of either process alone (see Figure 126.5). When obese patients lose weight and have a reduction in AHI, there is reduction of the volume of several upper airway soft tissues, in particular tongue fat.[113]

Mechanistically, crowding of the oropharynx, within a small rigid bony enclosure, may promote upper airway narrowing by virtue of increased collapsing surrounding tissue pressure around the upper airway lumen. The aforementioned tonsillectomy data are consistent with this hypothesis; patients with residual OSA after tonsillectomy had a smaller mandibular size such that there was still oropharyngeal crowding after tonsillectomy; patients without residual OSA in theory had large mandibular areas and less oropharyngeal crowding.[79] Finally, in adolescents, Schwab and colleagues also found that the ratio of soft tissue volume to craniofacial dimensions was increased in adolescents with OSA.[108] The key question is whether individuals whose primary driver of upper airway obstruction is small bony enclosure will be more amenable to oral appliances advancing the mandible or surgical interventions targeting facial bony structures.

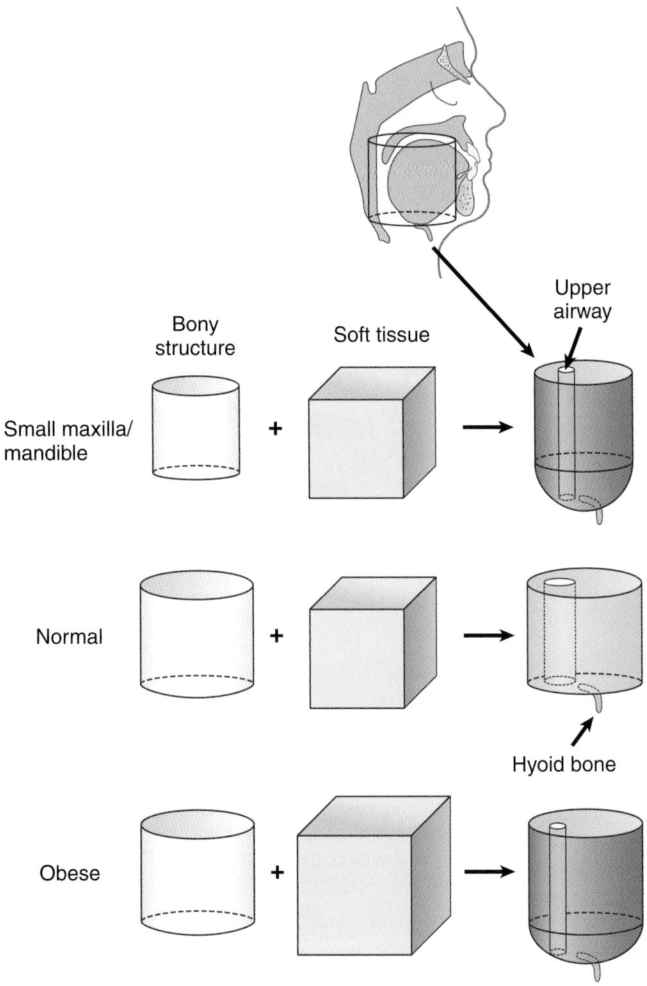

Figure 126.5 Schematic explanation of the interaction between upper airway bony enclosure and soft tissue contributing to the pharyngeal airway size as proposed by Ito and colleagues. Excessive soft tissue in relation to either a small maxilla/mandible (*upper part*) or obesity (*lower part*) results in pharyngeal airway narrowing and caudal displacement of the hyoid bone. (From Ito E, Tsuiki S, Maeda K, Okajima I, Inoue Y. Oropharyngeal crowding closely relates to aggravation of OSA. *Chest*. 2016;150:346–52.)

The importance of the relationship of upper airway craniofacial structure, obesity, and upper airway soft tissue has been well illustrated.[114] In this work, the authors performed a cluster analysis of a group of 89 adult OSA patients with moderate to severe OSA. The authors analyzed AHI, BMI, and cephalometric variables including craniofacial and soft tissue factors, hyoid bone, and pharyngeal space compartments. The group found three clusters. Cluster 1 had moderate OSA that was best explained by obesity alone. Cluster 2 had moderate OSA characterized by a hyperdivergent vertical pattern on cephalometry (with narrow velopharyngeal and oropharyngeal spaces) and lower BMI. Finally, cluster 3 had severe OSA characterized by obesity, displaced hyoid, large soft palate, and a hyperdivergent vertical pattern. The authors suggest that craniofacial modification may be a reasonable treatment alternative for patients in clusters 2 and 3. This study shows that different upper airway abnormalities may predominate as one of the etiologic mechanisms of a smaller upper airway, with some patients showing multifactorial causes with interactions between craniofacial structure, obesity, and soft tissue volume.

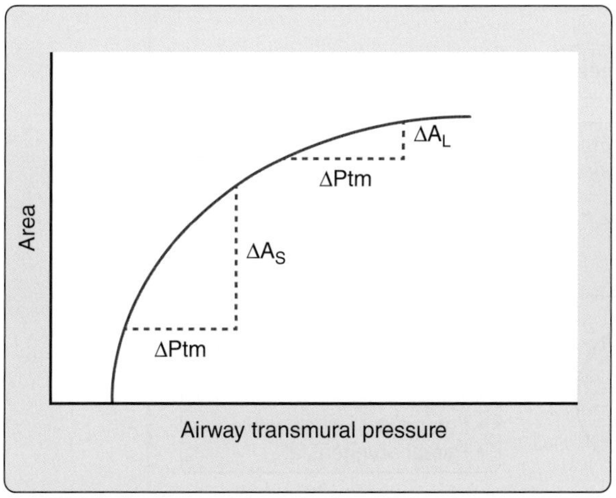

Figure 126.6 Illustration of the "tube law" of the pharynx. As transmural pressure (Ptm) increases, so does cross sectional area. The slope of the tube law represents compliance of the pharynx. Note that compliance decreases as the area of the pharynx increases.

Intrinsic Properties of the Upper Airway

The collapsing effect of transmural pressure on upper airway patency is subject to modification by the intrinsic compliance of the pharyngeal wall. In addition to the Isono and colleagues[115] data noted previously in this chapter, it has been shown that, in the isolated upper airway model of collapsibility, critical closing pressure is negative during complete paralysis, indicating that at normal atmospheric pressure, the normal upper airway remains open.[116,117] These studies suggest that the pharyngeal wall has an intrinsic "stiffness" or resistance to collapse. The determinants of such intrinsic stiffness have not been fully elucidated, but likely involve complex interactions among many of the pharyngeal components already discussed, including muscles (which may have different properties in a passive state compared with a stimulated state), bony structures (particularly in the nasopharynx), soft tissues, as well as vascular properties, with such interactions affecting pressure and cross-sectional area relationships.

In the passive or paralyzed nasopharynx, the relationship between pharyngeal transmural pressure and cross-sectional area is curvilinear, implying that the airway becomes more compliant as the cross-sectional area decreases, that is the "tube law" (Figure 126.6). Therefore baseline decreased airway cross-sectional area is itself likely a determinant of diathesis for upper airway obstruction, supported by evidence that the pharyngeal airway is smaller during wakefulness in patients with OSA relative to that of normal subjects.[118-120]

In association with such intrinsic properties of the upper airway, increased inspiratory lung volume is associated with increased upper airway caliber and decreased collapsibility. Potential mechanisms through which the increased caudal traction works include increased longitudinal tension, increased subatmospheric pressure through the trachea, and decreased transmural pressure.[30,121,122] Therefore, caudal traction appears to influence upper airway collapsibility by both dilating and stiffening the pharyngeal airway, as well as decreasing extramural tissue pressure. It is likely that patients with OSA are more dependent on such increased lung volume-associated dilatation and/or stiffening because of their relatively compliant upper airway.[123,124]

Vascular perfusion of the upper airway is also a potential determinant of intrinsic pharyngeal wall stiffness. Vasoconstriction and vasodilatation have been shown to cause a decrease and increase in upper airway resistance, respectively.[125-127] A series of experiments have investigated the relationship between rostral fluid shifts and upper airway properties, demonstrating an association between reduction in leg fluid volume and increased neck fluid volume and circumference.[128] In awake subjects, such rostral body fluid shift is associated with increased pharyngeal resistance,[129] decreased upper airway cross sectional area,[130] and increased upper airway collapsibility.[131,132] Conversely, preventing lower limb fluid edema during the day resulting in a small rostral body fluid shift and decreased snoring.[133] Similar results have been found in patients with drug-resistant hypertension[134] and end-stage renal dialysis,[135-137] two groups in which there is evidence of an increased prevalence of OSA.[138] Interestingly, despite similar changes in leg total fluid volume and neck circumference with lower body positive pressure, men have a larger increase in collapsibility than women,[132] suggesting that a differential response to fluid shifts between men and women could contribute to the difference in gender prevalence in OSA.

Once upper airway closure occurs, surface mucosal forces may impede subsequent upper airway opening.[44] In awake humans, surfactant and/or other topical lubricants have been shown to decrease the opening and closing pressures of the upper airway, and to decrease upper airway resistance in sleeping normal subjects.[139,140] Mucosal lining forces may be particularly important in patients with OSA with mucosal inflammation from repeated trauma[139] in whom the AHI in sleep decreases with the use of such soft tissue lubrication.[140,141]

In summary, upper airway patency is determined by multiple factors that are present during wakefulness and sleep, all typically further compromised during sleep compared with awake, leading to changes in upper airway function that contribute to sleep-related upper airway obstruction. The four primary factors include neuromuscular activity of the upper airway, craniofacial structure, tissues surrounding the upper airway, and the intrinsic properties of the airway (Figure 126.7). The following section reviews the sleep-specific effects on these factors and associated upper airway resistance and patency.

SLEEP EFFECTS ON UPPER AIRWAY PATENCY AND COLLAPSIBILITY

The sleep state is a challenge, rather than a period of rest, for the ventilatory system. In addition to the reduced activity of upper airway dilators discussed previously in this chapter, consequences of the loss of wakefulness on the upper airway include reduced upper airway caliber, increased upper airway resistance, increased pharyngeal compliance, and collapsibility. Ultimately, these changes lead to reduced tidal volume and hypoventilation.

Upper Airway Caliber and Resistance

The sleep state is associated with upper airway narrowing and a corresponding increase in upper airway resistance. Using nasopharyngoscopy during sleep in normal subjects, Rowley and colleagues[45,142] have shown that, during NREM sleep, both retropalatal and retroglossal cross-sectional area decreases to approximately 70% of awake cross-sectional area, with further narrowing of the retroglossal airway during REM sleep. Decreased cross-sectional area corresponds with the pattern of decreased upper airway dilator muscle

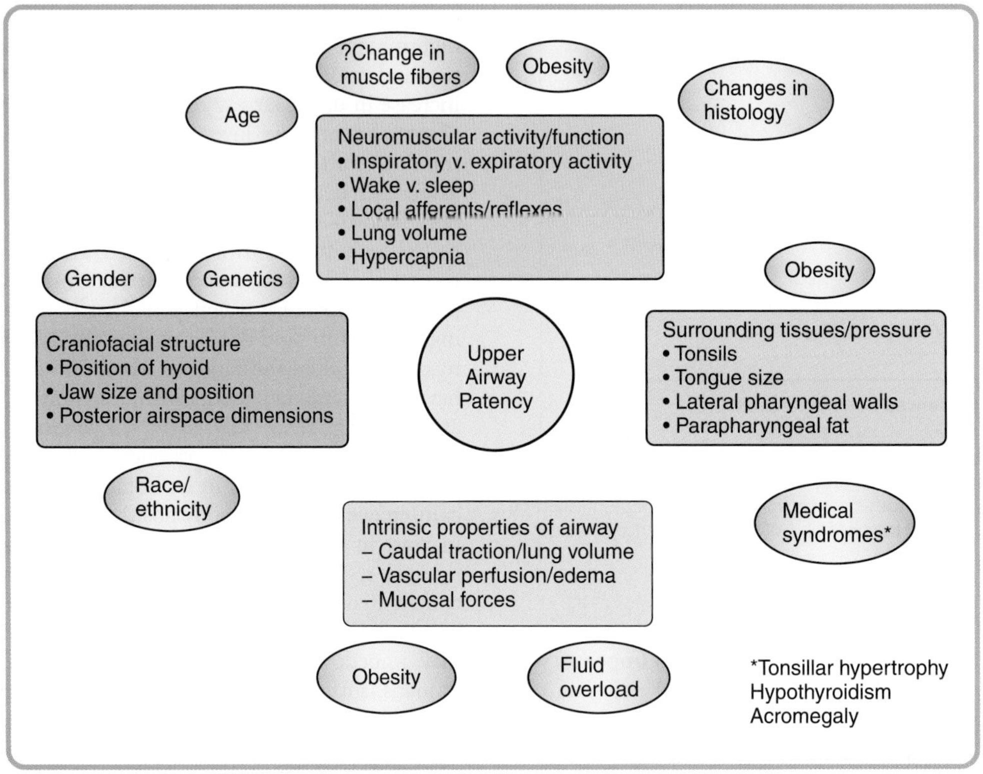

Figure 126.7 Summary showing the major determinants of upper airway patency and other factors that modify these main determinants.

activity during NREM sleep and further reduction of the genioglossus during REM sleep. In REM sleep, retroglossal but not retropalatal cross-sectional area decreases further, compared with NREM sleep.

The evidence for increased upper airway resistance during sleep is compelling, even in normal subjects.[45,142-144] In fact, increased upper airway resistance occurs as early as sleep onset and continues to increase, reaching highest values in sleep-wave sleep. The majority of evidence indicates that there are no further increases in upper airway resistance during REM sleep compared with NREM sleep in normal humans.[45,142,145] In summary, the sleep state is associated with upper airway narrowing, which manifests by increased upper airway resistance and decreased pharyngeal caliber.

It is important to note that upper airway resistance is not an independent measure of the dynamic behavior of the pharyngeal airway during sleep. Many subjects exhibit inspiratory-flow limitation, in which the pressure-flow graph demonstrates a changing relationship between driving pressure and inspiratory flow, culminating in complete dissociation between pressure and flow; that is pressure continues to decrease with no further increase in flow (Figure 126.8, *A*). Thus the optimal physiologically meaningful measurement of upper airway resistance is the slope of the linear portion of the pressure-flow loop, which likely reflects upper airway caliber at the narrowest point in the upper airway at the beginning of inspiration (Figure 126.8, *B*).

Measurements and Meanings of Compliance and Collapsibility

The walls of the pharyngeal airway consist of compliant soft tissue structures, amenable to changes in pressure during the respiratory cycle. During wakefulness, upper airway caliber is constant during inspiration, with a decreased caliber during expiration, returning to inspiratory values at end expiration. This finding has been observed in both normal subjects[146,147] and in patients with OSA[146] using either CT scanning or nasopharyngoscopy. Using nasopharyngoscopy, NREM sleep has been observed to be associated with significant dynamic within-breath changes in cross-sectional area, reaching a nadir at mid-inspiration,[146] with a rapid increase in cross-sectional area during expiration (Figure 126.9).[49] In addition, in subjects with OSA, there is progressive upper airway narrowing before the onset of apnea that is seen primarily during expiration.[148] BMI appears to be a determinant of the degree of airway narrowing seen in these studies.[45,49] The sleep reversal in the pattern of change in upper airway cross-sectional area is thought to be due to sleep-related increase in upper airway compliance, a decrease in pharyngeal caliber, and, subsequently, decreased (more negative) inspiratory intraluminal pressure.

The changes in upper airway patency during sleep can be investigated using compliance as a measurement. Compliance of the pharyngeal wall is an important modulator of the effect of pressure changes on upper airway patency. The occurrence of pharyngeal narrowing and flow limitation suggests, although does not prove, increased pharyngeal compliance during sleep. Using a methodology that measures changes in cross-sectional area at different levels of applied pressure, it has been demonstrated that compliance is increased as the pharyngeal caliber decreases[100,115,149] and that the upper airway of patients with OSA is more compliant than that of normal subjects,[100,123,149,150] consistent with an increased propensity to collapse. Using real-time MRI, Wu and colleagues confirmed that compliance is increased in subjects with OSA compared with subjects without OSA.[151] Using a methodology that combines measurement of cross-sectional area via

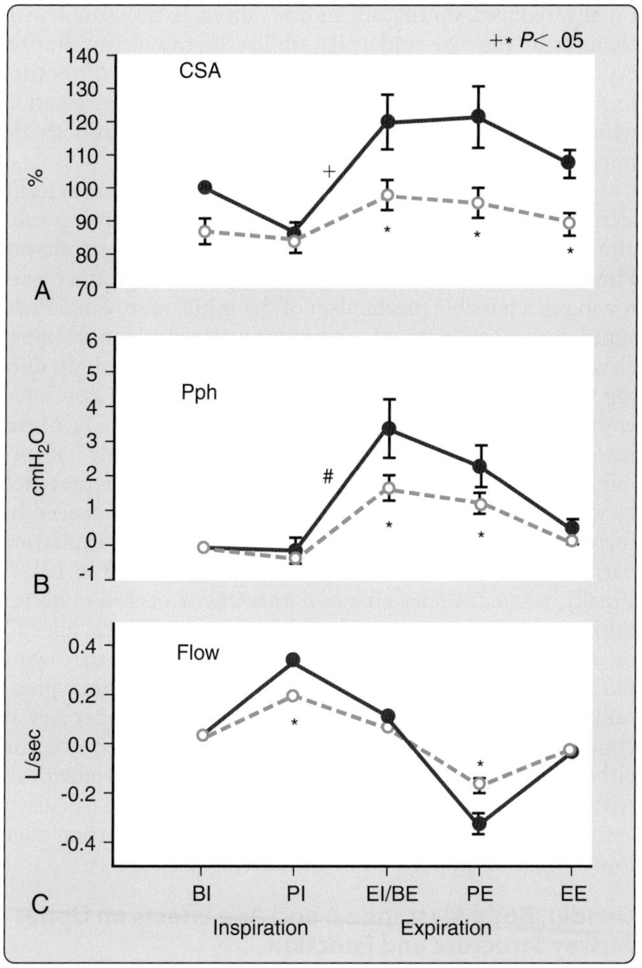

Figure 126.8 Retropalatal cross-sectional area (CSA) **(A)**, pharyngeal pressure **(B)**, and flow **(C)** during control (*closed circles*) and hypocapnic hypopnea (*open circles*). Note the significant CSA change throughout the respiratory cycle within the control breaths in comparison to the hypopnea breaths. BE, Beginning expiration; BI, beginning inspiration; EE, end expiration; EI, end inspiration; PE, peak expiration; PI, peak inspiration. (Modified from Sankri-Tarbichi AG, Rowley JA, Badr MS. Expiratory pharyngeal narrowing during central hypocapnic hypopnea. *Am J Respir Crit Care Med.* 2009;179:313–9.)

fiberoptic nasopharyngoscopy and measurement of intraluminal pressure at the same level in normal subjects has confirmed that retropalatal compliance is increased during NREM sleep compared with wakefulness with no difference between REM sleep and wakefulness.[45] At the retroglossal level, however, compliance is not increased during either NREM or REM sleep compared with wakefulness.[142] Marques and colleagues used a similar technique to compare retropalatal and retroglossal caliber and compliance in the same set of subjects with OSA.[152] They found that retropalatal caliber was smaller than retroglossal caliber and that retroglossal compliance was higher than retroglossal compliance.

Collapsibility, that is the propensity of the upper airway to collapse or obstruct under certain conditions, increases during sleep compared with awake, likely due to many of the factors discussed previously in this chapter. Upper airway collapsibility has been primarily measured using the critical closing pressure (P_{crit}) which is based upon the concept of the Starling resistor,[153] whereby maximal flow through the resistor is dependent on the resistance of the upstream segment and the pressure surrounding the collapsible segment (Figure 126.10). In humans, the critical closing pressure can be partitioned between its passive mechanical properties (passive P_{crit}) and active dynamic responses (active P_{crit}).[154,155] Applying this model to humans, it has been shown that across the spectrum of obstructive sleep-disordered breathing, active P_{crit} correlates with propensity for airway collapse.[101,102,156] For instance, P_{crit} in normal subjects is generally less than 10 cm H_2O whereas in patients with predominant hypopneas it is between 0 and -5 cm H_2O and in patients with predominant apneas it is greater than 0 cm H_2O. Although both active and passive P_{crit} are increased in patients with OSA compared with control subjects, the difference between active and passive P_{crit} is greater in non-OSA controls compared with those with OSA, likely associated with the greater ability of normal subjects to maintain airway patency.

The roles of mechanical loads and compensatory responses related to P_{crit} are summarized in Figure 126.11. As shown in the left hand bar with graded shading, approximate levels of P_{crit} measurements define a continuum of upper airway collapsibility

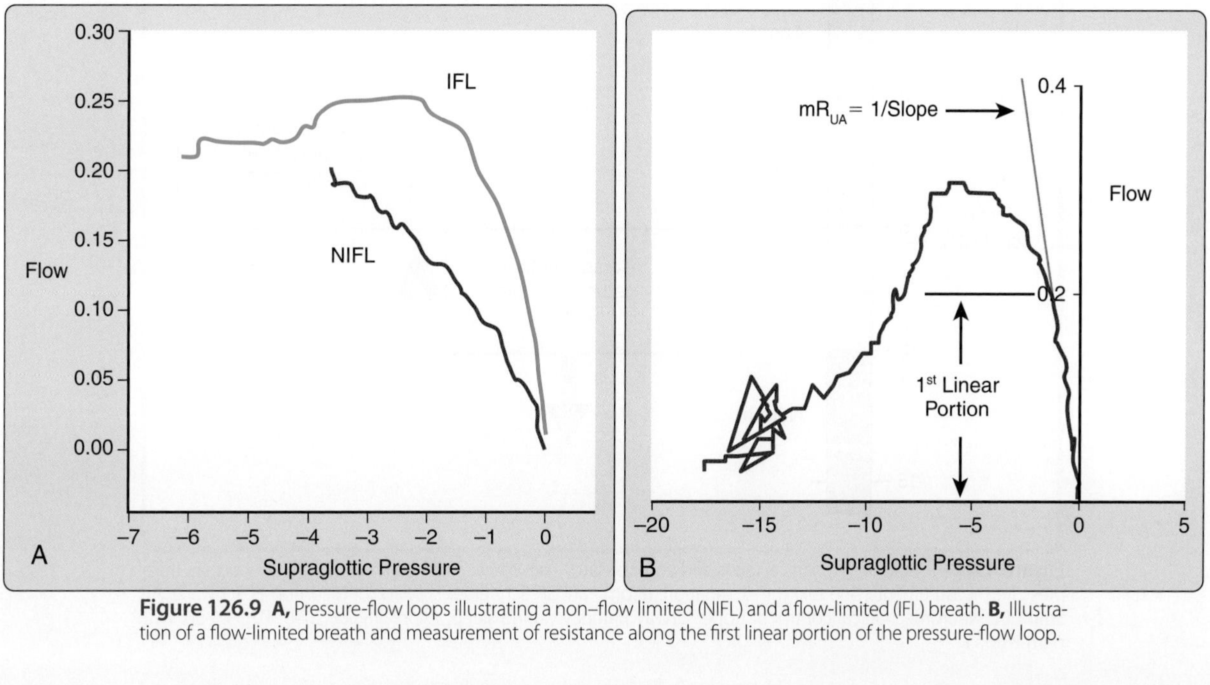

Figure 126.9 **A,** Pressure-flow loops illustrating a non–flow limited (NIFL) and a flow-limited (IFL) breath. **B,** Illustration of a flow-limited breath and measurement of resistance along the first linear portion of the pressure-flow loop.

from health to disease. A P_{crit} of approximately −5 cm H_2O represents the level above which obstructive hypopneas and apneas will occur. Structural characteristics of the upper airway impose mechanical loads and increase P_{crit}, predisposing the upper airway toward collapse. Intact dynamic neuromuscular responses decrease P_{crit} and maintain upper airway patency. In contrast, blunted neuromuscular responses increase P_{crit} and predispose the upper airway toward obstruction.

Upper Airway Narrowing and Ventilatory Motor Output

There is evidence that upper airway collapsibility is related to neurochemical drive and ventilatory motor output to the upper airway. Changes in ventilatory motor output are associated with reciprocal changes in upper airway resistance.[157,158] This is observed more strongly in individuals with a highly collapsible airway such as snorers with inspiratory flow limitation.[159]

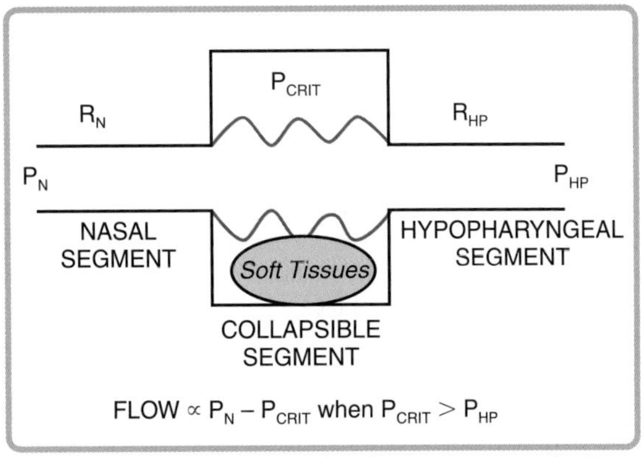

Figure 126.10 Starling resistor model of the upper airway. In this model, flow is proportion to the difference between P_N and critical pressure (P_{crit}) with P_{crit} is greater than P_{HP}. P_{HP}, hypopharyngeal (downstream) pressure; P_N, nasal (upstream) pressure; R_{HP}, resistance in the hypopharyngeal segment; R_N, resistance in the nasal segment.

Finally, reduced ventilatory motor output is associated with changes in the size and collapsibility of the airway during expiration.[148] When loop gain is used as a measure of ventilatory control, however, studies have found no clear association with upper airway collapsibility per se, even though both are important for the pathogenesis of OSA.[160,161]

Upper airway obstruction during sleep is characteristically attributed to inspiratory narrowing due to a collapsing subatmospheric pressure against a hypotonic pharyngeal airway. However, several lines of evidence implicate expiratory narrowing as a possible mechanism of the initial narrowing. First, ventilatory motor output is an important determinant of upper airway patency. Oscillation of ventilatory motor output, during the characteristic periodic breathing of OSA, is associated with pharyngeal narrowing or obstruction at the nadir of the motor output, especially in individuals with a highly collapsible airway.[162] Second, an obstructive apnea is often preceded by expiratory narrowing of the upper airway as evidenced by increased expiratory resistance[163] or progressive expiratory narrowing, detected by fiberoptic imaging (Figure 126.12).[148] Finally, whereas upper airway narrowing or occlusion occurs during a spontaneous or induced hypocapnic central apnea[99] or induced hypocapnic hypopnea,[49] pharyngeal narrowing during central hypopnea occurs during the expiratory phase only and is associated with increased expiratory upper airway compliance. Therefore upper airway obstruction may occur in either inspiration or expiration (Figure 126.13). Individuals with a high surrounding tissue pressure may be particularly susceptible to expiratory pharyngeal narrowing during such low ventilatory motor output and driving pressure.

Gender, Body Mass Index, and Age Effects on Upper Airway Structure and Function

Potential determinants of upper airway mechanics during sleep include many variables known to be associated with an increased prevalence of OSA, such as gender, BMI, and age.

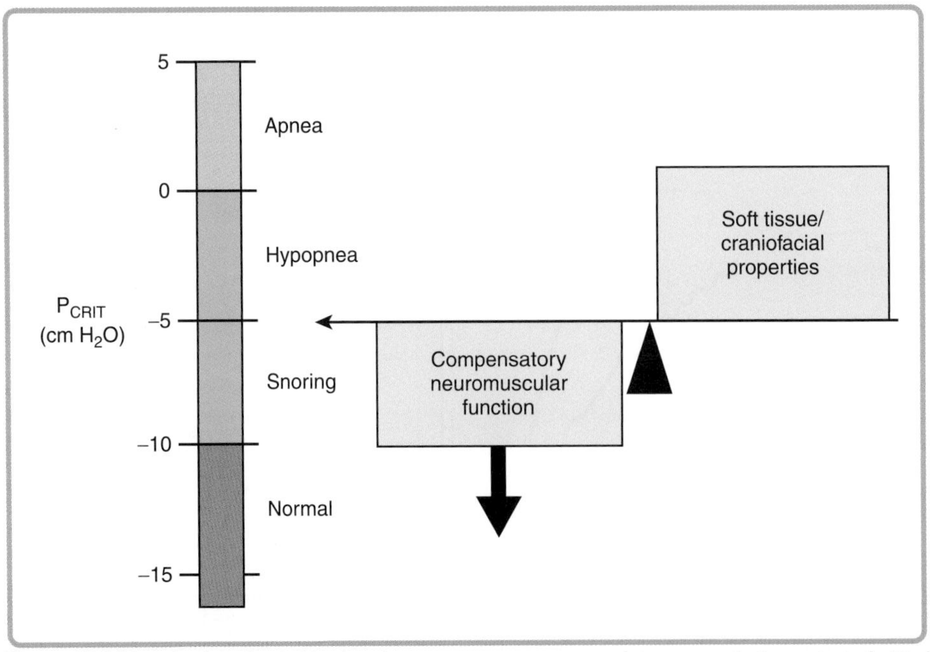

Figure 126.11 Role of mechanical loads and compensatory neuromuscular responses in the context of critical pressure measurements. See text for explanation. (From Patil SP, Schneider H, Marx JJ, Gladmon E, Schwartz AR, Smith PL. Neuromechanical control of upper airway patency during sleep. *J Appl Physiol.* 2006;102:547–56. With permission.)

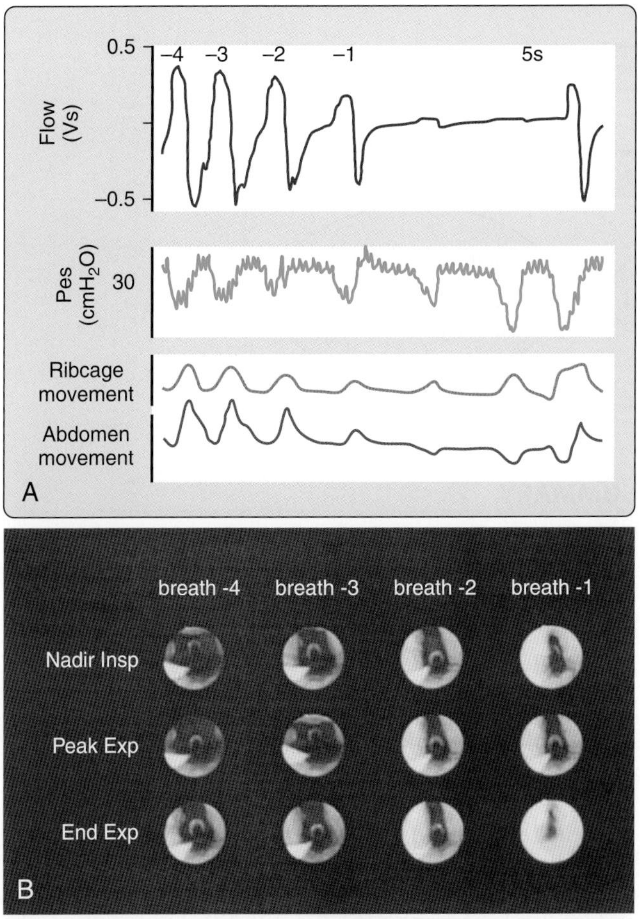

Figure 126.12 **A,** A recording of airflow (flow; inspiration positive), esophageal pressure (Pes), and rib cage and abdominal movements. Tracings show four breaths leading to an obstructive apnea (breaths-4, -3, -2, and -1). During the apnea, respiratory effort is indicated by the negative swings in the esophageal pressure and paradoxical rib cage and abdominal movements. **B,** Fiberoptic images of the retropalatal airway during the four breaths shown in **A** where breath-1 is the breath immediately preceding the apnea and breath-4 is the breath farthest away from the apnea. Within each breath the images selected correspond to the smallest cross-sectional area that occurred during inspiration (Nadir Insp), the largest CSA during expiration (Peak Exp), and the CSA at end-expiration (End Exp). Note that progressive narrowing is occurring in both inspiration and expiration. Within each image the dark area is the airway lumen, the lighter horseshoe shape is the epiglottis, and the white triangular shape in the bottom left corner is the esophageal pressure catheter. (From Morrell MJ, Arabi Y, Zahn B, Badr MS. Progressive retropalatal narrowing preceding obstructive apnea. *Am J Respir Crit Care Med.* 1998;158(6):1974–81.)

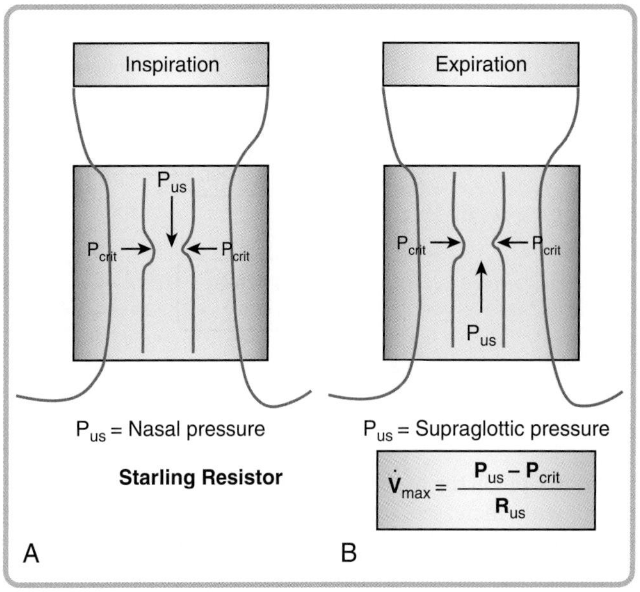

Figure 126.13 Schematic illustration for the collapsible segment of upper airway during hypocapnic hypopnea as a Starling resistor. In this model, flow is determined by the gradient between the upstream segment and critical closing pressure (P_{crit}). During inspiration **(A)**, when upstream pressure (P_{us}) (i.e., nasal pressure) is below the P_{crit}, the collapsible segment is closed, and no flow occurs. During expiration **(B)**, when P_{us} in the supraglottic area is below the P_{crit}, the collapsible segment is closed, and no flow occurs. During hypocapnic hypopnea, expiratory flow is limited, correlating with the gradient between the supraglottic pressure and P_{crit}. Hence, this pressure gradient is an important determinant of pharyngeal narrowing. Rus, Upstream resistance; V_{max}, maximal flow. Asterisk represents the site of retropalatal pressure measurement. (From Sankri-Tarbichi AG, Rowley JA, Badr MS. Expiratory pharyngeal narrowing during central hypocapnic hypopnea. *Am J Respir Crit Care Med.* 2009;179, 313–9.)

The majority of studies indicate no consistent difference in upper airway caliber, or compliance, between men and women without OSA. Upper airway resistance during NREM sleep is also similar in both genders,[145,164] although one study[165] demonstrated higher upper airway resistance in men during slow wave (delta) NREM sleep. REM sleep has not been similarly studied. Likewise, studies during wakefulness demonstrate no significant difference in upper airway cross-sectional area or smaller airway in women.[147,166-168] In addition, sleep-related narrowing is similar in men and in women (an approximately 40% decrease in cross-sectional area for both genders) from wakefulness to NREM sleep.[169] However, it appears that men have increased retropalatal compliance compared with women[169] because of gender difference in neck circumference, again indicating that factors other than gender itself are important in explaining such gender differences in upper airway function. Finally, there is no demonstrated gender difference in P_{crit} under active conditions in subjects without sleep disordered breathing.[164] Thus, the available studies taken together do not suggest a gender difference alone in upper airway mechanics during wakefulness or sleep, except for higher retropalatal compliance in men compared with women, in subjects without OSA. However, it should be noted that several studies have found lower collapsibility in women compared with men when subjects with OSA are studied.[161,170]

A few studies have examined the relationship between body mass index and P_{crit}. Genta and colleagues found that BMI, as well as other measures of obesity including neck and waist circumference, positively correlated with P_{crit} (more obese patients had a more collapsible airway).[90] Sands and colleagues found that P_{crit} was negative in normal weight subjects and positive in obese subjects with OSA.[26] However, Kirkness and colleagues found that gender modulates the effect of BMI on P_{crit}.[154] Although increasing BMI was associated with increased collapsibility in both men and women, the change in P_{crit} per change in BMI was higher in men than in women. In addition, the influence of BMI on P_{crit} was seen only in premenopausal women.[154]

The effect of age on upper airway resistance during sleep is variable across different studies. Browne and colleagues[171] and Thurnheer and colleagues[145] found no difference in upper airway resistance between young (<40 years) and older (>40 years) subjects. In contrast, in a group of 60 subjects without OSA, Rowley and colleagues found age to be the only independent predictor of upper airway resistance, with increased age associated with increased upper airway resistance. BMI

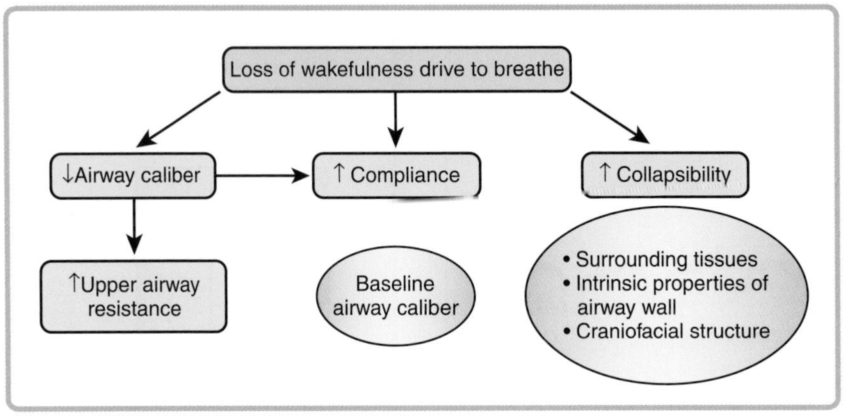

Figure 126.14 Effect of the loss of wakefulness drive to breathe on the upper airway.

was not a predictor of resistance.[164] Increasing age was associated with increased upper airway resistance during sleep in a linear fashion.[172] Overall, it appears that aging is associated with increased upper airway resistance, and thus possibly increased diathesis for pharyngeal narrowing, during sleep. However, as age does not appear to be a predictor of P_{crit} itself,[154] the significance of age-related increased upper airway resistance is unclear.

Hormonal Activity and Upper Airway Activity

There is also evidence that upper airway collapsibility can be influenced by hormonal activity, particularly leptin activity, in humans. For example, Shapiro and colleagues found in obese subjects that, although leptin levels were not associated with passive P_{crit} or the severity of sleep apnea (presumably OSA), increased leptin levels were associated with an increased difference between active and passive P_{crit}, independent of BMI and neck circumference.[173] Thus, leptin appears to be associated with a decreased propensity to upper airway collapse.

In summary, upper airway patency during sleep is compromised by the loss of wakefulness drive of breathing. The loss of the wakefulness drive to breathe results in decreased upper airway neuromuscular activity and reflex activity, leading to decreased upper airway caliber and increased in upper airway resistance. The loss of wakefulness drive to breathe also results in increased airway compliance and collapsibility. Figure 126.14 summarizes the important modifiers of upper airway patency during sleep.

CLINICAL PEARLS

The upper airway may be compromised, and an individual put an increased risk for OSA, because of enlargement of soft tissue structures such as the tonsils, tongue, and lateral pharyngeal walls due to disease or obesity. Craniofacial structure, which is determined by genetics, race, and ethnicity, is an important determinant of upper airway patency; clinically significant changes can include micro- and retrognathia, overjet, and a high arched palate. Obesity, through a decrease in lung volume (particularly functional residual capacity), infiltration of the tongue with fat, and fluid overload can each lead to changes in the intrinsic properties of the upper airway, increasing propensity to collapse. These factors, in association with sleep-related alterations in both neural control of the upper airway and central neural control of breathing, increase the propensity to upper airway obstruction and/or collapse in sleep in some individuals, leading to the clinical disorder of OSA.

SUMMARY

Upper airway patency is determined by multiple factors that are present during wakefulness and sleep, with sleep generally associated with compromise of these factors, leading to changes in upper airway function that contribute to upper airway obstruction. The four major determinants of upper airway patency are neuromuscular activity, craniofacial structure, tissues surrounding the upper airway, and the intrinsic properties of the airway itself. The relationship between craniofacial structure and tissues surrounding the upper airway relationship may lead to circumstances of oropharyngeal crowding, increasing the propensity to collapse. These determinants are themselves modified by other factors such as age, obesity, gender, ethnicity, fluid overload, and other medical disorders such as tonsillar hypertrophy (Figure 126.12). During sleep, the loss of the wakefulness drive to breathing results in decreased upper airway neuromuscular activity and reflex activity, leading to decreased upper airway caliber and increased upper airway resistance (Figure 126.13). In addition, there is associated increased airway compliance and increased collapsibility, both of which are influenced by factors that determine baseline upper airway caliber, such as surrounding tissues, craniofacial structure, and the intrinsic properties of the upper airway.

This chapter has discussed the important structural aspects of upper airway structure, function, and patency. It is, however, important to note that, although the upper airway narrows in humans during sleep, whether any given individual develops sufficient obstruction to develop the clinical disorder of OSA is likely an interplay between both upper airway structure and function and neural control of breathing during sleep.

SUGGESTED READINGS

Cori JM, O'Donoghue FJ, Jordan AS. Sleeping tongue: current perspectives of genioglossus control in healthy individuals and patients with obstructive sleep apnea. *Nat Sci Sleep*. 2018;10:169–179.

Gurgel M, Cevidanes L, Pereira R, et al. Three-dimensional craniofacial characteristics associated with obstructive sleep apnea severity and treatment outcomes [published online ahead of print, 2021 Jul 17]. *Clin Oral Investig*. 2021. https://doi.org/10.1007/s00784-021-04066-5.

Ito E, Tsuiki S, Maeda K, Okajima I, Inoue Y. Oropharyngeal crowding closely relates to aggravation of OSA. *Chest*. 2016;150:346–352.

Kirkness JP, Schwartz AR, Schneider H, et al. Contribution of male sex, age, and obesity to mechanical instability of the upper airway during sleep. *J Appl Physiol*. 2008;104(6):1618–1624.

Marcus CL, Keenan BT, Huang J, et al. The obstructive sleep apnoea syndrome in adolescents. *Thorax*. 2017;72:720–728.

Patil SP, Schneider H, Marx JJ, Gladmon E, Schwartz AR, Smith PL. Neuromechanical control of upper airway patency during sleep. *J Appl Physiol*. 2007;102(2):547–556.

Rowley JA, Sanders CS, Zahn BR, Badr MS. Gender differences in upper airway compliance during NREM sleep: role of neck circumference. *J Appl Physiol*. 2002;92(6):2535–2541.

Saboisky JP, Stashuk DW, Hamilton-Wright A, et al. Neurogenic changes in the upper airway of patients with obstructive sleep apnea. *Am J Respir Crit Care Med*. 2012;185(3):322–329.

Sankri-Tarbichi AG, Rowley JA, Badr MS. Expiratory pharyngeal narrowing during central hypocapnic hypopnea. *Am J Respir Crit Care Med*. 2009;179(4):313–319.

Schwab RJ, Pasirstein M, Kaplan L, et al. Family aggregation of upper airway soft tissue structures in normal subjects and patients with sleep apnea. *Am J Respir Crit Care Med*. 2006;173(4):453–463.

Schwab RJ, Pasirstein M, Pierson R, et al. Identification of upper airway anatomic risk factors for obstructive sleep apnea with volumetric magnetic resonance imaging. *Am J Respir Crit Care Med*. 2003;168(5):522–530.

Van de Perck E, Heiser C, Vanderveken OM. Concentric vs anteroposterior-laterolateral collapse of the soft palate in patients with obstructive sleep apnea. *Otolaryngol Head Neck Surg*. 2021: 1945998211026844. Epub ahead of print.

Wang SH, Keenan BT, Wiemken A, et al. Effect of weight loss on upper airway anatomy and the apnea-hypopnea index. The importance of tongue fat. *Am J Respir Crit Care Med*. 2020;201(6):718–727. https://doi.org/10.1164/rccm.201903-0692OC.

A complete reference list can be found online at ExpertConsult.com.

Chapter

127

Snoring and Pathologic Upper Airway Resistance Syndromes

Riccardo Stoohs; Avram R. Gold

Chapter Highlights

- Over the past 2 decades, knowledge of pathologic pharyngeal collapse during sleep has expanded from apnea and hypopnea to include even the mildest, silent inspiratory airflow limitation (IFL) during sleep. Both the clinical researcher and the sleep medicine practitioner of today must be able to recognize the mildest IFL on a polysomnogram and its clinical implications.
- Although habitual snoring is very common, the prevalence of isolated snoring (snoring in the absence of apnea and hypopnea, oxygen desaturations, arousals from sleep, and symptoms of obstructive sleep apnea) is unknown. Recent clinical investigation has led to uncertainty about whether such snoring can be considered benign.
- The paradigm of IFL during sleep leading to recurrent respiratory effort–related arousals is inadequate to explain the varied signs and symptoms of upper airway resistance syndrome (UARS) or to distinguish between patients with UARS and asymptomatic, healthy individuals whose polysomnograms are remarkably similar.

Snoring and upper airway resistance syndrome (UARS) represent obstructed breathing during sleep that is too mild to cause more than slight sleep fragmentation but with potential pathologic significance. There is growing evidence that mild inspiratory airflow limitation (IFL) during sleep, even in the absence of audible snoring or increased sleep fragmentation, may have a causative role in a variety of disabling somatic and affective disorders.

BACKGROUND

Glossary of Terms Central to This Chapter

The terms defined in the following are described in detail and in context in this chapter:

Inspiratory airflow limitation. IFL describes a state of the upper airway (UA, the pharynx) during sleep in which inspiratory airflow plateaus at a maximal level despite a continued increase in the pressure gradient between the nostrils and the hypopharynx. The failure of inspiratory airflow to increase despite the continued increase in the pressure gradient across the UA is caused by fluttering of the UA that prevents further increase in airflow. IFL can be divided into two subgroups based on whether it is *audible:* (1) *snoring* and (2) *silent IFL.*

Snoring or inspiratory snoring. Audible inspiratory fluttering of the UA. It can occur during obstructive hypopnea when hypopnea is associated with a decrease in inspiratory airflow by 30% lasting at least 10 seconds, accompanied by either an arousal from sleep or a 3% decrease in oxygen saturation. Alternatively, it can occur in the absence of the earlier criteria for hypopnea with higher levels of airflow or with shorter duration or absence of arousals or oxygen desaturation. The presence of inspiratory snoring *always indicates the presence of IFL.* Although expiratory snoring exists, and will be discussed later in this chapter, the term *snoring* used without a modifier in this chapter refers to inspiratory snoring. *Snoring* is further divided into two subgroups: (a) *habitual snoring* and (b) *isolated snoring.*

Habitual snoring: This term describes an observation (often a complaint) by a bed partner or roommate that a person consistently snores when asleep.

Isolated snoring: After polysomnography (PSG), if an otherwise healthy, asymptomatic, habitual snorer does not meet the current *International Classification of Sleep Disorders*, third edition[1] (ICSD-3) criteria for obstructive sleep apnea (OSA), the patient is described as having *isolated snoring.* Specific criteria for being "otherwise healthy" in the context of being a habitual snorer are described later in this chapter.

Silent inspiratory airflow limitation. Silent IFL is defined and characterized by the same *fluttering* of the UA that characterizes snoring; however, the frequency of the fluttering during silent IFL is, by definition, inaudible by humans.

Respiratory effort–related arousal (RERA): RERAs are transient arousals from sleep that follow a period of nonhypopneic IFL (either snoring or silent IFL) and are presumed to be caused by the inspiratory effort required to move air across a fluttering airway. Whether an arousal after a period of IFL is in fact caused by the IFL cannot be definitively ascertained during clinical PSG; it is a presumption. To label an arousal a RERA, the ICSD-3 requires 10 seconds of recognizable IFL preceding the arousal. A standard time requirement for IFL preceding a RERA, however, is not a consistent feature of RERAs in research; a single flow-limited inspiration before arousal is the definition in some research.

Respiratory disturbance index (RDI): ICSD-3 has replaced the apnea-hypopnea index (AHI) as a measure of the severity of OSA with the frequency of apneas, hypopneas, and RERAs. In this chapter this new measure of the severity of OSA will be termed the *RDI.*

Upper airway resistance syndrome: The UARS does not exist in the ICSD-3. It should be thought of as a syndrome described by Dr. Christian Guilleminault and used by researchers who have broken away from the paradigm that hypersomnolence in patients with sleep-disordered breathing requires the presence of sleep fragmentation by apneas and hypopneas.[2] In this chapter, UARS is defined as the symptom of either hypersomnolence or fatigue, together with the presence of IFL during sleep adjudicated by PSG and an AHI of less than 5 per hour; the latter is the threshold of an OSA diagnosis in the ICSD-3.

Upper Airway Resistance Versus Pharyngeal Collapse

Two terms used to describe the behavior of the UA (or pharynx) during sleep among snorers and patients with UARS are increased *UA resistance* and *UA collapse.* Many sleep researchers consider IFL during sleep to result from narrowing of the pharyngeal airway and increased resistance caused by the relaxation of pharyngeal dilator muscles, together with subatmospheric UA pressures during inspiration. As they measure increasingly negative esophageal or supraglottic pressures during inspiratory snoring, they think of *UA resistance* increasing. From this reasoning the clinical term *UARS* was derived (as discussed later).

In contrast to this intuitive model of increasing upper airway resistance during sleep is the experimentally validated Starling resistor model of IFL[3] (see Chapter 24). The Starling resistor model postulates that the pharyngeal airway during sleep is a collapsible tube that will collapse whenever the pressure within falls below a critical level, the pharyngeal "critical pressure" (Pcrit). It has been shown experimentally that as the severity of sleep-disordered breathing increases from isolated snoring to severe OSA, the pharyngeal Pcrit progressively increases from negative (subatmospheric) levels to positive levels.[4,5] Collapse of the pharynx, however, is not synonymous with apnea. When the pharynx collapses during sleep, one might experience either apnea (no inspiratory airflow) or IFL (inspiratory airflow that has reached its maximum). When the pressure at the *upstream* end of the pharynx (the nares during inspiration) falls below Pcrit, the pharynx collapses, with resulting apnea. When the pressure at the nares is above Pcrit, but the pressure at the downstream end of the pharynx (supraglottic pressure during inspiration) falls below Pcrit, as in a snorer, the pharynx also collapses. Because pharyngeal collapse leads to cessation of inspiratory airflow, pharyngeal pressure immediately equilibrates with nasal pressure opening the airway, with resumption of inspiratory airflow. The result is cyclical collapse and opening (fluttering) of the pharyngeal airway *limiting* inspiratory airflow to a fixed, maximal level, with the driving pressure fixed at nasal pressure minus Pcrit, no matter how low supraglottic pressure descends. Therefore, according to the Starling resistor model, the UA does not experience *increased resistance* during sleep, but a *fixed driving pressure* that limits airflow to a maximal level.

The language subsuming UA resistance and UA collapse therefore is derived from two different models of IFL. In this chapter we will allude to *pharyngeal collapse* in the section that follows, describing the polysomnographic appearance of IFL, but use the term *UA resistance* for the remainder of this chapter, which does not require modeling of IFL.

Upper Airway Resistance Syndrome

As introduced in the glossary, we use the term *UARS* in this chapter, and it is still found as a diagnosis in the medical literature. However, the ICSD-3 does not include UARS in its classification of sleep-related breathing disorders, but rather incorporates the polysomnographic manifestations of UARS into OSA. A brief discussion of the history of UARS will help the reader understand this dichotomy.

UARS came to public attention after the publication of a case series in 1993 by Dr. Christian Guilleminault and associates.[2] From among 48 patients with a diagnosis of idiopathic hypersomnolence, they selected 15 with the following characteristics: intermittent or continuous snoring with an AHI below 5 per hour, more than 10 arousals per hour of sleep (a threshold they chose), and arousals associated with *UA resistive events* identified using a pneumotachograph measurement of airflow and esophageal manometry to quantify effort.

Treatment of these 15 patients with nasal continuous positive airway pressure (CPAP) relieved the patients' hypersomnolence (measured objectively by the Multiple Sleep Latency Test). Because the patients did not meet diagnostic criteria for OSA, the investigators designated a new syndrome—UARS. They hypothesized that the hypersomnolence was related to sleep fragmentation by UA resistive events too mild to meet the diagnostic criteria of hypopnea. They further hypothesized that patients with UARS have increased sensitivity to the respiratory effort related to these resistive events, giving rise to repetitive arousals, compared with patients with OSA who typically arouse in response to higher degrees of obstruction, that is, apneas and hypopneas. The hypothesis that patients with UARS exhibit increased sensitivity to respiratory effort during sleep led to their arousals being termed *RERAs*.

Almost from the start, the establishment of a new syndrome of sleep-disordered breathing based on sleep fragmentation by RERAs created controversy.[6,7] To eliminate the need for an additional syndrome of sleep-disordered breathing based on sleep fragmentation by RERAs, the authors of ICSD-3 incorporated RERAs into the diagnostic criteria for OSA, creating diagnostic thresholds for OSA based on the combined frequency of obstructive events: apneas, hypopneas, and RERAs—the RDI. Therefore, by the clinical criteria of ICSD-3, UARS has been "absorbed" into OSA.

Investigators have since observed that the sleep of patients with UARS is characterized not only by the presence of RERAs but also by electroencephalographic differences and differences in sleep architecture that distinguish it from the sleep of healthy individuals. These *qualitative* differences in the sleep of patients with UARS resolve with treatments that eliminate IFL during sleep and the hypersomnolence of patients with UARS. Therefore, although the ICSD-3 clinical criteria for OSA will result in many patients being treated for OSA who previously were diagnosed with UARS, it is not established that these former patients with UARS are

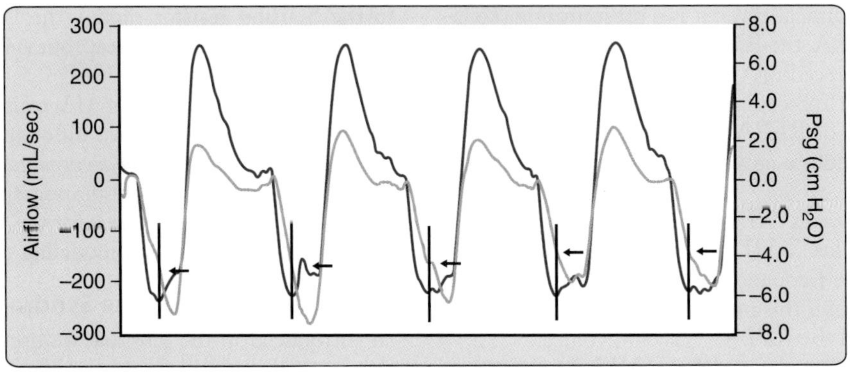

Figure 127.1 This figure illustrates inspiratory airflow limitation (IFL) in a sleeping research participant wearing a nasal mask attached to a pneumotachograph measuring airflow, with a pressure catheter placed through her nose to just above her vocal cords to measure supraglottic pressure (Psg). Airflow is the *blue tracing* with the units indicated on the left axis (inspiration is downgoing). Effort, represented by the Psg, is the *yellow tracing* with the units indicated on the right axis. For each inspiration, a plateau in airflow during early inspiration is intersected by a *vertical line*. Beyond the line, there is no further increase in inspiratory airflow despite the continued decrease in Psg and a continued increase in the inspiratory pressure gradient Patm—Psg. Indeed, not only does the inspiratory airflow not increase, but also, in the first four breaths it appears to decrease, a phenomenon known as *negative effort dependence* of airflow. IFL occurs when Psg decreases below this participant's pharyngeal critical pressure (Pcrit). The *horizontal arrows* mark the Psg at the onset of maximal flow (intersected by the *vertical line*) and suggest that this participant's pharyngeal Pcrit is approximately −4 cm H_2O, a common value for primary snorers or individuals who have upper airway resistance syndrome.[4]

hypersomnolent because of sleep fragmentation by RERAs. In consequence, UARS continues as a syndrome being studied by researchers examining alternatives to the OSA pathophysiologic paradigm of sleep fragmentation by apneas, hypopneas, and RERAs.

Inspiratory Airflow Limitation

Classically, the term *snoring*, the audible fluttering of the pharynx during inspiration, has been used to describe IFL during sleep. The term *snoring*, however, implies that pharyngeal fluttering is present only when it can be heard by a listener; the word *snore* itself resembles the sound of snoring. Hearing, however, is an insensitive means of detecting inspiratory fluttering of the pharyngeal airway during sleep. Because using the term *snoring* may lead one to believe that IFL is only present when audible, we have chosen to describe the characteristic inspiratory airflow through a fluttering UA during sleep as a state of *inspiratory airflow limitation* (as defined in the glossary earlier). The term *IFL* was first used by Schwartz and associates[8] in their study of pharyngeal collapsibility during sleep in healthy humans[8] and was derived from the parallel term *expiratory airflow limitation*, used to describe expiratory airflow from the lungs of patients with asthma, chronic obstructive bronchitis, and emphysema whose bronchi flutter on expiration, limiting airflow.[9]

Recognizing Inspiratory Airflow Limitation with Physiologic Testing

With the incorporation of RERAs into the diagnostic criteria for OSA, recognizing the presence of IFL preceding an arousal and differentiating its appearance from that of non-flow-limited breathing during PSG is an important skill. To visually identify IFL using a digitized airflow signal, one must sample the analogue signal adequately to see rapid oscillations of inspiratory airflow caused by fluttering of the airway. A sampling frequency of at least 100 Hz should be used for this purpose.[10] Furthermore, filtering of the airflow signal with a high-frequency filter can eliminate the oscillations of inspiratory airflow and should not be used during the collection of the airflow signal. The signal should be collected unfiltered and, ideally, analyzed without either high- or low-frequency filtering.[11] The airflow and pressure tracings that appear in the figures that follow were collected unfiltered with a sampling frequency of 128 Hz, and are displayed unfiltered.

Figure 127.1 illustrates five breaths during continuous non–rapid eye movement (NREM) stage 2 (N2) sleep at atmospheric pressure, all characterized by IFL. The individual being monitored is a 24-year-old woman with a body mass index (BMI) of 19.9 kg/m^2, does not snore, and has an AHI of 0.3 per hour. Because Figure 127.1 has both an airflow tracing and a supraglottic pressure tracing, it precisely demonstrates the presence of IFL. Specifically, it shows that inspiratory airflow is limited to a maximal level (intersected by the vertical lines), despite the observation that the pressure gradient across the pharyngeal airway (atmospheric pressure minus supraglottic pressure) continues to increase (atmospheric pressure remains the same while supraglottic pressure continues to decrease beyond the vertical line). This defines IFL.

Figure 127.2 demonstrates both IFL and non-flow-limited inspiration in the same individual diagnosed with UARS during nasal CPAP titration. Although the left panel of the figure clearly demonstrates IFL at atmospheric pressure like that observed in Figure 127.1, the right panel, recorded at the therapeutic nasal CPAP level of 4 cm H_2O, presents airflow and supraglottic pressure tracings that parallel each other through four inspiratory cycles. The parallel tracings demonstrate that inspiratory airflow is continuously proportional to the driving pressure, 4 cm H_2O minus supraglottic pressure, and thus, according to the earlier definition of IFL, is not flow limited.

Figures 127.1 and 127.2 illustrate that, when one is provided with both an airflow signal and a supraglottic pressure signal, recognizing IFL is not difficult. It is emphasized that IFL is not defined by any specific decrease in inspiratory airflow (e.g., a 30% or 50% decrease in airflow) relative to *non*-flow-limited inspiration. Rather, IFL is defined by a specific relationship of airflow to driving pressure (nasal pressure minus supraglottic pressure). IFL can be more difficult to recognize in the absence of a supraglottic pressure signal because one is then missing driving pressure; indeed, the presence of IFL can only be *assumed* in the

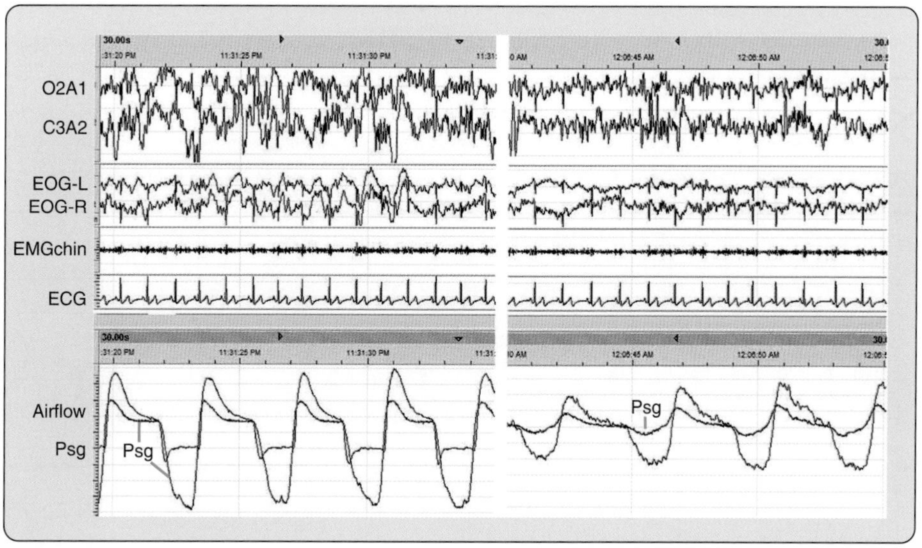

Figure 127.2 This figure demonstrates both inspiratory airflow limitation (IFL) and *non*-flow-limited inspiration in the same individual during nasal continuous positive airway pressure (CPAP) titration. The two polysomnographic tracings are obtained in stage N2 sleep, 1 hour apart. Below the sleep monitoring channels recording electroencephalograms (O2A1, C3A2), electrooculograms (EOG-L [left] and EOG-R [right]), superficial electromyograms of the chin (EMGchin), and electrocardiogram (ECG) are recordings of airflow (a pneumotachograph tracing) and supraglottic pressure (Psg). The *left panel* demonstrates four breaths at atmospheric pressure, whereas the *right panel* demonstrates four breaths with nasal CPAP at 4 cm H_2O. In each panel, airflow (*black tracing*) and Psg (*blue tracing*) are superimposed. The *left panel* demonstrates the plateau of inspiratory airflow (downgoing) at a maximal level occurring as Psg continues to decrease, which defines IFL. In the *right panel*, because pharyngeal pressure and Psg do not fall much below 4 cm H_2O (the CPAP applied to the nasal mask), Psg always remains above pharyngeal critical pressure, and the airflow and pressure tracings parallel each other (airflow is always determined by the pressure gradient: 4 minus Psg).

absence of a supraglottic pressure tracing. To enable clinicians to recognize IFL during clinical PSG without the recording of supraglottic pressure, researchers have investigated the possibility of identifying IFL from the airflow signal alone.

In 1998 two studies evaluated the utility of a plateau of inspiratory airflow measured as a nasal pressure signal (pressure transducer-generated airflow [PTAF]) to identify IFL.[12,13] One study[13] used a computer algorithm to classify each PTAF inspiration as non-flow-limited (sinusoidal in shape and resembling the airflow signal in the right panel of Figure 127.2), flow-limited (having a clear plateau and resembling the airflow signal in Figure 127.1 and the left panel of Figure 127.2), or intermediate (not sinusoidal but not fulfilling their program's criteria for an inspiratory plateau). The PTAF signal clearly separated their asymptomatic controls of patients without OSA from their patients with OSA, with the former having fewer flow-limited events. In a similar study of seven habitual snorers, Clark and associates[12] found that an inspiratory airflow plateau determined by PTAF identified flow-limited inspirations with a sensitivity and specificity of approximately 80%. Thus PTAF evidence of a clear inspiratory airflow plateau is a reasonably reliable method for identifying IFL during clinical PSG.

The ability to recognize IFL during diagnostic PSG, whether in-laboratory or during out-of-center sleep testing (OCST), can also be aided by the finding that the ratio of the inspiratory time to the time of the entire respiratory cycle (i.e., the "duty cycle") is prolonged.[14] This distinction is illustrated in Figure 127.2, where four flow-limited inspirations (left panel) take up a larger portion of the respiratory cycle time than the non-flow-limited inspirations (right panel), where expiratory time is more prolonged. During IFL, the inspiratory airflow increases rapidly and remains near maximum throughout most of inspiration (left panel), maximizing the tidal volume under the flow-limited conditions. During the *non*-flow-limited breaths (right panel), the increase in inspiratory airflow is more gradual, and airflow remains near maximum for a shorter portion of inspiration.

Figure 127.3 represents both IFL and *non*-flow-limited breathing in a single patient with UARS undergoing nasal CPAP titration. In the absence of a supraglottic pressure signal, IFL can be recognized by the change in the airflow tracing between the two left panels recorded at CPAP levels of 4 and 5 cm H_2O demonstrating IFL, and the right panel recorded at a CPAP of 6 cm H_2O illustrating non-flow-limited airflow at therapeutic CPAP. At 4 and 5 cm H_2O, the flow-limited inspiratory airflow tracing is characterized by a rapid increase in airflow to a maximum, followed by a prolonged plateau at maximal flow. At 6 cm H_2O, the non-flow-limited inspiratory airflow increases more gradually without a subsequent plateau but with a rapid decrease of airflow and a shorter ratio of inspiratory time to respiratory cycle time (exhalation is prolonged relative to flow-limited conditions). Thus, in the absence of a supraglottic pressure signal, both the shape and the relative duration of the inspiratory airflow tracing provide evidence for the presence of IFL.

In Figure 127.4, a 30-second epoch of sleep from a patient with UARS provides examples of overt IFL, more subtle IFL, and *non*-flow-limited breathing. Although several breaths in Figure 127.4 demonstrate the rapid increase in inspiratory airflow and long inspiratory airflow plateau of IFL, several (marked by an asterisk) demonstrate a less prolonged plateau of inspiratory airflow. The presence in these breaths, however, of a rapid increase in inspiratory airflow followed by a short plateau, as well as the accompanying snoring (recorded by microphone) for one of the breaths, can be used to identify all of these as examples of subtle IFL compared with the one *non*-flow-limited inspiration (marked by an arrow). Viewed from the perspective of respiratory cycle time, one can also appreciate that the non-flow-limited breath is preceded by the

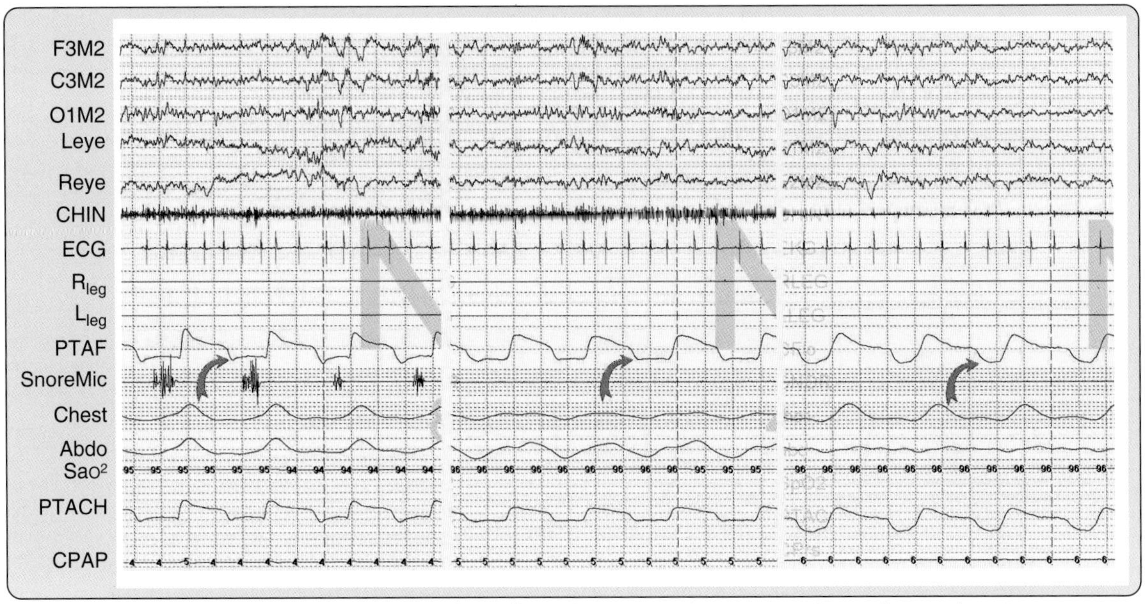

Figure 127.3 This figure's three panels, from left to right, represent three 12-second intervals at nasal continuous positive airway pressure (CPAP) levels of 4 cm H_2O, 5 cm H_2O, and 6 cm H_2O. Below the sleep monitoring channels recording electroencephalograms (F3M2, C3M2, O1M2), electrooculograms (L_{leg} and Reye), superficial electromyograms of the chin (CHIN) and right and left tibialis anterior (R_{leg} and L_{leg}), and ECG are several channels recording respiratory parameters. The respiratory channels include a pressure transducer-generated airflow (PTAF) signal, a microphone placed on the neck to record snoring (SnoreMic), impedance plethysmography of the chest and abdomen (Chest and Abdo; movement), oxyhemoglobin saturation (Sao_2), a pneumotachograph airflow signal (PTACH), and a pressure transducer-recorded CPAP level (CPAP). At 4 cm H_2O, the *left panel*, the patient's inspirations all demonstrate inspiratory airflow limitation (IFL) with audible snoring. Inspiratory airflow (downgoing) is seen to increase rapidly and then to plateau with a prolonged time spent at maximal inspiratory airflow (highlighted by the *arrow*). At 5 cm H_2O, IFL persists without snoring. Inspiratory airflow, again, increases rapidly and then demonstrates a prolonged plateau at maximal flow (highlighted by the *arrow*). At 6 cm H_2O, the airflow tracing no longer demonstrates IFL. Inspiratory airflow increases to its maximum more gradually and then immediately decreases, spending only a short time at maximal airflow. Expiratory time is prolonged relative to flow-limited conditions (the two *left panels*), and inspiration is a smaller percentage of the respiratory cycle.

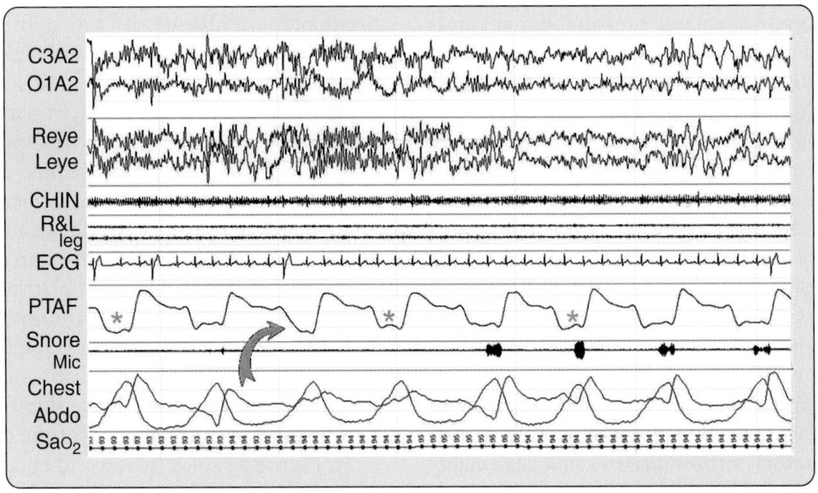

Figure 127.4 This figure demonstrates a 30-second epoch of non–rapid eye movement stage 2 (N2) sleep containing eight consecutive breaths representing both overt and subtle (*asterisks*) inspiratory airflow limitation and a *non*-flow-limited breath (*arrow*). The sleep parameters recorded include electroencephalograms (EEGs; C3A2, O1A2), electrooculograms (EOGs; Reye and Leye), superficial electromyogram of the chin (CHIN), superficial electromyograms of the right and left tibialis anterior (R_{leg} and L_{leg}), and electrocardiogram (ECG). The respiratory parameters recorded are labeled similarly to those in Figure 127.3. Refer to the text for a complete characterization of the breathing. PTAF, Pressure transducer-generated airflow.

longest exhalation, and the ratio of inspiratory time to respiratory cycle time for the breath is lower than for the flow-limited breaths in the figure.

To summarize, IFL can be recognized, using a nasal pressure signal, as a plateau in inspiratory airflow and a prolongation of inspiratory time relative to total respiratory cycle time. Inspiratory airflow can be observed to rise rapidly to a maximum and to remain there for most of inspiration. Snoring, the audible manifestation of the fluttering pharyngeal airway characterizing IFL, is not as sensitive an indicator of

IFL as the combined airflow and driving pressure criteria (Figures 127.1 and 127.2) or the airflow tracing alone. Figure 127.1, which in fact is a tracing of a lean female with no history of snoring, demonstrates definitive evidence of IFL determined by her airflow and supraglottic pressure recordings. In Figure 127.3, nasal CPAP of 5 cm H_2O resolves the patient's snoring before the airflow tracing demonstrates resolution of IFL at 6 cm H_2O. Figure 127.4 demonstrates five breaths clearly characterized by the airflow plateau associated with IFL, only four of which demonstrate snoring. For this reason, the presence of snoring should not be relied on to determine whether a patient with sleepiness or fatigue has sleep-disordered breathing. Even in the absence of apneas and hypopneas, silent IFL (defined in the glossary) associated with arousals (RERAs) may be prevalent enough to establish a diagnosis of OSA when using ICSD-3 criteria, or UARS, using the criteria of sleepiness or fatigue in the presence of IFL as presented in the glossary. Similarly, the absence of snoring should not be relied on to determine whether a nasal CPAP level is therapeutic (i.e., has eliminated IFL). Rather, the polysomnographic technologist and sleep medicine physician should differentiate IFL during sleep from non-flow-limited inspiration using an airflow signal generated by either a pneumotachograph or a PTAF signal and determine therapeutic nasal CPAP as the pressure that eliminates IFL (as demonstrated in Figures 127.2 and 127.3). A CPAP level that eliminates IFL will, of necessity, eliminate all apneas, hypopneas, and RERAs.

PATHOLOGIC UPPER AIRWAY RESISTANCE SYNDROMES: CLINICAL ASPECTS

Snoring

Habitual snoring, as described early in the glossary, can be observed in patients with OSA complaining of daytime sleepiness, fatigue, and insomnia. Habitual snoring may also occur in the absence of symptoms and signs of OSA and without an RDI (a frequency of apneas, hypopneas, and RERAs) adequate to establish a diagnosis of OSA in the absence of symptoms, that is, an RDI of 15 per hour. In the latter instance, according to the ICSD-3, it is regarded as "isolated snoring," listed in the category of sleep-related breathing disorders.

As already noted, snoring is a sleep-related sound caused by vibration of soft tissue in the UA under conditions of IFL. In most individuals with isolated snoring, the snoring is limited to inspiration, although early expiratory snoring or snoring throughout expiration can occur.[15] The presence of expiratory snoring with low mean oxygen saturation during sleep may indicate coexisting chronic obstructive pulmonary disease in patients with OSA, warranting further evaluation for pulmonary disorders.[16] Whether occurring during inspiration or expiration, snoring is generated by high-frequency opening and closing (fluttering) of UA structures, including the tongue base and soft palate, aided by the adhesive properties of mucosal secretions. Acoustic studies have shown that the major frequency content of snoring is below 2000 Hz, with peak power below 500 Hz.[17] Snorers experience increased total pulmonary resistance during sleep related to reduced UA muscle tone causing IFL and leading to increased inspiratory effort.[18]

There is considerable variation in the prevalence figures reported for habitual snoring, because of differences in subject selection and whether the snoring data is subjective (from patient or bed partner) or objective (measured or recorded) and how it was defined (isolated or habitual). In addition to differences in methodology regarding diagnoses and snoring assessment, differences in gender and obesity distribution between studies may affect snoring prevalence significantly. Both gender and obesity can affect UA resistance (alternatively, collapsibility, assessed as the pharyngeal Pcrit) either by structural changes or neuromuscular mechanisms. Thus the variability of study design is one reason for the varied prevalence figures for habitual snoring seen in the literature.

The severity of subjective snoring reported by the bed partner may not correspond with either objectively assessed snoring or the subjective assessment of the sleep technician monitoring the patient.[19] This may, in part, be due to considerable night-to-night variability of snoring intensity. The time spent snoring and snoring volume within one individual can vary from night to night, depending on factors such as sleeping position, medications, alcohol intake, and cumulative or acute sleep debt. Alternatively, the discrepancy observed between a bed partner's report of snoring severity and that observed during in-laboratory PSG could be due to allergens in the home environment altering UA pressure-flow relationships or even the bed partner's sensitivity to the noise or willingness to complain.[20]

In the 2011 Centers for Disease Control and Prevention report on unhealthy sleep behaviors, the study reports a snoring prevalence of 48% based on a telephone survey.[21] The report does not indicate how many of the snorers in this survey complained of hypersomnolence or other symptoms of OSA. Furthermore, the report does not specify the snoring severity of those individuals labeled as snorers: intermittent versus habitual. Based on data from the Sleep Heart Health Study, a sample of 5615 community-dwelling adults between the ages of 40 and 98 years, 13% of the participants had an AHI of less than 5 per hour and reported *habitual* snoring (3 to 7 nights/week).[22] These data estimate a prevalence of habitual snoring without OSA of less than 15% in a community sample. Symptom data, however, are not provided, and so one cannot determine a prevalence of isolated snoring. Of note, 29% of the 5615 men and women did not know whether they snored (perhaps because of not having a bed partner). Although the previous two examples illustrate the difficulty investigators have in determining the prevalence of habitual and isolated snoring, it remains clear that snoring is a common phenomenon that frequently prompts a referral for a sleep evaluation to establish a diagnosis of OSA.

When a habitual snorer presents for a sleep evaluation, PSG is warranted if witnessed apnea, hypersomnolence, fatigue, insomnia, somatic syndromes typically described among patients who have UARS (discussed in the next section), or comorbidities such as metabolic syndrome, cardiac dysrhythmia, or atrial fibrillation are present. In this case PSG may lead to treatment of OSA when the ICSD-3 diagnostic criteria for OSA are met. Habitual snoring in the absence of witnessed apnea, symptoms or syndromes, or comorbidities (after appropriate screening for comorbidities) does not automatically warrant a polysomnogram. Habitual snoring is a common occurrence among middle-aged, overweight men, and polysomnographic evaluations of *all* habitual snorers carries a very high cost-to-benefit ratio. A more practical approach would be to monitor asymptomatic, healthy, habitual snorers over time for the development of signs and symptoms that would support obtaining PSG. Alternatively, OCST can be used to rule out moderate to severe OSA in asymptomatic, healthy, habitual snorers in need of reassurance.

The rationale for not obtaining PSG in asymptomatic, healthy, habitual snorers extends beyond the issue of costs, to a consideration of benefit. Specifically, even if such an individual fulfills ICSD-3 criteria for OSA, the question is whether such an asymptomatic, healthy individual is in fact in need of treatment. To the contrary, cross-sectional polysomnographic data from a study by Pavlova and associates[23] of 163 asymptomatic, nonobese individuals screened for the absence of metabolic syndrome and cardiovascular disease (25% reporting "some" snoring) demonstrate that many such individuals have RDIs above 15 per hour, fulfilling ICSD-3 criteria for OSA. Indeed, the mean RDI for individuals older than 65 years was 22 per hour in Pavlova's study. Similar data exist in three studies comparing inspiratory airflow dynamics during sleep between patients with somatic syndromes[24,25] and UARS[26] with those of rigorously screened healthy control subjects. For the three studies, 4 (11%) of 35 healthy control subjects (14 men and 21 women) met the ICSD-3 threshold for OSA that would justify their treatment without symptoms or comorbidities (RDI ≥ 15/hour). Another 4 of the healthy control subjects had values of RDI between 10 per hour and 15 per hour, approximating the threshold for treatment.

Lee and associates[27] demonstrated that the amount of time spent snoring was correlated with the extent of asymptomatic carotid artery stenosis, independent of AHI and histories of other comorbidities. These findings suggest that in individuals predisposed to atherosclerosis (by smoking, hypertension, or hyperlipidemia), habitual snoring may be an *additional* risk factor for developing carotid artery atherosclerosis. On the other hand, a study with a 17-year follow-up of 380 community-dwelling adults failed to document a significant relationship between objectively measured nocturnal time spent snoring and all-cause mortality from cardiovascular disease.[28] In the absence of certainty about the effects of habitual snoring, one should evaluate, beginning with noninvasive methods, an asymptomatic, habitual snorer without metabolic syndrome or atrial fibrillation for evidence of atherosclerosis before deciding that the patient is not in need of treatment and can be followed over time.

Asymptomatic, healthy individuals seeking treatment for habitual snoring or isolated snoring (after PSG because of reports of witnessed or patient-perceived apnea) will usually do so because they are concerned about the disruption of their bed partner's sleep. Any treatment that will lower the pharyngeal Pcrit, reducing the occurrence of IFL, will also have a beneficial effect on audible snoring. A wide variety of over-the-counter remedies are available for snoring, but they are of limited efficacy. There are limited or absent benefits of products such as nasal dilators, lubricants, oral dietary supplements, and magnetic pillows and mattresses.[29] In contrast to these ineffective treatments, any effective treatment used for OSA will be effective for asymptomatic snoring. Among these treatments, few isolated snorers choose nasal CPAP, considering it a burden to use and to maintain.

Successful or partially successful treatment of isolated snoring has been reported using lifestyle modifications. A lifestyle modification such as weight reduction (by diet or bariatric surgery, see Chapter 139) can be an effective treatment for snoring because it can substantially lower pharyngeal Pcrit.[30] There is an independent, beneficial effect of physical activity on self-reported snoring in obese women.[31] Another lifestyle alteration that can decrease the intensity of snoring is avoiding alcohol consumption before going to bed.[32] Other lifestyle modifications that can reduce snoring include avoiding sleep deprivation and the use of sedative-hypnotic medications.

Oral mandibular advancement appliances have been used successfully for the treatment of mild to moderate OSA and asymptomatic snoring in patients with a healthy dentition. Good results can be achieved with 50% to 75% of maximal voluntary protrusion.[33,34] For patients with an insufficient number of healthy teeth, a tongue-retaining device may be a good alternative. Patients should be advised that snoring may not be completely abolished, but significant reductions in the time spent snoring and snoring intensity can be obtained. They should also be aware that mandibular and maxillary incisors may procline (mandibular) or retrocline (maxillary) significantly with long-term use of an oral appliance.[33]

Surgery can be performed for isolated snoring to decrease its occurrence and intensity. Surgical targets include the nasal turbinates and septum, the nasopharynx, oropharynx, tongue base, and hypopharynx. Sleep nasendoscopy with a flexible endoscope is increasingly used to perform a preoperative assessment of possible surgical targets. For this procedure, anesthesia is used to simulate sleep. At present, the data regarding the value of nasendoscopy before surgical treatment of snoring are indeterminate. The surgical method depends on the surgeon's preference and the availability of equipment, but procedures are performed using a scalpel, radiofrequency ablation, and yttrium-aluminum garnet laser. Studies assessing the efficacy of these procedures have typically shown good immediate- and short-term results. However, many of these studies have relied only on subjective assessments of snoring. A study on the subjective versus the objective improvement of snoring after palatal surgery published in 1994 did not find any objective improvement in snoring despite a subjective improvement in greater than 75% of the participants.[35] Palatal surgery for isolated snoring improved subjectively and objectively, but the objective improvement was short lived and correlated poorly with the subjective improvement on an individual basis.[36] A long-term study evaluating patients treated with palatal surgery found a substantial rebound of snoring even in the absence of weight gain. In addition, about a third of the patients continued to experience surgical side effects (swallowing dysfunction, altered voice, and pain) that left them dissatisfied with the decision to have palatal surgery.[37] Surgery intended to relieve nasal obstruction alone does not produce a significant improvement of objectively assessed snoring intensity and snoring time, nor does it decrease the AHI, despite improvement in nasal resistance.[38]

The consequences of leaving isolated snoring untreated relate specifically to the concern of whether untreated isolated snoring progresses to OSA over time. According to a study that followed individuals with isolated snoring over 5 years with PSG, isolated snoring does not progress to OSA over 5 years in the absence of a significant change in body weight.[39] Thus, to date, there is no evidence that isolated snoring progresses to OSA in the intermediate term.

In summary, isolated snoring is a diagnosis of exclusion reserved for habitual snorers who are otherwise asymptomatic, without metabolic syndrome and cardiovascular disease, and who do not meet polysomnographic or OCST criteria for OSA. The potential for adverse long-term cardiovascular outcomes in isolated snoring remains uncertain. Treatment of isolated snoring is currently limited to attempting to improve the sleep quality of the bed partner. Available treatments include lifestyle modifications, oral appliances, and soft tissue surgery. Most available treatment options lead to short-term success but fail in the long term.

Upper Airway Resistance Syndrome

UARS is defined as the symptom of either hypersomnolence or fatigue, together with the presence of IFL during sleep by in-laboratory PSG and an AHI of less than 5 per hour (see the glossary earlier in this chapter). ICSD-3 absorbs UARS into OSA by including RERAs into the severity assessment of sleep fragmentation in OSA. ICSD-3 criteria for OSA now classify any patient fulfilling the previously noted UARS definition with an RDI above 5 per hour as having OSA. Clearly a portion of UARS has been absorbed into OSA by the clinical criteria of ICSD-3. However, there are still patients meeting the definition of UARS elaborated in this chapter, with an RDI of less than 5 per hour who are not included within the ICSD-3 definition of OSA and are not considered, clinically, to have sleep-disordered breathing. Nevertheless, to investigators of UARS and to clinicians attempting to treat the hypersomnolence of a patient without a clear diagnosis because of too few RERAs, the recognition that sleep-disordered breathing may, in fact, exist outside the limits of the ICSD-3 is important and worthy of consideration. In this section we discuss the varied clinical presentation of UARS, its polysomnographic appearance, and its evolving paradigm. To facilitate this discussion, when we refer to OSA, we will use the ICSD-2 definition of OSA—an AHI of at least 5 per hour—to match the definition used in the research to be presented.

Anthropometric Features and Risk Factors

Compared with patients with OSA, those with UARS are younger, leaner, and more frequently female. Published studies of patients with UARS, as defined by the previous criteria, have established a mean age of 40 years, with the average BMI between 23 and 30 kg/m^2 (normal weight or overweight; less often, obese), and approximately 50% female.[40–42] Although craniofacial abnormalities, such as a narrow, elongated face characterized by a high arched palate, reduced upper and lower intermolar distances, and a narrow anterior nasal aperture (adenoid facies), have been reported in patients with UARS, these same findings are also commonly observed in patients with OSA[43] and so cannot be considered specific for UARS. The presence of these abnormalities suggests a disturbance of facial development caused by increased nasal resistance during early childhood with mouth breathing.[44]

Signs and Symptoms

The most observed polysomnographic feature of UARS patients is nonapneic, habitual snoring or silent IFL with relatively few adjudicated apneic or hypopneic events (AHI < 5/hour). In clinical practice, these patients will seek medical attention for their condition because they also suffer from nonrestorative sleep, fatigue, sleepiness, or insomnia. In fact, patients with UARS are more commonly referred to a sleep disorders center for their symptoms than for their snoring. Before referring these patients for cognitive behavior therapy (CBT) for insomnia, a careful sleep-related history revealing snoring without witnessed apnea will prompt polysomnographic investigation with documentation of IFL during sleep. It is emphasized that a report of witnessed apnea does not preclude a diagnosis of UARS because about one-third of patients with UARS are reported to have witnessed apnea but have an AHI below the threshold for OSA.[45] Similarly, the absence of audible snoring does not preclude a diagnosis of UARS because inaudible IFL is observed in about 10% of patients diagnosed with UARS.[45,46] Typically, these patients have been diagnosed with insomnia and, in the absence of a sleep-related history of habitual snoring, are referred for CBT without performing PSG. When CBT fails to improve their condition and PSG is performed to exclude an intrinsic sleep disorder, IFL in the absence of audible snoring can be demonstrated.[47]

The earliest reports of UARS emphasized the importance of hypersomnolence as a diagnostic criterion distinguishing it from isolated snoring.[2,15] Before those reports, PSG technology used a thermistor or thermocouple to generate a qualitative airflow signal that could not be used to recognize IFL. Thus the link between hypersomnolence and IFL could not be made, and patients with UARS often received a diagnosis of idiopathic hypersomnolence. The earliest reports of UARS substituted a pneumotachograph recording of airflow for the qualitative airflow signal, together with an esophageal pressure catheter measurement of inspiratory effort to establish the presence of IFL during sleep in patients with UARS.[2,15] With time and the growth of clinical experience evaluating patients with UARS, the diagnostic criteria for UARS have been expanded to include complaints of hypersomnolence or fatigue.[7,45]

Hypersomnolence indicates increased sleep pressure expressed by short sleep latency, a state that is inconsistent with a complaint of insomnia. Fatigue, on the other hand, is generally associated with longer sleep latencies, reflecting a state of hyperarousal commonly observed in patients with insomnia. About one-third of patients with UARS complains of sleep-onset insomnia, and nearly two-thirds reports sleep maintenance insomnia.[40] Characteristically, the complaints of fatigue and insomnia among patients with UARS are associated with the complaint of nonrestorative sleep.

Of interest, patients with UARS complain of more subjective sleep disturbance than patients with OSA who have much more disrupted sleep.[48] Patients with UARS can also experience a variety of parasomnias. Among these are sleep-related bruxism,[45] chronic sleepwalking in children,[49] and catathrenia.[50]

At present, there is not enough evidence to conclude that UARS is an independent cardiovascular risk factor. An increased prevalence of arterial hypertension among nonapneic snorers has been reported,[51] and borderline arterial hypertension has been lowered with nasal CPAP in a small series of patients with UARS.[52] Hypotension and orthostatic intolerance have also been documented in about 20% of patients with UARS.[53]

Psychiatric symptoms such as depression[41,42,54,55] and anxiety[54-56] have been demonstrated among patients with UARS and have responded dramatically to treatment using nasal CPAP and rapid palatal expansion in case reports.[54,55] Conversely, failure to diagnose and treat UARS is associated with a worsening of these symptoms over time.[41]

At present, there are limited data available regarding cognitive function among patients with UARS. Using a psychomotor vigilance task, Stoohs and associates[57] have reported increased reaction times among patients with UARS compared with patients who have OSA. Although those with UARS perceive themselves to have impaired cognitive function compared with healthy control subjects, objective testing fails to demonstrate such a difference.[58]

Patients with UARS also commonly present with a variety of findings characteristic of the functional somatic syndromes: headaches and functional gastrointestinal symptoms and alpha-delta sleep.[45] These functional somatic syndrome symptoms and signs (specifically, sleep-onset insomnia, headache, irritable bowel syndrome, and alpha-delta sleep) decrease in prevalence among sleep-disordered breathing patients as the

AHI increases.[45] Conversely, when patients with functional somatic syndromes undergo PSG, IFL during sleep is commonly observed (fibromyalgia, temporomandibular joint syndrome, Gulf War illness, and irritable bowel syndrome have been studied).[24,25,59,60] In this setting, nasal CPAP has been shown to relieve the symptoms of functional somatic syndrome patients by relieving their IFL during sleep[60,61] (see the section Pathophysiology and Clinical Correlates for a discussion of mechanism).

Polysomnographic Findings

Polysomnographic findings among patients with UARS can be subdivided into those characterizing breathing with associated arousals and those characterizing sleep architecture (electroencephalographic frequencies, sleep staging). Concerning sleep architecture, researchers have observed findings consistent with unstable, nonrestorative sleep among patients with UARS.

Polysomnographic Findings Characterizing Breathing. Breathing in UARS is, by definition, characterized by an AHI below 5 per hour of sleep and periods of IFL during sleep with flows greater than 50% of waking levels (exemplified in Figures 127.2 to 127.4) and terminated by arousals or changes in the background electroencephalographic rhythm associated with a return of airflow to a non-flow-limited state (i.e., RERAs).[41] In several large studies, the mean AHI for patients with UARS is consistently 2 per hour, and the frequency of RERAs is between 5 per hour and 20 per hour.[40–42] Oxyhemoglobin saturation generally remains greater than 90% throughout sleep.[40,42] One study that used a snore microphone to determine the prevalence of breaths associated with audible snoring among 424 patient with UARS observed a 21 ± 23% (mean ± standard deviation) prevalence of such breaths during sleep.[42] It is likely that if a study were performed that included both a snore microphone and a pressure transducer for airflow measurement to identify both snoring and inaudible IFL, the prevalence of such breaths would be considerably higher and not a sporadic occurrence.

The preceding description of breathing during sleep in UARS does not define the syndrome based on thresholds for IFL or RERAs. Empirically, periods of IFL during sleep in UARS may last a few breaths or be continuous for many PSG epochs. The presence of IFL has not been defined by a consensus frequency of *resistive* events, but it is a characteristic of breathing during sleep that can be described in a PSG report based on the sleep stages in which it occurs and an impression of the prevalence of flow-limited breaths in those sleep stages (e.g., continuous, intermittent, or uncommon; Figure 127.4 is one 30-second epoch of continuous IFL in a patient with UARS). Similarly, in the UARS literature, RERAs have not been defined by a consensus length of the preceding period of IFL, as has been done in the ICSD-3. Rather, the duration of IFL preceding a RERA has been undefined[2]: 10 seconds[41] or one flow-limited breath,[26] depending on the study. Because the diagnosis of UARS is not dependent on thresholds for resistive events or RERAs, UARS cannot be classified as mild, moderate, or severe based on these events. Indeed, there are no published data relating the severity of hypersomnolence among patients who have UARS to RERA frequency or prevalence of IFL. New techniques to analyze flow signals to document not only flow limitation but also recovery breaths may lead to more useful methods to characterize the abnormal breathing events.[62]

Polysomnographic Findings Characterizing Sleep Architecture. PSG of patients who have UARS demonstrates findings consistent with unstable, nonrestorative sleep. Among these findings is alpha frequency intruding into sleep, increased sleep stage shifts, and cyclic alternating pattern (CAP).

Patients with UARS experience increased alpha frequency, a frequency observed during quiet wakefulness, within their sleep electroencephalogram.[45,63] This increased alpha frequency may be seen in stage N3 sleep, where it has been termed *alpha-delta sleep*[45,64] (Figure 127.5) or in N1 and N2 sleep[55] (Figure 127.6; also observed in Figure 127.4). It is emphasized that this alpha frequency occurs during continuous sleep and is not the consequence of an electroencephalographic arousal. Resolution of this finding has been observed among adolescent patients with UARS when sleep quality improves after rapid palatal expansion[55] (Figures 127.5 and 127.6).

Patients with UARS also demonstrate sleep stage instability with frequent shifting from deeper to lighter sleep stages or to wakefulness, with decreasing depth of sleep designated as the stage sequence: REM, N3, N2, N1, and wake. The frequency of sleep stage shifting in patients who have UARS is decreased by treatment with nasal CPAP[61] (Figure 127.7) and rapid palatal expansion.[55] The mechanism by which nasal CPAP eliminates sleep stage shifts is not simply elimination of sleep fragmentation associated with RERAs. Although shifts between stages N2, N1, and wake require an intervening arousal, stage shifts between REM, N3, and N2 do not require an arousal. Indeed, the N3-to-N2 sleep stage shifts in Figure 127.7 that decrease in frequency with nasal CPAP all occur during continuous sleep, the difference between N3 and N2 being determined by the prevalence of delta waves, and do not represent the elimination of RERAs by nasal CPAP. The occurrence of frequent shifts from deeper to lighter sleep is hypothesized to be an adaptive response to a danger or *stressor*, lightening the individual's sleep and allowing a quicker response to an emergency.[65] Increased shifts from deeper to lighter sleep commonly occur in healthy people sleeping for the first night in a new location, such as a sleep laboratory.[66]

A second manifestation of sleep stage instability among patients with UARS is the occurrence of CAP, which is defined by a periodic disruption of NREM sleep by electroencephalographic events that do not meet the threshold for an arousal by conventional sleep staging criteria.[67] Among patients with UARS, increasing levels of these nonarousal electroencephalographic events correlate with increasing levels of sleepiness and fatigue.[67] Furthermore, the presence of CAP is a marker for increased sympathetic nervous system tone commonly found under conditions of stress.[68]

Pathophysiology and Clinical Correlates

Hypotheses concerning the pathophysiology of UARS continue to evolve as the manifestations of the disorder and the body systems affected increase in number. Initially it was hypothesized that the disorder as one of sleep fragmentation by RERAs associated with hypersomnolence that improved with nasal CPAP treatment.[2,15] Although this paradigm of UARS, henceforth termed the *RERA paradigm*, provided an explanation for the hypersomnolence associated with UARS, it did not provide an explanation for the somatic, cognitive, and affective complaints, such as insomnia, fatigue, body pain,

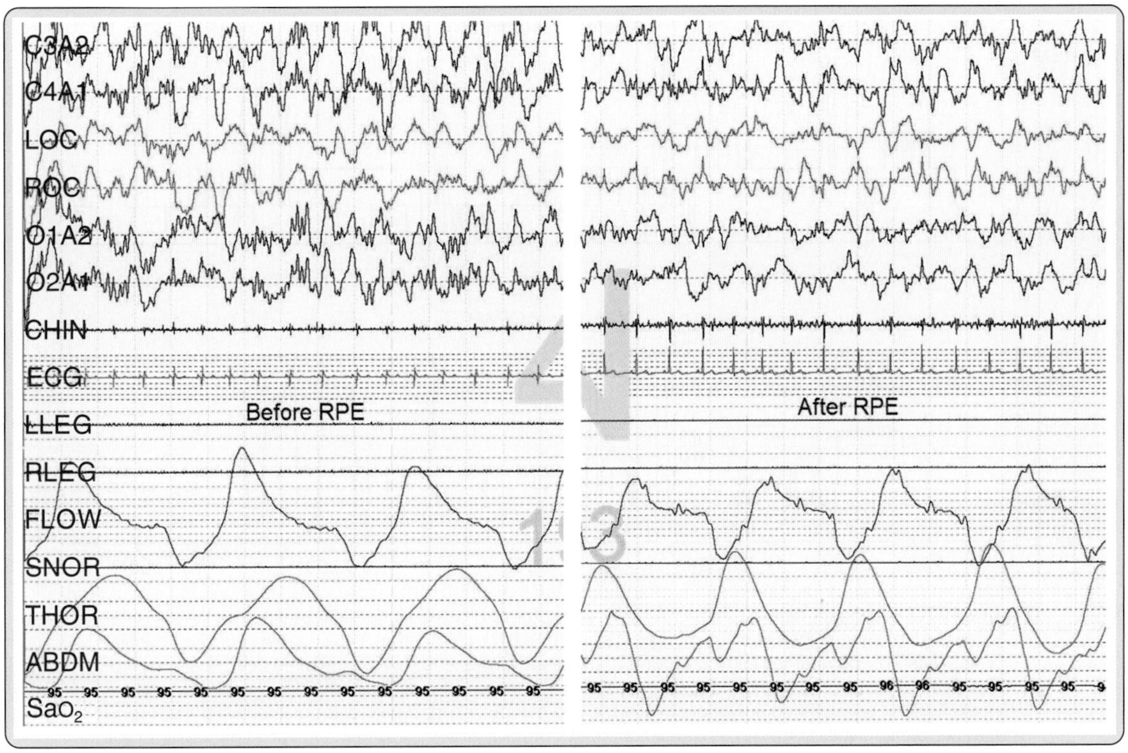

Figure 127.5 This figure demonstrates two 15-second periods of NREM stage 3 (N3) sleep recorded at the same time of night, before and after rapid palatal expansion (RPE; 13 months between studies) in a 16-year-old boy with severe chronic fatigue who was diagnosed with upper airway resistance syndrome. Recording includes four electroencephalographic channels (*purple*; C3A2, C4A1, O1A2, O2A1), left and right electrooculograms (*green*; LOC, ROC), electromyograms of the chin (CHIN) and left and right tibialis anterior muscle (LLEG, RLEG), and an electrocardiogram (ECG). Respiratory channels include pressure transducer airflow (FLOW), a snore microphone (SNOR), thoracic and abdominal wall movement (THOR, ABDM), and oxygen saturation (Sao_2). Before RPE, the patient demonstrates alpha-delta sleep characterized by low-frequency, high-amplitude delta waves with superimposed prominent 7- to 11-Hz alpha waves observed best in electroencephalographic leads C3A2 and C4A1. After RPE, the alpha frequency is greatly decreased in amplitude or gone. Associated with this change, the ECG demonstrates a decrease in heart rate between studies from 72/minute before RPE to 64/minute after RPE, suggesting decreased sympathetic nervous system tone between studies.

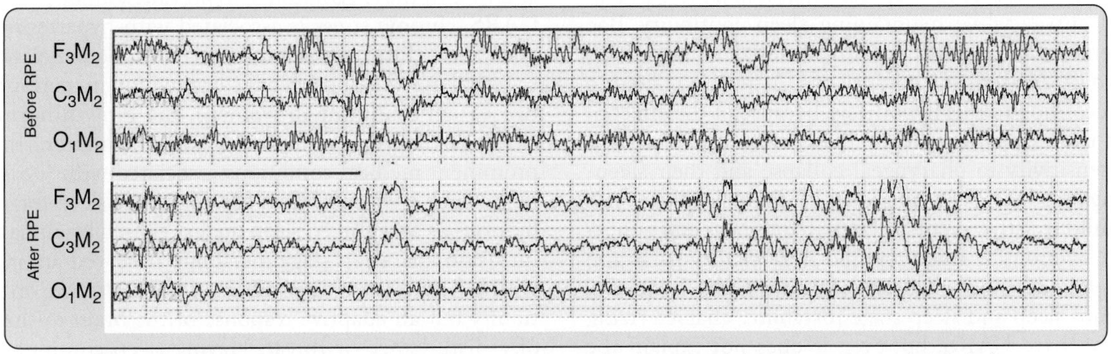

Figure 127.6 This figure demonstrates 30 seconds of stage N2 sleep recorded at the same time of night, before and after rapid palatal expansion (RPE), from an 18-year-old man with severe depression who was diagnosed with upper airway resistance syndrome. The two recordings each include three electroencephalographic channels (F_3M_2, C_3M_2, O_1M_2). As in Figure 127.5, the recording before RPE shows prominent alpha frequency (at approximately 7 Hz; seen well above the *orange line*). After RPE, the alpha frequency is greatly reduced in amplitude, and the underlying theta frequency of 3 to 5 Hz is seen more clearly. (Reproduced with permission from Miller P, Iyer M, Gold AR. Treatment resistant adolescent depression with upper airway resistance syndrome treated with rapid palatal expansion: a case report. *J Med Case Rep.* 2012;6[1]:415.)

depression, anxiety, cognitive dysfunction, and gastrointestinal dysfunction, or for the parasomnias, such as bruxism, sleepwalking, and catathrenia, that have subsequently been associated with UARS.*

*References 45, 49, 50, 54–56, 58, 69, 70.

As clinical experience with patients who have UARS increased, investigators came to postulate that the hypersomnolence of these patients is not simply the consequence of sleep fragmentation but also of altered sleep quality that affects its restorative properties. The alpha frequency intrusion into sleep[45,63] and the unstable sleep stages characterized by

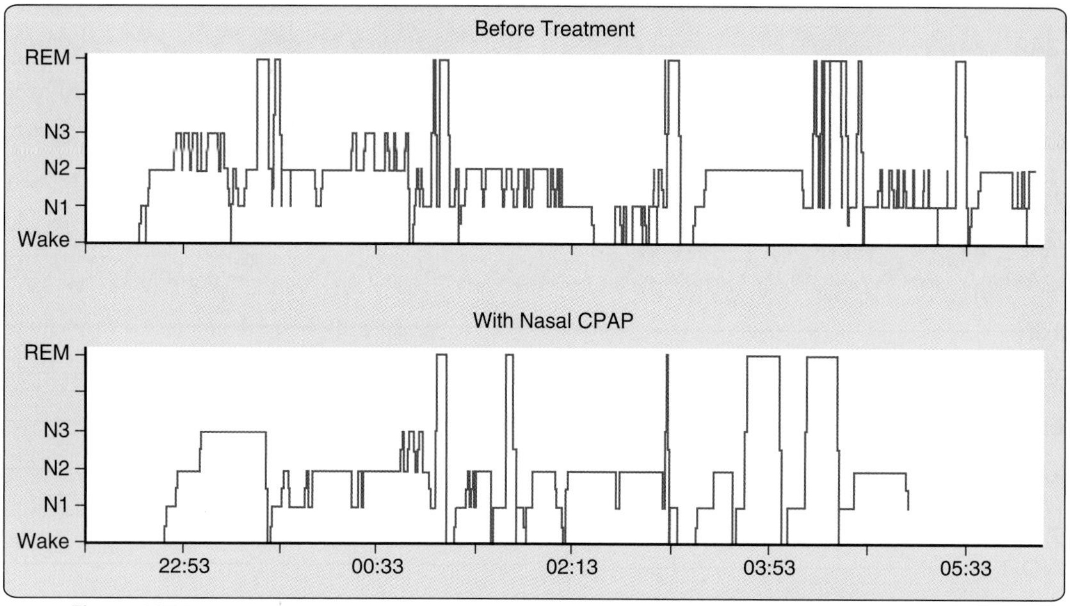

Figure 127.7 This figure demonstrates two hypnograms (plots of sleep stages against time of night, with increasing depth of sleep staged as wake, N1 [NREM stage 1], N2, N3, [REM]) from a 43-year-old veteran of the first Gulf War (1990–91) who returned with complaints of moderate fatigue and severely impaired sleep quality (symptoms of Gulf War illness) and was found to have an apnea hypopnea index of 5 per hour.[61] The upper hypnogram is derived from his polysomnogram before treatment, and the lower hypnogram was obtained from a polysomnogram performed (while sleeping with nasal continuous positive airway pressure [CPAP] at 9 cm H_2O) after the veteran slept with nasal CPAP nightly for 3 weeks and experienced improvement of his fatigue and sleep quality. The initial hypnogram demonstrates frequent shifts from deeper to lighter sleep stages throughout the night. The hypnogram obtained after symptomatic improvement demonstrates fewer sleep stage shifts. Frequent shifts from deeper to lighter sleep are thought to be an adaptive response to stress that enables the individual to respond more quickly to an emergency. NREM, Non–rapid eye movement; REM, rapid eye movement. (Reproduced with permission from Amin MM, Gold MS, Broderick JE, Gold AR. The effect of nasal continuous positive airway pressure on the symptoms of Gulf War illness. *Sleep Breath.* 2011;15[3]:579–87.)

increased shifts from deeper to lighter sleep[55,61] and CAP,[67]as described earlier, were considered alternative responses to pharyngeal collapse during sleep that maintain a more patent pharyngeal airway while maintaining sleep continuity. Bao and Guilleminault[71] have further hypothesized that UARS evolves into OSA over time because of UA trauma related to snoring. According to this hypothesis, because of the effect of snoring on the UA, patients with UARS eventually lose their increased sensitivity to pharyngeal collapse and their sleep-maintaining response. As a consequence, their sleep deepens, and their mild resistive events become hypopneas and apneas terminated by arousal. This proposed *sleep quality* paradigm of UARS provides an explanation for the alpha frequency intrusion into sleep and sleep stage instability characterizing patients who have UARS; however, it does not explain the spectrum of somatic, cognitive, and affective disorders also associated with UARS.

A third paradigm of UARS, the *chronic stress* paradigm, builds on the *sleep quality* paradigm of UARS and provides a more complete explanation for the varied symptoms associated with the syndrome.[72] The paradigm postulates that some individuals can become sensitized to UA resistance as a stimulus that activates the stress response (activation of the hypothalamic-pituitary-adrenal axis and sympathetic nervous system by the brain's limbic system) as if it were an existential threat. Because UA resistance during sleep occurs for at least several hours daily, in these individuals it constitutes a chronic stress with associated symptoms, including sleep-onset and sleep-maintenance insomnia, headaches, gastrointestinal and bladder irritability, body pain, anxiety, and depression. In addition to these symptoms, so prevalent among patients with UARS, chronic stress is associated with hypertension, type 2 diabetes mellitus, gonadotrophic hormone deficiency leading to sexual dysfunction (erectile dysfunction in men and polycystic ovarian syndrome in women), and growth hormone deficiency leading to diminished growth in children. These are all prominent medical conditions associated with OSA. According to such a chronic stress paradigm, the sleep fragmentation by arousals and altered sleep quality caused by alpha frequency intrusion and sleep stage instability observed among patients with UARS is not a direct effect of UA resistance on sleep continuity but an adaptive response of the brain to the existence of a disturbance or threat. Having sleep continuously interrupted or having a state of vigilance maintained during sleep through alpha frequency intrusion and sleep stage instability theoretically enables the individual to respond more quickly to a danger, an apparent survival advantage.[65] This advantage, however, is accompanied by the disadvantages of parasomnias and daytime sleepiness resulting from the chronically altered sleep. Two recent studies that used self-report somatic arousal (the symptoms of increased sympathetic nervous system activity) to quantify stress in sleep-disordered breathing patients support the chronic stress paradigm. The studies demonstrate that as the level of somatic arousal increases among patients with UARS and with OSA, the severity of sleepiness and fatigue and the prevalence of insomnia complaints, anxiety, and somatic syndromes increases.[73,74] The chronic stress paradigm of UARS explains not only the hypersomnolence associated with UARS, but also the somatic complaints, affective disorders, cognitive dysfunction, and parasomnias observed among patients with UARS.[72]

In summary, the pathophysiologic and associated clinical paradigm of UARS has evolved from sleep fragmentation by RERAs through altered sleep quality as a direct response to UA resistance, leading to milder resistive events than occur among patients with OSA, to recent consideration of UA resistance, provoking chronic stress with sleep-related, somatic, cognitive, and affective consequences. The pathophysiologic paradigms of UARS will continue to evolve as new data accumulate. However, the recognition that altered sleep *quality* contributes to the hypersomnolence and fatigue of patients with UARS supports the idea that UARS also exists below the RDI threshold for a diagnosis of OSA, an important possibility when one contemplates making the diagnosis of idiopathic hypersomnolence.

Treatment

The treatment of UARS uses the same treatments that have been discussed earlier for snoring. Chief among these treatments is nasal CPAP, which is highly effective and can be precisely titrated by the prescribing physician to eliminate IFL during sleep. To titrate nasal CPAP for patients with UARS, one must titrate to convert IFL during sleep into non-flow-limited breathing, as illustrated in Figures 127.2 and 127.3. The mean therapeutic level of nasal CPAP for 22 patients with UARS was found to be 7 cm H_2O with a range of 4 to 9 cm H_2O.[5] There is no published data using autotitrating positive airway pressure (PAP) in these patients. For patients unable (or unwilling) to use nasal CPAP, alternative forms of treatment, such as mandibular advancement appliances or tongue-retaining devices, weight loss, and surgical procedures, may be considered as previously described. Applying PAP through an oronasal mask may not be a reliable method for eliminating IFL during sleep[75,76] and anesthesia.[77] Among pediatric patients, rapid palatal expansion performed by an orthodontist has been used effectively to treat UARS (e.g., the patients in Figures 127.5 and 127.6[55]) and mild OSA.

Future Directions

An effort is underway to describe, more completely, the pathophysiology associated with increased UA resistance (IFL) during sleep. With the progress occurring in artificial intelligence and machine learning, an effort is underway to use technology to study the prevalence of IFL during sleep in large populations and to correlate its presence with signs and symptoms of sleep-disordered breathing. In 2017, under the auspices of the American Thoracic Society, a workshop was conducted to develop standards for the recording of airflow and the visual identification of IFL, to improve its clinical recognition and serve as a resource for technologic innovators using machine learning to quickly analyze PSG airflow signals for the presence of IFL.[11] Subsequently, studies have been published applying machine learning to IFL detection demonstrating high levels of sensitivity and specificity.[10,78] The effort appears to be underway to better define the role of IFL in isolated snoring and pathologic UARSs.

CLINICAL PEARLS

- Silent inspiratory airflow limitation (IFL) during sleep is characterized by either an inspiratory airflow plateau or an increase in the ratio of inspiratory time to the respiratory cycle time, with a prolongation of the time near maximal inspiratory airflow.
- In a patient consulting the clinician for habitual snoring that disturbs his or her bed partner, with normal alertness, no somatic or metabolic disorders, and no known cardiovascular disease, polysomnography (PSG) will likely reveal either isolated snoring or asymptomatic obstructive sleep apnea (OSA). Consider evaluating the results of a carotid ultrasound, looking for evidence of atherosclerosis, before foregoing specific OSA treatment in this setting.
- For patients with functional somatic syndromes complaining of insomnia, fatigue, headache, body pain, gastrointestinal or bladder irritability, and anxiety and depression, with or without audible snoring, consider performing PSG to diagnose upper airway resistance syndrome (OSA by ICSD-3 criteria) because prevention of IFL during sleep may be an effective treatment not only for fatigue and insomnia but also for somatic symptoms.

SUMMARY

Our understanding of pathologic pharyngeal collapse during sleep has progressed from recognizing obstructive apneas and hypopneas associated with arousal from sleep and oxygen desaturation (clinically, OSA) to recognizing the mildest IFL without audible snoring, arousal, or oxygen desaturation. At the same time, our understanding of the consequences of pathologic pharyngeal collapse during sleep has expanded from hypersomnolence and cardiovascular and metabolic disorders to include associations with somatic syndromes, affective disorders, and carotid artery atherosclerosis independent of metabolic syndrome. Underlying this evolution is a new paradigm of *sleep-related breathing disorders* (often referred to as "sleep-disordered breathing") in which pharyngeal collapse during sleep acts not only directly, causing oxygen desaturation and arousal from sleep, but also indirectly, with even the mildest IFL during sleep serving as a chronic activator of the body's stress response. In this context, one can appreciate the evolving understanding of what constitutes clinically significant sleep-related breathing disorders associated with sleep-related UA pathophysiology.

SELECTED READINGS

Broderick JE, Gold MS, Amin MM, et al. The association of somatic arousal with the symptoms of upper airway resistance syndrome. *Sleep Med.* 2014;15:436–443.

de Godoy LB, Palombini LO, Guilleminault C, et al. Treatment of upper airway resistance syndrome in adults: where do we stand? *Sleep Sci.* 2015;8(1):42–48.

Dubrovsky B, Raphael KG, Lavigne GJ, et al. Polysomnographic investigation of sleep and respiratory parameters in women with temporomandibular pain disorders. *J Clin Sleep Med.* 2014;10:195–201.

Gold AR, Dipalo F, Gold MS, et al. Inspiratory airflow dynamics during sleep in female fibromyalgia patients. *Sleep.* 2004;27:459–466.

Gold AR, Schwartz AR. The pharyngeal critical pressure: the whys and hows of using nasal continuous positive airway pressure diagnostically. *Chest.* 1996;110:1077–1088.

Guilleminault C, Kirisoglu C, Poyares D, et al. Upper airway resistance syndrome: a long-term outcome study. *J Psychiatr Res.* 2006;40:273–279.

Guilleminault C, Stoohs R, Clerk A, et al. A cause of excessive daytime sleepiness: the upper airway resistance syndrome. *Chest.* 1993;104:781–787.

Hosselet JJ, Norman RG, Ayappa I, et al. Detection of flow limitation with a nasal cannula/pressure transducer system. *Am J Respir Crit Care Med.* 1998;157:1461–1467.

Johnson KG, Johnson DC, Thomas RJ, et al. Flow limitation/obstruction with recovery breath (FLOW) event for improved scoring of mild obstructive sleep apnea without electroencephalography. *Sleep Med.* 2020;67:249–255. https://doi.org/10.1016/j.sleep.2018.11.014.

Kshirsagar RS, Harless L, Liang J, et al. The efficacy of surgery for upper airway resistance syndrome: a systematic review, meta-analysis and case series [published online ahead of print, 2021 Mar 29]. *Am J Otolaryngol.* 2021;42(5):103011.

Lee SA, Amis TC, Byth K, et al. Heavy snoring as a cause of carotid artery atherosclerosis. *Sleep.* 2008;31:1207–1213.

Marshall NS, Wong KK, Cullen SR, et al. Snoring is not associated with all-cause mortality, incident cardiovascular disease, or stroke in the Busselton Health Study. *Sleep.* 2012;35:1235–1240.

Schneider H, Krishnan V, Pichard LE, et al. Inspiratory duty cycle responses to flow limitation predict nocturnal hypoventilation. *Eur Respir J.* 2009;33:1068–1076.

So SJ, Lee HJ, Kang SG, et al. A comparison of personality characteristics and psychiatric symptomatology between upper airway resistance syndrome and obstructive sleep apnea syndrome. *Psychiatry Investig.* 2015;12(2):183–189.

Stoohs RA, Knaack L, Blum HC, et al. Differences in clinical features of upper airway resistance syndrome, primary snoring, and obstructive sleep apnea/hypopnea syndrome. *Sleep Med.* 2008;9:121–128.

A complete reference list can be found online at ExpertConsult.com.

Chapter 128

Obstructive Sleep Apnea: Heritable Phenotypes and Genetics

Logan Schneider; Susan Redline

Chapter Highlights

- For most of the characteristic features of obstructive sleep apnea syndrome (OSAS)—snoring, daytime sleepiness, and reported apneas—there is strong evidence for a family history, such that most patients with OSAS often have relatives (e.g., parents, siblings) who have similar symptoms, a diagnosis of obstructive sleep apnea (OSA), or both. The familial aggregation of objectively measured OSAS, quantified through use of twin- and family-based cohort studies, estimate that risk for OSA is increased by 25% to 200% in individuals with an affected first-degree relative.
- Using family studies, the heritability (the proportion of the variance in a trait attributable to genetic factors) for apnea-hypopnea index (AHI) is estimated to be between 0.30 to 0.40. Heritability estimates for specific features of sleep apnea, such as apnea duration, are estimated to be as high as 0.60, suggesting that variations in more specific features of sleep apnea are more heritable than summary count measures, such as the AHI.
- Although there is a strong correlation between OSA and obesity, only 35% of the genetic variance in the AHI may be accounted for by genes that influence obesity (with 65% of the genetic variance likely the result of genetic variants in other etiologic pathways). Other potentially inherited risk factors (or intermediate phenotypes) for OSA include craniofacial structural traits that influence upper airway patency; body fat distribution, including propensity for airway fat deposition; chemoreflex ventilatory control; and arousal responses to ventilatory stimuli.
- Pedigree studies analyzed using linkage analysis, association studies, and meta-analyses of candidate and genome-wide association studies of OSAS-related traits, including overnight hypoxemia—some analyzed in combination with linkage or admixture data—provide evidence for increased susceptibility to OSAS in persons who inherit variants for genes in pathways implicated in ventilatory control, pulmonary disease, inflammation, body fat distribution, craniofacial structure, and iron metabolism.
- There is a dynamic interaction between the genetic architecture of OSAS and its physiologic consequences. Most notably, both chronic intermittent hypoxia and inflammation from repeated collapse of the airway are associated with changes in the transcription and translation of genes that lie along pathways implicated in cardiovascular disease (e.g., inflammation and vascular reactivity). Consequently, the dysregulation of these pathways further contributes to the pathogenesis of sleep-disordered breathing.

INTRODUCTION

Obstructive sleep apnea syndrome (OSAS) is a disorder of breathing during sleep, affecting approximately 1 in 4 men and approximately 1 in 10 women,[1] with estimates of nearly 1 billion people affected worldwide.[2] The current obesity epidemic in the United States has increased OSAS prevalence by 14% to 55% over the last 2 decades, resulting in millions of untreated individuals.[1,3] OSAS is characterized by repeated complete (apnea) or partial (hypopnea) collapse of the upper airway, usually accompanied by a physiologic consequence, such as a surge in heart rate and peripheral vascular tone, cortical arousal, or oxyhemoglobin desaturation, leading to daytime sequelae such as excessive sleepiness. The variable clinical presentations and findings of a disease are *phenotypes*. The distinct mechanistic pathways playing a role in determining the phenotypes are *endotypes*.

Typical of a complex phenotype, OSAS is fully defined by a constellation of symptoms and physiologic data. Although this type of information is routinely integrated into clinical diagnostic and treatment pathways, it is more challenging to integrate these various types of phenotype data into research definitions of phenotypes for use in genetic studies. Moreover, the need for very large sample sizes to detect low-effect-size genetic variants requires that phenotypic assessments be feasibly measured using routinely collected clinical data or home-based measurements. To overcome these challenges, new phenotypic and analytic strategies have been employed to tease out the pathophysiologic mechanisms derived from and influencing the underlying genetic architecture of this complex disorder, using a range of approaches such as advanced signal processing of routinely collected polysomnography signals through multi-staged genetic association studies that leverage information on linkage, admixture, and pleiotropy to increase statistical power. This chapter summarizes the approaches for phenotype derivations relevant to genetic studies; the intermediate pathways or endotypic pathways that may shed light on the genetics of OSAS; and the current familial, genetic and genomic studies of OSAS in humans.

DEFINING OBSTRUCTIVE SLEEP APNEA SYNDROME PHENOTYPES FOR GENETIC STUDIES

In seeking to understand the genetic basis of a disorder, the first step is to identify the most appropriate phenotype measures. The choice of measurement should balance clinical/physiologic relevance, feasibility of measurement, and reliability. Genetic studies of OSAS typically focused on the apnea-hypopnea index (AHI), which is readily available from clinical and research polysomnograms (PSGs). However, additional features extracted from the PSG, including those derived from advanced signal processing, hold potential for further refining phenotypic assessment.

Apnea-Hypopnea Index

Despite the inherent limitations of the AHI recognized since the initial diagnostic criteria were outlined in the first edition of the *International Classification of Sleep Disorders* manual,[4] OSAS disease severity is typically quantified by the AHI, an estimate of respiratory event frequency (apneas + hypopneas) throughout the sleep period. The AHI historically has been used as a primary measure of severity resulting from relative ease of calculation and correlation with other indices of severity (e.g., oxygen desaturation index, sleep fragmentation), and night-to-night reproducibility (intra-class correlations of >0.80).[5] Although the AHI demonstrates modest heritability (>0.20), as a simple count of the number of respiratory disturbances per hour of sleep, it does not directly provide information on key physiologic processes that likely are heritable, such as airway collapsibility, breathing stability, and propensity for oxygen desaturation and sleepiness. Moreover, the mechanisms—and thus the genetic bases—for OSA predominance in rapid eye movement (REM) versus non–rapid eye movement (NREM) sleep differ. Genetic studies that do not separately consider state-specific event frequency measures may fail to identify genes influencing fundamental neuromuscular control mechanisms underlying OSAS.

State-Specific and Event-Specific Features of Obstructive Sleep Apnea Syndrome

Although the use of the AHI in genetic studies is supported by its moderate heritability, newer studies have begun to explore other features of sleep-disordered breathing (SDB) that quantify differences in the duration, clustering, and sleep stage distribution of respiratory events as promising phenotypes for genetic studies of OSAS. As such, a significant genetic heritability has been reported for AHI specific to REM and NREM sleep, average levels of event-related nocturnal oxygen desaturation, and average duration of sleep-related respiratory disturbances (which has heritability up to 0.60[6]). The utility of analyzing AHI specific to state is supported by emerging genome-wide association studies (GWAS) showing evidence for unique state-specific genetic variants[7] and genetic variants that associate with respiratory event duration.[8,9] Moreover, epidemiological data show that several of these measurements, such as event duration and event-associated desaturation, predict important clinical outcomes,[10,11] suggesting that genes identified for these traits are likely to have clinical relevance.

Physiologic Endotypes

Evidence from the fields of breast cancer, hearing loss, lipid metabolism, type 2 diabetes, and psychiatric illness highlights that the use of specific disease subtypes or mechanistic aspects of disease not only improves power of genetic association at lower sample size but does so in a biomechanistically informed way.[12-14] For OSAS, recent progress has been made in applying advanced signal processing to routinely conducted PSG to estimate *endotypes*, measures of disease subtypes characterized by distinct pathophysiologic mechanisms. These indices include arousal threshold, loop gain, neuromuscular compensation, and airway collapsibility.[15] Individual patients with OSAS identified by similarly elevated AHI levels will have variable combinations of abnormalities in these various physiologic traits. Therefore mechanistically defined endotypes may help identify genes more closely related to disease processes and help define subpopulations of patients with unique prognostic and treatment-response features. As the techniques for deriving detailed endotypes from routinely collected PSG data are further refined and validated, they will provide the means for scaling to the large numbers needed for genetic epidemiologic studies.

Multivariate Phenotypic Measures and Pleiotropy

An approach for phenotype derivations for complex chronic diseases is through use of summary measures that incorporate information from multiple related phenotypes that presumably share common genetic risk factors, or *pleiotropy*. Recent studies of hypertension, inflammatory pathways, psychiatric illness, as well as of OSAS have shown that this type of approach can reveal novel genetic signals and improve statistical power compared with single-trait analysis.[16-19] Methods that use both multivariate regression to model the correlation across traits as well as principal components (PC) analysis to provide summaries of linear combinations of traits have been used in genetic studies.[20] A systematic analysis compared heritability and linkage signals of single OSAS-related traits compared with multiple traits summarized as PCs.[20] The PCs, based on both questionnaire responses to snoring and excessive daytime sleepiness and PSG measures including AHI and measures of hypoxemia and event duration, showed stronger genetic signals than any single-trait analysis and were generalizable across populations. It is important to note that methods that combine phenotypes to boost heritability/genetic discovery assume underlying common genetic risk factors for these traits (or "pleiotropy") and are less informative for heterogeneous disease processes, with limited ability to identify distinct pathobiologic pathways contributing to disease.[21]

Intermediate Disease Pathways and Phenotypes

Multiple risk factors have been identified for OSAS (Figure 128.1). Some of these factors reflect environmental or social exposures, such as alcohol consumption, smoking, and nasal congestion, whereas others reflect biologic factors such as menopause/hormones, comorbidities, and fluid overload.[22,23] However, the strongest OSAS risk factors have an established inherited, or genetic, basis. As such, these latter traits may be considered intermediate phenotypes, and multiple genetic variants associated with these phenotypes may influence OSAS susceptibility. Key risk factors include those that influence airway anatomy, such as craniofacial structure (e.g., retrognathia, micrognathia) and airway soft tissue (parapharyngeal fat, macroglossia), and factors that influence airway neuromuscular activation and breathing patterns during sleep (airway collapsibility pressure, dilator reflexes, ventilatory control, arousal threshold, and autonomic activity).[24-29] Obesity influences both airway anatomy as well as physiology. Intermediate traits can reveal stronger associations with specific gene products, as a result of isolating underlying anatomic and pathophysiologic contributions to the downstream phenotype. However, even the most prominently associated comorbidity—obesity—is found in only 50% to 70% of cases of OSAS,[30-32] highlighting the multiplicity of mechanisms that influence individual susceptibility.[33]

A brief summary of key intermediate traits, and their genetic basis, is provided later, focusing on obesity-related traits, craniofacial structure, and physiologic traits, including influences associated with ventilatory control, circadian and sleep-wake rhythms, and inflammation. Although investigating genes in risk factor pathways may be fruitful, it is important to note that susceptibility genes for intermediate traits associated with OSAS may not be equivalent to the susceptibility genes for OSAS itself.

Obesity and Body Fat Distribution

The risk for OSA is increased by 2 to 10 times by the presence of obesity, with the strongest associations observed in middle age.[34] Multiple factors contribute to this association, including the direct effects of excessive fat on airway caliber and lung capacity, as well as metabolic effects of fat, including inflammation and insulin resistance, which may influence ventilatory control and neuromuscular function relevant to OSAS pathophysiology. The distribution of fat, such as in the neck and upper airway, is likely more relevant to the etiology of OSAS than a nonspecific measure, such as body mass index (BMI). Although AHI and BMI share only about 35% of their genetic variance,[35] further genetic overlap may emerge as more precise measures of body fat distribution are integrated into studies of OSAS genetics.

The last decade has seen an explosion of very large genetic studies of obesity. Heritability estimates for obesity-related traits, including BMI, skinfold thickness, regional body fat distribution, and fat mass, range from 40% to 70%.[34,36,37] It is likely that many obesity loci contribute to OSAS but have effects that are too small to detect in studies of only modest sample sizes. Nonetheless, large GWAS have identified and replicated hundreds of genetic variants for these traits,[38] including more than 50 genomic regions associated with measures of body fat distribution.[39] Genetic loci for BMI seem to map to genes within hypothalamic-pathways, whereas genes for body-fat distribution seem to more frequently associate with adipocyte biology, influencing the local deposition of fat and metabolic activity.[40] It is plausible that genetic variants

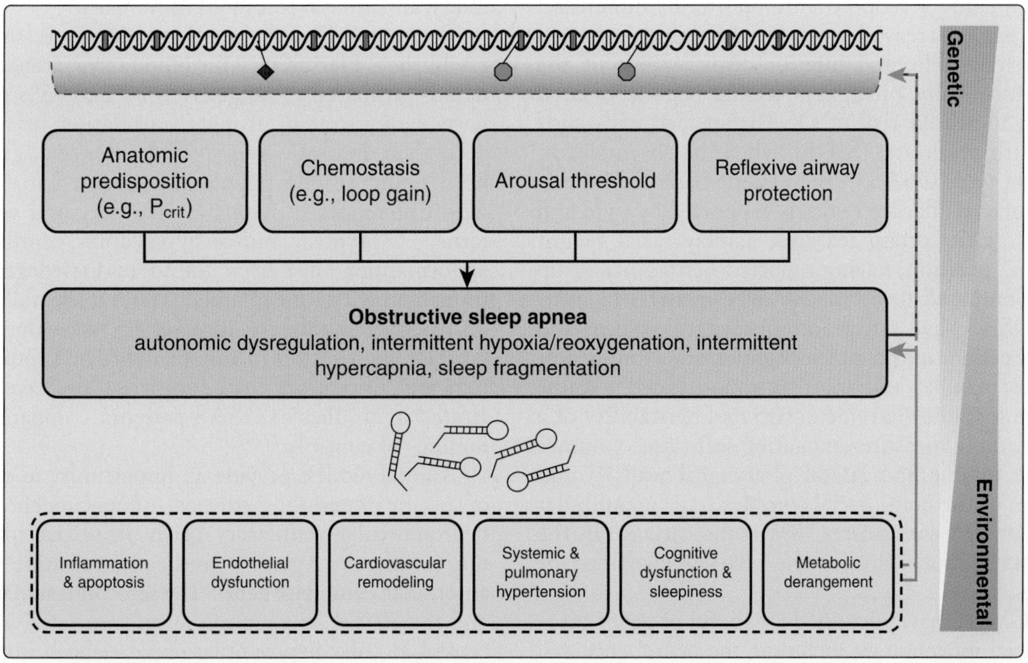

Figure 128.1 A framework for understanding the interplay of genetic and environmental influences in obstructive sleep apnea syndrome (OSAS). The main phenotypic contributions to OSAS pathophysiology have genetic underpinnings, some of which are modulated by epigenetic modification and posttranscriptional regulation, both of which result in and are influenced by the consequences of sleep-disordered breathing. P_{crit}, Passive critical closing pressure of the upper airway.

for specific fat depots may predispose to OSAS-related upper airway collapse, especially if they influence pharyngeal fat pads and tongue fat deposits,[41,42] or waist circumference (reducing lung capacity). Genetic variants that influence local fat deposition may also be relevant for OSAS, as many of these variants also associate with increased blood pressure and abnormal lipid levels[39]—traits common in OSAS—and because they show sexual dimorphism, a feature of OSAS.[43] Despite the promise of interrogating obesity-related genes in OSAS genetics, it is important to note that other than for rare, monogenic forms of obesity, most effects for common variants for any obesity trait are small; for example, less than 5% of the phenotypic variation for BMI is explained by all known alleles combined. As such, the connection between the genetic underpinnings of obesity and the complex phenotypic traits of obstructive sleep apnea (such as the AHI) has expectedly been difficult to elucidate through current methods of genetic analysis, even using such pointed investigations as candidate gene analyses (see the section Candidate Gene Studies). Nonetheless, a few obesity-related genetic risks have been identified by a few studies employing varied genetic-analysis strategies, from the respiration-influencing adipokine leptin to a few multifunctional genes (such as *GRP83*, *HK1*, *SELENOP*, and *HIP/PAP*) that are related to maintaining energy balance. The hope is that, with larger sample sizes and more refined phenotypes (with links to obesity), the complex bidirectional relationship between the shared heritability of OSA and obesity will come to light.

Craniofacial Morphology

Similar to adiposity, upper airway anatomy—from soft tissue structures to craniofacial morphometry—also plays a critical role in heritable OSAS risk.[44,45] Imaging of the upper airway has demonstrated larger lateral pharyngeal wall and tongue size among patients with OSAS.[46] Cephalometric markers of OSAS include a reduced anteroposterior dimension of the cranial base, increased lower facial height, shortened and retracted mandible, and inferior displacement of the hyoid.[47-49] Additionally, brachycephaly has been associated not only with increased risk of OSAS but also with sudden infant death syndrome (SIDS), which has been shown to co-aggregate with OSAS.[50] The genetic basis for inheritance of craniofacial characteristics is supported by twin and family studies, with certain features, namely facial height and mandibular position, having reported heritability of up to 80%.[51,52] Compared to normative data, relatives of individuals with OSAS have a decreased pharyngeal volume and smaller airway caliber in the glottic region from a longer soft palate, smaller maxilla, and more retropositioned mandible.[53,54] Imaging studies have demonstrated heritability of a number of anatomic measures, including soft tissue volumes (including the tongue and lateral pharyngeal walls)[51] and bony structures of the craniofacial complex (e.g., mandibular length and width),[44] with nearly 30% of the variance in the minimum cross-sectional area of the pharynx explained by genetic factors.[55]

Although GWAS have identified a handful of genes associated with facial morphology, including the neural crest cell transcription factor, *PAX3,* important to development,[56] there are at least 50 congenital syndromes with associated maxillary and/or mandibular dysgenesis and SDB, such as Pierre-Robin syndrome and Treacher-Collins syndrome, that provide insights into the genetics of OSAS-associated craniofacial development. Implicated pathways include those associated with fibroblast growth factor (e.g., *FGFR1, FGFR2, FGFR3*), transforming growth factor-β (e.g., *TGFBR1, TGFBR2*), homeobox (e.g., *MSX1, MSX2*), and sonic hedgehog (e.g., *PTCH, SHH*). Other genes essential to proper craniofacial development include those in the endothelin pathway (e.g., *ECE1, EDN1, EDNRA*),[57-59] and *TCOF1*, which is the cause of Treacher-Collins syndrome.[60]

Ventilatory-Related Risk Factors

Although anatomic factors undoubtedly contribute significantly to airway obstruction, there is growing evidence that the pathophysiology of OSAS reflects contributions beyond the simple collapsing pressure of the upper airway (P_{crit}), including loop gain, a measure of instability of the overall ventilatory control system; brain arousal thresholds to hypoxia, hypercapnia, and/or ventilation; and upper airway muscle dilator reflex responses to increased ventilatory load.[61] When severe anatomic compromise is not playing a pivotal role in airway collapse, individualized interactions among these other physiologic entities likely explain the phenotypic variation evident within OSAS populations.[62] Certain factors play a more significant role than others, depending upon the individual. For example, reductions in central inspiratory drive result in greater increases in upper airway resistance in those individuals with an anatomic predisposition to OSAS.[63] Conversely, obese individuals without OSAS may be protected by a less collapsible airway (i.e., more negative collapsing pressure, P_{crit}) and a more robust airway dilator reflex.[64] However, like structural imaging, these physiologic features are challenging to measure at scale but may be amenable to exploration in animal models (e.g., chemosensitivity). However, recent advances in physiologic modeling hold promise for using routinely collected PSG data to estimate loop gain, neuromuscular collapsibility, and arousal threshold in humans.[65]

The genetic basis for many ventilatory-related traits is well established. Heritability for blood oxygen chemoresponsiveness is estimated to range from 30% to 75%.[66] Twin studies have demonstrated stronger correlation between monozygotic than dizygotic twins.[67-70] Evidence of genetic drift has been found among populations adapted to life at altitude, with differences in hypoxic sensitivity and ventilatory patterns.[71,72] Hypoxic and/or hypercapnic ventilatory response abnormalities have been found in first-degree relatives of probands with unexplained respiratory failure,[73] chronic obstructive pulmonary disease,[74,75] or asthma.[76] Similarly, familial aggregation of impairments in hypoxic responsiveness and respiratory load compensation have been demonstrated in families of OSAS patients, compared with that of families of controls.[77-81]

Animal models provide an opportunity to explore the role of specific proteins in pathways influencing chemoreflexes and neuromuscular ventilatory drive. As expected, chemoreceptors for blood oxygen[82-84] and carbon dioxide[85,86] levels were among the candidate genes. The serotonin signaling pathway[87] and the *PHOX2B* gene mutation associated with congenital central alveolar hypoventilation[88,89]—both implicated in not only OSAS but also SIDS—were found to be important. Finally, endothelin pathway genes important to craniofacial development have also been found to play a role in hypoxic response in knockout and transgenic models.[90,91]

Circadian Rhythms

Circadian genes influence multiple physiologic and metabolic processes, including propensity for obesity[92] and lung disease.[93] The most obvious connection between OSAS and circadian rhythm is in the distribution of REM and NREM sleep and variations in neuromuscular responses over the sleep period. It appears that NREM-related apneas and hypopneas may be rooted in physiologic instability of ventilatory control associated with sleep state changes, while anatomic aspects of OSAS are more evident during REM as a result of muscle hypotonia, predisposing to more severe and prolonged oxyhemoglobin desaturations.[94-96] Recent GWAS report associations between OSAS and variants in circadian genes,[97] supporting a role for circadian control in OSAS pathogenesis. These studies also reported unique genetic associations between AHI measured in REM versus NREM.[7]

Respiratory Arousal Threshold

Genetic differences in the accumulation of and response to homeostatic factors can result in changes to the arousal threshold, which when low can result in propagation of apneas, and when high can result in prolonged airway obstruction. Women and African Americans have lower arousal thresholds than men and those of European ancestry, respectively, suggesting that genes that influence this endotype may differ by sex and race/ethnicity. Hypocretin (orexin) levels are noted to be reduced in OSAS,[98] suggesting a role for these genes in OSAS, because of their relationship to arousal and muscle tone, as well as appetite regulation and weight.[99,100] Apnea event duration, reflecting variations in arousal threshold,[9,101] has been associated with four variants in *RP11-96H17.1*, a gene that is largely expressed in brain tissue.[9] Further identifying genes that influence arousal threshold—a pharmacologic target—may inform precision medicine approaches for OSAS.

Inflammation and Metabolic Dysfunction

An augmented inflammatory milieu present in OSAS patients, such as elevated levels of interleukin 6 (IL-6) and tumor necrosis factor-α (TNF-α),[102] is well described. Most of the literature has focused on the consequences of OSAS-related chronic intermittent hypoxia (CIH) on adverse cardiovascular disease, believed to be mediated by the proinflammatory effects of reactive-oxygen species triggering activation of the Toll-like receptor-NFκB signaling pathway, resulting in acute phase reactant and cytokine release, which in turn results in atherosclerotic plaque growth as well as lung and renal injury.[103-106] However, there is also evidence suggesting that chronic inflammation may predispose to, or exacerbate, OSAS, possibly through effects on chemoresponsiveness[107,108] and respiratory muscle strength.[109] A bidirectional association between insulin-resistance or metabolic syndrome and OSAS also has been reported,[110,111] consistent with inflammation and metabolic dysfunction also operating as antecedent risk factors for OSAS.

There are multiple GWAS of various inflammatory phenotypes, including CRP and IL-6,[112] as well as diabetes.[113] Genetic risk factors for inflammatory pulmonary diseases also have been reported.[114] The identification of genetic associations between various genes regulating inflammation, particularly those that are expressed in lung tissues, and sleep-related hypoxemia,[97,115] suggests that inflammatory processes may influence the extent to which individuals become more or less hypoxic with respiratory disturbances. Growing evidence that many inflammatory and metabolic disorders may be mediated by epigenetic changes also suggests that manifestations of OSAS may be mediated by changes not only in DNA coding but in DNA methylation. For example, the inflammatory imbalance induced by CIH is likely regulated at the epigenetic level, as a number of studies have reported DNA methylation changes in regulatory regions for genes (e.g., *FOXP3*, *IRF1*, *IL1R2*, and the like) in primary inflammation pathways.[116,117]

DEMOGRAPHIC CONSIDERATIONS

Sex

There is clear evidence for sexual dimorphism for OSAS,[118] with women and men reporting different symptoms and showing differences in the distributions of the AHI in NREM but not in REM sleep.[101] In particular, NREM AHI levels are about twice as high in middle-aged and older men compared with women, while in REM, the average AHI is the same in men and women. OSAS endotypes also differ by sex: women have a lower arousal threshold, lower loop gain, and less collapsibility than men, and these differences account for as much as 30% of the sex-related difference in average NREM AHI.[101] Given differences in pathophysiologic mechanisms, it is not surprising that the genetic factors that influence OSAS differ by sex. Specifically, a GWAS identified 13 significant statistical interactions between sex and single-nucleotide polymorphisms (SNPs); 12 GWAS associations with OSAS were observed only in men.[7] The most significant GWAS association in this study was for AHI in NREM sleep in men only, for an SNP overlapping the *RAI1* gene and encompassing genes *PEMT1*, *SREBF1*, and *RASD1*. These findings highlight the importance of considering sex as a biologic variable in genetic analysis, which can be explored through sex-stratified analyses and testing for interactions. This need also underscores the necessity for studies of large size with representation of both men and women.

Age

OSAS also markedly varies with age, with evidence of age-by-sex interactions. In particular, OSAS increases in prevalence from early adulthood through senescence, with marked increases in women after menopause. Therefore genetic analyses need careful adjustment for age and possibly for age-by-sex interactions.

OSAS affects 2% to 4% of children,[119] and is most commonly associated with adenotonsillar hypertrophy. However, similar to adults, obesity in children is associated with an increase in OSAS prevalence and severity.[120] Pedigrees have been reported with evidence of intergenerational transmission of OSAS from parent to child, suggesting that there are common genetic risk factors that influence both pediatric and adult OSAS.[121,122] Residual OSAS after tonsillo-adenoidectomy is more common among children of parents with OSAS than children with un affected parents,[123] further pointing to a central role for genetic contributions to the pathophysiology of OSAS beyond an anatomic predisposition in the members of these multiply affected families.[124]

Race and Ethnicity

It is important to appreciate the potential for race- and ethnic-specific effects of genetic mutations. Associations with several OSAS risk factors (or *intermediate phenotypes*) with OSAS vary by race/ethnicity. For example, in the Multi-Ethnic Study of Atherosclerosis, smaller increases in BMI resulted in larger increases in AHI in Chinese than in non-Hispanic whites, Hispanics, and African Americans.[125] In the Cleveland Family study, AHI levels were associated with both bony (e.g., intermaxillary distance and head form) and soft tissue (e.g., tongue volume and soft palate length) characteristics among European descendants.[126] However, among African Americans, although soft tissue factors associated with OSAS severity, bony anatomic feature associations with OSAS were weak.[126] In analyses adjusted for BMI, prevalence and severity of OSAS also appear to vary by continental ancestry. Analyses from Brazilian[127] and U.S.-based admixed populations have shown that global African ancestry is associated with a lower AHI, while the US study also showed that Amerindian ancestry was associated with more severe OSA.[9] This highlights not only the importance of inclusion of diverse racial and ethnic groups in analyses but also the need for stratified analyses to identify population-specific genetic risk factors, some of which may reflect differences in anatomic risk factors, whereas others may reflect differences in evolutionary factors responding to environmental stressors leading to differences in ventilatory and other traits relevant to OSAS. Consistent with race-specific genetic associations for other chronic diseases,[128] initial multi-ethnic GWAS studies have reported a number of unique genetic associations for OSAS-related traits across racial and ethnic groups.[7,8,97] However, these findings have been difficult to replicate, reflecting differences in allele frequencies across populations and availability of replication samples.

FAMILIAL AGGREGATION OF OBSTRUCTIVE SLEEP APNEA SYNDROME

The initial evidence for a genetic basis for OSAS was from studies reporting family clustering of the disorder and epidemiologic data highlighting the importance of a positive family history in defining the risk of OSAS. This familial aggregation, for both disease severity (as measured by AHI) and associated symptoms, has been reported in adults and children as well as obese and nonobese subjects. More important, the heritability of AHI and OSAS symptoms has been consistently demonstrated via various study designs (cohorts, small and large pedigrees, twins, and case-control studies) in populations of varying ethnic and racial backgrounds.[53,54,129-131] The odds of a person with OSAS in a family with affected relatives to that for someone without an affected relative has been reported to be anywhere from 2:1 to 46:1.[19,53,54,131] This risk seems to increase as the number of affected relatives increases (Table 128.1).[19]

Analyses from both pedigree and twin studies have provided heritability estimates of the main OSAS severity measure, the AHI, ranging from 35% to 73%.[132-135] One study from a small sample of 48 monozygotic and 23 dizygotic Hungarian twins identified high heritability of a number of OSAS-related features: 55% for apnea index, 69% for respiratory disturbance index, 75% for respiratory arousal index, 83% for oxygen desaturation index (ODI), 96% for nadir SpO_2, and 97% for time spent with $SpO_2 < 90\%$.[135] Pedigree analyses have also shown significant sibling and parent-to-offspring correlations (approximately 0.21) for AHI, which are greater than those between unrelated spouses.[19] Although genetic correlations and heritability estimates are likely lower in general population cohorts, the existing data support a significant role for genetic factors in influencing the AHI level.

In addition to studies of the heritability of the AHI, signs and symptoms of the disorder have been found to be heritable. The concordance of snoring is significantly higher among monozygotic twins than dizygotic twins.[130,136] Sleepiness, a cardinal feature of OSAS, is heritable and associated with multiple genetic variants.[135,137] Of particular interest is the finding from a very large population-based GWAS of excessive daytime sleepiness that demonstrated that variants for sleepiness associate with two phenotypic subclasses: one characterized by high sleep propensity and the other by sleep fragmentation.[137] Given that OSAS is associated with sleepiness and sleep fragmentation, further investigation may help to understand whether the reported sleep fragmentation-sleepiness variants reflect a susceptibility to sleepiness directly attributable to OSAS-related sleep fragmentation, versus a susceptibility to sleep fragmentation that leads to both sleep-related breathing disturbances and sleepiness. An overlapping genetic basis has been found in models of genetic correlations with daytime sleepiness and snoring, supporting the possibility of pleiotropic pathways (where one or a set of genetic variants influence several phenotypes).[130]

As summarized earlier, pedigree studies have demonstrated transmission of OSAS across generations, suggesting OSA susceptibility among adults and children may be influenced by a common underlying genetic architecture.[138] Additionally, within pediatric populations, both OSAS and its primary risk factor—adenotonsillar hypertrophy[139]—have been shown to be more prevalent in siblings of children with OSAS than in controls. Although familial aggregation of tonsillar hypertrophy may reflect common exposures to household irritants, it is

Table 128.1 Likelihood of Sleep-Disordered Breathing as a Function of Degree of Familial Multiplicity of Sleep Apnea

	One Affected Relative	Two Affected Relatives	Three Affected Relatives
Increased apneic activity	1.30 (1.03, 1.65)	1.70 (1.05, 2.73)	2.21 (1.08, 4.52)
Sleep apnea syndrome	1.58 (1.02, 2.45)	2.51 (1.05, 6.01)	3.97 (1.07, 14.7)

Increased apnea activity was defined as an RDI that exceeded the following age-specific threshold levels: 5, 10, 15, 20, and 25, for the age categories <15 years, 15–24 years, 25–44 years, 45–64 years, and >65 years, respectively. Sleep apnea syndrome was defined as an RDI ≥15 and subjectively reported sleepiness. Odds ratios (with 95% confidence intervals) adjusted for age, sex, race, and body mass index.

also possible that this finding is due to genetic similarities in immune responses to environmental exposures.

Several studies have reported on coaggregation of OSAS with acute life-threatening events and SIDS.[131,140,141] SIDS research has highlighted the fundamental role that serotonin plays in respiratory drive, possibly suggesting overlapping biologic mechanisms between SDB and the widespread abnormalities in brainstem serotonergic signaling among SIDS victims.[142]

Genetic Analyses

Candidate Gene Studies

Candidate gene approaches were among the first methods of genotype-phenotype association. In these studies, the frequency of genetic variants within genes thought a priori to relate to disease susceptibility are compared between groups with and without a phenotype of interest (e.g., OSAS) or are assessed in relation to a quantitative phenotype (e.g., AHI) via generalized linear models. Relative to other genetic analyses, candidate gene studies tend to have high statistical power but are incapable of discovering new genes or gene combinations. A number of plausible candidate genes derived from some of the aforementioned intermediate pathways have been studied in this way (Box 128.1).

One early candidate gene study of about 1500 individuals of European and African descent assessed key intermediate pathways screening more than 1000 SNPs from 53 candidate genes.[143] Among European Americans, C-reactive protein (CRP) and glia-derived neurotrophic factor were significantly associated with OSAS; whereas, among Blacks, significant associations were found within the serotonin receptor 2a (*HTR2A*) gene, conferring a nearly twofold risk of OSAS.[143] Additional, suggestive associations for 5-HT_2a receptor and endothelin-1 as well as for the leptin receptor and hypocretin receptor 2 were noted for the European Americans and African Americans, respectively.[143] Although such findings necessitate replication, a number of subsequent, confirmatory genetic analyses or physiologic studies have supported these findings.

Serotonin's role in respiration is suggested through the presence of receptors in the carotid body and brainstem regions in close proximity to chemoreceptive ventilatory control centers and hypoglossal nuclei. In animal models, upper airway reflexes and ventilation appear to rely, in part, upon serotonergic signaling at many levels, from the carotid body to the hypoglossal nerve to medullary respiratory centers.[87] Moreover, arousal and sleep-wake neurocircuitry appear to rely, in part, upon serotonergic signaling.[144] Replication of associations with serotonergic genes has been reported in several meta-analyses that pooled data for 500 to 700 cases and controls across multi-ethnic populations from Japan, China, Turkey, and Brazil.[145-147] As a result of these studies, multiple serotonin-related mutations have been identified: a 5-HTT gene-linked polymorphic region conferring triple the risk of OSA, the 148G/A allele of the *HTR2A* gene conferring a nearly doubled risk of OSAS, and a 5-HTT intron 2 variable number tandem repeat conferring a 20% increased risk of OSAS.[145-147] Although these findings, too, necessitate replication and functional follow-up, they nonetheless add weight to the plausible role of serotonin signaling in OSAS.

Acting on the nucleus tractus solitarius and hypoglossal motor nucleus, the appetite- and energy-balance–regulating adipokine leptin appears to also influence ventilatory drive.[148,149] In support of this pathway, increased serum levels

Box 128.1 CANDIDATE GENES FOR INTERMEDIATE PHENOTYPES FOR OBSTRUCTIVE SLEEP APNEA

Obesity

FTO (fat mass and obesity–associated gene)
- Melanocortin-4 receptor
- Leptin
- Pro-opiomelanocortin
- Melanocyte-stimulating hormone
- Neuropeptidase Y
- Prohormone convertase
- Neutrophic receptor TrkB
- Insulin-like growth factor
- Glucokinase
- Adenosine deaminase
- Tumor necrosis factor-α

Glucose regulatory protein
Agouti signaling protein
β-Adrenergic receptor
Carboxypeptidase E
Insulin-signaling protein
Resistin
Ghrelin
Adiponectin
Gamma-aminobutyric acid transporter
Orexin

Ventilatory Control

RET protooncogene
PHOX2B
HOX IIL2
KROX-20
Receptor tyrosine kinase
Neurotrophic growth factors
- Brain-derived neurotrophic factor
- Glia-derived neurotrophic factor
- Neurotrophic factor-4
- Platelet-derived growth factor

Neuronal synthase
Acetylcholine receptor
Dopaminergic receptor
Substance P
Glutamyl transpeptidase
Endothelin-1
Endothelin-3
Leptin
EN-1
GSH-2
Hypocretin (orexin)

Craniofacial Structure

Class I homeobox genes
Growth hormone receptors
Growth factor receptors
Retinoic acid
Endothelin-1
Collagen types I and II
Tumor necrosis factor-α

of leptin in obese women were shown to correlate with compensatory upper airway neuromuscular responses to experimental airway occlusion.[85] Similarly, leptin knockout mice hypoventilate and have a diminished hypercapnic ventilatory response, both of which improve in response to leptin replacement.[130] This hypercapnic response appears to be mediated by melanocortin, a derivative of pro-opiomelanocortin, which has been demonstrated by others to have strong links to OSAS and serum leptin levels, suggesting a role for the hypothalamus and pituitary in OSAS susceptibility.[132,151] Finally, a number of candidate gene studies have reported associations between OSAS and the leptin receptor.[143,152]

Inflammation as an intermediate phenotype was described earlier, and effects on OSAS may be mediated through pharyngeal edema, tonsillar hypertrophy, respiratory muscle weakness, upper airway neuropathic changes, and effects on the glomus cells.[153] A number of cytokines (TNF-α[154,155] and IL-6[156]) and acute phase reactants (CRP[143]) have been linked to OSAS through candidate gene studies. Among children with OSAS (compared with snoring controls), nitric oxide synthase (NOS) and endothelin also are reportedly elevated.[157] Given the importance of inflammation in cardiovascular disease, these findings suggest individuals with OSAS and a genetic inflammatory diathesis may be at increased risk of cardiovascular disease. Recent findings suggest that a proinflammatory phenotype may predispose individuals to both OSAS and cardiovascular disease. Studies implicating inflammatory gene pathways in sleep-associated hypoxemia (reviewed later) further suggest another possibility: genetic predisposition to pulmonary inflammation may increase the severity of hypoxemia resulting from a given hypopnea or apnea. This may lead both to an increased likelihood of recognizing OSAS (which depends on associated hypoxemia to identify hypopneas) and to a more severe OSAS phenotype.

The apolipoprotein E (*APOE*) allele associated with increased Alzheimer disease risk, *APOEε4*, was reportedly associated with increased OSAS risk; however, these findings were not replicated in subsequent studies.[158-161] Further exploration of the region of association suggests that the closely approximated hypoxia-inducible factor 3 (*HIF3*) may be the actual gene of interest. Nonetheless, among individuals with OSAS, the presence of at least one copy of the *APOEε4* risk allele may result in increased risk of cognitive impairment, possibly as a result of greater susceptibility to oxidative stress or neuroinflammation.[162-164]

Angiotensin II is the vasoconstrictive end product of the renin-angiotensin system. However, its ability to modulate afferent neuronal activity from the carotid body implicates a role in ventilatory drive as well. The angiotensin-converting enzyme (*ACE*) gene has been associated with OSAS in Chinese cohorts.[165-169] This effect was most notable among individuals with hypertension.[165-169] Although a primary association between OSAS and *ACE* was not replicated in either the Wisconsin Sleep Cohort or the Cleveland Family Study, *ACE* genotype modulated the relationship between OSAS and hypertension.[170,171] Together these findings suggest that ACE's role in OSAS pathophysiology may be as a moderator of cardiovascular disease risk, potentially akin to inflammatory pathway genes.

Linkage Analysis

Linkage analysis examines family genetics in an effort to identify and quantify the co-segregation of a marker locus with a disease locus. Even though this method lacks the ability to identify specific disease-causing variants, the co-segregated alleles among related individuals help identify genomic regions with high probability of harboring risk alleles. An additional benefit of this strategy is the identification of rare, large-effect mutations that may be disproportionately represented in families with multiple affected members. Notably, in one linkage study of African Americans, the *HTR2A* gene was implicated by a nearby linkage peak on chromosome 13 associated with both AHI and BMI,[172] lending further support for the role that serotonin plays in OSA pathobiology.

A promising strategy is to use linkage data to restrict the analytic window used when conducting genome-wide analyses of potentially millions of genetic single-nucleotide variants, thus increasing statistical power by reducing the multiple comparison burden. Using a multi-phased approach that began with linkage analysis and then used association analysis for variants under the linkage peak, weighted for functional evidence in independent cohorts, multiple functional rare variants in *DLC1* were identified to associate with overnight levels of oxygen saturation.[115] *DLC1* was previously implicated in lung-related diseases, and this study suggested that its effects on pulmonary endothelial cell function and smooth muscle contractility also may influence severity of OSAS-related hypoxemia. A similar combined linkage-association analysis approach also identified associations between overnight hypoxemia with variants in angiopoietin-2 (*ANGP2*), a gene also involved in lung injury syndromes.[173]

Admixture Mapping

Another strategy to increase statistical power is to combine admixture mapping with association testing. Admixture mapping is typically used in recently admixed populations who have different ancestral disease distributions and allele frequencies. Similar to linkage analysis, the area under a local admixture peak is analyzed for genetic variants that associate with the trait of interest. This approach was applied to an analysis of the US-based Hispanic Community Health Study/Study of Latinos.[9] Admixture mapping analysis identified local African ancestry at the chromosomal region 2q37 as genome-wide significantly associated with AHI, as well as European and Amerindian ancestries at the chromosomal region 18q21 as suggestively associated with both AHI and percentage time $SpO_2 < 90\%$ (T90). Subsequent combined ancestry-SNP association analyses identified novel variants in ferrochelatase (*FECH*) to associate with both AHI and hypoxemia, findings which were replicated in independent samples. An association with variants in the iron/heme metabolism pathway was potentially identified because of the power of admixture mapping to identify variants that differ by ancestry, which is not unexpected for genes influencing red blood cell biology. These findings suggest a novel role for iron metabolism in influencing OSAS but require further replication and functional assessments.

Next-Generation Sequencing

With the advent of next-generation sequencing technologies, the ability to incorporate genetic markers that reasonably cover the whole genome has become feasible, at scale. GWAS have played a pivotal role in elucidating the pathobiology of complex diseases, such as macular degeneration[174] and inflammatory bowel disease,[175] which would not have been discoverable through traditional candidate-gene approaches, defined a priori. Additionally, discovery beyond the gene-centric approaches of the past is critical for understanding the genetic architecture of complex disorders, because coding regions account for only 11% of the GWAS discoveries, whereas 43% of associations are intergenic and 45% are located in introns.[176] However, the multiplicity of tests performed on the millions of genetic variants, SNPs, necessitates statistical adjustments for the high risk of false positives, resulting in low statistical power to detect the often low-effect variants. This ultimately requires huge sample sizes, on the order of hundreds of thousands of individuals, and demands replication of any findings because of the possibility of the "winner's curse" (i.e., false positives). Strategies that used linkage or admixture mapping to maximize statistical power for GWAS were described earlier. Several other studies focusing on more precise pathophysiologic phenotypes of OSAS have yielded promising results (Table 128.2).

Several novel loci were identified in one study that included 3551 participants from three cohorts.[177] One variant, the lysophosphatidic acid receptor (*LPAR1*) gene, associated with the AHI at a liberalized significance threshold, was replicated in independent cohorts.[177] This proinflammatory gene is expressed in embryonic cortex and was observed to cause craniofacial abnormalities in a mouse knockout model. A different variant, this one in the prostaglandin E2 receptor (*PTGER2*), was also replicated.[177] Another study explored multiple phenotypes—AHI, average nocturnal oxyhemoglobin saturation, and respiratory event duration—in three Hispanic/Latin-American cohorts totaling more than 10,000 individuals.[6] Of the two genome-wide significant loci identified, one (in the G-protein receptor *GPR83*) was associated with AHI and the other (near the pseudogenes *C6ORF183/CCDC162P*) with respiratory event duration in the initial discovery study.[6] However, the availability of comparable data in independent cohorts with similar ancestry was limited, and these results could not be replicated. *GPR83* is expressed in multiple OSAS-relevant brain regions, such as the hypoglossal nuclei, dorsal motor nucleus of the vagus nerve, and the nucleus of solitary tract,[178] and appears to play a role in energy balance[179] and sleep-wake neurotransmission,[180] based on mouse models. A more recent, combined discovery and replication GWAS of 10 ethnically diverse cohorts comprising nearly 23,000 individuals explored a number of measures of nocturnal oxygen status: average SpO_2, minimum SpO_2, and percentage of the night with SpO_2 below 90%.[97] Minimum SpO_2 demonstrated significant associations with the interleukin-18 receptor (*IL18R1*) region that were predominantly driven by associations in males, highlighting the inflammatory aspects of OSAS and sex-specificity of findings.[97] The hexokinase 1 (*HK1*) region was associated with average SpO_2 (and percentage of the night with SpO_2 < 90% among European Americans),[97] which may be explained through bidirectional pathophysiologic links to OSA: hypoxia-inducible factor 1a-regulated glycolysis[181] and *HK1*-regulated inflammation.[182]

Building upon this refined phenotypic framework, 10 cohorts with whole-genome sequencing or imputed genotype data were analyzed, representing more than 21,000 individuals of multiple ancestries.[183] The analyses assessed genetic associations with four measures of nocturnal hypoxia with clinical relevance, high heritability, or prior significant GWAS findings: average oxyhemoglobin saturation, minimum oxyhemoglobin saturation, the percent of the sleep recording with SpO_2 < 90%, and the average desaturation per hypopnea event. Using gene-based association methods across cohorts, *ARMCX3* and the accompanying antisense gene (*ARMCX3-AS1*) were found to associated with OSAS-triggered intermittent hypoxia, suggesting a role for neuronal dysfunction and/or reactive oxygen species (ROS) and carotid body sensitization.[183] GWAS in the multi-population analyses also replicated a prior association,[97] between both of the interleukin-18 receptor subunits (*IL18RAP*) and two oxygen saturation phenotypes (average event desaturation and minimum SpO_2), pointing to a potential influence of pulmonary inflammation on gas exchange. Finally, in population-specific mechanistic analyses, a number of genes in inflammatory (e.g., *NRG1*),

Table 128.2 Functional Significance of Genetic Associations from Next-Generation Sequencing Analyses

Gene	Associated Phenotype	Functional Significance
Redox		
[183]*ARMCX3* & *ARMCX3-AS1* (antisense gene)	Average desaturation	Mitochondrial trafficking and aggregation affecting CNS neuronal function and survival
Inflammation		
[177]*LPAR1*[a]	AHI	Proinflammatory through monocytic proliferation; possible neuromuscular developmental influences
[6]*GPR83*	AHI	Regulatory T-cell development; possible CNS sleep-wake, metabolic, and thermoregulatory activity
[183]*IL18RAP*[a]	Minimum SpO_2 and average desaturation	Macrophage-related, proinflammatory cytokine pathway
[97]*IL18R1*[a]	Minimum SpO_2	Macrophage-related, proinflammatory cytokine pathway
[97]*HK1*	Average SpO_2 and T90	Carbohydrate metabolism regulator interacting with hypoxia-inducible factor 1a in inflammatory cascades
Other		
[9]*FECH*	AHI and T90	Iron homeostasis and heme biosynthesis
[6]*C6ORF183/CCDC162P*	Event duration	Pseudogenes associated with red blood cell traits

[a]Indicates a replicated finding.
AHI, Apnea-hypopnea index; CNS, central nervous system; T90, % time spent with SpO_2 < 90%.

vascular (e.g., *ATP2B4*), and hypoxia-response (e.g., *ETV4*) pathways were found.[183] One important aspect to note regarding these next-generation sequencing studies is that few findings for rare variant associations have been replicated, reflecting the challenges of using this technology, especially for conditions where population-specific effects may drive associations or where there are limited available independent data with the appropriate phenotypic and genomic resolution.

-Omics Approaches

Epigenomics

Epigenetics encompasses heritable biochemical changes that alter gene activity through modifications to deoxyribonucleic acid (DNA) (e.g., addition of a methyl group) that do not impact the primary DNA sequence/code. Modifications such as histone acetylation, DNA methylation, and chromatin remodeling, affect the accessibility of the DNA for transcription, whereas noncoding ribonucleic acids (RNAs) tend to affect gene expression at the translational level. Many DNA modifications happen outside of genes in regulatory regions, resulting in changes in expression levels of genes.[184,185]

A number of plausible links between the pathophysiology of OSAS and epigenetics have been made. For one, cyclic hypoxia tends to be more cytotoxic than chronic hypoxia, because the repeated deoxygenation-reoxygenation leads to the production of ROS and the activation of a number of transcription factors, including NF-κB and hypoxia-inducible factor-1 (HIF-1). Nonetheless, a causal relationship between OSAS and epigenotypes is difficult to establish because of the bidirectional relationship that exists. For example, inherited and environmentally induced DNA methylation patterns may affect the development of OSAS. Some small studies have sought to infer causality by studying potential reversibility of epigenetic changes in the setting of OSAS treatment and/or in vitro induction of intermittent hypoxia, but there are many confounding factors that must be accounted for in these studies. Moreover, the OSAS-induced changes to DNA expression may not necessarily result in increased OSAS severity but may instead affect the clinical outcomes of the disorder.

Histone Modification

In general, histone acetylation results in more accessible DNA, promoting transcription of these regions, whereas deacetylated histones tend to result in gene silencing through a less accessible heterochromatin. Comparatively, histone methylation can variably result in transcriptional activation or suppression, dependent upon the number and position of the methyl moieties. In vivo and in vitro experiments have demonstrated changes in expression patterns of histone-modifying enzymes. In OSAS patients, *SIRT1* underexpression highlighted potential links to cardiovascular dysfunction that can result from suppressed endothelial nitric oxide synthetase (NOS) activity.[186,187] The overexpression of *HDAC2* in animal models of intermittent hypoxia can mediate interferon-stimulated gene expression.[188] Moreover, the primary role of inflammation resulting from chronic intermittent hypoxia is highlighted by the overrepresentation of activating (H3K9ac) and repressing (H3K27me3) histone marks in proinflammatory/oxidative-stress-signaling pathways and antiinflammatory/antioxidant pathways, respectively.[189] Nonetheless, coupling of candidate histone modifications to specific modifying enzyme changes has not yet been demonstrated in either OSAS or models of intermittent hypoxia.

DNA Methylation

As with histone methylation, DNA methylation can have either activating or repressing effects on gene expression, through controlling the accessibility of DNA as a result of changes in the chromatin state. The site of DNA methylation is usually in regions enriched with cytosine-guanine dinucleotides (CpG). The pattern of CpG methylation across the genome is heritable.[190] Various in vitro and in vivo models of chronic intermittent hypoxia have demonstrated DNA methylation changes affecting redox, inflammatory, and other pathways in patterns consistent with primary genomic analyses (Table 128.3).

DNA methylation changes have been reported in association with excessive daytime sleepiness, including in *C7orf50* (associated with diabetes), *KCTD5* (associated with shortened and fragmented sleep in flies), and *RAI1* (associated with circadian and sleep disorders, including AHI in NREM sleep in men).[191] Interestingly, more associations were observed in the African-American sample, suggesting the possibility of an interaction between adverse environmental exposures and genetic architecture mediating sleepiness, one of the most clinically impactful manifestations of OSAS.

Transcriptomics

Generally, changes in gene expression can be assessed through assays of the messenger RNA transcripts (the "transcriptome"). One small study found differential upregulation of a number of genes when comparing postsleep to presleep gene expression in OSAS patients and controls, with pathophysiologically relevant genes involved, such as the antioxidant enzyme catalase.[192] In an analysis of postsleep gene transcription in individuals with OSAS before and after successful CPAP adherence, one study demonstrated changes in expression patterns of pathways involved in cancer neogenesis after CPAP.[193] In an effort to isolate the consequences of OSAS-related hypoxia, a study explored the transcriptome of individuals abruptly withdrawn from CPAP and supplied with either supplemental oxygen or room air.[194] In contrast to the individuals withdrawn onto supplemental oxygen, who had no significant differential gene expression patterns, the individuals withdrawn to room air had 25 upregulated genes of which a handful (*HPSA8, HSPA1A, ITGAX, PPP4C, TRAFD1*, and *ZFAND3*) are part of the IH-driven NF-κB-signaling pathway.[195] Similarly, among the 15 upregulated pathways uniquely identified in the withdrawal to room air group, two pathways—the interferon alpha and gamma pathways—are upstream modulators of NF-κB, further highlighting the specific role that SDB-related hypoxia may play in inflammation-mediated cardiovascular disease.[196] Comparatively, eight upregulated pathways overlapped among the groups withdrawn to room air and supplemental oxygen.[194] Although the mechanisms underlying the upregulation of pathways relating to oxidative stress are unclear, the common link to inflammatory pathways, specifically TNF-α and IL-6/JAK/STAT3 signaling pathways, underscores the consequences of repeated airway collapse and vibration from turbulent airflow.[194]

Noncoding RNAs

Posttranscriptionally, gene expression can be modified through a plethora of noncoding RNAs. Most studied in OSAS are the microRNAs (miRNAs), which are duplexes of approximately 22 nucleotides that inhibit messenger RNA (mRNA)

Table 128.3 Methylation Status Changes in Select Genes Associated with Various Models of Sleep-Disordered Breathing Pathophysiology

Genes	Methylation Status	Clinical/Pathophysiologic Association
Redox		
[198,199]Sod1, Sod2, Txnrd2, Prdx4	Hypermethylated promoter	Chronic intermittent hypoxia with increased ROS
[200]Ace1	Hypomethylated promoter	Chronic intermittent hypoxia with diminished vasodilatory response and increase ROS
[200]Atg	Hypomethylated enhancer	Chronic intermittent hypoxia with diminished vasodilatory response and increase ROS
Inflammation		
[116]*FOXP3*	Hypermethylated intron 1	Pediatric OSA with elevated hsCRP
[117]*IL1R2*	Hypomethylated promoter	Oxygen desaturation index with increased *IL1R2* expression
Other		
[201]*Rab3a*	Hypomethylated promoter	Chronic intermittent hypoxia with tumor growth and invasion
[202]*eNOS*	Hypermethylated promoter	Pediatric OSA with decreased *eNOS* expression
[117]*NPR2*	Hypomethylated promoter	Less sleepiness in OSA with increased *NPR2* expression
[117]*SP140*	Hypermethylated promoter	More sleepiness in OSA with increased *SP140* expression

hsCRP, High-sensitivity C-reactive protein; OSA, obstructive sleep apnea; ROS, reactive oxygen species.

Table 128.4 Differential Regulation among Select microRNAs Associated with Sleep-Disordered Breathing Pathophysiology

miRNA	Effect of Chronic Intermittent Hypoxia	Clinical/Pathophysiologic Association
[203]miR-378a-3p	Upregulation	CPAP-related blood pressure reduction
[203]miR-100-5p	Upregulation	CPAP-related blood pressure reduction
[203]miR-486-5p	Downregulation	CPAP-related blood pressure reduction
[204]miR-664a	Downregulation	AHI-associated atherosclerosis marker
[205]miR-130a	Upregulation	OSA-associated pulmonary hypertension (via *GAX*)
[206]miR-630	Downregulation	OSA-associated endothelial dysfunction (via *Nrf2, AMP kinase*, and tight junction pathways)
[207]miR-223	Downregulation	Chronic intermittent hypoxia-associated pulmonary hypertension
[208,209]miR-21	Upregulation	Chronic intermittent hypoxia-associated atrial remodeling and fibrosis
[210]miR-155	Upregulation	Chronic intermittent hypoxia-associated kidney injury (via *FOXO3a*)
[211]miR-31	Upregulation	Chronic intermittent hypoxia-associated cardiac hypertrophy (via *PKCε*)
[212]miR-145	Downregulation	Chronic intermittent hypoxia-associated aortic remodeling (via *Smad3*)
[213]miR-365	Downregulation	Chronic intermittent hypoxia-associated inflammation (via *IL6*)
[214]miR-218	Upregulation	Chronic intermittent hypoxia-associated aortic apoptosis (via *Robo1*)
[215]miR-26b	Upregulation	Chronic intermittent hypoxia-associated cognitive dysfunction
[215]miR-207	Downregulation	Chronic intermittent hypoxia-associated cognitive dysfunction
[216]miR-452	Downregulation	Chronic intermittent hypoxia-associated insulin resistance (via *RETN, TNF-α*, and *CCL2*)
[217]miR-203	Downregulation	Chronic intermittent hypoxia-associated insulin resistance (via *SELENOP* and *HIP/PAP*)

AHI, Apnea-hypopnea index; CPAP, continuous positive airway pressure; miRNA, microRNA; OSA, obstructive sleep apnea.

translation through promoting degradation or silencing of select mRNAs. Although the preponderance of pathobiologically associated miRNAs that have been reported to date are outlined in Table 128.4, similar to other genetic associations with OSAS, no candidate miRNA has demonstrated consistent association across the translational continuum from in vitro models of intermittent hypoxia to in vivo animal models of chronic intermittent hypoxia to cohort studies. Nonetheless, among the findings to date, OSAS-associated markers of elevated cardiovascular risk—from endothelial dysfunction, hypertension, and atherosclerosis—may be associated with upregulated miR-130a and miR-574, as well as downregulated miR-107, miR-199, miR-485, miR-630, and miR-664a.[197] Furthermore, connections to the multisystem sequelae of chronic intermittent hypoxia, from neurocognitive dysfunction to cardiovascular remodeling and from insulin resistance to chronic kidney injury, may be moderated through interactions with the activity of hypoxia-inducible factors (HIFs) and their responsive genes. As such, many miRNAs that are upregulated by hypoxia are direct targets of HIF-1α, HIF-2α, NF-κB, or their responsive genes, resulting in a positive feedback loop that serves to stabilize HIF-1α; whereas hypoxia appears to downregulate miRNAs that generally protect against injury through suppression of inflammatory signaling or HIF.[197]

CLINICAL PEARL

A positive family history of OSAS (or of related symptoms) is useful in identifying patients at increased risk for the disorder. Craniofacial abnormalities and obesity can each have a genetic basis and are easily recognized risk factors for OSAS. Clinicians should ask about OSAS symptoms in family members, including offspring. Individuals from families with more than one affected member may harbor genetic variants for OSAS and may benefit from close follow-up after interventions such as surgery to ensure their OSAS is adequately treated. Individuals with family histories of lung disease also may be at increased risk for OSAS-related hypoxemia.

SUMMARY

As a result of advances in genetic technologies and growth of datasets with polysomnographic measurements, there has been much progress in understanding the complex phenotype of obstructive sleep apnea. This field will continue to evolve through methodological advances that promote better phenotyping at scale in conjunction with the accumulation of large cohorts of individuals, deeply phenotyped with biometric, diagnostic, and genetic data such as in the National Heart Lung Blood Institute's *Transomics in Precision Medicine Program*, as well as through less deep but very large cohorts such the *UK Biobank* and the *All of Us* programs.

To date, the most consistent genetic signals from candidate gene studies appear to involve serotonin pathways, whereas unbiased genome-wide analyses suggest the importance of genes, particularly those impacting overnight hypoxemia, in inflammatory pathways. Use of state-specific, sex-specific, and race/ethnicity-specific analyses have suggested novel genetic variants not evident in analyses of more heterogenous phenotypes or samples. More precise phenotype definitions and a further understanding of sex-specific and population-specific differences in pathophysiology, and their association with genetic and molecular etiologies, promise to inform precision-medicine approaches for linking information on genetic pathways to targets for therapeutic interventions. The relatively small fraction of the genetic heritability identified to date highlights the complexity of the bidirectional influence of genetics and environment. Further investigations into the interplay between the genetic and environmental contributions to OSAS, and incorporation of genomic mediators such as epigenetic markers into genetic studies, will provide a means of better understanding its pathogenesis and persistence, with the goal of improving screening/preventive strategies, diagnostic tools, and personalized therapeutics.

ACKNOWLEDGMENT

This chapter is dedicated to Peter Tishler, MD, a clinical geneticist and dedicated mentor, who inspired much of the early work of the genetics of OSAS, generously imparting his wisdom and knowledge of human genetics together with his demand for rigor in research and clarity in communications.

SELECTED READINGS

Cade BE, Chen H, Stilp AM, et al. Genetic associations with obstructive sleep apnea traits in Hispanic/Latino Americans. *Am J Respir Crit Care Med*. 2016;194(7):886–897. https://doi.org/10.1164/rccm.201512-2431OC.

Chen H, Cade BE, Gleason KJ, et al. Multiethnic meta-analysis identifies *RAI1* as a possible obstructive sleep apnea–related quantitative trait locus in men. *Am J Respir Cell Mol Biol*. 2018;58(3):391–401. https://doi.org/10.1165/rcmb.2017-0237OC.

Chen Y-C, Hsu P-Y, Hsiao C-C, Lin M-C. Epigenetics: a potential mechanism involved in the pathogenesis of various adverse consequences of obstructive sleep apnea. *Int J Mol Sci*. 2019;20(12):2937. https://doi.org/10.3390/ijms20122937.

Eckert DJ, White DP, Jordan AS, et al. Defining phenotypic causes of obstructive sleep apnea: identification of novel therapeutic targets. *Am J Respir Crit Care Med*. 2013;188:996–1004.

Jeong HH, Chandrakantan A, Adler AC. Obstructive sleep apnea and dementia-common gene associations through network-based identification of common driver genes. *Genes (Basel)*. 2021;12(4):542.

Larkin EK, Patel SR, Goodloe RJ, et al. A Candidate gene study of obstructive sleep apnea in European Americans and African Americans. *Am J Respir Crit Care Med*. 2010;182:947–953.

Liang J, Cade BE, He KY, et al. Sequencing analysis at 8p23 identifies multiple rare variants in DLC1 associated with sleep-related oxyhemoglobin saturation level. *Am J Hum Genet*. 2019;105(5):1057–1068. https://doi.org/10.1016/j.ajhg.2019.10.002.

Liu Y, Zhang X, Lee J, et al. Genome-wide association study of neck circumference identifies sex-specific loci independent of generalized adiposity. *Int J Obes (Lond)*. 2021;45(7):1532–1541.

Maierean AD, Bordea IR, Salagean T, et al. Polymorphism of the serotonin transporter gene and the peripheral 5-hydroxytryptamine in obstructive sleep apnea: what do we know and what are we looking for? A systematic review of the literature. *Nat Sci Sleep*. 2021;13:125–139.

Malhotra A, Ayappa I, Ayas N, et al. Metrics of sleep apnea severity: beyond the apnea-hypopnea index. *Sleep*. 2021;44(7):zsab030.

Pack AI. Application of personalized, predictive, preventative, and participatory (P4) medicine to obstructive sleep apnea. A roadmap for improving care? *Ann Am Thorac Soc*. 2016;13(9):1456–1467. https://doi.org/10.1513/AnnalsATS.201604-235PS.

Patel SR, Goodloe R, De G, et al. Association of genetic loci with sleep apnea in European Americans and African-Americans: the Candidate Gene Association Resource (Care). *PLoS ONE*. 2012;7:e48836.

Redline S, Tishler PV, Tosteson TD, et al. The familial aggregation of obstructive sleep apnea. *Am J Respir Crit Care Med*. 1995;151:682–687.

Schwab RJ, Pasirstein M, Kaplan L, et al. Family aggregation of upper airway soft tissue structures in normal subjects and patients with sleep apnea. *Am J Respir Crit Care Med*. 2006;173:453–463.

Wang H, Cade BE, Sofer T, et al. Admixture mapping identifies novel loci for obstructive sleep apnea in Hispanic/Latino Americans. *Hum Mol Genet*. 2019;28(4):675–687. https://doi.org/10.1093/hmg/ddy387.

A complete reference list can be found online at ExpertConsult.com.

Chapter 129

Deep Phenotyping of Sleep Apnea

Bradley A. Edwards; Magdy Younes; Eric Heckman; Melanie Pogach; Robert Joseph Thomas

Chapter Highlights

- Sleep-disordered breathing (SDB) demonstrates a wide range of recognizable patterns with specific pathophysiologic implications.
- SDB patterns may be overt, suggesting specific driver phenotypes, or may need to be "extracted" using mathematical/computational means.
- SDB patterns of high loop gain and sleep fragmentation are recognizable on routine polysomnography, but a vast array of other clinically meaningful patterns is also seen.
- SDB patterns change with therapy; therapy patterns also provide insight into pathophysiology.
- It is important to recognize that sleep modifies SDB in important and recognizable ways.
- Optimal identification of SDB phenotypes will be necessary to provide endotype-targeted therapies as part of personalized sleep apnea care.

INTRODUCTION

The scoring manual of the American Academy of Sleep Medicine (AASM), accessible through the internet,[1] is a living volume that undergoes updates and provides a commonly used standard. The standard scoring guidelines generate sleep stage, heart rate, breathing, and motor activation metrics. However, sleep signals, individually or in combination, are rich in biologic information with value beyond that of the standard metrics. For example, besides the standard stages (see Chapter 197), alternative methods of characterizing sleep include a continuous sleep depth measure called the odds ratio product (ORP), cyclic alternating pattern (CAP) of non–rapid eye movement (NREM) sleep (see Chapter 198),[2] and cardiopulmonary coupling (high-, low-, and very low-frequency coupling of autonomic and respiratory drives, modulated by cortical delta power).[3] NREM stage N3 is usually associated with stable breathing. However, such periods frequently occur outside N3, during a stable form of N2, when the electroencephalogram (EEG) usually shows a non-CAP morphology. Arousals are traditionally scored as an all or none event but show a wide range of perturbation and recovery kinetics and individual differences, which may amplify or dampen the progression of respiratory events.[4-8] In the following sections, we will present concepts and methods to recognize and determine phenotypes and endotypes.

ENDOTYPES AND PHENOTYPES

The term *endotype* refers to the pathophysiologic mechanisms of disease. Abnormalities in upper airway anatomy and physiology, control of breathing, and interaction of these with state (sleep, wakefulness) are the pathophysiologic mechanisms involved in sleep breathing abnormalities.[9,10] The term *phenotype* refers to the consequences of the pathophysiologic mechanisms. These include physiologic abnormalities, clinical features, and response to therapy. Understanding these concepts may lead to more personalized treatment of sleep breathing disorders.

The Sleep State and Sleep-Breathing Phenotypes

Airflow patterns and arousal thresholds are modulated by sleep macrostructure (rapid eye movement [REM] and NREM sleep, stages of NREM sleep), sleep microstructure (CAP and non-CAP), homeostatic sleep drive, medications, and age. Data suggest that NREM sleep is bimodal rather than graded, with stable and unstable regimes (Figure 129.1), or alternatively conceptualized as effective and ineffective.[3] Thus rather than thinking in terms of grades of NREM sleep (N1 to N3) of progressive depth, the stability domain has only two forms of NREM sleep: stable and unstable. N3 is usually stable, N1 is always unstable, but N2 may be stable or unstable. These periods of stability intrinsic to NREM sleep can determine the instantaneous presence or absence of sleep apnea. Cardiopulmonary analysis shows stable breathing periods result in high-frequency coupling of respiration and heart rate variability, simultaneously associated with high EEG delta power. Such periods are not restricted to N3 but make up most of N2 in health. Intermittent periods of stable breathing are well recognized in patients with even severe obstructive sleep apnea, during both N3 and N2.[11] Flow limitation can be prominent, and both hypoxia and hypoventilation may occur during these obstructed but stable periods with prolongation of inspiratory time with minimal breath-to-breath variability of tidal volume. These periods do have an impact on the EEG, but visual determination is not possible, and computational

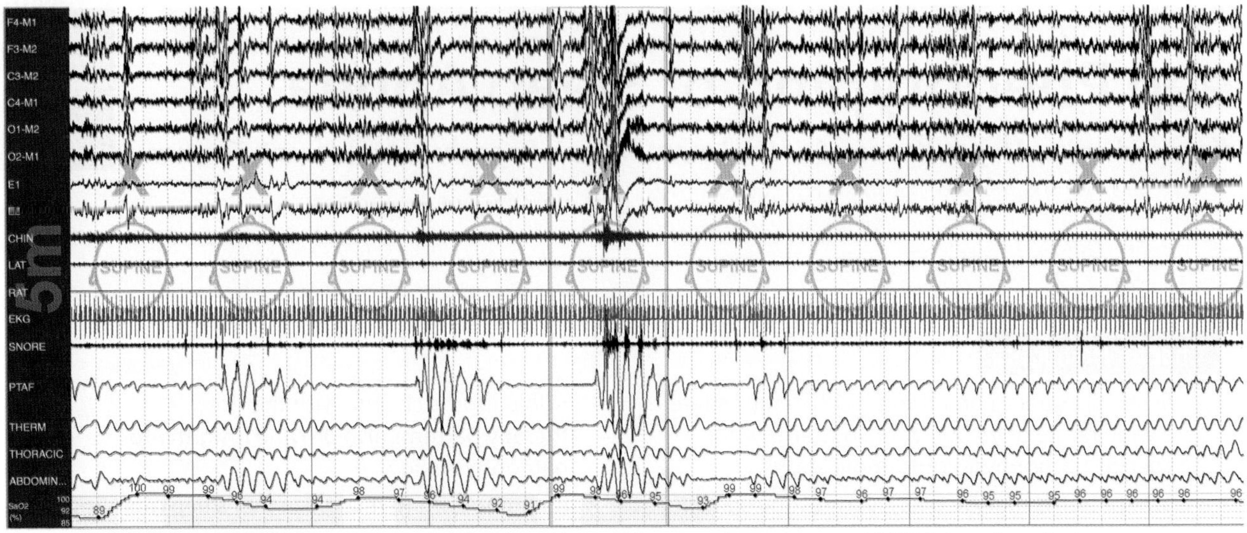

Figure 129.1 Spontaneous switch from unstable to stable non–rapid eye movement (NREM) sleep. Five-minute polysomnogram snapshot of stage N2, showing the relatively abrupt switch from a state of respiratory events and arousals to a state with stable breathing and absence of arousals.

methods such as the respiratory cycle–related EEG change are required.[12,13] The persistence of CAP-type features on the EEG may also occur during slow wave sleep associated with severe persistent flow limitation, suggesting the presence of concomitant disruptive influences from hypoxia, hypercapnia, excessive respiratory effort, and upper airway stimulation.

Excessively unstable NREM sleep disproportionate to disruptive pathology on the polysomnography (PSG) may be recognized by a sleep fragmentation phenotype. This phenotype can be suggested by prolonged sleep-wake transitional instability (>10 minutes), low sleep efficiency (<70%), persistently high N1 stage during positive airway pressure (PAP) titration (>15%), and poor evolution of slow wave sleep (<1 Hz).[14] Chin electromyography (EMG) tone elevations during NREM sleep are not part of the conventional arousal definition, but the duration and degree of elevation vary markedly between individuals and stay consistent within individuals. The same concept can be applied to the EEG (arousal duration or return to sleep) and heart rate responses to arousal—interindividual variability is contrasted with intraindividual stability.[15]

Sleep Depth, Network Strength, and Cohesion

The continuity of sleep during individual sleep cycles across a typical night requires networking, cohesion, and reciprocal interactions of NREM and REM sleep processes. Intuitively, stable periods of NREM sleep are deeper, but both stable and unstable NREM sleep can have varying degrees of depth. Conventional stages do not effectively capture sleep depth, even if in most instances N3 is deeper and more stable than N2.

One established method of assessing continuous sleep depth is the ORP.[16-18] The currently accepted method (described in greater detail later in the chapter) of measuring arousal threshold in patients with obstructive sleep apnea (OSA) is to determine the peak negative pharyngeal pressure immediately preceding arousals that occur at the time of upper airway (UA) opening and averaging the results over the obstructive events. Apart from being invasive, this approach assumes that there is only one arousal threshold in a given patient. There is, however, no single arousal threshold in any individual. Arousability changes continuously as state progresses from wake to deep sleep within each sleep cycle and following sporadic brief arousals and awakening. Furthermore, arousal threshold can be measured only during periods of recurrent events; it is not possible to measure the threshold in this way during periods of stable breathing, and this is quite important for determining the increase in sleep depth required to achieve stability.

ORP is calculated every 3 seconds from the power spectrum of the EEG. It represents the EEG powers in four different frequency bands relative to each other, with higher values representing increased propensity for an arousal. It has an excellent correlation ($r^2 = 0.98$) with arousability, defined as the probability of an arousal or awakening occurring within 30 seconds. It also changes appropriately in response to sleep deprivation, sleep restriction, and brief acoustic stimuli and increases across the night, as may be expected from the decrease in homeostatic sleep pressure.

Figures 129.2 and 129.3 illustrate some of the information that can be provided using the ORP. Figure 129.2A shows the progressive decrease in ORP and, by extension, arousability within each sleep cycle. Furthermore, it shows that whenever ORP was above 1.0 (light sleep; horizontal dotted line) there were recurrent respiratory events. As OSA treatment results in unstable breathing converting to stable breathing, the ORP decreased below 1.0 (vertical dotted lines). Often, stage N3 was scored as ORP decreased further. However, it is important to note that in this patient, transition from an oscillatory pattern to a stable pattern occurred prior to the appearance of stage N3 in all four respiratory cycles where ORP decreased below 1.0. This indicates that measures to increase sleep depth beyond light sleep may be helpful for this patient.

By contrast, Figure 129.2B shows that recurrent respiratory events continued despite ORP being near zero (deepest sleep). Such behavior suggests that measures to increase sleep depth in this patient might be ineffective. Furthermore, the occurrence of arousals along with these events, despite very deep sleep, suggests that the arousal stimulus at the end of the events was strong. Titration of continuous positive airway

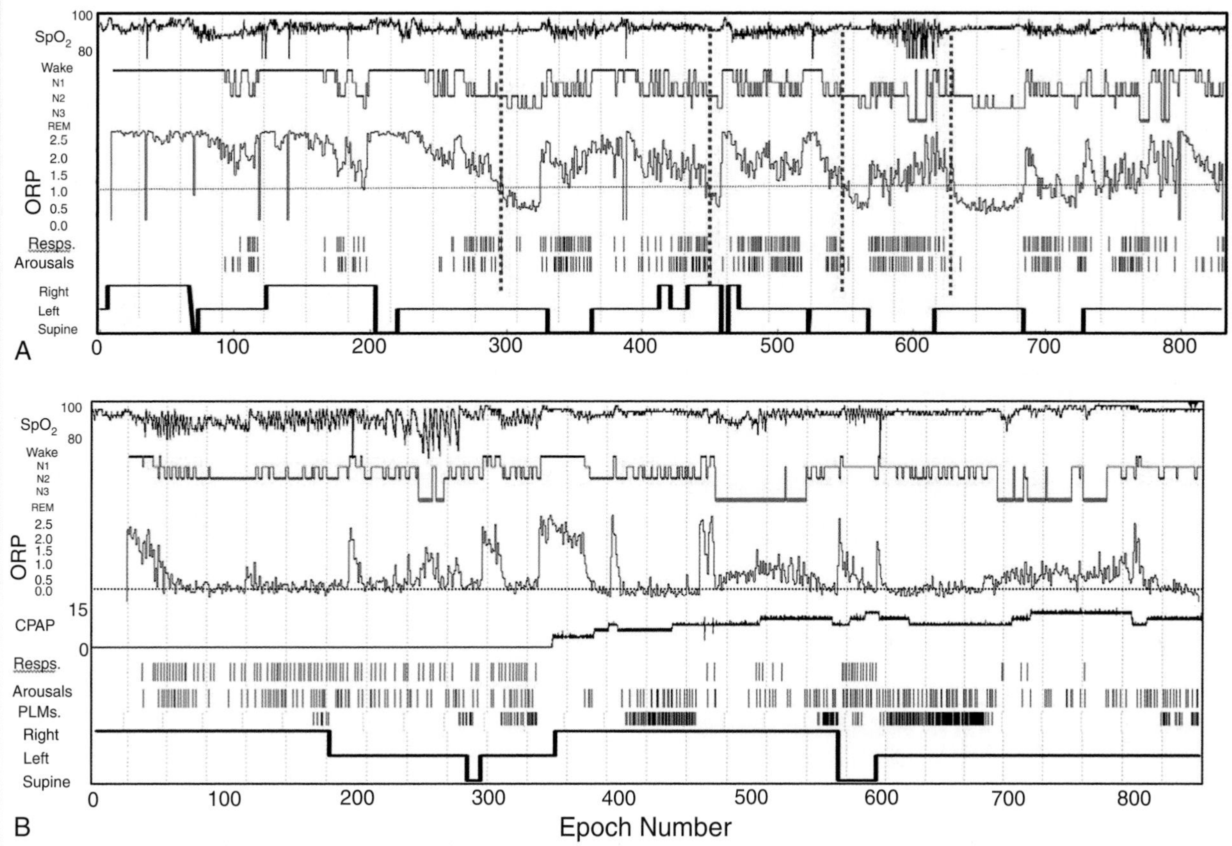

Figure 129.2 Odds ratio product (ORP) dynamics across a night. Tracings showing the relation between the ORP and repetitive obstructive events in two patients with obstructive sleep apnea (OSA). Tracings represent, from top to bottom, oxyhemoglobin saturation (SpO_2), sleep stages, ORP, continuous positive airway pressure (CPAP) (**B** only), respiratory events (Resps), arousals, and body position. Note that ORP undergoes cyclic changes throughout the night. **A,** Recurrent events occur only when ORP is above 1.1 (light sleep, *horizontal dotted line*) and stop abruptly as soon as ORP decreases below that level (four *vertical dashed lines*). The change occurs within stage N2. Stage N3 appears at an even lower ORP. **B,** Recurrent events occur despite very deep sleep (ORP ≈0.1). When CPAP was applied, OSA was eliminated except for a brief period in the supine position, but excessive arousals continued during non–rapid eye movement (NREM) sleep. These were, however, associated with intense periodic limb movements (PLMs). In this patient N3 was not scored before or during CPAP.

pressure (CPAP) in this split study eliminated OSA except for a brief period in the supine sleep. ORP remained very low on CPAP except during REM sleep, where ORP is typically higher than in NREM sleep.

When ORP is high during recurrent events, it is not clear whether light sleep is the result of recurrent OSA preventing sleep from progressing to deeper levels or is independent of it and the result of abnormal central regulation of sleep depth. Figure 129.3 shows two patients with severe OSA in whom ORP was quite high prior to the application of CPAP. In both cases, CPAP essentially eliminated OSA and markedly reduced arousals. Panel A shows that elimination of OSA was followed by a reduction in ORP to deep levels (compare the horizontal dotted lines before and on CPAP), indicating that the high arousability before CPAP was a consequence of OSA. By contrast, in the patient in panel B, ORP remained high throughout. Thus a brief CPAP titration can determine whether the high arousability is OSA-related or the result of abnormal regulation of sleep depth. This has two potential applications that require experimental validation. First, finding that high arousability is inherent to the patient may help direct therapy. Second, by indicating sleep remains light on CPAP, a high ORP may foretell future intolerance to CPAP once sleep deprivation is ameliorated.

Interaction of Respiratory Event Termination and Electrocortical Responses

The standard teaching is that an arousal from sleep is necessary for airway opening. There is new information that only a proportion of respiratory recovery is arousal dependent and that blood gas changes can drive airway opening without an electrocortical arousal.[6] Although the degree of arousal does amplify associated autonomic features roughly proportional to the degree of alpha/beta intrusion,[19] stage and state modulation are also important. It is conceptually useful to consider NREM sleep as manifesting bimodal stable versus unstable characteristics.[7] For example, when sleep drive is high and NREM state is stable, airway opening can likely occur without a classic electrocortical arousal, the high sleep drive masking EEG arousal recognition or simply preventing an arousal. This allows the brainstem and chemoreceptor or mechanoreceptor-based respiratory reflexes to open the airway.[6] When NREM sleep is in an unstable mode, the networked driving of state couples nearly all prevalent physiology and pathology. Thus

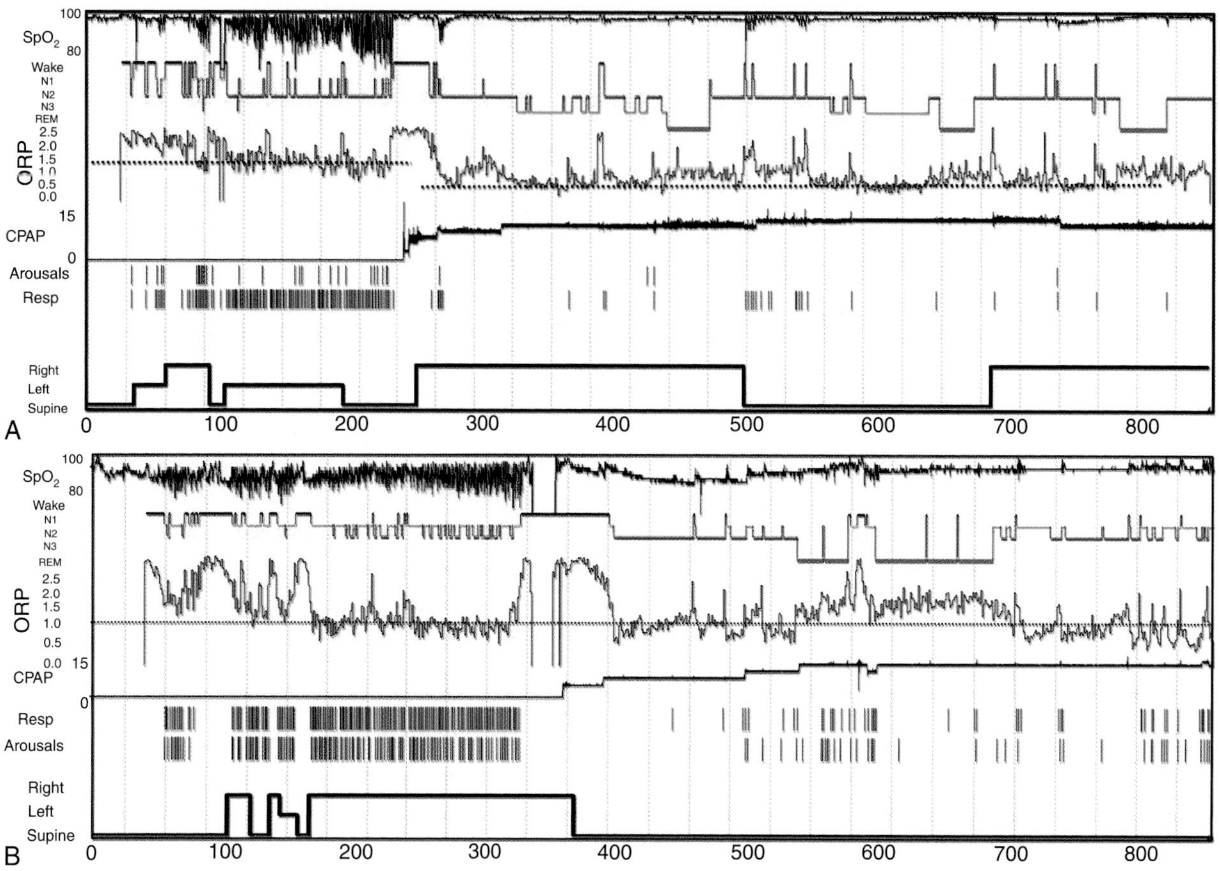

Figure 129.3 **A,** Odds ratio product (ORP) response to continuous positive airway pressure (CPAP). Elimination of obstructive sleep apnea (OSA) was followed by reduction in ORP to deep levels (compare the *horizontal dotted lines* before and on CPAP), indicating that the high arousability prior to CPAP was a consequence of OSA. **B,** ORP response to CPAP. Tracings showing different ORP responses to application of CPAP. Format as in Figure 129.2. Both patients had severe OSA and ORP was quite high prior to CPAP (>1.0; very light sleep). ORP failed to decrease after elimination of OSA, suggesting that light sleep prior to CPAP was unrelated to OSA.

tidal volume fluctuations, EEG arousals, heart rate change, hemodynamic/autonomic oscillations, and even periodic motor activation are all coupled and occur nearly simultaneously. During such a condition, it is hard to be sure arousal is *necessary,* but arousals certainly *occur,* in close temporal relationship, to respiratory recovery. K-complexes are frequent accompaniments of respiratory recovery and may reflect the interplay and interaction of sleep disruptive and restorative forces.[20,21] Medications that increase slow wave, such as atypical antipsychotics, can obscure the faster components of arousals, when clusters of slow waves may be the only visually evident marker of respiratory-related arousal. During REM sleep, respiratory fluctuations occur as part of the REM sleep state and independent of arousals (increase in EMG tone), and it is unknown if these tidal volume and flow fluctuations, when exaggerated but without EMG increases, disrupt REM sleep. When REM without atonia is also present, respiratory-related arousal and REM sleep scoring can be difficult and sometimes impossible.

Sleep depth postarousal varies substantially among patients with OSA from being very light to very deep. The ORP fluctuates after an arousal, rising to wake levels and then decreasing as sleep resumes and stabilizes. ORP-9 is the ORP 9 seconds after the start of the arousal.[22] If the ORP remains high several seconds after the arousal, it suggests that the “glue” (network cohesion) of sleep is poor, and this high ORP-9 would indicate that the high arousability is much more likely to be the result of abnormal central regulation of sleep depth. In patients with high ORP-9 (highly arousable soon after a previous arousal), arousal is likely to occur soon after the obstruction and interrupt the recruitment of pharyngeal dilators, leading to recurrence of events. Conversely, subjects in whom sleep becomes quite deep immediately after arousal (low ORP-9) can tolerate the obstruction for a longer time, allowing the reflex recruitment of dilator muscles, thereby increasing the probability of resolving the obstruction without arousal. ORP-9 was found to be the main determinant of average sleep depth and to be invariably high in patients with a very high apnea-hypopnea index (AHI). Furthermore, ORP-9 is quite reproducible even when remeasured after 5 years, suggesting that it is a trait (Younes M; unpublished observations).

Easy Arousability (Low Arousal Threshold)

As noted, early investigations into the mechanism of OSA suggested that the UA would not open unless arousal occurred.[20] Most sleep apnea patients are capable of opening their airway without classic electrocortical arousal[9,21,22] and, rather than being an essential compensatory mechanism,[23] arousal

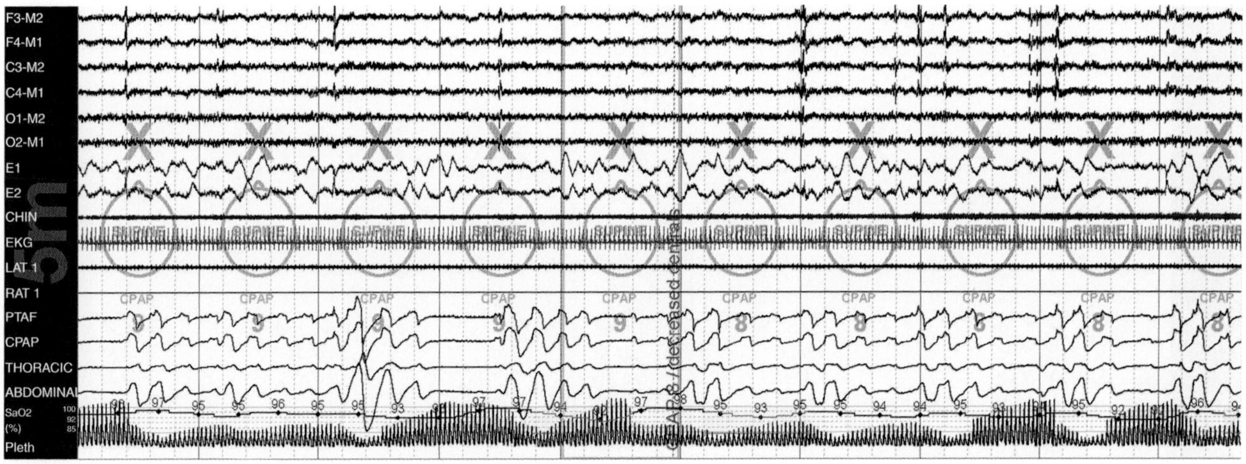

Figure 129.4 Effect of continuous positive airway pressure (CPAP) on high loop gain sleep apnea. CPAP opens the airway, but the underlying rhythm continues.

is an important contributor to the recurrence of events and a high AHI in many patients.[21,22] Unlike the patients that were investigated in the 1970s (long events with severe hypoxemia and, often, hypercapnia),[20] in most current patients events are brief with generally mild hypoxemia and no hypercapnia.

There is much evidence that in many patients arousals occur with minimal, nonthreatening, increases in respiratory drive (i.e., easy arousability); that pharyngeal dilators can open the airway without arousal if given the time to respond; and that opening without arousal is often followed by stable sleep and breathing:

1. It was estimated that the changes in $Paco_2$ at the chemoreceptor at the time of arousal in most patients is no more than 2 to 3 mm Hg and the average change in SpO_2 is only 3.1 ± 3.5%.[21]
2. Consistent with these estimates, in recent studies that evaluated arousal threshold from the negative pharyngeal pressure immediately preceding UA opening, the threshold negative pressure was in the range of −10 to −30 cmH_2O with an average of ≈20 cmH_2O.[24-27] This is less than twice the pressure generated during the first obstructed breath in healthy subjects during eupnea (range 8–22 cmH_2O).[28] Doubling of respiratory output in patients with OSA is achieved within five breaths when SpO_2 decreases by ≈4% along with an increase in end-tidal Pco_2 of ≈3.0 mm Hg.[17]
3. UA opening occurs without arousal in an average of 17% of obstructive events and before arousal in another 25%, and events without arousal or terminating before or after arousal occur in the same patient, all indicating that opening without or before arousal is common in most patients.[21]
4. Most patients develop periods of stable breathing without arousal at the same P_{crit},[11] and it has long been observed that OSA tends to disappear if the patient enters stage N3, where arousability is low.[28] Stable sleep in patients with OSA is associated with higher genioglossus activity,[29] consistent with the idea that a higher arousal threshold affords the dilators more time to respond before arousal occurs and that this leads to more stable breathing.

Impact of easy arousability on loop gain. The premature occurrence of arousal at minimally impaired blood gas tensions should in theory reduce the chemical drive at the time of UA opening, which would tend to reduce loop gain and the ventilatory overshoot. However, arousal is associated with ventilatory stimulation independent of chemical drive.[30] Importantly, the ventilatory overshoot correlates with the intensity of arousal.[21] Higher postevent ventilation associated with high intensity arousals is not the result of a greater arousal stimulus (more negative pharyngeal pressure), suggesting that arousal intensity is a trait.[31] Studies have even shown that arousal intensity is a highly heritable trait.[32] Thus arousal intensity may be considered an independent phenotype that modulates the ventilatory response to arousal.

Assessing Event Significance in Stable NREM Sleep: Periods of Stable Breathing

Respiration is stable during conventional slow wave sleep. Increased genioglossus tone and increases in CO_2 occur during periods of stable breathing,[11] with overt hypoventilation and hypoxia if flow limitation is severe. Spontaneous periods of stable breathing do not occur during REM sleep. The central problem with associating stable breathing phenomenon exclusively with slow wave sleep by any definition is that such stable periods occur predominantly in N2, including those with no N3. Figures 129.4 through 129.7 demonstrate the impact of these periods in creating stable periods as a component across a dynamic range of pathology. Stable periods dominate the rebound effects of successful PAP titration and the majority of the time is usually N2. Some clues to the nature of this phenomenon can be gained from the concept of NREM sleep bimodality. The first clue came from the description of CAP and non-CAP from Italian researchers in the mid-1980s.[23] CAP and non-CAP periods occur across NREM sleep; non-CAP occurs in N2 or N3.[2] Subsequently, the autonomic and respiratory associations of CAP/non-CAP were described.[24] Finally, the description of the cardiopulmonary coupling technique showed that NREM sleep has bimodal characteristics in health and disease. High-frequency coupling is associated with high delta power, non-CAP EEG, stable breathing, strong sinus arrhythmia, and blood pressure dipping.[3] Low-frequency coupling is associated with unstable breathing (reaching scorable thresholds of sleep apnea in disease), cyclic variation in heart rate, CAP EEG, and blood pressure nondipping. Thus stable breathing periods reflect natural integrated network states of the brain and are amplified and

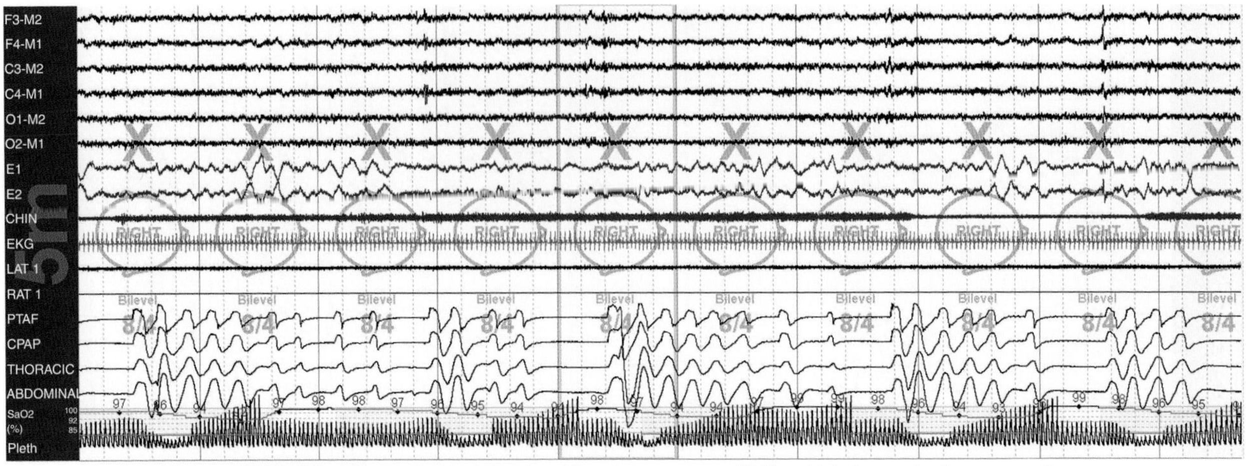

Figure 129.5 Effect of nonadaptive bilevel positive airway pressure (PAP) on high loop gain sleep apnea. Same subject as in Figure 129.4. The cycle times prolong, likely because of worsening of hypocapnia. Events during titration often show minimal oxygen desaturation, or even signal reductions reaching thresholds for hypopnea, and may show atypical long, short, or ataxic patterns.

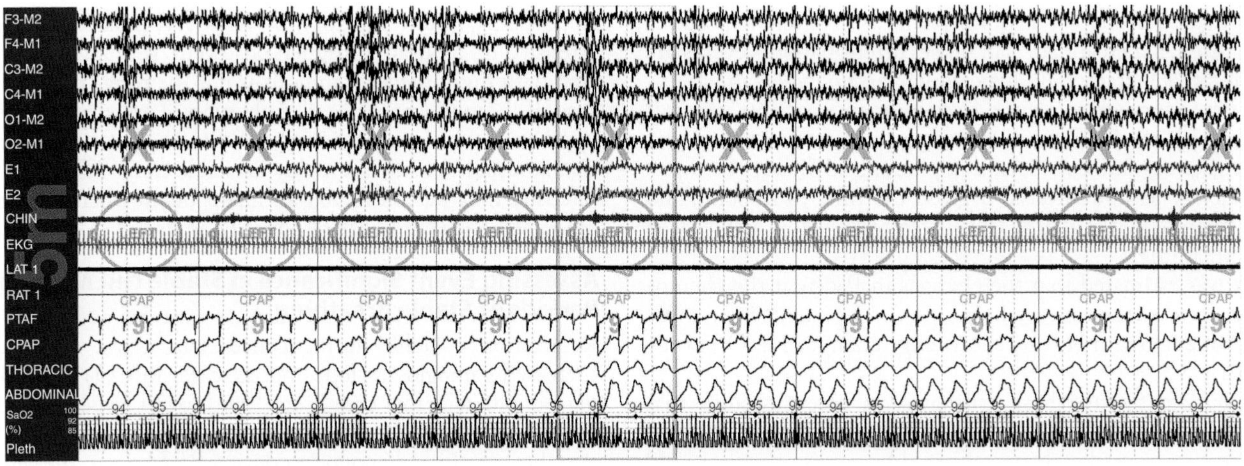

Figure 129.6 Stabilizing effect of "stable non–rapid eye movement (NREM)" sleep on sleep apnea. Same subject as in Figure 129.4. Conventional stage is N3.

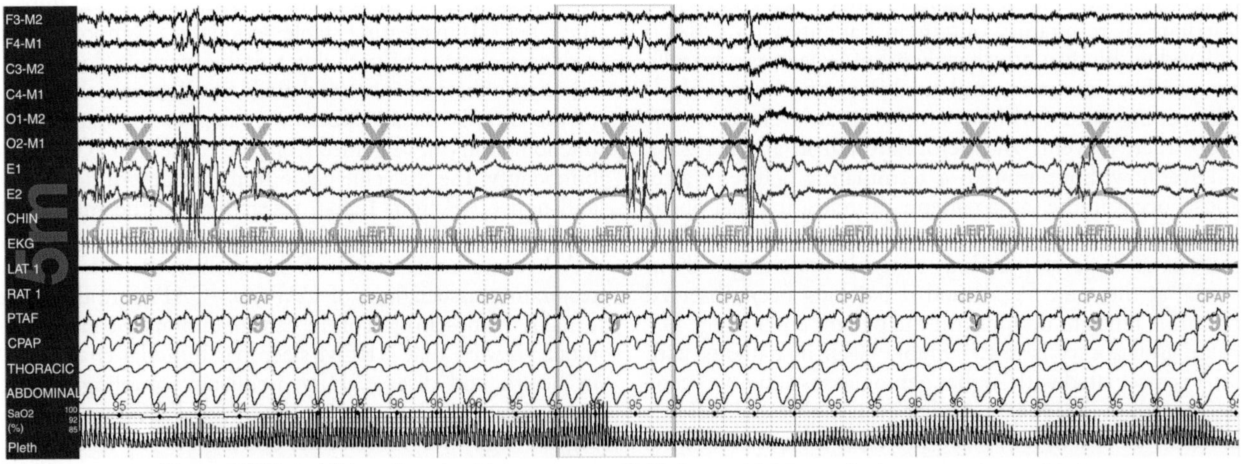

Figure 129.7 Stabilizing effect of rapid eye movement (REM) sleep on high loop gain sleep apnea. Same subject as in Figure 129.4.

readily recognizable in sleep apnea patients, as the two states are markedly different on visual inspection. Benzodiazepines and related drugs increase stable EEG periods[25,26] and may be expected to increase stable breathing periods. Zolpidem increases blood pressure dipping[27] and could do so through the induction of stable NREM periods.

Loop Gain: A Concept Relevant to Understanding Scoring, Classic Phenotype Limitations, and Therapy

Whether UA opening is followed by stable breathing or recurrent cycling depends on loop gain, an engineering term that describes the relationship between the magnitude of a response to the magnitude of an instigating perturbation (▲ output / ▲ input) by any system. For the respiratory system, the loop represents the connection between the sensors of respiratory stimuli, the control centers, and the mechanical/chemical pump that executes the breathing. Simplistically, a loop gain above 1.0 is associated with respiratory event cycling and a loop gain below 1.0 with stable breathing. In sleep apnea, high loop gain reflects a ventilatory response to hypopnea that overcorrects the changes in blood gas tensions produced by that hypopnea. This overcorrection leads to a second hypopnea (from reduced drive to UA and lung muscles), and the cycle repeats.

Loop gain varies between individuals and with disease states.[28] High loop gain is found in systems with large swings in blood gases and ventilation (e.g., periodic breathing in congestive heart failure, severe sleep apnea). Low loop gain indicates a stable system but also one that may not respond adequately to a reduction in ventilation (e.g., obesity hypoventilation). A loop gain above 1, however, does not indicate the reason(s) for the instability or what needs to be corrected to eliminate the cycling.

The "controller" converts the signal from the chemoreceptors into a ventilatory drive for the plant (anticipated ventilation for a given $Paco_2$). The "plant" refers to the lungs, blood, and tissues where CO_2 is stored. The plant produces the change in $Paco_2$ for a given change in ventilatory stimulus, and its performance depends on the mechanical and biochemical properties of its components (e.g., lung compliance, ventilation-perfusion matching, hemoglobin concentration, etc.). For most awake individuals, eupneic $Paco_2 \approx 40$ mm Hg, and for sleeping individuals, it is ≈45 mm Hg. The "mixer" represents the time it takes for the capillary blood from the lungs to reach the chemoreceptors and is primarily a function of cardiac output. The sensitivity of each of the system's components to a change in input represents its "gain." The controller gain is the ▲ Ve / ▲ $PaCO_2$, where ▲ Ve is change in ventilation, plant gain is ▲ $PaCO_2$ / ▲ Ve, and the mixing gain determines the speed with which changes in $PaCO_2$ and PaO_2 from the plant are detected by the controller.[29] The overall loop gain (Ve disturbance / Ve response) is the product of controller, plant, and mixing gains and determines how stable the respiratory system is.

The metabolic respiration control system active during sleep is exquisitely sensitive and designed to maintain $PaCO_2$ homeostasis rather than oxygenation. Two levels of $PaCO_2$, the apneic and eupneic thresholds, are critical to its operation. As elegantly demonstrated by Bulow in the 1960s,[30-32] *apneic threshold* represents a level of $PaCO_2$ below which breathing stops. *Eupneic threshold* is the $PaCO_2$ at which stable breathing occurs. Below the eupneic threshold, ventilatory drive is reduced, whereas above it is increased.[33] During sleep, the apneic threshold is usually 2 to 6 mm Hg below the eupneic sleeping $PaCO_2$ level but only 1 to 2 mm Hg below the wakefulness eupneic $PaCO_2$ level.[34,35] This small difference between awake eupneic and sleep apneic $PaCO_2$ is one reason behind the instability of the respiratory system during sleep. When loop gain is too high, periodic breathing, hypocapnic central apneas, and NREM dominance of sleep apnea emerge. When loop gain is too low, hypoventilation results. High loop gain protects respiration during REM sleep and may explain why NREM mixed periodic breathing with obstruction improves or "disappears" during REM sleep.

Quantitative polysomnogram analysis has also been used to differentiate cardiac-related periodic breathing from noncardiac causes and may help predict the effectiveness of CPAP for central sleep apnea with Cheyne-Stokes breathing (CSA-CSB). In brief, a surrogate of loop gain can be estimated from the ratio of ventilation length (VL) divided by the apnea length (AL) or (VL/AL). VL/AL greater than 1[36] and cycle duration/length (CL = VL + AL) longer than 45 seconds[37] are suggestive of CSA of a cardiac cause. Loop gain (LG) can also be derived by the means of a duty ratio (DR = VL / CL) of periodic breathing, $LG = 2\pi / (2\pi DR - \sin 2\pi DR)$.[38] In a pilot study of 14 patients with congestive heart failure and Cheney-Stokes breathing (CHF-CSB), LG was significantly higher among the nonresponders, and a value of greater than 1.2 predicted lack of response to CPAP in 7 out of 7 patients.[38] High loop gain also predicts residual apnea on CPAP.[39] Although simple to determine and encouraging from pilot data, such findings are limited to patients with already clear periodic breathing and should be validated in a larger, prospective manner.

Event Cycle Characteristics

Event Cycle Length

The cycle length (Figures 129.8 and 129.9) of a respiratory event reflects the time to arousal, respiratory drivers, effects of phasic suppression of muscle tone for REM sleep events, and intrinsic network properties of the sleeping brain. The time to arousal is dependent on the input to brainstem arousal centers, which may be from within (respiratory effort), somatic afferents from the UA, or visceral afferents (including respiratory chemoreflex sensing of O_2 in the carotid body and CO_2 in the carotid body and ventral brainstem surface). The nucleus of the solitary tract in the medulla is a major convergence point for these afferents,[40] and the lateral parabrachial complex may have a specific role in hypercapnic arousal.[41]

Respiratory driving may be reactive (response to UA obstruction) or active, when the respiratory chemoreflex arc is hyperactive as in CHF,[24] at high altitude,[42] and after exposure to hypoxia (sensory long-term facilitation).[43] Phasic effects of REM sleep can cause obstructive, central-looking, or pseudo-periodic patterns, the latter when eye movements occur with similar interphasic intervals. This latter phenomenon can be incorrectly characterized as periodic breathing, especially if EEG is not available, as with in-home sleep testing.

Event cycle length is entrainable. The best examples are high altitude (short, less than 30 seconds, often 15–20 seconds) and CHF (long, most characteristically 60 seconds or longer) cycles (Figures 129.8 and 129.9). Adaptive ventilation can convert a short cycle to a long cycle; the authors have never seen this therapy convert a long to a short cycle, but if cardiac function improves, such a conversion may be possible. Cycle length can also increase with supplemental oxygen or use of a

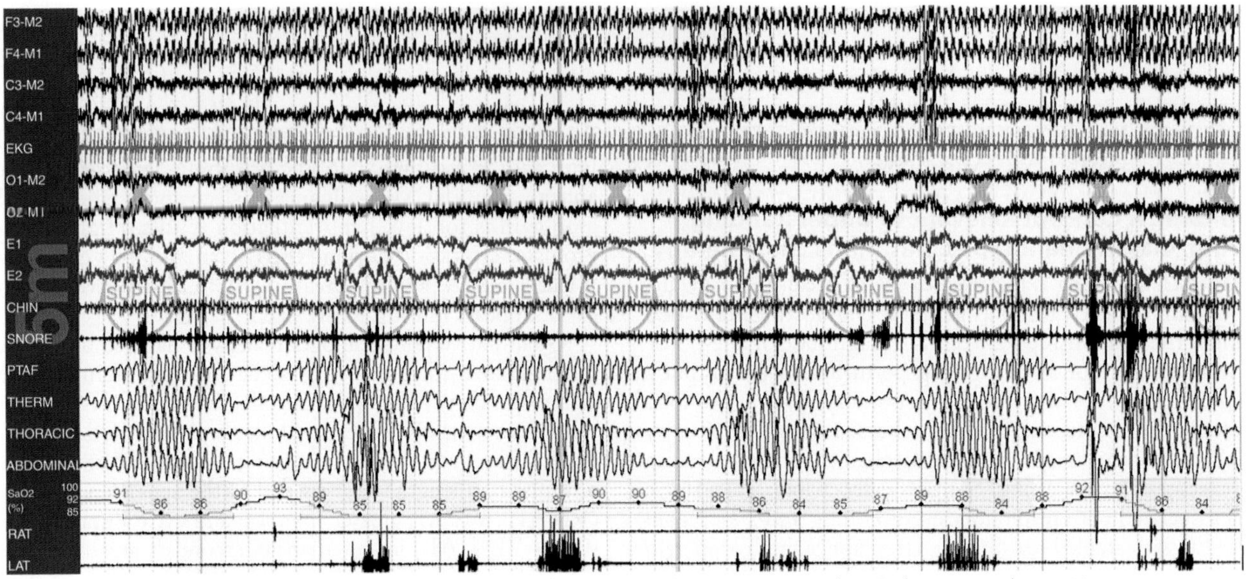

Figure 129.8 Long-cycle periodic breathing. Five-minute polysomnogram snapshot. Cycle times are close to 50 seconds in this patient with congestive heart failure.

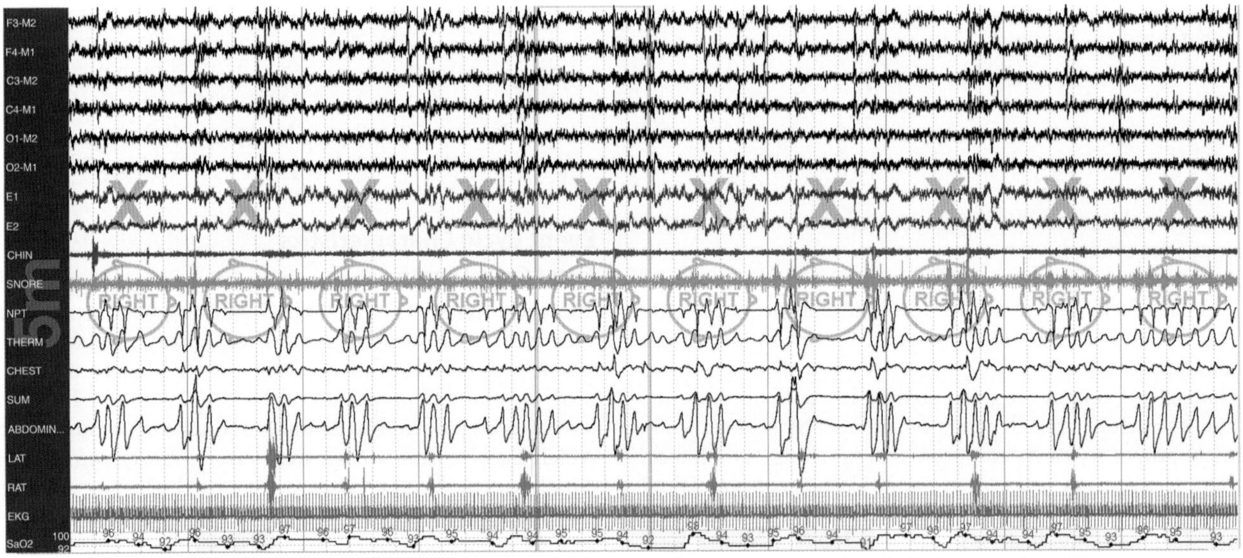

Figure 129.9 Short-cycle periodic breathing. Five-minute polysomnogram snapshot. Cycle times are about 30 seconds.

nonvented mask to minimize hypocapnia[44] by prolonging the time to arousal. It is plausible that other rhythmic and repetitive arousing stimuli such as experimental auditory arousals can entrain "CAP," but there will be biologic constraints on frequencies that can entrain sleep state. Too frequent arousing stimuli will wake up the subject, but too infrequent stimuli will likely only transiently arouse the subject without entrainment to the cycle time of the arousing stimulus.

Ultrashort Respiratory Events

The typical respiratory event evolves over 30 to 40 seconds. When respiratory chemoreflex driving is strong in the setting of normal cardiac function, cycle times shorten and can be as short as 20 seconds. This pattern strongly resembles that seen at high altitudes. Travelers to high altitudes often experience restlessness, frequent brief arousals, and unrefreshing sleep,[45] at least in part due to periodic breathing. In contrast to heart failure, the cycle times are 15 to 25 seconds, characterized by two to five large tidal volume breath clusters followed by apneas of 5 to 15 seconds in duration. There is a marked increase in arousals and reduction of slow wave sleep likely related to the hypoxemia narrowing the $Paco_2$ reserve and increasing controller gain.[46] A male predominance has been reported.[47] In idiopathic CSA, similar to high altitude, cycles of central apneas are shorter (20–40 seconds) and not as gradual and smooth as in classical CSR.[48,49] Although 10 seconds is the standard minimum event length for scoring, shorter events with biologic consequences should reasonably be tagged.

Ultralong Respiratory Events

Two types of long events are seen. In one pattern, there is prolonged and progressive flow limitation that is terminated by

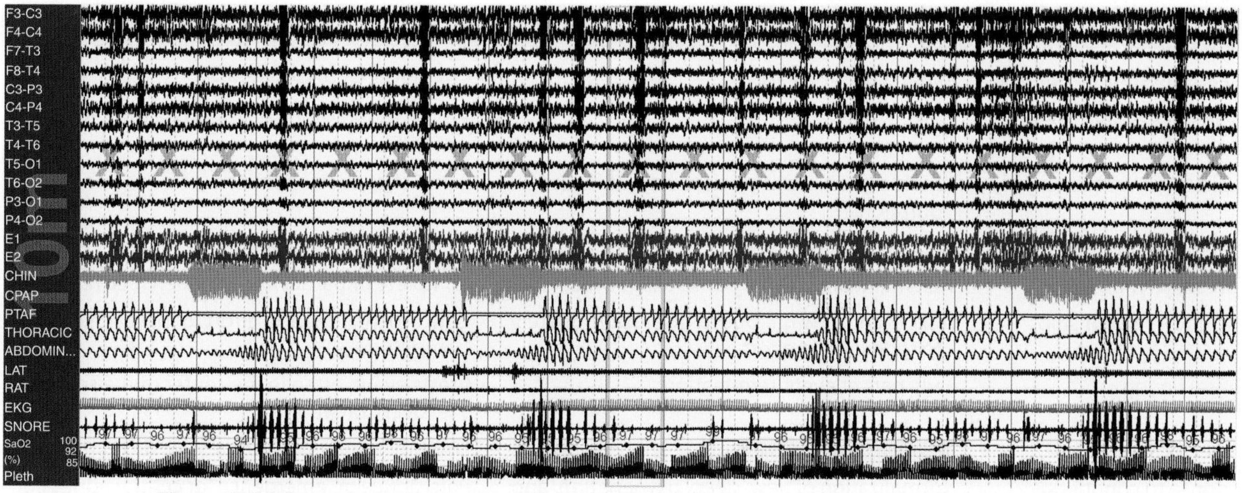

Figure 129.10 Pseudoperiodic breathing from external driving. Ten-minute polysomnogram snapshot. Patient using a vagal nerve stimulator for refractory epilepsy. The blocklike chin tone increase is a stimulation artifact. During the stimulation phase, there is respiratory suppression.

an arousal; this pattern is typical of the pattern called *upper airway resistance syndrome.*[50-52] Though this entity has been folded into OSA, the pattern is distinctive enough. The second pattern is seen in patients with CHF: long-cycle (>60 seconds) periodic breathing/Cheyne-Stokes respiration.[53-55] One consideration when the event duration is long is that the apnea-hypopnea index/respiratory disturbance index (AHI/RDI) may underestimate severity, as there are fewer but longer events.[56]

Event Cycle Rhythm

External driving of sleep respiration can occur with neurostimulators (e.g., vagal, nerve stimulator for epilepsy; Figure 129.10). These stimulation pulses will have a metronomic timing and can cause respiratory suppression with precise repeated timing.

Prolongation of the Inspiratory Phase of Obstructed Breaths

The inspiratory phase normally occupies less than half the duration of the breath (duty cycle <0.5).[57] The inspiratory phase is often prolonged during mild-to-moderate obstructive events and during steady flow limitation.[42,43] This takes place to different extents in different patients,[42,44] and there is evidence that the ability to increase the duty cycle in the face of airway obstruction may be genetically determined.[44]

Audible snoring or recordable UA vibrations are frequently noted. The pattern of flow limitation (the shape of the flow-limited breath) may have individual characteristics (similar within the same individual). Analysis of respiratory cycle–related EEG changes during such periods shows an impact on electrocortical activity.[12]

Flow Shapes and Site of Upper Airway Obstruction

Simultaneous UA video recordings with PSG show that specific flow-limitation shapes correlate with specific sites or mechanisms of UA collapsibility. Although these patterns may be dynamic across a night or change with body position in a given individual, a predominance of a single shape suggests a dominant site of obstruction. These shapes include flat or plateau-shaped (tongue base), increased negative effort dependence (progressive worsening of flow limitation from start to termination of inspiration), abrupt sharp dips (epiglottic collapse), and a "pinch" at the end of inspiration (soft palate prolapse). Shape analysis can predict oral appliance therapy response,[58] and epiglottic collapse patterns seem to predict a poor response to CPAP.[59]

NREM Versus REM Dominance and Relation to Loop Gain

For practical purposes, periodic breathing and hypocapnic central apnea do not occur in REM sleep (the exception is a patient with CHF who demonstrates periodic breathing during the wake state). NREM dominance is well described in idiopathic CSA,[6], periodic breathing associated with heart failure or stroke,[61] opiate-induced sleep apnea,[62] and high-altitude periodic breathing.[63] NREM dominance is also a feature of complex apnea/treatment-emergent CSA, regardless of the exact definition used.[64]

The simplest method to establish NREM dominance is the NREM versus REM AHI/RDI. However, to be useful, the comparisons should (1) be made at the same body position and (2) consider the stage and state of sleep. Determining sleep state dominance of sleep apnea can be difficult in those with substantial obstruction, where two distinct patterns can coexist: periodic (nonobstructive) breathing during NREM sleep and obstructive events during REM sleep. The use of PAP usually clarifies the situation—REM disease is readily eliminated, whereas NREM disease is not. Patterns of oximetry that are characteristic of REM versus NREM dominance are described in the section Photoplethysmography and Oximetry.

Respiratory events both at sea level (often) and high altitude (always) and in patients with positive pressure–induced or amplified respiratory instability have short cycles that are less than 30 seconds. By the conventional scoring guidelines, flow limitation excludes a "central hypopnea" in the scoring manual, yet this idea has been conclusively shown to be false from the following data: (1) at high altitude, a pure chemoreflex

Table 129.1 Recognition of Strong Chemoreflex Modulation of Sleep Breathing

Polysomnographic Feature	Relatively Pure OSA	Chemoreflex-Modulated SA
Periodic breathing, Cheyne-Stokes	Rare	Typical (often short cycle, <30 seconds in absence of CHF)
Respiratory event timing	Variable (each event tends to have different durations)	Self-similar/metronomic
Severity during sleep state	Greater severity in REM	Minimal severity in REM
Effort signal morphology	Well maintained during obstructed breath	Complete or partial loss between recovery breaths
Flow-effort relationship	Discordant: flow is reduced disproportionately to reduction in effort	Concordant: flow and effort follow each other in amplitude
Arousal timing	Early part of event termination	Crests event, often in the center of the sequence of recovery breaths
Oxygen desaturation	Irregular, progressive drops, V-shaped contour	Smooth, symmetric, progressive drops rare
Response to continuous positive airway pressure	Normalization of flow, sleep, oxygenation, and ventilation	Persistence or "emergence" of central apneas or periodic breathing

The key difference of this schema from that proposed by Randerath et al. (*Sleep*. 2013;36:363-368) and evaluated by Dupuy-McCauley et al. in relation to the American Academy of Sleep Medicine (AASM) criteria (*J Clin Sleep Med*. 2021;17[6]:1157-1165) is that flow limitation is NOT used as an absolute triage point, as this feature of airflow may be seen in central hypopneas.
CHF, Congestive heart failure; OSA, obstructive sleep apnea; REM, rapid eye movement; SA, sleep apnea.

form of sleep apnea, flow limitation, occurs frequently; (2) heart failure patients with otherwise classic Cheyne-Stokes respirations (CSRs) can demonstrate flow limitation; (3) the airway can close during polysomnographic central apnea;[65,66] and (4) central hypopneas demonstrate flow limitation.[67] In clinical practice, snoring can be seen in association with CSR but usually occurs associated with the arousal, whereas in more purely obstructive events, the snoring occurs during the event and transiently resolves during the arousal.

A consistent feature of hypocapnic, heightened chemoreflex-mediated central apnea is the predominance of metronomic self-similar events during NREM sleep, especially during non–slow wave stages.[14,61,68-72] Self-similarity can be mathematically quantified and predict acute emergence of central apneas during positive pressure titration.[73] The use of cardiopulmonary coupling analysis to estimate self-similarity is described in Chapter 202. In contrast to hypocapnic CSA, in OSA and in many cases of hypercapnic CSA, the disease worsens markedly during REM sleep, especially if the motor neurons of the diaphragm are involved.[29,69] Notable exceptions are congenital central hypoventilation syndrome (CCHS) and opioid-induced CSA, where the disease is worse in NREM sleep.

High loop gain predisposes to the phenomenon of complex apnea (treatment-emergent CSA [TE-CSA] in the *International Classification of Sleep Disorders* [ICSD] third edition).[74] TE-CSA is merely an *outcome* of airway opening alone in those with high loop gain apnea. If there is hypoxic carotid body sensitization, then TE-CSA can be expected to improve over time, but if hypoxia is mild and high loop gain is present, long-term persistence could be expected. The key feature is NREM-dominant central hypopneas or periodic breathing with obstruction, resolving spontaneously during REM sleep. Table 129.1 summarizes some of the differentiating features of obstructive and chemoreflex driving of respiratory events.

Ataxic Respiration

When there is continuous variability of rate, volume, and rhythm of breathing during NREM sleep (nearly looking like respiration in REM sleep), often admixed with obstructive or central apneas of variable duration, the term *ataxic respiration* may be used. The events may be so short and the respiratory abnormality so devoid of predictable fluctuations that the standard rules may overscore or underscore events. Opiate use is the most common cause,[75,76] but any brainstem neurologic abnormality, such as multiple sclerosis, brainstem stroke, craniovertebral junctional anomalies, and Parkinson disease, may also exhibit these features. Opiate-associated ataxic breathing (Figure 129.11) is usually accompanied by mild hypercapnia, and in general, ataxic breathing is sensitive to reductions in CO_2 by increasing ventilation, such as by applying CPAP.

Respiratory Patterns during Adaptive Ventilation Therapy

Adaptive servo-ventilation (and ventilators [ASVs]) provides expiratory support, inspiratory pressure support, and backup supportive responses guided by measures of ventilation or flow averaged over several minutes.[77,78] There are specific challenges in assessing the response to adaptive ventilation therapy.[79] Current adaptive ventilators estimate residual disease using the tidal volume signal (typically requiring 50% reduction to tag events). This signal is the combination of patient + machine; thus a relative contribution of 10% to 90% looks identical to a 90% to 10% but might represent different hemodynamics and arousal status. The tidal volume signal only reaches thresholds of "event detection" when this compensation fails. Thus there can be severe ongoing periodic breathing, reflected by the pressure waveform ("pressure cycling"), whereas the AHI detection algorithm yields a minimum or even a zero value. With an analogy to auditory noise cancellation, the device is canceling the variations in tidal volume, but the driving "noise," the high loop gain–based periodic breathing, continues unabated. Moreover, adaptive ventilation can cause substantial patient-ventilatory desynchrony,[80] which remains unidentified. In the SERVE-HF trial, up to a device detected AHI_{TIDAL} 10/hour of use was taken as a success, which likely overlooked a large degree of ongoing

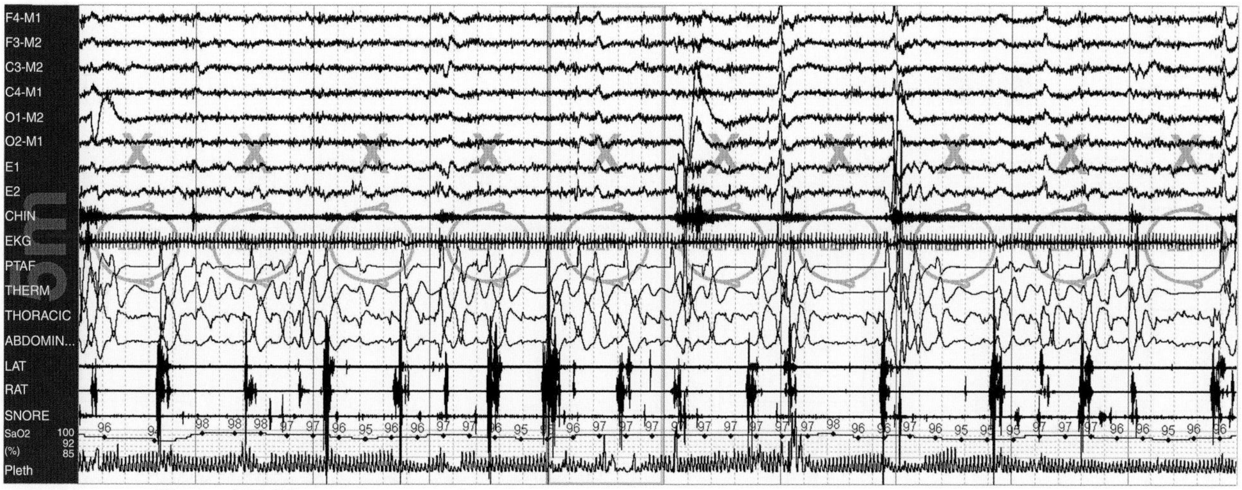

Figure 129.11 Ataxic respiration from opiate use. Five-minute polysomnogram snapshot. Note (1) relatively mild oxygen desaturation; (2) short but variable-length central apneas; (3) arousals and periodic motor activation.

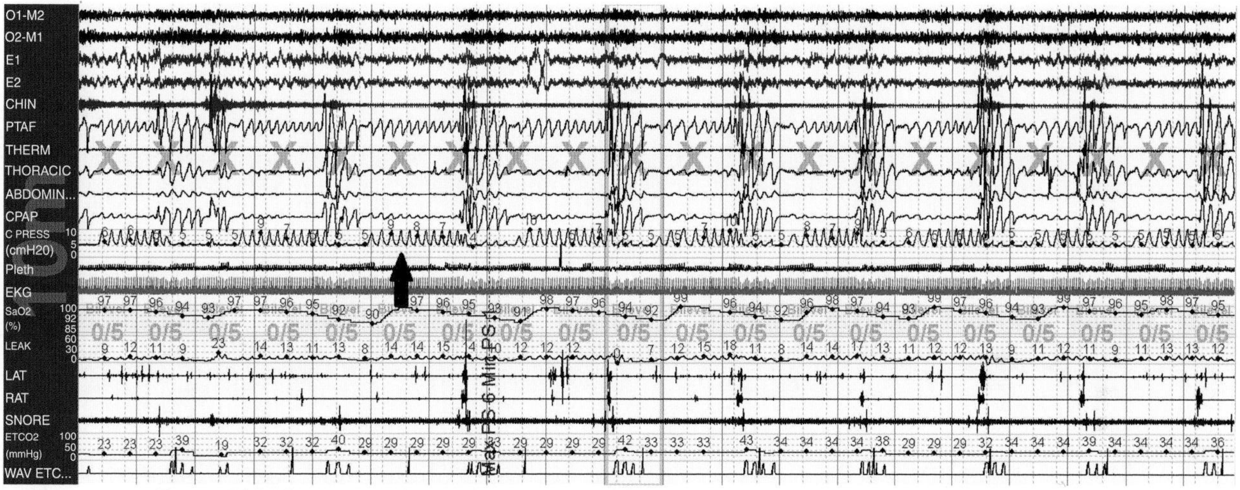

Figure 129.12 Pressure cycling with adaptive ventilation. Five-minute snapshot. The *arrow* points to typical pressure cycling of failing adaptive ventilation (C-PRESS trace).

unrecognized periodic breathing in addition to the basic scoring issues already mentioned. See Figure 129.12 for excessive "pressure cycling," which is the response of an adaptive ventilator to ongoing periodic breathing. When pressure cycling persists, sleep fragmentation can be severe even if respiration is "improved." Speeding or slowing of the native respiration rate, hypocapnia, breath stacking (rapid ventilator-delivered breath on top of the spontaneous breath), and variability of expiratory duration mimicking an opiate effect are all patterns of patient-ventilator asynchrony. When the ventilator enables stable respiration, cycling between the minimum and maximum pressure support zone is minimal. These patterns can be seen both on laboratory polysomnograms and from analysis of raw data from devices during use.

Home Sleep Testing: Cardiopulmonary Recordings or Autonomic Activation-Based Approaches

Respiratory signal amplitude reduction, oxygen desaturation associations, event cycle time, periodic breathing, and stable breathing periods are readily identifiable on home sleep apnea testing, allowing the generation of metrics very close to conventional PSG. Cardio-acceleration and finger plethysmographic amplitude reduction can be useful event tags (arousal equivalents), along with abrupt flow recovery of previously flow-limited breaths.

Recognizing REM sleep– and NREM sleep–dominant apnea is possible on home sleep apnea testing by using oximetry patterns and event self-similarity, despite the absence of EEG. V-shaped oxygen desaturation with variable duration events reflects REM dominance, and band-like oxygen desaturation with self-similar events reflects NREM-dominant/high loop gain apnea. "Sagging" oxygen saturations that do not return to baseline suggest, but do not prove, hypoventilation, as various forms of impaired cardiopulmonary reserve, including ventilation-perfusion mismatch, can cause disproportionately severe sleep hypoxia. These patterns are shown in Figures 129.13 through 129.16.

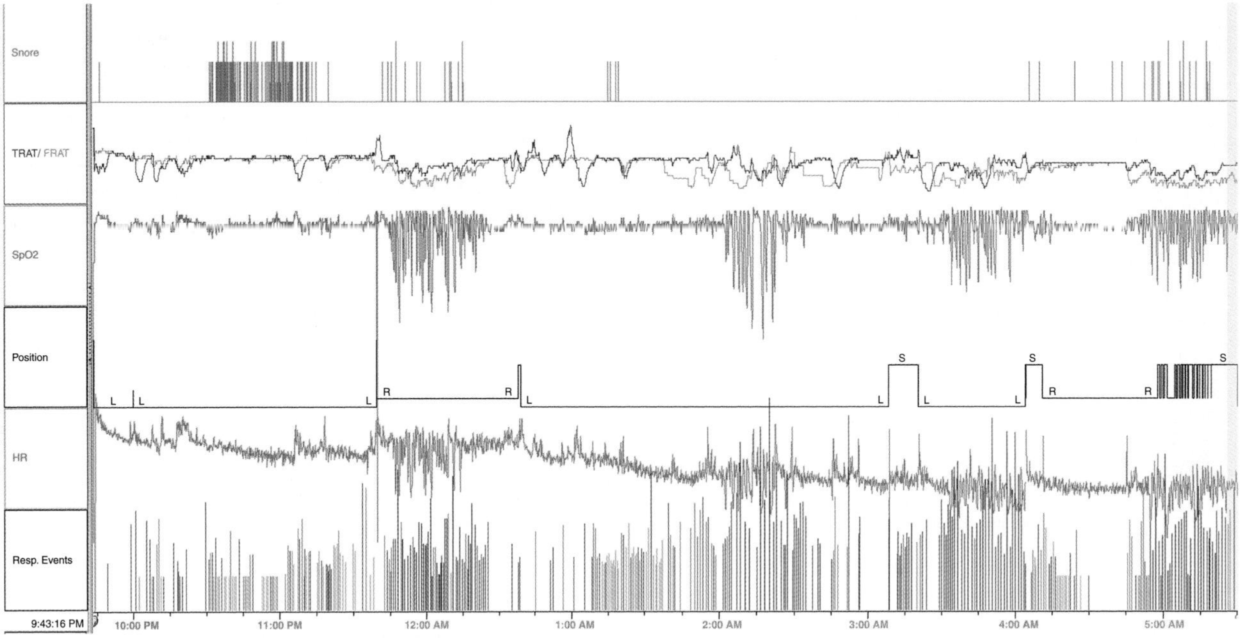

Figure 129.13 Obstructive sleep apnea. V-shaped oxygen desaturation (as discussed further in the section Oximetry and REM Apnea) is virtually diagnostic of rapid eye movement (REM)-dominant obstructive sleep apnea.

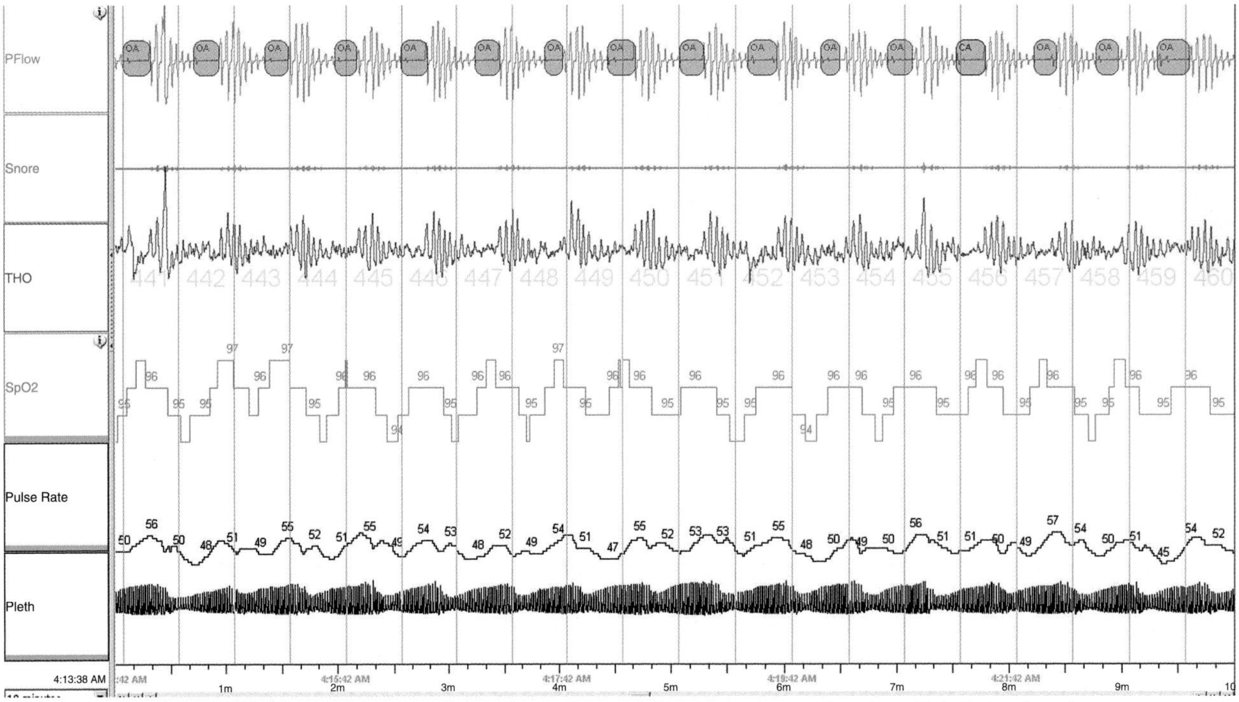

Figure 129.14 High loop gain on home sleep apnea study. Note the waxing and waning self-similarity of nearly all measured signals, flow, effort, pulse rate, oximetry, and plethysmographic signal amplitude.

High Loop Gain Phenotype and Presumptive Endotype in Home PAP Waveform Data

Modern PAP devices measure and store airflow and pressure data but display only automated charts of residual event and compliance indices.[81] This allows for tracking of presumed efficacy and adherence.[82] However, vendor algorithms vary, and there are no specific guidelines or standards for capturing, measuring, or scoring the data.[82] High-resolution flow data can also be reviewed directly, enabling visual/manual assessment of events. Several studies have examined the relationship between device-detected events and device-reported AHI based on flow measurements (AHI_{FLOW}) and findings on PSG.[81,83-88] The findings mostly demonstrate good correlation,[84-87] with one study showing device overestimation.[83] Event-by-event analysis in one study showed that the automatic detection had high specificity but only modest sensitivity (for a cutoff of AHI >10/hour, sensitivity was 0.58 and specificity 0.94), with good agreement for apneas but less

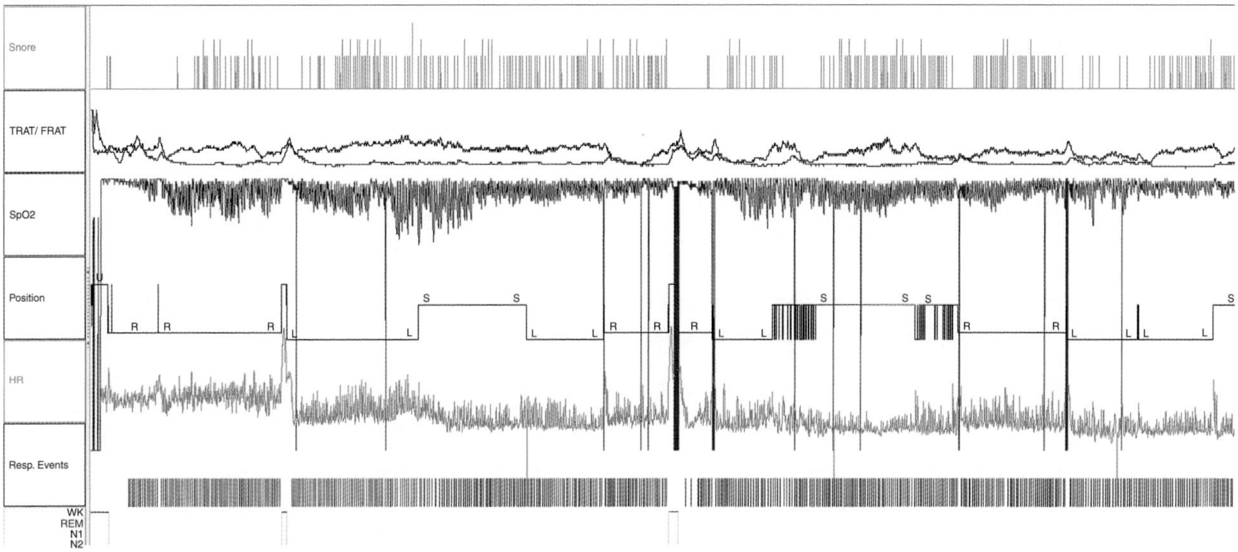

Figure 129.15 Mixed obstructive and high loop gain physiology. Note periods of bandlike oxygen desaturation, scored as obstructive *(red)* and central *(blue)* apneas.

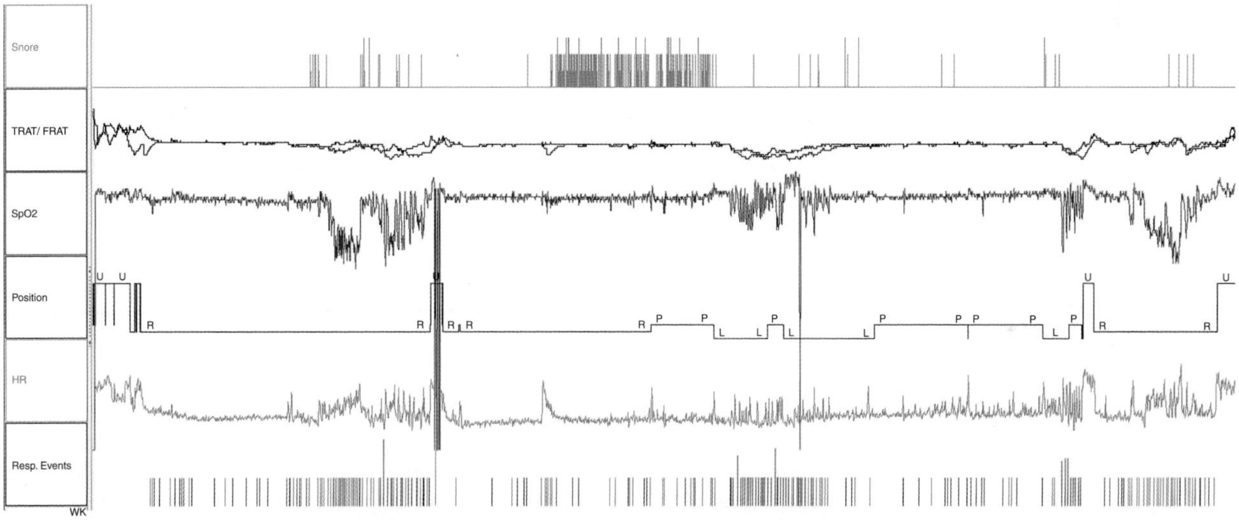

Figure 129.16 Plausible hypoventilation on a home sleep apnea study. Note the low baseline oximetry and the lack of return to baseline of oxygen saturations during rapid eye movement (REM) sleep.

so for detecting hypopneas,[81,85,88] Thus there is concern that efficacy can be overestimated by machine downloads. High accuracy of device detection was reported,[89] but the study has limited application, in our opinion, to general practice because besides using the summed machine autodetection events, (1) hypopneas on the validating PSGs were scored with 4% desaturation, which makes little sense when contrasting with a treatment tracking device, as desaturations are readily minimized even by subtherapeutic CPAP and (2) patients with difficult or incomplete CPAP titrations (inability to normalize) were explicitly excluded,[89] yet such individuals are exactly the population for whom we depend most urgently on reliable device performance. In an analysis from an academic center cohort not limited to straightforward cases manually/visually evaluating flow patterns, residual AHI_{FLOW} >5, 10, and 15/hour was seen in 32.3%, 9.7%, and 1.8% versus 60.8%, 23%, and 7.8% of subjects, respectively, based on automated versus manual scoring of waveform data.[90] This suggests a substantial subset of patients may be incompletely treated despite reassuring machine values.

Approaches to Positive Pressure Therapy Data

Flow based and derivatives of flow data are readily available from positive pressure therapy devices.[82] Direct visualization of data from CPAP machines can readily identify periods of stable and unstable breathing (an example is shown in Figure 129.17). Periodic breathing is readily recognized, as are overt obstructive events. Differentiation of obstructive from CSA can be aided by device determination of open and closed airway apnea using forced oscillation. The SomnoNIV group has proposed criteria for the assessment of respiratory polygraphy in ventilator-dependent patients.[91,92] Leak effects are critical in volume and adaptive ventilation more than standard continuous or bilevel ventilation. Abnormal triggering, patient-ventilator desynchrony, overventilation, induction of CSA, and atypical patterns of muscle activation (accessory

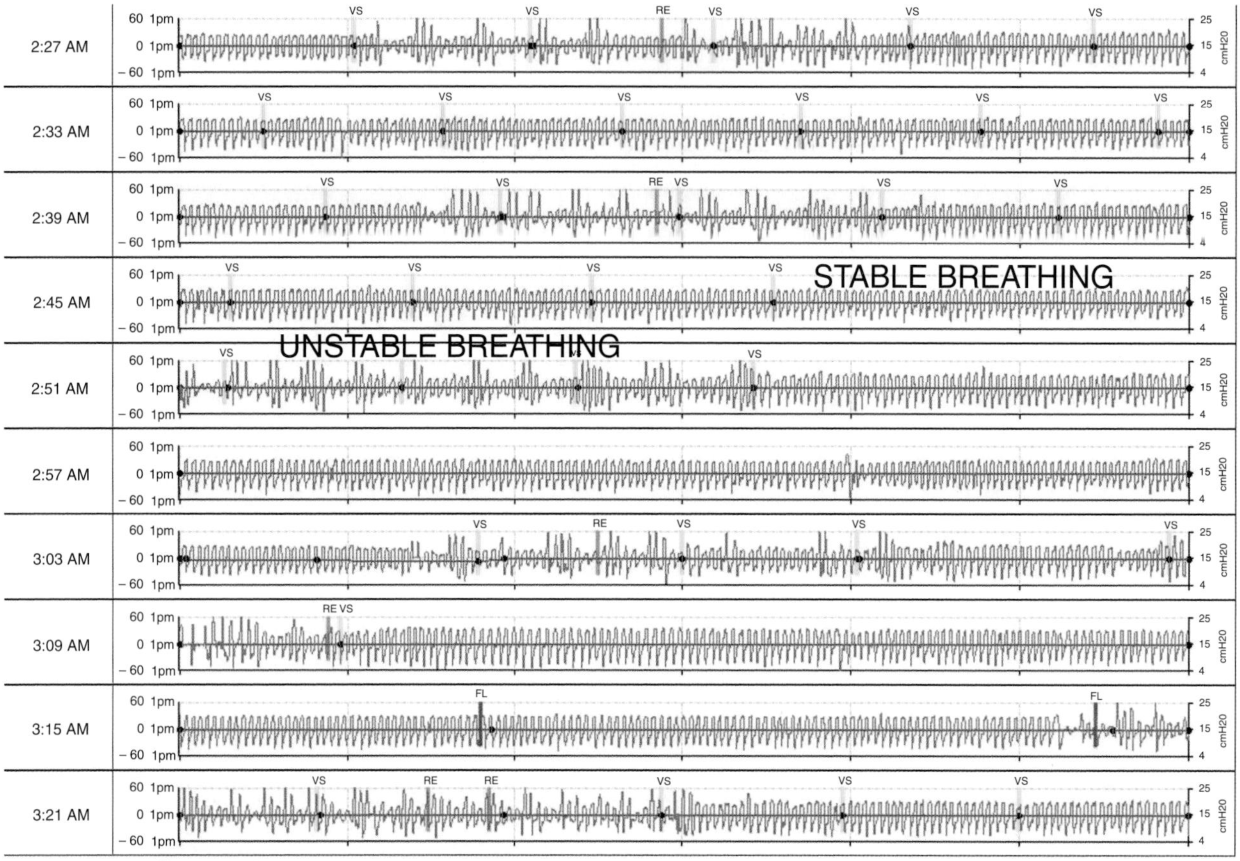

Figure 129.17 Stable versus unstable breathing on home therapy waveforms. Each horizonal line is 6 minutes on continuous positive airway pressure (CPAP). Stable and unstable breathing periods are marked on the sample snapshot. Stable breathing is recognized as prolonged periods of minimal tidal volume variability. Flow limitation may or may not be present.

muscle use) are only some of the challenges in this population. Several respiratory measures are likely stable in a given individual across nights. These include respiratory rate, interbreath interval, inspiratory and expiratory time, duty cycle, and in the case of modes with a backup rate, percentage of machine- or patient-triggered breaths. Examples of abnormal waveform data during home positive pressure ventilation are shown in Figures 129.18 through 129.23.

Photoplethysmography and Oximetry

Pulse oximetry is derived from photoplethysmography (PPG), which uses the characteristics of light absorption as it is transmitted through tissues to comment on the local blood volume. Different aspects of the plethysmogram can detect venous versus arterial flow and is leveraged to detect oxygen desaturation. Besides pulse, a respiratory pattern can be detected, as can neural activity in the form of sympathetic and vagal tone.[93]

The Oximetry Signal

The detected signal of the PPG includes a large DC (direct current, nonpulsatile) and AC (alternating current, pulsative components). The pulsatile AC signal is largely responsible for generating the "normal" PPG waveform, with the time frame between intervals representing the cardiac cycle. The detail provided on the PPG waveform is significant, with a second peak representing a dicrotic notch correlating with the closure of the aortic valve and the end of systole. Cardiovascular parameters such as stroke volume and vasomotor tone can predictably affect the amplitude and shape of the PPG signal. (Figure 129.24A).[94] The PPG signal can be used as a triage tool to try to differentiate true hypoxia from artifactual values attributable to poor signal quality. This is particularly useful in sleep studies where equipment must be worn for prolonged periods, often without close monitoring from technicians (Figure 129.24B and *C*). Although a change in amplitude can occur with fluctuating neuronal tone, a lack of clear peaks on the PPG signal should raise the question of signal loss instead of plummeting hemoglobin-oxygen saturation. Treating mild OSA could be helpful for hypertension,[95] and as sympathetic activation is one mechanism for OSA-linked hypertension, the plethysmographic signal could help identify which patients might benefit. An autonomic risk indicator can be generated from the signal and its components, with predictive value for cardiovascular events.[96]

Oximetry and Peripheral Perfusion

The pulsatile strength of the PPG can serve as an indirect measure of peripheral perfusion. Although many factors can contribute to changes in pulsatile strength in the critically ill (temperature, vasoactive drugs, stroke volume) in the setting of the sleep laboratory, over short periods, this is largely influenced by vasomotor tone. Pulsatile strength can be quantified

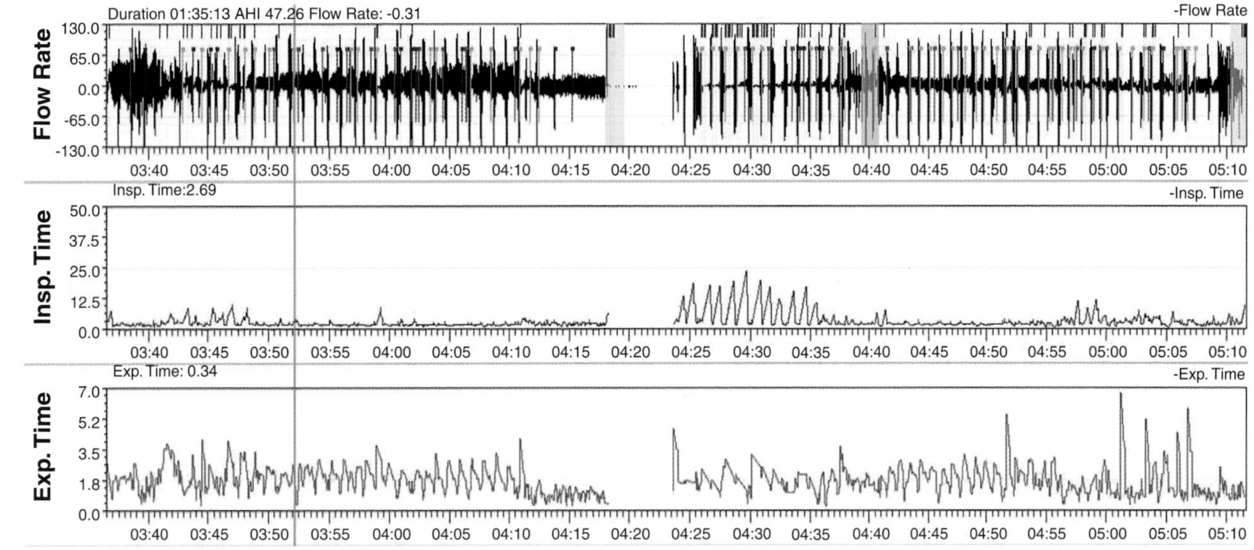

Figure 129.18 Periodic breathing on CPAP, home therapy data. About 145 minutes of data. From top: airflow, inspiratory time, and expiratory time. Note repeated flow oscillations with a self-similar timing and marked variability of expiratory time across the entire period.

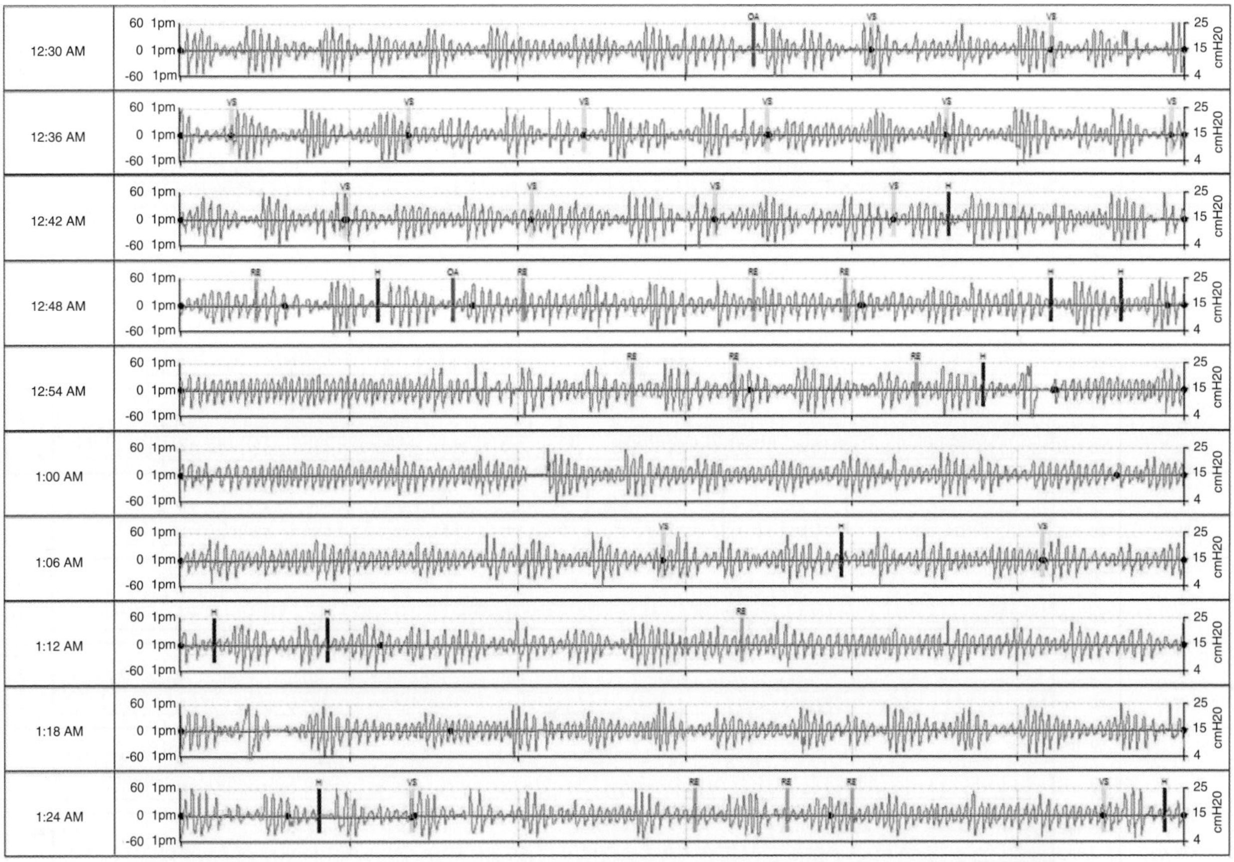

Figure 129.19 Residual short-cycle periodic breathing on continuous positive airway pressure (CPAP). Residual sleepiness and fatigue. EncoreAnywhere (Philips-Respironics) data; each horizontal line is 6 minutes. Note persistent short-cycle respiratory events almost entirely undetected by the algorithm; *arrows* identify two examples.

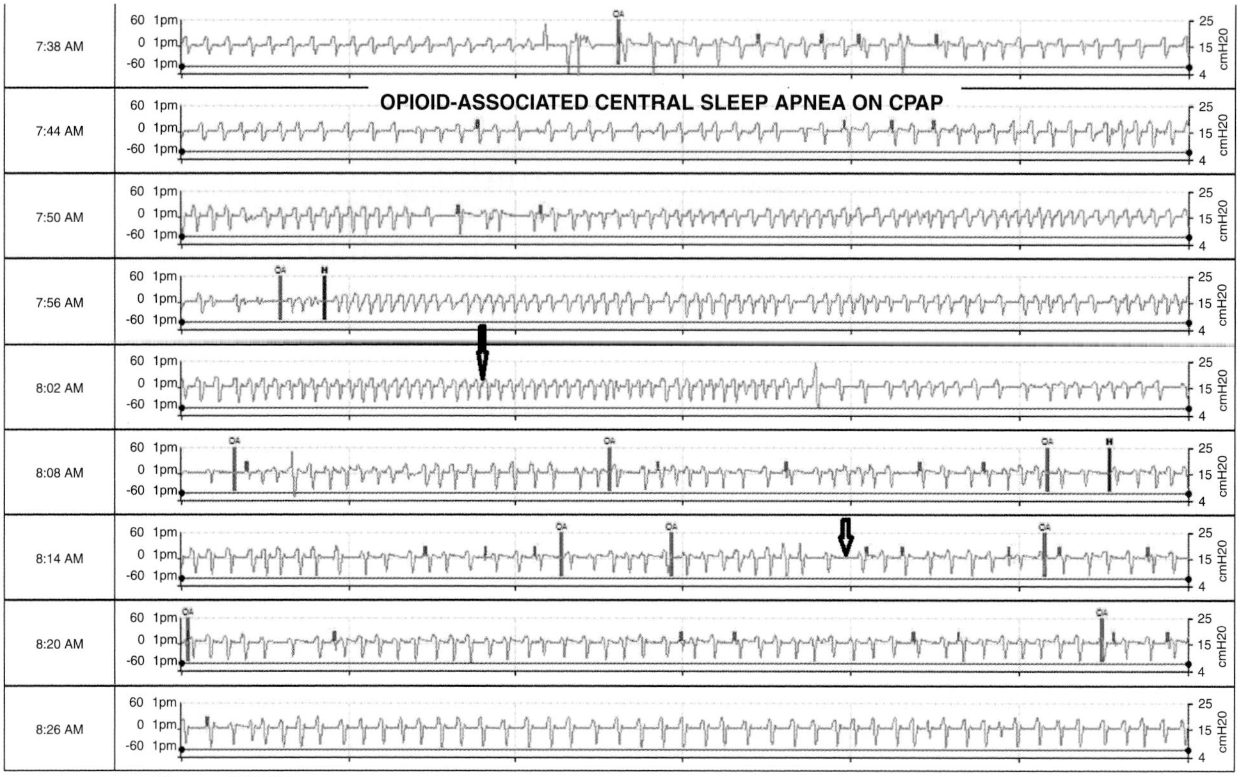

Figure 129.20 Opiate-associated sleep apnea. Snapshot from EncoreAnywhere (Philips-Respironics) in a patient who uses high-dose opiates and is treated with continuous positive airway pressure (CPAP), acetazolamide, and enhanced expiratory rebreathing space (dead space, EERS). Each horizontal line represents 6 minutes. *Note:* (1) Variability of expiratory duration, the typical opiate effect. (2) Variable respiratory rates, including bradypnea. (3) False detection of obstructive events, with tags falling on all parts of the respiratory cycle, expiratory and inspiratory, suggesting that the detection algorithm is unable to accurately process ataxic breathing patterns. The machine-detected apnea-hypopnea index (AHI) was 22, though the patient noted refreshing sleep. *Long arrow* identifies a short expiratory duration, *short arrow* a long duration. H, hypopnea; OA, obstructive apnea.

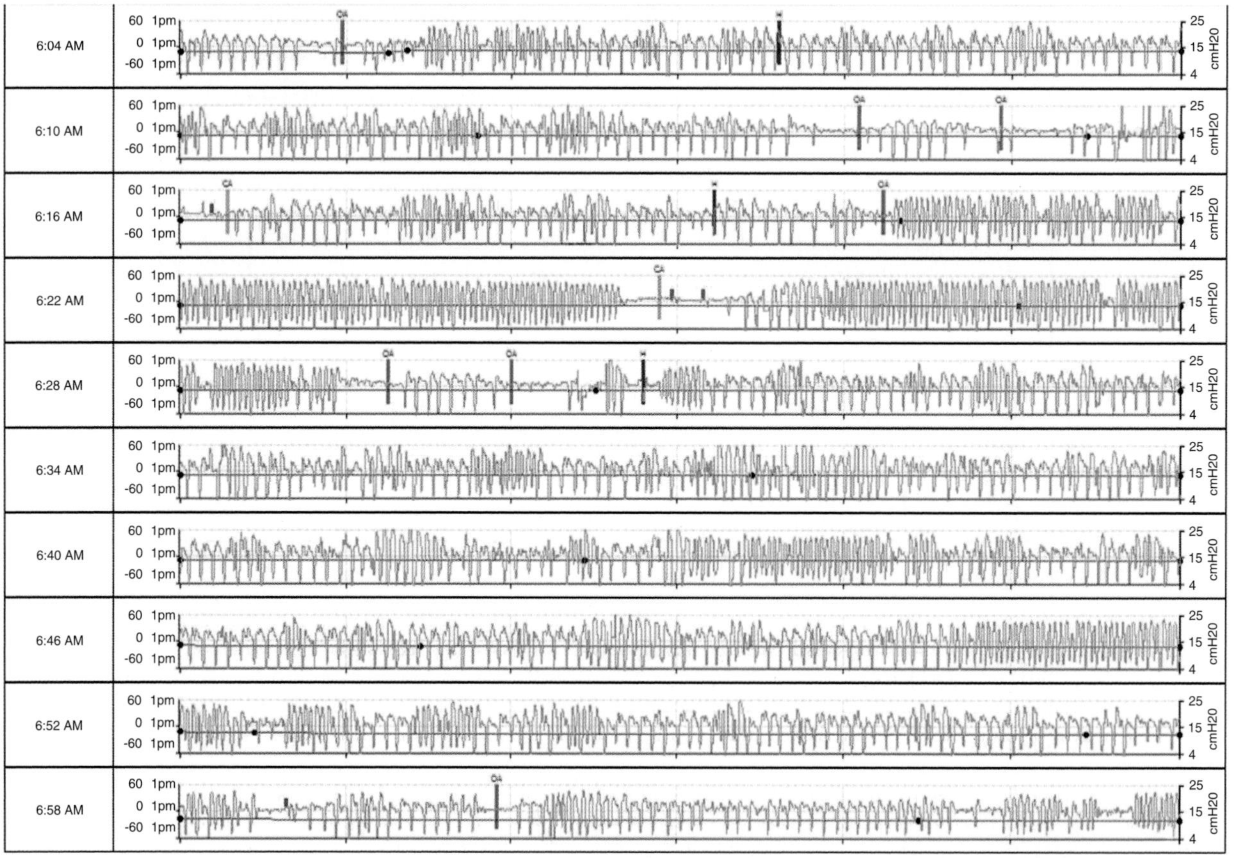

Figure 129.21 Complex respiratory waveforms and software detection limitations. Snapshot from EncoreAnywhere (Philips-Respironics) in a 52-year-old male patient not using opiates but with uncertain cause of ataxic respiration. Brain and high spinal magnetic resonance imaging (MRI) was normal. Note the substantially pathologic respiratory patterns (apneas, ataxic rhythm, clusters of tachypnea) largely undetected by the software. Six minutes per horizontal line of flow. CA, Central apnea; H, hypopnea; OA, obstructive apnea.

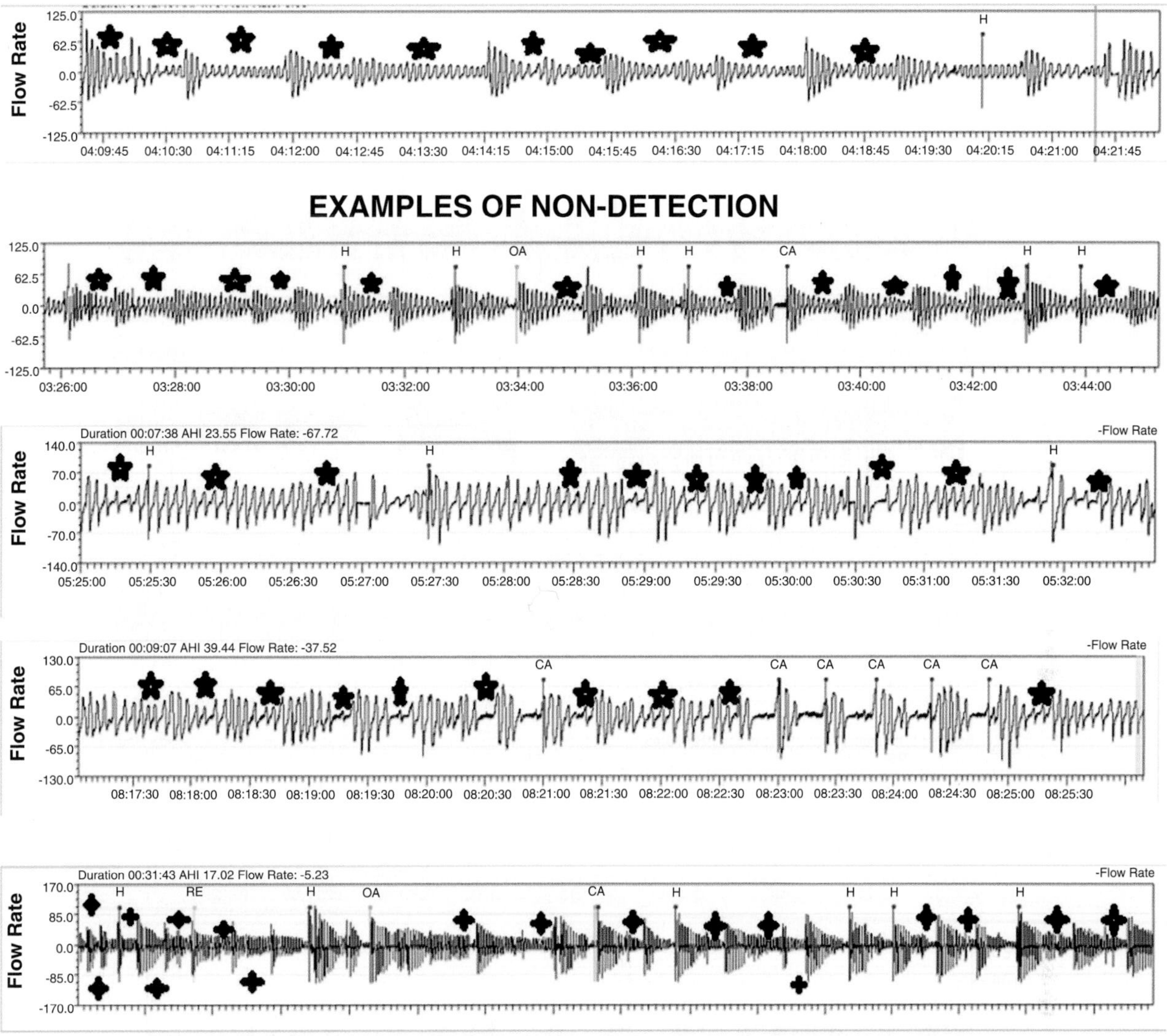

Figure 129.22 Missed event during CPAP use. Various samples, each from different patients, at different compressions to show events tagged and missed autodetection via the algorithms. The missed events are tagged with *star* symbols. CA, Central apnea; H, hypopnea; OA, obstructive apnea.

in terms of a perfusion index (AC / DC × 100%); however, this is not commonly monitored by sleep studies. In addition, many pulse oximetry devices clean and alter the raw PPG data (often inverting it) intended to ease the interpretation by the clinician.[94] Yet this cleaned pattern of change of the plethysmography amplitude can provide useful insights to changes in sympathetic tone.[97,98] Amplitude changes in the PPG associated with events hint at the physiologic consequences for the individual patient. Given the spectrum of severity of symptoms associated with mild sleep apnea, such patterns can help hint at the burden of sleep disruption associated with mild events. Given that excessive sympathetic activation is hypothesized to be a mechanism for cardiovascular comorbidities in sleep apnea, this information has direct clinical relevance (Figure 129.25).[99] This can be particularly helpful in the setting of a type III sleep study, where EEG arousals are not tracked but arousals can be suggested by associated fluctuations in the plethysmography tracing.

Respiration Sculpts Oximetry/PPG

Intrathoracic pressure changes during respiration affect cardiac output, and this change can be seen by changes in the local blood volume measured by PPG. This pattern, termed *respiratory-induced intensity variations (RIIVs)*, makes it possible to track not only pulse but respirations.[93] The ability to extract this information from a single signal allows insight into the autonomic nervous system dynamics and application of alternative modes of sleep analysis, such as cardiopulmonary coupling, as an alternative measure of inherently stable versus unstable sleep.[3,100,101]

Oximetry and REM Apnea

An extensive literature exists for alternative measures from oximetry ranging from desaturation characteristics to alternative time series statistics and power spectral density analysis.[102] OSA is often REM dominant, thought to be related to the maximal UA muscle relaxation and decreased

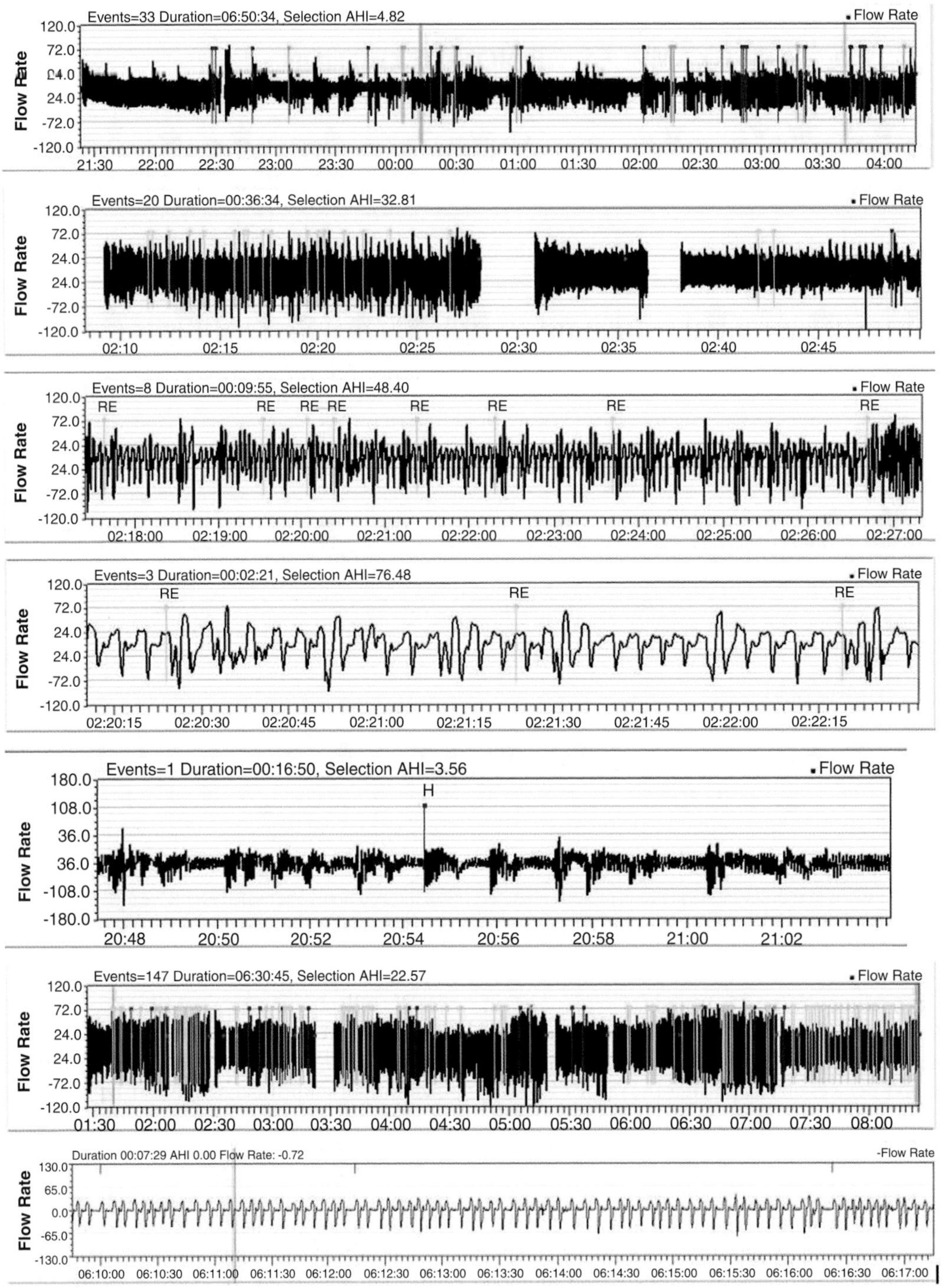

Figure 129.23 Phenotype at a glance. Various types of patterns noted from home positive airway pressure (PAP) devices. Variable degrees of self-similarity, irregularity, and tidal volume variance. The lowest graph is possibly normal rapid eye movement (REM) sleep. Various compressions offer complementary views, all from different patients. The only stable breathing sample is the lowest. The pattern seen in the third sample from the top shows abrupt tidal volume increases, and this pattern may be induced by periodic limb movements with arousals.

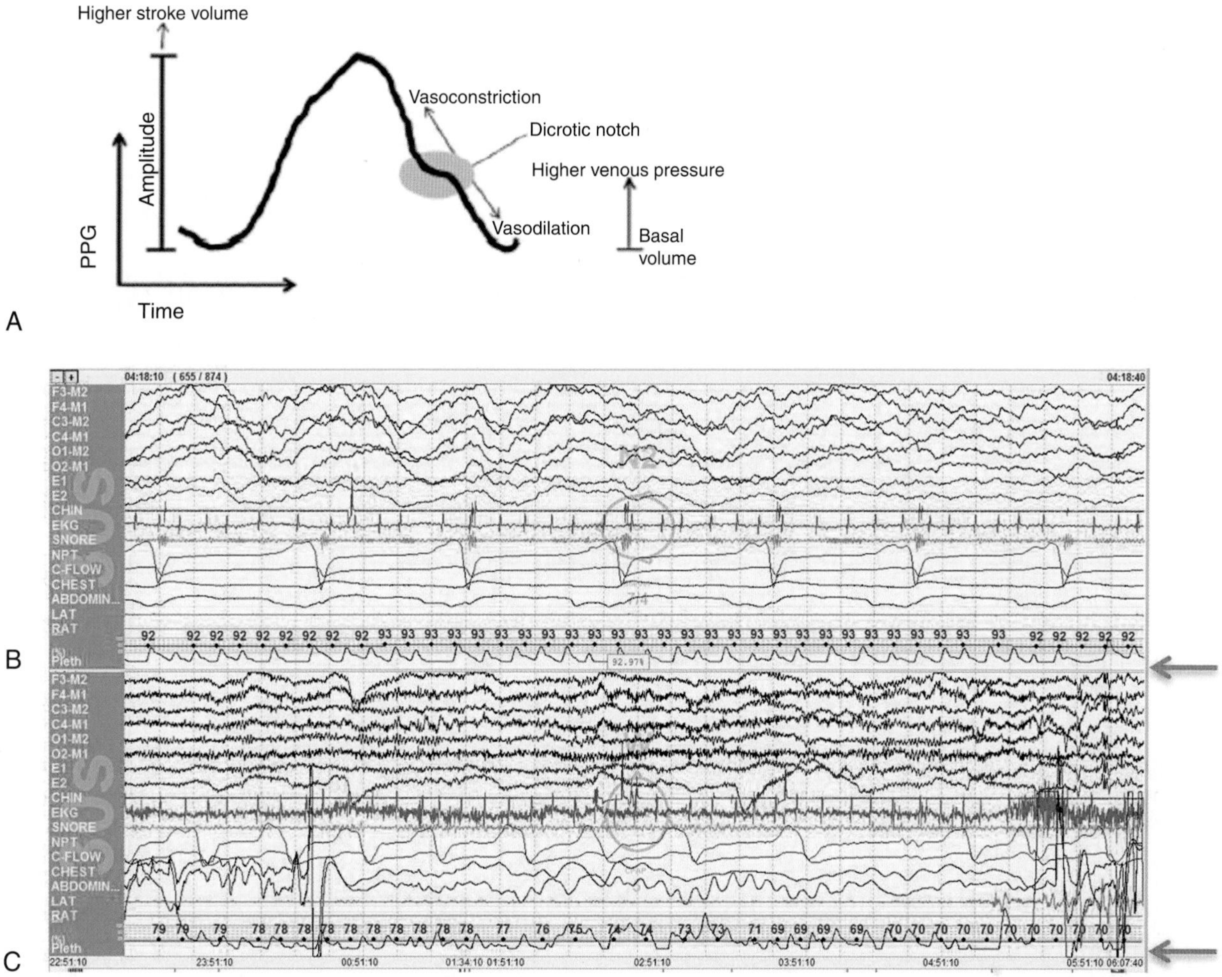

Figure 129.24 The photoplethysmography (PPG) waveform. **A,** The PPG waveform and morphologic changes associated with hemodynamic changes. **B,** The photoplethysmography signal *(arrow)* clearly demonstrates a double-peaked shape with an irregular rate associated with the patient's atrial fibrillation. The amplitude also clearly varies, likely given the beat-to-beat stroke volume changes associated with atrial fibrillation. **C,** The PPG signal *(arrow)* demonstrates an unstable baseline with flattened waveforms. These changes suggest that the significant hypoxia indicated by Spo_2 is likely from poor signal quality, a conclusion further bolstered by the lack of significant respiratory events to correlate with the hypoxia. (A, from Sahni R. Noninvasive monitoring by photoplethysmography. *Clin Perinatol.* 2012; 39:573-583.)

chemosensitivity to trigger respiratory drive.[103] Apnea duration and severity of hypoxia are worse in sleep apnea patients during REM,[104] and severe cases can lead to progressive oxygen desaturation without complete interval oxygen recovery to baseline in between events. This stacking of events leads to a characteristic V-shaped oxygen desaturation during REM sleep with prolonged desaturation duration and greater desaturation area, defined as the area between the baseline and the SpO_2 trace during desaturation. This pattern is suggestive of relative REM-related hypoventilation (Figure 129.26).

Oximetry and NREM Apnea

The power spectral density is a way of examining the frequency content of an oximetry signal, with sleep apnea patients characteristically having peaks in the 0.014- to 0.03-Hz band.[102] This technique has been proposed as a novel way for screening for OSA by oximetry.[105,106] However, characteristics of this band can vary with sleep apnea subtypes, with differences in variance, skewness, and kurtosis.[102] CSRs have been shown to have particularly stable changes in oxygen saturation with central events, given the self-similar nature of periodic breathing.[107] CSR has been shown to have a distinct SpO_2 power spectral density with a narrow and high peak compared with typical OSA patients.[108] Periodic breathing has similarly demonstrated a uniquely identifiable power spectral density analysis of respiratory flow signals.[109]

A bandlike pattern on oximetry can be seen on the hypnogram during NREM sleep, which indicates prolonged segments of periodic breathing producing a repetitive pattern in the oximetry (Figure 129.27). CSA is typically associated with high loop gain states.[110,111] Hypoxia burden (event-linked) may be a better marker of cardiovascular risk.[112,113] Sleep apnea endotypes of direct clinical relevance, especially loop gain analysis, are likely to be commercially available.[114]

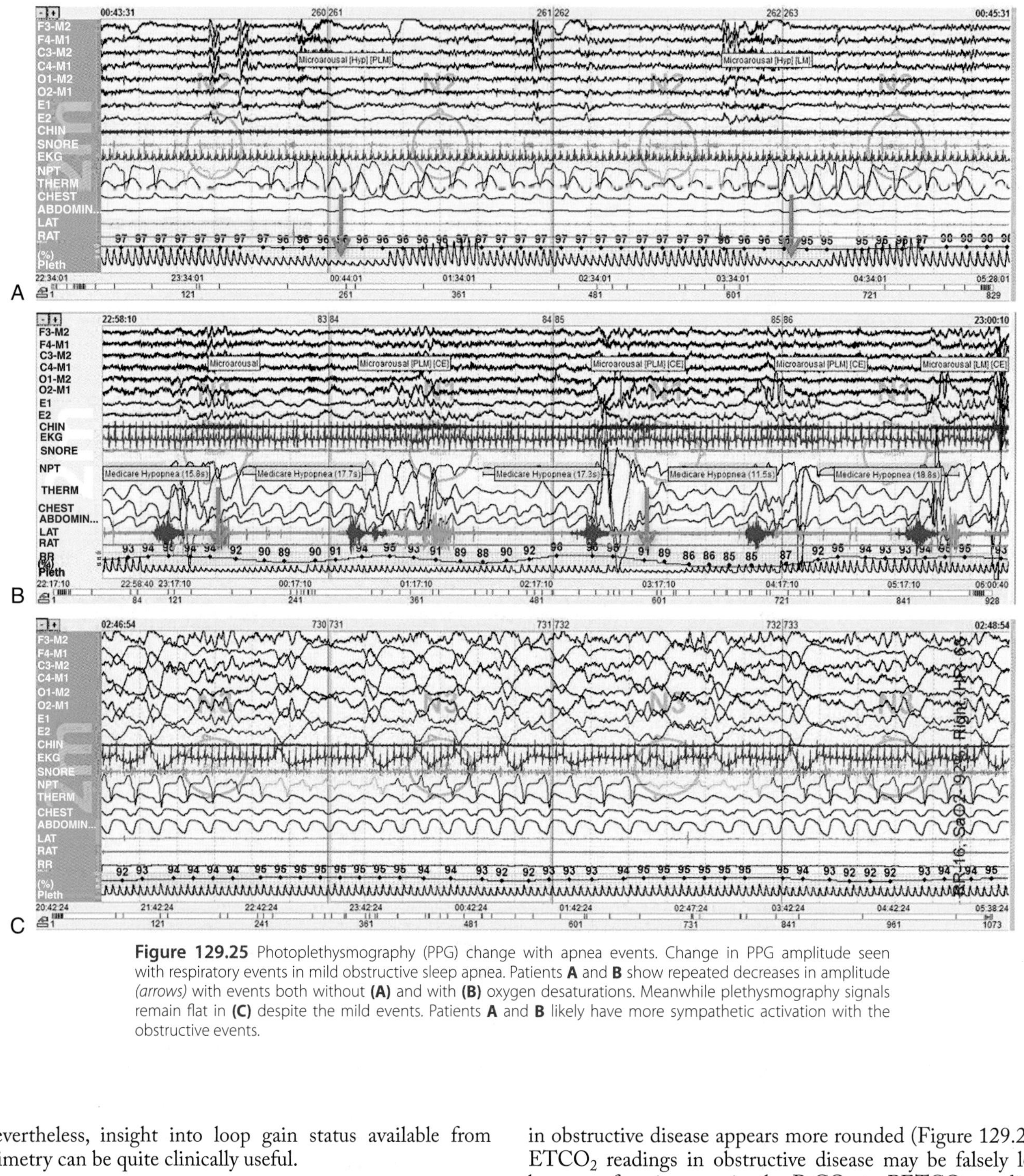

Figure 129.25 Photoplethysmography (PPG) change with apnea events. Change in PPG amplitude seen with respiratory events in mild obstructive sleep apnea. Patients **A** and **B** show repeated decreases in amplitude *(arrows)* with events both without **(A)** and with **(B)** oxygen desaturations. Meanwhile plethysmography signals remain flat in **(C)** despite the mild events. Patients **A** and **B** likely have more sympathetic activation with the obstructive events.

Nevertheless, insight into loop gain status available from oximetry can be quite clinically useful.

Insights from Carbon Dioxide/Capnometry and Ventilator Desynchrony

Suspected abnormalities of ventilation can be gleaned from continuous oxygen plethysmography during sleep. But oximetry is not a substitute for CO_2 measurement. CO_2 data can confirm abnormalities suspected from oximetry and may unveil overlooked or unsuspected pathology. The end-tidal capnography waveform provides a graphic measurement of exhaled CO_2, is affected by alveolar dead space (V_{DA}) and tidal volume (V_T) [$P_{ET}CO_2 = PaCO_2\ (1 - V_{DA} / V_T)$], and is typically 2 to 5 mm Hg lower than arterial CO_2. The normal $ETCO_2$ waveform has a distinct plateau, whereas the waveform seen in obstructive disease appears more rounded (Figure 129.28). $ETCO_2$ readings in obstructive disease may be falsely low because of an increase in the $PaCO_2$ to $PETCO_2$ gradient as a result of incomplete alveolar emptying. CO_2 has high tissue solubility and diffuses through the skin. Capnometers, which increase skin permeability to diffusion by "arterializing" capillary blood, are used to measure transcutaneous CO_2. The devices are fragile and expensive, and recalibration and sensor replacement at a different site every 4 hours are recommended with most monitors. Although $TcCO_2$ readings are typically very close to $PaCO_2$,[115] differences can emerge at higher CO_2 levels.[116]

Persistently low sleep SpO_2 out of proportion to airflow obstruction is suggestive of, but not diagnostic for, sleep hypoventilation. Low sleep SpO_2 that exceeds what might be

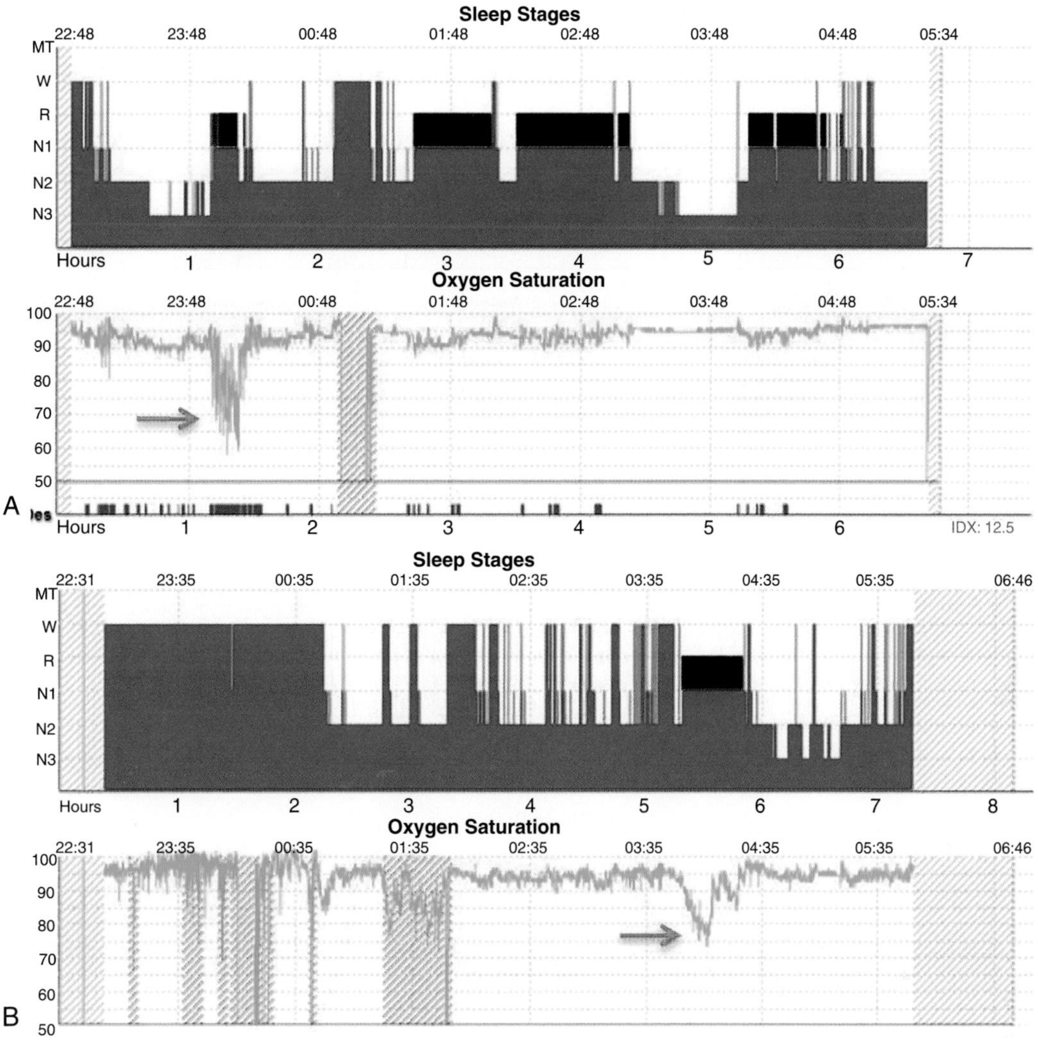

Figure 129.26 Oximetry in rapid eye movement (REM)-dominant apnea. REM V (or spear tip) shaped desaturation *(arrows)*. **A,** Stacked REM obstructive events leads to cyclic oxygen desaturations on top of a V-shaped progressive oxygen desaturation in the first REM block. This is prevented in the following REM blocks with continuous positive airway pressure (CPAP) titration. **B,** A clearer V-shaped desaturation is seen during the sole REM block.

expected based on airflow limitation alone can also be seen in shunt physiology from atelectasis or obesity or V/Q mismatch from underlying cardiopulmonary pathophysiology, without associated hypoventilation. A "sagging" oxygen desaturation profile, where the return to baseline is progressively impaired, can be seen with hypoventilation and is often REM stage specific. Examples of hypoventilation are in Figures 129.29, 129.30, and 129.31.

Asynchrony with Noninvasive Ventilators

Noninvasive ventilator devices are often initiated with empirical settings, without the guidance of sleep CO_2 or PSG data, which often limits detection of asynchrony. Even when noninvasive ventilator devices are assessed and titrated in the sleep laboratory, the vast majority of patient-ventilator asynchrony goes unrecognized. The SomnoNIV group (a multicenter work group from eight university or general hospitals from France, Belgium, and Switzerland) has proposed criteria for the assessment of respiratory polygraphy in ventilator-dependent patients.[91] Abnormal triggering (Figure 129.32), patient-ventilator desynchrony, overventilation and induction of CSA, atypical patterns of muscle activation (accessory muscle use, UA obstruction leading to switch to backup respiratory rate in assist control mode), and leak effects and impact of different body positions and sleep stages all must be considered.

INTEGRATED PHYSIOLOGIC ENDOTYPING AND ITS CLINICAL IMPLICATIONS FOR PERSONALIZED MEDICINE

OSA is a heterogeneous and complex disorder, and a "one-size-fits-all" approach fails to take into account the multiple "endotypes" now recognized to comprise OSA. The previous sections discuss various approaches to identify individual phenotypes and the possible driver endotypes. However, what may be more useful is the simultaneous assessment of multiple endotypes, which usually requires mathematical/computational analysis.

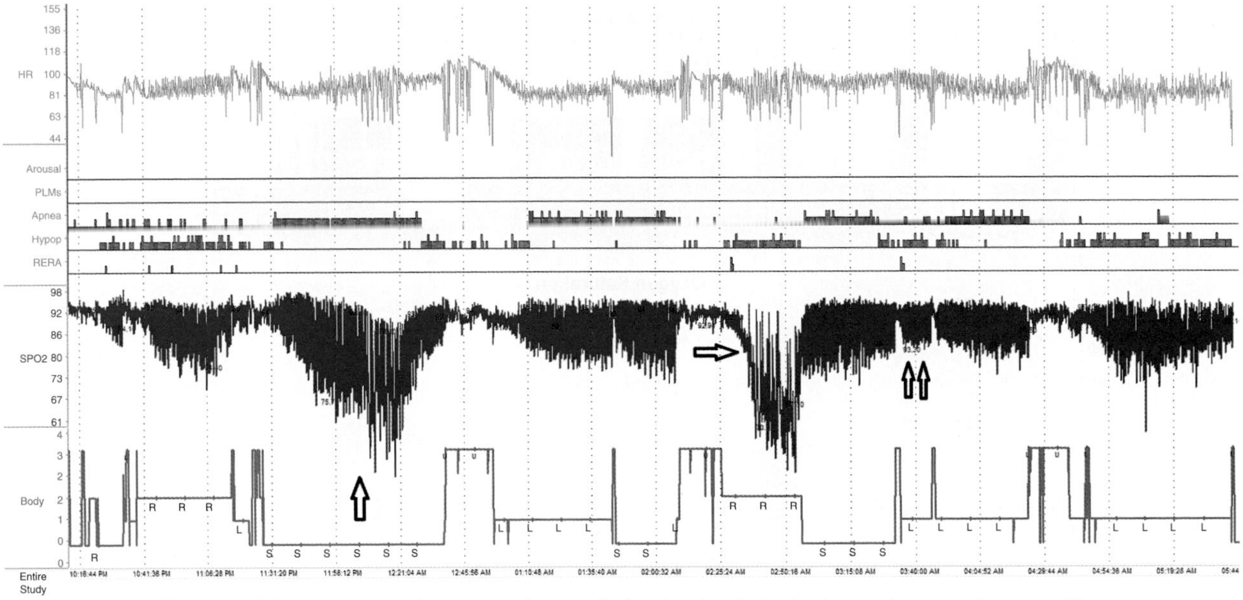

Figure 129.27 Oximetry analysis. Home sleep study. Besides the obviously abnormal oxygenation, note **(1)** V-shaped desaturation virtually pathognomonic of rapid eye movement (REM) sleep–related sleep apnea *(vertical single arrow)*; **(2)** possible REM sleep hypoventilation *(right-pointing arrow)*: V-shaped desaturation AND failure of return to baseline of oximetry; **(3)** bandlike oxygen desaturation typical of periodic breathing *(double vertical arrows)*. In this instance, the concomitant obstructive features resulted in greater desaturations than are typically seen with periodic breathing.

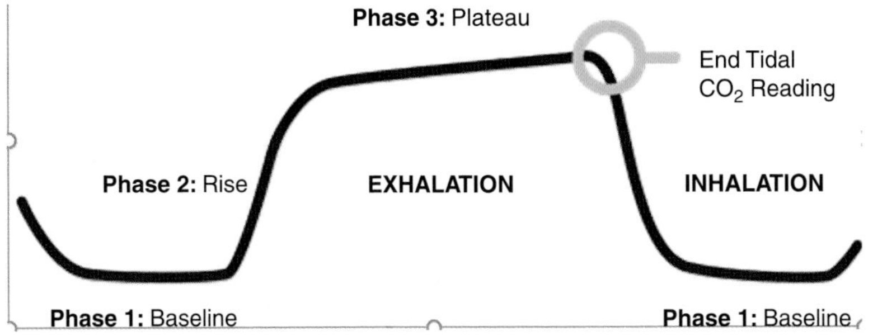

Figure 129.28 Basic capnometry profile. Using a mainstream $ETCO_2$ sensor, $ETCO_2$ can be measured with a nonvented mask interface while on positive pressure ventilation. When there is a leak in the system, the capnography waveform plateau is lost and the $ETCO_2$ readings become low and nonphysiologic.

Multiple Endotypes Responsible for OSA

OSA is a multifactorial disorder caused by a combination of anatomic and nonanatomic endotypes.[117] Although poor or compromised pharyngeal anatomy is the key driver in whether an individual will develop OSA, it is now recognized that the majority (≈69%) of patients also have additional nonanatomic endotypes that contribute to OSA. These include:

1. Ineffective upper airway dilator muscles: The upper airway has a range of muscles capable of dilating/reopening the airway in response to airway collapse. Thirty-six percent of OSA patients have particularly weak compensatory muscle responses that are incapable of reopening the airway.
2. Low respiratory arousal threshold: Patients with a low arousal threshold typically arouse easily and quickly in response to airway collapse. This pattern of rapid awakening reduces the ability for compensatory muscle responses to reopen the airway during sleep and may induce ventilatory instability that can potentiate further collapse. Approximately 37% of patients have abnormally low thresholds for respiratory arousal.
3. Unstable ventilatory control (high loop gain): Thirty-six percent of patients with OSA have ventilatory control systems that are hyperresponsive. Such high loop gain systems are counterproductive and produce greater breathing instability that often potentiates further airway collapse.

Importantly, each of these endotypes contributes to OSA in all patients, but to different degrees, such that OSA occurs for different reasons in different people[117] and is affected by age,[118,119] gender,[120-123] obesity,[124] and ethnicity/race.[125,126] The relative importance of each of the nonanatomic endotypes appears dependent on the degree of anatomic compromise/UA collapsibility.[127] That is, nonanatomic endotypes play a larger role if the UA is moderately collapsible as opposed to if there is high or minimal anatomic compromise (Figure 129.33). Ultimately, whether an individual will develop OSA depends on the interaction of these endotypes. For example, an individual

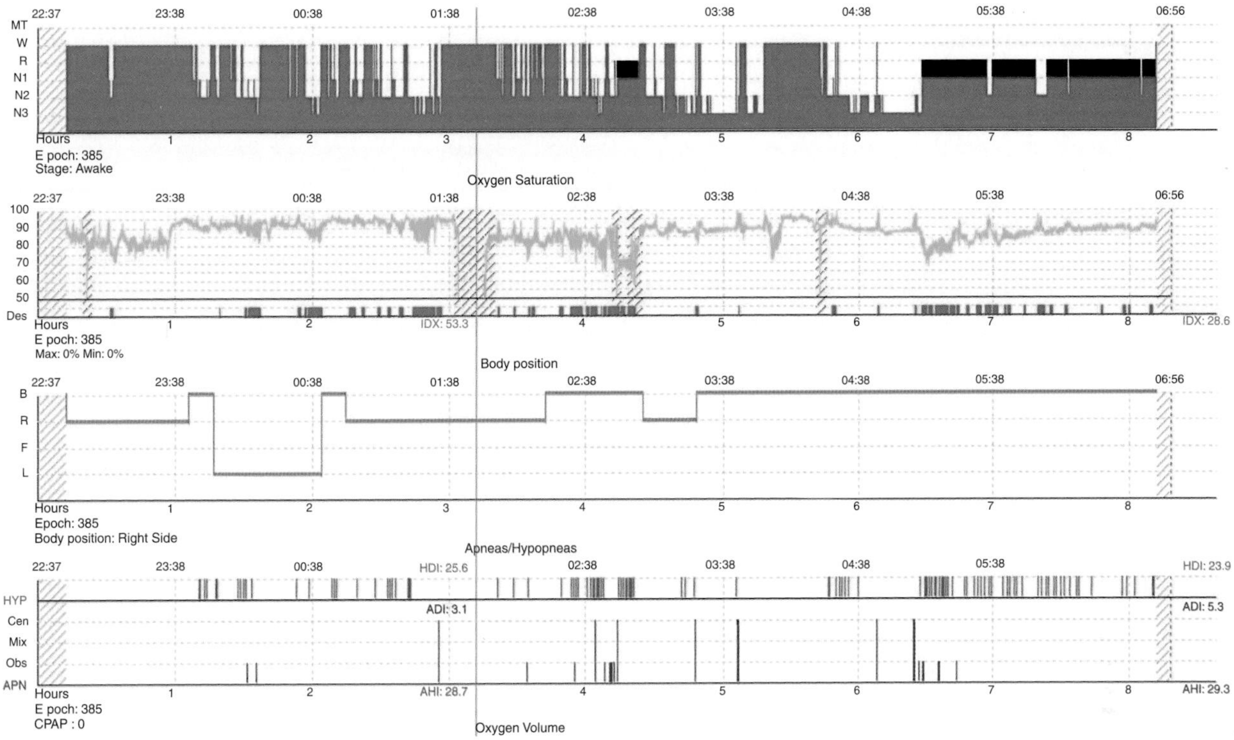

Figure 129.29 Hypoxia pattern suggesting hypoventilation. "Sagging" of the oximetry despite relative paucity of respiratory events could signify hypoventilation, ventilation-perfusion mispatch, or hypoventilation.

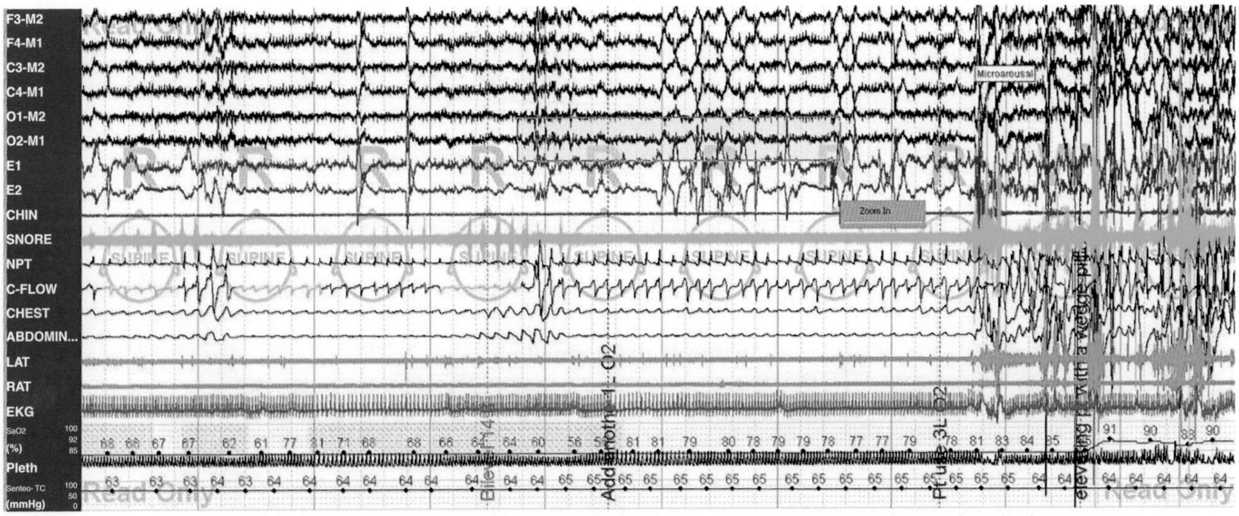

Figure 129.30 Hypoventilation as determined by transcutaneous capnometry. Severe hypoxia but also hypercapnia in rapid eye movement (REM) sleep (Tcco$_2$ is 64–65 mm Hg).

with a vulnerable airway (mild-to-moderate anatomic impairment) can be protected from developing OSA if they have a robust UA muscle response that can reopen the airway and prevent collapse (Figure 129.34). Similarly, another individual with the same degree of anatomic impairment can develop OSA if they have any combination of poor muscle response, high loop gain, or low arousal threshold.

Measuring the Endotypes

The current "gold standard" methods to quantify all four OSA endotypes require complex protocols involving the manipulation of CPAP where participants are often required to sleep while heavily instrumented (e.g., pressure catheters in the airway/esophagus, EMG wires into key pharyngeal muscles, etc.).[117,128-132] Although the protocols used by researchers are varied and have evolved, they first typically involve placing participants on a level of CPAP that abolishes all respiratory events and flow limitation during sleep. Once stable non-flow-limited breathing is established, the investigators periodically perform a series of short (≈5 breaths) or long (≈3 minutes) drops in the CPAP to varying subtherapeutic levels. The changes that occur in airflow, respiratory effort, and pharyngeal muscle activity in response to these "controlled" periods of obstruction are then used

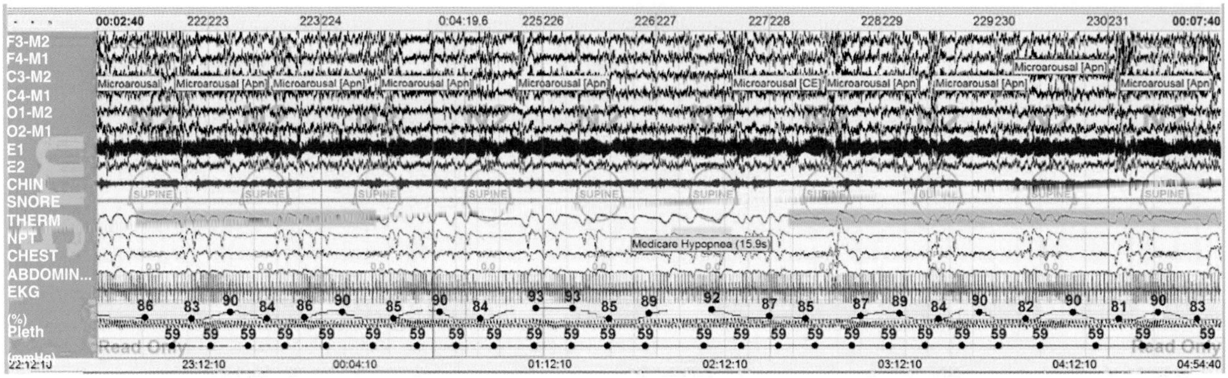

Figure 129.31 Ataxic breathing with hypercapnia. Ten-minute snapshot. An ataxic periodic breathing pattern with repeated central apneas and persistent hypercapnia (transcutaneous CO_2 reading of 59 mm Hg. This patient has long-standing quadriplegia and uses a baclofen pump for spasticity.

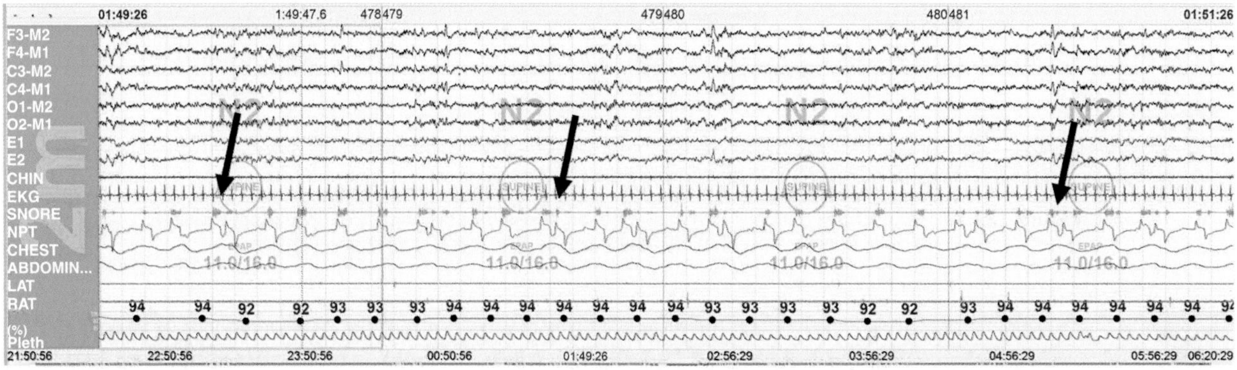

Figure 129.32 Patient-ventilator desynchrony. Titration polysomnography (PSG), 2-minute window. Demostrates patient-ventilator asynchrony in a patient with amyotrophic lateral sclerosis (ALS) undergoing titration using a volume-targeted mode. The image demonstrates intermittent double triggering *(black arrows)* because of the patient's (or neural) inspiratory time exceeding the ventilator inspiratory time, so essentially 1 patient breath = 2 ventilator breaths. The ventilator sensed that the patient's inhalation flow had stopped when the inhalation was incomplete. This issue is commonly encountered in neuromuscular disorders (NMDs) and can be resolved by increasing the inspiratory time or changing the cycle sensitivity (decreasing it) so that the ventilator senses late termination of inhalation.

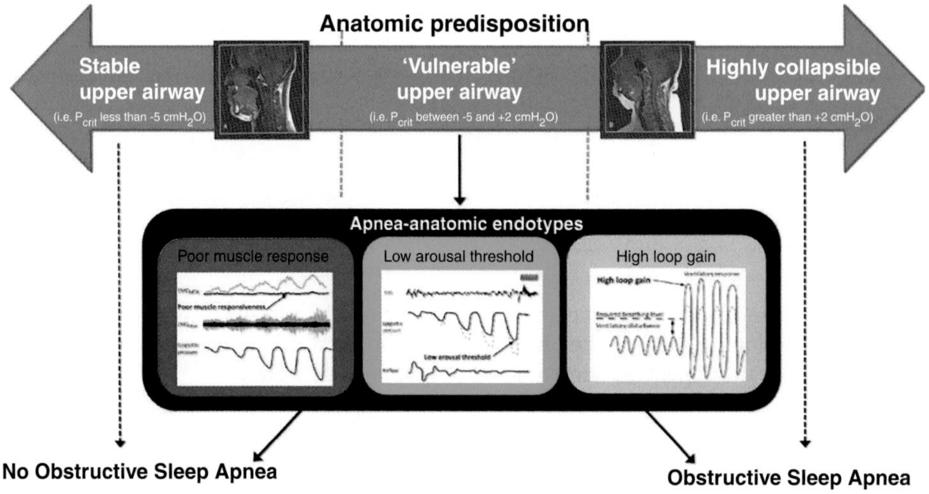

Figure 129.33 Relationship between the obstructive sleep apnea (OSA) endotypes. In order to have OSA, an individual needs to have some degree of anatomic predisposition. Those with a stable upper airway will never develop OSA, whereas those with a highly collapsible airway will always develop OSA. For those individuals who are in the vulnerable upper airway space (defined as those with a P_{crit} of −5 to +2 cmH_2O), whether they develop OSA is dependent on the presence of one or more abnormal nonanatomic endotypes. (Adapted from Refs. 117, 150, and 151.)

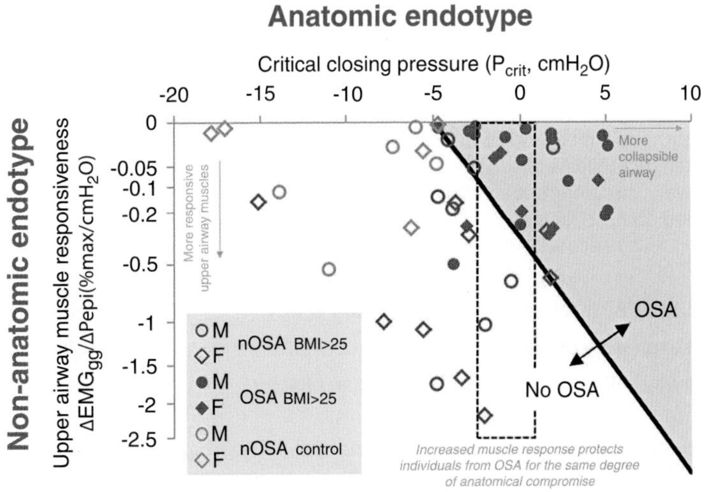

Figure 129.34 The combination of how both anatomic and nonanatomic endotypes interact to predispose toward obstructive sleep apnea (OSA) in overweight/obese individuals with and without OSA (nOSA). Here the anatomic endotype was assessed by measuring the critical closing pressure or P_{crit}, whereby a more positive number indicates a more collapsible airway. Upper airway muscle responsiveness is assessed by measuring the slope of the relationship between genioglossus muscle activity (EMG_{gg}) against epiglottic pressure (P_{epi}). Note that when comparing those at similar degrees of anatomic compromise, whether individuals have robust or poor muscle responsiveness helps explain whether they are likely to have OSA *(gray shaded area)* or be protected from it, despite being overweight or obese. Each of these endotypes influence the clinical presentation of OSA and have major implications for whether certain treatments will be effective in a given patient. Thus targeted, individualized treatment approaches are likely to be essential if we ever want to effectively treat OSA with non continuous positive airway pressure (CPAP) therapies. BMI, Body mass index; F, Female; M, Male. (Adapted from[124].)

to derive estimates of the four endotypes. These techniques to measure the endotypes are too complex and resource-dependent, making their translation into the clinical environment a significant challenge.

As such, intensive research effort has been put into developing simpler techniques that can measure or estimate the OSA endotypes (either in isolation or simultaneously) from tests, many of which could be easily performed in the clinical environment (Table 129.2).

Of all of these simplified noninvasive techniques, one that is drawing a lot of attention is the ability to quantify all four key OSA endotypes using data collected from routine diagnostic clinical PSG.[133-135] More specifically, this technique fits a mathematical model to the observed fluctuations that naturally occur in a patient's breathing during sleep to derive a breath-by-breath assessment of ventilatory drive, from which the endotypes can be derived. Notably, these PSG-derived endotypes correlate well with the same variables derived using the "gold-standard" measures. The main challenges of measuring the OSA endotypes using this technique is its rather heavy reliance on high-quality signals (especially nasal pressure), technical expertise to process the signals, and accurate sleep staging and respiratory events/arousal scoring according to set criteria. Furthermore, given that the criteria used to score PSGs has evolved, recent work has highlighted that the scoring criteria employed can have a significant impact on not just the measurement of the endotype[136,137] but also its ability to predict response to treatment.[136] To overcome the hurdle of variable scoring (both from interscorer differences and scoring criteria used), inclusion of recent work on automating the identification of UA obstruction[138] and sleep stage/arousal scoring[139] will likely be required to ensure clinical uptake. Furthermore, recent work has also been focused on providing a cloud-based version of the software to enable greater implementation in both research and clinical settings.[114]

Evidence that the OSA Endotypes Predict Response to Treatment

The recognition that multiple endotypes are responsible for the development of OSA helps explain why CPAP-alternative interventions such as oral appliances, UA surgery, and agents/pharmacologic interventions (i.e., supplemental oxygen or sedatives) have to date shown only a modest improvement in OSA severity when administered to unselected patients. Such interventions are typically only targeting one endotype, and whether the intervention reduces OSA severity will likely depend on both (1) how much that intervention improves the endotype and (2) whether additional endotypes are contributing to their OSA. A summary of studies that have assessed whether knowledge of the OSA endotype can predict treatment response is shown in Table 129.3.

Although some of the studies have shown good predictive capability when using one OSA endotype, it seems at this early stage that knowledge of more than one endotype allows for greater accuracy with predictions. For example, early physiologic studies suggested that measures of a patient's anatomic compromise alone were insufficient to identify those that showed a good response in terms of improvement in OSA severity with an oral appliance.[140-142] The first study to assess the impact that oral appliance therapy had on all four endotypes (measured using the "gold standard" techniques), albeit in a small physiologic study, reported that those who benefited the most from the therapy were those individuals with a mildly

Table 129.2 Summary of Simple, Clinically Applicable Tools to Measure OSA Endotypes

OSA Endotype	Clinical Variable	Study	Performed in Sleep/Wake	Requires an Additional Test
Anatomic compromise/ airway collapsibility	Combination of clinical and PSG characteristics (NREM-OAI/AHI >0.44, waist circumference >106 cm, mean obstructive apnea duration >22.1 seconds and REM-AHI >39.9)	Genta et al.[152]	Sleep	No
	Therapeutic CPAP level	Landry et al.[153]	Sleep	Yes/No
	Negative expiratory pressure	Hirata et al.[154]	Wake	Yes
	Upper airway collapsibility index (UACI)	Osman et al.[155]	Wake	Yes
	Flow or nasal pressure signal from a clinical PSG	Sands et al.,[133] Azarbarzin et al.,[156,157] Genta et al.[158]	Sleep	No
	Upper airway visualization (e.g., Mallampati, Friedman, MRI-derived imaging)	Islam et al.,[159] Li et al.,[160] Smith et al.,[161] Chi et al.,[162] Schwab et al.[163]	Wake	Yes/No
	Craniofacial characteristics	Sutherland et al.,[164] Schwab et al.[165]	Wake	Yes
Muscle compensation	Nasal pressure signal from a clinical PSG	Sands et al.[133]	Sleep	No
Respiratory arousal threshold	3 PSG characteristics (AHI <30 events/hr, nadir SpO_2 >82.5%, and hypopneas >58.3%)	Edwards et al.,[166] Thomson et al.[137]	Sleep	No
	Nasal pressure signal from a clinical PSG	Sands et al.[134]	Sleep	No
Loop gain	Breath hold duration	Trembach et al.,[167] Messineo et al.[168]	Wake	Yes (but could be done during consult)
	Chemoreflex test	Wang et al.[169]	Wake	Yes
	Nasal pressure signal from a clinical PSG	Terill et al.[135]	Sleep	No

Adapted from Edwards et al.[170]

AHI, Apnea-hypopnea index; CPAP, continuous positive airway pressure; MRI, magnetic resonance imaging; OAI, obstructive apnea index; OSA, obstructive sleep apnea; PSG, polysomnography; SpO_2, peripheral capillary oxygen saturation.

collapsible airway and a low/normal loop gain at baseline.[143] That is, if an intervention is given that targets improving the anatomy/collapsibility (i.e., oral appliance), those who gain the greatest benefit are those whose OSA is primarily caused by a mild anatomic issue (and have favorable nonanatomic endotypes). More recently, two independent studies[144,145] in larger sample sizes that estimated the endotypes using the noninvasive tools have confirmed that this particular combination of favorable traits is largely repeatable, which is promising for the field.

The presence of a low arousal threshold has been linked to poor short- and long-term CPAP adherence in several studies.[119,146-149] These findings suggest that one way to improve CPAP adherence might be to raise the arousal threshold in these individuals with a sedative. In line with this, Schmickl and colleagues[147] demonstrated that eszopiclone improves CPAP usage overall, especially in those with a low arousal threshold.

CLINICAL IMPLICATIONS AND FUTURE DIRECTIONS

Overall, this collective body of evidence has provided great promise that the personalization of OSA treatment may not be too far away. However, many hurdles still need to be overcome before they can be made available for mainstream use. Many of the studies conducted to date are relatively small physiologic studies. The morphologic patterns described earlier in the chapter have not been validated prospectively, even something as simple as REM versus NREM dominance or cycle length of respiratory events. More studies measuring the OSA endotypes in much larger sample sizes (with greater diversity) will be required. Furthermore, showing that the findings and prediction thresholds are repeatable will be important in providing clinicians with a framework to make physiology-based treatment recommendations.

Table 129.3 Summary of Studies that Have Assessed Whether Knowledge of the OSA Endotypes Predicts Treatment Response

OSA Endotype(s) Targeted	Treatment Intervention	Study	N	Duration of Intervention	Responder Definition Used	OSA Endotypes Measured	Key Findings Predicting Response
Anatomy/collapsibility	Weight loss (via dietary/lifestyle measures)	Schwartz et al.[171]	13	≈17 months	Correlation with ΔAHI[a]	C	Those with milder collapsibility at baseline experienced greater reduction in their AHI with weight loss.
	Oral appliance	Ng et al.[140]	10	Single night	AHI_{Post} <5/hr	C	Collapsibility alone was not a predictor of response.
		Chan et al.[141]	69	Single time point after 6–8 acclimatization periods	50% ↓AHI	Anat	No differences at baseline between responders/nonresponders in the volumes of the airway and soft tissue structures, skeletal class, or cephalometric measurements.
		Sutherland et al.[142]	18	Single time point	50% ↓AHI	Anat	No differences in upper airway structure between groups.
		Edwards et al.[143]	14	Single night	50% ↓AHI and AHI_{Post}<10/hr	C, A, L, M	The combination of loop gain and collapsibility predicted response to therapy with 100% sensitivity and 87.5% specificity.
		Marques et al.[172]	25	Single night	70% ↓AHI	Anat, C	Posteriorly located tongue and mild collapsibility at baseline were associated with greater treatment efficacy.
		Bamagoos et al.[144]	93	Varied	50% ↓AHI	C, A, L, M (n)	Greater oral appliance efficacy was associated with lower loop gain, higher arousal threshold, lower response to arousal, moderate (nonmild, nonsevere) pharyngeal collapsibility, and weaker muscle compensation.
		Vena et al.[58]	81	Varied	50% ↓AHI and AHI_{Post}<10/hr	Anat surrogate (n)	Depth of respiratory events and presence of expiratory "pinching" (validated to reflect palatal prolapse) were predictors of response.
		Op de Beeck et al.[145]	36	3 months	50% ↓AHI	C, A, L, M (n)	Responders exhibited lower loop gain at baseline compared with nonresponders, a difference that persisted after adjustments for baseline AHI, BMI, and collapsibility.
		Jugé et al. (2020)	72	>9 weeks	50% ↓AHI and AHI_{Post} <10/hr or AHI <5/hr	Anat	When mandibular advancement alters inspiratory tongue movement, therapeutic response to oral appliance therapy was more common among those who convert to a beneficial movement pattern.
	Upper airway surgery	Schwartz et al.[173]	13	>2 months	50% ↓NREM AHI	C	Collapsibility alone was not a predictor of response.
		Joosten et al.[174]	46	≈3 months	50% ↓AHI and AHI_{Post} <10/hr	L (n)	A low loop gain at baseline predicted surgical response.
		Li et al.[175]	31	≈4 months	Predicted post-treatment AHI	L (n)	A low loop gain at baseline predicted surgical response.
	Hypoglossal nerve stimulation	Schwab et al.[176]	13	12 months	50% ↓AHI and AHI_{Post} <20/hr	Anat	Smaller soft palate volumes at baseline and greater tongue movement anteriorly predicted response.
		Vanderveken et al.[177]	21	6 months	50% ↓AHI and AHI_{Post} <20/hr	Anat	The absence of complete concentric collapse at the level of the palate was a predictor of response.
		Op de Beeck et al.[178]	91	12 months	50% ↓AHI and AHI_{Post} <10/hr	C, A, L, M (n)	In adjusted analysis, a favorable response to therapy was independently associated with higher arousal threshold, greater muscle compensation, and lower loop gain (in milder collapsibility).

Continued

Table 129.3 Summary of Studies that Have Assessed Whether Knowledge of the OSA Endotypes Predicts Treatment Response—cont'd

OSA Endotype(s) Targeted	Treatment Intervention	Study	N	Duration of Intervention	Responder Definition Used	OSA Endotypes Measured	Key Findings Predicting Response
Muscle compensation	Desipramine	Taranto-Montemurro et al.[179]	12	Single night	20/hr ↓AHI	C, A, L, M	Those with poor muscle compensation at baseline experienced greater reduction in AHI on therapy.
	Atomoxetine + oxybutynin (ATOX)	Taranto-Montemurro et al.[180]	17	Single night	50% AHI reduction	C, A, L, M (n)	Patients with lower AHI, mild collapsibility, and higher fraction of hypopneas over total events had a complete response with ATOX.
Respiratory arousal threshold	Triazolam	Berry et al.[181]	12	Single night	N/A	A	N/A
	Eszopiclone	Eckert et al.[182]	17	Single night	Compared ΔAHI in patients with low vs. high arousal threshold	A	Patients with a low arousal threshold showed greater reduction in AHI (43%↓).
	Trazodone	Eckert et al.[183]	7	Single night	Correlation with ΔAHI[a]	A	Arousal threshold alone did not predict treatment response.
	Trazodone	Smales et al.[184]	13	Single night	Upper 50th percentile of subjects based on the %ΔAHI between groups	A	Arousal threshold alone did not predict treatment response.
	Zopiclone	Carter et al.[185]	12	Single night	Correlation with ΔAHI[a]	A	Arousal threshold alone did not predict treatment response.
Loop gain	Carbon dioxide	Xie et al.[186]	26	Single night	30% ↓AHI	C, L	No difference in collapsibility between groups. Responders had a higher loop gain (driven by ↑controller gain).
	Hyperoxia	Wellman et al.[187]	12	Single night	N/A	L	Patients with higher loop gain showed greater reduction in AHI (46%↓ vs 16%↓).
		Xie et al.[186]	26	Single night	30% ↓AHI	C, L	No difference in collapsibility or loop gain between groups.
		Wang et al.[169]	20	2 months	Correlation with ΔAHI	L	Controller gain (awake) was lower in those who experienced greater reductions in the AHI.
		Sands et al.[188]	36	Single night	50% ↓AHI	C, A, L, M (n)	The combination of elevated loop gain, less severe collapsibility, and greater muscle compensation at baseline predicted response.
Respiratory arousal threshold and loop gain	Eszopiclone and oxygen (hyperoxia)	Edwards et al.[189]	20	Two nights (placebo vs. treatment), 1-week washout period	50% ↓AHI and AHI_{Post} <15/hr	C, A, L, M	Combination therapy lowered AHI, ventilation associated with arousal, and loop gain. Responders had less severe OSA, a less collapsible upper airway, and greater upper airway muscle effectiveness.[a] A lower therapeutic CPAP requirement (as a surrogate for collapsibility) was also a significant predictor of response.[190]

Adapted from Edwards et al.[170]

A, Arousal threshold; AHI, apnea-hypopnea index; AHI_{Post}, treatment AHI; Anat, anatomy; C, collapsibility; CPAP, continuous postive airway pressure; L, loop gain; M, muscle responsiveness; N/A, not assessed; NREM, non–rapid eye movement; OSA, obstructive sleep apnea.

[a]Analysis not reported in original publication; performed post hoc using data included in tables and figures.

(n) = measured noninvasively from a standard clinical polysomnogram (PSG).

CLINICAL PEARLS

- Sleep state data contain information about causative mechanisms, which is not captured by conventional scoring.
- The propensity to sleep fragmentation/easy arousability and respiratory control instability (high loop gain) are two important features that may be extracted from the PSG and even home sleep apnea tests. This information can aid management strategies.
- NREM sleep dominance of apnea is correlated with high loop gain, and REM-dominant apnea with collapsible airways.
- Specific oximetry patterns may suggest high-loop-gain, REM-dominant obstruction.
- A number of mathematical/computational approaches are now available to phenotype sleep apnea, which raise optimism that personalized sleep apnea care is a practical option and not just a research exercise.

SUMMARY

The rich information inherent in sleep state signals enables a number of methods of phenotyping. Such analysis is done with the premise that patterns reflect biology and thus driver endotypes and individual differences of clinical and therapeutic significance. Methods of phenotyping range from the visual analysis of patterns to mathematical/computational analysis. Specific respiratory, oximetry, and capnometry patterns are examples of visual analysis, and mathematical estimation of self-similarity (consecutive respiratory events with identical timing and morphology), bandwidth of cardiopulmonary coupling, continuous sleep depth, and estimation of loop gain from disturbance/response analysis are examples of computational applications to phenotyping. The collective body of data on phenotyping sleep signals has provided great promise that the personalization of sleep apnea treatment may not be too far away. Ideally, multiple complementary methods would be used to generate a composite score that would "weight" the different driver components and the response of the individual to perturbations, and estimate a success or failure probability. Such a score would reasonably integrate disease severity, prior therapy history, and individual medical and social factors known to hamper optimal medical management across multiple dimensions.

SELECTED READINGS

Amatoury J, Azarbarzin A, Younes M, Jordan AS, Wellman A, Eckert DJ. Arousal intensity is a distinct pathophysiological trait in obstructive sleep apnea. *Sleep*. 2016;39:2091–2100.

Dutta R., Delaney G., Toson B., et al. A novel model to estimate key obstructive sleep apnea endotypes from standard polysomnography and clinical data and their contribution to obstructive sleep apnea severity. *Ann Am Thorac Soc.* 2021;18(4):656–667.

Eckert DJ, White DP, Jordan AS, Malhotra A, Wellman A. Defining phenotypic causes of obstructive sleep apnea. Identification of novel therapeutic targets. *Am J Respir Crit Care Med.* 2013;188(8):996–1004.

Gilmartin GS, Daly RW, Thomas RJ. Recognition and management of complex sleep-disordered breathing. *Curr Opin Pulm Med.* 2005;11:485–493.

Malhotra A, Mesarwi O, Pepin JL, Owens RL. Endotypes and phenotypes in obstructive sleep apnea. *Curr Opin Pulm Med.* 2020;26(6):609–614.

Op de Beeck S., Wellman A., Dieltjens M., et al. Endotypic mechanisms of successful hypoglossal nerve stimulation for obstructive sleep apnea. *Am J Respir Crit Care Med.* 2021;203(6):746–755.

Thomas RJ, Terzano MG, Parrino L, Weiss JW. Obstructive sleep-disordered breathing with a dominant cyclic alternating pattern-a recognizable polysomnographic variant with practical clinical implications. *Sleep*. 2004;15;27:229–234.

Wellman A, Edwards BA, Sands SA, et al. A simplified method for determining phenotypic traits in patients with obstructive sleep apnea. *J Appl Physiol (1985)*. 2013;114(7):911–922.

Younes M. Pathogenesis of obstructive sleep apnea. *Clin Chest Med.* 2019;40:317–330.

Younes M, Hanly PJ. Immediate postarousal sleep dynamics: an important determinant of sleep stability in obstructive sleep apnea. *J Appl Physiol.* 2016;120:801–808.

Younes M, Schweitzer PK, Griffin KS, Balshaw R, Walsh JK. Comparing two measures of sleep depth/intensity [published online ahead of print, 2020 Jul 6]. *Sleep*. 2020:zsaa127. https://doi.org/10.1093/sleep/zsaa127.

Zinchuk A, Yaggi HK. Phenotypic Subtypes of OSA: a challenge and opportunity for precision medicine. *Chest*. 2020;157:403–420.

A complete reference list can be found online at ExpertConsult.com.

Chapter

130

Clinical and Physiologic Heterogeneity of Obstructive Sleep Apnea

Grace W. Pien; Lichuan Ye

Chapter Highlights

- Heterogeneity in the physiologic factors and range of clinical presentations contributing to the development of obstructive sleep apnea (OSA) is increasingly recognized. Investigators have sought to distinguish subtypes or phenotypes of OSA based on characteristic pathophysiologic or clinical attributes.
- Anatomic and physiologic subtypes have been used to identify individuals likely to have OSA and to determine whether particular subgroups respond better to some therapies than others, especially based on underlying pathophysiology and mechanism of treatment.
- A range of clinical OSA phenotypes have been differentiated by traits including age, sex, and presenting symptoms. Recent studies using unsupervised approaches, such as cluster analysis, have expanded our understanding of clinical phenotypes in OSA, differences in how they respond to therapy, and relationships to outcomes, such as cardiovascular disease.
- This chapter reviews anatomic and physiologically focused and clinically oriented OSA phenotypes and explores their implications for pathogenesis, treatment, and clinical outcomes.

Heterogeneity in the physiologic factors leading to the development of obstructive sleep apnea (OSA) and the wide range of clinical presentations have long been recognized. However, when describing the disease, OSA has frequently been reduced to a single attribute, the apnea-hypopnea index (AHI). Although AHI quantifies the frequency of abnormal breathing occurrences during sleep and is associated with clinical outcomes, including daytime sleepiness, hypertension, stroke, and all-cause mortality, it overlooks many properties that characterize OSA, such as dominance in rapid eye movement (REM) or non-REM sleep, the magnitude and duration of associated reductions in oxygen saturation, or the total hypoxic burden associated with apneic events. AHI also fails to convey which pathophysiologic traits may underlie the development of OSA in a given individual or group of patients, or to consider patients' symptoms and their severity. As we increasingly recognize the complex and multisystem effects of OSA, knowledge of these and other specific clinical or pathophysiologic attributes are likely to be critical to determining whether some therapies are more appropriate for specific patients when compared to others.

Investigators have used a number of approaches to describe the disease heterogeneity observed in patients with OSA. Numerous studies have identified homogeneous subtypes or phenotypes of OSA based on unique pathophysiologic or clinical characteristics.[1–7] An OSA phenotype has been operationally defined as "*a category of patients with OSA distinguished from others by a single or combination of disease features, in relation to clinically meaningful attributes (symptoms, response to therapy, health outcomes, quality of life).*"[8] This definition offers flexibility for recognizing clinically relevant phenotypes even when the underlying mechanisms of categorization remain to be understood. Identification of OSA phenotypes can advance understanding of disease mechanisms, optimize participant selection for clinical trials, improve prognostication, and ultimately achieve more personalized treatment.[8,9]

Approaches and analytic methods for identifying clinical and pathophysiologic phenotypes in OSA have been reviewed.[8,10–12] Briefly, these methods can be categorized into supervised and unsupervised approaches. Supervised analyses evaluate predetermined phenotypes based on single or multiple features and generally assume that the features categorizing subjects represent underlying biologic or mechanistic differences. Unsupervised methods, such as cluster analysis, are data driven and aim to classify subjects into relatively homogeneous subgroups based on multiple disease features. The unsupervised approach has the advantage of identifying new phenotypes and generating new hypotheses. However, the relevance of newly described phenotypes needs to be established by anchoring them to relevant patient outcomes using supervised analyses.[8]

In this chapter we review clinically relevant OSA phenotypes based on single or multiple disease features, including anatomic and physiologically focused and clinically oriented features (e.g., demographics, polysomnography, symptoms, and comorbidities) and their implications for pathogenesis, treatment, and clinical outcomes, if known.

ANATOMIC AND PHYSIOLOGIC PHENOTYPES UNDERLYING OBSTRUCTIVE SLEEP APNEA

Anatomic Phenotypes

Defining Phenotypes Using Craniofacial and Soft Tissue

The development of OSA depends on anatomic and physiologic factors that differ from person to person. Phenotyping can be used to delineate variations in craniofacial morphology leading to anatomic compromise of the upper airway in several ways (see Chapter 168).

Cephalometric measurements obtained from direct measurement, radiographs, and computerized tomography and magnetic resonance imaging (MRI) techniques have been used to characterize differences in soft tissue and bony craniofacial attributes between individuals with and without OSA. Skeletal characteristics that are common among patients with OSA include maxillary deficiency,[13] mandibular retrusion,[14] inferior displacement of the hyoid bone,[15,16] and abnormalities of the cranial base.[17] Shorter mandibular length[18] and lower facial height[19] have also been observed in patients with OSA. Although craniofacial abnormalities are more common among nonobese persons with OSA, obese individuals with OSA often have enlargement of the soft tissue structures, including the tongue and soft palate.[20,21]

Combinations of bony craniofacial and soft tissue characteristics that lead to OSA have been examined in largely White samples using facial phenotyping,[22,23] a digital photography technique that is highly correlated with MRI and compares favorably given its lower cost, greater availability, and greater simplicity.[23] Characteristics such as smaller mandibular triangular area, wider and flatter mid and lower face, and shorter, retruded jaw may predict OSA independent of obesity.[22] Nevertheless, although skeletal and soft tissue attributes have had some success in describing anatomic subtypes at risk for OSA, to date, there is little data to suggest that they predict clinical manifestations of OSA or clinically important outcomes, such as cardiovascular events or death.

Instead, they may be more suited for determining whether some anatomic subtypes are better candidates for specific therapies for OSA compared to others. The ability of cephalometric measures to predict successful deployment of mandibular advancement devices (MAD) has recently been reviewed.[24,25] A smaller hyoid-to-mandibular plane distance was the most consistent predictor across studies, with a shorter anterior cranial base and shorter soft palate also associated with MAD response.[24] However, small samples, methodologic differences across studies and conflicting results led the authors to conclude that, on balance, the data were "relatively weak and somewhat inconsistent," and should not be used in isolation to make clinical decisions.

Cephalometric parameters alone have also been deemed insufficiently reliable for predicting treatment outcomes after uvulopalatopharyngoplasty or multilevel salvage soft tissue surgery for OSA.[1] Although individual studies have identified a range of traits associated with successful treatment, overall, given a lack of consistent results, anatomic subtypes do not appear to reliably predict surgical outcome after these procedures.[1]

A number of studies have explored racial and ethnic differences in the anatomic characteristics of OSA patients, finding that variations in skeletal and soft tissue dimensions may help to explain disparities in OSA prevalence (reviewed by Dudley and Patel[26]). For instance, soft tissue factors such as the tongue area are more important for predicting OSA risk in African Americans,[26] whereas among Asians, craniofacial features have better predictive value.[27,28] Differences in anatomic phenotypes between males and females with OSA may also exist,[29,30] but these data are relatively sparse.

Other Ways of Defining Anatomic Subtypes

The site or degree of upper airway obstruction in patients with OSA has been used to define subgroups and examined to determine whether this characteristic predicts the response to non–positive airway pressure (PAP) therapies. To date, these studies have demonstrated variable results.[31,32] Tongue base collapse has been associated with better odds for successful response to treatment with an MAD[33]; however, other investigators have concluded that identifying the site of collapse does not adequately predict oral appliance outcome.[3,4] Using drug-induced endoscopy, a method for directly visualizing dynamic upper airway collapse, complete concentric collapse at the level of the palate predicted poorer response to upper airway stimulation therapy.[34] At present, patients with concentric collapse are generally excluded from consideration for implanted hypoglossal nerve stimulators.

Differences in inspiratory and expiratory airflow shapes may also help to identify the site of airway collapse and have been used to describe anatomic subtypes among patients with OSA, including individuals with isolated palatal and lateral wall collapse and those with tongue-based obstruction.[35,36] However, whether these subtypes can predict clinical outcomes or treatment response has not yet been examined. Alternatively, upper airway collapsibility, measured by passive upper airway critical closing pressure (passive P_{Crit}), has been used as a global measure of anatomic upper airway compromise.[2,37]

Phenotyping Based on Physiologic Subtypes

Physiologic factors, including ventilatory control stability, the respiratory arousal threshold, and pharyngeal dilator muscle effectiveness or responsiveness, have been identified as important contributors to the development of OSA in up to two-thirds of patients.[2] Specific subtypes of each trait influence the development of OSA and may determine the response to therapy. These include an oversensitive ventilator control system (i.e., ventilator control instability or high loop gain), a low respiratory arousal threshold, and poor pharyngeal dilator muscle effectiveness/responsiveness during sleep.[2]

Ventilatory Control System

The stability and responsiveness of the ventilatory control system during sleep are often described using the concept of loop gain, a term borrowed from the engineering literature to characterize the magnitude of changes in ventilation in response to a disturbance of the negative feedback loop regulating ventilation.[38] Systems with high loop gain react with larger ventilatory changes to a given perturbation (e.g., an apnea or hypopnea) and are more likely to become unstable due to small disturbances. In contrast, low loop gain systems respond with smaller changes in ventilation and are more inherently stable.

High and low loop gain phenotypes may respond differently to various therapies for OSA. For example, individuals with OSA and high loop gain are more likely to develop complex sleep apnea, that is, PAP-emergent central sleep apnea,[39] and to have a larger reduction in AHI in response to oxygen administration compared to patients with low loop gain.[40] Individuals with low loop gain may be more likely to benefit from upper airway surgery for OSA.[41]

Respiratory Arousal Threshold

The respiratory arousal threshold, or level of ventilatory drive needed to precipitate an arousal from sleep, varies between individuals and can also play a role in the development of sleep apnea events. Individuals who have a lower arousal threshold are more likely to awaken from sleep due to small changes in ventilatory drive, before pharyngeal reflexes that activate upper airway dilator muscles to maintain airway patency and promote periods of stable breathing are activated, as occurs in individuals with higher respiratory arousal thresholds.[42] Low arousal threshold predicted poor long-term continuous positive airway pressure (CPAP) adherence among nonobese individuals in a cohort of nearly 1000 male veterans with OSA,[43] illustrating how understanding a patient's physiologic phenotype might identify individuals more likely to need targeted interventions to use CPAP successfully. Secondary analyses of data from a trial assessing the effect of eszopiclone on CPAP adherence[44] suggest that sedatives may improve longer-term CPAP usage (>1 month) among those with a low arousal threshold,[45] but prospective validation of these results is needed. Sedative hypnotics have also been examined as standalone treatment for OSA. In one small study, eszopiclone administration to OSA patients with a low arousal threshold resulted in a 43% decrease in AHI, suggesting that increasing the arousal threshold in such patients may offer a therapeutic benefit.[46] However, arousal threshold alone did not predict treatment response in similar subsequent studies.[47–49]

Upper Airway Muscle Responsiveness

Variability in the magnitude of the response of pharyngeal dilator muscles to negative intraluminal pressure, the threshold at which this response is activated and the resulting change in ventilation also influence the likelihood of developing sleep apnea events.[50,51] In a group of 75 men and women with OSA who were carefully characterized by physiologic phenotype, approximately one-third of patients with OSA were observed to have poor upper airway muscle responsiveness or effectiveness,[2] that is, a limited ability to activate the pharyngeal dilator muscles during sleep in response to negative collapsing pressure. Significantly lower muscle compensation was noted at baseline among individuals in a small study who experienced the largest improvements in AHI after receiving desipramine, a drug that stimulates upper airway muscles.[52] Other studies examining the effect of pharmacologic agents that target serotonergic, noradrenergic, and cholinergic pathways contributing to reductions in upper airway muscle activity during sleep have not attempted to differentiate patients with poor pharyngeal dilator muscle responsiveness, and such drugs have generally either failed to improve OSA severity or have demonstrated only modest success.[53,54] Nevertheless, a recent small trial in which a median decrease in AHI of 63% was noted after administration of atomoxetine (a norepinephrine reuptake inhibitor) and oxybutynin (an antimuscarinic agent) to nonphenotyped OSA patients[55] has generated interest in whether such therapies may be effective specifically for patients with poor upper airway muscle responsiveness. To date, trials of other therapies that target the genioglossus muscle, including surgical treatments such as hypoglossal nerve stimulation therapy[34] and noninvasive myofunctional therapy, have not sought to identify patients with reduced upper airway dilator muscle responsiveness who might be most responsive to muscle-focused treatments.[56]

Using Physiologic Phenotypes in an Integrative Approach

As our understanding of the contributions of different pathophysiologic processes to sleep apnea development has grown, an appreciation that different individual physiologic subtypes interact with each other and with the patient's anatomy to impact OSA risk has likewise deepened. Integrative models that incorporate information from the three aforementioned physiologic traits—loop gain, respiratory arousal threshold, and pharyngeal muscle dilator responsiveness—and include a measurement of anatomic predisposition (summarized using the pressure at which the passive upper airway collapses as a surrogate) have been proposed to predict how different phenotypic combinations would interact along these key biologic pathways, resulting in the presence or absence of OSA. For instance, good passive upper airway anatomy may offset low arousal threshold to protect against development of obstructive apneas, or low arousal threshold may preclude upper airway muscle recruitment, leading to apneic events.[57] How individuals might respond to trait-specific non-PAP interventions singly and in combination has also been examined both hypothetically and to a limited degree, in practice (e.g., in a small study, patients with a combination of lower loop gain and a less collapsible upper airway experienced the largest reduction in sleep-disordered breathing events using oral appliance therapy).[58]

Although these models are intriguing, additional work is needed to determine whether observed results are durable beyond a single night, as tested in many studies, and to internally and externally validate the findings before they can be deployed clinically. Methods for assessing physiologic phenotypes using simple and easily obtainable surrogate measures that can differentiate relevant variations are being developed[59–62]; however, most studies examining physiologic traits have relied on technically challenging, time-consuming protocols that cannot be performed in the average clinical sleep laboratory.[61]

Furthermore, whether these physiologic phenotypes represent expressions of the genetic variants associated to date with increased risk for sleep apnea remains to be understood. A number of studies have established that there is a strong genetic component to sleep apnea.[63–65] Genome-wide association studies have identified several gene loci that influence apnea characteristics, including respiratory event length and frequency and mean oxygen saturation during sleep.[66–68] However, more work needs to be done to identify a wider range of traits associated with OSA, to clarify how these gene loci may interact, and to determine whether they result in anatomic and pathophysiologic phenotypes for OSA as described in the existing literature.

CLINICAL PHENOTYPES OF OBSTRUCTIVE SLEEP APNEA

Phenotyping Based on a Single Feature

Race and Ethnicity

A growing body of evidence supports the existence of racial disparities in the prevalence, risk factors, clinical presentation, diagnosis, and treatment of OSA.[69] For example, a meta-analysis and recent review both reported a higher prevalence and more severe OSA in African Americans compared to US Whites.[26,70] Obesity and craniofacial factors may contribute differently to OSA in different ethnic groups. At the same level of disease severity, for instance, Chinese patients have been found to be less obese, with more craniofacial restriction, and smaller tongue size compared to Whites.[27] In addition, the association between body mass index (BMI) and AHI has been found to be strong in South Americans but weak in African Americans. That is, for a similar BMI increase, South Americans show a greater increase in AHI compared to African Americans.[71]

Although there is substantial evidence that African Americans are at higher risk of hypertension and other cardiovascular consequences, whether OSA explains some of this disparity remains unclear. Blood pressure normally falls or "dips" at nighttime, but older African American adults with OSA are more likely to have a "nondipping" blood pressure pattern compared to their White counterparts. The association between this "nondipping" pattern and OSA severity appears to vary by race and use of antihypertensive medication.[72] With regard to treatment, African Americans may experience poorer outcomes from OSA therapies. For example, although African American children have a higher prevalence of OSA, they are less likely to undergo adenotonsillectomy, which is the first-line treatment for pediatric OSA.[73] Evidence also suggests that adherence to CPAP treatment is inferior in minority groups compared to Whites, with significantly lower adherence observed in African Americans.[74]

Age

With increasing age, airway collapsibility increases and may play a greater role in OSA pathogenesis, suggesting that OSA in older individuals may represent a distinct physiologic phenotype.[75] There is a clear age-related increase in the prevalence of OSA.[76] The clinical presentation of OSA in older adults can be subtle, leading to challenges for clinical diagnosis.[77] For example, older adults with OSA may present with less sleepiness at the same level of AHI,[78] and they are less likely to endorse snoring but more likely to suffer cognitive impairment.[77] OSA has been found to be associated with increased all-cause mortality, especially that due to coronary artery disease, but this relationship was only observed in individuals younger than 70 years.[79] Similarly, there is a lack of association between OSA and hypertension[80] or atrial fibrillation among older adults[81] compared to younger adults. Regarding treatment, because the importance of obesity as a risk factor of OSA decreases with age[76] and the potential benefit of higher BMI on mortality in older adults,[82] weight loss cannot be universally recommended for elderly patients, as it is for younger people.[77] When used consistently, CPAP can be highly effective in older adults, with demonstrated cognitive benefits in those with impaired cognitive function.[83] Untreated OSA significantly contributes to higher cardiovascular mortality in older adults, but adequate CPAP treatment may reduce this risk.[84]

Sex

Epidemiology studies have confirmed that OSA is two to three times more prevalent in men than in women.[85,86] Substantial sex differences exist in OSA physiology, clinical presentations, and health consequences, suggesting sex-specific mechanisms and the need for sex-specific clinical recognition and management in OSA.[85,87–90] When viewing OSA against a wide range of lifestyle and comorbidity factors, a recent epidemiologic study reported a stronger association with hypertension, daytime sleepiness, and physical inactivity in females, whereas there was a stronger association with witnessed apnea and waist circumference in males.[85] Similarly, OSA has been reported to have a stronger association with heart failure[91] and endothelial dysfunction[92] in females than in males, suggesting that females may be more vulnerable to OSA cardiometabolic comorbidities. On the other hand, central or abdominal obesity in males with OSA may contribute to greater insulin resistance and inflammation and play a more important role in OSA pathogenesis in males.[93,94] Although females with OSA showed more impairment in daytime functioning and symptoms than males, both sexes benefit from CPAP treatment.[95] There appear to be no sex differences in satisfaction with the CPAP interface,[96] but female patients may require lower pressures of CPAP pressure, even considering OSA severity.[97]

Excessive Daytime Sleepiness

Approximately 60% of OSA patients report excessive daytime sleepiness (EDS), with a higher prevalence of EDS seen in individuals with more severe OSA.[98] It is believed that EDS is caused by the sleep fragmentation and nocturnal hypoxemia characteristic of OSA.[99] CPAP treatment can significantly improve EDS, with a strong dose-related response observed between hours of CPAP use and improvement in EDS.[100,101] However, some patients continue to experience EDS, even after adequate treatment with CPAP. The prevalence of residual sleepiness, defined as an Epworth Sleepiness Scale (ESS) score greater than 10, after 1 year of CPAP treatment was 12% in a French multicenter study.[102] Of note, EDS is not a symptom exclusive to OSA. Hormonal, metabolic, and inflammatory mechanisms, independent of OSA, can all contribute to EDS.[103]

OSA with and without EDS may be distinct clinical phenotypes.[104,105] The presence of EDS has been shown to modify the relationship between AHI and mortality,[106] hypertension,[107] and insulin resistance,[108] with stronger associations seen in OSA patients with EDS. In a recent review, Garbarino and colleagues[105] summarized the studies examining differences between EDS and no-EDS patients with OSA. They found that male gender, younger age, and higher BMI were predictors of EDS. Furthermore, the positive effects of CPAP treatment on blood pressure, insulin resistance, cardiovascular diseases, and endothelial dysfunction, as demonstrated in OSA patients with EDS, have not been consistently observed in those without EDS.[105] For example, in the MOSAIC trial, which included OSA patients who were minimally symptomatic with an average ESS score less than 10 at baseline, CPAP treatment did not improve the 5-year calculated vascular risk.[109] In a recent study in post–myocardial infarction patients, those with EDS had significantly higher rates of reinfarction and major adverse cardiac events compared to those without excessive sleepiness, even after adjusting for clinically relevant factors such as age, left ventricular ejection fraction, and AHI.[110] Although EDS is commonly viewed as a classic symptom of OSA, more investigation is needed to understand why EDS occurs in some patients but not others and whether patients without EDS benefit from CPAP treatment.

Phenotyping Based on Multiple Features

Recent studies using an unsupervised approach, such as cluster analysis, have expanded our understanding of phenotypes in OSA. In this section we primarily review the established clinical phenotypes, based on symptom presentations that have been confirmed in both clinical- and population-based cohorts,[4,6,111] and their implications for treatment and cardiovascular outcomes.

Identification of Distinct Symptom Phenotypes of Obstructive Sleep Apnea

The first study to apply cluster analysis to identify distinct OSA clinical phenotypes used data from the Icelandic Sleep Apnea Cohort (ISAC), which included patients with newly diagnosed moderate to severe OSA.[6] The analyses included a total of 23 variables representing prevalent and clinically significant symptoms and comorbidities in the OSA population. Three clinical subtypes were revealed: a *disturbed sleep* group, including members with the highest probability of experiencing insomnia-related symptoms; a *minimally symptomatic* group, whose members were relatively asymptomatic and more likely to feel rested upon waking up; and a *sleepy* group, whose members presented with classic OSA symptoms, including EDS, and witnessed nighttime breathing pauses. No significant differences were observed in terms of sex, BMI, or AHI among the three groups.[6]

The same three subtypes were replicated in the Korean Genomic Cohort,[111] a population-based cohort with a lower prevalence of the sleepy group but higher prevalence of minimally symptomatic individuals compared to the original Icelandic clinical cohort. This is consistent with the observation that OSA is prevalent with a relatively low symptom burden in the general public.[112] This cluster analysis was also replicated in the Sleep Apnea Global Interdisciplinary Consortium (SAGIC), which included nine academic sleep centers worldwide.[113,114] In addition to the three subtypes previously reported,[6] two additional clusters were identified, including one with moderate sleepiness and one with predominantly upper airway symptoms, such as snoring and witnessed apneas.[4] Data from both clinical- and population-based cohorts around the world confirm that distinct clinical phenotypes of OSA exist,[115] with three major subtypes, including disturbed sleep or insomnia, asymptomatic, and excessively sleepy groups.[9]

Obstructive Sleep Apnea Clinical Subtypes and Treatment Outcomes

Data from the Icelandic Sleep Apnea Cohort was used to examine whether clinical subtypes respond differently to PAP therapy.[116] Changes in symptoms, demographics, and comorbid conditions within and across the three subtypes were evaluated after 2 years of PAP treatment. In the disturbed sleep group, PAP nonusers and users demonstrated similar changes in insomnia-related symptoms. Many patients continued to complain of insomnia-related symptoms even after effective treatment for OSA. Although the minimally symptomatic group continued to be relatively asymptomatic, they demonstrated significant improvements in sleepiness and fatigue, with more improvements among PAP users. Not surprising, the sleepy group showed the most improvement in symptoms, with greater changes in almost all symptoms in PAP users than nonusers. Therefore patterns of OSA treatment response may differ by initial clinical phenotype and treatment adherence. In some OSA patients with difficulty sleeping, insomnia symptoms may be due to mechanisms other than OSA and may require therapies targeted specifically at these symptoms.[116]

Obstructive Sleep Apnea Clinical Subtypes and Cardiovascular Outcomes

Data from the Sleep Heart Health Study (SHHS) were used to examine the relationship between OSA clinical phenotypes and cardiovascular outcomes.[5] Although the questionnaires for symptoms used in the SHHS were different from those in ISAC or SAGIC, unsupervised cluster analysis identified the same three phenotypes (disturbed sleep, minimally symptomatic, excessively sleepy) in individuals with an AHI of more than 15 events per hour. This study identified a fourth subtype, which was labeled a moderately sleepy group. Over the median follow-up time of 11.8 years, survival analyses suggested that the excessively sleepy group had a higher rate of subsequent coronary artery disease, heart failure, and all cardiovascular events compared to the other three groups and to the control group without OSA. The excessively sleepy group was the only group that had significantly increased rates of these cardiovascular events compared to the control group without OSA. Therefore the increased cardiovascular risk in individuals with OSA was seen primarily in the excessively sleepy group.[5]

The role of EDS in cardiovascular risk has also been highlighted in other studies.[107,110,117] The mechanism of the effect of EDS on cardiovascular risk remains unknown and needs to be further investigated. Nevertheless, the finding of different risks for cardiovascular events in OSA clinical subtypes has important implications. It may partly explain the negative finding from the large, randomized controlled Sleep Apnea Cardiovascular Endpoints (SAVE) trial, which examined whether CPAP prevents major cardiovascular events in moderate to severe OSA.[118] OSA patients with severe sleepiness with an ESS greater than 15 were excluded from the SAVE trial, given ethical concerns that randomization of these patients to no treatment could lead to sleepiness-related crashes. However, this decision may have excluded the subgroup of patients with the highest risk for cardiovascular events. Future studies are needed to examine the effect of CPAP on cardiovascular outcomes in studies that include patients who are excessively sleepy. Alternative study designs could be considered given the safety concerns regarding randomization for these individuals with EDS. For example, propensity score matching, which was used in a study to examine the effect of CPAP on fasting lipid levels, could be considered to replicate covariate balance associated with randomizations and to reduce causal inference.[119]

Other Clinical Phenotypes Based on Multiple Features

Other groups around the world have also applied cluster analysis to identify clinical phenotypes in OSA, based on multiple features, including polysomnography (PSG) characteristics,[7] comorbidities,[120] or a combination of demographics, comorbidities, and clinical presentations.[121–123] Given differences in available variables and what was included in the cluster analysis, it is difficult to compare these clinical phenotypes, which need to be further replicated in additional populations. Some of the studies have linked the identified clinical phenotypes to outcomes including cardiovascular events[7] and CPAP treatment success.[123] For example, physiologic phenotypes were examined using routine PSG data and their association with cardiovascular outcomes. Seven clusters were identified based on PSG features. Among them, three clusters—the "hypopnea and hypoxia," "periodic limb movements of sleep" (PLMS), and "combined severe" groups—demonstrated increased risk for adverse cardiovascular events.[7]

CLINICAL PEARLS

- Skeletal and soft tissue attributes have been used with some success to describe anatomic subtypes at risk for obstructive sleep apnea (OSA). However, there is little data to date to suggest that they reliably predict clinical or treatment outcomes.
- Although physiologic factors, including ventilatory control stability, the respiratory arousal threshold, and pharyngeal dilator muscle responsiveness, influence OSA development and may determine treatment response, streamlined assessment techniques and further validation are needed before they can be deployed clinically.
- Our understanding of the heterogeneity of OSA has been expanded recently by identification of distinct clinical phenotypes using symptoms, comorbidities, polysomnographic features, and other characteristics. Several studies have demonstrated that subgroups of individuals with OSA, such as those with excessive sleepiness, are at greater risk for adverse cardiovascular outcomes.
- Recognizing individual variability in the underlying pathophysiology, clinical presentation, and outcomes of different phenotypes of OSA forms the basis for developing personalized sleep apnea treatment that will change how we approach the care of patients with this common disorder.

SUMMARY

Over the last 2 decades, our understanding of the complex physiologic and multidimensional clinical heterogeneity of obstructive sleep apnea has grown remarkably, building upon a foundational understanding of anatomic and basic clinical OSA phenotypes. Use of innovative data analytic techniques and sophisticated physiology protocols has yielded descriptions of clinical and pathophysiologic phenotypes or subgroups that are becoming more widely recognized. Evidence that these phenotypes may be associated with differential risk for clinical outcomes and may respond differently to specific therapies continues to accumulate.

Individual variability in the underlying pathophysiology, clinical symptoms, and outcomes of different OSA phenotypes forms the basis for the development of personalized sleep apnea treatment. Although this is in its early stages, leveraging phenotypic data has great potential for more confidently predicting which therapies may best suit an individual patient. Further work is needed to delineate distinct disease endotypes or subtypes defined by a specific pathobiology with identifiable genetics and biomarkers, and consistency in clinical presentation, physiologic characteristics, natural history, patient outcomes, and response to specific therapies.[8,124] Although existing phenotypes generally incorporate some of these characteristics, they lack others. Nevertheless, clinical and physiologic phenotyping may offer a transitional step toward personalized sleep apnea treatment until we have a deeper understanding of how endotypes propel the phenotypic expression of OSA.

SELECTED READINGS

Chen H, Eckert DJ, van der Stelt PF, et al. Phenotypes of responders to mandibular advancement device therapy in obstructive sleep apnea patients: a systematic review and meta-analysis. *Sleep Med Rev*. 2020;49:101229.

Denolf PL, Vanderveken OM, Marklund ME, Braem MJ. The status of cephalometry in the prediction of non-CPAP treatment outcome in obstructive sleep apnea patients. *Sleep Med Rev*. 2016;27:56–73.

Dudley KA, Patel SR. Disparities and genetic risk factors in obstructive sleep apnea. *Sleep Med*. 2016;18:96–102.

Eckert DJ, White DP, Jordan AS, Malhotra A, Wellman A. Defining phenotypic causes of obstructive sleep apnea. Identification of novel therapeutic targets. *Am J Respir Crit Care Med*. 2013;188(8):996–1004.

Edwards BA, Wellman A, Sands SA, et al. Obstructive sleep apnea in older adults is a distinctly different physiological phenotype. *Sleep*. 2014;37(7):1227–1236.

Loewen AH, Ostrowski M, Laprairie J, Maturino F, Hanly PJ, Younes M. Response of genioglossus muscle to increasing chemical drive in sleeping obstructive apnea patients. *Sleep*. 2011;34(8):1061–1073.

Malhotra A, Mesarwi O, Pepin JL, Owens RL. Endotypes and phenotypes in obstructive sleep apnea. *Curr Opin Pulm Med*. 2020;26(6):609–614.

Mazzotti DR, Keenan BT, Lim DC, Gottlieb DJ, Kim J, Pack AI. Symptom subtypes of obstructive sleep apnea predict incidence of cardiovascular outcomes. *Am J Respir Crit Care Med*. 2019;200(4):493–506.

Owens RL, Edwards BA, Eckert DJ, et al. An integrative model of physiological traits can be used to predict obstructive sleep apnea and response to non positive airway pressure therapy. *Sleep*. 2015;38(6):961–970.

Peppard PE, Young T, Barnet JH, Palta M, Hagen EW, Hla KM. Increased prevalence of sleep-disordered breathing in adults. *Am J Epidemiol*. 2013;177(9):1006–1014.

Ye L, Pien GW, Ratcliffe SJ, et al. The different clinical faces of obstructive sleep apnoea: a cluster analysis. *Eur Respir J*. 2014;44(6):1600–1607.

Younes M, Ostrowski M, Atkar R, Laprairie J, Siemens A, Hanly P. Mechanisms of breathing instability in patients with obstructive sleep apnea. *J Appl Physiol (1985)*. 2007;103(6):1929–1941.

Zinchuk A, Yaggi HK. Phenotypic subtypes of OSA: a challenge and opportunity for precision medicine. *Chest*. 2020;157(2):403–420. https://doi.org/10.1016/j.chest.2019.09.002.

A complete reference list can be found online at ExpertConsult.com.

Chapter 131

Obstructive Sleep Apnea: Clinical Features, Evaluation, and Principles of Management

Harly Greenberg; Matthew T. Scharf; Sophie West; Preethi Rajan; Steven M. Scharf

Chapter Highlights

- Obstructive sleep apnea (OSA) is the most common respiratory disorder of sleep, with a high prevalence that is linked to the increase in obesity in the general population.
- OSA is frequently comorbid with cardiovascular, cerebrovascular, and metabolic diseases and is commonly observed in populations with these comorbidities.
- The clinical presentation of OSA is heterogeneous, with some patients exhibiting excessive daytime somnolence, whereas others exhibit disturbed nocturnal sleep and some reporting minimal symptoms.
- The pathogenesis of OSA is complex, with contributions from anatomic and mechanical factors that increase collapsibility of the upper airway, as well as factors that lead to instability of ventilatory control and arousals from sleep that promote apneas and hypopneas.
- Clinical assessment, in addition to various screening questionnaires, is useful to identify patients at risk for OSA. However, accurate diagnosis requires monitoring of sleep.
- In-laboratory polysomnographic testing for OSA and various technologies for ambulatory or out-of-center-sleep testing are presented. The utility and limitations of these techniques are discussed.
- An individualized treatment approach emphasizing chronic disease management that improves sleep-related health outcomes is necessary to optimize care.

DEFINITION

Obstructive sleep apnea/hypopnea syndrome (OSAHS) is the most common form of sleep-disordered breathing, consists of recurrent episodes of upper airway (UA) obstruction or narrowing at night, and may be associated with recurrent hypoxia, sleep fragmentation, and elevation of sympathoadrenal tone. There is general agreement that OSAHS is associated with substantial increase in overall use of health care resources.[1,2] Most studies agree that treatment of OSAHS reduces the overall cost of health care.[2]

Classic signs and symptoms of OSAHS include loud snoring, excessive daytime sleepiness (EDS), snorting and gasping at night (associated with apnea/hypopnea termination), disordered breathing events witnessed by bed partners, nocturia, and insomnia. OSAHS is often, but not always, associated with obesity, large neck circumference, and crowding of the oropharynx. Signs/symptoms of important comorbid conditions, such as hypertension, heart failure, cerebrovascular accidents, and pulmonary hypertension, may be present as well.

BRIEF HISTORY

Burwell and colleagues[3] are often given credit for the first medical description of a patient with probable OSAHS. These authors described an obese, sleepy, hypercapnic patient demonstrating periodic breathing, who reminded them of the character Joe in the Charles Dickens 1836 novel *The Posthumous Papers of the Pickwick Club.* However, others had used this term previously.[4] Although the prevailing thought was that hypoventilation, possibly owing to excess weight, contributed to somnolence, Kuhl[5] described breathing cessations at night during polysomnography (PSG) and attributed sleepiness to the resultant sleep fragmentation. As a result of these findings, Gastaut and colleagues[6,7] added measurements of airflow and chest wall motion to other PSG measures to document obstruction of the UA at night. The Bologna group of Lugaresi and Coccagna[8] demonstrated large swings in systemic and pulmonary artery pressures during apneas, thus documenting that nocturnal breathing disorders had major adverse consequences and required treatment. After the observation of Kuhl, the Bologna group reported that tracheostomy improved symptoms in a group of "Pickwickian" patients.[8,9] It was subsequently shown that obese patients with repetitive UA obstruction during sleep, in contrast to those with the Pickwickian syndrome, did not necessarily have awake hypercapnia,[10] and indeed, most did not. The term *obstructive sleep apnea* (OSA) is used to describe the disorder.

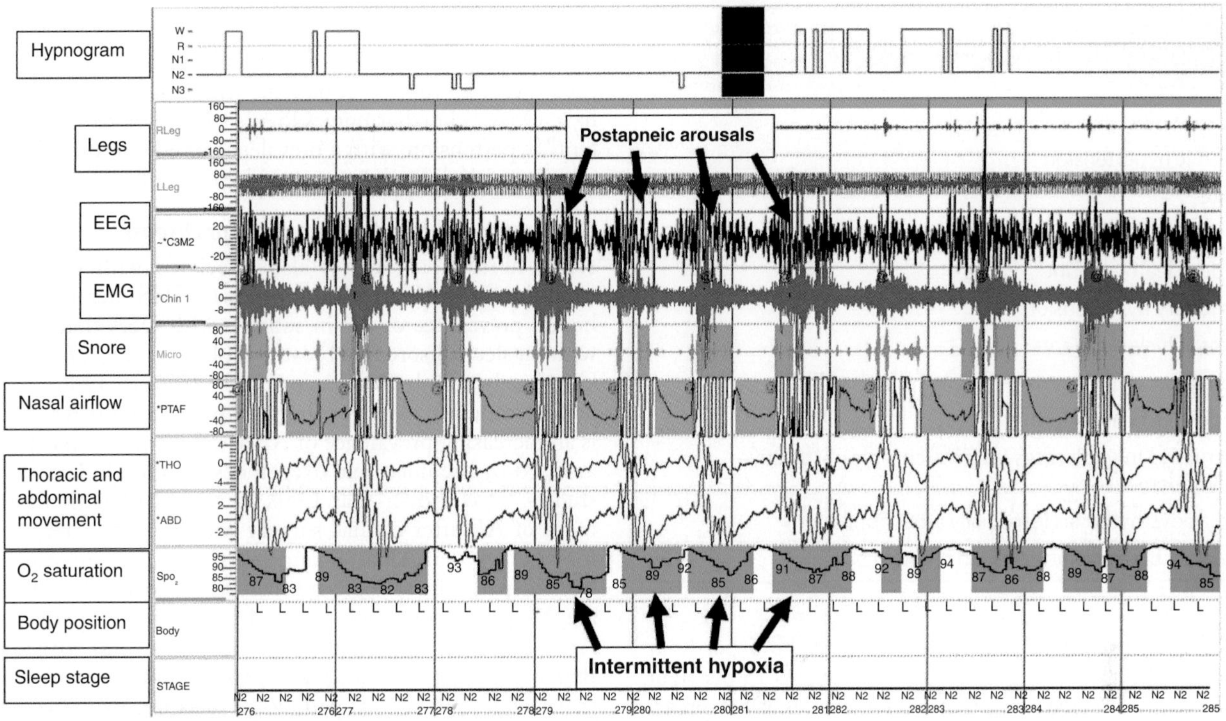

Figure 131.1 Repetitive obstructive apneas in a patient with severe obstructive sleep apnea. The *vertical lines* represent 30 seconds. Cessation of airflow is associated with continuation of ribcage motion, substantial intermittent reductions in oxygen saturation, and postapneic arousals. This tracing was taken with the subject in stage 2 sleep. ABD, Abdomen; EEG, electroencephalogram; EMG, electromyogram; PTAF, pressure transducer-generated airflow; Spo_2, saturation of peripheral oxygen; Thor, thoracic.

In 1981 Sullivan and colleagues[11] reported that nasally applied continuous positive airway pressure (CPAP) could alleviate UA obstruction in OSA. Additional therapies have been developed: UA surgery, mandibular advancement, and stimulation of the hypoglossal nerve. The physician is able to offer a variety of therapies tailored to the individual patient.

As the awareness of the importance of OSA as a major causative risk factor for numerous important medical conditions spread, novel methods of diagnosing OSA were developed. Classically, OSA was diagnosed in a laboratory setting, performed overnight, where PSG was performed. To reduce the complexity, discomfort, and costs, over the last 15 to 20 years, devices that incorporate a smaller number of channels for diagnosis and management of OSA were introduced. These devices are often suitable for home use and in many areas have been standard of practice for diagnosis and management of OSA in many patients.

PHYSIOLOGIC EFFECTS

It is now well established that OSA has a number of acute physiologic effects that are thought to contribute to adverse multisystem consequences.[12] These include intermittent hypoxia (IH) occurring as a result of apneas and hypopneas, exaggerated negative swings in intrathoracic pressure (ITP), and arousals associated with apnea termination. IH leads to increased sympathoadrenal tone,[13,14] oxidant stress in the brain[15] and in the myocardium,[16,17] and endothelial dysfunction.[18] Further, arousals associated with termination of apneas, hypopneas, and periods of inspiratory flow limitation contribute to heightened sympathetic tone.[19] Exaggerated swings in ITP, primarily during inspiration against an occluded airway, lead to increased venous return and stress on the right ventricle.[20] The latter appears to be primarily responsible for pulmonary hypertension, a common finding in OSA. Sleepiness is thought to be, at least in part, a result of the terminal arousals and associated sleep fragmentation. Figure 131.1 shows an example of a subject with very severe OSA who demonstrates intermittent hypoxia associated with apneas, postapneic arousals, and severe sleep fragmentation.

OSA is an independent major risk factor for a number of associated medical conditions (Table 131.1). Severe OSA is a risk factor for all-cause mortality.[21,22] However, it is unclear whether mild to moderate sleep apnea is associated independently with all-cause mortality. Chief among specific causes of mortality/morbidity are cardiovascular disease, including hypertension, stroke, myocardial infarction, and congestive heart failure, as well as insulin resistance and type 2 diabetes mellitus, depression, and sleepiness, leading to work- and automobile-related accidents. Heightened sympathoadrenal tone, oxidant stress, and proinflammatory cytokines appear to be involved in the pathogenesis of these conditions.

EPIDEMIOLOGY

There are varying estimates of the prevalence of OSA, largely owing to differences in diagnostic methods, definitions of disease, and differences in age, gender, and body mass index (BMI). In a recent systematic review, the prevalence of OSA ranged from 9% to 38% overall, using an apnea-hypopnea

Table 131.1 Medical and Mental Health Conditions for Which Obstructive Sleep Apnea is an Associated or Risk Factor

All-cause mortality
Systemic hypertension
Stroke
Myocardial infarction
Sudden death at night
Pulmonary hypertension
Motor vehicle accidents
Depression
Congestive heart failure
Obstructive lung diseases (asthma/chronic obstructive pulmonary disease)
Cardiac dysrhythmias (especially atrial fibrillation)
Type 2 diabetes mellitus/insulin resistance

index (AHI) cut-off of greater than or equal to 5 per hour. With an AHI cut-off of greater than or equal to 15 per hour, the prevalence ranged from 6% to 17% overall. OSA prevalence was higher with older age, male gender, and higher BMI.[23] Although female gender is associated with a lower prevalence of OSA, OSA risk increases substantially in women after menopause.[24,25]

Prevalence in Ethnic Cohorts/Racial Differences in Obstructive Sleep Apnea

There are disparities in the prevalence of OSA, as well as risk factors that may contribute to sleep-disordered breathing among different racial and ethnic populations.[26] Among African Americans, Native Americans, and Hispanics, OSA prevalence is increased, which may be due in part to increased obesity rates.[27] Other studies suggest that OSA severity is higher in African American compared to White men, even when controlling for BMI.[28] In the Jackson Heart Sleep Study, a high prevalence of moderate or severe OSA (24%) was found among African Americans living in the southern United States. In this population, male sex, snoring, BMI, and neck circumference were strong predictors of OSA.[29] Limited data also suggest that African Americans may be more susceptible to hypertension in association with OSA than other populations. OSA is also more prevalent in Asian populations compared to Whites. Craniofacial structure among Asians appears to confer an elevated risk of OSA despite lower rates of obesity.[26] Anatomic features, including differences in craniofacial structure or soft tissues of the UA, fat distribution, or the physiologic response to UA obstruction, may differ among ethnic groups and could modify OSA risk. However, obesity remains a risk factor for OSA across ethnic groups.[30]

Prevalence in Disease-Specific Cohorts

As OSA is associated with cardiac, cerebrovascular, pulmonary, metabolic, and other comorbid diseases, it is worthwhile to consider the prevalence of OSA in relevant disease-specific cohorts. Other chapters in this volume deal with these comorbidities in greater detail.

Hypertension

One of the most studied cardiovascular comorbidities of OSA is systemic hypertension. Most observational studies have shown that up to 50% of patients with systemic hypertension have OSA.[31] Furthermore, OSA is a common cause of "resistant" hypertension, with a prevalence of 64% in one cohort of patients with difficult-to-control hypertension.[32]

Cardiovascular and Cerebrovascular Disease

Atrial fibrillation (AF) is also associated with OSA. Data from the Sleep Heart Health Study (SHHS) demonstrated a higher prevalence of AF in subjects with OSA than in those without sleep-disordered breathing (4.8% vs. 0.9%; $P = .003$).[33] Conversely, a high prevalence of OSA (32% to 49%) has been demonstrated in various cohorts of patients with AF.[34] There is an increasing prevalence of AF as OSA severity increases as assessed by the nocturnal oxygen desaturation index.[35] Other studies have shown that OSA is associated with development of AF after cardiac surgery and with an increased risk for recurrence of AF after cardioversion or ablation therapy.[36] Several pathophysiologic mechanisms associated with OSA are thought to contribute to development and perpetuation of AF, including large intrathoracic pressure swings with apneas that increase atrial transmural pressure, intermittent hypoxemia, alteration in sympathovagal balance, oxidative stress, and systemic inflammation.[37] It is also evident that central sleep apnea (CSA) and Cheyne-Stokes respiration (CSR) are associated with incident atrial fibrillation, particularly in older patients. A causal association is plausible as CSA is often associated with increased chemoresponsiveness, hypocapnia, and augmented autonomic activity that may contribute to AF. Alternatively, CSA may be sign of underlying heart disease that leads to AF.[38]

OSA is also common in congestive cardiomyopathy and may adversely affect outcomes. In a cohort of systolic heart failure patients, 61% were found to have sleep-disordered breathing; approximately half had OSA, whereas CSA was present in the remainder.[39] OSA is also an independent risk factor for cerebrovascular disease, with threefold to fourfold increased odds of incident stroke in moderate to severe OSA (AHI > 20/hour).[40,41] In conjunction with this, the prevalence of OSA in post–cerebrovascular accident cohorts is notably high, ranging from 38% to 74%.[42]

Type 2 Diabetes Mellitus

The association of OSA with type 2 diabetes mellitus is also well described. Cross-sectional data from the SHHS demonstrated that OSA is independently associated with glucose intolerance and insulin resistance (odds ratio [OR], 1.27; range, 0.98 to 1.64 for AHI >15/hour).[43] A prospective study of 1453 nondiabetic subjects showed that severe OSA (AHI > 30/hour) was associated with an increased risk of incident type 2 diabetes mellitus over a 13-year follow-up period even after adjustment for BMI and waist circumference (OR, 1.71; range, 1.08 to 2.71).[44]

Chronic Obstructive Pulmonary Disease

Although some studies have suggested that the occurrence of OSA in chronic obstructive pulmonary disease (COPD) is not greater than expected based on the prevalence of each disease in the general population,[45] others have shown an increased prevalence of COPD among OSA patients compared with matched control subjects.[46] A case-control study of 1497 patients with PSG-proven OSA compared with 1489 age- and gender-matched control subjects showed that COPD was more prevalent in the OSA group (7.6% vs. 3.7%; $P < .0001$).[47] OSA was also found to be highly prevalent among a cohort of patients with moderate to severe COPD referred for pulmonary rehabilitation.[48] Regardless of whether the concomitant prevalence of COPD and OSA is greater than can be expected by chance occurrence, the coexistence of these disorders, termed the *overlap syndrome*, is associated with more severe nocturnal hypoxemia, hypoventilation, pulmonary hypertension, comorbid obesity, and diabetes mellitus than that observed in isolated OSA or COPD.

Asthma

Several studies have suggested that the prevalence of OSA is approximately double in asthma cohorts compared with the general population.[49] Asthma severity, BMI, gastroesophageal reflux, and female gender have been associated with increased OSA risk in asthma. Further, data from the Wisconsin Sleep Cohort showed that a diagnosis of asthma was associated with increased risk for incident OSA.[50] Most common, OSA is seen in obese patients with severe asthma. Potential mechanisms linking OSA with asthma include apnea-associated elevation of parasympathetic tone that contributes to airway hyperresponsiveness and intermittent hypoxia/reoxygenation, leading to oxidative stress and systemic inflammation.[51]

Chronic Kidney Disease

OSA is also frequently observed in patients with chronic kidney disease, with prevalence rates as high as 50% in end-stage renal disease (ESRD).[52] An increasing prevalence of OSA has been associated with declining kidney function, ranging from 41% in patients with chronic kidney disease to 48% in those with ESRD.[53] The relationship between renal dysfunction and OSA also may be bidirectional. OSA might contribute to renal dysfunction by exacerbating hypertension, diabetes mellitus, endothelial dysfunction, sympathetic neural activity, systemic inflammation, and oxidative stress.[54,55] Conversely, renal dysfunction may contribute to OSA, possibly owing to fluid overload that may increase UA edema. Support for a bidirectional relationship comes from data that demonstrate improvement in the AHI with intensive nocturnal hemodialysis in ESRD.[56] In addition, removal of fluid by ultrafiltration, without affecting uremia, was shown to improve the AHI in association with a decline in fluid volume of the neck.[57]

RISK FACTORS

Upper Airway Anatomy

Abnormal UA anatomy, resulting in smaller cross-sectional area, is an important factor contributing to OSA.[58] Although adiposity and elevated BMI are important risk factors, when matched for BMI, OSA subjects still demonstrate smaller minimum cross-sectional area of the UA than control subjects, indicating that factors other than BMI contribute to UA narrowing.[59] Magnetic resonance imaging (MRI) volumetric analyses demonstrated the importance of soft tissue factors, including increased volume of the lateral pharyngeal walls, soft palate, tongue, and parapharyngeal fat pads, that compromise the airway lumen in OSA.[60]

Pharyngeal collapse during sleep occurs most commonly in the retropalatal region. This portion of the UA is most susceptible to collapse because it is the narrowest segment of the airway and has the greatest compliance. Airway obstruction may also occur in the retroglossal, hypopharyngeal, and epiglottic regions.[61] MRI studies also demonstrated the role of increased tongue fat content in OSA subjects, which is mostly localized to the posterior region of the tongue and is a correlate of OSA severity. The increase in tongue fat may contribute to airway obstruction during sleep, not only by narrowing the airway but also by adversely affecting genioglossal function as a pharyngeal dilator.[62] Obesity may also indirectly contribute to UA collapsibility by reducing lung volume. Lower lung volume is associated with reduced tracheal caudal traction on the UA, which decreases stiffness of the lateral pharyngeal walls and promotes airway collapse.[63]

In addition to decreased cross-sectional area, differences in the shape and length of the UA are evident. An increased anterior-posterior dimension decreases efficiency of UA dilator muscles. Increased UA length contributes to its collapsibility.[60] Decreased size of the maxilla with a narrowed and high palatal arch and a small retropositioned mandible can narrow the UA.[64] The relationship of tongue volume to jaw size or craniofacial restriction has been shown to correlate with severity of OSA in both obese and nonobese subjects.[65]

UA collapse may also occur at the level of the epiglottis in up to 30% of subjects, which may contribute to a poor therapeutic response to CPAP or oral appliances. Epiglottic collapse may be related to aging-induced decreased collagen and elastin content of structures supporting the UA.[66]

Other factors that contribute to a narrow airway lumen in OSA include edema and inflammation of UA soft tissue, possibly owing to vibratory trauma from snoring.[67] In addition, rostral shift of blood volume and edema fluid from the lower extremities during recumbancy has been associated with increased neck circumference, elevated UA resistance, and increased AHI.[68] Normal males have increased pharyngeal length compared with age- and BMI-matched females, which may increase the propensity to UA collapse.[69]

Upper Airway Mechanics and Other Pathophysiologic Mechanisms Leading to Inspiratory Flow Limitation and Upper Airway Obstruction

The UA can be modeled as a collapsible tube through which air flows (Starling resistor) (Figure 131.2). The collapsibility of the airway is determined by the compliance and elastic properties of the airway, as well as tonic and phasic activity of the UA dilator muscles. During inspiration the pressure within the pharyngeal lumen becomes more negative with increasing inspiratory effort and/or narrowing of the lumen. The intraluminal pressure at which the UA collapses and zero airflow (obstructive apnea) occurs is termed the *critical closing pressure* (Pcrit) of the airway.[70] Pcrit of the passive oropharynx can vary widely: Pcrit in normal subjects was reported to be to be at -4.35 ± 4.15 cm H_2O, near atmospheric pressure in mild to moderate OSA at 0.56 ± 1.54 cm H_2O, and above atmospheric pressure in severe OSA at 2.23 ± 2.96 cm H_2O. When Pcrit is at or above atmospheric pressure, pharyngeal dilator muscle activity is required to maintain airway patency.[70]

Partial UA collapse may result in inspiratory flow limitation demonstrated by a flattened inspiratory flow-time waveform, Figure 131.3, *B*. However, although some patients exhibit a flat inspiratory flow-time curve when flow limited, others demonstrate a sharp reduction in flow from a peak at the onset of inspiration to mid-inspiration as driving pressure increases, a phenomenon termed *negative effort dependence* (NED), Figure 131.3, *C*.[71] More

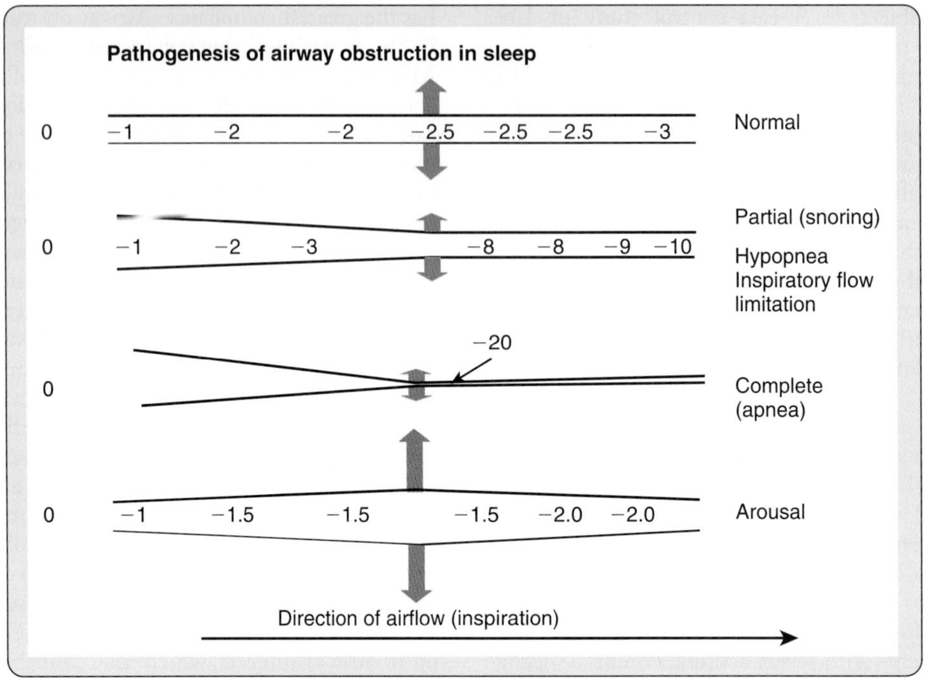

Figure 131.2 Pathogenesis of upper airway (UA) closure in obstructive sleep apnea (OSA). The UA is depicted as a tube. With inspiration, there is a small gradient of pressure in the direction of flow (*upper panel*). Even though pressure is slightly negative, the airway is held open by UA dilator muscles (*orange arrow*, force represented by length of the *arrow*). With narrowing of the UA and some decrease in abductor force, the gradient of airway pressure is greater; flow may become limited. Vibrations in the airway produce snoring. With complete closure of the UA, no air can flow. Pressure in the airway is negative and will be equal to intrathoracic pressure (no flow condition). Closure of the UA occurs because of decreased activity of UA dilator muscles. When brainstem and other appropriate receptors sense no airflow, with hypoxia and hypercapnia, UA dilators are activated and open the airway (*bottom panel*).

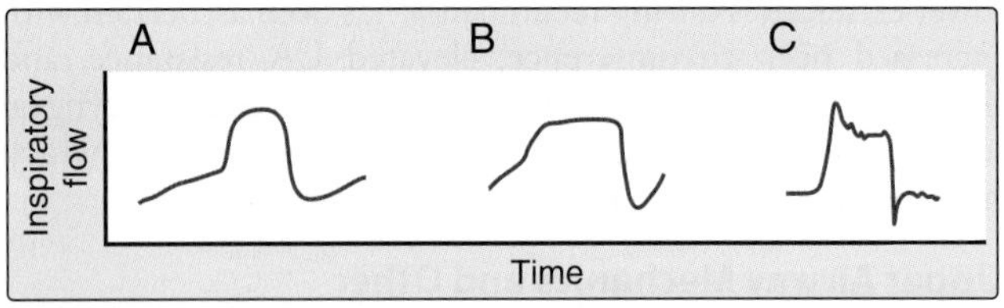

Figure 131.3 Inspiratory flow-time curves. **A,** Unobstructed breath. **B,** Inspiratory flow limitation: note flattened inspiratory flow-time curve where flow is independent of inspiratory effort or driving pressure. **C,** Negative effort dependence: Note abrupt reduction in flow from onset of inspiration to mid-inspiration.

compliant regions of the UA, such as the retropalatal area, rapidly collapse with increasing negative driving pressure leading to NED, whereas less compliant structures, such as the tongue base, typically do not obstruct further with increasing negative driving pressure and produce minimal or no NED.[61,71]

Physiologic traits other than anatomic or mechanical properties of the UA contribute to the occurrence and severity of OSA.[70,72] Understanding these traits may ultimately lead to targeted personalized multimodality therapy (see Chapter xx). Physiologic traits that contribute to OSA, aside from *UA collapsibility* (high Pcrit), have been identified.[73] These include:

- *Loop gain*: Loop gain quantifies response of the ventilatory system to decrements in ventilation, such as those induced by UA obstruction. High loop gain results in excessive ventilatory response to apnea or hypopnea, contributing to ventilatory instability and perpetuates back-to-back apneas.
- *Arousal threshold*: A low arousal threshold, with frequent arousals resulting from ventilatory disturbances, can destabilize sleep and ventilation by causing rapid changes in the sleep-wake ventilatory set point for carbon dioxide (CO_2), with reduction in ventilatory drive to the UA dilator muscles when sleep resumes after arousal and wakefulness ventilatory drive is lost.
- *Upper airway dilator muscle responsiveness/effectiveness*: In some patients, inadequate activation of UA dilator muscles in response to obstruction is a predominant pathophysiologic feature. In others, UA dilators do not effectively open the airway.

CLINICAL IDENTIFICATION AND ASSESSMENT

Signs and Symptoms of Obstructive Sleep Apnea

Snoring, nocturnal choking or gasping, reported apneas, dry mouth in the morning, sleepiness, and restless sleep are common symptoms in OSA. Most patients with OSA will report snoring, but many patients who do not have OSA will also report snoring. Nocturnal choking/gasping may be the most useful individual complaint suggesting OSA.[74] The other symptoms taken individually may have a limited utility in diagnosing OSA. A morning headache has a low sensitivity for detection of OSA but high specificity.[74] Therefore caution should be exercised in diagnosing OSA solely on the basis of individual reported symptoms; rather, the number and pattern of symptoms should be considered.

Dry mouth in the morning, reported by about a third of OSA patients, may be due to mouth breathing during sleep. Of interest, a response of almost always having a dry mouth upon awakening increased linearly from 22.4% to 34.5% to 40.7% in those with mild, moderate, or severe OSA, respectively.[75]

Nocturia may be a symptom of OSA.[76] This may be due to atrial natriuretic peptide, which has been shown to increase during sleep in OSA.[77,78] With CPAP treatment, both the frequency of nocturia and urine volume are decreased.[79]

Gastroesophageal reflux disease (GERD), particularly at night, may be a symptom of OSA.[80] Nocturnal reflux symptoms were associated with severity of OSA[81] and with worse sleep efficiency.[82] Treatment with CPAP improved GERD symptoms and reduced 24-hour acid contact time in the esophagus.[81,83,84] OSA was associated with an increased risk of Barrett esophagus, which is a pathologic finding in patients with long-standing GERD.[85] The common association of OSA with GERD may be a result of large decreases in intrathoracic pressure coupled with increases in intraabdominal pressure occurring during obstructed inspiratory efforts. This altered pressure gradient may facilitate movement of gastric acid across the lower esophageal sphincter into the esophagus. Alternatively, obesity, which increases risk for hiatal hernia, may be the primary factor leading to this association.[86]

About 20% of OSA patients complain of a morning headache.[87] Possible mechanisms of headache include hypercarbia, hypoxia, or poor sleep. Such headaches usually resolve within 4 hours.[88] To qualify as a sleep apnea–related headache, symptoms have to resolve with OSA treatment. Morning headache has a relatively high sensitivity but poor specificity for OSA.

Sleepiness and Sleep Disturbance

Patients with OSA can present with sleepiness, fragmented sleep/insomnia, or may have minimal sleep complaints. Sleepiness in OSA is thought to arise from sleep disruption and sleep deprivation associated with frequent apneas or hypopneas. EDS is a term often used to describe a high degree of sleepiness. To quantify subjective sleepiness, the Epworth Sleepiness Scale (ESS) is a commonly used scale that asks the patient to fill out his or her likelihood of dozing in eight different situations. The ESS is high in OSA patients and increases with OSA severity.[89] However, sleepiness is not universally present in patients with OSA, and some do not complain of sleepiness and have a normal ESS. It has been reported that less than 50% of patients with moderate to severe OSA had EDS.[90] Thus the presence or absence of sleepiness should not be used to rule OSA in or out.

It is still important to assess EDS in patients with OSA because EDS is associated with a number of deleterious outcomes, including an increased risk for motor vehicle crashes,[91] occupational injury,[92] cognitive impairment in the elderly,[93] and worse quality of life among academic physicians.[94] The presence of EDS has also been shown to be predictor of long-term CPAP use in patients with OSA.[95]

Deficits in Cognition

A wide range of objectively documented cognitive deficits have been associated with OSA.[96,97] Subjective cognitive complaints, such as a sense of impaired concentration and worsening memory, are commonly reported by OSA patients.[98] Cognitive deficits could be due to intermittent hypoxia, sleep fragmentation/frequent arousals, or excessive daytime somnolence. Neuropsychological function can be broadly divided into attention, executive functioning, sensory motor processing, language, and mood/emotion/personality domains. Patients with OSA demonstrate impairments in many categories, although studies have often yielded inconsistent results on the types of impairments and whether there are impairments in specific domains.[97,99]

One meta-analysis of cognitive improvements with CPAP therapy for OSA showed a small improvement in attention but not in other cognitive domains.[100] However, another meta-analysis focusing on different subdomains of executive function showed improvements in executive function with CPAP.[101] Of interest, in a large randomized, sham-controlled trial, CPAP treatment improved executive function, but not other domains, at 2 months, but it did not show improvements in any cognitive domain at 6 months.[102] Nonetheless, these results support the notion that deficits in attention and executive function may be observed in OSA and may improve with treatment.

Patients with OSA have an increased risk of motor vehicle accidents,[103] including among commercial drivers.[104] CPAP treatment reduces the motor vehicle accident rate.[104] The higher motor vehicle accident rate in patients with OSA could be due to sleepiness, impaired attention, or other cognitive deficits.[105] In fact, patients with OSA performed far worse than control subjects in a simulated driving task and even worse than subjects impaired by alcohol. Objective sleepiness measured by a Multiple Sleep Latency Test and the AHI explained little of the variance in impaired driving performance, making individual prediction difficult.[106] These results highlight the importance of screening OSA patients for cognitive problems and assessing driving and occupational safety.

Depression

About a quarter of OSA patients are reported to have clinical depression.[107] Newly diagnosed OSA patients are twice as likely to develop depression within 1 year compared with control subjects.[108] The incidence of depression was found to be increased with increasing OSA severity.[109] CPAP therapy results in sustained improvement in depression scores, particularly in patients with moderate to severe OSA.[110,111] Although CPAP treatment typically improves depression-related symptoms, unresolved EDS was associated with persistence of depressive symptomatology, as was comorbid cardiovascular disease and female gender, highlighting the complexity of the association between depression and OSA.[112] Of note, although treatment with CPAP was shown to improve depression compared to oral placebo, randomized controlled trials comparing therapeutic CPAP to sham CPAP have not shown a benefit of CPAP in resolving depression.[113]

Physical Findings

The most commonly reported risk factor for OSA is obesity, especially if the BMI is more than 30 kg/m^2.[114] Patients with OSA have a larger neck circumference than normal subjects. The average neck circumference, measured at the superior border of the cricothyroid membrane in the upright position, was 43.7 ± 4.5 cm in patients with OSA and 39.6 ± 4.5 cm in normal subjects (P = .0001).[115] A neck circumference of at least 40 cm has a sensitivity of 61% and a specificity of 93% for OSA, regardless of gender.[116]

Examination of the UA should assess nasal patency, oropharyngeal anatomy, and craniofacial structure. Increased nasopharyngeal resistance, due to nasal septal deviation, turbinate hypertrophy, polyps, or other obstructing lesions, is associated with OSA.[117] The soft palate, uvula, base of tongue, and tonsils should be observed with attention to their size, length, and overall volume in relation to the oropharynx. A low-lying or redundant soft palate and uvula, often with edema or erythema due to vibratory trauma and inflammation from snoring, are frequently present in OSA. Both the Mallampati classification, which assesses oropharyngeal anatomy with the tongue protruded, and the Friedman classification, which is a similar assessment but without tongue protrusion, are commonly used to stage oropharyngeal crowding.[118] In addition, tonsil size should be assessed.

Retrognathia, or retrusion of the mandible, narrows the posterior air space and can increase the propensity for airway collapse during sleep. A high arched and narrow hard palate may also predispose to OSA. Assessment of dentition, in particular, the presence of overjet, defined as displacement of the mandibular teeth posteriorly compared with the maxillary teeth, is indicative of a small oral cavity that may result in posterior displacement of the base of the tongue, which can narrow the retroglossal airway.[119] Assessment of the condition of the molars is helpful, if oral device therapy is contemplated.

The association of OSA with a range of different ophthalmic conditions is increasingly recognized.[120] As the population prevalence of OSA is high, it can be expected that people with coexistent OSA will be found in any ophthalmic disease population studied. It is difficult to establish direct causation from OSA with the current evidence, but damage to the retinal vasculature could be caused by many of the pathophysiologic aspects of OSA, including apneas, intermittent hypoxia, increased respiratory efforts with intrathoracic pressure swings, arousals from sleep, sleep fragmentation, sympathetic activation with blood pressure surges, heart rate rises, and hypertension.

Anyone therefore presenting to the sleep clinic with a history of diabetic retinopathy (particularly diabetic macular edema), glaucoma, floppy eyelid syndrome, nonarteritic ischemic optic neuropathy (NAION), keratoconus, and age-related macular degeneration should have further evaluation for OSA in the context of other supporting symptoms. NAION, in particular, seems to have direct potential associations with OSA, as people wake up with a visual defect, which raises the question of the potential nocturnal impact of OSA on the eye.

Floppy eyelid syndrome, commonly seen in OSA,[121] may be apparent by observing easily turning and floppy eyelids, papillary conjunctivitis, and corneal epithelial erosions, but it is much more likely that the patient or medical record will provide the diagnosis. Fundoscopy can be helpful in diagnosing NAION, but the signs can be subtle. Acute disc swelling may be seen, which can progress over several months to optic disc pallor due to atrophy. An altitudinal field defect in the affected eye may be picked up (loss of the upper or lower hemifield) in confrontational field testing in clinic or with automated field testing.

ASSESSMENT

Questionnaire-Based Assessment

A number of standardized tools for screening for OSA have been developed. A recent task force[122] was commissioned by the American Academy of Sleep Medicine to review some 29 available screening tools for OSA in adults, to determine reliability, efficacy, and feasibility for use in clinical settings. Many tools have been developed to screen for OSA. No single tool is recommended.[122] However, a number of screening tools are currently in use and, although not perfect, are helpful when combined with clinical criteria for assessing risk for OSA in adults. In addition to screening for excessive sleepiness (ESS), a questionnaire, the STOP-BANG,[123] may be useful for screening for OSA in adult patients.

The mnemonic STOP-BANG includes the following:

- S: "Do you snore loudly, loud enough to be heard through a closed door?"
- T: "Do you feel tired or fatigued during the daytime almost every day?"
- O: "Has anyone observed that you stop breathing during sleep?"
- P: "Do you have a history of high blood pressure with or without treatment?"
- B: BMI > 35 kg/m^2
- A: Age > 50 years
- N: Neck circumference > 43 cm (17 in)
- G: Gender, male

When more than three items are positive, the sensitivity and specificity for OSA are 87% and 31%, respectively.

DIAGNOSTIC TESTING

Types of Sleep Studies

Sleep testing is currently classified into levels of complexity. Type 1 is the classic in-laboratory full PSG as discussed previously, including measures of airflow, respiratory effort, oxygenation, electroencephalogram, electrooculogram, and electromyogram, to allow for sleep staging. Type 2 is an out-of-laboratory portable study essentially equivalent to the in-laboratory study (minimum of seven parameters). Type 3 is an unattended portable recording measuring at least four channels: heart rate, oxygen saturation, airflow, respiratory effort, but no sleep staging. Type 4 is an unattended portable study, measuring a minimum of three channels, such as heart rate, oxygen saturation, and respiratory analysis.

In-Laboratory or Full Polysomnographic Sleep Testing

The diagnosis of sleep apnea should be confirmed objectively by sleep testing. The gold standard test is PSG (see Chapter 200), a multichannel assessment of physiologic variables performed in a laboratory equipped with proper sensors, trained personnel, and a standardized way of recording results, with a qualified individual to interpret the study. Many laboratories also record continuous video imaging of the patient, both for medical-legal reasons and to observe parasomnias. Table 131.2 contains a list of some of the most common variables recorded during in-laboratory PSG testing; typical PSG epochs with recordings of these parameters are presented in Figures 131.1 and 131.4.

Technical specifications and acceptable derivations for in-laboratory PSG testing are specified in the *American Academy of Sleep Medicine (AASM) Scoring Manual*,[124] as well as elsewhere in this volume, as are the visual rules for sleep staging, respiratory events, limb movement events, and other "events" of note.

The *AASM Scoring Manual*[124] recommends that the primary means for detecting apnea is absence of the oronasal thermistor signal, although alternatives are suggested. The manual recommends that the primary method for identifying hypopnea should be nasal pressure, although alternatives are also suggested. During PAP titrations, it is recommended to use the change in PAP mask pressure as the primary flow signal. The manual recommends the use of esophageal manometry or respiratory impedance plethysmography thoracoabdominal belts as the primary measure of respiratory effort. For detection

Table 131.2 Variables Commonly Recorded during In-Laboratory Polysomnography

Variable Recorded	Purpose	Comment
Electroencephalogram (EEG) (several channels) Electromyogram (EMG) of submentalis muscle (or other facial as indicated) Electrooculogram (EOG)	Sleep staging	Use standard 10/20 system for EEG. Fewer channels are generally recorded for sleep staging than for seizure focus localization. If nocturnal seizure foci are suspected, consider using a suitable montage. Epochs recorded for sleep are generally 20 to 30 sec long, whereas shorter epochs are generally used for seizure detection
Oronasal airflow	Sleep-related changes in airflow	Nasal air pressure to detect apneas, hypopneas, flow limitation. Thermistor for backup for apneas
Microphone	Snore detection	Some systems use airflow perturbations as a measure of snoring
End-tidal carbon dioxide (CO_2) measures Transcutaneous CO_2 measures	Assessment of alveolar ventilation	Transcutaneous CO_2 generally suitable for thin-skinned individuals, such as infants and children, may also be used in adults
Pulse oximetry	Assessment of changes in pulse and oxygen saturation	Some definitions of DBEs incorporate criteria for event-related desaturation (3% or 4%). The extent to which oxygen saturation falls during a DBE will depend on the length of the event, underlying oxygen stores, and underlying lung function
Respiratory effort	Determination if DBEs are related to obstruction of the upper airway (obstructive) or cessation of central neurologic respiratory output (central)	Most commonly used are measures of respiratory system movement (rib cage, abdomen). Measures of respiratory effort used in research or special situation include respiratory muscle EMG (diaphragm, parasternal) and esophageal pressure
Body position	Record changes in body position and correlate these to respiratory events	
EMG: anterior tibialis	Detect movement of the legs	In special circumstances the EMG of other muscle groups, such as the deltoid, may be recorded
Electrocardiogram	Abnormalities of cardiac rate and rhythm	Generally a single lead, sometimes not standardized

DBEs, Disordered breathing events.

of snoring, microphones, piezoelectric sensors, or perturbations in nasal air pressure are all considered acceptable. The reader is referred to this publication for more detailed analysis.

The severity of sleep apnea is usually defined in terms of frequency of respiratory "events." These include "apneas" (cessation or near-cessation of airflow), and "hypopneas" (reduction in airflow with accompanying physiologic changes) (see later). In general, a greater frequency of such events per hour of sleep is associated with a more severe clinical syndrome. However, many patients with a "severe" respiratory event index have minimal symptoms, and many with a "mild" index have severe sleepiness. In general, severity of OSA, as estimated from accepted techniques of respiratory event indexes, appears to be a reliable predictor of neurocognitive changes, such as sleepiness and vigilance.

Sleep-related respiratory events have been defined in various ways. In adults a respiratory event must last at least 10 seconds, usually equivalent to at least two breaths for the average adult.[5,6,8,9] "Apneas" are universally defined as airflow decreased to less than 10% of the baseline. They are further characterized as "obstructive," "central," or "mixed." Obstructive apneas are characterized by cessation or near-cessation of airflow, with continued evidence of respiratory effort (Figure 131.5). This is related to obstruction of the UA while respiratory effort continues. Central apneas are characterized by cessation or near-cessation of airflow with absence of respiratory effort (Figure 131.6). That is, breathing stops because of loss of neurologic respiratory output. Mixed apneas are characterized by cessation and near-cessation of airflow for at least 10 seconds. The early part of the event appears central, whereas the latter appears obstructive (Figure 131.5).

Partial reductions in inspiratory airflow or hypopneas also occur. The current requirement (AASM) is for a 30% to 90% reduction in airflow, accompanied a physiologic consequence. In the United States the current recommendations for hypopneas for adults generally follow the AASM definitions. However, the Centers for Medicare and Medicaid Services (CMS) continues to use the definitions of disordered breathing events from an earlier version of the AASM criteria. See Table 131.3. Many insurance providers have specific guidelines for authorizing treatment for OSA depending on severity. Most older individuals will qualify for treatment based on either set of criteria. However, many younger patients judged eligible for treatment by AASM criteria are not eligible according to CMS criteria.[125]

Definitions for disordered breathing events in adults and children are shown in Tables 131.3 and 131.4. Because the respiratory rate in children is more rapid than in adults, most events in children incorporate a recommended length of at least two respiratory cycles. However, there are exceptions (see Table 131.4).

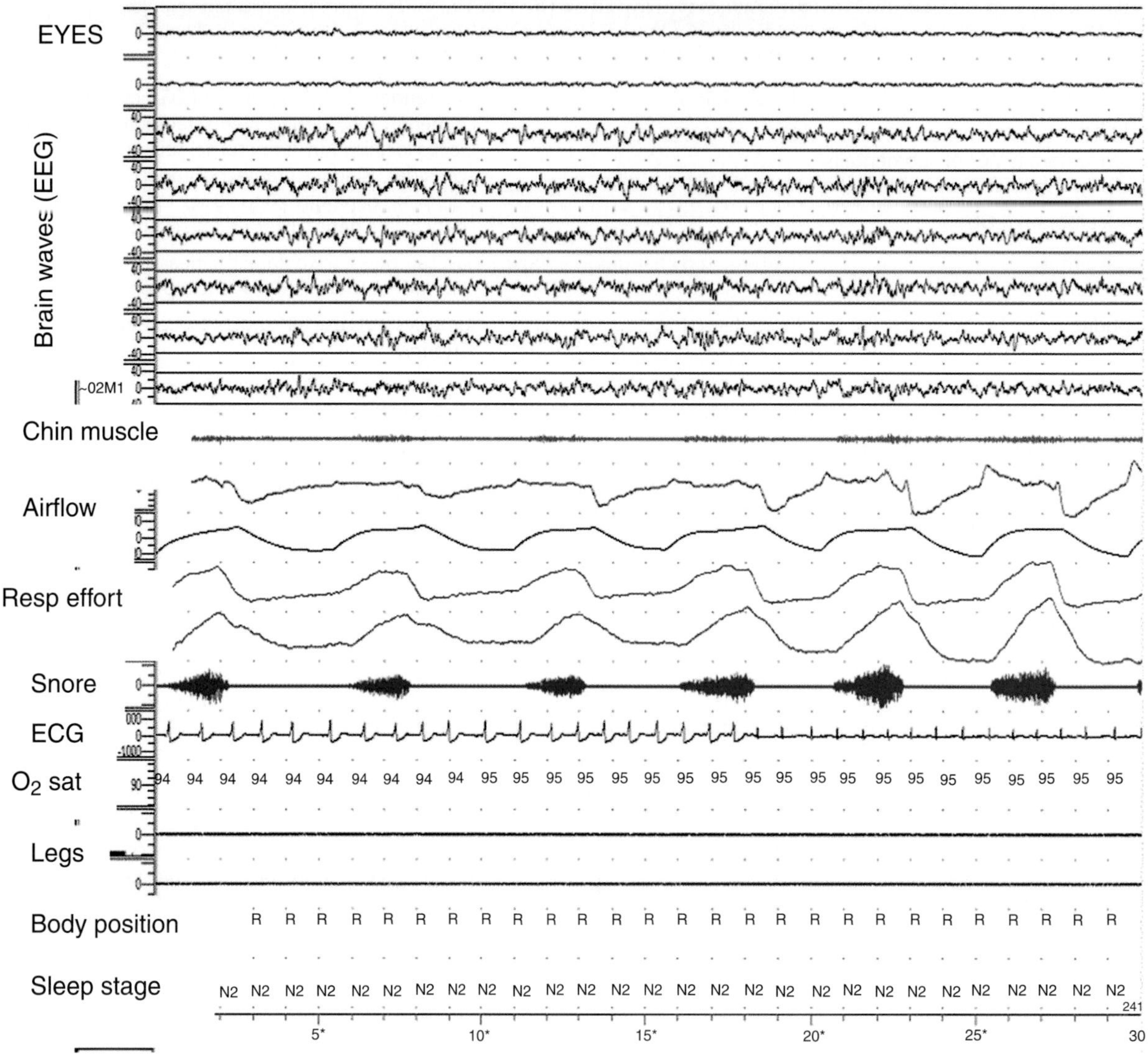

Figure 131.4 Sample montage for polysomnography: "Eye" movements for left and right eyes (*upper* and *lower trace,* respectively); "EEG" (electroencephalogram) for six selected leads; "Chin": submentalis electromyogram (EMG) to aid in staging rapid eye movement; airflow: measured by thermistor and nasal air pressure (*upper* and *lower trace,* respectively); "Resp (respiratory) effort" recorded from impedance pneumography belts from rib cage and abdomen (*upper* and *lower traces,* respectively); snore is measured from a microphone taped to the neck; "ECG" (electrocardiogram); "O_2 sat" (oxygen saturation) is measured from a pulse oximeter; "Legs": anterior tibialis EMG measured from right and left legs (*upper* and *lower trace,* respectively); "Body position" from a position sensor (patient is in the right lateral position); "Sleep stage" is scored by a technologist. This epoch is 30 seconds long.

Severity criteria: For adults, most definitions apply the term *mild* if the AHI is 5 to 14.9 events per hour of sleep; the term *moderate* is applied if the AHI is 15 to 29.9 per hour of sleep, and the term *severe* is applied if the AHI is greater than or equal to 30 per hour of sleep. For children (≥1 year of age) the term *mild* is applied for AHI 1 to 4.9 per hour of sleep; the term *moderate* is applied for AHI 5 to 9.9 per hour of sleep, and the term *severe* is applied for AHI greater than or equal to 10 per hour of sleep. When does an individual transition from childhood to adulthood? The AASM suggests age 18 years being the onset of adulthood. However, recognizing the ambiguity and uncertainty of this, the laboratory director is allowed to specify the onset of "adulthood" as greater than or equal to 13 years.

There is a type of disordered breathing event that does not quite meet the criteria for apneas or hypopneas but nevertheless has a physiologic consequence, primarily leading to sleep fragmentation due to postevent arousals. These are called "respiratory event–related arousals" (RERAs) and are associated with flow limitation (Figure 131.7). Detection of flow limitation is not possible with thermistors or any other sensor that simply records the presence or absence of flow (e.g., tidal CO_2 monitoring). Therefore preference should be given to using nasal air pressure recording.

Finally, "hypoventilation" is defined for adults when the end-tidal or transcutaneous partial pressure of carbon dioxide (Pco_2) is greater than 55 mm Hg for greater than or equal to 10 minutes. For children, "hypoventilation" is scored when

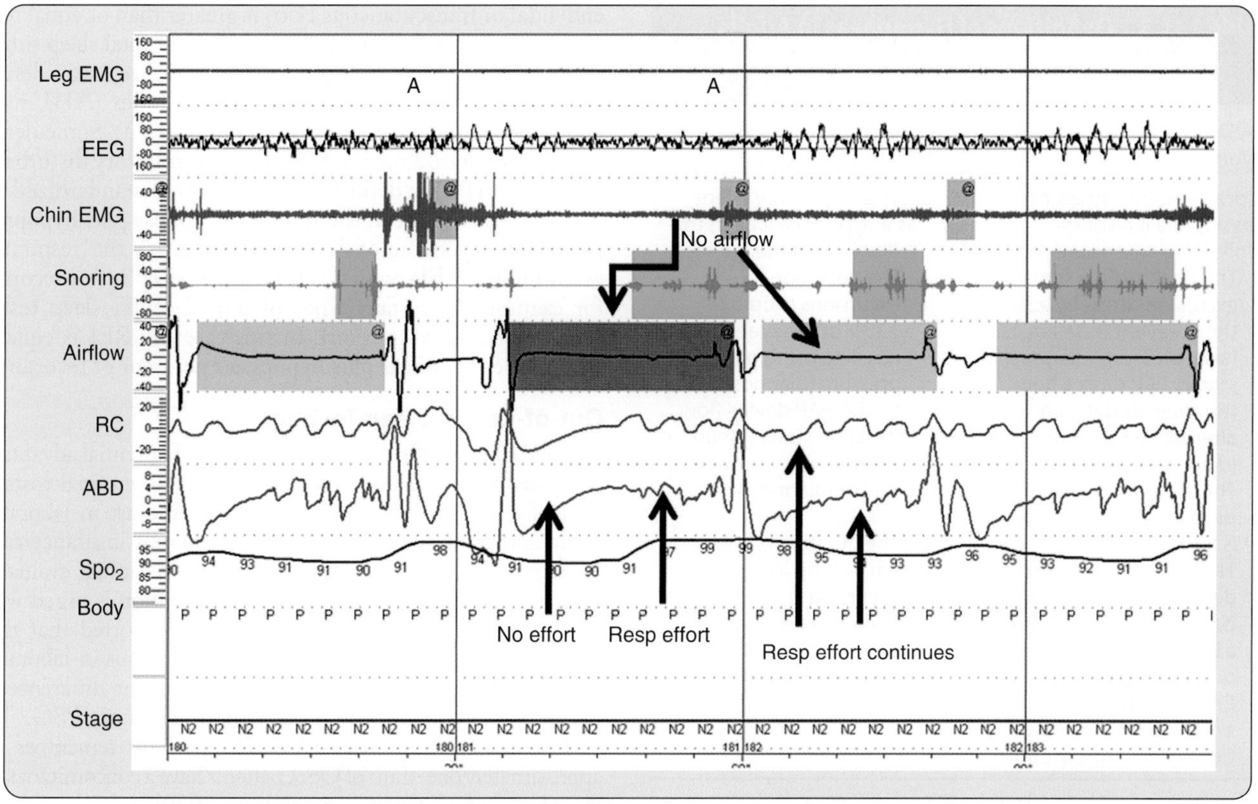

Figure 131.5 Examples of "obstructive" and "mixed" apneas. See text for definitions. ABD, Abdomen; EEG, electroencephalogram; EMG, electromyogram; RC, rib cage; Resp, respiratory; Spo_2, saturation of peripheral oxygen.

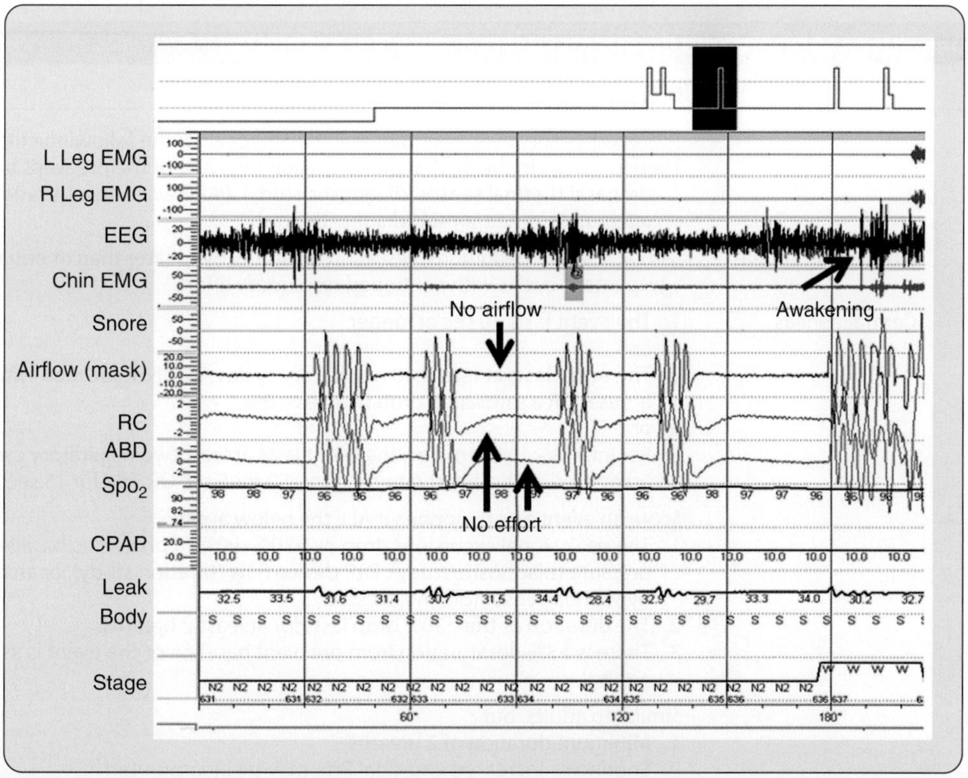

Figure 131.6 Example of central apneas in an adult. See text for definitions. ABD, Abdomen; CPAP, continuous positive airway pressure, EEG, electroencephalogram; EMG, electromyogram; RC, rib cage; Spo_2, saturation of peripheral oxygen.

Table 131.3 Definitions of Hypopneas in Adults According to AASM and CMS: Duration of Event: 10 Seconds

AASM Criteria for Scoring Hypopneas	CMS Criteria for Scoring Hypopneas
Score a respiratory event as hypopnea if all of the following criteria are met: 1. The peak airflow signal excursion drops by ≥30% of the preevent baseline using nasal pressure (diagnostic study), PAP device flow (titration study), or an alternative hypopnea sensor (diagnostic study). 2. The duration of the >30% drop in signal excursion is >10 sec. 3. There is a >3% oxygen desaturation from preevent baseline and/or the event is associated with an arousal. *or* Criteria 1 and 2 and there is a >4% oxygen desaturation from preevent baseline.	Score a respiratory event as a hypopnea if all of the following criteria are met: 1. The peak signal excursions drop by >30% of the preevent baseline using nasal pressure (diagnostic study), PAP device flow (titration study), or an alternative hypopnea sensor (diagnostic study). 2. The duration of the >30% drop in signal excursion is >10 sec. 3. There is a >4% oxygen desaturation from preevent baseline.

AASM, American Academy of Sleep Medicine; CMS, Centers for Medicare and Medicaid Services; PAP, positive airway pressure.
For both sets of scoring criteria, "apneas" are scored when there is a reduction of airflow by ≥90% for at least 10 sec compared to baseline. Classification into obstructive, central, or mixed apnea is explained in the text.

end-tidal or transcutaneous P_{CO_2} is greater than or equal to 50 mm Hg for greater than or equal to 25% of total sleep time.

Regarding other measures of severity, we have defined severity in terms of the apnea-hypopnea index (AHI: number of apneas plus hypopneas per hour of sleep). Some definitions incorporate a measure called the "respiratory disturbance index" (RDI). This definition is not as well standardized but has been used to mean the number of apneas plus hypopneas plus RERAs per hour of sleep. Another term is the "respiratory event index" (REI), which is used when sleep is not recorded, for example, in certain types of out-of-center sleep testing (OCST) (see next section). In this case the REI is equal to the number of apneas plus hypopneas per hour of recording.

Out-of-Center Sleep Testing

Limited-channel OCST offers a number of potential advantages compared with in-laboratory PSG.[126] First, the initial costs are generally less than those of the state-of-the-art in-laboratory study, and primarily for this reason, numerous insurance carriers require OCST for reimbursement in the initial evaluation of many patients with suspected OSA. Caution is urged when using OCST. However, two studies have reported that there was no long-term cost saving using OCST versus in-laboratory PSG.[127,128] There are apparently no significant differences in health outcomes between OCST and in-laboratory PSG.[129]

In considering the use of OCST, one must remember that approximately one-third of OSA patients have a concomitant sleep disorder,[130] of which approximately two-thirds require treatment. Thus patients need to be evaluated by a professional skilled in the evaluation and management of sleep disorders, whether OCST, in-laboratory PSG, or both are used in the diagnostic assessment.

Table 131.4 Definitions of Disordered Breathing Events during Sleep: Children

Event Type		Definition
Apneas		Score respiratory events as apneas if they meet all of the following criteria: There is a drop in the peak signal excursion by ≥90% of the preevent baseline using an oronasal thermal sensor (diagnostic study), PAP device flow (titration study), or an *alternative* apnea sensor (diagnostic study)
	Obstructive apneas	Similar to adult definitions, cessation of airflow by greater than or equal to two respiratory cycles with continued respiratory effort.
	Central apneas	1. The event lasts 20 sec or longer. *or* 2. The event lasts at least two respiratory cycles AND is associated with postapneic arousal OR a saturation drop of at least 3%. *or* 3. For infants <1 year of age, the event lasts at least two respiratory cycles and is associated with a heart rate drop to <50 for 5 sec OR <60 for 15 sec.
Hypopneas		Score an event as a hypopnea if ALL the below apply: 1. The peak signal excursions drop by ≥30%–90% of preevents baseline using nasal pressure (diagnostic study), PAP device flow (titration study), or an *alternative* hypopnea sensor (diagnostic study). 2. The duration of the ≥30% drop lasts for at least 2 breaths. 3. There is ≥3% desaturation from preevent baseline or the event is associated with an arousal.
RERAs (optional)		Similar to adults, but 1. Minimum duration of 2 breaths 2. Snoring or increased end-tidal P_{CO_2} may be incorporated

PAP, Positive airway pressure; P_{CO_2}, partial pressure of carbon dioxide; RERAs, respiratory event-related arousals.
Age: Children are defined as <18 years old. However, the laboratory director or other sleep specialist has the option of defining children as <13 years old.

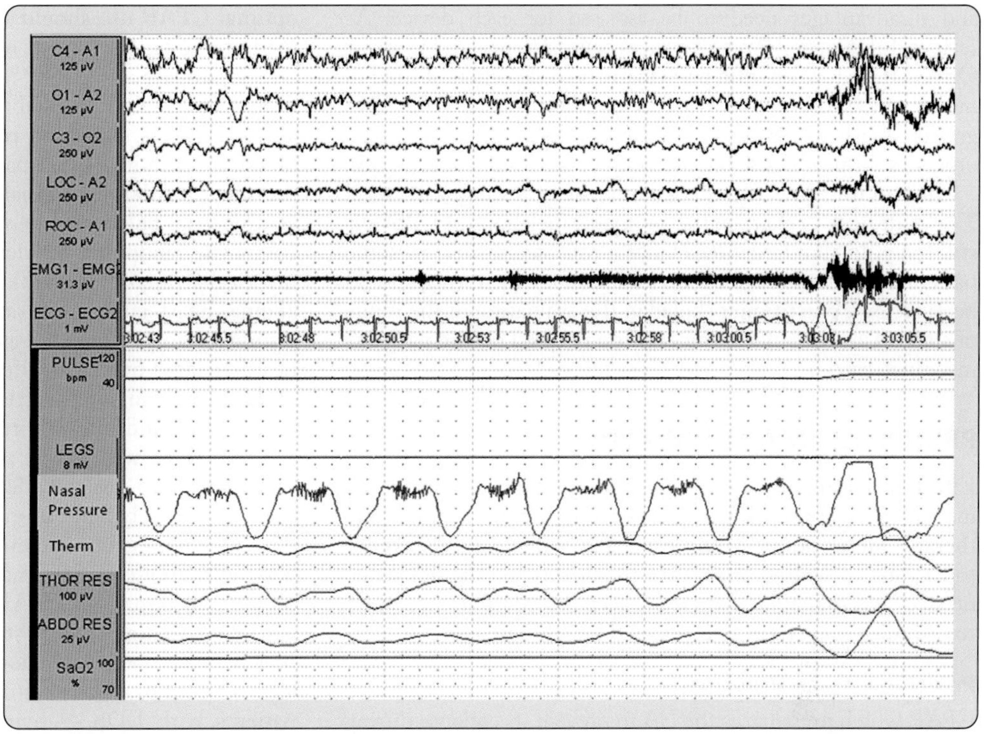

Figure 131.7 Example of inspiratory flow limitation or a respiratory event–related arousal (RERA). Compare airflow measured by oronasal thermistor (Therm), with that measured by nasal pressure (NP). For the NP signal, the inspiratory direction is up, expiratory direction down. Note that with the NP transducer, inspiratory flow limitation (flattening of the signal and snoring) is readily detected. Note the arousal after this event (electroencephalogram [EEG] and electromyogram [EMG]). The first three channels are EEG, left electrooculogram (EOG; left electrooculogram [LOC], and right EOG (right electrooculogram [ROC]). ABDO, Abdominal; ECG, electrocardiogram; EMG, submentalis EMG; Legs, pretibial EMG; pulse is derived from the pulse oximeter; RES, respiratory effort; Sa_{O_2}, oxygen saturation; THOR, thoracic.

Because of the limitations of OCST for detection of nonrespiratory sleep disorders, many insurance carriers prefer to authorize OCST for initial evaluation but will allow exceptions to OCST in certain patients and allow in-laboratory sleep disorders. Most of these will be suspected based on a careful and thorough sleep history. Table 131.5 lists common reasons for *not* performing OCST in patients suspected of OSA. However, individual insurance providers have specific reasons for allowing in-laboratory studies to be performed, and the requirements of each carrier should be determined.

Attempts at simplified screening for OSA based on recording one or a limited number of variables includes oximetry,[131] sophisticated analysis of an electrocardiogram,[132] and peripheral arterial tonometry (PAT). The latter is a device placed on the finger and measures pulse oximetry and volume of the finger.[133] The abrupt arousals associated with termination of obstructive events are associated with bursts of sympathetic discharge causing vasoconstriction that decreases the volume of the digit. In addition to PAT and standard oximetry, the device records pulse rate and movement (actigraphy). The RDI measured using PAT was highly correlated with RDI measured during in-laboratory PSG. The area under the receiver-operating curve was 0.82 and 0.87 for thresholds of RDI = 10 per hour and RDI = 20 per hour, respectively. The photoplethysmograph (PPG) measures pulse, oxygen saturation, and peripheral digital volume, which are analyzed by proprietary algorithms that generate clinically relevant respiratory waveforms and approximation of the sleep-wake state. A study using the AASM 2012 apnea-hypopnea detection scoring parameters validated this device against standard in-laboratory PSG and showed excellent correlation between the PPG- and PSG-derived AHI.[134]

Table 131.5 Some Reasons for NOT Doing OCST for Diagnosis of OSA

Age <18 years	
Patient lacks cognitive or physical ability to put on equipment	
Chronic obstructive pulmonary disease	
Congestive heart failure	
Neuromuscular disorders	Parkinson disease
	Amyotrophic lateral sclerosis
	Spina bifida
Comorbid sleep disorders	Periodic limb movement disorder/ restless legs syndrome
	Parasomnia
	Central sleep apnea
	Nocturnal seizures
	Narcolepsy
Previous OCST is negative despite high clinical suspicion for OSA	
Previous home study technically inadequate to establish Dx of OSA	
Super obesity (BMI >40 or 50)	

BMI, Body mass index; Dx, diagnosis; OSA, obstructive sleep apnea; OCST, out-of-center sleep testing.
Note: the requirements for individual insurance providers should be clarified when ordering studies for particular patients.

There has been an explosion in development of devices for sleep apnea detection in the home environment. A thorough review of many devices was published in 2018.[135] The advantages and disadvantages need to be assessed for each device. As reviewed elsewhere,[136] type 3 devices have false-negative rates for OSA of 13% to 20%, with particularly poor detection of mild to moderate OSA. Type 4 devices (lacking sleep staging) may have greater false-negative rates. Further, when concomitant sleep disorders are suspected, OCST will not give the complete diagnosis.

The bottom line regarding home sleep testing with level 3 or 4 devices is that, at the moment, in-laboratory PSG is still the gold standard. OCST has a role (see earlier) in some patients, but the decision as to which mode of testing should be made by a practitioner skilled in the evaluation of the range of sleep disorders. Often the decision is based on the patient's insurance carrier.

PRINCIPLES OF MANAGEMENT

Effective treatment requires a patient-centered chronic disease management approach that goes beyond initial diagnosis and therapy prescription. Monitoring and enhancing adherence to therapy, providing alternative therapeutic modalities when needed, and managing comorbid sleep disorders are necessary to optimize long-term sleep-related health outcomes.

Positive Airway Pressure

CPAP, which pressurizes the UA to prevent its collapse during sleep, remains the mainstay of therapy for OSA (see Chapter 132). Initiation and prescription of CPAP may be accomplished by in-laboratory PSG with CPAP titration, which determines CPAP pressure requirements for all stages of sleep in all sleep positions. Alternatively, autotitrating positive airway pressure (APAP) devices may be used to initiate therapy. Data supporting APAP for initiation of CPAP therapy are limited but show noninferiority with regard to adherence and impact on daytime somnolence.[137,138] Patients with comorbid cardiopulmonary disorders, especially those with obesity hypoventilation syndrome, nocturnal hypoventilation due to neuromuscular disorders, CSA, and Hunter-Cheyne-Stokes breathing are not candidates for APAP therapy.

Most placebo-controlled studies demonstrated improvement in subjective measures of daytime somnolence, whereas data are mixed with regard to objective measures.[139] A systematic analysis demonstrated that CPAP improves both subjective and objective measures of daytime sleepiness, especially in severe OSA (AHI > 30/hour).[140] Similarly, clinical trials of the effects of CPAP on neurobehavioral and cognitive performance, as well as on overall quality of life, are mixed, with some studies demonstrating benefit.[102] A randomized placebo-controlled clinical trial in patients with mild to moderate OSA with a complaint of daytime somnolence showed an improvement in functional outcomes, including quality of life, subjective daytime sleepiness, and mood, compared with sham CPAP.[141]

In a multicenter effectiveness study that used both subjective and objective measures of daytime somnolence and quality of life as outcome measures, a greater percentage of patients achieved improvements in both subjective and objective measures of daytime somnolence and quality of life with longer nightly duration of CPAP use, up to 7 hours per night. Although the mean nightly duration of CPAP use in this trial was 4.7 ± 2.2 hours, a substantial minority of patients demonstrated benefit with a shorter duration of nightly CPAP use, although some subjects exhibited residual sleepiness with more than 7 hours of use per night. Thus assessment of optimal CPAP use should rely not only on hours of nightly use but also on assessment of relevant treatment outcomes.[142]

The impact of CPAP on cardiovascular outcomes has been more difficult to establish in randomized controlled trials. CPAP was shown to reduce morning, but not evening, blood pressure in a OSA patients with well-controlled blood pressure.[143] A large multinational randomized secondary prevention trial failed show an effect of CPAP on the primary composite endpoint of death from cardiovascular causes, myocardial infarction, stroke, or hospitalization for unstable angina, heart failure, or transient ischemic attack, although significant improvement was noted in daytime sleepiness and health-related quality of life.[144] It is worth noting that most of the participants in this trial were men who had moderate to severe OSA and minimal to moderate sleepiness (ESS ≤15) and that those with severe sleepiness and hypoxemia (oxygen saturation [Sa_{O_2}] values <80%) were excluded. Thus patients most likely to benefit from CPAP were excluded from the trial. Further, mean adherence to therapy was only 3.3 hours per night. These factors may have contributed to failure to observe an impact of CPAP on cardiovascular and cerebrovascular outcomes. Such studies are also difficult to interpret because specific phenotypes of OSA may predispose to adverse cardiovascular outcomes. Such phenotypes include patients with EDS,[145] hypoxic burden,[146] rapid eye movement–associated sleep apnea,[147] and other PSG features.[148] It has been suggested that future clinical trials should focus on these subgroups of OSA patients to better assess the impact of treatment.[149]

The efficacy of CPAP is limited by suboptimal adherence. Many measures have been introduced to improve adherence to CPAP therapy: technologic improvements in PAP delivery, educational and supportive efforts, and cognitive behavioral therapy. An approach using automated CPAP adherence telemonitoring with patient feedback via text messaging improved CPAP adherence without additional provider intervention.[150]

Central apneas may emerge during CPAP therapy and disrupt sleep, limiting efficacy and tolerability of CPAP. *Treatment-emergent CSA* may occur in 4% to 20% of OSA patients treated with CPAP. In many cases treatment-emergent CSA will resolve over weeks to months, although it may persist in approximately one-third of cases.[151] Hunter-Cheyne-Stokes respiration, which is also not well treated with CPAP, is common in patients with systolic heart failure and may also contribute to failure of CPAP therapy in this population. Reassessment of sleep-disordered breathing in patients intolerant of CPAP may identify the emergence of these forms of sleep-disordered breathing that may require alternative therapeutic modalities.

Oral Appliances

Mandibular advancement oral appliances can be considered either as first-line therapy for mild to moderate OSA or as an alternative for patients intolerant of CPAP. Mandibular protrusion increases the retropalatal airway by lateral expansion and augments the oropharyngeal and retroglossal airway by anterior movement of the tongue base.[152] Although not as effective as CPAP in eliminating disordered breathing events, improvement in functional outcomes and systemic hypertension achieved with oral appliances is similar in magnitude to that seen with CPAP, which may reflect better adherence to therapy.[153,154] However, because of the variable response to oral appliances, it is important

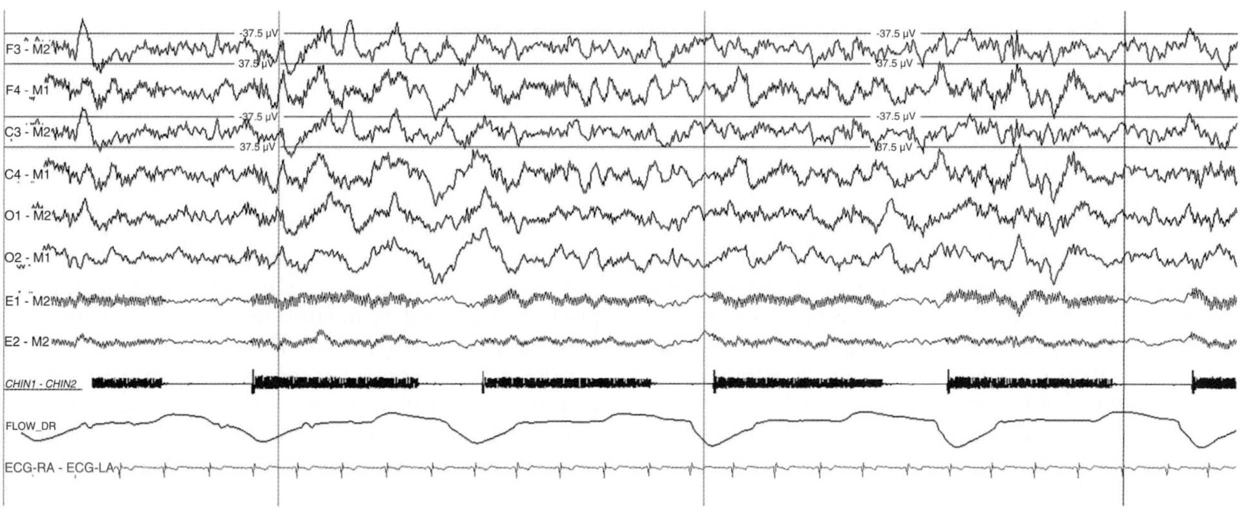

Figure 131.8 Polysomnographic segment during hypoglossal nerve stimulation (HGNS). Note increased genioglossal inspiratory activation in response to HGNS. ECG-LA, Electrocardiogram at left arm; ECG-RA, electrocardiogram at right arm.

to perform follow-up PSG or OCST to assess efficacy of the appliance because subjective reports may not reliably predict improvement in the AHI. In a study of patients with mild to severe OSA, only 65% of the cohort who had subjective symptomatic improvement with oral appliance therapy achieved an AHI of less than or equal to 10 per hour on follow-up PSG. The degree of mandibular advancement was then increased in the incomplete responders. An additional 30% of the cohort achieved an AHI of less than or equal to 10 per hour after this secondary adjustment, indicating the importance of the follow-up PSG.[155] Better predictors of response to oral appliances and accurate determination of the optimal degree of mandibular advancement may improve utility and efficacy of this modality.

Features associated with oral appliance efficacy include a moderately, but not highly, collapsible pharynx (as assessed by measures of Pcrit), weaker UA dilator muscle compensation for airway obstruction, lower loop gain (reflecting greater ventilatory stability), and higher arousal threshold (reflecting greater sleep stability). These findings are plausible because oral appliances may be unable to correct more severe pharyngeal collapsibility; in addition, ventilatory control and sleep instability may not be resolved with a structural intervention. To identify optimal settings for oral appliances, the following approaches have been used: remote titration of oral appliances during PSG,[156] visualization of velopharyngeal widening with mandibular advancement during awake nasopharyngoscopy, or drug-induced sleep endoscopy (DISE).[157] These are seldom used clinically. Mandibular advancement devices have been associated with dental occlusive changes with prolonged use, suggesting the importance of extended dental follow-up.[158]

Surgical Therapy

Electrical stimulation of the hypoglossal nerve was developed in response to the observation that inadequate neural activation of the UA dilator muscles is a key factor in the pathophysiology of OSA.[159] The most commonly used device delivers phasic electrical pulses to the hypoglossal nerve at the onset of inspiration, augmenting genioglossal inspiratory activity (Figure 131.8). Surgical implantation of the device is described in Chapter 175. Current guidelines limit this therapy to adult patients with moderate to severe OSA, AHI 15 to 65 per hour, and BMI less than or equal to 32 kg/m^2. In addition, drug-induced sleep endoscopy is performed to exclude patients with concentric retropalatal collapse, which may indicate UA fat and soft tissue distribution that limits efficacy. There is a durable clinical response, with approximately 70% of patients achieving greater than 50% improvement in the AHI and an AHI less than 20 per hour, with improvement in daytime sleepiness and quality of life. Average therapy usage is 5.6 ± 2.1 hours per night after 12 months, which is greater than that reported in most trials for CPAP. Adverse effects are minimal and mostly relate to stimulation-induced discomfort.[160]

Other sleep surgical procedures, with the goal of reducing UA collapsibility during sleep, can reduce the burden of sleep-disordered breathing and play a role in chronic disease management when other options have failed. In the era of precision medicine, targeted UA examination using fiberoptic nasopharyngoscopy, DISE, and radiologic imaging offers important tools to identify predominant sites of obstruction in the nasopharynx, velopharynx, lateral pharyngeal walls, base of the tongue, and the epiglottis.[161] Details of surgical management can be found in Chapter 175. Evaluation of the nasopharynx is especially important because treating nasal obstruction with septoplasty, inferior turbinate reduction, or nasal valve stabilization may improve PAP adherence and reduce pressure requirements; it may also improve acceptance of oral appliance therapy.[162] Assessment of UA soft tissue, including tonsils, velopharynx, lateral pharyngeal walls, and tongue base, is important for targeted surgery. A clinical staging system based on observation of the oropharynx, such as that offered by Friedman and colleagues,[118] and which classifies palate position, tonsil size, and BMI, can be a useful predictor of outcome of palatal surgery and tonsillectomy. These authors showed that the best response is achieved when the inferior border of the palate is above the base of the tongue, with enlarged tonsils and BMI less than 40 kg/m^2. Other palate and pharyngeal surgical procedures have been developed to spare tissue and reduce lateral pharyngeal wall collapse. These include expansion pharyngoplasty,[163] tongue base reduction and genioglossus advancement,[164] and maxillomandibular advancement

(MMA). The latter is especially useful in the setting of a dentofacial deformity, such as bimaxillary hypoplasia and retrognathia, and may also be useful in patients without dentofacial deformity who exhibit complete lateral pharyngeal wall collapse because MMA can improve lateral pharyngeal wall stability. MMA may be used as a first-line surgical procedure in selected cases.[161]

Weight-reduction programs and bariatric surgery are valuable treatment modalities (see Chapter 139). Although most studies have shown that bariatric surgery is associated with improvement in AHI and BMI, it is important to recognize that OSA can persist after substantial weight loss.[165] Follow-up PSG, rather than reliance on symptoms, is important to determine whether further OSA therapy is needed.

Positional therapy may also be useful in selected patients in whom disordered breathing events occur predominantly during supine sleep. Positional OSA patients tend to be younger, with lower BMI, smaller neck and waist circumference, and lower AHI than non–position-dependent subjects. Avoidance of supine sleep can lead to reduction in the AHI, particularly with use of positioning devices, which are typically worn around the chest or waist and prevent inadvertent supine sleep. Newer devices sense supine positioning and initiate vibrations until the subject changes to a nonsupine position.[166]

In the era of personalized medicine, future therapeutic approaches may be individualized based on symptom phenotypes that may predict long-term cardiovascular and cerebrovascular risk, as well as pathophysiologic endotypes that may guide selection of therapeutic modalities (see Chapters 128–130). Thus thinking about OSA as a heterogeneous disorder with multiple "phenotypes" and "endotypes" might facilitate development of new individualized therapies that aim at "treatable traits" to optimize therapeutic outcome.[73]

CLINICAL PEARL

Obstructive sleep apnea (OSA) is highly prevalent, particularly in patients with comorbid cardiovascular, cerebrovascular, and metabolic disease. Because OSA independently contributes to morbidity and mortality, with multisystem consequences, clinical suspicion for OSA should be a priority for clinicians, especially in patients with these comorbidities. However, it should be recognized that the clinical presentation of OSA is heterogeneous, with distinct patterns of symptomatology that include not only the classically recognized complaint of excessive daytime somnolence but also encompasses patients with a primary complaint of disturbed nighttime sleep and even those who are minimally symptomatic. Clinical assessment and sleep testing with in-laboratory polysomnography or out-of-center sleep testing in appropriately selected patients is necessary for accurate diagnosis. Effective treatment of OSA and any comorbid sleep disorders requires a focus on optimizing sleep-related health outcomes using a chronic disease management approach.

SUMMARY

The clinical presentation of OSA is heterogeneous, with distinct patterns of symptomatology that include not only the classical complaint of excessive daytime somnolence but also encompassing patients with a primary complaint of disturbed nighttime sleep and those with minimal symptoms. Further, new research has recognized that the pathophysiologic basis of OSA is also heterogeneous, with anatomic and mechanical factors that increase UA collapsibility playing a major role in some individuals, whereas ventilatory control and sleep instability are more important factors in others.

OSA is highly prevalent and is overrepresented in populations with cardiovascular, cerebrovascular, and metabolic disease. The acute, repetitive physiologic perturbations during sleep that occur as a result of obstructive apneas and hypopneas include sleep fragmentation, large swings in intrathoracic pressure, increased sympathoadrenal tone, and intermittent hypoxia and reoxygenation. These factors lead to multiple adverse systemic consequences, including excessive sleepiness and impairment of cognitive function, mood, vigilance, and performance, including driving ability. OSA has been shown to be an independent risk factor for multiple cardiovascular, cerebrovascular, and metabolic disorders.

Although clinical presentation and questionnaire-based tools can identify patients at risk for OSA, diagnosis requires objective monitoring. In-laboratory PSG testing remains the gold standard for accurate identification of OSA; however, OCST using ambulatory technology is useful in selected patients. Skilled assessment and management of this chronic disorder is necessary to ensure optimal long-term outcomes. Most studies have demonstrated improvement in daytime somnolence and quality of life with CPAP therapy. Other therapeutic modalities, including mandibular advancement oral appliances and surgical approaches to the UA, including hypoglossal nerve stimulation, are useful alternative modalities. Investigational approaches that define the predominant pathophysiologic basis for OSA in an individual patient may ultimately lead to a personalized or precision approach to treatment.

SELECTED READINGS

Ayappa I, Norman RG, Krieger AC, Rosen A, O'Malley RL, Rapoport DM. Non-invasive detection of respiratory effort-related arousals (RERAs) by a nasal cannula/pressure transducer system. *Sleep*. 2000;23(6):763–771.

Azarbarzin A, Sands SA, Stone KL, et al. The hypoxic burden of sleep apnoea predicts cardiovascular disease-related mortality: the Osteoporotic Fractures in Men Study and the Sleep Heart Health Study. *Eur Heart J*. 2019;40(14):1149–1157.

Caples SM, Anderson WM, Calero K, Howell M, Hashmi SD. Use of polysomnography and home sleep apnea tests for the longitudinal management of obstructive sleep apnea in adults: an American Academy of Sleep Medicine clinical guidance statement. *J Clin Sleep Med*. 2021;17(6):1287–1293.

Carberry JC, Amatoury J, Eckert DJ. Personalized management approach for OSA. *Chest*. 2018;153(3):744–755.

Edwards BA, Andara C, Landry S, et al. Upper-airway collapsibility and loop gain predict the response to oral appliance therapy in patients with obstructive sleep apnea. *Am J Respir Crit Care Med*. 2016;194(11):1413–1422.

Gottlieb DJ, Punjabi NM. Diagnosis and management of obstructive sleep apnea: a review. *JAMA*. 2020;323(14):1389–1400.

Kushida CA, Nichols DA, Holmes TH, et al. Effects of continuous positive airway pressure on neurocognitive function in obstructive sleep apnea patients: The Apnea Positive Pressure Long-term Efficacy Study (APPLES). *Sleep*. 2012;35(12):1593–1602.

Kylstra WA, Aaronson JA, Hofman WF, Schmand BA. Neuropsychological functioning after CPAP treatment in obstructive sleep apnea: a meta-analysis. *Sleep Med Rev*. 2013;17(5):341–347.

Liu SY, Wayne Riley R, Pogrel A, Guilleminault C. Sleep surgery in the era of precision medicine. *Atlas Oral Maxillofac Surg Clin North Am*. 2019;27(1):1–5.

Mazzotti DR, Keenan BT, Lim DC, Gottlieb DJ, Kim J, Pack AI. Symptom subtypes of obstructive sleep apnea predict incidence of cardiovascular outcomes. *Am J Respir Crit Care Med*. 2019;200(4):493–506.

National Institute for Health and Care Excellence. Obstructive sleep apnoea/hypopnoea syndrome and obesity hypoventilation syndrome. Published: 20 August 2021. https://www.nice.org.uk/guidance/ng202.
Patil SP, Ayappa IA, Caples SM, Kimoff RJ, Patel SR, Harrod CG. Treatment of adult obstructive sleep apnea with positive airway pressure: an American Academy of Sleep Medicine systematic review, meta-analysis, and GRADE assessment. *J Clin Sleep Med.* 2019;15(2):301–334.
Rapoport DM, Sorkin B, Garay SM, Goldring RM. Reversal of the "Pickwickian syndrome" by long-term use of nocturnal nasal-airway pressure. *N Engl J Med.* 1982;307(15):931–933.
Schwab RJ, Pasirstein M, Pierson R, et al. Identification of upper airway anatomic risk factors for obstructive sleep apnea with volumetric magnetic resonance imaging. *Am J Respir Crit Care Med.* 2003;168(5):522–530.
Strollo PJ, Soose RJ, Maurer JT, et al. Upper-airway stimulation for obstructive sleep apnea. *N Engl J Med.* 2014;370(2):139–149.
Testelmans D, Spruit MA, Vrijsen B, et al. Comorbidity clusters in patients with moderate-to-severe OSA [published online ahead of print, 2021 May 3]. *Sleep Breath.* 2021. https://doi.org/10.1007/s11325-021-02390-4.
Weaver TE, Maislin G, Dinges DF, et al. Relationship between hours of CPAP use and achieving normal levels of sleepiness and daily functioning. *Sleep.* 2007;30(6):711–719.
White DP, Younes MK. Obstructive sleep apnea. *Compr Physiol.* 2012;2(4):2541–2594.
Wickwire EM, Albrecht JS, Towe MM, et al. The impact of treatments for OSA on monetized health economic outcomes: a systematic review. *Chest.* 2019;155(5):947–961.
Ye L, Pien GW, Ratcliffe SJ, et al. The different clinical faces of obstructive sleep apnoea: a cluster analysis. *Eur Respir J.* 2014;44(6):1600–1607.
Zinchuk A, Yaggi HK. Phenotypic sub-types of obstructive sleep apnea: a challenge and opportunity for precision medicine. *Chest.* 2020;157(2):403–420.

A complete reference list can be found online at ExpertConsult.com.

Chapter 132

Positive Airway Pressure Treatment for Obstructive Sleep Apnea

Neil Freedman; Karin Johnson

Chapter Highlights

- Continuous positive airway pressure (CPAP) therapy is indicated for patients with moderate to severe obstructive sleep apnea (OSA) with or without symptoms, and for patients with mild OSA with associated symptoms or comorbid illnesses. Autotitrated positive airway pressure (APAP) used in an unattended setting, either to determine a fixed CPAP pressure or as a primary treatment, is reasonable therapy for most patients with uncomplicated moderate to severe OSA. Titration studies to determine the optimal therapy are recommended if there are comorbid illnesses that increase the incidence of central sleep apnea or hypoventilation that CPAP or APAP may not fully treat, or if there is a suboptimal response with CPAP or APAP that cannot be fixed using adherence or waveform data.
- CPAP consistently improves or resolves respiratory events across the spectrum of disease severity and improves symptoms of daytime sleepiness, especially for patients with moderate to severe OSA. Improvements in blood pressure (BP) are relatively small, with reductions in BP tending to be greatest in patients with untreated hypertension, daytime sleepiness, and in those patients with better adherence with therapy. Improvements in other outcomes are inconsistent across the spectrum of disease severity.
- Adherence with positive airway pressure (PAP) therapy is far from perfect. Systematic education via several approaches, with or without behavioral therapy, has been the only intervention that has been associated with consistent improvements in adherence with PAP therapy. APAP therapy has been shown to result in similar adherence and improvements in other important outcomes when compared with conventionally titrated CPAP therapy. The role of telemedicine and virtual monitoring have shown promise in some studies, although further research is required to better define their roles in the management of PAP therapy for OSA. The roles of other interventions, including heated humidification, prescription hypnotics, direct patient engagement, and sleep specialist care, for most patients with OSA are not clear.
- Advanced PAP technologies, including bilevel PAP and expiratory pressure relief (EPR) settings, have not been consistently associated with better adherence or improvements in other important outcomes in the treatment of OSA when compared to standard CPAP therapy. Based on the outcomes data, the roles for bilevel PAP and devices with EPR technology in the management of most patients with OSA are not clear.
- In appropriate OSA patients, an ambulatory approach using home sleep apnea testing and APAP therapy with adjustments based on PAP device data analysis should lead to reductions in the cost of management of OSA, while not adversely affecting patient outcomes. Telemedicine and online monitoring is also expected to have a growing role in patient management driven by technologic advances and research on its benefits, as well as for the COVID-19 pandemic.

INTRODUCTION

Treatment with positive airway pressure (PAP) remains the primary therapy for most patients with obstructive sleep apnea (OSA), especially those with moderate to severe OSA. This chapter will review various forms of PAP therapy for the treatment of OSA, highlighting the indications for treatment, methods for determining an effective pressure prescription, treatment outcomes, and methods that may improve adherence with therapy. The initial part of the chapter will focus on how continuous positive airway pressure (CPAP), autotitrated CPAP (APAP), bilevel PAP (BPAP), and expiratory pressure relief (EPR) work and how adherence data can be used to optimize treatment. The latter portion of the chapter will review CPAP's effects on important patient outcomes in OSA patients and approaches to improve adherence with therapy.

CONTINUOUS POSITIVE AIRWAY PRESSURE FOR THE TREATMENT OF OBSTRUCTIVE SLEEP APNEA

CPAP therapy was initially described as a treatment for OSA by Sullivan and colleagues in 1980.[1] Since its initial description, CPAP has become the predominant therapy for the treatment of patients with OSA as it has been demonstrated to resolve sleep-disordered breathing events and improve several clinical outcomes.[2–5] Treatment with CPAP is typically indicated for patients with moderate to severe OSA as defined by an apnea hypopnea index (AHI) greater than or equal to 15 events per hour, with or without associated symptoms or comorbid diseases, and for patients with mild OSA (AHI ≥ 5 to ≤ 14 events/hour) with associated symptoms or comorbid diseases (Figure 132.1).

CPAP is conventionally delivered via a nasal mask at a fixed pressure that remains constant throughout the respiratory cycle. The proposed mechanism of action of CPAP therapy is that it acts as a pneumatic splint that maintains the patency of the upper airway in a "dose-dependent" fashion. It does not exert its effects by increasing upper airway muscle activity and acts only as a treatment, but not a cure, for the disorder.[6] Several studies have demonstrated that withdrawing CPAP therapy in patients with OSA across the spectrum of disease severity results in the recurrence of OSA and associated daytime symptoms in most patients within 1 to several days.[7–9]

Basics in the Delivery of Positive Airway Pressure

PAP equipment involves three basic parts, including a device with a motor, a mask that covers either the nose and/or the mouth, and a tube that connects the device to the mask.[10] PAP has improved greatly since Colin Sullivan invented CPAP in June 1980 in Australia, using a vacuum cleaner motor attached to pool tubing and a mask made from a plaster cast glued to the patient's face. Current PAP units are much more complex and may include an air filter, sensors (motor speed, gas volumetric flow rate, pressure, snore transducer), microprocessor-based controller, data storage, multilingual displays, internal modem for data transfer, and humidifiers with heated tubing.

Motor/Flow Generator and Transducers

To provide a constant desired pressure at the patient's airway, adjustments in flow must be made to account for several factors, including the loss of pressure between the flow generator and the patient's airway, fluctuations in breathing, and excessive air leak. Transducers monitor the motor speed, flow, and pressure at a fixed point downstream from the flow generator. Because the sensor is within the device and not in the mask, the device must calculate the predicted pressure at the mask based on the flow measurements at different points in the system. The length and diameter of the tubing and mask characteristics may affect the pressure and flow; thus the technician must take into account the tube type, and in some cases mask type, in order for the microprocessor to make the correct calculations. The mask air leak flow can also be calculated by subtracting the estimated flow through the exhaust of the device from the flow through the tubing.

To maintain a stable mask pressure, the microprocessor must adjust the turbine speed in response to deviations in pressure that occur from leak or normal swings in air pressure from breathing. The flow signal is sent through low- and high-pass filters to separate the respiratory flow signal from artifacts. Low-pass filters exclude large, quick deviations in flow (e.g., coughs or sneezes). Some devices have high-pass filters that exclude fast frequencies, including cardiogenic fluctuations. Feedback limits determine if expected flow or pressure is beyond the expected range of flow variation at a particular motor speed (e.g., break in the tubing) and prevent the device from delivering too much or too little pressure. With increasing altitude, fan speed needs to be increased to maintain the same pressure. Most newer devices adjust automatically to altitude.

Leak Compensation

Unlike invasive ventilation, managing excessive air leak is an important factor that must be compensated to optimize therapy. Leak affects aspects of performance, including pressure delivered, cycle and trigger thresholds, and respiratory event determination. Leak is pressure, flow, and mask dependent and can be determined from the flow rate at the end of exhalation. Air leak falls into two categories including intentional, or expected, leak that includes air leak from exhalation ports on the mask and varies by mask type, and unintentional, or excessive, leak that typically occurs from the mouth or around the mask. In general, unintentional leak should be less than 24 L per minute with nasal masks and less than 36 L per minute with full-face masks. Most PAP devices have inputs for the mask style to know what range of leak to expect and to adjust for expected leak on adherence data; however, given the variation between different mask styles, there is still a range.

Most devices can compensate for excessive leak by constantly monitoring flow, looking for deviations from the expected respiratory flow, and adjusting the motor speed to minimize excessive air leak. Because there are normal variations in the patient's breathing cycle, the expected leak is usually averaged over several breaths. If leak is high, APAP algorithms may compensate by lowering the pressure, which may reduce unintentional leak and reduce or resolve excessive mask leak. The lips and tongue sometimes act like a one-way valve opening during exhalation when the pharyngeal pressure is highest. This is called valve leak or expiratory puffs. Expiratory puffs may falsely imply flow limitation, which can cause APAP algorithms to increase pressures unnecessarily. Some algorithms place less reliance on flow limitation when a large leak is present.

Respiratory Cycle Determination

Determination of the inspiratory and expiratory cycles is essential not only to provide BPAP but also for EPR and

Typical indications for CPAP therapy for OSAS

Moderate to severe OSAS (≥15 events per hour of sleep) with or without associated symptoms or comorbid diseases

Mild OSAS (≥5 – ≤14) *with* symptoms *or* associated comorbid diseases:
- Symptoms:
  - Excessive daytime sleepiness, impaired cognition, mood disorders or insomnia
- Comorbid diseases:
  - Hypertension, ischemic heart disease or history of stroke

Figure 132.1 Typical indications for continuous positive airway pressure (CPAP) therapy for obstructive sleep apnea syndrome (OSAS).

determination of inspiratory flow limitation (IFL) in APAP algorithms. The initiation of inspiration is marked by a switch from negative to positive flow (relative to baseline). The point at which the flow signal switches from positive to negative flow is the start of expiration. Because the sensor is removed from the airway, altering cycle and trigger sensitivities farther from nonzero value can help synchronize the machine with the patient's breathing pattern.

Expiratory Pressure Relief

A common complaint in many patients with OSA using CPAP is the uncomfortable feeling of exhaling against positive pressure. This consequence is one potential barrier to the long-term acceptance of CPAP therapy. Several PAP manufacturers have developed EPR systems in an attempt to remedy this potential problem. EPR device technologies allow pressure relief during exhalation with the goal to make CPAP therapy more comfortable and ultimately to improve adherence to therapy. EPR technologies briefly reduce the PAP pressure up to 3 cm H_2O during exhalation before returning the pressure to its set PAP setting before the initiation of inspiration. Certain EPR technologies monitor the patient's airflow during exhalation and reduce the expiratory pressure in response to the airflow and patient effort. The amount of pressure relief varies on a breath-by-breath basis, depending on the actual patient's airflow and is also dictated by the patient's preference setting on the device.

Although several PAP manufacturers have developed EPR devices for the market place, only the Philips Respironics (Philips Respironics, Murraysville, PA) technology (CFLEX) has been evaluated in the peer-reviewed literature.[11–14] Several randomized controlled trials have evaluated the role of CFLEX technology compared with standard CPAP therapy in patients with uncomplicated, predominantly moderate to severe OSA. Overall, the use of CFLEX technology at fixed pressure relief settings has not been associated with improved adherence in either the parallel or crossover trials. In addition, improvements in other commonly measured outcomes (subjective sleepiness, objective alertness, vigilance, or residual OSA) were similar to, but not better than, standard CPAP therapy. CFLEX therapy has not been shown to offer significant benefits in that subgroup of patients that require CPAP pressures of greater than or equal to 9 cm H_2O. Based on these data, the routine use of CFLEX technology is not recommended as a method to improve adherence or other major outcomes compared with fixed CPAP therapy. Further randomized controlled trials are necessary to determine if this technology offers any objective advantages over fixed CPAP therapy in select groups of patients.

In our experience, EPR may be beneficial for some patients and prevents the need to convert to BPAP for tolerance. Some patients only need EPR during the ramp period. In other patients, the drop in pressure may induce more treatment-emergent central events and intolerance, so we recommend that the patient be treated with and without EPR on setup to determine what is most comfortable rather than be set for all patients. Similarly, some patients find starting at low pressures suffocating (often elicited by asking if they feel they have to suck in air) and prefer to start with no ramp or a higher start ramp setting, which can be tested on setup.

Autotitrated Positive Airway Pressure

Autotitrated (also known as auto–, automated, autoadjusting or automatic) positive airway pressure (APAP) incorporates the ability of the PAP device to detect and respond to changes in upper airway flow and or resistance in real time. This review will focus on how APAP works and the literature related to APAP in the treatment of patients with previously diagnosed OSA, as there is currently little evidence to support the use of APAP technology for the diagnosis of OSA.[4,5,15]

Currently available APAP algorithms use proprietary algorithms to noninvasively detect and respond to variations in patterns of upper airway inspiratory flow and/or resistance.[10] Most APAP machines monitor a combination of changes in inspiratory flow patterns, including IFL, snoring (indirectly measured via mask pressure vibration), reductions of airflow (hypopnea), and absence of flow (apneas), using a pneumotachograph, nasal pressure monitors, or alterations in compressor speed. The algorithms use different methods to process the flow signal, which can result in differences in event detection. The flow is sampled many times per second, scaled with a low-pass filter to remove artifact, and then a mean flow is determined for a given period of time. Peak flow can be a poor measure of breath volume, which can lead to over- or underestimation of an apnea or hypopnea. Of importance, different device manufacturers use different algorithms to both determine if sleep-disordered breathing events are present and how they respond to resolve these events. Philips Respironics uses a weighted peak flow (WPF) method to estimate ventilation, whereas ResMed (ResMed, San Diego, CA) uses a scaled, low-pass, filtered absolute value of respiratory flow and a root mean squared technique (RMS) of the variance of the flow from the mean to compare one moving time period to another Figure 132.2).

Philips Respironics' WPF method first determines the inspiratory period, then the inspiratory volume and the points on the inspiratory flow curve that correspond to the 20% and 80% volume. The average flow of all points between the 20% and 80% points is used as the WPF, a measure of ventilation. The model uses WPF values over the prior 2 minutes and determines the average of values between the 80th and 90th percentiles. This baseline is then used to compare to the current WPF to assess for decreases in amplitude that would indicate apnea, hypopnea, or other sleep-disordered breathing events.

ResMed's APAP algorithm uses a RMS method that determines ventilation from variance of the flow throughout the entire breath by comparing individual flow points to the mean airflow over a defined time period. The mean airflow is the zero-point between inspiration and expiration; thus variance from this mean divided by two equals the amplitude of the inspiratory flow. By taking the square root of the variance squared, outlying values receive less weight. A moving short time period (e.g., one breath or 2 seconds) can be compared to a moving longer period (e.g., 5 minutes) to evaluate for sleep-disordered breathing events.

Most currently available devices detect flow limitation via proprietary algorithms using flow versus time profiles to detect apneas and hypopneas, but fewer devices evaluate flow limitation. To evaluate flow limitation, Philips Respironics determines roundness, flatness, skewness, and WPF to rate the most recent four breaths as better, worse, or the same compared to baseline. Roundness is determined by the

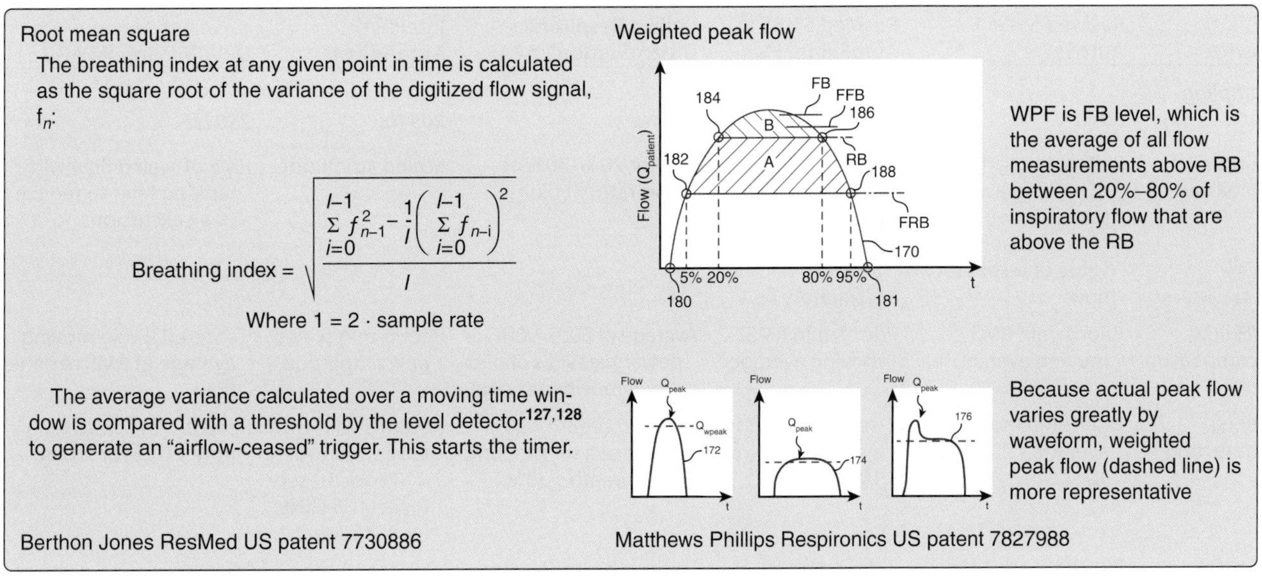

Figure 132.2 Signal processing methods. FB, Flatness baseline; FFB, flatness flat baseline; FRB, flatness round baseline; RB, round baseline, weighted peak flow.

similarity of the WPF between 5% and 95% values to a sine wave. Flatness is determined by the absolute value of the variance between 20% and 80% of inspiratory flow from the average of all the values in the same period and dividing by the 80% volume point. Skewness is determined by dividing the average of the highest 5% of flows in the middle third of the breath by the average of the highest 5% of flows in the first third of the breath.

ResMed also determines flow limitation. For S9-S1 For S9-S11 Autoset models, flow limitation is calculated using a combination of flatness index, breath shape index, ventilation change, and breath duty cycle. Ventilation change is the ratio of the current breath ventilation to recent 3-minute ventilation. Breath duty cycle is the ratio of current breath time of inspiration to total breath time of recent 5 minutes. When a breath is severely flow limited, the flow limitation index will be closer to 1, as opposed to when the breath is "normal" or round, the flow limitation index will be 0.

There are several studies that have evaluated the reliability of sleep-disordered breathing event detection, specifically the apnea-hypopneas index (AHI), based on the device flow measurements compared to polysomnography (PSG).[16–9] Most found reasonable correlation between the AHIs, with some studies showing device overestimation and others demonstrating underestimations of the AHI.[18,19] Most studies demonstrate a stronger correlation between the PAP- and PSG-defined AHIs at higher AHI levels.

One potential shortfall of APAP technology is their ability or inability to detect and differentiate obstructive from central sleep-disordered breathing events. The inability to clearly differentiate types of events has clinical ramifications for APAP devices as inappropriately increasing pressure in response to central events could lead to overtitration, with worsening of central events and sleep fragmentation. Different manufacturers use different technologies to better determine the types of sleep-disordered breathing events. Several devices use the forced oscillation technique (FOT) to determine airway patency to differentiate central from obstructive apneas.[20,21] FOT is a technology that assesses changes in airway resistance to define upper airway patency. When a reduction in flow is detected, the device provides a small oscillation in the flow, for instance, 1 cm H_2O at 4 to 5 Hz, which is only reflected back to the flow sensors if the airway is closed. Low resistance in the absence of flow (open airway) is interpreted as a central event, and increased resistance in the absence of flow (closed airway) is interpreted as an obstructive event. Philips Respironics APAP algorithm uses pressure pulses rather than oscillations to test for airway patency throughout an apnea. A mixed apnea can be determined if the airway is open for only part of the flow cycle. In general, FOT is a better technology for differentiating between central and obstructive apneas. Although some devices detect periodic breathing, there are no devices that can reliably distinguish between central and obstructive hypopneas. Thus, in the absence of full central apneas, most devices will increase pressure in response to periodic breathing, and it may be difficult to differentiate whether residual hypopneas on adherence data are central in nature.

Table 132.1 summarizes the differences between the algorithms for several different APAP devices, including ResMed AutoSet devices, ResMed AutoSet for Her, Philips Respironics DreamStation 2 APAP (essentially the same algorithm as Philips Respironics System One REMstar Auto), and DeVilbiss IntelliPAP AutoAdjust and IntelliPAP 2 AutoAdjust.

Once upper airway flow or impedance changes have been detected, the APAP devices use proprietary algorithms to automatically increase the pressure until the flow or resistance has been normalized. Once a therapeutic pressure has been achieved, the APAP devices typically reduce pressure until flow limitation or increases in airway resistance resume. Most devices have a therapeutic pressure range between 4 cm H_2O and 20 cm H_2O, giving the clinician the ability to adjust the upper and lower pressure limits based on the clinical conditions and the patient's response to therapy. This should be differentiated from BPAP or auto-BPAP (discussed later), in which a separate inspiratory positive airway pressure (IPAP) and expiratory positive airway pressure (EPAP) are set with

Table 132.1 Auto-CPAP Algorithms

Device	ResMed S9-S11 AutoSet	ResMed S10-S11 AutoSet for Her	Philips Respironics DreamStation2 APAP	DeVilbiss IntelliPAP AutoAdjust	DeVilbiss IntelliPAP 2
Sampling Rate	***50 Hz***	***50 Hz***	***100 Hz***	***205 Hz***	***250 Hz***
Ventilation measure	RMS of the variance of moving average, scaled, low-pass, filtered absolute value of respiratory flow	RMS of the variance of moving average, scaled, low-pass, filtered absolute value of respiratory flow	WPF of 20%–80% of inspiratory volume	Scaled amplitude	RMS of scaled flow with ranking filter to reduce peak excursions
A/H flow comparison	Prior 1-min RMS moving average	Prior 1-min RMS moving average	Average of 80th–90th percentile WPFs of prior 4-min moving average	Prior 5-min scaled flow amplitude	Centered 3-min moving average of RMS of patient flow
Apnea detection	2-sec RMS moving average <25% for 10 sec	2-sec RMS moving average <25% for 10 sec	WPF per breath <20% for 10 sec, terminating with breath >30%	Recent 1-min with flow amplitude <10% for 10 sec (or set 0%–20% for 6–150 sec)	Recent 1-min with RMS flow <10% for 10 sec
Non-OA detection	S9-S10: 1-cm 4-Hz FOT throughout apnea with mixed apnea detection	1-cm 4-Hz FOT with mixed apnea detection	During the apnea, one or more pressure test pulse. Non-OA if pulse generates a significant amount of flow, otherwise OA	<5% for 10 sec	Microoscillating pressure (nominally 0.07 cm) modulated frequency detecting stable airway resistance characteristics during event
Hypopnea detection	Above with at least one obstructed breath	12-sec RMS scaled average 25%–50% for 10 sec with at least one obstructed breath	20%–60% for 10 sec and either 60-sec timeout or a terminating breath over 75% of recent WPF	10%–50% for 10 sec (or set 30%–70% for 6–150 sec)	RMS flow 10%–40% default (upper limit adjustable between 30%–50%) for 10 sec
Flow limitation detection	Breath by breath flow limitation index from breath shape index, RMS flatness index, and ventilation change and breath duty cycle	Breath by breath flow limitation index from breath shape index, RMS flatness index, and ventilation change and breath duty cycle	Relative changes in the peak, flatness, roundness, shape (skewness) of inspiratory wave form. Evaluated over short period (4 breaths) and over long period (several minutes). Statistical measures are used to help minimize false event detection	NA	Breath by breath detection of relative flatness of inspiratory waveform, detecting positive, negative, or zero slope. Score averaged over 12 sec, Score averaged over 12 sec and graded as none, mild, moderate, or severe
Other events detection	Unknown apnea: Apnea with leak >30 L/min	Unknown apnea: Apnea with leak >30 L/min	Variable breathing: Standard deviation/ adjusted mean flow over 4-min window above threshold	Report exhale puff index: Number of expiratory puffs/h	Exhale puff graded as none, mild, moderate, or severe. Time with exhale puff reported. Reported time with exhale puffing:
OA/ hypopnea response	Increases pressure based on starting pressure for every 10 sec of apnea. When starting pressure is 4, pressure change is 3. Pressure change drops linearly down to 0.5 when starting pressure is 20.	Increases pressure based on starting pressure for every 10 sec of apnea. When starting pressure is 4, pressure change is 2.5. Pressure change drops linearly down to 0.5 when starting pressure is 20.	If two apneas or one apnea/one hypopnea or two hypopneas: Increases 1 over 15 sec and holds for 30 sec. NRAH logic limits max pressure to 11 or 3 higher than preapnea baseline. If more apneas within 8 min decrease pressure by 2 for 30 sec, then down to 1 over level that prevents snore, then holds pressure for 15 min. Pressure will continue to increase in response to two hypopneas	Increases 1/min for OA. If other events in last 6 min, increases 0.5/min for one hypopnea in last minute and 1 cm/min if > one hypopnea in last minute	Increases 1/min for OA. If other events in last 6 min, increases 0.5/min for one hypopnea in last minute and 1 cm/min if > one hypopnea in last minute; less response if expiratory puffs

Continued

Table 132.1 Auto-CPAP Algorithms—cont'd

Device	ResMed S9-S11 AutoSet	ResMed S10-S11 AutoSet for Her	Philips Respironics DreamStation2 APAP	DeVilbiss IntelliPAP AutoAdjust	DeVilbiss IntelliPAP 2
Sampling Rate	*50 Hz*	*50 Hz*	*100 Hz*	*205 Hz*	*250 Hz*
Flow limitation response	S9: Uses 3-breath average FL index. Increment typically around 0.6/breath for severely flow limited breaths. Lower increment if lower FL index, high leak, or as pressure increases further above 15. S10: Increment max 0.6/breath, otherwise same as S9	Uses single-breath FL index: Increment max 0.5/breath for severely flow-limited breaths. Lower increment if lower FL index, high leak, or as pressure increases further above 10	Pressure increases by 0.5/min in response to FL. Intermittent upward scans by 1.5 over 3 min to see if improvement in FL, then deceases if no improvement. If pressure not held by snore, A/H, or VB logic, then enters testing protocol that collects 3- to 5-min data, then P_{crit} and Popt search[a]	NA	Max increment 0.5 cm of 0.5/min determined by severity and duration of flow limitation. Lower increment if high leak, expiratory puffs, or if no A/H/snore in last 8 min. Pressure response determined by severity and duration (15 sec/min) to evoke response: 0.5 cm
Vibratory snore response	S9: Increment max 1/breath. Lower increment if snore is less severe, high leak or as pressure increases further above 10. S10-S11: Increment max 0.6/breath for a loud snore, otherwise same as S9	Increment max 0.5/breath. Lower increment if snore is less severe, high leak, or as pressure increases further above 10	If 3 snores within 60 seconds, with no more than 30 seconds between snores, increase 1 cm H_2O over 15 seconds then hold for 1 min with higher snore threshold at higher pressures	1 cm H_2O/min for 3 snores per 6-min window	If moderate-severe snore increases 0.5/min
Other pressure changes	Gradual decrease to Pmin over 40 min after apnea, over 20 min after FL or snoring	Gradual decrease to Pmin over 40 min after apnea and over 20 min after snore and 60 min after flow limitation as soon as breathing is stable	1. If high variable breathing is noted, then if recent (5 min) pressure was stable, then pressure stays same; if recent pressure decrease then increases by 0.5/min up to 2, and if recent pressure increase, then decreases by 0.5/min up to 2 2. If large leak, reduces pressure by 1 over 10 sec and holds pressure for 2 min	Decreases 0.6 every 6 min until either lowest pressure or events occur	If no events in 6-min window, decreases 0.6 every 6 min until either lowest pressure or events occur. If central apnea in 6-min period: pressure decrease and no increase for 6 minutes. If periodic breathing in 6-min window no increase in pressure, then decreases in pressure depending upon level of PB detection
High leak detection	95th percentile leak > 24 L/min	95th percentile leak > 24 L/min	Leak level exceeds flow limit for a given pressure	95 L/min	Leak level exceeds flow limit for a given pressure
Ramp	S9: 0–45 min ramp. S10-S11: 0–45 min ramp or AutoRamp starts ramping when sleep onset if inferred	0–45 min ramp or AutoRamp starts ramping when sleep onset if inferred	Smart ramp increases faster if obstructive events or FL occur. RampPlus allows patient to set starting ramp pressure	0–45 min ramp	0–45 min ramp
Pressure relief	EPR off, 1–3 cm	EPR off, 1–3 cm	Flex off, 1–3	SmartFlex off, 1–3 cm	SmartFlex off, 1–3 cm

[a]Downward search sequence for P_{crit} begins ramping down 0.5/min until Pmin as long as no worsening in FL. If worsening, Pcrit is set and pressure quickly increases by 1.5 and held for 10 min. Then Popt search increases pressure by 0.5/min for at least 2.5 min to test if FL improves, worsens, or stays the same. If improvement, continues 0.5/min pressure increase; if no improvement, pressure decreases by 1.5 and sets Popt and holds for 5 min. FL or other events end all holds.

A/H, Apnea/hypopnea; EPR, expiratory pressure relief; FL, flow limitation; FOT, forced oscillation technique; Hz, hertz; max, maximum; NA, not applicable; NRAH, nonresponse apnea hypopnea logic; OA, obstructive apnea; PB, periodic breathing; Pcrit, critical pressure; Pmax, maximum pressure; Pmin, minimum pressure; Popt, optimal pressure; RMS, root mean squared; VB, variable breathing; WPF, weighted peak flow.

All pressures in cm H_2O. Data from Kushida CA, Chediak A, Berry RB, et al. Clinical guidelines for the manual titration of positive airway pressure in patients with obstructive sleep apnea. *J Clin Sleep Med* 2008;4:157-171.

changes in pressure across each respiratory cycle. Similar to CPAP, expiratory relief and other pressure delivery modifications are available for APAP technologies, although these additional pressure modifications have not been shown to consistently improve several APAP-related outcomes, including in-laboratory titration success, PAP adherence, or other outcomes, such as daytime sleepiness.[22,23] Because pressure changes occur throughout the sleep period, some have postulated that APAP devices may actually increase sleep fragmentation.[24] This concern has not been substantiated in studies evaluating changes in sleep structure or in clinical trials that have measured subjective sleepiness as a main outcome. Specifically, the frequency of microarousals and sleep fragmentation induced by APAP devices appears to be small, and clinical outcomes related to subjective sleepiness also show no significant differences compared with conventional CPAP therapy.[25–30]

Currently available APAP machines have several potential limitations. As previously discussed, the inability to accurately distinguish obstructive and central events may lead to unintentional overtitration. Additionally, most APAP algorithms are limited in their ability to recognize flow limitation and respiratory events in the setting of large mask leaks.[31–34] This may lead some, especially older, algorithms to "interpret" decreased flow from leak as an event and increase pressure, which may further worsen leak. Also, the ability of the APAP devices to respond to sustained hypoventilation in the absence of upper airway obstruction is unclear as most APAP studies have excluded patients at high risk for hypoventilation, including those patients with obesity hypoventilation syndrome and/or chronic respiratory diseases.

Given these potential limitations in technology and the exclusion of patients with many comorbid diseases from the randomized trials comparing APAP to in-laboratory–titrated CPAP therapy, the previous and current professional society guidelines regarding the use of APAP recommend that APAP devices only be used for patients with uncomplicated moderate to severe OSA.[4,5,15] APAP devices typically should not be used without an attended in-laboratory titration study to define pressure ranges in the patients with comorbid medical conditions that could potentially affect their respiratory patterns during sleep (complicated OSA), including (1) congestive heart failure; (2) lung diseases, such as chronic obstructive pulmonary disease (COPD); and (3) patients expected to have nocturnal arterial oxyhemoglobin desaturation due to conditions other than OSA (e.g., obesity hypoventilation syndrome and other hypoventilation syndromes). Patients who do not snore (either due to palatal surgery or naturally) should not be titrated with an APAP device that relies on vibration or sound in the device's algorithm.[4,5,15] Finally, APAP devices are not recommended for split-night titrations, given the lack of data to support such a practice.

Autotitrated Positive Airway Pressure Outcomes. There have been several randomized controlled trials that have compared APAP technology to conventionally titrated CPAP therapy for the treatment of uncomplicated OSA.[26-30,35–44] Compared with standard fixed CPAP therapy, APAP devices as a group are almost always associated with a reduction in mean pressure across a night of therapy in the range of 2 to 2.5 cm H_2O, although peak pressures during the night tend to be higher than fixed CPAP therapy. Similar leak levels were found comparing automatic to fixed settings with ResMed, Philips Respironics, and Weiman devices.[45] Aside from these differences, APAP and standard CPAP are similar with regard to improvements in several outcomes, including objective adherence, ability to eliminate respiratory events, and subjective daytime sleepiness as measured by the Epworth Sleepiness Scale (ESS).[46,47] These findings have been consistently demonstrated for APAP therapy used as a primary chronic therapy and for APAP used for a short therapeutic trial to determine a fixed CPAP setting for ongoing CPAP therapy. There are few data regarding improvements in blood pressure (BP) with APAP therapy and no long-term data regarding any cardiovascular outcomes.[48]

It should be noted that the majority of the literature concerning APAP technology as a treatment for OSA has evaluated patients with uncomplicated, predominantly moderate to severe OSA (AHI ≥ 15 events/hour), and therefore the results and recommendations that have been reviewed predominantly apply to this group of patients. The data comparing efficacy of APAP versus attended in-laboratory–titrated CPAP in patients with mild OSA (AHI = 5 to 14) are more limited.[43,46] Based on the available information, there appear to be similar improvements in important outcomes, including resolution of sleep-disordered breathing, daytime sleepiness, and adherence with therapy between APAP and CPAP even in patients with more mild disease, although it is difficult to make reliable recommendations concerning the use of APAP for this subgroup of patients.

Although the use of APAP as a therapy, with or without changing the patient to a fixed CPAP device, has also been well described, the optimal method for determining treatment success is controversial. Most of the newer PAP devices calculate several parameters, including device use time, an AHI, and leak data. Although adherence with PAP therapy can be reliably determined using the various PAP tracking systems, the validity of the PAP-calculated AHI data are not as easy to interpret as the various PAP manufacturers define respiratory events differently from each other and differently from the standard scoring definitions used by the American Academy of Sleep Medicine (AASM) (Table 132.1).[49,50] In general, PAP-calculated AHIs less than 10 events per hour tend to correlate with adequately treated sleep-disordered breathing events and have been associated with improved outcomes in randomized controlled trials.[51] This is especially true when these findings are associated with the resolution of nighttime snoring and daytime symptoms.

In summary, APAP technologies appear to be as effective as conventional fixed CPAP therapy when used for treatment in attended and unattended settings in patients with moderate to severe uncomplicated OSA.[4,5] Although APAP technologies as a group reduce the mean treatment pressure across the night, they appear to result in similar objective adherence and improvements in other important clinical outcomes when compared with in-laboratory–titrated CPAP therapy. Although APAP therapy has demonstrated some shortcomings in the peer-reviewed literature, the technology is rapidly advancing. The main benefits of APAP technology is the ability to provide more rapid treatment to patients with uncomplicated OSA and possibly the saving of health care dollars by eliminating some attended in-laboratory sleep studies that are typically required for CPAP titrations.[52]

Bilevel Positive Airway Pressure Therapy

BPAP therapy's potential benefits in treating patients with OSA were first described in 1990.[53] As opposed to CPAP, which delivers a fixed pressure throughout the respiratory cycle, BPAP therapy allows the lower EPAP and higher IPAP to be set separately. Pressures generally range from an EPAP minimum of 4 cm H_2O to an IPAP maximum of 25 to 30 cm H_2O. Most devices use a flow trigger to determine when to change from IPAP to EPAP and vice versa. The trigger is set above zero flow to sense a significant patient effort. Different methods that use flow, shape, and volume algorithms are used to cycle from IPAP to EPAP in efforts to minimize desynchrony. A flow cycle algorithm changes to EPAP when the flow drops below a percentage (e.g., 25%) of the peak flow, so the patient will not encounter resistance to exhalation. A shape-cycling algorithm uses shape of flow, and a volume-cycle algorithm uses exhaled volume to cycle to EPAP. There can be significant variation between devices in terms of how quickly pressurization levels are met and whether a device has a delay or premature cycle, especially in the setting of excessive unintentional leak. If there is a mismatch between the patient's respiratory cycle and the device control cycle, there can be patient discomfort or intolerance. In older BPAP devices, the motor was braked at the transition point from higher to lower pressures, and the motor was accelerated when the device transitioned from lower to higher pressure, which affected synchrony and tolerability. Newer devices allow for a smoother transition in pressure changes.

Some BPAP devices include cycle, trigger, inspiration time, and rise time settings that can be adjusted to enhance effectiveness and patient comfort, especially for patients with COPD, obesity hypoventilation, or neuromuscular disorders. Depending on the device, these settings may apply only to triggered breaths (Philips Respironics BiPAP ST) or also to spontaneous breaths (ResMed BPAP S and BiPAP ST). Use of rise time, trigger and cycle sensitivity, inspiration time and back-up rate is discussed further in other chapters.

In its initial description, BPAP therapy demonstrated that obstructive events could be eliminated at a lower EPAP compared to conventional CPAP pressures. However, in our experience, because of the delay in detecting the onset of inspiration and for the pressure adjustment to be delivered to the patient, it is common for the inspiratory pressure needed for BPAP settings to prevent obstruction during early inspiration to be higher than the CPAP pressure needed to prevent the same. For example, a patient requiring CPAP at 8 cm H_2O may require BPAP at 10/6 cm H_2O so that a pressure of 8 is reached early enough in the inspiration to maintain airway patency.

Autobilevel Positive Airway Pressure Therapy

Autobilevel therapy has also been developed, which, using proprietary algorithms, automatically adjusts both the EPAP and IPAP in response to sleep-disordered breathing events. Limited data indicate that, compared with CPAP, auto-BPAP therapy results in similar adherence and other important outcomes in patients who have had poor initial experiences with CPAP therapy.[54,55] There is currently no peer-reviewed literature evaluating outcomes with auto-BPAP therapy for OSA in PAP-naïve patients. Thus, unlike non–auto-BPAP therapy, no recommendations can be made for auto-BPAP therapy for treating patients with OSA.

Determining the Optimal Positive Airway Pressure Setting for Obstructive Sleep Apnea Patients

The optimal PAP settings for home use may be defined as the minimal pressure required to resolve all apneas, hypopneas, snoring, prolonged partial airflow limitations, and arousals related with these events in all stages of sleep and in all sleep positions.[2,56–58] Simply, the optimal PAP setting should resolve all sleep-disordered breathing in supine rapid eye movement (REM) sleep, to account for the effects of gravity and changes in muscle tone that may occur in different sleep stages and positions.[59] The optimal pressure should also maintain oxygen saturation at or above 90% and should minimize mask leak, allowing and maintaining only the intentional mask leak that is appropriate for the given pressure. The pressure should be as low as possible to also minimize pressure intolerance, which can include awakenings, discomfort, air swallowing, and periodic breathing or treatment-emergent central apneas.

Older versions of the AASM practice parameters recommended a full night of attended CPAP titration based on the criteria outlined previously, with repeat titrations recommended for patients in whom symptoms of OSA reappear despite adherence with CPAP therapy, for patients who sustain a significant weight loss either through diet or bariatric surgery, or if CPAP adherence and benefits remain suboptimal by current standards.[56,57] More recent clinical practice guidelines from the AASM recommend either unattended APAP or attended CPAP titrations to determine an adequate CPAP setting for longer-term therapy.[4,5]

The use of home sleep apnea testing (HSAT) is currently not recommended for the titration of CPAP or other PAP therapies as there are few data evaluating the reliability of home sleep testing for this indication. Given the absence of data regarding HSAT for CPAP titration, the Centers for Medicare and Medicaid Services and commercial insurance companies in the United States typically will not reimburse providers who use HSAT for this indication. Similarly, because various proprietary APAP algorithms are far from perfect for detecting and resolving all sleep-disordered breathing events, when a patient is having difficulty with unattended APAP therapy, and/or residual awakenings, nocturia, or daytime symptoms persist, even if the residual AHI suggests adequately treated obstructive sleep apnea syndrome (OSAS), further adjustments can be made based on adherence data, but if optimal settings cannot be found, in-laboratory titration is indicated.[17]

Titrating Bilevel Positive Airway Pressure Therapy for Obstructive Sleep Apnea

BPAP therapy is typically titrated during an attended in-laboratory sleep study, but auto-BPAP can be started empirically like APAP for uncomplicated OSA and may be guided by the pressures needed to prevent obstruction with CPAP. As is the case for CPAP titrations, the current guideline recommendations for BPAP titration strategies are based on consensus opinion.[59] EPR is available with some BPAP systems.

The Philips Respironics BiFlex device differs from conventional bilevel systems in two major respects. First, the inspiratory pressure is reduced slightly near the end of inspiration, and the expiratory pressure is slightly reduced near the beginning of expiration. Although the data regarding the use of traditional bilevel and BiFlex therapies do not demonstrate any advantages over CPAP therapy in patients with newly diagnosed OSA, one study has demonstrated a potential role for BiFlex therapy in patients who are noncompliant with CPAP therapy.[13] Although intuitively one would predict that BPAP would increase adherence by reducing expiratory pressure-related discomfort and side effects, there are in fact no objective outcomes studies that show BPAP therapy improves adherence and or daytime sleepiness when compared with CPAP therapy for patients with uncomplicated OSA.[4,5,57] This may be partly related to the induction of treatment-emergent central sleep apnea in some patients with BPAP.[60]

Overall, BPAP therapy remains a reasonable option for CPAP-intolerant patients, OSA with concurrent COPD, and in those with the obesity hypoventilation syndrome.[3–5,61] The role of BPAP therapy and its variants in otherwise uncomplicated OSA remains unclear.

Finding Optimal Positive Airway Pressure Settings

Titration Studies. Although there are current recommendations to guide clinicians on how to manually titrate PAP therapy in an attended laboratory-based setting, these recommendations largely serve as guidelines as they are principally based on the consensus of expert opinion and not on randomized trials demonstrating their superiority over other methods of manual titration.[59] The AASM guidelines classify the adequacy of a CPAP titration as delineated in Table 132.2.

Most patients with only OSA do not require an initial titration, and there is a growing trend for in-laboratory attended CPAP titrations to be reserved for patients with OSA and concomitant cardiac and/or respiratory disease, those with obesity hypoventilation syndrome, and for those who are having difficulty with CPAP initiated in an unattended setting. As these trends continue to evolve, patients with OSA may benefit by realizing shorter waiting times for CPAP therapy, and health care dollars should be saved by reducing the need for unnecessary PSG.[52]

Table 132.2 Adequacy of CPAP Titration Definitions

Adequacy of Titration	Definition
Optimal	Reduces the RDI to <5 for at least a 15-min duration and should include supine REM sleep at the selected pressure that is not continually interrupted by spontaneous arousals or awakenings
Good	Reduces the RDI to ≤10 or by 50% if the baseline RDI < 15 and should include supine REM sleep that is not continually interrupted by spontaneous arousals or awakenings at the selected pressure
Adequate	Does not reduce the RDI to ≤ 10 but reduces the RDI by 75% from baseline (especially in severe OSA patients), or one in which the titration grading criteria for optimal or good are met, with the exception that supine REM sleep did not occur at the selected pressure
Inadequate	A titration that does not meet any one of the earlier given grades

CPAP, Continuous positive airway pressure; OSA, obstructive sleep apnea; RDI, respiratory disturbance index; REM, rapid eye movement.
Modified from Kushida CA, Chediak A, Berry RB et al. Clinical guidelines for the manual titration of positive airway pressure in patients with obstructive sleep apnea. *J Clin Sleep Med.* 2008:4;157–71.

Split-Night Studies. For patients who require an in-laboratory baseline study, a "split-night" sleep study, in which the initial portion of the study is used to objectively document an individual's sleep-disordered breathing, followed by a CPAP titration during the second portion of the night, may be indicated in certain situations.[57,59,62] A split-night sleep study may be considered when the following criteria have been met: (1) an AHI of more than 40 events per hour is recorded during the initial 2 hours of the PSG and (2) at least 3 hours remain during the PSG to conduct an adequate CPAP titration. Split-night studies can also be considered for individuals who demonstrate less severe OSA, with an AHI of 20 to 40 events per hour or minimal criteria of AHI greater than or equal to 5 for requalification during the initial 2 hours of a sleep study, although data suggest that CPAP titrations in this subgroup of patients may be less accurate when performed in the split-night protocol setting. In our experience, if no optimal setting is found, unless it is clear that the patient requires a different PAP type that would require an additional in-laboratory titration, the patient may be empirically started on an APAP or auto-BPAP setting and then further adjusted based on adherence data.

Continuous Positive Airway Pressure Prediction Formulas

Although current recommendations warrant that CPAP titrations occur during a full overnight in-laboratory PSG or via home APAP therapy, some data suggest that a fixed-pressure CPAP can be successfully initiated in an unattended home setting using alternative approaches. Specifically, several studies confirm that CPAP therapy initiated in an unattended home setting, without HSAT/PSG monitoring or a PAP adherence download to confirm the efficacy of treatment, can be successful in many patients with uncomplicated OSA (OSA without associated COPD, congestive heart failure [CHF], or hypoventilation syndromes) when CPAP settings are determined either by a clinical prediction formula or by CPAP self-adjusted to resolve snoring and daytime symptoms[28,63,64] (Table 132.3).

It is important to note that all of these methods typically offer only a starting pressure for initiating CPAP therapy. As observed in several of the study protocols, many patients may require pressure adjustments based on symptoms and problems with therapy. Given the supporting data from several clinical trials and recommendations from clinical practice guidelines that support the expanded use of APAP for patients with uncomplicated OSA, there is a growing trend for PAP therapy, either fixed CPAP or via APAP, to be initiated in the home for many patients with uncomplicated OSA.[4,5] Thus there is little utility to using prediction formulas for the initiation or adjustment of PAP therapy.

Retitration versus Empirical Adjustments Based on Clinical Response and Adherence Data

The AASM guidelines currently recommend considering a repeat titration study for patients who do not achieve an optimal or good PAP titration. There are actually few data evaluating the quality or efficacy of PAP titrations, as defined by the AASM clinical guidelines, in clinical practice. Specifically, few data exist on how often patients actually achieve an optimal PAP titration, despite having their PAP pressures determined in an attended setting. Furthermore, there are few data examining the outcomes of patients who are initiated on CPAP therapy after undergoing PAP titrations that are less than optimal. Many of the randomized controlled trials evaluating the effect of CPAP on various outcomes have shown a mean residual AHI or respiratory disturbance index of 5 or greater, indicating that greater than 50% of these patients underwent CPAP titrations that did not achieve optimal results. Of the limited existing data from clinical settings, only approximately 50% to 60% of patients with OSA achieve an "optimal" titration, and up to 30% to 40% achieve only an "adequate" or "inadequate" titration.[65,66] Thus many patients on CPAP therapy, even those who undergo attended in-laboratory titrations, may currently be treated with suboptimal pressures settings. More data are needed to better define the optimal clinical and physiologic benchmarks for the various levels of PAP titration adequacy and to determine the outcomes and proper management for patients who do not achieve optimal or good PAP titrations during an in-laboratory titration study. The important point is that the clinician should not assume that a given patient is on an adequate CPAP setting simply because their CPAP pressure was determined during an in-laboratory titration study.

Table 132.3 Clinical Prediction Formulas Used to Determine an Effective CPAP Setting

Study	Clinical Prediction Formula
Miljeteig and Hoffstein, 1993	P(eff) = 0.13 (BMI) + 0.16 (NC) + 0.04 (RDI) − 5.12
Nahmias, 1995	P(eff) = 8.7 + 0.028 (% IBW) + 0.015 (RDI) − 0.071(nadir Sao_2)
Lin et al., 2003	P(eff) = 0.52 + 0.174 (BMI) + 0.042 (AHI)
Stradling, 2004	P(eff) = 2.1 + 0.048 (ODI) + 0.128 (NC)
Hukins, 2005	BMI < 30 = 8 cm H_2O BMI 30–35 = 10 cm H_2O BMI > 35 = 12 cm H_2O
Loredo, 2007	P(eff) = 30.8 + 0.03 (RDI) − 0.05 (nadir Sao_2) − 0.2 (mean Sao_2)

AHI, Apnea-hypopnea index; BMI, body mass index; CPAP, continuous positive airway pressure; IBW, ideal body weight; NC, neck circumference; ODI, oxygen desaturation index; P(eff), effective CPAP pressure; RDI, respiratory disturbance index; Sao_2, arterial oxygen saturation.

Whether or not pressures are originally found on a titration study or started empirically, it is our practice to closely follow both our patient's clinical response and adherence data and, if needed, waveform analysis. Signs of suboptimal treatment may be obvious, such as the inability to tolerate PAP pressure setting or residual sleepiness, or signs may be subtle, such as residual nocturia or multiple awakenings despite other signs of adherence and benefit. As previously discussed, the algorithms used to determine residual AHI may be inaccurate and do not reflect all types of events that may lead to suboptimal treatment, so even patients with AHI of less than 1.0 may still need adjustments (Figure 132.3).

Our approach starts with analysis of mask leak because mask leak often drives intolerance and suboptimal response, especially with APAP or auto-BPAP, whose algorithms are affected by leak. We will request or perform a mask fitting, even if the patient does not complain about leak bothering them, if there is otherwise a suboptimal response. In general, before making other changes we fix the mask leak and then reevaluate; however, if pressures are high, we may lower the pressure at the same time. For nonbothersome leak in setting of low residual AHI and optimal clinical response, we may assure the patient to not worry about high leak that may be due to higher pressures, facial hair, or other factors that can increase leak.

After addressing leak, we assess clinical response, including both nocturnal symptoms of number of awakenings and nocturia, as well as daytime symptoms and the ability to use PAP therapy throughout the night. Our goal is not to use the device for more than 4 hours or have residual AHI of less than 5 or normal ESS. Instead, our usage goal is the ability to use CPAP for the entire sleep period, preferably at least 6 to 8 hours with minimal or no awakenings. Our symptom goal is to relieve nocturnal and daytime symptoms; so even if the residual AHI is normal, we consider mask or pressure changes or further assessment for residual hypoxia or hypoventilation with overnight oximetry or measures of carbon dioxide control. If a patient's use is optimal and symptoms are controlled, but residual AHI is elevated to greater than 5, we may attempt a pressure change based on whether we think the residual

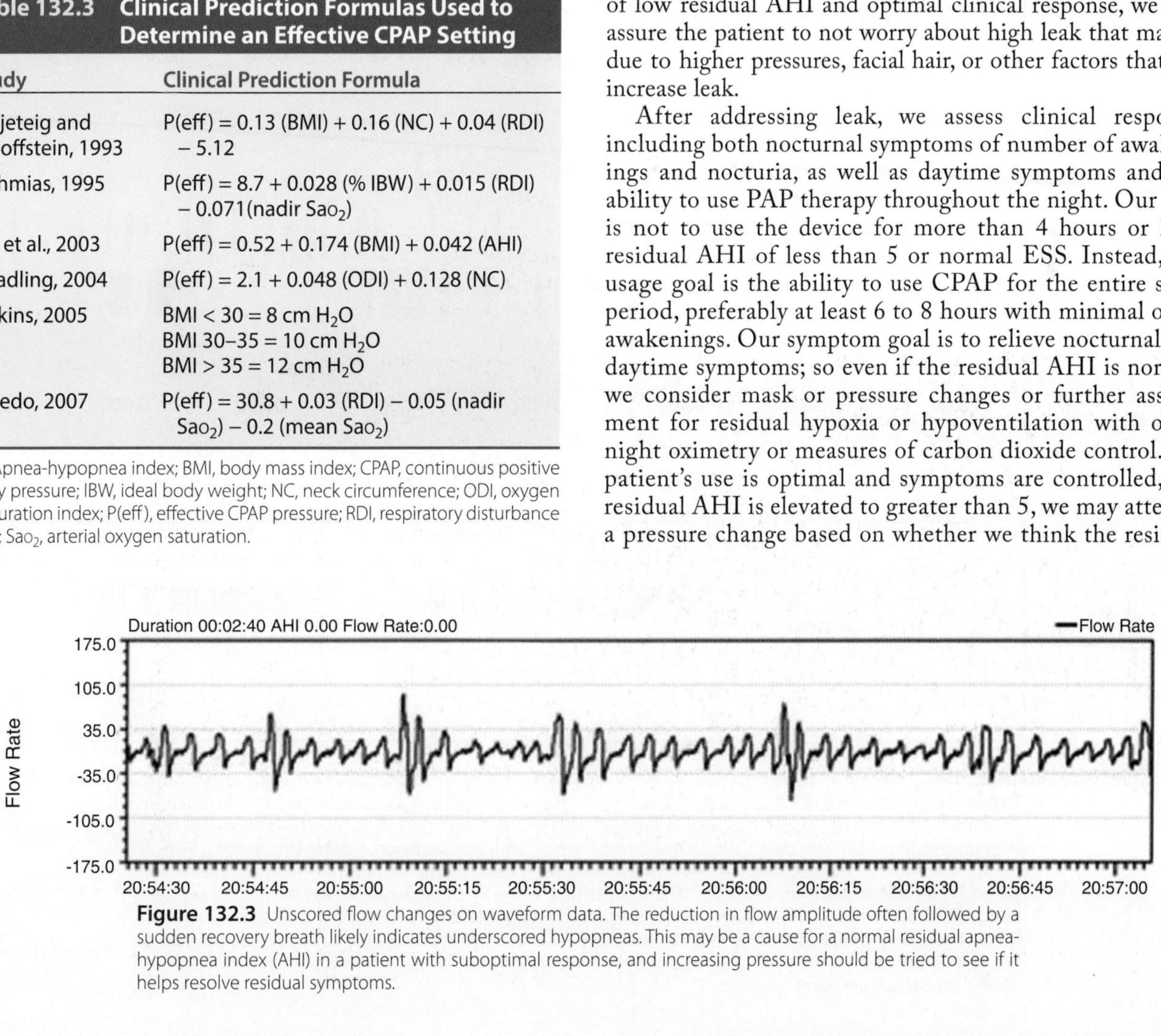

Figure 132.3 Unscored flow changes on waveform data. The reduction in flow amplitude often followed by a sudden recovery breath likely indicates underscored hypopneas. This may be a cause for a normal residual apnea-hypopnea index (AHI) in a patient with suboptimal response, and increasing pressure should be tried to see if it helps resolve residual symptoms.

events are obstructive or central in nature or check overnight oximetry on treatment, but we may allow for persistent elevated AHI, especially if oximetry shows stable oxygen saturations.

The pattern of events on detailed data (Figure 132.4) and waveform analysis can often be helpful in determine whether events, especially hypopneas but also obstructive apneas, are actually more central in nature (Figure 132.5; Table 132.4)

Four of the most common fixable patterns that are often overlooked are suboptimal response despite low AHI due to REM-related events (Figure 132.6); treatment-emergent central sleep apnea or periodic breathing; high leak causing the device to automatically turn on and off, resulting in lower use than patient reports (Figures 132.7 and 132.8); and residual hypoxia or hypoventilation. Recognition of these clinical and data patterns can guide PAP adjustments. It is important to follow the response to the adjustments to determine whether they had the desired effect. Some residual symptoms may be due to other factors, such as insufficient sleep time, insomnia, medications, or other disorders. So if adjustments are not resulting in the desired improvements, we may revert to previous settings. In addition, if an adjustment in one direction leads to a worsening response, it may suggest that other either adjustments in another direction should be tried or there is a need to switch to another modality, such as servo-ventilation or volume-assured pressure support for treatment-emergent central sleep apnea.

Summary data can also be used to suggest the presence of other sleep disorders, such as delayed sleep phase, insufficient sleep from shift work, poor sleep hygiene with napping, or irregular sleep times (Figure 132.8).

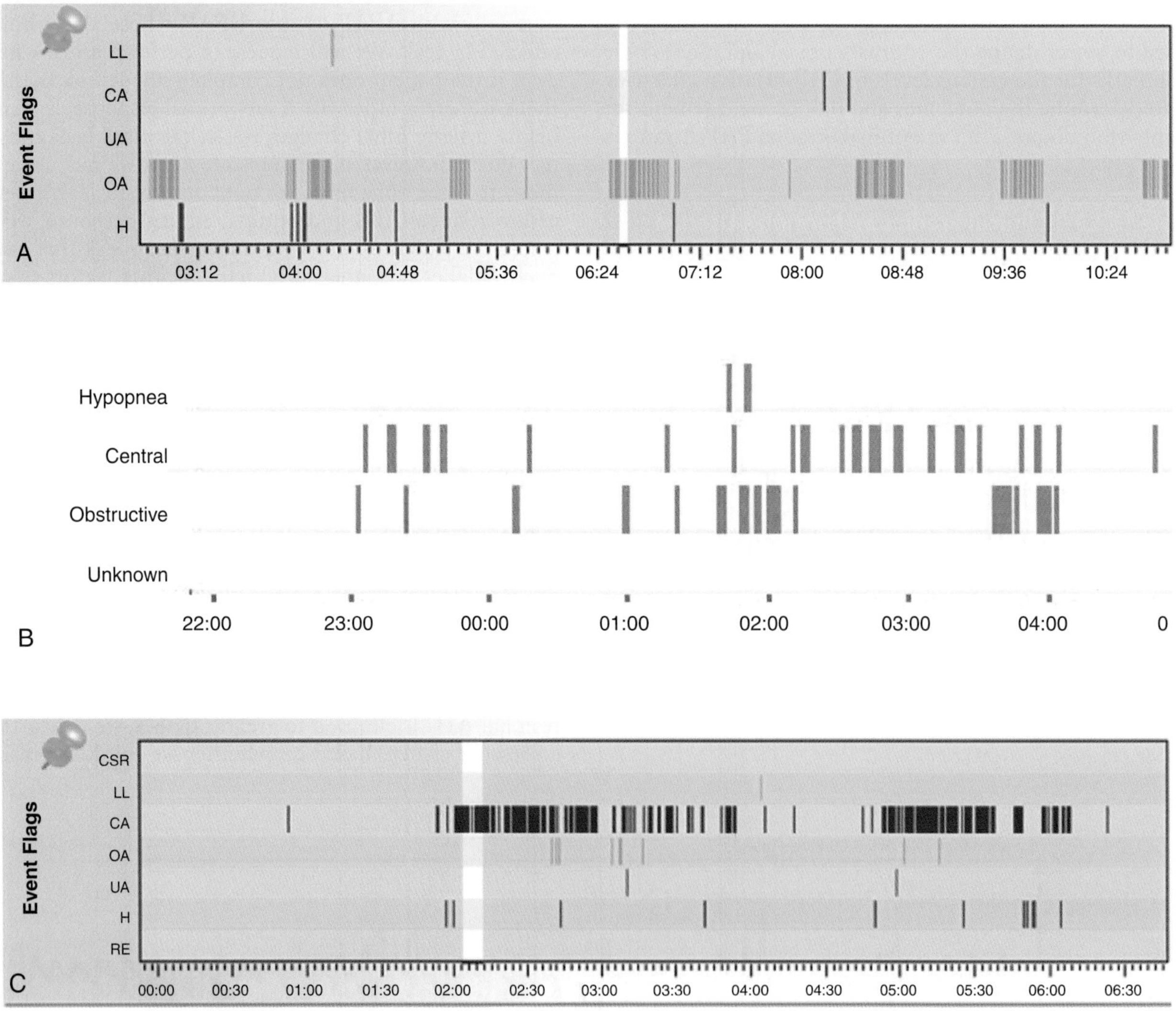

Figure 132.4 Detailed data patterns. **A,** Obstructive events clustering throughout the night, likely in rapid eye movement (REM) periods, suggest increasing pressure will help. **B,** Obstructive events primarily in two clusters likely representing REM, with mostly central events in between, consistent with non–rapid eye movement (NREM) events, which further suggests that increasing pressure will likely help obstructive but worsen central events, and lowering pressures will likely inadequately treat obstructive events in REM, so advanced positive airway pressure modalities should be considered. **C,** Reverse REM pattern with gaps between recurrent central events throughout NREM that resolve in REM suggests that lower pressure should be tried first because are primarily central events. CA, Central apnea; CSR, Cheyne-Stokes respiration; H, hypopnea; OA, obstructive apnea; RE, respiratory effort related arousal; UA, unknown apnea.

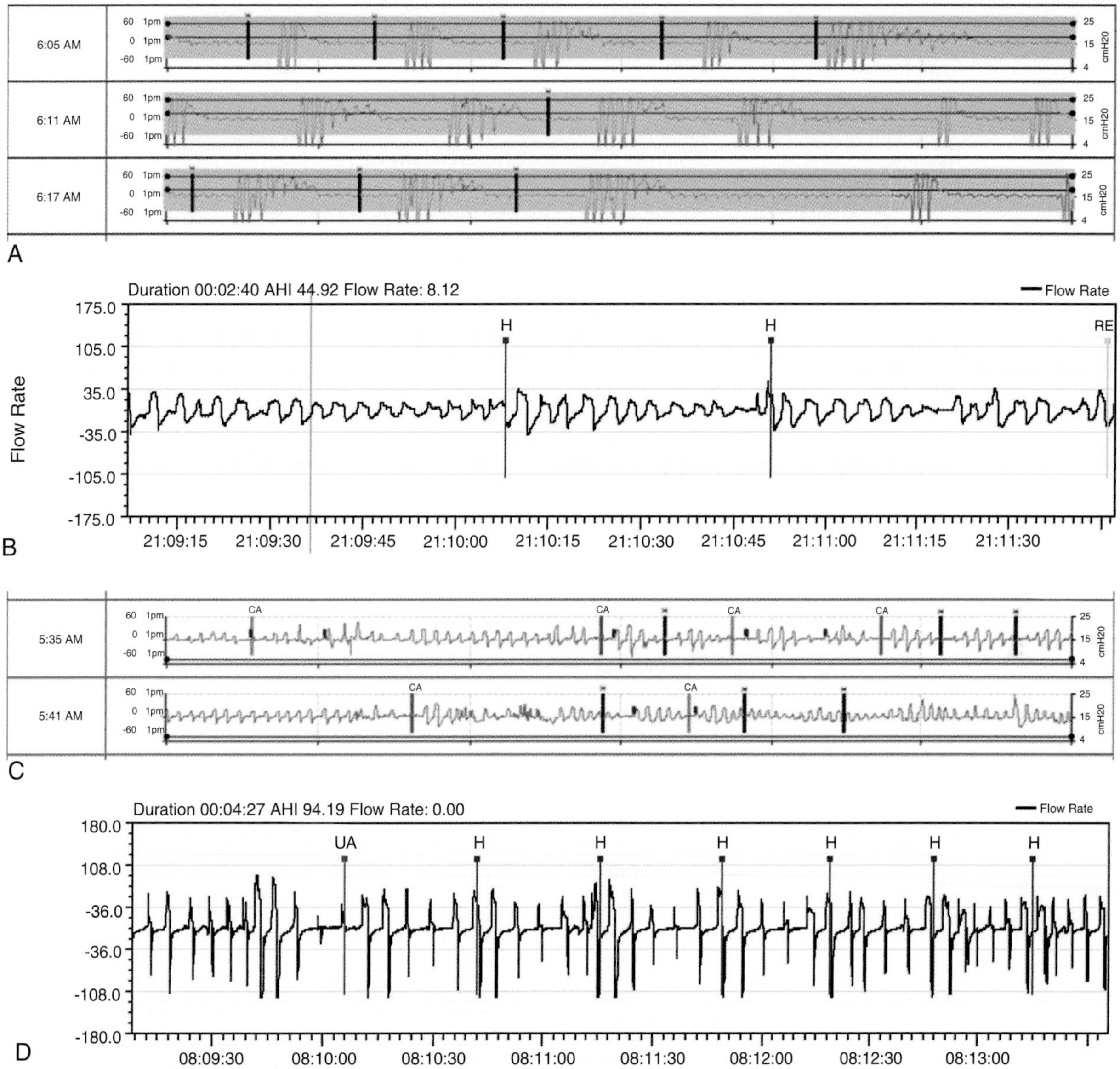

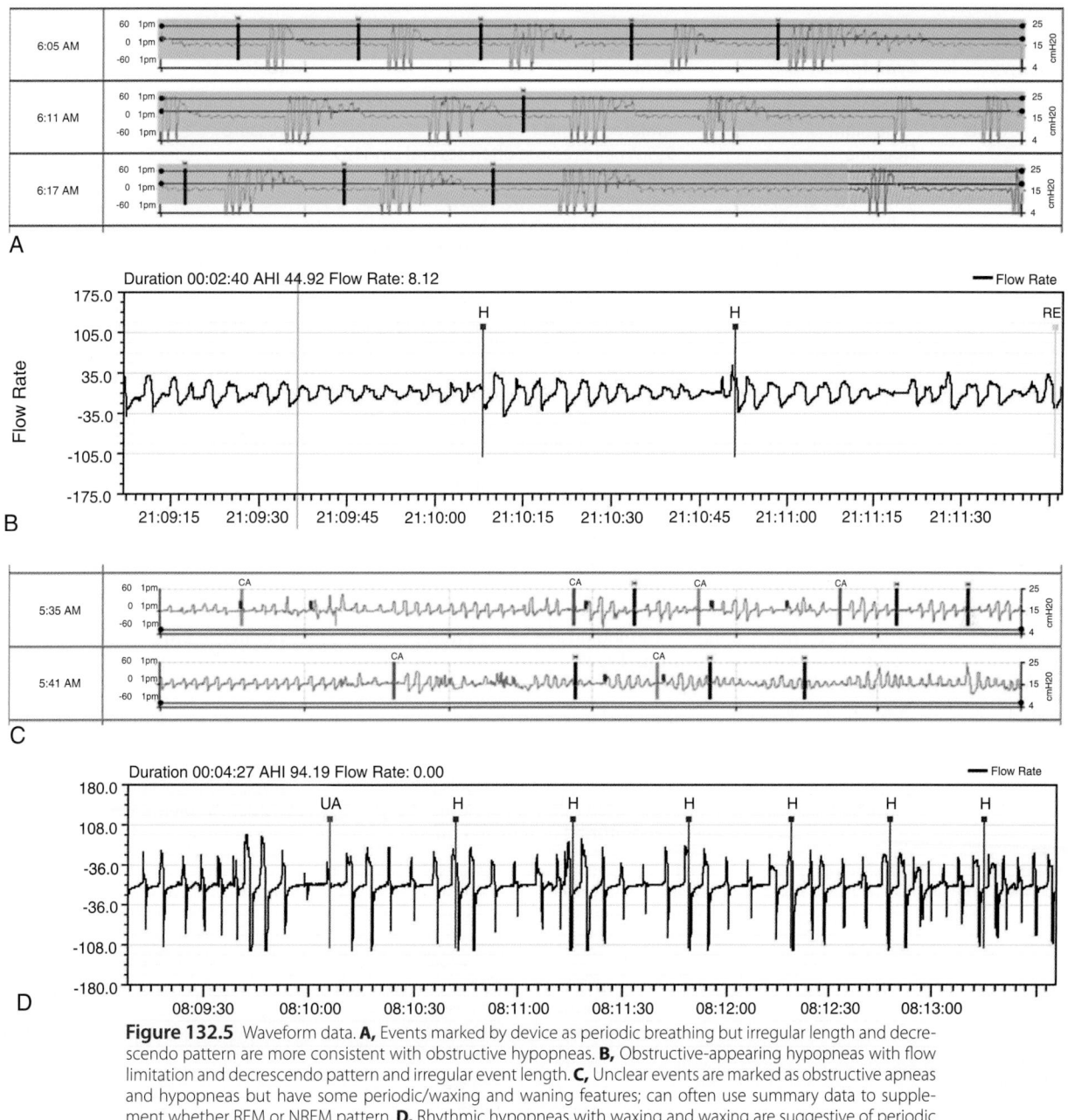

Figure 132.5 Waveform data. **A,** Events marked by device as periodic breathing but irregular length and decrescendo pattern are more consistent with obstructive hypopneas. **B,** Obstructive-appearing hypopneas with flow limitation and decrescendo pattern and irregular event length. **C,** Unclear events are marked as obstructive apneas and hypopneas but have some periodic/waxing and waning features; can often use summary data to supplement whether REM or NREM pattern. **D,** Rhythmic hypopneas with waxing and waxing are suggestive of periodic breathing. AHI, Apnea-hypopnea index.

BENEFITS OF CONTINUOUS POSITIVE AIRWAY PRESSURE THERAPY

It is the perception of many nonsleep practitioners and the lay public that CPAP treatment consistently resolves or improves several important outcomes, including sleep architecture, daytime sleepiness, neurocognitive function, mood, quality of life, and cardiovascular disease in all patients with OSA. When titrated appropriately, CPAP therapy has been demonstrated to resolve most sleep-disordered breathing across the spectrum of disease severity and has been demonstrated to be superior to placebo, conservative management, and positional therapy with regard to this outcome.[4,5,61] Randomized controlled trials have also shown CPAP therapy to be superior to placebo at increasing the percentage and total time in stages N3 (non–rapid eye movement sleep [NREM] stage 3) and REM sleep. CPAP's effects on other sleep parameters, including stages N1 and N2 sleep (NREM stages 1 and 2, respectively), total sleep time, and the arousal index, have been inconsistent across studies.[57,61]

Continuous Positive Airway Pressure Treatment and Daytime Sleepiness

Several randomized controlled studies have shown that CPAP therapy significantly improves or resolves subjective symptoms of daytime sleepiness in OSA patients who suffer from this complaint, predominantly in those who suffer from severe OSA (AHI > 30 events/hour).[4,5,28,67–74] The minimal and optimal amounts of nocturnal use necessary to improve symptoms of daytime sleepiness are, however, not well defined, as

Table 132.4 Common Symptoms and Data Patterns That Support Adjustment

Physiology	Symptoms	Data	Adjustment
Residual REM-related events	Awakenings 2 h or later in the night Nocturia Short use around 2–3 h Intolerance often with difficulty tolerating pressure or feeling short of breath or not enough air in middle of night	Residual AHI often normal if only REM-related events 95%/max pressure often several cm/H_2O higher than median pressure Detailed data shows clustered events with REM timing Waveform data may not have classic obstructive flow limitation	Increase EPAP or EPAPmin to ~95% pressure
Treatment-emergent central apnea/periodic breathing	Residual daytime symptoms Short use Intolerance often with difficulty tolerating pressure at sleep onset	Residual AHI often elevated but may be <5 Residual events often have more central apneas than obstructive apneas, but most events may be hypopneas representing periodic breathing Detailed data may show events throughout night that stop with REM pattern or events at sleep onset Waveform data may show periodic breathing or recurrent central apnea pattern	Make sure no leak issues Change to fixed pressure Lower pressure unless patient is having treatment onset events and says feeling in need of more air Turn off EPR Lower PS or change BPAP to CPAP Consider titration with advanced PAP therapy or other treatments discussed in Chapter 125
High leak with auto-on/off	Patient says they have the machine on much longer than the data reports Complains of mask leak	Night summary data shows machine turning on and off repetitively. High mask leak	Mask fitting Lower maximum pressures
Comorbid hypoxia or hypoventilation	Suboptimal clinical response that could include morning headaches, fatigue, awakenings at night	Residual AHI often normal Overnight oximetry on treatment with low baseline oxygen saturations Elevated bicarbonate levels ≥27 or elevated ABG P_{CO_2} or home TC_{CO_2} monitoring despite treatment	Titration study using TC_{CO_2} monitoring If already on BPAP or volume-assured pressure support, increase pressure support or goal volumes Consider supplemental oxygen after hypoventilation is treated

ABG, Arterial blood gas; AHI, apnea-hypopnea index; BPAP, bilevel positive airway pressure; CPAP, continuous positive airway pressure; EPAP, expiratory positive airway pressure; EPAPmin, minimum expiratory positive airway pressure; EPR, expiratory pressure relief; max, maximum; PAP, positive airway pressure; P_{CO_2}, partial pressure of carbon dioxide; REM, rapid eye movement; PS, pressure support; REM, rapid eye movement; TC_{CO_2}, transcutaneous carbon dioxide.

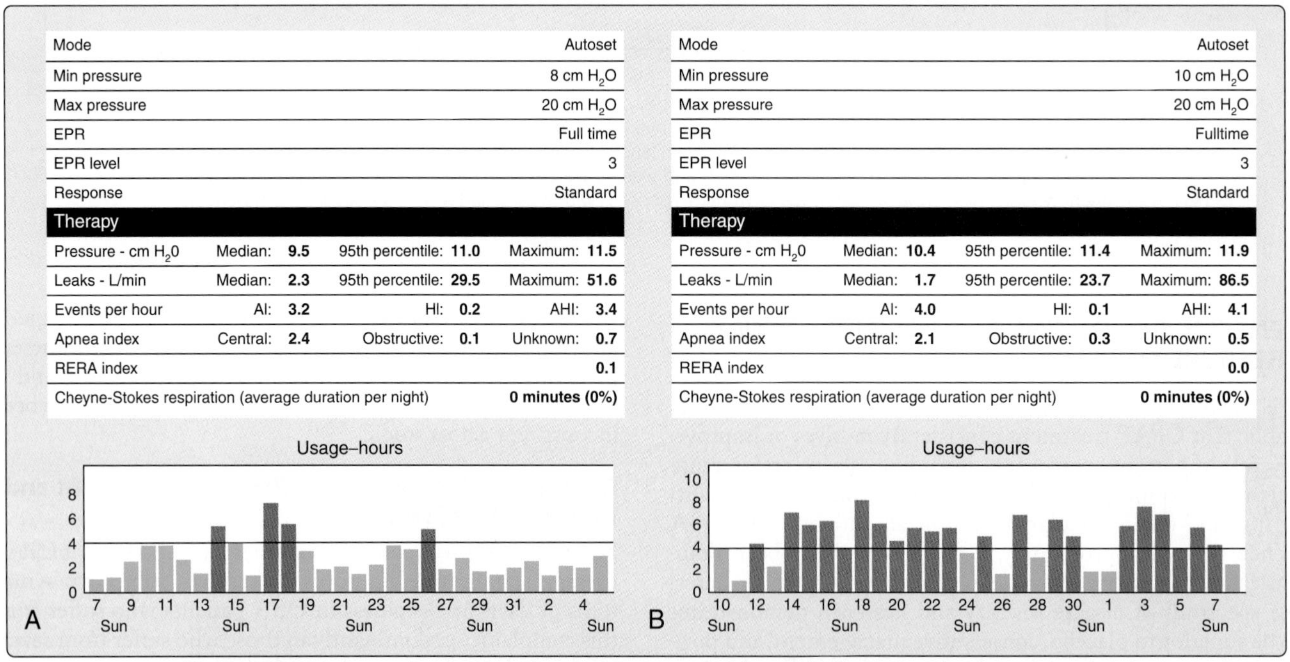

Figure 132.6 Summary data. **A,** Before pressure change, patient felt in need of more air and was mouth breathing when awakened after 1 to 2 hours of sleep. **B,** After expiratory positive airway pressure (EPAP) minimum increased closer to 95% pressure, patient was able to sleep longer. AI, Apnea index; AHI, apnea-hypopnea index; HI, hypopnea index; max, maximum; min, minimum; RERA, respiratory effort-related arousal.

AirCurve 10 VAuto					
Serial number					23191915264
Mode					**Spont**
EPAP/IPAP					**9.0 / 17.0 cm H_2O**
Easy-Breathe					**On**
Statistics					
Usage					3 h 18 min
Leak–L/min			Median: **57.6**		95th %: **66.0**
Events per hour	AHI: **37.2**		AI: **37.2**		HI: **0.0**
	Central: **0.0**		Obstructive: **0.0**		Unknown: **37.2**

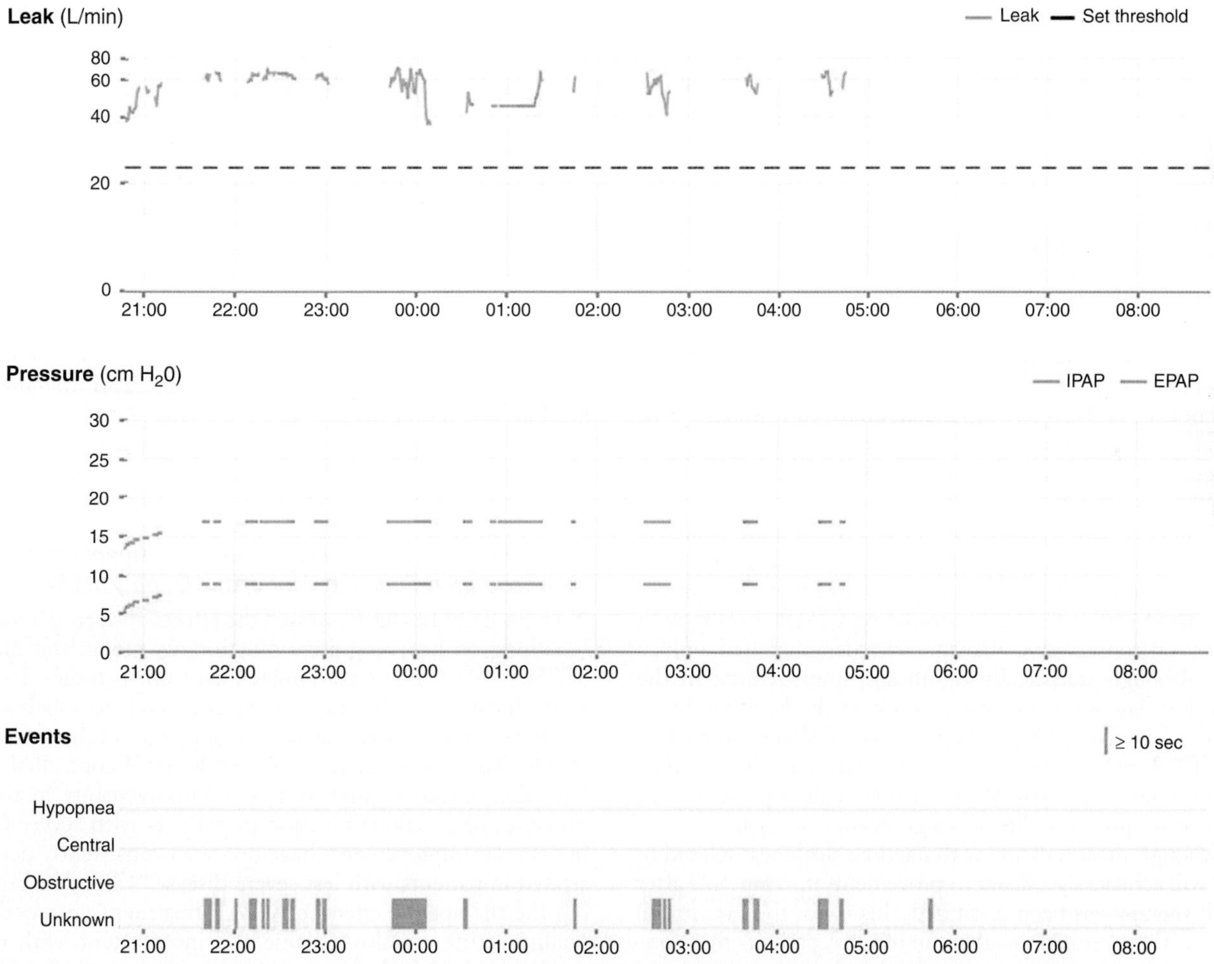

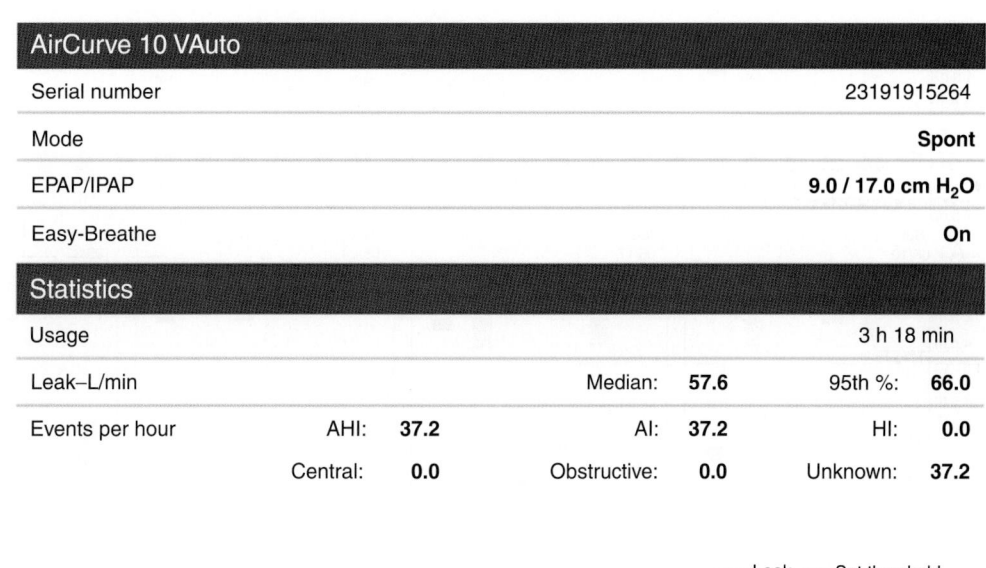

Figure 132.7 Auto-stop/start in the setting of high leak causing short usage. Note the very frequent starting and stopping of pressures in the night in the setting of high leak. The machine marked all events as unknown due to the high leak. Mask fitting should be performed, and if needed, pressures or pressure support may need to be reduced. AI, Apnea index; AHI, apnea-hypopnea index; EPAP, expiratory positive airway pressure; HI, hypopnea index; IPAP, inspiratory positive airway pressure.

even partial nocturnal use (as little as 2 hours/night) has been associated with significant improvements in daytime symptoms in some patients.[75,76,81] Although the minimal amount of time required on a nightly basis to improve symptoms of daytime sleepiness is not well established, it is clear that CPAP therapy is required for a least a portion of each night as symptoms of daytime sleepiness reappear when CPAP therapy is discontinued for as little as 1 to 2 nights.[8,77,78] Reoccurrence of daytime symptoms upon CPAP withdrawal has been observed across the spectrum of OSA severity. As mentioned

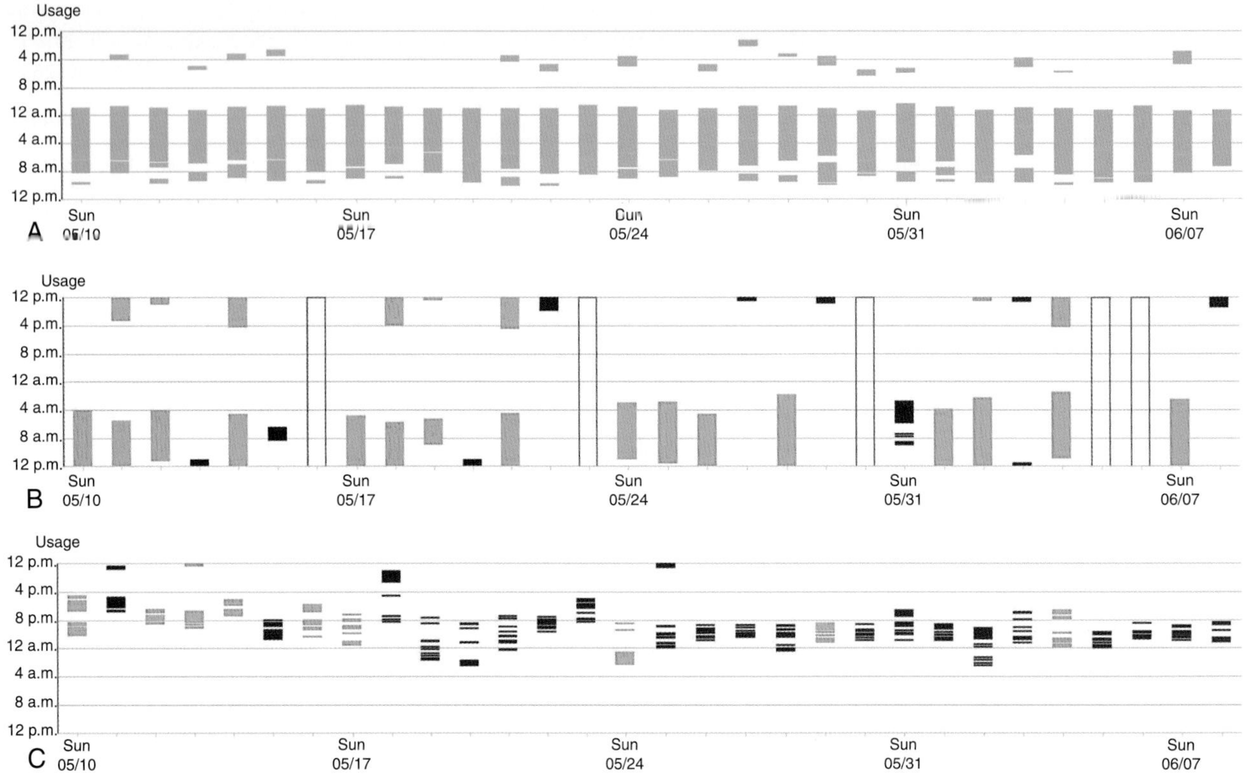

Figure 132.8 Summary data. **A,** Napping around 4 p.m. **B,** Shift work leading to short use 2 days per week. **C,** Auto-stop/start due to high leak causing underreporting of usage hours.

previously, a specific threshold for nightly use of CPAP, in terms of improvements in symptoms of daytime sleepiness, does not exist and is likely dependent on the individual.[75,76] In general, greater adherence to CPAP therapy on a nightly basis has been associated with greater improvements in symptoms of daytime sleepiness.

The data regarding the effects of CPAP on more objective measures of daytime sleepiness are more inconclusive across the spectrum of disease severity.[61,72] A large meta-analysis of randomized controlled trials comparing CPAP therapy with placebo or conservative management demonstrated only a small, although statistically significant, improvement in the mean sleep latency as measured on either the Multiple Sleep Latency Test (MSLT) or Maintenance of Wakefulness Test (MWT). Across all studies, the mean sleep latency improved by 0.93 minutes ($P = .04$). Whether this small improvement in objective sleepiness is clinically significant is unclear.

Although most patients with daytime sleepiness related to OSA will achieve significant improvements in symptoms after CPAP therapy has been instituted, this is not the case for all patients. There remains a subgroup of OSA patients that continue to suffer from symptoms of residual daytime sleepiness despite adequate adherence with CPAP therapy, although the actual prevalence of residual daytime sleepiness in CPAP-compliant patients remains undefined.[75,76,79–81] Prospective observational data have demonstrated that as many as 20% to 30% of those patients who are compliant with their CPAP therapy for greater than or equal to 7 hours per night may still complain of subjective sleepiness (ESS score > 10) after 3 months of treatment.[75,76] In addition, many patients also may not achieve normal levels of objective alertness (as defined by the MSLT or MWT) or associated functional outcomes (as defined by the Functional Outcomes of Sleep Questionnaire), despite seemingly adequate nightly use of CPAP therapy. The mechanisms responsible for this syndrome of residual daytime sleepiness also remain unclear but may in part be related to the oxidative injury effects of long-term intermittent hypoxemia on the sleep-wake–promoting regions in the brain.[82]

Continuous Positive Airway Pressure Treatment Effect on Neurocognitive Function, Mood, and Quality of Life

Numerous studies have assessed the effects of sleep-disordered breathing on neurocognitive functioning, mood, and quality of life.[57,69,83–95] Most randomized controlled studies demonstrate inconsistent improvements in several neurobehavioral performance parameters across the spectrum of disease severity.[4,5,61] For example, large-scale randomized controlled trials have demonstrated mild, transient improvements in several measures of executive function in patients with severe OSA, but similar improvements have not been consistently demonstrated in patients with less severe disease.[96] The data regarding the therapeutic effects of CPAP treatment on mood and quality of life are also variable and inconsistent, with many randomized trials demonstrating no clear benefits of CPAP therapy compared with placebo or conservative treatments in these parameters.

One reason for the inconsistent improvements in neurocognitive function demonstrated with CPAP therapy is that the impact of OSA on neurocognitive function for the majority of patients with OSA may be relatively small across the spectrum of disease severity. The Apnea Positive Pressure Long-term Efficacy Study (APPLES) trial demonstrated that most patients with OSA did not demonstrate significant neurocognitive deficits and that the degree of deficit was only weakly associated with the degree of oxygen desaturation and not associated with the AHI.[97] Treatment with CPAP in the APPLES trial was associated with improved long-term sleep duration, quality, and architecture but not memory.[95] Another possible explanation for the inconsistent effect of CPAP in improving outcomes associated with neurocognition, mood, and quality of life is the use of multiple, different measures of function to assess similar parameters. For example, there is near-universal use of the ESS when assessing improvements in subjective sleepiness, yet there are multiple tests that are used across several studies to assess for improvements in mood, neurocognitive function, and quality of life. Further research is required to better define the role of CPAP therapy in alleviating these symptoms and deficits in susceptible OSA patients.

Despite the inconsistent data regarding improvements in neurocognitive function with CPAP use, several observational studies support a significant reduction in the incidence of motor vehicle accidents in patients with OSA after the initiation of CPAP therapy.[98] Although the actual time course to improved driving performance in real-life situations is not clear, driving-simulator performance can improve in as little as 2 to 7 nights of therapy. Similar to other aspects of neurobehavioral performance that may be adversely affected by OSA, many patients with OSA may continue to demonstrate impaired driving-simulator performance despite several months of high adherence to CPAP therapy.[99] The explanation for this last finding is not completely clear, although it is likely that many patients may still not be adhering to PAP therapy enough on a nightly basis and/or achieving enough sleep on a regular basis to normalize their driving skills. Unfortunately, there is no specific threshold of CPAP use or duration of treatment that can accurately predict a given individual's fitness to safely drive a vehicle. Because the severity of OSA alone is not a reliable predictor of motor vehicle accident risk, the clinician must take into account several factors, including improvements in subjective symptoms and adherence with therapy before determining a driver's ability to safely operate a motor vehicle.

Continuous Positive Airway Pressure Treatment and Cardiovascular Disease

Although untreated OSA has been associated with an increased risk for hypertension and other cardiovascular diseases in certain populations, the literature and outcomes data supporting the beneficial effects of CPAP on cardiovascular outcomes have been inconsistent.[57,61,100–104] Several randomized clinical trials and meta-analyses have assessed the effects of CPAP on BP.[105–108] Overall, CPAP treatment appears to attenuate the adverse effects of untreated OSA on daytime and nocturnal systolic and diastolic BP and on 24-hour mean BP. These data demonstrate that, compared with placebo, sham CPAP, or supportive therapy alone, CPAP treatment is associated small (−1.8 to −3.0 mm Hg), but statistically significant, improvements in diurnal mean arterial systolic and diastolic BPs. When considering pooled data, improvements in systolic and diastolic BPs have been observed both during the daytime (2.2 ± 0.7 mm Hg and 1.9 ± 0.6 mm Hg, respectively) and nighttime (3.8 ± 0.8 mm Hg and 1.8 ± 0.6 mm Hg, respectively).[107] One study found the largest improvements in morning BP and more at 2 months than after 6 months of treatment.[108] In general, improvements in BP with CPAP therapy have been associated with greater severity of baseline OSA (higher AHI), the presence of subjective daytime sleepiness, younger age, and greater adherence with CPAP use on a nightly basis.

One of the main limitations of the current studies evaluating the effect of CPAP use on BP in patients with OSAS is that, although these studies evaluated BP as an outcome measure, several of the studies either did not include patients with hypertension or included patients with hypertension who were already adequately controlled on antihypertensive medications. More robust reductions and clinical improvements in BP with CPAP therapy have been observed when evaluating data from studies that included patients with uncontrolled hypertension.[109] In patients with uncontrolled hypertension at baseline, the use of CPAP has been associated with significantly greater reductions in awake systolic and diastolic BP (7.1 mm Hg and 4.3 mm Hg, respectively) compared to placebo or sham PAP therapy. These improvements have been observed even after controlling for several potential confounders, including severity of disease, daytime sleepiness, patient demographics, use of antihypertensive medications, CPAP adherence, and duration of CPAP therapy. Other studies in patients with refractory hypertension and untreated OSA support improvements in various parameters of BP measurement with CPAP therapy.[110]

Few studies have compared the effects of CPAP against antihypertensive medication on BP reduction in patients with OSA and hypertension. In one randomized controlled trial, medical treatment with valsartan (160 mg daily) alone without CPAP therapy reduced several parameters of BP significantly more than CPAP therapy alone over an 8-week period.[111] Specifically, valsartan therapy demonstrated superior reductions in 24-hour mean arterial pressure (24-hour mean BP: −2.1 mm Hg with CPAP vs. 9.1 mm Hg with valsartan, $P < 0.001$), as well as mean arterial BPs during the daytime and throughout the night when compared with CPAP therapy. Other studies have demonstrated similar results.[112,113]

As noted previously, the presence of subjective daytime sleepiness has generally been associated with a more robust improvement in BP with CPAP therapy. There is some bias in these data, as most of the studies that have evaluated various outcomes have in fact predominantly assessed patients with OSA and such associated daytime sleepiness. Because more than half of all patients with OSA, including those with severe disease (AHI ≥ 30), do not have associated daytime sleepiness, it would be important to determine if treating patients with OSA who do not complain of subjective sleepiness improves BP and/or reduces the incidence of hypertension and other cardiovascular morbidities. Several randomized controlled trials have assessed the effect of CPAP on BP and other cardiovascular outcomes in patients without daytime sleepiness.[102,114] One of these large randomized controlled trials assessing CPAP therapy compared with conservative therapy in patients with moderate to severe OSA without daytime sleepiness found that CPAP therapy did not result in a statistically significant reduction in incident hypertension or cardiovascular events (nonfatal myocardial infarction or stroke, transient ischemic attack, CHF, or cardiovascular death) over a period of 4 years of follow-up.[114] When the data were stratified by CPAP adherence, however, patients using prescribed CPAP therapy for more than 4 hours per night did demonstrate a small, but statistically significant ($P = .04$), reduction in the incidence of hypertension over the 4-year study period.

Results from the *S*leep *A*pnea cardio*V*ascular *E*ndpoints (SAVE) Trial, which included a large number of patients without daytime sleepiness, also demonstrated that therapy with CPAP plus usual care, as compared with usual care alone, did not prevent cardiovascular events in patients with moderate to severe OSA and established cardiovascular disease.[102] Thus the benefit of treating patients with moderate to severe OSA who do not have symptoms of daytime sleepiness or cardiovascular disease remains to be better defined regarding the risk of future cardiovascular morbidity and mortality.[103]

The role of CPAP therapy as an adjunctive therapy to resolve or reduce the occurrence or reoccurrence of cardiac arrhythmias is also uncertain. Several observational studies have demonstrated an association between OSA and atrial fibrillation, as well as a higher risk of recurrence of atrial fibrillation after electrical cardioversion or catheter ablation therapy. Although some observational studies have shown an association between increased adherence with CPAP therapy and a lower reoccurrence rate of atrial fibrillation after these procedures, other studies have demonstrated no benefit of CPAP use on the recurrence of atrial fibrillation after intervention.[115–120] One small randomized controlled trial also demonstrated no effect of CPAP on the recurrence of atrial fibrillation after cardioversion for atrial fibrillation, although the generalizability of the results are limited, given the relatively small sample size.[119] Because most of the current data regarding CPAP therapy and atrial fibrillation are based on observational studies, the role of CPAP as an adjunct treatment to prevent or improve atrial arrhythmia control remains uncertain. Finally, although there may be an increased risk of ventricular arrhythmias (tachycardia and fibrillation) in some patients with untreated OSA, there are limited data evaluating the effect of PAP therapy for reducing the incidence and prevalence of these events.[121] Thus the role of PAP therapy for reducing ventricular arrhythmias in patients with OSA is not clear.

There are several possible explanations for why CPAP therapy has not been demonstrated to result in more consistent and greater improvements in BP and other cardiovascular outcomes in patients with OSA. First, much of the literature assessing the effects of CPAP on BP have been based on small trials of relatively short duration (3 months or less). This duration of treatment, even in patients with underlying hypertension, may not be a long enough treatment time to improve BP. Second, as mentioned previously, although several of the studies used BP as an outcome measure, many of the studies included in the meta-analyses enrolled patients without hypertension at baseline. Thus one would not necessarily expect to observe a change in BP if hypertension was not present at the initiation of the studies. Also, most of the patients who had hypertension at enrollment were on antihypertensive medications during most of the studies, which is likely to attenuate the effect of CPAP on BP.[122] Third, although improvements in BP tend to be associated with better CPAP adherence, overall adherence in most studies have typically averaged between 4 and 5 hours per night. In the SAVE Trial, the long-term PAP adherence for study participants was only 3.3 hours per night.[102] Thus inadequate nighttime CPAP use, especially when not used during the later parts of the night when REM sleep is more likely to occur, may limit the beneficial effect of therapy on BP in those with and without hypertension.[123] Fourth, even though OSA is found to be an independent risk factor for hypertension in many populations, hypertension is typically associated with several comorbid conditions that are also related to OSA. Thus treating OSA without treating the other comorbid conditions may not result in significant improvements in BP or other cardiovascular outcomes. Fifth, it is possible that many patients with long-standing hypertension have fixed disease, which CPAP therapy may not improve. Finally, not all untreated OSA patients are necessarily at similar risk for the development of hypertension and other cardiovascular diseases. There are emerging data that suggest that certain phenotypes of patients with OSA, specifically those without daytime sleepiness, may be at lower risk for cardiovascular problems than those with daytime sleepiness.[124] Thus trials that are unable to stratify patients deemed to be at higher risk for hypertension may only demonstrate mean results across a given population. When, and if, biomarkers are discovered that may identify patients at higher risk for hypertension and other cardiovascular diseases, therapies such as CPAP may be targeted to at-risk populations that would be deemed to derive greater benefits from therapy.

There are currently limited long-term randomized controlled data evaluating the effect of CPAP on any cardiovascular outcomes, including mortality. Previous long-term observational data supported the potential beneficial effects of CPAP therapy on cardiovascular outcomes comes.[125] Marin and colleagues[125] followed a large group of male OSA patients with a spectrum of OSA severity and associated daytime sleepiness in a prospective observational study over a period of 10 years. Their results demonstrated two important findings: (1) Compared with normal nonsnoring control subjects, patients with untreated severe OSA (defined as an AHI >30 events/hour) had a significantly increased incidence of both fatal and nonfatal cardiovascular events and (2) CPAP treatment (>4 hours/night) in patients with severe OSA (AHI ≥ 30 events per hour) reduced the incidence of adverse cardiovascular outcomes and improved survival, demonstrating outcomes similar to normal control subjects. Similar improvements in outcomes with CPAP therapy were not observed in OSA patients with less severe disease, as untreated mild to moderate OSA was not observed to be associated with increased risks of cardiovascular morbidity or mortality in this study. Another observational study also demonstrated improvements in cardiovascular mortality across a spectrum of OSA severity, although the data are limited by absence of a control group.[126] These results were not supported by the SAVE Trial data as noted previously. When reviewing the relevant literature, the use of PAP, compared with no treatment or sham, has not been associated with reduced risks of cardiovascular outcomes or death for patients with OSA.[103]

Given the inconclusive nature of CPAP therapy on cardiovascular outcomes in general, the AASM clinical practice guidelines have recommended CPAP therapy only as an adjunctive treatment to lower BP in hypertensive patients with OSA.[4,5] Several other authorities and professional societies have recommended that further supporting data are required to better determine the role of CPAP therapy on improving cardiovascular outcomes before making recommendations for its use in various populations.[100,101,103]

Continuous Positive Airway Pressure Therapy in Patients with Mild Obstructive Sleep Apnea

Most of the literature assessing the effects of CPAP on various outcomes has predominantly evaluated OSA patients with moderate to severe disease. Although approximately 28% of patients with mild disease (AHI = 5 to 14 events/hour) complain of subjective daytime sleepiness, it remains unclear whether treating this group of patients with CPAP therapy improves their daytime symptoms.[127] Results from the CPAP Apnea Trial North American Program (CATNAP) Trial demonstrated that CPAP therapy significantly improved daytime symptoms as measured by the Functional Outcomes of Sleep Questionnaire (FOSQ) when compared with sham CPAP therapy in patients with mild to moderate OSA over an 8-week period of follow-up.[128] The APPLES trial was a large multicenter randomized controlled trial comparing the neurocognitive effects of therapeutic CPAP with sham CPAP across the spectrum of OSA severity.[96] As expected, subjective daytime sleepiness and objective alertness as assessed by the MWT was improved by CPAP therapy at 6 months, but significant improvements in both of these parameters were only observed in patients with severe OSA (AHI ≥ 30). In patients with moderate disease (AHI = 15 to 29), improvements in subjective sleepiness, but not objective alertness, were observed after 6 months of therapy. In patients with mild disease, there were no significant improvements in objective alertness or subjective sleepiness after 2 and 6 months of CPAP therapy. Other studies have also demonstrated limited benefits in patients with more mild disease.[129] Thus the role of CPAP therapy for this indication in patients with mild disease remains unclear based on the current data. It appears reasonable to initiate CPAP therapy in patients with daytime symptoms, but the decision to continue chronic therapy in this patient group should be based on a response to therapy. For patients with mild disease without daytime symptoms, it is not clear that treating these patients is beneficial or should be recommended based on the current data. Patients with mild obstructive sleep-disordered breathing, which includes mild OSA, but also upper airway resistance syndrome and prolonged partial airflow limitation are more likely to present with atypical symptoms, such as insomnia, somatic symptoms such as depression, fibromyalgia, or chronic fatigue or headaches, so it is reasonable to try CPAP to see if treatment improves these types of symptoms.[58]

The Role of Continuous Positive Airway Pressure Therapy in Patients with REM-Predominant Obstructive Sleep Apnea

The prevalence of REM–sleep-related or REM-predominant OSA is unclear, in part due to the absence of a standard definition for this entity. This OSA variant tends to be more common in women, although it may affect adult patients of both genders across the age spectrum.[66,130] The association of this OSA variant with daytime or nighttime symptoms is not clear, but it appears that a subgroup of patients is affected. Of importance, sleep-disordered breathing during REM sleep appears to be independently associated with hypertension and other cardiovascular disease.[131] For those patients who demonstrate this type of OSA and complain of daytime symptoms and or nighttime sleep disturbance, it is unclear if treatment with CPAP consistently improves daytime or nighttime symptoms. Limited observational data of CPAP therapy in symptomatic patients with such REM-predominant OSA has demonstrated significant improvements in daytime sleepiness, fatigue, and the FOSQ. These improvements with CPAP therapy were similar to patients with OSA not limited to REM sleep.[49] However, there are no randomized controlled data assessing any outcomes in this subgroup of patients, including cardiovascular disease.

Obstructive Sleep Apnea and Comorbid Diseases

CHF is a common disease with an estimated prevalence of concomitant OSA of approximately 33%. Small randomized controlled and observational trials initially demonstrated a beneficial effect of CPAP therapy on left ventricular ejection fraction (LVEF) in patients with concomitant OSA and CHF with systolic dysfunction.[132,133] Compared with optimal medical management alone, CHF patients with moderate to severe OSA showed LVEF improvements of 5% to 9% over 1 to 3 months.[132,133] Since these earlier studies, several additional randomized controlled studies have assessed the effects of CPAP therapy on LVEF in CHF patients with and without systolic dysfunction.[134] Overall, CPAP therapy has shown statistically significant improvements in LVEF in patients with OSA and concomitant systolic dysfunction, with an average improvement in LVEF across studies of approximately 5%. In patients with diastolic CHF and concomitant OSA, CPAP therapy has not been associated with significant improvements in LVEF (1%). For patients with CHF and systolic dysfunction, one would expect this degree of improvement in LVEF to be associated with improvements in other outcomes based on trials of medical therapies for CHF. However, it is uncertain if the improvements in LVEF in patients with OSA and concomitant CHF translate into improvements in other important outcomes, such as reductions in hospitalizations and mortality.[103,135] Most of the studies evaluating this patient population have been limited by small sample sizes and relatively short durations of follow-up (typically 12 weeks or less).

The "overlap syndrome" refers to the coexistence of OSA with COPD. The prevalence of OSA in patients with COPD appears to be similar to that of the general population. Prospective observational and retrospective studies have shown that untreated OSA in this patient group is associated with an increased risk for death and severe COPD exacerbations leading to hospitalizations compared to groups of COPD patients without concomitant OSA.[136,137] Observational data have also shown that CPAP therapy in OSA patients with COPD has been associated with significant reductions in both acute exacerbations of COPD, such as requiring hospitalizations and death, with outcomes similar to COPD patients without OSA. Increased adherence to CPAP therapy has been independently associated with reduced mortality in this patient population, whereas decreased CPAP adherence and increased age have been independently associated with increased mortality.[137] Observational data would suggest that adherence to CPAP therapy for as little as 2 hours per night has been associated with a reduction in mortality in this group of patients. Given the current observational data, it is reasonable to recommend CPAP therapy in patients with the overlap syndrome, although, given the absence of randomized controlled data in this patient population, the role of CPAP therapy to reduce exacerbations or improve mortality remains undefined.

The role of CPAP therapy in improving important outcomes in patients with associated diabetes mellitus (short-term and long-term glucose control) and concomitant OSA is unclear as most of the trials evaluating the use of CPAP in this patient population have yielded inconsistent results.[138–140] The role of CPAP as an adjunct therapy to improve weight loss is also uncertain, and adequate treatment of OSA has not been observed to result in enhanced weight loss in the majority of studies.[141,142]

COMPARISON OF CONTINUOUS POSITIVE AIRWAY PRESSURE TO OTHER OBSTRUCTIVE SLEEP APNEA TREATMENTS

Oral appliances (nonadjustable, mandibular advancement devices, and tongue retaining devices) are typically recommended for patients with mild to moderate OSA and for patients with severe disease who fail or do not tolerate CPAP therapy. In general, CPAP therapy results in greater improvements in the AHI and degree of oxygen desaturation when compared with oral appliance treatment. Despite these findings, improvements in daytime sleepiness tend to be similar between the two therapies. This may be related to greater overall adherence with oral appliance therapy compared to CPAP.[143,144] Comparisons of CPAP with oral appliance therapy for improvements in BP are difficult. Although most of the pooled data suggest a favorable effect of oral appliance therapy on many parameters of BP, most of the studies have been observational, with few head-to head-comparisons between the two treatments.[145,146] Thus, based on the current data, it is difficult to draw conclusions or make recommendations between the two therapies concerning the outcome of BP.

Oxygen Therapy Compared to Continuous Positive Airway Pressure for Obstructive Sleep Apnea

The risk of cardiovascular disease related to untreated OSA is dependent on numerous factors, including the severity of disease, as defined by the AHI, and the degree of associated oxygen desaturation. Several small studies have shown that nocturnal oxygen therapy alone can in fact improve both the AHI and degree of oxygen desaturation, although such therapy may be associated with a prolongation of apneas and hypopneas. CPAP, however, has been associated with greater improvements in the AHI when compared with nocturnal oxygen therapy alone.[147] Further, a short-term (12 weeks) randomized controlled trial has shown that CPAP results in greater reductions in 24-hour mean arterial BP when compared with nocturnal oxygen (2 L/minute) or supportive therapy without CPAP in patients with moderate to severe OSA, cardiovascular disease, or multiple cardiovascular risk factors. Similar to other studies, decreases in BP with CPAP therapy were relatively small compared with baseline or the control group (−2.4 mm Hg).[148] Oxygen therapy alone was not associated with any changes in BP compared to baseline or the control group over the study period. Thus, based on the limited literature, oxygen therapy alone should not be recommended as a primary treatment for OSA.

OUTCOMES SUMMARY

CPAP consistently improves or resolves OSA events across the spectrum of OSA severity and improves symptoms of daytime sleepiness predominantly in patients with moderate to severe OSA. Improvements in other outcomes are inconsistent. Treatment with CPAP has been associated with small reductions in BP, with greater reductions being observed in patients with poorly controlled or resistant hypertension and in those patients with associated daytime sleepiness. The role of CPAP therapy in reducing long-term cardiovascular risk or mortality in OSA is uncertain based on the current data, but the current literature does not support the use of CPAP therapy to reduce cardiovascular disease based on typical adherence patterns. Finally, the role of CPAP for patients without daytime symptoms with or without cardiovascular disease or cardiovascular risk factors across the spectrum of OSA severity is undefined with most results demonstrating little or no benefit.

ADHERENCE AND PROBLEMS WITH CONTINUOUS POSITIVE AIRWAY PRESSURE THERAPY

In a perfect world, all patients with OSA would use their CPAP therapy all night, every night. Unfortunately, just like many therapies associated with other chronic diseases, adherence with CPAP therapy for OSA is far from ideal. Willingness to initiate CPAP and ongoing adherence with treatment are both issues. Although there are no formal definitions of what constitutes adherence with CPAP therapy, most studies have arbitrarily defined the minimal adherence threshold as use of CPAP at greater than or equal to 4 hours per night for 70% of the observed nights.[77] Using this definition, subjective adherence ranges between 65% and 90%, whereas objective measures of CPAP adherence have demonstrated use in the range of 40% to 83%.[149] Most studies have shown that patients usually overestimate their CPAP usage by approximately 1 hour per night, a pattern that is observed in both new and long-term OSA patients.[77,150] Because many patients do not use CPAP for their entire sleep period, apnea burden has been suggested as a measure to represent the true effectiveness of using PAP. By calculating (device AHI × on-PAP time) + (sleep study AHI × off-PAP time), a better representation of PAP effectiveness may allow for better comparison to efficacies of other therapies and may better explain disparities in clinical and research findings.[151]

Short-term follow-up of OSA patients demonstrates that CPAP usage patterns typically fall into two groups: (1) use of CPAP for greater than 90% of the nights, with an average usage time of greater than 6 hours per night, and (2) use of CPAP intermittently, with an average usage of less than 3.5 hours per night.[152] Early follow-up for patients newly initiated on CPAP therapy is important as these patterns of use can typically be identified within the first several days to several months of CPAP therapy.[145–148] Long-term objective follow-up has demonstrated that approximately 68% of OSA patients continue to use their CPAP therapy after 5 years.[150] A study of nonsleepy patients with OSA found 64% adherence at 4 years.[153]

Some studies have suggested certain parameters that may predict greater short- and long-term adherence to therapy. In some studies, improved adherence has been associated with symptoms of subjective sleepiness (ESS > 10), severity of OSA (AHI > 30), and average nightly adherence within the first 3 months of therapy. Reduced short- and long-term adherence has been observed in patients reporting problems during their initial night with CPAP therapy in the sleep laboratory.[150,154] Of interest, although one might expect higher levels of CPAP pressure to predict poorer adherence, neither high nor low CPAP pressures have been shown to reliably predict CPAP use. Several studies have also associated African American race and lower socioeconomic status with poorer adherence with CPAP therapy, even in patients with standardized access to care and treatment.[155–159] The reasons for these last observations are not clear, although many other studies have not found factors such as race/ethnicity, gender, smoking status, or age to be consistent predictors of adherence.

ROLE OF OBJECTIVE ADHERENCE MONITORING AND LIMITATIONS WITH CURRENT TECHNOLOGY

Unfortunately, when taken together, most studies have not been able to identify factors that consistently predict short- and or long-term adherence with CPAP therapy. The SAVE Trial found that higher initial adherence, loud snoring, and fixed CPAP pressure had the greatest predictive value for 24-month adherence.[160] Because adherence with PAP therapy tends to be suboptimal, subjective adherence tends to overestimate objective PAP use, there are no consistent early predictors of PAP adherence, and PAP adherence patterns tend to be determined early in most patients, professional societies currently recommend, and many payer policies require, objective adherence data review to document adherence with therapy and identify problems that can be addressed.[3,4] Although most randomized controlled trials have used objective adherence data to monitor outcomes related to PAP therapy, the overall impact of assessing objective adherence data for all patients on PAP therapy is uncertain.

Most of the PAP manufacturers have developed sophisticated online software and smartphone-based programs for monitoring several parameters of PAP therapy, including nightly adherence, efficacy of therapy (residual AHI, including central vs. obstructive events), and problems with mask fit (primarily amount of air leak). Although there are several potential advantages to these programs, the technologies also have several potential limitations, including how different devices define the AHI, abnormal leak, and periodic breathing, and how different manufacturers differentiate between central and obstructive sleep-disordered breathing events.[18] Furthermore, the PAP-calculated AHI and leak thresholds have not been found to predict adherence.[51,161] To improve the impact of these technologies on meaningful patient outcomes, several improvements will be required, including (1) standardization of respiratory event and leak definitions among manufacturers, as well as validation of the device outputs compared with PSG; (2) improved access of PAP adherence data for frontline providers, including determining ways to more easily integrate PAP adherence data into the various electronic medical record software programs; and (3) education of nonsleep specialists on interpretation of the available adherence information.

INTERVENTIONS TO PROMOTE CONTINUOUS POSITIVE AIRWAY PRESSURE ADHERENCE

Typical problems that may lead to reduced adherence with CPAP therapy include claustrophobia, nasal congestion, pressure intolerance, and poor mask fit. Several interventions have been proposed and instituted in an attempt to improve adherence with CPAP therapy (Table 132.5).

The most consistent intervention that has been associated with improved CPAP adherence in most, but not all, PAP naïve patients is systematic education. Several approaches, including provider and home-based education of the patient and spouse, supportive care at therapy initiation or follow-up, phone calls, home-based videos, and daylong educational programs have been associated with improved adherence, although no one intervention has been demonstrated to be consistently beneficial in all patient groups. In general, increased intensity of patient education and/or frequency of health provider contact have been associated with improved CPAP adherence.[162] Overall, these educational interventions tend to improve CPAP adherence by approximately 35 to 50 minutes per night, although the effects of these interventions on other important outcomes, such as daytime sleepiness, quality of life, and cardiovascular disease and risk are unclear. Several behavioral approaches have also been associated with improved adherence. In general, these behavioral approaches, including motivational interviewing and cognitive behavioral therapy delivered in individual or group settings, have been associated with average improvements in adherence of 1.5 hours per night. The overall impact of these behavioral approaches on CPAP adherence is not well defined, as the data supporting these approaches are of lower quality than the data supporting the previously discussed educational interventions. Electronic patient engagement through CPAP devices and applications with systems such as ResMed MyAir and Philips Respironics DreamMapper have shown significant increases in short-term adherence rates and usage, but longer-term data are not as clear. Patients may also use these platforms to monitor their response to treatment and alert their provider if changes are noted Figure 132.9).

The data evaluating the effects of heated humidification on adherence to CPAP therapy remain controversial. Although there are some studies that demonstrate that the addition of heated humidification can improve adherence to CPAP therapy, there are several studies demonstrating no improvement in adherence with this intervention.[57,163–167] Patients who tend to benefit the most from the addition of heated humidification are those with symptoms of nasal congestion or rhinitis. Limited data evaluating the role of heated tubing to heated humidification have shown no improvements in adherence in patients with and without nasopharyngeal complaints.[168] The role of nasal steroids with or without heated humidification therapy, especially in unselected CPAP naïve patients with OSA, remains unclear as many studies have demonstrated little benefit for this intervention in improving CPAP use.[166,169]

CPAP delivery interfaces, or masks, come in several shapes and sizes, including nasal masks, full-face (oronasal) masks that cover both the nose and the mouth, nasal pillows that fit into the nostrils, and oral interfaces that fit into the mouth. Some studies have observed a negative impact of oronasal masks on CPAP adherence, whereas other studies have not confirmed these findings, and there are few data on the newest generation of masks.[170] Oronasal masks may be better for patients with chronic nasal congestion or obstruction, for those patients who are predominantly mouth breathers, and for patients requiring higher CPAP pressures when mask leak is an issue. Nasal pillows typically have not been recommended for CPAP settings of greater than 12 cm H_2O due to the potential for interface leak, although select patients may do well with a nasal pillows interface even with higher PAP settings.[171] Overall, although proper mask fit may be crucial to the initial and ongoing acceptance of CPAP therapy, the optimum form and type of CPAP delivery interface remains

Table 132.5 Effects of Interventions on PAP Adherence

Intervention	Effect on PAP Adherence	Comments
Education/supportive care	Beneficial	Various approaches helpful, including phone calls, office and home visits, individual and group sessions Best intervention, or combination, unclear
Behavioral therapies	Beneficial	Various therapies helpful, including motivational interviewing and CBT Most interventions studied in addition to education Best intervention, or combination, unclear
Heated humidification	Beneficial for some patients	Most, but not all data, support improved adherence Most helpful for patients with nasal congestion or rhinitis Addition of nasal steroids not helpful The role of heated tubing is not clear based on limited studies
Advanced PAP (bilevel, EPR, and APAP)	No benefit	Not associated with improved adherence for OSA BiFlex, may be the exception in CPAP noncompliant patients ASV may be beneficial in some patients with treatment-emergent central sleep apnea with high residual AHI on CPAP
Mask type	Unclear	Best mask type unclear Limited data show better adherence with nasal pillows and nasal masks Changing masks may alter effective PAP pressure
Direct patient engagement applications	Unclear	Significant improvements in 90-day adherence rates and hours of use in short-term studies, but no long-term data Limited to data to base recommendations
Telemedicine	Unclear	Limited data suggests benefit, whereas other data do not support approach Overall, there are no data demonstrating worse outcomes with this approach Further research is required to better define its roles in the management of PAP therapy for OSA
Adherence monitoring	Unclear	Objective adherence monitoring recommended, but no clear data that the intervention itself improves compliance
Sleep specialist care	Unclear	Observational studies support approach RCTs show no advantage in uncomplicated OSA
Hypnotics	Controversial	Eszopiclone (short term) may improve PAP titration efficacy and 6-month adherence Data do not support other hypnotics

AHI, Apnea-hypopnea index; APAP, autotitrated positive airway pressure; ASV, adaptive servo-ventilation; CBT, cognitive behavioral therapy; OSA, obstructive sleep apnea; PAP, positive airway pressure; RCTs, randomized controlled trials.

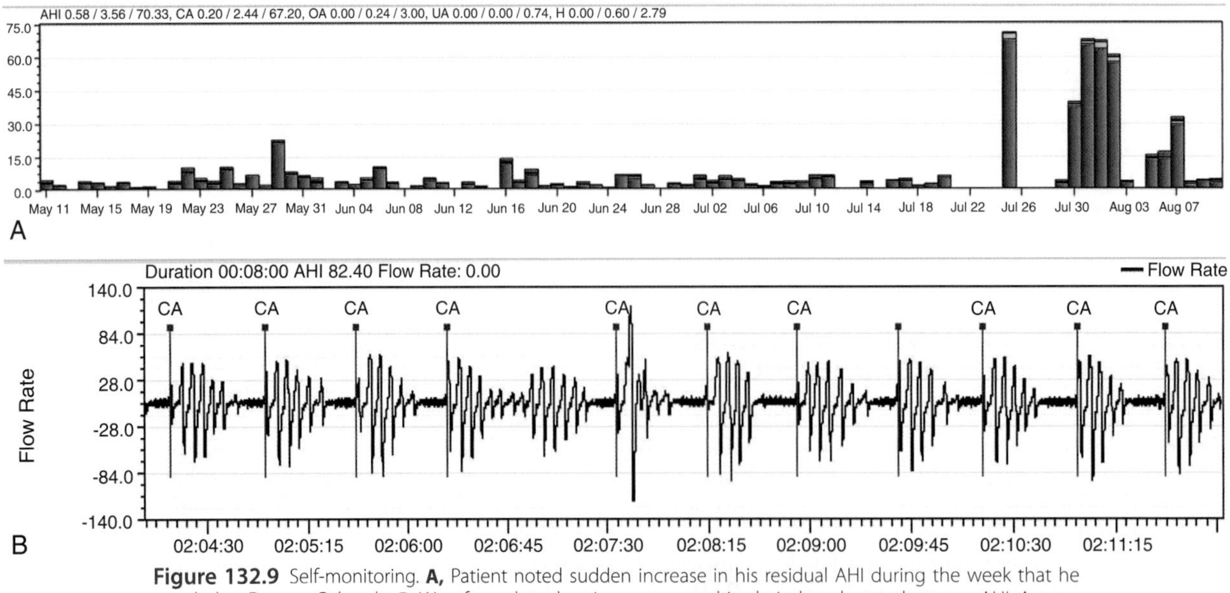

Figure 132.9 Self-monitoring. **A,** Patient noted sudden increase in his residual AHI during the week that he traveled to Denver, Colorado. **B,** Waveform data showing recurrent altitude-induced central apneas. AHI, Apnea-hypopnea index; CA, central apnea; H, hypopnea; OA, obstructive apnea; UA, unknown apnea.

unclear.[172,173] In general, the best interface for a given patient, which tends to correlate to the best adherence with therapy, is the one that the patient is most comfortable wearing.

Changing interfaces once a problem arises has not been shown to consistently improve long-term adherence in various studies, although from a clinician's standpoint, attention to mask complaints and changing masks when problems arise can improve adherence in select patients. The provider should be aware that changing the mask type from nasal to oronasal or vice versa might change the necessary effective treatment pressure that was initially identified during an in-laboratory titration.[174] Thus, for those patients on fixed PAP therapy, the clinician should consider the need for adjusting the pressure and/or having the patient perform an in-laboratory PAP titration if problems arise or persist after a mask change has been instituted.

Because many patients may complain of sleep disruption and/or difficulty initiating sleep during the first few days to weeks of CPAP therapy, several studies have evaluated the use of prescription hypnotics to improve adherence to CPAP treatment, either in the sleep laboratory during a PAP titration study or during the first few weeks of therapy. Although some studies have demonstrated that, in newly diagnosed patients with severe OSA, treatment with eszopiclone (3 mg) before an overnight titration study or during the first 14 days of PAP therapy has been associated with improved quality of CPAP titrations (greater proportion of patients with optimal or good titrations) and improved adherence to CPAP therapy over the first 6 months of treatment, respectively, these results are not typical of most of the literature regarding the use of hypnotics as adjunctive therapies to improve adherence.[65,175] When compared with placebo or usual care, other randomized controlled studies have demonstrated no significant benefits, although no significant adverse effects of other hypnotic therapies (zaleplon or zolpidem) on CPAP adherence.[176,177] As with most studies, the data evaluating the effects of hypnotics on CPAP adherence have looked at relatively short-term adherence in specialized centers of care. The ability to generalize these data to a typical clinical population and office setting is uncertain based on the current literature, and care should be used when applying this approach to a given patient or population. Given the limited data, the use of short-term or chronic hypnotics should generally be avoided in patients with OSA.

The Role of the Sleep Specialist in Improving Continuous Positive Airway Pressure Adherence

Several retrospective and observational studies have shown that sleep specialist consultation, before an in-laboratory sleep study and/or during the initiation and follow-up of CPAP therapy, has been associated with improved CPAP adherence and other important outcomes, such as patient satisfaction and timeliness of care.[149,178] Alternatively, three randomized controlled trials in symptomatic patients with a high clinical suspicion of uncomplicated moderate to severe OSA demonstrated that management by either a specially trained nurse, nurse–primary care physician team, or primary care physician resulted in outcomes (CPAP adherence and improvements in daytime sleepiness) that were similar to management by sleep specialists.[179–181] In addition to similar CPAP adherence, all of these studies demonstrated a significant cost savings in the non–sleep specialist group. Thus the data supporting the role of the sleep specialist in the treatment and overall management of all patients with uncomplicated moderate to severe OSA are not well defined based on the current literature. More research is necessary to better determine which groups of patients with OSA may receive the most benefit from sleep specialist management of CPAP therapy.

Current recommendations, based predominantly on expert opinion, suggest that patients should have initial office follow-up during the first few weeks of prescribed CPAP therapy. Thereafter patients using CPAP should be followed on an annual basis and as needed to troubleshoot problems as they arise.[4,5] These recommendations for office and face-to-face follow-up may change as we learn more from the expansion of telemedicine use and online data monitoring, which we expect the COVID-19 pandemic to rapidly increase. Government and commercial payers have defined rules and policies that regulate how and when patients on CPAP should have office follow-up and objective adherence monitoring. Based on the current outcomes literature, the optimal method or schedule for short- or long-term follow-up is not clear. Clinicians must determine appropriate follow-up based on a given patient's response to therapy and payer policies that may guide requirements to continue treatment.

Technology to Improve Continuous Positive Airway Pressure Adherence

Several additional applications of technology have been used in an attempt to improve PAP adherence. Interventions include the use of online PAP adherence monitoring software as described earlier, telemedicine, and patient interactive technologies. As noted previously, most patients overestimate their adherence with therapy, and thus objective monitoring of CPAP therapy is typically recommended.[3–5] Although the literature supports the concept that CPAP usage can be reliably determined by CPAP tracking systems, the role of objectively measuring PAP adherence and its impact on improving adherence in all patients are uncertain.[51,161] A Japanese randomized controlled trial found that telemedicine was noninferior to 1- and 3-month face-to-face visits in terms of long-term adherence rates.[182] Other limited data suggest that online monitoring of PAP adherence and the use of a telemedicine management strategy result in similar, and in some cases improved, adherence when compared to traditional face-to-face evaluations. Given the limited data and inconsistent outcomes, more data are required to better define the role of this approach.[183–187]

Finally, although several PAP device manufacturers have developed software (smartphone and computer-based applications) aimed at improving patient involvement with their CPAP therapy, there are currently no randomized trials evaluating these interventions on long-term PAP adherence. Observational data evaluating more than 100,000 patients using ResMed MyAir found significantly higher adherence rates (87% vs. 70%) and hours of use (5.9 vs. 4.9 hours) than patients with usual monitoring. A white paper evaluating 40,000 patients using Philips Respironics DreamMapper also reported improved 90-day adherence when comparing active to standard care groups. Overall, given the limited data, it is unknown whether these programs improve long-term adherence. In addition, more standardization around the privacy and security of these online data are needed as these technologies advance.[188]

COVID-19 and Positive Airway Pressure Therapy for Obstructive Sleep Apnea

Due to the risk of aerosolization of virus from PAP therapy, the COVID-19 pandemic has affected the treatment of OSA. The pandemic led to at least temporary reductions in in-laboratory testing[188a] that have caused more patients, even with comorbidities, to be diagnosed with home testing and empirically started on treatment. Use of other data sources to optimize therapy has become more important as, especially, titration studies are limited and hopefully will provide the opportunity to collect data on their benefit. Virtual mask fittings using facial analysis technology may be able to supplement the need for face-to-face mask fittings. The pandemic has also brought to light the risk of exposure to bed partners and potential contamination of humidifiers and devices that may be reduced with nonvented masks and viral filters.[189,190]

CLINICAL PEARLS

- Continuous positive airway pressure (CPAP) is the first-line therapy for patients with moderate to severe obstructive sleep apnea (OSA), especially for those with daytime symptoms.
- CPAP therapy consistently resolves sleep-disordered breathing events and improves symptoms of daytime sleepiness in symptomatic patients, especially for patients with moderate to severe disease. There are inconsistent data concerning the benefits of CPAP therapy with regard to neurocognitive function, mood, quality of life, and cardiovascular outcomes across the spectrum of disease severity. The data regarding the benefits of CPAP therapy in patients with more mild disease is even more controversial, especially in those without daytime symptoms or underlying cardiovascular disease.
- The role of CPAP therapy for patients without associated daytime symptoms across the spectrum of OSA severity is unclear based on the current data. Most randomized controlled trials (RCTs) in this patient group have failed to demonstrate improvements in important outcomes, including blood pressure, cardiovascular morbidity and mortality, neurocognitive function, and/or quality of life.
- Adherence with CPAP therapy is suboptimal for many patients, although improvements in adherence have been consistently associated with systematic education with and without behavioral therapy. The roles of other interventions, including heated humidification, hypnotics, and telemedicine, to improve adherence to CPAP therapy are unclear based on the current outcomes data from observational and RCTs.
- The roles of advanced PAP technologies, including (expiratory pressure relief and bilevel PAP pressure devices are not clear, as they have typically not been associated with improved adherence, daytime sleepiness, or quality of life in patients with OSA when compared to CPAP alone.
- Autotitrated positive airway pressure used in an unattended setting, either to determine a fixed CPAP setting or as a primary treatment, is reasonable therapy for patients with moderate to severe OSA without underlying comorbidities. Understanding the differences between devices from different companies may help optimize their utility.

SUMMARY

CPAP therapy remains the mainstay of treatment for patient with moderate to severe OSA, especially in those patients with daytime sleepiness. The role of PAP therapy in patients with OSA in the absence of daytime sleepiness or for cardiovascular outcomes has not been confirmed by clinical trials, but in our experience, patients' other symptoms and, especially, somatic comorbidities may benefit from PAP therapy for all severities of OSA. Despite its potential to improve several clinical outcomes, including daytime sleepiness, neurocognitive dysfunction, quality of life, and BP, long-term adherence with therapy remains suboptimal. Newer technologies, such as APAP, especially when fully utilizing adherence and waveform data to manage therapy, have the potential to improve the treatment of OSA with most data, demonstrating that this technology is as effective as in-laboratory–titrated CPAP in patients with uncomplicated moderate to severe OSA. Based on the outcomes data, current clinical guidelines have evolved to the point that APAP is recommended as reasonable first-line therapy for patients with uncomplicated moderate to severe OSA. As more practitioners adopt an ambulatory management approach through the use of HSAT and APAP treatment, patients with uncomplicated OSA may benefit in several ways, including through reduced wait times to initiating therapy and potentially via reduced health care spending. Other technologic advancements, such as EPR and BPAP devices, are supported by limited data and appear to offer no advantages over conventionally titrated CPAP therapy or APAP in the majority of patients with OSA.

SELECTED READINGS

Anttalainen U, Tenhunen M, Rimpila V, et al. Prolonged partial upper airway obstruction during sleep—an underdiagnosed phenotype of sleep-disordered breathing. *Eur Clin Respir J.* 2016;3:31806.

Fava C, Dorigoni S, Dalle Vedove F, et al. Effect of CPAP on blood pressure in patients with OSA/hypopnea a systematic review and meta-analysis. *Chest.* 2014;145(4):762–771.

Holmqvist F, Guan N, Zhu Z, et al. Impact of obstructive sleep apnea and continuous positive airway pressure therapy on outcomes in patients with atrial fibrillation—results from the Outcomes Registry for Better Informed Treatment of Atrial Fibrillation (ORBIT-AF). *Am Heart J.* 2015;169(5):647–654.e642.

Hwang E, Chang J, Benjafield A, et al. Effect of telemedicine education and telemonitoring on continuous positive airway pressure adherence. The Tele-OSA randomized trial. *Am J Respir Crit Care Med.* 2018;197:117–126.

Javaheri S, Gottlieb DJ, Quan SF. Effects of continuous positive airway pressure on blood pressure in obstructive sleep apnea patients: the Apnea Positive Pressure Long-term Efficacy Study (APPLES). *J Sleep Res.* 2020;29(2):e12943.

Johnson KG, Johnson DC. Treatment of sleep disordered breathing with positive airway pressure devices: technology update. *Med Devices (Auckl).* 2015;8:425–437.

McEvoy R, Antic N, Heeley E, et al. CPAP for prevention of cardiovascular events in obstructive sleep apnea. *N Engl J Med.* 2016;375:919–931.

Patil S, Ayappa I, Caples S, et al. Treatment of adult obstructive sleep apnea with positive airway pressure: an American Academy of Sleep Medicine systematic review, meta-analysis, and GRADE assessment. *J Clin Sleep Med.* 2019;15:301–334.

Phillips CL, Grunstein RR, Darendeliler MA, et al. Health outcomes of continuous positive airway pressure versus oral appliance treatment for obstructive sleep apnea: a randomized controlled trial. *Am J Respir Crit Care Med.* 2013;187(8):879–887.

Thomas RJ, Bianchi MT. Urgent need to improve PAP management: the devil is in two (fixable) details. *J Clin Sleep Med.* 2017;13(5):657–664.

Weaver TE, Mancini C, Maislin G, et al. Continuous positive airway pressure treatment of sleepy patients with milder obstructive sleep apnea: results of the CPAP Apnea Trial North American Program (CATNAP) randomized clinical trial. *Am J Respir Crit Care Med*. 2012;186(7):677–683.

Yu J, Zhou Z, McEvoy R, et al. Association of positive airway pressure with cardiovascular events and death in adults with sleep apnea: a systematic review and meta-analysis. *J Am Med Assoc*. 2017;318:156–166.

A complete reference list can be found online at ExpertConsult.com.

Chapter 133

Pharmacologic Treatments for Obstructive Sleep Apnea

Abigail L. Koch; Susheel P. Patil

Chapter Highlights

- This chapter organizes a discussion of pharmacologic treatments for obstructive sleep apnea (OSA) based on pathophysiologic mechanisms (e.g., anatomic, neuromuscular, and neuroventilatory control) that the medications generally target.
- Stratifying treatments based on pathophysiologic targets may be useful in personalizing therapy for patients with OSA.
- Despite otherwise effective treatment for OSA, some patients may experience persistent sleepiness despite adequate sleep time and may be appropriate candidates for adjunctive stimulant therapy.

Therapy for obstructive sleep apnea (OSA) has traditionally included continuous positive airway pressure (CPAP) therapy, oral appliances, upper airway surgeries, and weight reduction.[1] Given the difficulties with adherence or sustaining the effects of conventional therapies in treating OSA, investigation of alternative and/or adjunctive therapies is an active area of interest, particularly pharmacotherapies. Selecting and studying pharmacologic targets that might successfully treat OSA in humans constitutes a challenging endeavor because of the complexity of respiratory control, the multiple neurochemical pathways that drive respiration, interactions with sleep state, and limitations in animal models of OSA.[2,3] An ideal pharmacologic agent for OSA would need to possess the ability to (1) maintain normal airway patency and respiratory drive during both non–rapid eye movement (NREM) and rapid eye movement (REM) sleep and (2) mitigate the effects of intermittent arousals and hypoxemia.[4]

Current pharmacologic approaches for the management of OSA are best described as alternative therapy in patients for whom other primary, adjunctive, or even other alternative therapies have not been beneficial. However, given the current evidence, such an alternative therapy approach should be considered investigational with perhaps few exceptions, until appropriate clinical trials have been completed.

Potential OSA treatments can be considered based on the mechanisms identified to be important in the pathogenesis of OSA (Figure 133.1). Therapeutic approaches for OSA targeting anatomic features (e.g., excess pharyngeal mucosal tissue, upper airway edema, and mucosal congestion), neuromuscular (e.g., muscle responsiveness), and neuroventilatory (e.g., arousal threshold, apnea threshold, and loop gain) mechanisms are potential targets. The objective of this chapter is to organize a discussion of pharmacotherapies for OSA based on the pathophysiologic mechanisms that the interventions target. Stratifying treatments based on pathophysiologic targets may be useful in personalizing optimal therapy for patients with OSA,[5] while taking patient preference into account.[6] The chapter concludes with reviewing management of residual excessive sleepiness in patients despite adequate control of OSA and adherence to therapy.

PHARMACOTHERAPY FOR OSA TARGETING ANATOMY

Most patients with OSA have an anatomic predisposition to upper airway collapse.[7] The interactions between soft tissues within a fixed craniofacial structure are major determinants of the propensity for collapse[8] and are often regarded as fixed and heritable traits.[9] Beyond surgical treatments which, in certain instances, can directly address craniofacial and soft tissue features that contribute to OSA, pharmacotherapies that can modify upper airway anatomy are quite limited. However, medications that primarily reduce soft tissue mass through assisting weight loss, decreasing airway edema, and improving chronic rhinosinusitis (CRS) can improve upper airway anatomy and potentially improve OSA severity (Table 133.1).

Weight Loss

Obesity, particularly central obesity, clinically assessed by increased neck and waist circumferences, is associated with an increased prevalence of OSA (see Chapter 139). Lifestyle modifications, pharmacotherapy, and surgical treatment for weight loss are associated with reductions in OSA severity and sometimes resolution.[10,11] Several studies have investigated medical management of weight loss and its effect on OSA with sibutramine, a monoaminergic reuptake inhibitor that reduces reuptake of serotonin, norepinephrine, and dopamine, thus suppressing appetite. In these participants, sibutramine did result in weight loss; however, mixed results were observed with respect to improvement of the apnea-hypopnea index (AHI).[12,13] Liraglutide, a glucagon-like peptide-1 (GLP-1) agonist used to treat type 2 diabetes and obesity, has been shown to reduce weight by 4.2% and OSA severity by 6.1 events/hour in obese individuals with

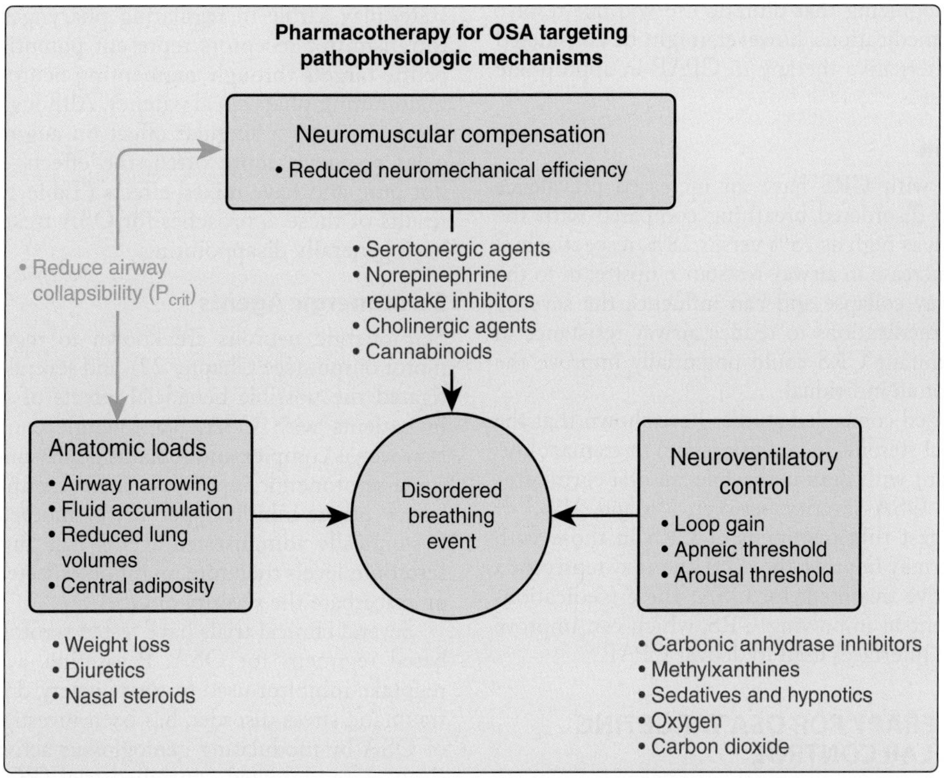

Figure 133.1 Pharmacotherapies for obstructive sleep apnea (OSA) targeting pathophysiologic mechanisms. Certain therapies can be considered on the basis of the pathophysiologic mechanisms targeted. OSA is a consequence of increases in anatomic loads on the upper airway, impairments in neuromuscular compensation, and/or alterations in neuroventilatory control. Different pharmacologic treatments may target the root pathophysiologic impairments contributing to OSA and alleviate the disorder.

Table 133.1 Pharmacotherapy for Sleep Apnea Targeting Anatomy

Class	Generic Name	Influence on OSA Severity	Study Design
Weight Loss			
	Sibutramine	7% ↓[a], 36%↓	Open label,[12] open label[13]
	Liraglutide	25% ↓	RCT[13]
Airway Edema			
	Spironolactone	45% ↓	Open label[16]
	Spironolactone + Metolazone	17% ↓[b]	Open label[17]
	Spironolactone + Furosemide	14% ↓	RCT[18]
Nasal Congestion			
	Fluticasone	5% ↓	RCT[21]
	Tramazoline + Dexamethasone	21% ↓	RCT[22]

[a]Not statistically significant.
[b]Non–rapid eye movement (NREM) only; rapid eye movement (REM) difference not statistically significant.
OSA, Obstructive sleep apnea; RCT, randomized controlled trial.

moderate-to-severe sleep apnea.[14] Although weight reduction is essential in the treatment of OSA, pharmacotherapies for weight loss should be considered adjunctive to other OSA therapies as part of a multidisciplinary approach to the treatment of OSA.

Airway Edema

Rostral fluid shifts from the legs to the neck, which occur when sleeping in a recumbent position, have been demonstrated to increase the severity of OSA, particularly in those in a fluid overload state such as heart failure or end-stage renal disease.[15] These fluid shifts may increase neck circumference or parapharyngeal edema, which can increase upper airway collapsibility and OSA severity. Diuretic medications and sodium-restricted diets have been studied as a method to improve fluid retention and minimize the fluid shifts that may affect the upper airway. Several studies of varied participants with either uncontrolled or resistant hypertension and OSA evaluated the use of spironolactone in combination with a diuretic (e.g., thiazide, metolazone, or furosemide) and showed a decrease in hypertension and OSA severity.[16,17] However, none of the interventions decreased the AHI to fewer than 5 events/hour.[18] Recognizing that diuretic use will not resolve OSA alone, these medications, however, might be considered as adjunctive or alternative therapy to CPAP in appropriate patient populations.

Nasal Congestion

Individuals living with CRS have an increased prevalence of comorbid sleep-disordered breathing compared with the general population, as high as 75% versus 18%, respectively.[19] CRS leads to an increase in airway resistance upstream to the site of upper airway collapse and can influence the severity of OSA.[20] Using medications to reduce airway resistance in those with concomitant CRS could potentially improve the severity of OSA for an individual.

A few randomized controlled studies have shown that the use of inhaled nasal steroids (e.g., fluticasone) or tramazoline, a nasal decongestant with dexamethasone, an oral corticosteroid, can improve OSA severity between 5% and 21%.[21,22] These studies suggest that treatment of CRS in those with concomitant OSA may improve the AHI and may represent a reasonable adjunctive treatment for OSA. These medications have another benefit in improving CRS, which can improve adherence to nasal interfaces used to deliver CPAP.

PHARMACOTHERAPY FOR OSA TARGETING NEUROMUSCULAR CONTROL

Pharyngeal muscle activation maintains upper airway patency during wakefulness. With sleep onset, pharyngeal muscles relax, increasing a person's susceptibility to upper airway collapse. A reduced capacity to recruit pharyngeal dilator muscles in the setting of partial upper airway collapse can contribute to the pathogenesis of OSA. Specific neurotransmitters, including serotonin, norepinephrine, and acetylcholine, which vary as a function of the sleep-wake state, play a role in regulating pharyngeal tone. Thus neurotransmitter receptors represent potential pharmacotherapeutic targets through augmenting neuromuscular tone and maintaining pharyngeal patency. Although some pharmacotherapies have a singular effect on augmenting neuromuscular response, more often, the effects of most drugs are not pure and have mixed effects (Table 133.2). Overall, the results of these approaches for OSA treatment to date have been generally disappointing.

Serotonergic Agents

Serotonergic neurons are known to regulate upper airway motor output (see Chapter 22), and several studies have investigated the possible beneficial effects of serotonergic agents in patients with OSA. Serotonergic control of respiration, however, is complex and remains poorly understood. Whereas some serotonergic inputs are excitatory and facilitate respiration,[23] others inhibit upper airway motor neuron function.[24] Systemically administered agents that augment or attenuate serotonin levels therefore might be expected to either improve or exacerbate the severity of OSA.[25]

Several clinical trials have tested serotonergic medication–based regimens for OSA. Paroxetine, a selective serotonin reuptake inhibitor used to treat anxiety, depression, and post-traumatic stress disorder, has been investigated for treatment of OSA by modulating genioglossus activity during NREM sleep. A randomized controlled trial (RCT) in severe OSA showed that peak inspiratory genioglossus muscle activity during NREM sleep significantly increased with paroxetine compared with placebo; however, the AHI was not significantly different between the two.[26]

Mirtazapine, an antidepressant with both 5-hydroxytryptamine (serotonin; 5-HT)$_1$ agonist and 5-HT$_3$ antagonist effects, has been more widely investigated as a medication for OSA treatment.[25] The results to date have

Table 133.2 Pharmacotherapy for Sleep Apnea Targeting Neuromuscular Control

Class	Generic Name	Influence on OSA Severity	Study Design
Serotonergic Agents			
	Paroxetine	2% ↓[a]	RCT (crossover)[26]
	Mirtazapine	49% ↓, 55% ↑	RCT,[27] RCT[28]
	Fluoxetine + Ondansetron	40% ↓	RCT[29]
Norepinephrine Reuptake Inhibitor			
	Protriptyline	48% ↓, 7% ↓[b]	RCT,[30] open label[32]
	Atomoxetine	9% ↑[a]	Open label[34]
	Atomoxetine + Oxybutynin	63% ↓	RCT (crossover)[35]
Cholinergic Agents			
	Physostigmine	24% ↓	RCT[121]
	Donepezil	51% ↓, 22% ↓, 3% ↓	RCT,[36] RCT,[37] RCT[38]
Cannabinoids			
	Dronabinol	29% ↓, 50% ↓	Proof of concept,[41] RCT[42]
Other			
	Salmeterol	11% ↓[a]	RCT[43]

[a]Not statistically significant.
[b]Apnea index only; apnea-hypopnea index (AHI) not reported.
OSA, Obstructive sleep apnea; RCT, randomized controlled trial.

been disappointing without a consistent improvement in OSA severity or subjective sleepiness and with a potential for weight gain.[27,28] Weight gain and sedation are relatively common side effects of mirtazapine, two problems linked with OSA.

Investigators have also compared placebo, fluoxetine (a central 5-HT_2 agonist), ondansetron (a peripheral 5-HT_3 antagonist), and combined fluoxetine and ondansetron in a short-term RCT in adults with mild-to-severe OSA. Combined high-dose therapy with fluoxetine and ondansetron showed some efficacy. The regimen reduced the mean AHI significantly compared with baseline after 2 and 4 weeks, compared with no changes with placebo.[29] However, no subsequent confirmatory trials have been performed. Common side effects observed with these medications include headache, constipation, dry mouth, and hypersomnolence, although these side effects were not seen during this 4-week clinical trial.

Norepinephrine Reuptake Inhibitors

Protriptyline, a nonsedating tricyclic antidepressant, acts as both a serotonin and norepinephrine reuptake inhibitor and has also been shown to have partial treatment effects in OSA at doses up to 30 mg. Mechanisms that contribute to improvements in OSA severity include reduction in REM sleep duration[30] and increased hypoglossal and recurrent laryngeal nerve activity with increased upper airway motor tone.[31] In at least two small clinical trials, use of protriptyline for severe OSA (mean AHI range, 71–75/hour) was associated with reductions in AHI by 21% to 33%.[30,32] Furthermore, improvements in subjective sleepiness were seen in most patients despite significant residual disordered breathing, suggesting that protriptyline may have independent alerting effects.[30] Documentation of significant residual disordered breathing and hypoxemia, however, has diminished enthusiasm for this treatment. Side effects of protriptyline include dry mouth, urinary hesitancy, constipation, confusion, and ataxia, all of which may limit the use of medications in this class.[33]

Atomoxetine, a selective norepinephrine reuptake inhibitor, has been studied alone and in combination with oxybutynin, an anticholinergic agent. When studied as a single-agent therapy in a small, open-label trial over 4 weeks, atomoxetine improved daytime sleepiness as assessed by the Epworth Sleepiness Scale (ESS); however, no improvement in the mean respiratory disturbance index (RDI) was seen, and there was some evidence of an increase in disturbed sleep.[34] A more recent RCT evaluated the use of atomoxetine in combination with oxybutynin compared with placebo on separate nights and reported a substantial decrease in OSA severity. The mean AHI decreased by 63% from 28.5 to 7.5 events/hour; however, no improvement in subjective sleepiness was observed. When administered separately on a second night, neither atomoxetine nor oxybutynin alone decreased the AHI. Side effects of the combined treatment included difficulty initiating micturition, dry mouth, headache, and insomnia.[35] Larger and longer prospective studies are needed before this combination of pharmacotherapy might be considered a suitable treatment option for patients with OSA.

Thus specific serotonergic and norepinephrine reuptake inhibitors in combination with anticholinergic medications may have modest effects on OSA severity and should continue to be considered as investigational. Use of serotonergic medications could be considered as an alternative therapy in OSA patients intolerant of other forms of OSA treatment, particularly in patients in whom these medications are already planned to be used for comorbid disorders such as depression (mirtazapine or protriptyline), anorexia (mirtazapine), migraine (protriptyline), attention deficit hyperactive disorder (atomoxetine), and cataplexy (protriptyline or fluoxetine). Improvements in OSA severity with these medications should not be assumed based on symptoms and should be monitored by sleep testing.

Cholinergic Agents

Acetylcholine, a cholinergic neurotransmitter active primarily during REM sleep, is involved in the modulation of upper airway motor tone and has been shown to increase hypoglossal and phrenic nerve activity in experimental animals and improve respiratory drive.[36] Donepezil, a reversible inhibitor of the acetylcholinesterase enzyme often used to treat memory impairment in Alzheimer disease (AD), has been tested as a potential treatment for OSA in patients with and without AD. An initial study was performed in 23 patients with AD and mild-to-moderate OSA. This RCT demonstrated that at 3 months, donepezil improved the mean AHI from 20.0 to 9.9 events/hour, whereas placebo demonstrated no improvement in AHI. As would be expected with a cholinergic medication, increased REM sleep was observed in the donepezil group at 3 months.[36] Another RCT of donepezil was conducted in 21 male patients with OSA but without AD. This study also found donepezil to improve mean AHI at 1 month, although the effects were more modest, with a mean AHI reduction of 23% (pretreatment mean of 42.2 events/hour versus ontreatment mean of 32.8 events/hour) versus a mean AHI increase of 14% (pretreatment mean of 26.4 events/hour versus ontreatment mean of 31.0 events/hour) in the placebo group.[37] This study found no differences in REM sleep between the groups. A third small RCT evaluated whether a single dose of donepezil lowered the AHI by changing the arousal threshold or loop gain. No difference in posttreatment AHI (51.8 events/hour versus 50.0 events/hour), arousal threshold, or loop gain was observed between placebo and donepezil, respectively; however, sleep efficiency and total sleep time were decreased with donepezil.[38] The single-night study results differ from the long-term treatment studies described, which suggests that any potential benefits with donepezil for OSA severity may be related to the duration of treatment. Side effects observed with donepezil included dizziness, nausea, headaches, vivid dreams, and nightmares. Although donepezil should be considered an investigational treatment for OSA, patients with AD and OSA in whom donepezil is already being considered for memory-related conditions may benefit.

Cannabinoids

Cannabinoid agonists have been investigated as a candidate target for OSA therapy.[39] Dronabinol, a nonselective cannabinoid type 1 (CB1) and type 2 (CB2) receptor agonist, is hypothesized to inhibit afferent vagal nerve activity, which may result in disinhibition of upper airway motor neurons.[40] In an early trial,[41] participants with moderate OSA treated with CPAP were withdrawn from their CPAP treatment for 1 week and given dronabinol in an escalated dose over 3 weeks up to 10 mg. The pretreatment mean AHI was reduced by 29% from the pretreatment mean AHI of 48.8 events/hour. Side effects noted during the study included somnolence and increased appetite without weight increase. Subsequently an RCT of dronabinol was conducted to treat moderate-to-severe

OSA. Treatment for 6 weeks with dronabinol 2.5 mg or 10 mg nightly resulted in a dose-response decrease in mean AHI by 6.6 and 8.5 events/hour from a mean baseline AHI of 28.2 and 26 events/hour, respectively. Dronabinol 10 mg daily significantly decreased the mean ESS score by 3.8 and 2.3 compared with baseline and placebo, respectively. Reported adverse effects included drowsiness (8%), headache (8%), nausea/vomiting (8%), and dizziness (4%). Neither dose of dronabinol was associated with weight gain.[42] Additional controlled studies are still needed on the potential effects of dronabinol in OSA; thus this treatment should continue to be considered an investigational therapy.

Other

Salmeterol is a long-acting beta-agonist (LABA) that has been investigated as a treatment to improve OSA by relaxing pharyngo-constricting muscles. In one RCT, polysomnography (PSG) was done on 3 nights: baseline, with placebo, and with salmeterol 50 μg in 20 participants without obstructive lung disease. No difference in sleep architecture or OSA severity was observed between nights. A small increase in heart rate and decrease in time spent with the oxygen saturation below 90% was seen on the salmeterol night.[43] Thus treatment with a LABA is not indicated for treatment of OSA.

Pharmacotherapies for OSA Targeting Primarily Neuroventilatory Mechanisms

Neuroventilatory mechanisms play an influential role in the expression of OSA severity. Physiologic parameters such as the arousal threshold, apnea threshold, CO_2 reserve, and circulatory time determine an individual's response to reduced ventilation from any cause whether mediated centrally (central hypoventilation) or peripherally (obstruction). Globally, these measures determine the degree of ventilatory instability (loop gain) and whether disordered breathing will be mitigated or perpetuated (see Chapter 23). Neuroventilatory mechanisms therefore present a potential pharmacotherapeutic target for OSA treatment. Although more often considered as potential treatments for central sleep apnea (see Chapter 125), some of these pharmacologic approaches have been examined in the setting of OSA (Table 133.3).

Carbonic Anhydrase Inhibitors

Acetazolamide, a carbonic anhydrase inhibitor (CAI) that induces a metabolic acidosis, thereby increasing ventilation, has been studied primarily in patients with central sleep apnea resulting from high altitude or heart failure, who often have unstable ventilatory control (high loop gain). Similarly, some patients with OSA have also been shown to have an elevated loop gain.[44] An early 1-week study of acetazolamide showed a mild improvement in the apnea index from mean pretreatment to ontreatment (25 events/hour and 18 events/hour, respectively).[45] Subsequently, an RCT evaluated patients with OSA on CPAP treatment at varied altitudes (490, 1860, and 2590 meters), during which CPAP was replaced with acetazolamide. Treatment with acetazolamide at higher altitudes mildly improved the AHI compared with placebo (at 1860 meters: ontreatment AHI 47.8 versus 52.8 events/hour; at 2590 meters: AHI 54.9 versus 72.7 events/hour, respectively).[46] In one study of OSA patients treated with CPAP, acetazolamide after 7 days reduced the mean loop gain by 41% and the mean AHI by 41%.[47] In another RCT, participants with hypertension and OSA were assigned to acetazolamide, CPAP, or both for 2 weeks. The AHI improved in all three arms, with the largest decrease seen in the arm assigned to combination therapy with acetazolamide and CPAP (mean

Table 133.3 Neuroventilatory Control

Class	Name	Influence on OSA Severity	Study Design
Carbonic Anhydrase Inhibitors			
	Acetazolamide	28% ↓, 29% ↓, 61% ↓	Open label,[45] RCT,[46] RCT[48]
	Zonisamide	33% ↓	RCT[49]
	Topiramate + Phentermine	68% ↓	RCT[50]
Methylxanthines			
	Aminophylline	10% ↓[a]	RCT[122]
Opioid Antagonists			
	Naltrexone	12% ↓	RCT[54]
Dopamine Agonists			
	Bromocriptine	↔	Open label[53]
Sedatives and Hypnotics			
	Zolpidem	12% ↓[a]	Open label[60]
	Zopiclone	20% ↓[a]	RCT[61]
	Eszopiclone	23% ↓, 3% ↓[a]	RCT,[57] RCT[58]
	Trazodone	0% ↓[a], 26% ↓	Open label,[64] RCT[65]
	Gabapentin	92% ↑	RCT[66]
	Sodium oxybate	35% ↓[a], 25% ↓[a]	RCT,[70] RCT[62]

[a]Not statistically significant.
OSA, Obstructive sleep apnea; RCT, randomized controlled trial.

AHI reduction: acetazolamide 15 events/hour, CPAP 31 events/hour, combined 39 events/hour).[48] However, difficulties with tolerability of acetazolamide may preclude long-term use, as patient-reported side effects included paresthesias, altered taste, nocturia, and hypokalemia.

Two other medications, which have weak CAI activity, have been investigated for the treatment of OSA: zonisamide and topiramate. These medications are traditionally used as antiepileptic pharmacotherapy and have complex mechanisms of action in addition to CAI activity. Both zonisamide and topiramate also augment weight loss, two properties that may improve OSA. Zonisamide at 100 mg nightly for 4 weeks decreased the mean AHI by 33% in an RCT; however, there was no difference in weight or subjective sleep quality between the three groups (zonisamide, CPAP, placebo). Mean ontreatment AHI was lower in the zonisamide group compared with the placebo group (mean AHI decreased by 8.8 versus 0.5 events/hour, respectively), though CPAP decreased the mean AHI by 42.5 events/hour.[49] In addition, an RCT of topiramate combined with phentermine for the treatment of OSA was performed in obese adults. The combined treatment resulted in weight loss and improved AHI compared with placebo (weight loss 10.2% versus 4.3%; AHI decrease 31.5 events/hour versus 16.6 events/hour). Adverse events most frequently reported included dry mouth (50%) and dysgeusia (27%).[50] However, whether the reduction in OSA severity was the result of weight loss, a drug effect, or both remains unknown. Pharmacotherapy with a CAI, particularly acetazolamide, may be useful as an adjunctive treatment to CPAP when CPAP-emergent central apneas are a persistent issue. The use of alternative weaker CAIs such as zonisamide or topiramate should be considered investigational as a primary treatment for OSA, though they may have beneficial effects in those with seizure disorders and comorbid OSA intolerant of other primary or alternative OSA therapies.

Methylxanthines, Opioid Antagonists, and Medroxyprogesterone

Theophylline, an oral methylxanthine, has been evaluated in the treatment of OSA. A small RCT evaluated theophylline for the treatment of OSA and demonstrated a slight reduction in the AHI by 18%; however, participants experienced worsened sleep quality.[51] Another RCT of theophylline demonstrated a 27% reduction in AHI compared with placebo.[52] However, given the minimal-to-modest treatment effects, methylxanthines should be considered investigational therapy in the treatment of OSA, though there may be beneficial effects in those with obstructive lung disease and comorbid OSA intolerant of other primary or alternative OSA therapies.

In recognition of the effects of opiate agonists on respiratory depression, another early investigation tested multiple medications, including naloxone (an opioid antagonist), theophylline, and bromocriptine mesylate (a dopamine agonist). None of these agents had any significant beneficial effects on the frequency or duration of obstructive apneas and hypopneas or oxygen desaturation indices.[53] Naltrexone 50 mg was compared with placebo in a double-blind crossover study. Compared with control, mean AHI 32.9 events/hour, and placebo, AHI 37.6 events/hour, naltrexone significantly decreased the mean AHI to 29.1 ± 26.2.[54] However, given incomplete treatment effects, these medications should not be considered appropriate for use as primary therapy in the treatment of OSA.

Medroxyprogesterone acetate, a respiratory stimulant, has been studied as a potential treatment for OSA.[55] Thirteen men with OSA and no hypercapnia during wakefulness were treated with 60 mg/day of medroxyprogesterone acetate for 4 weeks in an open-label study, and no difference in OSA severity was seen. Thus medroxyprogesterone acetone cannot be recommended as primary, adjunctive, or alternative treatment for OSA.

Sedatives and Hypnotics

The use of sedatives and hypnotics in the treatment of OSA appears counterintuitive, given concerns of worsening of OSA as a result of the myorelaxant and central nervous system (CNS) sedative effects of many of these medications.[56] However, a low arousal threshold in a patient with OSA may result in a premature arousal before compensatory neuromuscular mechanisms have sufficient time to restore upper airway patency. A premature arousal, when combined with an underlying state of ventilatory instability, may result in persistent disordered breathing during sleep. One study[44] demonstrated that 37% of OSA patients have a low arousal threshold, raising the possibility that increasing the arousal threshold using sedatives/hypnotics might represent a therapeutic target.

Clinical studies testing this possibility have looked at the use of eszopiclone, zopiclone, and zolpidem, nonbenzodiazepine gamma-aminobutyric acid (GABA) receptor modulators. One study randomized 17 subjects with OSA and a nadir Sao_2 >70%, to one night of eszopiclone 3 mg and one night of placebo.[57] The arousal threshold, quantified by the nadir epiglottic pressure level associated with electroencephalogram (EEG) arousal, was observed to increase by 18% in stage N2 sleep and the mean AHI was reduced by 23% (from 31 events/hour to 24 events/hour) in the eszopiclone condition compared with the placebo condition. No significant difference in hypoxemia severity was seen between the two groups. However, in another RCT, participants with mild-to-moderate OSA who received either eszopiclone or placebo for two consecutive nights demonstrated no significant difference in AHI between the groups.[58] Both studies examined the effects of eszopiclone over only a few nights; thus the long-term effects of this medication on OSA are unknown.

Zolpidem and zopiclone, medications with similar mechanisms of action, have also been tested for their effects on OSA. In general, it appears that nonbenzodiazepine GABA receptor modulators do not appear to substantially improve or worsen OSA severity, gas exchange, or sleep parameters in uncomplicated patients with OSA.[59-62]

Medications that are not classically considered sedatives or hypnotics have also been examined for their effects on OSA. Several studies have examined the use of trazodone, an antidepressant medication with serotonergic, antihistaminergic, and antiadrenergic effects, to treat OSA.[63-65] Trazodone given at 100 mg for one night was reported to increase the arousal threshold by 32% but did not reduce the AHI.[64] A subsequent study of 15 severe OSA patients given trazodone 100 mg or placebo had conflicting results, demonstrating no significant changes in arousal threshold, but mild improvements in AHI with trazodone compared with placebo (28.5 events/hour versus 38.7 events/hour, respectively).[65]

Gabapentin, an analgesic and anticonvulsant medication, was shown to increase the AHI in older men.[66] Another anticonvulsant medication, tiagabine, which increases slow wave activity during sleep, in an RCT did not change the duration of slow wave sleep, OSA severity, or arousal threshold.[67] Sodium oxybate, the sodium salt of gamma-hydroxybutyrate, is traditionally used for treating excessive daytime sleepiness and cataplexy in narcolepsy and is associated with central nervous system depression. Studies have primarily focused on the safety of this medication in patients with OSA. Two single-night studies demonstrated no significant effects on OSA severity.[68,69] In contrast, a randomized, placebo-controlled trial where patients with OSA used sodium oxybate or placebo for 2 weeks showed a reduction in AHI compared with placebo (mean difference −8.2 versus −0.8 events/hour, respectively).[70]

These data suggest that, at the very least, certain sedatives and hypnotics may not exacerbate OSA, as conventional wisdom would hold, and could be used in patients with comorbid insomnia when indicated. However, given the noted conflicting results and the lack of long-term safety studies, the use of sedatives and/or hypnotics to treat OSA, whether as adjunctive or alternative therapy, should be considered investigational.

Supplemental Oxygen

Many of the consequences of OSA are attributable to nocturnal hypoxemia. Studies done before the widespread use of CPAP reported that supplemental oxygen administration in OSA patients during sleep significantly increased the oxygen saturation of hemoglobin (Sao_2), but also lengthened apneas with associated hypercapnia and respiratory acidosis.[71-73] These early studies found no improvement in subjective or objective measures of daytime sleepiness with nocturnal oxygen treatment.[20,74] Thus oxygen therapy alone during sleep is not recommended as a primary or alternative therapy for most OSA patients.

However, improvements in OSA severity with oxygen therapy alone may depend on whether a patient has stable or unstable ventilatory control (low or high loop gain, respectively). In a study of subjects with severe OSA, oxygen reduced the AHI by 53% in the high loop gain group compared with 8% in the low loop gain group.[75] An RCT that compared 1 night of oxygen to placebo suggested that oxygen reduced the OSA severity by approximately 30% (mean AHI: pretreatment mean, 58 events/hour versus ontreatment, 41 events/hour), of which 25% of participants were considered responders, defined as an AHI reduction by more than 50% of pretreatment values.[76] The presence of high versus low loop gain did not predict which participants responded to oxygen therapy. However, prediction models using multivariable regression analysis showed that elevated loop gain in the setting of less severe airway collapsibility and greater compensation increased the likelihood of identifying who would respond to treatment with supplemental oxygen (positive predictive value [PPV] 69 ± 13% and negative predictive value [NPV] 100 ± 0%).[76] Therefore the use of supplemental oxygen may improve OSA severity in patients with specific combinations of physiologic endotypes.

Patients with significant cardiovascular disease (e.g. coronary artery disease or cerebrovascular disease) and only a marginally elevated frequency of abnormal breathing events during sleep, but who have severe oxyhemoglobin desaturation during those events, might benefit from reduced risk of myocardial ischemia from oxygen supplementation.[77,78] The use of oxygen therapy could be considered as alternative therapy in those with OSA and significant intermittent hypoxemia that are intolerant of a primary therapy such as CPAP to minimize potential cardiovascular and metabolic risks. However, although hypoxemia may resolve, in some instances, disordered breathing events could be lengthened and predispose to hypercapnia in at-risk patients. In the absence of any high-grade evidence, such use should be considered controversial, particularly because oxygen administration is not without risks (e.g., hypercapnia, fire risk). An attended sleep study to document the optimal minimal oxygen dose for efficacy in OSA patients in preventing hypoxemia and minimizing hypercapnia should be considered.

Oxygen may also be added as adjunctive therapy to positive airway pressure (PAP) in patients in whom CPAP or bilevel PAP is effective in treating the abnormal respiratory events, but hypoxemia persists because of V/Q mismatching or hypoventilation.[79] Patients with OSA who require supplemental oxygen therapy during wakefulness will almost always require supplemental oxygen during sleep, even if PAP therapy maintains a patent upper airway.[80] However, it should be determined whether persistent oxygen desaturation with the patient using CPAP is related to hypoventilation,[10] because bilevel positive pressure in this population may obviate the need for added oxygen.

Oxygen therapy instead of CPAP may be considered in patients with mild OSA who have a transmissible infection (e.g., COVID-19) in whom there is concern that PAP may disseminate pathogen into the atmosphere.[81] High-flow oxygen has been used in COVID-19–infected OSA patients while in a state of hypoxemic respiratory failure.[82]

Transtracheal Oxygen Delivery

Several reports have described the use of transtracheal oxygen administration in patients with OSA who are intolerant of CPAP.[83-85] One study described the use of this modality as salvage therapy in a patient with chronic obstructive pulmonary disease and OSA overlap syndrome with persistent hypoxemia despite CPAP and in-line oxygen.[86] These data are too limited to recommend this mode of oxygen delivery, and thus transtracheal oxygen use in OSA should be considered investigational.

Carbon Dioxide Modulation

Relative hypocapnia, particularly in the presence of a reduced CO_2 reserve (i.e., the difference in CO_2 during eucapnia and the apnea threshold), is known to destabilize breathing and result in periodic breathing. Although this mechanism is of concern in those with central sleep apnea, it can play a role in those with OSA, particularly those with forms of complex sleep apnea. In physiologic studies, elevations of CO_2 through introduction of increased CO_2 gas content or increases in dead space have been shown to stabilize periodic breathing. This has led to investigation of these approaches as an adjunctive approach for the clinical treatment of patients with OSA, particularly those with complex sleep apnea.

Inspired CO_2. Several studies have shown some benefit with the use of inspired CO_2 in patients with and without heart failure. Some have used CO_2 tanks with a tightly fitted mask;[87-90] and some have bled CO_2 through a CPAP device.[91]

Others have reported no improvement in sleep quality or arousals with the use of inspired CO2.[87,92] The combined use of CO_2 with CPAP used lower concentrations of CO_2 than in the studies that did not use positive pressure support. A small proof-of-concept study using a precisely controlled CO_2 flow modulator delivering 0.5% to 1.0% concentration of CO_2 in a PAP circuit improved the AHI from 43 events/hour while on CPAP to 4.5 events/hour.[93] However, further studies are needed before use can be clinically recommended and should be considered investigational.

CO_2 rebreathing. Rebreathing of CO_2 through the addition of 400 to 600 mL of dead space without a continuous-bias flow has been shown to decrease AHI and arousals and improved sleep quality in patients with heart failure and central sleep apnea; however, adverse events limit its use. Reported adverse events included fatigued respiratory muscles, vasoconstriction, tachycardia, and increased cardiac contractility.[94] With the implementation of PAP, relative hypocapnia is not uncommon, which can contribute to CPAP-emergent central apneas. In a retrospective review of CPAP-resistant OSA with mild hypocapnia during wakefulness (mean $ETco_2$ 38.1 ± 3.1 mm Hg), a lower volume of dead space (100–150 mL) using a non-vented mask and small sections of respiratory tubing to raise the $ETco_2$ by 2 to 3 mm Hg demonstrated improvements in sleep apnea severity without tachypnea or tachycardia as an adverse effect.[95] This approach can be implemented with appropriate planning and coordination in the home setting, though additional studies are needed to verify consistency.

Other Pharmacotherapy for OSA Not Targeting Neuromuscular or Neuroventilatory Control

Clonidine, an alpha-2-adrenergic agonist with REM-suppressing properties, has been investigated as a treatment for OSA in at least one small RCT in which participants received 2 consecutive nights of clonidine 0.2 mg and placebo in a randomized order. Clonidine compared with placebo resulted in both decreased REM sleep duration and obstructive apnea index (20.6 versus 19.3 events/hr). No difference in NREM or overall AHI and no improvement in daytime sleepiness was observed.[96] Because of the minimal decrease in REM-related AHI and small study size, clonidine should not be considered as a treatment for OSA.

Medication for "Residual" Excessive Daytime Sleepiness in OSA

Even with objectively documented successful treatment of OSA, including acceptable adherence to therapy, it has been estimated that as much as 10% of OSA patients continue to report significant excessive daytime sleepiness (EDS).[97] The significance of EDS cannot be understated, given its role in contributing to motor vehicle accidents, impaired psychological functioning, and reduced work performance.[45] The cause of such "residual" EDS, however, can be difficult to definitively ascertain.[98]

As part of the clinical management of patients with appropriately treated OSA but persistent EDS, other conditions such as insufficient sleep time, insomnia, medication-related side effects, or other comorbid sleep disorders should be carefully ruled out. Successful treatment of OSA should be documented by objective adherence to therapy and a normal AHI, with the prescribed CPAP regimen based on a sleep study or adherence data. Objective documentation of EDS with a multiple sleep latency test (MSLT) or Maintenance of Wakefulness Test (MWT) could be considered, although it is not a requirement for most third-party payers, and such testing is typically performed when there are concerns of primary CNS hypersomnolence disorders such as narcolepsy. If EDS persists despite adequate OSA treatment, the use of nonsympathomimetic stimulants (i.e., caffeine) or psychostimulant medications (i.e., nonamphetamine or amphetamine derivates) could be used as part of an overall management strategy to improve daytime alertness (Table 133.4).[99]

Traditionally, amphetamine-class medications have been used to treat residual EDS in OSA patients, based on data available in narcolepsy and sleep-restricted individuals (see Chapter 112). The use of these medications is not discussed further in this section because of the potential for harmful cardiovascular consequences and potential negative mood- and sleep-related effects and the paucity of data regarding their use in the treatment of residual EDS in OSA patients.

Modafinil and armodafinil, the *r*-isomer of modafinil, are nonamphetamines currently Food and Drug Administration (FDA)-approved for the treatment of residual hypersomnolence in adequately treated OSA patients.[100] The wake-promoting effects of the medication are incompletely understood, but are primarily the result of dopaminergic-mediated pathways.[101] Several relatively large, randomized placebo-controlled clinical trials have demonstrated that modafinil[102-105] and armodafinil[100,106-109] can safely reduce EDS based on subjective and objective measures[110] and improve quality of life in patients with OSA adequately treated with CPAP.[104,105] For example, an RCT of modafinil versus placebo reported normalization of the ESS in 51% of the modafinil group versus 27% in the placebo group.[103] Although the mean sleep latency on an MSLT was improved in the modafinil group compared with placebo group, normalization of the MSLT (>10 minutes) was similar between the groups (29% versus

Table 133.4 Excessive Daytime Sleepiness

Name	Influence on EDS	Study Design
Modafinil + CPAP	32% ↓, 26% ↓	RCT,[103] RCT[102]
Armodafinil + CPAP	36% ↓, 41% ↓	RCT,[107] open label[108]
Solriamfetol + CPAP	5% ↓, 58% ↓	RCT,[114] RCT[115]
Pitolisant	23% ↓	RCT[117]

CPAP, Continuous positive airway pressure; EDS, excessive daytime sleepiness; RCT, randomized controlled trial.

25%, respectively). A subsequent RCT evaluated the effects of placebo compared with modafinil at a 200- or 400-mg dose. Improvements in ESS scores and mean sleep latency on the MWT were reported, with similar improvements for the 200- and 400-mg modafinil dose groups. No change in CPAP adherence was reported in these two studies.[102,103] However, in a separate 12-week open-label continuation of modafinil from the study by Pack and colleagues,[103] mean CPAP use was observed to decline from 6.3 hours/night to 5.9 hours/night,[111] suggesting that such agents may in fact reduce adherence to the primary therapy used by a patient for their OSA. Clinicians therefore should continually remind their patients to be adherent to their primary OSA therapy to maximize the wake-promoting effects of both therapies.

A similar literature base is available regarding the efficacy of armodafinil for residual EDS in patients with treated OSA. Armodafinil has a duration of action that is 10% to 15% longer than modafinil. Data from a pooled analysis[107] of two RCTs[105,112] found that adjunctive treatment in CPAP-adherent OSA participants with residual EDS with armodafinil significantly improved wakefulness, long-term memory, and patients' ability to engage in activities of daily living. Armodafinil also reduced patient-reported fatigue, evaluated separately from sleepiness, and was well tolerated.[107] Treatment with armodafinil showed no effect on subsequent CPAP adherence.[109] A multicenter, flexible-dose, open-label study found that armodafinil remained effective for more than 12 months in patients with residual EDS and treated OSA.[108]

The most commonly reported adverse events in the studies as reported, which were associated with both medications, included headache (≈15%–20%), nausea (≈10%–20%), insomnia (≈5%–10%), and anxiety (≈5%–15%). Up to 15% of patients in one study discontinued medications because of such adverse events. A rare but serious adverse event that clinicians should be aware of involves serious rashes, including Stevens-Johnson syndrome or toxic epidermal necrolysis, which typically occur within 5 weeks of the initiation of therapy, but in rare cases occurs later than that. Rare cases of multiorgan hypersensitivity presenting as fever, rash, and organ system dysfunction have been reported with modafinil and armodafinil, in addition to anaphylactoid reaction with armodafinil. Modafinil and armodafinil may decrease the effectiveness of hormonal birth control; thus women should be advised of this possibility, with consideration of nonhormonal contraceptive approaches.

Solriamfetol, a selective norepinephrine/dopamine reuptake inhibitor, was approved by the FDA to improve wakefulness in patients with EDS associated with OSA and narcolepsy. The medication has a lower binding affinity to dopamine and norepinephrine receptors than modafinil/armodafinil and does not have the monoamine-releasing effect of amphetamines.[113] In theory, solriamfetol may have a more modest side effect profile than even modafinil and armodafinil.

Two studies have focused on solriamfetol to treat residual EDS in the setting of adequately treated OSA.[114,115] In one RCT, the effect of placebo and solriamfetol at doses of 37.5, 75, 150, and 300 mg on EDS was studied.[114] Participants had OSA with current or prior primary treatment and EDS determined by an ESS greater than or equal to 10 and were not required to be adherent to their primary OSA treatment. All doses of solriamfetol were associated with improved subjective sleepiness measured by ESS as early as the first week and extending through the 12 weeks of the study. ESS scores at 12 weeks decreased by greater than or equal to 7 points with higher doses (150 and 300 mg) compared with a mean decrease of 3.3 points in the placebo group.[114]

In another study, investigators conducted an RCT of solriamfetol for people with OSA and EDS.[115] ESS and the MWT sleep latency were improved at week 4 compared with baseline and remained improved in those that continued solriamfetol compared with those that were given placebo for the final 2 weeks.[115] This effect appears to be sustained to 1 year, as suggested in the open-label phase of another study,[116] where approximately 80% of OSA participants maintained an ESS below 11 through 52 weeks. Adverse effects reported in those receiving solriamfetol included headache (10.1%), nausea (7.9%), decreased appetite (7.6%), anxiety (7.0%), and nasopharyngitis (5.1%).[116]

Pitolisant is a selective histamine H3-receptor antagonist/inverse agonist with wake-promoting effects that is used in the treatment of narcolepsy. It has been studied as an alternative to primary treatment in those with moderate-to-severe OSA that do not tolerate CPAP and have EDS (ESS ≥12). One RCT found that ESS was decreased (mean difference 2.8; 95% CI [−4.0, −1.5]) ontreatment compared with placebo.[117] During 12 weeks of use, adverse events included headache, insomnia, nausea, and vertigo; however, these had similar frequency between treatment and placebo groups (24% versus 19.4%, $P = 0.377$).

In summary, the use of stimulant therapy in patients with OSA should be considered adjunctive therapy in the treatment of residual EDS in patients with adequately treated OSA with CPAP, including with documentation of acceptable adherence to CPAP, and after excluding other causes of EDS. More controversial is whether stimulants should be considered as an alternative therapy for patients with EDS because of OSA who are intolerant of treatments for their OSA. At least two studies suggest that modafinil during a 2-day CPAP withdrawal or for 2 weeks in patients with mild-to-moderate untreated OSA demonstrates significant improvements in driving performance in a driving simulator, subjective sleepiness, and attention and vigilance on the psychomotor vigilance test.[118,119] A randomized, placebo-controlled study evaluating the use of armodafinil to improve driving performance and weight loss in sleep apnea showed no difference in driving performance but did have an increased weight loss compared with placebo at 6 months on treatment.[120] In patients in high-risk situations where alertness and performance are critical (e.g., professional drivers, military personnel) and are unable to use their primary PAP therapy (e.g., unreliable electrical source while traveling), there may be a role for stimulants as sole treatment for brief periods. However, continued reinforcement of adherence to the patient's prescribed OSA treatment, in addition to monitoring for medication side effects, is necessary to avoid potential long-term adverse effects of stimulants.

CLINICAL PEARLS

Despite the efficacy of traditional primary treatments such as CPAP, oral appliance therapy, and upper airway surgery for OSA, these treatments can have suboptimal adherence or result in incomplete therapy. Alternative pharmacotherapies have been studied for the treatment of OSA; however, most remain investigational as a primary treatment for OSA and have not been approved in this role by regulatory agencies. In patients with certain comorbid conditions with OSA, some pharmacotherapies may be considered alone when a patient is intolerant of a primary therapy for OSA or as adjunctive treatment with other OSA treatment options. In patients with OSA and residual sleepiness, adjunctive stimulant therapy can be considered, but only after ensuring that the patient has adequate OSA treatment and sleep time and that no other sleep disorders may explain the residual sleepiness.

SUMMARY

In light of traditional primary treatment modalities for OSA, including CPAP, oral mandibular advancement devices, and upper airway surgeries, often having poor adherence rates and/or insufficient long-term outcomes, adjunctive and alternative treatment options for OSA continue to be investigated. There has been a long-standing attempt to identify pharmacologic agents that may treat OSA, though none to date have demonstrated sufficient effectiveness to obtain regulatory agency approval. There may be reason for promise in the future as our understanding of the pathophysiologic basis of OSA improves and approaches to identify mechanisms that are most important in a particular patient are being developed to personalize the treatment of OSA. At this time, most pharmacotherapies do not have proven efficacy and should currently be considered as investigational or adjunctive therapy rather than primary therapy for OSA. Despite effective treatment for OSA, some patients may experience persistent sleepiness despite adequate sleep time and may be appropriate candidates for adjunctive stimulant therapy. Given the challenges that some patients experience with primary therapies for OSA, continued investigation into alterative and adjunctive OSA treatment options will continue.

SELECTED READINGS

Aishah A, Lim R, Sands SA, et al. Different antimuscarinics when combined with atomoxetine have differential effects on obstructive sleep apnea severity. *J Appl Physiol (1985)*. 2021;130(5):1373–1382.

Avellar AB, Carvalho LB, Prado GF, Prado LB. Pharmacotherapy for residual excessive sleepiness and cognition in CPAP-treated patients with obstructive sleep apnea syndrome: a systematic review and meta-analysis. *Sleep Med Rev*. 2016;30:97–107.

Hudgel DW, Patel SR, Ahasic AM, et al. The role of weight management in the treatment of adult obstructive sleep apnea. An official American Thoracic Society clinical practice guideline. *Am J Respir Crit Care Med*. 2018;198(6):e70–e87.

Liu HM, Chiang IJ, Kuo KN, Liou CM, Chen C. The effect of acetazolamide on sleep apnea at high altitude: a systematic review and meta-analysis. *Therap Adv Respirat Dis*. 2017;11(1):20–29.

Mitchell LJ, Davidson ZE, Bonham M, O'Driscoll DM, Hamilton GS, Truby H. Weight loss from lifestyle interventions and severity of sleep apnoea: a systematic review and meta-analysis. *Sleep medicine*. 2014;15(10):1173–1183.

Mulchrone A, Shokoueinejad M, Webster J. A review of preventing central sleep apnea by inspired CO2. *Physiol Measurem*. 2016;37(5):R36–R45.

Nigam G, Camacho M, Riaz M. The effect of nonbenzodiazepines sedative hypnotics on apnea-hypopnea index: a meta-analysis. *Annal Thoracic Med*. 2019;14(1):49–55.

Schweitzer PK, Rosenberg R, Zammit GK, et al. Solriamfetol for excessive sleepiness in obstructive sleep Apnea (TONES 3). A randomized controlled trial. *Am J Respir Crit Care Med*. 2019;199(11):1421–1431.

Taranto-Montemurro L, Messineo L, Sands SA, et al. The combination of atomoxetine and oxybutynin greatly reduces obstructive sleep apnea severity. A randomized, placebo-controlled, double-blind crossover trial. *Am J Respir Crit Care Med*. 2019;199(10):1267–1276.

Taranto-Montemurro L, Messineo L, Wellman A. Targeting endotypic traits with medications for the pharmacological treatment of obstructive sleep apnea. A review of the current literature. *J Clin Med*. 2019;8(11).

A complete reference list can be found online at ExpertConsult.com.

Chapter 134

Alternative Strategies to Management of Sleep-Disordered Breathing

Robert Stansbury; Patrick J. Strollo, Jr.

Chapter Highlights

- Commonly used treatments such as CPAP, oral appliance therapy, and upper airway surgery will remain important considerations in the management of SDB but these traditional interventions lead to suboptimal outcomes in many individuals.
- Important progress has been made toward developing new treatments for SDB including pharmacotherapy and neurostimulation.
- Future management will depend heavily on integration of multiple data levels for SDB to effectively manage this common disease. For instance, a patient with moderate symptomatic SDB that tended to worsen when supine and who wishes to avoid a permanent device may be managed with a combination of pharmacologic agents and head of bed elevation.

INTRODUCTION

Sleep-disordered breathing (SDB) syndrome is a common clinical problem that is underdiagnosed and represents a spectrum of disease ranging from sleep disruption related to increased airway resistance to profound daytime sleepiness in conjunction with a multitude of health consequences.[1,2] SDB manifests in various ways including obstructive sleep apnea (OSA); central sleep apnea (CSA), both with and without Cheyne-Stokes respiration; and sleep-related hypoventilation. Epidemiologic data, in part because of the obesity epidemic, suggest that the prevalence of OSA is increasing in the population.[3,4] Providers should be familiar with treatment options available for the care of these individuals.

Historically a one size fits all approach was applied to the management of OSA, with patients being managed almost exclusively with positive airway pressure (PAP) therapy. PAP adherence data demonstrate a significant number of patients with OSA are intolerant of this therapy and will not be successfully treated.[5] As we move into an era of personalized medicine, tailoring therapy to individuals' clinical and physiologic phenotype will likely improve treatment of OSA. Importantly, patient preferences should also weigh heavily on therapy decisions.[6] In this chapter we review considerations for a personalized approach to OSA followed by a discussion of various treatment modalities based on the underlying pathophysiologic mechanism(s) driving recurrent upper airway obstruction.

CONSIDERATIONS IN THE PERSONALIZED MANAGEMENT OF OBSTRUCTIVE SLEEP APNEA

The current management paradigm for patients with OSA usually involves a diagnostic sleep study followed by a trial of PAP therapy. Alternative therapies are normally not discussed/initiated until PAP therapy has failed (in many instances multiple times). This current management paradigm is driven by multiple factors such as lack of familiarity with alternative treatments, third-party reimbursement policies, and ease of PAP initiation. Little is done in clinic to personalize OSA treatment, and many patients are likely lost to follow-up after PAP failure. With increased recognition of OSA heterogeneity and the understanding that the apnea-hypopnea index (AHI) is not a particularly effective way to cohort individuals, the field is primed to make progress toward precision medicine in the management of SDB. Although there are various approaches to OSA phenotyping, integration of these different models will most likely progress the field toward personalized management of OSA. OSA is a complex and heterogeneous disorder with multiple levels of data that require integration to predictively model disease expression and response to therapy (Figure 134.1).[7] An exhaustive review is beyond the scope of this chapter; however, we will briefly review key clinical and physiologic phenotypes described in OSA as these topics are becoming increasingly important considerations in the current management of OSA.

Clinical Phenotypes

Although clinicians have long recognized the heterogeneity in the presentation of OSA, clinical phenotypes were formally characterized recently by the work of Ye and colleagues.[8] These researchers used cluster analysis based on response to questionnaires to identify clinical phenotypes in the Icelandic Sleep Apnea Cohort (ISAC). Three distinct clinical presentations of OSA were identified based on symptom experiences and the existence of major comorbidities. These included (1) disturbed sleep, (2) excessive daytime sleepiness, and (3) minimal symptomatology. Follow-up work supports this clinical phenotyping and may have important implications for OSA therapy. For

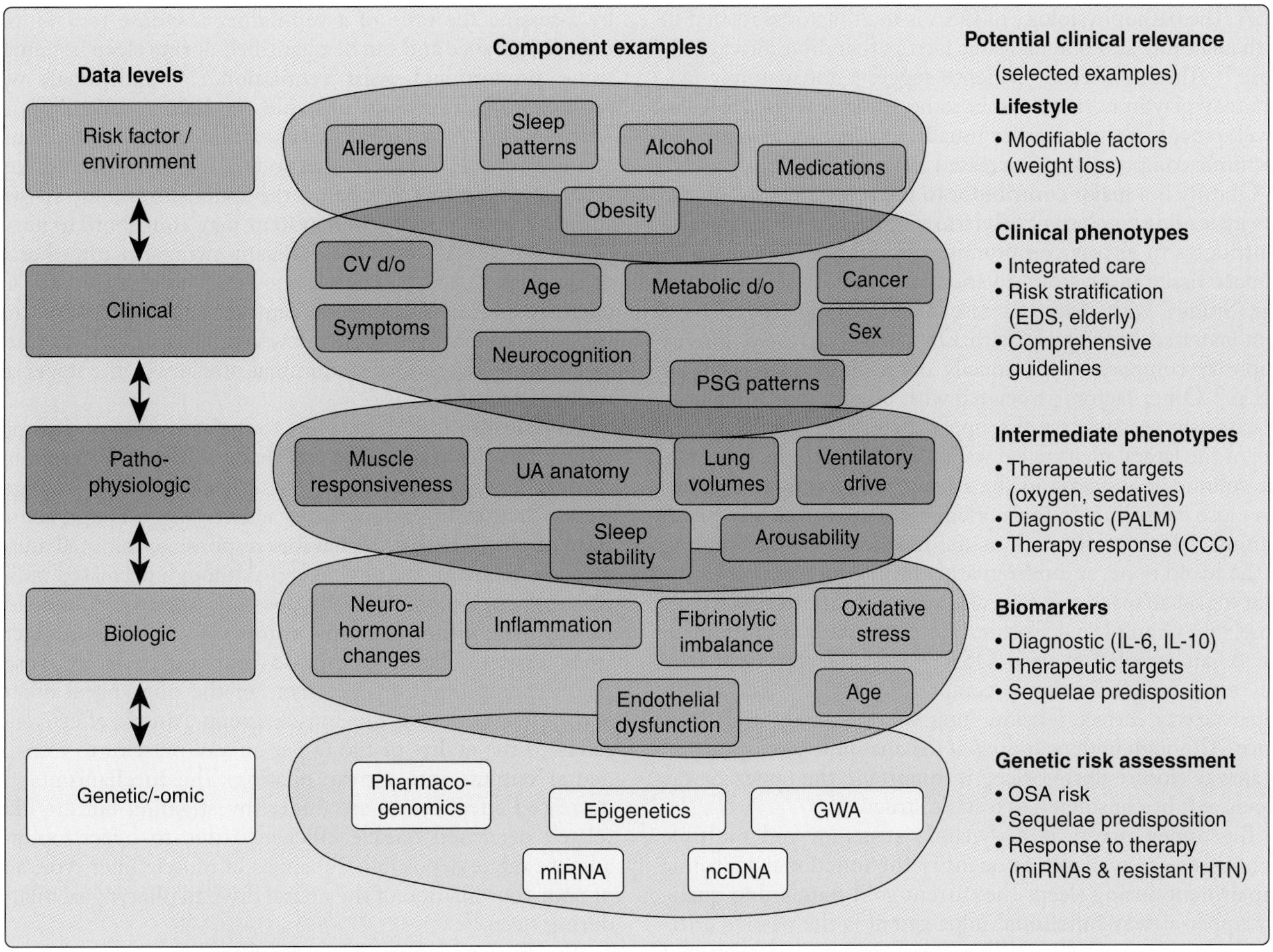

Figure 134.1 Data levels of sleep-disordered breathing and clinical relevance to diagnosis and treatment. Current data levels of phenotyping in sleep-disordered breathing with examples of components being studied. This research will likely lead to improved diagnostic and treatment paradigms for sleep-disordered breathing.

instance, a 2-year follow-up study of the ISAC demonstrated that the excessive daytime sleepiness cohort had a particular robust response to therapy for OSA.[9]

Clinical phenotyping may also be an important consideration when evaluating cardiovascular risk in an individual with OSA. Epidemiologic data strongly support an association between OSA and morbidity/mortality, including coronary heart disease, congestive heart failure (CHF), stroke, and atrial fibrillation.[10-13] Yet large trials assessing continuous positive airway pressure (CPAP) therapy for individuals with OSA have found no cardiovascular benefit of CPAP treatment in intention to treat analyses.[14,15] These results are likely in part due to lower than expected CPAP adherence in the trials, but are also likely driven by a focus on participants who were not excessively sleepy. Credence to this argument is forthcoming. Mazzotti and colleagues recently characterized OSA symptom subtypes and assessed their association with prevalent and incident cardiovascular disease (CVD) in the Sleep Heart Health Study.[16] Using latent class analysis they observed four subtypes of symptoms: disturbed sleep, minimally symptomatic, excessively sleepy, and moderately sleepy. In adjusted models, the "excessively sleepy" subtype was associated with a more than threefold increased risk of prevalent HF compared with each of the other subtypes. They identified a significant association between the "excessively sleepy" subtype and coronary heart disease ($P = .015$). These findings have potential implications. Individuals with the excessively sleepy subtype were at increased risk of CVD compared not only with participants without OSA, but also relative to participants in other clinical subtypes with sleep apnea and a similar AHI.

This clinical phenotyping may inform routine clinical practice by developing appropriate and validated clinical support tools for clinicians in identifying the subtype at increased risk for adverse outcomes that would have a significant effect on therapy decisions. For instance, a clinician may feel more comfortable recommending a patient with a history of coronary artery disease and no significant sleep complaints who is found to have a mildly elevated AHI to forgo aggressive interventions to normalize the AHI and to adopt simple lifestyle modifications.

Physiologic Phenotypes

Another important consideration in determining treatment interventions for OSA is physiologic traits that contribute to

OSA. The pathophysiology of OSA is multifactorial related to both anatomic and nonanatomic factors that drive airway collapse.[17] Although recent evidence suggests nonanatomic factors may play important role in some patients with OSA, the development of this disorder usually requires some degree of anatomic compromise or increased airway collapsibility.[18-20]

Obesity is a major contributor to the anatomic load on the airway leading to pharyngeal narrowing and collapse. Obesity contributes to airway compromise through the deposition of adipose tissue in or around various regions of the upper airway. Studies with magnetic resonance imaging (MRI) have demonstrated individuals with OSA have increased tongue adiposity compared with equally obese individuals without OSA.[21] Other factors associated with obesity that contribute to extrinsic pressure on the upper airway include increased size of the lateral pharyngeal walls and increased total soft tissue volume in and around the airway.[22,23] Craniofacial structures also contribute to the anatomic load on the airway. Small craniofacial structures such as the mandible, low positioning of the hyoid bone, and retrognathia lead to a reduction in the pharyngeal airspace and a greater susceptibility to airway collapse.[24,25] Craniofacial features are particularly important in the Asian population with OSA.[26] Other factors that may play a minor role in airway compromise include fluid shifts, upper airway surface tension, lung volumes, and nasal resistance. Although understanding of the anatomic predisposition to airway closure during sleep is important, the upper airway should not be considered as a static structure.

The upper airway is a dynamic structure and multiple techniques are available to quantify the functional anatomic impairment during sleep. The current gold standard to quantify upper airway functional impairment is the passive critical closing pressure (P_{crit}). This measurement is determined while individuals are on CPAP and estimates the pressure at which the upper airway collapses and airflow ceases.[27] In normal individuals the upper airway structures prevent closure during sleep and negative pressures below -5 cm H_2O are required to collapse the airway. Individuals with anatomic abnormalities will have airway collapse at more positive pressures ($P_{crit} \geq +5$ cm H_2O); however, there is marked variation in P_{crit} and apnea severity.[18,28] For instance, some individuals with significant sleep apnea have only mild-to-moderate anatomic impairment (-2 cm $H_2O \leq P_{crit} \leq +2$ cm H_2O) that can also be seen in the non-OSA population.[29] The development of OSA is clearly related to more than the anatomic load on the upper airway; however, this factor remains a key therapeutic target.

In recent years there has been significant progress in our understanding of the nonanatomic physiologic mechanisms of OSA.[30] This understanding is predicted to have significant implications in terms of risk stratification and treatment decisions for individuals with OSA. To date three important nonanatomic factors have been described: (1) ventilatory control instability (high loop gain), (2) low respiratory arousal threshold, and (3) decreased pharyngeal dilator muscle responsiveness/effectiveness.

Loop gain is an engineering term used to describe the stability of a system controlled by a negative feedback loop. When applied to breathing it refers to the response of the respiratory system to fluctuations in CO_2 levels. Individual responses to CO_2 fluctuations are important in the pathogenesis of both OSA and CSA.[31] In OSA, loop gain is quantified by assessing the ratio of a ventilatory response to a ventilatory disturbance and can be quantified during sleep in humans using proportional assist ventilation.[32-34] Individuals with high loop gain have an unstable ventilatory control system whereby they have an excessive ventilatory response to small changes in CO_2 followed by periods of low ventilatory drive as CO_2 drops precipitously below the apneic threshold. An oversensitive ventilatory control system may contribute to airway closure in OSA through significant swings in intrathoracic pressure that occur in response to small changes in CO_2 and decreased output from neural centers to the pharyngeal dilator muscles during periods of low ventilator drive.[17] The latter significantly decreases intraluminal pressure in the upper airway, promoting collapse.

Muscle responsiveness refers to the activation of the upper airway muscles responsible for airway dilation to respiratory stimuli (i.e., hypercapnia or pharyngeal pressure changes). Research assessing genioglossus activity suggests that about a third of people with OSA have no response or minimal muscle response to airway narrowing.[17,35] Although decreased muscle responsiveness alone typically does not cause OSA, individuals with significant anatomic compromise may be protected from airway collapse through a potent muscle response.[36] Another important characteristic of the pharyngeal dilators is the effectiveness of this muscle group. Muscle effectiveness refers to the ability of the upper airway muscles to translate neural outputs into airway dilation. The mechanism(s) for decreased effectiveness are under investigation but are likely related decreased muscle efficiency (due to hypertrophy or adipose tissue deposition), changes in muscle fiber type, and/or poor coordination of the neural drive to pharyngeal dilators during sleep.[37]

The final nonanatomic factor found to be an important physiologic mechanism in OSA pathogenesis is termed respiratory arousal threshold. The arousal threshold refers to the level of ventilatory drive that leads to awakening (cortical arousal) during sleep. Historically this was thought to be a protective mechanism to restore airflow during a respiratory event. Subsequent work has shown that cortical arousals are not necessary to restore airflow and contribute to worsening apnea severity through a destabilized breathing pattern, as well as inadequate recruitment of the pharyngeal dilators.[38,39]

THERAPIES PRIMARILY TARGETING AIRWAY ANATOMIC LOADS/AIRWAY COLLAPSIBILITY

OSA is a heterogeneous disorder; however, in most cases the development of airway obstruction is driven by some degree of anatomic compromise or increased airway collapsibility. The cornerstone of treatment has historically focused on therapies that reduce the anatomic load on the upper airway including PAP therapy, mandibular advancement devices, and upper airway surgeries. Although these can be effective, a number of other interventions targeting the anatomic loads are available and may be important options in a personalized approach to OSA.

Hypoglossal Nerve Stimulation

In 2014 the Food and Drug Administration approved the first (and only commercially available) hypoglossal nerve stimulator (HNS) for the treatment of OSA. See also Chapter 175 that reviews surgical aspects of this therapy. The HNS device directly addresses airway collapsibility related to inadequate muscle activation through unilateral stimulation of the hypoglossal nerve (CN XII) synchronized with ventilation. The HNS is a pacemaker-like pulse generator with a sensing lead, implanted between the intercostal muscles to sense changes in thoracic pressure during respiration and a stimulation lead that is implanted submentally on the distal branches of the hypoglossal nerve to stimulate protrusion of the genioglossus muscle (Figure 134.2). Airway patency is maintained not only directly through genioglossal protrusion, but also indirectly through mechanical coupling of the velopharyngeal airway wall and palatoglossal muscles.[40,41] The STAR trial is the largest HNS trial to date and enrolled 126 patients, with 124 patients included in the 12-month follow-up.[42] At 12 months, mean AHI decreased 52%, from 32.0 to 15.3 events per hour, while the median AHI decreased 68%. This trial also reported significant improvements in secondary quality-of-life endpoints, including the Epworth Sleepiness Scale (ESS), Functional Outcomes of Sleep Questionnaire (FOSQ), and snoring as reported by bed partner. Follow-up of this patient cohort demonstrates this device is safe and durable with reasonable effectiveness compared with the absence of effective therapy before the availability of HNS.[43,44] As HNS therapy has become more widely adopted, additional outcome data outside of the STAR cohort have become available and reported equally significant results.[45]

HNS is currently indicated in patients 22 years or older with body mass index (BMI) ≤32 and moderate to severe OSA (AHI range 15–65) who are intolerant of CPAP therapy. If an individual qualifies a drug-induced sleep endoscopy (DISE) is performed to assess the pattern of upper airway obstruction.[46] Individuals with concentric collapse of the velopharynx during DISE do not respond to HNS while subjects with predominate anterior-posterior collapse respond well to this therapy. Contraindications to HNS therapy include central + mixed apneas >25% of the total AHI, anatomic findings that would compromise the performance of upper airway stimulation, conditions or procedures that have compromised neurologic

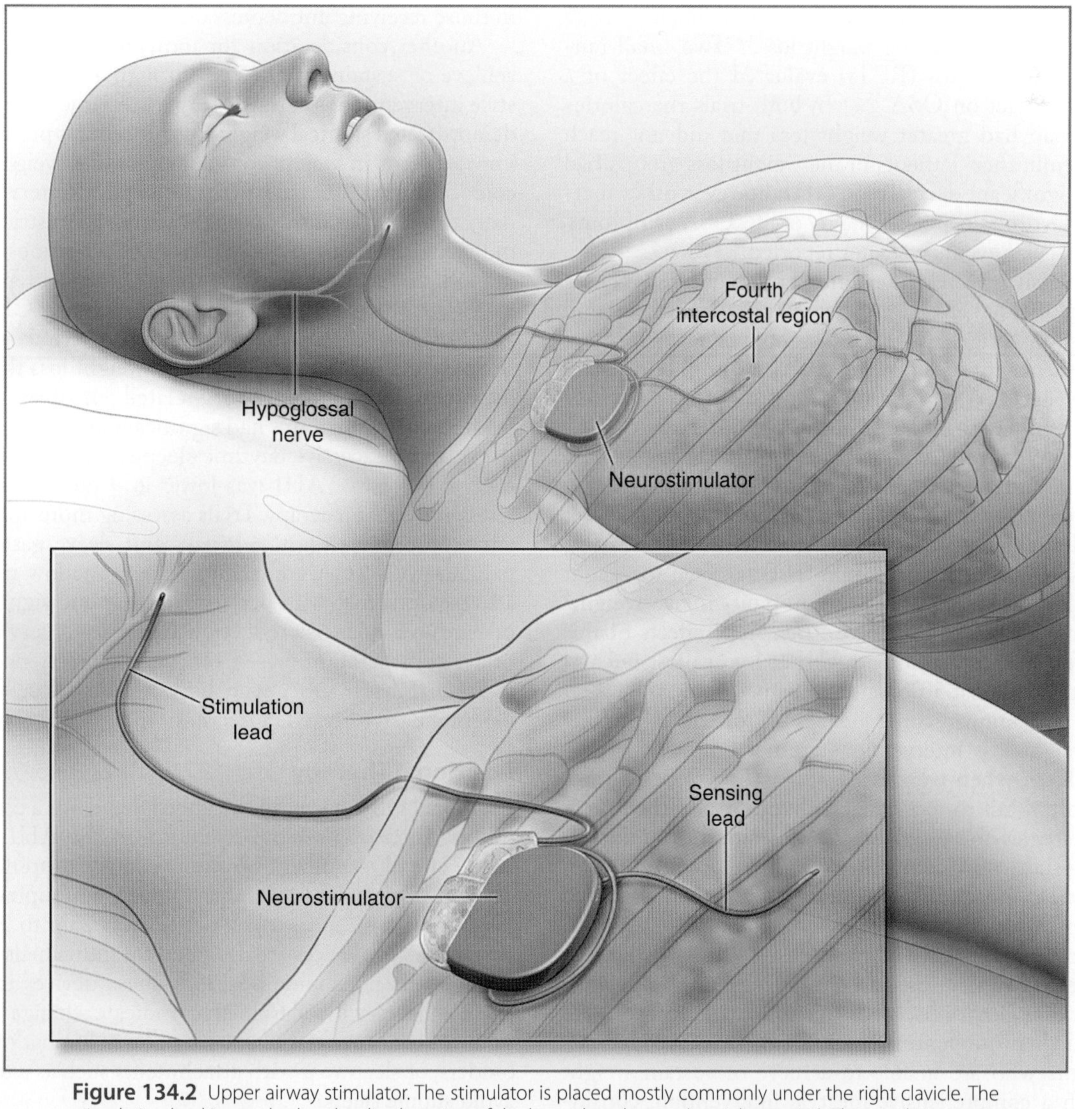

Figure 134.2 Upper airway stimulator. The stimulator is placed mostly commonly under the right clavicle. The stimulation lead is attached to the distal portion of the hypoglossal nerve (cranial nerve XII). The ventilation sensing lead is placed between the external and internal intercostal muscles with the sensing lead facing the pleura. (From Strollo PJ, Soose RJ, Maurer JT, et al. Upper-airway stimulation for obstructive sleep apnea. *N Engl J Med.* 2014;370:139-149.)

control of the upper airway, and individuals who are pregnant or plan to become pregnant. Follow-up studies have reported minimal adverse events and none to be life threatening. The most common complication related to the device has been tongue weakness, reported in 17% of participants. The majority of these cases resolved spontaneously.[47]

Medical/Surgical Weight Loss

Excess weight is a well-established predictor of OSA.[48] Consequently, weight loss is an important strategy for the management of OSA and supported by professional societies.[49,50] As outlined earlier in this chapter, obesity-related impairments of upper airway function are mediated through several direct mechanisms. Central obesity can also indirectly encourage airway collapse through decreasing functional residual capacity and thus reducing tracheal traction on the upper airway.[51] Regardless of the weight loss intervention, remission of OSA is achievable, with those losing more weight and having a less severe degree of sleep apnea at baseline being more likely to achieve disease resolution.[52,53]

Weight loss through reduced-calorie diets has been extensively studied, with diets restricted to approximately 1000 kcal/day successfully inducing weight loss.[54] Two small randomized controlled trials (RCTs) evaluated the effect of a reduced-calorie diet on OSA.[55,56] In both trials the calorie-restricted group had greater weight loss that did not reach statistical significance. Patients in the weight loss groups had statistically significant decreases in AHI; however, other metrics such as daytime sleepiness, quality of life, OSA symptoms, and cardiovascular events were not reported.

Comprehensive lifestyle intervention programs that include a reduced-calorie diet, exercise/increased physical activity, and behavioral counseling likely have the most beneficial effects in terms risk/benefit balance for medical weight loss and improvement in OSA.[57-59] Results from the Sleep AHEAD study demonstrated that intensive lifestyle intervention was associated with reduced OSA severity, quantified as a decrease in the AHI compared with diabetes support and education.[60] This study cohort is an ancillary group from a multicenter randomized clinical trial (n = 5145) to determine the effects of an intensive lifestyle intervention (ILI) targeted to weight loss on cardiovascular morbidity and mortality in overweight/obese patients with type 2 diabetes. Beneficial effects of this intensive lifestyle intervention on AHI at 1 year persisted at 4 years, despite an almost 50% weight regain.

Despite the known consequences of obesity, in many instances weight loss interventions are not initiated by providers.[61,62] Even when weight loss counseling is performed, physicians often fail to recommend the most effective interventions/strategies for weight loss.[63] Specific recommendations for a successful comprehensive lifestyle intervention targeting weight loss are available and should be implemented when caring for obese patients with sleep apnea.[54,64] Unfortunately, some patients fail a comprehensive lifestyle intervention program for weight loss and have persistent obesity with the complications that arise with this disease. In appropriate situations further interventions may be necessary.

In patients who are unable to achieve or sustain weight loss through a comprehensive lifestyle intervention, consideration should be given to pharmacotherapy. Available agents include phentermine, orlistat, lorcaserin, liraglutide, naltrexone/bupropion, and phentermine/topiramate extended release. Two small studies to date have examined the effect of weight loss medication in obese adults with OSA. Winslow and colleagues randomized 45 subjects to phentermine/topiramate versus placebo for 28 weeks.[65] Both groups received lifestyle-modification counseling during the trial period. Polysomnography (PSG) data were obtained at baseline, week 8, and week 28. At week 28, the group receiving phentermine 15 mg plus extended-release topiramate 92 mg experienced a mean weight loss of −10.8 kg, whereas the group receiving placebo experienced a mean weight loss of −4.7 kg. There were also significant improvements in AHI, mean overnight oxygen saturation, Pittsburgh Sleep Quality Index, and systolic blood pressure in the intervention group. Another placebo-controlled trial using liraglutide showed similar findings in weight loss and sleep indices, as well as sleep/health-related quality of life end points.[66] This study also implemented lifestyle counseling in both groups. Limited randomized trial data support the idea that the addition of a weight-loss medication to a behavioral weight-loss program. Practitioners should use caution when considering these medications in patients with underlying cardiovascular disease or seizure disorder, as well as in those receiving antidepressant therapy.

Another consideration for individuals who are unable to achieve or sustain weight loss through a comprehensive lifestyle intervention is bariatric surgery. A large Cochrane review demonstrated surgical weight loss procedures produced greater improvement in weight loss outcomes and weight associated comorbidities compared with nonsurgical intervention.[67] To date, three RCTs have specially evaluated gastric banding in individuals with OSA.[68-70] Interestingly, the most recent trial randomized individuals with severe OSA and a BMI of 35 to 45 kg/m^2 to gastric banding (n = 14) versus CPAP therapy (n = 20 CPAP).[70] Similar to results of previous studies, gastric banding had a greater effect on weight loss than alternate interventions but not on OSA-related outcomes. The research team found both groups had significant and similar reductions in AHI and excessive daytime sleepiness at 18 months; however, the effective AHI was lower at 9 months in the group receiving CPAP therapy. Trials assessing more aggressive bariatric procedures (gastric bypass and sleeve gastrectomy) in patients with OSA are lacking. Given the low risk of severe adverse outcomes with bariatric surgery and significant effect on cardiovascular risk reduction, bariatric surgery is an appropriate consideration, based on patient preferences, in obese individuals with OSA who have failed to lose weight with comprehensive lifestyle intervention.

Positional Therapy

Positional OSA has been variably defined but a common definition is a 50% or more reduction in the AHI while lying in the lateral recumbent position versus the supine position.[71] The prevalence of OSA that appears on supine sleep and resolves with sleep in other positions is 25% to 30%.[72] Positional therapy devices are designed for individuals to maintain sleep in the nonsupine position. These devices include electrical sensors with alarms that indicate change in position, semirigid backpacks, full-length pillows, lumbar or abdominal binders, or sleepwear with attachments such as a tennis ball to avoid supine sleep.

Limited studies to date have evaluated positional therapy as a primary treatment for OSA. Jackson and colleagues studied individuals with moderate positional OSA on routine diagnostic PSG with a parallel group design trial of 4-week treatment using a sleep position modification device (active) or sleep hygiene advice (control).[73] Outcomes were measured at baseline and after a 4-week treatment period. There was a significant reduction in the amount of supine sleep in the active group (mean ± SD change from baseline, active group 99.5 ± 85.2 minutes, control group 68.6 ± 103.2 minutes, $P = .002$), and an improvement in AHI (active reduced by 9.9 ± 11.6 versus control group reduced by 5.3 ± 13.9, $P = .01$). There were no significant differences in quality of life, daytime sleepiness, mood, symptoms, neuropsychological measures, or blood pressure between the groups. A recent Cochrane review included eight studies with 323 participants and concluded positional therapy was less effective than CPAP for reducing AHI, but individuals may be more adherent to positional therapy compared with CPAP.[74] Positional therapy was shown to be better than inactive control for AHI and ESS. No conclusion could be drawn regarding the superiority of a specific in terms of treatment effectiveness.

There have been attempts to define a clinical phenotype of positional apnea, but because of limited data positional devices are currently not recommended as a primary therapy in any specific OSA subtypes. However, positional therapy can be an effective alternative or secondary treatment option for individuals with positional sleep apnea. As with other treatments this therapy should be guided by patient preferences, objective data, and clinical response.[75]

Expiratory Nasal Resistors

Expiratory nasal resistors (ENRs) or nasal expiratory positive airway pressure (EPAP) devices are disposable one-way resister valves that operate by creating positive end-expiratory pressure during a patient's normal breathing while causing minimal resistance during inspiration (Figure 134.3). ENRs primarily relieve mechanical loads on the upper airway. These resistors support airway patency not only through an increase in the end-expiratory airway size, but also by augmenting lung volumes and tracheal traction.[76,77]

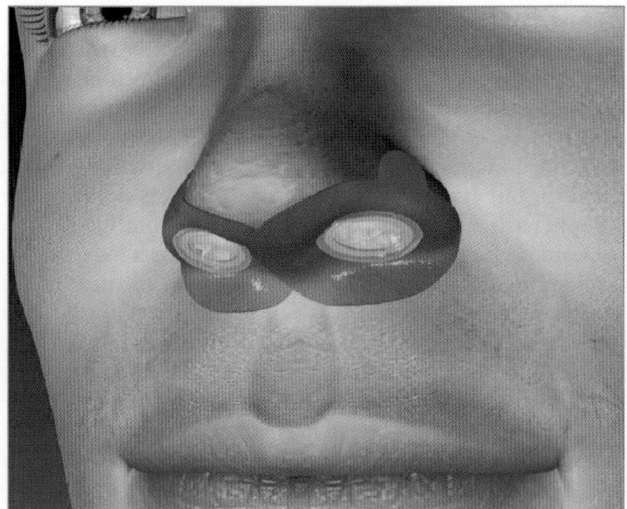

Figure 134.3 Expiratory nasal valve/nasal expiratory positive airway pressure. These devices consist of single-use valves inserted in the nostrils before sleep and are held in place by adhesive. The valve has minimal inspiratory resistance but creates significant resistance during exhalation leading to the development of back pressure supporting airway patency. (From Kryger MH, Berry RB, Massie CA. Long-term use of a nasal expiratory positive airway pressure [EPAP] device as a treatment for obstructive sleep apnea [OSA]. *J Clin Sleep Med.* 2011;7(5):449-53B.)

The largest ENR study to date was a prospective multicenter, parallel group, randomized, placebo-controlled, double-blind trial performed across 19 sites with 3-month follow-up.[78] PSG was performed on two separate nights (random order: device-off and device-on) at week 1 and after 3 months of treatment. The research team found the following: at 3 months, the percentage decrease in the AHI was 42.7% (ENR) and 10.1% (sham), $P < .0001$. A follow-up study on subjects who met adherence and efficacy criteria and were instructed to continue nightly use of ENR for 12 months was performed.[79] At 6 and 9 months, participants completed the ESS and daily diary for compliance, and at 12 months, they underwent PSG with EPAP treatment. Median AHI was reduced from 15.7 to 4.7 events per hour. There was also significant improvement in subjective daytime sleepiness and reported snoring after 12 months of treatment.

Although there is suggestion that ENRs may be effective therapy for some patients with OSA (mild disease or positional OSA), currently there no clear characteristics or patient phenotypes that predict a favorable response to these devices.[80] ENRs may be considered in individuals who have failed conventional treatments such as PAP therapy or a mandibular advancement device.

Nasopharyngeal Stents

Nasopharyngeal stents have been studied as a potential therapeutic modality for OSA. These devices are inserted through the nares and into the nasopharynx, preventing airway obstruction, and are typically used in the acute setting to maintain airway patency. No RCTs have been completed assessing the efficacy of these devices in OSA. Small uncontrolled studies have had conflicting results, with some studies demonstrating limited effectiveness and low tolerability of nasopharyngeal airway stenting devices, while other studies have shown a significant benefit in treating OSA, with a high level of patient acceptance. A systematic review of 16 small studies including 193 patients demonstrated the mean AHI decreased from 44.1 ± 18.9 to 22.7 ± 19.3 episodes per hour ($P < .00001$).[81] The mean lowest oxygen saturation, increased from 66.5% ± 14.2% to 75.5% ± 13.9% ($P < .00001$). Until controlled studies on nasopharyngeal stents are completed, they cannot be recommended in the management of OSA.

THERAPIES TARGETING NEUROVENTILATORY AND NEUROMUSCULAR MECHANISMS

Phrenic Nerve Stimulation

A recent technology used in the care of individuals with SDB is phrenic nerve stimulation. The current device consists of a neurostimulator that is placed in either the left or right pectoral region; a stimulation lead placed in either the left pericardiophrenic or right brachiocephalic vein to unilaterally stimulate the phrenic nerve; and a sensing lead that is placed in a thoracic vein, such as the azygos vein, to sense respiration by thoracic impedance (Figure 134.4).[82] The system aims to stimulate diaphragmatic contraction producing changes in CO_2 concentrations and tidal volumes similar to normal breathing. Fluctuations in CO_2 are important in the pathogenesis of OSA and CSA.[31] Currently, the primary role of this device is treatment of CSA that occurs when there is a recurrent transient reduction in the respiratory control center's generation of breathing rhythm.

FDA approval for this device was based on a multicenter trial in which 151 patients with moderate-to-severe CSA (AHI >20 events per hour, ≥50% central apneas) underwent device implantation and were randomly assigned to active stimulation or no stimulation for 6 months.[83] At 6 months, the stimulation group was more likely to achieve 50% or greater reduction in AHI from baseline (51% versus 11%). Secondary outcomes were also improved in the stimulation group compared with controls, including mean AHI, arousal index, oxygen desaturation index, as well as quality of life and daytime sleepiness. These improvements persisted at 12 months in a follow-up study.[84]

This device may be considered in selected patients with symptomatic CSA who fail or do not tolerate other therapies. However, cardiovascular outcomes and long-term safety data are not yet available. The majority of patients in the study cohort were men (89%) with a mean age of 65 years and more than half of these individuals had heart failure. This technology has also not been compared with other treatments of central apnea. Further work is required to define patients who would benefit from this device, and further assessment of long-term safety is necessary.

Pharmacotherapy

A number of mechanisms have been proposed by which drugs could mitigate SDB. Medication targets include an increase in ventilatory drive, an increase in tone of upper airway dilator muscles, a reduction in the proportion of rapid eye movement (REM) sleep, an increase in cholinergic tone

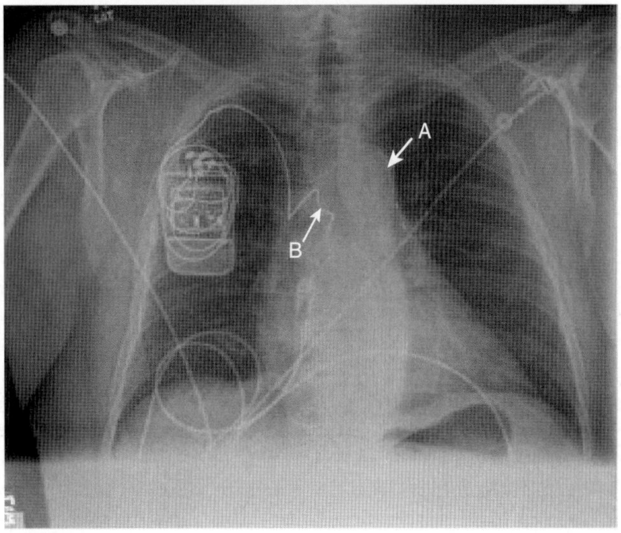

Figure 134.4 Chest imaging of implanted phrenic nerve stimulator. This image demonstrates the neurostimulator in the right pectoral region with the stimulation lead (A) in the left pericardiophrenic vein and the sensing lead (B) in the azygous vein. (From Abraham WT, Jagielski D, Oldenburg O, Augostini R, et al. Phrenic nerve stimulation for the treatment of central sleep apnea. *JACC Heart Fail.* 2015;3(5):360-369.)

during sleep, an increase in arousal threshold, a reduction in airway resistance, and a reduction in surface tension in the upper airway.

Historically, serotonergic mechanisms were considered as the main mechanism for loss of neuromuscular input during sleep. This hypothesis led to studies evaluating the effect of serotonergic agents such as mirtazapine, protriptyline and fluoxetine on OSA.[85-89] In general, studies evaluating medications targeting serotonergic mechanisms have had limited success in preclinical models and clinical trials. Research also suggests that serotonergic mechanisms are less important in the development of apnea in both animal models and in humans. At best, the data suggest these medications have a modest effect of OSA and are not currently recommended as primary therapy for OSA.

Interest in increasing cholinergic tone with medication has also been evaluated to treat SDB. Early work evaluated anesthetized, paralyzed, vagotomized, and artificially ventilated cats. These researchers examined the effects of changes in respiratory drive produced by activation of cholinergic and GABAergic (gamma-aminobutyric acid) receptors at the ventrolateral aspects of the medulla oblongata on phasic intrabreath discharge patterns of hypoglossal and phrenic nerves.[90] Application of cholinergic agents to the ventral medullary surface increased hypoglossal activity. This work led to small studies evaluating the effect of donepezil, a reversible inhibitor of acetylcholinesterase, on SDB. The first study enrolled 23 patients with mild-to-moderate Alzheimer disease and AHI greater than 5/hour.[91] Subjects were allocated into two groups: donepezil treated (n = 11) and placebo treated (n = 12). PSG and cognitive evaluation using Alzheimer disease assessment scale-cognitive (ADAS-cog) subscale were performed at baseline and after 3 months. In the group treated with donepezil AHI decreased from 20.0 to 9.9 events per hour while no significant change was noted in the placebo group. Lowest oxygen saturation and time spent with oxygen saturation less than 90% were also improved in the group treated with donepezil. Another small, placebo-controlled trial was conducted in 21 men with OSA but no Alzheimer disease.[92] Although this study also showed improvement in AHI, the results were less dramatic. Currently there are inadequate data to recommend donepezil as a primary or alternative treatment for SDB, but it may be an appropriate consideration for patients with Alzheimer disease and comorbid OSA.

Despite a large number of potential pharmacologic targets for OSA there is currently no FDA-approved medication for the treatment of obstructive sleep and there is insufficient evidence to recommend the use of medications in the treatment of OSA.[93,94] However, recent insights into pathways involved in the development of OSA and improved understanding of clinical, as well as physiologic phenotypes opens the possibility for the first effective pharmacotherapy of OSA.[95-97]

Taranto-Montemurro and colleagues investigated the efficacy of the combination of a noradrenergic (atomoxetine) and an antimuscarinic (oxybutynin) agent on OSA severity.[98] This randomized, placebo-controlled, double-blind crossover trial included 20 individuals with mild-to-moderate OSA. Participants underwent two overnight sleep studies performed approximately 1 week apart. Participants received either placebo (two pills) or 80 mg atomoxetine plus 5 mg oxybutynin 30 minutes before their study. The intervention led to a decreased AHI from 28.5 to 7.5 events/hour and was accompanied by an increase in the oxygen saturation nadir. Genioglossus muscle responsiveness was greater in the intervention group compared with those in the placebo group. These striking results are encouraging but more work is required to assess the safety profile, specific indications, and contraindications for the proposed combination in patients with OSA.

Given our improved understanding of the multifactorial nature of SDB, it is not surprising that research to date, which has not targeted specific phenotypes, has failed to identify a single pharmacologic agent that effectively treats sleep apnea. Future research selecting patients based on clinical and physiologic phenotype and likely using combination therapy may have more success in identifying pharmacologic interventions to address SDB.

Myofunctional Therapy/Training

Myofunctional therapy (MT) has been suggested as a treatment for OSA since the 1990s and entails exercises that target oropharyngeal structures that are crucial to the maintenance of pharyngeal patency.[99-101] An early study recruited 20 chronic snorers in the United Kingdom.[102] These subjects underwent a week of recording their snoring followed by a one-on-one session with a therapist who taught singing techniques, including appropriate use of the diaphragm, and specific singing exercises that involved activity in the soft palate. After this session the participants were provided with instructional handouts and asked to practice these exercises 20 minutes per day. After 3 months snoring recorded in the same way was found to be significantly reduced in duration.

Subsequent work in myofunctional training has been promising but reports to date have been small and highly selective. For instance, a meta-analysis from 2015 found only 9 adult studies (120 patients) that reported PSG, snoring, and/or sleepiness outcomes.[103] These data suggest myofunctional therapy may have promise in treating adults with OSA. Analysis demonstrated a significant decrease in AHI from a mean of 24.5 to 12.3 events per hour with improvement in oxygenation saturation, as well as improvement in other subjective outcomes. This same analysis also demonstrated statistically significant improvement in AHI for the pediatric population, and work by Villa and colleagues demonstrated myofunctional therapy could be successfully applied to children with OSA who had residual symptoms after adenotonsillectomy.[104] Although preliminary work has been encouraging, currently there are inadequate data to recommend myofunctional therapy as a primary treatment for OSA.[105]

Supplemental Oxygen

Early work using supplemental oxygen to address hypoxemia associated with SDB demonstrated worsening of hypercapnia with respiratory acidosis, longer apneic spells, and no improvement in symptoms.[106-109] Currently oxygen therapy alone is not recommended as a primary treatment for SDB; however, research has identified specific subgroups who may respond robustly to supplemental oxygen.

Wellman and colleagues evaluated the effect of oxygen on the AHI in six individuals with OSA with a relatively high loop gain and six with a low loop gain.[110] Loop gain was determined by a validated proportional assist ventilation model. In the high loop gain group, AHI decreased from 63 ± 34 episodes/hour to 34 ± 30 episodes/hour (P = .03) while there was no significant change in AHI on oxygen (44 ± 34 episodes/hour on air, 37 ± 28 episodes/hour on oxygen, P = .44). In the high loop gain group supplemental oxygen was found to stabilize ventilation (lower loop gain).

A subsequent study used PSG to identify elevated loop gain and assessed the predictive value of elevated loop gain in combination with other physiologic traits (post hoc analysis) in terms of response to oxygen. These traits (collapsibility, compensation and arousability) were quantified using a recently developed automated technique for estimating the four key traits through analysis of routine clinical sleep studies (PSG).[111] Elevated loop gain was not a significant univariate predictor of responder/nonresponder status (primary analysis). In post hoc analysis, a logistic regression model based on elevated loop gain had better collapsibility and compensation had 83% accuracy in predicting responders to supplemental oxygen. Responders exhibited an improvement in OSA severity (ΔAHI 59% ± 6% versus 12% ± 7% in predicted nonresponders, P = .0001) plus lowered morning blood pressure and "better" self-reported sleep. This study illustrates the potential implications of physiologic phenotyping and how clinicians may identify patients whose condition is treatable using supplemental oxygen, as well as identifying those individuals who should consider other therapies.

The addition of supplemental oxygen to PAP therapy should also be considered in patients whose respiratory events are well controlled with treatment but continue to have hypoxemia. During titration studies supplemental oxygen may be added during PAP titration when the oxygen saturation persists at 88% or less for 5 minutes or more in the absence of obstructive respiratory events.[112] Persistent hypoxemia may occur in patients with cardiopulmonary comorbidities, severe obesity and in individuals currently using daytime supplemental oxygen. Optimally, supplemental O_2 should be entrained to the PAP device through the tubing outlet using a T-connector rather than directly into the mask.[113]

SUMMARY

Improvements in physiologic and clinical phenotyping for SDB have primed the sleep medicine field to enter an era of personalized care. Research into simpler techniques to identify these phenotypes that are scalable to clinical care is required but will likely change the landscape of SDB diagnosis and management in the near future. Moving forward, therapy decisions for SDB will be based on clinical presentations, susceptibility to future health risks related to SDB, underlying pathophysiology, and health outcomes (Figure 134.5).[114] PAP alternatives discussed in this chapter and elsewhere may well play a larger role in the management of sleep breathing disorders as we enter an era of precision medicine.

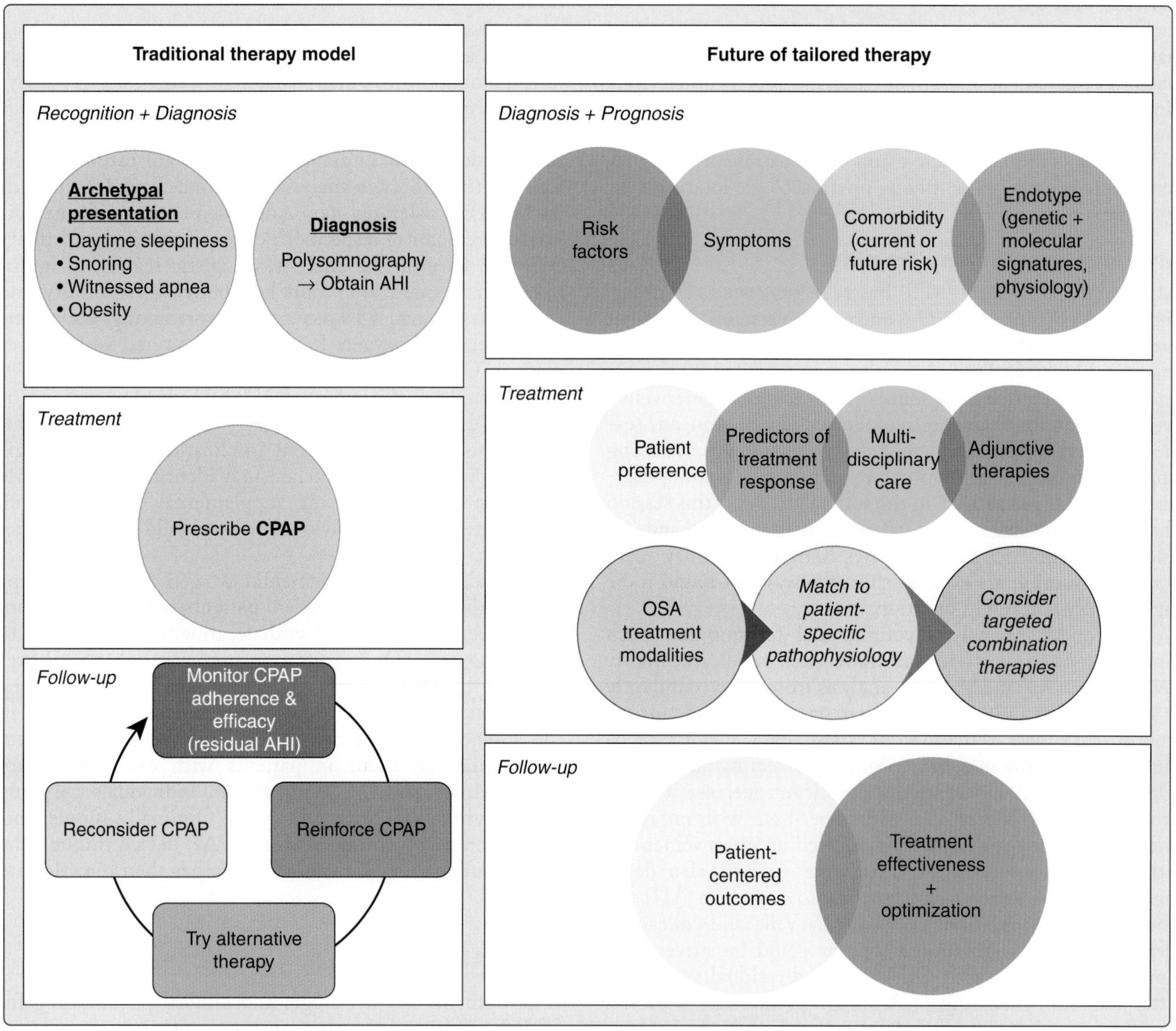

Figure 134.5 Classic therapy model of CPAP for all versus personalized (tailored) therapy for the management of sleep-disordered breathing as the sleep medicine field moves into an era of precision medicine practitioners will evaluate multiple areas of data in the evaluation and management of sleep-disordered breathing to tailor therapy while following important patient centered outcomes. (From Sutherland K, Kairaitis K, Yee BJ, Cistulli PA. From CPAP to tailored therapy for obstructive sleep apnoea. *Multidiscip Respir Med.* 2018;13:44.)

CLINICAL PEARLS

DISE involves evaluation of the pattern of airway closure during flexible laryngoscopy while a patient is given sedation monitored by an anesthesiologist. This procedure has been demonstrated to be helpful in determining candidacy for HNS treatment of OSA. DISE may have other roles in evaluation and treatment of sleep apnea. DISE may aid in the identification of airway obstruction when the awake examination is not consistent with sleep testing (i.e., no apparent airway obstruction but severe sleep apnea). DISE may also help predict surgical treatment success of certain airway procedures.

In the assessment of a patient's appropriateness for bariatric surgery, many preoperative clinics include a specific OSA screening questionnaire such as the STOP-BANG that incorporates an assessment of **s**noring, **t**iredness/fatigue, **o**bserved apnea, self-reported high blood **p**ressure, **b**ody mass index, **a**ge, **n**eck circumference, and **g**ender/sex. Those identified as high risk of having OSA are then typically referred for confirmatory tests, such as PSG or home sleep apnea test (HSAT). If significant SDB is identified, surgery may be delayed until therapy for the patient's OSA is optimized. Although many patients will have resolution of their OSA after bariatric surgery, OSA may persist in some patients and postoperative follow-up with objective sleep testing (PSG or HSAT) is indicated to ensure adequate improvement of OSA.

SELECTED READINGS

Aishah A, Lim R, Sands SA, et al. Different antimuscarinics when combined with atomoxetine have differential effects on obstructive sleep apnea severity. *J Appl Physiol (1985)*. 2021;130(5):1373–1382.

Berry RB, Kryger MH, Massie CA. A novel nasal Expiratory Positive Airway Pressure (EPAP) device for the treatment of obstructive sleep apnea: a randomized controlled trial. *Sleep*. 2011;34(4):479–485.

Colquitt JL, Pickett K, Loveman E, Frampton GK. Surgery for weight loss in adults. *Cochrane Database Syst Rev*. 2014.

Costanzo MR1, Ponikowski P2, Javaheri S3, Augostini R4, Goldberg LR5, Holcomb R6, Kao A7, Khayat RN4, Oldenburg O8, stellbrink C9, Abraham WT4; remedē system pivotal trial study group. *Am J Cardiol*. 2018;121(11):1400–1408.

De Felício CM, Da Silva Dias FV, Voi Trawitzki LV. Obstructive sleep apnea: focus on myofunctional therapy. *Nat Sci Sleep*. 2018;10:271–286.

De Vito A, Carrasco Llatas M, Vanni A, Bosi M, Braghiroli A, Campanini A, de Vries N, Hamans E, Hohenhorst W, Kotecha BT, Maurer J, Montevecchi F, Piccin O, Sorrenti G, Vanderveken OM, Vicini C. European position paper on Drug-Induced Sedation Endoscopy (DISE). *Sleep Breath*. 2014;18(3):453–456.

Eckert DJ. Phenotypic approaches to obstructive sleep apnoea - New pathways for targeted therapy. *Sleep Med Rev*. 2018;37:45–59.

Edwards BA, Redline S, Sands SA, Owens RL. More than the sum of the respiratory events: personalized medicine approaches for obstructive sleep apnea. *Am J Respir Crit Care Med*. 2019;200(6):691–703.

Foster GD, Borradaile KE, Sanders MH, Millman R, Zammit G, Newman AB, et al. Sleep AHEAD research group of look AHEAD research group. a randomized study on the effect of weight loss on obstructive sleep apnea among obese patients with type 2 diabetes: the sleep AHEAD study. *Arch Intern Med*. 2009;169:1619–1626.

Gaisl T, Haile SR, Thiel S, Osswald M, Kohler M. Efficacy of pharmacotherapy for OSA in adults: a systematic review and network meta-analysis. *Sleep Med Rev*. 2019;46:74–86.

Mazzotti DR, Keenan BT, Lim DC, Gottlieb DJ, Kim J, Pack AI. Symptom subtypes of obstructive sleep apnea predict incidence of cardiovascular outcomes. *Am J Respir Crit Care Med*. 2019;200:493–506.

Sands SA, Edwards BA, Terrill PI, et al. Identifying obstructive sleep apnoea patients responsive to supplemental oxygen therapy. *Eur Respir J*. 2018;52(3):1800674. Published 2018 Sep 27.

Srijithesh PR, Aghoram R, Goel A, Dhanya J. Positional therapy for obstructive sleep apnoea. *Cochrane Database Syst Rev*. 2019;5:CD010990.

Strollo PJ, Soose RJ, Maurer JT, et al. Upper-airway stimulation for obstructive sleep apnea. *N Engl J Med*. 2014;370:139–149.

Taranto-Montemurro L, Messineo L, Azarbarzin A, et al. Effects of the combination of atomoxetine and oxybutynin on OSA endotypic traits. *Chest*. 2020;157(6):1626–1636.

Taranto-Montemurro L, Messineo L, Sands SA, Azarbarzin A, Marques M, Edwards BA, Eckert DJ, White DP, Wellman A. The combination of atomoxetine and oxybutynin greatly reduces obstructive sleep apnea severity. a randomized, placebo-controlled, double-blind crossover trial. *Am J Respir Crit Care Med*. 2019;199(10):1267–1276.

Taranto-Montemurro L, Messineo L, Wellman A. Targeting endotypic traits with medications for the pharmacological treatment of obstructive sleep apnea. A review of the current literature. *J Clin Med*. 2019;8(11):1846.

Ye L, Pien GW, Ratcliffe SJ, Björnsdottir E, Arnardottir ES, Pack AI, Benediktsdottir B, Gislason T. The different clinical faces of obstructive sleep apnoea: a cluster analysis. *Eur Respir Jour*. 2014;44(6):1600–1607.

A complete reference list can be found online at ExpertConsult.com.

Chapter 135

Brain Health in Sleep Apnea: Cognition, Performance, Mechanisms, and Treatment

Michael W. Calik; Mary J. Morrell; Terri E. Weaver

Chapter Highlights

- Impact: Some patients with obstructive sleep apnea (OSA) demonstrate cognitive, emotional, and performance deficits.
- OSA is increasingly recognized as one of the potentially modifiable risk factors for mild cognitive impairment and dementia; its multiple effects on the central nervous system are acknowledged, albeit their nature and prognosis are yet to be fully understood.
- Mechanisms: During nocturnal apnea-hypopnea episodes and sleep fragmentation, both maladaptive and adaptive pathways are likely to be initiated in the brain of OSA patients; the net result will depend on the chronicity of process and characteristics of each patient.
- Treatment: OSA treatment with continuous positive airway pressure (CPAP) results in consistent improvement in cognition and performance, although the magnitude of improvement is variable.
- Some patients experience residual sleepiness using optimal nightly duration of CPAP, which may be related to white matter compromise.
- The role of CPAP and its long-term effectiveness for cognitive and performance deficits needs further study.

Obstructive sleep apnea (OSA) is one of the potentially modifiable risk factors for mild cognitive impairment and dementia,[1–6] and it is commonly associated with serious cardiovascular and metabolic comorbidities.[7–9] Nocturnal episodes of complete or partial pharyngeal obstruction in patients with OSA result in intermittent hypoxia, hypercapnia, and sleep fragmentation, followed by reoxygenation.[10,11] An increase in respiratory effort, in association with hypoxemia or hypercapnia, triggers the frequent sleep arousals that usually terminate the apneic episodes but also contribute to abnormal sleep architecture and lighter and less restorative sleep.[12] Progressive changes in sleep quality and structure, changes in cerebral blood flow, neurovascular and neurotransmitter changes, and the cellular redox status in OSA patients all may constitute contributing factors to cognitive decline.[10,13–15]

Increased road traffic accidents, reduced quality of life, excessive daytime sleepiness, labile interpersonal relationships, and decreased work and school efficiency have all been documented in OSA patients.[15–17] These impairments and deficits are not always reversed with treatment.[16–18] Beneficial effects of treatment on cognitive performance, sleepiness, and neural injury in OSA (Figure 135.1) are documented in a meta-analyses[19,20] and a meta-review.[21] Three studies also suggest beneficial effects of continuous positive airway pressure (CPAP) therapy in minimally symptomatic and older OSA patients, respectively.[22–24] In a study of a well-characterized longitudinal cohort (the Alzheimer's Disease Neuroimaging Initiative cohort), the self-reported presence of untreated sleep-disordered breathing, including OSA and "sleep apnea," was associated with an earlier age at cognitive decline, up to a decade.[4] This association was found to be significant even when accounting for possible confounding factors, such as sex, apolipoprotein ε4 status, diabetes mellitus, depression, body mass index, cardiovascular disease, hypertension, age at baseline, and education of participants. Moreover, this link appeared significantly attenuated in patients who used CPAP, suggesting that use of CPAP may delay progression, or onset, of cognitive impairment.[4] However, the effect of CPAP on delay in age of Alzheimer disease dementia onset was not demonstrated in this study.[4]

The current dearth of fully effective treatments for the central nervous system (CNS) sequelae of OSA is likely to be a reflection of an as yet poorly understood intricate interplay of both adaptive and maladaptive processes with the hypoxemia, reoxygenation, hypercapnia or hypocapnia, and sleep fragmentation that occur in the CNS of OSA patients.[15,25] The overall net result of ongoing neuroinflammatory processes and ischemic preconditioning for each particular patient depends on the stage of this OSA-induced dynamic process, effects on other body systems, cognitive reserve, and idiosyncratic susceptibility.[13,15,26,27] Thus different therapeutic approaches might benefit different stages and conversely might aggravate

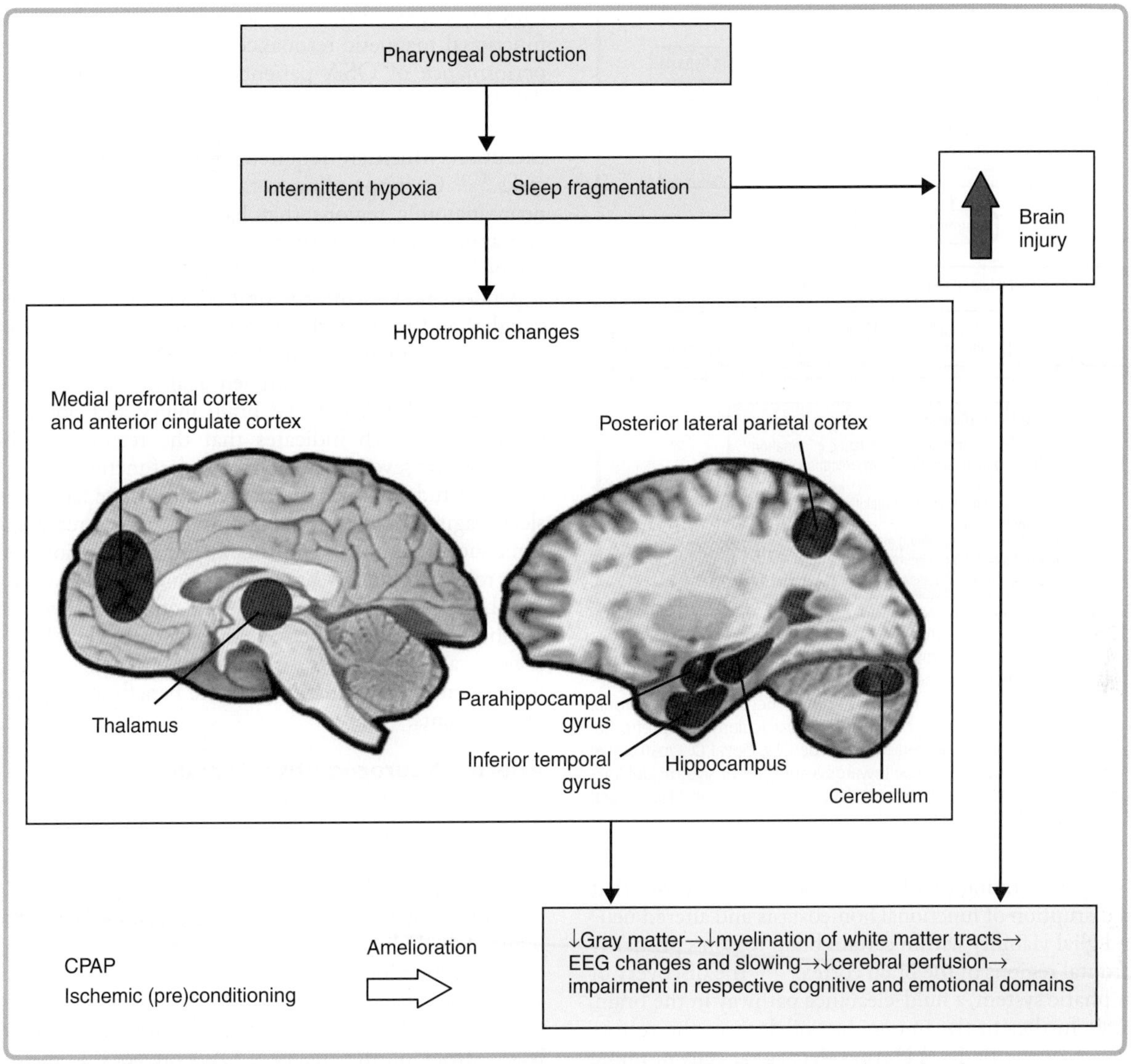

Figure 135.1 Brain regions and mechanisms involved in sleep apnea injury. The nocturnal episodes of complete or partial pharyngeal obstruction result in intermittent hypoxia and sleep fragmentation. Both intermittent hypoxia and sleep fragmentation can aggravate brain injury (*red arrow*) and cause hypotrophic changes in several brain regions shown.[164] Ensuing neurophysiologic and neurochemical changes can also manifest in cognitive and emotional deficits that can be ameliorated (*white arrow*) with continuous positive airway pressure therapy (CPAP) and/or ischemic preconditioning. EEG, Electroencephalography. (From Rosenzweig I, Glasser M, Polsek D, et al. Sleep apnoea and the brain: a complex relationship. *Lancet Respir Med.* 2015;3:404–14.)

damage in some patients.[13,15,26] This chapter addresses recent findings regarding the impact of OSA on cognition and performance, describing possible mechanisms and the impact of treatment.

NEUROPATHOLOGY OF OBSTRUCTIVE SLEEP APNEA

Changes in cerebral blood flow that occur during obstructive apneas[28] and apnea-induced hypoxemia, combined with reduced cerebral perfusion, likely predispose patients to nocturnal cerebral ischemia.[29,30] In addition, an altered resting cerebral blood flow pattern in several CNS regions has been shown in OSA, along with hypoperfusion during the awake states.[31] Numerous clinical studies have demonstrated changes in the electroencephalogram of OSA patients compared with healthy individuals, including aberrant cortical excitability[32–34] and an associated array of neurocognitive deficits, including sustained attention, memory, vigilance, psychomotor execution, and executive function.[5,12,35,36] Taken collectively, such studies have delineated a putative neurocircuitry "fingerprint" of OSA-induced brain injury and have suggested a disconnection of the frontal regions (Figure 135.2) and a disruption of the (cerebellar)-thalamocortical oscillator, with involvement of the hippocampal formation.[11,12] It has been previously suggested that the constellation of symptoms frequently encountered in OSA patients, such as depression, disturbances in attention, dysmetria of thought and affect, and executive and verbal memory deficits,[37–39] point to similarities with two other recognized neurologic clinical syndromes—frontal lobe syndrome and the cerebellar cognitive affective syndrome.[12,40]

The prefrontal model suggests that the sleep disruption, intermittent hypoxemia, and hypercapnia experienced by OSA patients alter the normal restorative process that occurs

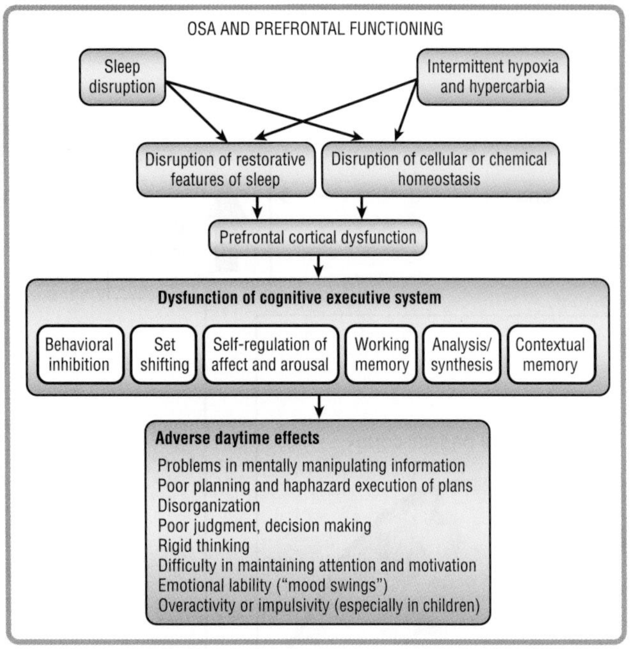

Figure 135.2 The proposed prefrontal model. In this model, obstructive sleep apnea (OSA)-related sleep disruption and intermittent hypoxemia and hypercarbia alter the efficacy of the glymphatic system to clear harmful metabolites during sleep and disrupt the functional homeostasis and neuronal and glial viability within particular brain regions, particularly the prefrontal regions of the brain cortex. (Modified from Beebe DW, Gozal D. Obstructive sleep apnea and the prefrontal cortex: towards a comprehensive model linking nocturnal upper airway obstruction to daytime cognitive and behavioral deficits. *J Sleep Res.* 2002;11:1–16.)

during sleep, generating cellular and biochemical stresses that result in disruption of functional homeostasis and altered neuronal and glial viability within certain brain regions, primarily the prefrontal regions of the brain cortex.[41,42] The discovery of the glymphatic system, a fluid-clearance pathway in the brain, contributes further to the importance of sleep to the restorative process of the brain.[43] During sleep, glial cells promote the flow of cerebrospinal fluid (CSF) in between interstitial space, thus clearing away harmful metabolites, such as beta-amyloid. In OSA patients, clearance of these metabolites has been shown to be decreased, suggesting impaired clearance of these metabolites from the interstitial space.[44] This model has been proposed as a theoretical framework for the relationship between sleep fragmentation and nocturnal hypoxemia and predominantly frontal deficits (Figure 135.2).[42] OSA-induced neuropathologic alterations can lead to destabilization of the executive system, causing behavioral disturbance in inhibition, maintenance of performance, self-regulation of affect and arousal, working memory, analysis and synthesis, and contextual memory.[41,42] Alterations in the executive system can adversely affect cognitive abilities, resulting in maladaptive types of behavior as depicted in Figure 135.2.[41,42] Nonetheless, unlike some other neurologic disorders, the impairments associated with OSA are more likely to produce inefficient performance rather than inability to perform.[42] For example, when memory- or divided attention–related neuronal circuitry is incapacitated, other CNS systems and circuitries may be recruited in an effort to compensate.[41,42] However, if such systems are themselves affected by sleep fragmentation or hypoxemia, their compensatory contributions might be suboptimal. This may account for the increased activation of the prefrontal cortex under conditions of sleep deprivation documented by functional magnetic resonance imaging.[41,42] Impairments in performance of OSA patients can be further explained by deficits in elementary cognitive functions, specifically, sensory transduction, feature integration, and motor preparation and execution, which are required, even in simple response-time tasks.[42,45] Corresponding to the deficits in OSA patients, the neuroanatomic regions that have been reported in clinical and animal studies as affected in OSA suggest that both the cerebellar modulation of neural circuits and the normal state-dependent flow of information between thalamus (and basal ganglia) and frontoparietal cortex are likely to be affected in susceptible patients (Figure 135.1).[12,25,46–52]

Some clinicians have argued against such a reductionist approach to OSA-induced brain injury and point out that emerging research indicates that the relationship between OSA disease severity and cognitive dysfunction is the product of a multitude of susceptibility and protective factors and that sleep fragmentation, hypoxemia, and cognitive reserve are only three such aspects.[11,12,20] Other factors are duration of the disease, role of the blood-brain barrier, presence of hypertension, metabolic dysfunction, systemic inflammation, levels of cerebral blood flow, and genetic vulnerability.[20,53] Further research is necessary to provide a clear understanding of the risk for neurocognitive dysfunction and the benefit and optimization of treatments.

Affected Neurocognitive Domains

Despite contradictory results and ongoing polemics in the field, most studies to date agree that patients with OSA can have deficits in attention and vigilance, long-term visual and verbal memory, visuospatial and constructional abilities, and executive function.[15,21,37] Several associations have been recognized, including the association between worsening global cognitive functioning and the severity of hypoxemia, as well as the association between attention and vigilance dysfunction and the degree of sleep fragmentation.[15,21,53] Consensus is less strong on the effects of OSA on working memory and short-term memory.[21] In some studies, language ability and psychomotor functioning have been shown to be largely unaffected by OSA,[21] whereas others have pointed to psychomotor slowing as the most vulnerable cognitive domains and also the least responsive to treatment with CPAP.[54] Similarly, several studies showing impairments in language abilities in patients with severe OSA have not shown agreement on whether phonemic or semantic domains have the greatest effect.[55] Neurodevelopmental stages of adolescents and children with OSA appear to dictate a higher risk for this deficit.[56] A recent meta-analysis of 19 studies investigated the cognitive functioning of OSA patients before they received any treatment and revealed significant negative effect sizes in the cognitive domains of nonverbal memory, concept formation, psychomotor speed, construction, executive functioning, perception, motor control and performance, attention, speed of processing, working and verbal memory, verbal functioning and verbal reasoning, thus corroborating the mounting evidence that neuropsychological functions are impaired in OSA.[57]

In children with OSA the results of studies assessing cognitive performance and effects of treatment are similarly divergent.[58,59] In a recent study of children 7 to 12 years of age with sleep-disordered breathing (SDB), who were followed for 4 years, treatment of the SDB led to improvements in several aspects of neurocognition, collectively categorized as performance intelligence quotient (IQ).[58] Performance IQ represents fluid intelligence that is reflective of incidental learning, and it describes one's ability to adapt to new situations.[60] In this study, improvements were recorded in tasks associated with spatial visualization, visuomotor coordination, abstract thought, and nonverbal fluid reasoning.[58] However, overall improvements in academic ability or behavior were less clear. Furthermore, tendency to worsening of verbal IQ, which, unlike performance IQ, is more likely to be affected by formal education and learning experiences, was noted in a treated group.[58] A definitive explanation for this finding was not provided, and no statistically significant association between the reduction in verbal IQ performance and treatment was demonstrated.[58] Conversely, in another influential study, younger children with SDB followed for 12 months of treatment showed significant improvements in academic performance.[59] The different neurodevelopmental ages of children and different test parameters used provide a complex clinical data set against which no finite conclusions can be drawn. Nonetheless, patterns and associations seem to be emerging from this and earlier work, among which the association between performance IQ and slow wave activity (SWA) during non–rapid eye movement (NREM) sleep is perhaps the strongest one.[58,61]

It has been argued that cognitive improvements in treated OSA may reflect increased stability of brain activity during sleep, allowing crucial synaptic repair and maintenance to occur and counteracting toxic effects of arousal and hypoxic effects of OSA.[58,62] This argument is concordant with findings showing that the neurochemical and gene environments of sleep and sleep activity patterns present crucial window periods during which the brain can restore cellular homeostasis, increase signal-to-noise ratio, and reinforce neuronal circuitry for subsequent cognitive processing demands.[14,63,64]

PROPOSED MECHANISTIC ROLE FOR PERTURBED SLEEP IN PATIENTS WITH OBSTRUCTIVE SLEEP APNEA

Sleep and sleep deprivation alter molecular signaling pathways that regulate synaptic strength, plasticity-related gene expression, and protein translation in a bidirectional manner.[64] Moreover, sleep deprivation can impair neuronal excitability, decrease myelination, lead to cellular oxidative stress, misfolding of cellular proteins, and impair the glymphatic clearance of brain macromolecules.[64–66] Frequent brief awakenings lead to fragmented sleep that negatively affects the next day's cognitive and emotional functioning, in a manner similar to that of total sleep deprivation.[2]

Several studies have attempted to assess whether OSA patients are more vulnerable to sleep loss–induced performance deficits, with special emphasis on driving performance variables, with varied results.[67–70] From the practical point of view, it is of major interest to develop reliable and practical bedside tests to help clinicians advise patients on their individual risk for traffic accidents.[15,53] Animal studies suggest that sleep fragmentation independently affects similar brain regions to those affected by intermittent hypoxia, as occurs in OSA.[10] Also, clinical studies of the effects of sleep deprivation on cognition in the general population suggest comparable cognitive impairments to those seen in OSA.[71]

Frequent partial arousals during sleep in OSA patients contribute to abnormal sleep architecture and symptoms of excessive daytime somnolence (i.e., sleepiness).[10,11,72] An independent association between excessive daytime somnolence and cognitive impairment has been demonstrated, and several prospective studies have shown that excessive daytime somnolence is associated with an increased risk for cognitive decline and dementia.[1] Further, in a prospective cohort study of Japanese American men in the Honolulu-Asia Aging Study, lower nocturnal oxygenation and reduction in stage 3 (slow wave) NREM sleep were associated with the development of microinfarcts and brain atrophy.[73] Conversely, men with longer slow wave sleep time showed slower cognitive decline.[73]

The relationship between OSA and its effect on selected sleep stages merits particular attention, given that each of the sleep stages, with its attendant alterations in neurophysiology, is associated with facilitation of important functional learning and memory processes[14] (also see Chapter 29). In OSA patients the proportion of stage 2 NREM sleep (N2) has been shown to be increased, whereas proportions of stages 1 and 3 NREM sleep (N1, N3) and rapid eye movement (REM) sleep are decreased.[55] Limited experimental studies conducted to date have shown specific impairments of sleep-dependent consolidation of verbal declarative information in patients with OSA.[74] Furthermore, several clinical studies suggest disturbed spatiotemporal evolution of sleep spindles in patients with OSA during the night.[75,76]

However, dynamic analysis of sleep architecture is required to fully gauge the neurophysiologic effect of sleep fragmentation on sleep in OSA patients.[15] For example, in one study of mild OSA the exponential decay function of SWA was demonstrated to be significantly slower in OSA patients compared with control subjects.[77] This was due to the more even distribution of SWA throughout the night, without significant decrease in total slow wave and REM sleep time. These results show that mild sleep fragmentation can alter the dynamics of SWA, without significantly decreasing the amounts of slow wave and REM sleep and emphasizing the need to perform SWA decay analysis in sleep fragmentation disorders.[77] In the same study a decrease in spindle activity was observed in N2 and N3 sleep that was not attributed to an increase of SWA.[75,77] Such a reduction in total spindle density has also been reported in sleep maintenance insomnia and is likely to be related to sleep fragmentation.[75–77]

The model proposed by Landmann and colleagues[78] suggests an integrative framework for the qualitative reorganization of memory during sleep. It further builds on studies that have shown that sleep facilitates the abstraction of rules and the integration of knowledge into existing schemas during slow wave sleep.[63,64,78] REM sleep, on the other hand, has been shown to benefit creativity, which requires the disintegration of existing patterns.[78] Both respective sleep stages have been commonly reported as reduced or fragmented in patients with OSA, and their dysregulation could underlie some of the frequently reported cognitive and performance deficits in OSA patients.[33,55] In line with this argument, one study that investigated the neurocognitive deficits in OSA found that the number of microarousals during the night was the best predictor of episodic memory deficit.[79] Traditionally, obstructive events during NREM sleep have been viewed as associated with greater cognitive deficits or impaired quality of life, whereas REM sleep events have been shown to be associated with greater sympathetic activity, arterial hypertension, and cardiovascular instability in patients with OSA.[80,81]

The role for fragmented REM sleep in spatial navigational memory in OSA patients has been addressed with a physiologically relevant stimulus.[82] During this study, patients spent two different nights in the laboratory, during which they performed timed trials, before and after sleep, on one of two unique three-dimensional spatial mazes.[82] Normal consolidation of sleep was achieved with use of therapeutic CPAP throughout the first night, whereas, during the second night, CPAP was reduced only during the REM stages. Patients showed improvements in maze performance after a night of normal sleep, but those improvements were significantly reduced after a night of isolated REM disruption, without changes in psychomotor vigilance. Noted cognitive improvements were positively correlated with the mean REM run duration across both sleep conditions.[82]

It has been argued that the sense of excessive daytime sleepiness and of feeling unrefreshed in the morning in some OSA patients could be due to the inability to augment NREM SWA or REM sleep. Moreover, in some OSA patients, reduction of REM sleep can lead to dissociation of REM traits with other sleep stages, further affecting critical sleep windows for memory formation and consolidation.[14] Equally, it has been shown that when high homeostatic demands are not fully met during sleep, in the subsequent wake period microsleeps can occur in highly active regions of the brain[83] and can lead to concomitant disability for the function subserved by that region.[63,83] To what extent this takes place in OSA patients and whether this also contributes to attention-vigilance dysfunction and the higher frequency of traffic accidents noted for this patient group are yet to be fully defined.[15] Previously reported retarded SWA decay throughout the night, even in patients with mild OSA, further supports the notion of nonrestorative sleep in OSA.[77]

Several studies have aimed to discern the role of sleep in cognition and cognitive decline, with potential effect on the way we consider sleep in patients with OSA. For example, as depicted in Figure 135.3, *A*, it has been suggested that the amount of atrophy in the medial prefrontal cortex (mPFC), predicts the extent of disrupted slow wave (N3) sleep in older people and consequent impaired overnight episodic hippocampal memory consolidation.[64,84] The mPFC area has been shown to be independently affected by OSA (Figure 135.1) and has been known to be involved in the generation of slow waves.[15,84] It has been proposed that improving slow wave sleep in older adults (irrespective of their OSA status) may represent a novel treatment for minimizing cognitive decline in later life.[84]

The importance of sleep spindles in cognition has also gained interest over the past several years.[15,85] It has been shown that, during the night, OSA patients, unlike healthy control subjects, display a significant proportion of slow spindles in the frontal, central, and parietal regions.[75] One recent study has shown that older adults who express fewer prefrontal fast sleep spindles also exhibit a proportional impairment in hippocampal functioning during the subsequent wake periods and, with that impairment, a deficit in the ability to form new episodic memories.[86] Fast sleep spindles represent part of a coordinated NREM sleep–dependent memory mechanism, and it is thought that hippocampal sharp-wave ripples provide feedback excitation, which initiates neuroplasticity in spindle-activated cortical neurons.[64] Relative to slow sleep spindles, fast sleep spindle activity is associated with greater hippocampal activation and greater hippocampal-cortical functional connectivity.[2,86] The sleep architecture of even mild OSA patients shows a high degree of sleep fragmentation, which results in a different time course of SWA and a decreased sleep spindle index compared with control subjects.[77] Whether this deregulated spindle formation and activity present another contributory facet to cognitive complaints in patients in OSA, however, remains a conjecture at this point (Figure 135.3, *A*).[1–3,39,84]

Mental Health and Sleep Associations in Obstructive Sleep Apnea Patients

A bidirectional relationship between sleep and the function of the brain circuitry involved in emotions is increasingly supported by studies that further build on long-standing clinical observations of co-occurring mood and sleep disorders.[15,87] Not surprising then, a variety of mental health issues, such as affective disorders, emotional lability, anxiety, and depression, have been reported as highly prevalent in individuals with OSA,[88] with a systematic meta-analysis reporting that 35% and 32% of OSA individuals are affected with depression or anxiety,[89] respectively, despite considerable heterogeneity and a high risk for bias in these studies.[15] Evidence from various studies is particularly suggestive of a role for REM sleep in selective emotional memory processing and sleep-dependent emotional memory depotentiation (Figure 135.3, *B*).[87] Moreover, REM sleep is suggested to play a role in recalibrating the sensitivity and specificity of the brain's response to emotional events, both positive and negative.[87] This recalibration effect likely occurs, at least in part as a result of modulation of noradrenergic brainstem activity and the responsive profiles of the amygdala and mPFC, two regions critically involved in detecting emotional salience.[15,87]

Of the psychiatric disorders, the evidence for increased prevalence of OSA is particularly strong in major depressive disorder and posttraumatic stress disorder (PTSD),[89–91] both independently associated with REM sleep disturbance.[15] Specifically, PTSD is independently associated with decreases in the total time spent in REM sleep. It is also associated with marked fragmentation of REM sleep, indicative of arousal-related awakenings from REM sleep linked to adrenergic surges.[87] CPAP adherence has been shown to be reduced in veterans with PTSD and comorbid OSA.[90] Based on the current knowledge of OSA-induced sleep deficits, it can be argued that in PTSD patients with comorbid OSA, the additive effect of sleep disturbances associated with the OSA can further impair the quantity and quality of REM sleep. This would likely also affect the REM noradrenergic "housekeeping" function because it has been shown that REM sleep reduces, and thus likely restores, concentrations of CNS noradrenaline to baseline, allowing for optimal awake-state functioning.[15,87]

More specifically, several studies suggest that quiescence of locus coeruleus activity, a brainstem structure that is a source of noradrenergic input during REM sleep throughout the night, restores the appropriate next-day tonic-phasic response specificity within the emotional salience network (e.g., locus coeruleus, amygdala, mPFC).[87] It is hence feasible that OSA-induced REM fragmentation could further

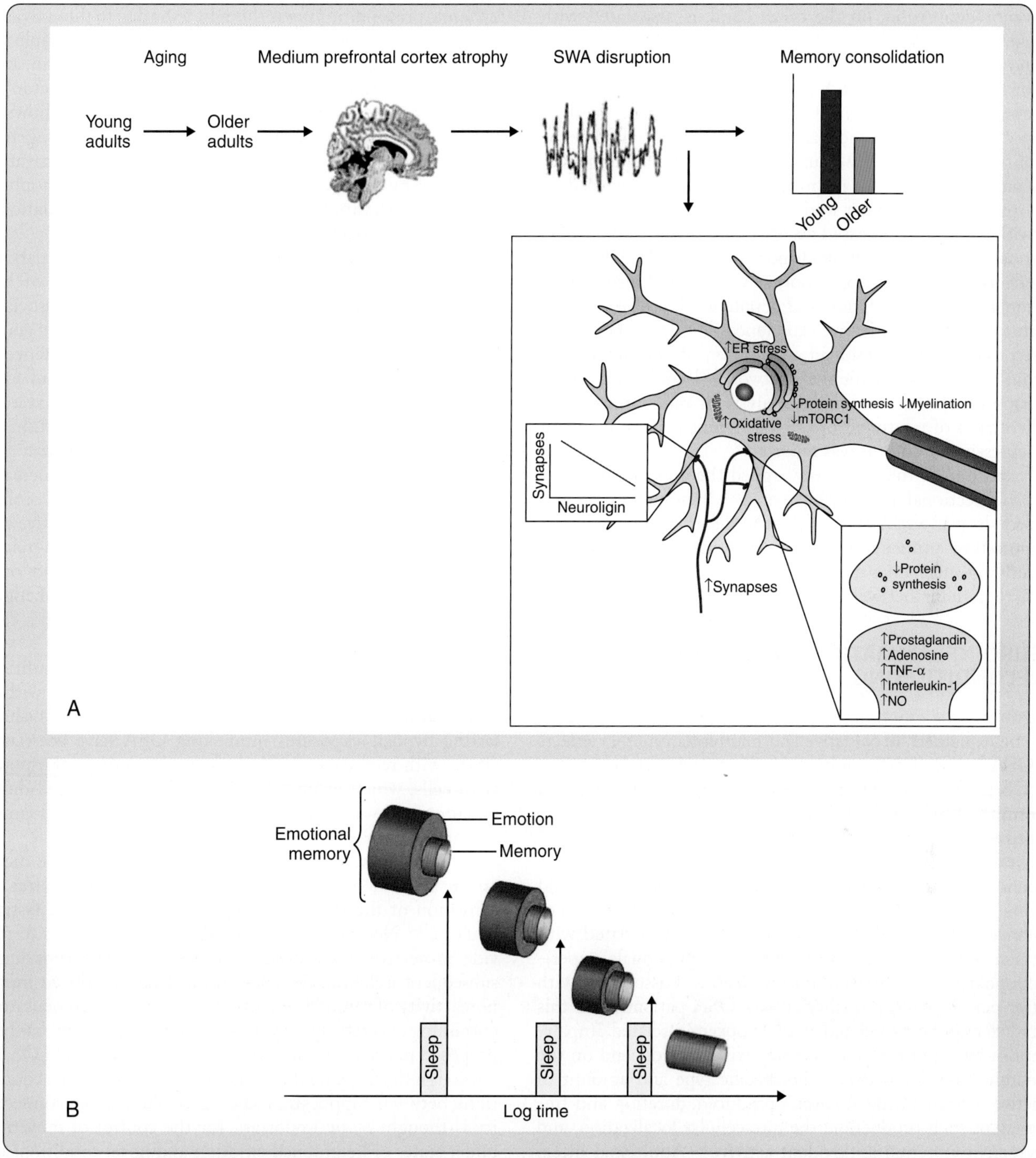

Figure 135.3 The proposed role for sleep in cognition and emotions. **A,** *Cognitive sleep:* Sleep apnea and aging can independently cause gray matter atrophy in the prefrontal cortex. Atrophy can mediate the degree of slow wave activity (SWA) disruption, whereas SWA in turn can mediate the degree of impaired memory retention.[84] SWA activity disruption likely also leads to cellular stress.[65] **B,** *Emotional sleep:* Conceptual schematics of "the sleep to forget and sleep to remember" model are shown, as described by Goldstein and Walker.[87] Over one or several nights and numerous repetitions of this rapid eye movement mechanism, sleep transforms an emotional memory into a memory of an emotional event that is no longer emotional.[87] ER, Endoplasmic reticulum; mTORC1, mammalian target of rapamycin contact 1; NO, nitric oxide; TNF-α, tumor necrosis factor-α. (From Rosenzweig I, Glasser M, Polsek D, et al. Sleep apnoea and the brain: a complex relationship. *Lancet Respir Med.* 2015;3:404–14.)

aggravate the hyperadrenergic state of some PTSD patients and lead to decreased connectivity between the PFC and amygdala and thus exaggerated amygdala reactivity.[87] The functional outcome may be an aggravated disease course and worse prognosis.[15,87] Of note, in the prospective Honolulu-Asia Aging Study, in which men (n = 3801) aged 71 to 93 years at baseline (1991) were followed until their death, higher nocturnal oxygenation during REM sleep was associated with less gliosis and neuronal loss in the locus coeruleus.[73]

Major depression, on the other hand, is associated with exaggerated REM sleep qualities and deficiency in monoamine activity.[87] The bidirectional-dual relationship between major depression and OSA has been suggested by findings of several studies.[39] In some OSA patients, fragmented REM sleep can precipitate a vicious cycle of impaired REM regulation and rebound REM augmentation.[15] This, along with concomitant changes in neurotransmitter systems caused by hypoxemia, could further lead to reduced monoamine activity, with associated increased negative rumination and ensuing depression, in genetically predisposed individuals.[15] Through its effects on REM sleep, comorbid OSA might also lead to dysfunctional consolidation and depotentiation of emotional memory from prior affective experiences.[15,87] It has been proposed that this may result in a condition of chronic anxiety within autobiographic memory networks (Figure 135.3, *B*).[87] In support of this, in a meta-analysis of randomized controlled trials of treatment of OSA a significant improvement in depressive symptoms was reported.[92]

Even though the previously argued theoretical constructs of a bidirectional relationship between fragmented or disturbed sleep in OSA and psychiatric disorders are indirectly supported by animal and neuroimaging studies of sleep,[87] the underlying mechanics are likely to be more complex and, as such, require further well-designed studies.[15]

NEUROINFLAMMATION AND ISCHEMIC PRECONDITIONING

Cognitive and emotional complaints of OSA patients may also be explained by oxidative and neuroinflammatory effects of OSA on the CNS emotional salience network.[12,15,35,36,39] In OSA, repetitive occlusions of the upper airway lead to intermittent hypoxia and recurrent hypoxemia, typically characterized by short cycles of hypoxemia and reoxygenation.[26] However, the patterns vary greatly among patients, and, depending on the characteristics of each individual, the end results might be either adaptive or maladaptive.[25,26,93,94] For instance, oxygen desaturation during sleep is associated with decision-making deficits.[93] In contrast, individuals experiencing oxygen desaturation during sleep was associated with better perceived sleep quality among OSA patients, and this paradox may be associated with hypoxemia-related impairment of perception.[94] The outcome will likely depend on the dynamic interplay between the specific type and amount of reactive oxygen-nitrogen species produced, duration and frequency of such production, the intracellular localization, and microenvironmental antioxidant activity.[13] Additional interplay depends on factors such as genetic makeup, nutrition, and other lifestyle-related variables, all of which affect the redox status.[13,26] A variety of studies to date suggest that the severity of hypoxia, its duration, and its cycle frequency are fundamental determinants of outcomes (Figure 135.4, *A*).[95,96] For example, it has been acknowledged that short, mild, and lower cycle frequencies of intermittent hypoxia may generate beneficial and adaptive responses in the brain, such as ischemic preconditioning.[26] Conversely, chronic, moderate to severe, and high-frequency intermittent hypoxia can induce maladaptive disruption of homeostatic mechanisms, leading to dysfunction and sterile neuroinflammation.[13,26]

Ischemic preconditioning represents a generalized adaptation to ischemia by a variety of cells.[27,97] In OSA, induction of ischemic preconditioning is thought to be due to the activation of several gene programs, including the hypoxia inducible factor-1, vascular endothelial growth factor, erythropoietin, atrial natriuretic peptide, and brain-derived neurotrophic factor.[98,99] Various end mechanisms and pathways have been shown to play a role in preconditioning, including those of long-term facilitation of phrenic motor output, chemoreflex activation, vascular remodeling, neoangiogenesis, productive autophagy, reactive gliosis, various synaptic alterations, and modulation of adult hippocampal neurogenesis.[13,100,101]

CPAP treatment of OSA has been shown to partially reverse structural imaging changes in gray matter of hippocampal regions and to ameliorate some of the associated cognitive deficits, possibly also by modulating adult neurogenesis.[102] Neuroimaging studies show the coexistence of hypotrophic and hypertrophic changes in the brain of OSA patients, which were taken to reflect the evolving nature of OSA-associated brain injury.[25,46] It has been proposed that, at any given time, ongoing maladaptive neuroinflammatory processes likely exist alongside adaptive mechanisms of increased brain plasticity and ischemic preconditioning.[15] As a corollary to these findings, in a study that compared the cognitive performance of patients with high and low levels of OSA-related hypoxemia, controlling for demographic factors and other aspects of OSA severity, an unexpected advantage of higher levels of hypoxemia on memory was demonstrated in a carefully matched clinical cohort.[103]

Several studies also suggest that, under certain conditions, intermittent hypoxia can increase immune defenses without exacerbating inflammation.[13,26] Moreover, in animals, short-lasting hypoxic exposures mimicking OSA have been associated with recruitment of bone marrow–derived pluripotent stem cells, which exhibited upregulation of stem cell differentiation pathways, particularly involving CNS development and angiogenesis.[26]

Another powerful central neuroprotective adaptive mechanism for ischemic events has been demonstrated after the activation of the intrinsic neurons of the cerebellar fastigial nucleus.[104] Neurostimulation of these nuclei appears to provide "protective" reduced excitability of cortical neurons during subsequent ischemic episodes and to lead to reduced immunoreactivity of cerebral microvessels.[12] Also, a "compensatory" entraining of cerebellum by hypertrophic hippocampi has been proposed to occur in some younger patients with mild OSA.[46] Although there are no direct monosynaptic anatomic connections between hippocampi and cerebellum, their connectivity is thought to be important for the control of movement under states of heightened emotion and novel conditions and for associative learning.[12,15] Failed adaptation of cerebellar networks to injury, of any etiology, has been shown to lead to cognitive deficits and hyperactivity, distractibility, ruminative behaviors, dysphoria, and depression in some patients.[12,40]

Neuroinflammation in Obstructive Sleep Apnea

There are, however, relevant maladaptive effects of intermittent hypoxia.[15,105] These include neuroinflammation, and although the exact neurocellular sources for associated processes are still incompletely defined, activation of astroglia is likely to be important.[13,15,96] In addition, oligodendrocytes, myelin-producing cells of the CNS, have been shown to be selectively sensitive to hypoxia and sleep fragmentation.[106,107] The subsequent loss of buffering functions can ultimately contribute

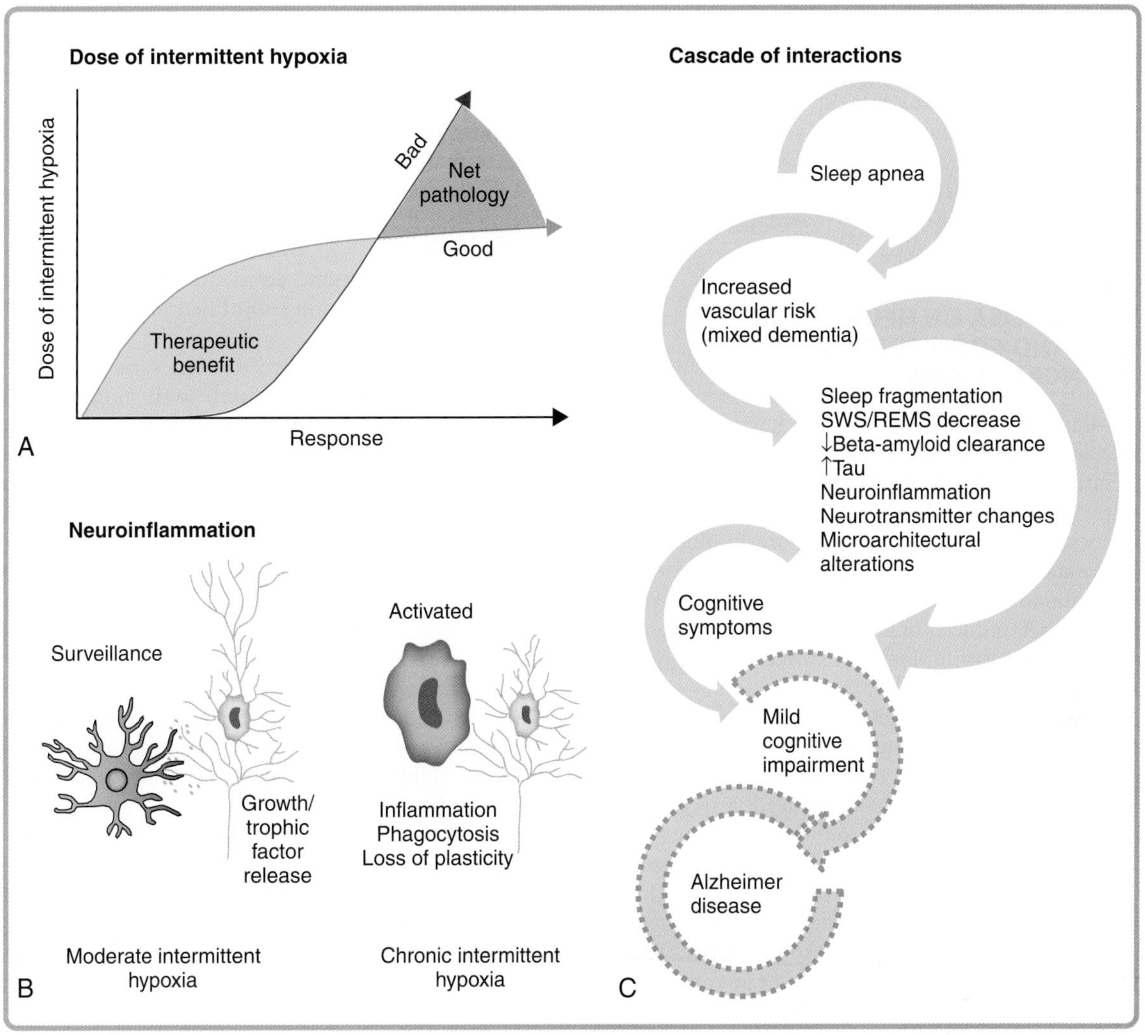

Figure 135.4 Adaptive and maladaptive processes induced by intermittent hypoxia. **A,** Conceptual presentation of the net effect of cycles of intermittent hypoxia, of varied length and frequency, over a period of time (minutes to days to weeks), as described by Dale and colleagues.[96] High doses still elicit neuroadaptive mechanisms, but the balance is shifted and maladaptive processes, such as neuroinflammation **(B),** are likely to be instigated. Finding an optimal dose is key to developing effective treatment.[96] **C,** Possible cascade of interactions between sleep apnea and Alzheimer disease. REMS, Rapid eye movement sleep; SWS, slow wave sleep. (From Rosenzweig I, Glasser M, Polsek D, et al. Sleep apnoea and the brain: a complex relationship. *Lancet Respir Med.* 2015;3:404–14.)

to pathologic processes, such as increased glial proliferation and microglial activation (Figure 135.4, *B*).[15,96] Astroglial and microglial cells play critical roles in regional blood flow regulation and inflammatory processes in the brain, as well as critical coordination of bioenergetics through lactate transport.[96] Under normal conditions, microglia in the healthy CNS exhibit a surveillance phenotype that synthesizes and releases neuroprotective growth and trophic factors.[96] However, severe and prolonged hypoxia can activate microglia toward a toxic, proinflammatory phenotype that triggers pathology, including hippocampal apoptosis, impaired synaptic plasticity, and cognitive impairment.[96] Neuroinflammation has been shown to independently increase the brain's sensitivity to stress, resulting in stress-related neuropsychiatric disorders, such as anxiety and depression.[15,108]

Dynamic changes in transcription of inflammatory genes have been demonstrated after exposure to intermittent hypoxia.[15,96] Increased prostaglandin E_2 neural tissue concentrations have also been demonstrated in hippocampal and cortical regions, accompanied by lipid peroxidation of polyunsaturated fatty acids.[96] Similarly, it has been shown that increased carbonylation- and nitrosylation-induced oxidative injury emerges in susceptible brain regions after exposure to intermittent hypoxia and promotes excessive daytime somnolence.[13,96] Toll-like receptor 4 (TLR4) expression and activity have also been shown to be increased on monocytes of patients with OSA.[109] Similarly, ligands for TLR4 have been shown to be increased in the serum of children with OSA.[15,109] The microglia of the cortex and brainstem exhibit TLR4 expression after chronic intermittent hypoxia, when it is postulated to play a region-specific and differential (adaptive or maladaptive) role.[15,52,109] This finding is of particular interest because TLR4 has also been strongly implicated in several inflammatory and neurodegenerative disorders, including vascular dementia and Alzheimer disease.[109] In cognitively healthy adults, intermittent hypoxia has been correlated with increases in phosphorylated and total tau and beta-amyloid[54] concentrations in CSF, key components of Alzheimer pathology.[1,15] Similarly, cerebral amyloidogenesis and tau phosphorylation, along with neuronal degeneration and axonal dysfunction, have been demonstrated in the cortex and brainstem of animals exposed to intermittent hypoxia.[2] Taken together, these findings support the role for neuroinflammatory processes in cognitive and emotional deficits of OSA patients. They further suggest a close association between hypoxemia-induced maladaptive processes and dementia (Figure 135.4, *C*).[6,15,110]

THE IMPACT OF OSA ON NEUROLOGIC DISORDERS AND COGNITIVE AND PERFORMANCE DEFICITS

Several neurologic disorders have been associated with OSA.[12] For example, adults with epilepsy appear at increased risk for OSA.[111] Conversely, OSA is a recognized independent risk factor for stroke (see also Chapter 103 and 150).[12,112] OSA has been associated with seizure exacerbations in older adults with epilepsy, and treatment with CPAP may represent an important avenue for improving seizure control in this population.[12,113,114] OSA-induced brain injury is believed to exacerbate neural damage during incident stroke and to increase the risk for a subsequent stroke.[115,116]

In addition, an increasing body of evidence from animal studies suggests that cerebral amyloidogenesis and tau phosphorylation, two cardinal features of Alzheimer disease, can be triggered by intermittent hypoxia.[2] Indeed, a recent large longitudinal study of data obtained from the Alzheimer's Disease Neuroimaging Initiative showed that normal cognitive and mild cognitive individuals with OSA had increased florbetapir positron emission tomography uptake (i.e., a measure of amyloid burden) and decreased CSF Aβ42 levels, as well as increased CSF total tau and phosphorylated tau compared to individuals without OSA.[117] Other smaller studies have also shown higher amyloid burden, decreased CSF Aβ42 and Aβ40 levels, and increased blood tau in OSA patients compared to individuals without OSA,[118–123] and that treatment of OSA with CPAP was associated with increases in with Aβ,[120,122] suggesting improvement in the glymphatic clearance of brain macromolecules.[66] Thus current evidence suggests a causal relationship between OSA and Alzheimer pathogenesis that may be treated with CPAP. However, whether CPAP may delay the onset of cognitive impairment in Alzheimer disease needs to be further investigated.[4]

Intermittent hypoxia and associated generation of reactive oxygen species, known to occur during nocturnal apneic episodes, have been shown to initiate neuronal degeneration and axonal dysfunction in the cortex and brainstem of animals.[2,12] Also, oligodendrocytes, myelin-producing cells of the CNS, are selectively sensitive to hypoxia and sleep fragmentation.[12,107] However, it is not clear to what extent this particular vulnerability contributes to the widely reported hypotrophic white matter changes in the brains of some OSA patients, including the fornices and corpus callosum.[12,124,125] Impaired learning capabilities have been documented in children with OSA, along with increased hyperactivity and incidence of attention deficit disorders.[10] On the other end of the age spectrum, as noted earlier, several clinical studies have suggested that older patients with OSA might suffer accelerated brain atrophy, cognitive decline, and the onset and severity of dementia.[11,95,126–128]

It has been estimated that approximately 80% of OSA patients complain of both excessive daytime sleepiness and cognitive impairment, and half also report personality changes.[42] One in four patients with newly diagnosed OSA has appreciable neuropsychological impairments.[42,129] Studies suggest that memory impairments can be found in up to 9% of OSA subjects; 2% to 25% have problems with sustained attention, and 15% to 42% demonstrate difficulties with executive functioning.[42,130] Moreover, the increased frequency of work-related and traffic accidents in OSA patients may be taken as a surrogate indicator of neurobehavioral performance deficits.[42,131,132]

Patients with OSA are 37 times more likely to complain of sleepiness compared with nonsnoring healthy control subjects.[104] Work limitation in terms of difficulties with time management, mental tasks, interpersonal relationships, and work output have all been associated with excessive daytime sleepiness.[42] OSA patients are 7.5 times more likely to have difficulties with concentration at work, have a ninefold increase in difficulty learning new tasks, and are 20 times more likely to have problems performing monotonous tasks.[42,133] In addition, occupational accidents have been reported to occur in 50% of male OSA patients, whereas the risk for occupational accidents in women with OSA has been reported as 6 times greater than in control subjects.[42,131,134]

Of particular note is the finding that motor vehicle drivers, regardless of OSA status, do not always perceive their impairment and continue to drive while sleepy.[42,135] Overall, compared with normal control subjects, OSA patients are 2 to 13 times more likely to experience a driving-related traffic accident.[136] Such accidents are more likely to occur in those who manifest greater daytime sleepiness.[42,136] However, OSA has also been associated with motor vehicle crashes independent of daytime sleepiness.[137] Sleepiness due to work schedules and sleepiness due to OSA are independent risk factors for accidents.[42] For example, in commercial vehicle drivers, in whom both of these sleepiness-promoting conditions coexist, those with the highest level of sleepiness have a twofold increase in multiple accidents.[138] The data for OSA and automobile crashes are numerous and consistent: As a group, OSA patients' risk for motor vehicle collisions is increased twofold to fourfold (Videos 135.1 and 135.2).[42]

On driving simulators, OSA patients hit more obstacles, have increased error in tracking and visual search, have increased response time to secondary stimuli, and drive out of bounds more times compared with non-OSA control subjects.[139] Still, not all OSA patients who drive have accidents, and as many as two-thirds never have a collision.[135,139] A means to identify OSA patients at greatest risk for motor vehicle collisions is still not clear based on available literature, and this complicates decision making from a medical and legal perspective.[42]

ASSESSMENT OF COGNITIVE AND NEUROBEHAVIORAL PERFORMANCE DEFICITS IN OBSTRUCTIVE SLEEP APNEA

To understand the cognitive and neurobehavioral performance deficits that affect patients with OSA, it is helpful to consider these from a categorical perspective.[42] The effects of

Box 135.1 DEFINITION AND ASSESSMENT OF COGNITIVE AND NEUROBEHAVIORAL DEFICITS ASSOCIATED WITH OBSTRUCTIVE SLEEP APNEA

Cognitive Processing

Behavior

Decreased ability to digest information

- Slowing on task
- Increased errors
- Decline in total number correct and/or completed per unit of time

Measures Commonly Used to Assess Deficit

Self-paced tasks of short duration (1–5 min), including arithmetic calculations, communication, or concept attainment

- Paced Auditory Serial Addition Task (PASAT)
- Trail Making Test parts A and B: sequencing numbers (A) or letters and numbers (B)
- Category Test: six sets of items organized around different principles, with a seventh set comprising previously shown items
- Digit Symbol Substitution Test: supplying matching symbol, given the corresponding number
- Digit Backward: stating verbally provided numbers in reverse order
- Letter Cancellation: cancellation of target alphabets from presentation of randomized alphabets

Memory

Behavior

Decreased ability to register, store, retain, and retrieve information

Measures Commonly Used to Assess Deficit

Short-term memory: timed tasks of up to 10 min that require free recall of words, numbers, paragraphs, or figures

- Probed, Recall Memory Task (words)
- Digit Span Forward (numbers)
- Wechsler Memory Scale Story Task (paragraph)
- Rey Auditory-Verbal Learning Test (figure)

Long-term memory: presenting the subject with lists of items that are longer than the seven-item memory capacity

- California Verbal Learning Test

Procedural memory: gradual acquisition and maintenance of motor skills and procedures

- Mirror Tracing Task
- Rotary Pursuit Task

Sustained Attention or Vigilance

Behavior

- Inability to maintain attention over time.
- Slowing of response time (time on task)
- Increased errors
- Reduction in the fastest optimal response times
- Periods of delayed or no response (lapses)
- Response to stimuli when none presented (false responses)

Measures Commonly Used to Assess Deficit

Short-duration tasks (30 minutes)

- Psychomotor Vigilance Task
- Four-Choice Reaction Time Test
- Steer Clear
- Continuous performance tests

Divided Attention

Behavior

Inability to respond to more than one task or stimuli, such as with driving

Measures Commonly Used to Assess Deficit

Divided Attention Driving Test: mimics vigilant-related behavior essential to driving

- Tracking (the ability to stay within the driving lane)
- Visual search (looking for and avoiding obstacles, traffic lights, etc.)

Executive Functioning

Behavior

Problems with manipulating and processing information

- Inadequate planning and execution of plans
- Disorganization: poor judgment, decision making
- Inflexible: emotional lability
- Impulsivity
- Difficulty maintaining motivation

Measures Commonly Used to Assess Deficit

Volition component or intentional behavior

- Assessed by asking the patients' preferences, what they like to do, or what makes them angry

Planning component

- Porteus Maze Test
- Tower Tests: Tower of London, Tower of Toronto, Tower of Hanoi
- Wisconsin Card Sorting Test

Purposive action

- Tinkertoy Test

Effective performance

- Random Generation Task

Modified from Dinges D. Probing the limits of functional capability: the effects of sleep loss on short-duration tasks. In: Broughton R, Ogilvie R, eds. *Sleep, Arousal, and Performance*. Birkhäuser; 1992:177–88.

sleep loss on performance include changes in cognitive performance, difficulty with working memory, slowing of response or inability to sustain attention across the duration of the task, declines in best effort or fastest response, lapses, and false responses.[42,140] As noted earlier, in OSA, hypoxemia-reoxygenation cycles with attendant biochemical and cellular alterations cause dysfunction of the prefrontal cortex, among other CNS regions.[42] This results in impaired executive function manifesting as false responses, problems with working memory and contextual memory, problems with cognitive processing in addition to deficits in the pattern of responses, and self-regulation of affect and arousal.[41,42] A description of the performance deficits and commonly used assessment techniques in OSA patients is given in Box 135.1.[34]

Tests that can be performed in the clinical setting include the Digit Symbol Substitution Task (90-second test) to assess cognitive processing and the Psychomotor Vigilance Task to evaluate the ability to sustain attention.[42] Summary information regarding the neurobehavioral tests has been reviewed, and the difficulty in selecting the most appropriate test, plus the heterogeneity of tests used, is highlighted.[53,141] The effects of OSA on cognitive processing, memory, sustained attention,

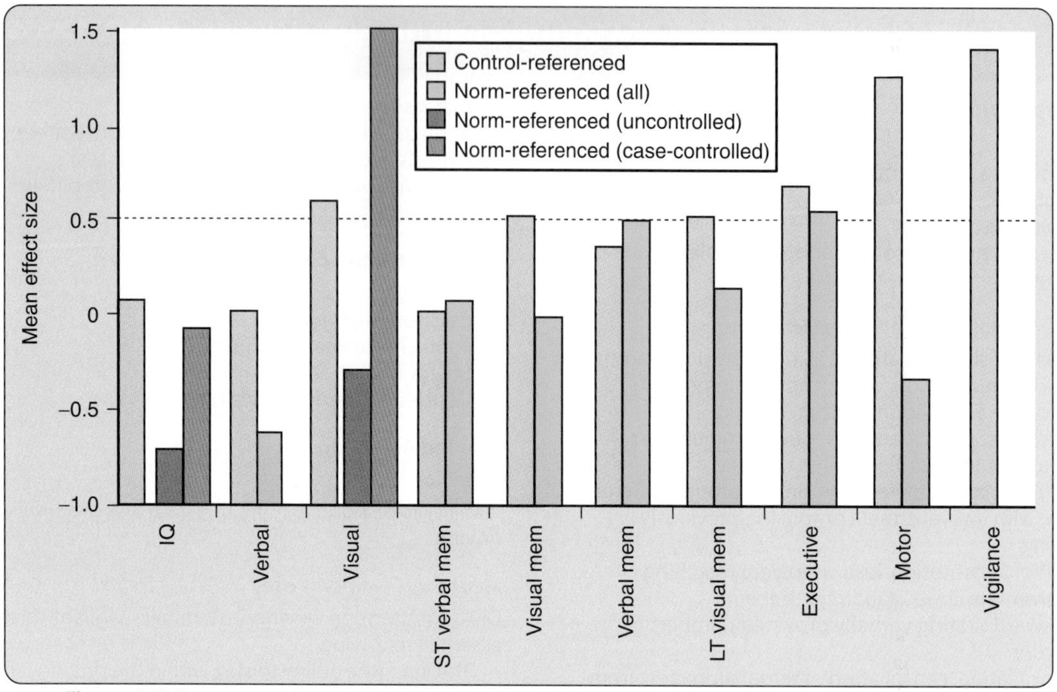

Figure 135.5 Summary of mean effect sizes across domains and data sets. Positive values indicate deficits relative to healthy adults, and negative values indicate strengths relative to healthy adults. The data set for moderate intelligence and visual functioning is split into case-controlled and uncontrolled samples for domains where study design (case-controlled vs. uncontrolled) moderated the data. IQ, Intelligence quotient; LT mem, long-term memory; ST mem, short-term memory. (Modified from Beebe DW, Groesz L, Wells C, et al. The neuropsychological effects of obstructive sleep apnea: a meta-analysis of norm-referenced and case-controlled data. *Sleep.* 2003;26:298–307.)

and executive and motor functioning are further shown in Figure 135.5, which reports the effects of OSA in patients relative to healthy adults.[42]

An additional issue to consider when assessing patients with OSA is their subjective cognitive and emotional complaints.[15] A detailed analysis of important studies in the field has suggested only a weak correlation between (subjective) cognitive complaints in patients with OSA and their objective cognitive functioning.[15,142] Divergent results of subjective versus objective complaints have been recognized in other medical populations, and several possible explanations for this in OSA patients have been suggested.[15] For example, an insufficient specificity of current tests for deficits documented in OSA is evident and largely acknowledged.[53] Currently used and validated objective tests for cognition are frequently designed to assess deficits found in patients with traumatic brain injury and as such do not specifically assess impairments in OSA-induced brain injury.[15,142] Cognitive domains are not unitary constructs, and only the carefully deconstructed analysis of their different subcapacities and their vulnerabilities to a range of risks and protective factors specific to OSA can provide a more realistic assessment of an individual's disability.[15,20,53] Similarly, a number of impairments may be secondary to other symptoms of OSA, such as sleepiness itself, or they can be a sign of psychological distress.[142,143]

Subjective cognitive complaints are linked to the quality of life, work productivity, and health care utilization of patients.[142] A meta-analysis of 13 randomized controlled studies showed no significant differences in overall and psychological quality of life comparing values of CPAP-treated patients with control subjects; however, there were improvements in physical quality of life.[144] It is important that future randomized controlled trials studies account for subjective cognitive complaints.[142]

EFFECT OF OBSTRUCTIVE SLEEP APNEA TREATMENT ON ASSOCIATED NEUROCOGNITIVE DEFICITS AND DISORDERS

Nonpharmacologic and pharmacologic treatments for OSA have been shown to improve cognitive outcomes in OSA patient subpopulations, as described in Chapter 131 to 134. The results of several meta-analyses suggest that CPAP treatment reduces sleepiness complaints and mood problems and that it improves objective cognitive functioning in OSA pati ents.[18,19,142,145,146] However, many questions regarding treatment with CPAP remain and need to be clarified, the most fundamental of which are when to start treatment and what is the optimal adherence.[15,147] The optimal treatment protocols, likely in combination with other lifestyle or pharmacologic approaches, may only be achieved once the full spectrum of the neuropathology of OSA is understood.[11,12,15] For example, it has been shown that, in some treatment-compliant patients, the beneficial effect of CPAP on symptoms of sleepiness and sleep quality can be obtained after only few days of treatment. On the other hand, the effects on other subjective and objective cognitive symptoms are less well defined, and to provide similar therapeutic effects, much longer duration of treatment may be required.[139,148]

Two studies suggest that prolonged treatment might in fact be required in patients with severe OSA.[149,150] In one of these, an almost complete recovery of white matter tract pathology in patients with severe OSA was demonstrated in association with significant improvement in memory, attention, and executive functioning, only when 1 year of CPAP adherence was achieved.[149] The functional neuroanatomy of OSA has been highlighted in a study that documented that 3 months of treatment with CPAP improved cognitive function in several domains that corresponded to gray matter volume increases in frontal and hippocampal regions.[102] Most studies investigating treatments for OSA, however, fail to account for incomplete reversal of tissue damage or deficits in cognition, suggesting that early initiation of a prolonged treatment regimen might be necessary to optimize improvements in the neurocognitive disease process associated with OSA.[151–153]

The need for a longer duration of treatment with CPAP in elderly patients compared with younger patients has been suggested by the findings of a small pilot study that found that treatment of severe OSA in Alzheimer disease patients of mild to moderate severity was associated with significantly slower cognitive decline over 3 years;[150] although, 1 year of CPAP treatment has been shown to improve sleepiness and quality of life in older people with OSA.[23]

Less striking, limited evidence with drugs such as donepezil, physostigmine, and fluticasone also points to better cognitive outcomes in treated patients, likely necessitating longer treatments.[154,155] Pharmacologic treatment may also be required in patients with OSA who, despite adequate CPAP use, continue to complain of residual sleepiness.[156] It has been suggested that, among the most common explanations for persistent sleepiness in OSA patients, low CPAP compliance, inadequate CPAP titration leading to residual respiratory events and sleep fragmentation, mask or mouth leaks, treatment-emergent central sleep apnea, behaviorally induced insufficient sleep syndrome, comorbid psychiatric disorders, sedative medication use, and undiagnosed coexisting sleep disorders predominate.[157] However, it has been recognized that some compliant CPAP users can still experience excessive daytime somnolence even after sleep hygiene improvement, optimization of CPAP treatment, and comorbid disorders management, and those patients are then considered as suffering from true residual sleepiness.[157] Although its pathophysiologic mechanisms remain unclear based on retrospective studies, the prevalence of such residual sleepiness can be estimated at approximately 10%.[16,17,157]

In clinical cases, in which there is residual sleepiness despite levels of nightly use greater than 5 hours per night and deemed severe enough to require treatment with an alerting drug, an objective evaluation at baseline should be done. This will allow proper assessment of vigilance on treatment.[157] Of alerting drugs commonly used in other sleep disorders, modafinil, armodafinil, and solriamfetol have been shown to have some effects on CPAP-resistant sleepiness[157,158] (see also Chapter 53). Solriamfetol has shown improvements in both objective and subjective daytime sleepiness, as well as enhanced daily functioning and work productivity.[158–161] A meta-analysis of the effect of modafinil and armodafinil in patients with residual sleepiness suggested improved objective and subjective measures of sleepiness, wakefulness, and patients' perception of disease severity, with overall good tolerance and minimal side effects.[156] Moreover, a trend toward decreased CPAP after treatment with these agents was also observed.[156] Methylphenidate,[157] dexamphetamine, venlafaxine, and atomoxetine are yet to be tested specifically for this indication. Similarly, pitolisant, a selective histamine H_3 receptor antagonist with wake-promoting effects used to treat narcolepsy,[162] significantly reduced self-reported daytime sleepiness and fatigue and improved patient-reported outcomes in OSA patients refusing or nonadherent to CPAP.[163] Future large prospective studies are required to better define predictive baseline characteristics and possible causal mechanisms for residual sleepiness, as well as to inform and guide clinicians in choosing the most appropriate pharmacologic treatments.

CLINICAL PEARLS

Obstructive sleep apnea is increasingly recognized as one of the potentially modifiable risk factors for cognitive and performance deficits and dementia in adults. During untreated apnea-hypopnea episodes, intermittent hypoxemia and hypercapnia occur, along with sleep fragmentation and changes in cerebral blood flow and subsequent reoxygenation. These may, independently, and in combination, result in cognitive deficits and reduced daytime performance, with functional consequences for work and school efficiency. Clinician awareness of these impairments and their prompt treatment will reduce the burden of illness on the individual patient with OSA, as well as the public health risks.

SUMMARY

Patients with OSA demonstrate variable cognitive and performance deficits. Such deficits are more easily identified in those with more severe OSA.[42] The long-term effectiveness of CPAP with regard to reducing performance deficits in patients with mild OSA needs further exploration.[42,43] The disruption of normal sleep physiology by OSA has been increasingly recognized as an underappreciated factor regarding such deficits, which, together with hypoxemia and other already recognized factors, may further aggravate age-related memory deficits in patients with OSA.[2,3,6,84,86] Clinically, this dynamic interplay underscores numerous subjective and objective cognitive and emotional complaints in some patients.[15,39,87] Moreover, there are many contributing factors in the relationship between OSA and cognitive dysfunction (Figure 135.6).[53] An understanding of the proportional effect of these factors in each individual OSA patient is a major challenge because they typically occur simultaneously and, in all likelihood, target similar neurocircuitry.[15] Persistent deficits, even after prolonged treatment with CPAP in some patients, suggest that early detection of the CNS sequelae in OSA is vital so that appropriate treatment can be administered before irreversible atrophic and metabolic changes occur. However, the optimal timing of initiation of treatment and the duration of optimal treatment are still unclear. Studies discussed in this chapter suggest that ameliorating the acute and chronic effects of neuroinflammation may offer legitimate therapeutic targets in OSA.[2,13,96] Similarly, although they are in their infancy, studies of clinical approaches that target the sleep disturbance factors of this intricate equation advocate a significant future treatment intervention potential.[15]

Despite the need for more evidence regarding cognitive and performance deficits in community-acquired samples in sham CPAP-controlled studies, there is significant documentation that untreated and CPAP-nonadherent OSA patients are at risk for traffic and occupational accidents.[42] Recent findings also raise valid questions about the mechanics of associations between OSA and dementia and further highlight the public health importance of detecting and targeting patients with OSA at highest risk for cognitive decline.

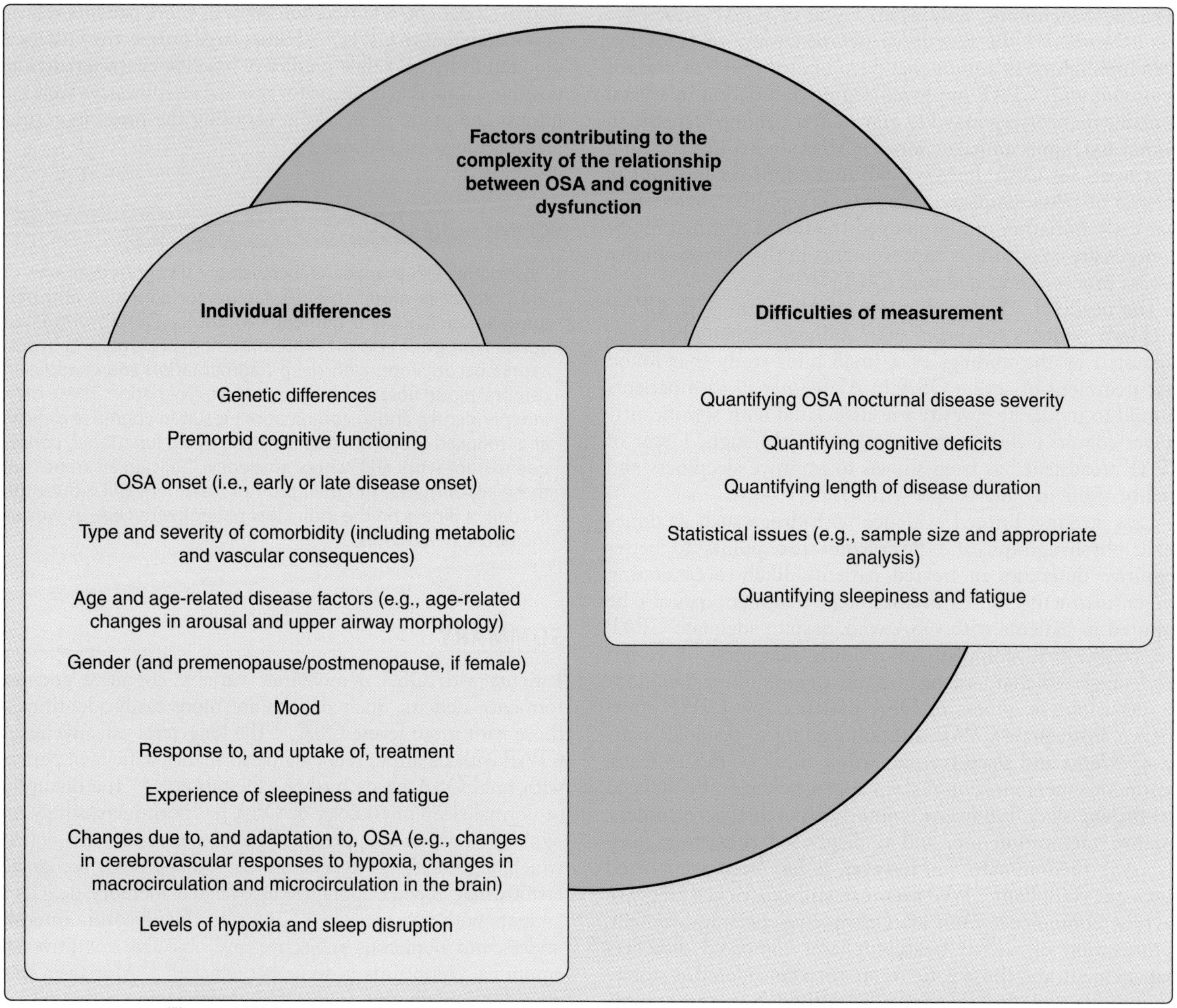

Figure 135.6 Summary of individual differences and measurement factors contributing to the complexity of the relationship between obstructive sleep apnea (OSA) severity and cognitive dysfunction. (Modified from Bucks RS, Olaithe M, Rosenzweig I, Morrell MJ. Reviewing the relationship between OSA and cognition: where do we go from here? *Respirology*. 2017;22(7):1253–61.)

ACKNOWLEDGMENTS

The author was supported by the National Institute for Health Research Respiratory Biomedical Research Unit at the Royal Brompton and Harefield National Health Service Foundation Trust, Imperial College, London.

SELECTED READINGS

Bucks RS, Olaithe M, Rosenzweig I, Morrell MJ. Reviewing the relationship between OSA and cognition: where do we go from here? *Respirology*. 2017;22(7):1253–1261.

Dalmases M, Solé-Padullés C, Torres M, et al. Effect of CPAP on cognition, brain function and structure among elderly patients with obstructive sleep apnea: a randomized pilot study. *Chest*. 2015;148(5):1214–1223.

Dauvilliers Y, Verbraecken J, Partinen M, et al. Pitolisant for daytime sleepiness in patients with obstructive sleep apnea who refuse continuous positive airway pressure treatment. *A randomized trial Am J Respir Crit Care Med*. 2020;201(9):1135–1145. [Published correction: *Am J Respir Crit Care Med*. 2020;202(1):154-155.]

Ferini-Strambi L, Marelli S, Galbiati A, et al. Effects of continuous positive airway pressure on cognition and neuroimaging data in sleep apnea. *Int J Psychophysiol*. 2013;89(2):203–212.

Kheirandish-Gozal L, Yoder K, Kulkarni R, et al. Preliminary functional MRI neural correlates of executive functioning and empathy in children with obstructive sleep apnea. *Sleep*. 2014;37(3):587–592.

Kilpinen R, Saunamäki T, Jehkonen M. Information processing speed in obstructive sleep apnea syndrome: a review. *Acta Neurol Scand*. 2014;129(4):209–218.

Lal C, Siddiqi N, Kumbhare S, Strange C. Impact of medications on cognitive function in obstructive sleep apnea syndrome. *Sleep Breath*. 2015;19(3):939–945.

Liguori C, Maestri M, Spanetta M, et al. Sleep-disordered breathing and the risk of Alzheimer's disease. *Sleep Med Rev*. 2021;55:101375.

Lim DC, Pack AI. Obstructive sleep apnea and cognitive impairment: addressing the blood-brain barrier. *Sleep Med Rev*. 2014;18(1):35–48.

Macchitella L, Romano DL, Marinelli CV, et al. Neuropsychological and socio-cognitive deficits in patients with obstructive sleep apnea [published online ahead of print, 2021 Jul 2]. *J Clin Exp Neuropsychol*. 2021:1–20.

Maierean AD, Bordea IR, Salagean T, et al. Polymorphism of the serotonin transporter gene and the peripheral 5-hydroxytryptamine in obstructive sleep apnea: what do we know and what are we looking for? A systematic review of the literature. *Nat Sci Sleep*. 2021;13:125–139.

Malhotra A, Shapiro C, Pepin JL, et al. Long-term study of the safety and maintenance of efficacy of solriamfetol (JZP-110) in the treatment of excessive sleepiness in participants with narcolepsy or obstructive sleep apnea. *Sleep*. 2020;43(2):zsz220.

McCloy K, Duce B, Swarnkar V, Hukins C, Abeyratne U. Polysomnographic risk factors for vigilance-related cognitive decline and obstructive sleep apnea. *Sleep Breath*. 2021;25(1):75–83.

Owen JE, Benediktsdottir B, Cook E, Olafsson I, Gislason T, Robinson SR. Alzheimer's disease neuropathology in the hippocampus and brainstem of people with obstructive sleep apnea. *Sleep*. 2021;44(3):zsaa195.

Polsek D, Gildeh N, Cash D, et al. Obstructive sleep apnoea and Alzheimer's disease: in search of shared pathomechanisms. *Neurosci Biobehav Rev*. 2018;86:142–149.

Ylä-Herttuala S, Hakulinen M, Poutiainen P, et al. Severe obstructive sleep apnea and increased cortical amyloid-β deposition. *J Alzheimers Dis*. 2021;79(1):153–161.

Zhu Y, Fenik P, Zhan G, et al. Degeneration in arousal neurons in chronic sleep disruption modeling sleep apnea. *Front Neurol*. 2015;6:109.

A complete reference list can be found online at ExpertConsult.com.

Chapter 136

Obstructive Sleep Apnea and Metabolic Disorders

Mary Ip; Daniel J. Gottlieb; Naresh Punjabi

Chapter Highlights

- With the common risk factor of obesity, obstructive sleep apnea (OSA) and metabolic disorders often coexist. Obesity itself is considered a metabolic disease. With global escalation of obesity trends, the current and future health care burdens of these conditions are of immense concern.
- OSA produces intermittent hypoxia and sleep disruption, with evidence for downstream cascades of sympathetic activation, oxidative stress, and inflammation—pathways that align with the pathogenetic mechanisms in metabolic disorders.
- Growing epidemiological and clinical evidence suggests that OSA may modulate metabolic outcomes. The confounding effects of obesity on metabolic disorders have, however, been difficult to dissect. Of greater clinical relevance may be potential synergistic effects between OSA and obesity, mediated partly through exacerbation of adipose tissue dysfunction.
- Animal and cell-based studies, mostly using intermittent hypoxia regimens as a surrogate model of OSA in humans, have provided evidence for deleterious effects on various tissues and cells in the pathogenesis of metabolic dysfunction and have elucidated relevant molecular pathways.
- Despite suggestive data from human observational studies, no definitive evidence has yet emerged to indicate that controlling OSA would result in improvement in metabolic function of significant clinical impact. Future studies must address the challenges of small heterogeneous samples, diverse methodology for metabolic evaluation, and issues regarding withholding treatment for OSA for substantial periods in randomized controlled studies.

INTRODUCTION

Normal daytime function is determined by the quantity and quality of nocturnal sleep, which also play a vital role in general health. Observational and experimental research has shown that, in addition to the associated daytime impairments, sleep restriction can perturb normal glucose homeostasis and increase the risk for type 2 diabetes mellitus.[1,2] Concurrent with expansion of our understanding of metabolic implications of sleep quantity and quality, evidence has also accumulated linking obstructive sleep apnea (OSA) to alterations in glucose metabolism.[3,4] The potential of a causal effect of OSA on the development of insulin resistance, glucose intolerance, and type 2 diabetes has led to research on the mechanisms that may explain the observed association. This chapter reviews the available evidence on the means through which OSA could lead to abnormalities in glucose metabolism examining the potential effects of sleep fragmentation and intermittent hypoxemia. The effects of OSA on autonomic activity, corticotropic function, generation of oxygen reactive species, and adipocytokines potentially represent some of the possible intermediary mechanisms that explicated the observed associations. In addition, the impact of OSA on disorders of lipid metabolism is reviewed. Before the discussion of the metabolic implications of OSA, a brief summary of the terminology used in the chapter is provided.

DEFINITIONS

Diabetes Mellitus, Glucose Intolerance, and Insulin Resistance

The American Diabetes Association consensus guidelines divide diabetes mellitus into four distinct clinical and pathophysiologic types and outline the criteria for defining diabetes mellitus and other categories of hyperglycemia (Table 136.1).[5] Type 1 diabetes mellitus results from cell-mediated autoimmune destruction of the pancreatic beta cells. It usually occurs in young, non-obese people and accounts for approximately 5% to 10% of those diagnosed with diabetes mellitus. Type 2 diabetes mellitus (formerly known as non–insulin-dependent diabetes mellitus) reflects a state of insulin resistance in peripheral tissues (e.g., skeletal muscle, fat, and liver) that is accompanied by an inadequate compensatory increase in insulin secretion. It usually occurs among overweight and obese

Table 136.1 Criteria for Diabetes Mellitus, Impaired Fasting Glucose, and Impaired Glucose Tolerance

		Glucose Criteria	
Condition	Test	mg/dL	mmol/L
Diabetes mellitus	Fasting	≥126 mg/dL	≥7.0
	Random	≥200	≥11.1
	2 hours after glucose load	≥200	≥11.1
Impaired fasting glucose	Fasting	100–125	6.1–6.9
Impaired glucose tolerance	2 hours after glucose load	140–199	7.8–11.0

adults and accounts for more than 90% to 95% of people with diagnosed diabetes mellitus. Gestational diabetes mellitus is the third category of diabetes and is defined as the occurrence of glucose intolerance during pregnancy. Gestational diabetes complicates approximately 4% of the pregnancies in the United States, resulting in 135,000 cases annually. The fourth type of diabetes mellitus includes other secondary types of diabetes mellitus, which result from genetic defects of beta-cell function and insulin action, other endocrinopathies (e.g., Cushing syndrome), and pancreatic destruction by specific drugs or toxins.

In addition to the definitions provided for diabetes mellitus, the American Diabetes Association consensus statement also provides a definition for prediabetes, which includes impaired glucose tolerance and impaired fasting glucose. Impaired fasting glucose is defined as a fasting glucose level between 100 mg/dL and 125 mg/dL. Impaired glucose tolerance is defined as a 2-hour post-challenge glucose level between 140 mg/dL and 200 mg/dL during the oral glucose tolerance test. Not only is prediabetes a risk factor for type 2 diabetes,[6] it also increases the risk of nephropathy, chronic kidney disease,[7] small fiber neuropathy,[8-10] retinopathy,[11,12] and macrovascular disease.[13-16] Risk factors for prediabetes include older age, male sex, higher body mass index, central obesity, and a family history of type 2 diabetes.[17]

Studies relating OSA to altered glucose metabolism have employed fasting glucose values and results of the oral glucose tolerance test as the primary outcomes. Several studies have also examined other, more direct measures of insulin sensitivity. The gold standard technique for assessing insulin sensitivity is the hyperinsulinemic euglycemic clamp.[18] During the euglycemic clamp, exogenous insulin is administered at a rate designed to maintain a stable level of hyperinsulinemia, while exogenous glucose is infused to maintain or "clamp" the serum glucose concentration. At steady state, the exogenous glucose infusion rate represents the amount of glucose uptake by the tissues and provides a measure of insulin sensitivity. To maintain euglycemia, insulin-sensitive subjects require high glucose infusion rates, whereas insulin-resistant subjects require low glucose infusion rates. Because the hyperinsulinemic euglycemic clamp method is invasive and time consuming and imposes a substantial burden on the subject, several alternative and simpler measures of insulin sensitivity have been proposed. These include the insulin suppression test and the intravenous glucose tolerance test. Fasting and post-glucose challenge levels of serum insulin are also commonly used as they are least burdensome but provide crude estimates of insulin sensitivity. Finally, the product of fasting insulin (I_0) and glucose levels (G_0), also known as the homeostasis model assessment (HOMA) index,[19] is also a widely used proxy measure of insulin sensitivity particularly in large epidemiologic studies (Table 136.2).

Metabolic Syndrome

A number of definitions of the metabolic syndrome have been put forth from various international agencies. Although there are subtle differences across the proposed definitions, insulin resistance is common to all and is considered the core defect. According to criteria proposed by the National Cholesterol Education Program (NCEP) Adult Treatment Panel III,[20] metabolic syndrome is diagnosed in the presence of three or more of the following: (1) abdominal obesity with waist circumference exceeding 40 inches in men and 35 inches in women; (2) serum triglycerides > 150 mg/dL; (3) high-density lipoprotein (HDL) cholesterol < 40 mg/dL in men and < 50 mg/dL in women; (4) blood pressure > 130/85 mm Hg; (5) fasting glucose > 110 mg/dL (Table 136.3). Proponents of the metabolic syndrome argue that clustering of risk factors is helpful for assessing the risk for type 2 diabetes mellitus and cardiovascular diseases such as stroke.[21] However, it has also been argued the need to define metabolic syndrome given the limited evidence that cardiovascular disease risk associated with this syndrome is no greater than the risk imparted by its individual components.[22,23] Despite this ongoing controversy, the NCEP definition of the syndrome is used in this chapter.

Dyslipidemia and Fat Metabolism

Lipids circulate in blood in the form of lipoproteins, of which there are five types. These include chylomicrons, very low–density lipoproteins (VLDL), intermediate-density lipoproteins (IDL), low-density lipoproteins (LDL), and HDL. Chylomicrons, the largest of the lipoproteins, are primarily responsible for transporting dietary lipids from the intestine to the liver. VLDL particles, which are produced in the liver, are triglyceride-rich lipoproteins that contain 10% to 15% of the total serum cholesterol. VLDL particles serve as precursors of LDL cholesterol, which constitutes 60% to 70% of the total serum cholesterol. LDL cholesterol is the primary atherogenic lipoprotein associated with an increased risk for cardiovascular disease.[24,25] Triglyceride-rich VLDL can also be atherogenic independent of LDL, especially when serum triglyceride levels exceed 200 mg/dL. In contrast, HDL cholesterol is protective against cardiovascular disease with low levels increasing the risk for coronary heart disease.[20] Atherogenic dyslipidemia can be defined as an LDL cholesterol level greater than 100 mg/dL and/or triglyceride levels ≥ 150 mg/dL, and/or an HDL cholesterol < 40 mg/dL. Thresholds for abnormal HDL levels in men and women are as follows: <40 mg/dL in men and <50 mg/dL in women.[20]

Table 136.2 Assessment Tools for Glucose Metabolism in Clinical Practice and Research

Test	Brief Methodology	Parameter(s) Measured	Comments
Blood glucose	Fasting venous blood sample for plasma glucose level Interstitial blood glucose monitoring	Fasting glucose level Glucose level in subcutaneous interstitial tissue	Conventional test for diagnosis of DM/impaired fasting glucose Used selectively in clinical practice, only shows trends of glycemia, and not direct blood glucose levels. Relatively expensive device
Hemoglobin A_{1c} (HbA_{1c})	Spot venous blood sample for glycated hemoglobin level	Glycemic status over past 2–3 months	Used in clinical practice to assess glycemic control in past 2–3 months in DM HbA_{1c} ≥6.5% is used for diagnosis of DM (ADA/WHO) HbA_{1c} of 5.7%–6.4% is used for diagnosis of prediabetes (ADA) Higher levels predict worse diabetic complications
Oral glucose tolerance test (OGTT)	Oral glucose loading (75 g) followed by evaluation of 2-hour post–blood glucose loading	Impaired glucose tolerance (IGT)	2-hour glucose ≥11.1 mmol/L for diagnosis of DM 7.8–11 mmol/L for diagnosis of IGT
	Oral glucose loading followed by evaluation of glucose every 30 minutes; simultaneous insulin levels measured	Insulin sensitivity	May be reflecting insulin secretion in response to glucose loading rather than insulin sensitivity Poor test reproducibility resulting from variability of gastrointestinal absorption and other factors
Hyperinsulinemic euglycemic clamp	A dose-response curve for data on exogenous insulin is generated by measuring the variable infusion rate of glucose required to maintain euglycemia	Insulin sensitivity	Gold standard for assessing insulin sensitivity The steady-state rate of peripheral glucose utilization (M value) is measured as milligrams of glucose used per kilogram of body weight per minute Labor-intensive investigation
Homeostasis model assessment (HOMA)	Fasting venous blood sample with glucose and insulin measurements		First derived from epidemiologic studies
	HOMA-IR: insulin (μU/mL) × glucose (mmol/L)/22.5	Insulin resistance: HOMA-IR	Measures basal insulin resistance and insulin secretion
	HOMA-β: [20 × insulin (μU/mL)]/[glucose (mmol/L) − 3.5]	Insulin secretion: HOMA-β	Reflects mainly hepatic insulin resistance
Frequently sampled intravenous glucose tolerance test (FSIGT, FSIVGTT)	Fasting baseline blood glucose (and insulin), followed by frequent sampling after glucose injection (for insulin sensitivity, insulin is injected 20 minutes later) for 3 hours. A computer model describing plasma dynamics (minimal model) is applied for deriving metabolic parameters	Assesses both pancreatic beta cell secretory capacity and peripheral glucose uptake in response to the bolus IV glucose Additional information on insulin sensitivity is gained by administration of insulin 20 minutes after the glucose load	Validated for insulin sensitivity against hyperglycemic euglycemic clamp No need for on-line measurements or external control of infusion Reflects whole-body insulin sensitivity
Short insulin tolerance test (SITT)	Administration of exogenous insulin followed by monitoring of fall in blood glucose over the next 30 minutes to derive the glucose disappearance rate	Insulin sensitivity	Validated for insulin sensitivity against hyperglycemic euglycemic clamp No need for on-line measurements or external control of infusion

OBSTRUCTIVE SLEEP APNEA AND GLUCOSE METABOLISM

It has been about 3 decades since the original descriptions relating OSA and abnormalities in glucose metabolism. Since then a number of clinical and epidemiologic studies have identified an independent association between OSA, insulin resistance, glucose intolerance, and type 2 diabetes mellitus. In addition, some endocrine disorders that affect glucose metabolism (polycystic ovarian syndrome,[26] Cushing syndrome,[27] acromegaly[28]) have been strongly associated with sleep apnea. Available studies on the topic of OSA and glucose homeostasis have been categorized into three major groups based on method used to assess OSA. The first group of studies has characterized the association between symptoms of OSA (e.g., snoring) and various parameters of altered glucose metabolism. These studies have shown that symptoms or signs of OSA such as snoring are associated with a higher prevalence and incidence of type 2 diabetes mellitus independent of confounders such as age, body mass index, smoking, physical activity, family history of type 2 diabetes mellitus, and habitual sleep duration.[29-42] These associations have been noted in diverse samples, including various racial and minority subgroups as well as in women during pregnancy. Although such studies have provided cross-sectional and longitudinal data and suggest a causal effect of OSA, defining dose-response associations and characterizing the putative roles of intermittent hypoxemia and sleep fragmentation is not possible given the lack of polysomnographic data.

The second group of studies addresses the limitations of the first group and has used either polysomnography or respiratory polygraphy to examine whether OSA severity and the degree of nocturnal hypoxemia and sleep fragmentation are associated with abnormalities of glucose metabolism. In these studies, the apnea-hypopnea index and the degree of measures of intermittent hypoxemia have been consistently associated with the degree of insulin resistance, glucose intolerance, and prevalent type 2 diabetes mellitus independent of factors such as obesity.[43-65] The collective body of cross-sectional and longitudinal data, which have included a wide repertoire of outcomes ranging from measures of insulin sensitivity to variability of glycemic control in those with type 2 diabetes, support the notion that intermittent hypoxemia has a central role in altering normal glucose homeostasis. In fact, epidemiologic data show that disordered breathing events associated with even mild degrees of oxyhemoglobin desaturation (i.e., 2% and 3%) are associated with fasting hyperglycemia.[66]

The third group of studies represents interventional trials that have examined changes that occur in glucose homeostasis after the institution of positive airway pressure (PAP) to treat OSA. The consistency of available data from clinical and epidemiologic studies on the causal association between OSA and insulin resistance, glucose intolerance, and type 2 diabetes initially led to the expectation that treatment of OSA with PAP therapy would have a favorable impact on glycemic

Table 136.3 Definition of Metabolic Syndrome of the National Cholesterol Education Program Adult Treatment Panel III (NCEP-ATIII)

Risk Factor	Defining Level
Abdominal obesity (waist circumference)	
Men	>102 cm
Women	>88 cm
Triglycerides	≥150 mg/dL
High-density lipoprotein cholesterol (HDL cholesterol)	
Men	<40 mg/dL
Women	<50 mg/dL
Blood pressure	≥130/≥85 mm Hg
Fasting glucose	≥110 mg/dL
Asian criteria for abdominal obesity[a]	
Men	≥90 cm
Women	≥80 cm

[a]Asian abdominal obesity criteria: data from *The IDF consensus worldwide definition of the metabolic syndrome.* Brussels: International Diabetes Federation; 2006. http://www.idf.org/webdata/docs/IDF_Meta_def_final.pdf

Data from National Cholesterol Education Program (NCEP) expert panel on detection, evaluation, and treatment of high blood cholesterol in Adults (Adult Treatment Panel III). Third report of the National Cholesterol Education Program (NCEP) Expert Panel on Detection, Evaluation, and Treatment of High Blood Cholesterol in Adults (Adult Treatment Panel III) final report. *Circulation* 2002;106:3113–421.

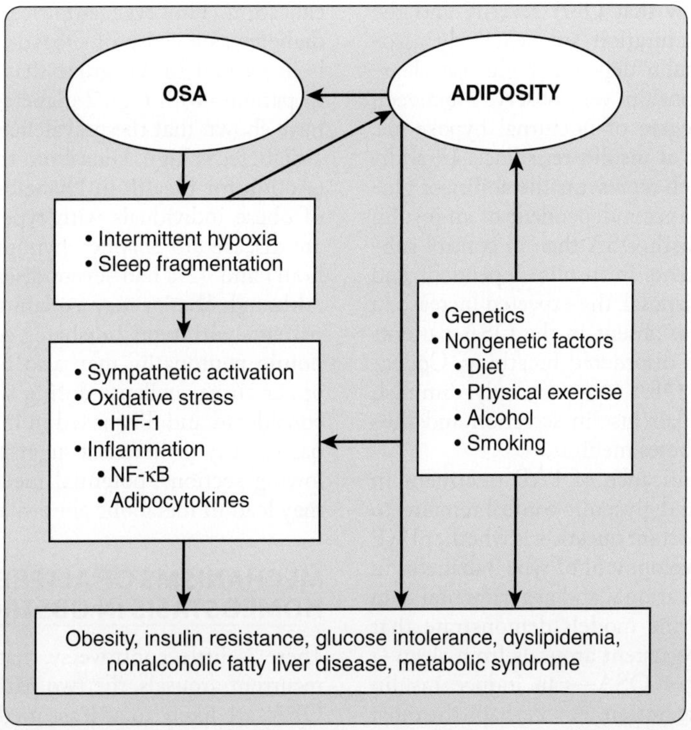

Figure 136.1 Proposed mechanistic links of obstructive sleep apnea and metabolic disorders. HIF-1, Hypoxia-inducible factor-1; NK-κB, nuclear factor kappa B.

control in patients with type 2 diabetes. Initially, small, uncontrolled studies showed such an effect; however, the results of a 2019 meta-analysis[67] conducted by the American Academy of Sleep Medicine identified four randomized clinical trials with a relatively modest collective sample size of 238 patients and concluded that there was insufficient evidence to suggest efficacy of PAP therapy for improving glycemic control as assessed by glycosylated hemoglobin (HbA1C). A similar conclusion was reached in a previous systematic review,[68] which used different selection criteria and identified 10 studies of PAP therapy in patients with type 2 diabetes. The lack of improvement in HbA1C in randomized treatment trials of OSA in type 2 diabetes could be due to the limited sample size, the inclusion of patients with relatively well-controlled type 2 diabetes[69] with limited further potential for additional improvement, or suboptimal adherence to PAP therapy. Alternatively, treatment of OSA may have little impact on glycemic measures in established type 2 diabetes, in which pancreatic beta-cell function is already significantly impaired with limited potential for recovery. Experimental data from murine models have shown that alterations in glucose metabolism induced by intermittent hypoxia are in fact not reversible even after the exposure to intermittent hypoxia has been removed.[70]

Although a majority of the available studies have employed steady-state measures of glucose metabolism (e.g., fasting glucose or insulin), available data indicate that OSA may also impair glucose and insulin dynamics. It is well established that a decrease in peripheral insulin sensitivity is fed back to the pancreatic beta cell, which increases insulin output to maintain normal glucose tolerance.[71] A defect in this compensatory response in the face of insulin resistance is central to the pathogenesis of glucose intolerance and type 2 diabetes mellitus.[18] The frequently sampled intravenous glucose tolerance test (FSIVGTT) has been used to model glucose and insulin kinetics and characterize insulin-dependent and insulin-independent mechanisms of glucose disposal.[72] Although limited, the available data show that OSA severity and the degree of oxyhemoglobin desaturation are negatively associated with the degree of insulin-dependent glucose clearance. A dose-response relationship was observed between the apnea-hypopnea index, degree of nocturnal hypoxemia, and FSIVGTT-derived index of insulin resistance. In addition, glucose effectiveness, which represents the ability of glucose to influence its own clearance independent of an insulin response, is lower in subjects with OSA than in control subjects. Finally, despite impairments in insulin-dependent and insulin-independent glucose disposal, the expected increase in pancreatic insulin secretion was absent in the OSA patients with moderate to severe sleep disordered breathing. Collectively, these findings suggest OSA may not only diminish insulin sensitivity but also impair insulin secretion and thus increase the risk for type 2 diabetes mellitus.

Although the clinical significance of PAP treatment in patients with type 2 diabetes and glycemic control remains to be determined, an equally important question is whether PAP treatment can mitigate the development of type 2 diabetes in those with prediabetes. Observational and experimental data collected in humans and murine models demonstrate that intermittent hypoxemia and recurrent arousals from sleep—the pathognomonic features of OSA—can induce insulin resistance and impair insulin secretion.[73-75] Perhaps the most interesting observation has been that the deleterious effects of intermittent hypoxia on insulin sensitivity and insulin secretion persist long after the exposure to intermittent hypoxia has ceased.[70] The potentially irreversible effects of intermittent hypoxia on insulin secretion, an effect mediated through an increase in pancreatic oxidative stress, provide a strong biologic argument for considering early intervention for OSA before there is a substantial loss in beta-cell mass. A recent retrospective study showed that patients with untreated moderate or severe disease have a higher risk of developing type 2 diabetes (adjusted hazards ratio of ~2.0–2.6) independent of obesity.[76] Regular PAP use was associated with a reduction of type 2 diabetes incidence from 3.41 to 1.61 per 100 person-years with an adjusted hazard risk equivalent to that of patients without OSA. Controlled randomized data on a small cohort of patients with OSA have also shown that PAP treatment leads to improvements in insulin sensitivity and glucose disposal.[77] Thus the presence of untreated OSA in patients with prediabetes may further exacerbate β-cell failure through a variety of additional mechanisms, including the effects of oxidative stress, systemic inflammation, sympathetic nervous system hyperactivity, and alterations in certain cytokine profiles. Alleviating the pathophysiologic stress imposed by OSA may not only preserve beta-cell function but also concurrently decrease β-cell workload by improving insulin sensitivity. Studies on the effects of PAP therapy in prediabetes are limited. A proof-of-concept study characterized the effects of nightly PAP therapy for 2 weeks in a sleep laboratory and found improvements in insulin sensitivity and glucose tolerance.[77] In the only other randomized trial of adults with OSA and prediabetes, PAP therapy was associated with improvements in insulin sensitivity but only in those with severe OSA,[78] an observation that motivates the focus on assessing those with moderate to severe disease.

Although much of the previous discussion focused on whether OSA precedes type 2 diabetes and associated abnormalities, it is important to recognize the potential of reverse causation. However, empirical evidence implicating type 2 diabetes as a cause of OSA is, at best, weak. Nonetheless, it is important to recognize that OSA is a common condition in patients with type 2 diabetes. Indeed, a number of studies have shown that the prevalence of OSA in patients with type 2 diabetes is high. Data from the multicenter Sleep AHEAD (Action for Health in Diabetes) study show that in a cohort of obese individuals with type 2 diabetes, 34% had moderate disease ($15 \leq$ apnea-hypopnea index [AHI] < 30 events/hour) and 42% had severe disease (AHI ≥ 30 events/hour).[79] Although obesity may explain the high prevalence of OSA in patients with type 2 diabetes, some have suggested that autonomic neuropathy may also increase the predisposition for upper airway collapse during sleep.[80-82] Thus OSA should be considered and diagnosed in individuals with type 2 diabetes, particularly if there is a suggestive clinical history. In the following sections, potential mechanisms through which OSA may lead to metabolic abnormalities are reviewed.

MECHANISMS OF ALTERED GLUCOSE HOMEOSTASIS IN OBSTRUCTIVE SLEEP APNEA

There is little controversy that intermittent hypoxemia and recurrent arousals, the two pathophysiologic concomitants of OSA, are likely to at least mediate the metabolic abnormalities observed in OSA. Several animal and human studies have shown that exposure to intermittent hypoxia can alter glucose homeostasis. Exposure to sustained or intermittent hypoxia has been shown to increase fasting insulin levels in various rodent models.[83-87] Similarly, experimental studies in humans corroborate the notion that hypoxia can adversely affect glucose metabolism. Normal subjects demonstrate impairments in insulin sensitivity when exposed to either sustained or intermittent hypoxia.[88-90] Furthermore, disruption of normal sleep continuity resulting from recurrent arousals in OSA may also adversely affect glucose metabolism.[73-75] Potential mechanisms that may explicate this association include (1) activation of the sympathetic nervous system; (2) formation of reactive oxygen species (ROS); and (3) increases in inflammatory cytokines (i.e., interleukin-6 and tumor necrosis factor-α and adipocyte-derived factors such as leptin, adiponectin, and resistin).

It is well established that intermittent hypoxemia and sleep fragmentation in OSA can independently activate the sympathetic nervous system,[91] which has a central role in regulating glucose metabolism. Sympathetic nervous system activation and resulting catecholamine release can reduce insulin-mediated glucose uptake, decrease insulin sensitivity, promote beta-cell apoptosis, and impair insulin secretion. Catecholamines can also inhibit insulin-mediated glycogen synthesis, increase glycogenolysis, and diminish the ability of glucose to stimulate its own disposal.[92-101] Moreover, an increase in sympathetic activity has lipolytic effects resulting in the release of free fatty acids (FFAs) from adipocytes,[99] which, in turn, can worsen insulin sensitivity.[95,99] Finally, catecholamine-mediated vasoconstriction can shunt glucose and insulin from skeletal muscle to less metabolically active areas and decrease net glucose uptake.[95] In fact, numerous studies have shown that medications causing vasoconstriction induce insulin resistance and, notably, certain medications causing vasodilation increase insulin sensitivity.[102-104] In addition to the hemodynamic effects, chronic sympathetic activation can alter skeletal muscle morphology to a more insulin resistant type,[105] inhibit insulin signaling, and decrease insulin-mediated glucose uptake by adipocytes.[106] Thus sympathetic nervous system activation in OSA could certainly accelerate the progression from prediabetes to type 2 diabetes.

Oxidative stress and the increased production of ROS represent another mechanism through which OSA may accelerate the progression from prediabetes to type 2 diabetes. Hypoxemia followed by re-oxygenation in OSA increases ROS production, similar to what has been observed with ischemia-reperfusion injury. In fact, lipid peroxidation, protein carboxylation, and markers of DNA oxidation are higher in patients with OSA than in normal subjects.[107] Excessive ROS concentrations can inhibit insulin-stimulated substrate uptake in muscle and adipose tissue[108-111] and damage the beta cell, given its constitutively low levels of antioxidant enzymes such as catalase, glutathione peroxidase, and superoxide dismutase.[112-114] Thus, hypothetically, decreasing oxidative stress by treating OSA with PAP therapy in prediabetes could protect the beta cell against ROS-induced injury and the accompanying loss of function. Consequently, OSA treatment in prediabetes may well provide a clinically useful strategy to attenuate the progression from prediabetes to type 2 diabetes.

Subclinical inflammation and adipocyte-derived factors have also been implicated in the pathogenesis of prediabetes and type 2 diabetes.[115-118] Higher levels of inflammatory markers (e.g., high-sensitivity C-reactive protein, hs-CRP; interleukin-6, IL-6) and alterations in adipokine profiles have also been reported in OSA.[119-121] Given that exposure to hypoxia can increase cytokine production[122-126] and that sleep loss can activate the cellular immune response and induce inflammatory cytokines,[127,128] OSA may hasten the progression from prediabetes to type 2 diabetes through low-grade systemic inflammation. By obviating nocturnal hypoxemia and improving sleep quality, PAP therapy may decrease or delay the conversion from prediabetes to type 2 diabetes.

The effects of intermittent hypoxemia in OSA on glucose metabolism are likely related to changes induced at the level of transcriptional regulation with an increase in hypoxia inducible factor-1 (HIF-1).[129,130] Activation of HIF-1 with intermittent hypoxia may occur either because of hypoxia itself or because of increased formation of ROS.[131] HIF-1 is a master regulator of oxygen homeostasis and controls a variety of physiologic responses to hypoxia, including erythropoiesis, angiogenesis, glucose metabolism, and lipid metabolism.[132] HIF-1 increases circulating endothelin-1,[133] which can also influence insulin sensitivity. In vitro studies show that endothelin-1 acutely decreases insulin-stimulated glucose uptake,[134] stimulates glycogenolysis, causes a dose-dependent increase in hepatic glucose production, and increases plasma glucose levels.[135] In humans, endothelin-1 infusion at non-pressor doses diminishes insulin secretory response to glucose.[136] Finally, HIF-1 has been implicated in activation of sympathetic nervous system during intermittent hypoxia, which will be discussed further.[137] The metabolic significance of HIF-1 is further highlighted by transgenic studies that show that mice with partial deficiency of HIF-1α do not exhibit an increase in serum insulin levels with intermittent hypoxemia.[129]

Intermittent hypoxia can increase activity of a major pro-inflammatory transcription factor, nuclear factor κB (NF-κB).[138,139] Although the mechanisms of NF-κB activation with intermittent hypoxia are not well defined, it is likely that enhanced production of ROS has an important role. Activated NF-κB translocates to the nucleus, where it increases the expression of multiple inflammatory genes for inflammatory cytokines, including tumor necrosis factor-α (TNF-α), interleukin-1β (IL-1β), and IL-6.[140] TNF-κ and IL-6 disrupt insulin signaling pathways and worsen insulin sensitivity. Thus intermittent hypoxia may lead to insulin resistance via activation of transcription factors HIF-1 and NF-κB in the liver and other insulin-sensitive tissues.

OBSTRUCTIVE SLEEP APNEA AND FAT METABOLISM

Adipose tissue or fat deposited in organs is active endocrine tissue, regulated in the expression and release of adipocytokines that modulate body metabolism. Sleep apnea is reported to be independently associated with the serum levels of several adipokines, including adiponectin and adipocyte-fatty acid–binding protein, which are also closely related to glucose metabolism.[141,142] In this association, body fat is always a difficult confounder to completely exclude. The effect of treatment of OSA, usually with CPAP for limited durations, in restoring adipokine levels to that of nonapneic control subjects has shown controversial and mostly negative results.[141-143]

FFAs, primarily released from adipose tissue, are the primary energy source in states of prolonged fasting when insulin levels are at their lowest.[144] An increase in adipose tissue lipolysis and higher circulating FFA levels have been associated with the development of insulin resistance.[145] FFAs also impair secretion of insulin from the pancreatic beta cell.[146] Factors that regulate adipose tissue lipolysis include the autonomic nervous system, neuroendocrine hormones (e.g., growth hormone and cortisol), and various adipocytokines such as leptin, adiponectin, interleukin-6, and tumor necrosis factor-α.[147] Because OSA demonstrates increase in sympathetic nervous system activity and is also associated with alterations of several factors that regulate lipolysis (e.g., adipocytokines, growth hormone), there is good biologic basis to speculate that OSA could negatively impact regulation of FFA metabolism.

In a recent study, the severity of OSA was independently associated with alterations in FFA metabolism.[148] Specifically, increasing AHI, as was the degree of oxygen desaturation during sleep, was associated with adipocyte insulin resistance and impairments in FFA kinetics after a glucose challenge. Furthermore, the amount of stage N3 sleep was negatively associated with FFA suppression after the glucose challenge and a delayed recovery phase after that suppression. These findings indicate nocturnal hypoxemia and poor sleep quality in OSA impair FFA metabolism, which may, in turn, contribute to perturbed insulin and glucose homeostasis.

Although the underlying mechanisms have not been fully elucidated, FFAs could induce insulin resistance by activating several serine kinases that inhibit insulin activity[149,150] and interfere with insulin receptor signaling.[151] FFAs also activate inflammatory signaling pathways by increasing secretion of cytokines, such as tumor necrosis factor-α and interleukin-6, and by interacting with members of the Toll-like receptor (TLR) family.[152,153] In healthy volunteers, exposure to intermittent hypoxia decreases whole-body insulin sensitivity and increases TLR2 expression in peripheral mononuclear cells.[154] In addition to peripheral insulin resistance, FFAs decrease hepatic insulin sensitivity, stimulate gluconeogenesis, and inhibit insulin- and glucose-dependent suppression of endogenous glucose production from the liver.[155] Acute exposure to FFA increases insulin secretion and stimulates beta-cell expansion, while prolonged exposure leads to beta-cell apoptosis,[156,157] and via the TRL2/TLR4 signaling pathway, perpetuates inflammatory processes, eventually leading to beta-cell failure.[158] Thus abnormalities in FFA metabolism can elicit the two "hits" (i.e., insulin resistance and beta-cell dysfunction) needed for the development of type 2 diabetes in OSA.

Against the background of the potential role of OSA in altering FFA kinetics, there is also evidence that total cholesterol and LDL cholesterol levels are high in OSA not only in adults but also in children.[159,160] Experimental models show that the severity of hypoxia is an important determinant of the degree of dyslipidemia.[161] Intermittent hypoxia likely induces dyslipidemia through lipid biosynthesis in the liver because of upregulation of HIF-1, SREBP-1, and stearoyl coenzyme A desaturase 1, a key enzyme of lipid biosynthesis and lipoprotein secretion in the liver.[162,163] As with the impact of PAP therapy on glucose homeostasis, there are studies[164,165] that show a favorable effect of PAP therapy, but large randomized trials are lacking on whether it improves total and LDL cholesterol.

THERAPEUTIC IMPLICATIONS

As shown previously and elsewhere in this volume, the relationship between sleep apnea and metabolic abnormalities is complex.[162] Increased body weight and in particular truncal distribution (neck and abdomen) of adipose tissue play direct roles on respiratory mechanics predisposing to upper airway collapse. At the same time, obesity and visceral obesity share various intermediary pathways of fat and glucose dysmetabolism with OSA, culminating in interrelated and complex networks (Figure 136.1). Insulin resistance, secondary leptin resistance, and other hormonal dysregulations are frequently present in patients with obesity, type 2 diabetes, and sleep apnea. It is suggested that the treatment of each of the associated clinical conditions, including bariatric surgery, anti-obesity/anti-diabetic drugs, or PAP, may positively influence not only their specific primary target condition but also the others.[166] Ultimately, the crucial balance may hang between the contributions of sleep apnea and other well-established metabolic determinants toward the emergence of clinical disease. Thus a great deal of research remains to be done.

CONCLUSIONS

The last 3 decades have seen an enormous growth in the evidence of the potential impact of OSA on insulin resistance, glucose intolerance, type 2 diabetes, and dyslipidemia. Abnormalities in glucose and lipid metabolism increase the risk for coronary heart disease and type 2 diabetes. Thus the metabolic implications of OSA have major implications from a clinical and public health perspective. Clearly, there are major gaps in our knowledge of the impact of OSA on glucose metabolism. Thus research is clearly needed to provide additional evidence on whether treatment of OSA has favorable effects on glucose and fat metabolism and to better define the mechanisms through which intermittent hypoxemia or sleep fragmentation impact upon metabolic function, and determine whether adverse metabolic effects of OSA mediate some of the associated cardiovascular risk observed with this condition.

CLINICAL PEARL

Strong associations are recognized between OSA and various metabolic disorders, notably obesity, type 2 DM, dyslipidemia, and NAFLD. Despite abundant suggestive evidence for independent associations between OSA and metabolic dysfunction, a causal or aggravating role for OSA in dysmetabolism is not yet delineated, and treatment of OSA has not been definitively shown to prevent or improve metabolic dysfunction. A reasonable holistic clinical approach mandates high vigilance regarding the clustering of these conditions, with relevant screening and specific management considered accordingly. The need for appropriate body weight control measures is particularly relevant in this regard.

All patients with polycystic ovarian syndrome, Cushing syndrome, or acromegaly should be considered at risk for OSA.

SUMMARY

Continuing evidence indicates that OSA is associated with insulin resistance, glucose intolerance, type 2 diabetes mellitus, dyslipidemia, and metabolic syndrome and other related disorders. Experimental and observational data from human studies indicate that OSA, through the pathophysiologic effects of intermittent hypoxemia and recurrent arousals, can negatively influence insulin sensitivity and glucose tolerance. Data from experimental studies show that intermittent hypoxia can induce insulin resistance and lead to hepatic steatosis and steatohepatitis. Increase in sympathetic nervous system activity, generation of oxidative reactive species, and an increase in low-grade systemic inflammation are some of the putative mechanisms linking OSA to metabolic dysfunction. There is evidence implicating OSA and its concomitants of sleep fragmentation and intermittent hypoxia to metabolic abnormalities. In addition, there are data suggesting that type 2 diabetes mellitus is a risk factor for OSA. Understanding the associations between OSA and alterations in glucose metabolism has clinically relevant implications for all health care professionals in the clinical and research arena.

SELECTED READINGS

Adderley NJ, Subramanian A, Toulis K, et al. Obstructive sleep apnea, a risk factor for cardiovascular and microvascular disease in patients with type 2 diabetes: findings from a Population-Based Cohort Study. *Diabetes Care.* 2020;43(8):1868–1877.

Arnardottir ES, Lim DC, Keenan BT, et al. Effects of obesity on the association between long-term sleep apnea treatment and changes in interleukin-6 levels: the Icelandic Sleep Apnea Cohort. *J Sleep Res.* 2015;24(2):148–159.

Bonsignore MR, McNicholas WT, Montserrat JM, et al. Adipose tissue in obesity and obstructive sleep apnoea. *Eur Respir J.* 2012;39(3):746–767.

Chirinos JA, Gurubhagavatula I, Teff K, et al. CPAP, weight loss, or both for obstructive sleep apnea. *N Engl J Med.* 2014;370(24):2265–2275.

Imes CC, Bizhanova Z, Sereika SM, et al. Metabolic outcomes in adults with type 2 diabetes and sleep disorders [published online ahead of print, 2021 Jun 9]. *Sleep Breath.* 2021. https://doi.org/10.1007/s11325-021-02408-x

Kent BD, Grote L, Bonsignore M, et al. Sleep apnoea severity independently predicts glycaemic health in nondiabetic subjects: the ESADA study. *Eur Respir J.* 2014;44(1):130–139.

Pamidi S, Wroblewski K, Stepien M, et al. Eight hours of nightly CPAP treatment of obstructive sleep apnea improves glucose metabolism in prediabetes: a randomized controlled trial. *Am J Respir Crit Care Med.* 2015;192(1):96–105.

Pugliese G, Barrea L, Laudisio D, et al. Sleep apnea, obesity, and disturbed glucose homeostasis: epidemiologic evidence, biologic insights, and therapeutic strategies. *Curr Obes Rep.* 2020;9(1):30–38.

Rogers AJ, Kaplan I, Chung A, McFarlane SI, Jean-Louis G. Obstructive sleep apnea risk and stroke among blacks with metabolic syndrome: results from Metabolic Syndrome Outcome (MetSO) registry. *Int J Clin Res Trials.* 2020;5(1):143.

Simon S, Rahat H, Carreau AM, et al. Poor sleep is related to metabolic syndrome severity in adolescents with PCOS and obesity. *J Clin Endocrinol Metab.* 2020;105(4):e1827–e1834.

Stelmach-Mardas M, Brajer-Luftmann B, Kuśnierczak M, Batura-Gabryel H, Piorunek T, Mardas M. Body mass index reduction and selected cardiometabolic risk factors in obstructive sleep apnea: meta-analysis. *J Clin Med.* 2021;10(7):1485.

Strand LB, Carnethon M, Biggs ML, et al. Sleep disturbances and glucose metabolism in older adults: the cardiovascular health study. *Diabetes Care.* 2015;38(11):2050–2058.

Vacelet L, Hupin D, Pichot V, et al. Insulin resistance and type 2 diabetes in asymptomatic obstructive sleep apnea: results of the PROOF cohort study after 7 years of follow-up. *Front Physiol.* 2021;12:650758.

Wei R, Gao Z, Xu H, et al. Body fat indices as effective predictors of insulin resistance in obstructive sleep apnea: evidence from a cross-sectional and longitudinal study : BFI as Predictors of IR in OSA [published correction appears in Obes Surg. 2021 Mar 22;:]. *Obes Surg.* 2021;31(5):2219–2230.

A complete reference list can be found online at ExpertConsult.com.

Chapter 137

Overlap Syndromes of Sleep and Breathing Disorders

Jose M. Marin; Santiago Carrizo; Marta Marin-Oto

Chapter Highlights

- Sleep depresses the central control of breathing and muscle tone. These changes have no adverse effects in healthy subjects. However, in patients with pulmonary diseases such as chronic obstructive pulmonary disease (COPD), asthma, interstitial lung diseases, and pulmonary hypertension, these changes may worsen gas exchange and induce significant hypoxemia and hypercapnia, especially during rapid eye movement sleep.
- As COPD, asthma, and sleep-related breathing disorders (SRBD) are very prevalent disorders in adults, overlap of SRBD, particularly obstructive sleep apnea, and either COPD or asthma is frequent in clinical practice. Such overlap, termed overlap syndrome, carries an excessive risk for worsened sleep and awake-related outcomes than any one of these conditions alone, including increased risk of COPD exacerbations and mortality.
- Practitioners should identify the coexistence and severity of SRBD in patients with COPD or asthma, and the presence and severity of the overlap syndrome, and establish a personalized treatment in each case. A sleep study should be considered in any patient with COPD or asthma with signs and symptoms of SRBD, such as snoring and excessive daytime sleepiness, or with inappropriate awake hypoxemia.
- The specific treatment of each SRBD in patients with overlap syndrome must be carried out individually. In-laboratory polysomnography will be the study of choice to establish the type of ventilatory support and the need for supplemental oxygen.

INTRODUCTION

The respiratory system shows normal physiologic changes during sleep, including decreased central breathing output, decreased lung volumes, increased airway resistance, and ventilation-perfusion mismatching. Overlap syndromes are defined as the coexistence in the same patient of sleep-related breathing disorders (SRBD), particularly obstructive sleep apnea (OSA), and one or more of the following chronic respiratory conditions: chronic obstructive pulmonary disease (COPD), asthma, interstitial lung disease (ILD), and pulmonary hypertension (PH). The clinical relevance of identifying the coexistence of an SRBD in patients with these chronic respiratory disorders lies not only in the diagnosis of an overlap syndrome but also in the worse prognosis for these coexistent respiratory diseases and the resultant need for specific treatment of the concomitant sleep-disordered breathing.

CHRONIC OBSTRUCTIVE PULMONARY DISEASE

The latest version of the Global Initiative for Chronic Obstructive Lung Disease (GOLD) document defines COPD as a common, preventable, and treatable disease that is characterized by persistent respiratory symptoms and airflow limitation that is due to airway and/or alveolar abnormalities usually caused by significant exposure to noxious particles or gases and influenced by host factors, including abnormal lung development. The definition also states that "significant comorbidities may have an impact on morbidity and mortality."[1] Of specific relevance to sleep medicine, the importance of coexistence of morbidities for the patient's prognosis is recognized.

Sleep Complaints and Sleep-Related Breathing Disorders in Chronic Obstructive Pulmonary Disease

Sleep disturbance is common in COPD without other coexistent primary sleep disorders. In a large survey done in North America and Europe, 40% of patients reported problems with their sleep.[2] In a recent European survey, 78.1% of patients with COPD reported some degree of nighttime symptoms, including one or more of the following: dyspnea, cough with increased sputum production, wheezing, and difficulty with the maintenance of sleep. The prevalence of such nighttime symptoms was positively correlated with the severity of spirometrically measured airflow obstruction.[3] Polysomnographic studies have shown that these patients have problems initiating or maintaining sleep, reduced rapid eye movement (REM) sleep, and frequent microarousals. This poor sleep quality increases in parallel with the frequency of nocturnal respiratory symptoms such as cough and wheezing[4] and COPD severity.[5]

SRBD can be grouped into four clinical entities: sleep-related hypoxemia or nocturnal hypoxemia (NH), hypoventilation during sleep (HVS), OSA, and respiratory effort–related arousals (RERAs). A patient is considered to develop isolated NH when SaO_2 during sleep falls below 90% without coexisting hypercapnia. There is no agreed-upon criterion to diagnose NH in terms of percentage of total sleep time with SaO_2 below 90% (CT90). NH is prevalent in COPD. NH defined as at least 10% in CT90 is present in 66% of patients with COPD with daytime SaO_2 above 90% on breathing room air, and without concomitant OSA,[6] with severe NH (e.g., CT > 30) in 23%. The prevalence of NH increases with COPD severity as defined by GOLD classification (Figure 137.1). Reduced rib cage contribution to breathing during sleep with a subsequent reduction in functional residual capacity and augmented ventilation-perfusion mismatching can explain in part NH in COPD.[7] Daytime gas exchange abnormalities are, however, somewhat predictive of sleep oxygen desaturation among patients with COPD.[8] Given the shape of the oxyhemoglobin dissociation curve, patients on the steep portion of the curve (e.g., $PaO_2 < 60$ mm Hg breathing room air during daytime) would be expected to have a greater fall in SaO_2 during sleep, particularly during REM sleep.

Sleep-related HVS in COPD is the result of an accentuated physiologic hypoventilation. This happens in these patients as a consequence of decreased central respiratory drive response to chemical and mechanical inputs,[9] increased upper airway resistance resulting from a loss of tone in the upper pharyngeal muscles,[10] and reduced efficiency of diaphragmatic contraction resulting from lung hyperinflation.[11] To define HVS, sleep arterial tension carbon dioxide ($PaCO_2$) or expiratory end-tidal tension ($etCO_2$) must be measured. Values of $PaCO_2$ or $etCO_2$ during sleep above 50 mm Hg

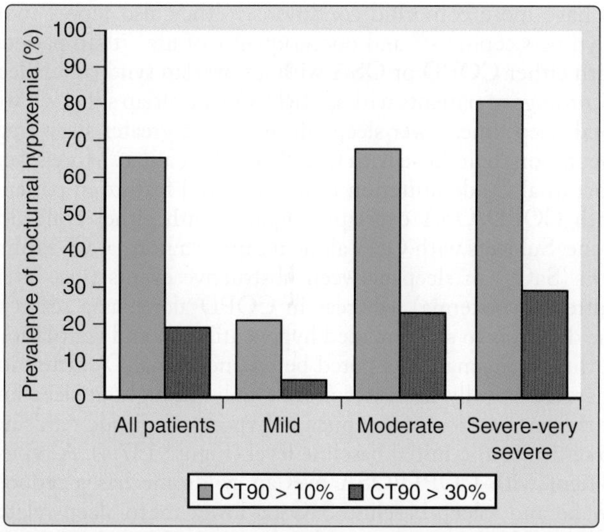

Figure 137.1 Prevalence of nocturnal hypoxemia (NH) in chronic obstructive pulmonary disease (COPD). Patients are sorted according to severity of COPD as indicated by their forced expiratory volume in the first second in % predicted (FEV_1%): mild COPD (> 80%), moderated COPD (50 – 80%) and severe to very severe COPD (< 50%). Prevalence of NH is presented using two cut-offs of percent of recording time with an SaO_2 < 90% (CT90): > 10% (*teal*) and > 30% (*red*).

for more than 10 minutes are consistent with HVS. Most hypercapnic patients with COPD also develop HVS during sleep; however, in normocapnic patients, HVS may occur in REM sleep.[12] The prevalence of RERAs in COPD is unclear. However, COPD is characterized by lower airway abnormalities and collapsibility that can contribute to RERAs, so more studies are warranted to evaluate the clinical significance of COPD-RERAs overlap.

Chronic Obstructive Lung Disease and Obstructive Sleep Apnea Overlap Syndrome

Definitions and Classifications

OSA causes repetitive decrease or absence of inspiratory and expiratory airflow, sympathetic activation, and intermittent oxyhemoglobin desaturation and hypercapnia.[13,14] Severity grades of mild (apnea-hypopnea index [AHI] ≥ 5 and < 15 episodes/hour), moderate (AHI ≥ 15 and < 30 episodes/hour), and severe (≥ 30 episodes/hour) have a progressive impact on outcomes.[15-19]

The coexistence of COPD and OSA was first described as the overlap syndrome by David Flenley almost 30 years ago.[20] He believed that the clinical course and prognosis of such "overlap patients" were worse than patients suffering from COPD or untreated OSA alone. These opinions remain valid today. Nevertheless, at present, the term *overlap syndrome* is not a formal diagnostic designation for patients suffering from OSA and COPD. A classification of severity for this entity is not available, and health outcomes appear to depend on the severity of OSA and COPD independently.

Epidemiology of Chronic Obstructive Pulmonary Disease/Obstructive Sleep Apnea Overlap Syndrome

In pulmonary clinics, OSA and COPD are two of the most prevalent chronic respiratory disorders. It is estimated that 10% of the general population has moderate to severe COPD as defined by an FEV_1/FVC ratio of less than 0.7 plus an FEV_1 of less than 80% predicted.[21] The prevalence of COPD increases with age and is directly related to the prevalence of tobacco smoking, but outdoor and indoor air pollution are also major COPD risk factors. In 2020 COPD was the third leading cause of death worldwide.[1]

Among men and women between the ages of 30 and 60 years, 20% and 9%, respectively, had an AHI of at least 5 events/hour in the Wisconsin Sleep Cohort Study,[22] with an increase in moderate to severe SDB (AHI ≥15 events/hour) over the last 2 decades.[23] The sex disparity of OSA ends around age 55 years, with a sharp rise among postmenopausal women.[23-25]

There are, however, no studies that directly assess the prevalence of the COPD/OSA overlap syndrome. Because COPD and OSA are each increasing throughout the world in association with an aging population, presumably the overlap syndrome is becoming more prevalent. In clinical series, it has been noted that approximately 11% of patients with at least moderate OSA, as defined by an AHI of more than 20 events/hour, have airflow limitation on spirometry.[26] In a European population study of patients with predominantly mild COPD, the coincidence of OSA syndrome (AHI > 5 events/hour accompanied by excessive daytime sleepiness) occurred in 1% of the total population.[27] The Sleep Heart Health Study found that 19% had airway obstruction (defined as $FEV_1/FVC < 0.7$) that was predominantly mild. The prevalence of OSA, defined as a respiratory disturbance index of more than 10 events/hour, was not higher in subjects with airway obstruction (defined as $FEV_1/FVC < 0.7$) compared with the nonobstructed population.[28] There were 254 participants (4.3%) who had both characteristics: obstructive airway disease and sleep apnea. As expected, the respiratory disturbance index increased with higher body mass index (BMI) in participants with and without airway obstruction. An age effect was not specifically addressed in this study. In short, the few available population studies of the association between COPD and OSA (i.e., overlap syndrome) show great variability in the prevalence of this association.

Sleep in Patients with Chronic Obstructive Pulmonary Disease/Obstructive Sleep Apnea Overlap Syndrome

In the Sleep Heart Health Study, patients with COPD/OSA overlap syndrome had a lower total sleep time, lower sleep efficiency, and higher daytime sleepiness as assessed by the Epworth Sleepiness Scale[29] than did patients with COPD alone. They were also more likely to have greater sleep-related oxygen desaturation compared with participants with OSA or airway obstruction alone.[28] Most importantly, patients with overlap syndrome, compared with patients with either COPD or OSA alone, display more profound oxygen desaturation during sleep, as well as worse daytime hypoxemia and hypercapnia.[26]

Risk Factors for Chronic Obstructive Pulmonary Disease/Obstructive Sleep Apnea Overlap Syndrome

Using comorbidities network analysis, we have reported that, in the general population, individuals carrying the diagnosis of COPD are more predisposed at an earlier age to diseases characteristically seen in the elderly.[30] Some of the comorbid conditions such as obesity, smoking, opioid use, and heart disease are also specific OSA risk factors. Active smoking,[31] and both pharyngeal and lower extremity edema associated with episodic use of oral corticosteroids or impaired cardiac output, may contribute or aggravate OSA.[32] There is also evidence that patients with advanced COPD who lose weight may show reduced upper airway obstruction. Thus the typical patient with COPD, overweight-obese and sleepy ("blue bloater") has a high probability of suffering from COPD/OSA overlap syndrome (Figure 137.2). In contrast, the emphysematous phenotype ("pink puffer") has a much lower risk of suffering from OSA. This has been confirmed in the COPDGene project, an American prospective cohort study of smokers with/without COPD. In a subgroup of smokers who had both a chest CT scan and a sleep study, investigators found an inverse relationship between AHI and the percentage of emphysema. They also found that those with COPD/OSA had higher upper airway collapsibility.[33]

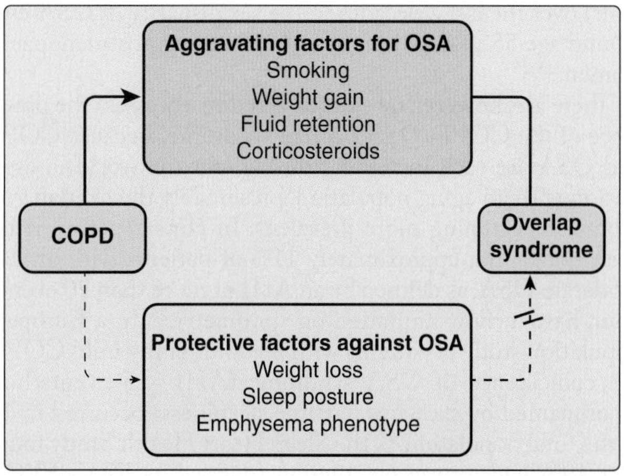

Figure 137.2 Interactions between chronic obstructive pulmonary disease and obstructive sleep apnea (OSA) contributing to asthma/OSA overlap syndrome. COPD, Chronic obstructive pulmonary disease.

Sleep and Breathing Pathophysiology of Chronic Obstructive Pulmonary Disease/Obstructive Sleep Apnea Overlap Syndrome

Because obesity also reduces FRC during sleep, overweight/obese patients with COPD/OSA overlap syndrome are particularly subject to a reduction of alveolar volume and greater gas exchange abnormalities during sleep apneas and hypopneas (Figure 137.3). Further, respiratory control center output is reduced during sleep, especially during REM sleep,[34] including blunted ventilatory responses and mouth occlusion pressure responses to CO_2.[35] During obstructive apneic episodes, to overcome the upper airway resistance and to maintain adequate airflow to the lung, increased diaphragmatic and abdominal muscle effort is required. This can be particularly difficult in patients with COPD who already have increased intrathoracic airway resistance and lung hyperinflation at baseline. When patients with COPD develop such obstructive apnea episodes, the compensatory response of the respiratory center is slower, apneas are longer, and changes in PaO_2 and PaO_2 are more intense compared with non-COPD subjects. Patients with COPD/OSA overlap syndrome who have awake hypoxemia are especially prone to nocturnal oxygen desaturation by being on the steep portion of the oxyhemoglobin dissociation curve.

Clinical Features of Chronic Obstructive Pulmonary Disease/Obstructive Sleep Apnea Overlap Syndrome

Compared with patients with COPD alone or OSA alone, overlap patients of similar ages tend to be more obese and to have more comorbid conditions.[36] They also report more daytime sleepiness[28] and poorer quality of life[37] than patients with either COPD or OSA without overlap syndrome. Sleep recordings of patients with COPD/OSA overlap show a lower total sleep time, lower sleep efficiency, and greater sleep fragmentation than those with COPD or OSA alone. More severe nocturnal O_2 desaturation is also a typical feature in patients with COPD/OSA overlap compared with either condition alone. Subjects with OSA alone return to a normal O_2 saturation (SaO_2) in sleep between obstructive events (i.e., intermittent hypoxemia), whereas in COPD alone, as a result of the diathesis to sleep-related hypoventilation and ventilation-perfusion mismatch as noted before, nocturnal O_2 saturation characteristically decreases more evenly throughout sleep and at the termination of an apnea or hypopnea episode tends not to return to the initial baseline level (Figure 137.4). A typical patient with COPD/OSA overlap syndrome has a reduced awake and asleep baseline SaO_2, a lower mean sleep-related SaO_2, and a longer time with hypoxemia than patients with OSA or COPD alone.

The majority of patients with OSA alone do not develop significant sleep-related hypercapnia because of interapnea hyperventilation. However, if the patient also has COPD, the abnormal mechanical and chemical ventilatory responses

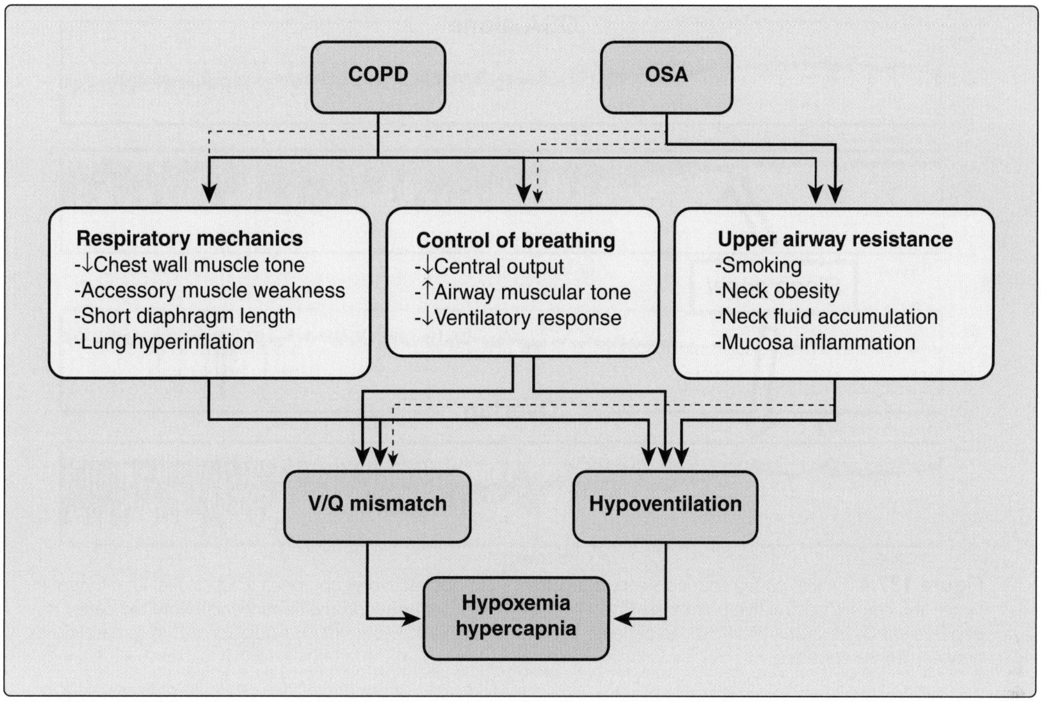

Figure 137.3 Pathways involved in producing sleep-related hypoxemia and hypercapnia in chronic obstructive pulmonary disease (COPD)/obstructive sleep apnea (OSA) overlap syndrome.

as noted before may result in post-apnea CO_2 levels that do not return to baseline. Over time, progressive desensitization of the respiratory center in response to OSA-related hypoxic-hypercapnic episodes develops, such that patients with COPD/OSA overlap syndrome can remain hypercapnic during sleep.[38] Of note, continuous positive airway pressure (CPAP) treatment for the OSA (see Diagnosis and Management of COPD/OSA Overlap Syndrome) can partially reverse this phenomenon.[39] Although daytime hypercapnia can develop in OSA without COPD, awake hypercapnia is much more frequent in the patient with overlap syndrome.[40] Both daytime hypoxemia and hypercapnia are predictors of right-sided heart failure in patients with COPD,[41] and therefore these should be considered potentially treatable markers of otherwise poorer prognosis in COPD/OSA overlap.

Excessive sleepiness in patients with OSA alone is associated with decrements in school and work performance.[42] Further, there is also a strong association between OSA severity, as measured by the AHI, and the risk of traffic accidents.[43] It is reasonable to expect that in patients with COPD/OSA overlap syndrome, such performance decrements and risks reflect the sum of the severity of the sleep disorders of both entities, but such consequences of the COPD/OSA overlap syndrome have not been evaluated specifically. Similarly, whereas OSA is considered an independent risk factor for insulin resistance, with OSA severity predicting risk for incident diabetes,[44] neither COPD alone nor COPD/OSA overlap has been specifically linked with risk of metabolic disorders.

Both OSA and COPD alone are associated with an increased risk of cardiovascular morbidity and mortality.[45] In COPD alone, however, arterial hypertension prevalence is similar to that of the general population, and patients with COPD/OSA overlap appear to have the same prevalence rates as patients with OSA alone.[36] Untreated OSA patients are also particularly susceptible to the development of atrial fibrillation,[46] as are patients with COPD alone, likely related to nocturnal O_2 desaturation.[47,48] A community-based retrospective cohort analysis, including data collected on 2873 patients older than 65 years, confirmed an increased risk of new-onset atrial fibrillation in COPD/OSA overlap syndrome compared with OSA or COPD alone.[49]

Epidemiologic data indicate that incidence of coronary artery disease, stroke, and heart failure is increased in OSA[15,16,50] and COPD[51]; no such incidence data are available for COPD/OSA overlap. However, Chaouat and colleagues demonstrated that patients with COPD/OSA overlap syndrome have increased daytime pulmonary vascular resistance compared with patients with OSA alone,[26] whereas Sharma and colleagues recently documented a higher right ventricular mass and remodeling indices in overlap syndrome compared with patients with COPD alone.[52] In addition, arterial stiffness, a surrogate marker of subclinical atherosclerosis, has also been found to be significantly higher in subjects with COPD/OSA overlap than in those with OSA alone.[53] Finally, whereas increased oxidative stress is associated with both COPD and OSA, with evidence of increased circulating proinflammatory cytokines and leukocytes in both disorders, no specific data exist regarding COPD/OSA overlap syndrome and risk and prevalence of such oxidative stress compared with COPD or OSA alone. Key risk factors for endothelial dysfunction, atherosclerosis, and ultimately cardiovascular diseases are depicted in Figure 137.5.

In both COPD alone and OSA alone, the risk of excess all-cause mortality increases in association with increasing severity of these disorders. The excess of mortality is most marked in younger individuals with OSA[54] and in more elderly patients with COPD.[55] Overall, evidence indicates that mortality is increased in patients with COPD/OSA overlap. For

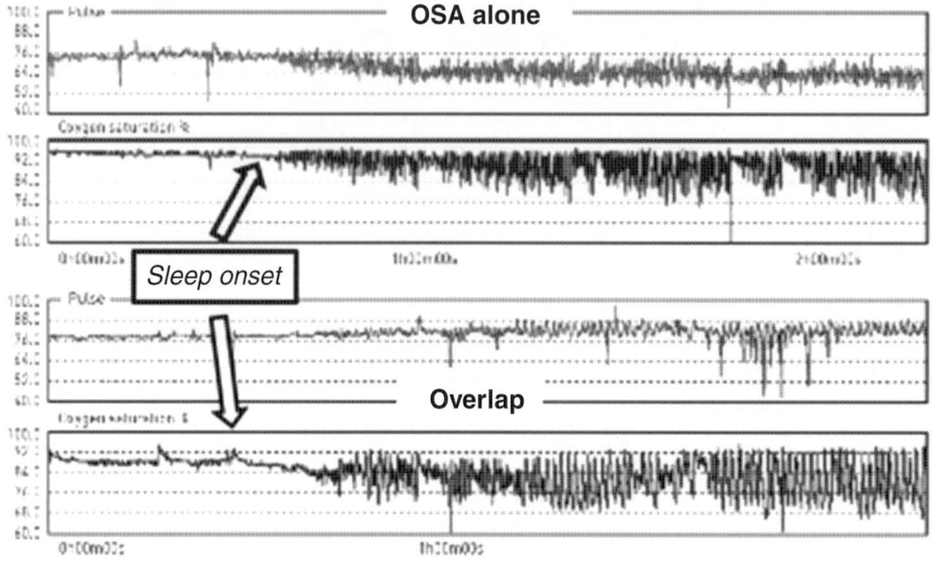

Figure 137.4 Typical pattern during sleep of a patient with obstructive sleep apnea (OSA) alone: OSA (*upper panel*) and chronic obstructive pulmonary disease (COPD)/OSA overlap syndrome (*lower panel*). Note the pattern of persistent O_2 desaturation in overlap patients, in contrast to the OSA patients O_2 saturation return to baseline between apnea episodes.

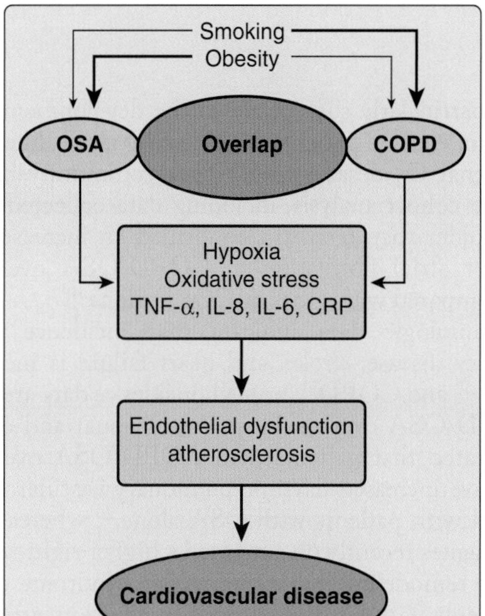

Figure 137.5 Schematic that illustrates potential pathways involved in producing accelerated cardiovascular disease as a result of obstructive sleep apnea (OSA), chronic obstructive pulmonary disease (COPD), and COPD/OSA overlap syndrome. CRP, C-reactive protein; IL, interleukin.

example, in patients with OSA studied at sleep clinics, the coexistence of COPD has been found to increase the risk of death compared with patients with OSA alone.[56] We have recently confirmed this in a large cohort of patients with an average age of 57 years, referred with suspected SDB. In addition to polysomnography (PSG), all patients underwent spirometry as a routine procedure,[36] During a median follow-up period of more than 9 years, all-cause mortality was higher in the overlap group untreated for OSA (42.2%) than in the COPD-only group (24.2%) (Figure 137.6). In the patients with COPD, comorbid untreated OSA remained a risk factor for death even after adjustment for FEV_1 percentage predicted as a surrogate of COPD severity. There was a significantly higher number of cardiovascular deaths in patients with COPD only and untreated overlap syndrome compared with overlap patients treated appropriately for their OSA with CPAP. Interestingly, the second most frequent cause of death was cancer in patients with both OSA and COPD alone.[57,58]

Nocturnal death risk appears to be increased in COPD compared with the general population, mainly during COPD exacerbations.[59] NH, an important pathophysiologic feature of OSA, is associated with sudden cardiac death (SCD). Gami and colleagues[60] reported on 10,701 consecutive adults undergoing diagnostic PSG and sought to identify the risk of SCD associated with OSA. During an average follow-up of 5.3 years, 142 patients had resuscitated or fatal SCD. Independently of well-established risk factors, SCD was best predicted by age older than 60 years, AHI above 20, mean nocturnal SaO_2 below 93%, and nadir nocturnal SaO_2 below 78%. No data are available in this study regarding the risk of nocturnal death in patients with COPD/OSA overlap versus COPD or OSA alone. Nevertheless, the report by McNicholas and FitzGerald[59] documented that nocturnal death was higher among patients admitted for acute exacerbation of chronic bronchitis or emphysema than in patients admitted for other causes. It is possible that increased sympathetic activity along with a reduction in the delivery of oxygen to the myocardium can increase the risk of arrhythmias and mortality during nighttime hours in patients with COPD. Whether the coexistence of OSA (i.e., COPD/OSA overlap) increases this risk remains unknown.

Diagnosis and Management of Chronic Obstructive Pulmonary Disease/Obstructive Sleep Apnea Overlap Syndrome

In the absence of overlap-specific symptoms, the diagnosis of COPD/OSA overlap syndrome requires PSG and spirometry. PSG should be considered in patients with COPD "when OSA is suspected because of either symptoms or the development of hypoxemic complications—cor pulmonale and polycythemia—with daytime PaO_2 greater than 60 mm Hg."[61] In-laboratory all-night PSG is the preferred sleep study for COPD patients and suspected SRBD to accurately capture both non–rapid eye movement and rapid eye movement pathology.

The therapeutic management of identified COPD/OSA overlap syndrome patients should, in general, be based on optimizing treatment for both conditions (COPD and OSA) following corresponding clinical recommendations.[1,43] The goal of such therapy includes improvement in subjective outcomes, such as sleep fragmentation, sleep quality, and daytime sleepiness, as well as optimization of more objective data regarding daytime alertness and function and COPD- and OSA-specific cardiopulmonary outcomes, such as frequency of COPD exacerbation.

Positive airway pressure (PAP) delivery with a nasal or face mask, is the most effective treatment for OSA. Continuous PAP (CPAP) is the optimal PAP therapy for most patients with OSA; bilevel PAP, which delivers a higher pressure during inspiration than during expiration, may also be used if a pressure gradient that increases alveolar ventilation is necessary, effective, and tolerated.

In COPD, noninvasive ventilation (NIV) in a specifically ventilatory mode (usually bilevel PAP) is consistently shown to be highly effective in the setting of acute and acute-on-chronic hypercapnic respiratory insufficiency. In contrast, data regarding the effects of NIV on quality of life, lung function, gas exchange, and long-term survival have been contradictory when it is used in the chronic setting in patients with COPD, in part because of the absence of studies of sufficient power and duration,[62] In the United States, NIV is reimbursed for patients with severe COPD and all the following criteria: (1) OSA has been ruled out; (2) awake $PaCO_2$ is 52 mm Hg or higher; and (3) sleep oximetry shows SaO_2 of 88% or less for 5 minutes or more while breathing supplemental O2 at 2 L/minute or at the patient's prescribed FiO_2.[63]

Data have now accrued specific to COPD/OSA overlap syndrome regarding nocturnal PAP, specifically CPAP. In a long-term cohort study, overlap syndrome patients not treated with CPAP demonstrated both an increased risk of death from any cause and an increased risk of hospitalization for COPD exacerbation compared with overlap patients who were treated with and adhered to CPAP.[36] In another observational study, the use of CPAP added to long-term oxygen therapy improved survival among overlap patients with chronic respiratory failure.[64] Finally, a retrospective analysis of 227 patients with COPD/OSA overlap syndrome treated with CPAP revealed that greater time on CPAP was associated with a reduced risk of death after controlling for common risk factors.[65]

The choice between CPAP (preferred for OSA) and bilevel PAP (possibly preferred for hypoventilation) can be determined during the titration session, based on the pattern of SDB. Nevertheless, there is no specific evidence in the literature of the superiority of CPAP or bilevel PAP for the treatment of patients with COPD/OSA overlap syndrome regarding long-term outcomes. Supplemental oxygen should be added to the mask or the PAP circuit if the otherwise optimal-appearing PAP regimen (whether CPAP or bilevel PAP) alone fails to provide satisfactory oxygenation. The ideal setting in which to adjust these parameters is the sleep laboratory, and such "titrations" should be conducted by well-trained technicians with the design, guidance, and interpretation of clinicians with sleep breathing expertise. Transcutaneous CO_2 tracking during titration is ideal.

In most patients with COPD alone, NH, when present, is corrected with supplemental O_2 through a nasal cannula. Nevertheless, alveolar ventilation of such patients is particularly dependent on the peripheral stimulant effect of hypoxemia. Therefore, to minimize the tendency toward CO_2 retention, particularly during sleep hours, such O_2 supplementation should be titrated carefully. The emergence of morning headache after O_2 initiation in patients with COPD is an indication to perform a PSG study to exclude the coexistence of OSA or to investigate the development of CO_2 retention. In OSA, supplemental oxygen treatment without PAP can eliminate or reduce NH, but it does not reduce the AHI, daytime hypersomnolence,[66] or nocturnal blood pressure.[67] The role of oxygen supplementation as a solo nocturnal therapy in COPD/OSA overlap syndrome has not been sufficiently explored.

No specific studies have been conducted on sleep quality, SDB, or long-term clinical outcomes to evaluate the effects of pharmacologic treatment in patients with COPD/OSA overlap syndrome. The most common drugs currently prescribed in stable COPD, such as long-acting anticholinergics and long-acting beta-agonists, have been shown to improve nocturnal O_2 saturation but not the quality of sleep.[68,69] Theophylline, potentially useful for patients with COPD and SDB as a central respiratory stimulant with enhancement of the activity of the respiratory muscles,[70] is currently not clearly shown to be efficacious in improving COPD-related sleep breathing disorders or perturbed quality of sleep. Inhaled corticosteroids used in patients with stable COPD have not been specifically linked with either enhanced or decreased sleep continuity. Benzodiazepine sleep aids are typically avoided in patients with COPD and OSA. There is evidence that nonbenzodiazepine hypnotics do not decrease respiratory drive and do not cause daytime drowsiness.[71]

The role of surgery in the treatment of COPD/OSA overlap, as well as the need for special precautions regarding preoperative and postoperative evaluation and care in such patients undergoing surgery for treatment of their COPD or OSA, including lung transplant, lung volume reduction, upper airway surgery, and bariatric surgery, also remains to be established.

ASTHMA

The Global Initiative for Asthma (GINA) in its last version of 2021, defined asthma as a heterogeneous disease, usually characterized by chronic airway inflammation. It is defined by a history of respiratory symptoms such as wheeze, shortness of breath, chest tightness, and cough that vary over time and in intensity, together with variable expiratory airflow limitation (https://ginasthma.org/wp-content/uploads/2021/05/GINA-Main-Report-2021-V2-WMS.pdf).[71a] Asthma and OSA have links in common. If bronchial inflammation is a hallmark of asthma, inflammation of the upper airway plays an important role in the pathogenesis of OSA.[72] According to a report from the National Health and Nutrition Examination

Survey, in 2011-2014, current asthma prevalence was 8.8% among adults in the United States. Of interest, it was higher among adults with obesity (11.1%) compared with adults of normal weight (7.1%).[73]

Sleep has a deep impact on the morbidity and mortality of patients with asthma. Classical studies linked nocturnal asthma to an increased risk of mortality, with 70% of deaths and 80% of respiratory arrests caused by asthma occurring during nocturnal hours.[74] The normal physiologic changes that affect the lung during sleep and how those changes may contribute to nocturnal asthma have been reviewed in depth.[75] Nocturnal asthma is characterized by coughing, wheezing, or dyspnea that interrupts and disturbs sleep, with such patients complaining of frequent arousals and poor sleep quality.[76] Nocturnal asthma generally indicates poor control of asthma and the need to modify overall asthmatic treatment. Sleep studies done when current asthma treatment was not available showed lower sleep efficiency, more awakenings, and less stage 3 to 4 sleep in subjects with asthma compared with those without.[77] Cognitive performance, as tested by psychometric testing, has also been shown to be impaired in patients with nocturnal asthma.[78] Circadian peak expiratory flow variation of 20% or more, a surrogate parameter of asthma instability, has been associated with poorer daytime cognitive performance compared with healthy control subjects.[79] Effective asthma treatment resulted in the recovery of cognitive impairment to a level of performance comparable to that of the healthy control subjects, paralleled by a reduction of circadian peak expiratory flow variation below 10% and by the resolution of nocturnal asthma symptoms.

Asthma and Obstructive Sleep Apnea Overlap Syndrome

Epidemiology

The occurrence of OSA in patients with asthma shows a prevalence of OSA two to three times higher than patients without asthma both in larger population studies using sleep questionnaires and in cross-sectional studies using PSG.[80-81] Of interest for clinicians, as asthma worsens, patients are at greater risk of OSA. PSG-diagnosed OSA is present in most patients with severe asthma.[81] Conversely, OSA increases asthma burden and is associated with poor asthma control. It appears that OSA aggravates asthma through non-eosinophilic inflammatory pathways independent of obesity and other confounders.[82] Thus OSA may be a contributor to neutrophilic asthma and PSG should be considered in this asthma phenotype. On the other hand, the GINA initiative recommended investigation for the coexistence of OSA (i.e., asthma/OSA overlap syndrome) in all patients with asthma, especially in those with severe asthma, difficult to control asthma, and asthma with associated obesity.

Pathophysiology and Risk Factors for Asthma/Obstructive Sleep Apnea Overlap Syndrome

Obesity is a risk factor for both asthma and OSA and therefore for asthma/OSA overlap syndrome. There is a "dose-response" effect of increasing BMI on increasing the risk of incident asthma, especially in women.[83] Many patients with nonatopic asthma and most patients with atopic asthma suffer from nasal obstruction resulting from rhinitis and chronic sinusitis, which cause nasal congestion and airflow resistance, and nasopharyngeal polyps, which reduce airway caliber. These lead to increasing intrathoracic and pharyngeal negative pressure, which promotes upper airway collapse during inspiration, snoring, and obstructive apnea.[84] Similarly, in patients with chronic asthma, persistent mucosal inflammation affects the upper airway by decreasing the cross-sectional area of the pharynx, promoting upper airway collapse.[85]

Inhaled corticosteroids are the most effective and most widely used drugs in asthma. Their long-term effects on the collapsibility of the pharynx remain unknown. However, the effects of oral corticosteroids on the upper airway are well known and are generally adverse, including myopathy of the muscles of the pharynx, fatty infiltration of the pharyngeal wall, and accumulation of liquid in the neck. In asthma clinics, patients with asthma requiring frequent bursts or consistent use of oral corticosteroids were found to have a high prevalencc of OSA (>90%) after adjustment for BMI and neck circumference.[86]

Factors potentially effective in reducing the risk and severity of OSA in patients with asthma include the same factors as in the case of patients with COPD/OSA overlap: weight loss, sleep in the lateral decubitus position, and smoking cessation. The effect of adjusting asthma medications to improve concomitant OSA has not been studied. In nonasthmatic patients with OSA, there is both molecular and clinical evidence of the ability of inhaled corticosteroids to reduce upper airway inflammation and to improve AHI in a subgroup of patients with concomitant allergic rhinitis.[87] Nasally inhaled corticosteroids and oral anti-leukotrienes may reduce snoring and obstructive apneas in children with asthma and OSA. Figure 137.7 shows these complex interactions.

The potential mechanisms by which OSA may worsen asthma are also multifactorial. Obstructive apneic episodes are associated with repetitive arousals from sleep, perturbations in

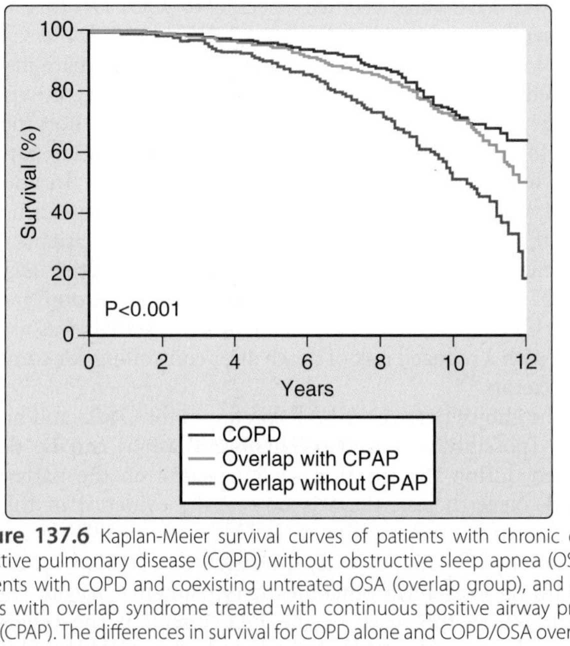

Figure 137.6 Kaplan-Meier survival curves of patients with chronic obstructive pulmonary disease (COPD) without obstructive sleep apnea (OSA), patients with COPD and coexisting untreated OSA (overlap group), and patients with overlap syndrome treated with continuous positive airway pressure (CPAP). The differences in survival for COPD alone and COPD/OSA overlap syndrome treated with CPAP are statistically different compared with patients with untreated overlap syndrome ($P < 0.001$).

autonomic activity, and intermittent hypoxemia.[43] Increased vagal tone during obstructive apnea episodes can contribute to nocturnal asthma through stimulation of muscarinic receptors of the central and upper airways. Negative intrathoracic pressure during obstructive events leads to intermittent loss of lower esophageal sphincter tone; associated gastroesophageal reflux is associated with bronchial microaspiration of gastric acid, potentially promoting nocturnal asthma.[88] By stimulation of carotid body receptors, intermittent hypoxia can enhance bronchial responsiveness through vagal pathways.[89] Chronic intermittent hypoxia in OSA may also induce a low-grade systemic inflammation characterized by the elevation of serum proinflammatory cytokines and chemokines. Local inflammatory changes of the upper airways similar to those noted in asthma are also prominent in OSA. Such inflammatory changes may reduce airway caliber and at the same time increase underlying bronchial hyperresponsiveness, thus representing a potential asthma trigger.

Clinical Outcomes and Treatment in Asthma/Sleep-Disordered Breathing Overlap Syndrome

There are no long-term studies of comorbid OSA and asthma and thus no current specific guidelines. However, in patients with asthma/COPD overlap, OSA treatment with CPAP has important potential pathophysiologic beneficial effects for patients with asthma, including reducing gastroesophageal reflux, airway and systemic inflammation, and airway smooth muscle contractility.[89] Data do exist documenting that CPAP treatment for comorbid OSA improves asthma symptoms, decreases the use of rescue medication, and improves asthma-specific quality of life.[90-93] Further, in a short-term randomized trial, CPAP use decreased airway reactivity in patients with asthma without OSA, possibly through reducing bronchial inflammation.[94]

Second-line treatments for OSA, such as mandibular advancement devices and upper airway surgery, have not been prospectively evaluated in patients with asthma/OSA overlap. However, bariatric surgery for patients with OSA and morbid obesity may be effective not only for OSA resolution but also for improving asthma.[95] There are no published studies assessing clinical outcomes related to the use of asthma medications in asthma/OSA overlap syndrome. At this time, therefore, it appears that asthma in patients with OSA should be treated according to current asthma treatment guidelines in addition to optimizing treatment of the comorbid OSA.

INTERSTITIAL LUNG DISEASE

ILD comprises over 200 nonmalignant, noninfectious lung entities. All ILD are characterized by cellular inflammatory proliferation and fibrotic changes affecting alveolar and airspaces. The term idiopathic pulmonary fibrosis (IPF) is defined when no cause of ILD is identified. IPF is the most common ILD, affecting primarily older adults, and has the worse prognosis of all ILD.[96] Most patients present with exertional dyspnea, dry cough, or Velcro-like crackles on chest examination. Frequent physiologic findings include low vital capacity and reduce the diffusing capacity of the lung for carbon monoxide and resting hypoxemia or exertional desaturation. The incidence and mortality of IPF appear to be increasing mainly because of improvements in the ability to diagnose the condition because of advances in chest imaging.[97]

Sleep quality is poor in patients with ILD, mainly because of cough, and breathlessness that disrupts the normal sleep architecture and ultimately contributes to daytime fatigue in this population.[98] Esophageal dysmotility and reflux, also prevalent in ILD, and the pulmonary fibrotic process itself are the main intermediate mechanisms that explain the nocturnal cough. In a short and old study, and compared with control subjects, Perez-Padilla and colleagues reported worse sleep quality in patients with ILD, with more time in stage N1 (33.7% of total sleep time versus 13.5%), less time in REM sleep (11.8% versus 19.9% of total sleep time), and more fragmentation of sleep.[99] In this study, patients with awake hypoxemia ($SaO_2 < 90\%$) had greater abnormalities in sleep structure than did those with SaO_2 above 90%. Recently, in a cross-sectional analysis, 101 patients with a diagnosis of ILD were evaluated with the Pittsburgh Sleep Quality Index (PSQI) as a sleep quality tool.[100] It was found that sleep quality was very poor and independently associated with increasing symptoms of depression and sleepiness.

Hypoxemia during sleep is also common and tends to be worse in those with more severe daytime hypoxemia.[99] During REM sleep, O_2 desaturation is often more severe than that occurring during exercise.[101] The role of nocturnal desaturation on health outcomes in patients with ILD has been evaluated retrospectively in a large cohort of patients with ILD.[102] In this study, the desaturation index (DI) was defined as the number of desaturation events above 4%/hour. Desaturation was present in 37% of patients, and 31% of them had PH on echocardiography. Increased DI was associated with higher mortality independent of age, gender, BMI, and PH. If NH is detected, it is reasonable to treat these patients with oxygen therapy.

Interstitial Lung Disease and Obstructive Sleep Apnea Overlap Syndrome

OSA is prevalent in ILD but underrecognized. In a sample of 50 patients with stable ILD, OSA was confirmed with PSG in 88%.[103] Of those, 68% were moderate to severe (AHI >15 events per hour of sleep). It appears that the severity of OSA, as indicated by AHI, inversely correlates with total lung capacity and, interestingly, poorly correlates with BMI.[103] Observational data have implicated OSA in ILD. In the Multi-Ethnic Study of Atherosclerosis (MESA), community-dwelling adults underwent PSG and CT scan; 32% had an AHI greater than 15.[104] Moderate to severe OSA was associated with subclinical ILD and with evidence of alveolar epithelial injury and extracellular matrix remodeling. These findings support the hypothesis that OSA may contribute to early ILD. Treatment of OSA with CPAP appears to improve health status in patients with ILD. In a single study with newly diagnosed IPF and moderate-to-severe OSA, there was a significant improvement in the Epworth Sleepiness Scale (ESS), PSQI in those patients treated with CPAP.[105]

PULMONARY HYPERTENSION

PH is defined as an increase in mean pulmonary artery pressure (mPAP) at least 25 mm Hg at rest, measured by right heart catheterization. The current classification of PH consists of five categories: (1) primary pulmonary arterial hypertension; (2) PH resulting from left-sided heart disease; (3) PH associated with chronic pulmonary diseases, such as COPD and OSA; (4) chronic thromboembolic PH; and (5) PH resulting from various disorders, such as sarcoidosis or systemic vasculitis.[106]

Pulmonary Hypertension and Sleep-Disordered Breathing Overlap Syndrome

Epidemiology

There are limited data evaluating the association between OSA and PH. One study conducted to determine the prevalence and significance of nocturnal oxygen desaturation in patients with PH, using home oximetry studies, showed that 69.7% of patients spent more than 10% of sleep time with SaO_2 below 90%.[107] NH correlates with advanced PH and right ventricular dysfunction. Interestingly, 60% of this subgroup with NH had no exertional hypoxemia. In a small study of patients with idiopathic PH who had full PSG, Schulz and colleagues found that 30% of these patients had periodic breathing, defined as a crescendo-decrescendo pattern of hyperventilatory phases alternating with central apneas or hypopneas of at least three consecutive cycles.[108] Most of these patients, however, had normal nocturnal oximetry. In another study of 38 patients with PH who had ambulatory cardiorespiratory sleep studies, 18 (47%) had an AHI exceeding 10 events per hour.[109] A subgroup of 22 patients also had in-laboratory PSG. Among patients who underwent both studies, home sleep studies accurately predicted an AHI of 10 events or more during PSG (area under the receiver operating characteristic curve, 0.93; $P = .002$). However, the corresponding value for pulse oximetry was 0.63 (P = not significant). Therefore, when SDB is suspected among patients with PH, evaluation should include full PSG or modified cardiorespiratory sleep studies rather than pulse oximetry alone.

In the largest series of patients with confirmed precapillary PH by right heart catheterization, home cardiorespiratory sleep studies demonstrated that, among 169 patients, 26.6% had an AHI of more than 10.[110] Of these, 27 patients (i.e., 16%) had OSA and 18 patients (i.e., 10.6%) had central sleep apnea. High-altitude pulmonary hypertension (HAPH) is a particular kind of PH that affects permanent residents at altitudes greater than 2500 m. The prevalence of SRBD and clinical characteristics of highlanders with and without HAPH in comparison to those in healthy lowlanders has been recently studied.[111] In a case-control study of highlanders living at altitudes exceeding 2500 meters without polycythemia, those with HAPH had a higher AHI (mean: 33.8 events/hour) and spent a greater percentage of the nighttime with an O_2 saturation below 90% (mean: 78%) than highlanders without PH (9.0 events/hour, and 33% O_2 saturation < 90%, respectively). Multivariable regression analysis confirmed an independent association between mPAP and both AHI and CT90, when controlled for age, gender, and body mass index. That is, intermittent hypoxemia resulting from OSA is an important determinant of PH in high-altitude residents. From all of these studies, it seems that the prevalence of PH/SDB overlap appears to be higher in PH patients than that in the general population.

Clinical Features of Pulmonary Hypertension/Sleep-Disordered Breathing Overlap Syndrome

The extent to which SDB contributes to the PH patient's symptoms and disease progression is unclear. In a retrospective review of 52 consecutive patients with PH referred for assessment of possible SDB, 71% had SDB.[109] Patients with PH only and those with PH/SDB overlap showed no differences in cardiopulmonary hemodynamics at baseline assessed by right-sided heart catheterization. After a median follow-up of 4.7 years, no differences in survival between those with and without SDB were observed. There are no specific clinical features in patients with PH/SDB overlap syndrome compared to patients with PH alone. Similar to heart failure, there was a lack of subjective daytime sleepiness as assessed by the Epworth Sleepiness Scale in patients with PH/SDB overlap,[107,109,111] possibly explained by elevated sympathetic nervous activity in both heart failure and PH that can act as an adrenergic cortical alerting mechanism.[112,113] Predictors of SDB in patients with PH do not differ from those of the general population, being mainly older age and BMI.[107-111]

Pathophysiology and Outcomes in Pulmonary Hypertension/Sleep-Disordered Breathing Overlap Syndrome

Coexistent OSA may contribute to the worsening of underlying PH. During obstructive events, negative intrathoracic pressures result in right ventricular overload.[114] This could be aggravated by intermittent hypoxia and elevated sympathetic nervous activity that typically occurs during sleep in patients with OSA. However, although dysfunction of the autonomic nervous system modulation assessed by heart rate variability was demonstrated in patients with PH and OSA, the presence of OSA in patients with PH did not appear to further reduce vagal modulation.[115] In addition to weight gain or use of oral steroids, patients with PH are more predisposed to the development of OSA if they accumulate fluid in the neck during sleep.[116] Such a rostral shift of fluid from the legs during the daytime to the neck at night has been demonstrated in patients with left ventricular failure[117] (Figure 137.8).

No studies have evaluated the prognosis of PH/SDB overlap. However, the presence of PH may have prognostic importance in patients with OSA; for example, an observational study of 83 patients with OSA (AHI > 5) who underwent pulmonary artery catheterization for unspecified reasons documented 1-, 4-, and 8-year survival rates that were lower among patients with PH (mean pulmonary artery pressure > 25 mm Hg at rest) than among those without PH.[118] Kusunose and colleagues examined the predictive

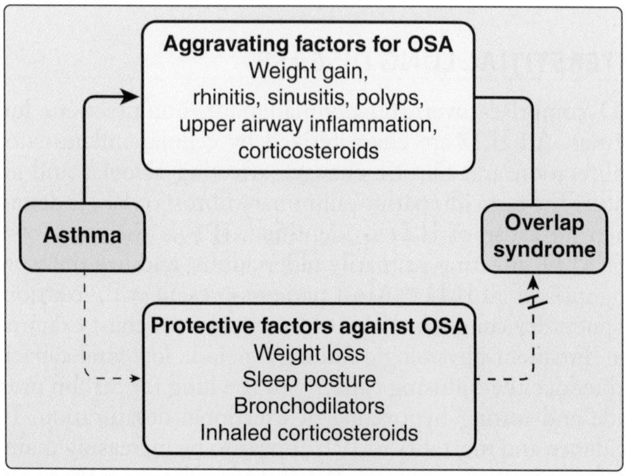

Figure 137.7 Interactions between asthma and obstructive sleep apnea (OSA) contributing to asthma/OSA overlap syndrome.

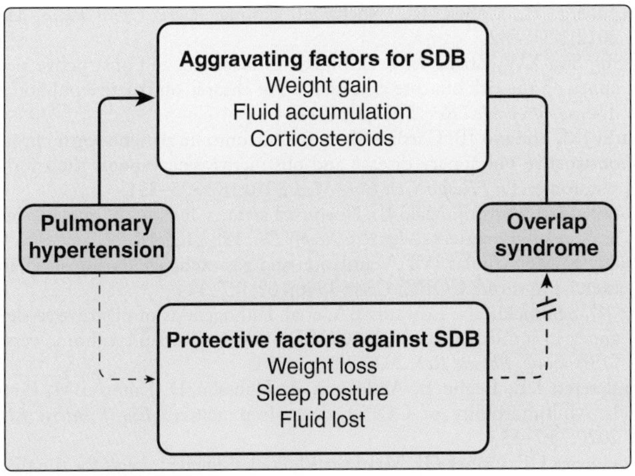

Figure 137.8 Interactions between pulmonary hypertension and sleep-disordered breathing (SDB).

value of right-sided cardiac functional alterations on echocardiography in SDB patients with preserved left ventricular ejection fraction.[119] They found that after a mean follow-up of 3.1 years that the presence of right heart dysfunction at baseline predicted the composite outcome of heart failure or death. No studies have systematically evaluated the effect of SDB treatment on PH/SDB overlap syndrome outcomes. Patients with PH should be evaluated by PSG when presenting with symptoms that suggest the coexistence of SDB and treated per standards.

Despite known limitations, the AHI has dominated research on OSA/respiratory disease overlap. Machine learning and clustering approaches currently being applied to OSA[120] may provide novel and clinically meaningful insights or biomarkers.

INSOMNIA IN PULMONARY DISEASES

According to the American Academy of Sleep Medicine (AASM), insomnia is defined as a history of frequent difficulty in initiating or maintaining sleep and significant disruption of daytime functioning for at least 1 month.[121] Despite being considered a serious public health problem that affects 10% of the general population,[122,123] there has been little interest in the study of insomnia in pulmonary disorders. Specifically, there are no data on the prevalence and burden of insomnia in patients with PH or ILD. In COPD older studies reported a high prevalence of self-reported insomnia that appears related to the severity of the respiratory symptoms compared with subjects without COPD.[124,125] Using the AASM criteria, Budhiraja and colleagues interviewed 183 patients with COPD about their sleep.[125] Insomnia was present in 27.3% of participants. The severity of COPD as assessed by pulmonary function test ($FEV_1 < 50\%$ predicted) or by the Medical Research Council dyspnea scale was not different among participants with insomnia or without insomnia. Interestingly, the presence of insomnia was associated with increased daytime sleepiness and worse quality of life. There are no studies that have evaluated the causality of factors associated with insomnia in patients with COPD or that have evaluated the insomnia as a determinant of health outcomes in COPD.

Treating chronic insomnia in patients with COPD is challenging. Because of the prevalence of insomnia, it is common that patients with COPD request medicines to improve their quality of sleep. Benzodiazepines should be avoided if possible in patients with COPD because they may reduce alveolar ventilation, decrease arousal response, and increase apnea frequency, and therefore they can worsen hypoxemia and hypercapnia.[126] Some non-benzodiazepine hypnotics such as zolpidem[127] and melatonin receptor antagonists, such as ramelteon,[128] have been reported to have no adverse effects on gas exchange in patients with COPD. Suvorexant, up to twice the maximum recommended dose, did not cause sleep breathing disorders in a multicenter, randomized, double-blind, placebo-controlled, cross-over study, in patients with mild-moderate COPD.[129] Physicians managing patients with COPD and insomnia should use preferably non-benzodiazepine hypnotics.

Studies indicate that the prevalence of insomnia among patients with asthma ranges from 44% to 70%.[130,131] The risk of insomnia increased with the severity of asthma.[131] Among adolescents from the general community, a survey reported that almost twice as many adolescents with severe asthma had clinically significant insomnia than adolescents with mild or no asthma.[132] Daytime sleepiness was frequent in this population, and 28% of its variance was accounted for by insomnia severity, whereas only 2% was accounted for by asthma severity. Conversely, in the Nord-Trøndelag Health Study, an ongoing health survey of the adult population (aged >20 years) in Norway, the risk of developing asthma in those with chronic insomnia was three times higher than in those without insomnia.[133] No specific treatment of insomnia for patients with asthma have been evaluated in clinical trials. In summary, insomnia remains a common problem among patients with asthma that should be addressed in any patient as part of his or her comprehensive treatment.

CLINICAL PEARLS

- Overlap of obstructive sleep apnea (OSA) with chronic obstructive pulmonary disease (COPD), the COPD/OSA overlap syndrome, affects more than 1% of adults. The prevalence of OSA overlap with asthma, the asthma/OSA overlap syndrome, and the prevalence of sleep-disordered breathing (SDB) overlap with pulmonary hypertension (PH), the SDB/PH overlap syndrome, are not well defined. Nevertheless, the coexistence of OSA in asthma and PH increases with increasing severity of both pulmonary disorders.
- Obesity increases the risk of OSA in populations with COPD and with asthma.
- Untreated OSA in COPD/OSA overlap is associated with worsened clinical outcomes for both the OSA and the comorbid pulmonary disorder. Conversely, effective identification and treatment of OSA reduces diurnal and nocturnal symptoms and improves clinical outcomes in patients with COPD/OSA overlap.

SUMMARY

OSA and COPD, each prevalent and clinically important conditions in adults, carry numerous common risk factors, including obesity and smoking. The COPD/OSA overlap syndrome affects more than 1% of the general population and carries a risk of more adverse diurnal and nocturnal physiologic and clinical outcomes, including greater sleep fragmentation, more severe NH, and increased overall mortality. Effective identification and treatment of the comorbid OSA, and the other features of SDB in the COPD/OSA overlap syndrome, improve overall clinical outcomes in the condition.

Asthma, ILD, and PH are also linked with OSA, and in the case of PH other types of SDB such as central sleep apnea and sleep-related hypoventilation, by common risk factors and mutually exacerbating pathophysiologic and clinical features. The prevalence of asthma overlap with OSA and PH overlap with SDB is not well defined but increases as the severity of both asthma and PH increases. Effective treatment of the comorbid OSA improves asthma-related and overall pathophysiologic and clinical outcomes of the asthma/OSA overlap syndrome, including airway and systemic inflammation, asthma control, and asthma-specific quality of life.

SELECTED READINGS

Chaouat A, Weitzenblum E, Krieger J, et al. Association of chronic obstructive pulmonary disease and sleep apnea syndrome. *Am J Respir Crit Care Med*. 1995;151:82–86.

Flenley DC. Sleep in chronic obstructive lung disease. *Clin Chest Med*. 1985;6:651–661.

Greenberg H, Cohen RI. Nocturnal asthma. *Curr Opin Pulm Med*. 2012;18:57–62.

Li SQ, Sun XW, Zhang L, et al. Impact of insomnia and obstructive sleep apnea on the risk of acute exacerbation of chronic obstructive pulmonary disease. *Sleep Med Rev*. 2021;58:101444.

Marin JM, Soriano JB, Carrizo SJ, et al. Outcomes in patients with chronic obstructive pulmonary disease and obstructive sleep apnea: the overlap syndrome. *Am J Respir Crit Care Med*. 2010;182:325–331

Montplaisir J, Walsh J, Malo JL. Nocturnal asthma: features of attacks, sleep and breathing patterns. *Am Rev Respir Dis*. 1982;125:18–22.

Mulloy E, McNicholas WT. Ventilation and gas exchange during sleep and exercise in severe COPD. *Chest*. 1996;109:387–394.

Orr JE, Schmickl CN, Edwards BA, et al. Pathogenesis of obstructive sleep apnea in individuals with the COPD + OSA Overlap syndrome versus OSA alone. *Physiol Rep*. 2020;8(3):e14371.

Vanfleteren LE, Beghe B, Andersson A, Hansson D, Fabbri LM, Grote L. Multimorbidity in COPD, does sleep matter? *Eur J Intern Med*. 2020;73:7–15.

Vogelmeier CF, Criner GJ, Martinez FJ, et al. Global strategy for the diagnosis, management, and prevention of chronic obstructive lung disease 2017 report. GOLD Executive Summary. *Am J Respir Crit Care Med*. 2017;195(5):557–582.

A complete reference list can be found online at ExpertConsult.com.

Chapter 138

Obesity-Hypoventilation Syndrome

Babak Mokhlesi; Renaud Tamisier

Chapter Highlights

- Obesity-hypoventilation syndrome (OHS) has been conventionally, and to some extent arbitrarily, defined by the combination of obesity and daytime hypercapnia during wakefulness occurring in the absence of an alternative neuromuscular, mechanical, or metabolic explanation for hypoventilation. This syndrome is also invariably accompanied by sleep-disordered breathing (e.g., obstructive sleep apnea or sleep hypoventilation) with a wide range of severity. Therefore sleep-disordered breathing is included as one of the diagnostic criteria in some definitions of OHS.
- During the last 3 decades the prevalence of extreme obesity has markedly increased in the United States and other countries. With such a global epidemic of obesity the prevalence of OHS is likely to increase.
- Patients with OHS have a lower quality of life with increased health care expenses and are at higher risk of developing pulmonary hypertension and early mortality as a result of cardiopulmonary complications, compared with similarly obese eucapnic patients with obstructive sleep apnea.
- OHS often remains undiagnosed until late in the course of the disease. Early recognition is important, as these patients have significant morbidity and mortality if left untreated. Effective treatment can lead to significant improvement in patient outcomes, underscoring the importance of early diagnosis.

HISTORICAL PERSPECTIVE

The association between obesity and hypersomnolence has long been recognized. Of historical interest, obesity-hypoventilation syndrome (OHS) was described well before obstructive sleep apnea (OSA) was recognized in 1969.[1-3] In 1955 Auchincloss and colleagues described in detail a case of obesity and hypersomnolence paired with alveolar hypoventilation.[4] One year later, Bickelmann and colleagues described a similar patient who finally sought treatment after his symptoms caused him to fall asleep during a hand of poker, despite having been dealt a full house of aces over kings.[5] Although other clinicians made the comparison some 50 years earlier,[6] Bickelmann popularized the term "Pickwickian syndrome" in his case report by noting the similarities between his patient and the boy Joe (Figure 138.1), Mr. Wardle's servant in Charles Dickens' *The Posthumous Papers of the Pickwick Club*.

DEFINITION

OHS has been conventionally, and to some extent arbitrarily, defined by the combination of obesity (body mass index [BMI] ≥ 30 kg/m^2) and daytime hypercapnia (partial pressure of arterial CO_2 or $Paco_2 \geq 45$ mm Hg at sea level) during wakefulness occurring in the absence of an alternative neuromuscular, mechanical, or metabolic explanation for hypoventilation. This syndrome is also invariably accompanied by sleep-disordered breathing (SDB), and therefore SDB is included as one of the diagnostic criteria in some expert definitions of OHS.[7]

Approximately 90% of patients with OHS have OSA defined by an apnea-hypopnea index (AHI) of at least five events per hour. In fact, close to 70% of patients have severe OSA with an AHI above 30.[8] The remaining patients have nonobstructive sleep hypoventilation. The American Academy of Sleep Medicine has arbitrarily defined sleep hypoventilation in adults by the following criteria: the $Paco_2$ (or surrogate such as end-tidal CO_2 or transcutaneous CO_2) is above 55 mm Hg for more than 10 minutes, or there is an increase in the $Paco_2$ (or surrogate) above 10 mm Hg compared to an awake supine value to a value exceeding 50 mm Hg for more than 10 minutes.[9] This point is relevant because, although the definition suggests a diurnal pathology, overnight polysomnography is required to determine the pattern of nocturnal SDB including hypoventilation (obstructive or nonobstructive) and to individualize therapy, particularly the optimal mode of positive airway pressure (PAP).

It is important to recognize that OHS is a diagnosis of exclusion and should be distinguished from other conditions that are commonly associated with hypercapnia (Box 138.1). A recent European Respiratory Society task force has proposed severity grading for OHS, including early stages defined by elevated bicarbonate level and/or sleep hypoventilation. The highest grade of severity was defined by daytime hypercapnia plus cardiovascular and metabolic comorbidities.[10] Such a statement suggests that comorbidities are of major importance because they impact health care resource utilization[11] and compromise the outcome of these patients.[12,13]

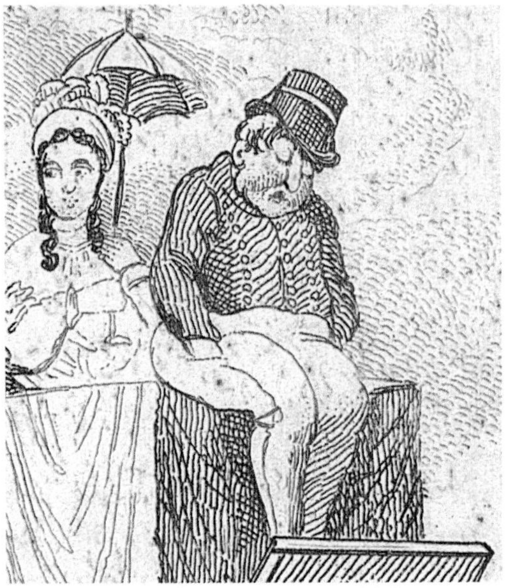

Figure 138.1 Joe the "Fat Boy," as depicted in Charles Dickens, *The Posthumous Papers of the Pickwick Club.* (London: Chapman and Hall, 1836.)

Box 138.1 DIAGNOSTIC FEATURES OF OBESITY-HYPOVENTILATION SYNDROME

Obesity

- Body mass index ≥ 30 kg/m^2

Chronic Hypoventilation

- Awake daytime hypercapnia (sea-level arterial P_{CO_2} ≥ 45 mm Hg)

Sleep-Disordered Breathing

- Obstructive sleep apnea (apnea-hypopnea index [AHI] ≥ 5 events/hour)
- Nonobstructive sleep hypoventilation is defined by AHI <5 events/hour and $PaCO_2$ (or a surrogate such as end-tidal PCO_2 or transcutaneous PCO_2) above 55 mm Hg for more than 10 minutes or an increase in the $PaCO_2$ (or surrogate) above 10 mm Hg compared to an awake supine value to a value exceeding 50 mm Hg for more than 10 minutes

Exclusion of Other Causes of Hypoventilation

- Severe obstructive airways disease (e.g., COPD)
- Severe interstitial lung disease
- Severe chest-wall disorders (e.g., kyphoscoliosis)
- Severe hypothyroidism
- Neuromuscular disease
- Congenital hypoventilation syndromes

EPIDEMIOLOGY

An "obesity epidemic" is present in many parts of the world and is associated with a myriad of comorbidities, including OHS. Severe obesity is a major risk factor for the development of OHS. In recent decades, the prevalence of obesity and severe obesity (Class III or BMI ≥ 40 kg/m^2) has increased worldwide.[14] The Centers for Disease Control and Prevention estimated that 7.6% of the adult United States population has a BMI of at least 40 kg/m^2.[15] Between 1987 and 2010 the prevalence of severe obesity increased by sixfold in the United States, affecting 1 in every 33 adults. Similarly, the prevalence of BMI at or exceeding 50 kg/m^2 has increased by 12-fold in the United States, affecting 1 in every 230 adults.[16] With such epidemic obesity, the prevalence of OHS is likely to increase.

Thirteen studies have reported a prevalence of OHS between 8% and 20% in patients referred to sleep centers for evaluation of SDB.[17-19] A meta-analysis of 4250 outpatients with obesity and OSA (mean BMI range between 30 and 44 kg/m^2 and mean AHI range between 40 to 60 events/hour)—who did not have chronic obstructive pulmonary disease—reported a 19% prevalence of awake hypercapnia.[20] Based on these data, approximately 19% of obese patients with OSA have OHS. East Asian populations are known to have OSA at a lower BMI compared with other populations, likely because of cephalometric differences.[21] Therefore, in these populations, OHS may be more prevalent at a lower BMI range than in non-Asian populations.[18,21-23] The prevalence of obesity-associated hypoventilation among consecutive patients with BMI exceeding 35 kg/m^2 hospitalized on medicine wards (excluding critical care units) has been reported to be 31%.[24] Although it remains unclear why the prevalence of obesity-associated hypoventilation in this hospitalized cohort was higher than the reported prevalence in outpatient obese patients with OSA, it may be related to the facts that the investigators enrolled subjects with a higher BMI (>35 kg/m^2 as opposed to >30 kg/m^2), and there was high prevalence of diuretic use (64% of the patients).

Prevalence estimates for OHS vary significantly across studies, owing partly to differences in sample characteristics, differences in disease definitions, and differences in assessment procedures.[17] In populations of patients with concomitant OSA, as the degree of obesity increases, the prevalence of OHS increases (Figure 138.2).[17] Laaban and colleagues[25] reported an OHS prevalence of 11% in a cohort of 1141 patients with OSA with a mean BMI of 30 kg/m^2, whereas Mokhlesi and colleagues[26] reported a prevalence of 24% in patients with OSA and a mean BMI of 44 kg/m^2. Among patients with OSA with BMI of 30 to 35 kg/m^2, the prevalence of OHS is 8% to 11% among non-Asian populations and increases to 18% to 31% among patients with OSA with BMI at or exceeding 40 kg/m^2.[25-28] The prevalence of OHS in the general population is unknown but can be estimated. The most recent report from the Centers for Disease Control and Prevention has estimated that approximately 6% of the general US adult population has morbid or severe obesity (BMI ≥ 40 kg/m^2).[29] If we conservatively estimate that half of patients with this degree of obesity have OSA and that approximately 20% of these patients with OSA have OHS, the prevalence of OHS can be estimated as roughly 0.6% (approximately 1 in 160 adults in the US population). In a general French population of mildly obese ambulatory patients (mean BMI approximately 35 kg/m^2) referred for routine blood tests, the estimated prevalence of OHS was 1.10% (95% CI 0.51, 2.27).[30] OHS may be more prevalent in the United States than in other nations because of its obesity epidemic. With such an epidemic, the prevalence of OHS is likely to increase. Therefore there is a need for a high index of suspicion on the part of clinicians to optimize early recognition and treatment of this syndrome.

CLINICAL PRESENTATION AND DIAGNOSIS

OHS is typically diagnosed either when an afflicted patient reaches a high state of acuity, in the form of acute-on-chronic

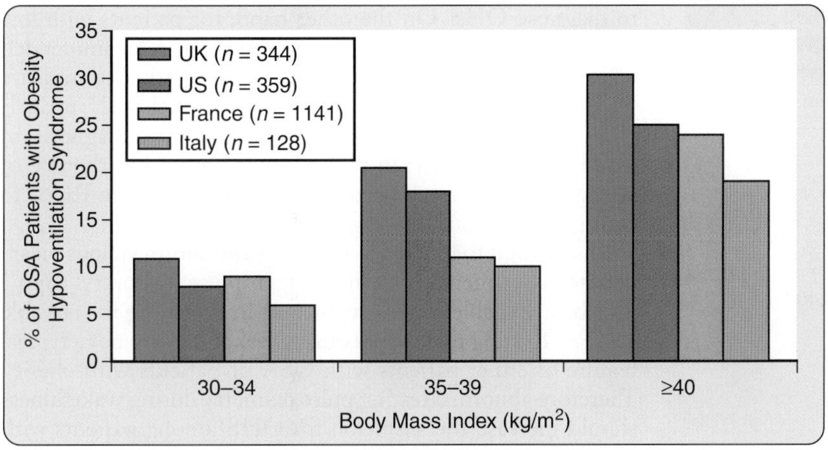

Figure 138.2 Prevalence of obesity-hypoventilation syndrome in patients with OSA, sorted by body mass index (BMI). In the UK study, the mean BMI was nearly 40 kg/m^2 and 38% of subjects had a BMI > 40 kg/m^2.[28] Similarly, in the US study, the mean BMI was 43 kg/m^2, and 60% of subjects had a BMI > 40 kg/m^2.[26] In contrast, the mean BMI in the French study was 34 kg/m^2, and only 15% of subjects had a BMI > 40 kg/m^2.[25] OSA, Obstructive sleep apnea. Italian data were provided by Professor Onofrio Resta, personal communication.[38]

hypercapnic respiratory failure,[31] or alternatively, when ambulatory care is escalated to include evaluation by pulmonary or sleep specialists.[27] Unfortunately, a delay in diagnosis is common; the diagnosis typically occurs during the fifth and sixth decades of life, and during this delay, patients with OHS use more health care resources than comparably obese normocapnic patients.[24,31-33] In one study, 8% of all admissions to a general intensive care unit met diagnostic criteria for obesity-associated hypoventilation (BMI > 40 kg/m^2, $Paco_2$ > 45 mm Hg and no evidence of musculoskeletal disease, intrinsic lung disease, or smoking history). All of these patients presented with acute-on-chronic hypercapnic respiratory failure.[34] Of these patients, nearly 75% were misdiagnosed and treated for obstructive lung disease (most commonly chronic obstructive pulmonary disease [COPD]) in spite of having no evidence of obstructive physiology on pulmonary function testing.

Patients with OHS tend to be morbidly obese (BMI ≥ 40 kg/m^2), have severe OSA (≥30 obstructive respiratory events/hour of sleep), and are typically hypersomnolent. Compared with patients with eucapnic OSA and similar BMI, patients with OHS are more likely to report dyspnea and manifest cor pulmonale. Table 138.1 provides the typical portrait of a patient with OHS, based on the clinical features of a large combined cohort of patients with OHS reported in the literature.[23-26,33,35-43] Although severe obesity (BMI ≥ 40 kg/m^2) is a predominant risk factor for OHS, not all patients with severe obesity develop OHS. It is worth noting that there are significant physiologic differences between obese patients who have OHS compared with similarly obese patients without OHS as summarized in Table 138.2.[44]

The two tests required to diagnose OHS are a sleep study (polysomnography or respiratory polygraphy) to establish the presence of SDB and a measurement of arterial blood gases during wakefulness to establish the presence of hypercapnia. The diagnosis of OHS can be delayed because measurement of arterial blood gases is not a standard practice in the management of patients with SDB.[45,46] Moreover, clinicians may misattribute hypercapnia to COPD.[47] Therefore, in obese patients suspected of having SDB, simple tests to screen for OHS are needed. Although the definitive test for alveolar hypoventilation is a room air arterial blood gas, an elevated serum bicarbonate level resulting from metabolic compensation of respiratory acidosis is supportive of OHS.[26]

Commonly used tests to identify patients likely to have OHS assess consequences of hypoventilation, namely elevated serum bicarbonate levels (i.e., total serum CO_2, which equals bicarbonate plus dissolved CO_2) and hypoxemia. The term *serum bicarbonate* is not strictly accurate because the chemical methods measure all CO_2 liberated from the serum. Some laboratories use the more correct term *total serum CO2* to describe measured serum bicarbonate. It is important to note that bicarbonate represents 96% of total serum CO_2, and the remainder is mostly dissolved CO_2. The kidneys respond to chronic respiratory acidosis by increasing the serum bicarbonate level. Mokhlesi and colleagues first demonstrated that a venous serum bicarbonate threshold of 27 mEq/L—suggestive of chronic respiratory acidosis—could be used for OHS diagnosis in obese patients with diagnosed OSA.[26] Their data demonstrated that among patients who were obese with OSA and normal renal function, serum bicarbonate level below 27 mEq/L had a 97% negative predictive value for excluding a diagnosis of OHS. Macavei and colleagues assessed earlobe capillary blood gas samples from patients referred to a sleep center and determined that bicarbonate values calculated from the Henderson-Hasselbach formula have similar predictive values.[28] A calculated serum bicarbonate level of at least 27 mEq/L had a sensitivity of 85% and a specificity of 89% for the diagnosis of OHS among their patient sample. Two additional studies have confirmed serum bicarbonate to be an independent and reliable predictor of OHS.[19,48] Therefore, in the absence of alternative causes (e.g., use of loop diuretics), an increased serum bicarbonate level suggests the presence of a raised $Paco_2$. Hypoxemia, another consequence of hypercapnia as dictated by the alveolar gas equation, can also serve as a surrogate marker for hypercapnia. Pulse oximetry, which is noninvasive and accessible, is an attractive tool for identifying obese patients who are likely to be hypercapnic. However, hypoxemia can occur in morbidly obese patients without hypercapnia because of other reasons.

Figure 138.3 shows the prevalence of OHS in obese patients with OSA (BMI ≥ 30 kg/m^2 and AHI ≥ 5) using a serum bicarbonate level combined with other readily available measures such as severity of obesity, impairment of respiratory mechanics, and severity of OSA.[26] Indeed, several investigators have suggested incorporating serum venous bicarbonate (HCO_3^-) levels into the definition of OHS, particularly because using a single measurement of arterial Pco_2 for OHS diagnosis is susceptible to a number of confounding factors, including the impact of periprocedural patient anxiety leading to hyperventilation.[49] However, one study showed that

Table 138.1 Clinical Features of Patients with Obesity-Hypoventilation Syndrome

Clinical Features	Mean (Range)
Age (years)	52 (42–61)
Male (%)	60 (49–90)
Body mass index (kg/m^2)	44 (35–56)
Neck circumference (cm)	46.5 (45–47)
PH	7.38 (7.34–7.40)
Arterial PCO_2 (mm Hg)	53 (47–61)
Arterial PO_2 (mm Hg)	56 (46–74)
Serum bicarbonate (mEq/L)	32 (31–33)
Hemoglobin (g/dL)	15
Apnea-hypopnea index	66 (20–100)
SpO_2 nadir during sleep (%)	65 (59–76)
Percent sleep time $SpO_2 < 90\%$	50 (46–56)
FVC (% predicted)	68 (57–102)
FEV_1 (% predicted)	64 (53–92)
FEV_1/FVC	0.77 (0.74–0.88)
Medical Research Council dyspnea class 3 or 4 (%)	69
Epworth Sleepiness Scale score	14 (12–16)

Features are based on aggregated sample of 757 patients from 15 studies. Data taken from *Respir Care* 55(10):1347-62, 2010.

Table 138.2 Physiologic Differences between Eucapnic Morbidly Obese Patients and Those with Obesity-Hypoventilation Syndrome

	Eucapnic Morbid Obesity	Obesity-Hypoventilation Syndrome
Waist : Hip ratio	↑	↑↑
FEV_1/FVC	Normal	Normal/↓
Total lung capacity	Normal	Slight ↓
Functional residual capacity	↓	↓
Vital capacity	Normal or ↓	↓↓
Expiratory reserve volume	↓	↓↓
Work of breathing	↑	↑↑
Hypercapnic/hypoxic ventilatory drive	Normal	↓
Inspiratory muscle strength	Normal	↓

FEV_1, Forced expiratory volume in first second; FVC, forced vital capacity.

with adequate local anesthesia and sufficient technical expertise, radial artery puncture to obtain arterial blood gases did not alter end-tidal CO_2.[50] Recent guidelines published by the American Thoracic Society recommend that in obese patients with SDB who are strongly suspected of having OHS, a $PaCO_2$ rather than serum bicarbonate or SpO_2 be obtained to diagnose OHS. On the other hand, for patients with low to moderate probability of having OHS, it is recommended to use serum bicarbonate level to decide whether to measure $PaCO_2$: in patients with serum bicarbonate below 27 mEq/L clinicians may forgo measuring $PaCO_2$, as the diagnosis of OHS is very unlikely; in patients with serum bicarbonate of at least 27 mEq/L, clinicians may need to measure $PaCO_2$ to confirm or rule out the diagnosis of OHS.[51]

In addition to blood gas sampling and serum venous bicarbonate assessments, daytime finger pulse oximetry (SpO_2) may be a valuable tool for clinicians in screening for possible OHS.[52] Resting hypoxemia during wakefulness is not a typical feature of either patients with OSA or patients with obesity. Therefore abnormal resting pulse oximetry during wakefulness should increase the suspicion for OHS among patients with obesity and OSA.[26,53,54] Similarly, significant sleep-associated hypoxemia, defined as oxygen saturation below 85% for more than 10 continuous minutes, in an obese patient with OSA should raise suspicion for presence of sleep hypoventilation and possibly OHS.[55] In a meta-analysis, the mean difference of percentage of total sleep time with SpO_2 spent below 90% was 37.4% (56.2% for OHS, 18.8% for eucapnic obese patients with OSA) with very little overlap in the 95% confidence intervals.[20] However, recent guidelines recommend to not use SpO_2 to decide when to measure $PaCO_2$ in patients suspected of having OHS until more data about the usefulness of SpO_2 in this context become available.[51]

Ultimately, a rise in carbon dioxide levels (≥45 mm Hg) during wakefulness is necessary to define hypoventilation. There are a variety of techniques to measure carbon dioxide, such as daytime arterial blood gases, arterialized capillary blood gases, venous blood gases, end-tidal carbon dioxide, and transcutaneous carbon dioxide monitoring. Each of these techniques has its advantages and disadvantages.[56,57] The most reliable and practical method for identifying sleep hypoventilation is to measure carbon dioxide levels continuously during sleep by end-tidal or transcutaneous monitoring.[54] Improving technologies should greatly expand our ability to identify and quantify nocturnal hypoventilation in sleep laboratories, or even at home.

MORBIDITY AND MORTALITY

As already noted, the majority of patients with OHS are severely obese and have severe OSA.[18] Although severe obesity[58] and severe OSA are independently associated with increased risk of morbidity and mortality,[59-63] OHS may contribute further.[13] Systemic hypertension is highly prevalent in patients with OHS, ranging from 55% to 88%.[8,19,64-68] Metabolic and cardiovascular diseases are the most prevalent comorbidities and usually diagnosed before the recognition of OHS.[69,70] These comorbidities reinforce the frailty of patients with OHS; indeed, among the two clinical presentations commonly encountered in OHS, patients who are diagnosed during an acute exacerbation of chronic respiratory failure present more often with heart failure, coronary heart disease, and pulmonary hypertension (PH) than patients referred to a sleep specialist for suspected OSA.[12]

The morbidity associated with a diagnosis of OHS can vary, as illustrated by Jennum and colleagues, who evaluated 755 patients with a diagnosis of OHS (using International Classification of Disease-10 diagnostic codes) from a Danish national patient registry: in the 3 years before OHS diagnosis

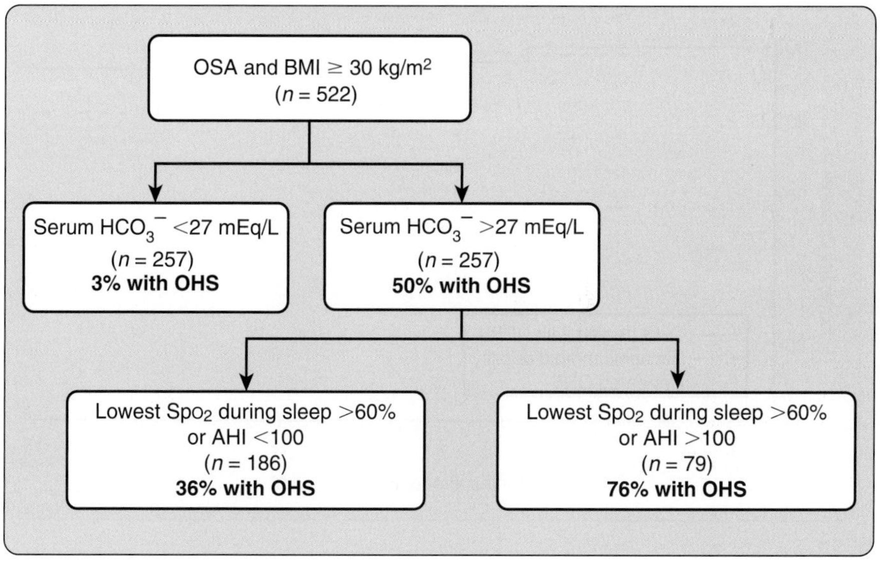

Figure 138.3 Decision tree to screen for obesity-hypoventilation syndrome based on observation in 522 obese patients with OSA (BMI ≥ 30 kg/m² and AHI ≥ 5). Among those with a serum bicarbonate > 27 mEq/L, OHS was present in 50% of patients. Very severe OSA (AHI > 100 events/hour or Spo_2 nadir during sleep less than 60%) increased the prevalence of OHS to 76%.[26] AHI, Apnea-hypopnea index; BMI, body mass index; OHS, obesity-hypoventilation syndrome; OSA, obstructive sleep apnea.

these patients were more likely than age- and sex-matched controls to be diagnosed with a variety of medical conditions, including cellulitis, carpal tunnel syndrome, type 2 diabetes, congestive heart failure, obstructive lung disease, and arthritis of the knee.[69] It remains unclear if these conditions would be more prevalent than in an obese-matched cohort with uncomplicated OSA. Furthermore, quality of life ratings among OHS patients appear to be lower than those with hypoventilatory respiratory disorders such as obstructive lung disease.[71]

Cardiovascular morbidity is of particular concern in OHS.[13] Kessler and colleagues found a PH prevalence of 58% among a cohort of 34 OHS patients, compared with just 9% among a sample of similar OSA patients.[72] Similarly, Berg and colleagues reported on 20 OHS patients from a Canadian health registry, comparing them to obese-matched controls.[41] OHS patients in their study were nine times more likely to have a diagnosis of cor pulmonale and nine times more likely to have a diagnosis of congestive heart failure. Moreover, hospitalized patients with obesity-associated hypoventilation are at increased risk of admission to the intensive care unit and need for invasive mechanical ventilation compared with hospitalized patients with eucapnic obesity.[24] PH is the condition likely to be directly linked to chronic hypoventilation; it is highly prevalent: about half of patients with OHS exhibit PH.[13,33,73,74]

In addition to significant comorbidities, patients with OHS also have elevated mortality. Three observational studies that enrolled patients at the time of hospitalization for acute-on-chronic hypercapnic respiratory failure reported all-cause mortality of 18% at 1 year and 31% and 35% at 3 years.[75-77] In these three studies the proportion of patients who were treated with long-term PAP therapy remains unknown. Another study enrolling hospitalized patients with stable hypercapnic respiratory failure from the medicine wards reported no mortality during the index hospitalization, but an all-cause mortality of 23% at 1½ years in patients with untreated OHS.[24] In a more recent retrospective study of 202 hospitalized patients with hypercapnic respiratory failure, 61 (30%) were due to OHS and/or hypercapnic OSA. Only one patient died during the index hospitalization. However, 30-day readmission was 17% and at 30 months, 35% of patients had died.[77] Unfortunately, data on PAP prescription and adherence are not available in this study either.

In contrast, Budweiser and colleagues conducted a retrospective analysis of 126 patients with OHS enrolled during hospitalization who were highly adherent to noninvasive ventilation (NIV) during sleep, with the NIV modality initiated in pressure support mode and after an adaptation period switched to pressure-cycled assist controlled mode. They found that the 1-, 2- and 5-year survival rates to be 97%, 92%, and 70%, respectively.[42] An individual patient data meta-analysis of 1162 patients with acute-on-chronic hypercapnic respiratory failure resulting from OHS who survived hospitalization revealed that patients discharged on empiric NIV had a significantly lower mortality at 3 months compared with patients discharged without any PAP therapy.[78] Given that hospitalized patients suspected of having OHS, who develop an acute-on-chronic hypercapnic respiratory failure, have higher short-term (1 to 2 years) mortality than ambulatory patients with OHS,[76] the recent guidelines from the American Thoracic Society recommended that hospitalized patients suspected of having OHS be started on NIV therapy before being discharged from the hospital and continued on empiric NIV therapy until they undergo outpatient workup and titration of PAP therapy in the sleep laboratory, ideally during the first 3 months after hospital discharge.[51] More research is needed on the optimal timing of the sleep study after a hospitalization for acute-on-chronic hypercapnic respiratory failure. Last, the role of autotitrating NIV devices in lieu of in-laboratory PAP titration requires further investigation, although a few small studies have suggested feasibility.[79,80]

In a retrospective study, 110 ambulatory patients with stable OHS treated with NIV in the form of bilevel PAP (mean inspiratory PAP of 18.5 ± 2.5 cm H_2O and mean expiratory PAP of 8.4 ± 1.9 cm H_2O) were matched with 220 patients with OSA treated with continuous positive airway pressure (CPAP, mean pressure of 8.9 ± 1.7 cm H_2O).[13] Despite similar rates of adherence to PAP therapy (mean bilevel PAP use of 6.2 ± 3.0 hours/night versus mean CPAP use of 5.8 ± 3.2 hours/night, $P = .29$), the 5-year mortality rates were 15.5% in the OHS cohort and 4.5% in the OSA cohort ($P < .05$). Patients with OHS had a twofold increase (OR 2; 95% CI: 1.11–3.60) in the risk of mortality compared with those with OSA. Using bilevel PAP less than 4 hours per night emerged as the strongest independent predictor of mortality in patients

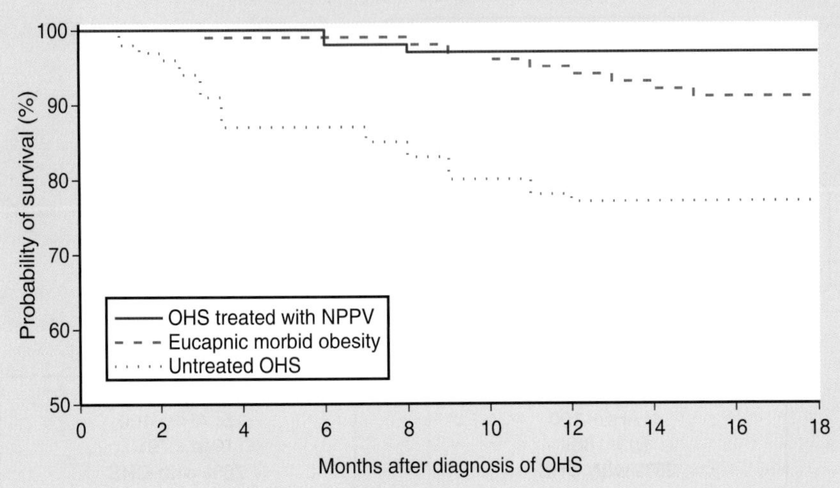

Figure 138.4 Survival curves for patients with untreated obesity-hypoventilation syndrome (OHS, *n* = 47; mean age 55 ± 14; mean body mass index [BMI] 45 ±9 kg/m^2; mean $Paco_2$ 52 ± 7 mm Hg) and eucapnic obese patients (*n* = 103; mean age 53 ± 13; mean BMI 42 ± 8 kg/m^2) as reported by Nowbar and colleagues[24] compared to patients with OHS treated with nocturnal positive pressure ventilation (NPPV) therapy (*n* = 126; mean age 55.6 ± 10.6; mean BMI 44.6 ± 7.8 kg/m^2; mean baseline $Paco_2$ 55.5 ± 7.7 mm Hg; mean adherence with NPPV of 6.5 ± 2.3 hours/day). Data for OHS patients treated with NPPV was provided courtesy of Dr. Stephan Budweiser and colleagues from the University of Regensburg, Germany.[42] (Reprinted from reference 8 with permission of the American Thoracic Society. Copyright American Thoracic Society.)

with OHS.[13] Together, these studies suggest that treatment with PAP therapy may lower the short-term mortality of patients with OHS (Figure 138.4).[7,42]

Indirect evidence from prospective observational studies suggests that long-term survival may be better in patients with OHS treated chronically with home NIV (most commonly in the form of bilevel PAP therapy) compared with CPAP therapy.[81] However, the largest randomized clinical trial with long-term follow-up (the Pickwick trial) found that in ambulatory patients with stable OHS and concomitant severe OSA (i.e., the great majority of patients with OHS), there was no significant difference in mortality in patients randomized to CPAP or NIV.[82]

Identifying patients with OHS in a timely manner is important, and treatment with PAP therapy should be initiated and monitored without delay to avoid adverse outcomes such as readmission to the hospital, acute-on-chronic respiratory failure requiring intensive care monitoring, or death. More important, adherence to therapy should be emphasized and monitored objectively.[83]

PATHOPHYSIOLOGY

The partial pressure of CO_2 in the arterial blood ($Paco_2$) is determined by the balance between CO_2 production and elimination. Although the main reason for reduced CO_2 elimination is reduced alveolar ventilation resulting from an overall decreased level of ventilation (i.e., minute ventilation), maldistribution of ventilation with respect to pulmonary capillary perfusion (i.e., an increase in physiologic dead space) may contribute as well. Further, the rate of CO_2 production in OHS is of particular physiologic concern: severely obese patients, with or without OHS, have increased work of breathing, increased oxygen cost of breathing, and increased CO_2 production compared with lean individuals.[84-86] The majority of individuals with severe obesity maintain homeostasis by increasing alveolar ventilation and associated CO_2 elimination, thereby averting progression to OHS. This is achieved by tight compensatory mechanisms, which require an intact integration between respiratory control and acid-base regulatory systems. Ultimately inadequate elimination of CO_2 relative to CO_2 production leads to chronic hypercapnia in patients with OHS. In addition to the differences as illustrated in Table 138.2, there are a variety of physiologic differences between patients with OHS and those with eucapnic obesity with or without OSA, such as increased upper airway resistance,[87] decreased respiratory system compliance compared with similarly obese subjects without OHS,[88] ventilation/perfusion mismatching secondary to pulmonary edema[89] or low lung volumes/atelectasis,[90] and, most important, impaired central response to hypoxemia and hypercapnia. Although these mechanisms contribute in varying degrees to the gas exchange abnormality observed in patients with OHS, the combination of SDB, a blunted central response to hypercapnia and hypoxia, and renal buffering can explain the progression from sleep hypoventilation to chronic daytime hypoventilation.[91-94]

Severe obesity (BMI ≥ 40 kg/m^2) increases the work of breathing because of the excess weight on the thoracic wall and abdomen.[88,95] However, it is unclear what role, if any, these altered mechanics have in the pathogenesis of OHS. The lung compliance of patients with OHS is less than equally obese controls (0.122 versus 0.157 L/cm H_2O). This can be explained by the lower functional residual capacity (1.71 versus 2.20 L). There is an even greater difference in chest wall compliance between the two groups (OHS 0.079 L/cm H_2O versus obese controls 0.196 L/cm H_2O).[88] Patients with OHS also have a threefold increase in lung resistance that has also been attributed to a low functional residual capacity.[88,96] The changes in lung mechanics are frequently demonstrated on spirometry by a low forced vital capacity (FVC) and forced expiratory volume in 1 second (FEV_1) and a normal FEV_1/FVC ratio. The spirometric abnormalities may be related to the combination of abnormal respiratory mechanics and weak respiratory muscles.[37,38,97,98] The abnormal respiratory system mechanics in subjects with severe obesity imposes a significant load on the respiratory muscles and leads to a significant increase in the work of breathing, particularly in the supine position.[88,95] As a result, morbidly obese patients dedicate 15% of their oxygen consumption to the work of breathing compared with 3% in nonobese individuals.[85]

The maximal inspiratory and expiratory pressures are normal in eucapnic morbidly obese patients but are typically reduced in patients with OHS.[99-101] Patients with mild OHS, however, may have normal inspiratory and expiratory pressures.[102] Further, the role of diaphragmatic weakness in the pathogenesis of this disorder remains uncertain because patients with OHS can generate similar transdiaphragmatic pressures at any level of diaphragmatic activation compared with eucapnic obese subjects.[100] In a study by Sampson, patients with OHS were able to generate equivalent transdiaphragmatic pressures (Pdi) as eucapnic obese patients during hypercapnia-induced hyperventilation, suggesting that respiratory muscle weakness may not play a role in the development of OHS. In addition, the OHS group showed no evidence of acute diaphragmatic fatigue (or neuromuscular uncoupling) throughout the hypercapnic trial when measured by the ratio of peak electrical activity of the diaphragm to peak Pdi, which theoretically eliminates the variable of patient cooperation.[100] Potentially more accurate assessments of diaphragmatic strength, for example, by cervical magnetic stimulation, have not been performed in patients with OHS.[103]

Patients with OHS are able to voluntarily hyperventilate to eucapnia,[104] evidence for a defective, "blunted," central respiratory drive. Further, patients with OHS do not hyperventilate to the same degree as eucapnic morbidly obese patients when rebreathing CO_2.[98,100,102] This deficit improves in most patients after PAP therapy.[102,105,106] In addition, patients with OHS do not augment their minute ventilation to the same degree as eucapnic obese OSA patients when breathing a hypoxic gas mixture.[102,106] This blunted hypoxic drive also improves with PAP therapy,[102,106] suggesting that such blunted drive is a secondary effect of the syndrome (and necessary for its persistence), but not the origin of it. Obesity, genetic predisposition, SDB, and leptin resistance have all been proposed as mechanisms for the blunted response to hypercapnia. Such blunted respiratory response to hypercapnia is unlikely to be genetic because the ventilatory response to hypercapnia is similar between first-degree relatives of patients with OHS and control subjects.[107]

Leptin, a satiety hormone produced by adipocytes, stimulates ventilation.[108-111] Obesity leads to an increase in CO_2 production and load.[84,86,108] Therefore, with increasing obesity the excess adipose tissue leads to increasing levels of leptin to increase ventilation to compensate for the additional CO_2 load. This is likely the reason that most severely obese individuals do not develop awake hypercapnia. Patients with OHS and OSA have significantly higher leptin levels compared with lean or BMI-matched subjects without OSA. Although the independent contribution of OSA or OHS to leptin production remains unclear, the data suggest that excess adiposity is a much more significant contributor to elevated serum leptin levels than the presence of OSA or OHS.[112-115] Patients with OHS, however, have a higher serum leptin level than eucapnic subjects with OSA matched for percent body fat; AHI and serum leptin levels each drop after treatment with PAP.[114,116,117] These observations suggest that patients with OHS may be resistant to leptin. For leptin to affect the respiratory center and increase minute ventilation it has to penetrate the cerebrospinal fluid (CSF). The leptin CSF-to-serum ratio is fourfold higher in lean individuals compared with obese subjects (0.045 ± 0.01 versus 0.011 ± 0.002, $P < .05$).[118] Individual differences in leptin CSF penetration may explain why some obese patients with severe OSA develop OHS and others do not.

OSA may well contribute to the ventilatory control defect because treatment with CPAP or bilevel PAP typically improves the response to hypercapnia.[102,105,106] The $P_{0.1}$ response to hypercapnia (a sensitive measure of respiratory drive) improves as early as 2 weeks and reaches normal levels after 6 weeks of therapy with PAP in patients with OHS who demonstrate an awake $Paco_2$ between 46 and 50 mm Hg. The response of minute ventilation to hypercapnia improves by the sixth week of PAP therapy but does not completely normalize.[102] Although such findings are not universal,[105,119,120] OSA appears well established in the pathophysiology of OHS by the resolution of hypercapnia in most patients after treatment with either tracheostomy or PAP therapy.*

Norman and colleagues have proposed an elegant mathematical model that explains the transition from acute hypercapnia during OSA to chronic daytime hypercapnia.[91] In most patients with OSA, the hyperventilation after an apnea eliminates all CO_2 accumulated during the apnea.[124] But if the interapnea hyperventilation is inadequate or the ventilatory response to the accumulated CO_2 is blunted, it could lead to an increase in $Paco_2$ during sleep.[92] Even in this acute setting during sleep the kidneys can retain small amounts of bicarbonate to buffer the decrease in pH. If the time constant for the excretion of the small amount of accumulated bicarbonate is slow, then the patient will have a net gain of bicarbonate, which may blunt the respiratory drive and lead to CO_2 retention during wakefulness to compensate for the retained bicarbonate.[91] Further, the combination of a decreased response to CO_2 and a slow rate of bicarbonate excretion rate will lead to a blunted respiratory drive for the next sleep cycle. Indeed, obese eucapnic individuals with an elevated serum bicarbonate level exhibit a blunted response to hypercapnic and hypoxic stimulation tests compared to equally obese eucapnic individuals with normal serum bicarbonate level.[52] Further research is needed to elucidate whether these individuals represent a subgroup of "early OHS" and whether they are at increased risk of progressing to overt daytime hypercapnia over time.

Many studies have tried to identify risk factors associated with hypercapnia in patients with OSA, but the results have been mixed.† In a large meta-analysis of 15 studies, Kaw and colleagues identified three factors that were significantly associated with chronic hypercapnia in obese patients who do not have COPD but do have OSA: (1) severity of obesity as measured by the BMI; (2) severity of OSA measured by either the AHI or hypoxemia during sleep; and (3) degree of restrictive chest physiology.[20]

TREATMENT

Treatment modalities for patients with OHS are based on different aspects of the underlying pathophysiology of the condition: reversal of sleep-disordered-breathing (OSA and/or nonobstructive sleep hypoventilation), weight reduction, and possibly pharmacotherapy.[126] Nocturnal PAP therapies are considered first-line treatment and are effective in improving patient outcomes.[127,128] However, treatment strategies that include weight reduction and physical activity should also be offered to patients with OHS to improve their metabolic and cardiovascular risk profiles.[65,129,130]

Positive Airway Pressure Therapy

PAP, in the form of CPAP was first described in the treatment of OHS in 1982.[121] Although subsequent studies confirmed

*References 18, 35, 40, 83, 102, 121-123.
†References 23, 25, 26, 33, 36-39, 125.

its efficacy, failure of CPAP in some cases has led to uncertainty whether CPAP should be attempted initially or if NIV (most commonly in the form of bilevel PAP) is a better modality.[25,83,119,121,131] In one prospective study of outpatients with severe OHS, 57% of patients were successfully titrated with CPAP alone. In these patients CPAP was titrated to treat OSA, and the mean pressure required was 14 cm H_2O.[55] The remaining 43% of patients failed CPAP titration because of persistent hypoxemia at therapeutic or near therapeutic pressures that had successfully treated OSA. In these patients the oxygen saturation remained below 90% for more than 20% of total sleep time. Because this was a single-night titration study, the question of whether residual hypoxemia would resolve with long-term CPAP treatment was not systematically evaluated.[67]

Observational studies and RCTs have reported improvements in awake respiratory failure, symptoms, and quality of life to a similar degree in both CPAP- and NIV-treated individuals with OHS.* Although CPAP does not increase alveolar ventilation, it can improve awake respiratory failure by facilitating the unloading of CO_2 accumulated during complete or partial airflow obstruction during sleep.[92,93]

Because more than 73% of people with OHS have concomitant severe OSA,[135] CPAP may be effective in improving nocturnal and awake gas exchange in at least a subset of these individuals. Thus far, three medium-term randomized clinical trials[134-136] and one long-term randomized clinical trial have compared NIV to CPAP.[82] Patients in these trials were ambulatory and in chronic stable hypercapnic respiratory failure. Participants in all three trials demonstrated concomitant OSA in addition to OHS, with mean AHI exceeding 60 events/hour. On average, adherence to CPAP and NIV were similar (5 to 6 hours/night, with CPAP used only 7 minutes/night less than NIV, 95% CI 43 minutes less to 29 minutes more). One clinical trial compared CPAP to bilevel PAP in spontaneous mode,[136] another compared CPAP to bilevel PAP ST mode (with a backup rate),[134] and the Spanish Pickwick trials compared CPAP to volume-targeted pressure support.[82,135] The duration of these RCTs was either medium term, for up to 2 to 3 months[134-136] or long term, for up to 5 years.[82] The resolution of hypercapnia (i.e., awake Pa_{CO_2} < 45 mm Hg) occurred to a similar extent in both NIV- and CPAP-treated patients. During short-term follow-up, 46.6% of individuals treated with NIV and 36.3% treated with CPAP had a Pa_{CO_2} below 45 mm Hg (11 more per 100 NIV-treated patients, 95% CI 2 fewer to 28 more; RR 1.29; 95% CI 0.94 to 1.77).[134-136] During long-term follow-up, 51.9% treated with NIV and 40.7% treated with CPAP had a Pa_{CO_2} below 45 mm Hg (11 more per 100 NIV-treated patients, 95% CI 4 fewer to 32 more; RR 1.28; 95% CI 0.91 to 1.79).[82] There was no difference in the degree of improvement in Pa_{O_2} between NIV and CPAP. Moreover, the need for oxygen supplementation, based on an awake Pa_{O_2} below 55 mm Hg, was not different during both short-term[134-136] and long-term follow-up.[82] Similarly, resolution of daytime sleepiness as assessed by an Epworth Sleepiness Score below 10 after therapy, occurred at similar rates in NIV and CPAP groups, in both short-term[134-136] (RR 1.04, 95% CI 0.87 to 1.23) and longer-term (RR 1.04, 95% CI 0.86 to 1.26) follow-up.[82] Changes in quality of life from three short-term trials[134-136] and one long-term were not different.[82] No deaths were recorded in three short-term studies, which included 311 patients treated with either NIV or CPAP.[134-136] After 5 years of following 204 participants, mortality rates were similar between NIV- and CPAP-treated groups (NIV 11% versus CPAP 15%; [adjusted hazard ratio of 0.82, 95% CI 0.36 to 1.87; $P = 0.631$]). Similarly, there was no difference in composite cardiovascular events (RR 1.17, 95% CI 0.56 to 2.44) between NIV and CPAP groups during long-term follow-up.[82] Moreover, in the long-term Pickwick clinical trial of patients with OHS and severe OSA who had echocardiographic evidence of PH at baseline (defined as pulmonary systolic pressure ≥ 40 mm Hg), both CPAP and NIV were equally effective and significantly decreased pulmonary artery systolic pressure by approximately 11 mm Hg.[74] As such, the difference in outcomes between NIV and CPAP in stable ambulatory patients with OHS and concomitant severe OSA is trivial.

Based on these findings, recent guidelines recommended CPAP rather than NIV as the initial treatment of stable ambulatory adult patients with OHS and concurrent severe OSA (AHI ≥ 30 events per hour) presenting with chronic stable respiratory failure.[51] Importantly, more than 70% of patients with OHS have severe OSA. Therefore this recommendation is applicable to the majority of patients with OHS. However, there is less certainty in patients with OHS who do not have concomitant severe OSA. It is important to note that improvements in awake hypercapnia may be achieved more slowly with CPAP than with NIV during the initial weeks of treatment. Patients presenting with a greater degree of initial ventilatory failure, poorer lung function, advanced age, or less severe OSA may be less likely to respond to CPAP.[83,134,137] The variation in response to therapy requires close monitoring of the patient, especially during the first 2 months of treatment to ensure improvement is achieved and sustained, with adjustment of therapy as appropriate. This particularly applies to OHS patients without severe OSA who are prescribed CPAP.

There are also moderate cost implications around the choice of PAP therapy, with NIV being substantially more expensive than CPAP.[82] A recent analysis of the Pickwick trial, in which 202 patients with OHS and severe OSA were randomized to CPAP or NIV and followed for a median of 3 years, demonstrated that NIV cost per patient was €857.6±105.5 higher than CPAP therapy each year.[138] In addition, NIV may require more resources for titration and equipment training. These considerations may delay access to NIV in comparison to CPAP, particularly in areas where skills necessary for more complex NIV devices are limited or where economic resources are a consideration. Similar levels of adherence are reported with CPAP and NIV, of 5 to 6 hours per night. Previous work has suggested adherence is an important modifiable predictor of hypercapnia in OHS.[83,132] The only long-term clinical trial to date that examined the role of NIV in patients with OHS without concomitant severe OSA revealed that NIV was superior to lifestyle changes in improving hypercapnia and quality of life and reducing daytime sleepiness. Patients adherent to NIV also had a reduction in hospitalization.[139] However, no studies to date have compared CPAP and NIV in patients with OHS without severe OSA.

The American Academy of Sleep Medicine has proposed guidelines for the titration of NIV in patients with chronic alveolar hypoventilation syndromes, although not specifically

*References 82, 83, 120, 125, 129, 132-136.

for OHS.[140] The most common mode of NIV used in clinical practice is bilevel PAP. During in-laboratory titration, expiratory positive airway pressure (EPAP) is increased until obstructive apneas are resolved.[141] If hypoxemia is persistent and/or estimated tidal volumes are lower than expected for the patient's ideal body weight, then pressure support must be increased.[140] Pressure support is the difference between inspiratory positive airway pressure (IPAP) and EPAP. Most patients with OHS require a pressure support level of at least 8 to 12 cm H_2O (i.e., an IPAP pressure setting that is at least 8 to 12 cm H_2O above EPAP) to achieve effective ventilation.[35,40,142,143]

Some patients with OHS may experience central apneas during NIV therapy. Central apneas could occur in OHS during CPAP or NIV titration because of decreased respiratory drive, heart failure, or unstable ventilatory control (high loop gain).[144] Advanced modes such as bilevel PAP with a backup rate can help alleviate central apneas in OHS. In the spontaneous-timed or timed mode, a backup respiratory rate of 10 to 12 breaths per minute should be initiated and titrated upward by one to two increments, generally not exceeding 16 breaths per minute. The backup respiratory rate should be initiated when a patient with hypoventilation syndrome manifests central apneas or inappropriately low respiratory rate and consequent low minute ventilation. Therefore, to perform an adequate NIV titration during sleep in patients with OHS, it is important to monitor several parameters during polysomnography such as mask flow, delivered pressure, air leak, estimated exhaled tidal volume, and triggered backup mechanical breaths.[140] Transcutaneous CO_2 monitoring, if available, provides useful information regarding the effectiveness of NIV or CPAP titration. Scoring respiratory events during NIV titration can be challenging, and a systematic description of these events has been proposed.[145]

In the minority of patients with OHS who do not have OSA, EPAP can be set at 5 cm H_2O and IPAP can be titrated to improve ventilation.[142,143] Switching to NIV should also be considered if the $Paco_2$ does not normalize or if there is persistent hypoxemia during sleep after 3 months of CPAP therapy with objective evidence of adherence to prescribed therapy.

Earlier studies suggested that sleep hypoventilation can be better controlled by NIV settings that optimize delivery of nocturnal ventilation with either the use of a higher mandatory backup respiratory rate of the ventilator[146] or the use of pressure-volume hybrid modes.[147] Two of these hybrid modes of volume-targeted pressure support are average volume assured pressure support (AVAPS) or intelligent volume assured pressure support (iVAPS). These modes of pressure support deliver a more consistent tidal volume. With volume-targeted pressure support modes, the pressure support or assistance delivered during the inspiratory phase aims to ensure a certain tidal volume that is calculated as a function of predicted body weight (usually 8 to 10 mL/kg ideal body weight or at 110% of patient's tidal volume). The AVAPS and iVAPS devices assess the preset tidal volume or minute ventilation over a variable time window of 1 to 5 minutes. The operating IPAP (or pressure assist) level is then allowed to fluctuate between a minimum and maximum pressure support level to ensure the target tidal volume. If a patient's tidal volume or minute ventilation decreases below a certain threshold, the device responds by increasing the IPAP and restores the tidal volume to approximately the preselected target volume. Such devices have an EPAP-minimum and EPAP-maximum range that must be preset as well. Although higher inspiratory pressures achieved with volume-targeted hybrid modes may also optimally relieve dyspnea, they may be more disruptive to sleep in some patients.[148] However, two studies that compared AVAPS to bilevel PAP/ST did not find any difference in sleep quality between the two ventilatory modes.[149,150] Additional settings may include spontaneous or timed respiratory rate settings, and newer technology has automated the respiratory rate selection based upon patient's minute ventilation and proportion of breaths that are triggered versus spontaneous over a period of time.

Two randomized controlled trials (RCTs) of patients with OHS have compared volume-targeted pressure support mode with fixed bilevel PAP/ST mode (with a backup respiratory rate).[149,150] In one trial of 50 patients, AVAPS was compared to bilevel PAP/ST, and patients were followed for 3 months.[149] In the other trial, 56 patients were randomized to either AVAPS-AE (automatic EPAP) or bilevel PAP/ST, and patients were followed for 2 months.[150] In both studies there was no significant difference between the two advanced PAP modes. Both PAP modalities significantly improved daytime $Paco_2$, sleep hypoventilation (as measured by transcutaneous CO_2), hypoxemia during sleep, and quality of life. The lack of such demonstrable difference between AVAPS and fixed bilevel PAP/ST in these trials may be due to the carefully "optimized" bilevel PAP/ST setting in these clinical research conditions.

There was no significant difference in the levels of PAP delivered between the two groups. In the first trial, patients randomized to AVAPS received mean pressures of IPAP 22 ± 5/EPAP 9 ± 1 cm H_2O with a backup rate of 14 breaths per minute verus bilevel PAP S/T mode with mean pressures of IPAP 23 ± 4/EPAP 10 ± 4 cm H_2O with a backup rate of 14 breaths per minute.[149] Despite these high pressure settings, the mean adherence to therapy was reasonable and not different between the two groups (AVAPS 4.2 hours/day, bilevel PAP S/T 5.1 hours/day). Comparative post hoc analysis revealed that in patients in whom more than 50% of the breaths were delivered as the backup respiratory rate experienced a greater control of nocturnal carbon dioxide by transcutaneous CO_2 monitoring, improved daytime $Paco_2$, and enhanced health-related quality of life at 3 months,[149] which supports the hypothesis that controlled NIV, which minimizes patient ventilatory effort in sleep, may help unload the respiratory muscles and provide optimal nocturnal ventilatory control and improved patient outcomes. However, most recent long-term Spanish Pickwick trial that compared CPAP to NIV in volume-targeted pressure support mode showed no difference in important patient-centered outcomes between these two modes after 5 years of follow-up.[82]

There are numerous technical difficulties with applying NIV in OHS. Advanced PAP modalities such as volume-targeted pressure support technology rely heavily and function properly when unintentional air leak from noninvasive mask remains low.[151] Although bench studies have shown that most NIV devices underestimate air leak and exhaled tidal volume, there is significant variability among manufacturers.[152]

The most common reason for persistent hypercapnia and hypoxemia in patients with OHS treated with PAP is lack of adherence to the PAP therapy. In a retrospective study of

75 outpatients with stable OHS, patients who used CPAP or bilevel PAP therapy for more than 4½ hours per/day had a considerably greater improvement in blood gases than less adherent patients ($\Delta Paco_2$ 7.7 ± 5 versus 2.4 ± 4 mm Hg, $P < .001$; ΔPao_2 9.2 ± 11 versus 1.8 ± 9 mm Hg, $P < .001$).[83] The degree of improvement in ventilation and gas exchange, which can be seen as early as 2 to 4 weeks after therapy,[83,102,153] may allow discontinuation of daytime oxygen supplementation in many patients with OHS.[83] However, the improvement in chronic daytime gas exchange abnormalities (i.e., hypercapnia and hypoxemia) even in patients that are adherent to PAP therapy is neither universal nor complete.[52,102]

Other possibilities behind persistent hypercapnia include inadequate CPAP pressure or insufficient NIV support, CPAP failure in OHS patients who do not have significant OSA, other causes of hypercapnia such as COPD, or metabolic alkalosis resulting from high doses of loop diuretics. In two studies,[83,136] the $Paco_2$ did not improve significantly in approximately a quarter of patients who had undergone successful PAP titration in the laboratory and were highly adherent (> 6 hours/night) with either CPAP or bilevel PAP therapy. It is conceivable that volume-targeted pressure support or higher levels of pressure support with fixed bilevel PAP in the ST mode would be more effective in normalizing ventilation and gas exchange. Reports of persistent hypoventilation after tracheostomy[35] highlight the need for aggressive nocturnal mechanical ventilation in addition to support of upper airway patency in at least a subset of OHS patients.

Early follow-up is imperative and should include assessment of adherence to PAP therapy; patients with OSA, although not specifically with OHS, frequently overestimate CPAP adherence.[154-156] Changes in serum bicarbonate level, improvements in resting room air pulse oximetry and end-tidal CO_2 measurements during wakefulness could be used as less invasive surrogates of ventilation if the patient is reluctant to undergo follow-up measurement of arterial blood gases. The majority of patients with OHS and concomitant severe OSA who demonstrate stability on NIV therapy can be safely switched to CPAP therapy and will not develop daytime hypercapnia.[157]

Oxygen Therapy

In some patients with OHS oxygen supplementation is necessary after the resolution of apneas and hypopneas during PAP titration, both CPAP and NIV, to keep Spo_2 above 88% to 90%. In two studies, the percentage of OHS patients requiring supplemental oxygen after adequate CPAP titration (i.e., resolution of obstructive apneas and hypopneas) was as high as 43%.[55,83] In contrast, in a relatively comparable group of patients with OHS, only 12% undergoing aggressive NIV titration with relatively high levels of pressure support (~13 cm H_2O above an average EPAP of 10 cm H_2O) required such oxygen supplementation.[149] This finding suggests that higher levels of pressure support during PAP titration must be considered to achieve adequate oxygenation and ventilation during sleep in a large proportion of patients with OHS. Oxygen supplementation as monotherapy without resolution of upper airway obstruction with CPAP or adequate ventilatory support with NIV is strongly discouraged. Two well-controlled clinical trials have reported that in a significant proportion of patients with OHS who were tested during wakefulness and in steady state, supplemental oxygen at high[158] and medium concentrations[159] worsened hypercapnia (because of a drop in tidal volume and minute ventilation). The Spanish Pickwick trial reported that in ambulatory patients with stable chronic hypercapnic respiratory failure, the addition of low-flow oxygen supplementation to PAP therapy or oxygen used during sleep without PAP did not increase hospital resource utilization after 2 months of follow-up.[160] It is plausible, however, that the risk of CO_2 retention with low-flow oxygen supplementation is higher during an acute-on-chronic hypercapnic respiratory failure in OHS.[161]

Weight Reduction

Weight loss interventions can have several benefits, including improvements in SDB and OHS, as well as improved cardiovascular and metabolic outcomes. Many strategies are available to achieve weight loss. Commercially available programs designed for weight loss tend not to be effective in the long term.[162] Very intensive lifestyle interventions have been proven to be successful in achieving weight loss of approximately 10 kg in obese patients with type 2 diabetes or prediabetes but do not improve long-term cardiovascular outcomes, as patients often regain weight.[163,164] Not surprisingly, bariatric interventions are more effective than lifestyle interventions in achieving significant and sustainable weight loss that can ultimately improve cardiovascular and metabolic outcomes. Three commonly performed bariatric surgery procedures in the United States are sleeve gastrectomy, Roux-en-Y gastric bypass, and laparoscopic adjustable gastric banding.[165,166] Sleeve gastrectomy has become the most common bariatric surgical intervention[166]; it was originally considered the first component of a two-stage biliopancreatic diversion with duodenal switch procedure, but it has proven to be an effective stand-alone bariatric procedure. The Roux-en-Y gastric bypass is the second most commonly performed bariatric surgery. Laparoscopic gastric banding is the least common; it is associated with lower perioperative morbidity, but more modest weight loss at both short- and medium-term follow-up. Biliopancreatic diversion is another bariatric procedure that is reserved for the extremely obese (BMI > 60 kg/m^2) and for those who have failed other bariatric operations. The safety of bariatric procedures has improved over time.[167] Clinical trials have reported improvements in metabolic[168-170] and cardiovascular morbidities,[171] and reductions in all-cause and cardiovascular mortality in patients undergoing laparoscopic sleeve gastrectomy or gastric bypass surgery.[172,173] It is more challenging to assess the impact of bariatric surgery on OHS given that many studies either did not assess for OHS, or excluded patients with OHS entirely.

Bariatric surgery has variable long-term efficacy in treating OSA.[174] A meta-analysis that included 12 studies with 342 patients that underwent PSG before bariatric surgery and after maximum weight loss reported a 71% reduction in the AHI, from baseline of 55 (95% CI 49 to 60) to 16 (95% CI 13 to 19).[175] Although only 38% achieved cure defined by AHI below 5, this drastic improvement in the severity of SDB would likely be enough to normalize daytime blood gases in most patients with OHS. It is also known that in the 6 to 8 years after weight reduction surgery OSA patients experience approximately 7% weight gain, which may lead to an increase in the AHI.[171,176]

There is an overall paucity of evidence, with two randomized clinical trials, no nonrandomized comparative studies, and four nonrandomized studies without a comparator.[177-182]

The results suggest that a comprehensive weight loss program (including motivational counseling, dieting oversight, and an exercise program) reduces body weight but confers no clinically significant effects compared with standard care (diet and exercise advice during a routine outpatient visit). In contrast, bariatric surgery is associated with more significant weight loss, resolution of OHS, reduction of OSA severity, and improvement in gas exchange, daytime sleepiness, and pulmonary artery pressure.

Bariatric surgery in OHS was associated with adverse effects in roughly one-fifth of patients in the only study that reported adverse outcomes published in 1986.[179] However, more recent data suggest a better safety profile for bariatric surgery. A prospective observational cohort study of 4776 patients undergoing bariatric surgery reported a 30-day mortality of 0.3% and incidence of major adverse events of 4.3%.[183] A recent retrospective observational cohort study of 65,093 undergoing bariatric surgery in the United States between 2005 and 2015 reported a 30-day mortality rate of 0.1% and 30-day adverse event of 3.8%. The overall 30-day complication rate by procedures was 5% after gastric bypass, 2.6% after sleeve gastrectomy, and 2.9% after band procedure.[184] The independent risk factors associated with mortality are intestinal leak, pulmonary embolism, preoperative weight, and hypertension. Depending on the type of the surgery, intestinal leak occurs in 2% to 4% of patients, and pulmonary embolism occurs in 1% of patients.[185] Ideally, patients with OHS should be treated with PAP therapy before undergoing surgical intervention to decrease perioperative morbidity and mortality. Moreover, PAP therapy using the patient's preoperative settings should be initiated immediately after extubation to avoid postoperative respiratory failure,[186-189] particularly because there is no evidence that PAP therapy initiated postoperatively leads to anastomotic disruption or leakage.[187,190]

Based on the limited available evidence, recent guidelines recommended using weight loss interventions in patients with OHS.[51] To achieve resolution of OHS, a long-term sustained weight loss of at least 25% to 30% of actual body weight is needed. Weight loss of this magnitude is more likely to be achieved with surgical interventions such as laparoscopic sleeve gastrectomy, Roux-en-Y gastric bypass, or biliopancreatic diversion with duodenal switch and not with laparoscopic gastric banding.[191] The choice of surgical procedure should be based on weighing potential risks of surgery against the maximum possible anticipated weight loss. OSA may persist despite the resolution of OHS after weight reduction surgery.[192]

Tracheostomy

Tracheostomy was the first therapy described for the treatment of OHS.[193] In a retrospective study of 13 patients with OHS, tracheostomy was associated with significant improvement in concomitant OSA. However, in seven patients the AHI remained above 20. Residual respiratory events were associated with persistent respiratory effort, suggesting that disordered breathing was caused by obstructive hypoventilation through an open tracheostomy rather than central apneas. Occasionally excessive neck skin folds can intermittently obstruct the tracheostomy orifice. However, the overall improvement in the severity of SDB after tracheostomy leads to the resolution of hypercapnia in the majority of the patients with OHS.[194] Currently, tracheostomy is generally reserved for patients who are intolerant of or not adherent to PAP therapy. Patients with tracheostomy may require additional nocturnal ventilation, as tracheostomy alone does not treat any central hypoventilation that may be present.[195] A polysomnogram with the tracheostomy open is necessary to determine whether nocturnal ventilation is required, and to specifically titrate the mode and levels of ventilation necessary.[35]

Respiratory Stimulation

Respiratory stimulants can theoretically increase respiratory drive and improve daytime hypercapnia, but such data in patients with OHS are extremely limited. Medroxyprogesterone acts as a respiratory stimulant at the hypothalamic level.[196] The results of treatment in patients with OHS have been contradictory. In a series of 10 men with OHS who were able to normalize their $Paco_2$ with 1 to 2 minutes of voluntary hyperventilation, treatment with 60 mg/day of oral medroxyprogesterone for 1 month resulted in normalization of the $Paco_2$ (from 51 mm Hg to 38 mm Hg) and improvement in the Pao_2 (49 mm Hg to 62 mm Hg).[197] In contrast, medroxyprogesterone did not improve $Paco_2$, minute ventilation, or ventilatory response to hypercapnia in three OHS patients that remained hypercapnic after tracheostomy.[119] Further, medroxyprogesterone may increase the risk of venous thromboembolism, particularly in this population whose mobility is limited.[198,199] In addition, high doses of medroxyprogesterone can lead to breakthrough uterine bleeding in women and to decreased libido in men.

Acetazolamide induces metabolic acidosis through carbonic anhydrase inhibition, which decreases serum bicarbonate, shifts the CO_2 response to the left, and increases minute ventilation.[119,200] Acetazolamide may also favorably impact OSA by improving loop gain.[201-203]

Most, but not all, patients with OHS can normalize their $Paco_2$ with 1 minute of voluntary hyperventilation.[104] The inability to eliminate CO_2 with voluntary hyperventilation may be due to mechanical impairment. In one study the ability to decrease the $Paco_2$ by at least 5 mm Hg with voluntary hyperventilation was the main predictor of a favorable response to respiratory stimulants.[204] Ideally, however, respiratory stimulants should not be used in patients who cannot normalize their $Paco_2$ with voluntary hyperventilation—because of limited ventilation and/or mechanical impairment—since it can lead to an increase in dyspnea or even worsening of acidosis with acetazolamide. Overall, pharmacotherapy with respiratory stimulants cannot be currently recommended as monotherapy in patients with OHS.

Hyperviscosity impairs oxygen delivery and can counteract the beneficial effects of erythrocytosis. Phlebotomy has not been systematically studied in patients with OHS who develop secondary erythrocytosis. In adult patients with congenital cyanotic heart disease phlebotomy has been recommended if the hematocrit is above 65% only if symptoms of hyperviscosity are present.[205] However, it is difficult to extrapolate this recommendation to patients with OHS because many symptoms of hyperviscosity are similar to the symptoms of OHS. Reversing hypoventilation and hypoxemia with PAP therapy eventually improves secondary erythrocytosis, and therefore phlebotomy is not needed in patients with OHS.[206]

CLINICAL PEARLS

- Approximately 8% to 20% of obese patients referred for polysomnography for suspicion of OSA have OHS. The prevalence of OHS is even higher in severely obese patients with OSA and in hospitalized patients with severe obesity. Unfortunately, OHS is typically underrecognized and undertreated. Delay in diagnosis and treatment leads to significant health care resource utilization and increased morbidity and mortality. Therefore a high index of suspicion is required to diagnose OHS in a timely fashion to improve patient outcomes.
- Nocturnal PAP therapies are considered first-line treatment and are effective in improving patient outcomes. Importantly, in ambulatory patients with stable OHS and concomitant severe OSA (i.e., nearly 70% of patients with OHS), there is no significant difference in outcomes between CPAP and NIV.
- Although significant advances have been made in the delivery of PAP therapy, adherence remains suboptimal in many patients with OHS. Therefore a comprehensive management should include strategies to improve PAP adherence.
- Although PAP therapy improves nocturnal and daytime hypoventilation and quality of life, weight reduction and increase in physical activity should be included as part of comprehensive treatment strategies to improve the metabolic and cardiovascular risk profiles of patients with OHS.

SUMMARY

With the current global epidemic of obesity, the prevalence of OHS is likely to increase. Despite the significant morbidity and mortality associated with the syndrome, it is often unrecognized and treatment is frequently delayed. A high index of suspicion can lead to early recognition of the syndrome and initiation of appropriate therapy. Significant advances have been made in the delivery of PAP therapy and NIV. Clinicians should encourage adherence to PAP therapy to avert the serious adverse outcomes of untreated OHS.

SELECTED READINGS

Berger KI, Rapoport DM, Ayappa I, et al. Pathophysiology of hypoventilation during sleep. *Sleep Med Clin*. 2014;11:289–300.

Borel JC, Tamisier R, Gonzalez-Bermejo J, et al. Noninvasive ventilation in mild obesity hypoventilation syndrome: a randomized controlled trial. *Chest*. 2012;141(3):692–702.

Gudivada SD, Rajasurya V, Spector AR. Qualifying patients for noninvasive positive pressure ventilation devices on hospital discharge. *Chest*. 2020;158(6):2524–2531.

Howard ME, Piper AJ, Stevens B, et al. A randomised controlled trial of CPAP versus non-invasive ventilation for initial treatment of obesity hypoventilation syndrome. *Thorax*. 2017;72(5):437–444.

Huttmann SE, Windisch W, Storre JH. Techniques for the measurement and monitoring of carbon dioxide in the blood. *Ann Am Thorac Soc*. 2014;11(4):645–652.

Kaw R, Wong J, Mokhlesi B. Obesity and obesity hypoventilation, sleep hypoventilation, and postoperative respiratory failure. *Anesth Analg*. 2021;132(5):1265–1273.

Masa JF, Corral J, Alonso ML, et al. Efficacy of different treatment alternatives for obesity hypoventilation syndrome. Pickwick study. *Am J Respir Crit Care Med*. 2015;192(1):86–95. https://doi.org/10.1164/rccm.201410-1900OC.

Masa JF, Corral J, Caballero C, et al. Non-invasive ventilation in obesity hypoventilation syndrome without severe obstructive sleep apnoea. *Thorax*. 2016;71(10):899–906. https://doi.org/10.1136/thoraxjnl-2016-208501.

Masa JF, Mokhlesi B, Benítez I, et al. Long-term clinical effectiveness of continuous positive airway pressure therapy versus non-invasive ventilation therapy in patients with obesity hypoventilation syndrome: a multicentre, open-label, randomised controlled trial. *Lancet*. 2019;393(10182):1721–1732. https://doi.org/10.1016/S0140-6736(18)32978-7.

Mokhlesi B, Masa JF, Brozek JL, et al. Evaluation and Management of Obesity Hypoventilation Syndrome. An Official American Thoracic Society Clinical Practice Guideline [published correction appears in Am J Respir Crit Care Med. 2019 Nov 15;200(10):1326]. *Am J Respir Crit Care Med*. 2019;200(3):e6–e24.

Mokhlesi B, Tulaimat A, Faibussowitsch I, Wang Y, Evans AT. Obesity hypoventilation syndrome: prevalence and predictors in patients with obstructive sleep apnea. *Sleep Breath*. 2007;11(2):117–124.

Mokhlesi B, Won CH, Make BJ, Selim BJ, Sunwoo BY; ONMAP Technical Expert Panel. Optimal noninvasive medicare access promotion: patients with hypoventilation syndromes: a technical expert panel report from the American College of Chest Physicians, the American Association for Respiratory Care, the American Academy of Sleep Medicine, and the American Thoracic Society. *Chest*. 2021;S0012-3692(21)01484–7 .

Murphy PB, Davidson C, Hind MD, et al. Volume targeted versus pressure support non-invasive ventilation in patients with super obesity and chronic respiratory failure: a randomised controlled trial. *Thorax*. 2012;67(8):727–734.

National Institute for Health and Care Excellence. Obstructive sleep apnoea/hypopnoea syndrome and obesity hypoventilation syndrome. 2021. https://www.nice.org.uk/guidance/ng202.

Wearn J, Akpa B, Mokhlesi B. Adherence to positive airway pressure therapy in obesity hypoventilation syndrome. *Sleep Med Clin*. 2021;16(1):43–59.

A complete reference list can be found online at ExpertConsult.com.

Chapter 139

Obstructive Sleep Apnea, Obesity, and Bariatric Surgery

Eric J. Olson; Anita P. Courcoulas; Bradley A. Edwards

Chapter Highlights

- Excessive body weight is a global health issue. In the United States, two of every three adults weigh more than their ideal body weight. Obesity (defined as a body mass index ≥30 kg/m^2) predicts increased morbidity and mortality. One of the health conditions that obesity has a significant effect on is obstructive sleep apnea.
- Inconsistent results from dietary, behavioral, and pharmacologic weight loss therapies have led to increasing interest in bariatric surgery, a variety of abdominal operations that restrict caloric intake and/or absorption and also likely affect neuroendocrine aspects of weight control.
- Bariatric surgery results in loss of approximately 60% of excess body weight or 30% of initial body weight. Notably, the weight loss achieved varies by the type of procedure.
- Bariatric surgery results in significant improvements on obstructive sleep apnea, but most patients have residual sleep-disordered breathing after surgical weight loss.
- Familiarity with the principles and applications of bariatric surgery is a requirement for sleep medicine practitioners, in view of the frequency with which coexistent obesity and sleep-related breathing disorders, obstructive sleep apnea, and obesity hypoventilation syndrome are encountered in clinical practice.

DEFINITIONS AND SYNOPSIS

In adults and children, overweight and obesity traditionally have been defined by the *body mass index* (BMI), which is the quotient of the weight in kilograms divided by the height in meters squared. Table 139.1 depicts the National Heart, Lung, and Blood Institute's weight classification system for adults, in which *overweight* is defined as a BMI 25 to 29.9 kg/m^2 and *obese* is defined as a BMI 30 kg/m^2 or greater.[1] Table 139.2 shows the weight classification system for children based on the Centers for Disease Control and Prevention growth charts.[2] Severe obesity in children is defined by the American Heart Association as a BMI greater than 120% of the 95th percentile for age and sex or a BMI 35 kg/m^2 or greater, whichever is lower.[3]

Obesity is one of the most important risk factors for obstructive sleep apnea (OSA).[4] Excessive body weight may increase propensity for upper airway narrowing during sleep by altering the function and the geometry of the pharynx.[4] In addition, obesity may alter ventilatory control and respiratory muscle function, leading to the obesity hypoventilation syndrome (OHS), which is characterized by obesity, chronic hypercapnia, and often sleep-disordered breathing (see Chapter 138).[5] Treatment for OSA includes continuous positive airway pressure (CPAP), oral appliances, upper airway surgeries, and risk factor modifications, including weight loss.

For patients desiring to lose weight, initial interventions include dietary modifications to reduce energy intake, enhanced physical activity to increase energy expenditure, and behavioral therapies to overcome barriers to compliance. Table 139.3 summarizes guideline recommendations for diet, exercise, and behavioral counseling for weight loss.[6] Pharmacotherapy may be considered for patients with a BMI 30 kg/m^2 or greater, or for those with a BMI of 27 kg/m^2 or greater and obesity-related disease who fail to achieve their weight loss targets after 6 months of diet and lifestyle changes. Currently approved therapies in the United States for adults include orlistat (also approved for children and adolescents), phentermine, lorcaserin, liraglutide, phentermine-topiramate, and naltrexone-buproprion.[7]

Surgical therapy for obesity, or bariatric surgery, is indicated for people with a BMI 35 to 39.9 kg/m^2 with associated health conditions such as OSA and a BMI 30 to 34.9 kg/m^2 if the associated condition is diabetes mellitus that is poorly controlled, and for BMI 40 kg/m^2 or greater even without associated comorbid conditions for whom other attempts at nonsurgical approaches to weight control have failed. Some bariatric surgery procedures restrict food intake by gastric resection, and others induce malabsorption or maldigestion.[8] The number of bariatric procedures being performed has increased in the past 10 years as a result of the rise in prevalence of severe obesity and refinement of operative techniques.

This chapter considers the epidemiology of obesity, potential mechanisms linking overweight and obesity with OSA, indications for bariatric surgery, technical aspects of common

Table 139.1 Classification of Overweight and Obesity in Adults by Body Mass Index

Category	Body Mass Index (kg/m²)
Underweight	<18.5
Normal	18.5-24.9
Overweight	25-29.9
Obesity	
Class 1	30-34.9
Class 2	35-39.9
Class 3 (extreme)	≥40

From North American Association for the Study of Obesity and the National Heart, Lung, and Blood Institute. The practical guide: identification, evaluation, and treatment of overweight and obesity in adults. NIH publication 00-4084. Bethesda, MD: National Institutes of Health; 2000. <http://www.cdc.gov/nccdphp/dnpa/obesity/defining.htm>.

Table 139.2 Classification of Overweight and Obesity in Children by Body Mass Index

Category	Percent Range in Body Mass Index
Underweight	Less than 5th percentile
Normal	5th percentile to <85th percentile
Overweight	85th to <95th percentile
Obese	95th percentile or greater

From https://www.cdc.gov/obesity/childhood/defining.html.

Table 139.3 Guideline Recommendations for Diet, Exercise, and Behavioral Counselling for the Management of Overweight and Obesity

Counsel overweight and obese patients on the benefits of weight loss.

Diet

- Pursue reduced caloric intake as part of a comprehensive lifestyle intervention, preferably with counseling input from a nutrition professional.

Targets

- 1200–1500 kcal/day for women and 1500–1800 kcal/day for men
- 500 kcal/day or 750 kcal/day energy deficit
- No specific dietary composition has proven to be more successful for weight loss; base the calorie-restricted diet on patient's preferences and health status

Physical activity

- Aim for increased aerobic physical activity (such as brisk walking) for ≥150 minutes/week.
- Higher levels of physical activity, approximately 200–300 minutes/week recommended to maintain lost weight or minimize weight regain in the long term.
- Tailor the activity to patient preference.

Lifestyle intervention and counseling

- Participate in ≥14 sessions for ≥6 months in a group or individual comprehensive program by a trained interventionist or trained nutritional professional who assists in adhering to a lower-calorie diet and increasing physical activity through use of behavioral strategies.
- For weight loss maintenance, prescribe face-to-face or telephone-delivered weight loss maintenance programs that provide at least monthly contact with a trained interventionist who helps participants consume a reduced-calorie diet, engage in high levels of physical activity, and monitor body weight at least weekly.

Modified from Jensen MD, Ryan DH, Apovian CM, et al. 2013 AHA/ACC/TOS guideline for the management of overweight and obesity in adults: a report of the American College of Cardiology/American Heart Association Task Force on Practice Guidelines and The Obesity Society. *Circulation*. 2014;129(Suppl 2):S102-S138.

bariatric procedures, perioperative management of patients with OSA, and outcomes of bariatric surgery, including its impact on OSA.

EPIDEMIOLOGY

Epidemiology of Obesity

Obesity prevalence is increasing worldwide. Per the Global Burden of Disease study data, global obesity prevalence has doubled in more than 70 countries since 1980, with youth obesity prevalence increases outpacing those in adults in many countries.[9] According to the National Health and Nutrition Examination Survey (NHANES), from 2015 to 2016, 39.8% of US adults, or approximately 93 million Americans, were obese and 7.7% had class 3 obesity.[10] Among US youth, 18.5% were obese and 5.6% had severe obesity.[10] From 1999–2000 through 2015–2016, there were significantly increasing trends in obesity in adults and youth.[11] Figure 139.1 shows the prevalence of adult obesity in 2018 per US state and territory per the Behavioral Risk Factor Surveillance System.[12] Adult and youth obesity prevalence is highest in non-Hispanic Blacks and Hispanics and lowest in non-Hispanic Asians.[11]

The increasing proportion of people who weigh more than their ideal body weight has formidable medical consequences including a reduction in life expectancy, with the increased mortality primarily from cardiovascular disease.[9,13,14] Furthermore, it is estimated that 20% of US national medical expenditures are spent on obesity-related illnesses.[15]

Epidemiologic Association Between Overweight/Obesity and Obstructive Sleep Apnea

Cross-sectional analyses of clinical and population samples have demonstrated notable colocalization of OSA and obesity.[4] OSA has been found in 50% to 80% of obese patients seen in clinical settings,[4] and 60% to 90% of adults with OSA may be overweight.[16] In the Wisconsin Sleep Cohort, an increase of 1 standard deviation (5.7 kg/m² BMI) was associated with a fourfold risk of an apnea-hypopnea index (AHI) of 5 or more events per hour.[17] Additionally, the Sleep Heart Health Study reported a dose-dependent relationship between increasing BMI and OSA: The prevalence of an AHI of 15 or more events per hour was 10% in the lowest BMI quartile (16–24 kg/m²), as opposed to 32% in the highest quartile (32–59 kg/m²).[18]

Longitudinal population and clinical samples also indicate that weight and AHI change congruently. In the Wisconsin Sleep Cohort, each 1% increase (or decrease) in weight was associated with a 3% increase (or decrease) in AHI, and in patients with mild OSA (AHI 5–15 events/hour) at baseline, a 10% weight gain led to a sixfold risk for developing moderate to severe OSA (AHI ≥15 events/hour).[19] In the

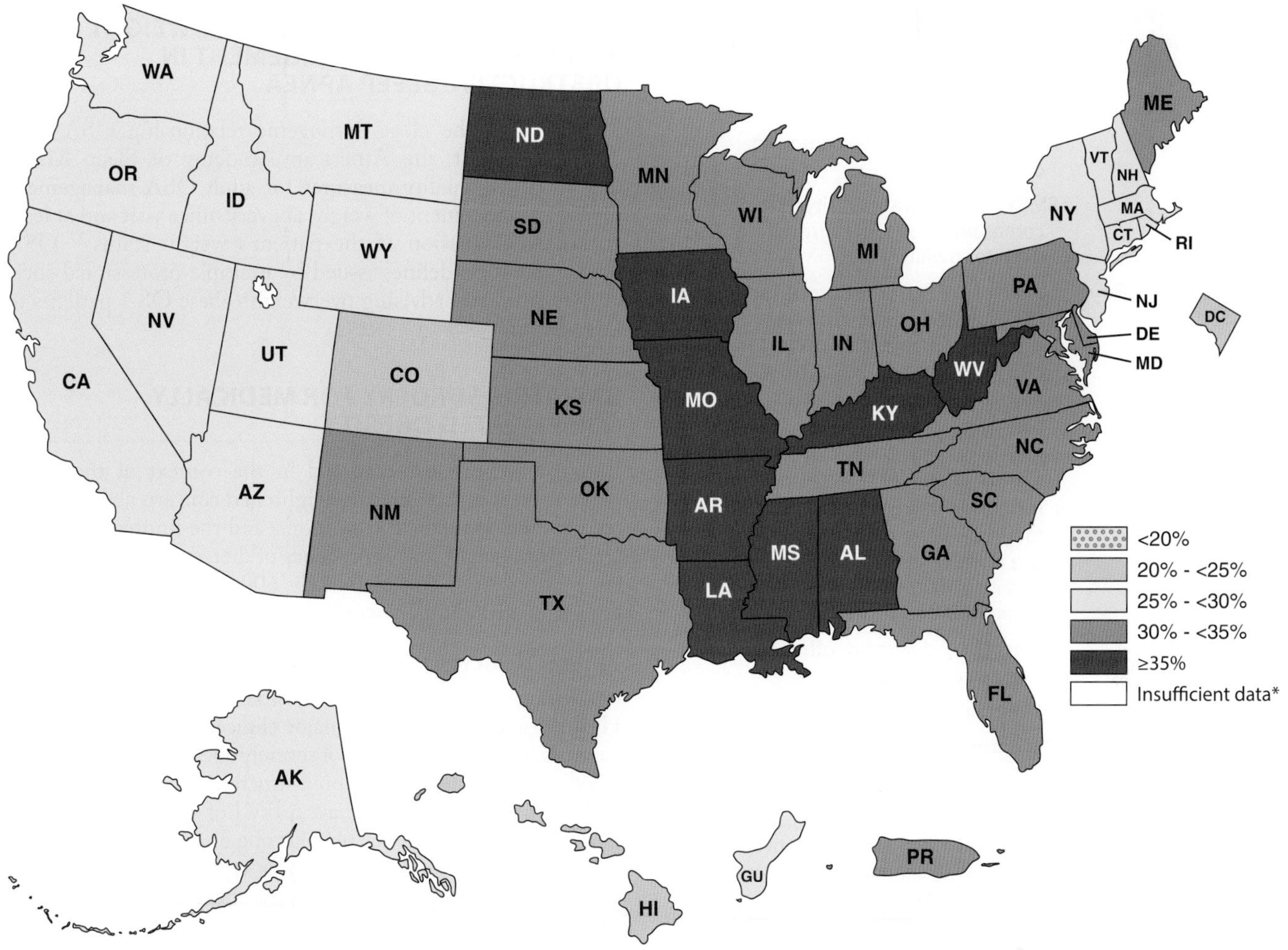

Figure 139.1 Prevalence of self-reported obesity among adults in the United States by state and territory per the Behavioral Risk Factor Surveillance System (BRFSS), 2018. No state or territory has an obesity prevalence of less than 20%. Nine states have an obesity prevalence of 35% or greater. The South (33.6%) and the Midwest (33.1%) have the highest prevalence of obesity, followed by the Northeast (28%), and the West (26.9%). (From Centers for Disease Control and Prevention. Obesity Prevalence Maps, 2018. https://www.cdc.gov/obesity/data/prevalence-maps.html#overalll.)

Sleep Heart Health Study, parallel changes in weight and AHI were similarly found over a 5-year follow-up period, but AHI increased more with weight gain than it decreased with weight loss.[20] Men tend to suffer a greater increase in AHI with weight gain than women,[20] whereas BMI has a greater effect on AHI in postmenopausal women than in premenopausal women.[4] Increasing age may attenuate the association of BMI and AHI.[18]

PATHOGENESIS

Mechanisms Linking Obesity to Obstructive Sleep Apnea Risk

Upper airway anatomic and neuromuscular factors may be influenced by parapharyngeal fat accumulation in several ways.[21] In obesity, upper airway size may be compressed by the deposition of adipose tissue, especially in the lateral pharyngeal fat pads, intraluminal structures (tongue, soft palate, uvula), and neck.[22-24] During wakefulness, increased pharyngeal dilator muscle activity provides compensation; the state-dependent attenuation of pharyngeal muscle activity with sleep, by contrast, leaves the upper airway vulnerable to collapse.[25] Overweight/obese individuals without OSA rely on enhanced upper airway dilator muscle responsiveness during sleep to allay the effect of compromised upper airway structure.[26] Accrual of fat around the upper airway may alter soft tissue properties, thereby heightening the propensity to collapse by increasing upper airway compliance,[27] or may change upper airway geometry, with a consequent decrease in the ability of pharyngeal muscles to dilate the airway.[28]

Obesity, a chronic inflammatory state itself, may contribute to increasing upper airway tissue inflammation[29] or to upper airway neuropathic damage through the pathophysiologic changes of diabetes mellitus.[30] Increased levels of proinflammatory cytokines in obesity may indirectly impair pharyngeal dilator muscle activity via their somnogenic effects, which may depress central nervous system upper airway muscle control.[31]

Thoracoabdominal viscera fat accumulation, typical in men, is also of likely pathogenetic importance in OSA, as suggested by population surveys reporting a two- to threefold increase in prevalence of symptomatic OSA in men compared with women.[17,32,33] The interaction of hormonal changes and accompanying increases in central fat deposition may contribute to the increased prevalence of OSA in postmenopausal

Table 139.4 Adult Patient Selection Criteria for Bariatric Surgery

Factor	Criteria
Weight	BMI ≥40 kg/m² with no comorbid conditions
	BMI ≥35 kg/m² with obesity-associated comorbidity (30–34.9 kg/m² if diabetes mellitus)[a]
Weight loss history	Failure of previous nonsurgical attempts at weight reduction, including nonprofessional programs (e.g., Weight Watchers)
Commitment	Expectation that the patient will adhere to postoperative care, including follow-up visits with physician(s) and team members; recommended medical management, including use of dietary supplements; and instructions regarding any recommended procedures or tests
Exclusions	Reversible endocrine or other disorders that can cause obesity
	Current drug or alcohol use
	Uncontrolled, severe psychiatric illness
	Severe cardiac disease
	Lack of comprehension of risks, benefits, expected outcomes, alternatives, and lifestyle changes required with bariatric surgery

From Mechanick JI, Youdim A, Jones DB, et al. Clinical practice guidelines for the perioperative nutritional, metabolic, and nonsurgical support of the bariatric surgery patient—2013 update: cosponsored by American Association of Clinical Endocrinologists, The Obesity Society, and American Society for Metabolic and Bariatric Surgery. Obesity. 2013;21:S1–S27.
[a]Aminian A, Chang J, Brethauer SA, Kim JJ; for the American Society for Metabolic and Bariatric Surgery Clinical Issues Committee. ASMBS updated position statement on bariatric surgery in class I obesity (BMI 30-35 kg/m²). *Surg Obes Rel Dis*. 2018; 14:1071-1087.

women.[4] Central obesity–induced reduction in lung volume[32] decreases "tracheal tug," a caudally directed, pharyngeal-stabilizing, lung volume–dependent traction force directed along the trachea.[34] Reduced lung volume may also destabilize breathing by altering the sensitivity of the negative feedback control loop, thereby increasing loop gain.[35] The reduction in lung volumes coupled with globally increased oxygen demand also may intensify the oxygen desaturation accompanying obstructive apneas and hypopneas.

Leptin, a hormone produced mainly by adipose tissue that has regulatory roles in energy intake, metabolism, inflammation, and sympathetic nerve activity, has an unclear role in OSA pathogenesis.[36] There may be a bidirectional relationship between obesity and OSA.[31] The intermittent hypoxia, sympathetic activation, and sleep fragmentation caused by repeated episodes of obstructive apnea and hypopnea produce metabolic alterations that provide biologically plausible means by which OSA also may exacerbate overweight and obesity (see Chapter 136).

RECOMMENDATIONS REGARDING WEIGHT ASSESSMENT AND MANAGEMENT IN OBSTRUCTIVE SLEEP APNEA

Underscoring the close pathogenic relationship OSA with excessive weight, the American Academy of Sleep Medicine (AASM) quality measures for adult OSA management include measurement of weight at every office visit and at least an annual discussion of the patient's weight status.[37] OSA management guidelines issued by multiple professional societies recommend advising overweight/obese OSA patients to lose weight.[38-42]

BARIATRIC SURGERY FOR MEDICALLY COMPLICATED OBESITY

Bariatric surgery has emerged in the context of the rising prevalence of severe obesity, heightened concern about associated comorbid medical conditions, and the limited success of traditional weight loss approaches of diet, exercise, and behavior modification. Approximately 600,000 bariatric surgeries are performed annually worldwide.[43]

Patient Selection

Guidelines originally issued by the National Institutes of Health[44] and reaffirmed by major clinical societies[45] state that bariatric surgery is an option for severely obese adult patients who failed to achieve weight loss on a structured, monitored exercise and diet program and who have a BMI of 40 kg/m² or greater, or a BMI of 35 to 39.9 kg/m² plus one or more obesity-related severe comorbid conditions, such as type 2 diabetes mellitus, hypertension, dyslipidemia, coronary artery disease, pseudotumor cerebri, asthma, venous stasis, severe urinary incontinence, debilitating arthritis, gastroesophageal reflux disease (GERD), nonalcoholic fatty liver disease, OSA, and OHS.[45] The International Federation for the Surgery of Obesity and Metabolic Disorders[46] and American Society for Metabolic and Bariatric Surgery (ASMBS)[47] also recommend that bariatric surgery may be offered to patients with class I obesity (BMI 30–4.9 kg/m²) and type 2 diabetes who have glycemia that is difficult to control, a position endorsed by the American Diabetes Association.[48]

Patients preparing to undergo bariatric surgery must complete a comprehensive nutritional and psychological screening for untreated depression, substance abuse, or eating disorders. The bariatric surgery candidate must demonstrate a complete understanding of the risks and benefits of the operation as a weight loss "tool," recognize the necessity after surgery to limit portion size and food types, and agree to follow a postoperative vitamin supplementation regimen. Patients are ineligible for surgery if they cannot understand or will not commit to the dietary changes and lifestyle modifications necessary to complement the procedure. In addition, poor surgical or anesthetic risk status (advanced congestive heart failure or suboptimally controlled angina pectoris), older age (>65–70 years), reversible endocrine or other disorders that might cause obesity, and active addiction behaviors are contraindications to bariatric surgery. Selection criteria for adult bariatric surgery are summarized in Table 139.4.[45] Recently revised ASMBS guidelines for bariatric surgery in adolescents (patients age 10–19 years; but "younger children who meet the other criteria could be considered when benefit outweighs risk") are shown in Table 139.5.[49]

Table 139.5 Adolescent Patient Selection Criteria for Bariatric Surgery

Factor	Criteria
Weight	BMI ≥40 kg/m² or 140% of the 95th percentile (whichever is lower)
	BMI ≥35 kg/m² or 120% of the 95th percentile with clinically significant comorbid conditions such as obstructive sleep apnea (AHI >5 events/hour), type 2 diabetes mellitus, idiopathic intracranial hypertension, nonalcoholic steatohepatitis, Blount's disease, slipped capital femoral epiphysis, gastroesophageal reflux disease, or hypertension
Commitment	The patient and family have the ability and motivation to adhere to recommended therapies pre- and postoperatively as determined by a multidisciplinary team.
Exclusions	Reversible endocrine or other disorders that can cause obesity
	Ongoing substance abuse problem (within the preceding year)
	Medical, psychiatric, psychosocial, or cognitive condition that prevents adherence to postoperative dietary and medication regimens
	Current or planned pregnancy within 12-18 months of surgery

From Pratt JSA, Browne A, Brown NT, et al. ASMBS pediatric metabolic and bariatric surgery guidelines, 2018. *Surg Obes Rel Dis*. 2018;14:882-901.

Rationale for Patient Assessment for Obstructive Sleep Apnea Before Bariatric Surgery

High OSA prevalence has been consistently reported among patients being considered for bariatric surgery and therefore screening for sleep breathing disorders is indicated.[50] In one large series of consecutive patients undergoing bariatric surgery the prevalence of OSA (defined as an AHI ≥5 events/hour) was 77%; 19% had moderate (AHI 15–30 events/hour) and 27% had severe OSA (AHI >30 events/hour).[51] Concurrent OSA may complicate endotracheal intubation and/or increase the difficulty of mask ventilation in obese patients. Commonly used perioperative drugs have inhibitory influences on central ventilatory drive, protective upper airway reflexes, and arousal mechanisms, which may further jeopardize the airway of the severely obese patient. Upper airway edema associated with endotracheal intubation and forced supine positioning also can acutely aggravate OSA risk after bariatric surgery. Episodes of desaturation associated with postoperative obstructive apneic episodes or hypoventilation may be exaggerated by the interaction of obesity-related reduction in pulmonary functional residual capacity with factors in the postoperative milieu. OSA may increase risk for and/or destabilize comorbid conditions in the obese patient, such as hypertension, atrial fibrillation, heart failure, and diabetes mellitus, and these conditions may require attention preoperatively or adversely affect the postoperative course. Therefore, close collaboration among the sleep specialist, the anesthesiologist, the bariatric surgeon, and the patient is crucial for proper planning to mitigate OSA-related complications perioperatively.

Preoperative Assessment for Bariatric Surgery in the Patient Without Known Obstructive Sleep Apnea

The AACE-TOS-ASMBS clinical practice guidelines[45] stipulate that the possibility of OSA should be considered in *all* bariatric surgery candidates. Screening for OSA was also deemed mandatory per the first international consensus conference on the perioperative management of OSA in bariatric surgery in 2016.[52] However, uncertainties exist regarding the specifics of the extent of the preoperative OSA evaluation.

Discernment of OSA status begins in all bariatric surgery candidates with a sleep-focused history and physical exam by the bariatric surgery team. The diagnostic features of OSA are discussed in Chapters 128 and 131. No cardinal symptom of OSA, such as snoring or excessive daytime sleepiness, is singularly sufficient to predict the presence of OSA or its severity in bariatric surgery candidates. Furthermore, no single best metric of body habitus for predicting OSA has been identified.[4] Instead, a combination of symptoms and signs is more discriminatory, so many prediction formulas combining clinical parameters have been created to hone clinicians' detection of OSA. One OSA screening tool extensively studied in preoperative patients is the STOP-BANG questionnaire.[53] This questionnaire poses "yes-or-no" questions about **S**noring, **T**iredness, **O**bserved apneas, blood **P**ressure, **B**MI greater than 35 kg/m², **A**ge greater than 50 years, **N**eck circumference greater than 40 cm, and male **G**ender, with OSA likelihood increasing with more affirmative responses. Sensitivity (proportion of patients with OSA correctly identified by STOP-BANG to have OSA) and specificity (proportion of patients without OSA correctly identified by STOP-BANG to not have OSA) for moderate to severe OSA (AHI > 15 events/hour) in patients with BMI 35 kg/m² or greater preparing for nonbariatric operations depends on the cutpoints selected: score 3 or greater: 97% (sensitivity) and 7% (specificity); 4 or greater: 86% and 28%; 5 or greater: 65% and 65%; and 6 or greater: 42% and 86%[54] These figures highlight the tradeoff inherent in OSA prediction tools: As the threshold for the number of required OSA features is increased, those incorrectly labeled as having OSA (false positives) decreases, but detection of patients with OSA (true positives) also decreases. In general, most OSA prediction tools are more sensitive than specific, favoring detection of true positives (presence of OSA in patients identified as having the disorder) and thereby minimizing false negatives, at the expense of false positives (designating many patients as having OSA when in fact they do not). Severe OSA is unlikely to be missed by OSA prediction tools, but reported sensitivities and specificities for a given screening tool have varied in the hands of different investigators.[55]

Guidelines emerging from the anesthesiology literature[50,56-58] recommend incorporating an OSA prediction tool or checklist in the preoperative assessment of patients preparing for any surgery. The STOP-BANG questionnaire is highlighted in several of these strategies; the American Society of Anesthesiologists guideline for the perioperative management of patients with known or suspected OSA contains its own OSA prediction checklist.[56] Patients judged low risk for OSA by the screening instrument are cleared to proceed to surgery without further sleep testing, whereas those deemed intermediate or high risk should proceed either to a formal sleep assessment or to surgery, with adjustment of their perioperative care for presumptive OSA, depending on the clinical status and urgency of the surgical issue.

In bariatric surgery programs in which neither polysomnography (PSG) nor home sleep apnea testing (HSAT) is uniformly performed in all candidates, use of an OSA screening tool is recommended to stratify high-risk OSA.[52] This practice will ensure that the surgical team deliberately contemplates OSA in an organized manner and will enhance detection of the most severe OSA cases. Because the best OSA screening tool is not known, the decision about which tool to use must be made locally by the bariatric surgery team, ideally with guidance from their sleep medicine colleagues. The designation of OSA status by the screening tool output must be integrated with other pertinent information, such as collateral observations about the patient's breathing during sleep from their bed partner, history of airway difficulties with previous anesthetics, anticipated surgical approach (open versus laparoscopic), and comorbidity burden. Those patients deemed to be high risk for OSA through integration of clinical information should proceed to formal sleep apnea testing as OSA cannot be diagnosed on clinical grounds alone.[59]

A routine role for pre–bariatric surgery sleep testing (PSG or HSAT) continues to be debated. Proponents cite the high prevalence of OSA among severely obese patients, the significant potential for perioperative complications from unrecognized OSA, and the limited accuracy of clinical impression alone in OSA diagnosis. Opponents point to the lack of data demonstrating improved postoperative outcomes with preoperative initiation of CPAP in patients undergoing bariatric surgery, the uncertainty regarding the relative contribution of OSA to postoperative complications in this population, challenges accessing timely sleep medicine testing and care, and potential clinical overuse of such testing in patients deemed to be at low risk by clinical impression or OSA screening tool.

Performing sleep studies in all bariatric surgery candidates without exception seems overly rigid. The reality is that if any OSA screening tool is systematically implemented, most patients will face the prospect of sleep testing before bariatric surgery because they will be judged to be at high risk by the OSA screening tool. For instance, in the study examining the performance of STOP-BANG in obese patients,[54] just 5% of preoperative patients with a BMI 35 kg/m^2 or greater scored 2 or greater. Additionally, sleep testing may be needed to establish OSA as a weight-related comorbid condition in building a justification for bariatric surgery, or if therapy for OSA is desired regardless of whether bariatric surgery is ultimately performed. In those patients without collateral sleep history or who are suspected of downplaying OSA symptoms, overnight oximetry monitoring may be an intermediate step between OSA screening by history and physical examination and a formal sleep study. In bariatric surgery programs in which preoperative PSG or HSAT is not routinely performed in every patient, preoperative consultation with a sleep specialist about the need for further sleep testing often is appropriate and is specifically recommended in situations of ambiguity about OSA status or its perioperative importance. Private insurers are increasingly mandating HSAT in cases of suspected OSA, and the adult bariatric surgery candidate with a high pretest probability of having moderate to severe OSA and without significant comorbid cardiopulmonary disease may be an appropriate candidate for HSAT followed by initiation of autoadjusting CPAP.[60] However, laboratory-based PSG is indicated and typically is covered by insurance carriers for the very obese suspects with OSA (BMI >45–50 kg/m^2) or those with suspected OHS, because of the possible need for attended titration of modalities other than CPAP, such as bilevel positive airway pressure (BPAP) and supplemental oxygen.

A high index of clinical suspicion in all potential bariatric surgery candidates must be maintained for OHS, because affected patients require more careful presurgical consideration, as patients with OHS would be expected to be at higher risk than eucapnic obese patients with OSA during bariatric surgery. The diminished ventilatory responsiveness to hypoxia and hypercapnia in OHS leads to increased sensitivity to sedatives and opioids, potentially greater problems with weaning from mechanical ventilation, and development of life-threatening obstructive apnea events, as well as acute worsening of hypercapnia with supplemental oxygen therapy unaccompanied by any ventilatory support such as BPAP.[61] Rates of comorbid conditions such as systemic hypertension, pulmonary hypertension, cor pulmonale, and angina are higher in patients with OHS than in eucapnic obese patients.[62] Accordingly, patients with OHS unrecognized before undergoing elective noncardiac surgery were more likely to have postoperative respiratory failure, heart failure, ICU transfers, and longer lengths of stay compared with OSA patients without OHS in a retrospective analysis.[63] OHS is also a risk factor for development of venous thromboembolic (VTE) disease, which is a leading cause of postoperative death in bariatric surgery.[64]

OHS can be challenging to diagnose before bariatric surgery because patients may not always appear dramatically different than eucapnic obese patients with OSA. Patients with OHS more commonly have lower extremity edema, report moderate to severe dyspnea on exertion, exhibit higher AHIs and more profound minimum oxyhemoglobin saturations during sleep, spend greater time with an oxyhemoglobin saturation lower than 90% during sleep, have lower awake oxyhemoglobin saturations, are afflicted with higher BMIs, demonstrate greater restrictive changes on pulmonary function testing, and use more health care resources compared with eucapnic obese patients with OSA (see Box 138.3 in Chapter 138). Preoperative serum bicarbonate measurement is recommended in all bariatric surgery candidates[52] because a value of 27 mEq/L or greater (reflecting metabolic compensation for chronic respiratory acidosis) is a sensitive but not specific marker for OHS in the obese patient with OSA.[65] If OHS is suspected, the following tests are recommended: arterial blood gas (hypoventilation manifests as hypercapnia, the severity of which should be determined), pulmonary function tests and chest radiograph (to search for other causes of chronic hypoventilation), echocardiogram (to assess the right heart pressures and function), complete blood count (to detect erythrocytosis), thyroid function tests (to rule out hypothyroidism, if not already done as part of routine testing of the obese patient), and PSG ideally with carbon dioxide monitoring.

Positive airway pressure (PAP) therapy for moderate to severe OSA (AHI ≥15 events/hour) should be initiated preoperatively.[52] Case-by-case decisions about CPAP are necessary in milder forms of OSA (e.g., position-dependent OSA); CPAP may be recommended preoperatively for a patient with mild OSA who also is hypersomnolent or in whom the degree of desaturation during obstructive apneas/hypopneas is of greater clinical concern, perhaps in the presence of comorbid conditions such as pulmonary hypertension. The elective nature of bariatric surgery should allow for follow-up assessment of newly initiated PAP therapy before surgery. In many bariatric surgery centers, adherence to PAP preoperatively is a mandatory prerequisite. The minimal preoperative PAP trial duration for achieving PAP acclimatization and garnering improvement in physical status is not known, but because patterns of PAP use may be established within the first week of therapy,[66] close follow-up monitoring in the first month to document adherence, address problems, and assess response is advised. In the patient with OHS, a repeat arterial blood gases analysis after 4 weeks of PAP therapy[5] may allow discontinuance of supplemental oxygen with confirmation of an adequate therapeutic response or may indicate the need for tracheostomy with or without ventilation if PAP fails to effect improvement.

Preoperative Assessment for Bariatric Surgery in the Patient with Established Obstructive Sleep Apnea

Patients with a known diagnosis of OSA already on an established therapy (usually PAP) as they explore bariatric surgery should be queried about adherence, technical difficulties, persistent symptoms despite therapy, and increases in weight since therapy initiation. Identification of any of these issues should prompt referral to a sleep specialist. Follow-up sleep apnea testing is indicated for patients with substantial weight gain (i.e., greater than or equal to 10% of body weight since treatment was initiated), change in their cardiovascular status, recurrent OSA symptoms, and/or unexplained PAP device download data.[67] Asymptomatic, PAP-adherent patients generally can proceed to surgery. They should be advised that PAP use will be required postoperatively so they should bring their equipment to the hospital. Preoperative settings for PAP with or without supplemental oxygen usually are maintained postoperatively, although acute adjustments may be necessary for factors such as opioid administration and postoperative pulmonary disorders (e.g., VTE, pneumonia). Patients with OSA treated previously with upper airway surgery who remain symptomatic, or in whom objective evidence of sleep-disordered breathing resolution is lacking, should be assumed to remain at risk for residual OSA and may benefit from a pre–bariatric surgery sleep evaluation.[68] Such patients should be advised that temporary application of PAP may be necessary in the immediate postoperative period if upper airway obstruction occurs. Bariatric surgery candidates who use an oral appliance for OSA should be instructed to continue therapy perioperatively.[52]

Common Bariatric Surgical Procedures

Bariatric surgical procedures have been historically grouped into three categories based on anatomic components: predominately malabsorptive procedures, predominately restrictive procedures, and procedures with both malabsorptive and restrictive components.[69] A majority of these operations are now performed by a less invasive, small-incision, laparoscopic approach. There has been evolution in the utilization of bariatric procedures with a recent shift to vertical sleeve gastrectomy (VSG).[70]

Roux-en-Y gastric bypass (RYGB) (Figure 139.2) combines creation of a small gastric pouch with modest intestinal or small bowel bypass to produce weight loss through both

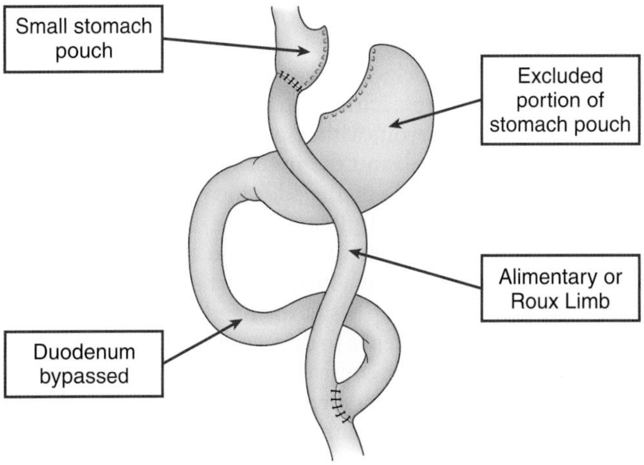

Figure 139.2 Roux-en-Y gastric bypass. (From https://www.nhlbi.nih.gov/sites/default/files/media/docs/obesity-evidence-review.pdf.)

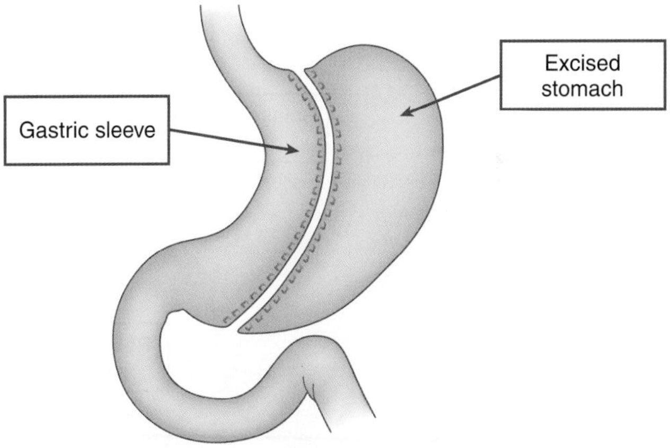

Figure 139.3 Vertical sleeve gastrectomy. (From https://www.nhlbi.nih.gov/sites/default/files/media/docs/obesity-evidence-review.pdf.)

restrictive and malabsorptive means. A traditional RYGB consists of transection of a small (15-mL) proximal gastric pouch along the lesser curvature of the stomach from the larger gastric segment, combined with a modest (encompassing 60–150 cm) intestinal bypass. The Roux-en-Y configuration allows biliopancreatic secretions and digestive juices to pass through the bile duct into the duodenum and then merge with the alimentary stream passing down from the stomach at the Y-type connection. The lengths of both the Roux and biliopancreatic limbs can be varied to produce more malabsorption. Most weight is lost in the first year. Approximately 80% of patients typically experience weight stabilization, usually slightly above weight nadir, approximately 3 years after surgery. The remaining 20% of patients slowly regain excess weight over longer-term follow-up, and risk regaining much of the lost weight.

VSG (Figure 139.3) is now the most commonly performed major bariatric procedure.[70] This operation restricts intake via a 70% vertical gastric resection, creating a long and narrow tubular gastric reservoir with no intestinal bypass. In many ways, VSG is intermediate between bypass and banding in terms of surgical complexity, postoperative risk, and weight loss results. The higher-pressure character of the tubular stomach after surgery might predict the development or persistence of GERD after VSG, yet this issue remains controversial. Like RYGB, the majority of weight loss occurs in the first 12 months postoperatively.

The *laparoscopic adjustable gastric band* is an inflatable silicone prosthetic device that is placed around the top portion of the stomach, just below the esophagus (Figure 139.4) and restricts the upper stomach size to a small volume. The band is attached to a reservoir, with a port placed under the skin on the abdominal wall, and the inner lining of the band is a balloon that is adjustable by the addition or removal of saline from the reservoir port. Inflation of the band increases the restriction of gastric outlet size and food flow. Postoperative management for patients who have undergone this procedure entails frequent follow-up visits for band adjustments/reservoir fills and strict adherence to dietary guidelines and lifestyle modification to achieve consistent weight loss. The weight loss trajectory after banding procedures is more gradual, with less weight lost than after either RYGB or VSG. The favorable aspects of this procedure are that it is less invasive and requires less operating time, and that the band is both adjustable and removable. Use of the band procedure has declined dramatically.

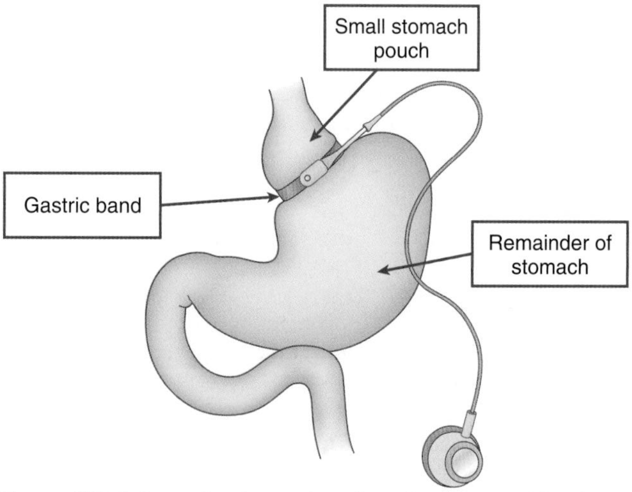

Figure 139.4 Gastric band procedure. (From https://www.nhlbi.nih.gov/sites/default/files/media/docs/obesity-evidence-review.pdf.)

The less commonly used *biliopancreatic diversion* (BPD) and *BPD with duodenal switch* (BPDDS) procedures (Figure 139.5), which result in an extreme degree of malabsorption, are reserved for the treatment of "superobese" patients. BPD combines a partial, subtotal gastrectomy and a very long Roux-en-Y anastomosis with a short common channel for nutrient absorption. With this procedure, patients can eat much larger quantities of food and still achieve and maintain weight loss. Disadvantages include higher postoperative surgical risks, loose and foul-smelling stools, intestinal ulcers, anemia, vitamin and mineral deficiencies, and possible protein-calorie malnutrition. Because of these potential problems, patients who undergo BPD require lifelong dietary supplementation and close follow-up monitoring. With weight loss and complications to those with BPD, the BPDDS is a hybrid operation that combines a gastric sleeve resection with a long intestinal bypass in the Roux-en-Y configuration. This procedure reduces ulcer rate, and dumping syndrome (the constellation of nausea, vomiting, abdominal pain or cramping, diarrhea, bloating, fatigue, palpitations, lightheadedness, sweating, and anxiety beginning within 15 to 30 minutes after eating) is eliminated by leaving intact the first portion of the intestine in the alimentary stream. BPD and BPDDS procedures are the most major and technically difficult bariatric procedures and consequently should be offered only by experienced surgeons and to patients able to undertake lifelong follow-up.

Two intragastric balloon systems are currently approved in the United States for adults with class I and II obesity and weight-related comorbidities who have failed to lose weight through diet and lifestyle modifications.[71-73] The balloon system (Figure 139.6) is either placed endoscopically or swallowed in a capsule and resides in the stomach for up to 6 months before being retrieved endoscopically, resulting in weight loss through satiety promotion, delayed gastric emptying, and caloric intake restriction. Potential adverse consequences, usually experienced in the first week of adaptation to the device, include nausea, vomiting, burping, abdominal pain, and gastric reflux that may require antiemetics and proton pump inhibitors. Later complications potentially include distal migration of the balloon into the intestine and possible

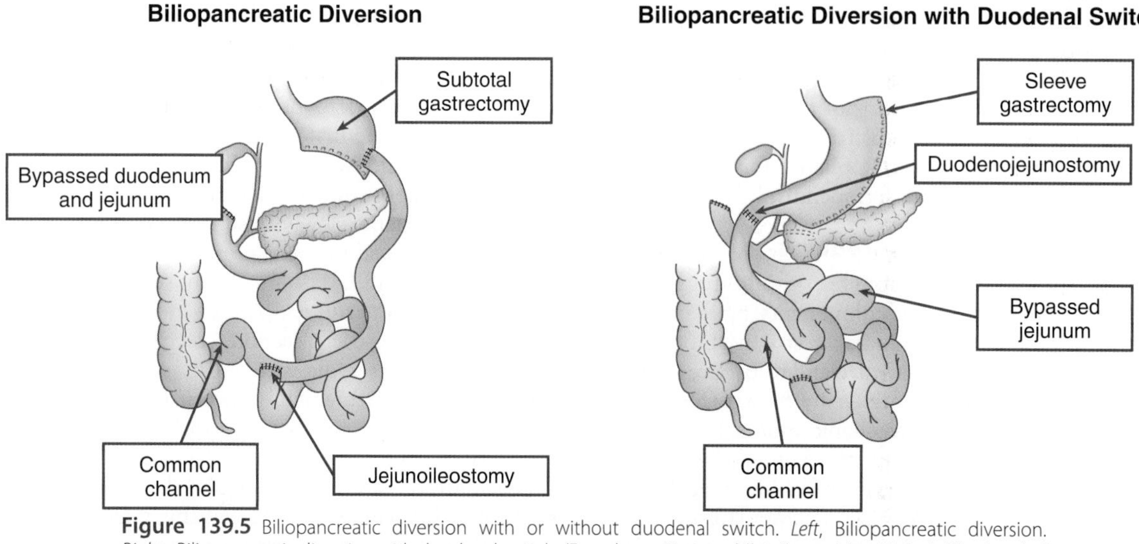

Figure 139.5 Biliopancreatic diversion with or without duodenal switch. *Left*, Biliopancreatic diversion. *Right*, Biliopancreatic diversion with duodenal switch. (From https://www.nhlbi.nih.gov/sites/default/files/media/docs/obesity-evidence-review.pdf.)

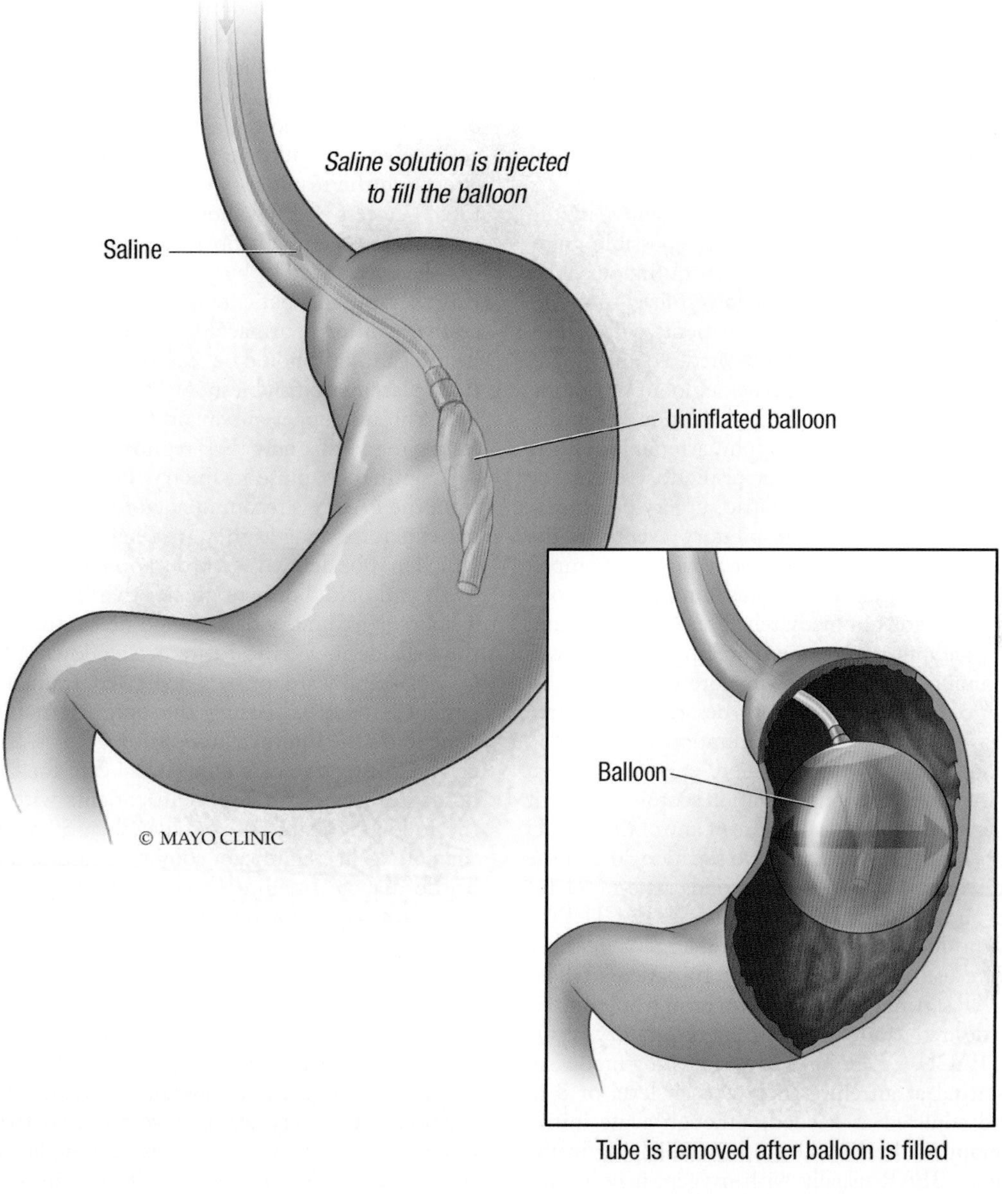
Saline solution is injected
to fill the balloon
Saline
Uninflated balloon
© MAYO CLINIC
Balloon
Tube is removed after balloon is filled

Figure 139.6 Intragastric balloon. (Used with permission of Mayo Foundation for Medical Education and Research, all rights reserved.)

bowel obstruction, pressure-related gastric ulcers, and persistent gastrointestinal symptoms resulting in early removal. Intragastric balloon therapy is contraindicated in patients with previous gastric surgery, a bleeding lesion in the upper gastrointestinal tract, coagulopathy, or pregnancy/desire to become pregnant. Weight loss is typically 10% to 15% of initial weight with much variability between individuals. Given the temporary intent of intragastric balloon therapy and need for balloon removal, patients cannot be lost to follow-up and behavioral modifications are crucial adjuncts. Intragastric balloon therapy might also be a bridging option before more definite bariatric surgery in the severely obese, but this has not been well studied.[73]

Most bariatric surgeons advocate a high-quality shared decision-making conversation with prospective patients with respect to the choice of bariatric procedure. Patients share their values and concerns while physicians provide general guidelines about the different potential mechanisms of action, percent weight loss over time, and morbidity profile among procedures. The optimal choice of procedure also depends in part on the expertise of the surgeon and the clinical facility, patient preference, and risk stratification.[45]

CLINICAL COURSE

Management of Known or Suspected Obstructive Sleep Apnea Immediately After Bariatric Surgery

Many details regarding optimal care of the patient with OSA immediately after bariatric surgery remain unclear. The following general recommendations are based on experience, consensus expert opinion for generic surgical care,[52,56-58,68] and the limited peer-reviewed literature.

Airway extubation after bariatric surgery should be performed only when the patient is fully awake and alert and has demonstrated evidence of return of neuromuscular function (as evidenced by sustained head lift for more than 5 seconds) and adequate vital capacity and peak inspiratory pressure.[56] Removal of the endotracheal tube should take place in the operating room, postanesthesia care unit (PACU), or special care unit so that airway control can be monitored closely and expertly addressed if lost.[56]

In the PACU, the patient should be maintained in the semiupright or lateral, not supine, position, if possible. Supplemental oxygen typically is provided under continuous pulse oximetry monitoring and titrated to the lowest level to maintain adequate oxygenation, especially in patients with OHS. Ventilation also must be specifically monitored, as supplemental oxygen may maintain adequate oxyhemoglobin saturation despite medication-exacerbated hypoventilation. Ventilation monitoring may include capnography, arterial blood gas testing, and scheduled assessments for respiratory events by PACU staff. In a study of a non–bariatric surgery perioperative patient population, recurrent respiratory events in the PACU powerfully predicted postoperative respiratory complications.[74] Respiratory events were scored during three consecutive 30-minute periods immediately after extubation and were defined as bradypnea (three or more episodes of fewer than 8 breaths/minute), apnea (one or more episodes of 10 seconds or longer of breathing cessation), desaturations (three or more episodes of oxyhemoglobin saturation below 90%), and pain-sedation mismatch (one or more episodes of high pain score and simultaneously high sedation score). Recurrent respiratory events meant that one or more of any of the PACU respiratory events occurred in at least two separate 30-minute time blocks and were associated with an odds ratio of 21 for postoperative respiratory complications.[74] In the PACU, PAP is instituted at the level prescribed before surgery in those patients who were using it preoperatively. In patients whose preoperative CPAP settings are not known or in whom initiation of CPAP is desired to address recurrent respiratory events emerging in the PACU, CPAP in the autoadjusting mode can be applied or started at an empirically chosen level of 8 to 10 cm H_2O and adjusted as needed, although acute initiation of such therapy in the PACU can be challenging in the PAP-naive patient. BPAP, usually with oxygen, may be initiated to address acute hypoventilation. PACU staff must be capable of monitoring and managing PAP therapy, including addressing interface leaks and observing diligently for signs of breakthrough upper airway obstruction despite PAP, such as snoring, choking, witnessed apneas, cardiac dysrhythmias, or repetitive oxygen desaturation.

In the first 24 postoperative hours after bariatric surgery, patients are likely to be the most vulnerable to potential OSA-related complications,[75] although OSA propensity may be increased for at least several days after bariatric surgery because of the aggregate effects of ongoing sleep deprivation, rapid eye movement sleep rebound, and medication synergies.[68] Fortunately, the length of hospital stay usually is short (3.5 days and 1.6 days for gastric bypass and restrictive procedures, respectively).[76] Clinicians must consistently keep the possibility of OSA in mind in all patients as they consider postoperative analgesia, monitoring, oxygenation, and patient positioning[56] for the duration of the hospitalization. Systemic opioids should be used cautiously because of their ability to depress the respiratory drive and cause subsequent oxygen desaturation. The use of patient-controlled analgesia is controversial, although it may be an option if used without a basal rate and with restricted dosing. Nonsteroidal antiinflammatory agents may help decrease opioid dosing as recovery progresses but should be used cautiously in the postsurgical patient because of the enhanced potential for bleeding complications. Benzodiazepines should be avoided because of their negative effects on the respiratory control and upper airway musculature.[56] Access to PAP should be available at all times during recovery—a seemingly obvious recommendation but one that may be overlooked by busy house staff, nurses unfamiliar with this therapy, and patients distracted or impaired by postoperative pain or pharmacologic obtundation. Properly trained health care staff should be readily available to assist patients in PAP placement, troubleshoot interface problems, observe for breakthrough upper airway obstruction, and reassure patients struggling with a new PAP regimen.

Continuous pulse oximetry monitoring after discharge from the PACU is recommended for all post–bariatric surgery patients for as long as they are deemed to be at increased risk, which may be defined as the duration of intravenous opioid use or an oral opioid dose of greater than 60 mg of codeine every 4 hours.[58] Oximetry data should be continuously observed at the bedside in a critical care or stepdown unit, by telemetry on a hospital ward, or by a dedicated, trained observer in the patient's room. Choosing the optimal monitoring site will depend on the interplay of multiple factors. It is reasonable to consider intensive care unit (ICU) care for the first 24 to 48 hours after bariatric surgery in patients with one or more of the following features: age older than 50 years, BMI greater than 60 kg/m^2, significant comorbid cardiopulmonary disease, brittle diabetes mellitus, severe OSA/OHS with worrisome record of suboptimal PAP compliance, sluggish emergence from anesthesia, and intraoperative complications. In the University HealthSystem Consortium evaluation, a review of the bariatric programs at 29 academic medical centers in the United States, 7.7% of patients undergoing gastric bypass required ICU support postoperatively.[76] Operative approach to bariatric surgery also must be considered. Case series from experienced surgery teams have reported that patients with established and treated OSA undergoing laparoscopic bariatric procedures do not require routine postoperative admission to the ICU.[77,78]

Incentive spirometry should be encouraged. If oxygen desaturations occur despite an appropriate PAP regimen, supplemental oxygen should be added while the provider searches for an explanation, such as transient worsening of upper airway obstruction requiring adjustment of PAP settings, VTE event, atelectasis, aspiration, pneumonia, or anastomotic leak. Caution with the use of supplemental oxygen without PAP during sleep is advised, because this strategy provides no protection against upper airway obstruction and will blunt detection of a disordered breathing event by oximetry monitoring. Postoperative supine positioning also should be avoided; instead, the head of the bed should be kept elevated in a semi-Fowler position (to at least 30 degrees) at all times. All post–bariatric surgery patients should be considered to be at moderate to high risk for VTE events; accordingly, thromboprophylaxis with low-molecular-weight heparin or low-dose unfractionated heparin, plus application of intermittent pneumatic compression stockings, is indicated in all patients.[64] The frequency of VTE after bariatric surgery with thromboprophylaxis is greater than 1%.[64] Because most VTEs occur after hospital discharge, the AACE-TOS-ASMBS advises extended chemoprophylaxis (duration unspecified) for patients at higher risk for such events, such as those with a history of VTE or reduced activity level.[45] Prolonged respiratory failure after bariatric surgery is uncommon, occurring in fewer than 1% of cases, according to data from the American College of Surgeons' National Surgical Quality Improvement program encompassing approximately 32,000 patients who underwent bariatric surgery between 2006 and 2008; the impact of OSA on the rate of respiratory failure is not known, because OSA was not a risk factor assessed in the analysis.[79]

Laparoscopic bariatric surgery is performed in some patients in an ambulatory setting. A consensus statement from the Society for Ambulatory Anesthesia[57] warns against use of outpatient surgical procedures in patients with OSA if it is accompanied by a nonoptimized comorbid condition; if an inability to control pain predominantly with nonopioid analgesic techniques can be anticipated; or if the patient is PAP nonadherent. Patients on PAP should be advised to bring their device to the ambulatory care facility for use during recovery. Discharge should not occur until the patient is observed to maintain adequate oxygenation (on PAP if necessary, if used preoperatively) in an unstimulated environment, preferably while sleeping.[57] Patients not on PAP should be advised to sleep exclusively in the nonsupine position, and PAP users should wear their device whenever sleeping, including naps, for "several days" after surgery. All are advised to minimize use of opioids.

Benefits of Bariatric Surgery

Postoperative weight loss may be stated in a number of ways. In earlier literature, post–bariatric surgery weight loss is reported as the mean percentage of excess weight loss, defined as

$$(\text{Weight loss}/[\text{preoperative weight} - \text{ideal weight}]) \times 100$$

In a review of 136 studies involving 22,000 bariatric surgery patients, Buchwald[80] reported the mean percentage of excess weight loss with bariatric surgery was 61.2%: 47.5% for gastric banding, 68.2% for gastric bypass (principally RYGB), and 70.1% for BPD and BPDDS. In general, these weight loss outcomes did not differ significantly between those studies reporting assessments at 2 years or more versus less than 2 years, but longer term follow-up was more limited.[80] Percentage of excess weight loss with sleeve gastrectomy has been reported to be 50% to 61% and approximately 33% with an intragastric balloon system.[81-83] In the Buchwald review, the mean decreases in weight and BMI were 28.64 kg and 10.43 kg/m^2 for gastric banding, 43.48 kg and 16.70 kg/m^2 for RYGB, and 46.39 kg and 17.99 kg/m^2 for BPD and BPDDS.[80]

Weight loss with bariatric procedures is now also reported as a percentage of initial body weight, calculated as

$$([\text{Weight at desired postsurgery time point} - \text{weight at surgery}]/\text{weight at surgery}) \times 100$$

Per the National Patient-Centered Clinical Research Network, the estimated mean percent of total weight lost at 5 years was 25.5% for RYGB, 18.8% for sleeve gastrectomy, and 11.7% for adjustable gastric banding.[84]

Many comorbid conditions correspondingly decrease in severity with weight loss. The Longitudinal Assessment of Bariatric Surgery (LABS) Study revealed mean diabetes remission rates of 71.2%, 69%, 64.6% , and 60.2% at 1, 3, 5, and 7 years after RYGB.[85] Bariatric surgery has demonstrated greater efficacy over medical therapies for meeting preselected glycemic targets[86] and reducing rates of diabetic macrovascular[87] and microvascular complications.[88] Hypertension lessened in severity or resolved after bariatric surgery in 78.5% per the Buchwald analysis.[80] Similarly, in the GATEWAY (Gastric Bypass to Treat Obese Patients with Steady Hypertension) randomized trial, remission of hypertension was achieved in 51% of surgical patients versus 0% in the control group.[89] Bariatric surgery–induced weight loss results in lower mean total, low-density lipoprotein, and very-low-density lipoprotein cholesterol and triglyceride levels and eliminates the need for lipid lowering medications in approximately 80%.[90] Improvement with respect to comorbid conditions are generally similar for RYGB and for VSG when performed laparoscopically.[82] Cancer risk also appears to be favorably impacted by bariatric surgery. In a large retrospective review, bariatric surgery was associated with a 33% lower risk of developing any cancer during a mean follow-up of 3.5 years.[91] Accordingly, overall, all-cause mortality appears to be lower after bariatric surgery. A retrospective cohort study demonstrated a 40% reduction in adjusted long-term mortality with bariatric surgery during a mean follow-up of 7.1 years.[92]

Weight loss and improvement in weight-related comorbidities with bariatric surgery have also been demonstrated in adolescents. RYGB or sleeve gastrectomy resulted in weight reductions of 28% and 26%, respectively after 3 years in a prospective cohort of 242 adolescents with a mean age of 17 years at surgery[93] and at 5 years there was no significant difference in percent weight change between adolescents and adults.[94] Diabetes remitted in 95% and prediabetes in 76%, abnormal kidney function resolved in 86%, elevated blood pressure abated in 74%, and dyslipidemia resolved in 66%. Adolescents were significantly more likely than adults to have remission of type 2 diabetes and of hypertension.

The greater impact of bariatric surgery versus usual care in various obesity-related parameters is demonstrated by the Swedish Obesity Study,[95] a large, prospective, nonrandomized, controlled trial that compared outcomes for 2010 obese subjects treated with bariatric surgery and for 2037 contemporaneously matched obese control subjects treated conventionally. At 2 years, weight decreased by 23.4% in the surgery group and increased by 0.1% in the control group, and after 10 years, weight increased by 16.1% over presurgical weight in the surgery group but had increased by 1.6% in control subjects ($P < .001$ at both time points). Improvements in clinical indices of diabetes, hypertriglyceridemia, and hypertension were more favorable in the surgery group, and the surgery group exhibited lower 2- and 10-year incident rates of diabetes than those for the control group. Randomized clinical trials have also indicated greater weight loss and improvements in weight-related comorbidities with surgical versus nonsurgical interventions.[96]

Long-Term Impact of Bariatric Surgery on Obstructive Sleep Apnea

Weight loss induced by bariatric surgery is consistently associated with reductions in AHI.[97] Tongue fat reduction appears to be the primary upper airway mechanism for improvement in AHI with weight loss after bariatric surgery.[98] Buchwald's meta-analysis[80] of selected bariatric surgery outcomes reported that OSA resolved or decreased in severity in 83.6%. The weighted (i.e., weighting results by sample size) mean change in the AHI was 40 events/hour, with a range of 16 to 52.8. Enthusiasm over these results must be tempered by several methodologic concerns. *Improvement* and *resolution* with respect to OSA were not explicitly defined. The studies included in the meta-analysis are not entirely specified, but a review of studies from the inclusion period (1990 to June 2003) revealed that reduction in OSA symptoms probably was sufficient in some studies to assess OSA response (i.e., postoperative PSG was not required in all subjects), the timing of PSG after surgery was nonuniform, and the results were variably reported (e.g., only preoperative and postoperative apnea indices were described, not AHIs).

More contemporary studies corroborate earlier series reporting that surgically induced weight loss is associated with symptomatic improvement in OSA when reassessment occurs approximately 1 year or longer after surgery. However, many patients have residual OSA. For example, even though gastric banding resulted in a mean AHI reduction of 23.4 events/hour, Lettieri and colleagues[98] found that 96% of patients still met criteria for OSA (AHI >5 events/hour), 83% had continued transient nocturnal hypoxia (oxyhemoglobin saturation below 90%), and 54% had persistent sleepiness (Epworth Sleepiness Scale [ESS] score >10) despite an average weight loss of 54 kg at a mean of 418 days postoperatively. Importantly, persistent OSA after bariatric surgery may attenuate the cardiovascular benefits of bariatric surgery.[99]

Three meta-analyses[100-102] demonstrate significant reductions in BMI and AHI with bariatric surgery (Table 139.6), yet many patients remain obese with mildly to moderately increased AHIs postoperatively. The mean residual AHI values per these meta-analyses were typically 12 to 15 events/hour. Per Greenburg, only 44% attained an AHI less than 10 events/hour.[101] The number of randomized controlled trials for analysis is very limited; just three such studies[103-105] were included in the most recent meta-analysis by Wong.[100] Between-study heterogeneity is consistently large because of diverse inclusion criteria, small sample sizes, marked differences in time between bariatric surgery and follow-up sleep apnea testing, different types of sleep apnea tests employed, different hypopnea definitions employed, high dropout rates, and failure to control for differences in sleep stages and positions in pre- and postsurgical sleep apnea testing.[100]

The latest meta-analysis[100] also provides some new insights. Bariatric surgery was associated with a significant reduction in the ESS score (weighted mean difference −5.5) and improved the nonsupine AHI to a greater degree than the supine AHI. There was a nonlinear relationship between weight loss and reduction of AHI that could be a result of heterogeneity in how weight loss impacts nonanatomic susceptibility traits for OSA such as ventilatory control sensitivity (i.e., loop gain), the respiratory arousal threshold, and upper airway muscle reflexes/responsiveness. Accordingly, health care providers must remain vigilant for persistent OSA with a systematic postoperative follow-up program, because even dramatic changes in weight do not guarantee objective cure of OSA.

The optimal timing for postoperative PSG is not clear but depends in part on the patient's weight loss evolution. The CPAP requirement for residual OSA is likely to fall by at least 2 to 4 cm H_2O in the year after surgery.[106] Autotitrating CPAP after surgery may bridge the patient to PSG and obviate subjective pressure reductions or serial sleep studies.

The AASM concluded that bariatric surgery may be adjunctive in the treatment for OSA, but rated this recommendation as an option, meaning that bariatric surgery is of uncertain clinical use in the management of OSA.[39] This designation was based on the lack of high-quality data and the potential for perioperative complications.

Risks and Complications of Bariatric Surgery

The LABS Consortium, a prospective, observational study of outcomes of bariatric surgical procedures at 10 clinical sites in the United States from 2005 to 2007, revealed operative mortality rates, defined as death within the first 30 days, of 0.3% for RYGB or laparoscopic adjustable gastric banding (4610 patients), 0% for laparoscopic adjustable gastric band procedure (1198 patients), 0.2% laparoscopic RYGB (2975 patients), and 2.1% open RYGB (437 patients).[107] A composite end point of death, deep vein thrombosis or venous thromboembolism, reintervention, and failure to be discharged by 30 days after surgery occurred in 4.1% of patients: 1% with laparoscopic adjustable gastric banding, 4.8% with laparoscopic RYGB, and 7.8% with open RYGB. Factors independently associated with an increased risk of the composite end point were a history of venous thromboembolic disease, an inability to walk 61 meters (approximately 200 feet), and extreme (approximately 55 kg/m^2 or greater) values of BMI. Box 139.1 lists the postoperative adverse events from bariatric surgery, which can be grouped as early and late. A dreaded complication is anastomotic leak that occurs in 1.6% per the University HealthSystem Consortium evaluation.[76]

The extent to which OSA is linked to complications after bariatric surgery is not fully known. In a review of more than 3000 patients, OSA, older age, male sex, and revision gastric bypass were found to be independent predictors for anastomotic leak.[108] In another study, OSA, hypertension, and less surgeon experience were identified by multivariate analysis as predictors of postoperative complications in a series of

Table 139.6 Meta-Analyses of the Impact of Bariatric Surgery on Obstructive Sleep Apnea

	Weighted Mean Difference in BMI (kg/m^2)	Weighted Mean Difference in AHI (events/hour)	Mean Residual AHI (events/hour)
Greenburg, 2009[100]	−17.9	−38.2	15.8
Ashrafian, 2015[101]	−14.0	−29.0	15
Wong, 2018[102]	−13.2	−25	12.5

AHI, Apnea-hypopnea index; BMI, body mass index.

nearly 200 patients undergoing laparoscopic RYGB.[109] In the LABS analysis, OSA also was independently associated with increased risk for the composite end point of a 30-day major adverse outcome.[107] Accordingly, OSA has been linked to increased cost of postoperative care[110] and higher risk for prolonged postoperative hospital stay.[111] In other studies, however, investigators have not identified OSA as an independent predictor of complications after bariatric surgery,[112-114] or the findings have been mixed.[115] Analysis of 91,000 adult bariatric surgery patients in the Nationwide Inpatient Sample database revealed that sleep-disordered breathing was independently associated with increased risk for emergent intubation and atrial fibrillation but decreased mortality, total charges, and length of stay.[115] These reports are challenging to interpret and compare because of differences in procedures used and uncertainty over how aggressively OSA was pursued preoperatively and managed postoperatively. Furthermore, many reports are single-center and possibly underpowered retrospective reviews, thus providing a lower grade of evidence. PAP initiated immediately after bariatric surgery does not appear to increase risk for anastomotic leaks.[116-118]

Box 139.1 COMPLICATIONS OF BARIATRIC SURGERY

Complications Common to All Bariatric Procedures

Early (up to 30 days after surgery)

Venous thromboembolic disease
Bleeding
Anastomotic leaks
Wound infections
Persistent nausea/vomiting, dehydration
Regional abdominal organ trauma
Incisional and internal hernias
Bowel obstruction
Atelectasis
Pneumonia
Cardiac dysrhythmias
Urinary tract infection
Death

Late (beyond 30 days after surgery)

Incisional hernias
Bowel obstruction from adhesions
Nutritional deficiencies
Anastomotic strictures, ulcers, or erosions
Cholelithiasis
Anemia
Persistence or recurrence of obstructive sleep apnea
Need for body contouring
Weight regain

Procedure-Unique Complications/Adverse Effects

Roux-en-Y Gastric Bypass

Dumping syndrome
Marginal ulcer
Internal hernias

Vertical Sleeve Gastrectomy

Refractory reflux
Hiatal hernia
Stricture at incisura

Laparoscopic Adjustable Gastric Banding

Band slippage or erosion
Port or device malfunction

Biliopancreatic Diversion

Loose, foul-smelling stools
Protein-calorie malnutrition

Pitfalls and Controversy

Controversy remains about the impact of OSA on bariatric surgery complications and thus to what extent OSA must be sought and treated preoperatively. Definitive data are not available. Bariatric surgery clinical practice guidelines[52] stipulate that OSA should be considered in all bariatric surgery candidates—but does that mean sleep apnea testing is mandatory and that if it yields a positive result, PAP is required? The answer to both of these questions is likely to be "no." Instead, the history and physical findings pertinent to OSA, perhaps initially organized by a screening tool sensitive to OSA in this population so that the search is consistent and systematized, must be combined with consideration of a host of other factors, both patient-related (comorbidity burden; OSA symptom severity; OHS likelihood) and procedure-related (open versus laparoscopic; inpatient versus ambulatory; anticipated postoperative opioid requirements), in deciding how to proceed. Those patients judged to be at low risk for having OSA as indicated by the collective clinical information (e.g., STOP-BANG score <3) can proceed directly to bariatric surgery without further sleep testing[50] *provided that* comorbidities are controlled, there is no untreated hypercapnia or hypoxemia, postoperative precautions are in place (e.g., careful monitoring in the PACU; minimization of opioid/sedative use; head of bed elevation; incentive spirometry), and the bariatric team is prepared to address OSA should it manifest during the immediate postoperative period. Patients deemed to be at intermediate or high risk for having OSA should proceed to a formal sleep assessment, with the sleep specialist guiding the ordering of sleep testing and the interpretation of findings.[50] PAP is started preoperatively for treatment of moderate to severe OSA (AHI ≥15 events/hour) and OHS. Preoperative PAP initiation allows the patient to begin accruing its neurobehavioral and cardiovascular benefits while working through other preparatory steps typically required for bariatric surgery. Furthermore, retrospective data suggest that it may decrease the risk of post–bariatric surgery complications[119,120] and is a consensus recommendation.[52]

CLINICAL PEARLS

- The sleep clinician should be mindful that bariatric surgery candidates are likely to have OSA or OHS, which require careful consideration during the preoperative evaluation and in the postoperative period.
- Post–bariatric surgery patients should be expected to lose 20 to 50 kg by 1 to 2 years postoperatively, which current studies indicate should be accompanied by a 50% to 75% reduction in AHI and a drop in required PAP levels.
- Autotitrating CPAP may be a useful management modality as weight decreases after surgery.
- Reduction in tongue fat appears to be an important mediator of AHI reduction after bariatric surgery.
- Despite dramatic weight loss, OSA may persist in many patients, so follow-up OSA testing is advised to reassess for this condition and to guide decisions about longer term PAP use.

SUMMARY

The prevalence of obesity, a leading cause of preventable disease and death, is increasing. Two-thirds of Americans currently are overweight or obese. Excess weight is the strongest risk factor for OSA because of its adverse effect on upper airway neuromuscular function and anatomy. Bariatric surgery, comprising a variety of procedures that limit food absorption or restrict intake (or both), is indicated for obese patients in whom an adequate exercise and diet program has failed to achieve results and who have either a BMI 40 kg/m^2 or greater, a BMI 35 to 39.9 kg/m^2 in conjunction with one or more obesity-related severe comorbid conditions, or a BMI 30 to 34.9 kg/m^2 and type 2 diabetes who have glycemia that is difficult to control. The mean percentage of excess weight loss with bariatric surgery is approximately 60%, and in patients with major obesity-related conditions, such as diabetes mellitus and hypertension, consistent improvement in clinical indices is to be expected. Thirty-day mortality rate for bariatric surgery is less than 1%. OSA is almost universally present in bariatric surgery candidates, sometimes in the context of OHS. The immediate post–bariatric surgery setting may exacerbate OSA, whereas OSA and its associated conditions may exacerbate challenges to the patient's immediate postoperative well-being. Systematic screening for OSA should therefore be a required component of preparation for bariatric surgery, with addition of a formal sleep evaluation for patients deemed to be at higher risk for OSA. Symptomatic improvement follows, but the OSA does not usually resolve with bariatric surgery–induced weight loss. The sleep clinician plays an important role in the bariatric surgery process, in preoperatively collaborating with the surgical team to identify OSA and by helping to define its significance, determining which patients need OSA treatment, introducing the possibility of bariatric surgery in their obese OSA patients as up to one-third may be interested,[121,122] and initiating or optimizing OSA therapy to postoperatively determining the degree of residual OSA and the need for additional treatment.

SELECTED READINGS

Ali M, El Chaar M, Ghiassi S, Rogers AM. For the American Society for Metabolic and Bariatric Surgery Clinical Issues Committee. American Society for metabolic and bariatric surgery updated position statement on sleeve gastrectomy as a bariatric procedure. *Surg Obes Relat Dis.* 2017;13:1652–1657.

Ali MR, Moustarah F, Kim JJ. On behalf of the American Society for Metabolic and Bariatric Surgery Clinical Issues Committee. American Society for metabolic and bariatric surgery position statement on intragastric balloon therapy endorsed by the society of American gastrointestinal and endoscopic surgeons. *Surg Obes Relat Dis.* 2016;12:462–467.

Aminian A, Chang J, Brethauer SA, Kim JJ. For the American Society for Metabolic and Bariatric Surgery Clinical Issues Committee. ASMBS updated position statement on bariatric surgery in class I obesity (BMI 30-35 kg/m^2). *Surg Obes Rel Dis.* 2018;14:1071–1087.

Arterbarn DE, Courcoulas AP. Bariatric surgery for obesity and metabolic conditions in adults. *BMJ.* 2014;349:g3961.

Busetto L, Dixon J, DeLuca M, Shikora S, Pories W, Angrisani L. Bariatric surgery in class I obesity: a position statement from the International Federation for the Surgery of Obesity and Metabolic Disorders (IFSO). *Obes Surg.* 2014;24:487–519.

Courcoulas AP, King WC, Belle SH, et al. Seven-year weight trajectories and health outcomes in the Longitudinal Assessment of Bariatric Surgery (LABS) Study. *JAMA Surg.* 2018;153(5):427–434.

de Raaff CA, Gorter-Stam MA, de Vries N, et al. Perioperative management of obstructive sleep apnea in bariatric surgery: a consensus guideline. *Surg Obes Relat Dis.* 2017;13:1095–1109.

The GBD 2015 Obesity Collaborators. Health effects of overweight and obesity in 195 countries over 25 years. *N Engl J Med.* 2017;377(1):13–27.

Hudgel DW, Patel SR, Ahasic AM, American Thoracic Society Assembly on Sleep and Respiratory Neurobiology, et al. The role of weight management in the treatment of adult obstructive sleep apnea. *Am J Respir Crit Care Med.* 2018;198(6):e70–e87.

Inge TH, Courcoulas AP, Jenkins TM, et al. Weight loss and health status 3 years after bariatric surgery in adolescents. *N Engl J Med.* 2016;374:113–123.

Inge TH, Corcoulas AP, Jenkins TM, et al. Five-year outcomes of gastric bypass in adolescents as compared with adults. *N Engl J Med.* 2019;380:2136–2145.

Jensen MD, Ryan DH, Apovian CM, et al. 2013 AHA/ACC/TOS Guideline for the management of overweight and obesity in adults: a report of the American College of Cardiology/American Heart Association task force on practice guidelines and the obesity society. *Circulation.* 2014;129(suppl 2):S102–S138.

Kent D, Stanley J, Aurora RN, et al. Referral of adults with obstructive sleep apnea for surgical consultation: an American Academy of Sleep Medicine clinical practice guideline [published online ahead of print, 2021 Aug 5]. *J Clin Sleep Med.* 2021. https://doi.org/10.5664/jcsm.9592.

The Longitudinal Assessment of Bariatric Surgery (LABS) Consortium. Perioperative safety in the longitudinal assessment of bariatric surgery. *N Engl J Med.* 2009;361:445–454.

Mechanick JI, Youdim A, Jones DB, et al. Clinical practice guidelines for the perioperative nutritional, metabolic, and nonsurgical support of the bariatric surgery patient—2013 update: cosponsored by American Association of Clinical Endocrinologists, The Obesity Society, and American Society for Metabolic and Bariatric Surgery. *Obesity.* 2013;21:S1–S27.

Ong CW, O'Driscoll DM, Truby H, Naughton MT, Hamilton GS. The reciprocal interaction between obesity and obstructive sleep apnoea. *Sleep Med Rev.* 2013;17:123–131.

Pratt JSA, Browne A, Browne NT, et al. ASMBS pediatric metabolic and bariatric surgery guidelines 2018. *Surg Obes Rel Dis.* 2018;14:882–901.

Schwartz AR, Patil SP, Laffan AM, et al. Obesity and obstructive sleep apnea: pathogenic mechanisms and therapeutic approaches. *Proc Am Thorac Soc.* 2008;5:185–192.

Wong A-M, Barnes HN, Joosten SA, et al. The effect of surgical weight loss on obstructive sleep apnoea: a systematic review and meta-analysis. *Sleep Med Rev.* 2018;42:85–99.

A complete reference list can be found online at ExpertConsult.com.

Chapter 140

Advanced Modes of Positive Pressure Therapy for Sleep-Disordered Breathing

Bernardo Selim; Babak Mokhlesi; Winfried J. Randerath; Shahrokh Javaheri

Chapter Highlights

- Knowledge of the basic working principles of noninvasive ventilation (NIV) and adaptive servo-ventilation (ASV) modes is helpful to select and customize the device's settings to match patient's respiratory needs (pathophysiology).
- NIV modes are bilevel positive airway pressure modes designed to deliver pressure-supported breaths. ASV devices are anticyclic ventilator pressure support devices. Built-in sensors and advanced computational capability (microprocessors) allow some of these modes (e.g., volume-assured pressure support [VAPS], ASVs in general) to automatically self-adjust ventilatory settings to match patient's needs.
- In NIV modes, three mechanical phases of breath delivery will determine the breath cycle (inhalation-exhalation): (1) the "trigger" that defines the beginning of inhalation, (2) the "inspiratory time" (Ti) that defines the time the device spends in inhalation, and (3) the "cycling" variable that defines the end of inhalation and therefore the beginning of exhalation.
- ASV modes adjust expiratory pressure, maximum and minimum inspiratory support, and a backup rate. The degree of control given to the algorithm is manufacturer specific.
- The presence of an unintentional (uncompensated) pressure-mask leak may interfere with both ASV and NIV mode performance. In a large leak, initiation of inhalation (trigger) may be delayed or missed, and the time required to reach inspiratory pressure (rise time [RT]) and remain in inhalation (Ti) may be inconsistent. Clinically, this may translate into desynchronies with the patient and insufficient ventilatory support (NIV) or excessive pressure cycling and sleep disruption (ASV).
- Synchrony between the patient and ventilation mode will be achieved once the patient's neural time (respiratory drive), respiratory system mechanics (compliance and resistance), and the device's settings (trigger sensitivity, RT, Ti, and cycle sensitivity) are matched. In some patients, manual customization of advanced NIV settings, such as trigger sensitivity, RT, Ti, and cycling, may be needed to reach synchrony and therefore successful ventilation.
- Based on the dynamic and complex nature of central sleep apnea/high loop gain or sleep-related hypoventilation disorders, the process of setting the parameters and adaptation of advanced ASV or NIV modes to the individual patient's requirements will rely on a close patient follow-up by experienced sleep physicians.

PART A: NONINVASIVE VENTILATION

Bilevel positive airway pressure (BiPAP), volume-assured pressure support (VAPS), and adaptive servo-ventilation (ASV) are advanced modes of noninvasive ventilation (NIV) positive airway pressure (PAP) introduced for the treatment of complicated sleep-related breathing disorders (SRBDs).[1] Widespread use of this technology is limited by high costs, scant clinical data, and incomplete understanding of propriety algorithms used to assess and respond to patient's respiratory breathing disorder. In this section we will delineate similarities and differences in technical aspects and settings of BiPAP in spontaneous mode (BiPAP-S) and spontaneous-timed mode (BiPAP-ST), as well as VAPS in spontaneous-timed mode (VAPS-ST) and pressure assist-controlled mode (VAPS-PAC), focusing on the bench literature assessing their technical performances when available. Clinical effectiveness of each device will be addressed in the therapeutic section of each respective SRBD.

MECHANICAL ANATOMY (HARDWARE) OF A POSITIVE AIRWAY PRESSURE BREATHING SYSTEM

NIV modes are delivered by PAP devices to the patient by a noninvasive interface (mask). The three essential components of this breathing system are (1) the flow generator ("blower" or turbine), (2) the tubing (single- or double-limb circuit), and (3) the mask (Figure 140.1).

In current devices, flow is generated by a "dynamic blower system" (direct current brushless motors) that changes speed to reach a preset target flow/pressure output. Based on input from sensors inside the device, a central controller (microprocessor) containing flow/pressure equations (propriety algorithms) adjusts the turbine speed in response to flow/pressure deviations (e.g., compensation for mask pressure leak). This closed feedback loop system permits the maintenance of a constant flow/pressure output.[2]

Usually, positive pressure is delivered by the device to the patient through a single-limb tubing system connected to a mask. Because the same tube is used for inhalation and exhalation, avoidance of carbon dioxide (CO_2) rebreathing is reached by calibrated leaks at the mask level (built-in exhalation port for intentional leak) and a minimal expiratory positive airway pressure (EPAP) of 4 cm H_2O to ensure an effective washout of exhaled CO_2. In addition, oronasal masks (e.g., full-face masks and total-face masks) contain a "safety expiratory valve" (antiasphyxiation valve) that opens in case of an unexpected device failure or breathing tube disconnection, allowing the patient to spontaneously breathe ambient air.

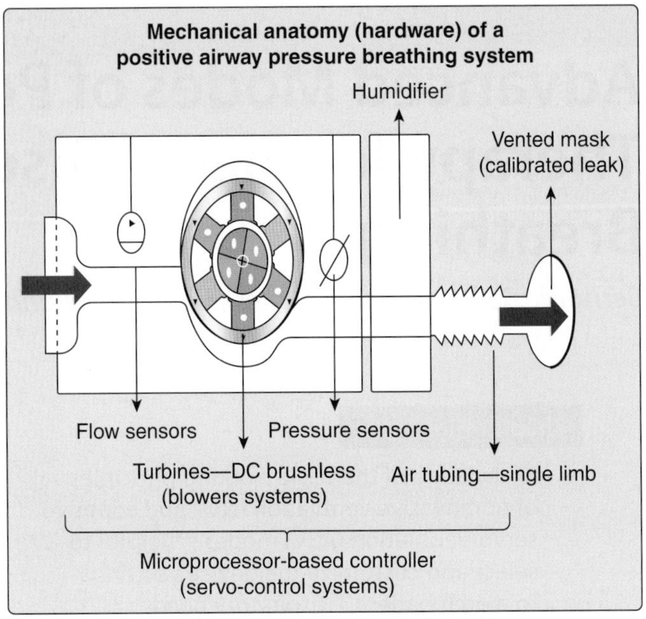

Figure 140.1 Mechanical anatomy (hardware) of a positive airway pressure (PAP) breathing system. The three essential components of PAP breathing systems are (1) the flow generator, a dynamic turbine, (2) the tubing (single or double-limb circuit), and (3) the mask (vented mask with calibrated leak). DC, Direct current.

PRINCIPLES OF NONINVASIVE MODES: ALGORITHMS (SOFTWARE) AND SERVO-MECHANISM (NEGATIVE FEEDBACK SYSTEMS)

Conceptually, all NIV modes share a common BiPAP platform that enables delivery of two different PAPs: inspiratory positive airway pressure (IPAP) during inhalation and EPAP during exhalation. The difference between the two pressures—pressure support (PS) level—determines the tidal volume (Vt) based on patient's respiratory system mechanics (compliance and resistance) (Figure 140.2, *A*). Beyond this basic function, NIV modes start to differentiate among each other by the way in which these PAPs are delivered and by the capability (or not) to "respond" (self-adjustment) to patient's dynamic respiratory variations. These differences are governed by undisclosed propriety algorithms (software) defining each mode.

At large, NIV modes are designed to either deliver a fixed BiPAP with or without backup rate (e.g., BiPAP-S or BiPAP-ST mode) or a variable BiPAP "responsive" to patient's respiratory disturbance (e.g., VAPS or ASV). In the latter group, VAPS mode has the capability to self-adjust its respiratory controlled settings (e.g., PAP, respiratory rate [RR]) to reach a preset target ventilatory support by adapting in real time to patient's respiratory disturbances. This "adaptive" response is based on a sophisticated negative feedback control system called servo-mechanism (Figure 140.3).

TYPES OF NONINVASIVE MODES USE FOR SLEEP-RELATED BREATHING DISORDER THERAPY

Due to an exponential increase of commercially available NIV devices, a wide variety of terminologies describing NIV modalities exists without standardization. Manufacturers continue to develop devices incorporating distinctive and proprietary algorithms for new modes of ventilation with adaptive facilities based on variants and combinations of the classical pressure control modes (Table 140.1). In this context, trademark names of modes (software) and devices (hardware) containing these modes are often confusing and wrongly used interchangeably.[3]

BILEVEL POSITIVE AIRWAY PRESSURE MODES

In 1990 Sanders and Kern[1] published the first paper to describe the treatment of obstructive sleep apnea (OSA) by "independently adjusted inspiratory and expiratory positive airway pressures" via a nasal mask. By introducing a flow sensor in the output circuit of the blower, the device was able to correctly detect the breath phase (inspiratory vs. expiratory) to modulate the degree of pressure (IPAP vs. EPAP) generated by the blower in spontaneous breathing.[1] With the evolution of digital processing of the flow signal, current NIV devices may also rely on timing parameters to initiate and/or terminate inhalation (timed breath) if a preset period of time passes without detection of spontaneous inhalation from the patient.

Pressure-Time Waveforms and Bilevel Positive Airway Pressure (BiPAP) Mode Settings: BiPAP-Spontaneous, BiPAP–Spontaneous-Timed, and Pressure Assist-Controlled

BiPAP is a pressure target ventilation mode delivering pressure-supported breaths. Although the delivery of IPAP (or the sum of EPAP and the PS level) supports (and/or augments) the patient's inhalation by a fixed PS, the delivery of EPAP during exhalation maintains an open upper airway by "pressure splinting."

In the inhalation-exhalation cycle of the device, inhalation may be initiated ("triggered") by patient's respiratory effort and/or time, resulting in the switch from EPAP to IPAP.

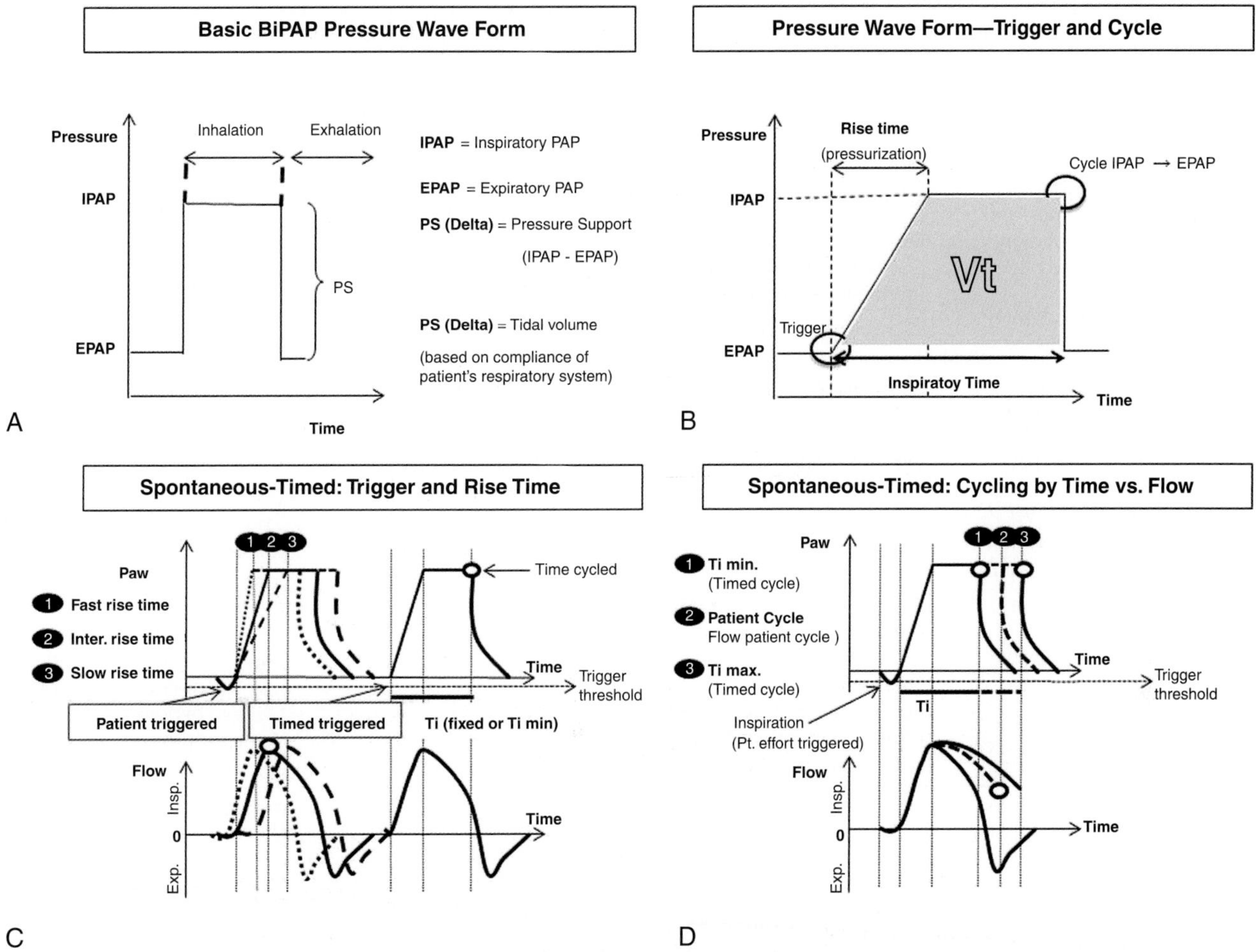

Figure 140.2 Bilevel positive pressure system (BiPAP) wave forms. **A,** BiPAP system delivers inspiratory positive airway pressure (IPAP) during inhalation and expiratory positive airway pressure (EPAP) during exhalation. The difference between the two pressures—pressure support (PS) level—determines the tidal volume (Vt) based on patient's respiratory system mechanics (compliance and resistance). **B,** Pressure wave form: trigger (initiation of inhalation), rise time (RT, pressurization time), inspiratory time (time spent in inhalation supported by IPAP) and cycle (termination of inhalation). **C,** Spontaneous-timed breath: trigger and RT. **D,** Spontaneous-timed breath: cycling by time versus flow. Exp., Expiratory; Insp., inspiratory; Inter., intermediate; max., maximum; min., minimum; Paw, airway pressure; Pt, patient.

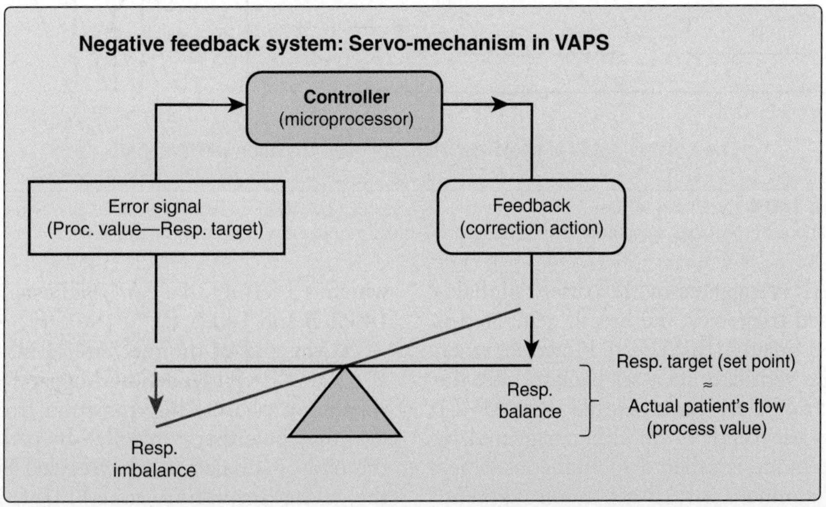

Figure 140.3 Negative feedback system: servo-mechanism in volume-assured pressure support (VAPS). Proportional negative feedback systems are based on the difference between the required respiratory target (set point) and the actual patient's flow (process value). This difference is called error signal. If the controller finds that the difference (error signal) is minimal, no changes in positive airway pressure (correction action) will be applied by feedback mechanism (*gray bar*). However, if the difference (error signal) is large (*red bar*), the controller will proportionally change the positive airway pressure needed to match the actual patient's airflow (process value) to the respiratory target (set point). Proc., process; Resp., respiratory.

Table 140.1 Types of NIV Modes: Nomenclature and Indications

NIV Devices	Indications	Pathophysiology Match	Action(s)
BPAP: Device that delivers a higher inspiratory pressure (IPAP) and a lower expiratory pressure (EPAP), potentially increases tidal volumes, and hence, alveolar ventilation. • S: **S**pontaneous (no back up rate) • ST = **S**pontaneous–**T**imed (back up rate)	• Alveolar hypoventilation syndrome (BPAP-S or BPAP-ST mode). • Primary central sleep apnea (BPAP-ST mode) • Second line treatment for CSA related to CHF (CSR-CHF) (generally BPAP-ST mode)	• Stabilization of upper airways • Hypercapnic respiratory failure (alveolar hypoventilation)	• Pneumatic splinting of upper airways • Support ventilation
Volume assured pressure support (VAPS): Feedback control system with self-adjustable pressures that target: • Target tidal volume (Vt) • Target alveolar ventilation (VA)	• Alveolar hypoventilation due to neuromuscular disease • OHS with failure to CPAP or without predominant OSA.	• Stabilization of upper airways • Hypercapnic respiratory failure (alveolar hypoventilation)	• Pneumatic splinting of upper airways • Support ventilation
Adaptive Servo Ventilation (ASV): Feedback control system with self-adjustable pressures that target an average ventilation or inspiratory flow.	• Systolic (EF ≥ 45%) or diastolic CSR-CHF • Primary sleep apnea • Treatment emergent central sleep apnea unresponsive to CPAP • CSAS due to long acting opioids with no carbon dioxide retention	• Hypocapnic or normocapnic respiratory failure	• Breathing pattern correction (it is not designed to provide ventilatory support in hypoventilation syndromes)

BiPAP, Bilevel positive airway pressure; CHF, congestive heart failure; CPAP, continuous positive airway pressure; CSA, central sleep apnea; CSAS, central sleep apnea syndrome; CSR, Cheyne-Stokes respiration; EF, ejection fraction; NIV, noninvasive ventilation; OHS, obesity hypoventilation syndrome; OSA, obstructive sleep apnea.

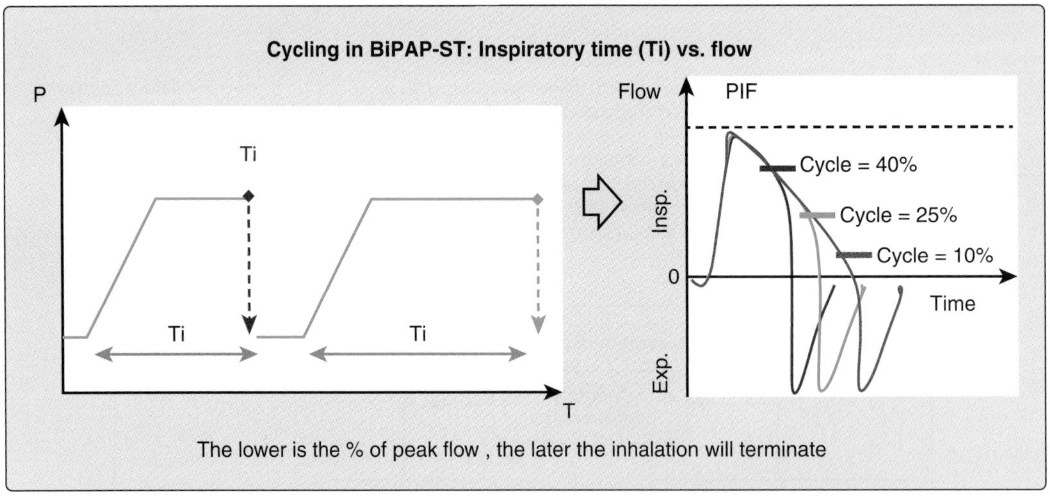

Figure 140.4 Cycling in BiPAP-ST: inspiratory time (Ti) versus flow. BiPAP-ST, Bilevel positive airway pressure–spontaneous-timed; Exp., expiratory; Insp., inspiratory; P, pressure; PIF, peak inspiratory flow; T, time.

When the switch to IPAP is triggered by the patient's inhalation (generally flow-based triggered), the breath generated is a "*s*pontaneous-triggered breath" (BiPAP-**S**). However, when IPAP is triggered by the ventilator at a set backup rate, the breath generated is a "*t*imed-triggered breath" (BiPAP-T). When the mode allows the IPAP to be either triggered by the patient or time, the mode is called a *s*pontaneous-*t*imed breath (BiPAP-ST). In summary, BiPAP-ST mode augments any breath initiated by the patient (*s*pontaneous) and supplies additional "mandatory" breaths should the patient's breath rate fall below the set backup rate (*t*imed). Once the inhalation is initiated, the time required for the pressure to rise from EPAP to IPAP (pressurization time) is called rise time (RT), which is a setting that can be adjusted in some devices (Figure 140.2, *B* and 140.2, *C*).

At the end of the mechanical inhalation, the switch from IPAP to EPAP is called cycling, and it marks the initiation of exhalation phase. This transition from inhalation to exhalation may be either controlled by patient's decrease in flow at the end of inhalation (flow-cycled breath) or by time set in the device (inspiratory time [Ti]) (Figure 140.2, *D* and Figure 140.4). In summary, when the patient retains control of the inhalation length and depth by determining the beginning (spontaneous trigger) and end of inhalation (flow cycled), it is called a "spontaneous breath." When the patient controls the onset of inhalation (spontaneous trigger) but the inhalation

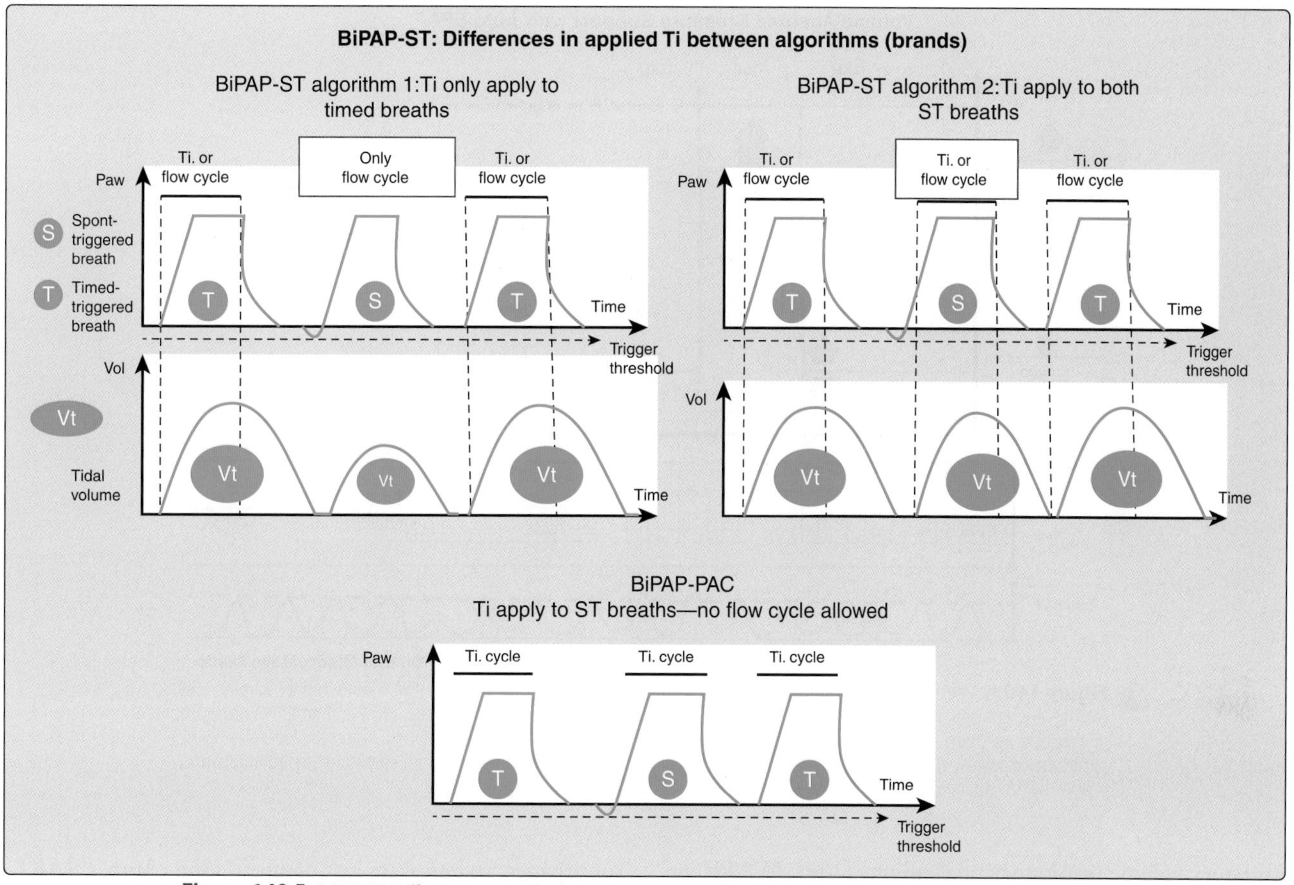

Figure 140.5 BiPAP-ST: Differences in applied inspiratory time (Ti) between algorithms (brands). Algorithm 1: BiPAP-ST mode will only apply to Ti to timed-triggered breaths but not to spontaneous-triggered breaths, resulting in more variable tidal volume (Vt) and minute ventilation. Algorithm 2: BiPAP-ST mode will only apply Ti to both timed-triggered breath and spontaneous-triggered breaths, resulting in more homogenous Vt. BiPAP in pressure assist-controlled (PAC) mode accommodates timed-trigger breath and spontaneous-triggered breaths, but cycling is always determined by a preset Ti. BiPAP-ST, Bilevel positive airway pressure–spontaneous-timed; Paw, airway pressure; Vol, volume.

length is regulated by time (Ti), then the breath is "assisted," otherwise the breath is "controlled," when all phases of the respiratory cycle are paced by the device's settings. Therefore, in assisted and controlled breaths, it is the Ti setting together with PS that will determine Vt based on patient's respiratory mechanics (Figure 140.2, *C*).

Due to propriety algorithm differences, the application of Ti in some BiPAP-ST modes may depend on the type of triggered breath. In general, Ti is applied to all time-triggered breaths; however, some BiPAP-ST modes may (or not) apply Ti to spontaneous-triggered breaths. Therefore, in those BiPAP-ST modes without a minimal Ti applied to spontaneous breaths, the duration of inhalation will exclusively depend on patient's respiratory effort, resulting clinically in a higher variability of Vts and minute ventilation (MV) in comparison to those modes applying Ti to all breaths (spontaneous and timed). To prevent such potential variability of Vt and MV, an alternative pressure-supported BiPAP mode may be considered: PAC mode. As in BiPÁP-ST mode, inhalation in PAC mode is either initiated by the device at a set rate (time-triggered breath) or the patient (spontaneous-triggered breath). However, different from ST mode, there is no spontaneous/flow cycling determined by the patient. The end of inspiration is controlled by the ventilator by applying a fixed Ti (time-cycled breath)[4] (Figure 140.5).

VOLUME-ASSURED PRESSURE SUPPORT MODES

At present, the VAPS mode can be applied by two different propriety algorithms patented under two different trademarks: Average Volume-Assured Pressure Support (AVAPS, Philips Respironics, Murrysville, PA) and Intelligent Volume-Assured Pressure Support (iVAPS, ResMed, San Diego, CA). Several commercially available devices containing the VAPS mode are approved by the U.S. Food and Drug Administration as medical devices intended to provide NIV support to treat adult and pediatric patients (≥66 lb/30 kg for VAPS mode) with respiratory insufficiency or respiratory failure, with or without OSA, either at home or in hospitals. In sleep medicine, NIV support may be indicated in certain sleep-related hypoventilation disorders, such as obesity hypoventilation syndrome (OHS) with predominant hypoventilation phenotype (true pickwickian syndrome), overlap syndrome (OSA and chronic obstructive pulmonary disease) unresponsive to continuous positive airway pressure (CPAP) and neuromuscular diseases (NMDs), among others.[5–13]

General Principles of a Volume-Assured Pressure Support Mode for Ventilatory Support in Sleep

In general, VAPS mode are available in bilevel ventilatory support devices that proportionately self-adjust inspiratory positive pressure to maintain either a consistent preset (target)

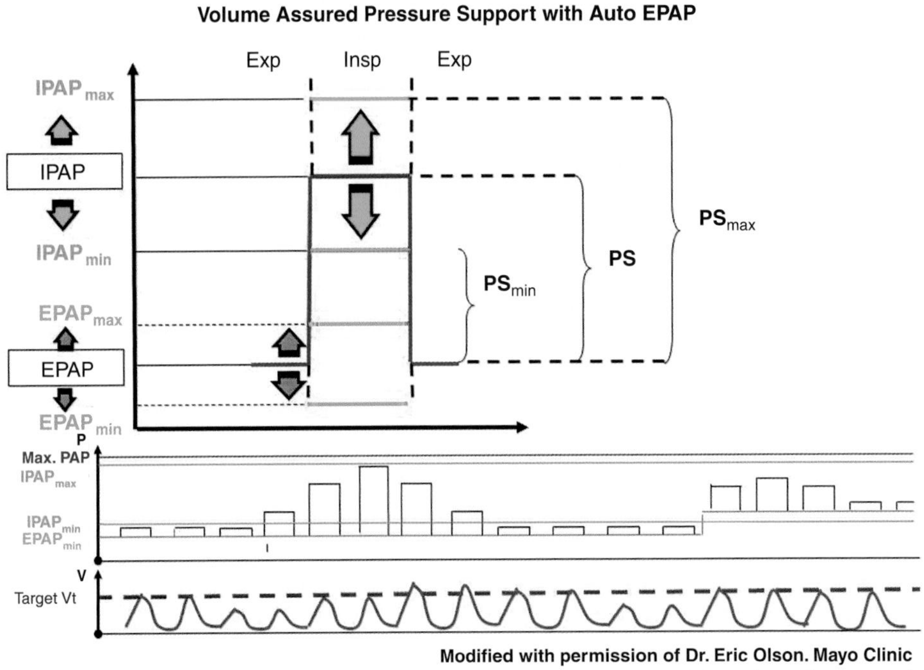

Figure 140.6 Volume-assured pressure support with auto-EPAP. Pressure support (PS) is adjusted by varying the IPAP level between the minimum (IPAP min) and maximum (IPAP max) settings. Auto-EPAP adjust EPAP pressure to stabilize an open upper airway in case of increased resistance. EPAP, Expiratory positive airway pressure; Exp., expiratory phase; Insp, inspiratory phase; IPAP, inspiratory positive airway pressure; max, maximum; min, minimum; V, volume; Vt, tidal volume.

respiratory volume (expiratory tidal volume [Vte], AVAPS) or ventilation (target alveolar ventilation [V_A], [iVAPS]) depending on the device's propriety algorithm applied. By servo-controllers (microprocessors), this mode continuously tracks patient's spontaneous respiratory flow and autoadjusts its respiratory settings. PS is adjusted by varying the IPAP level between the minimum (IPAP min) and maximum (IPAP max) settings, augmenting patient's inhalation when needed to reach a target volume (Vte) or ventilation threshold (V_A). This mode will also adjust the RR to treat hypoventilation and apply auto-EPAP to stabilize an open upper airway in case of increased resistance (e.g., OSA [Figure 140.6]).

The proportionate self-adjustment of each ventilatory parameter will respond to different respiratory events, and it varies by undisclosed propriety algorithms. In general, IPAP/PS and RR are reported to be proportionally adjusted to drops in Vte or V_A (hypoventilation), or flow limitation related to upper airways resistance (hypopneas, respiratory effort–related arousals, and snoring), whereas EPAP adjustments primarily respond to flow cessation from an upper airway obstruction (apnea).

Differences of Modes by Respiratory Targets and Settings

The VAPS algorithm patented in the Average Volume-Assured Pressure Support trademark (AVAPS) adjusts PS by varying the IPAP or PS level between the minimum (IPAP min or PS min) and maximum (IPAP max or PS max) settings to match a target Vte preset by the provider. The rate at which IPAP self-adjusts to achieve this targeted volume may be slow (by 1 cm H_2O/min), or fast (by up to 5 cm H_2O/min), and it can be set in certain devices by the provider (VAPS rate). This particular propriety algorithm analyzes the patient's spontaneous-airflow to calculate the Vte), automatically adjusting trigger, cycle sensitivities, and pressure leak compensation (Auto-TRAK). In some devices, Auto-TRAK is optional, allowing manual adjustment of trigger, RT, and cycle. In VAPS mode with autoadjusting EPAP capability, the device also monitors the patient's upper airway resistance and automatically regulates the EPAP required to maintain upper airway patency. When the breath rate is set to "auto," the device will adjust the backup breath rate based on the patient's spontaneous RR, remaining two breaths below detected average spontaneous breathing until a higher backup rate is needed to keep ventilation (Table 140.2).

Different from Vte target by AVAPS, iVAPS (ResMed) targets a preset V_A, adjusting for anatomic dead space calculated from patient's height.[14] By analyzing the patient's actual ventilation and respiration rate, PS and backup rate are continuously and proportionally self-adjusted to achieve and maintain the target V_A. In this mode the backup rate is factored in the V_A calculation, and it is designed to be at two-thirds of the "baseline spontaneous patient's rate" (target patient rate) during spontaneous ventilation. However, during apneic events or decreased MV, the backup rate may escalate to "target patient rate." In VAPS mode with autoadjusting EPAP capability, the device will automatically regulate the EPAP required to maintain upper airway patency. The device may also contain a "learn target" feature that allows the device to identify the patient's V_A and spontaneous RR and use these data as input in the device settings (Table 140.2).

In general, VAPS mode can be activated in ST or PAC mode. As in ST mode, inhalation in PAC mode is either initiated by the ventilator at a set rate (time-triggered breath) or the patient (spontaneous-triggered breath). However, different from ST mode, there is no spontaneous/flow cycling determined by the patient. The end of inspiration is controlled by the ventilator (time-cycled breath) by applying a fixed Ti.

Table 140.2 Differences of VAPS between Brands

Settings	AVAPS-AE (Philips Respironics)	iVAPS (ResMed)	VAPS (Breas) PCV
Target	Target tidal volume	Target alveolar ventilation (V_A)	Target tidal volume
VAPS modes	S, ST, PC, T	ST	ST
Backup rate	Option: "auto" (2 breaths below detected average spontaneous breath) Rate can be fixed	Is a target, not a fixed value "Target patient rate," in apnea Background rate ⅔ of target in spontaneous breathing It is a factor in the V_A calculation	Rate is fixed
EPAP	Auto-EPAP (AE) Fixed	Auto-EPAP (AE) Fixed	Fixed

AVAPS-AE, Averaged volume assured pressure support with auto-EPAP; EPAP, expiratory positive airway pressure; iVAPS, intelligent volume-assured pressure support; PC, pressure control; S, spontaneous; ST, spontaneous-timed; T, timed; VAPS, volume-assured pressure support.

SYNCHRONY, THE INTERPLAY BETWEEN PATIENT AND NONINVASIVE VENTILATION MODES

If properly set, NIV unloads ventilatory muscles and reduces the work of breathing by delivering pressure-supported breaths.[15] For this to occur, the interaction between the NIV mode and the patient should achieve synchrony by matching the patient's neural time (respiratory drive), respiratory system mechanics (compliance and resistance), and the device's settings.[15,16] For this to happen, the NIV flow and pressure delivery must synchronize with patient effort during all three mechanical phases of breath delivery: breath initiation (trigger), flow delivery (RT and Ti), and breath termination (cycling). In some NIV modes the trigger and the cycle are automatically adjusted by the device (based on propriety flow shape signal analysis) in an attempt to reach maximal synchrony with patient.[17] In other NIV modes, manual adjustment of the trigger is possible by adjusting the "trigger sensitivity," which is the inspiratory flow set above which the device triggers in spontaneous mode. In the case of flow-cycled breath, "cycle sensitivity" can also be manually set in the device by assigning a level of decadence of inhaled flow below which the device changes out of IPAP[18,19] (Figure 140.4).

Desynchronies occur when the timing set on the NIV does not match that of patient's respiratory efforts. Desynchrony between the patient and the NIV mode may overload ventilatory muscles (respiratory load), compromise respiratory ventilation, disrupt sleep patterns, and cause patient discomfort with subsequent poor compliance. The most frequent asynchrony results from pressure leak from the interface, compromising triggering (delayed or autotriggering), RT, Ti, and cycling.[20–24] Once the mask pressure leak is resolved, if residual trigger asynchrony is identified, the sensitivity should be a compromise between trigger difficulty and autotriggering. Similarly, cycle asynchrony can occur if the Ti is set too short (double triggering) or too long (active exhalation). This asynchrony can be addressed by appropriately setting the Ti[18] (Figure 140.7).

As in the presence of unintentional (uncompensated) pressure leak, the presence of increased resistance in the upper airway (e.g., OSA or glottic closure induced by hyperventilation) may compromise the effective delivery of Vt. As a consequence, increasing the delivered inspiratory pressure or Ti during NIV will not necessarily result in increased effective ventilation reaching the lungs until an appropriate EPAP is set to keep patency of upper airways.[25,26]

BENCH TEST ANALYSIS OF VOLUME-ASSURED PRESSURE SUPPORT

A bench test analysis is designed to determine the actual device performance when subjected to well-known simulated patients. Although the VAPS mode is servo-controlled and theoretically must apply the demanded pressure, target achievement may be compromised in strenuous conditions, such as (1) pressure leaks at the noninvasive interface (unintentional leak), (2) very high/low values of resistance and/or compliance of patient's respiratory system, or (3) inspiratory/expiratory pressure induced by the patient muscles is particularly intense.[27,28]

Testing leak compensation during NIV is essential to assure patient comfort and to reach a target lung volume and/or ventilation. The ability to trigger and cycle the breath in the face of a leak avoids asynchrony and improves patient's ventilatory support. In a single bench study published by Oscroft and colleagues,[29] VAPS mode targeting V_A was challenged to maintain a target ventilation over a range of lung compliance and resistance imposed by an artificial lung (Dual Training and Test Lung, Michigan Instruments, Grand Rapids, MI). This VAPS mode was noticed to deliver a slighter higher ventilation than prescribed (e.g., for a target ventilation of 10 L/min, the device delivered a median pressure of 10.2 to 12.4 L/min), even when additional leak was added to the system (between 8 and 33 L/min).[29] Contrary to those findings, Lujan and colleagues[30] found that unintentional dynamic inspiratory leaks (single-limb circuit with a leak port) in VAPS modes targeting Vt and V_A resulted in a reduction in pressure support without a guarantee of delivered Vt. The reduction in the delivered Vt for the highest inspiratory leak ranged between 21% and 40%, corresponding to a decrease in pressure support between 3.09 and 10.15 cm H_2O compared with those values without unintentional leak.[30] Therefore, in volume-targeted pressure support mode, it may be reasonable to set a minimum PS level, corresponding to a minimum safe volume for ventilation. Independent bench testing comparing different VAPS technology responses to changes in breath pattern are urgently needed.

PHYSIOLOGIC PARAMETERS TO HELP MATCH NONINVASIVE VENTILATION MODE TO PATIENT'S SLEEP-DISORDERED BREATHING

The *International Classification of Sleep Disorders,* third edition, has grouped the SRBDs into obstructive sleep apnea syndromes (OSASs), central sleep apnea syndromes

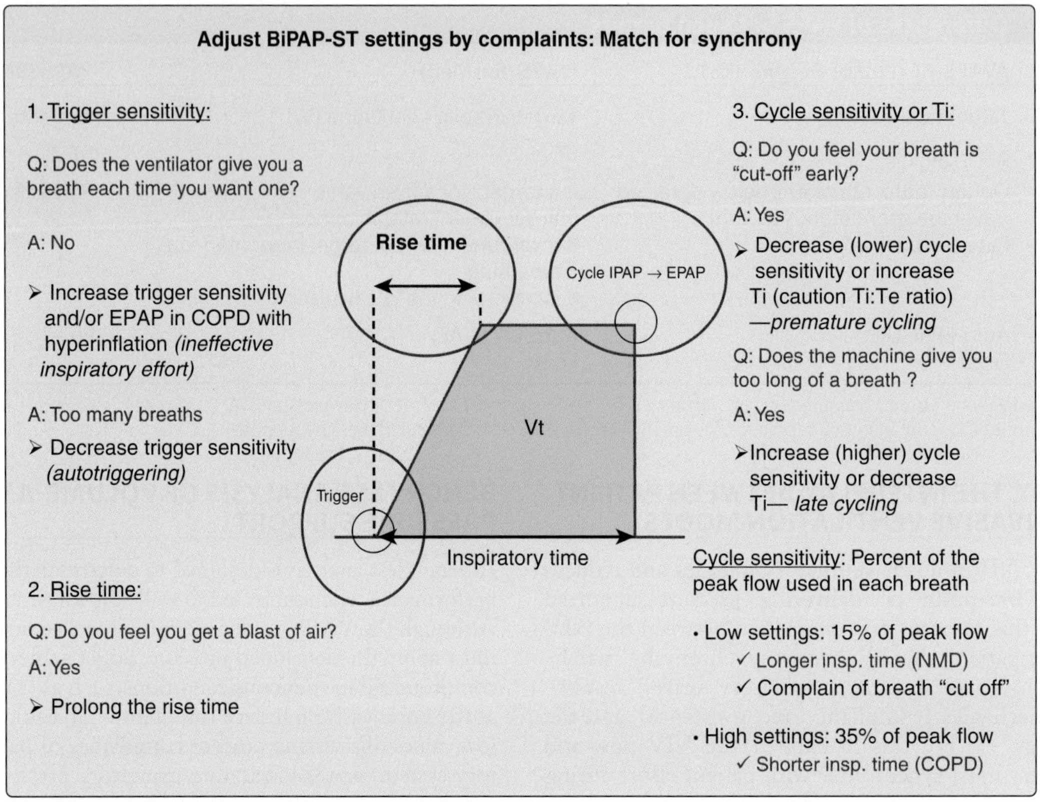

Adjust BiPAP-ST settings by complaints: Match for synchrony
1. Trigger sensitivity:
Q: Does the ventilator give you a breath each time you want one?
A: No
➤ Increase trigger sensitivity and/or EPAP in COPD with hyperinflation (ineffective inspiratory effort)
A: Too many breaths
➤ Decrease trigger sensitivity (autotriggering)
Rise time
Cycle IPAP → EPAP
Vt
Trigger
Inspiratory time
2. Rise time:
Q: Do you feel you get a blast of air?
A: Yes
➤ Prolong the rise time
3. Cycle sensitivity or Ti:
Q: Do you feel your breath is "cut-off" early?
A: Yes
➤ Decrease (lower) cycle sensitivity or increase Ti (caution Ti:Te ratio) —premature cycling
Q: Does the machine give you too long of a breath ?
A: Yes
➤ Increase (higher) cycle sensitivity or decrease Ti— late cycling
Cycle sensitivity: Percent of the peak flow used in each breath
• Low settings: 15% of peak flow
✓ Longer insp. time (NMD)
✓ Complain of breath "cut off"
• High settings: 35% of peak flow
✓ Shorter insp. time (COPD)

Figure 140.7 Adjust BiPAP-ST settings by complaints: match for synchrony. *1,* Mismatch between patient's inspiratory effort and ventilator triggering (ineffective inspiratory effort, double triggering and autotriggering). *2,* Pressurization time. *3,* Ventilator cycling does not coincide with end of patient's effort (premature cycling, before patients ends inhalation and late cycling when the patient ends inhalation before the machine cycle out of IPAP). BiPAP-ST, Bilevel positive airway pressure–spontaneous-timed; COPD, chronic obstructive pulmonary disease; EPAP, expiratory positive airway pressure; IPAP, inspiratory positive airway pressure; NMD, neuromuscular disease; Ti, inspiratory time; Vt, tidal volume.

(CSASs), and sleep-related hypoventilation-hypoxemic disorders (alveolar hypoventilation).[31] These disorders encompass a heterogeneous group of SRBDs with diverse pathophysiologic mechanisms. Conceptually, they may be divided into two main groups based upon their effect upon CO_2 balance, as reflected in arterial carbon dioxide tension ($Paco_2$). Sleep-related hypoventilation disorders are associated with hypercapnia ($Paco_2 \geq 5$ mm Hg) as a result of a predominant increased respiratory load (chest wall and lung elastic loads), decreased respiratory drive (ventilation control abnormalities), and/or inadequate respiratory muscle strength (neuromuscular unit impairment, neuromuscular disorders) (Figure. 140.8). In contrast, CSASs are eucapnic ($Paco_2 \leq 45$ mm Hg) or even hypocapnic ($Paco_2 < 40$) SRBDs characterized by intermittently diminished or absent respiratory efforts (central hypopneas or apneas). These two differentiated groups of SRBDs may guide the initial selection of an NIV mode to apply. In general, BiPAP and VAPS are modes usually recommended for patients with predominant alveolar hypoventilation in need of ventilatory support, whereas ASV mode is indicated for patients with CSA and preserved ventilation (Table 140.1). However, phenotypic variance in SRBDs and the individual response to NIV should be considered in the final decision of the best matching mode and settings (precision sleep medicine).

PART B: ADAPTIVE SERVO-VENTILATION

Constant and automatic PAP devices (CPAP and automatic positive airway pressure [APAP], respectively) deliver fixed or variable pressure throughout the entire breathing cycle, whereas BiPAP applies two different PAP levels for inspiration and expiration. These algorithms primarily prevent upper airway collapse. Although hypoventilation syndromes require augmentation of native ventilation as described earlier, complex breathing patterns of periodic breathing (PB), ataxic breathing, and treatment-emergent CSA (TECSA) require stabilization of respiratory rhythm. The ASV devices are designed to target respiratory rhythm and involve complex pathophysiologic and technical concepts,[32] and there are controversies regarding clinical efficacy.[33]

CENTRAL SLEEP APNEA/HYPOPNEA, PERIODIC BREATHING WITH HIGH LOOP GAIN

In contrast to OSA, central SRBDs are characterized by complete interruption (CSA) or partial diminishment (central hypopnea) of the respiratory drive to breathe.[34] A central apnea is characterized by a flat line in nasooral airflow and thoracoabdominal excursions, whereas a central hypopnea is characterized by proportional changes in airflow, thoracoabdominal excursions, and intrathoracic pressure, when

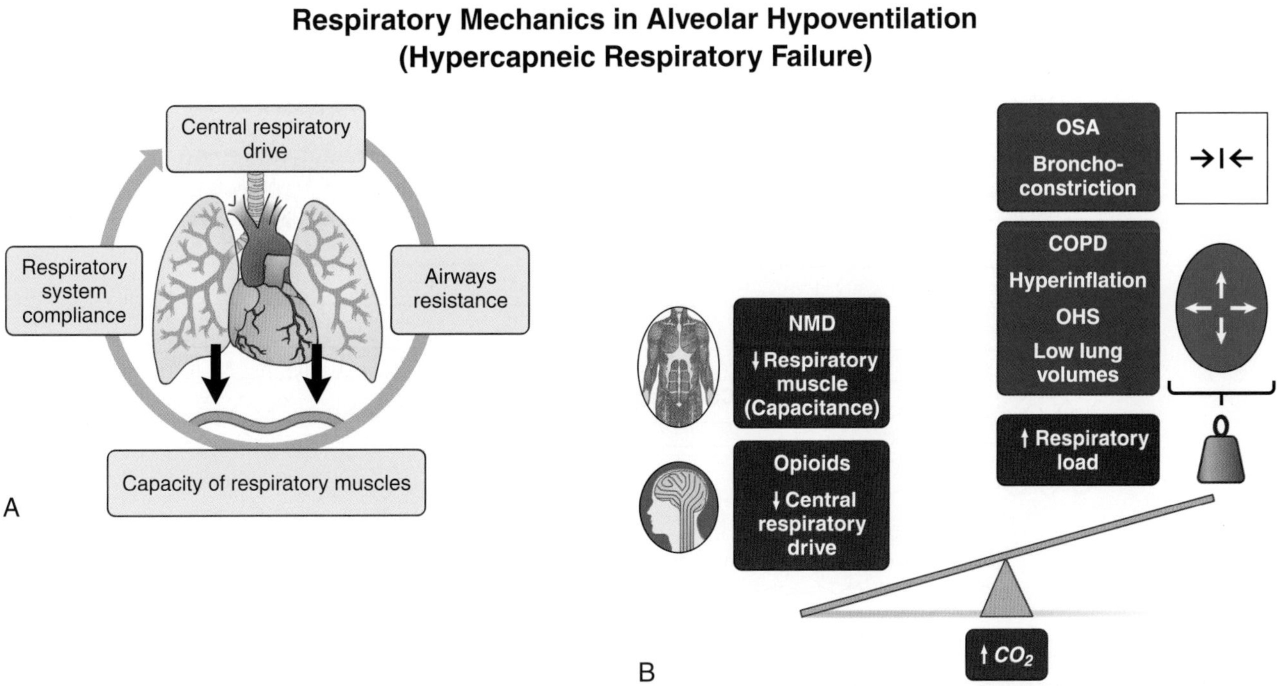

Figure 140.8 Respiratory mechanics in alveolar hypoventilation (hypercapnic respiratory failure). **A,** Normal respiratory balance is when the effort the individual has to exert to generate a breath (load imposed on the respiratory system), the strength of the respiratory muscles (capacity), and the central drive are in equilibrium. **B,** A decrease in central drive (e.g., opioids) causes a decrease in the activity of the respiratory muscles and, subsequently, a reduction in alveolar ventilation (V_A). Likewise, a weakness of the respiratory muscles (e.g., NMD) or an increase in respiratory load (e.g., overlap syndrome: COPD + OSA, OHS) causes an increase in work of breathing. V_A occurs when the imbalance exceeds a specific threshold. CO_2, Carbon dioxide; COPD, chronic obstructive pulmonary disease; NMD, neuromuscular disease; OHS, obesity hypoventilation syndrome; OSA, obstructive sleep apnea.

available in polysomnography (PSG) or cardiorespiratory polygraphy. Monitoring intrathoracic pressure by a balloon in the esophagus represents the gold standard to differentiate accurately central apneas and hypopneas from their obstructive counterparts. With CSA, there is a lack of any change in the esophageal pressure during the apnea (Figure 140.9), whereas central hypopnea (Figure 140.10) is characterized by proportional changes in respiratory drive, seen in pressure and airflow signals.[35–37] The hypercapnic phenotype of CSA is discussed elsewhere and is beyond the scope of this chapter.[34,38] In general, ASVs are not used for hypercapnic CSA.

The term *periodic breathing* in heart failure (HF) describes the waxing and waning pattern of airflow, Vt, and effort in the PSG (Figure 140.11). This breathing pattern was originally described by Hunter[39] almost 4 decades before the description by Cheyne and Stokes. If an acronym is used, it is best to refer to it as Hunter-Cheyne-Stokes breathing (HCSB) in the specific clinical situations of left ventricular dysfunction and HF. The European Respiratory Society Task Force on Central Sleep Apnea recommends describing the breathing pattern (PB) and adding the specific clinical situation (e.g., PB in HF).[38] However, this breathing pattern is as prevalent in asymptomatic subjects with left ventricular systolic dysfunction,[40] as in those with the syndrome of congestive heart failure (CHF).

PB is best explained by an upregulation of the ventilatory loop gain (LG), consisting of various components.[34] The chemical component of the LG reflects the upregulation of the peripheral and central chemoreceptors with an exaggerated response to variations of partial pressure of oxygen (Po_2) and partial pressure of carbon dioxide (Pco_2). With regard to the latter, Pco_2 sensitivity is augmented both above and below eupnea, both of which are the consequence of upregulation of the chemoreceptors.[34,41–45] Therefore a high LG produces ventilatory overshoot (hyperventilation) and undershoot (hypoventilation, apnea) in responses to breathing disturbances. High LG underlies PB in left ventricular systolic dysfunction and high-altitude PB.

Other examples of high LG are PB at high altitude (see Chapter 141) and TECSA when OSA is treated, particularly with CPAP. TECSA is part of the clinical syndrome of complex sleep apnea (high LG OSA),[46] but it also occurs after non-CPAP therapy of OSA,[47] for which reason TECSA best describes the appearance of CSA after treatment of OSA. True classic CSA persistence with continued CPAP use is less common, relative to persistent respiratory instability of lesser degrees and is seen as high residual apnea on CPAP. Due to its transient character, one view is that TECSA does not require a change of PAP therapy within the first 2 months after initiation. However, PAP-persistent CSA or preexisting CSA before PAP initiation may cause clinicians to focus on specific options, such as ASV.

TREATMENT OF CENTRAL SLEEP APNEA/ PERIODIC BREATHING ASSOCIATED WITH LEFT VENTRICULAR SYSTOLIC DYSFUNCTION

Left ventricular dysfunction is by far the most relevant cause of central respiratory disturbances as (see Chapter 149).[34,39–41,48] Non-PAP therapies of CSA are discussed in detail in Chapter 134.[39] Here, we briefly review PAP therapy in CSA

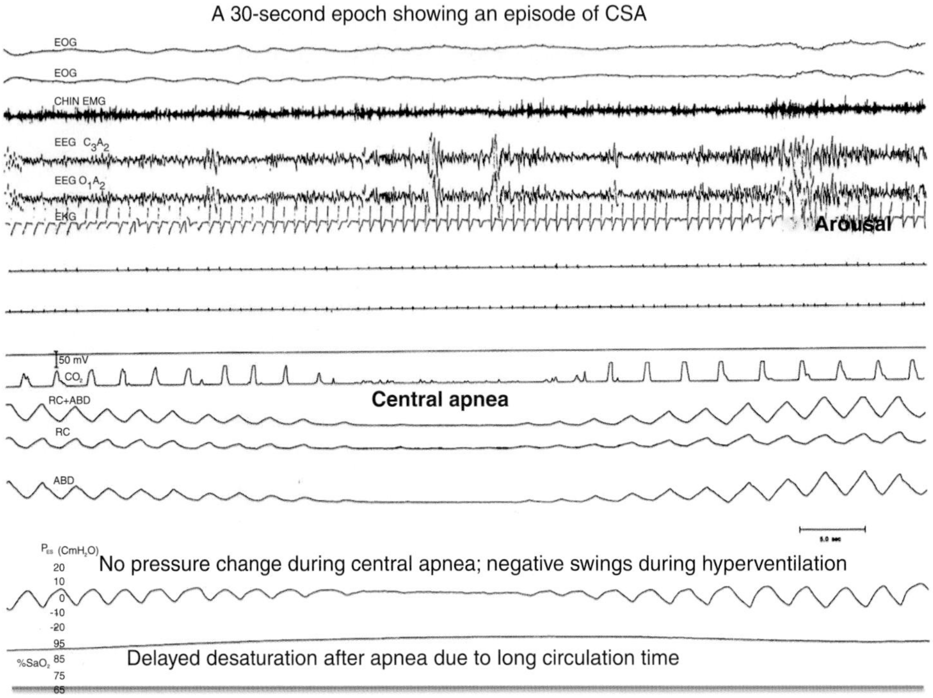

Figure 140.9 Polysomnographic example of central sleep apnea (CSA). Tracings are electro-oculogram (EOG), chin electromyogram (EMG), electroencephalogram (EEG), electrocardiogram (ECG), airflow measured by thermocouple (ninth row), carbon dioxide (CO_2), combined rib cage and abdominal excursions (RC + ABD), rib cage excursions (RC), abdominal excursions (ABD), esophageal pressure (ES), oxygen saturation (%SaO_2). Airflow is absent in the effort channels observed on RC, ABD, and esophageal pressure tracings. Note the smooth and gradual changes in the thoracoabdominal excursions and esophageal pressure in the crescendo and decrescendo arms of the cycle. The arousal occurs at the peak of hyperventilation.

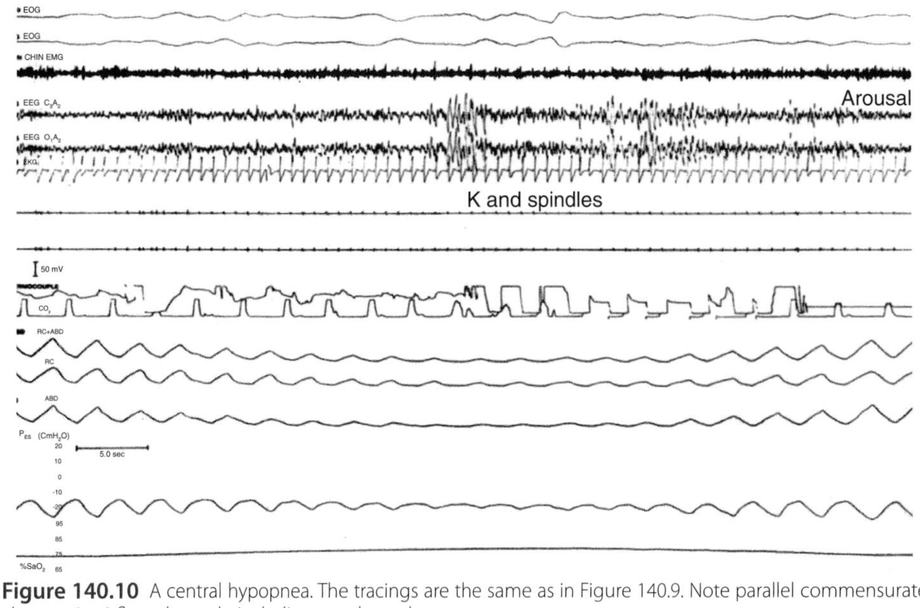

Figure 140.10 A central hypopnea. The tracings are the same as in Figure 140.9. Note parallel commensurate changes in airflow channels, including esophageal pressure.

and what motivated ASV development as the treatment of choice for CSA.

Continuous Positive Airway Pressure (CPAP, APAP, BiPAP)

PAP devices elevate the intraluminal pressure within the airways. PAP stabilizes the upper airway, increases the intraalveolar pressure, and improves work of breathing, ventilation-perfusion matching, interstitial fluid accumulation, and left ventricular afterload. Depending on central hemodynamics, when used in HF, CPAP suppresses CSA in only some patients. By increasing intrathoracic pressure, as venous return, right ventricular (RV) stroke volume and pulmonary blood volume decrease, and along with reduced afterload, pulmonary capillary pressure decreases, thus improving PB in a subset of patients who are responsive to CPAP.[37,49]

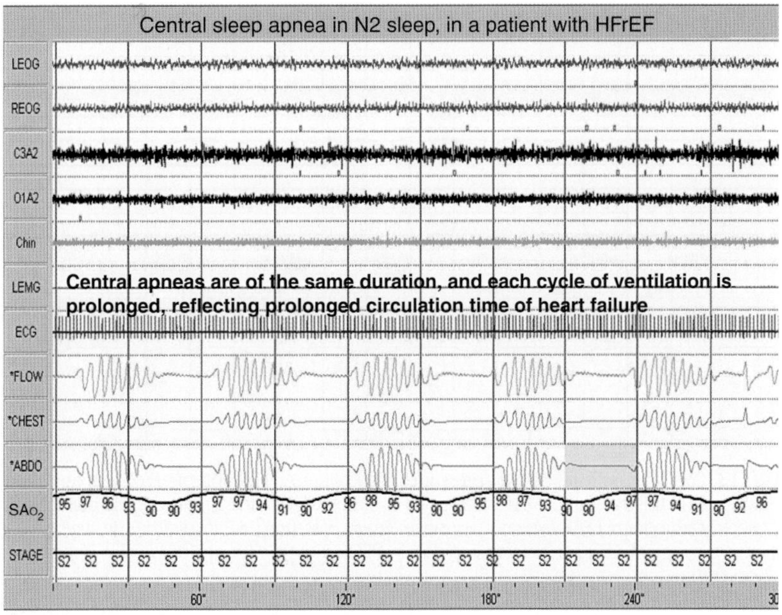

Figure 140.11 Classic Hunter-Cheyne-Stokes breathing (HCSB)/Hunter-Cheyne-Stokes respiration. A 10-minute polysomnographic example of HCSB. Tracings are: left electrooculogram (LEOG); right electrooculogram (REOG); electroencephalogram (C3A2); electroencephalogram (01A2); chin electromyogram (Chin); leg electromyogram (LEMG); electrocardiogram (ECG); chest excursions (chest); abdominal excursions (ABDO), oxygen saturation (SAO_2), and sleep stage (STAGE). HFrEF, Heart failure reduced ejection fraction.

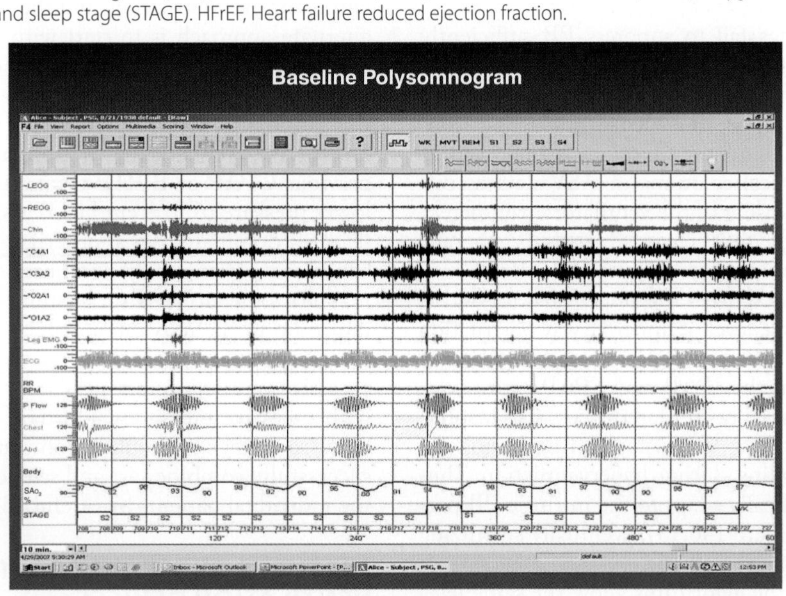

Figure 140.12 Pretreatment Hunter-Cheyne-Stokes breathing in heart failure. Tracings are: Left electrooculogram (LEOG); right electrooculogram (REOG); chin electromyogram (Chin); electroencephalogram (C4A1); electroencephalogram (C3A2); electroencephalogram (O2A1); electroencephalogram (O1A2); leg electromyogram (Leg EMG); electrocardiogram (ECG); respiratory rate (RR BPM); flow (pressure transducer; PFlow); chest excursions (chest); abdominal excursions (ABD); body position (body); oxygen saturation (SAO2); sleep stage (STAGE).

Overnight application of CPAP reduces central breathing disturbances by about 50%, and in these subjects ventricular arrhythmias decrease, presumably due to reduced sympathetic activity.[50] However, there were no significant changes in nocturnal arrythmias in CPAP nonresponsive patients. The lack of uniform suppression of CSA was confirmed in the Canadian Continuous Positive Airway Pressure for Patients with Central Sleep Apnea and Heart Failure (CANPAP) trial, in which CPAP failed to impact the primary end points, including death and hospitalizations. The CANPAP trial demonstrated that CPAP significantly improved respiratory disturbances in some subjects: 6-minute walking distance, sympathetic activation, and left ventricular ejection fraction (LVEF), but it failed to show an overall survival benefit.[51] In fact, therapy with CPAP was associated with early excess mortality, one reason the trial was terminated prematurely. Based on our earlier studies, it was suggested that the reason for early mortality was twofold[50,52]: CPAP was unable to uniformly suppress CSA, and in those subjects, adverse hemodynamic effects of CPAP on RV function could have contributed to excess mortality. Indeed, a later post hoc analysis concluded that in those patients, whose CSA was suppressed, survival improved.[53] At present, we suggest a CPAP trial as one option in the therapeutic approach to CSA/PB.[54] A reduction in AHI below 15 per hour is considered CPAP responsiveness based on the CANPAP trial. We generally do not recommend APAP or bilevel for treatment of CSA. Figures 140.12 and 140.13 show classic Hunter-Cheyne-Stokes respiration and lack of CPAP response, respectively.

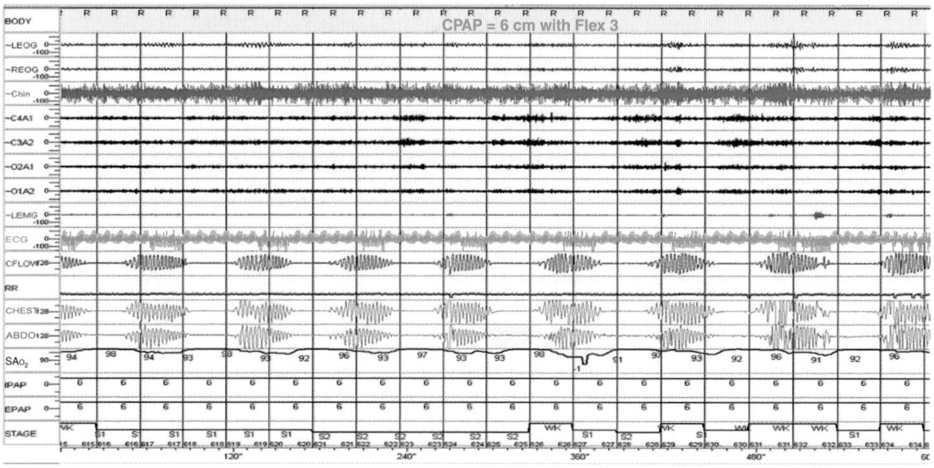

Figure 140.13 Continuous positive airway pressure (CPAP) failure. An example of CPAP incapable of suppressing central sleep apnea. In this patient, CPAP was increased to almost 18 cm of H_2O without any benefit. ABDO, Abdomen; ECG, electrocardiogram; EPAP, expiratory positive airway pressure; IPAP, inspiratory positive airway pressure; LEMG, left electromyogram; LEOG, left electrooculogram; REOG, right electrooculogram; RR, respiratory rate; SAO_2, alveolar oxygen saturation.

PRINCIPLES AND TECHNICAL ASPECTS OF ADAPTIVE SERVO-VENTILATION

As continuous PAP modes fail to suppress PB sufficiently, the unique algorithms of ASV were designed.[32] The ASV technology is provided in devices of three manufacturers in the United States and Europe (ResMed; Philips Respironics; Löwenstein Medical, Hamburg, Germany) (Table 140.3). Although the exact technical solutions of ASV devices differ in target parameters, sensing of the ventilatory parameters, and patterns of reaction, the most recent algorithms generally use three self-adjusting components (Figure 140.14).[32]

- The automatic EPAP stabilizes the upper airways and is changed according to the level of upper airway obstruction comparable to APAP.
- The difference between the IPAP and EPAP varies continuously and automatically. It determines the inspiratory pressure support (IPS, Vt): rising during periods of hypoventilation and falling during hyperventilation. Thus the algorithms anticyclically adapt to the intrinsic PB patterns of the subject (Figure 140.15), eventually stabilizing and eliminating PB (Figure 140.16).
- The actual versions of the algorithms allow the same level for the inspiratory and expiratory pressures. Thus, in the new versions of ASV devices, the IPS can be set to zero in the case of stable breathing detection. This is one way to prevent overventilation.
- In case of central apneas, the algorithms apply mandatory breaths to abort impending central apneas.

Given the algorithm for choosing the settings, the EPAP range, minimum and maximum IPS range, and breath rate (available in some ASV devices, but automatic in others), and expiratory pressure relief (available in some, but not others), the demographics, cause of CSA, and medications should be considered, as one size does not fit all.

For patients with reduced chest wall compliance, such as in obesity, a minimum IPS of 3 to 5 cm H_2O is reasonable to facilitate tonic ventilation. For the start of titration or therapy, a maximum IPS may be set at least about 8 to 10 cm H_2O above the minimum IPS and adjusted later as necessary during titration. If pressure cycling associated with arousals or distortion of respiratory patterns emerge, it suggests desynchrony or overventilation, and the IPS should be reduced. An alternate approach is to start with a lower IPS, such as 3 to 5 cm as allowed by the device, and then increase later. We normally choose EPAP between 5 and 15 cm H_2O and let the automatic algorithm respond appropriately to alleviate obstructive events. Other options include using data from a previous CPAP or BiPAP titration or simply starting with a lower pressure (6 to 8 cm H_2O) and increasing if obstruction features dominate. An appropriate level of EPAP is critical, because a patient with significant upper airway obstruction may not be ventilated successfully even when the algorithm ramps up to the maximum of IPS, in an attempt to open the closed upper airway. At the same time, when the airway opens, excessive ventilation may persist for some time, and this along with excessive pressure could have adverse consequences (as discussed later). It should be obvious that using ASV devices successfully combines art and science, with personalization to the individual patients by careful adjustments.

FEATURES OF SPECIFIC ADAPTIVE SERVO-VENTILATION DEVICES

ResMed Adaptive Servo-Ventilation

In all ResMed ASV devices (VPAP SV, VPAP Adapt Enhanced, VPAP Adapt, and AirCurve 10 in the United States; AirCurve 10 CS-A and AirCurve 10 CS in Europe), instantaneous inspiratory airflow is monitored and integrated to calculate the Vt. The device also monitors the patient's breathing rate by computing a moving average in a manner similar to that for calculating Vt, although over several breaths rather than 3 minutes. Minute ventilation (MV) is calculated as the product of breathing rate × Vt. A low-pass filter with a time constant of 3 minutes provides an average weighted minute ventilation, giving higher weight to more recent ventilation and progressively less weight to earlier values. Typically, three time constants encompass most of the necessary information reflecting recent ventilation. Using this continuously updated value, a target of 90% to 95% of the recent average ventilation is calculated. When the

Table 140.3 An Overview of the Algorithms of the Three Adaptive Servo-Ventilation Devices

Parameter	United States: AirCurve 10 Europe: AirCurve 10 CS-A PaceWave; AirCurve 10 CS Pacewave	DreamStation BiPAP autoSV	PrismaCR
Manufacturer	ResMed	Philips Respironics	Löwenstein Medical Technology
Target parameter of the algorithm	MV	Peak inspiratory flow	Relative MV
Calculation of target parameters	MV in 3-min moving window	Average peak flow calculated in 4-min moving window	Breath-by-breath MV compared to short-term MV average
Target for inspiratory pressure support	Target MV is set to 90% of recent 3-min average MV. Target MV is continually adjusted to reflect changes in the patient's own MV during the night and through various sleep stages	90%–95% of peak flow in absence of SRBD 60% percentile during SRBD	No threshold, regulation intends to stabilize relative MV, but not on a predefined level
Maximum inspiratory pressure (cm H_2O)	30	30	30
Maximum pressure support	20	30 minus prevailing EPAP	30 minus prevailing EPAP
Minimum pressure support	0	0	0
EPAP range, EPAP mode	ASV auto, ASV mode: 4–15 CPAP mode: 4–20	4–25 (default) automatic	4–20, default 5–8 in "Scope CSR," 7–13 in "Scope mixed" setting
	ASV mode: EPAP set manually at a fixed level	Can also be set manually to a fixed level up to 25	Can also be set manually up to 20
	ASV auto automatically adjusts to maintain upper airway patency		
EPAP responds to	Apnea, flow limitation and snoring	Apnea, hypopnea, flow limitation and snoring	Closed apnea, obstructive hypopnea, RERA, flow limitation, snoring
Early expiratory pressure relief	No	Yes	Yes
Definition of apnea	Respiratory flow decreases by more than 75% for at least 10 sec	Flow reduction 80%	Flow remains within apnea corridor, range of which is adjusted depending on current EPAP/IPS, leakage and average flow
Definition of hypopnea	Respiratory flow decreases to 50% for at least 10 sec	Flow reduction 50%	Reduction of MV 40% for 2 breaths
			PIF < 50% compared with average PIF
Backup frequency	Auto mode: adjust the timed backup rate from one that matches the patient's own recent rate towards the built-in default 15 BPM backup rate	Auto mode: default	Automatic backup frequency continuously adapted between 10 BPM and 20 BPM, depending on filtered spontaneous rate and patient's relative respiratory MV
	Adaptation to patients breathing in a moving window of 3 min weighted by most recent breath	Adaptation in moving window (12 breaths)	Fixed backup frequency possible, minimum 8/min
		Typical rate 3–5 breaths below patient's respiration	
		Minimum 8/min (up to 10/min)	
		Fixed backup frequency possible: Between 4 and 30 BPM in steps of 1	

Continued

Table 140.3 An Overview of the Algorithms of the Three Adaptive Servo-Ventilation Devices—cont'd

Inspiration time, expiration time, RT	Automatic application of inspiration time and RT	3 levels of rise time from end EPAP to maximum IPAP	Depending on current IPS, volume and breathing rate application of inspiration time and RT
Ramp	+ (while ramping, the rise in EPAP is a linear function)	+ (while ramping, EPAP rises more quickly than otherwise if obstructed events occur)	+ (while ramping, EPAP can already respond to obstructive events, but less dynamically)
SD card	+	+	+

ASV, Adaptive servo-ventilation; BPM, breaths per minute; EPAP, expiratory positive airway pressure; IPS, inspiratory pressure support; MV, minute ventilation; PIF, peak inspiratory flow; RERA, respiratory effort–related arousals; RT, rise time; SD, secure digital; SRBD, sleep-related breathing disorder.

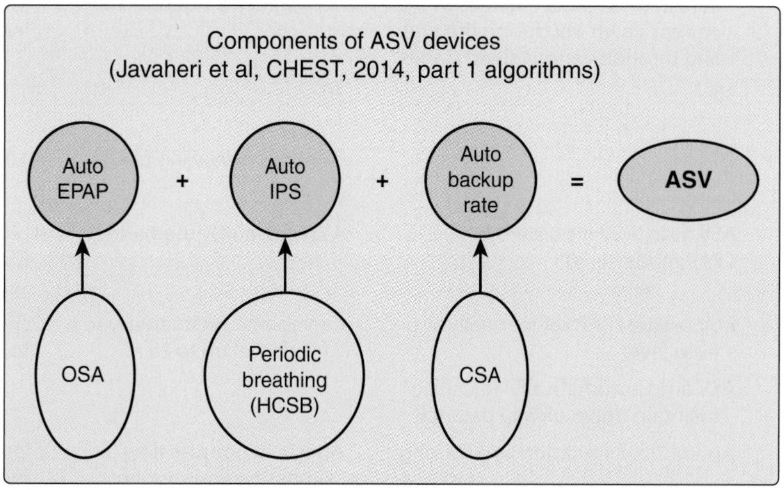

Figure 140.14 Various conceptual components of adaptive servo-ventilation (ASV). CSA, Central sleep apnea; EPAP, expiratory positive airway pressure; HCSB, Hunter-Cheyne-Stokes breathing; OSA, obstructive sleep apnea.

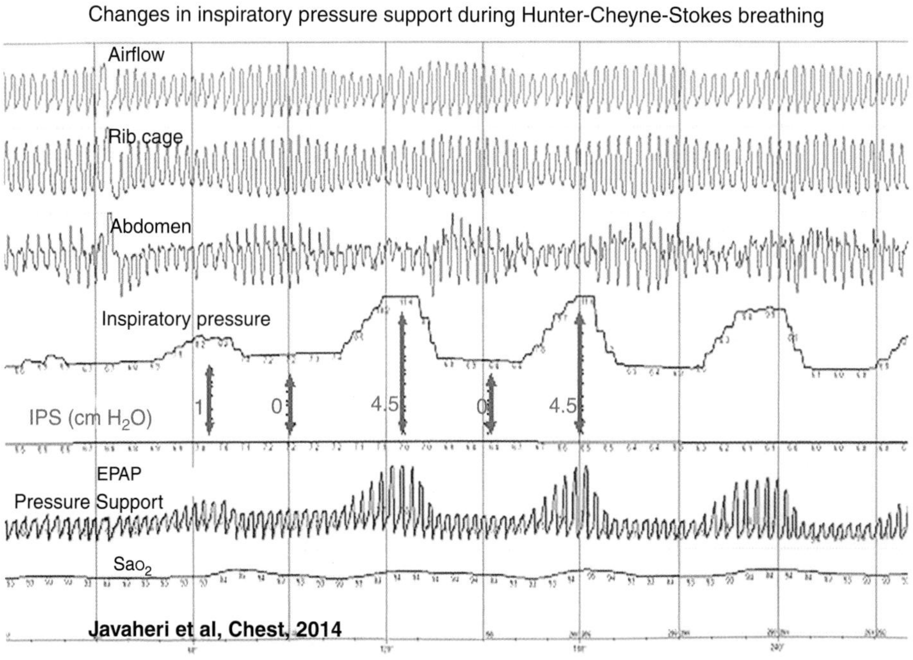

Figure 140.15 Various algorithmic outputs of an adaptive servo-ventilation machine as seen during polysomnography. EPAP, Expiratory positive airway pressure; IPS, inspiratory pressure support; Sao_2, arterial oxygen saturation.

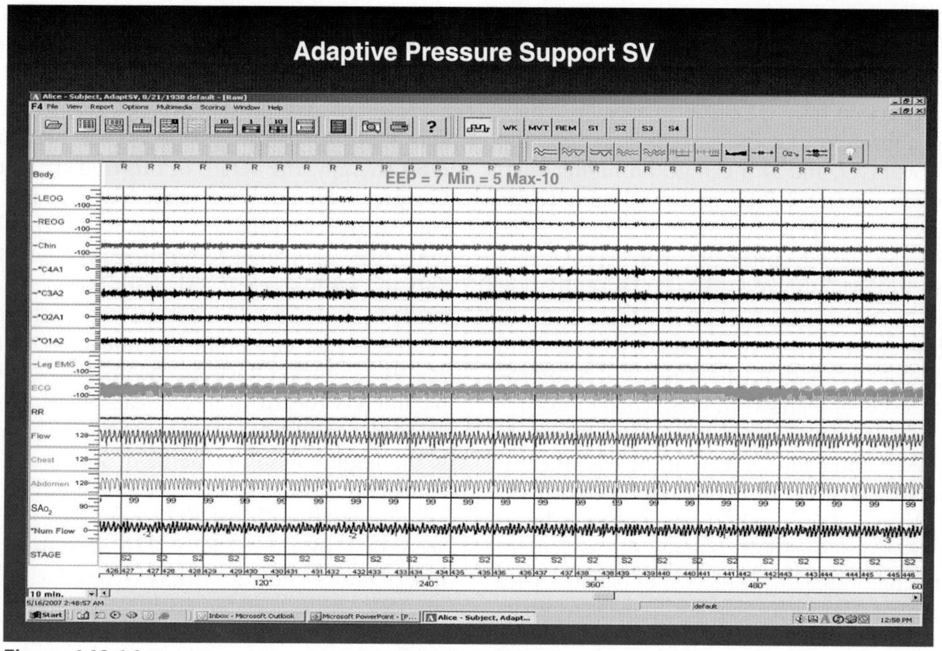

Figure 140.16 The figure shows successful application of adaptive servo-ventilation, same patient as in Figure 140.13. ECG, Electrocardiogram; EEP, end-expiratory pressure; EMG, electromyogram; LEOG, left electrooculogram; REOG, right electrooculogram; RR, respiratory rate; SAo_2, alveolar oxygen saturation; SV, servo-ventilation.

actual ventilation decreases below the target, an integral controller increases IPS proportional to the amount ventilation is below the target. Vice versa, when actual ventilation increases above the target, IPS decreases proportionally to the amount exceeding the target. Maximum inspiratory pressure is 30 cm of H_2O in the Air Curve series, and 25 cm H_2O in the remaining devices. Maximum IPS is constrained between maximum inspiratory pressure minus the prevailing EPAP.

The ResMed ASV device can be set to one of three modes: auto-ASV (engaging the automatic EPAP algorithm), ASV (fixed EPAP), or CPAP. Compared to previous versions, the devices allow IPS values of zero, a less aggressive IPS paradigm, and automatic EPAP. These advancements are relevant in the discussion of the SERVE-HF (Adaptive Servo-Ventilation for Central Sleep Apnea in Systolic Heart Failure) trial results, in which an old-generation ASV device was used, as detailed in Chapter 149.[32] In all ResMed ASV devices, the backup rate default is 15 breaths per minute. The device also monitors the patient's breathing rate by computing a moving average of the breathing period in a manner similar to that for calculating Vt, although over several breaths rather than 3 minutes, and can adapt to prevailing breathing rates. When ventilation is inadequate despite maximum support, or if excessive leak or other factors lead to failure in maintaining an adequate detectable MV, the backup rate will move toward 15 breaths per minutes by default.

Philips Respironics Adaptive Servo-Ventilation

The most recent Dream Station BiPAP autoSV servo-ventilation device by Philips Respironics is designed for effective treatment with minimal intervention. The device monitors peak inspiratory flow using a pneumotachograph in a 4-minute moving window. In theory, this peak flow should correlate with Vt and, when multiplied by breathing rate, MV. Two primary statistics are computed that set the target ventilation limits of the controller. The low ventilation limit is derived by computing 95% of the moving window mean peak inspiratory flow value and is used in the absence of sleep-disordered breathing (SDB). In the presence of SDB, the high limit tracks a value 60% above the moving window mean peak inspiratory flow. The algorithm determines these values repeatedly over time; IPS increases when measured flow is below the target, and IPS is decreased when flow is above the target. The DreamStation BiPAP autoSV algorithm is capable of withdrawing IPS entirely, a feature shared with the current ResMed VPAP Adapt (AirCurve) and may benefit some patients during parts of the night when breathing is normal and no support is needed. Maximum IPS levels are 30 cm H_2O minus the prevailing EPAP. To determine EPAP, DreamStation BiPAP autoSV analyzes the airflow signal to assess airway patency in a manner similar to the Philips Respironics current autotitrating PAP devices. The airflow response to a machine-triggered breath distinguishes obstructed versus open airway apneas. The backup rate may be set to two different modes: auto or fixed rate. If auto mode is enabled, the device synchronizes with the patient's intrinsic rate. In the ResMed device, the rate is always auto. Another difference between the ResMed and Philips Respironics devices is the expiratory pressure relief (biflex) algorithm in the Philips Respironics ASV.

Löwenstein Medical Technology Adaptive Servo-Ventilation

The AntiCyclic Servo Ventilation (ACSV) of prismaCR (Löwenstein Medical Technology) is regulated based on flow monitored by a pneumotachograph and integrated to compute current MV. IPS automatically varies to counterbalance changes in MV, whereas EPAP automatically varies to eliminate obstructive events. Unless set to a fixed value, the prismaCR adjusts EPAP in a manner similar to that of other APAP devices. In case of upper airway obstruction, EPAP automatically increases, remains on the new level for a certain waiting period, and then decreases given that no further obstructions occur. If needed, EPAP can be set manually from 4 up to 20 cm H_2O. For each current breath, actual MV is related to a short-term average MV of the last breaths. IPS reacts anticyclically with decreasing IPS when MV increases and increasing support when MV falls. This regulation principle targets stability of ventilation rather than bringing ventilation to a certain level derived from a long-term average, which might no longer be appropriate in the current situation. The maximum IPAP is 30 H_2O, and IPS can go no higher than the difference between current EPAP and maximum IPAP. Minimum IPS is always 0 cm H_2O in phases of hyperventilation; a baseline IPS can be set optionally, which provides a predefined pressure support in phases with stable ventilation (not applied during hyperventilation phases), for instance, to improve baseline oxygen saturation or to relieve dyspnea and thus reduce overall hyperventilation. The prismaCR also provides three optional levels of comfort modes, wherein expiratory pressure is varied between a lower level at the first part of expiration (early EPAP) and a higher level at the end of expiration to prevent airway obstructions effectively. As with the Philips Respironics device, this capability may allow a lower overall mean airway pressure level, which may enhance patient comfort and preserve hemodynamic function in patients with CHF. During apneas, mandatory breaths are applied automatically; the operator can manually choose a fixed backup rate. The optional automatic backup rate generates a first mandatory breath at 80% of the average spontaneous breathing rate, but it will not undercut 10 breaths per minute. If ventilation is successful (at least 80% relative MV), the automatic backup rate is decreased by 5% to allow the resumption of spontaneous breathing. The device also provides a ramp function for sleep onset, monitoring of leakage, AHI, and various additional parameters, as well as telemonitoring and telesetting via a global system for mobile (GSM) communication modem.

EFFICACY OF ADAPTIVE SERVO-VENTILATION

The efficacy of ASV on breathing disturbances, cardiac function, quality of life (QoL), and survival in different underlying conditions has been studied in cohort studies, case-control studies, and prospective randomized controlled trials (RCTs) (Table 140.4).[55–69] Teschler and colleagues[70] published the first acute RCT consisting of five arms, comparing oxygen, CPAP, BiPAP, and ASV for 1 night each. Consistent with later trials, they found a reduction of central disturbances with oxygen and CPAP by half. Although the effect of BiPAP varied widely, ASV almost uniformly normalized the central apnea index. Sharma and colleagues[63] performed a systematic review and meta-analysis of studies comparing ASV to subtherapeutic ASV, CPAP, BiPAP, oxygen, or no specific treatment. The weighted mean difference in AHI and LVEF both significantly favored ASV. ASV also improved the 6-minute walk distance but not other parameters of exercise or QoL. In addition, it has been demonstrated that the use of ASV is associated with a reduction in hypercapnic ventilatory response.[60] If confirmed, the downregulation of chemoreceptor hyperactivity could decrease chemical LG,[34] with further improvement in PB. One study suggests ASV decreases the burden of atrial fibrillation.[71] It can be summarized that with appropriate EPAP algorithm (auto-EPAP, not fixed EPAP; see discussion later), ASV effectively improves obstructive components, and with appropriately set IPS, it is superior to any other option in counterbalancing PB. Yet, in spite of the aforementioned studies, the largest RCT with ASV (SERVE-HF) was neutral in its primary outcome.

SERVE-HF Trial: Main Findings and Controversies on Technical and Pathophysiologic Concepts

In 2015 the publication of the results of the SERVE-HF trial, a multinational, prospective RCT,[72] stimulated an intensive and controversial discussion on the benefit or even harm of ASV therapy. The details of this trial are extensively covered in Chapter 149, and previously.[73] Briefly, the SERVE-HF trial studied the combination of optimum medical HF treatment with ASV compared to optimum medical treatment alone in patients with severe CHF with reduced LVEF (<45%) and predominant CSA.[72] Of importance, the primary combined cardiovascular end point did not differ significantly between the two groups. However, the analysis of secondary outcome parameters (death from any cause and cardiovascular death) showed unfavorable results in the ASV group. To date, this is the largest RCT in the field, and the results have led to a contraindication of ASV in cardiac failure with HF reduced ejection fraction (HFrEF) below 45% *and* predominant CSA, according to the SERVE-HF trial inclusion criteria. The investigators came up with two hypotheses to explain why use of ASV was associated with excess mortality: (1) CSA is a compensatory adaptive mechanism, implying, its treatment could be associated with excess mortality, and (2) the adverse hemodynamic effects of ASV was associated with excess mortality. Additional post hoc subanalyses of the SERVE-HF trial have been published. Eulenburg and colleagues[74] reported a significant difference between the ASV and control group in the subgroups with LVEF less than 30% and Cheyne-Stokes respiration (CSR) greater than 50%. Of importance, the risk of cardiovascular mortality did not increase with adherence to ASV use.

We have expressed concerns regarding the algorithm of the device used in the study and its pitfalls, which may account for the failings of the SERVE-HF trial.[73,75] The study results have been challenged due to a high percentage (23%) of substantial protocol violations, low ASV adherence (40% of patients used the ASV device <3 hours/day, 26.7% used the ASV device 0 hours/day) and unbalanced use of antiarrhythmic drugs between the two arms.[72,75] Most important, the ASV used was set at a fixed EPAP level and was unable to effectively treat upper airway obstruction, a phenotype that predominated with time.[72] For a critical discussion, see references 32 and 39. In consequence, there were significant amounts of desaturation, which persisted during the whole period of follow-up, potentially contributing to arrhythmias and premature mortality.[76] Regarding the hypothesis of CSA being compensatory, we have scientifically and critically discussed the pathophysiologic reasons why CSA is maladaptive and not compensatory.[77] The reanalysis[78] of the SERVE-HF trial showed that increased use of ASV was not associated with additional mortality, thus not demonstrating a dose-response relationship that would be expected were CSA protective, as suggested by the SERVE-HF trial investigators. For further discussion on this topic see Chapter 149. There are plausible biologic mechanisms involved in ASV failure, including patient-ventilator desynchrony, excessive pressure cycling and the associated hemodynamic surges, and induced hypocapnia.[79] These effects may be less likely with the current generation of ASVs but more likely when interacting with sleep fragmentation and variable degrees of upper airway obstruction.

Table 140.4 Summary of Adaptive Servo-Ventilation Studies

Study	Design	Population	Intervention	Outcome	Median or Average Follow-up Treatment Period	Results
Randomized Controlled Trials						
Pepperell, 2003[62]	Prospective, randomized, controlled, double-blind, monocenter	CHF (NYHA II–IV), stable drug therapy, ODI > 10/hr (3%)	15 ASV, 15 subtherapeutic ASV (11 completed trials)	Change in sleepiness (OSLER test)	1 mo	ASV reduced excessive daytime sleepiness, wakefulness +7.9 min vs. baseline, control: −1.0 min vs. baseline, between-group difference 8.9 min (95% confidence interval, 1.9–15.9 min)
Javaheri, 2011[56]	Prospective, randomized, controlled, crossover, multicenter	Baseline AHI ≥ 15/h and CAI ≥ 5/hr on CPAP titration (TECSA)	37 pts assigned to randomized order of 2 consecutive nights with BiPAP autoSV and BiPAP autoSV advanced	PSG parameters	N/A	BiPAP autoSV Advanced more effective than conventional BiPAP autoSV in treatment of SDB in pts with CSA
Randerath, 2012[55]	Prospective, randomized, controlled, monocenter	CHF (NYHA II–III, LVEF ≥ 20%), AHI ≥ 15/hr, coexisting OSA (20%–50%) and CSA (≤80%), optimal medication	35 pts on ASV (26 compliant at 12 months), 34 pts on CPAP (25 compliant at 12 mo)	Central AHI on treatment at 12 months	12 mo	ASV improved CSA and BNP over a 12-mo period more effectively than CPAP, central AHI 11/hr (CPAP) vs. 6/hr (ASV), $P < .05$
Arzt, 2013[92]	Prospective, randomized, controlled, monocenter	Stable chronic HFrEF (LVEF ≤ 40%), stable optimal medication, AHI ≥ 20/hr	37 pts assigned to ASV plus optimal medication (ITT analysis set 32 pts), 35 pts assigned to control group with optimal medication alone (ITT analysis set 31 pts)	Change of LVEF within 12 weeks of treatment	12 wk	Modest improvement in LVEF in both, ASV and control group (2.8 ± 5.5 vs. 2.3 ± 6.5%; $P = .767$)
Dellweg, 2013[59]	Prospective, randomized, controlled, monocenter	TECSA (AHI ≥ 15/hr with predominant OSA during initial PSG, AHI ≥ 15/hr with predominant CSA on CPAP after 6 wk)	19 pts assigned to NPPV, 18 pts assigned to ASV (15 pts in each group with completed follow-up)	AHI after 6 wk of therapy	6 wk	NPPV inferior to ASV in terms of suppressing central events (central AHI 10 vs. 2/hr, $P < .05$) as well as oxygen desaturations (21 vs. 5/hr, $P < .05$)
Galetke, 2014[64]	Prospective, randomized, crossover, monocenter	CV disease, AHI > 15/hr with >20% central respiratory events, optimal CV medication	39 pts using ASV and CPAP in randomized order for 4 wk each with 1 wk washout in between	Total, obstructive, central AHI	2 × 4 wk	ASV superior to CPAP in reduction of obstructive and central respiratory events (AHI 3 vs. 14/hr, obstructive AHI 0 vs. 4/hr, central AHI 3 vs. 9/hr, all $P < .001$)

Continued

Table 140.4 Summary of Adaptive Servo-Ventilation Studies—cont'd

Study	Design	Population	Intervention	Outcome	Median or Average Follow-up Treatment Period	Results
Morgenthaler, 2014[89]	Prospective, randomized, controlled, multicenter	TECSA (CAI ≥ 10/hr on CPAP initiation or residual CSR pattern), CHF NYHA III–IV excluded	33 ASV (17 evaluable) vs. 33 CPAP (19 evaluable)	Treatment efficacy (goal: AHI ≤ 10/hr, meaningful AHI difference ≥ 10/hr)	90 days	Treatment success: ASV 90%, CPAP 65%, $P = 0.02$; CAI: ASV 0.7/hr, CPAP 4.4/hr. ASV more reliably effective than CPAP in relieving TECSA,
Monomura, 2015 (SAVIOR-C study) [99]	Prospective, randomized, controlled, multicenter	Mild to severe CHF	102 ASVs + guideline-directed medical treatment (GDMT) vs. 103 GMDT only (control)	LVEF	24 wk	LVEF significantly improved vs. baseline in both groups. ASV not superior to GDMT in cardiac function improvement but improved clinical status (NYHA class + HF deterioration)
Khayat, 2015[100]	Prospective cohort study, monocenter	Hospitalization for AHF with LVEF ≤ 45%, no prior SDB diagnosis and PAP/NPPV treatment-naïve	PAP, modality not defined (276 CSA untreated, 58 CSA treated, 390 OSA untreated, 103 OSA treated), 245 no/mild SDB	Postdischarge all-cause mortality	3 yr	Newly diagnosed CSA or OSA are both independently associated with postdischarge mortality in patients with systolic CHF who are hospitalized for AHF
Cowie, 2015 (SERVE-HF)[72]	Prospective, international, multicenter, randomized, controlled	HFrEF (LVEF ≤ 45%), stable guideline-based medication, predominant central sleep apnea (AHI ≥ 15/hr, central AHI ≥ 10/hr)	666 pts assigned to ASV, 659 pts assigned to control group	Composite endpoint of all-cause death, lifesaving cardiovascular intervention, or unplanned hospitalization for worsening chronic heart failure	31 mo	Incident rate of primary end point did not significantly differ between groups (ASV: 54%, control: 51%). All-cause mortality and cardiovascular mortality were higher in the ASV group (35% vs. 29% and 30% vs. 24%). No beneficial effect on quality of life or symptoms of heart failure in ASV group
Eulenburg, 2016[74]	Secondary multistate modelling analysis of individual components of the primary SERVE-HF end point	See SERVE-HF	See SERVE-HF	See SERVE-HF	See SERVE-HF	Mortality risk is increased for cardiovascular death in patients not previously admitted to hospital, presumably due to sudden death, and in patients with poor left ventricular function.

Study	Design	Population	Intervention	Outcome	Median or Average Follow-up Treatment Period	Results
Hetzenecker, 2016[66]	Prospective, randomized, controlled, multicenter (subanalysis of study Arzt, 2013[92])	See Arzt, 2013[92]	See Arzt, 2013[92]	Arousals, sleep efficiency, and sleep stages (PSG), sleep fragmentation and sleep efficiency (actigraphy)	12 wk	ASV reduced arousal frequency (PSG), ameliorated sleep fragmentation and improved sleep efficiency (actigraphy)
FACE study, 2016[101]	Prospective multicenter observational cohort, France, up to January 31, 2013	CHF with reduced LVEF (HFrEF < 40%), midrange (HFmrEF 40%–49%), preserved (HFpEF: >50%)	361 CHF patients with CSA eligible for ASV therapy (258) vs. controls (133): refused/not compliant with ASV (<3 hr/night) (ResMed, AutoSet CS) 66% compliant to ASV therapy	All-cause death, hospitalization for worsening HF, heart transplant or ventricular assist device	21.6 mo	ASV improved prognosis in HFmEF in nonischemic HF; trend to increase in event rate in HFmrEF in ischemic heart disease; improved prognosis in HFpEF CHF with severe desaturations
ADVENT-HF trial, recruiting 2017[102]	Multicenter, multinational, randomized, parallel-group, open-label trial	Chronic HFrEF (≤45%) and SDB (OSA or CSA) with AHI ≥ 15 via PSG	Estimated >800, still recruiting 524 pts (31% CSA, 69% OSA) randomised till February 2018 on medical therapy alone or ASV (AutoSet-CS; ResMed, Australia) with nasal mask	All-cause mortality, first hospitalization for CV diseases, new-onset AF/flutter requiring anticoagulation but not hospitalization, or ICD shock not requiring hospitalization	Every 6 mo	Awaited
Toyama, 2017[68]	Prospective, randomized, controlled, monocenter	CSA/PB, LVEF ≤ 40%, NYHA II–III, stable medication	15 ASV, 15 no ASV (control)	Cardiac sympathetic nerve activity,(^{123}I-metaiodobenzyl-guanidine imaging)	6 mo	ASV improves CSA/PB, cardiac sympathetic nerve activity, cardiac symptoms/function and exercise capacity as opposed to control group
CAT-HF study, 2017[82]	Prospective, randomized, controlled, multicenter clinical trial, United States and Germany; 2013–2015	Hospitalised HF (HFrEF: EF >45% or HFpEF EF ≥ 45%) and SDB (OSA or CSA) with AHI ≥ 15 via PG	126 of 215 patients assigned on ASV plus optimized medical therapy (OMT): 65 vs. OMT alone (control): 61	Composite global rank score (death, CV hospitalizations, and percent changes in 6-min walk distance) Secondary endpoints: sleep apnea parameters, functional capacity, cardiovascular and all-cause death, days alive and out of the hospital, biomarkers, QoL, sleep parameters, imaging parameters, and NYHA functional class	6 mo	Neutral No improvement in 6-mo cardiovascular outcomes; however, a positive effect of ASV in patients with HFpEF Study was stopped after publication of SERVE-HF

Continued

Table 140.4 Summary of Adaptive Servo-Ventilation Studies—cont'd

Study	Design	Population	Intervention	Outcome	Median or Average Follow-up Treatment Period	Results
Knitter, 2019[103]	Prospective, randomized, controlled, crossover, monocenter	Complex sleep apnea pts adherent to ASV with LVEF > 45%	14 pts underwent consecutive PSG nights in random order with ResMed S7 VPAP Adapt, ResMed S9 VPAP Adapt, Philips Respironics BiPAP autoSV System One, Philips Respironics DreamStation autoSV	MV, QTc interval	N/A	Significant differences in MV and sleep architecture between different ASV devices higher MV was associated with small but statistically nonsignificant QTc prolongation
Prospective Cohorts, Case-Control Studies						
Oldenburg, 2011[60]	Prospective, cohort, monocenter	CHF (LVEF ≤ 40%), AHI ≥ 15/hr (>80% periodic breathing)	56 ASV, 59 control (ASV not initiated or noncompliant)	Treatment effects on periodic breathing, cardiac function, respiratory stability	6.7 mo	In contrast to controls, NYHA class, LVEF, oxygen uptake, 6-min walking distance, and NT-proBNP improved significantly
Imamura, 2016[104]	Case-control study, 2008–2014, Tokyo, Japan	HF NYHA III or IV (71% NYHA IV, LVEF 33 ± 17%) with ASV irrespective of SDB	85 patients receiving ASV 1 month vs. guideline-directed medical therapies (GDMT) (AutoSet-CS; ResMed, Australia) with full face mask (ResMed)	All-cause mortality and cardiac deaths	2-year follow-up	Continued ASV significantly lower all-cause mortality and cardiac death rate
Gorbachevski, 2020[105]	Prospective, interventional, monocenter	Pts with and without CHF (LVEF < 50%), AHI ≥ 15/hr, >50% central respiratory events, with ongoing PAP therapy, optimal CV medication	17 pts with CHF, 20 pts. without CHF, 3-part split night (random order of no treatment, automatic CPAP, ASV), analysis of selected 10-min segments of stable N2 sleep	Sympathovagal balance (SVB), hemodynamics	N/A	In subjects with CHF and CSA, neither automatic CPAP nor ASV favorably altered sympathetic drive at night. Conversely, treatment of heart-healthy subjects with CSA without CHF with automatic CPAP, but not ASV, favourably altered nocturnal SVB by decreasing the low frequency component and increasing the high frequency component of heart rate variability
Retrospective Studies						
Farney, 2008[94]	Retrospective, monocenter	AHI ≥ 20/hr, daily opioid intake for nonmalignant pain for ≥6 mo	22 pts with in-lab sleep PSG under ASV	Respiratory PSG parameters	N/A	ASV modulates the breathing patterns but does not eliminate ataxic breathing or hypoxemia, and does not consistently reduce apneas and hypopneas. Baseline AHI 67/hr, ASV AHI 54/hr

Study	Design	Population	Intervention	Outcome	Median or Average Follow-up Treatment Period	Results
Ramar, 2012[97]	Retrospective, monocenter	61 pts with CHF (HFrEF and HFpEF), 47 pts with chronic opioid use >6 months, all pts with AHI ≥ 5/hr, AHI > 5/hr or CSA persistence on CPAP	ASV titration (short term)	Treatment efficacy (goal: AHI ≤ 10/hr, TECSA abolishment)	N/A	ASV successful in 28 (60%) and 43 (71%) of opioid and CHF group, respectively (not significant). Higher BMI, HCO_3 and PB associated with decreased likelihood of ASV success
Javaheri, 2014[42]	Retrospective, monocenter	Chronic opioid use, CSA (CAI ≥ 5/hr, *n* = 16) or TECSA (CAI ≥ 5/hr on CPAP, *n* = 4)	All 20 pts on ASV, 9/20 pts with 2 prior CPAP titrations	PSG parameters	Up to 6 years (retrospective)	Chronic opioid use is associated with severe CSA which remains resistant to CPAP therapy. ASV effective in CSA treatment and over the long run, most patients remain compliant with the device
Hetzenecker, 2016[67]	Retrospective, monocenter	CHF (LVEF ≤ 50%), CSA, AHI ≥ 15/hr, CPAP responders and CPAP nonresponders switched to ASV	48 pts on CPAP therapy, 34 pts. on ASV therapy	Sleep quality based on PSG parameters	47 days	ASV reduces sleep fragmentation and improves sleep structure to a significantly greater extent than changes seen in CPAP responders
Hetland, 2016[106]	Retrospective observational study, 2007–2012, Østfold, Norway	HF NYHA class II-IV, LVEF ≤ 45%; CSR pattern ≥25% of sleeping time and dominant central sleeping pattern via PG	75 patients treated with ASV (31 patients with ASV for >3–18 months vs. 44 controls) (AutoSet-CS; ResMed, Australia)	Mortality and hospital admission of any cause and number of days in hospital in total	18 mo	ASV did not significantly affect CV death or combined CV death or hospital admissions after 18 mo; trend toward better CV event-free survival for ASV usage
Brill, 2017[107]	Retrospective, observational, monocenter	Pts on current ASV therapy	126 pts (51 TECSA, 27 coexisting OSA/CSA, 48 CSA), ASV discontinuation in patients "at risk," partly initiation of alternative therapies	Risk class according to SERVE-HF criteria, clinical course over 1 yr	Retrospective 1-yr clinical course	17 pts "at risk" (14%), SDB symptoms reappearing in most patients after short-term ASV discontinuation, further treatment: 6 ASV continuation, 4 CPAP, 3 none, 4 oxygen, 15 pts alive after 1 yr, no significant change in cardiac function

Continued

Table 140.4 Summary of Adaptive Servo-Ventilation Studies—cont'd

Study	Design	Population	Intervention	Outcome	Median or Average Follow-up Treatment Period	Results
Allam, 2017[86]	Retrospective data analysis, monocenter	Pts who underwent PSG on ASV	100 pts (CompSAS; 63%, CSA, 22%; CSA/Cheyne-Stokes breathing, 15%) receiving ASV, study segments that were included in the analysis consisted of 93 diagnostic studies, 92 ASV titrations, 69 CPAP titrations, 22 BiPAP-S/T, 11 CPAP + O_2, and 5 BiPAP-S. Therapeutic intervention trials <60 min in duration were not included	Change of AHI	N/A	Diagnostic AHI (median) 48/h, CPAP AHI 31/hr (P = .02), BiPAP-S AHI 75/hr, (P = .055), BiPAP-S/T AHI 15/hr (P = .002), ASV decreased AHI to 5/hr vs. baseline and vs. CPAP (P < .0001). ASV also increased REM sleep vs baseline and CPAP (18% vs. 12% and 10%, respectively; P < .0001). Overall, 64 patients responded to ASV treatment with mean AHI < 10/hr
Malfertheiner, 2017[108]	Retrospective, bicentric	Historical ASV use (91 in cardiac and 194 in respirology setting)	ASV	Clinical ASV use, patient distribution, proportion of patients with ASV contraindication as per SERVE-HF results	N/A	82% of pts with severe SDB, 33% predominant CSA, 65% periodic breathing, 20% LVEF ≤ 45%, 41% with CHF in cardiac setting, 80% with TECSA in respirology setting, 16% with ASV contraindication (CSA and LVEF ≤ 45%)
Randerath, 2017[109]	Retrospective, monocenter	Pts on ASV per clinical routine (period from 1998–2015)	293 pts on ASV	CV diseases, LVEF, PSG, SERVE-HF criteria	N/A	87% of pts with CV disease, 40% CHF, 16% LVEF ≤ 45%, SERVE-HF criteria present in 10% of pts
Javed, 2019 [110]	Retrospective, multicenter (subanalysis of SERVE-HF substudy)	See SERVE-HF, subananalysis of 280 pts	See SERVE-HF	Cheyne-Stokes respiration cycle length (CL), lung-to-periphery circulation time (LPCT), time to peak flow (TTPF), possibly reflecting cardiac function	12 mo	Pts who experienced serious adverse events (SAEs) had longer CSR CL, LPCT and TTPF as opposed to pts who did not experience SAE
Bordier, 2019[111]	Retrospective study, 2006–2018	Patient from the sleep unit of the CV department treated with ASV for sleep apnea: C/M/O apneas (PG)	32 patients with ASV: 8 deaths	CV mortality	Survival	CV deaths not predominant. No relation between SA or ASV and death

Study	Design	Population	Intervention	Outcome	Median or Average Follow-up Treatment Period	Results
Mansukhani, 2019[112]	Population-based study, using the Rochester Epidemiology Project database	CSA (AHI 41.6 ± 26.5/hr), with ASV therapy (65% ≥ 4 hr/night on ≥70% nights in their first month), and had ≥1 mo of clinical data before and after ASV initiation	309 CSA pts under ASV vs. health care utilization	Rates of hospitalizations, emergency department visits (EDV), outpatient visits (OPV) and medications prescribed per year (mean ± standard deviation)	2 yr pre-ASV and post-ASV initiation	ASV did not change health care utilization
Huseini, 2020[113]	Retrospective, monocenter	CSA (48% TECSA, 30% opioid use, 20% AF, 14% HF, 11% CKD) who trialled ASV	125 pts ASV vs. baseline, 106 pts ASV vs. prior CPAP	Clinical and PSG characteristics, adherence	4 wk	ASV effective and superior to CPAP in controlling central sleep apnea and improving symptoms. Only small proportion of HF pts. Early ASV treatment may improve long-term adherence

AF, Atrial fibrillation; AHF, acute heart failure; AHI, apnea-hypopnea index; ASV, adaptive servo-ventilation; BiPAP, bilevel positive airway pressure; CAI, central-apnea index; CHF, congestive heart failure; C/M/O, central/mixed/obstructive apnea; CompSAS, complex sleep apnea syndrome; CPAP, continuous positive airway pressure; CSA, central sleep apnea; CSR, Cheyne-Stokes respiration; CV, cardiovascular; HCO_3, bicarbonate; HFrEF, heart failure reduced ejection fraction; HFmrEF, heart failure midrange ejection fraction; HFpEF, heart failure preserved ejection fraction; ITT, intention to treat; LVEF, left ventricular ejection fraction; MV, minute ventilation; N/A, not applicable NP, natriuretic peptide; NPPV, noninvasive positive pressure ventilation; NT-proBNP, N-terminal pro–B-type natriuretic peptide; NYHA, New York Heart Association; OMT, optimal medical therapy; OSA, obstructive sleep apnea; OSLER, Oxford Sleep Resistance (Test); PAP, positive airway pressure; PB, periodic breathing; PG, polygraphy; PSG, polysomnography; pts, patients; QoL, quality of life; SDB, sleep-disordered breathing; SERVE-HF, Adaptive Servo-Ventilation for Central Sleep Apnea in Systolic Heart Failure (trial); TECSA, treatment-emergent central sleep apnea; VPAP, variable positive airway pressure.

Heart Failure with Preserved Left Ventricular Ejection Fraction

ASV has also been used in heart failure with preserved left ventricular ejection fraction (HFpEF). The FACE study is a French prospective observational cohort study that included various ASV indications and disease entities and was subject to cluster analysis. Of importance, it focused on different phenotypes of HF (HF < 40% [HFrEF]), 40% to 49% (midrange LVEF), and >50% (HFpEF). Patients with an AHI greater than 15 per hour were included and divided into the CSA group, if central events exceeded 50% and patients had coexisting CSA-OSA with greater than 20% central events or OSA with greater than 20% central events. Patients with CSA or CSA-OSA were treated primarily with ASV, whereas OSA patients received ASV if CPAP failed. The primary outcome parameter was the time to the first severe cardiovascular event (all-cause death, unplanned hospitalization, unplanned prolongation of a planned hospitalization for worsening of HF, cardiovascular death or unplanned hospitalization for worsening of HF, and all-cause death or all-cause unplanned hospitalization).[80] Patients who refused therapy or were not compliant with ASV (<3 hours/day) served as control subjects (n = 133) and were compared to 258 patients who accepted and were compliant with ASV.[49] The mean follow-up period was 21.6 months. Due to the nonrandomized character of the cohort, the treatment and control group differed in several aspects, including having a higher AHI, obstructive AHI, oxygen desaturation index (ODI), and time of saturation less than 90%. The authors did not find any significant difference between ASV patients and control subjects in HFrEF. However, ASV significantly improved the prognosis in patients with HFpEF and with severe oxygen desaturation. Moreover, ASV improved outcome significantly in HF with midrange LVEF in nonischemic HF, whereas there was no significant difference in ischemic HF.[81]

In the prospective randomized multicenter "cardiovascular improvement with MV-targeted ASV therapy in heart failure" (CAT-HF) trial, O'Connor and colleagures[82] studied the effect of ASV or optimal medical therapy (OMT). The authors included 126 patients hospitalized for acute decompensated HF with reduced or preserved ejection fraction and an AHI greater than or equal to 15 per hour. A global rank composite end point of death, cardiovascular hospitalizations, and 6-minute walking distance represented a primary end point. Inclusion criteria were acute HF based on reduced or preserved ejection fraction with dyspnea at rest or minimal exertion, elevated natriuretic peptide levels greater than or equal to 300 µg/mL, or N-terminal pro–B-type natriuretic peptide (NT-proBNP) greater than or equal to 1.200 µg/mL, together with other signs or symptoms of acute decompensation (orthopnea, rails, congestion, chest radiograph, or pulmonary capillary wedge pressure ≥25 mm Hg. The patients did not differ in anthropometric parameters, comorbidities, and characteristics of HF. The mean AHI was 36 ± 17 in the ASV group and 35 ± 17 in the control group. CSA was predominant in 72% of the patients in the ASV group and 79% in the control group. ASV was significantly superior to the control group in terms of AHI and ODI. The trial was stopped after the publication of the SERVE-HF trial data. After 6-month follow-up, there was no difference in the primary end point, whereas ASV was significantly superior in the subgroup of patients with HFpEF.[82] The findings of the CAT-HF study did not show differences in major outcome parameters in general but suggested beneficial effects in patients with HF with HFpEF. However, caution should be exercised, as the number of HFpEF patients was small and the study was terminated earlier than planned. Furthermore, details of sleep metrics with use of ASV were not reported.

Piccini and colleagues[71] performed a prospective subanalysis of patients with pacemakers or cardioverter-defibrillators in the CAT-HF study. The primary end points were the burden of atrial fibrillation and the occurrence of ventricular arrhythmia. The burden of atrial fibrillation was defined as the time in atrial tachycardia/atrial fibrillation. Ventricular arrhythmia included appropriately treated ventricular tachycardia (VT), ventricular fibrillation (VF), monitored VT/VF or nonsustained VT. Patients in the atrial fibrillation and in the VT/VF cohorts presented predominantly with reduced LVEF and predominantly combined CSA and OSA. The authors found a 39% reduction in atrial fibrillation burden under ASV therapy compared to OMT. There was no difference in the occurrence of ventricular arrhythmias between the two groups. These data are in contrast to the SERVE-HF trial, which suggested an increase in sudden cardiac death (death due to ventricular arrhythmias) in the ASV group. However, the study populations differ substantially due to the mixed character of the included patients in the CAT-HF subtrial versus predominantly central events in the SERVE-HF trial.

Daubert and colleagues[83] performed another reanalysis of the CAT-HF data, focusing on echocardiography to analyze cardiac remodeling. Imaging was performed at baseline and after 6 months of treatment. In patients with HFrEF, LVEF improved significantly in both groups (OMT vs. ASV plus OMT).[24] patients suffered from HFpEF, of which 13 had been randomized to receive ASV plus OMT and 11 to receive OMT alone. Nine patients in each group had paired baseline and 6-month echocardiograms. Patients with HFrEF and HFpEF showed trends toward improvement in diastolic indices, not reaching statistical indices.[83]

These findings confirmed data from Yoshihisa and colleagues,[84] a prospective observational study in 109 patients with symptomatic stable HFpEF in New York Heart Association (NYHA) stages II to IV and AHI greater than or equal to 15 per hour. The primary outcome was improvement in right heart function, pulmonary function, and exercise capacity, as well as mortality in HFpEF patients. Symptomatic HF patients with LVEF greater than or equal to 50% in a stable clinical situation and under OMT were included. CPAP was offered to the OSA-dominant and ASV to the CSR-CSA–dominant SDB patients[31] (CPAP, 16; ASV, 15) who were treated with PAP, whereas 78 formed the non-PAP group. There was a significant improvement of NYHA stage, systolic and diastolic blood pressure, right heart function, lung function, exercise performance, and survival under PAP therapy compared to those without PAP therapy.[84] However, the nonrandomized character and small number of included patients could have affected the results.

D'Elia and colleagues[85] performed a small prospective case-control study in patients with acute HFpEF and CSA. They were in an NYHA class greater than or equal to III, had LVEF greater than or equal to 45%, BNP greater than 200 pg/mL, and AHI greater than 15 per hour up to greater than 50% CSA. Ten patients were randomized to receive ASV (n = 5) in addition to optimal cardiac therapy or optimal cardiac therapy alone (n = 5). ASV significantly improved total AHI and CSA, as well as parameters of diastolic function (E/E′), pulmonary artery pressure, RV function, and BNP; these parameters changed nonsignificantly under optimal cardiac treatment alone. The aforementioned trials should set the stage for a large, well-powered, systematic RCT in subjects with HFpEF.

ASV IN COEXISTING OSA AND CSA, TREATMENT-EMERGENT CSA, AND SDB ASSOCIATED WITH USE OF OPIOIDS

The efficacy of ASV has been studied in coexisting OSA and CSA, opioid-induced CSA, or treatment-associated CSA. Allam and colleagues[86] studied the efficacy of different positive pressure modes in patients with various phenotypes of CSA. ASV normalized SDB in all subgroups and was superior to CPAP, CPAP plus oxygen, BiPAP-S and BiPAP-ST. Morgenthaler and colleagues.[87] compared ASV with NIV positive pressure ventilation in different phenotypes of CSA. Although both options sufficiently improved respiratory disturbances, ASV was more effective than noninvasive positive pressure ventilation. ASVs may be better at normalizing CSA than improving subjective or objective sleep quality.[67,88,89] At high altitude, supplemental oxygen is superior to ASV.[90] The cycle length of respiratory events is short at high altitude, whereas the ASV algorithms are designed to target long-cycle PB, which may be one explanation.

In coexisting OSA and CSA/PB, ASV was equally effective in suppressing obstructive disturbances as CPAP but was significantly superior regarding central events and BNP as a marker of cardiac function.[55,91] Arzt and colleagues[92] confirmed the data on the efficacy of ASV for SDB and BNP. Morgenthaler and colleagues[89] performed a multicenter RCT comparing optimized CPAP with ASV over 90 days in treatment-associated CSA. The patients suffered from a variety of underlying comorbidities, including cardiovascular disorders, insomnia and restless legs syndrome, or chronic opioid use. The efficacy of CPAP improved substantially over time, suggesting that the population was mixed with patients with treatment-persistent and TECSA. ASV was superior in terms of respiratory disturbances, both at the initial titration and after 90 days. In an accompanying editorial, Orr and colleagues[93] emphasized that the differences were not clinically significant, with similar adherence to both devices and similar QoL outcomes.

Dellweg and colleagues[59] conducted a trial comparing ASV and BiPAP-ST in patients with predominant obstructive AHI greater than or equal to 15 per hour at baseline and who had a predominant central AHI greater than or equal to 15 per hour after 6 weeks of CPAP therapy (CPAP-persistent CSA). CPAP reduced the AHI from 42 ± 15 per hour to 28 ± 8 per hour, mainly due to a reduction in obstructive disturbances. Both BiPAP-ST and ASV reduced the AHI significantly and substantially during the first night of treatment. However, after 6 weeks of treatment, the effect of BiPAP-ST was minimized, whereas it was stable under ASV.[59]

In trials of ASV, appropriate pressure settings is the key to success, as noted in the SERVE-HF trial.[32] This is also the case in opioid-induced sleep apnea. Farney and colleagues[94] failed to show sufficient efficacy with CPAP and ASV in a retrospective analysis of 22 patients. In contrast, Javaheri and colleagues[95] proved a good suppression of all types of respiratory disturbances with ASV compared to CPAP in a case series of 5 patients. These authors applied substantially higher PS. More recently, Javaheri and colleagues[96] prospectively studied ASV in severe opioid-induced CSA. The patients presented with overwhelming central disturbances. Before treatment with ASV, 16 of 20 patients had undergone a CPAP trial showing a 50% reduction in the breathing disturbances. However, ASV normalized AHI, oxygen saturation, and arousals. Ramar and colleagues[97] retrospectively investigated CPAP nonresponders with central breathing disturbances due to chronic HF or opioid use. They found that ASV enabled sufficient therapy in the majority of patients in both groups. A systematic review put together the data from 127 patients who used opioids for at least 6 months and were treated with different PAP algorithms. CPAP was mostly ineffective, whereas BiPAP and ASV achieved elimination of central apneas in 62% and 58%, respectively.[98] However, the question remains why 30% to 40% of patients with opioid-induced sleep apnea could not be treated optimally.

What Is Next for Adaptive Servo-Ventilation Devices?

ASV has proven to suppress, most effectively, PB in non-hypercapnic CSA. In addition, the backup frequency counterbalances any central apneas with open airways. Last, not least, the automatic EPAP component of the algorithms eliminate any accompanying upper airway obstruction in coexisting OSA and CSA. Therefore ASV might be the treatment of choice in various phenotypes and clinical presentations of central breathing disturbances. However, although CSA is at least a marker of poor outcome in some disease entities, especially in HF, the scientific data on outcome of ASV treatments are currently inconclusive. Despite its beneficial effects on pathophysiologic components (hyper-responsiveness of chemoreceptors), breathing disturbances, and LVEF, the negative prognostic results in the SERVE-HF trial require further evaluation. Having this in mind, the impact of ASV on HFpEF in small-sized studies, in acute or chronic situations, urgently needs confirmation in long-term, prospective RCTs.

CLINICAL PEARLS

- Noninvasive ventilation (NIV) bilevel positive airway pressure (BiPAP) modes are designed to either deliver a fixed pressure support (PS) with or without backup rate (e.g., spontaneous BiPAP or spontaneous-termed [ST] BiPAP mode) or a variable one "responsive" to patient's respiratory disturbance (e.g., volume-assured pressure support [VAPS]) in ST or pressure assist-controlled mode.
- VAPS delivers autoadjusting (variable) PS to reach a preset target lung volume or ventilation (i.e., expiratory tidal volume [Vt] or alveolar ventilation).
- The mechanical breath cycle (inhalation-exhalation) in a BiPAP mode can be defined by (1) the trigger variable that defines the beginning of inhalation, (2) the inspiratory time (Ti) that defines the duration of inspiratory PAP support, and (3) the cycling variable that defines the end of inhalation (initiation of exhalation). In an assisted or controlled breath, the Ti setting together with PS will determine Vt based on the patient's respiratory mechanics.

CLINICAL PEARLS—Cont'd

- Adaptive servo-ventilation (ASV) devices are fundamentally anticyclic pressure support devices with complex manufacturer-specific algorithms that variably target Vt or flow. The typical variables manipulated are expiratory PAP (auto or fixed), minimum and maximum PS, and an auto or prescribed backup rate.
- ASV devices suppress central sleep apnea (CSA) and periodic breathing effectively, but patient-ventilator desynchrony can occur.
- The increased risk of mortality seen in the SERVE-HF study has several plausible explanations.
- The interaction between ASV or NIV modes and the patient should achieve synchrony by matching the patient's neural time (respiratory drive) and rhythm, respiratory system mechanics (compliance and resistance), and the device's settings to achieve effective supported breaths to stabilize CSA (ASV devices) or hypoventilation (NIV).

SUMMARY

In the last 3 decades, the field of PAP devices has dramatically changed after the introduction of highly sophisticated ASV and NIV modes with algorithms capable to adapt and support a wide variety of complex SRBD patterns. It is expected that these devices with servo-ventilation controllers may play an important role in titration and therapy of selected group of complex patients (e.g., PB, CSA, OHS, NMD disorders, ataxic breathing from opioids). However, predicting and interpreting the actual performance of these modes in clinical application requires understanding their functioning principles and assessing their performance under well-controlled bench test conditions with simulated patients. Furthermore, large RCTs with long follow up are needed to better understand the proper role of this technology in the management of complex SRBDs presenting a wide range of pathologic phenotypes.

SELECTED READINGS

Brown LK, Javaheri S. Positive airway pressure device technology past and present: what's in the "Black Box"? *Sleep Med Clin.* 2017;12(4):501–515.

Farré R, Navajas D, Montserrat JM. Technology for noninvasive mechanical ventilation: looking into the black box. *ERJ Open Res.* 2016;2(1):00004–2016.

Gregoretti C, Navalesi P, Ghannadian S, Carlucci A, Pelosi P. Choosing a ventilator for home mechanical ventilation. *Breathe.* 2013;9:394–409.

Javaheri S, Brown LK, Randerath WJ. Clinical applications of adaptive servo-ventilation devices: part 2. *Chest.* 2014;146(3):858–868.

Javaheri S, Brown LK, Khayat RN. Update on apneas of heart failure with reduced ejection fraction: emphasis on the physiology of treatment: part 2: central sleep apnea. *Chest.* 2020;157(6):1637–1646.

Javaheri S, Brown LK, Randerath W, Khayat R. SERVE-HF: more questions than answers. *Chest.* 2016;149(4):900–904. https://doi.org/10.1016/j.chest.2015.12.021.

Randerath W, Schumann K, Treml M, Herkenrath S, Castrogiovanni A, Javaheri S, Khayat R. Adaptive servoventilation in clinical practice: beyond SERVE-HF? *ERJ Open Res.* 2017;3(4):00078–2017.

Selim B, Ramar K. Sleep-related breathing disorders: when CPAP is not enough. *Neurotherapeutics.* 2021;18(1):81–90.

Selim BJ, Wolfe L, Coleman 3rd JM, Dewan NA. Initiation of noninvasive ventilation for sleep related hypoventilation disorders: advanced modes and devices. *Chest.* 2018;153(1):251–265.

Voigt J, Emani S, Gupta S, Germany R, Khayat R. Meta-analysis comparing outcomes of therapies for patients with central sleep apnea and heart failure with reduced ejection fraction [published correction appears in *Am J Cardiol.* 2020 Nov 1;134:162]. *Am J Cardiol.* 2020;127:73–83.

Wang J, Covassin N, Dai T, et al. Therapeutic value of treating central sleep apnea by adaptive servo-ventilation in patients with heart failure: a systematic review and meta-analysis. *Heart Lung.* 2021;50(2):344–351.

A complete reference list can be found online at ExpertConsult.com.

Chapter 141

Sleep and Breathing at High Altitude

Edward Manning; Konrad E. Bloch; Jerome A. Dempsey; Shahrokh Javaheri; Vahid Mohsenin

Chapter Highlights

- Exposure to high altitude imposes significant strain on the entire body, in particular on the cardiopulmonary system and the brain. As a consequence, sojourners to high altitude frequently experience sleep disturbances, often reporting restless and sleepless nights.
- At altitudes above 3000 meters, almost all healthy subjects develop periodic breathing, especially during non–rapid eye movement sleep.
- The major change in sleep architecture after rapid ascent to high altitude consists of a reduction in deep sleep stages, that is, in slow wave activity.
- The primary reason for periodic breathing at altitude is a hypoxia-induced increase in chemoreceptor sensitivity to changes in Pa_{CO_2}—both above and below eupnea, leading to periods of apnea and hyperpnea.
- Carbonic anhydrase inhibitors improve periodic breathing through attenuation of the respiratory alkalosis induced by hypoxic stimulation of ventilation at altitude. This promotes hyperventilation and reduces the tendency to develop central sleep apnea by decreasing the plant gain of the respiratory feedback control system.
- Benzodiazepines and other gamma-aminobutyric acid receptor antagonists such as zolpidem improve sleep without affecting breathing pattern or cognitive function.
- Other modalities to improve high-altitude periodic breathing, including noninvasive ventilation and increasing dead space breathing, remain to be further investigated in humans.

EXPOSURE TO HIGH ALTITUDE

Each year several million people worldwide travel from areas of low elevation to altitudes over 2500 meters. Empirically, and because of higher risk for altitude illnesses, 2500 meters has been used as the threshold for high-altitude illnesses. However, polysomnography (PSG) at altitudes of both 1630 meters and 2590 meters shows decreased non–rapid eye movement (NREM) stage N3 sleep (slow wave sleep) and an increased apnea-hypopnea index (AHI) in the form of periodic breathing compared with the altitude of 490 meters. Interestingly, these healthy male subjects reported no changes in their total sleep time, excessive sleepiness, or acute mountain sickness (AMS) symptoms.[1]

With the increasing popularity of mountain sports such as skiing, climbing, and snowshoeing, and the latest trend in adventure travel to places such as the Andes and Himalayas, it is expected that the incidence of high-altitude exposure will continue to grow. These often-rapid ascents of unacclimatized individuals place them at an increased risk for AMS, insomnia, and sleep-disordered breathing.

This chapter focuses on the effect of high altitude on sleep and respiratory control systems, the clinical disorders associated with such effects, and the optimal treatments. Relevant features of acute physiologic adjustment to high altitude are summarized; then the characteristics of the sleep disturbance at high altitude, its pathogenesis, and therapeutic interventions are reviewed. Although much of the focus is on sleep after acute ascent to high altitude, alterations in sleep during long-term altitude exposure are also mentioned. Information in this chapter may also be relevant to the pathophysiology of central sleep apnea at low altitude.

PHYSIOLOGIC RESPONSES TO HIGH ALTITUDE

Primary among the changes in physical environment that attend the ascent to high altitude is a decrease in barometric pressure such that, although the fractional concentration of O_2 is similar to that at sea level, O_2 tension—the product of fractional concentration and barometric pressure—is reduced (Figure 141.1). This decreased O_2 tension of ambient air presents a threat to arterial and tissue oxygenation and elicits a series of responses that act to minimize tissue hypoxia. These responses consist of early increases in ventilation and cardiac output and, during more prolonged exposure, rise in circulating red cell concentration and adaptive changes in peripheral tissue, including increased spatial density of capillaries and mitochondria.

Increased Ventilation

The earliest and one of the most important of these responses is increased ventilation, which acts to minimize the extent of alveolar hypoxia and arterial hypoxemia in the face of

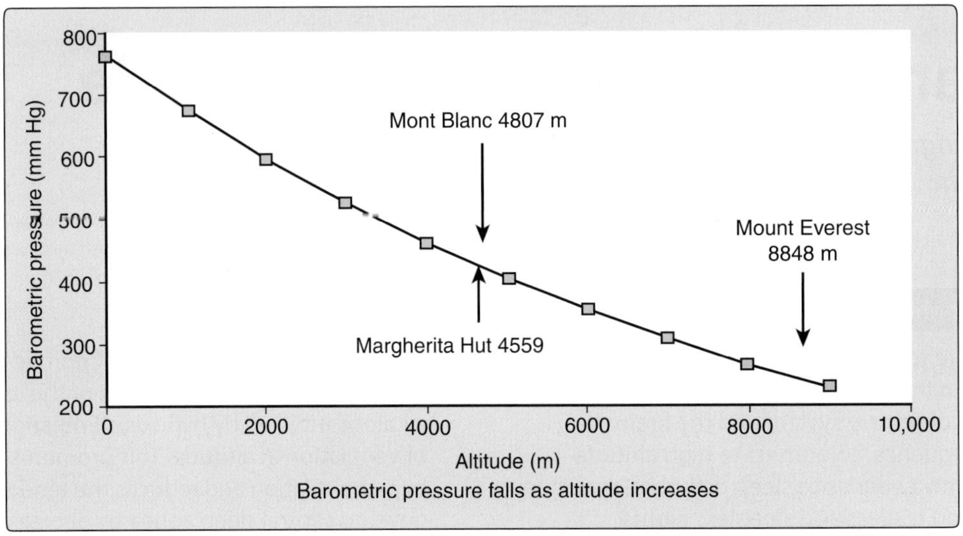

Figure 141.1 Relationship between altitude and barometric pressure. Inspired oxygen pressures at Margherita Hut, Italy, on the summit of Mont Blanc France, and Mount Everest are 84, 82, and 43 mm Hg, respectively.

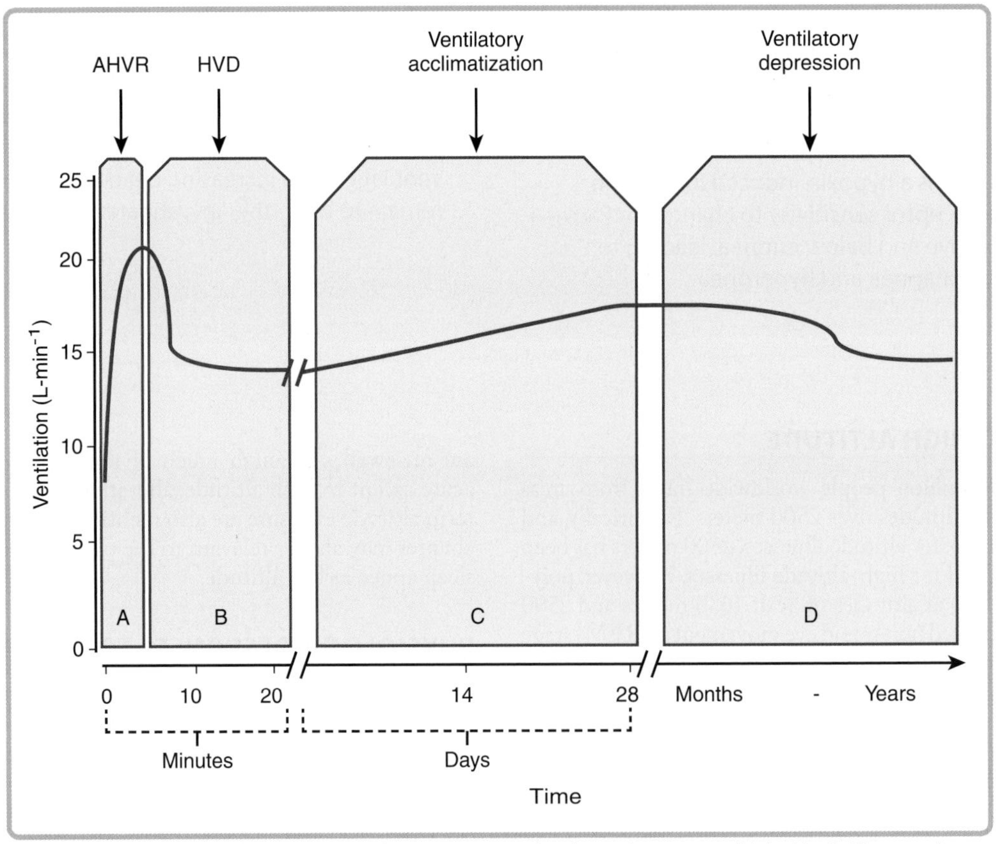

Figure 141.2 Temporal changes in ventilation on acute and prolonged exposure to high altitude. The acute hypoxic ventilatory response (AHVR) is followed within minutes by hypoxic ventilatory decline (HVD) before ventilatory acclimatization to hypoxia occurs. (From Ainslie PN, Lucas SJ, Burgess KR. Breathing and sleep at high altitude. *Respir Physiol Neurobiol.* 2013;188:233–56.)

a decrease in ambient O_2 tension (Figure 141.2). The acute hypoxic ventilatory response (AHVR) is followed within minutes by hypoxic ventilatory decline (HVD) before ventilatory acclimatization to hypoxia occurs. The exact mechanisms causing HVD are uncertain; however, its occur-rence could result from elevations in cerebral blood flow (CBF) increasing CO_2 and hydrogen ion (H^+) washout, resulting in decreased central chemoreceptor sensitivity and/or neural stimulus response.[2,3] The development of HVD has also been attributed, at least in part, to an increased peripheral chemoreflex threshold to the isocapnic hypoxic stimulus.[4] The magnitude of the ventilatory response to hypoxia increases with increasing altitude, but it also varies considerably among individuals at a fixed altitude. This variability, in part, reflects intrinsic, interindividual differences in the strength of the basal (pre-ascent) ventilatory response to hypoxia.[5]

Ventilation progressively increases over several days after ascent to high altitude (Figure 141.2). This gradual increase occurs despite the fact that the increasing ventilation is lessening hypoxia, the presumed stimulus to breathing, as well as increasing hypocapnic alkalosis, which is a ventilatory inhibitor. This is the phenomenon of ventilatory acclimatization to high altitude, which is manifested as a progressive decrease in arterial P_{CO_2} (Pa_{CO_2}) with increasing ventilation over several days. On restoration of normoxia, hyperventilation continues but slowly dissipates over several days.[6] Although the mechanism of such acclimatization is debated, studies in humans and animals suggest that increased hypoxic sensitivity of the carotid body may be a major contributor.[7] In any case, it is during the early phase of altitude adjustment, shortly after ascent, that sleep disturbances appear to be most marked; they tend to improve during the period of acclimatization.

Periodic Breathing

In the mid-19th century, Cheyne and Stokes described the crescendo-decrescendo breathing pattern that now bears their names in patients with cardiac problems and strokes. This type of periodic breathing, which is frequent during sleep in normal individuals at high altitude was observed shortly thereafter by others,[8] and it continues to be a consistent finding in current studies of sleep after ascent to high altitude.[9,10]

The major effects of sleep on ventilatory control include removal of the "wakefulness stimulus"—which is specifically associated with inhibition of motor output to dilator musculature of the pharyngeal airway, resulting in significant increases in upper airway resistance; critical dependence of ventilatory control on Pa_{CO_2} and the unmasking of an apneic threshold for P_{CO_2} residing within a few millimeters of mercury (mm Hg) below waking levels of eupneic Pa_{CO_2}; and a propensity for periodic breathing in the form of ventilatory overshoot and undershoot.[11] The temporal pattern of periodic breathing and its linkage to sleep stages show night-to-night variation and considerable intersubject differences.[12-19] Periodicity is usually evident early in sleep, during light sleep stages (NREM sleep N1 to N2), and can persist despite improvement in sleep architecture with increases in slow wave sleep, rapid eye movement (REM) sleep, and a reduction in the arousal index (Figure 141.3).[20] Periodic breathing at high altitude may also

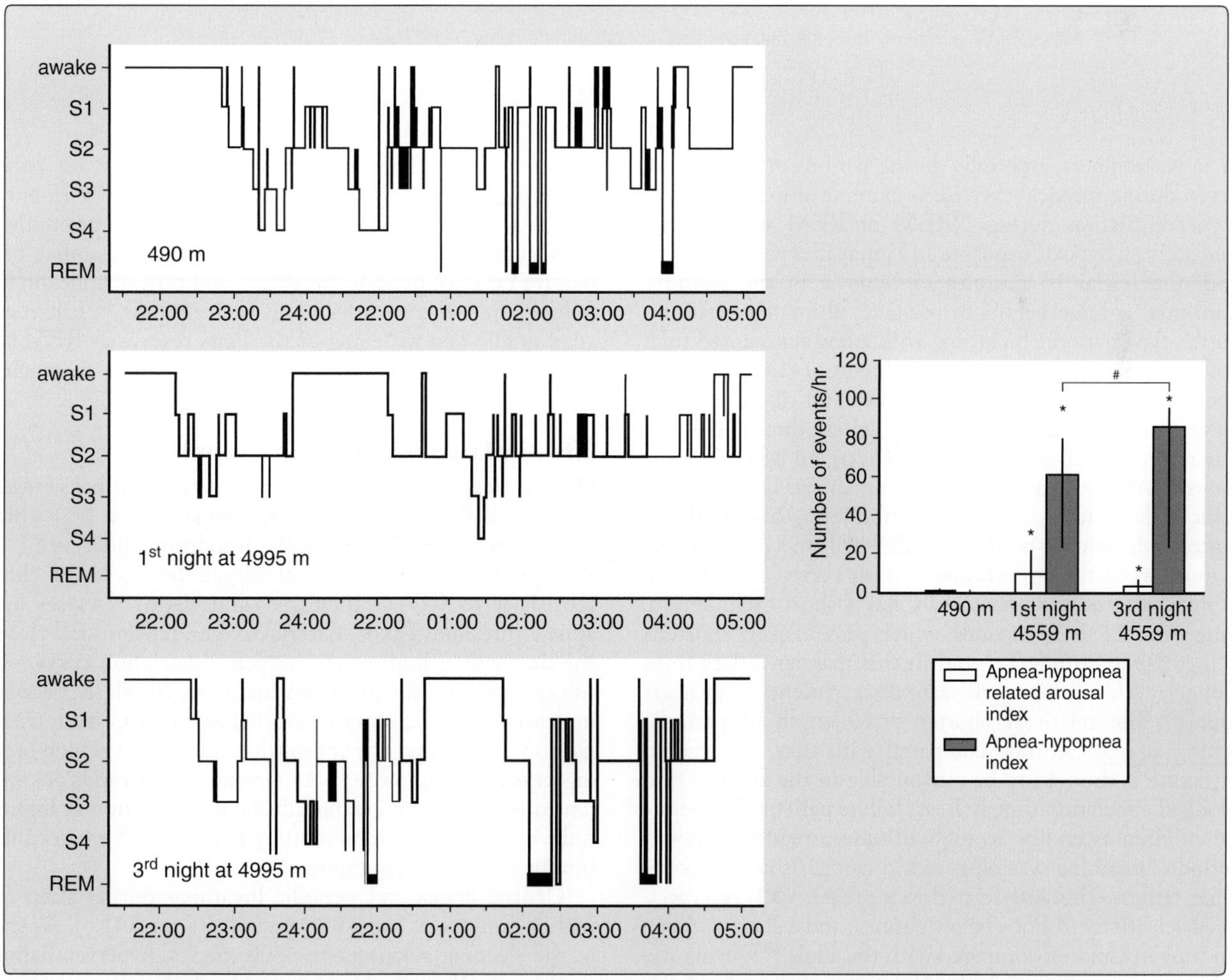

Figure 141.3 A normal subject who climbed to Regina Margherita Hut at 4995 meters within 24 hours had a reduction in total sleep time, slow wave sleep, and REM sleep and an increased number of arousals on polysomnography during the first night at 4995 meters compared with 490 meters. Three days of acclimatization resulted in improvement in sleep architecture, including increases in slow wave sleep and REM sleep and a reduction in the arousal index despite a further increase in apneas and hypopneas (*inset*), suggesting that periodic breathing was not the predominant cause of the sleep disturbances at altitude. (From Nussbaumer-Ochsner Y, Ursprung J, Siebenmann C, et al. Effect of short-term acclimatization to high altitude on sleep and nocturnal breathing. *Sleep.* 2012;35:419–23.)

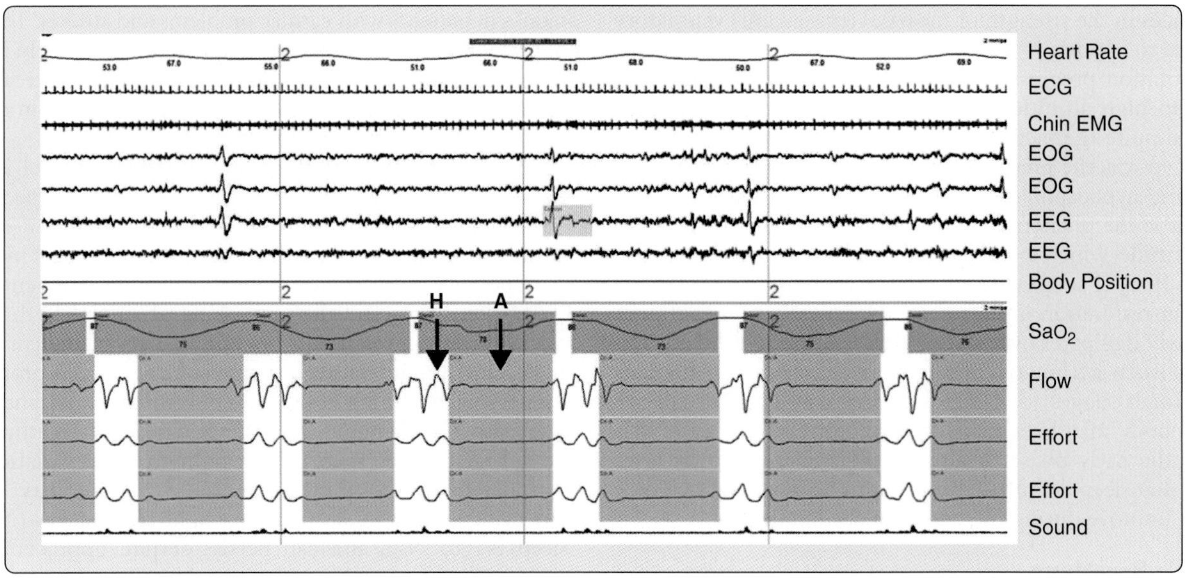

Figure 141.4 A 2-minute epoch from a polysomnogram from one subject during sleep at 5050 meters, showing periodic breathing with central sleep apnea. *Arrow H* indicates the period of hyperpnea, and *arrow A* the period of apnea. Of note, not all apneas were followed by electroencephalogram (EEG) arousals. Arterial oxygen saturation (Sao_2) reading showing periods of desaturation. Nasal airflow was measured by pressure transducer. Respiratory effort readings by piezoelectric bands. ECG, Electrocardiogram; EMG, electromyogram; EOG, electrooculogram. (From Ainslie PN, Lucas SJ, Burgess KR. Breathing and sleep at high altitude. *Respir Physiol Neurobiol.* 2013;188:233–56.)

occur in wakefulness, especially during periods of drowsiness, and even during physical exercise at extreme altitude.[21,22]

Hyperventilation during NREM or REM sleep begins immediately on hypoxic exposure and intensifies with time.[23,24] Within the initial 10 minutes of hypoxia in the sleeping human, tidal volume begins to oscillate, ultimately resulting in cluster-type periodic breathing with a few augmented tidal volumes interspersed with apneas (Figure 141.4). Hypoxia augments CO_2 chemosensitivity below and above eupnea. Consequently, $Paco_2$ is closer to the apneic threshold Pco_2, and therefore a small transient fall in $Paco_2$, for example, after an arousal with hyperpnea, results in an apnea. During these periodic cycles, arterial oxygen saturation (Sao_2) also oscillates and often—depending on the altitude—falls to a point on the steep portion of the oxygen dissociation curve. The periodic breathing pattern characteristically has a short cycle length, ranging from 12 to 34 seconds, which progressively shortens with increasing altitude[25-27] and in this manner differs from the longer cycles of 40 to 90 seconds in patients with heart failure.[28,29] The relatively shorter cycle length of periodic breathing at high altitude compared with that observed in heart failure is thought to be attributable to the absence of a pro-longed circulation time in heart failure patients. In prepubertal children ascending to high altitude, a reduced amount of periodic breathing was observed in comparison to accompanying fathers. This was related to a greater CO_2 reserve, a reduced sensitivity to Pco_2 below eupnea, and a shorter circulation time in children compared with the adult.[30] During the breathing clusters, the most obvious aspect of the periodicity is the oscillation of tidal volume, with a less obvious change in breathing frequency.[22,25] Like periodic breathing at sea level, periodicity at altitude is often initiated by movement, arousal, or a deeper breath with a resultant transient decrease in the prevailing $Paco_2$.

The most striking influence of sleep stage on periodic breathing at high altitude observed in most,[13,20,31] but not all,[18,32] studies is that the breathing periodicity promptly and consistently decreases in REM sleep. This is similar to the relative rarity of periodic breathing and central apnea in heart failure[33] and also in association with opioids.[34] This may be attributable to a widening of the Pco_2 reserve in REM sleep, making it less likely for the prevailing $Paco_2$ to reach the apneic threshold Pco_2.[33]

Effects of Hypoxia and Hypercapnia

During sleep, ventilation and oxygenation fall below waking values, and these relative changes are similar at high altitude and at sea level.[35] However, the important difference is that at high altitude, basal (awake) oxygenation is lower, chemosensitivity to CO_2 is increased, and $Paco_2$ is closer to the apneic threshold $Paco_2$. Arterial oxygen tensions fall closer to the descending limb of the oxygen dissociation curve, where values exponentially increase ventilation. Similarly, because of increased CO_2 chemosensitivity below eupnea, $Paco_2$ tensions fall to values nearer the apnea threshold, below which breathing ceases during sleep.[36] As a result, small variations in gas tensions have much greater effects on ventilation at high altitude, with greater stimulation by hypoxia and greater inhibition by transient hypocapnia.

Central apnea and periodic breathing during sleep occur within minutes of hypoxic exposure (Figure 141.5). As shown in the sleeping sojourner to 4300 meters, hyperventilation in response to the reduced Pao_2 occurs first, followed by oscillations in tidal volume and minute ventilation ($\dot{V}E$) between hypopnea and hyperpnea and then—usually following a single augmented inspiration—full-blown periodic breathing occurs with clusters of large breaths interspersed with apneas at regularly occurring cycle lengths averaging about 20 to 25 seconds.

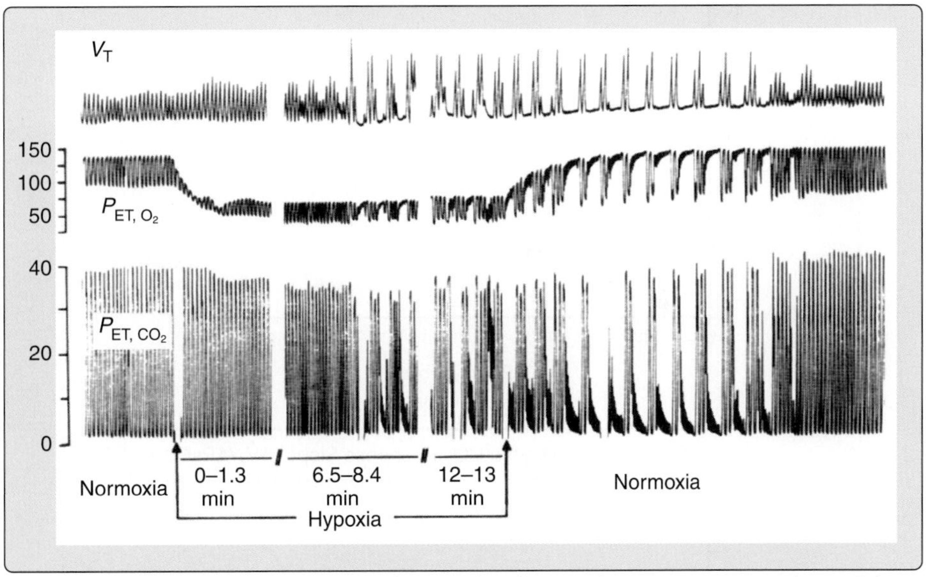

Figure 141.5 Time course of development of periodic breathing on abrupt exposure to simulation of the environmental hypoxia present at 4300 meters altitude during NREM sleep and its relief on restoration of normoxia (see description in text). (From Berssenbrugge A, Dempsey J, Iber C, et al. Mechanisms of hypoxia-induced periodic breathing during sleep in humans. *J Physiol.* 1983;343:507–24.)

This periodic pattern continues over several nights at high altitude. If normal oxygenation is suddenly restored (via increased inspired oxygen concentration, FIo_2), periodicity continues for a brief period with prolonged apneic length; then, as hyperventilation abates and $Paco_2$ rises, periodicity resolves, and a rhythmic, stable breathing pattern is restored. The causes of this hypoxia-induced cluster-type periodic breathing pattern involve responsiveness to CO_2 in both the ventilatory overshoot and undershoot portions of the periodic pattern. First, as described earlier (Figure 141.5), variations in $Paco_2$ correlate highly with the development of apnea and periodic breathing with hypoxia and its relief on restoration of normoxia. Second, if inspired fraction of CO_2 ($FIco_2$) is raised at hypoxia onset to prevent hypocapnia, periodic breathing is prevented, and if $Paco_2$ is raised during periodic breathing to elicit 1 to 2 mm Hg increases in $Paco_2$, rhythmic breathing is restored.[23]

The theoretical basis for the importance of $Paco_2$ changes depends on the effect of hypoxia on two types of "gains" that are the key determinants of the tendency toward ventilatory instability[33,37]: chemosensitivity (or controller) gain, defined by the slope of the ventilatory increase or decrease in response to hypercapnia or hypocapnia, respectively ($\Delta\dot{V}E/(\Delta Paco_2)$; and plant gain, or the efficiency with which changes in ventilation eliminates CO_2 ($\Delta Paco_2/(\Delta\dot{V}E)$ (Figure 141.6). Hypoxic exposure affects these gains in opposite directions; steady-state hypocapnic hyperventilation reduces plant gain, which by itself promotes ventilatory stability, whereas hypoxemia increases CO_2 chemosensitivity both above and below eupnea and narrows the difference between eupneic and apneic threshold $Paco_2$ (Figure 141.6). The latter mechanism is quite pronounced, overwhelming the former and therefore increasing the likelihood of periodic breathing.

During ventilatory bursts of periodic breathing, the oxygen dissociation curve is shifted to the left, favoring O_2 uptake by the lungs; alternately, during apneas the curve is shifted to the right, favoring O_2 release to the tissues. These findings indicate that satisfactory gas exchange may persist during periodic breathing.

At altitudes above 3000 meters and with Sao_2 less than 90%, almost all healthy subjects have sufficiently increased chemosensitivity to cause periodic breathing, especially during NREM sleep. With increased duration of hypoxic exposure and ventilatory acclimatization, plant gain is further reduced, and chemoreceptor sensitivity further increased. Thus a major—but not the only (see later)—determinant of whether longer durations of hypoxic exposure will result in periodic breathing is the balance struck between further changes in plant versus controller gains. Reports are mixed concerning the question of whether duration of hypoxic exposure increases, decreases, or has no effect on periodicity of breathing.[38] The stabilizing effect on respiratory rhythm of adding $FIco_2$ in hypoxia—even if $Paco_2$ is increased by only 1 to 2 mm Hg[23]—is likely attributed to reductions in plant gain[37] as is the effect of adding such ventilatory stimuli as acetazolamide[39] or progesterone, so long as these added stimuli do not increase chemoreceptor gain.[34] Thus we propose that the net effect of changes in chemosensitivity versus plant gain is the major determinant of periodic breathing in hypoxia at high altitude.[33] However, other important secondary modulators of periodic breathing are also likely to contribute, as outlined later.

Secondary Modulators of Periodic Breathing

CBF changes in response to hypoxia, and especially in response to transient changes in $Paco_2$ during periodic breathing (averaging approximately 3% ΔCBF/mm Hg $\Delta Paco_2$).[40] This highly sensitive cerebral vascular reactivity serves to regulate the Pco_2 difference between arterial blood and brain or cerebrospinal fluid, thereby minimizing changes in cerebral extracellular fluid Pco_2 and $[H^+]$ for any given change in $Paco_2$. On arrival to high altitude (5050 meters) the CBF velocity increases during NREM sleep compared with before sleep onset, with large oscillations secondary to varying cerebrovascular reactivity to $Paco_2$ and periodic breathing (Figure 141.7).[38] After 2 weeks of acclimatization the mean

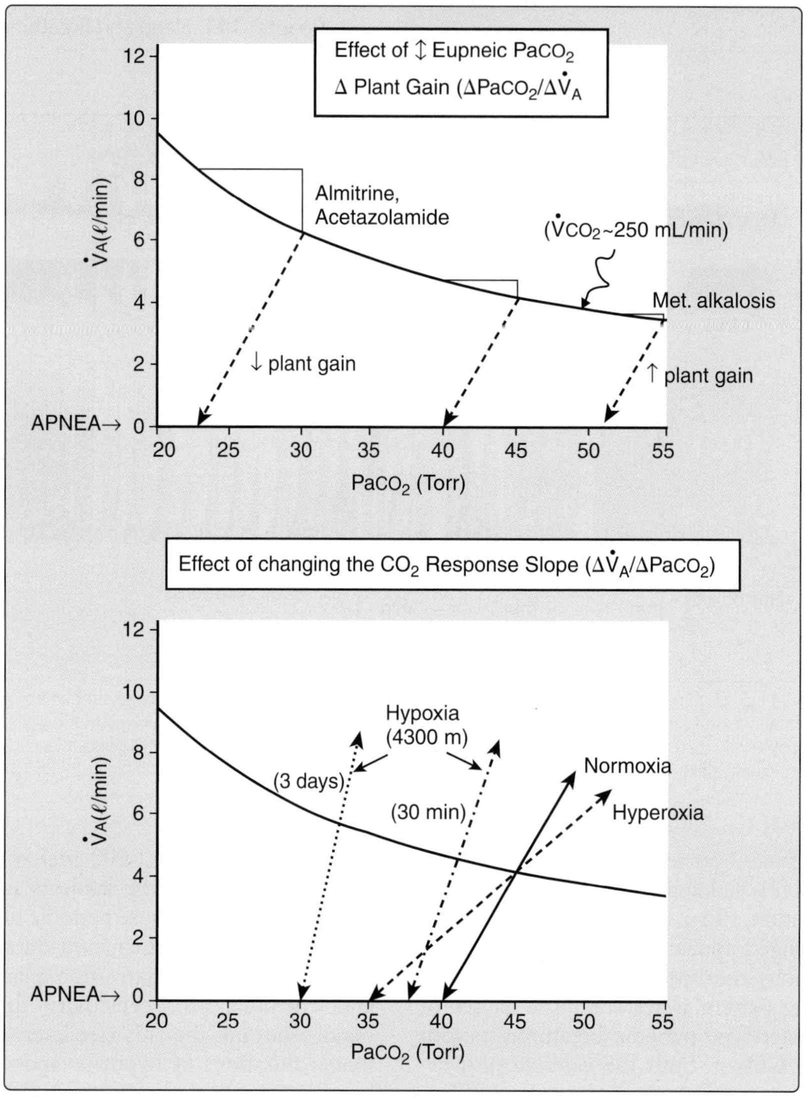

Figure 141.6 Graphic presentation of the relationship of $\dot{V}_A$ to $Paco_2$ at a fixed resting Vco_2 to illustrate how alterations in plant gain or controller gain effect the CO_2 reserve (eupneic $Paco_2$ – apneic threshold $Paco_2$) and the propensity for apnea and instability. *Top panel*: Changing plant gain by stimulating or reducing eupneic ventilation displaces $Paco_2$ along the isometabolic line relating $\dot{V}_A$ to $Paco_2$, thereby altering the $\Delta Paco_2/\Delta \dot{V}_A$ ratio and changing the CO_2 reserve and the susceptibility to apnea/periodicity. *Bottom panel*: Altering controller gain ($\Delta \dot{V}_A/\Delta Paco_2$ slopes) via acute hyperoxia or by acute and chronic hypoxia in normal subjects changes CO_2 reserve and susceptibility to apnea and breathing periodicity. Note that in hypoxia, controller and plant gains will change together. The hyperventilation and increased slope of the CO_2 response observed within the initial 30 minutes of hypoxia are each increased after 3 days in hypoxia. The stabilizing effect of reduced plant gain (decreased eupneic $Paco_2$) is outweighed by the increased controller gain, and the CO_2 reserve is markedly reduced, leading to breathing instability and apnea. $\dot{V}_A$, Alveolar ventilation; Vco_2, CO_2 production. (From Dempsey JA, Smith CA, Blain GM, et al. Role of central/peripheral chemoreceptors and their interdependence in the pathophysiology of sleep apnea. *Adv Exp Med Biol.* 2012;758:343–9.)

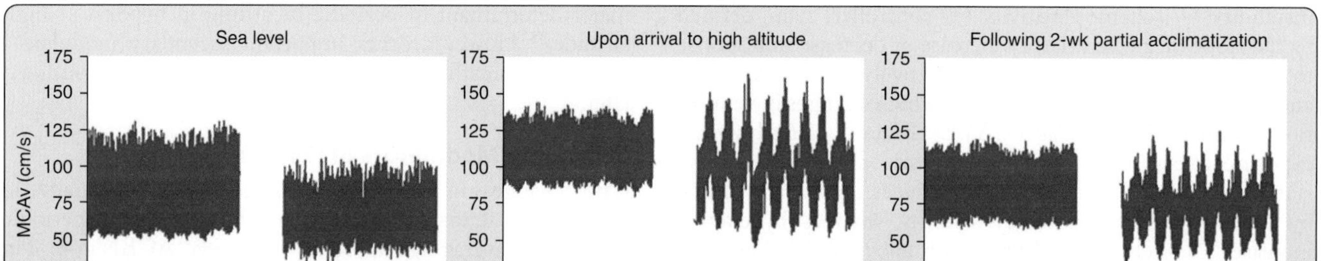

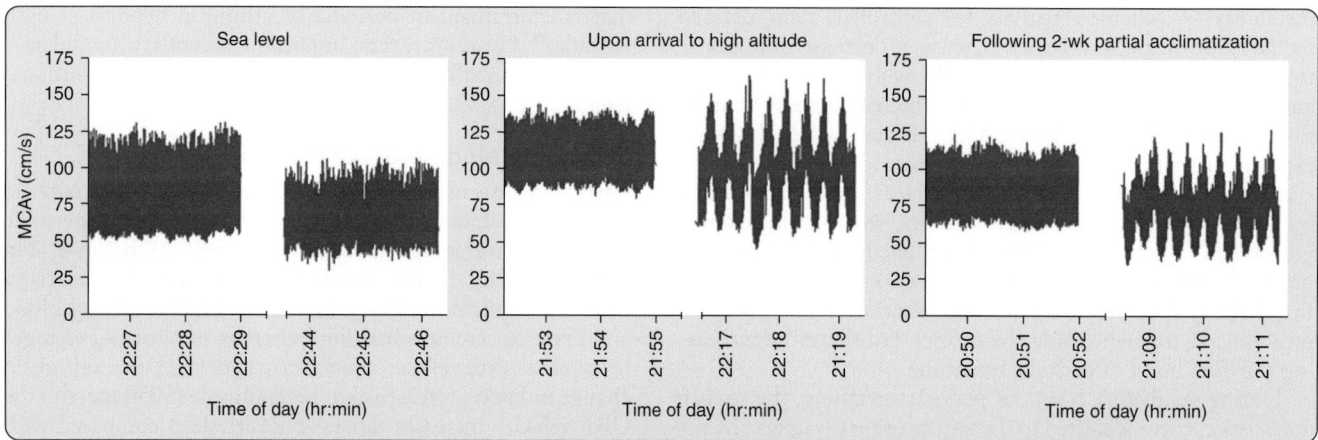

Figure 141.7 The changes in middle cerebral artery blood flow velocity (MCAv) on arrival to high altitude (*middle graph*) and after 2 weeks of partial acclimatization. The decrease in MCAv from wakefulness (left-hand trace) to stage N2 sleep (right-hand trace) was similar on arrival and following partial acclimatization to high altitude compared with sea level (≈10 cm/second). However, both awake and asleep MCAv levels were elevated on arrival to high altitude with marked oscillations compared with sea-level values. (From Burgess KR, Lucas SJ, Shepherd K, et al. Worsening of central sleep apnea at high altitude—a role for cerebrovascular function. *J Appl Physiol.* 2013;114:1021–8.)

CBF returns to that seen at sea level but continue to have large oscillations because of the persistent periodic breathing. When the sensitivity of the cerebrovascular response to CO_2 is reduced experimentally (via cyclooxygenase inhibition), the slope of the $Paco_2$ versus $\dot{V}E$ response is increased and the CO_2 reserve reduced[41]; at high altitudes periodic breathing is enhanced.[38] Conversely, acute (via intravenous acetazolamide) elevations in CBF velocity and reactivity to $Paco_2$ are related to improvements in breathing stability at high altitude during wakefulness[42] and sleep.[38]

Experimental increases in left atrial and pulmonary vascular pressures in the naturally sleeping canine model in normoxia will stimulate breathing, enhance the CO_2 response gain and controller gain, and reduce CO_2 reserve.[43] It is not known whether these same influences contribute to ventilatory control instability as pulmonary vascular resistance increases in humans with altitude-related hypoxia.

A powerful stabilizing influence on breathing occurs through the phenomenon of short-term potentiation (STP) of phrenic nerve and respiratory motor output, which occurs after abrupt removal of a chemoreceptor (or other types) of ventilatory stimuli. This results in a gradual dissipation of ventilatory drive back to control levels.[44,45] When apnea occurs during NREM sleep after a transient ventilatory overshoot, this is likely a manifestation of hypocapnic inhibition as well as vagal influences from lung stretch, which have overridden the stimulatory effect of STP.[45,46] Acute systemic hypoxemia also has the effect of reducing STP, thereby contributing to apnea and periodicity during sleep in hypoxia.[45] A recent study revealed changes in cardiac autonomic regulation in children who live at high altitudes in South America compared with controls who reside at low altitude. This suggests that exposure to chronic hypoxia in high altitude could recalibrate the autonomic nervous system, resulting in vasculature changes.[47]

The modulating roles of sex hormones on sleep-disordered breathing have been suggested by their protective roles against obstructive sleep apnea (OSA).[48,49] Sex hormones may directly con-tribute to ventilatory control through their effects on central respiratory centers, upper airways structure and function, lung dynamics, modulation of chemoreflex sensitivity, and plant gain.[50-52] The potential protective roles of sex hormones on periodic breathing at high altitude were tested in 23 men and 14 premenopausal women who had a sleep study at sea level and then at 3400 meters and 5400 meters. At sea level, a normal breathing pattern was observed in all subjects throughout the night. At 3400 meters there was a significant and large difference in the mean AHI between men (AHI = 40/hour: central apneas 77.6%, central hypopneas 22.4%) and women (AHI = 2/hour: central apneas 58.2%, central hypopneas 41.8%). However, with further ascent to the altitude of 5400 meters, AHI increased in both men and women (AHI = 87/hour: central apneas 60.0%, central hypopneas 40.0%; AHI = 41/hour: central apneas 73.2%, central hypopneas 26.8%, respectively). Interestingly, there was no difference in nocturnal Sao_2 between the genders in these data despite the large differences in the central respiratory event indexes.[53] However, methodological weaknesses prevent definitive conclusions from this investigation. In another study, at an altitude of 4559 meters, men more frequently than women exhibited increased nocturnal periodic breathing. Increased periodic breathing directly correlated with heightened hypoxic chemosensitivity that had been assessed at sea level.[54] These data suggest gender differences in hypoxic chemosensitivity and periodic breathing at high altitude, with men being at higher risk for the latter.

In summary, the pathogenesis of periodic breathing in altitude-related hypoxia is clearly multifaceted, although the key element appears to be hypoxia-induced increased chemosensitivity to CO_2, likely involving both primary carotid body stimulation and secondary effects of enhancing the central chemoreceptor CO_2 response.[55,56]

Sleep at High Altitude

In a comprehensive evaluation of normal subjects ascending to higher elevations (4995 meters), altitude-induced hypoxemia during the first night at this altitude was associated with a reduction in total sleep time, N3 sleep, REM sleep, and an increased number of arousals.[20,57] Breathing during sleep was characterized by increased minute ventilation, periodic breathing, and cyclic oxygen desaturation. Three days of acclimatization resulted in partial improvements of Sao_2 and of alterations in sleep architecture on the third night at 4559 meters, despite a further increase in central apneas and hypopneas, suggesting that periodic breathing was not the predominant cause of sleep disturbances at high altitude (Figure 141.3). In healthy young men, analysis of central and frontal sleep electroencephalography (EEG) recordings, obtained at 490, 1650, and 2590 meters, revealed an altitude-induced reduction in slow wave activity (0.8 to 4.6 Hz) quantified by spectral power density estimates (Figure 141.8).[58] Moreover, in the same study, changes in slow wave derived measures of neuronal synchronization were associated with psychomotor learning impairments at the higher altitudes. These data suggest a potential role of altitude-induced alterations in sleep structure in causing psychomotor and cognitive performance impairments during daytime.[59]

In patients with OSA, arousal correlates closely with the airway negative pressure, to a lesser degree to the level of hypercapnia, and least with the level of hypoxia.[60] This variable arousal response to peripheral stimuli may explain the disparity between improvement in sleep architecture and persistence of periodic breathing in high altitudes. Although the mechanisms of improvement in sleep architecture during acclimatization is not known, it is possible that there may be changes in arousal neural circuitry as elucidated in animal models. Parabrachial (PB) nucleus, located in rostral pons of mice relay node for visceral sensory information from the brainstem to the forebrain, receives chemosensory information from retrotrapezoid nucleus and the nucleus of the solitary tract, which sense hypercapnia and hypoxia, and from the upper airway afferents that respond to pulmonary negative pressure associated with apneas.[61] Mice with inhibition of PB neurons through optogenetic manipulation failed to wake up to hypercapnia and increased the latency to arousal by fourfold in response to the CO_2.[61]

There seems to be no consistent change in the amount of REM sleep at high altitude, which is variably found to be either unchanged (field study),[13,31,62] increased (field study),[63,64] or decreased (hypobaric chamber or field studies).[14,18,20] The inconsistencies of the effect of altitude on REM sleep among these studies are likely related to differences in settings (hypobaric chamber versus field studies), rate of ascent, and degree of physical exertion (being transported versus climbing) and sleeping altitude. There is a disparity between subjective evaluation of sleep quality and the objective findings of normal sleep

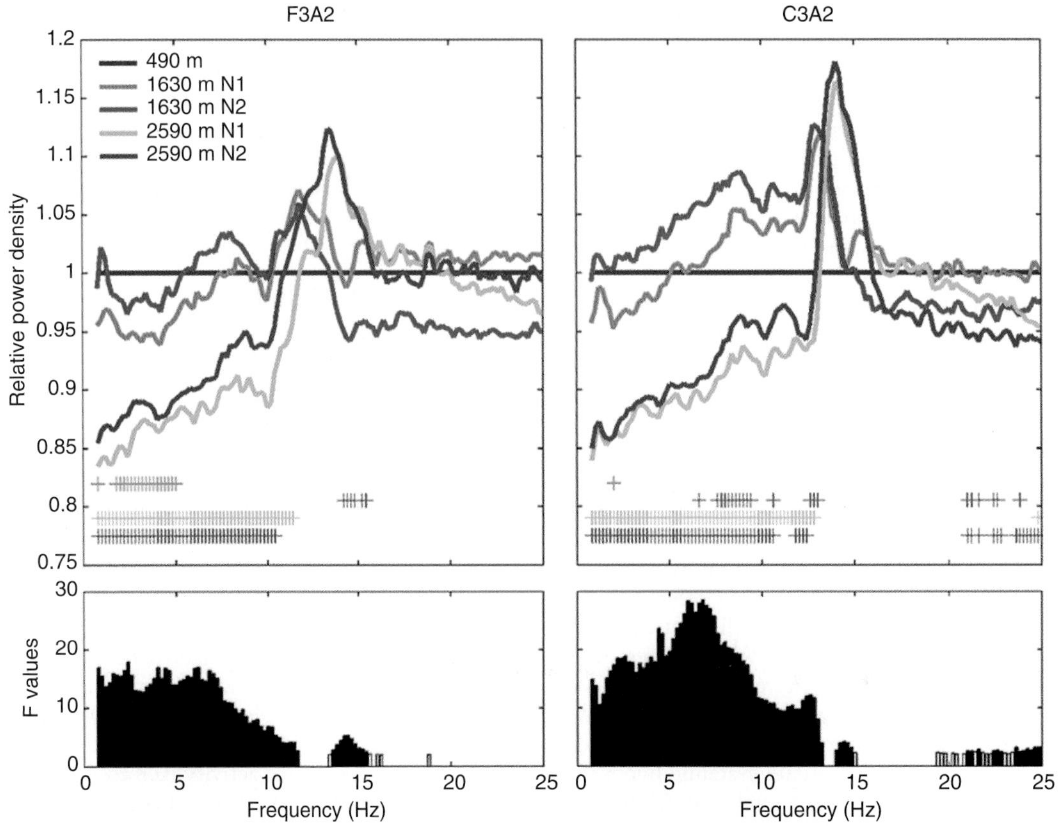

Figure 141.8 Relative NREM sleep EEG power density spectra at moderate altitude. *Upper panels:* Spectra at altitude (1630 meters and 2590 meters, N1 [first night] and N2 [second night]) are plotted relative to baseline sleep (490 meters; line at 1). Significant differences ($P < 0.005$, post hoc paired t-test) between baseline and altitude are indicated by "+" ($n = 44$). Frequency resolution: 0.2 Hz. *Lower panels:* F values of the frequency bins with significant P values for factor *condition* (490 meters N1, 1630 m N1, 1630 m N2, 2590 m N1, and 2590 m N2) of mixed model analysis of variance (ANOVA) with factors were incomplete and these 2 nights were excluded from the analysis. (Reproduced with permission. From Stadelmann K, Latshang TD, Nussbauer-Ochsner Y, et al. Impact of acetazolamide and CPAP on cortical activity in obstructive sleep apnea patients. *PLoS One.* 2014;9:e93931. doi: 10.1371.)

duration. After few nights at high altitude, there is improvement in total sleep time and sleep architecture; however, the subjects continue to complain about sleeplessness. This is most likely due to sleep fragmentation at altitude despite normal cumulative sleep duration that produces the impression of sleeplessness in that setting.[13,65,66]

In summary, on the first 2 nights after ascent to altitude, sleep is typically of near-normal duration or of decreased duration, with increases in NREM sleep stages N1 and N2 ("light" sleep) and decreases in stage N3 ("deep" sleep). Sleep quality seems to improve after the third night at the same altitude, with increased slow wave sleep and REM sleep, but this requires further study. Periodic breathing is present in a substantial proportion of sleep, with frequent arousals and disruption of sleep continuity. Of note, sleep architecture improves over 2 to 3 nights at the same altitude, but periodic breathing persists, suggesting that periodic breathing is not the predominant cause of sleep disturbances at high altitude.

Sleep at High Altitude after Long-Term Adaptation

In the Andes, South America at an altitude of 4330 meters, healthy natives have sleep duration and distribu-tion of stages comparable to those of subjects at lower altitude.[67] However, these native Aymara highlanders have periodic breathing with cyclic oxygen desaturation and elevated hematocrit.[68] Similar observations have been made in Sherpas native to high altitude but not in Sherpas native to low altitude.[69] It is possible that Sa_{O_2} induced by high altitude shifts Sa_{O_2} during sleep to the steeper portion of the dissociation curve and thereby amplifies the influence of ventilatory dysrhythmia on Sa_{O_2}. In Kyrgyz highlanders, with and without high-altitude pulmonary hypertension, a chronic altitude-related illness, a similar sleep structure was reported compared to Kyrgyz lowlanders.[70] However, highlanders had a significantly higher AHI with mostly obstructive events than lowlanders. The potential contribution of ethnic or genetic differences is suggested by a study comparing Tibetan and Chinese Han residents of 4000 meters. Sleep was studied in a hypobaric chamber at simulated altitudes of 2261 and 5000 meters. At the higher altitude, Tibetans had more periodic breathing, higher Sa_{O_2}, and better sleep structure than did the Han subjects.[71]

HIGH-ALTITUDE ILLNESSES

Physiologic Effects Resulting from Decreased Barometric Pressure

A study comparing sleep-disordered breathing in individuals exposed to hypobaric hypoxia (sleeping at altitude) and normobaric hypoxia (sleeping at sea level in a hypobaric chamber) reported that hypobaric hypoxia has larger effects on sleep-disordered breathing with poorer sleep architecture than normobaric hypoxia. Thirteen healthy, young males (average age 34 +/- 9 years) were observed by PSG in simulated altitude (hypobaric chamber with FIo_2 13.6% and barometric pressure 715 mm Hg, simulating altitude of 3450 meters) or real altitude (high altitude research station at 3450 meters with FIo_2 21% and barometric pressure 482 mm Hg) as well as a control condition (nonworking hypobaric chamber with FIo_2 21% and barometric pressure 718 mm Hg, normal atmospheric conditions). N3 sleep, REM, and mean Sao_2 were significantly decreased in hypoxic conditions but significantly decreased further in hypobaric hypoxic condition. AHI, oxygen desaturations, and heart rate significantly increased in the hypobaric hypoxic population. Although this sample size is relatively small, the study suggests that, in addition to hypoxia inducing sleep-disordered breathing, there is a role played by decreased barometric pressure that remains unclear and warrants further investigation.[72] The assumption that physiologic effects are solely a function of partial pressure of oxygen (PIo_2), regardless of the combination of ambient pressure and fraction of inspired oxygen (FIo_2) is referred to as the equivalent air altitude (EAA) model. Many trials attempt to simulate high altitudes during experiments using a hypobaric chamber (at normobaric pressure) because of logistic ease.[73] Such experimental designs rely on the EAA model, which is likely invalid at altitudes above 2000 meters.[74]

Although it is difficult to compare physiologic studies performed at high altitude resulting from multiple confounders such as length of time exposed to altitude and hypoxia, temperature variation, and small sample sizes resulting from logistical burdens of experimentation in high-altitude environments, there is evidence that decreased barometric pressure has an independent effect on human physiology, the pathophysiology of which remains unclear.[73]

Acute Mountain Sickness and High-Altitude Pulmonary Edema

Rapid altitude ascent is associated with a well-recognized clinical syndrome of acute altitude maladaptation: AMS. Depending on the definition, study setting, and population, the prevalence of AMS is around 20% at 3000 meters and around 50% at 5000 meters.[75] Typical symptoms are headache, loss of appetite, nausea, vomiting, and decreased mental acuity. Some studies found an association among AMS and high-altitude periodic breathing.[76] Whether insomnia is part of AMS or represents an independent type of altitude maladaptation is currently debated, and insomnia has been removed from the Lake Louise questionnaire, a common instrument to assess AMS.[77,78] Clearly, headache and the other mentioned symptoms of AMS may prevent a refreshing sleep at high altitude, and insomnia is very common in mountain tourists and climbers alike.

There is evidence from only few studies evaluating cognitive performance at high altitude. One investigation suggested a cognitive decline at high altitude in unacclimatized climbers, as a facet of AMS, which most likely reflected in part the central nervous system effects of hypoxemia compounded by the cerebral vasoconstrictor effects of hypocapnia and sleep fragmentation.[79,80] In healthy individuals ascending to 5050 meters without symptoms of clinically relevant AMS, a delayed psychomotor reaction time and impairments in a comprehensive battery of cognitive tests have been observed.[81,82] Data in acclimatized climbers are very scant, and one study found no evidence for significant cognitive impairment even at extreme altitudes of 7500 meters.[83]

High-altitude pulmonary edema (HAPE), another type of altitude maladaptation, is much less common than AMS, that is, it is rarely observed at altitudes below 3000 meters, and the prevalence at 4559 meters is estimated at 5% of unacclimatized mountaineers. The pathophysiology of HAPE is related to an excessive increase in pulmonary artery pressure in response to hypoxemia at high altitude, an uneven distribution of lung perfusion, and an increased pulmonary capillary permeability and resultant leakage of plasma proteins and red blood cells into the alveolar air space.[84,85] Although these are most common in the early post-ascent period when sleep disturbance and respiratory periodicity are also most pronounced, it is currently not clear whether the characteristic periodic breathing in sleep is correlated with the development or severity of these syndromes. However, periodic breathing was found to be common in mountaineers developing HAPE compared with control subjects.[86,87]

The adverse effects of high-altitude exposure on physiologic systems are complex but primarily involve the central nervous system and cardiopulmonary regulation. The rate of ascent and hence the degree of hypoxia exposure is the main determinant for the development of AMS, sleep disturbances, periodic breathing, and the risk for HAPE. With acclimatization AMS and sleep archi-tecture improve but periodic breathing persists with minimal effects on sleep continuity. Acclimatization to high altitude does not completely return the physiologic functions to sea level or low altitudes, even in long-term high-altitude dwellers.

Chronic Mountain Sickness

Natives and long-term residents of high altitude may exhibit chronic mountain sickness or Monge disease, a syndrome of excessive polycythemia with headache, dizziness, breathlessness, and sleep disturbance. The pathophysiology of the syndrome is debated, but it likely is induced by increased hypoxemia reflecting the combined effects of altitude, decreased ventilatory drive, and lung dysfunction. Compared with normal subjects, individuals with chronic mountain sickness exhibit exaggerated hypoxemia during sleep without an increase in respiratory disturbance index.[88-90] These subjects also exhibit greater daytime hypoxemia, and thus the primary role of sleep-associated desaturation in development of cor pulmonale in these patients remains uncertain.

Pre-existing Cardiopulmonary Disorders and High Altitude

As more low-altitude dwellers ascend to high altitudes, the number of individuals with comorbidities, such as patients with OSA, chronic obstructive pulmonary disease (COPD), long COVID,[90a] and heart failure, also ascend to higher altitudes to travel, sleep, and live. The high altitude exposure tends to worsen the cardiopulmonary function in these individuals.

Sleep Apnea

The respiratory pauses and hypopneas in sleep at high altitude are mainly of central origin, unassociated with snoring or other evidence of sleep-related upper airway obstruction, and accompanied by decreased rib cage and abdominal activity.[12,16,23,31,32] One study of subjects with moderate OSA with AHI of 26 events/hour at low altitude (60 meters) showed, in fact, that at a simulated altitude of 2750 meters obstructive events were entirely replaced by central apneas. The authors believed that the OSA resolved because of an increased respiratory rate and an increase in upper airway tone, whereas central sleep apneas developed because of hypocapnia.[63] Another crossover study to compare sleep disorders between normobaric hypoxia and hypobaric hypoxia revealed that hypobaric hypoxia induces greater disordered breathing and alterations to sleep architecture than normobaric hypoxia.[72] In a study of patients with moderate to severe OSA using a randomized crossover design, it was shown that a moderate altitude exposure (up to 2590 meters) in these untreated patients aggravated hypox-emia and increased the frequency of central apneas and hypopneas, but obstructive apneas persisted.[91] The transformation of OSA to central type at high altitude in some studies likely reflects an increase in hypoxic ventilatory drive, which may augment the activity of muscles of the upper airway.[92] Conversely, sleep studies of subjects living at moderate altitude (above 2400 meters) that were conducted at a lower altitude (1370 meters) in comparison to the altitude of residence, show that at the lower altitude the AHI was reduced. This was likely largely due to a decrease in central events; there was no change in frequency of obstructive apneas, although the latter were more prolonged at a low altitude.[93]

Because continuous positive airway pressure (CPAP) therapy is not feasible nor inconvenient during altitude travel, many patients with the OSA discontinue the treatment during an altitude sojourn. Studies have shown that these patients may experience pronounced hypoxemia and an exacerbation of sleep apnea with predominantly central events already at moderate altitude (1650 or 2590 meters).[91] In addition, the patient's driving simulator performance was impaired, and there was an elevation of blood pressure, an increased incidence of cardiac arrhythmias, and a prolongation of the QT time.[94] Randomized, placebo-controlled trials have shown that autoCPAP therapy in combination with acetazolamide normalized breathing disturbances and significantly improved oxygenation in OSA patients at altitude.[95] Acetazolamide therapy alone was superior than no treatment at all.[96] Based on these studies, it seems advisable that patients with OSA continue to use their CPAP therapy during altitude travel. If CPAP therapy is not feasible, patients may benefit from acetazolamide when traveling to the mountains.[97]

Chronic Obstructive Pulmonary Disease

A recent randomized crossover study comprising 40 participants demonstrated that individuals diagnosed with moderate to severe COPD (as defined by 2017 Global Initiative for Obstructive Lung Disease [GOLD] guidelines for grades 2 to 3, by clinician assessment of patient history and clinical examination or by FEV_1/FVC ratio < 0.7, $FEV_1 \geq 30\%$ and $\leq 80\%$ predicted) were found to have decreased Sa_{O_2} and higher AHI (mostly because of increased frequency of central apneas/hypopneas) during sleep studies at higher altitudes (1650 and 2590 meters) compared with lower altitudes (490 meters). At the higher altitude, participants experienced less slow wave sleep, spent more time awake, had higher AHI, and felt less alert after sleep.[98]

Heart Failure

A study in individuals with stable heart failure (average left ventricular ejection fraction, LVEF, 29% and a peak $\dot{V}O_2$ > 50% of the predicted) showed that they tolerated a short exposure to an altitude of 3454 meters well, even during exercise.[99] A different study characterized sleep-disordered breathing in individuals with decompensated heart failure at an altitude of 2640 meters by analyzing PSG findings of 16 patients in the first 48 hours of hospitalization for decompensated heart failure (average LVEF < 24%, NYHA class III–IV, clinical signs of decompensated heart failure, and elevated brain-natriuretic peptide) revealed sleep apnea (average AHI 45 events/hour) in all cases despite no known prior diagnosis of sleep apnea or CPAP use. Most patients had severe obstructive and central sleep apnea, nocturnal hypoxemia, and nearly half displayed Cheyne-Stokes respiration.[100] Although there is a theoretical concern for acute decompensation of right heart failure at high altitudes, more research is needed in this area. Altitude-induced increase in pulmonary pressure does not appear to increase right ventricular afterload enough to warrant clinical concern. Risk of hypoxic vasoconstriction may be a concern but may occur in less than 1% of cases.[101]

PREVENTION AND TREATMENT OF HIGH-ALTITUDE ILLNESSES

The prophylaxis and treatment of sleep abnormalities at high altitude and AMS in otherwise healthy altitude travelers are similar. Staged, gradual ascent to high altitude is an effective way to blunt sleep-related symptoms and to prevent AMS, but this may be inconvenient or not possible, as in flying to high-altitude research facilities. Pharmacologic approaches include carbonic anhydrase inhibitors and hypnotic agents. Noninvasive positive pressure ventilation or dead space breathing masks have also been evaluated as possible treatments; however, these are impractical and inconvenient for mountain climbers or those other than the recreational tourists at altitude.

Sleep Disturbances

Several studies suggest the safety and potential utility of temazepam for the treatment of sleep disturbance of high altitude.[102-105] Temazepam shortened sleep latency, decreased arousals, increased sleep efficiency, and increased REM sleep, with subjectively better quality sleep in climbers sleeping above 4000 meters.[103,105] The nonbenzodiazepine sedative agents zolpidem and zaleplon have each been found to be effective in improving sleep architecture and consolidation at high altitude. A study of these agents at a simulated altitude of 4000 meters and another in trekkers at 3613 meters showed that, compared with placebo, both agents increased sleep efficiency and decreased wakefulness and that zolpidem increased slow wave sleep. Neither drug, however, had an effect on nocturnal respiratory pattern or Sa_{O_2} nor decreased daytime cognitive or physical performance.[106,107] Importantly, zolpidem altered cognitive function and postural control during early awakenings in mountaineers, likely related to its long duration of action, which raises safety concerns regarding the use of this drug in alpine settings.[108]

Periodic Breathing

Acetazolamide, a carbonic anhydrase inhibitor, improves both the mean level and the stability of arterial oxygenation during sleep at high altitude and markedly reduces the proportion of sleep time during which periodic breathing occurs.[109-111] Because acetazolamide improves both high-altitude periodic breathing and AMS, it may contribute to an improved sleep quality in mountaineers. The beneficial effect of acetazolamide on periodic breathing is seen in both men and women but is more pronounced in men.[54] Acetazolamide is a respiratory stimulant that causes metabolic acidosis and hyperventilation by increasing renal excretion of bicarbonate.[39] These changes mimic the natural process of acclimatization. An effective prophylactic dose (for AMS prevention) of acetazolamide is 125 mg twice daily to be taken a day before ascent and con-tinued throughout the ascent and for 2 additional days after the highest sleeping altitude. As mentioned previously temazepam (7.5 mg or 10 mg) improves sleep but has neither beneficial nor adverse effects on breathing at high altitude. Methazolamide, a lipophilic analogue of acetazolamide, has fewer side effects than acetazolamide and has been used to treat high-altitude illnesses.[112]

Oxygen supplementation improves periodic breathing by widening the P_{CO_2} reserve as mentioned earlier. However, the issues with logistics of using oxygen at high altitude preclude its routine use except for the treatment of HAPE and high-altitude cerebral edema. Effects of other modalities to improve high-altitude periodic breathing, including noninvasive ventilation and increasing dead space breathing, have been shown to improve periodic breathing. Increasing prevailing CO_2 by adding dead space breathing significantly improved AHI in normobaric hypoxia experiments.[112] The field applications of this method should be further investigated before recommendations can be made to support its benefit for travel to high altitude.

CONCLUSIONS

Ascent to high altitude is characterized by frequent awakenings from sleep, which in part reflects sleep fragmentation from high-altitude periodic breathing. This ventilatory pattern comprising central apneas and hypopneas alternating with periods of hyperventilation is induced by hypoxic stimulation of the peripheral chemoreceptors at high altitude, coupled with enhanced CO_2 chemosensitivity, which facilitates the development of central apneas when Pa_{CO_2} falls below the eupneic threshold.

Sleep disruption decreases with time (acclimatization) at altitude. Therapies that have been shown to improve the periodic breathing of high altitude and the clinical syndrome of AMS include pretreatment with acetazolamide, an inhibitor of carbonic anhydrase that attenuates respiratory alkalosis, opposing the effects of hypoxia on the peripheral chemoreceptors. Short-acting benzodiazepines and other hypnotic agents may improve sleep quality without apparent beneficial or adverse effects on breathing in sleep.

CLINICAL PEARLS

- Sleep at high altitude is initially disturbed by the hypoxic stimulation of the peripheral chemoreceptors, resulting in widening of the P_{CO_2} reserve and proximity of the prevailing P_{CO_2} to the apneic threshold. This leads to periodic breathing, central apneas, hypopneas, and frequent arousals.
- Sleep disturbance at high altitude is characterized by a decrease in deep sleep stages and a reduced spectral density in the slow wave range. During acclimatization, sleep architecture improves but periodic breathing persists.
- Effective treatment for high-altitude periodic breathing includes acetazolamide, and certain benzodiazepines may improve sleep disturbances at high altitude.

SUMMARY

Exposure to high altitude imposes significant strain on the entire body, in particular on the cardiopulmonary system. Sojourners to high altitude may perceive a feeling of suffocation or shortness of breath on awakening from sleep. Objective observations show that sleep stages are generally shifted from deeper toward lighter sleep, along with a characteristic waxing and waning breathing pattern known as periodic breathing that accompanies sleep at high altitude. Such periodicity typically consists of two to four breaths, separated by a central apnea from the next period of hyperventilation.

The principal reason for apnea and periodic breathing during sleep in hypoxic environments is believed to be elevations in controller or feedback gain, as evidenced by the steep increase in the ventilatory-CO_2 response slope above and below eupnea. Periodic breathing at altitude seems to reflect the respiratory dilemma of acute altitude ascent in which the stimulatory effects of hypoxia are opposed by the inhibitory action of hypocapnic alkalosis. The outcome is respiratory oscillation. With an apnea, P_{CO_2} rises; this in turn lessens alkalotic inhibition and augments hypoxic stimulation. This triggers hyperpnea, which lessens respiratory stimulation by decreasing hypoxia and increasing alkalosis, leading to recurrent apnea. The occurrence of altitude-related apnea with lessening of ventilatory stimuli is enhanced during sleep.

The poor subjective quality of sleep at high altitude seems to reflect the reduction in deep sleep demonstrated by conventional staging and spectral analysis of the sleep EEG. In addition, fragmentation of sleep by frequent arousals occurs in part related to the periodic breathing pattern but also occurring spontaneously. Acclimatization to altitude is associated with a better-quality sleep.

The most common treatment for periodic breathing of high altitude and its associated syndrome of AMS is prophylactic administration of acetazolamide, an inhibitor of carbonic anhydrase, which likely works by reducing the setpoint for P_{CO_2} and the plant gain of the respiratory control system. The results of recent studies suggest that benzodiazepines and other sleep-promoting agents may improve sleep quality without apparent beneficial or adverse effects on breathing but with possible undesirable effects on cognitive performance during early awakenings.

ACKNOWLEDGMENTS

We thank Dr. Shahrokh Javaheri and Dr. Jerome Dempsey for contributing to this chapter in the previous edition of this work. It served as the foundation for the current chapter.

SELECTED READINGS

Ainslie PN, Lucas SJ, Burgess KR. Breathing and sleep at high altitude. *Respir Physiol Neurobiol.* 2013;188:233–256.

Bloch KE, Buenzli JC, Latshang TD, Ulrich S. Sleep at high altitude: guesses and facts. *J Appl Physiol.* 2015;119:1466–1480.

Dempsey JA, Smith CA, Blain GM, et al. Role of central/peripheral chemoreceptors and their interdependence in the pathophysiology of sleep apnea. *Adv Exp Med Biol.* 2012;758:343–349.

Furian M, Flueck D, Scheiwiller PM, et al. Nocturnal cerebral tissue oxygenation in lowlanders with chronic obstructive pulmonary disease travelling to an altitude of 2,590 m: Data from a randomised trial [published online ahead of print, 2021 Apr 26]. *J Sleep Res.* 2021:e13365.

Ju JD, Zhang C, Sgambati FP, et al. Acute altitude acclimatization in young healthy volunteers: nocturnal oxygenation increases over time, whereas periodic breathing persists. *High Alt Med Biol.* 2021;22(1):14–23.

Luks AM, Grissom CK. Return to high altitude after recovery from Coronavirus disease 2019. *High Alt Med Biol.* 2021;22(2):119–127.
Mohsenin V. Common high altitude illnesses. A primer for healthcare provider. *Brit J Med Med Res.* 2015;7:1017–1025.
Oliveros H, Lobelo R, Giraldo-Cadavid LF, et al. BASAN index (Body mass index, Age, Sex, Arterial hypertension and Neck circumference) predicts severe apnoea in adults living at high altitude. *BMJ Open.* 2021;11(6):e044228.
Shah NM, Hussain S, Cooke M, et al. Wilderness medicine at high altitude: recent developments in the field. *J Sports Med.* 2015;6:319–328.
Sydykov A, Mamazhakypov A, Maripov A, et al. Pulmonary hypertension in acute and chronic high altitude maladaptation disorders. *Int J Environ Res Public Health.* 2021;18(4):1692.

A complete reference list can be found online at ExpertConsult.com.

Chapter 142

Evolution of Sleep-Disordered Breathing across the Adult Years

Andrew W. Varga

Chapter Highlights

- Obstructive sleep apnea (OSA) prevalence increases with aging across adult populations, but the precise prevalence depends on how OSA is defined.
- The evolution of OSA with age differs between men and women, with the loss of sex hormones associated with menopause creating specific factors that can augment the development of OSA in women.
- Factors that influence OSA severity with aging include reduced slow wave sleep, reduced arousal threshold, increased pharyngeal collapsibility, and increased pharyngeal resistance.
- Although OSA prevalence increases with aging, in late life, individual severity of OSA may be influenced more by fluctuations in body mass index rather than continued advancing age.
- Sleepiness is a common consequence of OSA, but sleepiness is a less common consequence in older individuals compared with younger and middle-aged individuals.
- Evidence suggests OSA can accelerate the accumulation of beta-amyloid and tau, proteins associated with the pathogenesis of Alzheimer disease, and may hasten cognitive decline. Whether treatment of OSA can slow or reverse such changes remains unclear.
- Coronary vascular disease is an established consequence of OSA in middle age, but this risk appears diminished in the elderly. Conversely, the risk for cerebrovascular disease from OSA appears to remain elevated in the elderly.
- Evidence suggests that OSA with sleepiness is a risk factor for depression in middle age, but this risk appears to decrease in the elderly.

PREVALENCE OF OBSTRUCTIVE SLEEP APNEA WITH AGING

Obstructive sleep apnea (OSA), characterized by repetitive partial or complete closures of the upper airway during sleep, can occur at any age, even in infancy, but the prevalence and physiology of OSA in children, particularly before adolescence, differs from adults. Pediatric sleep-disordered breathing is covered in Chapter 178, and Chapter 192 is dedicated to apnea in the elderly. The prevalence of OSA is thought to increase with aging across adulthood, but ascertaining this is complicated by several factors, including how precisely OSA is defined and whether the condition is defined solely by meeting a minimum number of events per hour. The seminal Wisconsin Sleep Cohort Study[1] focused solely on middle-aged individuals 30 to 60 years old and found that 24% of men and 9% of women had an apnea-hypopnea index (AHI) ≥ 5/hour, in which hypopneas were defined as those terminating in at least a 4% drop in blood oxygen saturation (AHI4% ≥ 5/hour). By defining OSA syndrome as having an AHI4% ≥ 5/hour along with daytime hypersomnolence, 4% of men and 2% of women qualified.

A number of subsequent large, epidemiologic studies included individuals across a variety of ages. A large study of community-recruited individuals, HypnoLaus, used the AASM 2012 hypopnea definition (≥30% drop of airflow lasting at least 10 seconds with either an arousal or ≥3% oxygen saturation drop) and reported an AHI3A. When subjects were dichotomized by age (ages 40 to 60 years and ages 60 to 85 years), the proportion of subjects with AHI3A ≥ 15/hour was 26.8% in the younger group (39.6% in men, 13.9% in women) and 48.7% in the older group (64.7% in men, 35.2% in women).[2] This highlights that OSA prevalence is increased in both men and women with aging, although overall prevalence is higher in men. Interestingly, the prevalence of excessive daytime sleepiness with OSA, defined as a score on the Epworth Sleepiness Scale (ESS) of more than 10, was higher in younger subjects with the lowest levels of OSA (AHI3A 5–15/hour) in both men and women, but this difference was minimal in subjects with greater levels of OSA (AHI3A > 15/hour). This primary finding of increased OSA prevalence with aging has been consistent across a number of studies that examined a wide age range of individuals, with the degree of difference likely attributable to the different ways in which OSA was measured and defined. OSA prevalence was 5.7 times greater in 60-year-old versus 30-year-old Danish individuals,[3] 5.5 times greater in Australian individuals in their late 60s versus in their late 30s,[4] 2.9 times greater in Polish individuals older than 70 versus individuals in their 40s,[5] 5.8 times greater in Spanish individuals in their 60s versus in their 30s,[6] 3.1 times greater in American men age 65 to 100 versus age 20 to 44,[7] 11.7 times greater in American women age 65 to 100 versus age 20 to 44,[8] 7.2 times greater in Indian individuals ages 60 to 64 versus ages 30 to 39,[9] 5.3 times greater in Brazilian men in their 70s versus men in their 30s,[10] and 7.9 times greater in Brazilian women in their 70s versus women in their 30s.[10]

PATHOPHYSIOLOGY OF OBSTRUCTIVE SLEEP APNEA WITH AGING

Loss of sex hormones associated with menopause in women may have some specific contributions toward the development of increased OSA prevalence.[11-13] In postmenopausal women, fat mass is increased,[14] and the distribution of fat changes to favor increased deposition in the trunk with increased android fat proportion.[15] In postmenopausal women, increased waist circumference, indicative of truncal fat, was associated with greater OSA severity.[16] Sex hormones can also affect upper airway pharyngeal dilator muscles. Postmenopausal women were found to have reduced peak phasic and tonic genioglossus tone versus premenopausal women, a phenomenon not observed in those postmenopausal women on hormone replacement therapy.[17] Drug-induced sleep endoscopy showed evidence for greater anatomic obstruction in postmenopausal women versus premenopausal women, particularly at retropalatal and retrolingual levels.[18] Although adult women with OSA were found to have lower levels of serum progesterone, estradiol, and 17-OH progesterone,[19] a small randomized controlled trial of hormone replacement therapy did not improve the AHI, although blood oxygen saturation was improved and arterial carbon dioxide tension was lower.[20] Although menopause may have specific exacerbating effects on OSA, given that prevalence of OSA in men also increases with aging, it is clear that there are additional factors intrinsic to aging that play into this.

One of the prominent features of sleep architecture that changes with aging is a reduction in and increased fragmentation of slow wave sleep (non–rapid eye movement stage 3).[21-23] Slow wave sleep is a stage of sleep in which it is difficult to elicit apneas and hypopneas[24] owing to several features, including increased arousal threshold,[25] increased genioglossus tone,[26] and reduced collapsibility evidenced by reduced critical closing pressure (Pcrit)[27] in slow wave sleep versus other non–rapid eye movement sleep stages. Irrespective of sleep stage, several upper airway features in older individuals predispose to apnea or hypopnea occurrence. Several studies concur that the oropharynx lengthens with aging (although possibly differentially in men and women),[28-30] but with somewhat less consensus on changes in width of the upper airway. Although one study showed narrowing of nearly all upper airway dimensions with aging,[31] other studies showed increased upper airway cross-sectional area.[30,32] Pharyngeal collapsibility[33,34] and resistance[33,35] appear to increase with aging with a greater fall in genioglossus tone at sleep onset in elderly[36] and reduced upper airway reflex sensitivity with age.[37] Aging was associated with reduced genioglossus response to hypoxia,[38] although the same was not true for hypercapnia.[39] Arousal threshold has been reported to decrease with age in individuals without OSA.[40,41] This could potentially increase the frequency of respiratory events during sleep but may simultaneously reduce individual event severity (e.g., event length or associated oxygen desaturation). The observation that loop gain was reduced in older versus younger individuals[34,42] suggests that ventilatory control sensitivity is less likely to be a strong contributor to increased OSA prevalence with aging.

Although OSA prevalence is thought to increase with aging, severity of OSA within individual subjects may not worsen beyond a particular age. A longitudinal study of older adults with a mean age of 72.5 years at initial evaluation, assessed for OSA severity every 2 years for 18 years, showed that changes in OSA severity were independent of age and largely dependent on change in body mass index (BMI).[43] Other longitudinal studies with average entry age over 60 years and follow-up lasting on average three,[44] five,[45] or seven[46] years showed slight worsening of OSA severity in those with the least initial OSA severity and slight improvement in OSA severity in those with the greatest initial OSA severity. OSA severity was less related to BMI in these studies.

CONSEQUENCE OF OBSTRUCTIVE SLEEP APNEA WITH AGING: SLEEPINESS

Understanding the consequences of OSA in older subjects is complicated by a number of factors. Many of the health-associated consequences of OSA become significantly more common with aging and are driven by several aging-dependent factors and interactions, which ultimately might minimize the contribution of OSA independently. One of the more common immediate consequences of OSA is daytime sleepiness and cognitive dysfunction, predominantly in the attention and executive function domains. However, sleepiness as a function of OSA may actually decrease in older subjects. In a study of more than 200 community-dwelling older subjects, OSA was very common, with more than 50% of individuals having an AHI4% > 5/hour.[47] However, sleepiness by ESS scores was not significantly different between groups with increasing OSA severity and ranged from 4 to 6 across no OSA, mild OSA, and moderate to severe OSA groups. In a number of studies directly comparing younger and older subjects with age cut-offs in the 60- to 65-year range who had matched levels of moderate to severe OSA,[48-52] ESS scores in older individuals were consistently equal or less than those in younger individuals, and a meta-analysis[53] suggested ESS scores were significantly less in older subjects with OSA. Differences in sleepiness from OSA with aging may have to do with a number of factors, including higher overall arousal index in older individuals[41,54] and the degree to which depression drives sleepiness, which was more common in younger subjects.[55]

RISK FOR COGNITIVE DECLINE AND ALZHEIMER DISEASE

In spite of such reduced impact of OSA on sleepiness, older individuals with OSA may nonetheless be at risk for cognitive decline and risk for development of dementia, particularly Alzheimer disease (AD).[56] A meta-analysis found that AD patients have a fivefold increased risk of presenting with OSA compared with age-matched controls,[57] setting up the possibility that OSA constitutes a risk factor for AD and/or that AD pathophysiology contributes to the development of

OSA. Because accumulation of amyloid-beta and tau, the proteins that aggregate to form neuritic plaques and neurofibrillary tangles in AD respectively, as well as synaptic changes are thought to occur years to decades before the development of overt change in memory,[58] much focus has been placed on understanding the impact of OSA in cognitively normal older individuals on development of preclinical AD pathology and risk for future cognitive decline. Older women enrolled in the Study of Osteoporotic Fractures with objectively measured OSA were nearly twice as likely to develop mild cognitive impairment or dementia than age-matched women without OSA.[59] Older subjects in the Alzheimer disease Neuroimaging Initiative with a self-reported diagnosis of OSA had evidence for greater accumulation of both amyloid and tau over a 2.5- to 3-year period,[60] and developed mild cognitive impairment at an age that was on average 11 years earlier than those without self-reported OSA.[61] Increasing AHI in cognitively normal older subjects was associated with increased amyloid and tau at cross section[62,63] in a way that was dependent on ApoE genotype,[64] and increasing AHI was associated with longitudinal increases in amyloid burden even when cognition remained unchanged.[47]

The effects of OSA treatment in older subjects, particularly with positive airway pressure (PAP), have been understudied. A few studies indicate PAP treatment may be beneficial. In subjects with mild AD, although no clear cognitive benefits were observed between subjects randomized to 3 weeks of PAP versus 3 weeks of sham PAP,[65] subjects that continued using PAP for 1 year showed less cognitive decline than subjects who did not continue PAP.[66] In individuals with mild to moderate AD and severe OSA, median annual cognitive decline (by mini-mental status exam score) was significantly slower in continuous positive airway pressure (CPAP) users than in the non-CPAP users over a 3-year period.[67] In cognitively normal older individuals, although the number of people with a self-reported diagnosis of OSA and CPAP treatment was low, the average age of onset mild cognitive impairment was 10 years later than those with a self-reported diagnosis without treatment (and similar to individuals reporting no known OSA diagnosis).[61] Although adherent PAP treatment for at least 30 days in subjects with at least mild OSA (AHI4% > 5/hour) did not result in significant changes in cerebrospinal fluid (CSF) tau or amyloid-beta in cognitively normal middle-aged subjects, significant correlations existed between change in AHI on PAP and change in both CSF tau and amyloid-beta,[68] suggesting potentially greater benefit for those with more severe OSA. A small randomized clinical trial of CPAP on cognition in older subjects with severe OSA at 3 months showed improvements in executive function and episodic and short-term memory.[69] This differed from an earlier randomized clinical trial of CPAP in older subjects with OSA, in which no impact on cognition was observed at 3 months, although in this case improvements in sleepiness were observed.[70] Differences in these findings may be related to different inclusion criteria with regard to OSA severity or differences in PAP adherence in subjects randomized to CPAP therapy.

RISK FOR CEREBROVASCULAR DISEASE

In older individuals, risk to brain health from OSA may also stem from cerebrovascular disease. In a sample of individuals seeking sleep testing with an average of 60 years, OSA was associated with increased risk for stroke or death over 4 years, even after adjusting for numerous established additional stroke risk factors.[71] These findings were echoed in two studies of even older individuals with mean age in the late 70s. In the first, severe OSA (AHI4% > 30/hour) was associated with increased risk for stroke over a 6-year period,[72] while in the latter, severe nocturnal hypoxemia (≥ 10% of the night with SpO_2 levels below 90%) was associated with increased risk of incident stroke over a 7-year period.[73] Notably, the increased stroke risk observed in individuals 70 years of age on average with severe OSA was significantly mitigated in those with OSA adherent to PAP treatment.[74] In older individuals with a first stroke or transient ischemic attack, adherence to PAP in those with OSA was associated with decreased risk for subsequent stroke[75] or death.[76] A meta-analysis of several randomized controlled trials of PAP in subjects with identified OSA after an initial stroke showed an overall improvement in neurofunctional outcomes, albeit with high heterogeneity across the studies.[77]

RISK FOR CORONARY VASCULAR DISEASE

The risks of OSA regarding coronary vascular disease in older individuals appear less than those for cerebrovascular disease. Although increased risk for coronary vascular disease with OSA has been reasonably established in middle-aged subjects,[78-80] no increased risk was observed in men over 70 years old. Relatedly, a study showing increased risk of stroke in older individuals with OSA failed to show increased risk of coronary heart disease.[74] Although OSA was shown to be associated with increased cardiovascular mortality in older individuals with OSA,[81] this risk was attributable to deaths from stroke or heart failure, but not ischemic heart disease. The apparent differences in risk from OSA between cerebrovascular disease and coronary vascular disease in older individuals may be related to the pathophysiologic heterogeneity of stroke,[82] which has hemorrhagic and embolic etiologies in addition to local thrombosis. The risks of OSA toward hypertension appears to largely mimic risk for coronary vascular disease, where risk is clearer in middle-aged individuals, but less so in the elderly. Although one longitudinal study of individuals with a mean age of 68 years showed that severe OSA was associated with incident hypertension over 3 years,[83] no adjusted association between AHI and systolic/diastolic hypertension was found in individuals over 60 years[84] or over 65 years[85] of age in two other longitudinal studies.

RISK FOR DEPRESSION

Rates of depression are highest in middle age, but depression remains a significant problem among the elderly, and in both age groups, depression is more common in women.[86] In a study encompassing both middle-aged and older subjects aged 54 to 93 years, OSA with sleepiness was significantly associated with depression.[87] Although a study assessing OSA risk by Berlin scores found increased OSA risk in older individuals with depression than in those without,[88] other studies suggested no increased risk for depression across OSA severity groups in older individuals,[89] and associations between OSA risk and depression were attenuated in individuals after age 70 years.[90] Although depression scores were not a primary outcome in the Sleep and Vascular Endpoints (SAVE) study, a large randomized controlled trial of PAP for secondary prevention of cardiovascular disease with a mean age of 61 years, it is nonetheless noteworthy that individuals randomized to PAP showed significantly greater reductions in depression scores than individuals in the control group.[91,92]

CLINICAL PEARLS

- Although OSA prevalence increases with aging, OSA severity is most commonly mild in older subjects, which opens a wide array of effective treatment of treatment options.
- Aging is associated with several physiologic factors that increase OSA severity. However, these factors plateau in late life, such that in elderly, OSA severity does not increase with additional aging but may change as a function of changes to BMI.
- OSA may accelerate the accumulation of beta-amyloid and tau, proteins associated with the pathogenesis of AD, and hasten cognitive decline. Whether treatment of OSA can slow or reverse such changes is unknown.

SUMMARY

The prevalence of OSA increases with aging in the adult, but the precise prevalence estimates depend on how OSA is defined, with variability stemming from the definition of hypopnea, the number of events per hour that qualify as disease, and whether associated daytime symptoms are required. Aging is associated with several changes to upper airway physiology and neurophysiology that likely contribute to the increased prevalence of OSA with aging, including reduced slow wave sleep, reduced arousal threshold, increased pharyngeal collapsibility, and increased pharyngeal resistance. Additionally, in women, the loss of sex hormones stemming from menopause leads to both increased fat mass and fat redistribution favoring the trunk, as well as reduced peak phasic and tonic genioglossus tone, all of which can contribute to the onset or worsening of OSA. Although daytime sleepiness is a very common consequence of OSA, sleepiness is less common in elderly individuals versus young and middle-aged individuals with equivalent OSA severity. Depression and cardiovascular disease, broadly defined, are risks associated with OSA in middle age. With further aging into late adulthood, specific risk for coronary vascular disease from OSA appears to diminish, whereas risk for cerebrovascular disease remains elevated. In late life, OSA is associated with increased accumulation of beta-amyloid and tau, pathogenic proteins in AD, and may accelerate the pace of cognitive decline.

SELECTED READINGS

Alcantara C, et al. Sleep disturbances and depression in the multi-ethnic study of atherosclerosis. *Sleep*. 2016;39:915–925.

Bubu OM, et al. Obstructive sleep apnea, cognition and Alzheimer's disease: a systematic review integrating three decades of multidisciplinary research. *Sleep Med Rev*. 2020;50:101250.

Catalan-Serra P, et al. Increased incidence of stroke, but not coronary heart disease, in elderly patients with sleep apnea. *Stroke*. 2019;50:491–494.

Dancey DR, Hanly PJ, Soong C, Lee B, Hoffstein V. Impact of menopause on the prevalence and severity of sleep apnea. *Chest*. 2001;120:151–155.

Díaz-Román M, Pulopulos MM, Baquero M, et al. Obstructive sleep apnea and Alzheimer's disease-related cerebrospinal fluid biomarkers in mild cognitive impairment. *Sleep*. 2021;44(1):zsaa133.

Heinzer R, et al. Prevalence of sleep-disordered breathing in the general population: the HypnoLaus study. *Lancet Respir Med*. 2015;3:310–318.

Iannella G, et al. Aging effect on sleepiness and apneas severity in patients with obstructive sleep apnea syndrome: a meta-analysis study. *Eur Arch Otorhinolaryngol*. 2019;276:3549–3556.

Malhotra A, et al. Aging influences on pharyngeal anatomy and physiology: the predisposition to pharyngeal collapse. *Am J Med*. 2006;119:72.e79–14.

Marin JM, Carrizo SJ, Vicente E, Agusti AG. Long-term cardiovascular outcomes in men with obstructive sleep apnoea-hypopnoea with or without treatment with continuous positive airway pressure: an observational study. *Lancet*. 2005;365:1046–1053.

Sforza E, Hupin D, Pichot V, Barthelemy JC, Roche F. A 7-year follow-up study of obstructive sleep apnoea in healthy elderly: The PROOF cohort study. *Respirology*. 2017;22:1007–1014.

Sharma RA, Varga AW, et al. Obstructive sleep apnea severity affects amyloid burden in cognitively normal elderly. a longitudinal study. *Am J Respir Crit Care Med*. 2018;197:933–943.

Wellman A, et al. Chemical control stability in the elderly. *J Physiol*. 2007;581:291–298.

Yaggi HK, et al. Obstructive sleep apnea as a risk factor for stroke and death. *N Engl J Med*. 2005;353:2034–2041.

A complete reference list can be found online at ExpertConsult.com.

Section 16

Cardiovascular Disorders

Chapter 143

Introduction

Shahrokh Javaheri; Luciano F. Drager; Geraldo Lorenzi-Filho

Chapter Highlights

- Cardiocerebrovascular disorders, including systemic hypertension, coronary artery disease, congestive heart failure, stroke, and transient ischemic attacks, are prevalent and associated with excess morbidity and mortality as well as huge economic costs.
- One of the most significant developments in the field has been the recognition that sleep disorders such as sleep apnea are extremely common among patients with established cardiovascular disease and, when present, could contribute to a worsening outcome.
- Importantly, sleep disorders are also a potential cause of various cardiovascular diseases. This bidirectional relationship is well established for congestive heart failure and stroke, which can cause sleep disorders such as insomnia and sleep apnea. This chapter provides an overview of this section consisting of several chapters of sleep and cardiovascular diseases.
- Stroke is the most common downstream consequence of obstructive sleep apnea (OSA), and a sensitivity analysis of a randomized clinal trial has shown a reduction in stroke with positive airway pressure (PAP), but no significant improvement in other cardiovascular end points.
- In general, the negative studies suffer from methodological issues: patients used PAP less than 4 hours a night; exclusion of sleepy patients; exclusion of patients with severe OSA. Use of multiple coprimary, rather than single outcome, specifically cerebral consequences, and short duration.

Cardiovascular disease (CVD) has a high prevalence and is associated with excessive morbidity and mortality and huge economic costs. Annually, the American Heart Association, together with the Centers for Disease Control and Prevention, the National Institutes of Health, and other government agencies, update statistics on the impact of CVD. According to the 2021 update,[1] the prevalence of CVD (comprising coronary heart disease [CHD], heart failure [HF], stroke, and hypertension) in adults of 20 years of age or older is 49.2% overall (126.9 million in 2018) and increases with age in both males and females. However, excluding hypertension, the prevalence of CVD (CHD, HF, and stroke only) is 9.3% (26.1 million in 2018). In 2018 the estimated number of individuals who died of CVD was 868,662, with an associated huge economic impact of $363.4 billion.

Many of these individuals with cerebrocardiovascular disorders suffer from insomnia, obesity, sleep-disordered breathing events, and related consequences such as diabetes, depression, and hyperlipidemia, all of which could contribute to morbidity and mortality of these subjects, along with their huge health-related cost, noted previously.

This section on sleep and cardiovascular disorders focuses on the bidirectional relation between sleep disorders (sleep breathing disorders and insomnia) and CVD (cardiac failure, acute myocardial infarction, cardiac rhythm disorders, hypertension, stroke, and transient ischemic attack [TIA]).

IMPACT OF INADEQUATE SLEEP ON THE CARDIOVASCULAR SYSTEM

It is estimated that about 35% of adults get inadequate sleep, defined as less than 7 hours (see Chapter 5).[1] Short sleep duration has been associated with several cardiovascular and metabolic health outcomes, including prevalent and incident obesity, and all-cause cardiovascular mortality.[2,3] In this regard, we also emphasize the potential for bidirectional relationship with poor sleep contributing or causing CVD, and vice versa.

Future Directions

It remains to be determined, in a randomized controlled trial (RCT), if increasing total sleep time or treatment of insomnia would reverse the aforementioned adverse consequences.

IMPACT OF SLEEP-RELATED DISORDERED BREATHING ON THE CARDIOVASCULAR SYSTEM

The prevalence of obstructive sleep apnea (OSA) is on the rise, in part related to obesity.[4] The explosion of basic science and physiologic studies in both experimental animals and humans, as well as epidemiologic and clinical studies, support the bidirectional linking of sleep apnea to a variety of cardiovascular disorders,[5] similar to insomnia and CVD, noted previously (see Chapter 151).

There is plethora of evidence that OSA is extremely common among patients with established cardiocerebrovascular and metabolic disease.[5] For instance, among patients with hypertension, coronary artery disease, atrial fibrillation, type 2 diabetes, and metabolic syndrome, the prevalence of OSA ranges from 30% to 83% (Figure 143.1). On the other hand, OSA is largely underdiagnosed and undertreated. In addition to the low awareness of the medical community, there is also evidence that the typical symptoms associated with OSA observed in patients referred to the sleep specialist, such as excessive daytime sleepiness, are frequently not present among patients with established cardiocerebrovascular disease.[6-8]

Interesting, however, when such individuals are tested objectively in the laboratory, multiple sleep latency could be abnormal.[9]

Acutely, OSA is associated with a number of adverse consequences (Figure 143.2), including alterations in PO_2 and PCO_2, large negative swings in intrathoracic pressure and arousals, collectively imposing hemodynamic consequences, neurohormonal activation, oxidative stress, biochemical and cellular abnormalities, release of inflammatory mediators such as cytokines, and increased expression of adhesion molecules, resulting in attachment of white blood cells to endothelial cells and their transmigration.[5] These reactions underlie the pathologic processes involved in endothelial dysfunction syndrome, the underlying pathophysiologic mechanism for atherosclerosis, hypertension, stroke, HF, and coronary artery disease.

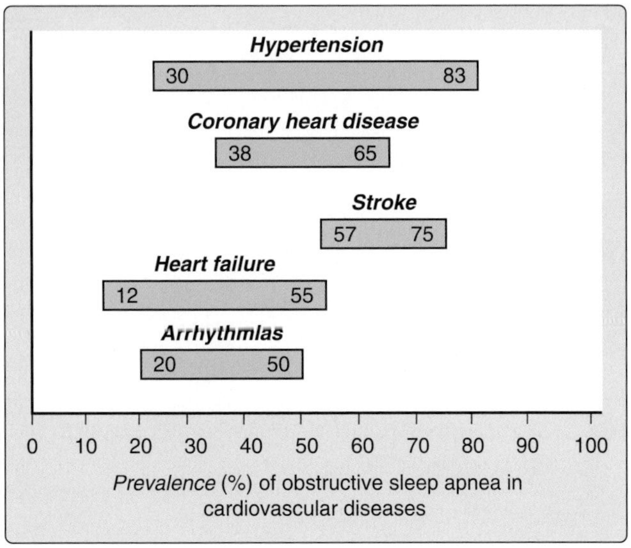

Figure 143.1 Prevalence (%) of obstructive sleep apnea in various cardiovascular disorders. The lower limit is invariably using an apnea-hypopnea index of at least 15/hour, indicating presence of moderate to severe OSA. (With permission from Javaheri S, Barbe F, Campos-Rodriguez F, et al. Sleep apnea: types, mechanisms, and clinical cardiovascular consequences. *J Am Coll Cardiol*. 2017;69[7]:841–58.)

Because of the aforementioned abnormalities, and along with cyclic changes in blood pressure resulting in wall stress, changes in coronary and cerebral blood flow, and diminished oxygen delivery, OSA could play a causative role or contribute to the development of atherosclerosis, and treatment of OSA with nasal continuous positive airway pressure (CPAP) attenuates surrogate markers of atherosclerosis.[10] Furthermore, a number of RCTs, some using 24-ambulatory blood pressure monitoring, demonstrate that the treatment of OSA with CPAP results in a reduction in systemic hypertension[5] (see Chapter 147), a major cause of downstream cerebrocardiovascular disorders. The most beneficial therapeutic effects on elevated blood pressure are observed in patients with severe OSA and resistant hypertension who are compliant with CPAP[5] (see Chapter 147). Although the fall in blood pressure is frequently small, it has been shown that even small reductions in blood pressure over the long term significantly decrease the incidence of cerebrovascular and cardiovascular diseases. Therefore, in patients with OSA, even a small drop in blood pressure, which could be maintained with long-term use of CPAP, is meaningful from a clinical and a public health point of view. Furthermore, treatment of OSA with CPAP may result in additional protection against vascular disorders because OSA may contribute to cardiovascular and cerebrovascular disease by a variety of mechanisms other than hypertension. Regardless of the precise mechanisms, observational studies consistently suggest that OSA is independently associated with increased cardiovascular mortality and treatment of OSA with CPAP is associated with decreased cardiovascular mortality.

In spite of the aforementioned studies, the SAVE trial[10] (Sleep Apnea Cardiovascular Endpoints), the largest RCT to examine the effect of CPAP on incident CVD, was neutral. In

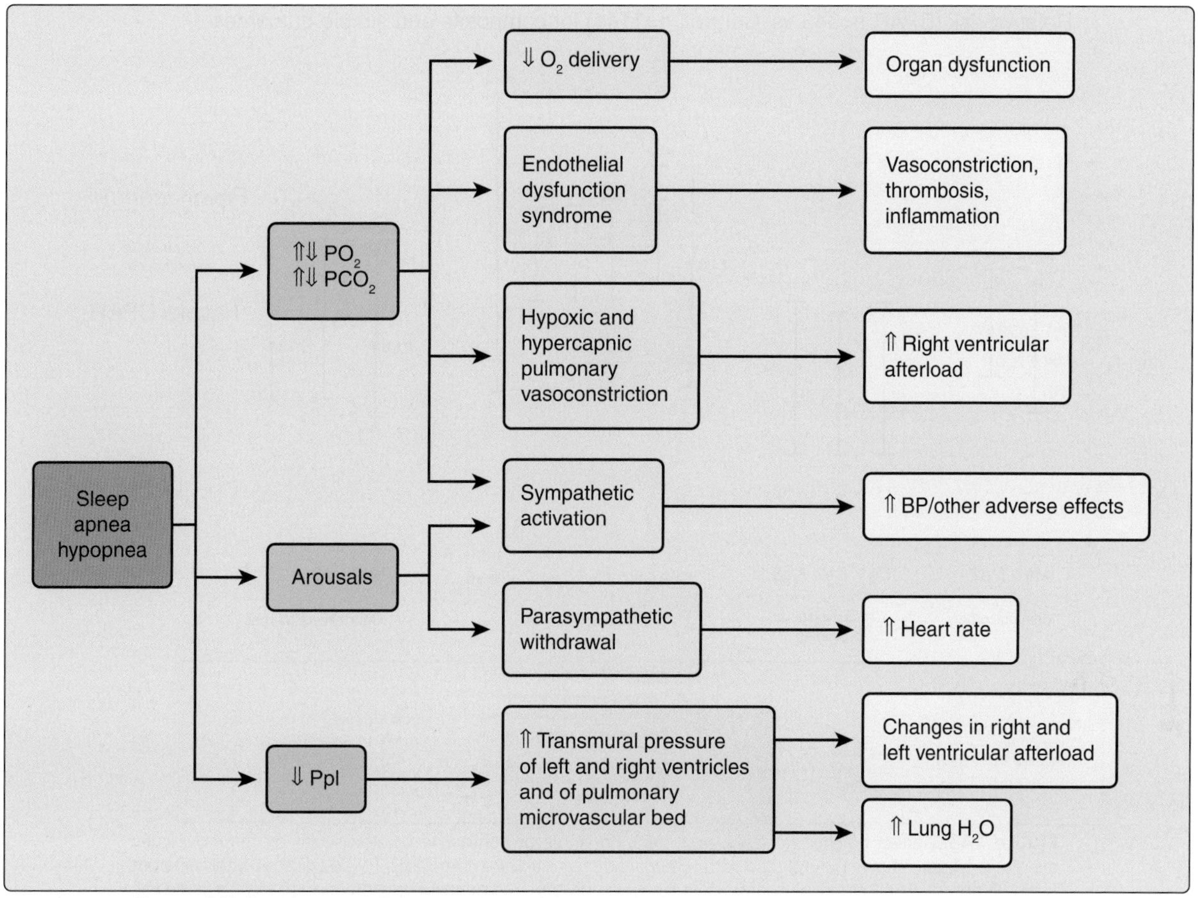

Figure 143.2 Pathophysiologic consequences of sleep apnea and hypopnea mediating adverse cardiovascular consequences. Pleural pressure (Ppl) is a surrogate of the pressure surrounding the heart and other vascular structures. ↑, Increased; ↓, decreased; BP, blood pressure; O_2, oxygen; PCO_2, partial pressure of carbon dioxide in the blood; PO_2, partial pressure of oxygen in the blood. (With permission from Javaheri S. Cardiovascular diseases. In: Kryger MH, Avidan AY, Berry RB, editors. *Atlas of Clinical Sleep Medicine.* 2nd ed. Saunders; 2014:316–28.)

this trial, 2687 patients with OSA and established cardiovascular disorders were randomized to CPAP or usual care. After a mean follow-up of 3.7 years and a mean CPAP use of 3.3 hours per day, the intention-to-treat analysis showed lack of benefit of CPAP therapy for the composite end point (death from any cardiovascular cause, myocardial infarction, stroke, hospitalization for HF, unstable angina, or TIA).

The results of the recent Spanish RCT has also been disappointing. In the ISAACC trial,[11] 1868 nonsleepy (Epworth Sleepiness Scale [ESS] < 10) patients with acute coronary syndrome with OSA (apnea-hypopnea index [AHI] ≥15 events/hour) and without OSA (AHI < 15 events/hour) were randomized to CPAP or, usual care. During a follow-up period of 3.4 years, similar to the SAVE trial, the rate of the composite of end point consisting of cardiovascular death, acute myocardial infarction, nonfatal stroke, hospital admission for HF, and new hospitalizations for unstable angina or TIA was similar in the CPAP and no-CPAP group. The average CPAP adherence was 2.8 hours/night in the CPAP group, less than 3.4 hours in the SAVE trial. The ISAACC trial is discussed in Chapter 149.

Future Directions

We have learned a lot from the SAVE trial, as detailed elsewhere.[12-14] The ISAACC trial has similar pitfalls. In a meta-analysis of 5 RCTs, we reported that among CPAP users, only the incidence of cerebrovascular, not cardiovascular, consequences of OSA improved (Figure 143.3). We suggest that a future trial should not exclude subjects with severe OSA, based on AHI threshold, severity of hypoxemia, or excessive daytime sleepiness; in both trials such subjects were excluded. Based on epidemiologic studies, and the pathophysiologic consequences of OSA, stroke (not cardiac pathology) is the most common downstream consequence of OSA. Therefore we suggest, for the first trial, cerebral consequences of OSA (TIA and stroke, death from stroke) should be considered as an only outcome (rather than combination of multiple cardiocerebrovascular coprimary end points that could dilute the positive effect of treatment on cerebral outcomes). In both trials multiple OSA consequences were packed together. Furthermore, because adherence to any therapy (drug or PAP) in any trial is the most critical determinant of a potentially favorable outcome, a negative outcome could be potentially related to poor adherence. We suggest a long pre-randomization use of CPAP and only randomize subjects who used CPAP for at least 5 hours for 2 months or so. We must emphasize that such pre-randomization strategy has been frequently used in drug therapy in HF trials.

Another approach is phenotypically oriented therapy, as there appear to be different phenotypes of OSA. However, such approach depends on finding an effective therapy for a specific phenotype as detailed elsewhere for OSA in HF.[15]

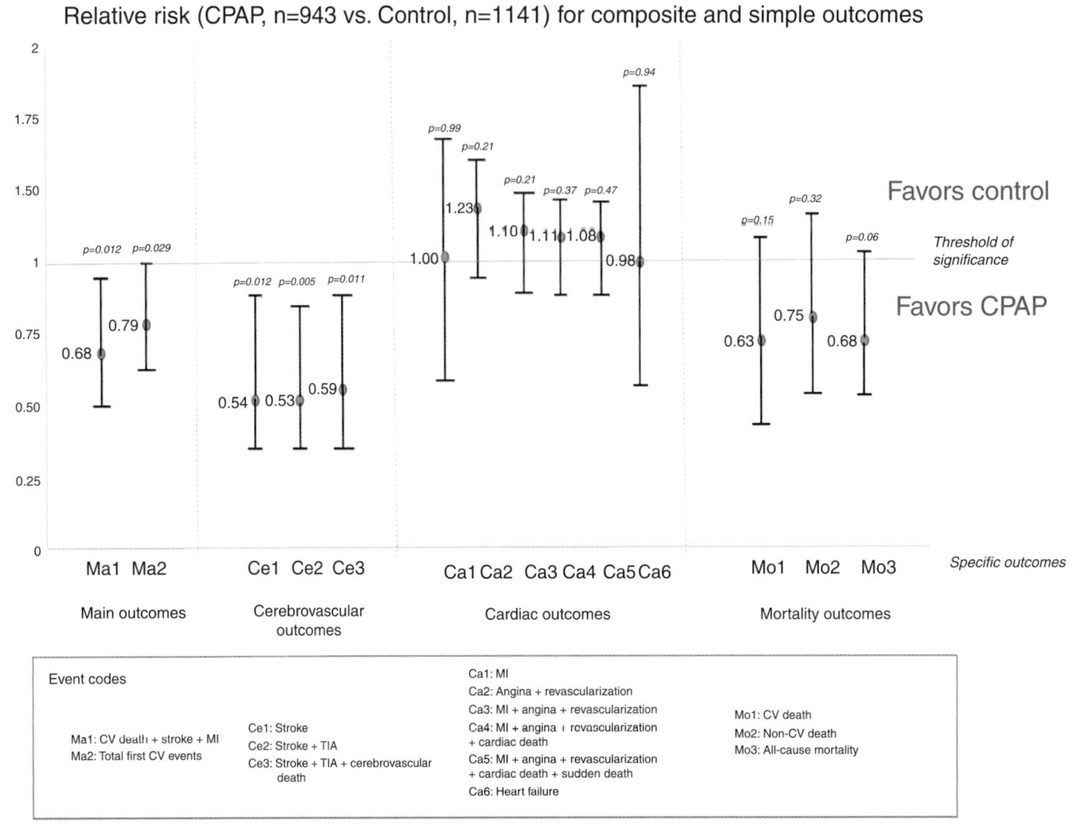

Figure 143.3 Effect of effective CPAP treatment on single or composite cardiovascular or cerebrovascular events. This figure shows the risk ratio with 95% confidence interval in the Y-axis. The X-axis shows the different types of individual and composite cardiovascular events divided into groups corresponding to (*from left to right*): primary outcome of the study, secondary outcome of the study, cerebrovascular outcomes, cardiac outcomes, and mortality outcomes. (With permission from Javaheri S, Martinez-Garcia MA, Campos-Rodriguez F, Peker Y. Continuous positive airway pressure adherence for prevention of major adverse cerebrovascular and cardiovascular events in obstructive sleep apnea. *Am J Respir Crit Care Med*. 2020;201[5]:607–10. doi:10.1164/rccm.201908-1593LE.)

IMPACT OF SLEEP-RELATED DISORDERED BREATHING IN HEART FAILURE

Over the last several years, we have recognized that both obstructive and central sleep apnea (CSA) are common in patients with both asymptomatic and symptomatic left ventricular dysfunction. Symptomatic patients with congestive heart failure, particularly those with reduced left ventricular ejection fraction, have the highest prevalence of both OSA and CSA, particularly the latter[8] (see Chapter 149).

Multiple studies have shown that presence of both OSA and CSA is associated with increased sympathetic activity in patients with HF who already suffer from hyperadrenergic state,[5] and RCTs show that treatment of CSA decreases sympathetic overactivity. Furthermore, observational studies suggest that both OSA and CSA are associated with increased readmission to the hospital and with excess premature mortality.

We note that so far there has been no RCT showing that treatment of OSA improves mortality of patients with HF. However, two large RCTs have been performed in HF with CSA: the first with CPAP and the second with adaptive servo-ventilation device.[16] These trials are discussed in detail in Chapter 149.

Given the algorithm of adaptive servo-ventilation, we had predicted that treatment of the CSA with this device[17] would improve mortality of patients with HF and this sleep disorder. Unfortunately, this large RCT with adaptive servoventilation showed a negative outcome with treatment.[15] We have also learned from this trial,[17] as we did from the SAVE trial, discussed previously (see Chapter 149 for details).

Future Directions

Currently clinical trials are ongoing. One trial uses an ASV with an improved algorithm. Specifically, algorithmic improvements include variable end-expiratory pressure, an algorithm similar to auto-titrating PAP, and capability to set inspiratory pressure support at desired levels chosen by the physician rather than the default settings of the device.

A phase 3 RCT, using nocturnal low-flow oxygen (provided by a concentrator, matched by a similar flow rate providing room air from an identical concentrator) to treat CSA in HF is ongoing, with the coprimary end point of HF re-admission and mortality combined (see Chapter 149).

Additionally, most recently, the unilateral phrenic nerve stimulation pacemaker has been approved by the U.S. Food and Drug Administration and is used to treat CSA of various causes, including CSA associated with HF.[18,19] This is exciting because the pacemaker is placed intravenously by a cardiologist and primes the phrenic nerve according to a set algorithm to eliminate central apnea during sleep. Adherence should be virtually complete, in contrast to mask therapy with PAP devices (for details see Chapter 149). A large RCT with this device to determine if treatment of CSA improves mortality of patients with HF is badly needed.

Finally, in the next few years, as we deeply understand the underlying mechanisms of various pheno- and endotypes of OSA[15] and CSA[20] in HF, tailored therapy may be applied, hoping to decrease the morbidity and mortality of patients.

CLINICAL PEARLS

- RCTs conclude that treatment of OSA with CPAP does not improve downstream cardiovascular consequences of OSA.
- A meta-analysis of randomized controlled trials show that treatment of OSA has decreased the incidence of stroke but not cardiac disorders.
- Routine treatment of HF with adaptive servo-ventilation when left ventricular ejection fraction is less 45% is contraindicated.
- Two randomized controlled trials to treat sleep apnea in HF, one with oxygen and the other with adaptive servo-ventilation, are ongoing.

SUMMARY

There is a bidirectional relationship between sleep disorders (sleep breathing disorders and insomnia) and CVD (cardiac failure, acute myocardial infarction, cardiac rhythm disorders, hypertension, stroke, and TIAs). Although treating improvement of sleep-disordered breathing has been hypothesized to reduce cardiovascular risk, randomized clinical trials to date have shown only reducing the risk of stroke. The RCTs to date have had methodological flaws, including exclusion of the very sleepy; exclusion of the most severe cases of OSA; and short duration of the studies. PAP adherence in the trials has been generally suboptimal.

SELECTED READINGS

Cowie MR, Linz D, Redline S, Somers VK, Simonds AK. Sleep disordered breathing and cardiovascular disease: JACC state-of-the-art review. *J Am Coll Cardiol.* 2021;78(6):608–624.

Cowie MR, Woehrle H, Wegscheider K, et al. Adaptive servo-ventilation for central sleep apnea in systolic heart failure. *N Engl J Med.* 2015;373(12):1095–1105. https://doi.org/10.1056/NEJMoa1506459.

Fox H, Oldenburg O, Javaheri S, et al. Long-term efficacy and safety of phrenic nerve stimulation for the treatment of central sleep apnea. *Sleep.* 2019;42(11):zsz158. https://doi.org/10.1093/sleep/zsz158.

Javaheri S, Barbe F, Campos-Rodriguez F, et al. Sleep apnea: types, mechanisms, and clinical cardiovascular consequences. *J Am Coll Cardiol.* 2017;69(7):841–858. https://doi.org/10.1016/j.jacc.2016.11.069.

Javaheri S, Brown LK, Abraham WT, Khayat R. Apneas of heart failure and phenotype-guided treatments: Part One: OSA. *Chest.* 2020;157(2):394–402. https://doi.org/10.1016/j.chest.2019.02.407.

Javaheri S, Brown LK, Khayat RN. Update on apneas of heart failure with reduced ejection fraction: emphasis on the physiology of treatment: part 2: central sleep apnea [published online ahead of print, 2020 Jan 17]. *Chest.* 2020;S0012-3692(20)30044-1. https://doi:10.1016/j.chest.2019.12.020.

Javaheri S, Brown LK, Randerath W, Khayat R. SERVE-HF: more questions than answers. *Chest.* 2016;149(4):900–904.

Javaheri S, Martinez-Garcia MA, Campos-Rodriguez F. CPAP treatment and cardiovascular prevention: we need to change the design and implementation of our trials. *Chest.* 2019;156(3):431–437.

Javaheri S, Martinez-Garcia MA, Campos-Rodriguez F, Muriel A, Peker Y. Continuous positive airway pressure adherence for prevention of major adverse cerebrovascular and cardiovascular events in obstructive sleep apnea. *Am J Respir Crit Care Med.* 2020;201(5):607–610. https://doi.org/10.1164/rccm.201908-1593LE.

McEvoy RD, Antic NA, Heeley E, et al. CPAP for prevention of cardiovascular events in obstructive sleep apnea. *N Engl J Med.* 2016;375(10):919–931.

Sánchez-de-la-Torre M, Sánchez-de-la-Torre A, Bertran S, et al. Effect of obstructive sleep apnoea and its treatment with continuous positive airway pressure on the prevalence of cardiovascular events in patients with acute coronary syndrome (ISAACC study): a randomised controlled trial [published online ahead of print, 2019 Dec 12]. *Lancet Respir Med.* 2019;S2213-2600(19)30271-1.

Virani SS, Alonso A, Aparicio HJ, et al. Heart disease and stroke statistics-2021 update: a report from the American Heart Association. *Circulation.* 2021;143(8):e254–e743.

Yin J, Jin X, Shan Z, et al. Relationship of sleep duration with all-cause mortality and cardiovascular events: a systematic review and dose-response meta-analysis of prospective cohort studies. *J Am Heart Assoc.* 2017;6(9):e005947. Published 2017 Sep 9.

A complete reference list can be found online at ExpertConsult.com.

Chapter 144

Sleep-Related Cardiac Risk

Reena Mehra; Richard L. Verrier

Chapter Highlights

- The brain, in subserving its need for periodic reexcitation during rapid eye movement sleep and dreaming, imposes significant demands on the heart by inducing bursts of sympathetic nerve activity, which reaches levels higher than during wakefulness. Juxtaposition of these sympathetic surges occurs on a background of enhanced parasympathetic tone. In patients with cardiac disease, such neural activity may compromise coronary artery blood flow, as metabolic demand outstrips supply and may trigger sympathetically mediated life-threatening arrhythmias in response to functional myocardial ischemia.
- An additional challenge is presented by non–rapid eye movement sleep, when hypotension relative to wakefulness may lead to malperfusion of the heart and brain as a result of a lowered blood pressure gradient through stenosed vessels.
- Impairment of ventilation by sleep-related breathing disorders, including obstructive sleep apnea (OSA) and central sleep apnea, which afflict millions of Americans, can generate reductions in arterial oxygen saturation and other pathophysiologic sequelae. OSA has been strongly implicated in the etiology of hypertension, myocardial ischemia, arrhythmias, myocardial infarction, heart failure, and sudden death in individuals with coexisting ischemic heart disease. Similarly, central sleep apnea has been associated with heart failure, stroke, and a variety of atrial and ventricular arrhythmias.
- Atrial fibrillation may be triggered by autonomic or respiratory disturbances during sleep in certain patient populations.
- Medications that cross the blood-brain barrier may alter sleep structure and provoke nightmares with severe cardiac autonomic discharge.

INTRODUCTION

In healthy individuals, sleep is usually salutary and restorative. Cardioprotective characteristics are primarily attributable to the enhanced parasympathetic tone, overall reduction in sympathetic nerve activation, and reduced arrhythmogenicity inherent in sleep compared to wakefulness (Figure 144.1).[1] Ironically, during sleep in patients with respiratory or heart disease, the brain can precipitate breathing disorders, myocardial ischemia, arrhythmias, and even death. Our observation that 20% of myocardial infarctions and 15% of sudden deaths occur during the period from midnight to 6:00 a.m. projects to an estimated 211,000 nocturnal myocardial infarctions and 55,000 nocturnal sudden deaths annually in the US population.[2] Thus sleep is not a fully protected state. Factors contributing to morning provocation of cardiac events, including myocardial infarction and stroke (Figure 144.2), include rapid eye movement (REM)-related autonomic fluctuations, diurnal patterning of hypercoagulable biomarkers, and rises in cortisol levels.[3] Furthermore, the nonuniform distribution of deaths and myocardial infarctions during the night is consonant with provocation by pathophysiologic triggers. The two main factors implicated in nocturnal cardiac events are sleep-state–dependent surges in autonomic activity[4] and depression of respiratory control mechanisms with ensuing hypoxemia,[5] which affect a vulnerable cardiac substrate. Precise characterization of their interaction in precipitating nocturnal cardiac events is, however, incomplete.

Although sudden death during sleep can be presumed to be painless, in many cases it is premature because it occurs in infants and adolescents and in adults with ischemic heart disease, for whom the median age is 69 years. Populations at risk for nocturnal cardiorespiratory events include several large patient groups (Table 144.1). For example, arrhythmias, including paroxysmal atrial fibrillation and nonsustained ventricular tachycardia, during sleep are triggered shortly after a sleep-disordered breathing event.[6]

It is an insidious component of the problem of nocturnal risk that many people are unaware of their respiratory or cardiac distress at night and therefore take no corrective action. Thus sleep presents unique autonomic, hemodynamic, and respiratory challenges to the diseased myocardium that cannot be monitored by daytime diagnostic tests. The importance of nocturnal monitoring of patients with cardiac disease extends beyond identifying sleep-state–dependent triggers of cardiac events because nighttime myocardial ischemia, arrhythmias, autonomic activity, and respiratory disturbances carry predictive value for daytime events (Box 144.1).

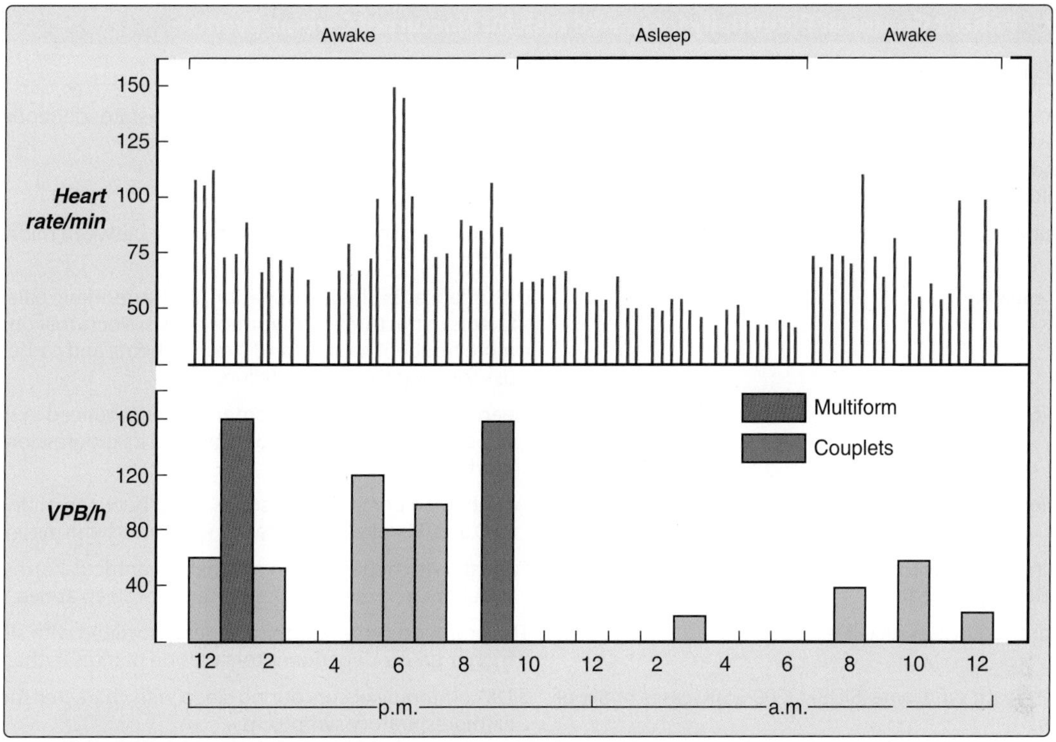

Figure 144.1 Tachogram showing ventricular premature beat (VPB) rate in a 43-year-old man with an old diaphragmatic transmural infarction. With onset of sleep, grade 2 VPBs were abolished. There was a progressive slowing in heart rate during the night, consistent with known enhanced parasympathetic tone during sleep. Upon awaking, there was a recurrence of VPBs. (From Lown B, Tykocinski M, Garfein A, et al. Sleep and ventricular premature beats. *Circulation.* 1973;48:691–701, published with permission from the American Heart Association.)

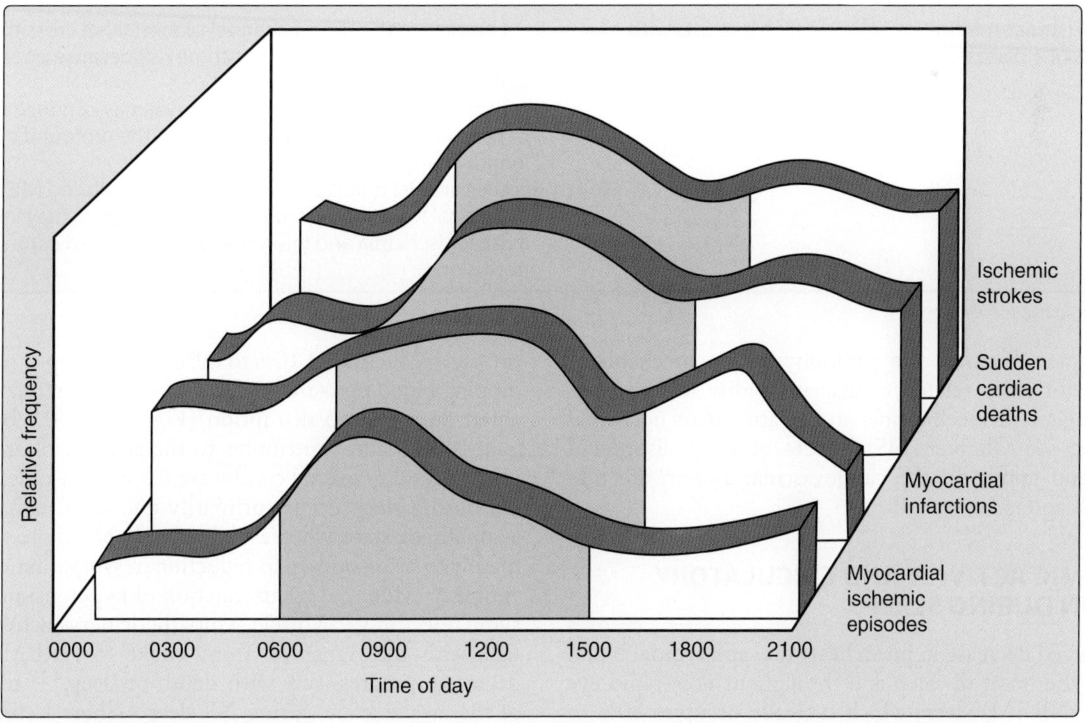

Figure 144.2 Myocardial ischemia, infarction, out-of-hospital sudden cardiac death, and stroke exhibit consistent circadian variation in time of onset. Incidents peak between 6 a.m. and noon, within several hours of awakening. The rationale for this event distribution is likely multifactorial, that is, peak cortisol levels, circadian variation of increases in circulating prothrombotic biochemical mediators, and lingering effects of rapid eye movement sleep, a stage that predominates in the later morning. (From Shepard JW Jr. Hypertension, cardiac arrhythmias, myocardial infarction, and stroke in relation to obstructive sleep apnea. *Clin Chest Med.* 1992;13:437–58, published with permission.)

Table 144.1 Patient Groups at Potentially Increased Risk for Nocturnal Cardiac Events

Indication (US Patients per Year)	Possible Mechanism
Angina, myocardial infarction (MI), arrhythmias, ischemia, or cardiac arrest at night; 20% of myocardial infarctions (211,000 cases/yr) and 15% of sudden deaths (55,000 cases/yr) occur between midnight and 6:00 a.m.[96]	The nocturnal pattern suggests a sleep-state–dependent autonomic trigger or respiratory distress.
Unstable angina, Prinzmetal angina	Nondemand ischemia and angina peak between midnight and 6:00 a.m.
Acute MI (1.1 million)[96]	Disturbances in sleep, respiration, and autonomic balance may be factors in nocturnal arrhythmogenesis. Nocturnal onset of MI is more frequent in older and sicker patients and carries a higher risk for congestive heart failure.
Heart failure (6.5 million)[96]	Sleep-related breathing disorders are pronounced in the setting of heart failure and may contribute to its progression and to mortality risk.
Atrial fibrillation (>6 million)[96]	Twenty-nine percent of episodes occur between midnight and 6:00 a.m. Respiratory and autonomic mechanisms are suspected.
Sleep apnea in patients with coronary disease (5–10 million patients with sleep apnea)	Patients with hypertension or atrial or ventricular arrhythmias should be screened for the presence of sleep apnea.
Long QT syndrome (1 case/2000 live births)[96]	The profound cycle-length changes associated with sleep may trigger pause-dependent torsades de pointes in these patients.
Sudden infant death syndrome (SIDS) (2000-2500 cases or 8% of infant deaths)	SIDS commonly occurs during sleep with characteristic cardiorespiratory symptoms.
Brugada syndrome in Western populations; Asians with warning signs of sudden unexplained nocturnal death syndrome (SUNDS)	SUNDS is a sleep-related phenomenon in which night terrors may play a role. The Brugada syndrome is genetically related to the long QT syndrome.
Patients with epilepsy (3.4 million)[97]	Sudden unexpected death in epilepsy (SUDEP) occurs primarily at night and in patients with a history of nocturnal seizures. Annual toll is 3600 deaths.[98]
Patients on cardiac medications (16.5 million patients with cardiovascular disease)[96]	Beta blockers and calcium channel blockers that cross the blood-brain barrier may increase nighttime risk because poor sleep and violent dreams may be triggered. Medications that increase the QT interval may conduce to pause-dependent torsades de pointes during the profound cycle-length changes of sleep. Because arterial blood pressure is decreased during NREM sleep, additional lowering by antihypertensive agents may introduce a risk for ischemia and infarction due to lowered coronary perfusion.

NREM, Non–rapid eye movement.

This chapter discusses the pathophysiologic mechanisms responsible for sleep-related cardiac morbidity and mortality. For a review of mechanisms and treatment of nocturnal arrhythmias, see Chapter 145. Effects of sleep-disordered breathing and apnea on the cardiovascular system are discussed in Chapters 146 to 149.

AUTONOMIC ACTIVITY AND CIRCULATORY FUNCTION DURING SLEEP

The generalized decrease in mean heart rate and arterial blood pressure at the onset of sleep and throughout non–rapid eye movement (NREM) sleep, which typically occupies 80% to 85% of sleep time, has prompted the assumption that sleep is a period of relative autonomic inactivity. NREM sleep, the initial stage, is characterized by marked stability of autonomic regulation with coupling of respiratory and cardiorespiratory centers in the brain, resulting in a high degree of parasympathetic tone and prominent respiratory sinus arrhythmia.[4,7] Blood pressure reduction of 10% to 20% during sleep is referred to as dipping blood pressure profile; however, this reduction is mitigated during sleep disruption (Figure 144.3).[8] Baroreceptor gain is high and contributes to the stability of arterial blood pressure and to overall cardiovascular homeostasis.[9] Bradycardia during sleep occurs primarily due to an enhanced parasympathetic state, whereas reduction in blood pressure appears mainly to be secondary to reduction in sympathetic nerve activation as evidenced by attenuation of hypotension by surgical sympathectomy.[10] Muscle sympathetic nerve activity is stable, falls with the transition from awake to NREM sleep, and decreases progressively with depth of sleep,[4,11] reaching half of the awake value during N3 sleep.[4] Short-lasting increases in muscle sympathetic nerve activity, heart rate, and arterial blood pressure accompany the appearance of high-amplitude K-complexes during N2 sleep.[4,11] Heart rate accelerations may even precede the electroencephalographic (EEG) arousals of N2 and rapid eye movement (REM) sleep.[12] Systemic vascular resistance, blood pressure, and heart rate oscillate markedly

Box 144.1 PREDICTIVE VALUE OF NOCTURNAL CARDIORESPIRATORY STATUS

- Because parasympathetic nerve activity is elevated during sleep in healthy individuals, lack of circadian pattern of heart rate variability and baroreflex sensitivity may be readily monitored for increased risk for cardiac events.
- Nondemand nocturnal ischemic episodes may disclose a critical underlying coronary lesion, coronary vasospasm, or transient coronary artery stenosis.
- In elderly subjects, nighttime multifocal ventricular ectopic activity predicts increased mortality from cardiac causes independent of clinically evident cardiac disease.
- Sleep apnea, which may be screened by heart rate variability analysis, conduces to hypertension, left ventricular remodeling, myocardial ischemia, and atrial and ventricular arrhythmias and is a risk factor for lethal daytime cardiac events, including myocardial infarction.
- Hypertensive patients with less than a 10% nocturnal decline in blood pressure (remaining higher than 101/65 mm Hg) are at increased risk for total and cardiovascular mortality and all cardiovascular end points, myocardial ischemia, frequent or complex ventricular arrhythmias, cerebrovascular insult, and increased organ damage, including left ventricular hypertrophy.
- Elevated nocturnal heart rates are associated with increased cardiac mortality.

during REM sleep in concert with the phasic and tonic periods of REM sleep. During transitions from NREM to REM sleep, bursts of vagus nerve activity may result in pauses in heart rhythm and frank asystole. Transitions between REM and NREM sleep elicit posture shifts that are associated with varying degrees of autonomic activation and attendant changes in heart rate and arterial blood pressure.[13] These shifts in body position increase in frequency as individuals age, and sleep becomes fragmented.

Autonomic nervous system activity is dramatically altered when REM sleep is initiated (Figure 144.4).[4] REM sleep is marked by profound muscle sympathetic nerve activation, in terms of both frequency and amplitude,[4,9] which attains levels significantly higher than during wakefulness.[4] Sympathetic nerve activity is concentrated in short, irregular periods that are most striking when accompanied by intense eye movements.[4] These bursts trigger intermittent increases in heart rate and arterial blood pressure to levels similar to those in wakefulness, with increased variability.[4,11,12] Significant surges and pauses in heart rate during REM sleep have been described in several species, including humans.[11,12] Cardiac efferent vagal tone and baroreceptor regulation[9] are generally suppressed during REM sleep, and breathing patterns may become highly irregular and may lead, in susceptible individuals, to oxygen desaturation. Thus, although subserving the neurochemical functions of the brain, REM sleep can disrupt cardiorespiratory homeostasis. The brain's increased excitability during REM sleep can also trigger major surges in sympathetic nerve activity to the skeletal muscular beds, accompanied by muscular twitching,[4] which interrupts the generalized skeletal atonia of REM.[13] The peripheral autonomic status characterized by muscle sympathetic nerve recording is compatible with reduced neuronal activity in the brainstem and other regions of the brain and reduced cerebral blood flow during NREM sleep and, during REM sleep, with increased brain activity in several discrete regions to levels higher than waking values.[14] Such breathing disturbances during REM sleep are increasingly recognized as triggers of cardiovascular events superseding overall sleep apnea not specific to REM sleep.[6]

The decline in autonomic activity during sleep is also evident in peroneal muscle sympathetic nerve activity[4,11] and peripheral levels of epinephrine and norepinephrine and mirrors the generalized sleep-induced decline in heart rate and arterial blood pressure.[15] A nocturnal nadir in plasma catecholamines is evident at 1 hour after sleep onset. Plasma cortisol is also depressed during sleep; increased levels are initiated at 5:00 a.m. Loss of sleep is accompanied by higher blood pressure and heart rate compared to control subjects attributable to enhanced sympathetic nerve activation.

In the absence of readily achieved, direct measures of cardiac-bound nerve activity, analysis of heart rate variability (HRV) has emerged as a widely accepted method for measuring cardiac sympathetic versus parasympathetic nerve dominance. High-frequency (HF) HRV is a general indicator of cardiac parasympathetic tone and includes the effects of respiration. The low- to high-frequency (LF/HF) ratio is widely accepted as an approximation of cardiac-bound sympathetic nerve activity, as validated by studies involving beta-adrenergic receptor–blocking agents. Decreased HRV, associated with a decline in parasympathetic nerve activity, is an established indicator of risk for sudden cardiac death after myocardial infarction. HRV analysis reveals a generalized increase in vagus nerve activity and a decrease in cardiac sympathetic nerve activity across the sleep period,[16,17] probably reflecting the dominance of total sleep time by NREM sleep. HRV studies using 5-minute intervals provide results consistent with muscle nerve recording, indicating increased HF and decreased LF (or parasympathetic nerve dominance) in NREM sleep but decreased HF and increased LF (or predominant sympathetic nerve activity) in REM sleep and during wakefulness.[12] In healthy individuals the increase in HRV measures of cardiac sympathetic nerve activity at onset of REM sleep is initiated before the transition from NREM sleep, as classically defined from the polysomnographic record.[12,17]

The typical circadian pattern of decreased nocturnal cardiac sympathetic nerve activity as described by heart rate[18] and HRV studies is altered in patients with coronary artery disease,[19,20] myocardial infarction,[16,21] and diabetes mellitus,[22] suggesting either increased nocturnal cardiac sympathetic nerve activity or decreased parasympathetic nerve activity compared with healthy subjects. The HF component has been observed to decrease approximately 10 minutes before onset of nocturnal myocardial ischemia.[21] In unmedicated patients with a recent myocardial infarction, the LF/HF ratio was significantly increased during both REM and NREM sleep, in contrast to healthy subjects, in whom this ratio during REM sleep is similar to awake levels and higher than during NREM sleep (Figure 144.5).[16] The conclusions were reached that myocardial infarction decreases the capacity of the vagus nerve to be activated during sleep, resulting in unbridled cardiac sympathetic nerve activity,[16] and that loss of rise in the HF component is characteristic of patients after an myocardial infarction and with residual myocardial ischemia.[21]

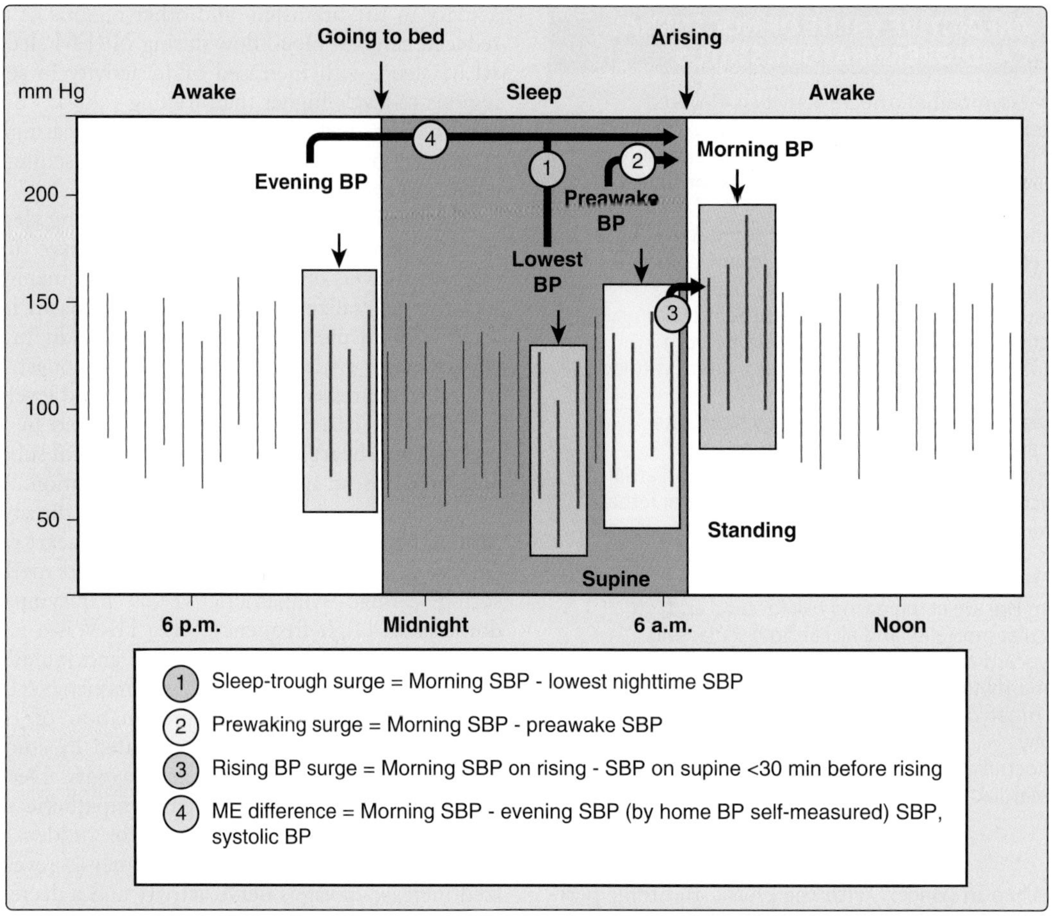

Figure 144.3 Definition of morning surge in blood pressure characterizing time-dependent measures, that is, sleep-trough surge, prewaking surge, and rising BP surge. Clinical relevance is underscored by increased stroke incidence in those with exaggerated morning blood pressure surges relative to those without this exaggerated morning surge. BP, Blood pressure; ME, morning-evening; SBP, systolic blood pressure. (From Kario K. Morning surge in blood pressure and cardiovascular risk: evidence and perspectives. *Hypertension*. 2010;56:765–73, with permission from the American Heart Association.)

These sleep-state–dependent profiles of autonomic activity have significant potential to affect coronary function and cardiac electrical stability in patients with ischemic heart disease.

Nocturnal Myocardial Ischemia and Angina

Accurate assessment and treatment of nocturnal angina has been a subject of concern for more than 2 centuries. In 1768 Heberden described angina that "will often oblige [the patients] to rise up out of their bed every night for many months altogether." John Hunter, the well-known 18th-century surgeon, reported chest pains that "seized him in his sleep so as to awaken him."[23] As early as 1923, MacWilliam[24] postulated that the mechanisms of nocturnal ventricular fibrillation and angina were stimulation of sympathetic nerves and increased arterial blood pressure. He described "reflex excitations, dreams, nightmares, etc., sometimes accompanied by extensive rises of arterial blood pressure (hitherto not recognized), increased heart action, changes in respiration, and various reflex effects" and noted "the suddenness of development of the functional disturbances in arterial blood pressure, heart action, etc., in the dreaming state." He documented greater stress on the circulatory system during dreaming than during wakefulness, with arterial blood pressures reaching 200 mm Hg. In the middle of the 20th century, the renowned cardiologists Paul Dudley White and Samuel Levine remarked on the frequency of myocardial infarction and angina in sleep and suggested an association with dreaming.

Ischemic activity is an important prognostic marker in patients with cardiac disease, and characteristics of both REM and NREM sleep may conduce to nocturnal myocardial ischemia and angina. The few studies in patients with cardiac disease that have used sleep staging have concluded that in the absence of significant depression of left ventricular function, nocturnal ischemic events occur primarily during REM sleep,[25,26] which is characterized by increased sympathetic nerve activity, metabolic demands, and heart rate surges. In patients with stable coronary artery disease, myocardial ischemia is largely attributable to bouts of sympathetically mediated surges in heart rate and resultant metabolic demands in flow-limited, stenotic coronary arteries.[6,20,26–30] Nowlin and coworkers[26] attributed nocturnal angina to heightened blood pressure after performing detailed, multisession polysomnographic analysis of four patients with advanced coronary artery disease and nocturnal angina pectoris. They established that attacks of nocturnal angina occurred predominantly during REM sleep (32 of 39 recordings) and were associated with heart rate acceleration. Dream content, in patients who could describe it, included awareness of chest pain and involved strenuous physical activity or emotions of fear, anger, or frustration.

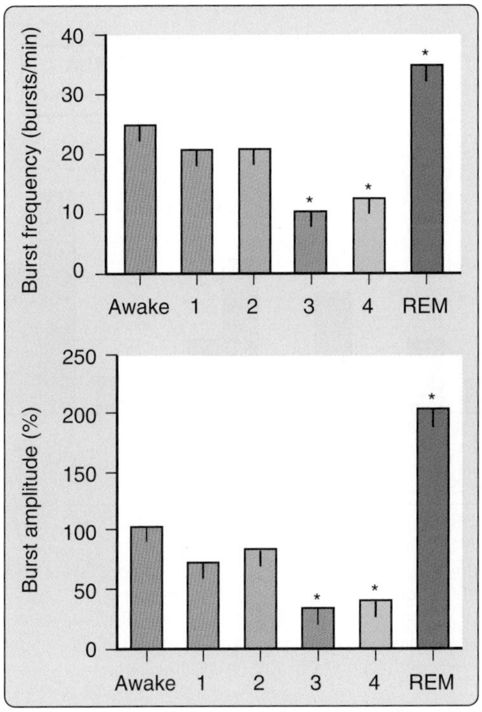

Figure 144.4 Sympathetic nerve burst frequency and amplitude during wakefulness, non–rapid eye movement sleep (eight subjects), and rapid eye movement (REM) sleep (six subjects). Sympathetic nerve activity was significantly lower during stages 3 and 4 ($P < .001$). During REM sleep, sympathetic nerve activity increased significantly ($P < .001$). Values are means ± standard error of the mean. *Asterisks* indicate statistically significant differences. (From Somers VK, Dyken ME, Mark AL, et al. Sympathetic nerve activity during sleep in normal subjects. *N Engl J Med.* 1993;328:303–7, with permission from the Massachusetts Medical Society. All rights reserved.)

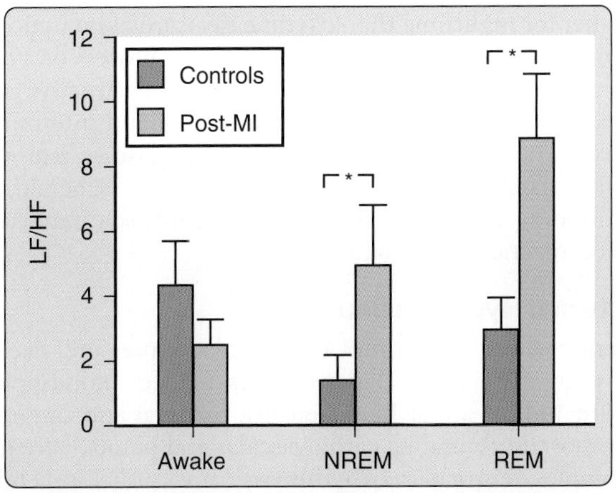

Figure 144.5 Bar graphs indicating low- to high-frequency (LF/HF) ratio of heart rate variability during the awake state (*left*), during non–rapid eye movement (NREM) sleep (*middle*), and during rapid eye movement (REM) sleep (*right*) in healthy subjects and in post–myocardial infarction (MI) patients ($P < .01$, when comparing control subjects and post-MI patients). Values are means ± standard error of the mean. *Asterisks* indicate statistically significant differences. (From Vanoli E, Adamson PB, Ba-Lin, et al. Heart rate variability during specific sleep stages: a comparison of healthy subjects with patients after myocardial infarction. *Circulation.* 1995;91:1918–22, published with permission from the American Heart Association.)

Nocturnal myocardial ischemia may be generated by mechanisms in addition to sympathetic nerve activity and unsatisfied metabolic demands. This possibility is suggested by the finding that nighttime ischemic events remain, although they are less frequent, in patients receiving beta-adrenergic receptor blockade therapy, the primary therapy that effectively reduces the overall incidence of and suppresses the morning peak in cardiac events by containing sympathetic nerve activity and demand-related myocardial ischemia.[30,31] The main factors that may contribute to nondemand-related myocardial ischemia during NREM sleep are decreased coronary perfusion pressure as the result of hypotension[6,26–33] and increased coronary vasomotor tone.[32] These influences decrease the metabolic threshold for induction of nocturnal myocardial ischemia, which has a nadir between 1:00 a.m. and 3:00 a.m.[28,32,34] During these hours in patients with stable coronary disease, Benhorin and colleagues[32] observed that myocardial ischemia can be provoked at heart rates of 83 beats per minute, in contrast to 96 beats per minute during midday, and that its incidence was not affected by beta-adrenergic receptor blockade. Patel and colleagues[31] noted that nocturnal myocardial ischemia is attended by heart rate elevations of 6 beats per minute or less in patients with unstable angina receiving beta-adrenergic receptor–blocking agents. Mancia[7] hypothesized that the hypotension of NREM sleep is a major contributor to nocturnal myocardial ischemia and myocardial infarction because it "reduces the volume and velocity of blood flow, favoring the development of thrombi and embolic and ischemic phenomena before and after arousal." It has also been postulated that myocardial ischemia provoked by transient thrombus formation is attributable to the nocturnal nadir in endogenous fibrinolytic activity and to peaks in serum levels of plasminogen activator inhibitor and tissue plasminogen activator antigen, increasing blood viscosity or hypercoagulability at night, and free-radical generation.[35]

Nondemand nocturnal myocardial ischemia is prevalent among patients with more severe coronary disease,[30,34,36] acute coronary syndromes,[21] or diabetes mellitus, populations with significant endothelial dysfunction. Indeed, it has been concluded that nondemand nocturnal ischemic episodes disclose a critical underlying coronary lesion, coronary vasospasm, or transient coronary artery stenosis.[31] Patel and colleagues[31] documented a nocturnal peak in ischemic events in their study of 256 hospitalized patients with the acute coronary syndromes of unstable angina and non–Q-wave myocardial infarction (Figure 144.6). Electrocardiograms (ECGs) were recorded within hours after patients" admission for chest pain to the coronary care unit for new-onset angina, sudden acceleration of previously stable angina, or angina within 1 month after myocardial infarction. In the hospital they received optimal medical therapy aimed at containing demand-related myocardial ischemia. It is important to note, however, that the peak in out-of-hospital onset of the syndromes followed the usual circadian pattern, as reported by Cannon and coworkers[37] in the Thrombosis in Myocardial Infarction (TIMI) III Study of 3318 patients. By contrast, in patients with longstanding diabetes mellitus or with documented autonomic nervous system dysfunction, there is no nocturnal decrease in myocardial ischemia or onset of acute myocardial infarction.

Demand-related ischemic episodes can be effectively contained by beta-adrenergic receptor blockade,[31] but antihypertensive treatment does not reduce the nocturnal incidence of nondemand-related myocardial ischemia.[38] The use of vasodilators to treat nondemand episodes resulting from endothelial dysfunction is the subject of debate. The lack of sleep staging and arterial blood pressure monitoring in patients with nocturnal myocardial ischemia leaves unidentified any contribution by autonomic and hemodynamic activity dictated by sleep states. Such monitoring would also disclose the prevalence of

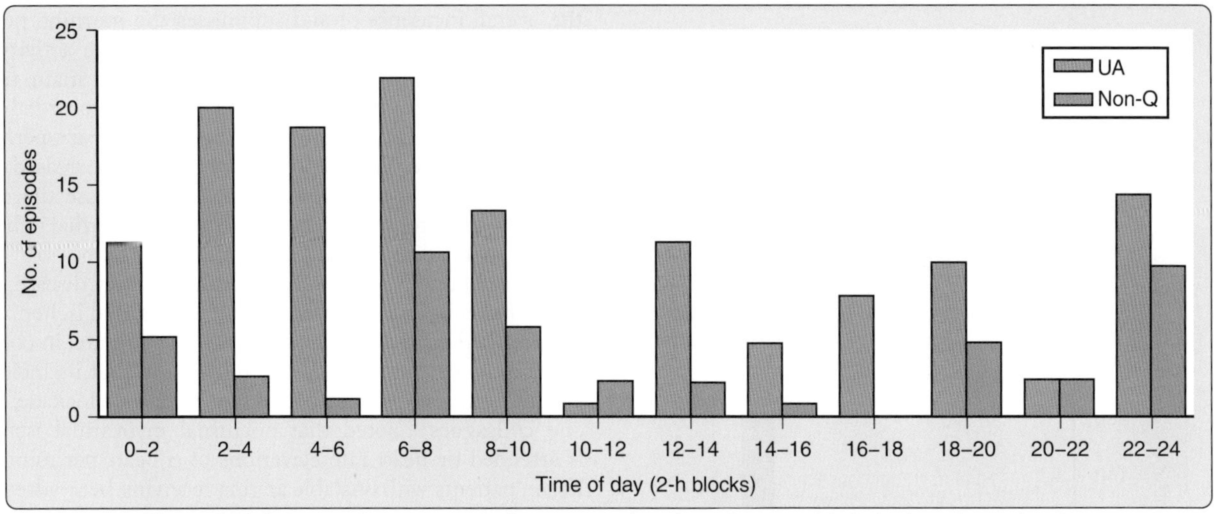

Figure 144.6 The circadian variation of ischemic activity based on 2-hour time blocks for the in-hospital study population. There is a single peak of ischemic activity at night between 10:00 p.m. and 8:00 a.m., and no morning peak in ischemic activity is apparent. Greater than 64% of episodes occurred during this period ($P < .001$, compared with daytime). The circadian distribution of ischemic episodes in unstable angina (UA) and non–Q-wave myocardial infarction (Non-Q) is similar to the overall pattern of ischemic activity. (From Patel DJ, Knight CJ, Holdright DR, et al. Pathophysiology of transient myocardial ischemia in acute coronary syndromes: characterization by continuous ST-segment monitoring. *Circulation.* 1997;95:1185–92, published with permission from the American Heart Association.)

the established proischemic influences of nocturnal arousal and rising from bed.[19,39]

Nocturnal Myocardial Infarction

Although only 20% of myocardial infarctions occur between midnight and 6:00 a.m., their nonuniform distribution implicates pathophysiologic triggers.[2] The dynamic perturbations in autonomic nervous system activity, both independent of and in conjunction with apnea,[40] are likely to constitute important triggers of myocardial infarction at night. REM-induced surges in sympathetic nerve activity have the potential to provoke tachycardia and hypertension, alterations that carry the potential for inducing myocardial infarction secondary to coronary artery plaque rupture and to inappropriate decreases in the myocardial oxygen supply-demand relationship or alpha-adrenergically mediated coronary vasoconstriction.

Alternatively, in a starkly opposite manner, the hypotension of slow wave sleep may lead to malperfusion of the myocardium because of reduced coronary perfusion pressure through stenotic vessel segments (Figure 144.7).[41] Several investigators[31,42,43] have attributed nocturnal myocardial infarction and myocardial ischemia to the relative hypotension of NREM sleep, which "reduces the volume and velocity of blood flow, favoring the development of thrombi and embolic and ischemic phenomena before and after arousal."[7] Mancia[7] therefore advocated avoiding drugs that enhance the hypotension of NREM sleep and prescribing antihypertensive medications only for daytime therapy.[7] He echoed the argument of Floras,[38] who observed that antihypertensive treatment did not reduce the incidence of nocturnal myocardial infarction and ischemia. Further evidence of the risk for hypotension-induced infarction has been provided by Kleiman and colleagues,[42] who reported that the incidence of subendocardial myocardial infarction clustered at 2:00 a.m. to 4:00 a.m., simultaneously with the nadir in arterial blood pressure. Other factors known to contribute to myocardial infarction are operative during sleep, including increased ventricular diastolic pressures and volumes caused by the fluid shifts resulting from assuming a supine posture, unfavorable alterations in the balance of fibrinolytic and thrombotic factors,[35] and chronic or episodic oxygen desaturation.[33,44–47]

Specific patient groups experience an increased incidence of nighttime myocardial infarctions, particularly those with poor ventricular function, advanced age, or diabetes mellitus.[48,49] The risk for development of congestive heart failure is higher for nighttime than daytime myocardial infarctions,[50] potentially because of either the pathologic process or a delay in obtaining high-quality care. Although obstructive sleep apnea (OSA) via sympathetic nerve surges and intermittent hypoxia is a risk factor for coronary heart disease and myocardial infarction, it has been proposed that ischemic preconditioning as a result of intermittent hypoxia may confer cardioprotection.[51]

Nocturnal Hypertension

Patients whose nighttime arterial blood pressure declines less than 10% from day to night (called "nondippers") (Figure 144.3)[8] are at increased risk for total and cardiovascular mortality[52] and all cardiovascular end points,[53] frequent or complex ventricular arrhythmias,[54] myocardial ischemia,[55] cerebrovascular insult,[56] and increased organ damage, including cardiac hypertrophy.[57] The sleep-trough morning surge in blood pressure leads to subclinical end-organ damage, including alterations in left ventricular and atrial morphology and in carotid intimal thickness.[58] The absence of a nocturnal decline in blood pressure is seen in OSA[59] and may be an important marker of complications among patients with type 1 diabetes mellitus,[60] and it may be reflected in the significant incidence of death at 2:00 a.m. to 4:00 a.m. among hypertensive women, reported by Mitler and colleagues[61] (Figure 144.8). Faulty baroreceptor activation may account for the fact that arterial blood pressure during sleep remains significantly elevated in these hypertensive patients, who typically show evidence of central hypersympathetic nerve activity

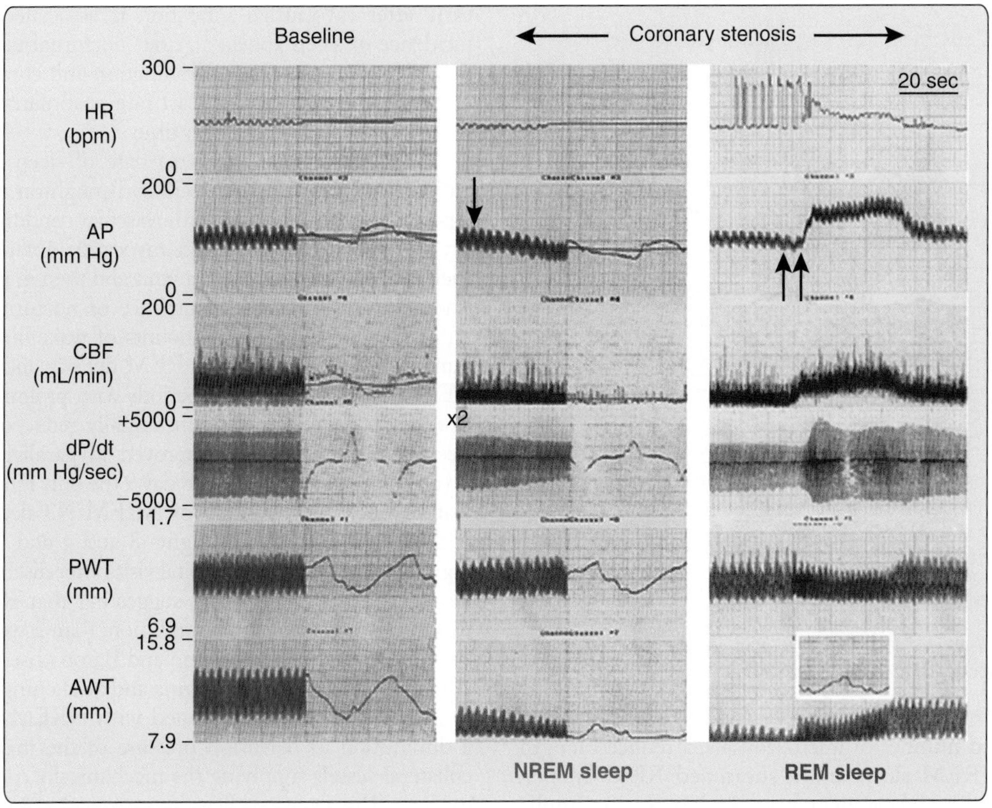

Figure 144.7 Representative tracings for hemodynamic variables at baseline (before stenosis) and during non–rapid eye movement (NREM) (*single arrow*) and rapid eye movement (REM) (*double arrow*) sleep in the presence of coronary stenosis. NREM sleep initiated a decrease in arterial pressure (AP), resulting in akinesis in the anterior wall (stenotic region). REM sleep induced a rapid increase in heart rate (HR), AP, and dP/dt_{max} (rate of change of left ventricular pressure). The onset of REM sleep increased coronary blood flow, which returned anterior wall function to the poststenotic condition before the onset of NREM sleep. (See expanded tracing in inset box.) AWT, Anterior wall thickness; bpm, beats per minute; CBF, coronary blood flow; PWT, posterior wall thickness. (From Kim SJ, Kuklov A, Kehoe RF, et al. Sleep-induced hypotension precipitates severe myocardial ischemia. *Sleep.* 2008;31:1215–20, published with permission from the Sleep Research Society and the American Academy of Sleep Medicine.)

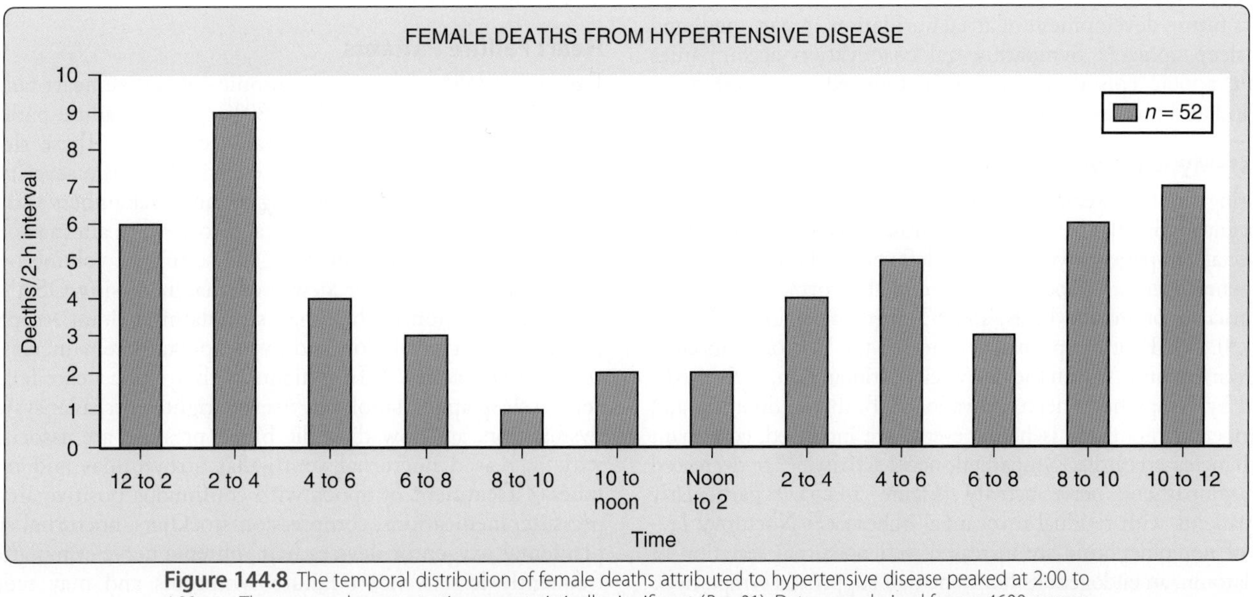

Figure 144.8 The temporal distribution of female deaths attributed to hypertensive disease peaked at 2:00 to 4:00 a.m. The temporal concentration was statistically significant ($P < .01$). Data were derived from a 4600-person (>8%) sample of deaths due to disease in New York City in 1979. (From Mitler MM, Hajdukovic RM, Shafor R, et al. When people die: cause of death versus time of death. *Am J Med.* 1987;82:266–74, published with permission from Excerpta Medica.)

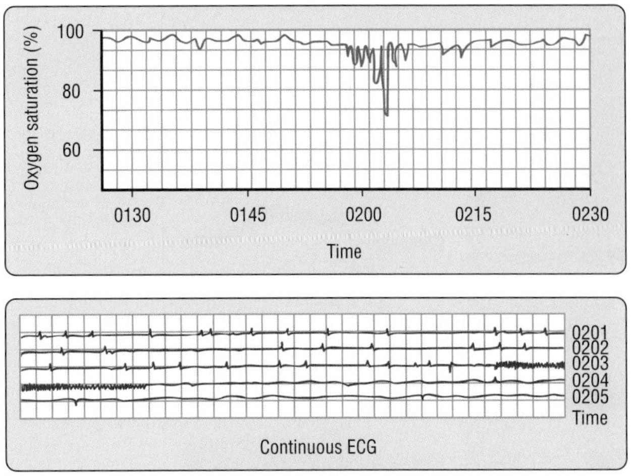

Figure 144.9 Importance of monitoring nocturnal oxygen saturation in patients who have sustained a myocardial infarction. Nonsustained ventricular tachycardia (*bottom*) and hypoxemia measured by pulse oximetry (*top*) occurred simultaneously in a patient on the third night after infarction. The patient died on the following day of cardiogenic shock. ECG, Electrocardiogram. (From Galatius-Jensen S, Hansen J, Rasmussen V, et al. Nocturnal hypoxemia after myocardial infarction: association with nocturnal myocardial ischaemia and arrhythmias. *Br Heart J.* 1994;72:23–30, published with permission from the British Cardiac Society.)

with an increased number of microarousals, a reduced length and depth of NREM sleep, and a shortened REM latency. Blunted endothelium-dependent vasodilation is also implicated. Molecular clock mechanisms are increasingly recognized to play an important role in blood pressure regulation, thus informing understanding of inherent susceptibilities and chronotherapeutics.[62]

Effects of Apnea on Cardiac Status

Sleep apnea is associated with periodic hypoxia, oxidative stress, increased sympathetic nerve activity, endothelial dysfunction, and enlarged atrial area,[63] factors that increase hypertension, coronary artery disease, arrhythmia, and heart failure.[64] Parasympathetic nerve dominance during sleep predicts future development of atrial fibrillation, in part mediated by sleep apnea.[65] Sympathovagal coactivation accompanies acute apneic episodes, resulting in reduced atrial refractory period and increased likelihood of atrial fibrillation.[66,67]

Post–Myocardial Infarction Patients

During the first weeks after myocardial infarction, sleep is significantly disturbed,[33,44] and nocturnal oxygen desaturation, especially in patients with impaired left ventricular function, may be generalized or episodic and may directly provoke tachycardia, ventricular premature beats, and ST-segment changes (Figure 144.9).[44–47] Poor sleep quality increases the risk of ventricular tachyarrhythmia within the first week postinfarction, likely mediated by sympathetic nerve activation.[68] Both the duration and number of nighttime ischemic events are increased, consonant with increased cardiac sympathetic nerve activity[31,69] or decreased parasympathetic nerve activity (Figure 144.5),[16] particularly in patients with residual myocardial ischemia.[21] Nocturnal levels of norepinephrine are increased, and nocturnal secretion of melatonin, an endogenous hormone that suppresses sympathetic nerve activity, is impaired.[70] These symptoms become normal over time so that within the first 6 months, ventricular tachycardia during sleep is relatively rare. Improved cardiac function early after myocardial infarction is associated with decreased incidence of sleep apnea.[71] A flat nocturnal tachogram, indicative of cardiac autonomic dysfunction and consisting of limited changes in instantaneous heart rate postinfarction, is associated with increased mortality over time.[72]

The most detailed study to date of sleep in postinfarction patients was performed in 1978 by Broughton and Baron,[33] who reported on the sleep and cardiovascular condition of 12 patients, age 33 to 70 years, after severe myocardial infarction, first during their stay in the intensive care unit and then in the hospital ward. They noted a "marked disturbance of nocturnal sleep patterns ... characterized by high amounts of wakefulness, stage 1, and number of awakenings, and REM density and low amounts of REM sleep, shorter REM periods with prolonged REM latencies. Sleep efficiency was substantially reduced."[33] All of these sleep-quality parameters improved in parallel with time after myocardial infarction until on day 9 the only remaining abnormal feature was a high content of NREM N3 sleep. REM density peaked on postinfarction nights 3 and 4 and NREM sleep on night 4. On subsequent hospital visits after discharge, the patients described terrifying dreams, suggesting that REM suppression was followed by REM rebound more than 2 weeks after the crisis. Of importance, Broughton and Baron observed that NREM sleep provoked nocturnal angina and awakening. They postulated that the hypotension associated with NREM sleep resulted in a diminution in perfusion pressure of the major coronary and collateral vessels supplying the mechanically compromised myocardium. The decreased heart rates typical of NREM sleep, however, were not observed, and heart rates were higher in NREM sleep than in wakefulness on half the nights recorded, indicating enhanced cardiac sympathetic nerve activity even in NREM sleep. In half of the cases the ECG amplitude decreased during anginal attacks. In the context of nighttime monitoring, it is of interest that T-wave alternans, an ECG phenomenon indicating vulnerability to lethal arrhythmias,[73] was documented in the nighttime ECG of a patient with left dysfunction enrolled in the ambulatory ECG arm of the Eplerenone Post-Acute Myocardial Infarction Heart Failure Efficacy and Survival Study (EPHESUS) (Figure 144.10).[74]

Heart Failure Patients

Excess mortality risk attends chronic congestive heart failure, particularly among the 40% to 80% of heart failure patients with either obstructive or central sleep apnea. These sleep-related breathing disorders may contribute to the severity of disease, specifically to remodeling of cardiac chambers and left ventricular diastolic dysfunction and to T-wave alternans.[73,75] Overnight rostral fluid shifts in the setting of volume overload contribute to upper airway edema, increasing OSA and fluid accumulation in the lungs, stimulating irritant receptors to incite hyperventilation and hypocapnia, thereby increasing central sleep apnea.[76] In patients with systolic heart failure, central sleep apnea, smoking,[77] severe right ventricular systolic dysfunction, and low diastolic blood pressure are associated with increased nocturnal ventricular arrhythmias and mortality.[78] Treatment of apnea with continuous positive airway pressure, medications, compression stockings, nocturnal supplemental oxygen or devices (e.g., phrenic nerve stimulation) frequently lessens heart failure symptoms and may reduce mortality risk. Trials are underway to test the effectiveness of many of these interventions.[79] Diagnostic and treatment strategies are discussed in Chapter 149.

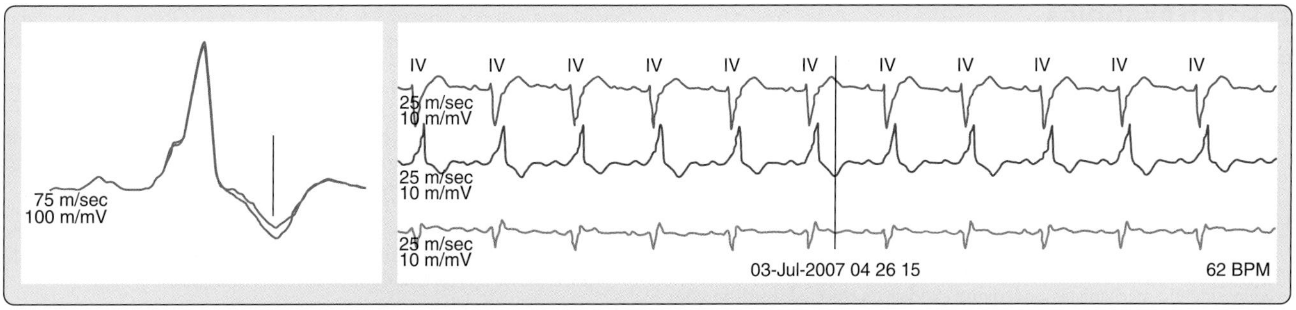

Figure 144.10 High-resolution template showing T-wave alternans (65 μV) in precordial lead V_3 in superimposed electrocardiographic (ECG) waveforms from a nighttime ambulatory ECG recording of a patient with heart failure and left ventricular dysfunction enrolled in the ambulatory ECG substudy of the Eplerenone Post-Acute Myocardial Infarction Heart Failure Efficacy and Survival Study (EPHESUS). The associated ECG strip is also provided. BPM, Beats per minute. (From Stein PK, Sanghavi D, Domitrovich PP, et al. Ambulatory ECG-based T-wave alternans predicts sudden cardiac death in high-risk post-MI patients with left ventricular dysfunction in the EPHESUS Study. *J Cardiovasc Electrophysiol.* 2008;19:1037–42, published with permission from Wiley.)

Patients with Epilepsy

Whereas most patients with epilepsy exhibit a low incidence of seizure at night,[80] sudden unexpected death in epilepsy (SUDEP) occurs primarily in patients with a history of nocturnal seizures and in the prone position.[81–83] SUDEP typically follows generalized tonic-clonic seizures with SUDEP events sequentially characterized by hyperventilation, apnea, bradycardia, and postictal generalized EEG suppression before the terminal asystole.[84] Greater than 99% of nocturnal seizures arise in NREM sleep.[85] The majority of genetic variants in those with SUDEP are related to cardiac sodium and potassium ion channel subunits, suggesting lethal cardiac arrhythmia and sudden cardiac death as a likely contributor to mortality.[86] Sleep disorders are common among patients with epilepsy; sleep apnea worsens seizures, and its treatment improves seizure control.[85,87] Sleep in patients with epilepsy is discussed in Chapter 106.

Elderly Patients

Elderly individuals' (particularly women's) reports of daytime sleepiness, suggesting poor quality of sleep, are associated with mortality, cardiovascular morbidity and mortality, myocardial infarction, and congestive heart failure.[88] Depression, poor health, daytime angina, a limited activity level, and cardiac arrhythmias may accompany disturbed sleep in elderly individuals. Initiating a moderately intense exercise program significantly improves sleep quality[89] and autonomic status[90] in formerly sedentary older people. Nocturnal myocardial ischemia is not uncommon in older patients with vascular disease who experience regular episodes of oxygen desaturation and increased heart rate. Ventricular tachycardia provoked by sleep apnea appears to be reduced with increasing age, a finding that is likely due to survivorship bias. However, it may also reflect altered nodal pathophysiology rendering protection in the elderly.[91] Conflicting evidence has been presented of increased risk for nighttime, compared with daytime, myocardial infarction and sudden cardiac death in elderly people.[44,48,92] Impaired baroreceptor sensitivity,[93] a measure of the capacity for reflex vagus nerve activation,[9] and increased LF power of HRV[94] are evident at night in susceptible elderly patients. Given this autonomic background, it is not surprising that nighttime multifocal activity in elderly patients is a predictor of cardiac mortality.

CLINICAL PEARLS

- Sleep exerts a major impact on the health of the patient with cardiac disease through both direct cardiovascular influences and sleep-disordered breathing.[95] In a sense, the diseased heart and lungs are unwitting victims of the needs of the sleeping brain, which commands dramatic alterations in autonomic and respiratory activity.
- A sizeable population experiences cardiac events during sleep, with identifiable high-risk groups (Table 144.1).
- Sleep presents unusual opportunities to monitor the patient with cardiac disease because there is growing appreciation of the fact that nighttime heart rate, blood pressure, myocardial ischemia, arrhythmias, and respiratory disturbances carry predictive value for daytime events (Box 144.1).
- Daytime tests cannot substitute for nighttime monitoring of the patient with cardiac disease because exercise treadmill testing and daytime ambulatory monitoring cannot replicate the autonomic, hemodynamic, or respiratory challenges that uniquely accompany sleep.
- Improved identification of the precise triggers of nocturnal cardiac events may be anticipated when technologies are integrated for monitoring sleep state, respiration, oxygen desaturation, and cardiovascular variables.

SUMMARY

Specific patient groups exhibit elevated sleep-related cardiac risk, including those with a history of cardiac arrhythmias, myocardial infarction, angina, heart failure, or sleep apnea; family members of an infant who died from sudden infant death syndrome; and patients with Brugada syndrome, long-QT syndrome, or epilepsy. Improved risk assessment is possible through noninvasive monitoring of autonomic variables and repolarization abnormalities.

ACKNOWLEDGMENTS

The authors thank Sandra S. Verrier for her editorial contributions.

SELECTED READINGS

Broughton R, Baron R. Sleep patterns in the intensive care unit and on the ward after acute myocardial infarction. *Electroencephalogr Clin Neurophysiol.* 1978;45:348–360.

Cerrone M. Controversies in Brugada syndrome. *Trends Cardiovasc Med.* 2018;28(4):284–292.

Hung J, Whitford EG, Parsons RW, et al. Association of sleep apnoea with myocardial infarction in men. *Lancet.* 1990;336:261–264.

Mancia G. Autonomic modulation of the cardiovascular system during sleep. *N Engl J Med.* 1993;328:347–349.

Purnell B, Murugan M, Jani R, Boison D. The good, the bad, and the deadly: adenosinergic mechanisms underlying sudden unexpected death in epilepsy. *Front Neurosci.* 2021;15:708304.

Purnell BS, Thijs RD, Buchanan GF. Dead in the night: sleep-wake and time-of-day influences on sudden unexpected death in epilepsy. *Front Neurol.* 2018;9:1079.

Shamsuzzaman AS, Somers VK, Knilans TK, et al. Obstructive sleep apnea in patients with congenital long QT syndrome: implications for increased risk of sudden cardiac death. *Sleep.* 2015;38:1113–1119.

Somers VK, Dyken ME, Mark AL, et al. Sympathetic nerve activity during sleep in normal subjects. *N Engl J Med.* 1993;328:303–307.

Trimer R, Cabiddu R, Mendes RG, et al. Heart rate variability and cardiorespiratory coupling during sleep in patients prior to bariatric surgery. *Obes Surg.* 2014;24:471–477.

Verrier RL, Klingenheben T, Malik M, et al. Microvolt T-wave alternans: physiologic basis, methods of measurement, and clinical utility. Consensus guideline by the International Society for Holter and Noninvasive Electrocardiology. *J Am Coll Cardiol.* 2011;44:1309–1324.

A complete reference list can be found online at ExpertConsult.com.

Chapter 145

Cardiac Arrhythmogenesis during Sleep: Mechanisms, Diagnosis, and Therapy

Reena Mehra; Murray Mittleman; Richard L. Verrier

Chapter Highlights

- The pronounced sleep state–dependent changes in autonomic nervous system activity and respiration can provoke both atrial and ventricular arrhythmias in patients with cardiovascular disease.
- Mortality due to ventricular arrhythmias is most frequent during sleep in the distinct syndromes of sudden infant death, sudden unexplained nocturnal death, and Brugada syndrome, each of which has been linked to genetic abnormalities. The proarrhythmic potential of class III antiarrhythmic agents (potassium channel blockers) for patients with significant heart rate pauses and the sleep-disrupting effect of medications must be considered. Reduced responsiveness to antiarrhythmic medications occurs in severe sleep-disordered breathing independent of the degree of hypoxia and rapid eye movement sleep.
- Cardiac arrhythmias are prevalent in the 16.5 million Americans with heart disease, with potentially severe consequences. Approximately 15% of sudden cardiac deaths, which result from lethal ventricular arrhythmias, occur during sleep, and most atrial arrhythmias in patients younger than 61 years have their onset at nighttime. Sleep apnea profoundly alters autonomic nervous system activity and increases risk of arrhythmia, hypertension, and myocardial infarction.
- Although emerging data support the clinical utility of the electrocardiogram (ECG) and sleep monitoring parameters derived from sleep study signal extraction in prediction of incident cardiac arrhythmia, electrocardiograms (ECGs) are currently not standardly collected for in-home sleep apnea testing with lack of systematic arrhythmia recognition of attended sleep studies of the more than 1.1 million overall sleep studies conducted annually.

We will review the current state of knowledge regarding epidemiology, risk factors, pathogenesis, and treatment options for each nocturnal arrhythmia type in relation to sleep and to sleep disruption attributable to sleep disorders.

VENTRICULAR ARRHYTHMIAS

Malignant ventricular arrhythmias are usually suppressed during sleep, as is evidenced by the nocturnal trough in incidence of myocardial infarction, sudden cardiac death, implantable cardioverter–defibrillator discharge, myocardial ischemic events, and arrhythmias, not only in the general population, but also in at-risk patients with ischemic heart disease.[1,2] This decrement coincides with lessened metabolic demands during non–rapid eye movement (NREM) sleep, which occupies approximately 80% of sleep time. However, sleep is not entirely free of risk, because the nocturnal incidence of sudden cardiac death, which is attributable to ventricular fibrillation, has been calculated at approximately 15%,[3] or 55,000 cases annually in the United States alone. Moreover, the nonuniformity of the nighttime distribution of these events (Figure 145.1)[3] suggests physiologic triggering that may be amenable to monitoring for improved diagnosis and therapy. Molecular pathways governing cardiac ion channel expression and myocardial repolarization identified by QT interval duration involve a clock-dependent oscillator, Krüppel-like factor 15 (*Klf15*), thus providing emerging insights into circadian influences contributing to ventricular arrhythmia and sudden nocturnal cardiac death.[4] Surges in cardiac sympathetic nerve activity during rapid eye movement (REM) sleep superimposed on a background of enhanced parasympathetic tone have been implicated in nocturnal ventricular arrhythmias and myocardial ischemia[5–8] (Chapter 144). The specific mechanisms of REM-induced cardiac events include direct effects on electrophysiologic status or indirect consequences of heart rate and arterial blood pressure accelerations, which may disrupt plaques and lead to intraarterial platelet aggregates, releasing proarrhythmic constituents such as thromboxane A_2.[9]

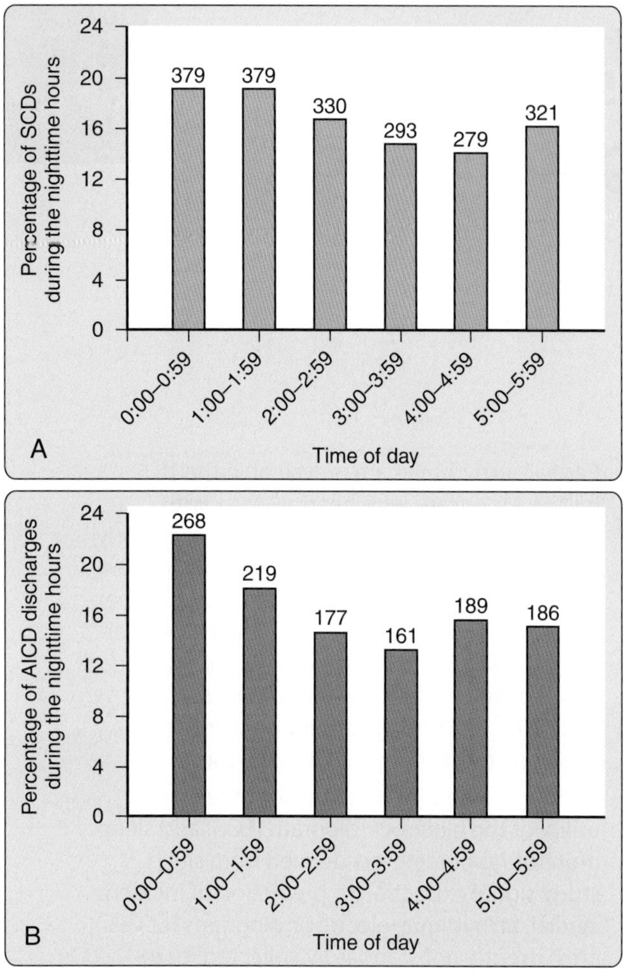

Figure 145.1 **A,** Hourly incidence of sudden cardiac death (SCD) onset between midnight and 5:59 a.m. from 12 studies enrolling 1981 patients. The number of sudden cardiac deaths observed each hour is indicated above each bar. **B,** Hourly incidence of automatic implantable cardioverter–defibrillator (AICD) discharge between midnight and 5:59 a.m. from seven studies enrolling 1197 patients, who experienced 1200 discharges during the nocturnal period. The number of discharges observed each hour is indicated above each bar. (From Lavery CE, Mittleman MA, Cohen MC, et al. Nonuniform nighttime distribution of acute cardiac events: a possible effect of sleep states. *Circulation.* 1997;5:3321–7.)

Myocardial ischemia or other changes in cardiac substrate and mechanical function resulting from cardiovascular disease,[10] myocardial infarction,[11] or aging[12] can amplify nocturnal cardiac electrical instability. Oxygen desaturation may trigger nighttime ventricular tachycardia in patients with cardiac disease in the subacute phase after myocardial infarction[11] or in those with heart failure.[10] Hypoxemia and tachycardia frequently occur together during sleep after major surgery to promote myocardial ischemia.[13] Frequent or complex arrhythmias are also characteristic of hypertensive patients in whom the typical nocturnal trough in blood pressure is not observed.[14] The nocturnal increase in QT-interval dispersion among survivors of sudden cardiac death,[15] acute myocardial infarction,[16] and heart failure[16] provides evidence of their increased vulnerability to cardiac arrhythmias at night.

REM-related nocturnal ventricular arrhythmogenesis may have a significant affective component. REM sleep dreams, which may be vivid, bizarre, and emotionally intense, commonly generate the emotions of anger and fear. Because these emotions have been linked in wakefulness to the onset of myocardial infarction and sudden death,[17] it is reasonable to hypothesize that when these affective states are evoked during dreaming, they may trigger lethal events. This possibility is illustrated by a case report of recurrence of ventricular fibrillation in a 39-year-old man with normal coronary arteries and cardiac function while sleeping. A subsequent sleep study determined that ventricular premature beats were substantially increased during REM and that dreams at the same hour that fibrillation had occurred were emotionally charged.[18]

Pathognomonic to REM sleep is blunting of hypoxic and hypercapnic responsiveness leading to more pronounced hypoxia relative to NREM sleep, often in an undulating pattern. Intermittent hypoxia, as observed in sleep apnea, doubled the incidence of myocardial ischemia-related arrhythmias (66.7% vs. 33.3%), particularly ventricular fibrillation, in an experimental model.[19] Chronic exposure to intermittent hypoxia in myocardial ischemia is a major risk factor for sudden cardiac death via mechanisms of sympathoactivation and alterations in ventricular monophasic repolarization, transmural ventricular action potential duration gradient, and endocardial calcium channel expression.[19] In some cases, arrhythmia frequency may be enhanced during NREM sleep, when latent automatic foci are exposed by the generalized reduction in heart rate after withdrawal of overdrive suppression, or when hypotension exacerbates impaired coronary perfusion.

Epidemiologic data identify a twofold higher odds of nocturnal ventricular arrhythmia in relation to sleep apnea that peaks during the midnight to 6 a.m. hours, highlighting sleep apnea-related propensity to trigger nocturnal sudden cardiac death.[20] This is independent of confounding influences, including obesity and self-reported underlying cardiac disease, and driven by nocturnal hypoxia[21] and propensity to trigger nocturnal sudden cardiac death in patients with sleep apnea. The case of a 65-year old male with ischemic cardiomyopathy and newly discovered sleep apnea, who experienced transient episodes of nonsustained polymorphic ventricular tachycardia, culminating in ventricular fibrillation with torsades de pointes in the morning hours and resulting in sudden nocturnal cardiac death, was discovered during assessment of more than 16,000 in-laboratory polysomnograms (Figure 145.2).[22] Other disorders of sleep, such as periodic limb movements associated with microarousals, have immediate temporal relationships with nonsustained ventricular tachycardia, implicating a role for accompanying surges in sympathetic nerve activity that are suggestive of causality (see Chapters 121, 144, and 146).

Therapy

In most cases an electrically unstable cardiac substrate underlies the propensity to develop nocturnal ventricular arrhythmias, and treatment is similar to that for daytime arrhythmias. If surges in sympathetic nerve activity, which typically occur during REM sleep and dreaming, are suspected, beta-adrenergic receptor blockade therapy may prove helpful, with careful attention to avoiding medications that disrupt sleep.[23]

In treating hypertensive patients, it is important to appreciate Mancia's[24] suggestion that pharmacologic therapy that exacerbates the hypotensive effect of NREM sleep may introduce the potential risk of thrombosis and embolism in patients with stenotic lesions in the heart or brain. Floras[25] determined that the nocturnal incidence of myocardial infarction was not diminished in patients treated with antihypertensive agents and suggested that the agents induced nocturnal hypotension.

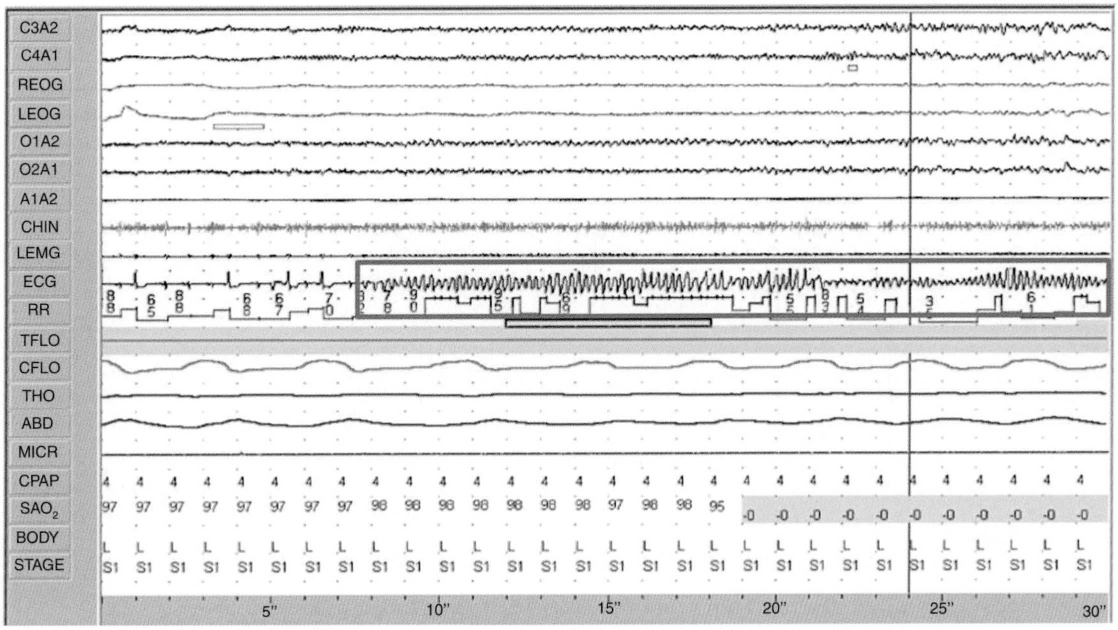

Figure 145.2 The record shows the terminal episode of polymorphic sustained ventricular tachycardia/ fibrillation with torsades de pointes on the electrocardiogram channel in stage 1 sleep in a patient with dilated cardiomyopathy and severe obstructive sleep apnea undergoing a split night study on continuous positive airway pressure. ABD, Abdominal effort; BODY, body position; C3A2, C4A1, O1A2, and O2A1, refer to electroencephalogram channels; CFLO, airflow; CPAP, continuous positive airway pressure; ECG, electrocardiogram; LEMG, left electromyogram; MICR, microphone; REOG and LEOG, right and left electrooculogram; RR, heart rate; SAo_2, alveolar oxygen saturation; STAGE, sleep stage; THO, thoracic effort. (From Mehra R, Strohl KP. Incidence of serious adverse events during nocturnal polysomnography. *Sleep.* 2004;27:1379–83.)

Thus special attention should be given to the hemodynamic effects of antihypertensive drugs and vasodilators to avoid precipitating cardiac events by inducing profound hypotension. The importance of ruling out "white coat" hypertension is underscored because greater than 30% of individuals with elevated blood pressure readings in the physician's office or hospital prove to be normotensive during daily life, as documented by ambulatory blood pressure monitoring.[26]

Nighttime onset of ventricular arrhythmias may also indicate provocation by disturbed breathing, which can be treated by continuous positive airway pressure (CPAP).[27] For example, sleep-disordered breathing provokes ventricular arrhythmias and appropriate firing of implantable cardioverter–defibrillators, suggesting apnea screening and therapy to reduce these events.[28] Reduction in ventricular ectopy burden in response to CPAP treatment of sleep apnea in heart failure patients is supported by randomized controlled trial data indicating salutary effects of sleep apnea reversal on ventricular arrhythmogenesis in the compromised heart.[29] Risk of apnea-induced cardiac events is not limited to the nocturnal period and can be monitored from continuous ECGs by T-wave alternans,[30] a marker of risk for lethal ventricular arrhythmias.[31]

The important deficiency in ECG monitoring during the 1.1 million at-home sleep studies conducted annually in the United States limits analysis of the effects of sleep-disordered breathing on the spectrum of atrial and ventricular arrhythmias.[32,33]

CONDUCTION DELAY: NOCTURNAL ASYSTOLE, ATRIOVENTRICULAR BLOCK, AND QT-INTERVAL PROLONGATION

Sinus pauses of less than 2 seconds, prolonged atrioventricular (AV) conduction, Wenckebach AV block, and bradycardia are well documented in normal populations during sleep and are attributed to effects of increased parasympathetic activity on AV node conduction.[34,35] These asystoles are more frequent in individuals who are young[36,37] or physically fit, such as athletes[38,39] and heavy laborers.[40] More extreme cases were observed by Guilleminault and colleagues,[41] who reported periods of sinus arrest of up to 9 seconds during REM sleep in young adults with apparently normal cardiac function. It was concluded that the nocturnal asystoles were the result of exaggerated, if not abnormally elevated, vagal tone because muscarinic receptor blockers significantly reduced the duration of the nocturnal asystoles but did not prevent them. No further therapeutic intervention was warranted.

However, in patients with cardiac disease, especially those taking class III antiarrhythmic drugs (potassium channel–blocking agents), nocturnal asystolic events can set the stage for ventricular arrhythmias. Such prolongation of cycle length can facilitate the development of early afterdepolarizations and the lethal arrhythmia torsades de pointes. In patients with damaged endothelium resulting from coronary atherosclerosis, the acetylcholine released by surges in vagus nerve activity could result in vasoconstriction rather than vasodilation because of impaired release of endothelium-derived relaxing factor.[42]

Hypoxia and sleep apnea are recognized precipitants of conduction delay and bradyarrhythmias; however, after adjustment for these factors in statistical analyses, REM sleep remains a significant driver of bradyarrhythmia, thereby implicating REM-specific influences underlying bradyarrhythmia, even independent of sleep apnea.[43] When apneic events occur in REM sleep, the combined influences can exert significant conduction delay resulting in higher degree atrioventricular block in those who are predisposed (Figure 145.3).[44] Hypoxia

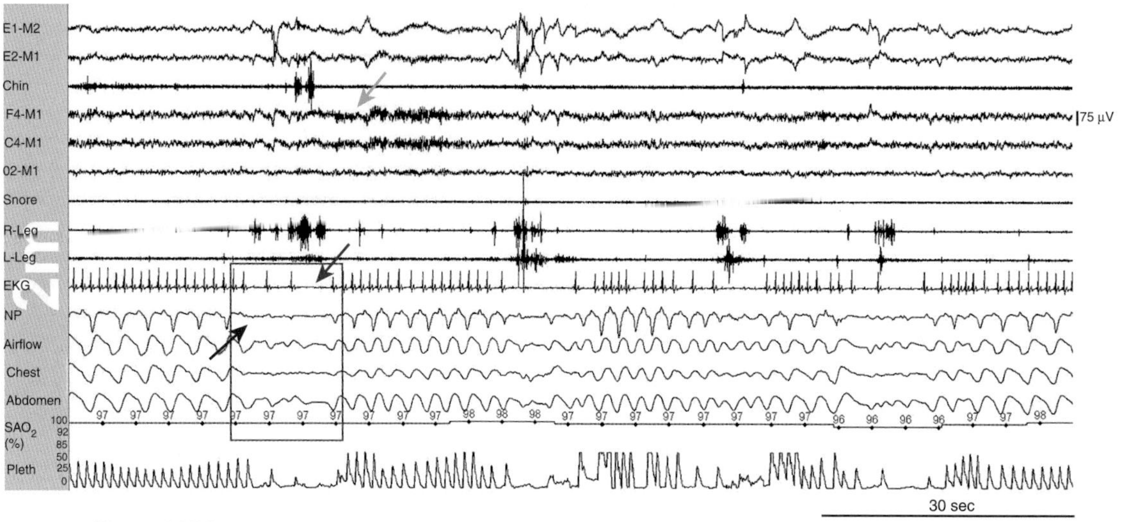

Figure 145.3 This 120-sec recording demonstrates a period of rapid eye movement sleep during which there were rhythm abnormalities on the lead II ECG (*red arrow*). These abnormalities are temporally related to respiratory events (*navy blue arrow*) in the absence of significant hypoxia via oximetry monitoring but in the presence of an EEG arousal (*yellow arrow*). (From Kaur S, Alsheikhtaha Z, Mehra R. A 48-year-old athletic man with bradycardia during sleep. *Chest*. 2018;154:e139–42.)

is a sympathetic stimulus leading to increased heart rate; however, in the absence of lung inflation, hypoxia leads to bradycardia, such as during an apneic event, and is prevented by vagolytic agents such as atropine.[45] Moreover, supplemental oxygen administered during apneic episodes mitigates bradyarrhythmia.[45] Atrioventricular conduction delay and asystole for up to 13 seconds have been identified in patients with severe sleep apnea.[46] Although epidemiologic studies identify first- and second-degree atrioventricular block patterns as more prevalent in patients with than without sleep apnea, these differences were not statistically significant.[47] Disparate findings in clinic-based versus epidemiologic studies are likely due to a lesser degree of sleep apnea severity observed in population-based studies.

Nocturnal heart rate pauses may be particularly arrhythmogenic in subsets of patients with the long QT syndrome (LQTS), a familial arrhythmogenic cardiac channelopathy, specifically LQT2 and LQT3 patients, who have mutations on the sodium channel, voltage-gated, type V, alpha gene (*SCN5A*).[48] The lethal arrhythmias occur almost exclusively at rest or during sleep, when the QT interval is typically prolonged.[49] Severe sleep apnea is associated with increased QT dispersion and represents an important therapeutic target to improve outcomes in LQTS.[50,51]

Therapy

Ascertaining whether patients exhibit nocturnal heart rate pauses is important when treating individuals for whom class III antiarrhythmic drugs (potassium channel blockers) are the primary option. Given diurnal patterning and circadian variation of conduction delay arrhythmias, chronotherapeutics, that is, the timing of medications to enhance beneficial outcomes and/or attenuate or avert adverse effects, is important to consider.

ATRIAL FIBRILLATION

In the more-than–6 million US patients with atrial fibrillation, which has serious consequences in terms of increased morbidity and mortality,[52] it is likely that 10% to 25% of the arrhythmias are facilitated by vagal influences. This has been termed *vagally mediated atrial fibrillation*. Several investigators have reported nocturnal peaks in onset of paroxysmal atrial fibrillation.[53–55] A significant midnight to 2:00 a.m. peak in atrial fibrillation onset and a higher average nocturnal incidence were documented by Rostagno and colleagues[53] in their review of records from 10 years of responses by mobile coronary care units staffed by cardiologists in Florence, Italy. This arrhythmia was also found to exhibit a peak in frequency of onset at midnight in a Japanese population of 60 years of age or younger. The maximal duration of the arrhythmia (77 ± 27 minutes per episode) was greatest between midnight and 6:00 a.m. (Figure 145.4).[54] Other investigators characterized a 4:00 a.m. to 5:00 a.m. peak in onset of paroxysmal atrial fibrillation that was refractory to antiarrhythmic drugs in a 3-month study of 67 patients with implantable cardioverters.[55] The 514 recorded episodes with an atrial rate greater than 220 beats per minute lasted more than 1 minute before termination by pacing or spontaneous reversion. A potential contribution of sympathetic nerve activity is implicated by the timing of these bouts of atrial fibrillation, which occurred during a period of sleep when REM typically emerges. However, the potential of REM sleep to trigger the arrhythmia was not discussed.

Patients with more frequent atrial tachycardia are more likely to develop atrial tachycardia/fibrillation at night.[56] Records of concurrent monitoring of sleep and nocturnal onset of atrial fibrillation are rare (Figure 145.5).[57] In the case illustrated, disruption of the nocturnal trough in heart rate disclosed sleep-related atrial fibrillation. Available evidence indicates that nocturnal atrial fibrillation is provoked during periods of intense vagus nerve activity, as indicated by heart rate variability studies,[58,59] and the presence of bradycardia,[60] in individuals with structurally normal hearts. Enhanced adrenergic activity may interact in a complex manner with changes in vagal tone to affect atrial refractoriness and dispersion of repolarization and to alter intraatrial conduction, thus increasing the propensity to develop this arrhythmia.[52,60] The high level of vagus nerve tone maintained during slow

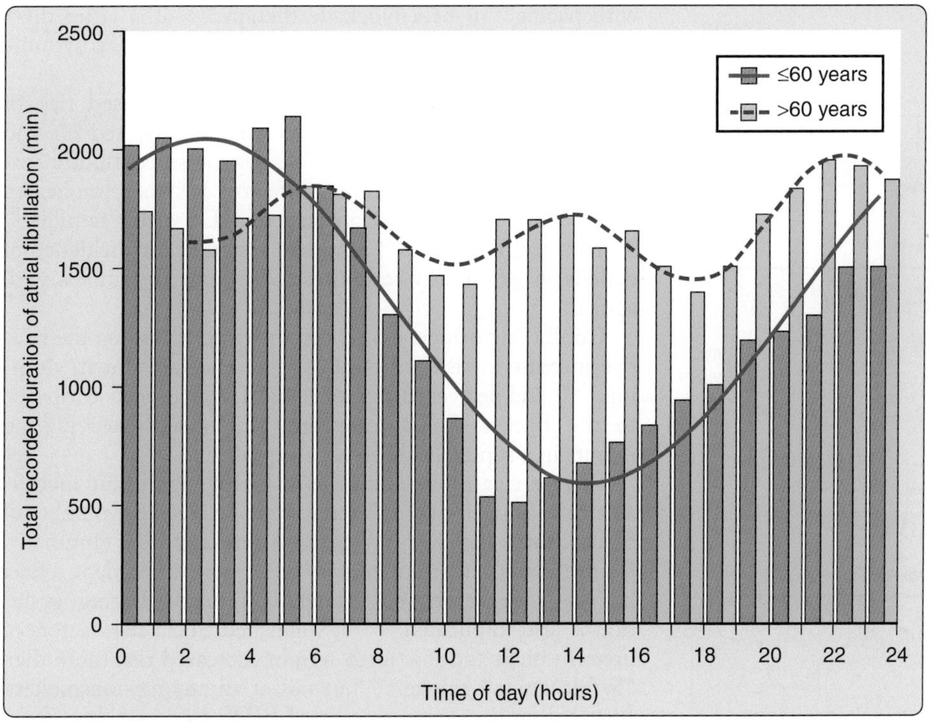

Figure 145.4 Hourly total duration of paroxysmal atrial fibrillation in younger (<60 years; *red bars*) and older patients (*green bars*). The single harmonic fit of the data from the younger patients is shown by the *unbroken line*. The triple harmonic fit in the older patients is shown by the *broken line*. A prominent monophasic circadian rhythm is present in younger patients, in contrast to a toneless triphasic rhythm in older patients. (From Yamashita T, Murakawa Y, Hayami N, et al. Relation between aging and circadian variation of paroxysmal atrial fibrillation. *Am J Cardiol*. 1998;82:1364–7.)

wave sleep has the capacity to exacerbate atrial fibrillation in patients whose atria are particularly prone to the arrhythmogenic influence of acetylcholine.[52]

Risk of atrial fibrillation is doubled if breathing during sleep is disordered[61] because apnea can provoke nocturnal hypoxemia, sympathetic nerve activity, and hemodynamic stress.[27,61] Obstructive apnea–induced surges in blood pressure and alterations in intrathoracic pressures distend atrial chambers and can activate stretch receptors. Intermittent hypoxia, more so than sleep fragmentation, results in modification and remodeling of atrial connexin-40 and connexin-43 in response to reactive oxygen species generated by nitric oxide.[62] The autonomic nervous system clearly plays a role, as experimental canine data show abolition of apnea-induced atrial fibrillation after ablation of the pulmonary arterial ganglionated plexus[63] and cardiac denervation.[64] In a retrospective clinic-based investigation, incidence of atrial fibrillation was strongly predicted by nocturnal oxygen desaturation in subjects younger than 65 years and by heart failure in older subjects.[61] Central sleep apnea and Cheyne-Stokes respiration have been identified as significant, high magnitude predictors of atrial fibrillation in two independent prospective epidemiologic cohorts.[65,66] Moreover, ablation for atrial fibrillation is effective in patients appropriately treated for sleep-disordered breathing but of limited value in patients whose apnea is not treated.[67] Furthermore, patients with atrial fibrillation and severe sleep apnea are less likely to respond to antiarrhythmic medical therapy, independent of the degree of hypoxia and sleep stage.[68]

Therapy

Medical therapy is similar to that for patients whose arrhythmias occur during the day, including therapy to control rate or terminate the arrhythmia pharmacologically or with an atrial cardioverter–defibrillator. Because nighttime atrial fibrillation is classified as *vagally mediated*, anticholinergic agents, such as disopyramide and flecainide, are sometimes helpful to prevent recurrences; adrenergicblocking drugs or digitalis sometimes worsen symptoms.[69] In addition, individuals with nocturnal onset of atrial fibrillation should be monitored for the presence of sleep-disordered breathing, which can be effectively treated by CPAP. Weight loss and cardiac risk factor interventions, including sleep apnea management, reduce atrial fibrillation burden and have favorable impacts on cardiac remodeling.[70] Treatment of sleep apnea in atrial fibrillation may also result in conversion of atrial fibrillation to normal sinus rhythm (Figure 145.6).[71] Anter and colleagues[72] recommended that, given the high prevalence of obstructive sleep apnea in patients with atrial fibrillation coupled with the increased incidence of extrapulmonary vein triggers, a sleep study should be performed in all patients with atrial fibrillation, and an ablation strategy should be adopted that incorporates targeting of extrapulmonary vein triggers.

SUDDEN INFANT DEATH SYNDROME

Sudden infant death syndrome (SIDS), the leading cause of mortality in infants between 1 week and 1 year of age, occurs during sleep.[73] The syndrome is a diagnosis of exclusion; that is, it includes all causes that remain unexplained after a thorough case investigation, including an autopsy, examination of the death scene, and review of the clinical history. Thus SIDS, which took a toll of 2234 infants in 2001 in the United States[74] or 8.1% of infant deaths, may be attributable to a variety of etiologies that challenge the developing cardiorespiratory system. The fatal event in SIDS victims is characterized by hypotension and bradycardia[75] and appears to be attributable to a deficit in the normal reflex coordination of heart rate, arterial blood pressure, and respiration during sleep.[76] This failure to respond to cardiorespiratory challenges during sleep may result from a binding deficit in the arcuate nucleus of SIDS infants[76] because muscarinic cholinergic activity in this

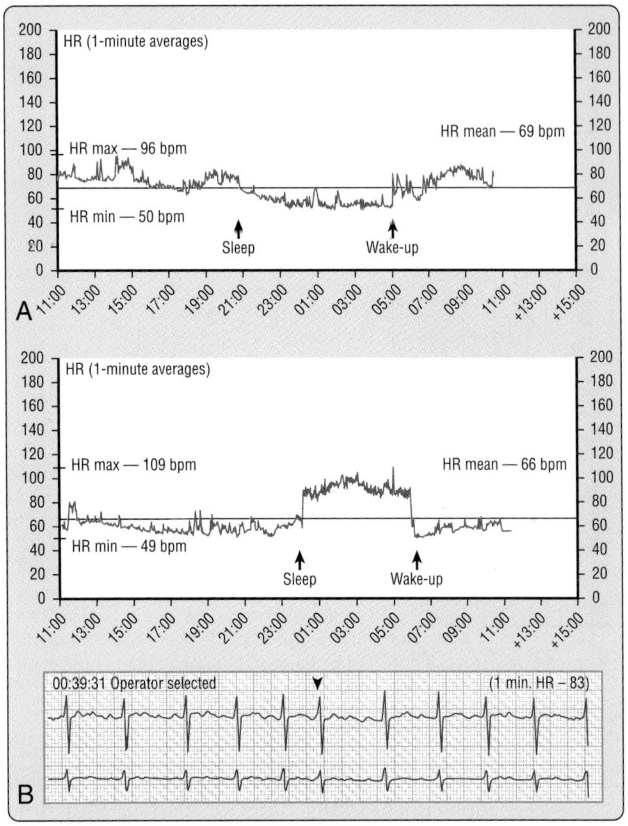

Figure 145.5 A, Heart rate (HR) trend from an ambulatory electrocardiogram (AECG) showing a normal circadian rhythm with a sleep-induced decrease in heart rate. **B,** HR trend from an AECG in our patient shows a nocturnal increase in HR caused by paroxysmal atrial fibrillation at the onset of sleep and a drop in HR after awakening, resulting from spontaneous conversion to sinus rhythm. The ECG (*lower*) documents atrial fibrillation during the sleep period. bpm, Beats per minute. (From Singh J, Mela T, Ruskin J. Images in cardiovascular medicine: sleep [vagal]-induced atrial fibrillation. *Circulation.* 2004;110:e32–3.)

structure at the ventricular medullary surface is postulated to be involved in cardiorespiratory control. Heart rates in infants who later died of SIDS are generally higher and exhibit a reduced range, suggesting altered autonomic control.[77] Autonomic instability has also been documented in NREM sleep in infants with aborted SIDS events.[78]

Repolarization abnormalities have also been observed. Evidence from a 19-year, prospective, multicenter observational study of 34,442 infants determined that significant prolongation (35 milliseconds or more) of the QT interval characterized the 24 (0.07%) infants who died of SIDS within the first year of life.[79] These results suggest that some SIDS cases may be attributed to a genetic defect that produces a developmental abnormality in cardiac sympathetic innervation and alters repolarization to increase the risk of ventricular arrhythmia. These repolarization abnormalities typify infants and children with the long QT syndrome genotype linked to chromosome 3 (LQT3). Mutations in the sodium channel gene *SCN5A* are the most common causes of long QT syndrome and are responsible for the arrhythmias and reduced heart rates. The genetic locus of the defect and the length of the QT interval are independent predictors of risk.[80] T-wave alternans, an electrocardiographic indicator of heightened vulnerability to sudden cardiac death,[25] has been reported in infants who became SIDS victims[81,82] or who were successfully treated with pacing[83] or beta-blockade therapy.[84,85] The latter therapy diminished T-wave alternans, indicating antiarrhythmic efficacy.

Among environmental influences, the increased risk of SIDS during the winter season is well documented[86,87] and is not related to bronchiolitis.[88] A genetic susceptibility that may interact with environmental factors has been implicated by a 5.8-fold increase in recurrence of SIDS within families.[89] Tishler and colleagues[90] reported a significant incidence of deficits in ventilatory responses to hypoxia in families with apnea.

Conflicting evidence has been provided regarding the relative increase in risk attributable to prone (face-down) sleeping,[91–95] and decreased incidence of SIDS has been attributed to the Back-to-Sleep campaign, which advocates placing infants in a supine position for sleeping.

Passive cigarette smoking is a highly significant modifiable risk factor in SIDS. A reduction of 61% in the number of SIDS deaths has been projected if smoking were eliminated from infants' environments.[92–96] A dose-dependent effect has been demonstrated. Maternal smoking during gestation is also implicated.[96–98] Established SIDS risk factors of preterm birth and low birth weight increased risk more than 15-fold among smokers[98] but not at all among nonsmokers. Illegal drug use increases risk of SIDS by more than fourfold.[99] The mechanisms may include impairment in chemoreceptor responsiveness, as a result of decreased sensitivity to carbon dioxide in infants of substance-abusing mothers.[99] The increase in SIDS due to passive smoking may be attributable to nicotine's adverse effect on chemoreceptor activation of respiration,[100] dulling the arousal response to hypoxia.[101] Nicotine and its metabolites have been found at autopsy in the pericardial fluid of SIDS infants.[102,103] Epicardial nicotine is associated with hypopnea[104] and affects the sinoatrial node and epicardial neural fibers to induce hypotension and bradycardia,[105,106] the documented symptomatology of the final event in SIDS infants.[75]

Therapy

This profile suggests some straightforward opportunities for intervention, including placing infants in a supine (face-up) position for sleeping and avoidance of maternal smoking during gestation and passive smoking during infancy. Theoretically, sodium channel blockade[48] or cardiac pacing[48,83] might be useful in treating infants diagnosed with the long QT3 syndrome, but prospective studies are required. Beta-blockade is the current treatment of choice.[48,84,85] Assessment of vulnerability to arrhythmias by QT-interval prolongation has been suggested in a prospective study[79] and by reports of T-wave alternans in ambulatory electrocardiographic (AECG) recordings.[84,85]

THE BRUGADA SYNDROME AND SUDDEN UNEXPLAINED NOCTURNAL DEATH SYNDROME

The striking phenomenon of sudden death during sleep has been reported in Western adults diagnosed with the Brugada syndrome, which strikes men almost exclusively, and in young, apparently healthy Southeast Asian men with the sudden unexplained nocturnal death syndrome (SUNDS). The latter syndrome is named *lai-tai* ("sleep death") in Laos, *pokkuri* ("sudden and unexpected death") in Japan, and *bangungut* ("to

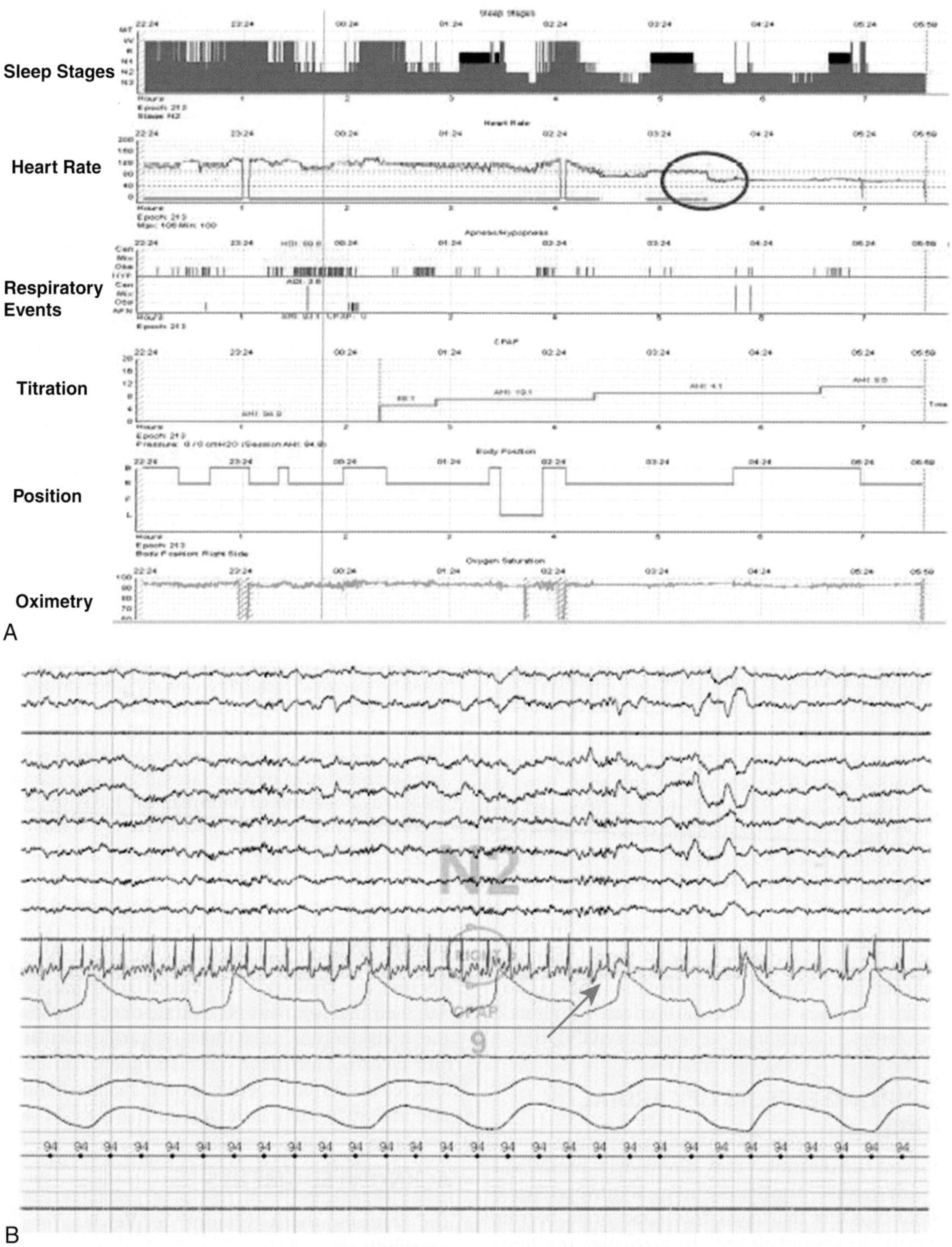

Figure 145.6 The hypnogram demonstrates (*from top to bottom*) sleep stages, heart rate, respiratory events, diagnostic portion and continuous positive airway pressure therapy, body position, and oxygenation. The *circle* shows when atrial fibrillation was reverted to normal sinus rhythm. **(B)** A 30-sec epoch is shown when the conversion of atrial fibrillation to normal sinus rhythm occurred with continuous positive airway pressure at 9 cm H_2O. (From Walia HK, Chung MK, Ibrahim S, et al. Positive airway pressure-induced conversion of atrial fibrillation to normal sinus rhythm in severe obstructive sleep apnea. *J Clin Sleep Med.* 2016;12:1301–3.)

rise and moan in sleep") in the Philippines. These syndromes probably represent the same disorder, which is characterized by right precordial ST segment elevation.[80,107] Deaths are due to lethal ventricular arrhythmias.

The Brugada syndrome is considered responsible for 4% to 12% of all sudden cardiac deaths and for approximately 20% of deaths in patients with structurally normal hearts.[80] The ECG abnormality is estimated to be present in approximately 5 per 10,000 inhabitants, and, apart from accidents, in geographic regions where it is widespread, this inherited syndrome is the leading cause of death of men younger than 50 years. A single sodium channel mutation in the *SCN5A* gene identified in an eight-generation kindred with a high incidence of nocturnal sudden cardiac death, QT-interval prolongation, and Brugada-like ECG characterizes 20% of Brugada patients; other mutations are suspected. Genetic defects in the sodium channel are also associated with progressive conduction system disease attended by bradycardia. A mechanistic link with enhanced presynaptic norepinephrine recycling was described.[108] Presynaptic sympathetic cardiac dysfunction was hypothesized, based on abnormal iodine-123 metaiodobenzylguanidine uptake, with bradycardia-dependent QT prolongation, intrinsic sinus node dysfunction, conduction abnormalities, and absence of ventricular ectopy.[109] The Brugada syndrome is genetically related to the long QT syndrome, which shares risk for lethal nocturnal ventricular arrhythmias,[110] a period when these patients exhibit abnormal levels of T-wave alternans.[31,111]

In the United States 117 SUNDS deaths were registered among male Southeast Asian immigrants or their descendants from 1981 to 1988.[112] Autopsies of those who died of SUNDS have established that cardiovascular disease is absent, but, in some instances, conduction pathways are developmentally abnormal.[107] Companions have reported that the immediate symptoms are onset of agonal respirations during sleep, along with vocalization; violent motor activity; nonarousability; rapid, irregular, deep breathing; perspiration; heart rate surges; and severe autonomic discharge. Several victims revived by vigorous massage reported sensations of airway obstruction, chest discomfort or pressure, and numb and weak limbs. When these symptoms recurred within weeks to months, they culminated in death.[113] Three victims who had been resuscitated from ventricular fibrillation then experienced recurring fibrillation in the hospital during sleep, accompanied by similar moaning vocalizations. In these three patients there was no evidence of atherosclerosis or structural abnormalities and no sleep apnea, but creatine kinase levels were markedly elevated, and potassium was depressed. Vagal tone is lower in SUNDS survivors than in healthy individuals, particularly at night.[114]

Therapy

Development of effective therapy for these syndromes has been particularly challenging. Currently, implantation of cardioverter–defibrillators appears to be the most effective approach in patients with Brugada syndrome[80] or at risk of SUNDS.[107]

SLEEP-DISRUPTING EFFECTS OF CARDIAC MEDICATIONS

Several important medications that are widely prescribed for patients with cardiac disease, including antihypertensive agents and beta blockers that cross the blood-brain barrier, have the potential to disrupt sleep.[23] In particular, the lipophilic beta blockers (pindolol, propranolol, and metoprolol) increase the total number of awakenings and total wakefulness compared with placebo and with the nonlipophilic atenolol. Penetration of the blood-brain barrier occurs with prolonged therapy, when these distinctions may become less apparent. In addition, pindolol, which has intrinsic sympathomimetic activity, increases REM latency and, as a result, decreases REM sleep time. Sleep disruption may provoke daytime fatigue and lethargy, symptoms widely reported by patients taking beta blockers, which may prompt discontinuation of the medication or noncompliance. It has been postulated that the mechanism of sleep disruption by beta-blocking agents is their well-known tendency to deplete endogenous melatonin,[115] a key sleep-regulating hormone that modulates sympathetic nerve activity. An additional important side effect of these beta blockers[23] is their potential to provoke nightmares. Despite these effects, it is the lipophilic beta blockers (propranolol, metoprolol, carvedilol) that have been shown to reduce the risk of sudden cardiac death.

Sleep disturbance has also been documented in conjunction with the widely used antiarrhythmic agent amiodarone.[116,117] Neurologic side effects were attributed to amiodarone in 20% to 40% of patients. Optimal antiarrhythmic management with this agent to minimize side effects dictates prescription of lower dosages and close patient monitoring and follow-up.

CLINICAL PEARL

Diagnosing and treating patients with nocturnal arrhythmias have been hampered by a paucity of information about concurrent autonomic nervous system activity, cardiac electrical instability, oxygen desaturation, and breathing disturbances. It is now possible to assess autonomic nervous system activity by ambulatory electrocardiographic monitoring of noninvasive markers, such as heart rate variability, a measure of autonomic nervous system tone, and heart rate turbulence, an indicator of baroreceptor function based on the pattern of heart rhythm recovery after a ventricular premature beat.[118] Simultaneous measurement of these indicators on continuous electrocardiographic monitoring, along with clinical history and analysis of cardiac electrical instability with QT-interval dispersion[15,16] or T-wave alternans,[31] promises to provide valuable information regarding vulnerability to nocturnal arrhythmias and potential provocation by the autonomic nervous system. Concurrent monitoring of oxygen saturation and respiratory patterns will provide essential information. Increased survival from in-hospital nighttime cardiac arrest can be anticipated with improved monitoring.[119]

SUMMARY

Because the etiology of nocturnal arrhythmias is multifactorial, their management necessitates a comprehensive approach and consideration of a host of cardiovascular and respiratory factors. Treatment must be tailored to contain neurally induced arrhythmias while avoiding exacerbation of hypotension and myocardial ischemia during NREM sleep.

ACKNOWLEDGMENTS

The authors thank Sandra S. Verrier for her editorial contributions.

SELECTED READINGS

Bitter T, Fox H, Gaddam S, et al. Sleep-disordered breathing and cardiac arrhythmias. *Can J Cardiol.* 2015;31:928–934.

Delisle BP, Stumpf JL, Wayland JL, et al. Circadian clocks regulate cardiac arrhythmia susceptibility, repolarization, and ion channels. *Curr Opin Pharmacol.* 2021;57:13–20.

Guilleminault CP, Pool P, Motta J, et al. Sinus arrest during REM sleep in young adults. *N Engl J Med.* 1984;311:1006–1010.

Huang B, Liu H, Scherlag BJ, et al. Atrial fibrillation in obstructive sleep apnea: neural mechanisms and emerging therapies. *Trends Cardiovasc Med.* 2021;31(2):127–132.

Javaheri S, Barbe F, Campos-Rodriguez F, et al. Sleep apnea: types, mechanisms, and clinical cardiovascular consequences. *J Am Coll Cardiol.* 2017;69(7):841–858.

Kinney HC, Filiano JJ, Sleeper LA, et al. Decreased muscarinic receptor binding in the arcuate nucleus in sudden infant death syndrome. *Science.* 1995;269:1446–1450.
Lin GM, Colangelo LA, Lloyd-Jones DM, et al. Association of sleep apnea and snoring with incident atrial fibrillation in the Multi-Ethnic Study of Atherosclerosis. *Am J Epidemiol.* 2015;182:49–57.
Linz D, Nattel S, Kalman JM, Sanders P. Sleep Apnea and Atrial Fibrillation. *Card Electrophysiol Clin.* 2021;13(1):87–94. https://doi.org/10.1016/j.ccep.2020.10.003.
Maan A, Mansour M, Anter E, et al. Obstructive sleep apnea and atrial fibrillation: pathophysiology and implications for treatment. *Crit Pathw Cardiol.* 2015;14:81–85.
Mancia G. Autonomic modulation of the cardiovascular system during sleep. *N Engl J Med.* 1993;328:347–349.
Marcondes L, Crawford J, Earle N, et al. Long QT molecular autopsy in sudden unexplained death in the young (1-40 years old): Lessons learnt from an eight year experience in New Zealand. *PLoS One.* 2018;13(4):e0196078.
May AM, Van Wagoner DR, Mehra R. OSA and cardiac arrhythmogenesis: mechanistic insights. *Chest.* 2017;151(1):225–241.
Priori SG, Wilde AA, Horie M, et al. HRS/EHRA/APHRS expert consensus statement on the diagnosis and management of patients with inherited primary arrhythmia syndromes: document endorsed by HRS, EHRA, and APHRS in May 2013 and by ACCF, AHA, PACES, and AEPC in June 2013. *Heart Rhythm.* 2013;10:1932–1963.
Schwartz PJ, Stramba-Badiale M, Segantini A, et al. Prolongation of the QT interval and the sudden infant death syndrome. *N Engl J Med.* 1998;338:1709–1714.
Smolensky MH, Hermida RC, Geng YJ. Chronotherapy of cardiac and vascular disease: timing medications to circadian rhythms to optimize treatment effects and outcomes. *Curr Opin Pharmacol.* 2021;57:41–48.
Verrier RL, Klingenheben T, Malik M, et al. Microvolt T-wave alternans: physiologic basis, methods of measurement, and clinical utility. Consensus guideline by the International Society for Holter and Noninvasive Electrocardiology. *J Am Coll Cardiol.* 2011;44:1309–1324.

A complete reference list can be found online at ExpertConsult.com.

Chapter 146

Cardiovascular Effects of Sleep-Related Breathing Disorders

Virend K. Somers; Shahrokh Javaheri

Chapter Highlights

- The cycle of apnea and recovery causes hypoxemia and reoxygenation, hypercapnia and hypocapnia, changes in intrathoracic pressure, and arousals. These consequences of sleep apnea, both obstructive and central apnea, adversely affect cardiovascular function. The cardiovascular effects of sleep apnea may be mediated by redox-sensitive gene activation, altered autonomic nervous system activity, oxidative stress, and release of inflammatory mediators. Pathophysiologic consequences of sleep apnea elicit acute and chronic cardiovascular changes.
- Hypoxemia has direct (decreased myocardial oxygen delivery and impaired diastolic dysfunction) and indirect (activation of sympathetic nervous system, promotion of endothelial cell dysfunction, and pulmonary arteriolar vasoconstriction) cardiac and vascular effects. Reoxygenation may cause additional damage through further production of free radical species. Hypoxemia-reoxygenation, with intermittent alterations in the partial pressure of oxygen (Po_2), may occur hundreds of times during sleep.
- Because of potentiated chemoreflex responses to hypoxemia-hypercapnia, the sympathetic and consequent presser responses to hypoxemia-hypercapnia and arousals, particularly in the absence of inhibitory effects of breathing, are marked. Nighttime sympathetic activation carries over into daytime wakefulness.
- Large negative intrathoracic pressures are generated during episodes of obstructive apnea, to a less extent during hyperventilation after central apnea, particularly in the presence of a poorly compliant respiratory system, which increases the transmural pressure (pressure inside minus pressure outside) of the intrathoracic vascular structures, including aorta, pulmonary vascular bed, atria, and ventricles.
- Bradycardias may be especially severe and are elicited because of activation of the diving reflex by the combination of hypoxemia and apnea. Episodes of up to 10 seconds or more of sinus arrest may occur because of chemoreflex-mediated vagal activation.
- Sleep apnea has been implicated in systolic and diastolic heart failure, ventricular arrhythmias, and atrial fibrillation. Whether treating obstructive sleep apnea prevents heart failure and arrhythmias or improves survival remains to be determined from randomized controlled trials.
- The largest randomized controlled trial of continuous positive airway pressure (CPAP) in patients with established cardiovascular disease (the SAVE trial) did not show cardiovascular benefit of CPAP on intention-to-treat analysis. Adaptive servo-ventilation therapy for central sleep apnea has been associated with increased cardiovascular mortality (SERVE-HF). However, there are important pitfalls in both aforementioned trials.

Sleep breathing disorders are characterized by cyclic changes in tidal breathing with intervening episodes of obstructive or central apnea or hypopnea. These disordered breathing events result in three basic pathophysiologic consequences: (1) intermittent arterial blood gas abnormalities characterized by hypoxemia-reoxygenation and hypercapnia-hypocapnia, (2) arousals and a shift to light sleep stages, and (3) large negative swings in intrathoracic pressure (Figure 146.1).[1-3] These pathophysiologic consequences of apnea and hypopnea, both obstructive and central, adversely affect cardiovascular function, acutely and chronically.

ARTERIAL BLOOD GAS ABNORMALITIES AND THEIR CONSEQUENCES

Periodic breathing consists of cyclic changes in breathing pattern that include episodes of apnea and hypopnea, resulting in hypoxemia and hypercapnia. After apnea and hypopnea,

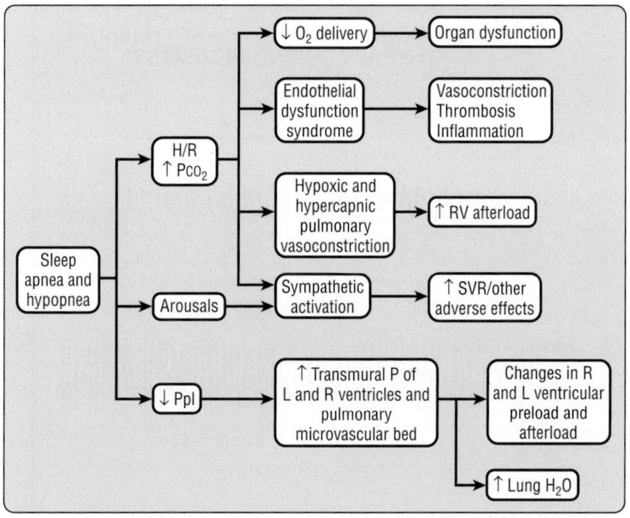

Figure 146.1 Pathophysiologic consequences of sleep apnea and hypopnea. Pleural pressure (Ppl) is a surrogate of the pressure surrounding the heart and other vascular structures. H/R, Hypoxia-reoxygenation; L, left; P, pressure; R, right; RV, right ventricular; SVR, systemic vascular resistance; ↑, increased; ↓, decreased. (Modified from Javaheri S. Sleep-related breathing disorders in heart failure. In: Mann DL, ed. *Heart Failure: A Companion to Braunwald's Heart Disease.* Saunders; 2003:478.)

hyperpnea ensues, resulting in reoxygenation and hypocapnia. These alterations in blood gases affect the cardiovascular system in different ways.

Hypoxemia and Reoxygenation

Hypoxemia has direct (decreased myocardial oxygen delivery) and indirect (activation of sympathetic nervous system, promotion of endothelial cell dysfunction, and pulmonary arteriolar vasoconstriction) cardiac and vascular effects. Hypoxemia with reoxygenation may be analogous to ischemia with reperfusion, and reoxygenation may cause additional damage through further production of free radical species. Biochemical injury resulting from hypoxemia-reoxygenation has considerable relevance to sleep apnea-hypopnea, where intermittent and profound alterations in the partial pressure of oxygen (Po_2) may occur hundreds of times during sleep.

Direct Effects of Hypoxia on Myocardium

Decreased myocardial oxygen delivery may result in an imbalance between myocardial oxygen consumption and demand, resulting in myocardial hypoxia, particularly if there is already coronary artery disease. At the same time, myocardial oxygen demand may be elevated because of concomitant tachycardia. Potential clinical consequences of myocardial hypoxia include nocturnal angina, nocturnal myocardial infarction,[4] arrhythmias, and even nocturnal sudden death.[5] Hypoxia may also impair myocardial contractility and cause diastolic dysfunction.[6]

Hypoxemia-Reoxygenation and Coronary Endothelial Dysfunction

Coronary vessel endothelial cells play a central role in vasoregulation, coagulation, and inflammation.[7] Blood flow and coagulation are modulated by production and release of vasoactive substances that include vasodilators and platelet deaggregators (e.g., nitric oxide, prostacyclin) and vasoconstrictors and platelet aggregators (e.g., endothelin and thromboxane). The balance between vasoregulatory agents is important in modulating coronary blood flow and coagulation status in both health and disease.

Through activation of certain transcription factors such as hypoxia-inducible factor-1 and nuclear factor-κB,[8,9] hypoxia increases the expression of a number of genes such as those encoding endothelin-1, a potent vasoconstrictor with proinflammatory properties, vascular endothelial growth factor, and platelet-derived growth factor. In contrast, it suppresses the transcriptional rate of endothelial nitric oxide synthase,[10] resulting in decreased production of nitric oxide, which is vasodilatory and has antimitogenic properties. Hypoxia also enhances expression of adhesion molecules and promotes leukocyte rolling and endothelial adherence,[11] and it is involved in induction of endothelial and myocyte apoptosis.[12]

Some of the aforementioned adverse effects of sustained hypoxia have also been observed with intermittent hypoxia (i.e., hypoxia-reoxygenation).[13-23] In this context, intermittent hypoxia has been proposed to be more deleterious than sustained hypoxia.[18,19] Reoxygenation through delivery of oxygen molecules provides a substrate for additional production of oxygen radicals and may contribute to oxidative stress.

The pathophysiologic consequences of hypoxemia-reoxygenation could lead to vascular inflammation and remodeling, similar to atherosclerosis.[7,23] Endothelial dysfunction has been demonstrated in a number of cardiovascular disorders, including hypertension, myocardial infarction, and stroke, and has also been reported in healthy young subjects who have been sleep deprived.[24] Interestingly, these cardiovascular disorders have been also associated with obstructive sleep apnea (OSA). It is therefore conceivable that endothelial dysfunction caused by sleep-related breathing disorders may contribute to worsening of atherosclerosis, atherothrombosis, and left ventricular dysfunction.[1,25]

The inflammatory and neurohormonal (see Obstructive Sleep Apnea and Systolic Heart Failure, later) consequences of altered blood gas chemistry have been best studied in patients with OSA, which is associated with increased sympathetic activity, high concentrations of endothelin, adhesion molecules, inflammatory cytokines, activation of white blood cells, oxidative stress, endothelial dysfunction, and hypercoa gulopathy.[1,22,25-40] These autonomic, biochemical, and functional alterations may be reversed with use of nasal continuous positive airway pressure (CPAP) to treat OSA. However, such systematic studies are lacking for central sleep apnea, with the exception of studies showing increased overnight and morning sympathetic activity and increased concentration of endothelin and brain natriuretic peptide in patients with heart failure with central sleep apnea compared with those without central sleep apnea (for details, see Chapter 149).[41]

Hypoxemia-Hypercapnia and the Autonomic Nervous System

Sleep apneas and hypopneas, both obstructive and central (Figures 146.2 and 146.3), increase sympathetic activity through complex mechanisms. Hypoxemia stimulates the peripheral arterial chemoreceptors in the carotid bodies, triggering reflex increases in sympathetic activity.[42,43] Hypercapnia stimulates the peripheral and the central chemoreceptors located in the region of the brainstem, also increasing sympathetic activity.

Both hypoxemia and hypercapnia increase ventilation, which, acting through thoracic afferents, buffers the increases in sympathetic drive during hypoxemia and to a lesser extent

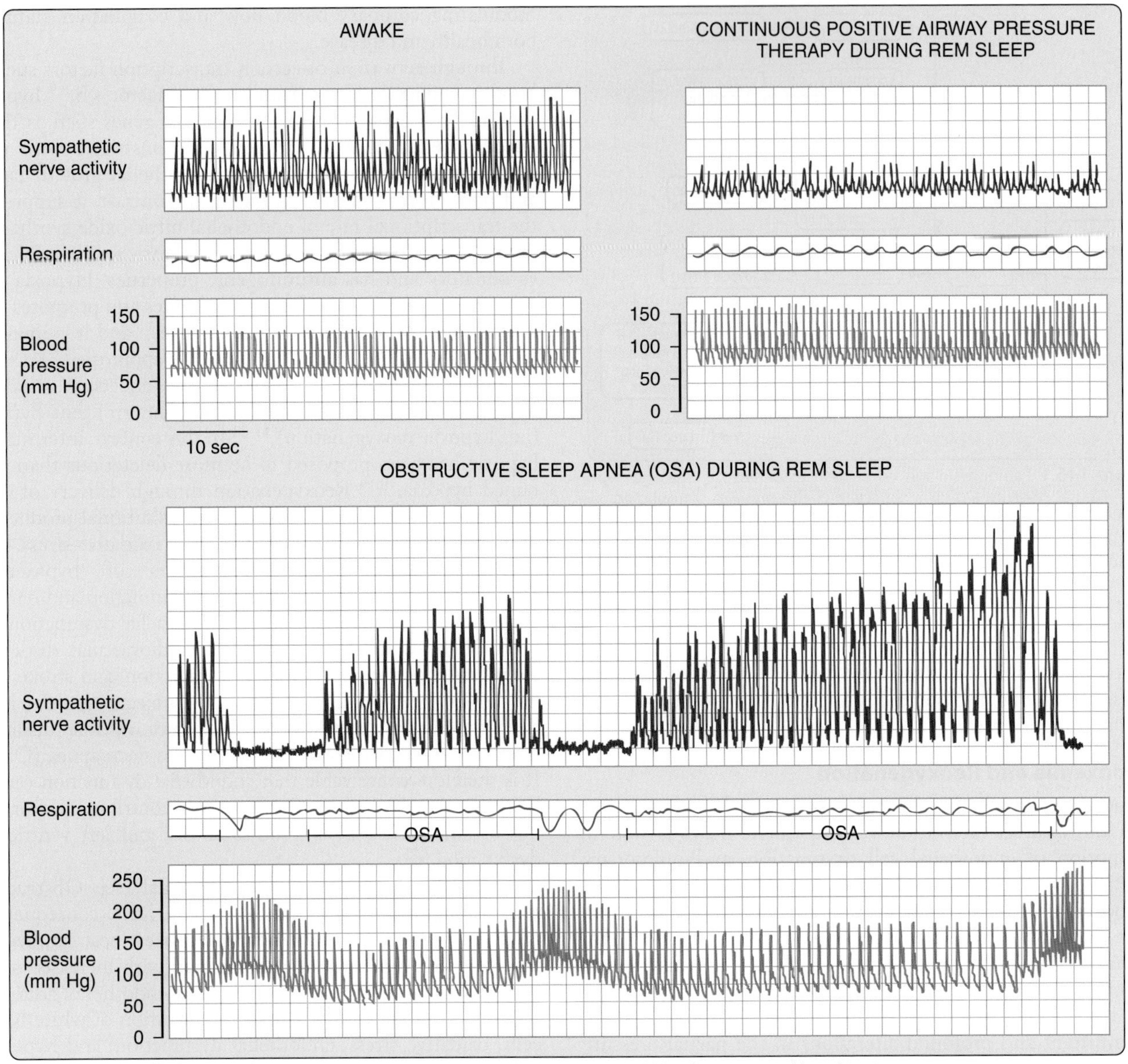

Figure 146.2 Recordings of sympathetic nerve activity, intraarterial blood pressure, and breathing in a normotensive patient with obstructive sleep apnea (OSA) during resting normoxic wakefulness (*top left*). The patient was free of any other overt cardiovascular disease and on no medications. Note the high levels of sympathetic nerve traffic even in the absence of apneic events. During rapid eye movement (REM) sleep (*bottom*), the repetitive hypoxemia and hypercapnia elicit chemoreflex-mediated sympathetic activation and vasoconstriction. At the end of apneas, with increases in cardiac output and severe vasoconstriction, intraarterial blood pressure can reach levels from 130/60 mm Hg during wakefulness to a peak of 220/130 mm Hg during apneas. At the end of apneas, there also is abrupt inhibition of sympathetic traffic because of the increase in blood pressure acting through the baroreflexes and the sympathetic inhibitory effects of the thoracic afferents. After treatment of OSA with continuous positive airway pressure (*top right*), there is a marked reduction in sympathetic traffic and in blood pressure. (From Somers VK, Dyken ME, Clary MP, et al. Sympathetic neural mechanisms in obstructive sleep apnea. *J Clin Invest.* 1995;96:1897–904.)

during hypercapnia.[42,43] Thus, when hypoxemia or hypercapnia occurs during apnea, the absence of ventilatory inhibition results in a potentiation of sympathetic activation and consequent vasoconstriction and blood pressure surges. In this context, and especially when there are potentiated chemoreflex responses to hypoxemia-hypercapnia,[44,45] the sympathetic and consequent pressor responses to hypoxemia-hypercapnia, particularly in the absence of inhibitory effects of breathing, are marked.

Nighttime sympathetic activation carries over into daytime wakefulness. Repetitive hypoxemia may be implicated because after 2 weeks of chronic intermittent hypoxemia, healthy normal subjects manifested an increase in sympathetic outflow, together with increased chemoreflex gain and blunted baroreflex function.[46]

Alveolar Hypoxia-Hypercapnia and Pulmonary Arteriolar Vasoconstriction

Alveolar hypoxia, in part through release of endothelin, and hypercapnia cause pulmonary arteriolar vasoconstriction and hypertension, which could adversely affect right ventricular function (see Chapter 147).

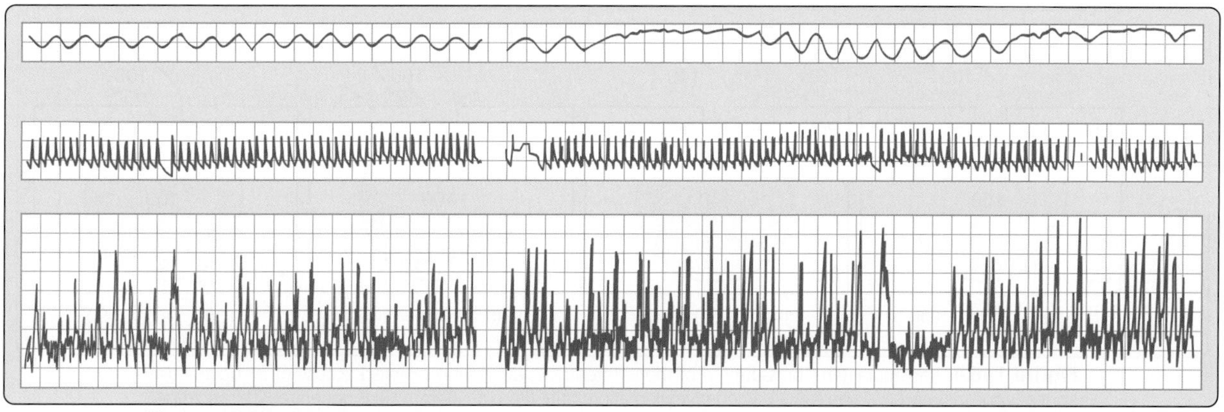

Figure 146.3 Recordings of breathing (*top*), beat-by-beat blood pressure (*middle*), and muscle sympathetic nerve activity (MSNA) (*bottom*) in a patient with severe congestive heart failure, during normal breathing on the *left* and during Cheyne-Stokes breathing on the *right*. Oxygen saturation was 94% during normal breathing and oscillated between 97% and 90% during Cheyne-Stokes breathing. MSNA total burst amplitude increased from 1533 arbitrary units per minute during normal breathing to 1759 arbitrary units per minute during Cheyne-Stokes breathing. Mean blood pressure was 70 mm Hg during normal breathing and peaked at 82 mm Hg during the hyperventilation that followed central apnea. Patients with heart failure have high levels of sympathetic drive even during normal breathing. During central apneas, there is a modest but significant further increase in sympathetic activity. (From Van de Borne P, Oren R, Abouassaly C, et al. Effect of Cheyne-Stokes respiration on muscle sympathetic nerve activity in severe congestive heart failure secondary to ischemic or idiopathic dilated cardiomyopathy. *Am J Cardiol.* 1998;81:432–6.)

Hypocapnia

Episodes of hyperpnea after apneas and hypopneas result in hypocapnia. Hypocapnia may impair myocardial oxygen delivery and uptake by coronary artery vasoconstriction[46] and shifting of the oxygen-hemoglobin dissociation curve to the left. Hypocapnia may also contribute to arrhythmogenesis.

AROUSALS, SHIFT TO LIGHT SLEEP STAGES, AND THE AUTONOMIC NERVOUS SYSTEM

Compared with wakefulness, the balance of activity of sympathetic and parasympathetic nervous system reverses in normal sleep.[47,48] Normally, there is a progressive reduction in sympathetic nerve traffic, heart rate, and blood pressure during the deepening stages of non–rapid eye movement sleep, such that sympathetic activity, heart rate, and blood pressure in stage 4 sleep are substantially lower than during supine resting wakefulness.[47,48] During phasic rapid eye movement (REM) sleep, there is an abrupt increase in sympathetic activity, resulting in intermittent and brief surges in blood pressure and heart rate. On average, blood pressure and heart rate during REM sleep are similar to levels recorded during wakefulness. Thus, during normal sleep, there is a well-regulated pattern of alteration in autonomic and hemodynamic measures, modulated by changes in sleep stage. These organized responses to normal sleep are disrupted in patients with sleep-related breathing disorders, both obstructive and central sleep apnea. Sleep architecture is dramatically altered in patients with OSA-hypopnea and in patients with heart failure and central sleep apnea. There is a shift to light sleep stages. Most important, however, apneas and hypopneas commonly result in arousals that are also associated with an increase in sympathetic activity and a decrease in parasympathetic activity,[48,49] and increasing blood pressure and heart rate. In OSA, arousals occur at the end of the apnea and with resumption of breathing. In patients with central sleep apnea and Hunter-Cheyne-Stokes breathing pattern, arousals occur at the peak of hyperventilation.

In addition to arousals, sleep-related breathing disorders may increase sympathetic activity by hypoxemia, hypercapnia, and changes in ventilation, as noted previously.

There are multiple adverse cardiac consequences of sympathetic activation. These include increased systemic vascular resistance and left ventricular afterload, venoconstriction with increased right ventricular preload, increased myocardial contractility, hypertrophy, tachycardia, and arrhythmias. Furthermore, increased myocardial norepinephrine may cause myocyte toxicity and apoptosis.[50,51]

Central sleep apnea and OSA increase sympathetic activity as measured by either microneurography or blood and urinary norepinephrine levels.[52-57] Treatment of obstructive[55-57] and central sleep apnea[53,58] decreases sympathetic activity, with important implications. First, with regard to central sleep apnea in heart failure, increased sympathetic activity is associated with poor survival; therefore a reduction in sympathetic activity should have favorable prognostic implications. OSA causes nocturnal increases in sympathetic activity and blood pressure, which carry over into the daytime. OSA is a known cause of hypertension, and in some patients blood pressure decreases relatively quickly with effective treatment of OSA with CPAP (see Chapter 130).

In summary, pathophysiologic consequences of sleep-related breathing disorders, such as increased periods of wakefulness (interruption insomnia), arousals, hypoxemia, and hypercapnia, collectively contribute to increased sympathetic activity.

EXAGGERATED NEGATIVE INTRATHORACIC PRESSURE AND ITS CONSEQUENCES

Large negative intrathoracic pressures are generated during episodes of obstructive apnea. In central sleep apnea, relatively large negative pressure deflections occur during hyperpnea, particularly in the face of less compliant (stiff) lungs (resulting from heart failure). However, pleural pressure changes are

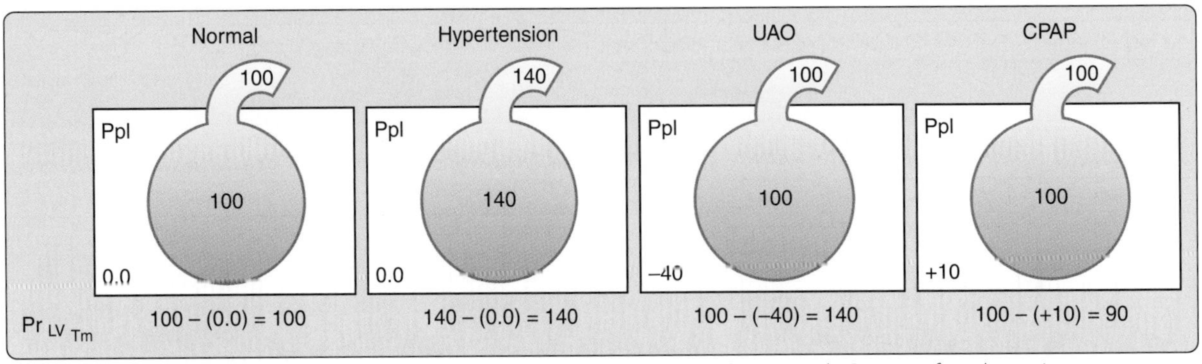

Figure 146.4 Transmural (Tm) pressure (Pr) of the left ventricle (LV) during systole. Because of an obstructive apnea (upper airway occlusion [UAO]), a negative pleural pressure (Ppl) of –40 mm Hg is generated. This increases left ventricular transmural pressure from 100 to 140 mm Hg, which is equivalent to an increase in systolic aortic blood pressure from 100 to 140 mm Hg. Note the reduction in left ventricular transmural pressure with application of nasal continuous positive airway pressure (CPAP). (Modified from Javaheri S. Sleep-related breathing disorders in heart failure. In: Mann DL, ed. *Heart Failure: A Companion to Braunwald's Heart Disease.* Saunders; 2003:480.)

usually more pronounced in obstructive than in central sleep apnea.

A number of studies have addressed the cardiovascular consequences of both negative and positive pressure deflections affecting right and left ventricular function.[59,60] Negative intrathoracic pressure increases the transmural pressure (pressure inside minus pressure outside) (Figure 146.4) of the intrathoracic vascular structures, including aorta, pulmonary vascular bed, atria, and ventricles. Larger-than-normal negative swings in intrathoracic pressure also occur during hyperventilation after central apnea, particularly in subjects with heart failure with a less compliant respiratory system.

According to Laplace's law, increased transmural myocardial pressure increases wall tension and myocardial oxygen consumption. Furthermore, negative intrathoracic perivascular pressure could increase extravascular lung water by favoring fluid transudation across the pulmonary microvascular bed and by diminishing lymph outflow from the lung.[61] This may account in part for cases of flash pulmonary edema reported in OSA, and sleep apnea may contribute to excess lung water and pulmonary edema in congestive heart failure. In addition, decreased intrathoracic pressure increases venous inflow, resulting in increased right ventricular diastolic filling, which in turn may decrease left ventricular compliance and volume, a phenomenon called ventricular interdependence. Application of nasal CPAP to treat sleep apnea, both obstructive and central, reduces transmural pressure by two mechanisms. First, and most important, it decreases or eliminates apneas, desaturation, and arousals, which, as noted previously, collectively increase sympathetic activity and result in cyclic surges in arterial blood pressure. Second, nasal CPAP not only attenuates steep surges in intrathoracic pressure but also actually increases the pleural pressure, thus decreasing transmural pressures across intrathoracic structures (Figure 146.4).

ACUTE HEMODYNAMIC EFFECTS OF SLEEP APNEA

The circulatory responses to individual apneas and hypopneas are governed by the interaction of stresses and physiologic consequences described previously.[62,63] Hemodynamic changes are related to development of hypoxemia, hypercapnia, presence or absence of breathing, changes in intrathoracic pressure, and the consequent mechanical effects.

Hemodynamic changes have been best studied in human OSA.[62,64,65] The evolution of a cycle of apnea and recovery is complex and represents an unsteady hemodynamic state. For these reasons, hemodynamic changes occur during the course of an apnea, and these changes are different from those occurring during the immediate or late postapneic periods. During recovery, arousals and ventilation further affect hemodynamics. Cyclic changes in heart rate and systemic and pulmonary arterial blood pressure paralleling periodic breathing occur commonly.[62,64-67] In some patients, there is a very clear and progressive bradycardia toward the end of apnea, with abrupt development of tachycardia with resumption of breathing, because of the vagolytic effects of lung inflation and arousals. This manifests as a pattern of repetitive bradycardias or tachycardias during sleep, which may be evident on Holter monitoring and may signify the presence of OSA. In experimental sleep apnea, decreases in heart rate are more severe during central than obstructive apnea, reflecting lack of activation of thoracic afferents.[63]

The bradycardias may be especially severe,[66,67] and they are elicited because of activation of the diving reflex by the combination of hypoxemia and apnea. Episodes of up to 10 seconds or more of sinus arrest may occur because of the chemoreflex-mediated vagal activation. The consequent absence of perfusion, because of asystole, may have implications for patients with preexisting severe cerebral or cardiac ischemia.

At the termination of obstructive apneas, there are surges in blood pressure. This cyclic change in blood pressure is one of the most consistent hemodynamic findings in patients with OSA. Multiple mechanisms are involved. During apnea, the increased hypoxemia and hypercapnia, acting through the chemoreflexes, progressively elicit sympathetic activation and vasoconstriction.[54] With resumption of breathing, because of the inspiratory increase in right ventricular filling, stroke volume may increase. Vagolytic effects of inspiration result in tachycardia. The increased stroke volume and heart rate result in an increased cardiac output entering a vasoconstricted peripheral circulation, with consequent acute increases in blood pressure.[54] However, just after termination of an obstructive apnea, there is abrupt inhibition of sympathetic activity to the peripheral blood vessels, in part because the deep breathing inhibits sympathetic activity through thoracic afferents and in part because of baroreflex inhibition of sympathetic activity secondary to the postapneic blood pressure surge. Nevertheless, despite the interruption in sympathetic nerve traffic, vasoconstriction persists for several seconds after termination of the sympathetic nerve discharge because of the kinetics of norepinephrine uptake, release, and washout at the neurovascular junction.

Another consistent finding is a mild reduction in stroke volume during obstructive apnea, which has been documented using noninvasive techniques for measuring beat-to-beat cardiac output.[62] This probably results from a decrease in left ventricular preload and an increase in afterload. Changes in stroke volume after termination of the apnea depend on where in the recovery cycle it is being measured.[62]

OBSTRUCTIVE SLEEP APNEA, LEFT VENTRICULAR DYSFUNCTION, AND HEART FAILURE

The relationship between central sleep apnea and heart failure is discussed in Chapter 149. In this section, we review OSA as a cause of heart failure.

Obstructive Sleep Apnea and Systolic Heart Failure

In a canine model mimicking severe OSA,[68] within a 1- to 3-month period of exposure to apneas during sleep, left ventricular systolic dysfunction developed. Left ventricular ejection fraction, measured during the daytime, decreased significantly because of an increase in left ventricular systolic volume.

In humans, there are two kinds of studies relating left ventricular systolic dysfunction and OSA—first, studies in which patients with OSA have been assessed for the presence of left ventricular dysfunction,[69-72] and second, studies in patients with established left ventricular systolic dysfunction who have been assessed to determine the prevalence of OSA.[73,74] In some studies,[75-77] changes in left ventricular ejection fraction in response to treatment for OSA have also been described.

Results of studies assessing left ventricular systolic function in OSA patients are conflicting.[69-71] However, in the two studies[70,71] in which technetium-99m was used to assess left ventricular systolic function, OSA was associated with left ventricular systolic dysfunction. Use of radionuclide ventriculography to assess left ventricular function is important because in obese subjects, echocardiography, which has been used in some studies, may be associated with technical difficulties.

Alchanatis and colleagues[70] studied 29 patients with severe OSA (apnea-hypopnea index [AHI] greater than 15/hour; mean AHI, 54/hour; lowest arterial oxygen saturation, 62%) and 12 control subjects (AHI, 9/hour; lowest saturation, 92%). The subjects were without known cardiovascular disease. The mean left ventricular ejection fraction was significantly lower in patients with OSA compared with the control group (53% versus 61%; $P < .003$). Six months after treatment with CPAP, left ventricular ejection fraction increased significantly to 56% ($P < .001$). Left ventricular diastolic dysfunction also improved significantly (see later).

In a large study[71] of 169 patients with OSA (AHI greater than 10/hour; mean AHI, 47/hour), 13 subjects (8%) had left ventricular systolic dysfunction (range, 32% to 50%). Left ventricular systolic dysfunction was not the result of ischemic disease as evidenced by echocardiography and dipyridamole stress testing. In seven patients who were treated for OSA (six with CPAP and one with upper airway surgery), 1 year after therapy, mean left ventricular ejection increased significantly from 44% to 63%.[71]

In the cross-sectional analysis of more than 6000 patients enrolled in the Sleep Health Heart Study,[72] the presence of OSA increased the likelihood of having a history of heart failure by an odds ratio of 2.5. Furthermore, there was a significant dose-dependent correlation between AHI and the prevalence of heart failure.

In studies of patients with established left ventricular systolic dysfunction undergoing polysomnography (reviewed in Chapter 149), the prevalence of OSA, defined as an AHI of at least 15/hour, ranged from 12% to 32%.[77] This wide range is not particularly surprising. The prevalence depends on a number of factors, including the number of obese patients with heart failure enrolled in each study and the different polysomnographic criteria used by various investigators for diagnosis of OSA. Another important issue is the difficulty in accurately classifying hypopneas into central versus obstructive, which is a determinant of prevalence of the phenotype of sleep-disordered breathing.

In a prospective study[73] of 81 patients with known systolic dysfunction and in whom no question was asked regarding snoring or other symptoms associated with OSA, 11% had OSA, with a mean AHI of 36/hour and lowest arterial oxygen saturation of 72%. In a retrospective study[74] of 450 patients with systolic dysfunction who were referred for a sleep study because of snoring and other symptoms of sleep apnea, 32% had OSA. From the aforementioned studies, however, it cannot be determined whether OSA preceded heart failure. Yet, as is discussed later, treatment of OSA with nasal CPAP increases left ventricular ejection fraction,[75,76] indicating that OSA contributes to worsening of left ventricular systolic dysfunction.

The mechanisms by which OSA may impair left ventricular systolic function are multiple. Hypoxemia plays a critical role, both by impairing myocardial contractility and through a host of neurohormonal mechanisms. In addition, increases in left ventricular wall stress and transmural pressure occur because of additive effects of the excess negative juxtacardiac pressure (during obstructive apneas) and development of hypertension.

The effects of positive airway pressure therapy on left ventricular ejection fraction in patients with OSA and systolic heart failure have been reported in five randomized clinical trials, two of which were double blind (Table 146.1). In three of the studies in which CPAP was used, including the only two double-blind randomized clinical trials, the rise in left ventricular fraction was minimal or not at all. It should be noted, however, that in at least two of these studies compliance with CPAP was also limited. In the two open studies in which compliance hours with CPAP were more than those in the double-blind studies, ejection fraction increased between 5% and 9%. In one open randomized clinical trial of CPAP versus a bilevel device, the ejection fraction increased significantly only with bilevel therapy.

Obstructive Sleep Apnea and Diastolic Heart Failure

Isolated left ventricular diastolic heart failure with relative preservation of left ventricular systolic function is the most common form of heart failure in elderly subjects. The pathophysiologic consequences of this form of heart failure relate

Table 146.1 Effects of Positive Airway Pressure Therapy on Left Ventricular Ejection Fraction in Patients with Obstructive Sleep Apnea and Systolic Heart Failure

Variable	Kaneko Open	Mansfield Open	Egea DB	Smith DB	Khayat Open	Khayat Open
n	12	19	20	23	11	13
AHI (*n*/hr)	40	25	44	36	30	34
LVEF (%)	25	35	29	30	29	26
Increase in LVEF (%)	9[a]	5[a]	2.2[a]	0.0	0.5	8.5[a]
Duration	4 wk	3 mo	3 mo	6 wk	3 mo	3 mo
PAP titration	CPAP yes	CPAP yes	CPAP yes	Auto CPAP	CPAP yes	Bilevel yes
Compliance (hr)	6.2	5.6	NR	3.5	3.6	4.5

[a]Indicates a statistically significant change.
AHI, Apnea-hypopnea index; CPAP, continuous positive airway pressure; DB, double blind; LVEF, left ventricular ejection fraction; NR, not reported; PAP, positive airway pressure.
Data from Kaneko Y, Flores JS, Usui K, et al. Cardiovascular effects of continuous positive airway pressure in patients with heart failure and obstructive sleep apnea. *N Engl J Med.* 2003;348:1233–41; Mansfield DR, Gollogly, NC, Kaye DM, et al. Controlled trial of continuous positive airway pressure in obstructive sleep apnea in heart failure. *Am J Respir Crit Care Med.* 2004;169:361–6; Egea CJ, Aizpuru F, Pinto JA, et al. Cardiac function after CPAP therapy in patients with chronic heart failure and sleep apnea: a multicenter study. *Sleep Med.* 2008;9:660–6; Schmidt LA, Vennelle M, Gardner RS, et al. Autotitrating continuous positive airway pressure therapy in patients with chronic heart failure and obstructive sleep apnea: a randomized placebo controlled trial. *Eur Heart J.* 2007;28:1221–7; Khayat RN, Abraham WT, Patt B, et al. Cardiac effects of continuous and bilevel crowded airway pressure for patients with heart failure and obstructive sleep apnea: a pilot study. *Chest.* 2008;134:1162–8.

to a hypertrophied, noncompliant left ventricle, shifting the pressure-volume curve upward and to the left. Therefore, for a given left ventricular volume, left ventricular end-diastolic pressure increases, resulting in elevated left atrial and pulmonary capillary pressure and in pulmonary congestion and edema.

As noted previously, hemodynamic studies[64,65] of patients with OSA have documented that pulmonary capillary pressure increases during the course of an obstructive apnea, indicating development of diastolic dysfunction. During obstructive apnea, left ventricular transmural wall tension increases because of an increase in aortic blood pressure and a simultaneous decrease in juxtacardiac pressure. Furthermore, hypoxemia may impair left ventricular relaxation, further impairing diastolic function.[78] Repeated exposure to nocturnal hypertension and hypoxemia and consequent development of OSA-induced systemic hypertension and increased left ventricular mass may also contribute to left ventricular diastolic dysfunction.

Most studies show that OSA is associated with an increase in left ventricular mass[79-82] and suggest that the OSA-related cardiac structural changes may resolve with CPAP treatment.[81] An early study[79] reported that OSA may cause left ventricular hypertrophy even in the absence of daytime systemic hypertension. This finding was later supported by another study[80] comparing patients with OSA (AHI > 20/hour) and those without OSA (AHI < 20/hour).

In the largest study,[82] consisting of 2058 Sleep Heart Health Study participants, left ventricular mass was associated with both apnea-hypopnea and hypoxemia indexes after adjustment for age, sex, ethnicity, study site, body mass index, smoking, systolic blood pressure, antihypertensive medication use, diabetes mellitus, myocardial infarction, and alcohol consumption. Although there are considerable data[73,74,83] regarding the prevalence of sleep apnea in patients with systolic heart failure (reviewed by Javaheri[77]), the prevalence of OSA in diastolic heart failure has been studied only in one large systematic study.[84] Bitter and colleagues evaluated 244 consecutive patients (87 women) with heart failure with a preserved ejection fraction (HFpEF). All underwent polygraphy, right heart catheterization, and echocardiography. The two major causes of HFpEF were systemic hypertension (44%) and coronary artery disease (33%). Forty-eight percent had an AHI of 15 or more per hour, a prevalence similar to that seen in patients with heart failure with a reduced ejection fraction (HFrEF). Among patients with an AHI of 15/hour or more, 23% had central sleep apnea. Consistent with the observation in HFrEF, patients with HFpEF and central sleep apnea had lower P_{CO_2} and higher left ventricular end-diastolic and pulmonary capillary wedge pressure than patients with OSA.

As noted earlier, isolated diastolic heart failure is highly prevalent in elderly subjects. Furthermore, elderly subjects have a high prevalence of OSA. It is speculated that OSA could be the cause of diastolic heart failure, or the presence of OSA could contribute to the worsening of left ventricular diastolic dysfunction. In this regard, a preliminary study reported that treatment of OSA improves left ventricular diastolic dysfunction,[70] an observation confirmed by the only randomized, placebo (sham CPAP)-controlled trial[81] showing that after 12 weeks on effective CPAP therapy, there was a significant increase in E/A ratio (the ratio of early to late diastolic filling) and a significant decrease in isovolumic relaxation and mitral deceleration. These observations are similar to the improvement seen in systolic function when patients with heart failure and OSA are treated with CPAP (Table 146.1).[75-77]

ARRHYTHMIAS IN OBSTRUCTIVE SLEEP APNEA

Obstructive Sleep Apnea Predisposing to an Arrhythmogenic Substrate

Repetitive nocturnal apneas elicit severe derangements in cardiovascular homeostasis. Hypoxemia, hypercapnia, acidosis, adrenergic activation, increased afterload, and rapid fluctuations in cardiac wall stress would reasonably be expected to be conducive to tachycardia-brachycardia oscillations and atrial and ventricular arrhythmias (Figures 146.5 and 146.6). A variety of atrioventricular arrhythmias, including complete heart block and ventricular asystole during sleep, have been

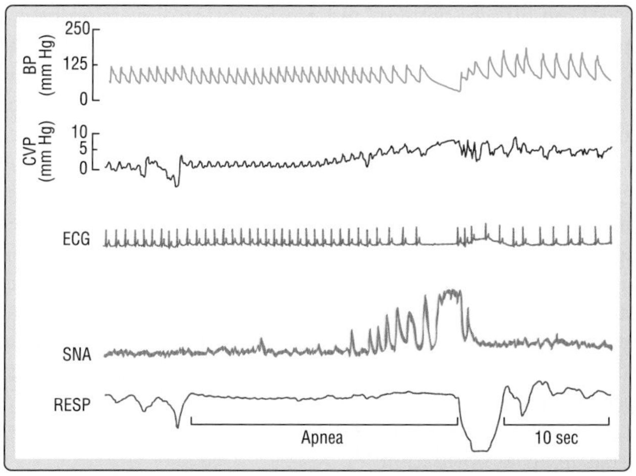

Figure 146.5 Recordings of intraarterial blood pressure (BP), central venous pressure (CVP), electrocardiogram (ECG), sympathetic nerve activity (SNA), and respiratory patterns (RESP) in a healthy subject during voluntary end-expiratory apnea. During apnea, there is a progressive increase in the RR interval on the ECG with eventual sinus pause and atrioventricular block. Accompanying this is increased sympathetic activity. The simultaneous sympathetic activation to peripheral blood vessels and vagal activation of the heart is characteristic of the diving reflex. Note the rapid increase in heart rate and sympathetic inhibition during resumption of breathing. This occurs in part because thoracic afferents activated by inspiration inhibit both sympathetic traffic and vagal cardiac drive. (From Somers VK, Dyken ME, Mark AL, Abboud FM. Parasympathetic hyperresponsiveness and bradyarrhythmias during apnea in hypertension. *Clin Auton Res.* 1992;2:171–6.)

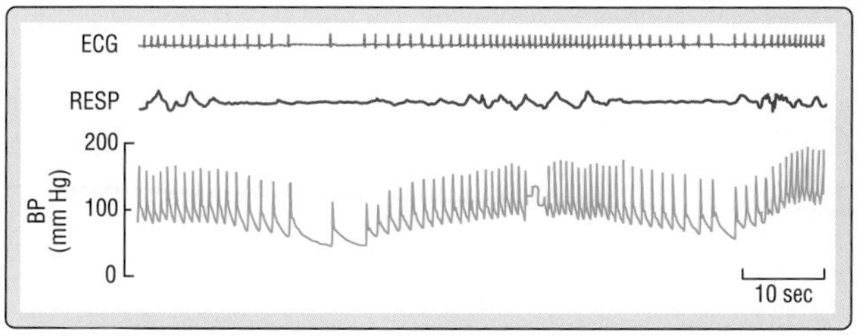

Figure 146.6 A patient with sleep apnea manifesting prolonged and profound bradyarrhythmias with absence of either atrial or ventricular contraction. The beat-by-beat blood pressure (BP) recording confirms the absence of any perfusion during the bradycardia. ECG, Electrocardiogram; RESP, respiratory pattern. (From Somers VK, Dyken ME, Mark AL, Abboud FM. Parasympathetic hyperresponsiveness and bradyarrhythmias during apnea in hypertension. *Clin Auton Res.* 1992;2:171–6.)

observed in patients with OSA[85-87] and have been eliminated by either tracheostomy or use of nasal CPAP.[85,86] Profound OSA-induced arrhythmias can occur in the absence of any major structural abnormalities in the conduction system.[88]

Although the normal heart would be less likely to manifest malignant arrhythmias in the setting of severe obstructive apnea, the ischemic, hypertrophied, or failing heart may be more susceptible.[89] Nevertheless, activation of the diving reflex[67,90] during apneas can often elicit severe bradyarrhythmias, even in the setting of a normal myocardium and normal cardiac electrophysiologic function.

Tachycardia-Bradycardia Oscillations

Patients undergoing Holter monitoring may be noted to have repetitive cyclic episodes of tachycardias and bradycardias during the night.[91,92] These cyclic fluctuations may be attributable to obstructive apneas, although this cannot be confirmed because standard Holter monitoring does not incorporate simultaneous measurements of either breathing pattern or oxygen saturation.

These oscillations in cardiac rate are for the most part explained by changes in cardiac autonomic drive related to breathing pattern. During the course of apnea, incremental hypoxemia elicits the diving reflex so that bradycardia becomes progressively more marked. With termination of apnea, hyperpnea occurs with consequent activation of thoracic afferents, which is vagolytic.[93] Thus, with resumption of breathing, abrupt lung inflation interrupts vagal drive to the heart, resulting in rapid-onset tachycardia. Furthermore, increased cardiac-bound sympathetic drive and withdrawal of parasympathetic activity because of arousals should also contribute to the tachycardia seen with termination of obstructive apnea. It is interesting that tachycardia persists even though blood pressure increases strikingly with termination of apnea. The vagolytic effects of inspiration and the arousal-associated changes in the autonomic nervous system not only interrupt the chemoreflex-mediated cardiac vagal drive but also blunt the expected cardiac vagal drive that would occur secondary to baroreflex activation by the postapneic surge in blood pressure.

Because of the repetitive nature of nocturnal apneas, Holter or other electrocardiographic monitoring at night manifests as a tachycardia-bradycardia pattern. This cardiac rate oscillation is less apparent in patients with autonomic dysfunction, such as patients with long-standing diabetes or cardiac transplant recipients with denervated hearts. Although the changes in cardiac rate are predominantly reflex mediated, breathing-related changes in cardiac filling, as well as rapid changes in cardiac transmural pressures resulting from the Müller maneuver, also modulate heart rate by variations in stretch of cardiac conduction tissue.

Bradyarrhythmias

The primary response to hypoxia is bradycardia.[90] When hypoxia is accompanied by the action of breathing, the bradycardic response is masked because of inhibition of cardiac vagal drive by ventilation.[67] The sympathetic response to hypoxemia, although evident to some extent during breathing, is also attenuated by ventilation and is therefore potentiated during apnea.[94,95] Patients with OSA may be particularly susceptible to hypoxia-induced bradyarrhythmias because their peripheral chemoreflex is heightened, so that even during voluntary apneas, hypoxemia elicits greater bradycardia than is seen in closely matched control subjects.[96] The arterial baroreflexes serve as an important buffer to diminish chemoreflex gain.[97] Impaired baroreflex sensitivity, such as is seen in hypertension[98] and heart failure,[99] may be associated with further increased chemoreflex drive. Thus patients with hypertension or heart failure who have OSA may manifest even greater sympathetic, and perhaps bradycardic, responses to obstructive apneas.

Profound bradyarrhythmias may have important consequences, particularly in patients with underlying cardiovascular disease. As an example, in the absence of recognition of OSA as a potential cause of the bradyarrhythmia, patients may receive pacemaker implantation, even though their cardiac conduction system may be completely normal and the bradyarrhythmias could be abolished by effective treatment with CPAP.[84,85,100] Second, prolonged episodes of asystole result in absence of perfusion (Figure 146.6). Absence of perfusion in the setting of apnea-induced hypoxemia, occurring repetitively through the night, may have important implications for ischemic damage to end organs in which there may already be preexisting circulatory compromise.

Ventricular Arrhythmias

There is an extensive literature on sleep apnea inducing nocturnal angina and cardiac ischemia evidenced by ST-segment depression.[101,102] Thus there is a potential contribution of OSA to ventricular arrhythmias through ventricular ectopy during profound bradycardia as well as polymorphic ventricular tachycardia resulting from cardiac hypoxia-ischemia. These episodes occur primarily with severe desaturation,[84,85] are more common in patients with coronary heart disease,[87] and are virtually eliminated with treatment.[84,85,100] The prevalence of these arrhythmias is low in patients without premorbid cardiorespiratory disease or severe desaturation.[103]

Atrial Fibrillation

In patients cardioverted for atrial fibrillation, those with polysomnographically proven OSA who were not receiving effective CPAP treatment had a 12-month recurrence rate of 82% compared with a 42% recurrence rate in patients with OSA receiving effective CPAP.[104] In patients cardioverted for atrial fibrillation in whom no sleep study had been done, the recurrence rate was 53%. This risk for recurrence in the patients with atrial fibrillation without a previous sleep study suggests that undiagnosed OSA may be present in a large proportion of patients with atrial fibrillation. In addition, among the untreated patients with OSA, those experiencing a recurrence of atrial fibrillation had more severe nocturnal hypoxemia than those without a recurrence. Furthermore, the increased recurrence in patients with untreated OSA could not be explained by factors such as antiarrhythmic medication, body mass index, hypertension, cardiac function, or atrial size.

Mooe and colleagues[105] observed that after coronary artery bypass surgery, patients with OSA were more likely to experience postoperative atrial fibrillation. However, it is not clear whether this was explained by other variables in the patients with OSA.

In a longitudinal study of several thousand patients, those with OSA had an increased risk for developing new-onset atrial fibrillation compared with those who did not have OSA. This risk was evident in patients aged 65 or younger, and it was especially marked in those with more severe nocturnal hypoxemia.[106] One study suggested that atrial fibrillation was more likely to occur in non-obese patients with severe OSA.[106a]

There are many reasons that OSA may be conducive to atrial fibrillation. Hypoxemia, presser surges, and sympathetic activation are all potential mechanisms leading to atrial fibrillation. High levels of C-reactive protein may also independently predict the development of atrial fibrillation.[107] Patients with OSA may have increased levels of C-reactive protein.[108-111] Furthermore, abrupt and dramatic changes in intrathoracic negative pressures may especially affect the atria because of their relatively thin walls compared with the ventricles. Increased pressure gradients with consequent increased atrial wall stretch, occurring repetitively through the night, may be expected to induce mechanical and electrical changes that are also conducive to atrial fibrillation.[112-114] Autonomic mechanisms may be pivotal. Animal models suggest that ganglionated plexus ablation may profoundly inhibit the development of atrial fibrillation in response to hypoxemia and apnea.[115]

About 50% of patients presenting for cardioversion have a high risk for sleep apnea compared with 30% of patients from a general cardiology clinic.[116] Even in patients with comorbid OSA undergoing pulmonary vein isolation, recurrence of atrial fibrillation is more than twofold greater in those not treated with CPAP compared with those receiving CPAP therapy.[117]

Technological advances, including in pacemakers, are enabling continuous monitoring and detection of both sleep apnea and of atrial fibrillation,[118] thus enabling dynamic simultaneous assessment of apnea as a trigger for atrial fibrillation, and whether atrial fibrillation begets apnea.[119] In any event, despite the promising data from observational studies of treating OSA on likelihood of atrial fibrillation, the unexpected findings of both the SERVE-HF[120] and SAVE[121] studies speak strongly to the need for randomized controlled trials in atrial fibrillation.[122]

Central Sleep Apnea and Heart Failure

The subject is covered in detail in Chapter 149. Even though central apneas are most pronounced during sleep, few studies have shown presence of oscillatory periodic breathing during wakefulness, and this carries a poor prognosis. The presence of periodic breathing in the upright awake position has been reported to be an important predictor of mortality in patients with heart failure. However, in none of the studies showing periodic breathing during wakefulness, were brain waves recorded. Without such information, it cannot be presumed definitively that central apnea during this time frame is synonymous with central apnea occurring during wakefulness.[123]

CLINICAL PEARLS

- Apnea and recovery cycles result in three basic abnormalities: alterations in blood gases, arousals, and changes in intrathoracic pressure.
- Hypoxemia-reoxygenation has deleterious effects on the cardiovascular system. This activates redox-sensitive genes, resulting in synthesis of vasoconstrictor and inflammatory mediators; increases sympathetic activity; and causes oxidative stress. These alterations have been best studied in patients with OSA.
- Untreated OSA may increase the risk for recurrence of atrial fibrillation after cardioversion.
- Sleep apnea can induce severe bradyarrhythmias, including prolonged periods of asystole and heart block, even in the setting of a normal myocardium and cardiac electrophysiologic function.
- OSA should be considered in patients who have ST-segment depression or angina occurring primarily at night.
- Heart failure may be significantly linked to the presence of either central sleep apnea or OSA.

SUMMARY

Sleep-related breathing disorders affect cardiovascular function in a variety of ways. OSA and central sleep apnea act through multiple mechanisms to elicit acute circulatory responses, which have implications for the development of chronic vascular and cardiac dysfunction. The acute responses to apnea are mediated in large part by the effects of apnea on blood gas chemistry, which exerts important cardiovascular effects directly on the myocardium and blood vessels and also acts through reflex mechanisms. Acute neural, circulatory, endothelial, inflammatory, and other responses to repetitive nocturnal hypoxemia and hypercapnia may act to induce long-term damage to the myocardium and to the coronary and other vascular beds. With the development of functional and structural cardiovascular disease, the consequences of acute apneas are magnified. For example, severe hypoxemia in the setting of sleep apnea is more easily tolerated by an overtly healthy cardiovascular system compared with one in which myocardial ischemia or left ventricular dysfunction is present, with consequent diminished cardiovascular reserve. Small, short-term studies have suggested that effective prevention of recurrent apneas may favorably affect surrogates of cardiovascular disease outcome, such as sympathetic activity, blood pressure, and left ventricular ejection fraction. The importance of large randomized controlled trials in establishing the benefits, if any, of treating sleep apnea in patients with heart failure is highlighted by the negative results of the recently completed SERVE-HF[120] study (examining effect of ASV in heart failure) and the SAVE[121] study (examining the effect of CPAP in OSA). Both these trials had important short fallings, which are reviewed in more detail in Chapter 149. It is important to note that the findings of the SERVE-HF cannot be extended to patients with heart failure with preserved ejection fraction, or other noncardiac causes of CSA.

SELECTED READINGS

Cowie MR, Linz D, Redline S, Somers VK, Simonds AK. Sleep disordered breathing and cardiovascular disease: JACC state-of-the-art review. *J Am Coll Cardiol.* 2021;78(6):608–624.

Cowie MR, Woehrle H, Wegscheider K, et al. Adaptive servo-ventilation for central sleep apnea in systolic heart failure. *N Engl J Med.* 2015;373(12):1095–1105.

Giannoni A, Gentile F, Sciarrone P, et al. Upright Cheyne-Stokes respiration in patients with heart failure. *J Am Coll Cardiol.* 2020;75:2934–2946.

Javaheri S, Barbe F, Campos-Rodriguez F, et al. Sleep apnea: types, mechanisms, and clinical cardiovascular consequences. *J Am Coll Cardiol.* 2017;69(7):841–858.

Javaheri S, Brown L, Abraham W, Khayat R. Apneas of heart failure and phenotype-guided treatments. Part one: obstructive sleep apnea. *Chest.* 2020;157:394–492.

Javaheri S, Brown L, Khayat R. Update on apneas of heart failure with reduced ejection fraction: emphasis on the physiology of treatment part 2: central sleep apnea. *CHEST.* 2020;157:1637–1646.

Javaheri S, Brown LK, Khayat R. Con: persistent central sleep apnea/hunter-cheyne-stokes breathing, despite best guideline-based therapy of heart failure with reduced ejection fraction, is not a compensatory mechanism and should be suppressed. *J Clin Sleep Med.* 2018;14(6):915–921.

Javaheri S, Brown LK, Randerath W, Khayat R. SERVE-HF: more questions than answers. *Chest.* 2016;149:900–904.

Javaheri S, Martinez-Garcia MA, Campos-Rodriguez F. CPAP treatment and cardiovascular prevention: we need to change our trial designs and implementations. *CHEST.* 2019;156(3):431–437.

Javaheri S, Martinez-Garcia MA, Campos-Rodriguez F, Muriel A, Peker Y. Continuous positive airway pressure adherence for of major adverse cerebrovascular and cardiovascular events in obstructive sleep apnea. *Am J Respir Crit Care Med.* 2020;201:607–610.

Mansukhani MP, Wang S, Somers VK. Sleep, death, and the heart. *Am J Physiol Heart Circ Physiol.* 2015;309(5):H739–H749.

McEvoy RD, Antic NA, Heeley E, et al. CPAP for prevention of cardiovascular events in obstructive sleep apnea. *N Engl J Med.* 2016;375(10):919–931.

Picard F, Panagiotidou P, Tammen AB, et al. Nocturnal blood pressure and nocturnal blood pressure fluctuations: the effect of short-term CPAP therapy and their association with the severity of obstructive sleep apnea. *J Clin Sleep Med.* 2021. https://doi.org/10.5664/jcsm.9564. [published online ahead of print, 2021 Jul 27].

Somers VK, Dyken ME, Clary MP, et al. Sympathetic neural mechanisms in obstructive sleep apnea. *J Clin Invest.* 1995;96:1897–1904.

Somers VK, Dyken ME, Mark AL, et al. Sympathetic-nerve activity during sleep in normal subjects. *N Engl J Med.* 1993;328:303–307.

Somers VK, Karim S. Upright Cheyne-Stokes respiration in heart failure. *J Am Coll Cardiol.* 2020;75; 2947-2949.

Somers VK, White DP, Amin R, et al. Sleep apnea and cardiovascular disease: an American Heart Association/American College Of Cardiology Foundation Scientific Statement from the American Heart Association Council for High Blood Pressure Research Professional Education Committee, Council on Clinical Cardiology, Stroke Council, and Council On Cardiovascular Nursing. In collaboration with the National Heart, Lung, and Blood Institute National Center on Sleep Disorders Research (National Institutes of Health) [published correction appears in Circulation. 2009 Mar 31;119(12):e380]. *Circulation.* 2008;118(10):1080–1111.

Stafford PL, Harmon EK, Patel P, et al. The Influence of obesity on the association of obstructive sleep apnea and atrial fibrillation. *Sleep Med Res.* 2021;12(1):50–56.

A complete reference list can be found online at ExpertConsult.com.

Chapter

147

Systemic and Pulmonary Hypertension in Obstructive Sleep Apnea

Francisco Campos-Rodriguez; Miguel A. Martínez-García; Vahid Mohsenin; Shahrokh Javaheri

Chapter Highlights

- There has been increased scientific interest in the cardiovascular effects of obstructive sleep apnea (OSA) and, among them, systemic hypertension has been identified as the most common cardiovascular consequence of OSA.
- There is enough high-quality evidence to support that OSA is an independent risk factor for the development of systemic hypertension, and for resistant hypertension.
- Although there is much less evidence, the hypoxia associated with OSA may cause pulmonary hypertension, which may affect the morbidity and mortality of these patients.
- If OSA is associated with hypertension, adequate treatment of the sleep disorder would be expected to improve blood pressure measurements and facilitate a better blood pressure control. Similarly, a potential beneficial effect would be anticipated for pulmonary artery pressure values.
- This chapter thoroughly addresses different aspects of the pathophysiology, epidemiology, and clinical association, as well the beneficial effect of OSA therapy on systemic and pulmonary hypertension.

PATHOPHYSIOLOGIC LINKS BETWEEN OBSTRUCTIVE SLEEP APNEA AND SYSTEMIC HYPERTENSION

The pathophysiologic mechanisms by which obstructive sleep apnea (OSA) contributes to blood pressure (BP) elevation are multifactorial. OSA consists of repetitive episodes of upper airway obstruction during sleep that trigger direct and intermediate mechanisms that may lead to an increase in BP levels, including negative intrathoracic pressures, repetitive arousals with sleep fragmentation, and episodes of hypoxia-reoxygenation, which lead to intermittent hypoxia, inflammation, oxidative stress, and increased sympathetic activity. Among these mechanisms, acute and chronic increased sympathetic activity seems to play a major role in the association between OSA and systemic hypertension (HTN). Intermittent hypoxia, a hallmark of OSA, may stimulate peripheral arterial chemoreceptors. Hypoxic stimulation of the carotid body leads to a reflex increase sympathetic activity, resulting in acute peripheral vasoconstriction and acute increases in BP.[1]

There is a great deal of evidence, both in animal models as well as in humans, showing that OSA increases muscle sympathetic nerve activity (MSNA) and can acutely elevate BP via sympathetically mediated vasoconstriction. In a canine model, OSA induced by intermittent airway occlusion during nocturnal sleep resulted in acute transient increases in nighttime BP and eventually produced sustained daytime HTN. Surgical denervation of peripheral chemoreceptors in rats prevented this increase.[2] In humans, MSNA directly measured by microneurography is elevated, not only during sleep, but also through the day. Similarly, plasma catecholamine levels, as well as nocturnal and 24-hour urinary catecholamines, are elevated in awake patients with OSA, independent of obesity.[1,3]

Although intermittent hypoxia mediates an increase in chemoreflex function, it decreases baroreflex function. In the long term, baroreceptor resetting and persistently increased sympathetic activity may induce vascular remodeling, leading to persistent elevation of BP, not only during sleep, but also during the waking time.[4]

Intermittent hypoxia, inflammation, and oxidative stress may also promote endothelin-1 production and downregulation of vasodilators such as nitric oxide, increasing arterial peripheral resistance, resting vascular tone, and BP. In the long term, these mechanisms may lead to endothelial dysfunction and subsequent development of atherosclerosis and HTN.

OSA patients have increased renin generation induced by efferent renal sympathetic nerve activation, which leads to elevations in plasma angiotensin II and aldosterone. This may cause vasoconstriction and sodium-water retention. Although primary hyperaldosteronism is prevalent in subjects with OSA, it has been more associated with resistant HTN.

Owing to the increase in vascular resistance resulting from sympathetic activation, patients with OSA usually present with predominantly diastolic HTN.[5] The sympathetic activation associated with obstructive events during sleep confers a nocturnal predominance of HTN, so it may be mostly unrecognized in daytime BP measurements, unless 24-hour ambulatory BP monitoring (ABPM) is ongoing, the so-called "masked HTN."

Conversely, HTN can also affect OSA severity. Fluid retention from increased renal- and aldosterone-mediated sodium retention may shift upward from the legs to the neck during the overnight recumbent position, increasing peripharyngeal edema and neck circumference, augmenting upper airway resistance and OSA severity.[6]

Epidemiologic and Clinical Association of Obstructive Sleep Apnea and Hypertension

Obstructive Sleep Apnea and Prevalent Hypertension

There is a close association between OSA and HTN. About 30% of patients suffering from HTN have OSA,[7] and conversely, 50% of patients with OSA have HTN.[8,9] Most cross-sectional studies analyzing the relationship between these two disorders have yielded an increased prevalence of HTN in OSA patients in a dose-response manner. In a study involving 2677 adults who were referred to a sleep clinic, the adjusted odds of HTN increased by 1% for every unit increase in the apnea-hypopnea index (AHI), with prevalence levels for HTN of 22.8%, 36.5%, 46%, and 53.6% in subjects with no, mild, moderate, and severe OSA, respectively.[10] In another cross-sectional study of 1741 community-dwelling subjects with suspected OSA, both mild and moderate-to-severe OSA were significantly associated with the presence of HTN, with adjusted odds ratios of 2.29 and 6.85 for mild and moderate-to-severe OSA, respectively.[11]

The Wisconsin and the Sleep Heart Health Study (SHHS) population-based cohorts have also provided data on this topic, both showing statistically significant associations between OSA and prevalent HTN.[8,9] The increase in the risk of HTN in the Wisconsin cohort was 4% for every unit increase in AHI, and a dose-response relationship between OSA severity and the prevalence of HTN was observed. The European ESADA cohort analyzed 11,911 adults referred for suspected OSA and observed that the oxygen desaturation index (ODI), but not the AHI, was independently associated with prevalent HTN, which supports the role that chronic intermittent hypoxia plays in OSA-related HTN.[12]

Obstructive Sleep Apnea and the Risk of Incident Hypertension

Although cross-sectional studies show a clear association between OSA and HTN, they are unable to demonstrate causality. There have been several longitudinal cohort studies that have examined the incidence of HTN in patients with OSA (Table 147.1). The Wisconsin population-based cohort followed 709 participants for 4 years.[13] After adjusting for multiple confounders, researchers found that patients with an AHI of at least 5 had a twofold higher risk of developing HTN, compared with participants without OSA at baseline (AHI < 1). In a Spanish clinical-based cohort of 1889 participants without HTN who were studied for OSA suspicion and followed for 10.1 years, the adjusted risk for developing new-onset HTN was significantly greater among patients with nontreated OSA (including patients who were not prescribed, declined, or were noncompliant to continuous positive airway pressure [CPAP] therapy), with adjusted hazard ratios between 1.33 and 1.78, compared with non-OSA controls.[14]

Two other prospective studies, however, failed to find any association between the presence of OSA and incident HTN. The SHHS studied 2470 participants, and after a follow-up of 5 years, incident HTN increased with increasing OSA severity, but this association did not reach statistical significance after adjustment for body mass index (BMI).[15] The authors, however, acknowledged that the small number of severe OSA cases, who accounted for only 4% of the whole cohort, may have biased the results. Another Spanish study, the Vitoria Sleep Cohort, assessed hypertensive status after a follow-up 7.5 years in a population-based cohort composed of 1180 subjects aged 30 to 70 years.[16] The risk of developing HTN was no longer significant after adjustment for age and other confounders. Differences in the population features (older in the SHHS compared with the Wisconsin cohort, and higher BMI and male prevalence in the Wisconsin cohort compared with the Vitoria cohort) and the procedure used to diagnose OSA (conventional polysomnography in the Wisconsin, compared with simplified respiratory polygraphy in the Vitoria cohort) have been advocated as relevant disparities that may explain the different findings observed in these studies.

Circadian Pattern of Blood Pressure in Patients with Obstructive Sleep Apnea

In healthy individuals, sleep is associated with a roughly 10% decrease in BP compared with wakefulness. This circadian pattern is referred to as "dipping pattern" and is attributable to the sympathetic withdrawal and subsequent parasympathetic predominance that occurs during non–rapid eye movement (NREM) sleep. Sleep-related BP dipping is paramount for cardiovascular health, and there is evidence that patients with hypertension with a nighttime decrease in BP lower than 10% (the so-called "nondippers") and those who increase their BP at night ("risers") exhibit greater organ damage and worse cardiovascular outcomes.

The sympathetic activation associated with obstructive respiratory events during sleep may blunt the normal nocturnal lowering of BP and result in a higher occurrence of nondipping or riser patterns in patients with OSA. Several studies using 24-hour ABPM have confirmed that OSA induces a high prevalence of nondipping or riser circadian patterns that can reach 84% of the patients with mild to severe OSA.[17] Additionally, OSA has also been shown to be a risk factor for nondipping incidence. The Wisconsin cohort examined a subsample of 328 adults followed for 7.2 years and observed a dose-response relationship between increased odds of developing a nondipping systolic BP and OSA severity at baseline (Table 147.1). Compared with an AHI below 5, adjusted odds ratio (OR), (95% confidence interval [CI]) of incident systolic nondipping for baseline AHI 5 to 14.9 and AHI of at least 15, were 3.1 (1.3–7.7) and 4.4 (1.2–16.3), respectively (P-trend = .006).[18]

REM Obstructive Sleep Apnea and Hypertension

Rapid eye movement (REM) sleep is associated with higher sympathetic activity and cardiovascular instability than NREM sleep in healthy individuals and in patients with OSA. Using beat-to-beat BP measurements and recordings of sympathetic nerve activity, it has been shown that sympathetic activity and mean BP were significantly higher in REM sleep, compared with NREM sleep and quiet wakefulness.[1] Furthermore, respiratory events during REM sleep are usually longer in duration. They are associated with more

Table 147.1 Studies That Have Investigated the Association between Obstructive Sleep Apnea and Incident Systemic Hypertension or Incident Nondipper Blood Pressure Pattern

Studies	Patients (*n*)	Age, BMI	Follow-up (Years)	Type of BP Measure	Type of Sleep Study	Main Findings
Peppard, 2000	709 (45% women) Population-based cohort	46 (7) years 29 (6) kg/m^2	4 years	Office BP	PSG	Compared with participants without OSA at baseline (AHI < 1), the adjusted OR for the incidence of hypertension were 1.42 (95% CI 1.13–1.78) for an AHI of 0.1–4.9, 2.03 (95% CI 1.29–2.17) for an AHI of 5.0–14.9, and 2.89 (95% CI 1.46–5.64) for an AHI ≥ 15.0.
Marin, 2012	1889 (20% women) Clinical-based cohort	49 (10) years 30 (3) kg/m^2	12.2 years	Office BP	PSG	Compared with controls (AHI < 5), the adjusted HRs for incident hypertension were greater among patients with OSA ineligible for CPAP therapy (1.33; 95% CI, 1.01–1.75) among those who declined CPAP therapy (1.96; 95% CI, 1.44–2.66), and among those nonadherent to CPAP therapy (1.78; 95% CI, 1.23–2.58). Compared with controls (AHI < 5), the adjusted HRs for incident hypertension were lower in patients with OSA who were treated with CPAP therapy (0.71; 95% CI, 0.53–0.94). There was no association between Epworth Sleepiness Scale score and incident hypertension.
O'Connor, 2009	2470 (55% women) Population-based cohort	59 (10) years 28 (5) kg/m^2	5 years	Office BP	PSG	Although the risk of developing hypertension significantly increased with increasing baseline AHI, this relationship was attenuated and no longer statistically significant after adjustment for confounders. Compared to participants without OSA at baseline (AHI < 5), the adjusted OR for the incidence of hypertension were 0.94 (95% CI 0.73–1.22) for an AHI of 5–14.9, 1.09 (95% CI 0.77–1.54) for an AHI of 15.0–29.9, and 1.50 (95% CI 0.91–2.46) for an AHI ≥ 30.0. Given that the number of participants with an AHI ≥ 30.0 was very small (only 97, 3.9%), the authors could not exclude a possible association in this subgroup of severe OSA.
Cano-Pumarega, 2011	1180 (51% women) population-based cohort	47 (10) years 25 (4) kg/m^2	7.5 years	Office BP	Respiratory polygraphy	The crude odds ratio for incident hypertension increased with higher AHI category with a dose–response effect ($P = .001$), but was not statistically significant after adjustment for age ($P = .051$). Adjustments for other further reduced the strength of the association between AHI and hypertension
Hla, 2008	328 (38% women) population-based cohort	49 (10) years 29 (4) kg/m^2	7.2 years	24-hr ABPM	PSG	There was a dose-response increased odd of developing systolic nondipping in participants with OSA categories (P or trend = .006). Compared to baseline AHI < 5, the adjusted odds ratios (95% CI) of incident systolic nondipping for baseline AHI 5 to < 15 were 3.1 (1.3–7.7), and for AHI ≥ 15 were 4.4 (1.2–16.3). There was not any association between an incident diastolic nondipping and OSA categories.

Continued

Table 147.1 Studies That Have Investigated the Association between Obstructive Sleep Apnea and Incident Systemic Hypertension or Incident Nondipper Blood Pressure Pattern—cont'd

Studies	Patients (*n*)	Age, BMI	Follow-up (Years)	Type of BP Measure	Type of Sleep Study	Main Findings
Mokhlesi, 2014	1451 (48% women) Population-based cohort	52 (10) years 29 (6) kg/m^2	24 years	24-hr ABPM and Office BP	PSG	There was a statically significant association between REM-AHI categories and the development of hypertension (*P* for trend = 0.017). Patients with a REM-AHI ≥ 15 had a greater risk of developing hypertension compared with those with REM-AHI < 1 (adjusted OR 1.77; 95% CI 1.08–2.92).
Mokhlesi, 2015	269 (38% women) population-based cohort	49 (8) years 29 (5) kg/m^2	6.6 years	24-hr ABPM	PSG	The authors observed a dose–response greater risk of developing systolic and diastolic nondipping BP with greater REM-OSA severity (*P* for trend = .021 for systolic and 0.024 for diastolic nondipping). Compared with patients with REM-AHI < 1, those with REM-AHI ≥ 15 had higher relative risk of incident systolic nondipping (2.84, 95% CI 1.10–7.29) and incident diastolic nondipping (4.27, 95% CI 1.20–15.13).
Appleton, 2016	739 men Population-based cohort	59 (10) years 28 (4) kg/m^2	6.6 years	Office BP	PSG	Severe REM-OSA (defined as an AHI ≥ 30 in REM) showed independent adjusted associations with recent-onset hypertension (OR 2.24; 95% CI 1.04–4.81).
Cano-Pumarega, 2017	1155 (56% women) Population-based cohort	44 (37–52) years 25 (22–27) kg/m^2	7.5 years	Office BP	Respiratory polygraphy	Compared with a control group without OSA (AHI < 3), men with an AHI ≥ 14 had a statistically significant greater risk of developing stage 2 hypertension (adjusted OR 2.54; 95% CI 1.09–5.95), whereas women did not show any association (adjusted OR 2.14; 95% CI 0.40–11.36).
Vgontzas, 2019	744 (52% women) Population-based cohort	47 (12) years 27 (5) kg/m^2	9.2 years	Self-report or receiving antihypertensive medication	PSG	Compared to non-OSA (AHI < 5), mild OSA (AHI 5–14.9) as well as moderate OSA (AHI 15–29.9) was significantly associated with increased risk of incident hypertension (adjusted HR 3.24; 95% CI 2.08–5.03 for mild OSA and HR 2.23; 95% CI 1.10–4.50 for moderate OSA). The association between OSA and incident hypertension was limited to young and middle-aged adults (adjusted HR 3.62; 95% CI 2.34–5.60) but was lost in adults older than 60 years (HR 1.36; 95% CI 0.50–3.72).

ABPM, Ambulatory blood pressure monitoring; AHI, apnea-hypopnea index; BMI, body mass index; BP, blood pressure; CI, confidence interval; CPAP, continuous positive airway pressure, HR, hazard ratio; OR, odds ratio; OSA, obstructive sleep apnea; PSG, polysomnography; REM, rapid eye movement.

significant oxygen desaturation, which may confer a higher cardiovascular risk than OSA during NREM sleep. Data from the Wisconsin cohort observed that REM OSA was cross-sectionally and longitudinally associated with HTN (Table 147.1).[19] The increased risk of prevalent HTN was most evident for REM-AHI values of 15 or higher, and a twofold increase in REM-AHI was associated with 24% higher odds of HTN. In this same cohort, the longitudinal analysis revealed a significant association between REM-AHI categories and the development of HTN. In contrast, NREM-AHI was not a significant predictor of incident HTN. In another substudy from the same cohort, the authors found a dose-response greater risk of developing systolic and diastolic nondipping BP with greater severity of OSA in REM sleep (Table 147.1).[20] Compared with individuals with REM AHI of less than 1, those with REM AHI of at least 15 had a nearly threefold higher risk of incident systolic and fourfold risk of diastolic nondipping. Finally, the MAILES study (Table 147.1) analyzed 739 community-dwelling men and found that severe REM OSA defined as a REM-AHI of at least 30, showed independent adjusted associations with prevalent (OR 2.40, 95% CI 1.42 to 4.06), and recent-onset HTN (OR 2.24, 95% CI 1.04 to 4.81).[21] As happened in the Wisconsin cohort, associations between NREM AHI and HTN were not seen.

All this evidence supports the role of REM OSA in the development of HTN, especially for REM-AHI greater than 15 events/hour.

Obstructive Sleep Apnea and Hypertension in Women and the Elderly

As happens with other cardiovascular consequences of OSA, the association with HTN has mostly been addressed in middle-aged males, whereas the relationship in special populations such as women and the elderly has barely been investigated.

Obstructive Sleep Apnea and Hypertension in the Elderly

According to the findings reported in several studies, it seems that the association between OSA and HTN is stronger in younger patients and declines with age, with several cohorts not showing any relationship between OSA and prevalent HTN in individuals older than 50 to 60 years.[11,22] A recent publication in 744 adults without HTN or severe OSA from the Penn State cohort who were followed for 9.2 years observed that mild-to-moderate OSA (AHI between 5 and 29.9) was significantly associated with incident HTN only in patients under 60 years (adjusted HR 3.62, 95% CI 2.34 to 5.60), but not in those older than 60 years (adjusted HR 1.36, 95% CI 0.50 to 3.72) (Table 147.1).[23]

There are no clear reasons for the lack of association between OSA and hypertension in the elderly. Survival bias and higher prevalence of HTN in the elderly may require larger samples to detect an effect of OSA on this disorder.

In contrast to these findings, a study in 470 subjects with an average age of 68 years who underwent 24-hour ABPM reported that HTN was more frequently encountered in subjects with an AHI of at least 15, and severe OSA (AHI ≥ 30) was independently associated with systolic HTN (OR 2.42, 95% CI 1.1 to 5.4).[24]

In summary, although the strongest association between OSA and HTN occurs in young and middle-aged individuals, the relationship in the elderly is controversial but cannot be discarded.

Obstructive Sleep Apnea and Hypertension in Women

There is controversy as to whether OSA is a risk factor for HTN in women as it is in men. Preliminary retrospective and cross-sectional studies have observed that this association was limited to men. More recently, the Vitoria Sleep Cohort prospectively followed 1155 normotensive individuals for 7½ years and showed that, for men, an AHI of at least 14 was associated with a significantly increased risk of developing stage 2 HTN. In contrast, no association was found in women (Table 147.1).[25] On the other hand, a study in 641 elderly subjects observed that the presence of HTN was significantly associated with OSA risk in females (OR 1.52, 95% CI 1.00 to 2.30), compared with males.[26] Another study that evaluated 277 perimenopausal women using 24-hour ABPM found that compared with women without OSA (AHI < 5), those with moderate-to-severe OSA (AHI ≥ 15) had a higher prevalence of HTN, were prescribed more antihypertensive medications, and had higher awake and nocturnal BP measures and more arterial stiffness.[27] Finally, data from the large European Sleep Apnea Database (ESADA) cohort that analyzed 7646 men and 3303 women reported that AHI and ODI had similar effects on prevalent HTN in both men and women.[12]

Thus, although the available evidence is small, OSA should not be disregarded as a potential risk factor for HTN in women. In fact, there is evidence showing that the endothelial function may be more impaired in women than in men with OSA, that OSA is associated with arterial stiffness and nondipping BP in patients with HTN regardless of sex, or that severe OSA during REM sleep is independently associated with early signs of atherosclerosis in women, all of which are pathophysiologic mechanisms that support the involvement of OSA in HTN in women.

In summary, although the association between OSA and HTN may not be as strong as initially suspected, all the evidence mentioned previously has led the scientific community to consider OSA as an important independent contributing factor to HTN. In this sense, in 2003 the Seventh Report of the Joint National Committee on Prevention, Detection, Evaluation, and Treatment of High Blood Pressure included OSA as one common identifiable cause of hypertension.[28]

Treatment of Hypertension in Patients with Obstructive Sleep Apnea

Lifestyle Changes

Evidence explicitly addressing the effects of lifestyle changes on HTN associated with OSA is scant. In a randomized controlled trial (RCT) of obese patients with moderate-to-severe OSA that investigated the effect of a weight loss intervention, CPAP, or a combination of both for 24 weeks showed similar efficacy to reduce systolic BP in all three study groups.[29] However, in patients with good adherence to CPAP, this reduction was more significant in the combined intervention group (14.1 mm Hg) than in either intervention alone (decrease of 6.8 mm Hg in the weight loss group, and 3.0 mm Hg in the CPAP group). These results highlight an interesting interaction effect between lifestyle modifications, weight loss measures, and CPAP in the control of BP.

Continuous Positive Airway Pressure Therapy

CPAP is the treatment of choice for severe and symptomatic OSA. CPAP has consistently been shown to avoid respiratory events and its consequences, including arousals, sleep fragmentation, oxygen saturation drops, and intermittent hypoxia. In this sense, CPAP has demonstrated to counter and normalize the elevated sympathetic activity observed in patients with hypertension and OSA. These effects suggest that CPAP treatment would decrease BP measures in patients with hypertension and OSA.

The effect of CPAP therapy on HTN has been widely investigated in multiple RCTs and several meta-analyses that have shown that CPAP significantly reduces BP in patients with OSA (Figure 147.1).[30-37] Studies using 24-hour ABPM consistently report drops of 2 to 2.5 mm Hg and 1.5 to 2 mm Hg in systolic and diastolic BP, respectively, compared with subtherapeutic or conservative treatment. The improvement in BP levels is usually greater for nocturnal than for diurnal measures.[38] Moreover, withdrawal studies have confirmed that when CPAP therapy is discontinued, there is a relapse of symptoms that are accompanied by a clinically relevant increase in BP.[39] In addition to the improvement in BP measures, CPAP has also shown to reverse the nondipper nocturnal BP pattern in patients with OSA.[40] Because long-term reductions of 2 to 3 mm Hg in systolic BP are associated with a 4% to 8% reduction in the future risk of stroke, and coronary heart disease, long-term treatment of OSA in patients with hypertension could eventually reduce the cardiovascular burden.

In spite of this beneficial effect of CPAP, the question that arises is why the effect on BP is so modest. Considering that CPAP avoids respiratory events and its adverse consequences, a much greater improvement in BP measures would be expected. Different reasons could be argued to explain this limited effect, in addition to the short-term follow-up of most trials and some methodological limitations or differences between studies. CPAP is not an antihypertensive therapy and thus may not decrease BP if the underlying cause of HTN is unrelated. In this sense, other pathophysiologic mechanisms underlying HTN, such as those associated with obesity, salt intake, and volume overload, may be unaffected by CPAP. Moreover, OSA and HTN are chronic disorders, and if OSA-induced HTN has been longstanding, with the consequent remodeling of the vascular bed and/or resetting of prevailing BP regulatory mechanisms (e.g., baroreflex), CPAP may not be able to reduce BP much, at least in the short term.[41] Unfortunately, and because of ethical reasons, most RCTs are limited to 3 to 6 months, so it is unknown whether CPAP therapy may increase or decrease its effect on BP in the long term. Although not explicitly designed to address BP, a recent post hoc analysis of the large SAVE trial with 2381 participants has reported a significant decrease in mean systolic and diastolic BP in the CPAP compared with the control group across the first 24 months of this RCT, supporting a long-term beneficial effect of CPAP on BP.[42]

Additionally, several factors can affect the degree of BP decrease with CPAP therapy, including OSA severity,[33,35] baseline BP levels (as is discussed later for resistant hypertension),[37,38] and CPAP adherence.[34,37,38] Hence, depending on these features, some study patients may have achieved greater or smaller antihypertensive benefits from CPAP.

As happens with any other treatment, adequate adherence to CPAP is paramount to obtain a beneficial effect of the therapy. Although the minimum threshold of adherence is unknown, at least 4 hours per night would be needed to decrease BP. Studies have also reported a dose-response effect, suggesting that greater CPAP adherence would be associated with better BP control.[33,34] In this sense, one of these meta-analyses estimated that 24-hour mean BP would decrease by 1.39 mm Hg for each 1-hour increase in effective nightly use of the CPAP device.[34]

Whether the presence of excessive daytime sleepiness in OSA is associated with a more significant reduction in BP is a matter of debate. Although some authors have observed that in nonsleepy patients with hypertension, CPAP did not achieve a reduction in BP measures, excessive daytime sleepiness has

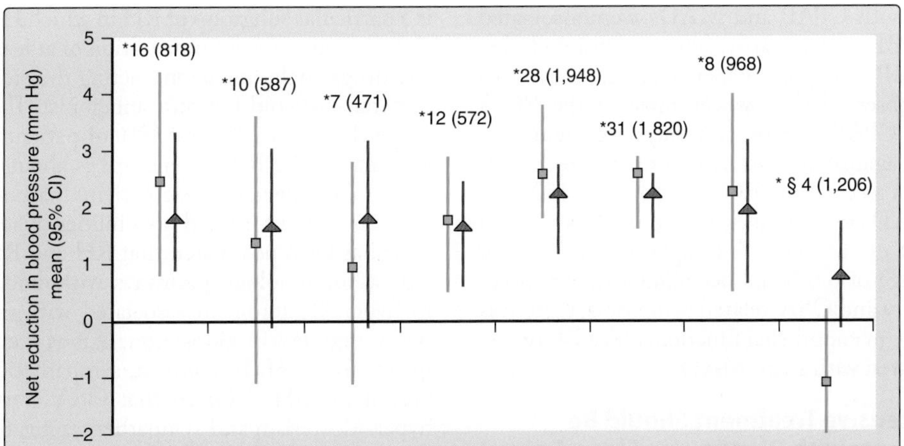

Figure 147.1 Effect of CPAP therapy on blood pressure in patients with systemic hypertension. Summary of different meta-analyses of randomized controlled trials. Positive figures mean improvement in BP level with CPAP treatment (net changes). *Number of studies included (number of patients included). § Patients without daytime hypersomnia. (Reprinted with permission from Javaheri S, Barbe F, Campos-Rodriguez F, et al. Sleep apnea. Types, mechanisms, and clinical cardiovascular consequences. *J Am Coll Cardiol.* 2017;69:841–58.)

not been identified as a variable related to BP changes in most meta-analyses. Remarkably, a Spanish RCT conducted in 359 hypertensive nonsleepy OSA patients found that a significant decrease in BP was achieved after 12 months of follow-up, but only in those subjects who used CPAP for more than 5.6 hours per night.[43] Similarly, one meta-analysis found no effect of CPAP on BP in nonsleepy patients, but when those with CPAP adherence more than 4 hours per night were separately assessed, a significant improvement in diastolic BP was observed.[32] These data suggest that CPAP may improve BP in nonsleepy patients, although they may require more hours of use of the device.

Hence different patterns of CPAP use, as well as OSA and HTN severity, may significantly influence the drop on BP achieved with CPAP treatment.

Continuous Positive Airway Pressure Therapy in Women and Elderly

Very few RCTs have analyzed the effect of CPAP on BP in women and the elderly. None of the RCTs conducted in elderly patients with OSA did observe any effect of CPAP on office BP.[44,45] However, BP was a secondary objective in all three studies, and none of them used 24-hour ABPM.

The only RCT specifically conducted in women did include subjects with and without HTN at baseline and analyzed only office BP.[46] However, after 3 months of follow-up, the CPAP group achieved a statistically significant decrease of 2.04 mm Hg in diastolic BP, and a near significant decrease of 1.90 mm Hg in mean BP, compared with the conservative control group, suggesting that this treatment may be equally effective in women as it has been shown to be in predominantly male cohorts.

Mandibular Oral Appliances

Mandibular advancement devices (MADs) improve OSA by moving the jaw and the tongue forward, thereby preventing pharyngeal collapse. The evidence regarding the effect of MAD on BP is scant, and the results of different studies are controversial. In a recent meta-analysis including 51 studies and 4888 patients, both CPAP and MADs were associated with reductions in BP, and a statistically significant difference between the BP outcomes associated with these two therapies was not observed.[47] However, most of the RCTs included comprised CPAP therapy, and only 7 of them analyzed MADs, either against an inactive control and/or CPAP. On the other hand, a recent large RCT randomized 150 subjects to effective MAD or sham device for 2 months with an objective assessment of adherence.[48] Despite effective use of MADs for an average of 6.6 hours per night with improvement in OSA severity and OSA-related symptoms, there was no significant change in endothelial function, office BP, or 24-hour ABPM, compared with sham MAD.

Which Antihypertensive Treatment Should Be Prescribed in Patients with Obstructive Sleep Apnea?

Antihypertensive drugs induce a larger decrease in BP compared with CPAP or MAD. However, few studies have addressed the topic of antihypertensive medication for patients with OSA and HTN, so the available evidence is weak. Theoretically, and according to the physiopathologic links between OSA and HTN, antihypertensive drugs that modulate sympathetic activity and the renin-angiotensin-aldosterone axis may be the best treatment options for hypertensive OSA patients. Among these, the most promising class of antihypertensive drugs would be diuretics, especially spironolactone. By reducing para-pharyngeal edema and secondary upper airway obstruction, these drugs would improve OSA severity and also reduce BP.

Among the most salient studies, an RCT that compared five commonly used antihypertensive drugs on office BP and ABPM in patients with HTN and OSA observed that all drugs had similar effects on daytime BP. However, the beta blocker atenolol reduced the nocturnal pressure slightly more than the other drugs.[49] In another RCT, valsartan achieved a fourfold greater reduction than CPAP in lowering 24-hour BP in patients with OSA.[50] Remarkably, in a subset of patients whose BP remained uncontrolled, the use of a combination of CPAP plus valsartan demonstrated significant additive effects of the two treatments, which suggests that the combined effect of both therapies may be additive on BP control.

A recent trial conducted in patients with newly diagnosed HTN and never-treated OSA has highlighted the different circadian effects of antihypertensive medication. Evening administration of antihypertensive medication compared with morning dosing further reduced nighttime systolic and diastolic BP, increased the dipper BP pattern, and induced a more significant decrease in office systolic BP.[51]

Based on the results of the available clinical studies, however, there is no definitive evidence about the best antihypertensive regimen for patients with OSA and HTN, and more trials are still needed to clarify this topic.

Resistant and Refractory Hypertension and Obstructive Sleep Apnea

Within the spectrum of patients with hypertension, there are some phenotypes characterized by an incomplete response to antihypertensive therapy, which involves resistant hypertension (RH) and refractory hypertension (RfH). RH is defined as those forms of idiopathic HTN in which BP levels remain uncontrolled despite the use of at least three antihypertensive drugs (including a diuretic) prescribed at optimal doses. RfH is a particular subgroup of RH in which HTN remains uncontrolled despite the administration of at least five antihypertensive drugs, including a long-acting thiazide-like diuretic and a mineral-corticoid receptor antagonist. The prevalence of RH ranges between 12% and 15% of patients with hypertension, and that of the RfH phenotype is about 3% of patients with RH.[52] As expected, these patients have an increased cardiovascular risk but limited possibilities of additional treatments.

It has been postulated that RH and RfH may have different pathophysiologic pathways, with fluid retention secondary to hyperaldosteronism associated with overactivation of the renin-angiotensin-aldosterone axis as the primary mechanism involved in RH. In contrast, sympathetic overactivity would prevail in RfH.[52] Given that OSA is associated with both hyperaldosterism and sympathetic activation, a close relationship between OSA and RH/RfH would be therefore expected.

Clinical and Epidemiologic Associations between Resistant/Refractory Hypertension and Obstructive Sleep Apnea

The association between OSA and RH was first described in 2001.[53] Since then all studies on the topic have concurred to report a high prevalence of OSA among patients with RH, ranging from 60% to 90% (Table 147.2).[54-61] OSA was the

Table 147.2 Studies That Have Investigated the Association between Resistant or Refractory Hypertension and Sleep Apnea

Studies	Patients (*n*)	Age (Years)	Type of BP Measure SBP/DBP (mm Hg)	Type of Sleep Study (AHI Threshold to Define OSA)	OSA Prevalence / AHI
Logan, 2001	41 pts with resistant HTN (24 men, 17 women)	57.2 (1.6) men 54.6 (1.8) women 58.3 (3.0)	24-hour ABPM SBP: 149.0 (2.6) in men, 150.6 (3.7) in women DBP: 86.3 (2.0) in men, 83.7 (1.9) in women	PSG (AHI ≥ 10)	82.9% (96% in men, 65% in women) Mean AHI: 32.2 (4.5) in men, 14.0 (3.1) in women
Gonçalves, 2007	63 pts with resistant HTN (21 men, 42 women) and 63 pts with controlled HTN (23 men, 40 women)	59 (7) in both the resistant and controlled HTN groups	24-hour ABPM SBP: 141 (17) in the resistant HTN group versus 121 (10) in the controlled HTN group DBP: 84 (12) in the resistant HTN group versus 74 (7) in the controlled HTN group	RP (AHI ≥ 10)	71% in the resistant HTN group versus 38% in the controlled HTN group (*P* < .001) Men: 86% versus 52% (*P* = .016) Women: 64% versus 30% (*P* = .002)
Prat-Ubunama, 2007	71 pts with resistant HTN	56.0 (9.9)	Office BP measurement SBP: 155.8 (27) DBP: 88.3 (15)	PSG (AHI ≥ 5)	85% (90% in men, 77% in women) Mean AHI: 24.1 (24.7) (men 20.8, women 10.8)
Lloberes, 2010	62 pts with resistant HTN (67.3% men)	59 (10)	24-hour ABPM SBP: 139.1 (1.6) DBP: 80.9 (1.2)	PSG (AHI ≥ 5)	AHI ≥ 5: 90.3% AHI ≥ 30: 70% Mean AHI: 47.8 (23.4)
Pedrosa, 2011	125 pts with resistant HTN (43% men)	52 (10)	24-hour ABPM SBP: 176 (31) DBP: 107 (19)	PSG (AHI ≥ 15)	AHI ≥ 15: 64% AHI ≥ 30: 32% Median AHI: 18 (interquartile range, 10–40)
Florczak, 2013	204 pts with resistant HTN (123 men, 81 women)	48.4 (10.6)	24-hour ABPM Daytime SBP: 145 (19), DBP: 90 (13) Nighttime SBP: 132 (19), DBP: 79 (12)	PSG (AHI ≥ 5)	AHI ≥ 5: 72.1% AHI ≥ 30: 26.5%
Ruttanaumpawan, 2009	42 pts with resistant HTN and 22 pts with controlled HTN, matched for age, sex and BMI	56.5 (1.6) in resistant HTN group, 60.1 (1.8) in controlled HTN group	24-hour ABPM in the resistant HTN group SBP: 149 (2) DBP: 85 (1)	PSG (AHI ≥ 10)	81% in the resistant HTN group versus 55% in the controlled HTN group (*P* = .03) Mean AHI: 24.9 (3.2) in the resistant HTN group versus 16.5 (2.7) in the controlled HTN group (*P* = .13)
Johnson, 2019	664 Black participants with HTN (205 men), of whom 96 (14.5%) had resistant HTN	64.9 (10.6)	Office BP measurement	RP (AHI ≥ 15)	25.7% of all HTN patients. Patients with resistant HTN were 1.92 times more likely (95% CI 1.15–3.20) to have OSA, compared to those with controlled HTN
Martinez-Garcia, 2018*	229 pts with resistant HTN (63% men). Of these, 42 (18.3%) had refractory HTN	58.3 (9.6) for the resistant HTN group and 58.4 (8.5) for the refractory HTN group	24-hour ABPM Resistant HTN SBP: 141.6 (11.2) DBP: 82.2 (10) Refractory HTN SBP: 152.4 (13.9) DBP: 85.6 (11.8)	RP (AHI ≥ 5)	AHI ≥ 5 Resistant HTN: 89.3% Refractory HTN: 100% (*P* = .027) AHI ≥ 30: Resistant HTN: 48.6% Refractory HTN: 64.3% (*P* = .044)

Only those studies that have used a sleep test (either respiratory polygraphy or conventional polysomnography) have been included. Studies that assessed sleep apnea risk based on screening questionnaires have not been included.
*This study investigated the association between OSA and refractory hypertension.
ABPM, 24-hour ambulatory blood pressure monitoring; AHI, apnea-hypopnea index; BMI, body mass index; DBP, diastolic blood pressure; HTN, hypertension; OSA, obstructive sleep apnea; PSG, polysomnography; RP, respiratory polygraphy; SBP, systolic blood pressure.

most common condition associated with RH in several studies.[58] This evidence has led the international guidelines to acknowledge OSA as an important contributing factor to RH.[62]

Regarding RfH, however, the evidence is more limited, and only one study has investigated its association with OSA. In a multicenter cross-sectional study,[54] composed of 229 consecutive patients with RH, those with RfH had a twofold higher risk of having severe OSA (OR 1.9, 95% CI 1.02 to 3.8) compared with RH patients. Moreover, the prevalence of an AHI ≥ 15 and AHI ≥ 30 was significantly higher in the RfH than in the RH group (95.2% versus 81.8% and 64.3% versus 48.6%, respectively).

It is worth noting that patients with RH and OSA do not usually complain of excessive daytime somnolence and therefore are not usually referred to sleep labs. Given the high prevalence of OSA in this group, there is agreement that all patients with RH without a known etiology should undergo sleep study regardless of the presence of sleep-related symptoms.

Obstructive Sleep Apnea Treatment and Resistant Hypertension

Beyond the recommendations common to all patients with hypertension and OSA that include lifestyle changes, diet, and antihypertensive treatment, some other therapies appear to be more effective in these patients, such as renal denervation or some types of antihypertensive therapies, such as spironolactone and other mineral-corticoid drugs.

Along with these measures, CPAP may be an essential additional treatment to achieve the best BP control in OSA patients with RH. The results from the seven RCTs (Figure 147.2)[63-69] and several meta-analyses conducted on this topic[70-73] suggest a significant reduction in systolic BP and diastolic BP ranging between 4.7 and 7.2 mm Hg and 2.9 and 4.9 mm Hg, respectively. This decrease in BP is larger than that obtained for non-RH. The largest of these RCTs, the HIPARCO study, enrolled 194 patients with RH defined by 24-hour ABPM who were randomized to CPAP or no CPAP over 3 months.[69] The CPAP group achieved a greater decrease in 24-hour mean BP (3.1 mm Hg) and 24-hour diastolic BP (3.2 mm Hg), but not in 24-hour SBP (3.1 mm Hg), compared with the control group.

Remarkably, some of these studies have also observed a recovering of the normal dipping nocturnal BP pattern in 35.9% to 51.7% of the patients treated with CPAP, and the largest improvements in BP measures were achieved in those patients with better adherence to CPAP.[63,69] Moreover, one study has demonstrated that good long-term adherence to CPAP is feasible in this population.[74] After a median follow-up of 57.6 months, 74.5% of this population had a CPAP use of at least 4 hours/night with a median use of 5.7 (interquartile range 3.9 to 6.6) hours per night.

At present, only one study has analyzed the effect of CPAP treatment on RfH.[66] This RCT has reported a more significant decrease in BP levels in the RfH group than in the RH group in both 24-hour SBP (−9 versus −1.6 mm Hg, $P = 0.021$) and 24-hour DBP (−7.3 versus −2.3 mm Hg, $P = 0.074$), especially at night (−11.3 versus −3.8, $P = .121$ and −8.8 versus −2.2, $P = .054$).

Remarkably, in one of the few studies focused on personalized medicine in RH and OSA, the authors observed three miRNAs obtained from responders and nonresponders to CPAP treatment from the HIPARCO study, which provided a discriminatory predictive model for a favorable BP response to CPAP.[75] CPAP treatment also significantly altered a total of 47 plasma miRNAs and decreased aldosterone-to-renin ratios in the responder, but not in the nonresponder group.

In summary, OSA is an independent risk factor for RH and RfH and shows a very high prevalence in this population. It is the most common condition associated with RH. Adequate CPAP therapy achieves a significant reduction in BP levels, which is even greater than in nonresistant HTN. Because the relationship between RH/RfH and OSA has only recently been detected, there are still future challenges that

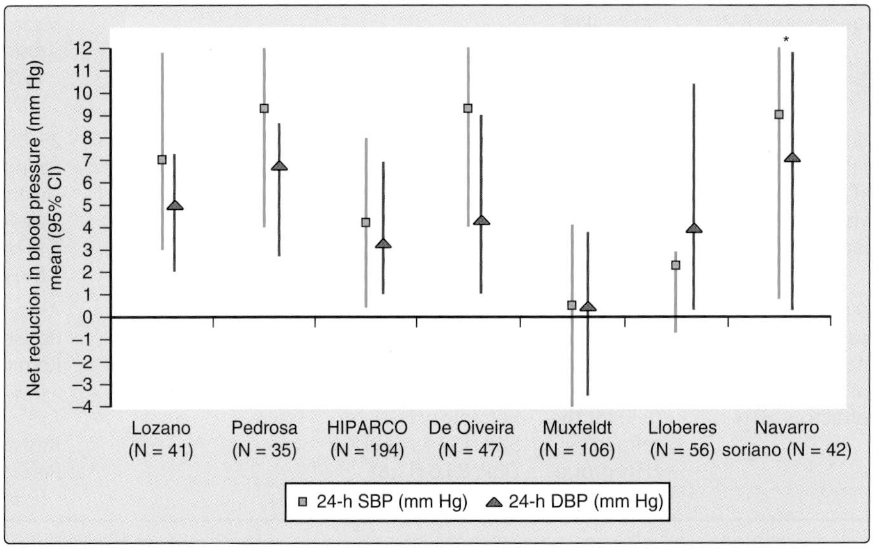

Figure 147.2 Effect of continuous positive airway pressure (CPAP) therapy on blood pressure (BP) in patients with resistant hypertension. The figure includes the results of the seven randomized controlled trials published to date. Positive figures mean improvement in BP level with CPAP treatment (net changes). *Refractory hypertension. DBP, Diastolic blood pressure; SBP, systolic blood pressure. (Modified from Javaheri S, Barbe F, Campos-Rodriguez F, et al. Sleep apnea. Types, mechanisms, and clinical cardiovascular consequences. *J Am Coll Cardiol.* 2017;69: *J Am Coll Cardiol.* 2017;69:841–58.)

must be addressed, mainly the long-term effect of treating OSA on the cardiovascular burden associated with RH/RfH.

PULMONARY HYPERTENSION

Obstructive Sleep Apnea as a Cause of Pulmonary Hypertension

In 1998 the second World Health Organization (WHO) conference on pulmonary arterial hypertension recognized sleep-disordered breathing as a secondary cause of pulmonary hypertension (PH). The classification of PH had been revised by World Symposium on Pulmonary Hypertension in 2013 and, more recently, in 2018.[76] There are five groups, each with several subgroups consisting of various causes of PH. The first group, pulmonary arterial hypertension, includes idiopathic pulmonary arterial hypertension. The second group is pulmonary venous hypertension, which is most commonly due to elevated left heart filling pressures such as left ventricular diastolic dysfunction. PH secondary to OSA falls into the third group, which also includes chronic obstructive pulmonary disease (COPD), interstitial lung diseases, and PH related to chronic exposure to high altitude. The primary pathophysiologic mechanism underlying PH in this group of disorders is hypoxia. However, as is emphasized later, OSA can cause PH through left ventricular diastolic dysfunction, as it occurs in group 2. Group 4 is PH resulting from thromboembolic pathologic disorders, and group 5 consists of different disorders that cannot be easily classified in the other four groups.

The gold standard for diagnosis of PH is right heart catheterization. The most recent recommendation for the hemodynamic definition of PH by the 6th World Symposium on Pulmonary Hypertension is resting mean pulmonary artery pressure (mPAP) of 20 mm Hg or higher instead of 25 mm Hg and greater.[77] Investigators in the field of sleep apnea have mostly used an mPAP of 20 mm Hg or higher, a threshold that is lower than the previous definition[78] but more relevant to the current definition. In this chapter, we defined PH according to the recently adopted criteria, which have become the rule independent of the cause of the PH. We also emphasized that right heart catheterization is essential for phenotyping PH, assessing its severity and the targeted therapy.

In patients with OSA, the prevalence of abnormal mPAP varies considerably, from 15% to 85%.[79-81] This variation in prevalence is, in part, due to the inclusion in some studies of patients with COPD, hypercapnic OSA (obesity-hypoventilation syndrome), and obesity, which contribute to increased frequency, prevalence, and severity of PH in OSA. In patients with OSA without comorbid disorders, PH is usually mild but could be severe, resulting in right heart failure.

Several studies have demonstrated the presence of PH in patients with OSA. Box 147.1 summarizes the six most extensive studies in which full-night PSG and right heart catheterization were performed.[70,80,82-85] In a French study[79] involving 220 consecutive patients with an AHI of greater than 20/hour, 37 patients (17%) had a resting mPAP of at least 20 mm Hg (range, 20 to 44 mm Hg), and in 17 patients (8%) the mPAP was 25 mm Hg or higher. Patients with a resting mPAP of

Box 147.1 STUDIES ON PULMONARY HYPERTENSION IN PATIENTS WITH OBSTRUCTIVE SLEEP APNEA

Chaouat A, Weitzenblum E, Krieger J, et al.[79]

220 consecutive French patients with AHI > 20 events/hour; AHI range, 24–179 events/hour in the PH group

1. 17% had mPAP > 20 mm Hg
2. Patients with mPAP > 20 mm Hg had more severe OSA, higher $PaCO_2$ and BMI, lower PaO_2, and a more obstructive and restrictive defect
3. $PaCO_2$ and FEV_1 were independent predictors of mPAP

Laks L, Lehrhaft B, Grunstein R, et al.[80]

100 consecutive Australian patients with AHI > 20 events/hour; AHI range, 21–105 events/hour

1. 42% had mPAP >20 mm Hg; range, 20 to 52 mm Hg
2. 5% had PH with mean PAP > 40 mm Hg
3. $PaCO_2$, PaO_2, and FEV_1 accounted for 33% of the variability in PH
4. Six patients (6%) with mPAP ranging from 20 to 52 mm Hg had normal PaO_2

Sanner BM, Doberauer C, Konermann M, et al.[85]

92 consecutive German patients with OSA and AHI >10; AHI range, 10–100 events/hour

1. COPD was an exclusion criterion
2. 20% had mPAP ranging from 20 to 26 mm Hg; two with PH had mean PAP ≥ 25 mm Hg
3. Eight patients had increased PAOP; all had systemic hypertension
4. PAOP and time spent at <90% saturation were independent predictors of mean PAP

Bady E, Achkar A, Pascal S, et al.[83]

44 patients with OSA and AHI > 5 events/hour; mean AHI 53.4 ± 25 events/hour in the PH group

1. COPD (FEV_1/FVC ratio < 60%) was an exclusion criterion
2. 27% had mPAP >20 mm Hg with mean pressure ≥ 28.5 mm Hg
3. All with PAOP ≤15 mm Hg
4. 18% had PH with mean PAP ≥ 25 mm Hg

Sajkov D, Wang T, Saunders NA, et al.[84]

32 patients with OSA and AHI > 10 events/hour; mean AHI 46.2 ± 3.9 events/hour

1. COPD (FEV_1/FVC ratio <75%) and any evidence of cardiovascular disease, including systemic hypertension were exclusion criteria
2. 34% had mPAP ≥ 20 mm Hg with mean PAP of 23.6 ± 1.1 mm Hg
3. Echocardiography did not show evidence for left ventricular or valvular heart disease

Alchanatis M, Tourkohoriti G, Kakouros S, et al.[82]

1. 29 patients with OSA and AHI > 15 events/hour; mean AHI 54 ± 19 events/hour
2. FEV_1/FVC ratio < 75% and left ventricular or valvular heart disease (echocardiography) were exclusion criteria
3. 21% of OSA patients had mPAP ≥ 20 mm Hg, range 22–30 mm Hg (right heart catheterization)

AHI, Apnea-hypopnea index; BMI, body mass index; COPD, chronic obstructive pulmonary disease; FEV_1, forced expiratory volume in 1 second; FVC, forced vital capacity; mPAP, mean pulmonary artery pressure; PAOP, pulmonary artery occlusion pressure; PH, pulmonary hypertension.

at least 20 mm Hg had more severe OSA, a higher $PaCO_2$, a higher BMI, and a lower PaO_2 than patients without PH. Furthermore, these patients had a higher prevalence of both obstructive and restrictive pulmonary defects. $PaCO_2$ and forced expiratory volume in 1 second (FEV_1) were the two significant predictors of high resting mPAP. When PH was defined as an mPAP of 30 mm Hg with exercise, virtually all patients met this criterion; in 23 patients (62%), the mPAP exceeded 40 mm Hg.

In an Australian study[80] of 100 consecutive patients with an AHI of 20 events/hour or more, 42% had elevated pulmonary artery pressure, with the mean pressure ranging from about 20 to 52 mm Hg. Some patients had overlap syndrome with COPD. In 24% of the patients, the mPAP was more than 25 mm Hg. In this study, $PaCO_2$, PaO_2, and FEV_1 accounted for about 33% of the variability in pulmonary artery pressure. Six patients with abnormal pulmonary artery pressure had normal PaO_2.

In a German study[85] of 92 consecutive patients with an AHI of greater than 10 events/hour and with COPD as an exclusion criterion, 20% had an mPAP of 20 to 25 mm Hg. Eight patients had increased pulmonary artery occlusion pressure (PAOP), and all of these patients had HTN that was presumably causing left ventricular diastolic dysfunction. PAOP and time spent with a saturation of below 90% were the independent variables predicting PH.

The presence of PH in patients with OSA without COPD was also confirmed in another French study.[83] In this study, however, COPD was defined by an FEV_1 of less than 70% predicted and a ratio of FEV_1 to forced vital capacity (FVC) of less than 60% predicted. The study involved 44 patients, 12 of whom (27%) had an mPAP higher than 20 mm Hg, all with PAOP of less than 15 mm Hg. The authors reported that mPAP was positively correlated with BMI and negatively correlated with PaO_2. Patients with elevated mPAP had significantly lower values for FVC and FEV_1. The mechanisms by which BMI positively correlated with PH could have been multifactorial and related to restrictive lung defect and hypoxemia.

Two other studies with the exclusion of patients with lung disease or left heart disease but with OSA showed PH in 34% of 32 patients[84] and 21% of 29 patients.[82]

Combining the results of the studies mentioned previously, with exclusion of lung and left heart diseases, using PSG to determine the presence of OSA, and right heart catheterization to define PH, 29 of 105 patients (28%) satisfy the current criteria (mPAP of 20 mm Hg or higher with a normal PAOP) for precapillary PH.

Prevalence of Obstructive Sleep Apnea in Patients with Pulmonary Hypertension

Four prospective studies examined the prevalence of OSA in patients with PH with diverse etiology and functional status, without evidence of left heart dysfunction, or lung diseases (Table 147.3).[86-89] The prevalence of OSA ranged between 11% and 89%, depending on the definition used to diagnose sleep-disordered breathing. Those studies using AHI of at least 5 events per hour to diagnose sleep-disordered breathing showed higher prevalence than those using AHI of more than 10 events per hour. All these patients had undergone right heart catheterization and had a PAOP of less than 15 mm Hg[86,87,89] and one study with PAOP of less than 18 mm Hg,[88] consistent with precapillary PH hemodynamics.[86-89]

In conclusion, PH is prevalent in patients with OSA and may occur in the absence of COPD, daytime hypoxemia, or left heart disease. Severe OSA, severe hypoxemia, hypercapnia (obesity-hypoventilation syndrome), obstructive or restrictive lung defects, and left heart disease are more commonly associated with PH and contribute to its severity. Conversely, OSA is also prevalent in patients with precapillary PHs, such as in idiopathic pulmonary arterial hypertension and chronic thromboembolic pulmonary hypertension, which may be part of pathophysiologic processes through perturbations of gas exchange, hemodynamics, and metabolic pathways.

Mechanisms of Pulmonary Hypertension in Patients with Obstructive Sleep Apnea

Intermittent nocturnal rises in the pulmonary artery pressure in association with upper airway collapse have been well documented. Multiple mechanisms mediate nocturnal rises in pulmonary artery pressure.[90] These include alterations in blood gases (i.e., intermittent hypoxemia and hypercapnia), cardiac output, lung volume, intrathoracic pressure, compliance of pulmonary circulation, and left ventricular diastolic dysfunction. With time and in the long run, nocturnal PH spills over to diurnal PH.

Diurnal PH in patients with OSA could be precapillary, capillary, or postcapillary, depending in part on comorbid disorders that may contribute to the development of PH. Postcapillary PH (pulmonary venous hypertension) is common

Table 147.3 Prevalence of Obstructive Sleep Apnea in Precapillary Pulmonary Hypertension

Studies	Study Type	No.	Age	BMI	RHC	PH Dx	AHI	Prevalence
Jilwan, 2013[87]	Prospective	46	53±13.6	25±4	mPAP > 25 PAOP < 15 mm Hg	IPAH (Group 1) or CTEPH (Group 4)	AHI ≥ 5/hour	89%
Dumitrascu, 2013[86]	Prospective	169	61.3±14.0	27±6	mPAP ≥ 25 PAOP < 15 mm Hg	IPAH (Group 1) or CTEPH (Group 4)	AHI > 10/hour	11%
Prisco, 2011[88]	Prospective	28	55.2±11.9	31±9	mPAP > 25 PAOP < 18 mm Hg	IPAH (Group 1) or Group 4, 5	AHI ≥ 5/hour	50%
Ulrich, 2008[89]	Prospective	38	61 (52-71)	25±1	mPAP ≥ 25 PAOP ≤ 15 mm Hg	IPAH (Group 1) or Group 3, 4	AHI ≥ 10/hour	11%

Data, mean ±SD or quartiles; AHI, apnea-hypopnea index; BMI, body mass index; CTEPH, chronic thromboembolic pulmonary hypertension; Dx, diagnosis; IPAH, idiopathic pulmonary hypertension; mPAP, mean pulmonary artery pressure; PAOP, pulmonary artery occlusion pressure; PH, pulmonary hypertension; RHC, right cardiac catheterization.

and results primarily from elevated left heart filling pressures, specifically because of their left ventricular hypertrophy, and diastolic dysfunction caused by diurnal HTN and nocturnal consequences of OSA. Regarding the latter, left ventricular hypertrophy could be present in patients with OSA even in the absence of daytime HTN,[91] presumably because of cyclic changes in systemic arterial BP and hypoxemia during sleep.[92] In the presence of a hypertrophied or noncompliant left ventricle, end-diastolic pressure increases, resulting in a backward passive increase in pulmonary venous, capillary, and pulmonary artery systolic and diastolic pressures. This acute postcapillary PH is reversible if the etiologic factor (e.g., OSA) is effectively treated. Otherwise, with persistent PH, remodeling of pulmonary vascular bed occurs, and vascular resistance increases, which in time may become irreversible even if the etiology of left heart disease is effectively treated.

Another mechanism for PH is alveolar hypoxia with or without associated hypercapnia— both of which have been shown to induce pulmonary arteriolar vasoconstriction and increasing pulmonary vascular resistance acutely. The combination of hypoxic-hypercapnic pulmonary arteriolar vasoconstriction and pulmonary venous hypertension could result in severe PH in patients with OSA.

Detailed molecular mechanisms underlying PH in OSA are beyond the scope of this chapter. However, the production of mediators ultimately results in endothelial cell damage, reduced nitric oxide production, vascular cell proliferation, and aberrant vascular remodeling.[93-94]

Loss of vascular surface area, as may occur in patients with COPD, is an important cause of capillary PH, and it may significantly contribute to PH in patients with OSA. Several studies have shown that COPD and a low FEV_1 are predictors of PH in patients with OSA.[79,80,95] COPD could also contribute to PH by way of arteriolar vasoconstriction resulting from hypoxemia and hypercapnia, as noted previously.

In summary, the consequence of OSA on the pulmonary circulation may vary from those of cyclic nocturnal PH, which occurs in virtually all patients, to diurnal PH, right ventricular dysfunction, and eventually cor pulmonale.[96]

Changes in Pulmonary Artery Pressure after Positive Airway Pressure Treatment

Because mechanisms of PH in OSA are multifactorial, the response of pulmonary circulation to therapy for OSA depends on several factors. For example, if the loss of vascular surface area resulting from the presence of COPD or other comorbid pulmonary disorders is contributing to PH in OSA, PH may not be fully reversible.[97] Similarly, if remodeling of the pulmonary vascular bed has occurred, long-standing effective therapy is necessary to affect any reversal component (reverse remodeling). Therefore, if CPAP is used to treat OSA, long-term compliance with therapy is critical and must be confirmed by objective adherence and efficacy monitoring. Effective treatment of OSA could improve PH. Here we review the studies that have implemented the right heart catheterization both at baseline as well as long term. In nonrandomized trials, CPAP treatment tended to decrease pulmonary artery pressure in only those with PH and not in those with normal mPAP.[82,98,99]

A randomized crossover trial in 23 patients with OSA (AHI 44 events/hour, or higher) and PH, 12 weeks of PAP therapy compared with sham CPAP, decreased mPAP from 28.9 ± 8.6 to 24.0 ± 5.8 mm Hg ($P < .0001$).[100] A more recent trial of positive airway pressure treatments (CPAP or respiratory assist device) in patients with obesity-hypoventilation syndrome and severe OSA showed marked improvement in systolic pulmonary artery pressure.[101] In this multicenter study, 196 patients were enrolled, 102 treated with CPAP, and 94 treated with respiratory assist device. Systolic pulmonary artery pressure decreased from 40.5 ± 1.5 mm Hg at baseline to 35 ± 1.3 mm Hg at 3 years with CPAP and from 41.5 ± 1.6 mm Hg to 35.5 ± 1.4 mm Hg with respiratory assist device. Positive airway pressure treatment decreased the prevalence of PH by 37% in the CPAP group and 52% in the respiratory assist device group based on right ventricular systolic pressure of less than 40 mm Hg on echocardiography. In the study, a large number of participants had echocardiographic evidence of left ventricular diastolic dysfunction, which improved with positive airway pressure therapy. It is therefore conceivable that improvement in PH was a consequence of improvement in diastolic dysfunction. Right heart catheterization could have delineated the mechanism but was unrealistic in this large study, although it could have been done in a subset.

The American College of Cardiology and American Heart Association expert consensus document recommends polysomnography to rule out OSA for all patients with PH. The recommendation is based on the idea that targeted therapy of OSA could either improve or prevent further deterioration in central hemodynamics.[102]

CLINICAL PEARL

HTN is the cardiovascular disease most closely associated with OSA. This association is even stronger in the case of RH. Current evidence supports that OSA is an independent risk factor for hypertension, based on the strength, consistency, and dose-response relationship shown across studies. RCTs and meta-analyses of these trials have demonstrated that OSA treatment with CPAP significantly reduces BP, with greater reduction in patients with higher BP levels. Although mild pulmonary arterial hypertension is common in patients with OSA, severe forms are usually associated with the presence of chronic lung disease, heart failure, or obesity-hypoventilation.

SUMMARY

HTN is the most common cardiovascular disorder associated with OSA. Prospective cohort studies support an independent role for OSA in the development of HTN, with a twofold greater risk of developing hypertension for patients with moderate-to-severe OSA. This association is even more robust in patients with RH, with OSA being the most common condition associated with RH in several studies. Patients with OSA also have a significantly greater risk of having a nondipping or riser circadian BP pattern, as well as nocturnal predominance of hypertension. The pathophysiologic links between OSA and HTN are multifactorial, but increased sympathetic activity mediated by intermittent hypoxia seems to be the main mechanisn involved, whereas fluid retention secondary to hyperaldosteronism would be the leading mechanisn in resistant hypertension. CPAP therapy significantly reduces BP by 2 mm Hg, although the effect may vary in different populations. This positive effect of CPAP is stronger in RH with drops of 3 to 5 mm Hg in BP measurements.

PH is also linked to OSA. Mild pulmonary arterial hypertension is common in OSA, usually because of hypoxia, whereas severe PH is usually associated with comorbidities such as chronic lung disease, heart failure, or obesity.

SELECTED READINGS

Bauters FA, Hertegonne KB, Pevernagie D, De Buyzere ML, Chirinos JA, Rietzschel ER. Sex differences in the association between arterial hypertension, blood pressure, and sleep apnea in the general population. *J Clin Sleep Med*. 2021;17(5):1057–1066.

Carlson JT, Hedner J, Elam M, et al. Augmented resting sympathetic activity in awake patients with obstructive sleep apnea. *Chest*. 1993;103:1763–1768.

Fava C, Dorigoni S, Dalle Vedove F, et al. Effect of CPAP on blood pressure in patients with OSA/hypopnea a systematic review and meta-analysis. *Chest*. 2014;145:762–771.

Javaheri S, Barbe F, Campos-Rodriguez F, et al. Sleep Apnea: types, mechanisms, and clinical cardiovascular consequences. *J Am Coll Cardiol*. 2017;69:841–858.

Jilwan FN, Escourrou P, Garcia G, et al. High occurrence of hypoxemic sleep respiratory disorders in precapillary pulmonary hypertension and mechanisms. *Chest*. 2013;143(1):47–55.

Marin JM, Agusti A, Villar I, et al. Association between treated and untreated obstructive sleep apnea and risk of hypertension. *J Am Med Assoc*. 2012;307:2169–2176.

Martínez-García M-A, Capote F, Campos-Rodríguez F, et al. Effect of CPAP on blood pressure in patients with obstructive sleep apnea and resistant hypertension: the HIPARCO randomized clinical trial. *J Am Med Assoc*. 2013;310:2407–2415.

Martínez-García M-A, Navarro-Soriano C, Torres G, et al. Beyond resistant hypertension. Relationship between refractory hypertension and obstructive sleep apnea. *Hypertension*. 2018;72:618–624.

Minai OA, Ricaurte B, Kaw R, et al. Frequency and impact of pulmonary hypertension in patients with obstructive sleep apnea syndrome. *Am J Cardiol*. 2009;104(9):1300–1306.

O'Connor GT, Caffo B, Newman AB, et al. Prospective study of sleep-disordered breathing and hypertension: the Sleep Heart Health Study. *Am J Respir Crit Care Med*. 2009;179:1159–1164.

Pedrosa RP, Drager LF, Gonzaga CC, et al. Obstructive sleep apnea: the most common secondary cause of hypertension associated with resistant hypertension. *Hypertension*. 2011;58:811–817.

Peppard PE, Young T, Palta M, Skatrud J. Prospective study of the association between sleep-disordered breathing and hypertension. *N Engl J Med*. 2000;342:1378–1384.

Sharma S, Stansbury R, Hackett B, Fox H. Sleep apnea and pulmonary hypertension: a riddle waiting to be solved. *Pharmacol Ther*. 2021;227:107935. [published online ahead of print, 2021 Jun 22].

Somers VK, Dyken ME, Clary MP, Abboud FM. Sympathetic neural mechanisms in obstructive sleep apnea. *J Clin Invest*. 1995;96:1897–1904.

Testelmans D, Spruit MA, Vrijsen B, et al. Comorbidity clusters in patients with moderate-to-severe OSA. *Sleep Breath*. 2021. https://doi.org/10.1007/s11325-021-02390-4. [published online ahead of print, 2021 May 3].

Xie J, Fan Z, Yisilamu P, et al. Hypoxemia and pulmonary hypertension in patients with concomitant restrictive ventilatory defect and sleep apnea: the overlap syndrome. *Sleep Breath*. 2021;25(2):1173–1179.

A complete reference list can be found online at ExpertConsult.com.

Chapter 148

Coronary Artery Disease and Obstructive Sleep Apnea

Yüksel Peker; Karl A. Franklin; Jan Hedner

Chapter Highlights

- Obstructive sleep apnea (OSA) is overrepresented in patients with coronary artery disease and occurs in about 56% of such patients, most of whom do not complain of excessive daytime sleepiness.
- OSA is even more prevalent during the presentation of myocardial infarction (MI) and may explain some cases of MI and sudden cardiac death around midnight and during early-morning hours.
- OSA may be an independent risk factor for atherosclerosis because of repeated apnea-induced hypoxemia and reoxygenation-induced oxidative stress with immediate and sustained sympathetic activation, endothelial dysfunction, and inflammation.
- Cohort studies report a reduction of nocturnal ischemia during elimination of obstructive events with continuous positive airway pressure (CPAP) treatment and lowering the risk for recurrent MI.
- Observational data suggest that CPAP may be beneficial in patients to prevent coronary artery disease, but there are also reports demonstrating that intermittent hypoxemia may favor the development of coronary collaterals, thus providing a protective effect.
- Randomized controlled trials examining the impact of CPAP treatment on long-term outcomes failed to show cardiovascular benefits in the intention-to-treat populations.
- Adequate use of CPAP, defined as at least 4 hours/day, was associated with improvement in major adverse cardiovascular and cerebrovascular events, with its most significant positive impact on the cerebrovascular outcomes.

Epidemiologic data suggest that obstructive sleep apnea (OSA) is overrepresented in patients with coronary artery disease (CAD). Experimental data demonstrates that OSA-related intermittent hypoxemia and reoxygenation may initiate a sequence of events involved in the development of atherosclerotic disease. However, interventional studies have not yet convincingly demonstrated increased survival after continuous positive airway pressure (CPAP) therapy of OSA in asymptomatic patients with CAD.

Sleep apneic events induce a state of increased cardiac oxygen demand, which occurs together with a reduction in oxygen supply due to lack of ventilation, which may trigger nocturnal angina in patients with CAD. Observational data suggest that elimination of OSA by CPAP can benefit patients at risk of CAD in the immediate and long term in sleep clinic cohorts with OSA-related symptoms, such as excessive daytime sleepiness. However, the majority of CAD patients with OSA do not report daytime sleepiness, and the recent randomized controlled trials (RCTs) have failed to demonstrate cardiovascular benefits of CPAP in intention-to-treat (ITT) populations, which may be explained by low adherence to CPAP. In addition, randomized trials have consistently included a non-sleepy OSA phenotype for ethical reasons. Hence the exact interaction between OSA and CAD awaits further insights on whom and when to treat.

The current chapter reviews the clinical and epidemiologic evidence behind the relationship between CAD and OSA and the impact of treatment on cardiovascular outcomes.

EPIDEMIOLOGY

The risk of experiencing angina pectoris or an acute coronary syndrome (ACS), such as unstable angina, acute myocardial infarction (MI), or sudden cardiac death (SCD), increases during the late hours of sleep or in the early morning hours soon after awakening.[1] It has been hypothesized that this is due to the occurrence of OSA.[2] This is supported by a previous study with simultaneous polysomnography (PSG) and electrocardiographic recordings demonstrating that episodes of nocturnal ischemia CAD in patients with OSA occur mainly during rapid eye movement (REM) sleep during episodes of high apnea activity and during sustained hypoxemia.[3] Moreover, a longitudinal observational study of 10,701 consecutive adults showed that 142 patients had been resuscitated or suffered a fatal SCD (annual rate, 0.27%) during an average follow-up of 5.3 years; the OSA severity indices (apnea-hypopnea index

[AHI] of at least 20 events/hour; hazard ratio [HR], 1.60; mean nocturnal oxygen saturation <93% [HR, 2.93], and a nadir oxygen saturation <78% [HR, 2.60]; all $P < .001$) were associated with SCD in a multivariate analysis.[4]

Prevalence of Obstructive Sleep Apnea and Coronary Artery Disease in the General Population

In the largest cross-sectional population study, the Sleep Heart Health Study,[5] including 6132 subjects who underwent unattended home PSG, there was a modest risk increase (odds ratio [OR], 1.27) for self-reported CAD when the highest and lowest AHI quartiles (11.0 vs. 1.3 events/hour) were compared.

Prevalence of Coronary Artery Disease in Sleep Clinic Cohorts

Most clinical studies of CAD in sleep clinic cohorts have included patients with OSA and with daytime symptoms. In consequence, compared with studies in the general population, these studies deal with symptomatic patients, those likely to suffer from more severe OSA, and, potentially, patients with excess comorbidities, such as obesity, diabetes mellitus, and cardiovascular disorders. The ongoing multicentric European Sleep Apnea Cohort (ESADA) study, which prospectively recruits adults with a new diagnosis of OSA, reported a CAD prevalence of 8.7% among 6616 patients in one study.[6] There was a dose-response relationship between AHI (no OSA [AHI < 5 events/hour], mild [AHI 5 to 15 events/hour], moderate [AHI 15 to 30 events/hour], severe OSA [AHI ≥ 30 events/hour]), and the occurrence of CAD (5%, 8%, 11%, and 12%, respectively; $P < .001$).[6]

Prevalence of Obstructive Sleep Apnea in Coronary Artery Disease Cohorts

Early uncontrolled and controlled studies from 1990 to 2010 conducted in CAD cohorts have shown a high occurrence of OSA and independent associations between these two conditions.[7–18] A later case-control study found OSA (based on AHI ≥15) in 35% of patients with acute MI compared with 15% in the control group ($P < .001$).[19] The adjusted OR for acute MI was 12.2 (95% CI, 2.0 to 72.6) applying the AHI cut-off value of 15 for OSA diagnosis. Moreover, the Sleep and Stent Study, which addressed the impact of OSA on prognosis of the CAD in five countries (Singapore, China, Brazil, Myanmar, and India), reported OSA (AHI of 15 or greater on cardiorespiratory polygraphy within 7 days of percutaneous coronary intervention [PCI]) in 45.3% of screened patients.[20] Baseline data of an RCT among revascularized CAD patients in Sweden (the *R*andomized *I*ntervention with *C*PAP in *C*oronary *A*rtery *D*isease and Obstructive *S*leep *A*pnoea [RICCADSA] Trial) revealed that 64% had an AHI greater than or equal to 15 (Figure 148.1), and most did not report daytime hypersomnolence.[21] Of note, OSA in this cohort was more common than hypertension, diabetes mellitus, obesity, and current smoking. The baseline data of another RCT, among CAD patients with ACS in Spain, the *I*mpact of *S*leep *A*pnea syndrome in the evolution of *A*cute *C*oronary syndrome Effect of intervention with *C*ontinuous positive airway pressure (ISAACC) Study, demonstrated that 45% had OSA (AHI ≥ 15 events/hour on cardiorespiratory polygraphy).[22] As shown in Table 148.1, 11 studies between 2011and 2019, totaling 6672 patients with CAD, demonstrated an OSA prevalence of about 56%.[19–29]

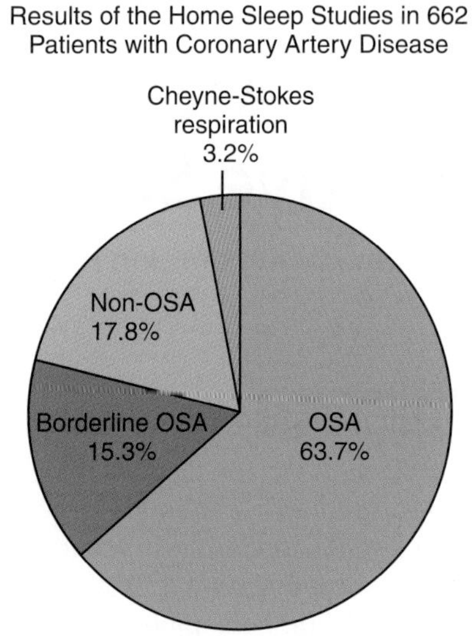

Figure 148.1 Classification of the groups based on the results of the unattended cardiorespiratory sleep recordings in patients with revascularized coronary artery disease. Obstructive sleep apnea (OSA) refers to apnea-hypopnea index (AHI) of 15 or more events/hour; borderline OSA, AHI 5.0–14.9 events/hour; non-OSA, AHI < 5 events/hour. (Modified from Glantz H, Thunström E, Herlitz J, et al. Occurrence and predictors of obstructive sleep apnea in a revascularized coronary artery disease cohort. *Ann Am Thorac Soc.* 2013;4:350–56.)

The Impact of Obstructive Sleep Apnea on the Prognosis of Coronary Artery Disease

Several studies during the first decade of the 21st century suggested a worse prognosis in CAD patients with concomitant OSA compared to those without OSA.[14,30–33] Conversely, neutral findings were also reported.[15,34] A meta-analysis addressing the impact of OSA on major adverse cardiac events (MACES) primarily focused on the CAD patients undergoing an acute or elective PCI, demonstrated a significantly increased risk for MACEs (OR, 1.52; 95% CI, 1.20 to 0.93) among 2465 patients from seven cohort studies with overnight sleep recordings within 1 month after the PCI.[35] These findings were supported by the above-mentioned Sleep and Stent Study,[20] demonstrating an increased crude incidence rate of MACEs among PCI patients with OSA compared with the patients with no OSA (3-year estimate, 18.9% vs. 14.0%) during a median follow-up of 1.9 years. The adjusted HR for OSA was 1.57 (95% CI, 1.10 to 2.24), independent of age, sex, ethnicity, body mass index (BMI), diabetes mellitus, and hypertension.[20] However, the rate of major adverse cardiac and cerebrovascular events (MACCEs) was similar in patients without OSA (90 events [15.1%]) and in the OSA group randomized to the no-CPAP group in the ISAACC cohort, with an HR 1.01 (95% CI, 0.76 to 1.35).[22] With a chosen AHI cut-off value of 15 events per hour for discrimination between OSA and no-OSA groups in a limited sleep study with cardiorespiratory polygraphy, the timing of the sleep studies within the first days of the ACS and the suboptimal adjustments for baseline comorbidities, as well as smoking status, have been regarded as important concerns regarding the null findings of the observational arm of the ISAACC trial.[36]

The prevalence of sleep apnea is also higher in patients with MI than in those with angina pectoris. This finding could be explained by the occurrence of central sleep apnea/Hunter-Cheyne-Stokes breathing (CSA/HCSB) as a result of reduced left ventricular ejection fraction (LVEF).[12] Indeed, the ideal timing for OSA screening after an acute MI remains unresolved. In a cohort study among 50 consecutive patients with ACS, an overnight PSG was conducted approximately 3 days after the acute event, and the patients with an AHI greater than or equal to 10 events per hour

Table 148.1 Prevalence of Obstructive Sleep Apnea in Patients with Coronary Artery Disease

First Author of Reference (Year)	Patients (No.)	Sex	Prevalence (%)	Diagnostic Criteria (Events/Hour)	Controlled
Sert Kuniyoshi[23] (2011)	99	Male, female	73	AHI ≥ 5	No
Schiza[24] (2012)	52	Male, female	54	AHI ≥ 10	No
Garcia-Rio[19] (2013)	192	Male, female	35	AHI ≥ 15	Yes
Glantz[21] (2013)	662	Male, female	64	AHI ≥ 15	No
Liu[25] (2014)	198	Male, female	45	AHI ≥ 5	No
Ben Ahmed[26] (2014)	120	Male, female	79	AHI ≥ 5	No
Loo[27] (2014)	68	Male, female	35	AHI ≥ 15	No
Ludka[28] (2014)	607	Male, female	66	AHI ≥ 5	No
Lee[20] (2016)	1311	Male, female	45	AHI ≥ 15	No
Jia[29] (2018)	529	Male, female	71	AHI ≥ 15	No
Sánchez-de-la Torre[22] (2019)	2834	Male, female	45	AHI ≥ 15	No
Total or mean	6672	—	56	—	—

at baseline were invited for a new investigation after 6 months.[37] Seventeen of 21 still had OSA, and there was a nonsignificant decrease in average AHI, whereas the patients with concomitant CSA/HCSR at baseline (n = 5) had no remaining central apneas at the follow-up.[37] Another study, published the same year, demonstrated OSA (AHI ≥ 10 events/hour) within the first 2 days after hospital admission in 54% of patients with ACSs and preserved LVEF, whereas 22 of 28 patients (79%) had residual OSA 1 month after the acute event, and only 6 of the 28 patients (21%) had OSA at 6-month follow-up.[38] A later study reported that 50% of CAD patients had an AHI greater than or equal to 15 at the time of acute presentation in the coronary care unit, whereas 28% had remaining OSA based on the same AHI cut-off at least 6 weeks after hospital discharge.[24] Thus not only CSA/HCSB, but also OSA, may be transient and, to some degree, related with the acute phase of the CAD, to the more supine position of patients in the coronary care units or to medications (sedatives and analgesics).

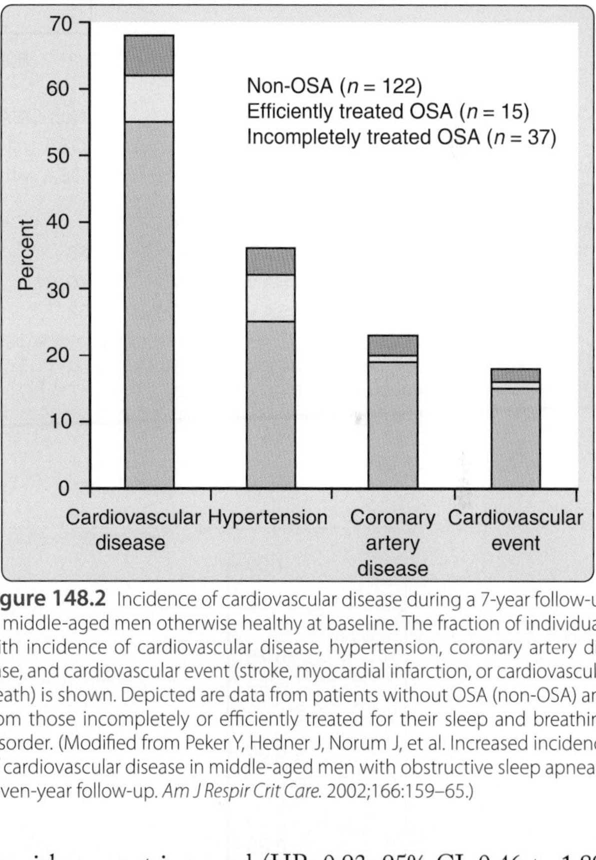

Figure 148.2 Incidence of cardiovascular disease during a 7-year follow-up in middle-aged men otherwise healthy at baseline. The fraction of individuals with incidence of cardiovascular disease, hypertension, coronary artery disease, and cardiovascular event (stroke, myocardial infarction, or cardiovascular death) is shown. Depicted are data from patients without OSA (non-OSA) and from those incompletely or efficiently treated for their sleep and breathing disorder. (Modified from Peker Y, Hedner J, Norum J, et al. Increased incidence of cardiovascular disease in middle-aged men with obstructive sleep apnea: a seven-year follow-up. *Am J Respir Crit Care.* 2002;166:159–65.)

Incident Coronary Artery Disease in Longitudinal Studies

After the first report on development of CAD among almost a quarter of untreated patients with OSA[39] and development of at least one cardiovascular disease (CVD) in greater than 50% of a normotensive sleep clinic cohort during a 7-year follow-up (Figure 148.2),[40] several larger studies from sleep clinic cohorts demonstrated increased risk of incident CVDs, CAD events, or cardiovascular mortality, with HRs ranging from 2.1 to 3.5.[41–44] Population-based longitudinal studies, the Wisconsin Sleep Cohort Study[45] and the Sleep Heart Health Study,[46] also demonstrated an increased risk for CVD mortality or incident CAD. However, the association was significant only in middle-aged men but not in the elderly or women.[46]

Impact of Obstructive Sleep Apnea Treatment on Patients with Coronary Artery Disease

Observational Studies

Several observational studies in the first decade of the 2000s suggested that treatment of OSA with CPAP was beneficial.[47–50] In a later prospective study of a consecutive cohort of elderly patients (≥65 years), the fully adjusted HRs for cardiovascular mortality were 2.25 (95% CI, 1.41 to 3.61) for the untreated severe OSA group compared with the control group, whereas the risk was not increased (HR, 0.93; 95% CI, 0.46 to 1.89) for the CPAP-treated group.[51] A similar study was performed among 1116 women in a sleep clinic cohort, demonstrating an HR of 3.50 (95% CI, 1.23 to 9.98) for untreated severe OSA compared with the control group, whereas the risk was not increased for the CPAP-treated group (HR, 0.55; 95% CI, 0.17 to 1.74).[43] More recently, the study of the observational arm of the RICCADSA cohort demonstrated no significant increase in MACEs in CAD patients with the sleepy OSA phenotype treated with CPAP compared with the CAD patients without OSA at baseline (adjusted HR, 0.96; 95% CI, 0.40 to 2.31).[52]

Evidence suggests that CPAP treatment reduces the number of ischemic events in patients with nocturnal angina and concomitant OSA in the short term.[53] The impact of CPAP on recurrent episodes in patients with acute MI and concomitant OSA in the long term has also been addressed.[19] After adjustment for confounding factors, treated OSA patients who were compliant with CPAP had a lower risk of recurrent MI and revascularization (adjusted HRs, 0.16 and 0.15, respectively) than untreated patients (Figure 148.3).[19]

Randomized Controlled Trials

The first RCT in a CAD cohort for MACCEs was the RICCADSA Trial,[54] which was a single-center study conducted in Sweden between 2005 and 2013. A consecutive population of 244 revascularized CAD patients with nonsleepy (Epworth Sleepiness Scale [ESS] < 10) OSA (AHI ≥ 15/hour) were allocated to autotitrating the CPAP or no-CPAP group, and the median follow-up period was 57 months. The primary composite cardiovascular end point (new revascularization, MI, stroke, or cardiovascular mortality) did not differ between the two groups (adjusted HR for CPAP, 0.62; 95% CI, 0.34 to 1.13) (Figure 148.4, *A*). However, on-treatment analysis showed a significant risk reduction when CPAP was used at least 4 hours per night (adjusted HR, 0.29; 95% CI, 0.10 to 0.86).[54]

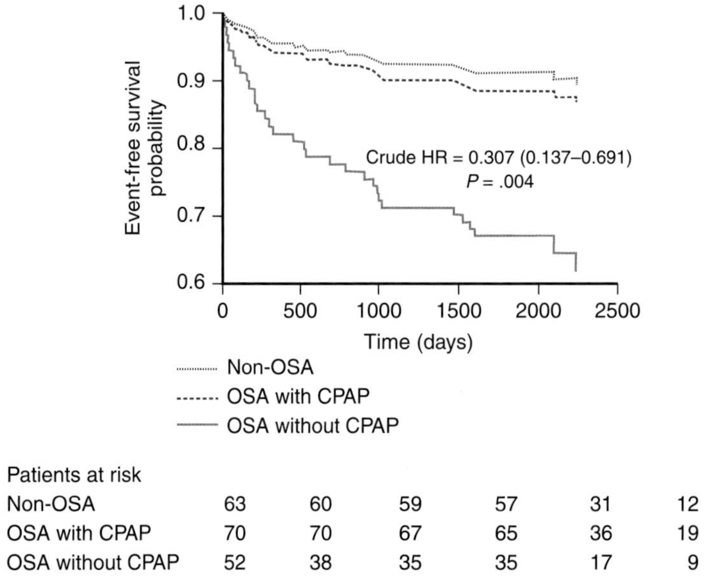

Figure 148.3 Time until first recurrent myocardial infarction in the three groups of patients with coronary artery disease. Crude hazard ratio (HR) of treated versus untreated obstructive sleep apnea (OSA) is presented. CPAP, Continuous positive airway pressure. (From Garcia-Rio F, Alonso-Fernandez A, Armada E, et al. CPAP effect on recurrent episodes in patients with sleep apnea and myocardial infarction. *Int J Cardiol.* 2013;168:1328–35.)

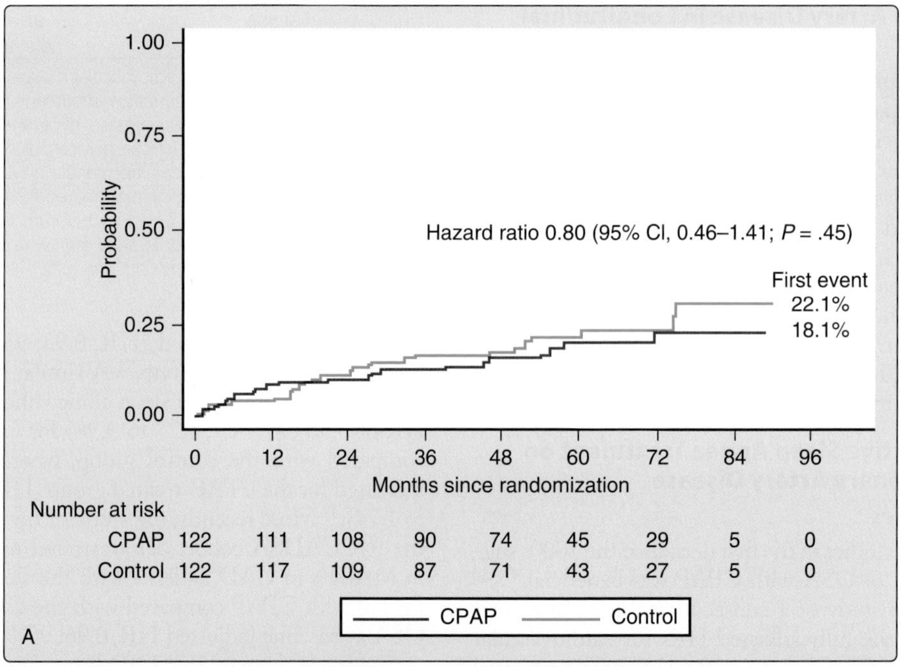

Figure 148.4 **A,** Cumulative incidences of the composite end point in the intention-to-treat population in the *R*andomized *I*ntervention with *C*PAP in *CAD* and *OSA* (RICCADSA) Trial.

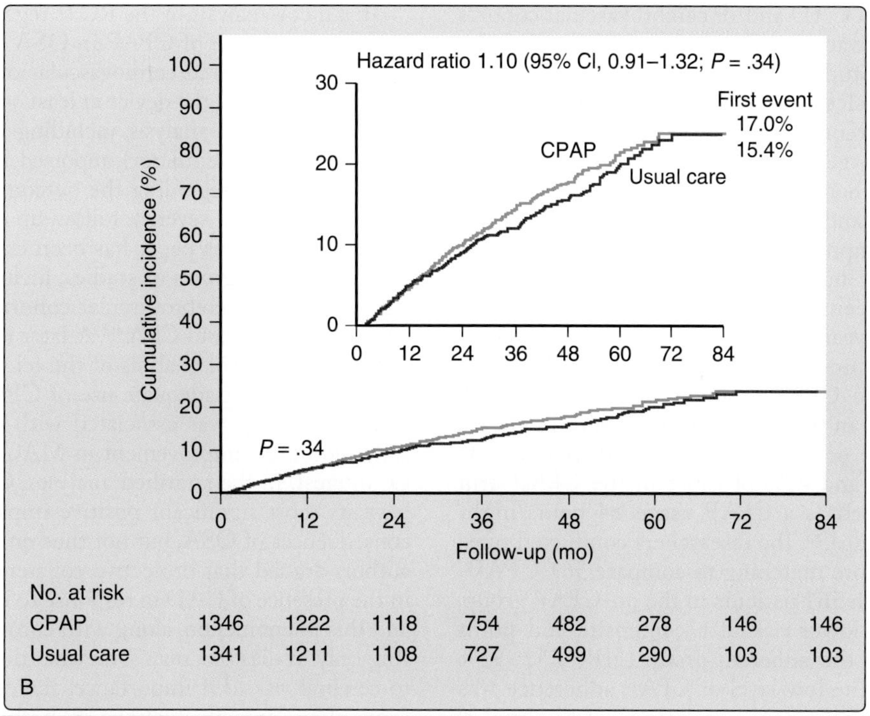

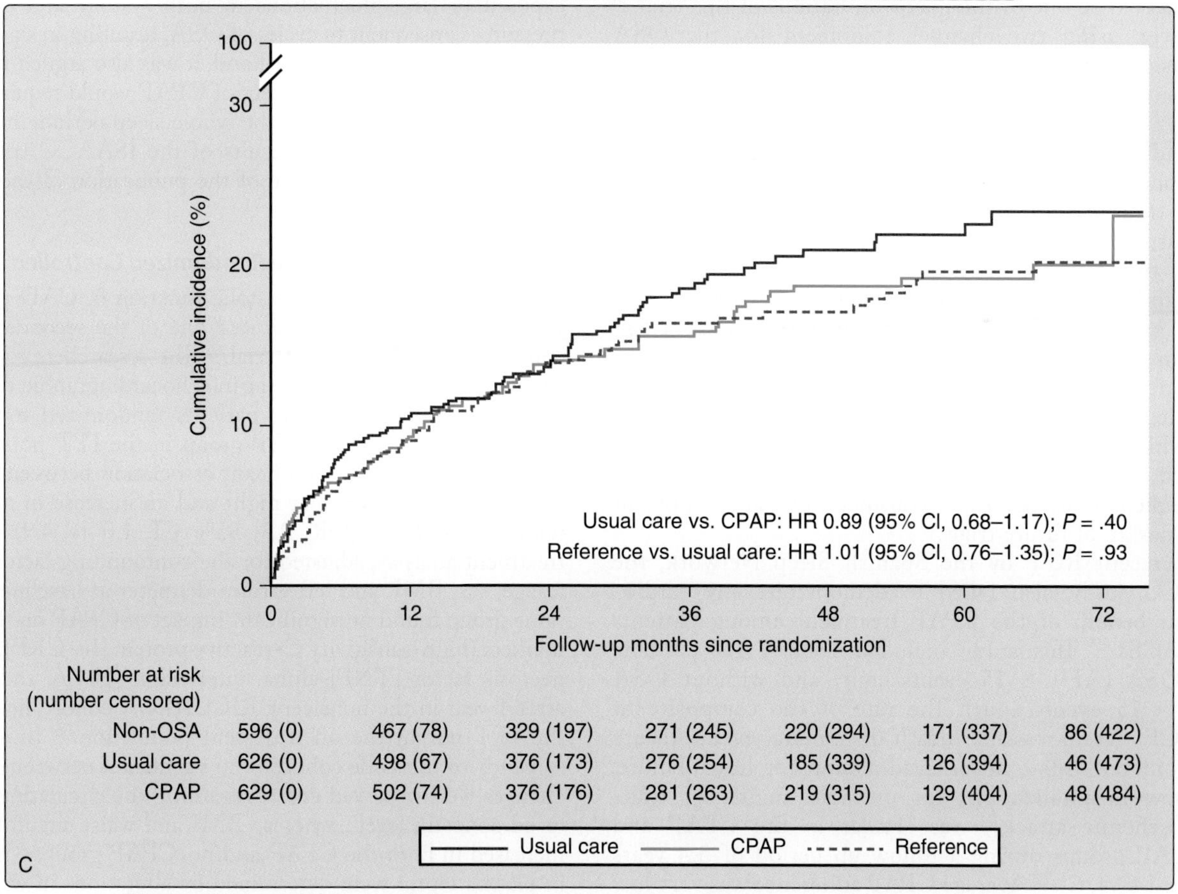

Figure 148.4 cont'd B, Cumulative event curve of the primary end point in the *S*leep Apnea cardio*V*ascular *E*ndpoints (SAVE) trial. **C,** Cumulative event curve of the primary end point in the CPAP group, the usual-care group, and the reference group. *Note:* The reference group is without obstructive sleep apnea. CPAP. Continuous positive airway pressure; HR, hazard ratio; OSA, obstructive sleep apnea. (**A** from Peker Y, Glantz H, Eulenburg C, et al. Effect of positive airway pressure on cardiovascular outcomes in coronary artery disease patients with non-sleepy obstructive sleep apnea. the RICCADSA randomized controlled trial. *Am J Respir Crit Care.* 2016;194:613–20); **B** from McEvoy RD, Antic NA, Heeley E, et al. CPAP for prevention of cardiovascular events in obstructive sleep apnea. *N Engl J Med.* 2016;375:919–31; **C** from Sánchez-de-la-Torre M, Sánchez-de-la-Torre A, Bertran S, et al. Effect of obstructive sleep apnoea and its treatment with continuous positive airway pressure on the prevalence of cardiovascular events in patients with acute coronary syndrome [ISAACC study]: a randomised controlled trial. *Lancet Respir Med.* 2020;8:359–67.)

The largest RCT in CAD and/or cerebrovascular cohorts hitherto conducted was the *S*leep *A*pnea cardio*V*ascular *E*ndpoints (SAVE) Study.[55] The researchers enrolled 2717 nonsleepy or mildly sleepy (ESS score <15) adults with a history of CAD or cerebrovascular disease and concomitant OSA, based on an oxygen desaturation index of at least 12 per hour on a two-channel home sleep recording device. The patients were randomized to CPAP or no CPAP, and the primary composite end point was cardiovascular death, MI, stroke, or hospitalization for unstable angina, heart failure, or transient ischemic attack. During an average follow-up of 3.7 years, the end-point event occurred in 17.0% of the patients in the CPAP group and in 15.4% of the patients in the no-CPAP group (HR for CPAP, 1.10; 95% CI, 0.91 to 1.32) in the ITT analysis (Figure 148.4, *B*). The average duration of adherence to CPAP therapy was 3.3 hours per night, and 42% of those in the CPAP-arm were adherent (defined as a CPAP usage ≥4 hours/night at the 2-year follow-up).[55] The researchers conducted one-to-one propensity-score matching to compare 561 CPAP-adherent patients with 561 patients in the no-CPAP group, and demonstrated a lower risk of a composite end point of cerebral events in the adherent group (HR, 0.52; 95% CI, 0.30 to 0.90).[55] The low level of CPAP adherence was suggested to be one of the major limitations of this trial.[56] Moreover, using two-channel equipment for the OSA diagnosis at baseline was a concern, given that this device has limitations in differentiating central and obstructive events.[57] It was argued that patients with CSA/HCSB may had been included, given that CSA/HCSB pattern is common in patients with stroke and heart failure enrolled in the trial.[57] Another major concern was the very high dropout rate (83%) from the primary consideration for eligibility to the end of the trial, and that some patients who were randomized to the control group had crossed over to CPAP group, possibly attenuating the effect of CPAP in ITT analysis.[58] Furthermore, subjects with moderate to severe desaturation and those with moderate excessive daytime sleepiness (ESS > 15 units) were excluded from the trial, which may have contributed to the negative results as detailed elsewhere.[59] We need to change our trial designs and implementations. These considerations are important in the design of future trials.

The recent RCT by the Spanish Sleep Network, the ISAACC study, also failed to demonstrate any cardiovascular benefit of the CPAP treatment among patients with ACSs.[22] This study included 1868 CAD patients with OSA (AHI ≥ 15 events/hour) and without OSA (AHI < 15 events/hour). The rate of the composite of MACCEs (cardiovascular death or nonfatal events [acute MI, nonfatal stroke, hospital admission for heart failure, and new hospitalizations for unstable angina or transient ischemic attack]) was similar in the CPAP and no-CPAP groups during a follow-up period of 3.4 years (Figure 148.4, *C*).[22] Average CPAP adherence was very low (2.8 hours/night) in the entire CPAP population, and there was no association between the MACCEs and CPAP compliance or OSA severity at baseline.[22] As aforementioned, assessment of the sleep studies within the first days of the ACS, the suboptimal adjustments for baseline comorbidities, and revascularization, in addition to the low adherence to CPAP, are discussed in a following commentary.[36]

In a meta-analysis of the RCTs regarding the cardiovascular outcomes,[60] use of CPAP in OSA patients was not associated with improved cardiovascular outcomes except in the subgroup that used the device at least 4 hours per night. However, another meta-analysis, including 10 trials (9 CPAP and 1 adaptive servo-ventilator), reported no evidence of benefit for PAP therapy regarding the outcomes adjusted for different levels of apnea severity, follow-up duration, or adherence to treatment.[61] This paper has been criticized for combining a heterogeneous group of studies, including both sleep clinic and cardiac and cerebrovascular cohorts, as well as including adults with OSA and CSA.[62] A later meta-analysis, focusing on the per protocol analysis of the relevant RCTs within the field, showed that adequate use of CPAP, defined as at least 4 hours per day, was associated with clinically and statistically significant improvement in MACCEs (Figure 148.5).[63] Of interest, in the stratified analyses, CPAP use appeared to have its most significant positive impact on cerebrovascular consequences of OSA, but not thus on cardiac outcomes. The authors argued that protective collateral vessels may develop in the presence of CAD in response to intermittent hypoxia,[64] and this phenomenon, along with coronary circulation occurring only in diastole, may somewhat diminish cardiac relative to cerebral risks. Of importance, the cerebral vascular bed is exposed to large fluctuations in both systolic and diastolic pressures consequent to cycles of OSA, resulting in significant vascular stress. On the other hand, it was also argued that the assumed cardioprotective effect of CPAP would require more than 4 hours of use, during the whole sleep period, including REM-sleep stages.[63] The results of the ISAACC trial were not yet available at the time of the publication of the aforementioned meta-analyses.[60,61,63]

Secondary Outcomes of the Randomized Controlled Trials

The impact of CPAP on diastolic function in CAD patients with nonsleepy OSA constituted one of the secondary outcomes in the RICCADSA trial.[65] The researchers found no significant changes after 1 year in echocardiographic diastolic function parameters among patients randomized to CPAP compared with the no-CPAP group in the ITT population. However, there was a significant association between CPAP use of at least 4 hours per night and an increase in diastolic relaxation velocity (OR, 2.3; 95% CI, 1.0 to 4.9) in on-treatment analysis, adjusted for the confounding factors such as age, sex, BMI, and left atrium diameter at baseline.[65] The same group found no significant impact of CPAP on the biomarkers (high-sensitivity C-reactive protein [hs-CRP], tumor necrosis factor [TNF]-alpha, interleukin [IL]-6, and IL-8) after 1 year in the nonsleepy RICCADSA cohort, neither in the ITT nor in the on-treatment population.[66] In another substudy of the same cohort,[67] no significant between-groups changes were observed either regarding the circulating leptin or adiponectin levels, whereas BMI and waist circumference increased in both the CPAP and no-CPAP groups. Changes in plasma leptin were determined by alterations in waist circumference (beta coefficient, 2.47; 95% CI, 0.77 to 4.40), whereas none of the analyzed parameters was predictive for alterations in circulating adiponectin levels.[67]

Among the other secondary outcomes addressed, depressive mood (defined as the Zung Self-rating Depressive Scale [SDS] score of 50 or more) was significantly improved among nonsleepy OSA patients in the CPAP group after 3 months

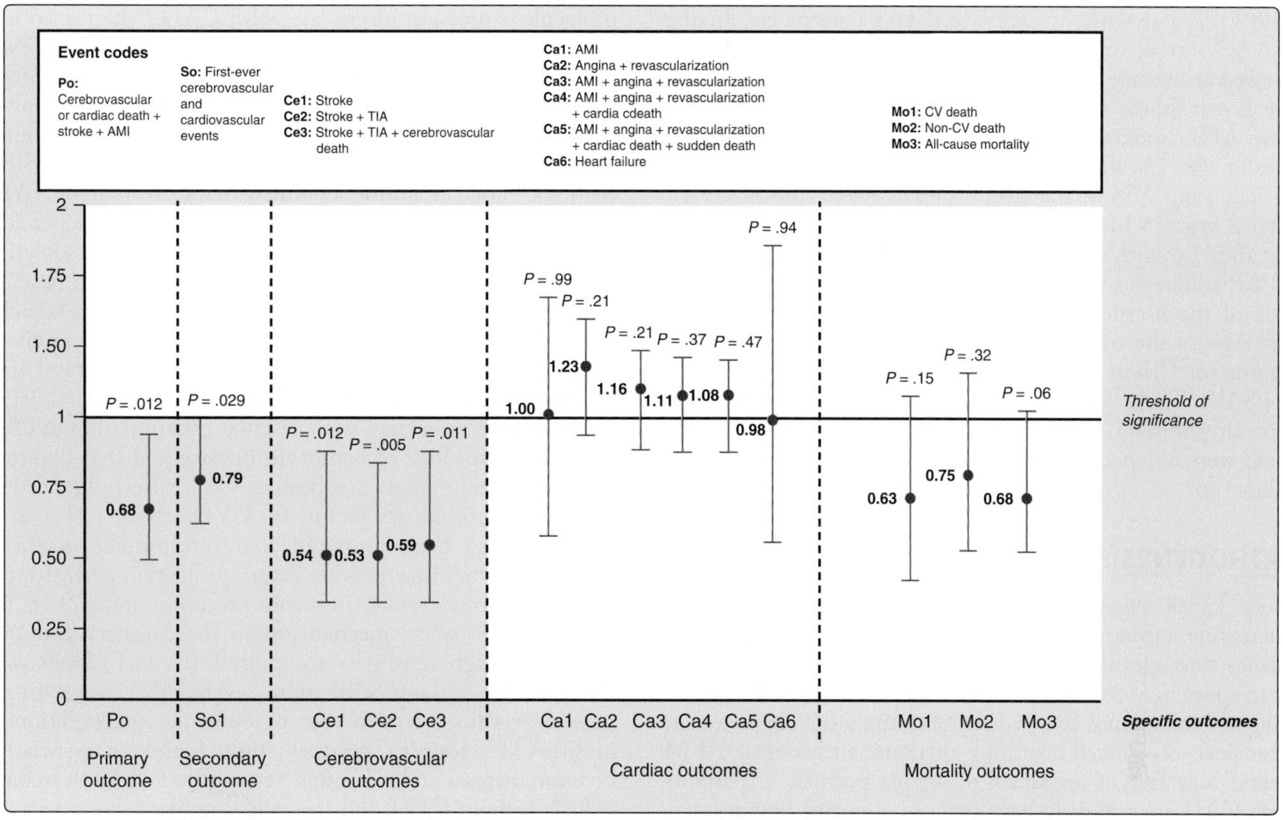

Figure 148.5 Summary of the main results on the effect of effective CPAP treatment on single or composite cardiovascular or cerebrovascular events. This figure shows the odds ratio with 95% confidence interval in the *y*-axis, whereas the *x*-axis shows the different types of individual and composite cardiovascular events divided into groups corresponding to (*from left to right*): primary outcome of the study, secondary outcome of the study, CV outcomes, cardiac outcomes, and mortality outcomes. AMI, Acute myocardial infarction; CPAP, continuous positive airway pressure; CV, cardiovascular; TIA, transient ischemic attack. (From Javaheri S, Martinez-Garcia MA, Campos-Rodriguez F, et al. CPAP adherence for prevention of major adverse cerebrovascular and cardiovascular events in obstructive sleep apnea. *Am J Respir Crit Care Med.* 2020;201:607–10.)

of treatment, which was stable up to 12 months, whereas no significant change was observed in the no-CPAP group in the ITT population.[68] Furthermore, CPAP adherence categories (CPAP usage, 3, 4, 5 hours/night) were significantly related with improvement in depressive mood (ORs 3.92, 4.45, and 4.89, respectively) in multivariate analyses adjusted for age, sex, BMI, LVEF, AHI, and ESS at baseline.[68] In the SAVE Trial, CPAP treatment was also associated with an improvement of depressive mood, defined according to the Hospital Anxiety and Depression Scale scores,[55] in the ITT population after 2 years. In the sleepy OSA phenotype, there were significant improvements in both SDS and ESS scores in the RICCADSA trial,[69] and the cut-off value of CPAP usage required for improvement in mood was 4 hours per night when change in ESS score from baseline was entered into the statistical model. In other words, the required "dose effect" of CPAP seems to be higher in sleepy apneic patients with a history of heart disease.[69]

An additional secondary outcome, the Health-Related Quality of Life (HRQoL), was also addressed in both RCTs.[55,70] In the SAVE Trial, CPAP treatment was associated with a minor, but statistically significant, improvement of the mean physical-component summary (from 45.4 to 46.9) and in the mental-component summary (from 52.6 to 53.6) of the Short-Form (SF)-36 questionnaires.[55] In the RICCADSA trial, 12 months of CPAP treatment had no significant effect on HRQoL as measured by the SF-36 in adults with CAD and nonsleepy OSA compared to those with no treatment. CPAP use was associated with a decrease in the physical component summary and an increase in the component summary. The latter was also dependent on decline in the ESS and the Zung Self-rating Depressive Scale scores.[70]

Adherence to Continuous Positive Airway Pressure Treatment in Coronary Artery Disease Patients with Obstructive Sleep Apnea

As mentioned earlier, excessive daytime sleepiness, a characteristic symptom of OSA, is often not reported in CAD patients. In one of the subprotocols of the RICCADSA trial, the impact of CPAP treatment on the Functional Outcomes of Sleep Questionnaire (FOSQ) was addressed among 105 patients without OSA matched with 105 OSA patients, of whom 80 were allocated to CPAP treatment.[71] The baseline FOSQ scores were similar in OSA and no-OSA groups, whereas excessive daytime sleepiness was almost fivefold higher in the OSA patients (OR, 4.8; 95% CI, 2.1 to 11.0). There was a significant improvement in the FOSQ score after 1 year in patients with excessive daytime sleepiness at baseline, notwithstanding suboptimal CPAP adherence.[71]

As pointed out in previous reviews and meta-analy ses,[60,61,63,72] CPAP adherence is challenging in CAD patients with OSA but without excessive daytime sleepiness. In the ISAACC trial, only 35% of the nonsleepy OSA patients showed an average CPAP usage of at least 4 hours per night at the 1-year follow-up.[73] The predictors of adherence at 1 year were AHI, smoking pack-years, long intensive care stay, and greater age.[73] In the RICCADSA trial, 60% of the nonsleepy patients, and 77% of the sleepy patients were still on CPAP after 2 years.[74] In the nonsleepy phenotype, age and CPAP use after 1 month were independently related with long-term CPAP adherence, suggesting that close supervision and support of the nonsleepy OSA patients during the first weeks and days of the treatment may increase adherence to CPAP treatment.[74] These findings were supported by the results of the SAVE Trial,[75] demonstrating that adherence during sham screening, initial CPAP titration, and the first month of treatment were independent predictors of adherence at the 2-year follow-up.

PATHOGENESIS

Sleep apnea causes recurrent hypoxia, reoxygenation, and fluctuating autonomic activity. Heart rate and blood pressure change through the apnea cycle, but the mechanisms by which sleep apnea may cause established CVD is unknown. Increased oxygen demand and reduced oxygen supply (i.e., hypoxemia) after sleep-disordered breathing, predominantly during REM sleep,[3] may trigger an attack of angina pectoris in patients with CAD, who already have reduced coronary flow reserve. Nocturnal periodic hypoxia may trigger mechanisms involved in the development of CAD and restenosis after PCI.[76] OSA is also associated with long-term alteration of cardiac structure, hemodynamic reflex function, and vascular structure or function. A report from the baseline echocardiographic investigations of the CAD patients with preserved LVEF in the RICCADSA cohort demonstrated a poorer diastolic function (OR, 1.9; 95% CI, 1.1 to 3.2) in patients with OSA after adjustment for traditionally recognized risk factors.[77] In OSA, baroreceptor and chemoreceptor responsiveness is modified[78]; along with sustained sympathetic activation,[79] vascular reactivity to hypoxemia or vasoconstrictors is elevated[80] while vascular endothelial function is reduced.[81] Some, but not all, of these changes appear to be specific to OSA in the sense that they are reversed by CPAP.[82–86]

The mechanisms responsible for functional vascular remodeling are incompletely understood, but oxidative stress after periodic hypoxia and reperfusion may play an important role.[87] Other steps in this process include compromised nitric oxide bioavailability, increased expression of adhesion molecules, and an acceleration of vascular inflammation, atherosclerosis, and vascular dysfunction. This hypothesis[87] is supported by data from patients with OSA demonstrating increased free radical production,[83] increased plasma-lipid peroxidation, increased adenosine and uric acid levels,[87] and increased levels of redox-sensitive gene expression products, including vascular endothelial growth factor[88] and inflammatory cytokines.[89] Of interest, there was an improvement of endothelial function in patients with OSA after inhibition of xanthine oxidase by allopurinol[90] or supplemental vitamin C.[91] Circulating levels of adhesion molecules[92] and adhesion molecule–dependent monocytes to endothelial cell avidity appear to be increased in OSA.[93] Finally, sleep apnea appears to provide an additive stimulus for adhesion molecule expression in patients with CAD.[94] Increased levels of circulating markers of inflammation, including TNF-alpha,[95] hs-CRP,[89,95] and IL-6,[89] have been inconsistently found to be increased in OSA. It is unknown whether one or several steps in this cascade are influenced by other comorbid conditions in OSA. A report from the Icelandic Sleep Apnea Cohort, including 454 untreated OSA patients (AHI ≥ 15), demonstrated that OSA severity was an independent predictor of levels of CRP and IL-6, but this association was found only in obese patients.[96] Although the baseline data of the RICCADSA cohort demonstrated an association between OSA and elevated CRP and IL-6, also in nonobese patients,[97] there was no significant improvement after 1 year of CPAP treatment.[66] This suggests that established CAD may be associated with vascular inflammation in OSA patients irrespective of comorbid obesity and that determinants of these markers are, besides OSA, also influenced by multiple comorbid risk factors for CVD.

It has also been proposed that intermittent nocturnal hypoxia in OSA may provide future protection against myocardial ischemic insults (ischemic preconditioning[98]) by the regulation of critical mechanisms in the coronary endothelium.[99,100] High-sensitivity troponin-T (hs-TnT) levels were lower in MI patients with more severe OSA, suggesting a possible cardioprotective role by ischemic preconditioning in OSA.[101] However, another study found an association between increasing AHI and increasing hs-TnT levels in individuals without CVD, and the follow-up data showed a relation between hs-TnT and risk for death or incident HF in all OSA categories, suggesting that subclinical myocardial injury caused by OSA may play a role for the future risk for cardiac disease.[102] Thus the short-term benefits of a possible ischemic preconditioning due to intermittent hypoxemia may be counteracted by other adverse outcomes in the long run.

The tentative association between OSA and CAD is supported by experimental data suggesting oxidative stress, endothelial dysfunction, and acceleration of vascular inflammation as a result of OSA. All these mechanisms facilitate the onset and progression of atherosclerosis. Presence of atherosclerosis in large arteries of OSA patients without other risk factors for CAD was associated with the severity of OSA.[103] Indeed, several studies have reported higher atherosclerotic plaque volume in the coronary vessels in OSA patients investigated with three-dimensional intravascular ultrasound.[104] The frequency of noncalcified or mixed plaques was much higher in patients with OSA investigated by noninvasive coronary computed tomography angiography.[105] Such plaques may jeopardize coronary flow reserve and generate symptoms of nocturnal angina during periods of increased flow demand. However, most heart attacks (i.e., acute MI, sudden cardiac death) stem from sudden rupture of less obtrusive plaques, which trigger thrombus formation in coronary vessels.[106]

CLINICAL COURSE AND PREVENTION

Early recognition and treatment of OSA may be beneficial in terms of CAD prevention. Patients with CAD and nocturnal angina should undergo sleep recording because nasal CPAP reduces angina attacks and nocturnal myocardial ischemia.[53] Although there is scientific support for a considerable effect of OSA on vascular structure and function, it is likely that development of CAD and other forms of vascular disease is determined by multiple genotypic and phenotypic factors. The absolute role of OSA in this concerted influence should evidently be better clarified. However, with the increasing recognition of OSA as an independent, additive, or even synergistic risk factor for CAD, we are facing a need for early identification of high-risk persons and a consensus on well-defined treatment strategies in such patients. Observational data suggest that elimination of sleep apneas by CPAP can benefit patients at risk of CAD in the immediate and long term in sleep clinic cohorts with OSA-related symptoms, such as excessive daytime sleepiness. However, the majority of CAD patients with concomitant OSA do not report daytime sleepiness, and recent RCTs have failed to demonstrate cardiovascular benefits of CPAP in ITT populations.[22,54,55] Adherence to CPAP seems to be the main challenge in CAD patients with a nonsleepy OSA phenotype.[74,75,106]

CLINICAL PEARLS

- Recurrent apneas during sleep lead to a sequence of events that, independently or in concert with other recognized risk factors, are likely to have adverse effects on vascular structure and function.
- Not only may phenomena such as hypoxemia, reoxygenation, and recurrent vascular wall stress induce coronary artery disease (CAD), but also the events themselves may aggravate already-existing compromised coronary artery flow reserve.
- The adverse health effects of obstructive sleep apnea (OSA) in terms of CAD development, progression, and proneness to complications are likely to depend on genotypic and phenotypic factors. Markers or predictors for identification of high-risk persons in this context are still lacking.
- Greater than 50% of patients with CAD have OSA, defined according to conventional criteria. A large fraction of these patients does not exhibit daytime sleepiness. Better characterization of specific phenotypes of OSA may provide means to investigate the role of limited adherence to CPAP and the importance of sleepiness on CAD development in patients with OSA.
- Recognition of the adverse effect of OSA on vascular disease will open a perspective of new primary and secondary prevention models for CAD that involve identifying and eliminating the sleep-disordered breathing.

SUMMARY

Recurrent apneas during sleep lead to a sequence of events that, independently or in concert with other recognized risk factors, are likely to have harmful effects on vascular structure and function. OSA-related phenomena, including hypoxemia, reoxygenation, and recurrent vascular wall stress, may induce CAD, and the events may aggravate already existing compromised coronary artery flow reserve. The epidemiologic support for a causal relationship between OSA and CAD is increasing, but is not fully, confirmed. This relationship is stronger in clinical cohorts than in the general population, which suggests that comorbid OSA in obese, hypertensive, smoking, and hyperlipidemic patients may provide an additive or synergistic risk factor for development of CAD.

Patients with CAD, including nocturnal angina, should therefore be considered for diagnostic sleep recording because elimination of apneas by nasal CPAP during sleep has been shown to reduce angina attacks and nocturnal myocardial ischemia. Likewise, prospective observational cohort data point to a reduction of recurrent MI and revascularization in CAD patients treated with CPAP. However, recent RCTs have failed to demonstrate cardiovascular benefits of CPAP in ITT populations. Per-protocol analyses of these trials suggest that adequate use of CPAP, defined as at least 4 hours per day, may reduce long-term cardiovascular and cerebrovascular events, with its most significant positive impact on the cerebrovascular outcomes.

The long-term tentative causal association between OSA and CAD is supported by experimental data suggesting endothelial dysfunction, acceleration of vascular inflammation, and development of atherosclerotic disease as a result of the breathing disorder. Increased recognition of the adverse effect of OSA phenotypes on vascular disease and improvement of adherence to CPAP treatment, as well as personalized treatment strategies, may open a perspective of new primary and secondary prevention models for CAD that involve identification and elimination of the OSA.

SELECTED READINGS

Celik Y, Thunström E, Strollo Jr PJ, Peker Y. Continuous positive airway pressure treatment and anxiety in adults with coronary artery disease and nonsleepy obstructive sleep apnea in the RICCADSA trial. *Sleep Med.* 2021;77:96–103.

Franklin KA, Nilsson JB, Sahlin C, et al. Sleep apnea and nocturnal angina. *Lancet.* 1995;345:1085–1087.

Gami AS, Olson EJ, Shen WK, et al. Obstructive sleep apnea and the risk of sudden cardiac death. *J Am Coll Cardiol.* 2013;62:610–616.

Garcia-Rio F, Alonso-Fernandez A, Armada E, et al. CPAP effect on recurrent episodes in patients with sleep apnea and myocardial infarction. *Int J Cardiol.* 2013;168:1328–1335.

Javaheri S, Martinez-Garcia MA, Campos-Rodriguez F, Muriel A, Peker Y. CPAP Adherence for prevention of major adverse cerebrovascular and cardiovascular events in obstructive sleep apnea. *Am J Respir Crit Care Med.* 2020;201:607–610.

Lu M, Fang F, Wang Z, et al. Association between obstructive sleep apnea and quantitative atherosclerotic plaque burden: a coronary computed tomographic angiography study [published online ahead of print, 2021 Jul 28]. *Chest.* 2021;S0012-3692(21):01489-6.

McEvoy RD, Antic NA, Heeley E, et al. CPAP for prevention of cardiovascular events in obstructive sleep apnea. *N Engl J Med.* 2016;375:919–931.

Peker Y, Glantz H, Eulenburg C, et al. Effect of positive airway pressure on cardiovascular outcomes in coronary artery disease patients with nonsleepy obstructive sleep apnea. The RICCADSA randomized controlled trial. *Am J Respir Crit Care.* 2016;194:613–620.

Querejeta Roca G, Redline S, Punjabi N, et al. Sleep apnea is associated with subclinical myocardial injury in the community: the ARIC-SHHS study. *Am J Respir Crit Care Med.* 2013;188:1460–1465.

Sánchez-de-la-Torre M, Sánchez-de-la-Torre A, Bertran S, et al. Effect of obstructive sleep apnoea and its treatment with continuous positive airway pressure on the prevalence of cardiovascular events in patients with acute coronary syndrome (ISAACC study): a randomised controlled trial. *Lancet Respir Med.* 2020;8:359–367.

Zinchuk AV, Chu JH, Liang J, et al. Physiological traits and adherence to therapy of sleep apnea in individuals with coronary artery disease [published online ahead of print, 2021 Jun 22]. *Am J Respir Crit Care Med.* 2021. https://doi.org/10.1164/rccm.202101-0055OC.

A complete reference list can be found online at ExpertConsult.com.

Chapter 149

Heart Failure

Shahrokh Javaheri

Chapter Highlights

- Multiple studies from across the globe show that about 50% of patients with heart failure, both heart failure with reduced ejection fraction and preserved ejection fraction, have moderate to severe sleep apnea with an apnea-hypopnea index exceeding 15/hour.
- Both obstructive and central sleep apneas may occur concomitantly in the same patient. Therapy will depend, in part, on predominant apnea type, which is determined by polysomnography.
- Multiple studies also indicate that both obstructive and central sleep apneas are independently associated with readmission to the hospital and excess mortality. Furthermore, observational studies suggest that effective treatment decreases the number of readmissions and premature mortality.
- The largest randomized trial of adaptive servo-ventilation in heart failure with reduced ejection fraction (HFrEF) was neutral, with increased cardiovascular mortality in the treated arm compared with the usual care. Therefore use of the device is not indicated for treatment of heart failure with reduced left ventricular ejection fraction. The device could be used in those with preserved ejection fraction.
- Phrenic nerve stimulation has been approved by the U.S. Food and Drug Administration for treatment of central sleep apnea of various etiologies. Sustained efficacy has been shown up to 5 years.
- Two ongoing randomized controlled trials are in process to evaluate oxygen and newer devices in HFrEF.
- For treatment of obstructive sleep apnea, continuous positive airway pressure therapy is the treatment of choice. Importantly, an observational study suggests that survival benefits are encountered only in those who are compliant with the device.

Heart failure (HF) has been known for more than 2 centuries to be associated with abnormal breathing patterns, and John Cheyne and William Stokes have been credited for its description—hence the eponym *Cheyne-Stokes breathing*.[1,2] However, 37 years earlier, John Hunter,[3,4] a British physician, was the first to describe this breathing pattern, which is characterized by gradual crescendo-decrescendo changes in tidal volume, commonly with an intervening central apnea (Figure 149.1).[5] We therefore refer to this pattern as *Hunter-Cheyne-Stokes breathing* (HCSB). Periodic breathing is a pattern of breathing characterized by cyclic fluctuations in the amplitude of airflow and tidal volume.[6] It consists of recurring cycles of apnea or hypopnea, or both, followed by hyperpnea. The apneas and hypopneas may be obstructive (i.e., the result of upper airway occlusion) or central.[6] Obstructive sleep apnea (OSA)–hypopnea is the most common form of periodic breathing in persons without HF. However, in patients *with* HF, both obstructive and central periodic breathing are common and frequently occur together, although one phenotype is predominant. As initially described, HCSB is a form of periodic breathing with central sleep apnea (CSA) and hypopnea that occurs in patients with HF, mostly those with reduced left ventricular ejection fraction (LVEF), and has a long cycle time.[7] The latter is an important feature of HCSB breathing and reflects the prolonged circulation time that is a pathologic feature of HF. Polysomnographic studies have reported a high prevalence of this disorder in ambulatory patients with stable HF.[8]

EPIDEMIOLOGY OF HEART FAILURE AND SLEEP-RELATED BREATHING DISORDERS

HF remains a major public health problem.[9] In 2017, 80,480 individuals died from HF; 809,000 with this diagnosis were discharged from the hospital. The American Heart Association has estimated that about 6.2 million Americans over 20 years of age have HF. Furthermore, it is projected that the prevalence will increase 46% from 2012 to 2030, resulting in more than 8 million people 18 years of age or older with HF. In 2030, 2.97% of the population will suffer from HF.

Left ventricular (LV) myocardial failure is the most common cause of HF in adults, and it could be predominantly diastolic, referred to as *heart failure with preserved ejection fraction* (HFpEF) when EF is greater than 50%, or manifested by combined systolic and diastolic dysfunction, referred to as *heart failure with reduced ejection fraction* (HFrEF) when EF is

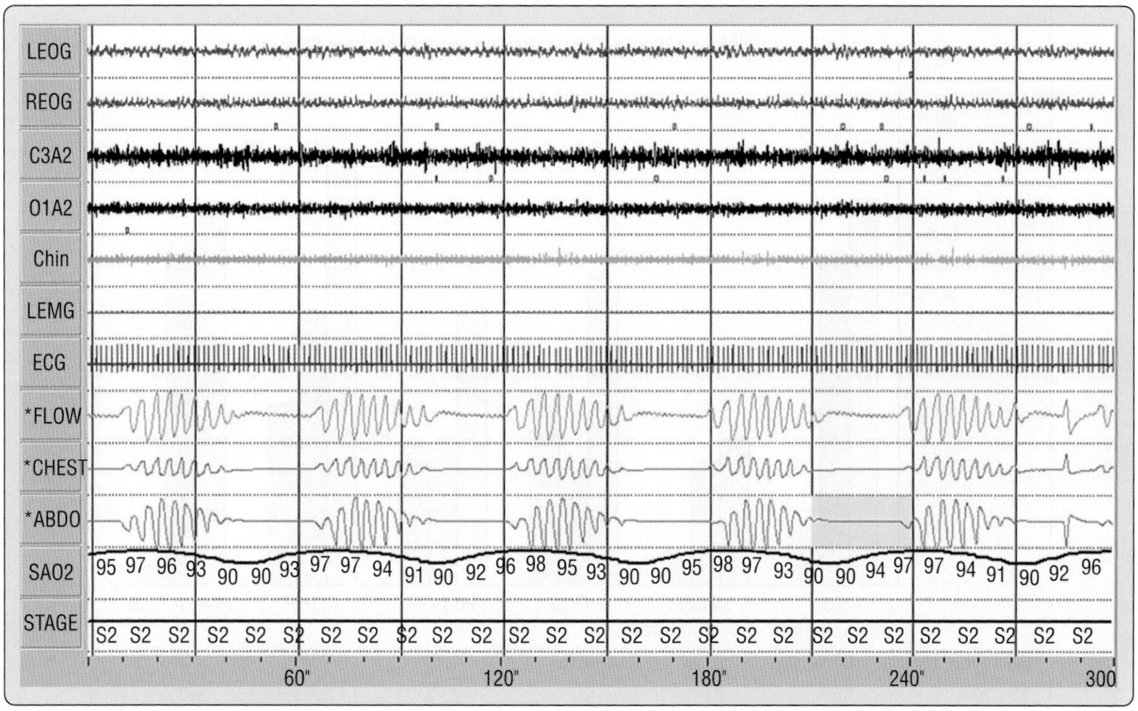

Figure 149.1 A 10-minute epoch of a patient with systolic heart failure and Hunter-Cheyne-Stokes breathing. Note recurrent hypoxia/reoxygenation as a result of central sleep apnea. (From Kryger MH. *Atlas of Clinical Sleep Medicine.* 2nd ed. Saunders; 2014.)

less than 40%. The principal hallmark of HFrEF is a depressed LVEF, which is commonly associated with an increase in end-diastolic and systolic volumes. The symptoms, which result from both diminished cardiac output and the concomitant diastolic dysfunction, include shortness of breath, orthopnea, nocturnal dyspnea, nocturia, fatigue, and exercise intolerance. Many of these symptoms overlap with those of sleep apnea, making it difficult to suspect sleep apnea when comorbid with HF.

Meanwhile, it is estimated that 20 million people may have asymptomatic LV systolic dysfunction, and, with time, these persons are likely to develop HFrEF. As is discussed later, overall about 50% of individuals with LV systolic dysfunction both asymptomatic or symptomatic suffer from moderate to severe sleep apnea.

The other phenotype, HFpEF, is the most common form of HF in elderly patients. The pathophysiologic consequence of LV diastolic dysfunction relates to a hypertrophied or a noncompliant left ventricle shifting the pressure volume curve upward and to the left. Therefore, for a given LV volume, LV end-diastolic pressure increases, resulting in elevated left atrial and pulmonary capillary pressures, pulmonary congestion, and edema. Similar to asymptomatic LV systolic dysfunction, which, with time, leads to HFrEF, asymptomatic LV diastolic dysfunction is also independently associated with incident overt HF and is predictive of all-cause death.[10]

SLEEP APNEA IN HEART FAILURE WITH REDUCED EJECTION FRACTION

Sleep-disordered breathing is prevalent in HFrEF, HFpEF, acute cardiogenic pulmonary edema, and asymptomatic LV dysfunction (Figure 149.2). The prevalence has been systematically studied in patients with HFrEF.[11] This has been shown both by polysomnography and respiratory studies.[5,7,12-16] One large study showed that about 50% of treated, stable patients with HF had an apnea-hypopnea index (AHI) of 15 events per hour or greater, a value much higher than that seen in the general population.[17]

SLEEP APNEA IN HEART FAILURE WITH PRESERVED EJECTION FRACTION

There is also a high prevalence of sleep apnea in HFpEF[18,19] (Figure 149.1). The largest prospective study[18] to date evaluated 244 consecutive patients (87 women). The two major causes of HFpEF were systemic hypertension (44%) and coronary artery disease (33%). Forty-eight percent had an AHI of 15 or more per hour, of whom 23% had CSA. Patients with CSA had lower Pco_2 but higher LV end-diastolic and pulmonary capillary wedge pressure. The latter finding is critical to the development of periodic breathing and CSA because increased wedge pressure and pulmonary congestion decrease the Pco_2 reserve, the major mechanism underlying CSA.[20]

There is a vicious cycle between HFpEF and sleep apnea. Hemodynamic studies show that pulmonary capillary pressure increases during the course of obstructive apnea, indicating the development of LV diastolic dysfunction (see Chapter 120). Chronic repetitive exposure to negative swings in intrathoracic pressure, cyclic nocturnal hypertension and hypoxemia, and diurnal systemic hypertension could eventually result in worsening the LV hypertrophy, dysfunction, and HF. OSA is associated with an increase in LV mass and dysfunction.[21-23] Furthermore, in an observational study, patients with OSA treated with continuous positive airway pressure (CPAP) experienced a reversal of diastolic dysfunction.[22] In another

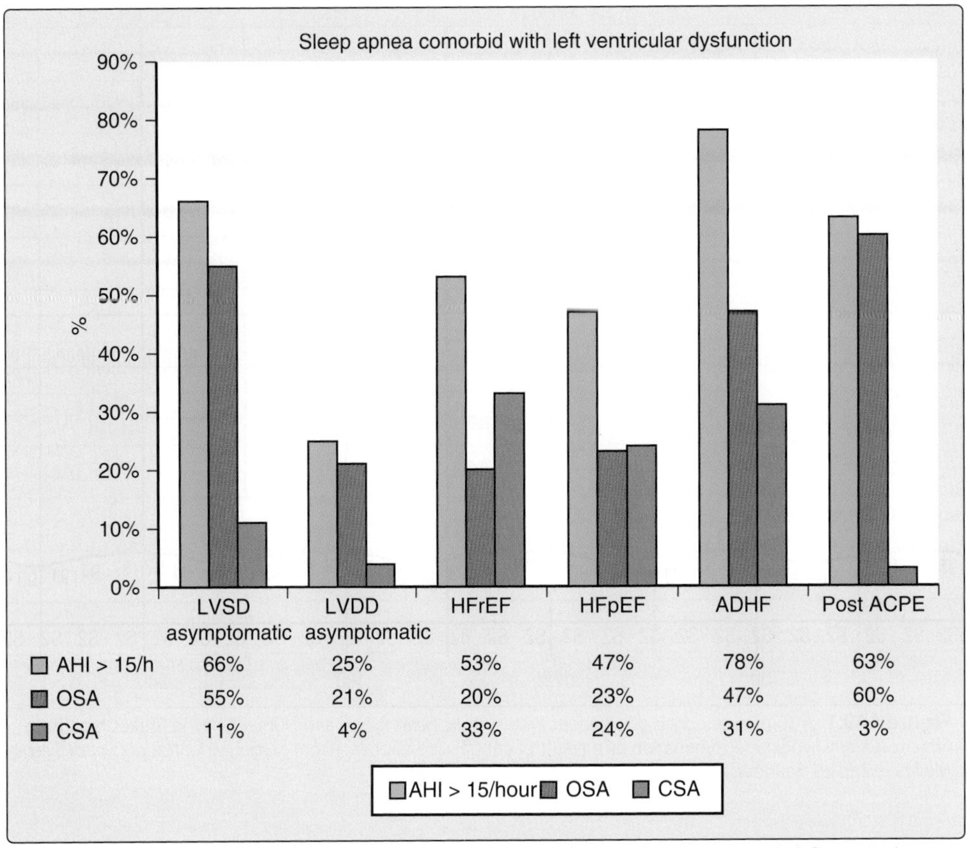

Figure 149.2 Prevalence (%) of moderate-to-severe sleep apnea (AHI ≥ 15) in asymptomatic left ventricular systolic dysfunction (LVSD) or left ventricular diastolic dysfunction (LVDD), heart failure with preserved ejection fraction (HFpEF) or heart failure with reduced ejection fraction (HFrEF), acutely decompensated heart failure (ADHF), and acute cardiogenic pulmonary edema. ACPE, acute cardiogenic pulmonary edema; AHI, apnea-hypopnea index; CSA, central sleep apnea; OSA, obstructive sleep apnea. (Modified from Javaheri S, Barbe F, Campos-Rodriguez F, et al. Sleep apnea: types, mechanisms, and clinical cardiovascular consequences. *J Am Coll Cardiol.* 2017;69[7]:841–858.)

observational study, an adaptive servo-ventilation (ASV) device was used to treat patients with HFpEF and HCSB and severe CSA. ASV treatment led to a significant decrease in left atrial diameter and early-to-atrial (E/A) filling velocity ratio, whereas the early filling–to–early diastolic mitral annular velocity ratio increased significantly.[21] It therefore appears that treatment of both OSA and CSA results in remodeling of the left heart structures. These observational findings have been confirmed by a randomized placebo (sham CPAP)–controlled trial, showing that, after 12 weeks on effective CPAP therapy, there was a significant increase in the E/A ratio and a significant decrease in isovolemic relaxation and mitral deceleration time.[24] The results of these studies have important therapeutic implications for HFpEF because, to date, there are no approved therapies to reduce hospitalization or mortality for this disorder, which is on the rise, and the growing elderly population in whom HFpEF is the predominant phenotype of HF guarantees additional burden.[25] In addition, similar to asymptomatic LV systolic dysfunction, which, as noted earlier, will eventually lead to HFrEF, it has been shown that LV diastolic dysfunction is a precursor to HFpEF.[10]

In summary, the prevalence of moderate to severe sleep apnea is about 50% in both forms of HF, HFrEF and HFpEF (Figure 149.2), and introduction of beta blockers in the therapeutic armamentarium of HF has had no impact on the prevalence of sleep apnea. In contrast to OSA (which is the predominant form of the disorder in the general population with a rare episode of central apnea in the pattern, in HF), central and OSA commonly occur together. Sleep physicians reviewing the polysomnogram therefore have to determine the predominant form of the disorder to determine therapeutic options. The predominant phenotype, obstructive versus central, is variable and in large part depends on the categorization of hypopneas into central or obstructive.

SLEEP-DISORDERED BREATHING IN ACUTE CARDIOGENIC PULMONARY EDEMA

Acute cardiogenic pulmonary edema (ACPE) is a life-threatening condition, and OSA is a frequent comorbidity.[26] In a longitudinal observational study of 104 patients, 61% of the patients had OSA defined as an AHI of 15 or higher per hour of recording. Incidence of recurrent ACPE and myocardial infarction was significantly increased in patients with OSA than in those without OSA, and all 17 deaths occurred in the OSA group. OSA was independently and significantly associated with ACPE recurrence, incidence of myocardial infarction, and death.[26] A randomized controlled trial (RCT) with CPAP is needed to determine if treatment improves aforementioned adverse outcomes.

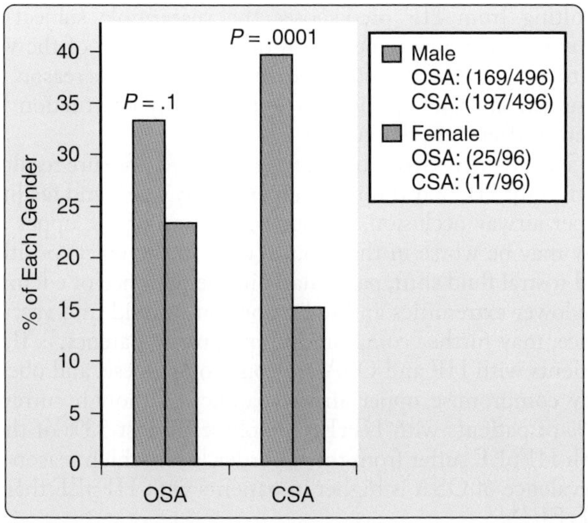

Figure 149.3 Prevalence of obstructive sleep apnea (OSA) and central sleep apnea (CSA) in men and women with systolic heart failure. The prevalence of CSA is much lower in women than in men. A similar trend is found in OSA, although it is not statistically significant. (From Javaheri S. Sleep related breathing disorders in heart failure. In: Mann DL, editor. *Heart Failure: A Companion to Braunwald's Heart Disease*. Saunders; 2004;471–87.)

GENDER AND SLEEP-RELATED BREATHING DISORDERS IN HEART FAILURE

In the general population, the prevalence of OSA is much higher in men than in women. This also holds true for CSA in HFrEF. Combining the results of several studies of patients with HFrEF, about 40% of the male patients and 18% of the female patients have CSA (Figure 149.3). A similar trend was found for OSA.

In women with congestive HF and systolic dysfunction, the risk of CSA was six times higher in those ages 60 years and older than in those younger than 60 years.[27] A similar difference was also reported for OSA–hypopnea before and after age 60 years. Thus female hormonal status plays a role in the development of sleep-disordered breathing in women with and without HF.

Progesterone is a known respiratory stimulant, and its effects on the respiratory system may, in part, explain the lower prevalence of central and OSA in menstruating women. Progesterone increases ventilation[28] and the tone of the dilator muscles of the upper airway.[29] Furthermore, premenopausal women have a significantly lower apneic threshold than men.[30] This should decrease the probability of developing central apnea during sleep in female subjects (see the following section on Mechanisms of Central Sleep Apnea in Heart Failure).

MECHANISMS OF SLEEP-RELATED BREATHING DISORDERS IN HEART FAILURE

Mechanisms of Central Sleep Apnea in Heart Failure

The mechanisms of periodic breathing and CSA in HF are complex and multifactorial (see Chapter 100).[20] In HF alterations occur in various components of the negative feedback system controlling breathing that increase the likelihood of developing periodic breathing, during both sleep and wakefulness. In addition, there are specific sleep-related mechanisms that explain the genesis of CSA and the reason periodic breathing becomes so prevalent during sleep.

Mathematical models of the negative feedback system predict that increased arterial circulation time (which delays the transfer of information regarding changes in Po_2 and Pco_2 from pulmonary capillary blood to the chemoreceptors, referred to as *mixing gain*), enhanced gain of the chemoreceptors, and enhanced plant gain (e.g., decreased functional residual capacity), which are the three components of the loop gain, collectively increase the likelihood of periodic breathing.[31]

Loop gain is the engineering term that defines the tendency of the negative feedback loop toward instability in response to a ventilatory disturbance. As an example, normally, a short pause in breathing, an apnea, or hypopnea causes a compensatory increase in ventilation. If the magnitude of the increase in ventilation is greater than or equal to the magnitude of the preceding respiratory disturbance, that is, loop gain is 1 or greater, the system becomes unstable and will fluctuate between underventilation and overventilation.

Delay in transfer of information resulting from prolonged circulation time, that is, increased mixing gain, plays a fundamental role in destabilization of a negative feedback system.[5,7,20,32] It has the potential to convert a negative feedback system to a positive feedback system. In HF, arterial circulation time may be increased for a variety of reasons, including dilation of cardiac chambers, increased pulmonary blood volume, and decreased cardiac output. However, patients with HF invariably have increased circulation time. Therefore, although increased circulation time is necessary to develop periodic breathing, it does not explain why only some patients with HF have periodic breathing. The second component of the loop gain that increases the likelihood of occurrence of periodic breathing (and also central apnea during sleep) is the gain of the chemoreceptors.[33] In persons with increased sensitivity to CO_2 (or hypoxia), the chemoreceptors elicit a large ventilatory response whenever the Pco_2 rises (or the Po_2 decreases). The consequent intense hyperventilation, by driving the Pco_2 below the apneic threshold, results in central apnea. As a result of central apnea, Pco_2 rises (and Po_2 falls), and the cycles of hyperventilation and hypoventilation (hypopnea) or central apnea are maintained. Differences in the gain of the chemoreceptors among patients with HF may, in part, explain why only some patients with HF develop periodic breathing and CSA.

The third component of the loop gain that may contribute to the development of periodic breathing in HF is decreased functional residual capacity, which results in underdamping.[20,34] This means that, for a given change in ventilation (e.g., a pause in breathing), changes in the controlled variables—namely Po_2 and Pco_2—will be augmented (referred to as *increased plant gain*). In turn, the augmented changes in Po_2 and Pco_2 result in a pronounced compensatory ventilatory response, and overcompensation tends to destabilize breathing. Patients with HF may have decreased functional residual capacity for a variety of reasons, including pleural effusion, cardiomegaly, and decreased compliance of the respiratory system. Functional residual capacity may decrease further in the supine position, facilitating the development of periodic breathing in this position.

The aforementioned mechanisms that collectively increase the loop gain and the likelihood of periodic breathing are present during both sleep and wakefulness. However, in the supine position and during sleep, further changes, such as a reduction in functional residual capacity, metabolic rate (another factor in the plant gain), and cardiac output, occur that will augment the likelihood of developing periodic breathing beyond that observed during wakefulness. Furthermore, loop gain, as described previously, differs from the dynamic loop gain during sleep when periodic breathing is present and steady state is absent.[20]

Meanwhile, like obstructive apnea, central apnea usually occurs during sleep or when a subject is awake but dozing. The genesis of CSA during sleep relates specifically to the removal of the nonchemical drive of wakefulness on breathing and to the unmasking of the apneic threshold—the level of Pco_2 below which rhythmic breathing ceases.[20] The difference between two Pco_2 set points—the prevailing Pco_2 minus the Pco_2 at the apneic threshold, referred to as *Pco_2 reserve*—is a critical factor for the occurrence of CSA. The smaller the difference, the greater the likelihood of occurrence of apnea.

Normally, with the onset of sleep, ventilation decreases and Pco_2 increases. As long as the prevailing Pco_2 is above the apneic threshold, rhythmic breathing continues. However, in some patients with HF, the awake prevailing Pco_2 does not significantly rise with onset of sleep.[35,36] Importantly, however, patients with HF who develop central apnea have increased CO_2 chemosensitivity below eupnea[37] while asleep, as well as above eupnea while awake, as discussed previously.[31] Because of increased CO_2 chemosensitivity below eupnea,[37] the prevailing Pco_2 and the apneic threshold Pco_2 are close together, increasing the likelihood of developing central apnea during sleep. The increased chemosensitivity above eupnea becomes particularly pathophysiologic during arousals occurring after apneas, when excessive ventilatory response lowers the prevailing Pco_2 toward or below the apneic threshold.

The reason for the lack of the normally observed rise in Pco_2 in some patients with HF is not clear. It could result from the lack of the normally observed sleep-induced decrease in ventilation. Conceivably, because of increased venous return in the supine position, and in the presence of a stiff left ventricle, pulmonary capillary pressure could rise. This results in an increase in respiratory rate and ventilation, preventing the normally observed rise in Pco_2. At the same time, the increase in pulmonary capillary pressure increases the chemosensitivity below eupnea and decreases the Pco_2 reserve, promoting the likelihood of developing central apnea. The mechanisms remain to be fully elucidated, although vagal afferents have been shown to have significant influences on the responsiveness of both carotid bodies as well as central chemoreceptors.[19] Patients with HF and low arterial Pco_2 have a high probability of developing central apnea during sleep. Predictive value of a low steady-state arterial Pco_2 (<35 mm Hg) is about 80%.[38] The reason for this association lies on the fact that a low arterial Pco_2 is caused by increased pulmonary wedge pressure, which, per se, sensitizes carotid bodies and the central chemoreceptors promoting CSA, as noted previously.[31] Meanwhile, although an awake low arterial Pco_2 is highly predictive of CSA, it is not a prerequisite. Many patients with HF and CSA have a normal awake arterial Pco_2. What is important is the proximity of the apneic threshold to the arterial Pco_2 and an increased CO_2 chemosensitivity below eupnea.

MECHANISMS OF OBSTRUCTIVE SLEEP APNEA IN HEART FAILURE

As noted earlier, OSA and hypopnea are also common in HF. The mechanisms are multifactorial. First, periodic breathing resulting from HF predisposes the susceptible subjects to develop upper airway occlusion during the nadir of the ventilatory cycles of periodic breathing.[39] For this reason, we observed multiple episodes of upper airway obstruction frequently after central apneas.[39]

Second, increased venous congestion and pressure resulting from right HF may diminish upper airway size[40] and facilitate upper airway occlusion. Venous congestion of the upper airway may be worse in the supine (than in the erect) position, and rostral fluid shift, particularly in the presence of edema in the lower extremities and redistribution of fluid into vascular space, may further compound upper airway patency.[41] Third, patients with HF and OSA are commonly obese, and obesity may compromise upper airway patency. Although currently 35% of patients with HFrEF are obese, almost 53% of those with HFpEF suffer from this disorder,[42] for which reason the prevalence of OSA is higher in patients with HFpEF than in HFrEF.[18,19]

In summary, decreased upper airway size resulting from both venous congestion and obesity may predispose patients with HF to develop upper airway occlusion during the nadir of the ventilatory cycles of periodic breathing, when the tone of the dilator muscles of the upper airway decreases the most.

PATHOLOGIC CONSEQUENCES AND PROGNOSTIC SIGNIFICANCE OF SLEEP-RELATED BREATHING DISORDERS

The cycles of apnea-hypopnea and hyperpnea, both obstructive and central, are associated with three adverse consequences. These include arterial blood gas abnormalities characterized by intermittent hypoxemia-reoxygenation and hypercapnia-hypocapnia, excessive arousals and shift to light sleep stages, and large negative swings in intrathoracic pressure (see Chapter 119). The pathophysiologic consequences of obstructive and central sleep apneas and hypopneas are qualitatively similar (but worse in OSA than in CSA), adversely affect various cardiovascular functions, and are potentially most detrimental in the presence of established coronary artery disease and LV systolic and diastolic dysfunction. In the long run, these adverse consequences result in excess morbidity, hospital readmission, and mortality of patients with HF.

EFFECTS OF OBSTRUCTIVE SLEEP APNEA ON SYMPATHETIC ACTIVITY, CARDIOVASCULAR FUNCTION, HOSPITAL READMISSION, AND MORTALITY

In patients with HF, the presence of OSA is associated with increased sympathetic activity[43] and reduced LVEF, which are reversed if sleep apnea is effectively treated with nasal CPAP. There are five randomized clinical trials of CPAP therapy for OSA in patients with HFrEF. In three of these studies,[44-46] LVEF increased significantly (when compared with the control group) by about 10%, 5%, and 2%. In two[44,47] of these five studies, sham CPAP was used in the control group; in one,[44] LVEF increased significantly but slightly (2%), and, in the other one,[47] ejection fraction did not increase. In the latter study, auto-CPAP was used, and the adherence hours to CPAP were less than in the two previous studies,[45,46] which had demonstrated 10% and 5% increases in ejection fraction.

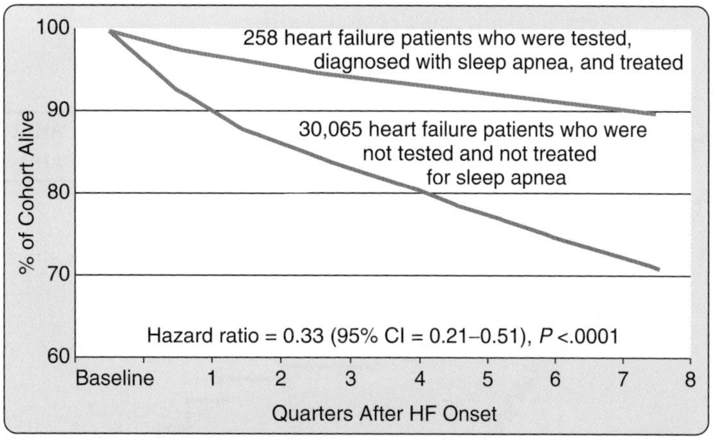

Figure 149.4 Data were from Medicare beneficiaries who were diagnosed with new heart failure. The 2-year survival of the 258 patients who were tested, diagnosed, and treated for sleep apnea was much better than the survival of the 30,065 patients who were not tested for sleep apnea. The survival was adjusted for age, gender, and Charlson Comorbidity Index. (Modified from Javaheri S, Caref B, Chen E, et al. Sleep apnea testing and outcomes in a large cohort of Medicare beneficiaries with newly diagnosed heart failure. *Am J Respir Crit Care Med.* 2011;183:539–46.)

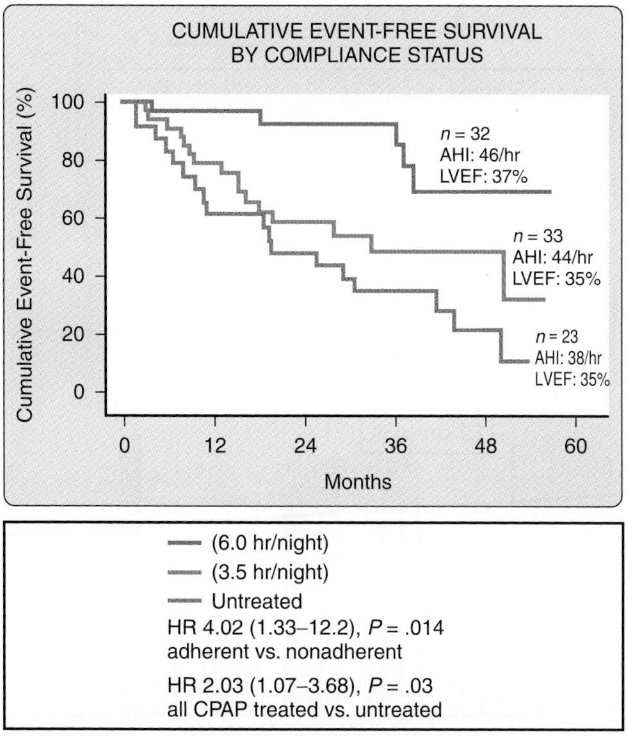

Figure 149.5 Probability for hospitalization and mortality of patients with heart failure and obstructive sleep apnea decrease if they are treated with continuous positive airway pressure (CPAP) and adhere to therapy. AHI, Apnea–hypopnea index; HR, hazard ratio; LVEF, left ventricular ejection fraction. (From Kryger MH. *Atlas of Clinical Sleep Medicine.* Elsevier; 2010; modified from Kasai T, Narui K, Dohi P, et al. Prognosis of patients with heart failure and obstructive sleep apnea treated with continuous positive airway pressure. *Chest.* 2008;133:690–6.)

In one study, 45 patients with OSA (mean AHI = 27/hour of sleep) and HFrEF (mean LVEF = 36%) were randomized to CPAP (n = 22) or no CPAP (n = 23) for 6 to 8 weeks. In comparison of the two groups, there were no significant changes in LVEF.[47]

In HF, OSA is an independent predictor of mortality,[48] and two observational studies (Figure 149.4) confirm this association and further suggest that therapy with CPAP improves survival, particularly in those who are most compliant with it (Figure 149.5).[49,50] This latter observation in patients with HF is similar to that in patients with hypertension, as studies indicate that the reduction in blood pressure is most prominent in those who are most adherent to CPAP therapy (see Chapter 120 and Figure 149.4).

OSA is independently associated with excess hospital readmission and that treatment of sleep apnea could lower the rate of readmissions. In one study from a heart hospital, Khayat and colleagues[51] demonstrated that severe OSA was independently associated with 1.5 times higher readmission when compared to patients with HF but without OSA. Meanwhile, two studies have shown that treatment with CPAP decreases the rate of readmission.[49,52]

EFFECTS OF CENTRAL SLEEP APNEA ON SYMPATHETIC ACTIVITY, CARDIOVASCULAR FUNCTION, HOSPITAL READMISSION, AND MORTALITY

Like OSA, CSA is associated with increased sympathetic activity and reduced LVEF, which is reversed by effective therapy with CPAP[53] and oxygen.

Most studies have suggested that presence of CSA decreases survival among patients with HFrEF.[53-59] We followed 88 patients with HF with (n = 56) or without (n = 32) CSA with a median follow-up of 51 months.[57] After controlling for 24 confounding variables, we found that CSA was associated with excess mortality (hazard ratio, 2.14; P = .02; Figure 149.6). The average survival of patients with HF but without CSA was 90 months compared with 45 months for those with CSA. That CSA contributes to excess mortality in HF is supported by the observation that effective treatment of CSA with CPAP in HFrEF[60] and with ASV in HFpEF[61] improves survival. The first study[60] was based on the post-hoc analysis of the Canadian randomized clinical trial, and the second one was a randomized trial involving a small number of patients with HFpEF.[61] The results of a relatively large observational study[62] of patients with predominantly CSA who agreed to use ASV are consistent with those of the aforementioned randomized trials.

Similar to findings in OSA, CSA has been found to be an independent predictor of hospital readmission within 30 days after discharge.[51] Further, treatment of CSA has been shown to be associated with decreased hospital readmission.[63-65] Virtually all of these studies from Japan are observational; the end points were a combination of premature mortality and readmission resulting from HF, and ASV devices were used to treat CSA, or when mixed with OSA.[63-65]

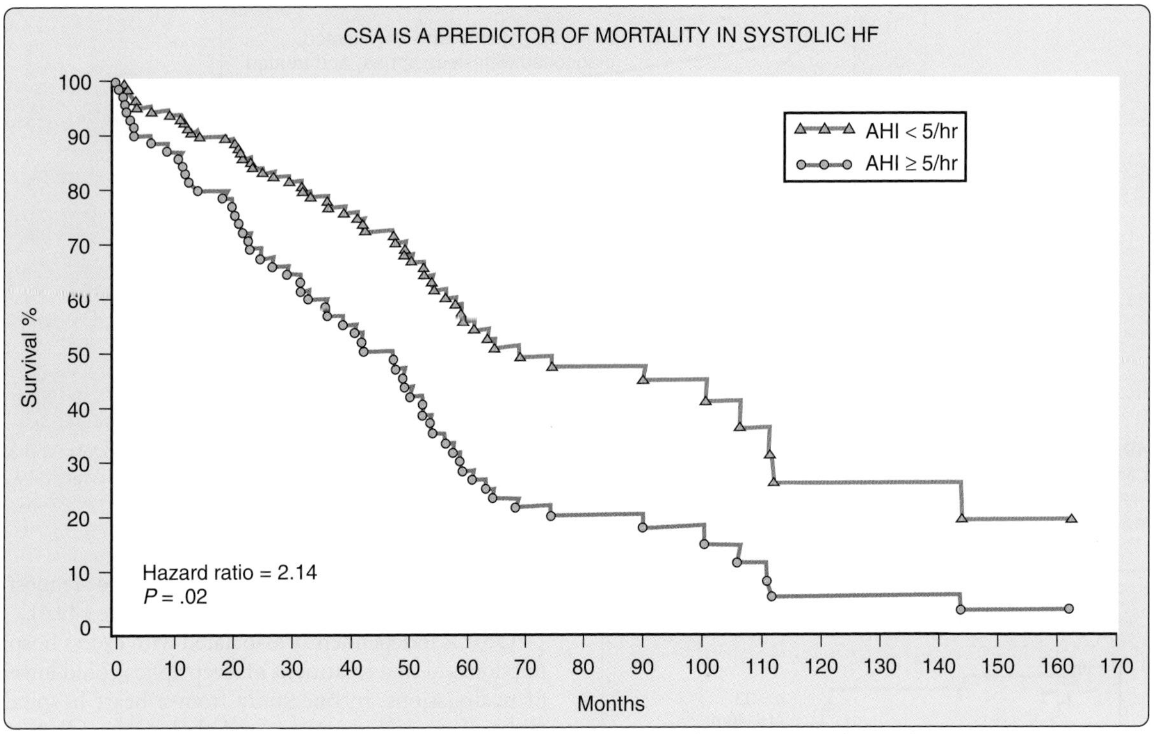

Figure 149.6 Probability of survival in patients with systolic heart failure (HF) according to the presence or absence of central sleep apnea (CSA). AHI, Apnea-hypopnea index. (From Kryger MH. *Atlas of Clinical Sleep Medicine*. Elsevier; 2010; modified from Javaheri S, Shukla R, Zeigler H, Wexler L. Central sleep apnea, right ventricular dysfunction, and low diastolic blood pressure are predictors of mortality in systolic heart failure. *J Am Coll Cardiol.* 2007;49:2028–34.)

CLINICAL PRESENTATION OF OBSTRUCTIVE AND CENTRAL SLEEP APNEAS IN PATIENTS WITH HEART FAILURE

Obesity is an important risk factor for development of OSA in patients with HF,[66-68] as it is for patients without HF. Patients with HFrEF and OSA are significantly heavier and snore habitually (Figure 149.7). They may also have a higher systemic arterial blood pressure than subjects with CSA. Aside from obesity and habitual snoring, it is often difficult to clinically suspect the presence of sleep apnea in patients with HF because (1) the prevalence of sleepiness is similar in HF patients with and in those without sleep apnea[8,10] (Figure 149.7) and (2) the symptoms of HF and sleep apnea overlap. The overlapping symptoms of sleep apnea and HF include sleep-onset and maintenance insomnia, nocturia, waking up with shortness of breath (orthopnea, paroxysmal nocturnal dyspnea, hyperpnea resulting from periodic breathing), unrefreshed sleep, and daytime fatigue. The overlapping of the symptoms of HF and sleep apnea undoubtedly contributes to the underdiagnosis of sleep-related breathing disorders in patients with HF. CSA, in particular, is most difficult to diagnose,[33] because obesity and habitual snoring, which are the two hallmarks of OSA (Figure 149.7), are commonly absent in patients with HF and CSA.[8,33] However, there are some clues that, when present, should increase the probability of the presence of CSA. These include a high-numbered class in the New York Heart Association classification, low LVEF, and low steady-state arterial Pco_2, atrial fibrillation, and nocturnal ventricular arrhythmias (Figure 149.8). Even when there is no subjective daytime sleepiness, such patients score 10 or less on the Epworth Sleepiness Scale (ESS) when tested objectively by multiple sleep latency, short sleep latencies, even below 5 minutes, are observed.[69]

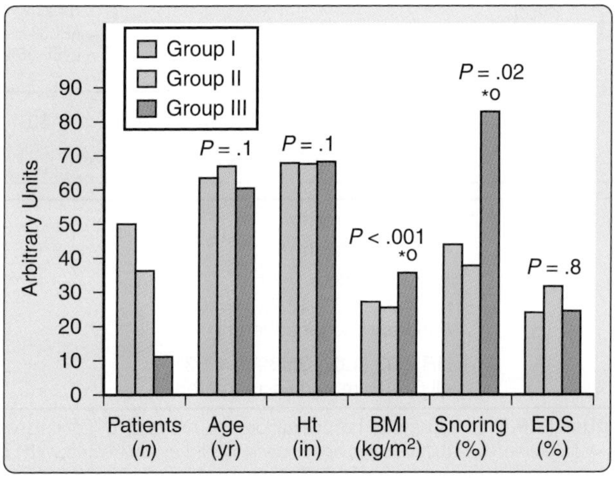

Figure 149.7 Demographics, historical data, and physical examination findings in patients with heart failure without sleep apnea, with central sleep apnea (CSA), and with obstructive sleep apnea (OSA). Patients with OSA were more obese and had a higher prevalence of habitual snoring than patients with CSA. There was no difference in prevalence of excessive daytime sleepiness between the patients with heart failure and the patients without sleep apnea. BMI, Body mass index; EDS, excessive daytime sleepiness; Ht, height. (From Kryger MH. *Atlas of Clinical Sleep Medicine*. Elsevier; 2010; modified from Javaheri S. Sleep disorders in systolic heart failure: a prospective study of 100 male patients—the final report. *Int J Cardiol.* 2006;106:21–8.)

INDICATIONS FOR POLYSOMNOGRAPHY IN HEART FAILURE

As noted, patients with HF and sleep apnea do not generally present with symptoms that distinguish them from patients with HF without sleep apnea. Furthermore, because HF is common, it is not possible to perform sleep studies on all

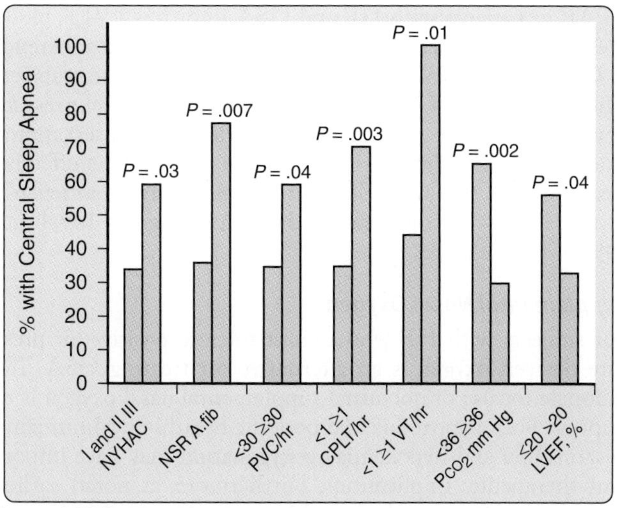

Figure 149.8 Clinical and laboratory characteristics that are more likely to be associated with central sleep apnea. A. fib, Atrial fibrillation; CPLT, couplets; LVEF, left ventricular ejection fraction; NSR, normal sinus rhythm; NYHAC, New York Heart Association Class; PVC, premature ventricular contractions; VT, ventricular tachycardia. (From Javaheri S. Sleep disorders in systolic heart failure: a prospective study of 100 male patients—the final report. *Int J Cardiol.* 2006;106:21–8.)

patients with HF. However, there are a number of clinical and laboratory findings that, when present in patients with HF, should increase clinical suspicion for sleep apnea. These markers are different for OSA and CSA.

Risk factors for OSA-hypopnea in patients with HF are similar to those in patients without HF. They include obesity, increased neck size, habitual snoring, and hypertension. These risk factors and others, such as witnessed apnea, waking up unrested, and excessive daytime sleepiness, when present, should increase the level of suspicion for the presence of OSA. The following are symptoms that should alert the clinician to the possibility of apnea in patients with HF:

- *Nocturnal angina*—substernal chest pain that awakens the patient—should increase suspicion for sleep apnea in the general population and for patients with coronary heart disease and HF.
- *Paroxysmal nocturnal dyspnea* characteristically awakens the patient with shortness of breath, which is relieved with resumption of an erect position. However, this symptom may be a perception of shortness of breath occurring during the hyperpneic phase of periodic breathing, suggesting presence of sleep apnea.
- *Restless sleep, maintenance insomnia,* and *leg movements* may reflect periodic arousals and movements after apneas and hypopneas. Periodic limb movement, however, is also found in patients with systolic HF.[70,71]

Patients with HF and progressive ventricular systolic or diastolic dysfunction or patients who remain in New York Heart Association classes III or IV, despite intensive medical therapy, should have a diagnostic sleep study.

As noted earlier, several studies[52-54] have shown that patients with HF with low arterial P_{CO_2} have a high prevalence of CSA. The predictive value of low P_{CO_2} (<35 mm Hg) is about 80%.[38] However, many patients with HF have CSA apnea without daytime hypocapnia.[54,55]

Several studies have shown that patients with HF and sleep apnea have a higher prevalence of atrioventricular arrhythmias, especially atrial fibrillation[72] and nocturnal ventricular arrhythmias.[73] The presence of these arrhythmias should increase suspicion for the presence of CSA.

When the previously mentioned risk factors for obstructive and CSA are present, polysomnography should be performed for diagnosis and response to therapy. Such an approach has been shown to decrease hospital readmission and improve survival, as discussed previously.

Box 149.1 TREATMENT OF OBSTRUCTIVE SLEEP APNEA IN PATIENTS WITH HEART FAILURE OPTIMIZATION OF CARDIOPULMONARY FUNCTION

- To eliminate or improve periodic breathing
- To decrease right atrial and central venous pressure upper airway congestion/edema, which may increase upper airway size
- To improve functional residual capacity, which may increase upper airway size as lung volume increases
- Avoidance of benzodiazepines, opioids, alcoholic beverages, and Viagra
- Weight loss if applicable
- Nasal positive airway pressure devices:
  - Continuous positive airway pressure (CPAP)
  - Bilevel positive airway pressure (see Chapter 107)
- Oral appliances (see Chapter 109):
  - Supplemental nocturnal nasal oxygen to minimize desaturation and to decrease periodic breathing
- Upper airway procedures:
  - Uvulopalatopharyngoplasty (see Chapter 108)
  - Laser surgery (see Chapter 108)
  - Based on the basis of NHANES 2013 to 2016 data, the prevalence of CVD (comprising CHD, HF, stroke, and hypertension in adults ≥20 years of age is 48.0% overall (121.5 million in 2016) and increases with age in both males and females. CVD prevalence excluding hypertension (CHD, HF, and stroke only) is 9.0% overall (24.3 million in 2016).

TREATMENT OF SLEEP-RELATED BREATHING DISORDERS IN PATIENTS WITH HEART FAILURE

The choice of therapy for OSA or CSA is based on the type of sleep apnea.[74,75]

Treatment for Obstructive Sleep Apnea

In general, treatment of OSA–hypopnea is similar in patients with and without HF, although there are some differences (Box 149.1). In the presence of cardiovascular disease, every attempt should be made to treat OSA with positive airway pressure devices.

Optimization of Cardiopulmonary Function

Optimal treatment of HF by improving both periodic breathing and lower extremity edema may decrease the likelihood of developing upper airway occlusion. Furthermore, in biventricular HF, elevated right atrial and central venous pressure may result in pharyngeal congestion and edema, which along the fluid from lower extremities translocated cephalad in supine position could result in narrowing of the upper airway. Therefore therapeutic measures to decrease the lower extremity edema and venous pressure[41] are advisable. Also, optimal treatment of HF to decrease lung water and pleural effusion could increase lung volumes, which should increase upper airway size, which is dependent on lung volume.

Weight Loss

In the general population, obesity is a major risk factor for OSA, and weight reduction improves OSA (see Chapter 139). Similarly, obesity is associated with increased risk of a new-onset cardiovascular disease, including HF.[66,67] In spite of these aforementioned relationships between obesity, OSA, and HF in the general population, studies of patients with HF have consistently demonstrated an obesity paradox, indicating that obesity is a strong independent predictor of improved outcomes for patients with chronic HF.[66,67] However, many patients with HF and OSA are obese,[8] and OSA per se has been shown to be a risk factor for the development of HF.[76] Thus we generally advise weight loss for obese patients with OSA, irrespective of HF. However, studies are needed to determine optimal body weight and whether purposeful weight loss in congestive HF comorbid with OSA improves cardiac function.

Exercise

AHI has been reported to decrease with supervised exercise, CPAP, or exercise plus CPAP.[77] These results are similar to effects of exercise in OSA in the general population.[78] Multifactorial mechanisms could include decreased rostral fluid redistribution, stabilization of chemoreceptor sensitivity, improved nasal resistance, sleep quality, weight loss (if it occurs), and strength of pharyngeal dilator muscles.

Avoidance of Alcoholic Beverages, Benzodiazepines, Opioids, Smoking, and Phosphodiesterase-5 Inhibitors at Bedtime

The use of alcoholic beverages and benzodiazepines may increase the likelihood of upper airway occlusion by promoting the relaxation of the muscles of the upper airway. Opiates may induce CSA and contribute to OSA, and withdrawal improves both.[79] We also advise patients that phosphodiesterase inhibitors used to treat erectile dysfunction (e.g., sildenafil [Viagra], vardenafil [Levitra], and tadalafil [Cialis]) may worsen OSA. In a randomized double-blind placebo-controlled study,[80] it was shown that 50 mg of sildenafil significantly increased the obstructive AHI and desaturation in a group of patients with OSA.

Smoking, via mechanisms mediated by nicotine, the active chemical in tobacco, increases efferent sympathetic activity (at least, in part, because of stimulating peripheral chemoreceptors in the carotid bodies, which contain excitatory nicotinic receptors) and plasma catecholamine resulting in increases in blood pressure, heart rate, and myocardial oxygen consumption.[81] In addition, nicotine decreases oxygen availability and causes coronary vasospasm, all promoting ventricular tachyarrhythmia. This is not surprising because excessive adrenergic overactivity is the underlying mechanism of arrhythmias, and HF, in particular, when comorbid with sleep apnea, is already a hyperadrenergic state.

Positive Airway Pressure Devices

Positive airway pressure devices are the treatment of choice and have been most successfully used to treat OSA in the general population and in patients with HF. Short-term use of CPAP in patients with HF and OSA improves LVEF, blood pressure, and ventricular systolic volume,[44-46] but adherence to CPAP is a critical factor. For CPAP-noncompliant subjects who complain of a high expiratory pressure, bilevel pressure devices should be tried. As noted earlier, two observational studies[49,50] of patients with HF have shown that effective treatment of OSA with CPAP improves survival, particularly in those who are compliant with CPAP (Figures 149.4 and 149.5).[50]

Supplemental Nasal Oxygen

For subjects with HF who cannot tolerate positive air pressure devices, oxygen is an alternative for treating OSA. The rationale for use of nocturnal supplemental nasal oxygen is to improve both hypoxemia and periodic breathing. Minimizing desaturation and hypoxemia-reoxygenation may have important therapeutic implications. Furthermore, as noted earlier, improvement in periodic breathing may decrease in obstructive disordered-breathing events that occur at the nadir of ventilation. We emphasize, however, that there are no systematic long-term studies treating OSA of patients with HF with oxygen.

Upper Airway Surgical Procedures

Upper airway surgical procedures are performed for treatment of OSA in the general population, but there are no data in patients with HF.

Oral Appliances

Oral appliances are used to treat OSA, particularly in patients who cannot tolerate CPAP (see Chapter 109). Limited data are available in HF.[82,83] We speculate that efficacy of these devices in patients with HF and OSA is similar to that in the general population. After application, a sleep study is recommended to ensure effectiveness.

Treatment for Central Sleep Apnea

Figure 149.9 shows our approach to treatment of patients with CSA in HF.

Optimization of Cardiopulmonary Function

Intensive therapy for HF with diuretics, angiotensin-converting enzyme inhibitors, beta blockers, and cardiac resynchronization therapy (CRT) can improve periodic breathing. Because pulmonary congestion and edema are associated with narrowing of P_{CO_2} reserve,[84] reduction in wedge pressure should be associated with widening of P_{CO_2} reserve and improvement in CSA. Furthermore, with therapy, arterial circulation time decreases (as stroke volume increases and cardiopulmonary blood volume decreases), and functional residual capacity may increase (because of a decrease in cardiac size, pleural effusion, and intravascular and extravascular lung water). These changes contribute to the stabilization of breathing.

Beta blockers, by increasing stroke volume and decreasing pulmonary capillary pressure, should be particularly helpful in improving periodic breathing in systolic HF. An additional beneficial effect of beta blockers may relate to their counterbalancing of nocturnal cardiac sympathetic hyperactivity, resulting from repetitive arousals and desaturation. The reduction in cardiac sympathetic activity may have contributed to improved survival in trials of beta blockers in patients with HF. One particular side effect of beta blockers, however, is related to their effect on

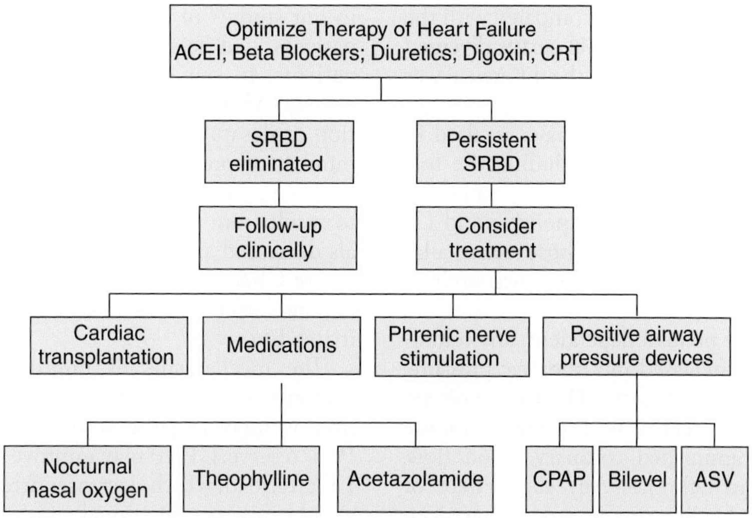

Figure 149.9 Treatment of central sleep apnea in patients with systolic heart failure. ACEI, Angiotensin-converting enzyme inhibitor; ASV, adaptive servo-ventilation; CRT, cardiac resynchronization therapy; CPAP, continuous positive airway pressure; SRBD, sleep-related breathing disorder. (Modified from Javaheri S. Sleep-related breathing disorders in heart failure. In: Mann DL, editor. *Heart Failure: A Companion to Braunwald's Heart Disease*. Saunders; 2004:482.)

melatonin. Melatonin, a sleep-promoting chemical, is secreted via the cyclic adenosine monophosphate–mediated beta-adrenergic signal transduction system. Some beta blockers (exceptions include carvedilol), by inhibiting this process, decrease melatonin secretion[85] and could potentially contribute to worsening of sleep.

Regarding improvement in cardiac function and CSA, a few studies of CRT[86] showed some improvement in CSA, particularly noticeable in those with CRT-induced hemodynamic improvement. However, CRT devices are ineffective for OSA; although, in one study,[87] OSA improved, and improvement correlated with a decrease in circulation time.

If periodic breathing persists after cardiopulmonary function is optimized, several approaches are possible (Figure 149.9).

Cardiac Transplantation

After cardiac transplantation, CSA is virtually eliminated.[88] However, with time, a large number of cardiac transplant recipients develop OSA.[88] OSA developed in those who had gained the most weight after transplantation, and it was associated with habitual snoring, poor quality of life, and systemic hypertension. Cardiac transplantation was also associated with a high prevalence of restless legs syndrome and periodic limb movements (Figure 149.10).[88]

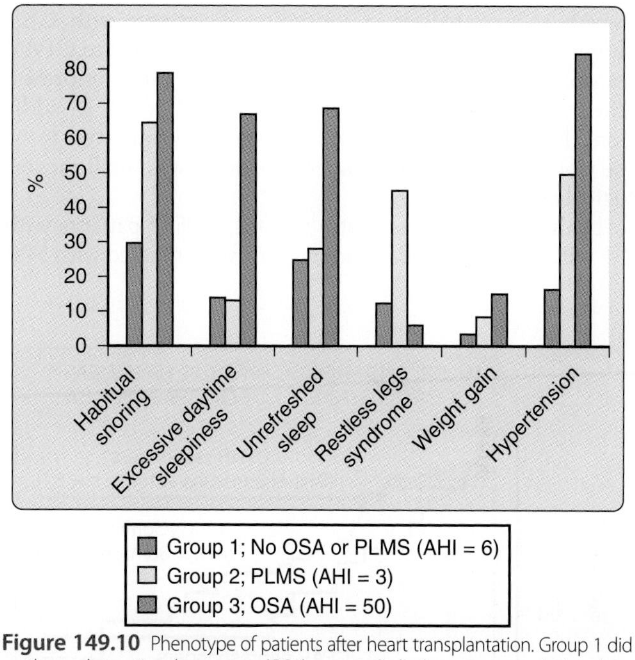

Figure 149.10 Phenotype of patients after heart transplantation. Group 1 did not have obstructive sleep apnea (OSA) or periodic limb movements during sleep (PLMS), Group 2 had PLMS, and Group 3 had OSA. Weight gain is in kilograms since the transplantation. AHI, Apnea–hypopnea index. (Modified from Javaheri S, Abraham W, Brown C, et al. Prevalence of obstructive sleep apnea and periodic limb movement in 45 subjects with heart transplantation. *Eur Heart J*. 2004;25:260–6.)

Positive Airway Pressure Devices

Continuous Positive Airway Pressure. Several devices, including CPAP, bilevel pressure, and ASV, have been used to treat CSA in patients with HF.

In contrast to treatment of OSA, where application of nasal CPAP invariably results in virtual elimination of obstructive disordered-breathing events, treatment of CSA in patients with HF is difficult, and response to therapy is not uniform.[89] In our study,[90] first-night CPAP titration was effective in improving CSA in 43% of the patients (57% were considered CPAP nonresponsive). In the multicenter Canadian trial,[91] 43% of the patients were considered CPAP nonresponsive at 3 months. In this trial, 132 patients were randomized to the control group and 128 to the CPAP arm. The baseline features were similar in the two randomized groups. The patients in the therapeutic arm were adapted to CPAP over 1 to 3 nights (without formal titration), and the maximum pressure was set at 10 cm H_2O or lower at whatever was tolerated.

A second polysomnography was performed at 3 months in both groups. There was no significant change in AHI in the control group. In the CPAP arm, the average AHI decreased by 50%, with considerable improvement in desaturation. Furthermore, the average plasma norepinephrine level decreased, and LVEF increased (all statistically significant). These measurements remained unchanged in the control group. However, after an interim analysis was performed, the safety-monitoring committee recommended termination of the study. This, in part, was related to worsened transplantation-free survival (primarily because of increased number of deaths from progressive HF and sudden death) of the CPAP-treated patients compared with the control group (P = .02). Although the survival curves diverged after about 3 years (favoring the CPAP arm), the difference was not statistically significant (P = .06).

We speculated that CPAP therapy could have resulted in excess early mortality for several reasons, including the following[92]: (1) those who died were patients with HF and CSA whose periodic breathing was CPAP nonresponsive and (2) those who died were patients with HF whose ventricular function (according to the Frank-Starling curve) was preload dependent.

If RV and LV function are preload dependent, any reduction in venous return by the increased intrathoracic pressure, with application of CPAP, could decrease RV stroke volume and return to the left ventricle, decreasing LV stroke volume and causing hypotension, diminished coronary blood flow, myocardial ischemia, and arrhythmias. Any such effect of CPAP on blood pressure is further augmented during sleep when blood pressure normally decreases.

The aforementioned assumptions that, in the Canadian trial, excess cardiovascular death resulting from CPAP occurred primarily in CPAP nonresponders were confirmed by a post-hoc analysis of mortality of patients with CSA (Figure 149.11).[60] In those whose CSA responded to CPAP, transplantation-free survival was significantly improved when compared with the untreated control group. In addition, the mortality of CPAP nonresponders appeared to be the worst, although the number of patients was small for statistical significance.

In the Canadian trial[91] at 3 months, 43% of patients with HF with CSA were CPAP nonresponsive, compared with 57%

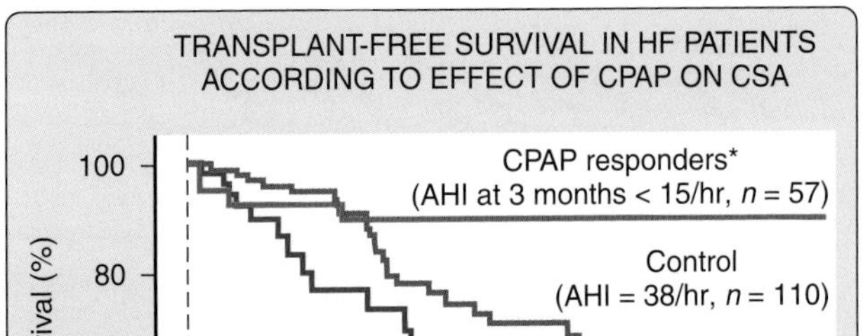

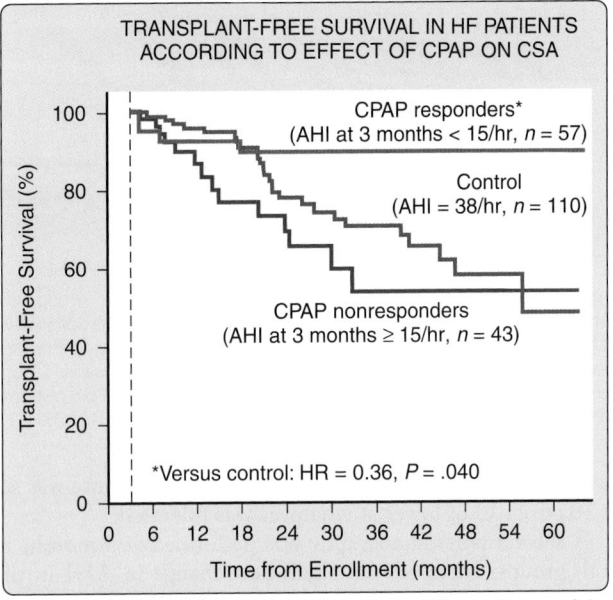

Figure 149.11 Probability of survival in patients with systolic heart failure (HF) comparing continuous positive airway pressure (CPAP) responders to a control group (patients with systolic heart failure and similar apnea–hypopnea index [AHI]) and to CPAP nonresponders. CPAP responders had a significantly increased probability of survival compared with the control group. CPAP nonresponders tended to have a poor survival when compared with the control group, although this was not significant. CSA, Central sleep apnea; HR, hazard ratio. (From Kryger MH. *Atlas of Clinical Sleep Medicine*. Elsevier; 2010; modified from Artz M, Floras JS, Logan AG, et al. Suppression of central sleep apnea by continuous positive airway pressure and transplant-free survival in heart failure. *Circulation*. 2007;115:3173–80.)

in our study[90] of first-night use. Typically, CPAP-responsive patients had less severe CSA than CPAP-nonresponsive patients. In our study,[93] in CPAP-responsive patients, the average AHI decreased from 36 to 4 per hour, with elimination of desaturation. An important observation was that the number of premature ventricular contractions, couplets, and ventricular tachycardia decreased. This effect was presumed to result from decreased sympathetic activity, because arousals decreased and saturation improved. Patients with HF and severe CSA (57% of the patients) did not respond to CPAP, and use of CPAP had no significant effect on ventricular irritability.

The mechanisms of improvement in CSA in CPAP-responsive patients are multifactorial. One may relate to improvement in pulmonary congestion, which should widen P_{CO_2} reserve. CPAP may improve stroke volume by decreasing LV afterload, which decreases arterial circulation time. CPAP should increase functional residual capacity, which decreases underdamping, and CPAP opens the upper airway, which is a benefit for those patients with CSA in whom upper airway closure occurs.

Adaptive Servo-Ventilation. However, as noted earlier, 43% to 57% of patients with HF and CSA are unresponsive to CPAP.[89,90] For these patients, and those who are intolerant to CPAP, until recently ASV devices were recommended (see end of this section). These devices provide varying amounts of anticyclic inspiratory pressure support during different phases of periodic breathing, augmenting ventilation when the patient's minute ventilation decreases below a target and withdrawing support when the patient's ventilation is above the target. In this way, periodic breathing is eliminated while on the device. In addition, the device initiates a breath on a timely basis, preventing development of a central apnea. Finally, the new generation of these devices is equipped with automatic end expiratory positive pressure algorithms[94] that operate to eliminate obstructive disordered breathing events. Having this benefit, these devices were expected to be advantageous for treatment of complex sleep-related breathing disorders when CSA and OSA and hypopneas are all present. Specifically, in patients with HF, such complex breathing events are frequently observed during polysomnography. In addition, the phenotype of sleep apnea may vary during progression of HF and during acute decompensation when excess fluid from the lower extremities translocates to the neck area in supine position. Under such circumstances, upper airway obstruction could occur, and a fixed end expiratory positive airway pressure with either a CPAP or bilevel device is inadequate to eliminate obstructive events.

ASV devices had been used in many studies to treat CSA in patients with congestive HF, generally with favorable results until 2015, when it was reported that ASV treatment could increase mortality in patients with HFrEF in a large randomized study (see later).[95]

Meanwhile, as noted previously, with automatic variable end expiratory positive pressure algorithms, ASV devices are effective in treating both CSA and OSA. In the three trials[96-98] that compared CPAP versus ASV in patients with HF and coexistent OSA and CSA, ASV was significantly more effective in improving LVEF than CPAP. Because both obstructive and central sleep disorders commonly occur together, and the phenotype may change with time (e.g., obstructive events becoming prominent during acute decompensation of the HF), ASV devices with automatic end expiratory positive pressure rhythm can be effective under such circumstances.

In spite of many nonrandomized studies, a large multisite international clinical trial (SERVE-HF)[95] that evaluated the effect of treating CSA with an ASV device in patients with HF and reduced ejection fraction (HFrEF) raised serious concerns about the safety of ASV in these patients. Not only was ASV ineffective, but post-hoc analysis found excess cardiovascular mortality in treated patients. The cause of the excess mortality is unknown; the authors hypothesized that CSA may be a compensatory mechanism with a protective effect in HFrEF. Based on pathophysiologic consequences of CSA, we have critically discussed the evidence that in HFrEF, CSA is maladaptive rather than protective.[99,100]

In addition, there are several other (perhaps more) plausible explanations for the excess cardiovascular mortality in the trial as discussed in detail elsewhere.[101] These include methodological issues, the use of an old generation ASV device, which is no longer manufactured by the sponsor of the trial, residual sleep-disordered breathing with significant oxygen desaturation, patient selection, data collection, and treatment adherence as well as group crossovers as potential confounding factors.[101] Only the device-related issues are briefly reviewed here.

The data from the trial[95] show that the device was ineffective in a number of patients. There could be multiple reasons for these residual events. Two important issues regarding the algorithm of the first-generation ASV device used in SERVE-HF could have been contributory: First, it allows for only fixed expiratory positive airway pressure, and second, there were flaws in the inspiratory pressure support algorithm that were addressed and improved considerably in the later-generation models.[97,102] Other factors that collectively with aforementioned variables could have contributed to long-term arrhythmias and premature mortality are arousals and oxygen desaturation. In this regard, in the largest mortality study so far reported, more than 900 patients with well-treated HF were followed for 10 years.[103] The degree of overnight desaturation below 90% was among several variables significantly associated with mortality, and there was a dose-dependent relationship between time below 90% and premature death.

Independent of the reasons why the trial failed, manufacturers of ASV devices have declared that ASV devices are contraindicated for patients with HF and CSA when LVEF is 45% or less.[104] Clinical trials evaluating device treatment of these patients continue.

A Suggested Clinical Approach to the Treatment of Central Sleep Apnea in Patients with HFrEF

The first step is to first make sure that HF is maximally treated, both pharmacologically and device-wise, when indicated.[105,106] This could improve or eliminate periodic breathing. Otherwise choices include therapy with CPAP or phrenic nerve stimulation[107] as depicted in the figure with assessment of responsiveness and consideration of adding other therapies (Figure 149.12, see also Chapter 129).

Cardiac Pacing

There are scant data suggesting that atrial overdrive pacing improves periodic breathing in patients with symptomatic sinus bradycardia.[108] The mechanism remains unclear, but it could have been the improved cardiac output. However, if cardiac pacing improves CSA, biventricular pacing[109] should be more effective than atrial pacing overdrive,[86,110] as discussed earlier. In one study,[109] CRT decreased central AHI from 31/hour to 17/hour. There was no effect on obstructive disordered breathing events.

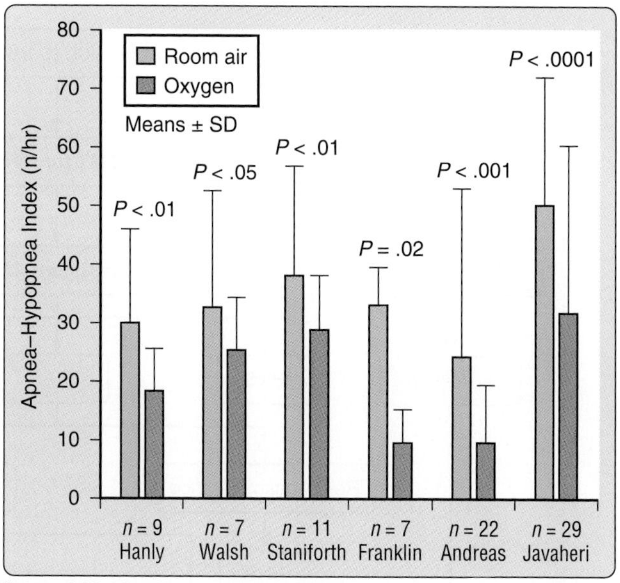

Figure 149.12 Effects of supplemental nasal oxygen on apnea–hypopnea index in patients with systolic heart failure.

Transvenous Unilateral Phrenic Nerve Stimulation

Transvenous unilateral phrenic nerve stimulation has been used to stimulate the phrenic nerve to treat CSA. In the acute study,[111] 16 patients underwent 2 successive nights of polysomnography—1 night with and 1 night without phrenic nerve stimulation from either the right brachiocephalic vein or the left pericardiophrenic vein. Stimulation resulted in significant improvement in the AHI, Central Apnea Index, arousal index, and oxygen desaturation index 4%. No significant changes occurred in the Obstructive Apnea Index or AHI. This approach may represent a novel therapy for CSA and warrants further study.

The pivotal RCT showed significant improvement in CSA, reduction in arousals, and improved oxygen desaturation index.[112] Persistent efficacy has been demonstrated up to 5 years with improved ESS and quality of life.[113-115]

Medications

Nasal Nocturnal Oxygen. Systematic studies in patients with systolic HF[116,117] have shown that nocturnal therapy with supplemental nasal oxygen improves CSA (Figure 149.13). Oxygen therapy may also decrease arousals and improve the hypnogram by shifting sleep structure to deep sleep stages. In addition, randomized placebo-controlled, double-blind studies have shown that short-term (1 to 4 weeks) administration of nocturnal supplemental nasal oxygen improves maximal exercise capacity[118] and decreases overnight urinary norepinephrine excretion.[119]

Three randomized clinical trials of nocturnal nasal oxygen therapy[120-123] for 9-, 12-, and 52-week periods reported that, when compared with the control group, oxygen therapy

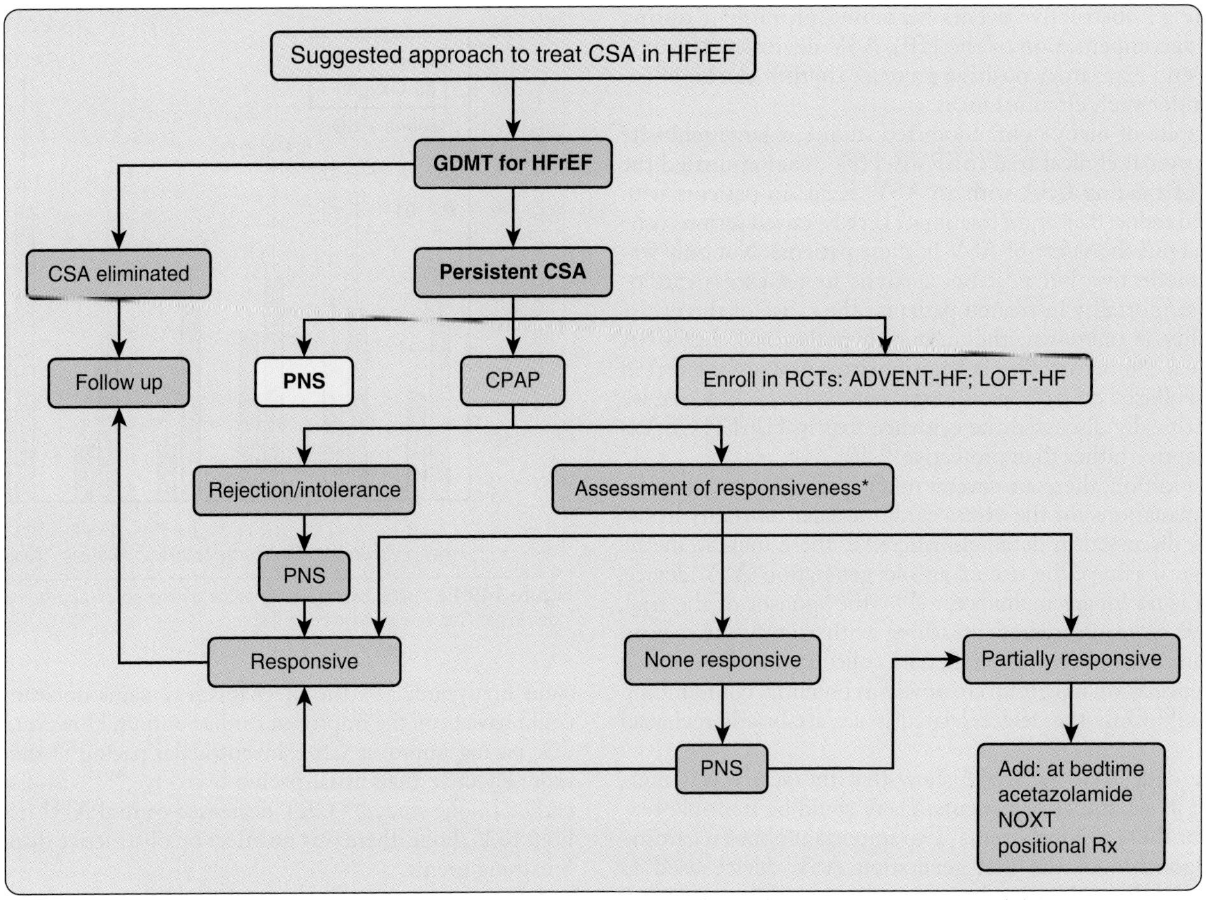

Figure 149.13 A suggested clinical approach to the treatment of central sleep apnea in patients with heart failure with reduced ejection fraction. Phrenic nerve stimulation (PNS) is available in the United States. In countries where PNS is not available, the clinician may proceed directly to the therapies in the partially responsive category. Responsiveness is defined as apnea-hypopnea index < 15 events/hour on therapy, based on CANPAP post-hoc analysis showing association with decreased mortality at this level. ADVENT-HF, Effect of Adaptive Servoventilation on Survival and Hospital Admissions in Heart Failure (NCT01128816); CSA, central sleep apnea; GDMT, guideline-directed medical therapy for heart failure; HFrEF, heart failure with reduced ejection fraction; LOFT-HF, Impact of Low-Flow Oxygen Therapy on Hospital Admissions and Mortality in Patients With Heart Failure and Central Sleep Apnea (NCT03745898); NOXT, nocturnal oxygen therapy; RCT, randomized controlled trial. (Modified from Javaheri S, Brown LK, Abraham WT, Khayat R. Apneas of heart failure and phenotype-guided treatments: part one: OSA. *Chest.* 2020;157[2]:394–402.)

improved CSA and desaturation and significantly increased LVEF and quality of life of patients with HF. In the oxygen-treated group, LVEF increased 5% (versus 1% in the control group) in the 12-week study,[123] and 5.5% (versus 1.3% in the control group) in the 52-week study.[121]

Supplemental administration of nasal oxygen may decrease periodic breathing by several mechanisms. These include an increase in the difference between the prevailing Pco_2 and the Pco_2 at the apneic threshold; a reduction in the ventilatory response to CO_2 and perhaps to hypoxemia; and an increase in body stores (e.g., lung contents) of oxygen, which increases damping. Prospective placebo-controlled long-term studies, however, are necessary to determine whether nocturnal oxygen therapy has the potential to decrease mortality of patients with systolic HF.

Recently, the National Heart, Lung, and Blood Institute (NHLBI) approved a phase III RCT evaluating nocturnal oxygen (NOX) for the treatment of CSA in patients with HF with reduced ejection fraction. The trial is a multisite randomized, double-blinded, controlled pragmatic clinical trial to test the hypothesis that nocturnal low-flow oxygen therapy (NOXT) will reduce HF-related hospital admissions and all-cause mortality rates (primary composite outcome). A secondary aim of the trial is to test the hypothesis that NOXT will improve sleep quality, quality of life, mood, and exercise capacity.

This 5- to 6-year trial has begun recruiting patients.

Theophylline. Several studies[124,125] have shown the efficacy of theophylline in the treatment of CSA in HF. In a double-blind randomized placebo-controlled crossover study of 15 patients with treated, stable systolic HF, oral theophylline at therapeutic plasma concentration (11 μg/mL, range 7 to 15 μg/mL) decreased the AHI by about 50% and improved arterial oxyhemoglobin saturation.[124]

Mechanisms of action of theophylline in improving central apnea remain unclear. At therapeutic serum concentrations, theophylline competes with adenosine at some of its receptor sites. In the central nervous system, adenosine is a respiratory depressant, and theophylline stimulates respiration by competing with adenosine. Conceivably therefore an increase in ventilation by theophylline decreasing the plant gain could decrease central apnea during sleep. Theophylline does not increase ventilatory response to CO_2.

Potential arrhythmogenic effects and phosphodiesterase inhibition are common concerns with long-term use of theophylline in patients with HF. Therefore further controlled studies are necessary to ensure its safety. If theophylline is used to treat CSA, frequent and careful follow-ups are necessary.

Acetazolamide. Acetazolamide improves CSA by decreasing the plant gain in patients with HF with CSA.[126-128] In a double-blind placebo-controlled crossover study[129] of 12 patients with HF, acetazolamide, administered at about 3 mg/kg one-half hour before bedtime, decreased the central AHI significantly from about 57/hour (in the placebo arm) to 34/hour. Acetazolamide improved arterial oxyhemoglobin desaturation significantly. Furthermore, patients reported improved subjective perceptions of the following: overall sleep quality, feeling rested on awakening, falling asleep unintentionally during daytime, and fatigue. Acetazolamide therefore could have other advantageous effects when used in patients with HF and CSA, including acting as a mild diuretic and also normalizing the alkalemia (caused by loop diuretics) commonly present in patients with HF. In our patients, arterial blood pH decreased from 7.43 to 7.37.[129]

Benzodiazepines. Benzodiazepines, by decreasing arousals, may decrease CSA. However, a placebo-controlled double-blind study[130] showed a reduction in arousals but failed to show any improvement in CSA in patients with systolic HF. Although benzodiazepines do not increase the number of central apneas, their use may increase the likelihood of developing obstructive apneas in some patients with HF.

Inhaled Carbon Dioxide and Addition of External Dead Space

Several studies have shown that low-level inhalation of CO_2 and addition of external dead space (by increasing Pco_2) improve CSA.[131-134] However, studies[132,133] show that CO_2 inhalation increases spontaneous arousals, which are associated with increased sympathetic and decreased parasympathetic activity. One study[134] also showed that addition of dead space was associated with increased arousals. Because of the adverse cardiovascular effects of increased sympathetic overactivity in HF, use of CO_2 and external dead space to treat CSA in HF should be avoided. However, dynamic CO_2 inhalation,[135] when it can be inhaled intermittently within a part of breathing cycle, could eventually prove useful.

Phenotypic Treatment of Sleep-Disordered Breathing in Heart Failure

In HF, both CSA and OSA are heterogeneous syndromes, with varied pathophysiologic mechanisms, clinical presentations, and predisposing factors. Several physiologic phenotypes/endotypes exist, and each one could become a target of therapy (see also Chapter 129). This approach is in its infancy.[134,135]

CLINICAL PEARLS

- Because of the increased average life span and improved therapy of ischemic coronary artery disease and hypertension, the prevalence of HF remains high.
- Periodic breathing is common in HF and is characterized by apnea, hypopnea, and hyperpnea, which cause sleep disruption, arousals, hypoxemia/reoxygenation, hypercapnia/hypocapnia, and changes in intrathoracic pressure. Periodic breathing includes both obstructive and central sleep-related breathing disorders. All of these adversely affect sleep and cardiovascular function.
- Periodic breathing may contribute to the remodeling of LV dysfunction and to the progressively declining course of HF.
- Several studies have demonstrated that both CSA and OSA are associated with increased mortality of patients with HF and systolic dysfunction.
- There are only a few long-term studies on the treatment of sleep apnea in systolic HF. These show that effective treatment of both CSA and OSA with CPAP improves mortality of patients with HF.
- At this time ASV is not recommended in CHF when LVEF is less than 45%.

SUMMARY

HF is a common disorder that has a significant economic impact and is associated with excess morbidity and mortality. Because of increased average life spans and improved therapy for hypertension and ischemic coronary artery disease, the incidence and prevalence of HF remain high.

One factor that may contribute to the progressively declining course of HF, hospital readmission, quality of life, and premature mortality is the occurrence of periodic breathing, with repetitive episodes of apnea, hypopnea, and hyperpnea. Episodes of apnea, hypopnea, and the following hyperpnea collectively cause hypoxemia and reoxygenation, hypercapnia and hypocapnia, changes in intrathoracic pressure, and sleep disruption and arousals. These pathophysiologic consequences of sleep-related breathing disorders have deleterious effects on the cardiovascular system, and they may be most pronounced in the setting of established HF and coronary artery disease.

Multiple studies have demonstrated increased readmission and premature mortality independently associated with obstructive and CSA comorbid with HF. In addition, multiple studies have also demonstrated that effective treatment of both obstructive and CSA decreases hospital readmission and improves survival, particularly in those patients who are most adherent to therapy.

ASV devices with automatic inspiratory pressure support and automatic end-expiratory positive pressure algorithms, along with a backup rate, are effective in the treatment of hybrid sleep-related breathing disorders consisting of both CSA and OSA but are not recommended when LVEF is less than 45%. The best approach for patients with low LVEF is not clear, and future research is needed to guide the management of these patients.

SELECTED READINGS

Bitter T, Faber L, Hering D, et al. Sleep-disordered breathing in heart failure with normal left ventricular ejection fraction. *Eur J Heart Fail.* 2009;11:602–608.

Carlisle T, Ward NR, Atalla A, et al. Investigation of the link between fluid shift and airway collapsibility as a mechanism for obstructive sleep apnea in congestive heart failure. *Physiol Rep.* 2017;5(1):e12956. https://doi.org/10.14814/phy2.12956.

Coniglio AC, Mentz RJ. Sleep breathing disorders in heart failure. *Heart Fail Clin.* 2020;16(1):45–51. https://doi.org/10.1016/j.hfc.2019.08.009.

Cowie MR, Woehrle H, Wegscheider K, et al. Adaptive servo-ventilation for central sleep apnea in systolic heart failure. *N Engl J Med.* 2015;373:1095–1105.

Javaheri S. Sleep disorders in systolic heart failure: a prospective study of 100 male patients. The final report. *Int J Cardiol.* 2006;106:21–28.

Javaheri S, Barbe F, Campos-Rodriguez F, et al. Sleep apnea: types, mechanisms, and clinical cardiovascular consequences. *J Am Coll Cardiol.* 2017;69(7):841–858. https://doi.org/10.1016/j.jacc.2016.11.069.

Javaheri S, Brown LK, Abraham WT, Khayat R. Apneas of heart failure and phenotype-guided treatments: Part One: OSA. *Chest.* 2020;157(2):394–402. https://doi.org/10.1016/j.chest.2019.02.407.

Javaheri S, Brown LK, Khayat RN. Update on apneas of heart failure with reduced ejection fraction: emphasis on the physiology of treatment: part 2: central sleep apnea. *Chest.* 2020;157(6):1637–1646.

Javaheri S, Caref B, Chen E, et al. Sleep apnea testing and outcomes in a large cohort of Medicare beneficiaries with newly diagnosed heart failure. *Am J Respir Crit Care Med.* 2011;183:539–546.

Jilek C, Krenn M, Sebah D, et al. Prognostic impact of sleep disordered breathing and its treatment in heart failure: an observational study. *Eur J Heart Fail.* 2011;13:68–75.

Kasai T, Narui K, Dohi T, et al. Prognosis of patients with heart failure and obstructive sleep apnea treated with continuous positive airway pressure. *Chest.* 2008;133:690–696.

Murtaza G, Turagam MK, Akella K, et al. Pacing therapies for sleep apnea and cardiovascular outcomes: a systematic review. *J Interv Card Electrophysiol.* 2021;61(1):11–17.

Nayak HM, Patel R, McKane S, et al. Transvenous phrenic nerve stimulation for central sleep apnea is safe and effective in patients with concomitant cardiac devices [published online ahead of print, 2020 Jun 30]. *Heart Rhythm.* 2020;S1547-5271(20)30622-30626. https://doi.org/10.1016/j.hrthm.2020.06.023.

Wang J, Covassin N, Dai T, et al. Therapeutic value of treating central sleep apnea by adaptive servo-ventilation in patients with heart failure: a systematic review and meta-analysis. *Heart Lung.* 2021;50(2):344–351.

Wongboonsin J, Thongprayoon C, Bathini T, et al. Acetazolamide therapy in patients with heart failure: a meta-analysis. *J Clin Med.* 2019;8(3):349. https://doi.org/10.3390/jcm8030349. Published 2019 Mar 12.

Yancy CW, Jessup M, Bozkurt B, et al. 2017 ACC/AHA/HFSA focused update of the 2013 ACCF/AHA Guideline for the Management of Heart Failure: a report of the American College of Cardiology/American Heart Association Task Force on Clinical Practice Guidelines and the Heart Failure Society of America. *Circulation.* 2017;136(6):e137–e16.

Zhang J, et al. Exploring quality of life in patients with and without heart failure. *Int J Cardiol.* 2016;202:676–684.

A complete reference list can be found online at ExpertConsult.com.

Chapter 150

Sleep-Disordered Breathing and Stroke

Claudio L.A. Bassetti

Chapter Highlights

- Sleep-disordered breathing (SDB) and stroke are common and intertwined problems; each may cause the other, and they can arise from similar predisposing factors.
- SDB doubles the risk of stroke, and treatment with continuous positive airway pressure (CPAP) may reduce the risk of stroke in patients compliant with this treatment.
- Severe SDB is present in 30% of patients with stroke, worsens stroke outcome, and increases the risk of recurrence.
- CPAP in patients with poststroke SDB is feasible and may have a beneficial effect on stroke outcome.

HISTORY

John Cheyne recognized periodic breathing after stroke in 1818, and Broadbent recognized sleep apnea symptoms with stroke in 1877.[1,2] It is, however, only since the 1990s that the association between sleep and stroke has been increasingly studied and recognized.

STROKE

Stroke is a focal neurologic deficit of acute onset and vascular origin; about 65% of patients have ischemic stroke, 15% intracerebral hemorrhage, and 20% transient ischemic attacks (TIAs) in which neurologic deficits resolve within 1 hour.

Stroke has an estimated lifetime risk for those aged 25 years or older of 25% and represents worldwide the second most common cause of mortality and disability-adjusted life years.[3] Despite a declining stroke incidence related to improvement in prevention and treatment measures, the number of strokes is anticipated to increase in the next few decades because of the population aging.[4]

Risk factors for stroke include atrial fibrillation, arterial hypertension, dyslipidemia, disorders of glucose metabolism, overweight (abnormal waist-to-hip ratio), excessive alcohol consumption, cigarette smoking, and physical inactivity. Patients with heart disease, asymptomatic carotid stenosis, history of TIA, depression, psychosocial stress, and age older than 65 years are also at higher risk for stroke.[5] Primary prevention of stroke includes treatment of risk factors, regular physical exercise, reduction of body mass index to less than 25, anticoagulation for atrial fibrillation, and endarterectomy in patients with at least 70% carotid stenosis. Emergency treatment includes the systemic use of fibrinolytic agents and endovascular treatment (thrombectomy). Management of acute stroke includes placement of patients in a stroke unit, early recognition of medical complications, and prescription of agents that inhibit platelet aggregation. Surgery may be considered in patients with accessible (e.g., cerebellar) hemorrhages and malignant middle cerebral artery strokes. After stroke, treatments include neurorehabilitation and the prevention of further events with platelet antiaggregants, blood pressure–lowering medications, statins, management of other risk factors, and, in selected patients, anticoagulation and endarterectomy.

Sleep-Disordered Breathing and Stroke Risk

Epidemiology

Habitual snoring, a symptom of sleep-disordered breathing (SDB), was studied since the 1990s and found to represent an independent risk factor for stroke with a pooled risk of about 1.5.[6] In the last 20 years an increasing number of studies assessed the association of polygraphic/polysomnographic assessed SDB and risk of stroke. Three studies first drew attention to this topic. In an observational US cohort study of 1022 patients published in 2005, obstructive sleep apnea (OSA) was associated with an increased odds ratio (OR) of 2.0 for stroke and death, even after adjusting for multiple cardiovascular risk factors. The risk was higher (OR = 3.3) in patients with severe OSA (apnea-hypopnea index [AHI] > 36/hour).[7] In a single-center study published also in 2005 from Spain of 1387 male patients with OSA followed for up to 10 years, patients with severe OSA (AHI > 30/hour) had a significantly higher incidence of fatal and nonfatal cardiovascular events including stroke compared with patients with mild to moderate OSA, patients with OSA treated with continuous positive airway pressure (CPAP), 377 simple snorers, and 264 controls.[8] In a US population-based cohort study of 5422 participants at least 40 years of age followed up over 9 years and published in 2010, OSA predicted ischemic stroke in multivariable regressions adjusted for age, sex, and vascular risk factors in men (OR = 2.9) but not women.[9]

A statement paper of the European Neurology (EAN), Respiratory (ERS), Sleep (ESRS), and Stroke Society (ESO) societies published in 2020 reviewed the current scientific evidence on this topic.[10] A total of 9 systematic reviews with meta-analysis and 14 additional primary studies (published after the SR/MA) were found (publications until January 2019 were included). The authors concluded that OSA doubles the risk of stroke (with a relative risk ranging from 2.02 to 2.24 over a follow-up period of 3 to 10 years), especially in young to middle-age patients, without differences between women and men.[10] This risk may be related to the association of OSA with atrial fibrillation and coronary heart disease, but evidence was considered to be still insufficient. Current knowledge suggests that SDB is also linked with white matter disease and silent strokes.[11,12] In a study of 503 elderly individuals who were free of previously diagnosed cardiovascular and neurologic diseases, moderate to severe OSA (AHI ≥15) was independently associated with the presence of white matter changes (OR: 2.08; 95% CI: 1.05–4.13) compared with no OSA even after adjustment for hypertension.[13]

Pathophysiology

Several acute and chronic consequences of nocturnal respiratory events may explain the link between SDB and increased risk for stroke. Sympathetic hyperactivation, intermittent hypoxemia with oxidative stress, and inflammation likely increase the risk for atherosclerosis and cardiovascular morbidities. However, this link has been difficult to prove because sleep apnea and stroke share many of the same risk factors such as obesity and diabetes.

1. **Acute effects.** Acutely, apneas and hypopneas during sleep can be accompanied by decreased cardiac output, cardiac arrhythmias, systemic hypotension or hypertension, vasodilation resulting from hypoxia and hypercapnia, and increased intracranial pressure. These factors lead to a roughly 15% to 20% reduction in cerebral blood flow velocities during respiratory events.[14] Large fluctuations in cerebral blood flow may be particularly detrimental because patients with SDB have been shown to have diminished vasodilator reserve and impaired cerebral autoregulation.[15] Type, duration, and timing of respiratory events affect hemodynamic consequences. Near-infrared spectroscopy (NIRS) studies have shown that SDB can disrupt autoregulatory mechanisms and cause brain hypoxia, particularly with severe SDB (AHI > 30) (Figure 150.1).[16] These effects are particularly detrimental to the ischemic region (penumbra) bordering the stroke.[17] Transcranial Doppler studies have shown that both obstructive and central apneas can alter cerebral blood flow.[15,18,19] Paradoxical embolization resulting from right-to-left shunting in patients with patent foramen ovale during long apneas is another potential mechanism of stroke.[20] In light of these observations, it is not surprising that snoring and SDB have been associated (in some but not all studies) with the onset of cerebrovascular events at night and strokes that are apparent on awakening (so-called "wake-up strokes").[20-24]
2. **Chronic effects.** Patients with significant SDB (AHI > 30/hour) have an increased long-term mortality that is partially the result of cardio- and cerebrovascular events and explained by multiple potential mechanisms.[25] Chronically, SDB (and even habitual snoring) are associated with hypertension, which is a major risk factor for stroke. In the Wisconsin sleep cohort, an AHI of greater than 15 was independently associated with a threefold increased risk for developing new hypertension within a 4-year period.[26] In a prospective cohort study of 1889 participants without hypertension, Marin and colleagues found an increased risk for incident hypertension within a 12-year period in patients with an AHI of 5 or greater who were ineligible for CPAP therapy, among those who declined CPAP therapy, and among those nonadherent to CPAP therapy, whereas the risk was lower in patients with AHI of 5 or greater who were treated with CPAP therapy.[27] SDB is associated also with coronary heart disease, myocardial infarction,

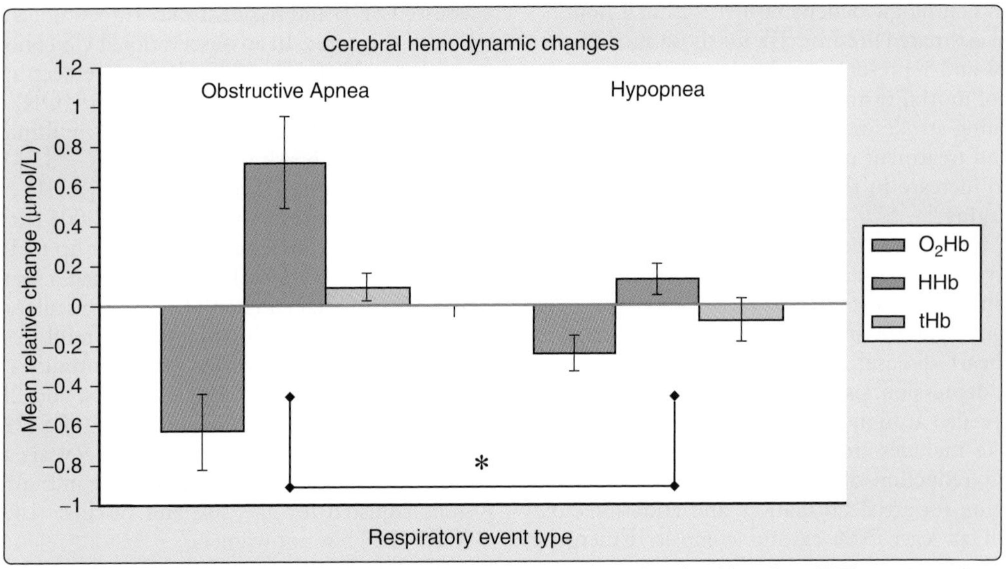

Figure 150.1 Cerebral hemodynamic alterations in patients with sleep-disordered breathing (SDB) as estimated by near-infrared spectroscopy (NIRS). Patients with snoring (*n* = 7, apnea-hypopnea index [AHI] = 2 ± 2/hour); mild SDB (*n* = 7, AHI = 14 ± 8/hour, range); and severe obstructive sleep apnea syndrome (*n* = 5, AHI = 79 ± 20/hour) were studied. NIRS data associated with different respiratory events (obstructive apnea and hypopnea) were averaged for each patient. Subsequently, corresponding cerebral hemodynamic (and peripheral oxygen saturation, Sp_{O2}) relative changes were assessed via integrals adjusted for duration. The relative changes in brain tissue parameters (concentrations of oxyhemoglobin [O_2Hb], deoxyhemoglobin [HHb], and total hemoglobin [tHb]) were significantly larger during obstructive apneas than during hypopneas.[42]

heart failure, and atrial fibrillation, all of which are risk factors for stroke.[28,29] Several observations also support the hypothesis that SDB worsens atherogenesis. The intima media thickness of the common carotid artery is increased in patients with SDB compared with controls matched for age and vascular risk factors.[30] Patients with SDB have also an increased arterial stiffness, a recognized marker of cardiovascular risk and long-term morbidity.[31] Finally, large negative intrathoracic pressure swings impose a mechanical stress on the heart, aorta, and carotid arteries.[32]

Treatment of Sleep-Disordered Breathing and Reduction of Stroke Risk

Treatment of SDB was shown to have positive effects on multiple cardiovascular risk factors. A few studies have shown that CPAP produces reductions in mean arterial blood pressure. Pepperell and colleagues[33] reported that therapeutic CPAP levels reduced mean arterial blood pressure by 2.5 mm Hg, whereas subtherapeutic CPAP levels increased blood pressure by 0.8 mm Hg. Such an effect could reduce stroke risk by about 20%.[33] Although the effects of CPAP on hypertension and cardiovascular events are debated, CPAP has been shown to reduce blood pressure in patients with OSA and cardiovascular disease or multiple cardiovascular risk factors.[34,35] Treatment with CPAP also can improve other detrimental hemodynamic, neural, and molecular effects of SDB such as factor VII clotting activity, fibrinogen levels, and platelet activation or aggregation.[36]

There have been important observational studies reporting the positive effect of SDB treatment on risk of stroke. Marin and colleagues first reported in 2005 a decrease of fatal and nonfatal cardiovascular events including stroke in which patients were treated with CPAP.[8] Later studies confirmed this observation of a positive effect of treatment on subsequent risk of stroke, particularly in patients with severe SDB who were adherent to CPAP with use of 4 or more hours/night.[37-39] The multicenter SAVE trial assessed the effect of CPAP for prevention of cardiovascular effects on 2717 adults between 45 and 75 years of age with moderate to severe OSA and coronary or cerebrovascular disease. After a mean follow-up of 3.7 years no difference was observed in stroke incidence between the CPAP and the usual care group.[40] However, the inclusion of mainly Asian patients, the exclusion of patients with excessive daytime sleepiness and recent stroke, and the poor adherence to treatment (<4 hours/night) in the majority (58%) of patients limit the generalizability of the results.

In a meta-analysis of 5 randomized controlled studies that reported results from participants with an average use of CPAP of at least 4 hours/night and a follow-up period of at least 12 months, 943 users and 1141 controls were included. Sufficient CPAP use was found to prevent stroke (risk reduction: 0.68; 95% confidence interval [CI]: 0.50 to 0.92; $P = .01$) but not cardiac events.[41]

The current scientific evidence on this topic was reviewed in a statement paper of the EAN, ERS, ESRS, and ESO published in 2020.[10] A total of four systematic reviews with meta-analysis and four additional primary studies were found. The authors concluded that CPAP treatment may reduce the stroke risk in patients adherent to CPAP treatment (>4 hours per night) but that further randomized controlled trials are needed.

Sleep-Disordered Breathing after Stroke

Epidemiology

Between 1996 and 1999, three large, systematic studies demonstrated for the first time a very high frequency of SDB in patients with stroke and TIA and characterized the type of disturbances that can be seen in this clinical setting.[42-44]

In a recent meta-analysis of 89 studies (for a total of 7096 patients with stroke and TIA) the frequency of SDB was systematically reviewed. Fifty-four studies were performed in the acute phase of stroke (within 1 month), 23 studies in the subacute phase (after 1 to 3 months), and 12 studies in the chronic phase (after more than 3 months). The mean AHI was 26.0/hour (standard deviation [SD] 21.7–31.2). The frequency of SDB with an AHI greater than 5 was 71% and with an AHI greater than 30 was 30%. Males had a higher percentage of SDB (AHI >10/hour) than females (65% vs. 48%; $P = .001$). Overall, the severity and prevalence of SDB were similar in all examined phases after stroke, irrespective of the type of sleep apnea test performed. The heterogeneity between studies was considered high.[45]

Only few studies assessed the prevalence of SDB in stroke subtypes. Patients with TIA were found to have lower values of AHI, while patients with hemorrhagic, brainstem, nocturnal/wake-up, and recurrent strokes were reported (in some but not all studies) to have higher AHI.[24,46-51]

In the previously mentioned meta-analysis of 89 studies, the severity and prevalence of SDB were overall similar in all examined phases after stroke.[45] However, single studies had suggested an improvement over time particularly of central events and in patients with hemorrhagic strokes.[21,45,52] However, only three studies assessed intraindividually and with full polysomnography the evolution of SDB from the acute to subacute-chronic phase of stroke.[21,53,54] In the largest study so far conducted and published in 2020, a total of 166 patients with stroke were evaluated by full polysomnography within the first week after stroke and 105 of them were re-examined after 3 months.[54] At baseline AHIs of more than 5/hour and AHI of more than 30/hour were found in 81% and 25% of patients, respectively. OSA was more prevalent than central sleep apnea (CSA; 84% vs. 13%). The initial AHI was 21 ± 18 and decreased significantly at follow-up to 18 ± 16 ($P = .018$). In 68% of patients the predominant type of SDB remained unchanged (79% in patients with OSA and 44% in patients with CSA).

Clinical Features

1. **Breathing disturbances during sleep.** The most common form of SDB in patients who have had a stroke is OSA (Figure 150.2). Occasionally, patients may present with both OSA and Cheyne-Stokes breathing (CSB) (Figure 150.3). OSA is often worse in rapid eye movement (REM) sleep, whereas CSB is usually worse in light non–rapid eye movement (NREM) sleep.[42] In the first few days after stroke, CSA and other forms of central periodic breathing are present during at least 10% of the recording time in about one-third of patients.[52,55-57]
2. **Breathing disturbances during wakefulness.** Hemispheric strokes in the frontal cortex, basal ganglia, or internal capsule may cause respiratory apraxia, with impaired voluntary modulation of breathing amplitude and frequency, leaving patients unable to take a deep breath or hold the breath.[58]

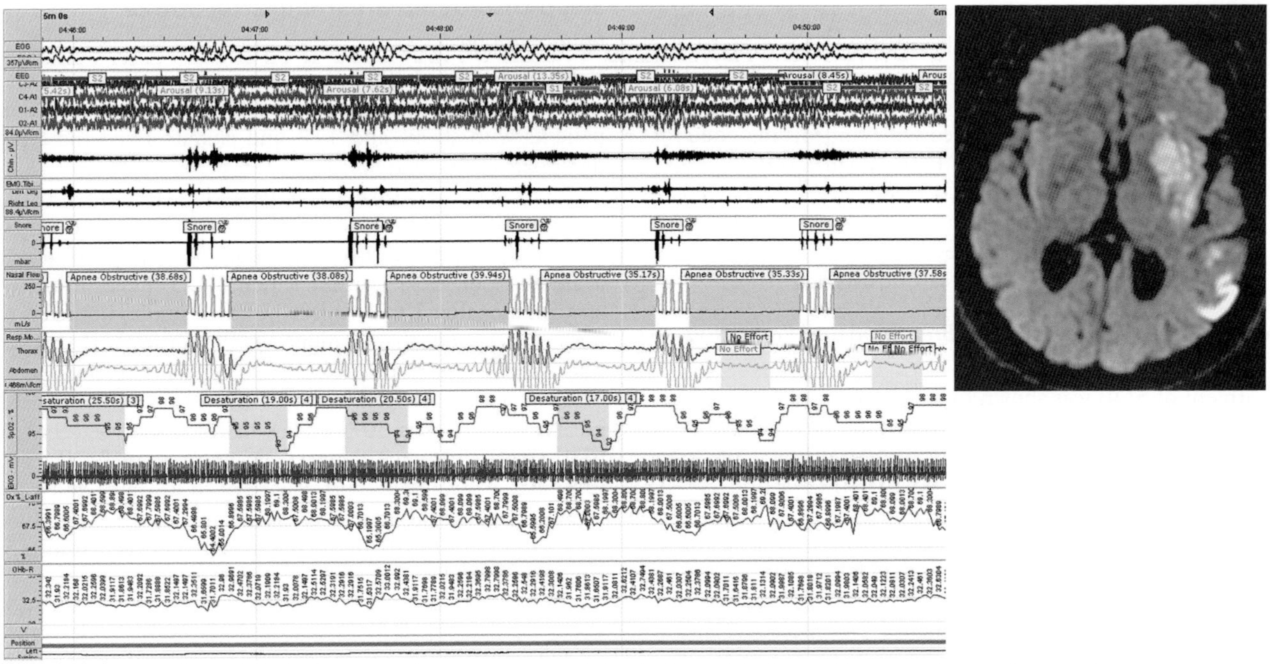

Figure 150.2 Obstructive sleep apnea in acute ischemic stroke. This 70-year-old man has left middle cerebral artery stroke, carotid artery occlusion, and atrial fibrillation. He has habitual snoring but no excessive daytime sleepiness. Aphasia and severe hemiparesis are clinically apparent. National Institutes of Health stroke score is 16, and there are no signs of heart failure. Polysomnography 2 days after stroke onset shows an apnea-hypopnea index (AHI) of 79 and minimum oxygen desaturation of 85%. The AHI normalized (<5/hour) with continuous positive airway pressure. (MRI courtesy Professor A. Valavanis, Institute of Neuroradiology, University Hospital, Zürich, Switzerland.)

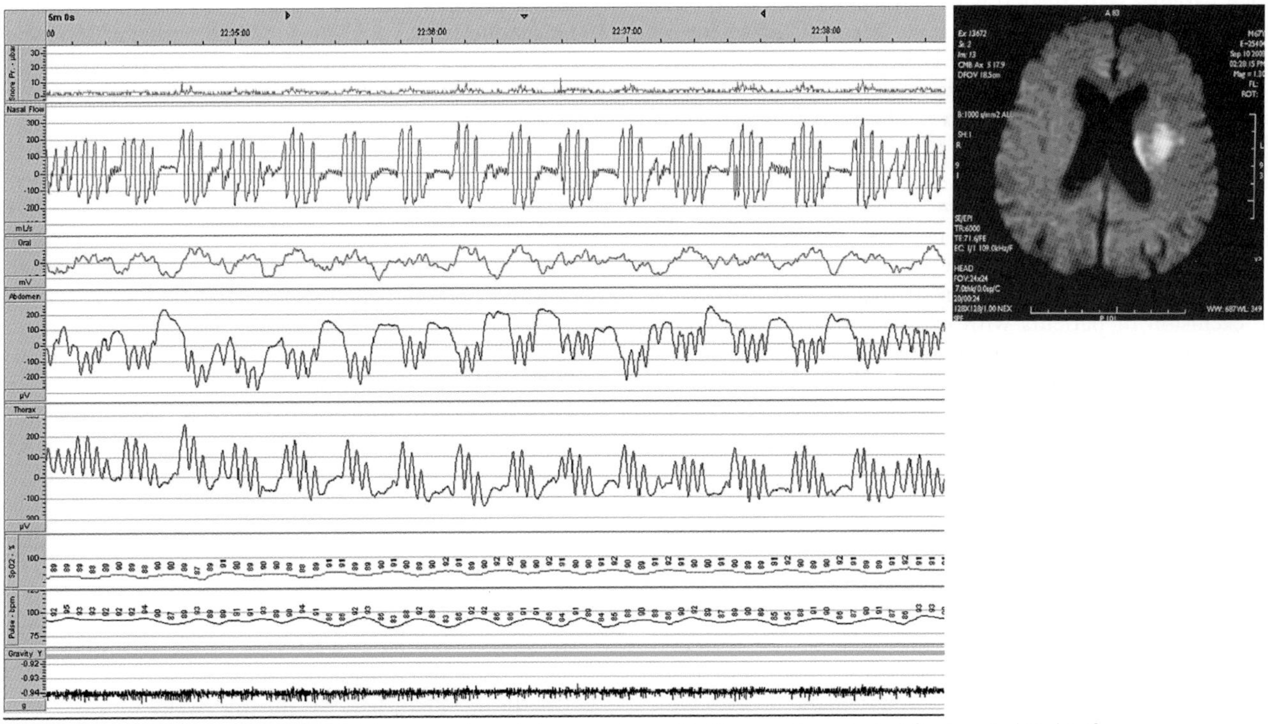

Figure 150.3 Central sleep apnea in acute ischemic stroke. This 63-year-old man had a left subcortical stroke of unknown origin, with arterial hypertension and habitual snoring but no excessive daytime sleepiness. He had a mild hemiparesis, with a National Institutes of Health stroke score of 8 and no signs of heart failure (cardiac ejection fraction, 55%). Polysomnography the first night after stroke onset showed an apnea-hypopnea index (AHI) of 53 (mainly central apneas). The patient spontaneously improved after 1 week (AHI = 16). (MRI courtesy Professor G. Schroth, Institute of Neuroradiology, University Hospital, Bern, Switzerland.)

Sustained respiratory rates above 25 to 30 per minute in the absence of hypoxemia (neurogenic hyperventilation) were originally described in six comatose patients with ventrotegmental pontine strokes but were subsequently attributed to pulmonary edema (and stimulation of lung and chest wall afferent reflexes).[59] Neurogenic hyperventilation after stroke can be seen also in awake patients without pulmonary edema, with brainstem as well as subcortical strokes, and typically (but not invariably) indicates a poor prognosis.[60,61]

Inspiratory breath holding (apneustic breathing), originally described in two patients with bilateral ventrotegmental mediocaudal (infratrigeminal) pontine stroke, is rare and usually secondary to basilar artery occlusion.[62]

Erratic variations in breathing frequency and amplitude (ataxic or Biot breathing) and failure of automatic breathing (central sleep apnea or Ondine's curse) usually imply a lateral medullary stroke, often bilateral.[63,64] Damage to the medullary reticular formation and nucleus ambiguous may cause a loss of automatic breathing, whereas a lesion that includes the nucleus of the solitary tract is necessary to cause failure of both automatic and voluntary respiration.[65]

Volitional breathing can be impaired by brainstem strokes involving corticobulbar and corticospinal pathways at pontine and medullary levels.[58] Spinal cord stroke can impair both automatic and voluntary breathing. Anterior spinal artery strokes can affect reticulospinal pathways, located anteriorly in the lateral columns of the first three cervical segments, which are crucial for automatic breathing.[66] In contrast, posterior spinal artery strokes can damage corticospinal pathways in the dorsolateral spinal cord and impair voluntary control of breathing.[67] Strokes that extend up to the C1 level usually cause severe respiratory insufficiency and necessitate ventilatory support. Repetitive yawning can accompany hypersomnia (e.g., in patients with thalamic or posterior hypothalamus stroke) and can also occur as a release phenomenon in patients with brainstem and supratentorial lesions. Yawning can also occur with insular and caudate lesions.[68]

Pathophysiology

1. **SDB preceding stroke.** Overall, stroke severity, topography, and etiology do not correlate with the presence and type of poststroke SDB.[69,70] The preexistence of SDB in most patients with poststroke SDB is suggested also by two other observations: (1) the prevalence of SDB is similar in patients with TIA and stroke and (2) patients with poststroke SDB frequently report a history of snoring preceding stroke.[42,52,71]
2. **Worsening or de novo SDB after stroke.** Some patients develop (or worsen preexisting) SDB after stroke. This has been shown in isolated patients examined before and after stroke.[72] The hypothesis that SDB can appear de novo after stroke is supported also by the observation that SDB can improve to a great extent or even normalize in the days or weeks that follow the acute event.[54,73] Several factors can explain the worsening (or appearance de novo) of SDB after stroke.

First, CSA with CO_2 hypersensitivity can be seen after bilateral and severe strokes but also with unilateral and small hemispheric strokes as well as after rostrolateral medullary lesions also in the absence of heart failure.[57,74,75] Strokes in these areas can also cause acute cardioautonomic changes, including atrial fibrillation, suggesting the possibility that the appearance poststroke of CSA may refect in patients with a lesion in the central autonomic network, a change in the sympathetic-parasympathetic balance.[76] Nonneurogenic factors, including older age, left ventricular failure, coronary heart disease, acute caudorostral fluid shifts related to the nocturnal recumbent body position, and carotid stenosis, may also contribute to the appearance of CSA.[57,77,78] CSA in the context of asymptomatic carotid stenosis (in 39% of patients in one study) was associated with a shift in sympathicovagal balance secondary to an increased baroreflex and chemoreflex sensitivities in the carotid body.[79]

Second, patients with stroke may develop or worsen OSA from weak upper airway muscles or poor coordination between upper airway, intercostal, and diaphragmatic muscles resulting from brainstem or hemispheric strokes that impair cranial nerve function.[49,80] Accordingly, dysphagia and hypoglossal nerve dysfunction are associated with poststroke SDB.[81,82]

Third, acute brain damage may affect respiratory drive (see previous).

Finally, other factors such as hypoxemia resulting from aspiration or respiratory infections, reduction of voluntary chest movements on the paralyzed side, supine position, and sleep fragmentation secondary to stroke or stroke complications can also worsen breathing control during sleep.[83]

Diagnosis

Despite the high frequency of SDB, its cost effectiveness, and the fact that treatment may have a positive effect (see later), the American Heart Association and the American Stroke Foundation recommend routine screening for SDB.[84,85]

The suspicion of SDB should be particularly high in obese male patients with a history of habitual snoring, witnessed apneas, hypertension, diabetes mellitus, and sleep-onset/wake-up stroke.[21,44,86] In this clinical setting, however, asking for typical clinical symptoms and using SDB questionnaires validated in the general population appear to be of limited utility.[87]

For this reason, various approaches are recommended to assess for the presence of SDB in patients with stroke. Different forms of unattended respirography or polysomnography were shown to be sufficiently accurate to diagnose SDB and estimate its severity.[21,49,88,89] Full polysomnography is needed only in a minority of patients.

The optimal timing of sleep studies after stroke or TIA is unknown. Although studies within days of a stroke may be less representative of the patient's baseline, treatment of SDB soon after stroke could potentially minimize further brain injury and improve outcome.

Effects on Stroke Outcome and Recurrence

Effects on Stroke Outcome. The first study to report a negative effect of SDB on stroke outcome was published in 1996; in patients undergoing rehabilitation, OSA was associated with a higher mortality and poorer functional outcome at 1 year.[90] Subsequent studies suggested also an association of poststroke SDB with early neurologic worsening, longer hospitalization, poorer outcome, and higher long-term mortality.[21,86,88,91-95] Detrimental effects of SDB on blood pressure, cerebral oxygenation, and fibrinogen levels were documented and considered as potential explanations for the negative effects on acute stroke evolution.[17,96,97]

In a statement paper of the EAN, ERS, ESRS, and ESO published in 2020, the current scientific evidence on this topic was reviewed.[10] A total of two systematic reviews with meta-analyses and five additional primary studies (published after the SR/MA) were found (publications until January 2019 were included). The authors concluded that, although current evidence is inconclusive, OSA may be associated with a worse clinical outcome and an increase in all-cause mortality.

Two recent studies support this conclusion. A study of 995 patients with ischemic stroke reported an association between SDB (which was assessed with a portable device and found in 63% of patients) and a worse functional and cognitive (but not overall stroke) outcome at 90 days poststroke.[98] A second study using full polysomnography in 165 patients with stroke found an association between initial AHI and neurologic outcome (as assessed by the modified Rankin Scale) at 3 months.[54]

Effects on Stroke Recurrence. Studies on the effect of SDB on stroke recurrence appeared in the last 15 years and showed first contradictory results.[21,93,99] A meta-analysis published in 2014 suggested, however, a dose-response relationship between severity of poststroke SDB and risk of both recurrent events and mortality.[95] More recently, a study of 842 patients with ischemic stroke found an association between the presence of SDB (as assessed by a portable device) and recurrent ischemic stroke (but not mortality) after a median follow-up time of 591 days.[51]

Treatment

Treatment of SDB in patients with stroke can be a clinical, technical, and logistical challenge. Treatment strategies should always include prevention and early treatment of secondary complications (e.g., aspiration, respiratory infections, pain) and cautious use or avoidance of alcohol and sedatives that may worsen breathing during sleep. Patient positioning in the acute phase can improve oxygen saturation and reduce severity of OSA by 20%.[83,100,101] In patients with heart failure, a lateral sleeping position was shown to reduce the severity of central sleep apnea.[102]

The effect of supplemental oxygen in nonhypoxemic patients with stroke is unclear.[103] Even the most recent stroke guidelines, while pointing to the necessity to keep oxygen saturations above 92% to 94%, do not specify how to measure or correct nocturnal oxygen saturation.[85] In a trial of patients with SDB, oxygen was found to be inferior to CPAP in reducing blood pressure levels in patients with high cardiovascular risk.[35]

Treatment of Obstructive Sleep-Disordered Breathing (Obstructive Sleep Apnea). CPAP is usually the treatment of choice for OSA, but CPAP compliance can be a challenge because most patients with stroke and SDB lack excessive daytime sleepiness and may not perceive much benefit from CPAP. In addition, patients with stroke may have trouble using CPAP if they have dementia, delirium, aphasia, anosognosia, pseudobulbar or bulbar palsy, or severe motor impairment.

The first two studies on treatment of poststroke SDB were published in 2001. In a study of 105 patients with stroke treated in a rehabilitation unit, CPAP was accepted by 70%, and poor acceptance was associated with aphasia and severe stroke. CPAP use over 10 days led to an improvement of subjective well-being and lower nighttime blood pressure values.[104,105] Subsequent studies found, however, a low CPAP compliance in patients with acute stroke, which ranged from 12% to 22% over a follow-up of 2 to 60 months.[21,53,104,106,107] Over time, the number of reports on acceptable compliance and positive effects of CPAP in patients with stroke who tolerated treatment increased.[81,108] These better results may have arisen from careful selection of patients, the use of new respiratory devices (including adaptive servo-ventilation [ASV] machines) and headgears, higher motivation and instruction of the treating teams, and frequent contact with patients.[109,110] In 45 patients with acute TIA, auto-CPAP had acceptable adherence and reduced the risk for recurrent stroke 82% over a treatment period of 90 days.[110] In patients with stroke treated within 24 hours with CPAP, stroke severity was improved in those using CPAP more than 4 hours/night.[111] Parra and colleagues reported an improved 1-month neurologic recovery and fewer cardiovascular events by 24 months in 71 patients with moderate to severe SDB (AHI ≥ 20) started on CPAP within the first 3 to 6 days after stroke onset compared with 69 untreated patients with SDB.[89] At 5 years, the patients with treated SDB also had better survival than the untreated SDB stroke group.[112]

In a meta-analysis published in 2019, 10 randomized controlled trials with CPAP as intervention were analyzed. The mean CPAP use across the trials was 4.5 hours/night (95% CI: 3.97 to 5.08) with an odds ratio of dropping out with CPAP of 1.8 (95% CI: 1.05 to 3.21; $P = .033$). The combined analysis showed an overall neurofunctional improvement with CPAP with considerable heterogeneity across the studies. Long-term survival was improved in only one trial.[113]

After this meta-analysis three additional randomized controlled trials have been published in patients with poststroke SDB. The first studied included 30 patients with CPAP and 40 patients without CPAP; at 1 year no difference was found in recurrent cardiocerebrovascular events, but the CPAP group were less sleepy and had a better functional outcome.[114] The second study included 168 patients with CPAP and 84 patients without CPAP; at 1 year 59% patients of the CPAP group had the best neurologic symptom severity versus 38% of controls ($P = .038$) with an absolute risk reduction of 21% (number needed to treat, 4.8).[115] The third study included nonsleepy patients, 41 randomized to CPAP and 22 to standard care; no differences were found over 2 years in terms of recurrent cardiocerebrovascular events or neurologic outcome.[116]

Two studies are currently running to assess weather CPAP for poststroke SDB may have a positive effect on acute infarct growth (as assessed by MRI, eSATIS trial), improve functional outcome, and reduce stroke recurrence (eSATIS trial, sleep SMART trial).[117,118]

Treatment of Central Sleep-Disordered Breathing (Central Sleep Apnea). In patients with CSA, breathing disturbances can be improved with oxygen and possibly also lateral sleeping position.[100,119] Clinical experience and a few studies suggest that ASV may be effective in poststroke patients with CSA and CSB, including those nonresponsive to conventional CPAP.[120]

Tracheostomy and mechanical ventilation may become necessary in patients with central hypoventilation, central apneas, and ataxic breathing.

CLINICAL PEARLS

- Clinicians should consider SDB and sleep-wake disorders as potential risk factors for stroke as well as modulators of its outcome.
- The study of SDB in patients poststroke offers a unique opportunity to expand our knowledge about the brain mechanisms involved in breathing control.

SUMMARY

SDB independently doubles the risk for stroke, while CPAP may reduce the risk of stroke in patients adherent to treatment (at least 4 hours/night). Severe SDB (AHI > 30) is found in 30% of patients with stroke and TIA. After the acute phase of stroke, SDB can improve. Severe SDB worsens stroke outcome and increases the risk of stroke recurrence. Treatment of SDB is feasible even in the acute phase and may improve stroke outcome.

SELECTED READINGS

Bassetti C, Aldrich M, Chervin R, Quint D. Sleep apnea in the acute phase of TIA and stroke. *Neurology*. 1996;47:1167–1173.

Bassetti CLA, Randerath W, Vignatelli L, et al. EAN/ERS/ESO/ESRS statement on the impact of sleep disorders on risk and outcome of stroke. *Eur J Neurol*. 2020;27(7):1117–1136.

Bravata DM, Sico JJ, FRagoso CA, al e. Diagnosing and treating sleep apnea in patients with acute cerebrovascular disease. *JACC*. 2018;7:e008841. DOI: 008810.001161/JAHA.008118.008841.

Brown DL, Shafie-Khorassani F, Kim SK, et al. Sleep-Disordered Breathing is associated with recurrent ischemic stroke. *Stroke*. 2019;50:571–576.

Lisabeth LD, Sanchez BN, Lim DC, et al. Sleep-disordered breathing and poststroke outcomes. *Ann Neurol*. 2019;86:241–250.

Liu X, Lam DC, Chan KPF, Chan HY, Ip MS, Lau KK. Prevalence and Determinants of Sleep Apnea in Patients with Stroke: a meta-analysis. *J Stroke Cerebrovasc Dis*. 2021;30(12):106129. [published online ahead of print, 2021 Sep 30].

Tanayapong P, Kuna ST. Sleep disordered breathing as a cause and consequence of stroke: a review of pathophysiological and clinical relationships. *Sleep Med Rev*. 2021;59:101499.

Yaggi H, Concato J, Kernan WN, Lichtman JH, Brass LM, Mohsenin V. Obstructive sleep apnea as a risk factor for stroke and death. *New Engl J Med*. 2005;359:2034–2041.

A complete reference list can be found online at ExpertConsult.com.

Chapter 151

Insomnia and Cardiovascular Disease

Sogol Javaheri; Daniel J. Buysse; Martica H. Hall

Chapter Highlights

- Insomnia is a highly prevalent sleep disorder that has increasingly been associated with incident cardiovascular morbidity and mortality.
- Potential mechanisms underlying the association between insomnia and cardiovascular disease include increased sympathetic nervous system activity, dysregulation of the hypothalamic pituitary adrenal axis, and increased inflammation. Depression and anxiety, which are associated with both insomnia and cardiovascular disease, may also serve as biobehavioral mediators in this relationship.
- Mechanistic studies and randomized trials are needed to better understand the biobehavioral mechanisms through which insomnia contributes to cardiovascular disease and whether insomnia treatment could reduce cardiovascular morbidity or mortality.

INTRODUCTION

Insomnia is the most prevalent sleep disorder in the United States and worldwide. Approximately 30% of Americans suffer from insomnia symptoms, and 10% meet criteria for a diagnosis of insomnia. Insomnia symptoms include self-reported difficulty falling or staying asleep or waking too early despite having adequate opportunity to sleep.[1] A diagnosis of insomnia is made if these symptoms are persistent, occurring at least three times a week, and coupled with perceived daytime impairment, such as problems with concentration, memory, or attention, fatigue, lethargy, errors at work, impaired driving, any other form of vocational or social dysfunction, headaches or gastrointestinal symptoms resulting from sleep loss, daytime sleepiness, changes in mood, or specific worrying about sleep.[2] Up to 40% of individuals with insomnia have symptoms that last for 3 years or more.[3]

Both insomnia symptoms and insomnia disorder are increasingly recognized as potential risk factors for cardiovascular disease (CVD), including hypertension, heart failure (HF), coronary heart disease, subclinical CVD, and CVD mortality.[4] These risks appear to be particularly high when insomnia occurs with objectively measured short sleep duration of less than 6 hours.[5] Although dissatisfaction with sleep quality or quantity is a diagnostic criterion for insomnia disorder, no specific sleep duration defines this condition.[2] Insomnia accounts for only approximately 20% of individuals with self-reported short sleep duration,[6,7] whereas approximately 50% of individuals with insomnia have objectively short sleep duration.[6] Thus insomnia coupled with short objective sleep duration may represent a distinct phenotype with additive adverse effects on cardiometabolic health. Given variation in how insomnia is defined and measured, however, heterogeneity in the literature may contribute to conflicting data and difficulty interpreting results.

Insomnia and CVD are highly comorbid, and the presence of insomnia may increase CVD risk, including incident disease, risk for cardiovascular events, and mortality in patients with CVD.[8,9] However, data have not established that insomnia is causally related to CVD, either via pathogenesis or modification of the clinical course of disease. In this chapter we summarize the relationship between insomnia and manifestations of CVD, address several biobehavioral mechanisms through which insomnia may increase cardiovascular risk and outcomes, and describe programmatic research that could test these mechanisms and the extent to which treatment of insomnia may alter cardiovascular morbidity or mortality.

PUTATIVE PSYCHOBIOLOGIC MECHANISMS LINKING INSOMNIA TO CARDIOVASCULAR DISEASE MORBIDITY AND MORTALITY

Insomnia may contribute to the development and clinical course of CVD through a number of psychobiologic pathways, including psychological and physiologic arousal, stress, major depressive disorder (MDD), inflammation, and hypothalmic-pituitary-adrenal (HPA) axis dysregulation. Putative psychological mechanisms linking insomnia with CVD are depicted in Figures 151.1 and 151.2.

Psychological and Physiologic Arousal

Patients with insomnia report increased psychological and physiologic arousal.[10] Increased indices of physiologic arousal observed in patients with insomnia have included increased heart rate and decreased heart rate variability during sleep, increased fast-frequency electroencephalographic activity during non–rapid eye movement sleep (i.e., 16 to 32 Hz, known as beta activity), impaired inhibitory processes in the brain during sleep, increased 24-hour whole-body metabolic rate, and decreased ability to initiate polysomnography-assessed sleep during the daytime multiple sleep latency test. Yet it is important to note that not all studies show evidence of increased physiologic arousal in patients with insomnia.[11] These discrepancies likely reflect the heterogeneous and waxing and waning nature of the disorder.

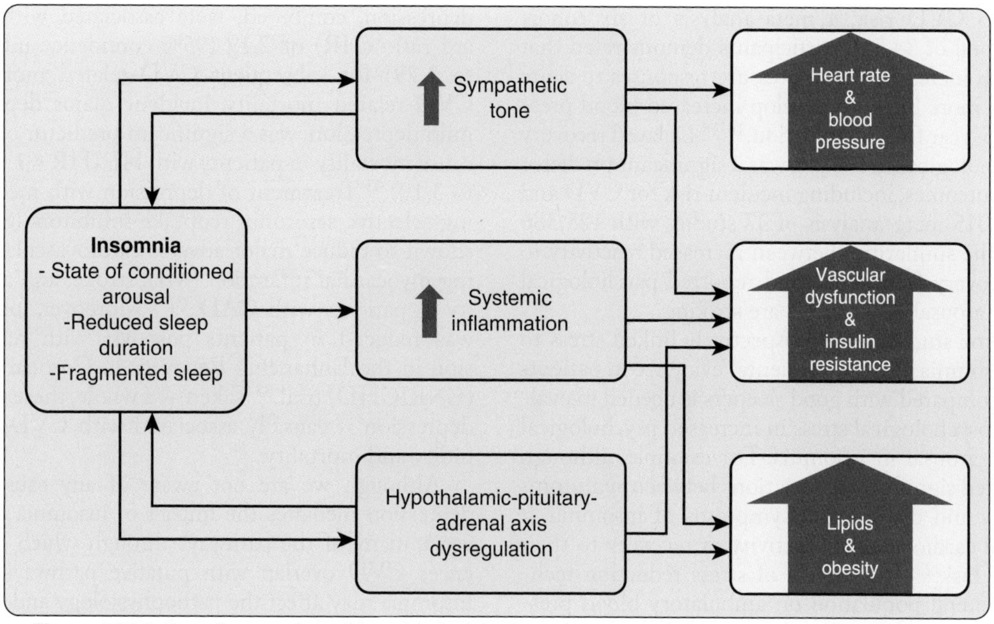

Figure 151.1 Flow diagram of possible pathophysiologic mechanisms underlying association between insomnia and adverse cardiovascular sequalae.

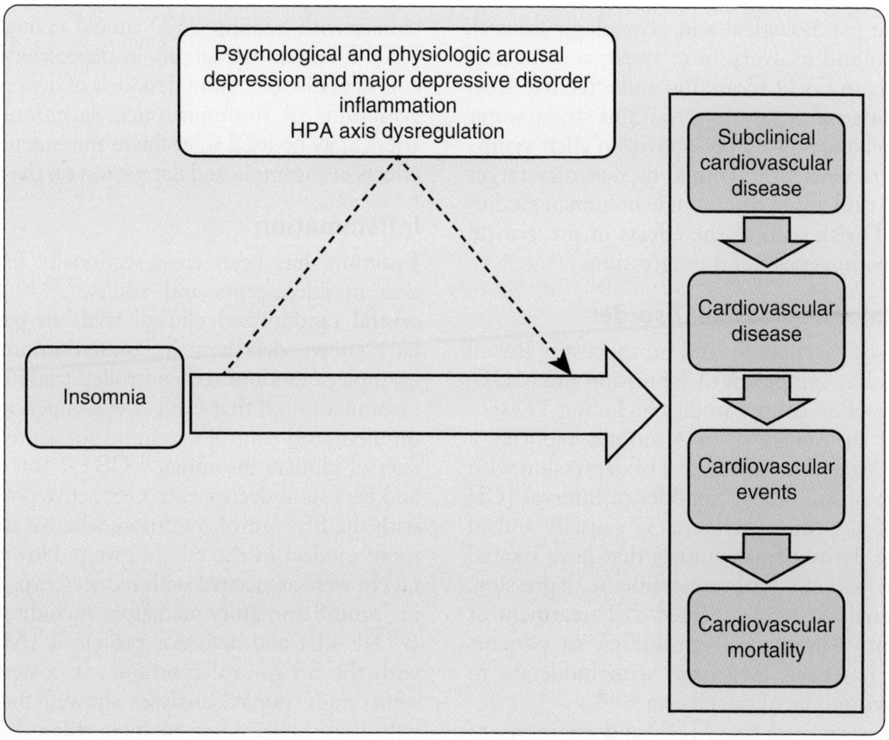

Figure 151.2 Conceptual model of putative psychobiologic mechanisms linking insomnia and cardiovascular morbidity and mortality.

Considerable evidence has demonstrated that psychological stress is associated with increased cardiovascular reactivity and CVD morbidity and mortality. Both observational and laboratory stressors can induce increased heart rate and decreased heart rate variability, increases in blood pressure and arterial stiffness, and increased circulating levels of norepinephrine and cortisol. For example, a 2014 meta-analysis of 186 studies reported that cardiovascular reactivity to acute psychological stress in adult men and women was associated with key indices of cardiovascular risk including increased heart rate and blood pressure, increased circulating levels of catecholamines, shortened pre-ejection fraction, and cardiac parasympathetic nervous system deactivation.[12] Beyond acute laboratory stressors, other meta-analyses have similarly shown that chronic stressors such a low socioeconomic status,[13] job strain,[14,15] acculturation to Western society,[16] and perseverative intrusive thoughts[16,17] are associated with increased cardiovascular reactivity and/or delayed recovery from stress.

With respect to CVD risk, a meta-analysis of six cohort studies with a total of 34,556 participants demonstrated that participants with increased blood pressure responses to acute stress were 21% more likely to develop increased blood pressure over an 11.5-year follow-up period.[16-18] Delayed recovery from acute psychological stress, too, was a significant predictor of adverse CV outcomes, including incident risk for CVD and mortality in a 2015 meta-analysis of 37 studies with 125,386 participants.[19] The similarities between increased reactivity to and delayed recovery from stress and reported psychological and physiologic arousal in insomnia are striking.

Although some studies have prospectively linked stress to symptoms of insomnia,[19-21] experimental evidence in patients with insomnia compared with good sleepers is needed to evaluate the role of psychological stress in increased psychological and physiologic arousal in insomnia. For example, although one study reported significant associations between symptoms of social anxiety and distress and symptoms of insomnia, it did not evaluate cardiovascular reactivity or recovery to their social exclusion task.[22] The success of stress reduction techniques in the general population on ambulatory blood pressure, although modest,[23] suggests that these approaches may be used to reduce psychological and physiologic indices of stress and their downstream consequences to CVD morbidity and mortality in patients with insomnia. Animal models, too, may be used to probe psychological and physiologic arousal, including reactivity to and recovery from stress, as a mechanism linking insomnia to CVD. Common and effective stress paradigms such as maternal separation, restraint stress, water aversion, and cage exchange have been shown to elicit symptoms of insomnia in rodents.[23-25] Animal models may target key questions that are difficult to disentangle in human studies of insomnia and CVD risk such as the effects of sex, critical periods, and disease pathogenesis and progression.

Depression and Major Depressive Disorder

Insomnia has been cross-sectionally and prospectively linked with depression, including symptoms of depression and MDD. A 2016 meta-analysis of 34 cohort studies including 172,077 participants followed an average of 60.4 months reported a large effect for insomnia and increased risk of depression with a pooled relative risk of 2.27 (95% confidence interval [CI] = 1.89–2.71).[26] Evidence that insomnia is causally linked to depression may be derived from studies that have treated insomnia disorder in patients with concomitant depression. Two separate meta-analyses have reported that treatment of insomnia with cognitive-behavioral approaches in patients with both disorders has been associated with moderate to large effect sizes on symptoms of depression.[26-28]

Prospective evidence suggests that MDD and symptoms of depression are significant risk factors for CVD. For example, clinical and subclinical depression have been associated with hypertension, arterial stiffness, decreased endothelial function, cardiac ischemia, hospitalized angina, peripheral vascular disease, cardiovascular events, and CVD-related mortality,[29-31] although prospective studies are lacking. In contrast, strong, consistent evidence suggests that incident depression is a frequent outcome of CVD, with twice as many female patients with coronary artery disease (CAD) developing MDD compared with male patients.[32] Depression in patients with CAD is not without consequence. A meta-analysis of nine studies with 4012 patients with HF reported that mild and major depression, combined, were associated with a pooled hazard ratio (HR) of 2.19 (95% confidence interval [CI], 1.46 to 3.29) for subsequent CVD-related mortality.[33] Beyond CVD-related mortality, incident major depression, but not mild depression, was a significant predictor of subsequent all-cause mortality in patients with HF (HR = 1.98, 95% CI, 1.23 to 3.19).[33] Treatment of depression with medication, including selective serotonin reuptake inhibitors (SSRIs), has been shown to reduce major adverse cardiovascular events, including myocardial infarction (MI), stroke, and all-cause mortality in patients with CAD.[33,34] Moreover, long-term survival was reduced in patients post-MI with refractory depression in the Enhancing Recovery in Coronary Heart Disease (ENRICHD) trial.[35] Taken as a whole, these data suggest that depression is causally associated with CVD, including morbidity and mortality.

Although we are not aware of any causal evidence that depression mediates the impact of insomnia on CVD or vice versa, many of the pathways through which depression influences CVD overlap with putative pathways through which insomnia may affect the pathophysiology and clinical course of CVD.[4,36] As already noted, future studies of cognitive behavioral therapy for insomnia (CBT-I) for reducing depression in individuals with insomnia and MDD should evaluate indices of CVD risk pre- and posttreatment. In addition, studies in individuals with existing CVD should evaluate the extent to which CBT-I–related reductions in depression attenuate the clinical course of disease. Animal models of depression known to induce symptoms of insomnia, such as chronic unpredictable mild stress, may be used to evaluate the independent and interactive effects of insomnia and depression on the pathogenesis of CVD.

Inflammation

Insomnia has been cross-sectionally linked with inflammation in adolescents and adults.[32,37,38] Moreover, data from several randomized clinical trials in patients with insomnia have shown decreased inflammation after treatment.[38,39] For example, a randomized controlled trial in 123 older adults with insomnia found that CBT-I was superior to tai chi and a sleep seminar (SS) control condition for acute and persistent remission of clinical insomnia.[40] CBT-I was associated with acute and persistent decreases in C-reactive protein (CRP) compared with the SS control condition, whereas decreases in CRP were more modest in the tai chi group. However, both CBT-I and tai chi were associated with reduced expression of genes encoding proinflammatory mediators, including nuclear factor-kappa B (NF-κB) and activator protein-1 (AP-1), when compared with the SS control condition. In a separate report from the same study, pooled analyses showed that among participants with high multisystem biologic risk at baseline (e.g., increased glucose, insulin, HbA1c, lipids, CRP, and fibrinogen) for cardiometabolic disease, clinically significant improvements in sleep in the CBT-I and tai chi groups reduced the likelihood of being in the high-risk group at a 1-year follow-up.[40,41] These data suggest that insomnia is causally related to inflammation, at least in mid- to late-life adults.

Data linking insomnia symptoms and disorder to inflammation is important in the context of CVD. A large and consistent body of evidence has shown that systemic inflammation and/or expression of genes mediating inflammation are associated with CVD risk, including vascular remodeling, arterial stiffness, atherosclerosis, atherosclerotic plaque destabilization, intracranial aneurysm, HF, and mortality.[42-44] Moreover, a meta-analysis of studies including 7472 patients with multisystem chronic inflammatory disorders reported elevated CVD risk (HR 1.32, 95% CI, 1.16 to 1.50), with evidence suggesting that increased severity of inflammation was associated with greater CVD risk.[45] The extent to which inflammation mediates the association between insomnia and CVD morbidity and mortality remains untested. Randomized trials focused on inflammation and insomnia may also include markers of subclinical CVD, such as arterial stiffness, that may plausibly change over the longitudinal study period. Animal models of stress and depression, which are associated with symptoms consistent with insomnia, are also appropriate in this context. In addition, animal models are especially well suited for identifying key moderators of the insomnia-inflammation-CVD relationship, including age, sex, and environmental factors that induce insomnia-like symptoms.

HPA Axis Dysregulation

In light of the central role of psychophysiologic arousal in insomnia, it is not surprising that stress hormones, especially cortisol, are elevated in patients with insomnia.[46] Vargas and colleagues hypothesized that ultradian cortisol pulsatility, which is normally decreased during sleep, may be elevated as a result of conditioning in patients with insomnia.[47] A recent study that compared daytime and nighttime cortisol levels in patients with insomnia randomized to CBT-I or an attention control condition provides some support for this novel hypothesis. Improvements in sleep pre- to posttreatment were associated with a statistically significant increase in the day-to-night ratio of urinary-free cortisol. Although intriguing, more research is needed to evaluate the causal impact of insomnia on HPA axis dysregulation.

Dysregulation of the HPA axis has long been implicated in the pathophysiology and clinical course of CVD, including hypertension, acute coronary syndromes, stroke, and cardiovascular mortality.[47-51] Similar to the other psychobiologic mediators reviewed in this chapter, the extent to which HPA axis dysregulation mediates the association between insomnia and CVD morbidity and mortality remains untested. Insomnia trials in patients who have undergone preventive cardiology procedures or who have experienced acute cardiovascular events may be used to evaluate the extent to which HPA axis dysregulation (or stress reactivity, depression, inflammation) is associated with the clinical course of disease. As with the other putative mediators, animal models of insomnia may be used to model the impact of HPA axis dysregulation on CVD risk factors such as blood pressure regulation and arterial stiffness.

Insomnia and Hypertension

Multiple large prospective and cross-sectional studies support an association between insomnia and hypertension, particularly when insomnia is coupled with short sleep duration.[7,52-55] The Penn State Cohort followed 786 individuals from a random community sample who had a complaint of insomnia for at least 1 year and who were free of baseline hypertension for 7½ years. Chronic insomnia was associated with increased risk of hypertension after adjusting for confounders (adjusted odds ratio [OR] 2.24 [95% CI, 1.19 to 4.19], P =.010). The risk was higher among individuals with insomnia who had polysomnographic sleep duration less than 6 hours (OR 3.75 [95% CI, 1.58 to 8.95], P =.012).[7] A prospective study of middle-aged male Japanese workers followed for 4 years showed that persistent complaints of difficulty initiating (n = 192) or difficulty maintaining sleep (n = 286) measured by a questionnaire was associated with increased risk of incident hypertension after adjusting for confounders (OR 1.96 [95% CI, 1.42 to 2.70] and OR 1.88 [95% CI, 1.45 to 2.45], respectively).[52] Finally, a meta-analysis of 11 prospective studies assessed both short sleep duration and insomnia symptoms and risk of incident hypertension.[55] Of the 11 studies, one used actigraphy to measure sleep duration, one used polysomnogram, and the remainder used self-reported habitual sleep duration. Objectively measured sleep duration was more strongly associated with incident hypertension than self-report, but statistically significant results were observed only after omitting one study that incorporated both daytime and nighttime sleep (OR 1.25 [95% CI, 1.09 to 1.44], P =.04). Insomnia symptoms, specifically difficulty maintaining sleep, early morning awakening, and the combination of all insomnia symptoms, were also significantly associated with increased risk of hypertension (OR 1.20 [95% CI, 1.06 to 1.36], OR 1.14 [95% CI, 1.07 to 1.20], and OR 1.05 [95% CI, 1.09 to 1.44], respectively).[55] Another systematic review of insomnia and hypertension identified 64 studies of insomnia and hypertension and found that chronic insomnia (both with and without objective short sleep duration) is strongly associated with elevated blood pressure and hypertension. Additionally, presence of hypertension was predictive of future insomnia among older but not middle-aged adults.[53]

Given the cross-sectional and prospective data suggesting an association between insomnia symptoms and hypertension, mechanistic studies and randomized controlled trials are needed to determine potential proximal and distal mechanisms and therapeutic targets. The importance of chronicity also remains a question, as the effects of insomnia treatment on hypertension risk may differ early and later in the course of disease.

Use of animal models to examine pathophysiologic mechanisms linking insomnia to elevated blood pressure remains a challenge as there is no widely accepted mammal model of chronic insomnia. A small randomized controlled trial has investigated the impact of pharmacologic insomnia treatment on blood pressure among hypertensive patients. Li and colleagues randomized 402 patients with hypertension to either estazolam (n = 202) or placebo (n = 200) and at 28 days found improvement in subjective sleep quality and mood based on validated questionnaires (P <.001) as well as reductions in sedentary systolic and diastolic blood pressure (P <.001) in the treatment arm compared with control.[5] Limitations of this study include lack of home or 24-hour ambulatory blood pressure monitoring and short-term follow-up. Additionally, CBT-I is considered first-line therapy for treatment of insomnia. Ultimately, randomized controlled trials are needed to shed light on the extent to which insomnia is causally linked to elevated blood pressure and risk for hypertension.

Insomnia and Heart Failure

Insomnia is frequently comorbid with HF, with an estimated prevalence of 22% to 73% according to observational studies.[1,57] Patients with HF may suffer from insomnia symptoms for a number of reasons, including use of diuretics that can cause nocturia, sleep-disordered breathing and Hunter-Cheyne-Stokes breathing, mood disorders, paroxysmal nocturnal dyspnea, or orthopnea. Historically, Harrison noted that patients with HF may have difficulty sleeping because of the presence of periodic breathing and that treatment with oxygen subjectively improved these symptoms.[58] Longitudinal data from two studies have reported that insomnia symptoms may precede onset of HF,[59,60] raising the possibility that insomnia contributes to the development of HF. Additional studies have demonstrated that the presence of insomnia among patients with HF may worsen outcomes.[57] This is not surprising because pathophysiologic consequences of insomnia, such as aggravated sympathetic activity, could adversely affect the failing heart. It remains to be determined if treatment of insomnia could improve HF, or treatment of HF and sleep apnea improve insomnia. It is also plausible that effective treatment of insomnia may reduce some of the symptoms of HF and its treatment. For instance, one study of older adults with insomnia, but without HF, found reduced nocturia after brief behavioral therapy for insomnia,[61] but it is not clear if this would benefit patients with HF, in whom nocturia may be iatrogenic or related to sleep apnea.

In the Nord-Trondelag Health study (HUNT), the largest prospective study to date, 54,279 individuals in a Norwegian population without HF were followed for a mean of 11.3 years. Baseline insomnia symptoms were collected by questionnaire. The number of insomnia symptoms was associated with increased risk of incident HF in a dose-dependent manner after adjusting for confounders. Those with three insomnia symptoms had a fivefold increased risk of incident HF (OR 5.25 [95% CI, 2.25 to 12.22]). Of the individual symptoms, difficulty initiating sleep was most strongly associated with incident HF.[57,59] In another prospective cohort of 2322 middle-aged men, self-reported insomnia symptoms were associated with a 1.5-fold increased risk of incident HF after adjusting for confounders (HR 1.52 [95% CI, 1.16 to 1.99]).[60] However, neither of these studies measured other potentially relevant sleep characteristics (e.g., sleep duration) or sleep-related symptoms (e.g., daytime impairment).

Insomnia may also increase risk for cardiac events in patients with existing CVD. A prospective observational study of 1011 consecutive, symptomatic patients with HF in Japan assessed presence (n = 519) or absence of insomnia (n = 492) and followed for cardiac events over a 2+-year period. After adjusting for known CVD risk factors, the presence of insomnia was an independent predictor of cardiac event rates (HR 1.90, P <.001). Follow-up analyses suggested that decreased exercise capacity (P =.002) and activation of the renin-angiotensin-aldosterone system, but not echocardiographic or neuroendocrine factors, increased event risk in patients with insomnia.[57] Increased activation of the renin-angiotensin-aldosterone system correlates with worse outcomes in patients with acute decompensated HF,[62] and lowered exercise tolerance (measured by peak exercise oxygen consumption) is an independent marker of survival[63,64] among patients with HF. Future studies are needed to determine whether insomnia itself is associated with adverse outcomes or whether it is a potential marker of increased risk as the result of other mechanisms among patients with HF.

In addition to mechanistic studies to understand the direction and nature of the relationship between insomnia and HF, randomized studies investigating effect of insomnia treatment on quality of life and other outcomes are also needed. To this end, a small pilot study randomized 23 patients with HF to BBTI or sleep monitoring and found clinically significant improvement in insomnia symptoms, quality of life, and mood compared with the control group, suggesting that insomnia treatment is well tolerated and beneficial to patients with HF.[63] Larger trials are needed to determine whether insomnia treatment could result in reduced hospitalizations or length of stay, HF exacerbations, and other cardiovascular end points in this population.

Insomnia and Coronary Heart Disease

Insomnia is highly prevalent among patients with coronary heart disease (CHD), estimated at approximately 36% (as estimated with the Insomnia Severity Index) among individuals with recent MI[65] and 37% among those hospitalized with acute coronary syndrome.[66,67] In addition to the possibility of independently contributing to pathogenesis of CHD, insomnia may also increase depressive symptoms,[66] which also contribute to worsening CVD risk, as summarized later. Multiple prospective, observational studies have shown associations between insomnia symptoms or insomnia disorder and increased risk of CHD, recurrent ACS, and mortality.[67-72] A meta-analysis of 13 prospective studies including 122,501 men and women showed that self-reported insomnia was associated with a 45% increased risk of cardiovascular morbidity or mortality over a 3- to 20-year follow-up.[73]

Prospective analysis of 52,610 men and women in the HUNT study cohort followed for an average of 11.4 years found that insomnia symptoms, including difficulty initiating sleep, difficulty maintaining sleep, and having nonrestorative sleep, were associated with a 27% to 45% increased risk of incident MI, after adjusting for key CVD risk factors. A dose-response association was demonstrated between the number of insomnia symptoms and incident MI.[70] A large study (n = 22,040) from the Taiwan National Health Insurance Research database reported a 68% increased risk of incident MI (95% CI, 1.31 to 2.16) over a 10-year follow-up period in individuals with an insomnia diagnosis, compared with age- and gender-equated individuals without a diagnosis of insomnia.[74] Importantly, these data suggest that the link between insomnia and CVD is observed in different racial/ethnic groups with different diets and sociocultural characteristics.

Short sleep duration is also associated with CHD mortality. A large prospective observational study from Taiwan followed 392,164 individuals who reported sleep duration at a general health visit and demonstrated a U-shaped relationship between self-reported sleep duration and CHD mortality. Specifically, those sleeping less than 4 hours had a 34% increased risk of CHD death (95% CI, 1.11 to 1.65) compared with those sleeping 6 to 8 hours, although collection of sleep duration by a single question was a major limitation. A meta-analysis pooling data from 24 cohorts of 474,684 men and women also demonstrated a U-shaped association between sleep duration and CVD death, with a 48% increased risk of developing or dying from CHD among those sleeping less than 5 to 6 hours.[75,76] These studies did not address insomnia specifically, but it seems plausible that insomnia coupled with short sleep duration further increases risk of CHD, as evidence suggests with hypertension. To this end, a study of 41,192 adults from the Swedish National March Cohort collected information on habitual sleep duration, difficulty falling asleep, maintaining sleep, early morning awakening, and nonrestorative sleep and followed participants for 13.2 years for MI, stroke, HF, and CVD death. A 42% increased risk of MI (95% CI, 1.15 to 1.76) was observed among those sleeping less than 5 hours. Risk was attenuated after adjustment for

BMI and depressive symptoms, but higher risk was observed among those with short sleep and insomnia symptoms.[75]

A few small studies suggest that insomnia treatment may serve as a novel therapeutic target for reducing CHD morbidity and mortality. A small pilot study randomized 29 patients with insomnia (defined by Insomnia Severity Index >10) to web-based CBT-Ior sleep hygiene recommendations and demonstrated a clinically but not statistically significant reduction in the Insomnia Severity Index and blood pressure in the treatment arm.[77]

FUTURE DIRECTIONS AND POTENTIAL THERAPEUTIC TARGETS

Examining different phenotypes of insomnia—for example, insomnia with short objective sleep duration—may help to better characterize the role of insomnia as a risk marker or pathogenic agent in incident CVD and CVD events. Experimental studies can also evaluate pathophysiologic mechanisms, such as activation of renin-angiotensin-aldosterone and sympathetic nervous systems or alterations in cortisol regulation. Distinguishing the independent and combined effects of insomnia and mood disorders, particularly depression, on incident and prevalent CVD should also be addressed. Finally, the role of insomnia among those with arrythmias is a relatively unstudied area; even cross-sectional and observational data are lacking.

Remaining challenges include consistently applying diagnostic criteria for insomnia and its various phenotypes to provide more uniformity in current research. Variation in the precise definition of insomnia in the current literature may introduce heterogeneity and requires caution when interpreting results. Nonetheless, present data overall suggest that there is a high prevalence of insomnia among patients with a variety of CVD, and in some cases symptoms of insomnia may predate and predict incident CVD. Presence of insomnia may also serve as a marker for worse outcomes among those with comorbid CVD. Additionally, insomnia coupled with short sleep duration may be a distinct phenotype that confers additional CVD risk. Small studies have demonstrated that CBT-I and its variants are well tolerated among individuals with comorbid insomnia and CVD and can improve both insomnia symptoms[63,77] and quality of life.[63] Larger studies addressing whether insomnia treatment may also improve CVD outcomes are needed.

CLINICAL PEARL

Insomnia is a highly prevalent sleep disorder, and a number of prospective studies show an association between insomnia and increased risk of incident hypertension, coronary heart disease, and HF. Increased sympathetic nervous system activity, elevated inflammatory markers, and dysregulation of the hypothalamic-pituitary-adrenal axis are potential mechanisms underlying the relationship between insomnia and CVD. Insomnia symptoms combined with objective short sleep duration may reflect a more severe phenotype that could further increase risk of adverse cardiovascular health.

SUMMARY

Insomnia is the most prevalent sleep disorder worldwide and has a wide public health impact. Both cross-sectional and prospective studies have demonstrated associations with insomnia and hypertension, coronary heart disease, and HF. Potential pathophysiologic mechanisms include elevations in sympathetic nervous system activity, inflammation, and dysregulation of the hypothalamic-pituitary-adrenal axis. Small randomized controlled studies have generally shown safety and efficacy of insomnia treatment in these populations in improving insomnia symptoms and quality of life, but larger randomized controlled trials are necessary to address whether insomnia treatment may also improve CVD outcomes and to better characterize pathophysiologic mechanisms underlying these relationships.

SELECTED READINGS

Bathgate CJ, Edinger JD, Wyatt JK, Krystal AD, et al. Objective but not subjective short sleep duration associated with increased risk for hypertension in individuals with insomnia. *Sleep*. 2016:39 1037–1045.

Bertisch SM, Pollock BD, Mittleman MA, et al. Insomnia with objective short sleep duration and risk of incident cardiovascular disease and all-cause mortality: Sleep Heart Health Study. *Sleep*. 2018;41(6):zsy047. https://doi.org/10.1093/sleep/zsy047.

Cappuccio FP, Cooper D, D'Elia L, Strazzullo P, Miller MA. Sleep duration predicts cardiovascular outcomes: a systematic review and meta-analysis of prospective studies. *Eur Heart J*. 2011;32(12):1484–1492. https://doi.org/10.1093/eurheartj/ehr007.

Fernandez-Mendoza J, He F, Calhoun SL, Vgontzas AN, Liao D, Bixler EO. Objective short sleep duration increases the risk of all-cause mortality associated with possible vascular cognitive impairment. *Sleep Health*. 2020;6(1):71–78. https://doi.org/10.1016/j.sleh.2019.09.003.

Fernandez-Mendoza J, He F, Vgontzas AN, Liao D, Bixler EO. Interplay of objective sleep duration and cardiovascular and cerebrovascular diseases on cause-specific mortality. *J Am Heart Assoc*. 2019;8(20):e013043. https://doi.org/10.1161/JAHA.119.013043.

Fernandez-Mendoza J, Vgontzas AN, Liao D, et al. Insomnia with objective short sleep duration and incident hypertension: the Penn State Cohort. *Hypertension*. 2012;60(4):929–935.

Jarrin DC, et al. Insomnia and hypertension: a systematic review. *Sleep Med Rev*. 2018;41:3–38.

Javaheri S, Redline S. Insomnia and risk of cardiovascular disease. *Chest*. 2017;152:435–444.

Johnson KA, Gordon CJ, Chapman JL, et al. The association of insomnia disorder characterised by objective short sleep duration with hypertension, diabetes and body mass index: A systematic review and meta-analysis [published online ahead of print, 2021 Jan 23]. *Sleep Med Rev*. 2021;59:101456. https://doi.org/10.1016/j.smrv.2021.101456.

Laugsand LE, Strand LB, Platou C, Vatten LJ, Janszky I, et al. Insomnia and the risk of incident heart failure: a population study. *Eur Heart J*. 2014;35:1382–1393.

Laugsand LE, Vatten LJ, Platou C, Janszky I, et al. Insomnia and the risk of acute myocardial infarction: a population study. *Circulation*. 2011;124:2073–2081.

Manolis TA, Manolis AA, Apostolopoulos EJ, Melita H, Manolis AS. Cardiovascular complications of sleep disorders: a better night's sleep for a healthier heart / from bench to bedside. *Curr Vasc Pharmacol*. 2021;19(2):210–232. https://doi.org/10.2174/1570161118666200325102411.

Meisinger C, Heier M, Löwel H, Schneider A, Döring A. Sleep duration and sleep complaints and risk of myocardial infarction in middle-aged men and women from the general population: the MONICA/KORA Augsburg cohort study. *Sleep*. 2007;30(9):1121–1127. https://doi.org/10.1093/sleep/30.9.1121.

A complete reference list can be found online at ExpertConsult.com.

Other Medical Disorders

Chapter 152

Introduction

Christine Won; John Park; Lisa F. Wolfe

Most sleep and other medical professionals agree that sleep quality and sleep disorders impact all facets of health and biology. Initially, it was the impact of sleep disorders on cardiovascular health that prompted attention. More recently, there is growing evidence that poor sleep and sleep disorders can affect other seemingly unrelated organ systems. In these chapters we discuss the role of sleep and sleep disorders, specifically in endocrine, renal, and gastrointestinal systems. Moreover, we discuss the relationship between sleep and pain, pain disorders, and sedation. Finally, this chapter delves into the role of sleep in patients with life-threatening conditions, including cancer. This section aims to unravel the bidirectional relationship between sleep and these other medical conditions.

Hormones affect sleep and vice versa. The intricate pathways that regulate human physiology can often be perturbed by insufficient or irregular sleep. Moreover, disturbed sleep may disrupt the synchrony of biologic rhythms that dictate hormone peaks and troughs. The chapter on endocrine disorders discusses the complex relationship between sleep and thyroid function, adrenal disease, glucose metabolism, sex hormone regulation, and obesity. It also relates the different endocrine disorders to sleep disturbances. The impact of thyroid disease and its association with sleep-disordered breathing is critically evaluated. Finally, the endocrinopathies of obesity (fat being our largest endocrine organ) as they relate to lethargy, sleepiness, and sleep breathing disorders is thoroughly described.

The role of sleep in end-stage renal disease and hemodialysis patients is rarely considered. Chapter 157 describes the often-neglected relationship between sleep-related movement, breathing disorders, and renal disease. In addition, the chapter explains the impact of metabolic derangements related to end-stage renal disease and the effect of hemodialysis on sleep quality, architecture, and rhythm.

The impact of gut flora on sleep has been a recently evolving science. How our gut microbiome can impact sleep and sleepiness is discussed. Sleep disturbance is also discussed in less-thought-of conditions, such as gastroesophageal reflux, liver disease, and bowel syndromes. Seemingly unrelated organ dysfunctions can be closely tied to mechanisms of sleep and sleepiness.

This section also discusses other emerging areas in sleep medicine, that is, sleep in critical illness and cancer. In these morbid conditions, healthy sleep is often not considered a priority. However, as these chapters demonstrate, sleep is integral to the mind and body's healing processes. Therefore healthy sleep may be more than a luxury, but an impactful necessity for recovery and long-term health. Simple, but often overlooked, interventions for improving sleep in the intensive care unit, such as controlling light and noise, may also improve delirium and recovery. Although we are just beginning to understand the relationship between sleep and inflammation or tissue injury and healing, there is potential for sleep interventions to improve outcomes in even the most morbid conditions.

Finally, in this section the relationship between sleep and pain is discussed. Pain is a subjective experience that in part may be shaped by sleep. Bidirectionally, pain can disrupt sleep, leading to subsequent detriments in quality of life and health. The chapter analyzes interesting experiments that involve sleep deprivation and pain tolerance. The connection between the two seems undeniable in chronic pain syndromes, such as fibromyalgia or chronic myalgic encephalitis. There is robust data to suggest that poor sleep may exacerbate these diseases, and achieving good-quality and sufficient sleep may be as essential as good nutrition and exercise in treatment approaches.

Anesthesiologists are becoming increasingly aware of the pain-sleep-sedation connection. The appropriate management of perioperative patients may hinge on the patient's sleep quality or sleep disorders. The intersection of anesthesiology and sleep medicine is even more critical, with evidence suggesting improved perioperative outcomes when managing sleep disorders.

These chapters pertaining to "other medical conditions," are no less important in their impact on sleep medicine. Emerging science supports the role of sleep in the pathophysiology and the treatment of endocrine, renal, and gastrointestinal disorders; in the critically ill; in patients with cancer and pain syndromes; and in the perioperative scenario.

Chapter 153

Sleep and Cancer across the Life Span

Sheila N. Garland; Eric Zhou; Marie-Hélène Savard; Sonia Ancoli-Israel; Josée Savard

Chapter Highlights

- Sleep disturbances and insomnia are common in patients with cancer before treatment, while undergoing cancer treatment, and long into survivorship.
- Actigraphy data show disrupted rest-activity patterns in patients with cancer, especially during chemotherapy.
- Several cancer-specific factors may trigger or worsen sleep disturbances, including adjuvant treatments, medication side effects, nocturnal hot flashes, fatigue, pain, psychological disturbances (e.g., depression, anxiety), and behavioral factors.
- There is accumulating evidence supporting the efficacy of nonpharmacologic interventions (cognitive behavioral therapy in particular), mindfulness-based therapies, and physical activity to treat cancer-related sleep disturbances.
- Increasing survival rates for children diagnosed with cancer have resulted in a growing population of survivors who require attention for their sleep; the related intervention must be age appropriate.
- Cancer caregivers are often overlooked in the context of clinical care but suffer from poor sleep at rates comparable to the patients for whom they provide care.
- Patients with advanced cancer have complex sleep presentations, characterized by both insomnia and hypersomnia and complicated by medication or treatment-related side effects.
- Increased clinical and research attention is needed to develop and test prevention strategies to mitigate the potential impact of insomnia on cancer recovery and long-term survivorship.

INTRODUCTION

Patients with cancer complain of sleep disturbance before treatment; during chemotherapy, radiation therapy, or maintenance therapies (e.g., hormonal therapy); and after the completion of treatment,[1,2] which contributes to decreased long-term quality of life.[3,4] This chapter reviews the evidence on cancer-related sleep disruption and its treatment across the life span, with specific sections devoted to sleep disruption in children and adolescent patients with cancer, adult survivors of childhood cancer, patients with advanced cancer, and cancer caregivers. Considering that most people diagnosed with cancer will spend more time in survivorship recovering from the consequences of the disease than being treated for it, it is important to identify and treat problems with sleep to promote long-term overall health.

SLEEP DISTURBANCE IN ADULTS WITH CANCER

The majority of research in cancer has focused on the identification and treatment of insomnia symptoms and disorder with less attention on other aspects of sleep health.[6] The literature is also hampered by a lack of definitional clarity, which negatively affects our overall understanding of sleep in cancer. For the purposes of this chapter, we specify the aspect of sleep being discussed (e.g., insomnia symptoms or disorder) and use the terms *sleep disturbance* or *sleep difficulties* to refer to general alterations when further specificity is not possible.

Prevalence of Cancer-Related Sleep Disturbance and Insomnia

The earliest studies of cancer-related sleep disturbance and insomnia were cross-sectional and conducted mainly in the posttreatment phase. This research identified that between 30% and 50% of patients with cancer report sleep difficulties and that nearly 20% met the diagnostic criteria for an insomnia disorder[7-14] but were limited by the use of small, convenience samples, and single-item sleep measures. Moreover, sleep was often assessed several months and even years after the completion of treatment. Because of their cross-sectional nature, these studies also did not provide information on the natural course of sleep impairments (incidence, remission, persistence) throughout the cancer care trajectory and beyond.

More recently, two large-scale longitudinal studies assessed the evolution of sleep impairments over time in heterogeneous cancer samples. Close to 1000 patients awaiting surgery were assessed at baseline during the perioperative phase and 2, 6, 10, 14, and 18 months later.[15,16] At baseline, 59% had insomnia symptoms, including 28% with an insomnia disorder.[17] Although these rates steadily decreased over time, 36% of the sample still suffered from insomnia symptoms, whereas

21% met the criteria for insomnia disorder 18 months later. Moreover, the general persistence rate (i.e., insomnia present at two consecutive time points on 2- to 4-month intervals) was 51%, whereas 35% of patients had insomnia persisting for at least three consecutive time points. Insomnia disorder was a particularly enduring condition, with persistence rates varying from 69% to 80%.

Another large-scale prospective study assessed the presence of insomnia in 823 patients scheduled to receive at least four cycles of chemotherapy for various types of cancer of all stages.[18] Sleep difficulties were assessed on day 7 of cycle 1 and cycle 2 of chemotherapy. At cycle 1, 80% of patients exhibited insomnia symptoms, including the 43% meeting the criteria for an insomnia disorder, rates that decreased to 68% and 35%, respectively, at cycle 2. Among good sleepers at cycle 1, 35% developed insomnia symptoms at cycle 2, of whom 10% developed an insomnia disorder.

The prevalence of sleep disturbances appear to vary as a function of cancer site, being more frequent in patients with breast and ovarian cancer, and less frequent in patients with prostate cancer.[19-21] Analyses in patients with urinary and gastrointestinal cancer show no difference between men and women, which suggests that the higher rates found in women with breast and gynecologic cancer are not solely attributable to sex.[16] A meta-analysis of 29 studies, with a total sample of 2315 patients diagnosed with head and neck cancer, reported an insomnia prevalence rate of 29% before treatment, 45% during treatment, and 40% after treatment.[22-25] Using a DSM-5-based diagnosis of insomnia disorder, the prevalence of insomnia before and after treatment was 21% and 23%, respectively.[5]

Cancer-Related Sleep Disturbance and Insomnia in Long-Term Cancer Survivors

Sleep disturbance and insomnia appear to be among the longest-lasting symptoms reported by cancer survivors. As with the studies mentioned previously that documented high rates of sleep disturbance during and in the posttreatment period for breast cancer survivors, several studies provide evidence that this disturbance is long lasting.[26] Further, although other symptoms tend to resolve, once established, sleep disturbance persists. In a 5-year follow-up study of 190 women diagnosed with breast cancer compared with healthy controls, quality-of-life ratings improved to be equal to or better than peers, whereas sleep problems and cognitive function remained significantly impaired.[27] High rates of long-term sleep disturbance have also been documented with other cancer types. In a sample of 77 patients with head and neck cancer who had survived at least 3 years after surgery, 83% of patients reported poor sleep.[28] A case-control study at 5 years postdiagnosis reported that 56.6% of lung cancer survivors had poor sleep as compared with only 29.5% of noncancer controls.[29] Further, 49% of the participants who did not have sleep difficulties before their lung cancer diagnosis would go on to develop these problems over the average 8-year survival time. Given that sleep disturbance is associated with impaired neurocognitive function,[30] as well as an increased risk of developing, and worsened recovery from, many mental health disorders,[31] the persistence of sleep disturbance in cancer survivors has significant implications for overall recovery.

Objective Characterization of Sleep Disturbance in Individuals with Cancer

Although objective measures are not recommended for the diagnosis of insomnia,[32] they can be used to characterize and/or quantify the type of disturbance that cancer survivors experience. Actigraphy, a noninvasive, continuous, ambulatory measure of circadian rest-activity rhythms, has been used to objectively characterize the sleep and rhythms of patients with cancer.[33-35] Studies comparing patients with cancer to healthy controls have consistently shown less contrast between daytime and nighttime activity in patients with cancer, a pattern indicative of circadian disruption.[36-42] Among patients with advanced cancer, objective data from actigraphy have shown high sleep fragmentation despite normal sleep duration.[43]

A few studies have used polysomnography (PSG) to assess sleep disturbances in patients with cancer.[44] The earliest study using PSG compared the sleep of patients with breast or lung cancer without sleep complaints, patients with insomnia, and healthy sleeping volunteers. It showed that patients with insomnia had the shortest total sleep time, but patients with lung cancer had the longest sleep-onset latency, lowest sleep efficiency, and greatest wake time during the night.[45] In a sample of 56 women treated with chemotherapy, radiotherapy, and hormone therapy for early-stage breast cancer, sleep-onset latency, rapid eye movement sleep latency, wake after sleep onset, sleep efficiency, and distribution of sleep stages were similar to those found in healthy women of the same age.[46] Similarly, when sleep was assessed using PSG in 26 breast cancer survivors an average of 4½ years posttreatment, half of whom were poor sleepers, their average sleep efficiency was 86%, with a sleep-onset latency of 13 minutes, and wake after sleep onset of 48 minutes.[47] There were no significant differences in PSG-measured sleep between good and poor sleepers in this study; however, women who were poor sleepers had significantly more periodic leg movements (122 versus 24 per hour). In contrast, when PSG was used to assess sleep in 114 patients with advanced cancer, it showed reduced sleep quantity and quality, with an average sleep efficiency of 77% and virtually no slow wave sleep compared with normative data.[48] However, the objective characterization of sleep in patients with cancer is challenging, and studies have failed to recruit sufficient samples because of study refusal, poor compliance, or ongoing symptoms.[48,49]

Prevalence of Sleep Disorders Other than Insomnia in Patients with Cancer

The available literature, although limited and mainly conducted in patients with head and neck, lung, brain, and breast cancer, suggests the presence of sleep disorders other than insomnia in patients with cancer. Prevalence rates of obstructive sleep apnea (OSA), ranging from 12% to 92%, were found in small-scale studies (17 to 33 patients) conducted among patients with head and neck cancer.[50,51] There is also some evidence suggesting that OSA may be associated with treatments such as surgery and radiotherapy among these patients,[52] but prospective studies are warranted to investigate to what extent OSA is caused or exacerbated by the cancer itself or by cancer treatment. In a meta-analysis of 29 studies with a total sample of 2315 patients diagnosed with head and neck cancer, the prevalence of OSA was 71% when an apnea-hypopnea index (AHI) cut-off score of 5 was used, 47% with an AHI cut-off score of 15, and 37% when OSA was defined as snoring. With respect to treatment modality, the pooled prevalence rate was 67% among patients who underwent surgery in addition to chemoradiotherapy, 58% among patients who underwent surgery alone, and 50% among patients who underwent chemoradiotherapy only. This same meta-analysis also examined the prevalence of hypersomnia, defined as excessive daytime sleepiness or drowsiness. The prevalence rate of hypersomnolence during curative and palliative treatment was 35% and 86%, respectively; however, this was measured in only two studies. When defined with the Epworth Sleepiness Scale[53] cut-off of 10, the pooled prevalence of sleepiness was 39%.

Sleep-disordered breathing also appears to be frequent in patients with lung cancer. The Sleep Apnea in Lung Cancer Screening (SAILS) study assessed a cross-sectional sample of 66 patients with lung cancer using home sleep apnea testing.[54] The majority (80%) had OSA (AHI ≥ 5 events/hour), and 50% had moderate to severe OSA (AHI ≥ 15 events/hour). Daytime sleepiness and significant nocturnal hypoxemia were also significant concerns. In patients with brain tumors, tumor removal resulted in a significant decrease in the AHI.[44] Rates of OSA have also been found to be high in women with breast cancer who had completed chemotherapy, with almost half of the patients (48%) having at least five respiratory events per hour of sleep.[55] In the same study, the prevalence of periodic limb movements (PLM) defined as a PLM index exceeding 5 was 36%.[56] Both of these sleep disorders were substantially more frequent than in age-comparable women without cancer. These high prevalence rates of PLM and OSA may help explain some of the sleep disturbance found in this population. However, others reported no difference in the amount of sleep-disordered breathing among patients with cancer, patients with insomnia, and healthy volunteers.[45] Clearly, larger studies are needed to better estimate the prevalence of OSA and PLM in various types of cancer.

PATHOGENESIS OF CANCER-RELATED SLEEP DISRUPTION

Specific Contributors to Sleep Disruption and Insomnia

Cancer Treatments

Cancer treatment typically involves a combination of surgery, chemotherapy, radiation therapy, targeted therapies, immunotherapy, and/or hormone therapy, all of which have the potential to provoke or to intensify sleep disturbances because of their emotional impact, their direct physiologic effects, or their side effects.[57] Chemotherapy is thought to be particularly disruptive to sleep.[3,58] Patients report more subjective sleep disturbance (lower sleep quality and duration, total sleep time) during the active phases of chemotherapy compared with rest periods.[59] Longitudinal studies using subjective measures have also shown gradual increases in sleep impairment with this treatment[60] as well as persistence of elevated insomnia rates across chemotherapy cycles.[18] Conversely, another study found no change in sleep with the introduction of chemotherapy for breast cancer as measured prospectively with a sleep diary, but most participants already had poor sleep before the initiation of this treatment.[61] Of note, studies that included PSG data have not observed a significant deterioration of sleep parameters with the introduction of chemotherapy.[62,63]

Chemotherapy appears to be particularly disruptive for rest-activity circadian rhythms,[3,64,65] although radiation therapy was also found to have a detrimental effect.[65,66] In a study of 85 women with breast cancer, 72-hour actigraphy showed that the first administration of chemotherapy was associated with short-term disruption of sleep-wake rhythm, whereas repeated administration resulted in progressively worse and more enduring impairments.[64] In patients with early-stage breast cancer, there are some data suggestive of improvement of the rest-activity patterns back to precancer treatment levels once the active phase of cancer treatment is over, but the disturbance remains worse than in matched controls.[36] A recent study, conducted among 49 patients with advanced cancer assessed with actigraphy, found 45% of patients showing a sustained deterioration of their rest-activity pattern after chemotherapy administration, with both increased nighttime activity level and decreased diurnal activity level.[67] Similarly, repeated administration of chemotherapy in 180 patients with breast cancer was associated with progressive impairment in nocturnal melatonin production.[69] Some recovery was observed for actigraphy assessed sleep duration, time spent awake during the night, and sleep efficiency; however, these values were still not equivalent to baseline.[69]

Data from a prospective analysis of sleep-wake cycles assessed via actigraphy in patients undergoing allogeneic hematopoietic cell transplant and quality of life at 6 months showed robust associations between longer durations of activity during the day and earlier declines of activity in the evening with better overall recovery of quality of life.[68]

Sociodemographic Factors

Older age has been found to be associated with a decreased risk for cancer-related insomnia[2,19,70]; however, what constitutes "younger" or "older" age is not used consistently. In self-reported survey data from 861 breast cancer survivors, body mass index was not associated with daytime sleepiness or short sleep duration.[71] Additionally, being female or belonging to a racial or ethnic minority group (specifically Black or non-Hispanic White) is associated with an increased likelihood of sleep disturbance.[21]

Other Physical Symptoms and Comorbidities

Many cancer-related somatic symptoms may affect sleep negatively. Dyspnea, urinary symptoms (e.g., because of radiation therapy in the urogenital area), gastrointestinal symptoms (e.g., chemotherapy-induced nausea), and pain (e.g., associated with use of aromatase inhibitors) in both men and women are all very likely to impair sleep.[65,72] In addition, medications that are commonly administered with chemotherapy, such as opioids, antiemetic medications, and corticosteroids, are also known to disrupt sleep.[73-75] The occurrence or exacerbation of menopausal symptoms appears to be another important contributor to cancer-related sleep disturbances.[76] Indeed, the estrogen deficiency induced by chemotherapy and hormone therapy, the abrupt cessation of hormone replacement therapy at cancer diagnosis, or an ovary removal may trigger or exacerbate preexisting hot flashes. Change in self-reported vasomotor symptoms is significantly associated with parallel changes in insomnia complaints.[77] Greater PSG-measured sleep disturbances are also associated with nocturnal hot flashes in women with breast cancer.[78,46]

Fatigue is one of the most frequent and disturbing complaints of patients with cancer,[79,80] with 70% to 100% of patients during active treatment and approximately 30% after the treatment phase reporting feeling weak and tired.[81] Cancer-related fatigue has been defined as a "persistent, subjective sense of tiredness related to cancer and cancer treatment that interferes with usual functioning."[82] The relationship between sleep disruption and fatigue appears to be bidirectional. Patients typically report fatigue as the main consequence of their poor sleep.[85,86] Accordingly, there is evidence that sleep disturbance is a significant predictor of fatigue,[87-90] but the reverse may also hold true. A longitudinal study showed that fatigue significantly predicted a subsequent increase in insomnia symptoms during the cancer care trajectory, whereas insomnia was not found to predict subsequent fatigue.[91] The impact of fatigue on sleep could be due to behavioral changes occurring with fatigue. Indeed, fatigued individuals tend to nap more during the day and extend their sleep periods during the night, which may in the long run impair their circadian rhythm and make their nighttime sleep less consolidated and lighter.[92,93] This may be particularly the case during cancer treatments, when patients suffer from higher levels of fatigue and are very likely and often encouraged to rest to recuperate.[94,95]

Pain has often been thought to be the cause of sleep disruption, not only in patients with cancer but also in patients with a multitude of other medical conditions.[96] In a sample of 2862 cancer outpatients, the risk of reporting insomnia symptoms was 2.7 times higher for those having pain,[97] which is consistent with other empirical evidence showing that cancer-related pain significantly predicts the incidence or exacerbation of sleep difficulties.[98,99] Sleep disturbance has also been demonstrated to mediate the relationships between posttraumatic stress disorder symptoms and pain intensity and pain-related interference[100] in cancer survivors. There are also data showing increased objectively assessed sleep disturbances and rest-activity rhythm impairments measured with actigraphy among men, but not women, with pain.[101] One hypothesis explaining the association between pain and insomnia comorbid with cancer is that pain may be the initial cause of the frequent awakenings, but psychological distress prevents the patient from falling back to sleep.[102] A second hypothesis explains that whereas sleep leads to recovery and repair of tissue and may offer a temporary cessation of the awareness of pain, poor sleep leads to difficulty in managing pain.[103] In this way, a cycle of pain and poor sleep may become self-perpetuating positive feedback loop.

Other Psychological Symptoms or Disorders

Insomnia rates in patients with cancer can be as high as rates in depressed patients; therefore clinicians should not overlook the possibility that poor sleep in patients with cancer may indicate some psychological distress. Patients with cancer and high levels of psychological distress were 4.5 times more likely to report sleep difficulties than those with low levels.[97] Further, in 213 patients undergoing chemotherapy, insomnia was only correlated with anxiety/depression scores and not with individual participant characteristics or cancer- or treatment-related factors.[104] In one sample of patients with newly diagnosed breast cancer, insomnia was the most frequent symptom, reported by 88% of patients, and was correlated with high levels of psychological distress and anxiety.[105] However, contrary to the belief that disturbed sleep before treatment is attributable to the increased stress and anxiety resulting from a recent diagnosis of a potentially life-threatening illness, insomnia and fatigue were rated high even in those patients who rated themselves low on anxiety. Similarly, another study revealed that 46% of prostate cancer survivors with an insomnia disorder did not have clinical levels of anxiety or depressive symptoms.[106] Thus there is evidence that, although insomnia and psychological distress are interrelated, there are still a significant proportion of patients who have isolated insomnia.

CLINICAL MANAGEMENT OF SLEEP DISTURBANCES

Assessment of Sleep Disturbance in Patients with Cancer

A systematic review and meta-analysis outlined the best practices for the assessment and management of insomnia in adults with cancer.[81,107] It is recommended that all patients with cancer be screened for sleep disturbances at initial diagnosis, start of treatment, regular intervals during treatment, end of treatment, posttreatment survivorship, upon recurrence or progression, at end of life, or during times of personal transition (e.g., family crisis). The assessment process typically begins with a brief screening instrument[108] or questions such as, "Are you having problems falling asleep or staying asleep? Are you experiencing excessive sleepiness? Have you been told that you snore frequently or stop breathing during sleep?" Individuals who screen positive are then recommended to complete a more focused assessment consisting of a semistructured clinical interview and validated measures.

Clinical Interview

A semistructured clinical interview should cover the following content areas:

1. **Characterization of the sleep complaint:** The event (or events) that they believe to have precipitated their sleep problems, the nature of the difficulty (i.e., difficulty falling asleep, staying asleep, or waking up too early), the frequency and duration of the problem, the success, or lack thereof, of any previous attempts at treatment; ensure that adequate opportunity is available for sleep
2. **Typical sleep-wake pattern:** A characterization of a typical sleep-wake schedule consisting of the following: typical time to bed at night and wake in the morning; time they actually fall asleep and wake up; number of awakenings and how long these awakenings last; activities they engage in when they are awake at night (e.g., checking social media, lying in bed, and trying harder to sleep); napping frequency, timing, and duration; change in routine on weekends
3. **Individual and family history:** Useful to identify factors that may predispose an individual to experience insomnia or other sleep disorders; patients often report that themselves or one or more of their immediate family members have past or present experience with insomnia[109] or other sleep disorders
4. **Behavioral, cognitive, and environmental presleep conditions:** An examination of what activities the individual engages in before bed, such as watching television, working on the computer, or keeping busy with other tasks or going to bed earlier and trying harder to "force" sleep, and how the patient feels emotionally before bed

5. **Perceived impact of sleep disturbances, next day function, and compensatory behaviors:** Patients may report difficulty concentrating or paying attention, sleepiness and/or fatigue, affective disturbances, or a worsening of comorbid physical or psychiatric conditions as consequences of their sleep problems. They may also engage in, or discontinue, activities to try and cope with their daytime dysfunction. This may include daytime napping, stimulant use (e.g., caffeine), and canceling physical activity or social engagements
6. **Presence of other sleep disorders:** A number of other sleep disorders may account for (or exacerbate) the presenting insomnia symptoms or represent an additional comorbidity to be considered. To assess for these disorders, especially for clinicians less familiar with the signs and symptoms of the various intrinsic sleep disorders, it is recommended that a screening questionnaire be used. Although many such instruments exist,[110] only two are considered brief,[111,112] and only one is both brief and comprehensive.[112] If the patient presents with symptoms suggestive of one or more of these disorders, a sleep study (PSG) may be warranted. If a patient has restless legs syndrome, the clinician should make sure that the patient does not have iron deficiency, which commonly occurs in gastrointestinal carcinomas. If the patient has developed movement disorders secondary to a chemotherapeutic agent, a trial of a dopaminergic agent should be initiated. If a patient has developed OSA, for example, secondary to enlarged lymph nodes in the pharynx, as may occur with lymphoma or with nasopharyngeal carcinoma, continuous positive airway pressure treatment as well as specific treatment directed at these areas should be initiated.
7. **Medical and psychiatric history:** A number of medical and psychiatric conditions, along with their treatments, can contribute to and complicate sleep disturbances.[113] Hypoxemia caused by spread of cancer to the lung or the development of lung fibrosis in response to chemotherapy or radiation therapy may require treatment, as patients with hypoxemia are known to have disturbed sleep. If the patient has clinical depression along with insomnia, concurrent therapy for the mood disorder as well as for insomnia should be initiated. If the cancer is causing pain that is disturbing sleep, the pain must be treated concurrently with the insomnia. A thorough review of medications (both prescribed and over the counter) is necessary to identify any potential substances that may be contributing to their dysfunction. Attention should be paid to whether these are taken in the morning or evening depending on whether they impair or promote sleep. Anxiolytic medications are often used as a hypnotic/sedative to reduce presleep arousal, but this is not recommended as a long-term solution for reasons of tolerance, dependence, and the potential for other negative outcomes.[114,115]

Measurement Instruments

A standard sleep diary has been developed and is recommended for use[116]; however, should alternate versions be used, they should include, at minimum, information on time to bed and wake time (which provide information on time spent in bed), sleep latency, frequency of nightly awakenings, wake time after sleep onset, total sleep time, early morning awakenings, nap frequency and duration, fatigue ratings, stimulant consumption (e.g., caffeine intake), and medication usage. It is recommended that patients complete 1 to 2 weeks of sleep diaries to allow for a more representative evaluation of baseline sleep patterns and the Insomnia Severity Index (ISI).[117] In the absence of another possible comorbid sleep disorder, the diagnosis of insomnia does not require the use of laboratory-based assessments (i.e., PSG) or ambulatory assessment (i.e., actigraphy).

TREATMENT OF CANCER-RELATED SLEEP DISTURBANCES

The treatment of cancer-related sleep disturbances should employ a combined approach that targets any contributing factors (e.g., hot flashes, pain, fatigue, nocturia) and the factors that are believed to maintain the sleep difficulties over time (i.e., maladaptive sleep behaviors, dysfunctional beliefs about sleep).[118] Although sleep disturbances may have been initially triggered by factors such as hot flashes or pain, it is likely not sufficient to treat only those factors to address the sleep difficulty because insomnia becomes rapidly self-reinforced. It is recommended that cognitive behavioral interventions be used as first-line treatments before pharmacologic treatment. However, patients may require short-term use of pharmacologic interventions until cognitive behavioral therapy takes effect or is available.[119] A person-centered and stepped-care approach is recommended for the nonpharmacologic management of sleep disturbance in patients with cancer.[81]

Evidence-Based Treatments for Cancer-Related Sleep Disturbances

Pharmacotherapy

Hypnotic medications, particularly benzodiazepines, are by far the most commonly prescribed treatment for sleep disturbances in patients with cancer. A study conducted among 1984 cancer survivors found that 41% had received a prescription for a sleeping medication since their cancer diagnosis and that 23% were currently using one.[120] The median duration of use was 34 months, which considerably exceeds the recommendations from the 2005 National Institutes of Health state-of-the-science conference on insomnia of using hypnotic medications for no longer than 4 to 6 weeks.[121] A recent position statement by the American Academy of Sleep Medicine (AASM) reviewed the available literature on prescription and over-the-counter insomnia treatments (behavioral approaches were not evaluated).[122] Although not specific to cancer, this statement evaluated a wide range of potential pharmacologic insomnia treatment options. According to this guideline:

- No pharmacologic agent was rated as being supported by more than "weak" evidence.
- No pharmacologic agent was recommended as superior to any other approach.
- No over-the-counter approaches were recommended for insomnia treatment.

Short-term (less than 2 weeks) or occasional (less than 3 nights per week) utilization of pharmacotherapy may be indicated in times of stress (e.g., before surgery) in patients who are very ill or unable to complete behavioral interventions. Guidelines agree that the choice of a medication should be informed by patient-specific factors, including age, proposed length of treatment, primary sleep complaint, history of drug or alcohol abuse, side effect profiles of the medications, tolerability of treatment, including the potential for interaction with other current medications, response to prior treatment, and patient preference.[118,119] Patients should be warned of any potential harm or adverse effects; however, these may not be completely known as few trials have evaluated the efficacy and potential to counteract with cancer treatment. The National Comprehensive Cancer Network has reviewed the agents available to aid with sleep initiation, sleep maintenance, or total sleep time.[119]

Cognitive Behavioral Therapy

In 2021, the American Academy of Sleep Medicine released a clinical practice guideline recommending cognitive behavioral therapy for insomnia (CBT-I).[123] This supports that all adult patients should receive cognitive behavioral therapy for insomnia (CBT-I) as the initial treatment for chronic insomnia disorder. It was further recommended that clinicians should use a shared decision-making approach, including a discussion of the benefits, harms, and costs of short-term use of medications, to decide whether to add pharmacologic therapy in adults with chronic insomnia disorder in whom CBT-I alone was unsuccessful.[123a] The National Institutes of Health state-of-the-science conference on insomnia also concluded that CBT-I is the most effective treatment for insomnia.[121]

Guidelines for the treatment of sleep disturbances and insomnia in cancer have also concluded that CBT-I should be the first-line treatment.[81,107,124] Meta-analytic findings compiled from 8 studies (published before 2015) of cancer survivors ($n = 752$) were consistent in demonstrating that CBT-I (combining stimulus control, sleep restriction, cognitive restructuring, sleep hygiene, and sometimes relaxation) was associated with clinically and statistically significant improvements in multiple insomnia outcomes, including sleep efficiency, sleep-onset latency, wake after sleep onset, and insomnia symptom severity, as measured by the ISI, as compared with usual care, waitlist control, or active comparator conditions.[125] Further, observed effects were found to persist at 6-month follow-up, which demonstrates that CBT-I is durable.

Since that meta-analysis, a number of other randomized controlled trials have been published that further support the efficacy of CBT-I in cancer. In a trial with a heterogeneous group of 99 cancer survivors, CBT-I had benefits that were not further augmented by the addition of a stimulant medication.[126,127] Further, in addition to improvements in insomnia outcomes, CBT-I improves depression[128] and overall quality of life in cancer survivors.[129] There is also some evidence that cancer-related fatigue may be improved after CBT for insomnia[130-133]; however, nonsignificant results have also been found in other studies.[134,135] This may be due, in part, to the lack of sensitivity to change of some fatigue measures, but it still indicates that the relationship between sleep and fatigue is a complex one.

Because a lack of access to CBT-I has limited its dissemination,[136] efficacy of CBT-I delivered via alternative delivery models has been examined. Internet delivery of CBT-I versus a waitlist control[137] showed clinically and statistically significant reductions in insomnia severity, sleep-onset latency, number of awakenings, and overall fatigue (all with medium to large effect sizes) in breast cancer survivors. Self-led and video formats of CBT-I have also demonstrated efficacy; however, the effects of face-to-face sessions appear to be larger than less interactive mediums.[132,138-140] Whether internet CBT-I is inferior to in-person CBT-I has not yet been tested in cancer survivors. A recent RCT found that a stepped care CBT-I, beginning with an internet-based intervention for patients with less severe symptoms, was not statistically inferior to a standard 6-session face-to-face CBT-I. This supports the view that stepped care models of CBT-I are valuable alternatives to make this treatment more readily available.[140a]

Mindfulness-Based Therapies

Mindfulness-based therapies (MBTs) are increasingly being investigated for their potential to improve sleep disturbances and insomnia in cancer survivors. MBTs typically come in the form of standardized programs such as Mindfulness-Based Stress Reduction, Mindfulness-Based Cancer Recovery, or Mindfulness-Based Cognitive Therapy.[141-143] These programs share a focus on the cultivation of mindfulness, typically defined as an open, nonreactive, and nonjudgmental awareness of the present moment. A variety of meditation practices (e.g., body scan, sitting, walking) are introduced to allow the participant to practice mindful awareness with a gradual increase in time spent in meditation over the course of the program.

No meta-analysis of the efficacy of MBTs for insomnia in cancer populations has been conducted, although a narrative review of six randomized controlled trials (RCTs) of MBTs in survivors of cancer noted that the majority of studies failed to select persons with sleep disturbance as an enrollment criterion, with the majority using a waitlist or treatment as usual control.[144] As such, effects observed on sleep may be due to nonspecific effects or a consequence of improvement in comorbidities such as depression, anxiety, and distress. A systematic review concluded that MBTs are likely to be effective, but that evidence was limited by small sample sizes, lack of attention control groups, unknown adherence, and a wide range of interventions across studies.[124] One of most rigorous studies to date, which used a noninferiority research design, was conducted among 111 patients with various types of cancer and compared an eight-session CBT with a mindfulness-based cancer recovery intervention (MBCR, an adaptation of Mindfulness-Based Stress Reduction).[145] Short-term outcomes of MBCR on insomnia severity were inferior to those of the CBT-I condition but became noninferior at the 3-month follow-up, suggesting that CBT-I is associated with faster improvements. Further evaluation of efficacy of MBTs for insomnia in cancer is needed, taking into account insomnia selection criteria, active comparator conditions, and efforts to target sleep with greater precision independent of effects on psychological stress or mood.

Physical Activity

An increasing number of studies have specifically evaluated the effect of physical activity on sleep quality and quantity among patients with cancer.[146-152] A systematic review of 15 controlled and uncontrolled studies of exercise interventions (including yoga) in 1691 women with breast cancer reported that exercise interventions generally improved sleep outcomes.[153] In contrast, a meta-analysis including 21 studies (experimental and quasi-experimental) of exercise interventions (excluding yoga) to improve sleep in 1595 people diagnosed with cancer did not suggest a significant effect of exercise interventions on subjective or objective sleep.[154] In an aggregated meta-analysis of individual patient data from 17 RCTs with a total sample of 2173 patients, exercise was associated with a small, but significant, decrease in sleep disturbances but not sleep quality.[155] A major criticism of these reviews was that most of the trials did not select patients on the basis of minimal insomnia severity or sleep disturbance at baseline. Thus it is not clear if physical activity is potent enough to treat a clinically significant sleep disorder. In addition, questions regarding the optimal type, frequency, and dosage of exercise needed to improve sleep have yet to be answered. Objective measures, such as actigraphy movement counts and inflammatory biomarkers, will aid in understanding the underlying biologic mechanisms of these interventions and provide a more robust explanation of their relationship to sleep outcomes.

SLEEP AND CANCER IN SPECIAL POPULATIONS

Children and Adolescents

Childhood cancers are rare, with fewer than 16,000 new cases diagnosed annually in the United States.[156] As a result, the literature studying sleep among pediatric patients with cancer is hampered by limited sample sizes, coupled with the diversity of cancers (and their associated treatments) in this population. Further complicating matters is the potential for discrepancies between children's actual sleep and their parents' reporting of their sleep.[157] Clinicians working with this population are advised to assess sleep during a period that includes both weekdays (typically school days) as well as weekends, given the potential for variability in their sleep.[158]

Up to 25% of healthy children experience problems with their sleep.[159] Therefore, when children are diagnosed and subsequently treated for their cancer, it may be exacerbating a preexisting problem that the family is already dealing with. There are known direct effects of a child's cancer treatment that impair their sleep and circadian activity rhythms, which can include the use of corticosteroids,[160,161] a core component of treatment for the most common childhood cancer (e.g., acute lymphoblastic leukemia). Further, treatments for brain cancers may cause excessive daytime sleepiness, despite sufficient sleep.[162] There are also indirect effects of a child's cancer treatment that influence sleep. For example, inpatient hospitalizations require that the child sleep in an unfamiliar environment with elevated noise and light levels and medical staff room interruptions, which results in decreased total sleep duration and increased nighttime awakenings.[163] One final factor that requires attention is the role that parent behaviors have with respect to a child's sleep in the context of cancer. Disrupted sleep in the treatment phase does not have to result in long-term sleep disturbances years after treatment has ended. However, this can be the case when parents of children with cancer are more accommodating with respect to maladaptive sleep-related behaviors (e.g., screen use in bed), possibly because of the difficulty they experience limit setting in the context of a child with a life-threatening illness.[164,165]

Considerable data suggest that behavioral interventions for pediatric insomnia are effective.[166] However, few of these studies have examined children with special needs, including pediatric cancer. Limited data suggest that CBT-I can be adapted for adolescents who have survived cancer, with attention paid toward both developmental (e.g., delayed sleep phase) and cancer-related (e.g., fatigue) issues that may impair their sleep.[167]

There has been scant research examining the prevalence of sleep disorders other than insomnia in children with cancer. There was one study reporting that 19% of pediatric cancer survivors were at risk for sleep-disordered breathing[168] compared with less than 5% in healthy children.[169] This may be due to the fact that children who have prolonged exposure to corticosteroids during treatment and those with central nervous system tumors that affect the hypothalamic-pituitary-adrenal axis are at increased risk for obesity.[170]

Adult Survivors of Childhood Cancer

With more than 80% of children diagnosed with cancer surviving at least 5 years,[171] a number that is increasing as treatments improve, greater attention is being paid to managing the long-term sequelae of cancer, including poor sleep. Their sleep issues have an impact on their health. Adult survivors of childhood cancer reporting poor sleep quality are five times more likely to be depressed.[172,173] The prevalence of disturbed sleep in this population is possibly best understood through the lens of national cohort studies, including the Childhood Cancer Survivor Study (CCSS). From CCSS data, we see that an estimated 17% of adult survivors of childhood cancer report disrupted sleep.[173] Further, adult survivors of childhood cancer were more likely to report poor sleep efficiency, daytime sleepiness, and sleep supplement use than their siblings.[174] Survivors who are female, unmarried, depressed, or have a history of radiation therapy were more likely to be fatigued.[173] Data from smaller studies show even greater rates of sleep disruptions, with approximately 28% of adult survivors of childhood cancer reporting a sleep efficiency below 85%.[175] From this study, it is notable that investigators also reviewed the medical note for these survivors on the day that they completed the questionnaires that indicated poor sleep efficiency, revealing that only one out of three patients with poor sleep had a discussion about sleep documented. This underscores a consistent issue in this group and across all cancer groups: sleep is underdiscussed and often overlooked in the context of cancer.

Patients with Advanced Cancer

Nearly all patients with advanced cancer report some degree of sleep disruption. From about half to three-quarters of outpatients attending cancer or palliative care clinics report some sleep disturbance,[43,176,177] with some estimates suggesting that up to 96% of patients with advanced cancer have sleep difficulties.[178-181] When assessed using a structured clinical interview, 69% of a sample of 51 community-dwelling patients receiving palliative care for cancer had some sleep-wake difficulties, including 22% with an insomnia disorder (+10% with subsyndromal symptoms) and 22% with a hypersomnolence disorder (+8% with subsyndromal symptoms).[182] In a study of patients with metastatic breast cancer, 63% reported sleep disturbances. Difficulty falling asleep was associated with both depression and pain, whereas increased awakenings during the night was associated with only depression.[183] Similarly, another study conducted among 101 patients with advanced cancer (any type) found that sleep difficulties were associated with increased pain, depressive and anxiety symptoms, and a poorer sense of well-being.[184] In a prospective study, 15% of terminally ill patients with cancer had sleep disturbance (insomnia or hypersomnia), and 29% had subclinical disturbance at the moment of registration to a palliative care unit. These rates increased to 26% and 37%, respectively, at the time of admission. There was a change in sleep status in 67% of patients between the two time points; sleep deteriorated (46%) more frequently than it improved (21%).[185] Another study found that patients with advanced lung cancer reported poorer sleep and more daytime sleepiness than healthy controls and that their sleep disturbances were characterized by breathing difficulties, cough, nocturia, and frequent awakenings, all of which may be suggestive of sleep-disordered breathing.[186] Estimates suggest that half (52%) of patients with head and neck cancer undergoing palliative care experience insomnia.[22] Finally, a study suggested that poor sleep quality and use of sleep medications were, along with hopelessness and depression, the best predictors of desire for hastened death in 102 terminally ill patients attending a palliative care unit,[187] thus emphasizing the importance of offering appropriate sleep management to these patients.

Despite the high needs, research to date has largely overlooked patients with advanced cancer. The lack of routine screening and appropriate screening measures has hampered the assessment of sleep disturbance in patients with advanced cancer. Additional reasons that patients with advanced cancer have received comparatively less attention include the complex medical needs of this group, the belief that sleep disruption is an expected side effect of disease or treatments, the routine use of pharmacotherapy to manage sleep problems, and the difficulty adapting current nonpharmacologic therapies. One of the few studies to assess interventions for this population developed and piloted a Cognitive Behavioral and Environmental Intervention to improve insomnia and hypersomnolence in community-dwelling patients receiving palliative care.[182] The intervention consisted of one individual 60-minute session that identified the most relevant behavioral (e.g., limiting napping, stimulus control), cognitive (e.g., challenging beliefs about the need to limit activity to preserve energy), and environmental (e.g. reducing bedroom noise, ensuring daytime light exposure) strategies, and the patient was provided with a booklet to help them apply the strategies over the following 3 weeks. The authors reported considerable challenges with recruitment for the intervention particularly because of existing limitations or rapidly declining function, a prompt prescription of a new hypnotic or psychostimulant medication, and a high rate of participant refusal. Despite variable adherence, patients with insomnia reported satisfaction and sleep improvements. Other brief, sleep-focused interventions have also reported challenges with recruitment despite efforts to minimize participant burden[188] and lower-than-expected treatment effects.[189] These factors highlight some of the challenges in providing interventions to this population. Additional research is needed to find the right balance of treatment efficacy with participant burden.

Cancer Caregivers

The burden for someone caring for a patient with cancer is tremendous. Cancer caregivers are often invisible patients because there is someone in their lives with a life-threatening disease that requires attention. As such, ongoing sleep disruptions are mostly overlooked, despite their prevalence. Insufficient or poor-quality sleep is commonly reported by those providing care for pediatric and adult patients with cancer.[164,190] Estimates suggest that up to 40% of caregivers report at least one sleep problem such as short sleep duration, nocturnal awakenings, wake after sleep onset, or daytime dysfunction. An overarching theme of the cancer caregiving experience is the idea that they sleep "with one eye open" at all times because of the need to remain vigilant in case the patient needs them.[191] The cancer patient's poor sleep appears to affect the caregivers' sleep, and vice versa.[192] Unfortunately, there are limited studies examining behavioral interventions for sleep disturbances among cancer caregivers.[193]

FUTURE DIRECTIONS

Given the prevalence and perniciousness of sleep problems in cancer, there is an urgent need for prevention and early intervention programs to improve the overall experience and recovery of the 17 million individuals diagnosed with cancer worldwide.[194] More research is warranted on children, adolescents, and young adults with cancer, survivors of childhood cancer, patients with advanced cancer, and cancer caregivers, including clinical studies investigating the efficacy of nonpharmacologic interventions for sleep disturbances, as it is unclear whether the same treatment modalities can be offered to these patients. The mechanisms through which these interventions are effective also deserve investigation. Finally, attention is needed to develop and test interventions to prevent development to and/or exacerbation of sleep disturbances at the time of cancer diagnosis and during treatment to preserve overall quality of life.

CLINICAL PEARLS

- Sleep disturbances are among the most common and most distressing complaints of patients with cancer. When left untreated, these symptoms can significantly impair patients' quality of life.
- Those at highest risk appear to be those who are female, younger age, and receiving chemotherapy and who have other physical and psychological symptom burden.
- Clinicians should screen routinely for sleep disturbances and administer evidence-based treatment strategies.

SUMMARY

There is strong evidence to support a higher prevalence of sleep disturbances and insomnia in patients diagnosed with cancer beginning before treatment and lasting well into survivorship. Certain cancers may increase the likelihood of other sleep disorders such as sleep apnea, hypersomnia, and sleep-related movement disorders. Some demographic and clinical characteristics appear to be associated with higher prevalence including being female, younger age, receiving chemotherapy, and other physical and psychological symptom burden. Assessment of sleep is recommended at diagnosis, at regular intervals, at periods of transition/stress during cancer, and into survivorship. Nonpharmacologic interventions are recommended over pharmacologic, which should only be used for brief periods, intermittently, or in situations and populations where nonpharmacologic interventions are not available or desirable. The nonpharmacologic treatment with the strongest evidence of efficacy in cancer is CBT-I. Other treatments that may be helpful include mindfulness-based and exercise interventions.

SELECTED READINGS

Christodoulou G, Black DS. Mindfulness-based interventions and sleep among cancer survivors: a critical analysis of randomized controlled trials. *Curr Oncol Rep*. 2017;19(9):60.

Howell D, Keller-Olaman S, Oliver TK, et al. A pan-Canadian practice guideline and algorithm: screening, assessment, and supportive care of adults with cancer-related fatigue. *Curr Oncol*. 2013;20(3):e233–e246.

Johnson JA, Rash JA, Campbell TS, et al. A systematic review and meta-analysis of randomized controlled trials of Cognitive Behavior Therapy for Insomnia (CBT-I) in cancer survivors. *Sleep Med Rev*. 2016;27:20–28.

Kotronoulas G, Wengstrom Y, Kearney N. Sleep patterns and sleep-impairing factors of persons providing informal care for people with cancer: a critical review of the literature. *Cancer Nurs*. 2013;36(1):E1–E15.

Lee S, Narendran G, Tomfohr-Madsen L, Schulte F. A systematic review of sleep in hospitalized pediatric cancer patients. *Psychooncology*. 2017;26(8):1059–1069.

Ma Y, Hall DL, Ngo LH, Liu Q, Bain PA, Yeh GY. Efficacy of cognitive behavioral therapy for insomnia in breast cancer: a meta-analysis. *Sleep Med Rev*. 2021;55:101376.

Mercier J, Savard J, Bernard P. Exercise interventions to improve sleep in cancer patients: a systematic review and meta-analysis. *Sleep Med Rev*. 2017;36:43–56.

Savard J, Ivers H, Savard MH, et al. Efficacy of a stepped care approach to deliver cognitive-behavioral therapy for insomnia in cancer patients: a noninferiority randomized controlled trial. *Sleep*. 2021:zsab166. [published online ahead of print, 2021 Jul 6].

Savard J, Ivers H, Savard MH, Morin CM. Cancer treatments and their side effects are associated with aggravation of insomnia: results of a longitudinal study. *Cancer*. 2015;121(10):1703–1711.

Savard J, Ivers H, Villa J, Caplette-Gingras A, Morin CM. Natural course of insomnia comorbid with cancer: an 18-month longitudinal study. *J Clin Oncol*. 2011;29(26):3580–3586.

Savard J, Liu L, Natarajan L, et al. Breast cancer patients have progressively impaired sleep-wake activity rhythms during chemotherapy. *Sleep*. 2009;32(9):1155–1160.

Zhou ES, Recklitis CJ. Insomnia in adult survivors of childhood cancer: a report from project REACH. *Support Care Cancer*. 2014;22(11):3061–3069.

Zhou J, Jolly S. Obstructive sleep apnea and fatigue in head and neck cancer patients. *Am J Clin Oncol*. 2015;38(4):411–414.

A complete reference list can be found online at ExpertConsult.com.

Chapter 154

Fibromyalgia and Chronic Fatigue Syndromes

Vivian Asare; Douglas Kirsch; Christine Won

Chapter Highlights

- Sleep-related complaints and sleep disturbances are principal features of fibromyalgia (FM) and CFS. Sleep quality affects patients' pain and fatigue symptoms as well as quality of life. The pathophysiologic role of sleep disturbances in FM and CFS is currently poorly understood despite the recognition of poor sleep quality as a frequent symptom.
- Several polysomnographic findings have been described in patients with FM and CFS. The relevance of sleep electroencephalogram (EEG) findings to daytime symptoms of FM and CFS are not well understood. Conventional methods for sleep-stage scoring or quantifying EEG may not be sensitive enough to detect relevant sleep changes in patients with FM or CFS.
- Comorbid sleep disorders may affect sleep quality of patients with FM and CFS, and treating these sleep disorders may augment primary therapies for these syndromes. Targeted therapy toward sleep disorders or sleep complaints includes pharmacologic and nonpharmacologic approaches.

FIBROMYALGIA AND SLEEP

Fibromyalgia (FM) is characterized by generalized pain, chronic fatigue, and nonrestorative sleep. In 2016 the American College of Rheumatology revised diagnostic criteria to include physician tender-point criteria and patient-reported survey of pain, with symptoms occurring for at least 3 months.[1–3] The global prevalence of FM is approximately 3% to 8%. Approximately 75% of patients with FM are women, and most patients are age 30 to 50 years.[4]

Although current diagnostic criteria for FM do not include specific sleep abnormalities, sleep disturbances and complaints of poor sleep quality and daytime fatigue are common. In fact, the only thing more common than sleep-related complaints is symptoms of pain.[5] Nonrestorative sleep correlates closely with somatic symptoms and pain severity. A night of reported nonrestorative sleep often translates to higher perceived morning pain, intensified afternoon pain severity, and ultimately greater activity interference at the end of the day.[6] A specific etiology for FM is unknown, although it is speculated that disturbances in central nervous system (CNS) function likely contribute. The pathophysiologic role of sleep disturbances in FM is currently unknown despite the recognition of this as a frequent symptom.

Polysomnographic Features of Fibromyalgia

Patients with FM compared with healthy individuals demonstrate greater disturbances during sleep on polysomnography (PSG). Sleep-onset latency, arousal index, awakenings, and length of awakenings tend to be increased in patients with FM, whereas total sleep time and sleep efficiency are reduced[7] and have an increased number of sleep-stage shifts and a shorter duration of N2 sleep stage.[8] In addition, PSG data suggest that patients with FM have reduced total rapid eye movement (REM) and slow wave sleep time corrected for age, and these changes are associated with increased musculoskeletal and mood symptoms. The best predictor of subjective sleep quality in FM patients is time spent awake in bed, as measured by PSG data.[9] These PSG findings suggest that patient-reported sleep complaints are not fully explained by sleep misperception, as previous authors have suggested.[10]

Several sleep electroencephalography (EEG) microstructure findings have been described using power spectral and frequency domain analysis. Beta frequency (14 to 38 Hz) is generally considered to reflect arousal; it is associated with lightened sleep perception and is linked with depression. When muscle and joint pain are experimentally provoked during sleep, beta power and alpha (8 to 13 Hz) frequency bands are increased on spectral analysis, whereas delta (0.5 to 4 Hz) and sigma (12 to 14 Hz) power is reduced.[11] Sigma frequency (reflecting sleep spindles) is generated from corticothalamic networks, appears to be responsible for lack of perceptual awareness and unresponsiveness during sleep, and it is associated with perception of greater sleep depth. Patients with FM demonstrate fewer sleep spindles per minute of stage N2 sleep and reduced spindle frequency even when controlling for age, depression, and psychiatric diagnosis. Reduced spindle number and spindle frequency activity in stage N2 sleep may affect sensory processing in the thalamus and is associated with a lower pain threshold.[12]

Occipital alpha frequency (8 to 13 Hz), which is associated with relaxed wakefulness with eyes closed in healthy individuals, has been found to intrude on the sleep EEG in patients with FM.[13,14] Alpha intrusion has been identified in 70% of patients with FM compared with 16% of control subjects.[14] Two patterns of alpha activity during sleep have been described: (1) a phasic alpha pattern or alpha-delta sleep, which describes a pattern of alpha activity superimposed on delta waves of slow wave sleep (found in 71% of patients with FM with alpha intrusion); (2) a tonic alpha pattern, in which the alpha frequency occurs throughout non–rapid eye movement (NREM) sleep (found in 29% of patients with FM with alpha intrusion). Alpha-delta sleep is associated with worse sleep efficiency, perception of lighter sleep, longer pain duration, and increased morning stiffness and pain. In patients with FM, but not in healthy control subjects, the alpha-delta ratio increases exponentially through the night.[15] Nonrestorative sleep has been described in 100% of patients with FM with the alpha-delta pattern, 25% with the tonic alpha pattern, and 58% of patients with FM without significant alpha intrusion. Alpha intrusion is also associated with symptoms of vigilance during sleep manifested as an increased tendency to wake to an external response and the perception of shallow or unrefreshing sleep.[16] There is no association between the occurrence of depressed mood or memory complaints in patients with FM and any of the alpha frequency patterns.[17]

Whether alpha intrusion causes or results from chronic pain is unclear. When painful stimuli to muscles and joints are applied during slow wave sleep, an arousal effect with decreased delta waves and increased alpha activity is observed. Stimulation of superficial pain to the skin, on the other hand, does not elicit the same EEG response during sleep, suggesting that deep, but not superficial, pain alters sleep architecture.[11] Alternatively, alpha sleep may predispose the individual to increased arousability because of pain or other stimuli.

Not all investigators agree that the alpha EEG findings during sleep are significant because they also occur in 15% of normal individuals and in 40% of patients with other pain syndromes, such as rheumatoid arthritis.[18] Most subjects exhibiting this pattern have a non-pain-related medical or psychiatric condition.[19] In normal individuals, alpha intrusion may be elicited by auditory or deep pain stimuli during slow wave and is associated with subjective complaints of disturbed sleep.[20]

The alpha EEG findings, although not specific to FM, correlate with the subjective feeling of nonrestorative sleep. The amount of this rhythm correlates with objective measurements of pain, and decreasing the amount of alpha intrusion with medications results in perceived improvement in sleep and pain. The biochemical and cellular processes that occur with this EEG finding are unknown and warrant further study.

Cyclic alternating pattern (CAP) describes a phenomenon whereby the EEG activity is periodic within NREM sleep. CAP is characterized by sequences of transient electrocortical events that are distinct from background EEG activity and recur at up to 1-minute intervals. This periodic activity, originally thought to be arousals, is now theorized to be the process of sleep maintenance and sleep fragmentation. CAP phase A1 pattern is considered to be an index of sleep stability, whereas CAP phases A2 and A3 are markers of sleep instability or poor sleep quality.[21] CAP A2 and A3 are increased in patients with FM compared with controls. Greater frequency of these subtypes are associated with increased number of tender points in patients with FM.[22] Furthermore, when A2 and A3 subtypes are pharmacologically decreased, patients with FM describe improvements in fatigue and in the Hospital and Anxiety and Depression Scale (HADS) score.[23] Some scientists hypothesize that excessive phasic EEG activity may reflect enhanced or abnormal activity within the insula, anterior cingulate cortex, and ventromedial prefrontal cortex, areas responsible for modulating abnormal nociceptive processing. However, it remains unclear whether CAP EEG findings reflect disturbed sleep processes and are pathogenic in FM, or whether they are consequences of pain and other syndromes found in patients with FM.

Pathophysiologic Correlates of Altered Sleep in Fibromyalgia

Neurologic mechanisms that regulate sleep and are in turn affected by sleep disturbances may play a role in the etiology and maintenance of FM. Several studies have shown that patients with FM have decreased levels of serotonin and the serotonin metabolite 5-hydroxyindole-3-acetic acid in the cerebrospinal fluid and blood serum.[24,25] Serotonin modulates pain transmission, and decreased serotonin synthesis induces a hyperalgesic state and insomnia. The precursor to serotonin, 5-hydroxytryptamine, is released at axonal nerve endings in the basal hypothalamus as a neurotransmitter during wakefulness and is important in the sleep state–dependent modulation of the nociceptive process of pain. A reduction in serotonin may be partially responsible for reducing delta sleep and predisposing to an alpha EEG rhythm. High levels of substance P are found in the cerebrospinal fluid of patients with FM and may contribute to serotoninergic deficiency.[26] Substance P appears to be a biologic marker for the presence of chronic pain and the stress response.[27,28] Studies suggest that some individuals have a genetic predisposition for FM through the elevated frequency of polymorphisms in the serotonin transporter, dopamine D4 receptor, and catechol-*O*-methyltransferase genes.[29,30] Together, these findings suggest serotonin plays a role in promoting both analgesia and sleep.

Serotonin is transformed into melatonin in the pineal gland. The decrease in serotonin in patients with FM has been speculated to result in decrease melatonin synthesis, leading to abnormal sleep patterns. Some studies have described low nocturnal melatonin peak levels and a decrease in overall melatonin secretion in patients with FM.[31] Recent data asserts that there is a nocturnal disruption to melatonin, while an increase in daytime melatonin levels is present in patients with FM compared to healthy control subjects. This overall dysregulation of melatonin secretion correlates with perceived pain, depressive symptoms, and poor sleep quality.[32] Melatonin has been used successfully to treat sleep-wake cycle disturbances in some patients with FM and has resulted in improved pain, mood, anxiety, and quality of life.[33] However, other studies demonstrate no difference in melatonin levels and a lack of association between melatonin and disease duration, sleep disturbances, fatigue, and pain scores.[34,35]

There is substantial evidence indicating that sensitization of the CNS pain pathway plays a crucial role in the pathophysiology of FM.[36] Neuroimaging studies show that patients with FM may exhibit abnormal perception of painful stimuli through central changes that result in increased pronociception or through decreased activity in descending pain inhibitory pathways, such as the anterior cingulate cortex and thalamus.[37] There is altered regional cerebral blood flow to the thalamic areas where encoding and inhibiting pain transmission occurs and to areas where ablation has been shown to result in persistent insomnia in cats.[38,39] Altered thalamic regional cerebral blood flow may cause loss of growth hormone (GH) secretion during slow wave sleep and result in sleep alterations in patients with FM. Somatomedin C or insulin-like growth factor-1, which regulates GH production, is low in about one-third of FM patients,[40] and exogenous GH may improve their sleep quality.[41]

Fibromyalgia may be considered a stress-related disorder. Stressors such as physical trauma, hormonal alterations, and emotional stress play an important role in triggering the development of FM and its somatic symptoms, including widespread chronic pain. Stress may directly affect the hypothalamic-pituitary-adrenal axis and the autonomic system, which induces central alterations that blunt cortisol, lead to abnormal regulation of GH, and cause heart rate variation and sensitivity to orthostatic changes on tilt-table tests.[42,43] Stress may directly affect sleep, causing sleep disruption, especially during slow wave sleep, and further modulate the hypothalamic-pituitary-adrenal axis and exacerbate musculoskeletal pain and fatigue symptoms. Sleep disturbances are also related to disturbances in mood and cognition and may affect coping mechanisms to stress.

Common Sleep Complaints and Sleep Disorders in Fibromyalgia

One of the most prevalent and clinically challenging complaints in this patient population is unrefreshing or nonrestorative sleep, which is present in greater than 75% of patients with FM.[44] Patients often report feeling unrested or worse after a night of sleep. In addition, patients with FM commonly report sleep fragmentation, early-morning awakenings, and insomnia.[45] Despite reporting significant subjective sleepiness and fatigue, however, patients with FM demonstrate less objective daytime sleepiness on Multiple Sleep Latency Tests (MSLTs) than healthy control subjects.[46]

Primary sleep disorders, such as sleep apnea, restless legs syndrome (RLS), and periodic limb movements of sleep (PLMS), may be found in patients with FM. It has been reported that approximately 2% of women presenting to a rheumatology clinic with a new diagnosis of FM will have sleep apnea.[47] Women with FM are more likely to have sleep-related breathing disorders, such as hypoxemia, inspiratory airflow limitation, and upper airway resistance syndrome, rather than frank sleep apnea. Treatment of sleep-disordered breathing with positive airway pressure (PAP) therapy improves functional outcomes in women with FM.[48] In contrast, 44% of men presenting to a rheumatology clinic with a new diagnosis of FM have been purported to have sleep apnea,[49] although this finding has not been consistently supported. Therefore sleep-disordered breathing may be found in select patients with FM, but current evidence is not convincing for a direct association between sleep apnea and FM.

RLS has been described to be more frequent in female patients with FM (20% to 64%) compared with women in the general population (2% to 15%).[50–52] Genetic studies suggest a common genetic background and coheritability of FM and RLS.[53,54] The occurrence of RLS in patients with FM leads to worse sleep quality and quality of life.[55] The reason for the high prevalence of RLS in this population is unknown but may result from common central processes, such as dysfunction of the dopaminergic system. There are emerging data suggesting that the experience of pain among patients with FM may be in part due to dysfunction in the release of dopamine within the CNS. When subjected to deep muscle pain, normal subjects release dopamine in the basal ganglia, whereas FM patients do not. In normal subjects, the amount of dopamine release correlates with the amount of perceived pain; however, there is no such correlation in FM patients.[56]

Approach to the Management of Sleep Disturbances in Fibromyalgia

The general goal of FM treatment is to develop an individualized therapeutic program that involves various approaches. FM symptoms of pain and sleep disturbances affect quality of life, including the patient's ability to work, to participate in everyday activities, and to maintain relationships. For these reasons, therapies directed at alleviating sleep symptoms are integral to the treatment plan of patients with FM.

At present, only three drugs (pregabalin, duloxetine, and milnacipran) are approved by the U.S. Food and Drug Administration to reduce FM symptoms.[57] Pregabalin is an anticonvulsant that downregulates presynaptic excitatory neurotransmitter release through its action on an $\alpha_2\beta$ receptor that regulates flow of calcium channels.[58] It is found to be effective in reducing the severity of the two major FM symptom domains: pain and sleep disturbance.[59] Duloxetine and milnacipran, serotonin-norepinephrine reuptake inhibitor antidepressants, increase the availability of serotonin and norepinephrine at CNS synaptic clefts. They have the potential to reduce pain by correcting the functional deficit of 5-hydroxytryptamine and norepinephrine neurotransmission in the descending inhibitory pain pathway.[60]

In addition, several pharmacologic agents have been tested specifically for their potential to improve sleep in patients with FM. These medications include chlorpromazine, amitriptyline, suvorexant, fluoxetine, mirtazapine, trazodone, and cyclobenzaprine. Chlorpromazine has been shown to decrease alpha-delta EEG frequencies, while reducing pain and trigger point tenderness.[61] Suvorexant has been shown to increase total sleep time, reduce wake after sleep onset, and reduce next-day pain sensitivity in patients with FM and comorbid chronic insomnia.[62] Tricyclic antidepressant medications, such as amitriptyline, which affect serotonin metabolism in the CNS, reduce alpha-delta sleep time and promote restorative sleep in patients with FM, although effects appear to decline after 6 months of therapy.[63,64] Fluoxetine has been shown to help sleep and depressed mood in women with FM.[65] Amitriptyline and fluoxetine combined have resulted in significant improvement among patients with FM in general sleep scores and appeared to be superior to either drug alone.[66] Mirtazapine has a pharmacologic profile that includes serotonergic and antihistaminic properties, which lead to antidepressive and sedative effects. Mirtazapine has been shown to reduce pain and fatigue and to improve sleep quality in most patients with FM.[67] Trazodone has been shown to markedly improve sleep duration, sleep efficiency, and sleep quality based on the Pittsburgh Sleep Quality Index in patients with FM. Improvements with the use of trazodone were also observed on the Fibromyalgia Impact Questionnaire, the Beck Depression Inventory, the HADS, and pain interference with daily activities.[68] Trazodone plus pregabalin administered over 12 weeks showed significant improvement in sleep quality, depression, pain, and global fibromyalgia severity.[69] Very low-dose cyclobenzaprine (1 to 4 mg) at bedtime resulted in improvement in CAP sleep EEG and improved FM symptoms. Responding patients showed lower frequency of CAP A2 and A3 and reported improved fatigue and HADS depression score. CAP changes appeared to be a useful biomarker that predicted treatment benefit.[23] These findings underscore the clinical benefit of primarily treating sleep complaints and normalizing sleep architecture in FM.

Sodium oxybate has been evaluated in double-blind, randomized, placebo-controlled trials for treatment of FM. Sodium oxybate has been noted to reduce tender points and fatigue symptoms and to improve sleep quality. Six of seven pain and fatigue scores (overall pain, pain at rest, pain during movement, end-of-day fatigue, overall fatigue, and morning fatigue) were relieved for approximately one-third of subjects treated with sodium oxybate compared with 6% to 10% in the placebo group.[70,71] Sodium oxybate also led to improved scores on the Epworth Sleepiness Scale, Jenkins Scale for Sleep, Functional Outcomes of Sleep Questionnaire, and Short Form-36 health questionnaire. Doses of both 4.5 and 6 g split into two doses (bedtime and 2.5 to 4 hours later) improved outcomes, although only the 6-g dose improved sleep efficiency, stage N2 sleep, and slow wave sleep.[72] This pharmacologic therapy also significantly decreased alpha intrusion, sleep latency, and REM sleep. However, sodium oxybate is not approved as a labeled treatment for FM by the U.S. Food and Drug Administration.

Nonpharmacologic therapies for improving sleep have been explored. Spinal and extremity joint manipulation or mobilization, massage, and various soft tissue techniques improve pain intensity, FM symptom impact, depressive symptoms, and sleep quality. Sex differences were observed in response to these treatments, with women having a greater reduction in pain and FM symptoms, although sleep quality improved equally in men and women.[73]

Screening for primary sleep disorders, such as sleep-disordered breathing, RLS, and circadian disorders, is important. Even mild inspiratory flow limitation is associated with sleep fragmentation, fatigue, and excessive daytime sleepiness in women with FM. Nasal PAP therapy in patients with sleep-disordered breathing may improve fatigue, pain, sleep fragmentation, disability, and Rheumatology Distress Index scores.[48] When patients with FM and RLS are treated with pramipexole, a dopamine-3 receptor agonist, they experience significant improvement in measures of pain, fatigue, and functional and global status.[74]

In conclusion, screening for and treating primary sleep disorders, implementing good sleep hygiene recommendations, and pharmacologic management of FM may improve sleep quality and directly affect FM symptoms.

CHRONIC FATIGUE SYNDROME AND SLEEP

Chronic fatigue syndrome (CFS) is a disabling condition characterized by severe fatigue lasting for more than 6 months and the presence of at least four out of eight minor criteria. The term *CFS* was first introduced in the 1980s after a clear viral etiology could not be definitively found.[75] At the 2011 International Consensus Report meeting, advocates adopted the term *myalgic encephalitis* to better reflect an underlying disease process involving neuropathology and widespread inflammation.[76] Most recently, in 2015, the Institute of Medicine proposed a new name, systemic exertion intolerance disease (SEID), that described both the central elements of the disease and the debilitating physical and cognitive effects of the condition.[77] In this chapter we will use the term *CFS* for consistency.

CFS may overlap with other chronic somatic syndromes, such as FM syndrome and irritable bowel disorder. Diffuse muscular pain, fatigue, and sleep disturbances are part of the definitions of both CFS and FM. As a result, 20% to 70% of patients with FM meet criteria for CFS, and 35% to 70% of those with CFS have coexistent FM.[1,78,79] These conditions may constitute continuums of the same physiologic and psychosocial processes, with varying degrees of pain, fatigue, and disturbed sleep. Patients who are SARS-CoV-2 survivors may report long-term symptoms that resemble CFS. Thus, it is possible we may be seeing an increase in CFS in the future[79a] (see also Chapter 213).

Complaints of unrefreshing or nonrestorative sleep are very common in patients with CFS.[80] Disturbed sleep is a known cause of fatigue and may play a role in the pathogenesis of CFS. However, the nature of the sleep impairment in CFS remains unknown. Although complaints of unrefreshing sleep are pervasive, there are no apparent neurophysiologic correlates of dysfunctional sleep in CFS, and there are no PSG findings that discriminate between subjects with CFS and normal control subjects. These observations suggest that psychosocial factors may affect the perception of poor sleep quality. Primary sleep disorders occur often in patients with CFS and may contribute to the presence of daytime dysfunction. However, there is currently little evidence to indicate that treating primary sleep disorders improves fatigue associated with CFS. Therefore primary sleep disorders are likely comorbid rather than an associated condition of CFS.

Polysomnographic Findings in Chronic Fatigue Syndrome

Despite the fact that sleep complaints are frequently reported in patients with CFS, there are no specific or consistent PSG findings that characterize sleep in patients with CFS. PSG EEG may show increased number and duration of awakenings.[81,82] Reduced total sleep time and sleep efficiency, both in in-laboratory PSG and in-home studies, have been described.[83,84] Sleep-onset latencies are often longer in patients with CFS compared with healthy control subjects.[85] It has been reported that patients with CFS may have altered parasympathetic activity. A recent study found that CFS subjects compared to healthy control subjects have diminished nocturnal parasympathetic activity, suggesting hypervigilant sleep. This alteration in parasympathetic activity is particularly diminished during slow wave sleep and was associated with reports of poor sleep quality and well-being in CFS patients.[86] This finding may also reflect poor sleep hygiene or daytime napping, which decrease nocturnal sleep drive. Based on limited data, there appear to be very few differences or mixed findings in sleep architecture between CFS patients and healthy individuals. Shorter durations of N2 sleep have been shown in those with CFS and FM, but not in those with CFS alone. Although total N3 sleep time has been shown to be unchanged in monozygotic twins discordant for CFS, when the twin with CFS is intentionally sleep delayed by 4 hours, there is decreased slow wave activity during the first NREM period, suggesting a potential deficiency in sleep homeostasis.[87] Some studies have reported reduced REM sleep,[84] whereas others have observed a higher percentage of REM in patients with CFS.[88–90] Rates of sleep state transitions between wake, N1, and REM into N2 sleep, and transitions from N3 into wake or N1, may also be greater in those with CFS and comorbid FM. In those with CFS without FM, sleep-state transitions from REM to wake may be greater.[91] CAP

EEG has not been explored extensively in CFS; existing limited data suggest possibly an increase in CAP during NREM sleep in patients with CFS compared with healthy control subjects.[85] Therefore a single-night PSG performed with traditional technology does not appear useful for discriminating individuals with CFS from healthy control subjects or from other chronic pain or fatigue conditions, nor do these subtle differences in sleep architecture and EEG findings provide a correlate for sleep complaints in patients with CFS.[92]

Power spectrum analysis of the EEG does not seem to provide strong evidence for abnormal alpha intrusion in NREM sleep in subjects with CFS. No significant differences in spectral power in any frequency band have been found between cotwins with and without CFS.[93] In fact, some studies showed a reduction in alpha power by spectrum analysis during N2, N3, and REM sleep in CFS subjects.[85,94] Analysis of other spectral bands (theta, delta, beta) shows inconsistent results. For example, delta power has been reported to be increased, decreased, or no different in CFS groups compared with normal control subjects.[94,95] Therefore conventional methods for sleep-stage scoring or quantifying EEG have failed to identify specific findings or may not be sensitive enough to detect sleep changes in patients with CFS.

Biochemical Correlates of Altered Sleep in Chronic Fatigue Syndrome

The pathogenesis of CFS remains unknown. Abnormalities of the central and autonomic nervous systems, and in some cases infections, have been hypothesized.[96] Adolescent patients with CFS often have findings of postural orthostatic tachycardia syndrome, suggesting autonomic dysfunction and a potential neutrally mediated cause of chronic fatigue.[97] The cognitive behavior model for CFS suggests predisposing and perpetuating factors. The onset may be related to an infection or other CNS abnormalities, but the perpetuation of the condition may be determined by psychosocial factors, such as maladaptive behavior or negative conditioning.[98] Maladaptive responses include reduced physical activity, leading to autonomic dysfunction, increased nervous system sensitivity, and increased CFS symptom burden.

Common Sleep Complaints and Sleep Disorders in Chronic Fatigue Syndrome

Unrefreshing or nonrestorative sleep, even after a night of sufficient sleep duration, is a frequent complaint occurring in 87% to 95% of CFS patients.[99,100] Nocturnal neurophysiologic disturbances that result in the nonrestorative sensation after sleep in CFS patients are not detected by traditional sleep monitoring, suggesting current measurements may not be sufficiently sensitive to detect subtle disturbances in sleep in this population.

Subjects with CFS with complaints of nonrestorative sleep have a very high co-occurrence of daytime dysfunction. Objective testing has shown cognitive impairments in attention, motor functioning, information processing, and executive functioning.[101] Pathologic sleepiness, however, is not objectively demonstrated on MSLT despite CFS patients reporting greater subjective sleepiness and poorer sleep quality than healthy control subjects.[102,103] One potential reason for this may be that CFS patients may suffer from sleep quality misperception. Poor self-rated health and depressive symptoms have been found to be associated with overreporting of sleep difficulties and underestimation of sleep efficiency.[104] Alternatively, current measures may not reliably differentiate between fatigue and sleepiness, resulting in discordances between subjective and objective sleep-related measurements.[105]

Actigraphy studies in children with CFS report a sleep pattern consisting of more than 10 hours of continuous sleep.[106] Impaired daily sleep-wake rhythms and disturbed sleep were observed only in some children with CFS. Most actigraphy studies to date have shown mixed findings relating to circadian rhythm disturbances.[107–109]

PSG studies on population-based subjects have shown the presence of a primary sleep disorder in approximately 18% of patients with CFS compared with 7% of control subjects.[91] In the clinical setting, 46% to 95% of patients with CFS have comorbid sleep disorders, such as primary insomnia, obstructive sleep apnea, PLMS, or narcolepsy.[82,110–112] Sleep disorders were once considered exclusionary for the diagnosis of CFS. This concept is challenged; it has been found that there are no significant differences between patients with CFS in the presence or absence of OSA with regard to CFS symptoms, indexes of anxiety and depression, subjective sleep variables, and Short Form-36 quality-of-life measures.[113] Currently, there is no evidence to suggest that treatment of sleep-related breathing disorders with PAP therapy will reduce fatigue and increase vigor in CFS.[114] However, because of their high frequency and their potential compounding of symptoms in patients with CFS, a thorough evaluation for underlying organic sleep disorders and aggressive treatment are warranted.

Approach to the Management of Sleep Disturbances in Chronic Fatigue Syndrome

CFS patients tend to have an exacerbation of daytime fatigue symptoms after a night of perceived poor sleep.[115] Therefore treating sleep complaints may benefit CFS symptoms. Cognitive behavioral therapy (CBT) and graded exercise therapy (GET) are recommended treatments for CFS.[116,117] Both treatment modalities decrease fatigue and improve physical function and may improve sleep quality.[118–120] GET has been found to improve perceived sleep quality in patients suffering from insomnia by helping to decrease muscle tension and improve general mood and anxiety management.[121,122] Similarly, CBT improved sleep perception by improving anxiety management, mood, and by helping to modify unhelpful beliefs. Whether targeted therapy for sleep complaints, such as insomnia or sleep disruption, improves CFS outcomes is unknown. More studies in this area are required because sleep disturbances perpetuate CFS and affect quality of life.

CLINICAL PEARLS

- Sleep-related complaints, such as poor sleep quality and nonrestorative sleep, are pervasive in fibromyalgia (FM) and chronic fatigue syndrome (CFS) and may be associated with complaints of pain and fatigue.
- Patients with FM demonstrate greater sleep disturbances on polysomnography, such as reduced total sleep time, sleep efficiency, rapid eye movement and slow wave sleep, and increased arousals and alpha intrusion.
- Decreased serotonin levels in the central nervous system may contribute to altered nociception and sleep disturbances in FM.
- Therapies targeted at improving sleep, including treating comorbid sleep disorders, are important adjuncts to treatment of FM and CFS.

SUMMARY

Sleep disturbances, sleep complaints, and comorbid sleep disorders are common in patients with FM and CFS. Many characteristic daytime symptoms, such as chronic pain and fatigue, may be related to nonrestorative sleep patterns associated with the diseases. Pain and sleep disturbances interact reciprocally—pain affects sleep processes, and sleep disturbances affect pain threshold—to influence disease severity and chronicity. Sleep disturbances therefore may contribute to fatigue, psychological disturbances, and impaired quality of life. To the extent that nonrestorative sleep may exacerbate fibromyalgia or chronic fatigue symptoms, treatments that directly improve sleep quality may improve daytime symptoms of these disorders.

SELECTED READINGS

Ahmed M, Aamir R, Jishi Z, Scharf MB. The effects of milnacipran on sleep disturbance in fibromyalgia: a randomized, double-blind, placebo-controlled, two-way crossover study. *J Clin Sleep Med.* 2016;12(1):79–86.

Çetin Buğra, Sünbül Esra Aydın, Toktaş Hayal, Karaca Merve, Özgür Ulutaş Hüseyin Güleç. Comparison of sleep structure in patients with fibromyalgia and healthy controls. *Sleep Breath.* 2020;(4):1591–1598.

Diaz-Piedra C, Catena A, Sánchez AI, Miró E, Martínez MP, Buela-Casal G. Sleep disturbances in fibromyalgia syndrome: the role of clinical and polysomnographic variables explaining poor sleep quality in patients. *Sleep Med.* 2015;16(8):917–925.

Fatt SJ, Beilharz JE, Joubert M, et al. Parasympathetic activity is reduced during slow-wave sleep, but not resting wakefulness, in patients with chronic fatigue syndrome. *J Clin Sleep Med.* 2020;16(1):19–28.

Haney E, Smith ME, McDonagh M, et al. Diagnostic methods for myalgic encephalomyelitis/chronic fatigue syndrome: a systematic review for a National Institutes of Health Pathways to Prevention workshop. *Ann Intern Med.* 2015;162(12):834–840.

Jason LA, Kot B, Sunnquist M, et al. Chronic fatigue syndrome and myalgic encephalomyelitis: toward an empirical case definition. *Health Psychol Behav Med.* 2015;3(1):82–93.

Jung Chung Mun, Davis Mary C, Campbell Claudia, Finan Patrick, Howard Tennen. Linking non-restorative sleep and activity interference through pain catastrophizing and pain severity: an intra-day process model among individuals with fibromyalgia. *J Pain.* 2020;21(5-6):546–556.

Liedberg GM, Björk M, Börsbo B. Self-reported nonrestorative sleep in fibromyalgia—relationship to impairments of body functions, personal function factors, and quality of life. *J Pain Res.* 2015;8:499–505.

Maksoud R, Eaton-Fitch N, Matula M, Cabanas H, Staines D, Marshall-Gradisnik S. Systematic review of sleep characteristics in myalgic encephalomyelitis/chronic fatigue syndrome. *Healthcare (Basel).* 2021;9(5):568.

Mantovani E, Mariotto S, Gabbiani D, et al. Chronic fatigue syndrome: an emerging sequela in COVID-19 survivors?. *J Neurovirol.* 2021:1–7. [published online ahead of print, 2021 Aug 2].

Smith ME, Haney E, McDonagh M, et al. Treatment of myalgic encephalomyelitis/chronic fatigue syndrome: a systematic review for a National Institutes of Health Pathways to Prevention workshop. *Ann Intern Med.* 2015;162(12):841–850.

Vijayan S, Klerman EB, Adler GK, Kopell NJ. Thalamic mechanisms underlying alpha-delta sleep with implications for fibromyalgia. *J Neurophysiol.* 2015;114(3):1923–1930.

Wagner JS, DiBonaventura MD, Chandran AB, Cappelleri JC. The association of sleep difficulties with health-related quality of life among patients with fibromyalgia. *BMC Musculoskelet Disord.* 2012;13:199.

Wolfe F, Clauw DJ, Fitzcharles MA, et al. 2016 Revisions to the 2010/2011 fibromyalgia diagnostic criteria. *Semin Arthritis Rheum.* 2016;46(3):319-329.

A complete reference list can be found online at ExpertConsult.com.

Chapter 155

Endocrine Disorders

Neesha Anand; Octavian C. Ioachimescu

Chapter Highlights

- The hypothalamus plays a major role in integrating sleep and various metabolic functions.
- Most hypothalamic and pituitary hormones exert important effects on sleep-wake homeostasis.
- Sleep-disordered breathing is very common in acromegaly (both obstructive and central sleep apnea).
- The association between hypothyroidism and obstructive sleep apnea remains controversial.
- The hypothalamic-pituitary-adrenal axis plays a significant role in stress coping, with major influences on sleep homeostasis.
- Low testosterone levels and obesity play important roles in obstructive sleep apnea.
- Androgens appear to exacerbate obstructive sleep apnea, and there is some evidence of a protective effect of female sex steroids on upper airway patency during sleep.

INTRODUCTION

The endocrine system can be conceptualized as an array of hypothalamus-pituitary-target organ axes, with the target organs being represented by the "effector" endocrine glands (e.g., thyroid, adrenal, gonads, adipose tissue; Figure 155.1). These effects are important in sleep neurobiology because some of these hormones are neuropeptides and may have significant effects. We discuss here mainly the endocrine effects of these hormones, whereas the paracrine, autocrine, and local neuromodulating effects of these factors are beyond the scope of this chapter. We do not address in great detail here the endocrine physiology in relation to sleep or sleep deprivation, which are reviewed thoroughly in Chapter 27. Physical exam findings are reviewed in Chapter 67.

HYPOTHALAMIC DISORDERS AND SLEEP

Since the initial description of encephalitis lethargica or von Economo's "sleepy sickness" because of lesions of the dorsal part of the hypothalamus, and our understanding that lesions of certain anterior hypothalamic areas lead to severe insomnia, the role of hypothalamus in sleep-wake regulation has become more evident. The hypothalamic regions could be damaged by locoregional tumors or their treatment and by inflammatory or infiltrative conditions. Several studies have documented that the suprachiasmatic nucleus, the master circadian pacemaker, and peptidergic cell populations of the lateral hypothalamus (the wake-promoting orexin neurons and the sleep-promoting melanin-concentrating hormone neurons) are targeted by African trypanosomiasis or by human immunodeficiency virus infection.[1]

Damage to the hypothalamus may be associated with a variety of symptoms, including sleepiness, fatigue, and disturbances in the sleep-wake regulatory systems or circadian rhythms. Many case reports or short series illustrate that pathology of the lateral hypothalamus can lead to hypersomnia or narcolepsy, whereas involvement by infiltrative, inflammatory, or neoplastic conditions of the anterior hypothalamus may disrupt the circadian clock of these patients or lead to severe insomnia. Inflammatory infiltrates were also observed in the hypothalamus of two patients who died with Kleine-Levin syndrome.[2,3] Although the exact biochemical changes or hormonal changes occurring in this disorder are still unclear, it is conceivable that an autoimmune insult at the level of the thalamus or the hypothalamus is involved in the pathogenesis. Further, there are data supporting the concept that narcolepsy type 1 is a hypothalamic disorder, mediated entirely or not by hypocretin or orexin and involving not only the sleep-wake frontier but also motor, psychiatric, emotional, cognitive, metabolic, and autonomic functions.[4]

PITUITARY DISORDERS AND SLEEP

The anterior pituitary hormones are part of the following endocrine axes: hypothalmic-pituitary-adrenal (HPA), hypothalmic-pituitary-thyroid (HPT), and hypothalamic-pituitary-gonadal (HPG) as well as somatotropic (hypothalamic-pituitary–growth hormone) and lactotrophic (hypothalamus-pituitary-prolactin) systems. Vasopressin and oxytocin are synthesized and released from posterior hypophysis; they exert many autocrine, paracrine, or neuropeptidergic actions but have less known endocrine effects relevant to sleep or involvement in sleep disorders. Similarly, less is known about the physiologic roles of pituitary adenylate cyclase–activating polypeptide (PACAP), which may be involved in the homeostatic regulation of sleep, possibly in a circadian entraining mechanism via the retinohypothalamic tract or in some pathway involved in the control of respiration.[5-7]

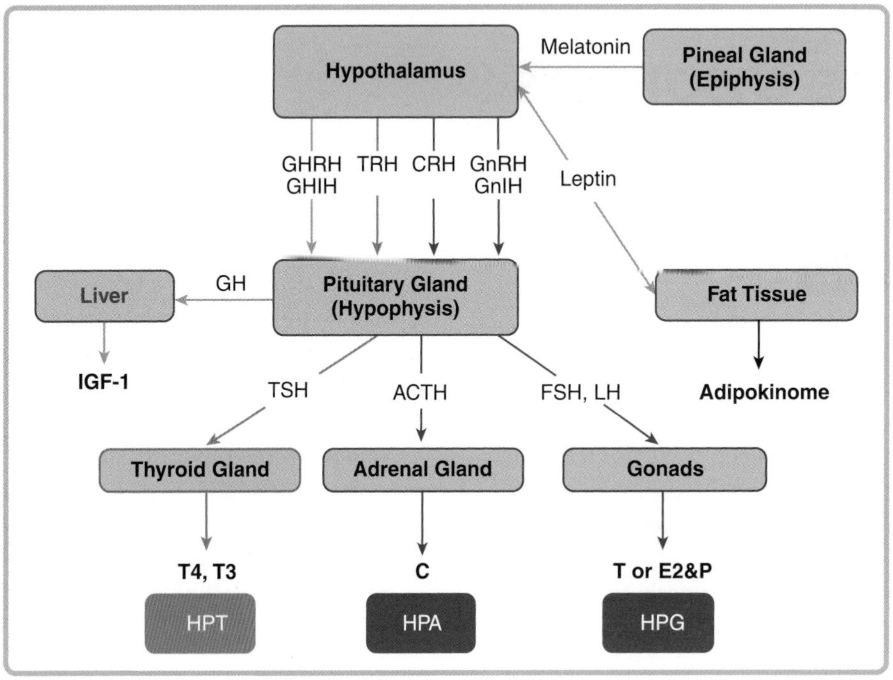

Figure 155.1 Diagram represents the main hypothalamic-pituitary-target gland axes: somatotropic axis (on the left, in *light blue*, via growth hormone [GH], growth hormone–releasing hormone [GHRH], growth hormone–inhibiting hormone [GHIH], and insulin-like growth factor-1 [IGF-1]), hypothalamic-pituitary-thyroid axis (HPT, in *green*, via thyrotropin-releasing hormone [TRH], thyroid-stimulating hormone [TSH], thyroxine [T4], and triiodothyronine [T3]), hypothalamic-pituitary-adrenal axis (HPA, in *dark blue*, via corticotropin-releasing hormone [CRH], adrenocorticotropic hormone [ACTH], and cortisol [C]), and hypothalamic-pituitary-gonadal axis (on the *right*, in *red*, via gonadotropin-releasing hormone [GnRH], gonadotropin-inhibiting hormone [GnIH]; follicle-stimulating hormone [FSH]; luteinizing hormone [LH], and testosterone [T] or estradiol [E2]/progesterone [P]). Additional interactions illustrated here are the interactions between the fat tissue, which secretes adipokines or so-called adipokinome, and the interaction between pineal gland and hypothalamus, via melatonin. Not illustrated here are the negative feedback loops exerted by the effector hormones (IGF-1, T3, C, T, E2/P) on the hypothalamus and the pituitary gland; additionally, for purpose of simplicity, prolactin pathways were omitted.

Growth Hormone–Secreting Tumors (Acromegaly and Gigantism) and Sleep Apnea

The neuroendocrine condition of growth hormone (GH) excess leads to acromegaly in adults and gigantism in children. The GH and insulin-like growth factor-1 (IGF-1) excess lead to acral enlargement, coarse facial features, and growth of the synovial tissues and articular cartilages (with acromegalic arthropathy in up to 75% of cases).[8] Sleep-disordered breathing (SDB) is very common in acromegaly; up to 70% of patients diagnosed with acromegaly have sleep apnea, even after correction for obesity.[9-12] In a study of 53 consecutive referrals of patients with acromegaly, almost all had severe snoring.[13] Thirty-one patients (93%) referred because of suspected SDB had sleep apnea, compared with 12 patients (60%) referred without suspected sleep apnea. Central sleep apnea (CSA) was the predominant type of apnea in 33% of patients.

Excessive daytime sleepiness and fatigue are common symptoms in patients with acromegaly. The currently accepted explanations are represented by coexistent obstructive sleep apnea (OSA; most of the cases), direct effects of GH in promoting sleep (still unclear in humans), effect of prior cranial radiotherapy, coexistent hypogonadism or hypothyroidism, and hypothalamic GH-secreting tumors affecting somnogenic hypothalamic areas (rarely).

The pathophysiologic mechanisms of SDB in acromegaly are still unclear. Several hypotheses have been proposed. OSA may result from macroglossia, hypertrophy of the submaxillary salivary glands, soft tissue thickening (especially of the soft palate and uvula), changes in the bone architecture of the upper airway (dorsocaudal rotation of the mandibular angle or reduced lingual "enclosure"), leading to smaller cross-sectional area and higher collapsibility of the hypopharynx. OSA may also result from altered neuromuscular control of the upper airway, dysfunction of the upper airway dilators such as sternohyoid myopathy, or obesity (if present). A study conducted in the Han and Hani Chinese population suggested an association between specific single-nucleotide polymorphisms in the *GHR* gene and OSA syndrome; rs12518414 genotype frequency was associated with OSA, whereas the A allele frequency was lower in the OSA group compared with controls.[14] The CSA in patients with acromegaly may be the result of abnormalities in the control of breathing that result from left ventricular (systolic or diastolic) dysfunction, central pathways disinhibiting respiratory control, increased response to hypercapnic hypoxic drive, or direct or indirect effects exerted by GH on respiratory control centers.

The presence of OSA may confer additional cardiovascular risk for patients with acromegaly. GH and IGF-1 excess lead to left ventricular hypertrophy, systolic and diastolic myocardial dysfunction and cardiac dysrhythmias, and glucose intolerance and diabetes mellitus. Hypertension is highly prevalent in patients with acromegaly (up to 50% of cases), whereas cardiomyopathy is present in most patients. Hypertension is related to chronic hypervolemia (GH and IGF-1 increase sodium reabsorption by acting directly on the distal tubules epithelial cells' sodium channels),[15] endothelial dysfunction, insulin resistance, or coexistent sleep apnea.[9] Most acromegaly patients die from cardiovascular disease.[16] OSA improves in many patients with acromegaly after GH tumor resection surgery. Nevertheless, prospective studies show that OSA persists in approximately 40% of cases cured of acromegaly, requiring periodic reassessment.[9,17-22]

Growth Hormone–Secreting Tumors and Restless Legs Syndrome

About 21% of patients with acromegaly have restless legs syndrome (RLS) or Willis-Ekbom disease.[23] Patients with active disease had worse acromegaly-related quality of life (QoL), higher severity of RLS symptoms by the International RLS Rating Scale, longer sleep latencies and wake after sleep onset, higher arousal and periodic limb movements during sleep indexes, and worse sleep efficiency.[23] The prevalence of RLS was not correlated with serum GH or IGF-1 levels, and the relationship stood even after exclusion of patients with OSA.[23] Interestingly, Taylor-Gjevre and colleagues[24] showed that the prevalence of RLS was almost as high (24.4%) in patients with osteoarthropathy, a condition frequently associated with acromegaly, so it would be interesting to parse out how many patients with acromegaly with and without osteoarthropathy have RLS.

Prolactin-Secreting Tumors (Prolactinoma)

Prolactinomas are prolactin (PRL)-secreting tumors and account for approximately 40% of pituitary adenomas. In patients with untreated prolactinoma, secondary hypogonadism is the most frequent endocrine abnormality. Patients with prolactinoma spend more time in slow wave sleep (SWS) than healthy controls (on average, 79 versus 37 minutes in controls), whereas REM sleep does not seem to differ between the two groups. The current working hypothesis is that PRL stimulates both SWS and REM sleep, although the exact mechanism is still unclear. These findings are concordant with reports of good sleep quality in patients with prolactinoma and discordant with the abnormal sleep of patients with other endocrinopathies.[25]

Adrenocorticotropic Hormone–Secreting Pituitary Tumors (Cushing Disease)

Excess adrenocorticotropic hormone (ACTH) secretion by pituitary tumors (Cushing disease, most frequently caused by pituitary microadenomas) or ectopically (by extrapituitary ACTH-secreting or corticotropin-releasing hormone [CRH]–secreting tumors such as small cell lung cancer and atypical bronchial carcinoids) presents with manifestations resulting from the systemic effects of hypercortisolism.[26] When nocturnal cortisol secretory profile was analyzed in a group of patients with Cushing disease, adrenal activity was found to start predominantly during periods of non–rapid eye movement (NREM) sleep, similarly to matched healthy controls. Thus, even when the typical pituitary-adrenal axis nocturnal oscillation pattern is lost or blunted (such as in Cushing disease), the link between the endocrine activity and the ultradian rhythmicity of NREM and rapid eye movement (REM) sleep seems to be preserved.[27]

Nonfunctioning and Gonadotropin-Secreting Pituitary Adenomas

Nonfunctioning macroadenomas (NFMAs) are pituitary tumors without systemic hormonal hypersecretion. Several authors reported that patients with resected NFMAs have sleep complaints and circadian alterations, as well as objective PSG or actigraphy changes.[28] In one study, patients with NFMAs had reduced sleep efficiency, less REM sleep, more N1 sleep, and more awakenings in the absence of associated apneas or periodic limb movements (compared with controls). Actigraphy revealed longer rest durations, more awakenings at night, and less activity during the day. Patients with treated NFMAs reported more fatigue and impaired QoL.[29] In another study, Joustra and colleagues[30] found melatonin secretion abnormalities in a significant percentage of patients with NFMAs and pituitary craniopharyngiomas, likely owing to either suprachiasmatic clock abnormalities induced by suprasellar extension or the treatment instituted for the pituitary tumor.

Craniopharyngioma

Large, suprasellar tumors tend to extend micropapillae into surrounding structures, which can cause hypothalamic damage. Similarly, attempted gross total resection can lead to local damage with subsequent hypothalamic obesity, thirst alterations and dysregulation of temperature, visual field defects, panhypopituitarism, sleep-wake disturbance, or increased daytime sleepiness.[31,32] The latter was associated with decreased nocturnal melatonin levels and higher body mass index (BMI); as such, further studies on the possible beneficial effects of melatonin substitution on daytime sleepiness and weight control in these patients are needed. Compared with healthy controls, patients successfully treated for craniopharyngiomas may report impaired QoL, excessive fatigue,[33] increased daytime sleepiness,[26,34,35] or severe sleepiness despite normal sleep patterns.[35,36] In one study,[37] craniopharyngioma patients presented with significantly decreased area-under-the-curve melatonin concentrations compared with healthy controls and with a strong association between low midnight melatonin and reduced total sleep time (TST), reduced time of night sleep, impaired sleep efficiency, and reduced physical activity. Patients with craniopharyngioma were sleepier and more likely to have RLS than control individuals of similar age.[38] All subjects showed normal CSF hypocretin-1 levels.[38]

Growth Hormone Deficiency

Numerous animal[39,40] and human[41-43] studies have showed that growth hormone–releasing hormone (GHRH) has soporific effects, increasing TST and SWS, even in the absence of GH.[39,44] Furthermore, studies in humans[45,46] indicate that GH itself may stimulate REM sleep. Untreated growth hormone deficiency (GHD) of primary pituitary origin, because of the GH negative feedback loop (i.e., lack of GH leads to compensatory increase in GHRH) leads to an enhanced hypothalamic GHRH activity, which could lead in turn to increased sleep pressure and excessive daytime fatigue. The sleep disturbances in GHD may differ according to the origin of the disease, that is, either pituitary (with overactive hypothalamic GHRH neurons) or hypothalamic (with reduced GHRH activity).

Several studies have evaluated sleep in GHD.[47-50] Adults with GHD often complain of fatigue, fatigability, or impaired overall QoL.[51] One study found that patients with GHD had worse QoL scores, with tiredness being the most affected domain, irrespective of etiology. Patients with pituitary GHD spent more time in SWS and had a higher intensity of SWS than their controls. In contrast to pituitary GHD, patients with hypothalamic GHD had lower intensity of SWS than their controls. In the same study, older patients with pituitary GHD had more fragmented sleep and overall less REM sleep.[52] Insufficient REM sleep may in turn be linked to the emergence of memory disturbances.[53,54]

Interestingly, patients with OSA appear to have a relative GH deficiency, which is likely related to hypoxia and abnormal sleep architecture, possibly reversible after continuous positive airway pressure (CPAP) therapy.[55,56] A study by Xu and colleagues[57] suggested that serum GHRH levels in patients with moderate-severe OSA may, in fact, play a protective role for the cognitive function. Contrary to earlier observations, more recent data suggest that GH therapy administered to patients with GHD does not induce or aggravate OSA.[58] Twelve weeks, but not 6 weeks, of CPAP therapy increased IGF-1, with a further increase after 24 weeks. Total and pulsatile GH secretion, secretory burst mass, and pulse frequency were also increased by 12 weeks. Therefore CPAP therapy seemed to improve GH-IGF-1 axis in a time-dependent manner.[59]

Oliveira and colleagues[60] described a cohort of 21 adults with isolated GHD resulting from GHRH resistance caused by a homozygous null mutation in the GHRH receptor gene, and 21 age- and sex-matched controls. The GHD subjects showed polysomnographic evidence of poorer sleep with reduced sleep efficiency, TST, duration of N2 and REM in minutes; increased duration of N1, wake, and wake-time after sleep onset. As such, the authors' conclusion was that GHRH resistance had a significant role in the observed alterations of sleep quality in these subjects.

PINEAL DISORDERS AND SLEEP

The pineal gland is constituted by pinealocytes, which secrete melatonin (derived from serotonin), with important regulatory roles of the circadian and infradian rhythms. The pineal gland melatonin acts on numerous peripheral tissues, in concert with the melatonin in the retina, bone marrow, platelets, and gastrointestinal tract. Although the complete surgical excision of the pineal gland leads to very few endocrine disturbances (which could point toward a vestigial aspect or a nonessential role), pineal pathology may occasionally have some consequences on sleep-wake homeostasis (Table 155.1). Pineal gland tumors are relatively rare but are the most frequent pineal pathology seen in clinical practice. These tumors may lead to signs and symptoms attributable to local mass effect, involvement of adjacent anatomic structures, and rarely endocrine effects.

There are inconsistent data about the effects of hypermelatoninemia or hypomelatoninemia in certain types of tumors. Recent studies show that serum melatonin levels are generally very low or absent (rather than elevated) in both treated and untreated pineal tumors.[61] Nevertheless, two clinical presentations that have been reported in the past deserve to be briefly mentioned here. First, rare cases of pineal tumors can present with clinical manifestations indistinguishable from narcolepsy ("secondary narcolepsy"), although they may also be due to concurrent hypothalamic involvement.[62,63] Second, cases of circadian-timed headaches, excessive daytime fatigue, and severe insomnia have been reported and posited to be related to a pineal endocrine insufficiency because exogenous melatonin administration improved or resolved the presenting clinical symptoms.[64,65]

THYROID DISORDERS

Disturbances of the HPT axis such as altered thyroid function or abnormal thyroid-stimulating hormone (TSH) levels may affect the arousal-promoting system. Overall, the effects of thyroid hormones are more likely activating than soporific. So far, there have been only a few studies that shed light on the association between HPT axis and neural pathways involved in generating or maintaining alertness. Thyrotropin-releasing hormone (TRH) and its receptors are widely distributed in the central nervous system (CNS). Aside from its TSH-releasing effect, TRH exerts many other neuromodulatory actions, including stimulative, antidepressant, and neurotrophic effects. An open-label study[66] examined the effects of a small dose of oral levothyroxine (25 mcg) on sleep and daytime somnolence of nine patients with idiopathic hypersomnia. The authors found that after 4 weeks of levothyroxine administration, TST and hypersomnolence improved significantly, effects that were maintained at 8 weeks. Unfortunately, posttreatment thyroid function testing was not available in most of the subjects.[66] Mechanistically, it is possible that small doses of levothyroxine reduce TSH production or that patients with idiopathic hypersomnia may have intrinsic alteration of the HPT axis.

Hyperthyroidism and Restless Legs Syndrome

Reduced levels of dopamine (DA) in certain areas of the brain seem to play an important role in the pathophysiology of RLS, either as a primary biochemical disturbance or as a secondary condition, as in iron deficiency (because iron is a cofactor for tyrosine hydroxylase, a key enzyme in the synthesis of DA). The DA agonists effectively alleviate RLS symptoms, and they typically are the first line of therapy. Currently, there is an accumulating body of evidence showing that DA may suppress the activity of the HPT axis.[67-69] First, the 24-hour profile of TSH resembles the typical circadian variation in clinical symptoms for RLS patients; levels of TSH increase in the evening, as does the severity of RLS symptoms (interestingly, dopaminergic tone seems also to increase in the evening[68]). Second, DA modulates thyroid hormones by enhancing the biochemical functions of the cytochrome P-450 (CYP-450, heme, and iron containing) liver enzymes that metabolize them and by inhibiting directly the pituitary TSH secretion. In addition, low iron levels diminish the available catalytic units of CYP-450 capable of degrading thyroid hormones.

One interesting theory posits that the main cause of RLS is an imbalance between the dopaminergic system and the HPT axis.[70] This theory stems from several observations: (1) thyroid hormone levels seem to follow DA levels[67,68]; (2) TRH regulates TSH synthesis by stimulating transcription and translation of the TSH β-subunit gene, while DA inhibits this process[71]; (3) antidopaminergic agents (e.g., metoclopramide, neuroleptics) tend to worsen RLS complaints,[72] whereas DA agonists diminish RLS symptoms; (4) reduced levels of iron in the brain diminish the DA system activity, which in turn aggravates RLS; (5) the HPT axis increases its activity during sleep restriction,[73] which could also aggravate RLS; (6) some of the effects of elevated thyroxine

Table 155.1 Main Neuropeptide Hormones in the Central Nervous System with Important Actions on Sleep-Wake Homeostasis

Source	Neuropeptide Hormone	Role in Sleep-Wake Homeostasis	Other Regulatory Roles
Hypothalamus	Hypocretin	Consolidates sleep Suppresses REM sleep	Feeding (+); mood; thermoregulation and energy expenditures; reward
	Melanin-concentrating hormone (MCH)	Promotes sleep	Feeding (+); memory
	Galanin	Promotes NREM sleep Promotes REM sleep	Anxiety; neuroregeneration; pain
	Growth hormone–releasing hormone (GHRH)	Promotes NREM sleep	Growth hormone (GH) release (+)
	Thyrotropin-releasing hormone (TRH)	Promotes wakefulness Inhibits NREM sleep	Feeding (−); energy homeostasis; locomotion
	Corticotropin-releasing hormone (CRH)	Promotes wakefulness Modulates REM sleep	Anxiety; depression; stress
	Cholecystokinin (CCK)	Promotes wakefulness Promotes NREM sleep	Anxiety; feeding (−); pain
	Somatostatin (SST)	Promotes wakefulness Promotes REM sleep Inhibits NREM sleep	GH release (−)
	Corticostatin (CST)	Promotes NREM sleep Inhibits REM sleep	GH release (−); learning; memory; pain (−)
	Brain-derived neurotrophic factor (BDNF)	Promotes NREM sleep (?) Inhibits wakefulness	Feeding (−); synaptic plasticity (+)
	Dynorphin	Promotes NREM sleep	Pain
	Melanocyte-stimulating hormone (MSH)	Promotes NREM sleep (?)	Stress regulation; feeding (−); motivation; pain; reward
	Neuropeptide Y	Modulates both NREM and wakefulness	Feeding (+); anxiety; addiction
	Vasoactive intestinal peptide (VIP)	Promotes REM sleep	Circadian regulation; feeding (−)
Anterior pituitary	GH	Promotes REM sleep Inhibits NREM sleep (?)	Cell growth (anabolic effects)
	Adrenocorticotropic hormone (ACTH)	Promotes wakefulness	Feeding (−); motivation; pain; reward
	Prolactin (PRL)	Promotes REM sleep	Lactation; stress modulation
	Pituitary adenylate cyclase–activating polypeptide (PACAP)	Promotes REM sleep	Circadian regulation; feeding (+); memory; stress; pain
Posterior pituitary	Vasopressin (AVP)	Circadian regulation (present also in the hypothalamus, including suprachiasmatic nucleus)	ACTH secretion (+); thirst and water excretion
	Oxytocin	Circadian regulation (?)	Lactation; anxiety; mood
Pineal gland	Melatonin	Promotes sleep	Circadian regulation; reproduction
Stomach (and hypothalamus)	Ghrelin	Promotes wakefulness	Feeding (+)
Adipose tissue (and hypothalamus)	Leptin	Promotes NREM sleep Promotes wakefulness (?)	Feeding (−); energy expenditure (+); thermogenesis (+)

levels, as seen in hyperthyroidism, resemble some symptoms of RLS; (7) opioids, the first class of drugs used to treat RLS, are also known to depress the HPT axis[74,75]; (8) several drugs known to alleviate RLS symptoms, such as carbamazepine, phenobarbital, and valproic acid, are inducers of CYP-450 system; and (9) conversely, tricyclic antidepressants, antihistaminic agents, selective serotonin reuptake inhibitors, and neuroleptics are CYP-450 inhibitors, and they all have the potential to worsen RLS symptoms.[70] Support of this theory comes from an earlier report of a patient with RLS and hypothyroidism on thyroid replacement therapy, who had a low serum ferritin level (iron deficiency). On successive challenge and withdrawal of L-thyroxine, there was significant worsening in the International Restless Legs Syndrome Study Group (IRLSSG) severity score, periodic limb movement index, and sleep efficiency.[76,77] A study by Tan and colleagues[77] found a strong association between hyperthyroidism and RLS symptoms, despite the fact that the overall prevalence of RLS was very low (0.2%).

Hypothyroidism and Obstructive Sleep Apnea

OSA and hypothyroidism share a few similarities: (1) they are very prevalent disorders, (2) both have subclinical phenotypes that can go on undetected for years, (3) their exact prevalence in a particular population is often unknown and inviting for wrongful extrapolations, (4) both are defined with somewhat fluid diagnostic criteria (e.g., hypopnea definition, apnea-hypopnea index [AHI] threshold, technology employed for diagnosis, TSH assays, threshold for subclinical hypothyroidism), and (5) they have common clinical manifestations and major comorbidities; for all these reasons, clinically they could be very easily confused with each other. For example, OSA is characterized by snoring, excessive daytime sleepiness, fatigue, apathy, frequent headaches, and memory impairments and is often associated with obesity or depression; these manifestations are nonspecific and are frequently seen in hypothyroidism. Furthermore, large goiters can also cause upper airway compression, ventilatory impairment, and possibly OSA.[78,79] Given these considerations, it is not surprising that a number of investigators found these conditions to coexist in 1.2% to 11% of the population studied.[79-81]

The evidence for a relationship between hypothyroidism and OSA has been inconsistent. In one analysis of the US National Health and Nutrition Examination Survey (NHANES), the authors studied 5515 adult subjects newly diagnosed with hypothyroidism and found a significant association between hypothyroidism and sleep apnea, even after adjusting for demographics and BMI.[82] Moreover, Bozkurt and colleagues[83] found that obese women with OSA had higher prevalence of Hashimoto thyroiditis, in parallel with OSA severity. In contrast, a cross-sectional study[84] did not show significant differences on thyroid ultrasonography and found a similar prevalence of Hashimoto thyroiditis in OSA and control groups. Similarly, Bahammam and colleagues[85] failed to detect a significant difference in the prevalence of hypothyroidism in patients with or without a diagnosis of OSA. However, they found subclinical hypothyroidism in 11.1% of patients with OSA compared with 4% in patients without OSA and concluded that subclinical hypothyroidism was more frequent in OSA.[85] Interestingly, a large study showed that, compared with euthyroid patients, those with subclinical hypothyroidism had poorer sleep based on the Pittsburgh Sleep Quality Index, longer sleep latency and shorter sleep duration; younger age, lower BMI, and female sex were independent risk factors for poor sleep quality in subclinical hypothyroidism.[86] However, thyroid replacement therapy of subclinical hypothyroidism did not change prevalence or severity of OSA.[87] Several studies have found similar results and suggest that routine thyroid function testing is not necessary in OSA patients,[81,88,89] whereas others disagree.[90,91]

Sleepiness, obtundation, and ultimately coma seen in advanced myxedema could be the result of either (1) a very reduced rate of basal metabolism, or (2) undiagnosed and untreated hypoxic (and possibly hypercapnic) OSA. Several mechanisms explaining the association between OSA and hypothyroidism have been posited: reduced cross-sectional area of the upper airway resulting from infiltration with mucopolysaccharides and water (e.g., macroglossia), myxedema-related upper airway myopathy, or reduced respiratory drive (as hypothyroidism blunts both hypoxic and hypercapnic ventilatory responses).[92,93] The downstream effects of the respiratory drive blunting on OSA likely vary by disease phenotype. As such, in patients with high loop gain or a tendency for ventilatory overshoot, blunted sensitivity may lead to relative stability of the airway and a decrease in OSA severity[94,95]; similarly, the impact of thyroid replacement therapy on SDB may also vary by phenotype.

The effect of thyroid hormone replacement therapy on OSA coexistent with hypothyroidism has been variable and based on rather small cohorts.[92] One study suggested that OSA was a secondary phenomenon in many of the hypothyroid patients and that it may be reversible.[96] Thyroxine replacement therapy was associated with improvement in macroglossia, myxedema, and facial puffiness, suggesting that changes in upper airway anatomy seen in hypothyroidism may contribute to the development of OSA in these patients. Furthermore, several studies suggested the possibility of a stronger connection between OSA and cardiovascular complications in the initial phase of thyroid hormone replacement therapy because rapid restoration of the euthyroid state in these patients may confer additional cardiovascular risks.[92,97]

In summary, the association between OSA and hypothyroidism is unclear, possibly because hypothyroidism nowadays is diagnosed at a much milder severity than the myxedema observed in earlier investigations.

Hypothyroidism and Restless Legs Syndrome

The relationship between hypothyroidism and RLS is not clear. Banno and colleagues[98] analyzed the comorbidities of RLS and found a trend toward a prior diagnosis of acquired hypothyroidism in female patients with RLS (within 5 years before PSG). Interestingly, women were twice as likely to be on thyroid replacement therapy at the time of evaluation. For some reasons, patients with pulmonary hypertension were found to have a very high prevalence of RLS (43.6%), with moderate to severe symptoms. Among these patients, those with a history of hypothyroidism (67%) and those on opioids for relief of leg pain (69%) were more likely to have RLS.[99] Again, of interest is the fact that most of these patients were on thyroid replacement therapy.

Sleep Quality in Hypothyroidism

Excessive daytime sleepiness and fatigue are frequent symptoms in hypothyroidism. Although at times other sleep disorders (e.g., OSA, RLS) may be the cause of these symptoms, a primary CNS effect is also possible. Marked reductions in SWS have been described in patients with hypothyroidism, which are reversible with thyroid replacement therapy. Increased movements in sleep and reduced REM sleep have been described in patients with congenital hypothyroidism. One study concluded that neither subclinical hypothyroidism nor hyperthyroidism was significantly associated with decreased sleep quality in elderly men.[100]

ADRENAL DISORDERS AND SLEEP

The relationship between OSA and HPA axis activity in humans is unclear. An earlier study[101] looked at cortisol awakening response (CAR) in obese male subjects newly diagnosed with severe OSA compared with obese nonapneic matched

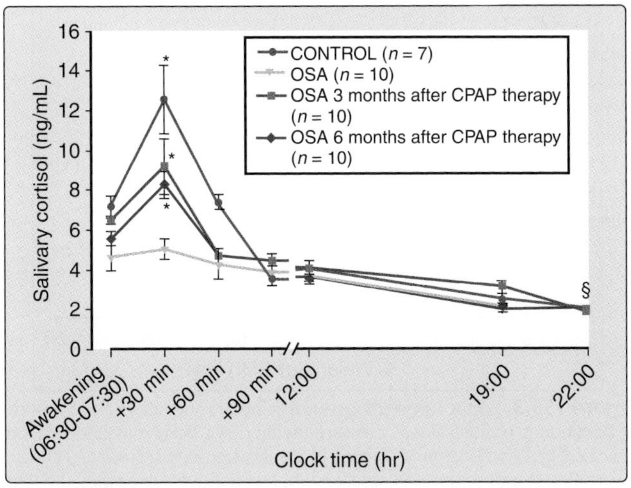

Figure 155.2 Effect of weight loss on testosterone (T) levels, as shown in different studies. Each *circle* represents a study, and its diameter is directly proportional to the study size. (From Fui MN, Dupuis P, Grossmann M. Lowered testosterone in male obesity: mechanisms, morbidity and management. *Asian J Androl.* 2014;16[2]:223–31, which was modified after Grossmann M. Low testosterone in men with type 2 diabetes: significance and treatment. *J Clin Endocrinol Metab.* 2011;96[8]:2341–53, Figure 155.1. Copyright of Endocrine Society, *The Journal of Clinical Endocrinology & Metabolism.*)

controls and found the following: (1) a flattening of the CAR in OSA, (2) lower levels of cortisol at awakening in patients with OSA, (3) preserved circadian activity of the HPA axis, (4) that 3 to 6 months of CPAP therapy led to significant restoration of the sleep architecture and the pattern of CAR (Figure 155.2),[101] and (5) CPAP therapy reduced the morning cortisol differences between patients with OSA and controls. In summary, the authors found a significant dysregulation of HPA axis activity in adult patients with OSA, as shown by the flattening of the diurnal pattern of cortisol production, seen mostly in the first hour after awakening, which was restored after 3 or 6 months of CPAP therapy.[101] Later, the same investigators[102] characterized the diurnal variations of salivary free testosterone, free cortisol, and their ratio in 10 subjects newly diagnosed with OSA and 7 matched controls. The main finding was that OSA subjects displayed hypocortisolism upon awakening and a significant reduction in testosterone concentration in the evening versus controls. The OSA subjects had higher free testosterone: free cortisol ratios in the morning and significantly lower ratios in the evening versus controls. Others did not find significant differences in the total and free testosterone levels between normal sleepers without SDB and three subtypes of OSA.[103] However, the authors suggested that there was an association between HPA axis activity in patients with severe OSA but not in the mild and moderate disease subtypes. The results showed significantly higher levels of cortisol in the severe OSA group as compared with normal sleepers and mild or moderate OSA. In addition, the testosterone:cortisol ratio was significantly lower in the severe OSA group compared with moderate OSA. In addition, a negative correlation was observed between minimal SpO_2 and AHI, and a positive correlation between cortisol and AHI.[103]

Cushing Syndrome

Patients with Cushing syndrome (CS) typically have truncal or central obesity, diabetes mellitus, hypertension, androgenic hirsutism, psychiatric manifestations such as depression, and cognitive impairments. Most of these patients also have sleep complaints and sleep disorders. SDB appears to be common in patients with CS. In one study 32% of patients had at least mild sleep apnea.[104] Considerable snoring and obesity were found in both apneic and nonapneic patients. Nonapneic patients with Cushing disease differed strikingly from healthy volunteers, having lighter and more fragmented sleep.[104] A large longitudinal study found that patients with CS were associated with an increased likelihood of OSA.[105] Patients with CS had a 2.82-fold higher risk of developing OSA later in life. Serum cortisol was found to be an independent predictor of AHI after controlling for BMI and Homeostatic Model Assessment for insulin resistance score.[106]

Specific polysomnographic features of sleep have been described in patients with CS. In a study of patients with pituitary ACTH-dependent Cushing disease or ACTH-independent CS, patients with major depressive disorder, and normal healthy controls, there were substantial PSG similarities: All three patient groups demonstrated poorer sleep continuity, shorter REM latency, and increased first REM period density compared with normal subjects.[107] Furthermore, patients with ACTH-independent CS and major depressive disorder had elevated REM activity and density.

Adrenal Insufficiency

Adrenal insufficiency is caused by primary adrenal dysfunction (Addison disease, characterized by both mineralocorticoid and glucocorticoid secretion insufficiency and increased ACTH) or secondary adrenal dysfunction (i.e., a hypothalamic or pituitary dysfunction resulting in reduced cortisol levels but normal levels of mineralocorticoids). Very few systematic assessments of sleep have been done in patients with untreated Addison disease. One single-center, cross-sectional study[108] found that fatigue was a frequent complaint in patients with adrenal insufficiency (between 41% and 50% of patients, depending on the etiology) and that fatigue is influenced by the cortisol levels; additionally, salivary cortisol levels were not correlated with the instantaneous fatigue. Acute administration of exogenous cortisol can improve the daytime fatigue significantly not only in patients with Addison disease but also in healthy women.[109]

SEX HORMONE DISORDERS AND SLEEP

Testosterone in Sleep Restriction

Impaired sleep quality, reduced TST, circadian rhythm disruptions, and SDB may be associated with reduced testosterone levels. (See Chapter 27 for discussion on the role of sex hormones on sleep in men.) Although studies confirm the effect of total sleep deprivation[110,111] on lower testosterone, data on the effect of sleep restriction on the hypothalamus-pituitary-gonadal (HPG) axis remain somewhat contradictory. The effect of sleep deprivation on testosterone levels seems to be age dependent[112]; other factors explaining discrepancies in the literature may be confounding factors, such as time of the day spent asleep,[110,113] circadian shifts, changes in sex hormone–binding globulin (SHBG) levels, circadian rhythm disruptions, stress, depression, medications, and methodologies used (e.g., self-reported versus objective TST). For example, although the physiology described previously suggests that it is the first 3 to 4 hours of sleep that are critical to determining the increase in testosterone, a study has shown that partial sleep restriction to 4½ hours was associated with a lower morning testosterone level when sleep was permitted in the first half rather than the second half of the night.[110] This was not unexpected because testosterone levels have been shown to decrease with increasing time awake.[114] One study showed a marked reduction (10% to 15%) in circulating testosterone levels in young healthy men after 8 days of partial sleep restriction of 5 hours per day (00:30 to 05:30 hours)[115]; in this study, SHBG levels were not measured. In a subsequent study in which sleep was restricted during the first part of the night and permitted from 04:00 to 08:00 hours for 5 nights, there was no significant change in testosterone levels, whereas SHBG decreased.[116] Similarly, serum concentrations of testosterone, luteinizing hormone, and PRL were reduced after only 24 to 48 hours of total sleep deprivation.[117-119] Patel and colleagues[120] studied a large cohort of men (as part of NHANES), demonstrating again that older age, impaired sleep, and higher weight were associated with low testosterone: serum levels decreased by 0.49 ng/dL per year of age, by 5.85 ng/dL per hour of sleep loss, and by 6.18 ng/dL per unit of body mass index (BMI, kg/m^2) increase. Further, nonstandard shift workers with shift-work sleep disorder (SWSD) had worse hypogonadal symptoms and lower testosterone levels than daytime workers and nonstandard workers without SWSD, suggesting again that poor quality sleep and circadian rhythm disruption have a reciprocal relationship with testosterone levels.[121]

Sleep Apnea Effects on Testosterone

Low testosterone levels have been reported in men with OSA,[55] and this appeared to be independent of age, degree of obesity, and presence of awake hypoxemia or hypercapnia. Subsequently, in a study of 89 obese men (BMI ≥ 35 kg/m^2), the severity of OSA was inversely correlated with the free testosterone levels, even after correction for age and BMI.[122] In a case-control study of 15 men with OSA and 15 matched controls, both total and free testosterone levels were lower in patients with OSA, and testosterone was inversely correlated with the OSA severity, as defined by the oxygen desaturation index (ODI), and independent of obesity.[123] Triglyceride and uric acid levels were also significantly higher in patients with OSA. A negative correlation between testosterone and uric acid levels and a positive correlation between testosterone and high-density lipoprotein cholesterol levels were also found, independent of BMI and waist circumference. This study suggested that, in patients with obesity and OSA, the severity of hypoxia during sleep may be an additional contributing factor to reduced testosterone levels, regardless of BMI or central obesity. A similar association between hypoxia and reduced testosterone has also been shown in nonobese men with OSA.[124] In addition to hypoxia, sleep fragmentation may contribute to reduced testosterone levels.[125] Conversely, there is a body of literature that supports the idea that the age-related decline in testosterone in men with OSA is primarily related to obesity.[126-128] Moreover, weight loss has shown to result in an increase in plasma total testosterone levels in obese men[129,130] (Figure 155.3).

Although older data suggested that treatment of OSA by CPAP therapy or uvulopalatopharyngoplasty results in increases in morning plasma testosterone levels at 3 months,[55,131] most studies[56,132,133] showed that CPAP therapy used for a single night[134] or up to an average of 10 months[135] is generally without effects on follicle-stimulating hormone,

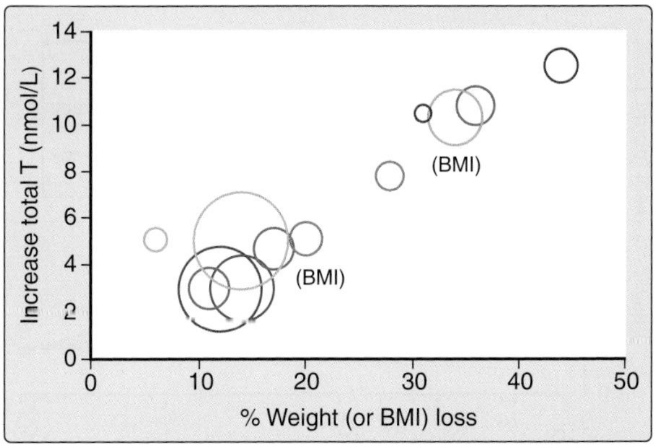

Figure 155.3 Cortisol awakening response before and after 3 and 6 months of continuous positive airway pressure therapy. BMI, Body mass index. (From Ghiciuc CM, Dima Cozma LC, Bercea RM, et al. Restoring the salivary cortisol awakening response through nasal continuous positive airway pressure therapy in obstructive sleep apnea. *Chronobiol Int.* 2013;30[8]:1024–31. Copyright Informa Healthcare USA, Inc.)

luteinizing hormone, or testosterone, even when good compliance is ensured. Madaeva and colleagues monitored the effect of CPAP therapy on spontaneous nocturnal erections in men with age-related androgen deficiency and disruptive pattern of nocturnal penile tumescences (NPT). The study found that not only did CPAP therapy produce a rebound of SWS and "fast-sleep phase" but it also resulted in NPT recovery.[136] However, as noted in previous studies, there was not a significant change in testosterone levels with CPAP therapy.[136] Cignarelli and colleagues[137] conducted a systematic review and meta-analysis to evaluate the effects of CPAP on testosterone and gonadotropins in male patients with OSA. The authors found that, out of 10 prospective cohort and 2 randomized controlled studies (for a total of 388 patients), CPAP use was not associated with a significant change in total testosterone levels. Therefore OSA may not have a direct effect on testosterone levels. Although CPAP therapy has not shown to consistently increase testosterone levels, weight loss does so in a linear fashion.

Testosterone Effects on Sleep Apnea

A number of reports have described the development of OSA after testosterone therapy in both sexes, although these reports or small studies used mainly supraphysiologic doses of intramuscular testosterone.[138-140] Although the evidence is still rather anecdotal, exogenous testosterone administration has been considered deleterious enough in OSA that clinical guidelines contraindicate the therapy in the presence of untreated OSA.[141,142] In a study of obese men with OSA, testosterone undecanoate versus placebo was administered intramuscularly at baseline, at 6 weeks, and at 12 weeks. The authors used the modified Duffin rebreathing method in isohyperoxic and isohypoxic conditions and assessed the changes in minute ventilation versus CO_2 concentrations or $PaCO_2$.[143,144] Testosterone administration was associated with a slightly worse ODI at 7 weeks, but not at 18 weeks. There were no correlations between ODI and testosterone levels,[145] but positive correlations were noted between changes in serum testosterone and hyperoxic ventilatory recruitment threshold and hypoxic burden at 6 to 7 weeks, but not at 18 weeks.[146] The authors suggested that time-dependent alterations in ventilatory recruitment threshold may mediate the changes in respiration during sleep observed with testosterone. In summary, according to the current evidence and apart from transient adverse effects, testosterone treatment at normal doses may not lead to SDB.

Testosterone and Sleep Quality

Both insufficient and excessive testosterone levels have been shown to affect sleep architecture. In men aged 65 years or older, those with lower testosterone levels had reduced sleep efficiency, increased nocturnal awakenings, and less time in SWS.[128] The administration of testosterone and the abuse of androgenic or anabolic steroids have been reported to be associated with reduced TST, insomnia, and increased awakenings.[138,147,148] Administered acutely, methyltestosterone increases arousal and diminishes sleep changes attributed to activation of the brain serotonergic system.[149] In a study of patients with drug-induced hypogonadism[150] with and without gonadal steroid replacement, hypogonadal males had reduced 24-hour PRL levels and a reduced percentage of deep sleep in the hypogonadal state compared with those receiving testosterone replacement. Melatonin secretion was found to be increased in male patients with GnRH deficiency and in low-testosterone hypergonadotropic hypogonadal patients.[151]

Sex Hormones and Sleep-Disordered Breathing in Women

Lower estradiol levels have been associated with poor sleep quality in 45- to 49-year-old women.[152] Sleep disruption during pregnancy and after birth is well recognized, and menopause is often associated with insomnia (see Chapter 159). The latter is likely related to several factors, including hot flashes, mood disorders, and development or worsening of SDB, in parallel with a higher propensity to have central or android obesity (versus gynoid) type.[153]

Estrogens and progesterone seem to be protective factors against development of OSA in women, thus explaining some of the sex-based differences in disease prevalence and severity. The evidence comes from studies in which sleep was evaluated during different phases of the menstrual cycle,[154,155] menopause,[156] hormone replacement therapy (postmenopausally),[156] or pregnancy.[157,158] Some authors found that upper airway resistance is lower during the luteal compared with follicular phase.[154] Progesterone is thought to promote its effects through direct stimulation of respiratory drive by increased ventilatory responses to hypercapnea and hypoxia[159,160] and by enhancing upper airway dilator muscle activity[161] (and consequently, reduced upper airway resistance).

Lower estradiol levels have been associated not only with abnormal sleep architecture but also with a higher severity of OSA across a broader age spectrum (24- to 72-year-old women).[155] Conversely, postmenopausal subjects who received estrogen replacement therapy seem to have less severe SDB compared with those taking placebo.[156,162] Currently it is still unclear whether hormonal therapy has an advantageous risk-to-benefit ratio for SDB in women.[163,164] Similarly, although progesterone levels fall after menopause, no consistent therapeutic effect of progesterone administration in OSA has been demonstrated[163] (Table 155.2).

Androgens could also explain the observed sex-based dimorphisms in sleep architecture and SDB severity. O'Connor and colleagues[165] performed a retrospective analysis of 830 patients with PSG-diagnosed OSA and found that the total AHI was significantly higher in men compared with women. However, women with SDB tended to have more frequent respiratory events during REM sleep compared with men and to have a higher prevalence of OSA that occurs mostly in REM sleep. Koo and colleagues[166] also found among 221 subjects, REM-related SDB was more prevalent in women than men and more prevalent in younger individuals of both sexes, suggesting that differences may depend also on age (or duration of OSA).

Several studies showed that testosterone influences both neural control of breathing[167] and upper airway mechanics.[139] For example, Zhou and colleagues[168] examined the effect of transdermal testosterone (5 mg/day, administered during the follicular phase of the menstrual cycle) on hypocapnic apneic threshold during sleep in eight healthy premenopausal women. The authors concluded that testosterone increases hypocapnic apneic threshold in premenopausal women, thus leading to breathing instability during sleep.

Sleep and Polycystic Ovary Syndrome

Polycystic ovary syndrome (PCOS) affects up to 10% of women of reproductive age and of all ethnic extractions, making it the most common endocrine disorder of women in this age group. PCOS is defined by four components: oligomenorrhea, clinical and biologic features of hyperandrogenism, polycystic ovaries by ultrasonography, and exclusion of other causes of androgen excess.

Several studies showed that PCOS is strongly associated with increased central adiposity and with OSA, in direct relationship with the degree of androgen excess.[169-173] Patients with PCOS are olig ovulatory or anovulatory (by definition); thus they have low circulating levels of progesterone, which may contribute to the high prevalence of SDB in this condition. Furthermore, studies in adults with PCOS have found various strengths of association between PSG measurements and serum androgens and parameters of glucose metabolism. For example, the AHI of obese PCOS patients correlated with total and free testosterone levels.[169] However, others[172] found a correlation between the risk for or severity of SDB and insulin levels or other measures of glucose tolerance. The strongest risk factor for OSA in women with PCOS was fasting insulin levels and glucose-to-insulin ratio, a measure of insulin resistance.[170] In addition, there is a difference in circadian melatonin rhythms between obese adolescent participants with PCOS and controls. Girls with PCOS had later clock-hour of melatonin offset, later melatonin offset relative to sleep timing, and longer duration of melatonin secretion than control subjects, even after adjusting for age, activity level, and BMI.[174]

ADIPOSE TISSUE

The adipose tissue represents one of the largest and most active endocrine organs, known to be secreting a plethora of hormones. White adipocytes are secretory cells, releasing lipid products such as fatty acids resulting from lipolysis, cholesterol, prostaglandins, endocannabinoids, fat-soluble vitamins such as alpha-tocopherol and active form of vitamin D_3, glucocorticoids (converting cortisone to cortisol), estrogens, and others. Several major protein hormones are

Table 155.2 Known Associations between Neuroendocrine Abnormalities and Major Sleep Conditions

Sleep Disorder/ Endocrine Abnormality Associated	Somatotropic Axis	HPT Axis	HPA Axis	HPG Axis	Other
OSA	Reduced GH and IGF-1 levels (correlated with severity of SDB)	Controversial (hypothyroidism is a risk factor for OSA)	Unclear (exaggerated response of corticotrophs to CRH, not explained by obesity alone)	Low testosterone (males), elevated androgens, and reduced progesterone (females) are risk factors for OSA (obesity is a confounder)	Increased sympathetic activity, changes in adipokinome (increased leptin, leptin resistance, decreased adiponectin), decreased hypocretin, higher incidence of diabetes mellitus, hyperinsulinemia, and metabolic syndrome Activated RAAS
Insomnia	Unclear	Hyperthyroidism	Hypercortisolism	In perimenopausal women: reduced sleep quality, sleep maintenance insomnia ("hot flashes") Abnormal CAR?	Unclear
RLS	Acromegaly patients have higher rates of RLS	Hyperthyroidism and hormone replacement for hypothyroidism are associated with RLS	Unclear	Unclear	Unclear

CAR, Cortisol awakening response; CRH, corticotropin-releasing hormone; GH, growth hormone; HPA, hypothalamic-pituitary-adrenal; HPG, hypothalamic-pituitary-gonadal; HPT, hypothalamic-pituitary-thyroid; IGF-1, insulin-like growth factor-1; OSA, obstructive sleep apnea; RAAS, renin-angiotensin-aldosterone system; RLS, restless legs syndrome; SDB, sleep-disordered breathing.

synthesized and secreted by adipocytes, the most prominent of which are leptin and adiponectin, which are produced primarily (not exclusively) in the fat cells. The circulating level of leptin is generally directly related to the body mass or the amount of fat; by contrast, circulating adiponectin levels are reduced in obesity. Leptin is involved in regulation of appetite, angiogenesis, and insulin secretion, whereas adiponectin is mainly insulin sensitizing, antiinflammatory and proangiogenic.

Obesity and Sleep

In obesity, secretion of a number of adipokines is dysregulated and associated with fat tissue inflammation and with several obesity-associated complications (versus pure surrogate, "innocent bystander" biomarkers). There is a solid body of literature showing that, as obesity worsens and fat tissue grows disproportionately to its vascular supply, local hypoxia develops, and other downstream biologic changes converge to generate more robust local and systemic inflammation (Figure 155.4).

The relationship between quantity of sleep (TST) and obesity has been extensively examined.[175-182] Most of the studies found a significant association between obesity and short sleep in children and some even in adults (although the latter was weaker).

To date, there are few studies on the relationship between sleep quality and obesity. One study[182] examined the link between obesity and three sleep characteristics (duration, quality, and stability) in a family medicine setting. The authors found significant associations between sleep quality, duration or bedtime stability, and obesity. The association between sleep quality and obesity was negative and linear, while the association between sleep duration and obesity was U-shaped (as seen in multiple other studies). Less stable bedtimes during the week (OR = 2.3) or on weekends (OR = 1.8) were also associated with obesity. The association between sleep quality and obesity was not explained by patient demographics or snoring.[182]

What is the pathogenic connection between obesity and poor-quality or short sleep? First, short sleep, poor-quality sleep, or unstable bedtimes may provide more opportunities to eat and could activate downstream a metabolic cascade that increases appetite, reduces satiety, and worsens the fatigue, leading to adverse behavioral changes (e.g., curtailed levels of exercise, increased intake of hypercaloric, concentrated sweets) and more fat mass deposition. Conversely, obesity is an inflammatory condition that leads to release of biologically active cytokines, which could activate the HPA axis, with subsequent reduced TST or impaired sleep quality, which perpetuates this vicious cycle.

Indeed, both TST reduction (with preserved SWS) and SWS suppression (with normal TST) have been linked to insulin resistance (without compensatory hyperinsulinemia), resulting in impaired glucose tolerance and increased risk for developing type 2 diabetes mellitus. Furthermore, sleep restriction is also associated with decreased serum leptin (an anorexigenic hormone) levels and increased levels of ghrelin

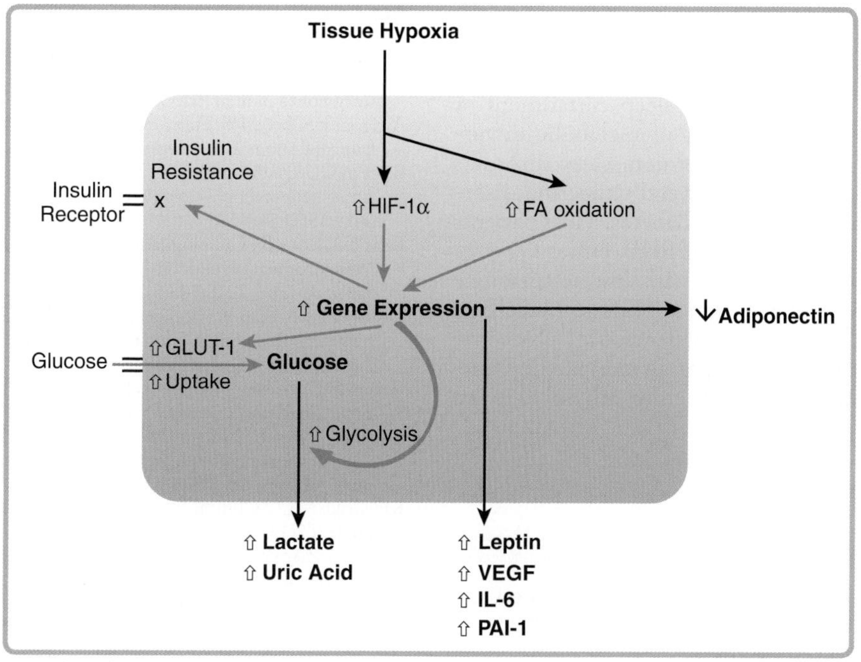

Figure 155.4 Diagram illustrates the effects of intermittent hypoxia at the level of a white adipocyte: activated transcription factor (hypoxia-induced factor-1α [HIF-1α]) leads to expression of more than 1000 genes; fatty acid (FA) oxidation in the mitochondria; increased glucose uptake through the cell membrane, mainly resulting from increased availability of glucose transporter-1 (GLUT-1); blocking of the insulin receptor, with subsequent insulin resistance; and activation of the glycolysis, which leads to increased production of lactate, which will be released into the circulation. In terms of adipokines, low oxygen tension at the level of the adipose cell leads to reduced adiponectin and increased leptin, vascular endothelial growth factor (VEGF), and plasminogen activator inhibitor-1 (PAI-1).

(orexigenic), hunger, exacerbated appetite, and craving for hypercaloric foods. Further evidence suggests that reduced TST may represent a permissive environment for the activation of multiple genes that may be involved in the development of obesity. Indeed, the heritability of BMI is higher in short sleepers. Therefore it is conceivable that chronic and progressive sleep curtailment seen so often in modern Western society could contribute to the current obesity, diabetes, and metabolic syndrome epidemics seen in both adults and children.

Besides the general link between obesity and sleep, central, android-type obesity is also a powerful and consistent epidemiologic predictor of OSA.[183,184] Conversely, significant weight loss leads to improvement in SDB severity and associated metabolic abnormalities.[185] Because association does not necessarily mean causality, the reverse is also possible, that is, that OSA promotes the development of obesity. Although the data are limited for the latter directionality,[185] several mechanisms are possible. For example, chronic intermittent hypoxia and sleep fragmentation of SDB could alter the central control of energy regulation and general metabolism (e.g., trough-altered serotonergic activity in the hypothalamus[185] through leptin, insulin resistance, or hyperinsulinemia) and increase appetite and oral intake. As such, selective serotoninergic agonists and antagonists have been tried as treatments for central obesity[184] and for OSA, but with limited effects.[186] The low circulating testosterone and GH levels noted in OSA also seem to occur in some patients with central obesity.[55,184] In obesity, recombinant GH administration appears to reduce central body fat, whereas CPAP therapy for OSA may restore the GH secretion during sleep.[187] If, indeed, OSA causes central obesity, it would be expected that treatments that reverse SDB result in weight loss. Some studies of patients with OSA suggested that CPAP therapy reduces visceral fat mass, even without significant changes in BMI,[187,188] but large, controlled, and randomized studies specifically addressing this issue are lacking. As mentioned previously, central obesity is also associated with hyperinsulinemia and insulin resistance, but their exact links with OSA are still under investigation. Hyperinsulinemia has been found in patients with OSA, independent of weight, BMI, or central type of obesity.[189] Nevertheless, the questions of whether and to what extent CPAP improves insulin resistance or diabetes control remain controversial. Further discussion on the interrelationships between obesity, diabetes, or metabolic syndrome and SDB can be found in Chapters 26 and 114.

Both OSA and obesity are associated with poor quality sleep. Kim and colleagues[190] demonstrated that sleep quality in patients with OSA was significantly affected by the degree of obesity (negative correlation), but not by the severity of OSA. Another recent study investigating the impact of obesity on cognitive function and memory impairment in patients with moderate-to-severe OSA found that obese patients had delayed reaction times during psychomotor vigilance testing and decreased working memory as compared to nonobese patients with OSA, suggesting again a correlation between obesity and memory or other cognitive domains, independent of SDB.[191] Therefore weight-loss management should also be emphasized to improve quality of sleep and memory/cognition in addition to reducing severity of OSA.

SUMMARY

In a general conceptual framework, sleep is under both neural and hormonal control. The neural control is exerted via a complex network of nuclei or neuronal groups that highly interconnected and multifunctional, whereas hormones exert many autocrine, paracrine, or endocrine effects. There is a strong connection between sleep and metabolic processes.

Disorders of the hypothalamus-pituitary-target organ axes frequently present with sleep symptoms and occasionally with frank comorbid sleep disorders. Accumulating evidence suggests an important role played by sleep curtailment or specific disorders in the pathogenesis of metabolic disturbances associated with obesity. Furthermore, sleep disorders such as OSA are very common in several endocrine disorders, such as acromegaly, obesity, and diabetes. Most patients with acromegaly have some degree of SDB, either OSA or CSA. OSA seems to be associated with low testosterone levels, while androgen administration appears to exacerbate OSA. Furthermore, there is some evidence of a protective effect of female sex steroids on upper airway patency during sleep. It is still controversial whether hypothyroidism is a distinct risk factor for SDB.

CLINICAL PEARLS

- Endocrine derangements may lead to or are associated with hypersomnia, OSA, RLS, insomnia, circadian disorders, and other sleep disorders.
- Endogenous or exogenous excess of GH, cortisol, or androgens may predispose to development of OSA.
- Excess of catecholamines, cortisol, or thyroxine is associated with insomnia.
- OSA may be associated with low testosterone (direct effect or mediated by aging, obesity, fragmented sleep, and intermittent hypoxia).
- Adipose tissue is one of the largest and most active endocrine gland and secretes a very complex set of factors that constitute the "adipokinome."

SELECTED READINGS

Akatsu H, Ewing SK, Stefanick ML, et al. Association between thyroid function and objective and subjective sleep quality in older men: the osteoporotic fractures in men (MrOS) Study. *Endocr Pract.* 2014;20(6):576–586.

Arrigoni E, Chee MJS, Fuller PM. To eat or to sleep: that is a lateral hypothalamic question. *Neuropharmacology.* 2019;154:34–49.

Bassetti CLA, Adamantidis A, Burdakov D, et al. Narcolepsy - clinical spectrum, aetiopathophysiology, diagnosis and treatment. *Nat Rev Neurol.* 2019;15(9):519–539.

Bhasin S, Brito JP, Cunningham GR, et al. Testosterone therapy in men with hypogonadism: an endocrine society clinical practice guideline. *J Clin Endocrinol Metab.* 2018;103(5):1715–1744.

Giustina A, Barkan A, Beckers A, et al. A consensus on the diagnosis and treatment of acromegaly comorbidities: an update. *J Clin Endocrinol Metab.* 2019.

Green ME, Bernet V, Cheung J. Thyroid dysfunction and sleep disorders. *Front Endocrinol (Lausanne).* 2021;12:725829.

Kahal H, Kyrou I, Uthman OA, et al. The prevalence of obstructive sleep apnoea in women with polycystic ovary syndrome: a systematic review and meta-analysis. *Sleep Breath.* 2020;24(1):339–350.

Klibanski A. Clinical practice: prolactinomas. *N Engl J Med.* 2010;362(13):1219–1226.

Massumi RA, Winnacker JL. Severe depression of the respiratory center in myxedema. *Am J Med.* 1964;36:876–882.

McGinty DJ, Sterman MB. Sleep suppression after basal forebrain lesions in the cat. *Science.* 1968;160(3833):1253–1255.

Melmed S, Casanueva FF, Klibanski A, et al. A consensus on the diagnosis and treatment of acromegaly complications. *Pituitary.* 2013;16(3):294–302.

Richter C, Woods IG, Schier AF. Neuropeptidergic control of sleep and wakefulness. *Annu Rev Neurosci.* 2014;37:503–531.

Tesoriero C, Del Gallo F, Bentivoglio M. Sleep and brain infections. *Brain Res Bull.* 2019;145:59–74.

Young T, Finn L, Austin D, Peterson A. Menopausal status and sleep-disordered breathing in the Wisconsin Sleep Cohort Study. *Am J Respir Crit Care Med.* 2003;167(9):1181–1185.

A complete reference list can be found online at ExpertConsult.com.

Chapter 156

Pain and Sleep

Anthony G. Doufas; Elissaios Karageorgiou

Chapter Highlights

- Chronic pain and poor sleep hygiene are major public health challenges with great economic and societal impact. Pain disturbs sleep, and recent evidence from longitudinal cohorts indicates that impaired sleep may in turn promote and/or exacerbate chronic pain.
- Experimental and epidemiologic evidence supports a bidirectional relationship between pain and common pain-related comorbidities, such as insomnia and mood disorders, in patients with chronic pain. This chapter presents current evidence regarding potential mechanisms mediating the development and maintenance of this interactive nexus of comorbidities in patients suffering from chronic pain and sleep disorders.
- A diligent diagnostic approach is considered essential to comprehensively manage patients with chronic pain and comorbid insomnia. The chapter describes sleep assessment instruments that are in wide use in clinical and research practice in both pain and sleep medicine.
- Evidence from randomized controlled trials provides support for comprehensive, multimodal management of the patient comorbidities associated with chronic pain, including insomnia and depression. This chapter examines recent evidence for the effectiveness of modern pharmacologic and cognitive behavioral therapies in the treatment of chronic pain patients.

Sleep and pain are critical processes of life with great biologic and evolutionary value. In the normal state, pain perception and sleep regulation operate via a sensitive and well-orchestrated physiologic balance, which primarily serves to protect sleep function. When pain is excessive or deregulated, it disturbs sleep and diminishes its capacity to provide the necessary physiologic and mental homeostatic recovery for the individual. Although a comprehensive physiologic link between sleep and pain remains elusive, clinical and experimental evidence supports a bidirectional, dynamic influence between the two. Steadily accumulating evidence from observational microlongitudinal and macrolongitudinal studies, as well as randomized controlled interventions, suggests that inadequate or disrupted sleep may exacerbate an existing pain condition or mediate the development of a new pain condition, which in turn may worsen sleep disturbance.

EPIDEMIOLOGY OF PAIN AND COMORBID SLEEP DISORDERS

Chronic pain and impaired sleep are two major, yet unmet, public health challenges that are associated with enormous economic and societal cost because of their sheer prevalence and significant impact on morbidity.[1–5] According to the 2016 National Health Interview Survey, chronic pain affects approximately 50 million US adults (20.4%), and high-impact chronic pain (i.e., interfering with work or life most days or every day) affects approximately 19.6 million US adults (8%).[6] On the other hand, the 2015 Sleep in America Poll showed that a large fraction of the US adults who suffer from chronic pain reported a significant impact of the latter on their daily activities (46%) or mood (55%).[7,8] International large population surveys have estimated similar 1-year prevalence for chronic pain conditions (up to 40%) in both developed and developing countries, with joint-related (17.5%) and low back (18.5%) pain being the most frequent.[9] Large epidemiologic cross-sectional observations in general and clinical populations suggest a close connection between impaired sleep, physical pain, and mood disturbances, such as anxiety and depression disorder.

Community-based studies estimate that greater than 40% of people who suffer from chronic insomnia do so in the context of physical pain,[10] whereas moderate to severe sleep disturbances and comorbid depression occur in up to 80% of patients with chronic pain.[11–13] Although cross-sectional studies are important in characterizing the various morbidity phenotypes in patients suffering from chronic pain and disturbed sleep,[14] they cannot shed light in the causal mechanisms underlying the commonly observed associations. Instead, longitudinal observational cohorts are better fit to evaluate potential causal factors or modifiers of the relationship between sleep, pain, and mood dysfunction in patients suffering from chronic pain.

Insomnia as a Risk Factor for Chronic Pain

Evidence from large prospective longitudinal studies (Table 156.1), with follow-up periods ranging from 1 to 13 years, have demonstrated that disturbed sleep in pain-free subjects could

Table 156.1 Prospective Longitudinal Studies Evaluating the Relationship between Impaired Sleep and Pain[a]

Baseline Condition	Author	Population	Follow-up	Sleep Metrics	Pain Condition	Pain Metrics	Outcome	Results
Impaired sleep	Cavinet et al., 2008[15]	Middle-aged healthy population (N = 3767)	1 yr	Insomnia questionnaire (4-item)	Musculoskeletal pain	Frequency of pain symptoms	New-onset pain	For men: adjusted OR, 1.8; 95% CI, 1.2–2.9; for women: adjusted OR, 1.9; 95% CI, 1.3–2.8
	Odegard et al., 2011[21]	Headache-free population (HUNT-2 and HUNT-3, N = 15,060)	11 yr	Sleep onset and terminal insomnia (composite score)	Headache (all types)	ICHD-2 criteria	New-onset headache	Adjusted RR, 1.4; 95% CI: 1.2–1.7
	Mork et al, 2012[168]	Unselected CWP-free women (N = 12,350)	11 yr	Sleep problems (ordinal variable)	CWP and musculoskeletal pain	CWP and musculoskeletal pain (yes/no)	New-onset CWP	Adjusted RR, 3.4; 95% CI, 2.3–5.2
	Sanders et al., 2013[23]	Healthy TMD-free (OPPERA, N = 3263)	3 yr	PSQI (7-item, composite score)	TMD	Questionnaire and clinical examination	First-onset TMD	Adjusted HR, 1.3; 95% CI, 1.2–1.5
	McBeth et al., 2014[19]	Middle-aged free of CWP (N = 4326)	3 yr	Sleep problems (4-item ordinal scale)	CWP	CWP (ACR criteria)	New-onset CWP	Adjusted OR, 1.8; 95% CI, 1.2–2.8
	Generaal et al., 2017[17]	Women (N = 1860) participating in the Netherlands Study of Depression and Anxiety (NESDA)	6 yr	Insomnia (Women's Health Initiative Insomnia Rating Scale; [IRS] ≥9) and short sleep duration (≤6 h)	Chronic multisite musculoskeletal pain	Chronic pain grade (CPG)	Chronic pain onset	For insomnia: Adjusted HR, 1.6; 95% CI, 1.3–2.0; for short sleep duration: HR, 1.5; 95% CI, 1.2–1.9
	Sivertsen et al., 2017[22]	Women giving birth at Akershus University Hospital in Norway (N = 1480)	2 yr	BIS	Bodily pain	Bodily pain (yes/no) subscale of PRIME-MD	Postpartum bodily pain	Adjusted RR, 1.8; 95% CI: 1.3–2.5
	Blagojevic-Bucknall et al., 2019[169]	Participants (aged ≥50 years) with joint pain lasting ≥3 mo and no pain interference (N = 1878)	3 yr	Jenkins Sleep Scale	Joint pain	MOS 12-item short form health survey (SF-12)	Joint pain with pain interference	Adjusted RR, 1.2; 95% CI, 1.0–1.5
	Halonen et al., 2019[18]	Working age population from the Swedish Longitudinal Occupational Health Survey (N = 12,222)	6 yr	Karolinska Sleep Questionnaire ("sleep problems": yes/no)	LBP	Pain affecting daily activities	Incident LBP	Adjusted RR, 1.3; 95% CI, 1.3–1.5

	Huang et al., 2019[20]	Patients with CWP (N = 17,920) with (N = 5466) and without (N = 12,454) comorbid insomnia	13 yr	Primary or secondary insomnia diagnosis (ICD-9-CM)	CWP (ICD-9-CM)	CWP (ICD-9-CM)	Increase in the medications and ambulatory care services for CWP	For antidepressants: OR,3.8; 95% CI, 3.6–4.1; for muscle relaxants: OR, 3.1; 95% CI, 2.4–3.8; for pregabalin: OR, 1.8; 95% CI, 1.0–3.2; for gabapentin: OR, 1.7; 95% CI, 1.4–2.0 for ambulatory care visits: $\beta = 1.8$; 95% CI, 1.6–2.0; $P < .001$[b]
Pain	Odegard et al., 2013[24]	Insomnia-free population (HUNT-2 and HUNT-3, N = 19,279)	11 yr	Sleep onset and terminal insomnia (composite score)	Headache and chronic musculoskeletal pain	ICHD-2 criteria; Nordic questionnaire and ACR criteria	New-onset insomnia	For headache: adjusted OR, 2.2; 95% CI, 1.9–2.6; for chronic musculoskeletal pain: adjusted OR, 1.8, 95% CI: 1.6–1.9
	Tang et al., 2015[25]	Older adults (N = 6676)	3 yr	Jenkins Sleep Scale	Musculoskeletal pain	ACR criteria	New-onset insomnia	For "some pain": adjusted[c] OR,1.46; 95% CI, 1.21–1.75; for CWP: 1.80; 95% CI; 1.47–2.22

[a]This list presents in chronologic order major prospective longitudinal cohorts that were published in the last 10 years.
[b]The association between insomnia and ambulatory care visits was examined using multivariate generalized linear models after adjustment for the propensity score.
[c]Statistical model adjustment included the present of sleep disturbances at baseline.
ACR, American College of Rheumatology; BIS, Bergen Insomnia Scale; CI, confidence interval; CPG, clinical practice guidelines; CWP, chronic widespread pain (new name for fibromyalgia, FM); HR, hazard ratio; HUNT: Nord-Trøndelag Health Study, Norway; ICD-9-CM, *International Classification of Diseases: Clinical Modification,* ninth revision; ICHD, *International Classification of Headache Disorders;* LBP, low back pain; MOS: Medical Outcomes Study; OPPERA, Orofacial Pain, Prospective Evaluation, and Risk Assessment; OR, odds ratio; PACE, Paracetamol for Low-Back Pain Study; PRIME-MD: Primary Care Evaluation of Mental Disorders; PSQI: Pittsburgh Sleep Quality Index; RR; risk ratio; TMD, temporomandibular disorder.

significantly increase the risk (odds ratios [ORs] and relative risk ratios ranging from 1.3 to 3.8) for different chronic pain conditions, including musculoskeletal pain,[15–18] chronic widespread pain,[19,20] headaches,[21] postpartum bodily pain,[22] and temporomandibular joint disorder.[23]

Pain as a Risk Factor for Insomnia

Evidence from a large-scale prospective longitudinal Norwegian cohort (Nord-Trøndelag Health Study, *N* = 19,279) has shown that, compared with pain-free control subjects, insomnia-free subjects who were suffering from headache or chronic musculoskeletal pain at baseline, were twice as likely to develop insomnia 11 years later (OR, 1.8; 95% confidence interval [CI], 1.8 to 2.2).[24] Similarly, various types of chronic pain complaints among older adults were associated with an increased risk of insomnia of up to four times for the next 3 years. Of interest, the combination of physical limitations and reduced social participation explained greater than 65% of the effect of pain on insomnia onset.[25]

Mood Disorder as a Comorbid Link between Pain and Sleep

Abnormal sleep is a primary symptom of affective diseases and has also been incriminated as a risk factor for the development of depression.[26] In addition, mood disorders are quite common among patients suffering from chronic pain.[27] Evidence from the World Mental Health Surveys[9,28,29] and the National Comorbidity Survey,[30] two large cross-sectional cohorts, showed that chronic pain conditions increased the odds for developing depression and anxiety disorders by up to four times, with approximately 20% of pain patients reporting symptoms of depression and 35% of them reporting an anxiety disorder in the past year.[30]

The close relationship between mood disorders and insomnia in the context of pain has also been demonstrated in a large community-based sample of 18,980 European participants, where pain conditions such as backache and joint/articular disease were as strongly associated with symptoms of insomnia as they were with depression and bipolar disorders (ORs ≅5).[10] Although pain-related insomnia shares several mood, cognitive, and behavioral characteristics with primary insomnia,[13,31,32] insomnia due to pain seems to last longer and is associated with more daytime impairment[33] compared with primary insomnia.[10] This points to a possible interactive effect of impaired sleep and pain on the daily function, a hypothesis that has received support from two separate cohorts of Norwegian (*N* = 6892) and Finnish (*N* = 6060) employees, where pain and insomnia at baseline synergistically predicted objective health outcomes and disability retirement in these populations.[34]

A longitudinal investigation of patients with pain found that anxiety and depression increased the likelihood for persistence of insomnia over the course of a year,[16] whereas a bidirectional association between anxiety and chronic pain has recently been suggested by two other cohorts.[35,36] Among the 614 participants in the Netherlands Study of Depression and Anxiety, who were free of depression and anxiety at baseline, those with multiple locations of joint-related pain, were at higher risk for first-onset mood disorder during the 4-year follow-up period (adjusted hazard ratio of 2.9; 95% CI, 1.7 to 4.8).[36] Conversely, in the same study population, both baseline depression and an increase in the depressive symptoms have been shown to mediate the effect of insomnia on the development of multisite musculoskeletal pain in 1860 participants, during a 6-year follow-up period.[17] Alternatively, feelings of anxiety experienced in the early phase after lower extremity trauma predicted the presence of pain up to 24 months later.[35]

The above epidemiologic evidence suggests that, in conjunction with somatosensory information processing, emotional and cognitive networks are critical components of the so-called *pain matrix*[37] (Figure 156.1, *A*), by evolving a noxious stimulus into a painful percept, and demonstrate aberrant resting activity and somesthetic reactivity in sleep disorders (Figure 156.1, *B*). From a clinical perspective, these data point to the role of the pain matrix as a central agent in associations between sleep disorders, pain, and emotional-cognitive disorders (Figure 156.1, *C*). The neuroscience and the clinical implications of the pain matrix are discussed below.

PAIN PROCESSING FROM SENSATION TO PERCEPTION ACROSS WAKEFULNESS AND SLEEP

Bodily pain is a multimodal percept defined as an unpleasant somatosensory experience integrating sensory, cognitive, and emotional processes. Thus all clinical and research taxonomy systems that classify pain[38] explain this experience as a synthesis of sensory, cognitive, and emotional processes, involving precise spatiotemporal dynamics of the respective brain networks from which the pain percept arises. Indeed, and in keeping with evidence from scientific studies of experimental pain and analgesia, as well as pathologic conditions of hyperalgesia or insensitivity to pain, a painful percept is associated with differential activity of somatosensory, emotional, and cognitive neural networks.[39,40]

Neural Processing of Nociceptive Stimuli across Wakefulness and Sleep

Figure 156.1 depicts the brain networks involved in the genesis of pain perception during wakeful rest, along with their relative metabolic activity across sleep stages. Intact and precise spatiotemporal functional connectivity among these pain matrix networks is critical for the perception of pain.[37] Distinct somatosensory information is transmitted from the periphery to the central nervous system (CNS) for further processing via the thalamus, where information is gated dependent on a person's brain state during sleep and wakefulness.[41] Once the sensory information reaches the cortex, it is processed at progressively higher-order somatosensory network areas (SI and SII), followed by association cortex emotion and cognitive processing networks. Emotion networks will give rise to the *negative feeling* of pain and involve anterior temporal, insular, and, to an extent, medial frontal nodes. On the other hand, cognitive networks allow for *awareness* and *attention* to painful stimuli, as well as *motivational reactivity* and *pain avoidance*, by combining learned responses with a plan for action, predominantly involving dorsal frontal networks.[37,39] Pain perception thus is not limited within primary somatosensory cortices and somesthesia networks.

Beyond this initial perception, pain is dynamically processed over time. Circadian and ultradian rhythms allow us to create and solidify a memory of what it *feels* to have and how we *thought* about having pain, beyond the memory of *sensing* a specific painful experience. For example, contextual episodic memory consolidation across ultradian cycles[42] is optimal during non–rapid-eye movement (NREM) sleep, when the hippocampus is relatively more active and in synchronization with

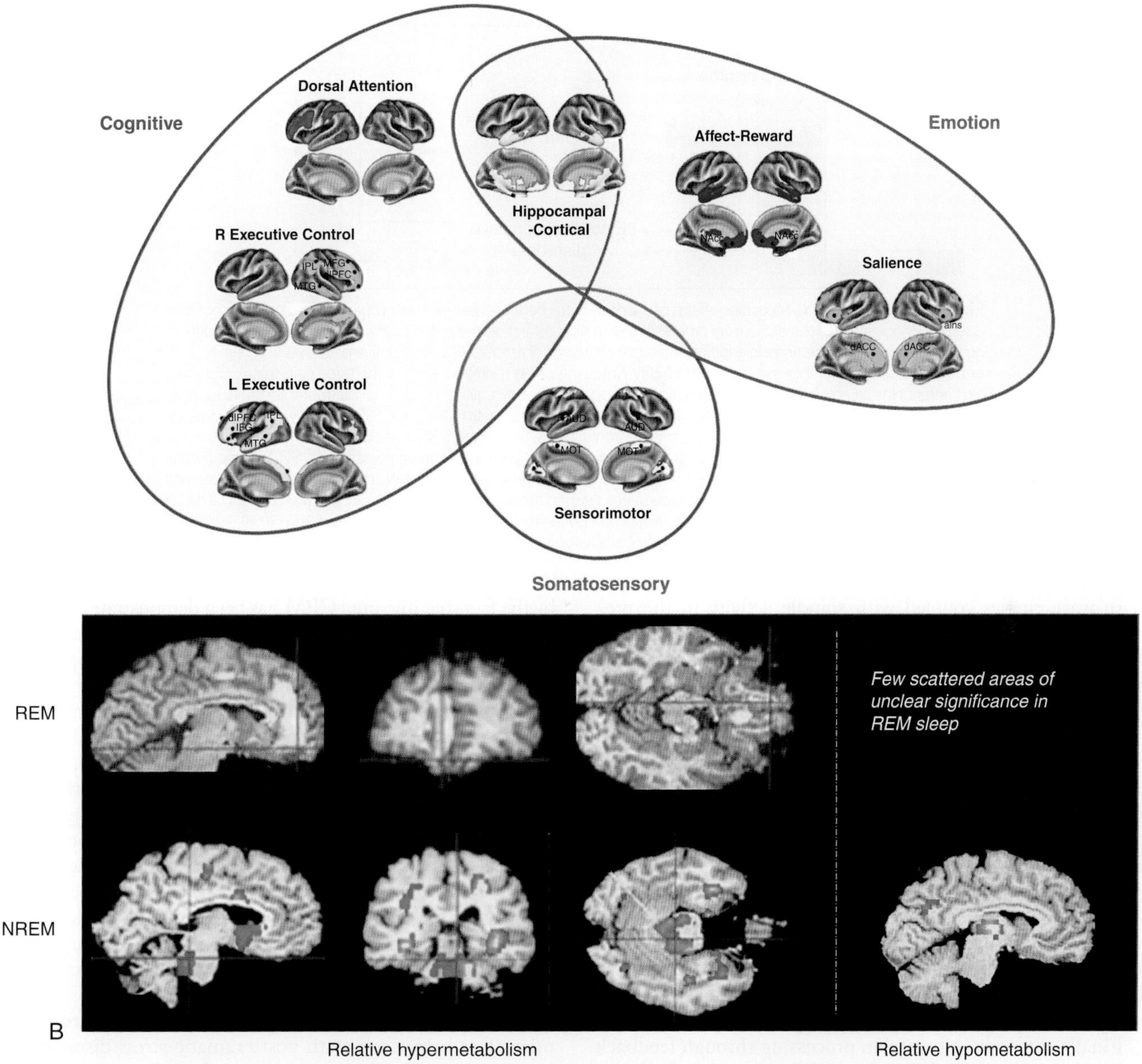

Figure 156.1 The pain matrix: brain networks, sleep-wake metabolic dynamics, and mediating roles between sleep, pain, and emotional-cognitive disorders. **A,** Select networks of the brain derived through independent component analysis contributing to the pain matrix: These networks are involved in processes combining somatosensory, cognitive, and emotional modalities, including pain information processing, and clustered according to their contribution in the three core components of the pain matrix (i.e., somesthesia, cognition, and emotion). The predominant forward flow of information from somesthesia to cognitive and emotion modular networks is further enriched by feedback flow within and between clusters, thus optimizing pain information consolidation. **B,** Relative metabolic brain activity during sleep states compared to wakefulness: Emotion networks are more active in rapid eye movement (REM) sleep, explaining the preferential emotional and procedural information consolidation during REM. *Cognitive networks* receive information from hippocampal structures during non–rapid eye movement (NREM) sleep, as represented by sharp-wave ripple hippocampal activity, translated into cortical spindle activity via thalamic relay; yet overall cortical activity remains relatively decreased in NREM sleep, in contrast to its relatively increased hippocampal activity. Finally, lower-level *primary somatosensory and primary association cortical sensory networks* remain relatively hypoactive across sleep stages, in line with the observed increased threshold required for sensory stimuli to induce a behavioral response during sleep.

Continued

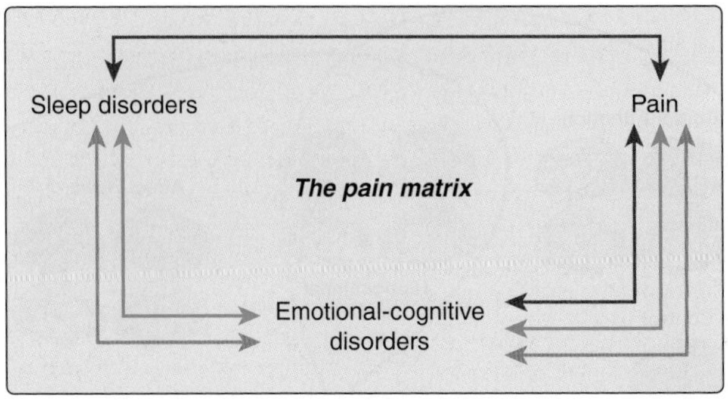

C

Figure 156.1 cont'd **C,** Mediating effects of the pain matrix networks between sleep, pain, and emotional-cognitive disorders: Modulation of somatosensory processes have a direct effect on the comorbidity of sleep and pain disorders, in both acute and chronic settings. In addition, indirect modulation of emotional and cognitive processes from either sleep or pain disorders further increase their comorbidity. *Note*: Line colors represent each of the three pain matrix networks. aIns, anterior insula; amHipp, anterior medial hippocampus; Amyg, amygdala; aPFC, anterior prefrontal cortex; AUD, auditory cortex; dAcc, dorsal anterior cingulate cortex; dlPFC, dorsal lateral prefrontal cortex; FEF, frontal eye field; IPL, inferior parietal lobule; IPS, intraparietal sulcus; MFG, middle frontal gyrus; MOT, motor; MTG, middle temporal gyrus; NAcc, nucleus accumbens; SFG, superior frontal gyrus; vlPFC, ventral lateral prefrontal cortex; VIS, visual; vmPFC, ventral medial prefrontal cortex. (Combined and modified from Nofzinger EA, Buysse DJ, Miewald JM, et al. Human regional cerebral glucose metabolism during non-rapid eye movement sleep in relation to waking. *Brain*. 2002;125:1105–15; Nofzinger EA, Mintun MA, Wiseman M, et al. Forebrain activation in REM sleep: an FDG PET study. *Brain Res*. 1997;770:192–201; and Weng TB, Pierce GL, Darling WG, et al. The acute effects of aerobic exercise on the functional connectivity of human brain networks. *Brain Plast*. 2017;2:171–90.)

sharp-wave ripples coupled with spindle activity in the prefrontal cortex,[43–45] whereas affective memories are consolidated best during REM sleep through relational associations when emotion networks are metabolically active (Figure 156.1).[45,46] Furthermore, studies indicate that both episodic and emotional memory consolidation are also achieved across longer circadian cycles through modulation of the respective brain networks and with some studies suggesting that emotional memory consolidation is more sensitive to circadian disruptions compared to episodic memory consolidation.[47–50] Cortisol attenuation seems to have a central role in these effects being primarily caused by circadian and not ultradian disruptions.[51,52] It is worth noting, however, that in most experimental designs it is difficult to completely control for ultradian processes when studying circadian-mediated memory consolidation. Overall, these cognitive-emotional network-state associations, although not specific to pain, are integral in pain processing.[53]

Finally, dynamic information processing through feedback pathways explains the descending inhibitory control of pain processing, which is best achieved in deep sleep, allowing even peripheral pathways to modulate their responsiveness to pain stimuli over time and across sleep-wake states.[54–56]

Sleep Disruption Leading to Conditioned Pain Modulation

Studies in human volunteers have demonstrated that sleep disruption alters pain processing by activating major inflammatory pathways[57] and promoting the expression of proinflammatory cytokines, such as tumor necrosis factor-α (TNF-α), interleukin-1β (IL-1β), and interleukin-6 (IL-6), in the peripheral blood[58] and/or by impairing central mechanisms of pain-inhibitory control (namely, conditioned pain modulation [CPM]),[59] thus leading to hyperalgesia with musculoskeletal sensitization and spontaneous pain symptoms.[60] Proinflammatory cytokines eventually promote homeostatic sleep induction via mechanisms that, among others, include IL1β-mediated gamma-aminobutyric acid-A ($GABA_A$) receptor agonism,[61] thus leading to tissue restoration.[62,63] In contrast, CPM is invariably associated with sleep disruption. Specifically, the mechanistic effect of sleep disruption in relevance to clinical practice is highlighted further by the fact that impaired CPM has been demonstrated in several chronic pain conditions, including chronic widespread pain,[64] temporomandibular joint disorder,[65,66] and low back pain,[67] in which sleep disturbances are highly prevalent.

With regard to the cognitive network of pain matrix that is involved in attention and arousal, the dorsal prefrontal cortex is least active and "rests" during NREM sleep,[68] in support with evidence that sleep deprivation leads to blunted attentional modulation of painful stimuli.[69] Furthermore, emotional memory consolidation is critically dependent on both hippocampal-amygdalar theta activity during REM[70] and spindle activity during slow wave sleep (SWS).[71] Specifically, experimental sleep deprivation in humans enhances amygdala-dependent recollection of emotionally negative memories,[72] supporting the hypothesis that sleep deprivation facilitates chronicity of negative emotions via salience-emotional networks. In contrast, allowing consolidation of REM stages during sleep minimizes fear in patients with posttraumatic stress disorder.[73] A recent study evaluating experimental sleep deprivation, as well as real-world total sleep time over a period of time, in relation to pain perception, revealed that sleep deprivation decreased pain thresholds, an effect mediated through somatosensory network hyperreactivity, and striatal and insular cortex hyporeactivity to pain, the latter being key nodes of emotional brain networks (see also Figure 156.1).[74] This evidence seems to contradict findings from studies on neurodegenerative disorders and chronic hyperalgesia, where emotional and cognitive network hyperreactivity and thalamic hyporeactivity to stimuli is observed, yet highlight how poor sleep modifies brain function in addition to structural changes, when compared to neurodegeneration, as well as the long-term differential modulating effect of chronic conditions on the pain matrix networks,[37,75,76] when compared to hyperalgesia syndromes.

CLINICAL IMPLICATIONS OF THE BIDIRECTIONAL RELATIONSHIP OF SLEEP AND PAIN

In line with evidence that physiologic sleepiness due to chronic sleep loss increases sensitivity to pain,[77,78] primary sleep disorders, such as insomnia[79] and restless legs syndrome,[80] are associated with hyperalgesia. The observed effects are attributed to impairment of central pain-inhibitory[79] or amplification of descending pain-facilitatory[80] pathways. Moreover, treatment with continuous positive airway pressure in subjects suffering from sleep-disordered breathing (SDB) can reverse the observed hyperalgesia, although it is not clear whether this effect was due to restoration of sleep continuity or resolution of nocturnal hypoxemia.[81] That said, analyses of the Cleveland Family Study demonstrated a significant positive association between recurrent nocturnal hypoxemia and pain complaints in subjects with SDB[82] and, along with other findings from humans[83–85] and in vitro[86] experiments, there is compelling evidence that intermittent hypoxia with its associated inflammation is an additional mechanism to sleep disruption for altering pain perception.[87] In contrast, a recent survey of patients referred to an academic sleep center showed that, although SDB comorbid with insomnia was related to more pain compared to either SDB or insomnia alone, no polysomnography (PSG) measures of SDB severity (e.g., number or arousals, or amount of hypoxia) mediated this effect.[88] A recent systematic review of the literature concludes that, due to the highly variable findings across different studies, more research is needed to clarify the relationship between the various SDB phenotypes and pain processing,[89] ideally by streamlining protocols.

In addition to the above primary sleep disorders, there is evidence that disrupted circadian rhythms also impact pain perception. Patients with knee osteoarthritis pain, for example, were more likely to have aberrant circadian rest-activity rhythms if comorbid insomnia was present.[90] Expanding this observation on the treatment venue, when patients with chronic back pain were treated with morning bright light, not only did they have increased pain thresholds, but also had improved cognitive and emotional aspects of pain perception, as well as quality of sleep, and about a fourth of the effect size of pain interference could be explained by circadian phase advancement.[91] The extent to which such treatment effects are mediated primarily through improved circadian rhythms, rather than from improved sleep duration and consolidation, or even are the result of the mood-stimulating effect of light on the emotional networks of pain matrix, remains to be established. It is reasonable to hypothesize a combination of the above is at play; however, controlled experiments are needed to establish the relative contribution of each process.

The observed cognitive and emotional changes in patients suffering from pain or insomnia could also act as mediators or potential confounders on the relationship between sleep and pain.[92] For example, the ability of attention to modulate pain perception is an important mechanism to cope with pain,[93] and insomnia with short sleep duration has been shown to impair the control of executive attention function.[94] Of interest, attentional bias toward pain and pain-related information reduced distraction from the painful stimuli,[95] undermined sleep,[31] and strengthened the association between pain severity and disability in patients with chronic pain.[96] Moreover, pain catastrophizing[97] has been shown to magnify pain experience, possibly through a detrimental effect on sleep.[98] Presleep cognitive arousal in patients with chronic pain was found to be a more reliable predictor of subsequent sleep quality than was presleep pain.[99] Combined, these intriguing findings point to the hyperarousal hypothesis for insomnia[100] as a potential underlying mechanism linking insomnia to mood disorders and pain. Specifically, certain patients either have a biologically driven cortical state of hyperarousal or fail to achieve adequate slow wave activity in the dorsal frontal lobes during sleep, whereas others become so after a maladaptive response to stimuli,[101] thus conceptually linking chronic insomnia and its relation to pain via the 3P model (i.e., predisposing, precipitating, and perpetuating factors in the development of chronic syndromes) (Figure 156.2).[102]

ASSESSMENT OF SLEEP IN THE CONTEXT OF CHRONIC PAIN

The development of reliable instruments for assessing sleep and pain phenotypes is an essential prerequisite for accurately characterizing the relationship between pain and comorbid insomnia, hence effectively managing this patient population.

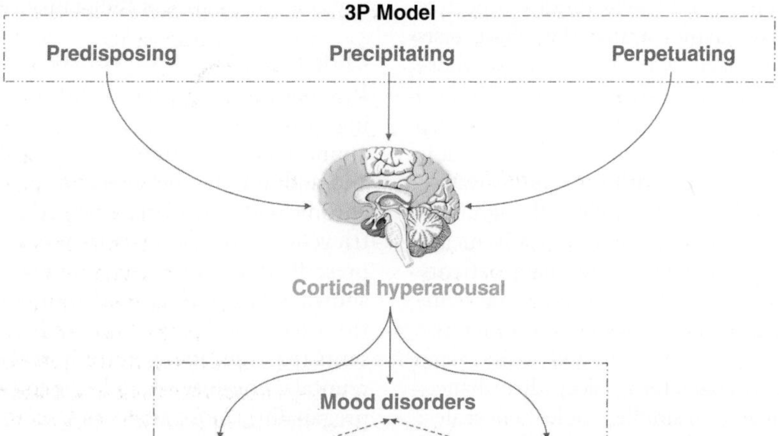

Figure 156.2 The 3P model (predisposing, precipitating, and perpetuating factors) in the development of cortical hyperarousal toward the chronicity of insomnia, pain, and mood disorders. According to the 3P model, predisposing factors, such as genes and brain development, provide a substrate for precipitating factors, such as bodily injury or social stressors, to introduce a hyperaroused cortical state, which can become chronic through perpetuating factors, such as maladaptive behaviors. This cortical hyperarousal can contribute directly to the chronicity of pain and sleep disorders, as well as indirectly through the mediating effects of comorbid mood disorders.

In contrast to pain, which can be assessed only by patient's questioning, sleep can be evaluated both by objective and subjective measures. Overnight attended PSG (i.e., the evaluation of quantitative and qualitative parameters of sleep with the use of electroencephalographic, respiratory, and electrocardiographic monitoring modalities) is considered a gold standard for the objective assessment of sleep. Actigraphy monitoring, another objective method for indirectly estimating sleep duration, although having less specificity than PSG,[103] has been validated in large longitudinal cohorts of patients with chronic pain.[104]

The significance of combining objective and subjective measures of sleep is highlighted in chronic insomnia, which is characterized by *negative sleep discrepancy*; that is, patients experience greater sleep disturbance than is measured objectively. In patients with chronic widespread pain who are treated with opioids, the discrepancy between actigraphy and self-reported assessments of sleep is both magnified and of high night-to-night variability with both negative and positive estimates.[105] Pain intensity and treatment with opioids tend to increase the discrepancies between diary- and actigraphy-based assessments, with age being an important modifier of these effects. Patients with less severe pain show the greatest sleep disruption at higher doses of opioids, whereas in those with more intense pain, opioids may even prove beneficial by increasing the amount of SWS.[106] On the other hand, in younger patients, high doses of opioids have led to a subjective overestimation of sleep quality (i.e., positive sleep discrepancy), whereas the opposite is true for older patients who are treated with opioids.[107] The above observations highlight the need for objective real-world measures of sleep duration and quality. That said, quality of life is highly subjective, depending on a person's values, desires, and personality in general, as well as developmental and environmental factors, thus indicating that symptom evaluation for disease burden also requires subjective markers of symptom severity and treatment response.

Scoring instruments for evaluation of sleep consist of either a simple, one-item scale assessing "sleep quality," in general, or more complex and extended questionnaires looking at several aspects of sleeping behavior, that is, sleep initiation and maintenance, number of awakenings, and the restorative aspect of sleep. Validation studies have demonstrated that these tests can discriminate between subjects with insomnia and those with normal sleep. Certain instruments, such as the Medical Outcomes Study Sleep Scale,[108–110] the Chronic Pain Sleep Inventory,[111] and the Insomnia Severity Index,[112,113] are able to detect changes in sleep associated with the administration of analgesia in pain patients. It is still not clear, though, how such tests should be constructed to have a clinically meaningful impact on the management of chronic pain patients. Are more elaborate scoring tools and those containing pain-specific components (e.g., Brief Pain Inventory Interference Scale,[114] Chronic Pain Sleep Inventory,[111] and Daily Sleep Diary[115]) better equipped to characterize sleep disturbances in the context of pain, compared to simple, single-item scales? A validation study of the Sleep Quality Scale (11 points; 0 for *best possible sleep* to 10 for *worst possible sleep*) showed that in patients treated for chronic widespread pain, the simple instrument correlated closely with the Medical Outcomes Study Sleep Scale and was also sensitive enough to detect improvement in sleep quality after pain treatment.[116] In the same patient population, actigraphy has also shown a good agreement with diary-based assessment of sleep, with both methods being able to detect sleep improvement as a result of cognitive behavioral therapy for insomnia.[117]

Since the 2008 IMMPACT (Initiative on Methods, Measurement, and Pain Assessment in Clinical Trials) consensus on clinically important outcomes in chronic pain trials, when the need for assessing the interference of pain with sleep was originally introduced,[114,118,119] sleep is increasingly included in the overall evaluation framework of patients with chronic pain.[120] As a consequence, more trials now include sleep pattern among the core phenotyping domains of chronic pain patients, with Pittsburgh Sleep Quality Index,[121] Brief Pain Inventory,[114] Medical Outcomes Study Sleep scale,[108] and Insomnia Severity Index[112] being the most commonly used assessment instruments.[120,122]

An outcomes-based research approach might be necessary to determine the type of sleep assessment that could add clinical value to the management of patients with chronic pain (e.g., objective vs. subjective tests, extended and more complex questionnaires vs. shorter and simpler ones, combination of objective and subjective methods) (Figure 156.3).

MANAGEMENT OF PATIENTS WITH CHRONIC PAIN AND COMORBID SLEEP DISORDERS

Because of the physiologic and phenotypic complexities associated with the interaction of pain, comorbid sleep disorders, and mental illness, the therapeutic management of chronic pain patients is a challenging task. In this context it is encouraging that sleep outcomes are being incorporated into randomized controlled trials (RCTs) designed to evaluate treatments for chronic pain. The inclusion of sleep assessments in such trials might also provide indirect evidence for the physiologic basis of the comorbid relationships among pain, disturbed sleep, and mental illness. Tables 156.2 and 156.3 present a list of important RCTs evaluating pharmacologic and nonpharmacologic interventions for various types of pain conditions, where both pain and sleep outcomes have been assessed. Considering the mechanism of action of most pain pharmacotherapies, it follows that insomnia or excessive daytime sleepiness are the main sleep outcomes studied.

Pharmacologic Interventions Targeting Pain

Pharmacologic analgesic interventions in patients suffering from chronic pain of various etiologies include acetaminophen,[123] antiinflammatory drugs,[124,125] opioids,[126,127] and sodium channel blockers.[128] In patients suffering from chronic widespread or neuropathic pain, tricyclic[129] and nontricyclic[130] antidepressant and anticonvulsant[104,131] drugs, prescribed as adjuvants or even monotherapies, have also shown relative success in improving pain outcomes. With the exceptions of acetaminophen and modern antidepressants (e.g., selective serotonin and serotonin-norepinephrine reuptake inhibitors) and anticonvulsants (e.g., gabapentin, pregabalin), most analgesics seem to alter sleep in a manner quite similar to that of pain, that is, by disrupting sleep continuity and/or suppressing both REM and SWS.[132] It is thus not surprising that effective opioid analgesia, may not be associated with a complete restoration of normal sleep architecture, despite improving subjective sleep assessment outcomes.[106,107,133] However, due to the lack of systematic longitudinal assessments of the sleep-disrupting effects of

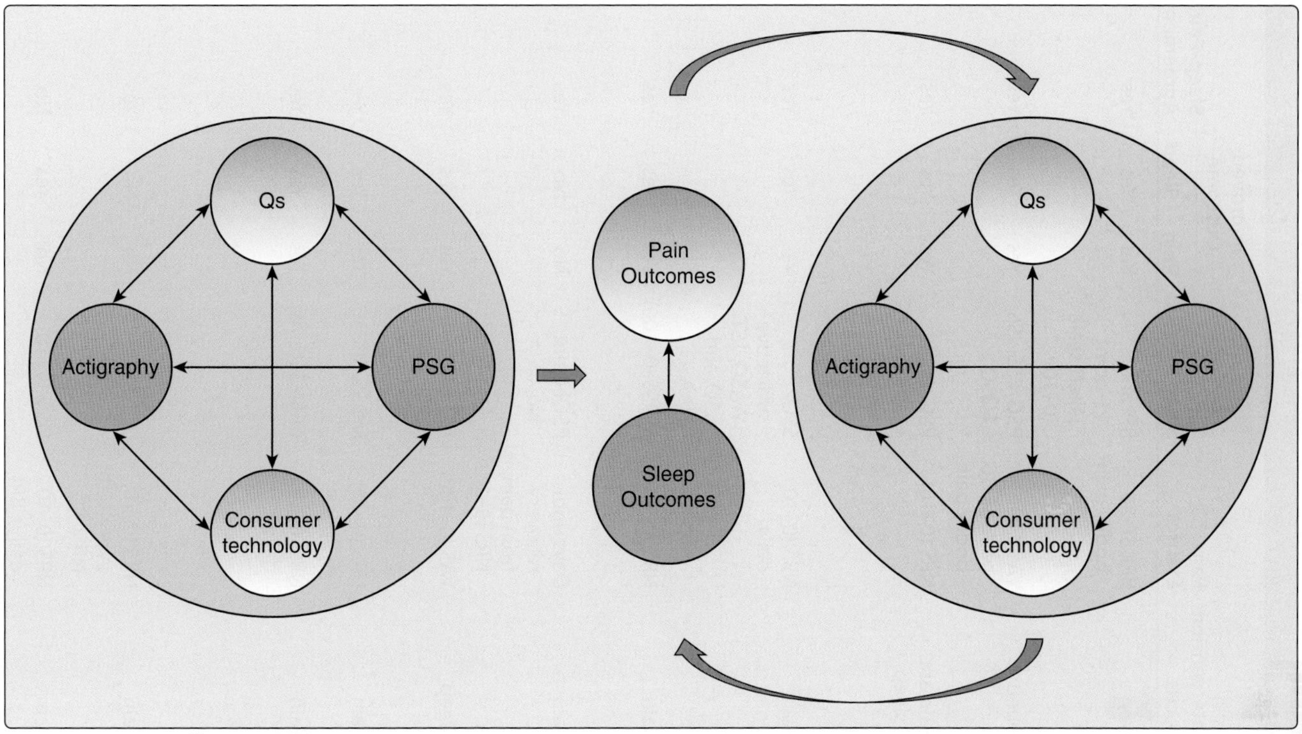

Figure 156.3 Outcomes-based algorithm in the assessment of comorbid sleep and pain disorders. Outcomes-based algorithms can help in identifying better assessment protocols in the diagnosis and treatment response of comorbid sleep and pain disorders. Starting from a comprehensive assessment, objective and subjective measures can be selected and weighted according to sleep and pain outcomes and, after a few iterations of the process, define an optimal comprehensive protocol. PSG, Polysomnography; Qs, questionnaires.

analgesics, it is unclear whether a sole disturbance of sleep architecture (i.e., not associated with subjective complaints) constitutes a physiologic potential for altering pain outcomes or changes the natural course of pain disease in the long term. This issue directly relates to the yet unanswered question about the clinical meaning of the various sleep phenotypes evaluated by different assessment methods.

Pharmacologic Interventions Targeting Insomnia

Several double-blinded RCTs have demonstrated the efficacy of novel CNS depressants and nonbenzodiazepine hypnotics that specifically target sleep function, in reducing pain and improving overall function in patients suffering from chronic widespread and low back pain.

Sodium oxybate is the sodium salt of γ-hydroxybutyrate, an endogenous metabolite of GABA with CNS-depressant properties.[134] Administration of sodium oxybate in patients suffering from chronic widespread pain significantly improved subjective sleep, pain, and functional outcomes, whereas it also increased sleep stability and the amount of SWS.[134,135] Similarly, the administration of eszopiclone, a nonbenzodiazepine hypnotic,[136] in patients suffering from chronic low back pain, was associated with a significant increase in total sleep time, a reduction in pain, and an improvement in the ratings of depression.[137]

Although rigorous consensus criteria[118,122] may question the meaningfulness of the improvement in pain and other functional outcomes demonstrated by the small analgesic effects of these interventions,[134,137] these findings are important RCT evidence that targeting sleep physiology may alter pain perception and improve functional outcomes in patients suffering from chronic pain.

Pharmacologic Interventions Targeting Both Pain and Comorbid Insomnia or Circadian Disorders

Melatonin is a pineal gland hormone with a circadian pattern of secretion and well-known sleep-wake circadian regulation, antiinflammatory, and antihyperalgesic effects. Although melatonin has demonstrated efficacy both in treating pain and improving sleep quality when administered in patients with temporomandibular joint disorder[138] or endometriosis-associated chronic pelvic pain,[139] the small sample size of these trials does not allow evaluations of interactions between its pain-relieving and sleep-restoring effects. Instead, improved pain perception through optimization of circadian rhythms was best achieved after a counterpoint approach, where 1-hour bright morning light therapy for 13 days was sufficient to improve pain, pain sensitivity, and sleep in patients with chronic low back pain, and for which, advancement of circadian phase might be a possible mediating mechanism.[91] Whether combination of melatonin and bright light therapy will achieve more than an additive effect in improving pain via optimization of circadian rhythms remains to be established.

Pregabalin, an anticonvulsant agent with voltage-dependent calcium channel $\alpha_2\delta$ subunits ligand properties,[140] has been effective both in treating pain and restoring sleep quality in patients with neuropathic conditions, and it is one of first-line therapies for neuropathic pain.[141,142] Both the analgesic and sleep-enhancing effects of pregabalin are presumably mediated by the same mechanism, that is, a

Table 156.2 Randomized Controlled Trials Evaluating the Effects of Pharmacological Interventions on Pain and Sleep Outcomes in Patients with Chronic Pain and Comorbid Insomnia[a,b]

Condition	Study	Population	Blinding	Control	Follow-up	Intervention	Intervention Focus	Pain Metrics	Sleep Metrics	Improved Outcome: Pain	Improved Outcome: Sleep	Sleep-Pain Agreement
Chronic widespread pain	Arnold et al., 2010[130]	CWP ($N = 507$)	Double	Placebo	12 wk	Duloxetine (SNRI)	Pain	BPI, SF-36 bodily pain	BPI and 11-point Likert scale (0–10)	Yes	Yes	Yes
	Moldofsky et al., 2010[134]	CWP ($N = 151$)	Double	Placebo	8 wk	Sodium oxybate (γ-hydroxybutyric acid)	Sleep	VAS, FIQ pain, SF-36 bodily pain	PSG, ESS, JSS, FOSQ	Yes	Yes	Yes
	Roth et al., 2012; Roth, 2012 #1634	CWP ($N = 206$)	Double	Placebo	4 wk	Pregabalin (anticonvulsant)	Pain and sleep	NRS (0–10)	PSG, self-reported sleep assessment	Yes	Yes	Yes
	Arnold et al., 2015[131]	CWP with comorbid depression ($N = 155$)	Double	Placebo (crossover)	6 wk	Pregabalin (anticonvulsant)	Pain	NRS (0–10, daily)	SSQ, subjective WASO, TST, LSO, and NAASO	Yes	Yes	Yes
Low back pain	Steiner et al., 2011[126]	CLBP ($N = 539$)	Double	Placebo	84 days	Buprenorphine (partial agonist of the μ-opioid receptor)	Pain	NRS (0–10)	MOSS (0–100)	Yes	Yes	Yes
	Williams et al., 2014[123]	Acute low back pain ($N = 1596$)	Double	Placebo	3 mo	Paracetamol (mild analgesic)	Pain	Days until recovery from pain, NRS (0–10)	PSQI (item No. 6)	No	No	Yes
	Goforth et al., 2014[137]	CLBP ($N = 52$)	Double	Placebo	1 mo	Eszopiclone (nonbenzodiazepine hypnotic)	Sleep	VAS (0–100)	TST (sleep diary)	Yes	Yes	Yes
	Yarlas et al., 2016[127]	CLBP ($N = 660$)	Double	Placebo	12 wk	Transdermal Buprenorphine	Pain	NRS (0–10)	MOSS, SPI	Yes	Yes	Yes
	Christoph et al., 2017[170]	CLBP ($N = 360$)	Double	Placebo and active (tapentadol)	26 wk	Cebranopadol and tapentadol (nociceptin/orphanin FQ peptide receptor and opioid peptide receptor agonists)	Pain	NRS (0–10, daily)	CPSI (5 items)	Yes	Yes	Yes
Neuropathic pain	Kalliomäki et al., 2013[124]	Posttraumatic neuralgia (N=133)	Double	Placebo	1 mo	Chemokine receptor 2 (CCR2) antagonist (anti-inflammatory)	Pain	NRS (0–10, every 12 h), NPSI	SI (NRS, 0–10)	No	No	Yes
	Huffman et al., 2015[171]	PDPN ($N = 352$)	Double	Placebo (crossover)	6 wk	Pregabalin (anticonvulsant)	Pain	NRS (0–10, daily), BPI	DSIS (0–10)	No	Yes	No

	Raskin et al., 2016[172]	PDPN ($N = 147$)	Double	Placebo (crossover)	6 wk	Pregabalin on NSAID background	Pain	NRS (0–10), BPI	SI (0–10)	Yes	Yes	Yes
	Andresen et al., 2016[173]	Spinal cord injury neuropathic pain ($N = 58$)	Double	Placebo	12 wk	Palmitoylethanolamide (PEA, endocannabinoid potentiator)	Pain	NRS (0–10, daily)	ISI, sleep disturbance (NRS 0–10)	No	No	Yes
	Merante et al., 2017[146]	PDPN ($N = 452$)	Double	Active: pregabalin	5 wk	Mirogabalin (anticonvulsant)	Pain and sleep	VAS (0–10), BPI, SF-MPQ	DSIS (0–10)	Yes	Yes	Yes
	Liu et al., 2017[174]	Postherpetic neuralgia ($N = 220$)	Double	Placebo	8 wk	Pregabalin (anticonvulsant)	Pain and sleep	NRS (0–10), SF-MPQ	DSIS (0–10)	Yes	Yes	Yes
	Kato et al, 2019[175]	Postherpetic neuralgia ($N = 765$)	Double	Placebo	14 wk	Mirogabalin (anticonvulsant)	Pain and sleep	ADPS, VAS (0–10, SF-MPQ)	DSIS (0–10)	Yes	Yes	Yes
	De Greef et al., 2019[128]	Nav 1.7 mutations-related small fiber neuropathy ($N = 23$)	Double	Placebo (crossover)	13 wk	Lacosamide (sodium channel blocker)	Pain	NRS (0–10, daily)	DSIS (0–10)	Yes	Yes	Yes
Other types of chronic pain	Schwertner et al., 2013[139]	Endometriosis ($N = 36$)	Double	Placebo	8 wk	Melatonin	Pain and sleep	VAS (0–10, daily)	Sleep quality (VAS, 0–10, daily)	Yes	Yes	Yes
	Vidor et al., 2013[138]	Myofacial TMD pain ($N = 32$)	Double	Placebo	4 wk	Melatonin	Pain and sleep	VAS (0–10, daily)	Sleep quality (VAS, 0–10, daily)	Yes	Yes	Yes
	Strand et al., 2016[125]	Rheumatoid arthritis ($N = 556$)	Double	Placebo	12 mo	Tofacitinib (Janus kinase [JAK] inhibitor) or adalimumab (tumor necrosis factor inhibitor)	Pain	Patient assessment of arthritis pain (VAS, 0–10)	MOSS	Yes	Yes	Yes
	Maarrawi et al., 2018[129]	Chronic neck pain	Double	Placebo	2 mo	Amitriptyline (tricyclic antidepressant)	Pain	VAS (0–10)	BIS	Yes	Yes	Yes

[a]Emphasis is given on the agreement between the changes in the pain- and sleep-related outcomes as a result of interventions targeting sleep, pain, or both sleep and pain functions.
[b]This list presents in chronologic order randomized controlled trials that were published in the last 10 years. Investigations with no clear prospectively defined hypotheses regarding the examined outcomes, studies with conclusions based on exploratory and/or subgroup, unplanned analyses, and those studies that were not preregistered at ClinicalTrials.gov, or an equivalent national database, were not included.
ACR, American College of Rheumatology; ADPS, average daily pain score; BPI, brief pain inventory; BIS, Bergen insomnia score; CBT, cognitive behavioral therapy; CLBP, chronic low back pain; CPSI, chronic pain sleep inventory; CWP, chronic widespread pain (new name for fibromyalgia, FM); DSIS, daily sleep interference scale; ESS, Epworth Sleepiness Scale; FIQ, Fibromyalgia Impact Questionnaire; FOSQ, Functional Outcomes of Sleep Questionnaire; IBS, irritable bowel syndrome; ISI, insomnia severity index; JSS, Jenkins Sleep Scale; LSO, latency to sleep onset; MOSS, Medical Outcomes Study Sleep Scale; NAASO, number of awakenings after sleep onset; NPSI, neuropathic pain symptom inventory; NRS, numerical rating scale; NSAID, nonsteroidal antiinflammatory drugs; PDPN, painful diabetic peripheral neuropathy; PSG, polysomnography; PSQI: Pittsburgh Sleep Quality Index; SE: sleep efficiency; SI: sleep interference; SNRI, serotonin-norepinephrine reuptake inhibitor; SPI, Sleep Problems Index; TMD, temporomandibular disorder; TST, total sleep time; SF-36, 36-item medical outcomes study short-form health survey; SF-MPQ, Short-Form McGill Pain Questionnaire; VAS, visual analogue scale; WASO, wake after sleep onset.

Table 156.3 Randomized Controlled Trials Evaluating the Effects of Nonpharmacologic Interventions on Pain and Sleep Outcomes in Patients with Chronic Pain and Comorbid Insomnia[a,b]

Condition	Study	Population	Blinding	Control	Follow-up	Intervention	Intervention Focus	Pain Metrics	Sleep Metrics	Improved Outcome: Pain	Improved Outcome: Sleep	Sleep-Pain Agreement
Arthritis	Vitiello et al., 2013[158]	Elderly (>60 yr) patients with osteoarthritis ($N = 367$)	Double	Education-only	9 mo	CBT for pain and insomnia	Pain and sleep	Chronic pain scale (6 items; 0–10)	ISI, SE (actigraphy)	No	Yes	No
	Smith et al., 2015[154]	Knee osteoarthritis ($N = 73$)	Double	Active: behavioral desensitization	6 mo	CBT for insomnia	Sleep	VAS (0–100 mm)	WASO, TST, SOL, SE (Diary, PSG, actigraphy), ISI	Yes	Yes	Yes
	Ward et al., 2017[161]	Rheumatoid arthritis ($N = 25$)	Single	Active: "usual care"	13 wk	Yoga intervention	Pain and sleep	VAS (0–100 mm)	ISI	Yes	Yes	Yes
Chronic wide-spread pain	Kashikar-Zuck et al., 2012[176]	Juvenile CWS, ($N = 112$)	Single	CWP education	6 mo	CBT	Pain	VAS (0–10 cm)	VAS (0–10 cm)	No	No	Yes
	Van Gordon et al., 2017[163]	CWS ($N = 85$)	Double	Active: cognitive behavior theory	6 mo	Meditation awareness training (MAT)	Pain and sleep	SF-MPQ	PSQI	Yes	Yes	Yes
	Wang et al., 2018[162]	CWS ($N = 85$)	Single	Active: aerobic exercise	52 wk	Tai chi (Yang style)	Pain and sleep	FIQR (0–100)	PSQI	Yes	No	No
	McCrae et al., 2019[153]	CWS comorbid with insomnia ($N = 74$)	Single	"Usual care"	6 mo	CBT for insomnia	Sleep	VAS (0–10 cm)	Sleep diary (WASO, TST, SOL, SE)	No	Yes	No
						CBT for pain	Pain			No	Yes	No
Other types of chronic pain	Slangen et al., 2014[177]	PDPN ($N = 33$)	No	No intervention: "best medical treatment"	6 mo	Spinal cord stimulation plus "best medical treatment"	Pain	Pain Severity Index	MOSS	Yes	No	No
	Palermo et al., 2016[178]	Adolescents with chronic pain and their parents ($N = 269$)	Single	Active: Internet-delivered education	6 mo	Internet-delivered CBT	Pain and sleep	NRS (0–10)	ASWS	No	Yes	No
	Smitherman et al., 2016[155]	Chronic migraine and comorbid insomnia ($N = 31$)	Single	Sham: "lifestyle modification"	6 wk	CBT for chronic migraine	Sleep	Headache diary	PSQI	Yes	Yes	Yes

[a]Emphasis is given on the agreement between the changes in the pain and sleep outcomes as a result of interventions targeting sleep, pain, or both sleep and pain functions.
[b]This list presents in chronologic order main randomized controlled trials that were published in the last decade. Investigations with no clear prospectively defined hypotheses regarding the examined outcomes, studies with conclusions based on exploratory and/or subgroup, unplanned analyses, and those studies that were not preregistered at ClinicalTrials.gov, or an equivalent national database, were not included.
ASWS, Adolescent sleep wake scale; BPI, brief pain inventory; CBT, cognitive behavioral therapy; CWP, chronic widespread pain (new name for fibromyalgia, FM); FIQR, Fibromyalgia Impact Revised Questionnaire; ISI, Insomnia Severity Index; LSO, latency to sleep onset; MOSS, Medical Outcomes Study Sleep Scale; NRS, Numerical Rating Scale; PDPN, painful diabetic peripheral neuropathy; PSG, polysomnography; PSQI, Pittsburgh Sleep Quality Index; SE, sleep efficiency; SI, sleep interference; SOL, sleep-onset latency; TST, total sleep time; SF-MPQ, Short-Form McGill Pain Questionnaire; VAS, visual analogue scale; WASO, wake after sleep onset.

reduction in the influx of calcium ions into oversensitized neurons, followed by a subsequent reduction in the synaptic activity of the latter.[140]

Studies in volunteers[143] and patients suffering from chronic pain[104,144] have demonstrated the beneficial effects of pregabalin on sleep function. The fraction of SWS is increased, and there is an associated improvement in self-assessed sleep quality, whereas a high degree of association between improvement in sleep and pain relief has been observed in patients with diabetic and postherpetic neuralgia, suggesting that the analgesic action of pregabalin might be mediated via its sleep-restoring effects.[145] Recently, mirogabalin, an agent with selective affinity for the $\alpha_2\delta$-1 subunit of the voltage-dependent calcium channels and significantly more potent than pregabalin, has also been used to treat patients with diabetic and postherpetic neuropathic pain.[146]

Nonpharmacologic Interventions for Pain and Comorbid Insomnia

Cognitive behavioral therapy (CBT) has been a successful psychological intervention for primary insomnia.[147] The recognition of pain as an emotionally charged experience has prompted the development and application of such psychological interventions in the management of patients with chronic pain. However, two large meta-analyses of RCTs, comparing cognitive behavioral therapy for pain (CBT-P) with active or passive control treatments, have shown that CBT-P had only a small, short-lived effect on pain outcomes.[148,149]

On the other hand, although insomnia-specific cognitive behavioral therapy (CBT-I) has been quite effective in treating insomnia comorbid with psychiatric and medical conditions, its positive impact on psychiatric symptoms per se was much stronger than the improvement noted in medical outcomes, including pain.[150] This evidence agrees with the findings of a recent meta-analysis of 11 RCTs assessing nonpharmacologic treatments of sleep in patients with chronic pain and comorbid insomnia, where the effect of CBT-I on pain was modest and approximately half of that exerted on insomnia.[151] The observed resistance to CBT that specifically focuses on pain, emphasizes the complex psychophysiology of chronic pain and has recently spurred the combination of CBT-P, with treatments aiming at the psychological aspects of the disease, by improving sleeping behavior (i.e., a *hybrid* psychological intervention).[152–155]

The first pilot applications of hybrid CBT in patients with chronic pain showed that, although not effective in reducing pain intensity, CBT-PI did have a positive effect on sleep and significantly reduced pain interference, depression, and fatigue.[156,157] In another application, the *Lifestyles* RCT tested a hybrid intervention (CBT-PI) against CBT-P and an education-only control in older patients with osteoarthritis pain and comorbid insomnia.[158] Hybrid CBT-PI significantly improved sleep, but not pain, over a 9-month assessment period, whereas a post hoc secondary analysis showed that a subset of patients with more severe pain and insomnia at baseline did experience significant improvement for both pain and sleep at 18 months.[159] Of interest, regardless of the treatment arm, the presence of a clinically significant sleep benefit at 2 months after therapy initiation, predicted an improvement for both sleep and pain at 18 months, suggesting that a sustained improvement in sleep quality is necessary before a clinical benefit for pain emerges.[160] These observations are supported by recent RCTs, which indirectly emphasize the important role of CBT-I in achieving a significant and lasting effect on pain in a subset of patients, not only in the context of hybrid therapy, but also when CBT-I is applied as a sole intervention.[153–155]

Although it is early to conclude about the effectiveness of hybrid therapy for treating chronic pain in general, steadily accumulating evidence shows that a properly engineered hybrid therapeutic framework, possibly including other forms of mind-body interventions, such as yoga,[161] tai chi,[162] meditation,[163] or bright morning light therapy,[91] may enhance the therapeutic effect of pain-specific modalities. The fact that only a small fraction of patients enjoy a larger benefit from hybrid interventions makes precision medicine phenotypic characterization of patients with chronic pain an important focus for future research. Factors such as emotional and cognitive ailments,[92] other medical conditions, and drug treatments with the potential for promoting insomnia[164] also need to be taken into account because they may mediate or confound the clinical picture.

As shown in Tables 156.2 and 156.3, for a variety of chronic pain conditions, an agreement between treatment-induced changes in pain and sleep outcomes is common, independent of how effective is the therapy under evaluation. This observation confirms previous findings from a systematic review of Cochrane meta-analyses, showing that changes in sleep and pain outcomes of various interventions tend to be in the same direction.[165] Although these findings indicate a strong link between sleep and pain, and even general well-being,[166,167] it is evident that, when used alone and independent of targeted function (i.e., sleep or pain), no current pharmacologic or CBT modality is both sufficiently safe and effective to improve pain in the long term.

CLINICAL PEARLS

- Pain disturbs sleep, and impaired sleep might exacerbate responses to pain. Sleep disorders, depression, and impaired cognitive coping mechanisms are highly prevalent among patients with chronic pain; sleep disorders such as sleep deprivation, insomnia, and sleep apnea have been associated with various phenotypes of pain complaints.
- The sleep medicine physician should be aware of the complex epidemiology of chronic pain and follow a diagnostic approach that includes a comprehensive evaluation of both pain and sleep phenotypes, as well as a thorough assessment of patient's mental health.
- Different types of chronic pain benefit from different pharmacologic approaches (e.g., modern antidepressants, sodium oxybate, anticonvulsants for chronic widespread pain, and anticonvulsants for neuropathic pain), but all interventions are uniformly associated with improvement in both sleep and pain functions independent of therapeutic target.
- Hybrid cognitive behavioral psychotherapies that are targeting both pain and comorbid insomnia in the same individual have the potential not only to further improve patient outcomes but also to initiate a new paradigm in the understanding of pain-sleep conundrum.

SUMMARY

Chronic pain and poor sleep hygiene are major public health challenges with great economic and societal impact. A reciprocal relationship between the two is slowly being established, based on micro longitudinal and macro longitudinal studies in both volunteers and patients with chronic pain. Activation of major inflammatory pathways and impairment of central pain matrix network and descending pain-inhibitory signals seem to be important candidate mechanisms for the hyperalgesic effect of both acute and chronic sleep loss. Patients with chronic pain, mood disorders, and cognitive changes associated with preoccupation with pain- or sleep-related information, seem to potentiate the bidirectional influence between pain and comorbid insomnia. In the context of pain, several self-administered sleep assessment instruments have demonstrated reasonable discriminatory capacity to distinguish patients with sleep disorders from normal sleepers. In addition, when applied to pain patients, these tests can detect improvement in sleep quality associated with analgesia interventions. In patients with chronic pain, pharmacologic therapies targeting either pain or sleep outcomes significantly improve both. More recent evidence suggests that the effect sizes of such interventions on pain or comorbid sleep disorders may be further increased by CBTs and mind-body interventions that simultaneously address sleep- and pain-related symptoms.

SELECTED READINGS

Afolalu EF, Ramlee F, Tang NKY. Effects of sleep changes on pain-related health outcomes in the general population: a systematic review of longitudinal studies with exploratory meta-analysis. *Sleep Med Rev*. 2018;39:82–97.

Chan WS, Levsen MP, Puyat S, et al. Sleep discrepancy in patients with comorbid fibromyalgia and insomnia: demographic, behavioral, and clinical correlates. *J Clin Sleep Med*. 2018;14:1911–1919.

Curtis AF, Miller MB, Rathinakumar H, et al. Opioid use, pain intensity, age, and sleep architecture in patients with fibromyalgia and insomnia. *Pain*. 2019;160:2086–2092.

Dahlhamer J, Lucas J, Zelaya C, et al. Prevalence of chronic pain and high-impact chronic pain among adults—United States, 2016. *MMWR Morb Mortal Wkly Rep*. 2018;67:1001–1006.

Eccleston C, Palermo TM, Williams AC, et al. Psychological therapies for the management of chronic and recurrent pain in children and adolescents. *Cochrane Database Syst Rev*. 2014;5:CD003968.

Generaal E, Vogelzangs N, Penninx BW, Dekker J. Insomnia, sleep duration, depressive symptoms, and the onset of chronic multisite musculoskeletal pain. *Sleep*. 2017;40(1). https://doi.org/10.1093/sleep/zsw030.

Huang CJ, Huang CL, Fan YC, Chen TY, Tsai PS. Insomnia increases symptom severity and health care utilization in patients with fibromyalgia: a population-based study. *Clin J Pain*. 2019;35:780–785.

Krause AJ, Prather AA, Wager TD, Lindquist MA, Walker MP. The pain of sleep loss: a brain characterization in humans. *J Neurosci*. 2019;39:2291–2300.

Mathias JL, Cant ML, Burke ALJ. Sleep disturbances and sleep disorders in adults living with chronic pain: a meta-analysis. *Sleep Med*. 2018;52:198–210.

Miettinen T, Mäntyselkä P, Hagelberg N, Mustola S, Kalso E, Lötsch J. Machine learning suggests sleep as a core factor in chronic pain. *Pain*. 2021;162(1):109–123.

Peyron R, Fauchon C. Functional imaging of pain. *Rev Neurol (Paris)*. 2019;175:38–45.

Tang NK, Fiecas M, Afolalu EF, Wolke D. Changes in sleep duration, quality, and medication use are prospectively associated with health and well-being: analysis of the UK Household Longitudinal Study. *Sleep*. 2017;40(2). https://doi.org/10.1093/sleep/zsw079.

Tang NK, Lereya ST, Boulton H, Miller MA, Wolke D, Cappuccio FP. Nonpharmacological treatments of insomnia for long-term painful conditions: a systematic review and meta-analysis of patient-reported outcomes in randomized controlled trials. *Sleep*. 2015;38:1751–1764.

Tang NK, McBeth J, Jordan KP, Blagojevic-Bucknall M, Croft P, Wilkie R. Impact of musculoskeletal pain on insomnia onset: a prospective cohort study. *Rheumatology (Oxford)*. 2015;54:248–256.

Tang NKY. Cognitive behavioural therapy in pain and psychological disorders: towards a hybrid future. *Prog Neuropsychopharmacol Biol Psychiatry*. 2018;87:281–289.

Treede RD, Rief W, Barke A, et al. Chronic pain as a symptom or a disease: the IASP classification of chronic pain for the International Classification of Diseases (ICD-11). *Pain*. 2019;160:19–27.

Whibley D, AlKandari N, Kristensen K, et al. Sleep and pain: a systematic review of studies of mediation. *Clin J Pain*. 2019;35:544–558.

A complete reference list can be found online at ExpertConsult.com.

Chapter 157

Sleep and Chronic Kidney Disease

Melissa C. Lipford; Kannan Ramar

Chapter Highlights

- Sleep disturbances, such as insomnia, restless legs syndrome, periodic limb movements of sleep, and obstructive sleep apnea, are common across the wide spectrum of chronic kidney disease (CKD) patients. CKD is linked to an increased risk for sleep disorders through various pathophysiologic mechanisms. The occurrence of CKD continues to rise, and as a result, the prevalence of comorbid sleep disorders in this population is likely to grow. Similarly, sleep disorders may increase risks associated with development of CKD and contribute to the rising prevalence of CKD.
- Comorbid sleep disorders add significant burden to the quality of life, health care costs, and morbidity and mortality of patients with CKD.
- Changing from conventional to nocturnal hemodialysis results in improved cardiovascular function and improvement of sleep-disordered breathing
- This chapter provides an up-to-date review of the current available literature regarding sleep disturbances in patients with CKD and discusses the associated clinical implications and treatment options for the various sleep disorders common to this population.

Chronic kidney disease (CKD) is defined as abnormalities of kidney structure or function (defined by estimated glomerular filtration rate [eGFR] <60 mL/minute per 1.73 m^2) that is present for 3 or more months, with negative implications on health.[1] CKD is a common but serious condition associated with an increasing incidence and prevalence (16.8%) in the United States, particularly with the increasing prevalence of diabetes mellitus, metabolic syndrome, and hypertension, all being significant risk factors for CKD.[2,3] CKD is associated with increased mortality, decreased quality of life, and increased health care costs. CKD is also linked to an increased risk for sleep disorders. This chapter discusses the various sleep disorders across the spectrum of CKD patients and reviews the consequences and treatment options in this specific population.

OVERVIEW AND EPIDEMIOLOGY

Sleep disorders, such as insomnia, sleep-disordered breathing, restless legs syndrome, and excessive daytime sleepiness, occur in 45% to 80% of patients with end-stage renal disease (ESRD) requiring dialysis. In non–dialysis-dependent CKD patients, the prevalence of sleep disorders also varies widely, between 14% and 85%.[4–6] The reasons for this wide variation are multifactorial and may be related to the use of subjective versus objective data to assess sleep quality, the type of sleep disorder that is being evaluated, and the stage of CKD. Ezzat and Mohab[7] prospectively studied 90 patients split equally into the following groups: ESRD patients on regular hemodialysis (HD), CKD patients, and normal control subjects. Sleep disorders, including insomnia, obstructive sleep apnea, and excessive daytime sleepiness, were all more common in the ESRD and CKD patients compared to control subjects. The study group found an inverse correlation between hemoglobin, albumin, creatinine clearance, and the presence of sleep disorders.

The type of dialysis in the treatment of ESRD can impact clinical outcome. Changing from conventional to nocturnal hemodialysis results in improved blood pressure control, requiring fewer medications, regression of left ventricular hypertrophy, improved left ventricular function, and improvement of sleep apnea.[8]

Sleep quality indices are poor in many patients with CKD and appear to worsen with declining kidney function. Sabbatini and colleagues[9] found progressive worsening of sleep quality as measured by the Pittsburg Sleep Quality Index (PSQI), with progression of renal disease based on CKD stage. Similarly, a 4-year prospective cohort study in Japan found shorter sleep duration and worsened sleep quality (based on the PSQI) were associated with ESRD in patients with CKD.[10] Poor sleep quality on the PSQI has been noted in 84.6% of CKD patients compared with 59.5% of patients with the chronic disease hepatitis C.[11] The large-scale study Dialysis Outcomes and Practice Patterns demonstrated a 49% prevalence of sleep disorders in HD patients. Common elements in the clinical phenotype of HD patients (elevated body mass index [BMI], heart failure, diabetes mellitus, peripheral nerve disease, etc.) were all associated with poor sleep ($P < .05$).[12] Restless legs syndrome (RLS) symptoms and sleeping pill use were more frequent in CKD stages 3 and 4 compared with stages 1 and 2 or no CKD.[13] Poor sleep quality, when measured by the Kidney Disease Quality of Life survey, has been reported in approximately 57% of patients with CKD and was more common in advanced CKD stages (mean eGFR, 24.9 ± 10.6 mL/minute per 1.73 m^2).[14]

Reduced sleep efficiency and greater sleep fragmentation, as measured by wrist actigraphy, have been noted in CKD compared with non-CKD patients.[15] Patients with CKD stages 4 and 5 had shorter, more fragmented sleep, resulting in total sleep time and sleep efficiency being worse than patients on HD.[16] Patients with non–HD-dependent CKD had a higher prevalence (54.3%) of sleep-disordered breathing and periodic limb movement disorder (30%) compared with the general population.[17]

Although further studies are needed to clarify the heterogeneity of the results, the overall evidence points toward a far higher prevalence of sleep disorders in CKD patients compared with the general population.[4–6] CKD itself appears to promote sleep disturbances. CKD-associated anemia may result in development of RLS and periodic limb movements of sleep (PLMS). The volume overload that occurs in CKD may result in sleep-disordered breathing. The sleep associations may also be bidirectional. For example, long-standing sleep-disordered breathing may result in hypertension, which can be a factor leading to development of and worsening of CKD.[18] Identification and treatment of sleep disorders in CKD patients is exceedingly important. Chronic sleep disruption in CKD patients is associated with significant quality-of-life burden, and sleep disorders may also be associated with increased morbidity and mortality in this complex patient population.

INSOMNIA

Insomnia is defined as a persistent difficulty with sleep initiation, duration, consolidation, or quality that occurs despite adequate opportunity and circumstances for sleep and results in some form of daytime impairment (*International Classification of Sleep Disorders: Diagnostic and Coding Manual,* second edition).[19] Insomnia complaints include difficulty initiating sleep, maintaining sleep, or both. Although the mechanism is not entirely understood, insomnia-related poor sleep quality appears to increase the mortality risk among patients with CKD.[12]

Insomnia symptoms are more common in patients with CKD compared to the general population. About 60% of subjects on HD have insomnia, ranging from difficulty falling asleep in nearly one-half of patients to difficulty maintaining sleep or having early-morning awakening in one-fourth of patients.[20] In a multicenter trial involving more than 11,000 patients on maintenance HD, approximately 50% reported insomnia symptoms.[12] A comparison of 46 conventional hemodialysis patients to 137 control subjects from the Sleep Heart Health Study demonstrated a higher prevalence of short sleep (<5 hours) (odds ratio [OR], 3.27; 95% confidence interval [CI], 1.16 to 9.25) and decreased sleep efficiency (OR, 5.5; 95% CI, 1.5 to 19.6).[21] It is likely that both psychological and physiologic factors are responsible for the insomnia complaints in patients with CKD. Higher prevalence of anxiety, stress, and depression is reported in patients with CKD, and these are well-known risk factors for insomnia.[22] Rapid fluid, electrolyte, and acid-base changes that occur during HD are often associated with central nervous system symptoms, such as drowsiness and fatigue during or immediately after treatment.[23,24] In addition, blood reactions with the biocompatible equipment used in HD may lead to increased cytokine production; these cytokines have somnogenic properties.[25,26] Thus

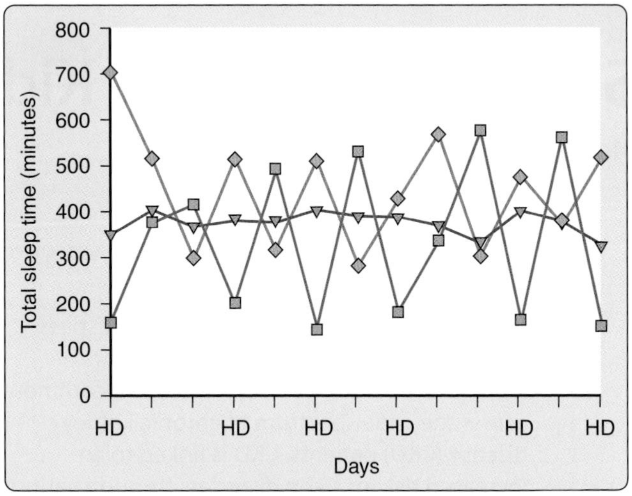

Figure 157.1 Total sleep time (TST) on hemodialysis (HD) treatment and non-HD nights. *Diamonds* represent subjects with longer TST on post-HD nights. *Squares* represent subjects with shorter TST on post-HD nights. *Triangles* represent subjects with a stable sleep pattern on pre-HD and post-HD nights.

HD patients may be more prone to sleep during the daytime hours, resulting in poor nighttime sleep efficiency. Changes in melatonin levels and patterns of melatonin secretion are also associated with HD. These may play a role in disrupting the circadian cycle of HD patients.[27] HD sessions are typically scheduled during the daytime hours. A prolonged period of rest during the day may affect circadian systems by altering exposure to zeitgebers, such as sunlight exposure, sleep-wake patterns, meal times, and social activity (Figure 157.1).

Treatment of Insomnia

There is very little evidence to guide treatment of insomnia among CKD patients. The main goals of treatment are to improve sleep quality and reduce daytime impairments, such as daytime fatigue and sleepiness. This can be accomplished by either pharmacologic, nonpharmacologic, or a combination of both of these approaches. The evidence, efficacy, and safety profile of these approaches are well discussed specifically in the chapters devoted to insomnia. However, studies using these approaches specifically in CKD patients are very limited.

Given the frequency of insomnia in CKD patients, it is not surprising the prevalence of routine use of sleep hypnotics in this population is 25.8%.[20] In a small randomized study comparing zaleplon with placebo, using the PSQI to assess for sleep quality, zaleplon reduced sleep latency and improved sleep efficiency and sleep quality without significant side effects in HD patients.[28] In another randomized crossover study comparing the effects of clonazepam with zolpidem, both drugs improved PSQI in HD patients; clonazepam was more effective in decreasing PSQI scores than zolpidem, whereas the latter was better tolerated.[29] However, caution should be exercised as these agents may have adverse interactions with other medications CKD patients are taking and may result in side effects, such as daytime sleepiness or increased risk of falls. Hypnotic-related side effects may be more common in this population, particularly if the agents are renally metabolized. Renal dosing and dose alterations with respect to HD schedule may be necessary with many medications frequently used to optimize sleep, such as gabapentin or benzodiazepine agents.

Nonpharmacologic approaches, such as sleep hygiene, stimulus control, and cognitive behavior therapy (CBT), have been well studied as treatments for insomnia in the general population; however, there are limited data for CKD patients with insomnia. In a study of patients on peritoneal dialysis, CBT has shown to improve fatigue as measured by the Global Fatigue Severity Scale (GFSC) and decrease inflammatory cytokines.[30] In patients on HD, CBT results in improved PSQI, GFSC, and Beck Depression and Anxiety Inventory scores, along with reduced inflammatory markers and oxidative stress.[31] When the benefit of exercise during dialysis was evaluated, it was noted that aerobic activity, with moderate intensity during the first 2 hours of a dialysis session, could improve sleep quality as measured by the PSQI.[32] The effect of acupressure to improve sleep quality and fatigue in renal patients on HD was evaluated in a randomized controlled trial of 1 month. Patients who received acupressure had significantly lower levels of fatigue, better sleep quality, and less depression compared with control subjects. In addition, HD induces a heat load, and patients often respond with an increase in body temperature of approximately 0.5° to 1.0° C; this increase in body temperature may result in insomnia on the nights after treatment.[33] The use of cool dialysate during HD has been shown to improve nocturnal sleep (i.e., shorter sleep latency, longer sleep duration, and longer rapid eye movement latencies) by decreasing sympathetic activation.[34]

Despite the overall limited data of nonpharmacologic approaches to treat insomnia in CKD patients, it is reasonable to consider these approaches as first line because their side effects and complications are relatively minor.

In summary, nonpharmacologic methods, such as behavioral techniques and cognitive therapy, as well as pharmacologic approaches and combinations of these methods, may be used for the treatment of insomnia in patients with CKD, noting the previous caveats. There remains a need for further studies assessing efficacy and safety of long-term therapies for chronic insomnia in CKD patients.

RESTLESS LEGS SYNDROME AND PERIODIC LIMB MOVEMENTS DURING SLEEP

Although the pathogenesis is not well understood, CKD is one of the secondary causes of RLS and PLMS (see Chapter 121 for comprehensive discussion of RLS and PLMS). Prevalence of RLS in CKD patients not on dialysis is reported to be 11% to 26% based on structured interview studies.[35,36] In nondialyzed CKD patients, it has been reported that approximately 11% fulfilled the RLS criteria of the International Restless Legs Syndrome Study Group[37] compared with 3% in healthy control subjects.[35] Looking at RLS across different stages of renal dysfunction, the prevalence among CKD patients may be as high as 26%[36] compared with what has been described in the general population (3% to 15%).[38–40] An increased prevalence of RLS also has been described in a Japanese study; 3.5% of Japanese patients with CKD had RLS compared with 1.5% of healthy control subjects.[41] The occurrence of RLS is also greater in children with CKD (15.3%) compared with healthy control subjects (5.9%) and may be underdiagnosed.[42–44] In children RLS did not seem to be associated with stage of CKD, etiology, duration, dialysis, or transplant status. Children with RLS are likely to rate their sleep quality as poor and report using sleep medications.

Among patients with ESRD requiring HD, RLS is present in 14% to 58%.[45–47] Some of the earlier studies suggested even higher prevalence rates, but these may have been limited by inconsistent criteria used for RLS or use of surveys without a structured clinical interview to validate symptoms.[48] The wide range of prevalence may also be due to small sample size in some studies and the location of patient recruitment (dialysis vs. sleep centers). Most of the studies suggest prevalence rates of 20% to 30% among ESRD patients requiring HD.

PLMS are reported in 42% of CKD patients on the transplant waitlist compared with 27% of patients after kidney transplantation.[49] A study using 48-hour, seven-channel, ambulatory polysomnogram (PSG) that included electromyogram signals from bilateral anterior tibialis muscles found PLMS (defined by periodic limb movement index [PLMI] ≥5/hour of sleep) to be present in 85.4% of HD subjects.[47] Defining "clinically relevant" PLMS as PLMI greater than or equal to 25 per hour, 71% met that criterion. They also noted that those who also had RLS had a much higher PLMI (median PLMI of 87/hour in those with coexisting RLS vs. 16/hour in those without RLS).[47]

These data suggest that the overall rate of RLS and PLMS are much more frequent in patients with CKD and ESRD than in the general population. The exact mechanism of how CKD may give rise to RLS remains elusive, but some proposed theories associate the sleep-related movement disorder to uremia[50] and low intact parathyroid hormone,[51] whereas the association with reduced serum ferritin has been much less robust compared to studies on subjects without CKD. There also appears to be a strong genetic influence in single-nucleotide polymorphisms that may influence the development of RLS among CKD patients.[52]

Clinical Characteristics of Restless Legs Syndrome in the Chronic Kidney Disease Population

Similar to the general population, RLS appears to be more prevalent among females with CKD, but the mean ages between those with and without RLS do not differ.[35,36,45] The prevalence of RLS does appear to increase with worsening eGFR.[41,42] Molnar and colleagues[53] looked at a group of 176 CKD patients on a waitlist for renal transplantation and found the prevalence of RLS to be 1.8%, 5.1%, 6.5%, and 23.5% in patients with eGFRs greater than 60, 30 to 59, 15 to 29, and less than 15 mL per minute per 1.73 m^2, respectively (Figure 157.2). In HD patients there are inconsistent findings regarding RLS association with sex, age, iron, hemoglobin, and ferritin.[45,46,54] One study concluded the only difference in laboratory values between HD patients with or without RLS was the level of C-reactive protein.[55] Compared with idiopathic RLS subjects, those with RLS and ESRD had much a higher PLMI (103.6 ± 74.4 vs. 22.0 ± 18.9; $P < .001$) and a much longer suggested immobilization test index (PLMS per hour of immobility tested during wakefulness) (127.9 ± 82.3 vs. 13.8 ± 29.0; $P < .001$).[56] These findings suggest some physiologic differences between uremic RLS and idiopathic RLS.

Morbidity and Mortality

Not unexpectedly, RLS is independently associated with a multitude of sleep-related complaints, reduced quality of life, and increased mortality. In patients with CKD and ESRD, RLS is independently associated with greater fatigue.[57] Compounding this increased fatigue may be the increased risk for

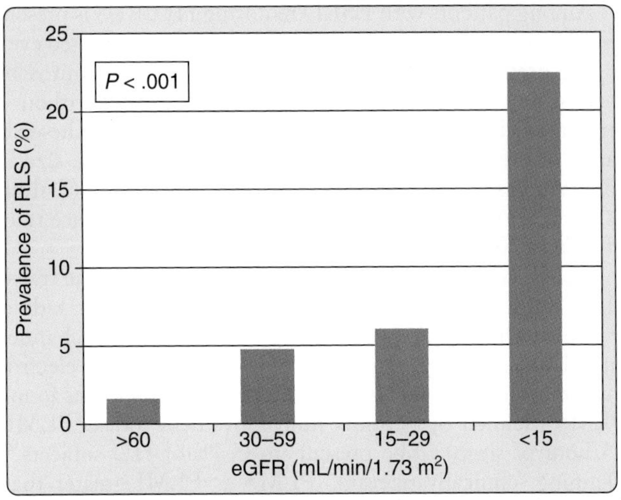

Figure 157.2 Association between presence of restless legs syndrome (RLS) and severity of chronic kidney disease based on estimated glomerular filtration rate (eGFR). (From Molnar MZ, Novak M, Ambrus C, et al. Restless legs syndrome in patients after renal transplantation. *Am J Kidney Dis.* 2005;45[2]:388–96, used with permission.)

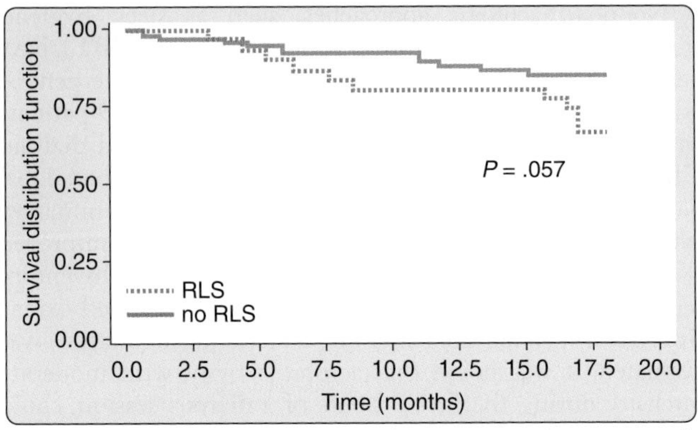

Figure 157.3 Kaplan-Meier estimates of all-cause mortality at 18 months in patients with and without restless legs syndrome (RLS). (From La Manna G, Pizza F, Persici E, et al. Restless legs syndrome enhances cardiovascular risk and mortality in patients with end-stage kidney disease undergoing long-term haemodialysis treatment. *Nephrol Dial Transplant.* 2011;26[6]:1976–83, used with permission.)

other sleep disorders, such as sleep apnea (see section Sleep-Related Breathing Disorders) and insomnia in CKD patients with RLS.[47,58,59] RLS is also independently associated with depression in patients on HD and after renal transplantation, even after adjusting for the presence of insomnia or use of antidepressants (antidepressants may cause/worsen RLS symptoms).[60,61] These findings likely explain the worse quality of life reported by patients with CKD and RLS compared with those with RLS and intact renal function.[62] RLS remains independently associated with lower quality-of-life assessments, even after adjusting for insomnia, age, gender, and comorbid conditions.[59,63,64]

Although the data on RLS and PLMS contributing to cardiovascular morbidity in the general population are inconclusive, there are some data suggesting that RLS in ESRD patients may increase cardiac morbidity. The incidence of new cardiovascular events (myocardial infarction, cerebral stroke, or peripheral artery occlusion) in patients with CKD and RLS is 64.5% compared with 39.1% in patients without RLS and likely contributes to the higher 18-month mortality seen in this group[65] (Figure 157.3). In a follow-up study over 30 months, ESRD patients with RLS have increased adjusted hazard ratio of mortality (adjusted for age, sex, comorbid conditions, functional status, and clinic location) of 1.39 (CI, 1.08 to 1.79) compared with ESRD patients without RLS.[63] Increased PLMS seem to predict mortality. Survival rate at 20 months among ESRD patients with a PLMI of more than 20 per hour is 50% compared with 90% in ESRD patients with a PLMI of less than 20 per hour.[66]

Treatment of Restless Legs Syndrome

Based on a limited number of studies addressing the needs of CKD patients, the overall treatment approach to RLS does not appear to be different from that of non-CKD patients.[67] Few small trials have shown the benefit of exercise in reducing RLS symptoms, including exercise during dialysis.[68,69] In CKD patients the treating clinician must keep in mind that most of the medications currently used to treat RLS are renally excreted. Therefore it would be advisable to start at the lowest dose possible and uptitrate the dose at a slower rate than for those with normal renal function. In patients who are on dialysis, it would be advisable to give a dose after dialysis. There are few comparative studies of different agents, and those studies are significantly limited by small sample size such that one class of medication cannot be recommended over another as the initial agent. Medications such as iron supplements, alpha-2 delta ligands (gabapentin, pregabalin, or gabapentin enacarbil), dopamine agonists (pramipexole, ropinirole, or the rotigotine patch), and benzodiazepines could be considered. In those with severe, refractory symptoms, opiates may also be a consideration.[67,70]

Kidney transplantation is reported to have some benefit in improving RLS symptoms. Resolution of RLS symptoms is reported to occur between 1 and 38 days after undergoing renal transplantation, and symptoms may recur in 10 to 60 days in those whose transplantation fails.[71,72] In a follow-up period of up to 3 years, patients whose transplanted kidneys are still functioning have continued resolution of RLS.[72] These findings suggest that normalizing renal function can improve RLS symptoms, but the specifics of this mechanism remain elusive.

SLEEP-RELATED BREATHING DISORDERS

There appears to be a strong association between CKD and sleep apnea, of which the most common form is obstructive sleep apnea (OSA)[73] (see Section 14 [Sleep Breathing Disorders] of this book for a comprehensive discussion). The hypoxemia of sleep apnea is associated with increased risk of death among advanced chronic kidney disease and end-stage kidney disease.[74] Its prevalence in CKD and HD patients ranges from 30% to 73%.[17,32,73,75–79] This wide range of reported prevalence is due to the variable cut-off value of the apnea-hypopnea index (AHI) or respiratory disturbance index (RDI) that was used to define the presence of OSA and the varying degree of renal dysfunction. For example, in a study of 1624 subjects who were diagnosed with OSA (based on AHI ≥5 events/hour), 30.5% had CKD.[75] The prevalence of CKD has been shown to be as much as threefold higher in an OSA group compared to control subjects (prevalence of 9.1%).[75] In a much smaller study of 63 subjects on HD, 51% had OSA, defined as RDI of 15 or more.[80] It is, however, worthwhile to note that a cross-sectional study of patients enrolled in the Kaiser Permanente health care system found that, among 85,376 patients with a diagnosis of CKD, only 3.3% had sleep apnea, based solely on diagnostic codes or positive airway pressure device prescriptions.[81] This low prevalence rate may have been confounded by the number of patients with sleep apnea who are undiagnosed, as it seems inconsistent with other studies, and in fact the 3.3% prevalence rate is even lower than the rate of sleep apnea seen among the non-CKD population.[82,83]

Despite the wide variability in the prevalence studies mentioned previously, a more consistent finding is the association with increasing prevalence of OSA with worsening renal function.[21,84,85] Using an RDI of 15 or greater, 38% of subjects with CKD were shown to have OSA, whereas 51% of subjects with ESRD had OSA.[80] It has been demonstrated that for each 10 mL per minute per 1.73 m^2 decrease in eGFR, the OR for OSA is 1.42, even after adjustment for age, BMI, and presence of diabetes mellitus.[86] Similarly, it has been shown that patients on HD have an OR of 4.14 for having an AHI of more than 15, compared with 2.19 in CKD patients (eGFR ≤ 40 mL/minute per 1.73 m^2).[85] OSA also appears to have a causal role in worsening CKD; untreated sleep-disordered breathing may result in hypertension, which secondarily worsens CKD.[18]

Few studies specifically address central sleep apnea (CSA; generally defined by a central apnea index ≥5/hour) in CKD. The number of CSA events may be six times higher, and with greater resultant desaturations, in those with CKD than those with normal renal function.[76] Compared with those with eGFR of 90 mL per minute per 1.73 m^2 or greater, the percentage of total RDI that is due to CSA events is three times greater in those with eGFR of 60 mL per minute per 1.73 m^2 or less (14.9% of total RDI compared with 4.9%).[16] Patients on HD with sleep apnea often have CSA-predominant sleep apnea (the majority of breathing events are central in etiology).[87] In these CSA-predominant subjects, there is a greater incidence of atrial fibrillation. Of interest, the central apnea indices are lower on the night after HD, suggesting that volume overload may contribute to the development of CSA in susceptible patients.[87]

Identifying CKD patients with OSA requires a high index of suspicion because these patients seem to present with less severe or atypical sleep-related complaints.[88–90] A history of snoring and witnessed apneas are reported less often in ESRD subjects than in control subjects without ESRD.[90] Similarly, complaints of unrefreshing sleep and morning headaches are less frequent in ESRD subjects.[90] The mean maximal snoring intensity during PSG is reduced in ESRD subjects compared with control subjects.[90] Furthermore, subjects with ESRD have lower BMI and neck circumference compared with control subjects with comparable AHI.[90] When compared with CKD subjects without OSA, CKD patients with OSA less frequently report increased sleepiness as measured by the Epworth Sleepiness Scale.[89]

Pathophysiology

CKD may potentiate the likelihood of sleep apnea through mechanisms of volume overload, fluid redistribution, and altered chemoresponsiveness. Internal jugular vein volume and upper airway mucosal water content, rather than upper airway cross-sectional area, correlate with AHI in subjects undergoing HD.[91] This correlation remains significant even after adjusting for age, sex, height, BMI, and percent reduction of urea. This is consistent with the finding that even a 0.5-L rostral fluid shift during recumbency can lead to significant increase in neck circumference and upper airway resistance.[92,93] The findings that nocturnal HD can reduce AHI and that AHI may increase back to baseline when off of nocturnal HD support the fluid-shift theory further. Nocturnal HD can mitigate nocturnal fluid shifts by extracellular fluid removal at night and by improved ultrafiltration owing to longer dialysis periods.[4]

Another contributing mechanism toward sleep apnea in CKD patients may be altered chemosensitivity. Unstable chemosensitivity leads to destabilization of respiratory control and may contribute to the severity of OSA.[94] Subjects with ESRD and coexisting OSA have higher ventilatory sensitivity to arterial partial pressure of carbon dioxide than those without OSA.[78] This relationship is independent of age, sex, or BMI. By switching from conventional HD to nocturnal HD, chemoresponsiveness to hypercapnia may be reduced and lead to a decrease in AHI.[95]

Although chronic uremia has also been proposed to result in upper airway muscle dysfunction, there have not been convincing data to confirm this theory. Rather, it is more likely that multiple factors are ultimately responsible for the increased likelihood of OSA in CKD. For any given individual, one factor may have a greater influence over another, leading to the variable expression of OSA in these patients.

Influence of Sleep Apnea on Outcomes in Chronic Kidney Disease Patients

OSA and CKD share many comorbidities, including hypertension, diabetes mellitus, and obesity. Therefore it is difficult to independently associate worsening kidney function in CKD patients to OSA alone. However, there is some evidence to suggest that the coexistence of OSA in patients with CKD may worsen microalbuminuria and eGFR and be associated with increased levels of cystatin C (a sensitive biomarker that reflects impaired renal function and is associated with latent CKD).[96,97] Furthermore, being at high risk for OSA, as defined by scoring positively in two of three main domains in the Berlin Sleep Apnea Questionnaire, may be an independent risk factor for kidney graft loss, particularly in female transplant recipients.[60] Potential mechanisms by which OSA contributes to worsening renal function may include intermittent hypoxemia, sympathetic surges associated with arousals, and systemic inflammation, which may lead to endothelial dysfunction and tubulointerstitial injury.[73,98,99]

OSA also contributes to worse quality of life, as it does in those without CKD. Those with both OSA and CKD score worse in vitality, social functioning, and mental health measures on the Short Form-36 Health Survey.[100] Patients with CKD and moderate or severe OSA (AHI ≥ 15) have greater complaints of excessive daytime sleepiness and impairment in verbal memory, working memory, attention, and psychomotor speed compared with those without OSA.[101]

Treatment of Sleep-Related Breathing Disorders

With OSA and CKD both independently increasing cardiovascular morbidity and mortality, it is crucial to treat OSA to mitigate these consequences. Unfortunately, although there is an exhaustive literature confirming the benefits of continuous positive airway pressure (CPAP) therapy in treatment of OSA,

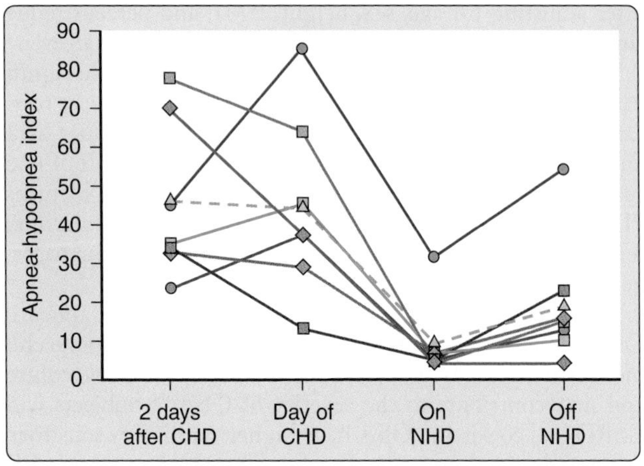

Figure 157.4 Apnea-hypopnea index (AHI) in seven patients with a baseline AHI of ≥15 events/hour. Mean values are represented by the *broken line.* CHD, Conventional hemodialysis; NHD, nocturnal hemodialysis.

there is a limited literature regarding treatment outcomes specifically in CKD patients.[102] Some studies have shown the efficacy of CPAP in improving glomerular hyperfiltration and eGFR in subjects with OSA but with normal baseline renal function.[61,103] Adaptive servo-ventilation (ASV) therapy in CKD patients with moderate to severe obstructive and central sleep apnea and heart failure (mean ejection fraction of about 45%) may result in improvement in eGFR; New York Heart Association functional class; and serum levels of brain natriuretic peptide, creatinine, cystatin C, C-reactive protein, and noradrenaline.[104,105] It should also be recalled that based on the recently published Servo Ventilation in Patients with Heart Failure (SERVE-HF) trial, ASV is not currently recommended for patients with primary central sleep apnea if the ejection fraction is less than 45%.[106]

Beyond positive airway pressure devices, changing the timing of dialysis in renal failure patients has been shown to improve sleep apnea. As mentioned earlier, nocturnal HD compared with conventional HD may improve AHI severity[4] (Figure 157.4). Nocturnal HD may also lead to a decrease in percentage of sleep time spent at oxygen saturation less than 90%, a decrease in heart rate, and an increase in vagal tone.[107] Nocturnal HD may also result in a decrease in chemoreflex response and an improvement in AHI.[95]

Nocturnal peritoneal dialysis (NPD) may also result in improvements in OSA compared with continuous ambulatory peritoneal dialysis (CAPD). When subjects matched for demographics, BMI, comorbidities, adequacy of dialysis, and peritoneal transport properties are converted from NPD to CAPD, AHI worsens markedly.[108] It appears that NPD lessens OSA because of its greater efficacy in fluid removal based on greater reduction in total body water.[108] Magnetic resonance imaging assessment of the upper airways confirms significant reductions in nasopharyngeal and oropharyngeal volumes, minimal pharyngeal cross-sectional area, and tongue volume enlargement after converting to NPD from CAPD.[109]

Several studies report improvements in OSA after renal transplantation. Since earlier reports of resolution of OSA after transplantation,[110] there have been conflicting results reported by others. Several studies suggest that not all patients undergoing transplantation had resolution of their OSA, with some suggesting that less than half of their study patients had resolution.[111–113] The small sample sizes of these reports and varying durations between the pretransplantation and posttransplantation PSG, which may result in BMI increase due to immunosuppressives, may account for the conflicting results. However, taken together these reports suggest that some patients with OSA may significantly improve after transplantation.

CPAP should still be considered the initial therapy of choice for patients with OSA and CKD because of its proven efficacy. For CKD patients, additional considerations may include converting from conventional to nocturnal HD or from continuous ambulatory peritoneal dialysis to NPD. Furthermore, transplantation may potentially improve OSA, but this effect may be counterbalanced by the potential weight gain associated with medications required as part of the antirejection regimen.

CLINICAL PEARL

Concurrent sleep disorders are common in patients with chronic kidney disease (CKD), and the prevalence of various sleep disorders seems to increase with worsening kidney function. Because of coexisting comorbidities in CKD patients, symptoms of sleep disorders may be atypical or initially attributed to other conditions. Thus it is important for the clinician to specifically inquire about sleep disorders, such as insomnia, RLS, or sleep apnea. When using pharmacologic therapies for sleep disorders, clinicians must carefully consider renal excretion of some medications and anticipate the need to appropriately adjust the dose or timing of the medication. Treating coexisting sleep disorders in CKD patients can substantially improve quality of life and, particularly in the case of sleep apnea, may be associated with reduced morbidity and mortality. Changing from conventional to nocturnal hemodialysis results in improved cardiovascular function and improvement of sleep-disordered breathing.

SUMMARY

Sleep disturbances, such as insomnia, RLS, PLMS, and OSA, are common across the spectrum of CKD. The pathophysiologic mechanisms that drive these sleep disorders in CKD patients are complex and incompletely understood. What is appreciated is that sleep disorders have significant effects on morbidity, quality of life, functional status, and possibly mortality in this population. Therefore an assessment of sleep-related complaints and sleep disorders should be pursued in all CKD patients. Treatment of sleep disorders may be complex and unique to this population because of the nature of their underlying medical disease.

SELECTED READINGS

Abuyassin B, et al. Obstructive sleep apnea and kidney disease: a potential bidirectional relationship? *J Clin Sleep Med.* 2015;11(8):915–924.

Al Mawed S, Unruh M. Diabetic kidney disease and obstructive sleep apnea: a new frontier? *Curr Opin Pulm Med.* 2016;22(1):80–88.

Elder SJ, et al. Sleep quality predicts quality of life and mortality risk in haemodialysis patients: results from the Dialysis Outcomes and Practice Patterns Study (DOPPS). *Nephrol Dial Transplant.* 2008;23(3):998–1004.

Hui L, Benca R. The bidirectional relationship between obstructive sleep apnea and chronic kidney disease. *J Stroke Cerebrovasc Dis.* 2021;30(9):105652.

Jhamb M, Ran X, Abdalla H, et al. Association of sleep apnea with mortality in patients with advanced kidney disease. *Clin J Am Soc Nephrol.* 2020;15(2):182–190.

Lee J, et al. The prevalence of restless legs syndrome across the full spectrum of kidney disease. *J Clin Sleep Med.* 2013;9(5):455–459.
Lee JJ, et al. Improvement of sleep-related breathing disorder in patients with end-stage renal disease after kidney transplantation. *Clin Transplant.* 2011;25(1):126–130.
Lin CH, Lurie RC, Lyons OD. Sleep apnea and chronic kidney disease: a state-of-the-art review. *Chest.* 2020;157(3):673–685.
Lindner AV, Novak M, Bohra M, Mucsi I. Insomnia in patients with chronic kidney disease. *Semin Nephrol.* 2015;35(4):359–372.
Molnar MZ, Novak M, Ambrus C, et al. Restless legs syndrome in patients after renal transplantation. *Am J Kidney Dis.* 2005;45(2):388–396.
Owada T, et al. Adaptive servoventilation improves cardiorenal function and prognosis in heart failure patients with chronic kidney disease and sleep-disordered breathing. *J Card Fail.* 2013;19(4):225–232.
Puckrin R, Iqbal S, Zidulka A, et al. Renoprotective effects of continuous positive airway pressure in chronic kidney disease patients with sleep apnea. *Int Urol Nephrol.* 2015;47(11):1839–1845.
Roumeliotis A, Roumeliotis S, Chan C, Pierratos A. Cardiovascular benefits of extended-time nocturnal hemodialysis. *Curr Vasc Pharmacol.* 2021;19(1):21–33.
Sabbatini M, et al. Zaleplon improves sleep quality in maintenance hemodialysis patients. *Nephron Clin Pract.* 2003;94(4):c99–c103.
Szentkiralyi A, et al. High risk of obstructive sleep apnea is a risk factor of death censored graft loss in kidney transplant recipients: an observational cohort study. *Sleep Med.* 2011;12(3):267–273.
Voulgaris A, Bonsignore MR, Schiza S, Marrone O, Steiropoulos P. Is kidney a new organ target in patients with obstructive sleep apnea? Research priorities in a rapidly evolving field [published online ahead of print, 2021 Aug 12]. *Sleep Med.* 2021;86:56–67.

A complete reference list can be found online at ExpertConsult.com.

Chapter 158

Sleep in the Critically Ill Patient

Melissa P. Knauert; Gerald L. Weinhouse; Margaret A. Pisani; Brent E. Heideman; Paula L. Watson

Chapter Highlights

- Sleep deficiency, including poor sleep quality, insufficient sleep duration, and irregular circadian rhythms, is common in critically ill patients. Sleep in the intensive care unit (ICU) is characterized by shortened overnight sleep, severe fragmentation, decreased stages N3 and rapid eye movement sleep, and circadian disruption.
- Efforts to study sleep in critically ill patients are currently labor intensive, expensive, and limited by electroencephalographic abnormalities caused by neuropathology and frequently used psychoactive medications.
- Factors that affect sleep quality in the ICU include patient-care–related interventions, the ICU environment, pain, anxiety, and critical illness itself.
- Efforts to promote improved sleep may result in a positive impact on patient outcomes, such as patient satisfaction, delirium incidence, time on mechanical ventilation, and both in-hospital and postdischarge recovery.
- Improving the sleep of critically ill patients may best be achieved by a multicomponent protocol designed to optimize environmental factors and minimize use of medications known to disrupt sleep.

INTRODUCTION

More than four million adults are cared for in US intensive care units (ICUs) each year, with approximately 800,000 requiring mechanical ventilation.[1] On a single day (January 11, 2021), during the peak of the second wave of the SARS CoV-2 infections in the US, there were about 29,000 COVID patients in US ICUs.[1a] Sleep deficiency, including poor sleep quality, insufficient sleep duration, and irregular circadian rhythms, during critical care illness has been extensively described.[2–4] In addition, ICU patients have been shown to experience atypical sleep, characterized by delta waves without cyclic organization and by the absence of K-complexes and sleep spindles, and pathologic wakefulness—delta and theta waves in behaviorally awake patients.[5–7] The causes of sleep deficiency are multifactorial and include the patient's underlying illness, emotional state, pain, the ICU environment, and medications. For decades, decreased sleep quality was perceived as an unavoidable effect of ICU management, and attention was focused on addressing the patients' disease process, organ dysfunction, and hemodynamic management. More recently, sleep promotion has been recognized as a critical element in critical care delivery, although the need to support circadian function remains underrecognized.[8] Furthermore, as more patients survive their critical illness, significant efforts are now being directed toward optimizing modifiable risk factors, such as poor-quality sleep, that can further improve ICU outcomes.

ICU patients rank sleep disruptions as one of the chief causes of distress during their ICU stay.[9,10] In addition to emotional distress, sleep deprivation may also contribute to impaired immune function, metabolic abnormalities, prolongation of mechanical ventilation, impaired participation with physical therapy, delirium, and cognitive dysfunction. The management of ICU patients should include a team-based and interdisciplinary approach to minimize disruptive factors that prevent patients from achieving consolidated sleep. At present, no pharmacologic agent is approved for use as a sleep aid in the ICU. In this chapter we will review the methods available to evaluate sleep, the characteristics of sleep in ICU patients, causes of sleep disruption, clinical outcomes that might be adversely affected by poor sleep quality, and methods to improve sleep in critically ill patients.

ASSESSMENT OF SLEEP IN THE INTENSIVE CARE UNIT

Sleep can be measured by both subjective and objective means, using the metrics of quantity, quality, and pattern of distribution (Figure 158.1). All methods of sleep measurement have been found to have limitations when applied to critically ill patients. And although polysomnography (PSG) remains the gold standard method for measuring sleep in ICU patients, it is labor intensive, expensive, and impractical to perform in routine clinical practice. Other measurement modalities may provide valuable information toward our efforts of quantifying and improving sleep in the critically ill.

Subjective Methods

Various subjective measurements, including nursing logs, visual observation by health care staff, and patient report, have been studied and used. The sleep observation tool is the most valid

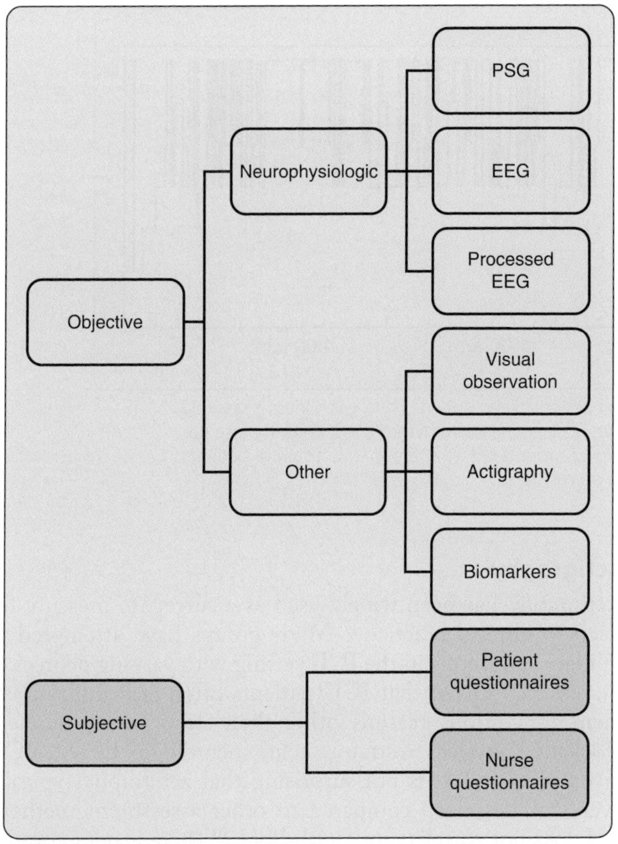

Figure 158.1 Objective (*blue*) and subjective (*pink*) sleep measurement methods used in the intensive care unit. (Modified from Jeffs DL, Darbyshire JL. Measuring sleep in the intensive care unit: a critical appraisal of the use of subjective methods. *J Intensive Care Med.* 2019;34(9):751–60.)

measurement tool for nurse-observed sleep but is impractical for routine use.[11–13] Other tools, such as the Richards-Campbell Sleep Questionnaire (RCSQ) have been specifically developed for use in critically ill patients.[14] The RCSQ has been compared to PSG and is considered to be the most valid and reliable patient questionnaire for this group of patients.[12] The RCSQ includes five to six visual analogue scales (Box 158.1) and has been demonstrated to have a moderate correlation to PSG ($r = 0.58$).[14] A simple numerical rating scale of 0 to 10 (0 indicating worst sleep, 10 indicating best sleep) has been proposed as a more feasible method to measure ICU patients' sleep. This correlated well with the RCSQ score.[15] Unfortunately, the use of self-report instruments for ICU sleep assessment is limited due the impaired consciousness, inadequate memory recall, and delirium that is frequently present in critically ill patients.[16–18] Despite the inherent limitations, sleep survey questionnaires can be a practical, inexpensive method to assess patients' sleep.

Polysomnography

PSG is regarded as the most reliable method for measuring sleep in critically ill patients. Studies have shown that electroencephalographic (EEG) electrodes and leads do not interfere with routine patient-care needs and that electrical interference from other patient-care devices does not affect PSG quality significantly.[4,19] However, several important factors make widespread use of PSG impractical in this population. First, PSG in the ICU is expensive, time consuming, poorly tolerated by patients, and requires trained personnel to perform the initial setup and maintain electrode signal quality throughout the study. Of note, critically ill patients frequently experience as much sleep time during the day as during the night (Figure 158.2).[5] Therefore, if a full assessment of a patient's sleep is to be obtained, 24-hour recordings are necessary.

Box 158.1 RICHARDS-CAMPBELL SLEEP QUESTIONAIRE

Patients are asked to rate the following statements regarding the quality of their sleep last night on a visual analogue scale of 0–100. Lower scores indicate worse sleep. Question 6 is optional; it was not part of the original questionnaire but has been added and is used to evaluate overnight noise.[14]

1. My sleep last night was: light ... Deep
2. Last night, the first time I got to sleep, I: just never could fall asleep ... Fell asleep almost immediately
3. Last night, I was: awake all night ... Awake very little
4. Last night, when I woke up or was awakened, I: couldn't get back to sleep ... Got back to sleep immediately
5. I would describe my sleep last night as: a bad night's sleep ... A good night's sleep
6. I would describe the noise level last night as: very noisy ... Very quiet

The greatest challenge with examining sleep in the ICU stems from the atypical sleep patterns frequently present in ICU patients. The original Rechtschaffen and Kales (R&K)[20] scoring system and even the current American Academy of Sleep Medicine (AASM)[21] guidelines for scoring are not reliable in critically ill patients. The interpretation of EEG data in this population is complicated by the effects of both the underlying illness and the numerous psychoactive medications that these patients receive during their ICU stay.[22–24] Cooper and colleagues[5] were the first to note the difficulty in applying standard scoring criteria to this population, finding that electrophysiologic sleep was not identifiable in 12 of the 20 ICU patients in their study. Further evidence of the limitations of R&K criteria was noted by Ambrogio and colleagues[25] who compared manual sleep assessment to spectral analysis. They found that the interobserver reliability of R&K methodology was poor ($\kappa = 0.19$). Two other research groups have also evaluated the limitations of R&K criteria in critically ill patients and have proposed new scoring criteria. Drouot and colleagues,[6] recommend the addition of two new states: "atypical sleep" and "pathologic wakefulness." Watson and colleagues[7] encountered similar limitations of the standard scoring and proposed comprehensive scoring criteria that incorporated both stages of encephalopathy (based on previous neurology literature[26]) and typical sleep (Figure 158.3, *A* and *B*). This approach allowed the coevaluation of sleep state and level of consciousness in critically ill patients throughout the course of their illness. Although there is controversy on whether this approach should be called a *sleep* staging method,[27] there is evidence that monitoring for the absence of K-complexes and sleep spindles (a feature of atypical sleep) and for the presence of other pathologic brain waves (e.g., burst suppression) can lead to information regarding prognosis and outcomes (Figure 158.4).[28–30]

The problems mentioned earlier led researchers to explore the use of computerized methods of scoring. Spectral analysis of EEG data analyzing the proportion of spectral frequency of theta, alpha, delta, and beta power, as well as the spectral edge frequency (the frequency below which 95% of spectral power

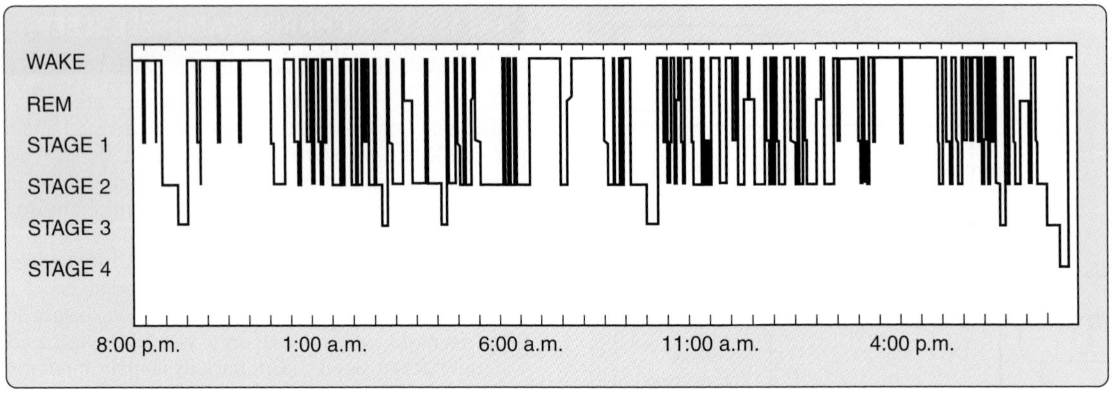

Figure 158.2 A 24-hour hypnogram of an intensive care unit patient. Sleep during critical care illness is severely fragmented and distributed evenly across 24 hours. Oftentimes, a clear circadian rhythm is not seen in these patients. REM, Rapid-eye movement. (From Cooper AB, Thornley KS, Young GB, et al. Sleep in critically ill patients requiring mechanical ventilation. *Chest* 2000;117:809–18, with permission.)

resides, low values indicating sleep and high values indicating wakefulness), has been used as a measure of sleep in critically ill patients.[2,3,25] Although this method has a higher rate of agreement compared to visual scoring, limitations for this method include inconsistencies in the selection of epochs to include for analysis. Other advanced analytic methods, such as the odds ratio product (ORP)[31] can distinguish between different levels of wakefulness and therefore may improve the characterization of atypical sleep and pathologic wakefulness when compared to visual scoring. Further, higher average ORP and less variation between right- and left-sided ORP values are associated with improved likelihood of successful extubation from mechanical ventilation, which highlights the potential for novel PSG analysis to predict outcomes in the critically ill.[32] Limited channel recording may also be beneficial, as an automated single-channel EEG sleep staging algorithm[33] has shown a good correlation with visual scoring in non-ICU patients but has not been validated in the critically ill.

Processed Electroencephalographic Monitors

The limitations of PSG in critically ill patients have led to interest in the use of processed EEG (pEEG) devices to monitor sleep in the ICU. pEEG monitoring tools, such as the bispectral index (BIS) monitor and the patient state index, were developed to monitor levels of sedation in patients undergoing anesthesia. These devices record brain activity via two to four leads placed on the forehead and report a numerical value, calculated from analysis of the EEG waveforms, which correlates with clinical depth of anesthesia in healthy volunteers.[34] Efforts have been made to evaluate the utility of BIS in assessing the level of sedation outside of the operating room, including various ICU settings.[35–40] BIS has been compared to PSG as a measure of sleep in healthy volunteers. BIS values decreased (decreased consciousness) with an increasing depth of sleep, but there were notable overlaps between BIS values and sleep stages, making conclusive stage assignment impossible.[41,42] Two studies to date have aimed to use BIS in the evaluation of sleep rather than sedation or consciousness levels in critically ill patients[43,44]; however, both studies relied on previously published BIS values for sleep identification that had been established in healthy volunteers,[45,46] In summary, no study to date has validated BIS measurement of sleep in ICU patients by comparing BIS to PSG as a standard.

Actigraphy

Actigraphy has been widely used as a surrogate measure for sleep in clinical practice.[47] Many groups have attempted to validate actigraphy in the ICU setting with varying degrees of success.[48,49] Given that ICU patients often lack limb movement for various reasons other than sleep (neuromuscular blockade, physical restraint, acute neurologic deficit, ICU myopathy, etc.), it is not surprising that actigraphy typically overestimates sleep compared to other assessment methods and does not correlate well with PSG.[50] There is poor correlation between wrist and ankle actigraphy in this setting.[51] The relatively unobtrusive nature and cost-effectiveness of this tool make it appealing for use in carefully selected ICU subjects to allow longer-term follow-up of ICU or hospital sleep.

Summary

At present, PSG remains the gold standard to assess sleep in the ICU. However, it is notable that the atypical EEG of ICU patients, coupled with changes in guidelines from R&K to AASM, have resulted in a heterogeneous landscape of reported data. Despite these limitations, some consistent patterns are evident when evaluating sleep in the ICU. In the next section we will review the characteristics of sleep in critically ill patients.

CHARACTERISTICS OF SLEEP IN THE INTENSIVE CARE UNIT

Studies reporting subjective sleep in critically ill patients reveal a consistent perception of poor sleep quality.[52–55] Patients specifically complain about trouble initiating sleep, experiencing lighter sleep, and frequent awakenings with significant difficulty returning to sleep. Despite the knowledge that sleep in the ICU patients is poor, only 32% of ICU providers reported having a sleep-promoting protocol in their ICUs.[56]

Increased daytime sleep, decreased nighttime sleep, severe sleep fragmentation, circadian rhythm disruption, an increase in light sleep (stages N1 and N2), along with a decrease in stages N3 and rapid eye movement (REM) sleep, as well as atypical sleep are common. The mean total sleep time (TST) in critically ill patients is generally reported to be in the normal range but with great variability. TST has been shown to vary between 1.7 and 19.4 hours, with a mean TST that was normal (8.8 ± 5 hours) in one study.[57] Other studies report a

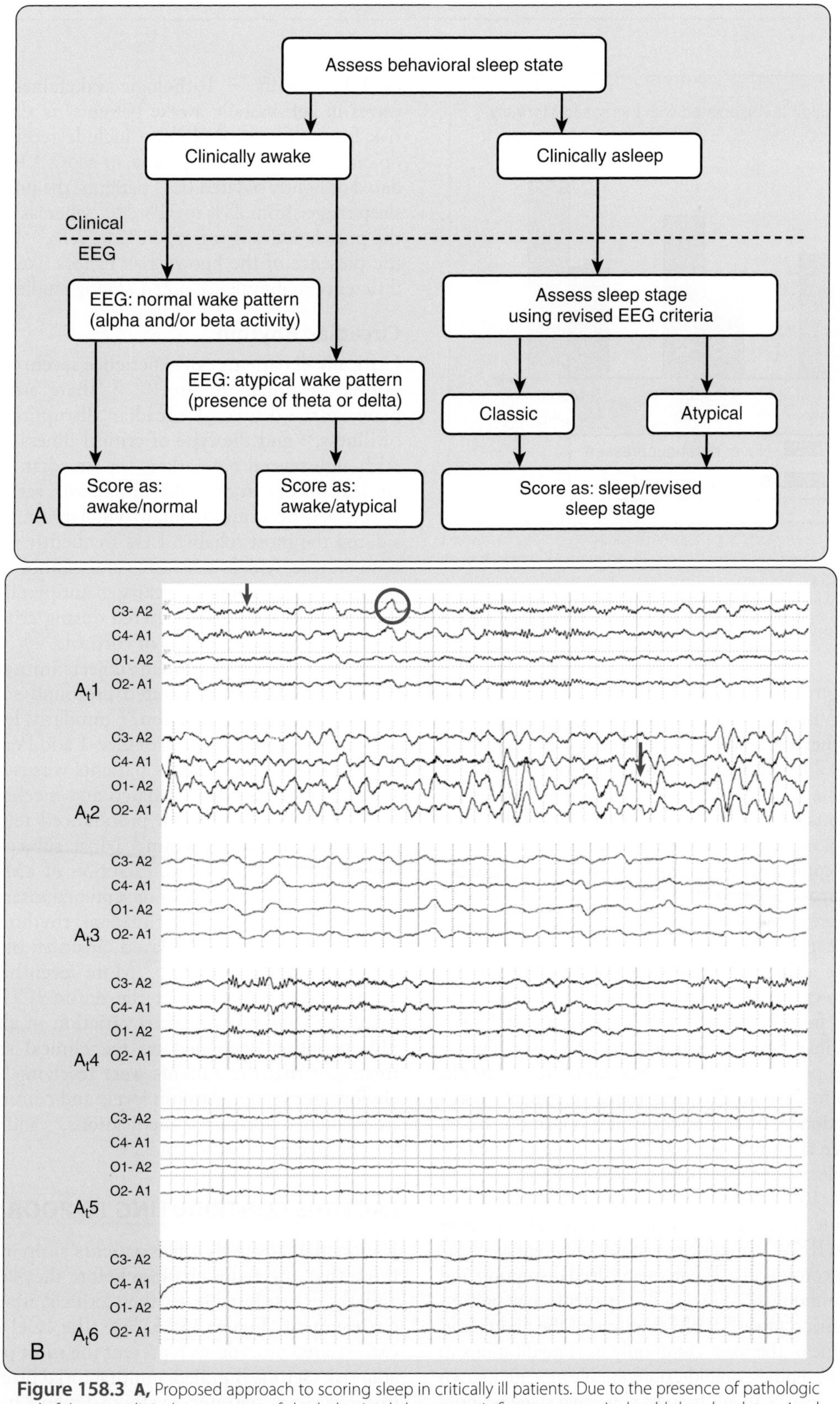

Figure 158.3 **A,** Proposed approach to scoring sleep in critically ill patients. Due to the presence of pathologic wakefulness, a clinical assessment of the behavioral sleep state is first necessary. It should then be determined whether the EEG pattern is normal. If normal, classic sleep stages can be used. If the EEG pattern is abnormal, atypical stages as demonstrated in (**B**) should be used. **B,** Six proposed atypical sleep stages noted on EEG obtained during 24-hour illness. A_t1 (atypical stage 1), characterized by having at least 10% alpha and/or theta activity (indicated by the *arrow*) but may also include delta activity (indicated by the *circle*). A_t2 (atypical stage 2), characterized by the presence of polymorphic delta but with the presence of background beta, alpha, or theta activity (indicated by the *arrow*). A_t3 (atypical stage 3), characterized by a polymorphic delta activity without the presence of background beta, alpha, or theta activity. A_t4 (atypical stage 4), defined by a burst-suppression pattern, intermittent EEG activity alternating with periods of isoelectric EEG activity is classified as atypical stage 4. A_t5 (atypical stage 5), defined by a suppression pattern EEG; a very low-voltage EEG activity (<20 μV amplitude) is classified as atypical stage 5. A_t6 (atypical stage 6), characterized by a complete lack of EEG/cortical activity as shown. EEG, Electroencephalogram. (From Watson PL, Pandharipande P, Gehlbach BK, et al. Atypical sleep in ventilated patients: empirical electroencephalography findings and the path toward revised ICU sleep scoring criteria. *Crit Care Med.* 2013;41:1958–67, with permission.)

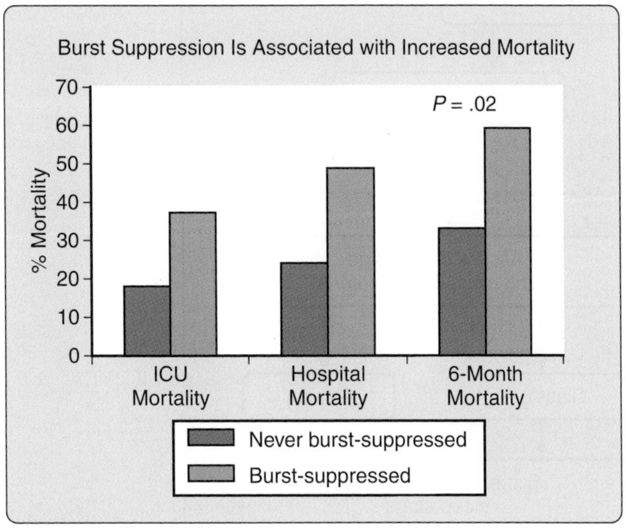

Figure 158.4 Presence of burst suppression is associated with increased mortality. ICU, Intensive care unit. (From Watson PL, Shintani AK, Tyson R, et al. Presence of electroencephalogram burst suppression in sedated, critically ill patients is associated with increased mortality. *Crit Care Med.* 2008; 36:3171–7, with permission.)

median TST ranging from 5 to more than 8 hours, with wide variability.[4,58,59] When interpreting TST data, it is important to consider whether data was collected only nocturnally or through an entire 24-hour cycle, as often greater than 40% of sleep in these patients occurs during day.[5,57,58,60] Not unexpectedly, in patients receiving sedative medications, the total "sleep" time is prolonged (10.09 to 18.9 hours).[61]

ICU patients commonly experience severe sleep fragmentation and an increase in sleep stages N1 and N2, along with decrease in the more restorative stages N3 and REM. In studies of ICU patients, stage N1 and N2 sleep are markedly increased and may comprise as much as 96% ± 6% of TST.[4,5,57–60] The majority of data in critically ill patients show a decrease in stage N3 sleep, ranging from less than 1%[58,59] to 9 ± 18% of TST.[57] Conversely, other investigations demonstrate normal or higher-than-expected proportions of stage N3 sleep; for example, increased N3, up to 25% of TST, was found in patients post–myocardial infarction.[62] In the critically ill population, REM sleep is reduced across all ICU settings. Studies have shown anywhere from a moderate decrease (10% to 15% of TST),[53,62,63] to a severe decrease (<10% of TST),[7,59,64] to even a total absence of REM sleep in some critically ill patients.[3,57] Although the cause for this decrease in REM is unknown, a couple of potential explanations are worth considering. The frequent sleep disruption and fragmentation commonly observed in ICU patients may prevent the natural progression toward REM throughout the night. And of importance, some of the most commonly used medications in ICU (e.g., benzodiazepines, opioids, norepinephrine) are known to suppress REM sleep.[65] In addition to abnormal stage proportions, critically ill patients' sleep is also severely fragmented into short periods and is distributed throughout the day and night (Figure 158.3).[5,57] Studies report more than 25 awakenings per hour in a variety of critically ill patient cohorts.[57,58,63]

Many critically ill patients experience "atypical sleep" characterized by delta waves without cyclic organization, the absence of K-complexes and sleep spindles, and unusual sleep-stage transitions, such as the progression from stage N1 directly to REM sleep. K-complexes and sleep spindles, features of stage N2 sleep, are frequently absent from long periods of recordings in ICU patients.[7,28] Pathologic wakefulness (delta and theta waves in behaviorally awake patients) is also common.[6,7] The risk factors for atypical sleep include receiving sedatives and opioids, having delirium, coma, or sepsis.[5] In conscious nonsedated or lightly sedated ICU patients, the prevalence of atypical sleep ranges from 23% to 31%,[4,6,57] whereas in sedated patients, the prevalence ranges from 50% to 97%.[5,7,66] The variability in the presence of the known risk factors likely accounts for the difference in prevalence noted among studies.

Circadian Rhythm

Critically ill patients can experience severe disruptions in their normal circadian rhythm.[3,67–71] There are also associations between the degree of circadian disruption and the severity of illness,[72] and the type of critical illness (brain injury).[67,73] Although several biomarkers for circadian rhythm have been studied for use in critically ill patients, serum melatonin and its metabolite urine 6-sulfatoxymelatonin (aMT6s) are considered the most reliable. Less frequently used are core body temperature, which is invasive and cannot be used for febrile patients or for patients receiving antipyretics,[74] and cortisol levels, which are notably altered during critical illness due to changes in the metabolism of cortisol.[75,76]

A study of normal human subjects infused with endotoxin to mimic sepsis demonstrated profound suppression of circadian clock gene expression.[77] Similarly, levels of melatonin and messenger RNA levels of Cry-1 and Per-2 are reported to be decreased in septic ICU patients versus nonseptic control subjects.[78] In a study of sedated and mechanically ventilated ICU patients, there was a pronounced temporal disorganization of circadian rhythm.[3] Most subjects exhibited preserved, but phase-delayed, excretion of aMT6s. In a similar study, when compared to nonseptic counterparts, septic ICU patients have decreased circadian rhythm periodicity and amplitude, as well as a delayed circadian phase (as measured by urinary aMT6s levels).[79] More recently, in a study measuring aMT6s throughout the entire ICU stay of patients (median, 10 days), a marked variation in aMT6s was noted. This variation depended on the clinical state and medical treatment that the patients were receiving.[69] There are associations between melatonin levels and common ICU medications, such as adrenergic medications,[69] and sedatives, such as benzodiazepines and opioids.[69,80]

FACTORS CONTRIBUTING TO POOR SLEEP

Factors that adversely affect patients' sleep in the ICU include those that affected their sleep before they arrived in the ICU and those attributable to their critical illness and the ICU environment (Figure 158.5).[81,82] The ICU environment and care-related procedures represent the most potentially modifiable risk factors. Bundled, multifactorial protocols designed to improve sleep (see later) for these patients typically target several of these areas for improvement. There are numerous other ICU and illness-related factors that variably affect patients; these include pain, anxiety, discomfort from ICU equipment or procedure, and delirium.

Noise

High sound levels (i.e., noise) can produce physiologic changes similar to a generalized stress reaction, and these effects can prevent patients from initiating or maintaining sleep.[83] Studies that have measured noise levels in the ICU usually find them

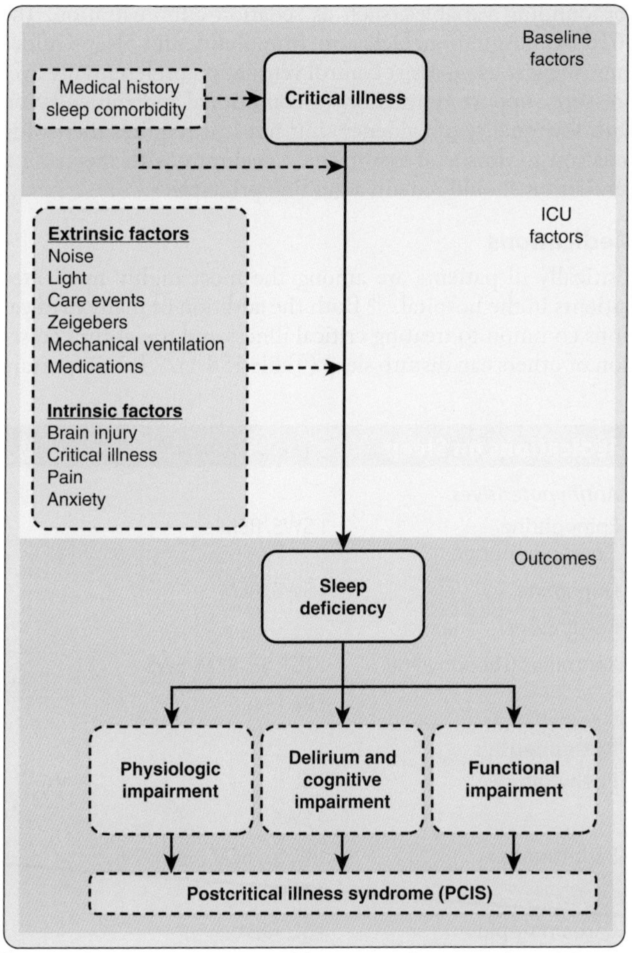

Figure 158.5 Summary model of factors contributing to sleep deficiency and poor outcomes in critically ill patients. ICU, Intensive care unit.

to be in violation of the World Health Organization recommendation for hospital average and peak sound levels of 30 and 40 dBA, respectively.[84] ICU-based investigations have demonstrated average sound levels between 43 to 66 dBA[58,83,85,86] and peak sound levels between 80 to 90 dBA.[83,85–92] Noise has been the most commonly cited external sleep-disruptive factor, with talking and alarms being the most common type of disruptive sounds.[81] The cause of high sound levels in the ICU is under investigation. Whereas some authors have implicated noise from equipment and hardware in the room,[93,94] patients have identified hearing people (i.e., health care staff) talking as the most "annoying" impedance to their sleep.[95,96] Some experts suggest that compliance with overnight sound guidelines may not be possible in modern hospitals due to unavoidable machine noise inside patient rooms.[86,92,97] Of interest, when noise levels were measured while ICU patients were monitored with PSG, noise accounted for only 10% to 11.5% of arousals, 17% of awakenings, and 8% to 14% of the fragmentation index, highlighting that noise is only one of many ICU sleep-disrupting factors.[57,63,98,99] Some studies designed to reduce noise exposure, that is, use of earplugs, have demonstrated modest success in improving patients' perceived sleep, but most studies bundle the use of earplugs with other interventions, such as eye masks to limit light exposure.[100–102] Objective measures of sleep improvement with noise reduction alone have been less consistent.[103]

Light

Day-night light patterns are the primary external cue (zeitgeber) for the entrainment of circadian rhythms, which in turn direct the timing and quality of sleep. Approximately one-third of patients report that nighttime light is disruptive to their sleep, and it is second only to noise for its impact among disruptors from the ICU environment.[81] Studies of light measurements in the ICU demonstrate problems with both overnight and daytime light levels. During the overnight period, investigations suggest a pattern of dim overnight light punctuated with multiple, brief exposures to bright light. During the day, light levels are low and insufficient to promote normal circadian entrainment.[3,69,104–108] Median light levels in the morning can be especially low, and peak light intensity appears to be delayed occurring in the late afternoon.[109] This may contribute to the circadian phase delay previously mentioned. Early sleep interventions focused on lowering overnight light levels have shown some promise.[110,111] However, these protocols may also result in more light peaks or more light variability, the effects of which are unknown.[112]

In acutely hospitalized non-ICU patients, daytime bright light interventions aimed at normalizing circadian alignment have demonstrated improved sleep in elderly patients,[113,114] delirious elderly patients,[115] and in cardiology patients,[116] but not in cirrhotic patients.[117] A small pilot study indicates that the use of timed light exposure (enhanced light exposure from 9 a.m. to noon) administered by lightbox may be able to entrain circadian rhythms of critically ill patients, but a larger study is needed to confirm these findings.[118]

Patient-Care Events

Frequent bedside care with hands-on assessment is a characteristic and often necessary part of ICU care. Overnight care events cause primary disturbance and increase local sound and light levels. In addition, these care events may act as nonphotic zeitgebers and further circadian disruption in critically ill patients.[119] The number of direct patient contact events has been reported to range from 40 to 60 per night.[110,120,121] A study of nighttime patient interactions estimated that 14% of nocturnal interactions were not time critical.[122] The institution of a clustered-care sleep-promotion protocol resulted in an increase in the average time between staff entering patients' rooms from 26 to 46 minutes.[8,110] Although efforts should be made to coordinate care in such a way that allows for consolidated sleep times, only about 10% of arousals and awakenings have been shown to be attributable to patient-care activities.[123]

Nonphotic Zeitgebers

Nonphotic zeitgebers are present in the ICU care environment and may also directly cause irregular circadian rhythms and indirectly contribute to both shortened sleep and poor-quality sleep. Although less influential than light, timing of feeding is a relatively strong zeitgeber; this is especially true for entrainment of peripheral circadian clocks, including the gastrointestinal system, liver, and pancreas.[124,125] Feeding has been shown to uncouple peripheral tissue circadian oscillators from the master clock.[126] Patients in the ICU are most commonly fed on a continuous basis 24 hours a day; this can be expected to have circadian effects.[127] Similarly, physical activity has a role in entraining peripheral clocks.[128–130] It could be hypothesized that the immobility of the ICU deprives patients of the exercise-related zeitgeber signals and deprives patients of other important zeitgebers associated with exercise, such as light exposure and social interaction.

Mechanical Ventilation

The relationship between mechanically supported ventilation and sleep is complex. Several studies have compared spontaneous modes of ventilation (i.e., pressure support ventilation) with controlled modes and concluded that controlled modes, such as assist control and proportional assist ventilation, are favorable for sleep in their specific cohort.[63,131–135] One observational study found that the presence of an artificial airway had the largest positive effect on sleep after controlling for other variables, including noise and light.[2] It may not be reasonable, however, to draw broad conclusions based on the available literature, considering the enormous heterogeneity among patients, the small size of most studies, and confounding variables, such as sedation administration. The 2018 Pain, Agitation, Delirium, Immobility, and Sleep Guidelines suggest using assist control ventilation preferentially over pressure support ventilation (a conditional recommendation with low quality of evidence) but not if it requires increasing sedation to do so.[8] Comfort and synchrony with mechanical ventilation should remain a guiding principle.

Medications

Critically ill patients are among the most highly medicated patients in the hospital.[136] Both the addition of many medications common to treating critical illness and the abrupt cessation of others can disturb sleep (Table 158.1).[65] It is important

Table 158.1 Effect of Commonly Used Intensive Care Unit Medications on Sleep

Sedatives/Hypnotics	
Benzodiazepines	↓W, REM, SWS, SL ↑TST, Stg II
Propofol	↓W, SL ↑TST
Alpha$_2$ agonists (dexmedetomidine)	↓SL, REM ↑SWS
Analgesics	
Opioids	↓TST, REM, SWS ↑W, Stg II
NSAIDs	↓TST, SE
Antipsychotics	
Typical (haloperidol)	↓W, SL ↑SE, Stg II
Atypical (olanzapine)	↓W, SL ↑TST, SE, SWS
Antidepressants	
Tricyclics	↓W, REM ↑TST
SSRIs	↓TST, SE, REM ↑W
Trazodone	↓W, SL, REM ↑TST, ±SWS
Cardiovascular	
Antihypertensives	
Beta antagonists	↑W, SL ↓REM (variable, depends on lipid solubility)
Alpha$_2$ agonists	↓REM
Calcium antagonists	NA
ACE inhibitors	No effect on sleep
Diuretics	NA
Amiodarone	Nightmares
Antihypotensives	
Epinephrine/norepinephrine	↓SWS, REM
Dopamine	↓SWS, REM
Respiratory	
Xanthines (theophylline)	↓TST, SE, REM, SWS ↑W
Antiepileptics	
Phenytoin	↓SL ↑SWS
Barbiturates	↓W, SL, REM ↑TST
Carbamazepine	↓SL, REM ↑SWS
Valproic acid	↓W ↑TST
Gabapentin	↓W ↑TST, REM, SWS
H$_2$ Antagonists	
Cimetidine?	↑SWS
Corticosteroids	↓REM, SWS ↑W, Stg II
Substances of Abuse	
Ethanol	↓SL, REM (first half of the night) ↑REM (second half of the night), nightmares
Cannabis	↓REM ↑SWS (if acute use; tolerance if long-term use)
Nicotine	↓TST, REM ↑SL

Although individual reactions may vary, some of the known effects on sleep architecture should be considered whenever possible to decrease the incidence of sleep disturbance during critical care illness.

↓, Decreased; ↑, increased; ACE, angiotensin-converting enzyme; NA, not available; NSAIDs, nonsteroidal antiinflammatory drugs; REM, rapid eye movement; SE, sleep efficiency; SL, sleep latency; SSRIs, selective serotonin reuptake inhibitors; Stg II, stage II sleep; SWS, slow wave sleep; TST, total sleep time; W, wakefulness.

From Weinhouse GL. Pharmacology I: effects on sleep of commonly used ICU medications. *Crit Care Clin*. 2008;24(3):477–91, reproduced with permission.

to note, however, that studies of medications' effect on sleep architecture have been done on healthy volunteers rather than the critically ill, who are often in a state of inflammation, on multiple other medications, have potentially altered drug metabolism and bioavailability and potentially could have a compromised blood-brain barrier. Therefore the true effect of these medications on sleep is unquantifiable under these circumstances.

Sedatives and analgesics have perhaps received the most attention in this regard, as they may contribute to the risk of ICU delirium, which may also intersect with the risk of poor sleep.[8] Benzodiazepines and analgesics have been shown to decrease N3 sleep in favor of increasing N1 and N2 sleep, whereas propofol increases N3 and decreases REM sleep.[137] Dexmedetomidine, an alpha$_2$ agonist, may induce a state more physiologically like naturally occurring sleep but still lacks key sleep features.[138] Patients are more arousable when sedated with dexmedetomidine compared to benzodiazepines and propofol. Although this can be beneficial for various clinical situations, such as ventilator weaning, it may lead to more sleep fragmentation in a noisy ICU. In one survey of patients who underwent elective heart surgery, difficulty resting and sleeping was reported more commonly with dexmedetomidine than with propofol. Dexmedetomidine has been shown to increase N2 sleep and decrease N1 sleep in critically ill patients sedated with an infusion overnight.[139,140] Fewer episodes of delirium are reported under sedation with dexmedetomidine than with benzodiazepines, which is a very important outcome.[141] For this reason, dexmedetomidine is recommended for use overnight if a sedative infusion is needed, although it is not recommended for the sole purpose of inducing sleep.[8]

Acute medication withdrawal in ICU patients may be an important issue affecting their sleep.[142] Medications taken by patients at home are often discontinued when they are admitted for a critical illness because they have potentially undesirable effects, are considered nonessential, and potentially contribute to the adverse effects of polypharmacy, or because of loss of enteral access or function. Withdrawal of some medications (e.g., opioids, benzodiazepines, nicotine, and antidepressants) can lead to insomnia and sometimes an increase in REM percentages. In cases when REM-suppressing medications, such as benzodiazepines and opioids, are abruptly discontinued, the recovery sleep may have a disproportionately high percentage of REM sleep.[143] In the critically ill, this may play a more important physiologic role, as cardiac and respiratory instability are greatest during REM sleep. Therefore a gradual withdrawal of these agents whenever possible may reduce disruption of sleep neurophysiology.

Some commonly used medications in the ICU may affect patients' sleep by their effect on preexisting sleep disorders. Opioids, for example, are the mainstay of analgesia in critical care units but may worsen airway obstruction in those with obstructive sleep apnea.[144] Physical restraints and medications, such as beta blockers, antiemetics, and neuroleptics may worsen periodic limb movements (PLMs) and restless legs syndrome symptoms.[145]

Patient Factors That Disrupt Sleep in the Intensive Care Unit

Sleep disruptions are not always clearly attributable to external causes. Pre-illness factors, such as psychological disorders (e.g., anxiety, posttraumatic stress disorder, panic attacks), poor sleep habits, and inconsistent bedtime routines, have been associated with disturbed sleep quality during acute hospitalization.[54,146] The ICU-acquired risk factors most frequently cited by patients as disruptive to sleep quality are pain and discomfort, immobility/restricted movement, and worry/anxiety/fear.[8,17,55,147] A qualitative study of patients, surrogates, and clinical staff in the ICU found that more than half the participants indicated that psychological factors, emotional and cognitive factors, affected sleep more than the ICU environment.[148] Factors inherent to critical illness itself have been suggested as possible sleep-disruptive forces. Those that have been shown to correlate with sleep disruption in univariate analysis include illness severity, delirium, hypoxemia, and alkalosis.[64,99,149]

Summary

There are multiple external and patient factors that disturb sleep in critically ill patients. Recognizing and minimizing these factors is important to both the comfort and the clinical outcomes of patients.[150] However, some causes of sleep disruption may be unavoidable in the setting of acute critical illness and its treatment. More research is needed to determine how best to address these sleep-disrupting factors and which factors are associated with undesirable sleep-related ICU outcomes.

SLEEP-RELATED INTENSIVE CARE UNIT OUTCOMES

Sleep and circadian disruption in the ICU are relatively new fields of investigation; therefore robust long-term ICU outcomes are not yet available. There is, however, growing evidence that disrupted sleep during the ICU negatively affects outcomes both during and after critical illness.[28,111,151–153] Of importance, although studies in critically ill patients are needed, data from non-ICU subjects and animal studies indicate that sleep deprivation is associated with impairments in immune, metabolic, respiratory, and cardiovascular function.[154–156]

Patients' Intensive Care Unit Quality of Life

Perhaps the best-established outcome of ICU sleep disturbance is the effect it has on patients' ICU quality of life. Those patients who survive critical illness often remember their poor sleep and assign a high degree of stress to their sleep disturbance.[9,10,157] Self-report questionnaires, however, are subject to recall bias and are limited to those who are conscious and stable; therefore patients who are most sick and/or have cognitive impairment, for example, would be excluded. Problems with generalizability notwithstanding, available data suggests that patients recall their ICU sleep as being worse than their sleep before the ICU, and for many it has an impact on their ICU quality of life and a potential impact on their sleep and quality of life beyond the ICU.

Participation with Physical Therapy

The importance of early mobilization during the ICU in improving overall outcomes, such as critical illness neuromyopathy and delirium, has been highlighted in recent years.[8] Sleep loss often leads to decreased energy and activity levels and can thereby negatively impact physical recovery. Poor sleep is associated with decreased physical performance in older community-dwelling men and women.[158,159] However, its effect on ICU patients has not been proven, and a recent study failed to show an association between subjective sleep quality and participation with physical therapy the following day.[160] Wakefulness-enhancing medications, such as modafinil, have been used in the ICU both to try to improve cognition and facilitate physical rehabilitation, but it has not been studied systematically.[161,162] Although data remains very limited in critically ill patients, the interaction of sleep disruption and physical recovery remains a promising avenue of future investigation.

Intensive Care Unit Delirium

There has been considerable interest in understanding the relationship between sleep disturbance and the development of ICU delirium, and it is believed that causality may be bidirectional. ICU delirium is an acute syndrome characterized by poor attention, cognition, and awareness, and it is an independent risk factor for mortality, longer days on mechanical ventilation, longer length of ICU and hospital stay, and risk of developing post-ICU syndrome. Its defining features can all be replicated under experimental conditions of sleep deprivation, fueling the interest in a possible link. REM sleep deprivation has been shown to be associated with an increase in delirium.[64] Several studies of sleep-promotion interventions have also demonstrated reductions in delirium.[64,111,163] Furthermore, one study showed that the number of days of delirium during an ICU stay was significantly associated with postdischarge sleep disturbance.[153] There are many possible underlying pathophysiologic mechanisms. Two possibilities that have been studied include abnormalities of functional network connectivity in prefrontal cortical areas[164–166] and circadian/melatonin dysregulation.[167]

Respiratory Outcomes

Mechanical ventilation may affect sleep and, conversely, sleep quality may affect the success or failure of liberation from mechanical support. The poor sleep experienced by patients maintained on both invasive and noninvasive mechanical ventilation has been associated with several negative outcomes, including prolonged mechanical ventilation itself and mortality.[29,168] Late noninvasive ventilation failure has been correlated with increased daytime sleep and decreased REM.[149] Similarly, abnormal wakefulness and poor correlation between sleep depth between right and left brain hemispheres has been demonstrated in patients who were not ready to be extubated from invasive mechanical ventilation.[32] In a cohort of invasively ventilated patients, the presence of atypical sleep and the absence of REM sleep were independently associated with prolonged weaning.[29] Although there has been some data to suggest that sleep deprivation can directly affect inspiratory muscle endurance and upper airway function, these study results suggest that it is the brain dysfunction rather than muscle weakness associated with poor sleep that may contribute to a delay in extubation.

Immune Function

Sleep loss has been demonstrated to affect both innate and adaptive immunity in healthy volunteers.[169] Abnormalities in T-helper and natural-killer cell number and their function have been noted in association with sleep deprivation.[170,171] Under experimental conditions, vulnerability to infection created by sleep deprivation has been demonstrated in subjects' weak response to vaccination and greater likelihood of developing clinical viral illness.[172,173] Important to critical illness, the proinflammatory cytokines, tumor necrosis factor-α and interleukin-6, are increased in association with poor sleep quality.[174] No study has yet established the relationship between sleep and outcomes after infection, such as sepsis. However, it is at least plausible, if not likely, that poor sleep during critical illness has adverse effects on immune function and therefore on clinical outcomes.

Disruption of Glucose Metabolism

All three elements of sleep deficiency have been associated with alteration in glucose metabolism.[175] Healthy human subjects exposed to sleep restriction of 4 hours per night over 5 nights and tested for intravenous glucose tolerance show a –25% decrease in insulin sensitivity and a –30% decrease in the acute insulin response to intravenous glucose.[156] Subsequent studies in healthy human subjects who were similarly sleep restricted have confirmed these findings.[176–178] Poor sleep quality in the form of sleep fragmentation without accompanying loss of TST has also been associated with decreased insulin sensitivity in two different studies.[179,180] Finally, in a study of circadian misalignment we see that eating and sleeping out of normal circadian phase is associated with an increase in glucose levels.[181] Although these studies used healthy human subjects, it is again likely that the effects of sleep deficiency are equally or more impactful during critical illness.

Prognosis

The electrophysiologic features of sleep have been used as a biomarker for prognosis. The loss of normal sleep architecture and specifically the absence of sleep spindles and K-complexes is a marker of poor prognosis in ICU patients with respiratory failure, acute encephalopathy, posttraumatic coma, and subarachnoid hemorrhage.[28,151,168,182,183]

PROMOTION OF SLEEP IN THE INTENSIVE CARE UNIT

Clinical staff, patients, and patient surrogates value sleep and agree that sleep is important to recovery; however, there is a significant gap between such beliefs and the prioritization and/or implementation of sleep-promotion protocols.[56,148,184] In the ICU, clinical staff may be overly focused on overnight environmental causes of sleep disruption while neglecting daytime elements of sleep promotion, such as the provision of appropriate photic and nonphotic zeitgebers.[185] As noted earlier, less than a quarter of sleep arousals are attributable to environmental stimuli.[53,57] In addition, sleep may be disrupted by stress, anxiety, and pain, which can be underappreciated by clinical staff.[8,148] There is pressure, at times, to try to improve sleep with medications, but that can be harmful. Appropriate control of pain and anxiety should be considered as a supportive measure for sleep and should follow societal guidelines to minimize the negative side effects of the relevant medication classes.[8] And although there may be a limited role for medication, the most effective strategy to promote sleep in the ICU is a multicomponent approach predicated on creating an environment conducive for sleep to occur naturally while optimizing patients' comfort, both physically and psychologically.

Nonpharmacologic Sleep Promotion

Nonpharmacologic hospital-based sleep-promotion protocols combine one or several of the following components: sound control, light control, rescheduling of routine patient care to provide a sleep opportunity, provision of eye masks, provision of ear plugs, sleep education, treatment of anxiety, promotion of relaxation, and when applicable, adjustment of ventilator settings.[186,187] ICU sleep-promotion interventions most commonly include overnight environmental sound and light reduction via "quiet time" protocols and clustering of patient-care activities.[8,110–112,186,188] These interventions are inherently complex and require broad stakeholder involvement because of the myriad sources of environmental disruption.[189] Improvement in sleep has been demonstrated with nonpharmacologic interventions, although results have been inconsistent, likely due to methodologic differences between studies and the difficulty measuring sleep in the ICU.[190]

Strategies to create physical and psychological relaxation and thus promote sleep may be particularly challenging in the ICU. Nonpharmacologic relaxation approaches have included massage, guided imagery/virtual reality, a warm or weighted blanket, music, aromatherapy, and acupressure.[191–194] Patient preferences, within the limitation of available resources, should guide which techniques are offered. It is sometimes the case, however, that the adjunctive use of pharmacologic anxiolysis, analgesia, and sedation will have to be considered if these measures are insufficient.

Knowing patients' normal sleep patterns and sleep-related comorbidities may also be important to individualizing their sleep-care plan but may be overlooked when attention is focused on a life-threatening illness. A sleep assessment at time of admission to the ICU and daily reassessment has been proposed to document patients' sleep hours, use of sleep aids, sleep-related comorbidities, and preferences for environmental conditions; for example, some ICU patients have reported feeling more comforted by hearing voices nearby, whereas others prefer quiet.[195] A complete understanding of preexisting sleep disorders is particularly important because some common ICU medications and procedures may worsen preexisting sleep conditions.

Pharmacologic Sleep Promotion

Although sleep disruption is common in ICU patients, there is a paucity of randomized controlled trials of pharmacologic agents for treatment in this patient population. Hypnotics have not been studied for use in the ICU, and their known adverse effects may contribute to ICU delirium. Several other medications, however, have begun to be studied for this indication. There is no currently recommended pharmacologic sleep aid for critically ill patients.[8]

Melatonin has been studied for the promotion of sleep in ICU patients in several small investigations (Table 158.2). A recent Cochrane review of these studies, however, did not find enough evidence to support a recommendation for its use.[196] Ramelteon, a melatonin-receptor agonist, has not been well studied for sleep promotion in the critically ill, and two recent studies have yielded conflicting results regarding its efficacy to reduce ICU delirium.[197,198]

Selected pharmacotherapy to help treat pain and anxiety, thereby supporting sleep, may be at times necessary. Analgesics should be used to target pain control rather than sedation or "sleep," and benzodiazepines should be avoided aside from very specific clinical scenarios (e.g., alcohol withdrawal, seizures).[8] Sedatives have sometimes been given under the mistaken belief that sedation and sleep are equivalent. Both propofol and benzodiazepines have been shown to suppress identifiable deep non–rapid eye movement and REM sleep in the critically ill and are not recommended for sleep promotion.[199–201] Dexmedetomidine, discussed earlier, is known to promote biomimetic N3 in healthy volunteers and cause a compensatory reduction in REM sleep.[202,203] Although it has been shown to increase N2 sleep and decrease N1 sleep, it does not increase either N3 or REM sleep in studies of the critically ill.[139,140,204]

Table 158.2 Clinical Trials Evaluating the Effects of Exogenous Melatonin Replacement in Critically Ill Patients

Author (Year)	Study Design	Reported Results	Comments
Shilo (2000)[212] *N* = 8	Double-blind placebo controlled 3 mg controlled-release melatonin or placebo given at 22:00	Treatment dramatically improved both the duration and quality of sleep Melatonin in ICU patients may help sleep induction and resynchronization of the "biologic clock"	Wrist actigraphy was used to measure "sleep" and disruptions Half of the ICU patients were on a ventilator Control group included general medicine ward patients
Ibrahim (2006)[213] *N* = 32	Double-blind, randomized, placebo-controlled 3 mg oral melatonin or placebo given at 20:00	Melatonin was well absorbed, and a standard dose increased blood levels approximately 1000-fold Failed to increase observed nocturnal sleep	Sleep was assessed by bedside nurse observation only Use of "extra sedation" and haloperidol was nonsignificantly higher in control group
Bourne (2008)[80] *N* = 24	Double-blind, randomized, placebo-controlled 10 mg oral melatonin or placebo given at 21:00 for 4 nights	Nocturnal sleep quantity was severely compromised in both groups at the start of the study. Melatonin use was associated with increased nocturnal sleep efficiency.	"Sleep" monitoring was done by bispectral index (BIS) and actigraphy, nurse and patient survey. Proposed that 10-mg dose is too high and may lead to carryover of effects. Suggested 1–2 mg immediate-release dose

All patients in these studies had undergone tracheostomy placement and were not receiving continuous sedation at the time of study.
ICU, Intensive care unit.

Many other medications, including antidepressants, typical and atypical antipsychotics, and antihistamines, have been used to try to improve the sleep of critically ill patients. Sedating antihistamines should be avoided due to possible antimuscarinic effects associated with ICU delirium. Antipsychotics have been used as hypnotic agents due to their sedating properties. However, when administered in the absence of documented mental disorder, they are associated with higher ICU and hospital length of stay, as well as increased hospital mortality.[205,206] The use of these medications must therefore be weighed against their many potential adverse effects.

Multicomponent Bundles

A bundled approach to the problem of poor sleep in the ICU that combines many of the previously listed interventions stands as the recommended sleep-promotion strategy.[8] Most of the protocols studied have included environmental control, clustering of care, eye masks, and ear plugs. One of the larger, more complex, protocols included a guideline that emphasized nonpharmacologic measures and specifically discouraged the use of sedating medications but provided an approach to the judicious use of either zolpidem or antipsychotics to promote sleep.[111] Some of these protocols have not been able to demonstrate improved sleep by objective measures, which may be a reflection of the difficulty of measuring sleep in this patient population. Studies have reported subjective improvements in sleep and reductions in ICU delirium.[207] Although the specific elements of a multicomponent protocol that should be included are not clear and may be dictated by resource availability, this approach is considered low risk and with the potential for very significant benefit for critically ill patients.[8]

SLEEP POST–INTENSIVE CARE UNIT

For patients who survive their critical illness, sleep problems may persist well beyond the ICU and take days or months to resolve.[62,208–211] A systematic review of 22 studies of sleep after hospitalization and critical illness found that the prevalence of sleep disturbances, usually insomnia and sleep-disordered breathing, ranged between 50% to 67% in the first month.[152] These studies, which varied considerably in methodology, also found a prevalence of 22% to 57% after 3 to 6 months and 10% to 61% after 6 months· Fortunately, both subjective and objective assessments concluded that improvement was likely over time. Some COVID patients who survived ICU stays were reported to have sleep disorder symptoms for long periods after discharge.[214,215] This was especially true in those in those with neurologic complications[216] (see also Chapter 213).

Risk factors for post-ICU sleep disturbances include prehospital, in-hospital, and posthospital factors. Prehospital insomnia, poor self-reported sleep during hospitalization, and poor physical- and mental health–related (including anxiety, depression, and posttraumatic stress) quality of life after discharge were risk factors for poor post-ICU sleep in cardiothoracic and neurosurgical ICU patients.[208] Other studies have also concluded that chronic comorbidities, severity of illness, female sex, and older age were risk factors as well; however, these results have been less consistent.[152] Posthospital factors associated with poor sleep after ICU discharge include pain, depression, anxiety, posttraumatic stress disorder, and the use of hypnotic drugs.[153] Further research is needed to clarify and quantify the impact of sleep deficiency on post-ICU sleep. Studies should be undertaken to understand the interactions between sleep and the post-ICU syndrome symptoms, including pain, depression, posttraumatic stress disorder, and cognitive impairment. Future work should also include developing strategies to prevent and treat post-ICU sleep disturbances.

CONCLUSION

Sleep plays an integral role in our overall health and is vital to our ability to recover from illness. Critically ill patients frequently experience multiple aspects of sleep deficiency, including poor sleep quality, insufficient sleep duration, and irregular circadian rhythms. Sleep is difficult to measure in the ICU. Nevertheless, emerging evidence links ICU sleep deficiency with poor critical illness outcomes, including increased mortality. There is limited evidence for effective sleep promotion in the ICU, but to date, multicomponent, nonpharmacologic interventions are the most promising intervention.

CLINICAL PEARL

Sleep in critically ill patients is extremely fragmented and divided between day and night. Patients experience a significant decrease in the restorative sleep stages—N3 and REM. Multiple factors can disrupt sleep in the intensive care unit (ICU); they include pain, anxiety, noise, around-the-clock care, abnormal light patterns, mechanical ventilation, medication effect, and critical illness itself. Circadian disruption also plays a role in ICU sleep disruption. Of importance, sleep deprivation during critical illness is an independent risk factor for worse clinical outcomes. A team-based, interdisciplinary approach toward implementation of nonpharmacologic measures to improve sleep should be considered whenever possible. At present, no pharmacologic agent has been approved specifically for treating sleep disturbances in critically ill patients.

SUMMARY

Millions of patients are treated in ICUs each year and are known to suffer poor sleep during their critical care illness. Recently, increased focus on the intersection of sleep and critical care medicine has elucidated better understanding of the importance of sleep quality in this population. Sleep is best evaluated with PSG, although some alternative techniques have been used. During critical illness, patients experience increased N1 and N2 sleep and decreased N3 (slow wave sleep) and REM sleep. In the ICU, sleep is likely to be fragmented and distributed in brief interrupted periods over 24 hours, not following a normal circadian pattern. Common sleep-disrupting factors in the ICU are patient-care activities, noise, light levels, deleterious medication effects, and critical illness itself. The management of ICU patients should include a team-based and interdisciplinary approach to minimize disruptive factors that prevent patients from achieving consolidated sleep. Efforts should be made to address pain and anxiety, and to reduce avoidable noise while trying to cluster the delivery of patient care outside of dedicated sleep periods. At present, no pharmacologic agent is approved for use as a sleep aid in the ICU.

ACKNOWLEDGMENTS

Dr. Melissa P. Knauert received career development funds from the National Center for Advancing Translational Science

(KL2 TR000140); National Heart, Lung, and Blood Institute (K23 HL138229); and the American Academy of Sleep Medicine Foundation. Dr. Paula L. Watson received support from the National Institutes of Health (MO1 RR-00095) and the Vanderbilt Clinical and Translational Science Award grant UL1 RR024975-01 from the National Center for Research Resources/National Institutes of Health.

SELECTED READINGS

Altman MT, Knauert MP, Murphy TE, Ahasic AM, Chauhan Z, Pisani MA. Association of intensive care unit delirium with sleep disturbance and functional disability after critical illness: an observational cohort study. *Ann Intensive Care.* 2018;8(1):63.

Bourne RS, Mills GH. Sleep disruption in critically ill patients—pharmacological considerations. *Anaesthesia.* 2004;59:374–384.

Cooper AB, Thornley KS, Young GB. Sleep in critically ill patients requiring mechanical ventilation. *Chest.* 2000;117:809–818.

Devlin JW, Skrobik Y, Gelinas D, et al. Clinical practice guidelines for the prevention and management of pain, agitation/sedation, delirium, immobility, and sleep disruption in adult patients in the ICU. *Crit Care Med.* 2018;46(9).

Freedman NS, Gazendam J, Levan L. Abnormal sleep/wake cycles and the effect of environmental noise on sleep disruption in the intensive care unit. *Am J Respir Crit Care Med.* 2001;163:451–457.

Frontera JA, Yang D, Lewis A, et al. A prospective study of long-term outcomes among hospitalized COVID-19 patients with and without neurological complications. *J Neurol Sci.* 2021;426:117486.

Gao CA, Knauert MP. Circadian biology and its importance to intensive care unit care and outcomes. *Semin Respir Crit Care Med.* 2019;40:629–637.

Gehlbach BK, Chapotot F, Leproult R, et al. Temporal disorganization of circadian rhythmicity and sleep-wake regulation in mechanically ventilated patients receiving continuous intravenous sedation. *Sleep.* 2012;35(8):1105–1114.

Hu RF, Jiang XY, Chen J, et al. Non-pharmacological interventions for sleep promotion in the intensive care unit. *Cochrane Database Syst Rev.* 2015;10:CD008808.

Kamdar BB, King LM, Collop NA, et al. The effect of a quality improvement intervention on perceived sleep quality and cognition in a medical ICU. *Crit Care Med.* 2013;41:800–809.

Kaplan PW. The EEG in metabolic encephalopathy and coma. *J Clin Neurophysiol.* 2004;21:307–318.

Lutchmansingh DD, Knauert MP, Antin-Ozerkis DE, et al. A clinic blueprint for post-coronavirus disease 2019 recovery: learning from the past, looking to the future. *Chest.* 2021;159(3):949–958.

Thille AW, Reynaud F, Marie D, et al. Impact of sleep alterations on weaning duration in mechanically ventilated patients: a prospective study. *Eur Respir J.* 2018;51(4).

Vassallo P, Novy J, Zubler F, et al. EEG spindles integrity in critical care adults. Analysis of a randomized trial. *Acta Neurol Scand.* 2021. https://doi.org/10.1111/ane.13510. [published online ahead of print, 2021 Jul 26].

Watson PL, Pandharipande P, Gehlbach BK. Atypical sleep in ventilated patients: empirical electroencephalography findings and the path toward revised ICU sleep scoring criteria. *Crit Care Med.* 2013;41:1958–1967.

Weinhouse GL, Schwab RJ, Watson PL. Bench-to-bedside review: delirium in ICU patients—importance of sleep deprivation. *Crit Care.* 2009;13(6):234–241.

A complete reference list can be found online at ExpertConsult.com.

Chapter

159

Perioperative Sleep Medicine

Vivian Asare; Jean Wong

Chapter Highlights

- With the rise of obesity, the prevalence of obstructive sleep apnea (OSA) has also increased. In the surgical population, OSA is more prevalent, and patients are at increased risk for postoperative complications.
- About 80% of cases of OSA are undiagnosed, and the importance of screening protocols preoperatively can serve a role in identifying an especially vulnerable surgical population.
- Sleep efficiency, rapid eye movement sleep, and slow wave sleep decrease the first night after surgery and then slowly recover to preoperative baseline by postoperative night 7.
- Preoperative and postoperative application of continuous positive airway pressure (CPAP) significantly decrease postoperative apnea-hypopnea index and shows a trend toward decreased length of hospital stay. Patients diagnosed with OSA and initiated on CPAP before surgery may have significantly reduced risk for postoperative cardiovascular adverse events, compared with patients with undiagnosed OSA.

OVERVIEW: PREVALENCE OF OSA IN THE GENERAL AND SURGICAL POPULATION

Obstructive sleep apnea (OSA) is the most common breathing disorder during sleep and is categorized by repetitive upper airway collapse and associated sleep fragmentation leading to numerous deleterious pathophysiologic changes.[1] These changes include endothelial dysfunction, sympathetic nervous system activation, nocturnal hypoxemia, and hypercapnia, and in turn increase risk for cardiovascular complications,[2] arrhythmias, stroke,[3] and sudden cardiac death.[4] Four major prevalence studies of patients with an apnea-hypopnea index (AHI) of greater than or equal to 15 found that 7% to 14% of men and 2% to 7% of women have OSA.[5–8] With the rise of obesity, the prevalence of OSA has also increased since these studies were published. Trends of increased prevalence of sleep-disordered breathing in the United States over the time periods of 1988 to 1994 and 2007 to 2010 have shown percentage increases of OSA in different age groups and genders ranging from 12.2% to 54.8%. The largest increases are in the 30- to 49-year-old range.[9] The prevalence of mild OSA (AHI, 5 to 15 per hour) is as high as 22% of men and 9% of women.[10] Even with the well-documented rise of OSA, reports estimate that about 80% of cases of moderate and severe OSA remain undiagnosed and subsequently untreated.[11] Awareness of the prevalence of OSA in the surgical population is exceedingly important given increased risk for complications. This chapter discusses (1) prevalence of OSA in various surgical populations, (2) reported perioperative risks, (3) changes in sleep architecture in the postoperative period, (4) the most common and effective validated screening tools recommended in this population, and (5) perioperative clinical management of patients with suspected or known OSA.

PREVALENCE OF OBSTRUCTIVE SLEEP APNEA IN SURGICAL POPULATIONS

The prevalence of OSA in surgical patients varies based on the type of surgery. In patients undergoing orthopedic surgery, OSA prevalence ranges from 5.5%[12] to 6.7%.[13] In a general surgical population, about 3% of patients had a diagnosis of OSA.[12] In their surgical population–based study from 1998 to 2007, using the National Inpatient Sample database, general and orthopedic surgical patients with a discharge diagnosis using *International Classification of Diseases: Clinical Modification,* ninth revision (ICD-9-CM) of OSA were evaluated. These patients were compared to demographic-matched control subjects without OSA, and the perioperative risk for pulmonary complications was analyzed. The prevalence of OSA steadily increased from 1998 to 2007, and in 2007, 2.7% of general surgical patients and 5.5% of orthopedic patients held a diagnosis code of sleep apnea.[12] This method of estimating prevalence in a population, as expected, can lead to underestimation, especially in patients who have undiagnosed OSA or improperly documented diagnostic codes. In a historical cohort study, the proportion of surgical patients with undiagnosed moderate to severe OSA were analyzed. Surgical patients were initially screened using the STOP-BANG (snoring, tiredness, observed apnea, blood pressure, body mass index, age, neck size, gender) questionnaire and then underwent confirmatory polysomnography (PSG) with results blinded to anesthesiologists and surgeons. In this cohort study, 38% of surgical patients who had a sleep study were found to have moderate to severe OSA (AHI ≥ 15). In those with a preexisting diagnosis of OSA, 15% were not identified as having OSA by anesthesiologists, and 58% were not identified by surgeons. Surgeons and anesthesiologists did not diagnose

93% and 65% of patients with moderate OSA and 90% and 53% of patients with severe OSA, respectively.[14]

In a recent study, as high as 80% of patients with severe carotid artery stenosis undergoing elective surgery were found to have OSA with a mean AHI of 14.5 ± 12.9 (22, mild; 16, moderate; and 6, severe cases of OSA).[15] Another well-documented surgical population with a high prevalence of OSA is patients undergoing bariatric surgery. A retrospective study that evaluated consecutive patients undergoing preoperative evaluation for bariatric surgery found that 71.4% of patients had OSA. Furthermore, 83% of these patients were not diagnosed with OSA before their bariatric surgery.[16] Overall, in patients undergoing elective surgery, 24% of patients are found to be at high risk for OSA using the Berlin Questionnaire as a screening tool during preoperative evaluations.[17] Despite the high prevalence of OSA in the surgical population, especially in patients undergoing cardiovascular procedures and bariatric surgery, there exists a disparity in rates of clinical recognition in the perioperative period. Multiple studies have shown that OSA increases risk for perioperative complications, including pulmonary, cardiovascular, and subsequently increased length of stay and risk for transfer to critical care units. These risks make diagnosing OSA in the preoperative assessment period important and may predict outcomes.

PERIOPERATIVE RISKS ASSOCIATED WITH OBSTRUCTIVE SLEEP APNEA

The overall prevalence of OSA is higher in the surgical population compared to the general population.[9] Moreover, increases of surgical volume along with prevalence of OSA[18] has galvanized interest in clearly elucidating the effects that sleep-disordered breathing has on perioperative outcomes. In this section we will discuss several large-scale analyses and single-center studies that have investigated the association between OSA and clinical outcomes in the perioperative period. Certain key pathophysiologic mechanisms of OSA are important to understand and help to explain the increased susceptibility to adverse events during the perioperative period in this patient population. Potent respiratory depressants, such as general anesthesia, sedatives, and analgesics, can impair ventilatory response systems and may predispose patients to postoperative complications.[1] The main components of OSA affected are the caliber of the upper airway, responsiveness of the dilator muscles to pharyngeal collapse, threshold of arousal from sleep during hypoxemia and hypercapnia, and the overall stability of the ventilatory control system. Opioids and other sedatives during the perioperative period decrease the respiratory drive to hypoxia and hypercapnia, which then decrease neural output to upper airway dilating muscles. These changes in neural output increase upper airway collapsibility and can also impair arousal.[1] With known deleterious physiologic changes during the perioperative period in OSA patients, it is no surprise that there is an increased risk for cardiopulmonary adverse events, with the literature describing up to a twofold to threefold increase.[19]

Postoperative pulmonary complications in patients with OSA have been well described by researchers over the years. Most studies, including a large national database evaluation of effects of OSA on pulmonary outcomes in patients undergoing both elective and nonelective orthopedic and general surgery, reveal worse outcomes in this surgical population.[12] OSA patients in the perioperative period are at increased risk for acute respiratory distress syndrome, aspiration pneumonia, bacterial pneumonia, respiratory failure, difficult intubation, and emergent endotracheal intubation.[12,20–22] Compared to matched control subjects, OSA patients have increased rates of hypoxemia, intensive care unit transfers, and subsequent increased mean length of hospital stay.[23,24]

In the general population it is well established that OSA increases risk for various cardiovascular complications,[2] including hypertension,[25] arrhythmias, stroke,[3] sudden cardiac death,[4] myocardial ischemia, and heart failure.[26] Reports suggest that during the perioperative period, and even 30 days postoperatively, OSA patients are at increased risk for adverse cardiovascular events. In a recent multicenter prospective cohort study in patients undergoing major noncardiac surgery, unrecognized severe OSA was found to be associated with increased risk of 30-day postoperative cardiovascular complications.[27] The primary cardiovascular outcomes being myocardial injury, congestive heart failure, atrial fibrillation, thromboembolism, and stroke. Rates of adverse cardiovascular events in patients with severe OSA was 30% compared with 19% in patients without OSA. Age, renal impairment, peripheral vascular disease, and OSA are all known independent risk factors for postoperative cardiovascular events.[27] Specifically, the risk of myocardial ischemia in the perioperative period has been correlated with the severity and duration of hypoxemia.[28] In patients with known OSA it has been determined that severity of sleep apnea and hypoxemia worsens compared to their preoperative baseline, and furthermore, 26% of patients develop de novo OSA in the postoperative period, placing patients at increased risk for adverse cardiac events.[29,30]

Sleep apnea is a known predictor of atrial fibrillation. The mechanisms associated with OSA and atrial fibrillation are well documented, and intermittent hypoxia and atrial remodeling play a primary role in the pathogenesis.[31] In patients undergoing cardiac surgery, reports have shown 6% increased odds of new-onset atrial fibrillation for every five-unit increase in AHI.[32] Postoperatively, patients undergoing coronary artery bypass grafting (CABG) are at increased risk for atrial fibrillation,[33] and in this population the prevalence of OSA is as high as 47%.[34] In a single-center prospective study of patients undergoing CABG, patients at high risk for OSA and confirmed OSA were found to have an increased risk for postoperative CABG atrial fibrillation compared to those without OSA (odds ratio [OR], 1.98).[34] Similarly, in the bariatric population, a large database analysis show that OSA is independently associated with a significantly increased OR of atrial fibrillation (OR, 1.25; 95% confidence interval [CI], 1.11 to 1.41; $P < .001$), emergent endotracheal intubation, and mechanical ventilation.[16]

OSA severity as measured by the AHI has been confirmed to be associated with increased risk of postoperative complications; however, other parameters have been proposed to also assist in measuring risk of adverse events in surgical patients.[35] Nocturnal hypoxemia is a common occurrence in patients with OSA, and recent studies have shown specific parameters, such as the oxygen desaturation index (ODI), cumulative sleep time percentage with oxyhemoglobin saturations less than 90% (CT90), and minimum and mean oxyhemoglobin saturation, can provide supplementary clinical data about the severity of OSA and risk for postoperative complications.[35]

In patients undergoing elective surgery with clinical features of OSA, nocturnal oximetry preoperatively showing an ODI of 4% oxygen desaturation with greater than or equal to five events per hour, compared to patients with an ODI of 4% with less than five events, have increased rates of postoperative complications.[36] The rates of postoperative complications increase from 2.7% in patients with ODI of 4% with less than five events to 15.3% in patients with an ODI of 4% with greater than or equal to five events.[36] The postoperative pulmonary complications observed include hypoxemia requiring supplemental oxygen, atelectasis, pneumonia, pulmonary embolism, and bronchospasm. Cardiac complications included chest pain and a junctional arrhythmia. Other adverse postoperative events include intraperitoneal and gastrointestinal bleeding. Hwang and colleagues[36] determined that an ODI of 4% with greater than or equal to five events is associated with increased rate of postoperative complications and that this risk increases with increasing severity of ODI.

Along with the ODI, CT90 and mean pulse oximetry oxygen saturation (Spo_2) are significant predictors for postoperative adverse events. In patients undergoing general surgery, Chung and colleagues[37] demonstrated that the optimal predictive cut-off for high risk of postoperative complications was an ODI greater than 28.5 events per hour, mean preoperative overnight Spo_2 less than 92.7%, and a CT90 greater than 7.2%. In OSA patients undergoing upper airway surgery, a minimum Spo_2 less than or equal to 80% is associated with postoperative complications, including postextubation desaturations, tongue edema, negative pressure pulmonary edema, and upper airway obstruction requiring reintubation.[38] These reports suggest that overnight oximetry could be used as an adjunct tool to further stratify patients at risk for hypoxemia in OSA patients and assess risk of postoperative adverse events.

CHANGES IN SLEEP ARCHITECTURE AND SLEEP-DISORDERED BREATHING IN THE POSTOPERATIVE PERIOD

The perioperative period has increased risk for adverse events in patients with OSA, as described earlier. Anesthetics and analgesics have been found to profoundly alter normal sleep architecture postoperatively and worsen sleep-disordered breathing in patients with and without OSA. As established, OSA patients have an increased risk for upper airway collapsibility,[39,40] and this vulnerability of airway obstruction increases during the postoperative period. These critical dynamic physiologic changes may increase perioperative adverse events. Creating perioperative protocols to help mitigate risks for adverse events, necessitates a clear understanding of the timing of physiologic changes during the postoperative period.

Studies suggest that, depending on the type of surgery, the extent of sleep architecture disturbance can vary postoperatively. During the postoperative period in healthy patients undergoing elective abdominal surgery, rapid eye movement (REM) sleep was found to be initially suppressed, followed by a week of REM rebound.[41] Slow wave sleep in this same population tends to decrease 2 nights postoperatively.[42] Laparoscopic procedures, compared to open surgeries, have less pronounced sleep architecture changes.[43]

In patients with OSA these sleep architectural changes are more pronounced, and sleep-disordered breathing becomes more severe in the postoperative period. Researchers have found that when evaluating OSA patients using portable PSG on postoperative nights (PNs) 1, 3, 5, and 7, patients experience significant sleep fragmentation and worsening of AHI and oxygen saturation.[44]

A balanced anesthesia technique of general anesthesia—with propofol, an opioid, an inhalational agent, and muscle relaxant in patients with OSA—significantly increases AHI on PN3.[44] In non-OSA patients this increase is seen on both PN1 and PN3. The median AHI in OSA patients increases from preoperative baseline AHI of 18 to 29 per hour on PN3. This increase is from 2 to 8 per hour in non-OSA patients, and this increase in AHI is sustained in both patient populations above preoperative baseline on PN5 and does not return completely to baseline until PN7.[44] This pattern of change in sleep architecture is not the same during REM sleep.

In REM sleep, REM-AHI decreases by 91% in patients with OSA on PN1, compared to preoperative baseline.[44] The increase in REM-AHI in OSA patients on PN3 is not statistically significant, compared to the non–rapid eye movement AHI increase pattern seen on PN3. In non-OSA patients, REM-AHI significantly increases from preoperative baseline on PN3. There does not appear to be a correlation between opioid requirements and AHI postoperatively in OSA patients; however, the central apnea index and obstructive apnea index on PN1 were correlated with the first 24-hour opioid requirement.[44] Oxygen saturations, along with AHI severity, also change during the postoperative period. In OSA patients the ODI improves on PN1 but then increases on PN 3, 5, and 7 compared to preoperative ODI baseline. The CT90 significantly increases on PN 3 and 5 for OSA patients. In non-OSA patients, the CT90 increase is only observed on PN3.[44]

Not surprising, sleep architecture is also disrupted during the postoperative period. Sleep efficiency, REM sleep, and slow wave sleep decrease the first night after surgery and then slowly recover to preoperative baseline by PN7. REM sleep decreases by 18% on PN1 and slowly recovers to preoperative baseline by PN7. Slow-wave sleep decreases by about 10% in OSA patients on PN1 but then has a quick recovery by PN3 to baseline, and it then surpasses baseline values by 4% by PN7.[44]

In summary, sleep-disordered breathing worsens, and there are profound sleep architecture changes in the postoperative period in OSA patients. In OSA patients, when observed for 7 nights postoperatively, there is a 61% increase in AHI on PN3, which is accompanied by an increase in ODI by 60%, a fourfold increase in percentage sleep time below Spo_2 90%, and a worse oxyhemoglobin saturation nadir. Postoperative changes in sleep architecture also correlate with worsening hypoxemia and AHI. Postoperative REM rebound may account for severity of oxygen desaturations and AHI changes on PN3.[42,44]

SCREENING FOR OBSTRUCTIVE SLEEP APNEA IN THE PREOPERATIVE PERIOD

In the postoperative period, 80% of death or near-death events in patients with OSA occur within the first 24 hours after surgery.[45] Most of these events occur on hospital floors without significant monitoring.[46] Identifying patients who are at risk for OSA in the preoperative period is clinically important and allows for implementation of risk mitigation measures and appropriate precautions and monitoring. Based on consensus of the American Society of Anesthesiologists (ASA) Task Force, Society of Anesthesia and Sleep Medicine, and the American Academy of Sleep Medicine, all patients with risk factors or suspicion of having underlying OSA should undergo appropriate preoperative evaluation, including medical record review, patient and family interview, screening protocol, and physical examination. Screening protocols or questionnaires to assess for OSA have sensitivity values ranging from 36% to 86% and specificity values ranging from 31% to 95% for AHI scores of greater than or equal to 5.[47] Preoperative evaluations should be performed in advance of surgery to allow adequate time for anesthesiologists and surgeons to decide on clinical management of patients suspected of having OSA. They can decide to manage the patient perioperatively based on clinical information or can plan to conduct further testing with referral for sleep study testing and initiation of OSA treatment before or after scheduled surgery.[47,48]

Feasibility and reliability are major considerations when choosing appropriate screening tools in the preoperative period. Recommended screening tests with comparable accuracy and validation in surgical patients include the STOP-BANG tool, Berlin Questionnaire, ASA checklist, and the Perioperative Sleep Apnea Prediction (P-SAP) score.[48]

The STOP-BANG tool is a widely used screening tool and has been validated in surgical patients, sleep clinic patients, and the general population.[49] It is an eight-item screening tool with questions about snoring, tiredness, observed pauses in breathing, hypertension, body mass index greater than or equal to 35 kg/m^2, age greater than or equal to 50 years, neck size (≥17 inches in men, ≥16 inches in women), and male gender. Each item is scored yes (1) or no (0), giving a range of scores from 0 to 8, with a score between 0 to 2 being low risk, 3 to 4 intermediate, and 5 to 8 being considered high risk for having moderate to severe OSA. The sensitivity of a STOP-BANG score greater than or equal to 3 to detect moderate to severe OSA (AHI ≥ 15) and severe OSA (AHI ≥ 30) is 93% and 100%, respectively.[50]

The Berlin Questionnaire was initially developed to detect patients with OSA in primary care settings. It is an 11-item questionnaire with three categories, the first being snoring history, daytime sleepiness, and history of hypertension or obesity. When two of the three categories are found to be positive, then a patient is considered high risk for OSA. In the general population, the sensitivity and specificity of the questionnaire to predict an AHI greater than or equal to 15 was 58.8% and 77.6%, respectively. The sensitivity and specificity when used to detect severe OSA, with AHI greater than or equal to 30, is 76.9% with a small decrease in specificity to 72.7%.[51]

The ASA checklist is a routine screening tool for OSA in surgical patients. It consists of 12 items for adults and 14 items for children. The checklist combines three categories: physical characteristics, history of airway obstruction, and daytime sleepiness. Patients are considered high risk of having OSA if two or more categories are scored as positive. Patients are considered low risk if only one or no categories are scored as positive.[52] The sensitivity for predicting OSA is 72.1%, and the specificity is 38.2%.[48]

The P-SAP score validates six of the eight elements of the STOP-BANG questionnaire and evaluates upper airway characteristics (Mallampati and thyromental distance < 6 mm) and includes a question about diabetes mellitus diagnosis. The elements of the P-SAP score were first described in a typical university hospital surgical population. The sensitivity is 93.9%, and the specificity is 32.3% in predicting risk for having OSA.[53]

The purpose of the above-mentioned screening tools is to detect high-risk patients for OSA in the preoperative period, to allow for clinical planning and management to help mitigate risks for postoperative adverse events.

PERIOPERATIVE MANAGEMENT OF PATIENTS WITH SUSPECTED OR KNOWN OBSTRUCTIVE SLEEP APNEA

Patients who screen positive for being high risk for moderate to severe OSA in the absence of diagnostic confirmatory PSG should be treated as having OSA and considered at increased risk for perioperative complications.

Preoperative and postoperative application of continuous positive airway pressure (CPAP) significantly decreases postoperative AHI and is associated with a trend toward decreased length of hospital stay.[54] Patients diagnosed with OSA and initiated on CPAP before surgery have significantly reduced risk for postoperative cardiovascular adverse events, compared with patients with undiagnosed OSA.[55] Both myocardial infarctions and unplanned reintubations are increased in untreated OSA patients.[20,56] CPAP therapy is recommended preoperatively when OSA is severe and continued postoperatively when feasible, especially if postoperative monitoring reveals evidence of airway obstruction. Patients should continue use of CPAP on their home settings during sleep and when sedated while hospitalized. Similarly, patients using alternative treatments, such as an oral appliance, positional therapy pillows, or hypoglossal nerve stimulators, should continue their use in the perioperative setting. If there are questions or concerns about effectiveness of therapy, a referral before surgery to their sleep specialist is recommended.[47,48]

If patients have known OSA, but either decline therapy or are noncompliant before surgery, there are sparse data supporting that delaying surgery in those cases is recommended. However, in patients with comorbid conditions, such as uncontrolled systemic disease, pulmonary hypertension,[57] hypoventilation,[58] or resting hypoxemia,[59] the risk of postoperative complications has been found to be increased, and further preoperative assessment for disease optimization is warranted.

Patients with untreated OSA with optimized comorbid conditions, under the discretion of surgeons and anesthesiologists, may proceed with surgery if postoperative strategies for mitigation of adverse events are implemented and patients are counseled on the increased risks of complications posed by OSA in the perioperative period.[48] The urgency of the surgery, availability of postoperative monitoring, and the type of surgery may all play a role in the decision to proceed with surgery or to refer to a sleep specialist for further evaluation and treatment. A referral to a sleep medicine specialist has been found to reduce the rate of discontinuation of CPAP therapy[60] and improve overall PAP adherence.[60,61]

Institutions should implement protocols for patients with known or suspected OSA to help clinicians manage these patients with respect to the type of anesthesia, analgesic regimen, and postoperative monitoring to help reduce the risk of adverse outcomes.[48]

The ASA Task Force recommends minimizing opioid use, using multimodal short-acting agents for analgesia and considering local and/or regional anesthesia where appropriate in high-risk patients. Although there is no clear consensus on monitoring parameters or location for OSA patients postoperatively, continuous pulse oximetry or capnography may provide important clinical warnings about patients with postoperative events that may possibly require escalation of care and early intervention. The ASA Task Force recommends considering monitored settings in high-risk patients from the post–anesthesia care unit with severe OSA, a STOP-BANG score greater than or equal to 5, postoperative parenteral opioids, or significant comorbid conditions.[47]

CLINICAL PEARLS

Obstructive sleep apnea (OSA) increases risk for adverse outcomes in the perioperative period. Changes in sleep architecture postoperatively may contribute to pathophysiologic changes that alter the caliber of the upper airway and respiratory arousal threshold, subsequently worsening apnea-hypopnea index and oxygen saturations postoperatively. Using screening tools during preoperative evaluations allows for identifying patients at risk for OSA and appropriately managing them to allow for optimization, treatment, and risk mitigation.

SUMMARY

OSA is the most common sleep disorder and has been found to increase the risk for cardiovascular complications,[2] arrhythmias, stroke,[3] and sudden cardiac death.[4] Intermittent hypoxia, hypercapnia, sympathetic activation, and associated arousals that characterize sleep-disordered breathing have been found to increase risk for adverse outcomes in the postoperative period.[20,21,27,28] There are profound sleep architecture changes, and sleep-disordered breathing worsens in the postoperative period in OSA patients.[44] Studies suggest preoperative initiation of CPAP therapy may help decrease risks.[55] Screening tools are recommended to help identify patients at risk for OSA in the preoperative period, with the goal of optimizing patients before surgery and instituting perioperative risk mitigation strategies to reduce risk for postoperative complications.

SELECTED READINGS

Chung F, Abdullah HR, Liao P. STOP-Bang Questionnaire: a practical approach to screen for obstructive sleep apnea. *Chest*. 2016;149(3):631–638.

Jonsson Fagerlund M, Franklin KA. Perioperative continuous positive airway pressure therapy: a review with the emphasis on randomized controlled trials and obstructive sleep apnea. *Anesth Analg*. 2021;132(5):1306–1313.

Kaw R, Chung F, Pasupuleti V, Mehta J, Gay PC, Hernandez AV. Meta-analysis of the association between obstructive sleep apnoea and postoperative outcome. *Br J Anaesth*. 2012;109:897–906.

Kaw R, El Zarif S, Wang L, Bena J, Blackstone EH, Mehra R. Obesity as an effect modifier in sleep-disordered breathing and postcardiac surgery atrial fibrillation. *Chest*. 2017;151(6):1279–1287.

Kaw R, Wong J, Mokhlesi B. Obesity and obesity hypoventilation, sleep hypoventilation, and postoperative respiratory failure. *Anesth Analg*. 2021;132(5):1265–1273.

Luo JM, Zhang DM, Xiao Y, et al. Perioperative evaluation of obstructive sleep apnea in bariatric surgery population. *Zhongguo Yi Xue Ke Xue Yuan Xue Bao*. 2018;40(5):617–624.

Memtsoudis S1, Liu SS, Ma Y, Chiu YL, et al. Perioperative pulmonary outcomes in patients with sleep apnea after noncardiac surgery. *Anesth Analg*. 2011;112(1):113–121.

Nahorecki A, Postrzech-Adamczyk K, Święcicka-Klama A, Skomro R, Szuba A. Prevalence of sleep apnea in patients with carotid artery stenosis. In: Cruzio WE, Dong H, Radeke HH, et al., eds. *Advances in Experimental Medicine and Biology*. New York, NY: Springer; 2019.

Peppard PE, Young T, Barnet JH, Palta M, Hagen EW, Hla KM. Increased prevalence of sleep-disordered breathing in adults. *Am J Epidemiol*. 2013;177:1006–1014.

Seet E, Nagappa M, Wong DT. Airway management in surgical patients with obstructive sleep apnea. *Anesth Analg*. 2021;132(5):1321–1327.

Singh M, Liao P, Kobah S, Wijeysundera DN, Shapiro C, Chung F. Proportion of surgical patients with undiagnosed obstructive sleep apnoea. *Br J Anaesth*. 2013;110(4):629–636.

Subramani Y, Singh M, Wong J, Kushida CA, Malhotra A, Chung F. Understanding phenotypes of obstructive sleep apnea: applications in anesthesia, surgery, and perioperative medicine. *Anesth Analg*. 2017;124(1):179–191.

Suen C, Clodagh R, Talha M, Chung F, et al. Sleep study and oximetry parameters for predicting postoperative complications in patients with OSA. *Chest*. 2019;155(4):855–867.

A complete reference list can be found online at ExpertConsult.com.

Chapter 160

Sleep and Gastrointestinal Health

Steve M. D'Souza; Ronnie Fass; Fahmi Shibli; David A. Johnson

Chapter Highlights

- Gut function occurs in an independent circadian fashion and is regulated mainly by timing of food intake. Gastrointestinal (GI) flora exhibit daily oscillation in abundance, and alterations in the circadian rhythm can shift this oscillation and lead to dysbiosis.
- Sleep-related dysbiosis is associated with increased microbe-immune interactions and downstream proinflammatory effects.
- Reflux symptoms adversely affect normal sleep, and gastroesophageal disease is associated with worsening of sleep dysfunction. Sleep disturbances and functional dyspepsia are closely related.
- Alcohol consumption increases gut epithelial permeability and leads to an inflammatory reaction that is worsened by circadian dysfunction and can lead to hepatic fat deposition.
- An inflammatory hepatic reaction seen in obesity is associated with increased fat deposition causing nonalcoholic fatty liver disease and may explain the association with sleep apnea.
- Circadian dysrhythmia, such as that seen in night-shift workers, is associated with irritable bowel syndrome. Sleep disruption increases the frequency of inflammatory bowel disease (IBD) flares and is associated with disease severity. IBD therapeutics such as TNF-α inhibitors may improve sleep dysfunction in these patients. Melatonin may also improve IBD symptoms and sleep disturbances.
- Circadian clock genes may act as tumor suppressors and mutations can contribute to carcinogenesis in the GI tract.

INTRODUCTION

Normally the gastrointestinal (GI) system has a unique expression of circadian oscillation, and disruption of this rhythm or dissociation from the central circadian rhythm can have a profound effect on disease pathogenesis.

GASTROINTESTINAL FUNCTION IN NORMAL SLEEP

Circadian Rhythm

The circadian clock plays a role in the majority of physiologic systems, including the GI tract.[1] Daily variation of gut motility, endocrine and exocrine gut function, and microbial barrier integrity are among the many functions affected by the circadian clock and are primarily modified by timing of food intake.[2] Perturbations to suprachiasmatic nucleus function as well as to gut circadian function can lead to a mismatch between the two rhythms.[3] Changes in light and dark exposure can modify pineal gland melatonin secretion and thus affect sleep habits.[4-6] Likewise, alterations in the timing and quantity of meal intake can adversely affect gut circadian rhythm.[7-10] Sleep disturbances can affect GI tract function and, conversely, GI disease can negatively affect sleep quality. There is clearly an intricate relationship between the GI tract and the circadian rhythm.

Gene Expression

Daily circadian oscillation of gene expression is heavily regulated by the master circadian genes *CLOCK* and *Bmal1*, the expression of both being vital for normal circadian metabolic activity.[11] Downstream from *CLOCK* and *Bmal1*, the cryptochrome circadian regulator (CRY) and period circadian protein homolog (PER) groups of genes act as circadian regulators of protein expression associated with the light-dark cycle.[12,13] See Chapter 13 for more detail.

MICROBIOME VARIATION IN NORMAL AND ALTERED SLEEP

Major bacterial species in the GI tract of rodents demonstrate variations in levels that are present only in the context of a functional circadian clock.[14] Additionally, shifting feeding pattern to primarily during the light or dark portions of the daily light-dark cycle shows a compensatory shift in the oscillatory microbial abundance.[15]

Various factors can alter the circadian oscillation expression and abundance of gut flora. Frequent shifts in day-night feeding are associated with loss of this daily variation, although it is not clear if this is a microbially or physiologically initiated change.[15] Sleep fragmentation is associated with decreased microbial diversity in the ileum and colon, which may be a contributing factor.[16] Food content is also related to the adaptability of the circadian microbial oscillatory pattern. High-lipid, high-carbohydrate, and alcohol-containing diets decrease the resilience of the microbial variation to shifts in the light-dark feeding cycle and may contribute to the deleterious reorganization of the intestinal microbiota with consequent dysbiosis.[9,17,18] In addition, diet-related dysbiosis appears to directly affect microbial influence on gene expression, which is possible mechanism for direct contribution of the microbiome to circadian disruption.

The composition of gut microbiota is closely tied to energy absorption and retention.[19,20] Translating this to sleep dysbiosis, it is likely that fluctuations in gut bacterial composition associated with abnormal sleep are directly linked to states of pathologic energy metabolism, including metabolic syndrome and fatty liver disease.

In addition to affecting energy extraction, sleep-related dysbiosis upsets a key balance in the interaction between gut flora and the native immune system. Bacterial products interact with host immune receptors, including Toll-like receptors (TLRs).[21] Activation of these receptors leads to increased downstream upregulation and expression of inflammatory cytokines, including interleukin-6 (IL-6) and tumor necrosis factor-α (TNF-α), chemokines, as well as proinflammatory transcription activators such as NF-κB.[22,23] Murine studies of sleep-dysfunction demonstrate upregulation of proinflammatory cytokines.[24-26] Thus increased bacterial product translocation suggests that microbial variation, as seen in altered sleep, can contribute to a proinflammatory state that is associated with many GI disorders.

SLEEP AND GASTROINTESTINAL DISEASE

Gastroesophageal Reflux Disease

Gastroesophageal reflux disease (GERD), which affects about 20% of the US adult population, involves primarily the esophagus but may also affect adjacent organs, such as the oropharynx, larynx, and pulmonary system.[27] However, GERD may also have a systemic effect, leading to sleep disturbances.

There is a bidirectional relationship between GERD and sleep, in which GERD adversely affects sleep by awakening patients from sleep during the night or more commonly causing multiple, short, amnestic arousals that lead to sleep fragmentation.[28] In turn, poor sleep may adversely affect GERD by enhancing perception of intraesophageal stimuli, such as acid (centrally mediated sensitization) and increase in esophageal acid exposure, possibly by altering the normal relationship between ghrelin and leptin.[29,30] This relationship, if not interrupted, creates a vicious cycle, whereby GERD leads to poor sleep and bidirectional, poor sleep exacerbates GERD (Figure 160.1).

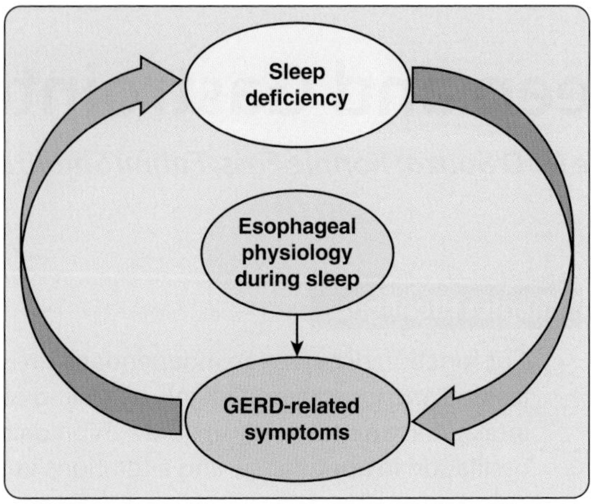

Figure 160.1 The vicious cycle between gastroesophageal reflux disease (GERD) and sleep.

Box 160.1 PHYSIOLOGIC CHANGES IN UPPER GUT DURING SLEEP

Oropharynx
- Decreased salivary secretion and flow
- Decreased swallowing rate

Esophagus
- Decreased primary and secondary esophageal peristalsis
- Decreased esophageal acid clearance
- Decreased upper esophageal sphincter pressure
- Decreased perception of intraesophageal stimuli

Stomach
- Increased gastric acidity
- Decreased gastric emptying

Epidemiology

Epidemiologic studies have demonstrated that about 65% of patients with GERD experience both daytime and nighttime symptoms.[31-34] Approximately 13% of patients with GERD experience only nighttime symptoms, whereas 50% of patients with GERD report that heartburn awakens them from sleep.[27,33,34] In the general population, 25% report having heartburn symptoms during sleep time.[35]

In general, sleep disturbances in patients with GERD are poorly recognized and rarely elicited during clinic visits, despite the significant impact of these disturbances on quality of life and perception of disease severity. About 50% of patients with nonerosive reflux disease reported that GERD symptoms were responsible for difficulty getting a good night's sleep.[36] The prevalence of sleep disturbances increases with the frequency of nighttime heartburn episodes during the week. Frequent nocturnal heartburn is associated more strongly with impaired health-related quality of life and work productivity as compared with patients with GERD without nighttime symptoms.[37]

Nocturnal reflux may lead to insomnia, snoring, tossing and turning, and even nightmares. GERD may also affect patients' sleep experience by causing nocturnal cough, choking, wheezing, sore throat, and breathlessness.[38,39] Unfortunately, sleep disturbances resulting from GERD are rarely recognized in clinical practice and commonly not elicited by physicians despite their profound effect on patients' quality of life and work productivity.[37,40]

Pathophysiology

Esophageal defense mechanisms are pivotal for preventing mucosal injury during acid reflux events. The accentuated noxious effects of nocturnal reflux are driven primarily by a decrease in saliva production, swallowing rate, primary and secondary esophageal peristalsis, gastric emptying, and conscious perception of reflux events (Box 160.1).[41]

Sleep impairs esophageal acid clearance in both patients with GERD and healthy controls.[42] Acid clearance during sleep time occurs predominantly in association with arousals from sleep.[43,44] Furthermore, esophageal clearance time during sleep remains prolonged regardless of the pH level or the volume of the refluxate.[43,44] Sleep, but not body position (supine), is a significant factor for acid migration to the proximal esophagus for even minute volumes of acid reflux and markedly prolongs acid clearance.[45]

During wakefulness, the contact of esophageal mucosa with acid results in enhanced salivary bicarbonate secretion and flow and increased swallowing frequency, which propel the refluxate from the distal esophagus into the stomach as well as neutralize the pH of the esophageal lumen. However, during sleep, salivary secretion and flow are virtually absent,[46] and swallowing frequency is markedly reduced from 25 swallows per hour during the awake state to approximately 5 swallows per hour during sleep.[47] Upper esophageal sphincter pressure progressively declines with deeper stages of sleep, resulting in an increased risk of reflux reaching the larynx, pharynx, and pulmonary system.[48,49] Transient lower esophageal sphincter (LES) relaxation and gastroesophageal reflux occur primarily during transient arousals from sleep or when patients are fully awake.[50] Furthermore, acid reflux events may occur during either prolonged periods of wakefulness or brief arousals from sleep.[51] Overall, LES basal pressure is not affected during sleep.

Esophageal acid clearance and airway protection are dependent on secondary esophageal peristalsis and the esophago–upper esophageal sphincter contractile reflex.[52-54] The rate of secondary esophageal peristalsis decreases progressively with deeper sleep stages and is absent in slow wave sleep.[50,55] The sleep related changes to gastric emptying may also promote nocturnal reflux.

Alteration in esophageal physiology during sleep may accentuate the effect of gastroesophageal reflux on esophageal mucosa. This leads to a more severe disease and sleep disturbances. Patients with nighttime reflux are more likely to develop severe erosive esophagitis, peptic stricture, esophageal ulceration, extraesophageal manifestations, Barrett's esophagus (BE), and adenocarcinoma of the esophagus.[56-58]

Sleep Disturbances

The main mechanisms causing sleep disturbances in patients with GERD are conscious awakenings that may be associated with symptoms and short, amnestic arousals that are not associated with symptoms but still can lead to sleep fragmentation.[59] Acid reflux events are more commonly associated with short amnestic arousals, which tend to occur during stage 2 sleep and rarely during the rapid eye movement (REM) period.[60]

Interestingly, when patients with GERD transition from sleep to awakening in the morning, it is associated with marked increase in the number of gastroesophageal reflux events immediately after awakening and before any meal consumption.[61] This phenomenon termed "risers' reflux" is not dependent on body position (recumbent or upright) and may explain patients' report of GERD-related symptoms immediately after waking up in the morning.

Although studies were able to demonstrate differences in sleep architecture among the different GERD phenotypes or before and after instituting antireflux treatment in patients with GERD, spectral analysis of sleep has demonstrated a shift in the electroencephalogram (EEG) power spectrum toward higher frequencies in patients with heartburn and erosive esophagitis as compared with those with functional heartburn and thus no GERD, despite similar sleep architecture.[62]

Overall, studies have demonstrated that GERD may lead to sleep disturbances and thus sleep deprivation. However, an intriguing line of research studies have suggested that sleep deprivation per se may exacerbate GERD through two mechanisms, centrally mediated esophageal hypersensitivity and an increase in the degree of esophageal acid exposure. Acute sleep deprivation (3 hours) has been shown to significantly reduce perception thresholds for esophageal pain as compared to good sleep (at least 7 hours).[63] In addition, acute sleep deprivation may lead to abnormal esophageal acid exposure in normal healthy subjects, probably through alteration in the relationship between ghrelin (increase) and leptin (decrease), leading to increase in craving feelings and thus food consumption.[30,64]

Some patients lack typical or atypical manifestations of GERD but report sleep disturbances and poor quality of sleep ("silent reflux").[65] Thus sleep disturbances can be the sole manifestation of GERD in a subset of patients.

Sleep Apnea

The relationship between obstructive sleep apnea (OSA) and GERD remains controversial. Some investigators have suggested that GERD is associated with OSA and that there may be a potential causal link between the two disorders.[66] Kerr and colleagues have demonstrated that precipitous drops in pH were frequently preceded by arousals (98.4%), movement of the patient (71.9%), and swallowing (80.4%).[67] Arousal and movement may trigger gastroesophageal reflux by causing transition alteration in the pressure gradient across the lower esophageal sphincter (LES). Additionally, the lowered intrathoracic pressure that accompanied OSA may by itself predispose the patient to gastroesophageal reflux by exacerbating the LES pressure gradient. Treatment with nasal continuous positive airway pressure (CPAP) showed reduction in the frequency of gastroesophageal reflux by elevating intrathoracic pressure.[67] However, other studies have failed to demonstrate a causal relationship between OSA and GERD. Patients subjectively report that the quality of sleep is affected by the severity of GERD; however, objective correlation between GERD and OSA is lacking, suggesting that maybe both are common entities that share similar risk factors but may not to be causally linked.[66] OSA is not influenced by severity of GERD.

Only a few small studies have evaluated the effect of nasal continuous positive airway pressure therapy (nCPAP) on gastroesophageal reflux (GER) in patients with OSA. Kerr and colleagues demonstrated that nCPAP reduced the percentage of total recording time that esophageal pH was less than 4.0 from 6.3% to 0.1%.[67] Tawk and colleagues showed that nCPAP normalized the esophageal acid exposure in 81% of patients with OSA and GERD.[68] However, Ing and colleagues demonstrated that nCPAP reduced the GER parameters in patients with OSA and those without OSA, suggesting that the effect of nCPAP was likely nonspecific.[69]

Complications

Nocturnal GERD is associated with increased risk of severe gastroesophageal disease, such as erosive esophagitis, peptic stricture, BE, and adenocarcinoma of the esophagus.[57]

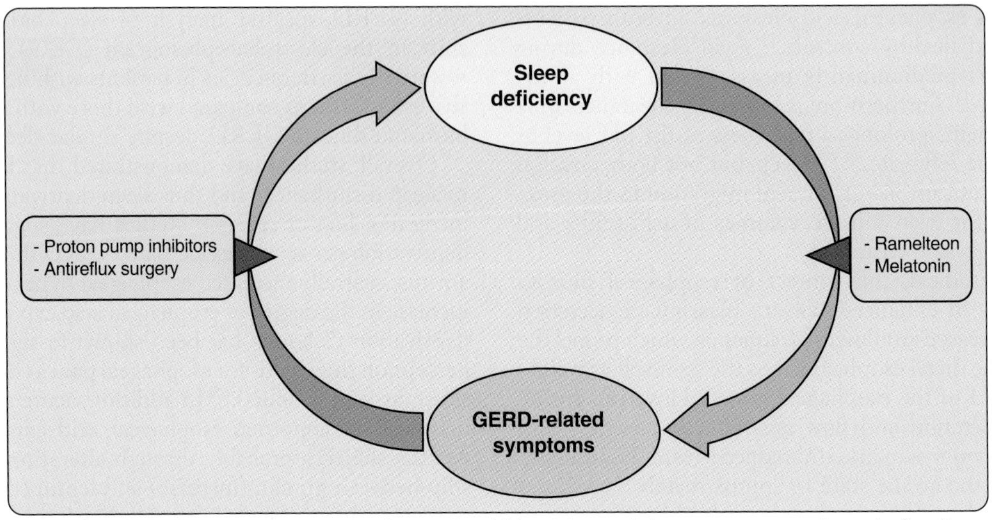

Figure 160.2 Therapeutic interventions that can "break" the vicious cycle between gastroesophageal reflux disease (GERD) and sleep.

Box 160.2 LIFESTYLE MODIFICATION FOR NIGHTTIME REFLUX

- Elevate the head of the bed
- Avoid the right decubitus position
- Avoid late-night meals or snacks (last meal at least 3 hours before bedtime)
- Improve sleep hygiene (minimizing disturbances to normal sleep)

The risk of esophageal adenocarcinoma is eight times higher among patients with weekly reflux symptoms compared with asymptomatic subjects. The risk is even higher in patients reporting nocturnal heartburn.[56,57]

Treatment

Treatment of nighttime GERD initially requires lifestyle modifications, such as avoiding food consumption at least 3 hours before bedtime, elevating the head of the bed, avoiding the right decubitus position, which is more associated with reflux events than the other sleep time positions, and improving sleep hygiene by minimizing disturbances to normal sleep.[70]

The bidirectional relationship between GERD and sleep provides an opportunity for two completely different lines of therapy that will "break" the vicious cycle (Figure 160.2). Obviously, the focus has been and remains on improving GERD and consequently restoring normal sleep. Proton pump inhibitors (PPIs) are effective in reducing sleep disturbances and improving sleep quality and thus quality of life in GERD patients with nighttime symptoms.[71-74] Most of the aforementioned studies assessed only subjective sleep parameters using patients' report diaries or validated questionnaires. However, demonstrating improvement in objective sleep parameters using polysomnography in PPI trials has proven to be a more difficult task.

In patients with GERD, who failed once-a-day PPI, optimization of GERD treatment that targets nighttime reflux is currently recommended (Box 160.2). Beside the aforementioned lifestyle modifications, other intervention may include the following: change PPI administration before dinner if symptoms are primarily during nighttime, split PPI dose (before doubling it) to be given before breakfast and dinner, or add a histamine 2 antagonist (H2RA), Carafate or Gaviscon, before bedtime. The effect of antireflux surgery on sleep quality has been rarely examined, but several small studies suggested marked improvement.[75]

Another approach is to provide treatment that improves sleep, which may result in improvement of GERD-related symptoms. Zolpidem use in patients with GERD reduced arousals associated with reflux events by more than 50% as compared with placebo but resulted in a significantly longer esophageal acid clearance time.[76] Ramelteon improved daytime and nighttime GERD symptoms, sleep efficiency, and sleep latency in patients with nonerosive reflux disease compared with placebo.[77]

Improvement in sleep disturbances related to GERD remained a priority in drug development; thus it is highly plausible that a better therapeutic approach may require a combination of both antireflux medication and a sleeping pill.

Barrett's Esophagus

As previously described, patients with BE have the highest esophageal acid exposure during nighttime as compared with other GERD phenotypes.[78] Furthermore, patients with BE have marked increase in the frequency of spontaneous gastroesophageal reflux during sleep but demonstrate faster acid clearance times, during both waking and sleep as compared with healthy volunteers.[78] Overall, it appears that patients with BE can adequately clear acid from the distal esophagus but experience considerable acid mucosal contact time because of repeated episodes of spontaneous reflux during sleep.[78]

Although not clearly demonstrated, it has been hypothesized that melatonin can potentially prevent the sequence from erosive esophagitis to BE to esophageal adenocarcinoma.[79] Melatonin (besides its effect on circadian rhythm and sleep) is a free radical scavenger, which activates several antioxidative enzymes and mechanisms.

There are several studies demonstrating an association between BE and obstructive sleep apnea (OSA).[80-83]

Sleep and Functional Dyspepsia

Sleep disturbances are common in patients with functional dyspepsia, and functional dyspepsia is very common in subjects with sleep disturbances. In general, almost two-thirds of patients with functional gastrointestinal disorders report some type of sleep abnormality. By far, sleep deprivation is the most common, affecting almost half of these patients.[84] The most commonly reported sleep abnormalities in functional dyspepsia included waking up repeatedly during the night and waking up in the morning feeling tired or not rested. Importantly, half of the patients reported that functional dyspepsia symptoms awakened them from sleep during the night.

Among shift workers or subjects with sleep disturbances, functional bowel disorders, such as functional dyspepsia and irritable bowel syndrome (IBS) are very common.[85,86] Gender, body mass index, number of night shifts worked, work-related stress, and dietary patterns were shown to be significantly related to functional dyspepsia and insomnia in shift-working nurses.[87] The prevalence of sleep disorders was similar when patients with functional dyspepsia and postprandial distress symptoms (PDS) subtype were compared with those with the epigastric pain syndrome (EPS) subtype.[88] Sleep disturbances in functional dyspepsia have been shown to reduce sleep efficiency, increase arousals, and result in abnormal amounts of REM sleep.[89]

Treatment with H2RA, such as nizatidine, has been shown to significantly improve gastroesophageal reflux symptoms, gastric emptying, and sleep disorders in patients with functional dyspepsia.[90] Psychological intervention may improve functional dyspepsia and consequently related sleep disturbances.[91]

Alcohol-Related Liver Disease

Circadian Rhythm

Alcohol use is closely tied to sleep cycles and dietary intake, with alcohol use disorder being linked to timing of intake.[92] Liver circadian function is independent of central light-dark regulated circadian function and is more closely tied to dietary intake.[3,93] Disruption between the two systems, such as that seen in overnight shift workers or chronically late-night eaters, leads to mismatch between the two rhythms and alters liver metabolism.[93]

The inflammatory reaction after alcohol consumption can disrupt the normal metabolism of the liver and over time can develop into the steatosis and impaired function that is seen in alcohol-related liver disease (ALD). This disruptive process is amplified by discordance between central and liver circadian function.[94-97]

Another factor related to both ALD and circadian rhythm is gut dysbiosis.[98] Alcohol consumption adversely affects the gut microbial barrier and promotes microbial proliferation and a subsequent inflammatory reaction.[98,99] Similarly, sleep alteration and central circadian disruption is also related to decreased gut barrier function and microbial proliferation.[15,98,100] These effects appear to be additive, and alcohol consumption in those with central circadian disturbances is associated with an increased inflammatory reaction and increased gut permeability compared to alcohol consumption in those with normal central circadian function.[18,101]

Cytokine Expression

The expression of inflammatory cytokines in a circadian dysrhythmic state follows drinking of alcohol even in patients without liver disease. Sleeping after binge alcohol consumption increases expression of cytokines IL-2 and interferon (IFN)-γ.[102] Patients with chronic alcoholism exhibit both loss of REM sleep and variation in inflammatory cytokine expression.[103]

In addition to direct effect on cytokine expression, alcohol consumption also indirectly promotes cytokine expression through increased intestinal epithelial permeability to bacterial products. This increase in permeability allows molecules such as lipopolysaccharide to bind to TLRs and promote downstream expression of interleukins.[21] This effect is pronounced in a disrupted circadian state.

Microbiome Effects

Alcohol consumption is linked to various intestinal epithelium changes, including increased permeability.[104] This leads to translocation of bacterial products such as lipopolysaccharide and subsequent proinflammatory cytokine upregulation. Studies of pathologic sleep states demonstrate that circadian disruption further increases alcohol-related intestinal barrier permeability.[18] Night-shift workers who consume alcohol are at higher risk for gut hyperpermeability and endotoxemia compared with their day-shift counterparts.[97] They are also at higher risk for hepatic steatosis.

Circadian dysrhythmia is also one of the factors that directly lead to dysbiosis that contributes to hepatic steatosis.[98,105-107] Disruption in the daily circadian microbial variation, through poor sleep, high-caloric diet, and altered timing of food consumption can contribute to increased bacterial overgrowth, translocation, and subsequent endotoxemia, as well as decreased bile acid metabolism, which are all associated with increasing the pathogenesis of alcohol-related hepatitis and increased hepatic fat deposition.[9,106]

Nonalcoholic Fatty Liver Disease

Circadian Rhythm

Nonalcoholic fatty liver disease (NAFLD) is associated with obesity and metabolic syndrome and lack of alcohol consumption; it results in increased hepatic lipid deposition.[108] Both the gut circadian rhythm as well as the central rhythm directly affect fat metabolism, storage, and energy expenditure.[109-111] Disruption in synchrony between central and gut circadian rhythms impairs the synergistic effect on lipid catabolism and promotes lipid storage.[112,113]

Similar to what is seen in ALD, circadian fluctuation in microbial permeability and proliferation is related to obesity and NAFLD.[114] Sleep disorders such as sleep apnea are also associated with NAFLD.[115]

Liver fat deposition is promoted by variation and disruption of a normal sleep cycle, more specifically disruption of central and peripheral circadian rhythms. Murine models of *CLOCK* mutation result in hyperglycemia, hyperlipidemia, and obesity.[116]

Microbiome Effects

Gut flora is essential in the absorption and metabolism of micronutrients, and sleep disturbance and dietary changes can contribute to obesity under certain microbiome states. In addition, high-fat diet and sleep disruption affect the central circadian rhythm in part because of alterations in the composition of intestinal flora. This manifests through variations in concentrations of microbial products and altered metabolism of short-chain fatty acids.

Disease Implications

Studies of melatonin on murine models demonstrated reduction in oxidative stress markers and reversal of reactive oxygen species (ROS) upregulation from hyperlipidemia with improvement in hepatocyte survival.[117,118] Studies of probiotics and synbiotics have yielded mixed results.[119,120]

Irritable Bowel Syndrome

Circadian Rhythm

Functional bowel disorders, such as IBS, are related to abnormal motility, inflammation, hypersensitivity, and gut dysbiosis, all of which are related to circadian disruption. Because of circadian regulation of gastrointestinal motility, disruption between central and gut circadian regulation, such as that seen in shift workers, is a predisposing factor for dysmotility and IBS.[121-125] Additionally, as described earlier, gut dysbiosis is associated with increased systemic inflammation, and this is believed to influence functional dysmotility.

A circadian model may offer opportunity for therapeutics for IBS as well. Because of decreased pineal secretion of melatonin during circadian imbalance,[4-6] melatonin supplementation has been trialed as a potential modulator for IBS symptom relief with some success.[126]

Cytokine Expression

Sleep deprivation can result in overexpression of inflammatory cytokines, including IL-6 and TNF-α and cytokines, can also be expressed after increased interaction between gut immune cells and bacteria.[127] Increased symptom severity, especially pain, is associated with poor sleep and increased stress hormone secretion, as well as elevated inflammatory cytokine expression, and about a third of patients with IBS have a sleep disorder.[128]

Microbiome Effects

IBS and microbiome alterations are closely linked. Postinfectious IBS is a well-recognized phenomenon. It is also likely that microbial antigen recognition may potentiate the inflammatory cascade that contributes to development of IBS-like symptoms. Microbial products, such as lipopolysaccharide, induce a host inflammatory response, and expression of cytokines such as TNF-α and IL-6 in conditions with high intestinal permeability.[22,129] Indeed, these proinflammatory products are increased in chronically sleep-deprived or altered states, and this effect likely contributes to increased IBS symptomatology.

Disease Implications

There are several potential targets for treatment of sleep disorders with meaningful benefit for IBS. One potential therapy is melatonin supplementation, which has been demonstrated to have efficacy in reducing both sleep dysfunction and IBS symptoms in patients with inflammatory bowel disease (IBD).[126] Another theory of disease pathogenesis and trigger suggests that circadian dysrhythmia may play a role in triggering new onset disease or flares.

Inflammatory Bowel Disease

Circadian Rhythm

Circadian disruption and subsequent colonic inflammation are believed to be contributors to pathogenesis of IBD.[130] A Western diet and lifestyle, including night-shift work, are known risk factors for Crohn's disease and ulcerative colitis. Experimental studies in shift workers and sleep-deprived patients find similar increased inflammatory marker production.[131]

Circadian disruption is also directly linked to IBD manifestation. Patients with IBD are more likely to have acute flares and are at higher risk for hospitalization when sleep is disrupted.[132] Conversely, patients with IBD report poor sleep,[133,134] often as a consequence of their disease, suggesting a pattern for disease progression.[129] Additionally, active IBD may contribute to dysregulation of circadian *CLOCK* genes, suggesting a possible route for potentiation of disease through a circadian pathway.[135,136]

Cytokine Expression

Pathogenesis and relapse of IBD is heavily linked to the presence of inflammatory markers, including TNF-α and interleukins. Current treatment strategies are targeted at reducing inflammatory cytokine expression, especially TNF-α. Sleep deprivation and dysrhythmia can contribute to overexpression of IL-6 and subsequently TNF-α.

A variety of hormonal stimuli also affect the expression of inflammatory cytokines. The adrenal steroid hormone cortisol is tied to stress response and is modulated by depth and length of sleep.[137] Cortisol and other corticosteroids have multiple downstream effects, including alterations in circadian immune cell activity and gut permeability.[138,139] Low levels of circulating cortisol have been associated with increased IL-6 and TNF-α production, whereas high levels are associated with suppression of inflammatory gene expression.[140] Other steroid hormonal stimuli include estrogens, which promote mucosal barrier integrity, and estrogen receptor expression is downregulated in IBD.[141,142] Estrogen therapy has been demonstrated to improve sleep in murine models and in in situ studies of postmenopausal women.[143,144]

Catecholamines such as epinephrine are secreted in a circadian fashion and in correlation with the stress response. Sympathetic innervation of the enteric nervous system plays a key role in maintaining tolerance of microbial stimulation within dendritic cells in the gut, having both proinflammatory and inhibitory effects.[145,146]

Gut circadian function can affect cytokine expression through the modulation of ghrelin and leptin. Ghrelin is an intestinally secreted orexigenic hormone that is secreted in response to systemic inflammation and sleep deprivation.[147] Patients with IBD demonstrate a compensatory rise in serum ghrelin levels.[148] Additionally, patients with IBD and poor sleep have increased levels of proinflammatory cytokines including resistin and a decrease in anorexigenic hormone leptin and catabolic hormone adiponectin.[149]

Microbiome Effects

Gut dysbiosis is a known contributor to pathogenesis and exacerbation of IBD. Many environmental factors, such as stress, are associated with thinning of the colonic mucus layer. This enables increased interaction between lumen-associated microbes with the mucosal epithelium and can lead to an increased inflammatory response. Although lumen-associated and mucosal-associated flora are typically different taxa in healthy patients, patients with IBD demonstrate variation in mucosal-associated flora, implying disruption in the protective mucus layer. The binding of microbe-associated molecular patterns (MAMPs) and pathogen-associated molecular patterns (PAMPs) to microbial pattern-recognition receptors associated with the colonic mucosal epithelium subsequently leads to inflammatory cytokine expression and pathogenesis and has been observed in Crohn's disease.

Disease Implications

Dysbiosis, circadian imbalance, and inflammatory cytokine overexpression can contribute to IBD and thereby may present therapeutic targets for disease mitigation. Medications used in IBD, such as TNF-α inhibitors, have been successfully used in other inflammatory conditions, including rheumatoid arthritis and ankylosing spondylitis, with improvement in sleep quality in addition to the primary disease management.[150,151] This effect has been demonstrated in patients with IBD as well, although it is unclear if this improvement is due to successful treatment symptoms during disease flares.[152]

Gastrointestinal Cancer

Circadian Rhythm

Although many of the aforementioned disease states predispose patients to carcinogenesis, altered circadian rhythm may also predispose to gastrointestinal malignancy. This linkage has been found primarily in colorectal cancer (CRC) and pancreatic cancer.[153,154]

CRC has been found to be especially affected by circadian dysrhythmia. A number of studies have linked gut dysbiosis to CRC.[155,156] This linkage is evident in studies of night-shift workers, who are at increased risk of developing CRC.[157] This risk is time dependent, with direct increase in risk by approximately 3.2% for every 5 years spent in night-shift work.[158]

Gut dysbiosis and systemic inflammation are secondary effects of circadian disruption that are related to pathogenesis of CRC; however, circadian disruption can primarily affect pathogenesis.[159,160] Decreased expression of circadian *CLOCK* genes has been found in neoplastic tissue. This change is found across tumor staging and affects metastatic tissue as well.[161]

Although this change can result in carcinogenesis, it may also be a part of the disease process. Circadian *CLOCK* genes can act as tumor suppressors, in that mutations can lead to colon neoplasia.[161,162] Since circadian genes alter normal tissue metabolism, cancerous tissues that alter circadian gene expression can shift into more proliferative pattern.[163,164] This is sometimes accomplished by direct oncogene effect.[162]

Cytokine Expression

Sleep dysfunction can promote GI carcinogenesis. Many cell types, including cancer cells, demonstrate circadian function.[165] Modulation of proliferation of these cell types is directly affected by central circadian genes. Inhibition or mutation of central circadian genes or downstream products, such as period genes, is associated with carcinogenesis.[166] Inflammatory genes, such as TNF-α, can act as tumor suppressors or can promote an inflammatory cascade. Sleep dysfunction greatly increases TNF levels and IL-6 and C-reactive protein levels.[167]

Microbiome Effects

Gut dysbiosis is strongly implicated in the pathogenesis of GI-related cancers, especially CRC.[168] Dietary factors, such as low-fiber and high-fat intake, are associated with dysbiotic changes.[169] Fermentation of dietary fiber into short-chain fatty acids by obligate anaerobes leads to colonic luminal acidification and decreased conversion of primary to secondary bile acids.[170,171] Secondary bile acids are associated with increased oncogene transcription and ROS formation that lead to carcinogenesis.[172] This mirrors changes associated with poor sleep and could serve as a possible mechanism for the increased CRC rate among night-shift workers and those with altered sleep schedules.

Disease Implications

Improving sleep hygiene and optimizing night-shift worker schedules present possible targets for both intervention in and prevention of CRC. Bright light therapy and melatonin have been used to improve sleep quality in patients with cancer.[173] Additionally, there are other potential direct targets for therapy that may be promising, including drugs that modify the clock genes or regulators of clock genes. Several drugs that target central circadian components have been demonstrated to have clinical benefit.[174] There are also regulators of clock genes that are under investigation, modulators of casein kinase and Fbxw7, which alter expression of clock components.[175-177] Both paradigms of new treatment targets offer potential for future enhanced therapeutic regimens.

CLINICAL PEARLS

- Disordered sleep, as well as abnormal timing or intake of food, can alter the composition of GI flora and contribute to disorders of energy storage, metabolism, and inflammation.
- Naps have also been associated with greater esophageal acid exposure time and symptoms as compared with nocturnal sleep.
- Disordered sleep upregulates cytokine expression associated with IBD activation.
- Alteration of circadian gene expression as well as proinflammatory changes in the microbiome promote carcinogenesis.

SUMMARY

The circadian rhythm is an important mediator of daily metabolism and the healthy physiologic state, and this is accomplished through a cyclic variation in gene expression. Alterations in circadian gene expression or separation between the central and gut circadian rhythm, mainly through a disconnect between light-dark cycle and food intake, can lead to various GI disease states, including GERD, BE, functional dyspepsia, ALD and NALD, IBS, IBD, and cancer. These pathologic states may bidirectionally contribute to circadian dysrhythmia perpetuating and likely increasing disease effects. Meaningful targets for therapy for this spectrum of GI disease may be found in restoration to or maintenance of a synchronous circadian rhythm. An expanded use of melatonin for inflammatory diseases associated with sleep is provocative and warrants more focused study.

SELECTED READINGS

Conley S, Jeon S, Lehner V, Proctor DD, Redeker NS. Sleep characteristics and rest–activity rhythms are associated with gastrointestinal symptoms among adults with inflammatory bowel disease. *Dig Dis Sci*. 2020. https://doi.org/10.1007/s10620-020-06213-6.

Fass R. The relationship between gastroesophageal reflux disease and sleep. *Curr Gastroenterol Rep*. 2009;11(3):202–208. https://doi.org/10.1007/s11894-009-0032-4.

Matenchuk BA, Mandhane PJ, Kozyrskyj AL. Sleep, circadian rhythm, and gut microbiota. *Sleep Med Rev*. 2020;53:101340.

Mody R, Bolge SC, Kannan H, Fass R. Effects of gastroesophageal reflux disease on Sleep and Outcomes. *Clin Gastroenterol Hepatol*. 2009;7(9):953–959. https://doi.org/10.1016/j.cgh.2009.04.005.

Oldfield EC, Dong RZ, Johnson DA. Non-alcoholic fatty liver disease and the gut microbiota: exploring the connection article history. *Gastro Open J*. 2015;1(2):30–43. https://doi.org/10.17140/GOJ-1-107.

Orr WC, Fass R, Sundaram S, et al. The effect of sleep on gastrointestinal functioning in common digestive diseases. *Lancet Gastroenterol Hepatol*. 2020;5:616–624.

Parekh PJ, Oldfield Iv EC, Challapallisri V, Ware JC, Johnson DA. Sleep disorders and inflammatory disease activity: Chicken or the egg? *Am J Gastroenterol*. 2015;110(4):484–488. https://doi.org/10.1038/ajg.2014.247.

Rosselot AE, Hong CI, Moore SR. Rhythm and bugs: circadian clocks, gut microbiota, and enteric infections. *Curr Opin Gastroenterol*. 2016;32(1):7–11. https://doi.org/10.1097/MOG.0000000000000227.

Smith RP, Easson C, Lyle SM, et al. Gut microbiome diversity is associated with sleep physiology in humans. *PLoS One*. 2019;14(10). https://doi.org/10.1371/journal.pone.0222394.

Voigt RM, Forsyth CB, Green SJ, et al. Circadian disorganization alters intestinal microbiota. *PLoS One*. 2014;9(5). https://doi.org/10.1371/journal.pone.0097500.

A complete reference list can be found online at ExpertConsult.com.

Psychiatric Disorders

Section 18

Introduction

Chapter 161

Eric A. Nofzinger

This section, entitled Psychiatric Disorders, is a timely collection describing state-of-the-art research related to the relationships between sleep and psychiatric disorders. The work described represents the cumulative integrated knowledge to date from several key developments in science over the past 6 decades.

First, since the 1950s, fueled by seminal findings in the explorations of the nature of sleep, basic science research has led to an incredibly rich understanding of the neural underpinnings of the global states of consciousness defined largely by the electroencephalogram, including waking and non–rapid eye movement (NREM) and rapid eye movement (REM) sleep. As a result of this research, sleep is no longer a mysterious state of being, impervious to scientific study, but now is understood to be a rich tapestry and integration of discrete behavioral states, each with well-defined interactions in neural circuitry that overlap with those involved in the generation and perpetuation of psychiatric disorders.

Second, at the human level, sleep has been shown to play a fundamental role in human behavior, involving interactions between homeostatic, circadian, and cognitive functions, all of which are related to psychiatric disorders.

Third, a clinical field of sleep medicine has evolved that has defined how sleep is disrupted in humans, leading to significant detrimental impacts on function that result in human suffering. Much of this pathology and its manifestations involves how the brain functions either normally or abnormally in psychiatric disorders, a group that is disproportionately recognized in sleep clinics.

Fourth, sleep and psychiatric disorders are associated in several ways. From a sleep disorders perspective, many cases of insomnia will be associated with a psychiatric disorder that may cause the insomnia complaints. From a psychiatric perspective, a large number of psychiatric disorders are associated with disruptions in sleep. These are recognized at both the subjective level and the polysomnographic level. Many of the medications used to treat sleep disturbances overlap with those that treat psychiatric disorders. Many of the interventions used to treat psychiatric disorders have distinct effects on sleep, either subjectively or objectively.

Fifth, a field of cognitive neuroscience has flourished in which the brain is now understood, at its highest level of organization, to have regional brain specificity for particular behaviors and cognitive processes, such as motor behavior, sensory processing, thought, and emotion.

Finally, there have been enormous technical developments in ways to "image" the human brain at both the structural and functional levels, such as magnetic resonance imaging (MRI), positron emission tomography, and functional MRI, making possible the testing of hypotheses at a regional brain level in relation to human behavior, health, and pathology. This section represents an overview of the wisdom generated from these cumulative scientific developments toward the study of sleep and psychiatric disorders.

This section begins with the chapter Emotion and Sleep. Historically, most of the literature on the relationships between sleep and psychiatric disorders had focused on defining sleep in specific psychiatric disorders based on diagnostic criteria. Although interesting observations were found, an emphasis on studying discrete disorders was found to have some limitations when matched with the heterogeneity of psychiatric symptoms in a large population, which often cut across disorders but may be better defined by dimensions of abnormal behavior. The Research Domain Criteria (RDoC) initiative project, launched by the National Institute of Mental Health (NIMH) in 2009, was a response to the growing awareness of these issues. RDoC is a research framework for investigating mental disorders. It integrates many levels of information, from genomics and circuits to behavior and self-report, to explore basic dimensions of functioning that span the full range of human behavior, from normal to abnormal. RDoC is not meant to serve as a diagnostic guide, nor is it intended to replace current diagnostic systems. The goal is to understand the nature of mental health and illness in terms of varying degrees of dysfunction in general psychological/biologic systems. In this spirit the new chapter on the domain of emotion is an attempt to represent research more along the lines of this NIMH initiative.

The chapter on Anxiety Disorders shows the bi-directional relationships between mental disorders and sleep. Effective management of the anxiety disorder relies on an assessment and treatment of underlying sleep disorders, and in the assessment of sleep disorders an assessment and management of the anxiety disorders is required. And in the case of PTSD it is often necessary to screen for and treat any co-morbid mental or physical disorders that may be present.

The chapter on Mood Disorders is an overview of a long history of research in the area of sleep and mood disorders showing how the biology of sleep has been used as a tool to further understand the mechanisms and treatments of mood disorder patients.

The next chapter, Schizophrenia and Sleep, is written in more of the traditional view of a distinct psychiatric disorder, and in the case of schizophrenia (SCZ), which is likely less of a dimensional disorder as described, this view is still appropriate. As the authors describe,

> *"Schizophrenia is thought to reflect an aberrant neurodevelopmental trajectory that evolves into a brain dysconnectivity syndrome, through cumulative risk factors such as migration, urbanicity, childhood social withdrawal or trauma. The pathogenesis of SCZ has yet to be fully established. However, aberrant synaptic activity, structural and functional brain imaging abnormalities, and more recently, altered NREM sleep oscillations have been reported in SCZ patients."*

In the final chapter in this section, Substance Abuse, the relationships between sleep and substance abuse are defined by a state-of-the-art understanding of the changes in neurocircuitry underlying disorders of abuse and their overlaps with the circuitry involved in sleep-wake regulation. Of importance, the roles of sleep and sleep regulation in drug addiction relapse and a role for sleep in treatment of addiction disorders are explained.

Chapter 162

Emotion and Sleep

Louise Beattie; Andrew Gumley

Chapter Highlights

- Emotional health and mental well-being are closely connected to sleep health. Although this is perhaps axiomatic, a better understanding of the nuances of these relationships could open up new routes through which to improve health and well-being and treat psychiatric conditions.
- A burgeoning literature is beginning to disentangle and delineate the relationships between sleep and emotion. Although sleep-emotion research has historically largely employed self-report measures, these are increasingly being used in tandem with experimental, neuroimaging, or physiologic measures and methods, to add value.
- The relationships between sleep and emotion are applicable to the development and maintenance of psychiatric conditions. Key recent models incorporating both sleep and emotion are identified and synthesized, providing an overview as to this landscape and its salient features.
- As sleep and emotion combined have only fairly recently begun to be investigated with modern methodologies, there is much yet to be understood and integrated with cognate fields. To conclude this chapter, salient gaps in current knowledge are highlighted and clinical implications discussed, alongside potential future directions.

INTRODUCTION

Sleep disturbances are common within a range of psychiatric presentations and may predate psychiatric illness and/or exacerbate symptoms. One way in which sleep and psychiatric disorders are connected is via emotion. Emotional dysregulation occurs across psychiatric diagnoses and overlaps with sleep disruption; even outside of a diagnosable disorder, sleep disturbances can be associated with poorer mental health and well-being. As poor sleep can often be successfully treated, sleep interventions have the potential to mitigate or ameliorate psychiatric symptoms and improve well-being. An enhanced understanding of the connections between sleep and emotion could help improve interventions and outcomes within psychiatry, notwithstanding potential benefits to mental health and well-being outside of psychiatric disorders.

Yet although sleep and emotion have long been associated, research is only beginning to disentangle and delineate these relationships with modern methodologies. These have added value over and above more traditional methods, such as (retrospective) self-report, in terms of ascertaining the underlying distal and proximal causes and mechanisms. Indeed, within affective neuroscience fundamental questions, such as how to define and investigate fear, are debated.[1] A more comprehensive understanding of relevant mechanistic processes could then drive better, more efficacious treatments.

First, some key terms and technical language are defined. The term "affect" is used to indicate any subjective feeling or emotion.[2] Emotions are more than subjective experiences; they also involve behavioral and physiologic reactions.[3,4] This difference is not always clearly demarked in the literature.[5] Moods differ from emotions in that they can lack an object, that is, they are less situationally dependent.[6] Emotionality also comprises conceptualizations as to the self and others that may be longstanding, with potential implications for metacognition.

The conceptual relationships between sleep and emotion, and their roles within psychiatric disorders, are the focus of this chapter and these are viewed psychologically. Emotion is primarily considered in terms of its phenomenological experience and associated constructs; pain and fatigue are not included. Although a limited number of biologic pathways are incorporated as appropriate, a detailed account of all potentially relevant biologic factors are beyond the current scope, and there are many potential regions of overlap yet to be fully elucidated. In this chapter sleep is considered broadly, encompassing circadian and homeostatic processes, sleep architecture, sleep disturbances, and sleep disorders. To focus on current understandings, modern methodologies, and emergent trends, this chapter concentrates on review evidence published between 2010 and 2020.

A biomedical database (https://pubmed.ncbi.nlm.nih.gov/) was searched to identify relevant review articles that included transparent and explicit theorizing of sleep-emotion in the form of clear pathways or models. Identified articles included book chapters, narrative reviews, and meta-analyses, and theorizing could be based on an existing framework from a cognate field. It should be noted that the same evidence base could feature across different accounts. From these articles, salient features were identified and synthesized.

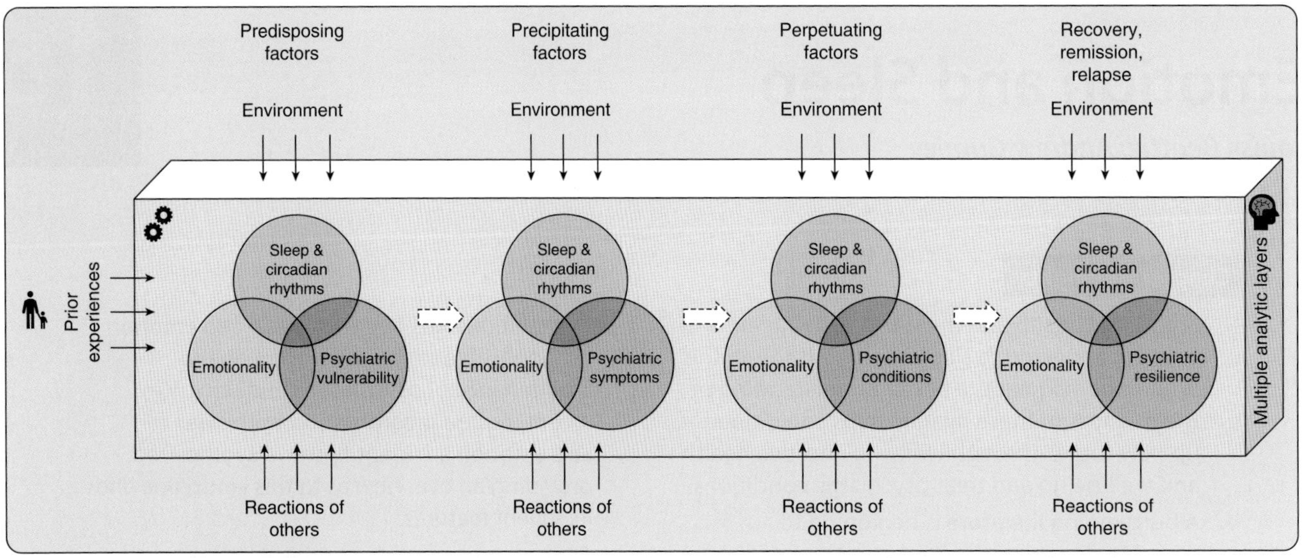

Figure 162.1 An overview of salient processes and factors that are relevant to the sleep, emotionality, and psychiatric symptom associations.

OVERVIEW OF KEY APPROACHES

Although sleep and emotion are connected outside of psychiatric illness, a number of authors aim to understand the sleep-emotion relationship in the context of either a specific disorder, or psychopathology in general. Emotional dysregulation is often mentioned; likewise sleep is often couched in phrases such as sleep disruption, sleep disturbance, sleep deficit, sleep problem, and poor sleep quality. Such terminology can lack clarity and precision. For example, some terms may appear to be equivalent but mask real differences in understandings as to the biologic underpinnings. In contrast, apparently dissimilar phrases may refer to similar processes. Language usage is therefore worthy of cognizance.

A number of authors considered sleep-emotion relationships through the lens of a psychiatric disorder, notably depression, bipolar disorder, posttraumatic stress disorder (PTSD), and insomnia.[7-42] It should be noted that insomnia and nightmare disorder feature within the *Diagnostic and Statistical Manual of Mental Disorders,* fifth edition (DSM-5). Three connections were often made, between (1) PTSD, fear learning, rapid eye movement (REM) sleep and nightmares, as well as (2) bipolar disorder, mood disruption and circadian factors, and 3) depression, hyperarousal, stress reactivity, and insomnia. Other authors considered psychiatric factors transdiagnostically, and presented shared mechanisms which may be relevant across a range of disorders.[30,43-58] Although some authors assessed concurrent mechanistic pathways, others considered the evolution of factors and relationships over time or at a specific timepoint.[11,21,28,40,49,59-61]

Figure 162.1 provides an overview and extension as to how a tripartite balance between sleep, emotionality, and psychiatric conditions (and their mutual relationships) may be related across predisposing, precipitating, and perpetuating stages, as well as in relapse, remission, and recovery. The biologic underpinnings of these can be understood at multiple levels of analysis (e.g., genetics, neurotransmission, functional activity). These relationships are constrained by three factors: (1) prior experiences and learning (including from childhood), (2) environmental factors (e.g., circumstances, setting), and (3) the reactions of others (e.g., supportive, normalizing, or invalidating), and these may have a positive or negative influence on any ultimate psychiatric trajectory.

Putative and candidate mechanisms discussed to date have been collated and are presented in Figure 162.2. Sleep-related factors are broadly grouped under circadian factors, sleep homeostatic, sleep architecture, and sleep medicine. Chronodisruption, sleep reactivity, and insomnia complaints may be especially important concepts, with clinical relevance; sleep architecture alterations (including REM sleep) may become more readily translatable to applied clinical settings in future. Emotionality is arguably a more diffuse area with blurred boundaries across varied brain and body systems. However, negative affect features prominently. A common cluster of mechanisms broadly relates to stress system functioning, hyperarousal, fear learning, and psychosocial events or trauma. Another cluster relates to reward systems and positive affect (and/or anhedonia).

Two pathways are of particular relevance. First, corticolimbic dysregulation is relevant to capacity to cope and adaptive emotional responding, threat perception, and cognitive biases. A seminal article reported a lack of prefrontal-amygdala connectivity and hyperamygdala responsivity to increasingly aversive images following sleep deprivation.[62] This raises the possibility that certain types of sleep disturbances may alter emotional brain processing, suggesting both a neural pathway and a potential treatment mechanism of action. Second, is the potential for (REM) sleep to "recalibrate" the emotional brain of particular relevance to fear processing, nightmares, and PTSD. However, the directionality of emotion effects with REM sleep, at different etiologic timepoints, is equivocal and requires further research before firm conclusions can be drawn.

COMMON STRANDS

It is clear from the accounts of published articles that sleep and emotion are connected at multiple levels in myriad ways.

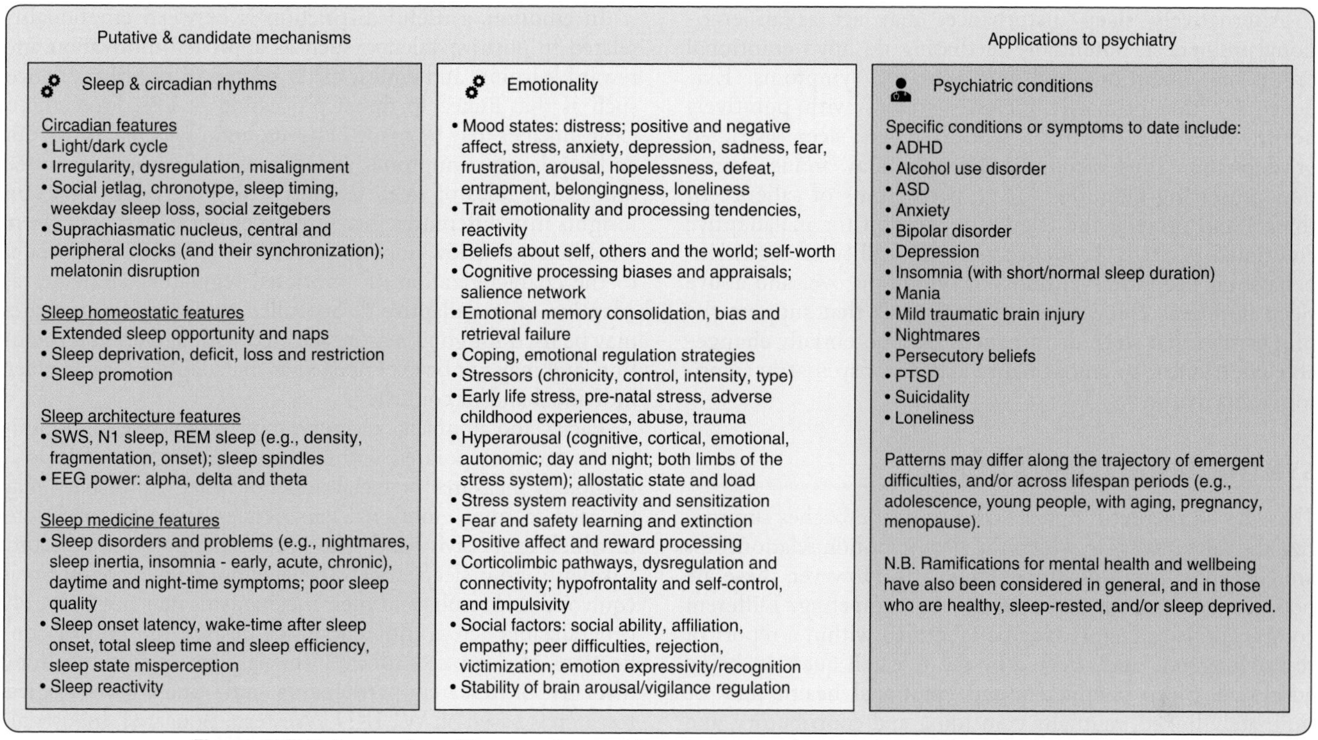

Figure 162.2 An overview of factors and potential mechanisms, and psychiatric conditions, that have been reviewed in the context of the associations between sleep, emotionality, and psychiatric symptoms to date.

These connections encompass 24-hour relationships over the diurnal sleep-wake activity patterns found in humans that are linked to how individuals feel and function throughout the day. These relationships can be considered as a facet of emotional well-being, or within the terms of psychiatric symptoms and disorders, and some common overarching features are apparent across a range of accounts. A role of sleep in emotionality opens up the possibility that cognitive-behavioral sleep interventions may be employed within psychiatric conditions to helpfully address additional (non-sleep) symptoms and facilitate treatments. The contribution of sleep within emotionality and psychiatric etiology is the focus of the next section.

Sleep Disturbances Within Complex Emotion Systems

Various pathways and cycles of relevance to emotionality, and psychiatric conditions, have been detailed. These include factors implicated in sleep, emotionality, and psychiatric symptoms to create nuanced and highly detailed understandings of (overlapping) pathways and mechanisms. Some of these factors may then be assumed to have influences on phenomenology, and this approach may yield important insights of relevance to pharmaceutical interventions and their mechanism(s).

The contributions of factors to the development and maintenance of psychiatric symptoms or disorders have also been a focus. Depictions detailed pathways and cycles that can be autoreinforcing, cascading, and escalating. The influential 3P model developed by Spielman, of the relative influences of **P**redisposing, **P**recipitating, and **P**erpetuating factors over time, has also been employed to frame potential factors.[59] As such, the ultimate development of a psychiatric disorder is influenced by the preceding and subsequent milieu, and a number of accounts feature some form of stressor. Clinical staging models are a potentially useful point of reference in this context, as they describe how different patterns of symptoms and their severity may evolve over time.[63]

Somewhat discrete from these perspectives, other authors have adopted external frameworks of emotional processing. Emotion regulatory processes and mechanisms can be detected across a range of accounts. Cognitive appraisals of events and reactions to them will be influenced by extraneous factors and prior experiences, and some individuals will have a greater likelihood than others of responding in a manner that initiates symptomatic pathways. Related to this is what individuals notice within their environment and its processing stages. As such, emotional regulatory processes will likely influence different stages of emotional responding, at different times, and these will be important to further unpack and incorporate into future models.

Sleep Disturbances as a (Modifiable) Emotional Exacerbator

In terms of how a psychiatric condition develops over time, sleep disturbances may contribute toward emotional alterations, and potentially psychiatric symptoms, by making them worse. Here, sleep is not considered as any nonconsequential epiphenomenon of emotional alterations or psychiatric difficulties. As such, sleep disturbances can be taken as a tipping point, increasing the likelihood of negative emotionality and difficulties with adaptive coping. Sleep disturbances could potentially amplify emotional alterations, acting as a moderator. They may thus ultimately affect divergences in symptom manifestations by providing fuel for maladaptive patterns of emotionality.

Alternatively, sleep disturbances may act as an emotional influencer, potentially mediating de novo emotional processing alterations and/or psychiatric symptoms. Evidence for this primarily includes studies with putatively healthy research participants who have been sleep restricted or deprived. Thus sleep disturbances may induce emotion processing alterations (e.g., perceptions of salience or threat) and provide the trigger or ignition for maladaptive emotional patterns. Evidence as to the utility of cognitive-behavioral sleep interventions for symptoms over and above sleep problems comes from clinical trials that support the proposition that sleep disturbances are a potentially changeable contributor to emotionality and/or a psychiatric symptom exacerbator.[64]

SYNTHESIS AND LIMITATIONS

These broad theoretical perspectives and approaches summarize the salient ways in which the sleep-emotion relationships are conceptualized, sometimes implicitly. However, these are not necessarily mutually exclusive or competing. Different combinations of factors may be identified within a report or research agenda and affected by the research question being addressed. Sleep parameters and emotional health may be intimately linked, mutually coinciding and contributory, and yet separable—with associated implications for the preferred first-line treatments. A number of converging factors influence the reciprocal ways in which sleep affects mental health, including those that individuals shape themselves.

There are some caveats to this synthesis. Other factors relevant to emotionality and insomnia have been identified and could be incorporated into future conceptual models and hypothesis-driven research.[65,66] By necessity, the reviewed articles are limited by the sheer volume of relevant factors that could be discussed at different levels of explanation. Indeed, mechanistic accounts indicate the overlap of sleep and emotional factors at multiple levels and facets of biology and (neuro)cognition, notwithstanding the number of potential psychiatric disorders and associated features in existence. By design, this synthesis emphasizes the common, transdiagnostic features that are represented across a range of accounts. While attempting to be parsimonious, it is important to emphasize that the relative balance and weightings of different factors in specific symptom patternings and trajectories have yet to be fully elucidated. This "lumping" approach has, however, highlighted some common strands, and a more fine-grained diagnostic "splitting" approach may yield additional insights in future.

MECHANISTIC CONSIDERATIONS

While the preceding sections focus on common theoretical themes across accounts, the underlying mechanistic processes warrant further attention. However, it is apparent that although common building blocks can be identified, these can be assembled in different fashions and viewed from different perspectives. The current National Institute of Mental Health (NIMH) Research Domain Criteria (RDoC) framework is worth mentioning in this respect.[67] This is an agenda by NIMH to refocus attention on such building blocks, outside of current diagnostic nosologies, to advance the understanding, etiology, and treatment of psychiatric conditions.

In emotion, a useful distinction is between emotionality related to positive valence, such as approach motivation and reward learning, and emotionality related to negative valence, such as that linked to threat processing or loss. From these, clear linkages may be made between brain systems, behaviors, and psychiatric symptoms, and this could highlight potential differential roles of sleep features. This may yield important insights into differences in symptom profiles, such as between anhedonia and low mood. A further consideration relates to the characterization of emotional regulatory strategies as adaptive or maladaptive.[68] So-called maladaptive strategies may be used for good reason, selected with agency and intention, and may not be experienced as maladaptive for any given individual and/or context.

Facial and nonfacial receptive and productive communication are incorporated within the social domain of RDoC. Although measures of facial and nonfacial expressivity may be used to infer emotional experiences, there are occasions in which expressivity and emotional experiences can discord. Likewise, how sleep affects facial emotional recognition is equivocal and results and their mechanisms may not be highly generalizable across different tasks, despite the known connections of sleep and affect.[69] This is relevant to the cultural diversity of research participants and much psychological research is based on WEIRD (Western, Educated, Industrialized, Rich and Democratic) samples.[70,71]

It is also notable that the cognitive domain of RDoC comprises factors implicated within emotional regulation processes, such as attention, cognitive control, and memory processes, as well as language. There is a large body of literature focused on the different cognitive effects of sleep deprivation and sleep restriction.[72] Furthermore, in the RDoC, arousal, sleep/wakefulness and circadian rhythms are considered as modulators of arousal and regulation. Recent research indicates that arousal comprises three aspects: wakeful, autonomic, and affective.[73] Although research studies consider a small number of factors in great detail, a comprehensive understanding of sleep and emotion, and its roles in psychiatric conditions, will ultimately encompass a panoramic view inclusive of the full brain and body. Identifying which neural systems are involved and how, in who, and when, will be a forthcoming research focus. For example, individual differences in the effects of sleep deprivation are known.[74]

KNOWLEDGE GAPS

The literature summarized in this chapter considers relationships between sleep and emotion, with applicability to psychiatric conditions. However, there is clear scope to enhance the understanding of these relationships in different directions and some clear knowledge gaps are evident. One such potential research direction relates to participant characteristics. Although some studies have focused on children and adolescents, other notable characteristics that could be studied further include gender and sex, race and culture across the lifespan. In addition, studies of induced sleep deprivation typically sample healthy adults who have been carefully screened, and this approach may not entirely mirror naturalistic sleep disturbances or indeed emergent mental illnesses. Similarly, the disambiguation of sleepiness, fatigue, and tiredness; insomnia from poor sleep; and insomnia from an (objective) loss of sleep are worth bearing in mind. For example, induced sleep loss is not necessarily equivalent to self-assessed judgments of inadequate total sleep duration, and self-rated sleep is susceptible to bias in insomnia and time in bed can be elongated. Indeed, induced sleep restriction over a period of days is associated with a disconnect of neurocognitive task performance and sleepiness judgments.[75] To the extent to which sleep loss is present and analogous to induced sleep deprivation, functional brain changes could be linked to characteristic alterations.[72] However, causal inferences are more challenging within naturalistic sleep studies, as is differentiating between potential proximal or more distal etiologic or maintaining mechanisms.

Different fields under the broad umbrella of sleep research have developed somewhat independently of each other, and there is scope for further cross-pollination here. Similarly, theoretical integration with established cognitive models of other psychiatric disorders could offer additional etiologic understandings and opportunity for treatment. Sleep and emotional disturbances could also be relevant to disorders beyond those considered to date, and to add further complexity, diagnostic comorbidities are common and important to consider. For example, even within a single disorder, multiple symptom conceptualizations are possible.[76]

A clear knowledge gap relates to the precise role of REM sleep. It has been proposed that this sleep stage weakens the experienced emotional resonance of emotional memories. REM sleep has also been implicated in enhanced experienced emotionality and PTSD etiology. Prospective and longitudinal research designs are needed to directly test potentially competing hypotheses using a range of assessment measures and participant samples. Research questions could include different parameters of REM sleep, such as its duration, density, onset, and/or fragmentation. Well-defined research participants would also help delineate the role of (subjective) trauma and nightmares, and other putative markers of sleep health and emotional well-being.

FUTURE DIRECTIONS

Technological innovation will play an increasing role in our daily lives going forward. Three ways in which this may exert influences on sleep, emotion, and psychiatric conditions immediately stand out. First is the increasing use of activity monitors and wearables to monitor sleep patterns and health in general. However, the accuracy of some of these models has been queried, and the increased focus and attention to sleep may prove deleterious for the sleep of some individuals. The second relates to social media platforms and other such software to facilitate connectedness between individuals who are physically distant. These may influence mental health and well-being and shape the structure of our daily lives. Third, digital interventions are attractive due to their potential scalability, and may fit readily within a stepped care model of health care provision.[77] A further promise of technology relates to its potential to empower individuals (including those with serious and enduring mental illness) to promote their own health and well-being, and independence and autonomy. For example, through promoting sleep health how individuals feel and function throughout the day may be improved.

CLINICAL PEARLS

- Sleep and emotionality are closely linked and relevant to psychiatric disorders. Sleep and chrono-disturbances, nightmares and insomnia, mood disruption, stress responses and threat perceptions, and mood disorders and PTSD, and are commonly considered. A rapidly expanding literature is increasingly unpacking these relationships.
- The relationships between sleep, emotionality, and psychiatric symptoms are complex. Some authors have honed in on biologic pathways, while others have proposed models as to interrelationships and cycles, taken an etiologic perspective, and/or segmented the processes involved in emotional processing. Ultimately a comprehensive and holistic model will encompass specific features of emotionality, sleep and psychiatric symptoms, and their interrelationships, across their etiologic development, at multiple levels of comprehension.
- Of particular interest is the suggestion that sleep disturbances are a modifiable factor by which quality of life could be enhanced and prognostic outcomes improved. A large body of evidence has demonstrated the effectiveness of cognitive behavioral interventions for poor sleep and insomnia. Sleep disturbances could therefore be an acceptable route by which to instigate treatment.

SUMMARY

Sleep and emotionality are closely connected and relevant to psychiatric conditions. Commonly considered psychiatric symptoms and conditions include depression, bipolar disorder, insomnia, alcohol use disorders, PTSD and nightmares, as well as mental health and well-being in general. Through such a lens, sleep homeostatic and circadian factors, sleep architecture, and sleep disturbances have been considered and associated with emotionality. Emotionality incorporates mood, emotional regulation, trait emotionality, trauma, stress reactivity, fear learning, significance appraisals, and reward processes. These associations have been considered etiologically and in terms of a range of biologic layers. Thematic clusters relate to insomnia, depression, stress reactivity, and hyperarousal; fear learning, REM sleep, nightmares, and PTSD; and bipolar mood disruption, circadian rhythms, and bipolar disorder.

Some authors consider these relationships in terms of complex emotion systems, which can span biologic processes, more (neuro)cognitive models as to relationships, etiologic perspectives, and emotion processing frameworks. Another approach relates to sleep disturbances as a potentially modifiable influencer of emotionality, and this may open up new avenues for treatments. This could occur via moderation or mediation. Of note, are indications that corticolimbic connectivity alterations can be induced with sleep deprivation in healthy research participants; however, it is unclear to what extent this type of sleep disturbance is manifest within naturalistic sleep disturbances, or their equivalence. An important focus of future research relates to clarifying the role of REM sleep in experienced emotionality over time, and its role both in nightmares and PTSD. Technology, including activity monitors, social media platforms, and digital interventions, will play an increasing role in assessing and treating sleep disruption going forward, the effects of which remain to be seen.

SELECTED READINGS

Blake MJ, Trinder JA, Allen NB. Mechanisms underlying the association between insomnia, anxiety, and depression in adolescence: implications for behavioral sleep interventions. *Clin Psychol Rev*. 2018;63:25–40.
Cacioppo JT, Hawkley LC. Perceived social isolation and cognition. *Trends Cogn Sci*. 2009;13(10):447–454.
Colvonen PJ, Straus LD, Acheson D, Gehrman P. A review of the relationship between emotional learning and memory, sleep, and PTSD. *Curr Psychiatry Rep*. 2019;21(1):2.
Freeman D, Garety P. Advances in understanding and treating persecutory delusions: a review. *Soc Psychiatry Psychiatr Epidemiol*. 2014;49(8):1179–1189.
Goldstein AN, Walker MP. The role of sleep in emotional brain function. *Annu Rev Clin Psychol*. 2014;10:679–708.
Gruber R, Cassoff J. The interplay between sleep and emotion regulation: conceptual framework empirical evidence and future directions. *Curr Psychiatry Rep*. 2014;16(11):500.
Harvey AG, Murray G, Chandler RA, Soehner A. Sleep disturbance as transdiagnostic: consideration of neurobiological mechanisms. *Clin Psychol Rev*. 2011;31(2):225–235.
Kahn M, Sheppes G, Sadeh A. Sleep and emotions: bidirectional links and underlying mechanisms. *Int J Psychophysiol*. 2013;89(2):218–228.
Littlewood D, Kyle SD, Pratt D, Peters S, Gooding P. Examining the role of psychological factors in the relationship between sleep problems and suicide. *Clin Psychol Rev*. 2017;54:1–16.
Malhi GS, Kuiper S. Chronobiology of mood disorders. *Acta Psychiatr Scand Suppl*. 2013;(444):2–15.
Palmer CA, Alfano CA. Sleep and emotion regulation: An organizing, integrative review. *Sleep Med Rev*. 2017;31:6–16.
Riemann D, Krone LB, Wulff K, Nissen C. Sleep, insomnia, and depression. *Neuropsychopharmacology*. 2020;45(1):74–89.

A complete reference list can be found online at ExpertConsult.com.

Chapter 163

Anxiety Disorders and Posttraumatic Stress Disorder

Soo-Hee Choi; Murray B. Stein; Andrew D. Krystal; Steven T. Szabo

Chapter Highlights

- Anxiety and trauma-related disorders are associated with complaints of disturbed sleep. This chapter provides a review of the diagnostic criteria, sleep features, and treatment of sleep-related problems in patients with panic disorder, generalized anxiety disorder, social anxiety disorder (social phobia), and posttraumatic stress disorder.
- Abrupt nocturnal awakenings are often encountered in anxiety and trauma-related disorders, such as panic disorder and posttraumatic stress disorder, in which non–rapid eye movement and rapid eye movement sleep abnormalities have been implicated, respectively.
- Treatments that target sleep can improve outcomes in patients with anxiety and trauma-related disorders and will be discussed where possible.

Anxiety and trauma-related disorders are the most common group of mental disorders, affecting more than 18% of the general population in a 1-year period.[1] The National Comorbidity Survey Replication, a large, cross-national epidemiologic survey conducted in 2001 to 2003, found that 28.8% of adults 18 years and older had a diagnosis of an anxiety disorder at some point in their lifetime.[2] Up to one-third of the population experiences insomnia at any given time,[3–5] and insomnia is often comorbid with mental disorders.[3,6] Although insomnia is often a preexisting condition in individuals who experience both insomnia and an anxiety disorder, and some evidence suggests that disturbed sleep is likely a risk factor for the development of anxiety disorders, the most typical pattern is for insomnia to begin concurrent with or after the onset of an anxiety disorder.[3,7–10] Thus onset of an anxiety disorder often heralds the onset of a sleep problem, which suggests that a sizable portion of the burden of insomnia in the general population is associated with—and perhaps even etiologically attributable to—anxiety disorders.

Anxiety disorders are commonly seen in primary care settings, where patient complaints of sleep problems are often prominent.[11] Sleep disturbances are included among the diagnostic features of generalized anxiety disorder (GAD), separation anxiety disorder, and posttraumatic stress disorder (PTSD). Treatments targeted to sleep problems and worry, tension, and other manifestations of anxiety are often similar (e.g., cognitive or behavioral techniques, benzodiazepine medications, relaxation). The antihypertensive prazosin, which in some studies has shown to be a treatment option for nightmares and sleep disturbance in patients with PTSD, can also be added to this set of therapies. Thus it is important to consider the diagnosis and treatment of anxiety disorders when caring for a patient with prominent sleep complaints. The converse is equally true: Attention to sleep problems is integral to the management of patients with anxiety disorders. Whereas sleep dysregulation has been extensively studied in depressive disorders, the polysomnographic (PSG) study of anxiety disorders is less well developed, but given the comorbidity of anxiety disorders and depression there are likely to be some common features. PSG studies of anxiety disorders indicate that there are abnormalities in initiating and maintaining sleep and in sleep-stage distribution. Such studies are one of the primary foci of the material reviewed in this chapter.

There has been relatively little work on the origin of these dysregulations of sleep. However, there are well-documented neurobiologic links between anxiety and sleep dysfunction. This includes circadian gene abnormalities in individuals with anxiety disorders.[12] There is also elevated cortical and peripheral arousal in both anxiety and insomnia patients. In both groups there appears to be activation of arousal systems.[13,14] In anxiety, limbic structures, such as the amygdala and hippocampus, are activated in response to emotion-provoking stimuli. These structures in turn stimulate systems mediating arousal, including lateral hypothalamic hypocretin-orexin neurons, noradrenergic neurons in the locus coeruleus, and serotoninergic neurons in the raphe nuclei, which promote wakefulness.

This chapter provides a review of sleep features in patients with panic disorder, GAD, social anxiety disorder (social phobia), and PTSD. As sleep disturbances related to specific phobias have been seldom investigated, and obsessive-compulsive disorders are now a distinct category apart from anxiety disorders in the *Diagnostic and Statistical Manual of Mental* Disorders, fifth edition (DSM-5), they are not included here. In the cases of PTSD, which has also been moved to a separate chapter in the DSM-5 but nonetheless will be considered

Box 163.1 DSM-5 CRITERIA FOR PANIC DISORDER

Diagnostic Criteria: 300.01 (F41.0)

Recurrent unexpected panic attacks. A panic attack is an abrupt surge of intense fear or intense discomfort that reaches a peak within minutes and during which time four (or more) of the following symptoms occur:

Note: The abrupt surge can occur from a calm state or an anxious state.

- Palpitations, pounding heart, or accelerated heart rate
- Sweating
- Trembling or shaking
- Sensations of shortness of breath or smothering
- Feelings of choking
- Chest pain or discomfort
- Nausea or abdominal distress
- Feeling dizzy, unsteady, lightheaded, or faint
- Chills or heat sensations
- Paresthesias (numbness or tingling sensations)
- Derealization (feelings of unreality) or depersonalization (being detached from oneself)
- Fear of losing control or "going crazy"
- Fear of dying

Note: Culture-specific symptoms (e.g., tinnitus, neck soreness, headache, uncontrollable screaming or crying) may be seen. Such symptoms should not count as one of the four required symptoms.

- At least one of the attacks has been followed by 1 month (or more) of one or more of the following:
  1. Persistent concern or worry about additional panic attacks or their consequences (e.g., losing control, having a heart attack, "going crazy")
  2. A significant maladaptive change in behavior related to the attacks (e.g., behaviors designed to avoid having panic attacks, such as avoidance of exercise or unfamiliar situations)
  3. The disturbance is not attributable to the physiologic effects of a substance (e.g., a drug of abuse, a medication) or another medical condition (e.g., hyperthyroidism, cardiopulmonary disorders).
  4. The disturbance is not better explained by another mental disorder (e.g., the panic attacks do not occur only in response to feared social situations, as in social anxiety disorder; in response to circumscribed phobic objects or situations, as in specific phobia; in response to obsessions, as in obsessive-compulsive disorder; in response to reminders of traumatic events, as in posttraumatic stress disorder; or in response to separation from attachment figures, as in separation anxiety disorder).

DSM-5, *Diagnostic and Statistical Manual of Mental Disorders*, fifth edition.

here, and panic disorder, an additional focus relates to the core paroxysmal events that can manifest in relation to sleep (e.g., nightmares, nocturnal panic attacks). This chapter also reviews current pathophysiologic concepts for sleep disturbances in anxiety and related disorders, and it reviews the types of treatments and their outcomes that target or indirectly influence sleep in these conditions.

PANIC DISORDER

Epidemiology and Clinical Features

Panic disorder has a 12-month general population prevalence of 2% to 3%, is more common in women than men, and has a typical age of onset in late teens or early 20s, although it can start earlier in life.[1,2] Onset is rare in older adulthood.[2] The characteristic feature of panic disorder is recurrent unexpected panic attacks (Box 163.1), which are acute episodes of severe anxiety associated with a wide array of somatic symptoms, such as chest pain, tachycardia, shortness of breath, psychosensory disturbances (i.e., changes in sound or light intensity, alterations in the perception of time, derealization), and lightheadedness. Classic panic attacks reach peak severity quickly and last only seconds to minutes in most cases. Panic attacks are well documented to be able to occur during sleep; in this chapter, the terms *nocturnal panic* and *sleep panic* are synonymous and refer to the same phenomenon.

Panic disorder is diagnosed when a person experiences recurrent unexpected panic attacks (Box 163.2). Some persons experience infrequent panic attacks for years without conspicuous changes in their health. More often, however, panic attacks are complicated by anticipatory anxiety (i.e., apprehension about future attacks) or worry about possible underlying medical disorders (e.g., heart disease). Such concerns, if lasting for 1 month or longer after the panic attack or attacks, satisfy criteria for the diagnosis of panic disorder. Alternatively, behavioral change (e.g., frequent visits to the emergency department, avoidance of places where attacks have occurred in the past) subsequent to the attacks also justifies this diagnosis. Patients also may become frightened of places or situations in which unexpected panic attacks have occurred.

Marked distress in, or the actual avoidance of, places (e.g., bridges, tunnels, airplanes) or situations (e.g., driving, shopping, traveling) in which unexpected panic attacks or panic-like symptoms have occurred in the past is referred to as *agoraphobia*. Although agoraphobia is frequently a consequence of panic disorder, it can also occur independently of panic disorder and is separately diagnosable in DSM-5. When not tied to panic disorder, agoraphobia (i.e., fear and avoidance of particular situations owing to fear of incapacitation or embarrassment) may be a complication of illness and the repercussions thereof, such as vertigo or other forms of physical incapacity.

Sleep Features

At least two-thirds of patients with panic disorder report moderate to severe sleep difficulties, including difficulty initiating and maintaining sleep, nonrestorative sleep, and nocturnal panic attacks.[15–17] Sleep difficulties and sleep deprivation can lead to worsening of anxiety symptoms, including panic attacks, in patients with panic disorder.[18] Most PSG studies have found decreased sleep efficiency and total sleep time and increased sleep-onset latency in panic disorder patients,[19–24] although some studies have not found such disturbances.[20] Because panic disorder and major depression are often comorbid, it is possible that comorbid depression may be partially

Box 163.2 PANIC ATTACK SPECIFIER

Note: Symptoms are presented for the purpose of identifying a panic attack; however, panic attack is not a mental disorder and cannot be coded. Panic attacks can occur in the context of any anxiety disorder, as well as other mental disorders (e.g., depressive disorders, posttraumatic stress disorder, substance use disorders) and some medical conditions (e.g., cardiac, respiratory, vestibular, gastrointestinal). When the presence of a panic attack is identified, it should be noted as a specifier (e.g., "posttraumatic stress disorder with panic attacks"). For panic disorder, the presence of panic attack is contained within the criteria for the disorder, and panic attack is not used as a specifier.

An abrupt surge of intense fear or intense discomfort that reaches a peak within minutes and during which time four (or more) of the following symptoms occur:

Note: The abrupt surge can occur from a calm state or an anxious state.

- Palpitations, pounding heart, or accelerated heart rate
- Sweating
- Trembling or shaking
- Sensations of shortness of breath or smothering
- Feelings of choking
- Chest pain or discomfort
- Nausea or abdominal distress
- Feeling dizzy, unsteady, lightheaded, or faint
- Chills or heat sensations
- Paresthesias (numbness or tingling sensations)
- Derealization (feelings of unreality) or depersonalization (being detached from oneself)
- Fear of losing control or "going crazy"
- Fear of dying

Note: Culture-specific symptoms (e.g., tinnitus, neck soreness, headache, uncontrollable screaming or crying) may be seen. Such symptoms should not count as one of the four required symptoms.

DSM-5, *Diagnostic and Statistical Manual of Mental Disorders*, fifth edition. Modified with permission from the American Psychiatric Association. *Diagnostic and Statistical Manual of Mental Disorders*. 5th ed. American Psychiatric Association Press; 2013. Copyright 2013, American Psychiatric Association.

responsible for sleep disturbances in panic disorder; however, some of these studies have excluded subjects with comorbid depression.[21,23,25] Of those excluding comorbid depression, some still found evidence for sleep disturbance in persons with panic disorder.[21,23]

One type of sleep disturbance reported to occur in panic disorder is isolated sleep paralysis, a transient gross motor paralysis that can occur at sleep onset or offset. Although common in those with narcolepsy, it can also occasionally occur in those without this condition. It appears to arise when the involuntary immobility characteristic of rapid eye movement (REM) sleep intrudes into the waking state. This may relate to brainstem norepinephrine neurons in the locus coeruleus being quiescent in REM sleep and failing to revert to spontaneous pacemaker-like firing activity on waking, which is thought to lead to cortical arousal.[26,27] In addition to being unable to move during isolated sleep paralysis, some patients report anxiety, chest pressure, and other somatic sensations. Isolated sleep paralysis has not only been reported in association with panic disorder, it can also occur in other anxiety and trauma-related disorders, such as PTSD.[28–32] One study investigating the prevalence of isolated sleep paralysis found that the prevalence of isolated sleep paralysis in subjects with a primary diagnosis of panic disorder (20.8%) did not seem differentially higher than that in PTSD (22.2%) or GAD (15.8%).[33]

Several surveys and studies of populations with panic disorder have documented the occurrence of panic attacks emerging from sleep as a not uncommon feature of the disorder. These episodes are often described as being awakened abruptly from sleep, usually with physical symptoms, such as shortness of breath, that also characterize the person's panic attacks in awake states. Sleep panic attack episodes appear to be non–rapid eye movement (NREM) sleep phenomena that occur at the transition between sleep stages N2 and N3 (NREM sleep stages 2 and 3), and thus they are not associated with dream mentation.[19,34,35] Approximately one-half of patients with panic disorder report experiencing sleep panic attacks at some point during the course of their illness.[15,36] Some studies estimate that up to one-third of patients experience recurrent nocturnal panic.[15,16,36,37] There is some evidence to suggest that nocturnal panic attacks are associated with higher suicidality in individuals with panic disorder.[38,39] Individuals with nocturnal panic may also experience more frequent daytime panic attacks and greater somatic symptoms during daytime attacks than individuals with panic disorder without nocturnal panic.[36] Although it has been suggested that nocturnal panic may itself be a marker of more severe panic disorder,[36,40] this has not consistently been found across studies.[37,41,42] Nocturnal panic appears to be associated with states of diminished arousal, such as sleep and relaxation.[15,42–44] Although greater motor activity during sleep, as evidenced by increased epochs of movement time, has been reported with panic disorder, patients might actually move *less* on the nights when they experience sleep panic attacks,[45] leading the authors to suggest that movement during sleep may serve as a temporary protective mechanism against the episodes.

Several authors have suggested that the occurrence of panic attacks during NREM sleep implicates a more endogenous, physiologic (rather than cognitive or attributional) explanatory mechanism. Specific mechanisms that have been proposed include sensitivity to subtle increases in blood carbon dioxide levels,[46] irregular breathing during slow wave sleep,[47] and abnormalities in autonomic activity.[19,20,44] In addition, these symptoms may also be mediated through activation of locus coeruleus activity.[35] Furthermore, sodium lactate administered during sleep was found to be associated with increased cardiac and respiratory reactivity in panic disorder patients relative to control subjects,[48] and pentagastrin administered during sleep resulted in abrupt awakenings accompanied by panic symptoms in patients with panic disorder.[49] These findings have been cited as evidence for a physiologic explanation for nocturnal panic because during sleep the influence of cognitive factors is purportedly less.

However, several studies suggest that cognitive factors also play a role. In an investigation using caffeine administration during sleep, more fully elaborated panic attacks were preceded by a period of lighter sleep before awakening, providing support for a mixture of physiologic and cognitive influences on sleep panic.[50] In another study, participants with recurrent nocturnal panic attacks who were primed to expect intense physiologic changes during sleep, as indicated by an auditory signal, were less likely to awaken with panic symptoms than those for whom such a signal was unexpected, highlighting a role for presleep attributions.[51] Physiologic differences in those with nocturnal panic have also been found to normalize with cognitive behavior therapy (CBT).[52] Based on this evidence, it has been argued that although physiologic differences exist for those with nocturnal panic, they should be seen as a function of panic disorder psychopathology rather than as an explanatory mechanism.[44]

Treatment

The aim of drug treatment is to block panic attacks (waking and nocturnal panic attacks) and to eliminate secondary fears and avoidance activities (e.g., sleep phobias). The removal of exogenous stimulants (e.g., caffeine, amphetamine, catecholamine enhancers) and the correction of maladaptive behavior (e.g., sleep deprivation) that often exacerbate panic disorder should also be an integral part of the drug treatment program. If a thorough medical assessment has not recently been performed, this should be conducted, including, routine thyroid-stimulating hormone measurement to rule out most thyroid problems, before proceeding with specific antianxiety treatments.

Both pharmacologic and psychological interventions are used as treatments for panic disorder and are often used in combination.[53,54] Among several classes of medication that have shown efficacy for symptoms of panic disorder (frequency of panic attacks, anticipatory anxiety, and phobic avoidance), selective serotonin reuptake inhibitors (SSRIs) and serotonin-norepinephrine reuptake inhibitors (SNRIs) are considered first-line treatment for panic disorder.[55] SSRIs approved by the U.S. Food and Drug Administration (FDA) for the treatment of panic disorder include paroxetine, sertraline, and fluoxetine. Initial adverse effects of SSRIs include insomnia and jitteriness, as well as drowsiness, lightheadedness, nausea, and diarrhea, but many of them improve with continued use.[55] Initial activating properties of fluoxetine can especially mimic panic symptoms, resulting in poor tolerability, so clinicians should start with low doses and titrate up slowly. In comparison, paroxetine initially has sedative effects and tends to calm patients, which may lead to greater adherence, but its potential for weight gain should also be considered.[56] The SNRI venlafaxine is also FDA approved for the treatment of panic disorder. Tricyclic antidepressants (e.g., clomipramine and imipramine) and monoamine oxidase inhibitors (e.g., phenelzine and tranylcypromine) are considered to have equal efficacy as SSRIs and SNRIs in the treatment of panic disorder but are used as second-line treatments because of their adverse event profiles, such as dietary restrictions (for monoamine oxidase inhibitors) and anticholinergic side effects (for tricyclic antidepressants).[54,55] High-potency benzodiazepines (alprazolam, extended-release alprazolam, and clonazepam are approved by the FDA for this purpose) have also been widely used to treat panic disorder, although they are recommended as second-line treatment due to risk of dependence.[54] Because of their rapid onset of action, benzodiazepines can be useful as concomitant short-term treatment to reduce or prevent panic attacks, reduce anticipatory anxiety, and alleviate initial adverse effects of the antidepressant (e.g., insomnia, jitteriness).[55] After 4 to 12 weeks, benzodiazepine use can be slowly tapered while the serotonergic medication is continued. Benzodiazepines can be effective for as-needed use when patients are faced with panic attacks or phobic stimuli.[55,56] Although the noradrenergic and specific serotonergic antidepressant mirtazapine has not been extensively studied in anxiety disorders, it may be useful as an adjunctive agent due to its beneficial effect on sleep.[55] Some medications (e.g., propranolol, buspirone, hydroxyzine) used often in the management of other forms of anxiety have been shown to be ineffective in the treatment of panic disorder.[57,58] Although there has been little pharmacologic research on the treatment of sleep disturbances associated with panic disorder, preliminary observations suggest that sleep-panic attacks are responsive to antidepressant-antipanic medications.[59,60]

Research has shown CBT to be at least as beneficial as first-line drug treatments.[61] CBT involves challenging irrational thoughts about panic symptoms and their consequences, the elimination of avoidance behavior, and gradual exposure to feared interoceptive sensations and agoraphobic situations. CBT also has the benefit of yielding long-lasting effects.[61] It is unclear whether standard CBT for panic disorder is beneficial in improving sleep, although one study suggests that combined pharmacologic treatment and CBT was insufficient in eliminating objective and self-reported sleep disturbances.[23] One CBT study included modifications targeted to nocturnal panic, such as psychoeducation about normal physiologic changes during sleep, challenging of catastrophic thoughts about nocturnal panic, interoceptive exposure to relaxation conditions, and sleep hygiene.[52] Compared with waitlist controls, participants who received this intervention fared better on measures of physiologic and self-reported anxiety and sleep quality, including nocturnal panic specifically. There is otherwise little information to guide the specific treatment of patients with panic disorder who have nocturnal panic attacks.[62]

In the absence of empirical data in this regard, it is recommended that patients with significant sleep disturbance, including nocturnal panic attacks, be treated with an antipanic agent or with CBT and that they undergo CBT for insomnia or sleep-targeted pharmacotherapy. Human subjects experiencing panic anxiety have been found to have elevated levels of the peptide hypocretin-orexin in their cerebrospinal fluid compared with subjects not experiencing it.[63] Based on the large body of evidence indicating that hypocretin-orexin activity promotes wakefulness, there is reason to believe that panic anxiety–related sleep disturbance might be mediated by this system.[64] As such, agents that block hypocretin-orexin receptors, which have recently become available in the United States (e.g., suvorexant), may be particularly useful in disorders of sleep associated with a panic anxiety component. Future research is needed to test this hypothesis.

GENERALIZED ANXIETY DISORDER

Epidemiology and Clinical Features

GAD is typified by chronic anxiety and excessive, pervasive worry (Box 163.3). In community surveys, the 12-month prevalence of GAD is approximately 3%,[1] with lifetime rates being higher (≈6%).[2] As is the case for all of the anxiety disorders, the prevalence is higher in women than in men, with GAD showing an approximate 2:1 female-to-male ratio. The natural course of GAD can be characterized as chronic, with few complete remissions, a waxing and waning course of symptoms, and the substantial depressive comorbidity.

GAD, it might be argued, has been poorly named. This has led to a tendency to consider it a generic form of anxiety and to make the diagnosis inappropriately and pervasively. Many anxiety (and depressive) disorders are characterized by chronic

Box 163.3 DSM-5 CRITERIA FOR GENERALIZED ANXIETY DISORDER

Diagnostic Criteria: 300.02 (F41.1)

1. Excessive anxiety and worry (apprehensive expectation), occurring more days than not for at least 6 months about a number of events or activities, such as work or school performance.
2. The individual finds it difficult to control the worry.
3. The anxiety and worry are associated with three (or more) of the following six symptoms (with at least some symptoms having been present for more days than not for the past 6 months):
   Note: Only one item is required in children.
   - Restlessness or feeling keyed up or on edge
   - Being easily fatigued
   - Difficulty concentrating or mind going blank
   - Irritability
   - Muscle tension
   - Sleep disturbance (difficulty falling or staying asleep, or restless, unsatisfying sleep)
4. The anxiety, worry, or physical symptoms cause clinically significant distress or impairment in social, occupational, or other important areas of functioning.
5. The disturbance is not attributable to the physiologic effects of a substance (e.g., a drug of abuse, a medication) or another medical condition (e.g., hyperthyroidism).
6. The disturbance is not better explained by another mental disorder (e.g., anxiety or worry about having panic attacks in panic disorder, negative evaluation in social anxiety disorder [social phobia], contamination or other obsessions in obsessive-compulsive disorder, separation from attachment figures in separation anxiety disorder, reminders of traumatic events in posttraumatic stress disorder, gaining weight in anorexia nervosa, physical complaints in somatic symptom disorder, perceived appearance flaws in body dysmorphic disorder, having a serious illness in illness anxiety disorder, or the content of delusional beliefs in schizophrenia or delusional disorder).

DSM-5, *Diagnostic and Statistical Manual of Mental Disorders*, fifth edition. Modified with permission from the American Psychiatric Association. *Diagnostic and Statistical Manual of Mental Disorders.* 5th ed. American Psychiatric Association Press; 2013. Copyright 2013, American Psychiatric Association.

anxiety and tension; these features alone are therefore insufficient to make this diagnosis. It is the presence of excessive and uncontrollable worry about multiple factors, such as work, health, and the well-being and safety of family members, that defines GAD. Patients with GAD often present to their primary care practitioner, where somatic complaints (e.g., headache, back or shoulder pain due to chronic muscle tension, chronic gastrointestinal distress) might predominate.

Sleep Features

Insomnia and GAD are highly overlapping, frequently comorbid disorders. Sleep disturbance, defined as difficulty initiating or maintaining sleep, or sleep that is restless and unsatisfying, is one of the six features (with a minimum of three needed to establish the diagnosis) associated with chronic worry in the DSM-5 criteria for GAD. Three of the other five features—fatigue, irritability, and difficulty concentrating—are also possible consequences of sleep loss. The core cognitive feature of GAD, excessive worry ("apprehensive expectation"), is commonly implicated in the genesis and maintenance of insomnia problems, in that patients often report their worry as most uncontrollable and bothersome at bedtime, interfering with their ability to fall asleep. In a study of comorbid psychiatric disorders in an insomnia sample, GAD was the most commonly diagnosed anxiety disorder.[65] Conversely, difficulty sleeping has been reported in 56% to 75% of persons with GAD,[66,67] although empirical data are largely lacking on the prevalence of sleep disturbance in GAD samples. One difference between GAD and primary insomnia may be the foci of worry at night; in primary insomnia the focus of worry is typically the insomnia itself, whereas in GAD the worry is focused on areas that are also preoccupations during the day (e.g., career, finances, relationships).

A systematic review reported that objective studies of sleep have found evidence for decreased total sleep time, increased sleep-onset latency, and variations in NREM sleep architecture in individuals with GAD compared to healthy control subjects, whereas the evidence for differences in sleep efficiency and REM parameters is mixed in GAD.[24] Furthermore, the sleep architecture findings in GAD are unremarkable, and the conclusion is that GAD is characterized by a nonspecific sleep-onset and sleep-maintenance insomnia that compromises sleep quality.[68] Of note, these studies provide evidence that GAD can be differentiated from major depression: The classic reduction in REM sleep latency seen in endogenous major depression is usually not seen in nondepressed patients with GAD.[69–71] However, given that most patients with GAD, particularly those encountered in general medical settings, also suffer from major depression, it should be expected that more classic depression-related sleep problems (e.g., early-morning awakening) also will be seen. It is doubtful that differentiation of GAD from other anxiety or depressive disorders can be made on the basis of differences in sleep symptoms or PSG findings.

Treatment

Treatment for this chronic condition is, not surprisingly, often prolonged (i.e., several years). The combined intervention of psychotherapeutic, pharmacotherapeutic, and supportive approaches is considered the most effective treatment for GAD.[56]

Clinical experience suggests that improvement in insomnia parallels the overall benefits associated with pharmacologic treatment of GAD; however, studies often do not report sleep findings in GAD. SSRIs (fluoxetine, sertraline, paroxetine, fluvoxamine, citalopram, and escitalopram) and SNRIs (venlafaxine, desvenlafaxine, duloxetine, milnacipran, and reboxetine) are considered as first-line pharmacotherapies for GAD. Tricyclic antidepressants are also effective; however, their use has largely been supplanted by SSRIs and SNRIs due to adverse event profiles. Benzodiazepines (e.g., alprazolam, clonazepam) are used extensively in the management of GAD, although they are recommended for second-line treatment and short-term use. The available evidence suggests that the antianxiety effects of these compounds persist indefinitely in most cases and are not associated with dosage escalation in the long term.[72] However, a substantial advantage of antidepressants over benzodiazepines is the fact that the former treat comorbid depression, whereas the latter do not. The nonbenzodiazepine anxiolytics buspirone and pregabalin are also considered as second-line treatment for GAD.[73] Buspirone, a 5-hydroxytryptamine 1A (5-HT_{1A}) receptor partial agonist, has efficacy limited to the treatment of GAD.[74] However, it usually takes at least several weeks to reach therapeutic efficacy, and its common side effects include insomnia, dizziness, sweating, and nausea.[55,56,73] One approach is to initiate buspirone concomitant with benzodiazepine and then taper the benzodiazepine use after several weeks, at which point the buspirone should have reached its full therapeutic effects.[56] Pregabalin, a structural analogue of gamma-aminobutyric acid, has been shown to be efficacious for GAD both in acute treatment and prophylaxis from several randomized clinical trials. It has also been reported to alleviate sleep disturbances and depressive symptoms associated with GAD.[55,75]

Clinicians can also consider using other medication classes. Low doses of the atypical antipsychotic quetiapine have been shown to be effective in the treatment of GAD.[76] A randomized-withdrawal, double-blind, placebo-controlled study showed that extended-release quetiapine (50 to 300 mg daily) monotherapy was effective at maintaining improvements in functioning and sleep quality in GAD.[77] However, guidelines recommend quetiapine as a second-line treatment due to metabolic adverse effects.[73,78] Although limited data have suggested the efficacy of the antihistamine hydroxyzine in the treatment of GAD, the long-term efficacy of this agent is unknown.[73,79] One placebo-controlled study found that adding the hypnotic eszopiclone to the SSRI escitalopram was beneficial for both insomnia symptoms and daytime anxiety associated with GAD.[80] However, when this study was repeated with zolpidem CR, improvement with sleep, but not anxiety, symptoms was observed, suggesting that eszopiclone may have direct anxiolytic effects.[81] A recent systematic review and network meta-analysis reported that escitalopram, venlafaxine, and pregabalin were more efficacious than placebo, with relatively good acceptability in the treatment of GAD.[82] Fluoxetine, sertraline, buspirone, mirtazapine (noradrenergic and specific serotonergic antidepressant), and agomelatine (antidepressant acting as an agonist for melatonin MT1 and MT2 receptors and as an antagonist for serotonin 5-HT_{2C} receptors) were also found to be efficacious and well tolerated, but these findings were limited by small sample sizes. Paroxetine, benzodiazepines, and quetiapine were effective but poorly tolerated when compared with placebo.[82]

CBT is highly effective in treating GAD,[83] and such treatments have also been shown to be effective for insomnia complaints.[84] In older adults, in whom benzodiazepines may be relatively contraindicated because of concerns about adverse effects (e.g., falls leading to fractures), psychosocial treatments may be particularly appealing.[85] The potential efficiency of integrated psychotherapeutic interventions that target both excessive generalized worries and worries about sleep warrants further exploration[86]; however, empirical investigation of such treatment approaches is not yet available.

SOCIAL ANXIETY DISORDER (SOCIAL PHOBIA)

Epidemiology and Clinical Features

The term *social anxiety disorder* is synonymous with *social phobia,* and the two terms may be used interchangeably. Social anxiety disorder can be described as excessive fear of being judged negatively, embarrassed, or humiliated in one or more social situations (Box 163.4). Anxiety in social situations can

Box 163.4 DSM-5 CRITERIA FOR SOCIAL ANXIETY DISORDER (SOCIAL PHOBIA)

Diagnostic Criteria: 300.23 (F40.10)

1. Marked fear or anxiety about one or more social situations in which the individual is exposed to possible scrutiny by others. Examples include social interactions (e.g., having a conversation, meeting unfamiliar people), being observed (e.g., eating or drinking), and performing in front of others (e.g., giving a speech).
   Note: In children, the anxiety must occur in peer settings and not just during interactions with adults.
2. The individual fears that he or she will act in a way or show anxiety symptoms that will be negatively evaluated (i.e., will be humiliating or embarrassing; will lead to rejection or offend others).
3. The social situations almost always provoke fear or anxiety.
   Note: In children the fear or anxiety may be expressed by crying, tantrums, freezing, clinging, shrinking, or failing to speak in social situations.
4. The social situations are avoided or endured with intense fear or anxiety.
5. The fear or anxiety is out of proportion to the actual threat posed by the social situation and to the sociocultural context.
6. The fear, anxiety, or avoidance is persistent, typically lasting for 6 months or more.
7. The fear, anxiety, or avoidance causes clinically significant distress or impairment in social, occupational, or other important areas of functioning.
8. The fear, anxiety, or avoidance is not attributable to the physiologic effects of a substance (e.g., a drug of abuse, a medication) or another medical condition.
9. The fear, anxiety, or avoidance is not better explained by the symptoms of another mental disorder, such as panic disorder, body dysmorphic disorder, or autism spectrum disorder.
10. If another medical condition (e.g., Parkinson disease, obesity, disfigurement from burns or injury) is present, the fear, anxiety, or avoidance is clearly unrelated or is excessive.

Specify if:
Performance only: If the fear is restricted to speaking or performing in public.

Specifiers

Individuals with the performance-only type of social anxiety disorder have performance fears that are typically most impairing in their professional lives (e.g., musicians, dancers, performers, athletes) or in roles that require regular public speaking. Performance fears may also manifest in work, school, or academic settings in which regular public presentations are required. Individuals with performance-only social anxiety disorder do not fear or avoid nonperformance social situations.

DSM-5, *Diagnostic and Statistical Manual of Mental Disorders*, fifth edition.

take the form of a panic attack, marked by extreme discomfort and physical symptoms, such as heart racing, shaking, sweating, blushing, and other symptoms. In other cases the symptoms are less acute but last longer, especially in anticipation of or before an upcoming social situation (e.g., worrying for days or weeks ahead of time about having to attend a dinner party).

Overt signs of discomfort (blushing, tremor in voice, sweating, motor tics) that might be apparent to another person are extremely distressing to the social phobic patient. One of these symptoms ("I sweat too much"; "I have the shakes") might be the chief and exclusive complaint of the social phobic patient when seeking treatment from his or her family physician. Public speaking may also be endorsed as a prominent source of anxiety, although further inquiry often reveals social fears and avoidance in many more socially routine situations, such as speaking to small groups, interacting with authority figures, and relating to peers. DSM-5 encourages the use of the specifier "performance-only type" for the subset of individuals whose social fears and anxiety truly are limited to public speaking or other performance situations.

Social anxiety disorder and the associated avoidance can significantly interfere with daily functioning and reduce quality of life.[85] Many patients report that they always have been "shy"; onset of the disorder is in early childhood (i.e., it has "always been there") in approximately half of cases, whereas in the other half it appears to develop de novo in adolescence among those without a background of pathologic shyness. Social anxiety disorder affects slightly more women than men, although men more commonly present to mental health treatment settings for its treatment.

Sleep Features

Complaints of insomnia are not uncommon in patients with social anxiety disorder if the clinician specifically elicits them, although it is rare for a patient with social anxiety disorder to present with sleep disturbances as his or her chief complaint. Anecdotally, persons with social anxiety disorder are somewhat more likely to experience sleep difficulties, particularly increased sleep latency, when experiencing anticipatory anxiety in advance of a highly feared social event (e.g., job interview, oral presentation).

Although no evidence has been found for the presence of objective sleep disturbance in social anxiety disorder, a small body of research indicates a link between subjective sleep problems and social anxiety symptoms.[24] In one study that specifically focused on subjective sleep in patients with social phobia, 60% of participants could be categorized as poor sleepers compared with only 7% of healthy control subjects.[87] Furthermore, self-reported sleep impairment in patients with social anxiety disorder was associated with the symptom severity.[88] Meanwhile, poor sleep quality was shown to diminish the effects of CBT for social anxiety disorder.[89]

The results of PSG are largely normal in social anxiety disorder, with sleep latency and sleep efficiency being similar in patients and healthy control subjects. REM sleep latency, REM sleep distribution, and REM sleep density are also normal in social anxiety disorder.[90] An actigraphy assessment of sleep also showed no differences between adolescents with social anxiety disorder and healthy control adolescents.[91]

Treatment

There is a solid evidence base for managing social anxiety disorder with either pharmacotherapy or CBT.[92] Evidence from previous studies suggests that all SSRIs, venlafaxine, pregabalin, and clonazepam have strong evidence for benefit and are recommended as first-line treatments for social anxiety disorder.[55,93] Although monoamine oxidase inhibitor antidepressants (e.g., phenelzine, moclobemide) are also efficacious for social anxiety disorder, they are used as second-line for refractory cases because of their relatively poor adverse event profiles.[56,93] Other secondary options include mirtazapine and gabapentin, as well as the benzodiazepines bromazepam and alprazolam. Due to negative findings, tricyclic antidepressants, buspirone, and quetiapine are not recommended.[55] Clinical experience suggests that some patients with the performance-only specifier of social anxiety disorder (e.g., public speaking or anxiety limited to other performance situations, such as playing a musical instrument in public) may respond to beta blockers on an as-needed basis, whereas individuals with more generalized, pervasive social anxiety symptoms require regular dosing—to *prevent* the occurrence of symptoms in situations that occur so commonly that as-needed medication cannot be used—with either a benzodiazepine or one of the aforementioned antidepressants.

Individual and group CBT are also effective, and their duration of effects is longer than that for medication treatments.[94–96] A combination of psychosocial and drug therapies may be considered to achieve an optimal response; often, rather than starting CBT and medications together, a stepped approach can be used, starting with one modality and adding the other if needed.[97] Whereas there had been initial excitement about the possibility of speeding or otherwise facilitating the effects of CBT with D-cycloserine for social anxiety disorder,[98] a recent study failed to show benefits of such an approach over CBT alone.

Of interest, poorer pre-CBT sleep quality has been noted as a predictor of poorer response to subsequent CBT, with the concomitant suggestion that sleep problems should be addressed before starting CBT. The impact of successful social anxiety disorder treatment on sleep symptoms has not been ascertained. For transient insomnia symptoms, a short course of hypnotics may be beneficial.

POSTTRAUMATIC STRESS DISORDER

Epidemiology and Clinical Features

PTSD encompasses emotional, cognitive, and behavioral symptoms that persist for more than 1 month after exposure to one or more serious psychological traumatic events.[99] PTSD, previously included within the anxiety disorders, in now included in a separate trauma-related disorders chapter in the DSM-5. PTSD is characterized by the recurrent, unwanted mental and emotional reexperiencing of a previous traumatic event. The trauma is one that would be experienced by almost anyone as profoundly disturbing, usually falling into the category of an event that was life-threatening (e.g., violent attack with physical injury, sexual assault, serious motor vehicle collision) or profoundly and abruptly life-altering (e.g., sudden death of a loved one from accidental or unanticipated medical causes). Traumatic experiences that yield PTSD, such as military combat or domestic violence (i.e., intimate partner abuse), often occur as repeated episodes and not single events.

After exposure to severe traumatic experiences, it is the norm to experience brief (lasting several days) periods of anxiety, recurrent thinking about the event, and insomnia. In cases in which these symptoms persist more than 3 days and cause functional impairment, accompanied by prominent feelings of unreality or memory problems (i.e., dissociative symptoms), a diagnosis of acute stress disorder may be appropriate. In most such cases the symptoms wane over the ensuing weeks, but when they do not, which is the pattern in 10% to 30% of cases, depending on the nature and severity of the traumatic event, and the symptoms interfere with functioning or cause great distress, a diagnosis of PTSD may be applied. To qualify for a PTSD diagnosis, characteristic symptoms must be noted in four domains: reexperiencing symptoms (e.g., nightmares or daytime intrusive thoughts or images, including flashbacks), avoidance of trauma reminders, negative cognitions and mood, and hyperarousal symptoms (e.g., insomnia or increased startle response) (Box 163.5).

Lifetime prevalence of PTSD is reported to be as high as 7% to 8%, with a 12-month prevalence in the range of 2% to 3%.[1,2] PTSD is approximately twice as prevalent in women as men in the general population. Common sources of PTSD in men (although increasingly in women) are military combat and physical assault; in women, intimate partner violence and violent injury, often associated with sexual assault, are common sources. Like many other anxiety and related disorders, PTSD is often encountered comorbid with major depression, both in general population samples and in clinical settings.

Sleep complaints are virtually ubiquitous in patients with PTSD.[100] Patients sometimes report not having slept well for decades, with these reports corroborated by their bed partners. Extreme hypervigilance, sometimes bordering on paranoia, but evidently linked to habits learned during combat experiences, may take the form of a combat veteran with PTSD spending several hours each evening "patrolling" the perimeter of his home to ensure that it is protected from intruders. Nightmares, often accompanied by vivid recall on wakening, are commonplace, as is extreme motor activity, according to companions' reports. It is not uncommon to encounter patients who have tried numerous over-the-counter and prescription medications to help with their sleep, to no avail. Many patients also have alcohol abuse problems, which can complicate the clinical picture and make determining the nature of the sleep disorder even more difficult. In some cases, other risk factors for disturbed sleep, such as obstructive sleep apnea (OSA), are present, making an informed evaluation by a sleep expert, with a particular focus on possible sleep-disordered breathing, of considerable value.

Individuals suffering with PTSD are afflicted with hyperactivity of the norepinephrine system during waking and sleep.[101,102] Exaggerated noradrenergic signaling is associated with sleep fragmentation and nightmares, which are common in PTSD.[103] Preclinical work has implicated changes in the amygdala, which leads to activation of the locus coeruleus through corticotropin-releasing hormone receptors as a key mechanism mediating hyperarousal, hypervigilance, and sleep disturbances in PTSD.[104] These considerations support the use of agents that enhance serotonin tone, such as most of the antidepressants, because this inhibits locus coeruleus norepinephrine neurons and is also thought to inhibit amygdala activity.[105–107] They also suggest the use of alpha-adrenergic antagonists, such as prazosin, which block locus coeruleus outputs that have hyperarousing effects (see later).

Sleep Features

Previous studies of subjective and objective sleep have demonstrated the presence of sleep disturbance in PTSD.[24] Subjective sleep complaints in PTSD often include the two sleep symptoms listed in the diagnostic criteria: nightmares, which are viewed as reexperiencing phenomena, and insomnia (i.e., impairment in initiating and maintaining sleep). A survey of male Vietnam War veterans with PTSD confirms that insomnia complaints are very common symptoms of PTSD, although nightmares are more specific to the disorder.[108] In a community survey, PTSD was often (in ≈70% of cases) associated with sleep complaints, including insomnia and other types of sleep disturbance, such as violent or injurious activities during sleep, sleeptalking, or hypnagogic and hypnopompic hallucinations.[109] These rates seem very high and need to be replicated, but they do point to the usefulness of a thorough sleep assessment in conjunction with diagnostic assessment of PTSD and other trauma-related disorders. Heightened arousal during sleep has also been reported by patients with PTSD, including excessive motor activity and fearful awakenings with somatic anxiety symptoms.[110,111] Isolated sleep paralysis is also associated with PTSD and with trauma exposure even in the absence of PTSD, although its specificity to PTSD relative to other anxiety disorders is unclear (see also Panic Disorder, earlier).[108,112,113] Furthermore, subjective sleep impairment has been shown to be linked to PTSD symptom severity, and baseline sleep problems may contribute to the development of PTSD after the traumatic event. These findings suggest that subjective sleep disturbances may play a role in the development, maintenance, and treatment of PTSD and indicate a particular need to address sleep problems in the treatment of PTSD.[24]

Subjective reports of sleep disturbance are often discrepant with the findings of PSG. Findings on objective sleep disturbances in PTSD are inconsistent. A systematic review has shown particular disturbances in sleep efficiency and sleep maintenance in PTSD, as well as shorter total sleep time and increased sleep-onset latency. Furthermore, several studies indicate various alterations in REM parameters in individuals with PTSD compared to healthy controls subjects.[24] However, the findings from studies comparing individuals with PTSD to trauma-exposed control subjects are mixed, although individuals with PTSD report more sleep disturbance than trauma-exposed control subjects. These preclude any conclusion on the role of sleep disturbance in trauma exposure. Future research is needed to better understand the role of perceived sleep disturbance in PTSD.[24]

However, the authors of a meta-analysis of 20 PSG studies found that overall, PTSD patients had increased stage 1 sleep, decreased slow wave sleep, and increased frequency of eye movements during REM sleep periods (REM sleep density).[114] Moreover, they found that several moderating variables—age, sex, comorbid depression, and substance use—affected the relationship between PTSD and sleep disturbances. A possible factor that can contribute to the lack of significant findings in individual studies, as raised in a review,[115] is that some persons with PTSD (and other psychiatric conditions, such as primary insomnia) might sleep better in the laboratory environment because of the perception that it is a "safe" setting, thus making evidence of objective sleep

Box 163.5 DSM-5 CRITERIA FOR POSTTRAUMATIC STRESS DISORDER

1. In posttraumatic stress disorder, the person has been exposed to actual or threatened death, serious injury, or sexual violence in one (or more) of the following ways:
   - Directly experiencing the traumatic event(s).
   - Witnessing, in person, the event(s) as it occurred to others.
   - Learning that the traumatic event(s) occurred to a close family member or close friend. In cases of actual or threatened death of a family member or friend, the event(s) must have been violent or accidental.
   - Experiencing repeated or extreme exposure to aversive details of the traumatic event(s) (e.g., first responders collecting human remains; police officers repeatedly exposed to details of child abuse).

   Note: This criterion does not apply to exposure through electronic media, television, movies, or pictures, unless this exposure is work-related.
2. The person has one (or more) of the following intrusion symptoms associated with the traumatic event(s), beginning after the traumatic event(s) occurred:
   - Recurrent, involuntary, and intrusive distressing memories of the traumatic event(s).

   Note: In children older than 6 years, repetitive play may occur in which themes or aspects of the traumatic event(s) are expressed.
   - Recurrent distressing dreams in which the content and/or affect of the dream are related to the traumatic event(s).

   Note: In children, there may be frightening dreams without recognizable content.
   - Dissociative reactions (e.g., flashbacks) in which the individual feels or acts as if the traumatic event(s) were recurring. (Such reactions may occur on a continuum, with the most extreme expression being a complete loss of awareness of present surroundings.)

   Note: In children, trauma-specific reenactment may occur in play.
   - Intense or prolonged psychological distress at exposure to internal or external cues that symbolize or resemble an aspect of the traumatic event(s).
   - Marked physiological reactions to internal or external cues that symbolize or resemble an aspect of the traumatic event(s).
3. The person persistently avoids stimuli associated with the trauma and has numbing of general responsiveness (not present before the trauma), as indicated by three (or more) of the following:
   - Avoidance of or efforts to avoid distressing memories, thoughts, or feelings about or closely associated with the traumatic event(s).
   - Avoidance of or efforts to avoid external reminders (people, places, conversations, activities, objects, situations) that arouse distressing memories, thoughts, or feelings about or closely associated with the traumatic event(s).
4. The person has negative alterations in cognitions and mood associated with the traumatic event(s), beginning or worsening after the traumatic event(s) occurred, as evidenced by two (or more) of the following:
   - Inability to remember an important aspect of the traumatic event(s) (typically due to dissociative amnesia and not to other factors such as head injury, alcohol, or drugs).
   - Persistent and exaggerated negative beliefs or expectations about oneself, others, or the world (e.g., "I am bad," "No one can be trusted," "The world is completely dangerous," "My whole nervous system is permanently ruined").
   - Persistent, distorted cognitions about the cause or consequences of the traumatic event(s) that lead the individual to blame himself/herself or others.
   - Persistent negative emotional state (e.g., fear, horror, anger, guilt, or shame).
   - Markedly diminished interest or participation in significant activities.
   - Feelings of detachment or estrangement from others.
   - Persistent inability to experience positive emotions (e.g., inability to experience happiness, satisfaction, or loving feelings).
5. The person has marked alterations in arousal and reactivity associated with the traumatic event(s), beginning or worsening after the traumatic event(s) occurred, as evidenced by two (or more) of the following:
   - Irritable behavior and angry outbursts (with little or no provocation) typically expressed as verbal or physical aggression toward people or objects.
   - Reckless or self-destructive behavior.
   - Hypervigilance.
   - Exaggerated startle response.
   - Problems with concentration.
   - Sleep disturbance (e.g., difficulty falling or staying asleep or restless sleep).
6. Duration of the symptoms is longer than 1 month.
7. The disturbance causes clinically significant distress or impairment in social, occupational, or other important areas of functioning.
8. The disturbance is not attributable to the physiological effects of a substance (e.g., medication, alcohol) or another medical condition.

Specify whether the person has **dissociative symptoms** of depersonalization or derealization: The individual's symptoms meet the criteria for posttraumatic stress disorder, and in addition, in response to the stressor, the individual experiences persistent or recurrent symptoms of either of the following:
- **Depersonalization:** Persistent or recurrent experiences of feeling detached from, and as if one were an outside observer of, one's mental processes or body (e.g., feeling as though one were in a dream; feeling a sense of unreality of self or body or of time moving slowly).
- **Derealization:** Persistent or recurrent experiences of unreality of surroundings (e.g., the world around the individual is experienced as unreal, dreamlike, distant, or distorted).

Note: To use this subtype, the dissociative symptoms must not be attributable to the physiological effects of a substance (e.g., blackouts, behavior during alcohol intoxication) or another medical condition (e.g., complex partial seizures).

Specify if the symptoms have **delayed expression**: If the full diagnostic criteria are not met until at least 6 months after the event (although the onset and expression of some symptoms may be immediate).

DSM-5, *Diagnostic and Statistical Manual of Mental Disorders*, fifth edition.
Modified with permission from the American Psychiatric Association. *Diagnostic and Statistical Manual of Mental Disorders.* 5th ed. American Psychiatric Association Press; 2013.

disturbance less discernible. Other sleep disturbances objectively observed in some studies of PTSD include movement abnormalities and sleep-disordered breathing,[116–119] although one report found reduced movement time during sleep in patients with PTSD compared with control subjects.[120] The prominence of nightmares in PTSD, which most typically arise from REM sleep, has focused interest on REM sleep variables. Previous findings suggest that sleep in PTSD is characterized by REM sleep abnormalities and increased noradrenergic activity during REM sleep that may contribute to the development of PTSD.[121–123] For a detailed discussion, see Chapter 61.

Treatment

As noted previously, thorough assessment of sleep complaints is integral to the overall management of PTSD. Although the absolute rates of sleep disturbances such as OSA or parasomnias in patients with PTSD remain to be determined, clinical experience suggests that these are commonly encountered in this clinical population and should be seriously considered in most cases. In cases in which the suspicion is high, patients should be referred to a sleep physician for assessment. Patients with PTSD are also likely to have comorbid mental disorders, such as major depression, and other anxiety disorders, such as panic disorder. Treatment therefore needs to encompass these clinical entities, as well as comorbid alcohol or other substance abuse or dependence, which are also often encountered in patients with PTSD.

There is a strong and growing evidence base for particular pharmacologic and psychological treatments for PTSD. Pharmacologic treatments with support for efficacy in the treatment of PTSD include the SSRIs (sertraline and paroxetine are approved by the FDA for this indication, and strong evidence also exists for fluoxetine), the SNRI venlafaxine, and, to a lesser extent in terms of strength of evidence, tricyclic antidepressants imipramine and amitriptyline.[124–126] SSRIs are known to be effective in reducing severity of the full range of PTSD symptom clusters and improving symptoms unique to PTSD, not just symptoms attributable to depression.[56] However, none of these antidepressants has been demonstrated to have therapeutic effects on sleep in PTSD patients.

The alpha$_1$-adrenergic receptor antagonist prazosin has been investigated in the treatment of nightmares or sleep disturbance associated with PTSD. Six randomized placebo-controlled clinical trials involving veterans, active-duty service members, and civilian participants showed moderate to large effects of prazosin in alleviating PTSD-related nightmares and sleep disturbance and in improving overall clinical status.[127–132] However, in contrast to previous trials, a recent randomized placebo-controlled study with a much larger sample of military veterans with long-standing and chronic PTSD reported negative results of prazosin for distressing dreams or sleep quality.[133] This recent study stands in contrast to a previous study in active duty military personnel, where prazosin robustly outperformed placebo.[131] These divergent data suggest that there may be a role for the use of prazosin in some patients with PTSD, such as those with more recent onset or with marked abnormalities in autonomic nervous system activity.[133] Although supporting evidence of efficacy is weak, low doses of atypical antipsychotics may also be considered clinically for patients with unique secondary clinical manifestations of PTSD, such as extreme agitation, violence, or hypervigilance, in those who have not responded to treatment with other medications. Also, in some studies, adjunctive risperidone yielded improvements in sleep quality in veterans with chronic military-related PTSD.[134] Due to insufficient evidence of efficacy, anticonvulsants are typically not recommended for use in PTSD.[125,135] Evidence for the effectiveness of benzodiazepines in the treatment of PTSD is lacking, despite their continued use in clinical practice.[124,135] Benzodiazepines are to be avoided in individuals with PTSD due to their theoretical risks of interference with extinction learning.[125]

More than in any of the other anxiety and related disorders, the use of evidence-based psychotherapy is critical either as primary or adjunctive treatment for PTSD.[136–138] There is accumulating evidence that psychosocial treatments that focus on sleep aspects of PTSD, such as nightmares, can have strong therapeutic effects across the full spectrum of PTSD symptoms.[139,140] Few studies have used psychotherapeutic interventions to treat PTSD and examined their effects on sleep quality. In one small study, 5-week treatment using eye movement desensitization reprocessing therapy improved sleep consolidation and reduced wake time after sleep onset.[141] Another study reported the safe and effective use of CBT for insomnia in patients with comorbid insomnia and PTSD, and improved sleep was reported to facilitate entry into exposure therapy for PTSD.[142] Additional studies that incorporate psychotherapeutic techniques with medication strategies are needed to formally evaluate their benefits.[143]

CLINICAL PEARLS

- Effective treatment of anxiety and trauma-related disorders includes assessing and managing sleep disturbances.
- Clinical experience suggests that education and encouragement about behavioral factors that disturb sleep can be helpful as an adjunct to treatment in nearly all cases.
- If sleep disturbances persist after the successful treatment of the primary anxiety disorder, the patient should be reevaluated for other possible medical or sleep disorders.
- In the case of posttraumatic stress disorder, where there is reason to suspect that comorbid medical, psychiatric, and sleep disorders (e.g., alcohol or substance abuse, obstructive sleep apnea) are especially common, a high index of suspicion should be maintained, and a thorough medical and sleep evaluation may be considered early in the course of assessment and treatment.

SUMMARY

Anxiety and trauma-related disorders are extremely common and often associated with disturbances of sleep. These disturbances vary across the anxiety disorders and related conditions and consist of difficulty falling asleep, difficulty staying asleep, early-morning awakening, and nightmares. Patients with GAD can have increased sleep latency and significant reductions in total sleep time and variations in NREM sleep architecture. Clinical experience suggests these disturbances are tightly linked to pathologic worry, and improvement in insomnia closely parallels the successful amelioration of core anxiety symptoms. PTSD and, to a lesser extent, panic disorder are often characterized by recurrent frightening arousals from sleep. Sleep complaints are so prevalent in PTSD that it could be argued that every assessment of sleep disturbance should include taking a thorough history of traumatic events. Conversely, every assessment of a patient with PTSD should include a thorough assessment of sleep symptoms and additional investigation and follow-up as warranted. Available evidence suggests that the predominant sleep pathologic process in PTSD relates to REM sleep, whereas that in nocturnal panic relates to NREM sleep. However, reports of high rates of sleep-related breathing disorders and parasomnias in PTSD suggest that a more complex etiology for sleep disturbance might exist in some individual patients with this disorder. Although these sleep disturbances were long believed to be symptoms of the anxiety disorders, the available evidence increasingly suggests that the relationship of sleep problems and anxiety disorders may be more complex and in some cases bidirectional. This evidence strongly speaks for the need to target treatment specifically to the sleep problems in patients with anxiety-related conditions. Some, but clearly not all, evidence-based pharmacologic and psychosocial treatments for anxiety disorders seem to improve sleep as part of their spectrum of therapeutic effects. However, sleep outcomes are not often reported in clinical trials, leaving some uncertainty as to a given treatment's efficacy for sleep disturbances. In some instances, preferred medications with good evidence of efficacy for anxiety disorders (e.g., SSRIs) can actually worsen sleep while they ameliorate daytime and phobic anxiety. As a result, a specific sleep-targeted therapy is needed in many patients with anxiety difficulties. There is a growing set of evidence-based pharmacologic and behavioral interventions available for treating the sleep problems of anxiety patients. Addressing the sleep problems of patients with anxiety and trauma-related disorders using these interventions promises to improve outcomes.

SELECTED READINGS

American Psychiatric Association. Practice Guideline for the Treatment of Patients with Panic Disorder; 2009. Available at https://www.psychiatry.org/psychiatrists/practice/clinical-practice-guidelines.

Cox RC, Olatunji BO. A systematic review of sleep disturbance in anxiety and related disorders. *J Anxiety Disord.* 2016;37:104–129.

Cusack K, Jonas DE, Forneris CA, Wines C, Sonis J, Middleton JC, et al. Psychological treatments for adults with posttraumatic stress disorder: a systematic review and meta-analysis. *Clin Psychol Rev.* 2016;43:128–141.

Holder N, Woods A, Neylan TC, et al. Trends in medication prescribing in patients with PTSD from 2009 to 2018: a National Veterans Administration Study. *J Clin Psychiatry.* 2021;82(3):20m13522. https://doi.org/10.4088/JCP.20m13522. Published 2021 May 4.

Ipser JC, Stein DJ. Evidence-based pharmacotherapy of post-traumatic stress disorder (PTSD). *Int J of Neuropsychopharmacol.* 2012;15:825–840.

Monti JM, Monti D. Sleep disturbance in generalized anxiety disorder and its treatment. *Sleep Med Rev.* 2000;4(3):263–276.

Moore BA, Pujol L, Waltman S, Shearer DS. Management of post-traumatic stress disorder in Veterans and Military Service Members: a review of pharmacologic and psychotherapeutic interventions since 2016. *Curr Psychiatry Rep.* 2021;23(2):9. https://doi.org/10.1007/s11920-020-01220-w. Published 2021 Jan 6.

Raskind MA, Peskind ER, Chow B, et al. Trial of prazosin for post-traumatic stress disorder in military veterans. *N Engl J Med.* 2018;378(6):507–517.

Richards A, Kanady JC, Neylan TC. Sleep disturbance in PTSD and other anxiety-related disorders: an updated review of clinical features, physiological characteristics, and psychological and neurobiological mechanisms. *Neuropsychopharmacology.* 2020;45(1):55–73.

Stein MB. Attending to anxiety disorders in primary care. *J Clin Psychiatry.* 2003;64:35–39.

VA/DOD Clinical Practice Guidelines for the Management of Posttraumatic Stress Disorder and Acute Stress Reaction. 2017. Available at. https://www.healthquality.va.gov/guidelines/MH/ptsd/.

A complete reference list can be found online at ExpertConsult.com.

Chapter 164

Affective Disorders

Christoph Nissen; Elisabeth Hertenstein

Chapter Highlights

- Comorbidity with insomnia is highly frequent in patients with affective disorders. Insomnia represents a predictor for the de novo onset of an affective disorder, and insomnia persisting after remission is a predictor for relapse.
- Targeted treatment with cognitive behavioral therapy for insomnia is a window into treatment and, potentially, the prevention of affective disorders.
- The close link between sleep and affective disorders is of high scientific interest. Recent work suggest that homeostatic changes in synaptic plasticity and chronobiologic factors seem to be important mechanisms in the development, maintenance, and treatment of affective disorders.
- Noninvasive brain stimulation is a promising tool for basic research and treatment. For instance, sleep slow waves can be modulated through closed-loop auditory stimulation during sleep, with potential effects on mood, cognition, and underlying mechanisms, such as alterations in synaptic plasticity.

INTRODUCTION

Affective disorders are a group of disorders characterized by marked changes in mood and energy, mostly taking an episodic course. The human affective state can change between two poles, depression and mania. Depression is defined as a state of low mood, anhedonia, loss of energy, fatigue, reduced psychomotor drive, insomnia, mental rumination, self-doubt, guilt, and suicidality lasting for 2 weeks or longer. Mania describes a state of elevated mood, irritability, increased psychomotor drive, distractibility, logorrhea, elevated sexual drive, reduced sleep need, and delusions of grandiosity lasting for 1 week or longer. To be diagnosed as depression or mania, the affective state has to be clearly different from a person's usual state and not an adequate reaction to a present situation.

Of interest, whereas depression and mania represent two opposing poles in almost every domain, they are both characterized by reduced sleep duration. Most patients in a depressive episode suffer from disturbed sleep continuity and daytime tiredness (insomnia). Hypersomnia can, in some patients, also be a symptom of depression, but is much less prevalent. In a manic episode, sleep duration is often shortened over an extended period, but patients typically do not feel tired. On the contrary, they often report being full of energy with only a few hours of sleep per night.

Depressive episodes are divided into three degrees of severity: mild, moderate, and severe. Whereas patients with mild depression are still able to cope with everyday life with some difficulties, patients with severe depression are unable to cope with everyday life. Severe episodes can occur with or without psychotic symptoms. Frequent psychotic symptoms within a severe depressive episode comprise delusions regarding impoverishment or guilt and hypochondriacal delusions. Psychotic symptoms typical for schizophrenia, such as bizarre delusions or intense hallucinations, are not characteristic for a depressive episode. Whereas single depressive episodes can occur, more than half of the patients who go through one depressive episode will have another episode. Major depressive disorder, characterized by recurrent episodes of depression and full remission between episodes, is the most frequent affective disorder. A minority of patients suffer from chronic depression. Dysthymia is a chronic state of mild depression lasting for at least 2 years. Double depression is a chronic form of depression with dysthymia plus recurrent episodes of major depression, or, in other words, major depressive episodes without full remission between episodes. In seasonal affective disorder, depressive episodes occur only (primarily) during wintertime and might come along with atypical symptoms, such as increased appetite, weight gain, and hypersomnia.

Besides the described unipolar affective disorders (with depressive episodes only), there is bipolar disorder with both depressive and manic episodes. Bipolar disorder is less frequent and often associated with a more severely reduced level of functioning compared to unipolar depression. Manic episodes are divided into two degrees of severity: hypomania (less severe) and mania. Bipolar disorder with only hypomanic without full manic episodes are referred to as bipolar II disorder. Disorders with a chronic cycling between hypomanic and depressive phases, without clear remission, are referred to as cyclothymia. Patients with cyclothymia are typically less severely affected than patients with bipolar disorder and are mostly able to cope with everyday life.

SLEEP AS A WINDOW TO THE BRAIN

Polysomnography

In ancient Greek medicine, melancholia was one of the four temperaments, characterized by prolonged sadness, irritability, agitation, and sleeplessness. Melancholia is, in some aspects, a predecessor of depressive disorder. Strikingly, sleeplessness is already mentioned as one of the core symptoms of melancholia in one of the earliest systematic descriptions in Hippocrates' "Aphorisms," written in the 4th century before Christ.

In later times, researchers made efforts to use sleep as a "window to the brain," with the idea that specific patterns of sleep disturbances correspond to specific mental disorders. For instance, Emil Kraepelin, a prominent German psychiatrist of the 19th century, distinguished two types of affective disorders: endogenous and neurotic. Endogenous depression was assumed to result from biologic causes and included syndromes that would nowadays be classified as depression with somatic syndrome (*International Classification of Sleep Disorders,* 10th edition [ICD-10]) or melancholic features (*Diagnostic and Statistical Manual of Mental Disorders,* fifth edition [DSM-5]). Particularly, disturbances of sleep continuity in the form of early-morning awakening were considered to be indicative of endogenous depression. Neurotic (or reactive) depression, on the other hand, was assumed to have psychosocial conflicts as a cause. Difficulties falling asleep were considered typical for patients with neurotic depression. However, the allocation of specific patterns of sleep difficulties to specific mental disorders is not scientifically tenable. Rather, work over the past decades has shown that various forms of sleep continuity difficulties (sleep-onset problems, sleep-maintenance problems, and early-morning awakening) are highly prevalent across diagnostic entities of mental disorders[1] and do not reliably distinguish between disorders. In addition, insomnia subtypes are variable within one person over time.[2]

One step further, sleep architecture was researched using polysomnography (PSG), with the aim of illuminating the nature of and ways to treat affective disorders. One prominent hypothesis is the rapid eye movement (REM) sleep disinhibition hypothesis, postulating that disinhibition of REM sleep (shortened REM sleep latency, high REM density, and increased REM sleep duration, indicative of high REM sleep pressure) represents a biomarker of major depression. In a cholinergic REM sleep induction test, REM sleep is experimentally induced with a cholinergic substance. This effect is pronounced in patients with acute depression, compared to healthy control subjects, patients with other psychiatric diagnoses, and patients with remitted depression.[3] Effective antidepressant agents, such as selective serotonin reuptake inhibitors, venlafaxine, or clomipramine, suppress REM sleep and prolong REM sleep latency. Researchers thus hoped that PSG could be used to inform differential diagnosis, predict the course of the disorder, and serve as a predictor for response to a specific drug. This hope, however, has largely been dissipated. REM sleep disinhibition is not specific for depression but is also frequently observed in patients with other mental disorders, including schizophrenia, borderline personality disorder, and substance dependency.[1] In addition, REM sleep latency decreases markedly with age, a confounding factor that may have biased earlier results.[4] Besides limitations in scientific validity, an implementation of PSG for diagnostic purposes is hindered by low practicability because PSG would be only valid after a drug washout period of 14 days or longer. The effect of medications used in depression on sleep architecture have also been evaluated with PSG.[5]

Brain Circuits

Both insomnia and depression are characterized by a 24-hour hyperactivity in the ascending reticular arousal system (ARAS).[6,7] This finding has been associated with a cognitive, emotional, and physical hyperarousal that is characteristic for both disorders and manifests in rumination, anxiety, and difficulties falling asleep both during the day and at night.[8] Patients with depression, in contrast to patients with insomnia only, also present with a hyperactivity of the emotional system, including the amygdala and the ventral anterior cingulate cortex during wake and during REM sleep.[9] Patients with insomnia, in contrast, show heightened amygdala reactivity to sleep-related stimuli but no general hyperactivation of the emotional system.[10] Clinically, this could manifest in core symptoms of depression, such as low mood, anxiety, and low self-esteem, that are absent in primary insomnia. As a third finding, patients with depression suffer from reduced executive functions ("pseudodementia") that could be linked to a hypoactivity of the dorsal executive system.[11] Such profound cognitive deficits are absent in patients with insomnia.[12] Reduced cognitive function is associated with reduced slow wave sleep.[13]

Taken together, neuroimaging results can, in part, explain the similarities and close relationship between insomnia and depression because both are characterized by a hyperarousal of the ARAS. The findings might also explain differences between the two disorders because only patients with depression exhibit profound alterations in the emotional and cognitive system. If sleep disturbances that are typical for depression, namely impaired sleep continuity, increased REM sleep pressure, and reduced slow wave sleep, could be manipulated, this may allow for improvements in three core domains of depressive symptomatology, namely hyperarousal, mood, and cognitive deficits. Noninvasive brain stimulation methods currently under research may have the potential to achieve such targeted alterations of sleep continuity and sleep architecture.[14]

Synaptic Plasticity

Following the two process model, sleep is regulated through a homeostatic and a circadian process.[15] Homeostatic sleep pressure gradually builds up with increasing duration of wakefulness. This means that a sufficiently long period of wakefulness is required to allow sleep onset and sleep continuity. In accordance, sleep during the day will lead to a decrease in sleep pressure and impede night sleep. The circadian process is regulated by the nucleus suprachiasmaticus, the "master clock" of the brain, and determines the optimal time window for sleep. Partly independent of the homeostatic process, humans (in the absence of a circadian rhythm disorder or behaviorally induced circadian shifts) will sleep better during the night compared to the day. In addition, individual chronotypes determine whether someone is a "night owl" or a "morning lark." Besides endogenous rhythms, exogenous circadian zeitgebers, such as light exposure, physical activity, and food consumption, influence the circadian system and sleep. The two processes interact to determine an individual, adaptive window for sleep.

The synaptic homeostasis hypothesis, put forward by Giulio Tononi and Chiara Cirelli, posits that a critical function of slow wave sleep is to regulate synaptic plasticity.[16] According to the hypothesis, net synaptic strength increases during wakefulness because synaptic connections are strengthened and newly built during the daytime. Continued increase in synaptic strength, however, leads to saturation, a deterioration of the signal-to-noise ratio, and decreased information processing. The hypothesis posits that, during slow wave sleep,

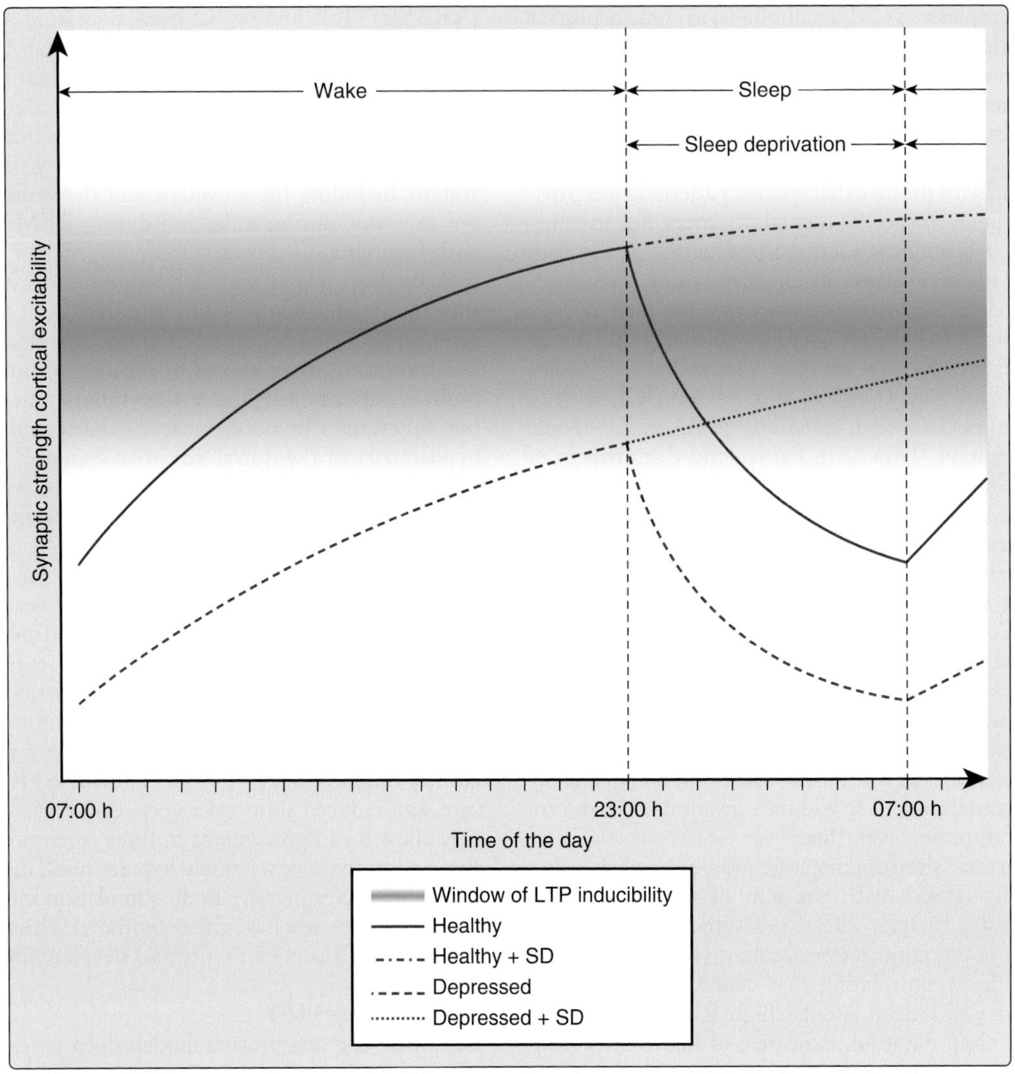

Figure 164.1 Synaptic plasticity model of therapeutic sleep deprivation in MDD. The figure depicts the proposed interplay between the time course of net synaptic strength (homeostatic plasticity; *solid* and *dotted lines*) and the inducibility of synaptic LTP (associative plasticity; *green window*). Wakefulness leads to an upscaling and sleep to a downscaling of net synaptic strength. Whereas in healthy control subjects SD eventually leads to synaptic saturation and deficient LTP inducibility, SD compensates for attenuated synaptic strength and evokes an antidepressant effect in patients with MDD via a shift into a window of more favorable LTP inducibility. LTP, Long-term potentiation; SD, sleep deprivation. (From Wolf E, Kuhn M, Normann C, et al. Synaptic plasticity model of therapeutic sleep deprivation in major depression. *Sleep Med Rev.* 2016;30:53–62.)

net synaptic strength decreases and synaptic homeostasis is restored, leading to a restoration of information processing.

In patients with unipolar depression, however, the opposite has been observed: A night without sleep is followed by a significant improvement of symptoms in 50% to 60% of patients.[17] After a nap, depressive symptoms reoccur in the majority of those who initially responded to sleep deprivation.[18] At first sight, this finding seems to be at odds with the synaptic homeostasis hypothesis. However, our research group has recently proposed a model integrating the synaptic homeostasis hypothesis of sleep-wake regulation and a synaptic plasticity hypothesis of depression to explain the therapeutic response to sleep deprivation.[19] Following the synaptic plasticity hypothesis of depression, decreased neuroplasticity is a critical pathomechanism of depression.[20] Indices of synaptic plasticity decrease with chronic stress in animals and with several episodes of major depressive disorder in humans.[21] Antidepressant drugs enhance neuroplasticity, ideally when combined with increased behavioral activity that can be boosted through psychotherapy.[20] The idea is that antidepressant drugs promote a window of plasticity, which needs to be shaped through meaningful interaction with the environment. As outlined earlier, prolonged wakefulness boosts synaptic plasticity similar to antidepressant drugs and psychotherapy. Given that patients with major depression appear to be in a state of reduced synaptic plasticity, extended periods of wakefulness might be necessary to shift the level of plasticity into an adaptive window.[19] In turn, sleep decreases synaptic strength and might thus eliminate the antidepressant effect of therapeutic sleep deprivation (Figure 164.1).

Although sleep deprivation could, in principle, be a valid alternative treatment, specifically for patients for whom pharmacologic treatment is not feasible, for instance, due to comorbidities, side effects, or pregnancy, it is not very commonly applied in clinical practice. A major reason is that 1 night of sleep deprivation has only short-term effects until the next sleep episode, and total sleep deprivation over an extended period of time is not feasible. However, for psychotherapy, a response to sleep deprivation can be used to demonstrate that improvement is possible, which may help patients to overcome feelings of hopelessness. Predictors for a response to sleep deprivation include a short REM sleep latency and a melancholic subtype of depression with worsening of symptoms in the morning, early-morning awakening, anhedonia, psychomotor inhibition, and loss of appetite and libido.[22] At present, the topic is mainly of scientific interest because it might inform further developments of rapid mechanisms of response and relapse, potentially related to basic synaptic processes in the brain.

Chronobiology

Following the two-process model of sleep-wake regulation described earlier, sleep is governed by a homeostatic sleep drive and circadian rhythm. Modifications of sleep behavior, such as total or partial sleep deprivation, often have effects on both systems. From a scientific perspective, it is often difficult to disentangle homeostatic and circadian effects. Whereas the effects of sleep deprivation in patients with depression might be explained through changes in synaptic plasticity, they can also be explained through circadian mechanisms. Likewise, sleep-related symptoms of depression, such as the typical morning low, can be explained through sleep homeostasis and the circadian rhythm. Other symptoms of mood disorders more clearly indicate an involvement of the circadian system, such as seasonal effects and strictly periodic mood switches in rapid cycling disorders. Compelling evidence suggests that internal circadian markers of patients with affective disorders, such as sleep, core body temperature, and cortisol, are out of synchrony with external cues.[23] Shifting the sleep phase forward by 6 hours, without changing total sleep duration, has short-term antidepressant effects comparable to those of total sleep deprivation.[24] The mechanism behind this effect could be a reset of the disregulated circadian system. To this date, the exact mechanisms behind the imposing effects of sleep deprivation and sleep phase advance are not sufficiently understood. With a combination of total sleep deprivation, sleep phase advance, and bright light therapy, effects can be sustained for a considerably longer period of time,[25] indicating that several mechanisms may act in concert.

Clinically, the efficacy of chronotherapy has primarily been shown for patients with seasonal affective disorder ("winter depression"). Regular circadian zeitgebers, such as bright light in the early morning, decrease of light intensity in the evening, regular meals and physical activity, and targeted administration of melatonin, are well researched and effective in seasonal affective disorder.[26,27]

TREATING INSOMNIA TO IMPROVE DEPRESSION CARE

Almost all patients with severe depression suffer from sleep continuity problems, and about 25% fulfil the criteria for insomnia disorder.[28] More severe sleep disturbances are associated with more severe depression, greater functional impairment, lower treatment response rates, and increased suicide risk.[28,29] Sleep disturbances can also be shown in PSG, where patients with depression exhibit disturbed sleep continuity, decreased deep sleep, and heightened REM pressure.[1] Most patients report a combination of sleep-onset problems and sleep-maintenance difficulties.[30] As insomnia (or hypersomnia) is listed as a symptom of depression according to the ICD-10[31] or DSM-5 criteria, the high prevalence of insomnia in this patient group has not received much attention in the past. It was assumed that the sleep problem is merely a symptom and would remit with successful treatment of the underlying affective disorder.

However, recent research has demonstrated that patients with insomnia (without a mental disorder) have an increased risk for the de novo onset of depression.[32,33] Insomnia often persists after remission of a depressive episode and increases the risk of relapse into depression.[34] Patients who remit from depression without persistent sleep disturbances have a higher probability to regain their premorbid functional level.[35] Taking these more recent insights into account, in the DSM-5, insomnia disorder can be diagnosed as a comorbidity of major depressive disorder.[36]

Cognitive behavioral therapy for insomnia (CBT-I) is effective not only in patients with "primary" insomnia but also in those with depression as a comorbidity.[37] CBT-I does not only improve sleep but also has small effects on depressive symptoms in patients with both disorders.[38] This effect is shown in Figure 164.2. Following international guidelines for the treatment of insomnia, CBT-I is recommended as a first-line treatment also for those with comorbid mental disorders.[39,40]

Clinically, the relevance of insomnia is best evaluated through the course of the illness. If insomnia is also present in phases when depression is remitted, it can be diagnosed as a comorbid disorder and treated with CBT-I. In addition, if insomnia is severe and associated with a high level of suffering, CBT-I may also be considered in patients who suffer from insomnia only within a depressive episode. In CBT for depression, patients learn strategies, such as increasing their level of activity and decreasing time in bed, that may already have a small effect on sleep. However, when insomnia is severe, these strategies are mostly not sufficient. CBT-I, a treatment package consisting of bedtime restriction, relaxation, and cognitive therapy, is feasible and effective for the improvement of insomnia in patients with comorbidity.[37]

Because insomnia is a predictor for the de novo onset of depression, CBT-I may also be effective for the prevention of affective disorders.[41] In a pilot trial, Harvey and colleagues[42] found evidence that CBT-I, administered in interepisodic patients with bipolar disorder and insomnia, has a phase prophylactic effect. Whereas only 14% of patients treated with CBT-I (n = 30) relapsed into a depressive or manic episode in the follow-up time frame of 6 months, the percentage was 42% in the control group that received only psychoeducation (n = 28). Besides, CBT-I effectively reduced insomnia in this patient group. In depression, no such preventive effect could be shown.[43] However, in this trial the relapse rate into depression was generally low in both groups in the follow-up time frame of 6 months (4% in both groups taken together). Whereas guidelines recommend disorder-specific treatment of insomnia in patients with affective disorders, with the aim of reducing insomnia severity, the efficacy of CBT-I as a preventive treatment still needs to be more thoroughly evaluated in larger randomized controlled trials with sufficiently long follow-up intervals.

If CBT-I is not available or not effective, guidelines recommend pharmacologic treatment of insomnia in patients with affective disorders.[40] In this patient group, sedating antidepressants, such as doxepine, trimipramine, trazodone, and mirtazapine, are often given in a low dose before bedtime to improve sleep. In contrast to benzodiazepines and benzodiazepine receptor agonists, sedating antidepressants have no relevant risk of tolerance and dependency. However, long-term studies on sedating antidepressants for the treatment of insomnia have not been conducted. Most antidepressants have marked effects on sleep continuity, sleep depth, and REM pressure. Those are summarized in Table 164.1.

Benzodiazepines and benzodiazepine receptor agonists cannot be recommended for widespread long-term use, first, because of the risk of tolerance and dependency, and second, because of their detrimental effects on synaptic plasticity.[44]

OUTLOOK

Noninvasive brain stimulation (NIBS) is a promising tool for basic research and treatment. In contrast to deep brain stimulation, where a stimulator is implanted into the brain during surgery, NIBS techniques work with electric current, sounds, or magnetic impulses in a noninvasive way.

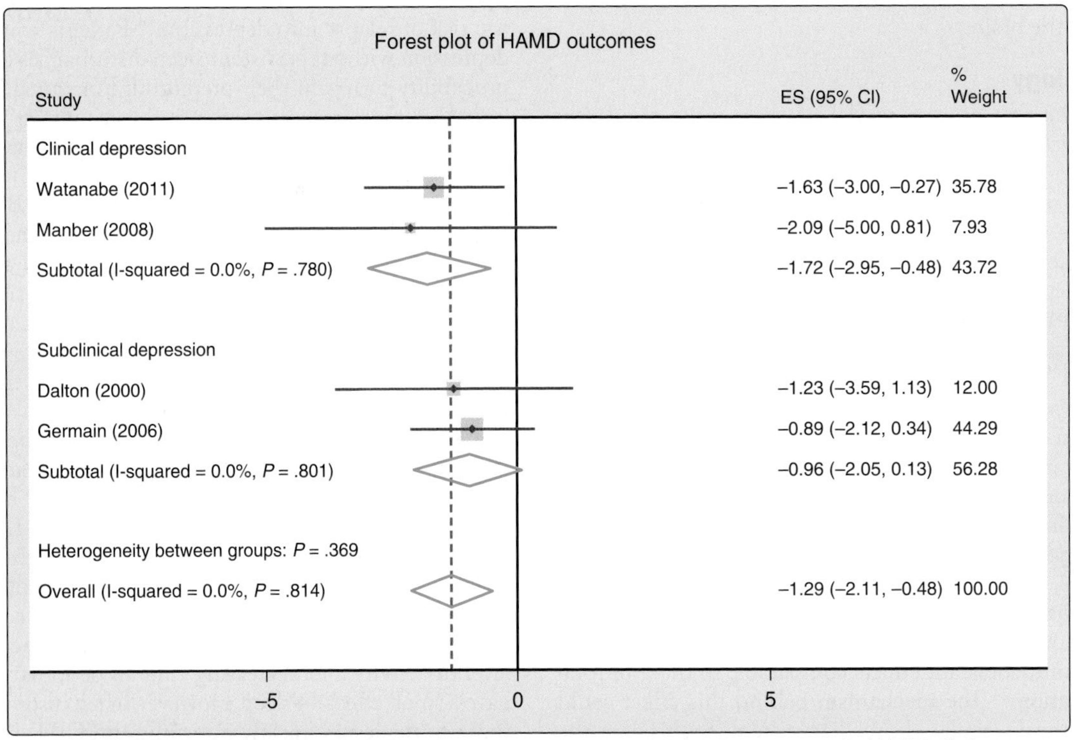

Figure 164.2 Forest plot showing effect of insomnia treatment on Hamilton Depression scale (HAMD). CI, Confidence interval; ES, effect size. (From Gebara MA, Siripong N, DiNapoli EA, et al. Effect of insomnia treatments on depression: a systematic review and meta-analysis. *Depress Anxiety.* 2018;35(8):717–31.)

Table 164.1 Impact of Antidepressants on PSG-Recorded Sleep[14]

Types of Antidepressants[a]	Sleep Continuity	Slow Wave Sleep	REM Sleep
Nonspecific Monoamine Reuptake Inhibitors (TCAs)			
Amitriptyline	↑	⇌SWS %	↓REM %, ↑REM latency
Doxepin	↑	⇌SWS %	↓REM %, ↑REM latency
Clomipramine	↑	↑	↓REM %
Desipramine	↑	↑	↓REM %
Nortriptyline	?	↑	↓REM %
Imipramine	?	?	↓REM %
Selective Serotonin Reuptake Inhibitors (SSRIs)			
Citalopram	?	?	↓
Fluvoxamine	↓	?	↓
Fluoxetine	↓	?	↓
Paroxetine	↓	?	↓

Continued

Table 164.1 Impact of Antidepressants on PSG-Recorded Sleep[14]—cont'd

Types of Antidepressants[a]	Sleep Continuity	Slow Wave Sleep	REM Sleep
Noradrenaline Reuptake Inhibitors (NRIs)			
Maprotiline	↑	?	↓
Viloxazine	↓	↓SWS %	↓
Norepinephrine-Dopamine Reuptake Inhibitors (NDRIs)			
Bupropion	?	↓	↑
Serotonin-Noradrenaline Reuptake Inhibitors (SNRIs)			
Venlafaxine	↓	?	↓REM %
Monoamine Oxidase Inhibitors (MAOIs)			
Moclobemide	↓	?	↓REM %
Phenelzine	↓	?	↓REM %
Other Mechanisms of Action			
Trimipramine	↑	⇌SWS %	⇌REM %
Mirtazapine	↑	⇌SWS %	⇌REM %
Trazodon	↑	↑SWS %	⇌REM % (↑ to ↓, individual studies)

REM, Rapid eye movement; SWS, sleep wave sleep; TCAs, tricyclic antidepressants.
From Riemann D, Krone LB, Wulff K, Nissen C. Sleep, insomnia, and depression. *Neuropsychopharmacology.* 2020;45(1):74–89.

Acoustic stimulation has been used successfully to modulate sleep slow waves. Guided by simultaneous electroencephalogram monitoring, tones are applied at the peak of a slow wave with the aim of boosting slow wave sleep and spindles.[14] The sounds are adapted to the individual hearing threshold of the participant so that they are processed by the brain but not consciously heard by the participant. In young adults this stimulation appears to have the potential to boost memory consolidation.[45] Slow waves can also be disrupted through acoustic stimulation.[46] Because total or partial sleep deprivation is an effective but, for long-term application, impractical treatment, disruption of slow waves through acoustic stimulation may be an alternative that is less burdensome for the patient and can be applied several nights in a row. However, the efficacy and safety of acoustic slow wave boosting and disruption has not yet been tested for the treatment of patients with affective disorders in clinical studies.

A new and interesting treatment option for depression is the anesthetic substance ketamine. Administered in a subanesthetic dosage, one application of ketamine has a rapid antidepressant effect.[47] It is assumed that its mechanism of action in patients with depression is a boost of synaptic plasticity.[47] Although ketamine itself is not sleep related, it is interesting in the context of sleep and affective disorders because its assumed mechanism of action might be similar to that of sleep deprivation.

CLINICAL PEARL

Insomnia with sleep-onset or sleep-maintenance difficulties is highly prevalent in patients with affective disorders. Around one-quarter fulfil the criteria for comorbid insomnia disorder. Insomnia needs disorder-specific treatment. The first-line treatment is cognitive behavioral therapy for insomnia, a treatment program that is also effective in patients with insomnia and mental or somatic comorbidity.

SUMMARY

Recurrent changes in mood, psychomotor drive, and cognition, most familiar in the form of major depression and mania, characterize affective disorders. In a long line of research, sleep has been investigated as a "window to the brain," with the idea that specific sleep disturbances correspond to specific forms of affective disorders and inform diagnosis and treatment. However, initial hopes have not been fulfilled; rather, sleep disturbances appear to represent transdiagnostic alterations. An interesting link between sleep and affective disorders is that sleep deprivation can trigger a switch out of a depressive episode and, in patients with bipolar disorder, a switch into mania. Changes in neuroplasticity may represent a critical underlying mechanism. All affective disorders have high comorbidity rates with sleep disorders, mostly insomnia. Novel work suggests that CBT-I might have the potential to prevent the de novo onset or improve the course of an affective disorder.

SELECTED READINGS

Ahmad A, Anderson KN, Watson S. Sleep and Circadian Rhythm Disorder in Bipolar Affective Disorder. *Curr Top Behav Neurosci.* 2021;48:133–147. https://doi.org/10.1007/7854_2020_150

Baglioni C, Nanovska S, Regen W, Spiegelhalder K, Feige B, Nissen C, et al. Sleep and mental disorders: a meta-analysis of polysomnographic research. *Psychol Bull.* 2016;142(9):969–990.

Berger M, Riemann D, Höchli D, Spiegel R. The cholinergic rapid eye movement sleep induction test with RS-86. State or trait marker of depression? *Arch Gen Psychiatry.* 1989;46(5):421–428.

Geiger-Brown JM, Rogers VE, Liu W, Ludeman EM, Downton KD, Diaz-Abad M. Cognitive behavioral therapy in persons with comorbid insomnia: a meta-analysis. *Sleep Med Rev.* 2015;23:54–67.

Geoffroy PA, Hoertel N, Etain B, et al. Insomnia and hypersomnia in major depressive episode: prevalence, sociodemographic characteristics and psychiatric comorbidity in a population-based study. *J Affect Disord.* 2018;226:132–141.

Hertenstein E, Feige B, Gmeiner T, et al. Insomnia as a predictor of mental disorders: a systematic review and meta-analysis. *Sleep Med Rev.* 2019;43:96–105.

Nofzinger EA, Buysse DJ, Germain A, et al. Alterations in regional cerebral glucose metabolism across waking and non-rapid eye movement sleep in depression. *Arch Gen Psychiatry*. 2005;62(4):387–396.
O'Brien EM, Chelminski I, Young D, Dalrymple K, Hrabosky J, Zimmerman M. Severe insomnia is associated with more severe presentation and greater functional deficits in depression. *J Psychiatr Res*. 2011;45(8):1101–1105.
Riemann D, Krone LB, Wulff K, Nissen C. Sleep, insomnia, and depression. *Neuropsychopharmacology*. 2020;45(1):74–89.
Wehr TA, Wirz-Justice A, Goodwin FK, Duncan W, Gillin JC. Phase advance of the circadian sleep-wake cycle as an antidepressant. *Science (New York)*. 1979;206(4419):710–713.
Wirz-Justice A, Benedetti F, Berger M, et al. Chronotherapeutics (light and wake therapy) in affective disorders. *Psychol Med*. 2005;35(7):939–944.
Wolf E, Kuhn M, Normann C, Mainberger F, Maier JG, Maywald S, et al. Synaptic plasticity model of therapeutic sleep deprivation in major depression. *Sleep Med Rev*. 2016;30:53–62.

A complete reference list can be found online at ExpertConsult.com.

Chapter 165

Schizophrenia and Sleep

Armando D'Agostino; Anna Castelnovo; Fabio Ferrarelli

Chapter Highlights

- Schizophrenia (SCZ) is arguably the most intensely researched psychiatric disorder due to the disruptiveness of its clinical presentation and its profound impact on the lives of affected individuals, their relatives, and the responding health system. Although typical symptoms include delusions, hallucinations, and diminished emotional expression, sleep disturbances have been reported extensively since the earliest descriptions of the disorder. Sleep disturbances can often be observed before the onset of psychosis in clinical high-risk individuals and are known to precede the reexacerbation of symptoms throughout the patient's life span. Chronically disturbed sleep can also negatively impact social function, mood, cognition, and quality of life in patients with SCZ.
- SCZ is thought to reflect an aberrant neurodevelopmental trajectory that evolves into a brain dysconnectivity syndrome through cumulative risk factors, such as migration, urbanicity, childhood social withdrawal, or trauma. The pathogenesis of SCZ has yet to be fully established. However, aberrant synaptic activity, structural and functional brain imaging abnormalities, and, more recently, altered non–rapid eye movement sleep oscillations have been reported in SCZ patients.
- Despite a recent growth of interest toward the study of sleep in SCZ, clinical sleep-related complaints are seldom addressed in those patients. Insomnia, sleep-related breathing disorders, and circadian sleep-wake rhythm disorders are highly prevalent in this population and should be adequately assessed and treated. Central disorders of hypersomnolence and sleep-related movement disorders also can be observed and tend to be more commonly associated to exposure to antipsychotic medications.
- This chapter emphasizes the major pathogenetic mechanisms that are currently thought to underlie SCZ and relates them to emerging evidence from sleep research. It also provides practical recommendations to address the complex interplay between wake- and sleep-related symptoms in everyday clinical practice. Finally, it highlights future directions of inquiry to further establish the relationship between sleep abnormalities and SCZ.

The phenomenologic similarity between dreams and psychosis fueled the interest of most pioneers in modern psychopathology. Eugen Bleuler, who coined the term *schizophrenia* (SCZ) from two ancient Greek words indicating a split (σχίζω, *skhízō*) mind (φρήν, *phrḗn*), wrote that "the modalities of thinking of schizophrenic subjects are very similar to dreaming" and that "most of the characteristics of schizophrenic thinking (particularly delusional thinking) are explained by the differences between the dreaming and the wakefulness way of thinking."[1] In the second half of the 20th century, several polysomnographic (PSG) studies based on such observations failed to identify neurophysiologic signatures of dream sleep intrusions into wakefulness to explain psychosis. However, those studies began revealing several sleep abnormalities and have built a solid foundation for the study of sleep in patients diagnosed with SCZ.

EPIDEMIOLOGY AND RISK FACTORS

Schizophrenia is a chronic disorder, with an estimated worldwide prevalence up to 1% and an incidence of approximately 1.5 per 10,000 people.[2] The World Health Organization Global Burden of Disease study identified SCZ among the 10 leading causes of years lived with disability in individuals between 25 and 54 years of age.[3] Indirect costs, such as unemployment and social support, account for this elevated burden, along with direct hospitalization costs. Age of onset is typically in young adulthood, although early-onset forms of the disorder have been described in children and adolescents. Childhood-onset SCZ (COS), diagnosed before the age of 12 years, is considered a rare disorder with an estimated prevalence of less than 0.04%,[4] whereas early-onset SCZ (EOS) is diagnosed between 12 and 18 years of age and has a cumulative incidence of 9.1 per 100,000 person-years at risk.[5] Several lines of evidence suggest that COS and EOS are generally more severe[6,7] and reflect a heavier genetic loading,[8] along with more severe premorbid neurodevelopmental abnormalities[9] than the typical onset form. The prevalence of SCZ is higher in developed countries and in migrants compared to native-born populations.[10] Age of onset is usually 3 to 5 years earlier in men than in women, regardless of culture and definition of illness.[11] All-cause mortality is generally considered twofold to threefold higher than the general population,[2] and life expectancy is reduced by 15 to 25 years.[12] Leading global mortality risk factors, which include smoking, physical inactivity, being overweight, and having high glucose and cholesterol levels, are commonly observed in SCZ patients. In the United States, cardiovascular disease and suicide are among the main causes of death for this population.[13] The estimated suicide rate for SCZ patients is 579 per 100,000 person-years, with a lifetime risk of death by suicide of approximately 5%.[14]

SCZ has a high estimated 70% to 85% heritability,[15] with a relevant polygenic component, which includes thousands of common alleles that contribute to disease risk. By sampling 36,989 patients and 113,075 control subjects worldwide, the SCZ Working Group of the Psychiatric Genomics Consortium identified 108 independent SCZ-associated genomic loci, which only explain 3.5% of the liability for the disorder.[16]

Among environmental risk factors, obstetric complications have been linked to an increased risk for SCZ, as well as to an earlier age of onset, a poorer course of the illness, and ventricular enlargement.[17]

An umbrella review of 55 meta-analyses or systematic reviews recently examined several putative risk factors for SCZ.[10] Whereas convincing evidence of association was found only for the ultra–high-risk (UHR) SCZ state and for Black Caribbean ethnicity in England, several other factors were suggestive, including being a first- or second-generation immigrant, belonging to an ethnic minority, urbanicity, having the trait anhedonia, low premorbid intelligence quotient, minor physical anomalies, olfactory identification impairment, winter/spring season of birth in the Northern Hemisphere, childhood social withdrawal or trauma, *Toxoplasma gondii* immunoglobulin G, and non–right handedness. Substance abuse—most prominently cannabis and alcohol but also hallucinogens, sedatives, and other substances—also significantly increases the overall risk of developing SCZ up to 10 to 15 years after a diagnosis of substance use disorder (SUD).[18]

DIAGNOSIS AND CLINICAL COURSE

SCZ is a heterogeneous disorder with a broad range of clinical manifestations, including positive symptoms (e.g., delusions, hallucinations) and negative symptoms (e.g., avolition), as shown in Table 165.1. Positive symptoms are generally present at illness onset and represent core features of psychosis, a syndrome characterized by altered reality testing that is classically associated with SCZ spectrum disorders.

SCZ is usually diagnosed after a prodromal, at-risk stage in which subthreshold psychotic symptoms begin to emerge. In the prodromal stage, women tend to be less socially isolated, have higher levels of education, and have more work experience compared to men, all functional advantages that are thought to depend on the neuroprotective effects of estrogen. However, some authors have argued that premorbid functioning depends on age of onset and negative symptoms, rather than gender.[19] After a full-blown first episode of psychosis (FEP) in patients with SCZ, acute exacerbations of psychosis recur in the context of (often) persistent negative and cognitive symptoms. Despite intensive clinical interventions, patients remain at risk of recurring psychotic crises throughout their lives. A meta-analysis of 14,484 cases indicates that SCZ features during an FEP are strong predictors of poor long-term outcome and higher risk of relapse at 3 years.[20] In this framework, some authors suggest it might be preferable to use the term *psychosis* rather than SCZ when communicating with patients, to better reflect the possibility of favorable outcomes. However, the view that patients with SCZ have a generally poor psychosocial outcome has recently been challenged. Although the majority of patients need continuous support throughout their lives, many individuals with SCZ live independently outside of health care facilities, and up to 50% have a positive outcome in prospective studies.[21] In the long term, when prominent psychotic symptoms subside, several patients continue to experience residual symptoms that include social and emotional withdrawal. The clinical course of SCZ is often complicated by medical and psychiatric comorbidities. Hepatitis, cardiovascular diseases, diabetes, obesity, sexual dysfunction, and obstetric complications are commonly observed.[22] SUD is one of the most frequently observed psychiatric comorbidities, with high prevalence of cannabis (26.2%), alcohol (24.3%), and stimulant (7.3%) use.[23] Smoking, poor eating habits, and lack of exercise also significantly contribute to physical morbidity, along with side effects from antipsychotic (AP) medications. Thus improving access to comprehensive health care services and promoting healthy lifestyle habits should be among the main objectives of treatment throughout the patient's life span.

ETIOPATHOGENETIC MECHANISMS

Despite several decades of brain imaging and neuropathologic, electrophysiologic, and pharmacologic studies, the neurobiology of SCZ has yet to be fully established. SCZ is highly polygenic, with common single nucleotide polymorphisms in more than 100 loci, contributing to slightly higher risk of disease, along with a few rare or de novo copy number variants that confer a significantly larger disease risk. Several of those risk genes encode proteins that have been involved in the pathogenesis of SCZ, including voltage-dependent calcium channels, as well as glutamate, gamma-aminobutyric acid (GABA), and dopamine receptors.[24]

In what follows, we present some of the hypothesized etiopathogenetic mechanisms of SCZ and related supporting findings in patients with this disorder.

Aberrant Synaptic Activity

Physiologic synaptic activity depends on molecular pathways that are influenced by a variety of environmental factors during neurodevelopment. Preclinical models of SCZ have begun to define the role of inflammatory and oxidative stress-response cascades in modulating synaptic development and maintenance, particularly during adolescence. In this period, aberrant myelination and plasticity are thought to interfere with physiologic pruning of synapses, intensifying the abnormal neurodevelopmental trajectory in individuals at risk for SCZ. Several neuronal subpopulations contribute to the pathogenesis of this disorder. The mechanism of action of AP medications, which involves blocking dopamine receptors, suggests that presynaptic dopamine dysregulation is a final common pathway to psychosis proneness.[25] According to an influential dopaminergic theory of SCZ, cognitive and perceptual distortions that lead to full-blown symptoms

Table 165.1 Comparison of Essential ICD-10 and DSM-5 Criteria for Schizophrenia

ICD-10	DSM-5
Either at least one of the syndromes listed under option 1 or at least two of the symptoms and signs listed under option 2 should be present for most of the time during an episode of psychotic illness lasting for at least 1 month (or at some time during most of the days). 1. At least one of the following: A. Thought echo, thought insertion or withdrawal, or thought broadcasting B. Delusions of control, influence, or passivity, clearly referring to body or limb movements or specific thoughts, actions, or sensations; delusional perception C. Hallucinatory voices giving a running commentary on the patient's behavior, discussing him between themselves, or other types of hallucinatory voices coming from some part of the body D. Persistent delusions of other kinds that are culturally inappropriate and completely impossible (e.g., being able to control the weather or being in communication with aliens from another world) 2. Or at least two of the following: E. Persistent hallucinations in any modality, when occurring every day for at least 1 month, when accompanied by delusions (which may be fleeting or half-formed) without clear affective content, or when accompanied by persistent overvalued ideas F. Neologisms, breaks, or interpolations in the train of thought resulting in incoherence or irrelevant speech G. Catatonic behavior, such as excitement, posturing or waxy flexibility, negativism, mutism, and stupor H. "Negative" symptoms, such as marked apathy, paucity of speech, and blunting or incongruity of emotional response; it must be clear that these are not due to depression or to neuroleptic medication	The presence of two (or more) of the following, each present for a significant portion of time during a 1-month period (or less if successfully treated), with at least one of them being option 1, 2, or 3: 1. Delusions 2. Hallucinations 3. Disorganized speech (e.g., frequent derailment or incoherence) 4. Grossly disorganized or catatonic behavior 5. Negative symptoms (i.e., diminished emotional expression or avolition) For a significant portion of the time since the onset of the disturbance, level of functioning in one or more major areas (e.g., work, interpersonal relations, or self-care) is markedly below the level achieved before onset; when the onset is in childhood or adolescence, the expected level of interpersonal, academic, or occupational functioning is not achieved Continuous signs of the disturbance persist for a period of at least 6 months, which must include at least 1 month of symptoms (or less if successfully treated); prodromal symptoms often precede the active phase, and residual symptoms may follow it, characterized by mild or subthreshold forms of hallucinations or delusions (e.g., odd beliefs, unusual perceptual experiences)
Most commonly used exclusion criteria: If the patient also meets criteria for a mood episode, the criteria listed earlier must have been met before the disturbance of mood developed; the disorder is not attributable to organic brain disease or to alcohol- or drug-related intoxication, dependence, or withdrawal	Schizoaffective disorder and depressive or bipolar disorder with psychotic features have been ruled out because either (1) no major depressive, manic, or mixed episodes have occurred concurrently with the active-phase symptoms or (2) any mood episodes that have occurred during active-phase symptoms have been present for a minority of the total duration of the active and residual periods of the illness
Clinical subtypes associated with prevalent symptoms: 1. Paranoid schizophrenia 2. Hebephrenic schizophrenia 3. Catatonic schizophrenia 4. Undifferentiated schizophrenia 5. Residual schizophrenia 6. Simple schizophrenia	Clinical subtypes (described in previous versions up to DSM-IV-TR) abandoned in DSM-5 due to perceived lack of heuristic value

Modified from the *International Statistical Classification of Diseases and Related Health Problems*, tenth revision (ICD-10) (World Health Organization, 2016) and from the *Diagnostic and Statistical Manual of Mental Disorders*, fifth edition (DSM-5) (American Psychiatric Association, 2013).

stem from the altered appraisal of stimuli, perhaps through a process of aberrant salience attribution. However, significant heterogeneity of striatal dopamine function has been reported in molecular imaging studies. Although elevated dopamine synthesis and release capacities appear widespread, receptor/transporter availabilities and synaptic levels are abnormal only in a subgroup of patients, thereby contributing to interindividual differences in treatment response to, and side effects from, AP medications.[26]

Several lines of evidence have recently suggested that disturbed glutamatergic transmission, likely mediated by parvalbumin-positive GABA interneurons, might contribute to the biologic processes underlying other clinical aspects of the disorder, such as cognitive dysfunction.[24] According to the "*N*-methyl-D-aspartate receptor hypofunction" hypothesis of SCZ, impaired glutamatergic signaling downregulates the function of cortical GABAergic interneurons, thereby reducing recurrent inhibition of pyramidal glutamatergic neurons.[27] In this context, SCZ is better viewed as a network disorder in which defective integration among brain areas reflects aberrant modulation of synaptic efficacy.[28]

Structural and Functional Brain Imaging Abnormalities

From a neuroanatomic point of view, reductions in gray matter thickness and volume, along with alterations of white matter integrity, have been consistently reported in patients with SCZ. Those structural brain abnormalities tend to progress during the course of illness and are likely affected by long-term exposure to AP medications.[29,30] Indeed, a meta-analysis of 246 magnetic resonance imaging (MRI) studies confirmed that cumulative AP dosage correlates with increased variability in patients' intracranial—especially lateral and third ventricle—volumes.[31] At the same time, brain imaging-based machine learning algorithms found that reduced medial prefrontal and temporo-parieto-occipital gray matter volume (GMV) and increased cerebellar and dorsolateral prefrontal GMV predicted 1-year social functioning outcomes in a group of 116 individuals at clinical high risk (CHR) for psychosis and SCZ.[32] This prediction outperformed expert prognostication and shows how neuroanatomic abnormalities can precede illness onset and may significantly affect the trajectory of this disorder. Regarding functional brain imaging abnormalities in SCZ, the inconsistent findings that emerged from a first wave of functional MRI (fMRI) studies led to the current stage of research, in which data are pooled together from large consortia. The North American Prodromal Longitudinal Study (NAPLS-2) consortium established thalamocortical dysconnectivity in 243 CHR individuals using baseline MRI.[33] A partially overlapping dataset also revealed an intrinsic cerebellar-thalamic-cortical (CTC) hyperconnectivity pattern in at-risk individuals, a pattern that can also be observed in patients diagnosed with SCZ.[34] The CTC connectivity correlated with level of disorganization and predicted time to conversion in those 182 CHR subjects, among which the 19 who converted to psychosis had the most pronounced hyperconnectivity. Data from 236 FEP patients who underwent fMRI resting-state or task-activated studies recently confirmed partial normalization of aberrant brain activation after AP treatment. Although heterogeneous, a predominant hypoactivation pattern of prefrontal cortices, amygdala, hippocampus, and basal ganglia was partially normalized at follow-up.[35] In summary, when compared to healthy individuals, resting-state thalamocortical networks have been found to be hypoconnected or hyperconnected in patients with SCZ and CHR individuals, respectively.[36]

Electrophysiologic Alterations in Wakefulness and Sleep

Compared to functional brain imaging, the exquisite temporal resolution of electroencephalogram (EEG) recordings has the advantage of capturing oscillatory brain activity of underlying neuronal systems. Abnormalities of neural oscillations have been described both during wakefulness and sleep in SCZ. The most extensively studied electrophysiologic alterations in this population are smooth pursuit eye movement, oculomotor antisaccades, deficits in P50 event-related potential inhibition, prepulse inhibition of the acoustic startle reflex, P3 event-related potentials, and mismatch negativity.[37]

More recently, sleep alterations have emerged as valuable readouts of underlying neuronal circuit dysfunctions that are not influenced by wakefulness-related confounders, including clinical symptoms.[38] In the past decade, several groups reported deficits of sleep spindle density in chronic, AP-medicated patients with SCZ,[39–45] with only few exceptions.[46–48] Spindle morphology was also affected in SCZ patients, which showed decreased amplitude and duration relative to healthy control (HC) subjects.[39–40] These results have been established using different methods, which include visual inspection of the band-pass filtered signal[42] and different automated spindle detection algorithms.[39–41,43,45]

Spindle impairments were also observed in early-course psychosis patients[49,50] and in unmedicated adolescents with early-onset SCZ.[51] In the former group, differences with HC subjects seemed to be specifically driven by the subgroup of psychotic patients diagnosed with SCZ.[50] Although their specificity for SCZ has yet to be established, spindle deficits are considered a promising marker of disrupted thalamocortical function in those patients[52] and a potentially treatable target linking risk genes to impaired cognition.[53] Among those risk genes, the *CACNA1I* gene encodes a calcium channel that is abundantly expressed in the thalamic reticular nucleus (TRN), known as the "spindle generator," and plays a critical role in spindle activity.[54] Intriguingly, spindle density has recently been found to inversely correlate with declarative and procedural memory consolidation in patients with SCZ.[55]

Findings on slow wave abnormalities are more heterogeneous, possibly due to methodological issues and to the influence of AP medications.[56] A reduced slow wave number and/or density in non–rapid eye movement (NREM) sleep was clearly identified in several studies on drug-free or drug-naïve patients compared to HC subjects.[47,57–59] More recently, reduced slow wave power and slow wave density were observed in early-course patients.[60]

CLINICAL SLEEP-RELATED FEATURES

Sleep disturbances are consistently reported by patients with SCZ[61] and are often present before illness onset.[62] Alongside other symptoms, it has been suggested that disturbed sleep may help predict those who will develop psychosis among high-risk individuals.[63,64] Moreover, chronically disrupted sleep has wide-ranging negative effects on social function, mood, cognition, and quality of life in people with SCZ.

Despite a growing interest in the research community about the role of sleep in psychotic disorders, clinical sleep problems are often left unaddressed in those patients. In a recent study, although clinicians believed that sleep disturbances may exacerbate psychotic experiences, up to 82% assessed sleep problems informally, rather than using standard assessment measures, and no intervention was recommended.[65] In a cohort of patients with early psychosis, half of which had diagnosed sleep disorders, only about a quarter received specific treatment, and less than 10% were found to be in line with clinical guidelines.[66]

In the following sections, after briefly presenting sleep disturbances that do not meet diagnostic criteria for a sleep disorder, as assessed with actigraphy and PSG or EEG recordings, we will examine the most commonly reported sleep disorders in patients with SCZ.

Actigraphy and Sleep Architecture Alterations in Schizophrenia

Actigraphy data indicate that patients with SCZ sleep more at night and have a poorer sleep efficiency (SE), a longer sleep latency (SL), and more nighttime awakenings compared to

HC subjects.[67] UHR youth display similar sleep disturbances, which are associated with clinical symptomatology.[68] Of interest, in UHR persons, increased sleep dysfunction was also associated with decreased bilateral thalamus volume.[69]

Sleep architecture is also altered in patients with chronic SCZ relative to healthy populations, as documented by several PSG studies. A recent meta-analysis of PSG findings confirmed actigraphy data, with the exception of total sleep time (TST), and also revealed a reduction in slow wave sleep (SWS) and a decrease in rapid eye movement (REM) sleep duration and latency in SCZ patients compared to HC subjects.[70]

Sleep-Wake Disorders in Schizophrenia

Sleep disorders have been scantily investigated in SCZ. A first detailed study carried out using structured diagnostic interviews, sleep diaries, and actigraphy in 60 outpatients with early nonaffective psychosis, revealed that 80% had at least one sleep disorder; comorbidity of sleep disorders was found to be high, with an average of 3.3 sleep disorders per patient, and the most common diagnoses were insomnia and nightmare disorder.[66]

Insomnia

Insomnia is a pervasive, yet often overlooked condition in SCZ, especially in the acute phase of the illness. Whether insomnia is precipitated by a hyperarousal state, as in healthy individuals,[71] sustained by positive symptoms, such as hallucinations and delusions,[72] or by specific mechanisms involving the dopaminergic system,[73] is yet to be elucidated. In addition, negative symptoms, such as avolition, and cognitive deficits may lead to excessive daytime inactivity and inadequate sleep hygiene, which in turn interferes with nighttime sleep.[71] The elevated rates of substance/drug use/abuse in patients with SCZ is also likely to contribute to the occurrence of substance-induced insomnia.

Sleep-Related Breathing Disorders

In patients with SCZ, rates of obesity and the metabolic syndrome are higher compared to the general population, mainly due to weight gain secondary to AP medications, physical inactivity and poor diet. As the primary risk factor for obstructive sleep apnea (OSA) is obesity, elevated rates of sleep apnea are expected in patients with SCZ. A recent review of the literature has revealed a paucity of quality research in this area.[74] Current available data suggest higher rates of sleep apnea in SCZ patients.[75] Despite this known association, OSA is underrecognized in people with SCZ in the clinical setting.[76] The diagnostic utility of OSA screening tools remains to be investigated. However, it has been proposed that OSA screening should be conducted with emphasis on neck circumference greater than 40 cm, body mass index greater than 25, male sex, age greater than 50 years, and witnessed apneas or loud snoring. In contrast, sleep symptoms should be considered as a subordinate criterion for PSG referral, given that most patients with SCZ lack partners to report snoring or nocturnal apnea, and they are unlikely to report symptoms of daytime sleepiness.[74]

Central Disorders of Hypersomnolence

Hypersomnolence in SCZ patients may emerge during AP treatment, especially with clozapine and, to a lesser extent, with olanzapine, quetiapine, or phenothiazines, such as chlorpromazine. However, prevalence of hypersomnia due to a medication/substance in those patients is largely unknown. When addressing hypersomnolence, clinicians should also carefully investigate patients' use of alcohol, given the known comorbidity with alcohol use disorder in this population.

An association between psychosis and narcolepsy has been suggested in both adults and children, with a prevalence ranging from 1% to 10%.[77,78] However, evidence is controversial,[79] and a study conducted on more than 500 adult subjects with narcolepsy type 1 (NT1) from two large European cohorts, pointed out that SCZ-like psychosis is rarely comorbid with NT1 (≈1.8%).[80]

In narcoleptic patients, SCZ-like symptoms may occur as a result of stimulant therapy.[81] Although this side effect is infrequent, literature on high-dose stimulants is not in full agreement.[82] Furthermore, primary symptoms of narcolepsy (e.g., sleep paralysis, hypnagogic/hypnopompic hallucinations, hypersomnolence, obesity)[78,81] can be confused with psychotic symptoms. When hallucinations and delusions are prominent, cases of narcolepsy can simulate SCZ. It is also possible an overlap between narcolepsy and SCZ, at least in terms of symptomatology, may reflect the abnormal activity of similar neuronal pathways.[83] For example, a sleep-wake instability may alter the sensory thalamic gateway, favoring the emergence of hallucinations. From a pathogenetic perspective, autoimmunity might play a role, although current data are too limited to draw a conclusion.

Circadian Rhythm Sleep-Wake Disorders

Patients with SCZ tend to have a more irregular, inconsistent sleep-wake schedule, with increased SL, longer time in bed, and more fragmented sleep.[67,84,85] Several studies have documented circadian rhythm sleep-wake abnormalities in those patients, ranging from delayed and advanced sleep phase to irregular and free-running rest-activity patterns. Altered rest-activity and light-exposure patterns have been assessed by clinical interviews and actigraphy[86,87] and confirmed by the study of secretion or excretion melatonin profiles.[84] Endogenous melatonin levels and sleep-promoting action seems to be compromised in SCZ,[88] to the extent that the correlations between melatonin levels and several sleep parameters observed in healthy subjects are absent in SCZ patients.[88a]

Circadian rhythm integrity has been strongly and repeatedly associated with outcome measures of cognitive performance and global functioning in patients with SCZ[86,89]; abnormal circadian rhythm is also associated with increased psychotic symptom severity in clinical high-risk subjects.[90]

The evidence linking brain disorders and circadian dysfunction is mostly correlational.[91] Disturbed circadian rhythm can be a byproduct of lifestyle, behavioral factors, and intensity of psychiatric symptoms. However, circadian abnormalities are also present in stable, nonacute SCZ patients following a fixed routine when compared to unemployed, healthy volunteers. Specifically, an actigraphy study found that sleep phase was out of synchrony with environmental nighttime in half of the patients with SCZ relative to none of the HC group.[84] Circadian desynchronization might also be related to medication status, as suggested by the observation that long-term treatment with high doses of AP medications was associated with decreased daytime alertness and less robust circadian activity rhythms in SCZ patients.[86] However, AP medications are known to globally improve sleep quality,[92] and the emergence of sleep and circadian rhythm disruptions often precedes the diagnosis of SCZ.[89] Finally, genome-wide association studies have suggested that several genes involved in the development of SCZ are linked to sleep and/or circadian regulation.[93,94] Thus abnormal circadian rhythms might affect the individual's adaptation to his/her environment, thereby facilitating the emergence of SCZ and other psychiatric disorders.

Parasomnias

Parasomnias are disorders characterized by abnormal behavioral or physiologic events occurring in association with both NREM and REM sleep. Four classes of drugs that are commonly used in the clinical practice have been implicated as triggers for NREM sleep parasomnias. They are (1) benzodiazepine receptor agonists and other GABA modulators, (2) antidepressant medications, (3) beta blockers, and (4) AP compounds.[95] The strongest evidence for medication-induced sleepwalking, an NREM sleep arousal disorder, exists for zolpidem, a GABA modulator. Two atypical AP medications, olanzapine[96,97] and quetiapine,[98] as well as several first-generation AP medications, including chlorprothixene, perphenazine, and thioridazine, have been associated with sleepwalking in several case reports.[99,100] A differential diagnosis to consider in sleepwalkers who on a regular basis get something to eat is nocturnal eating disorder, which some studies have reported to be more frequent in obese patients with SCZ and schizoaffective disorder, especially those affected with comorbid insomnia and depression.[101,102]

Higher prevalence of REM sleep without atonia (up to 12%) has been found in individuals on selective serotonin reuptake inhibitor and serotonin and norepinephrine reuptake inhibitor treatment.[103] In contrast, AP medications have not been noted to produce REM sleep behavior disorders, except for an isolated case report on quetiapine.[104] Furthermore, it has been suggested that nightmares are more common in patients with psychosis than in the general population and that the presence of nightmares is associated with increased daytime and nighttime impairment.[105]

Sleep-Related Movement Disorders

In patients with SCZ, a diagnosis of restless legs syndrome (RLS) may be particularly difficult to determine due to the inclusion of subjective sensory symptoms in their complex delusional system, along with the erroneous interpretation of motor symptoms ("legs seem to move by themselves"). Diagnosis can be even more challenging, as neuroleptic-induced akathisia can closely resemble RLS. In support of a neuroleptic-induced akathisia, there is the experience of inner restlessness that is constantly perceived throughout the day, whereas in support of RLS there is the experience of leg paresthesia and the worsening of symptoms at night, as well as while resting. Although both akathisia and RLS are characterized by an increased number of awakenings and decreased SE, in neuroleptic-induced akathisia, sleep disturbances are usually milder.[106]

TREATMENT

Treatment of Clinical Symptoms: Antipsychotic Medications

After the serendipitous discovery of chlorpromazine's AP properties almost 70 years ago, several successful compounds were developed that exerted their effect primarily through dopamine receptor D2 (DRD2) blockade and were called first-generation antipsychotics (FGAs). More recently, atypical, or second-generation, antipsychotics (SGAs) were introduced, which, in addition to DRD2, interact with other neurotransmitter systems and especially serotonin receptors 2 (5HT-2R). Clozapine, arguably the most effective available AP, has a unique receptor binding profile characterized by low DRD2 affinity, high dopamine receptor D4 affinity, and effects on serotonin, acetylcholine, histamine, and glutamatergic neurotransmission.[107] More recently, AP compounds with partial agonism at dopamine receptor sites, including aripiprazole and cariprazine, were introduced. A list of the most commonly prescribed AP compounds, along with their known pharmacologic effects, is presented in Table 165.2.

Pooled data from 53,463 patients confirmed the effectiveness of AP compounds compared to placebo, with stronger effects for clozapine on overall symptoms and amisulpride for positive symptoms. Principal causes of discontinuation were sedation, extrapyramidal Parkinson-like motor symptoms, weight gain, prolactin elevation, and QTc prolongation.[108] In general, SGAs carry a lower risk of extrapyramidal symptoms, but they have a higher risk of cardiometabolic side effects compared to FGAs. These side effects contribute to the patients' poor adherence to treatment, largely due to the lack of illness insight.

Clozapine is considered a mainstay for treatment-resistant SCZ (TRS), diagnosed in approximately 30% of patients after an inadequate response to trials with at least two different AP medications.[109] Response rates up to 60% of TRS patients have been reported with clozapine. This drug also reduces the risk of suicide and aggression and has been associated with lower all-cause mortality compared to other AP compounds in SCZ patients.[110] Nonetheless, clozapine remains underprescribed, and it is administered only to patients who failed to respond to other AP drugs, largely due to the risk of inducing neutropenia and agranulocytosis that requires regular blood monitoring. Several prescribers have advocated for major access to this treatment, and the stronger association between clozapine and neutropenia relative to other AP drugs has been recently challenged.[111]

AP medications remain the gold standard of both acute and long-term pharmacologic treatment of SCZ due to their efficacy in improving patients' positive symptoms. However, those compounds are far less effective in ameliorating negative symptoms and cognitive dysfunctions, which appear to affect the overall functioning of SCZ patients more than the psychosis itself. Evidence about increased effectiveness when using more than one AP medication in SCZ is mixed. The combination of aripiprazole with clozapine has been associated with the lowest risk of rehospitalization.[112] Furthermore, recent meta-analyses appear to support AP polypharmacy over monotherapy, although significance of the effect disappears when evidence is limited to double-blind trials.[113] Thus clinical management of patients should cautiously consider the increased burden of side effects when AP medications are coadministered.[114]

Treatment Adherence and Long-Acting Injectables

Several long-acting injectable (LAI) formulations have been marketed for FGAs and SGAs to address the problem of nonadherence and perhaps decreasing side effects associated with more variable pharmacodynamics of oral formulations.

Table 165.2 Main Antipsychotic Drugs Prescribed for Schizophrenia, Listed by Progressive Date of FDA Approval

Antipsychotic Compound	Main Pharmacologic Effects[b]	Recommended Dose Range (mg/day)[c]	Long-Acting Injectable Formulation
First Generation			
Chlorpromazine	Dopamine, serotonin antagonism	400–800	Not available
Haloperidol	Dopamine antagonism	2–30	Available
Second Generation			
Clozapine	Dopamine, serotonin, norepinephrine antagonism	150–900	Not available
Amisulpride[a]	Dopamine antagonism	400–800	Not available
Risperidone	Dopamine, serotonin, norepinephrine antagonism	2–8	Available
Olanzapine	Dopamine, serotonin antagonism	10–30	Available
Quetiapine	Dopamine, serotonin, norepinephrine multimodal	400–800	Not available
Ziprasidone	Dopamine, serotonin antagonism	40–160	Not available
Aripiprazole	Dopamine, serotonin partial agonism and antagonism	10–30	Available
Paliperidone	Dopamine, serotonin, norepinephrine antagonism	6–12	Available
Asenapine	Dopamine, serotonin, norepinephrine antagonism	10–20	Not available
Iloperidone	Serotonin, dopamine antagonism	12–24	Not available
Lurasidone	Dopamine, serotonin antagonism	40–160	Not available
Cariprazine	Dopamine, serotonin partial agonism and antagonism	1.5–6	Not available
Brexpiprazole	Dopamine, serotonin partial agonism and antagonism	2–4	Not available

[a]Not approved by FDA, marketed in Europe since the early 1990s.
[b]FGAs and SGAs bind to a wide variety of central nervous system receptors; reported main effects are based on the Neuroscience-based Nomenclature (NbN2R), 2nd edition, project developed by European College of Neuropsychopharmacology (ECNP), American College of Neuropsychopharmacology (ACNP), International College of Neuropsychopharmacology (CINP), Asian College of Neuropsychopharmacology (AsCNP) and International Union of Basic and Clinical Pharmacology (IUPHAR); available at https://nbn2r.com, 2019.
[c]Ranges reflect lower effective dose for maintenance and maximum daily dose for oral treatment of schizophrenia in adult patients without significant comorbidity; dose adjustments are recommended in presence of strong/moderate inhibitors or inducers of cytochrome P-450 drug metabolism and for patients who are known poor/ultrarapid drug metabolizers.
FDA, US Food and Drug Administration; FGAs, first-generation antipsychotics; SGAs, second-generation antipsychotics.

The risk of rehospitalization is 20% to 30% lower during LAI treatment compared with equivalent oral formulations, and LAI medications have been associated with the highest rates of relapse prevention, together with oral clozapine.[115] However, conflicting findings on LAI's tolerability and efficacy led some authors to conclude that evidence in favor of those compounds over oral AP compounds is currently not sufficient,[116] so their use involves primarily patients with frequent relapses due to nonadherence.

Nonpharmacologic Treatment of Schizophrenia

When pharmacologic interventions are ineffective, electroconvulsive therapy may help a subgroup of TRS patients with catatonia, aggression, or suicidal behavior, particularly when a rapid improvement of symptoms is needed.[117] Low-frequency (1 Hz) transcranial magnetic stimulation over the temporal cortex has shown some effect on auditory hallucinations, whereas neither low- nor high-frequency (10 Hz) stimulation of the dorsolateral prefrontal cortex was better than sham stimulation in ameliorating negative symptoms in patients with SCZ.[118,119]

Other nonpharmacologic treatments include psychosocial interventions. Most available guidelines recommend cognitive behavioral therapy (CBT), cognitive remediation, psychoeducation, and supported employment services for all patients diagnosed with SCZ. In patients with low service engagement, which leads to frequent relapse or social deterioration, assertive community treatment can improve outcome. Interventions aimed at developing self-management skills and enhancing person-oriented recovery, social skills training, supportive psychotherapy, and family interventions are also recommended for the long-term treatment and rehabilitation of SCZ patients. Of note, CBT for insomnia has consistently shown success in the treatment of patients with psychosis, although future double-blind two-arm studies in larger groups of patients receiving AP medications are needed to establish better efficacy when compared to medication treatment alone.[72]

Effects of Antipsychotic Medications on Sleep in Schizophrenia

The majority of studies investigating the effects of AP medications on sleep support a role for these drugs in ameliorating subjective and objective sleep disturbances in patients with SCZ. Both FGAs and SGAs appear to improve sleep quality and increase TST and SE.[73,120] This effect is probably partially mediated by the reduction of psychotic symptoms and their related distress.[121] Furthermore, some of the low-potency FGAs (e.g., promazine and chlorpromazine) and most SGAs (e.g., olanzapine, clozapine, risperidone, paliperidone), but not high-potency FGAs (e.g., haloperidol), exert a direct effect on sleep, as confirmed by their sleep-promoting effects in healthy subjects.[121] Clozapine has been shown to increase TST and SE, as well as decrease SL and wake time after sleep onset. The sleep-promoting effects of olanzapine are also well known, with increases in both SE and SWS. Risperidone has been shown to increase SWS, whereas its active metabolite, paliperidone, increases TST, SE, stage N2, and REM, and it decreases SL, waking, and stage N1. The variability of effects on sleep architecture is most likely related to their receptor profiles, such as the high affinity for the histaminergic receptor of olanzapine and paliperidone, which have the largest impact on SWS.[122] Although FGAs and SGAs tend to improve overnight sleep, a disruption of the sleep-wake cycle has also been attributed to the sedative effects of those compounds during the daytime.[123] The sedative effect of low-potency agents, such as chlorpromazine, is likely related to increased slow wave and reduced alpha activity, whereas nonsedative, high-potency FGAs, such as haloperidol, increase alpha activity and have a minor impact on EEG slow activity during wakefulness.[124] Among SGAs, clozapine, olanzapine, and quetiapine are associated to the highest risk for sedation.

Antipsychotic Medications and Sleep Disorders

Although benzodiazepines have long been known to worsen sleep-disordered breathing, the impact of AP medications is less clear.[74] Because exposure to benzodiazepines appears to be bound by a dose-response relationship with mortality in SCZ,[125] long-term prescription of these compounds should be avoided. Data on central apneas are lacking, although the higher cerebrovascular and cardiometabolic risk profile associated with AP medication use suggests this population is at increased risk of central respiratory events.

Because the efficacy of AP medications largely relies on the blockade of D2 receptors, which appear to be specifically involved in the pathogenesis and treatment of RLS, their implication in sleep-related movement disorders has been hypothesized. Several case reports suggested a role for AP compounds in inducing RLS, especially olanzapine and quetiapine.[126] A large study on RLS in medicated SCZ patients (n = 182) and matched control subjects (n = 108) revealed that the incidence and prevalence of RLS symptoms was significantly higher in the SCZ group (21.4% and 47.8%, respectively) relative to the control group (9.3% and 19.4%, respectively).[127] However, no significant difference in age, duration of illness, cumulative exposure to neuroleptics, medication dose, or combination of therapy was found between individuals who were diagnosed with RLS and those who were not. The relationship between AP medications and periodic leg movement (PLM) has also been investigated. Although an initial association was reported in a sleep study on 10 SCZ patients,[128] only a small proportion (7 of 52 patients) had a PLM index greater than 5 in a more recent study on late-life psychosis.[129] Furthermore, a preliminary line of evidence is linking AP-induced RLS to polymorphisms located on several circadian genes or genes involved in SCZ pathogenetic pathways, such as dopamine receptors or dopamine metabolism.[130–132]

FUTURE DIRECTIONS

In this final section, we wish to provide a brief description of what we consider important areas of future inquiry to further establish the relationship between sleep abnormalities and SCZ. One of those areas concerns the investigation of sleep-related disturbances, and especially reduced sleep spindles and slow waves, as putative, predictive, diagnostic, and/or prognostic biomarkers of SCZ. Biomarkers are neurobiologic factors that are linked to the pathophysiology of major psychiatric disorders[133] and that can be assessed objectively and tend to be stable over time.[134] Furthermore, neurophysiologic biomarkers, such as EEG oscillations, offer exquisite temporal measures of neuronal circuits underlying clinical and cognitive characteristics of SCZ.[37] Thus it stands to reason that spindles and slow waves should be evaluated as putative biomarkers for SCZ spectrum disorders. To be predictive biomarkers, sleep EEG oscillations should be able to identify those individuals who will develop SCZ before the onset of illness. CHR individuals represent a unique group enriched for precursors of SCZ. Clinically, those individuals have different longitudinal courses, with one CHR subgroup experiencing a full remission of psychotic symptoms, a second subset with persistent subsyndromal symptoms, and a third subgroup with progression of psychotic symptoms and, eventually, a transition to full-blown SCZ.[135] Future sleep studies should therefore investigate the ability of spindles and slow waves to predict the clinical course of CHR individuals, and especially of those who will develop SCZ. Spindles and related sleep disturbances may also represent a diagnostic biomarker for SCZ. Indeed, several sleep EEG studies have reported that spindle deficits are present in chronic, early-course, and early-onset SCZ; are unrelated to AP medication exposure; and are not observed in patients with other psychiatric disorders.* However, given the relatively small sample sizes analyzed, these findings will need to be replicated in a larger cohort of patients, including those with SCZ and other major psychiatric disorders. In patients with SCZ, sleep spindles and slow waves also could be used as prognostic biomarkers. For example, SCZ patients with lower spindle and/or slow wave parameters at baseline assessments may have worse clinical prognoses, whereas those with higher spindles/slow waves may experience better clinical outcomes.

Future work should also investigate the implication of neural dysfunctions underlying sleep abnormalities in the neurobiology of SCZ. Slow waves, which occur primarily in frontal and prefrontal cortical (PFC) areas, are generated and coordinated by excitatory, glutamatergic cortical pyramidal neurons.[136] Sleep spindles are initiated by inhibitory, GABAergic neurons in the TRN. The TRN, which is also described as the spindle pacemaker, can generate spindle oscillations in isolation and after optogenetic activation,[137] although the interplay between TRN and other thalamic nuclei regulate and propagate sleep spindle activity within the thalamus. This intrathalamic activity

*References 39, 40, 44, 50, 51, 53, 54.

is then relayed through thalamocortical projections to the cerebral cortex, where spindle oscillations are synchronized, amplified, and sustained over time.[138] At the cortical level, spindles are particularly prominent in fronto-parietal and PFC regions. These cortical areas also show the largest spindle deficits in patients with SCZ,[40] as well as a reduction in slow wave density in FEP patients.[60] Decreased PFC activity, along with the mediodorsal thalamus, has been reported by resting-state fMRI connectivity in both chronic and early-course SCZ.[54] Furthermore, computational models have shown that alterations in the excitatory/inhibitory balance, which relies on glutamatergic and GABAergic inputs, may underlie thalamocortical neural dysfunctions in SCZ.[139] Altogether, these findings point to abnormalities in the thalamocortical network and in GABA and glutamate neurotransmission in patients with SCZ. Future studies should therefore focus on characterizing these neuronal and molecular underpinnings of spindle and slow wave abnormalities in SCZ. For example, a multimodal imaging approach that combines sleep EEG, resting-state fMRI, and magnetic resonance spectroscopy imaging in FEP patients could establish whether these abnormalities are present at illness onset and how they relate to clinical symptomatology and other core features of SCZ spectrum disorders.

Finally, ameliorating sleep abnormalities may contribute novel treatment interventions for SCZ. Several sleep studies from our and other research groups have shown that spindle and slow wave impairments are associated with worse clinical symptoms in SCZ patients.[56] In healthy subjects, increasing evidence indicates that sleep spindles[140–142] and slow waves[143,144] are implicated in learning, memory consolidation, and plasticity. Furthermore, recent work has linked deficits in spindles[43,49,145] and slow waves[146,147] to impaired cognitive performance in patients with SCZ. Because spindle and slow wave abnormalities appear to be associated to the clinical and cognitive dysfunctions of SCZ, reversing such sleep abnormalities could have a clear therapeutic potential. Slow waves and spindles can be increased using several approaches, including pharmacologic and nonpharmacologic interventions.[148–150] Future studies should therefore assess whether those interventions can reliably enhance sleep spindle and slow wave deficits in patients with SCZ, and whether such enhancement leads to an improvement in their functional impairments. This work could eventually pave the way to the development of novel, early treatment interventions in SCZ based on sleep neurophysiology.

CLINICAL PEARL

In individuals with schizophrenia (SCZ), including chronic and early-course patients, disrupted sleep patterns and sleep disorders are frequently present, although not routinely assessed. Besides insomnia, sleep-related breathing disorders and circadian sleep-wake rhythm disorders are the most common comorbidities that can negatively impact the SCZ patients' quality of life. Antipsychotic medications, currently the gold standard of treatment in SCZ, can also contribute to the emergence of hypersomnolence and/or sleep-related movement disorders in those patients. Thus, to provide optimal care to patients with SCZ, clinicians should always assess for the presence of sleep disturbances and sleep disorders and, when indicated, provide adequate treatment.

SUMMARY

SCZ is a highly disabling, chronic brain disorder that is estimated to affect almost 80 million people worldwide. Although SCZ is diagnosed based on a range of clinical symptoms, including delusions, hallucinations, and diminished emotional expression, sleep disturbances have been reported extensively since the earliest descriptions of the disorder. Sleep disturbances are known to precede the onset of SCZ and to predict symptom reexacerbations during its clinical course. Furthermore, in addition to aberrant synaptic plasticity and structural and functional brain imaging alterations, reduced NREM sleep oscillatory activities have been recently implicated in the neurobiology of SCZ. In everyday practice, patients' sleep complaints are highly prevalent but are often left unattended. Severe insomnia often impairs patients' global quality of life and must be discerned from circadian sleep-wake rhythm abnormalities or medication-induced, sleep-related movement disorders. Sleep-disordered breathing should also be routinely assessed, given the high prevalence of comorbid cardiovascular and metabolic syndromes in patients with SCZ. In addition, second-generation AP medications, the most widely prescribed pharmacologic treatments in SCZ, may induce hypersomnolence and facilitate the occurrence of sleep disorders in those patients. Thus adequately addressing sleep disturbances and sleep disorders in patients with SCZ can benefit their daytime symptomatology and significantly contribute to ameliorate their quality of life.

SELECTED READINGS

Castelnovo A, Graziano B, Ferrarelli F, et al. Sleep spindles and slow waves in schizophrenia and related disorders: main findings, challenges and future perspectives. *Eur J Neurosci.* 2018;48:2738–2758.

Ferrarelli F. Sleep abnormalities in schizophrenia: state of the art and next steps [published online ahead of print, 2021 Mar 17]. *Am J Psychiatry.* 2021. https://doi.org/10.1176/appi.ajp.2020.20070968. appiajp202020070968.

Ferrarelli F, Tononi G. Reduced sleep spindle activity point to a TRN-MD thalamus-PFC circuit dysfunction in schizophrenia. *Schizophr Res.* 2017;180:36–43.

Gardner RJ, Kersanté F, Jones MW, et al. Neural oscillations during non-rapid eye movement sleep as biomarkers of circuit dysfunction in schizophrenia. *Eur J Neurosci.* 2014;39:1091–1106.

Manoach DS, Pan JQ, Purcell SM, et al. Reduced sleep spindles in schizophrenia: a treatable endophenotype that links risk genes to impaired cognition? *Biol Psychiatry.* 2016;80:599–608.

Monti JM, Monti D. Sleep in schizophrenia patients and the effects of antipsychotic drugs. *Sleep Med Rev.* 2004;8:133–148.

Monti JM, Torterolo P, Pandi-Perumal SR. The effects of second generation antipsychotic drugs on sleep variables in healthy subjects and patients with schizophrenia. *Sleep Med Rev.* 2017;33:51–57.

Reeve S, Sheaves B, Freeman D. Sleep disorders in early psychosis: incidence, severity, and association with clinical symptoms. *Schizophr Bull.* 2019;45:287–295.

Robertson I, Cheung A, Fan X. Insomnia in patients with schizophrenia: current understanding and treatment options. *Prog Neuropsychopharmacol Biol Psychiatry.* 2019;92:235–242.

Woodward ND, Heckers S. Mapping thalamocortical functional connectivity in chronic and early stages of psychotic disorders. *Biol Psychiatry.* 2016;79:1016–1025.

Wulff K, Dijk DJ, Middleton B, et al. Sleep and circadian rhythm disruption in schizophrenia. *Br J Psychiatry.* 2012;200:308–316.

A complete reference list can be found online at ExpertConsult.com.

Chapter

166

Substance Abuse

Ian M. Colrain; George F. Koob

Chapter Highlights

- Addiction can be conceived of as a process mediated by changes in the activity of brain neurocircuitry. Acute intoxication effects eventually lead to allostatic modulation of brain circuits that result in hedonic withdrawal symptoms with cessation of use of the addictive substance and a compromised executive function.
- Sleep regulation involves many of the same neural circuits that are affected by addiction to alcohol, cannabis, and other drugs. Acute intoxication, especially with alcohol, can lead to abrupt changes in sleep architecture. Withdrawal syndromes often involve sleep disturbance as a prominent feature, and these can be a pathway to relapse. Sleep dysregulation can compromise executive function leading to addiction re-engagement.
- Erratic sleep patterns, altered circadian rhythms, and frank insomnia have been linked to an increased likelihood of alcohol and substance use in adolescents.
- Although effective treatment of addiction remains challenging, there is some emerging evidence that therapeutic interventions that also improve sleep may be helpful in reducing the likelihood of relapse.

INTRODUCTION

As outlined elsewhere in this volume, different states of sleep and transitions between sleep and wakefulness are supported by a complex set of patterns of neuronal activation and neurotransmitter release within specific neurocircuits (see Chapters 45 to 51). Many of these neurocircuits are also affected by alcohol or other addictive drugs.[1] Thus, unsurprisingly, acute intoxication from alcohol and other drugs affects sleep in several ways that vary based on their effects on the different neurocircuits activated by the drug. The tolerance to these effects that may develop with chronic use and the development of an alcohol use disorder (AUD) or other substance use disorder (SUD) are accompanied by adaptations of several neurotransmitter systems within such neurocircuits, either by modulating their release or modifying the sensitivity of their response mechanisms.[2] Hedonic withdrawal effects after cessation of use can also be associated with changes in sleep behavior and regulation resulting from the consequent neurochemical imbalance within specific neurocircuits. Over time, recovery can occur to restore a normal balance of neurocircuitry function (homeostasis), but some changes that are induced by alcohol and other drugs may be resistant to restoration, termed allostasis. Allostasis can be defined as stability through change and reflects an abnormal set point with significant allostatic load. This chapter outlines the effects of alcohol, cannabis, and opioid drugs on sleep in the context of what is known of the potential interactions between their neurophysiologic effects and those underlying sleep function. It is presented within a heuristic framework that has been developed to explain neuroadaptation associated with different phases of addiction and has recently been applied to alcohol's effects on sleep.[3] AUD is a major focus because of its much higher (29%) lifetime prevalence relative to other SUDs.[4] Cannabis remains the most commonly abused illegal drug worldwide, and opioids are the most common legally prescribed class of drugs leading to substance abuse disorders.[5]

DIAGNOSTIC FEATURES: DEFINITIONS AND CONCEPTUAL FRAMEWORK OF ALCOHOL AND OTHER SUBSTANCE USE DISORDERS

The Diagnostic and Statistical Manual of Mental Disorders, fifth edition, (DSM-5) diagnosis of an SUD is based on endorsement of 11 abuse and dependence criteria with the severity being determined by the number of criteria being endorsed.[6] The criteria are the following:

1. Substance often taken in larger amounts and/or over a longer period than intended
2. Persistent attempts or one or more unsuccessful efforts made to cut down or control substance use
3. A great deal of time spent in activities necessary to obtain the substance, use the substance, or recover from effects
4. Craving or strong desire or urge to use the substance
5. Recurrent substance use resulting in a failure to fulfill major role obligations at work, school, or home
6. Continued substance use despite having persistent or recurrent social or interpersonal problems caused or exacerbated by the effects of the substance
7. Important social, occupational, or recreational activities given up or reduced because of substance use
8. Recurrent substance use in situations in which it is physically hazardous

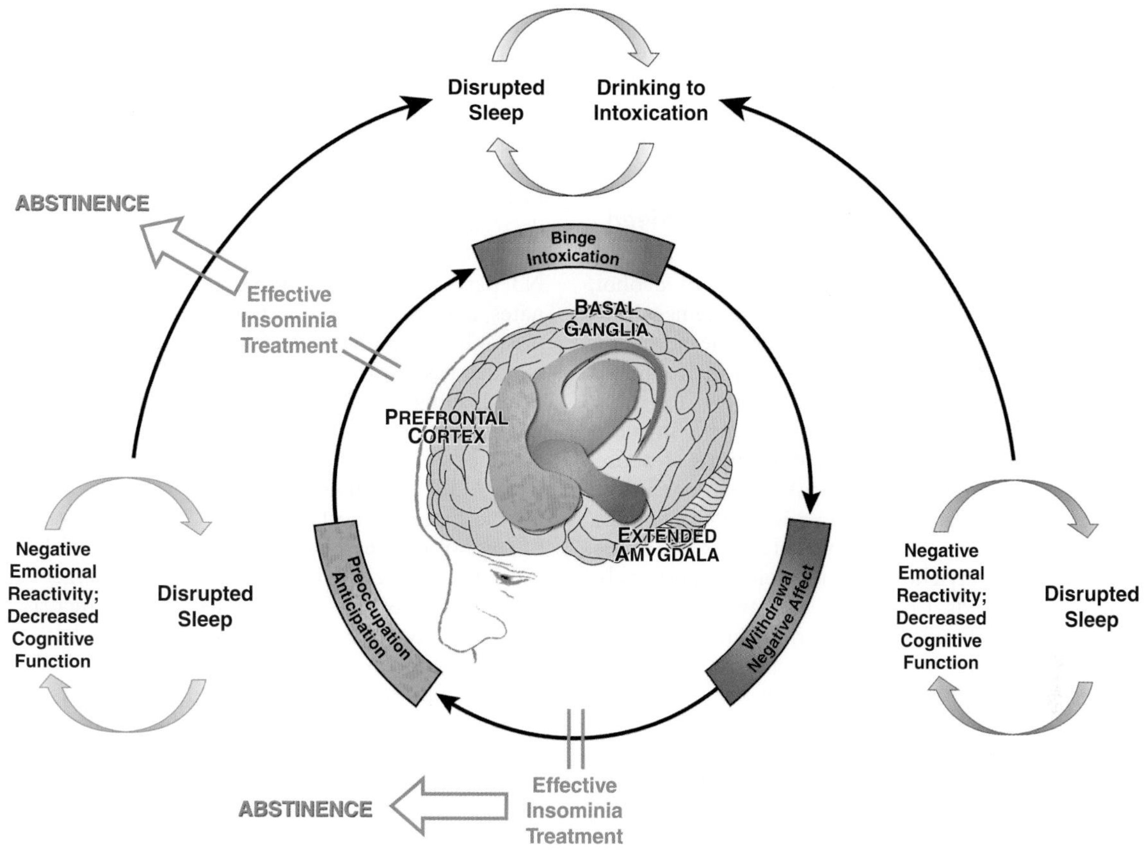

Figure 166.1 Framework for how sleep dysregulation is caused by alcohol use disorder (AUD) and how sleep dysregulation causes or exacerbates AUD with reference to the three-stage conceptual framework for the neurobiologic basis of addiction. In the binge/intoxication stage (which involves reward neurotransmitters and associative mechanisms in the nucleus accumbens shell and core and then engage stimulus-response habits that depend on the dorsal striatum), drinking to intoxication or binge drinking is hypothesized to disrupt sleep, and the consequent sleep disruption is hypothesized to drive further excessive alcohol drinking. In the withdrawal/negative affect stage (that may engage activation of the extended amygdala and its projections to the hypothalamus and brainstem), withdrawal disrupts sleep and may be a trigger for excessive drinking to provide relief from insomnia. In the preoccupation/anticipation stage (that involves the processing of conditioned reinforcement in the basolateral amygdala and the processing of contextual information by the hippocampus), residual sleep dysregulation may set up relapse, particularly when paired with stress- and/or alcohol-related cues. The treatment of sleep disturbances, particularly in the negative affect/withdrawal stage and preoccupation/anticipation stage, is hypothesized to help promote abstinence and treat AUD.

9. Substance use continued despite knowledge of having a persistent or recurrent physical or psychological problem that is likely to have been caused or exacerbated by the substance
10. Tolerance, as defined by either needing to use markedly increased amounts of the substance to achieve intoxication or experiencing a markedly diminished effect with continued use of the same amount
11. Withdrawal, as manifested by either the characteristic withdrawal syndrome for the substance or taking the substance or one that is closely related to relieve withdrawal symptoms

In each case, "mild" is defined as two or three symptoms, "moderate" as 4 to 5 symptoms, and "severe" as more than 6 symptoms out of the possible 11 listed.

In AUD and other SUDs, a pattern of drug taking evolves that is often characterized by binges that can be daily episodes or prolonged days of heavy drinking or use and is characterized by a severe emotional (hedonic) and somatic withdrawal syndrome. Many individuals with AUD or SUD continue with such a binge/withdrawal pattern for extended periods of time, but some individuals evolve into a situation in which they must have alcohol or their drug of abuse available at all times to avoid the negative consequences of abstinence. Here, intense preoccupation with obtaining alcohol or the drug (craving) develops that is linked not only to stimuli that are associated with obtaining the drug but also to stimuli that are associated with withdrawal and the aversive motivational state. A pattern ultimately develops in moderate to severe AUD/SUD in which the drug must be taken to avoid the severe dysphoria and discomfort of abstinence. Accompanying and contributing to this downward hedonic spiral is compromised executive function reflected in impaired cognitive function, which contributes to relapse and can be exacerbated by sleep disturbances.

Addiction has been heuristically framed as a three-stage cycle: *binge/intoxication*, *negative affect/withdrawal*, and *preoccupation/anticipation* ("craving")[7] (Figure 166.1). These three stages represent dysregulation in three functional domains (incentive salience/pathologic habits, negative emotional states, and executive function, respectively)[8,9] and are hypothesized to be mediated by three major neurocircuitry elements (basal ganglia, extended amygdala, and prefrontal cortex, respectively).[10] The three stages are conceptualized as interacting with each other, becoming more intense, and ultimately leading to the pathologic state that is known as addiction.[7]

Possible Neurochemical Interactions between Sleep and Addiction

The remainder of this chapter explores the effects of alcohol, cannabis, and opioids on the neurotransmitter systems within the neurocircuits that are considered key to the addiction cycle outlined previously. As recently reviewed in Koob and Colrain[3] for AUD and in Valentino and Volkow[1] for other SUDs, several neurotransmitter systems involved in sleep regulation are affected by alcohol and other drugs of abuse, where binge/intoxication can lead to acute alterations in the release or effects gamma-aminobutyric acid, opioid peptides, hypocretin, norepinephrine, 5-hydroxytryptamine, dopamine, glutamate, histamine, acetylcholine, mu-opioids, endocannabinoids, and glucocorticoids. Long-term use can produce allostatic modulation that then leads to aberrant function in the negative affect/withdrawal stage and may persist with long-term abstinence into *the preoccupation/anticipation stage.*[1,3]

Sleep and Alcohol

Evidence of the Impact of Drug Intoxication on Sleep: Alcohol

Alcohol is a central nervous system (CNS) sedative. Its impact on sleep varies as a function of dose, the time between drinking, and sleep onset, during which metabolism and some elimination will have occurred, age, sex, and somatic factors such as body fat percentage and genetic factors in the production of liver enzymes.[11] Reviews of acute alcohol effects on sleep and sleep in AUD can be found in Ebrahim and colleagues[12] and Colrain and colleagues.[13] A detailed review of the bidirectional links between alcohol and circadian rhythm disturbances can be found in Hasler and colleagues.[14]

The administration of intoxicating doses of alcohol to social drinkers in the laboratory leads to a reduction in sleep-onset latency (SOL), and when taken across the whole night, a small increase in wake after sleep onset (WASO). However, in split night studies, WASO is shown to decrease in the first half of the night and to increase in the second half of the night relative to placebo or nondrinking nights.[3] Other sleep continuity variables, such as the number of awakenings and sleep efficiency (i.e., minutes asleep as a proportion of time in bed), show similar trends[3] (i.e., improvement in the first half of the night and worsening in the second half, relative to control nights).

There is a generally held view in the literature that alcohol suppresses rapid eye movement (REM) sleep, with a rebound increase in REM sleep that occurs when blood alcohol levels decrease. As reviewed by Koob and Colrain,[3] doses of between 0.75 and 1.2 g/kg alcohol before bed led to decreases in REM in the first half of the night of up to 6.7% less than with no alcohol. However, although values in the second half of the night were sometimes higher than with a zero blood alcohol level, a rebound from a first half suppression was not always seen. This was notably the case in the two largest studies in which both men and women were investigated.[15,16] In studies that looked only at whole-night data, intoxicating doses of alcohol show variable results when data are collapsed over the entire night, but with a general trend for whole night REM to be modestly decreased.[3] This was also the case in the small number of studies from the 1970s in which alcohol administration was studied in patients with AUD.[3] As with social drinkers the acute effects of alcohol in AUD were largely an increase in N3 (or before[17] in slow wave sleep[18] [SWS]) and a decrease in REM.[3]

The consensus view in the literature is that alcohol increases N3, particularly early in the night when it typically predominates, and this was supported in recent reviews.[3,12,13] Unsurprisingly, in parallel to the first half of the night increase there is a decrease in the second half of the night relative to non-drinking nights, although when the data are collapsed across the whole night of sleep, a modest dose-related increase in N3 is still observed.[3] Studies of alcohol administration to patients with AUD also showed an increase in N3.[3] Consistent with the N3 findings, most studies that have investigated the effects of alcohol on sleep electroencephalography (EEG) show an increase in delta activity that appears to be larger earlier in the night[3] but may also be associated with an increase in frontal alpha activity,[16] possibly indicative of alpha-delta sleep.[19]

Unfortunately, very few studies have looked at repeated alcohol administration over multiple nights to enable a determination of the extent to which the effects observed from single-night studies may habituate over time. Gross and Hastey[20] studied 10 young male persons with AUD for at least 5 days of alcohol of up to 3.2 g/kg per day. No habituation appeared to occur for either SWS elevation or REM suppression with alcohol. In two studies of repeated administration of alcohol in non-AUD participants, effects on SOL, REM, and WASO in the first or second part of the night did not change over 3 drinking nights.[21,22] In a longer study of 9 nights of drinking, WASO in the first part of the night increased, the reverse of the pattern expected with habituation.[23] N3 sleep effects may, however, show some habituation. Although the decrease seen in the second half of the night did not appear to change, the first half increase appeared to decrease over 3 nights in studies by Feige and colleagues[21] and Rundell and colleagues[22] and at night 9 in a study by Prinz and colleagues.[23] In summary, it would appear from the limited evidence available that the major effects of alcohol on sleep do not demonstrate habituation with repeated intoxication with the possible exception of the increase in N3 early in the night.

Evidence of the Impact of Drug Withdrawal on Sleep: Alcohol

Sleep disturbances are extremely common in sober patients with AUD, and comorbid insomnia is highly prevalent.[24] Studies in which AUD were studied within 30 days of sobriety show substantial alterations in sleep architecture relative to controls. Although there is substantial variation between studies, on average SOL, WASO, N1, and REM are increased, and N3 is decreased in AUD relative to controls.[3] When reported data were analyzed as a function of time since drinking cessation, there was no apparent trend for normalization within 30 days.[3] AUD may also have impaired recovery from sleep deprivation.[25] Delta power in NREM sleep is also reduced in recently sober AUD compared with controls,[26,27] particularly in the first sleep cycle[28] and with a greater effect in African Americans than in Caucasians.[25] Evoked EEG delta responses also show reduced amplitude and incidence in recently sober AUD relative to controls.[29]

Evidence of the Impact of Long-Term Abstinence on Sleep: Alcohol

Longitudinal assessment of sleep in abstinent AUD has been conducted in a handful of studies.[30-32] These show persistent sleep problems with extended abstinence, including increased SOL, increased N1%, and increased WASO, with some evidence of partial recovery in the elevated REM and diminished N3 seen on withdrawal. However, N3 remains lower than in controls even after extended abstinence.[33] EEG effects seen in withdrawal also extend into long-term abstinence with NREM delta in particular being reduced[33,34] compared with controls. Evoked delta responses are diminished in long-term abstinent AUD[35,36] and, despite showing some evidence of showing partial recovery with abstinence,[29,37] remain at levels substantially less than controls even after several months of sobriety.[29] The long-lasting reduction of spontaneous and evoked delta activity may be related to the known, largely irreversible acceleration of brain shrinkage that is seen in AUD, especially in the frontal and prefrontal areas of the brain where delta activity is also predominant,[38] and the areas of the brain implicated in executive function deficits associated with AUD.

Relationship Between Alcohol Use Disorder and Insomnia

Patients with insomnia have around double the risk of having an AUD diagnosis than good sleepers,[39-41] and patients with AUD have a high prevalence of insomnia.[42,43] Although symptoms of insomnia can precede AUD,[39,44] insomnia is seen with withdrawal and for long periods of abstinence[43,45] and can be predictive of relapse.[43] The bidirectional relationship between insomnia is AUD is also present between insomnia and risky drinking, particularly in adolescence (see Hasler and colleagues[46] for review), and there is some evidence that addressing sleep issues in college students can lead to beneficial outcomes in terms of alcohol use.[47]

Although there is a clear bidirectional association between AUD and insomnia, treatment studies have shown that the comorbidities can be dissociated, and treatments that improve sleep may have little or no impact on drinking.[43,48] However, treatment of insomnia in AUD may nonetheless lead to subsequent benefits in drinking via symptom relief, improvement in overall quality of life, and improved cognitive functioning.[43,49] There are few studies that evaluated the opposite causal link, whether treating drinking in AUD leads to improvements in insomnia, largely because of the difficulty in finding treatment that are effective for AUD. Acamprosate may help normalize sleep.[50,51] There have been no studies of sleep effects in AUD being treated with naltrexone, but one study reported positive effects of topiramate on both sleep and drinking.[52] Recent studies have shown that immediate-release formulations of gabapentin, an anticonvulsant drug that has AUD a secondary indication, can improve sleep and reduce drinking in AUD.[53] Over a 12-week treatment program, gabapentin had a significant linear dose effect on drinking and Pittsburgh Sleep Quality Index total score relative to placebo.[53] It has also been shown to be effective in treating AUD-related insomnia.[54,55] However, a recent study of an extended release formulation of gabapentin did not show beneficial effects on drinking or on sleep.[56] Finally, hypocretin has been identified as a neuromodulator of both sleep-wake regulation (see Chapter 49) and as a potential therapeutic target for addiction.[57,58] Although there are no published studies of hypocretin antagonist therapies on AUD, an ongoing clinical trial may provide evidence of suvorexant as a possible treatment for AUD and AUD-related insomnia.[59] (See the work by Panin and Peana[60] for a more thorough review on sleep and pharmacotherapy for AUD.)

Summary of Alcohol Use Disorder and Sleep

Alcohol is ubiquitous in many societies as a legal substance and the most commonly abused substance. There is an immediate impact of alcohol intoxication on several neurotransmitter systems within reward and stress neurocircuits related to sleep and sleep regulation.[3] These lead to a biphasic response of sleep quality with some initial improvements followed by worsening of sleep as blood alcohol and metabolite levels drop over the course of a night. Allostatic modulation of the reward and stress neurocircuits then leads to hedonic withdrawal in dependent individuals, and the withdrawal syndrome includes substantially disturbed sleep. Many of the sleep changes, after cessation of alcohol use, last for an extended period, may affect executive function, and as a result may be a factor in relapse to drinking. There is some evidence to suggest that sleep may provide a therapeutic window for effective treatment of AUD and that future therapies for AUD should address the sleep issues associated with withdrawal and extended abstinence.

Cannabis

Possession of cannabis is currently illegal under United States federal law, and marijuana is the most prevalently used illegal drug by the federal law metric,[61] with evidence that the prevalence of e-cigarette use (vaping) of cannabinoids also is increasing.[62] However, at the time of publication, a majority of US states have legalized medical marijuana use, and around 20% have legalized recreational use. There is also a growing international trend for either legalization, decriminalization, or some allowance of restricted use. Recent data indicate that around 16% of the US population endorse past-year marijuana use, with evidence of a marijuana use disorder being present in 1.6% of the population overall and in 2.1% of adolescents.[63]

There are two cannabinoid receptors in the human central and peripheral nervous systems, CB1 and CB2. These respond to activation by endocannabinoids, which, at least in the case of those affecting CB1, have a role in the circadian regulation of the wake-sleep cycle.[64] Further the endocannabinoid anandamide displays a strong circadian rhythm.[65] The endocannabinoid system also responds to phytocannabinoids, the two most commonly used being delta-9-tetrahydrocannabinol (THC) and cannabidiol (CBD). THC has psychoactive effects and can be intoxicating; CBD may be psychoactive but does not produce intoxication. Both can be extracted from marijuana, and CBD can also be extracted from hemp. Synthetic versions of THC such as dronabinol and nabilone and of CBD such as Charlotte's web are also available, as well as combinations of THC and CBD such as nabiximols and Sativex.

As seen later in the chapter, given the legal, ethical, and regulatory challenges associated with administering an illegal substance, there is a general paucity of research into the effects of cannabis intoxication on sleep, the effects of cannabis withdrawal on sleep, and the relationship between sleep factors and cannabis relapse. However, particularly lacking are studies of those with a diagnosed cannabis-specific SUD, as opposed to cannabis users. The equivalent situation for alcohol would be if

Table 166.1 A Summary of the Early Studies Evaluating the Impact of THC or Marijuana on Sleep

Study	Subjects	Substance	Nights	Doses
Pivik, 1972[73]	4 young men	Oral THC	1 or 2	0.061 to 0.258 mg/kg
Cousens, 1973[72]	9 young men with mild insomnia	Oral THC	1 per dose	10, 20, and 30 mg
Pranikoff, 1973[77]	10 young men	Smoked marijuana	2	Subjective "high"
Barratt, 1974[74]	8 young men	Oral THC	10	0.2 mg/kg
Feinberg, 1975[76]	7 young men	Oral THC	3	210 mg/day
Karacan, 1976[78]	32 men	Smoked marijuana	2	Typical use (2.5 to 23 cigarettes)
Feinberg, 1976[75]	4 young men	Oral THC	3	210 mg/day
Freemon, 1982[86]	2 brothers	Oral THC	14	30 mg

THC, Delta-9-tetrahydrocannabinol.

almost all the studies had been conducted on "drinkers" rather than AUD. As with alcohol, however, there are data suggesting that the preexistence of sleep[66] or circadian problems[67] before cannabis use in adolescence can predict subsequent use, and that sleep and circadian factors may mediate the relationship between other risk factors such as family history, inhibition control, or externalizing and internalizing traits on marijuana use.[68] Drazdowski and colleagues[69] reported that 44% of the college student marijuana users who they studied reported using marijuana as a sleep aid. Path analysis also showed that using marijuana as a sleep aid significantly predicted marijuana use frequency and problems with use over both the past month and the previous year. A similar pattern was seen when using daytime dysfunction from the PSQI as the predictor variable.[69]

Evidence of the Impact of Drug Intoxication on Sleep: Cannabis

As reviewed in Babson and colleagues[70] and Gates and colleagues,[71] early work on the effect of cannabis on sleep from the 1970s produced mixed results. These studies tended to have very small subject numbers and varied substantially in terms of the doses administered and other methodological factors (Table 166.1).

Unsurprisingly, findings across these studies were inconsistent, but with some hints of increased SWS and decreased REM.[72-77] However, the relatively large Karacan 1976[78] study showed the marijuana users to have less REM than controls and no difference between marijuana users and controls for SWS. A later study by Nicholson and colleagues[79] studied eight young occasional marijuana users (four women) on doses of 15 mg of THC, 5 mg of THC + 5 mg of CBD, and 15 mg of THC + 15 mg of CBD. They reported no effects on sleep of the THC 15-mg dose. The combination of THC and CBD at 5 and 15 mg showed a modest decrease in stage 3 but not stage 4 or SWS with the 15-mg combined dose also demonstrating an increase in WASO. As reviewed in Gates and colleagues,[71] subjective findings from studies not using PSG measures are also variable, with some evidence of a perceived decrease in SOL, and no apparent effect of dose (to the limited extent that it has been studied).

A handful of studies have used validated sleep scales to assess the impact of medical marijuana use, with variable results. There is some evidence of a decrease in perceived sleep disturbance and/or increase in perceived sleep quality. In two studies using the Respironics Nightcap system, there was an improvement in sleep efficiency resulting from to an increase in NREM sleep and a decrease in wakefulness.[80,81] It is unclear as to whether any modest objective or subjective effects on sleep may be secondary to effects on the medical conditions for which the medicinal marijuana was being used (e.g., pain, human immunodeficiency virus). However, medical marijuana users have been shown to report "improving sleep" as a major reason for consumption, and this is particularly the case in those with posttraumatic stress disorder.[82] A recent analysis of people who use medical marijuana showed that 48% of those surveyed had insomnia as a major reason for use, and 25% reported improvement in insomnia as a primary benefit.[83]

Evidence of the Impact of Drug Withdrawal on Sleep: Cannabis

Withdrawal symptoms occur in the majority of those who demonstrate cannabis dependence. Sleep dysfunction and strange dreams are two of the more frequently reported symptoms, and trouble getting to sleep has been reported as being the most distressful symptom.[84] As indicated in a recent review by Gates and colleagues[85] other sleep-related withdrawal symptoms include waking up early and sleeping more than usual, although the proportion of dependent and nondependent cannabis users demonstrating sleep-related symptoms varied greatly across different studies.[85] The Freemon[86] study showed some evidence of increased SOL and WASO in the first couple of nights of withdrawal, with effects resolving by night 5. Bolla and colleagues[87] studied 17 marijuana users (5 who met DSM-IV[88] criteria for dependence and 1 who met criteria for abuse) who were selected based on self-report of prior sleep disturbance during prior periods of abstinence. Data from the first 2 nights after quitting were compared with matched controls. On the first night of abstinence marijuana users had less total sleep time (TST) and N3 sleep than controls. These differences persisted into night 2, which also showed them having lower sleep efficiency and increased SOL relative to controls. TST, socioeconomic status, SOL, and N3 were worse in night 2 than in night 1 for the abstinent marijuana group. The same authors[89] conducted a second study of 18 (13 men) daily users (40 to 210 joints per week), on nights 1, 2, 7, 8, and 13 after quitting. All data were reported relative to the first night of quitting, which were similar to those reported in their earlier study.[87] SE% continued to decline, was significantly worse on night 8, and was even more so at night 13. SOL continued to increase across the period of study. SWS showed an increase after 1 week of abstinence, and REM showed a trend to decrease over time, significantly so at night 13. Periodic leg movements (PLMs) also showed an increase over time and were significantly higher 1 week and 2 weeks after quitting, although this was largely due to a dramatic increase in four of the users.

The Relationship between Poor Sleep and Cannabis Use

There is emerging evidence that, as with alcohol, poor sleep can be a predisposing factor for marijuana use. However, the small number of studies that have looked at sleep issues as a predictor of relapse have produced variable results, with some evidence that increased SOL predicts the amount of marijuana used at relapse.[90] In a groundbreaking study, Mednick and colleagues[91] were able to show that short sleeping in adolescents had not only a social network effect but also an 11% increase in the likelihood that friends of a short-sleeping adolescent would also demonstrate short sleep. Marijuana use was more powerful, with friends of a user having a 110% increase in likelihood of use. Intriguingly, there was a 19% increase in the likelihood of drug use in the friends of adolescents who are short sleepers, with a substantial proportion of this variance being entirely due to the sleep effect. In summary poor sleep is associated with marijuana use, one's own poor sleep can influence sleep quality in one's social network (up to four degrees of separation), and one's own poor sleep can affect the likelihood of others using marijuana. This form of network analysis is a new analytic approach but clearly warrants more use in the sleep and substance use fields.

Several more traditional papers using longitudinal assessment have also shown predictive relationships between poor sleep and/or aberrant circadian rhythms and subsequent marijuana use. A school-based study of 4500 youth demonstrated that 9% of youth with insomnia were significantly more likely to use cannabis (and alcohol) at baseline and at 7-year follow-up than good sleepers.[92] A smaller sample of 95 youth studied at three time points (substance naïve at T1) revealed that known risk factors at T1 such as internalizing and externalizing behaviors, poor inhibitory control, and family history predicted subsequent marijuana (and other substance) use as did chronotype, daytime sleepiness, and erratic sleep behaviors. Importantly the pathway analysis also revealed that erratic sleep-wake behaviors was a significant mediator of the psychiatric factors on marijuana use.[68] Work emerging from major longitudinal studies funded by the National Institutes of Health is also supportive of poor sleep or circadian aberrations being predictive of subsequent marijuana use in adolescents. Hasler and colleagues[67] reported data from the National Consortium on Alcohol and Neurodevelopment in Adolescence (NCANDA) study. They found that increased levels of eveningness, later weekday and weekend bedtimes, and shorter weekday sleep duration at baseline predicted greater marijuana use at the 1-year follow-up, after covarying for baseline marijuana use.

A recent large study of more than 7000 college students focused on cannabis users approaching the threshold for hazardous use (43% of the sample) and possible cannabis use disorder (21% of the sample).[93] The authors were particularly interested in the relationship between insomnia symptoms and the likelihood of use of protective behavioral strategies to mitigate cannabis-related issues. They reported that a 1 standard deviation increase in insomnia symptoms increased the odds of cannabis use by 12% and the odds of a probable cannabis use disorder by 20%. Importantly more severe insomnia was associated with a decreased likelihood of protective behavioral strategy use, again showing a link of sleep disturbances with potential executive function deficits.

Given this and other studies that have shown relations between insomnia symptoms and cannabis use, and the evidence for sleep difficulties being associated with cannabis withdrawal, the same questions previously posed for alcohol can be asked for cannabis. That is, is there a relationship between treatments for marijuana withdrawal and sleep, and do these effects impact relapse?

A study using the Respironics Nightcap system[94] evaluated the impact of nonintoxicating doses of oral THC (Marinol) and 2.4 mg of lofexidine on withdrawal symptoms marijuana. THC alone did not decrease relapse and led to an increase in SOL. However, lofexidine alone and combined with THC increased total sleep, decreased SOL, improved subjective feelings about sleep, and significantly reduced relapse.[95] Another synthetic THC analogue, nabilone, has also been shown to both improve objective (Actiwatch Sleep Efficiency) and subjective measures of sleep during marijuana withdrawal and to reduce relapse.[96]

The antidepressant Remeron (30 mg, mirtazapine) improved sleep efficiency and the subjective feeling of falling asleep easily but did not improve objectively measured SOL and did not lead to improved relapse rates. The antipsychotic quetiapine decreased the intensity of several marijuana withdrawal symptoms, including subjective (but not objective) measures of sleep during withdrawal, but it increased craving and worsened relapse relative to placebo.[97] As with AUD, however, gabapentin shows some promise in addressing both sleep problems associated with withdrawal and relapse after abstinence. Mason and colleagues[98] reported that 1200 mg per day of gabapentin led to decreased use of marijuana over an extended period and significant improvements in sleep as measured by the Pittsburgh Sleep Quality Index in patients with diagnosed marijuana dependence.

Summary of Cannabis Use and Sleep

The literature relating sleep to cannabis use and misuse is nowhere near as extensive as that for alcohol and AUD, and there are no definitive findings on acute effects of marijuana intoxication on objective measure of sleep. However, there is a widely held belief among marijuana users that sleep is improved with use, and insomnia is often cited as a factor in why people use. There are more data available on withdrawal effects in users but relatively little on withdrawal effects in those with a cannabis use disorder. There is strong evidence that poor sleep, chronotype, and evidence of insomnia appear to have strong predictive relationships with later marijuana use in adolescents, a key population for this drug. With the possible exception of gabapentin and nonintoxicating doses of synthetic THC, there is little evidence of a beneficial effect of pharmacotherapy improving sleep and relapse in those withdrawing from marijuana use.

Given the increasing prevalence of marijuana use and its near ubiquitous presence in modern society, the sleep field must pay more attention to the relationship between marijuana use, cannabis use disorder, and sleep.

Opioids and Sleep

It has been estimated that opioid use disorders, involving natural and synthetic opioids, such as heroin, morphine, codeine, oxycodone, and fentanyl, affect more than 16 million people worldwide and over 2.1 million in the United States.[99] Although rates of nonmedical use of opioids declined 10.5% from between 2003 and 2005 and 2012 and 2014[100] (and has continued to decline since[63]), the rate of opioid analgesic abuse or dependence[88] increased 24.7% over the same period,[88] with all of the increase happening in men.[100] More recent data, however, show that the rate of opioid use disorder has not increased further.[63] For a detailed review of opioid use disorder, including treatment options, comorbidity risks and public policy implications see Blanco and Volkow.[101] For the recent AASM position paper on opioids and sleep see the work by Rosen and colleagues.[102]

Opioids have been associated with sleep since the first synthesis of morphine—named after Morpheus, the Roman god of sleep and dreams.[103] As with alcohol and cannabinoids, there is overlap between brain systems involved in opioid addiction and those underpinning sleep-wake regulation. Endogenous opioids innervate the locus coeruleus to exert an opposing effect to corticotropin-releasing factor and may play a role in modulating stress reactions.[1] Opioid tolerance has been hypothesized to thus enhance stress-induced activation of the LC and other noradrenergic brainstem systems and to increase arousal and stress reactions, with drug seeking and use motivated by the need to dampen the allostatic tone. The activation of locus coeruleus norepinephrine system during opioid withdrawal is thought to be the underlying reason for the commonly observed symptoms of hyperarousal and insomnia. However, the hyperarousal and insomnia may also be due to the upregulation of the hypocretin system that has been observed in animal studies and in postmortem histology of the brains of opioid addicts.[1] Interestingly, narcolepsy appears to be protective of opioid addiction, a fact hypothesized to be due to their downregulated hypocretin system.[104]

Evidence of the Impact of Drug Intoxication on Sleep: Opioids

Studies of sleep in acute opioid intoxication are rare. Kay and colleagues[103] studied 10 male federal prisoners who had in the past been addicted to opioids on three different doses of morphine sulphate for 1 night each separated by a week of nonuse. There was a strong dose response effect for REM suppression, with almost no REM in the 30-mg/70-kg dose. Wake increased and N3 decreased with increasing dose.[103] The same authors[105] studied six male federal prisoners before and after the induction of stable multinight doses of 240 mg of morphine. Relative to control nights before, nights when using had slightly lower levels of REM, similar levels of N3, and less wakefulness and N1 in the first 2 hours of sleep. In a pattern similar to that seen with alcohol, there was some evidence of alpha-delta sleep during N3.[105] A third study from this group also examined acute heroin intoxication at different doses for 1 night each and reported increased wake and decreased REM and N3 with the lowest dose (3 mg/70 kg), and highly significant dose-related increases in wake and decreases in N3 and REM.[106] Taken together these studies would suggest that opioid effects on sleep habituate and stabilize over time, a position supported in the review by Wang and Teichtahl.[107]

As outlined in the work by Blanco and Volkow,[101] treatment for opioid use disorder often involves administration of full or partial mu-opioid receptor agonists, with tapering doses to mitigate withdrawal. These have been commonly found to be associated with subjective reports of sleep disturbance, which in the case of methadone have been found to be in between 40% and 88% of patients undergoing treatment and result in elevated levels of daytime sleepiness.[108] Polysomnographic studies of opioid agonist treatment show highly variable results: TST, decreased[109-111] or not,[112] sleep efficiency being lower[109,110] or not,[112] REM being decreased[109,111,112] or not,[110] N3 being decreased[109-111] or not,[112] SOL being increased[111] or not,[109,112] and WASO being increased[110] compared with controls. A study comparing high (150 mg) to low (75 mg) methadone doses showed little differences in sleep parameters other than the high-dose group having less N3.[113] However, almost all sleep parameters were worse in the patients on methadone for chronic pain, and REM and N3 were reduced in those also using benzodiazepines.[113] These data highlight the need to consider comorbid conditions and drug use when interpreting opioid effects, factors that probably contribute to the variability in observed sleep effects between studies.

Opioids also have direct effects on the regulation of breathing and can alter hypercapnic and hypoxic ventilatory responses and suppress respiration.[107] Unlike alcohol or cannabis, opioid agonists have been reported to increase the rates of sleep-disordered breathing, in particular central events.[107] A study comparing chronic opioid users to nonusers referred to a clinic with suspected sleep apnea demonstrated that although the overall apnea-hypopnea index (AHI) was not significantly higher in the opioid group, the central apnea index was six times that of the controls. Morphine dose was significantly related to the rate of central apneas.[114] Similar results have been reported regarding those undergoing opioid replacement therapy. A study of 50 patients using methadone compared with 20 controls showed no difference in obstructive events, but an average central apnea index of 6.7 events per hour versus 0.25 for controls.[112] In a study of 10 patients on methadone (50 to 120 mg/day), 7 of the 10 exhibited an AHI of greater than 20 events per hour (24.9 to 52.6) with the majority of the events being central apneas in most cases. Four of the 10 had a central apnea index of greater than 10 events per hour (12.7 to 41.5), and 3 exhibited periodic breathing.[109] In a larger study of 70 patients who were otherwise at low risk for sleep-disordered breathing (young, low body mass index [BMI]) undergoing opioid detoxification on buprenorphine, moderate or severe apnea was present in one-third of the patients, and mild in another third, with more central than obstructive events.[115] However, a longitudinal study of methadone replacement therapy found no central apneas in 23 patients studied over 12 months. Obstructive events did increase over time, probably because of observed weight gain.[116] The same authors had previously reported an elevated respiratory disturbance index in methadone patients using a high dose versus those on a low dose, despite no group differences in BMI. No central events were reported as being observed.[113]

Evidence of the Impact of Drug Withdrawal on Sleep: Opioids

There are very few data available on the effects of acute withdrawal from opioids. Howe and colleagues studied 20 heroin users admitted for detoxification on average less than 2 hours since their last dose and five control subjects over 5 to 7 nights. On night 1, REM values were similar to controls,[117] but total wakefulness was reduced and N3 was significantly elevated.[118] Across the next 4 nights, REM showed an initial drop to half the night 1 levels with some small recovery.[117] Total wakefulness increased on night 1 and stayed high, and N3 decreased to substantially below control levels and remained low through night 5.

Lewis and colleagues studied four naïve heroin users (themselves) pre-use, during, and postuse of 7.5 mg of heroin. REM was suppressed on the first night of use but showed recovery to near baseline levels across the next 2 nights. There was a rebound to baseline levels on the first night of withdrawal. There was some evidence of increased wakefulness and N1 with heroin use but no alterations in N3. Differences between these studies, particularly. Differences between the results of the studies, particularly in REM effects, may reflect the habituation to chronic dosing in individuals with opioid addiction.

One recent study compared individuals with opioid addiction to controls after 1 week of detoxification, with no significant withdrawal symptoms at the time of study. Nonetheless the individuals with opioid addiction showed significantly lower TST and sleep efficiency, significantly greater WASO, and significantly longer SOL than controls, with no differences in REM or N3.[119]

Although it has been hypothesized that poor sleep during opioid replacement therapy may increase the likelihood of relapse,[108,111,120] few studies have actually investigated this. Indeed, studies that have evaluated sleep in those that complete detoxification versus those who do not have not found worse sleep in the noncompleters.[121,122] However, sleep latency and TST were significant predictors of relapse in a comparison of 10 days of tapering doses of methadone and 6 days of tapering doses of lofexidine, with 2 weeks of postdrug follow-up using diaries to estimate TST, sleep latency, and WASO,[123] yet again suggesting that sleep disturbances may affect executive function. In terms of treatment for sleep disturbance, although trazadone has been shown to be ineffective at improving sleep or relapse,[120] there are promising data showing a significant benefit of cognitive behavior therapy for insomnia related to methadone maintenance therapy.[124]

Summary of Opioids and Sleep

As reflected in the AASM position paper,[102] the major sleep concern with opioids is the high risk of sleep-disordered breathing, and central apneas in particular, resulting from the respiratory suppression effects. In addition, methadone maintenance therapy and other treatment approaches are characterized by long-lasting negative effects on sleep, including difficulty initiating and maintaining stable sleep.

CLINICAL PEARL

Alcohol and other substance use disorders can have negative impacts on sleep. When dealing with patients with sleep problems, take a detailed alcohol and drug use history and consider these before prescribing pharmacotherapy. Chronic opioid therapy can disrupt sleep and increase the risk for sleep-disordered breathing.

SUMMARY

Many abused substances affect the CNS by altering neurocircuits known to have a role in the normal regulation of sleep. Acute intoxication with these substances can lead to immediate sleep disruption and chronic use to allostatic modification of said neurocircuitry, bringing the system to a new normal, adapting to the presence of the drug. This allostasis may result in somewhat normalized sleep, depending on the substance being used. Nonetheless, withdrawal will almost inevitably destabilize the system, leading to disrupted and dysfunctional sleep. For some substances the withdrawal effects may be transient; for others, such as alcohol, they may persist for long periods. In such cases, the desire for relief from the symptoms may provide a pathway to relapse and thus provide motivation for continued drug misuse, executive function deficits, and further sleep dysregulation.

Alcohol, cannabis, and opioids, as the three most prominent in terms of health care costs and public policy implications, provide examples of how drugs can affect sleep in terms of the three-stage cycle of addiction.[7] Although sleep AUD is well understood, clearly more work is needed to understand the impact of cannabis intoxication and cannabis use disorder on sleep and subsequent daily function, given the increased prevalence of its use and the increased strength of more openly available products in states and countries in which at least medicinal use is legal. Opioid use disorder remains a major health problem in the Western world, and current treatments leave patients with inadequate sleep and elevated risk of sleep-related breathing disorders. Very little is known about the impact of polysubstance abuse on sleep.

SELECTED READINGS

Babson KA, Sottile J, Morabito D. Cannabis, cannabinoids, and sleep: a review of the literature. *Curr Psychiatry Rep*. 2017;19:23.

Blanco C Volkow ND. Management of opioid use disorder in the USA: present status and future directions. *Lancet*. 2019;393:1760–1772.

Brower KJ. Insomnia, alcoholism and relapse. *Sleep Med Rev*. 2003;7:523–539.

Colrain IM, Nicholas CL, Baker FC. Alcohol and the sleeping brain. *Handb Clin Neurol*. 2014;125:415–431.

Dokkedal-Silva V, Fernandes GL, Morelhão PK, et al. Sleep, psychiatric and socioeconomic factors associated with substance use in a large population sample: a cross-sectional study. *Pharmacol Biochem Behav*. 2021;210:173274. https://doi.org/10.1016/j.pbb.2021.173274.

Ebrahim IO, et al. Alcohol and sleep I: effects on normal sleep. *Alcohol Clin Exp Res*. 2013.

Ek J, Jacobs W, Kaylor B, McCall WV. Addiction and sleep disorders. *Adv Exp Med Biol*. 2021;1297:163–171. https://doi.org/10.1007/978-3-030-61663-2_12.

Gates PJ, Albertella L, Copeland J. The effects of cannabinoid administration on sleep: a systematic review of human studies. *Sleep Med Rev*. 2014;18:477–487.

Koob GF, Colrain IM. Alcohol use disorder and sleep disturbances: a feed-forward allostatic framework. *Neuropsychopharmacology*. 2020;45:141–165.

Koob GF, Le Moal M. Drug abuse: hedonic homeostatic dysregulation. *Science*. 1997;278:52–58.

Koob GF, Volkow ND. Neurobiology of addiction: a neurocircuitry analysis. *Lancet Psychiatry*. 2016;3:760–773.

Mason BJ, et al. Gabapentin treatment for alcohol dependence: a randomized clinical trial. *JAMA Intern Med*. 2014;174:70–77.

Walker JM, et al. Chronic opioid use is a risk factor for the development of central sleep apnea and ataxic breathing. *J Clin Sleep Med*. 2007;3:455–461.

Wang D, Teichtahl H. Opioids, sleep architecture and sleep-disordered breathing. *Sleep Med Rev*. 2007;11:35–46.

A complete reference list can be found online at ExpertConsult.com.

Section 19

Dentistry and Otorhinolaryngology

Chapter 167

Dentistry and Otorhinolaryngology in Sleep Medicine: Below the Brain and Above the Larynx

Gilles Lavigne; Meir Kryger

Dentistry and otorhinolaryngology are two complementary health care professions that play a role in the assessment and management of sleep-disordered breathing, sleep bruxism, and orofacial pain syndromes, all of which can negatively impact sleep.

Otorhinolaryngologists can identify anatomic abnormalities that cause sleep-disordered breathing and manage these conditions with various surgical treatments, including hypoglossal nerve stimulation (see Chapter 175).[1] The goal is to remove or correct anatomic or functional abnormalities that contribute to sleep-disordered breathing. The nasal-pharyngeal area also poses a challenge for anesthesiologists in diagnosing obstructive sleep apnea (OSA) and in administering anesthesia (see Chapter 174).

General dentists, who examine the mouth and craniofacial structures in patients of all ages, are ideally positioned to screen for sleep-disordered breathing. Early orthodontic intervention can correct narrow dental arches, retrognathia, and short lingual frenula (see Chapter 168). These abnormalities can negatively impact breathing and craniofacial growth. Maxillofacial surgeons can apply a series of surgical treatments to correct these defects and improve breathing (see Chapter 175). Oral medicine practitioners, prosthodontists, and general dentists with training in dental sleep medicine can prescribe oral appliances and mandibular advancement devices (MAD) to manage snoring and sleep apnea or occlusal splints to prevent tooth damage induced by sleep bruxism. Comorbid orofacial pain, including temporomandibular pain and tension-type headache, is another area of dental expertise (see Chapters 168 to 173, covering orthodontics, sleep bruxism, and orofacial pain in relation to apnea and insomnia, and oral appliances to manage OSA).

Not all patients agree to or can adhere to regular use of a continuous positive airway pressure (CPAP) or MAD device. Input from psychologists, respiratory therapists, and sleep educators can help motivate patients to use these devices. For some patients, behavioral therapy could be useful.

Two general endotypes are considered in sleep apnea: (1) anatomic (e.g., retrognathia, narrow and deep palate, narrow nose, airway obstruction, fatty tongue) and (2) physiologic, including low arousal threshold causing sleep instability, low muscle tone in muscles that preserve airway patency during sleep, and irregular breathing in patients with high loop gain (see Chapters 128 and 129).[2,3]

In the case of sleep bruxism, the role of anatomic and physiologic phenotypes is less clear. In a subgroup of patients, one putative phenotype is characterized by abnormal arousals associated with autonomic nervous system dysfunction.[4] More research is needed to clarify and delineate the sleep bruxism phenotypes to guide clinicians in patient management.

The challenges for dentistry and otorhinolaryngology include deciding (1) who will identify vulnerable individuals with clinically validated and user-friendly phenotyping tools and (2) who will select the best therapeutic approaches. Artificial intelligence applied to sleep medicine is a promising avenue to improve clinical diagnosis accuracy and treatment choice. Some patients benefit from combined therapies (e.g., CPAP plus an oral appliance; or either one plus a sleep positioner, diet control, or bariatric surgery). Complementary approaches to manage sleep bruxism (see Chapter 176) and sleep apnea (see Chapter 134) can be customized for individual patient needs, social reality, motivation, and adherence. We are making significant progress toward personalized sleep medicine, which is the optimal way to provide the most effective treatment to patients with sleep disorders.[5]

In summary, dentistry and otorhinolaryngology act as partners in two sleep medicine approaches: (1) early correction to prevent and/or guide the growth of upper airway anatomic structures and (2) correction of anomalies using surgery or appliances. Do we need to reiterate that the nose and mouth allow air to reach our lungs and oxygen to reach our brain?

A complete reference list can be found online at ExpertConsult.com.

Chapter 168

Oronasopharyngeal Growth and Malformations with Orthodontic Management

Stacey Dagmar Quo; Benjamin T. Bliska; Nelly Huynh

Chapter Highlights

- Sleep-disordered breathing (SDB) is marked by varying degrees of collapsibility of the pharyngeal airway. The hard tissue boundaries of the airway dictate the size and therefore the responsiveness of the muscles that form this part of the upper airway. Thus the airway is shaped not only by the performance of the pharyngeal muscles to stimulation but also by the surrounding skeletal framework.
- The upper and lower jaws are key components of the craniofacial skeleton and the determinants of the anterior wall of the upper airway. The morphology of the jaws can be negatively altered by dysfunction of the upper airway during growth and development. In turn, the altered morphology of the jaws can be positively influenced by orthodontic treatment.
- The association between altered dentofacial morphology and SDB has been well documented in children, adults, and patients with craniofacial syndromes. Whether this disease of childhood has the same origins as adult obstructive sleep apnea but more subtle manifestations has not been determined. The length and volume of the airway increase until the age of 20 years, at which time there is a variable period of stability, followed by a slow decrease in airway size after the fifth decade of life. The possibility of addressing the early forms of this disease with the notions of intervention and prevention can change the landscape of care.
- Correction of specific skeletal anatomic deficiencies can improve or eliminate SDB symptoms in both children and adults. It is possible that the clinician may adapt or modify the growth expression, although the extent of this effect is uncertain. These strategies seek to alter an abnormal facial growth pattern wherein SDB worsens over time. Future research should focus on determining in which individuals dentofacial morphology makes a significant contribution to the pathogenesis of SDB. This may bring clinicians one step closer to targeting specific treatments that more effectively treat the disorder.

This chapter provides an integrated vision to both the scientist and clinician dealing with growth and development of the oronasopharyngeal structures. The upper airway is a unified complex of three distinct but structurally integrated, dependent, and contiguous entities: the nasal cavity, the oral cavity, and the pharynx. The first part of this chapter reviews the fundamentals of growth of the craniofacial complex and the development of the upper airway. The second section outlines those characteristics based on current definitions of the sleep-disordered breathing (SDB) syndrome; that is, there is a broad range of anthropomorphic characteristics and obstructive sleep apnea (OSA) severity that needs to be better delineated. The last section reviews management and treatment strategies based on what is known about craniofacial development and anatomy.

CRANIOFACIAL GROWTH AND DEVELOPMENT OF THE UPPER AIRWAY

Early theories of craniofacial development were based on the belief that growth of the face and jaws was essentially immutable because of intrinsic regulation by inherited genetic traits. Research centered on finding the location or sites where these traits were expressed that drove normal form and function of the other surrounding structures. During the early twentieth century, it was believed that differential deposition and resorption on the surface of bones were largely responsible for growth of the craniofacial skeleton. This remodeling theory then gave way to one heralding the role of the sutures, which held that similar to the epiphyses of the long bones, it was the connective tissue and cartilaginous joints of the craniofacial skeleton that produced expansive proliferative growth forcing the bones and soft tissues away from each other.[1] Exemplifying this theory was the concept that the mandible was much like a horseshoe-shaped long bone, with the condylar cartilage acting like open-ended epiphyseal plates, pushing the mandible down and away from the rest of the head.

Several inconsistencies in the hypothesis that sutures alone could be the determinants of craniofacial growth surfaced. Sutural growth was more similar to periosteal apposition of bone than previously understood, and sutures acted as reactive sites of bone growth rather than growth centers. Scott, in 1953, proposed the nasal septum theory of growth, which held as its main tenet that the anterior and inferior growth of the nasal septal cartilage was the determining, driving force of facial growth.[2] Whereas Scott's theory contributed to the understanding that growth at the sutures and surface remodeling were essentially reactive sites of bone growth, it was still founded in the paradigm that craniofacial development and morphogenesis were genetically predetermined and unalterable.[1] In modern perspective, the nasal septal cartilage is considered an important growth center; however, the mechanism behind this growth has been appropriately updated as described here.

A fundamental shift in the field of craniofacial biology emerged with Moss's introduction of the functional matrix hypothesis in the early sixties.[3] Previous theories deemed craniofacial growth to be predetermined by genetic traits. The functional paradigm introduced the idea of plasticity of development and growth of the craniofacial skeleton.[1] According to this theory, (1) the role of our genes was to initiate the process by setting the initial context under which development could occur; and (2) extrinsic environmental and functional demands of the various craniofacial components determined all future aspects of growth. Subsequent research has shown much of the functional demands, described by Moss, lay in the nervous system and from control of the musculature, where aberrant neuronal function[4] or innervation[5] contribute to abnormal craniofacial growth and development. This theory revolutionized the field by introducing two important concepts. First, it brought the possibility of growth modification as a treatment option for malocclusions or facial malformations by changing the direction of facial development to a more desired outcome. Second and perhaps more important, the plasticity of development opened a new area of research, focusing on the critical time and specific factors that lead to the maladaptive plasticity of the form and function of the craniofacial complex.[6]

With the emergence of developmental molecular biology, the genetic and external or epigenetic regulation of craniofacial growth is now better understood, and the modern synthesis is that both genomic and epigenetic factors are necessary contributors to craniofacial development.[7,8] Several genes and gene products regulate the morphogenesis and intrauterine development of the craniofacial complex. There is an extremely complex interaction between these genetic factors and epigenetic influences of the maternal environment. Recent animal studies have demonstrated that prenatal exposure to nicotine,[9] excessive thyroxine,[10] and maternal stress[11] can have varying effects on subsequent craniofacial and/or mandibular morphology and growth. The plasticity of early craniofacial development and response to functional demands depends not only on the effects of certain environmental conditions on the underlying genetic code; previous environmental conditions may have directly upregulated or downregulated specific genetic regulatory factors and indirectly further influenced the response.

Prenatal Craniofacial Growth

The earliest form of the face appears in the fourth week of life with the enlargement and movement of the frontonasal prominence, as well as the paired maxillary and mandibular prominences stemming from the first branchial arch. These five prominences emerge to encircle the stomodeum, or primitive mouth. A critical aspect of this process is the migration of cranial neural crest cells into the developing facial prominences. Unlike in the rest of the body, these neural crest cells develop into the majority of the craniofacial hard tissues, including the bone, cartilage, and teeth of the craniofacial complex.[12] The specific end tissue into which these cranial neural crest cells develop is determined largely by the family of Homeobox or *HOX* genes. The variable expression of *HOX* transcription factors causes the groups of cranial neural crest cells in the distinct prominences to respond differently to the same growth factors.[13]

After rapid growth of the two mandibular prominences, there is midline fusion in the fifth week of development.[14] Initial mandibular development is dependent on tightly controlled molecular signaling between the oral ectoderm and the underlying core of cranial neural crest cells.[12] Further development is contingent on the formation and growth of Meckel cartilage, the first skeletal element of the mandible. The subsequent elongation of this rod of cartilage leads to promotion of outgrowth of the mandible, and the primary ossification of the mandible occurs as intramembranous bone formation along this cartilaginous core.[15] As the bony mandible further develops, Meckel cartilage largely disappears, eventually to persist only as small portions of the incus and malleus of the middle ear. In addition to the mandible, the mandibular processes also form the lower lip and the lower areas of the cheeks.

The lateral and medial nasal processes originate as ectodermal thickenings on the surface of the frontonasal process early in the fifth week of embryonic life. Subsequent broadening of the head and medial growth of the maxillary processes result in medial displacement of the early nasal processes. As the two medial nasal processes merge at the midline, the philtrum and columella of the nose are formed. Deeper aspects of the medial nasal processes will differentiate to form the nasal septum, which is a key growth center of the midface postnatally. Fusion of the medial nasal process with the maxillary process leads to formation of the majority of the upper lip, the zygomas, and the maxilla bilaterally. The lateral nasal processes go on to form the sides and alae of the nose as the subsequent 2 weeks sees the formation of the future nostrils and nasal cavity with the development of the primary and secondary palates.[16] Secondary palate formation relies on the coordinated growth and movement of the primordia of the tongue and both lower and upper jaws. During the sixth week of development, paired lateral palatal shelves arise as medial projections from each maxillary process. Critically, at this time, there is rapid anterior growth of the early mandible by proliferation of Meckel cartilage, which displaces the tongue forward, lowering it relative to the palatal shelves.[17] Once the tongue has descended, during the seventh week, the palatal shelves rotate from a vertical to a horizontal position directed toward the midline. Further growth of the shelves sees them fuse at the midline, as well as with the primary palate anteriorly and the nasal septum superiorly.[18]

By the ninth week of fetal development, the initial cartilaginous facial skeleton is well established, composed of the chondrocranium forming the skull base, the nasal capsule in the upper face, and the Meckel cartilage in the lower face. Within the 12th week of fetal growth, areas of ossification appear and bone begins to rapidly replace this cartilaginous template to form the early cranial base. At this same time, the bones of the cranial vault, as well as the mandible and maxilla, develop through intramembranous ossification.

Postnatal Craniofacial Growth

The general pattern of postnatal development is the cephalocaudal gradient of growth, in which there is an axis of increased growth that extends away from the head. Structures away from the brain tend to grow more and later than those structures closer to the brain. Mandibular growth begins later and continues longer than does the growth of the midface.[19] This pattern of growth continues until maturity and is exemplified in the proportionality of head size to total body length. At birth, the head makes up almost a quarter of the total body length, which decreases to around 12% in the adult. Facial growth can be summarized as being driven forward initially by growth of the cranial base, then the maxilla and mandible both grow back and up to fill in the space created as they are being pulled down and forward away from the cranial base by the soft tissues in which they are embedded.

During infancy and early childhood, the cranial base increases in length through endochondral ossification that occurs at important growth sites called synchondroses. The synchondroses push the growth of the face forward until around the age of 7 years, when they begin to become less active and later ossify and fuse. Much of the forward movement of the maxilla is due to the growth of the cranial base pushing it downward and forward from behind. Further forward displacement of the maxilla results from bone apposition at the sutures located posteriorly and superiorly that connect it to the cranial base. Unlike the forward displacement generated by the synchondroses, the bone formation at these sutures is instead responsive in nature to the downward and forward pull of the maxilla from the growth of the associated soft tissues and nasal septum. Much of the increase in size of both the nasal and oral cavities occurs from surface remodeling of the maxilla and not from sutural growth. As the maxilla is translated downward and forward, the periosteum acts to remove bone at the floor of the nose, while at the same time bone is formed on the roof of the mouth. Over time, this results in a hollowing out and widening of the nasal cavity.[20] In addition, the palatal vault deepens with age despite the bone apposition on its surface because of the increased growth of the alveolar process that accompanies tooth eruption. Transverse growth in maxillary width results from growth at the midpalatal suture and appositional remodeling along the lateral aspects of the posterior region of the maxilla and the maxillary tuberosity.[21] This bone deposition at the tuberosity allows sagittal lengthening of the maxilla. The midpalatal suture begins to fuse in early adolescence but stays amenable to orthopedic force required for maxillary expansion treatment until around the age of 14 years in most individuals.

Lacking open sutures necessary for suture apposition of bone, the mandible instead grows by endochondral ossification at the condyle, as well as by a combination of extensive surface bone remodeling. Unlike an epiphyseal plate or synchondroses, the growth of the condyle is responsive to translation of the mandible rather than driving it.[22] Transverse increases in the body of the mandible occur through surface apposition and remodeling of bone. The dentoalveolar structures develop with the eruption of the teeth, which continue to erupt throughout life to maintain occlusal contact, matching the vertical growth of the ramus.

First described in 1930,[23] the hard and soft tissues undergo different rates of growth throughout childhood development. This is evident in the upper airway of children and has important implications for obstructive sleep disorders. Because of the significance of suckling to the newborn infant, the epiglottis is located close to the soft palate, which facilitates separation of the pathways for respiration and deglutition.[24] Neonates are born as obligate or preferential nasal breathers, but this changes as the upper airway matures. Between the ages of 1 and 2 years, vertical growth allows the larynx to descend to the level of the fifth cervical vertebra, and the epiglottis descends, which accommodates the newly acquired function of speech for the child.[25] The hyoid bone descends to a lower position in the neck, and the posterior third of the tongue descends to form the anterior wall of the oropharynx. Mainly as a result of hypertrophy of the adenoids and tonsils that frequently can exceed the growth of surrounding skeletal structures, adenoid and tonsillar tissue is found to be largest relative to the surrounding anatomy between the ages of 4 and 6 years.[26-28] This not coincidentally is the same age range at which OSA is most frequently seen in children. The upper airway volume then increases in adolescence because of both the concurrent increase in vertical skeletal growth and involution of the lymphoid tissue, which decreases in size after 12 years of age.[27,29] During the adolescent years, the upper airway also becomes larger in the transverse dimension and more elliptical.[29] The length and volume of the airway increase until the age of 20 years, at which time there is a variable period of stability, followed by a slow decrease in airway size after the fifth decade of life.[30]

DENTOFACIAL MORPHOLOGY ASSOCIATED WITH SLEEP-DISORDERED BREATHING

Dentofacial morphology in children and in adults has been assessed by lateral and anterior-posterior cephalography, dental casts of the upper and lower teeth, digital photography, and three-dimensional magnetic resonance imaging (MRI).[31] Cephalography is limited by landmark identification, measurement variability, and two-dimensional assessment of a three-dimensional anatomy. In children, only a few studies assess three-dimensional dentofacial measures.[32,33] However, all these imaging methods are performed while the patient is either awake or sedated, which does not reflect upper airway volume and soft tissue sleep-related changes. Whereas dentofacial morphology is an important component to the multidisciplinary assessment and management of SDB, no single cephalometric measurement that can effectively predict OSA severity.[34] Only in a select few diagnosed patients can dentofacial morphology be considered the main cause of adult OSA.[35] Moreover, most phenotypic definitions of OSA underline the strong participation of the upper airway function in the pathophysiology (see also Chapters 128 and 129 on phenotyping in relation to sleep breathing disorders).[35]

Children

In children, although adenotonsillar hypertrophy and obesity often contribute to SDB, dentofacial morphology can further contribute to the narrowing of the upper airway. Furthermore, a recent study suggested that persistent SDB after adenotonsillar surgery was observed in children with compromised dentofacial morphology.[36] Behavioral or functional oral breathing in SDB is associated with altered craniofacial growth,[37] altered muscle recruitment in the nasal and oral cavities,[38] and change in posture.[39] These ideas will be further explored in this chapter, in the section on treatment strategies. For children between 6 and 8 years, dentofacial morphology is a stronger risk factor for SDB than obesity is.[40] Cephalometric studies suggest that a long and narrow face, transverse deficiency, and retrognathia are craniofacial morphologic factors associated with a narrow upper airway and SDB in children,[41] which are also particular to oral breathing.[42]

Studies measuring differences in position between the maxilla and mandible (ANB: A point, nasion, B point) show an increased ANB angle in children with OSA or with primary snoring compared with controls.[43,44] In the primary snorers, this was associated with a decreased SNB angle (sella, nasion, B point),[43] which is a measure of retrognathia. In children with OSA, a decreased SNB angle and lower hyoid bone position and mandibular volume[33] were observed with three-dimensional imaging.

An increased mandibular plane angle and increased lower anterior facial height are associated with OSA.[32,37,43,44] However, a meta-analysis showed significant heterogeneity across selected studies,[32,43-47] suggesting insufficient evidence of a strong association. Retrognathia creates a posterior displacement of the tongue base, which further narrows the upper airway and is associated with a high-arched (ogival) palate due to tongue position.[47] Although a narrow maxilla is associated with OSA and snoring, only a few studies have reported this from dental impressions of hard and soft tissues,[45,46] as this cannot be measured from lateral cephalograms. Moreover, orthodontic correction of a narrow maxilla (rapid maxillary expansion) has been reported to reduce respiratory indexes.[48,49] These earlier studies suggesting an association between morphology and sleep apnea do not fully explain causality of dentofacial morphology in the pathophysiologic process of SDB.

In children with OSA, it was suggested that 50% also have sleep bruxism, a concomitant sleep movement disorder[50] that can affect their dentofacial health, although no causal relationship has been established. Parents report tooth grinding twice more often in children who are habitual snorers than in nonsnorers and more often in younger children than in older ones.[51] Up to 60% of children with sleep bruxism but without sleep apnea have a retrusive mandible; 28% have short faces (brachyfacial type).[52] Adenotonsillectomy reduced sleep bruxism muscle activity in 75% of OSA children as reported by questionnaires.[53] A temporary maxillary occlusal splint of 3 mm in thickness was worn 3 months by children (aged 6–8 years) with a history of sleep bruxism, oral breathing, and snoring.[54] As reported by questionnaires, tooth-grinding noises were decreased in 89% of patients, whereas snoring was reduced in 55.5% of patients.[54] This could be explained by potentially restoring nasal breathing during sleep as all participants adapted from oral breathing to nasal breathing after treatment.[54] The associations between SDB and sleep bruxism in children need further investigation and objective data. A full description of sleep bruxism is found in Chapters 169 and 170.

Adults

In adults, obesity is the main anatomic risk factor for SDB. Like in children, dentofacial morphology can also contribute to a compromised upper airway, and this is more often observed in nonobese patients with OSA.[55]

Overall, studies have reported that a retrusive mandible, macroglossia, lowered hyoid bone position, and/or retrusive maxilla can be associated with the presence of OSA[31,55-57] and snoring.[57] A lower hyoid bone position is suggested to be a proxy of tongue shape, posture, and tone, which could increase upper airway collapsibility.[31] MRI studies in Asian and white populations observed a shorter and smaller mandible in patients with sleep apnea than in controls.[58] This was significant in men with sleep apnea and not reported in women.[31] Mandibular morphology seems to be a stronger risk factor than maxillary morphology for OSA in adults.[58] Taking into account the genetic influence on dentofacial morphology, comparison of a cohort of siblings with and without sleep apnea found a short mandible and a lower hyoid bone position to be the most important risk factors for sleep apnea.[59]

Palatal morphology and increased length and thickness of the soft palate are also risk factors for OSA and for snoring.[60] In addition, patients with sleep apnea are reported to have longer soft palates than snorers.[57] In comparing lateral cephalograms and dental casts of OSA adults with those of controls, an increased palatal depth was seen as measured at the first and second premolars and molars,[61] although this was not a consistent finding.[62] By anteroposterior cephalometric measurements and three-dimensional analyses, patients with OSA had narrower maxillas.[63]

Craniofacial Syndromes

Multiple craniofacial syndromes can have a higher incidence of SDB because of modified craniofacial morphology or hypertrophy of soft tissues. Outlined in Table 168.1, among the mandibular hypoplasia syndromes are Pierre Robin, Prader-Willi, Treacher Collins, and Marfan. Moreover, some syndromes can be associated with neuromuscular disorders, which can further negatively affect breathing during sleep. In children with craniofacial syndromes and SDB, the causes of obstruction or restriction of the upper airway can be at multiple levels, requiring multidisciplinary management and multiple treatments.[64-66]

SDB is often associated in children with midface hypoplasia; 50% of nonsyndromic and syndromic craniosynostosis children,[67] such as children with Apert, Crouzon, and Pfeiffer syndromes, develop SDB.[65] SDB improves during the first 3 years of life in the absence of midface hypoplasia.[68] However, this is not observed in children with syndromic craniosynostosis and midface hypoplasia (Apert or Crouzon/Pfeiffer).[68] Midface advancement surgery was successful in the short term with improved respiratory outcomes in 55% but was ineffective in 45% of children.[65] In this latter group, endoscopy and volume measurements showed obstruction of the hypopharynx.[65] After adenotonsillectomy, 60% of children with

Table 168.1 Syndromic and Craniofacial Morphology Associated with Obstructive Sleep Apnea

- Maxillary hypoplasia or mid-face hypoplasia, **such as syndromic craniosynostosis (Apert, Crouzon, Pfeiffer), achondroplasia, trisomy 21, and cleft palate**
- Mandibular hypoplasia, such as Pierre-Robin, Prader-Willi, Treacher Collins, and Marfant
- Mandibular hypoplasia or micrognathia, such as Pierre-Robin, Smith-Lemli-Opitz syndrome, and trisomy 21
- Orofacial hypotonia, such as Smith-Lemli-Opitz syndrome, and trisomy 21
- Cleft lip and palate, such as Pierre-Robin
- Maxillary and mandibular hypoplasia, such as Turner syndrome
- Neuromuscular disorders, such as Duchenne muscular dystrophy, myopathies, Guillain-Barré syndrome, and myasthenia gravis

syndromic craniosynostosis had less desaturation events (arterial blood oxygen saturation [Sao_2] 4%).[64] Achondroplasia, an autosomal dominant congenital disorder, is also characterized by midface hypoplasia, leading to increased risks for development of SDB. Approximately 35% of patients with achondroplasia have SDB,[69] associated with increased lower facial height and retrognathia.[70]

In addition to midface hypoplasia, patients with trisomy 21 also have micrognathia and orofacial hypotonia, which predisposes them to SDB,[71] as found in 50% of pediatric and adult cases.[66] Although suggested as the first-line treatment, adenotonsillectomy resolves SDB in only 27% to 34% of cases in patients with trisomy 21.[72,73] Other alternative treatments are positive airway pressure therapy, mandibular distraction osteogenesis, midface advancement, and oral appliances. Oral appliances with tongue-stimulating knobs have been shown to improve orofacial muscle function.[66]

Cleft lip and palate children showing midface hypoplasia have a significantly higher incidence of SDB (22%–37.5%)[74,75] than do healthy children (5%).[76] Furthermore, 34% of syndromic children with cleft lip and palate reported symptoms, whereas 17% of nonsyndromic children with cleft lip and palate did.[74] After various surgical interventions (e.g., adenotonsillectomy, flap takedown, tonsillectomy, and partial adenoidectomy), only 38.5% of patients had improved SDB.[74]

Syndromes characterized by micrognathia and orofacial hypotonia, such as Smith-Lemli-Opitz syndrome, or by smaller maxilla and mandible, such as Turner syndrome, can also have increased incidence of SDB.[77,78]

Pierre Robin sequence is characterized by a triad of craniofacial anomalies consisting of micrognathia, cleft palate, and glossoptosis leading to respiratory and feeding issues. Most infants with Pierre Robin sequence (85%) also have sleep breathing disorders.[79] Nonsurgical management of Pierre Robin sequence in infants includes positional therapy, placement of nasopharyngeal airway, and oral appliances with velar extension. Positional therapy is successful in 49% to 52% of cases.[80,81] Oral appliances with velar extension were reported in one study to effectively reduce OSA at hospital discharge and 3 months later, in the absence of any adverse events.[82] Surgical management includes tongue-lip adhesion or glossopexy, subperiosteal release of the floor of the mouth, mandibular distraction osteogenesis, and tracheotomy. Mandibular distraction osteogenesis is reported to have better outcome measures than tongue-lip adhesion in regard to oxygen saturation, apnea-hypopnea index (AHI), and number of post-procedure tracheostomies.[83] However, both surgeries had comparable complications.[83]

MANAGEMENT AND TREATMENT STRATEGIES

Management and treatment acknowledge that SDB can be a dysfunction that both affects and results from deficits in the upper and lower airways. There can be a cumulative positive feedback loop in which repetitive respiratory-related arousals cause changes to the properties of the upper airway, and this causes end-stage sequelae that exacerbate the initial stimulus.[84] This section focuses on the treatment strategies for the pediatric patient. For more information on adult SDB treatment, refer to Section 14 of this volume.

The indication for treatment underlies what is pathologic and what is normal. What constitutes abnormal breathing as a disease that necessitates treatment? Snoring carries consequences of cognitive impairments, suggesting that benign primary snoring, in specific cases, should be treated as a disease. The incidence of snoring is much higher than the incidence of OSA,[85] and snoring, as the start of the cascade of abnormal breathing, is now recognized as an abnormality in children.[86] Even with early intervention, the recurrence of SDB has been documented in studies of pediatric patients observed through adolescence.[87] So, although the timing of treatment is relevant, early detection and treatment of SDB children are only part of the solution because there can be a familial inheritance of both symptoms and anatomic risk factors.[88] Consequently, asymptomatic children with at-risk morphologic characteristics and a familial history of SDB should be monitored for further evaluation. Although much pediatric screening has traditionally focused on the presence of snoring, other nighttime breathing abnormalities associated with SDB have been described. These include flow limitations, tachypnea, thoracoabdominal asynchrony, obstructive cycling and oral breathing. However, only oral breathing is a readily witnessed symptom and will be the focus of this section.

There is not a linear relationship of symptoms to severity of the disease, and similarly, if there is a disproportion in anatomic structures, it may not necessarily correlate with the symptoms or the severity of the disease.[89] A study that observed SDB children 4 years after treatment showed that despite the improvement in respiratory parameters, complaints of daytime sleepiness persisted in the treated and untreated SDB group compared with asymptomatic, non-SDB controls. For the health care practitioner treating children, there are screening measures to decide if a child needs further care. Again, see Section 14 of this volume for more information on SDB and OSA diagnosis and management. These factors can be distilled down to the presence of daytime or nighttime symptoms, the orofacial anatomy, and the familial history of SDB (Box 168.1). The intent of early treatment is to ameliorate the disorder, halt the continued cycle of worsening OSA, and prevent early systemic complications. The consequences of neurocognitive deficits and cardiovascular changes are evident in children,[90] similar to the systemic changes seen

Box 168.1 SCREENING MEASURES FOR PEDIATRIC TREATMENT

Presence of daytime and nighttime symptoms
Orofacial anatomy
Familial history

Box 168.2 CURATIVE STRATEGIES FOR PEDIATRIC OBSTRUCTIVE SLEEP APNEA SYNDROME

Increase in airway size (nasal cavity, nasopharynx, oropharynx, hypopharynx)
Improvement in function
Alteration of craniofacial growth

in adults. It is possible that OSA in an adult could have begun in childhood or adolescence. Although there are no long-term outcome studies that demonstrate the progression of these changes from childhood into adulthood with end-organ morbidity, recent evidence suggests that early neural impairments of praxia and gnosia, both problems of higher order cortical processing, present in both children and adults as the same disorder.[91]

There are three general treatment strategies for SDB. The problem of collapsibility affecting airflow exchange in SDB can be primarily related to inadequate airway size creating airflow resistance, and the first line of treatment is directed at enlarging the airway. MRI studies of OSA children show a smaller upper airway cross-sectional area. However, children with normal oronasopharyngeal anatomy may suffer from OSA,[92] and the AHI has not been shown to directly correlate with airway volume.[89] First-line treatment approaches to increasing space in the nasal cavity, nasopharynx, oropharynx, and hypopharynx are reviewed. SDB may also encompass a component of muscle alteration that may be a primary (etiologic) or secondary effect.[84] The second component of therapy addresses the alterations in function as a consequence of muscle remodeling, myopathy and neuropathy that may be associated with SDB. The third strategy incorporates the challenge to complete care, and that raises the question of whether a cure or complete resolution of the disease is possible by changing the underlying facial growth pattern and modifying the anatomy to eliminate structure as an etiologic factor in the disease. This paradigm for care is summarized in Box 168.2.

Strategy 1: Increase in Airway Size

Although the area of greatest collapsibility is the soft tissue of the oropharynx, the properties along the entire upper airway will affect this collapsibility. Each part of the pharynx (i.e., nasopharynx, oropharynx, hypopharynx) serves different functional roles, and so treatments to increase airway size are reviewed according to location in the upper airway (Figure 168.1), at 4 anatomic sites: *nasal, nasopharynx, oropharynx*, and *hypopharynx.*

Nasal Cavity Site

It is obvious the entrance to the airway at the initial site of airflow is the nasal cavity. The nasal influences on snoring

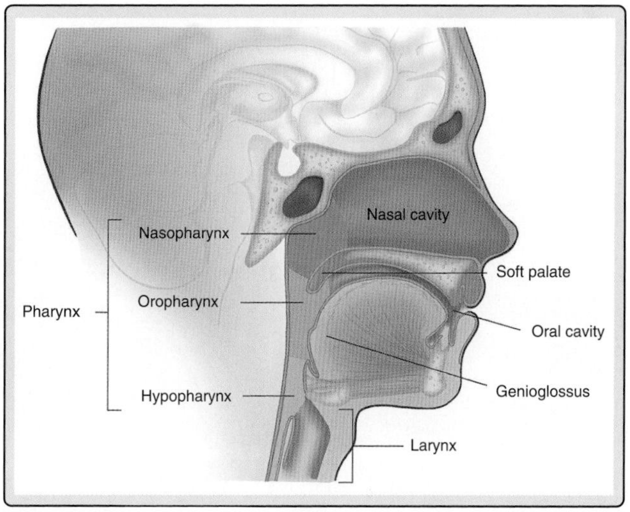

Figure 168.1 The upper airway: nasal cavity, nasopharynx, oropharynx, and hypopharynx.

and SDB are widely known because nasal obstruction can cause sleep disturbances that affect daytime performance. The degree of nasal obstruction does not correlate with the severity of OSA,[93] probably because the extent of nasal resistance does not correlate with the amount of nasal airflow.[94] This is evident in patients with choanal atresia who have nasal obstruction as a clinical feature. In this population, it was reported that 65% are diagnosed with OSA[95] versus the entire patient group. Systematic review of the relationship between nasal obstruction and OSA shows that nasal obstruction plays a modulating role in OSA but is not a direct causative factor.[96] Whereas the relationship between nasal obstruction and SDB is not linear, it is thought either to be linked to an increase in nasal resistance initiating unstable oral breathing or to result from impaired nasal reflexes that hinder continued ventilation. Increased nasal resistance depresses the critical closing pressure of the pharyngeal muscle walls, rendering the airway more collapsible. The critical closing pressure is correlated with the severity of SDB.[89] Pharyngeal compliance is impaired in a cycle in which SDB can both result from and be worsened by nasal obstruction.[97]

Orthodontic Expansion: Transverse Nasomaxillary Widening. Early studies of maxillary expansion, using an orthodontic screw type expander attached to the dentition, show that both dentoalveolar and craniofacial structural changes were created.[98] The amount, location, and rate of force application to the facial skeleton from expansion appliances create localized changes in the bony housing surrounding the teeth. This occurs with a potential effect at the sutural level of the maxilla. Rapid maxillary expansion (RME), which refers to a rate of expansion of at least 0.25 mm/day, was described in the medical literature dating back to 1975 as a therapy for medical ailments and referenced in the dental literature for medical problems since 1974.[99,100] This early work described maxillary expansion to treat problems such as enuresis, nasal congestion, and asthma. These conditions are also present in patients with OSA, although the term OSA syndrome was not coined until 1976.[101]

In 1980 surgical widening of the maxilla to increase the lateral dimension of the nasopharynx was first described as

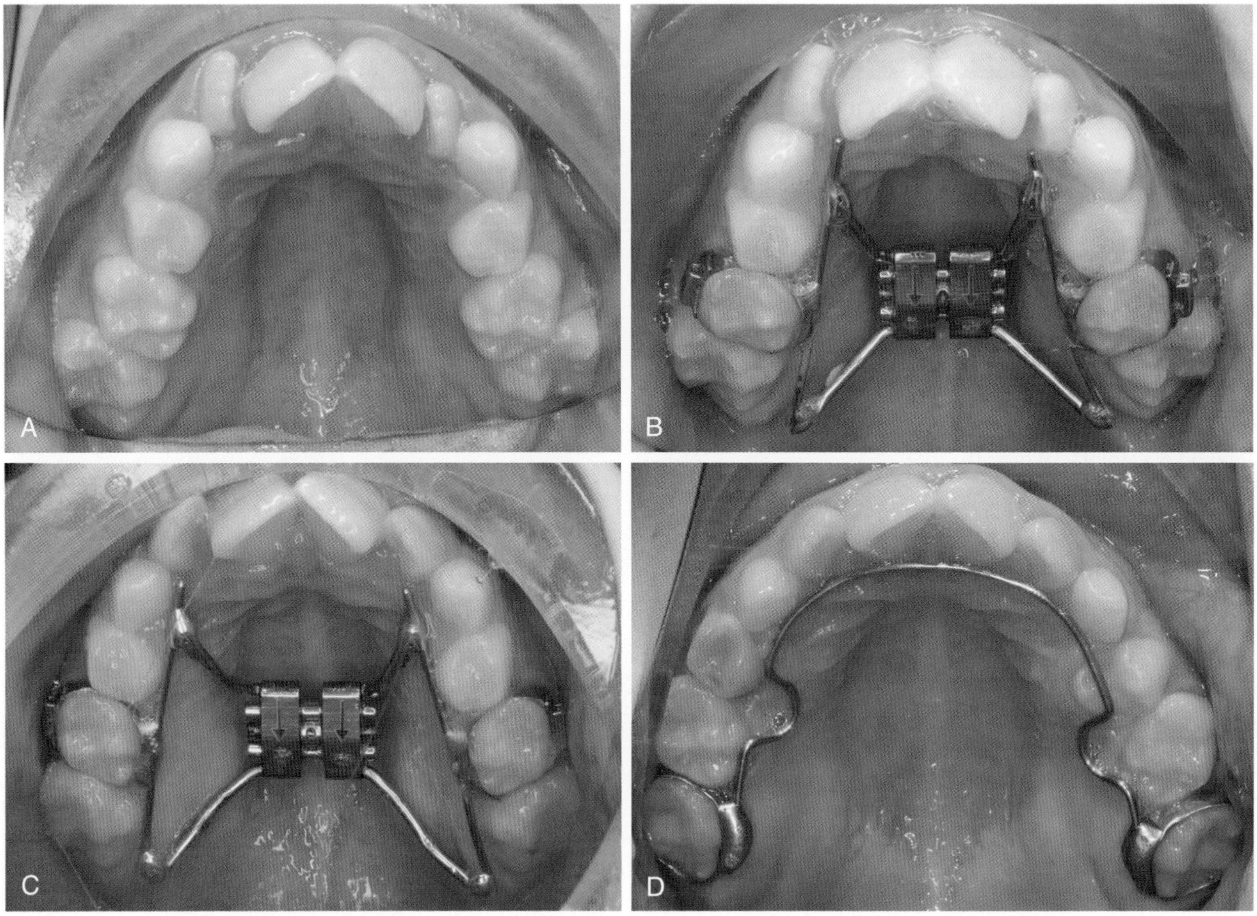

Figure 168.2 Rapid maxillary expansion. **A,** Initial shape. **B,** Insertion of first expander. **C,** Insertion of second expander. **D,** Retaining device to maintain the expansion.

a treatment for adult OSA. Nonsurgical rapid palatal expansion was first suggested as a therapy for OSA in 1998.[102] Pirelli and collaborators[103] published seminal work in 2004 using RME to successfully treat the OSA syndrome in children with a narrow maxilla. Several other groups have corroborated this work, and now other published studies also describe the effectiveness of maxillary expansion in treating children with or without narrow palates, with or without retrognathic mandibles. The general appliance design is depicted in Figure 168.2, *B*. In the maxilla, the applied force from the expansion appliance creates midpalatal (also called median palatal or palatal) suture separation. This results in distraction osteogenesis across the palate and it results in an increase in both the width of the maxilla and the transverse labio-nostril support (Figure 168.3).[104,105] Both the oral and nasal volume is increased as the triangular nasal fossa is enlarged by widening the nasal inlet, the nasal floor, and outward movement of the lateral nasal walls.[104] Because the functional space of two different structures is enlarged, nasomaxillary expansion is a more appropriate description, although the historical literature is cited as rapid maxillary expansion.[102]

Several studies show that maxillary expansion reduces nasal resistance, with a moderate level of evidence that RME therapy in a growing child causes increases in nasal cavity width and in

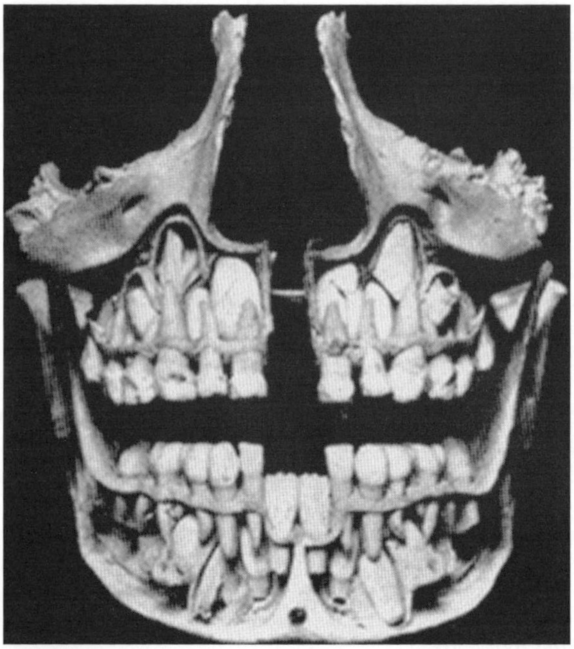

Figure 168.3 Maxillary expansion across the midpalatal suture and concurrent nasal cavity expansion. The erupting teeth provide transverse labionostril support.

the posterior nasal airway, associated with reduced nasal resistance and increased total nasal flow.[106] The stability of the results can be expected for at least 11 months after the orthopedic therapy.[107] In one study, nasal airflow measured by rhinomanometry improved in the supine position in 65% of the patients.[108] Changes in nasal geometry were evident with increases in intranasal width, nasal cross-sectional area, and nasal volume.[104] Airway properties were examined, showing decreases in nasal resistance measured by rhinomanometry[104] and acoustic rhinometry, along with changes in head position and decreases in the craniocervical angle.[109] RME therapy through sutural opening creates an increase in the nasal cavity width, area, and volume in children, allowing a reduction in nasal resistance.

The majority of children responded to expansion therapy, and OSA was eliminated in a few children.[110] Most expansion studies looked at children with narrow upper jaws (selection criteria for treatment) and malocclusions, including crossbites, dental crowding, and mandibular retrusion. Expansion as a first-line therapy was initiated in a few of the studies. Mandibular retrusion was not specifically a factor in selection of patients, although it was noted in more than half of the patients studied. Two of the studies used bimaxillary expansion.[111,112] Bimaxillary expansion was employed because of the dental compensation in both the maxilla and mandible from a narrowed maxilla. The dentition is tipped inward toward the tongue, which creates a narrowed intraoral space. Dental expansion of the lower dentition aids in achieving maximum skeletal expansion of the upper jaw. The effectiveness of bimaxillary expansion as a treatment option for pediatric SDB was first described a decade ago.[113] The overall expansion data of all studies are varied, but mostly with a general improvement in both sleep parameters and subjective symptoms of SDB. The therapeutic effects of nasomaxillary expansion include increasing space for dental crowding, increasing airway dimensions, and decreasing nasal resistance in addition to treating SDB.

Maxillary expansion is a common noninvasive orthodontic treatment that is well tolerated by children. Advantages as therapy for SDB include little or no risk of morbidity or discomfort, with treatment performed in an outpatient setting during a 4- to 6-month period. There is a high level of acceptance for initiating this type of therapy, especially because many children with SDB also have concomitant dental crowding. The reported risks of RME therapy include bite opening, relapse, microtrauma of the temporomandibular joint and the midpalatal suture, gingival recession, and root resorption.[107,114] Whereas these effects are not usually encountered, the incidence is also age dependent, seen more with maturation. There are no current guidelines for selection of patients, other than the studies that treated children with narrow palates and dental crossbites, in which teeth of the upper arch do not horizontally overlap teeth of the lower arch. Future work will help identity which types of patients will benefit most, how much expansion can be gained, and at what age to initiate expansion.

Whereas the expansion results for SDB are promising, these studies were not controlled or randomized and were limited to only a few groups that reported data. Few new therapies of pediatric SDB have been validated with randomized controlled trials. Current pediatric guidelines recommend referring children with maxillary transverse narrowing for orthodontic therapy and possible RME treatment for persistent OSA syndrome after adenotonsillectomy.[115] Orthodontic expansion therapy has three potential effects for the child with SDB. It can widen the intranasal volume to reduce nasal resistance, which improves airway collapsibility and SDB; it can facilitate other SDB treatments, such as positive pressure therapy or allergy management, by allowing improved nasal airflow; and it can facilitate the transition from oral to nasal respiration, which can have a secondary effect on oronasopharyngeal growth. The effect of RME on orofacial growth and facilitating nasal respiration is discussed in the next part of this chapter.

RME appliances use the dentition for force delivery, but there can be unwanted tooth movement side effects that accompany the skeletal change. Removable appliances that attach to the teeth to change the muscle tension on the underlying bone have been used with a small degree of success. More recently, palatal bone anchored expansion appliances offer greater nasal cavity expansion because the dentition is bypassed, which minimizes the side effects to the adjacent teeth and periodontium.[116] The dental movement precludes further skeletal expansion because the teeth move at a rate faster than that of the maxillary skeleton—a ratio of about 3:1 for older adolescents and 2:1 in children with primary or mixed dentition.[117] If the expansion appliance is anchored to the dentition, the amount of skeletal nasal cavity expansion is limited by the concurrent dental expansion.[118] There are now three types of maxillary transverse widening expansion devices, which are categorized by the site of attachment (Figure 168.4): The attachment can be anchored (1) solely to the teeth (Figure 168.4, *A*), (2) in hybrid attachment to both bone and teeth or bone and tissue (Figures 168.4, *B* and *C*), or (3) solely to the bone (Figure 168.4, *D*). The volumetric increase with RME is evident in the nasal fossa, but not posteriorly in the nasopharynx.[105] Recent work using bone borne transverse expansion shows greater promise in improving nasal airflow because increased expansion is evident in the posterior maxilla, suggesting a greater reduction in nasal resistance throughout the nasal cavity and extending to the nasopharynx (Figure 168.5); this yields improvement in SDB and associated symptoms. The same amount of posterior maxillary expansion, not evident in traditional tooth-borne expansion, has been seen in both children and adults.[116] Subsequently bone borne expansion with endoscopic bony surgical separation for the adult patient has been used as an adjunct in combination therapies and also as a stand-alone SDB treatment (Figure 168.6).

Because orthodontic expansion is easily tolerated by the pediatric patient, it can be used more than once during growth of a given individual, as seen in Figure 168.2. However, some type of holding or retaining appliance may be needed for many years and so there is long-term ongoing care. The length of this time is dependent on the eruption status of the dentition and the ability to sustain nasal respiration.

Greater changes in nasal width were evidenced when expansion was done early in maturation versus late in maturation.[119] This suggests that RME therapy should be considered as an early-stage treatment in pediatric SDB, as the intervention timing seems critical for predicting RME orthopedic outcomes. The emphasis on treatment "timing" is further described in Strategy 3 in this chapter.

Surgical Expansion: Removal of Soft Tissue. Turbinate hypertrophy and septal deviations may contribute to nasal

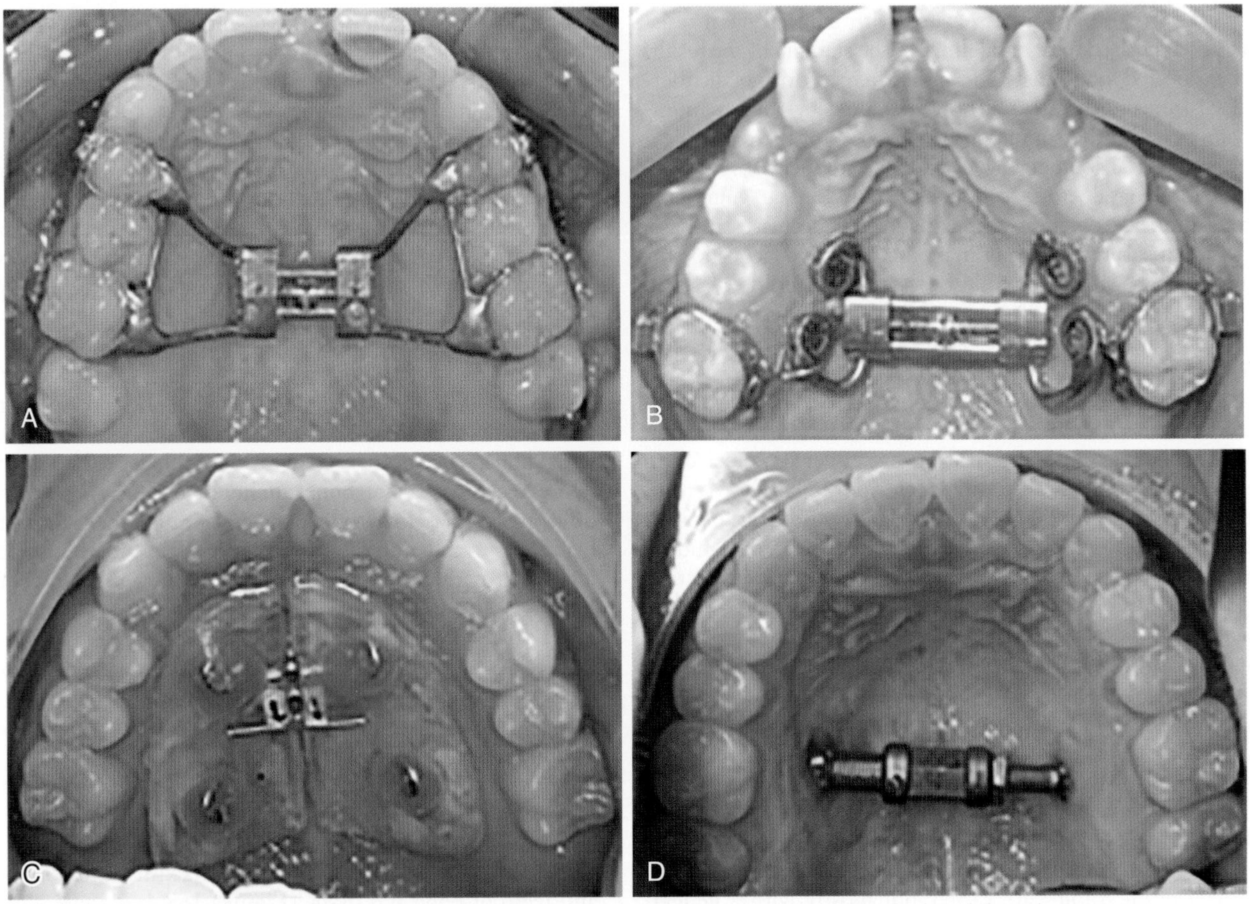

Figure 168.4 Maxillary transverse widening expansion devices. **A,** Tooth borne. **B,** Hybrid tooth/bone borne. **C,** Hybrid tissue/bone borne. **D,** Bone borne.

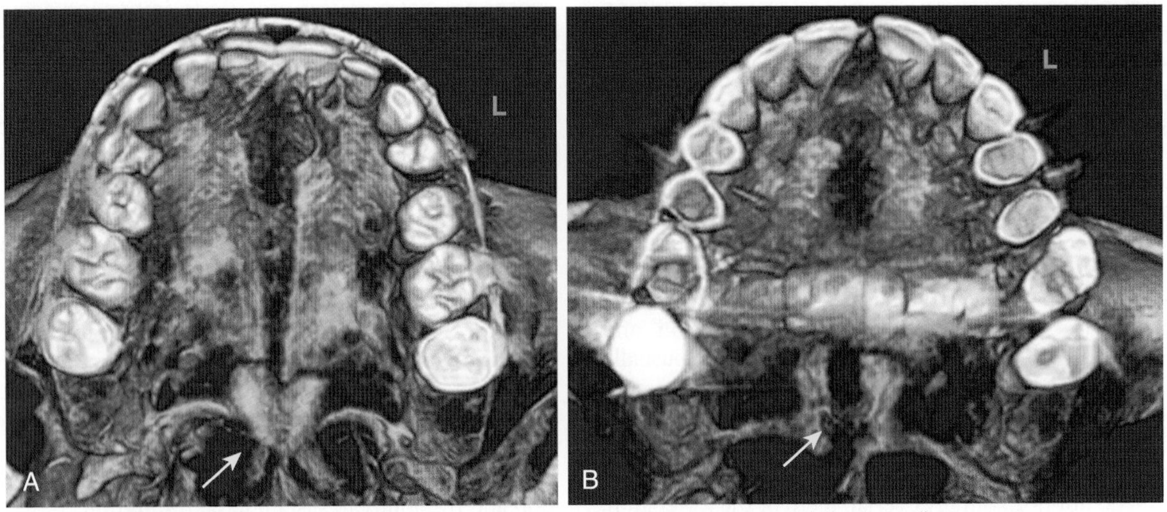

Figure 168.5 Palatal view of **(A)** pyramidal type of anterior expansion seen in tooth borne maxillary expansion. **B,** Palatal view of 62-year-old patient shown in Figure 168.6, showing greater posterior maxillary expansion as shown by comparing the yellow arrows.

obstruction. Although pediatric nasal surgery in isolation does not have a consistent improvement on the apnea-hypopnea index in SDB patients, it can improve snoring, subjective sleep quality, daytime sleepiness, and sleep-related quality of life measures, among other SDB outcome measures. In children, radiofrequency ablation and microdebrider-assisted reduction have been used to reduce turbinate volume.[120] Inferior turbinate hypertrophy, which has been described on the opposite side of a deviated septum, has been shown to reverse after septoplasty to correct the septal deviation.[121] In toddlers and young children, septal surgery is not often considered until closer to pubertal maturation as the septal

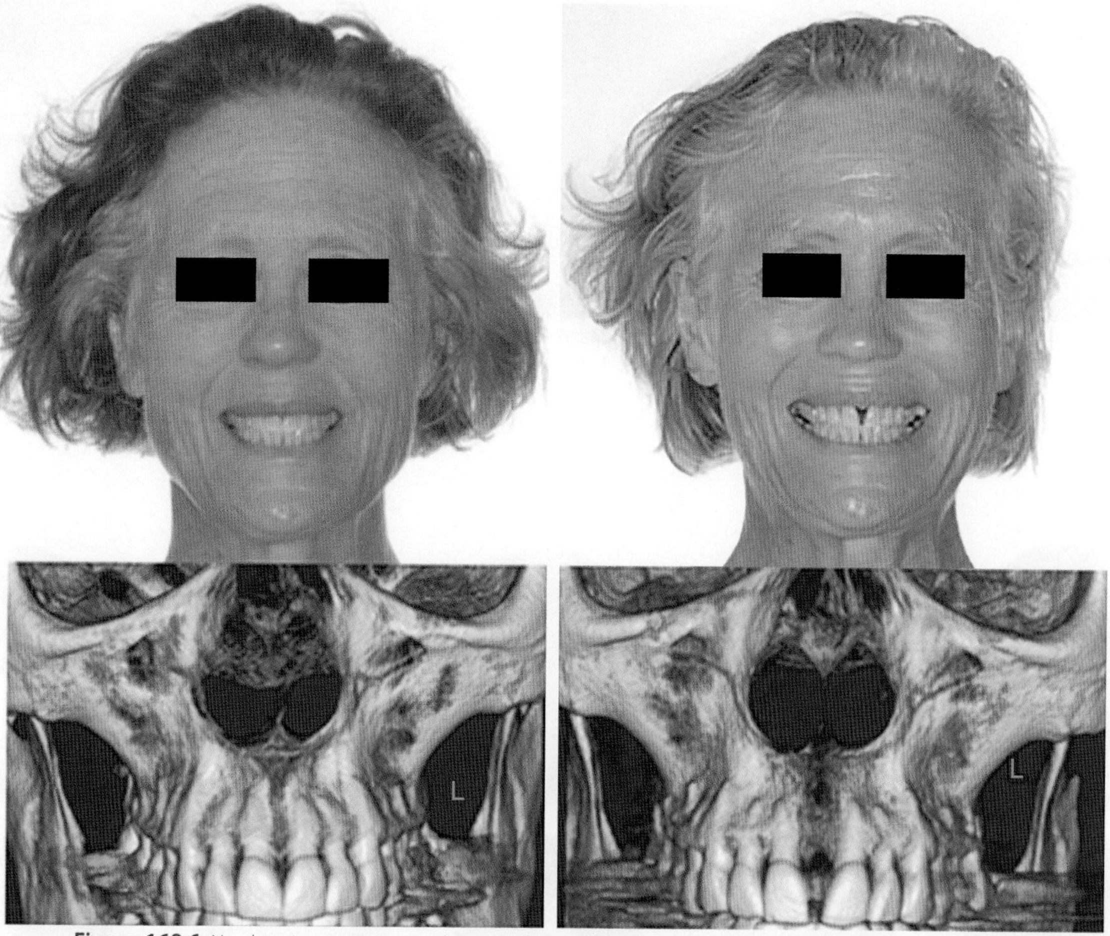

Figure 168.6 Nasal cavity expansion at the nasal floor and lateral nasal walls from the midline separation. Transpalatal distraction with endoscopically assisted surgical expansion. Sixty-two-year-old patient with severe obstructive sleep apnea (OSA).

cartilage is thought to be a growth mediator of the nasomaxillary complex. In recent years, successful nasal septal surgery has been performed in children with nasal obstruction without disturbing the development of the midface.[121] Removal of the septal obstruction was advocated before adolescence to avoid the growth distortions that ensue from the lack of nasal breathing and has been advocated in children at 6 years old[122] and even at birth, in cleft and noncleft children.[123]

Reduction of Inflammation and Medication Management. SDB is more prevalent in patients with allergic diseases.[124] Allergic rhinitis hinders nasal respiration by increasing nasal resistance and is considered a risk factor for SDB.[125] Allergic rhinitis is one of the major causes of impaired nasal function, affecting up to 40% of the general population in developed countries, with an increasing prevalence. Although the evidence generally supports a connection between SDB and allergic rhinitis, this connection is not definitive, and the mechanism linking these two diseases and the mechanism of how nasal inflammation causes SDB are unclear. The cause-and-effect link between allergic rhinitis and SDB is not fully understood, although allergic and nonallergic rhinitis are the most common causes of nasal congestion.[124] This topic is further described in Chapter 133.

Nasopharynx Site

Orthodontic Expansion by Sagittal Nasomaxillary Lengthening. Studies within the past decade show an improvement in maxillary length and airway size using tooth-borne and bone-borne maxillary protraction. A recent meta-analysis of six studies concluded that maxillary protraction appliances can lengthen the nasopharynx and the posterior pharyngeal airway behind the maxilla in the pediatric patient.[126] However, these results were not always stable over the long term, with reported dentoalveolar relapse in 25% to 30% of cases and little mention of the stability of the skeletal orthopedic effect of the protracted maxilla or the increase in posterior airway dimensions. The idea of anchoring traction directly onto the maxillary skeleton instead of the dentition was introduced in 2008.[127] A recent pilot study examined the use of bone-anchored dental implant maxillary protraction (see design in Figure 168.7) as a strategy to treat maxillary retrusion in children with SDB.[128] Improvements in maxillary length, nasopharyngeal size, and respiratory parameters were demonstrated. Dental, skeletal, and soft tissue alterations were noted, illustrating changes in facial growth (Figure 168.8) that may result from airway enlargement through skeletal traction. Although the sample size was small, the improvements in AHI suggest bone-anchored traction as another orthodontic/orthopedic therapy to treat pediatric SDB.

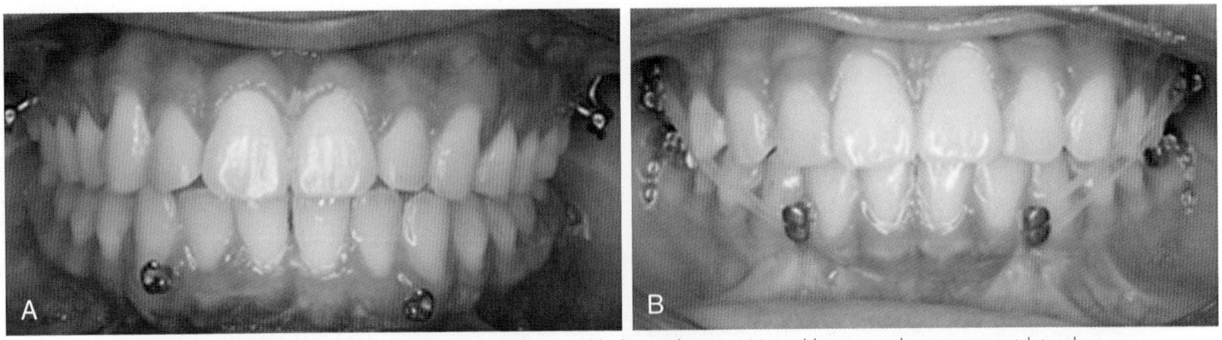

Figure 168.7 Placement of bone anchors. **A,** Mandibular anchors positioned between the permanent lateral incisor and cuspid and the maxillary anchor positioned under the zygoma but emerging at the upper first molar. Surgi-Tec type miniplate anchors. **B,** Elastic traction attaching the upper to the lower bone miniplate anchors, DePuy Synthes type.

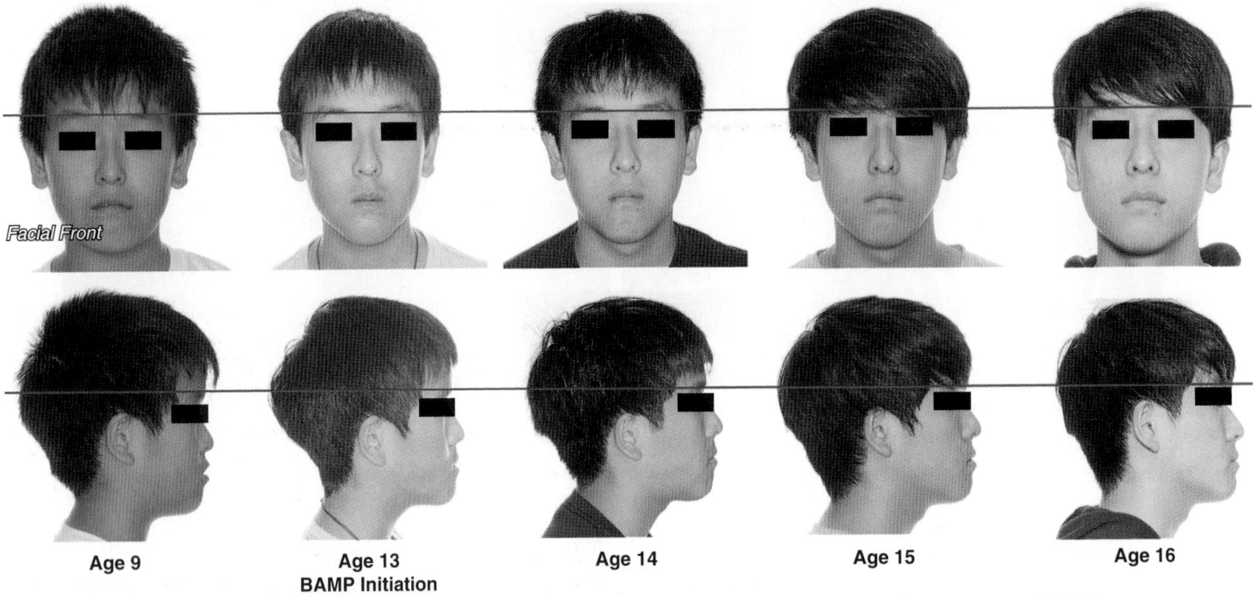

Figure 168.8 Facial growth from age 9 to age 16. Bone-anchored dental implant maxillary protraction (BAMP) treatment initiated at age 13. BAMP continued until age 16.

Surgical Expansion by Removal of Soft Tissue. An alternative mode of increasing airway size is through the surgical removal of structures or obstructions, further described in Chapter 175. In children these procedures may include reduction of the inferior nasal turbinates, sinus surgery, or adenoidectomy. There is a nonlinear relationship between the level of nasal resistance and the severity of SDB. This may explain why the reported cure rate of adenotonsillectomy for OSA in meta-analyses of children with a mean age of 6.5 years was only 59.8%, showing that adenotonsillectomy as the first-line and most common therapy for pediatric OSA may be insufficient.[129]

Oropharynx Site

The retropalatal area is represented here, which is often the site of greatest airway narrowing in children. SDB children have more fluctuation in airway size, with narrowing during inspiration that is more prominent in higher oropharyngeal levels.[130] Surgical adenotonsillectomy can enlarge this space. Whereas maxillary expansion increases the nasomaxillary space, imaging studies using cone beam computed tomography and lateral cephalography do not depict any changes at the oropharyngeal level with RME. Children with OSA have a narrowed space at this level compared with controls, but after RME therapy, there was no evidence of increased oropharyngeal airway volume.[131]

Surgical Expansion by Removal of Soft Tissue. Hypertrophy of the tonsils (pharyngeal and palatine) is the second major cause of respiratory obstruction in childhood, followed by allergic rhinitis, and is found to be associated with allergic rhinitis in many children, exacerbating the respiratory symptoms. As described earlier in this chapter, tonsils generally initiate hypertrophy within the first 3 years of life, the period of highest immunologic activity during childhood. Because tonsil growth outpaces craniofacial growth from 3 to 7 years of age, most symptoms are observed during this period, coinciding with the peak incidence of childhood OSA syndrome. Tonsil atrophy starts after 10 years of age and is completed in adulthood. The first-line therapy for pediatric SDB is adenotonsillectomy, which has been associated with a decline in the critical closing pressure of the muscles along the pharynx, rendering the upper airway less collapsible.[89] Surgical therapies are further described in Chapter 175.

Hypopharynx Site

Hypopharyngeal airway obstruction can be caused by the prominence or relaxation of the base of the tongue, the lateral pharyngeal wall, and, occasionally, the aryepiglottic folds of the epiglottis.

Use of Oral Appliances. Several case report studies show the effectiveness of oral appliances that hold the lower jaw forward in treating SDB and OSA in children. The use of oral appliances in the treatment of adults is well established, and the specific mechanics of how these appliances work is further discussed in Chapter 173. Oral appliances that advance the jaw forward are similar to the functional appliances used in orthodontics that address problems of pediatric mandibular deficiency through changes in the dentition and the growth of the maxillomandibular complex. As a result, oral appliances can affect the forward growth of the upper and lower jaw, which may be inappropriate for children unless there is retrognathia. The long-term side effects of this growth restraint on the pediatric developing airway warrant further examination.

Surgical Expansion by Skeletal Surgery. Orthognathic advancement surgery is not considered a treatment option for the pediatric patient until after jaw growth cessation. Because of the late-stage timing, other therapies would be enacted before orthognathic surgery is planned. Mandibular advancement surgery enlarges the hypopharyngeal space, whereas maxillary advancement surgery enlarges the nasopharyngeal and oropharyngeal cavities. Bimaxillary or maxillomandibular advancement surgery creates expansion across the entire pharynx. Again, expansion/advancement surgery is described in Chapter 175.

Continuous Positive Airway Pressure. Continuous positive airway pressure (CPAP) stents the pharyngeal airway open and prevents the muscular walls from collapsing. It is not a curative strategy as it does not increase the airway size or change the neuromotor properties of the surrounding musculature. Studies in children demonstrate the efficacy of CPAP therapy in reducing or eliminating symptoms and improving respiration but also acknowledge the challenges of restriction of nasomaxillary growth, along with compliance with and adherence to routine use. Consequently, CPAP is used as a secondary measure when adenotonsillectomy, bimaxillary expansion, or pharmacologic management has not improved SDB or as a primary option for obese children or children with craniofacial syndromes. This form of therapy, used primarily in adults, is further outlined in Chapter 132.

Strategy 2: Improvement in Function

Changing the Mode of Respiration

As described earlier in this chapter, the nasorespiratory pattern is critical in shaping the normal development of the upper airway. Initial SDB treatment strategies in children are targeted to promote and to sustain nasal respiration. Removal of nasal obstructions can promote nasal respiration during the day and night, but the relevance of establishing daytime nasal respiration in affecting nighttime upper airway properties is not known. If nasal obstruction is sufficiently severe, a transition to oral breathing may occur. Nasal breathing is the primary route of airflow, responsible for most inhaled ventilation during wake and sleep states. The transition from nasal to oronasal breathing at night increases with age. Transitioning to primarily oral airflow can be detrimental because it can change the upper airway properties. Open mouth breathing during sleep can create lengthening of the pharynx and lowering of the hyoid bone,[132] which increases upper airway resistance from increased collapsibility of the pharyngeal lumen and posterior retraction of the tongue. Upper airway resistance during sleep is significantly lower during nasal breathing than during oral breathing,[133] which may further compromise the airway and increase the work of breathing if oral breathing is sustained during sleep.

Oral breathing in children can also have a potentially dysmorphic effect on the developing orofacial complex. Based on the earlier described functional matrix theory of Moss, it is thought that nasal respiration provides continuous airflow through the nasal passage to induce a constant stimulus for the lateral growth of the nasal cavity and maxilla and for lowering of the palatal vault.[134] The laminar and turbulent airflow patterns are created by the nasal structures, which in turn shape the nasal structures. Nasal breathing allows the nose to smell, warm, humidify, and filter inspired air. Through humidification, nasal breathing allows for optimal thermoregulation through the heat transfer between inspired air and the nasal mucosa.[135] The position and shape of the bone are the result of air pressures and flow patterns through the nasal and oral cavities. The second effect of oral breathing on the facial skeleton is mediated by changes in muscle recruitment patterns, which result in an altered soft tissue and skeletal morphology and posture. Increased nasal resistance can yield a more collapsible airway, and it potentiates mouth breathing that can create the postural and thus muscular changes that lead to unfavorable jaw growth. So the oral breathing cycle is perpetuated once it is initiated. This suggests that one of the tenets of SDB therapy would be to change the respiratory mode from oral breathing to a predominantly nasal breathing mode. Nasal ventilation is the most important function for normal facial growth.

It is challenging to understand what oral breathing means to a given individual because there is not a standard well-accepted test to identify cause and treatment prognosis. The controversy stems from the inability to quantify nasal versus oral respiration or if spontaneous transitions from oral to nasal breathing occur and the lack of long-term data with growth maturation. Reliable tests to assess continuous airflow through the nose and mouth are lacking, and often the assessments are made on clinical presentation and subjective perceptions of the patient. Tests that measure airflow and nasal resistance, such as anterior rhinometry, acoustic rhinometry, nasal peak flow, rhinomanometry, pneumotachography, and the more recent computational fluid dynamics. The last are not routinely used because the testing results are operator dependent and do not consistently correlate with the patients' subjective complaints. Nasal congestion, as a marker of nasal /oral breathing has been extensively examined and the Nasal Obstruction Symptom Evaluation (NOSE) is a short, validated, disease-specific assessment of nasal obstruction symptom severity.[136] While the NOSE Scale may be a reliable assessment of alterations in nasal breathing in adults, its utility for children may not be applicable, especially because children's symptoms are often reported by the parent caregiver.

Oral breathing is thought to be an oral habit or a maladaptive response to a perturbation. Despite the associations to maxillomandibular growth, few studies explore how to cure oral breathing. The most common respiratory mode is a combination of simultaneous oral and nasal airflow[137] described as oronasal breathing.[123] During sleep, normal subjects without nasal disease or SDB are nasal breathers, with only 4% of total ventilation time spent breathing orally.[138] Neonates are born as obligate or preferential nasal breathers, but as outlined earlier in this chapter, this changes as the upper airway, neural development, and central neural control of breathing system mature (see Chapters 22 and 23). Even patients with severe nasal obstruction from either allergies or soft tissue enlargement display some measure of nasal respiration.[139]

Given the multifactorial nature of the nasorespiratory mode on the expression of SDB, facial growth, and the normal execution other rhythmic functions, relief of nasal obstruction using the therapies in Strategy 1 to facilitate nasal respiration is only part of the solution. Other multilevel variables in respiratory control should also be addressed, such as the development of nasal breathing at the habitual level and regaining nasal vasomotor control. Some children with adequate upper airways breathe through the mouth because of habit.[139] Nasal obstruction can be the stimulus for oral breathing, but removal of the obstruction to create nasal patency does not always induce a spontaneous change in the respiratory mode. Although RME therapy can enlarge the intranasal space and reduce nasal resistance, afterward the oral respiratory mode does not automatically revert, suggesting that a patterned mode of breathing develops. Even after surgical removal of enlarged tonsils in children, changes in airway muscle tone were variable after surgery,[140] demonstrating spontaneous but partial motor tone and posture improvement.

Muscle Rehabilitation

At sleep onset, pharyngeal muscle activity is reduced and becomes slightly atonic (i.e., hypotonic) during rapid eye movement sleep (see Chapters 22 and 23 for more information on muscle physiology and breathing). During adolescence, the dilating upper airway reflexes show a gradual reduction of responsiveness, and so the collapsibility of the upper airway increases. Some amount of airway reflex attenuation, or blunting, occurs with age. Normal healthy children and adolescents show neuromuscular compensations of increasing genioglossus electromyographic (EMG) activity in response to increased resistive loading, indicating that these children and adolescents have active upper airway neuromuscular reflexes during sleep. In opposition, some data support that some OSA syndrome children and adults show higher EMG activity during wake than normal controls and lower EMG activity during sleep.[141] These daytime increases in EMG activation impart a resistance to collapse,[142] and these mechanisms have been described in obese non-OSA adolescents as a neural compensation. Snoring may or may not be present in children, but over time it creates vibratory stress in the upper airway and is hypothesized to induce change or injury to the affected pharyngeal muscles.

The collapsible pharynx, as a tube composed of paired muscles with no bony perimeter, mediates airflow from the nose in the upper airway to the lungs of the lower airway. With repetitive collapse in OSA, the sustained pressure in the collapsible pharynx can result in myopathy from repetitive microtrauma to the pharyngeal muscles.[143] The pharyngeal muscle motor activation can become altered such that the sensory afferent response to neurochemical (hypoxemia or hypercapnia) or neuromechanical (respiratory effort) stimuli becomes diminished or absent. Over time, these insults can lessen neuromuscular control of the upper airway muscles that regulate airway opening and collapse, resulting in a neuropathy that interrupts the interplay of the airway dilating opening muscles against the airway contracting or closing muscles.

Upper airway patency during sleep is controlled by the ventilatory drive to the respiratory musculature. If OSA is modeled as a progressive disease, ideally a given treatment strategy would reverse these resultant muscular changes. Muscle (or neuromuscular) rehabilitation extends beyond the impairment to treat the functional consequences using exercise therapy to change muscle strength, posture, endurance, coordination, or responsiveness (see Chapter 134). Treatment targets three general pathways. One rationale is to restore the afferent sensory proprioception to the dilator muscles. Proprioceptive feedback is crucial to sensorimotor performance and is associated with neuroplastic reorganization within the sensorimotor cortex and the supplemental motor areas.[144] Transcutaneous electrical stimulation, transcranial magnetic stimulation, or myofunctional therapy (MFT) has been used to treat altered sensory input to the airway musculature. The second possible mechanism targets the efferent motor loop using electrical stimulation directly to the hypoglossal nerve[145] to improve the genioglossus response (see Chapter 175). Both these mechanisms are thought to reestablish the coordinated, synchronous, and synergistic muscle firing patterns of the upper airway dilator muscles. The third rehabilitation mechanism lies in restoring impairments in cortical processing. Physical exercise promotes motor skill learning in normal individuals. Cortical changes have been described as a reduction of volume in the limbic and frontal areas of the brain in OSA patients, with a reversal increase in volume after CPAP treatment, demonstrating neuroplasticity in adults.[146] One week of tongue task training induced a 23% reduction in AHI, enough time to induce neuroplastic changes in the primary motor cortex (M1) through an increase in the genioglossus motor area representation.[147,148] These same types of brain structural changes have been demonstrated for dysphagia rehabilitation in stroke patients using swallowing exercises.[149] Even proprioception and proprioceptive training as a muscle rehabilitation strategy necessitate a certain level of cognitive integration.

The physiologic mechanisms of neuromuscular rehabilitation have not been fully elucidated. Recent work in muscle physiology shows skeletal muscle as a secretory organ that secretes messenger molecules in contraction, called myokines.[150] Myokines act as an autocrine, paracrine, and endocrine signal, where the signal does not necessarily travel through the nervous system. As a hormone or neurotransmitter, it can directly affect humoral or neural regulation of several systemic functions, including breathing and bone growth. Indirectly, it has endocrine action on other organs, bypassing the central nervous system through cross-talk signaling pathways. Irisin, an exercise induced myokine, was found to be

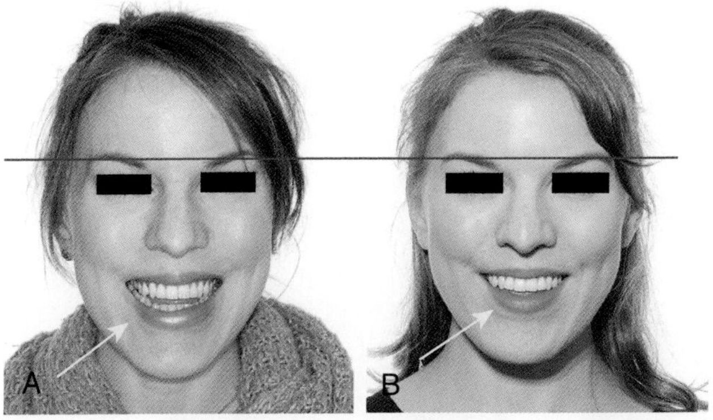

Figure 168.9 Effect of myofunctional therapy on muscle performance. **A,** Increased pull of facial muscles on the right side: depressors anguli oris and labii inferioris, causing soft tissue asymmetry, noted with the yellow arrow. **B,** Noted improvement in facial muscle symmetry after 3 months of myofunctional therapy.

inversely associated with the severity of sleep apnea in OSA males compared with healthy male controls[151] and serum levels of irisin were reversed with CPAP.[152] Irisin has been shown to induce the expression of another myokine, brain-derived neurotrophic factor (BDNF), involved in neurogenesis and neuronal development and linked to neuroplasticity and neuroprotection and circadian regulation. Compared with controls, adults with OSA have increased serum levels of BDNF[151] that some report is reversed with CPAP. Perhaps therapeutic muscle contraction stimulated myokine release provides a plausible pathway to improve OSA airway myopathy.

Myofunctional therapy has attracted much attention across different specialties, not all related to abnormal breathing. Since MFT was introduced as a therapy to improve OSA in adults, several studies examined MFT in adults and children for OSA therapy. Systematic reviews and meta-analyses conclude improvements in AHI, oxygen saturation, and symptoms, despite the challenges in comparing studies with varying treatment protocols.[151a] Studies cannot support MFT as a stand-alone therapy but suggest muscle training (see Figure 168.9) as adjunctive in a multitherapy/combination therapy modality.[153,154] Performance of these rehabilitation exercises during the day supposes that airway collapsibility during sleep will be reduced.

Future work in muscle rehabilitation will likely outline screening and treatment parameters and identify the most effective muscle rehabilitation techniques for managing SDB. The majority of studies highlight the genioglossus, but all the inspiratory and expiratory muscle groups have been targeted using rehabilitation: nasal, oral, cervical, pharyngeal, and pulmonary musculature. These same muscle groups are tightly coupled in other nonrespiratory reflexive functions, such as coughing and rhythmic actions such as mastication, swallowing. As abnormal swallowing was described in OSA patients, numerous studies look to improvements in swallowing to increase genioglossus tonicity and excitability. With little adverse effects of therapy, enough evidence supports MFT to treat SDB, but because therapy is heavily dependent on patient compliance, expedient muscle training must be identified. Muscle deficits in one function could affect other serial motor pathways that act in a coordinated, timed, synchronous, or rhythmic parallel function. A triptych of dysfunctions in resting posture, swallowing, and phonation has been targeted.[155] A more extensive rehabilitation of the entire muscular respiratory system has been proposed[156] but is such an extensive treatment needed if earlier dysfunction and subsequent intervention is identified? This is explored in the next section on treatment timing. Longer term studies can address questions of treatment timing, age, and severity appropriateness and lend more definition to the initiation, end point, and duration of muscle rehabilitation.

Strategy 3: Craniofacial Growth Modification

Does oral breathing cause abnormal orofacial development, and if so, does this cascade of altered growth exacerbate SDB or predispose a growing child to SDB? A simple cause-and-effect relationship between upper airway respiratory function and dentofacial and skeletal morphology has not yet been determined, despite the myriad studies in the clinical specialties of otolaryngology, oral surgery, and orthodontics—all areas that are specific to treating the upper airway, the jaws, or the teeth. However, there are associations between OSA syndrome, craniofacial anatomy, facial growth, jaw size and shape, and malocclusions as outlined earlier in this chapter. The genesis of these relationships stems from the hypothesis that oral breathing from dysregulation or impaired nasorespiratory function can affect craniofacial growth of the nasal cavity, maxilla, mandible, and consequently the pharyngeal airway. Although controversial, the relationship between nasal obstruction and facial growth has been demonstrated in animal experimental and human clinical trials.[157]

Timing

By the age of 4 years, the craniofacial skeleton has reached 60% of its adult size; by the age of 7 years, 75% total craniofacial growth is complete, and by the age of 12 years, 90% total craniofacial growth is reached.[158] The ability to modify an underlying growth pattern is age dependent, determined by the growth velocity. The midface, specifically the oronasopharyngeal area, represents the highest level of sensorimotor integration, where there is synchronous development and coordination of the nervous system, musculature, cartilage, and bony skeleton. The vital reflexive functions, such as respiration, mastication, and phonation, shape and direct craniofacial growth. These physiologic demands change as these functions mature and become more precise, which in turn direct morphogenesis. Abnormal functions, such as oral breathing, influence oronasopharyngeal morphology. These distortions or discoordinations can become exaggerated during periods of increased growth velocity, especially during puberty. In the pediatric patient, once the reflexive function becomes abnormal, the morphology of the developing skeleton and neuromusculature that support that function may change in a way that increases airway resistance causing exacerbation of the underlying dysfunction.

Passive Loading

In this section, we cover how to change the shape of nasal, upper jaw, lower face, and pharyngeal structures.

Shape Changes in the Nasal Cavity. As described earlier in this chapter, the muscle pattern exerts a passive tension on the developing airway through the force mediated on the nasomaxillary structure. The nasal cavity and the maxilla grown in unison, and their morphogenesis and physiology are tightly

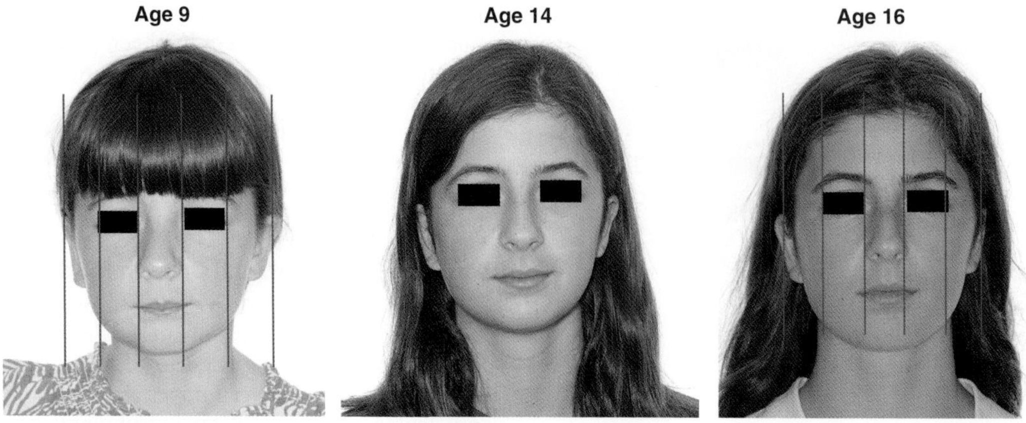

Figure 168.10 Narrowing nasal morphology with chronic nasal congestion, showing narrowing of nasal radix from age 9 to age 16.

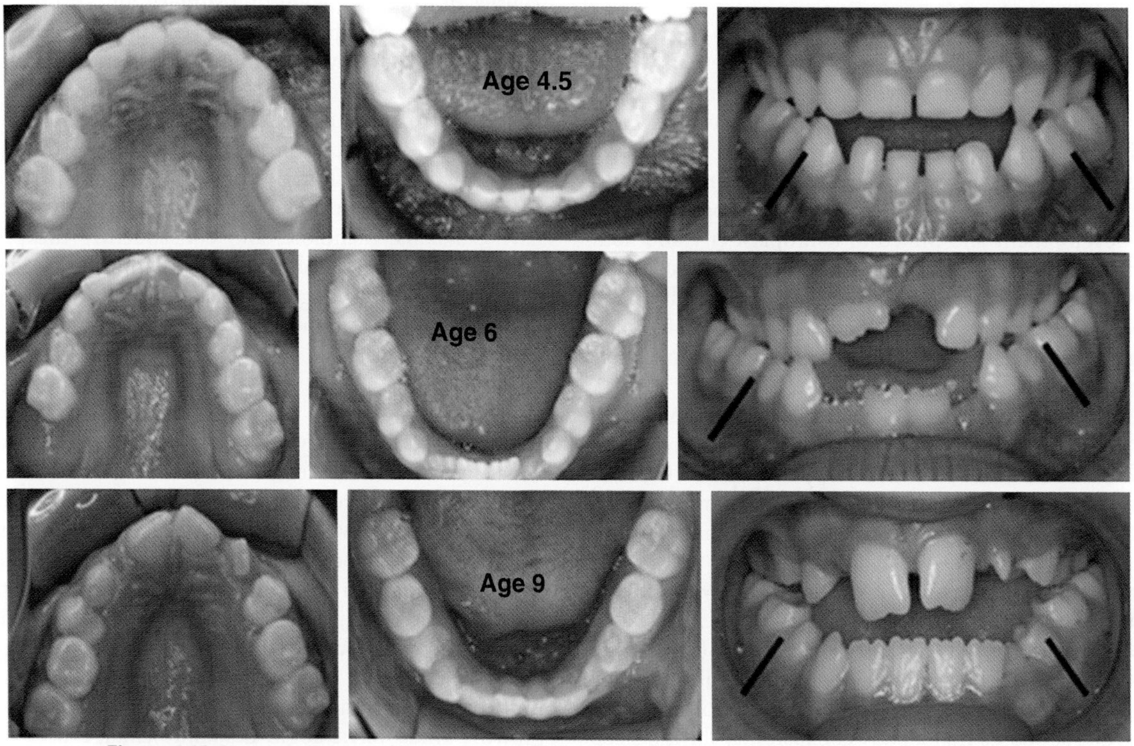

Figure 168.11 Natural growth of the maxillomandibular complex in response to nasal obstruction, leading to a malocclusion. Gradual narrowing of the maxilla from ages 4.5 to 9 years, while the lower archform shape remains intact. Note the lingual tipping of the lower dentition as a dentoalveolar compensation, as marked by the black lines.

coupled as the maxillary bone defines both entities. Advances in imaging now allow better visualization of the nasal cavity, though longitudinal descriptions of nasal cavity changes from nasal congestion are lacking. Nasal growth velocity parallels body height velocity. Figure 168.10 demonstrates the morphologic narrowing changes in the nasal aperture, radix and nasion areas that may develop in response to chronic nasal obstruction. As nasal volume decreases, nasal resistance increases, which can exacerbate upper airway collapsibility, causing a cycle of progressively worsening SDB. This induced distortion in morphogenesis could partly explain the pathogenesis of SDB.

Shape Changes in the Upper Jaw. Numerous studies have shown a relationship between nasal airway obstruction and aberrant facial growth. In children and adults, morphologic effects of impaired nasal respiration are evident, including narrowing of the maxilla, reduced development of the mandible, increased vertical growth of the lower face, dental crowding and malocclusion,[37] and altered head posture. A new posture compensates for the decrease in nasal airflow to allow respiration. However, these are not consistent phenomena in children or adults with oral breathing tendencies.

These changes are typified in Figure 168.11 and occur passively because there is no directly applied force or load to the bony skeleton, other than through the attached musculature. In response to chronic oral breathing, three distinct developmental changes may be manifested. The upper jaw narrows, suggesting that the volume of the nasal cavity becomes smaller as the upper jaw continues to narrow. The second

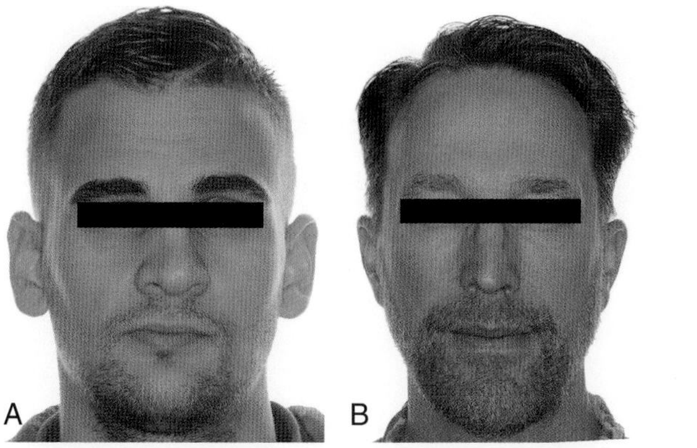

Figure 168.12 Facial morphologies associated with obstructive sleep apnea (OSA). **A,** Decreased lower facial height individual with a closed gonial angle and bimaxillary retrusion. **B,** Increased lower facial height individual with bimaxillary dental protrusion and an open gonial angle.

developmental change is seen in the dentition, as the teeth add a second layer of insult to this distortion by compensatory inward tipping in both the upper and lower jaws. This restricts the intraoral volume even more, which potentiates a postural and neuromuscular adaptation of the genioglossus muscle. It can be argued that aggressive efforts are needed to combat the inherent tendency for upper jaw narrowing in oral breathers, even after the obstacles to nasal airflow are removed, because of the muscle alterations. The subsequent effect on the mandible is the third level of passive distortion that intensifies the pharyngeal collapsibility as the hypopharynx narrows with the backward rotation of the mandible. This narrowing is specifically evident at the retroglossal area.

Shape Changes in the Lower Jaw. In a growing child, abnormal nasal resistance may affect the growth of the mandible.[159] During puberty, these deleterious changes can be magnified because of the growth velocity seen during teenage years. Deleterious effects of mouth breathing are the sensory stimulus that propagates abnormal tongue position and altered orofacial musculature tone. The muscle recruitment pattern is modified when nasal respiration changes to oral breathing.[160] Some of these growth responses can be exaggerated because of the concurrent effect of molar tooth eruption occurring at the same time. In oral breathers, it has been reported that mandibular growth is redirected posteriorly. Oral breathing that develops from nasal obstruction has an effect on the largest pharyngeal dilator muscle that keeps the airway open, the genioglossus. In an open mouth posture, the genioglossus adopts a low-lying position in the floor of the mouth. The relationship of breathing to airway problems shows a lowered position of the hyoid bone in OSA syndrome patients. In this dorsocaudal position, EMG activation of the tongue on experimental animals shows a weaker protrusive force, suggesting a possible mechanism for increased collapsibility, as decreased genioglossus tension led to an increased muscle length in experimental animals.[161] The increased size of the genioglossus would narrow the pharyngeal airway, and this increases collapsibility. Genioglossal activity is increased with nasal compared with oral breathing, with supine versus sitting body position, and during inspiratory resistive loading, probably because of an altered respiratory drive and reflex activation. This effect, coupled with the potential edema from the negative airway pressure generated during sleep, exacerbates the disorder, exemplifying the necessity to treat the sequelae of the root cause. A cyclic pattern of distortion develops in which the lower jaw rotates backward because of mode of breathing. This changed position narrows the retroglossal airway, which could potentiate increased repetitive activation stimuli to keep the airway open, leading to an increase in pharyngeal muscle mass. Further muscle injury can result from snoring, vibration, or increased airway resistance.

The term adenoid facies has historically been used to describe the long, narrow, flat face of the individual with oral hypotonia and protruding teeth and lips that are widely separated at rest, often accompanied by an open bite malocclusion.[37] The original work on experimental animals by Harvold and colleagues[157] demonstrated that there is a variable response to this insult of forced oral respiration. Oral breathing was not linked to a specific skeletal structure. Similarly, there is not a defined facial type or malocclusion that accompanies adenotonsillar hypertrophy in an oral breather. Several studies corroborate this conclusion because there is not a consistent relationship between nasal resistance and dentofacial morphology, as described earlier in this chapter. These differences are illustrated in Figure 168.12, which shows varied facial phenotypes with OSA.

The three cases illustrated in Figures 168.13 further demonstrate the variable response of mandibular growth to impaired nasal respiration. All three patients had therapy for their malocclusion, but the problem of allergies, nasal obstruction, and oral respiration persisted after bimaxillary expansion treatment. The records shown illustrate disproportionate jaw growth expressed during adolescence: a lack of forward upper jaw development and straight vertical mandibular descent with no forward growth (Figure 168.13, *C*), with forward mandibular growth rotation (Figure 168.13, *B*), versus backward mandibular growth rotation (Figure 168.13). The dentoalveolar development from tooth eruption can affect the forward (Figure 168.13, *B*) or backward rotation (Figure 168.13, *A*) of the mandible, and this important effect cannot be discounted. These are three different expressions of mandibular growth, from the same stimulus of increased airway resistance from nasal obstruction. However, medical intervention has not been shown to influence the pattern of facial growth in children with allergies. Surgical therapy to relieve nasal airway obstruction in children (whether adenoidectomy or turbinectomy) has not been shown to predictably affect ultimate facial form.[162]

The end point is an altered muscle recruitment pattern that changes muscle tone, function, and soft tissue adaptation, which influence the skeletal morphology. Thus the oral breather may present with a normal appearance to severe skeletal and dental irregularities. "Nasal obstruction presents the trigger factor, but it is the deviant muscle recruitment which causes maldevelopment."[157]

Shape Changes in the Pharyngeal Airway. The soft tissues that form the anterior border of the pharyngeal airway are attached to the maxilla and mandible. Consequently, the size of the pharyngeal airway is affected by the amount and direction of maxillomandibular growth. Whereas there is an inherited growth pattern that accounts for the familial tendency or inheritance in OSA, there can be different epigenetic expressions of craniofacial malformation overlaid on

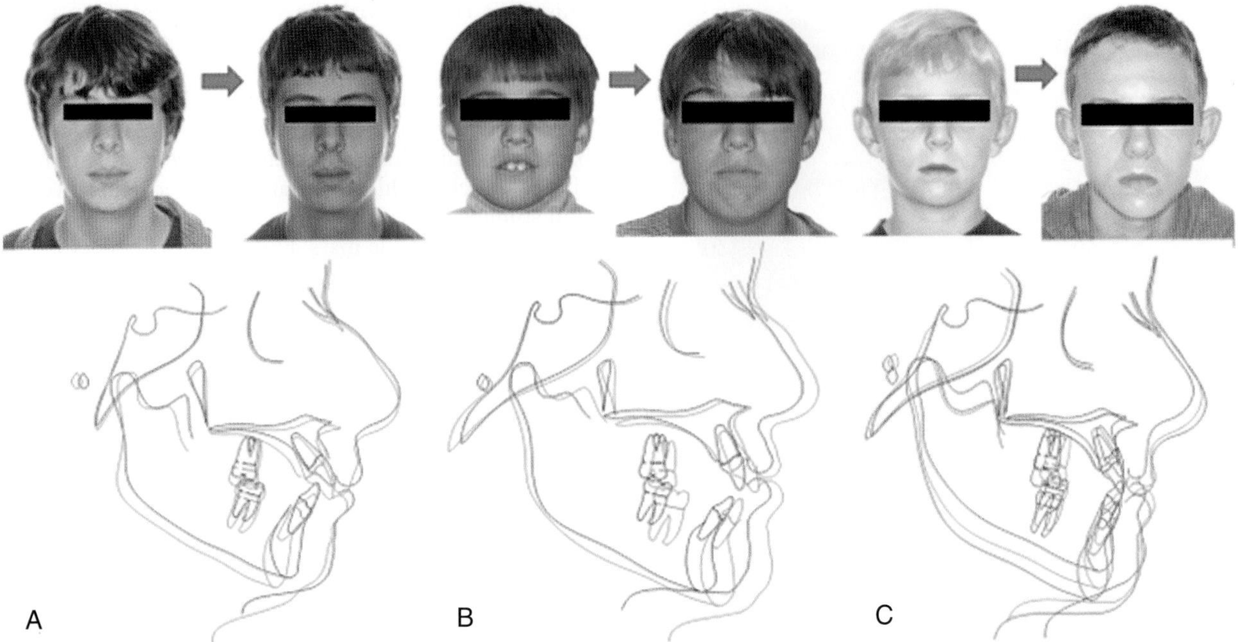

Figure 168.13 Variable maxillomandibular growth expression to allergic nasal obstruction. **A,** Backward/posterior maxillomandibular rotation. **B,** Minimal forward upper jaw growth, normal lower jaw growth. **C,** Minimal upper jaw growth, straight vertical maxillomandibular descent.

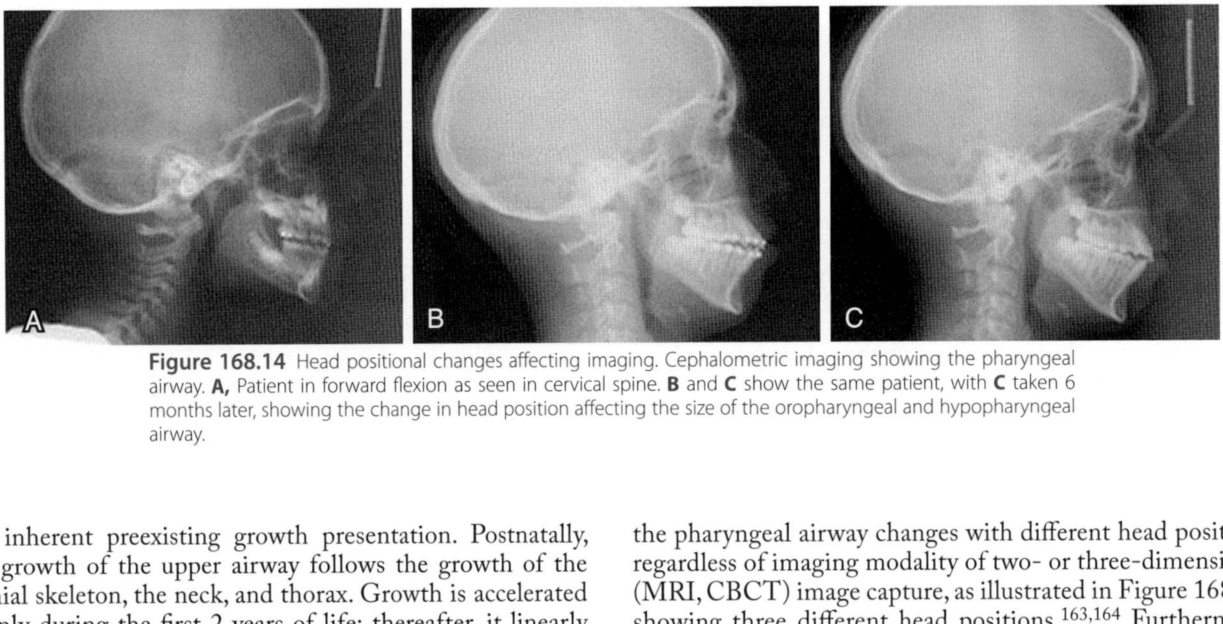

Figure 168.14 Head positional changes affecting imaging. Cephalometric imaging showing the pharyngeal airway. **A,** Patient in forward flexion as seen in cervical spine. **B** and **C** show the same patient, with **C** taken 6 months later, showing the change in head position affecting the size of the oropharyngeal and hypopharyngeal airway.

the inherent preexisting growth presentation. Postnatally, the growth of the upper airway follows the growth of the cranial skeleton, the neck, and thorax. Growth is accelerated mainly during the first 2 years of life; thereafter, it linearly follows the growth of the body. No large-scale, longitudinal characterization of the dimensional airway changes in children have been done. Airway size has been correlated with facial morphology, as described earlier in this chapter. Morphologic changes in the pharyngeal airway can be studied only through imaging and therein lies the dilemma. While there are numerous imaging studies using two- and three-dimensional techniques, the documentation of nasorespiratory function is lacking. Several novel imaging techniques that better characterize the airway are being used, and this is a growing field of study. The inherent difficulty of repeatable accurate characterization of a movable entity where there is fluidity in the walls of the upper airway is directly dependent on consistent patient positioning during imaging. The size of the pharyngeal airway changes with different head positions regardless of imaging modality of two- or three-dimensional (MRI, CBCT) image capture, as illustrated in Figure 168.14, showing three different head positions.[163,164] Furthermore, respiration is a dynamic action that may not be accurately depicted in a static three-dimensional image, especially when activation of the dilator muscles that govern the collapsibility is dependent on the sleep stage.[163] Airway imaging done while upright does not directly correlate with supine imaging, as there is a rostral shift of fluid while supine, nor does awake imaging correlate with imaging done during sleep. Imaging is a useful adjunct in diagnosis and treatment but cannot be a stand-alone measure as a cornerstone for determining the site of obstruction, especially because airway properties are dependent on pressures upstream and downstream from the pharyngeal site of collapse.[165] Importantly, airway size does not directly correlate with AHI severity,[93] as depicted in Figure 168.15.

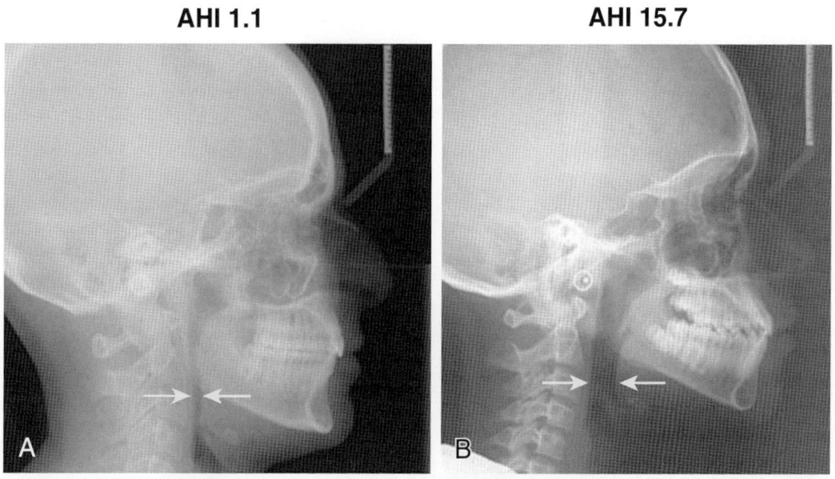

Figure 168.15 Airway size does not correlate with sleep-disordered breathing (SDB) severity. **A,** Patient with narrow pharynx and low apnea-hypopnea index (AHI) of 1.1. **B,** Patient with larger pharynx and higher AHI of 15.7. Note the differences in the postural cervical spine curvature.

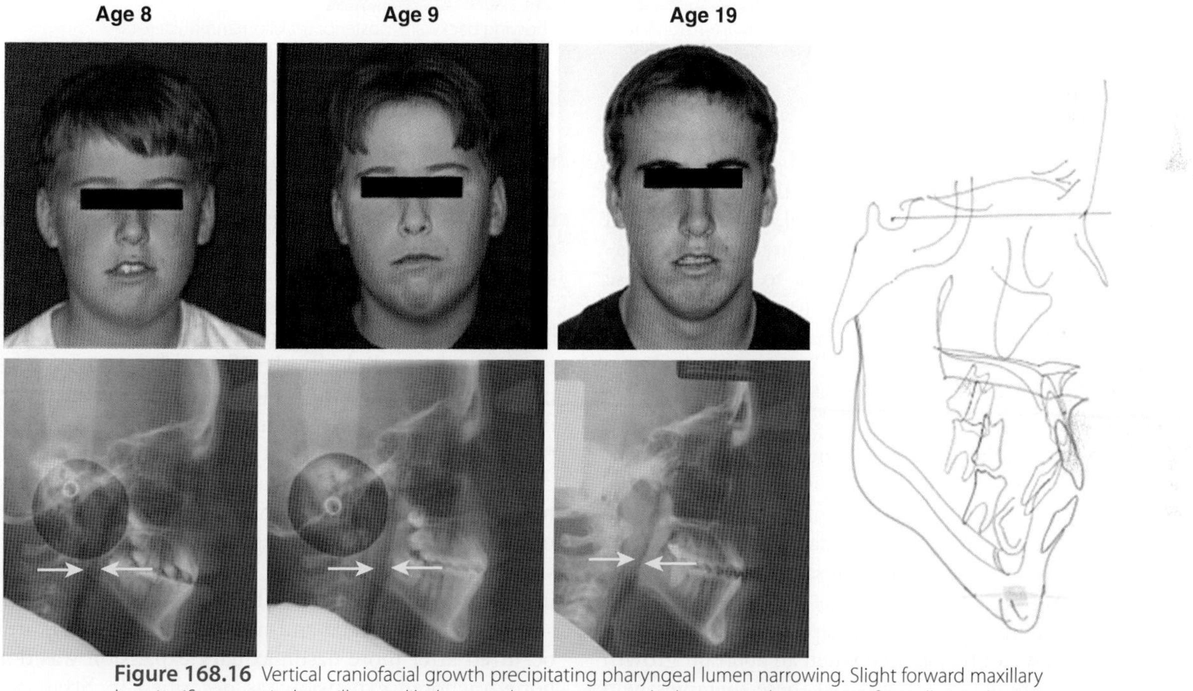

Figure 168.16 Vertical craniofacial growth precipitating pharyngeal lumen narrowing. Slight forward maxillary but significant vertical maxillomandibular growth in a patient with chronic nasal congestion from allergic disease. The lack of anterior maxillomandibular growth coupled with upper airway muscle edema could account for the concomitant pharyngeal lumen narrowing. Airway lengthening and lumen narrowing could be other factors contributing to sleep-disordered breathing (SDB).[169]

However, the edematous morphologic enlargement within the pharyngeal tissue has been well described, attributed to increases in the soft palate, tongue, and lateral pharyngeal walls[166] (see Section 14). The pharynx of OSA patients undergoes various histopathological changes, which may include tissue edema and inflammation created by the negative pressure in the upper airway during sleep, hypertrophy of mucous glands, changes in blood flow and capillary volume, fat and other tissue deposition in and around the pharynx, vascular dilatation, changes in connective tissue, increase in proinflammatory mediators, and muscle–nerve fiber derangement/loss.[167] These changes are typified in Figure 168.16, showing the increased thickness of the pharyngeal walls that developed over time in a patient with chronic nasal congestion.

In this example, there is slight forward maxillary but significant vertical maxillomandibular growth. The lack of anterior maxillomandibular growth coupled with upper airway muscle edema could account for the concomitant pharyngeal lumen narrowing. Airway lengthening is associated with vertical oropharyngeal growth and this aberrant growth direction could be another factor contributing to SDB.[168] Posterior rotational maxillomandibular growth can also precipitate a similar lumen narrowing as shown in Figures 168.16 and 168.17. Both of these aberrant growth patterns were expressed during adolescent growth.

These cases illustrate the answer to the question about disease propagation if craniofacial malformation is not only a cause but also a consequence of SDB. It is a variable response,

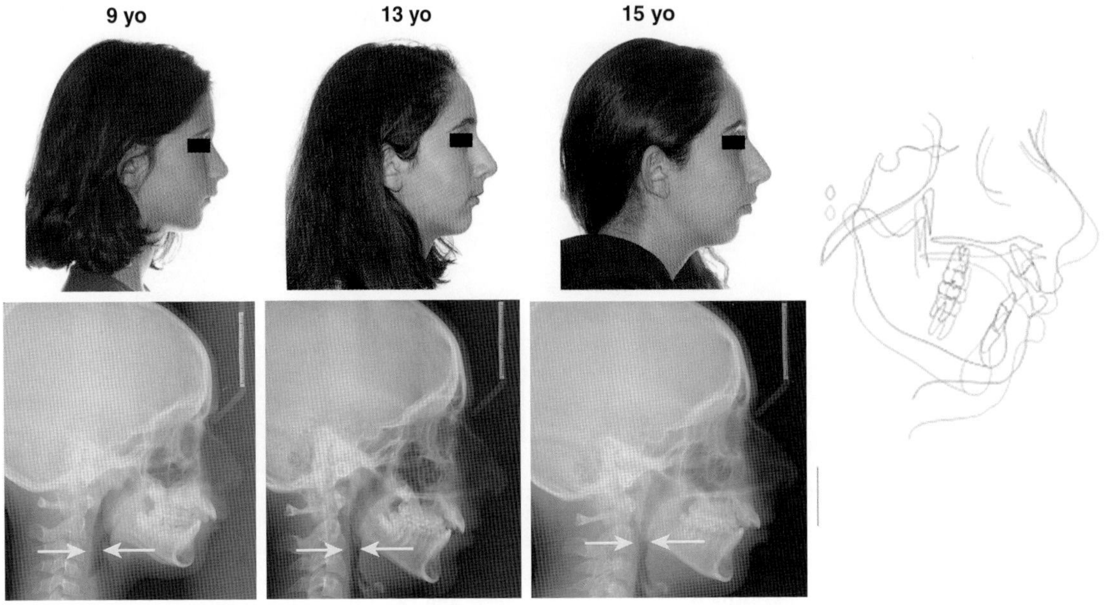

Figure 168.17 Maxillofacial growth from age 9 to age 15, showing backward/posterior maxillomandibular rotation leading to pharyngeal narrowing during adolescence, when the airway should be enlarging with pubertal growth.

depending on how the effect of impaired nasal respiration affects the muscle recruitment and activation at multilevel sites, affecting the interdependent structural, physiologic, and behavioral factors. For some patients, this paradigm of propagation would hold true. The challenge is to identify those patients who are more at risk for aberrant muscle alterations, and for these patients neuromuscular rehabilitation may be beneficial.

Active Loading

Induced Bone Remodeling. If bone remodeling is the result of passive force application, active force application as an epigenetic effect to direct bone development could be a strategy to increase airway size or to redirect unfavorable growth patterns, beyond the inherent genetic expression. Not all patients develop a dysmorphic growth pattern as a result of impaired nasal respiration, so interventional therapy to modify existing growth patterns may not be justified when an aberrant growth pattern cannot be predicted. However, if these therapies help improve the critical closing pressure, the pharyngeal collapsibility could ultimately be improved or even normalized.

The consideration for this direction of care lies in the shortcomings of current therapies. In adults, the "gold standard" for treatment of OSA is CPAP followed by oral appliance. Whereas, for children, adenotonsillectomy is the first-line therapy and nasal CPAP is considered after other therapies have not completely improved respiration. As listed previously in this chapter, CPAP is burdened with problems of compliance due to mask fit, comfort, or initiation of CPAP use. As an extraoral appliance, it may exert a molding force on the facial skeleton and the dentoalveolar bone. This force can cause remodeling and redirection of maxillomandibular jaw growth in the pediatric patient.[169] This retrusive remodeling force from the positive pressure from the mask or machine can create a skeletal jaw imbalance and negate all earlier efforts to enlarge the airway size. As increased nasal resistance is both a cause and consequence of SDB, an often prescribed treatment not only treats the problem but can also perpetuate it. However, induced bone remodeling through active force application can rectify these iatrogenic craniofacial alterations. There remains the question as to how long this imbalance is to be sustained.

Increases in the soft tissue greater alar cartilage and alar base width were evident post expansion, but these differences were not clinically significant[170] and were negligible 6 months posttreatment.[171] However, other work describes the integrated soft tissue stretching of the nasal, facial, and velopharyngeal muscles with expansion of the premaxilla and a continuous interaction that affects the underlying bony structure. This altered morphogenesis is predicated by the extent of nasomaxillary expansion, suggesting that inadequate expansion will not yield the shape change that potentiates a change in nasorespiratory function. These subtle alterations in soft tissue drape of the facial and nasal muscles (see Figure 168.18) occurred after more nasomaxillary expansion was done using bone anchored expansion (as described in Strategy 1). This illustrates Moss's functional matrix theory (described earlier in this chapter) as the increased expansion also coincided with improvement of SDB symptoms.

Through the combination of therapies, it may be possible to modify the inherent growth pattern. Efforts to target therapy at the site of greatest airway narrowing or obstruction may not be adequate because airway narrowing and collapse from sensorimotor dysfunction are thought to occur at multiple sites.[172] Several studies report combination therapy using several different treatment modalities. However, there are currently no studies that detail the effectiveness of a comprehensive and combined approach of treatments and growth modification to the nasal cavity, nasopharynx, oropharynx, and hypopharynx while also implementing muscle rehabilitation to address the concomitant neuromuscular adaptations of an impaired airway. This monumental effort would necessitate the collaboration of the multiple specialists involved in the treatment of upper airway disorders.

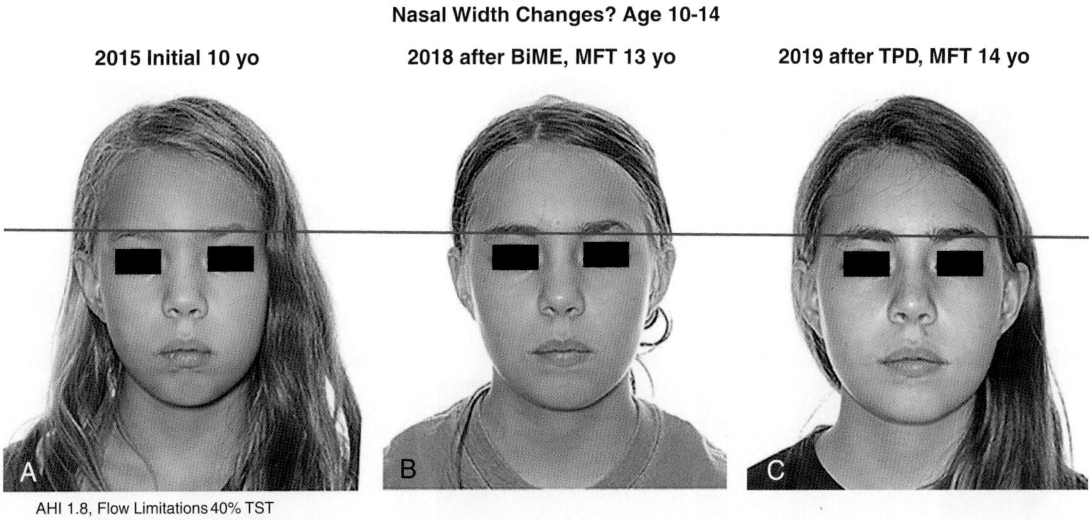

Figure 168.18 Morphologic changes in the nasal and facial muscles after nasomaxillary expansion. **A,** Initial presentation at 10 years old. **B,** After bimaxillary expansion at 13 years old. **C,** After bone anchored TPD expansion. The relaxation of the facial musculature and changes in nasal morphology were not achieved until more nasomaxillary expansion was rendered, suggesting improvement in nasorespiratory function will follow the change in nasal morphology.

Prophylactically treating the entire airway, instead of targeting the site of greatest obstruction or narrowest opening, may seem aggressive and extreme. However, children with SDB have blunted responses to hypercapnia,[173] demonstrating early neural deficits that are thought to be reversed with treatment, but it is not known if there is complete recovery. Reports of a high recurrence of SDB in later teenage years[87] suggest that some neural dysregulation persisted and perhaps worsened after previous treatment. Treatment is usually initiated from daytime or nighttime symptoms. The onset of symptoms may underlie a larger problem, as it is not known how long the primary cause needs to be present before symptoms develop. The most viable treatment may be consistent early screening to identify patterns before the onset of symptoms. By the time treatment is rendered, even if it is done at any early age, there may already be alterations in muscle recruitment and tone that initiate the development of a craniofacial malformation with subsequent lower airway deficits that could propagate the disease. A population-based longitudinal study observing children from 6 months to 7 years of age found that early symptoms of snoring, mouth breathing, and witnessed apneas had statistically significant effects on behavior in later childhood, suggesting that early symptoms warrant examination as early as the first year of life.[174] Herein lies the challenge of defining reliable screening patterns that are predictive of the disease in childhood becoming problematic in adulthood, as this prevention has not been established.

A stepwise evidence-based approach for the diagnosis and multitherapeutic management of childhood SDB has been recently presented.[175] This approach, starting with weight control followed in succession with nasal corticosteroids, adenotonsillectomy, dentofacial orthopedics such as mandibular advancement or maxillary expansion, CPAP, and maxillofacial surgery, is illustrated in Figure 168.19. This case demonstrates that despite early best efforts at recognition at age 9, diagnosis, and intervention of multiple therapies, including adenotonsillectomy, allergy management, multiple rounds of bimaxillary expansion, and nasal CPAP, the upper airway problems may still persist. For this particular case, problems of CPAP adherence rendered it ineffective as long-term treatment. Ultimately, on growth cessation, maxillomandibular advancement was the final treatment rendered, which normalized respiratory parameters and symptoms. Anatomic insufficiencies were improved to maximize the enlargement of the pharyngeal space. However, these gains cannot be maintained in the face of weight gain with subsequent pharyngeal narrowing, as symptoms returned as an adult.

SUMMARY

Many of the factors leading to pediatric SDB create secondary morphologic changes that exacerbate and perpetuate the syndrome. The approach to establish normal daytime and nighttime respiration is a multidisciplinary endeavor, involving the treatment of the upper airway (nasal cavity and all three components of the pharynx), the attendant surrounding musculature, and the lower airway. The directive would be to screen for the dysfunction before it becomes a disorder. Because of the shared anatomy, multiple treatments acting synergistically may yield improved outcomes, thus necessitating a greater degree of very early collaboration between specialists in sleep medicine, otolaryngology, allergy, surgery, speech, neurology, psychiatry, pulmonology, and orthodontics to manage effectively this multisystem disorder. To achieve successful treatment of upper airway breathing disorders, future efforts aimed at modifying the anatomy can hold the promise of prevention of problems of constricted size and impaired function because oronasopharyngeal malformation may be not only a cause but also a consequence of SDB.

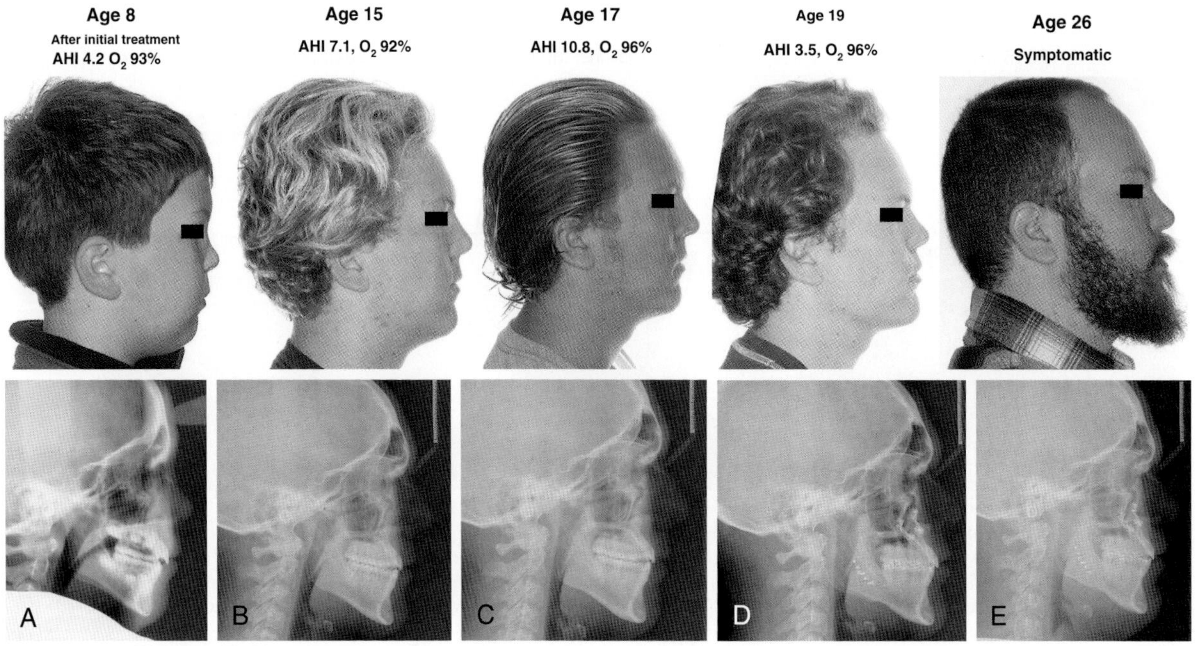

Figure 168.19 Craniofacial development from age 8 to age 19. **A,** Records at age 8 showing airway and facial proportions after adenotonsillectomy, indicating residual sleep-disordered breathing–obstructive sleep apnea (SDB/OSA) (apnea-hypopnea index [AHI]SD 4.2, residual symptoms). Bimaxillary orthodontic expansion initiated. Initial diagnosis of OSA at age 5 (AHI 2.9 with daytime symptoms). **B,** Age 15, after bimaxillary expansion was completed at age 8 and again at age 10. AHI increased to 7.1. **C,** Age 17, in preparation for maxillomandibular advancement (MMA). AHI increased to 10.8 with disproportionate increase in symptoms. **D,** Age 19 after MMA, with normalization of AHI and resolution of symptoms. Note the pharyngeal airway enlargement and accompanying facial soft tissue profile changes. **E,** Age 26, when patient developed daytime fatigue, but also with weight gain.

SELECTED READINGS

Camacho M, Chang E, Song S, et al. Rapid maxillary expansion for pediatric obstructive sleep apnea: a systematic review and meta-analysis. *Laryngoscope*. 2017;127:1712–1719.

Carrasco-Llatas M, O'Connor-Reina C, Calvo-Henríquez C. The role of myofunctional therapy in treating sleep-disordered breathing: a state-of-the-art review. *Int J Environ Res Public Health*. 2021;18(14):7291. https://doi.org/10.3390/ijerph18147291. Published 2021 Jul 8.

de Felício CM, da Silva Dias FV, Trawitzki LVV. Obstructive sleep apnea: focus on myofunctional therapy. *Nat Sci Sleep*. 2018;10:271–286. https://doi.org/10.2147/NSS.S141132. eCollection 2018.

Gurgel M, Cevidanes L, Pereira R, et al. Three-dimensional craniofacial characteristics associated with obstructive sleep apnea severity and treatment outcomes [published online ahead of print, 2021 Jul 17]. *Clin Oral Investig*. 2021. https://doi.org/10.1007/s00784-021-04066-5.

Marcus CL, Smith RJ, Mankarious LA, Arens R, Mitchell GS, Elluru RG, et al. Developmental aspects of the upper airway: report from an NHLBI Workshop, March 5-6, 2009. *Proc Am Thor Soc*. 2009;6(6):513–520.

Mediano O, Romero-Peralta S, Resano P. Obstructive sleep apnea: emerging treatments targeting the genioglossus muscle. *J Clin Med*. 2019;8(10):1754.

A complete reference list can be found online at ExpertConsult.com.

Chapter 169

Sleep Bruxism: Definition, Prevalence, Classification, Etiology, and Consequences

Peter Svensson; Taro Arima; Gilles Lavigne; Eduardo E. Castrillon

Chapter Highlights

- Sleep bruxism (SB) is a frequent oral behavior in healthy individuals that can be a sleep-related movement disorder. It is characterized by teeth grinding or clenching frequently but not exclusively associated with sleep arousal.[1]
- SB is masticatory muscle activity during sleep characterized as rhythmic (phasic) or nonrhythmic (tonic). SB has traditionally been considered an oral parafunction with nonfunctional gnashing, grinding, or chewing movements of the mandible, triggered by occlusal discrepancies, which then could lead to occlusal trauma and dysfunction of the stomatognathic system.
- Current research emphasizes central nervous system factors and regulation of the autonomic nervous system rather than occlusal and anatomic factors.
- SB forms a continuum of masticatory muscle activities ranging from normal physiologic behaviors ("normobruxism") to potentially detrimental consequences to the stomatognathic system ("pathobruxism").
- Understanding the definitions, physiology versus pathophysiology, and the underlying mechanisms of SB at the individual level impacts management of SB patients.

DEFINITIONS

Gnashing and clenching of the teeth have been reported since ancient times and even mentioned in the Old Testament of the Bible.[2] *Bruxism,* the preferred term to characterize these oral behaviors, originated from the Greek word *brygmos* (βϱυγμός), which means gnashing of the teeth. Bruxism has been the focus for many health professions and, more specifically, in dentistry for many years and was described for the first time in the scientific literature by Marie and Pietkiewicz in 1907.[3]

Historically, many definitions of bruxism have been proposed and used. An international expert group proposed the following new consensus-based definition[4]:

> Bruxism is a repetitive jaw-muscle activity characterized by clenching or grinding of the teeth and/or by bracing or thrusting of the mandible. Bruxism has two distinct circadian manifestations: It can occur during sleep (indicated as sleep bruxism [SB]) or during wakefulness (indicated as awake bruxism [AB]).[4]

A subsequent consensus report from the same group added that SB is masticatory muscle activity during sleep characterized as rhythmic (phasic) or nonrhythmic (tonic) and is not a movement or sleep disorder in otherwise healthy individuals.[1]

SB can range from a normal and physiologic behavior ("normobruxism") to a potentially detrimental condition with pathophysiologic consequences for the stomatognathic system ("pathobruxism"). Thus SB could be considered a normal behavior at the individual level or with some comorbidities (e.g., insomnia, sleep apnea, gastroesophageal reflux disorder, and rarer neurologic conditions, such as rapid eye movement [REM] sleep behavior disorder [RBD] or epilepsy). This chapter will focus on the phenomenon of SB in this context.

PREVALENCE

The prevalence of SB varies depending on the specific criteria used and the methods used to establish the diagnosis. Most of the literature available on the epidemiology of SB is based on self-reports, that is, simple questions such as "Are you aware of clenching or grinding your teeth during sleep?" or questionnaires (e.g., the Oral Behaviors Checklist)[5] (see also Chapter 172). Using such methodology, SB is reported to be present in 8% to 31% of the general population.[6] SB has been reported in the literature as occurring as "frequent as three times a week" with a prevalence of 9.3%, as "frequent" bruxism in 14%, and as "often" bruxism in 15.3%.[6] For comparison, AB is reported as "often" in 22.1% and "any AB during the last 6 months" in 31% of the population. Overall, these prevalence figures suggest that SB is very common. In summary, a reasonable

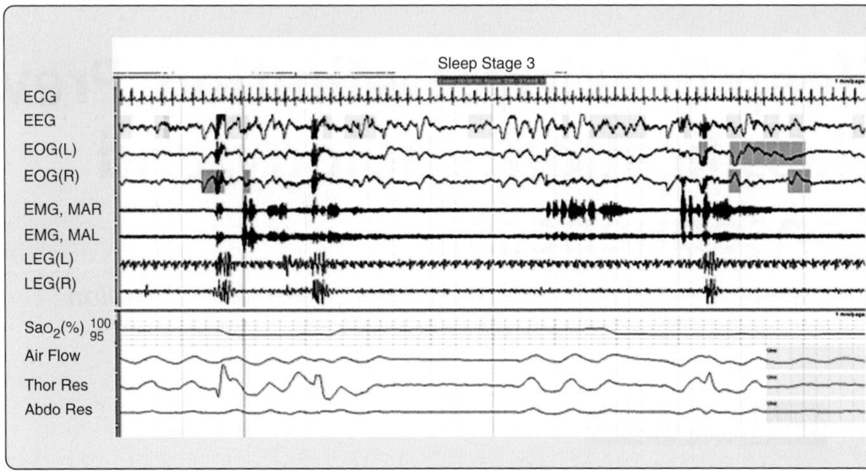

Figure 169.1 A typical polysomnographic (PSG) recording for the assessment of rhythmic masticatory muscle activity (RMMA). This recording includes electrocardiogram (ECG), electroencephalogram (EEG), electrooculogram (EOG), electromyogram (EMG) of the right masseter (MAR) muscle, EMG of the left masseter (MAL) muscle, movement recording of the right leg (LEG[R]), movement recording of the left leg (LEG[L]), oxygen saturation (Sao_2[%]), airflow, thorax expansion resistance (Thor Res), and abdomen expansion resistance (Abdo Res). Gold standard criteria for sleep bruxism demand that PSG recordings for RMMA also include synchronized audio and video recordings (not included in this figure). (Courtesy Faramarz Jadidi, PhD.)

estimate of self-reported SB prevalence is between 8% and 12%.[6,7]

There are nevertheless obvious limitations with prevalence data based on self-reports of SB; for example, if the patients sleep alone, they may not be aware of their SB behavior or, if their sleep partner sleeps very deeply, they may not be told. Furthermore, information from health care providers can cause bias. A classic example is that the majority of patients who may report SB have received the information from their dentist.[8]

The gold standard for an objective SB diagnosis is based on polysomnography (PSG), including audio and video recordings as described in Chapter 172[9] (Figure 169.1). Due to issues such as relatively high costs, there is not much epidemiologic information on SB using PSG criteria. One recent general population large-scale PSG study reported a prevalence of 7.4% SB in adults using exclusively PSG methodology.[10] Unfortunately, this report lacked the video and audio recordings that are needed to fulfill the gold standard requirements and remove false-positive events, for example, derived from body movements or scratching the skin/electrodes.[9,11] Furthermore, only 1 night was used due to the very large sample of that epidemiologic study.[10] It is still an open question if night-to-night variability may significantly interfere with the accuracy of rhythmic masticatory muscle activity (RMMA) scoring as a diagnosis criterion, a subject for further study and refinement with applications of ambulatory home recording devices.[12–16]

It has also been suggested that an overestimation of the SB prevalence is possible when only self-reports are used.[10,17] Of interest, SB prevalence appears not to differ between genders but to decrease with age.[6,18] The reason for the age dependency, so far, is not well understood but must await confirmation from PSG-based SB studies. As a less accurate but more manageable approach than PSG studies to determine definite SB in larger cohorts across age, gender, ethnicity/cultures, ambulatory single-channel electromyographic (EMG) devices may hold promise as technology continues to improve.[19–21] Despite the small amount of scientific information about genetics in SB, a recent review suggested that SB may, at least in part, be genetically determined and environmentally expressed (see the section Pathophysiology versus Physiology for more information).[22–25] However, it will be a complex task to identify specific candidate genes for SB, and more research in this field will be needed.

CLASSIFICATION

One of the most logical ways to classify bruxism is to use the circadian rhythm to divide this oral activity into AB and SB, recognizing it may overlap in some subjects[26] because the physiology/pathophysiology may differ.[6,27] There are, however, many additional possibilities to subclassify SB, given the definition of "repetitive jaw-muscle activity," for example, depending on the specifics of the EMG activity (type, duration, frequency, amplitude, total amount, etc.). One could speculate that concentric, short-lasting, infrequent, and low-intensity jaw-muscle contractions would have different clinical consequences (e.g., tooth wear, orofacial pain, and headache) than eccentric, longer-lasting, frequent, and high-intensity jaw-muscle contractions; further studies are obviously needed to test such hypotheses and better techniques to phenotype bruxism.[28] One of the first studies to use operationalized research criteria, derived from the literature, defined phasic, tonic, and mixed EMG bursts and episodes, and it established cut-off values for SB and non-SB.[9] These three types of EMG bursts are scored as an episode called RMMA. These research criteria subsequently have been refined in a follow-up study.[29] Before these criteria and specific cut-off points are extrapolated for clinical use, further validation is needed with various recording systems, full PSG or limited number of, EMG channels, taking into account that SB may form a continuum of masticatory muscle activities.[30–32] Furthermore, the specifics of such EMG criteria need to be elaborated, for example, to take into account the amplitude and total amount of jaw-muscle activity (area under the EMG curve, duty cycles, amplitude probability distribution function, gap analyses, etc.).

In the *International Classification of Sleep Disorders,* third edition (ICSD-3, 2014) SB was classified as a sleep-related movement disorder (www.aasmnet.org/store/product.aspx?pid=849). It should be noted that the proposed new updated consensus definition, described earlier, states that SB is not considered a movement disorder *in otherwise healthy individuals.*[1] Sleep-related movement disorders are characterized by simple and stereotypic movements that disturb sleep, although the patients may or may not be aware of such movements. A study showed that SB events and periodic limb movement (PLM) are time linked, suggesting that at least some of the underlying mechanisms may be in common.[33] (See also Chapter 121 for more information on restless legs syndrome (RLS) and PLMs during sleep.) In this way, the more mechanism-based ICSD classification of SB is entirely compatible with the consensus-based descriptive definition of SB.[1]

It should be recognized that the clinical diagnosis of SB is associated with considerable diagnostic uncertainty like most other medical diagnoses and, for example, neuropathic pain.[34] One approach is to use the grading system criteria proposed in the consensus report mentioned earlier.[1,4] This diagnostic grading system takes into account the methods and their validity to determine the presence of SB. Three levels were proposed: possible, probable, and definitive. Possible AB or SB is based on self-reports using the history or questionnaires. Probable AB or SB will be based on the outcome from the clinical examination, for example, tooth wear or hypertrophic jaw muscles and eventually also the self-report. Definitive (i.e., in the sense of final at a given time point in the life of the patient) will be based on the outcome from a PSG study following the gold standards for SB,[9] whereas for AB, it was proposed to use assessment of muscle activity or ambulatory EMG.[1,4] It is suggested to apply this grading system to better characterize and classify (phenotype) SB, which should allow better insights into both risk factors and pathophysiology of SB, but also to better understand the potential pathophysiologic consequences of SB.

PATHOPHYSIOLOGY VERSUS PHYSIOLOGY

Basically, the etiology of SB is still controversial, and it may be more appropriate to talk about risk factors that lead to, or are associated with, increased masticatory muscle activity instead of etiologic factors. Historically, SB has been associated with three major domains: anatomic, psychological, and central nervous system (CNS) factors. A short review of these topics is provided as follows.

In the dental community, the anatomic factor has for a long time been considered a main factor for SB because the prevalence of SB was much higher in population groups with malocclusion than in comparable groups with normal occlusion.[35] This tendency was also seen in patients with so-called occlusal discrepancies.[36] A classical mechanistic hypothesis was that SB would be caused by dental factors, for example, occlusal disharmony/supracontacts, which would "irritate" the CNS and trigger excessive jaw-muscle activity, that is, bruxism.[37] Logically, the adjustment or correction of occlusal disharmony therefore would result in the immediate disappearance of the habitual grinding of the teeth because the disharmony/supracontacts would be "equilibrated" by selective grinding or advanced dental restorative procedures.[36,38] Further support to this hypothesis was derived from the observation that SB is most prevalent in 8- to 15-year-old children, with mixed dentitions and more unstable occlusions.[39] However, these views are now downplayed because of a lack of good evidence to support any close relationships or causality between occlusal factors or craniofacial morphology and SB in well-designed studies.[27,40–42] Further, experimental studies with insertions of artificial and reversible supracontacts have shown a decrease, rather than an increase, in jaw-muscle activity during sleep, contradicting the occlusal-based hypothesis of SB.[43] In other studies it was shown that the elimination of interferences in occlusion and articulation did not influence jaw-muscle activity during sleep.[44,45] Today, therefore SB is considered to be mainly regulated and influenced by the CNS autonomic nervous system (CNS-ANS) with psychological-hyperarousal factors with little, if any, contribution from anatomic factors (occlusion, craniofacial morphology)[41,46–48] (see also Chapter 30).

Psychological factors such as anxiety,[49–55] neuroticism,[56] competitiveness,[57] emotional tension,[58] aggressiveness,[59] stress, and maladaptive/less positive coping strategies[60] have frequently been associated with SB, although some controversy remains on their specific contribution; a phenotype may be present in some individuals and not in others.[61] In particular, questionnaires and self-report data have linked SB to stress,[49,51,53,55,62–68] and some studies have also used excretion of urinary catecholamine or salivary chromogranin A as biomarkers of stress and found significant relationships.[62,69] It appears that a variety of psychological vulnerability factors may predispose, maintain, or exacerbate SB.

Finally, the role of comorbidities and CNS function should be considered in the search of understanding the pathophysiology of sleep motor anomalies. RLS[9,70] and another sleep-related movement disorder, such as RBD, are considered to be concomitant to SB and seem to be significant risk factors for SB in some individuals (see Chapter 172).[70,71] It remains to be demonstrated whether this co-occurrence is due simply to age—intersecting epidemiology, that is, prevalence of SB and RLS or RBD, merges with a higher probability of comorbidity across ages: SB in younger ages and RLS or RBD in older ages—or whether there are some common pathophysiologic bases.

Sleep apnea in some individuals may be a significant risk factor or comorbidity for SB.[72,73] Interest in the putative link between SB and sleep breathing disorders is growing; however, the strength of such an association is still debated, and causality is not yet fully proven.[74–79] Insomnia is also another sleep disorder that may be comorbid with SB, as found in two general population studies.[10,80]

Medications or neuroactive substances, such as selective serotonin reuptake inhibitors,[81,82] dopamine antagonists,[83] or recreational drugs (amphetamine, alcohol, nicotine, caffeine),[18,84] are also considered risk factors for some vulnerable SB patients; however, the level of evidence is often modest.

Genetic susceptibility, as mentioned previously, has been relatively little examined, but there is some evidence of a hereditary predisposition based on twin studies, but accounting only for 20% to 50% of the variance.[24,25,85,86] A recent study was also able to demonstrate specific associations between patients with probable AB, SB, and combined AB and SB and single nucleotide polymorphisms in dopaminergic pathway genes.[87] The lessons learned, for example, from pain genetics, would predict that it is highly unlikely to identify a single gene responsible for SB,[22] but rather that several genes and their haplotypes will interact in a complex manner with environmental, psychological, and endogenous factors.[88,89] Furthermore, genetic studies of SB will need a careful phenotyping of the patient and their individual levels of masticatory muscle activity rather than relying on patient reports and simple clinical assessment of the potential consequences of SB.

In general, SB patients are not bad sleepers; it is their sleep partners who are most sleep disturbed, by the grinding sounds. Comparisons between young and healthy patients with SB and control subjects have shown normal sleep organization and macrostructure.[71,90] Several critical parameters of sleep, such as sleep latency, total sleep time, percentage of time spent in the various sleep stages, and number of awakenings, are within normal limits in sleep bruxers.[29,90–92] They also report a normal amount of time spent awake during the sleep period, and they demonstrate sleep efficiency that falls within the usual range of good sleepers (>90%). Moreover, sleep bruxers without pain or insomnia rarely complain about poor sleep quality.

There is emerging evidence of a sequence of biologic events culminating with excessive jaw-muscle activity, that is, teeth grinding or clenching. First, SB may occur in all sleep stages, but it has been established that SB episodes are most frequently (>80% of the time) encountered in sleep stages 1 and 2 (N1 and N2), in the minutes before REM stage and not as previously suggested during REM sleep.[9,93–100] Furthermore, studies have now linked SB to a cyclic alternating pattern (CAP).[92,101] The CAP consists of a cyclic pattern of electroencephalographic (EEG), electrocardiographic, and EMG activation every 20 to 60 seconds,[102] and about 80% of SB episodes are observed in association with the CAP.[92] This may serve as a resetting mechanism for physiologic functions in relation to sleep environment or endogenous factors that act as a permissive window to allow the occurrence of otherwise inhibited motor activity, such as SB or other body or limb movements.[92,103] The association between SB and CAP is further supported by findings showing that greater than 50% of SB episodes occur in clusters (within 100 seconds) and that approximately 15% to 20% occur in the transition from deep sleep (stage N3) to REM sleep.[101] These findings are also consistent with the observation that SB is preceded by alpha EEG activity and is associated with a tachycardia.[104–107] Lavigne and colleagues[9,29] have made a series of important contributions to the understanding of the SB in the sequence of biologic events during sleep. The sequence seems to be initiated by a change in the autonomic-cardiac sympathetic and parasympathetic balance, which subsequently is followed by a rise in EEG activity with more delta activity. This arousal response is followed by tachycardia and increased jaw-opener muscle activity, with an increase in respiratory amplitude (one to breath breaths), and, finally, EMG activity in the jaw-closing muscles is often described as rhythmic jaw movements or as RMMA.[48,108] Also, surges in blood pressure are linked to RMMA episodes. These findings support the concept that SB is secondary to exaggerated transient motor and ANS activation in relation to microarousals.[109–111] The presence of RMMA and SB tooth grinding is frequent in young and healthy SB patients, but it is not always the case in the general population; older subjects may have concomitant sleep breathing disorders or insomnia.[10,72,73,78] The sleep arousal axis allows a better understanding of the integration between the ANS and the CNS; the sympathetic/parasympathetic balance during sleep may influence SB and also explain why cardiovascular/respiratory factors may interact with SB.[71,110,112] Microarousals seem to be important, although not the only factor contributing to the genesis of RMMA-SB, and, indeed, experimental studies with application of vibrotactile stimuli during sleep indicate that such stimuli may cause microarousal without awakenings but with activation of SB and RMMA.[109]

In summary, anatomic factors such as dental occlusion appear to have little, if any, influence on the genesis of SB. There appears to be no single etiologic factor that explains SB but, rather, a set of factors that may interact and exacerbate normal sleep-related bruxism. To avoid confusion, the term *etiologic factors* should be used cautiously and is better substituted by *risk factors*. So far, the most evidence supports the hypothesis that SB is centrally mediated and under the influence of autonomic system functions and brain arousal responses.

It is important to note that knowledge on pathophysiology and mechanism of SB is not only an academic exercise because there are important clinical consequences of the phenomenon. First, it should be recognized that the consequences of SB can form a continuum from no effects to significant and deleterious impact on oral structures and quality of life (e.g., severe tooth attrition, jaw-muscle soreness and pain, and headache). This means that SB should not be treated in each and every patient but rather should be based on a careful examination and analysis of the problems and needs in the individual patient. Second, oral appliances may reduce tooth wear and grinding sounds, but SB cannot be cured by occlusal rehabilitation procedures; the occurrence of sleep-related RMMA will persist. The use of psychological methods (relaxation and cognitive behavioral therapy) may help, although evidence is as yet scarce; in some cases medication may be justified to alleviate the ANS and CNS arousal-permissive influences on SB genesis. Subsequent chapters will address in more details the management of SB (see Chapters 172 and 173). It should also be kept in mind that SB has been proposed to serve normal physiologic purposes, by moving the mandible slightly forward and thereby increasing airway patency, and can be due to the tooth-contacts to activate secretion of saliva during sleep to keep oral tissues moist.[113] In this sense SB may also contribute to maintenance of the homeostasis of the stomatognathic system during sleep, which could be coined "normobruxism" to differentiate from "pathobruxism," where potential detrimental effects may occur, such as excessive tooth wear, pain in the stomatognathic system, headaches, and so forth.

CLINICAL PEARLS

- Sleep bruxism (SB) is a frequent condition and, based on self-reports, affects about 12% of the population.
- SB has a counterpart during awake states, but the pathophysiology and clinical consequences may differ.
- A diagnostic grading system is suggested as useful to distinguish between possible, probable, and definitive types of SB.
- SB cannot be explained by only dental factors, such as occlusion or craniofacial morphology, but is influenced by a range of psychological factors and the central nervous system function in combination with the autonomic nervous system.
- Natural microarousal responses, that is, a sequence of biologic events, may contribute to a permissive effect, leading to SB.

SUMMARY

SB is considered a common condition associated with activation of the masticatory muscles leading to teeth grinding or jaw clenching. The potential consequences of SB form a continuum from no deleterious effects, to severe tooth wear and tooth destruction, to headache upon awakening, and to craniofacial pain complaints. In addition, sleep partners can be disturbed by the noise from tooth gnashing, and SB can have a negative impact on the quality of life. It is a consistent finding that children (15%) more often report SB than adults (8%). There is a general consensus that there is no single cause of SB but that CNS and psychological factors, including stress, may contribute; in severe cases, excessive sleep arousal responses are influenced by autonomic factors. Diagnosis and clinical examination of the orofacial region are essential to be performed. A definite (i.e., final) diagnosis of SB, however, can be made with only PSG recordings of jaw-muscle activity, preferably together with audio-video signals. Due to the multifactorial etiology and complex pathophysiology of sleep bruxism, management is always symptomatic. In otherwise healthy individuals the approach should be reassuring and explanatory of the fact that SB may be a natural behavior.

SELECTED READINGS

Bornhardt T, Iturriaga V. Sleep Bruxism: An Integrated Clinical View. *Sleep Med Clin.* 2021;16(2):373–380.

Carra MC, Huynh N, Fleury B, Lavigne G. Overview on sleep bruxism for sleep medicine clinicians. *Sleep Med Clin.* 2015;10:375–384.

Lavigne GJ, Khoury S, Abe S, et al. Bruxism physiology and pathology: an overview for clinicians. *J Oral Rehabil.* 2008;35:476–494.

Lavigne GJ, Rompré PH, Montplaisir JY. Sleep bruxism: validity of clinical research diagnostic criteria in a controlled polysomnographic study. *J Dent Res.* 1996;75:546–552.

Lobbezoo F, et al. Bruxism defined and graded: an international consensus. *J Oral Rehabil.* 2013;40:2–4.

Lobbezoo F, Ahlberg J, Manfredini D, et al. Are bruxism and the bite causally related? *J Oral Rehabil.* 2012;39:489–501.

Lobbezoo F, Ahlberg J, Raphael KG, et al. International consensus on the assessment of bruxism: report of a work in progress. *J Oral Rehabil.* 2018;45:837–844.

Lobbezoo F, Visscher CM, Ahlberg J, et al. Bruxism and genetics: a review of the literature. *J Oral Rehabil.* 2014;41:709–714.

Mayer P, Heinzer R, Lavigne G. Sleep bruxism in respiratory medicine practice. *Chest.* 2016;149:262–271.

Rompré PH, Daigle-Landry D, Guitard F, et al. Identification of a sleep bruxism subgroup with a higher risk of pain. *J Dent Res.* 2007;86:837–842.

A complete reference list can be found online at ExpertConsult.com.

Chapter 170

Assessment of Sleep Bruxism

Frank Lobbezoo; Ghizlane Aarab; Kiyoshi Koyano; Daniele Manfredini

Chapter Highlights

- The main challenge in relation to sleep bruxism (SB) concerns its assessment. So long as consensus on how to assess SB is lacking, studies on the condition will lack comparability and global acceptance. The recent suggestion for a diagnostic grading system of "possible," "probable," and "definite" SB is an important step toward consensus.
- For a "possible" or " probable" diagnosis of SB, self-report and clinical approaches are indicated, whereas for a "definite" (i.e., final) diagnosis, instrumental assessments such as electromyography (EMG) or polysomnography (PSG), preferably in combination with audio-video recordings, are required.
- As yet, insufficient evidence has been accumulated to support the use of ambulatory EMG devices as stand-alone tools for the assessment of SB, as tested against full PSG recordings.
- In the absence of full consensus on the assessment of SB, an accurate differential diagnosis that considers oral-motor disorders, such as orofacial dyskinesia and oromandibular dystonia, and its distinction from normal orofacial activities that involve jaw, lip, and tongue movements will be difficult. Likewise, purported associations of SB, such as those suggested for rapid eye movement behavior disorder, obstructive sleep apnea, and gastroesophageal reflux disease, will be hard to interpret unequivocally.
- It will be a stimulating challenge for the near future to operationalize the foregoing suggestions for diagnostic grading, taking into consideration the important work that has already assessed this topic.

DEFINITION OF BRUXISM

In 2013 an international group of experts, led by the main author of this chapter, has defined bruxism as a repetitive jaw-muscle activity characterized by clenching or grinding of the teeth and/or by bracing or thrusting of the mandible. The condition has two distinct circadian manifestations: sleep bruxism (SB) and awake bruxism (AB).[1] The new consensus definition, which is suggested for clinical and research purposes in all relevant dental and medical domains, has already been included in leading documents, such as the orofacial pain guidelines of the American Academy of Orofacial Pain[2] and the third edition of the *International Classification of Sleep Disorders* (ICSD-3),[3] showing its emerging international acceptance.

Despite the successful introduction of the new definition of bruxism, the international group of experts decided in 2018 to formulate separate definitions for SB and AB in a second consensus paper, both conditions being generally considered as different behaviors (Box 170.1).[4] The authors of the second consensus paper stress that in otherwise healthy individuals, bruxism should be considered as a behavior rather than a disorder. This represents a true paradigm shift that was initiated in a recent commentary[5] on the first consensus definition paper of 2013.

This chapter reviews recent insights into the methodological aspects and the differential diagnosis for bruxism restricted to sleep. More details on the definition, epidemiology, consequences, and management of SB can be found in Chapters 169, 171, 172, and 176.

ASSESSMENT OF SLEEP BRUXISM

For the assessment of SB, multiple tools are available. Whether any of them, alone or in combination, is uncontestably valid, however, remains unknown and thus a matter of debate. In 2018 a grading system was suggested for SB: For a "possible" diagnosis, self-report of the condition or a proxy (such as a bed partner or a parent) report is sufficient.[4] For a diagnosis of "probable" SB, clinical features suggestive of SB should be present, with or without a positive self-report, whereas for a "definite" (i.e., final) diagnosis, positive findings on instrumental assessment (e.g., electromyography [EMG] or polysomnography [PSG]) are required, with or without a positive self-report and/or a positive clinical inspection.

Presented next are various approaches to the assessment of SB, elaborated in some detail.

Self-Report

For a possible diagnosis of SB, a self-report of the condition can be obtained by questionnaires and/or by oral history taking. Questionnaires can be used to obtain information about the

BOX 170.1 SEPARATE DEFINITIONS FOR SLEEP AND AWAKE BRUXISM PER INTERNATIONAL CONSENSUS

Sleep Bruxism

Sleep bruxism is a masticatory muscle activity during sleep that is characterized as rhythmic (phasic) or nonrhythmic (tonic) and is not a movement disorder or a sleep disorder in otherwise healthy individuals.

Awake Bruxism

Awake bruxism is a masticatory muscle activity during wakefulness that is characterized by repetitive or sustained tooth contact and/or by bracing or thrusting of the mandible and is not a movement disorder in otherwise healthy individuals.

From Lobbezoo F, Ahlberg J, Raphael KG, et al. International consensus on the assessment of bruxism: report of a work in progress. *J Oral Rehabil.* 2018;45:837–44.

BOX 170.2 BRUX SCALE OF THE ORAL PARAFUNCTIONS QUESTIONNAIRE FOR THE ASSESSMENT OF SELF-REPORTED BRUXISM

Questions

1. How often do you clench your teeth during sleep?
2. How often do you grind your teeth during sleep?
3. How often do you clench your teeth while awake?
4. How often do you grind your teeth while awake?

Response Options

Never (0)
Sometimes (1)
Regularly (2)
Often (3)
Always (4)

From van der Meulen MJ, Lobbezoo F, Aartman IH, Naeije M. Self-reported oral parafunctions and pain intensity in temporomandibular disorder patients. *J Orofac Pain.* 2006;20:31–5.

Table 170.1 Questionnaires for Assessment of Physical and Psychological Domains in Temporomandibular Disorders and Sleep Bruxism as Recommended by the Diagnostic Criteria for TMD (DC/TMD)

Domain	Questionnaire	Abbreviation
Pain intensity, physical function	Graded Chronic Pain Scale	GCPS
Pain locations	Pain drawing	N/A
Limitation	Jaw Function Limitation Scale	JFLS
Distress	Patient Health Questionnaire-4	PHQ-4
Depression	Patient Health Questionnaire-9	PHQ-9
Anxiety	Generalized Anxiety Disorder-7	GAD-7
Physical symptoms (somatization)	Patient Health Questionnaire-15	PHQ-15
Oral behaviors	Oral Behaviors Checklist	OBC

N/A, Not applicable.
From Schiffman E, Ohrbach R, Truelove E, et al. Diagnostic Criteria for Temporomandibular Disorders (DC/TMD) for clinical and research applications: recommendations of the International RDC/TMD Consortium Network and Orofacial Pain Special Interest Group. *J Oral Facial Pain Headache.* 2014;28:6–27.

condition itself and on its possible causes and consequences, as well as possible comorbid conditions and differential diagnostic considerations (see the section Differential Diagnosis). An example of a questionnaire for the assessment of SB that can be used in the research setting and in the clinic is the so-called BRUX scale, developed and tested for its psychometric properties by van der Meulen and associates.[6] The BRUX scale consists of four questions that can be answered on a five-item verbal scale (ranging from never to always), two of which deal with SB (Box 170.2). The BRUX scale is part of a more extensive tool, the Oral Parafunctions[a] Questionnaire (OPQ).[6] Apart from four bruxism questions (the BRUX scale), the OPQ inquires about chewing on pens or pencils, nail biting, and chewing gum (the BITE scale), as well as about vacuum sucking with the tongue, playing or pushing with the tongue, lip biting, sucking on lips/cheeks, and playing with a denture (the SOFT scale). In addition, the OPQ assesses behaviors that may strain the jaw, such as sleeping on the belly. Not only the latter behavior but also some of the other behaviors can occur during sleep, and their effects should thus be distinguished from SB.

Another comprehensive tool for the assessment of SB and other (possibly comorbid) oral behaviors is the Oral Behaviors Checklist (OBC).[7,8] This 21-item tool was composed based on expert opinions and on patient contributions. Like the OPQ, the OBC uses a 5-point scale for its responses (for sleep-related behaviors: none of the time, <1 night/month, 1 to 3 nights/month, 1 to 3 nights/week, 4 to 7 nights/week). Although the daytime behaviors were tested for reliability by means of EMG recordings, the sleep-related behaviors were not subjected to reliability assessments so far. Of importance, whereas the OPQ asks about the presence or absence of single behaviors, the OBC contains several questions that ask about the presence or absence of multiple behaviors in one and the same question, for example: "Based on the last month, how often do you clench or grind teeth when asleep, based on any information you may have?" Because clenching and grinding are commonly considered distinct conditions, this mode of inquiring yields less information than when single behaviors are being assessed.[9] Nevertheless, the OBC was well received by the international community (see later; see also Table 170.1).

Multiple self-report tools are available for the assessment of the possible causes and consequences of SB. For one of the

[a] By definition, a parafunction is a disordered function, which implies that a behavior like SB only has negative consequences. However, recent studies suggest that SB may also have positive physiologic functions, for instance, maintaining upper airway patency and stimulating salivary flow, which in turn aids to protect the health of the upper alimentary tract. Hence the term *parafunction* is to be avoided.[1]

most commonly suggested consequences, temporomandibular disorders (TMD), and for several possible causes of SB (see Chapters 169 and 172), the recently published Diagnostic Criteria for TMD (DC/TMD)[10] suggests a comprehensive protocol for the assessment of several physical and psychological domains by means of, in most cases, validated questionnaires. The domains and their respective assessment tools are shown in Table 170.1. Although the DC/TMD is a leading and largely evidence-based system, clinicians are free to select their own questionnaires for the assessment of SB and its possible causes and consequences.

When a questionnaire is completed and analyzed before the clinical consultation, the clinician knows better what to expect. In addition, patients usually have gained an improved awareness of their oral behavior, which helps improve the reliability of the oral history, the second way of obtaining self-reported data on SB. An important advantage of an oral history over the use of questionnaires is the way in which the questions are formulated: They can be adapted to the individual patient's knowledge and cognitive abilities. For research purposes, on the other hand, an oral history lacks standardization. Also, oral history taking may be influenced by the clinician's preconceived ideas about SB. A disadvantage of the use of questionnaires for the assessment of SB is that approximately 80% of bruxism episodes are free of grinding sounds.[11] In consequence, owing to lack of awareness for many such events, self-reports of the condition may be characterized by underscoring, with respect to the standard reference for a definite SB diagnosis (see further in the section Instrumental Assessment). An investigation reporting both PSG and self-reported SB assessment in a large general population sample showed PSG confirmation of SB in less than one-half of the patients self-reporting this behavior.[12] Likewise, in a group of female TMD-pain patients, poor concordance of self-reported SB with instrumental approaches was observed.[13] Furthermore, the occurrence and severity of SB fluctuate over time,[14] which further hampers the accuracy of self-reports of SB. Hence questionnaires should be interpreted with caution, and preferably, they should be used in combination with other assessment tools.[15]

As a final remark, it must be pointed out that, despite the aforementioned disadvantages, self-reported approaches to the assessment of SB have been used to collect data for several research purposes. The generalization of findings on most SB issues is thus limited.[16,17]

Clinical Examination

A clinical examination that assesses probable SB (as described previously) focuses on the extraoral assessment of masticatory muscle hypertrophy (see earlier) and on the intraoral assessment of hyperkeratosis (i.e., tooth-induced impressions in cheeks ["linea alba"], tongue ["indentations"], and/or lips),[18,19] tooth wear (Figure 170.1, *A* and *B*),[20] fracture or failure of restorations and implants,[18,21,22] and signs such as tooth mobility, pulp necrosis, and traumatic ulcers.[19] Of importance, all of those clinical features lack specificity in the assessment of SB. Masseter muscle hypertrophy, for example, should be distinguished from parotid salivary gland pathology, although it also can be associated with AB activities or other poor oral behavior.

Tooth wear can have multiple causes.[23] Whereas intrinsic mechanical tooth wear (attrition) is caused by tooth-tooth contacts as in sleep grinding, extrinsic mechanical tooth wear

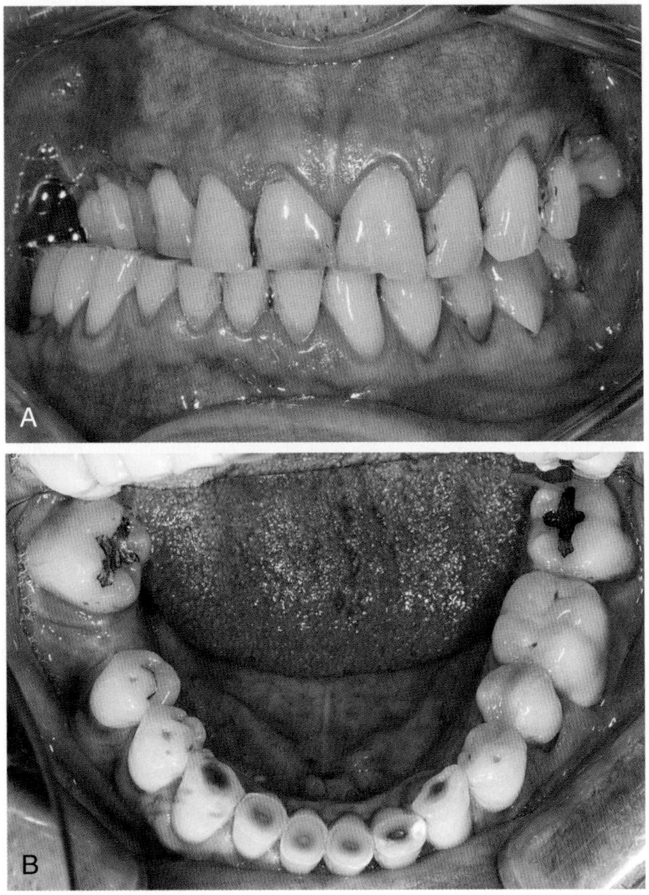

Figure 170.1 Example of sleep-related grinding damage. **A,** Frontal view. **B,** Occlusal view on the lower jaw.

(abrasion) is due to tooth contact with objects (e.g., toothbrushes, pens, or fingernails), and chemical tooth wear (erosion) is a chemically caused type of tooth wear (as with reflux of stomach contents [intrinsic type] or an acidic diet [extrinsic type]). The interpretation of tooth wear in SB recognition is not simple because no single cause is present, and the wear could have happened years before the examination. As a consequence, this complicates the interpretation of a worn dentition in terms of tooth-grinding activities as well. This is illustrated by a study in young adults,[20] in which it was concluded that although the presence of attrition is indeed associated with the presence of SB, the degree of attrition does not show a dose-response relationship with the severity (specifically, the frequency of jaw-muscle contractions per hour of sleep) of SB.

From a dental point of view, the direction of tooth grinding is an important factor to consider in restorative dentistry: A restoration should be loaded toward the central axis of the tooth and not away from the center to prevent fractures of the fillings. So long as the tooth wear is confined to the enamel, the direction of grinding can be established with the so-called "scratch test," whereby a small scratch is placed on the wear facet by means of a scalpel. At baseline and after a brief time interval of a few nights, dental precision impressions are made of the scratches and subsequently studied under scanning electron microscopy. Such scratches will show most microwear on their leading edge, that is, on the edge opposite to the grinding direction.[24] When extensive dental restorations are planned, this information can be taken into account.

Several reviews have been published on the effects of SB on dental implants and on implant-supported prostheses.[21,22,25] In short, SB seems to be unrelated to biologic complications (e.g., failing osseointegration of the implants), although some evidence suggests that bruxism causes mechanical complications (e.g., fractures of implants or suprastructures/prostheses). It should be noted that, despite this evidence, there is still a need for better understanding in general and specialist dental practices of the extent to which, and under which circumstances, SB can be seen as a causal factor for the occurrence of dental implant complications.[26]

Apart from the aforementioned aspects, the clinical examination may include a functional examination of the masticatory system, based on the paradigm that bruxism and TMD pain are potentially causally related. To that end the clinician may use the highly sensitive muscle and joint palpation tests, a negative outcome of which confirms the absence of TMD pain, and/or the highly specific dynamic/static pain tests, a positive outcome of which confirms the presence of TMD pain.[27,28] Whether or not SB and TMD are actually causally related, however, is highly debated in the literature. According to a review that was published almost 25 years ago,[29] the nature of this relationship is still unclear. A more recent systematic review[17] yields a slightly different, although not opposing, insight into the purported causal association between SB and TMD: Investigations based on self-report or clinical examination, or both, suggested a positive association between the two conditions, although these studies are characterized by some potential bias and confounders at the assessment level. By contrast, studies based on use of more quantitative and specific methods to assess SB (e.g., EMG or PSG; see later) showed much weaker associations with TMD symptoms. Apparently, the more precisely SB is defined, the less clear is its purported association with TMD. This was confirmed in a recent systematic review of the literature that was published during the past decade.[30] In consequence, the value of a TMD pain diagnosis is limited in the context of the assessment of SB.

A recent study assessed the correlation between questionnaire-based SB and a diagnosis of SB based on an oral history in combination with a clinical examination.[31] Using a brief questionnaire, both self-reported sleep-related grinding (*"Are you aware of the fact that you grind your teeth during sleep?"*) and proxy- (e.g., partner-) reported sleep-related grinding (*"Did anyone tell you that you grind your teeth during sleep?"*) were assessed, whereas the question to assess self-reported sleep-related clenching was formulated as follows: *"On morning awakening or on awakenings during the night, do you have your jaws thrust or braced?"* In addition, and preceded by an oral history during which the self-awareness of SB was reassessed, a brief clinical examination was performed focusing on the presence of shiny tooth wear spots for sleep-related grinding and on the presence of masseter muscle hypertrophy, "linea alba" on the cheek mucosa, tongue scalloping, and positive manual palpation of the masseter muscles for sleep-related clenching. Proxy-reported sleep-related grinding showed a high correlation between both approaches ($\Phi = 0.93$), whereas a lower (albeit still acceptable) correlation value was found for sleep-related clenching behavior ($\Phi = 0.64$). Of interest, the nonproxy self-report yielded a lower correlation value ($\Phi = 0.63$) than the proxy-based one, which underlines the importance of including proxy reports in dedicated questionnaires and oral history taking.

Of note, at present, data are lacking on the correlation between clinically established SB and the definite diagnosis of this condition obtained by instrumental techniques (as described next). Thus further research on this topic is strongly encouraged.

Instrumental Assessment

As described earlier, a definite (i.e., final) diagnosis of SB can be based on a positive PSG recording, preferably in combination with audio-video recordings and with bruxism outcome measures above a predefined threshold in concert with self-report of such episodes and expected clinical features on the physical examination. Because, as elaborated to follow, PSG is a rather complicated, inaccessible, and expensive tool, several alternative instrumental techniques have been developed over the years with the aim of objectifying the presence of SB in individual patients. To follow is an overview of the most commonly applied tools for the instrumental assessment of SB.

Intraoral Appliances

A commonly used technique to assess the presence and progression of sleep-related grinding is determining the wear of a hard occlusal stabilization appliance (Figure 170.2, *A* and *B*). This appliance (or "splint"), which is indicated for TMD pain and for SB, is worn over the upper or lower dental arch. A systematic review of the available randomized clinical trials demonstrated that the evidence is insufficient for a recommendation for or against the use of stabilization splint therapy for the treatment of TMD.[32] Likewise, for the treatment of SB, a systematic review concluded the following:

> There is not sufficient evidence to state that the occlusal splint is effective for treating sleep bruxism. Indication of its use is questionable with regard to sleep outcomes, but it may be that there is some benefit with regard to tooth wear.[33]

In other words, it is likely that in at least some patients with SB, the grinding behavior persists, thereby wearing down the stabilization splint. Hence the splint may function as a tool for the assessment of the presence and progression of grinding-type SB but not for that of clenching-type SB, which is associated with less material wear than the grinding type. In addition, quantifying splint wear is fraught with difficulties, both of a technical nature and in terms of interpretation.[19]

Another frequently used intraoral appliance for the assessment of SB is the Bruxcore plate (Bruxcore-Bruxism-Monitoring-Device [BBMD]; Bruxcore, Boston, Massachusetts), a thin (0.51-mm) polyvinyl chloride sheet with four layers of two alternating colors that is fitted to the dental arch. When worn during the night, sleep-related grinding activities will lead to wear of the colored layer(s), thus yielding a measure for the amount of SB. Unfortunately, as outlined in detail previously,[15] several drawbacks are attached to this method, the most important one being the finding that the Bruxcore plate scores do not correlate with jaw-muscle activities detected on the electromyogram (EMG) during sleep.[34] In all likelihood, this is due to the fact that bruxism is characterized not only by tooth grinding but also by clenching activities, the latter leading to less material wear than from grinding, as is also the case with splints (see earlier). Clearly, other methods are needed to establish a definite SB diagnosis.

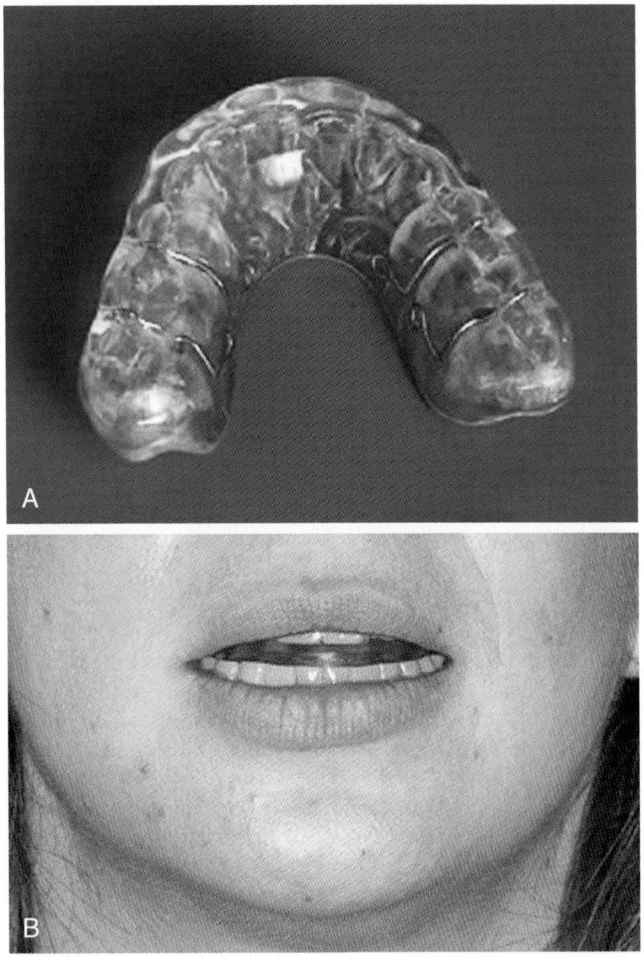

Figure 170.2 A, Example of a hard occlusal stabilization appliance indicated for the management of sleep bruxism and commonly used to assess the presence and progression of the condition based on wear patterns on the occlusal surface. **B,** In situ on the upper jaw.

Electromyography

From the preceding discussion, it can be gathered that an objective assessment of jaw-muscle activities is an essential step in the diagnosis of SB. To that end, EMG is commonly used. A vast number of EMG devices are available. Some of these have been developed specifically for the assessment of SB, sometimes in combination with a management option.[35] Although the devices have various differences in technical and practical characteristics, they all are easy to use, relatively cheap, and portable, thus allowing recording at home ("ambulatory recording"). A major drawback of most ambulatory EMG recorders (i.e., type IV) is that they do not provide the clinician with information about the sleep-wake state, nor do they allow the discrimination between SB activities on the one hand and other sleep-related/nocturnal orofacial activities on the other, thus potentially leading to overscoring of the number of "bruxism" events during the recording time. With that in mind, recent developments combine EMG recordings with one or more additional leads (e.g., heart rate[36] or multiple leads, including pulse wave intervals, actigraphy, and audio-video recordings[37]). These type III devices may yield the optimal combination between EMG alone (i.e., type IV) and full PSG recordings (i.e., type I in sleep laboratory and II if used at home) for the assessment of SB.

BOX 170.3 SLEEP BRUXISM EVENTS (BURSTS AND EPISODES), DEFINED BY THEIR CONSTITUENT RHYTHMIC MASTICATORY MUSCLE ACTIVITY CHARACTERISTICS

Phasic (Rhythmic) Episodes

At least three suprathreshold EMG bursts[a] in the masseter and/or temporalis muscles, lasting ≥0.25 second[b] and <2 seconds and separated by two interburst intervals of <2 seconds[c]

Tonic (Sustained) Episodes

One EMG burst of ≥2 seconds

Mixed Episodes

Both phasic and tonic characteristics

Nonclassified Bursts

Either one EMG burst lasting ≥0.25 second and <2 seconds or two EMG bursts lasting ≥0.25 second and <2 seconds and separated by one interburst interval of <2 seconds

[a]EMG threshold can be established in different ways: >20% of the maximum voluntary contraction (MVC) level,[39] >10% of the MVC level,[40] or a multiplication (e.g., three times) of the background (noise) level of the EMG signal.
[b]EMG events <0.25 second are considered twitches or myoclonic activities.
[c]When the time interval between two bursts is ≥2 seconds, a new event (burst, episode) starts.
EMG, Electromyogram.

Polysomnography

According to the ICSD-3,[3] PSG is needed for an accurate assessment of SB. Pioneer work on this topic has been performed by the research group of Lavigne and collaborators,[38–41] on whose work most of the following information is based. The repetitive jaw-muscle activities that are recorded with PSG are indicated as rhythmic masticatory muscle activity (RMMA). Traditionally, the characteristics of the RMMA recording are used to define SB events (i.e., bursts and episodes; see Box 170.3). Of note, although separate criteria were previously proposed for ambulatory recordings using one or only a few leads,[42] current equipment usually allows for sufficiently high sample rates to enable application of the criteria as described in Box 170.3 for ambulatory recordings as well.

Full PSG recordings can be obtained with ambulatory equipment in the home environment (i.e., type II), but the recordings can also be performed in a highly controlled (but rather unnatural) hospital-based sleep laboratory environment (i.e., type I). Specifically for the assessment of SB, PSG includes surface EMG recordings, obtained from at least one jaw-closing muscle (right and/or left masseter and/or temporalis muscle). The use of audio-video recordings is more feasible in the sleep laboratory environment than in the home milieu and contributes to the accuracy of a definite SB diagnosis.[43] These studies help in ruling out other orofacial activities that can be confused for SB events, such as swallowing, yawning, and sleep-talking.

As noted previously and described in Chapter 169, research diagnostic criteria have been developed and also have evolved over the years. The classical and current recommendations, including the total duration of SB events and the total duration of the intervals between SB events, are given in Box 170.4. An important limitation of the application of those criteria is the fact that the frequency and severity of SB are known

BOX 170.4 OUTCOME MEASURES AND CUT-OFF CRITERIA FOR SLEEP BRUXISM, BASED ON ANALYSES OF RHYTHMIC MASTICATORY MUSCLE ACTIVITIES DURING SLEEP

Sleep Bruxism Outcome Measures

Classical outcome measures[39]
- Number of sleep bruxism episodes/night
- Number of sleep bruxism episodes/hour (of sleep)
- Number of sleep bruxism bursts/hour (of sleep)
- Number of sleep bruxism bursts/episode

Additional outcome measures[77,78]
- Total bruxism time by total sleep time: bruxism time index
- Total duration of intervals between sleep bruxism events

Sleep Bruxism Cut-off Criteria

Classical criteria[39]
- >4 episodes/hour, *and*
- 6 bursts/episode and/or >25 bursts/hour, *and*
- At least 1 episode/night with grinding sounds

Adapted criteria[41,79]
- Low intensity: >1 and ≤2 episodes/hour
- Moderate intensity: >2 and ≤4 episodes/hour
- High intensity: >4 episodes/hour

to fluctuate considerably over time.[44] The diagnostic consequences of the time-variant nature of SB have been quantified by suggesting the use of 95% probability cut-off bands around the previously suggested cut-off points that are included in Box 170.4.[14] For example, with use of a cut-off point of four episodes occurring in each hour of sleep, to distinguish sleep "bruxers" from "nonbruxers," the 95% probability cut-off band suggests that only patients with at least seven episodes per hour are likely to be sleep bruxers, whereas persons with one or fewer episodes per hour are likely to be nonbruxers.[14] Of importance, the study authors indicated that because they worked with a mixture of previous data[45] and data that they collected themselves, the suggested cut-off bands should be considered an illustration of principle.

The accuracy of portable instrumental devices for the measurement of SB against PSG, assumed as the gold standard, was assessed in a systematic review.[45] Using several databases and a quality assessment tool (i.e., Quality Assessment of Diagnostic Accuracy, version 2), the reviewers identified only four studies evaluating three different devices—Bitestrip, EMG-telemetry recorder, and Bruxoff—that could be included. In a disappointing turn, the validity of the included instrumental approaches with respect to PSG recordings was not only scarce but also not solid enough to support use of those techniques as stand-alone tools for assessment of SB. The most promising device was the Bruxoff,[36] which assesses not only the increased EMG masticatory muscle events that are characteristic for SB but also electrocardiographic changes that have been shown to occur in association with SB events,[46] thereby improving the accuracy of the device over that of the other portable instruments. The outcome of a systematic review, however, implies that PSG is still the gold standard for the assessment of SB.[39] On the other hand, a recent commentary describes a plea to move on from the use of PSG cut-off points to a continuum spectrum.[47] This is related to the growing notion that scoring criteria that are based on cut-off points are of questionable clinical usefulness given the absence of a clear association between such points and the possible clinical consequences of SB (e.g., tooth wear, TMD pain, dental restoration failure, etc.). Therefore the authors suggest to increase the current knowledge base of the epidemiologic characteristics and natural course of self-reported and/or instrumentally assessed SB that is needed to identify risk factors for the clinical consequences of SB.

DIFFERENTIAL DIAGNOSIS

Dental sleep medicine is a growing domain that is defined as "...the [dental] discipline concerned with the study of the oral and maxillofacial causes and consequences of sleep-related problems."[48] Several so-called dental sleep disorders can be distinguished, namely, oral movement disorders (including SB), sleep-breathing disorders, oral moistening disorders (e.g., dry mouth, excess salivation), gastroesophageal reflux, and orofacial pain. In individual patients, these disorders can be associated with each other.[49] A broader knowledge of the whole range of dental sleep disorders and their associations is therefore imperative in the interest of providing the best possible management for every single one of our patients. Therefore a professional collaboration between medical doctors and dentists is crucial.[50,51]

In this section on differential diagnosis, SB is considered in the context of oral movement disorders, rapid eye movement (REM) behavior disorder (RBD), sleep-disordered breathing, and gastroesophageal reflux disease.

Movement Disorders

Oral movement disorders are common conditions.[52] In some cases the abnormal oral movement can be considered a focal manifestation of a generalized movement disorder, such as Gilles de la Tourette syndrome, Huntington disease, idiopathic torsion dystonia, and Parkinson disease (PD). The disorder also can be a side effect of medication taken for the generalized disorder.[53] In other cases the oral movement disorder, notably orofacial dyskinesia or oromandibular dystonia, is the sole disorder present.

Orofacial dyskinesia is characterized by involuntary, mainly choreatic (dance-like) movements of the jaw, and other structures, such as the face, lips, and tongue. The same structures can be affected by oromandibular dystonias, which consist of excessive, involuntary, and sustained muscle contractions. Both disorders have been reviewed extensively.[52,53] As possible causes, loss of inhibitory control of the basal ganglia, certain psychiatric diseases, excessive usage of dopaminergic medications, and the chronic use of antipsychotic drugs (neuroleptics) have been mentioned in the literature. When the disorder is caused by neuroleptics, it is indicated as a "tardive" condition. In addition, some anecdotal evidence from case studies suggests that certain dental conditions, such as edentulism and dentoalveolar trauma, also may play a causal role in the etiology of orofacial movement disorders. Peck and coworkers[54] have formulated a set of diagnostic criteria for this condition (see Box 170.5).

When orofacial movement disorders persist in sleep, they can easily be confused with SB. Of note, orofacial dyskinesias and oromandibular dystonias can be misdiagnosed as grinding

BOX 170.5 DIAGNOSTIC CRITERIA FOR OROFACIAL DYSKINESIA AND OROMANDIBULAR DYSTONIA

Orofacial Dyskinesia

History should be positive for the following:
- Neurologic diagnosis of dyskinesia in the orofacial region

Examination by neurologist should be positive for the following:
- Sensory and/or motor nerve conduction deficit, *and*
- Central and/or peripheral myopathic disease, *and*
- Muscular hyperactivity confirmed by intramuscular EMG

Oromandibular Dystonia

History should be positive for the following:
- Neurologic diagnosis of oromandibular dystonia

Examination by neurologist should be positive for the following:
- Sensory and/or motor nerve conduction deficit, *and*
- Central and/or peripheral myopathic disease, *and*
- Dystonia confirmed by intramuscular EMG

EMG, Electromyogram.
From Okeson JP, Phillips BA, Berry DT, et al. Nocturnal bruxing events in subjects with sleep-disordered breathing and control subjects. *J Craniomandib Disord.* 1991;5:258–64; Balasubramaniam R, Ram S. Orofacial movement disorders. *Oral Maxillofac Surg Clin North Am.* 2008;20:273–85, vii.

(phasic) or clenching (tonic) behavior, respectively, especially when the disorder is confined to the jaw. SB also needs to be differentiated from faciomandibular myoclonus; parasomnias such as abnormal swallowing, night terrors, confusional arousals; and, rarely, from sleep-related epilepsy.[3] This underlines the need for proper diagnostic procedures, including an extensive medical and dental history, the more so because the treatment of orofacial movement disorders differs from that of SB, with a primary role for medical specialists instead of dentists (see Chapters 106 on epilepsy and 122 on movement disorders for more information).

Rapid Eye Movement Behavior Disorder

RBD is a neurologic disorder that occurs during the REM phases of sleep and features abnormal, powerful body movements mimicking motor behavior in contrast with the muscle paralysis (atonia) that usually is observed during REM sleep (see Chapter 118). The disorder may lead to aggressive or complex behaviors, which may be accompanied by loud vocalizations related to the emotions experienced while dreaming. It essentially affects older men and may go undiagnosed for years before medical attention is sought. Diagnosis is confirmed with PSG, which typically shows absence of normal REM sleep atonia and sometimes abnormal behaviors. Treatment may be attempted with clonazepam.

Because of its frequent association with the alpha-synucleinopathies, such as PD, RBD is considered to be an important risk factor for later onset of neurodegenerative disorders, including dementia.[55,56] Pilot case studies reported that patients with RBD also may show tooth grinding.[57,58] In particular, a case-control study comparing data from 28 patients with idiopathic or PD-related RBD with those from 9 age- and sex-matched control subjects suggested that in the presence of high-frequency RMMA during sleep, RBD should be suspected.[58] Of interest, on the one hand, these findings support the hypothesis that different sleep disorders may co-occur in the same person as part of complex spectra of alterations of the normal sleep structure; on the other hand, they are in apparent contrast with currently available knowledge on idiopathic SB, which occurs mainly in non-REM sleep stages 1 and 2, as described in other chapters. Clearly, more research is needed to this topic. Future longitudinal studies monitoring RBD patient groups on the occurrence of SB and PD can further deepen our understanding of these conditions' correlations. In addition, such studies may facilitate identifying the early presentation of PD or other neurodegenerative disorders, such as dementia.

Sleep-Disordered Breathing

Sleep-related breathing disorders are a group of conditions related with alterations of the normal airflow and respiration during sleep. As described elsewhere in this book (see the section Sleep Breathing Disorders from Chapter 123 and more in this volume), they commonly are divided into five categories: (1) obstructive sleep apnea (OSA) syndromes, (2) central sleep apnea syndromes, (3) sleep-related hypoventilation syndromes, (4) sleep-related hypoventilation resulting from a medical condition, and (5) other sleep-related breathing disorders.[3] In this discussion the focus is on OSA, which has been called into consideration for its possible relationship with SB.[59]

OSA is a breathing disorder that is characterized by the occurrence of apneic-hypoapneic episodes during sleep. It is considered a primary sleep disorder, characterized by the collapse of the pharynx over the upper airways, which may cause their total (i.e., apnea) or partial (i.e., hypopnea) obstruction and may lead to oxygen desaturation and arousal, that is, awakening from sleep.[3] Among others, obesity, increasing age, male gender, menopausal state in women, and individual variability in lung volume and ventilation control have been identified as risk factors for OSA. Nevertheless, as in the case of SB, the pathophysiology of OSA is not yet fully understood because it is plausible that a combination of neuromuscular and anatomic characteristics and nonanatomic phenotypic traits play a role in the pathogenesis of obstruction.[60]

In the adult population, apneic episodes have been reported in greater than 30% of patients with possible bruxism.[61] Because SB is correlated with arousal episodes,[62] and a high number of short arousal episodes also have been observed in patients with OSA, a possible relationship between the two phenomena (i.e., airway obstruction and SB episodes) has been hypothesized.[59] In some PSG studies, an increase in the EMG activity of jaw muscles was observed in 40% to 60% of patients with OSA[63]; in some cases, a tonic or phasic activity of the masseter at the end of the apneic event has been described.[64–68] However, findings regarding the temporal relationship between the two phenomena are inconclusive yet and do not allow determination of important clinical questions: Does bruxism-like jaw-muscle activity actually follow or precede the apnea? Do they coincide, or are the events temporally unrelated?

Four hypothetical scenarios may be identified for the association between SB and OSA: (1) The two phenomena are unrelated with respect to temporal sequence, (2) the onset of the OSA event precedes the onset of the SB event within a limited time span, (3) the onset of the SB event precedes the onset of the OSA event within a limited time span, or (4) the onset of both phenomena occurs at the same moment.[69]

The most plausible hypothesis is that all four of these temporal relationships between an SB event and an OSA event are actually possible and that the relative predominance of one specific sequence of events may vary from patient to patient. For instance, the role of SB events may range from a protective activity against the apnea, in an attempt to protrude the relaxed mandible and restore airway patency,[59] to an OSA-inducing activity, as a consequence of the airways' mucosal swelling resulting from an SB-induced trigeminal cardiac reflex.[70] Interindividual differences, especially in the anatomic location of the airway obstruction, also may play a role in determining the nature of the SB-OSA relationship. To further clarify this relationship, studies exploring the underlying pathophysiologic mechanisms, large cohort studies for the assessment of risk indicators, and longitudinal clinical studies for causality are required.

Gastroesophageal Reflux Disease

Gastroesophageal reflux (GER) is the physiologic regurgitation of stomach contents into the esophagus and the mouth, which normally may occur after eating and is asymptomatic (see Chapter 161). When the frequency and duration of such reflux episodes increase, signs and symptoms may emerge, reflecting the development of pathophysiologic changes leading to GER disease (GERD). The predominant symptom is known as "heartburn" because of the classic painful chest sensation, and it can affect 7% to 10% of people in the general population during waking hours. GERD is more common during sleep owing to the facilitation of reflux in the supine position, but very little is known about its sleep-time prevalence.[71]

With respect to SB, GERD assumes importance because of the need for taking this condition into account during the differential diagnosis when tooth wear is detected (see the section Clinical Examination). Also, despite the absence of sound literature data on the issue, the possible coexistence of the two conditions may increase the risk for severe tooth damage. In particular, an interesting recent hypothesis suggested that SB-like RMMAs can be induced in healthy persons by experimental esophageal acidification.[72] This suggestion found support in early observations of an increase in the number of SB episodes with lowering of the pH of saliva and esophageal contents,[73] as well as in a more recent investigation describing a 73% prevalence of SB in patients with GERD.[74]

FINAL CONSIDERATIONS AND FUTURE DIRECTIONS

SB has been studied with increasing frequency over the past several decades. Notwithstanding the enormous effort, the condition is still not fully understood. An important development has been the formulation of new definitions by an international group of bruxism experts.[1,4] Because these definitions have been widely adopted by leading professional and scientific organizations, at least future studies can be expected to be comparable regarding the description of SB. The main challenge in relation to SB, however, is still its assessment. So long as consensus on how to assess SB is lacking, studies on this condition will lack comparability and global acceptance. The suggestion from the international consensus points[1,4] toward a diagnostic grading system (possible, probable, and definite SB, as defined earlier) and is only a small first step toward a solution. It should be noted that the assessment approach followed depends on the study aim. For example, for a large-scale epidemiologic assessment, a possible diagnosis may be sufficient, in that large numbers of participants will compensate for the lower accuracy. On the other hand, when associations of sleep-related events with SB phenomena are the aim of a study, a definite diagnosis with high accuracy will be necessary, with all of the possible drawbacks of limited availability and high costs attached to it. Of importance, in the absence of full consensus on the assessment of SB, a proper differential diagnosis that includes, for example, orofacial dyskinesia and oromandibular dystonia, will be difficult as well. Likewise, purported associations of SB, such as those suggested for RBD, OSA, GERD, and other dental sleep disorders, will be hard to interpret unequivocally in terms of their causal implications. It will be a challenge in the nearby future to operationalize the suggestions for diagnostic grading as formulated recently,[1,4] taking into consideration the important work that has already assessed this topic.[38,39,41,75–79]

CLINICAL PEARLS

- For a "possible" or "probable" sleep bruxism (SB) diagnosis, self-report and clinical approaches are sufficient, whereas for a "definite" diagnosis, electromyography or polysomnography,[80] preferably with audio-video recordings, is required.
- SB should be differentiated from several other sleep-related conditions, among which are orofacial movement disorders with manifestations that persist in sleep.
- Among others, rapid eye movement behavior disorder, obstructive sleep apnea, and gastroesophageal reflux disease are important comorbid conditions in patients with SB with possible causal associations.

SUMMARY

SB is a masticatory muscle activity during sleep that is characterized as rhythmic (phasic) or nonrhythmic (tonic) and is not a movement disorder or a sleep disorder in otherwise healthy individuals. For a diagnosis of possible or probable SB, self-report and clinical approaches constitute adequate confirmation; for a definite diagnosis, EMG or PSG, preferably with audio-video recordings, is required. As yet, the evidence is insufficient to support the use of ambulatory EMG devices as stand-alone tools for the assessment of SB, as tested against full PSG recordings. This is even more critical in differentiation of SB from several other sleep-related conditions, including orofacial movement disorders with manifestations that persist in sleep. RBD, OSA, and GERD are important comorbid conditions in patients with SB, with possible causal associations.

SELECTED READINGS

Abe S, Gagnon JF, Montplaisir JY, et al. Sleep bruxism and oromandibular myoclonus in rapid eye movement sleep behavior disorder: a preliminary report. *Sleep Med.* 2013;14:1024–1030.

Blanchet PJ, Rompré PH, Lavigne GJ, et al. Oral dyskinesia: a clinical overview. *Int J Prosthodont.* 2005;18:10–19.

Carra MC, Huynh N, Fleury B, Lavigne G. Overview on sleep bruxism for sleep medicine clinicians. *Sleep Med Clin.* 2015;10(3):375–384.

Lavigne G, Kato T, Herrero Babiloni A, et al. Research routes on improved sleep bruxism metrics: Toward a standardised approach [published online ahead of print, 2021 Mar 6]. *J Sleep Res.* 2021;e13320.

Lavigne GJ, Rompré PH, Montplaisir JY. Sleep bruxism: validity of clinical research diagnostic criteria in a controlled polysomnographic study. *J Dent Res.* 1996;75:546–552.
Lobbezoo F, Aarab G, Wetselaar P, et al. A new definition of Dental Sleep Medicine. *J Oral Rehabil.* 2016;43:786–790.
Lobbezoo F, Ahlberg J, Raphael KG, et al. International consensus on the assessment of bruxism: Report of a work in progress. *J Oral Rehabil.* 2018;45(11):837–844.
Maluly M, Andersen ML, Dal-Fabbro C, et al. Polysomnographic study of the prevalence of sleep bruxism in a population sample. *J Dent Res.* 2013;92:97S–103S.
Manfredini D, Ahlberg J, Aarab G, et al. Towards a Standardized Tool for the Assessment of Bruxism (STAB)—overview and general remarks of a multidimensional bruxism evaluation system. *J Oral Rehabil.* 2020;47(5):549–556.
Manfredini D, Ahlberg J, Castroflorio T, et al. Diagnostic accuracy of portable instrumental devices to measure sleep bruxism. A systematic literature review of polysomnographic studies. *J Oral Rehabil.* 2014;41:836–842.
Manfredini D, Ahlberg J, Wetselaar P, Svensson P, Lobbezoo F. The bruxism construct: from cut-off points to a continuum spectrum. *J Oral Rehabil.* 2019;46:991–997.
Manfredini D, Guarda-Nardini L, Marchese-Ragona R, Lobbezoo F. Theories on possible temporal relationships between sleep bruxism and obstructive sleep apnea events. *Sleep Breath.* 2015;19:1459–1465.
Paesani DA, Lobbezoo F, Gelos C, et al. Correlation between self-reported and clinically based diagnoses of bruxism in temporomandibular disorders patients. *J Oral Rehabil.* 2013;40:803–809.
Rompré PH, Daigle-Landry D, Guitard F, et al. Identification of a sleep bruxism subgroup with a higher risk of pain. *J Dent Res.* 2007;86:837–842.
Wieczorek T, Wieckiewicz M, Smardz J, et al. Sleep structure in sleep bruxism: a polysomnographic study including bruxism activity phenotypes across sleep stages. *J Sleep Res.* 2020:e13028. https://doi.org/10.1111/jsr.13028. [Epub ahead of print Mar 11, 2020].

A complete reference list can be found online at ExpertConsult.com.

Chapter 171

Management of Sleep Bruxism: Psychological, Dental, and Medical Approaches in Adults

Daniele Manfredini; Alberto Herrero Babiloni; Alessandro Bracci; Frank Lobbezoo

Chapter Highlights

- The main challenge in managing sleep bruxism (SB) in adults is to differentiate between the treatment of bruxism itself or of its possible consequences.
- A multimodal approach, including different conservative strategies, is the best available strategy to manage SB in the clinical setting. Such an approach may be identified with the acronym "Multiple-P," encompassing pep talk (i.e., counseling), physiotherapy, psychology (i.e., cognitive-behavioral treatments), plates (i.e., oral appliances), and pills/pharmacology.
- Even within this framework, it remains a challenge to identify the most effective protocol to reduce SB activity. This incomplete knowledge can be explained by factors related to the inclusion of different bruxism patients' phenotypes in the various treatment protocols. In addition, the management of potential SB consequences (e.g., tooth wear, jaw-muscle pain) is sometimes used as an indicator of treatment of bruxism itself, thus possibly generating confusion.
- With the emerging concept of bruxism as a muscle activity that must be viewed as the sign of underlying or comorbid conditions, future therapeutic studies targeting the etiology of such muscle activity will shed light onto the indications and effectiveness of any specific approach to SB reduction.
- Given their relative safety and nonharmful nature, it seems prudent to recommend the inclusion of cognitive-behavioral approaches in any SB treatment protocol to maximize the effects of a multimodal approach, even if they are not necessarily effective as standalone therapies.
- When medication is prescribed, this needs to be done by a qualified and licensed health care practitioner.

INTRODUCTION

Before discussing any management strategy or treatment plan for sleep bruxism (SB), one must consider that the risk factors and the mechanism(s) associated with SB are not fully understood. The relationship between etiology, clinical correlates, and, consequently, treatment need has to be considered. Current knowledge indicates a need for caution and avoidance of irreversible and one-size-fits-all approaches.[1] SB is not due to a single risk factor and single cause; psychosocial, neurologic, and physiologic factors that may be contributing to SB need to be examined when management plans for SB are developed.

Thus it is a clinical diagnostic challenge to determine when SB is just an oral behavior needing either no treatment or just mild counseling approaches, or when clinicians have to intervene with strategies to manage the possible negative consequences of SB, such as tooth wear or pain, or when SB is comorbid with other sleep or medical conditions (e.g., insomnia, sleep-disordered breathing, gastroesophageal reflux disorder [GERD], epilepsy, rapid eye movement [REM] behavior disorder [RBD]) that should be the real target for treatment (see Chapter 170). Unfortunately, the treatment of SB itself (i.e., the reduction in SB frequency and severity) versus the management of its potential consequences are frequently mixed together. Such overlap can generate confusion about the effectiveness of treatment modalities, complicates the interpretation of literature findings, and may confound research-driven therapeutic strategies in the clinical setting.

This chapter's objective is to focus on the management strategies in adults that might reduce the number of SB events and the amount of sleep-time masticatory muscle activity (MMA). Within this frame of reference, a common sense approach based on a combination of more global strategies (i.e., Multiple-P: pep talk, psychology, physiotherapy, plates, and pills) rather than the traditional dental ones is considered the best course of action for an otherwise healthy person (i.e., in the absence of any major psychological or medical disorders) (Table 171.1).[2] To follow is an overview providing the most common psychological, dental, and medical approaches, with the intent to guide the different categories of medical professionals (e.g., dentists, sleep doctors, psychologists, neurologists, general physicians) who are involved in this clinical field to better manage their SB patients. As seen in Table 171.2, some of these approaches are in need of further evidence to support their efficacy and safety with patients, as pointed out in a recent systematic review on bruxism management strategies.[2]

PSYCHOLOGICAL TREATMENT

Current evidence suggests that bruxism is a sign of some underlying or comorbid conditions. As such, bruxism is viewed as a muscle activity or behavior and not a disorder per se in otherwise healthy persons.[3,4] This implicitly supports the view that a behavioral approach may be pivotal to help patients more successfully manage their bruxism that is related to stress and emotional tension. In this context, assessment instruments and associated interventions within the framework of ecologic momentary assessment and intervention (EMAI) have recently been introduced for in-field use to enable patients to manage bruxism.[5] The potential effectiveness of this strategy for the reduction of jaw-muscle tension and overuse is quite intuitive for awake bruxism (AB). On the other hand, the etiologic complexity of SB, which is not necessarily related to

Table 171.1 Multiple-P Strategy for Sleep Bruxism Management within the Framework of a Common Sense Approach

Treatment	Description
Pep talk	Counseling patients by giving them explanations on the condition and the way to self-manage it
Psychology	Cognitive-behavioral approaches involving strategies to improve patients' cognitive awareness, possibly with the help of a professional
Physiotherapy	Treatment regime based on passive or active exercises aiming to stretch the jaw muscles and improve perception of relaxed condition
Plates	Oral appliances of different types, from protective mouth guards against tooth wear to mandibular advancement devices for breathing disorders
Pills	Pharmacologic treatment including the possible use of several drugs and medications (e.g., muscle relaxants, anxiolytics, botulinum toxin, clonidine)

The "Ps" acronyms were based on the original publication by Lobbezoo et al., 2008[8] and the successive elaboration by Manfredini et al., 2016.[2]

Table 171.2 Summary of Effectiveness (Efficacy and Safety) of Approaches to Reduce Sleep Bruxism: Empirically Rated as Weak, Moderate, or Strong[c]

Strategy	Effect	Level of Evidence	Notes
Behavioral[a]			
Counseling	Potential	Weak	For this group of modalities, the effects are likely mediated via possible reduction of awake bruxism and improvement of sleep hygiene (no concrete data on effectiveness)
Psychological	Potential	Weak	
Biofeedback (EMAI)	Potential	Weak	
Dental			
Oral appliances (no positional changes)	Positive (short term)	Strong	Transient effects, if present Risk to aggravate apnea if not enough maxillary space
Mandible repositioning	Potential	Moderate	Effect may be mediated via improvement in breathing and/or reduction of sleep breathing apnea
Occlusal adjustment	None	Strong for no effect	Risk for occlusal dysesthesia
Pharmacologic[b]			
Muscle relaxants	Neutral	Moderate	Doubtful effects on symptoms
Clonazepam	Positive	Low-moderate	Indications needed: risk addiction
Botulinum toxin	Positive	Strong	Reduce EMG power, not RMMA (and doubtful effects on symptoms): risk on TMJ bone density and toxin travel to CNS
Clonidine	Positive	Moderate	Risk for hypotension: dose dependent
Antidepressants (SSRIs)	Potentially negative	Weak (case reports)	Risk of sleep bruxism increase
Alternative			
Contingent electrical stimulation	Positive (short term)	Moderate	Preliminary data
Vibratory stimulus delivered by an oral appliance	Positive (short term)	Weak (case series)	Preliminary data
Transcranial magnetic stimulation[b]	Positive (short term)	Weak (case series)	Preliminary data

[a]Note that studies on behavioral modalities refer to the short-term use of such strategies as standalone treatment modalities. The findings do not diminish the role and importance of cognitive-behavioral approaches as part of multimodal management strategies.
[b]To be prescribed and administered by qualified health care providers (e.g., sleep physicians, neurologists, oral and maxillofacial surgeons, dentists). Please note that most medications listed are off label for sleep bruxism management (i.e., not approved for such indication by medical authorities of most countries).
[c]Whenever possible, treatment approaches of each group are ordered in terms of effectiveness and benefit-to-cost ratio.
CNS, Central nervous system; EMAI, ecologic momentary assessment and intervention; EMG, electromyogram; RMMA, rhythmic masticatory muscle activity; SSRIs, selective serotonin reuptake inhibitors; TMJ, temporomandibular joint.

psychological issues, indicates the importance of careful scientific evaluation of EMAI in the future.

In general, behavioral modalities encompass a wide variety of methods, ranging from counseling (i.e., "pep talk") to professional psychological support. Patients can play an active role in the self-care management of bruxism. For this reason, it is important to teach them some concepts about bruxism pathophysiology and principles of sleep hygiene instructions (e.g., reduction of caffeine, smoking, and alcohol intake; avoidance of vigorous exercise or late-night working). Among the strategies that have been proposed to manage SB, examples include biofeedback, psychoanalysis, hypnosis, progressive relaxation, meditation, sleep hygiene, habit reversal, and massed practice. Unfortunately, the literature on this topic is neither large nor consistent enough to support clear-cut statements regarding the clinical outcomes of such interventions. Some interesting data coming from researches on temporomandibular disorders patients suggest that biofeedback strategies are of valuable help in the clinical management of such conditions.[6] Although the potential benefit of biofeedback and cognitive-behavioral treatment to manage bruxism has always been advocated in the clinical setting, recent studies do not seem to fully support their effectiveness.

Two recent papers dealt with sleep hygiene and relaxation techniques compared with untreated participants[7] and with the effects of wake-time electromyogram (EMG) biofeedback on SB parameters.[8] The studies had similar duration (3 to 4 weeks) and had two and three observation points, respectively. The total number of recruited subjects amounted to just 29 individuals, and neither of these studies, however, followed up with patients after the end of treatment. Findings from one study suggest that a protocol comprising teaching sleep hygiene measures and muscle relaxation techniques is not effective for reducing SB.[7] Of interest, findings from the other paper suggest that a wake-time, EMG-based biofeedback program aiming to reduce AB may also reduce SB events.[8]

Such findings are not supportive of the earlier reports of positive effects associated with several cognitive-behavioral approaches, which led to the inclusion of psychologically based strategies as part of a common sense approach to bruxism management.[9] Notwithstanding, sleep medicine offers several other examples of potential usefulness for strategies of psychological support; for instance, the management of insomnia can be more effective when a series of cognitive and behavioral approaches are integrated. Likewise, it seems reasonable that, even if not effective as standalone therapies, adding psychologically based strategies to SB treatment protocols would enhance positive clinical outcomes. Thus, given their safety and nonharmful nature, it is recommended that cognitive-behavioral approaches are included in any multimodal treatment protocol thanks to the favorable cost-to-benefit ratio. Future studies exploring this issue for SB alone or with comorbidities are certainly warranted.

DENTAL INTERVENTIONS: ORAL APPLIANCES

Two different approaches should be distinguished in this category: (1) reversible, temporary modalities (e.g., oral appliances [OAs]), and (2) irreversible treatments (e.g., selective occlusal adjustments, oral rehabilitation, and orthodontics). The second category of approaches found its origin in some past beliefs about the role of occlusal abnormalities in the etiology of bruxism. On the other hand, given the consistency of literature showing an absence of relationship between SB and features of dental occlusion,[10] those approaches are not biologically supported, and cannot be considered an argument worthy of future investigations.[11] Conversely, OAs (i.e., "plates") are among the most common modalities used to manage symptoms of temporomandibular disorders (TMDs). Within the communities of orofacial pain practitioners, it is frequently accepted that the effects of OAs on symptom relief are not necessarily related to dental occlusion-mediated effects and are likely mediated by some transient changes in joint load area and muscle fibers recruitment.[12] Thus, in the instance of an OA as a proposed therapy, the question is whether they effectively reduce SB or not.

Over recent years, there have been several reports on the effectiveness of OAs, either with a before-after design or with a randomized controlled trial (RCT) design. The latter includes comparison groups treated with gabapentin,[13] with palatal appliances,[14] or adopting different protocols concerning intermittent versus continuous appliance wearing,[15] different vertical dimensions of occlusion (VDO),[16] or different appliance designs.[17,18] These papers generally have low sample sizes with nonhomogeneous recruitment strategies as far as the SB severity and the demographic features are concerned. Follow-up duration also varies across studies and ranges from very few nights in a short-term crossover investigation[17] to up to 3 months in an uncontrolled pre-poststudy.[19] Similarly, the observation points vary widely, with only a few studies having more than baseline and end-of-treatment assessments. In addition, inconsistency of recording settings across studies, namely, sleep laboratory versus home environment, is another factor that should be taken into account when interpreting the results.

Findings on the effects of treatment protocols on SB parameters are variable and thus difficult to interpret. The investigations comparing different OA designs and treatment regimens suggest that stabilization splints are better than palatal splints,[14] an intermittent use is superior to continuous wearing,[15] a 3-mm increase in VDO is more effective than a 6-mm increase,[16] a mandibular advancement appliance (MAA) with a robust advancement (75%) is only slightly superior to less marked (25%) advancement devices,[17] and the restriction of mandibular movements with oral appliances does not have any major influence on jaw-muscle activity during sleep.[18] Stabilization appliances are equally as effective as the neuroleptic drug gabapentin, which is only slightly superior to reduce SB events in subjects with poor sleep quality.[13] One before-after study concludes that a MAA providing a 50% to 75% advancement decreases the number of unspecific events of MMA.[19]

Despite the variability in the design of the earlier-described studies, some general remarks can be made. First, it seems that almost every type of OA is somehow effective in reducing SB activity. This may suggest the existence of a potential "novelty effect" associated with the use of an OA, which leads to a reduction in sleep-time MMA, possibly due to the transient need for reorganizing motor unit recruitment. This hypothesis may find support in the observation that intermittent OA use is more effective to reduce SB than continued use.[15] However, the actual existence, clinical meaning, and duration of this effect should be assessed in future studies that use longer follow-up time spans. Besides, early findings suggested an absence of significant effects between using full-coverage or palatal appliances on the rhythmic masticatory muscle activity (RMMA) index,[20,21] thus making it important to explore this issue in future research. Second, it seems that OAs that are designed to provide a high extent of mandible advancement (50% to 75%) are effective in reducing SB.[17,19] Such findings may be explained with the reduced contractile properties of masseter muscles when the mandible is advanced[22] and/or with the elimination of the amount of SB-like motor phenomena that are actually part of respiratory arousal.[23] Thus the potential mechanisms of action through which OAs may reduce SB are yet to be explored in detail for evidence-based recommendations to emerge.

A recent trial showed no effects of invisible orthodontic retainers (i.e., neither increase nor decrease) on the number of SB events in a population of healthy young adults.[24] Some preliminary reports suggest caution against the possible aggravation of breathing disorders with the use of stabilization OAs.[25,26] As for the dental and orthopedic issues, it must also be remarked that a prolonged use of MADs may expose patients to unwanted side effects related to the alteration of musculoskeletal homeostasis.[27] Further work is needed also to explore these issues.

MEDICAL THERAPY

Along with psychological approaches and oral appliances, management options include treatments that can be grouped under the umbrella of "medical therapies." Physiotherapy, even if belonging to the Multiple-P framework, is mainly oriented to the management of potential clinical consequences of bruxism, such as pain in the masticatory muscles and impaired jaw function. For AB, it is also used to reduce the jaw-muscle activity itself by means of specific strategies to control for muscle tension and activation (e.g., myofeedback).[28] On the other hand, given the paucity of data on the potential use of physiotherapy to reduce SB,[29,30] per the chapter's objective, it will not be discussed in this section.

Pharmacologic approaches (i.e., "pills") are to be considered the most relevant medical approach that may have a role in effectively reducing SB.

Because modern etiologic theories of SB focus on central nervous system factors interacting with the autonomic system, a pharmacologic treatment directed toward the underlying condition that is associated with SB might have plausible "curative" effects for SB itself. The uncertainties about the different types of bruxism activities that are related with the various comorbid conditions explains why, at present, no safe and/or definitive medication for SB has been identified. Indeed, although all the pharmacologic approaches that have been investigated in the research setting (i.e., botulinum toxin, clonazepam, and clonidine) seem to reduce either the intensity or the number of SB with respect to placebo, drugs are not indicated as a first-step approach. Indeed, all drugs should be tested for the potential side effects associated with long-term use. In addition, an identification of the causes of bruxism must be recommended before starting any one-fits-all pharmacologic approach for SB. A paper reviewing several RCTs on this topic best exemplifies the complexity and preliminary nature of current findings.[2]

Two of the papers included in the review deal with botulinum toxin injections of the jaw muscles, either in a controlled setting[31] or in an uncontrolled setting.[32] Two other papers had a crossover design, assessing the effectiveness of clonazepam[33] or clonidine[34] with respect to placebo. In total, 90 participants took part in those studies. In general, the findings from botulinum toxin studies are supportive of its effectiveness to reduce the intensity (i.e., strength of muscle activity) of SB episodes but not their frequency (i.e., the number of times muscle-related SB episodes are triggered). Follow-up assessments are provided for up to 12 weeks only, so it is not possible to draw conclusions on the longer-term duration of those effects.[35] In addition, emerging findings on the possible osteopenic-inducing effects of repeated botulinum toxin injections suggest caution before recommending its routine use. Similarly, the two placebo-controlled crossover studies suggest that both clonazepam and the antihypertension drug clonidine may have SB-reducing effects. On the other hand, the observation period in the protocol was limited to 3 nights, and there was no long-term evaluation of the potential side effects and/or risks associated with the medication protocol.[33,34] In addition, the earlier findings were not fully confirmed by a successive study, showing that clonidine has a 30% superior effect than clonazepam in reducing the number of RMMA episodes.[36]

Thus, based on presently available data, it seems that all tested pharmacologic approaches may reduce SB compared to placebo interventions. It is then reasonable to turn attention to their potential mechanisms of action and applicability in everyday life. Botulinum toxin's effects are not surprising, and they are in line with the expected pharmacologic properties of the drug. However, the fact that both studies using botulinum toxin show a reduced intensity of SB, but no effect on frequency of SB episodes, suggests that peripherally acting drugs do not affect the genesis of SB episodes. Such findings are consistent with clinical investigations showing that improvement in muscle pain levels after botulinum toxin injection is not unequivocally superior to placebo[37,38] or to physiotherapy.[39] On the other hand, centrally acting drugs (i.e., clonazepam and clonidine) have been reported to be potentially effective in reducing SB frequency in a few low-sample studies. The effects of clonazepam, which has sedative and muscle relaxant properties, were to a certain extent predictable, although the actual action mechanism of clonidine is possibly related with the prevention of sympathetic autonomic dominance.[40] One hypothesis is that, because clonidine is a selective alpha$_2$-agonist with sympatholytic effect and activation of the sympathetic autonomic nervous system precedes bruxism events, such medication probably interrupts the cascade of events that results in bruxism episodes.[40] Within this context, it must be noted that data on clonidine effects are interesting from an experimental perspective, but they are yet to be refined in terms of safety and cost-to-benefit ratio. High dose clonidine[40] induced hypotension in 20% of individuals; a low dose is better tolerated,[34] but the complexity of autonomic interactions suggests that it is prudent to recommend that medical doctors write the prescriptions and follow the patients for side effects.

Other studies suggest a potential, even if minor, role of dopaminergic medications (i.e., D2 receptor agonist bromocriptine; catecholamine precursor L-DOPA) to attenuate SB.[41,42] There are, however, emerging indications that antidepressants of the family of selective serotonin reuptake inhibitors may trigger SB in some individuals.[43] Thus the proof of concept associated with recently identified genetic dopamine and serotonin candidates will need evaluation to support their putative role in SB genesis. Until then, it can be said that there is limited evidence to draw definite conclusions concerning the efficacy and safety of various drugs on bruxism that could be prescribed by a dentist at this time. Obviously, more controlled research on this underexplored subject will be welcome in the near future.

Among the other medical approaches proposed over the years to treat bruxism, one paper reported an uncontrolled series of 10 patients receiving electrical stimuli to the masseter muscles.[44] The protocol provided a 3-night EMG recording under three conditions, namely, one without electrical stimuli versus 2 nights with stimuli provided at two different sensation thresholds immediately after the heart rate exceeded 110%. Findings are suggestive of the effectiveness of such electrical stimuli to suppress SB. This finding is in line with papers adopting different protocols of contingent electrical stimulation of the temporalis muscle, either with an RCT[45,46] or a before-after design.[47] All these data on the use of EMG-based stimulations must be reappraised when standardized strategies for the interpretation of the EMG signal will be available.[48] In future researches, the possibility of adding transcranial magnetic stimulation as another novel experimental treatment could be considered, although evidence is quite limited.[49,50] Similarly, adding more data on the possible usefulness of vibratory stimuli delivered by an intraoral device upon teeth touching on the appliance during sleep bruxism events is recommended.[51]

MANAGEMENT OF SLEEP BRUXISM WITH SLEEP COMORBIDITIES

As discussed in previous sections, SB can be concomitant to other sleep disorders (see Chapters 169, 170, and 172). This observation suggests that SB and the possible indications to treatment should always be assessed within the framework of sleep medicine. Sometimes, SB patients' complaints are suggestive of a possible comorbidity with other sleep disorders and conditions, thus making the request of a consultation with a sleep physician mandatory. If the sleep condition is already known, then dental, psychological, and medical collaborations are essential to achieve the best outcome with respect to any individual patient's belief, expectation, and social capacity to afford treatment.

As a summary of what can be found in other chapters, it must be remarked that:

- For insomnia, CBT and medication are the reference choices (see Chapters 95 to 100).
- For obstructive sleep apnea, continuous positive airway pressure, different types of oral appliances, and ear, nose, and throat or maxillofacial surgeries are among the approaches to be tailored according to the severity of the breathing condition (see Chapters 132 to 134 and 175). For sleep apnea, some alternative treatments may be considered and are summarized in Chapters 134 and 176.
- For gastroesophageal reflux disease, medication and a sleep positioner may be indicated (see Chapter 160).
- For neurologic conditions such as epilepsy, headache, and RBD, medical management is essential (see Chapters 106, 107, and 118, respectively).

CONCLUSIONS

Recommendations for SB management at the individual level are not yet the result of rigorous scientific evidence. Because SB is most often an oral behavior, in an otherwise healthy person, it is most likely a condition not requiring treatment until the relationship with clinical symptoms and consequences is fully clarified for each distinctly-identified motor activity. SB is not a one-size-fits-all activity. Thus, when treatment is needed, before deciding which therapeutic measure is the best for a given patient according to his/her medical and psychosocial presentation, the clinician should seek a definitive diagnosis with special emphasis on what factors contributed to the initiation and perpetuation of the SB activity. Such approach should include an assessment of the role of comorbidities, such as insomnia, sleep apnea, GERD, and RBD, which may require a special combination of treatment modalities. In addition to that, it must be remarked that the strategies to manage SB should be prescribed and administered by qualified health care providers (e.g., sleep physicians, neurologists, oral and maxillofacial surgeons, dentists).

CLINICAL PEARLS

- Sleep bruxism (SB) treatment is often confused with the management of its potential clinical consequences, such as tooth wear or orofacial pain.
- Health care providers must understand that a proper strategy for SB reduction has to take into account the different causes and comorbid conditions underlying or accompanying SB.
- Currently, there is not a one-fits-all approach to treat SB, but it can be suggested that positive effects on SB reduction may be achieved with a combination of strategies provided within the framework of a conservative (e.g., Multiple-P) approach.

SUMMARY

Management of SB focuses on reducing the number of SB events and time asleep with MMA. This should not be confounded with the need to manage and/or prevent possible clinical consequences of SB (e.g., tooth wear, orofacial pain). For an otherwise healthy person (i.e., in the absence of any major psychological or medical disorders), the best common sense approach is based on a combination of more global strategies (i.e., "Multiple-P": pep talk, psychology, physiotherapy, plates, and pills), rather than the traditional dental ones.

Because there is a paucity of outcomes research on SB management, recommendations for SB management at the individual level are not based on rigorous scientific data. Thus, in management of SB, one must consider the medical and psychosocial presentation, and seek a definitive diagnosis with special emphasis on what factors contributed to the initiation and perpetuation of the condition.

SELECTED READINGS

Bhattacharjee B, Saneja R, Bhatnagar A, Gupta P. Effect of dopaminergic agonist group of drugs in treatment of sleep bruxism: a systematic review [published online ahead of print, 2021 Jan 14]. *J Prosthet Dent*. 2021;(20):30752–30756. https://doi.org/10.1016/j.prosdent.2020.11.028. S0022-3913.

Bussadori SK, Motta LJ, Horliana ACRT, Santos EM, Martimbianco ALC. The current trend in management of bruxism and chronic pain: an overview of systematic reviews. *J Pain Res*. 2020;13:2413–2421. https://doi.org/10.2147/JPR.S268114. Published 2020 Sep 30.

Greene CS, Menchel HF. The use of oral appliances in the management of temporomandibular disorders. *Oral Maxillofac Surg Clin North Am.* 2018;30(3):265–277.
Landry-Schönbeck A, de Grandmont P, Rompré PH, Lavigne GJ. Effect of an adjustable mandibular advancement appliance on sleep bruxism: a crossover sleep laboratory study. *Int J Prosthodont.* 2009;22:251–259.
Lobbezoo F, Ahlberg J, Manfredini D, Winocur E. Are bruxism and the bite causally related? *J Oral Rehabil.* 2012;39(7):489–501.
Lobbezoo F, Ahlberg J, Raphael KG, et al. International consensus on the assessment of bruxism: report of a work in progress. *J Oral Rehabil.* 2018;45(11):837–844.
Manfredini D, Ahlberg J, Winocur E, Lobbezoo F. Management of sleep bruxism in adults: a qualitative systematic literature review. *J Oral Rehabil.* 2015;42(11):862–874.
Manfredini D, De Laat A, Winocur E, Ahlberg J. Why not stop looking at bruxism as a black/white condition? Aetiology could be unrelated to clinical consequences. *J Oral Rehabil.* 2016;43(10):799–801.
Manfredini D, Guarda-Nardini L, Marchese-Ragona R, Lobbezoo F. Theories on possible temporal relationships between sleep bruxism and obstructive sleep apnea events. An expert opinion. *Sleep Breath.* 2015;19(4):1459–1465.
Melo G, Duarte J, Pauletto P, et al. Bruxism: an umbrella review of systematic reviews. *J Oral Rehabil.* 2019;46(7):666–690. https://doi.org/10.1111/joor.12801.
Raphael KG, Santiago V, Lobbezoo F. Is bruxism a disorder or a behaviour? Rethinking the international consensus on defining and grading of bruxism. *J Oral Rehabil.* 2016;43(10):791–798.
Saletu A, Parapatics S, Anderer P, Matejka M, Saletu B. Controlled clinical, polysomnographic and psychometric studies on differences between sleep bruxers and controls and acute effects of clonazepam as compared with placebo. *Eur Arch Psychiatry Clin Neurosci.* 2010;260:163–174.

A complete reference list can be found online at ExpertConsult.com.

Chapter 172

Orofacial Pain/Temporomandibular Disorders in Relation to Sleep Bruxism and Breathing Disorders

Gregory Essick; Massimiliano DiGiosia; Aurelio Alonso; Karen Raphael; Anne E. Sanders; Gilles Lavigne

Chapter Highlights

- Among chronic orofacial pain conditions, temporomandibular disorders (TMDs) are the most common. The etiology of TMD is multifactorial. The role of sleep-disordered breathing (SDB) and sleep bruxism (SB) in the initiation and persistence of TMD pain is poorly understood.
- There is a higher prevalence of SDB or suspected SDB in patients with TMDs, and a higher prevalence of TMDs among patients with SDB. Respiratory effort–related arousals during sleep are more frequent in women with TMD than in control subjects. Signs and symptoms of SDB predict incident TMD.
- The premise that SDB leads in a dominant sequence to SB, and eventually to TMD, is not supported currently by scientific evidence.
- SB may help preserve or restore airway patency in certain patients with SDB; individuals with milder forms of SDB are more likely to exhibit SB than individuals with severe obstructive sleep apnea.
- There does not exist a causal relationship between SB and TMD.
- Phenotyping may be helpful in exploring the association between SB and myofascial TMD. It is hypothesized that high-background masticatory muscle activity during sleep may be of pathogenic significance to the TMD pain.

Temporomandibular disorders (TMDs) are a heterogeneous family of musculoskeletal disorders that represents the most common chronic orofacial pain condition.[1-3] TMD is characterized by persistent pain in the temporomandibular joint, the periauricular region, and the muscles of the head and neck, and by painful chewing and impaired oral function. The *Diagnostic Criteria for Temporomandibular Disorders* (DC/TMD) protocol, published by the International Research Diagnostic Criteria for Temporomandibular Disorders (RDC/TMD) Consortium, is used to guide diagnosis of TMD for research purposes.[4,5] Although criteria for TMD have changed over the years, prevalence of TMDs has been estimated historically at between 5% and 12%, with higher rates among women (of reproductive age) than among men.[1,6-9] Estimates suggest that TMD results in almost 18 million lost work days annually for every 100 million working adults in the United States.[3] In view of the considerable cost to work productivity and to health care, there is interest in identifying risk factors associated with the onset and maintenance of TMD.[10]

One plausible risk factor for TMD is sleep-disordered breathing (SDB).[11] A preliminary report suggested that as many as 75% of patients diagnosed with TMD have clinical characteristics suggestive of SDB.[12] This coexistence of disorders has suggested that SDB contributes to sleep bruxism (SB), a disorder characterized by rhythmic jaw muscle activity and grinding of the teeth during sleep (see Chapters 169 and 170). Furthermore, SB has been associated with and/or suggested to be the cause of TMD in susceptible persons through microtrauma to the temporomandibular joint or masticatory muscles from hyperactivity during sleep.[13-16] Against this background, the diagnosis and treatment of SDB, as well as SB, in patients with TMD are rationalized as efforts to reduce pain and correct dysfunction. However, no rigorous research has shown that treatment of SDB alters the likelihood of developing TMD or the natural course of existing TMD. For more information on sensory mechanisms, pain, and sleep interaction, readers are referred to Chapters 30 and 156; for SB etiology and mechanisms and SB diagnosis, they are referred to Chapters 169 and 170, respectively. Addressed in separate sections of this chapter are the association between SDB and SB and that between SB and TMD.

SLEEP-DISORDERED BREATHING AS A CAUSATIVE CANDIDATE FOR TEMPOROMANDIBULAR DISORDER

Remarkably few studies have shown an association between SDB and TMD. A study[17] of patients with mild or moderate obstructive sleep apnea (OSA) evaluated for signs and symptoms of TMD[2] revealed an estimated prevalence of TMD of 39% in patients with mild to moderate OSA, which was substantially greater than estimates for the general adult population.[17,18] The OSA-TMD study was limited by the lack of a control group, the relatively small sample size, and selection bias. Another small observational study[19] of patients diagnosed with TMD showed that 28% (50% of men and 23% of women in the study) met criteria for OSA and 43% for insomnia signs and symptoms.

Two TMD studies (one case-control, the other prospective) named OPPERA (Orofacial Pain: Prospective Evaluation and Risk Assessment) compared the strength of association between signs and symptoms of OSA and chronic TMD.[20] In OPPERA's chronic TMD case-control study, odds of TMD were elevated more than threefold (odds ratio, 3.6; 95% confidence interval, 2.0 to 6.5) in those at high risk for OSA, independently of demographic, autonomic, and behavioral characteristics. In the prospective cohort, OPPERA subjects at risk for OSA had 1.7 times the incidence of TMD over the median 2.8-year follow-up period, independently of demographic, autonomic, and behavioral characteristics. The association remained statistically significant with further adjustment for subjective sleep quality. Both OPPERA studies were limited by the absence of polysomnography (PSG) data and difference of the subject demographics compared with the general population.

Extending the OPPERA findings, a recent case-control study found a higher prevalence of TMD in subjects at high risk of OSA (30.7%) compared with subjects at no risk (18.5%).[21] It is possible that in such studies many participants classified by questionnaire as having OSA signs or symptoms in fact had milder forms of SDB such as upper airway resistance (UAR)[22] or respiratory effort–related arousal (RERA).[23]

That TMD may be associated with milder forms of SDB, such as respiratory effort–related arousal (RERA), was shown in a PSG study conducted on middle-age (mean of 39.2 years) female patients with TMD (n = 124) and demographically matched control subjects (n = 46).[24] The patients with TMD had lighter and more disrupted sleep, a higher percentage of stage N1 sleep, and more sleep instability as seen by a greater number of awakenings and stage shifts toward N1. Furthermore, arousals associated with all respiratory events (apneas, hypopneas, and RERAs) were almost twice as frequent in the patients as in control subjects; nevertheless, the mean AHI was similar for both groups at less than 4 (events/hour). The respiratory disturbance index showed a trend (P = .06) toward being higher in the TMD group (8.1/hour) than in the control group (5/hour) owing to a higher RERA frequency in the former.

The co-occurrence of TMD and upper airway resistance syndrome (UARS) has led investigators of other work to postulate a TMD-UARS phenotype that develops during growth in response to disordered breathing during wakefulness.[25] This case series of Southeast Asian people revealed a high respiratory disturbance index (mean RDI was 19.6 events/hour), yet normal apnea-hypopnea index (mean AHI was 3.9 events/hour), and excessive daytime sleepiness (mean Epworth Sleepiness Score was 14.8) and multiple functional somatic complaints in addition to those of the TMD pain. The extent to which this Southeast Asian phenotype is distinctive of all females with RDC/TMD remains unknown.

Not all studies investigating the relationship between SDB and TMD find a significant association.[15,26-28] The sample sizes of these studies were small and methods not rigorous. Most recently, a study that sought to identify clinical comorbid conditions in TMD failed to detect a significant difference in the proportion reporting sleep apnea in a cohort of persons claiming to be affected by TMDs and musculoskeletal disorders and in a control group.[29]

In summary, strength of the evidence for an association between SDB and TMD is moderate. (Table 172.1). Studies to date suggest a real or possibly elevated prevalence of SDB associated with TMD and an increased prevalence of TMD associated with SDB. The causal mechanisms underlying the relationship between SDB and TMD have not been elucidated.

SLEEP-DISORDERED BREATHING AS A CAUSATIVE CANDIDATE FOR SLEEP BRUXISM

Bruxism refers to either clenching or grinding of the teeth. It can occur during wakefulness and/or during sleep (more information is available in Chapters 169 to 171). Here we review the putative role of SDB in SB; in a later section of the chapter, we address the role of SB in TMD. It is believed and/or proposed, by a growing number of clinicians, that SDB plays a role in SB and that the dentist may be the first to suspect SDB based on the patient report or clinical signs suggestive of SB.[30] Consistent with this hypothesis, one study found that all but 2 of 30 patients with tooth wear who were being treated with an occlusal splint for bruxism had at least mild OSA and 37% had severe OSA.[31] The authors suggested that dentists use tooth wear as a tool in the identification of patients with OSA. However, another report concluded that the associations of tooth wear with sleep disorders, orofacial pain, dry mouth, gastroesophageal reflux disease, and SB are complex, thus making it difficult to disentangle the consequences of a single condition such as SDB.[32]

Self-Reports of Sleep Bruxism in Patients with Sleep-Disordered Breathing

Two studies found an association between self-reports of bruxism/tooth grinding and adults with SDB.[33,34] These findings, however, have to be interpreted with caution, because they are based solely on the reports of patients' sleep partners or parents.

Sleep Recordings of Sleep Bruxism in Sleep-Disordered Breathing

In contrast with studies that have used surveys and questionnaires to assess the SDB-SB relationship, investigations using overnight sleep recordings have not consistently found an increase in prevalence of SB motor activity among persons with SDB. One study found no difference in the frequency of "bruxing" episodes between those with and without SDB, although the frequency of sleep arousals was greater in the SDB group.[35] Bruxing episodes, defined as bursts of masseter EMG activity measured as greater than 40% of maximum during awake clenching, were mostly associated with respiratory events in the SDB group. A later PSG study reported that 54% of adults with mild and 40% with moderate OSA met empiric criteria for SB. These were based on the presence of two or more of the following: more than 2.5 rhythmic

Table 172.1 Observations Supporting an Association Between Sleep-Disordered Breathing (SDB) and Temporomandibular Disorders (TMDs)

Observation	Supporting Research	Comments	Nonsupporting Research	Comments
Increased prevalence of TMD in patients diagnosed with OSA	Cunali et al, 2009[17]	Observational study; no control group; small sample size; subject selection bias	Petit et al, 2002[26]	Studies limited by one or more of the following: use of self-report to identify TMD and/or OSA, small samples of participants; large variability in methodology and variance in findings
Increased prevalence of OSA in patients diagnosed with TMD	Smith et al, 2009[19]	Observational study; no control group; small sample size	Collesano et al, 2004[27]; Hoffmann et al, 2011[29]	
Increased odds of signs and symptoms of OSA in patients with chronic TMD	Sanders et al, 2013[20]	Large multicenter case-control study; no objective sleep data		
Increased odds of TMD in individuals with signs and symptoms of OSA	Kale et al, 2018[21]	Case-control study of individuals presenting for dental treatment; no objective sleep data		
Initially TMD-free subjects with signs and symptoms of OSA more likely to develop first-onset TMD	Sanders et al, 2013[20]	Large multicenter prospective cohort study; no objective sleep data		
Increased frequency of RERAs in patients with TMD compared with control subjects	Dubrovsky et al, 2014[24]	Large sample case-control study	Camparis and Siqueira, 2006[15]; Rossetti et al, 2008[28]	
Increased frequency of RERAs in patients with TMD	Tay and Pang[25]	Large observational sample; no controls		

OSA, Obstructive sleep apnea; RERAs, respiratory effort–related arousals; TMD, temporomandibular disorder.

jaw-movement episodes per hour as determined by EMG during PSG, clinical observation (attrition, masticatory muscle fatigue, or temporomandibular joint discomfort) or subjective report of tooth grinding or clenching on one or more nights per week.[36] Because the number of rhythmic jaw movement episodes per hour was greater in patients with mild than in those with moderate OSA and the episodes were rarely associated with respiratory arousals, the study authors attributed their presence to the disturbed sleep characteristic of OSA.

More recent work, however, argues more strongly for an association between SB and SDB and offers plausible explanations for disparate findings among studies.[37] The frequency of SB events was higher in the OSA group (7.0 events/hour) than in the control group (2.9 events/hour) and the frequency of phasic SB events correlated positively with respiratory events and microarousals. SB was found in 48% of the patients with OSA, and the odds of SB were four times as great for the OSA group than for the control group (odds ratio was 3.96). In the patients with OSA, the phasic SB events often occurred in association with respiratory-related microarousals. A subsequent study using PSG investigated SB in patients with OSA, about two-thirds of whom had severe sleep apnea.[38] Sleep bruxism was identified in one-third of the patients, was largely of the phasic form, and was not associated with indices of the severity of the OSA upon controlling for demographic and sleep factors. Other studies also showed a high prevalence of SB in subjects with confirmed OSA.[39-41] In the most recent of these studies, the frequency of bruxism episodes was 3.4 times as great in patients with mild to moderate OSA compared with patients with severe OSA (5.5/hour versus 1.6/hour) and increased with the AHI only for the former.[41] Thus, the majority of the self-report– and PSG-based studies support that SB is elevated among adults when SDB coexists as determined by the presence of symptoms suggestive of SDB or by PSG evidence of SDB.

Some evidence also suggests that treatment of OSA in adults can reduce SB. A small study and a case report demonstrated that the frequency of bruxism events is decreased by treatment with continuous positive nasal airway pressure or mandibular advancement devices, respectively.[42-44]

Sleep Recordings of Increased Masticatory Muscle Activity in Sleep-Disordered Breathing

Groups of investigators have observed increased masticatory muscle activity during sleep in patients with SDB that is thought to result in forward posturing and stabilization, or in elevation of the mandible to help maintain airway patency. It might be that these muscle activities, even in the absence of tooth contact, are interpreted by adults (or parents of children) with SDB as tooth grinding or clenching during sleep. The earliest studies, conducted 30 years ago, identified increased EMG activity of the masseter muscles during the inspiratory phase of sleep respiration in patients with OSA, but not in individuals with normal sleep respiration.[45,46] The activity in the masseter was accompanied by similarly timed phasic activity in the submental (genioglossus, geniohyoid, mylohyoid, and digastric) muscles, leading to periodic variations in the jaw gap from end inspiration to end expiration and variations between obstructed and nonobstructive breaths. However, the jaw was more open in patients with OSA than in persons with normal sleep respiration. The study authors surmised that activity in the masseter muscle stabilized the jaw, enabling the submental muscles to more effectively elevate and forwardly posture the hyoid bone, thereby improving airway patency overall in patients with OSA but promoting mouth breathing at the termination of apnea events.

The suggestion that increased activity in the masseter muscles can improve airway patency in patients with SDB received remarkably little attention until recently.[47-49] In open-label sleep studies reported by one group of investigators, esophageal pressure and multiple channels of EMG data from the masticatory muscles were recorded in addition to the standard PSG channels in patients with mild OSA and UARS.[48] The clinician investigators demonstrated that patients with UARS exhibit frequent periods of tonic contraction of the jaw-closing muscles (including the masseter), upon which esophageal pressure drops appreciably, indicating reductions in the respiratory effort needed to breathe. However, no objective monitoring of jaw position or of tooth contact was performed. Nor was it determined whether the patients met diagnostic criteria for bruxism based on a combination of self-report, clinical, and PSG criteria. Other investigators recently reported that the absence of respiratory events in adults with OSA during periods of prolonged clenching, may be consistent with an airway-protective effect, as suggested earlier, of tonic SB-related activity of the masseter.[47-49]

Some investigators have observed that most phasic SB episodes occur after rather than before respiratory events in adults with SDB.[37,38,50] Commonly there is also an increase in the activity of the suprahyoid muscles, which along with the contraction of the jaw closing muscles protrudes the mandible and tongue, thereby aiding the restoration of airway patency. Because the cascade of events leading to a SB episode differs from that observed in the absence of the respiratory event (see Chapter 170), this postrespiratory event bruxism has been referred to as a secondary form of bruxism.[38,49,50] Because bruxism might serve a physiologic role to restore and preserve the patency of the airway, it has been suggested that sleep bruxism be viewed as a condition or behavior rather than a disorder in otherwise healthy people.[51] It has also been suggested that airway-protective bruxism may occur only in certain individuals for whom the masticatory muscle activity is likely to restore or preserve the patency of the airway, based on the anatomic location, severity of the collapse or other factors.[41,49] This could explain the inconsistent relationship in the literature between the severity of the SDB and prevalence or severity of the SB, as these two factors would not necessarily correlate. Future phenotyping of patients with OSA according to anatomic differences and physiologic reactivity is mandatory to a better understanding of the relationship between SDB and SB (see Chapters 23, 128, and 129).[41,52-54]

Other investigators have noted that contraction of the masseter and temporalis muscles occurs as part of the sleep arousal response on a third or more of respiratory events in patients with SDB.[55,56] The contractions are dependent on the duration and intensity of the arousals and occur in patients who have no other clinical signs of SB or PSG evidence of SB—that is, of the typical rhythmic masticatory muscle activity (RMMA). It is suggested that these elevations in masticatory muscle activity represent a nonspecific, general motor manifestation of the arousal during sleep and also may contribute to the restoration of a patent upper airway.[49,55]

SLEEP BRUXISM AS A CAUSATIVE CANDIDATE FOR TEMPOROMANDIBULAR DISORDER

The beliefs that bruxism, sleep and/or awake, plays a role in the onset or maintenance of TMD is well-established clinical dogma (see also Chapters 169 and 170). Surveys confirm that dentists with expertise in management of TMD believe that "oral parafunctional habits" are important in the onset of TMD.[57-61] The oral parafunction most often linked with TMD is bruxism.[62] Many discussions, reviews, and research studies fail to clearly differentiate whether the bruxism activities are believed to occur during sleep or when awake. Nevertheless, bruxism during sleep is characterized mainly by tooth grinding, and bruxism during awake periods may be characterized mainly by clenching.

Self-Reports of Sleep Bruxism in Patients with Temporomandibular Disorders

In an older review, 21 studies were identified over a 10-year period (1998–2008), which relied on participant self-report or questionnaire to identify bruxers, sometimes using only a single item.[63] Self-report and clinical observation studies found a positive association for bruxism and TMD. However, a much weaker association between bruxism and TMD was suggested in studies with better and more detailed objective methodology. Furthermore, studies of anterior tooth wear and experimental jaw clenching failed to demonstrate a relationship between bruxism and TMD.[63]

A more recent 10-year systematic review similarly found that 33 of 39 studies, 21 of which were based on self-report of bruxism, established a positive relation between bruxism and TMD.[64] However, the authors concluded that PSG did not demonstrate strong evidence for the relationship. All considered, an overwhelming majority of the self-report-based studies support the common belief that the frequency of some form of bruxism is elevated among patients with TMD, but this belief is not strongly supported by studies employing more objective, laboratory-based measures of SB.

Sleep Recordings of Sleep Bruxism in Patients with Temporomandibular Disorder

In contrast with the large number of studies examining the SB-TMD relationship using less-than-optimal methods, PSG-based studies are rare but increasing in number. The 10-year systematic review cited earlier in this chapter (1998–2008), identified only four studies, two of which appear to represent partial overlap in sampling.[63] One study compared groups diagnosed with SB with and without pain,[65] thus begging the question of whether SB is elevated in patients with TMD. Another study reported that subjects without TMD with relatively low levels of SB were more likely to report transient morning masticatory muscle pain than those with no or high levels of SB,[66] as has also been reported.[67] The results, however, did not address the clinical syndrome of TMD or the myofascial pain of TMD, which tends to be worse in the late afternoon or evening.[68]

Two reports of a third study (one being a pilot report for the larger study) were distinguished by standardized definitions of SB events and inclusion of a control group without TMD pain.[28,69] The report with the larger sample[69] but not the smaller sample[28] found significantly higher rates of individuals meeting validated research criteria for SB[70] among participants meeting RDC criteria for TMD than among healthy control subjects. Concern about the study's recruitment methods must be raised, however, because one-third of control subjects met research criteria for SB, as did nearly two-thirds of subjects with TMD. By contrast, a large population study estimated the prevalence of SB as 5.5% using a combination of questionnaires and PSG, or as 7.4% on the basis of PSG alone.[71] Other experts estimate self-reported tooth grinding prevalence as high as 8%.[72] This suggests that the reported[69] finding of unusually high rates of SB in both groups may stem from either use of nonstandard scoring methods for RMMA episodes or oversampling of persons engaging in SB in both case and control samples.

In a study that explicitly sampled patients with TMD and control subjects on the basis of presence or absence of meeting RDC criteria for myofascial TMD, rather than presence or absence of beliefs about engaging in SB, laboratory PSG evaluations found similarly low proportions in both groups of participants meeting PSG-based research criteria for SB (i.e., 10% and 11%, respectively).[73] Of note, the rate of self-reported SB was markedly higher among patients with TMD than among control subjects in this same sample. A more recent study that employed PSG to assess the presence and frequency of bruxism events but used a validated screener to assess TMD pain, rather than RDC criteria, to classify TMD status[74] found no relation between TMD pain and the intensity of SB.

Sleep Recordings of Increased Masticatory Muscle Activity in Patients with Temporomandibular Disorder

A possible resolution to the contradiction between self-reports versus PSG-confirmed SB may lie in nighttime activity that is associated with jaw pain on waking, that is, masticatory muscle hypertonicity or elevated background sleep EMG activity occurring during nonbruxism periods. Patients with myofascial TMD have elevated levels of background sleep EMG activity compared with non-TMD control subjects.[75] Moreover, among the patients with TMD, background sleep EMG was positively associated with pain intensity ratings on morning waking, whereas the frequency of SB event–related EMG was negatively associated with the ratings, as has been observed in other investigations.[66,76] The finding of sustained elevation in background sleep EMG activity found in patients with TMD persisted after institution in the analyses of controls for numerous sleep parameters on which the groups did differ (e.g., RERAs, stage N1 shifts). These data were revisited recently using percent high background EMG activity as the outcome measure. Differences were found for myofascial TMD subjects, with muscle pain only upon palpation versus those with both muscle and joint pain upon palpation, suggesting two phenotypes of myofascial TMD.[77] Masticatory muscle EMG tone remained high during sleep (i.e., no drop or no dipping as expected normally during sleep) in a subgroup of female subjects with muscle pain only upon palpation (about 27% of the TMD subjects in the study). This was in contrast to female subjects with both muscle and joint pain upon palpation, as well as in contrast to control subjects. These new findings suggest that the difference observed earlier for the TMD cases and controls in background masticatory muscle activity during sleep was largely driven by a subgroup of TMD cases, that is those with muscle pain only upon palpation. Although the prevalence of SB was greater for the muscle pain only subgroup (26%) than the muscle and joint pain subgroup (3%), neither differed statistically from the prevalence observed in the control group (11%). Nevertheless, these findings merit additional investigation given their potential implications for a role of SB in the association between TMD and SDB for specific phenotypes of TMD and SDB patients.

The observations described in the preceding text indicate that patients who have elevated pain in the early morning may falsely attribute their pain to nighttime jaw muscle activity involving SB rather than "muscle tension" (elevated background masticatory muscle activity). Although jaw muscle activity may aggravate pain, low-level elevations of activity occurring outside of SB periods are more likely to be responsible for the morning pain aggravation. Of additional note, the increase in RMS EMG activity in the TMD group versus the control group occurring during background sleep EMG (outside of the period with RMMA) was approximately equal to the increase potentially attributable to regular tooth-to-tooth contact (within RMMA). This type of nonfunctional tooth contact during the awake state has been found to occur more often in individuals with TMD than in control subjects.[78-81] It is consistent with a body of experimental studies showing that low-intensity clenching (7.5% and 20% of maximum bite force) can cause pain, delayed muscle soreness, and fatigue in the masticatory muscles.[82,83] Obviously, the clinical significance of and mechanism underlying this finding require further analysis.

Thus on reviewing the evidence on the relation between intense SB muscle activity and TMD pain, the best-quality studies to date do not support a convincing relationship. The understanding of any relationship between SDB and TMD cannot be simplified to a single association with SB that is too often determined in the clinical milieu. Given that masticatory muscle EMG activity may be elevated during sleep in persons with SDB even in the absence of clinical or EMG evidence of SB,[12,45,46,48,55,56] as described earlier in this chapter, we entertain the possibility that this elevated activity, which is similar to low-intensity clenching or tooth-to-tooth contact during the day, is of pathogenic significance in the persistence of TMD pain (Figure 172.1). This hypothesis is consistent with the stress-hyperactivity model of Ohrbach and McCall[84]: It is not the magnitude per se of the muscle activity in pain patients that is responsible for the nociception that leads to pain complaints. Rather, it is a persistent pattern of muscle reactivity, in the form of holding muscles in a particular shortened position, such as a "braced jaw." (p. 61).[84]

However, the prevalence of increased background masticatory muscle EMG activity during sleep in patients with SDB is unknown, as well as whether patients with sustained high background EMG activity are more likely to develop or maintain TMD pain than patients who exhibit no increase.

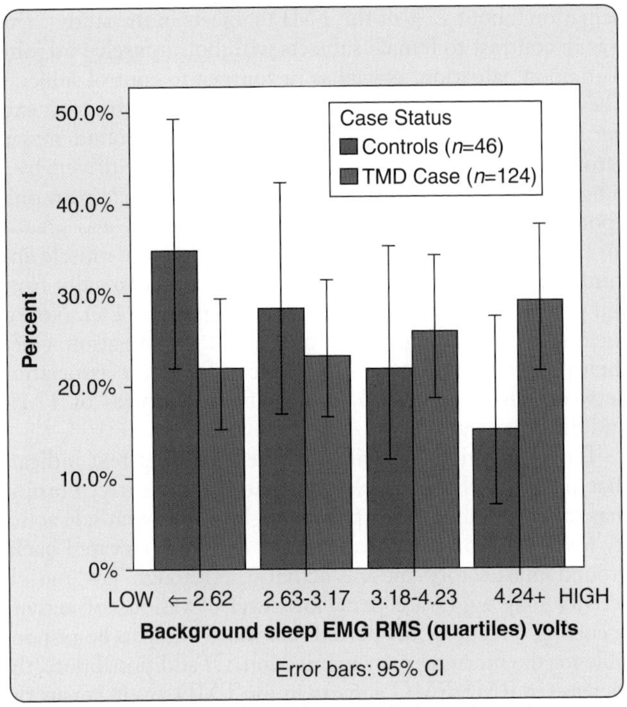

Figure 172.1 Hypothetical contributions of elevated masticatory muscle activity on the electromyogram (EMG) associated with sleep-disordered breathing (SDB) to temporomandibular disorders (TMDs). Some studies have reported increased EMG activity in the masticatory muscles of patients with SDB, and this increased activity could contribute to the elevation observed in patients with TMDs. Studies have suggested that the increased EMG activity of masticatory muscles of patients with SDB may be associated with mechanisms that maintain or restore airway patency or reflect a nonspecific increase associated with respiratory related arousals. However, further research is required to confirm a role for increased EMG activity observed in OSA and TMD subjects.

CLINICAL PEARLS

- In clinical populations, a high prevalence of SDB has been observed in patients with TMDs. These patients should be screened for SDB and treated as indicated.
- Both patients with SDB and those with TMD may report clenching or grinding their teeth during sleep. However, PSG that includes EMG of the masticatory muscles does not confirm the presence of SB in patients with TMD. SB might improve airway patency in some groups of patients with SDB; an hypothesis in need of evidence.
- Sustained (nondipping) background masticatory muscle activity during sleep, outside of SB periods, which is similar to low-intensity clenching or tooth-to-tooth contact during the day, may be of pathogenic significance in the persistence of TMD pain and thus represents a putative risk factor in a subgroup of TMD subjects with muscle pain.

SUMMARY

The widely held belief that bruxism, either sleep or awake, plays a major role in the development or persistence of TMD pain is not strongly supported by scientific evidence. Moreover, there is little evidence to support the premise of a cascade in time, in which SDB leads to SB, which in turns leads to TMD. Generalization of such beliefs, or a cause-and-effect relationship, does not stand in large population studies or in studies using optimal assessment methods.

A more complex interrelationship involving elevated background levels of activity in the masticatory muscles is emerging that may explain an association between SDB and TMD in some subgroups of patients. Phenotyping of differences among patients with OSA and with TMD will help clarify disparate clinical observation previously reported in the literature and will thus guide treatment selection in the future and better patient care.

SELECTED READINGS

Baad-Hansen L, Thymi M, Lobbezoo F, Svensson P. To what extent is bruxism associated with musculoskeletal signs and symptoms? A systematic review. *J Oral Rehabil.* 2019;46(9):845–861.

Balasubramaniam R, Klasser GD, Cistulli PA, et al. The link between sleep bruxism, sleep disordered breathing and temporomandibular disorders: an evidence-based review. *J Dent Sleep Med.* 2014;1(1):27–37.

Bussadori SK, Motta LJ, Horliana ACRT, Santos EM, Martimbianco ALC. The current trend in management of bruxism and chronic pain: an overview of systematic reviews. *J Pain Res.* 2020;13:2413–2421. https://doi.org/10.2147/JPR.S268114. Published 2020 Sep 30.

Dubrovsky B, Raphael KG, Lavigne GJ, et al. Polysomnographic investigation of sleep and respiratory parameters in women with temporomandibular pain disorders. *J Clin Sleep Med.* 2014;10(2):195–201.

Manfredini D, Guarda-Nardini L, Marchese-Ragona R, Lobbezoo F. Theories on possible temporal relationships between sleep bruxism and obstructive sleep apnea events. An expert opinion. *Sleep Breath.* 2015;19(4):1459–1465.

Martynowicz H, Gac P, Brzecka A, et al. The relationship between sleep bruxism and obstructive sleep apnea based on polysomnographic findings. *J Clin Med.* 2019;8(10):1–10.

Raphael KG, Janal MN, Sirois DA, et al. Masticatory muscle sleep background electromyographic activity is elevated in myofascial temporomandibular disorder patients. *J Oral Rehabil.* 2013;40:883–891.

Raphael KG, Sirois DA, Janal MN, et al. Sleep bruxism and myofascial temporomandibular disorders: a laboratory-based polysomnographic investigation. *J Am Dent Assoc.* 2012;143(11):1223–1231.

Sanders AE, Essick GK, Fillingim R, et al. Sleep apnea symptoms and risk of temporomandibular disorder: OPPERA cohort. *J Dent Res.* 2013;92(suppl 7):70S–7S.

Santiago V, Raphael K. Absence of joint pain identifies high levels of sleep masticatory muscle activity in myofascial temporomandibular disorder. *J Oral Rehabil.* 2019;46(12):1161–1169.

Schmitter M, Kares-Vrincianu A, Kares H, et al. Sleep-associated aspects of myofascial pain in the orofacial area among temporomandibular disorder patients and controls. *Sleep Med.* 2015;16(9):1056–1061.

Tay DKL, Pang KP. Clinical phenotype of South-East Asian temporomandibular disorder patients with upper airway resistance syndrome. *J Oral Rehabil.* 2018;45(1):25–33.

A complete reference list can be found online at ExpertConsult.com.

Chapter 173

Oral Appliances for the Treatment of Sleep-Disordered Breathing

Fernanda R. Almeida; Christopher J. Lettieri

Chapter Highlights

- Oral appliances (OAs) are an effective, well-tolerated, and easy-to-use treatment option for patients with snoring and/or obstructive sleep apnea syndrome (OSAS). They are indicated as first-line treatment for patients with mild to severe OSAS as an alternative to positive airway pressure (PAP) in patients who prefer this type of treatment or who are intolerant to a PAP device. OAs are most effective in younger, thinner patients with mild to moderate OSAS. They are less likely to be effective in obese patients.
- In general, and especially for moderate to severe disease, custom titratable devices offer superior treatment and a greater likelihood for successful therapy than other types of OAs. A successful outcome is more likely to be achieved with at-home progressive advancement of the mandible using a custom titratable/adjustable device. The result may be further enhanced by monitoring the therapeutic response.
- OAs are not as effective as PAP for reducing the apnea-hypopnea index and other objective sleep measures. However, improvements in daytime somnolence, quality of life, neurocognitive function, and cardiovascular outcomes (primarily blood pressure), appear to be similar with both treatments, likely due to the higher adherence to this therapy.
- OAs are generally well tolerated, and serious side effects or adverse consequences resulting in discontinuation of therapy are uncommon. Malocclusion is the most common long-term effect. However, this typically does not lead to discontinuation of treatment and may be mitigated by simple exercises each morning after removal of the device.

INTRODUCTION AND INDICATIONS

Oral appliances (OAs) are devices intended to treat obstructive sleep apnea (OSA) and primary snoring that can be used as primary therapy or as an adjunct to a positive airway pressure (PAP) device.[1] They are indicated as first-line treatment for selected patients with mild to severe obstructive sleep apnea-hypopnea syndrome (OSAS) as an alternate therapy for those who prefer this type of treatment, do not respond to or are unable or unwilling to tolerate PAP therapy. These devices have been proven to effectively improve the frequency and duration of obstructive events, oxygenation, nocturnal arousals, subjective sleepiness, neurocognitive function, blood pressure (BP), and quality-of-life (QoL) measures.

"Oral appliance" is a somewhat nonspecific term that has led to some confusion regarding its place in the treatment of sleep-disordered breathing. The two most common device types are mandibular advancement devices (MADs) (also referred to as mandibular repositioning devices or mandibular advancement splints) and tongue-retaining devices (TRDs). This chapter will focus exclusively on MADs as they are the most effective and widely used in clinical practice.

Although PAP remains the most common and most efficacious treatment for sleep-disordered breathing, poor acceptance of and adherence with these devices remains problematic. In addition, PAP is not the ideal treatment for all patients, and, like other medical disorders, an individualized approach to the treatment of OSAS is needed to optimize outcomes. As such, there remains a need for reliable and effective treatment alternatives. OAs offer effective therapy for many patients with sleep-disordered breathing and have become a proven, validated, and increasingly used treatment option. The American Academy of Sleep Medicine (AASM) published an updated clinical practice guideline for the use of OAs in the treatment of OSA and snoring in 2015.[2]

OAs offer several advantages over PAP. They are generally well tolerated in most individuals, and published reports have consistently shown that therapeutic adherence and patient preferences are superior to PAP.[3,4] In addition, these devices do not require a ready and reliable source of electricity or distilled water and thus may be easier to use, especially during travel.

This chapter provides a review of the different types of OAs, their mechanism of action, therapeutic effect, comparison between types of OAs and between OA and PAP treatment, patient and device selection, complications, and their role in the treatment of OSAS. This chapter will also highlight the role of the sleep physician and sleep dentist in proper patient and device selection and the need for an interdisciplinary approach to optimize outcomes for our patients.

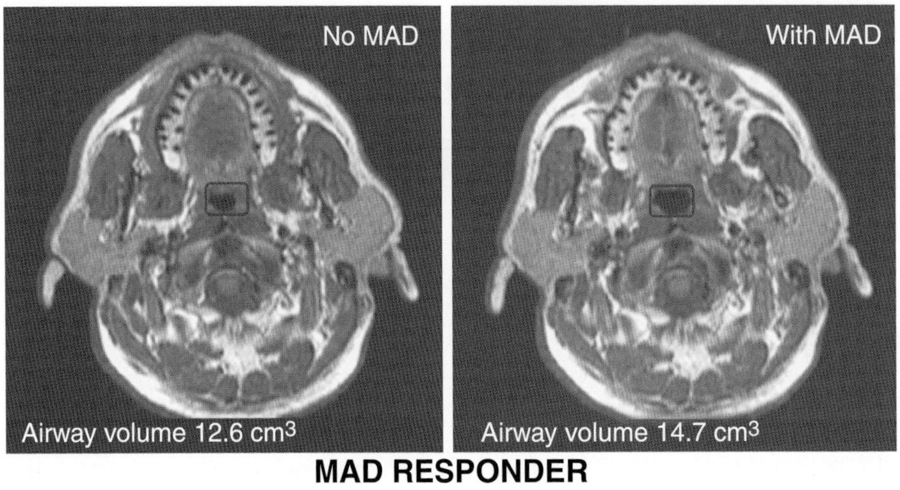

Figure 173.1 MADS responder. An increase in airway volume appears to result as seen in a magnetic resonance imaging axial view of a patient with and without the oral appliance.[1] MAD, Mandibular advancement device.

TYPES OF MANDIBULAR ADVANCEMENT DEVICES

MADs have numerous designs available, but these devices generally fall into either one-piece (monobloc) or two-piece (duobloc) configurations. They can differ substantially in size, type of material, degree of customization to the patient's dentition, and coupling mechanisms. In addition, the amount of occlusal coverage, adjustability of mandibular advancement, degree of mandibular mobility permitted (vertical and lateral), and allowance for oral breathing vary between the different available devices.

Two-piece MADs have become more commonly used in clinical practice and consist of a removable upper and a lower plate that are coupled to promote advancement of the mandible and mitigate mandibular retrusion during sleep. There are a variety of coupling modes between the upper and the lower plates, including elastic or plastic connectors, metal pins and tube connectors, hook connectors, acrylic extensions, or magnets. Duobloc splints offer advantages over monobloc devices by allowing a greater degree of lower jaw movements and, most important, allowing adjustability, which facilitates achievement to the most comfortable and efficient position of the mandible. MADs that permit lateral jaw movement or opening and closing while maintaining mandibular advancement may offer additional advantages by reducing the risk of complications and improving patient comfort and acceptance. Because patient tolerance to the amount of protrusion increases over time, splints capable of incremental advancement seem to have a clear practical advantage. These adjustable devices also facilitate improved efficacy as they can be titrated to a more optimal setting needed to ablate obstructive events. Although prefabricated appliances ("off the shelf") are commercially available, their efficacy and potential role as a "trial" device have been called into question.[5] New prefabricated devices have shown increased retention and improved effectiveness but are still inferior to custom-made devices.[6,7] The best retention, comfort, and efficacy are achieved with custom-made titratable OAs. Further comparisons between the different available types of OAs and potential advantages in the management of patients with sleep-disordered breathing are discussed later in this chapter.

MECHANISM OF ACTION

Current evidence suggests that the pathogenesis of OSAS reflects reduced upper airway size and altered upper airway muscle activity, resulting in diminished patency and airflow obstruction. Although it has been hypothesized that the primary mechanism of action of OAs arises from the anterior movement of the tongue and consequent increase in the anteroposterior dimensions of the oropharynx, it appears that this is an overly simplistic view. Many studies using a range of imaging modalities, including computerized tomography, magnetic resonance imaging (MRI), and nasendoscopy suggest that OAs induce more complex anatomic changes.[8,9] An increase in airway volume appears to result, in large part, by an increase in cross-sectional area of the velopharynx, in both the lateral and anteroposterior dimensions, and increases in the lateral dimension of the oropharynx as seen in an MRI axial view of a patient with and without the OA (Figure 173.1).

These changes are thought to be mediated through the palatoglossal and palatopharyngeal arches, which link the muscles of the tongue, soft palate, lateral pharyngeal walls, and the mandibular attachments. Interindividual variability in the airway configurational changes that occur with mandibular advancement may reflect variations in anatomy, and this is likely to have major relevance to the variable clinical response associated with this treatment modality. It is essential to understand that the efficacy of MAD is not solely associated with an increase in the upper airway size/volume. A well-designed trial using MRI to predict treatment outcomes failed to show a relationship between the amount of improvement in the apnea-hypopnea index (AHI) and the upper airway volume increase with the use of MAD.[10]

Anatomic imbalance has been proposed as an underlying mechanism in the pathogenesis of OSAS.[11] In this model, excess tissue within the bony enclosure must be present to generate sufficient tissue pressure to collapse the airway lumen. This extraluminal tissue pressure occurs in the context of either an excess of soft tissue within a normal bony enclosure size or by a normal amount of tissue compressed into a reduced bony enclosure. Mandibular advancement delivered by MADs effectively enlarges the bony enclosure and appears to improve anatomic balance.[12] Recent studies have focused on nonanatomic pathophysiologic traits of OSA, including poor pharyngeal muscle response, oversensitive ventilatory control, and low arousal threshold.[13] A small recent study has shown that patients with lower loop gain were more likely to respond to MAD treatment. Larger prospective studies are required to better understand the impact of MAD on non-anatomic components of OSA.[13,14]

The effects of OAs on upper airway neuromuscular pathways have not been well studied to date. Although some studies indicate that these devices stimulate genioglossus muscle activity,[15,16] studies using inactive, "sham" MADs have shown little change in sleep-disordered breathing.[17,18] This suggests that mechanical advancement of the mandible is the primary mechanism of action of these devices. This mechanical effect results in greater airway stability, which is evidenced by a reduced upper airway closing pressure during sleep.[19] This effect was demonstrated in a study of anesthetized OSA patients by Kato and colleagues,[20] who observed dose-dependent reductions in closing pressure of all pharyngeal segments with progressive mandibular advancement.

CLINICAL OUTCOMES AND MEASURES OF SUCCESS

Since the last published guidelines on the use of OAs in the treatment of OSAS, there has been a substantial increase in the quantity and quality of clinical trials evaluating the efficacy and effectiveness of OA therapy.[17,18,20–27] Several trials, including prospective designs using placebo arms and sham comparisons, have produced a high level of evidence and have allowed more robust treatment recommendations. In addition, trials assessing the treatment response between OAs and other primary therapies for OSAS, focusing on clinically meaningful outcomes, help better the understanding of appropriate patient selection and the expected therapeutic effect. In short, OAs have proven efficacy in improving polysomnographic (PSG) measures, daytime sleepiness, QoL, cardiovascular (CV) outcomes, and neurocognitive function for patients with both simple (primary) snoring and OSAS. The American Academy of Dental Sleep Medicine[28] has defined an effective OA as follows: "An oral appliance is custom fabricated using digital or physical impressions and models of an individual patient's oral structures. As such, it is not a primarily prefabricated item that is trimmed, bent, relined or otherwise modified. It is made of biocompatible materials and engages both the maxillary and mandibular arches. The oral appliance has a mechanism that allows the mandible to be advanced in increments of 1 mm or less with a protrusive adjustment range of at least 5 mm. In addition, reversal of the advancement must be possible. The protrusive setting must be verifiable. The appliance is suitable for placement and removal by the patient or caregiver. It maintains a stable retentive relationship to the teeth, implants or edentulous ridge and retains the prescribed setting during use. An oral appliance maintains its structural integrity over a minimum of 3 years."

Snoring

According to a Sleep in America Poll, habitual snoring is reported by about 60% of adults.[29] Snoring is a significant risk factor for OSAS. Still, not every snorer has OSAS, and the majority of individuals have primary snoring. Although snoring has been associated with an increased prevalence of CV disease, primary snoring, in and of itself, does not necessarily warrant therapy. However, snoring that interferes with social relationships or disrupts the sleep of bed partners should be addressed. Both prefabricated and customized OAs effectively reduce or eliminate snoring and have been shown to improve the QoL in patients with habitual snoring who do not have underlying OSAS or upper airway resistance syndrome. Snoring is an important factor in the treatment of OSAS, and in the *S*leep *A*pnea Cardio*v*ascular *E*ndpoints (SAVE) trial, very loud snoring before treatment was one of the best predictors of treatment adherence and therefore improvement in CV outcomes.[30]

Numerous therapeutic trials among patients with OSAS have found that OAs reduce, if not eliminate, snoring. However, several placebo-controlled trials have also found that OAs significantly improve both subjective and objective measures of snoring frequency and intensity compared to inactive control devices among nonapneic patients with habitual snoring.[5,23,24,26,27] In a trial exploring the effect that OAs had on snoring frequency, snoring intensity (average and peak loudness), and the anatomic site of snoring (palatal flutter or tongue base),[31] the investigators observed that all measured parameters were significantly improved with OA therapy. Of note, this study identified that OAs were more effective in reducing snoring originating from the soft palate than snoring originating from tongue base snoring. One trial has also observed that OAs reduced the frequency of snoring (odds ratio, 1.20; 95% confidence interval [CI], 1.89 to 0.51).[26] Other trials have also reported a similar reduction in snoring frequency with OA therapy.[27] In a subjective evaluation, 76% of OA users reported control of snoring compared to 43% of the nonusers, and 82% of the patients' partners were satisfied with the treatment.[32]

These devices have also been shown to improve QoL measures among nonapneic snorers. Similarly, the use of OAs produced a mean improvement in Functional Outcomes of Sleep Questionnaire (FOSQ) scores by 3.21 (95% CI, 2.82 to 3.60; $P < .001$) among patients with habitual snoring and mild OSA.[23]

Polysomnographic Variables and Reduction of the Apnea-Hypopnea Index

The effect of OAs on improvements in PSG variables and the AHI across the full spectrum of OSAS severities has been confirmed by several high-quality studies, including randomized controlled trials (RCTs), systematic reviews, and meta-analyses.[2,18,24,26,33,34]

OAs have been shown to significantly reduce the AHI in adult patients with OSAS. A meta-analysis of 34 RCTs, specifically exploring the effect of OAs on AHI, was conducted as part of the AASM's 2015 updated clinical practice guidelines for the use of OAs in the treatment of OSA.[2] Overall, OAs were found to be effective. In a weighted analysis the mean reduction in AHI was 13.60 events per hour. Successful therapy, as defined by a reduction of the AHI to less than 5 events per hour, is achieved in 36% to 70% of patients.[17,18,33,35] Using an AHI threshold of less than 10 per hour, OAs provide successful therapy in 30% to 86%.[20,36] Success rates appear to be inversely proportional to OSA severity, with the likelihood of successful treatment decreasing as the AHI increases.

OAs have also been shown to improve both nocturnal oxygenation and the oxygen desaturation index (ODI).[34,37–39] These improvements are more commonly observed with custom titratable devices. Similarly, OAs have been reported to improve nocturnal arousals, with several studies finding a greater than 50% reduction in arousal index.[39,40] Similar to PAP, OAs have not been shown to have a substantial impact on sleep architecture.

Daytime Somnolence and Quality-of-Life Measures

OAs have been shown to improve daytime sleepiness, function, and QoL in patients with OSAS. Numerous studies and clinical trials have established the benefits of OA therapy compared with no treatment or sham treatment. Various studies have shown that the improvement in daytime somnolence was significantly better with customized OAs compared with nontherapeutic devices.[39,41] After 3 months, the Epworth Sleepiness Score decreased from about 15 to 5 in those receiving OA therapy, compared with no change in the nontherapeutic group. Similarly, a long-term follow-up study reported similar findings.[24] OAs have been shown to improve objective measures of sleepiness using the Multiple Sleep Latency Test.[12] Two additional trials evaluating objective measures of wakefulness found that the improvements in the Maintenance of Wakefulness Test were similar between both PAP and OA therapy.[3,42] Across numerous published studies, the improvements in both subjective and objective measures of sleepiness achieved with OAs appear to be similar to that reported with PAP therapy. In a network meta-analysis comparing PAP, MAD, exercise training, and weight loss, there was no significant difference in the improvement of sleepiness between the treatments.[43] In contrast, a network meta-analysis of PAP and MAD[44] found a greater improvement of sleepiness with PAP. However, the authors caution the readers that there was a possibility of publication bias in favor of PAP that might have resulted in this difference. In a recent traditional meta-analysis, PAP and MAD showed similar efficacy in the improvement of sleepiness.[2] However, like PAP, although MADs are shown to improve daytime somnolence, residual sleepiness may persist despite otherwise adequate therapy. Therefore the addition of combination therapy may be recommended, such as the concomitant use of medication such as modafinil

OAs improve QoL measures in patients with OSAS. However, similar to PAP, these results are not uniformly consistent, vary between the different QoL end points, and are largely dependent on patient adherence. Compared with no treatment or nontherapeutic (sham) therapy, OAs produce significant improvements in QoL measures. As an example, one study found that overall FOSQ scores improved by 27.1% from baseline ($P < .001$; effect size, 0.90) in those using a customized OA, compared with a −1.7% decline in those using a similar sham device set at a nontherapeutic degree of mandibular advancement.[39] In a RCT comparing OA therapy to a placebo tablet, mandibular advancement produced superior improvements in QoL as measured by the FOSQ and Short Form-36 overall health score.[3] The magnitude of improvement was similar to that found with PAP. Similarly, Gauthier and colleagues[23] observed that mean overall FOSQ scores improved from 13.9 ± 0.8 to 17.2 ± 0.6 ($P \leq .01$) after 40.9 months of OA therapy. In a large randomized trial comparing MAD to PAP therapy, both treatments equally and significantly improved general QoL domains, although MAD was superior in the improvement of bodily pain, vitality, mental health, and mental component domains. A recent network meta-analysis comparing MAD to PAP found that MAD may be as effective as PAP, but further RCTs comparing the two treatments are required.[45]

The available evidence suggests that MADs are effective in improving QoL. Measured improvements are similar, or not inferior, to those reported with PAP therapy. These improvements are largely associated with custom titratable devices. Data regarding QoL outcomes with nontitratable (fixed) and prefabricated devices is limited.

Cardiovascular Outcomes

OSA is well recognized as an independent risk factor for CV disease, and its adverse effect on CV health and outcomes has been established. Intuitively, treatment of OSA should produce improvements in CV-related outcomes.

Similar to other modifiable or treatable cardiac risk factors, it is unreasonable to expect a complete reversal of underlying cardiac or endothelial dysfunction and elimination of future adverse events. With regard to OSA, irreversible or partially irreversible end-organ dysfunction may very well occur long before OSA is recognized and treated. OSA is typically not the sole cardiac risk factor present, and even optimal treatment of obstructive respiratory events does not address other potential confounding factors.

Effect of Oral Appliance Therapy on Blood Pressure

Numerous clinical trials and observational cohorts have accessed the impact of OA therapy on measures of BP.[3,4,24,46–52] Although the overall quality of the existing published literature is low, these studies have consistently found that OAs lead to modest reductions in systolic, diastolic, mean, and 24-hour BP recordings, and these improvements are similar to, if not superior to, those observed with PAP therapy. As stated, improvements in BP are modest, and similar to PAP, OAs may not provide adequate monotherapy for some patients with incident hypertension associated with OSA. They should be used in conjunction with lifestyle modifications and pharmacotherapy when needed. It should be noted that these studies are largely limited to custom, titratable devices, and the impact on BP on other device types is unknown.

Several studies have reported modest reductions in arterial BP.[23,34,47-50] Of interest, a study found that OA did significantly improve the number of nocturnal dippers, and this was not found with CPAP or placebo OA.[51] The effect of OA therapy on systemic BP was summarized in a recent meta-analysis.[52] In a pooled analysis of seven observational and RCT studies, OA therapy produced approximately a 2-mm reduction in systolic, diastolic, and mean arterial pressure.

The effects on BP between OA and PAP therapy have been directly compared in several studies, including three randomized trials.[3,4,34,47] A 3-month treatment trial of patients with mild to moderate OSAS comparing PAP, OA, and placebo pills found limited benefits of therapy on BP recordings, with only OA therapy producing reductions in nocturnal diastolic BP.[3] A noninferiority, randomized, crossover trial compared PAP and OA treatment among patients with moderate to severe OSA.[4] In a subgroup analysis of patients with known hypertension, both treatments performed similarly, with neither treatment having a superior effect. Specifically, 24-hour BP measures improved 2 to 4 mm Hg, and arterial stiffness was reduced by 1% to 2% from baseline.

Effect of Oral Appliance Therapy on Cardiovascular Morbidity and Mortality

The majority of the published literature related to OA therapy and CV outcomes is limited to the effect on BP. However, there has been a more recent focus on other markers of CV health and mortality that have shown small but significant improvements. Overall, studies demonstrate a significant improvement in cardiac function, CV event rates, microvascular endothelial function, and mortality with no substantial differences noted between treatment modalities.[34,51,53,54]

A small study measuring endothelial function and oxidative stress as markers for the development of CV disease found that treatment with an OA led to near-normalization of these markers, suggesting that OA therapy was effective in reducing the risk of CV disease.[55] A cohort of patients with untreated moderate to severe OSA, who did not have underlying CV disease, used changes in N-terminal pro–B-type natriuretic peptide (NT-pro-BNP) levels to assess CV function before and after randomization to either OA therapy or CPAP.[37] The investigators noted significant improvements in NT-pro-BNP values after OA therapy but not with CPAP.

A recent meta-analysis summarizing the CV effects of OA therapy[56] pooled data from 16 studies, including 11 RCTs, found significant improvements in both diastolic and systolic BP and improved daytime resting heart rate when compared with placebo or no treatment. Although several studies exploring the impact on heart rate variability, specific CV biomarkers, endothelial function, and arterial stiffness, there were too many limitations and heterogeneity in the findings to render a conclusive assessment. No included studies found any significant improvements in echocardiographic measures, and one observational study found the reduction in CV death seen with OAs was similar to that observed with PAP therapy.

Biomarkers and Metabolic Outcomes

OSAS leads to systemic inflammation that has been shown to increase the risk of developing several CV and metabolic consequences. Treatment with PAP has been shown to reduce levels of inflammation and metabolic biomarkers. However, OA therapy has not been shown to have a similar positive impact on these indices.[57] A randomized, sham controlled treatment trial study, failed to find improvements in inflammatory or metabolic biomarkers despite effective OA therapy.[34] Likewise, in a pilot study specifically designed to measure the effects of OA therapy on glucose control among patients with comorbid type 2 diabetes mellitus, the investigators did not find an improvement in hemoglobin A1c levels after 3 months of therapy.[58] One study found that OA therapy significantly improved C-reactive protein, interleukin-β, and tumor necrosis factor-α levels. Although some improvements were noted in those with severe OSA, the investigator found that improvements in these inflammatory markers were more commonly observed in patients with more moderate disease.[59] However, on balance the existing literature suggests OA therapy may not be appropriate for OSAS patients with comorbid diabetes mellitus or metabolic syndrome.

Neurocognitive Outcomes

Relatively few studies have explored the potential benefits of OA therapy on neurocognitive function. Similar to PAP, the existing literature shows mixed results with only modest or no improvements in cognitive measures.[3,60] In contrast, other trials have demonstrated some improvement in simulated driving performance,[61] divided attention, and executive functioning,[3] vigilance, and motor speed.[62] Although limited, the existing data suggests that the benefits of OA therapy are similar to those observed with PAP with regard to neurocognitive outcomes. For both treatment modalities, improvements are modest at best.

OUTCOME COMPARISON BETWEEN TYPES OF ORAL APPLIANCE DESIGNS AND POSITIVE AIRWAY PRESSURE THERAPY

There are numerous different types of oral devices available for the treatment of OSAS. The most commonly used devices are MADs, which typically attach to both dental arches and maintain the mandible in a forward position. Differences in design characteristics may impact patient comfort, treatment adherence, and the device's ability to provide successful treatment. In short, not all devices are equally effective or efficacious. Further, the nomenclature regarding OA therapy is nonuniform across the published literature. In addition, clinical trials frequently include a limited sample size and use one unique brand or type of device. This restricts the pooled understanding and measured benefits of OA therapy in the treatment of OSAS. As stated, this chapter will largely focus on OA therapy using mandibular advancement splints as they are the most commonly used, most effective, and most studied device in the management of sleep-disordered breathing.

Prefabricated MADs are available. These are often referred to as "boil and bite" or thermoplastic devices. They may be offered by some providers, such as dentists or physicians, and many are available over the counter. These can either be fitted by the patient themselves or molded to the patient's teeth in an office setting. There are a paucity of clinical data and outcome measures with this type of appliance. The current literature shows limited efficacy and lower acceptance rate compared with customized OAs.[5,25] Thus prefabricated devices are not recommended for clinical use in patients with OSAS. They may provide a reasonable and cost-effective treatment for simple snoring.

Fixed versus Adjustable Appliances

Customized, or individually fabricated devices, are either fixed (nonadjustable) or titratable (adjustable). Nonadjustable devices are monobloc, or single-piece appliances, where the degree of mandibular advancement is permanently fixed. Titratable appliances (adjustable or duobloc) allow adjustments in the degree of mandibular protrusion, with the intent that this allows greater optimization of treatment. This is an important distinction in both selection of the most effective treatment and in understanding the published literature. Due to selection biases, published studies using fixed or single-jaw-position appliances may underestimate the overall impact of OA therapy and introduce heterogeneity when understanding the potential benefits of titratable devices.[4,42,53,63]

There appears to be a dose-dependent relationship between the degree of mandibular advancement and the impact on AHI reduction.[64,65] In addition, the optimal protrusion required to stabilize the upper airways and ablate obstructive events varies between individuals.[7,66] Having the ability to adjust the degree of mandibular advancement allows for individualization of therapy, thus leading to a greater treatment effect. Titratable, or adjustable, appliances allow progressive protrusion of the mandible, and previous studies have shown that OA efficacy is related to the amount of mandibular advancement.[20,67,68] As such, determining the optimal degree of mandibular advancement is the most important factor influencing successful OA therapy.[69,70] This concept is analogous to the pressures used in PAP therapy. A systematic review of different types of OA devices concluded that there is no one device design feature that influences treatment efficacy, but rather treatment efficacy depends on the degree of mandibular protrusion and whether the device was a fixed or titratable appliance.[64]

Although titratable devices have been consistently shown to be superior to fixed devices, fixed devices may still have a role in the management of OSAS. These devices are typically less expensive, require a shorter period of adjustment, are more accessible, and may not require the same degree of provider expertise to fabricate and fit. However, because of their limited efficacy and higher failure rates, the use of these devices should be largely limited to those with milder forms of sleep-disordered breathing.

Oral Appliances versus Positive Airway Pressure Therapy

Several published RCTs and crossover studies have compared the efficacy of OAs to PAP in the treatment of OSAS, as seen in Table 173.1.[71]

Although both treatment options lead to improvements in both objective and subjective outcomes measures, the existing literature has consistently shown that PAP more efficaciously improves AHI, nocturnal arousals, and oxygenation. A meta-analysis of 15 RCTs, conducted as part of the AASM OA clinical practice guidelines, found that PAP more effectively improved the AHI.[72] In weighted analysis, the mean reduction in AHI was 6.24 events per hour (95% CI, 8.14 to 4.34) greater with PAP than with OAs. However, adherence with OAs are typically greater than those observed with PAP. As such, the greater efficacy of PAP may be negated by lower adherence, with some experts suggesting overall treatment effectiveness is similar between these two modalities. Both OAs and PAP have been shown to be superior to placebo or no treatment in improving QoL measures, with each treatment providing certain advantages in specific subcategories.[a] It should be noted that, although both treatments significantly improve numerous QoL domains, neither treatment option has consistently normalized these measures.

A large, retrospective study directly compared the efficacy of PAP to custom titratable OAs as primary therapy for all severities of OSA, that is, the OA group was not selected due to PAP failure or intolerance.[33] Overall, OA therapy reduced the mean AHI from 30.0 to 8.4. Using a definition of successful therapy as an on-treatment AHI of less than 5, OAs demonstrated similar efficacy relative to PAP among patients with mild OSA. Specifically, successful therapy was observed in 76% of the PAP and 62% of the OA group (P = .15). Rates of successful therapy were greater with PAP in those with moderate and severe OSA: 71% vs. 51% in the moderate group and 63% vs. 40% in the severe group. However, it should be noted that the magnitude of AHI reduction was only significant in those with severe OSA. Among these patients, PAP resulted in a 5.9 events per hour greater reduction in the AHI compared with OAs (P < .001). In those with mild and moderate OSA, the reduction in AHI differed by less than two events per hour between PAP and OA therapy.

Although no RCTs have assessed objective OA adherence rates compared with PAP, subjective patient reports of both adherence and preference clearly favor OA therapy. This was highlighted in the OA practice parameters, which concluded adherence with OAs is better overall than with CPAP in adult patients with OSA, although with a low quality of evidence.[72] Overall, OAs were used for 30% more hours per night compared with PAP. Given the relative equality in overall disease control, these findings challenge current practice parameters that recommend that OA treatment should only be considered in patients with mild to moderate OSA or in those who have failed or refuse PAP treatment. Long-term comparative effectiveness studies of these two treatment modalities are clearly needed.

PATIENT AND DEVICE SELECTION

There are multiple factors that should be considered when determining which patients are ideal candidates for OA therapy. Similarly, there are multiple different types, designs, and brands of OA devices, each with its own inherent advantages and limitations. Understanding these factors can aid clinicians in making appropriate treatment decisions.

Indications and Contraindications

The AASM practice parameters on OAs in the treatment of sleep-disordered breathing advocate the use of these devices in patients with mild, moderate, and severe OSA who prefer this form of treatment over PAP, or who do not respond to or are unable to tolerate PAP.[72] This guideline suggests that clinicians should use custom titratable OAs as first-line therapy or as an alternate to PAP as an effective and reliable means to improve physiologic sleep measures, daytime sleepiness, and QoL in adult patients with OSAS.

Selection of appropriate patients for OA therapy, based on the likelihood of successful treatment, remains a somewhat elusive goal at present. Although considerable research has attempted to identify the factors that predict a good response, the clinical utility of such approaches remains to be proven. In general, younger, thinner patients, with positional OSAS and an overall lower AHI appear to be the preferred candidate for OA therapy. However, in the absence of clear selection criteria, the clinician should rely on clinical judgment and patient preference when choosing the appropriate therapeutic approach.

Dentists experienced in dental sleep medicine have a prominent role in determining whether or not a patient is an ideal candidate for OA therapy. The evaluation includes a medical and dental history and a complete intraoral examination. This includes an assessment of the soft tissues, periodontal health, temporomandibular joint (TMJ) function, and dental occlusion. Patients require a sufficient number and location of healthy teeth to retain the device and promote mandibular advancement. Specifically, patients require a minimum of 6 teeth in the upper and in the lower jaw each, with at least 2 teeth in each quadrant. Other common clinically used criteria require a minimum of 10 teeth on the lower arch and a strong and retentive favorable maxillary ridge for an effective use of OA devices.[28] In addition, the patient should have the ability

[a]References 3, 4, 7, 22, 40, 42, 60, 61, 63, 72.

Table 173.1 Summary of Randomized Trials Comparing Oral Appliance to CPAP

Study	Design	Subject numbers (% Male) [Withdrawals]	Inclusion	Oral Appliance	Treatment (Washout) Duration	Baseline AHI	Treatment AHI		OA vs. CPAP		
							CPAP	OA	AHI	ESS	Patient Preference
Aarab (2011)[40]	Parallel *(placebo group included)*	57 (74%) (20 OA/18 CPAP) [7]	AHI 15–45 + ESS ≥ 10	Customized, two-piece, set 25.50, or 75% advancement depending on sleep study results at each level	24 wk	CPAP 20.9 ± 9.8 OA: 22.1 ± 10.8	1.41 ± 13.1	5.8 ± 14.9	↔ (*P* = .092)	↔	N/A—parallel groups
Barnes (2004)[3]	Crossover *(placebo group included)*	80 (79%) [24]	AHI 15–30	Customized, 4-wk titration to maximum comfortable advancement	3 × 12 wk (2 wk)	21.5 ± 1.6	4.8 ± 0.5	14.0 ± 1.1	CPAP	↔	CPAP
Engleman (2002)[42]	Crossover	48 (75%) [3]	AHI ≥ 5/h + ≥2 symptoms (including ESS ≥ 8)	Customized, one-piece, 80% maximal protrusion, two designs: (a) complete occlusal coverage or (b) no occlusal coverage, assigned randomly	2 × 8 wk (not reported)	31 ± 26	8 ± 6	15 ± 16	CPAP	CPAP	↔
Ferguson (1996)[22]	Crossover	25 (89%) [2]	AHI 15–50 + OSA symptoms	Snore-Guard (Hays & Meade), maximum comfortable advancement	2 × 16 weeks (2 wk)	24.5 ± 8.8	3.6 ± 1.7	9.7 ± 7.3	CPAP	N/A	OA
Ferguson (1997)[125]	Crossover	20 (95%) [4]	AHI 15–55 + OSA symptoms	Customized, two-piece appliance, titration starting at 70% maximum advancement over 3 mo	2 × 16 wk (2 wk)	26.8 ± 11.9	4.0± 2.2	14.2± 14.7	CPAP	↔	OA
Gagnadoux (2009)[7]	Crossover	59 (78%) [3]	AH 110–60 + ≥2 symptoms, BMI ≥ 35 kg/m²	AMC (Artech Medical), two-piece, advancement determined by single-night titration	2 × 8 wk (1 wk)	34 ± 13	2 (1–8)	6 (3–14)	CPAP	↔	OA

Continued

Table 173.1 Summary of Randomized Trials Comparing Oral Appliance to CPAP

Study	Design	Subject numbers (% Male) [Withdrawals]	Inclusion	Oral Appliance	Treatment (Washout) Duration	Baseline AHI	Treatment AHI: CPAP	Treatment AHI: OA	OA vs. CPAP: AHI	OA vs. CPAP: ESS	OA vs. CPAP: Patient Preference
Hoekema (2008)[37]	Parallel	103 (51 OA/52 CPAP) [4]	AHI ≥ 5	Thornton Adjustable Positioner type 1, titratable	8–12 wk	CPAP: ±27.6 OA: ±30.8	2.4± 4.2	7.8 ± 14.4	CPAP	↔	N/A—parallel groups
Lam (2007)[53]	Parallel *(placebo group included)*	101 (79%) (34 OA/34 CPAP) [10]	AHI ≥ 5–40 + ESS > 9 if AHI 5–20	Customized, non adjustable, set to maximum comfortable advancement	10 wk (83% referred for concurrent weight loss program)	CPAP: 23.8 ± 1.9 OA: 20.9 ± 1.7	2.8 ± 1.1	10.6 ± 1.7	CPAP	CPAP	N/A—parallel groups
Phillips (2013)[4]	Crossover	108 (81%) [18]	AHI ≥ 10 + ≥2 symptoms	Customized, two-piece appliance (SomnoMed), titrated to maximum comfortable limit in acclimatization period before study	2 × 4 wk (2 wk)	25.6 ± 12.3	4.5 ± 6.6	11.1 ± 12.1	CPAP	↔	OA
Randerath (2002)[126]	Crossover	20 (80%)	AHI 5–30 + OSA symptoms	ISAD (IST; Hinz, Herne, Germany), two-piece, nontitratable, set to two-thirds of maximum advancement	2 × 6 wk (not reported)	17.5 ± 7.7	3.2 ± 2.9	13.8 ± 11.1	CPAP	N/A	N/A
Tan (2002)[63]	Crossover	21 (83%) [3]	AHI 5–50	One-piece, 75% maximum advancement and Silensor (Erkodent) two-piece, titratable	2 × 8 wk (2 wk)	22.2 ± 9.6	3.1 ± 2.8	8.0 ± 10.9	↔	↔	N/A

AHI, Apnea-hypopnea index; BMI, body mass index; CPAP, continuous positive airway pressure; ESS, Epworth Sleepiness Scale; N/A, not applicable; OA, oral appliance; OSA, obstructive sleep apnea.

to protrude the mandible forward at least 3 mm to achieve a therapeutic result. Full upper and lower dentures likely preclude the use of an OA, but some edentulous patients may respond well to a TRD or to keep both upper and lower dentures connected in a forward position during sleep.

Not all patients are suitable candidates for the use of OAs due to associated medical or dental conditions and factors. In general, PAP affords a prompter initiation of therapy. A major clinical limitation of OA therapy is in circumstances where there is an imperative to commence more immediate treatment as there are inherent delays to attain optimal therapy using these devices. This includes situations involving severe symptomatic OSA (e.g., concern about driving risk or profound daytime impairments) and/or coexistent medical comorbidities, such as ischemic heart disease. Moreover, this treatment modality has no known role in treating central sleep apnea or hypoventilation states. In addition, some case reports have shown worsening of OSA severity in some patients using OAs.[22,73] This, together with the known potential for a placebo reponse, highlights the need for objective verification of treatment outcome using in-laboratory or home sleep testing with an OA in place at its prescribed, therapeutic position.[17,18]

The presence of periodontal disease may promote excessive tooth movement or worsening dental caries with an OA. One study has suggested that up to one-third of patients are excluded on the basis of such factors.[74] TMJ disorder, including joint dysfunction, pathology, and pain, are often a concern for patients and professionals involved in MAD therapy. Research suggests that there is no contraindication of MAD for the treatment of OSAS with concomitant TMD.[67,75]

Predictors of Successful Oral Appliance Therapy

Ultimately, the response to therapy is likely to be related to multiple patient factors, device features, and the clinical expertise of the treating provider. Clinical features reported to be associated with better outcomes and a greater likelihood of success include younger age, lower body mass index (BMI), supine-dependent OSA, lower AHI, smaller oropharynx, shorter soft palate, and smaller neck circumference.[76] In general, a favorable response is more likely in mild to moderate OSA, although benefits in severe OSA have been reported with a dose-dependent relationship. Although, achieving an AHI less than 10 per hour with OA therapy is less likely in patients with severe OSA.[4,33] Cephalometric measures, such as a shorter soft palate, longer maxilla, decreased distance between mandibular plane and hyoid bone, and larger mandibular plane to cranial base angle (sella-naison-mandibular plane; SNMP), either in isolation or in combination with other anthropomorphic and PSG variables, are thought to provide some predictive power regarding successful therapy with OAs.[17,77]

A variety of studies have assessed different methods of predicting OA treatment success. The sensitivity, specificity, positive predictive value, and negative predictive value show a wide variability, ranging from 36% to 100%, 25% to 100%, 38% to 100%, and 33% to 100%, respectively, and varied depending on definitions of treatment success (AHI or ODI <5 or 10/hour, respectively) and specific methods of prediction used.[78] The wide variability of these results makes it difficult to delineate the usefulness of OA therapy in routine clinical practice. Physiologic studies indicate that retroglossal, rather than velopharyngeal, collapse during sleep is highly predictive of OA success.[79] Physiologic measurements during wakefulness, including nasal resistance and flow-volume loops have been reported to differ between OA responders and nonresponders.[80,81] However, upper airway imaging and physiologic measurements have limited utility for a robust clinical prediction model during wakefulness and may aid in predicting the treatment response. Although in the research setting upper airway MRI studies and computational modeling techniques may be useful[8,82] the clinical utility of such approaches is limited due to cost and accessibility. Nasoendoscopy during wakefulness has inconsistent results; nasoendoscopy during drug-induced sleep[9,83] may be helpful, although costly and exposes the patient to risk of the procedure.[9,83,84]

Remotely controlled mandibular positioner (RCMP) devices have been introduced as a method of identifying individuals who will or will not respond to OA therapy during a single-night titration procedure.[85,86] The cost of this additional study would preclude its widespread adoption. More information on such device benefit is found later.

Recent studies have focused on nonanatomic pathophysiologic traits of OSA, including poor pharyngeal muscle response, an oversensitive ventilator control, and low arousal threshold.[87] A small study has shown that patients with lower loop gain were more likely to respond to MAD treatment, and another trial found that MADs reduce pharyngeal collapsibility in a dose-dependent manner.[88,89] However, larger and prospectively designed studies in this area are required to better understand the impact of MADs on nonanatomic components of OSA.

Appliance Selection

As discussed, there are multiple different OAs available, ranging from over-the-counter, prefabricated, fixed "boil and bite" devices, to customized adjustable duobloc mandibular advancement splints. It is the sleep dentist's role to determine the most appropriate type of appliance based on specific clinical features, to ensure the patient is provided the most efficacious and cost-effective therapy. Given the wide variability in the reported efficacy across different studies, there is a strong suggestion that OA design, in addition to both dental expertise and titration procedures, has an important influence on treatment outcomes. The appropriate design of the appliance needs to take into consideration the occlusal and dental health, hard and soft tissues, the number of anchorage teeth, and the need for sagittal adjustment and/or reactivation. These will often vary on a case-by-case basis. Duobloc OAs, consisting of upper and lower plates, offer the advantage of a greater degree of mandibular movement (vertical and lateral) and adjustability (advancement), permitting attainment of the most comfortable and efficient position of the mandible. It is generally considered that the best retention is achieved with OAs that are customized and individually fabricated from the patient's dental impressions.[28]

The treating dentist is responsible for teaching the patient how to appropriately use and care for the appliance. For adjustable (titratable) devices, patients must understand how to properly adjust the degree of advancement to ensure optimal treatment. As important, patients must be educated on potential side effects and complications and be instructed on exercises to mitigate this risk and avoid malocclusion of the bite.[90]

Associated dental conditions, such as bruxism, may influence the choice of appliance design. Patients who experience jaw discomfort after wearing a rigid monobloc OA may benefit from using an appliance that allows lateral and vertical jaw movement.

Duobloc designs are generally preferable because of greater comfort and the ability to titrate, allowing attainment of the most comfortable and efficient position of the mandible and greater degree of lower jaw movements. OAs that permit lateral jaw movement or opening and closing while maintaining mandibular advancement may confer advantages in terms of reduction of the risk of complications and better patient comfort and acceptance. However, monobloc devices, although typically more rigid and bulky, are sometimes used to resolve issues related to anchorage needs, dental conditions, and the occlusal relationship. Another important consideration is the vertical dimension of the OA. Minimum vertical opening depends on the amount of overbite. There are conflicting data on the effect of the degree of bite opening induced by OAs on treatment outcomes, although most patients appear to prefer minimal interocclusal openings.[35] In mouth-breathing patients, the selected OA design should have an anterior opening to permit comfortable breathing, and appliances should also have the ability to add elastics to decrease the mandibular opening and allow a large range of opening.[91] In the case of edentulous patients wearing partial dentures, the splint design selected for that patient should adapt to the remaining natural dental structures when the dentures are removed. Although TRDs have a very limited role in the treatment of OSAS, they may play a role in individuals with insufficient teeth who fail or are not tolerant of other therapies.

Several studies comparing the efficacy of different OA designs have found a higher treatment response using adjustable versus fixed devices.[23,36,92] A recent study assessing the addition of tongue protrusion using an anterior tongue bulb on an existing OA device showed further reductions in AHI compared to mandibular advancement alone.[93] There is a need for further research to differentiate the advantages of different OA designs.

The technique of impression and fabrication of appliances has become digital. Most OAs are now fabricated after digital scanning of the patient's teeth and adjacent tissues together with a scanned image of the proposed initial mandibular position. Some devices are three-dimensional printed or three-dimensional milled. The current digital protocols have decreased the manufacturing time and increased accuracy of the appliances, which will minimize chances of ill-fitting devices and improve comfort for the patient. It is important to note that cone beam computed tomography is not part of the digital workflow. The use of panoramic images is sufficient to assess patients' dentition and supporting structures before OA treatment. The imaging of the TMJ is not required before treatment because OAs are indicated in cases of mild to moderate temporomandibular disorders and does not affect the TMJ complex.

In summary, OA response is primarily related to three factors: (1) the patient (characteristics and pathophysiologic traits); (2) device design, which requires it to be custom made and allow further mandibular advancement; and (3) clinical expertise of the provider to ensure patient comfort and proper appliance titration.

OPTIMIZATION OF TREATMENT

The degree of improvement, particularly the AHI and objective PSG variables, varies greatly in the published literature. Many studies show a high residual AHI on therapeutic settings of these devices or use alternative definitions of successful therapy. However, other studies have found high rates of success while still using strict definitions of successful therapy, such as a residual AHI of less than 5 with improvement/resolution of symptoms. Although these differences may be confounded by the use of different device types or manufacturers, most experts agree that this variance is primarily driven by the different practices regarding how providers approach OA settings and the degree of mandibular advancement. Often, OAs are set at some percentage of the maximum degree of mandibular protrusion or based on patient comfort.

Although common in clinical practice, published reports show that this approach is commonly associated with higher AHIs and treatment failure rates. Like other medical therapies, an individualized approach to therapy is the most effective way to optimize treatment and outcomes. This is achieved by selecting the right type of appliance and determining the optimal degree of mandibular advancement needed to achieve sufficient ablation of obstructive respiratory events.

Models to predict OA success have limited accuracy. Although younger age, lower BMIs, and less severe OSA are often associated with greater success rates, no single variable has been consistently shown to predict who will benefit from OA therapy. This was highlighted in a recent review of OA therapy by Marklund,[94] who stressed that the lack of high-quality evidence, small sample sizes, variability in specific devices, consistency in measured variables, inconsistent definitions of successful therapy, and lack of external validation limit the validity of the published OA literature.

Overall, the optimization of OA treatment is similar in concept to the optimization of PAP therapy. The success of both treatment modalities is dependent on determining the settings (pressure or amount of mandibular advancement) needed to stabilize the upper airways. However, the practical application of determining this threshold is quite different. For PAP, the pressure required to ablate events and normalize sleep is typically easy to determine and can be performed either during an in-laboratory PSG or with an at-home automatic/autotitrating PAP platform. However, determining the optimal settings for OAs is not as straightforward and often requires more time.

Patients may not be able to initially tolerate the degree of mandibular advancement required to completely relieve obstructive events. This is typically not a treatment-limiting phenomenon, and tolerance is achieved in the majority of patients if they are allowed to slowly advance the device over time. And although there are a variety of studies that show the decrease in AHI is dependent on the amount of mandibular advancement, OAs cannot be easily tried for a single night to predict treatment success and may require several months of progressive mandibular advancement to achieve a therapeutic mandibular position.[20,67,70,95]

The determination of ideal mandibular advancement remains controversial.[96] Some practitioners advocate the use of a predetermined degree of mandibular advancement, typically set at 70% to 80% of maximum protrusion. This practice, however, is frequently associated with high residual AHIs and inadequate control of OSAS. Unfortunately, a persistence of events noted on the confirmatory sleep study may lead to a prescription of insufficient treatment, the need for further studies or additional devices (e.g., sleep positioner for supine position), or an inappropriate abandonment of OA. However, numerous studies have shown there is a dose-dependent relationship between the amount of mandibular advancement and improvements in both snoring and the AHI, although not an absolute one for all individuals. In addition, and similar to PAP pressures, the position at which an OA is most effective varies between patients. As such, the practice of using an arbitrary set point for mandibular protrusion should be discouraged, and instead, this setting should be found individually for each patient.

The use of a systematic, home-based titration, where patients incrementally advance their devices until subjective improvements in sleep quality and daytime symptoms are achieved, is significantly more likely to render more effective OA therapy. The follow-up PSG is conducted once subjective improvements are achieved. However, although beneficial, this relies on subjective measures of improvement, which are limited by night-to-night variations and the inaccuracies related to self-perception of sleep quality. The proper timing of this study and the use of adjunctive monitoring devices have further improved the likelihood of successful OA therapy. Using an AHI of less than 5 events per hour as the definition of successful therapy, investigators found this approach led to success rates of 70.3%, 47.6%, and to 41.4% of patients with mild, moderate, and severe OSA, respectively.[33]

Other investigators have shown that although 55% of patients achieve successful self-titration at home, another 32% can reach success with further PSG-guided titration.[97] Similarly, another study found an improvement in OA efficacy with the use of home oximetry to help titrate MADs.[69] Of interest, they found that 25% of the patients required additional mandibular advancement due to an abnormal ODI despite of resolution of symptoms. In addition, 20% of patients required further titration due to persistent symptoms, despite a normal ODI.

Further OA titration during the follow-up PSG can improve OA success by up to 35%.[70] This relatively simple protocol implemented in the sleep laboratory is similar in concept to in-laboratory PAP titrations. As directed by the sleep technologist, patients are directed to advance the appliance in 1-mm increments to eliminate snoring and persistent obstructive events (apneas, hypopneas, or arterial oxygen desaturation). However, sleep continuity should be preserved as much as possible, and patients should not be woken more than three times per night to achieve an adequate total sleep time.

Other titration protocols use a temporary appliance that can be adjusted with or without the need to wake the patient during the study. These protocols have mixed results and only a fair sensitivity in predicting the amount of mandibular advancement needed for successful OA therapy.[98] Studies, briefly listed earlier, have evaluated an remotely controlled mandibular protrusion, a protrusion device used during sleep to predict OA treatment outcomes.[85,86] The use of such a method is promising; independent studies and reproduceable findings are required to further assess their predictive value.[98] Combining RCMP with drug-induced sleep endoscopy might further improve prediction of MAD efficacy.[99] However, the additional substantial costs associated with such in-laboratory tests are an issue.

Similar to PAP, appropriate OA titration is vital to achieve optimum therapeutic efficacy. Successful therapy requires both a dentist with experience in OA treatment to ensure proper adjustments of these devices, as well as a sleep-disorder physician who should conduct follow-up evaluations and sleep testing to confirm effective treatment is achieved. The dentist should follow patients on a yearly basis and may advance/titrate the appliance further if symptoms reoccur. If maximum mandibular advancement is reached and symptoms are still present, the patient should be referred to the referring physician for further evaluation and consideration of adjunctive or alternative therapies.

SIDE EFFECTS AND COMPLICATIONS

The primary reasons for discontinuing OA treatment are an insufficient reduction of snoring, persistence of apneic events, and the development of treatment-related side effects.[100] The most common reasons patients discontinue OA therapy were device discomfort/cumbersomeness (46%) and limited perceived efficacy (36%).[32] Forty percent of nonadherence occurred within the first 6 months of therapy.

Most side effects caused by OA are mild and transient. The most frequently reported are excessive salivation, dry mouth, mouth or tooth discomfort, muscle tenderness, and jaw stiffness. Device adjustment can decrease short-term side effects by reducing pressure on the anterior teeth and excessive mandibular advancement. More persistent and severe side effects, including TMJ dysfunction (joint noise and pain) and dental crown damage, are uncommon.[21] One study using MRI found OAs to be innocuous to the TMJ in OSA patients.[67] Although existing TMJ disorders are typically considered a contraindication to OAs, a study of patients with known or prior TMJ dysfunction found that these patients can become eligible for OA therapy after simple physiotherapy exercises.[101] These exercises may be decisive in the use of OAs for patients with TMJ pain by reducing previous symptoms, promoting better compliance, and improving QoL. Although the occurrence of pain-related TMJ disorders was higher in patients using OAs (24%) compared to PAP (6%) in a randomized parallel study, there were no limitations in mandibular function in either group during the entire observational period.[102] Transient and nonserious TMJ pain occurred more frequently with OAs than PAP, but the risk of developing impairment of the temporomandibular complex was infrequent with long-term MAD use. Therefore pain related to the initial use of OAs is typically transient and not associated with a significant risk of long-term complications or functional limitations.

The use of titratable OAs over several years was found to have a significant impact on occlusal and dental structures.[103,104] Changes observed in craniofacial structures were mainly related to significant tooth movements. Of importance, the dental changes occurring from OA use are not limited to decreases in overbite and overjet but, rather, include a number of parameters of the dentition. Similarly, a study observed that the frequent use of a single-piece OA with full occlusal coverage for 5 years resulted in median reductions in overjet and overbite of 0.6 mm in patients with either snoring or OSA.[105] One study demonstrated clinically significant reductions of 2.3 mm and 1.9 mm in overbite and overjet, respectively, after an average of more than 11 years of treatment.[106] Of importance, overbite changes were observed to decrease less with time, whereas overjet continuously changed at a constant rate of 0.2 mm per year of OA use. Of interest, evaluating various studies on different commercial appliance designs, such as Herbst, Mobloc, Klearway, Somnomed, and TAP, it has been shown that the amount of change was related to the duration of therapy and not the type of appliance.[102–105,107,108] The one exception is the use of an appliance design that does not cover the lingual surface of the lower anterior teeth. These appliances would tend to increase lower incisor crowding, and therefore a full coverage of lingual and buccal surface of all present teeth is recommended.

It should be noted that changes in dentition are not restricted to OA therapy. In fact, nasal PAP masks have also been associated with dental side effects. One trial evaluated the side effects of nasal masks on the craniofacial structures.[109] After a mean PAP use of 35 months, there was a significant retrusion of the anterior maxilla, a decrease in maxillary mandibular discrepancy, a setback of the supramental and chin positions, a retroclination of maxillary incisors, and a decrease of convexity. However, these changes are more prominent in OA users compared with PAP users.[102]

Although changes in dental occlusion do occur, these are generally not a significant cause of treatment discontinuation. After a mean follow-up period of 5.8 years, the authors found that most individuals developed new occlusal contacts resulting from the development of a new occlusal equilibrium over time.[110] The patient's perceptions do not typically correlate with objective measurements, and occlusal changes often go unnoticed.[105] In addition, several reports have consistently found that patients perceive dental side effects to be less important than the benefits of improved daytime sleepiness and other sleep apnea symptoms. Therefore, despite the presence of irreversible long-term occlusal changes, OA therapy should be considered as a lifelong treatment for patients with OSA. However, patients managed with OAs should be educated on proper exercises to restore normal occlusion and mitigate some of these potential effects.

LONG-TERM ASSESSMENTS

After treatment optimization of MAD and objective follow-up by the referring physician, the dentist may advance/titrate the appliance further if symptoms reoccur. If maximum mandibular advancement is reached and symptoms are still present, the patient should be referred to the referring physician for further evaluation. On a yearly basis, the dentist should assess the integrity of the OA; it may need to be replaced, depending on usage and hygiene. OAs generally last approximately 2 to 3 years.

There is limited literature on long-term efficacy on OA. One study found that patients experienced a deterioration of OSA severity despite the use of OA and no weight gain; OA treatment had become less effective.[111] Therefore regular follow-up schedules with renewed sleep apnea recordings should be considered for these patients, to avoid suboptimal or a total loss of effects on sleep apneas, and patients should be referred to their referring physician every 5 years for continuing assessment.

Another important aspect of long-term assessments is the evaluation of side effects thorough clinical examination. Most of the patients are unaware of bite changes or find the changes unimportant compared to the benefits of the treatment. Also, after major proclination of lower incisors, the amount of mandibular advancement might diminish, lowering the efficacy of the device. As previously described, dental changes are progressive, and there is a need to assess if the lower incisor proclination does not affect the buccal alveolar bone in the area. An experienced dentist who works with sleep disorders should be responsible to explain and possibly ask patients to discontinue OA treatment if indicated.

As occlusal changes have been mainly associated with time of OA use and not amount of mandibular advancement or device type,[106] in milder cases of the disease, such as primary snoring or mild OSA with limited symptoms/comorbidities, patients may be advised to decrease usage of the device and not to use the OA for 1 to 3 days per week. This approach has been used and sounds plausible, but there has been no data to prove if it actually decreases side effects.

ADHERENCE AND PATIENT PERCEPTIONS

OSAS is a chronic disease, and treatment with either PAP or OAs requires cooperation from the patient. The limitations of effective OSAS treatment related to poor acceptance of and adherence with PAP therapy are well established. Both adherence and patient preferences are uniformly better with OAs compared with PAP, as seen in Table 173.1. Treatment adherence with OAs appears to be dependent on the type of the appliance, disease severity, and patient supervision.[112,113] For example, adherence rates are greater with custom-made MADs than tongue-retaining– or "boil and bite"–type appliances.[25,114] Self-reported use of OAs on greater than 75% of nights has been reported for as high as 96%, and 80% of patients use their device for greater than 75% of their sleep period.[21] Studies measuring long-term OA adherence (2 to 5 years) report adherence rates of 48% up to 90%.[15,100,115,116]

Adherence with OAs is consistently greater than that seen with PAP.[3] Although the existing literature strongly suggests that adherence with OAs is superior to PAP, the true difference in absolute use and long-term adherence between these therapies is unknown.[4,7] True assessments of OA use are limited by subjective reports, and it is common for patients to overestimate both total sleep time and compliance with medical therapies. Regardless, studies comparing objective measures with both modalities are needed to confirm these reports.

Recently, devices that provide a means to objectively monitor OA use have been developed. A 3-month prospective clinical trial, assessed the safety and feasibility of an embedded microsensor capable of objective recordings of OA use.[117,118] Several microsensors are currently available that can be integrated into OAs. The microsensors provide reliability and accurate wear-time and can be incorporated into OAs fabricated from different materials.[119,120] These microsensors are currently being used, and the initial research studies are ongoing. Studies using objective adherence have shown that OAs are used on average 6.4 hours per night, and after 3 and 12 months, the highest compliance was correlated to a more pronounced decrease in snoring.

It is hypothesized that the suboptimal efficacy of OA therapy is counterbalanced by the superior adherence relative to that for PAP. To explain this hypothesis, the concept of long-term effectiveness has been described as the mean disease alleviation (MDA), which takes into account the decrease in AHI and objective adherence. The MDA, expressed as a percentage, is calculated as (adjusted objective adherence × therapeutic efficacy)/100.[121–123] Mean OSA alleviation of PAP has been previously described as being 52%, whereas the mean OSA alleviation of OA was 51%.[122] In addition, a sleep-adjusted residual AHI (SARAH index) has been proposed as a more accurate assessment of treatment effectiveness and possibly a better indicator of long-term health benefits. It takes into account baseline disease severity, the time-on and time-off treatment relative to the total sleeping time.[123] The sole use of treatment AHI, or residual AHI to demonstrate therapeutic effectiveness, has failed to correlate to long-term health outcomes as it does not consider (1) the hours per night that the treatment is physically used; (2) if the treatment is being used only in the first 3 to 4 hours of the night, and most rapid eye movement sleep will occur later without a treatment; and (3) the long-term adherence rate, which is known to progressively decline with all therapies.

It is imperative to include the option of OA therapy as a choice for patients with OSA. Treatment plans involving and valuing patient participation in chronic disease management leads to improved treatment adherence and a higher QoL and life expectancy.[124]

FUTURE DIRECTIONS

OA therapy has emerged as the main alternative to PAP in the treatment of OSA. There is now a strong evidence base demonstrating the benefits of this therapy for improving physiologic sleep measures, daytime sleepiness, and QoL in OSA patients across the spectrum of disease severity. The existing literature suggests that the superior treatment efficacy of PAP is mitigated by inferior compliance relative to OA therapy, resulting in similar health outcomes. Long-term comparative effectiveness studies, using patient-centered and clinically important outcome measures, are required to verify this. The advent of objective compliance monitors for OA therapy is critical to such studies.[122] Cost-effectiveness studies are also warranted to appropriately inform and direct clinical care. In addition, prospective validation studies are required to evaluate predictors of treatment outcome, and more research is needed to determine optimal titration protocols to increase the effectiveness of OA and to decrease the time taken to attain optimal treatment.

Future studies are needed to compare the effectiveness of different types of appliances and different design features (e.g., the amount of vertical opening). Likewise, these studies ideally would help differentiate which patients should receive custom or titratable devices and identify those who could be appropriately managed with less expensive, fixed devices. Ongoing refinements and standardization of appliance design may eventually lead to improved outcomes and will be enhanced by a better understanding of the mechanisms of action of OA.

Snoring and sleep-disordered breathing are chronic and progressive conditions, raising the possibility that early intervention of snoring may retard the development of OSA. OA therapy would appear to have a major role in such a preventative approach, and further work is warranted to evaluate this possibility.

Finally, OSAS is increasingly recognized as a heterogeneous disorder with multiple pathophysiologic causes. However, new concepts in OSA pathogenesis and phenotypes have recently emerged and could help the field move toward a future "personalized medicine" approach, in which treatment is tailored to the patient.

CLINICAL PEARLS

OAs provide effective therapy for patients with OSAS and can be used as primary therapy for those with mild to moderate disease, or as an alternative treatment for individuals who fail or are intolerant to PAP. The nomenclature for this form of therapy is not standardized, and several different devices and designs are available, each with inherent advantages and limitations. This makes interpreting the published literature and understanding the role of OAs in clinical practice somewhat difficult. However, the data strongly suggest that custom and titratable OA devices offer the most advantageous therapy. Proper patient and device selection, in conjunction with appropriate means to determine the required degree of mandibular advancement, can optimize the therapeutic response and increase the likelihood of successful therapy.

SUMMARY

OAs increase the anterior-posterior diameter of the airway by advancing the mandible, tongue, and soft palate to a more anterior position, and they prevent posterior subluxation during sleep. However, there appears to be a more robust and complex mechanism of improved airway patency and stability of upper airway muscle activity provided by these devices.

OAs provide reliable and effective treatment for most individuals with OSAS, especially those with mild and moderate disease. Although they are approved as an alternative therapy for patients who fail or are intolerant of PAP, there is a growing body of literature that suggests OAs are effective across a wide range of OSA severity and should be considered as an additional first-line treatment option. Using titratable devices, a residual AHI is expected in greater than 50% of individuals. The likelihood of achieving successful ablation of obstructive events is enhanced by the use of titratable devices that are incrementally advanced to optimize both sleep continuity, ablation of obstructive events, and resolution of symptoms.

OAs are not as effective as PAP in reducing the AHI. However, they perform equally well when comparing other measured variables. In addition, the benefits of PAP with regard to clinical efficacy are offset by low adherence rates. OAs are more likely to be preferred by patients, and measures of adherence, although limited by subjective reports, are frequently superior to those seen with PAP. Given this, the overall effectiveness, as it relates to both disease alleviation and health outcomes, may be as good, if not better, compared with PAP.

These devices are generally well tolerated. Short-term side effects, such as excessive salivation, jaw and tooth discomfort, and occasionally TMJ discomfort/pain, are usually minor and not a reason for treatment discontinuation. Significant long-term side effects are rare, with malocclusion being the most common adverse consequences of OA therapy.

Treatment with OAs provide a unique opportunity for sleep dentists and physicians to collaborate in identifying appropriate patients, selecting the most beneficial devices, and individualizing care to optimize outcomes.

SELECTED READINGS

Barnes M, McEvoy RD, Banks S, et al. Efficacy of positive airway pressure and oral appliance in mild to moderate obstructive sleep apnea. *Am J Respir Crit Care Med.* 2004;170(6):656–664.

Bratton DJ, Gaisl T, Schlatzer C, Kohler M. Comparison of the effects of continuous positive airway pressure and mandibular advancement devices on sleepiness in patients with obstructive sleep apnoea: a network meta-analysis. *Lancet Respir Med.* 2015;3(11):869-878

Chan ASL, Cistulli PA. Oral Appliance treatment of obstructive sleep apnea: an update. *Curr Opin Pulmon Med.* 2009;15(6):591–596.

De Meyer MMD, Vanderveken OM, De Weerdt S, et al. Use of mandibular advancement devices for the treatment of primary snoring with or without obstructive sleep apnea (OSA): A systematic review. *Sleep Med Rev.* 2021;56:101407. https://doi.org/10.1016/j.smrv.2020.101407.

Ferguson KA, Cartwright R, Rogers R, Schmidt-Nowara W. Oral appliances for the treatment of snoring and obstructive sleep apnea: A review. *Sleep.* 2006;29:244–262.

Krishnan V, Collop NA, Scherr SC. An evaluation of a titration strategy for prescription of oral appliances for obstructive sleep apnea. *Chest.* 2008;133(5):1135–1141.

Marklund M, Stenlund H, Franklin KA. Mandibular advancement devices in 630 men and women with obstructive sleep apnea and snoring: tolerability and predictors of treatment success. *Chest.* 2004;125(4):1270–1278.

Ng JH, Yow M. Oral Appliances in the management of obstructive sleep apnea. *Sleep Med Clin.* 2020;15(2):241–250.

Phillips CL, Grunstein RR, Darendeliler MA, et al. Health outcomes of continuous positive airway pressure versus oral appliance treatment for obstructive sleep apnea: a randomized controlled trial. *Am J Respir Crit Care Med.* 2013;187(8):879–887.

Ramar K, Dort LC, Katz SG, et al. Clinical practice guideline for the treatment of obstructive sleep apnea and snoring with oral appliance therapy: an update for 2015. *J Clin Sleep Med.* 11(7):773–827.

Rangarajan H, Padmanabhan S, Ranganathan S, Kailasam V. Impact of oral appliance therapy on quality of life (QoL) in patients with obstructive sleep apnea - a systematic review and meta-analysis [published online ahead of print, 2021 Sep 13]. *Sleep Breath.* 2021. https://doi.org/10.1007/s11325-021-02483-0. 10.1007/s11325-021-02483-0.

Vena D, Azarbarzin A, Marques M, et al. Predicting sleep apnea responses to oral appliance therapy using polysomnographic airflow. *Sleep.* 2020:zsaa004.

A complete reference list can be found online at ExpertConsult.com.

Chapter 174

Anesthesia in Upper Airway Surgery

David Hillman; Peter R. Eastwood; Olivier M. Vanderveken

Chapter Highlights

- This chapter presents an overview of anesthetic considerations relating to upper airway surgery for patients with obstructive sleep apnea.
- Insightful anesthetic management of such cases requires an appreciation of the similarities and differences between the sleep and anesthetic states in relationship to their effects on upper airway and breathing function and on the arousal responses that help protect against disturbance of these essential physiologic functions.
- These issues are discussed in regard to both sedation for preoperative evaluation for obstructive sleep apnea surgery and perioperative management where surgery is undertaken.

OVERVIEW OF ANESTHESIA IN PATIENTS WITH OBSTRUCTIVE SLEEP APNEA

Although this chapter is concerned primarily with anesthesia for upper airway surgery to address problems related to obstructive sleep apnea (OSA), many of the considerations apply to anesthesia for patients with OSA undergoing surgery of any kind.

Sleep and anesthesia are associated with muscle relaxation, and patients with obstruction-prone airways are vulnerable to obstruction in either state. A critical difference between the states is that the arousal responses that protect against prolonged obstructive events during sleep are suppressed by sedative and anesthetic drugs, increasing vulnerability to asphyxia when under their influence.[1] Furthermore, the anatomic compromise of the upper airway in patients with OSA can cause difficulties with tracheal intubation or maintenance of airway patency during face mask ventilation under anesthesia.[2] These problems contribute to the well-documented increased risks of cardiopulmonary complications, unexplained intensive care unit admissions, and prolonged lengths of stay after surgery observed in patients with OSA.[3,4] Perioperative management principles to address these issues have been published by the American Society of Anesthesiologists[5] and other bodies[6-8] and include systematic preoperative identification of patients at risk of OSA, for example, by use of screening tools such as the STOP-BANG questionnaire (which was first developed for this purpose); choice of anesthetic technique to favor local or regional techniques where suitable, or ensure rapid return of consciousness after general anesthesia where circumstances permit; preparation for difficulties with tracheal intubation or airway management where sedation or general anesthesia is to be used; careful postoperative supervision, particularly when under the influence of sedatives or opioids, the use of which should be minimized where feasible; use of postoperative aids such as artificial airways or positive airway pressure therapy where airway compromise exists; and particular care after upper airway surgery.

Principles of Anesthesia in Upper Airway Surgery for Obstructive Sleep Apnea

Upper airway surgery is an undertaking that requires particularly close cooperation between surgeon and anesthesiologist. Patients presenting for these procedures do so because of compromised upper airway structure or function. In some circumstances upper airway obstruction is the presenting complaint, as may occur with tumors in the upper airway. In others the potential for obstruction may be great, as is the case for patients with OSA. Managing such airways is challenging in the perioperative period. In anesthesiology terms they are known as "difficult." A *difficult airway* has been defined by the American Society of Anesthesiologists as one that causes a conventionally trained anesthesiologist difficulty with face mask ventilation delivered to the upper airway, difficulty with tracheal intubation, or both.[9] Patients with OSA are vulnerable in both these respects. In addition, they are, of course, at increased risk of upper airway obstruction whenever asleep or sedated. Whereas the sleeping patient is naturally protected from prolonged asphyxia by a capacity to arouse and reactivate effective breathing function, mild sedation compromises arousal mechanisms and deep sedation or anesthesia abolish these responses.[10] Patients with OSA are therefore particularly vulnerable throughout the perioperative period because of their upper airway compromise, compounded by the effects of anesthetic, opioid, and other sedative drugs and the risk of postoperative hemorrhage or edema associated with aspects of upper airway surgery.

In keeping with this book's focus on sleep disorders, the focus of this chapter is on anesthetic considerations relating to upper airway surgery for OSA (see Chapter 175 for surgeries of upper airway). Surgery is frequently undertaken to treat OSA in children, of which tonsillar and adenoidal hypertrophy is a common cause.[11] Upper airway surgery is also regularly undertaken in adults for treatment of OSA, with several specific indications: removal of certain obstructing lesions in the upper airway; correction of abnormalities of the facial skeleton; unacceptability of nonsurgical treatments such as continuous positive airway pressure (CPAP) therapy and oral appliance therapy; and the need to relieve nasal obstruction to allow use of nasal masks for more comfortable, less intrusive delivery of CPAP than offered by face masks.[12] A variety of procedures are available, including nasal, palatal, and tongue base surgery; adenotonsillectomy (where hypertrophy exists); and a variety of orthognathic procedures.[13,14] The choice between them requires careful preoperative evaluation, often involving upper airway endoscopy, radiography (including cephalometry, conventional computed tomography [CT], and three-dimensional cone beam CT scans) and magnetic resonance imaging.[15]

Increasingly, preoperative evaluation for upper airway surgery has also involved use of sedation to simulate sleep-like conditions during endoscopy in a procedure known as drug-induced sleep endoscopy (DISE), occasionally termed drug-induced sedation endoscopy.[16,17] This is a test to evaluate suitability for and type of OSA-related surgery needed, as described further on in this chapter (see also Chapter 175 for surgeries of upper airway and Chapter 139 for bariatric surgery).

Hence sedation and anesthesia have roles in providing the conditions both for preoperative evaluation for upper airway surgery for OSA and for the surgical procedure itself. Insightful anesthetic management requires an appreciation of the similarities and differences between the sleep and anesthetic states in relationship to their effect on upper airway and breathing function and on arousal responses that act to protect against disturbance in these functions. This is required to facilitate production of sleep-like conditions during DISE and in clinical management during and after surgery, where several important factors must be taken into account: the shared influences of sedation, anesthesia, and sleep on upper airway behavior; how surgery can affect this behavior; the potential influences of OSA comorbid conditions including obesity and heart disease; the early postoperative challenges associated with emergence from anesthesia, pain, and its management; and the possibility of airway compromise from edema or hemorrhage.

Children present particular difficulties because of their small airway size and lung volumes relative to body size, predisposing them to upper airway obstruction and to rapid desaturation under such circumstances. Congenital problems associated with airway compromise, such as Down syndrome, also regularly manifest in childhood, further highlighting the challenges that confront pediatric anesthesiologists.[11] DISE has an increasing role in preoperative evaluation of pediatric patients with OSA, adding to these challenges.[18,19]

Preoperative Evaluation of Patients Presenting for Obstructive Sleep Apnea Surgery

Preoperative evaluation of patients presenting for general anesthesia of any kind should include consideration of the possibility of OSA given its wide prevalence and the associated perioperative risks.[3] Patients presenting for OSA surgery, however, usually have already had their OSA well characterized by a diagnostic home or laboratory-based sleep study. Often a trial of CPAP to treat the problem may have been undertaken, or be under way, or CPAP therapy may be a more-or-less established management component. Emergent or subsequent problems with compliance arising from difficulty in accepting or tolerating CPAP, usually because of its intrusive nature, are well documented as a common reason why adult patients with OSA require upper airway surgery.[20] Other patients may elect nasal surgery to allow easier application of CPAP via a nasal mask, rather than a more cumbersome oronasal face mask, as is required where there is nasal obstruction.

Often upper airway surgery for OSA is preceded by a surgeon-initiated investigation to determine the primary site of obstruction (velo-, oro-, or hypopharyngeal) and the nature of the obstructive process (lateral, anteroposterior, or concentric narrowing). It has been shown that the probability of multilevel upper airway collapse increases with increasing OSA severity and a greater degree of overweight and obesity.[21] This assessment allows the surgeon to determine the best procedure to counteract the problems identified by it, a so-called DISE-directed approach.

Apart from radiographic imaging (such as cephalometry and computed tomography [CT] scans), such evaluations usually involve endoscopic visualization of the upper airway under conditions conducive to obstruction. Early methods involved the performance of Müller maneuvers (inspiratory effort against an obstruction—the opposite of the Valsalva maneuver) during awake endoscopy or with the patient under mild sedation.[22] However, this is far removed from sleep-like conditions, in which the upper airway muscles are relaxed and obstruction occurs without exaggeratedly negative intraluminal pressures, so it has limited validity as an assessment of site and nature of upper airway collapse during sleep.[23]

Drug-Induced Sleep Endoscopy

To better simulate the conditions of sleep, DISE has evolved as a test to help determine suitability for surgery and the type of surgical procedure to be undertaken.[24,25] Its purpose is to help determine the level, degree, and pattern of upper airway collapse that underpins the patient's OSA. This procedure directly involves anesthesiologists because drugs are administered (usually intravenous propofol with or without midazolam or, increasingly, dexmedetomidine) to produce sedation and sleep-like muscle relaxation, which induces snoring and upper airway obstruction (partial or complete) in predisposed patients. The sedation technique used is integral to the validity of the assessment given the necessity to produce sleep-like patterns of upper airway behavior.[17]

Of note, with mild (wakeful) sedation, the upper airway muscles remain active, and sleep-like conditions cannot be assumed.[26] It is only if sleep itself supervenes or if sedation is deepened to a level where consciousness is lost through a direct drug effect that behavior of the relaxed upper airway is observed. Indeed, a step-like reduction in phasic genioglossus muscle activity, a major upper airway dilating force, is seen at the transition to unconsciousness at sleep onset and with anesthetic induction.[26,27] Hence establishing a predictable, consistent level of sedation is important. This is facilitated through use of intravenous agents delivered via infusion pumps at rates controlled according to depth of anesthesia. Depth of anesthesia is monitored using devices that continuously analyze frequency content of electroencephalographic signals, such as the bispectral index (BIS) monitor. This provides a numeric display ranging from a maximum awake score of 100 to a minimum (isoelectric) score of 0, which indicates the progression of electroencephalographic slowing with increasing levels of sedation. A BIS score below 60 is generally accepted as indicating a depth of sedation where unconsciousness is consistently present, with associated muscle relaxation; it has been suggested by some as the appropriate threshold for sedation for DISE.[28]

Although BIS monitoring has been best characterized for propofol, it appears to provide a valid measure of depth of sedation for other drugs commonly used for sedation for DISE, such as dexmedetomidine and midazolam. It should be noted that the rates of infusion required to produce specific depths of sedation can vary widely between individuals, which further underlines the desirability of depth monitoring for these procedures.[26] Choice of sedative agent is also a consideration. Although dexmedetomidine may offer greater hemodynamic stability, propofol has a more favorable pharmacokinetic profile, with quicker induction and emergence, and appears to demonstrate greater degrees of pharyngeal obstruction, which may more closely reflect conditions during rapid eye movement (REM) sleep, where muscle relaxation is profound.[29] These differences may reflect differences in the relationships between sedation levels and drug infusion rates, with a plateauing of sedative effect at higher dexmedetomidine infusion rates, while it progressively deepens with propofol.[30]

Observations made under the relaxed conditions of DISE will help determine suitability for non-CPAP treatment such as upper airway and skeletal surgery,[16,17] and for oral appliance therapy,[31] as well as guiding the choice of surgical procedure to be undertaken. Resolution of pharyngeal collapse at all levels of the upper airway is necessary to achieve successful treatment in the individual patient. Indeed, it has been demonstrated that multilevel collapse is present in a majority of patients with OSA and that the prevalence of complete collapse and multilevel collapse increases with increasing OSA severity and overweight and obesity.[21,32]

The use of DISE is based on the concept that upper airway behavior during drug-induced unconsciousness is similar to that in natural sleep with similar reductions in muscle activation, respiratory drive, and reflex gains at transition to the unconsciousness of each state.[26,27] However, a critical difference that is highly relevant to the considerations that follow (and to recovery after the DISE procedure) is that with natural sleep the capacity for spontaneous arousal is preserved, whereas with drug-induced sleep and sedation a dose-dependent depression of arousal responses prevails. This depression persists until physiologic drug elimination allows return of consciousness, so the deeply sedated or anesthetized patient is highly vulnerable to asphyxia if upper airway obstruction occurs and is not detected by and dealt with by attending medical or nursing staff.

Anesthesia for Surgery to Treat Obstructive Sleep Apnea

Patients with OSA present the anesthesiologist with many challenges. The problems they experience during sleep signify the presence of a narrow airway predisposed to obstruction when the upper airway (and other) muscles relax with onset of anesthesia. Obesity and presence of other comorbidities (such as hypertension—systemic and pulmonary, cardiovascular disease, cerebrovascular disease, metabolic syndrome, atrial fibrillation, or heart failure) may be contributing factors. If sufficiently severe, obesity may also predispose to atelectasis under anesthesia and to hypoventilation if spontaneous ventilation is preserved.[33,34]

A reduction in functional residual capacity (FRC) is another accompaniment of the muscle relaxation (in this case of chest wall muscles) that occurs with onset of anesthesia (and of sleep). The reduction can be profound in the morbidly obese with FRC decreasing to near residual volume.[34] This decrease in FRC is associated with atelectasis in the dependent parts of the lung with consequent shunt and hypoxemia. The loss of lung volume also is a significant contributor, along with upper airway muscle relaxation, to the increased airway collapsibility observed during anesthesia because of associated loss of longitudinal traction on the upper airway.[35] Conveniently, CPAP counteracts both problems, providing a pneumatic splint to the upper airway and increasing FRC, helping prevent or recruit atelectatic lung and offsetting the negative influence of volume loss on upper airway patency.

When hypoventilation is a prominent feature, bilevel ventilatory assistance is a preferred form of positive airway pressure therapy for obese patients, because it combines a background level of pressure to provide the benefits of CPAP with inspiratory pressure support to counteract the inadequate inspiratory flow.[36]

OSA is not restricted to the obese, however, and other pathogenetic factors are involved that are relevant to anesthesia. These include facial skeletal characteristics such as retrognathia and maxillary hypoplasia.[37] Such anatomic configurations, perhaps more than obesity itself, can present substantial challenges to the anesthesiologist. Potential problems include difficulty in performing endotracheal intubation and/or in maintaining airway patency during mask ventilation. Patients presenting such problems are said to have a "difficult airway." The presence of a difficult airway under anesthesia is an indicator of vulnerability to OSA.[38] Conversely, OSA is a risk factor for difficult intubation and/or difficulty with airway maintenance during the anesthetic procedure.[2] Hence the anesthesiologist should approach patients with OSA prepared for a difficult intubation. It is likely that, in the assessment of such patients, other factors indicating this possibility will be present, such as oropharyngeal crowding with high Mallampati scores, retrognathia with reduced thyromental distances and/or increased mandibular angulation, and increased neck circumference.[38] Increased neck circumference is a risk factor for OSA that is independent of obesity, although it reflects central fat deposition. Patients with large muscular necks are also at increased risk for OSA and may present additional airway management difficulties under anesthesia.[39] Apart from clinical evaluation, the anesthesiologist also should take advantage of the various radiographic and endoscopic preoperative investigations undertaken by the surgical team to assess upper airway structure and function in preparation for surgery (as outlined previously), to develop greater insights into the challenges ahead (Table 174.1).

Tracheal Intubation

Although some upper airway surgery procedures relevant to OSA can be done using local anesthesia (such as minor nasal surgery undertaken to improve the prospects of successful nasal CPAP delivery in patients with OSA and nasal obstruction or minimally invasive palatal surgery with modalities such as interstitial radiofrequency therapy), most cases require general anesthesia. In such cases, the patient is almost always tracheally intubated. The presence of an endotracheal tube allows the anesthesiologist to step back from immediate proximity

Table 174.1 Obstructive Sleep Apnea (OSA) and Perioperative Risk

Risk Factor	Potential Perioperative Consequences	Identification of Risk	Reducing Risk
OSA	• Upper airway obstruction with asphyxiation if unrecognized and untreated	• Clinical evaluation • Screening tools (e.g., STOP-BANG) • Sleep study when indicated	• Early identification • Preparation for potential difficulties with airway management (including intubation) • Techniques to minimize postoperative sedation, including caution with opioids • Perioperative use of CPAP therapy • Intensive monitoring until sentient and arousal responses are unimpaired • Referral for definitive diagnosis and treatment when OSA is first suspected perioperatively
OSA predisposing factors • Obesity • Familial • Craniofacial • Mandibular retrusion • Maxillary hypoplasia • Obstructing lesions in upper airway (e.g., tonsillar hypertrophy) • Other indicators of difficult intubation (e.g., elevated Mallampati score)	• OSA-related problems (see previous) • Difficult tracheal intubation • Difficult airway management • Delayed extubation/reintubation • Atelectasis, hypoventilation in morbidly obese	• Clinical evaluation • Endoscopy • Cephalometry • Upper airway imaging (CT, MRI)	• Awareness of predisposition and associated risks • Monitoring for these risks • Preparation for potential risks, including availability of appropriate equipment to manage them • Techniques to minimize postoperative sedation, including caution with opioids
OSA comorbidities • Hypertension • Cardiovascular/cerebrovascular disease • Metabolic syndrome • Depression	• Worsening of comorbid condition • Delayed recovery	• Clinical evaluation • Biochemical testing when indicated	• Optimize control preoperatively • Careful perioperative management

For further details see text.

to the head to allow surgical access while ensuring airway patency and, in addition, ensuring protection of the lower airway from aspiration of blood and other material during the procedure. The principal challenges in dealing with patients with obstruction-prone upper airways lie in placing the tracheal tube (intubation) at the start of the procedure and in ensuring airway patency after removal of the tube (extubation) on completion of anesthesia.

Airway Patency after Extubation

Several measures are required to ensure upper airway patency after extubation. First, apart from adequate reversal of any neuromuscular blockade if such drugs have been used, it is prudent to ensure the patient has regained consciousness before extubation. Early return of consciousness requires a choice of appropriate anesthetic drugs and titration of doses to facilitate this outcome. Second, extubation in the lateral posture should be considered where practicable, with the patient maintained in this position during sleep for the postoperative period in hospital. Third, CPAP or other positive airway pressure therapies should be readily available and used during sleep or sedation in patients with threatened or actual upper airway obstructive episodes. This is not a problem with CPAP-compliant patients, who expect the continuation of such therapy. It is more problematic in noncompliant patients, which is a good reason for preoperative induction of CPAP therapy where possible. Although the nose is the favored route of administration of CPAP for the majority of users, an oronasal face mask may be required perioperatively, particularly in the presence of edema or other conditions causing nasal obstruction. In the case of nasal surgery nasal packs should be avoided when possible. Furthermore, an important caveat is that CPAP therapy may be needed in the early postoperative period, even though the aim of surgery is to restore airway patency. This is because edema, secretions, blood, and clots can temporarily worsen airway patency despite surgical correction of the obstructing lesion. Although CPAP is a mainstay, use of other devices to improve airway patency, such as mandibular advancement or nasopharyngeal airway devices, may have a perioperative role beyond the postanesthesia care unit. Available literature to guide the perioperative use of these other devices remains limited at present, however.

Early Postoperative Care

Finally, the patient must be closely monitored while he or she remains at increased risk. Clinical care thus requires a higher nurse-to-patient ratio than in the general ward and continuous monitoring of oxygenation (oximetry) and ventilation (capnography, oronasal airflow). Such facilities are available in the postanesthetic care unit and other high-dependency areas. Oxygen therapy should be used with caution because it can conceal obstructive events, potentially leading to their prolongation. It is for this reason that monitoring oronasal airflow, either directly or with capnography, adds value to oximetry monitoring.[40] Attending staff members must be expert in the use of CPAP and noninvasive ventilation. Patients at increased risk of upper airway obstruction, such as those with OSA, often require prolonged stays in high-dependency areas postoperatively. Discharge of the patient from such an environment demands return of consciousness and subsequent unimpeded arousal responses to threatened airway compromise. To ensure this outcome, it is highly desirable to avoid opioids and other drugs with sedative potential whenever possible. Alternative analgesic techniques include use of nonsteroidal antiinflammatory drugs and acetaminophen, and analgesic-sparing strategies such as use of corticosteroids. There is also a place for use of topical anesthesia and nerve blocks in the perioperative setting.[5]

Postoperative edema and secretions can temporarily compromise airways in which procedures have been undertaken to ultimately improve patency. Hemorrhage is also a risk, particularly in the early postoperative period.

Postoperative Sleep

Because of the previously mentioned considerations, the perioperative period is one of vulnerability. Added to these potential airway and ventilatory impairments is the disruption to sleep that occurs during the first few days postoperatively. Sleep efficiency is reduced and sleep architecture distorted, with loss of REM sleep a feature.[41] Such sleep impairment increases the risk of postoperative delirium. Furthermore, as this early sleep disruption settles, REM sleep is restored, which is of relevance because it is the stage of sleep during which muscle activation and respiratory drive are most depressed and, consequently, risk of upper airway obstruction and hypoventilation is greatest.[42] Hence vulnerability to these events is not necessarily greatest on the first night or two postoperatively.

Discharge Requirements

The ideal circumstances for discharge of these patients from high-dependency care and from the hospital are achieved with the following clinical objectives: return of consciousness with no plan for subsequent use of opioids or sedatives that may impair arousal responses; resolution of edema and the particular risk of hemorrhage; and, where indicated, ability to self-administer CPAP, with willingness to use it when asleep. In some settings, these conditions may be met in the early postoperative period, depending on the nature of the procedure and the anesthetic technique used. If so, and if and comorbid conditions are well controlled, same-day discharge from hospital after surgery is possible.

These recommendations are consistent with current published guidelines for perioperative care of patients with OSA.[5,6] However, these guidelines are largely based on expert opinion and further study, and analysis of methods to improve perioperative outcomes is required to provide an objective evidence base and facilitate their ongoing development.[7,8]

CONCLUSIONS

Anesthesia for upper airway surgery to treat OSA is challenging. The surgery is often undertaken in patients who have been unable or unwilling to tolerate CPAP therapy or in those who have surgically correctable upper airway or craniofacial abnormalities. Sometimes it is undertaken to improve CPAP compliance by relieving nasal obstruction. Anesthetic management requires careful preparation, allowing for the possibility of difficult intubation, and careful management of extubation and emergence to ensure maintenance of airway patency, particularly in the period that precedes full return of consciousness and ability to promptly arouse from subsequent sleep in response to hypopneic or apneic events.

CLINICAL PEARLS

- The similar effects of anesthesia and sleep in reducing muscle activation and ventilatory drive mean that vulnerability to upper airway obstruction in one state indicates high risk of problems in the other.
- The anatomic features (e.g., retrognathia) that predispose to upper airway obstruction also increase difficulties with tracheal intubation and mask ventilation performed with the patient under anesthesia.
- A key difference between the states of sleep and anesthesia is suppression of the arousal responses that protect an individual during sleep by anesthetic agents, with increased risk of asphyxia in those with obstruction-prone airways, such as patients with OSA. Postoperative use of opioid and sedative drugs may extend these risks beyond the immediate postoperative period, and caution with use of these agents is mandatory.
- Postoperative edema further compounds potential early postoperative problems for patients who have undergone surgery for OSA.
- Close peri- and postoperative monitoring and management must take these matters into account.

SUMMARY

Anesthesia for upper airway surgery to treat OSA is challenging. Often such surgery is undertaken in patients who have been unable or unwilling to tolerate CPAP therapy. Sometimes it is undertaken to improve CPAP compliance by relieving nasal obstruction. Preoperative surgical evaluation often entails DISE to assess suitability for and type of surgery. This procedure requires an appreciation of the relationships between drug-induced sleep and sedation and natural sleep in terms of muscle relaxation, ventilatory depression, and reflex suppression to ensure that airway behavior is observed under sleep-like conditions. Anesthetic management for the upper airway surgery requires careful preparation, allowing for the possibility of difficult intubation, and careful management of extubation and monitoring of emergence and recovery to ensure maintenance of airway patency, particularly in the period that precedes full return of consciousness and the capability for prompt arousal from subsequent sleep in response to hypopneic or apneic events.

SELECTED READINGS

Albrecht E, Bayon V, Hirotsu C, Heinzer R. Impact of short-acting vs. standard anaesthetic agents on obstructive sleep apnoea: a randomised, controlled, triple-blind trial. *Anaesthesia*. 2021;76(1):45–53.

Brown KA. Outcome, risk, and error and the child with obstructive sleep apnea. *Paediatr Anaesth*. 2011;21:771–780.

Chung F, Liao P, Yegneswaran B, et al. Postoperative changes in sleep-disordered breathing and sleep architecture in patients with obstructive sleep apnea. *Anesthesiology*. 2014;120:287–298.

Chung F, Subramanyam R, Liao P, et al. High STOP-Bang score indicates a high probability of obstructive sleep apnoea. *Br J Anaesth*. 2012;108:768–775.

De Vito A, Carrasco Llatas M, Ravesloot MJ, et al. European position paper on drug-induced sleep endoscopy: 2017 Update. *Clin Otolaryngol*. 2018;43:1541–1552.

Hillman DR, Walsh JH, Maddison KJ, et al. Evolution of changes in upper airway collapsibility during slow induction of anesthesia with propofol. *Anesthesiology*. 2009;111:63–71.

Lechner M, Wilkins D, Kotecha B. A review on drug-induced sedation endoscopy - Technique, grading systems and controversies. *Sleep Med Rev*. 2018;41:141–148.

Leong SM, Tiwari A, Chung F, Wong DT. Obstructive sleep apnea as a risk factor associated with difficult airway management - A narrative review. *J Clin Anesth*. 2018;45:63–68.

Pelosi P, Croci M, Ravagnan I, et al. The effects of body mass on lung volumes, respiratory mechanics, and gas exchange during general anesthesia. *Anesth Analg*. 1998;87:654–660.

Practice guidelines for the perioperative management of patients with obstructive sleep apnea: an updated report by the American Society of Anesthesiologists Task Force on Perioperative Management of Patients with Obstructive Sleep Apnea. *Anesthesiology*. 2014;120(2):268–286.

Stewart M, Estephan L, Thaler A, et al. Reduced Recovery Times with Total Intravenous Anesthesia in Patients with Obstructive Sleep Apnea. *Laryngoscope*. 2021;131(4):925–931. https://doi.org/10.1002/lary.29216.

Vroegop AV, Vanderveken OM, Boudewyns AN, et al. Drug-induced sleep endoscopy in sleep-disordered breathing: report on 1,249 cases. *Laryngoscope*. 2014;124:797–802.

A complete reference list can be found online at ExpertConsult.com.

Chapter 175

Upper Airway Surgery to Treat Obstructive Sleep-Disordered Breathing

Olivier M. Vanderveken; Aarnoud Hoekema; Scott B. Boyd

Chapter Highlights

- Management with continuous positive airway pressure (CPAP) remains the standard treatment for moderate to severe obstructive sleep apnea (OSA). The effectiveness of CPAP is often limited by low patient acceptance, poor tolerance, and a suboptimal compliance. As a result, CPAP could result in less favorable effectiveness than required.
- Oral appliance therapy with custom-made mandibular advancement devices is a first-line, nonsurgical alternative for treatment of sleep-disordered breathing.
- In selected patients, alternative surgical treatment options for OSA are available: upper airway modifications, including upper airway surgery, neurostimulation therapy of the hypoglossal nerve, skeletal modifications, and tracheostomy.
- Objective sleep testing is always required before and after surgical treatment.

INTRODUCTION

Obstructive sleep-disordered breathing (OSDB) is a disorder with a high prevalence, and that is of increasing importance because of its neurocognitive and cardiovascular sequelae, leading to subsequent morbidity and mortality.[1] The main pathophysiologic feature of OSDB is upper airway narrowing (hypopnea) or collapse (apnea) occurring during sleep, resulting in intermittent hypoxemia and sleep fragmentation.[2] OSDB in adults spans a wide pathophysiologic continuum reflecting the various degrees of upper airway narrowing or collapse, ranging from intermittent snoring over the different levels of severity of the obstructive sleep apnea (OSA) up to the obesity hypoventilation syndrome, also referred to as the so-called pickwickian syndrome.[3,4] Abnormalities in the anatomy of the upper airway, the physiology of the upper airway muscle dilator, and the stability of ventilatory control are important causes of this repetitive upper airway narrowing and collapse occurring during sleep in these patients.[5] The recurrent upper airway obstructions cause repetitive episodes of hypoxia and hypercapnia and oscillations in heart rate and blood pressure. The recurrent arousals from sleep result in daytime sleepiness and increased risk of motor vehicle and occupational accidents.[6] Untreated or undiagnosed OSDB is an independent risk factor for hypertension, with consequent cerebrovascular and cardiovascular morbidity and high mortality.[7] As a result, OSDB has major socioeconomic consequences and should be approached as a chronic disease requiring long-term multidisciplinary management.[8,9]

THE NEED FOR NON–CONTINUOUS POSITIVE AIRWAY PRESSURE TREATMENT OPTIONS

General and conservative measures are essential steps in the management of patients with OSDB. These are reviewed in Chapters 132 and 140 (relevant to positive airway pressure devices), 133 (relevant to pharmacology), 134 (relevant to alternative strategies), and 139 (relevant to bariatric surgeries, a topic not covered in this chapter). Treatment with continuous positive airway pressure (CPAP), first described in 1981 by Sullivan and colleagues,[10] remains the treatment of choice for moderate to severe OSA. Adequate CPAP treatment improves hypertension, reduces the risk of nonfatal and fatal cardiovascular events, and has demonstrated that successful CPAP treatment prolongs survival.[11,12] Because of the high efficacy of CPAP, the therapeutic effectiveness of CPAP is potentially high. However, the clinical effectiveness of CPAP will often be hampered and limited by low patient acceptance, poor tolerance, and a suboptimal CPAP compliance, leading to significant residual disease burden during the time CPAP is not being used.[13,14] Therefore many OSA patients might remain inadequately treated due to inconsistent levels of CPAP compliance and usage.[13,15] As a result, CPAP could result in less favorable effectiveness than required.[13,14,16] When CPAP use is considered inadequate based on both symptom evaluation and objective monitoring data despite intensive efforts to improve CPAP use, alternative non-CPAP alternatives for the treatment of OSDB need to be considered (Table 175.1).[8,17,18]

Table 175.1 Non-CPAP Treatment Options for Patients with Obstructive Sleep-Disordered Breathing

Non-CPAP Treatment Options	
General measures	Avoidance of sedative drugs with myorelaxant effects Avoidance of alcohol consumption Sleep hygiene Weight loss in case of overweight or obesity Avoidance of supine position during sleep in case of positional sleep apnea
Specific therapeutic options	Oral appliance therapy Surgery • Upper airway bypass procedure: tracheotomy • Surgical upper airway modifications • Tongue suspension techniques • Upper airway neurostimulation therapy • Skeletal modifications • Bariatric surgery

CPAP, Continuous positive airway pressure.

Oral appliance therapy has gained growing interest and is increasingly prescribed as a noninvasive first-line alternative to CPAP[19] (see also Chapter 173). At present, custom-made, titratable mandibular advancement devices are recommended, preferably with objective measurement of compliance.[16]

One of the possible advantages of surgical management is that treatment efficacy is not as dependent on adherence as with device therapies, such as CPAP or oral appliance therapy.[19–21] It should however be noted that studies evaluating surgical interventions in OSA generally do not incorporate rigorous methods. Further, bias is introduced with the use of divergent criteria for surgical success. Therefore clinical practice surgical interventions for OSA are usually reserved for patients who are "nonresponsive" or "nonadherent" to noninvasive therapies, such as CPAP or oral appliance therapy.

Surgical modifications for OSDB fall into six main categories: upper airway bypass procedure, surgical upper airway modifications, tongue suspension techniques, upper airway neurostimulation therapy, skeletal modifications, and bariatric surgery (Table 175.1).

The severity of OSDB must be determined using objective testing before initiating non-CPAP treatment to identify those patients at risk of developing the complications of OSA, guide selection of appropriate treatment, and to provide a baseline to establish the effectiveness of subsequent treatment.[8] Follow-up sleep studies are routinely indicated to monitor the response to non-CPAP treatment options, including weight loss, positional therapy, oral appliance therapy, or surgery for OSDB. In patients undergoing CPAP treatment, follow-up sleep studies are not routinely indicated when the symptoms remain resolved with the treatment.[8]

Preoperative Evaluation

The comprehensive diagnostic workup of the OSDB patient should include a complete medical and thorough sleep history, evaluation of polysomnography (PSG) data, and previous OSA treatments. The PSG recording should not be older than 12 months and not be a split-night study.

It is helpful to also have a current assessment of the patient's level of subjective sleepiness and quality of life using the Epworth Sleepiness Scale (ESS) and the Functional Outcomes of Sleep Questionnaire (FOSQ) (see Chapters 68, 131, and 207).

Before proceeding with surgery, the medical workup should identify confounding factors that can increase the medical, anesthetic, and surgical risk of the surgical procedure. A thorough clinical examination should be performed with a clinical basic ear, nose, and throat (ENT) examination (CBE), including assessment of the nasal airway, the palatal region, the lateral pharyngeal walls, and the size and character of the tonsils. Within this CBE, patients need to undergo a laryngotracheoscopy using a flexible fiberoptic endoscope to visualize the tongue base, lateral pharyngeal walls, vallecula, pyriform sinuses, larynx, and epiglottis.[22] An intraoral examination is performed to assess dental status; soft tissues, including tongue and tongue base; malocclusions; and skeletal abnormalities.

The upper airway needs to be evaluated in detail. It has been demonstrated that the upper airway is significantly smaller in patients with OSDB compared to normal subjects, especially at the retropalatal and retroglossal levels.[23,24] In general the upper airway has rigid support in its proximal and distal segments but has a collapsible portion starting from the soft palate on to the larynx, with the size of its lumen being subject to the influence of surrounding pressures and the activity of dilator muscles. The potential collapse of the upper airway during sleep in OSDB patients will therefore occur in this so-called collapsible segment (Figure 175.1).

Before the introduction of CPAP, tracheotomy or "upper airway bypass surgery" offered effective treatment of OSA and patients with the pickwickian syndrome.[25] However, tracheotomy does not address the collapse in the collapsible segment of the vulnerable upper airway but successfully bypasses the obstruction, thereby eliminating OSA. Therefore tracheotomy is a highly effective treatment for OSA. On the other hand, tracheotomy is physically and socially very invasive and might substantially reduce quality of life.[26,27] At present the most often-used surgical procedures have greater acceptance but are generally less effective.

In the decision-making process toward the selection of the most appropriate surgical treatment option(s), other than tracheotomy, for the individual OSDB patient, the site(s), degree, and pattern of upper airway obstruction need to be determined (Figure 175.2).[17] Indeed, most of the specific non-CPAP approaches, apart from tracheotomy and bariatric surgery (Table 175.1), ideally strive to intervene at the specific anatomic region(s) that become obstructed during sleep.[22]

A variety of modalities, including pharyngeal pressure measurements and imaging and endoscopy techniques, can be used to identify therapeutic options.[28–31] Imaging techniques used for the preoperative evaluation include radiography, fluoroscopy, conventional computed tomography (CT), magnetic resonance imaging (MRI), and, increasingly, three-dimensional studies of the upper airway using cone beam CT scans.[32] In addition, cephalometric analysis can be performed.[33] Computational models of the upper airway based on CT or MRI have been introduced to simulate the effects of upper airway manipulations and predict success of non-CPAP treatment options.[24,34–36]

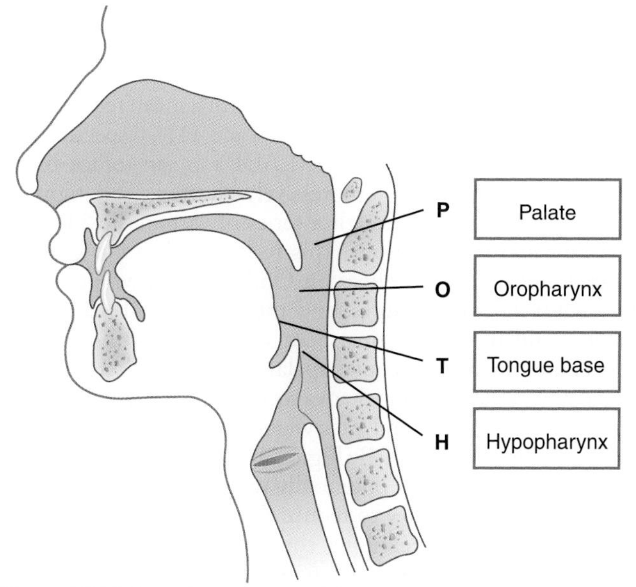

Figure 175.1 Sagittal cross-section of the upper airway with the "collapsible segment" depicted in *purple:* The upper airway has rigid support in its proximal and distal segments but has a collapsible portion extending from the soft palate to the larynx, with the size of its lumen being subject to the influence of surrounding pressures and the activity of dilator muscles. (Copyright Prof. Dr. Eric Kezirian, www.sleep-doctor.com.)

The different techniques for investigation of the upper airway all have their specific advantages and limitations.[28] Differences among the various techniques include aspects on invasiveness, exposure to radiation, costs related to the examination, and potential side-effects.[28,30,37] In addition, a crucial question on whether the upper airway behaves differently during wakefulness versus during natural sleep, remains unanswered up to this date in the literature.[38]

The technique of drug-induced sedation endoscopy (DISE; see also Chapter 174), first described as sleep nasendoscopy in 1991, has emerged as an alternative method to dynamically investigate the upper airway before non-CPAP treatment selection in patients with OSDB.[17,38–40] When comparing DISE with awake fiberendoscopy of the upper airway, identical findings were observed only in 25% of cases.[41] In addition, the treatment recommendations toward tongue base interventions and oral appliance therapy have the highest range of change, based on DISE compared to CBE.[42] DISE may not be predictive of surgical outcome[43] and lacks a uniform method of sedation.[38,44] No consensus exists on a standard DISE classification system[45]; in Figure 175.2 a generic scoring form is depicted.[46]

Several studies have reported that the most frequent site of upper airway obstruction in OSDB patients is the palatal level,[31,40,47] although, in a majority of OSDB patients, a multilevel collapse is observed within the collapsible segment of the upper airway.[31,48] The probability of multilevel collapse increases with increasing OSA severity and with an increased level of overweight or obesity.[31] Logically, resolution of pharyngeal collapse at all levels involved in the upper airway collapse during sleep will be necessary to achieve successful treatment in the individual OSDB patient undergoing one or more non-CPAP treatment option(s).

Surgical Upper Airway Modifications

An overview of the different techniques that aim to surgically modify the upper airway in OSDB patients is provided in Table 175.2.

Nasal Surgery

Depending on the anatomic deformity at the level of the septum, the turbinates, and/or, in case of alar collapse or nasal valve deformities, nasal surgery can be indicated to correct nasal obstruction.[22] However, nasal surgery, including septoplasty, septorhinoplasty, turbinoplasty, and/or radiofrequency ablation (RFA) volume reduction of the turbinates, cannot be recommended as a standalone procedure for the treatment of OSDB.[49,50] On the other hand, nasal surgery might be performed in patients with nasal obstruction, who experience

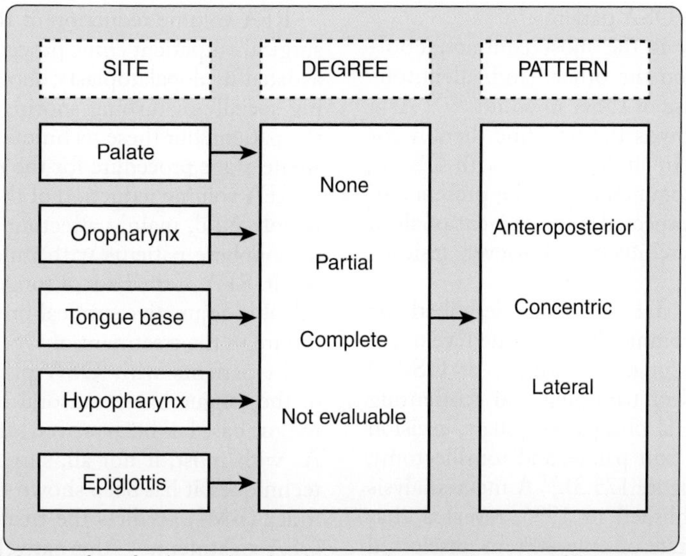

Figure 175.2 Scoring form for drug-induced sedation endoscopy: Reporting of the assessment of the level, the corresponding degree, and direction of upper airway collapse patterns. (From Vroegop AV, Vanderveken OM, Wouters K, et al. Observer variation in drug-induced sleep endoscopy: experienced versus nonexperienced ear, nose, and throat surgeons. *Sleep.* 2013;36:947–53.)

Table 175.2 Nonlimitative List of Surgical Upper Airway Modifications for the Treatment of OSDB

Surgical Upper Airway Modifications	
Nasal surgery	Septorhinoplasty
	RFA volume reduction turbinates
	Turbinoplasty
Pharyngeal procedures	RFA palate
	Adenotonsillectomy
	UPPP
	LAUP
	UPF
	ESP
	BRP
	Tongue base reduction ± epiglottoplasty
	• RFA tongue base
	• TORS
	• Coblation
	• Carbon dioxide laser
	Genioglossus advancement
	Hyoid myotomy ± suspension

BRP, Barbed reposition pharyngoplasty; ESP, expansion sphincter pharyngoplasty; LAUP, laser-assisted uvuloplasty; RFA, radiofrequency ablation; TORS: transoral robotic surgery; UPF, uvulopalatal flap; UPPP, uvulopalatopharyngoplasty.

problems with the use of CPAP or oral appliance therapy because of these nasal complaints, to improve adherence to treatment. Successful nasal surgery may also be associated with a reduction in therapeutic CPAP pressure required to alleviate OSA and may improve CPAP adherence.[51,52]

Pharyngeal Surgery

A surgical success with velopharyngeal and oropharyngeal surgical techniques as standalone treatment can only be anticipated when the upper airway collapse is limited to the retropalatal and/or oropharyngeal area, which is rarely the case in more severe OSA and/or obese OSA patients.[31,48]

Adenotonsillar hypertrophy is the most common etiology of OSA in children, but on the other hand, adenotonsillar hypertrophy is a rare cause of OSA in adults.[49,50] As a consequence, adenotonsillectomy is the first-line therapy for nonobese children with OSA. In adult patients with OSDB, adenotonsillectomy can be recommended in the presence of tonsillar hypertrophy, with an expected improvement of sleep respiratory disturbances and architecture; however, residual OSA will be common.

Uvulopalatopharyngoplasty (UPPP), first described by Fujita in 1987, is the most commonly performed velooropharyngeal surgical procedure in the treatment of OSA.[53] The UPPP procedure consists of trimming and reorienting the posterior and anterior lateral pharyngeal pillars, excision of the uvula and the posterior soft palate, and tonsillectomy, if not previously performed (Figure 175.3).[53] A meta-analysis by Sher and colleagues,[54] published in 1996, revealed that UPPP had an overall success rate of only 40% in unselected OSDB patients. However, when adding DISE to the diagnostic workup and preoperative evaluation for patient selection, it has been demonstrated that the success rate of UPPP increases compared to these historical control subjects.[55] The results of randomized controlled trials using the delayed design showed a significant reduction in OSA severity in the intervention group compared to the control group, with a mean reduction in apnea-hypopnea index (AHI) of 60% and 11%, respectively.[56]

Laser-assisted uvuloplasty (LAUP) is an office-based surgical procedure that progressively shortens and tightens the uvula and palate through a series of carbon dioxide laser incisions and vaporizations. This technique has not demonstrated any significant effect on OSA severity, symptoms, or on quality-of-life measures, and therefore LAUP cannot be recommended for the treatment of OSA.[57] Other palatal procedures include the uvulopalatal flap (UPF) technique, Z-palatoplasty, transpalatal advancement pharyngoplasty, palatal implants, and lateral pharyngoplasty.[58–62] The UPF is a modification of the UPPP (Figure 175.4).[22,59] The advantage of UPF is that it has a potentially reversible flap that can be taken down if necessary to reduce the risk of nasopharyngeal incompetence; the technique comes with less postoperative pain as there are no sutures along the free edge of the palate.[22]

Expansion sphincter pharyngoplasty (ESP) (Figure 175.5)[63] results in a repositioning of the palatopharyngeus muscle laterally, anteriorly, and superiorly. The effect of ESP may be mediated by three mechanisms: static opening of the lateral pharyngeal retropalatal recess, advancing the distal soft palate anteriorly, and reducing lateral wall compliance by mobilizing and repositioning the palatopharyngeus.[63] The results with this ESP procedure are promising, with demonstrated benefits in selected OSA patients (with severe palatal circumferential narrowing and bulky lateral pharyngeal tissue) with minimal complications.[63,64]

Barbed reposition pharyngoplasty (BRP)[65] mainly focuses on displacement of the posterior pillar (palatopharyngeal muscle) in a more lateral and anterior position, to enlarge the oropharyngeal inlet and the retropalatal space with suspension of the posterior pillar to the pterygomandibular raphe.[66] The results of a comparative study for single-level palatal surgeries suggest that BRP can be considered an effective procedure based on favorable postoperative outcomes, and both ESP and BRP proved to be superior to UPPP.[67]

RFA volume reduction of the palate, a minimally invasive surgical outpatient clinic procedure, as well as combined RFA-assisted uvulopalatoplasty, showed positive results in decreasing socially disturbing snoring as reported by the partner of the patient, but these techniques cannot be recommended as a single-stage procedure for the treatment of OSA.[68] The effect of RFA volume reduction of the tongue base on OSA severity is only mild, mainly affecting snoring complaints, especially in nonobese patients with mild to moderate OSA.[69,70] As a result, RFA of the base of tongue should be considered to be a valuable adjunctive surgical procedure and not a primary procedure in the treatment of OSA.[22,71,72]

In patients with OSA primarily related to hypertrophy of the tongue base, transoral robotic surgery (TORS) of the tongue base has been proven safe, feasible, and well tolerated.[73] As with most, if not all, surgical upper airway modification techniques, it has been shown that the preoperative body mass index (BMI) predicts the treatment success using TORS for OSA treatment.[74] Alternatively, cold ablation (coblation) or carbon dioxide laser techniques might be adopted, mainly in cases of tonsillar hypertrophy of the tongue base to perform lingual tonsillectomy.[22,75,76]

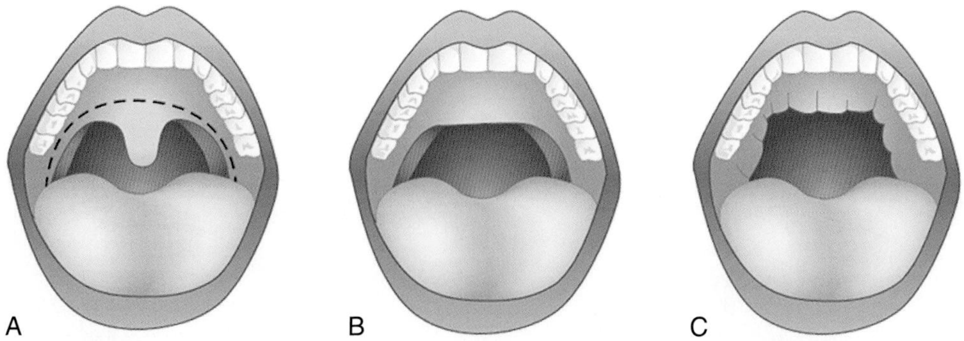

Figure 175.3 Uvulopalatopharyngoplasty technique. **A,** Redundant soft palate and tonsillar pillar mucosa are outlined. **B,** Tonsils, tonsillar pillar mucosa, and posterior soft palate have been excised. The extent of soft palate excision is determined by placing traction on the uvula and noting the position of the mucosal crease. **C,** Mucosal flaps of the lateral pharyngeal wall and nasal palatal muscle are advanced to the anterior pillar and oral mucosa of the soft palate. The wound is closed with 3-0 Vicryl braided suture. (From Troell RJ, Strom CG. Surgical therapy for snoring. *Fed Practitioner.* 1997;14:29–52.)

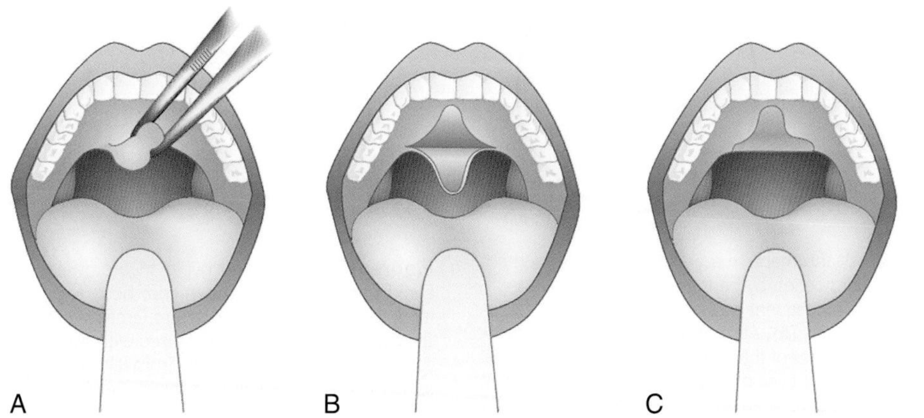

Figure 175.4 Reversible uvulopalatal flap (UPF) technique. **A,** Uvula reflected to identify mucosal crease of muscular sling. **B,** Knife removes mucosa on proposed flap site. **C,** Wound is closed with a half-buried suture of 3-0 Vicryl braided suture at the tip of the uvula and simple interrupted sutures along the mucosal closure. (From Troell RJ, Strom CG. Surgical therapy for snoring. *Fed Practitioner.* 1997;14:29–52.)

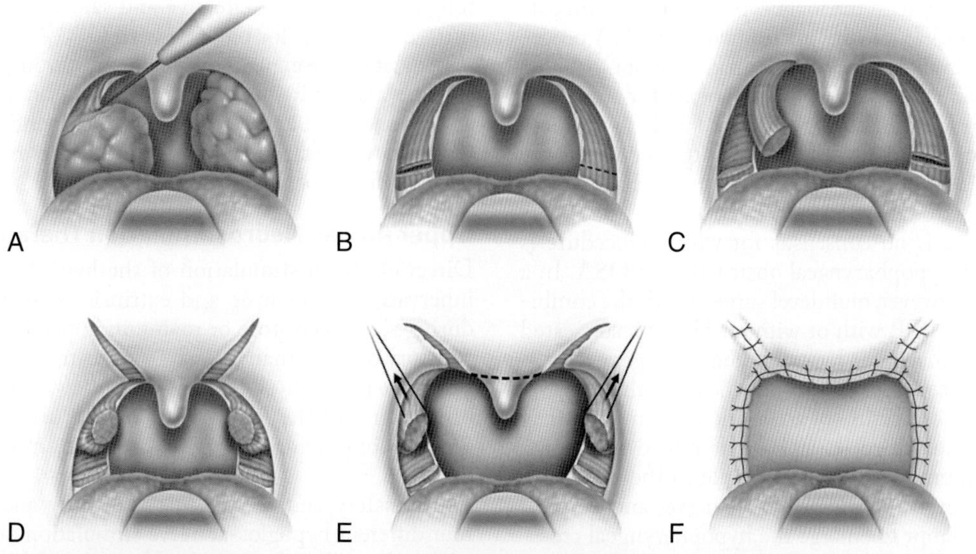

Figure 175.5 Surgical technique of the expansion sphincter pharyngoplasty. **A,** Tonsillectomy is performed. **B,** Horizontal incision is made to divide the inferior end of the palatopharyngeus muscle. **C,** The palatopharyngeus muscle is mobilized, although not completely, with care taken to leave its fascia attachments to the deeper horizontal constrictor muscles. **D,** Superolateral incision is made on the soft palate, revealing the arching fibers of the palatini muscles. **E,** Vicryl sutures are used to hitch up the palatopharyngeus muscle to the soft palate muscles superolaterally. **F,** Closure of the palatal incisions. (From Pang KP, Woodson BT. Expansion sphincter pharyngoplasty: a new technique for the treatment of obstructive sleep apnea. *Otolaryngol Head Neck Surg.* 2007;137:110–4)

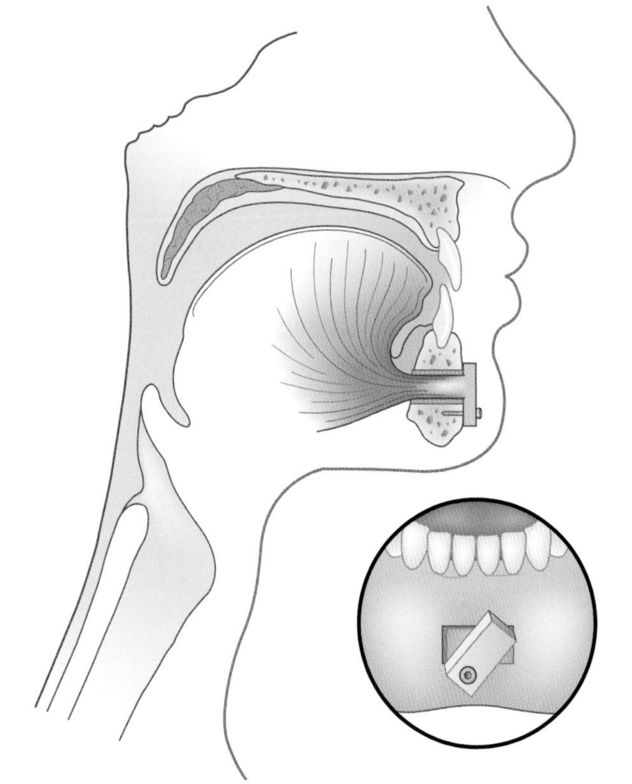

Figure 175.6 Genioglossal advancement. In a genioglossal advancement the tongue is put under anterior traction by performing a limited parasagittal mandibular osteotomy with subsequent advancement of the genial tubercle/genioglossus muscle complex **(A).** After removing the buccal cortex and medullary bone, the lingual cortex of the mandible, including the genial tubercle is fixated in its new anterior position **(B).** (Adapted from Riley RW, Powell NB, Guilleminault C. Obstructive sleep apnea and the hyoid: a revised surgical procedure. *Otolaryngol Head Neck Surg.* 1994;111:717–21.)

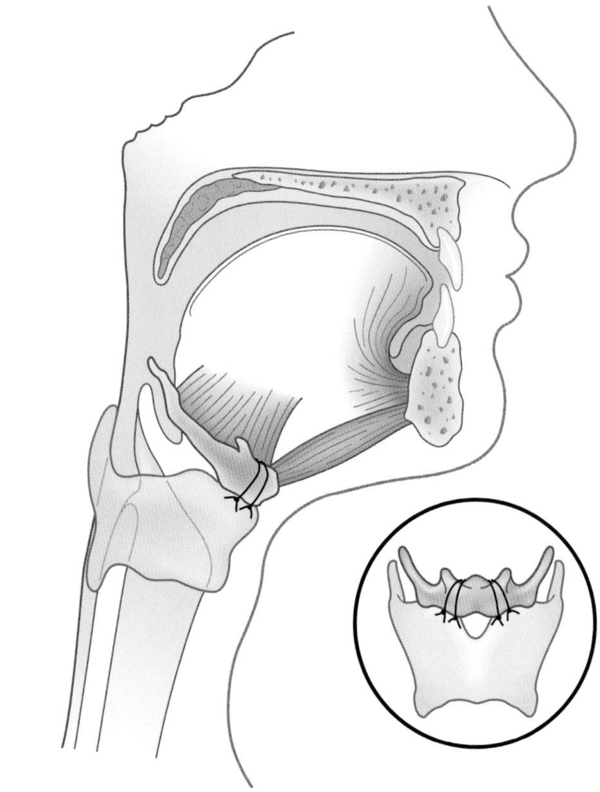

Figure 175.7 Modified hyoid myotomy and suspension procedure. The hyoid bone is isolated, the inferior body is dissected clean, and the majority of the suprahyoid musculature remains intact. The hyoid is advanced over the thyroid lamina and immobilized with sutures placed through the superior aspect of the thyroid cartilage. (From Riley RW, Powell NB, Guilleminault C. Obstructive sleep apnea and the hyoid: a revised surgical procedure. *Otolaryngol Head Neck Surg.* 1994;111: 717–21.)

Another treatment approach is genioglossal advancement (GA), which uses the forward placement of the geniotubercle to place sufficient tension on the tongue, preventing it from collapsing (Figure 175.6). It remains unclear whether a GA procedure is of additional value in the surgical treatment of OSA.[71,77]

Hyoid suspension (HS) or hyoid thyropexia for the treatment of OSA consists of securing the hyoid arch anteroinferiorly to the thyroid lamina, with or without hyoid myotomy (Figure 175.7).[22] An isolated HS treatment might be indicated in nonobese patients with moderate to severe OSA.[49,78]

At present, there is no consensus for which procedure is the best to address hypopharyngeal obstruction in OSA. In a systematic review, however, multilevel surgery with the combination of GA and UPPP, with or without HS, was suggested as the "accepted standard" for hypopharyngeal surgery.[79]

Tongue base procedures that do not focus on the removal of tissue and/or the correction of anatomic abnormalities can be divided into three categories and are described as follows: interventions that aim to tether the tongue to the mandible, electrical stimulation of the hypoglossal nerve, and surgical procedures that attempt to enlarge the hypopharyngeal cross-sectional area in the anteroposterior dimension by advancing the tongue via maxillomandibular osteotomies

Tongue Suspension Techniques

Suture-based tongue suspension procedures aim to tether the tongue to the mandible via sutures, ribbons, or barbs.[79] Tongue suspension should be considered in patients with OSA who demonstrate tongue base obstruction. As a stand-alone procedure, its success rate is only 36.6%.[79] In addition, tongue suspension is effective and safe as part of a multilevel surgical approach for patients with OSA.[79]

Adjustable tongue advancement, through placement of a tissue anchor in the tongue base and an adjustment spool at the mandible, and a tetherline to suspend the tongue, was reported to be feasible and safe, but further research is needed on the efficacy of this novel procedure.[80,81]

Upper Airway Neurostimulation Therapy

Direct electrical stimulation of the hypoglossal nerve, which innervates the intrinsic and extrinsic muscles of the tongue during sleep, to restore or maintain upper airway patency, has a history of more than 20 years of research and development.[82] From the pathophysiologic point of view, selective stimulation of branches of the hypoglossal nerve during sleep may treat OSA by improving upper airway dilator muscle activity during sleep.[83]

The safety and therapeutic feasibility and the efficacy of four different hypoglossal nerve stimulation devices have been explored in clinical trials: the Hypoglossal Nerve Stimulation (HGNS) system (Apnex Medical, St. Paul, MN [ceased operation in 2013]), the Aura6000 system (ImThera Medical, San Diego, CA), the Inspire Upper Airway Stimulation (UAS) device (Inspire Medical Systems, Maple Grove, MN), and the Genio system (Nyxoah, Mont-Saint-Guibert, Belgium).

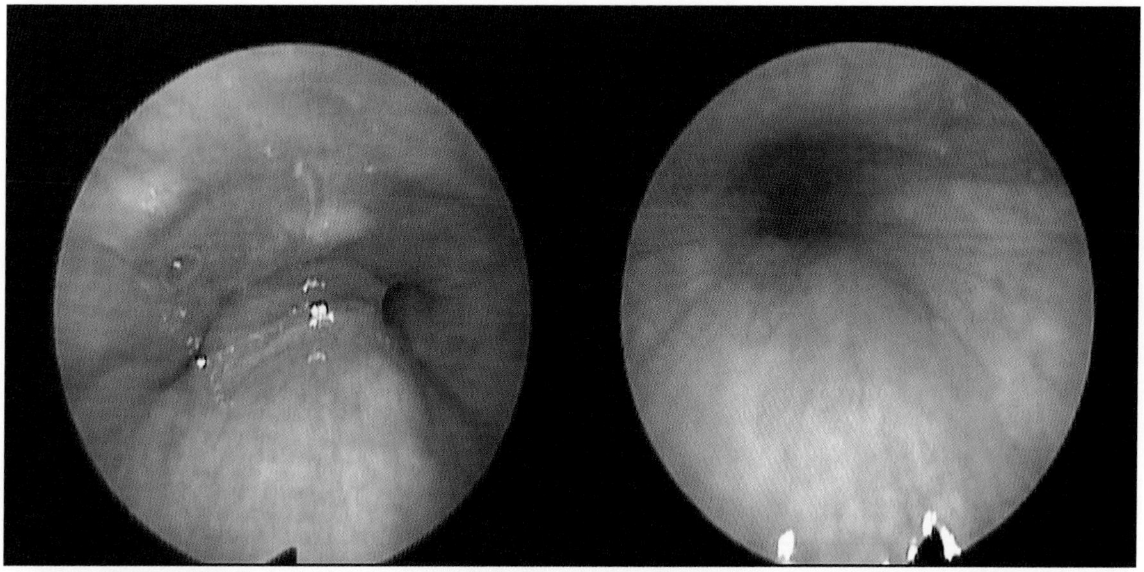

Figure 175.8 Example of anteroposterior (*left*) versus concentric (*right*) collapse at the palatal level during drug-induced sedation endoscopy. (From Vanderveken OM, Maurer JT, Hohenhorst W, et al. Evaluation of drug-induced sleep endoscopy as a patient selection tool for implanted upper airway stimulation for obstructive sleep apnea. *J Clin Sleep Med.* 2013;9:433–8.)

Results of these trials have been published and confirm the safety and feasibility of implantable systems for upper airway neurostimulation therapy for OSDB.[84–87] Three out of these four systems consist of an implantable pulse generator. Among these the main difference between the systems is that, with the Aura6000 system, the stimulation onto the body of the proximal hypoglossal nerve via the multielectrode lead will be continuous, obviating the need for respiration-sensing leads, whereas with the Inspire UAS device, the hypoglossal nerve stimulation is intermittent and synchronized with the respiration-sensing leads that measure the respiratory cycle.[83,85,88] Among other differences is the fact that during the surgical technique for the Inspire UAS system, the cuff section of the stimulation lead needs to be placed on the medial division of the distal hypoglossal nerve, thereby aiming at selective stimulation of the protrusor muscles of the tongue only.[89,90] Subsequently, appropriate placement of the stimulation lead needs to be confirmed by observing tongue protrusion during stimulation and by electromyographic monitoring during surgery.[89]

The Genio system is implanted submentally and stimulates the terminal branches of the hypoglossal nerve bilaterally via this implanted neurostimulator that will be activated externally.[87] The first results suggest that the relative noninvasiveness does not compromise its effectiveness relative to the other methods.[87]

The identification of OSA patients who are more likely to benefit from upper airway neurostimulation therapy has been an important part of their evaluation.[86,91] It is suggested that responders to upper airway neurostimulation therapy have a BMI less than or equal to 32 kg/m^2 and an AHI less than or equal to 50 events per hour sleep.[86] In addition, the absence of complete concentric collapse at the level of the palate, as documented during DISE, may predict therapeutic success with implanted upper airway neurostimulation therapy (Figure 175.8).[86,91] Therefore DISE can be recommended as a patient selection tool for implanted upper airway stimulation therapy for the treatment of OSA.[91]

The results of a large multicenter, prospective trial assessing the safety and effectiveness of upper airway neurostimulation therapy, using the Inspire UAS device (Figure 175.9) in 126 selected OSA patients, were published in 2014 (Stimulation Therapy for Apnea Reduction [STAR] trial).[89] The results of this pivotal trial demonstrated that hypoglossal nerve stimulation led to significant improvements in objective and subjective measurements of the severity of OSA.[89] Serious adverse events were uncommon, and the side effects were not bothersome to most patients.[89] In addition, the results of a randomized, therapy withdrawal part of the trial indicated that the reduction in the severity of OSA was maintained among those who continued the therapy, illustrating that the therapy effect is due to stimulation.[89]

Systematic reviews indicate that hypoglossal nerve stimulation for OSA is reported to be safe, with high rates of compliance and therapy adherence and stable outcome results over several years of follow-up.[82,88] Endoscopic findings in a subset of patients who underwent upper airway neurostimulation therapy, using the Inspire UAS device, revealed that responders to the therapy had larger retropalatal enlargement with stimulation than nonresponders and that the neurostimulation increased both the retropalatal and retrolingual areas.[92] This observation of multilevel enlargement induced by upper airway neurostimulation therapy may explain the sustained reductions of OSA severity in selected patients receiving UAS therapy.[89,92]

The 5-year follow-up data on the STAR trial confirm sustained improvements in sleepiness, quality of life, and respiratory outcomes during 5 years of upper airway stimulation therapy in these patients with moderate to severe OSA who have failed nasal CPAP, and serious adverse events were uncommon.[93] These results confirmed upper airway stimulation therapy with the Inspire device as a nonanatomic surgical treatment with long-term benefit for these patients.[93]

SKELETAL MODIFICATIONS

The combination of advancement of both maxilla and mandible to improve airway patency in obstructive sleep apnea syndrome (OSAS) patients is an approach to therapy in selected OSA patients. Although trial-based evidence is still

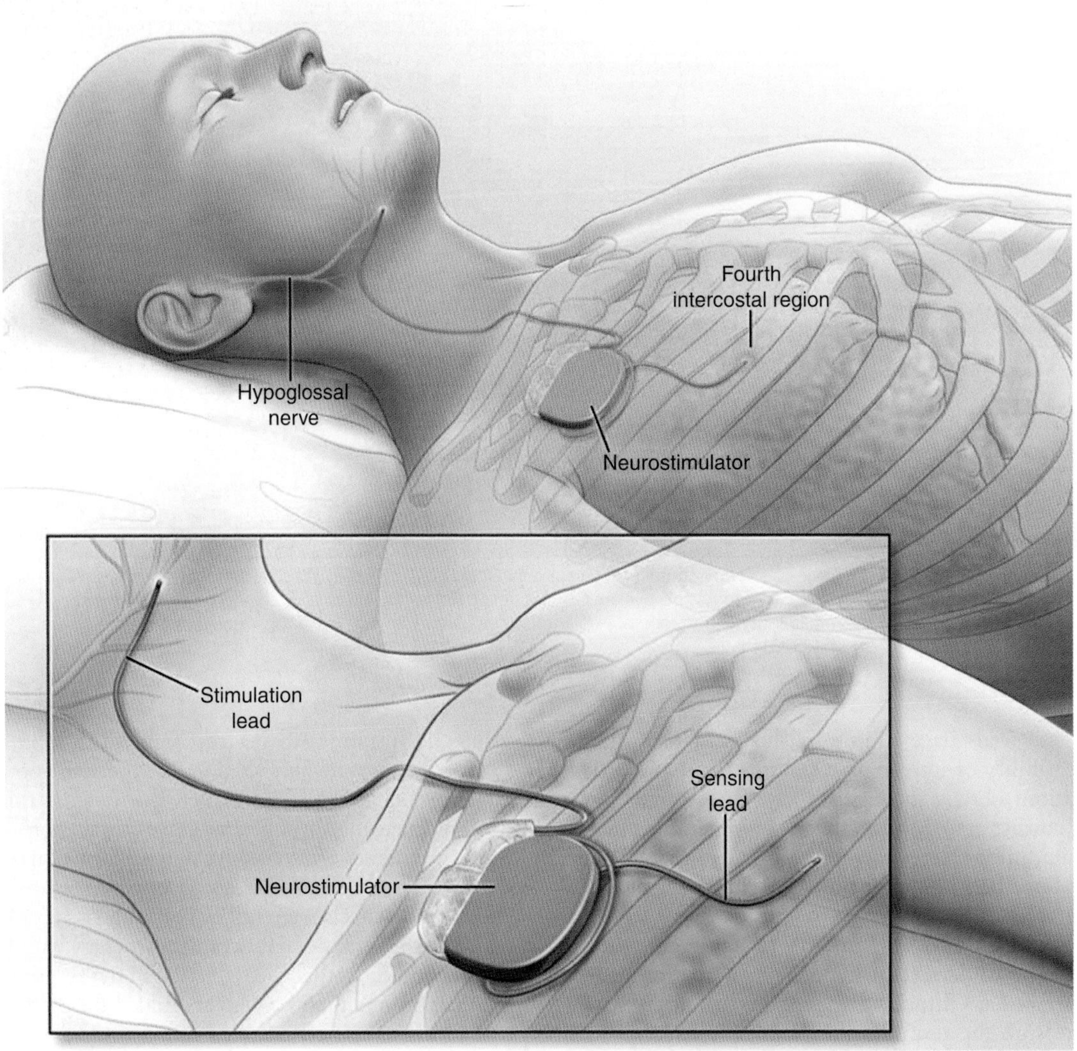

Figure 175.9 Upper airway stimulation using Inspire 2 implant (Inspire Medical Systems). The neurostimulator delivers electrical stimulating pulses to the hypoglossal nerve through the stimulation lead; the stimulating pulses are synchronized with ventilation detected by the sensing lead. For implantation of the device, the main trunk of the hypoglossal nerve (XII) was exposed by means of a horizontal incision in the upper neck at the inferior border of the submandibular gland. The nerve was followed anteromedially until it branched into a lateral and a medial (m-XII) division. The stimulation lead was placed on the m-XII branch. The cuff section of the stimulation lead includes three electrodes that can be arranged in a variety of unipolar or bipolar configurations for stimulation of the upper airway. Appropriate placement of the stimulation lead was confirmed by observing tongue protrusion during stimulation and by electromyographic monitoring during surgery. A second incision was made horizontally at the fourth intercostal region. The dissection was aimed at the upper border of the underlying rib. A tunnel was created posteroanteriorly between the external and internal intercostal muscles. The ventilatory sensor was placed in the tunnel, with the sensing side facing the pleura. A third incision was made horizontally, 2 to 4 cm inferior to the right clavicle. A pocket was created inferior to the incision and superficial to the pectoralis major muscle to accommodate the neurostimulator (implanted pulse generator). With a subcutaneous tunneling device, the leads of the stimulation electrode and the pressure sensor were led into the infraclavicular pocket and connected to the implanted pulse generator. Adequate functioning of the system was confirmed before closure. (From Strollo PJ Jr. Soose RJ, Maurer JT, et al. Upper-airway stimulation for obstructive sleep apnea. *N Engl J Med.* 2014;370:139–49.)

scarce, maxillomandibular advancement (MMA) surgery is currently regarded as a highly effective and safe surgical treatment modality for OSA.[94] MMA surgery in OSA patients consists of a bilateral sagittal split osteotomy of the mandible and a Le Fort 1 osteotomy of the maxilla (Figure 175.10). In OSAS patients, MMA surgery generally requires a minimum advancement of 10 mm of the mandible. In consequence, several upper airway muscles and ligaments are repositioned anteriorly, including the anterior belly of the digastric, mylohyoid, genioglossus, and geniohyoid muscles. The advancement of the maxilla pulls the soft tissue of the palate forward, tightens the palatoglossal and palatopharyngeal muscles, and increases tongue support. Moreover, "adding" the maxillary advancement also increases the amount of mandibular advancement that can be accomplished with surgery. To achieve additional improvements in oropharyngeal and hypopharyngeal airway patency, MMA surgery is frequently combined with a genioglossal advancement or a modified genioplasty[95,96] (Figures 175.6 and 175.11). To decrease the patient's cervical fat mass and further improve airway patency, cervicomental liposuction

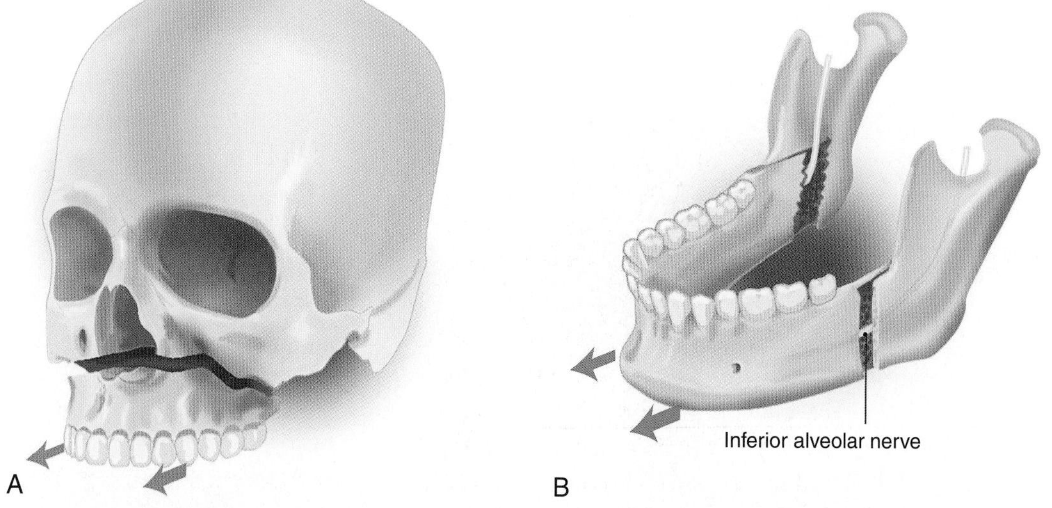

Figure 175.10 Maxillomandibular advancement (MMA) surgery. MMA surgery for obstructive sleep apnea syndrome provides enlargement of the upper airway by means of a Le Fort I advancement osteotomy of the maxilla **(A)** and a bilateral sagittal split advancement osteotomy of the mandible **(B).** (Adapted from Rosenberg AJ, Damen GW, Schreuder KE, et al. [Obstructive sleep-apnoea syndrome: good results with maxillo-mandibular osteotomy after failure of conservative therapy]. *Ned Tijdschr Geneeskd.* 2005;149:1223–6.)

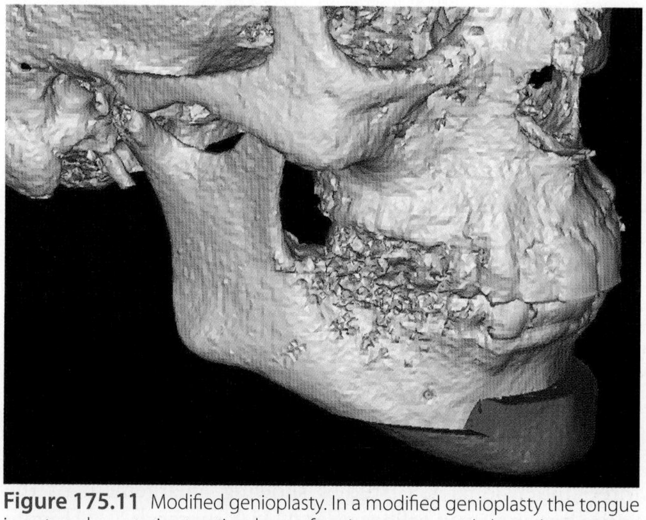

Figure 175.11 Modified genioplasty. In a modified genioplasty the tongue is put under anterior traction by performing a trapezoid-shaped osteotomy with advancement of the chin and the genial tubercle/genioglossus muscle complex.

may be added to the surgical plan in selected cases.[96] The resultant of this maxillary-mandibular-chin advancement is a structural enlargement of the nasoorohypopharyngeal airway and enhanced tension and decreased collapsibility of the pharyngeal dilator musculature. Because not primarily aimed at correcting dentofacial abnormalities, MMA surgery in OSA patients is sometimes also referred to as "telegnathic surgery." However, in some patients MMA surgery is used to concomitantly treat OSA and correct a dentofacial deformity.

Outcomes of Maxillomandibular Advancement Surgery for Obstructive Sleep-Disordered Breathing

OSA management after MMA surgery is generally successful in a high proportion of patients. A meta-analysis studying 627 patients from 22 studies demonstrated that the median surgical success, defined by a postoperative AHI of less than 20 with a greater-than-50% reduction in the AHI, is 86%.[97] Surgical cure, defined more stringently by a postoperative AHI of less than 5 per hour sleep, was observed in 43% of patients in this meta-analysis. After a mean follow-up of 5 months, a statistically and clinically significant reduction in the mean AHI from 63.9 to 9.5 and improvement in the lowest nocturnal oxyhemoglobin saturation from 71.9% to 87.7% is observed.[97] Similar improvements in most other PSG outcomes, such as sleep efficiency and sleep stages after MMA surgery, are observed. It should be noted that in about two-thirds of studies in this meta-analysis, previous or concurrent upper airway surgeries, such as UPPP, genioglossal advancement, and/or hyoid myotomy and suspension, have been performed. Of interest, patients who have had these previous upper airway surgeries performed were less likely to achieve a surgical cure with MMA surgery.[97] Another meta-analysis by Zaghi and colleagues[98] only included studies evaluating the outcomes of MMA surgery, excluding studies in patients who underwent adjunctive surgical procedures at the time of surgery (e.g., tonsillectomy, UPPP, or partial glossectomy). They included 45 observational studies evaluating the outcomes of MMA surgery in 518 OSAS patients. Surgical success and surgical cure were observed in 85% and 39% of patients, respectively. After a median follow-up of 6 months, a statistically and clinically significant reduction in the mean AHI, from 57.2 to 9.5, and improvement in the lowest nocturnal oxyhemoglobin saturation from 70.1% to 87.0% was observed.[98]

Although the number of studies evaluating long-term outcomes of MMA surgery is still limited, long-term results appear relatively stable over follow-up periods exceeding 2 to 5 years.[94,99] Studies have found statistically and clinically significant improvements in blood pressure after MMA surgery in OSA patients.[100,101] Finally, evidence for the medium to long-term stability of the skeletal advancements with MMA

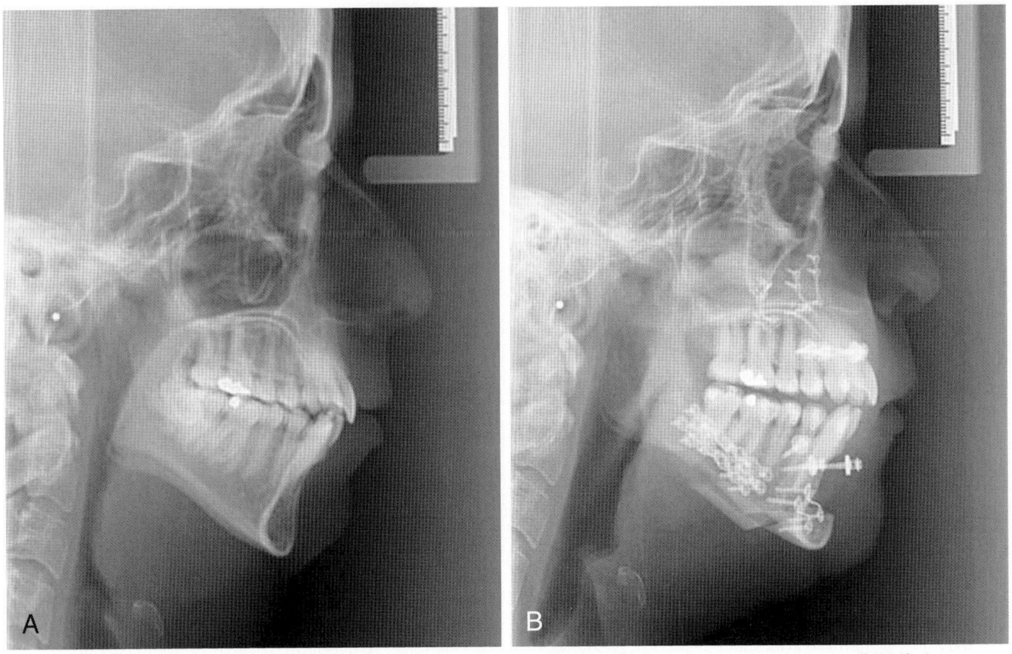

Figure 175.12 Two-dimensional airway changes after maxillomandibular advancement surgery (MMA). A preoperative **(A)** and postoperative **(B)** lateral cephalometric radiograph indicating the sagittal changes in upper airway space after MMA surgery combined with a modified genioplasty and cervicomental liposuction in a severe obstructive sleep apnea syndrome patient. (Adapted from Doff MH, Jansma J, Schepers RH, et al. Maxillomandibular advancement surgery as alternative to continuous positive airway pressure in morbidly severe obstructive sleep apnea: a case report. *Cranio.* 2013;31:246–251.)

surgery in OSA patients has been corroborated by several cephalometric studies.[102]

After MMA surgery for OSA, most patients report improvements in snoring; witnessed apneas; and excessive daytime sleepiness, morning headaches, memory loss, and impaired concentration.[97] The percentage of patients with elevated ESS values (i.e., >10) has been reported to decrease from 72% to 10%.[103] Also, the meta-analyses by Holty[97] and Zaghi[98] showed significant reductions in ESS values from 13.2 to 5.1 and from 13.5 to 3.2, respectively. Significant improvements in all domains of the FOSQ have also been reported.[100,104,105] Another study reported a 72% absolute reduction in subjective symptoms of depression or irritability after MMA surgery.[106] Most patients will be able to discontinue their CPAP after MMA surgery, with patients overall reporting that treatment was worthwhile and recommendable to others.[103]

As with many surgical interventions for OSA, randomized trials comparing MMA surgery with other interventions are scarce. There are, however, several cohort studies comparing the outcomes of MMA surgery with UPPP and CPAP, respectively.[106–111] When MMA surgery (n = 37) is compared with the results of a UPPP (n = 34), the mean change in AHI is significantly larger with MMA surgery (mean AHI reduction, 40.5 vs. 19.4).[109] This study could also not demonstrate an additional effect of a UPPP preceding MMA surgery on the final outcome.[109] When the AHI with CPAP therapy is compared with the AHI after MMA surgery, five cohort studies do not demonstrate significant differences between these two interventions.[97] To date, only one study performed a prospective randomized controlled trial that compared the therapeutic efficacy of MMA surgery with CPAP in 50 patients with severe OSAS (mean AHI, 56.8).[112] Although both CPAP and MMA surgery showed profound and significant improvements in AHI and ESS values after a 1-year treatment period, the degree of improvement was not clinical or statistical significantly different. The AHI reduced with CPAP from 50.3 to 6.3, whereas with MMA surgery, it was from 56.8 to 8.1, thereby suggesting equivalence of these treatments.

The effects of MMA surgery on the upper airway and surrounding structures have been extensively studied.[113] Two-dimensional cephalometric studies generally show a significant increase in velopharyngeal, oropharyngeal, and hypopharyngeal airway space after MMA surgery[104] (Figure 175.12). Furthermore, surgery may result in an increase in intermaxillary space, a decreased tongue proportion, and a more superior and anterior position of the hyoid bone.[104,113] These improvements in upper airway dimensions are confirmed by three-dimensional CT studies showing enlargement of the entire upper airway caliber after MMA surgery[113,114] (Figure 175.13). The increase in airway volume appears to be most pronounced in the velopharynx, followed by the oropharynx (Figures 175.14 and 175.15).[114] In addition, CT studies of the upper airway have also observed profound improvements in the lateral dimension and a considerable reduction of the upper airway length after surgery.[79,80] The latter phenomenon is suggested to contribute structurally to a decreased airway collapsibility after MMA surgery.[115] Many of the above-mentioned changes in upper airway dimensions and skeletal structures have been correlated with OSA improvements. However, at present there is insufficient data to support a relation between OSA improvements, such as AHI values and changes in the upper airway and its surrounding bony structures.[113]

Simultaneous advancement of the maxilla and mandible changes the skeletal framework of the face, thereby resulting in a possible rejuvenation of the middle and lower third of the face. This concept of a "reverse face lift," with positive effects on facial esthetics after MMA surgery in OSA patients, is observed in the majority of patients (Figure 175.16). Li and

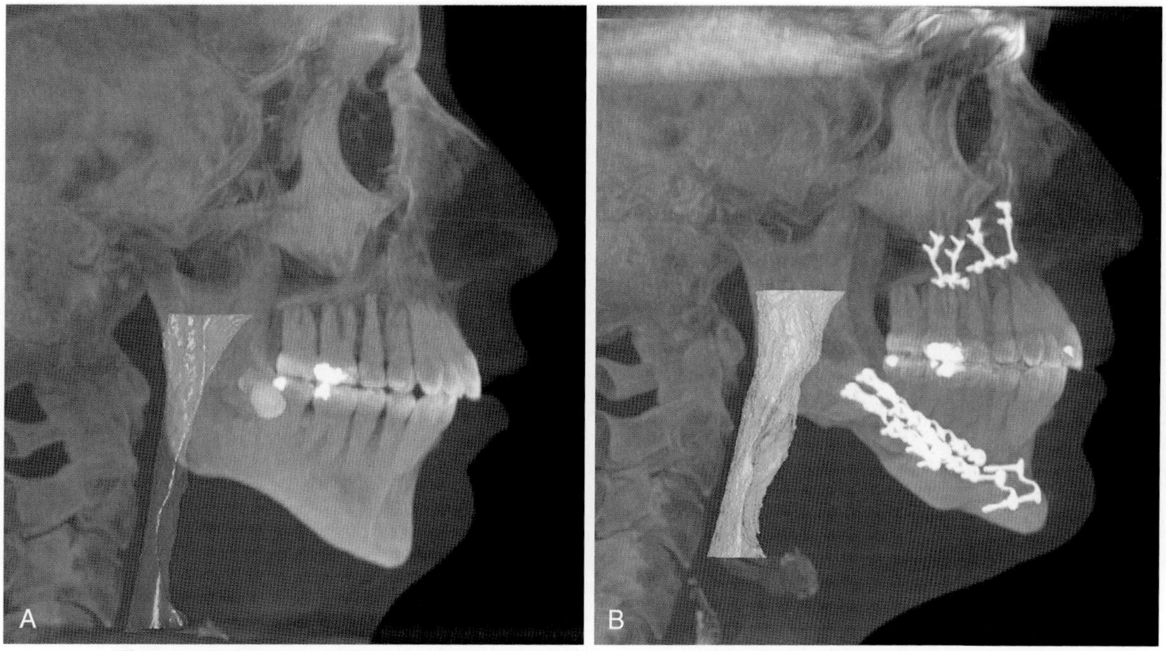

Figure 175.13 Three-dimensional airway changes after maxillomandibular advancement (MMA) surgery. A preoperative **(A)** and postoperative **(B)** cone beam computed tomography reconstruction of the upper airway, indicating the three-dimensional changes in upper airway space after MMA surgery combined with a modified genioplasty and cervicomental liposuction in a severe obstructive sleep apnea syndrome patient.

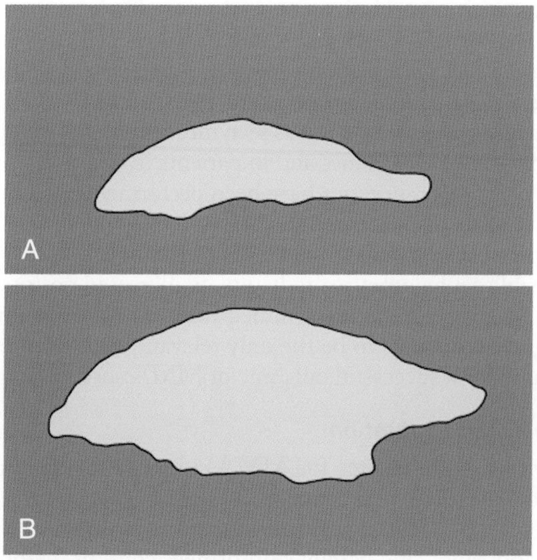

Figure 175.14 Velopharyngeal airway changes after maxillomandibular advancement (MMA) surgery. Enlargement of the minimal cross-sectional area of the velopharyngeal airway before **(A)** and after **(B)** MMA surgery combined with a modified genioplasty and cervicomental liposuction in a severe obstructive sleep apnea syndrome patient. (Adapted from Doff MH, Jansma J, Schepers RH, et al. Maxillomandibular advancement surgery as alternative to continuous positive airway pressure in morbidly severe obstructive sleep apnea: a case report. *Cranio.* 2013;31:246–51.)

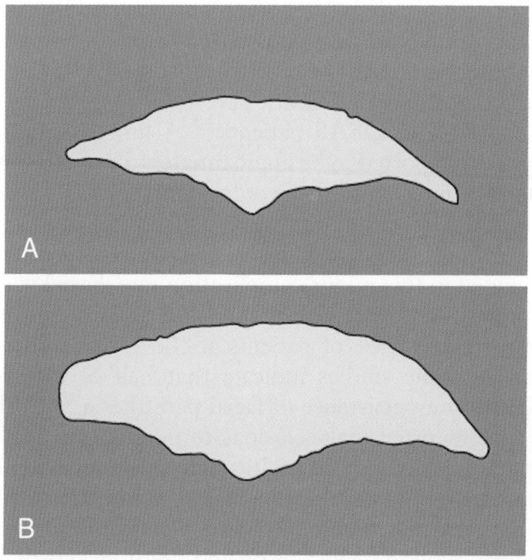

Figure 175.15 Oropharyngeal airway changes after maxillomandibular advancement (MMA) surgery. Enlargement of the minimal cross-sectional area of the oropharyngeal airway before **(A)** and after **(B)** MMA surgery combined with a modified genioplasty and cervicomental liposuction in a severe obstructive sleep apnea syndrome patient. (Adapted from Doff MH, Jansma J, Schepers RH, et al. Maxillomandibular advancement surgery as alternative to continuous positive airway pressure in morbidly severe obstructive sleep apnea: a case report. *Cranio.* 2013;31:246–51.)

colleagues[95,116] found that 6 months after surgery, 50% of patients reported a younger and 36% reported a more attractive facial appearance. It should be noted that 9% of patients in this study reported a less attractive facial appearance after surgery. Conversely, in another study, OSA patients indicated they were not to bothered by their appearance after MMA surgery.[117] Although patients seeking treatment for their OSA generally do not desire an esthetic facial improvement, it is important to communicate the anticipated facial changes before surgery. The magnitude of facial soft tissue changes of the lips and chin has been shown to correlate with 90% of the underlying dental and skeletal movement.[118] Because the majority of OSA patients exhibit normal craniofacial skeletal morphology, profound advancements should not result in an unacceptable deformity of facial esthetics. A surgical technique involving a so-called "counterclockwise" rotation of the occlusal plane, which has previously been used in correcting severe "bird-face" deformity, may be used to achieve both esthetic goals and to fulfill the main objective in the treatment of OSAS patients—an optimal increase in airway patency.[119]

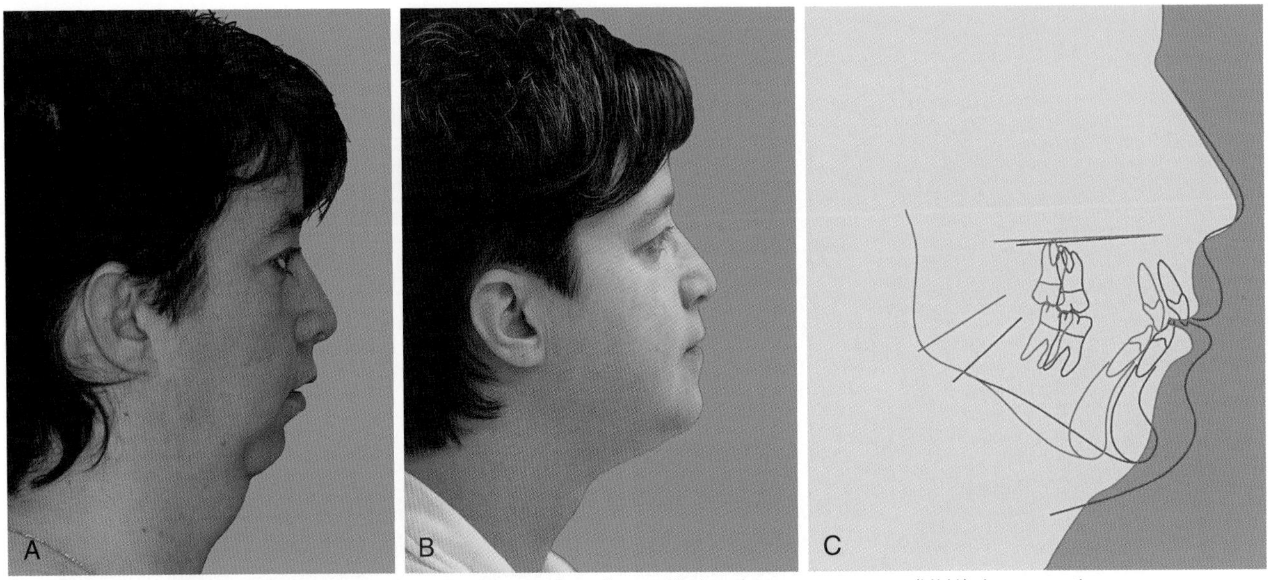

Figure 175.16 Effects on facial aesthetics of maxillomandibular advancement surgery (MMA). A preoperative **(A)** and postoperative **(B)** photograph illustrating the rejuvenation of the middle and lower third of the face after MMA surgery combined with a modified genioplasty and cervicomental liposuction in a severe obstructive sleep apnea syndrome patient. The profound advancement of the lower third of the patient's profile can be appreciated when the presurgical and postsurgical cephalometric radiographs are superimposed **(C).** (Adapted from Doff MH, Jansma J, Schepers RH, et al. Maxillomandibular advancement surgery as alternative to continuous positive airway pressure in morbidly severe obstructive sleep apnea: a case report. *Cranio.* 2013;31:246–51.)

Major complications after MMA surgery in OSA patients are rare.[97] Individual and nonfatal cases of cardiac arrest or dysrhythmia have been described after surgery.[120] No cases of immediate postoperative death have been reported after this type of surgery in OSAS patients.[97] A minor complication rate has been reported to be approximately 3%.[97] Minor complications include hemorrhage or local infections that are generally cured with either antibiotics or surgical drainage. The presence of postoperative malocclusions or facial paresthesia is not included in this minor complication rate. Facial paresthesia is present in almost all patients after surgery but resolves in approximately 85% of patients at the 1-year follow-up.[97] Conversely, some studies indicate that half of the patients treated report a persistence of facial paresthesia.[121] Although some have reported malocclusions to occur in up to 44% of patients after MMA,[120] a multicenter study reported only a few patients (6.7%) developed a malocclusion after MMA.[100] OSA patients may commonly have a concomitant dentofacial deformity, with malocclusion and presurgical orthodontic care followed by MMA surgery that will likely result in the correction of the preexisting malocclusion. Because increased age has been associated with an increased complication rate, older OSA patients appear more at risk of surgical complications.[122] Patients' perceived pain after MMA surgery is generally not profound and usually less when compared with the complaints after other upper airway surgeries.[122] An average hospital stay of 3.5 days is slightly longer after MMA surgery in OSA patients when compared with "conventional" orthognathic patients.[97] Most OSA patients are able to return to full work within 2 to 10 weeks after surgery.[106,122]

The most relevant patient characteristics and clinical factors predictive of a favorable outcome after MMA surgery in OSA patients include younger age and a lower preoperative BMI or AHI.[97] Also, the amount of advancement of the maxilla appears to correlate with the degree of reduction in AHI.[104] Patients with a surgical success are more likely to have their maxilla advanced 10 mm or more.[97] Conversely, the amount of mandibular advancement does not appear to correlate with a successful surgical outcome after MMA surgery in OSA.[97] A surgical cure (i.e., AHI < 5) was seen more often in patients with lower baseline AHI values and in patients in whom no preceding upper airway surgeries have been performed.[97,98] However, patients with higher baseline AHI values generally display a more pronounced reduction of AHI after surgery. With respect to possible cephalometric predictors, an increased postoperative posterior airway space, determined from lateral cephalometric radiographs, appears to be the only relevant variable of predictive value for a successful outcome of MMA surgery.[97]

Preoperative Evaluation

In general, prerequisites for MMA surgery include clinically "significant" OSA that is not susceptible to conservative management (e.g., CPAP), a medically and psychologically stable condition, and the patient's informed consent before surgery.[123] A lateral cephalometric head film and a preoperative PSG recording are mandatory to plan MMA surgery. Surgery may also be planned using three-dimensional imaging techniques, such as (cone beam) CT. Subsequently, virtual surgical planning can be conducted, which offers the surgeon valuable information on the anticipated skeletal, airway, and facial esthetic changes (Figure 175.17).[124] Finally, fiberoptic nasopharyngoscopy is also recommended before surgery. This can further help to identify nasal, retropalatal, or tongue base pathology that may affect the outcome of MMA surgery.

Postoperative Management

Medical surgical management of the postsurgical patient with OSA is more complicated than with conventional orthognathic patients, despite the profound postsurgical improvement in upper airway patency. Although the majority of

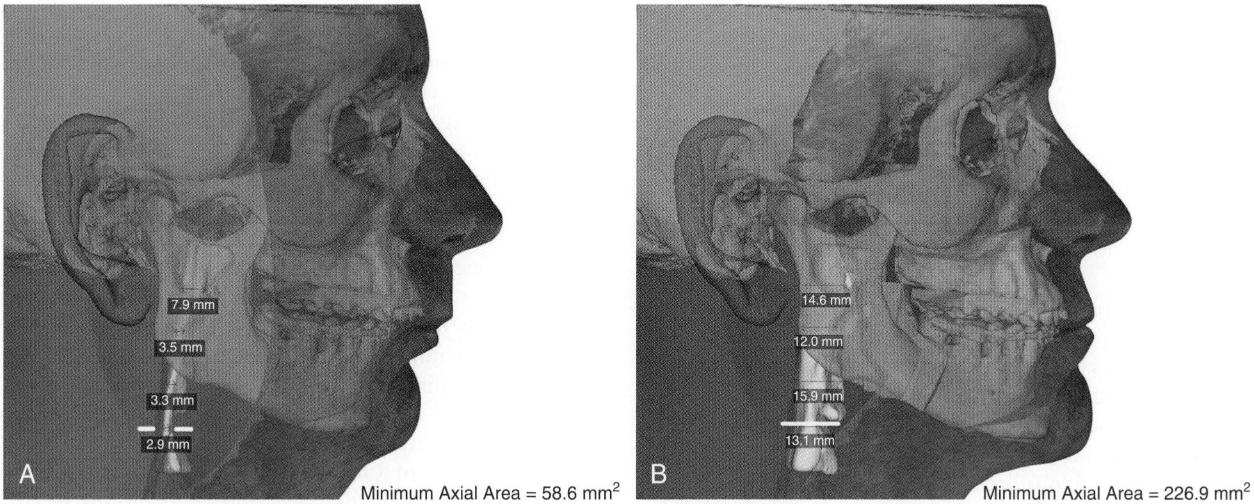

Figure 175.17 Three-dimensional planning of maxillomandibular advancement surgery (MMA). A preoperative **(A)** and postoperative **(B)** morph illustrating the anticipated skeletal, airway, and facial esthetic changes after MMA surgery with a genioplasty in a patient with obstructive sleep-disordered breathing. (Courtesy Mr. D. Brock; 3D Systems.)

OSA patients are stable when awake postoperatively, this may change dramatically with postoperative sedative medication or when the patient is asleep. Intensive care unit placement and the logical use of analgesic and hypertensive medication are therefore mandatory. If recovery is sufficient, discharge is up to the surgeon and patient but requires proper pain control and oral intake. Because younger patients tend to recover quicker, discharge is usually earlier in this patient category.

Follow-up of patients depends on the surgeon's individual protocol and the specific patient characteristics. It should be noted that postoperative edema will usually be maximal 72 hours after surgery. The effect of swelling after MMA surgery rarely compromises the upper airway because it is located more peripherally. However, swelling can sometimes be significant, which could worry patients. Frequent postoperative follow-up visits are recommended until patients are fully recovered. Because in sporadic cases patients may develop transient central sleep apnea after MMA surgery, PSG follow-up studies before the 6-month follow-up are not recommended.[125] Furthermore, it should be stressed to all overweight patients that weight loss is an important part of their pretreatment, but also posttreatment OSAS management, because even modest weight change will affect the outcome.

Treatment Algorithm for Maxillomandibular Advancement

MMA surgery is successful in a high proportion of patients and comparable to CPAP therapy in terms of effectiveness.[97] Several different treatment algorithms have been adopted for the selection of these surgical candidates for MMA surgery in OSA. Riley and colleagues[107] reported a phased protocol based on the specific site of upper airway obstruction. Depending on the level of airway obstruction (soft palate and/or base of tongue), patients are treated with a UPPP and/or a genioglossal advancement with hyoid myotomy and suspension in the first phase of this protocol. The second phase consists of MMA surgery and is generally reserved for phase-one failures. Because the majority of patients failing the first phase surgical phase tend to have more severe OSA, obesity, and mandibular deficiency,[107] others proceed with MMA surgery up front in patients with severe OSA and/or craniofacial dysmorphy.[122,126] Prinsell[106] adopts a "site-specific" approach in which OSA patients with "orohypopharyngeal narrowing caused by macroglossia with a retropositioned tongue base" are considered eligible for MMA surgery. Both Waite and colleagues[127] and Hochban and colleagues[111] adopt a protocol in which MMA surgery is considered a first surgical option in patients with specific "craniofacial deformities" (e.g., abnormal posterior airway space). Finally, the response to an oral appliance may also be used to select suitable candidates for MMA surgery.[128] Patients demonstrating a substantial reduction in baseline AHI (i.e., >50%) with oral appliance therapy appear as especially good candidates for MMA surgery.[128] Despite the variety of treatment protocols, a precise treatment algorithm for MMA surgery in OSA management is currently indefinite.

In conclusion, MMA surgery plays an important role in the correction of OSA that is refractive to noninvasive therapies. Because large advancements of the maxillomandibular complex are required in medically compromised patients, MMA surgery in OSA patients is generally more complex than "conventional" orthognathic surgery. With proper precautions it is, however, a safe and highly effective treatment modality for OSA. MMA surgery is probably the most effective surgical intervention in patients who are skeletally compromised (e.g., severe malocclusions, retrognathia, or bimaxillary retrusion). These patients should therefore be informed of MMA surgery as primary surgical treatment modality.

Combination Therapy, Including Multilevel Surgery

To reach the target, preferably an alleviation of the disease, it might be necessary to prescribe two or more therapies, with adjunctive therapies used as needed to supplement the primary treatment options.[8] In the treatment of OSDB, however, combining treatment options is somewhat undervalued.

Concerning the nonsurgical treatment options for OSDB, several possible combinations are reported, such as combining oral appliance therapy with a sleep position trainer or the combination of CPAP with oral appliance therapy.[129–131] In addition, positional treatment may also be an adjunct treatment in patients on CPAP who require high-pressure levels in the supine position to improve compliance with CPAP.[50]

The addition of oral appliance therapy has been shown to be an effective mode of combination therapy to control OSA after UPPP failure.[132] Combination of positional therapy and surgical upper airway modifications could result in a significant decrease in OSA severity in patients with positional OSA.[133,134]

Similarly, the combination of more than one surgical technique, either performed in one stage or staged, or so-called multilevel surgery, can be regarded as combination therapy for OSDB. For example, both UPPP or ESP can be part of a multilevel surgery for patients with more severe OSA.[135] The results of multilevel surgery, including UPPP with tonsillectomy and GA, with or without HS, have been described, and this particular combination has been suggested as the "accepted standard" for hypopharyngeal surgery.[79,136] Furthermore, combining transoral robot-assisted lingual tonsillectomy and UPPP in OSA patients results in a significant decrease in OSA severity, a significant improvement in daytime sleepiness, a high degree of patients' satisfaction, and an acceptable complication rate.[135,137,138]

Combining different treatment options for the alleviation of OSDB is undervalued and underinvestigated. Further research on the possible combinations is greatly needed.

CLINICAL PEARLS

- There is increasing evidence that untreated or undiagnosed obstructive sleep apnea (OSA) is an independent risk factor for hypertension, with consequent cerebrovascular and cardiovascular morbidity and high mortality. In consequence, OSA can lead to major socioeconomic consequences and should be approached as a chronic disease requiring long-term multidisciplinary management.
- Continuous positive airway pressure (CPAP) remains the standard to manage moderate to severe OSA. The clinical effectiveness of CPAP treatment, however, will often be limited by poor adherence. In consequence, there is a great need for non-CPAP treatment options alone or in combination, depending on the severity of OSA.
- To move away from "trial and error" empirical clinical paradigms, using drug-induced sedation endoscopy is suggested as an inherent part of the therapeutic decision-making process toward upper airway surgery and/or oral appliance therapy in patients with OSA.
- Nasal airway surgery complements most other surgical and nonsurgical treatments when the nose is obstructed. Site-directed upper airway procedures can be very effective, when combined appropriately, for addressing many combinations of obstruction. Upper airway neurostimulation appears promising for selected patients with multilevel soft tissue collapse and possibly in patients with particularly collapsible tissue, as opposed to structural abnormalities. Maxillomandibular advancement is a particularly useful option in selected patients. Tracheotomy is an important option for patients with severe comorbidities who cannot tolerate other less invasive treatment.
- It might be necessary to combine more than one option out of the available treatment options to achieve a successful outcome. Further research on the clinical effectiveness of the possible combinations is greatly needed because single treatments do not manage all OSA patients.

SUMMARY

OSDB has major socioeconomic consequences and should be approached as a chronic disease requiring long-term multidisciplinary management. Although CPAP is the more successful treatment for moderate to severe OSA when used properly and consistently, its clinical effectiveness will often be limited by poor patient and partner acceptance, which leads to suboptimal compliance. As many OSDB patients remain inadequately treated owing to inconsistent levels of adherence to CPAP, and as mild to moderate OSDB needs to be treated sufficiently to decrease morbidity and mortality, there is a great need for non-CPAP treatment options (Table 175.1). In addition, it might be necessary to combine more than one option out of the available treatment options to achieve a successful outcome targeting disease alleviation.

The spectrum of OSDB is quite diverse in nature and severity, and therefore the selection of the right treatment regimen for each individual patient will be of utmost importance. Among the different techniques that can be used for the preoperative upper airway assessment, DISE is increasingly performed for dynamic upper airway evaluation to select the proper non-CPAP treatment for patients with OSDB.

Surgical treatment of upper airway abnormalities, craniofacial deformations, or obesity may be applied in selected cases with OSDB. In general, sleep surgery procedures are directed at specific collapsible upper airway structures, and therefore preoperative upper airway investigation may add to a proper selection of a specific surgical procedure for an individual patient. Taking into account that in a majority of OSDB patients a multilevel collapse is observed within the collapsible segment of the upper airway, the treatment plan should aim at resolution of pharyngeal collapse at all levels involved in the upper airway collapse during sleep, to achieve successful treatment in the individual OSDB patient undergoing one or more non-CPAP treatment option(s).

The results of upper airway neurostimulation therapy in carefully selected OSDB patients are promising. Its safety, combined with its high rates of compliance and therapy adherence and sustained reductions of OSA severity, should sustain further research in this particular area.

SELECTED READINGS

Boyd SB, Upender R, Walters AS, et al. Effective apnea-hypopnea index ("effective AHI"): a new measure of effectiveness for positive airway pressure therapy. *Sleep*. 2016;39:1961–1972.

Boyd SB, Walters AS, Waite P, Harding SM, Song Y. Long-term effectiveness and safety of maxillomandibular advancement for treatment of obstructive sleep apnea. *J Clin Sleep Med*. 2015;11:699–708.

Camacho M, Noller MW, Del Do M, et al. Long-term results for maxillomandibular advancement to treat obstructive sleep apnea: a meta-analysis. *Otolaryngol Head Neck Surg*. 2019;160(4):580–593.

Lechien JR, Chiesa-Estomba CM, Fakhry N, et al. Surgical, clinical, and functional outcomes of transoral robotic surgery used in sleep surgery for obstructive sleep apnea syndrome: A systematic review and meta-analysis. *Head Neck*. 2021;43(7):2216–2239.

Kshirsagar RS, Harless L, Liang J, Durr M. The efficacy of surgery for upper airway resistance syndrome: A systematic review, meta-analysis and case series. *Am J Otolaryngol*. 2021;42(5):103011.

MacKay S, Carney AS, Catcheside PG, et al. Effect of multilevel upper airway surgery vs medical management on the apnea-hypopnea index and patient-reported daytime sleepiness among patients with moderate or severe obstructive sleep apnea: the SAMS randomized clinical trial. *JAMA*. 2020;324(12):1168–1179.

Pang KP, Baptista PM, Olszewska E, et al. Does drug-induced sleep endoscopy affect surgical outcome? A multicenter study of 326 obstructive sleep apnea patients. *Laryngoscope*. 2020;130(2):551–555. https://doi.org/10.1002/lary.27987.

Pang KP, Woodson BT. Expansion sphincter pharyngoplasty: a new technique for the treatment of obstructive sleep apnea. *Otolaryngol Head Neck Surg*. 2007;137:110–114.

Strollo Jr PJ, Soose RJ, Maurer JT, et al. Upper-airway stimulation for obstructive sleep apnea. *N Engl J Med*. 2014;370:139–149.

Vanderveken OM, Maurer JT, Hohenhorst W, et al. Evaluation of drug-induced sleep endoscopy as a patient selection tool for implanted upper airway stimulation for obstructive sleep apnea. *J Clin Sleep Med*. 2013;9:433–438.

Vicini C, Hendawy E, Campanini A, et al. Barbed reposition pharyngoplasty (BRP) for OSAHS: a feasibility, safety, efficacy and teachability pilot study. "We are on the giant's shoulders." *Ear Nos, Throat J*. 2015;272:3065–3070.

Vicini C, Montevecchi F, Pang K, et al. Combined transoral robotic tongue base surgery and palate surgery in obstructive sleep apnea-hypopnea syndrome: expansion sphincter pharyngoplasty versus uvulopalatopharyngoplasty. *Head Neck*. 2014;36:77–83.

Zhou N, Ho JTF, Huang Z, et al. Maxillomandibular advancement versus multilevel surgery for treatment of obstructive sleep apnea: A systematic review and meta-analysis. *Sleep Med Rev*. 2021;57:101471.

A complete reference list can be found online at ExpertConsult.com.

Chapter 176

Pharmacotherapy and Behavioral, Complementary, and Alternative Medicine for Sleep Bruxism

Ephraim Winocur; Luis F. Buenaver; Susheel P. Patil; Michael T. Smith, Jr.

Chapter Highlights

- Sleep bruxism is a common muscular behavior that can have harmful consequences, such as tooth damage and orofacial pain.
- Sleep bruxism may, in some cases that are not yet phenotyped, have protective benefits, including restoring the patency of the upper airway during flow limitation or increasing salivation to reduce chemically mediated tooth wear.
- The necessity to treat sleep bruxism should be decided on a case-by-case basis, weighing the balance of possible positive and negative consequences of the motor behavior against possible treatment-related side effects.
- Although conventional management approaches are efficacious (e.g., dental appliances to prevent tooth wear), they are often poorly tolerated, and alternative pharmacologic and complementary approaches are frequently sought.
- Pharmacotherapies and behavioral and complementary alternative medicine approaches are emerging for the management of sleep bruxism. The evidence base is preliminary; some promising interventions require systematic investigation. Potential side effects and the minimal/modest efficacy of many interventions limit their use at this time.

SLEEP BRUXISM

The nosology and conceptualization of bruxism is rapidly evolving. A recent international consensus meeting agreed to distinguish sleep bruxism (SB) from awake bruxism (AB),[1] because the etiologies are increasingly believed to be distinct. (See Chapters 169 to 172 for definition, comorbidities, and putative mechanisms.) According to the updated international consensus, SB is a masticatory muscle activity that occurs during sleep and is characterized as either rhythmic (phasic) or nonrhythmic (tonic). AB is a masticatory muscle activity occurring during wakefulness that is characterized by repetitive or sustained tooth contact and/or by bracing or thrusting of the mandible. It should be noted that neither SB nor AB is considered to be a movement disorder in otherwise healthy individuals (e.g., in absence of sleep-disordered breathing, epilepsy, or rapid eye movement behavior disorder [RBD], pain, insomnia, gastric reflux disorders, metal health disorders, addiction).

Both SB and AB may have positive, protective benefits, such as increasing salivation to minimize chemical tooth wear in the context of gastroesophageal reflux, or in the case of SB, preventing upper air collapse during flow limitation by restoring upper airway patency.[3,4] That said, both AB and SB may be a risk factor for negative oral health consequences. When SB can be linked to clinically significant deleterious outcomes such as the compromise of tooth integrity and fracture or orofacial pain, it can be conceptualized as a complex motor behavior with multifactorial pathophysiologies that should be properly managed. Another important conclusion reached by the consensus meeting was that standard cut-off points for establishing the presence or absence of bruxism should not be used in otherwise healthy individuals; rather, bruxism-related masticatory muscle activities should be assessed as a behavioral continuum. These new definitions are crucial for clinicians deciding which dental management approach is best or whether the patient should be referred to a sleep specialist or neurologist or otorhinolaryngology specialist before considering the dental consequences of SB.

In assessment of SB, it is critical to evaluate and consider that bruxism may be a sign of another underlying disorder requiring concurrent treatment, including obstructive sleep apnea, RBD, and epilepsy, as listed previously.[5] SB may also be a side effect of many medications, including antidepressants and antipsychotics[6] and recreational drugs such as 3,4-methylenedioxymethamphetamine (MDMA)/ecstasy[7] and nicotine.[8]

SB episodes are classified as either phasic (rhythmic), tonic (sustained), or a combination (mixed) of the two. Corresponding audible grinding noises are common, but variable.[2,9] In assessing management success, clinicians need to take into consideration that the frequency of SB episodes can vary in severity from nightly to intermittent in milder cases.[2,10] Treatment is typically sought for multiple reasons, including teeth-grinding sounds disruptive to a bed partner, teeth wear, facial pain, headaches, and teeth sensitivity. In addition, treatment planning must be designed according to comorbidities listed previously.

Pathophysiology

With respect to pathophysiology, modern evidence-based conceptualizations of SB emphasize central nervous system dysfunction and autonomic arousal as primary etiologies as opposed to peripheral mechanisms such as malocclusion, which have minimal empirical support. Multiple intrinsic factors, including genetics, aberrant autonomic sympathetic-cardiac activation, and neurotransmitter system dysfunction, have been implicated in the disorder.[11] Extrinsic factors such as medication side effects and tobacco/nicotine use are known to induce and/or exacerbate SB.[12]

Given the lack of a clear understanding between SB and various heterogeneous pathophysiologies, it is not surprising that there is no definitive cure for SB. Current conventional treatments focus on managing the harmful consequences of SB and protecting orofacial structures. The most frequently used interventions are dental appliances to prevent teeth wear, but caution is recommended with their use in presence of obstructive sleep apnea (see Chapter 171 for more information). These approaches, however, do not treat the underlying pathophysiology and are often poorly tolerated.[13] Medications, behavioral interventions, and complementary and alternative approaches for SB have received some preliminary research attention, but decisions to intervene with these approaches must be considered carefully, based on side effects, relatively sparse scientific evidence, and a potential unfavorable cost-benefit ratio.

Pharmacotherapies for Sleep Bruxism

Since SB is, based on the last 20 years' scientific evidence, most likely centrally mediated, best treatments would presumably involve neurotropic medications that regulate cerebral and autonomic hyperarousal. Pharmacotherapy for SB was briefly reviewed in Chapter 171, and because it is not a first-line treatment, we elected to cover its multidimensional putative benefit and risk.

A critical review intended to assess the exacerbating and ameliorating effect of drugs on bruxism in humans, however, found relatively more drugs that cause or aggravate SB than drugs that effectively reduce bruxism phenomenon.[8] Presently, there is a lack of strong evidence from which to draw firm clinical conclusions concerning the effects of drugs on SB.[14] The literature remains controversial and is based largely on anecdotal case reports.[8] Accordingly, no definitive recommendations can be made about the pharmacologic treatment of SB. Furthermore, all medications listed later are "off-label": that is, not recognized by governmental agencies as medications for SB. Clinicians must be extremely cautious in prescribing unapproved medication, and medical collaboration is recommended. See Table 176.1 for a summary of pharmacotherapies for SB in the literature.

Sedative, Anxiolytic, and Antidepressant Drugs

Psychosocial stress and psychopathology, particularly anxiety disorders, have traditionally been conceptualized as playing a pathophysiologic role in SB. However, this perspective has been questioned because of a lack of clear evidence linking these phenomena specifically to SB. A recent review identified mostly cross-sectional studies yielding mixed findings correlating SB with anxiety severity.[15] Some evidence, however, links AB with anxiety and psychosocial stress.[16] Nevertheless, benzodiazepines have been used clinically for SB because of their anxiolytic, muscle relaxant, and hypnotic properties. A placebo-controlled polysomnographic study found significant improvements in both the SB index and subjective sleep quality,[17] but a more recent polysomnography (PSG) study found clonazepam failed to significantly reduce SB activity compared with placebo.[18] Mixed findings may be due to differences between samples as the former study included patients with SB and comorbid sleep disturbances (e.g. insomnia, restless legs syndrome), whereas the latter excluded patients with comorbid sleep disorders. The benzodiazepine diazepam has also been reported to significantly reduce nocturnal masseter electromyographic (EMG) activity in patients suffering from clinical symptoms of masticatory hyperactivity.[19] Caution is warranted when prescribing benzodiazepines, especially for long periods because of potential adverse side effects, which include respiratory depression, tolerance, dependency, abuse, seizures upon abrupt withdrawal, somnolence, and occasionally muscular hypotonia and coordination disturbances. Respiratory depression is a particular concern in cases of comorbid sleep apnea, especially when combined with opioids.

Buspirone, an atypical anxiolytic, has been reported to relieve selective serotonin reuptake inhibitor–induced bruxism ("secondary bruxism") in some patients, to have no such effect in others, and possibly to cause bruxism in yet other patients.[19]

Sedating tricyclic antidepressants such as amitriptyline have been suggested as a treatment for SB, based on the presumed associations between depression and SB. However, insufficient evidence exists to support this assumption.[18] A recent comparative study aimed at investigating the short-term effects of occlusal splint therapy and tricyclic antidepressants (amitriptyline) on bite force and occlusal contact found that occlusal splint therapy may be more effective than tricyclic antidepressants in the treatment of bruxism.[20] Use of trazodone, another antidepressant medication, to manage SB is not evidence based, and so its possible benefits in some patients with obstructive sleep apnea and sleep arousal issues are unknown.[21,22] In general, available evidence suggests that drugs prescribed to treat anxiety and depression are relatively poor candidates for managing SB, particularly selective serotonin and serotonin-norepinephrine re-uptake inhibitors, which typically exacerbate SB.[23]

GABAergic Medications

Baclofen,[24] a gamma-aminobutyric acid (GABA) agonist, and tiagabine,[25] a GABA reuptake inhibitor, were found effective in the amelioration of SB. These studies suggest that SB, which has been categorized since 2005 by the International Classification of Sleep Disorders (ICSD-2 and ICSD-3)[26] as a movement disorder, may be successfully treated by the inhibitory neurotransmitter GABA, similar to other sleep-related movement disorders such as restless legs syndrome (RLS) and periodic limb movement disorder. This assumption, however, requires further investigation in well-designed studies.

Anticonvulsants

Gabapentin, an anticonvulsant, which is often used to treat neuropathic pain, chronic widespread pain disorder, and RLS, may also be effective in reducing rhythmic masseter muscle activity during sleep. A small study (n = 20) found that gabapentin significantly reduced hourly SB episodes,

Table 176.1 Drug Therapies for Sleep Bruxism (Unapproved Medication and No Clear Recommendation Extracted Because of the Paucity of Solid Evidence)

First Author (Year)[ref no.]	Study Design	Generic Name	Influence on Sleep Bruxism	Remarks
Saletu (2010)[17] Sakai (2017)[18]	Single-blind, placebo-controlled, nonrandomized, crossover PSG Randomized, double-blind, placebo-controlled, crossover trial	Clonazepam	↓ ↔	Possible serious adverse side effects. Risk of addiction
Montgomery (1986)[102]	Open trial (conducted on portable EMG)	Diazepam	↓	Possible serious adverse side effects
Winocur (2003)[8]	Case reports (described in critical review)	Buspirone	Mostly :↓ Few cases: ↑ or ↔	Possible serious adverse side effects Relieve SSRI-induced SB
Janati (2013)[24]	Single case report	Baclofen	↓	Possible serious adverse side effects
Kast (2005)[25]	Case reports	Tiagabine	↓	Possible serious adverse side effects
Ghanizadeh (2013)[28]	Randomized, double-blind, placebo-controlled trial	Hydroxyzine	↓	Pediatric sample; mechanism of action unclear
Huynh (2006)[19] Sakai (2017)[18]	Randomized, experimental[a] controlled, crossover studies with placebo and active treatments PSG Randomized, double-blind, placebo-controlled, crossover trial	Clonidine	↓ ↓	Possible serious adverse side effects
Winocur (2003)[8]	Crossover, double-blind (described in critical review)	Bromocriptine	↓ or ↔	Lobbezoo (1997) ↓ 4 out of 6 patients dropped out because of serious adverse side effects Lavigne (2001)[1] and Nishioka (1989) ↔
Lee (2010)[35] Tan (2000)[31] Zhang (2016)[34] Al-Wayli (2017)[33]	Randomized clinical trial Open-label prospective study Randomized clinical trial Randomized clinical trial	Botulinum toxin	↓ ↓ ↓ ↓	Reserved only to extreme severe cases of SB because of occasional complications and high cost. Mostly self-report outcomes
Madani (2013)[27]	Randomized controlled trial versus splint	Gabapentin	↓	Gabapentin was comparable to stabilization splint. Small sample size; $n = 20$

[a]Experimental trial as a proof of concept to challenge mechanism, not safety of medication.
↓ Ameliorate; ↔ no effect; ↑ exacerbate; EMG, electromyography; PSG, polysomnographic outcomes; SB, sleep bruxism.

comparable with the effects of stabilization splint management.[27] Gabapentin also significantly increased slow wave sleep; this was the mechanism of action hypothesized to account for its anti-SB effects. Completion of confirmatory and safety studies is necessary before that medication can be recommended.

Antihistamines

A recent randomized placebo-controlled clinical trial investigated the efficacy of hydroxyzine for treating parent-reported SB in 30 children.[28] Hydroxyzine is an H1 receptor antagonist with sedating properties that is typically used to treat itching and anxiety in children. Compared with placebo, hydroxyzine decreased the parental self-reported bruxism score without serious adverse effects. Although the mechanism of action is unknown, the authors speculated that the effects may be due to increased sleep depth, decreased anxiety, and muscle relaxation, although there is a lack of clear evidence linking anxiety and muscle tension with SB. Consequently, more research with objective measures is warranted and side effects must be controlled for their risk-benefit ratio.

Sympatholytic Medications

Sympatholytic medications have been suggested as having the potential to reduce SB by dampening sympathetic nervous system arousal during sleep. A promising randomized control study of 25 sleep bruxers found that clonidine, an alpha$_2$-adrenergic agonist, but not propranolol, a beta$_2$-adrenergic receptor antagonist, reduced SB activity by decreasing sympathetic tone in the 60-second period preceding the onset of SB events. The authors concluded that the diminution of paroxysmal sympathetic activation, which is typically observed before an SB event, reduced subsequent motor activation during SB.[19] A more recent, double-blind, randomized controlled crossover study replicated these findings.[18] Caution, however, should be taken when prescribing clonidine for SB because of its reported serious adverse side effects, including hypotension (observed in 20% of individuals with a mid dose), syncope, bradycardia, AV block, somnolence and fatigue, headache, sexual dysfunction, and so on.

Dopamine-Related Agents

A relationship between dopamine, the immediate precursor of norepinephrine, and SB has been hypothesized based on the role of dopamine in movement disorders such as Parkinson disease. The possible functional abnormalities of the central dopaminergic system in humans with SB was explored in a double-blind, placebo-controlled, neuroimaging study of the effects of bromocriptine, a dopamine agonist.[11] Unfortunately, four out of six subjects discontinued participation because of severe adverse effects. The two participants that completed the trial, however, demonstrated a 20% and 30% reduction in the number of hourly SB episodes measured polysomnographically compared with placebo.[11] A subsequent study by the same group,[29] as well as another study,[30] failed to demonstrate any significant effects of bromocriptine on SB.

The literature regarding the effects of dopamine antagonists on SB in humans is also conflicted. Some studies report exacerbating effects of haloperidol and other agonists; another study reported no impact; and at least one study found that risperidone improved SB.[8] The effect of dopamine-related medications on SB in humans remains unclear. More controlled, evidence-based research that identifies potential subgroups of responders and those at risk for dopamine related exacerbation is needed.

Botulinum Toxin Injections

Botulinum toxin (BT) injections are commonly used to treat cervical dystonia, blepharospasm, hemifacial spasm, tardive dyskinesia, and severe oromandibular dystonias, including SB. BT is a neurotoxin produced by the anaerobic bacterium *Clostridium botulinum*, which prevents the release of acetylcholine from presynaptic vesicles at the neuromuscular junctions, resulting in the blockade of motor fibers. Clinical effects are a temporary muscle contraction weakness, typically lasting 3 to 4 months.[23] Studies of BT injections for SB are limited and include a handful of case reports, an open-label prospective study,[31] and several small randomized controlled trials (RCT[32-34]), which primarily assessed pain, function, or self-reported bruxism. A single, pilot RCT (n = 12) used PSG to assess outcomes and reported that BT significantly decreased masseteric bruxism events compared with placebo saline injections over 12 weeks.[35] No subjects withdrew from the study, and no adverse events were reported. In an open-label study, 18 subjects diagnosed with severe bruxism were treated over 3 years.[31] Eighty-nine percent of the patients in this self-report study indicated a marked relief of grinding and functional improvement in chewing, swallowing, and/or speaking. The authors concluded that subjects required BT injections approximately every 5 months for effective, sustained relief.

A lack of placebo control and objective EMG measurement, however, limits conclusions that can be drawn. Two recent systematic reviews of BT that evaluated the four RCTs noted the extant literature is small and the methods subject to bias, but they concluded the BT appears to be relatively safe and can reduce the frequency of bruxism episodes and decrease pain and maximum occlusal force.[36,37] Despite the therapeutic potential of BT, the small number of studies and unresolved issues, including occasional complications related to local muscle weakness and high cost of treatment, indicate that BT injections should be reserved for severe cases of SB, in which all other therapies have failed and the clinical consequences of SB, including significant teeth wear, interference with dental rehabilitation, jaw muscle and/or temporomandibular joint pain, headaches, and social/marital conflicts, are evident. Further studies are awaited to elucidate if the animal and human observed temporomandibular bone damage is relevant (i.e., transient or pathologic in certain vulnerable individuals).[38]

Behavioral Interventions for Sleep Bruxism

Massed Practice Therapy and Habit Reversal for Bruxism

Massed negative practice and habit reversal are related behavioral therapies developed to reduce unwanted daytime behaviors, habits, compulsion, and tics. Early clinical approaches to bruxism failed to appreciate that SB and AB may be different problems requiring unique treatments. Both forms of bruxism were historically conceptualized as a tic-like habit[39] that may be reduced or even extinguished by enhancing the difference between the noxious aspects of bruxing or clenching, via conscious repetition of the behavior to induce muscle fatigue, and the absence of muscle fatigue resulting from cessation of the exercises.[40] One early study that compared such massed negative practice to relaxation training found that neither approach significantly reduced bruxism.[41] Some case reports, however, suggest a possible benefit of massed practice for AB.[39,42,43] Habit reversal is a related behavioral strategy designed to decrease maladaptive behaviors by increasing awareness of grinding and clenching and substituting a competing behavior such as jaw muscle relaxation, which is then reinforced. Habit reversal[44] has been effective in treating motor disorders (e.g., thumb sucking, nervous tics, nail biting), many of which are oral in nature.[45] A handful of studies of temporomandibular joint disorder (TMD) have found that habit reversal reduces facial pain[46-50] and associated maladaptive oral habits, which include AB and clenching.[46,48] There is minimal evidence, however, documenting that either massed practice or habit reversal interventions practiced during the daytime may generalize to or be effective for SB.

Arousal with Overcorrection

We are aware of at least one study that combined an arousal procedure with a behavioral intervention known as overcorrection to reduce SB behavior.[51] Overcorrection involves repeated practice of a positive substitute behavior (e.g., massage, teeth brushing, flossing, mouth rinsing) after punishment (awakening) for the targeted behavior. Arousal combined with overcorrection is an intervention based on operant conditioning, a principle posting that behavior is largely controlled by contingencies; punishment (i.e., arousal) and reinforcement (i.e., positive behavior). Arousal and overcorrection have been successfully used to treat nocturnal enuresis.[52] In a small, multiple baseline, multiple condition, behavioral experiment ($n = 2$),[51] each subject completed multiple baseline conditions, arousal-alone conditions (spouses awakened patients for 15 to 20 seconds), and arousals with overcorrection. In the overcorrection condition subjects were awakened and instructed to complete a 10-minute procedure, which included face and hand washing, brushing and flossing teeth, rinsing the mouth with water, then mouthwash, and repeating. The arousal with overcorrection condition was moderately effective in reducing the number of sleep bruxing episodes (>15 seconds) as observed and recorded by the subject's spouse during the 2-hour period immediately after sleep onset. Similar to other aversive conditioning studies, SB activity returned to baseline levels after cessation of treatment. With only one small study, the use of overcorrection for SB is unclear. Additional limitations of this approach include the feasibility of implementation with a partner, the lack of objective measures, and the ability to target only audible bruxing.

Nocturnal Biofeedback and Aversive Conditioning

Aversive conditioning is a type of behavioral conditioning in which a noxious stimulus is repeatedly paired with a maladaptive behavior targeted for extinction. EMG-activated alarms have been investigated as a form of aversive conditioning to treat SB. Typically, an audible tone is triggered during SB episodes with the purpose of waking a subject from sleep. Under this paradigm, for patients to avoid the noxious feedback and achieve consolidated sleep, they must learn to sleep without bruxing. Early studies using masseter and/or temporalis EMG activity thresholds to induce arousals consistently demonstrated reductions in SB duration, but not in frequency.[53,54] Moreover, most studies found that SB activity returns to baseline or is increased upon discontinuation of biofeedback.[55,56]

Subsequent efforts to sustain the treatment effects of EMG feedback have increased the aversive nature of the intervention by requiring that subjects become fully awake after an alarm. Two small ($n = 6$ and $n = 10$) studies employed an arousal task after auditory feedback. (One required subjects to perform a 3- to 5-minute task, and the other required subjects to get out of bed, cross the room, and record the time and sleep quality.) Both found significant reductions in SB lasting for up to 2 weeks upon discontinuation of the feedback.[57] A more recent single case study reported that reductions in bruxism frequency were maintained 6 months posttreatment.[58] Several additional one- and two-subject case studies of EMG feedback plus arousal, however, have yielded mixed results.[59-62]

More contemporary approaches have sought to improve biofeedback approaches by (1) delivering a stimulus that does not disrupt sleep and (2) improving upon SB detection algorithms to differentiate true bruxism episodes from benign parafunctional activities. A 5-night study ($n = 7$) explored afferent stimulation of the maxillary division of the trigeminal nerve using mild electrical stimulation of the lip during SB episodes.[63] The authors found significant reductions in SB event duration, but not frequency. Subjects did not report being awakened by the stimuli. Four small studies (sample sizes ranging from 11 to 19 subjects) have attempted to classically condition electrical stimulation to grinding and clenching behavior to extinguish SB. These studies, termed contingent electrical stimulation (CES), used a portable EMG device with advance signal processing features designed to differentiate grinding and clenching activity from other benign oral motor movements.[64-67] Patients precalibrate the device while awake by engaging in a variety of oral motor activities (e.g., grimacing, swallowing) and are able to adjust the level of the electrical stimulation so that it does not induce frank awakenings. Only one of the studies, however, used PSG to demonstrate that CES had no apparent effects on sleep architecture or continuity.[65]

These studies suggested that the device could discriminate between common parafunctional jaw muscle activity and SB and that feedback significantly reduced the number of SB episodes per hour. A 2014 systematic review of seven studies testing biofeedback treatments for SB, however, concluded that much of the literature was of poor quality, subject to bias, and found insufficient evidence that CES improved EMG measures of SB compared with controls.[68] A more recent (2018) meta-analysis, including six new studies (4 RCTs)[66,69-71] as well as two RCTs from the prior review, however, found that 5 nights of CES significantly reduced bruxism episode per hour, compared to control with no evidence that biofeedback substantially affected subjective sleep quality. Feedback in these studies included electrical, auditory, and vibratory stimuli. GRADE (Grading of Recommendations Assessment, Development and Evaluation)[72] analysis of the evidence quality ranged from low to moderate. Although there is mounting evidence supporting the short-term efficacy of CES, sustained long-term efficacy has yet to be investigated.

It should be noted that, although there are no evidence-based clinical diagnostic and management guidelines for ambulatory EMG-CES biofeedback, consensus-based guidelines recommend establishing a 2-week nonstimulus mode baseline followed by a 4-week active intervention phase. To promote long-term effects, the guidelines recommend a second 2-week baseline and 4-week active intervention phase.[73] Although the newer biofeedback approaches appear to have potential, larger and more rigorously designed longitudinal studies with long-term follow-up are needed.

Complementary and Alternative Interventions for Sleep Bruxism

Hypnotherapy

Hypnosis has been described as a state of focused attention involving intense concentration and inner absorption with a relative suspension of peripheral awareness.[74] Hypnotherapy often involves facilitating the patient's tendency to become engrossed in a perceptual or imaginative experience; promoting dissociation (mental separation of elements of experiences that would typically be processed together); and enhancing suggestibility (responding to subtle social and behavioral cues expressed by the patient, which increases likelihood of compliance with hypnotic suggestions).[74] Hypnotic procedures have been studied in the context of pain management,[75] the treatment of phobias,[76] and depression.[77]

There are a handful of published papers investigating the use of hypnosis in treating SB.[78-81] Most are case studies employing unstandardized methodology, self-report measures, and combined hypnotherapy with other intervention elements, precluding any conclusions about efficacy of hypnotherapy for SB. One uncontrolled study of eight subjects, however, incorporated EMG monitoring and found that SB activity was significantly reduced after a suggestive hypnotherapy intervention.[80] EMG data was not collected at follow-up assessment periods, so it is unclear whether the effects had any durability. Overall, because of the lack of methodological rigor and insufficient data, there is minimal evidence supporting hypnosis for SB.

Acupuncture, Physical Therapy, and Transcranial Magnetic Stimulation

Although the mechanism of action is unclear, acupuncture has been suggested as a potential treatment for bruxism. Acupuncture has been used to treat and ameliorate chronic facial pain related to TMD and mandibular dysfunction,[82-89] but there is a lack of evidence evaluating or demonstrating an effect of acupuncture on SB.

Physical therapy (PT) approaches for SB are varied, unstandardized, and include interventions such as electrotherapy, muscle exercises, muscle relaxation, postural procedures and awareness, and massage therapy. In addition to a lack of agreed-upon approaches, outcome measures are extremely heterogeneous, limiting the ability to draw conclusions across studies. Outcomes of physical therapy approaches range from muscle pain and activity, mouth opening, anxiety, stress, depression, sleep and oral health quality, and head posture assessed immediately after treatment or at other inconsistent follow-up periods. A recent review characterized the evidence supporting the efficacy of physical therapy for SB as very low because of poor methodological quality.[90] Although PT may have promise, its application with respect to SB requires development.

Repetitive applications of transcranial magnetic stimulation (rTMS) have been increasingly used for the management of depression, pain, and tinnitus.[91,92] A recent open-label pilot study (n = 12) used rTMS, applied bilaterally for 20 minutes daily for 5 consecutive days, to suppress corticobulbar pathways and inhibit jaw-closing muscle activity during sleep.[93] Participants used a portable, single-channel EMG recorder for 5 nights to establish baseline jaw-closing muscle EMG activity. During the intervention phase of the study, participants recorded jaw-closing muscle EMG activity during sleep on the nights after treatment. After the intervention phase, participants recorded jaw-closing muscle EMG activity during sleep for another 5 nights. The results showed that, compared to baseline, the intensity of jaw-closing EMG activity during sleep was suppressed both during and after rTMS. Decreases in clinical reports of jaw soreness were also demonstrated. Although the results are promising, further research, using randomized placebo controlled studies, are needed.[94]

Nutritional Supplements

Magnesium deficiencies have been associated with teeth grinding in sleeping and awake pigs.[95] Consequently, magnesium supplements have been suggested as a possible treatment for bruxism in humans[95,96]; however, these studies are small case reports; there are no RCTs. Studies investigating the efficacy of nutritional supplements[97-99] for bruxism are sparse and of insufficient scientific quality to support their use at this time.

CLINICAL PEARLS

- In general, there is insufficient evidence to strongly support pharmacotherapy for SB, but some medications, including anticonvulsants (gabapentin), alpha$_2$-adrenergic agonists (clonidine), GABAergic agents, and antihistamines (hydroxyzine, pediatric) warrant further study.
- The available evidence suggests that drugs prescribed to treat anxiety and depression are relatively poor candidates for treating SB, particularly selective serotonin and serotonin-norepinephrine reuptake inhibitors, which typically exacerbate SB.
- Botulinum toxin injections may be efficacious for SB (reduce amplitude of muscle activity, not its frequency) but should be reserved only for severe cases in which all other therapies have failed; the harmful consequences of SB are clear and outweigh the risks of adverse effects.
- With the exception of EMG biofeedback, many behavioral/psychosocial treatment approaches to SB are based on outdated conceptualizations of the pathophysiology of SB and, generally, lack strong empirical support for their efficacy.
- Currently, EMG-biofeedback devices vary in quality and capability. However, some studies support the efficacy of biofeedback treatment with or without arousal procedures. There is a need for larger RCTs that use standardized outcome measures to confirm and validate the efficacy of this treatment modality.
- CAM approaches to SB (i.e., hypnotherapy, acupuncture, physical therapy, nutritional supplements), in particular, are very limited and of insufficient scientific quality to support their use.
- Transcranial magnetic stimulation is a promising emergent approach to SB, which warrants attention but cannot be recommended at this early stage.

SUMMARY

To summarize the pharmacologic, behavioral, and complementary and alternative medicine (CAM) literature on SB, the general evidence base has been largely insufficient in terms of methodological rigor, and with some approaches the risk-to-benefit ratio must be carefully considered. None can be strongly recommended at this time.

With this said, with respect to pharmacologic approaches, BT is promising with a supportive preliminary evidence base. Clonidine is supported by two rigorous RCTs, but the potential serious side effect profile may limit its use to select cases, and medical collaboration is mandatory. Gabapentin is also promising, but limited to one RCT. Continued investigation of these pharmacotherapies is needed, and pharmacotherapy is obviously not a first-line approach in most individuals with SB. Furthermore, clinicians should exercise caution when using unapproved/unregulated medication (off-label use) for a specific condition and in presence of comorbidities (e.g., sleep apnea) or risk of addiction.

With respect to behavioral and CAM approaches, CES, EMG biofeedback, and TMS appear promising in terms of having plausible mechanisms of action and supportive preliminary data, especially CES because it is undergoing evaluation under rigorous protocols.

As the physiologic, behavioral, and psychological determinants of SB become well understood, novel pharmacologic, behavioral, and CAM interventions can be expected to be more readily developed and rigorously tested. This research gap is heightened by the fact that there is insufficient evidence for the effectiveness of standard oral splint treatment for SB.[100,101]

SELECTED READINGS

Bhattacharjee B, Saneja R, Bhatnagar A, Gupta P. Effect of dopalinergic agonist group of drugs in treatment of sleep bruxism: a systematic review [published online ahead of print, 2021 Jan 14]. *J Prosthet Dent.* 2021;(20):30752–30756.https://doi.org/10.1016/j.prosdent.2020.11.028. S0022-3913.

Carra MC, Huynh N, Lavigne G. Sleep bruxism: a comprehensive overview for the dental clinician interested in sleep medicine. *Dent Clin North Am.* 2012;56:387–413.

de Holanda TA, Castagno CD, Barbon FJ, Costa YM, Goettems ML, Boscato N. Sleep architecture and factors associated with sleep bruxism diagnosis scored by polysomnography recordings: A case-control study [published online ahead of print, 2020 Feb 19]. *Arch Oral Biol.* 2020;112:104685. https://doi.org/10.1016/j.archoralbio.2020.104685.

Huynh N, Lavigne GJ, Lanfranchi PA, Montplaisir JY, de CJ. The effect of 2 sympatholytic medications--propranolol and clonidine--on sleep bruxism: experimental randomized controlled studies. *Sleep.* 2006;29:307–316.

Lee SJ, McCall Jr WD, Kim YK, Chung SC, Chung JW. Effect of botulinum toxin injection on nocturnal bruxism: a randomized controlled trial. *Am J Phys Med Rehabil.* 2010;89:16–23.

Lobbezoo F, Ahlberg J, Raphael KG, et al. International consensus on the assessment of bruxism: report of a work in progress. *J Oral Rehabil.* 2018. https://doi.org/10.1111/joor.12663.

Manfredini D, Ahlberg J, Winocur E, Lobbezoo F. Management of sleep bruxism in adults: a qualitative systematic literature review. *J Oral Rehabil.* 2015;42(11):862–874. https://doi.org/10.1111/joor.12322.

Melo G, Duarte J, Pauletto P, et al. Bruxism: an umbrella review of systematic reviews. *J Oral Rehabil.* 2019;46:666–690.

Saletu A, Parapatics S, Anderer P, Matejka M, Saletu B. Controlled clinical, polysomnographic and psychometric studies on differences between sleep bruxers and controls and acute effects of clonazepam as compared with placebo. *Eur Arch Psychiatry Clin Neurosci.* 2010;260:163–174.

Winocur E, Gavish A, Voikovitch M, Emodi-Perlman A, Eli I. Drugs and bruxism: a critical review. *J Orofac Pain.* 2003;17:99–111.

A complete reference list can be found online at ExpertConsult.com.

From Childhood to Adulthood

Section 20

Chapter 177

Overview: Transition from Pediatric-Oriented to Adult-Oriented Health Care in Sleep Medicine

Stephen H. Sheldon

INTRODUCTION

Children are not just small adults. Anatomy, physiology, pathology, epidemiology, and pharmacology significantly differ. Therefore application of principles and practice of pediatric sleep medicine differs considerably when compared with adult sleep medicine. Comorbid factors also confound the practice of both disciplines. Children present a "moving target" through growth and development. Rapid changes occur during the first 2 years of life, settling into a more steady and regular pattern of maturation until puberty. After pubertal onset, again rapid changes occur in the growing adolescent. These changes then slow to mature into young adulthood.

Sleep-health concerns during childhood are addressed using developmental- and maturation-focused lenses. Transitioning from a child- or adolescent-centered approach to chronic medical conditions into a purposeful care model for adults is complex. Complexities of health care transition have been described by Reiss and colleagues.[1]

There have been significant advances in pediatric medical and surgical care. Children with complex disorders who, in the past, frequently did not survive the first decade of life, are now living productive lives into adulthood. Therefore there has become a significant need to transition care from child-oriented to adult-oriented practice.[2,3]

Transition has been defined as a purposeful, planned transfer of care from a pediatric-oriented to an adult-oriented health care provider/system in a timely, well-coordinated manner to provide continuous high-quality care. This effort should begin early, have clear coordination, and maintain focused lines of communication. Assessment of readiness of the patient and family for transition must be made and appropriately communicated.[4,5] Problems in transitional care exist, particularly lack of standardized practice guidelines and absence of evidence-based data. Barriers include methods of health care payment, absent mechanisms to ensure follow-up, and patient's lack of familiarity with adult-oriented systems of care.[6]

In sleep medicine, therefore, key elements required for successful transition have never been clearly defined. Nevertheless, professional organizations may take the lead in developing guidelines regarding professional and environmental support, decision making and consent, family support for transition, and professional sensitivity to psychosocial issues and disability. Successful transition programs may be modified from the adolescent young adult cancer programs. These may be embedded in an adult or pediatric institution, developed as a multidisciplinary program within a single city, created as a collaborative network partner model (hub and spoke), or be a single program that would cover multiple sites.[5]

Challenges are before us, particularly in sleep medicine. These include but are not limited to development of systems-level transitions; transition training for providers, families, and youth; and acknowledgment of factors affecting transition.[7] Three key elements seem to be required for successful transition. First, processes must be multifaceted and active. Timing must be individualized for each patient and condition (e.g., age of transition and length of the transition process). Finally, understanding transition to adult-oriented care (A-OC) for patients with severe functional limitations and complex medical conditions is more difficult and often requires more time and effort. The following examples may become a focus of discussion to develop appropriate guidelines.

PEDIATRIC OBSTRUCTIVE SLEEP APNEA

When a child is diagnosed with pediatric obstructive sleep apnea (OSA), diagnostic criteria, severity criteria, and primary therapeutic interventions differ considerably from those of the adult with OSA. Therefore professional environment and support require access of care to ensure A-OC is available in the community as well as assessing durable medical equipment needs and the differences between pediatric-oriented care (P-OC) and A-OC regarding reimbursement and follow-up. Partnerships must include the patient and family, the primary care provider, the pediatric sleep medicine specialist, and the adult-oriented sleep medicine specialist, as well as the DME provider. Coordination between professionals can focus on utilization and compliance as well as follow-up. Financing of the provision of treatment for OSA during and after transition requires sensitivity and understanding of the differences in reimbursement criteria for pediatric patients versus adult patients.

Decision making and consent suddenly shift from the parent/family to the patient, making access to care different. This would require partnerships in assessing the readiness of the young adult for transition as well as the practitioner's acceptance and understanding of this change in focus of decision making. Young adult and practitioner partnerships, careful concern regarding the timing of transition, and accountability for utilization of sleep medicine services and DME provisions. There must be continued coordination of monitoring and management of compliance and utilization and a refocus on financial responsibility because of reimbursement requirement differences. Because adolescents and young adults may have a significant change in their living situation, access to care may considerably change, and absence of family and support requires assessment. To successfully negotiate these changes, partnerships must be developed between family, primary care provider (PCP), pediatric sleep specialist, adult-oriented sleep specialist, and the school system. Coordination of insurance coverage by the family (and/or school or university) must include the sleep specialist and DME providers. Timing of transition requires considerable assessment of and individualization of the appropriateness for transition to adult-oriented care. Professional sensitivity to psychosocial issues and disability requires a shift and independence for use of positive airway pressure equipment and compliance. There is a significant shift of independence for responsibility of making and keeping follow-up appointments. Monitoring performance issues shifts from the school performance to work performance, driving, and other risky behaviors. There also is a considerable change in the assessment for responsibility for weight management.

NEUROMUSCULAR AND NEUROLOGICAL DISORDERS

Fulfilling the four factors of successful transition is much more difficult in children with neuromuscular disorders. Professional and environmental support are likely more available during the transition. However, access may be considerably variable. Additionally, A-OC professionals may be unfamiliar with pediatric diseases and disorders. Coordinators, particularly the PCP, may also not be familiar with the extent of these pediatric diagnoses (e.g., spinal muscular atrophy, mucopolysaccharidoses, Down syndrome and other chromosomal abnormalities, spina bifida with Chiari malformation). Decision making is also more difficult because of more profound developmental and maturational issues and competency in some patients. Nevertheless, there must be specific sensitivity to an underestimation of the abilities resulting from a particular medical disorder because many patients may be able to be competent in decision making regardless of disability. Family and support often include the extended family. Division of Services for Crippled Children has specific guidelines that should be understood by both the pediatric-oriented practitioner and adult-oriented practitioner. Social Security Administration as well as outside family support services should be available. Legal issues, such as power of attorney for health care, must be assessed and included in any transitional program. Health systems involvement is also essential. In patients with significant neuromuscular disorders, professional sensitivity to psychosocial issues and disability is clearly apparent. Many issues exist, and significant disability requires increased care coordination that may be best achieved with involvement of the PCP. Other involved professionals include but are not limited to specialists in sleep medicine, pediatrics, internal medicine, pulmonary medicine, neurology, surgery, physical therapy/occupational therapy, physiatry, otorhinolaryngology, and dentistry.

NARCOLEPSY

Although narcolepsy diagnosis most often occurs during adolescence, identification of narcolepsy (types 1 and 2) is occurring more frequently in the prepubertal child. Professional and environmental support must include education of adult-oriented professionals about the difference in diagnosis and management of pediatric narcolepsy. Many psychosocial differences occur. There must be a significant appreciation of differences in the approach to medication as well as differences in daytime responsibilities: there is a considerable shift between grade school, middle school, high school, college, and graduate school. This will then extend into the workplace. The locus of decision making and consent changes. This includes but is not limited to appointments and scheduling of follow-up visits, medication monitoring and ordering refills, and understanding school health services (school nurse within primary and secondary schools, university health services, and health care in the workplace). Changes in family and support can be significant. Health care professionals should involve understanding in the workplace with requests for accommodation for prophylactic naps, targeted benchmarks, and project timing. Responsibility and security for medications are also a focus of transitional care. Professionals must be sensitive to psychosocial issues and disability, driving and other hazardous behaviors, and participation in hazardous occupations. Further, they must understand medication changes and interactions between those that are typically prescribed for children and those that are prescribed for the adult patient.

CIRCADIAN RHYTHM DISORDERS

Professional and environmental support depends on the type of circadian rhythm disorder in neurologically normal children and those with other disabilities (e.g., those presenting with a free running circadian rhythm or an irregular sleep-wake cycle). This requires considerable understanding by the health professionals involved in the care of patients. Transfer from school, college, and workplace may be significant issues and may affect performance considerably. Circadian influences and behavioral and social influences must be considered.

Decision making and consent involves negotiating college and work schedules. Assessment of individual independence versus maturation and readiness for independence is crucial. Family and support typically involve continuation of health care insurance coverage with assessment of university health services and employee health services. There must be support of the school and workplace. Nap rooms may be a consideration. Continuation of phototherapy and lighting in the workplace is also important. Professional sensitivity to psychosocial issues and disability involve career choice guidance, counseling regarding sleep schedules on weekdays versus weekends, jet lag syndrome, and management of biologic rhythm variations. There also must be considerable attention paid to patients with vision impairment and other needs.

SUMMARY

There are four factors involved in successful transition programs: professional and environmental support and understanding, decision making and consent, family and support, and professional sensitivity to psychosocial issues and disability. Within each factor there must be assessment of appropriate access to care. Partnerships must be developed to facilitate transition. Coordination of care is essential for successful negotiation of systems, and appropriate timing of transitions requires particular assessment.

SELECTED READINGS

Cooley WC, Sagerman PJ. American Academy of Pediatrics; American Academy of Family Physicians; American College of Physicians; Transitions Clinical Report Authoring Group. Supporting the health care transition from adolescence to adulthood in the medical home. *Pediatrics.* 2011:182–200.

Gortmacher SL, Sappenfield W. Chronic childhood disorders: prevalence and impact. *Pediatr Clin North Am.* 1984;31:3–18.

Hobart CB, Phan H. Pediatric-to-adult healthcare transitions: current challenges and recommended practices. *Am J Health-Syst Pharm.* 2019;76:1544–1554.

Kirk V, Baughn J, D'Andrea L, et al. American Academy of sleep medicine position paper for the use of a home sleep apnea test for the diagnosis of OSA in children. *J Clin Sleep Med.* 2017;13(10):1199–1203. https://doi.org/10.5664/jcsm.6772. Published 2017 Oct 15.

Newacheck PW, Strickland B, Shonkoff JP, et al. An epidemiologic profile of children with special health care needs. *Pediatrics.* 1998;102:117–123.

Osborn M, Johnson R, Thompson K, et al. Models of care for adolescent and young adult cancer programs. *Pediatr Blood Cancer.* 2019:e27991.

Reiss J, Gibson R. Health care transitions: destinations unknown. *Pediatrics.* 2002;110:1307–1314.

Reiss JG, Gibson RW, Walker LR. Health care transition: youth, family, and provider perspectives. *Pediatrics.* 2005;115:112–120.

Chapter 178

Sleep-Related Breathing Disorders in Children

Tanvi H. Mukundan; Irina Trosman; Stephen H. Sheldon

Chapter Highlights

- As they approach adulthood, children with sleep-disordered breathing must be transitioned toward the care that will be provided by nonpediatricians. In this chapter, we review the unique nuances of this transition.
- There are additional challenges in the transition of care from pediatric to adult sleep medicine providers for medically complex patients with sleep disorders given their special needs.
- Sleep-disordered breathing in patients with Down syndrome, Prader-Willi syndrome, and congenital central hypoventilation syndrome is reviewed.
- We also outline the transition of care recommendations for patients with pediatric obstructive sleep apnea (from any cause), specifically those using positive airway pressure devices.
- Potential approaches and general principles for clinical transition are presented.

INTRODUCTION

The transfer of care for patients with chronic medical conditions from the pediatric to adult medical systems may present a significant challenge. This process typically occurs between the ages of 18 and 20 years and depends on the local jurisdiction, physician's office, institutional policies, the patient's and/or family's preferences, as well as insurance regulations. Pediatric patients often develop strong bonds with their pediatric sleep providers and may have difficulty transitioning to the adult providers, partially because of different practice styles between pediatric and adult clinicians.[1,2] Also, adult physicians often lack experience in treating childhood diseases and in dealing with adolescents and young adults with developmental disabilities.[3,4,5]

Change in insurance coverage, access to care, and, in the case of sleep medicine, different diagnostic criteria for pediatric and adult sleep disorders may create additional obstacles during this transition period. These challenges and the absence of a well-coordinated transition process may lead to a loss of follow-up, gaps in medical care, and subsequent detrimental outcomes. Thus the importance of an organized transition process cannot be understated, especially for patients with special needs and complex medical problems.

In 2002 the American Academy of Pediatrics, American Academy of Family Physicians, and American College of Physicians–American Society of Internal Medicine *Consensus Statement on Health Care Transitions for Young Adults With Special Health Care Needs* was released; it recommended clear and organized care transition guidelines for this vulnerable patient population.[6] Despite these clear guidelines, there is a paucity of well-organized transition process models and guidelines. The few models and guidelines that exist are primarily for patients with hemophilia, cystic fibrosis, congenital heart disease, and diabetes mellitus.[3,6] However, there are virtually no formal pediatric to adult care transition sleep programs in the United States. This is true even in academic practices and community clinics that have separate pediatric and adult specialists.

This chapter focuses on the transition of care of patients with obstructive sleep apnea (OSA). Congenital central hypoventilation syndrome is discussed, which can have a later onset and more mild symptoms; patients therefore survive well into adulthood. This chapter also covers care specific to patients with sleep disorders in the context of Down syndrome (DS), as this population represents a large and challenging portion of the pediatric sleep medicine population, as well as Prader-Willi syndrome (PWS).

TRANSITION OF CARE FOR OBSTRUCTIVE SLEEP APNEA

Pediatric OSA is part of the spectrum of pediatric sleep-disordered breathing, which also includes primary snoring. OSA can result in hypoxemia, hypercapnia, and sleep fragmentation, leading to daytime challenges and long-term health concerns. Pediatric conditions that often manifest OSA include DS and PWS and the neurologic conditions detailed in Chapter 179. Other disorders associated with OSA in the pediatric population that adult physicians may be unfamiliar with include achondroplasia, mucopolysaccharidoses (Hunter and Hurler syndromes), and rare conditions associated with craniofacial abnormalities (Table 178.1).

The presentation of OSA in the pediatric patient is wide and varied. The most common findings on history include frequent snoring, labored breathing during sleep, mouth

Table 178.1 Disorders with Anatomical Factors Contributing to Pediatric Obstructive Sleep Apnea[61,62]

Category	Syndromes	Anatomical features predisposing to OSA
Mucopolysaccharidoses	Hurler, Hunter syndromes	Upper airway soft tissue infiltration by macromolecules
Craniofacial clefts (lip and palate)	Pierre Robin sequence, Stickler, Treacher Collins, Goldenhar, and Nager syndromes	Short mandible, retrognathia, nasal deformity
Craniosynostoses	Apert, Cruzon, Pfeiffer, Muenke, and Saerthe-Chozen syndromes	Midface hypoplasia
Micrognathia	Pierre Robin sequence, Treacher Collins syndrome	Micrognathia, glossoptosis, midface hypoplasia
Achondroplasia	Short-limb dwarfism	Midface hypoplasia, retrognathia

Data from Shapiro J, Strome M, Crocker AC. Airway obstruction and sleep apnea in Hurler and Hunter syndromes. *Ann Otol Rhinol Laryngol.* 1985;94(5):458–61; Cielo CM, Marcus CL. Obstructive sleep apnoea in children with craniofacial syndromes. *Paediatr Respir Rev.* 2015;16(3):189–96.

breathing, gasping or snorting during sleep, sleep-related enuresis, sleeping upright, sleeping with the neck hyperextended, witnessed apneas, cyanosis, morning headaches, and behavioral concerns including difficulty with attention, learning, and focus.[7] Children have a greater ventilatory drive and thus have higher upper airway tone during sleep and can maintain greater airway patency.[8] An apnea-hypopnea index (AHI), or the frequency of obstructive apneas and hypopneas averaged per hour of sleep, of less than 1 per hour of sleep, is considered normal. An AHI of 1 to 5 per hour of sleep is classified as mild, 5 to 10 per hour is moderate, and an AHI of greater than 10 per hour is considered severe. Thus the criteria used to categorize the severity of OSA in children are markedly different from adults, in whom an AHI of 5 or more is considered abnormal.

The overall incidence of pediatric snoring is estimated between 10% and 25%, with pediatric OSA incidence between 1.2% and 5.7%.[7] It is likely that this value may be an underestimation of the true prevalence of OSA. This likely occurs as a result of multiple factors, including the common belief that children will simply grow out of snoring.

Untreated OSA has a variety of effects on children, both from a cognitive and metabolic standpoint. Early studies found that children with OSA who underperformed academically had a significant increase in the mean grades after OSA was treated compared with those children with OSA who were not treated.[9] Further evaluation revealed that worse cognitive outcomes were found in children with OSA who had a greater degree of inflammation assessed with high-sensitivity c-reactive protein.[10] Thus it was understood that the same inflammatory processes seen in adult OSA were also present in pediatric patients.

The most common pediatric OSA treatment is adenotonsillectomy (AT), because the most common etiology for pediatric OSA is adenotonsillar hypertrophy. The effectiveness of the AT in resolving pediatric OSA ranges from about 70% to 90%, depending on the study.[11] For those children who continue to have moderate to severe OSA after surgical intervention, or for whom surgical intervention is contraindicated or is inappropriate, positive airway pressure (PAP) should be considered.[7] Many children who have pediatric sleep apnea that starts earlier than age 10 will often outgrow their sleep apnea. However, those diagnosed after age 10 and children who are obese have a much higher risk of continuing to have sleep apnea as they age.[12] Unfortunately, at this time, there are no formal or well-described transitional care programs specifically for OSA. The transition of care need is most pronounced in patients being treated for OSA with PAP therapy. PAP is very effective at treating OSA; however, success rates are low, with most studies showing less than 50% PAP compliance.[13]

Down Syndrome

DS is the most common chromosomal disorder causing learning disability.[14,15] According to the Centers for Disease Control's 2008 data, more than 250,000 children, teens, and adults live with DS in the United States.[15a] The life expectancy of people with DS increased dramatically over the last few decades, and individuals with DS are now often living into their 60s.[16] This demographic change has been attributed to an overall increase in the number of babies with DS born to older mothers and a life expectancy prolongation for individuals with DS, especially in developed countries. The median age of patients with DS is 49 years, and the life expectancy of a 1-year-old child with DS is more than 60 to 65 years.[14] Thus pediatric providers see more patients with DS, and more adolescents with DS are now transitioning care from pediatric to adult medicine. OSA is more common in children with DS, with an estimated prevalence of 30% to 55% compared with otherwise healthy children (2%).[15-19] Risk factors for OSA in children with DS include hypotonia, macroglossia, tonsillar and adenoid hypertrophy, and anatomic features such as midfacial hypoplasia, an increased incidence of lower respiratory tract anomalies, and reduced tracheal diameter.[20,21]

Because of the high incidence of OSA in children with DS, the American Academy of Pediatrics (AAP) issued health supervision guidelines in 2011. These guidelines advocate for the creation of a medical home to facilitate pediatric providers in caring for children with DS, screen for sleep disorders (as well as other conditions commonly associated with DS), and facilitate their transition to adulthood. Pediatric providers should discuss symptoms of OSA (e.g., heavy breathing, snoring, uncommon sleep positions, frequent night awakening, daytime sleepiness, apneic pauses, and behavior problems) with parents at least once during the first 6 months of life and annually after that. Children with DS suspected to have an underlying sleep disorder should be referred to a physician with expertise in pediatric sleep disorders for further evaluation. In addition, an in-lab sleep study or polysomnogram (PSG) is recommended for all children with DS by 4 years of age to screen for OSA, as there is a poor correlation between parent report and PSG results.[22-24]

Like in the general population, PSG remains the gold standard for the diagnosis of OSA in patients with DS. Use of limited channel screening mechanisms such as pulse oximetry and capnography is not of sufficient sensitivity to diagnose OSA in patients with DS.[25]

Notably, PSG in patients with DS has revealed more severe degrees of OSA and greater rates of hypoventilation than in individuals without DS.[26] Hypoventilation correlated with elevated body mass index is considered to be obstructive in etiology; however, it may also be due to underlying restrictive lung disease or hypotonia. Additionally, patients with DS may have other pulmonary characteristics such as lower functional reserve capacity, pulmonary hypertension, recurrent pneumonia and/or aspiration, or interstitial lung disease, which may explain the increased prevalence of sleep-related hypoxemia in addition to OSA.[27,28] As patients with DS age, disorders such as hypothyroidism and obesity increase in prevalence.[29]

The prevalence of OSA in adults with DS is even higher than in the pediatric population and is estimated to be 78% to 90%. The increased prevalence may be related to obesity and hypothyroidism superimposed on the same predisposing factors for pediatric OSA. OSA in adult patients with DS is associated with hypoventilation, sleep disruption, decreased slow wave sleep, and greater intermittent hypoxemia.[16] These factors are thought to contribute to the mechanism of further deterioration of cognitive function and memory in individuals with DS, who are already at increased risk of Alzheimer disease.[30]

In addition, sleep in adults with DS is characterized by increased sleep fragmentation and circadian disruption.[31] Decreases in nocturnal total sleep time have been detected from polysomnographic data and are partially attributed to daytime napping as detected by daytime actigraphy.[32] Adults with DS may have severe sleep disorders that are not detected by self-reported sleep measures or reported by caregivers.[32] This may be related to questionnaires that reflect the caregivers' perceptions as opposed to the patient experience.

The DS population is also at increased risk for mental health problems, including depression, anxiety, obsessive-compulsive tendencies, developmental regression during adolescence, behavioral issues, and autism spectrum disease.[33] Subsequently, new behavioral sleep problems may emerge in addition to already existing sleep disorders. All the aforementioned conditions pose additional challenges for the management of sleep problems in this population.

The care of the patients with DS, as well as any pediatric patient with complex medical problems and sleep disorders, should be delivered through a multidisciplinary team, led by physicians educated and prepared to deal with the specific needs of this population. This team should include otolaryngologists, weight management specialists, psychologists, and sleep providers.

Otolaryngologists are more commonly involved in the care of patients with DS because of frequent middle ear disease and OSA. AT is still considered to be the first-line therapy for children with DS and OSA; however, the success level is lower than in the general population. Postoperatively, between 50% and 75% of patients with OSA and DS will have clinically significant residual sleep-disordered breathing.[34,35]

Other surgical interventions (supraglottoplasty in infants, tongue base reduction, lingual tonsillectomy, turbinate coblation, uvulopalatopharyngoplasty, and midface advancement in older patients) are frequently considered in individuals with DS and persistent considerable OSA. Drug-induced sleep endoscopy is often performed to determine which procedure(s) will be of greatest benefit.

Last, there have been new modalities developed for the treatment of refractory OSA in DS: for example, hypoglossal nerve stimulation (HNS). In a recent study performed by Diercks and colleagues, adolescents with comorbid DS and OSA demonstrated improvements in obstructive sleep apnea syndrome severity with an AHI (56% to 85% reduction) and quality-of-life scores after 6 to 12 months of HNS use.[36]

Patients with DS often require additional treatment with positive pressure ventilation (CPAP and bilevel PAP) for sleep-disordered breathing. Acclimation and compliance with PAP therapy are frequently very difficult. Behavioral interventions, desensitization programs, close relationships with durable medical equipment providers, and a close line of communication with the patient's family are extremely important. It is important to note that nonsurgical management of OSA in patients with DS requires significant support. Therefore the role of the sleep specialist is essential.

Obesity is frequently a major component of OSA, and weight management among patients with DS must be addressed by appropriate health providers.

The paucity of data on the transition process for youth with OSA translates to youth with DS and OSA.

Congenital Central Hypoventilation Syndrome

Congenital central hypoventilation syndrome (CCHS) is a rare congenital disorder of the autonomic nervous system that affects multiple body systems with a hallmark of disordered respiratory control. CCHS is typically identified in the neonatal period. About 20% of the cases will also have Hirschsprung disease; the combination is called Haddad syndrome. These children have abnormal ventilatory responses to hypoxemia and hypercapnia, leading to severe hypoventilation, which is most severe in non–rapid eye movement sleep. The patients have a normal respiratory rate but a reduced tidal volume.

CCHS is due to an abnormality of the *PHOX2B* gene, typically polyalanine repeat mutations (PARMs). The shorter PARMs may present with subtler findings. Therefore these individuals are diagnosed with late-onset central hypoventilation syndrome (LO-CHS) later during childhood or in adulthood and may present with symptoms or sequelae of untreated hypoventilation or difficulty weaning off of a ventilator in the setting of sedation or acute respiratory illness.[37]

There is no available cure for CCHS, and most patients require supportive care throughout the life span. Treatment is focused on maintaining ventilation. This can be accomplished with tracheostomy and mechanical ventilation. Diaphragm pacing by phrenic nerve stimulation is now used in some ambulatory children who require continuous ventilatory support. As with any rare disease with profound morbidity and mortality without therapeutic intervention, multidisciplinary care in a specialized center is most appropriate.[38] Because of the complexity of CCHS-related problems and the need for multispecialty involvement, care for patients with CCHS is usually provided at the pediatric tertiary care centers. Many issues must be addressed as a young person with CCHS begins the transition to adulthood, including transition preparation readiness assessment, transition plan, medical summary, discussion of living arrangement safety and home care, access to transportation, availability of medical providers with appropriate expertise in CCHS, and insurance coverage. Most of these issues are not unique to CCHS; however, the rarity of this genetic condition may present a significant challenge in finding appropriate care providers and a multidisciplinary team with appropriate expertise in CCHS. Thus, because of the underlying complexity of CCHS, most patients remain at CCHS specialty centers across the nation into adulthood.

Rapid-Onset Obesity With Hypothalamic Dysfunction

When hypoventilation takes place in the context of hyperphagia, rapid weight gain, and hypothalamic dysfunction, rapid-onset obesity with hypothalamic dysfunction (ROHHAD), a rare disorder, should be suspected as opposed to CCHS.[39] ROHHAD is not associated with the *PHOX2B* mutation and usually presents in early childhood (typically between ages 3 to 10 years) as opposed to during the neonatal period; however, the same subspecialized, multidisciplinary team is required given the presence of life-threatening hypoventilation. There is a high incidence of respiratory arrest, and many patients will require mechanical ventilation.

Prader-Willi Syndrome

PWS is a rare, complex genetic disorder associated with hypothalamic dysfunction, early morbid obesity with hyperphagia, short stature, intellectual deficiencies, and behavioral problems, endocrine dysfunction, and sleep disturbances. A multidisciplinary care approach is usually adopted to provide care for pediatric patients with PWS, including experts in genetics, endocrinology, nutrition, pulmonology and sleep, behavior, occupational and speech therapy, and social work.[40,41]

Sleep problems in PWS include altered sleep architecture, impairment in ventilatory control responses to hypoxemia and hypercapnia,[42] central sleep apnea (in children who are less than 2 years old),[43,44] OSA (in children older than 2 years old), and narcolepsy-like disorder.[45] OSA rates among children with PWS are as high as 44% to 100%,[43,46] as opposed to 2% to 3% of children in general community samples.[47] Risk of OSA in patients with PWS is mostly obesity related; however, other factors such as hypotonia, facial dysmorphism, restriction in lung volume secondary to obesity, and scoliosis are contributing factors.[44] OSA in patients with PWS may persist despite AT. Growth hormone therapy (GHT) is now considered to be a standard of care for patients with PWS. GHT increases lean body mass, improves linear growth,[48] and improves resting ventilation, ventilatory response to CO_2,[49] and behavioral problems.[50] GHT therapy risks include OSA resulting from accelerated growth of lymphoid tissues and a potential link to sudden death within the first 9 months of GHT initiation.[51] Therefore screening of adenotonsillar hypertrophy, hypothyroidism, and PSG are required before starting growth hormone. PSG is also repeated 8 to 10 weeks after initiating treatment.[41] However, sudden death in PWS has also been reported in the absence of GHT treatment and in patients treated with GHT with concurrent respiratory insufficiency or respiratory infection.[52,53]

Because of a variety of behavioral and mental health problems, including anxiety and obsessive-compulsive disorder, patients with PWS may be treated with psychotropic medications, including topiramate, selective serotonin receptor inhibitors, and antipsychotics. Side effects of these medications include weight gain, further contributing to obesity-related increased risks of OSA. In addition, patients with PWS may develop obesity hypoventilation syndrome.[54]

EDS and narcolepsy-like disorder have been reported in patients with PWS and may be related to obesity, OSA, and hypothalamic dysfunction.[55] Modafinil therapy has been reported to provide some benefits for the patients with PWS and EDS.[56,57]

The mortality rate of adult PWS is approximately 3% per year[58] as compared with that of 1% per year for the general population, and the average age of death was 33 years.[59] Because of the complexity of PWS, a multidisciplinary team of adult physicians, similar to the pediatric model, should be involved in the care of older patients with PWS. Adult sleep physicians should be aware of sleep problems in patients with PWS, including increased risks for persistent sleep-disordered breathing and EDS. Therefore we suggested sleep-disordered breathing screening and treatment as a standard of care for adult patients with PWS.

General Principles for a Clinical Transition Program

As children age into adulthood, it is imperative that conscientious choices are made about providing continuity of care for OSA treatment (Box 178.1). There are multiple challenges of the transition process from pediatric to adult sleep medicine providers. Adult sleep centers may have less multidisciplinary support staff, such as social workers and care coordinators in outpatient clinics. In addition, there may be a lack of sedation services, sleep psychologists, and/or child life specialists frequently available in large pediatric centers during procedures, sedation, and CPAP desensitization. For patients with complex medical disorders, including the patients whose life span dramatically increased in the last few decades, it may be very difficult to find an adult provider educated and prepared to take care of this unique population. Even when adult providers and services are identified, access to these is frequently limited, especially for patients with disabilities severe enough to be eligible for publicly funded insurance coverage.

Other barriers may include lack of accommodations for patients with autism, such as quiet waiting areas, reliance on adult caregivers to bring patients to medical appointments, and transportation issues. Many pediatric patients, especially those with special needs or complex medical conditions, are unprepared for the autonomy and ability to self-advocate that adult institutions expect. These issues are not unique to patients with sleep disorders and, unfortunately, are common among pediatric patients with special needs. Because of these reasons, pediatric sleep doctors and patients' families are frequently reluctant to transfer care to adult providers.

At the Hospital for Sick Children (Sick Kids) in Toronto, Canada, the sleep clinic created a formalized structure for care transitions that started well before adolescence. This

Box 178.1 GENERAL CONSIDERATIONS FOR THE TRANSITION FROM PEDIATRIC TO ADULT CARE

- Discussions regarding the transition to adult care should start in advance, ideally beginning at age 12 to 14.
- Medical providers, including the sleep medicine team, should create an institutional or department policy addressing the system's approach to the transition process. This policy should be discussed with the patients and families.
- Ideally, one sleep medicine team member (a nurse or a physician assistant) should oversee this transition process and assist the families.
- A list of adult medical providers with appropriate expertise in sleep disorders should be offered to the patients' families.
- The family should check adult providers' availability and insurance information in advance.
- Transfer of care should take place when the family is ready and the patient is stable and prepared for transfer of care.
- Parents and caregivers of children with intellectual disabilities should be advised to apply for legal guardianship.
- A package of detailed medical records and medical passport with a brief transition summary of a patient's diagnosis, evaluation, and interventions should be prepared. A transition summary should ideally also include the current treatment plan, relevant labs/test (i.e., sleep study results summary), PAP settings (for patients using PAP devices), and the patient's DME provider. The use of EMR can facilitate this process. This package should be sent to the identified adult provider, along with the pediatric provider's contact information.
- Pediatric sleep medicine providers should be accessible to adult providers until the transfer of care has been completed.

program was created because of very poor show rates when patients transitioned from their pediatric sleep provider to their adult sleep provider. This program focused on educating the parent and the patient and empowering patients early on to understand their diagnoses. The program then planned a transition over 6 to 9 months to ensure that the adult providers were also educated on the unique challenges of caring for young adults.[60] This provided both structure and education to help this vulnerable population. Similar programs and protocols should be developed by pediatric sleep centers in the United States.

Thus the main goal of any transition program is to create a seamless transfer of care. It is important to identify a time when it is possible to transition patients from pediatric to adult care. This is variable from patient to patient and can occur at many points during adolescence, depending on the maturity and autonomy level of the patient. The provider may consider having a list of adult providers for the patient. Ideally, sleep medicine providers would also partner with primary care providers to ensure that they are aware of the sleep issues and help to address any possible gaps in care. Because pediatric sleep apnea can be treated with PAP, it is important to ensure that medical equipment coverage continues to the new provider. Pediatric and adult sleep apnea have different scoring criteria; thus it is important to understand that there may be some financial and insurance reimbursement changes that occur during the transition period as well.

CLINICAL PEARLS

- The transfer of care for pediatric patients with chronic medical conditions and sleep disorders to adult medical providers may present a significant challenge.
- Patients and their families may be facing multiple barriers, including lack of appropriate communications among providers, insurance coverage limitations, and difficulties finding an adult provider with appropriate expertise.
- There are no existing guidelines nor well-organized transition process models for pediatric patients with sleep disorders in the United States.
- Each pediatric sleep center should strive to develop a well-organized transition program that should involve the current primary sleep provider, program coordinator, and social worker.
- Discussions and planning of transition to adult care should start in advance.
- The transition summary should ideally include the current treatment plan, relevant labs/tests, PAP settings (for patients using PAP devices), and the patient's DME provider. This information should be forwarded to the identified adult provider, along with the pediatric provider's contact information.
- Pediatric sleep medicine providers should be accessible to families and adult providers until the transfer of care has been completed.

SUMMARY

Transitions from pediatric to adult sleep medicine care must be further investigated. Different models may be adopted for private centers and academic institutions. We recommend a proactive, individualized, well-coordinated, multidimensional, and collaborative approach between patients, families, and providers. Appropriate medical documentation, effective transfer of medical records, communication with durable medical equipment companies, monitoring guidelines, attended sleep studies, actigraphy, and an interdisciplinary approach are extremely important, especially for complex medical patients, including patients with intellectual disabilities.

SELECTED READINGS

American Academy of Pediatrics, American Academy of Family Physicians, American College of Physicians -American Society of Internal Medicine. A Consensus statement on health care transitions for young adults with special health care needs. *Pediatrics*. 2002;110(6):1304–1306.

Cooley WC, Sagerman PJ. Supporting the health care transition from adolescence to adulthood in the medical home. *Pediatrics*. 2011;128:182–200.

Gozal D. Diagnostic approaches to respiratory abnormalities in craniofacial syndromes [published online ahead of print, 2021 Sep 17]. *Semin Fetal Neonatal Med*. 2021:101292. https://doi.org/10.1016/j.siny.2021.101292.

Health PCfMaC. Transition to Adult Healthcare Services Work Group Recommendations that Have Clinical Applicability. Available online: https://www.pcmch.on.ca/health-care-providers/paediatric-care/pcmch-stra.

Heffernan A, Malik U, Cheng R, Yo S, Narang I, Ryan CM. Transition to adult care for obstructive sleep apnea. *J Clin Med*. 2019;8(12). https://doi.org/10.3390/jcm8122120.

Heffernan A, Malki U, Cheng R, et al. transition to adult care for obstructive sleep apnea. *J Clin Med*. 2019;8:2120. https://doi.org/10.3390/jcm8122120.

McDonagh JE, Kelly DA. Transitioning care of the pediatric recipient to adult caregivers. *Pediatr Clin North Am* 2003;50:1561–1583.

Nagra A, McGinnity PM, Davis N, Salmon AP. Implementing transition: ready steady go. *Arch DisChild Educ Pract Ed*. 2015;100:313–320.

Prior M, McManus M, White P, Davidson L. Measuring the "triple aim" in transition care: a systematic review. *Pediatrics*. 2014;134:e1648–e1661.

Strategies-and-initiatives/transition-to-adult-healthcare-services/ (accessed on 1 November 2019).

White PH, Cooley C. Supporting the health care transition from adolescence to adulthood in the medical home. *Pediatrics*. 2018;142:1–22.

A complete reference list can be found online at ExpertConsult.com.

Chapter 179

Neuromuscular and Neurological Disorders

Craig Canapari

Chapter Highlights

- Improvements in the care of children with complex neurologic disorders have allowed many individuals with previously fatal disorders to survive into adulthood. Thus there is a growing need for transition programs to help these individuals and their families successfully move their medical care from the pediatric to the internal medicine world. Transition is a fraught period that may be associated with worsening medical status.
- Transition care is complicated by several factors, notably the variety of disorders that may be unfamiliar to internal medicine specialists; the complex needs of some individuals, especially those with more severe phenotypes of neuromuscular disease, epilepsy, and cerebral palsy; and the different structure of pediatric and internal medicine clinics.
- A structured transition program beginning in early adolescence and involving both the child and parents will help prepare the family for a successful transition. There are multiple dimensions to transition including medical, legal, financial, and social domains. The provision of a staff member to serve as a single point of contact may be very helpful. Research is very limited now as to what components of a transition program are most predictive of a successful transition.

BACKGROUND

Advances in the medical and surgical care of children with complex, chronic medical conditions have resulted in an increasing number of children with medically complex conditions surviving into adulthood, when previously they would have received all of their care in the pediatric health care system.[1,2] Every year, an estimated 500 to 750,000 young people with special health care needs become adults.[3–5] Many of these individuals have permanent disabilities.[6] Specifically, there has been an exponential increase in the survival of children requiring long-term ventilation.[7]

In spite of this, there is limited research on the best way to move these individuals from the pediatric to the adult health care system.[8] Most pediatric providers are not satisfied with the current transition programs at their institutions. Thirty percent of providers caring for children with neurologic problems were "not at all satisfied" with their current transition program.[9] When transition guidelines exist, relatively few providers are familiar with them.[10] Many institutions do not have written transition plans in place.[11,12] Of 17,000 adolescents with special needs, only 40% have discussed crucial transition topics such as finding an adult provider and transitioning insurance coverage with their current providers.[12a]

RATIONALE FOR TRANSITION OF CARE

The American Academy of Pediatrics recommends a coordinated approach to transitioning children to adult care, with the goals of helping young adults navigate health care, education, and employment successfully.[13] Transitioning adolescents to appropriate adult health care settings is a goal of Healthy People 2020.[14] Yet only about 17% of youth with significant health care needs are meeting very basic criteria for transition readiness, defined as having (1) spoken alone with their clinician at a visit, (2) worked with a clinician on self-care and understanding the health care transition that occurs at age 18, and (3) discussed transition care with their provider.[15] Pediatricians do not routinely discuss adult issues (e.g., adult sexuality, employment, or placement for disabled adults).[8] Children's hospitals lack support for issues such as job placements and have less experience with adult onset disorders.[3] Pediatric providers are typically used to having open communication with parents or guardians, whereas adult providers are more experienced in managing patient privacy by, say, obtaining permission to talk to parents. Adult providers are more experienced with guiding families through medicolegal issues such issues such as power of attorney, medical proxy, guardianship, and end of life care—key domains for youth with chronic disease and intellectual disability.[13]

Implementing appropriate transition planning is often difficult. There is a marked disparity in transition services between difference services. The transfer feels chaotic to many patients. In the adult system, there is limited multidisciplinary support.[13] All stakeholders involved may have some bias toward the status quo, leading to a delay in transition. Pediatric providers who have often cared for affected youth since the time of diagnosis often have difficulty letting go of patients, and youth often have little incentive to leave their comfortable care settings. Parents are reluctant to be sidelined in care decisions, which is more common in adult care settings. Finally, adult-centered providers often have received limited training or experience in dealing with pediatric onset disorders or transitional care.[16] Pediatric providers may have significant difficulty identifying adult providers well suited to caring for youth with unique needs rendered by significant neurodevelopmental compromise.[3] Therefore patients and their families may find it especially difficult to navigate adult transitions.[16] Additionally, special needs such as communication and physical limitations require additional time, space, and equipment (e.g., as lifts) that may not be readily available in some clinics.[17] Young adults with developmental disabilities often have depression, anxiety, stress, and poor self-esteem that result in poor social interaction and decreased coping skills.[18]

Implementing appropriate transition planning is critical for the continued success and health of patients, and is also important for pediatric institutions. Care of adults in children's institutions is frequently burdensome, both in terms of effects on hospital culture and in terms of cost. Adults are frequently readmitted and the cost of care may be higher than for children.[3,19] Decreased support at the time of transition can result in life-threatening illnesses, increased emergency room visits, more frequent hospitalizations, and distrust of the adult health care system. A lack of good services fostering independence can lead to increased health care needs and decreased participation in society.[20,21] The period of transition seems to be a vulnerable one, as deterioration in health is common.[22–26]

Navigating the transition in insurance and services can be particularly tricky for this patient population. Often, services such as physical therapy that are covered in the US public school system by the federally mandated Individuals with Disabilities Act may not be covered by medical insurance and end during the year of the individual's 21st birthday or upon high school graduation. After this, individuals become responsible for payment through insurance or out-of-pocket payments.[18,27] Adult Medicaid is not as comprehensive, and many patients may lose benefits.[28] Changing insurance can lead to changes in durable medical equipment providers and pharmacies.[29] Compounding this is the fact that many people with chronic disabilities are either unemployed or underemployed, making employer-sponsored health care unavailable.[30-32] The Affordable Care Act (ACA) has provisions to help with transitional care and improve access such as eliminating discrimination based on preexisting conditions. As a result, many Americans with disabilities continue to be covered under Medicaid, Medicare, or both.[18,33]

TRANSITION CARE BY CONDITION

The conditions covered in this chapter represent a range of neurologic disorders. Affected individuals have several common traits that may make it difficult for them to navigate the transition to adulthood. These conditions may be associated with variable degrees of cognitive and physical disabilities. Additionally, they may have complex medical needs across multiple domains and a dependence on other caregivers for activities of daily living.

Cerebral Palsy

Cerebral palsy (CP) is a group of chronic, lifelong conditions that affect body movement, muscle tone, and coordination in the context of static insult to one or more specific area of the brain during the fetal or perinatal period. Generally, CP is not progressive, although secondary conditions (e.g., scoliosis or contractures) may be.[34,35] CP is the most common motor disability of childhood, with 1 of 323 American children receiving the diagnosis.[36,37] In addition to motor limitations, CP can be associated with other developmental problems such as intellectual disability, epilepsy, and vision and hearing impairment.[38] Adults with CP are living longer, with an estimated population of 400,000 to 500,000 affected individuals in the United States.[39]

Increased longevity in individuals severely affected by CP has resulted in a need for more transitional care but difficulties in communication, learning, mobility, and feeding may hinder the ability of patients to navigate the adult-centered health care system. This is exacerbated by the lack of multidisciplinary services for adults with chronic illness, a dearth of adult providers interested in chronic disorders of childhood, and a lack of training opportunities for adult providers.[16] The combination of complex health needs superimposed on the fragmented adult health care system can result in significant difficulties for youth and their families.

The health of individuals with CP seems to worsen as they enter their twenties, with poor general health reported in 21% of individuals with CP between ages 20 and 22 years of age, versus 9% of children in the 15- to 18-year-old age group.[40] In spite of this, a survey of young adults with CP found that only 28% had assistance coordinating care, 29% had discussed transition care, and only 44% of their providers had discussed the changes in insurance that occurs at age 21.[41] Young adults have decreased access to care and rehabilitation and feel more isolated than they did in adolescence,[8,40] even as medical utilization increases over time.[42] At least some of this seems to be due to the fact that young people starting transition have a range of unmet health needs that tend to worsen worse during transition.[43] Minimal standardization is present for transition criteria. Age is the most common criteria for transition, although parent/caregiver initiation and the social/developmental status of the child is often taken into account.[8] Satisfaction by pediatricians of these transition practices is extremely low, with no physicians in a survey completely satisfied and 27% "not at all satisfied."[8]

A recent meta-analysis suggested that more than 20% of children with CP were affected by sleep disorders.[44] Sleep-disordered breathing is especially common. Multiple factors predispose CP patients to sleep problems, including

- Upper airway obstruction due to glossoptosis and poor pharyngeal muscle tone

- Visual impairment resulting in issues with sleep timing and maintenance
- Brainstem dysfunction, which may affect cardiac and respiratory control
- Postural limitations, which can cause pain and sleep discomfort
- Epilepsy treatment, which can disrupt normal sleep wake patterns
- Chronic pulmonary aspiration, which can decrease pulmonary reserve[45]

Little is known about the prevalence of these disorders in affected adults, but given the fact that it is a static disorder (albeit with progressive secondary complications), the prevalence is likely equal to or higher than that in children.

Spina Bifida

Spina bifida is the most common congenital neural tube defect, accounting for approximately 1500 births in the United States every year.[46] The mildest form is spina bifida occulta, which may occur in 5% of the population and is characterized by incomplete formation of one or more vertebral arches; it usually has no clinical sequelae. Spina bifida may be associated with meningoceles, outpouching of the meninges outside of the vertebral column. Myelomeningocele, in which the spinal cord is exposed, is always associated with Chiari II malformation, with herniation of the cerebellum and medulla into the spinal column.[47] A case series showed that 81% of children with myelomeningocele had sleep-disordered breathing (SDB). About 28% had predominantly central sleep apnea (CSA), with the majority having obstructive sleep apnea (OSA). After decompression surgery, the apnea-hypopnea indices improved overall but persistent CSA and OSA was common.[48] Hypoventilation may also occur. Critically, sleep apnea, along with female sex and a midbrain elongation 15 mm or greater on MRI, was associated with an increased risk of sudden death in young adults with myelomeningocele. It is unclear if treatment of sleep apnea reduces this risk given continuous positive nasal airway pressure (CPAP) use was noted in some of the patients who died.[49] Treatment options for SDB include oxygen, CPAP, otolaryngology evaluation, and invasive ventilation.[50,51] In addition to diagnosed SDB, spina bifida patients report poor sleep quality, reduced sleep, increased insomnia, and increased daytime fatigue more commonly than age-matched controls.[52]

One survey of pediatric neurosurgeons found that only 37% of SB clinics had a transition plan in place, with many surgeons following their patients into adulthood[53] given concerns surrounding the absence of coordinated multidisciplinary care for their adult patients. The providers noted that development of transition care guidelines, improved provider collaboration, and development of an advanced training pathway for adult providers would be helpful to improve transition.[54] One clinical model is a transition clinic staffed by a physicians treated in One transitional clinic model described in the literature included staffing by a physician trained in medicine and pediatrics, as well as a nurse and social worker, who would develop an individualized transition plan for patients.[55]

Conditions with Neuromuscular Weakness

Neuromuscular disorders encompass a range of diseases characterized by a genetic basis and progression of neuromuscular weakness. Some disorders, such as Duchenne muscular dystrophy and spinal muscular atrophy, have severe effects on the respiratory system and result in chronic respiratory failure. Other disorders, such as myotonic dystrophy, may have a milder respiratory course but other complications germane to the sleep physician. The advent of new treatments has resulted in increased lifespan for individuals who historically have died in childhood.

Duchenne Muscular Dystrophy

Duchenne muscular dystrophy (DMD) is an X-linked disorder due to mutations in the dystrophin gene that results in progressive destruction of muscle cells over time. The disorder typically presents with motor or developmental delay in early childhood and has an incidence of 1 in 5000 male births. DMD is associated with cognitive and learning disabilities in many individuals., with 27% of patients having IQs less than 70.[56] Learning disabilities, attention deficit hyperactivity disorder, and autism may occur. Cardiomyopathy is common, and currently due to advancements in the use of respiratory technology, cardiac issues are the primary cause of mortality.[57] Untreated individuals typically lose the ability to walk by 12 years of age and die by their mid-twenties. Medical treatments (specifically corticosteroid treatment) and respiratory therapies have greatly improved the survival of affected individuals.[58] A survival analysis showed that the mean age at death was 14.4 years in the 1960s, 25.3 years in the 1990s, and is now in the forties.[59]

Becker muscular dystrophy is also caused by mutations in the dystrophin gene but has a milder phenotype in terms of muscle weakness, typically with a loss of the ability to ambulate without assistance by 15 years of age. Cognition is usually spared.[60]

From a respiratory standpoint, forced vital capacity (FVC) tends to increase while patients are ambulating, plateau when they are starting to lose ambulation, and then decrease once using a wheelchair full time. There can be marked variation in the peak and rate of decline even in patients with the same genotype.[57,61]

Myotonic Dystrophy

Myotonic dystrophy (DM) is the most common muscular dystrophy among adults of European ancestry, with a prevalence of 1 in 7400 to 1 in 10,700 in Europe.[62–64] It comprises two major forms, DM1 and DM2. Both are clinically and genetically heterogeneous disorders inherited in an autosomal dominant fashion and associated with myopathy, cataracts, and cardiac conduction disease.[65] As DM2 tends to present in adulthood, with an age at onset typically in the third to sixth decade, transition is generally not a concern.[66] It is phenotypically milder as well.

In DM1, the severity of the disease is governed by an increasing severity with increasing numbers of trinucleotide repeats:

- Congenital DM1 is the most severe form. It presents in infancy with hypotonia, poor feeding, congenital joint contractures, and respiratory failure.[67] Up to 70% to 80% of patients may require mechanical ventilation. Mortality is up to 40% in severely affected infants.[68]
- Childhood DM1 presents before the age of 10 years, usually with cognitive and behavioral problems such as low IQ, attentional and executive problems, and mood problems.[69]

Muscle symptoms and physical disability develop over time.[67]

- Classic DM1 usually becomes symptomatic during the second, third, or fourth decade. Major associated problems include respiratory muscle weakness, myotonia, cataracts, cardiac arrhythmias, and excessive daytime sleepiness (EDS). Average lifespan is reduced.[67,70]
- Mild DM1 presents typically after age 40 with mild weakness, myotonia, and cataracts. Lifespan is normal.[70]

From a respiratory standpoint, restriction on lung function testing is common, as is alveolar hypoventilation. The observed respiratory dysfunction is not simply a function of muscle weakness[71] and is not completely understood. Testing of central respiratory drive has shown variable results, with some studies showing abnormalities[72,73] but other showing a normal CO_2 response.[74,75]

EDS is the most frequent nonmuscular complaint in DM1, being present in 70% to 89% of patients.[76] This seems to be due to a central dysfunction of sleep regulation and not simply SDB,[77] although it may be multifactorial. Methylphenidate[78] and modafinil[65,70] have both been shown to be effective in EDS in DM1. Polysomnography (PSG) should be performed in all patients with significant restriction on pulmonary function testing, EDS, or suspicion of apnea.[79]

Little is written about transition care in adolescents with DM1. Transition may be complicated by intellectual disability, communication problems, apathy, irritability, fatigue, and sleepiness, all of which are common in affected adolescents[80].

Mitochondrial Disorders

The primary mitochondrial disorders are caused by mutations in nuclear or mitochondrial DNA that cause metabolic issues with oxidative phosphorylation.[81] They may be spontaneous or heritable. True prevalence is difficult to determine given variable symptoms. Overall the prevalence is likely between 5 and 15 of 100,000 persons and reflects that these disorders are among the most common inherited metabolic and neurologic disorders.[81]

Developmental disabilities, myopathy, and epilepsy are common features in many mitochondrial disorders[82] and may affect sleep. Additionally, CSA, OSA, decreased ventilatory response to hypercarbia/hypoxia, and hypoventilation may all occur in mitochondrial disorders.[83,84] The current recommendations for patients with primary mitochondrial disease is that PSG be obtained based on clinical symptoms.[85]

Spinal Muscular Atrophy

Spinal muscular atrophy (SMA) is a group of genetic disorders all associated with degeneration of the anterior horn cells of the spinal cord, which results in muscle atrophy, weakness, and loss of deep tendon reflexes. The most common form is caused by a mutation in the *SMN1* gene and occurs with a frequent of 1 in 10,000 live births in the United States.[86] Subtypes range from type 0 (usually requiring invasive ventilation at birth with death occurring before 1 month of age) to type 4, with the diagnosis usually occurring in adulthood. Types 1 and 2 typically require ventilatory support in childhood due to progressive respiratory failure and recurrent pneumonia. In spite of the profound associated weakness, cognition is typically normal.[87] For type 1 infants, noninvasive ventilation is typically started at the time of diagnosis, as it improves both survival and quality of life.[12,88]

Understanding of the natural history of SMA, especially the more severe phenotypes, is in flux as a result of the advent of exciting new therapies for the treatment of this disorder. Historically, the majority of infants with type 1 would die before 2 years of age without continuous respiratory support.[89–91] Nusinersen, an antisense oligonucleotide given intrathecally, was approved by the U.S. Food and Drug Administration in 2016 as the first disease-modifying therapy for SMA. A double-blind trial showed a significant reduction in the risk of death or permanent ventilation.[92] Onasemnogene abeparvovec is a one-time gene replacement therapy approved in the United States in 2019 for infants less than 1 year of age. The initial trial showed that all treated subjects were alive and did not require permanent ventilation, compared with 8% of a historical cohort.[93] It is unclear what the long-term prognosis will be of treated children, but possible that adult clinics may be encountering treated young adults in the next few decades.

Myasthenia Gravis

The myasthenic syndromes are due to issues with transmission and the neuromuscular junction. Myasthenia gravis (MG) is an autoimmune disorder in which autoantibodies bind to acetylcholine receptors on the postsynaptic membrane on the neuromuscular junction, resulting in weakness of skeletal muscles.[94] The annual incidence is 8 to 10 cases per million, with a prevalence of 150 to 250 cases per million.[95] In children, the disorder takes three forms: transient neonatal myasthenia, congenital myasthenic syndromes, and juvenile myasthenia gravis (JMG).[96] The first occurs in infants born to mothers with MG and is usually self-limited and resolving, although affected infants may need respiratory support and/or treatment in early infancy. Congenital myasthenic syndromes are not autoimmune in origin. Rather, they are a group of disorders caused by alterations in the structure or function of proteins in the neuromuscular junction.[97] These disorders have a wide range of severity. Juvenile myasthenia gravis presents before the age of 19 years. Treatment options include acetylcholinesterase inhibitors, immunosuppressive agents, and thymectomy (if a thymoma is present). Respiratory insufficiency may occur as a result of diaphragmatic and intercostal weakness, especially during periods of stress such as surgery.[94] MG has been shown to be associated with poor sleep quality and excessive daytime sleepiness.[98] OSA is also common, with an estimated prevalence of 36% in adults.[99]

The Respiratory Care of Neuromuscular Patients

The use of non-invasive ventilation (NIV) and assisted cough has greatly reduced mortality and morbidity. Assisted cough is usually performed with a cough assist device several times a day and as needed. The benefits of NIV include normalizing gas exchange, lowering symptom burden, decreasing hospital admissions, and improving health related quality of life.[100] Nighttime NIV delays daytime hypercapnia, increases endurance and improves survival.[101] Newer guidelines[102] suggest an earlier start to NIV based on any of these criteria:

- Lung function testing findings of forced vital capacity (FVC) less than 50% predicted or maximum inspiratory pressures (MIP) less than 60 cm H_2O
- Awake baseline Spo_2 less than 95% or Pco_2 greater than 45 mm Hg
- Pulse oximetry abnormalities:
  - $ETCO_2$ or TCO_2 greater than 50 mm Hg for 2% or more of sleep time
  - Sleep-related increase in $ETCO_2$ or $TcCO_2$ of 10 mm Hg over awake baseline for 2% or more of sleep time
  - Spo_2 88% or less for 2% or more of sleep time or for at least 5 minutes continuously
  - Apnea-hypopnea index 5 or greater[61,103]

Overnight oximetry is not adequate to rule out hypoventilation in patients with neuromuscular weakness. Most patients have healthy lungs and are on the flat part of their oxyhemoglobin disassociation curve.[61] Annual PSG is recommended once an individual is using a wheelchair full time. It is unclear how frequently this should be monitored once a patient is using NIV at night.

There is little research comparing volume versus pressure ventilation in patients with neuromuscular weakness, although pressure ventilation will compensate better for mask leak, so it is probably a good first choice. Some patients with severe restriction will need volume ventilation.[105] Volume guaranteed pressure modes provide benefits from both volume and pressure controlled ventilation, although they are less studied and may result in more frequent arousals from sleep if there are large pressure swings.[106,107] Positive end expiratory pressure (PEEP) should be kept low unless absolutely necessary. High PEEP should be avoided, as it may reduce cardiac output and cause abdominal bloating.[105] Titration may be complex because of central apneas, glottic closure, asynchrony, and pseudocentral events, which may complicate finding appropriate settings.[106,107]

As neuromuscular disease progresses, daytime ventilation may be necessary as well, if oximetry is less than 95%, CO_2 is greater than 45 mm Hg, or if there is breathlessness during the day. In patients with DMD the disease will progress to this degree in all patients, usually in the third decade. Pressure or volume ventilation with a "sip and puff mode" delivered via a straw may greatly help with gas exchange, breathlessness, and even weight loss.[108,109] For many patients, continuing on NIV 24 hours a day, via mask or mask and mouthpiece, may be adequate. However, tracheostomy may be considered if the patient cannot manage secretions, cannot tolerate NIV, or failed to tolerate extubation after a critical illness. Of note, that patients who are dependent on NIV may still be extubated successfully after surgery or illness provided that they have clear lung fields on chest radiograph, are on room air, and are not sedated and able to cooperate with airway clearance and NIV.[110] Oxygen therapy without associated ventilation should be avoided in patients with neuromuscular weakness. Low oximetry is usually due to mucus plugging (best managed with airway clearance) or hypoventilation (best managed with ventilator support).[111]

Transition care presents special challenges in progressive neuromuscular disorders. During a time when most adolescents are moving toward independence, patients with progressive weakness are becoming more reliant on both family members and technology. In spite of this, there are no transition guidelines specific to neuromuscular disorders, nor do most centers have a standard protocol for transitioning technology-dependent patients to adult care.[29,112] Families and patients find the transition stressful, as they have often been seeing the same provider since early childhood and are often surprised by the degree of autonomy and self-advocacy expected in the adult system.[113]

Various countries have approached the problem of caring for these patients. In Japan, the majority of adults with DMD live in one of 27 specialized wards that provide comprehensive care, an arrangement that may not be acceptable in other communities or cultures.[114] For the past 10 years, a network of specialists in Paris have been voluntarily meeting monthly on a Saturday morning, without pay, to work out the transition needs of patients with complex neuromuscular disorders. Advances in these disorders is creating a large population of children with previously lethal disorders who are growing into adulthood. Spinal muscular atrophy, with the advent of gene therapy and small molecule therapy, may result in the first generation of patients with SMA type 1 surviving to adulthood.[115]

Organizations involved in the care of children and adults with neuromuscular disease have produced some tools to help with transition care. The Muscular Dystrophy Association has a detailed Road Map to Independence to help adolescents with the process of transition.[116] Parent's Project Muscular Dystrophy, another organization, has produced a detailed resource page for adolescents and young adults with DM,[117] as well as an emergency wallet card[118] and smartphone application.[119]

Epilepsy

Epilepsy is one of the most common chronic neurologic diseases of childhood.[120] It is characterized by recurrent, unprovoked seizures and is an umbrella term for multiple different seizure disorders. Some, such as benign Rolandic epilepsy, childhood idiopathic occipital epilepsy, and childhood absence epilepsy, tend to remit. Other disorders such as juvenile myoclonic epilepsy are lifelong conditions.[121] Depending on the type of epilepsy, developmental delay may occur. A full review of the classification of epilepsy types is beyond the scope of this chapter but a recent article provides a good overview.[122]

Seizures remit in about 50% to 80% of children with epilepsy.[123] The remainder will continue to require care for epilepsy and require transition to adult health care providers.[120] Significant comorbidities occur in adolescents with epilepsy, including attention deficit hyperactivity disorder, anxiety disorders, and depression—all disorders that may be associated with sleep disorders.[115]

There is a complex interplay between epilepsy and sleep. Good sleep hygiene is critical for seizure prevention. Non–rapid eye movement sleep and sleep-wake transitions are common times for seizures to occur.[124] EDS is a common complaint in epilepsy patients independent of seizure frequency, type of epilepsy syndrome, or presence of sleep-related seizures.[125] OSA is common in patients with refractory epilepsy.[126] Treatment with CPAP in affected individuals may help significantly with seizure control.[127] Other sleep disorders, such as central sleep apnea, restless legs syndrome/periodic limb movement disorder, and insomnia are also common in affected individuals.[128]

Transition care remains a work in progress in epilepsy, as in many of the other disorders noted in this chapter. One

Shared management model

Age and time	Provider	Parent/family	Youth
↓	Major responsibility	Provides care	Receives care
	Support to parent/family & child/youth	Manages	Participates
	Consultant	Supervisor	Manager
	Resource	Consultant	Supervisor/CEO

Kieckhefer GM., & Trahms CM. Supporting development of children with chronic conditions: From compliance toward shared management. Pediatric nursing 2000;26(4):354-363.

Figure 179.1 Shared management model.

survey of young adults with epilepsy showed than only 15% recall having discussed transition care with their pediatric provider.[129] Eighty percent of families felt that their child had had insufficient opportunities to develop autonomy.[22] Ideally, the idea of transitioning should be introduced between ages 12 and 16, with discussion of self-advocacy and educational/vocational training by age 16.[130,131] In Ireland, the Temple Star transition clinic is a transition group from adolescence that includes group discussions about disclosing epilepsy to peers, and lifestyle issues such as alcohol consumption, sleep hygiene, and stress management. Psychosocial support, negotiating driving regulation, and education and vocational goals and medication management are also addressed.[132] In Canada, a recent task force put together a seven-step process to prepare patients for transition, which included an assessment of risk factors for unsuccessful transition and a reassessment of the epilepsy diagnosis.[120]

BEST PRACTICES FOR TRANSITION CARE

Transition care for young adults with neurologic disorders requires a coordinated, stepwise approach. In the shared management model of transition care (Figure 179.1), the overall goal is to move youth from a model in which they are the passive recipient of care, through participation, management, and finally acting in a supervisory or "CEO" role.[120,133] The latter description is particularly apt for patients with disabilities, as learning to work with aides is a critical skill.

The key elements of a successful transition program will include consideration[16] of several key factors.

1. Timing: Will it occur at a given chronologic age, or based on developmental or social attainments such as graduating from high school or college?
2. Preparation: How long should this period be? The current thinking is that transition should be discussed in early adolescence, and that, ideally, time should be set aside at every visit to discuss transition program.
3. Coordination: Incorporation of feedback from the patient, his/her family, the patient's primary care provider, and adult providers who will be receiving the patient.
4. Involvement of both adult and pediatric services. Often, pediatric services handle the bulk of the burden of transitioning complex patients, with the result that crucial details may not be communicated clearly to the adult team. Better communication can help things go more smoothly for both parents and providers.
5. Developmentally appropriate health care. This means both assessing and tailoring approaches based on the cognitive ability of the patient, and also the patient's interaction style.[16,134,135]

The current guidelines for DMD highlight several important domains to consider during transition (Figure 179.2), all of which are worthy of consideration will all of the conditions described in this chapter.[136] It recognizes that the health care transition occurs in the context of potential changes in housing, transportation, education/employment, relationships with others, and activities of daily living. A recently published transition toolkit includes a transition readiness assessment, transition checklist, and medical summary form.[28]

FUTURE DIRECTIONS

The study of transition care for young adults with complex neurologic disorders is in its infancy. Although validated outcomes for transition care exist,[137] there is a lack of robust evaluation of transition care programs.[29] A recent Cochrane review showed only four small randomized control trials examining the efficacy of transitional care models.[23] Only one of the studies examined the conditions described in this chapter. This examined the efficacy of a 2-day transition preparation course for patients with spina bifida and showed no benefit in terms of the main end point of subjective well-being, role mastery, or self-care practice.[138]

In 2016 the UK's National Institute for Health and Clinical Excellence published a guideline identifying nine potential proposed beneficial features of transition clinics.[139] A cohort study of young adults in the United Kingdom with autism, type 1 diabetes, or cerebral palsy looked at these features and found that three of them were associated with improved outcomes. "Appropriate parental involvement" (both parent and patient happy with the degree of the parent's involvement in care), "promotion of health self-efficacy" (reflecting that the patient is satisfied with the help received in independently managing his or her condition), and "meeting the adult team prior to transfer" were all associated with increased well-being, satisfaction with services, and participation in care.[135]

CLINICAL PEARLS

Although the variety of neurologic disorders covered in this chapter are daunting, there are a few themes shared by them that should be focused on by the sleep physician. The primary one is the management of sleep-disordered breathing and/or hypoventilation. It is critical to use in-laboratory polysomnography with capnography to assess and manage these patients. Transcutaneous capnography can be particularly helpful if you are treating hypoventilation, as end tidal capnography cannula can interfere with mask fit. Additionally, patients may suffer from insomnia and/or hypersomnia. Given the complexity of some of these patients, nonmedical treatments and slow titration of any medications may be the best place to start.

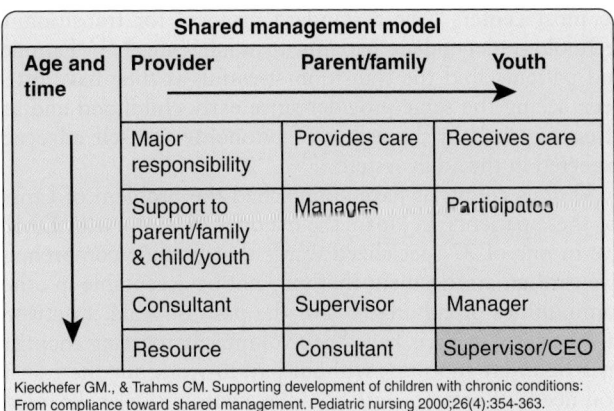

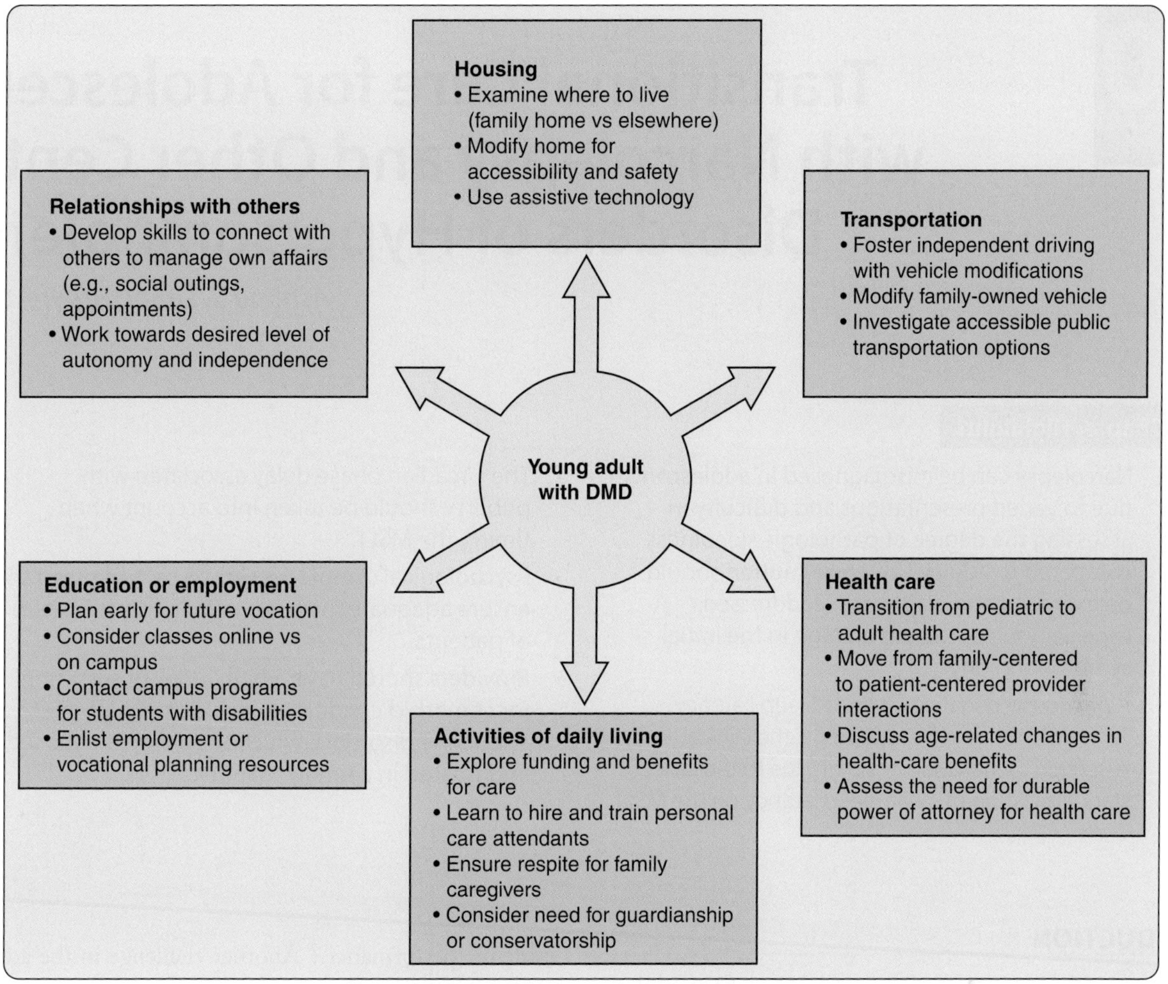

Figure 179.2 Duchenne muscular dystrophy transition.

SUMMARY

Implementing high-quality transition plans is potentially expensive and time consuming. It is clear from a review of the literature that are meaningful markers of successful transition programs need to be better defined for future study.[13] Additionally, transition care needs to be part of the residency curriculum for pediatric and adult residents.[13] The future is brighter than ever for many young adults suffering from chronic disease. Finding the best way to provide ongoing care and fostering health and independence is an exciting challenge.

SELECTED READINGS

Andrade DM, Bassett AS, Bercovici E, et al. Epilepsy: transition from pediatric to adult care. Recommendations of the Ontario epilepsy implementation task force. *Epilepsia*. 2017;58:1502–1517. https://doi.org/10.1111/epi.13832.

Binks JA, Barden WS, Burke TA, Young NL. What do we really know about the transition to adult-centered health care? A focus on cerebral palsy and spina bifida. *Arch Phys Med Rehabil*. 2007;88:1064–1073. https://doi.org/10.1016/j.apmr.2007.04.018.

Birnkrant DJ, Bushby K, Bann CM, et al. Diagnosis and management of Duchenne muscular dystrophy, part 3: primary care, emergency management, psychosocial care, and transitions of care across the lifespan. *Lancet Neurol.* 2018;17:445–455. https://doi.org/10.1016/S1474-4422(18)30026-7.

Burke L, Kirkham J, Arnott J, Gray V, Peak M, Beresford MW. The transition of adolescents with juvenile idiopathic arthritis or epilepsy from paediatric health-care services to adult health-care services: a scoping review of the literature and a synthesis of the evidence. *J Child Health Care*. 2018;22:332–358. https://doi.org/10.1177/1367493517753330.

Cheng PC, Panitch HB, Hansen-Flaschen J. Transition of patients with neuromuscular disease and chronic ventilator-dependent respiratory failure from pediatric to adult pulmonary care. *Paediatr Respir Rev*. 2019. https://doi.org/10.1016/j.prrv.2019.03.005.

Colver A, Rapley T, Parr JR, et al. *Facilitating the transition of young people with long-term conditions through health services from childhood to adulthood: the Transition research programme.* Southampton (UK): NIHR Journals Library; May 2019.

Crowley R, Wolfe I, Lock K, McKee M. Improving the transition between paediatric and adult healthcare: a systematic review. *Arch Dis Childhood.* 2011;96:548–553. https://doi.org/10.1136/adc.2010.202473.

Onofri A, Tan HL, Cherchi C, et al. Transition to adult care in young people with neuromuscular disease on non-invasive ventilation. *Ital J Pediatr.* 2019;45. https://doi.org/10.1186/s13052-019-0677-z.

Sheehan DW, Birnkrant DJ, Benditt JO, et al. Respiratory management of the patient with duchenne muscular dystrophy. *Pediatrics*. 2018;142:S62–S71. https://doi.org/10.1542/peds.2018-0333H.

Trout CJ, Case LE, Clemens PR, et al. A transition toolkit for duchenne muscular dystrophy. *Pediatrics*. 2018;142:S110–S117. https://doi.org/10.1542/peds.2018-0333M.

White PH, Cooley WC. Supporting the Health Care Transition From Adolescence to Adulthood in the Medical Home. 2018;142:22.

A complete reference list can be found online at ExpertConsult.com.

Chapter 180

Transitional Care for Adolescents with Narcolepsy and Other Central Disorders of Hypersomnolence

Ashima S. Sahni; Hrayr Attarian

Chapter Highlights

- Narcolepsy can be misdiagnosed in adolescents due to varied presentations and difficulty in assessing the degree of pathologic sleepiness compared to adults. Therefore caution should be exercised and diagnoses readdressed, especially when there is change in the initial symptomatology.
- A previously negative Multiple Sleep Latency Test (MSLT) should be repeated if the clinical suspicion for narcolepsy is high due to the lack of standardization of mean sleep latency on the MSLT.
- The circadian phase delay associated with puberty should be taken into account when timing the MSLT.
- Psychological symptoms should be addressed to ensure adequate mental health in this subgroup of patients.
- Providers should have a high index of suspicion for comorbid conditions, including metabolic/endocrine disorders, which should be diagnosed and treated in a timely manner.

INTRODUCTION

The American Academy of Pediatrics (AAP) defines adolescence as the decade spanning ages 11 to 21. Multiple international health organizations have recognized the unique health needs of adolescents during this pivotal phase of their lives. The AAP has also pointed out the vulnerability of this population because of a dearth of proper transitional care resources.[1] Hypersomnia is a serious condition, which impacts quality of life, including school performance and choice of employment, along with direct impact on health-related costs. Thus missed or late diagnosis with inadequate treatment carries greater social and economic burden. This chapter will discuss the challenges of transitioning care of adolescents with central disorders of hypersomnolence, pitfalls of misdiagnoses and erroneous treatments, and mitigation strategies.

Narcolepsy types 1 and 2 (NT1 and NT2, respectively), idiopathic hypersomnia, and Kleine-Levin syndrome are included in the central disorders of hypersomnolence, and this chapter will focus primarily on narcolepsy. For detailed discussions on epidemiology, pathophysiology, presentation, diagnosis, and treatment of each of the central disorders of hypersomnolence please refer to Chapters 111 to 114.

NARCOLEPSY

Clinical Symptomatology

Excessive Daytime Sleepiness

Excessive daytime sleepiness (EDS) is the hallmark of narcolepsy but is often overlooked by parents and only brought to attention when it starts adversely affecting mood, behavior, or academic performance.[2] Another challenge in the adolescent patient population is the variability in total sleep requirement per 24 hours across the 10 years of adolescence. In addition, the circadian phase delay that accompanies puberty results in sleep deprivation, which can complicate the evaluation of EDS in adolescents.

Compared to adults, sleep attacks are longer (Table 180.1) and manifest in a waxing and waning pattern of drowsiness in younger adolescents during passive activities.[3] Some individuals in this age group may exhibit restlessness, increased motor hyperactivity, aggressive behavior, inattentiveness, and increased emotional lability instead of drowsiness, which can be misleading at times, delaying the timely diagnosis of narcolepsy and management.[4,5] The modified Epworth Sleepiness Scale (ESS) and Pediatric Daytime Sleepiness Scale (PDSS) are age-specific tools to assist with the evaluation of sleepiness and are discussed in greater detail later in the chapter.

Illustrating the barriers to appropriate evaluation and treatment, a 2008 investigation of 290 adolescents with EDS found that only 34 (11.7%) were seen for this symptom over a period of 4 years. The average age in this Brazilian cohort was 13.5 ± 4.1 years, and the average duration of symptoms before seeking medical help was 3.0 ± 3.5 years. Narcolepsy was confirmed in 13 out of 34 (38%) with polysomnography (PSG) and the Multiple Sleep Latency Test (MSLT).[6]

Cataplexy

The presence of cataplexy differentiates NT1 from NT2 in the absence of a cerebrospinal fluid (CSF) assay for orexin levels, which is rarely pursued. Cataplexy has a polymorphic

Table 180.1 Clinical Presentation of Narcolepsy Features in Adolescents Compared to Adults

Clinical Features	Adolescents	Adults
Sleep attacks	1–180 sec but can have multiple episodes prolonging the total duration[9]	A few seconds up to 30 min
Cataplexy	Usually involves face May not have an emotional trigger Becomes less severe with age	Typically triggered by emotions
Hypnagogic/ hypnopompic hallucinations	Prevalence of 50%–66% Simple images and sounds, less frightening	Prevalence of 45%–60% Almost 95% are formed visual and frightening hallucinations
Sleep paralysis	Prevalence of 29%–60%	Prevalence of 38%–70%
Other features	Attention deficit and hyperactivity (31%) Neuropsychological problems in ≈62% (despite normal IQ) Prevalence of depression is 25%	When controlled of daytime sleepiness neuropsychological function is near normal in adults Prevalence of depression is 30%
REM sleep behavior disorder	Prevalence of RBD is 25%	Prevalence of RBD is 10%–15%

IQ, Intelligence quotient; RBD, REM sleep behavior disorder; REM, rapid eye movement.

presentation in adolescents, with 50% having late onset. The occurrence of cataplexy in childhood narcolepsy is reported between 60% and 75%[7] and up to 92% in adolescence.[6] The features distinguishing adolescent from adult cataplexy are detailed in Table 180.1.

"Cataplectic facies" are a common manifestation characterized by a droopy look involving facial grimace, tongue protrusion, mouth opening, and/or facial weakness, which can be easily mistaken for a seizure disorder.[8] A rostrocaudal progression of weakness has also been described in some children, starting from the face and then spreading to the trunk, arms, and lower limbs, eventually leading to a fall.[9] The severity of cataplexy may improve with age. Unlike adults, cataplexy in this age group can occur without an emotional trigger. Some authors have also described cataplexy in this population as a complex movement disorder with hypotonia (negative phenomena) and dyskinetic-dystonic movements (active phenomena), such as "tics."[10,11]

Hypnagogic Hallucinations/Sleep Paralysis

Like cataplexy, hypnagogic hallucinations and sleep paralysis are thought to represent episodic intrusion of rapid eye movement sleep (REM) into wakefulness.[12] However, hypnagogic hallucinations and sleep paralysis may be absent in many adolescent patients with narcolepsy and is distinct from the presentation recognized in adults (Table 180.1). For example, sleep paralysis and hypnagogic hallucinations were identified in 23% and 46% of patients, respectively, in a Brazilian cohort.[6]

Clinical Assessment Tools

There remains a dearth of validated measures for assessing cataplexy and EDS in the pediatric population. This need is usually filled by modification or adaptation of existing adult measures.

Modified Epworth Sleepiness Scale

The ESS was initially developed in 1990 to evaluate sleepiness in adults, but some questions are not applicable to adolescents. In the past, studies have used ESS as such for adolescents, some have modified the questions, and some have introduced new items, making it impossible to compare and validate. Adaptations included change in the question from "sitting quietly after a lunch without alcohol" to "sitting quietly after lunch"; "sitting inactive in a public place, for instance, a theater or meeting" to "sitting inactive at school"; or "in a car, while stopped for a few minutes in the traffic" to "doing homework or taking a test."[13–15] The modified questionnaire, the ESS-CHAD (the ESS for children and adolescents, Table 180.2) was found to have internal validity and a unidimensional structure with good model fit; however, internal validity for use in patients younger than 12 years has not been established, and external validity and cut-off values have not been determined.[16,16a] The PDSS can be found in Table 180.3, and

Table 180.2 Epworth Sleepiness Scale for Children and Adolescents

Scale

0 = Would never fall asleep
1 = Slight chance of falling asleep
2 = Moderate chance of falling asleep
3 = High chance of falling a sleep

Activities	Score
Sitting and reading	
Sitting and watching TV or a video	
Sitting in a classroom at school during the morning	
Sitting and riding in a car or bus for about half an hour	
Lying down to rest or nap in the afternoon	
Sitting and talking to someone	
Sitting quietly by yourself after lunch	
Sitting and eating a meal	

Modified from Janssen KC, Phillipson S, O'Connor J, Johns MW. Validation of the Epworth sleepiness scale for children and adolescents using Rasch analysis. *Sleep Med.* 2017;33:30–5.

Table 180.3 Pediatric Daytime Sleepiness Scale

Score 4 = Very often, always 3 = Often, frequently 2 = Sometimes 1 = Seldom 0 = Never					
Please answer the following questions as honestly as you can by circling one answer only:	4	3	2	1	0
How often do you fall asleep or get drowsy during class periods?					
How often do you get sleepy or drowsy while doing your homework?					
Are you usually alert most of the day?[a]					
How often are you ever tired and grumpy during the day?					
How often do you have trouble getting out of bed in the morning?					
How often do you fall back to sleep after being awakened in the morning?					
How often do you need someone to awaken you in the morning?					
How often do you think that you need more sleep?					

[a]Score this item in reverse order.
The Pediatric Daytime Sleepiness Scale was developed for middle-school children (age 11–15 years) but has not been directly compared to any existing questionnaires, although this scale has the ease of administration and robust psychometric properties. The eight questions are scored 0–4 by the child, with higher scores indicating greater sleepiness.
Modified from Drake C, Nickel C, Burduvali E, et al. The Pediatric Daytime Sleepiness Scale (PDSS): sleep habits and school outcomes in middle school children. *Sleep*. 2003;26(4):455–8.

other self-report tools to assist with the quantification of sleep and sleepiness are described in the left-hand column of Table 180.4.

Diagnostic Tools

Various tools can be used to provide objective data in support of a diagnosis of narcolepsy (Table 180.4) and are discussed more extensively in Chapters 112 and 207.

Pitfalls of the Multiple Sleep Latency Test in Pediatrics

The gold standard test to quantify daytime sleepiness remains the MSLT. The American Academy of Sleep Medicine (AASM) defines pathologic sleepiness as a mean sleep latency (MSL) of less than or equal to 8 minutes over five nap opportunities.[17] Studies, however, have shown that this cut-off may not always apply to the pediatric population, and if clinicians insist on this strict definition of pathologic sleepiness, then adolescents with narcolepsy or idiopathic hypersomnia may go undiagnosed. For instance, in a sample of 2498 MSLTs performed in patients with a suspected central disorder of hypersomnolence, the MSL in individuals less than or equal to 12 years of age was 11 minutes, and for the MSL of participants 13 to 20 years of age, it was 9 minutes. With use of the established cut-off for objective daytime sleepiness (MSL > 8 minutes), 27% of patients younger than 20 years had ambiguous MSLT results compared to only 9% to 10% among adults.[18] This raises the question of whether adolescents should have a different MSL cut-off when being evaluated for primary hypersomnia.

Specifically, in a group of patients ages 3 to 17 years (mean, 12 years) diagnosed with narcolepsy with cataplexy (NT1), Pizza and colleagues[19] suggested that greater than or equal to two sleep-onset REM periods (SOREMPs) *or* an MSL of less than or equal to 8.2 minutes were valid and reliable markers for pediatric NT1 diagnosis.

The MSLT protocol requires that an overnight PSG precede daytime testing and must record a minimum of 6 hours of sleep.[17] Therefore many sleep laboratories conclude the overnight portion of the study after 6 hours, although it is debatable whether 6 hours of sleep are sufficient for adults undergoing MSLT the next day. Adolescents typically require even more sleep. Short and colleagues[20] determined that healthy adolescents between the ages of 15 and 17 need 9 hours of sleep nightly, consistent with the National Sleep Foundation and the AASM's recommendations.[21,22] Even 1 night of partial sleep deprivation can significantly reduce MSL and increase the likelihood of false-positive MSLT results.[23]

Last, a circadian phase delay often accompanies puberty.[24] Approximately 1% to 4% of adolescents fulfill criteria for delayed sleep-wake phase disorder,[25] and another two-thirds have some degree of delay in their sleep wake cycles.[26] In a pediatric population with EDS, 13% had delayed sleep-wake phase disorder, and sleep was curtailed on school days compared to the weekends.[27] Therefore beginning the MSLT at an early clock time that coincides with the patient's usual sleep period may result in SOREMPs and short MSL.[28] In fact, when MSLTs were conducted with 10th graders, 16% showed two SOREMPs, and 48% had one SOREMP. Most of the SOREMPs occurred in the first two naps.[28a] SOREMPs were associated with later bedtimes, earlier rise times the day of the MSLT, and later circadian timing objectively measured by dim light melatonin onset. Therefore caution is advised in interpreting such results in adolescents without consideration of both their curtailed sleep and delayed sleep-wake cycles.

These findings demonstrate the need for careful conduct of in-laboratory testing, including sufficient time in bed during the overnight PSG, appropriate start time of the MSLT, and detailed documentation of sufficient sleep during the week leading up to testing.

Table 180.4 Diagnostic Tools Used in the Evaluation of Patients with Suspected Narcolepsy

Clinical History	Objective testing
Sleep diary	Actigraphy Overnight PSG followed by MSLT
Epworth Sleepiness Score–CHAD	CSF hypocretin
Pediatric Daytime Sleepiness Scale	HLA-DQB1*0602
Daily cataplexy diary	24-h PSG

CHAD, Children and adolescents; CSF, cerebrospinal fluid; HLA, human leukocyte antigen; MSLT, Multiple Sleep Latency Test; PSG, polysomnogram.
Modified from Nevsimalova S. The diagnosis and treatment of pediatric narcolepsy. *Curr Neurol Neurosci Rep.* 2014;14:469.

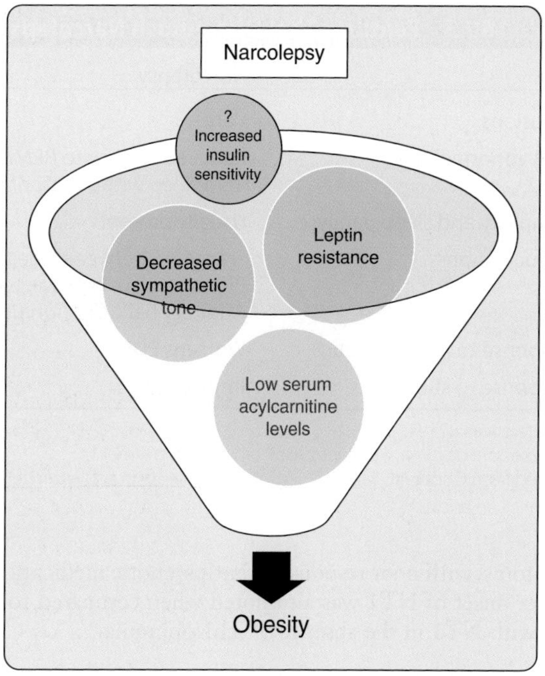

Figure 180.1 Proposed mechanisms relating to obesity and narcolepsy.

Other Tools

Hypocretin levels in the CSF could assist in differentiating NT1 from other causes of hypersomnia; however, given the invasiveness of lumbar punctures, CSF assays have not been widely adopted for clinical use in the evaluation of suspected central disorders of hypersomnolence.[29,30]

Neuroimaging may be warranted if secondary narcolepsy is suspected, especially in children. Some of the potential causes could be central nervous system tumors, such as occult neuroblastoma, inflammatory pathologies, demyelination, stroke, and neurometabolic disease, including Niemann-Pick disease.[31,32]

Overlap with Psychiatric and Behavioral Diagnoses

Childhood and adolescence are very vulnerable age periods in which global development takes place, and impairment in social interactions can have long-term mental health consequences. A complex interplay of biologic, psychological, sleep, and social factors contributes to various clinical outcomes in narcolepsy (Figure 180.2). A cross-sectional questionnaire survey of children with narcolepsy ages 4 to 18 years showed significantly higher Child Depression Inventory scores in patients compared to control participants, highlighting the increase in psychosocial problems encountered in this group.[4] In another matched case-control design, children with hypersomnia missed more days of school and had lower grades, as well as poorer quality of life, and engaged in fewer after-school activities.[33] A higher total score on social responsiveness scales was noted in patients with NT1 when compared to healthy control subjects (more prominently in girls) despite adequate narcolepsy treatment.[34] Some children may become introverted and spend greater time at home due to presence of narcoleptic symptoms, which further impacts their intellectual and social growth. Therefore it is imperative to screen these children earlier for psychological health with the help of questionnaires to provide appropriate care in a timely manner.[35]

The deficiency in orexin neurotransmission that underlies NT1 may explain the relationship between narcolepsy and psychiatric disorders. Orexin dysfunction has been implicated in various neuropsychiatric disorders, with the first evidence from the study by Taheri and colleagues (2001).[36] Mice models have shown that orexin plays a role in social behavior and sensory motor gating, in addition to roles in mood and anxiety. Orexin neurons also play role in social recognition memory.[37–39]

Of note, the symptoms of narcolepsy could be misdiagnosed as attention deficit/hyperactivity disorder (ADHD) or conduct disorder, leading to treatment with medication for wrong diagnoses. Sleep symptoms are very common in ADHD, and in a 2019 cohort of 538 adolescents with ADHD, the most common sleep disorders were sleep-disordered breathing and restless legs syndrome, as opposed to narcolepsy.[40]

Schizophrenia

The overlap of schizophrenia with NT1 has been reported between 5% and 13%.[41,42] This results in either a delay in NT1 diagnosis or a completely missed diagnosis, as highlighted in a case of a 12-year-old patient in whom the diagnosis of NT1 was delayed by 3 years.[43] Cavalier and Kothare[43] have compiled meaningful clues to differentiate the two conditions, which are highlighted in Table 180.5. Response to medication can also provide helpful information; for example, the onset of psychotic features after initiation of psychostimulants for sleepiness in NT1 or worsening of hypersomnia on initiation of psychotropic medications for schizophrenia may indicate misdiagnosis or overlap of the disorders.[44,45] From a pathophysiologic aspect, the two disorders have shared immune-mediated pathways. Furthermore, schizophrenia is a disorder of dopamine transmission in the mesocorticolimbic system. Because hypocretin regulates neurotransmission of dopamine activity within the ventral tegmental area, prefrontal cortex, and nucleus accumbens, pathophysiology of psychotic symptoms may be shared between both disorders.[46] Huang and colleagues[47] performed a case-control study comparing patients with both NT1 and schizophrenia to two control groups that included patients with only NT1 or schizophrenia. Patients with both NT1 and schizophrenia had higher body mass index (BMI), higher frequency of human leukocyte antigen–DQB1*03:01/06:02, and greater severity of psychotic

Table 180.5 Features That Distinguish Narcolepsy from Schizophrenia

	Narcolepsy	Schizophrenia
Delusions	Rare[a]	Core feature[a]
REM abnormalities	Reduced latency to REM sleep REM sleep without atonia	Some may have reduced latency to REM sleep
Cataplexy and sleep paralysis	Usually present	Sleep paralysis can be seen in very rare cases
Hallucinations	Transition between sleep and wakefulness Primarily visual (83%) Auditory hallucination uncommon[a]	During wakefulness Auditory (most prominent)[a]
Response to antipsychotics	Worsens EDS	Improves psychotic symptoms and hallucinations
Response to stimulants	Improves EDS	Worsens psychotic symptoms

[a]See references 82–84.
EDS, Excessive daytime sleepiness; REM, rapid eye movement.
Modified from Gupta AK, Sahoo S, Grover S. Narcolepsy in adolescence—a missed diagnosis: a case report. *Innov Clin Neurosci.* 2017;14(7–8):20–3.

symptoms, with poor response to antipsychotic medications.[47] Earlier onset of NT1 was also noted when compared to subjects with NT1 in the absence of schizophrenia.[47]

Cognitive Dysfunction in Adolescents with Narcolepsy

Cognitive problems may be observed in children and adolescents with narcolepsy. A Swedish study that assessed the performance of a verbal working memory task in adolescents with narcolepsy found an imbalance of cognitive resources, rather than deficit, in working memory. Narcolepsy patients had difficulty in monitoring and maintaining attention during the task when compared to healthy control subjects, and the authors concluded that dysfunction in the sustained attention system may be the origin behind self-reported cognitive difficulties in narcolepsy.[48]

However, a meta-analysis of all existing literature until 2018, which included 98 children and adolescents, did not find any specific deficits in Full Scale IQ (FSIQ) testing across the four studies included. In fact, the variance with the FSIQ score in this cohort was similar to that of the general population.[49]

A more extensive battery of tests that included perception and attention modules of the Vienna Test System demonstrated significant deficits among 36 adults with primary hypersomnias compared to 20 healthy control subjects. The deficits correlated with subjective sleepiness but not with MSL on MSLT.[50] In children and adolescents, more research is required to further address the prevalence, timing, and nature of cognitive deficits in primary hypersomnias in general and narcolepsy in particular.

Comorbidities of Narcolepsy Relevant in Adolescence

Precocious Puberty

Children with NT1 may also present with precocious puberty,[51] which may signify more general hypothalamic dysfunction.[52] Precocious puberty was found in 17% of patients with NT1, a 1000-fold increase compared to the general population and a 9-fold increase compared to obese adolescents.[52] The direct link between narcolepsy and precocious puberty, independent of obesity, may be explained by animal models that demonstrate close proximity of orexin immunoreactive (ORXIR) fibers to gonadotropin-releasing hormone (GnRH) cells. In fact, 75% to 80% of the GnRH cells in the preoptic nucleus of rats received direct innervation from these ORXIR fibers. In humans, hypocretin 1 (orexin-A) can suppress the firing frequency of the GnRH cells. Because the activity of GnRH cells is responsible for increasing luteal hormone (LH) secretion, one theory is that absent orexinergic inhibition results in an increase in secretion of LH and early puberty.[53-54]

Obesity

Overweight or obese body habitus was observed in 25% to 74% of patients with NT1 in a pediatric population.[55] In addition, 64.1% of this cohort experienced increased weight over the 3 to 4 years after diagnosis. The authors also demonstrated lower basal metabolic rate by 25% in NT1 patients compared to control subjects, even after controlling for food consumption and exercise.[55] Therefore, despite lower caloric intake, rapid and significant weight gain is common in the early course of the disease and directly impacts quality of life and school attendance.[56–61] There are also significant, BMI-independent increases in lipids, waist-hip ratio, waist circumference, and diastolic blood pressure in NT1 adolescents.[62]

Hypocretin is an appetite stimulant and regulator of fat metabolism; therefore a state of hypocretin deficiency is expected to reduce appetite and increase fat metabolism, causing weight loss. However, the contrary is seen in patients with narcolepsy and points to altered energy metabolism. Theoretical mechanisms linking obesity to narcolepsy have been proposed, as seen in Figure 180.1,[1] and hypocretin, physical activity, acylcarnitine, peripheral insulin sensitivity, and leptin resistance may also be implicated.[55,63–67]

Treatment with sodium oxybate has been associated with significant weight loss (3.4 kg in one investigation) in adult patients with narcolepsy; however, the systematic impact on weight in the pediatric population remains unknown.[68]

Obesity and precocious puberty may interact in a bidirectional manner in narcolepsy patients. Obesity results in excess leptin and aromatase levels, which influences sex hormones and pulsatile GnRH secretion, both of which are relevant for early puberty.[54] Precocious puberty itself can also lead to increased weight by direct action of estrogen on the hypothalamus and affecting both fat distribution and metabolism.[70]

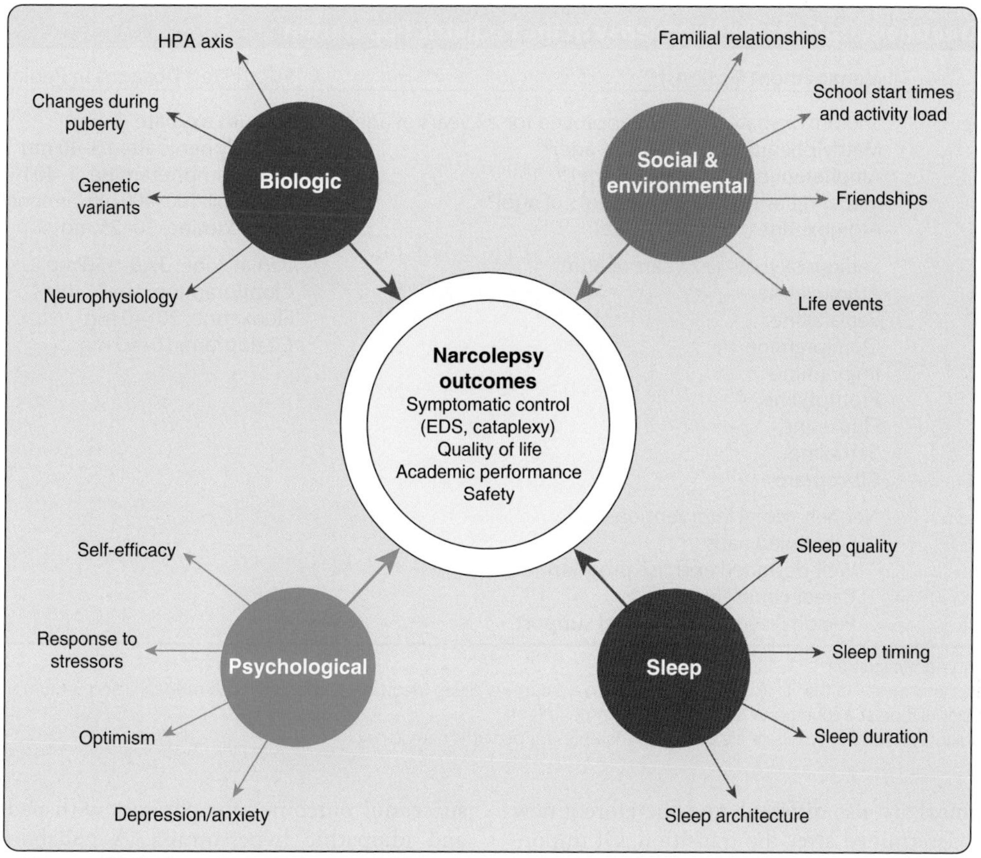

Figure 180.2 Biopsychosocial sleep model for pediatric narcolepsy as an interaction of biologic, psychological, sleep, and social interaction contributing to various clinical outcomes. EDS, Excessive daytime sleepiness; HPA, hypothalamic-pituitary-adrenal. (From Graef DM, Byars KC, Simakajornboon N, Dye TJ. Topical review: a biopsychosocial framework for pediatric narcolepsy and Idiopathic hypersomnia. *J Pediatr Psychol.* 2020;45(1):34–9.)

Polycystic Ovary Syndrome

Polycystic ovary syndrome (PCOS) is associated with obesity and OSA. Few case reports are described in literature in which the patients with PCOS were diagnosed with narcolepsy due to persistence of EDS independent of sleep-disordered breathing.[71–74] Low serum hypocretin was reported in 36 patients with PCOS when compared to a control group, but the value of serum hypocretin remains unclear,[75] and exact epidemiologic and etiologic pathways linking both the disorders is lacking.

Other Central Disorders of Hypersomnolence

Individuals with idiopathic hypersomnia experience profound EDS despite adequate and often prolonged nocturnal sleep durations. Idiopathic hypersomnia is distinct from narcolepsy, given the absence of abnormal intrusion of REM sleep, both clinically and during objective testing on PSG and MSLT. Issues related to navigation of the transition from pediatric to adult care can be addressed similarly to narcolepsy and are found later. Further content regarding the epidemiology, pathophysiology, presentation, diagnosis, and management of idiopathic hypersomnia is available in Chapter 113.

Providers caring for adult populations may be less familiar with Kleine-Levin syndrome (KLS).

KLS is a rare disorder mainly affecting adolescent males and usually has an unpredictable course but is self-limited.[76] The *International Classification of Sleep Disorders,* third edition diagnostic criteria for KLS require recurrent episodes of hypersomnia—at least 2 episodes that are days to weeks in duration, no more than 18 months apart.[76a] The hypersomnia period must be associated with one of the following ancillary symptoms: reduced cognition, altered perception, anorexia or hyperphagia, and behavioral disinhibition, which may be sexual in nature. There is normal alertness, cognition, behavior, and mood between the bouts. A more detailed discussion on KLS is available in Chapter 114.

Although KLS is considered a benign and self-limited disease, a recent large cohort study showed worse verbal memory and reduced processing speed on long-term follow-up, and therefore patients with KLS should undergo cognitive testing and be provided with academic support when necessary. Consideration of the academic ramifications of this disorder are essential during the transition of care from pediatric to adult clinics.[77] In addition, due to overlapping features of KLS with various psychiatric disorders, patients can be misdiagnosed, which may delay the correct evaluation and management to adulthood.[78]

TRANSITION OF CARE

History

As highlighted in the text earlier, symptomatology may change or evolve as the patient transitions from pediatric to adult clinics. After transition to adult care, extensive reevaluation of the history and clinical course is important, and diagnosis should be reestablished when in doubt. The tools

Table 180.6 Treatment Options for Narcolepsy in the Pediatric Population

Symptom	Management Options[a,b]	Suggested Dosages in Pediatric Patients[84]
Excessive daytime sleepiness	Sodium oxybate: U.S. FDA approved for ≥7 years of age[85] Methylphenidate (>6 years of age)[86] Amphetamines (>3 years of age)[87] Modafinil/armodafinil (>17 years of age)[87] Atomoxetine (>6 years of age)	Sodium oxybate: 2–6 g Methylphenidate: 10–40 mg Dextroamphetamine: 5–40 mg Modafinil: 100–400 mg, Armodafinil: 50-250 mg Atomoxetine: 10–25 mg
Cataplexy	Sodium oxybate (≥7 years of age) Atomoxetine Venlafaxine Clomipramine Imipramine Protriptyline Fluoxetine Sertraline Citalopram	Venlafaxine: 37.5–150 mg Clomipramine: 10–75 mg Fluoxetine: 20–40 mg Citalopram: 10–40 mg
General	Nonbehavioral interventions[32]: Scheduled naps Well-designed exercise program Career counseling Personalized psychological support	

FDA, US Food and Drug Administration.
[a]The most recent systematic review of the literature by the American Academy of Sleep Medicine supports the use modafinil and sodium oxybate to treat narcolepsy in the pediatric population at a conditional strength of recommendation.
[b]Only traditional stimulants and sodium oxybate are approved therapies for pediatric narcolepsy.

to quantify sleepiness are also different, and therefore a new baseline must be determined after the transition. Of importance, due to the strong association of obesity with narcolepsy and increased prevalence of sleep-disordered breathing in adulthood, OSA should be considered if sleepiness reemerges or worsens.

Diagnosis

The MSLT has various pitfalls in pediatric populations as emphasized earlier. Therefore providers may consider repeating the MSLT in the context of a previously inconclusive study or if the clinical presentation has changed during the transition of care. Repeat MSLT may be particularly relevant for NT2 and idiopathic hypersomnia, given the poor test-retest reliability of the MSLT outside of NT1. Measurement of CSF hypocretin levels could be considered to establish a previously missed diagnosis, as invasive procedures are generally withheld in pediatric patients.

Management

There is a paucity of randomized drug trials in pediatric narcolepsy patients, and therefore our understanding of safety, efficacy, and dosing of the medications is minimal. Some of the medications are not used due to long-term side effects relevant to children and adolescents (e.g., decreased growth with amphetamine and methylphenidate). In addition, monotherapy is encouraged in this age group. Medication pharmacokinetics are different when compared to adults. Therefore, during the transition from pediatric to adult clinic, sleep specialists should reevaluate medication regimens to ensure that the patients are adequately dosed and symptoms are well controlled. Table 180.6 details medication dosing in the pediatric population.[79]

Future Directions

As aptly highlighted in the review article by Graef and colleagues,[80] various biopsychosocial factors are implicated in successful outcomes for patients with pediatric narcolepsy and idiopathic hypersomnia. A collaborative multidisciplinary approach is required to manage patients transitioning from pediatric to adult care, and sustainable models that integrate pediatric behavioral sleep medicine specialists are needed. Greater education and more rigorous training is required to minimize diagnostic delays in patients with suspected central disorders of hypersomnolence, and psychosocial aspects require greater attention. Further research is required to evaluate the differences between patients who function well or poorly in the context of their hypersomnia.[80]

CLINICAL PEARLS

- The evaluation and management of central disorders of hypersomnolence and, specifically, narcolepsy is associated with a variety of complexities in pediatric and adolescent populations.
- Clinical presentation of narcolepsy is distinct from adults. Recurrent sleep attacks may prolong the total duration, hypnagogic hallucinations are less frightening, and cataplexy may occur without emotional trigger.
- Diagnostic confirmation of the central disorders of hypersomnolence with the Multiple Sleep Latency Test must take into account the circadian phase delay (and resultant sleep deprivation) during adolescence, which might produce false-positive results.
- Precocious puberty, obesity, and narcolepsy may have overlapping pathophysiologic mechanisms, and a high index of suspicion for comorbid metabolic and psychiatric disorders is required.
- Psychosocial factors, for example, academic issues, are essential to consider in the care of individuals with central disorders of hypersomnolence transitioning from pediatric to adult care.

SUMMARY

Adolescence generally is defined as the decade spanning ages 11 to 21 years and comes with unique health needs. However, at this time there are very few transitional care resources to bridge the gap between childhood and adulthood. The situation is no different when it comes to central disorders of hypersomnolence. Narcolepsy, the most well defined of these conditions, has unique clinical symptomatology that is very different from its presentation in adults. This includes the duration of sleep attacks, the features of hypnagogic hallucinations, the triggers of cataplexy, and the higher prevalence of dream enactment. In addition, there is significant overlap between narcolepsy and psychiatric syndromes in adolescence that may often lead to misdiagnosis. Last, narcolepsy, obesity, and precocious puberty share similar pathophysiologic substrates in this population. Already, evidence suggests higher health-related costs in this subgroup of patients due to increased prevalence of comorbidities before and after the diagnosis of narcolepsy, including metabolic/endocrine disorders, which include weight gain and diabetes mellitus; psychiatric disorders; epilepsy; and higher rates of upper airway infections.[38] Therefore appropriate transition of patients with narcolepsy and, more generally, central disorders of hypersomnolence from pediatric to adult care is required to ensure appropriate management.

SELECTED READINGS

Cairns A, Trotti LM, Bogan R. Demographic and nap-related variance of the MSLT: results from 2,498 suspected hypersomnia patients: clinical MSLT variance. *Sleep Med.* 2019;55:115–123.

Com G, Einen MA, Jambhekar S. Narcolepsy with cataplexy: diagnostic challenge in children. *Clin Pediatr.* 2015;54(1):5–14.

Ludwig B, Smith S, Heussler H. Associations between neuropsychological, neurobehavioral and emotional functioning and either narcolepsy or idiopathic hypersomnia in children and adolescents. *J Clin Sleep Med.* 2018;14(4):661–674.

Maski K, Trotti LM, Kotagal S, et al. Treatment of central disorders of hypersomnolence: an American Academy of Sleep Medicine clinical practice guideline. *J Clin Sleep Med.* 2021;17(9):1881–1893.

Palhano AC, Kim LJ, Moreira GA, Coelho FM, Tufik S, Andersen ML. Narcolepsy, precocious puberty and obesity in the pediatric population: a literature review. *Ped Endocrinol Rev.* 2018;16(2):266–274.

Pizza F, Barateau L, Jaussent I, et al. Validation of Multiple Sleep Latency Test for the diagnosis of pediatric narcolepsy type 1. *Neurology.* 2019;93(11):e1034–e1044.

A complete reference list can be found online at ExpertConsult.com.

Chapter 181

Congenital Heart Disease

Pnina Weiss

Chapter Highlights

- Over the last few decades, advances in the surgical and medical care of children with complex congenital heart disease (CHD) have led to a dramatic increase in their survival into adulthood. Studies on sleep disorders in adults with CHD are limited and are reviewed in this chapter.
- Cardiovascular complications of adult CHD (ACHD) are common. Heart failure may predispose patients to both obstructive and central sleep apnea. Conversely, sleep-disordered breathing may worsen heart failure, arrythmias, coronary artery disease, and pulmonary hypertension.
- Noncardiac complications of ACHD are prevalent and affect multiple organ systems, including pulmonary, renal, and hepatic. Neurocognitive and mental health problems are common. Genetic abnormalities occur in approximately 10% of individuals with CHD. How these factors increase the risk of sleep disorders is described in this chapter.
- Positive airway pressure to treat sleep apnea in adults with complex CHD has potential adverse sequelae on cardiovascular function and must be used cautiously, especially in patients with Fontan physiology. Considerations for using PAP therapy in this population are discussed.

EPIDEMIOLOGY

Over the last few decades, advances in the surgical and medical care of children with complex congenital heart disease (CHD) have led to a dramatic increase in their survival into adulthood.[1,2] CHD is reported in approximately 9.1 per 1000 live births.[3] In developed countries, more than 85% of children with CHD survive into adulthood and account for approximately two-thirds of all patients with CHD.[2,4,5] The prevalence of adult CHD (ACHD) in these countries has been reported as 1.7 to 4.1 per 1000 adults, increasing over the last decade to approximately 6.1 per 1000 adults.[2,6] In developing countries, where resources and medical care are limited, mortality rates are higher; it is estimated that worldwide there are 12 to 34 million adults with CHD, making up 22% to 26% of the total CHD population.[1] The distribution of lesion severity in the ACHD population varies by age and availability of health care resources. In developed countries, the number of adults with complex CHD has been rising and is close to 9%, most of whom have had surgical palliation.[1,2] Overall, the prevalence of CHD is similar in males and females. However, in ACHD the prevalence is higher in females, while the mortality rate is higher in males.[5,7] In African Americans, the incidence of CHD is overall lower, but the mortality rate is higher.[8] Further research is required to determine the causes of these disparities.

Genetic abnormalities occur in approximately 10% of children who have CHD[9]; examples include DiGeorge syndrome (22q11.2 deletion), Down syndrome (trisomy 21), Holt-Oram syndrome (TBX5), Klinefelter syndrome (47XXY), Noonan syndrome (PTPN11, KRAS, SOS1, RAF1, NRAS, BRAF, MAP2K1), Turner syndrome (45X), and Williams syndrome (7q11.23 deletion).[9] Many of these syndromes are associated with craniofacial and musculoskeletal abnormalities, intellectual disability, and mental health and behavior problems.

Classification of Congenital Heart Disease

Adults with CHD represent a heterogeneous population with respect to native anatomy, surgical repair, and physiology. They may have exercise limitation, hypoxemia, end-organ dysfunction, or other sequelae of their CHD. The physiologic variables used to classify ACHD by the American College of Cardiology/American Heart Association Taskforce on Clinical Practice Guidelines (Table 181.1) have value in prognosis, management, and association with quality of life.[9] Both anatomic and physiologic variables are used to classify the severity of ACHD (Table 181.2).

Lesions such as ventricular septal defect (VSD), atrial septal defect (ASD), and patent ductus arteriosus usually produce a left-to-right shunt, in which a portion of the pulmonary venous blood returns back to the lungs, reducing cardiac output by the amount of blood that was shunted.[10] With right-to-left shunts, which usually occur when pulmonary vascular resistance rises above systemic resistance, deoxygenated systemic venous blood is returned to the systemic arterial circulation without being oxygenated by the lungs, reducing oxygen content.[10] Obstructive lesions, such as valvular pulmonary stenosis or aortic coarctation, increase afterload, which can cause myocardial systolic dysfunction and decrease cardiac output.[11] Tetralogy of Fallot is the most common complex CHD[12]; it is characterized by the presence of a VSD, subpulmonary stenosis, overriding aorta, and right ventricular hypertrophy. Because of the high resistance to flow in the pathway between the right ventricle and the lungs, there is usually significant right-to-left shunting through the VSD. Single-ventricle physiology, characterized by absent or

Table 181.1 Physiologic Variables Used to Classify Adults with Congenital Heart Disease

Variable	Description
Aortopathy	Aortic enlargement occurs in some CHD or as a result of repair; it may be progressive Classified based on aortic diameter: *mild, moderate, severe*
Arrhythmia	Arrhythmias are common and can be cause of or worsen hemodynamics Classified by presence and response to treatment: *No arrhythmia, arrhythmia not requiring treatment, arrhythmia controlled with therapy, refractory arrhythmias*
Valvular heart disease	Severity defined as *mild, moderate, severe*
End-organ dysfunction	Clinical and/or laboratory evidence, including renal, hepatic, and pulmonary
Hypoxemia	Defined as oxygen saturation at rest on room air using pulse oximetry <90% • Severe: oxygen saturation < 85%
NYHA functional classification	Class I No limitation of physical activity II Slight limitation of physical activity III Marked limitation of physical activity IV Inability to perform physical activity without discomfort
Pulmonary hypertension	Defined as mean PA pressure by right heart catheterization≥25 mm Hg • Pulmonary artery hypertension is defined as mean PA pressure by right heart catheterization ≥25 mm Hg, PCWP ≤15 mm Hg and PVR ≥3 Wood units
Shunt (hemodynamically significant)	Considered *hemodynamically significant* if there is chamber enlargement distal to the shunt and/or sustained Qp:Qs ≥1.5:1
Venous and arterial stenosis	Examples include aortic recoarctation after repair, supravalvular aortic obstruction, branch PA, or pulmonary vein stenosis

ACHD, Adult congenital heart disease; CHD, congenital heart disease; NYHA, New York Heart Association; PA, pulmonary artery; PCWP, pulmonary capillary wedge pressure; PVR, pulmonary vascular resistance; Qp:Qs, pulmonary-systemic blood flow ratio.

Modified from Stout KK, Daniels CJ, Aboulhosn JA, et al. 2018 AHA/ACC Guideline for the management of adults with congenital heart disease: executive summary: a report of the American College of Cardiology/American Heart Association Task Force on Clinical Practice Guidelines. *J Am Coll Cardiol.* 2019;73:1494–1563.

hypoplastic pumping chambers or atrioventricular valves, had a high mortality, but because of improved surgical and medical care, patients are now living into adulthood.[12] Initially palliative procedures such as shunts or pulmonary artery banding were performed. However, long-term survival improved with the introduction of the Fontan operation, which results in systemic venous return being rerouted to bypass the right heart.[12] It requires a multistage approach, with the first stages characterized by mixing of systemic and pulmonary venous returns and hypoxemia. After the Fontan operation, flow from the systemic veins through the lungs and back to the ventricle is passive. Anatomic obstructions in the pulmonary vasculature, elevations of pulmonary vascular resistance or ventricular end-diastolic pressure, and dysrhythmias can decrease pulmonary flow and cardiac output.[12]

Complications of Adult Congenital Heart Disease

Mortality and morbidity associated with ACHD are most commonly a result of the cardiovascular complications of ACHD. Heart failure is the most common cardiovascular complication,[13] followed by arrhythmias,[14] coronary artery disease,[15] pulmonary hypertension, and infective endocarditis.[16] The development of heart failure and coronary artery disease is associated with worse outcomes.[17] The primary cause of death in adults with CHD is due to heart failure with a smaller number experiencing sudden cardiac death.[18,19] While previous studies indicated that simple CHD has a mortality similar to the general population,[19] a more recent study suggested that the risk of adverse cardiovascular events is actually increased.[20] However, it is clear that adults with complex CHD such as Eisenmenger syndrome and Fontan physiology have a worse long-term survival.[19] Cardiac transplantation has become increasingly more common in adults with complex CHD.[21]

Noncardiac complications are prevalent in adults with CHD and affect long-term outcomes, potentially contributing to the progression of heart failure.[22] Obesity, diabetes, hypertension, and renal disease appear to be more common in adults with CHD than the general population.[23-25] Renal and pulmonary disease in adults with CHD are associated with a worse survival rate.[26,27] Liver disease has been increasingly appreciated as a sequela of the Fontan procedure.[28] In addition, genetic abnormalities are common in patients with CHD, which can be associated independently with endocrine, immunologic, and neurologic disease.[29] Cyanotic CHD has extensive sequelae on multiple organ systems, including hematologic complications. After cardiovascular disease, the second most common cause of death in adults with CHD is pneumonia. Other causes of death include cancer, hemorrhage, infectious disease, and strokes.[18,19]

Mental health disorders are prevalent in patients with ACHD. Mood or anxiety disorders have been reported in approximately one-third of adults with CHD[30-32] and are associated with a higher mortality rate.[33] Posttraumatic stress disorder has also been reported.[34]

Adults with CHD are at risk for neurocognitive dysfunction. Neurodevelopmental problems are frequently seen in children with complex CHD,[35] which may be related to impaired cerebral oxygen delivery,[36] chronic disease, or underlying genetic abnormalities.[35] Children and adolescents have been reported to have neurodevelopmental disabilities, behavior problems, language and speech deficits, and attention-deficit/hyperactivity disorder.[35] In adults with CHD, there are limited data on long-term neurocognitive function. Deficits in executive functioning have been reported that appear to relate to the severity of CHD.[37,38]

Risk Factors for Sleep Disorders in Adult Congenital Heart Disease

Cardiovascular dysfunction can lead to both obstructive and central sleep apnea (Chapter 149), shifting based on the severity

Table 181.2 ACHD Classification Based on Anatomy and Physiologic Stage

Anatomy	Examples
I. Simple	
Native disease	Isolated small ASD or VSD, pulmonic stenosis
Repaired conditions	Ligated ductus arteriosus, repaired ASD or VSD without shunt or chamber enlargement
II. Moderate complexity	
Repaired or unrepaired conditions	Partial or total anomalous pulmonary venous connection, anomalous coronary artery arising from the pulmonary artery, AVSD, congenital aortic or mitral valve disease, aortic coarctation, Ebstein anomaly, ostium primum or moderate/large ASD, moderate/large ductus arteriosus, moderate/severe pulmonary valve regurgitation or stenosis, peripheral pulmonary stenosis, subvalvular aortic stenosis (excluding HCM), repaired tetralogy of Fallot, VSD with another abnormality and/or moderate/large shunt
III. Great complexity (or complex)	Cyanotic congenital heart disease, double outlet right ventricle, Fontan procedure, interrupted aortic arch, mitral atresia, single ventricle (including double inlet left ventricle, tricuspid atresia, hypoplastic left heart, or other abnormality functionally a single ventricle), pulmonary atresia, transposition of the great arteries, truncus arteriosus
Physiologic Stage	
A	NYHA Class I, no hemodynamic sequelae, no arrhythmias, normal exercise capacity, normal renal, hepatic, pulmonary function
B	NYHA Class II, mild hemodynamic sequelae, mild valvular disease, trivial or small shunt, arrhythmia not requiring treatment, objective cardiac limitation to exercise
C	NYHA Class III, moderate/severe valvular disease, moderate/severe ventricular dysfunction, moderate aortic enlargement, venous or arterial stenosis, mild/moderate hypoxemia, hemodynamically significant shunt, arrhythmias controlled with treatment, mild/moderate pulmonary hypertension, end-organ dysfunction responsive to therapy
D	NYHA Class IV, severe aortic root enlargement, arrhythmias refractory to treatment, severe hypoxemia, severe pulmonary hypertension, Eisenmenger syndrome, refractory end-organ dysfunction

[a]The "highest" relevant anatomic or physiologic feature is used to classify the severity of CHD.
ACHD, Adult congenital heart disease; ASD, atrial septal defect; AVSD, atrioventricular septal defect; CHD, congenital heart disease; HCM, hypertrophic cardiomyopathy; NYHA, New York Heart Association; VSD, ventricular septal defect.
Modified from Stout KK, Daniels CJ, Aboulhosn JA, et al. 2018 AHA/ACC Guideline for the management of adults with congenital heart disease: executive summary: a report of the American College of Cardiology/American Heart Association Task Force on Clinical Practice Guidelines. *J Am Coll Cardiol.* 2019;73:1494–1563.

of heart failure.[39,40] Elevated central venous pressure, associated with some CHD, can increase the cross-sectional airway of the upper airway, potentially contributing to obstructive sleep apnea (OSA).[41] In addition, in patients with heart failure, rostral shift of fluid from the legs when supine to the neck and lungs can also worsen both OSA and central sleep apnea (CSA).[42] Heart failure has also been associated with insomnia.[43]

In turn, sleep-disordered breathing can contribute to worsening cardiovascular function in ACHD. Heart failure and dysrhythmias could be worsened by the hypoxia, oxidative stress, endothelial dysfunction, and sympathetic activation associated with OSA.[44] Increases in pulmonary vascular resistance could contribute to morbidity and mortality in patients with lesions such as tetralogy of Fallot, in which long-term survival worsens with pulmonary insufficiency, deterioration of right ventricular function with associated ventricular arrhythmias, and sudden cardiac death.[45]

Some of the genetic abnormalities, common in patients with CHD, are associated with a higher risk of sleep disorders. Patients with Down syndrome,[29,46,47] DiGeorge syndrome,[48] and Turner syndrome[49] have craniofacial and musculoskeletal abnormalities that predispose them to OSA. Many of the genetic abnormalities are associated with intellectual disability, developmental delay, and mental health disorders that could contribute to sleep problems[50] (e.g., Down syndrome,[51,52] William syndrome[51,53,54]). In adults with Down syndrome, self-reported sleep measures such as Epworth Sleepiness Scale or Pittsburgh Sleep Quality Index may be normal despite the presence of OSA.[46]

Other comorbid conditions in adults with CHD can lead to sleep disorders. Obesity may be more common in adults with CHD[24,25] and can lead to OSA. Neurocognitive dysfunction and mental health disorders that are prevalent in adults with CHD, such as anxiety, depression,[30-32] and posttraumatic stress disorder,[34] can disrupt sleep (see Chapters 61, 163, and 164). Comorbidities, such as chronic kidney disease, can cause sleep disturbances such as insomnia, restless legs syndrome, periodic limb movements during sleep, and OSA.[55-57] Medications used to treat cardiac dysfunction or dysrhythmias (e.g., beta-adrenergic antagonists) can also contribute to sleep disruption.[58]

SLEEP DISORDERS IN CONGENITAL HEART DISEASE

Data on sleep disorders in children and adults with CHD are limited.

Children

In a small study, infants with CHD who underwent polysomnography demonstrated an apnea-hypopnea index (AHI) that was mildly increased (approximately 2.5/hour); apneas were primarily central. Sleep efficiency in those who were cyanotic was significantly decreased.[59] In hospitalized infants with CHD, sleep-disordered breathing, especially CSA, was associated with worse outcomes, including higher risk of mortality and longer stays.[60] In children with tetralogy of Fallot, sleep-disordered breathing, defined by a score of at least 8 in the Pediatric Sleep Questionnaire (PSQ), was identified in 38%, which is higher than the 5% to 11% reported in healthy children.[61] Sleep-disordered breathing in these children was associated with a worse cardiac symptom score, especially exercise tolerance and school performance.[62] Pulmonary hypertension in association with OSA in a child with Down syndrome and complex CHD has been described.[63]

Adults

In one study of 32 patients with d-transposition, who had undergone primarily Mustard and Senning procedures, 44% screened positive for sleep-disordered breathing, using the snoring, daytime tiredness, observed apneas, and high blood pressure (STOP) questionnaire.[64] In the study by Miles and colleagues, 22 adults with pulmonary valve incompetence after repair of tetralogy of Fallot or congenital pulmonary stenosis underwent overnight pulse oximetry to screen for sleep-disordered breathing.[65] Pulse oximetry was considered abnormal in 59% with an average 3% oxygen desaturation index (ODI) of 8.7/hour; 9% of the patients had severe abnormalities, defined as an ODI of more than 30/hour, oxygen saturation less than 90% for over 33% of the recording duration, and/or mean oxygen saturation less than 90%.[65] However, further confirmation of the presence and type of sleep-disordered breathing was not performed. In the study by Legault and colleagues, 10 adults with cyanotic CHD (resting oxygen saturations less than 90%) underwent a type III study; 6 patients demonstrated a decrease in their oxygen saturation during sleep (1% to 10%, mean 3.7%). None demonstrated sleep-disordered breathing or increased periodic limb movements; the average AHI was 1.1/hour.[66] In the study by Hjortshoj and colleagues, 20 adults with Eisenmenger syndrome, primarily resulting from VSD, underwent a type IV study; 3 patients (15%) had AHI exceeding 5, 1 with severe OSA and 2 with moderate OSA. OSA was significantly related to body mass index (BMI) and age but did not correlate with resting oxygen saturation, hemoglobin level, B-type natriuretic peptide concentration, or 6-minute walking distance.[67]

In a single-center retrospective study of 104 hospitalized adults with CHD, using type III sleep monitoring, 63% of the patients had sleep apnea, defined as a respiratory disturbance index (RDI) *of at least 5*.[68] Sleep apnea was classified as mild, moderate, and severe in 37%, 16%, and 10%, respectively. The majority of patients (92%) had OSA, while the remainder had CSA. The group of patients with moderate to severe sleep apnea had a higher proportion of males and higher BMI, norepinephrine concentration, and ascending aorta pressure than those who did not have sleep apnea. There was no difference between the two groups in B-type natriuretic peptide concentration, central venous pressure, cardiac index, presence of tachyarrhythmias (either atrial or ventricular), history of Fontan-type surgery, hypertension, or complex CHD. Patients suspected to have CSA had a higher New York Heart Association (NYHA) functional class. In multivariate analysis, NYHA functional class of at least II and BMI of 25 or greater were independent risk factors for RDI of at least 15. The study was limited by small study size and inclusion of patients with heterogenous CHD. Only hospitalized patients, the majority of whom had complex CHD and heart failure, were included, so applicability to an ambulatory population is unclear. In addition, the use of type III sleep monitoring, in which hypopneas were defined as a decrease in flow of 50% associated with 3% oxygen desaturation, could have under- or overestimated the severity of sleep apnea in the patients.

Data on subjective sleep quality and sleep disturbance in adults with CHD are also sparse. One study examined the association of exercise with a number of outcomes in 446 adults with CHD using survey and retrospective chart review. In the study, 84% of individuals had moderate or severe CHD. The average sleep duration was 7.0 hours, and delayed sleep onset and nocturnal awakenings were reported in 16% and 15% of subjects, respectively. Those who exercised frequently (twice or more per week) reported decreased nocturnal awakenings and sleep latency.[69]

POSITIVE AIRWAY PRESSURE IN ADULTS WITH CONGENITAL HEART DISEASE

Positive airway pressure (PAP) to treat sleep apnea in adults with complex CHD has potential adverse sequelae on cardiovascular function and must be used cautiously. PAP increases intrathoracic pressure and decreases venous return to the right side of the heart, which is of particular concern in patients with Fontan physiology, as it may decrease cardiac output. This has been demonstrated with levels of positive end-expiratory pressure as low as 6 cm H_2O.[70] In a study by Harada and colleagues, PAP therapy was used in eight hospitalized patients with ACHD; five received continuous positive airway pressure (CPAP) and three received adaptive servo-ventilation. In seven patients, symptoms such as sleepiness, sleep arousals, and headache improved. However, one patient with a repaired tetralogy of Fallot developed severe right ventricle dysfunction after receiving auto-adjusting PAP with a range of 4 to 16 cm H_2O.[68] There are few reports and no formal recommendations about the use of adaptive servo-ventilation (ASV) in adults with complex CHD.[68] ASV has been associated with excess cardiovascular mortality in patients with CSA, symptomatic, chronic heart failure (NYHA functional class II-IV), and reduced left ventricular ejection fraction (LVEF $< 45\%$); without further studies, its use should therefore be avoided in adults with complex CHD who meet these criteria.[71]

Monitoring of cardiovascular function to guide PAP therapy and prevent cardiac complications is important in adults with complex CHD. In a small study, four patients with complex CHD (single-ventricle physiology), history of Fontan repair, and severe OSA underwent CPAP titration under light conscious sedation in the cardiac catheterization laboratory. The maximal pressure that could be achieved without impairing cardiac function was determined, using measurements such as pulmonary capillary wedge pressure, mixed venous saturation, and cardiac index. Subjects then underwent polysomnography with CPAP titration in the sleep laboratory using the pressure obtained in the cardiac catheterization as the maximal pressure. In three subjects, sleep apnea was successfully treated with pressures that ranged from 6 to 8 cm H_2O, that were less than the maximal pressure, with improvement in subjective symptoms. One subject had persistent OSA and hypoxemia at the threshold pressure, requiring the addition of supplemental oxygen for adequate treatment.[72] However, this approach is not feasible for most patients. Initiation of PAP therapy with less invasive cardiac monitoring could be performed on an inpatient unit. Other facilities initiating PAP therapy in adults with complex CHD, especially with Fontan physiology, need to be aware of and have the capability to detect acute deterioration in cardiac function. Consultation with the patient's cardiologist is critical. Low levels of CPAP should be used; addition of supplemental oxygen could be considered for persistent OSA and hypoxemia. Longitudinal monitoring of cardiac function is necessary to detect any deterioration after initiation of PAP therapy.

RECOMMENDATIONS FOR CARE OF ADULTS WITH CONGENITAL HEART DISEASE AND RESEARCH

Despite the recognition that comorbidities have the potential to adversely impact long-term survival and outcomes of adults with CHD, the impact of sleep disorders in this population has not been adequately studied. As of 2019, neither screening for nor management of sleep disorders has been addressed in national or international guidelines on the management of adults with CHD.[1,9,22,73] It is recommended that adults with CHD be managed at regional ACHD programs with a multidisciplinary team and services; however, neither providers nor services with the expertise in diagnosing and managing sleep disorders were included.[9] In view of the fact that adults with CHD have multiple risk factors for sleep-disordered breathing, including a high prevalence of obesity,[24] it is imperative to include screening for OSA in the guidelines.

More research on the impact of sleep disorders in adults with CHD is needed. Potential areas include the prevalence of OSA and CSA in adults with complex CHD, as well as the presence of other disorders that disrupt sleep such as insomnia and restless legs syndrome. The impact of these disorders on as cardiovascular, psychological, neurocognitive, and endocrine outcomes must be studied. The effectiveness and safety of PAP therapy in treating sleep apnea in adults with complex CHD also merit further investigation.

CLINICAL PEARLS

- It is important to screen adults with CHD for sleep-disordered breathing and other disorders of sleep. Heart failure, the most common cardiovascular complication in adults with CHD, may predispose them to both OSA and CSA. Severe sleep apnea has been associated NYHA functional class of II or greater and BMI of at least 25.
- Cardiovascular complications of ACHD, such as heart failure, dysrhythmias, and pulmonary hypertension, could be worsened by the hypoxia, oxidative stress, endothelial dysfunction, and sympathetic activation associated with OSA if left untreated.
- Mood or anxiety disorders have been reported in one-third of patients with CHD and have the potential to cause sleep disorders.
- Frequent exercise (>2x/week) may help improve the sleep quality of adults with moderate or severe CHD as it has been associated with a decrease in nocturnal awakenings and sleep latency.
- PAP to treat sleep apnea in adults with complex CHD must be used cautiously, as it can decrease cardiac output in patients with Fontan physiology. Low levels of CPAP should be used; addition of supplemental oxygen could be considered for persistent OSA and hypoxemia. Consultation with the patient's cardiologist and monitoring of cardiovascular function with PAP therapy are important.

SUMMARY

Over the last decades, advances in the surgical and medical care of children with complex CHD have led to a dramatic increase in their survival into adulthood. Adults with CHD have many risk factors for sleep disorders, such as heart failure, elevated central venous pressure, obesity, genetic disorders with craniofacial and musculoskeletal abnormalities, mental health disorders, and neurocognitive deficits. In turn, sleep disorders, such as OSA, have the potential to worsen cardiovascular morbidity and mortality. However, studies on the prevalence, management, and treatment of sleep disorders are sparse. In hospitalized adults with CHD, a high prevalence of OSA was reported, which was independently associated with a higher NYHA functional class and body mass index *of at least 25*. The use of PAP to treat sleep apnea in adults with complex CHD, especially those with Fontan physiology, can worsen cardiovascular function. Low levels of CPAP should be used; addition of supplemental oxygen could be considered for persistent OSA and hypoxemia. Monitoring of cardiovascular function during PAP therapy is critical. Further research on the prevalence and impact of sleep disorders in adults with CHD is needed.

SELECTED READINGS

Baker-Smith CM, Isaiah A, Melendres MC, et al. Sleep-disordered breathing and cardiovascular disease in children and adolescents: a scientific statement from the American Heart Association. *J Am Heart Assoc.* 2021;10(18):e022427. https://doi.org/10.1161/JAHA.121.022427.

Diller GP, Kempny A, Alonso-Gonzalez R, et al. Survival prospects and circumstances of death in contemporary adult congenital heart disease patients under follow-up at a large tertiary centre. *Circulation.* 2015;132:2118–2125.

Harada G, Takeuchi D, Inai K, Shinohara T, Nakanishi T. Prevalence and risk factors of sleep apnea in adult patients with congenital heart disease. *Cardiol Young.* 2019;29:576–582.

Klouda L, Franklin WJ, Saraf A, Parekh DR, Schwartz DD. Neurocognitive and executive functioning in adult survivors of congenital heart disease. *Congenit Heart Dis.* 2017;12:91–98.

Legault S, Lanfranchi P, Montplaisir J, et al. Nocturnal breathing in cyanotic congenital heart disease. *Int J Cardiol.* 2008;128:197–200.

Miles S, Ahmad W, Bailey A, Hatton R, Boyle A, Collins N. Sleep-disordered breathing in patients with pulmonary valve incompetence complicating congenital heart disease. *Congenit Heart Dis.* 2016;11:678–682.

Moons P, Van Deyk K, Dedroog D, Troost E, Budts W. Prevalence of cardiovascular risk factors in adults with congenital heart disease. *Eur J Cardiovasc Prev Rehabil.* 2006;13:612–616.

Nanayakkara B, Lau E, Yee B, et al. Sleep disordered breathing in adults living with a Fontan circulation and CPAP titration protocol. *Int J Cardiol.* 2020;317:70–74. https://doi.org/10.1016/j.ijcard.2020.05.060.

Stores RJ. Sleep problems in adults with Down syndrome and their family carers. *J Appl Res Intellect Disabil.* 2019;32:831–840.

Stout KK, Daniels CJ, Aboulhosn JA, et al. 2018 AHA/ACC Guideline for the Management of Adults With Congenital Heart Disease: executive summary: a report of the American College of Cardiology/American Heart Association Task Force on Clinical Practice Guidelines. *J Am Coll Cardiol.* 2019;73:1494–1563.

Watson NF, Bushnell T, Jones TK, Stout K. A novel method for the evaluation and treatment of obstructive sleep apnea in four adults with complex congenital heart disease and Fontan repairs. *Sleep Breath.* 2009;13:421–424.

Webb G, Mulder BJ, Aboulhosn J, et al. The care of adults with congenital heart disease across the globe: Current assessment and future perspective: a position statement from the International Society for Adult Congenital Heart Disease (ISACHD). *Int J Cardiol.* 2015;195:326–333.

A complete reference list can be found online at ExpertConsult.com.

Chapter 182

Sleep in Intersex and Transgender Individuals

David de Ángel Solá; Meir Kryger

Chapter Highlights

- There is a growing body of literature on intersex and transgender sleep that has allowed clinical specialists to identify and attempt bridging medical knowledge gaps. High-level evidence remains scarce, however.
- Baseline sleep disturbances in these populations can arise from the experiences of feeling excluded from a predominantly binary society and difficulties understanding identity. Some data suggest early acceptance and social support could curb some of these difficulties.
- The medical and surgical treatments available for these communities are evolving and can directly or indirectly affect sleep. Neither type of treatment is necessarily pursued regularly, permanently, or in a specific order. Data acquisition from controlled cohorts to reach broad conclusions is therefore difficult.

INTRODUCTION

Sleep is often studied and reported on the basis of sexual dichotomy: patients are either female or male. There are many people who do not fit into this binary system and because of this might be systematically excluded from clinical studies and scientific investigation. The result has been a general knowledge gap in medicine that has become more evident in recent years. This chapter aims to bridge part of that gap with the limited evidence that exists on the topic within sleep medicine. We focus on two groups of people: intersex and transgender individuals. Although not always grouped together, many of the medical interventions sought by these individuals are similar: sex hormone therapy, genital or gender surgery, psychotherapy, among others. Given that many of the processes of transition, self-discovery, and change experienced in these communities mimic the challenges of and occur during adolescence, we have included this chapter in the section focusing on the transition from childhood to adulthood.

It is important to highlight that terminology used within these communities is complicated, at times controversial, and rapidly evolving. The specifics of such terminology are beyond the scope of this chapter; we use the most explicit terms encountered in recent medical literature. Nevertheless, understanding who makes up these communities is important.

Intersex is an umbrella term used to refer to those born with biological sex characteristics that do not fit the typical male-female binary and exist along a wide natural spectrum, being distinct from sexual orientation or gender identity. The prevalence of intersexuality depends heavily on the definitions used. In a seminal study quoted by the Intersex Society of North America, the prevalence appears as 1.7% of the human population.[1] However, the same study suggests that those who would require genital surgery to be recognizably classified as either male or female would be about 10 times lower. Additionally, the definition used in the study includes conditions most clinicians would categorize as male or female, such as vaginal agenesis or Turner syndrome. Exclusion of all those whose external genitalia match their chromosomal sex in infancy would bring the prevalence of intersex down to about 0.02% or less of the human population.[2]

Transgender is likewise an umbrella term but refers to people who do not identify (solely, partially, or completely) with the sex that was assigned at birth based on observable biological characteristics. The case definition will affect the perceived prevalence of transgenderism, but a good estimate based on a meta-analysis of 27 studies suggests it is 0.4% to 0.9% of the population with regard to identity, although less than 0.02% would seek any medical intervention or treatment.[3] Some people within this group fit the gender binary, such as natal males who identify as women (male-to-female, or MTF) or natal females who identify as men (female-to-male, or FTM). Others are *gender nonbinary* (GNB), identifying with both genders partially or completely, or with neither. It is possible for a person to be both intersex and transgender, and in fact the prevalence of transgenderism in the intersex community seems to be higher than in natal males and females.[4] In such cases, lower self-esteem along with higher levels of depression and anxiety have been reported.

Although little sleep-related research is available for either group, a growing body of evidence suggests they suffer from an abundance of sleep pathologies. The characterization and treatment of these disturbances, and their response to interventions, are poorly understood, but the available research has set a good starting point to develop protocols and identify investigational priorities. At this time there is a paucity of published data.

SLEEP QUANTITY AND QUALITY

Sleep quantity and quality vary throughout life for most individuals, and sleep problems are often reported. Sleep deprivation is particularly ubiquitous in society: roughly one-third of adults report sleeping less than the minimum recommended 7 hours a night.[5] This problem also has been documented in the transgender community, although there is a surprising degree of variation among the different groups with regard to severity. One survey that included 669 transgender individuals found that FTM transgender people reported similar sleep deprivation to the general population—32.7%, or roughly one-third. However, the MTF group had a greater proportion of sleep-deprived individuals—43.4%—while the GNB group fared worse, with 51.2% of people reporting sleeping 6 hours or less.[6] The finding for the GNB cohort is even worse when only extreme sleep restriction (i.e., reported sleep duration of 5 hours or less) is considered: 35.5% of GNB people fell within this group. No other LGBT+ or majority group reported a proprotion of more than 20% with extreme sleep restriction, showing an alarming degree of sleep deprivation specific to these individuals. The Pittsburgh Sleep Quality Index is a commonly used metric: as many as 80% of transgender individuals report poor sleep quality using this instrument.[7] No such studies were found for intersex individuals.

Both quality and quantity of sleep can be heavily influenced by a person's surroundings and mental health. Because of this, intersex and transgender communities are at risk with regard to sleep health. There are no studies at present that examine the general causes of sleep difficulties for these communities, but they are often discussed in the context of negative life experiences leading to self-acceptance problems.[8] Broadly speaking, transgender adults report a higher incidence than the general population for depressive symptoms, suicidality, interpersonal trauma, substance use, and anxiety disorders.[9] These findings are at least partly explained by exposure to stigma, discrimination, and bias events, while social support and community connectedness appear beneficial.

Unfortunately, obtaining social support and feeling they are part of their community have added difficulties within the transgender population, as some of their needs differ from those of the general public. These become more relevant in socioeconomically disadvantaged circumstances. For example, homeless shelters tend to segregate sleeping and hygiene arrangements by sex, leading transgender people to face difficulties in obtaining physically safe shelters that also provide adequate protection for their privacy.[10] Transgender youths can face similar problems because they are known to experience a higher proportion of adverse life events and substance abuse from an early age.[11] Within the foster care system, transgender youths also face challenges regarding their safety and privacy, similar to the aforementioned homeless adults.[12]

Fortunately, it seems that early intervention can be beneficial for children. Transgender children who feel supported in their identity have normal levels of depression and only minimally elevated anxiety.[13] Therefore ensuring these patients feel supported in their identity, including providing them with a safe personal space and privacy, can decrease the presence of stressors known to affect sleep.

Mental stressors seem to be less of a concern for intersex people,[14] although that can vary considerably depending on the baseline disorder of sex development diagnosed[15] and the medical trajectory with regard to their intersex condition.[16] Certainly there are reports of anxiety surrounding the diagnosis of intersexuality or disorders of sex development directly affecting bedtime routine, with patients crying themselves to sleep as they begin coping with the new information and its implications.[17] Theoretically, the problems described here should improve with treatment, as mental health does for transgender adolescents when they are allowed to live according to their gender identity. In practice, some of the treatment choices could themselves cause sleep disturbances.

HORMONAL TREATMENT

It has long been understood that there is a bidirectional relationship between sex hormones and sleep. Testosterone levels peak with the onset of sleep, are decreased by sleep deprivation, and can themselves trigger sleep disturbances if too low or too high.[18,19] Estrogen effects are best studied by observing diurnal and circadian rhythm variations seen throughout the menstrual cycle.[20] These variations can have effects on memory consolidation as related to sleep and other effects on female functioning.[21] As many transgender and intersex individuals choose to undergo hormonal therapy to suppress secondary characteristics of their natal sex or to develop characteristics of a different sex, concerns have been raised about how exogenous administration of these substances affects sleep.

For androgens, the main concerns are with regard to sleep-disordered breathing. One of the first cases to put forth this concern was documented in 1983 when a male receiving testosterone and human chorionic gonadotropin developed severe obstructive sleep apnea (OSA). It improved after 5 weeks off hormones but recurred 1 to 2 months after testosterone was reinitiated. It completely resolved once he was off hormones for 6 months.[22] Some studies have continued to support this impression, particularly in older men with hypogonadism in whom exogenous testosterone showed worsening apneas and hypoxemia, and decreased sleep duration.[23] The same study interestingly found that Functional Outcomes of Sleep Questionnaire and sleepiness (measured with the Epworth Sleepiness and Stanford scales) were not changed by the androgens. Despite these findings, in obese men with sleep apnea, testosterone administration only mildly worsened OSA in a time-limited fashion.[24] Nevertheless, the concern remains and has been recently echoed in the 2017 clinical practice guidelines published by the Endocrine Society on treatment of gender-dysphoric and gender-incongruent individuals.[25] The reference used to justify the concern is the same Society's guidelines for testosterone therapy in men with androgen deficiency. The latter guidelines recommend against starting androgen therapy in individuals with untreated sleep apnea and suggest monitoring hematocrit as an indirect marker for the development of OSA; they also list induction or worsening of OSA as an uncommon effect of testosterone therapy.[26] These latter recommendations would likely apply to the transgender community, although, lacking data, it is hard to be sure. One recent case series described one MTF individual whose sleep apnea resolved after starting androgen suppression and two FTM persons who developed sleep apnea upon starting androgens.[27] The possibility that testosterone may lead to sleep apnea is also an issue for intersex individuals when considering hormonal therapy.[28]

The potential deleterious effects of female sex hormones on natal males are less clear. Evidence from oral contraceptives, which alter sleep and raise core body temperature,[29] does suggest sleep would be affected. Furthermore, administration of female sex hormones to postmenopausal women seemed to reverse the electroencephalographic (EEG) changes induced by menopause[30] and clinically improve sleep quality.[31] Despite evidence suggesting changes are likely to happen, in one study administration of estrogen and anti-androgens in MTF patients had only a small influence on sleep EEG, with an increase in the duration of light sleep.[32] Another study contradicts this, with increased slow wave sleep and rapid eye movement sleep plus reported improved sleep quality in MTF subjects when sex hormones were started.[33] The reasons for this discrepancy could lie in the dosages of female sex hormones received, but because protocols are evolving, it is unlikely that a clear answer on how hormone therapy affects sleep for MTF will soon be elucidated.

The decision to pursue cross-sex hormonal therapy is never simple or straightforward and should always be guided by the patient's wishes with the aid of mental health professionals. In some cases, hormone therapy is either not pursued or postponed in favor of endogenous sex steroid suppression alone. This is often the case in children with extreme gender dysphoria. The case in children presents the added ethical difficulty of determining whether the sense of bodily autonomy has matured and whether the person has the capacity to consent to treatment. Decisions are made with the understanding that most children with gender dysphoria tend to outgrow this condition.[34] However, it can be exacerbated with the onset of puberty, which can lead to self-destructive behavior. In such cases, suppression of pubertal growth can be considered starting with Tanner stage 2.[35] Suppression can allow the patient to mature further and the team to be clearer on how to proceed. If the ultimate decision is to remove the suppressants, puberty usually resumes without issue.

SURGICAL TREATMENT

Feminization surgeries include augmentation mammoplasty, orchiectomy, penectomy, vaginoplasty, and others. Vaginoplasty is most commonly done through penile inversion, although the bowel may be used in certain cases. *Masculinizing surgeries* include mastectomy, oophorectomy, and hysterectomy to remove the female organs and then either phalloplasty (which requires skin grafting, urethral extension, and use of a penile prothesis) or metoidioplasty (whereby the clitoris is elongated and made to resemble a penis while keeping its erectile capabilities). Either procedure may be accompanied by scrotoplasty, using the labia majora, with or without testicular protheses. These transitions may take months or years, causing great stress and possibly resulting in poor sleep. The use of these procedures in intersex children and adolescents has recently come under scrutiny because there is a lack of evidence on benefits versus risks of these interventions early in life and a growing number of governments, and nongovernmental organizations have expressed their concern that such procedures could violate the human rights of children.[36] Many are hence advocating for these procedures to be postponed until later in life, partly with hopes that it will lead to less mental stress.

The previously described surgeries are complex and subject to numerous complications and pose the risk of the end result not fulfilling expectations of the patient. Although they have been described to improve many aspects of patients' lives, the areas of energy, fatigue, sleep, and rest seem to be negatively affected by the procedures.[37] Furthermore, individuals who have undergone feminizing or masculinizing surgeries remain at high risk of suicide compared with the general population, suggesting the effect on their well-being is not as robust as one would hope.

An important consideration in these cases is if an individual cannot continue hormone therapy after having had their gonads removed. This can occur for several reasons, from loss or change of health insurance, to poor tolerance of exogenous hormones, to personal choice. In these cases, there may be a neutralizing effect on sleep patterns and architecture, where these are not characteristic of the typical findings for males or females but result in a middle point between the two. This is supported by a study on murine models, in which observed diurnal sex differences on the sleep-wake cycle of mice was reduced or eliminated after gonadectomy.[38] It is also worth noting that some sex differences in sleep are not directly due to gonadal function, and these may persist even after hormonal therapy and gender surgery are pursued.

These interventions are relatively new and expanding. It is possible surgical interventions in the future will develop to include chronic medical complexities such as reproductive organ transplants. Indeed, the first transgender individual to attempt a uterine transplant was Lili Elbe (birth name, Einar Magnus Andreas Wegener) in 1931; the procedure resulted in the patient's death 3 months later.[39] The possibility has been revisited at present as a fertility option for MTF patients,[40] although currently the Montreal Criteria governing the ethics of the procedure require the recipient to be biologically female.[41] Nevertheless, the transplant has already been performed from female donor to female recipient, with the first successful live birth reported in 2015.[42] The recipient was medically immunosuppressed for a year before attempting conception with tacrolimus, azathioprine, and corticosteroids and remained so throughout the pregnancy. It is noteworthy that two of these agents (tacrolimus and corticosteroids) have been reported to cause sleep difficulties. Therefore, as treatment options for these individuals expand, it will be important to screen regularly for the emergence or recurrence of sleep disturbances.

CLINICAL PEARL

People who are intersex or transgender should regularly be screened for sleep disturbances, as these have been widely reported for them. Sleep disturbances can be present at baseline, sometimes resulting from mental stressors regarding their gender or sexual identity and their acceptance in their community. It can also result from treatments pursued, such as sex hormone administration or gender surgery. Male sex hormones could predispose to sleep-related breathing disorders and female sex hormones increase body temperature and may alter sleep architecture. Gender surgeries are a series of feminizing or masculinizing interventions that can happen over many years and may lead to complications, including mental and physical stress-related sleep deprivation.

SUMMARY

It is rapidly becoming clear that intersex and transgender individuals are particularly vulnerable to sleep pathologies, although this remains an understudied area of sleep medicine. Up to 80% of transgender individuals report poor sleep and some subgroups report severe sleep deprivation. The reasons for these sleep disturbances can be many and include mental stressors, which are less evident in intersex individuals compared with the transgender community and can be less common when intersex and transgender people feel supported in their identity. Sex hormone treatments can be sought by both groups and can affect sleep; the concern that exogenous androgens could cause or worsen sleep apnea is a particularly stressed concern in guidelines. Surgical options to feminize or marculinize the body are available for both groups. The multiple surgeries required over a long period of time can also directly or indirectly affect sleep. In the near future, it will be important to become familiar with the particular subgroups that make up these communities, as findings within these groups can be heterogenous. Sleep disturbances are already widely reported. As these individuals become more visible in our societies, it will be imperative to be at the forefront of treatment and closely follow or monitor these patients for a wide range of sleep disorders.

SELECTED READINGS

Auer MK, Liedl A, Fuss J, et al. High impact of sleeping problems on quality of life in transgender individuals: a cross-sectional multicenter study. *PLoS One*. 2017;12(2):e0171640.

Barrett-Connor E, Dam TT, Stone K, Harrison SL, Redline S, et al. The association of testosterone levels with overall sleep quality, sleep architecture, and sleep-disordered breathing. *J Clin Endocrinol Metab*. 2008;93:2602–2609.

Bowen AE, Staggs S, Kaar J, Nokoff N, Simon SL. Short sleep, insomnia symptoms, and evening chronotype are correlated with poorer mood and quality of life in adolescent transgender males. *Sleep Health*. 2021;7(4):445–450.

da Silva DC, Schwarz K, Fontanari AM, et al. WHOQOL-100 before and after sex reassignment surgery in Brazilian male-to-female transsexual individuals. *J Sex Med*. 2016;13(6):988–993.

Harry-Hernandez S, Reisner SL, Schrimshaw EW, et al. Gender dysphoria, mental health, and poor sleep health among transgender and gender nonbinary individuals: a qualitative study in New York City. *Transgend Health*. 2020;5(1):59–68.

Hembree WC, Cohen-Kettenis PT, Gooren L, et al. Endocrine treatment of gender-dysphoric/gender-incongruent persons: an endocrine society clinical practice guideline. *J Clin Endocrinol Metab*. 2017;102(11):3869–3903.

Hershner S, Jansen EC, Gavidia R, Matlen L, Hoban M, Dunietz GL. Associations between transgender identity, sleep, mental health and suicidality among a North American Cohort of College Students. *Nat Sci Sleep*. 2021;13:383–398. Published 2021 Mar 16.

Levenson JC, Thoma BC, Hamilton JL, Choukas-Bradley S, Salk RH. Sleep among gender minority adolescents. *Sleep*. 2021;44(3):zsaa185.

Warne G, Grover S, Hutson J, et al. Childrens' Research Institute Sex Study Group. a long-term outcome study of intersex conditions. *J Pediatr Endocrinol Metab*. 2005;18(6):555–568.

A complete reference list can be found online at ExpertConsult.com.

Sleep in Women

Section 21

Introduction

Chapter 183

Fiona C. Baker; Bei Bei

This section provides a foundation of knowledge about sleep in the context of women's health. There is growing recognition that health conditions in women and different reproductive stages of a woman's life cycle require unique considerations. There are differences between men and women in many aspects of sleep (behavior, physiology, sleep disorders), and within women, sleep varies according to reproductive stages and events, including across the menstrual cycle, during pregnancy, postpartum, and menopause. The prevalence and presentation of sleep disorders also vary according to reproductive stage, interacting with aging, and therefore the treatment of sleep disorders in women should be considered within the context of the reproductive cycle.

The first chapter in this section details sex differences in sleep. The subsequent chapters follow the reproductive stages across a woman's life cycle, focusing on characteristics of sleep and sleep disorders at each stage. To follow, are brief overviews of each chapter in the section about "sleep in women."

CHAPTER 184: SEX EFFECTS AND DIFFERENCES IN CIRCADIAN RHYTHMS AND SLEEP

Sex is a critical factor in sleep research and clinical sleep medicine. There are sex differences in circadian measures, with a generally shorter circadian period and more advanced phase in women. These differences have implications for how women cope with nighttime shift work and could also partly explain the higher prevalence of difficulty maintaining sleep or early awakenings in women. Women are more likely to report sleep difficulties and poor sleep quality than men, but objective measures of sleep tend to show better sleep in women than in men. This subjective-objective discordance is only partially explained by sex differences in psychosocial factors.

Being female is a risk factor for insomnia, even after controlling for mental and physical health factors; this risk progressively increases with age and changes with reproductive states. Women are more likely to be prescribed hypnotics, although recommended doses may differ from those for men, given sex differences in pharmacokinetics. In contrast, obstructive sleep apnea (OSA) is two times more common in men than women due to a combination of factors, including differences in regional body fat distribution, upper airway anatomy, respiratory control, and reproductive hormones. However, OSA may be underdiagnosed in women when presenting with nonspecific symptoms.

CHAPTER 185: THE MENSTRUAL CYCLE, SLEEP, AND CIRCADIAN RHYTHMS

There is a two-way interaction between the female reproductive system and sleep and circadian regulation. The menstrual cycle is associated with changes in sleep (increased spindle frequency electroencephalogram activity and a reduction in rapid eye movement sleep) and a higher body temperature with blunted circadian amplitude in the postovulatory luteal phase relative to the follicular phase. Self-reported sleep quality does not necessarily map onto these changes, with some women reporting difficulty sleeping midcycle, some premenstrually, and others reporting no change. Some women are more impacted by psychological and somatic symptoms, which can manifest with premenstrual syndrome or primary dysmenorrhea. Polycystic ovary syndrome is a risk factor for OSA, and OSA screening with follow-up polysomnography (PSG) is recommended for women with this condition.

The female reproductive system is influenced by sleep and circadian factors such that poor sleep quality, insufficient sleep, shift work, or the presence of a sleep disorder could impact reproductive function, with effects dependent on pubertal stage and age. Sleep, independent of time of day, has a major influence on pulsatile luteinizing hormone (LH) secretion in pubertal children, with higher LH pulse frequency during slow wave sleep. These sleep-related changes in LH and gonadotropin-releasing hormone secretion may help direct normal developmental changes in gonadotropin release across puberty. There is a change in the effect of sleep on LH pulse frequency in late puberty and in adult women in the follicular phase, with sleep-inhibiting LH pulse frequency and pulse initiation tending to follow brief awakenings.

CHAPTER 186: SLEEP AND SLEEP DISORDERS ASSOCIATED WITH PREGNANCY

Major physiologic changes that occur during the three trimesters of pregnancy are associated with significant changes to women's sleep. These changes are well documented in self-report, PSG, and actigraphy measurements in cross-sectional, longitudinal, and case-controlled studies. Sleep disturbances typically increase as pregnancy progresses, and significant sleep disturbances are reported by the majority of women toward the end of the pregnancy.

A number of sleep disorders, such as sleep-disordered breathing (SDB; see Chapter 187), restless legs syndrome, and insomnia increase in prevalence across pregnancy. Other pregnancy-related conditions, such as esophageal reflux and sleep-related leg cramps, add to the sleep challenges women face during pregnancy.

Although some degree of sleep disturbance is expected during pregnancy, sleep complaints need to be carefully assessed and managed. Untreated maternal sleep disorders are risk factors for adverse pregnancy and birth outcomes. Nonpharmacologic approaches are preferred and are effective for insomnia; pharmacologic treatments need to balance risk and benefits, taking into account drug safety profiles for pregnancy use.

CHAPTER 187: SLEEP-DISORDERED BREATHING DURING PREGNANCY

Multiple pregnancy-related physiologic changes that lead to anatomic narrowing and/or increased resistance within the respiratory system predispose women to increased risk for SDB, which worsens as pregnancy progresses. Risk factors for SDB in pregnancy may include habitual snoring, hypertension, higher body mass index, and older age and require further investigation. Excessive gestational weight gain is hypothesized to be a risk factor for developing SDB in pregnancy, but data supporting this relationship are currently lacking. SDB has a range of negative consequences on maternal outcomes, such as gestational hypertension, preeclampsia, and gestational diabetes, but causal mechanisms are not well understood. Although receiving less attention so far, SDB during pregnancy can also impact fetal outcomes (e.g., fetal mortality, miscarriages, preterm delivery, growth abnormalities). Fetal effects may be exerted directly or indirectly by exacerbation of underlying comorbid conditions that coincide with SDB.

Screening for SDB in pregnancy is not currently routinely carried out. Pregnancy-specific screening tools show promise but need further testing and development. When SDB is suspected in pregnancy, women should be evaluated and treated in line with standard guidelines. Positional therapy can be recommended as an adjunctive therapy to continuous positive airway pressure (CPAP). Patients with preexisting SDB that is already being treated should continue treatment during their pregnancy and postpartum; CPAP is safe and effective in the pregnant population. There is limited data on how the treatment of SDB could mitigate its impact on pregnancy and birth outcomes, and more research is needed.

CHAPTER 188: POSTPARTUM PERIOD AND EARLY PARENTHOOD

For most parents, early postpartum periods are associated with significant sleep disruptions, including reduced nighttime sleep, increased nighttime awakenings, decreased sleep efficiency, and altered sleep timing. Postpartum physical recovery, infant care, and life demands are all contributing factors. Although sleep generally improves over time, it often does not return to prepregnancy level by the end of the first postpartum year. It is important to recognize that many societal and cultural factors contribute to new parents' sleep during the postpartum period. There are significant ethnic and racial disparities in postpartum sleep health. Postpartum sleep and other dimensions of parental well-being are also influenced by policies such as return to work and paid parental leaves.

Significant sleep disturbances during the postpartum period are associated with a range of negative consequences, such as daytime sleepiness, fatigue, mood disturbances, and impairments to daily functioning. Low-intensity maternal sleep interventions (e.g., psychoeducation) showed limited benefits during the postpartum period. Promising findings have been reported where more intense interventions (e.g., residential services) were given to vulnerable women with significant sleep disturbances. Effective ways to support new parents' sleep during the postpartum period, especially increasing sleep duration and continuity during the early postpartum period, remain a major gap.

CHAPTER 189: SLEEP AND MENOPAUSE

Menopause is a major transitional process in women, consisting of complex and interactive changes in the central nervous and endocrine systems. Sleep can be negatively impacted by multiple factors before, during, and after menopause, including the emergence of sleep-disrupting hot flashes, changes in the hormone milieu, psychosocial factors, and the rise in sleep disorders and other clinical conditions that co-occur during this stage of life. Hot flashes are a cardinal symptom of the menopausal transition and may persist for several years postmenopause. Hot flashes are a major contributing factor to sleep disturbances and wake after sleep onset that are strongly associated with insomnia and depression. Hot flashes occur throughout the sleep period, appearing mostly in non–rapid eye movement sleep, and have varying degrees of impact on different women. Cognitive behavioral therapy for insomnia has been proven to successfully treat insomnia in midlife women, including in those who have frequent hot flashes.

As women proceed through the menopause transition and into postmenopause, they are at increased risk for developing OSA, attributed to aging and menopause-related factors, such as a preferential increase in intraabdominal or visceral deposition of fat. CPAP, along with weight loss and exercise, are the treatment of choice for these women. As women age, they are also at increased risk for other health conditions, including breast cancer, fibromyalgia, and thyroid dysfunction, which are all associated with sleep disruption that may be worsened by coincidental menopausal symptoms, such as hot flashes. The underlying causes of sleep problems in a midlife woman therefore can be complex, and consideration needs to be given to the combination of menopause-specific and age-related factors, as well as psychosocial factors (e.g., stress, depression, sociodemographic factors).

SELECTED READINGS

Baker FC, de Zambotti M, Colrain IM, Bei B. Sleep problems during the menopausal transition: prevalence, impact, and management challenges. *Nat Sci Sleep*. 2018;10:73–95.

Facco FL, Parker CB, Reddy UM, et al. Association between sleep-disordered breathing and hypertensive disorders of pregnancy and gestational diabetes mellitus. *Obstet Gynecol*. 2017;129(1):31–41.

Haddad S, Dennis C-L, Shah PS, Stremler R. Sleep in parents of preterm infants: a systematic review. *Midwifery*. 2019;73:35–48.

Kravitz HM, Janssen I, Bromberger JT, et al. Sleep trajectories before and after the final menstrual period in the Study of Women's Health Across the Nation (SWAN). *Curr Sleep Med Rep*. 2017;3(3):235–250.

Manber R, Bei B, Simpson N, Asarnow L, Rangel E, Sit A, Lyell D. Cognitive behavioral therapy for prenatal insomnia: a randomized controlled trial. *Obstet Gynecol*. 2019;133(5):911.

Miller MA, Mehta N, Clark-Bilodeau C, Bourjeily G. Sleep pharmacotherapy for common sleep disorders in pregnancy and lactation. *Chest*. 2020;157(1):184–197.

Neumann N, Lotze M, Domin M. Sex-specific association of poor sleep quality with gray matter volume. *Sleep*. 2020;43(9):zsaa035.

Pengo MF, Won CH, Bourjeily G. Sleep in women across the life span. *Chest*. 2018;154:196–206.

Sam S, Ehrmann DA. Pathogenesis and consequences of disordered sleep in PCOS. *Clin Med Insights Reprod Health*. 2019;13:1179558119871269.

Warland J, Dorrian J, Morrison J, O'Brien LM. Maternal sleep during pregnancy and poor fetal outcomes: a scoping review of the literature with meta-analysis. *Sleep Med Rev*. 2018;41:197–219.

Zhang B, Wing Y-K. Sex differences in insomnia: a meta-analysis. *Sleep*. 2006;29(1):85–93.

Chapter 184

Sex Effects and Differences in Circadian Rhythms and Sleep

Ari Shechter; Sean W. Cain

Chapter Highlights

- Morphologic differences between women and men in the suprachiasmatic nucleus, as well as the presence of sex hormone receptors there, suggest that sex may have a direct modulatory role on circadian rhythms and therefore sleep.
- Sex differences have been reported in human circadian physiology. Compared with men, women show earlier timing of melatonin and body temperature rhythms, as well as a shorter intrinsic circadian period.
- Women report more sleep complaints than men and are at increased risk of insomnia that begins at sexual maturation and persists throughout adulthood. Despite the higher prevalence of self-reported sleep difficulties and the perception of poor sleep, women often show better sleep quality than men when sleep is assessed objectively.
- Reasons for this discrepancy and more frequent self-reported poor sleep in women are unclear but may be due to sex-specific alterations in the circadian system, psychosocial factors, or sex differences in the homeostatic regulation of sleep.
- Obstructive sleep apnea (OSA) is reported to occur more frequently in men than women. However, recent work suggests that OSA may be underdiagnosed in women, and sex differences are less apparent when considering OSA in rapid eye movement sleep.

INTRODUCTION

Differences in body and brain morphology, biologic processes, and neurohormone secretion between women and men can influence the expression and regulation of behavioral and physiologic outcomes, including sleep and circadian rhythms. Biologic variables likely interact with psychosocial factors, further contributing to sex differences in sleep and/or circadian rhythms and susceptibility to the development of sleep disorders. Recent mandates have been put forth by research granting agencies to consider sex as a biologic variable in all funded research. These initiatives were established with the goal of further understanding sex influences on health and disease. As explained further later, sex is a critical factor to consider in sleep research and clinical sleep medicine practice. Understanding how sex differences affect sleep, circadian rhythms, and vulnerabilities to the adverse effects of disturbed sleep will have widespread ramifications for health, function, and well-being in both women and men.

SEX DIFFERENCES IN CIRCADIAN RHYTHMS

Sex Differences in Morphology of the Suprachiasmatic Nucleus

In humans (and all mammals), the suprachiasmatic nucleus (SCN) of the anterior hypothalamus is the master circadian oscillator. In the absence of this small piece of tissue (~50,000 neurons bilaterally in humans[1]), overt rhythms in behavior and hormone secretion cease.[2,3] When this tissue alone is transplanted into arrhythmic animals with an ablated SCN, circadian rhythms (measured with activity) return.[4,5]

The structure of the SCN in humans has long been known to be sexually dimorphic. The examination of postmortem tissue has shown that the shape of the SCN differs in women and men (elongated in women, spherical in men), although the overall volume, cell density, number of cells, and diameter of cell nuclei are the same.[6,7] Further study of the substructures in the SCN revealed that the most striking sex differences were in vasoactive intestinal polypeptide (VIP) neurons. Clear sex differences in the number of VIP neurons in the SCN developed by the age of 10, with girls and women having half of the number of VIP cells of men.[8,9] Women continue to have fewer VIP cells until the age of 40, when a decline in VIP cells was seen in men.[10] As VIP is a key modulator of light input to the clock,[11] such a sex difference could result in sex differences in circadian light sensitivity.

Sex Differences in Timing and Circadian Physiology

Although the functional consequences of these specific SCN structural differences in women and men remain unclarified, sex differences in circadian rhythms have been reported. In an early study by Rütger Wever, women tended to have a shorter circadian period (length of the endogenously generated day) under "free-running" conditions in which participants were able to choose their sleep-wake schedule.[12] Under such conditions, the sleep-wake cycle and body temperature rhythms can become desynchronized (showing different cycling periods). Wever found that when the sleep-wakefulness and body temperature rhythms remained synchronized, women exhibited shorter body temperature rhythm periods than the men (~18 minutes shorter; not a significant difference, likely because of low statistical power). After the sleep-wake and body temperature rhythms spontaneously desynchronized, temperature rhythms of women and men were virtually identical. Because of the trends toward a shorter day in women, Wever noted that "In the natural 24-hour day. . .the phase of the combined circadian rhythms relative to. . .local time, should be earlier in females than in males; i.e., females should tend more than males to be 'morning types,'" an idea later confirmed in large samples.[12-14]

More recently, a large study in 157 women and men (52 women, 105 men studied over more than 5000 days) demonstrated significant sex differences in circadian period as measured using a "forced desynchrony" protocol.[15] In this protocol, participants remain in windowless suites under dim light conditions (~3 lux) for approximately 1 month with sleep and wake times set, not freely chosen by participants (typically 20- or 28-hour "days" with one-third of the "day" set as a sleep opportunity). This protocol allows for underlying 24-hour rhythms in temperature and melatonin levels to be observed by removing the potential masking influences of the imposed sleep-wake schedule. Under these highly controlled conditions, circadian period was found to be significantly shorter in women (24 hours, 5 minutes) than in men (24 hours, 11 minutes). Furthermore, a significantly greater proportion of women had circadian periods shorter than 24.0 hours (35% versus 14%; Figure 184.1). These results are consistent with findings from nonhuman animals that demonstrated circadian period is shorter in females than in males.[16,17] Although approximately one-third the magnitude of the (nonstatistically significant) sex difference found by Wever (6 versus 18 minutes), such a sex difference has a significant impact; a period difference of a particular size is associated with a fourfold greater difference in circadian phase relative to the light-dark (LD) cycle. Thus a 6-minute difference in period becomes a 24-minute difference in clock alignment to the sleep-wake and LD cycle.[18]

The faster cycling of the circadian clock in women would be expected to result in a more advanced circadian timing relative to the LD cycle, and this has been demonstrated. Although early studies showed conflicting sex differences in circadian time (or none at all), this was likely due to the use of highly variable and masked temperature rhythms in ambulatory participants. Using dim light melatonin onset (DLMO; a more reliable measure of circadian time), it was reported that melatonin onset was approximately 1.5 hours earlier in women.[19] In that study, DLMO was defined as the point that melatonin levels reached twice the minimum detectable concentration. This advanced timing in women was later replicated, although to a lesser degree.[20] When defined using a fixed threshold (assuming sufficiently low light levels that do not cause melatonin suppression), melatonin onset is determined by both circadian phase and an individual's overall levels. That is, even with identical phase, an individual with high melatonin levels will appear to have an earlier phase using a fixed threshold. This was apparently happening at the group level when comparing women and men, as melatonin rhythm amplitude in women were found to be significantly higher than in men (approximately 50% higher)[20]; a result that was later nearly identically replicated.[21] When melatonin onset was adjusted for each individual's overall melatonin levels, women were found to have a difference of less than half the magnitude of that reported previously. Thus, by using the same fixed

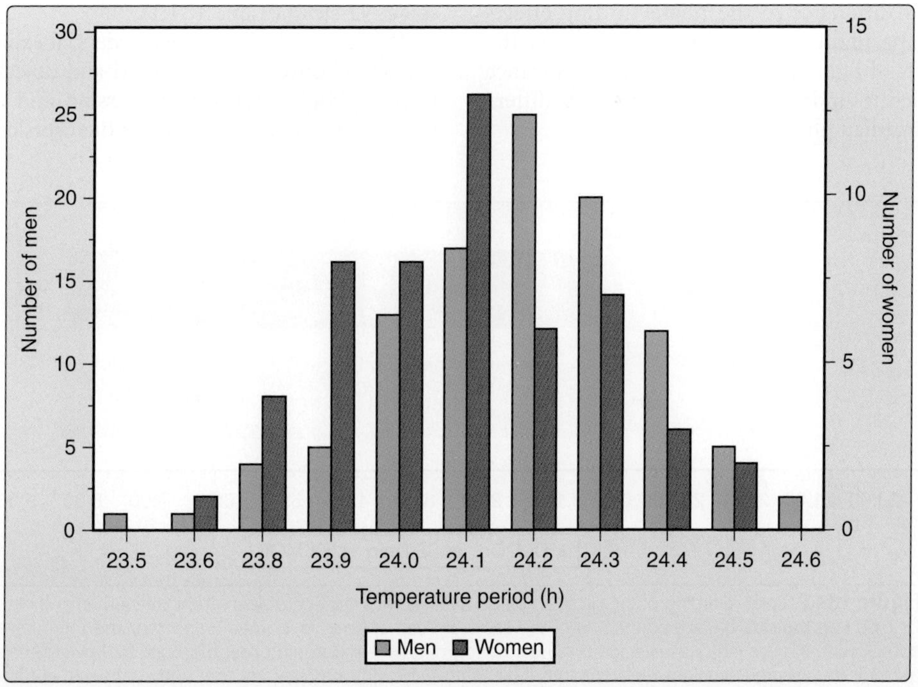

Figure 184.1 Histogram of circadian periods as assessed using core body temperature in men and women. The distribution of periods is more skewed to earlier times in women, relative to men. (Modified from Duffy JF, Cain SW, Chang AM, Phillips AJ, Münch MY, Gronfier C, Wyatt JK, Dijk DJ, Wright KP Jr, Czeisler CA. Sex difference in the near-24-hour intrinsic period of the human circadian timing system. *Proc Natl Acad Sci U S A.* 2011 Sep 13;108 Suppl 3:15602–8.)

threshold for women and men, the sex difference in biologic timing was exaggerated because of higher melatonin levels in women. Larger advances in women (~1.5 hours; Figure 184.2) were demonstrated in core body temperature rhythms under controlled conditions that reduce, or evenly distribute across the day, the masking effects of sleep/activity.[20,22]

A consistent result has emerged: women have advanced timing, relative to men. This has not only been shown using melatonin and temperature as phase markers but also circadian clock gene expression has been found to peak earlier in the dorsolateral prefrontal cortex of women than men.[23] Although advanced timing is expected based on the faster circadian period in women, the degree to which women are advanced is far greater than the difference in period would predict. Thus other mechanisms are likely contributing to this sex difference. One plausible mechanism is a sex difference in sensitivity of the circadian system to light: either a decreased sensitivity to delaying light in the evening, an increased sensitivity to advancing light in the morning, or both. Whether there are sex differences in circadian light sensitivity remains an open question. In a small study of 12 women and men, greater circadian sensitivity was found to bright light (2000 lux) in women than men.[24] However, other groups found no sex differences in light sensitivity and melatonin suppression at moderate to bright light intensities (200, 500, 1000, 1500, 2000, 2500, and 3000 lux).[25-27] Furthermore, in a study that generated individual dose response curves to light of intensities from 10 lux to 2000 lux, there was no sex difference found in the level of 50% melatonin suppression.[28] At least for melatonin suppression in the evening and night, there does not appear to be a large sex difference in light sensitivity. Although melatonin suppression in the evening has been reported to be very highly associated with the subsequent phase shift in circadian timing,[29] it is possible to dissociate melatonin suppression from phase shifting.[30] Thus a lack of difference between women and men in melatonin suppression does not necessarily preclude a sex difference in the phase-shifting effects of light in the evening/night. Studies directly measuring the phase shifting effects of light (in both the delay and advance directions) are needed to understand the observed sex difference in entrained circadian phase.

SEX DIFFERENCES IN SLEEP

Sex Differences in Sleep Behaviors and Sleep Physiology

Developmental Changes in Sleep Behaviors in Males and Females

A shift toward a more evening chronotype, or later preferred sleep timing, was noted as children progress into adolescence.[31] This delaying shift occurs in both males and females and is likely due to the changing hormonal milieu that accompanies sexual maturation. The delay in sleep timing occurs at a younger age in females compared to males, with the peak in eveningness seen earlier in girls (19.5 years) than in boys (20.9 years),[31] which is consistent with the earlier pubertal maturation seen in females versus males.[32] In adulthood, however, women prefer to go to bed earlier[33] and are earlier chronotypes than men (Table 184.1).[13,31] Sex differences in sleep timing disappear around the time of menopause.[31] This suggests a potential role of female gonadal hormones in influencing sleep timing preference.

Overview of Sleep Differences in Men and Women

Survey studies indicate that in adulthood, women have qualitatively different sleep than men (Table 184.1). Overall, women report more sleep complaints than men and are at increased risk of insomnia (described in further detail later).[34] In terms of self-reported sleep quality assessments, women reported shorter total sleep time, lower sleep efficiency, and worse global sleep quality than men.[35] In a large nationally representative British sample, women reported more difficulties in getting to sleep, remaining asleep, and getting enough sleep.[36] Despite the higher prevalence of self-reported sleep difficulties and the perception of poor sleep, women often show better sleep quality than men when assessed objectively. For instance, women have shorter sleep-onset latency, higher sleep efficiency, lower wake after sleep onset, and less light stage N1 sleep (Table 184.1).[37-40]

Psychosocial factors are a potential explanation for the discordance between self-reported and objective sleep quality in women. Higher rates of depression and anxiety observed in women are factors that may influence sleep quality ratings.[34]

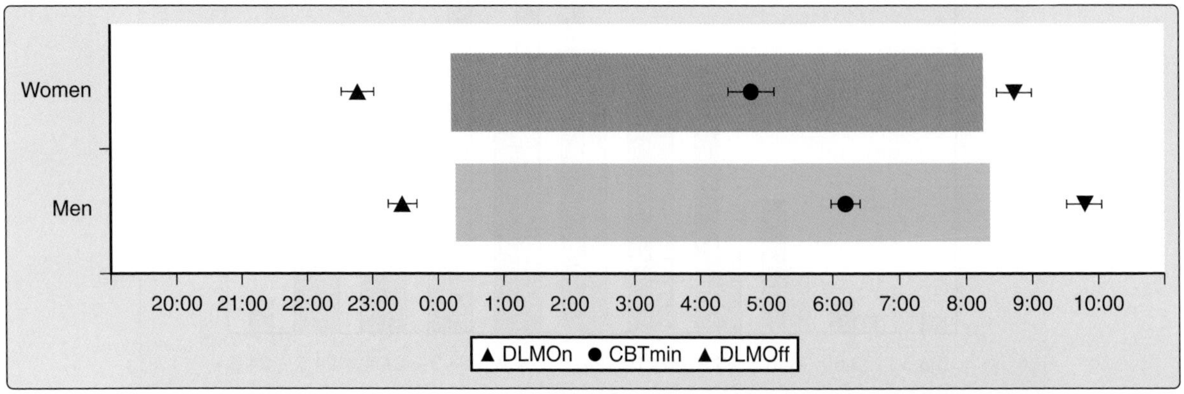

Figure 184.2 Relative timing of the circadian phase markers with respect to sleep timing in women and men. Colored bars indicate the average timing of the habitual sleep episode in women (*upper bar*) and men (*lower bar*). *Upward triangle* indicates average (±standard error) dim light melatonin onset (*DLMOn*). Downward triangle indicates average dim light melatonin offset (*DLMOff*). *Circle* indicates average core body temperature minimum. (Modified from Cain SW, Dennison CF, Zeitzer JM, Guzik AM, Khalsa SB, Santhi N, Schoen MW, Czeisler CA, Duffy JF. Sex differences in phase angle of entrainment and melatonin amplitude in humans. *J Biol Rhythms.* 2010 Aug;25[4]:288–96.)

Table 184.1 Sex Differences in Sleep in Adults

Variable	In Women versus Men
Self-Report	
Sleep timing/chronotype	Earlier
Sleep quality	Worse
Sleep difficulties	More
Objective	
Sleep-onset latency	Shorter
Sleep efficiency	Higher
Wake after sleep onset	Lower
Stage N1 sleep	Less
Stage N3 sleep	Higher
Slow wave activity	Greater response to sleep deprivation
Sleep Disorder	
Insomnia	More
Obstructive sleep apnea	Less
Narcolepsy	Less
REM sleep behavior disorder	Less
Restless legs syndrome	More

The effects of mood on sleep may also be sex dependent, because it has been reported that depressive symptoms were related to shorter self-reported total sleep time in women but not in men.[35] There may be other factors influencing this discrepancy, namely sex differences in the specific aspects of sleep that are considered when judging one's overall sleep quality. For instance, in a principal components analysis of the Pittsburgh Sleep Quality Index (PSQI), "sleep efficiency" and "sleep duration" were important determinants for men's ratings of sleep quality, whereas "daytime dysfunction" and "sleep disturbance" were important for women's ratings of perceived sleep quality.[41]

Evidence suggests that there may be sex differences in the homeostatic regulation of sleep. Levels of slow wave sleep (SWS) and slow wave activity (SWA)—physiologic markers of sleep homeostasis—are higher in women compared with men.[38,42-44] Some of these important sex differences in SWS emerge in adolescence. Specifically, a longitudinal polysomnographic study demonstrated that the typical decline in SWS/SWA that occurs in adolescence starts approximately 1.2 years earlier in girls than in boys.[45] Compared with girls, boys showed a larger age-related decline in SWS across adolescence.[46] A larger age-related decline in SWS is also noted in men versus women throughout adulthood, which suggests that this aspect of sleep is relatively less affected by aging in women.[44,47] Sex differences in sleep homeostasis were also demonstrated in a small study which assessed SWA after 40 hours of total sleep deprivation in men and women.[48] Compared with men, women had an enhanced SWA response to the sleep deprivation challenge, suggesting that sleep debt may accumulate more strongly in women.[48,49] The greater "need for sleep" reported in women may be indicative of this enhanced homeostatic sleep drive, and not sufficiently meeting this need may be an additional factor that contributes to worsened sleep perceptions in women versus men.

Recent work has explored sex differences in the circadian variation of sleep. The circadian timing of sleep propensity, sleep architecture, and alertness was assessed in men and women using an ultradian sleep-wake cycle procedure.[22] When expressed relative to habitual wake time, measures of sleep propensity and quality, and alertness, were phase-advanced by about 2 hours in women compared with men.[22] An advance in the circadian drive for sleep and alertness may help explain the higher prevalence of insomnia symptoms, and in particular difficulty maintaining sleep and early morning awakenings, reported in women versus men (further described later).[50,51]

Sex Differences in Sleep Disorders

The prevalence of several sleep disorders varies as a function of sex (Table 184.1). Insomnia and obstructive sleep apnea (OSA)—both among the most common sleep disorders—show sex differences, in which rates are higher and lower, respectively, in women versus men.[52] These conditions are discussed in further detail in the later sections.

In a population-based study, prevalence of narcolepsy was higher in men versus women (ratio of 1.8:1).[53] Because of the small number of cases, it remains unclear if this is a true sex effect or appears due to a referral bias.[54] Prior clinic-based studies found that rapid eye movement (REM) sleep behavior disorder is more common in men than women.[55-57] However, in a population-based cohort using polysomnography, there were no sex differences in prevalence of REM sleep behavior disorder.[58] The reported male predominance of REM sleep behavior disorder may therefore also be an artifact not representative of a true sex-based difference. Restless legs syndrome, on the other hand, has a prevalence in women that is approximately double that of men.[59] Restless legs syndrome appears to increase during pregnancy (see Chapter 186), with parous women showing heightened risk compared with men and nulliparous women.[60,61] This effect of pregnancy may therefore potentially account for the overall preponderance of the disorder in women versus men.[60]

Insomnia

Insomnia is the most common sleep disorder, and sex is one of the most important risk factors for the disorder.[62] A meta-analysis comprising 29 studies (n = 1,265,015 participants, 57% women) reported a significantly increased risk of insomnia in women versus men (risk ratio [RR] = 1.41).[63] When high-quality studies were considered (i.e., studies with sample size ≥ 5000, semi- or structured diagnostic interview, and diagnosis based on stringent operational criteria), the risk in women versus men was further increased (RR = 1.64).[63]

Insomnia is strongly related to affective disorders (e.g., depression and anxiety).[64,65] This may present another factor contributing to the sex-based differences in insomnia rates, because women also experience higher rates of depression and anxiety than men.[66] However, it appears that depression does not fully account for sex differences in insomnia. In the Penn State Sleep Cohort, female (versus male) sex was associated with two times the risk of insomnia (odds ratio = 2.05).[67] The heightened risk for insomnia in women remained but only slightly less so when controlling for mental health (including depression), sleep apnea, and physical health problems (odds ratio = 1.87).[67]

Hormonal, physiologic, and anatomic changes at key life stages throughout the female life span—such as puberty, the

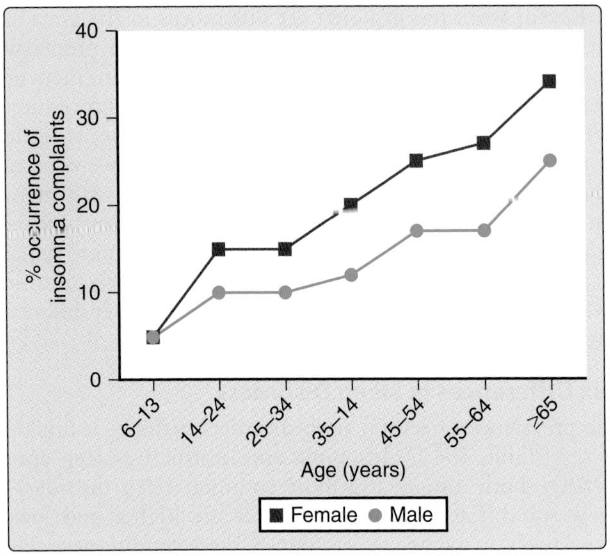

Figure 184.3 Sex differences in the prevalence of insomnia symptoms across the life span. Differences in the rates of insomnia between the sexes emerge after puberty and remain higher in women compared to men throughout adulthood. (Published with permission from Mong JA, Cusmano DM. Sex differences in sleep: impact of biological sex and sex steroids. *Philos Trans R Soc Lond B Biol Sci*. 2016; 371[1688]:20150110.)

menstrual cycle, pregnancy, and menopause—may contribute to the higher risk of insomnia in women compared with men. Differences in the rates of insomnia between the sexes appear to emerge after puberty and remain higher in women compared with men throughout adulthood (Figure 184.3).[49] In the aforementioned meta-analysis, the heightened risk of insomnia in women versus men was progressively increased when moving from young adulthood (15 to 30 years, RR = 1.28) to middle age (31 to 64 years, RR = 1.46) to old age (≥65 years, RR = 1.73).[63] Women often report disturbances in sleep quality across the menstrual cycle in response to fluctuations in gonadal hormones.[68] This is particularly true for women who experience premenstrual dysphoric disorder (PMDD), in which insomnia or hypersomnia is reported in up to 70% of cases (see Chapter 185 for more information).[69] In a survey study of 2427 pregnant women, 76% were found to be poor sleepers based on the PSQI, and 57% had at least subthreshold insomnia based on the Insomnia Severity Index.[70] Complaints of insomnia increase from 33% to 36% in premenopausal women to 44% to 61% in peri- and postmenopausal women.[71] (For a more detailed discussion on the effects of the menstrual cycle, pregnancy, and menopause on sleep, see Chapters 185, 186, 187, and 189).

Females are more likely to be prescribed hypnotic medications, and these medications affect sleep of males and females differently. A nationally representative prescription database study in Korea found that prescriptions for sedative-hypnotics was greater in women compared with men when tracked between the years 2011 and 2015.[72] Specifically, zolpidem prescriptions for insomnia were 1.6 times more frequent in women versus men.[72] Analysis of nationally representative data from the United States (i.e., the National Health and Nutrition Examination Survey) is consistent with this: Use of prescription medications commonly used for insomnia was higher in women versus men, and female sex was a significant predictor of use.[73] There are important sex differences in pharmacokinetics that have ramifications for pharmacologic approaches to insomnia. Recently, the FDA reduced the recommended dose of zolpidem in women by half, which was based on the finding that women metabolize the same dose of the drug slower than men.[74]

There have also been reported sex differences in the effects of pharmacologic sedative-hypnotic sleep aids on the sleep electroencephalogram. After administration of gaboxadol, an extrasynaptic $GABA_A$-receptor agonist, women have larger increases in SWA and theta activity compared with men.[75] Conversely, after administration of zolpidem, women have greater increases in sleep spindle activity compared with men.[75] These differences are thought to be related to the modulation of $GABA_A$-receptors by sex neurosteroids (e.g., estradiol, progesterone, testosterone), or sex differences in pharmacokinetics or $GABA_A$-receptor subtypes.[75]

From a psychological perspective, factors related to the causes and consequences of presleep hyperarousal may contribute to sex differences in insomnia etiology and treatment. In participants with psycho-physiologic insomnia, presleep arousal was associated with negative emotions in women, whereas in men, presleep arousal was associated with internal sleep locus of control (degree of perceived control over sleep).[76] Observations like this can potentially inform personalized cognitive therapeutic approaches for men and women.

Obstructive Sleep Apnea

The prevalence of OSA ranges from 9% to 38% in the general population.[77] Unlike insomnia, OSA is more common in men than women. A recent systematic review of 24 studies from around the world found that prevalence of OSA is 13% to 33% in men and 6% to 19% in women.[77] In adults 30 to 70 years old in the United States, the estimated male-to-female ratio is about 2:1 for OSA (apnea-hypopnea index [AHI] ≥15 events/hour) and closer to 3:1 for symptomatic OSA (AHI ≥ 5 events/hour plus symptoms of daytime sleepiness).[78] The male-to-female ratio increases further (5:1) when considering a clinical population.[79] The higher male-to-female ratio in clinical studies may occur because women are less likely than men to present with the classic symptoms of the disorder. For example, whereas men may present with symptoms such as loud snoring, gasping, and witnessed apneic events, women may present with nonspecific symptoms such as depression, lack of energy, sleepiness, and restless legs.[74] Accordingly, the disorder may be underdiagnosed in women. It was recently reported that when considering respiratory events in REM sleep and non–rapid eye movement (NREM) sleep separately, the prevalence of OSA in REM sleep (AHI ≥ 15 events/hour for events with at least 4% desaturation) does not differ between men and women.[80] The relatively higher rates of OSA in REM sleep versus NREM sleep in women is clinically relevant considering that REM sleep–related OSA may confer heightened cardiometabolic risk.[81] This sex difference in OSA in REM sleep may also contribute to the underdiagnosis/undertreatment of OSA in women, because total AHI predominantly reflects AHI in NREM sleep.

Differences in regional body fat distribution, upper airway anatomy, genioglossal muscle activity, craniofacial morphology, and respiratory control between men and women may account for sex differences in OSA.[79] Gonadal hormones may present another explanation. In women, key reproductive cycle events modulate the risk and expression of OSA. Whereas sex differences are not seen during the pre-/peripubertal time, adolescent males show worsened severity of clinical and polysomnographic markers of OSA than females after puberty.[82] The gonadal hormone progesterone increases genioglossal muscle activity, thereby reducing upper airway resistance,[52] and increases ventilatory response to hypercapnia and hypoxia.[83] The gonadal hormone testosterone, on the other hand, contributes to the development and worsening of OSA.[84,85] Thus higher levels of progesterone and/or lower testosterone may protect against the sleep-disordered breathing in premenopausal women.[79] The protective role of some female gonadal hormones on OSA is further emphasized by the finding that the incidence and severity of OSA increased substantially after menopause in women.[52] Increases in total body adiposity and, in particular, fat in the trunk and neck[86] after menopause may also contribute to increased OSA risk.

Polycystic ovary syndrome (PCOS) is considered one of the most common endocrine disorders in reproductive aged women. Sleep disturbances in general, including difficulty sleeping and restless sleep, are seen more frequently in women with PCOS versus controls.[87] PCOS also shows a strong relationship with OSA. A recent meta-analysis found that OSA is present in nearly a third of women with PCOS.[88] This association is likely due to the high rates of obesity in PCOS but may also occur because of low progesterone levels.[89]

Treatment approaches to OSA may also differ between the sexes. Men appear to require higher pressures for successful continuous positive airway pressure (CPAP) therapy than women, after adjusting for OSA severity.[90] In a longitudinal cohort study, weight loss was associated with a larger relative decrease in severity of sleep-disordered breathing in men than women.[91] In a randomized controlled trial of diet and physical activity targeting weight loss in individuals with obesity and type 2 diabetes, the intervention was more effective in reducing AHI in men versus women.[92]

SEX DIFFERENCES AND SHIFT WORK

Shift work (i.e., work that is scheduled to occur outside of the typical "9-to-5" day) is associated with several adverse physical and mental health consequences, including cardiovascular disease, metabolic dysfunction, obesity, cancer, and mood disorders.[93] These health effects are in part due to the combination of circadian misalignment and sleep disruption that are usually seen in shift workers. Accordingly, engaging in shift work may pose a different set of health risks for men and women, as might be expected considering the sex differences in the circadian system and sleep described previously.

Sex Differences in Shift Work Maladaptation

Most studies report that women have reduced tolerance to shift work than men, as demonstrated by more pronounced sleep problems, fatigue, and sleepiness.[94] Workplace accidents are more common among shift-working women, relative to men,[95] with accidents in the night being greater in women, despite nearly identical accident rates in the day.[96] The increased workplace accidents in shift-working women may partly reflect an enhanced effect of poor-quality sleep while engaged in shift work because of a greater sleep need in women. Sex differences in the vulnerability to acute sleep loss, however, have been demonstrated under controlled laboratory conditions in well-rested women.

Alertness has been shown to be more affected by acute sleep deprivation in women than in men both in the laboratory[97] and in the field settings.[98] The effect of sleep deprivation, however, appears to be hormone dependent. Progesterone (released during the luteal phase of the menstrual cycle) appears to mitigate the effects of sleep deprivation on cognitive performance in women.[99,100] Consistent with this, the adverse impact of sleep deprivation was recently shown only during the follicular phase of the menstrual cycle. In a 30-hour sleep deprivation protocol, when women were in the luteal phase, they performed similarly to men on sustained alertness, with a trend toward enhanced performance on long (3-second) lapses of attention (Figure 184.4).[101] Women in the follicular phase, however, performed poorly, with far slower reaction times and a higher proportion of long lapses of attention. These long lapses likely represent microsleeps and are of particular concern for workplace safety or commutes home after a night shift.

Sex differences in circadian rhythms contribute to the challenge of night-shift work in women. As mentioned previously, the shorter circadian period in women leads to a tendency for women to be more advanced in circadian timing and is a likely basis for more morning-type tendencies. Not surprisingly, those who are more morning type tolerate shift work less than evening types.[94]

Circadian amplitude may also play a role, as demonstrated in two studies that separated time awake and underlying 24-hour circadian rhythms. Using an ultradian sleep-wake cycle procedure consisting of 36 cycles of 60-minute wake episodes alternating with 60-minute nap opportunities, women were shown to have an increased amplitude of the diurnal and circadian variation of alertness than men.[22] This effect was mainly due to a larger decline in the nocturnal performance nadir. Similarly, using a 28-hour forced desynchrony protocol, the amplitude of the circadian modulation in performance was larger in women.[21] A common feature of these studies and the 30-hour sleep deprivation study mentioned previously is the demonstration of poorest performance in women in the early morning hours, close to the nadir in core body temperature. A greater vulnerability to performance failures during core body temperature minimum in women versus men may be why hyperthermic progesterone appears protective against performance decrements.

Sex-Specific Impacts of Shift Work on Health

Whereas male shift workers show increased risk of prostate cancer,[102] shift work in females is associated with increased breast cancer risk.[103] Endometrial cancer is an additional female-specific malignancy that was associated with night-shift work, particularly in females with obesity.[104]

Shift work has an impact on reproductive physiology in women, likely through circadian mechanisms. Studies in rodents have demonstrated that the circadian system is required for a regular reproductive activity. Estrus cycles and fertility are impaired by ablation of the SCN,[105] or clock gene mutations.[106] In humans, meta-analyses demonstrate that shift work is associated with menstrual cycle disruption.[107] Although a meta-analysis found an association of shift work with risk of miscarriage,[108] there is no evidence that shift work contributes to preeclampsia[109,110] or having babies small for gestational age.[109] Other meta-analyses report that shift work has either no association[111] or mild association with preterm delivery.[109] Overall, there is not sufficient evidence in the literature to recommend restricting shift work for females of reproductive age.[107]

It is likely that the disruption of menstrual cycles (and potentially fertility) in women shift workers reflects the disruptive effect of light at night on the biologic clock. Animal studies substantiate this idea. Mice exposed to chronic shifts of the LD cycle have been found to have severely impaired

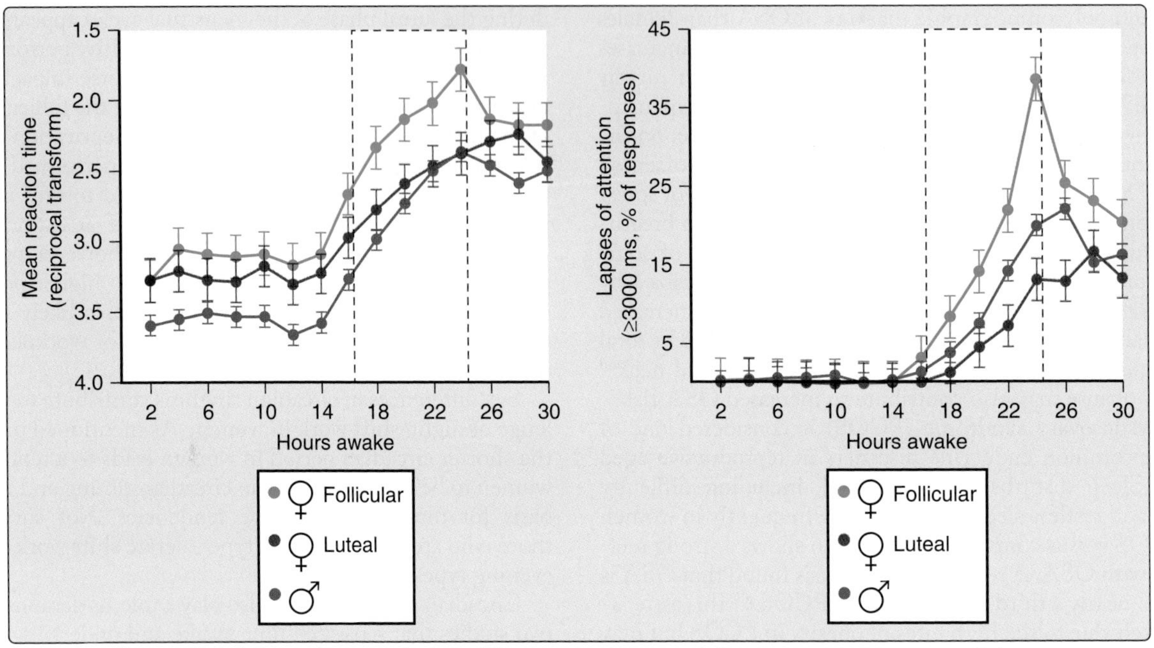

Figure 184.4 Sex and menstrual phase differences psychomotor vigilance test performance over 30 hours of wakefulness. In the follicular phase, women had longer reaction time (*left*) and a greater proportion of long (3-second) lapses of attention (*right*). Women in the luteal phase were not different from men in either measure, although there was a trend toward fewer long lapses than men. (Modified from Vidafar P, Gooley JJ, Burns AC, et al. Increased vulnerability to attentional failure during acute sleep deprivation in women depends on menstrual phase. *Sleep*. 2018; 41 [8]:zsy098.)

reproductive activity, reproductive success, and preovulatory luteinizing hormone surge.[112] Furthermore, repetitive reversal of LD cycles triggers irregular estrous cycles in mice that remain irregular for weeks after being returned to regular LD cycles. As humans have been shown to have more than 50-fold interindividual differences in the response of the circadian system to light at night,[28] some women may be more vulnerable to the disruptive effects of shift work on reproductive function.

CLINICAL PEARLS

- Women experience insomnia and self-reported sleep difficulties more frequently than men. Sex differences in circadian physiology, including a phase advance in rhythms and a shorter intrinsic circadian period in women versus men, may play a role in this. For instance, given similar bed and wake times, women may be sleeping at a later relative biologic time, which may contribute to difficulty maintaining sleep or premature awakenings.
- Psychosocial factors (e.g., depression, anxiety, hyperarousal) or alterations to sleep regulatory mechanisms (e.g., enhanced homeostatic sleep drive that is not being sufficiently met) may also disproportionately promote sleep difficulties in women.
- Often thought of as a predominantly male disease, OSA is found to occur more frequently in men versus women. However, OSA may be underdiagnosed and undertreated in women because of differences in clinical presentation, symptom reporting, and reliance on total apnea-hypopnea index for diagnosis.
- Compared to men, women show more maladaptation to nonstandard working hours, including more pronounced shift work–related sleep problems, fatigue, and work-related injuries and accidents.

SUMMARY

Various sex differences in circadian physiology, sleep behaviors, sleep quality, and sleep disorders are apparent throughout the life span. From adolescence through menopause, females have earlier sleep timing than males, suggesting a role of female gonadal hormones in influencing chronotype. This is mirrored by studies of circadian physiology conducted under controlled laboratory conditions that demonstrate that women have a phase advance in several circadian markers (e.g., melatonin). Women report poorer sleep quality overall and are at increased risk of insomnia compared with men, despite often showing better objective sleep quality. Women are at lower risk for OSA than men, potentially because of a protective effect of female gonadal hormones, or differences in upper airway anatomy or body fat distribution. However, emerging work suggests that OSA may be underdiagnosed in women and measures of OSA in REM sleep should be considered to more fully quantify risk profile in women. Sex differences in circadian rhythms of alertness, in the effects of sleep deprivation on vigilance, or in the response of the circadian system to light may help explain the lower tolerance to shift work and increased vulnerability to shift work maladaptation in women versus men.

SELECTED READINGS

Boivin DB, Shechter A, Boudreau P, et al. Diurnal and circadian variation of sleep and alertness in men vs. naturally cycling women. *Proc Natl Acad Sci U S A*. 2016;113(39):10980–10985.

Cain SW, Dennison CF, Zeitzer JM, et al. Sex differences in phase angle of entrainment and melatonin amplitude in humans. *J Biol Rhythms*. 2010;25(4):288–296.

Duffy JF, Cain SW, Chang AM, et al. Sex difference in the near-24-hour intrinsic period of the human circadian timing system. *Proc Natl Acad Sci U S A*. 2011;108(suppl 3):15602–15608.

Grant LK, Gooley JJ, St Hilaire MA, et al. Menstrual phase-dependent differences in neurobehavioral performance: the role of temperature and the progesterone/estradiol ratio. *Sleep*. 2020;43(2):zsz227.

Hrozanova M, Klöckner CA, Sandbakk Ø, Pallesen S, Moen F. Sex differences in sleep and influence of the menstrual cycle on women's sleep in junior endurance athletes. *PLoS One*. 2021;16(6):e0253376. Published 2021 Jun 17.

Lin CM, Davidson TM, Ancoli-Israel S. Gender differences in obstructive sleep apnea and treatment implications. *Sleep Med Rev*. 2008;12(6): 481–496.

Lindberg E, Janson C, Gislason T, et al. Sleep disturbances in a young adult population: can gender differences be explained by differences in psychological status? *Sleep*. 1997;20(6):381–387.

Mallampalli MP, Carter CL. Exploring sex and gender differences in sleep health: a Society for Women's Health Research Report. *J Womens Health*. 2014;23(7):553–562.

Mong JA, Cusmano DM. Sex differences in sleep: impact of biological sex and sex steroids. *Philos Trans R Soc Lond B Biol Sc*. 2016;371(1688): 20150110.

Rahman SA, Grant LK, Gooley JJ, Rajaratnam SMW, Czeisler CA, Lockley SW. Endogenous circadian regulation of female reproductive hormones. *J Clin Endocrinol Metab*. 2019;104(12):6049–6059.

Redline S, Kirchner HL, Quan SF, et al. The effects of age, sex, ethnicity, and sleep-disordered breathing on sleep architecture. *Arch Intern Med*. 2004;164(4):406–418.

Roenneberg T, Kuehnle T, Pramstaller PP, et al. A marker for the end of adolescence. *Curr Biol*. 2004;14(24):R1038–R1039.

van den Berg JF, Miedema HM, Tulen JH, et al. Sex differences in subjective and actigraphic sleep measures: a population-based study of elderly persons. *Sleep*. 2009;32(10):1367–1375.

Vidafar P, Gooley JJ, Burns AC, et al. Increased vulnerability to attentional failure during acute sleep deprivation in women depends on menstrual phase. *Sleep*. 2018;41(8).

Zhang B, Wing Y-K. Sex differences in insomnia: a meta-analysis. *Sleep*. 2006;29(1):85–93.

A complete reference list can be found online at ExpertConsult.com.

Chapter

185

The Menstrual Cycle, Sleep, and Circadian Rhythms

Fiona C. Baker; Christopher R. McCartney

Chapter Highlights

- Women's sleep varies across the menstrual cycle. The amount of N3 sleep remains constant, but rapid eye movement sleep is lower and spindle frequency activity is higher in the postovulatory luteal phase. The amplitude of the body temperature rhythm, but not the melatonin rhythm, is reduced in the luteal compared with the follicular phase.
- Sleep has a substantial impact on reproductive neuroendocrine function. In particular, luteinizing hormone (LH) pulse secretion—pulse frequency and amplitude—markedly increases during sleep in early pubertal subjects, whereas LH pulse frequency decreases during sleep in women during the follicular phase. Although the precise relevance of such sleep-related changes remains unclear, they may help explain the association between shift-work and menstrual disturbances.
- Menstrual-associated disorders are associated with altered sleep. Women with polycystic ovary syndrome have an increased risk of sleep-disordered breathing. Women with severe dysmenorrhea experience more wakefulness in association with their menstrual pain. Women with severe premenstrual syndrome have differences in sleep and circadian rhythms that are evident in both symptomatic and asymptomatic phases of the menstrual cycle.

INTRODUCTION

Women experience cyclic, approximately monthly, variations in reproductive hormones throughout their reproductive years, from menarche (first menstrual period) to menopause. When considering potential sex differences in sleep, it is important to understand that ovarian hormones can substantially influence various aspects of sleep. Sleep also has a prominent impact on reproductive physiology in pubertal girls and women, especially at the level of neuroendocrine systems that regulate ovarian function. The first part of this chapter is devoted to the important bidirectional interactions between sleep and reproductive function in women. The second part focuses on the apparent clinical implications of such interactions (e.g., menstrual disturbances in women shift workers), as well as sleep and circadian rhythms in the context of clinical reproductive disorders, such as polycystic ovary syndrome (PCOS).

FEMALE REPRODUCTIVE PHYSIOLOGY

Neuroendocrine systems, in particular the hypothalamic-pituitary-ovarian system, governs reproductive function in women.[1] Hypothalamic gonadotropin-releasing hormone (GnRH) stimulates pituitary gonadotrope cells to secrete the two gonadotropins—luteinizing hormone (LH) and follicle-stimulating hormone (FSH)—that govern ovarian sex steroid synthesis, ovarian follicular development, and ovulation. GnRH neuron cell bodies are located in the preoptic area and infundibular (arcuate) nucleus of the hypothalamus; GnRH neuronal projections extend to the median eminence, where GnRH is released into the hypophyseal portal system and subsequently gains access to pituitary gonadotropes. Of importance, GnRH release into the hypophyseal portal system is *pulsatile*. This episodic gonadotrope stimulation is mandatory for the maintenance of LH and FSH secretion as continuous GnRH agonism causes downregulation of both LH and FSH release. Moreover, faster GnRH pulse frequencies favor LH secretion, whereas slower GnRH pulse frequencies favor FSH secretion. In accordance, modulation of GnRH pulse frequency represents an important physiologic phenomenon in normal cyclic function.

The hypothalamic-pituitary-ovarian axis is quiescent during childhood, but toward the end of a female's first decade of life, neuroendocrine puberty is heralded by an increase in GnRH secretion initially restricted to sleep periods. The associated increase in LH secretion provokes ovarian sex steroid production and the emergence of secondary sex characteristics, whereas FSH secretion enhances ovarian follicular development. The complex hypothalamic-ovarian interactions governing cyclic reproductive function (e.g., periodic ovulation) are subsequently established over several years, although the mechanisms are poorly understood. Once fully established, ovulatory menstrual cycles are typically between 21 and 35 days, although menstrual cycle length tends to shorten as women enter their 40s.

By convention, the first day of menstrual bleeding is designated menstrual cycle day 1. Ovulation occurs around midcycle (e.g., cycle day 14 in a 28-day menstrual cycle), dividing the cycle

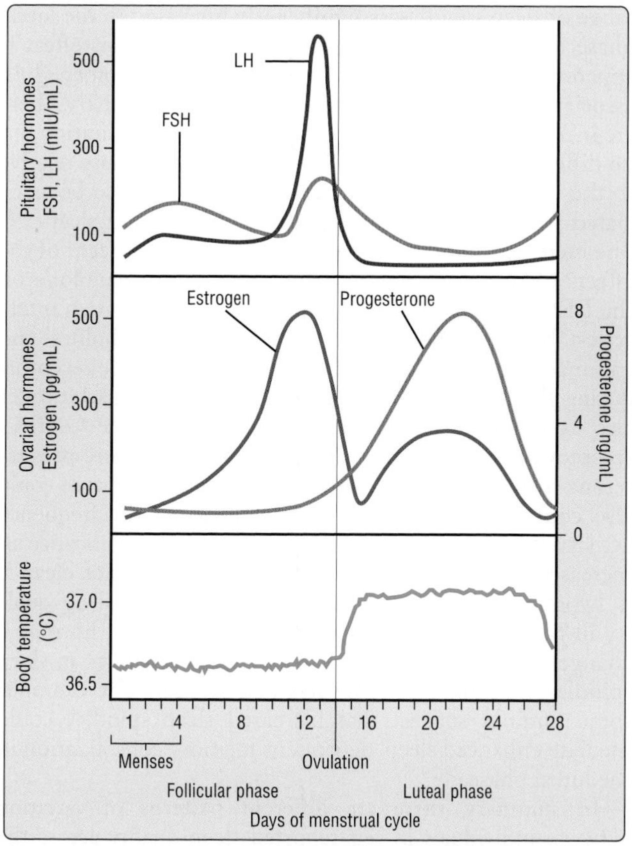

Figure 185.1 Mean daily plasma concentrations of estradiol, progesterone, follicle-stimulating hormone (FSH) and luteinizing hormone (LH), and basal body temperature throughout a "typical" 28-day ovulatory menstrual cycle. (Adapted from Pocock G, Richards CD. *Human Physiology: The Basis of Medicine.* New York: Oxford University Press; 1999:450.)

into two phases: the follicular phase, between the first day of menses and ovulation, and the luteal phase, between ovulation and the first day of menses (Figure 185.1).[2] During the follicular phase, FSH from pituitary gonadotropes stimulates ovarian follicular growth, with the eventual emergence of a dominant follicle. Follicular growth is accompanied by an increase in granulosa cell mass, with an associated rise in estradiol secretion. Circulating estradiol levels peak toward the end of the follicular phase, as the dominant follicle approaches full maturity. Threshold estradiol levels then provoke a marked increase in LH and FSH secretion from the anterior pituitary, the gonadotropin surge, which triggers ovulation about 36 hours later. The ruptured dominant follicle then transforms into a corpus luteum, which secretes both progesterone and estradiol during the luteal phase. In the absence of fertilization, the corpus luteum regresses approximately 14 days after ovulation: Associated hormone production drops precipitously, which leads to endometrial shedding (menstruation).

Menopause, which typically occurs in a woman's 40s or 50s, represents the cessation of cyclic reproductive function related to oocyte depletion. The reproductive hormone deficiency of menopause can be associated with significant vasomotor instability, hot flashes, night sweats, and sleep disturbance.[3,4]

INTERACTIONS BETWEEN THE FEMALE REPRODUCTIVE SYSTEM, SLEEP, AND CIRCADIAN RHYTHMS

Female reproductive hormones, specifically estrogen and progesterone, not only regulate reproductive tissue function during the menstrual cycle but also impact physiologic processes, such as sleep and circadian rhythms. The targets of sex steroid action within the neural circuitry that control sleep and wakefulness are not yet fully determined. However, evidence from rodent models suggests that estrogen can influence sleep-wake activity through its effects on arousal centers (e.g., the wake-promoting hypocretin/orexin system in the lateral hypothalamus), sleep centers (e.g., ventrolateral and median preoptic nuclei), and the suprachiasmatic nucleus (SCN, master pacemaker), to consolidate and enhance sleep-wake activity to the appropriate time of day.[5] Therefore the mechanistic framework is in place for ovarian sex steroids to influence sleep and circadian rhythms in women.

Sleep across the Menstrual Cycle

Surveys and studies based on self-reports have found that women across a wide age range (ages 18 to 50 years) are more likely to report sleep disturbances during the premenstrual week and during the first few days of menstruation compared to other times of the cycle.[6] For example, the Study of Women's Health Across the Nation (SWAN), which included women in their late reproductive years and women entering the menopausal transition, reported that self-reported sleep disturbance varied with cycle phase, being more likely to occur during the late luteal and early follicular phases of the menstrual cycle.[7] After controlling for cycle day and other confounders, poorer sleep quality was associated with hormonal factors, although relationships differed depending on reproductive stage: Higher levels of pregnanediol glucuronide (a progesterone metabolite) in urine were related to more troubled sleeping in the perimenopausal group, and higher urine FSH levels were related to more sleep complaints in the premenopausal group.[7] Another study that tracked daily sleep quality across the menstrual cycle in young women (21 ± 3 years) without significant menstrual-associated complaints also reported a small reduction in sleep quality around the time of menstruation.[8]

However, not all women report changes in their sleep across the menstrual cycle. Van Reen and Kiesner[9] identified three different variation patterns in sleep difficulty across the menstrual cycle: Some reported difficulty sleeping during midcycle, some reported difficulty during the premenstrual period, whereas in other women there was no clear relationship between the menstrual cycle and sleep difficulties. This interindividual variability might reflect different sensitivities of sleep centers to underlying hormone changes, or it may relate to interindividual differences in how psychological and somatic symptoms manifest across the menstrual cycle. As discussed later, women with menstrual-related problems, including dysmenorrhea and premenstrual dysphoric disorder, are between two and three times more likely than other women to report insomnia and excessive sleepiness during the day.[10]

Studies using objective measures of sleep (e.g., actigraphy, polysomnography [PSG]) have found variable effects of menstrual cycle phase on sleep.[6,11–13] Inconsistent findings may result from individual differences in how sleep, especially sleep quality, changes across the menstrual cycle, with small sample sizes in PSG studies and inherent methodologic challenges (e.g., variability in menstrual cycle length, difficulties with cycle-stage standardization, and confounding variables, such as the presence and timing of ovulation and age-related changes).[12] Although hormone levels were not measured, a large actigraphy study, which was a component of the SWAN study, found a 5% decline in sleep efficiency and a 25-minute decrease in total sleep time in the premenstrual week relative to the prior week in late-reproductive–age women,[14] matching other SWAN data showing poorer self-reported sleep quality in the premenstrual week in late-reproductive–age women.[7]

Studies using PSG, the gold standard method of sleep characterization, have generally involved small groups of women during a limited selection of menstrual cycle phases, such as midfollicular phase versus midluteal phase. An exception is the study by Driver and colleagues (1996),[15] in which nine women were tracked with PSG every other night across a menstrual cycle. They found no menstrual cycle–related changes in sleep-onset latency and sleep efficiency, or in percentage of slow wave sleep (SWS) and slow wave activity in non–rapid eye movement (NREM) sleep averaged across the night. These findings have generally been supported by most subsequent studies.

Across the menstrual cycle, although sleep homeostasis appears to be maintained, variations in rapid eye movement sleep (REM) sleep have been noted. For example, studies have found that the luteal phase is associated with earlier onset of REM,[16] shorter episodes of REM sleep,[12,17] and a tendency toward decreased percentage of REM sleep.[17] Using an ultra-rapid sleep-wake cycle procedure, Shechter and colleagues[18] reported that REM sleep was decreased (at circadian phase 0 degrees and 30 degrees) in the luteal phase, when body temperature was higher, compared with the follicular phase. Women with ovulatory cycles also have a shorter REM-onset latency in the luteal phase compared to women with anovulatory cycles.[19] In the absence of ovulation and corpus luteum formation, serum progesterone concentrations remain low; such women do not experience a true luteal phase, and core body temperature does not increase. Variation in the timing and amount of REM sleep during the menstrual cycle may be a consequence of direct steroid actions, altered circadian processes, and/or raised body temperature.[16,18] Limited correlational evidence links ovarian hormone levels or hormone dynamics with menstrual cycle PSG sleep measures.[17,20–22] For example, the amount of REM sleep was found to be negatively correlated with circulating progesterone and estradiol concentrations in the luteal phase in young women.[17] Also, a steeper rise in progesterone from follicular to luteal phase was associated with a greater amount of wakefulness after sleep onset in the luteal phase.[21] Within the follicular phase specifically, higher levels of FSH were associated with measures of wakefulness in both premenopausal and perimenopausal women without sleep complaints.[20] Although all these data are correlational, they suggest an interaction between the hypothalamic-pituitary-ovarian axis and the sleep-wake regulatory system in women.

Menstrual cycle–related changes may impact sleep more prominently with advancing age. A small PSG study found that women in the menopausal transition who were still cycling had more awakenings and arousals, as well as less N3 sleep, although there was no change in slow wave electroencephalogram (EEG) activity in the luteal phase compared to the follicular phase,[23] apparent effects that are not observed in most studies of younger women.[11]

The most dramatic menstrual cycle–related sleep changes are evident from spectral analysis of the sleep EEG and detailed analysis of sleep spindles. EEG activity in the 14.25- to 15.0-Hz band, which corresponds to the upper frequency range of sleep spindles, is significantly increased in the luteal phase compared with the follicular phase.[15,24] This effect is apparent in both young and perimenopausal women.[23] In association with increased spindle frequency activity, there are increases in both spindle density and spindle duration but no difference in spindle amplitude in the luteal phase relative to the follicular phase.[23] The luteal phase may also be associated with an increase in visually scored stage 2 sleep.[15,18] The increased spindle frequency activity is reminiscent of the effects of the progesterone metabolite allopregnanolone on the EEG in rats[25] and is hypothesized to represent an interaction between endogenous progesterone metabolites and gamma-aminobutyric acid A ($GABA_A$) membrane receptors during the luteal phase.[15] Benzodiazepines and barbiturates also exert their sedative effects by binding to the $GABA_A$ receptor but probably at a different site from where progesterone metabolites bind.[26] Increased body temperature could also contribute, in part, to the increased spindle frequency activity in the luteal phase.[27] Although the significance of increased spindle activity in the luteal phase is not clear, it is hypothesized to serve a role of maintaining sleep quality in the presence of substantial physiologic and hormonal changes in this phase.[13] Menstrual cycle variability in sleep spindles may have functional consequences. For example, some findings suggest that increased sleep spindles could mediate enhanced sleep-dependent memory consolidation in the luteal phase.[28,29]

In summary, there are different patterns of variation between individuals in self-reported sleep quality across the menstrual cycle, with the premenstrual phase and/or midcycle being linked with sleep difficulties in some women. PSG measures of sleep continuity and homeostasis appear to be relatively stable across the normal menstrual cycle, despite marked changes in hormone milieu. There are, however, some cycle-related changes in sleep, most notably an increase in upper spindle frequency activity, coincident with increased sleep spindle density and duration and a decrease in REM sleep during the luteal phase compared to the follicular phase.

Circadian Rhythms across the Menstrual Cycle

In women, circadian rhythms for hormone secretion, body temperature, and sleep-wake activity are superimposed on the menstrual cycle rhythm. As shown in Figure 185.2, men and women have the most similar body temperatures when women are in their follicular phase. In the luteal phase, body temperature is increased by 0.4° to 0.7° C compared to the follicular phase, due to the thermogenic action of progesterone secreted from the corpus luteum.[30] Studies of women in uncontrolled conditions have shown that the nocturnal decline in body temperature is blunted, reducing the amplitude of the temperature rhythm in the luteal phase compared to the follicular phase.[24] To study the true endogenous circadian rhythm, studies have used either a controlled ultra-short sleep-wake cycle or a constant-routine paradigm. The constant-routine paradigm includes maintenance of semirecumbent wakefulness in dim light and controlled food intake to limit influences from sleep-wake patterns, activity, light exposure, and meals. These studies have confirmed the existence of a blunted endogenous temperature rhythm in the luteal phase compared to the follicular phase.[18,24] Under controlled conditions, there is little difference in phase of the circadian temperature rhythm between follicular and luteal phases of the menstrual cycle.[18,31] The amplitude of the body temperature rhythm has been shown

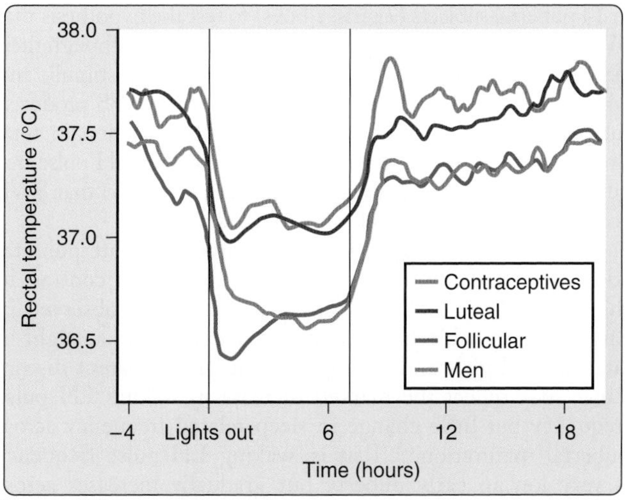

Figure 185.2 Mean diurnal rhythms in rectal temperature, plotted for 4 hours before lights-out and 20 hours thereafter in 8 young men, 8 young women taking monophasic oral contraceptives (active pill), and in 15 young women in the mid-follicular and mid-luteal phases of their ovulatory menstrual cycles. Vertical lines indicate average time in bed. Subjects followed their usual daytime schedules and spent the night in a sleep laboratory. (Published with permission from Baker FC, Driver HS. Circadian rhythms, sleep, and the menstrual cycle. *Sleep Med.* 2007;8:613–22.)

to be negatively related to circulating progesterone concentrations or the progesterone-to-estradiol ratio, suggesting that the balance of these two hormones may be important.[32] A decrease in the amplitude of the temperature rhythm may be mediated by progesterone acting either directly on the SCN or downstream of the SCN,[18] and/or it could reflect a modulation by progesterone of the hypothermic effect of melatonin.[33]

Based on ultra-short sleep-wake cycle or constant-routine studies, there are no differences in melatonin onset or offset, duration, or acrophase of the melatonin rhythm between the follicular and luteal phases of the menstrual cycle in young women.[18,31,34] Two of these three studies also found no difference in amplitude of the melatonin rhythm across menstrual phases,[18,31] suggesting that the changes in circadian rhythms in the luteal versus the follicular phase are limited to the body temperature rhythm, likely due to the effects of progesterone on thermoregulation.

Effects of Hormonal Contraceptives on Sleep

Studies investigating sleep in women taking hormonal contraceptives can provide important information about the effects of reproductive steroids beyond what is learned from observational studies in normally cycling women. Combined oral contraceptives are daily pill formulations that include both a low-dose progestin and a synthetic estrogen. The active hormone pills are typically taken for 21 consecutive days, followed by 7 days of hormone-free pills. These agents primarily act by preventing ovulation. Thus, although women taking combined oral contraceptives have vaginal bleeding during the hormone-free pill week, they do not have ovulatory menstrual cycles. Indeed, with hormonal contraceptives, endogenous hormone levels are low in the presence of high levels of synthetic hormones. Thus any apparent effects on sleep could reflect the effects from exogenous hormone and/or the suppression of endogenous hormone production.[35]

Sleep architecture is altered by oral contraceptives. Women taking oral contraceptives have less SWS than do women with ovulatory menstrual cycles.[12] Stage 2 sleep is significantly increased in women taking combined hormonal contraceptives compared to naturally cycling women in both menstrual cycle phases; further, stage 2 sleep is increased when women are taking their active hormone pills versus their hormone-free pills.[36] Also, the use of a synthetic progestin (medroxyprogesterone) alone is associated with a specific increase in upper spindle frequency activity in women.[37] Other sleep effects reported in combined hormonal contraceptive users include a shorter REM-onset latency and more REM sleep compared to women with ovulatory menstrual cycles.[12,38] Exogenous sex steroid hormones therefore appear to influence sleep differently than the variations in endogenous hormones across the menstrual cycle.

Diurnal and Circadian Rhythms in Reproductive Hormones

Diurnal rhythms are a common feature of the reproductive system. Animal studies suggest that molecular clocks are functional throughout the reproductive axis, including in GnRH neurons, gonadotropes, and cells within the ovary.[39] As a prominent example of a circadian rhythm in reproductive endocrinology, the timing of LH surge generation is restricted to the late afternoon in female rats,[40] which optimally coordinates ovulation with sexual opportunity and receptivity. This timing is under control of the master organismal clock in the SCN, and radiofrequency or electrolytic ablation of the SCN disrupts estrus cyclicity in female rats.[41,42] Although this stimulus to the rodent GnRH pulse generator is likely governed by the SCN on a daily basis, it is presumably relayed to the relevant GnRH neurons only in the setting of preovulatory estradiol concentrations. Similarly, as an interesting example of ovarian clock function in rodent reproduction, ovarian responsivity to exogenous LH, as measured by ovulation, is highest in the late afternoon.[43,44] However, the precise roles of circadian rhythms in primate ovulation remain unclear. In monkeys, for example, midcycle gonadotropin surges can be advanced by 12 to 18 hours with supraphysiologic estradiol administration,[45] suggesting that they are not rigidly constrained to a specific time of day. Similarly, although some studies in women suggest that LH surge initiation tends to occur in the morning,[46,47] another detailed study suggested that it may occur throughout the day or night.[48]

Outside of the midcycle window of the LH surge, cycling women exhibit diurnal changes in circulating gonadotropin and sex steroid concentrations. For example, cycling women demonstrate diurnal variations in mean serum LH concentrations, with peaks in the afternoon and nadirs at night, especially in the early follicular phase.[49–51] Serum FSH concentrations are also highest in the afternoon and lowest at night in both the early and late follicular phases.[52]

Studies of such diurnal rhythms can be significantly confounded by sleep and other environmental cues. For example, women studied in the early follicular phase demonstrated a reduction in sleep-related LH concentrations, regardless of whether they slept during nighttime or daytime hours.[53] Similarly, in normal women studied during the early follicular phase, LH responses to exogenous GnRH at nighttime were higher when asleep compared to when awake.[54] Controlling for such variables is necessary to determine if such patterns reflect an endogenous circadian rhythm.

Perhaps the most detailed studies of potential circadian rhythms in gonadotropin secretion were performed by Hall and colleagues.[55] In one such study of cycling women who remained awake for 24 hours in the early follicular phase, both mean LH and LH pulse amplitude, but not LH pulse frequency, increased in the evening hours (around hours 16:00 to 24:00). Although this study suggested a possible circadian rhythm of LH release, the investigators had not strictly controlled other potentially important environmental cues (e.g., posture, nutritional intake). In a subsequent study using a 32-hour constant-routine protocol in cycling women (early to midfollicular phase), the same investigators observed no time-related changes in estradiol, mean LH, mean FSH, mean free alpha subunit, LH pulse amplitude, free alpha-subunit pulse amplitude, LH pulse frequency, or free alpha-subunit pulse frequency; the latter two are surrogates for GnRH pulse frequency, despite seeing robust circadian rhythms in both core body temperature and thyroid-stimulating hormone.[56] Of note, similar findings were observed in postmenopausal (estrogen-deficient) women who remained awake for 24 hours under constant conditions.[57]

Overall, the aforementioned studies suggest the absence of a true circadian pattern of circulating gonadotropin concentrations. However, Rahman and colleagues[58] recently reported that circulating LH, FSH, estradiol, progesterone, and sex hormone–binding globulin (SHBG) concentrations demonstrated significant diurnal rhythms during the follicular phase under constant-routine conditions. In this particular study, hormone rhythmicity (peak timing and amplitude) was similar during standard sleep-wake conditions and during the constant-routine conditions, suggesting the presence of an underlying circadian pacemaker active in the follicular phase. In contrast to findings in the follicular phase, however, only FSH and SHBG exhibited significant diurnal rhythmicity during the luteal phase.[58]

Thus, although most studies suggest that reproductive hormones exhibit diurnal patterns in cycling adult women, results of detailed studies remain mixed regarding whether such changes represent true circadian rhythms.

Influence of Sleep on Gonadotropin-Releasing Hormone Pulse Generation in Pubertal Girls and Women

Although precise mechanisms are unclear, sleep has a major influence on pulsatile LH and, by inference, GnRH secretion in pubertal girls (and boys). In the 1970s, investigators discovered that the initial pubertal increase in LH secretion is restricted to nighttime. This nocturnal amplification of LH release usually manifests within an hour of sleep onset, and it occurs during daytime sleep periods.[59,60] These findings suggested that such nocturnal changes are specifically related to sleep rather than time of day.

LH and, by inference, GnRH pulse initiation is influenced by specific sleep stages in early pubertal subjects. Initial studies from the 1970s suggested that sleep-related LH pulses occur primarily during NREM sleep.[59,60] More recent studies confirm these findings but have expanded our understanding substantially. In particular, these newer studies of puberty suggest a strong relationship between SWS and LH pulse initiation during puberty.[61,62] An initial study by Shaw and colleagues,[61] performed in 5 pubertal boys and 4 pubertal girls, suggested that 52% of all sleep-related LH pulses were initiated during SWS, with 36% initiated during N2, 10% during REM, 2% during N1, and none during wake periods. When accounting for time spent in each sleep stage, LH pulse frequency was highest during SWS. Based on these findings, Shaw and colleagues[62] pursued a study in 14 pubertal subjects (7 girls, 7 boys) to test the hypothesis that SWS disruption can impact LH pulse initiation.[2] Although their experimental maneuvers (i.e., controlled auditory stimuli, and when necessary, shoulder shaking) used during SWS produced substantial SWS fragmentation and a 40% reduction in total time spent in SWS, these maneuvers did not alter LH pulse frequency. Sophisticated analysis of these data suggested that SWS accumulation predicted LH pulse initiation.

Sleep influences GnRH pulse generation in late pubertal adolescents and adult women as well. However, in contrast to the sleep-related LH pulse frequency increases observed in early pubertal subjects, LH pulse frequency slows at night in late pubertal girls and cycling women. This apparent discordance may reflect the marked increase in waking LH pulse frequency but little change in sleep-related frequency across pubertal maturation.[63] That is, waking LH pulse frequency is very low in early puberty but gradually increases across pubertal maturation such that by late puberty it exceeds sleep-associated pulse frequency.

Although LH pulse frequency slowing in women is most prominent in the early follicular phase,[49,51,64,65] it is also demonstrable in the late follicular phase.[66–69] This phenomenon in women specifically reflects an inhibitory influence of sleep as sleep is associated with slower LH pulse frequency during both nighttime hours (i.e., nighttime sleep vs. nighttime wake) and daytime hours (i.e., daytime sleep vs. daytime wake),[53,55] and LH pulse frequency slowing does not occur at night when subjects remain awake.[55,56] Hall and colleagues[56] discovered that, during the early follicular phase, LH pulses are uncommon during REM and SWS and more common after brief awakenings. Similar findings have been described in normal women studied in the midfollicular to late follicular phase.[70] Mechanisms underlying sleep-related reductions in LH pulse frequency during the follicular phase are unknown. However, naloxone administration appeared to prevent the sleep-associated decrease in LH pulse frequency in one study,[50] suggesting that such slowing is at least partly mediated by hypothalamic opioids. In contrast, other studies suggested that neither dopaminergic blockade (metoclopramide) nor serotonergic blockade (methysergide maleate) altered sleep-related LH pulsatility in the early follicular phase.[71,72]

Sleep likely interacts with other determinants of GnRH pulse generation. For example, a small study of early to mid-pubertal girls suggested that progesterone, the primary determinant of day-to-day GnRH pulse frequency in women, markedly suppresses LH pulse frequency while awake but not during sleep.[73] A larger, scientifically rigorous study of later-pubertal girls confirmed that progesterone acutely suppresses waking LH pulse frequency more so than sleep-associated LH pulse frequency.[74] A similar phenomenon pertains to adults: In normal women studied during the late follicular phase, dietary calorie restriction preferentially reduces daytime LH pulse frequency.[67,75] Taken together, these findings suggest differential control of GnRH pulse frequency depending on sleep status in both pubertal girls and adult women.

Mechanisms underlying the functional connection between sleep and altered GnRH pulse frequency remain unclear. Presumably, sleep's influence on GnRH pulse frequency reflects neuroanatomic connections between (1) sleep-generating and/or sleep-activated neurons and (2) GnRH neurons per se and/or the afferent neurons that directly impact pulsatile GnRH secretion, namely the infundibular (arcuate) neurons expressing kisspeptin, neurokinin B, and/or dynorphin.[76] Although specific neuronal connections have not been defined in humans, sleep-activated neurons in the hypothalamic ventrolateral preoptic area exhibit synaptic connections with GnRH neurons in mice.[77,78]

The physiologic relevance of sleep-associated changes in GnRH secretion also remains uncertain. However, because modulation of GnRH pulse frequency impacts LH versus FSH secretion, sleep-related changes may help direct the normal developmental changes in gonadotropin release across puberty,[79] and sleep-related slowing has been postulated to contribute to the early follicular prominence of FSH secretion in cycling women.[55] Limited indirect evidence supports these hypotheses. For example, untreated childhood obstructive sleep apnea (OSA) (i.e., sleep disturbance) appears to be associated with some delay in pubertal initiation (i.e., initial breast growth).[80] Although one might expect sleep duration and/or sleep quality and, by inference, sleep-related GnRH pulse frequency slowing to impact FSH secretion, results have been mixed in this regard. One study suggested that longer sleep duration (self-reported) correlates with higher urine FSH concentrations across the cycle,[81] but another study suggested that higher midfollicular serum FSH concentration correlates with lower sleep efficiency and greater wakefulness after sleep onset, but not with total sleep time.[20]

CLINICAL IMPLICATIONS

Shift Work and Menstrual Cycle Rhythms

Women shift workers who work on schedules that do not consistently conform to typical workdays have disrupted circadian rhythms and sleep schedules that can disrupt physiologic functions and negatively impact health. Such changes may include important alterations in reproductive function.[82,83]

In general, observational studies have provided evidence for reproductive disturbances, such as menstrual irregularity and subfertility in women shift workers.[84] For example, a 2014 meta-analysis of four studies involving 28,479 women suggested that shift workers—defined as those who work outside of usual working hours (hours 08:00 to 18:00)—experience higher rates of infertility, with an odds ratio (OR) of 1.80 (95% confidence interval [CI]: 1.01 to 3.20).[85] Similarly, meta-analysis of four studies involving 71,681 women suggested that shift workers experience higher rates of menstrual disruption (cycles <25 or >31 days) compared to non–shift workers, with an OR of 1.22 (95% CI: 1.15 to 1.29).[85] The latter findings primarily reflected a single study of 71,077 US women ages 28 to 45 years who had participated in the Nurses' Health Study II.[86] Compared to women who did not engage in rotating nighttime shift work, those who had the highest category of exposure demonstrated a 1.23 relative risk (95% CI: 1.14 to 1.33) of irregular menses after adjusting for age, age at menarche, parity, race/ethnicity, smoking status, alcohol consumption, physical activity, and body mass index (BMI). Shift-work nurses who report changes in menstrual function, compared to those who do not, report significantly more sleep disturbances, symptoms of shift-work intolerance, and longer sleep-onset latencies, suggesting an association between sleep disturbances and menstrual irregularities.[87]

Some evidence suggests that shift work, particularly nighttime shift work, may lead to fertility problems and increased risk for miscarriage; however, the effect size is uncertain.[88] Meta-analyses of the literature investigating the association between various working conditions and fetal and maternal health concluded that shift work poses minimal risk to the female reproductive system[89] and that there is insufficient evidence for clinicians to advise restricting shift work in reproductive-age women.[85] However, several professional bodies on health and safety state that shift work, particularly nighttime shift work, may increase risk for menstrual cycle disruption or pregnancy complications.[88]

The nature of the relationship between shift work and reproductive health remains unclear, but it could relate to increased stress, interruptions to daily routines and intimate relationships, as well as disrupted circadian rhythms and/or sleep,[88] which influence reproductive hormone secretion, particularly LH and FSH, as described in detail earlier.

Polycystic Ovary Syndrome

PCOS affects some 6% to 10% of women of reproductive age, and it is characterized by clinical and/or biochemical androgen excess (e.g., hirsutism), evidence of oligoovulation/anovulation (e.g., irregular or absent menstrual cycles), and polycystic ovarian morphology.[90] Common management goals include control of irregular menstrual bleeding (e.g., with combined oral contraceptives), treatment of hirsutism (e.g., by mechanical means, decreasing androgen production via combined oral contraceptives, and/or by blocking androgen action via spironolactone), and treatment of infertility.[91] PCOS is also associated with important comorbidities, such as obesity and insulin resistance[92]; dysglycemia, dyslipidemia, and other cardiovascular risk factors[93]; and depression, anxiety, and decreased quality of life.[94]

Women with PCOS are more likely to report poor sleep.[95] In community- and population-based studies, women with PCOS were significantly more likely to report difficulty falling asleep, even after adjusting for factors such as BMI and depressive symptoms.[96,97] PCOS has also been associated with alterations in sleep architecture: Obese adolescents and adult women with PCOS may exhibit longer sleep-onset latency,[98–100] reduced sleep efficiency,[98,99] and reduced time spent in REM sleep[98,99]; however, some of these latter findings may partly reflect differences in adiposity and/or underlying sleep-disordered breathing (SDB).

Women with PCOS are at increased risk for SDB.[101] In one early study, women with PCOS were 30 times more likely to suffer from SDB than control subjects.[100] A meta-analysis suggested that the risk of SDB is increased in adult women with PCOS (OR approaching 10), but not in adolescents with PCOS.[102] However, many such studies involved clinic-based patient cohorts, which tend to have greater numbers of women with more severe PCOS symptoms and greater adiposity; in accordance, these prevalence estimates should be interpreted cautiously.

Obesity is an important risk factor for SDB, but when compared with age- and weight-matched healthy control subjects, women with PCOS are more likely to have SDB during their reproductive years (Figure 185.3) and are more likely to report excessive daytime sleepiness (80% vs. 27% in control subjects), even after controlling for body weight.[103] Increased visceral obesity, which is common in women with PCOS, may be more closely associated with SDB risk compared to elevated BMI per se.[104]

The severity of SDB is associated with glucose intolerance and insulin resistance in women with PCOS, suggesting that SDB may contribute to the metabolic abnormalities in these women.[103] Although larger trials are needed, preliminary

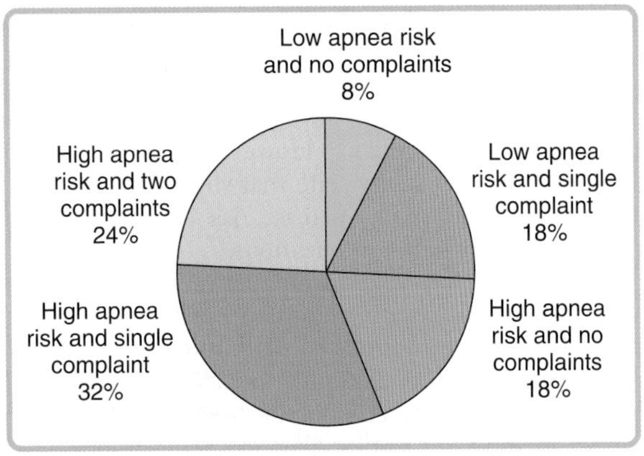

Figure 185.3 The frequency distribution of the risk for sleep apnea and sleep complaints in 40 women who have PCOS. (Published with permission from Tasali E, Van Cauter E, Ehrmann DA. Relationships between sleep disordered breathing and glucose metabolism in polycystic ovary syndrome. *J Clin Endocrinol Metab.* 2006;91:36–42.)

evidence suggests that successful treatment of SDB using continuous positive airway pressure (CPAP) therapy in extremely obese women with PCOS leads to a modest improvement in insulin sensitivity and a reduction in diastolic blood pressure.[105] According to current recommendations, medical providers caring for women with PCOS should consider screening for OSA using simple survey tools (e.g., the Berlin Questionnaire) with follow-up PSG as indicated.[91]

Beyond its effects on insulin sensitivity, it remains unclear whether sleep disturbances may otherwise contribute to the pathophysiology of PCOS. One study suggested that LH pulses tend to follow SWS in women with PCOS, similar to findings in normal puberty,[61,62] and were not appropriately inhibited by REM sleep.[70] In this same study, REM-associated LH pulse frequency was higher in PCOS compared to midfollicular to late follicular control subjects, and higher REM-associated LH pulse frequency was associated with higher testosterone levels, even after adjusting for other PCOS-related differences, such as BMI and cycle day during the study.[70] Thus elevated sleep-related LH pulse frequency in PCOS could partly reflect androgen-induced alterations in the relationships between sleep stages and LH pulse initiation.

Premenstrual Syndrome and Premenstrual Dysphoric Disorder

Premenstrual syndrome (PMS) is characterized by emotional, behavioral, and physical symptoms that occur in the premenstrual phase of the menstrual cycle, with resolution at the onset of menses or shortly thereafter. Although many women of reproductive age experience some premenstrual symptoms, up to 18% have more distressing symptoms that impact daily function.[106] Premenstrual dysphoric disorder (PMDD) is a severe form of PMS that occurs in 3% to 8% of women[106] and is classified as a depressive disorder in the American Psychiatric Association's *Diagnostic and Statistical Manual of Mental Disorders,* fifth edition.[107] A diagnosis of PMDD requires the occurrence of at least five specified symptoms (with at least one being a mood-related symptom) during the late luteal phase for at least two consecutive cycles. One of the potential PMDD-related symptoms is sleep disturbance (insomnia or hypersomnia). Pharmacologic management of severe PMS/PMDD includes selective serotonin reuptake inhibitors (the drug category of choice as recommended by the American College of Obstetricians and Gynecologists), anxiolytics, and agents that suppress ovulation.[108] Nonpharmacologic agents, such as calcium supplements, L-tryptophan, and cognitive/behavioral therapy have also been shown to be effective.[108]

Women with severe PMS typically report sleep-related complaints in the late luteal phase, such as insomnia, sleep disruption by body movements, awakenings, disturbing dreams, and poor sleep quality.[109] They also report sleepiness, fatigue, reduced alertness, and an inability to concentrate during the premenstrual phase.[109] In a sample of 265 young women, both poor sleep and ineffective emotion regulation were shown to mediate the relationship between greater depressive symptoms and premenstrual symptoms, suggesting that poor sleep may exacerbate the experience of premenstrual symptoms.[110]

Despite the just mentioned findings, studies using PSG have found little evidence of disturbed sleep in the symptomatic late luteal phase in women with severe PMS. For example, one study found that, although women with severe PMS/PMDD self-reported poorer sleep quality in the late luteal phase relative to the follicular phase, this did not correspond to poor PSG-assessed sleep quality as defined by sleep-onset latency, arousals, sleep efficiency, or quantitative EEG measures,[17] confirming findings from most earlier studies.[13,109] The perception of poorer sleep quality correlated with higher anxiety levels, suggesting that the mood state of women with severe PMS may impact self-assessment of sleep in the late luteal phase.[17]

Of interest, there is evidence for trait-like differences in sleep across the menstrual cycle between women with and without PMS/PMDD symptoms, although findings have varied between studies.[13,109] Two recent studies found that SWS was increased in both the follicular and luteal phases in women with severe PMS or PMDD compared to control subjects.[17,111] This was hypothesized to be functionally linked with decreased melatonin secretion, which was also evident in women with PMDD.[17,111,112]

There is also evidence of altered circadian rhythms in women with PMDD. High mean nocturnal temperatures, disturbances in melatonin, cortisol, and thyroid-stimulating hormone rhythms have been reported in women with severe PMS or PMDD compared with asymptomatic control subjects.[13,24,113] Under controlled conditions, a small group of women with PMDD, compared to women without PMS, symptoms were found to have lower nocturnal melatonin levels during both menstrual phases and decreased melatonin amplitude in the symptomatic luteal phase.[112] Given these disturbances in circadian rhythmicity, investigators have explored the possibility of treating PMDD by manipulating the timing of sleep with sleep deprivation protocols or with light therapy. Appropriately timed light therapy has shown some promise as a treatment for PMDD, possibly by altering nocturnal melatonin secretion.[114] However, a meta-analysis of clinical trials of bright light therapy concluded that larger trials are needed to define its role in PMDD.[115]

Studies have also investigated whether sleep deprivation during the symptomatic luteal phase is therapeutic for PMDD. In one study, 8 of 10 women with PMDD responded to sleep deprivation and maintained improved mood after a night of recovery sleep.[116] In a follow-up study, partial sleep deprivation had similar positive effects on mood in 60% to

67% of patients, although these effects were only significant after recovery sleep.[117]

Dysmenorrhea

Dysmenorrhea, defined as painful menstrual cramps of uterine origin, is the most common gynecologic complaint among women of reproductive age and is very severe in approximately 10% to 25% of women.[118] Primary dysmenorrhea is menstrual pain without organic disease, and secondary dysmenorrhea is associated with conditions such as endometriosis and pelvic inflammatory disease. Menstrual cramps may significantly impact productivity and quality of life and lead to activity restriction and absenteeism from work and school.[118,119]

PSG studies of women with primary dysmenorrhea found that the menstrual cramps were associated with disturbed sleep—poorer self-reported sleep quality, lower sleep efficiency, increased time spent awake, moving, and in stage 1 light sleep, and less REM sleep compared with both pain-free phases of the menstrual cycle and compared with women without menstrual pain.[120,121] Disturbed sleep, in turn, may exacerbate pain as sleep deprivation is associated with a decreased pain threshold.[122] Disturbed sleep may also lead to increased daytime sleepiness. In a large sample of adolescent girls, moderate (OR: 1.39; 95% CI: 1.12 to 1.72) and severe (OR; 1.46; 95% CI; 1.04 to 2.04) menstrual pain was significantly associated with increased risk of daytime sleepiness over the past month, with the relationship partially mediated by anxious/depressive symptoms, poor sleep quality, and insomnia.[123] However, given that menstrual pain is only evident for a few days each month, further studies are needed to determine whether daytime sleepiness in this group is evident across the menstrual cycle or only in association with days of menstrual pain.

In most women dysmenorrhea is effectively treated with analgesics and nonsteroidal inflammatory drugs (NSAIDs). Treatment of nocturnal pain with an NSAID restores both self-reported and objectively measured sleep quality in women with primary dysmenorrhea.[121] Treatment with melatonin was also shown to improve sleep and pain severity in a randomized controlled trial in women with primary dysmenorrhea.[124]

Sleep Disorders and the Menstrual Cycle

In the third edition of the ICSD (2014),[125] the only sleep disorder listed as being menstrual cycle–related is Kleine-Levin syndrome, or menstrual-related hypersomnia. This exceedingly rare condition is characterized by hypersomnolence in the week before and/or during menses, but such patients do not have persistent, excessive sleepiness at other times in the menstrual cycle.[109] In a review of 339 cases of recurrent hypersomnia,[126] 18 had menstrual-related hypersomnia; however, in the majority (13 of 18), menstruation was not the only precipitating factor. Patients with premenstrual hypersomnia have been successfully treated with either estrogen or combined oral contraceptives.[109]

There is little research about the variation in severity of sleep disorders, such as insomnia and OSA, according to the menstrual cycle phase. The severity of OSA may be greatest in the follicular phase; upper airway resistance is lowest in the luteal phase in healthy women.[127] However, women being evaluated with PSG for OSA in the self-reported follicular phase had a lower apnea-hypopnea index than women evaluated in their self-reported luteal phase.[128]

CLINICAL PEARLS

In some women the menstrual cycle impacts sleep quality, with sleep difficulties most likely before and during menstruation than at other times, depending in part on the presence of menstrual cycle–related psychological and somatic symptoms. Polysomnographic studies show that rapid eye movement sleep is reduced, and spindle frequency activity is increased, in the absence of a change in slow wave sleep amount in the luteal compared with the follicular phase. Assessment of sleep complaints in women should include an investigation of any association between symptoms and menstrual cycle phase or menstrual-related disorders. Sleep has a major influence on pulsatile luteinizing hormone secretion in pubertal girls and boys, which is thought to be important for the developmental changes in gonadotropin release across puberty. As such, alterations in sleep, such as in untreated childhood obstructive sleep apnea, may impact these normal developmental processes. Disruptions to circadian rhythms and sleep, such as with shift work, may also influence reproductive function in adult women, although further work is needed to clarify the relationship. Finally, given the high incidence of sleep-disordered breathing and its association with glucose intolerance in women with polycystic ovary syndrome, screening for sleep apnea and appropriate treatment with continuous positive airway pressure may be beneficial in these women.

SUMMARY

Menstrual cycle–related variations in reproductive hormones influence sleep and circadian rhythms. The amplitude of the body temperature rhythm is blunted, sleep spindle frequency activity is increased, and REM sleep is reduced in the luteal phase compared with the follicular phase. In turn, there are strong circadian and sleep influences on reproductive hormones that vary depending on pubertal stage and age. LH pulse initiation is uncommon during REM sleep; amplification of pulsatile LH secretion is strongly linked with sleep in pubertal girls (and boys), with SWS seeming to encourage LH pulse initiation. In contrast, LH pulse frequency slows with sleep in adult women during the follicular phase, with pulse initiation tending to follow brief awakenings.

The interaction between reproductive and sleep/circadian systems is apparent from studies in female shift workers, who are more likely to have menstrual-related disturbances. Menstrual-related disorders are also linked with altered sleep. Women with PCOS are at risk for SDB, which may contribute to insulin resistance and other metabolic abnormalities. Women with severe premenstrual syndrome or dysmenorrhea may have transient sleep disturbances or insomnia before/during menstruation. Assessment of sleep complaints in women should include an investigation of associations between symptoms and menstrual cycle phase or menstrual-related disorders.

SELECTED READINGS

Baker FC, Lee KA. Menstrual cycle effects on sleep. *Sleep Med Clin.* 2018;13(3):283–294.

Driver HS, Dijk DJ, Werth E, Biedermann K, Borbély AA. Sleep and the sleep electroencephalogram across the menstrual cycle in young healthy women. *J Clin Endocrinol Metab.* 1996;81:728–735.

Kervezee L, Shechter A, Boivin DB. Impact of shift work on the circadian timing system and health in women. *Sleep Med Clin.* 2018;13:295–306.

McCartney CR, Marshall JC. Clinical practice. Polycystic ovary syndrome. *N Engl J Med.* 2016;375:54–64.

Parry BL, Martinez LF, Maurer EL, Lopez AM, Sorenson D, Meliska CJ. Sleep, rhythms and women's mood. Part I. Menstrual cycle, pregnancy and postpartum. *Sleep Med Rev*. 2006;10:129–144.

Rahman SA, Grant LK, Gooley JJ, Rajaratnam SMW, Czeisler CA, Lockley SW. Endogenous circadian regulation of female reproductive hormones. *J Clin Endocrinol Metab*. 2019;104:6049–6059.

Sam S, Ehrmann DA. Pathogenesis and consequences of disordered sleep in PCOS. *Clin Med Insights Reprod Health*. 2019;13:1179558119871269.

Shechter A, Boivin DB. Sleep, hormones, and circadian rhythms throughout the menstrual cycle in healthy women and women with premenstrual dysphoric disorder. *Int J Endocrinol*. 2010:259345.

Soules MR, Steiner RA, Cohen NL, Bremner WJ, Clifton DK. Nocturnal slowing of pulsatile luteinizing hormone secretion in women during the follicular phase of the menstrual cycle. *J Clin Endocrinol Metab*. 1985;61:43–49.

A complete reference list can be found online at ExpertConsult.com.

Chapter 186

Sleep and Sleep Disorders Associated with Pregnancy

Bilgay Izci Balserak; Louise M. O'Brien; Bei Bei

Chapter Highlights

- In the first trimester, hormonal fluctuations and associated physiologic changes may disturb sleep. In the second trimester, subjective and objective sleep parameters improve compared to the first trimester. By the end of the second trimester, physical changes associated with a rapidly growing uterus, hormonal fluctuations, primary sleep disorders and anxiety associated with labor, delivery, and motherhood are the main reasons for sleep disturbances.
- Women can experience considerable daytime sleepiness and fatigue, as well as primary sleep disorders, such as sleep-disordered breathing (SDB) or restless legs syndrome (RLS), which may occur or worsen during pregnancy. SDB can result from added abdominal weight gain and changes in the respiratory system. Pregnancy-related RLS is a secondary form of RLS attributed to iron deficiency and hormonal changes. Complaints of nocturnal esophageal reflux and sleep-related leg cramps also occur and worsen as the pregnancy advances.
- Sleep disturbances may represent modifiable risk factors for adverse pregnancy outcomes, including preeclampsia and preterm birth. All sleep complaints need to be carefully monitored, and nonpharmacologic interventions for sleep disorders should be given priority, although, in severe conditions, pharmacologic treatment should be used with caution. Early identification and management of prenatal sleep disorders may prevent or minimize adverse maternal and fetal outcomes.

Sleep disturbance during pregnancy is common and multifaceted. With increasing gestation, sleep is significantly disturbed by the third trimester of pregnancy.[1–4] Sleep disturbances may result from internal and external factors that change the duration or structure of a normal sleep pattern and circadian rhythm.[5] Pregnancy-related anatomic, physiologic, hormonal, and psychological factors can occur in different stages of pregnancy and affect the degree and severity of sleep disturbances. Some of these pregnancy changes can also cause sleep disorders or exacerbate existing sleep disorders, which can impact maternal and fetal health. In accordance, clinicians need to identify pathologic sleep disturbance in pregnancy and provide timely management to reduce or prevent adverse maternal and fetal outcomes.

THE EFFECTS OF PREGNANCY-INDUCED HORMONAL CHANGES ON SLEEP

Pregnancy causes dramatic changes in melatonin, cortisol, estrogen, and progesterone, as well as pituitary hormones (gonadatropins, prolactin, growth hormone). These hormonal changes not only directly influence the sleep-wake cycles and sleep structure but also cause physiologic changes that increase the risk of sleep disorders (Figure 186.1). Sleep and circadian rhythms also have a role in regulating the secretion of these hormones.

Progesterone

The level of progesterone released from the placenta is 10 to 500 times higher at term than in the nonpregnant state.[6] Serum progesterone has a diurnal change, with higher concentrations in the evening.[7] Progesterone, intracellular progesterone receptors, and progesterone's metabolites acting on brain gamma-aminobutyric acid (GABA) receptors produce a soporific effect with a significant increase in non–rapid eye movement (NREM) sleep.[8] These effects may partly explain daytime sleepiness and fatigue in the first trimester when progesterone is steadily rising. Animal and human studies have demonstrated that exogenous progesterone administration shortens latency to sleep onset, lengthens latency to rapid eye movement (REM) sleep onset, and reduces total REM sleep.[8,9] Progesterone's soporific and thermogenic (temperature-raising) effects, and its inhibitory effect on smooth muscle (including gastrointestinal track, ureters, and bladder) also indirectly influence sleep.[5,6] Furthermore, increased respiratory rates caused by progesterone may protect the airway from occlusion, but complaints of feeling short of breath are common.

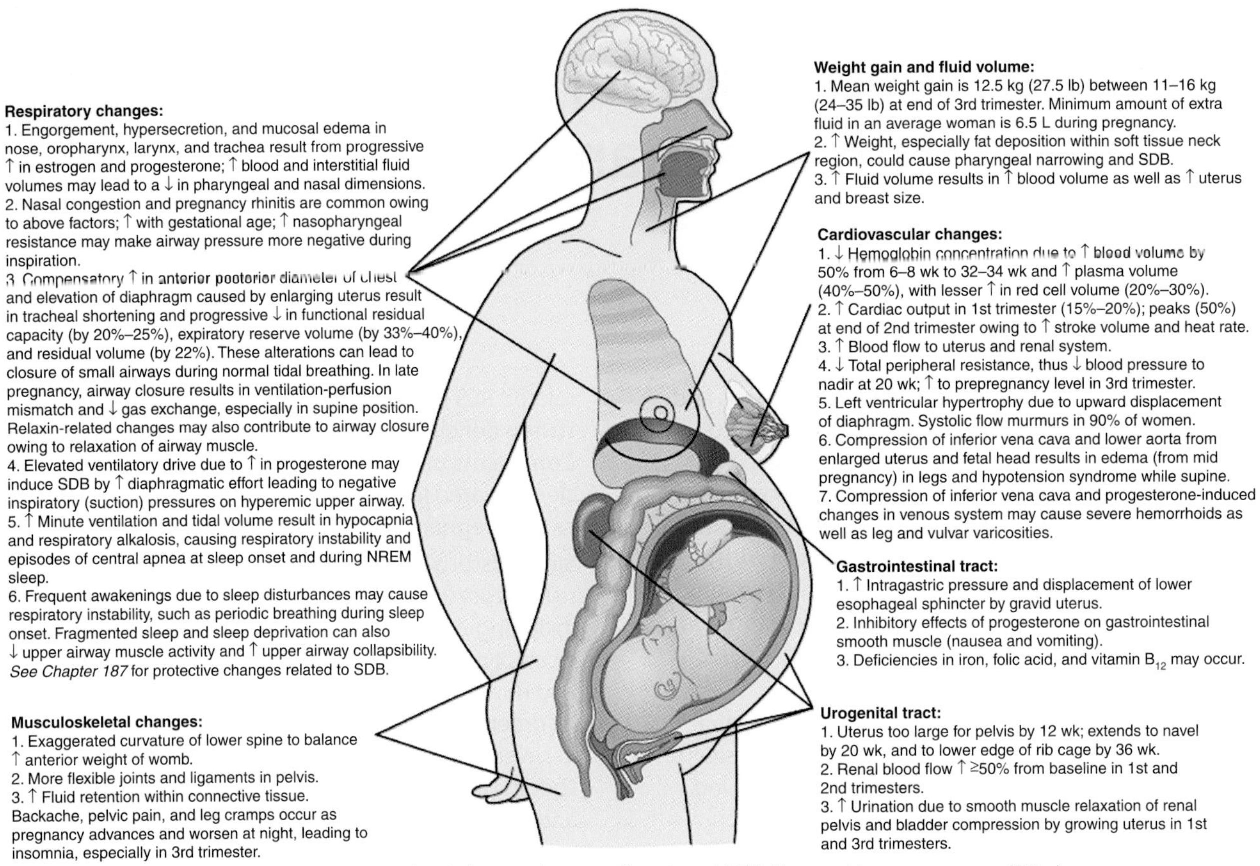
Respiratory changes:
1. Engorgement, hypersecretion, and mucosal edema in nose, oropharynx, larynx, and trachea result from progressive ↑ in estrogen and progesterone; ↑ blood and interstitial fluid volumes may lead to a ↓ in pharyngeal and nasal dimensions.
2. Nasal congestion and pregnancy rhinitis are common owing to above factors; ↑ with gestational age; ↑ nasopharyngeal resistance may make airway pressure more negative during inspiration.
3. Compensatory ↑ in anterior posterior diameter of chest and elevation of diaphragm caused by enlarging uterus result in tracheal shortening and progressive ↓ in functional residual capacity (by 20%–25%), expiratory reserve volume (by 33%–40%), and residual volume (by 22%). These alterations can lead to closure of small airways during normal tidal breathing. In late pregnancy, airway closure results in ventilation-perfusion mismatch and ↓ gas exchange, especially in supine position. Relaxin-related changes may also contribute to airway closure owing to relaxation of airway muscle.
4. Elevated ventilatory drive due to ↑ in progesterone may induce SDB by ↑ diaphragmatic effort leading to negative inspiratory (suction) pressures on hyperemic upper airway.
5. ↑ Minute ventilation and tidal volume result in hypocapnia and respiratory alkalosis, causing respiratory instability and episodes of central apnea at sleep onset and during NREM sleep.
6. Frequent awakenings due to sleep disturbances may cause respiratory instability, such as periodic breathing during sleep onset. Fragmented sleep and sleep deprivation can also ↓ upper airway muscle activity and ↑ upper airway collapsibility.
See Chapter 187 for protective changes related to SDB.
Musculoskeletal changes:
1. Exaggerated curvature of lower spine to balance ↑ anterior weight of womb.
2. More flexible joints and ligaments in pelvis.
3. ↑ Fluid retention within connective tissue.
Backache, pelvic pain, and leg cramps occur as pregnancy advances and worsen at night, leading to insomnia, especially in 3rd trimester.
Weight gain and fluid volume:
1. Mean weight gain is 12.5 kg (27.5 lb) between 11–16 kg (24–35 lb) at end of 3rd trimester. Minimum amount of extra fluid in an average woman is 6.5 L during pregnancy.
2. ↑ Weight, especially fat deposition within soft tissue neck region, could cause pharyngeal narrowing and SDB.
3. ↑ Fluid volume results in ↑ blood volume as well as ↑ uterus and breast size.
Cardiovascular changes:
1. ↓ Hemoglobin concentration due to ↑ blood volume by 50% from 6–8 wk to 32–34 wk and ↑ plasma volume (40%–50%), with lesser ↑ in red cell volume (20%–30%).
2. ↑ Cardiac output in 1st trimester (15%–20%); peaks (50%) at end of 2nd trimester owing to ↑ stroke volume and heat rate.
3. ↑ Blood flow to uterus and renal system.
4. ↓ Total peripheral resistance, thus ↓ blood pressure to nadir at 20 wk; ↑ to prepregnancy level in 3rd trimester.
5. Left ventricular hypertrophy due to upward displacement of diaphragm. Systolic flow murmurs in 90% of women.
6. Compression of inferior vena cava and lower aorta from enlarged uterus and fetal head results in edema (from mid pregnancy) in legs and hypotension syndrome while supine.
7. Compression of inferior vena cava and progesterone-induced changes in venous system may cause severe hemorrhoids as well as leg and vulvar varicosities.
Gastrointestinal tract:
1. ↑ Intragastric pressure and displacement of lower esophageal sphincter by gravid uterus.
2. Inhibitory effects of progesterone on gastrointestinal smooth muscle (nausea and vomiting).
3. Deficiencies in iron, folic acid, and vitamin B_{12} may occur.
Urogenital tract:
1. Uterus too large for pelvis by 12 wk; extends to navel by 20 wk, and to lower edge of rib cage by 36 wk.
2. Renal blood flow ↑ ≥50% from baseline in 1st and 2nd trimesters.
3. ↑ Urination due to smooth muscle relaxation of renal pelvis and bladder compression by growing uterus in 1st and 3rd trimesters.

Figure 186.1 Pregnancy-related changes that can affect sleep. NREM, Non–rapid eye movement; SDB, sleep-disordered breathing.

Estrogen

Estrogen secreted by the placenta increases significantly during pregnancy, peaks before birth, and declines after delivery.[6] Estrogen has excitatory effects on the nervous system and selectively decreases REM sleep activation of sleep-active neurons in the ventrolateral preoptic area.[10] Maternal plasma estriol has a 24-hour rhythm at 35 weeks' gestation, which occurs in the opposite direction of the cortisol rhythm.[7] However, the higher estrogen concentration during pregnancy causes vasodilation, and with the extra fluid that accumulates during pregnancy, women experience nasal congestion and ankle edema.[6] Estrogen also stimulates prolactin production and suppresses dopamine release, which may contribute to RLS.[11,12]

Cortisol

Cortisol starts to increase from the 25th week of pregnancy, with a twofold increase seen in late pregnancy that rapidly returns to normal levels after delivery.[6,7] This elevation is mostly due to placental secretion of corticotrophin-releasing hormone and adrenocorticotropic hormone (ACTH) and increased synthesis of cortisol-binding globulin (CBG) by the liver. Progesterone and cortisol also share binding sites on CBG.[7] Therefore an increase in the level of progesterone during pregnancy leads to higher levels of free cortisol. The normal diurnal cortisol rhythm includes a nadir level around midnight and marked elevation during early-morning hours.[7,13] In pregnant women, the morning peak is not obvious, probably due to the blunting effect of placental ACTH on maternal cortisol concentrations.[6,7] In the second trimester, women who reported long or short sleep and poor sleep quality had lower cortisol values during the day compared to women who reported sufficient sleep.[14] Poor sleep quality at 36 weeks' gestation has been linked to elevated evening cortisol concentrations.[15] Pregnant women with poor sleep in the third trimester have lower cortisol-melatonin ratios compared to good sleepers, as a result of a lower early-morning cortisol peak levels and a relatively higher concentration of melatonin.[7,13] A study found that maternal cortisol during pregnancy is mainly affected by biologic (e.g., age, body mass index [BMI], time of day, parity) and lifestyle (e.g., smoking, sleep sufficiency, employment) factors.[14]

Melatonin

Melatonin is synthesized by the pineal gland, secreted in response to darkness, and suppressed by light. Melatonin is involved in the regulation of circadian rhythms of reproductive hormones, with many peripheral tissues expressing melatonin and its receptors, including the ovaries.[16] The circadian rhythm of melatonin continues during pregnancy.[16] Melatonin's diurnal rhythm during the first and the second trimester is similar to a nonpregnant state, but levels increase in the third trimester.[13] In twin pregnancies, nocturnal melatonin levels are significantly higher after 28 weeks' gestation than in normal singleton pregnancies.[16]

Melatonin synergizes with oxytocin to promote the birth process, although its concentration does not change in either labor induction or cesarean delivery.[16] It is possible that altered rhythm or low levels of melatonin secretion might result in pregnancy complications because melatonin plays a role in fetal maturation and placenta/uterine homeostasis and is involved in correcting the pathophysiology of complications, such as preeclampsia and fetal brain damage.[16]

Prolactin

Prolactin is involved in immunoregulation, lactogenesis, and mammary tissue growth. Prolactin concentrations are 10-fold higher at term than in a nonpregnant state.[6] Prolactin secretion rhythms do not differ between pregnant good and poor sleepers.[13] Studies with small samples of pregnant women show episodic prolactin secretion and elevated levels during nocturnal sleep.[7] During a normal vaginal delivery, prolactin peaks for 4 to 6 hours and then descends to a normal circadian pattern; however, concentrations are significantly lower in women who have elective cesarean births compared with women who experience labor.[17] It is hypothesized that prolactin secretion may enhance slow wave sleep (SWS), as SWS is increased in patients with prolactinomas.[18]

Oxytocin

Oxytocin is secreted from the posterior pituitary gland. It promotes uterine contractions and lactation.[9] In late pregnancy it reaches the highest level at night, together with peaks in uterine activity rhythm.[19] In animals oxytocin promotes sleep in stress-free conditions, but it may induce wakefulness in high concentrations.[9] Oxytocin and melatonin act synergistically to assist in the process of labor and birth; this interaction during the night could explain the higher incidence of nocturnal births.[16,19]

Growth Hormone

Growth hormone (GH) prepares the maternal organism for the metabolic demands of the offspring and regulates food intake, fat retention, and the sensitivity to insulin and leptin in a cell-specific manner. Pituitary GH secretion is primarily regulated by growth hormone–releasing hormone and neurons in the arcuate nucleus of the hypothalamus. Maternal placental GH circulation levels increase in pregnancy from as early as the 8th week and peak around the 35th week.[20] Pituitary GH is released in a pulsatile manner, but the release of placental GH is continuous.[20] These hormones are closely associated with the maintenance of SWS and overall sleep regulation and thus are important for fetal development and maternal health.[6,18]

Leptin

Maternal serum leptin levels steadily increase, peak in late second trimester, and remain two to four times higher relative to the nonpregnant state. Leptin is produced and secreted by the placental and adipose tissues and has a key role in regulating body fat, energy expenditure, and fetal growth.[6] Extremes in either short or long sleep duration in early pregnancy are associated with altered leptin levels.[21]

Relaxin

The corpus luteum is the primary source of circulating relaxin during pregnancy. Serum relaxin peaks at the end of the first trimester and falls to an intermediate value until birth.[22] It contributes to connective tissue remodeling and relaxing pelvic ligaments to prepare for birth.[6] Although mechanisms remain unclear, relaxin can contribute to sleep disturbance due to relaxed airway, carpal tunnel syndrome from fluid retention, and low back pain due to relaxed ligaments.[6]

In summary, there is a bidirectional relationship between hormonal changes and altered sleep during pregnancy. Although these hormones have significant effects on sleep and circadian rhythms during pregnancy, altered sleep during pregnancy can also influence hormone levels. Further research is required, particularly for sleep-induced hormonal fluctuations and implications for adverse obstetrical outcomes.

PHYSIOLOGIC CHANGES IN PREGNANCY AND SLEEP IN NORMAL PREGNANCY

Pregnancy leads to a multitude of hormonal, anatomic, and physiologic changes, including changes in respiratory and cardiovascular systems that are detailed in Figure 186.1.[6] These changes are essential to maintain a healthy pregnancy, but some contribute to sleep problems, whereas others may have adverse effects on the fetus or the mother. Furthermore, circadian rhythms influenced by pregnancy-related changes are linked to sleep problems and mood disorders.

With the physical and hormonal changes in pregnancy, most women (66% to 97%) experience changes in sleep,[23–25] with nocturnal awakenings frequently reported in the third trimester.[2,26,27] Both objective and self-reported sleep measures show that sleep efficiency (SE) progressively decreases over pregnancy due to increased and longer nocturnal awakenings.[23–25,27] However, night-to-night and individual variability does exist.[28] Although numerous studies have attempted to describe sleep characteristics during pregnancy, findings are not always consistent due to different research designs (e.g., cross-sectional, longitudinal), settings (e.g., laboratory, home), assessment methods (e.g., self-report, polysomnography [PSG], actigraphy), sample sizes, data collection timing (e.g., different gestational periods), and comparisons (e.g., comparing women at various gestational ages with nonpregnant control subjects in different menstrual cycle phases). For example, studies comparing objective and self-reported measures find discrepancies in sleep-time estimates,[4,26] with self-reported total sleep time (TST) longer than PSG and actigraphic TST across trimesters.[29] These discrepancies may lead to spurious associations between sleep duration and adverse pregnancy outcomes. Further, most studies also failed to account for daytime naps.

First Trimester

Women report daytime sleepiness, fatigue, frequent naps, longer 24-hour TST and sleep-onset latency (SOL), and more wake after sleep onset (WASO).[a] A recent study reported that sleep onset timing was earlier during the first and second trimesters than before pregnancy and returned to the prepregnant state in the third trimester.[32] Sleep quality and SWS are lower compared to prepregnancy or nonpregnant state.[2,24,25,27]

[a]References 4, 24, 25, 27, 30, 31.

Dramatic alterations in hormone levels in the first trimester not only contribute to sleep disturbance[6,8] but also to fatigue and daytime sleepiness, morning sickness, waking with nausea, increased urinary frequency, physical discomforts (tender breasts or back pain), and mood changes.[2,30–33] Psychosocial stressors in unplanned pregnancies or the lack of psychosocial support, especially in first-time pregnancies,[29] could also lead to poor sleep quality in early pregnancy.[34]

Second Trimester

In most cases, self-reported and objective sleep parameters improve in the second trimester compared to the first trimester,[2,5,24,27,29] with lower fatigue and better sleep quality,[2,3,30,33] likely due to the stabilization of hormone levels. Compared to other trimesters, women in the second trimester have better SE and less WASO[27] (Table 186.1). However, a substudy of the Nulliparous Pregnancy Outcomes: Monitoring Mothers-to-Be (nuMoM2b; n = 782) study found that women spent a relatively long time in bed attempting to sleep, with WASO of more than 42 minutes.[35] By the end of the second trimester, the number of awakenings increases.[5] Women may experience disturbed sleep as a result of snoring, heartburn, irregular uterine contractions (Braxton-Hicks), fetal movements, leg cramps, or RLS.[1–3,36] Vivid dreams and pain in the back, neck, and joints were additional reasons for sleep disruption during the second trimester according to a National Sleep Foundation survey.[36] Although findings on PSG measuring SWS and REM sleep during second trimester are inconsistent,[24] a longitudinal study using at-home PSG showed that SWS slightly decreased, but REM sleep did not change relative to first trimester.[24]

Third Trimester

The majority (75% to 98%) of women report sleep disturbances with multiple nocturnal awakenings when approaching the 40th week of gestation.[2,30,36,37] Nocturnal sleep time is lower than the first two trimesters, but 24-hour TST may approach prepregnancy values,[2,25,26,30] likely due to more daytime napping. In fact, greater than 75% of women reported at least one nap each week in the third trimester.[30,36–38] Sleep in the third trimester features long SOL, low SE, and high WASO.[4,24–26] Most PSG studies showed less SWS and REM sleep when compared to previous trimesters or nonpregnant control subjects.[4,24,25,30] In exchange for this decrease, women have increased light sleep stages.[4,24,25,40] They also have decreased delta power during NREM sleep across pregnancy.[4,40]

Physical changes associated with a rapidly growing uterus, in addition to hormonal fluctuations, are the main causes of sleep disturbances in the third trimester.[3,26] Most women complain of urinary frequency, general physical discomfort, heartburn, leg cramps, spontaneous awakenings, and fatigue.[3,25,30,36,37] Fetal movements, difficulty maintaining sleep, shortness of breath, and other physical discomforts (breast tenderness, joint pain, backache, and itching) are often reported.[2,3,30,36] Women also attribute their sleep loss to internal factors (vivid dreams/nightmares, anxiety about labor/delivery, the fetus, and pregnancy complications) and external factors, such as their other children.[30,36,38] Employment schedules may also matter, as working women were less likely to nap and reported sleeping 1 hour less per night in the last month of pregnancy.[3,31,41] By the third trimester, women also often complain about difficulties with attention, concentration, and memory, and the risk of primary sleep disorders increases.[12]

Labor and Delivery

Pain, anxiety, uterine contractions, and administration of medications all affect sleep and result in sleep loss and low sleep quality during labor and immediately after delivery.[29,38,42] The rhythm of nocturnal uterine activity, presumably a result of peaks in oxytocin secretion patterns, may contribute to

Table 186.1 Sleep Pattern, Nocturnal Features, and Daytime Symptoms in Each Trimester, Labor, and Delivery

	First Trimester	Second Trimester	Third Trimester	Labor, Delivery
Pattern	↑TST ↑Number of naps ↑WASO ↓SE ↓SWS	↓TST ↑SE ↓SWS ↓WASO REM (no change)	↑TST ↑Number of naps ↑WASO ↑Sleep stage 1 ↓SE ↓SWS ↓REM	↓TST ↓SE ↓NREM ↓REM
Nocturnal features	Urinary frequency Physical discomfort (tender breasts/back pain)	At the end of the trimester: Snoring Restless legs syndrome Irregular uterine contractions Heartburn Vivid dreams Back, neck, and joint pain	Urinary frequency Physical discomforts Heartburn Irregular uterine contractions Fetal movements Muscle/leg cramps Shortness of breath Vivid dreams/nightmares Snoring Restless legs syndrome	Anxiety Forceful uterine contractions
Daytime symptoms	Fatigue Drowsiness Nausea Mood changes	Nasal congestion	Fatigue Drowsiness Impaired vigilance Nasal congestion	Fatigue Anxiety Pain

NREM, Non–rapid eye movement; REM, rapid eye movement; SE, sleep efficiency; SWS, slow wave sleep; TST, 24-hour total sleep time; WASO, wake (time) after sleep onset.

nocturnal awakenings, and most women experience spontaneous labor onset with forceful contractions at night.[16,19] In a longitudinal study of 35 women, sleep quality deteriorated progressively over the last 5 days of pregnancy and was lowest the night before contractions started and admission to the hospital for delivery.[42] In another study, a group of 20 women all reported being unable to sleep once contractions started.[43] As the latent phase of labor becomes prolonged, sleep is not possible even when sleep aids are used.[29,43]

Parity Differences in Sleep

Studies using objective sleep measures found that TST, SWS, and REM sleep during pregnancy were not significantly affected by parity,[4,24,25,28] but nulliparas (no prior birthing experience), especially employed women, were at higher risk for self-reported poor sleep quality,[29] possibly due to adjusting to a new role. Multiparas (with prior birthing experience) may be awakened during the night by older children[23,29,36,44] and report shorter sleep duration, longer SOL, and poorer sleep quality compared to nulliparas; however, when controlling for other children, multiparas have higher SE than nulliparas during pregnancy.[28,33] Nulliparous women were also sleepier from the first trimester to delivery compared to their multiparous counterparts.[31] During the third trimester, women younger than 30 years (also more likely to be nulliparas) had more TST than those older than 30 years,[2,29] whose sleep may be affected by other children or by a primary sleep disorder. For example, increasing age is recognized as a risk factor for RLS, SDB, and insomnia.[3,12,29]

Sleep Disparities in Pregnancy

There is a disproportionately high burden of poor pregnancy outcomes in Black women compared to other racial groups,[45] which may be explained by the weathering hypothesis on the cumulative effect of continuous exposure to social and economic inequalities.[46] Such chronic stressors overactivate the hypothalamic-pituitary-adrenal (HPA) axis and increase the risk for stress-related diseases, contributing to racial disparities in reproductive health. Chronic sleep loss further activates the HPA-axis and yields an abnormal immune/inflammatory cascade, which may subsequently impact pregnancy outcomes.[38]

Specific sleep characteristics, such as self-reported sleep quality, were poorer in African-American compared to White women during pregnancy.[23] The nuMoM2b study also reported that sleep duration in pregnant women varied by race/ethnicity and insurance status, and sleep continuity and timing varied by race/ethnicity, age, BMI, insurance status, and smoking history[35]; further, non-Hispanic Blacks and Asian pregnant women had the shortest sleep durations. However, it is yet to be elucidated how psychosocial stressors and racial/ethnic differences interact with maternal sleep to influence birth outcomes.[45]

In summary, most women experience sleep disturbance during pregnancy, with each trimester bringing different patterns of, and contributing factors to, sleep disturbance. If there is opportunity for napping, 24-hour TST can be higher in each trimester compared to nonpregnant women. Yet, nocturnal TST and SE decrease progressively during pregnancy, whereas sleep stage characteristics remain generally constant, although pregnant women tend to have more light sleep and less SWS. Nulliparity, being older than 30 years, and being employed are associated with poor sleep quality. There are discernible racial disparities in sleep disturbances during pregnancy.

SLEEP DISORDERS DURING PREGNANCY

The following sections outline the nature, epidemiology, risk factors, and management of common sleep disorders during pregnancy. Sleep-disordered breathing and its adverse effects in pregnancy are detailed in Chapter 187.

Insomnia during Pregnancy

During pregnancy, women may experience some or all of insomnia symptoms, ranging from acute to chronic insomnia[3,47,48] (see Chapter 93 on insomnia disorder). Careful evaluation of sleep complaints is needed so that symptoms of insomnia are distinguished from sleep disruption (e.g., physical discomfort, frequent urination). Insomnia during pregnancy may persist into postpartum periods; 68% and 50% of women with clinically significant insomnia at 32 weeks of pregnancy still meet diagnostic criteria for insomnia at 8-weeks and 2-years postpartum, respectively.[49]

Epidemiology

The prevalence of insomnia in the pregnant population is difficult to estimate owing to various definitions and assessment methods. Most existing studies used self-reported scales to measure insomnia symptoms and their response to treatment. These scales typically ask about difficulties with sleep but not the causes or contexts of sleep difficulties. For example, a woman reporting multiple nighttime awakenings due to urinations but who is able to fall back to sleep quickly may score high on these symptom-based scales, but her symptoms would be more consistent with sleep disruption and not insomnia. Based on these symptom scales, approximately 50% to 74% of women report symptoms of insomnia during pregnancy, and in 17% to 30% of women, these symptoms are clinically significant.[3,48,49] Prevalence of insomnia symptoms increases as pregnancy progresses, with the highest prevalence and most wake episodes in the third trimester.[3,47,48] In a prospective cohort study, insomnia status prevalence (95% confidence interval [CI]), based on an Athens Insomnia Scale score 8 or higher, was 6.1% (95% CI, 3.9 to 8.9) pregestational, 44.2% (95% CI, 39.3 to 49.6) in the first trimester, 46.3% (95% CI, 41.9 to 51.3) in the second trimester, and 63.7% (95% CI, 57.7 to 67.8) in the third trimester.[50]

Risk Factors

Risk factors for insomnia in pregnancy include being older than 30 years,[2,3] nulliparity,[47] single motherhood,[44] preeclampsia or pregnancy-induced hypertension,[3,51] prepregnancy affective disorders,[47,52,53] perinatal depression,[38,47,53] smoking,[48] negative body image,[54] and environmental factors, such as noise from other children, bed partners, or pets.[30,36] From cognitive behavioral perspectives, the 3P model (predisposing factors, precipitating factors, and perpetuating factors)[55] (see Chapter 91) is well suited to explain new onset or exacerbation of insomnia during pregnancy. The primary precipitating factors for prenatal insomnia are sleep disrupting physical changes (e.g., fetus growth, hormonal changes, urination, nausea) and voluntary sleep restriction due to employment and household responsibilities.[3,41] As women cope with these significant sleep disruptions, they may develop sleep-related thoughts and behaviors, such as "I will never get a good night sleep," spending more time in bed, or increasing caffeine intake.[3,48] These could perpetuate sleep problems and contribute to insomnia. This conceptualization allows treatments to be directed at modifiable precipitating and perpetuating factors to reduce and prevent insomnia in the perinatal periods.

Management

The diagnosis of insomnia requires adequate opportunity to sleep, with an inadequate ability to fall and stay asleep.[56] These criteria may be confused with multiple awakenings associated with pregnancy discomforts. Pregnant women also may have insomnia as a comorbid condition associated with SDB or depression. Untreated comorbid insomnia may reoccur even if the originating cause is treated.[57] In addition, insomnia in pregnancy can significantly affect physical and cognitive function and has implications for pregnancy outcomes.[58] Thus timely assessment and appropriate management (see Chapters 93 and 95 to 100) are essential.

Due to potential adverse effects of medication on the fetus during pregnancy, most couples and clinicians opt for nonpharmacologic therapies to treat insomnia. Behavioral and cognitive therapies[59,60] should be the initial treatment for women with insomnia during pregnancy after excluding other sleep disorders. Cognitive behavioral therapy for insomnia (CBT-I; see Chapters 95 to 97) is a well-established treatment for insomnia. It is also the preferred treatment option (compared to pharmacologic approaches) in about three-quarters of surveyed expecting couples.[61] A large randomized controlled trial (RCT) of CBT-I for women diagnosed with prenatal insomnia disorder reported a significant reduction in insomnia severity and higher remission rates compared to an active control condition.[59] Recent research effort is focusing on making CBT-I more widely accessible to the public and better integrated to the perinatal care system, attempting delivery of intervention via telephone, internet, and group formats.[62,63] A longitudinal RCT showed that a brief, therapist-assisted, digital cognitive behavioral intervention delivered during the perinatal transition not only reduced symptoms of insomnia at late pregnancy, but also had long-term benefits to sleep at 2 years postpartum.[63a]

Of note, many pregnant women do not seek treatment for insomnia because they either think it will naturally resolve after birth or wish to avoid medication. In the United States 11% of pregnant women used a sleep aid, including over-the-counter medications, at least a few nights a week, and 1% used alcohol at some point in pregnancy to help them sleep.[36] If nonpharmacologic therapies are not available, or persistent and severe insomnia is not responding, medications should be prescribed at the lowest effective dose for the shortest possible duration after discussion of potential risks and benefits with the patient. At present, histamine H_1 receptor antagonists, such as diphenhydramine and doxylamine, are widely used as over-the-counter sleep aids during pregnancy and are considered unlikely to cause harm to the fetus.[64,65] Unfortunately, most other hypnotic medications have either insufficient human data to evaluate risk during pregnancy or have been linked to increased fetal risk. Therefore prescribers should only consider hypnotic medication if nonpharmacologic approaches are unavailable and potential benefits outweigh the risk.

There is some evidence that insomnia symptoms during pregnancy may be alleviated via mindful yoga, acupuncture, massage, or exercise.[58,66] Herbal or dietary supplements, such as chamomile tea or lavender pillows, are also used as sleep aids,[60] but controlled studies are needed to assess the benefits and risks to fetal and maternal health.

Pregnancy-Related Restless Legs Syndrome (Willis-Ekbom Disease)

Pregnancy-related RLS is classified as a secondary form of RLS because symptoms typically resolve at the time of delivery.[11,12,67] Pregnancy-related RLS is a risk for RLS several years after pregnancy.[67,68] RLS may coexist with periodic leg movements in sleep (PLMS).[69] Arousals associated with repeated leg movements during sleep can significantly disturb sleep during pregnancy.[69,70] RLS symptoms are associated with shorter TST, more difficulty initiating and maintaining sleep, and more daytime sleepiness compared to pregnant women without RLS.[11,12,67,71] In extreme cases, symptoms are so disturbing that evening relaxation and falling asleep is almost impossible and creates a high risk for depression.[67,72] After delivery, the frequency of PLMS decreased by 50% to 100% in women with RLS based on leg actigraphy monitoring.[73]

Epidemiology

In 1940 Mussio-Fournier and Rawak made the first observation that RLS was exacerbated during pregnancy in German women.[12] Since 1940 numerous reports from around the world estimate prevalence at 3% to 36% in pregnant populations,[11,12,74] and all agree that RLS is two to three times more prevalent in pregnant than nonpregnant women,[11] even in ethnic groups where RLS is a rare condition. About half of pregnant women with RLS have moderate to severe symptoms, and there are dose-response relationships between the severity of RLS and poor sleep quality, poor daytime function, and daytime sleepiness.[74]

Most prospective studies report that prevalence rates of RLS increase as pregnancy progresses, peaking in the third trimester and resolving a few days before delivery.[11,12,71,73] A recent meta-analysis[75] reported that the frequency of RLS increased across the first, second, and third trimesters of pregnancy, with 8%, 16%, and 22%, respectively, of women reporting RLS symptoms, followed by a large decrease in RLS frequency to 4% after delivery. Variations in pregnancy-related RLS estimates can be attributed to differences in diagnostic criteria (earlier studies conducted before diagnostic criteria established by the International Restless Legs Syndrome Study Group [IRLSSG]), measurement issues, and associated risk factors (e.g., age, parity, ethnicity, regional variations, genetics). A recent meta-analysis[75] that included studies with a variety of methodologies for assessing prevalence of RLS, showed the pooled prevalence of RLS during pregnancy across all studies, compared to those using the IRLSSG criteria, was similar (21% and 22%, respectively).

In Western countries where studies used established diagnostic criteria for pregnancy-related RLS, prevalence ranges from 11% to 34%.[11,12,67,71,73] In Asian countries, prevalence varies from 3% to 20%.[11] In an epidemiologic study of 461 Taiwanese women interviewed using established criteria, the overall prevalence of RLS was 10.4%.[76] One of the first prevalence studies using international criteria and a structured clinical interview was performed in Italy with 642 pregnant women.[67] The RLS prevalence rate was 26.6%, and the mean onset of RLS symptoms was around the sixth month of pregnancy. Although 16.7% had never experienced RLS symptoms before pregnancy, about 10% had preexisting symptoms, and 15% had symptoms at least three times per week.[67] However, a recent prospective study in Switzerland found a lower prevalence (12%) and earlier onset (before the fifth month).[73] The pooled prevalence of RLS during pregnancy in the European, Western Pacific, Eastern Mediterranean, and the Americas regions has recently been reported as 22% (95% CI, 18% to 26%), 14% (95% CI, 5% to 22%), 30% (95% CI, 16% to 45%), and 20% (95% CI, 16% to 24%), respectively, with the Western Pacific region significantly lower than other regions.[75]

Pathophysiology

The pathophysiology of pregnancy-induced RLS has yet to be established. Potential factors include hormonal mechanisms, iron and folate metabolism, family history, depression, and multiparity.[11,12,71] Iron and folate deficiencies, often seen in pregnancy, are associated with RLS.[11,67,71] Earlier studies reported that women who developed RLS by the third trimester had lower folate and ferritin levels at preconception and lower folate, plasma iron, hemoglobin values and mean corpuscular volume throughout pregnancy in comparison with healthy control subjects.[11,67,71] A recent Czech study of 300 third-trimester women found that hemoglobin levels were significantly lower, and there was less hypochromic anemia in the RLS group compared to those without RLS.[77] However, these findings are not universally supported.[70,73,78]

Iron deficiency in the central nervous system (CNS), which results in the dysfunction of dopaminergic systems, may be responsible for RLS symptoms among women who have normal ferritin, an indicator of systemic iron storage. In this regard, cerebrospinal fluid (CSF) ferritin levels are informative, as RLS patients, even those with normal peripheral iron stores, have low CSF ferritin and high CSF transferrin.[12] Studies on CNS iron metabolism in pregnancy-related RLS are needed. However, the iron deficiency hypothesis cannot be supported for two reasons: (1) All pregnant women in the second half of pregnancy have similar hemoglobin and ferritin reductions, attributed to fetal growth and hemodilution, regardless of iron and vitamin supplementation.[67,71] (2) RLS symptoms resolve just before labor onset, even though the largest loss of blood and iron is at delivery, and it takes at least 3 months for iron storage to be restored.[6]

Hormones such as prolactin and estrogens may contribute to RLS in pregnancy. Prolactin may be involved due to its antidopaminergic feature.[12,70] However, there is no strong evidence for a causative role for prolactin in RLS[70] as its levels rise throughout pregnancy and continue to be elevated in breastfeeding women, yet RLS resolves with labor and delivery. In addition, RLS is not associated with diurnal rhythms of prolactin in the general population.[11,70] Elevated estradiol levels during pregnancy and its sudden decline with delivery of the placenta has been linked with RLS symptoms,[70] yet larger studies fail to confirm this.[11,73] Progesterone levels do not differ between women with and without RLS.[11,70] Thyroid hormone has also been speculated in the pathophysiology of RLS,[11] but levels were not found to differ between pregnant women with and without RLS in one recent study.[78] Thus more research is needed.

Family history of RLS and multiparity (especially closely-spaced pregnancies) may be independent risk factors for RLS.[11,67,68,73] RLS has been reported by 75% of multiparas who experienced RLS in a previous pregnancy[73] but had not experienced RLS between pregnancies.[2] The risk of RLS increases with the number of children in a dose-dependent way.[68] Other factors associated with RLS include older age, heavier maternal weight, smoking, peptic ulcer disease, varicosities, and concomitant SDB or depression.[11,67,73,76,78] Some medications, such as selective serotonin reuptake inhibitors (SSRIs), antihistamines, and antiemetics, may also trigger or exacerbate RLS symptoms.[11,12] Sleep deprivation, anxiety and stress, insomnia, and fatigue are also documented contributors to RLS in pregnancy.[11,12,67,68] In a prospective study of 1428 women, prepregnancy RLS was a risk factor for both antenatal and postnatal depression, whereas no added risk was seen in pregnant women with a new-onset RLS during pregnancy.[72] Nonetheless, studies that collected data via standard criteria failed to find associations with delivery outcomes.[74] Pregnancy may also act by unidentified mechanisms in women already genetically predisposed to RLS (e.g., a positive family history of RLS). Nonetheless, the genetic underpinning has yet to be elucidated.

Management

Pregnancy-related RLS is likely short term and highly symptomatic until delivery. Symptom severity and the impact on the individual are central in the decision to treat. As a first-line therapy (Figure 186.2), nonpharmacologic comfort strategies should be considered rather than medication that may affect the fetus. If sleep is severely disrupted by RLS, iron therapy may be warranted, or the lowest dose of pharmacologic therapy can be considered (also see treatment options in Figure 186.2 and Chapter 121)[68,90] but should be used with care, as no pharmacotherapies currently have a specific indication for RLS in pregnancy.

Sleep-Related Leg Cramps

Leg cramps are painful muscle contractions in the foot or leg and can mimic RLS. When they occur during sleep, there is a sudden awakening, and the pain can prevent a woman from returning to sleep. Nocturnal leg cramps increase in prevalence from 10% before pregnancy to 21% in the first, 57% in the second, and up to 75% in the third trimester.[1,71] Although mechanisms are unclear, leg cramps could be related to physiologic changes, including increased pressure on leg muscles, blood vessels, and nerves, or possibly an imbalance in nutrients. Risk factors may include exercise, electrolyte imbalances, salt depletion, renal dialysis, peripheral vascular disease, peripheral nerve injury, polyneuropathies, motor neuron disease, and certain drugs, including beta agonists and potassium-sparing diuretics.[79] There are only anecdotes and few studies on treatment to relieve or prevent nocturnal cramps. Interventions include hyperextension, massage, and reduction of phosphorous-containing substances, such as milk and meat.[1] Vitamin B was thought to be beneficial and is found in most perinatal vitamins. However, a systematic review of these treatments (magnesium, calcium, vitamin B, or vitamin C) involving 390 women did not suggest clear benefit.[79]

Nocturnal Gastroesophageal Reflux Disease

Gastroesophageal reflux disease (GERD) is a chronic disorder in which gastric contents enter the esophagus. GERD can worsen during pregnancy because of the additional abdominal weight and the anatomic and hormonal changes (Figure 186.1).[80] Nighttime symptoms include not only fragmented sleep but discomfort from injury to esophageal tissue caused by the acidic pH.[81] If reflux begins in pregnancy, the incidence typically peaks in late pregnancy and resolves after childbirth, when anatomy returns to normal. The incidence of GERD at

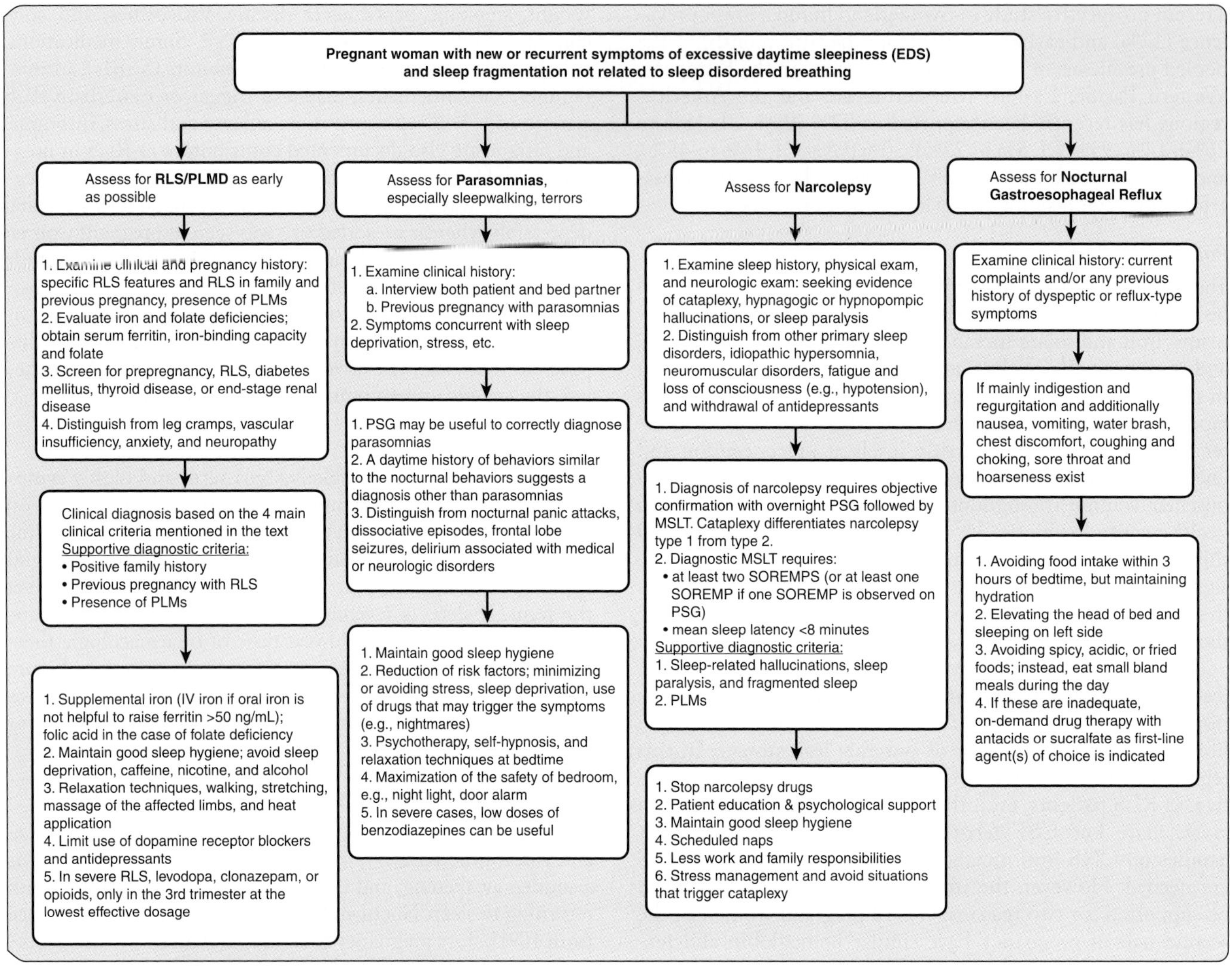

Figure 186.2 Management and treatment of non-sleep disordered breathing sleep-related disorders. IV, Intravenous; MSLT, Multiple Sleep Latency Test; PLMs, periodic leg movements; PLMD, periodic leg movement disorder; PSG, polysomnography; REM, rapid eye movement; RLS, restless legs syndrome; SOREMP, sleep-onset rapid eye movement sleep period.

any point in pregnancy ranges from 30% to 80%.[82] In a prospective longitudinal study, the prevalence of GERD symptoms doubled from 26% in the first trimester to 51% in the third trimester.[83] This is consistent with findings from another prospective study that showed 16.9% of GERD symptoms in the first, 25.3% in the second, and 51.2% in the third trimester, compared to 6.3% in nonpregnant women.[84] The pathophysiology of GERD in pregnancy may include elevated progesterone, with its inhibitory effect on smooth muscle[81,83]; repositioning of the stomach and intestinal tract as pregnancy progresses; increased intraabdominal pressure; and reduced esophageal sphincter pressure.[80]

Mild GERD symptoms can be managed with modifications to diet and lifestyle (Figure 186.2), such as no food within 3 hours of bedtime, smaller and more frequently meals, and sleeping upright or on the left side with head elevated.[67,81] Severe symptoms of GERD often are responsive to antacids, which have a low risk of harm to the fetus and have no documented adverse effects in animal studies.[80] Recently, a double-blind RCT on 100 symptomatic women showed comparable efficacy between alginate-based reflux suppressant and magnesium-aluminum antacid gel for treatment of heartburn at less than 36 weeks' gestation.[85] In a European prospective study of 553 cases of first-trimester exposure to histamine H_2 receptor antagonists (e.g., cimetidine) to treat GERD, a higher relative risk (RR) of preterm birth (8.9%) compared with control cases (5.6%) was noted, and two cases of neural tube defect in the offspring of women taking famotidine were reported.[86] H_2 receptor antagonists have low risk to the fetus, and although effective, may be best after the risk period of preterm birth (before 37 weeks).

Parasomnias during Pregnancy

Parasomnias in general populations are detailed in Chapters 115 to 120. No strong evidence supports increase in the incidence of parasomnias during pregnancy. In a longitudinal survey study of 325 women, sleep paralysis significantly increased in the second half of pregnancy (from 5.8% to 13.2%), but sleepwalking, sleeptalking, hypnagogic hallucinations, and sleep bruxism decreased in pregnancy compared to the 3 months preceding pregnancy.[87] Data on dreams and nightmares are inconsistent. Some reported increased frequency of dreams with gestational age,[88] although others noted that dream recall was equally prevalent among pregnant, postpartum, and nonpregnant women (88% to 91%).[89] Although comparable dream recall was found between women in their third trimester and nonpregnant women, pregnant women reported more disturbing dreams.[88] For example, 80% of new mothers reported particularly vivid, detailed, and disturbing dreams during pregnancy.[43] These dreams tend to involve anxiety about the infant and birth outcomes (especially in nulliparas), and often were accompanied by dream-associated behavior and confusional arousals.[89] When it comes to nightmares, one longitudinal survey showed that nightmares decreased from prepregnancy and throughout the three trimesters,[87] but another reported substantially higher incidence of moderately severe nightmares (more than one nightmare per week) among pregnant (21%) compared to nonpregnant (7%) women.[88]

Hormonal changes, fragmented sleep, and intense emotional stress may predispose pregnant women to frightening dreams, night terrors, or sleepwalking, especially in those with a genetic predisposition or previous history of parasomnia.[88,89] Cortisol levels may have a pivotal role in causation, with peaks occurring during the second half of the night, when REM sleep dominates and dream imagery and emotions are most intense.[6,7] Dreams and nightmares may be important indicators of the woman's psychological state. Parasomnia with complex, vigorous, or violent behavior are at risk for sleep-related injury and injury to the fetus. Data on treating parasomnias during pregnancy are scarce. In the general population, clonazepam is prescribed for some parasomnias, but due to its high risk for fetal harm, it is often discontinued during pregnancy.[90] In most cases no special treatment is necessary. Informing women about the likelihood of parasomnias, such as disturbing dreams, may reduce anxiety. Psychological and behavioral interventions should be considered (Figure 186.2 and Chapters 115 to 120).

Narcolepsy

Narcolepsy in the general population is detailed in Chapter 112. Differential diagnosis of narcolepsy during pregnancy may require consideration of pregnancy-related daytime sleepiness or vivid dreams. The prevalence of narcolepsy among pregnant women probably is similar to that in the nonpregnant population, but symptoms may be exacerbated or attenuated during pregnancy. In retrospective European cohort studies, women with narcolepsy symptoms before or during pregnancy tended to have a higher incidence of impaired glucose metabolism and anemia compared with asymptomatic women.[91,92] Reported rates of cesarean births were higher in women with narcolepsy-cataplexy than in women with narcolepsy and no cataplexy.[91] Cataplexy itself can be dangerous and stressful during pregnancy, and women may be concerned about their children inheriting narcolepsy. Women with narcolepsy are also prone to obesity, which may increase the risk of SDB and pregnancy complications.[92] In a recent animal study, an association between pregnancy and increased risk of maternal death was evident in the narcolepsy-cataplexy mice with complete hypocretin deficiency.[93]

Treatment of narcolepsy (see Chapter 112) is challenging in pregnant women. Most medications used in treating narcolepsy in nonpregnant populations should be used with caution, as human data are lacking to determine pregnancy risks.[94] Earlier studies reported prematurity, low birth weight, and withdrawal symptoms in infants of women taking amphetamines.[94,95] However, several large studies examining the use of methylphenidate or amphetamines for attention deficit hyperactivity disorder during pregnancy reported either no association or only a small association with a small increased RR of preeclampsia, preterm birth, congenital malformations, placental abruption, growth restriction (<1.5-fold) among exposed infants and mothers.[95] The safety of armodafinil and sodium oxybate in pregnancy awaits comprehensive human studies. However, a survey of 75 clinicians who treated narcolepsy during pregnancy found no evidence of teratogenicity with modafinil, sodium oxybate, methylphenidate, amphetamines, or SSRIs.[94]

In a retrospective study of 249 pregnant women with narcolepsy, symptoms did not change in 40%, worsened in 40%, and improved in 18% who withdrew from medication during the first trimester.[91,94] These types of studies are limited by recall bias and small numbers of pregnancies that occur in women taking antinarcolepsy medication.[86,90] A recent study of 123 women with narcolepsy who had previously been pregnant reported that one-third chose to discontinue therapy during pregnancy, whereas another third chose alternative management strategies, such as sleep extension and increased caffeine use.[96] No differences in fetal outcomes were observed between those who continued or discontinued pharmacotherapy. However, 37% of respondents indicated they had never received counseling about the risks of pharmacotherapy while pregnant, and 60% had not received counseling about contraceptive choices for women using narcolepsy pharmacotherapy.[96] On the basis of current evidence, medication as an option for managing narcolepsy should be carefully evaluated for conception and during pregnancy and prescribed only if potential benefit outweighs potential risk. If a woman requires medication during pregnancy or decides to continue medication while attempting to conceive, however, she can be reassured that evidence for considerable harm is lacking. With narcolepsy associated with cataplexy, an elective cesarean should be considered owing to the potential dangers for mother and newborn if a cataplexy episode occurs during labor.[94]

Patient education and psychological support are important for the woman and her family.[97] Good sleep hygiene and a supportive network are imperative to ensure adequate nocturnal sleep, adherence to scheduled daytime naps, and fewer role responsibilities. Behavioral interventions, including scheduled naps, stress management, and avoiding situations that trigger cataplexy are beneficial to decrease the risk of physical injury, as well as unpredictable sleepiness.

SLEEP DURING PREGNANCY WITH PREEXISTING MEDICAL AND PSYCHIATRIC CONDITIONS

Sleep in pregnant women with medical conditions, such as preeclampsia, affective disorders, asthma, and migraine headaches, has not been widely studied. These conditions may have a further impact on sleep during pregnancy. Studies using objective sleep measures report that women with gestational hypertension have impaired sleep quality and markedly altered sleep architecture, with significantly more SWS and less REM sleep.[98,99] These women also napped more frequently than healthy pregnant women.[99] In a large cohort study (n = 1332) during early pregnancy, women with a psychiatric diagnosis reported shorter sleep duration, increased frequency of exhaustion, and higher perceived stress levels compared with women without such diagnoses.[100] A systematic review of earlier studies also noted that sleep disturbance, fatigue, and stress were more frequent during pregnancy among women with anxiety disorders than among other pregnant women.[38] In a cross-sectional study of 1335 pregnant women, those with a history of asthma experienced more sleep disturbances and snoring than did nonasthmatic women.[101]

MATERNAL AND FETAL CONSEQUENCES OF EXTREME SLEEP DURATION AND POOR SLEEP QUALITY

Untreated sleep disorders or extremes of sleep duration (both short and long) are potential contributors to adverse health conditions in pregnancy, such as gestational diabetes mellitus, preeclampsia, fetal growth restriction, and preterm birth.[5,38,102] This section will discuss maternal and fetal outcomes associated with maternal sleep duration and sleep quality. Adverse outcomes associated with SDB are covered in Chapter 187.

Obesity or Excessive Weight Gain

Obesity affects two-thirds of reproductive-age women and is associated with pregnancy complications, such as gestational diabetes mellitus, hypertensive disorders, preterm birth, and stillbirth.[103] Although short and long sleep (≈<6 hours vs. ≈>9 hours) has been shown to be associated with weight gain and obesity in the nonpregnant population, there is limited evidence for a relationship between sleep duration and weight gain in pregnancy.[5,21,104]

Sleep loss associated with pregnancy discomforts may result in fatigue that leads to comfort eating, physical inactivity, and eventual obesity. Short sleep duration also allows additional time for food consumption and has been associated with an increase in gestational weight gain.[105] At the other end of the duration spectrum, data from a prospective, multicenter study of 1950 pregnant women found those who slept for more than or equal to 10 hours were nearly twice as likely to exceed the Institute of Medicine weight gain recommendations compared to women who reported less than 8 hours of sleep nightly.[106] Moreover, in a population-based cohort study of 710 pregnant women, sleeping less than 8 hours per day during the second or third trimester was found to be a risk for inadequate gestational weight gain.[107] Sleep disturbance may also lead to altered leptin levels and contribute to obesity. In a study of 830 women during early pregnancy, Qiu and colleagues[21] noted that short sleep (≤5 hours) and, to a lesser extent, long sleep (≥9 hours) were associated with elevated leptin levels if women were also overweight or obese. These data suggest that extremes of sleep duration have potential to play a role in weight management in pregnancy. Future studies should examine whether interventions to improve sleep hygiene have a positive impact on cardiometabolic measures. Optimizing weight before pregnancy and avoidance of excessive gestational weight gain may reduce the risk of developing sleep disorders and subsequent poor pregnancy outcomes.

Pregnancy-Induced Hypertension and Preeclampsia

Pregnancy-induced hypertension (PIH, gestational hypertension) is defined as repeated blood pressure recordings greater than 140/90 mm Hg, first diagnosed during pregnancy in a previously normotensive woman. Hypertensive disorders of pregnancy significantly increase the risk of maternal and perinatal morbidity; thus timely diagnosis and treatment are essential.[108] In a study of 161 pregnant women, longer SOL and WASO were associated with higher blood pressures after controlling for covariates, including BMI.[27] In a prospective cohort study of 1272 women, Williams and colleagues[51] found both short (<6 hours) and long (>9 hours) sleep durations in early pregnancy were associated with elevated mean blood pressure in the third trimester, with the highest risk of preeclampsia observed in women who slept less than 5 hours per night.[51] However, a study of more than 700 women using actigraphy did not support a link between short sleep, as defined as less than 7 hours with hypertension.[104]

Longitudinal studies of pregnant women indicate that poor sleep quality, fragmented sleep, and short sleep duration are associated with higher circulating inflammatory cytokines (interleukin [IL]-6, IL-8, and tumor necrosis factor) and C-reactive protein.[109] Nevertheless, given relatively small sample sizes and other limitations, these results should be interpreted with caution. The mechanisms of sleep disruption that affect cardiovascular morbidity in nonpregnant individuals are similar to the pathways for preeclampsia, with strong evidence for oxidative stress, inflammation, sympathetic nervous systemic activation, endothelial dysfunction, dyslipidemia, and obesity.[110]

Hyperglycemia and Gestational Diabetes Mellitus

Hyperglycemia (1-hour oral glucose tolerance test ≥140 mg/dL) can be detected at any time during pregnancy. Accumulating evidence links short sleep duration to risk of hyperglycemia,[104,111] but a causal relationship has not been established. Even mild hyperglycemia is associated with adverse maternal and fetal outcomes (i.e., preeclampsia, fetal growth restriction) and future development of type 2 diabetes mellitus, obesity, and cardiovascular disease in mother and child.[5] In a prospective cohort study of 1290 women before 20 weeks' gestation, women sleeping less than or equal to 4 hours per night had a fivefold increased (95% CI, 1.31 to 23.69) risk for gestational diabetes mellitus (GDM) compared to women sleeping 9 hours per night after adjusting for age and race; this association was, however, nonsignificant after adjusting for prepregnancy BMI.[112] A significant inverse relationship has been reported between sleep duration and 1-hour glucose values, with every 1 hour less sleep time linked to 4% increase in glucose levels; however, risk factors for GDM were not controlled.[113] Moreover, a prospective study of actigraphy in 782 pregnant women found that short sleep (<7 hours per night) and late sleep midpoint were associated with a twofold increased risk of GDM.[104]

A recent meta-analysis showed that extremes of sleep duration in early and midpregnancy were associated with GDM, although this association was only significant for long sleep (≥9 or ≥10 hours).[114] Another meta-analysis[111] that included an additional five manuscripts showed that short sleep was associated with a 1.7-fold increase in GDM; data from objective studies found that sleeping less than or equal to 6.25 hours per night was associated with a 2.84-fold increase in GDM. Further, sleeping more than 7 hours was not related to GDM; long sleep (e.g., >9 hours), was not examined.

Longer self-reported nap duration and severe daytime sleepiness have been associated with high glucose challenge test values.[115] Furthermore, a large study of more than 4000 women in China has provided evidence that poor sleep quality in early pregnancy predicts the development of GDM.[116]

Thus poor sleep may also have modulatory influences on glucose regulation, and improving sleep quality in early pregnancy may have clinical utility in reducing GDM risk.

Adverse Obstetric Outcomes

Short sleep duration in pregnancy can be considered a physiologic stressor, leading to longer labor and cesarean delivery.[38] In a prospective observational study of 131 nulliparas in their last month of pregnancy, those who slept less than 6 hours per night had a significantly longer labor duration and higher rate (4.5 times) of cesarean birth (controlling for infant birth weight) than nulliparas sleeping 7 hours or more by actigraphy measures.[117] A population-based study of 10,662 pregnant women supported these findings, indicating that short sleep in the last trimester is an independent risk factor for emergency cesarean birth (adjusted odds ratio [aOR], 1.57; 95% CI, 1.14 to 2.16).[118] These relationships between sleep and length of labor or type of delivery are also supported by a cross-sectional study of 457 pregnant women after excluding hypertension, gestational diabetes, or emergency cesarean, with poor sleep quality and sleeping less than 8 hours associated with longer labor and cesarean delivery.[119] Women with poor sleep, as identified by a Pittsburgh Sleep Quality Index (PSQI) score greater than 5, have been reported to be 20% more likely to have longer labor duration and to undergo cesarean delivery,[120] although another study suggested that cesarean delivery is associated with stress rather than sleep quality.[121] Daytime sleep may matter too. In a study of 120 women, longer daytime sleep duration was linked to shorter labor duration during vaginal delivery after controlling for maternal age but was not related to the risk of cesarean delivery.[122] More research is needed to investigate whether daytime naps can offset the risk of adverse obstetric outcomes associated with poor and short nocturnal sleep.

One mechanism for these adverse outcomes may be an increased perception of pain during labor. Beebe and colleagues[42] reported a greater pain perception being linked to shorter actigraphy sleep duration the night before hospitalization in women with spontaneous labor onset. Further, higher fatigue or increased stress during pregnancy may increase risk of cesarean birth.[121]

Fetal Complications

Maternal sleep is important for fetal growth because the secretion of growth hormone and uteroplacental blood flow are at their peak during sleep.[7,98] Fetal outcomes of maternal poor sleep are understudied, but most efforts have been focused on SDB (see Chapter 187). One challenge with studies of sleep duration is the inconsistency of a definition of short sleep, ranging from less than 4 hours to less than 8 hours per night, and that most studies used self-reported measures. In a case-control study of 734 pregnant women, those sleeping less than 8 hours per day were at high risk for first-trimester miscarriage (OR, 3.80; 95% CI, 1.01 to 14.3) or second-trimester miscarriage (OR, 2.04; 95% CI, 1.24 to 3.37).[123]

Findings on birth weight are mixed. Evaluation of birth weight data from over 1,000 singleton pregnancies did not demonstrate a statistically significant association between maternal short sleep (≤5 hours per night) and birth weight or prevalence of babies small for gestational age (SGA).[124] Similarly, Howe and colleagues[125] found no differences in birth weight or percentile in infants born to women reporting sleep less than 6 hours per night. However, other studies showed that both an SGA less than the 5th percentile and low birth weight are linked with sleeping less than 8 hours per night (OR, 2.2 and 2.8, respectively).[126,127] In a cohort study of more than 3500 women, compared to those sleeping 8 to 9 hours, women sleeping less than 7 hours in early pregnancy had infants with shorter birth length, by 2.4 mm, and a 42.7-g reduction in birth weight. The risk of low birth weight increased 83%, and the risk of SGA increased 56% in women sleeping less than 7 hours.[128] Similarly, a study of 176 Brazilian women found that first-trimester 24-hour sleep duration and its change throughout pregnancy were inversely associated with birth weight such that women with greater decreases in sleep duration gave birth to infants with lower birth weight Z-scores.[129] A meta-analysis suggests that findings are unclear in regard to whether short or long sleep duration impacts fetal growth, as the aORs for SGA and large for gestational age were 1.3 (95% CI, 0.9 to 2.0) and 1.5 (95% CI, 0.7 to 2.8), respectively.[102] However, it should be noted that the meta-analysis included both cross-sectional studies and longitudinal studies, all studies used subjective measures of sleep duration, and no consideration was given to daytime napping, environmental stressors, or racial differences.

Preterm Birth

A large prospective study found that short sleep (<5 hours) was associated with an increased risk of preterm birth (adjusted relative risk [aRR], 1.7, 95% CI, 1.1 to 2.8), and the highest risk was for medically indicated preterm birth (aRR, 2.4; 95% CI, 1.0 to 6.4).[124] Despite few studies, a tendency toward preterm birth has been suggested in women who sleep more than 10 hours per night compared to those sleeping 8 hours (aOR, 1.3; 95% CI, 0.9 to 1.9).[130] Overall, data from a meta-analysis suggests that short sleep duration is associated with preterm birth (aOR, 1.4; 95% CI, 1.0 to 2.1).[102]

Sleep quality also matters. In a study of 166 women, for every 1-point increase in PSQI score in early pregnancy, preterm birth increased by 25%.[131] Similarly, Blair and colleagues[132] reported that African-American women with poor sleep had a 10.2-fold increased risk of preterm birth compared with those with good sleep quality. IL-8 significantly mediated this association. The odds of preterm birth increased by 1.4 (95% CI, 1.2 to 1.6) with each unit increase in PSQI. In addition, shift work or jet lag has been associated with poorer fertility and early pregnancy loss via alterations in clock gene expression,[133] suggesting that circadian rhythm disruption may contribute to preterm birth.

Maternal Sleep and Stillbirth

Emerging data suggest that maternal sleep may play a role in stillbirth. It has long been recognized that posture in pregnancy has a profound impact on maternal hemodynamics, and pregnant women are often placed in a left lateral tilt position during labor and during cesarean section to avoid vena caval compression. Nonetheless, few people have extrapolated these practices beyond the delivery room. Data from several countries have shown that self-reported maternal supine going-to-sleep position is a significant risk factor for late-gestation stillbirth (at 28 weeks' gestation or longer). An individual patient data analysis that included five case-control studies demonstrated a 2.6-fold increased odds for supine sleep in women who experienced late stillbirth.[134] In the supine position, compression of the inferior vena cava occurs, with subsequent reduced blood flow and a reduction in cardiac output.[135] A cohort study of home sleep testing found no association between sleep position before 30 weeks' gestation and stillbirth,[136] which further suggests that it is the heavier gravid uterus later in the third trimester that conveys the risk. Maternal supine position appears to induce fetal quiescence,[137] an oxygen-conserving state observed during periods of fetal hypoxia, further evidence of biologic plausibility. Moreover, a small cross-sectional study suggested that maternal supine sleep was linked to a fivefold increase in low birth weight,[138] which was confirmed in a large individual patient data analysis of 1760 women that found a threefold increase in SGA outcomes.[139] Because most pregnant women spend at least some time in the supine position,[140] supine sleep is a potentially modifiable risk factor that could prevent up to 10% of late stillbirths.[141]

Other sleep behaviors, such as long sleep duration, non-restless sleep, and not waking in the night have also been associated with late stillbirth,[142] which raises the question of whether long periods of undisturbed sleep itncrease the risk of late fetal demise. Data are lacking on how the neuroendocrine and autonomic system pathways are regulated in pregnant women during sleep, and this is a fertile area for investigation.

EPIGENETICS AND FETAL OUTCOMES

The impact of maternal sleep on fetal health is a relatively new field, but it has been long known that the uterine environment can play a significant role in long-term health of the offspring (the Barker hypothesis)[143] via genetic, epigenetic, and environmental factors. Increasing evidence suggests that the epigenome is particularly susceptible to environmental exposures during the prenatal period, which can lead to long-term phenotypic alterations in the offspring.[144] Few studies have investigated maternal sleep as an environmental exposure, but evidence is emerging that epigenetic alterations occur after sleep deprivation.[145] Of particular relevance, animal studies suggest that epigenetic alterations appear to underlie increases in the susceptibility to obesity and metabolic dysfunction in the offspring of rats exposed to sleep fragmentation[146] and intermittent hypoxia.[147] The epigenetics of maternal sleep disruption is clearly a critical area for future investigation. In the future, alterations to the epigenome could be used as biomarkers of sleep loss or as therapeutic targets for sleep disorders.

MATERNAL PSYCHOSOCIAL CONSEQUENCES

Accumulated sleep loss, regardless of the cause during pregnancy, affects level of energy, mood, interpersonal functioning, concentration, and memory. As mentioned earlier, insufficient sleep may even trigger depression.[38] When sleep is measured using self-report, poor and short sleep during pregnancy is both concurrently and prospectively associated with worse mood and mental health. For example, in a population-based survey of more than 2800 women, depressive symptoms were strongly associated with insomnia during late pregnancy, especially when sleep duration was less than 5 or more than 10 hours, when SE was less than 75%, or when SOL was prolonged.[53] Poorer self-reported sleep quality during early pregnancy also predicted depressive symptoms in late pregnancy.[148] A prospective study on nearly 1400 women showed that poorer and shorter sleep in the third trimester was associated with higher depressive symptoms 3 months postpartum.[148] When sleep is measured using objective methods, however, the sleep-mood relationship is more mixed.[149] It is possible that sleep disturbance is a universal experience during pregnancy and that women's perception of sleep problems and their associated impact, rather than the disruption per se, plays a more important role in how sleep disruption affects their mental health and daytime functioning.

It is worth noting that the days leading up to childbirth and labor itself are usually associated with partial, sometimes total, sleep deprivation.[150] In vulnerable women, such as those with a history of bipolar disorder, this period of acute sleep deprivation could trigger episodes of severe psychiatric conditions, such as mania and postpartum psychosis.[52] Persistent sleep loss also is likely to interfere with the pregnant woman's ability to work efficiently, as a result of fatigue and sleepiness, especially by the third trimester.[29] In consequence, rates of absenteeism from the workplace may increase, and risk for accidents is higher at work and on the highway. Thus good sleep is essential to optimal maternal physical functioning and mental health. Early intervention to promote sleep may improve health outcomes for both mother and infant.

CLINICAL PEARLS

Sleep disturbance is common during pregnancy, and emerging evidence indicates a link between sleep disturbances and pregnancy complications. However, a clinical sleep assessment has not been part of routine prenatal care. Associations between sleep disturbance and pregnancy complications, the diagnosis and management of sleep disorders during pregnancy, cost-benefit analysis, and long-term benefits of treating sleep disorders during pregnancy have not been well studied. Future research focusing on understanding the biologic mechanisms of these associations and examining the impact of sleep-targeted interventions on perinatal outcomes are required to clarify these issues.

Recognition, management, and treatment of sleep disorders are beneficial for improving short- and long-term maternal and fetal health outcomes. Preferably, the obstetric clinician and the sleep specialist should communicate and share their clinical assessments and test results in an effort to prepare a successful management plan for pregnant women at risk. Clinical management of sleep disturbances during pregnancy should include education to inform women about the importance of sleep, the value of nonpharmacologic options as first-line therapeutic interventions, and the likely temporary nature of the disturbance during pregnancy. Women with a preexisting sleep disorder should be advised to take added precautions during pregnancy to maintain the health and well-being of both mother and fetus.

SUMMARY

Physical and hormonal changes during pregnancy can cause sleep disturbances and predispose women to develop a temporary sleep disorder, such as RLS, GERD, or SDB, or may worsen a preexisting disorder. These disorders are associated with adverse maternal and fetal outcomes. Although the many studies did not describe a temporal relationship between sleep disturbances and the development of adverse pregnancy outcomes, emerging evidence suggests that addressing sleep practices and treatment of sleep disorders both before and during pregnancy are critically important for optimal pregnancy outcomes. Large longitudinal studies are needed to examine prevalence and prospectively identify the gestational time frame for onset of a sleep disorder, to examine the dose-response relationship between severity of a sleep disorder and subsequent pregnancy complications, and to test interventions for these sleep disorders. Most important, validated screening tools to identify sleep characteristics and disturbances specific to pregnancy are needed.

ACKNOWLEDGMENT

We would like to thank Dr. Francesca Facco for providing helpful input regarding medication use for sleep disorders in pregnancy.

SELECTED READINGS

Cronin RS, Li M, Thompson JMD, et al. An individual participant data meta-analysis of maternal going-to-sleep position, interactions with fetal vulnerability, and the risk of late stillbirth. *E Clin Med.* 2019;10:49–57.

Facco FL, Kramer J, Ho KH, et al. Sleep disturbances in pregnancy. *Obstet Gynecol.* 2010;115(1):77–83.

Izci-Balserak B, Keenan BT, Corbitt C, et al. Changes in sleep characteristics and breathing parameters during sleep in early and late pregnancy. *J Clin Sleep Med.* 2018;14(7):1161–1168.

Ladyman C, Signal TL. Sleep health in pregnancy: a scoping review. *Sleep Med Clin.* 2018;13(3):307–333.

Lee KA, Zaffke ME, McEnany G. Parity and sleep patterns during and after pregnancy. *Obstet Gynecol.* 2000;95(1):14–18.

Lu Q, Zhang X, Wang Y, et al. Sleep disturbances during pregnancy and adverse maternal and fetal outcomes: a systematic review and meta-analysis. *Sleep Med Rev.* 2021;58:101436.

Manber R, Bei B, Simpson N, et al. Cognitive behavioral therapy for prenatal insomnia: a randomized controlled trial. *Obstet Gynecol.* 2019;133(5):911–919.

Miller MA, Mehta N, Clark-Bilodeau C, Bourjeily G, et al. Sleep pharmacotherapy for common sleep disorders in pregnancy and lactation. *Chest.* 2020;157(1):184–197.

O'Brien LM, Dunietz GL. Sleep in pregnancy. In: Duncan DT, Kawachi I, Redline S, eds. *The Social Epidemiology of Sleep.* Oxford University Press; 2019.

Picchietti DL, Hensley JG, Bainbridge JL, et al. Consensus clinical practice guidelines for the diagnosis and treatment of restless legs syndrome/Willis-Ekbom disease during pregnancy and lactation. *Sleep Med Rev.* 2014;22:64–77.

Reutrakul S, Anothaisintawee T, Herring SJ, Balserak BI, Marc I, Thakkinstian A, et al. Short sleep duration and hyperglycemia in pregnancy: aggregate and individual patient data meta-analysis. *Sleep Med Rev.* 2018;40:31–42.

Tsai SY, Lee PL, Lin JW, et al. Persistent and new-onset daytime sleepiness in pregnant women: a prospective observational cohort study. *Int J Nurs Stud.* 2017;66:1–6.

Warland J, Dorrian J, Morrison J, et al. Maternal sleep during pregnancy and poor fetal outcomes: a scoping review of the literature with meta-analysis. *Sleep Med Rev.* 2018;41:197–219.

Wilson DL, Fung A, Walker SP, et al. Subjective reports versus objective measurement of sleep latency and sleep duration in pregnancy. *Behav Sleep Med.* 2013;11(3):207–221.

A complete reference list can be found online at ExpertConsult.com.

Chapter 187

Sleep-Disordered Breathing in Pregnancy

Francesca Facco; Judette Louis; Melissa P. Knauert; Bilgay Izci Balserak

Chapter Highlights

- Pregnant women may be particularly predisposed to obstructive sleep apnea and other sleep-related breathing disorders due to the physiologic changes associated with the gravid state. In fact, sleep-disordered breathing (SDB) symptoms are common during pregnancy and worsen as the pregnancy progresses.
- In addition, outcomes that have been linked to SDB in the nonpregnant population, such as hypertension and insulin-resistant diabetes mellitus, have counterparts in pregnancy (e.g., gestational hypertension, preeclampsia, gestational diabetes mellitus).
- This chapter reviews several aspects of SDB, including its epidemiology, physiologic underpinnings, possible link to adverse pregnancy outcomes, and special considerations for screening and treatment in pregnancy.

PREGNANCY PHYSIOLOGY AND SLEEP-DISORDERED BREATHING

As reviewed in detail in Chapter 186, pregnancy is accompanied by alterations in physiology secondary to hormonal, mechanical, and circulatory changes characteristic of the gravid state. A clinician who examines a pregnant woman for potential sleep-disordered breathing (SDB) needs to be familiar with these pregnancy-related alterations; although some changes are risk factors to SDB, others may protect from it.

Respiratory System Changes That May Contribute to Sleep-Disordered Breathing

Multiple mechanisms lead to anatomic narrowing and/or increased resistance within the respiratory system during pregnancy. Increased levels of estrogen and progesterone induce capillary engorgement, hypersecretion, and mucosal edema of the upper airway.[1–3] These changes begin early in the first trimester and increase progressively throughout pregnancy. They may lead to a reduction in dimensions of the nasopharynx, oropharynx, and larynx with increased airflow resistance and an increase in the Mallampati score as pregnancy progresses.[3–6]

Furthermore, pregnancy rhinitis is nasal congestion of pregnancy without other signs of respiratory tract infection and with no known allergic cause.[3] This rhinitis results in difficulty breathing and resolves within 2 weeks after delivery. It occurs in up to 40% of women by the third trimester of pregnancy.[1,3,7] Increased nasal congestion may also cause increased nasopharyngeal resistance and produce more intrapharyngeal pressure during inspiration. Elevated intrapharyngeal pressure during inspiration contributes to pharyngeal airway narrowing,[8] which results in snoring, inspiratory flow limitation, and obstructed breathing during sleep.[9,10] Thus pregnant women are more likely to snore compared to nonpregnant women, and the prevalence of habitual snoring (≥3 nights/week) increases from the first to the third trimester of pregnancy.[5,11,12]

Increased fat deposition within the soft tissue regions of a woman's neck could also cause pharyngeal narrowing and predispose to snoring and SDB.[5,9,12,13] Pregnant women with a larger neck circumference during pregnancy and a higher baseline body mass index (BMI) report more symptoms of SDB than others.[4,5,14]

In addition, maternal blood volume peaks at a value 40% to 50% greater than prepregnancy by the third trimester.[15] The combination of increased blood volume, interstitial fluid, and recumbency during sleep result in displacement of fluid to a degree that could adversely affect upper airway patency.[2,3,15] Evidence also suggests that an increased tongue size relative to the oral cavity may lead to upper airway obstruction, possibly owing to fluid retention in the neck and tongue during pregnancy.[6,16] However, evidence regarding the nocturnal displacement of the fluid is conflicting. Although some studies indicated that nocturnal fluid shifting from the legs into the neck increases susceptibility or severity of pharyngeal obstruction,[17] other studies reported that such rostral fluid shifts do not increase the frequency of obstructed breathing events.[18]

A compensatory increase in the anterior–posterior and mediolateral diameters of the chest[19] and elevation of the diaphragm caused by the enlarging uterus result in tracheal shortening and progressive reductions in functional residual capacity by 20% to 25%, expiratory reserve volume by 15% to 20%, and residual volume by 22%, whereas oxygen consumption increases by 20%.[2,20] These alterations can lead to the closure of small airways during normal tidal breathing.[4,5,21] In late pregnancy, airway closure results in ventilation perfusion mismatch and reduced gas exchange,[22–24] especially in the supine position, due to gravity, intraabdominal pressure, and loss of muscle tone during sleep.[2,4,21,25]

During pregnancy, tidal volume and minute ventilation progressively increase by 40% and by 30% to 50%, respectively, as a result of respiratory stimulation by progesterone.[2,15,19] The elevated ventilatory drive of pregnancy may induce obstructive respiratory events by increasing diaphragmatic effort, which leads to negative inspiratory (suction) pressures on the hyperemic upper airway.[8] Furthermore, increased ventilatory drive, along with resultant respiratory alkalosis, may cause instability in respiratory control (loop gain) pathways, potentially increasing the likelihood of episodes of central apnea at sleep onset and during non–rapid eye movement sleep.[2,25,26] However, a recent study suggests that pregnancy does not increase the susceptibility to central apnea.[27]

Respiratory and Circulatory System Changes That May Protect against Sleep-Disordered Breathing

Several mechanisms of respiratory and cardiovascular change may lesson risk or the severity of apnea and hypopnea episodes. High levels of circulating progesterone during pregnancy may protect the upper airway from obstruction by increasing upper airway dilator muscle (genioglossal) activity and its responsiveness to chemical stimuli (carbon dioxide) during sleep.[28] Pregnancy-related increases in heart rate, stroke volume, and cardiac output with reductions in peripheral vascular tone may diminish the impact of apneic episodes.[28] Furthermore, as pregnancy advances, women tend to spend less time in the supine position during sleep.[29,30] This may decrease the rate of adverse respiratory events during sleep as the supine position is frequently associated with increased event rates.[31] However, O'Brein and colleagues[32] reported that greater than 80% of women spend some time sleeping in the supine position in the second and third trimesters of pregnancy.

EPIDEMIOLOGY OF SLEEP-DISORDERED BREATHING IN PREGNANCY

General population studies have estimated that SDB, most commonly obstructive sleep apnea (OSA), occurs in 2% to 25% of middle-aged adults in the community, but there are certain populations who are at greater risk.[33,34] For example, SDB may occur as much as 40% in obese and 70% to 90% of morbidly obese individuals.[35–37] In the general population of reproductive-aged women, epidemiologic studies suggest a 2% to 13% prevalence of SDB, but rates may be higher depending on the study population[37,38] and specifically within those seeking treatment. For example, among 420 premenopausal women referred for polysomnography (PSG) for sleep-related complaints, SDB was present in 70% of women younger than 30 years and in 83% of women older than 30 years. The younger group had less severe SDB (mean apnea-hypopnea index [AHI], 15.5 ± 22) than the older group (22.4 ± 34.6).[39]

During pregnancy, SDB is common and often worsens as pregnancy progresses.[31,40–42] Frequent snoring during pregnancy has been well characterized, and studies have consistently demonstrated that SDB symptoms, including snoring, increase as pregnancy progresses.[11,43,44] In general obstetric populations, the prevalence of prepregnancy or early pregnancy frequent snoring has been reported to be around 7% to 11%.[11,43,44] In the third trimester the frequency of snoring is increased, with reports ranging from 16% to 25%.[11,43–45] Using the Apnea Symptom Score from the Multivariable Apnea Prediction Index, one study found that symptoms of SDB increased significantly from the first trimester to the month of delivery; in addition, the increase in symptoms was not limited to snoring but included gasping, chocking, difficulty breathing, and apneic events.[31] In this study, 11.4% of subjects reported an increase in Apnea Symptom Score of 2 units or more, consistent with a clinically significant increase in symptoms; these women also experienced a significantly greater increase in subjective sleepiness than other subjects.[31]

Recent epidemiologic data based on objective sleep testing has provided better estimates on the prevalence and incidence of SDB in pregnancy. Olivarez and colleagues[46] performed sleep studies on 100 hospitalized pregnant women, admitted for a variety of obstetric and nonobstetric medical complications. The mean gestational age at the time of the sleep study was 32 weeks, and they reported a 20% incidence of SDB (AHI ≥ 5) with a mean AHI of 12.2.[46] When another group evaluated 175 obese pregnant women at 21 weeks' gestation with ambulatory sleep assessments, SDB prevalence was 15.4%.[47] The majority of cases were mild (AHI between 5 and 14.9), and the median AHI was 12.9.

Other studies have examined changes in SDB across pregnancy through serial assessments.[12,14,48–50] Pien and colleagues[49] studied 105 subjects, specifically recruiting 28% normal-weight, 24% overweight, and 50% obese subjects. SDB was present in 10.5% of women in the first trimester (median, 12.1 weeks). By the third trimester (median, 33.6 weeks), 26.7% of women had SDB. Women with third-trimester OSA were mostly obese (BMI ≥ 30) at baseline: Twenty of 50 (40.0%) obese women at baseline assessment had third-trimester OSA versus 8 of 55 (14.5%) normal or overweight women. Facco and colleagues[48] evaluated 128 high-risk pregnant women who had one or more of the following risk factors: obesity, chronic hypertension, presentational diabetes mellitus, prior preeclampsia, or twin gestation. Early-pregnancy SDB assessments were performed between 6 to 20 weeks' gestation (mean, 17 weeks), and late-pregnancy SDB assessments were performed between 28 to 37 weeks' gestation (mean, 33 weeks). In early pregnancy, the frequency of mild, moderate, and severe SDB was 12%, 6%, and 3%, respectively. These frequencies increased to 35%, 7%, and 5%, respectively, in late pregnancy. Twenty-seven percent of women (34/128) experienced a worsening of SDB during pregnancy, 20% (26/128) experienced new-onset SDB, whereas the other 6.25% (8/128) had SDB in early pregnancy that worsened in severity in late pregnancy.[48] Among the new-onset SDB, the majority were mild.[48]

The generalizability of the aforementioned studies is limited, as they studied high-risk populations. In contrast, Sleep-Disordered Breathing substudy of the Nulliparous Pregnancy Outcomes: Monitoring Mothers-to-Be (nuMoM2b) study, the largest epidemiologic study of objectively measured SDB in pregnancy to date, enrolled a group of demographically and geographically diverse nulliparous women. Participants in the nuMoM2b SDB substudy underwent in-home sleep apnea testing using a six-channel monitor that was self-applied by the participant for a single night at two time points: early pregnancy at 6 to 15 weeks of gestation and midpregnancy at 22 to 31 weeks.[6] More than 3700 women were enrolled, with 3264 having a valid sleep study in early pregnancy, 2512 in midpregnancy, and 2337 at both time points. SDB was found in 3.5 % of women in early pregnancy and increased to 8.2% in midpregnancy, with 5.2% of participants having new-onset SDB in midpregnancy. AHI distributions in early and mid-pregnancy are presented in Figure 187.1. In both early and midpregnancy, the majority of SDB cases were mild (5 ≤ AHI < 15). In women with SDB, the vast majority of apneic events were obstructive (Appendix 4 in[12]), indicating that almost all women identified as having SDB had OSA.

Risk factors for SDB in pregnancy include self-reported snoring, higher BMI, older age, and the presence of chronic hypertension, all of which are well-known risk factors for SDB outside of pregnancy.[14,48,49] Excessive gestational weight gain is theorized to be a risk factor for developing new-onset SDB in pregnancy, but epidemiologic data supporting this relationship are lacking at this time. Facco and colleagues[48] reported that carrying a twin gestation is associated with an increase in the risk of developing new-onset SDB in pregnancy. Although the twin pregnancies in this cohort, as expected, had greater maternal weight gain, in the cohort overall, weight gain did not differ significantly between women who developed new-onset SDB versus those who did not. Similarly, Pien and colleagues[49] reported that gestational weight gain was not associated with, or predictive of, third-trimester SDB. The nuMoM2b SDB study did report slightly increased rates of early-pregnancy weight gain among women found to have SDB; it was notable that pregnancy BMI and not pregnancy weight gain was predictive of prevalent and new-onset SDB.[14] Consistent with prior studies, the nuMoM2b SDB study found that frequent snoring, chronic hypertension, greater maternal age, and larger neck circumference were associated with an increased risk of SDB in pregnancy.

SLEEP-DISORDERED BREATHING AND ADVERSE PREGNANCY OUTCOMES

There is considerable heterogeneity in the definition of SDB among the studies examining SDB and pregnancy outcomes. In some of the largest cohorts, SDB was defined based on symptoms such as self-reported habitual snoring. The method of symptom assessments also varied, with some using interviews and others using questionnaires. Among the studies using objective testing, various laboratory and portable PSG assessments have been used, with varying AHI criteria for establishing a SDB diagnosis using prospective-longitudinal and cross-sectional methods. These differences between studies lead to difficulty in summarizing findings and their significance.

Potential Mechanisms for Adverse Maternal Outcomes

The underlying mechanisms linking sleep disturbances and adverse outcomes for the mother are likely multifactorial.[51,52] Dysregulation of pregnancy adaptations to the cardiovascular, metabolic, and immune systems can make women vulnerable to pregnancy complications.[52,53] Changes in sleep parameters, including even subtle obstructive respiratory events, could exacerbate these adaptations and increase the risk for adverse outcomes. SDB causes oxidative stress, autonomic

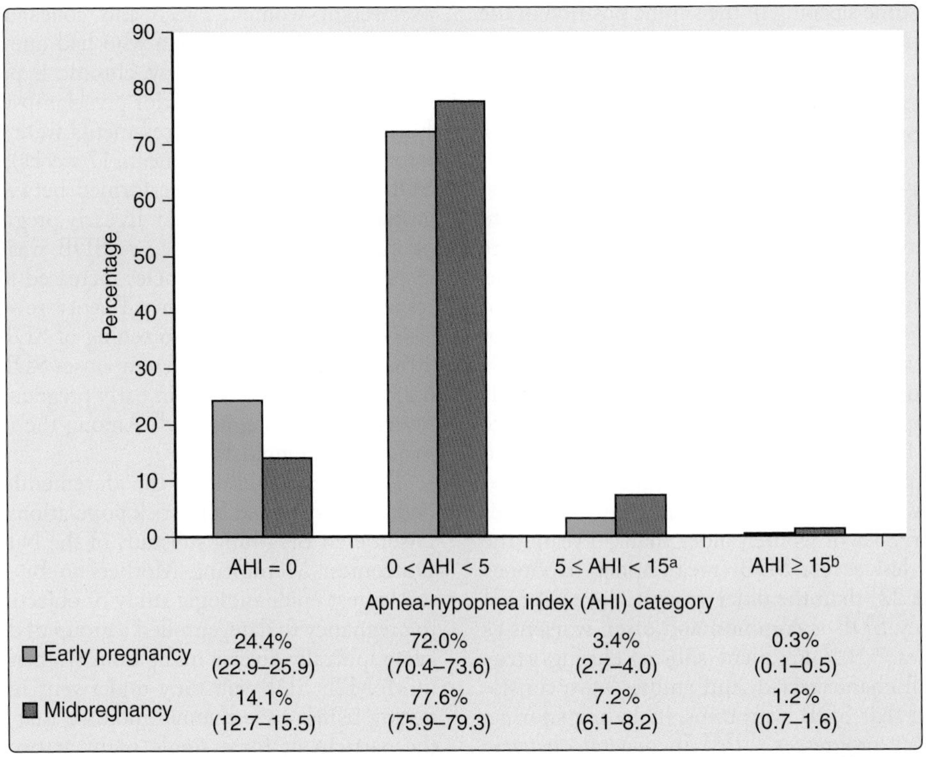

Figure 187.1 The distributions of women by apnea-hypopnea index (AHI) category in early and midpregnancy are presented, giving point estimate (95% confidence interval). [a]Mild sleep-disordered breathing; [b]Moderate or severe sleep-disordered breathing. (From Facco FL, Parker CB, Reddy UM, et al. Association between sleep-disordered breathing and hypertensive disorders of pregnancy and gestational diabetes mellitus. *Obstet Gynecol.* 2017;129(1):31–41.)

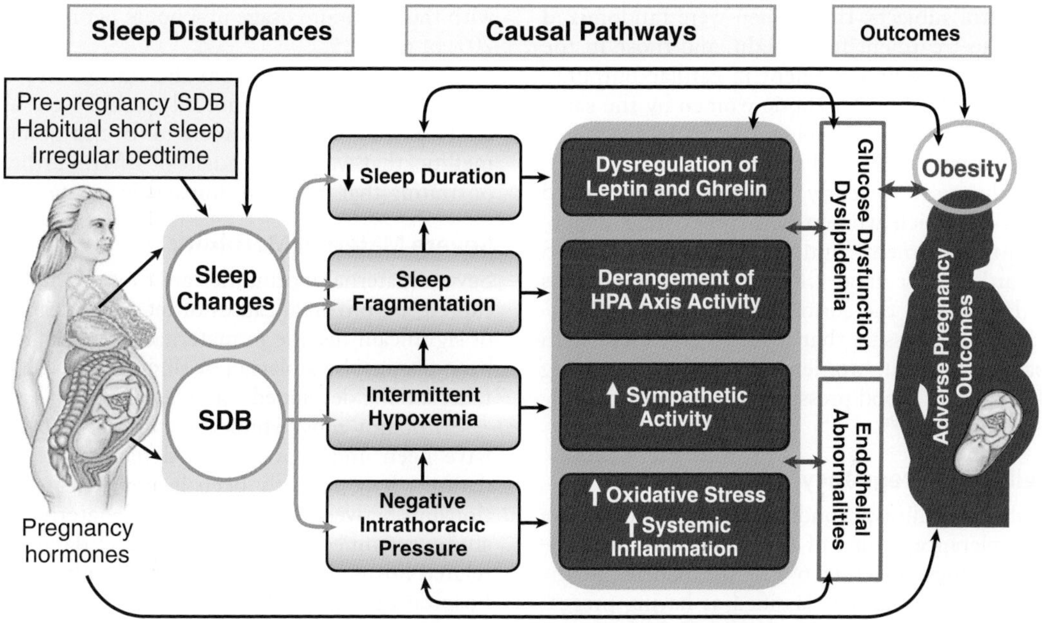

Figure 187.2 Schematic illustration of potential causal pathways linking sleep disturbances during pregnancy with adverse pregnancy outcomes. HPA, Hypothalamic-pituitary-adrenal; SDB, sleep-disordered breathing.

dysfunction, inflammation, and altered hormonal regulation of energy expenditure.[54] These same pathways are associated with adverse pregnancy outcomes.[55,56] Figure 187.2 is a conceptual model depicting potential pathways linking SDB and pregnancy complications.

Oxidative stress, a consequence of intermittent hypoxia-reoxygenation cycles in SDB, plays a pivotal role in development of hypertensive disorders of pregnancy, inducing proinflammatory cytokines that trigger further oxidative stress, sympathetic activation, and endothelial dysfunction.[56,57] Increased oxidative stress is also linked to development of gestational diabetes mellitus and preeclampsia.[58–60] Both animal and human studies observed that gestational exposure to intermittent hypoxia was associated with increased pancreatic beta cell proliferation, fetoplacental hypoxia, impaired fetal growth, hyperlipidemia, and epigenetic changes in offsprings.[61–64]

SDB-related sleep fragmentation could lead to increased sympathetic nervous system activity and derangement of hypothalamic-pituitary axis activity (e.g., blunted cortisol awakening response).[65–68] Disproportionate sympathetic activation then persists into the daytime, leading to increased peripheral vascular reactivity and catecholamine production, blunted baroreflex sensitivity, insulin sensitivity, and altered hepatic glucose release.[56,68,69] All these downstream SDB effects have been linked to processes seen in preeclampsia: endothelial dysfunction, elevated systemic arterial blood pressure, and decreased cardiac output.[70] SDB has also been strongly linked to systemic inflammation, including elevated interleukin (IL)-6, IL-8, tumor necrosis factor-α, C-reactive protein levels, and leukocyte counts.[56,71,72] Increased inflammation in early pregnancy is associated with adverse outcomes, particularly preeclampsia, gestational diabetes mellitus, and preterm birth.[55,73–75]

Slow wave sleep (N3) is disrupted as a consequence of SDB, which may also be a mechanism for adverse pregnancy outcomes.[76] Experimental studies of healthy subjects have demonstrated that disruption of N3 sleep can adversely alter insulin and glucose metabolism, sympathovagal balance, and cortisol.[76–78] Sleep loss and intermittent hypoxia have also been reported to induce changes in leptin and ghrelin hormones, which regulate appetite, satiety, and energy metabolism.[79–82] Evidence suggests that dysregulation of leptin and ghrelin may contribute to the pathophysiology of gestational diabetes mellitus and preeclampsia.[83,84]

Hypertensive Disorders of Pregnancy

Hypertensive disease complicates 5% to 10% of all pregnancies and remains one of the most proximate causes of perinatal morbidity and mortality.[85] Hypertension disorders of pregnancy are classified into subtypes according to clinical features: gestational hypertension, preeclampsia/eclampsia, and preeclampsia superimposed on chronic hypertension.[86] The risk factors for hypertensive disease include obesity and increased maternal age, which overlaps with some of the risk factors for SDB. This overlap makes it difficult to investigate the potential links between the diseases. However, a substantial body of evidence suggests a link between SDB and pregnancy-related hypertension, with most studies demonstrating a twofold increase in odds of gestational hypertension and preeclampsia in association with SDB.[43,47,87,88] In a large prospective study of 3306 women who underwent home testing for sleep apnea, women with sleep apnea in either early pregnancy (adjusted OR [aOR], 1.94; 95% confidence interval [CI], 1.07 to 3.51) or midpregnancy (aOR, 1.95; 95% CI, 1.18 to 3.23) were more likely to develop preeclampsia.[12] This relationship has been observed in other smaller epidemiologic and cohort studies.[87,89] However, some other studies have not been able to confirm this finding.[49,90,91]

To date, studies examining the effect of continuous positive airway pressure (CPAP) treatment of hypertension in pregnancy have been very limited in terms of sample sizes, duration of use, and in the scope of end points.[69,92–94] In the largest study, 24 women with severe preeclampsia had decrements in stroke volume and cardiac output compared with normal control subjects; the women were randomized to CPAP versus no treatment for 1 night, and those in the CPAP group showed an improvement in cardiac output.[69] In a different study of 10 preeclamptic women by the same authors, nasal CPAP was shown to increase fetal movements in patients studied with PSG and continuous ultrasound.[92] Poyares and colleagues[94] recently reported a randomized controlled study in which women with preexisting hypertension (receiving treatment) and snoring were allocated to either standard care or nasal CPAP in the first 8 weeks of pregnancy. Patients in the control group had a progressive increase in blood pressure that required treatment with α-methyldopa. In contrast, women allocated to receiving CPAP had decreases in blood pressure and in doses of antihypertensive medications.[94]

Diabetes Mellitus in Pregnancy

Gestational diabetes mellitus, a condition in women who have carbohydrate intolerance, is one of the most common complications of pregnancy, affecting 6% of pregnancies in the United States.[95] Women can be classified as having pregestational diabetes mellitus (i.e., having the disease before pregnancy) or gestational diabetes mellitus (i.e., disease diagnosed during pregnancy).[85] The incidence of diabetes mellitus–complicated pregnancies has increased in recent years in a manner parallel to the increase in maternal obesity.[96] Recognized complications of diabetes mellitus include gestational hypertension, preterm birth, malformations, fatal macrosomia, fetal growth restriction, stillbirth, and perinatal death.[90]

The studies that have examined the correlation between SDB and gestational diabetes mellitus have examined it both as an outcome and as a predictor. The relationship between SDB and insulin resistance/diabetes mellitus in the general population is well established and bidirectional. Although a causal link has not been proven, SDB is prevalent among patients with diabetes mellitus and is reported to precede the onset of diabetes.[97] Further, improved glucose control has been observed after initiating treatment of SDB with CPAP in the nonpregnant population.[97] Independent of other risk factors, individuals with SDB have an increased risk of developing type II diabetes mellitus, hyperinsulinemia, and metabolic syndrome (see Chapter 136). A systematic review of five observational studies (four assessed SDB via questionnaire, one via PSG) noted that pregnant women with SDB were at an increased risk of developing gestational diabetes mellitus (aOR, 1.86; 95% CI, 1.30 to 2.42).[91] This relationship was confirmed in a large prospective study: Among the participants of the nuMoM2b SDB study, SDB in early and midpregnancy was associated with gestational diabetes mellitus (early-pregnancy SDB: aOR, 3.47; 95% CI, 1.95 to 6.19 and midpregnancy SDB: aOR, 2.79; 95% CI, 1.63 to 4.77).[12] There is also some indication of a dose-response relationship: A prospective study using longitudinal, objective assessment of SDB demonstrated higher rates of gestational diabetes mellitus with increasing SDB severity; among women with no SDB, mild SDB, and moderate/severe SDB, the rates were 25%, 43%, and 63%, respectively.[90]

Intervention studies have shown limited effectiveness of SDB treatment in the management of gestational diabetes mellitus, possibly due to low compliance.[98] In a trial of CPAP versus no CPAP for 2 weeks in women with gestational diabetes mellitus, of the 15 women on CPAP, only 7 were adherent with the minimum usage of 4 hours per night for greater than 70% of nights.[98]

Conclusions drawn from the sum of this data must take into consideration that not all studies were able to demonstrate a relationship between SDB and gestational diabetes mellitus that was independent of BMI. Further, studies demonstrating that treatment impacts outcome are lacking.

Severe Maternal Morbidity

Severe maternal morbidities are those events that, if uninterrupted, are proximal causes of maternal death. After a period of significant decline in maternal mortality, recent years have been plagued by a plateau or slight increase in maternal mortality among developed countries.[99]

Although most studies regarding SDB and pregnancy have been underpowered to detect severe morbidity, large datasets have recently been leveraged to examine the relationship between SDB and severe maternal morbidity. One study examined data from a large database of delivery-related hospital discharges. In that study, among 55,781,965 hospital discharges, OSA was associated with an increased risk of in-hospital death (aOR, 5.28; 95% CI, 2.42 to 11.53), pulmonary embolism (aOR, 4.47; 95% CI, 2.25 to 8.88), and cardiomyopathy (aOR, 9.01; 95% CI, 7.47 to 10.87).[87] These relationships persisted and were exacerbated in the presence of obesity.

In another study, data from the Perinatal Center Database were used to identify women who had a delivery discharge from 2010 to 2014 at 95 different US hospitals. Among the 1,577,632 deliveries, 1963 women (0.12%) had a diagnosis code of OSA. A diagnosis of OSA was associated with cardiomyopathy (aOR, 3.59; 95% CI, 2.31 to 5.58), congestive heart failure (aOR, 3.63; 95% CI, 2.33 to 5.66), pulmonary edema (aOR, 5.06; 95% CI, 2.29 to 11.1), and maternal intensive care unit admission (aOR, 2.74; 95% CI, 2.36 to 3.18) in analyses adjusted for multiple covariates, including obesity, demographics, and maternal chronic medical conditions.[100]

Cesarean Delivery

In a large cohort study, women with pregnancies affected by snoring were more likely to undergo cesarean delivery, including both elective (OR, 2.25; 95% CI, 1.22 to 4.18) and emergency (OR, 1.68; 95% CI, 1.22 to 2.30) cesarean delivery.[101] This relationship has also been reported by other smaller observational studies that have used both symptom-based and PSG diagnosis of SDB.[45,47,88] Although the SDB-related causes for increased rates of cesarean delivery is not currently clear, it is postulated to be related to the high comorbidity of SDB with obesity, hypertension, and diabetes mellitus. These conditions increase the rate of pregnancy complications and induction of labor, which in turn can result in an increased rate of caesarean delivery.

Fetal and Infant Effects

To date, the potential effect of SDB on the fetus has received limited attention. Fetal effects may be exerted directly or indirectly by exacerbation of the underlying comorbid conditions that often track with SDB. Initial reports of fetal effects came from case reports in which fetal growth restriction and fetal heart rate decelerations were reported in pregnant women with SDB.[102] However, in many of those cases, confounding conditions such as hypertensive disease and diabetes mellitus coexisted, and therefore the association could not be assumed. More recent studies have attempted to examine that relationship more closely.

Fetal Mortality

Fetal mortality is the intrauterine death of any fetus at any gestational age. Fetal death at or beyond 20 weeks' gestation has been termed *stillbirth*.[85] There are limited studies examining the role of SDB in stillbirth. Recognized risk factors for stillbirth overlap with SDB risk factors and include advanced maternal age, African-American race, smoking, and maternal medical conditions such as diabetes mellitus and hypertension, obesity, growth restriction, and previous adverse pregnancy outcomes.[103] In data from a large perinatal database, the relationship between sleep apnea and stillbirth did not persist after controlling for hypertension and diabetes mellitus.[100] Although there is biologic plausibility for an association, further studies are needed to establish the role of SDB in stillbirth.

Miscarriages

Miscarriage or spontaneous abortion involves the loss of a pregnancy, usually within the first 3 months of conception. The estimated frequency of spontaneous abortion is between 12% and 24% of all clinically identified pregnancies. The risk factors for miscarriage include extremes of age, smoking history, increased BMI, previous miscarriage, hypertension, and diabetes mellitus. All of these are also risk factors for SDB. There is limited data linking SDB to miscarriage, and any discussions are mostly theoretical in nature. In a retrospective review of sequential clinic charts of 147 premenopausal women who had been referred to a sleep disorders clinic for an evaluation of sleep complaints, each with a history of at least one pregnancy, an association between SDB and number of miscarriages was demonstrated. In this study, overweight/obese women with SDB, especially those with moderate to severe SDB, had more miscarriages than women without SDB.[104]

Preterm Delivery

Preterm births are those births that occurred before 37 weeks of completed gestation. Although preterm birth occurs in approximately 10% of live births, it is responsible for a significant amount of neonatal morbidity and mortality.[105] Preterm birth may be classified as spontaneous in occurrence or medically indicated if it was precipitated by obstetric intervention, usually for maternal or fetal benefit.[85] The data on preterm birth and SDB has been inconsistent. Large cross-sectional studies of SDB in pregnancy have reported an increased risk of preterm delivery.[87,106] However, these studies did not differentiate between spontaneous and medically indicated preterm birth. One smaller retrospective study noted that there appeared to be an increase in medically indicated preterm delivery associated with preeclampsia among women with SDB.[88] In this study the rate of preterm birth among pregnant women with SDB compared with normal-weight control subjects was 29.8% versus 12.3% (aOR, 2.6; 95% CI, 1.02 to 6.6), and most cases of preterm birth were related to preeclampsia. Subsequent studies have continued to find an association between SDB and preterm delivery and neonatal intensive care unit admission.[107–109]

Fetal Heart Rate Abnormalities

The fetal nonstress test was initially introduced in 1975 as a method to describe fetal heart rate acceleration in response to fetal movement, a sign of fetal health.[85] It is currently the most commonly used form of fetal assessment in obstetrics. In the literature, a small number of studies have attempted to examine fetal well-being in response to nocturnal desaturations and have found conflicting results. In a small study, three of the four women with snoring had fetal heart decelerations that accompanied maternal desaturation; the type of fetal heart rate decelerations were not characterized.[110] In larger prospective studies with sample sizes of 20 women with PSG evidence of SDB, these findings were not confirmed.[46,111] In those studies, despite episodes of oxygen desaturation, no fetal heart rate decelerations were noted during SDB events. It is still unclear whether fetal hypoxia occurs during maternal apnea and, further, whether it is a primary contributor to the reported adverse pregnancy outcomes that are associated with SDB. In summary, the studies examining fetal heart rate decelerations and SDB are limited and inconclusive.[112]

Growth Abnormalities

Intrauterine growth restriction (IUGR) is defined as a fetus small for their gestational age, with most studies using less than the 10th percentile as a cut-off.[85] Findings from individual retrospective and observational studies of SDB and IUGR are mixed, with some failing to show an association. Using two nationwide databases in Taiwan, Chen and colleagues[89] examined the association between SDB and infant birth outcomes that included low birth weight and small-for-gestational-age (SGA) neonates. Women with OSA diagnosed in the year before pregnancy had approximately 30% higher odds of SGA neonates and 76% higher odds of low-birth-weight neonates compared to age-matched women without OSA. Conversely, in a study using data from the Perinatal Center Database, relationships between OSA and growth restriction did not persist after controlling for hypertension and diabetes mellitus.[100] Moreover, two recent meta-analyses did not confirm a relationship between SDB and birth weight or SGA.[113,114] However, a separate meta-analysis of moderate to severe SDB in pregnancy demonstrated an increased risk of fetal growth restriction (OR, 1.44; 95% CI, 1.22 to 1.71).[109]

Low birth weight, defined as a birth weight less than 2500 g, is an important cause of neonatal morbidity. Preterm delivery and growth restriction are two potential mechanisms leading to low birth weight. Regardless of the etiology, low birth weight is associated with increased short- and long-term morbidity, as well as health care costs.[85] Low birth weight was associated with SDB among pooled studies (OR 1.39; 95% CI, 1.14 to 1.65).[91] Most studies have not been able to report a difference in birth weight as a continuous number among women with and without SDB.[91] Two studies found a statistically significant difference between mean birth weights in women with and without SDB, with SDB-exposed neonates weighing 100 g less than unexposed neonates. However, clinically, this difference is of questionable significance.[88,115] In a multicenter pregnancy cohort study, 234 women were evaluated for SDB based on self-reported symptoms (snoring and/or witnessed apneas assessed using the Pittsburgh Sleep Quality Index questionnaire) and in-home PSG in the third trimester. Among this cohort, SDB was associated with delivering an infant that was SGA (aOR, 2.65; CI; 1.15 to 6.10).[116]

Growth abnormalities and SDB research has mostly focused on growth restriction. However, it is also important to consider that there may be an association with large-for-gestational-age (LGA) neonates due to obesity and diabetes mellitus among women with SDB. LGA neonates have higher rates of birth trauma, respiratory morbidity, as well as short- and long-term morbidity.[85] One study found more LGA neonates among obese women with SDB compared to obese and normal-weight control subjects (17% vs. 8% and 2.6%, respectively).[88] Bin and colleagues[117] found that antenatal or pregnancy-associated OSA (identified using *International Classification of Diseases,* 10th edition, Australian modification [ICD-10-AM] diagnosis codes) was associated with 27% higher odds of LGA neonates.

SCREENING FOR SLEEP-DISORDERED BREATHING IN PREGNANCY

Despite the growing prevalence of SDB and mounting evidence of worse maternal-fetal outcomes in pregnant women who have SDB, screening remains uncommon in routine practice.[118–120] Providers have identified a lack of institutional guidelines and effective screening tools as key barriers to screening and effective identification of patients at increased risk for SDB in pregnancy.[121]

As with all screening, tools for SDB in pregnancy need to be easily implemented, inexpensive, and aid practitioners in referring their patients for more definitive diagnostic testing without burdening patients with unnecessary testing. There are single-patient characteristics that have shown consistent associations with SDB in pregnancy. Snoring may be one of the most useful single symptoms for providers to query. In nonpregnant patients, habitual snoring has good correlation with PSG.[122,123] Frequent snoring has been shown to predict increased risk for SDB in pregnant women as well.[14,48,49] In a study using PSG to assess SDB in the first and third trimesters, maternal weight before pregnancy and maternal age were noted to be the major predictors of SDB risk.[124] In a large ($N = 3705$) prospective study of nulliparous women who underwent home PSG in early and midpregnancy, snoring, when combined with age and BMI, was predictive of prevalent and incident SDB.[14] This agrees with prior data demonstrating that older women and women entering pregnancy with a higher baseline BMI are at higher risk for preexisting and pregnancy-onset SDB.[43]

SDB screening tools specifically designed for the general population perform less reliably in the pregnant population. In a meta-analysis of six studies testing SDB screening tools, Epworth Sleepiness Scale (ESS) performance was poor, with a pooled sensitivity of 0.44 (95% CI, 0.33 to 0.56; heterogeneity statistic [I^2] = 32.8%) and a pooled specificity of 0.62 (95% CI, 0.48 to 0.75; I^2 = 81.55%).[125] In the same meta-analysis, the Berlin Questionnaire had a pooled sensitivity of 0.66 (95% CI, 0.45 to 0.83; I = 78.65%) and a pooled specificity of 0.62 (95% CI, 0.48 to 0.75; I^2 = 81.55%). Sensitivity decreased if screening was performed in early pregnancy (≤20 weeks' gestation, 0.47) and in high-risk pregnancy (0.44).[125] The STOP-BANG (snoring, tiredness, observed apnea, blood pressure, body mass index, age, neck size, gender) questionaire[126] has been less frequently studied in pregnant patients, but one study demonstrated acceptable predictive values, especially during the second and third trimesters.[125] The same study used multivariate analyses to show that predictors of OSA varied according to gestational age. In the first trimester, prepregnancy BMI was the only significant predictor of OSA; in the second trimester, "snore often" was the only significant predictor; and in the third trimester, weight gain and pregnancy BMI were significantly associated with OSA.[125] Finally, the Sleep Apnea Symptom Score, when combined with additional patient characteristics (age, BMI, and bed partner–reported snoring and breathing pauses), demonstrated improved sensitivity and specificity for predicting OSA in pregnant women.[127]

Several investigators have proposed pregnancy-specific tools for SDB screening. Facco and colleagues[128] reported on a four-variable model that included frequent snoring (yes or no), chronic hypertension (yes or no), maternal age, and baseline BMI as continuous variables. This tool performed well in predicting SDB in early pregnancy. Recent work by Izci-Balsarak and colleagues[16] compared several screening tools, including the Sleep Apnea Symptom Score of the Multivariable Apnea Prediction Questionnaire,[129] the Obstructive Sleep Apnea/Hypopnea Syndrome Score,[130] the ESS,[131] the model proposed by Facco and colleagues[128], and a novel BMI, age, and tongue enlargement (BATE) model. The four-variable model proposed by Facco and colleagues and the three-variable BATE model performed better than the nonpregnancy-specific tools. Although the sensitivity of the BATE algorithm (76% to 79%) was lower compared with the algorithm proposed by Facco and colleagues (86%), it had higher specificity (82% to 83% vs. 74%).[16] Similarly, investigators of the nuMoM2b study examined predictors of SDB and found that logistic regression models that included current age, current BMI, and frequent snoring in pregnancy predicted SDB in early pregnancy, SDB in midpregnancy, and new-onset SDB in midpregnancy with cross-validated area under the receiver-operating-characteristic curves of 0.870, 0.838, and 0.809, respectively.[14] As a supplement to their manuscript, the authors provide a predictive risk calculator based on their model that can be downloaded.[14] In summary, it appears that pregnancy-specific models that include age and snoring, plus key anthropomorphic measures (BMI, tongue size), may allow for effective SDB screening in pregnant patients.

DIAGNOSING SLEEP-DISORDERED BREATHING IN PREGNANCY

There is insufficient evidence to make strong recommendations regarding in-laboratory versus home-based diagnostic evaluation of SDB specific to pregnant patients. Therefore, when SDB is suspected during pregnancy, women should be evaluated in line with standard guidelines, that is, evaluation by a sleep specialist for a sleep-specific history, physical examination, and sleep testing.[132,133] Sleep testing can be reasonably accomplished via in-laboratory PSG[134] or technically adequate home testing.[47,133] There is growing evidence validating home sleep apnea testing in the gravid population.[135,136] Shorter wait time, increased access, increased convenience to patients, and lower cost make home-based testing an attractive first-test option.[133] The usual caveats regarding the decreased negative predictive value of home monitors apply to the gravid patient. Additional considerations include the possible need to repeat testing or convert to PSG and the need for PSG in the setting of comorbid cardiac, pulmonary, psychiatric, or neurologic disease.[133,137]

TREATMENT OF SLEEP-DISORDERED BREATHING IN PREGNANCY

Preexisting Sleep-Disordered Breathing

Patients with a preexisting SDB diagnosis and established treatment should continue treatment during their pregnancy. CPAP is considered safe and effective in the pregnant population.[93,94] Most patients are expected to require a pressure increase in the 1- to 3-cm H_2O range during the second trimester.[93,94] AHI increases appear relatively modest for most patients.[31] CPAP settings are now more easily monitored as devices become capable of functioning in an autoset mode, which will both adjust pressures within a designated range and will report compliance and residual AHI data. Pregnancy-induced changes in nasal congestion and weight may necessitate adjustments in mask fit and humidification.

Mandibular advancement devices in use with previously documented efficacy could be continued at least during the early part of pregnancy. However, at least one study has demonstrated autoset CPAP superiority versus such devices plus nasal strip in treating SDB in pregnant patients.[138] The effectiveness of mandibular advancement devices should be monitored during the pregnancy, and this may require a sleep study in the early third trimester, when women appear to demonstrate an increased AHI and a need for increased positive airway pressure (PAP) support.[93,94]

Positional therapy can be recommended as an adjuvant for all pregnant patients, in the absence of extenuating circumstances, as most patients have a positional component to their SDB disease, and nonsupine sleep is generally preferred for pregnant patients.[139] Postpartum, AHI levels can be expected to drop, possibly returning to prepregnancy levels.[140]

Patients with known preexisting SDB not undergoing treatment should be rapidly established on a PAP device. Autoset CPAP with data download is likely appropriate for these patients and will allow for rapid treatment, tracking, and adjustment as the pregnancy progresses. Initiation of treatment with a mandibular advancement device is not recommended as it generally takes several weeks to months to fit, adjust, and test the device.

Newly Diagnosed Sleep-Disordered Breathing

As with patients who have untreated preexisting SDB, it is recommended that newly diagnosed patients with SDB consider being rapidly initiated on treatment with a PAP device, presumably autoset CPAP in most cases. It is presumed that the benefits of improved sleep, daytime functioning, and reduction in motor vehicle accidents, all associated with CPAP treatment in the general population, would apply to pregnant women.[141]

However, as described earlier, data examining the effect of CPAP therapy on pregnancy outcomes are extremely limited. In small studies of preeclamptic women, CPAP was shown to improve cardiac output[69] and fetal movement.[92] In another study, early application of nasal CPAP in pregnant women at risk for preeclampsia (N = 12) alleviated sleep-related breathing disturbances but was not sufficient to prevent negative pregnancy outcomes.[94] In pregnant women with hypertension and chronic snoring (N = 16, n = 9 control subjects, n = 7 treatment), nasal CPAP use during the first 8 weeks of pregnancy combined with standard prenatal care was associated with better blood pressure control and improved pregnancy outcomes.[94] Finally, in a small randomized controlled trial (N = 36, 18/group) participants who were adherent to CPAP over 2 weeks had significantly improved insulin secretion compared to the control group. Regarding pregnancy outcomes, the CPAP group had significantly lower rates of preterm delivery, unplanned cesarean section, and neonatal intensive care unit admissions.[98]

Postpartum Considerations

Finally, when taking care of an obstetric patient with SDB, it is also important to consider the increased risk of perioperative complications associated with SDB.[87,142–145] An analgesic strategy that minimizes the need for systemic opioids should be considered. Opioids, when used, should be ordered as single doses rather than standing orders. Monitoring of maternal oxygen saturation should be considered for those getting systemic opioids, and women should wear their CPAP machine while in the hospital recovering from their delivery, as well as when they are discharged home. Predelivery consultation with an anesthesiologist to plan intrapartum and postpartum pain management should be considered.[141,146,147]

CLINICAL PEARLS

- Sleep-disordered breathing (SDB) prevalence and severity increase from the first to third trimester of pregnancy.
- Risk factors for SDB, specifically in pregnancy, have not been well characterized. Habitual snoring, chronic hypertension, maternal body mass index greater than 25 to 30 kg/m^2, and older maternal age are easily obtained elements that may effectively indicate risk of either preexisting SDB or pregnancy-onset SDB.
- Data suggest that SDB during pregnancy is associated with an increase in the incidence of adverse pregnancy outcomes, such as gestational hypertension, preeclampsia, and gestational diabetes mellitus. However, many studies did not define a temporal relationship between SDB and the subsequent development of adverse outcomes.
- Patients with a preexisting SDB diagnosis and established treatment should continue treatment during their pregnancy.
- In general, for patients without known preexisting SDB, there are not enough data at this time to support a strategy of universal screening for SDB in pregnancy.

SUMMARY

SDB in pregnancy is an ongoing area of research. It is clear that SDB prevalence and severity increase as pregnancy progresses, especially among high-risk women (e.g., with obesity). There are also data to suggest that SDB during pregnancy may increase the incidence of adverse pregnancy outcomes, such as gestational hypertension, preeclampsia, and gestational diabetes mellitus. However, many studies did not control for obesity, a strong risk factor for both SDB and adverse pregnancy outcomes, nor did they clearly define a temporal relationship between SDB and the subsequent development of adverse outcomes.

The optimal way to screen for SDB during pregnancy has yet to be determined, but data suggest that instruments routinely used in nonpregnant populations perform poorly in pregnancy. Recently, several investigators have proposed pregnancy-specific tools that perform better. Pregnant women in whom SDB is suspected should be evaluated and treated in line with standard guidelines; however, there are limited data at this time to suggest that treatment of SDB during pregnancy can alter pregnancy outcomes.

SELECTED READINGS

Bourjeily G, Danilack VA, Bublitz MH, et al. Obstructive sleep apnea in pregnancy is associated with adverse maternal outcomes: a national cohort. *Sleep Med*. 2017;38:50–57.

Bourjeily G, Danilack VA, Bublitz MH, et al. Maternal obstructive sleep apnea and neonatal birth outcomes in a population based sample. *Sleep Med*. 2020;66:233–240.

Chen YH, Kang JH, Lin CC, et al. Obstructive sleep apnea and the risk of adverse pregnancy outcomes. *Am J Obstetr Gynecol*. 2012;206(2):136. e131–e135.

Facco FL, Ouyang DW, Zee PC, et al. Development of a pregnancy-specific screening tool for sleep apnea. *J Clin sleep Med*. 2012;8(4):389–394.

Facco FL, Parker CB, Reddy UM, et al. Association between sleep-disordered breathing and hypertensive disorders of pregnancy and gestational diabetes mellitus. *Obstet Gynecol*. 2017;129(1):31–41.

Izci-Balserak B, Zhu B, Gurubhagavatula I, Keenan BT, Pien GW. A screening algorithm for obstructive sleep apnea in pregnancy. *Ann Am Thorac Soc*. 2019;16(10):1286–1294.

Liu L, Su G, Wang S, et al. The prevalence of obstructive sleep apnea and its association with pregnancy-related health outcomes: a systematic review and meta-analysis. *Sleep Breath*. 2019;23(2):399–412.

Louis J, Auckley D, Bolden N. Management of obstructive sleep apnea in pregnant women. *Obstet Gynecol*. 2012;119(4):864–868.

Louis JM, Koch MA, Reddy UM, et al. Predictors of sleep-disordered breathing in pregnancy. *Am J Obstet Gynecol*. 2018;218(5):521.e521–521.e512.

Newbold R, Benedetti A, Kimoff RJ, et al. Maternal sleep-disordered breathing in pregnancy and increased nocturnal glucose levels in women with gestational diabetes mellitus. *Chest*. 2021;159(1):356–365.

Pien GW, Fife D, Pack AI, et al. Changes in symptoms of sleep-disordered breathing during pregnancy. *Sleep*. 2005;28(10):1299–1305.

Romero R, Badr MS. A role for sleep disorders in pregnancy complications: challenges and opportunities. *Am J Obstetr Gynecol*. 2014;210(1):3–11.

A complete reference list can be found online at ExpertConsult.com.

Chapter 188

Postpartum Period and Early Parenthood

Robyn Stremler; Katherine M. Sharkey

Chapter Highlights

- Profound sleep changes—including shortened nighttime sleep, decreased sleep efficiency, multiple night awakenings, and altered sleep timing—are common during the postpartum period, resulting in daytime sleepiness, fatigue, and neurobehavioral decrements in new mothers, particularly in the first few months after delivery.
- Infant care demands drive the poor sleep and altered circadian rhythms experienced by postpartum women. Other factors that affect maternal sleep include the presence of other children in the home, support from partners and other family members, symptoms of anxiety and depression, return to work outside the home, infant feeding method, and infant sleep location.
- Postpartum depression is associated with maternal reports of sleep loss and infant sleep problems across a range of cultures with wide variations in sleep behaviors and practices.
- Interventions to preserve maternal sleep or prevent infant sleep problems in the early postpartum period seem to be of limited effectiveness, except among families of greater social disadvantage. Improvements in maternal report of sleep quality have been observed following interventions to reduce nighttime feeding and waking in the second half of the infant's first year.

OVERVIEW

It is likely that as long as there have been mothers, the experience of sleep disturbance and fatigue in the postpartum period has existed. However, sleep can be challenging to study during the first few months after birth. As may be expected, polysomnography (PSG) may be considered intrusive, and other methods such as actigraphy or questionnaires may be burdensome for women facing the demands of infant care. In addition, because sleep disturbance is expected in new mothers, sleep and circadian changes during this important life stage traditionally have not received ample attention, and early studies often included small, nondiverse samples of women at relatively low risk for postpartum complications.

Nevertheless, sleep and circadian rhythm changes during the postpartum period and their effects on maternal functioning and maternal-infant interactions are areas of intense interest. Multiple interacting physiologic, behavioral, and social factors affect postpartum sleep (Box 188.1), including hormonal changes, maternal age, type of delivery, type of infant feeding, infant temperament, return-to-work issues, previous birth experience, number of other children in the home, perinatal depression and anxiety, availability of nighttime support from the partner or others, and the pace at which the infant's sleep consolidates into longer, uninterrupted stretches.

Interventions to improve maternal sleep and fatigue in the early postpartum months have shown limited effectiveness, although one intervention study showed greater improvements in sleep in women at higher risk for sleep disruption, including those with worse baseline sleep and greater social disadvantage[1] (see the section Interventions to Improve Maternal Sleep). In addition, several studies aimed at decreasing infant nighttime awakenings in the second half of the first postpartum year demonstrated improvements in maternal report of sleep quality. To develop successful strategies to help those with debilitating sleep loss, additional research is needed to understand whether certain subgroups of new mothers are more vulnerable to postpartum sleep disturbances, what aspects of sleep and circadian rhythms should be targeted to reduce risk, and whether treatment improves long-term outcomes for women and their infants.[2]

POSTPARTUM SLEEP

The "postpartum period" can refer to different time frames, depending on context. For instance, maternal mortality is highest in the first 42 days after delivery, prompting both the American College of Obstetricians and Gynecologists and the World Health Organization to recommend a postpartum checkup within 3 weeks of delivery.[3] Other aspects of postpartum recovery extend beyond 6 weeks: indeed the first 12 weeks after delivery are often referred to as "the fourth trimester," and surveillance for other postpartum issues can last as long as 1 year. With respect to sleep disturbances, most

BOX 188.1 TYPICAL HORMONE, SLEEP, AND MENTAL HEALTH CONCERNS DURING THE POSTPARTUM PERIOD

Hormones

Abrupt drop in progesterone levels from those in pregnancy
Abrupt drop in estrogen levels from those in pregnancy
Prolactin levels fluctuate with lactation
Melatonin amplitude decreased

Sleep Patterns and Architecture

Sleep disrupted owing to infant care and feeding
Sleep more disrupted for first-time mothers than for experienced mothers
Tendency to sleep later into the morning hours
Increased slow wave sleep (delta sleep [i.e., N3 sleep stage])

Sleepiness and Sleep Challenges

Increased daytime sleepiness and neurobehavioral deficits
Difficulty with sleeping; new mothers may nap if not employed outside the home
Issues of infant sleep location emerge

Mental Health Concerns

Risk of postpartum depression
Risk of postpartum psychosis in women with bipolar disorder

women would say that the postpartum period continues from birth until infant sleep is consolidated with predictable day and night sleeping patterns.[4] Maternal sleep is poor immediately after childbirth. In one study of postpartum sleep in a hospital environment, first-time mothers logged an average total sleep duration of just 9.7 hours in the first 48 hours after delivery, with breastfeeding mothers obtaining more sleep, while environmental factors—such as hospital noise and room sharing—and type of delivery were not linked to sleep duration.[5] In the first week after delivery, sleep timing and duration are highly variable; new mothers typically have shorter nighttime sleep but longer daytime sleep than during pregnancy,[6] although there are striking individual differences, with some women showing marked deterioration and others showing preserved total sleep times.[7,8] Because of medical interventions for childbirth, most infants are born during morning and midday hours, with noninduced vaginal birth and home births both more likely to occur in the early morning.[9] Being in labor during the night has been associated with depressed mood during the first week after delivery[10] (see the section Postpartum Depression and Disturbed Sleep).

Several self-report and actigraphy studies have demonstrated that mothers experience disturbed sleep after childbirth and that they have more nighttime awakenings from disruptions during the first 4 weeks in comparison with the end of pregnancy and later postpartum months.[7,8,11-13] A handful of studies with relatively small samples have described sleep architecture in the postpartum period. Overall, new mothers have less N1 (stage 1) and N2 (stage 2) sleep and a significant increase in N3 slow wave (delta) sleep at 1 month postpartum compared to pregnancy.[1,11,14-17] These sleep pattern alterations may be related to increases in N3 mediated by prolactin[18] (see the section Breastfeeding versus Formula Feeding) or increased homeostatic drive from persistent insufficient sleep. A longitudinal polysomnographic study comparing first-time mothers to experienced mothers demonstrated that parity plays a role in sleep efficiency across the perinatal period: women with no children had significantly greater sleep efficiency than women who were already mothers before becoming pregnant and during all three trimesters. At 1 month postpartum, however, first-time mothers had more disrupted sleep than experienced mothers.[19] An actigraphy study also showed lower sleep efficiencies in nulliparous women compared to multiparas at postpartum weeks 1 and 6, but in this study first-time mothers also had greater sleep disruption during pregnancy.[8]

Improvements in postpartum sleep consolidation are gradual, and evidence suggests that, although sleep efficiency returns to a healthy range eventually, mothers' sleep quality does not revert all the way back to its pre-child baseline during the early years of parenting.[19,20] For instance, one study showed that nocturnal total sleep duration did not differ between postpartum women and controls during any of the first 13 postpartum weeks, but that the mothers' sleep was far more disrupted and less efficient at all time points.[20] The postpartum women in this sample spent more time in bed at night than nonpregnant women, and naps contributed a negligible amount of sleep, with an average of 0.4 naps per week ranging in duration from 3 to 19 minutes. As may be expected, mothers report that the majority of nocturnal awakenings are to provide infant care.[21] Sleep timing—particularly time of final morning awakening—is delayed during early postpartum recovery compared with pregnancy,[22] but by 3 to 4 months postpartum, women report earlier bedtimes and wake-up times, presumably because some women have returned to paid employment by that time.[13] Average maternity leave for employed women varies by region; for example, it is 12 months in Canada and around 10 weeks in the United States.[23] The impact of mothers' return to work on sleep in the context of the length of maternity leave has not been systematically studied.

Sleep disorders are prevalent during pregnancy and can affect birth outcomes in women and their infants (see Chapters 186 and 187). Sleep disorders that arise before or during pregnancy also affect new mothers' postpartum health. For instance, sleep-disordered breathing[24] and insomnia[25,26] frequently persist after pregnancy, and although restless legs syndrome often resolves after the birth of the infant,[27] it may herald postpartum depression (PPD).[28] Moreover, insufficient sleep, delayed sleep timing, and greater postpartum sleep disturbance all have shown associations with postpartum weight retention of 5 kg or more,[29-31] increasing women's risk for obesity and other chronic diseases later in life.[32,33] For example, Herring and colleagues examined associations between actigraphic sleep and postpartum weight gain changes in a sample of 159 Black and Hispanic mothers and found that women sleeping fewer than 7 hours at 5 months postpartum gained significantly more weight between 5 and 12 months postpartum than new mothers who slept at least 7 hours.[34] Strategies to decrease postpartum obesity could include interventions to improve maternal sleep.

SLEEP IN PARENTS OF PRETERM INFANTS

Mothers of premature and/or medically ill infants have different postpartum sleep challenges than mothers of healthy, full-term infants, with stress, anxiety, depression, prior sleep difficulties, delivery method, and feelings about the birth experience all playing a role in their sleep disturbances.[35,36] One actigraphy study of mothers of preterm infants in the first week after delivery showed an average of 2 hours more sleep at night after a vaginal birth compared with caesarean section, which may reflect more difficult birthing circumstances.[37] A study of mothers and fathers of preterm infants observed that new mothers reported more insomnia than fathers while the infant was hospitalized; moreover, these maternal insomnia ratings were associated with greater maternal report of infant sleep problems at the time of hospital discharge and 12 months later.[38] Mothers of preterm infants continue to report more sleep disturbances than those with full-term infants up to 20 weeks after delivery, a difference attributed to different brain maturation rates in preterm neonates when age is not corrected for prematurity.[39]

SLEEP IN NEW FATHERS

Although the sleep of new fathers has been understudied, it is starting to receive more research attention.[40] Perhaps in contrast to what may be expected, the scant data that exist indicate that some new fathers get even less sleep than new mothers in the early postpartum weeks.[41-43] Furthermore, although mothers report more fatigue,[41] fathers show higher levels of objective daytime sleepiness than mothers between 3 and 8 weeks postpartum.[43] Postpartum sleep disturbance appears to impact mood in fathers in a similar fashion as in mothers: in a study of 711 couples, depressive symptoms at 1 month postpartum were correlated with poorer subjective sleep quality on the Pittsburgh Sleep Quality Index (PSQI) at 6 months postpartum, and worse sleep quality predicted more depressive symptoms at 6 and 12 months postpartum in both parents.[44] Examination of societal trends shows that contemporary fathers spend significantly more time providing care for young children than in previous generations,[45] and this involvement may benefit both mothers and infants. A study that enrolled 57 mother-father-infant trios found that greater paternal caregiving at 3 months (during the day and at night) predicted better maternal and infant sleep consolidation at 6 months.[46]

POSTPARTUM NAPPING

New mothers may attempt to compensate for disturbed nighttime sleep with daytime napping.[47] Naps are more frequent and contribute more to total sleep duration over 24 hours in the earliest postpartum weeks compared with later postpartum periods.[8,11,12,41,48] Although women often are advised to "sleep when the baby sleeps," studies that have tracked napping behavior longitudinally across the postnatal period show that the majority of mothers no longer nap or only take occasional short naps from as early as 3 weeks postpartum onward.[8,49,50] Factors observed to predict more maternal napping at 3 months postpartum include maternal perception of greater sleep disturbance, longer duration of infant wake time at night, fewer other children at home, fewer employment hours outside the home, and availability of a partner to care for the infant during a nap.[47,50]

Although there is some evidence that mothers who nap during the day sleep less at night,[21,51,52] the interplay between postpartum napping, nighttime sleep, and daytime functioning has not been thoroughly explored. One exception is a study of first-time mothers at 3 to 6 months postpartum that assessed nighttime sleep as a predictor of next-day napping as well as the impact of napping on the subsequent night's sleep and found that longer daytime naps predicted longer sleep-onset latencies and more wakefulness during the night after the nap, but that sleep at night did not predict napping the next day.[21] Further research is needed to determine optimal timing and duration of napping and its effects on daytime alertness and cognitive function in the postpartum period, as well as to investigate any deleterious effects of napping, such as circadian disruption or insomnia.

DAYTIME FATIGUE AND MATERNAL FUNCTIONING

Daytime fatigue—defined as subjective feelings of exhaustion, tiredness, and/or loss of vitality—is a common experience for new parents.[41] Both biologic and psychosocial factors contribute to fatigue in new mothers. Reports of postpartum fatigue have been associated with reduced sleep time, low hemoglobin, and low ferritin levels, as well as employment and family responsibilities.[53,54] New mothers are at risk of developing anemia from iron demands of pregnancy and blood loss during delivery, infections (e.g., endometritis, urinary tract infections, mastitis), and thyroid dysfunction,[3] all of which may contribute to postpartum fatigue. Moreover, fatigue can be related to PPD, though they are separate constructs.[55] Thus women experiencing high levels of fatigue in the first few months after childbirth should be assessed for these issues and treated.[56]

Chronic insufficient sleep and postpartum fatigue are associated with worse daytime performance in new mothers on a psychomotor vigilance task (PVT).[20] In addition to short sleep duration and sleep fragmentation, later sleep timing[57] and depressed mood[12,58,59] have also been shown to be related to decreased PVT performance in new mothers. Postpartum sleep decrements can also lead to drowsy driving, potentially endangering families with young children.[60,61] For instance, in an anonymous survey of 72 parents (66 women, 6 men) with an infant 12 months of age or younger, 18.1% of the sample reported driving sleepy at least once per week and 8.3% reported falling asleep behind the wheel since the birth of their infant.[61] Compared to 52 parents in the study with no accidents, the 20 parents who reported a near-miss automobile accident did not differ in their reported sleep duration, snoring, number of night awakenings, or typical driving distance. Mothers' sleep disturbance can also impair more complex behaviors in the mother-infant dyad, such as maternal sensitivity to her infant in a free play interaction,[62] or during the infant's bedtime routine.[63] On the other hand, a study that explored links between maternal sleep disturbance/fatigue and mother-infant interactions found that maternal napping was associated with improved interactions related to fostering cognitive growth.[64] Individual differences and the time course over which women return to their baseline levels of sleep quality and daytime functioning after childbirth are poorly understood and deserve further study.[2]

HORMONAL CHANGES AND CIRCADIAN RHYTHMS

Women undergo substantial hormonal changes during pregnancy, parturition, and in the early postpartum period.

Delivery of the placenta reduces estriol and progesterone levels, with accompanying increases in oxytocin and prolactin.[65] The precipitous postpartum decline in progesterone and its derivative, the $GABA_A$ (gamma-aminobutyric acid receptor, class A) modulator allopregnanolone, has been implicated in perinatal anxiety[66] and may contribute to postpartum insomnia. Circadian patterns of hormone secretion also change across the perinatal period; for example, during pregnancy, the circadian rhythm of the hypothalamic-pituitary-adrenal (HPA) axis is blunted, circulating cortisol levels are two to five times higher than nonpregnant concentrations,[67] and lower levels of cortisol are associated with more subjective and objective sleep disturbance.[68] Although growth hormone, prolactin, melatonin, and thyroid-stimulating hormone also have distinct diurnal secretion patterns, less is known about circadian changes that occur in the postpartum period and associations with sleep and daytime sleepiness.

Melatonin levels and secretion patterns may be altered in postpartum women by increased nighttime light exposure during provision of infant care and decreased daylight exposure secondary to limited activity outside the home.[69] New mothers had higher levels of daytime melatonin excretion and blunted circadian rhythm amplitude at 4 and 10 weeks postpartum compared with nonpregnant nulliparous women,[70] and circadian shifts in dim light melatonin onset of up to 2.5 hours have been observed from the third trimester to 6 weeks postpartum.[69] Changes in circadian rhythms, including melatonin secretion patterns, may influence subsequent sleep quality and daytime fatigue. For instance, one small study showed a shortening of phase angle between melatonin onset and self-selected bedtime from the third trimester to 6 weeks postpartum, indicating that new mothers go to bed "earlier" in their biologic night during the postpartum period,[69] and another study showed that earlier sleep midpoint was associated with more predictable patterns of fatigue and fewer symptoms of stress and depression at 12 weeks postpartum.[71]

The most commonly dispensed advice regarding maternal sleep, the suggestion to "sleep when the baby sleeps," may not promote circadian rhythm entrainment. Entraining the mother's sleep to the infant's is less ideal than finding ways to more quickly facilitate the newborn's sleeping through the night. Although infants' endogenous circadian rhythms of cortisol, melatonin, and temperature develop between 8 and 18 weeks,[72] infant sleep-wake patterns are influenced by light-dark exposure and maternal sleep and have been observed to show a circadian pattern as early as 3 weeks.[73] Greater daytime light exposure in infants is associated with higher circadian amplitude, suggesting that manipulating ambient light may promote development of more consolidated sleeping patterns in infants.[74]

BREASTFEEDING VERSUS FORMULA FEEDING

Breastfeeding initiation rates range from 63% to 98% in high-income countries (HIC) and 89% to 99% in low-income to middle-income countries (LMIC), with 10% to 71% of women breastfeeding to some extent at 6 months postpartum in HIC and 62% to 99% in LMIC.[75] For lactating women, basal levels of prolactin are high, and a burst of prolactin secretion occurs at the onset of each breastfeeding event, regardless of when sleep occurs, although these bursts seem to be of a higher magnitude in the evening than in the morning.[76] Both basal levels and bursts of prolactin diminish to prepregnancy levels by approximately 3 months postpartum. Blyton and colleagues[18] studied 31 women in their home environment with portable PSG. Lactating women had less light sleep (N1 and N2), fewer arousals, and more deep sleep (N3), especially in the second half of the night, compared with nonlactating postpartum women. No difference was observed in the amount of rapid eye movement (REM) sleep or total sleep time between the two groups. Within 24 hours of weaning, prolactin levels return to low basal levels and to the circadian sleep–associated patterns found in healthy adults.[77]

Some parents choose to supplement infant feeding with formula in the hope that the infant will be better satiated, settle faster, and sleep longer at night so that they can obtain more nighttime sleep.[78] Studies examining the relationships between infant feeding method and parental sleep have found either no difference in subjectively rated sleep[79] and objectively measured total nighttime sleep[41,80] or increased amounts of sleep[78] for parents whose infants are breastfed compared to formula-fed. Because supplementation of breastfeeding with formula often is perceived as a strategy to increase infant sleep at night, parents should be made aware that research findings do not support a recommendation of formula feeding as a means to improve sleep. For women planning to breastfeed, it may be helpful to know that no existing study asking parents to report on the quality of their sleep has reported any difference between parents with breastfed and those with formula-fed infants.

Pharmacologic treatment for insomnia during lactation may be of concern because of potential effects of drug transmission through breastmilk on the newborn's growth and development,[81] as well as safety concerns regarding the mother's ability to awaken to respond to her infant at night. One observational study in 124 women, however, showed minimal sedation among infants breastfed by new mothers taking benzodiazepines, suggesting that breastfeeding need not be contraindicated when benzodiazepines are being used postpartum.[82] The World Health Organization has deemed occasional use of benzodiazepines during lactation as acceptable.[83] Similarly, use of zolpidem[84] and zopiclone[85] by small samples of women in the first week postpartum resulted in minimal transfer into breastmilk. Given their short half-lives, these hypnotics would be expected to be well tolerated in breastfed infants and should not be avoided in lactating women who would benefit from pharmacologic treatment for their insomnia.[86] (See Chapter 53 for a summary of common sleep-related medications and their ratings for potential harm to the newborn.)

BED SHARING AND ROOM SHARING

Bed sharing (also known as co-sleeping) is defined as an infant sleeping in the same bed with the caregiver. Room sharing refers to when the infant sleeps in the same room as, and in close proximity to, a parent or caregiver, but not occupying the same bed. Bed sharing is frequently implicated in sleep-related deaths among infants younger than 6 months of age; significant ethnic and racial disparities exist, with Black mothers more likely to report "ever" bed sharing and Black infants more likely to die of sudden infant death syndrome (SIDS) and accidental suffocation than White or Hispanic infants.[87,88] Thus, room sharing—rather than bed sharing—is the infant sleep arrangement recommended by the American

Academy of Pediatrics[89] and the Canadian Paediatric Society as a means to decrease risk of SIDS and accidental suffocation. Although few studies have examined the relationship between bed sharing or room sharing and mothers' sleep-wake patterns, bed sharing has become increasingly common during the postpartum period.[87,90-92] The proportion of usually bed-sharing infants in the United States rose from 5.5% in the period 1993 to 1994 to 12.8% in 1999 to 2000[92] and to 13.5% in 2010.[93]

It has been suggested that infants are at risk for SIDS because of an immature neurologic system and difficulty arousing from sleep. Older studies postulated that bed sharing may reduce the risk of SIDS, because a bed-sharing infant has more arousals from the mother's body heat, sounds, oxygen and carbon dioxide exchange, smells, movement, and touch.[90] However, greater risk of SIDS or asphyxiation for bed-sharing infants is likely directly related to overheating, the presence of pillows and soft surfaces, and exposure to adults who are smokers, extremely fatigued, intoxicated, or obese.[89,94] In contrast with risks imposed by bed sharing, room sharing may decrease risk of SIDS via increased sensory stimulation (e.g. noise, light, touch) of the infant with parental presence.[89]

Both room sharing and bed sharing impact maternal sleep. Mothers of predominantly room-sharing infants report more infant night awakenings than mothers of infants who sleep in separate rooms, and experience poorer self-rated and actigraphically measured sleep.[95,96] Bed-sharing mothers also have more disrupted sleep. Mosko and colleagues[91] assigned 20 usually bed-sharing and 15 usually separate-sleeping mother-infant dyads to bed-share for one night and then to sleep separately the following night. In this PSG study, bed sharing had no effect on REM sleep but increased the number of arousals and modestly reduced N3 deep sleep while increasing light sleep (N1 and N2) in the group of breastfeeding women. Women who routinely had their infant sleep in a separate room rated their sleep quality as lower on the night when they were assigned to bed-share, indicating that occasional bed sharing may be more disruptive to self-reported sleep quality than routine bed sharing. Given potential effects of bed sharing and room sharing on maternal sleep, discussions with parents related to safe infant sleep practices should also include acknowledgement of possible impact on parental sleep.

INTERVENTIONS TO IMPROVE MATERNAL SLEEP

Given that parent and infant sleep are inextricably linked, parental sleep disruption with a newborn is expected; hence interventions in the early postpartum months are usually aimed at prevention of significant infant sleep problems. As infant sleep is expected to consolidate and shift to a greater proportion of nighttime sleep, interventions delivered in the second half of the first postpartum year are typically focused on eliminating infant sleep problems that are persistent or significantly interfering with parent sleep. Many interventions to prevent infant sleep problems early in the postpartum period have focused on infant sleep outcomes without measuring parental sleep outcomes.[97-100] These interventions typically provided parents with information related to infant sleep and strategies to limit development of unwanted sleep associations, to increase the infant's self-soothing ability, and to facilitate day-night entrainment.

Two randomized controlled trials (RCTs) aimed at preventing early sleep problems through provision of information about infant sleep and settling strategies did assess parent sleep outcomes, although neither intervention specifically addressed maternal sleep behaviors.[101,102] Using single-item rating scales for sleep quality and quantity, researchers did not detect any effect of the interventions on infant or maternal sleep in the early postpartum period. An RCT of a behavioral-educational intervention designed to increase maternal and infant nighttime sleep and sleep continuity in the early postpartum period found no group differences in maternal or infant sleep as measured by actigraphy at 6 or 12 weeks postpartum.[103] Two samples of expectant parents, one socioeconomically advantaged and one low-income, were enrolled in an RCT of an antenatally delivered, modified sleep hygiene intervention to reduce parental nighttime sleep disruption in the early postpartum period.[1] In the socioeconomically advantaged sample, no group differences were seen in any sleep outcomes measured by actigraphy. In the low-income sample (in which the subjects reported worse sleep at baseline than socially advantaged participants), the intervention group attained significantly more nocturnal sleep (7.1 hours versus 6.5 hours), better sleep efficiency (80% versus 75%), and less wake time after sleep onset (19% versus 23%) than control subjects at 3 months postpartum. The few published intervention studies to improve parent sleep provide little support for universal delivery of antenatal or early postpartum strategies. Socially disadvantaged families may benefit most from advice regarding infant and maternal sleep, and future interventions should be tested in vulnerable populations.

Several RCTs conducted with older infants (6 months of age or older)[104-109] focused on providing parents with information on infant sleep and strategies to decrease night feeding and waking, but without provision of strategies to shape parent's sleep directly. Four of the studies[104,105,107,109] included maternal sleep outcomes and found reductions in problematic infant sleep behaviors and a concomitant improvement in self-reported sleep outcomes using the PSQI.

Given that the recent American College of Obstetricians and Gynecologists' Committee Opinion on Optimizing Postpartum Care[110] recommends a "discussion of coping options for fatigue and sleep disruption" as a key component of postpartum care yet offers no explicit advice or references to interventions, greater focus on the design and testing of interventions to improve maternal sleep is needed. Promising findings have been reported where postpartum care includes sleep and fatigue management. In Australia, for example, residential early parenting services are accessible to mother-infant dyads for addressing unsettled infant behaviors and maternal sleep disruption, fatigue, and distress. Intervention typically involves increasing maternal sleep opportunity, individualized "feed-play-sleep" routine and infant settling strategies, psychoeducation, and medical and psychological support. One such program found that after a 5-day admission, maternal distress (e.g., depression, anxiety, irritability) and insomnia symptoms, fatigue, daytime sleepiness, and objectively measured psychomotor vigilance improved significantly.[59,111] Further research is needed in understanding the treatment mechanisms and moderators to optimize care.

Strategies that have proved beneficial to sleep in other populations, such as mindfulness-based stress reduction, yoga, and tai chi, could also be tested in the postpartum period.[112] Cognitive-behavioral therapy for insomnia (CBT-I) may be a feasible and effective treatment for women with clinically significant postpartum sleep difficulties. In an open pilot study of CBT-I, Swanson and colleagues[113] treated 12 new mothers with comorbid PPD and insomnia. They adapted core CBT-I strategies to accommodate infant care and included components on facilitating infant sleep and requesting assistance with infant care. Participants demonstrated significant improvements in diary-reported sleep efficiency, sleep latency, and total sleep time, as well as a reduction in depressive symptoms. Future studies could examine this intervention in larger, randomized samples and test its efficacy as a preventive strategy.

The provision of postpartum care (including programs to improve maternal or infant sleep) is highly complex, dependent not only on the availability of empirically tested effective interventions but perhaps more so on policies and funding provisions to increase access by the community. Disparities exist with different lengths of parental leaves, varying levels of health care access, and other sociocultural factors (discussed later).

SOCIOCULTURAL FACTORS AND ETHNIC AND RACIAL HEALTH DISPARITIES

International and cross-cultural studies have described a wide range of mother-infant sleep behaviors in the postpartum period. This literature highlights significant cultural variation in the sleep environment, infant care practices, and, of course, the meanings attributed to them. Ethnographic data indicate that sleep is construed as a form of social behavior in many societies.[114] Whereas a solitary-sleeping infant is a common goal for many families in Western settings, close maternal-infant contact at night is the cultural norm in many other cultural groups.[115] Bed sharing is practiced in Malaysia, Brazil, Thailand, Japan, the Middle East, and among Māori and Pacific Islanders.[116-121] Culturally significant bed-sharing practices have been adapted to incorporate new information about the risk of SIDS while preserving important traditions. In New Zealand, for instance, Māori health workers use a novel sleeping space for infants, a shallow, flax-woven bassinet called a wahakura (from the words "waha," meaning *to carry*, and "kura," meaning *precious little object*), which provides a safe infant sleeping space in the mother's bed. Beginning in 2006, the wahakura, and a plastic version, called a Pēpi-pod, were distributed to families along with safe-sleeping education, and from 2009 to 2015 infant mortality rates dropped in New Zealand by 29%, mostly among Māori infants.[122] Bed sharing appears to have similar effects on maternal sleep in Western and non-Western cultures. For example, a recent actigraphy study in hunter-gatherer Hadza of Tanzania—a culture in which bed sharing is common among family members beyond spouses and the mother-infant dyad—showed that a higher number of individuals co-sleeping on the same surface was associated with more nighttime sleep disturbance in mothers, but that breastfeeding did not have a substantial impact on maternal sleep quality.[123] Outside of bed sharing at night, infant sleep may occur in other locations, such as outdoors, as practiced in Finland and other Northern European nations,[124] or while the infant is carried in a sling, as in African hunter-gatherer cultures while the mother works during the day.[125,126]

Many dimensions of sleep health are worse among women of ethnic and racial minority when compared with predominately White samples both in nonperinatal samples[127] and during pregnancy.[128,129] A few studies have documented sleep health disparities specifically among postpartum women.[1,130,131] Lee and Gay found that low-income women of racial/ethnic minority had shorter, more disrupted sleep compared with economically advantaged, mostly White women at 1 and 3 months postpartum.[1] Similarly, in their longitudinal study of low-income, mostly Black women, Doering and colleagues recorded average actigraphic nighttime sleep durations of just 5.5±1.4 hours at postpartum week 4 and 5.4±1.4 hours at postpartum week 8 with two-thirds of their sample obtaining mean sleep durations less than 6 hours at both time points.[130] In a qualitative study that explored the reasons behind these sleep disparities in a sample of low-income Black mothers, participants reported that worry, anxiety, and work and school responsibilities contributed to their poor sleep.[132] Black women in the United States are three to four times more likely to die from pregnancy complications than their White counterparts regardless of socioeconomic status.[133] Genetic and biologic differences do not explain this disparity; rather, systemic racism and bias from health care providers, substantial variations in care between hospitals that care for predominantly White versus Black populations, and physical consequences of chronic exposure to social stressors and racism have been identified as contributing factors.[134] Given these striking health inequities in maternal morbidity and mortality, and the possible contributions of poor sleep health to untoward outcomes for mothers, future work on postpartum sleep should examine race, ethnicity, and exposure to racism as factors for effective identification and treatment of perinatal sleep problems.

POSTPARTUM DEPRESSION AND DISTURBED SLEEP

Up to 50% to 60% of all new mothers experience postpartum "blues" in the 3 to 5 days after childbirth. The blues manifest as excessive and unpredictable crying episodes, labile mood, and sadness during a time that is expected to be joyful. These symptoms typically resolve within the first 2 postpartum weeks, and, although the "blues" often are attributed to rapid hormonal changes, increased time awake during the night and poor sleep quality are strongly associated with negative daytime mood, particularly in the first 4 weeks after childbirth.[12,13,78] Being in labor during the night and a history of sleep disruption during third trimester are also associated with a higher incidence of postpartum blues.[10] Postpartum psychosis is a psychiatric emergency that is associated with insomnia in the early postpartum period.[135-137] New mothers with a history of bipolar disorder may be at particular risk for development of postpartum psychosis consequent to sleep deprivation and require close monitoring for inability to sleep or decreased need for sleep.[138]

Approximately 10% to 20% of women experience a major depressive episode between 4 weeks and 12 months after delivery,[139,140] making PPD the most common complication of childbirth. Diagnostic criteria for PPD are the same as those of depressive episodes experienced at other times of life (see Chapter 164) but may also include difficulty sleeping when the baby is sleeping at night and worrying about hurting the baby, with considerable overlap with symptoms of anxiety during the postpartum period.[139,141] Mechanisms implicated in the development of PPD include changes in hormones and neurotransmitters, genetic factors, neuroinflammation, epigenetic changes, and perinatal changes in neurocircuitry.[142] Many environmental and psychosocial factors increase PPD risk, including poor social support, financial or marital stressors, adverse life events, impaired infant-mother interactions, and difficulties with labor and delivery or postpartum infant care. Several lines of evidence suggest that these stressors raise PPD risk through epigenetic changes and alterations in HPA axis function.[67,142] Insufficient sleep and disrupted sleep-wake patterns affect many of these pathways and likely contribute mechanistically to postpartum mood changes.

Poor sleep during pregnancy is associated with the development of postpartum depressive symptoms.[13,143,144] Wolfson and colleagues observed that mothers who developed depressive symptoms at 2 to 4 weeks postpartum had significantly different antenatal sleep patterns compared with nondepressed mothers, including later rise times, longer naps, and more total sleep at the end of their pregnancies.[13] A prospective study in expectant mothers found that self-report of disturbed sleep during third trimester predicted depression and anxiety scores during the first week postpartum, but actigraphic estimates of sleep during pregnancy were not related to mood.[7] In terms of sleep architecture, a polysomnographic study of 28 women showed that mothers who experienced negative postpartum mood (n = 9) had shorter REM latencies at third trimester and 1 month postpartum, a greater decrease in total sleep time from third trimester to 1 month postpartum, and lower sleep efficiencies at 1 month postpartum compared to nondepressed women.[145] Sleep difficulties in pregnancy have been shown to increase risk of developing PPD across a wide range of cultures including in China,[146] Greece,[147] and Korea.[148] Finally, the development of postpartum psychiatric symptoms other than depression, namely anxiety[149] and posttraumatic stress symptoms,[150] have also been linked to insomnia during pregnancy.

Self-reported sleep disturbance in the early weeks after delivery also heralds the onset of PPD at later postpartum time points (12 to 14 weeks postpartum), with longer sleep latencies, more daytime dysfunction, and worse perceived sleep quality predicting development of PPD.[151,152] In a sample at increased risk for postpartum mood disturbances, McEvoy and colleagues also found that use of sleep medications in the early postpartum period predicted development of PPD at 3 months postpartum.[152] Shortened sleep is ubiquitous in new mothers, and it appears that level of sleep disturbance, rather than sleep duration per se, plays an important role in perinatal depressive symptoms.[153] In a polysomnographic study, for example, the frequency of night awakenings, rather than a change in hormone levels or overall sleep duration, was related to negative mood at 1 month postpartum.[145] Worse postpartum sleep has been demonstrated to increase risk of depression in new fathers,[154] and in cultures in which new mothers receive substantial assistance with nighttime caregiving responsibilities.[155] CBT-I has been shown to improve sleep and reduce postpartum depressive symptoms in a small open trial.[113]

Circadian dysregulation across the perinatal period is related to PPD.[156]

A small study showed that later circadian phase in the third trimester of pregnancy was associated with more depressive symptoms at 2 and 6 weeks postpartum.[69] In a sample of high-risk expectant mothers, longer phase angle between dim light melatonin onset and sleep onset at 33 weeks' gestation was associated with more manic symptoms at postpartum week 2 and more obsessive-compulsive symptoms at week 6, and sleep-onset times later than approximately 11:30 p.m. during pregnancy predicted more manic and depressive symptoms at postpartum week 2.[157] Novel circadian rhythm–based interventions for PPD, including wake therapy,[158,159] bright light therapy,[160,161] and chronotherapy,[162] have shown promising results for reducing depressive symptoms and are worthy of further study.

The effects of infant sleep patterns on maternal sleep and development of PPD also are essential to consider. Mothers exhibiting major depressive symptoms at 4 and 8 weeks postpartum were more likely to report getting less than 6 hours of sleep in a 24-hour period during the previous week and being awakened by their baby three or more times between 10 p.m. and 6 a.m.[163] These findings suggest that infant sleep patterns and maternal sleep deprivation and fragmentation are significant contributors to the pathogenesis of PPD. Report of infant sleep problems at 6 to 12 months of age also is associated with maternal major depressive symptomatology, even after adjustment for known risk factors such as history of depressive illness.[164]

Because infant sleep problems in these studies were based on maternal report rather than on objective evaluations of infant sleep, depressed mothers may perceive their infant's sleep more negatively than nondepressed mothers or may be more likely to report sleep problems. In a study in which infant sleep was measured objectively, however, variability in infant sleep at 8 months predicted mothers' depressive symptoms at 15 months.[165] Furthermore, evidence indicates that treatment of infant sleep problems results in decreased incidence of maternal depression. Hiscock and colleagues performed two RCTs of brief behavioral interventions to reduce infant sleep problems that significantly decreased maternal reports of infant sleep problems and maternal symptoms of depression.[105,166] Parent training focused on developing healthy infant sleep patterns has also been shown to improve parental competence and marital satisfaction and to decrease parental stress.[99]

Perinatal depression in mothers may impact their children's sleep patterns. For instance, mothers with depression during pregnancy reported shorter sleep durations, longer sleep latencies, and more frequent night wakings in their children at age 3½ years.[167] Moreover, this impact appears to be long-lasting, as associations have been observed between maternal PPD and night waking at age 16 and overall sleep difficulties at age 18, even after controlling for depression and infant sleep problems in the child, socioeconomic variables, and antenatal depression.[168]

CLINICAL PEARLS

- If a specific sleep disorder such as restless legs syndrome, sleep apnea, or insomnia developed during pregnancy, evaluations during the postpartum period should determine if the difficulties have resolved.
- Reports of excessive sleepiness, fatigue, or sleep loss should be pursued and evaluated by health care providers because of increased morbidity and mortality in the mother, potential harm to the newborn, and their relationship to treatable medical conditions such as anemia, infection, thyroid dysfunction, and PPD.
- Evaluation for sleep disturbances and depression should be included in routine postpartum assessments; advice related to optimizing sleep in the postpartum period should be provided, taking into account cultural sleep practices.
- Severe sleep restriction in the postpartum period may contribute to retention of much of the pregnancy weight gain, development of depressive symptoms, and poor maternal-infant interactions, with potential risk to the health and safety of the newborn.

SUMMARY

The postpartum period is a time in a woman's life when sleep is greatly disturbed. The unpredictable sleep patterns of the newborn and intense infant care requirements contribute to the poor sleep and alteration of circadian rhythms in new mothers. New mothers attempt to counteract sleep loss at night through changes in their sleep schedules, including more frequent naps and sleeping later in the morning. Nevertheless, many women experience considerable daytime sleepiness and fatigue through the first few months. Socioeconomically disadvantaged women and racial and ethnic minorities—particularly Black mothers—have more postpartum sleep disturbances and experience higher rates of perinatal morbidity and mortality that must be addressed not only with targeted sleep interventions but also with systemic changes that address racism, bias, and differences in health care delivery. PPD affects between 10% and 20% of women, and those who report significant sleep loss and infant sleep problems are more likely to experience depression. Reports of excessive sleepiness, fatigue, or sleep loss should be evaluated by health care providers because of compromise in both maternal and infant well-being at a critical developmental phase and risk of PPD. Evaluation for sleep disturbance and depression should be a part of routine postpartum assessments, and advice related to optimizing sleep should be provided. Only a few studies have investigated the feasibility and efficacy of improving maternal sleep in the postpartum period, but results are promising. More work focused on improving sleep in new mothers and fathers is needed.

SELECTED READINGS

Doering JJ, Szabo A, Goyal D, et al. Sleep quality and quantity in low-income postpartum women. *MCN Am J Matern Child Nurs*. 2017;42:166–172.

Haddad S, Dennis C-L, Shah PS, et al. Sleep in parents of preterm infants: a systematic review. *Midwifery*. 2019;73:35–48.

Hall WA, et al. A randomized controlled trial of an intervention for infants' behavioral sleep problems. *BMC Pediatr*. 2015. https://doi.org/10.1186/s12887-015-0492-7.

Hiscock H, et al. Improving infant sleep and maternal mental health: a cluster randomised trial. *Arch Dis Child*. 2007;92:952–958.

King LS, Rangel E, Simpson N, et al. Mothers' postpartum sleep disturbance is associated with the ability to sustain sensitivity toward infants. *Sleep Med*. 2020. https://doi.org/10.1016/j.sleep.2019.07.017.

Lee KA, Gay CL. Can modifications to the bedroom environment improve the sleep of new parents? Two randomized controlled trials. *Res Nurs Health*. 2011;34:7–19.

Moon RY, Darnall RA, Feldman-Winter L, et al. SIDS and other sleep-related infant deaths: evidence base for 2016 updated recommendations for a safe infant sleeping environment. *Pediatrics*. 2016. https://doi.org/10.1542/peds.2016-2940.

Obeysekare JL, et al. Delayed sleep timing and circadian rhythms in pregnancy and transdiagnostic symptoms associated with postpartum depression. *Transl Psychiatry*. 2020. https://doi.org/10.1038/s41398-020-0683-3.

Okun ML, Mancuso RA, Hobel CJ, et al. Poor sleep quality increases symptoms of depression and anxiety in postpartum women. *J Behav Med*. 2018;41:703–710.

Signal TL, et al. Prevalence of abnormal sleep duration and excessive daytime sleepiness in pregnancy and the role of socio-demographic factors: comparing pregnant women with women in the general population. *Sleep Med*. 2014. https://doi.org/10.1016/j.sleep.2014.07.007.

Volkovich E, Bar-Kalifa E, Meiri G, et al. Mother-infant sleep patterns and parental functioning of room-sharing and solitary-sleeping families: a longitudinal study from 3 to 18 months. *Sleep*. 2018. https://doi.org/10.1093/sleep/zsx207.

A complete reference list can be found online at ExpertConsult.com.

Chapter 189

Sleep and Menopause

Fiona C. Baker; Massimiliano de Zambotti; Shadab Rahman; Hadine Joffe

Chapter Highlights

- The prevalence of sleep disturbances, especially difficulty maintaining sleep, escalates as women go through the menopause transition. Hot flashes are the most important contributor to the increase in sleep disturbances.
- Sleep disturbances during the menopause transition exhibit racial differences and affect quality of life, productivity, and health care utilization.
- Depression increases in prevalence as women approach menopause. It may contribute to poor sleep and/or develop secondarily to disrupted sleep.
- Cognitive behavioral therapy for insomnia improves insomnia symptoms in peri- and postmenopausal women, including those with hot flashes. In women with severe hot flashes, hormone and nonhormonal therapies, such as selective serotonin reuptake inhibitors, are effective at reducing hot flashes and in turn, may improve sleep.
- The prevalence of sleep-disordered breathing increases postmenopause, attributed to weight gain, changes in adipose tissue disposition, aging, and declines in reproductive hormones that can adversely affect the upper airway. The preferred treatment is continuous positive airway pressure along with weight loss and exercise programs.
- Coincident with the transition to menopause, as women age there is an increased prevalence of clinical conditions such as breast cancer, arthritis, fibromyalgia, and hypothyroidism. These clinical conditions or their treatments can adversely affect sleep. Sleep disturbances associated with these conditions may be further exacerbated by menopausal symptoms such as hot flashes.

PHASES OF THE MENOPAUSE TRANSITION

Menopause is the anchor point of a woman's transition during midlife to nonreproductive status and is confirmed to be present after 12 months of amenorrhea. The median age at onset of the menopause transition is 47 years, and the median age for the final menstrual period (FMP) is 51.4 years[1] but can range between 40 and 58 years of age. For many years, menopause was considered to be simply a consequence of depleted ovarian follicles (primary source of estrogen and progesterone). Today, however, menopause is recognized as a transitional process consisting of complex and interactive changes in the central nervous and endocrine systems, beginning years before complete cessation of menstruation and continuing for several years thereafter.[2]

The Stages of Reproductive Aging Workshop (STRAW) developed a menopause staging system to describe reproductive aging through menopause[3,4] (Figure 189.1). The menopause transition is divided into early (increased variability in menstrual cycle length) and late (amenorrhea for ≥60 days) stages.[3] The term perimenopause describes the menopause transition and first year of postmenopause. Vasomotor symptoms (VMS; hot flashes and night sweats) are more prominent during the late menopause transition. A hot flash is a sudden, transient sensation of moderate-intense heat that usually begins in the upper body. It is characterized by peripheral vasodilation and increased sweating and is primarily a thermoregulatory phenomenon.[5]

Postmenopause begins 1 year after the final menstrual period and is divided into an early stage lasting 5 to 8 years until levels of estradiol and follicle-stimulating hormone (FSH) stabilize, and a late stage when reproductive hormone changes are limited.[3] During the first 2 years postmenopause, FSH levels continue to increase, estradiol may rarely be produced, and VMS are most likely to occur. In postmenopausal women, VMS persist,[6] cumulatively burdening them for a median of 7 to 10 years across the menopause transition and postmenopause.[6,7]

Menopause is a universal phenomenon, but the timing and duration of these transitional stages and associated symptoms vary greatly between women and cannot be easily predicted. Midlife (middle age) is considered to be between 40 and 60 years of age, but there is no "generic" midlife woman.[8] In addition to the complexity of menopausal stages and hormonal fluctuations, midlife women may have young children at home, have grown children leaving home, and be caring for elderly parents or spouses. Other common challenges and new-onset problems in this age group include increasing career demands, changes in lifestyle, weight gain, and chronic health conditions. These scenarios all can adversely affect a woman's sleep during menopause.

Menarche (at start of stage −5) — FMP (0) (at start of stage +1a)

Stage	−5	−4	−3b	−3a	−2	−1	+1 a	+1b	+1c	+2
Terminology	**Reproductive**				**Menopausal transition**		**Postmenopause**			
	Early	Peak	Late		Early	Late	Early			Late
					Perimenopause					
Duration	*variable*				*variable*	1-3 years	2 years (1+1)		3-6 years	*Remaining lifespan*
Principal criteria										
Menstrual cycle	Variable to regular	Regular	Regular	Subtle changes in flow length	*Variable length* persistent ≥7-day difference in length at consecutive cycles	Interval of *amenorrhea* of ≥60 days				
Supportive criteria										
Endocrine										
FSH			Low	Variable*	↑ Variable*	↑ >25 IU/L**	↑ Variable*		Stabilize	
AMH			Low	Low	Low	Low	Low		Very low	
Inhibin B				Low	Low	Low	Low		Very low	
Antrial follicle count			Low	Low	Low	Low	Very low		Very low	
Descriptive characteristics										
Symptoms						Vasomotor symptoms *Likely*	Vasomotor symptoms *Most likely*			Increasing symptoms of urogenital atrophy

* Blood draw on cycle days 2-5 ↑ = elevated
** Approximate expected level based on assays using current international pituitary standard

Figure 189.1 The Stages of Reproductive Aging Workshop + 10 staging system for reproductive aging in women. The final menstrual period (FMP) is retrospectively confirmed after 12 months of no menstrual bleeding (amenorrhea) and a woman is considered to be early postmenopausal for the next 5 to 8 years (+1a, b, and c) before becoming late postmenopausal (+2) for the duration of her life. Before permanent cessation of menstrual cycles, women vary in the duration of their cycles during the stage known as the menopause transition. Early menopause transition is marked by increased variability in menstrual cycle length (persistent difference of ≥7 days in the length of consecutive cycles). The late menopause transition is marked by the occurrence of amenorrhea of 60 days or longer, usually accompanied by intermittent increases in follicle-stimulating hormone (FSH) level to greater than 25 IU/L. Perimenopause encompasses the menopause transition and first year postmenopause. Hot flashes and night sweats are most likely in the late menopause transition and early postmenopause. (From Harlow SD, Gass M, Hall JE, et al.; STRAW + 10 Collaborative Group. Executive summary of the Stages of Reproductive Aging Workshop + 10: addressing the unfinished agenda of staging reproductive aging. Menopause, 2012;19.)

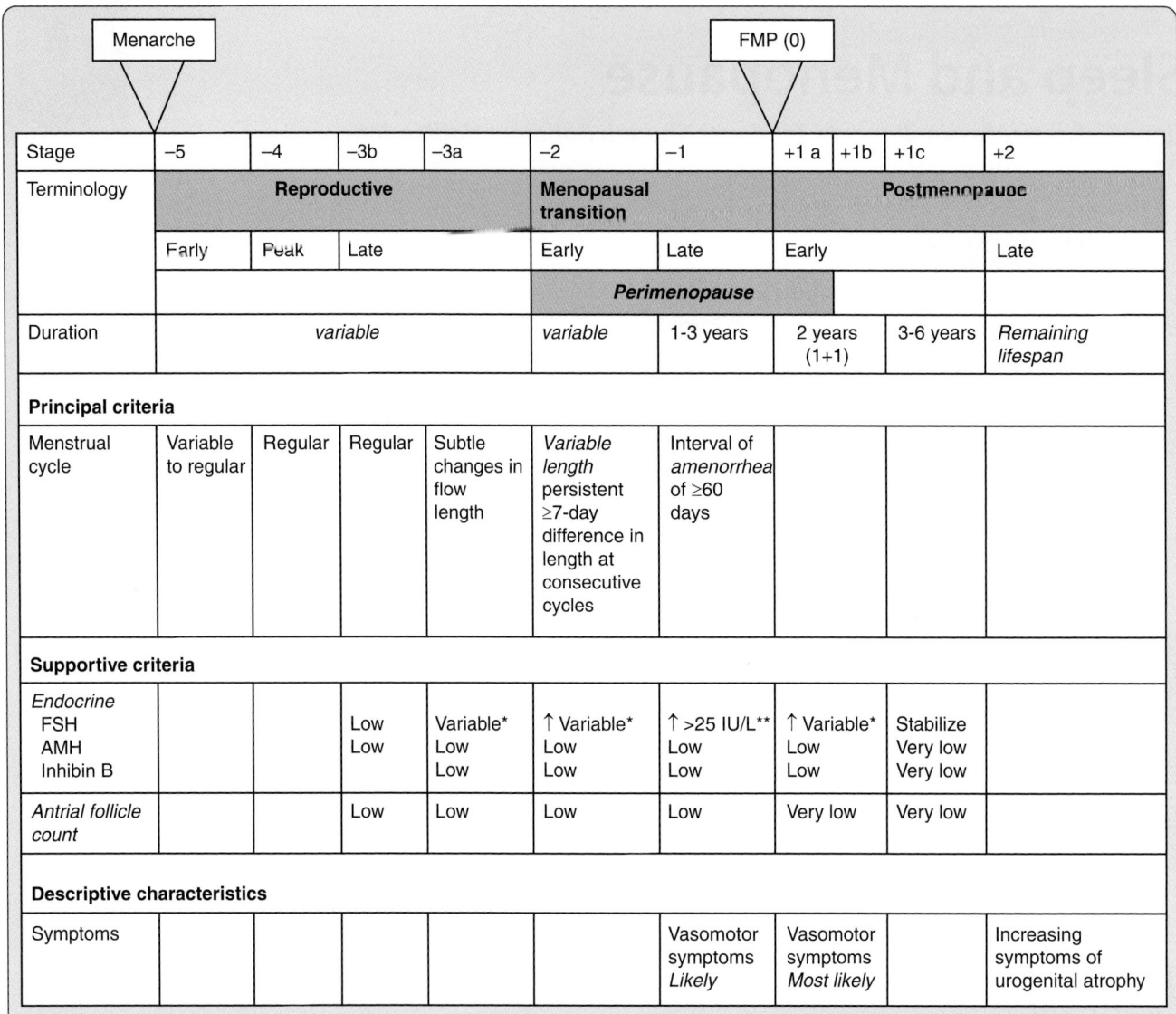

Surgical Menopause

Menopause can be induced by hysterectomy only when it is accompanied by a bilateral oophorectomy (removal of both ovaries). A bilateral oophorectomy induces an abrupt cessation of any ovarian hormone secretion, leading to a decline in estradiol and increased likelihood of menopausal symptoms. Although risk status for VMS may differ between women who undergo hysterectomy with ovarian conservation and those who have had a bilateral oophorectomy,[9] most studies have combined these two groups of women into a "surgical menopause" group and compared them with women who experience natural menopause.

SLEEP PATTERNS ACROSS THE MENOPAUSE TRANSITION

Surveys and Self-Reported Sleep Measures

Population surveys show that sleep problems are more common in midlife women during the menopause transition and postmenopause compared with premenopause.[10-14] Intermittent

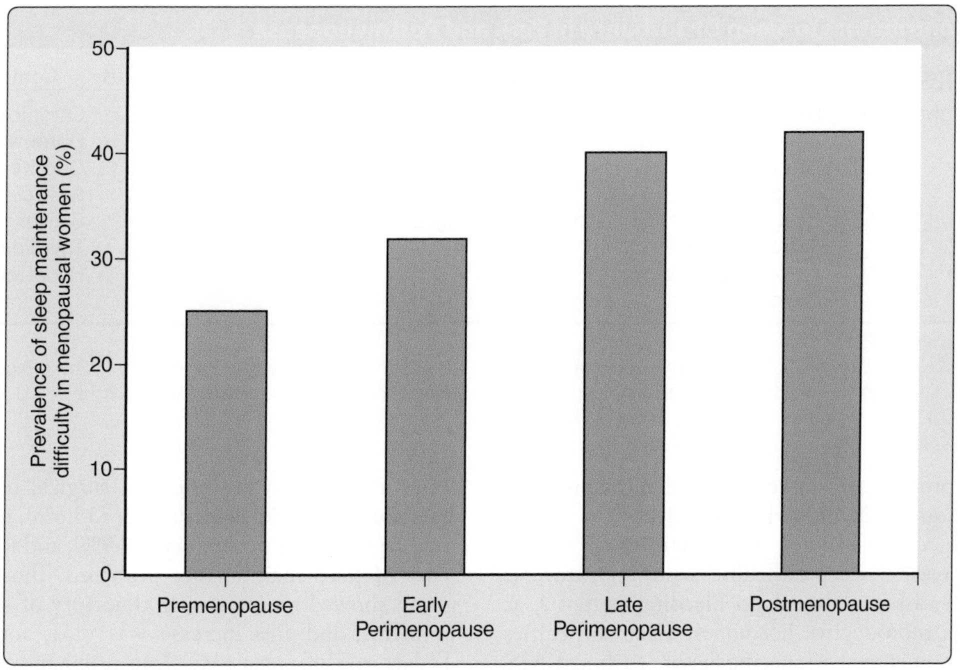

Figure 189.2 Percentage of women participating in the Study of Women's Health Across the Nation (SWAN) (*n* = 3045) reporting difficulty maintaining sleep at least three times per week in the preceding 2 weeks as they progress through the menopause transition. Women in transition from pre- to early menopause were more likely to have difficulty maintaining sleep than women who stayed premenopausal. Women in transition from early to late menopause also were more likely to have difficulty maintaining sleep. (Data from Kravitz HM, Zhao X, Bromberger JT, et al. Sleep disturbance during the menopausal transition in a multi-ethnic community sample of women. *Sleep.* 2008;31:979–90.)

awakenings are the most common sleep complaint and one of the most bothersome symptoms.[1,15] In the multicenter Study of Women's Health Across the Nation (SWAN), the perimenopausal state (compared with premenopause) was associated with greater odds of trouble sleeping, even after adjusting for age and ethnicity.[16,17] Results from cross-sectional analyses have been confirmed by longitudinal studies, which have shown an increase in sleep problems across the menopause transition.[1,18-20] SWAN found an increase in sleep difficulties, particularly due to frequent awakenings, as women transitioned from pre- to early peri-menopause and from early to late peri-menopause (see Figure 189.2).[21] Similarly, the Australian Longitudinal Study on Women's Health found that difficulty sleeping was associated with menopause status, but not age, after adjusting for several confounders including mental health score and night sweats.[18]

Some investigators have examined whether there are distinct symptom-based clusters of women or trajectories of symptom profiles, including sleep difficulties, across the menopause transition. Premenopausal sleep status predicts later poor sleep: women with moderate/severe poor sleep when premenopausal are approximately 3.5 times more likely to have poor sleep around the final menstrual period compared with those with no poor sleep at baseline.[22] Longitudinal analyses of SWAN data[23] showed four distinct trajectories for waking several times per night (at least three nights per week) across the menopause transition, with low (37.9%), moderate (28.4%), increasing (15.3%), and high (18.4%) prevalence trajectories. A low prevalence of waking several times per night before menopause, which accounted for 53% of the women, predicted a pattern of low prevalence into postmenopause. In contrast, sleep problems persisted into postmenopause in the groups of women with moderate and high trajectories.[23] Other sleep problems (trouble falling asleep, early morning awakening), as well as frequent VMS were strongly associated with frequent nocturnal awakenings that persisted into postmenopause.

In a different analysis of SWAN ratings of 58 symptoms (including mood, sleep, pain, hot flashes) collected over a 16-year period, using latent classes, six symptom classes emerged, ranging from highly to moderately symptomatic across most symptoms to moderately or mildly symptomatic for a subset of symptoms, to asymptomatic.[24] Sleep and fatigue symptoms were present in each symptom cluster, with varying degrees of severity, and tended to cluster with VMS. Overall, although symptoms improved or worsened for some women, most women remained in their same class from baseline (premenopausal), through the menopause transition, and into postmenopause.[24] Authors suggest that clustering of symptoms could reflect common underlying mechanisms.[24] Critically, women reporting financial strain had more than a fourfold increased odds of being in the moderate/severe symptom classes.

As described previously in this chapter, menopausal stages correspond with underlying changes in the reproductive hormone profile. SWAN tracked the relationship between hormone changes and reported sleep difficulties. Declining estrogen (estradiol) and increasing FSH levels were both associated with higher odds of frequent awakenings across the menopause transition[21] and a greater rate of change in FSH was associated with poorer sleep quality.[25] A steeper slope of decline in estradiol across menopause was also associated with

Table 189.1 Contributors to Sleep Disturbance in Peri- and Postmenopause

Menopause-Specific	General	Sleep Disorders	Mental Health Issues	Comorbid Illnesses
Hot flashes and night sweats ↓ Estradiol ↑ FSH ↓ Inhibin B ↑ Testosterone	Personal life stress Age-related factors Lifestyle factors (e.g., caffeine consumption) Socioeconomic and work-related factors (e.g., job strain)	Insomnia disorder Obstructive sleep apnea Periodic limb movement disorder Restless legs syndrome	Depression Anxiety	Chronic pain Fibromyalgia Obesity Gastroesophageal reflux Cancer Thyroid disease Hypertension

FSH, Follicle-stimulating hormone.
Data from Joffe H, Massler A, Sharkey KM. Evaluation and management of sleep disturbance during the menopause transition. *Semin Reprod Med.* 2010;28:404–21 and Baker FC, Lampio L, Saaresranta T, Polo-Kantola P. Sleep and sleep disorders in the menopausal transition. *Sleep Med Clin.* 2018;13:443–56.

more severe sleep problems in women enrolled in the prospective Melbourne Women's Midlife Health Project.[26]

Taken together, cross-sectional and longitudinal studies have found an increase in sleep difficulties as women traverse menopausal stages, assessed based on bleeding patterns, as well as changes in reproductive hormones. Sleep difficulties have been linked to menopause-specific factors such as VMS, as well as other factors including depressed mood, poor health, personal and work-related stress, and socioeconomic status (Table 189.1). Personality traits (e.g., neuroticism) have also been linked with insomnia symptoms that arise during the menopause transition.[27]

Sleep and Surgical Menopause

Surgical menopause (hysterectomy with or without bilateral oophorectomy) has been linked with poor sleep, as well as other menopausal symptoms.[1,19,28] In a cross-sectional analysis of the SWAN cohort, a sample of women who had a bilateral oophorectomy and who were not using hormone therapy had the highest prevalence of sleep difficulty, independent of age or years since surgery.[16] This effect was related to VMS. In a retrospective analysis of a different cohort of postmenopausal women, the group of women who had gone through surgical menopause had a greater likelihood of having insomnia symptoms (odds ratio: 2.1 [95% confidence interval: 1.06–4.3]) compared with the group who had gone through natural menopause.[29] Women who undergo bilateral oophorectomy are at increased risk for more severe VMS than women in natural menopause,[9] which could have a greater effect on sleep. Disturbed sleep and fatigue are common postoperative symptoms after hysterectomy[30]; however, women who had a hysterectomy (with or without oophorectomy) were still more likely than other midlife women to complain of trouble sleeping even years after surgery,[31] suggesting higher vulnerability to sleep difficulties in these women. Increased sleep disturbances after surgical menopause are not necessarily due only to abrupt changes in reproductive hormone levels but could also be related to a worse psychological health profile before menopause or worse health after hysterectomy compared with women with natural menopause.[19]

Longitudinal analysis of SWAN data from women tracked for a median of 5 years before and 7 years after surgical menopause (oophorectomy, at age 51.2 ± 4.0 years) supports the idea that at least some women may already have preexisting sleep problems before surgery: different trajectories were apparent for sleep maintenance problems (waking several times at night) in women with surgical menopause.[32] Four trajectories were identified: high (13.6%), moderate (33.0%), increasing during presurgery (19.9%), and low (33.5%) prevalence of sleep maintenance problems. Thus only 20% of the group showed an increasing trajectory of sleep maintenance problems, and this increase was most apparent presurgery. Trajectories of presurgery sleep problems continued postsurgery for all groups, with presurgery sleep maintenance problems persisting for years postsurgery.[32] Frequent VMS and early morning awakening were significantly associated with sleep maintenance problems postsurgery.

Racial and Ethnic Factors

There is some evidence that race and ethnicity influence the extent of sleep disturbances across the menopause transition. SWAN researchers showed that the prevalence of difficulty sleeping was lowest in midlife women of Japanese origin (28.2%) and highest in midlife Caucasian women (40.3%).[33] Also, a meta-analysis of 24 studies reported that peri-, post-, and surgical-menopausal White and Asian women, but not Hispanic women, have increased odds of sleep disturbance relative to premenopausal women.[34] In an analysis of racial/ethnic differences in sleep diary and actigraphy data from mostly postmenopausal SWAN participants, Whites slept the longest of all groups and had less wakefulness after sleep onset than Blacks and Latinx. They also reported a better sleep quality than Blacks, Chinese, and Japanese in America.[35] Major mediators of these associations were health problems, stress, financial hardship, and emotional well-being. Taking advantage of the longitudinal SWAN data set, investigators also explored mediators that changed from the premenopausal baseline assessment until the postmenopausal assessment, 18 years later. Increasing health problems was a significant mediator for the difference in wakefulness after sleep onset in Hispanics and Blacks, relative to Whites, and increasing number of stressors mediated differences in sleep duration for Hispanics or Japanese Americans, relative to Whites.[35] Midlife changes in health and stress may be a target for prevention of poor sleep postmenopause,[35] and are particularly relevant in minority women.

Objective Sleep Measures

Although there is strong evidence from epidemiologic studies showing an increase in self-reported sleep difficulties during menopause transition and early postmenopause, findings from objective polysomnographic (PSG) studies are mixed.[10]

Two large cross-sectional cohort studies (Wisconsin Sleep Cohort and SWAN), which controlled for several confounding factors, did not find evidence of poorer PSG-defined sleep in peri- or postmenopausal women. In fact, the Wisconsin Sleep Cohort Study found that peri- and postmenopausal women had better PSG sleep, including more slow wave sleep, than premenopausal women.[36] SWAN found no differences in PSG measures of sleep efficiency and sleep stages in peri- versus premenopausal women; however, women in late-perimenopause and postmenopause had more high-frequency beta electroencephalogram (EEG) activity during sleep (a marker of cortical hyperarousal), compared with premenopausal and early-perimenopausal women.[37] Increased beta EEG activity during sleep was partially related to higher frequency of self-reported VMS.[37]

Differences in PSG sleep parameters across midlife have been examined in relation to reproductive hormonal differences. A theoretical basis for the menopausal hormone changes having the potential to affect sleep structure comes from studies in animals showing that reproductive hormones, specifically progesterone and estradiol, affect sleep-wake regulation, although the precise mechanisms remain unclear.[38] SWAN data showed that a more rapid rate of change in FSH over a 5 to 7-year period was associated with higher percentage of slow wave sleep and a longer total sleep time.[25] At the same time, as described previously in this chapter, a greater rate of change in FSH was associated with a poorer subjective sleep quality.[25] Change in estradiol was unrelated to any PSG measures, although a lower estradiol/testosterone ratio (sampled 3–6 months before the sleep study) was associated with less wakefulness after sleep onset.[25] A cross-sectional analysis of premenopausal and early menopause transition women found a positive association between higher FSH levels and more wakefulness after sleep onset, but not with other sleep measures such as slow wave sleep.[39] These data, although not entirely consistent in the direction of the relationships found, support an interaction between the reproductive and sleep-wake regulatory systems.

In a longitudinal investigation, compared with the premenopausal visit 6 years prior, women in the menopause transition or postmenopause had a shorter total sleep time, lower sleep efficiency, and more awakenings, after adjusting for VMS, body mass index (BMI), and mood.[40] These changes in sleep were predicted by advancing age and not by an increase in FSH.[40] In contrast, increasing FSH was associated with a greater proportion of slow wave sleep (although not with slow wave EEG activity), which may reflect an adaptive change to counteract age-related sleep fragmentation.[40] Similarly, Kalleinen and colleagues showed that age had a greater effect on PSG recorded sleep than menopause status: although women in late-reproductive stage (age 45–51 years) and postmenopausal women had similar PSG measures, their objective sleep quality was much poorer than that of a group of young women.[41] SWAN reported that actigraphic sleep duration increased by 20 minutes and wakefulness after sleep onset decreased by 7.6 minutes across a 12-year period, spanning pre-/perimenopause into postmenopause, after adjusting for several covariates.[42] The severity of VMS, being postmenopausal, single, having some college education, and of Black race/ethnicity were all related to greater wakefulness after sleep onset. Of note, women as a group had short sleep duration at baseline (5.92 ± 1.0 hours). These data show that on average, women show some small improvements in objective sleep duration from midlife into early old age although there is heterogeneity in the changes of sleep patterns with age.

Taken together, objective data indicate subtle differences in sleep microstructure but few consistent differences in macrostructure according to menopausal stage and with postmenopausal aging. The presence of disruptive menopausal symptoms (e.g., VMS) rather than menopausal stage per se is a key factor in influencing objective sleep measures.

Circadian Rhythms during Menopause

One prominent theory of reproductive aging is that menopause results from the aging of multiple pacemakers in the brain and ovaries that control and coordinate a variety of circadian and other rhythms, including the sleep-wake cycle.[2] Numerous studies have shown estrogen's effect on circadian rhythms in female mammals.[38] These data suggest that circadian control of sleep might be perturbed by menopause, and preliminary data from studies in women suggest a change in the circadian system. For example, under constant routine conditions, postmenopausal women have an advanced melatonin acrophase time and tend to have an earlier melatonin onset compared with late-reproductive stage women, possibly as a consequence of menopausal hormone changes, although an effect of chronologic aging cannot be completely excluded.[43] An advanced circadian phase could contribute to more fragmented sleep or early morning awakening in postmenopausal women. As in other populations, markers of later circadian phase have been linked to higher anxiety[44] and depression[45] in menopausal women.

SLEEP DISTURBANCE ASSOCIATED WITH VASOMOTOR SYMPTOMS

Self-Reports of Sleep Disturbance

There is substantial individual variability in the frequency of hot flashes both between women, and within women over the course of the menopause transition and post menopause. This is likely a result of the variation between individuals in hypothalamic thermoregulatory activity and higher cortical activity in the insula.[46] Evidence suggests that inputs to the gonadotropin pulse regulator from KNDy (kisspeptin, neurokinin B, and dynorphin) neurons in the hypothalamus also contribute to VMS during the menopause transition.[47] A hot flash typically lasts a few minutes but can reoccur frequently throughout the day and night in some women. Perceived intensity of the flash can vary widely, from mild to severely disruptive. Some women have 20 or more hot flashes each day, whereas others report only 1 or 2 per week.

Longitudinal SWAN data showed the median duration of reported frequent VMS (≥6 days over the previous 2 weeks) is 7.4 years, with symptoms continuing a median of 4.5 years after the final menstrual period,[6] although there is substantial variability in timing and trajectories of VMS between subgroups of women.[48-50] In SWAN, women first reporting VMS in pre- or early perimenopause and Black women had the longest duration of frequent VMS.[6] Women with early onset of hot flashes have greater risk for subclinical cardiovascular disease.[51] Older age, changes in reproductive hormonal levels, surgical menopause, smoking, obesity, depression, anxiety, and heightened somatic attunement increase the likelihood of VMS.[52] The prevalence of VMS also varies by racial/ethnic groups, with SWAN data showing that Black women are most likely, and Chinese- and Japanese American least likely, to report VMS.[52] It is not clear whether these differences are the result of differences in lifestyle stressors, diet, cultural factors, or unidentified biologic factors,[51] although genetic variability plays a role.[54]

Self-reported VMS are consistently associated with poorer self-reported sleep quality and chronic insomnia.[1,16,17,55] Women with frequent and bothersome VMS, compared with those without, are more likely to report frequent nocturnal awakenings[33,56] and conversely, treatment that leads to a reduction of at least five hot flashes per day is associated with a clinically meaningful reduction in sleep problems.[57]

Objective Measures of Sleep

Although earlier studies investigating associations between hot flashes and objective sleep had mixed findings, more recent investigations with stronger designs showed a clear association between hot flashes and objectively measured poor sleep quality.[12] Inconsistencies in some studies are likely related to differences in methodology. For example, some studies related sleep with measures of hot flash frequency and severity recalled the following morning, which may be underreported. Others related sleep with objective measures of hot flashes (increased sternal skin conductance due to a sweat response), considered the gold-standard method of measuring hot flash frequency,[58] but differed in the way they analyzed windows of hot flashes and awakenings. Also, most studies have been observational, cross-sectional, and did not distinguish daytime from nighttime hot flashes. In a controlled model of new-onset hot flashes based on treatment of young premenopausal women with a gonadotropin-releasing hormone agonist (GnRHa) that simulates menopause, nocturnal hot flashes were definitively linked with more PSG awakenings, greater wake time after sleep onset, and more stage 1 sleep.[59] These results were seen when hot flashes were measured by both self-report in the morning and by physiologic changes in skin conductance during the night. These experimental data validate the subjective complaint of poor sleep quality associated with menopausal hot flashes. The magnitude of sleep fragmentation appears to be proportional to the number of nocturnal hot flashes, whereas daytime hot flashes show no association with objective or subjective sleep quality.[59] This finding suggests that interindividual variability in the link between hot flashes and sleep disruption may in part be explained by variability in the proportion of hot flashes experienced at night, as well as the absolute number of nocturnal hot flashes.

In a study of objective hot flashes and PSG sleep in women in the menopause transition, the majority of hot flashes (69%) were associated with awakenings.[60] Further, hot flash–associated wake time was responsible for more than 25% of objective total wakefulness at night, with substantial between-subject variability in the extent of this effect on sleep. Hot flash–associated wake time correlated with self-reported estimates of wakefulness.[60] Although individual nocturnal hot flash and wake pairs contribute to wakefulness, women with hot flashes also accrue wake time and sleep-stage transitions during periods of sleep when they do not have hot flashes,[61] indicating that sleep disruption is not entirely explained by nocturnal hot flash events.

PSG studies have investigated distribution of hot flashes according to sleep stages. Hot flashes are more likely to occur in non–rapid eye movement (NREM) than rapid eye movement (REM) sleep, possibly owing to the inhibition of thermoregulatory responses in this stage.[60,62,63] Also, hot flashes are less likely to be associated with an awakening in REM sleep than in NREM sleep.[64] Finally, by inducing hot flashes via GnRHa administration in premenopausal women, after accounting for time spent in each sleep phase, Bianchi and colleagues[65] showed that hot flashes occur primarily in association with N1 (19%) and wakefulness (51%), and to a less extent in N2 (12%), N3 (12%), and REM (6%).

Studies have examined the effect of hot flashes on aspects of sleep other than traditional PSG measures. Campbell and colleagues[37] reported that beta EEG activity during sleep was related to menopausal status, a relationship that was partly explained by self-reported hot flash frequency. Hot flashes are also associated with changes in autonomic nervous system activity.[66-68] Importantly, the physiology and effect of nocturnal hot flashes differs accordingly to whether hot flashes are associated with sleep disruption. Sudden transient increases in systolic and diastolic blood pressure, and heart rate (~20% increase) are evident in relation to hot flashes associated with awakenings/arousals.[64] In contrast, drops in systolic blood pressure, possibly reflecting the heat dissipation response, and marginal increases in heart rate are found in relation to hot flashes occurring in undisturbed sleep,[64] as is also evident for hot flashes recorded when women are awake in the day.[69,70] Sympathetic activity increased for both types of hot flashes but was more pronounced in those hot flashes associated with sleep disruption.[64]

Hot flashes are linked with measures of subclinical and clinical cardiovascular disease (e.g., endothelial dysfunction, higher carotid intima media thickness, high blood pressure).[51,71-74] It is possible that multiple hot flashes throughout the night disrupt nocturnal autonomic nervous system and cardiovascular balance and, consequently, the restorative aspects of sleep.

Nocturnal hot flashes constitute an important component of sleep disturbance during midlife but not all women who have menopause-related sleep problems complain of hot flashes.[12] Sleep in midlife women may potentially be affected by a sleep-disordered breathing (SDB) problem, mood disturbance, or medical condition. It is therefore critical to evaluate other causes of sleep disruption in midlife women, many of which may co-occur with hot flashes.

PSYCHOLOGICAL SYMPTOMS AND SLEEP DISTURBANCE IN MENOPAUSE

Depression and Anxiety

Longitudinal studies show that depressive symptoms increase during the menopause transition,[75] with a small number of women experiencing a major depressive episode.[76] The first onset of depression can rarely occur in the menopause transition[77-79]; however, the vast majority of women who experience depression during this phase have a prior history of depression, and their illness episode represents a recurrent depression episode.[76]

Depressive symptoms in menopausal women are strongly linked to VMS,[12,80,81] but the association is selective for nocturnal, and not daytime, hot flashes,[82] suggesting that mood is not affected by bothersome experiences during the day but by nocturnal vasomotor disturbance. This association is independent of the sleep disruption caused by nocturnal hot flash events, which also contributes to depressive symptoms.[82] Sleep parameters linked with depressive symptoms in this population include more NREM arousals, time in stage N1, transitions to wake, and reduced sleep quality.[82]

Although fragmented sleep contributes to depression, depression also has a significant negative effect on sleep in general (see Chapter 164), and this is equally the case during menopause. Peri- and postmenopausal women with depression report worse sleep quality[83] and have more objectively measured sleep disturbance.[84] Compared with nondepressed women with hot flashes, women with concurrent hot flashes and depression spend less time in bed and have longer sleep onset latency, shorter total sleep time, and lower sleep efficiency rather than more frequent awakenings.[84] Peri- and postmenopausal women with major depression also have increased levels of nocturnal melatonin, as well as a phase delay in their melatonin secretion.[36]

Few studies have investigated the association between anxiety and sleep disturbance in perimenopausal women, and it remains unclear whether there is an increase in anxiety symptoms or anxiety disorder in women transitioning to menopause.[85] However, higher levels of anxiety[86,87] and perceived stress[16] have been linked with complaints of poor sleep quality in midlife women, and anxiety is also associated with PSG-measured longer sleep latency and lower sleep efficiency.[88]

Midlife Stress

Financial strain, a chronic stressor associated with lower socioeconomic status, was found to be an independent correlate of sleep complaints and lower sleep efficiency in SWAN study participants; financial strain, as well as other stressors, could interfere with sleep via stress pathways including negative affect and autonomic/endocrine dysregulation.[89] There are multiple stressors for midlife women including jobs, family responsibilities, relationships, and caring for sick or elderly relatives,[90] and these stressors affect sleep. Midlife women may consider sleep a low priority that competes with many other demands of motherhood, career, marriage, and caring for aging parents.[91] Conversely, disrupted or poor sleep quality could affect a woman's ability to cope with life stressors. It has been suggested that being symptomatic during menopause transition is itself a unique stressor and may compound preexisting stressors.[90]

SLEEP DISORDERS

Insomnia Disorder

Many women experience an increase in insomnia symptoms during the menopause transition and these symptoms are severe, persistent, and affect daytime functioning in about 25% of women, qualifying them for a diagnosis of insomnia disorder. Based on a large cross-sectional survey, 26% of perimenopausal women qualified for a diagnosis of insomnia, a substantially higher prevalence than the rate of insomnia disorder found in premenopausal (13%) and postmenopausal (14.4%) women.[55] Also, 31.8% of perimenopausal and postmenopausal women reported that their insomnia was related to menopause, with difficulty maintaining sleep being the predominant complaint. However, sleep-onset insomnia complaints are also more common during early postmenopause.[92]

Hot flashes are a major factor in the increased prevalence of insomnia disorder in midlife women[55,93] and may precipitate the development of insomnia in vulnerable women. For those with preexisting insomnia, the approach to menopause may exacerbate symptoms, with hot flashes precipitating further sleep disruption and possibly worsening their insomnia. Although there are some unique factors related to insomnia that develops in the context of menopause (e.g., hot flashes[60] and the altered hormonal environment[39]), women with insomnia in the menopause transition seem to also share traits common to other populations with insomnia. For example, personality traits (e.g., neuroticism), physiologic hyperarousal, and depressive and anxiety symptomatology have been documented in menopausal insomnia.[27,93-95] In addition, insomnia-related symptoms (e.g., depression[96]) are exacerbated across the menopause transition, and potentially act as precipitating factors in the onset of insomnia.

Although objective sleep alterations do not always accompany sleep complaints in general populations, objective sleep deficits have been identified in women with insomnia disorder in the menopause transition. For example, PSG sleep alterations were evident in peri- and postmenopausal woman with insomnia, but not in premenopausal women with insomnia.[97] Women with insomnia disorder that developed in the menopause transition have more in-bed wakefulness and awakenings, reduced sleeping time, and lower sleep efficiency compared with controls, with about 50% of insomnia sufferers having fewer than 6 hours of sleep, as recorded during an overnight PSG laboratory assessment.[93] In women with menopause-associated insomnia, autonomic and cardiovascular profiles are altered at night[95,98,99] but not during the day.[94] These data are in line with the growing attention given to the combination of insomnia and objective short sleep duration, considered the most severe phenotype of the disorder, being associated with inflammatory and cardiovascular risk markers.[100-102] They highlight the need for combination treatments that target insomnia and menopause-specific symptoms. In contrast to those with insomnia, women with hot flashes occurring in the absence of insomnia are more likely to have lengthening rather than shortening of their PSG sleep time.[21,36,65]

Sleep-Disordered Breathing

As women proceed through the menopause transition and beyond, they are at increased risk for developing SDB,[92,103] attributed to aging, as well as menopause-related factors. In a cohort of approximately 6100, postmenopausal women had approximately 48% higher odds of screening positive for obstructive sleep apnea (OSA), compared with pre-/perimenopausal women.[92] Moreover, the risk of developing OSA has been associated with the severity of self-reported VMS in midlife women, an association that persisted after adjusting for age, BMI, smoking status, and self-reported hypertension, even in a subgroup restricted to BMI less than 25 kg/m^2.[104] Results of a longitudinal PSG study in midlife women showed that SDB severity was 21% higher in perimenopausal women and 31% higher in postmenopausal women, relative to premenopausal women.[103] Among those who started perimenopause, the apnea-hypopnea index (AHI) increased by 4% for each additional year in the menopause transition.[103] Given emergence of cardiovascular disease risk in perimenopausal women, associations of OSA with hypertension and increased

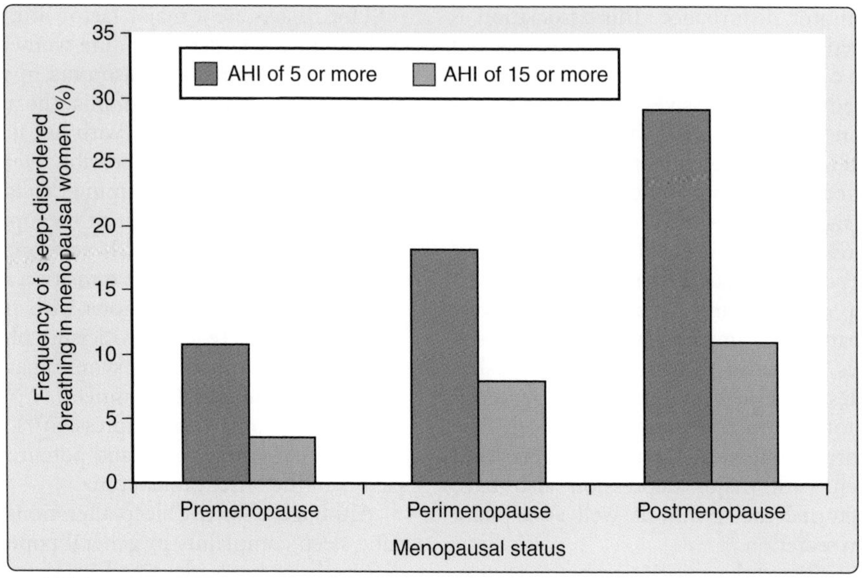

Figure 189.3 Prevalence of sleep-disordered breathing (SDB), indicated by apnea-hypopnea index (AHI) cut-off levels of 5 and 15 events/hour, in premenopausal (n = 498), perimenopausal (n = 125), and postmenopausal (n = 375) women who participated in the Wisconsin Sleep Cohort Study. Prevalence increased across menopausal groups. (Data from Young T, Finn L, Austin D, Peterson A. Menopausal status and sleep-disordered breathing in the Wisconsin Sleep Cohort Study. *Am J Respir Crit Care Med.* 2003;167:1181–5.)

arterial stiffness suggest that this treatable sleep disorder may affect cardiovascular health in women independent of physiologic changes associated with chronologic aging and the menopause transition.[105] These data highlight the importance of recognizing and treating SDB in midlife women.

The gender gap in prevalence of SDB is well documented,[106] although sex differences in clinical presentation of symptoms between men and women likely contribute to underdiagnosis in women.[107,108] Menopause has long been described as a risk factor for SDB[109] that may manifest as episodes of prolonged partial upper airway obstruction, with associated increases in carbon dioxide.[110] In studies with large samples of women that have controlled for important confounders influencing SDB severity, there is strong support for the hypothesis that menopause increases the risk of SDB.[111-113] Bixler and colleagues[111] found a ratio of one woman for every 3.3 men with apnea in their sample and this ratio fell to 1:1.44 when postmenopausal women were considered and matched with men by age and BMI. In an analysis of the women in the sample, the prevalence of mild SDB (defined as AHI 0–15, together with a self-report of moderate or severe snoring) and more severe SDB (AHI ≥15) was higher in postmenopausal women not using hormone therapy (HT) compared with premenopausal women, even after adjusting for age and BMI. In another large study, the prevalence of sleep apnea was higher in women over age 55 years, presumed to be postmenopausal (47%), compared with women under 45 years of age, presumed to be premenopausal (21%), even after controlling for BMI and neck circumference and confounding effect of age.[112] In addition to differential prevalence rates between men and women, there may be important disease comorbidities associated with each gender. For example, among a middle-aged to-older population, OSA severity, based on AHI, was associated with hypertension and depression exclusively in women, whereas diabetes was associated with OSA severity only in men.[114] These differences suggest that disease management plans may be further optimized based on sex.

Young and colleagues[113] examined cross-sectional and longitudinal PSG data collected on 589 middle-aged women participating in the Wisconsin Sleep Cohort Study. Results are shown in Figure 189.3. Postmenopausal women were 2.6 times more likely than premenopausal women to have SDB (AHI ≥5) and 3.5 times more likely to have more severe SDB (AHI ≥15). The odds of having SDB were not significantly higher for perimenopausal women compared with midlife premenopausal women. However, the data did suggest that the risk for SDB increases across the menopause transition. When women were stratified on years since last menstrual period, there was a significant linear trend toward increased risk for AHI of 5 or greater, with increasing postmenopause duration up to 5 years. Even when including known risk factors for SDB in analysis (age, BMI, smoking, and alcohol use), menopause status remained an independent risk factor for SDB.

Several factors could contribute to increased risk of SDB after menopause. An important factor is weight gain or a change in the distribution of adipose tissue, which progressively accumulates in the upper part of the body after menopause.[115] Nationally representative data from the US National Health and Nutrition Examination Survey (NHANES) found that nearly 70% of women in the perimenopausal age range (40–59 years) are either overweight or obese compared with approximately 52% of women in the premenopausal age range (20–39 years).[116] After menopause, there is also a preferential increase in intraabdominal or visceral deposition of fat relative to other areas of the body,[117] which may partially be due to menopause-related hormonal changes (HT decreases the shift to visceral adiposity and can lower serum lipid levels).[118,119] Both excess weight[120] and visceral fat have strong relationships with SDB, and visceral fat is believed by some to be the principal culprit leading to SDB.[121] Declining progesterone and estrogen levels could also contribute to increased incidence of SDB after menopause.[109] Progesterone increases ventilatory drive and affects upper airway dilatory muscles.[122] Popovic and White[123] found that genioglossus muscle activity was highest in the luteal phase of the menstrual cycle (high progesterone) in young women and lowest in postmenopausal women, although upper airway resistance did not differ between the groups. Muscle activity increased in the postmenopausal women following combined HT. Lower levels of estradiol are also associated with a greater risk of OSA after menopause.[124] Progesterone's stimulatory effect on respiration is thought to be mediated through estrogen-dependent receptors[125]; hence the menopausal-decline in both hormones could affect respiration.

Given the evidence of a protective role of progesterone on ventilation, together with epidemiologic evidence of the association between menopause and increased risk of SDB, it might be expected that HT would be effective at preventing or treating SDB. Indeed, in epidemiologic studies, HT has been associated with a lower prevalence of sleep apnea in postmenopausal women.[111,113] This relationship was confirmed in the Sleep Heart Health Study[126] even after controlling for well-documented healthy-user effect differences (e.g., education level, body weight, health awareness) between women who used HT and those who did not. However, clinical trials that evaluated effects of estrogens, progesterone, or both on SDB in postmenopausal women have produced conflicting results.[127] Although exogenous progesterone administration in postmenopausal women with SDB was associated with improved nocturnal ventilation in a number of studies, there was no significant change in the number of apneas or hypopneas.[124,128,129] The wide variability in responses to HT among individual women suggests that, if these hormones affect SDB, they do so through a specific mechanism that is not common to all cases of SDB. Given the health risks associated with using HT, continuous positive airway pressure remains the treatment of choice for SDB in peri- and postmenopausal women. Also, weight loss and exercise (specifically to reduce adiposity) should be strongly considered for any midlife or postmenopausal woman's SDB treatment plan.

Restless Legs Syndrome and Periodic Limb Movement Disorder

The prevalence of restless legs syndrome (RLS) and periodic limb movement disorder (PLMD) increases with age, and women are 37% more likely to report RLS symptoms compared with men.[130] Women are also more likely than men to report the early onset form of RLS (symptoms experienced younger than 45 years of age). While RLS and PLMD have been strongly linked with female reproductive life events such as pregnancy (see Chapters 186), an association between RLS or PLMD and the hormonal changes of menopause is less clear.[92]

Based on survey data, most female patients with RLS (69%) retrospectively reported a worsening of their symptoms after menopause.[131] However, the prevalence of RLS in women increases with age,[132] which makes it difficult to disentangle the relationship between RLS and menopause per se. In a population study of Swedish women, a strong association was found between VMS and RLS; however there was no relationship between use of HT and RLS.[132] The incidence of PLMD is high in postmenopausal women[133] and contributes to poor objective sleep quality in midlife women.[86] However, evidence from current studies does not support a strong link between PLMD and menopausal hormone changes. In a group of asymptomatic postmenopausal women, the incidence of periodic limb movements was unrelated to estradiol or FSH levels.[133] Further, short-term estrogen therapy did not alter the incidence or intensity of limb movements.[133] The increase in prevalence of RLS and PLMD after menopause may be related more to aging than to menopause transition.

MANAGEMENT OF SLEEP DIFFICULTIES IN MENOPAUSE

Estradiol levels fluctuate dramatically during the menopause transition and ultimately decline to very low levels postmenopause. With reduction in and ultimately cessation of ovulation, progesterone becomes less frequently produced. Consequently, estrogen therapy (ET) typically in combination with a progestin (together called hormone therapy, HT) was commonly prescribed for midlife and older women on a long-term basis in an effort to counter hormone deficiency and protect against osteoporosis, heart disease, and Alzheimer dementia. However, in 2003, the Women's Health Initiative clinical trial results abruptly reversed this practice by showing that use of a common HT regimen over an average of 7 years significantly increased risk of breast cancer, stroke, heart disease, and vascular dementia.[134]

Women are now being advised to avoid long-term exposure to HT and to use HT for only a short time to provide relief from hot flashes and improve quality of life during menopause transition. As a result, although historical data are available on the benefit of ET or HT for specific sleep conditions, hormonal treatments are rarely used as a first line of therapy for sleep conditions unrelated to VMS. In this section, we include information about the effects of HT, where available, on all sleep problems associated with menopause as these conditions may be concurrent and complicate hot flash-related sleep disturbance.

Hormone Therapy and Sleep

Multiple studies in midlife women without sleep complaints show that ET, with or without a progestin, as well as progestin therapy (PT) alone, improve perceived sleep quality[136] and, to a lesser extent, PSG indices of sleep quality.[15,16] When PSG measures were obtained in several small studies of midlife women without sleep complaints, some showed inconsistent and small benefits of ET or PT for sleep fragmentation measured, and others showed no benefit or a negative effect. There have been a limited number of investigations on effectiveness of HT for insomnia in midlife women, and some show improvement[137,138] while others show no effect[139] on perceived sleep quality and PSG measures. Inconsistent findings between studies may be attributed to differences in treatment duration, timing of treatment in relation to menopause transition, or even differences in HT formulations. Different preparations of HT improve sleep quality over placebo regardless of whether the estrogen is orally or transdermally administered.[136] Preliminary studies suggest benefit of natural progesterone over the synthetic progestin medroxyprogesterone on perceived sleep quality and selected PSG parameters.[12] One reason for these potential differences is that, unlike medroxyprogesterone acetate, micronized progesterone is metabolized to potent neurosteroids such as allopregnanolone and pregnanolone. These neurosteroids interact with the same brain gamma-aminobutyric acid (GABA) type A receptors as sedative-hypnotic medications, and they are soporific.[139]

When taken in the morning, natural progesterone can result in drowsiness,[140] particularly at higher doses. As a result, women on HT may be advised to take progesterone at night.

Mechanisms through which ET or HT may improve sleep are poorly understood. Animal models suggest that estrogen may increase homeostatic drive for sleep[141] and reduce synthesis of prostaglandins in the ventrolateral preoptic nucleus of the hypothalamus,[142] whereas the hypnotic effect of progestins is mediated through an effect on GABA-active metabolites.[143] As the greatest benefits of ET for sleep have been observed in women with co-occurring hot flashes, ET may improve sleep as an indirect consequence of its salutary effects on nocturnal hot flashes.[144]

In summary, ET and PT independently and together have positive effects on sleep quality in midlife and older women, independent of hot flashes. Data are more extensive and stronger for self-reported sleep problems than for PSG sleep measures, for which several small studies report mixed results. Data supporting the efficacy of HT for primary sleep disorders in midlife women are limited and do not support use of these interventions. Progesterone may also contribute potential adverse sedating effects as well. As a result, HT is not typically recommended for sleep problems unless hot flashes are thought to be the primary source of the sleep disruption.

Hormone Therapy for Sleep Disturbance Associated with Hot Flashes

Sleep disruption associated with hot flashes may be treated in several ways. ET has historically been the standard treatment. Numerous epidemiologic studies and several randomized clinical trials have shown that ET and HT reduce hot flashes and concurrently improve self-reported sleep quality,[12,13] although effect sizes have varied. PSG studies have generally replicated these findings. In women who experienced frequent hot flashes, ET decreased the number and duration of nighttime awakenings, increased REM sleep, and shortened sleep onset latency.[13] However, in several small studies of women with only mild or infrequent hot flashes, neither ET nor HT had a measurable effect on PSG measures of sleep. Recent data show efficacy of a novel treatment that combines estrogen therapy and a selective estrogen receptor modulator (SERM) for improved perceived sleep quality in women with hot flashes, particularly at lower doses of SERM.[145] Overall, HT can have a therapeutic effect on perceived sleep quality among women with hot flash–related sleep disruption.

Hormone Withdrawal

When HT is discontinued, it is commonly stopped abruptly. Sleep effects of withdrawal from HT are unknown, although abrupt estrogen withdrawal is shown to result in significant hot flashes[146,147] and would suggest sleep consequences with abrupt HT discontinuation. Among women who stop HT, sleep disturbance is an importance predictor of HT reinitiation.[148]

Selective Serotonin Reuptake Inhibitors, Serotonin and Norepinephrine Reuptake Inhibitors, and Gabapentin

Nonhormonal neuroactive pharmacotherapies have become established treatments for vasomotor symptoms, both in breast cancer patients and in healthy midlife women.[149] The vast majority of women enrolling in these hot flash clinical trials have comorbid insomnia symptoms, permitting investigation of the effects of these interventions on insomnia symptoms that commonly co-occur with hot flashes.[150] In recent trials, the serotonergic antidepressants escitalopram,[151] venlafaxine,[152] and paroxtine[153] have all been shown to be more effective than placebo in reducing insomnia symptoms and improving sleep quality. Although the magnitude of the beneficial effect on sleep symptoms is modest in some studies,[150] it was unexpected that sleep concerns would diminish, given that these agents can induce or exacerbate sleep problems in other populations receiving such treatments for mental illness.[154] Similar to serotonergic agents, gabapentin and pregabalin are neuroactive agents used to treat hot flashes, for which evidence also shows some benefit for sleep complaints.[155]

Hypnotics

Selective GABAergic agents (zolpidem, eszopiclone) improve sleep-onset[156,157] and sleep-maintenance[157,158] problems in women with vasomotor symptom–associated insomnia.[156-158] Randomized controlled trials show efficacy of zolpidem 10 mg[158] and eszopiclone 3 mg[156] for poor sleep quality and for sleep onset and sleep maintenance insomnia, resulting in improved quality of life. For those with hot flashes, eszopiclone also reduces the number of hot flashes reported at night, but not during the day,[157] suggesting that it helps women sleep through their hot flashes, although there may be a direct therapeutic benefit for hot flashes when drug levels are high. Zolpidem may augment the therapeutic effect of selective serotonin reuptake inhibitors (SSRI)/ serotonin and norepinephrine reuptake inhibitors (SNRIs) on sleep disruption in women with hot flashes, resulting in increased quality of life.[159] although these selective GABAergic therapies are effective, they should be dosed cautiously and the duration of their use minimized in midlife women. Women are more likely than men to have detectable zolpidem levels on the morning after ingestion, resulting in next-day slowed reaction time.[160]

Cognitive Behavior Therapy and Alternative Therapies

Randomized trials assessing the efficacy of cognitive behavioral therapy for insomnia (CBT-I) in menopause-related insomnia, including in women with hot flashes, show a robust benefit of CBT-I over behavioral control interventions,[161,162] and that CBT-I has a larger beneficial effect on insomnia symptoms in women with hot flashes than does ET, SSRI, SNRI, yoga, or exercise.[150] Cognitive behavioral therapy directed at hot flashes also shows improvement of sleep symptoms in breast cancer survivors.[163] Efficacy of these behavioral interventions has been demonstrated through online and telephone-based approaches to maximize access.[161,163] Although complementary and behavioral therapies may reduce hot flash frequency or severity in some women,[164,165] data from randomized clinical trials do not support the efficacy of treatments such as soy, black cohosh, omega-3, yoga, or exercise for VMS.[166-168] Exercise has a modest salutary effect on insomnia symptoms in women assigned to an exercise regimen to treat hot flashes.[169]

CLINICAL CONDITIONS WITH POTENTIAL EFFECTS ON SLEEP

As women age, coincident with the onset of menopause, health conditions are likely to develop, which can have an adverse effect on sleep. Cancer, neurologic disorders, cardiovascular or pulmonary disease, diabetes, hypothyroidism, gastroesophageal reflux disease, and musculoskeletal disease all are associated with sleep disruption.[13] Poor sleep could increase the risk of developing some of these conditions and/or exacerbate their severity.

Cancer

Sleep disturbance is a common correlate of cancers that women are more likely to develop with increasing age. As discussed in Chapter 153, determining the etiology of cancer-related sleep disruption can be complex, as multiple factors are likely to precipitate sleep problems. In a meta-analysis of data from breast cancer survivors, female-specific factors (hot flashes, menopause), other patient symptoms (pain, depressive symptoms, fatigue), and characteristics (race) were significantly associated with sleep disturbance.[170] In addition to the sleep-disrupting factors commonly experienced by most patients with cancer, women undergoing treatment for breast cancer are likely to experience hot flashes.[171] Hot flashes are a common precipitating factor in the development of insomnia in breast cancer survivors[172] and are associated with a less efficient, more disrupted sleep.[173] Hot flashes result from chemotherapy-induced ovarian disruption, and they also occur with the use of adjuvant antiestrogen therapy. Women with estrogen receptor–positive tumors are treated with the antiestrogens tamoxifen, aromatase inhibitors (e.g., anastrozole, letrozole, exemestane), and a GnRHa (e.g., leuprolide), or they undergo bilateral oophorectomy to prevent endogenous estrogens from stimulating growth of residual tumors or micrometastases. More than 50% of tamoxifen users experience hot flashes, which usually are more frequent and severe than those in natural menopause.[174]

HT is not indicated for treatment of hot flashes in women with a history of breast cancer,[175] making other therapies a necessity. SSRIs and SNRIs, clonidine, gabapentin, and pregabalin reduce the number and severity of hot flashes in women with a history of breast cancer.[176] Coadministration of a hypnotic, such as zolpidem, with an SSRI/SNRI improves sleep and quality of life more than use of an SSRI/SNRI alone in women with breast cancer who also have hot flash–associated sleep disturbance.[159] CBT is also beneficial, leading to improvements in subjective sleep, as well as mood and quality of life that are maintained over a year in women with insomnia secondary to breast cancer.[177] A randomized controlled trial[163] in breast cancer survivors comparing the efficacy of internet-based CBT with or without therapist support against a wait-list control group found that both types of CBT were significantly better in alleviating sleep disturbance associated with hot flashes (effect sizes ≥0.41) compared with the control group, suggesting that even a pragmatic, remote self-managed CBT program can be effective. Other interventions such as acupuncture, exercise, or melatonin have also shown some benefit for hot flashes and poor sleep quality, although larger clinical trials are needed.

Thyroid Dysfunction

The prevalence of thyroid disease, particularly hypothyroidism, increases with age and is far higher in women than in men. For midlife women living in iodine-replete areas, the prevalence of impaired thyroid function (i.e., thyroid-stimulating hormone [TSH] values outside the euthyroid range) is 9.6%.[178] Of these, the majority (6.2%) have elevated TSH, indicating clinical or subclinical hypothyroidism. Because hypothyroidism is typically characterized by tiredness and fatigue, and not sleepiness, such complaints by perimenopausal and postmenopausal women should be clinically evaluated in light of a TSH level. Women with hypothyroidism may be more likely than euthyroid women to have SDB (see Chapters 27 and 155), suggesting that hypothyroidism also may be a risk factor for SDB.[179] Midlife and older women with hypothyroidism also should be screened for clinical signs and symptoms indicative of SDB.

Hypertension

The prevalence of hypertension (HTN) rises sharply with onset of menopause. The etiology of this phenomenon is complex and still under investigation, but two factors strongly associated with HTN are obesity and SDB, conditions common in perimenopausal and postmenopausal women.[180,181] SDB is associated with HTN, as well as arterial stiffness, metabolic syndrome, and depression in peri- and postmenopausal women.[105,114] NHANES III documented a strong association between HTN and higher BMI in women.[180] For women in midlife, the prevalence of HTN was approximately 10% when BMI was less than 25, but rose to 39% when BMI was 30 kg/m^2 or greater. For women over 60 years of age, HTN occurred in 52% with a BMI less than 25 but was in more than 72% if BMI was 30 kg/m^2 or greater. Midlife women are at increased risk of HTN and SDB by virtue of their increased risk of obesity, rather than hormonal or menopausal factors per se. Sleep duration and efficiency were unrelated to HTN when controlling for several confounders in midlife women who participated in the SWAN study.[182]

Fibromyalgia

Sleep disturbance is a core symptom of fibromyalgia, which has a higher prevalence in women (3.4%) than in men (0.5%) and is more common in women over 50 years of age.[183] A link between reproductive hormone changes and fibromyalgia has been hypothesized[184] and there is some evidence that at least for some women, fibromyalgia symptoms start after the onset of menopause,[185] when estradiol levels decline. However, ET had no effect on pain thresholds or tolerance in postmenopausal women with fibromyalgia but the potential benefit for symptoms such as sleep disturbance and depression was not investigated.[186]

Neurodegenerative Disorders

Sleep disruption can be an early symptom of neurodegenerative conditions such as Parkinson or Alzheimer disease (see Chapters 102 and 105). These disorders occur more often in postmenopausal women than in age-matched men. Genetic factors and changes in biologic hormone milieu related to menopause may play an important role.[187] However, more research is needed to investigate possible associations among sleep disruption, estradiol decline, and development of neurodegenerative disorders in women.

CLINICAL PEARLS

Sleep difficulties are more common in midlife women transitioning to menopause compared with premenopause, with intermittent awakenings being the most common and bothersome complaint. Nocturnal hot flashes are an important component of sleep disturbance in midlife women, and both hormonal and nonhormonal therapies that alleviate hot flashes are associated with improvements in sleep quality.

Sleep-disordered breathing is more common in women after menopause, which may in part be attributed to a change in the distribution of adipose tissue, with an increase in intraabdominal fat, and to changes in reproductive hormones. Reports of fatigue or sleep complaints in postmenopausal women, possibly combined with hypertension and excessive weight, should prompt consideration of snoring and SDB in a clinical evaluation regardless of whether excessive daytime sleepiness is reported.

SUMMARY

Menopause is the physiologic centerpiece of a major developmental stage in the normal aging process, marking the transition from a reproductive to a nonreproductive stage of life. The menopausal transition, and the corresponding changes in the hormone milieu, are associated with an increased prevalence of sleep problems. A rise in sleep problems is strongly linked with vasomotor symptoms (hot flashes and night sweats) and can also coincide with mood symptoms, development of concomitant primary sleep disorders, chronic health conditions, and midlife stressors. Insomnia and fatigue are among the most frequent health complaints of perimenopausal women, including those who are not seeking treatment for menopausal symptoms. These sleep disturbances affect health-related quality of life, work productivity, and health care utilization across several years of the menopause transition. Clinical trials have shown that cognitive behavioral therapy for insomnia is effective in midlife women with menopausal insomnia, including those with hot flashes, presenting an alternative option to hormonal and nonhormonal pharmacologic treatments available for menopause-related sleep disruption. SDB increases in prevalence after menopause, which may be related to increased adiposity and centripetal weight gain, as well as hormonal changes and aging. Women suspected of having SDB should be evaluated and treated; continuous positive airway pressure remains the treatment of choice.

SELECTED READINGS

Baker FC, de Zambotti M, Colrain IM, Bei B. Sleep problems during the menopausal transition: prevalence, impact, and management challenges. *Nat Sci Sleep*. 2018;10:73–95.

Bianchi MT, Kim S, Galvan T, White DP, Joffe H. Nocturnal hot flashes: relationship to objective awakenings and sleep stage. *J Clin Sleep Med*. 2016.

Cheng YS, Tseng PT, Wu MK, et al. Pharmacologic and hormonal treatments for menopausal sleep disturbances: a network meta-analysis of 43 randomized controlled trials and 32,271 menopausal women. *Sleep Med Rev*. 2021;57:101469.

de Zambotti M, Colrain IM, Javitz HS, Baker FC. Magnitude of the impact of hot flashes on sleep in perimenopausal women. *Fertil Steril*. 2014;102:1708–1715.

Guthrie KA, Larson JC, Ensrud KE, et al. Effects of pharmacologic and nonpharmacologic interventions on insomnia symptoms and self-reported sleep quality in women with hot flashes: a pooled analysis of individual participant data from four MsFLASH Trials. *Sleep*. 2018;41(1).

Joffe H, Crawford S, Economou N, et al. A gonadotropin-releasing hormone agonist model demonstrates that nocturnal hot flashes interrupt objective sleep. *Sleep*. 2013;36(12):1977–1985.

Joffe H, Massler A, Sharkey KM. Evaluation and management of sleep disturbance during the menopause transition. *Semin Reprod Med*. 2010;28:404–421.

Kravitz HM, Janssen I, Bromberger JT, et al. Sleep trajectories before and after the final menstrual period in the Study of Women's Health Across the Nation (SWAN). *Curr Sleep Med Rep*. 2017;3(3):235–250.

Kravitz HM, Joffe H. Sleep during the perimenopause: a SWAN story. *Obstet Gynecol Clin North Am*. 2011;38:567–586.

Kravitz HM, Matthews KA, Joffe H, et al. Trajectory analysis of sleep maintenance problems in midlife women before and after surgical menopause: the Study of Women's Health Across the Nation (SWAN). *Menopause*. 2020;27(3):278–288.

Matthews KA, Hall MH, Lee L, et al. Racial/ethnic disparities in women's sleep duration, continuity, and quality, and their statistical mediators: study of Women's Health Across the Nation. *Sleep*. 2019;42(5).

Matthews KA, Kravitz HM, Lee L, et al. Does mid-life aging impact women's sleep duration, continuity, and timing? A longitudinal analysis from the Study of Women's Health Across the Nation. *Sleep*. 2019.

Mirer AG, Young T, Palta M, Benca RM, Rasmuson A, Peppard PE. Sleep-disordered breathing and the menopausal transition among participants in the Sleep in Midlife Women Study. *Menopause*. 2017;24(2):157–162.

A complete reference list can be found online at ExpertConsult.com.

Sleep Medicine in the Elderly

Section 22

Chapter 190

Introduction

Cathy Alessi; Jennifer L. Martin; Constance H. Fung

Sleep problems are common among older adults, particularly in those with coexisting psychiatric and medical conditions. In studies among older adults that compare good sleepers with poor sleepers, the poor sleepers were found to take more medications, make more clinician visits, and have poorer self-ratings of health, suggesting a strong relationship between comorbidities and poor sleep in older people. Evidence suggests sleep disturbance may be more strongly associated with these types of risk factors (e.g., medications, comorbidities), which are common in older adults, rather than aging alone. As described in other sections of this book, however, age-associated changes in sleep have been reported (e.g., decrease in N3 sleep, more nighttime awakenings); many of these changes begin earlier in adulthood and progress throughout life with notable changes occurring by middle age and a relative plateau in older age. The appropriate treatment of sleep problems in older adults must be guided by knowledge of likely contributing factors. When pharmacologic treatment is considered, risks and benefits must be carefully weighed. Generally pharmacotherapy should be considered only after nonpharmacologic approaches have been explored. However, this does not mean that advanced age, alone, should limit testing and treatment of sleep disorders, because addressing these problems in older adults can lead to significant improvements in health and quality of life.

What follows this introduction are brief overviews of the chapters making up this section on sleep medicine in older adults.

CHAPTER 191: PSYCHIATRIC AND MEDICAL COMORBIDITIES AND EFFECTS OF MEDICATIONS IN OLDER ADULTS

Because older age is often associated with multiple chronic conditions and polypharmacy, sleep problems in this population are often best addressed with a multifaceted and interprofessional approach. Mental health conditions, such as depression, anxiety, and bereavement, are prevalent in older adults and may contribute to sleep disturbance. Medical conditions that influence sleep are also common in older adults, and frequently there is a bidirectional relationship between sleep disturbance and these problems, such as chronic pain, cardiovascular disease, pulmonary disease, chronic kidney disease, gastrointestinal conditions, and endocrine and genitourinary problems. A systematic approach is often necessary to appropriately identify and manage sleep problems in older adults. Overall, the higher burden of illness and the greater number of medications used to treat these comorbidities play an important role in the quantity and quality of sleep in older adults. There is also significant concern about use of sedative hypnotics and certain other medications in older adults, particularly those who are frail, in whom the "number needed to treat" a condition is sometimes greater than the "number needed to harm" (i.e., risks of treatment may outweigh potential benefits). Deprescribing (the process of intentionally reducing or eliminating medications to improve health and/or decrease risk of adverse drug effects) is an important approach to address this polypharmacy and may, in fact, improve sleep quality for older patients.

CHAPTER 192: OBSTRUCTIVE SLEEP APNEA IN OLDER ADULTS

Sleep-disordered breathing is underdiagnosed and undertreated in older adults. Evidence suggests that one of the most common types of sleep-disordered breathing, obstructive sleep apnea (OSA), increases in prevalence to about age 70 years, then plateaus. Differences in the clinical presentation and manifestation of OSA in older adults may be a key factor explaining underrecognition. The male predominance in OSA appears to disappear with age, with evidence for a striking rise in OSA prevalence in women after menopause. Obesity also decreases in importance as a risk factor for OSA after age 60. Compared to younger people, older patients with OSA may be more likely to experience sleep complaints, nocturia, and cognitive dysfunction. Several physiologic mechanisms have been postulated to explain the relationship between OSA and nocturia in older adults. Many factors likely explain the susceptibility to cognitive dysfunction in older adults with OSA. Although OSA is strongly associated with cardiovascular disease in middle-aged people, there is also accumulating evidence that sleep-disordered breathing increases the risk of cardiovascular disease and stroke in older adults.

Increasing evidence indicates that positive airway pressure (PAP) therapy is associated with reduced cardiovascular morbidity, less cognitive dysfunction, and lower all-cause mortality in older adults with OSA. Older age itself does not appear to affect PAP adherence; however, treatment emergent central sleep apnea appears to be more prevalent in older compared with younger adults. Alternatives to PAP therapy can be considered in older adults, but upper airway surgery may not be particularly effective in older adults, and morbidity of surgery may be especially high in this population. Data are limited on positional therapy or other approaches for OSA in older adults.

CHAPTER 193: INSOMNIA IN OLDER ADULTS

Insomnia is common in older adults and is an important contributor to functional impairment and morbidity. Unfortunately, the assumption that insomnia is an inevitable consequence of aging may lead to insomnia remaining unrecognized, undiagnosed, and untreated by health care providers. Factors that have been implicated in the development of late life insomnia include psychiatric and medical comorbidities, medications, and other substances, and comorbid sleep disorders, in addition to age-related changes in homeostatic and circadian sleep/wake regulation. Insomnia symptoms are associated with an increased risk of falls in older adults, and sedative hypnotic medications also increase their risk of falls and fractures, therefore impacting the overall risk profile of sedative hypnotic agents in this population. Findings from studies of the potential effects of insomnia on cognitive function in older adults have been mixed in terms of whether insomnia is associated with cognitive impairment.

Nonpharmacologic treatments for insomnia are recommended before sedative-hypnotic use in adults. Cognitive behavioral therapy for insomnia (CBT-I) has been proven successful in older adults, including among those individuals with and without comorbid conditions, and for those with hypnotic dependency. Older adults should be offered CBT-I as first-line treatment for chronic insomnia. Current guidelines suggest caution in the use of sedative hypnotics in older adults. However, hypnotic medication use is highest and most often chronic in older adults despite evidence that benefits of these medications in older adults are lower compared to younger people.

CHAPTER 194: CIRCADIAN RHYTHMS IN OLDER ADULTS

One of the most prominent changes in 24-hour behavior with aging is a shift in sleep timing to earlier hours, characterized by going to bed earlier and waking up earlier. Although the period, or cycle length, of the circadian system has been reported to shorten with age in animals, studies using forced desynchrony protocols in humans have not shown a difference in period length between younger and older adults. Many circadian rhythms of biologic processes do shift earlier with age, including rhythms of cortisol, melatonin, and core body temperature. There is also a change in the shape of the circadian sleep–promoting signal, with older adults more vulnerable to sleep disruption in the latter half of the habitual sleep period. The response to light as a primary entraining signal for the human circadian timing system may also be altered, and a reduction in amplitude of some circadian rhythms, including cortisol, melatonin, and core body temperature, in addition to performance and gene expression in the suprachiasmatic nucleus (SCN) and prefrontal cortex, has been observed. The number of cells in the SCN of humans decreases with age, with more pronounced changes in patients with Alzheimer disease. Modest alterations in circadian rhythm timing may be an early sign of cognitive decline and potential development of neurodegenerative disease and is associated with increased risk of mortality. Rest-activity monitoring by actigraphy is commonly used to monitor sleep-wake rhythm in older adults, and many activity rhythm variables have been associated with cognitive changes as well.

CHAPTER 195: SLEEP IN LONG-TERM CARE SETTINGS

Sleep disturbance is very common and often disabling among residents in long-term care (LTC) settings, such as nursing homes, assisted-living facilities, dementia care units, and community-based homes for older people. Sleep disturbance also increases risk of LTC placement among community-dwelling older adults. Sleep disturbance in LTC residents is associated with impaired function, less functional recovery over time, social disengagement, increased risk of falls, frailty, agitation, and increased mortality. Examples of factors that contribute to sleep disturbance in LTC residents include advanced age, environmental factors (e.g., noise, light, room temperature, roommates), and nocturnal care activities (e.g., incontinence care) that disturb sleep. Lack of physical activity and social isolation with considerable periods of time spent in bed, extended daytime napping, and excessive daytime sleepiness are also common. Most LTC residents have multiple chronic medical and psychiatric conditions and/or receive medications that may disrupt sleep. Common sleep disorders in LTC residents include irregular sleep-wake rhythm disorder, chronic insomnia disorder, OSA, and restless legs syndrome. Because some LTC residents cannot recall their sleep problems because of memory impairment, information from family members and LTC caregivers should be sought. Polysomnography may be difficult to obtain in LTC residents, and many have cognitive impairment that may complicate sleep stage scoring. Wrist actigraphy has been used for sleep assessment in LTC residents with dementia. Pharmacologic treatment for insomnia is commonly used in LTC residents, but there is increasing evidence of risk of harm; nonpharmacologic interventions should be first-line therapy in this setting. There is some evidence for use of CBT-I in LTC residents who are cognitively intact. Bright light therapy may be beneficial for sleep disturbances in dementia. Morning sunlight exposure (30 to 60 minutes) and bright lights installed in common areas (e.g., dining rooms, activity areas) with time spent in these areas each day has been recommended. Social activity, physical activity, and exercise may also be beneficial. Multicomponent interventions that combine a variety of these nonpharmacologic approaches have been shown to maintain the circadian sleep-wake rhythm and improve sleep in several studies involving residents in LTC settings.

Chapter 191

Psychiatric and Medical Comorbidities and Effects of Medications in Older Adults

Steven R. Barczi; Mihai C. Teodorescu

Chapter Highlights

- Late-life sleep disturbances and insomnia are prevalent and typically multifactorial in etiology with significant potential to impact the quality of life of older persons. Insomnia in this age group frequently coexists with other geriatric syndromes and health problems, leading to the preferred nosology of comorbid insomnia. Because these clinical entities cross organ systems and transcend discipline-based boundaries, they pose a challenge in using traditional approaches to care.
- Management of sleep difficulties in the elderly therefore requires a multifaceted and interprofessional approach directed at treating behavioral, medical, and psychiatric factors while also addressing coexistent primary sleep disorders.

INTRODUCTION

Epidemiology and Nosology

The number of Americans ages 65 and older grew by a third in the last decade and is projected to nearly double to 95 million by 2060.[1] This group is more racially and ethnically diverse with higher percentages remaining in the workforce after age 65. Furthermore, advances in health care have extended life span with concurrent rise in multiple chronic conditions (multimorbidity) and patient complexity. Multimorbidity is of particular relevance to older age, as the number of morbidities and proportion of the population with multimorbidity have a strong association with age.[2] The specific prevalence of individual conditions varies based upon the age group, gender, and population sampled (e.g., community-based versus clinic cohort).

Geriatric syndromes are age-related disorders that have a multifactorial etiology and can lead to loss of functional reserve with reduced quality of life for an older person. They may present as a predominant symptom or symptom cluster (e.g., poor mobility and falling) that involves several distinct organ systems and can respond to a multifaceted intervention. Sleep disturbances and insomnia in older adults fit the typical profile of a geriatric syndrome with multiple contributing and alleviating factors. In fact, older age is one of the best predictors of change in sleep structure.[3] Prevalence of geriatric syndromes increases with age and can coexist: although 20% of cases in 60 to 69 years age group were not found to have any syndromes, 48% of cases in those over 80 years had more than four syndromes simultaneously.[4]

The prevalence of sleep difficulties increases with advancing age and health complexity with susceptibility to the disruptive effects of many endogenous and exogenous factors. These sleep changes appear more strongly associated with psychosocial and health factors rather than aging itself.[5,6] In a cohort of more than 300 community-dwelling seniors (mean age 72) followed for 3 years, sleep disturbances were related to physical, environmental, and health factors rather than to age-dependent sleep changes.[7] In a longitudinal study of sleep in later life, participants were followed for up to 27 years and identified a significant decrease in sleep efficiency with age (3.1% per decade, decreasing from 90% before age 50, to 80% with age between 60 and 80, and 72% to age >90).[3] In addition, sleep efficiency of females was 5% less than that of males. People whose general health rating was "very good" were found to have more efficient sleep than those whose general health rating was "very bad."

Multimorbidity and Sleep

Health problems appear to have additive effects when considering the likelihood of concomitant sleep complaints. The 2003 Sleep and Aging survey (part of the Sleep in America poll) reported that 36% of people age 65 years and older without comorbid illnesses had sleep problems, 52% with one to three comorbidities had sleep disturbances, and 69% of those with four or more comorbidities had disturbed sleep.[3] In addition, there was an inverse relationship between the self-perceived quality of these respondents' sleep and the number of comorbidities they had.[5] The number of comorbidities was higher in the low–sleep efficiency "cluster" compared to the high-efficiency "cluster" in a longitudinal followed cohort.[3]

Belonging to the high–sleep efficiency cluster was associated with having lower prevalence of hypertension, circulatory problems, general arthritis, breathing problems, and recurrent episodes of depression compared to the low-efficiency cluster. In a large study of 42,116 participants 50 years old and older, there was a dose-dependent relationship between the number of chronic conditions and the sleep disturbances-index variable.[8] Regarding sleep duration, short sleep duration seems to be associated with multimorbidity among women, but neither short nor long sleep duration was found to be related to multimorbidity among men in a large cross-sectional study.[9]

Polypharmacy

Closely related to cumulative disease burden is the use of multiple medications. Polypharmacy is generally defined as taking more than five medications. It increases incrementally in relationship to the number of coexisting age-associated diseases. Population-based surveys report between 89% and 94% of those over 65 years take prescription medications, with nearly 40% taking more than 5 medications and 12% taking more than 10 medications.[10,11]

Consequences of polypharmacy include adverse drug effects, drug-drug interactions, and medication cascade effects. The cascade effect refers to the use of medications to treat the side effects of other medications. The Drug Burden Index (DBI) tool quantifies individual exposure to anticholinergic and sedative medications. Prevalence of DBI exposure increases progressively with the number of drugs used, rising from 43% of those prescribed 0 to 4 chronic drugs to 95% of those on at least 12 chronic drugs (adjusted OR 27.8, 95% CI 26.7 to 29.0).[12] In a study analyzing the uniform data set from more than 37,000 participants enrolled at approximately 39 Alzheimer disease centers, taking one to four additional medications was associated with nine times higher odds of sedative hypnotics use, whereas use of five or more medications was associated with almost 14 times higher odds of sedative hypnotics use.[13]

Deprescribing

Older people are at high risk for adverse drug effects resulting from changes in renal function, liver clearance, physiologic reserve, body composition, and cellular metabolism. In frail older people the number needed to treat is sometimes greater than the number needed to harm.[14] Deprescribing is the process of intentionally reducing or discontinuing a medication to improve the person's health or reduce the risk of adverse drug effects. Risk-modifying medicines (aspirin, statins, antihypertensives, bisphosphonates, calcium, and vitamin D) appear to be more successfully deprescribed than symptom-modifying medicines (analgesics, laxatives, antidepressants, hypnotics, and anxiolytics).[14] In a longitudinal, prospective, nonrandomized study of poly-deprescribing (>3 drugs) in 122 subjects (compared with 55 nonresponders [NR]) followed for 3 years, nighttime sleep quality improved in 45% (versus 7% in NR), with only 4% sustaining a worsening in nighttime sleep quality after medication removal (versus 33% in NR).[15]

Comorbid Insomnia

In older adults with chronic illnesses, the terms *primary insomnia* and *secondary insomnia* do not adequately represent the complex interplay of cause and effect in determining etiology (Figure 191.1). Sleep difficulties in older persons can

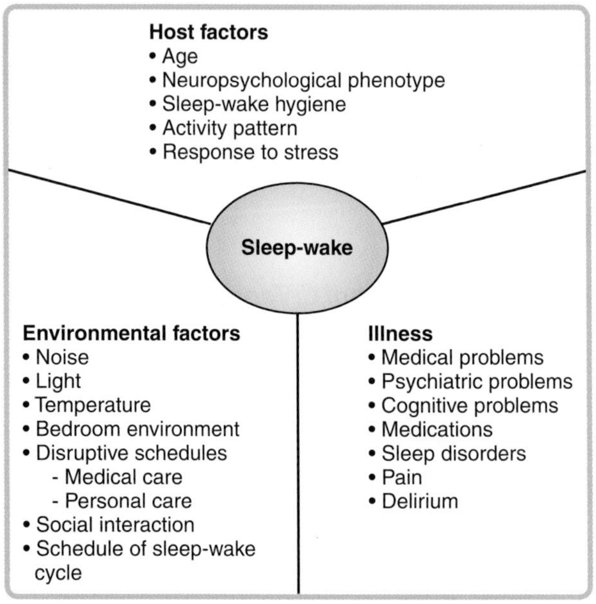

Figure 191.1 Sleep-wake symptomatic status depicted as a syndrome that results from dynamic interactions among genetic and phenotypic characteristics, illness as a function of comorbid conditions and polypharmacy, and environment, to include modulating nociceptive interactions with disruptors and zeitgeber qualities. This model could further identify predisposing, precipitating, and perpetuating factors, but it underscores the limited ability to establish a clear, consequential relationship in the context of the ever-changing interplay of these factors.

be conceptualized as a geriatric syndrome because they are attributable to multiple and interdependent predisposing, precipitating, and perpetuating factors.[16] Medical or psychiatric conditions may act as precipitating events and produce symptoms of discomfort and emotional distress that may lead to increased sympathetic drive, hypothalamic-pituitary-adrenal activation, and ultimately recruitment of neural systems to produce arousal.[10,11] In acute situations, pathophysiologic changes such as hypoxemia, metabolic derangements, fever, or systemic inflammatory responses can also lead to delirium with characteristic alterations in sleep-wake patterns.[11] Psychological factors of hyperarousal, stress response, predisposing personality traits, and maladaptive attitudes can perpetuate sleep changes seen during illness in later life.[17] In many situations, the interplay between underlying illnesses and their treatments, sleep hygiene, medications, and the sleep environment is contributing to the problem. The precise relationship between an illness and the neurophysiologic, biochemical, and hormonal sequelae that contribute to sleep disruption remains uncertain in most cases of insomnia in the older adults. For these reasons, establishing a clear, consequential relationship becomes a clinical challenge. Therefore the term *comorbid* is considered to describe insomnia more adequately. The 2005 National Institutes of Health State-of-the-Science Conference on Insomnia proposed using the diagnosis of comorbid insomnia when an illness coexists with sleep changes but the dynamics of cause and effect are not proven.[10]

Comprehensive Assessment of a Sleep Problem: The Star Method

Effectively addressing multiple co-occurring problems is a great challenge when treating geriatric populations. A systematic approach is necessary when identifying and managing multiple interacting medical, social, and mental health factors on sleep in older persons. Premature closure that occurs when rapidly identifying the most overt causative factor but neglecting other contributing issues can lead to incomplete diagnoses and less effective treatment plans. The Wisconsin Star Method is an example of a geriatrics model of care to understand and address complexity in geriatric care.[18] Further compounding these challenges is the high degree of variability from one older adult or population to the next, generated by multiple factors ranging from age-related physiologic heterogeneity to different sets of psychosocial experiences over the course of lifetimes. Under such circumstances, evidence-based guidelines, developed from studies of single problems in homogeneous populations, are of limited utility at best. We need to conceptualize sleep as part of a network of potentially interacting variables, with the links between them varying in strength, from very weak (i.e., negligible) to very strong (i.e., directly causal or interdependent). Some factors by themselves may not be sufficient to contribute to the sleep problem but become so by interacting synergistically with other factors (e.g., use of diuretic leads to nocturia, which in turn disrupts sleep). Obviously, the benefit of such an approach translates into generating hypotheses, prioritizing and sequencing interventions, and integrating clinical pearls with evidence-based guidelines.

Management

The management of comorbid insomnia is evolving. Historically, if a sleep problem was attributed to an associated physical or mental illness, then the primary focus was on optimizing treatment of that underlying health concern. This placed an emphasis on correcting neurochemical, metabolic, and physiologic derangement in illness with the hope that sleep would improve. Evidence from a series of controlled trials has demonstrated the efficacy of cognitive behavioral therapy (CBT) in managing insomnia complaints in a variety of different illnesses. On these grounds, there is a growing trend for all comorbid insomnia to be treated the same as primary insomnia with CBT and, when indicated, adjunctive hypnotic therapy.[19] This approach is supported by a study of CBT for insomnia in older adults with osteoarthritis, coronary artery disease, or pulmonary disease. Ninety-two participants (mean age 69 years) were randomly assigned to classroom CBT or stress management and wellness training (placebo condition). CBT participants had larger improvements on 8 out of 10 self-report measures of sleep; the type of chronic disease had no impact on these outcomes. These results challenge the dichotomy between primary and secondary insomnia and suggest that psychological factors are likely involved in insomnias that are presumed to be secondary to medical conditions.[20] Although more data are needed to determine the most effective approach, a multifaceted intervention appears most logical, including optimization of comorbid health issues and treatment of insomnia using CBT and/or pharmacotherapy.

PSYCHIATRIC CONDITIONS AND SLEEP IN THE OLDER ADULT

Mental health conditions are prevalent in the geriatric population and are often associated with complaints of difficulties related to sleep, which are a part of the diagnostic criteria of many psychiatric disorders. Therefore to be an independent diagnosis, insomnia has to constitute a distinct complaint and be more prominent than that typically associated with mental disorders.[21] Psychiatric and somatic symptoms, as well as the level of physical activity, significantly and independently increase the risk of insomnia in older clinic patients.[22] Acutely ill psychiatric patients show reduced sleep efficiency, prolonged sleep latency, decreased total night sleep, and increased arousals.[23] Conversely, those with sleep difficulties are associated with a higher prevalence of psychiatric disorders and symptoms compared to those without sleep complaints.[24-26] In a general population of elderly women (age over 65), short and long sleep duration groups have increased prevalence of mental health issues (66% and 26%, respectively).[27] Part of this clinical correlation may reflect the high overlap of mental health with physical health issues, including general health status, activity limitations, and chronic health conditions.

Depressive Disorders

Depression is associated with sleep disturbances in both elderly general populations[28] and clinical populations, with insomnia in the primary care setting showing a stronger association to depression than any other medical disorder.[29] In a large cross-sectional study (more than 700 subjects, mean age 80), approximately one-third of subjects endorsing depression symptoms (Geriatric Depression Scale score > 5) reported moderate/severe sleep onset/sleep maintenance difficulties, while almost another third reported mild ones.[30] Older adults with a history of depression show impairments in sleep quality and lower levels of health functioning; these impairments were at a gradient with declines in those with current depression.[31]

Sleep complaints also foreshadow the onset of depression in older adults, with insomnia a strong risk factor for future depression in elderly patients not currently depressed.[32] Insomnia at baseline and 1 year later increased eight times the risk of development of depression[33] in one elderly cohort. Clinical sleep disturbance (defined as a Pittsburgh Sleep Quality Index [PSQI] score >5) was found to be a powerful predictor of depression recurrence (adjusted hazard ratio nearly 5) in a 2-year longitudinal study of community-dwelling older adults.[34]

Objective and subjective sleep findings in depression have different implications and may not always correlate with each other.[35,36] Between 60% and 80% of depressed adults and older adults complain of difficulty falling or staying asleep, or being tired in the day.[37,38] These subjective sleep complaints may persist beyond the resolution of depressive symptoms.[39] Prevalence of symptoms is comparable between genders.[40] There appears to be an association between greater level of depressive symptoms and worse subjective sleep quality and more subjective daytime sleepiness, as well as objectively measured wake after sleep onset (WASO) and wake episodes longer than 5 minutes.[41]

Objective sleep findings in older adults with depression include prolonged time to sleep onset, decreased sleep efficiency, poor sleep continuity, and increased early morning awakening. Additionally, total sleep time is reduced with relative increases in stages 1 and 2 sleep with corresponding decreased slow wave sleep (SWS). There are also shortened rapid eye movement (REM) latency, a longer first REM period, and increased total REM sleep and REM density.[23,42,43] Although these patterns of sleep change are well described in depressed persons, no single sleep variable is currently specific enough to distinguish depression from other psychiatric disorders.[23] Further, longitudinal studies of electroencephalogram (EEG) sleep profiles in depression show state and trait characteristics, meaning some of these characteristics can change over time.[44] Such differentiation may play a role in identifying those at high risk for depression, predicting future episodes of depression, and assessing the response to pharmacologic and behavioral treatments.

Bipolar Affective Disorder

Over recent decades, there has been a large increase in numbers of older adults with bipolar affective disorder, thought to be due to overall population aging as well as the improving efficacy of pharmacotherapy.[45] Overall, individuals with bipolar spectrum disorders experience significantly more sleep loss and social rhythm disruption after both minor and major life events compared with normal populations, leading to disrupted biologic rhythms and affective symptoms.[46] Manic episodes usually involve a prolonged time of increased activity with minimal sleep. Insomnia can precede manic episodes as a first symptom in up to 77% of cases.[47] Although first-onset mania can occur in the elderly, this warrants suspicion of medical illness or drug effects as contributors. Of those with onset of mania in later life, many have a history of depression.[48] Moreover, sleep loss may trigger manic episodes, emphasizing a need to clinically monitor sleep changes and address sleep-disrupting factors in an attempt to decrease such exacerbations.[47] Sleep disturbance appears to predict suicide ideation indirectly via depressive symptoms, cognitive failures, and medication nonadherence. Poor sleep and cognitive failures augment depressive symptomatology, which, in turn, further increases suicide ideation.[49]

Bereavement and Grief

A systematic review looking at late-life spousal bereavement found a strong relationship between bereavement and nutritional risk and involuntary weight loss as well as evidence for impaired sleep quality and increased alcohol consumption.[50] The highest levels of grief are usually found within the first 4 months of bereavement, with recovery periods varying with the stress of the bereavement or coping skills and extending to 2 to 3 years. In 38 bereaved seniors (>2 months after the event), questionnaire and diary-based measures of sleep correlated with the level of depressive symptomatology. Sleep duration correlated with the level of grief severity, while no sleep measure correlated with days since loss.[51] In a cross-sectional survey of 170 women (mean age 66 years) assessed in average at 26 months from the loss event, insomnia was reported by 13% of subjects. Other sleep-related symptoms included an irregular sleep pattern, nightmares, and sleeping excessively.[52]

Sleeping 6.5 to 9 hours per night at baseline predicted better social functioning, better emotional health, and more energy during bereavement in older persons.[53] Baseline complicated grief scores of recently widowed elderly individuals were significantly associated with sleep difficulties at 18-month follow-up.[54] In a study of 28 bereaved older adults who lost their spouse, assessed at 4 months or later from the loss event, polysomnographic data demonstrated mildly prolonged latency to sleep and REM sleep and mildly reduced sleep time and sleep efficiency. Higher grief tended to be associated with less time spent asleep and reduced alertness at 8 p.m.[55] In summary, problems with sleep during bereavement may predict current and future depression and offer a potential target of treatment.

Anxiety Disorders

Common anxiety conditions in older adults include generalized anxiety disorder (GAD) and panic disorder. Most anxiety conditions in the elderly are continued disorders from earlier in their life, with the exception of some increased agoraphobia. Although not a specific anxiety disorder, many older adults can have increased anxiety when faced with chronic health conditions, functional limitations, or concerns about issues such as safety or finances, which in addition to certain medications used to treat them may contribute to neurochemical changes and/or increased adrenergic drive. This is reflected in the findings that even subclinical anxiety symptoms are associated with higher levels of WASO as measured by actigraphy and sleep log.[52]

GAD, a condition of overall hyperarousal, is the most prevalent condition of subjects complaining of insomnia who have a mental health diagnosis in the adult population.[56] Sleep disturbance is a core symptom in the diagnosis of GAD and is endorsed in about two-thirds of patients with this diagnosis.[44] In a cross-sectional sample derived from the Einstein Aging Study (702 participants, average age of 80), approximately 30% of subjects scoring in the anxiety range (Beck Anxiety Inventory score > 11) indicated moderate/severe sleep-onset/sleep maintenance difficulties, while approximately 50% endorsed mild difficulties.[30] Objective findings include more awakenings, longer time to fall asleep, and decreased sleep efficiency and time, with less consistent findings of more stage 2, and decreased SWS.[23,57]

About 80% of older adults with GAD also have a depressive disorder, making specific objective sleep findings difficult to interpret. However, anxiety symptoms were associated with poor sleep efficiency and greater time spent awake after sleep onset (i.e., sleep fragmentation) in a population of elderly women, even after accounting for significant depressive symptoms.[58] These findings suggest that untreated anxiety symptoms may account for poor sleep quality in older women that persists even after treatment of depressive symptoms.

Panic disorder is also associated with sleep complaints, including trouble falling sleep, disturbed and restless sleep, as well as nocturnal panic attacks. Nearly one-fourth of patients with panic disorder report either severe sleep restriction (≤5 hours) or increases (≥9 hours) in sleep duration.[59] Nocturnal panic attacks occur at least weekly in 18% to 45% of panic disorder patients.[60,61] These attacks are characterized by similar symptom severity and duration of daytime panic attacks and occur usually in the first few hours of sleep in transition from stage 2 to SWS.[62] People with nocturnal panic attacks have higher rates of insomnia and depression than people with panic disorder without nighttime episodes.[63,64] Sleep panic attacks can occur with parts of a clinical history similar to sleep apnea, parasomnias, gastroesophageal reflux disease (GERD), and posttraumatic stress disorder (PTSD), a consideration during the workup of sleep complaints.

In older adults with PTSD, many had symptoms for years with this condition continuing in later life. It appears that although the severity of PTSD seems similar among younger and older adults, the elderly report less reexperiencing but more symptoms of hyperarousal compared with younger people.[65] Sleep disturbance commonly occurs in PTSD with rates from 44% to 91%, including insomnia and nightmares.[66] The most specific findings in PTSD are recurrent awakenings and excessive body movement.[67] A meta-analysis of 20 polysomnographic studies comparing sleep in people with and without PTSD reported more stage 1 sleep, less slow wave sleep, and greater REM density; older PTSD patients had less SWS and REM sleep than age-matched control participants, with possible confounding by the time elapsed since traumatic experiences.[68]

Elders may also be more predisposed to exacerbations or new onset of symptoms in the context of worsening health conditions, confronted with death of friends/spouses, as well as their own mortality. In addition, previous mechanisms for coping may be affected by physical limitations (e.g., a man who works himself to fatigue, or runs to relieve tension, but now has retired or has pain that limits his exercise ability) or cognitive limitations (e.g., regular inhibition of intrusive thoughts leading to more effective coping may be impaired in a person with executive dysfunction such as mild cognitive impairment), which are more likely to occur with increased age.

MEDICAL CONDITIONS AND SLEEP IN THE OLDER ADULT

An individual medical illness may have several mechanisms that interfere with sleep, and it may have different effects on sleep architecture in its acute versus chronic state. The immediate physiologic derangements or distress of an illness may transiently disturb sleep. Chronic pain, cardiovascular disease, pulmonary disease, chronic kidney disease (CKD), gastrointestinal conditions, and endocrine and genitourinary conditions have been associated with poor sleep. Sleep disturbance may worsen symptoms in these disorders or even worsen the prognosis.

Pain

The overall prevalence of pain increases with advancing age to the point that it affects more than 50% of older persons living in the community and more than 80% of nursing home residents.[69,70] The relationship between pain and sleep is complex; pain can disrupt sleep, and poor sleep may increase perceived pain intensity.[71] In a population of adults aged 55 to 84, 19% reported that pain disrupted their sleep at least a few nights per week, and 12% reported almost nightly sleep fragmentation because of pain.[5] In referral populations of patients with chronic pain, prevalence rates of insomnia can range between 50% and 70%.[72] In a polysomnographic study of older adults with chronic pain, afflicted individuals spent significantly longer time in bed and had worse sleep-onset latency, sleep latency to N2, sleep efficiency, WASO, and number of awakenings compared with a control group; sleep duration and time spent in each sleep stage did not differ between the two groups. Investigators found also that older people with chronic pain had lower intensity in the delta frequencies (0.5 to 1.99 Hz and 2 to 4 Hz) throughout the whole night, especially in the first 6 hours.[73] Actigraphy recordings and sleep diary data seem to confirm these findings and showed subjects with chronic pain spending significantly more time in bed, resulting in a lower sleep efficiency.[74]

Arthritis

An estimated 52.5 million adults have physician-diagnosed arthritis, and 22.7 million report arthritis-attributable activity limitations. As the population ages, arthritis is expected to affect an estimated 67 million adults in the United States by 2030.[75] Evidence suggests that as many as 60% of those with arthritis experience pain during the night, mediating a substantial amount of the relationship between arthritis and sleep problems. Adults over age 65 with knee arthritis have been observed to have problems initiating sleep (31%), problems maintaining sleep (81%), and a tendency to awaken early in the morning (51%).[76] In a sample of approximately 600 older adults with osteoarthritis (mean age 78), correlates of poor sleep were greater arthritis severity, three or more comorbid conditions, depressed mood, and restless legs syndrome; poor sleep was significantly associated with greater fatigue.[77]

One-year longitudinal relationships of sleep difficulties with pain, depression, and functional disability have been studied in 288 older adults (mean age at inclusion 67.9 years) with knee osteoarthritis. Longitudinal analyses used baseline sleep disturbance to predict the 1-year change in pain, disability, and depression.[78] Cross-sectional analyses revealed a significant association of sleep disturbance with pain and depression, but not functional disability. The sleep-pain relationship was wholly explained by depressive symptoms; in contrast, depression was significantly and independently associated with both pain and sleep problems. Furthermore, sleep disturbance exacerbated effects of pain on depression, such that depressive symptoms were greatest among those with both significant sleep problems and higher-than-average pain. In 1-year longitudinal analyses, sleep problems predicted increases in depression and disability, but not pain. Cognitive-behavioral approaches demonstrated efficacy in improving self-reported measures of sleep.[20] At least one-third of respondents in a recent survey had clinically moderate to severe levels of pain and sleep symptoms, significant enough to lead almost half of these ultimately to participate in a randomized trial comparing three group-format behavioral interventions.[79]

Gastroesophageal Reflux Disease

Insomnia is frequently associated with the presence of GERD.[80] Up to 70% to 90% of individuals with GERD report nighttime symptoms and sleep disruption.[81,82]

The prevalence of daily reflux symptoms for those older than 50 years has been reported at 10%.[83] A survey including more than 14,000 respondents reported heartburn being more prevalent in elderly (approximately 62%) compared with younger people (59%), whereas prevalence of frequent symptoms (more than twice per week) was also higher in elderly (approximately 31%).[84] Sleep disturbance was present in 29% of the older adults compared with 19% in younger ones. The relationship between disturbed sleep and GERD is likely bidirectional: sleeping increases the likelihood of reflux, and reflux episodes often awaken the patient.[85,86]

Patients with nighttime acid reflux may underestimate the degree of sleep disruption that occurs when objective measurements of pH and EEG arousal are compared with patient recollection the next morning.[85] Ambulatory 24-hour esophageal pH monitoring obtained in 54 out of 313 consecutive patients

(>62 years old) from a primary care setting demonstrated 20% (11/54) of this subgroup exhibiting increased acid contact time; only 6 individuals (11%) exhibited both symptomatic and objective indications of acid reflux.[87] A pilot study enrolling 16 subjects with chronic insomnia found silent reflux in 25% of subjects, as evidenced by abnormal 24-hour pH testing. Aggressive treatment of these subjects resulted in normalization of sleep efficiency in three out of four subjects.[88]

Reviewing the patient history for nocturnal cough or wheezing as a surrogate for reflux is also important, because not all patients with overnight reflux experience classic chest pain, but their sleep may be disrupted nevertheless. Published evidence demonstrates that acid suppression therapy reduces nighttime heartburn symptoms, reduces GERD-associated sleep disturbances, and improves subjective sleep quality and next day's work performance.[89] Finally, a mechanical link between the phrenoesophageal ligament and the lower esophageal sphincter may explain the coexistence of sleep apnea and reflux.[86,90]

Heart Disease

Many relationships exist between cardiac disease and sleep. Nocturnal ischemia, nighttime arrhythmias, and sleep-disordered breathing are all linked to altered sleep in underlying heart disease. A well-described circadian pattern of myocardial ischemia or infarction occurs early to mid-morning and is ascribed to the catecholamine surge that accompanies awakening and upright status. In a retrospective analysis of more than 3300 adults presenting with acute coronary syndrome (ACS), 26% of the individuals were awakened from sleep[91]; older age and lower left ventricular ejection fraction were independent predictors of nocturnal ACS in this cohort. Chronic problems with sleep initiation correlate with an increased risk of death from coronary artery disease in male patients.[92] In a study of more than 1200 women experiencing initial myocardial infarction (MI), half reported new onset of or worsening sleep disturbance before MI, with a similar across racial groups. Women reporting prodromal sleep disturbance were more likely to be older, to be heavier, and to report cognitive changes, new or increasing anxiety, and unusual fatigue.[93]

Moderate or severe insomnia was reported by 37% of patients with ACS during hospitalization and was associated with 76 minutes more WASO measured by home PSG. Although depression and insomnia were strongly associated, about one in four patients with insomnia did not report significant depressive symptoms.[94]

Finally, coronary artery bypass surgery is associated with protracted sleep disturbance up to 2 years after the procedure.[95] The mechanism for this is unclear with occult heart failure, secondary mood issues, or brain microvascular ischemic changes as possibilities.

Heart failure is a major public health concern among older adults. Data from the National Institutes of Health Heart, Lung, and Blood Institute Framingham Heart Study indicate that heart failure incidence is about 10 per 1,000 population at an age over 65 years.[96] With increasing average life span, it is projected that the incidence and prevalence of congestive heart failure will continue to rise. In a cross-sectional study of 223 elderly patients with New York Heart Association classification of II to IV, consistent difficulties maintaining sleep were reported by 23% of men and 20% of women, and 25% of the subjects were awake 1 to 3 hours per night.[97] In a study of more than 600 older adults (mean age 78), cardiopulmonary symptoms (i.e., dyspnea and nighttime palpitations) and pain had significant direct associations with sleep disturbances.[98] Comorbid depression was also identified as a factor that increasingly contributes to sleep disturbance in elderly patients with congestive heart failure (CHF).[99] In a multisite randomized controlled trial including subjects with a heart failure hospitalization (in the prior 6 weeks), 45% of participants reported poor sleep (PSQI ≥ 5).[100] Improved sleep quality correlated with improved exercise capacity and reduced depressive symptoms, but not with changes in body mass index or resting heart rate.

The classic sleep maintenance disturbance associated with CHF includes orthopnea, paroxysmal nocturnal dyspnea, nocturia, and sleep-disordered breathing. Both central and obstructive sleep apnea are common in the CHF population. More than 50% of patients with moderate to severe congestive heart failure experience periodic breathing in the form of Cheyne-Stokes respiration. This may lead to increased sleep fragmentation and an increase in daytime sleepiness.[101,102]

Nocturia is common and often severe in patients with stable CHF. In a cross-sectional observational study of 173 patients (mean age 60 years; left ventricular ejection fraction of 32%) with stable chronic heart failure, a third of patients awakened three or more times per night to void.[103] This group has a nearly sevenfold increase in the odds of reporting insomnia symptoms. There were decreases in sleep duration and efficiency, REM, and stage 3 sleep, and physical function and increases in the percent of WASO, insomnia symptoms, fatigue, and sleepiness across levels of nocturia severity.

Chronic Lung Disease

In 2011 6.3% (15 million) of adults aged 18 years and older reported that they had chronic obstructive pulmonary disease (COPD).[75] Another estimated 15 million adults have impaired pulmonary function and COPD symptoms but are unaware of having COPD because the disease has not been diagnosed by their physician with the use of spirometry. Approximately 80% to 90% of identified COPD cases occur among persons aged at least 45 years.[75] COPD contributes to poor sleep continuity, as well as increased daytime sleepiness.[104] In a study of correlates of insomnia in Chinese patients aged 60 years and older (142 subjects), compared with sex- and age-matched controls, frequency of insomnia was 47.2% in patients and 25.7% in controls, with higher rates in frequencies of early, middle, and late insomnia.[105] Another study of 183 patients with COPD showed higher odds ratios (OR) for insomnia for current tobacco users (OR, 2.13), in those with frequent sadness/anxiety (OR, 3.57); oxygen use was associated with lower odds (OR, 0.35) of insomnia.[106]

Changes reported include increase in sleep stage changes, decreased total sleep time, and increased number of arousals.[107] Even individuals with mild to moderate COPD have lower sleep efficiency, a lower total sleep time, and lower mean overnight oxygen saturation compared with controls.[108] The sleep disturbance is frequently related to nocturnal cough, wheezing, and shortness of breath because of worsening of pulmonary mechanics and gas exchange during sleep. Hypoxemia, which is common in COPD during REM sleep, correlates with an increase in arousal and excessive daytime sleepiness. Although the use of oxygen therapy frequently corrects the underlying hypoxemia, it does not appear to improve sleep quality.[107] Use of inhaled ipratropium bromide improves sleep quality and duration presumably via improved airflow.[109] However, use of a long-acting bronchodilator, such as formoterol, although overall beneficial, may result in insomnia.[110]

The prevalence of insomnia symptoms in a sample of more than 1800 subjects with asthma, part of a 25,000-subject questionnaire, was significantly higher among people with asthma than those without (47% versus 37%).[111] In the subgroup reporting asthma and nasal congestion, 56% had insomnia symptoms. The risk of insomnia increased with the severity of asthma; nasal congestion (OR 1.50), obesity (OR 1.54), and smoking (OR 1.71) increased the risk. Nocturnal asthma symptoms resulting in nighttime awakenings may occur in more than 70% of persons with asthma. Other reported sleep symptoms include difficulties falling asleep, difficulties maintaining sleep, early morning awakenings, and daytime sleepiness. Asthma control correlates with quality of sleep.[112]

Diabetes and Endocrine Disorders

In a large study of more than 13,000 adults with diabetes mellitus, 24% reported insomnia.[113] In community-dwelling older adults (age > 60 years) with diabetes (n = 316), the prevalence of sleep disturbance was 25%. The sleep disturbance group had an average of 4.4 hours of sleep and used significantly more over-the-counter or prescription sleeping medications.[114] People with diabetes may have disrupted sleep resulting from advanced age, obesity, treatments for and complications of common comorbid diseases (e.g., depression, cardiovascular disease). Diabetes-specific complications, such as neuropathy, could directly interfere with sleep or contribute to restless legs and nocturnal leg cramps. In almost 10,000 adults participating in the National Health and Nutrition Examination Survey 2005-2008, diabetes was associated with increased odds of inadequate sleep, frequent daytime sleepiness, restless legs symptoms, sleep apnea, and nocturia.[115] All of these showed greater odds with increasing severity in a graded fashion. Diabetes duration was significantly associated with the same problems; risk increased 20% to 30% per 10 years since diagnosis.

A growing body of literature indicates a link between sleep and glycemic control. Thirty percent of patients with diabetes demonstrate sleep maintenance disturbances, with the severity of disruption correlating with the degree of hyperglycemia.[116,117] Interestingly, the likelihood of being insulin resistant increases linearly with co-occurring sleep complaints.[118] Consequently, high Hba1c was found to be associated with difficulty in maintaining sleep but also early morning awakenings.[119] In an ancillary study of the Coronary Artery Risk Development in Young Adults, among the 40 subjects with diabetes, 10% higher sleep fragmentation was associated with a 9% higher fasting glucose level, a 30% higher fasting insulin level, and a 43% higher insulin resistance estimated using the homeostatic model assessment (HOMA) method. Insomnia was associated with a 23% higher fasting glucose level, a 48% higher fasting insulin level, and an 82% higher HOMA level.[120]

One-third of patients with diabetes have problems with sleep fragmentation, with nocturia, leg cramps, leg pain, and cough as contributing factors. Likewise, patients with diabetes have an increased prevalence of both RLS and periodic limb movements of sleep (PLMS).[121] A growing body of epidemiologic and experimental evidence links sleep apnea and disorders of glucose metabolism; however, the cause-and-effect relationship remains to be determined.[122]

Among 6000 subjects (age > 65) participating in the Osteoporotic Fractures in Men study, no difference in sleep quality was found between subclinical hypothyroid and euthyroid men.[123] Compared to euthyroid men, subclinical hyperthyroid men had lower mean actigraphic total sleep time, lower mean sleep efficiency, higher mean WASO, and increased risk of sleep latency of at least 60 minutes.

Renal and Urologic Diseases

Sleep disruption is common in urologic and kidney diseases. Benign prostatic hyperplasia and prostate cancer are typically diseases of the aging male, steeply increasing with age. Overactive bladder is characterized by urinary urgency, frequency, nocturia, and sometimes incontinence. It increases markedly with advancing age in both men and women.[124]

Nocturia is a well-recognized etiology for sleep maintenance disturbance in later life, and nighttime urination is often associated with poor quality of sleep and increased fatigue in the daytime.[125] It is reported to be an independent predictor both of self-reported insomnia (75% increased risk) and reduced sleep quality (71% increased risk) based on a survey of more than 1400 elderly individuals.[126] In the National Health and Nutrition Examination Survey, prevalence of nocturia, defined as two or more voiding episodes nightly, followed a linear progression with age from 8.2% in men aged 20 to 34 years to 55.8% in men aged at least 75 years. Data also showed nocturia to be a strong predictor of mortality, with a dose-response pattern in increased mortality risk with increasing number of voiding episodes nightly.[127]

The severity of nocturia increased with advancing age. Urinary incontinence, recurrent cystitis, and diabetes mellitus were the strongest associated factors for nocturia of any degree.[128] Other etiologies include polyuria, low bladder capacity, sleep apnea, excessive fluid intake before bedtime, alcohol, caffeine, diuretics, and medical disorders such as hypertension, congestive heart failure, and prostatic disease. The nocturnal polyuria syndrome is characterized by an inappropriate nocturnal urine output, often an undetectable plasma antidiuretic hormone during the night, and increased thirst, particularly at night[129]; 24-hour urine output is normal or only moderately increased. In older adults with concurrent insomnia and nocturia, brief behavioral treatment for insomnia (instructions on reducing time in bed and setting a regular sleep schedule) may also improve self-reported nocturia.[130]

Approximately 40% of community-dwelling older adults report sporadic or chronic urinary incontinence,[131] with the most common cause being the overactive bladder syndrome. Urine loss is considered a geriatric syndrome insofar that it leads to a spectrum of physical, psychological, and social consequences that can be a detriment to a person's functioning and quality of life. The effects of incontinence on sleep are best studied in the nursing home population with both polysomnographic and actigraphy samples demonstrating sleep disruption with nocturnal wetting episodes. Interestingly 51% of these episodes occurred during or within 60 seconds of an abnormal sleep breathing event.[132] In those who are chronically incontinent, the relationship between urine loss and awakening is not as tight.[133]

CKD and end-stage renal disease have a steady increase over age 60 with a striking rise in prevalence beyond age 75.[134]

In a longitudinal study (up to 2 years) of patients with CKD who were on and not on dialysis, patients with CKD not on dialysis had disruption of sleep independent of several risk factors.[135] There are marked abnormalities seen in the sleep of patients with CKD with overall reduction in total sleep time, decreased sleep efficiency resulting from WASO, and reduced total REM.[136] Overall prevalence of insomnia in patients on hemodialysis (HD) was described to be between 45% to 86%.[137] Patients on HD had sleep disruption of much greater severity than that found among those with CKD not on dialysis. Missing or shortening the prescribed duration of dialysis appeared associated with greater severity of sleep disturbance.

Patients on HD have a 50% to 80% rate of sleep-wake complaints and a higher prevalence of OSA (which improves after dialysis), RLS, PLMS, early insomnia, and excessive daytime sleepiness.[136,138,139] Quality of sleep was associated with hemoglobin level, serum albumin, and depression in 89 patients on HD with a mean age of 60 years. In a study involving patients on HD with a mean age of 65 years, treatment of anemia of kidney disease with erythropoietin improved sleep quality by polysomnographic and subjective measures and reduced the numbers of periodic limb movements.[140] Over 50% of patients on HD endorse chronic pain, and this is felt to be significantly associated with insomnia and depression in this condition.[141]

Cancer

Cancer is very frequently a disease of older persons. Approximately 1.5 million new cases of cancer are diagnosed annually.[75] Approximately one in two males and one in three females will receive a diagnosis of cancer over their lifetime. The prevalence of sleep problems in individuals with cancer is difficult to determine with wide variance based upon type and stage of cancer. Large epidemiologic studies suggest that sleep problems are very common (55% to 87% of patients[142,143]) with approximately half of patients reporting onset within the period 6 months prediagnosis to 18 months postdiagnosis.[144] In a study of 867 elders (46% women) newly diagnosed with breast, colorectal, lung, or prostate cancer, insomnia remained present in almost of quarter of patients 1 year after their cancer diagnosis. Authors reported a lessening of reports of pain, fatigue, and insomnia over time; however, a high attrition rate was present.[145]

Persons with cancer may have a baseline history of insomnia or other sleep disorder, or they may have sleep effects from the cancer, its treatment, or the psychological response to the diagnosis.[143] In a meta-analysis of sleep across chemotherapy treatment, subjective and objective sleep quality was found to be poor and nocturnal awakenings frequent across chemotherapy treatment. Daytime sleepiness increases in the active phase of chemotherapy, and insomnia symptoms are common before and after chemotherapy treatment. In women with recurrent or metastatic breast cancer, difficulty falling asleep, nocturnal awakenings, difficulty awakening, and daytime sleepiness are problematic at different points in chemotherapy treatment.[146]

Most of the studies reported in the literature report on sleep changes in early-stage cancer.[144] Up to 44% of hospitalized cancer patients are prescribed hypnotic therapy.[147,148] In a large sample of approximately 2000 cancer patients, about 23% reported taking hypnotic medications. Factors associated with a greater utilization of hypnotic medication were older age, greater difficulties initiating sleep, more stressful life events experienced in the past 6 months, higher levels of anxiety, past or current psychological difficulties, greater use of opioids, and past or current chemotherapy treatments.[149]

MEDICATIONS IN OLDER ADULT AND IMPACT ON SLEEP

The use of prescription drugs and over-the-counter (OTC) drugs is common in older adults. A multitude of OTC and prescription medications are known to influence the sleep-wake cycle and produce comorbid insomnia (see Chapter 53). Their adverse effects are diverse but can be broadly categorized as those that produce drowsiness or daytime somnolence, those that are activating or stimulating to the brain, those that interfere with sleep by indirect mechanisms, those that may directly exacerbate primary sleep disorders, and those that influence sleep architecture via other affects. Adverse side effects and drug-drug or drug-disease interactions are more likely to occur in older adults. These effects can then lead to direct or indirect effects on overnight sleep quality and quantity. Many of these drugs can alter patterns of sleep and wakefulness both during periods of administration as well as during periods of withdrawal. It is especially important to avoid using hypnotics or stimulants as agents in the cascade effect (use of medications to treat sleep-related side effects of other medications), unless all other attempts at medication adjustment have been considered.

Medications That Promote Daytime Sleepiness

Drowsiness is an extremely common side effect of medications, with close to 600 medications cited as causing drowsiness in the side effects index of the *Physician's Desk Reference*.[150] Excessive daytime sleepiness is a frequent sleep complaint in the elderly with a baseline tendency for older adults to have shorter sleep latency during the day.[151] Many medications have the capacity to interfere with acetylcholine or histamine, both regulatory neurotransmitters for wakefulness. These anticholinergic agents are known to have somnogenic effects, waking drowsiness as well as negative cognitive, affective, and quality-of-life outcomes in older adults.[152] Antihistaminergic drugs appear to have variable central nervous system penetration and, binding with H1 antagonists such as diphenhydramine, have much greater likelihood for sedation and cognitive impairment than do tertiary antihistamines.[153] General classes of agents with these effects include antihistamines, antispasmodics, antipsychotics, antiemetics, and antiparkinsonian drugs. Notable specific examples include tricyclic antidepressants such as amitriptyline, doxepin, imipramine, cimetidine, mirtazapine, and oxybutynin.

Medications can also produce sleepiness via other mechanisms. In those individuals taking levodopa or dopamine agonists, there is an increased prevalence of excessive daytime sleepiness and sleep attacks.[154] Anticonvulsant agents such as gabapentin, lamotrigine, tiagabine, and levetiracetam frequently produce sleepiness in older adults. Morphine and other opiate analgesics can contribute to daytime somnolence and decreased alertness as well as disrupt overnight sleep efficiency and architecture.

Medications That Activate the Central Nervous System

A large number of medications disturb sleep via excitation or activation of the central nervous system. Sleep quality may be affected if these agents are taken before the patient's bedtime or have a sustained half-life that extends into the typical sleep period. Common OTC products for cold and flu contain pseudoephedrine, ephedrine, or other sympathomimetics. OTC analgesics employed for headache therapy contain caffeine. Agents used to manage chronic lung disease, such as inhaled and oral beta-agonists, corticosteroids, and theophylline, can contribute to sleep disruption. Activating antidepressants such as desipramine, bupropion, venlafaxine, reboxetine, and most selective serotonin receptor inhibitors (SSRIs) can sometimes adversely affect sleep initiation and maintenance. Insomnia has been reported as a frequent side effect with SSRI use with prevalence of 16.4% with sertraline, 15% with fluoxetine, and 14% with paroxetine.[155] With SSRIs, although individuals may appreciate an improvement in subjective sleep quality, objective sleep often worsens.[35] Activating medications such as methylphenidate, selegiline, and modafinil are often seen on geriatric medication lists. Careful evaluation of doses and times of administration for such medications may be considered to avoid interference with the desired sleep period.

Medications That Affect Sleep by Worsening Other Conditions

Medications can sometimes interfere with sleep by worsening an underlying medical or psychiatric condition that then affects sleep. Medications that worsen heart failure such as nonsteroidal antiinflammatory drugs, calcium channel blockers, or sodium complexed antibiotics have the potential to cause central sleep apnea, nocturia, or other sleep problems seen in this condition. Medications including nitrates and calcium channel blockers can decrease lower esophageal sphincter tone with resultant nocturnal gastroesophageal reflux. Amitriptyline and other anticholinergic medications, although potentially helpful with sleep because of sedation, can also contribute to confusion as well as urinary retention, with subsequent arousals from delirium or nocturia. Late afternoon or evening diuretic treatment may cause nocturia and sleep fragmentation. Antipsychotic medications can produce parkinsonian symptoms with accompanying adverse effects on sleep. Quetiapine may be least likely to cause this adverse effect. Hypoglycemic agents, if they produce nocturnal hypoglycemia, can increase nocturnal arousals.

Medications That Can Exacerbate Primary Sleep Disorders

A number of medications have been reported to exacerbate primary sleep disorders. Nocturnal movement disorders such as RLS and PLMS can worsen in the setting of a number of antidepressant medications. In a study of 274 consecutive patients on antidepressants as compared with 69 controls, those taking SSRIs or venlafaxine had an odds ratio greater than 5 for having a periodic leg movement index greater than 20, while bupropion was similar to controls.[156] Tricyclic antidepressants and lithium are also associated with a greater prevalence of nocturnal movement disorders. Caffeine, antihistamines, alcohol, and benzodiazepine withdrawal can all worsen RLS. Antipsychotic therapies are associated with greater PLMS prevalence.

Based on a series of small studies and case reports, opiate analgesia use, especially sustained release or long half-life formulations, is associated with increased central apneas, sustained hypoxemia, and prolonged duration of the abnormal breathing events.[157] These changes occur in the context of the well-established acute respiratory depressant effects. Benzodiazepines may worsen sleep-disordered breathing by increasing the arousal threshold, although preliminary studies suggest that some hypnotics (such as trazodone) may improve OSA in patients with a low respiratory arousal threshold.[158]

Medications That Affect Sleep Architecture via Other Mechanisms

Certain medications may directly affect the sleep architecture. Beta blockers are frequently prescribed in older adults in the context of hypertension and heart disease. The more lipophilic agents such as propranolol and some of the newer-generation beta blockers have been shown to suppress melatonin, increase sleep fragmentation, as well as increase nightmares in some people.[159] Other agents such as lithium, benzodiazepines, benzodiazepine receptor agonists, and GABA-hydroxybutyrate are associated with a worsening of disorders of non–rapid eye movement parasomnias. Tricyclic antidepressants, monoamine oxidase inhibitors, venlafaxine, and mirtazapine have been documented to induce REM sleep behavior disorder, a parasomnia very specific to older adults.

Oxybutynin is the most studied of the anticholinergic agents. Night terrors have been reported with this agent in case reports, in addition to mild sedation. Polysomnographic changes include a decrease in the amount of REM sleep of approximately 15%, increased REM sleep latency.[160] Reported effects of donepezil include an increase in REM sleep with a decrease in slow frequencies in REM sleep, decrease in stage 1, increase in stage 2.[161] An increase in REM sleep density, decrease in REM sleep latency, and nightmares have been reported in healthy elderly volunteers.[162] Changes observed with galantamine in healthy volunteers include a decrease in REM sleep latency, increase in REM sleep density, and a decrease in SWS.[163]

SUBSTANCE ABUSE IN OLDER ADULT AND RELATIONSHIP TO SLEEP

Legal substances of abuse (alcohol, nicotine, and caffeine) as well as illicit ones (stimulants, marijuana, opiates) can disrupt sleep. There is a large amount of substance use in older adults with comorbid psychiatric conditions and health problems, which further contribute and complicate sleep disturbances, and warrants clinical assessment and treatment as a potential route of improving sleep complaints. Among those with a mental disorder, the lifetime prevalence of an addictive disorder, not including nicotine or caffeine dependence, is 29%, mostly accounted for by alcohol.[164]

Alcohol Dependence

Community rates of alcohol dependence in the geriatric population are 2% to 3% of men and 1% of women.[165] In elderly clinical cohorts, rates are higher (4% to 23%), likely because of the increased comorbid medical disorders.[166] The direction of sleep disruption and alcohol dependence is likely bidirectional with 50% of alcoholics reporting sleep problems before the onset of alcohol dependence.[167] Quantity of drinking and depression appear to predict insomnia severity,[168] whereas sleep problems may increase the risk of an older adult developing alcohol problems.[169] Elderly people with an alcohol addiction may have other substance-related comorbidities, which may further impair their sleep, including nicotine dependence in 50% to 70% and dependence on prescribed sedatives, anxiolytics, and opioid analgesics (2% to 14%).[166]

Although acute ingestion may decrease sleep latency, subsequent sleep is of poorer quality and shorter duration. Increased arousals occur as the blood alcohol level falls in the hours after alcohol intake, with resultant sleep maintenance insomnia.[170] Acetylcholine, glutamate, GABA, norepinephrine, dopamine, and adenosine neurotransmitter systems are affected, as well as circadian cycle, body temperature, release of cortisol, and nocturnal release of growth hormone. Alcohol decreases pharyngeal muscle tone and lowers the arousal threshold, increasing the risk of apneas and more severe oxygen desaturations during apneas.

Chronic consumption results in long-term alterations of the neurotransmitter systems affected by alcohol. Although sleep complaints vary, difficulty falling asleep is reported as the most significant factor associated with substance use.[169] People over the age of 55 with an alcohol dependence have higher sleep latency, lower sleep efficiency, and lower delta sleep when compared with younger people with an alcohol dependence and those of both age groups without an alcohol dependence.[171]

An older person with alcohol dependence is likely to still have disrupted sleep even after having sustained abstinence, since alcohol dependence may result in permanent effects on the brain.[172] People with an alcohol dependency who have been abstinent for 3 to 6 weeks have worse sleep than those people without such a dependency as indicated by polysomnographic assessment,[173] with changes persisting at 2½ years.[169,174] During abstinence, insomnia and sleep architecture changes are significant factors predicting alcohol relapse.[171,175] In addition, 75% of above age 60 abstinent males with alcohol dependency had sleep-disordered breathing compared with 25% for 40 to 59 years of age.[176] Higher rates of PLMS have also been observed.[177]

Caffeine

Caffeine is consumed by 90% of the adult population in the United States.[178] There appears to be a curvilinear relationship between caffeine intake and age, with intake being greatest among individuals aged 50 to 70 years, and intermediate among those 70 to 79 years.[178] In a study of 1528 older adults, participants in the age group 60 to 69 years of age reported consuming 17.6 cups of caffeinated coffee per week, with a slight subsequent reduction over the next 2 decades of age to 12.8 cups of caffeinated coffee per week.[179] Because of the greater proportion of adipose tissue to lean body mass, a dose of caffeine expressed as mg/kg total body weight may result in higher plasma and tissue concentrations in elderly compared with younger individuals. Age and plasma caffeine concentrations significantly predict a poorer quality sleep.[180] Adults over 67 years old on caffeine-containing medications report significantly more trouble falling asleep after controlling for multiple factors.[181] Hospital-dwelling older adults with a higher serum caffeine concentration reported sleep problems more than those with lower levels.[180]

Tobacco and Nicotine

Tobacco use remains the leading preventable cause of death and disease in the United States, with approximately 480,000 deaths occurring annually because of cigarette smoking and exposure to secondhand smoke. Tobacco use is a chronic disease with multiple relapses, especially in older adults. Nearly 11% of the population age 65 and older smokes.[182] In a cohort of almost 500 women followed over 25 years, chronic heavy smoking subjects were more likely to report insomnia at mean age 65 (adjusted OR = 2.76).[183] Elderly smokers endorse more difficulties with sleep onset and staying asleep than nonsmokers. In all age groups, smokers drink more caffeine and are more likely to be depressed.[184] The overlap of nicotine dependence with other health-risk behaviors (such as drinking, unhealthy eating habits, insufficient leisure activities, and physical inactivity) was positively correlated with a higher risk of sleep disturbances in a cross-sectional study of almost 5000 Chinese older adults (age > 60).[185]

SPECIAL CONDITIONS

Caregiving

Elderly caregivers represent 13% of all caregivers and are more likely to be caring for a spouse, often with dementia. Caregivers identify barriers to health-promotion activities, including lack of time, decreased energy, and additional costs for providing care for the care recipient. Up to two-thirds of older adult caregivers have some form of sleep disturbance.[186] Predisposing factors for changes in the sleep of a caregiver include increasing age, female gender, and caregiver burden.[187] Caregiver burden encompasses the spectrum of physical, psychological or emotional, social, and financial problems experienced by the care provider.

In a study of community-dwelling spousal caregivers of patients with Alzheimer disease, caregivers objectively slept less than older noncaregivers and subjectively reported more sleep problems and functional impairment as a result of poor sleep.[188] Caregivers who could not leave their care recipient alone in an emergency, a greater number of hours per day providing care, and more frequent memory-related problems in the care recipient were related to higher WASO.[189] In the case of the vulnerable caregiver, it can be very difficult to fall back asleep after being awakened by a care recipient who needs assistance with toileting, administration of medication, redirection back into bed, orientation, or emotional reassurance, particularly when these nocturnal interactions are prolonged or emotionally charged.

Additional risks for poor sleep include fluctuations in the status of the care recipient, the need for vigilance to safeguard the care recipient at night, and worry about current and future events, which caused rumination.[190] The caregiver's situation is analogous to that of a rotating shift worker who must be alert at night and during the day, often on an inconsistent schedule.[186] The combination of depression and high-stress situations (e.g., caring for a spouse or a person with dementia, or living with the care recipient) increased the likelihood of sleep problems.[191] This situation puts the caregiver at risk for long-term partial sleep deprivation that may partially explain why one of the strongest factors in deciding to institutionalize a spouse or family member with dementia is poor overnight sleep of the affected individual.[192]

CLINICAL PEARLS

- Sleep complaints are often comorbid with chronic health issues as well as the associated changes in a person's lifestyle, sleep hygiene, and medication regimes that occur secondary to the illness. Furthermore, these health problems rarely exist in isolation and instead frequently coexist with psychiatric diagnoses, neurologic diseases, and primary sleep pathology.
- In view of the multiple pathways of disrupted sleep, a multifaceted management approach is best to improve symptoms. This includes optimizing the underlying illness and the environment, adjusting potentially offending medications, using cognitive-behavioral approaches, and employing judicious hypnotic therapy based on current evidence.
- Older adults are often in special situations (caregiving, hospitalization, end of life, abstinence after alcohol dependence) that make them particularly vulnerable to incident sleep disturbances. A heightened awareness and recognition of these situations is necessary.
- Many medications can alter patterns of sleep and wakefulness during periods of administration as well as periods of withdrawal. It is especially important to avoid using hypnotics or stimulants to treat sleep-related side effects of other medications unless all other options have been considered.
- Insomnia is a public health problem, but treating it with prescription sleep medications that are higher risk for older adults may increase rather than decrease health outcomes. Clinicians may wish to consider routine drug regimen reviews with patients. This may be particularly applicable to patients with cognitive impairment and those who cannot live independently. Specific medication cautions should be tailored to patients' age, health, living situation, and cognitive status.

SUMMARY

As the field of medicine continues to advance, people are living longer with more comorbid medical and psychiatric conditions. This higher burden of illness and the numbers of medications used to treat these conditions play an important role in the quality and quantity of sleep in older adults. In approaching sleep complaints in geriatric patients, it is essential that practitioners recognize the multidimensional mechanisms by which illness affects sleep. Equally important, a balanced management approach (Figure 191.2) that includes optimizing the underlying illness, adjusting medications, using cognitive-behavioral approaches, and using judicious hypnotic therapy seems justified based on the current evidence.

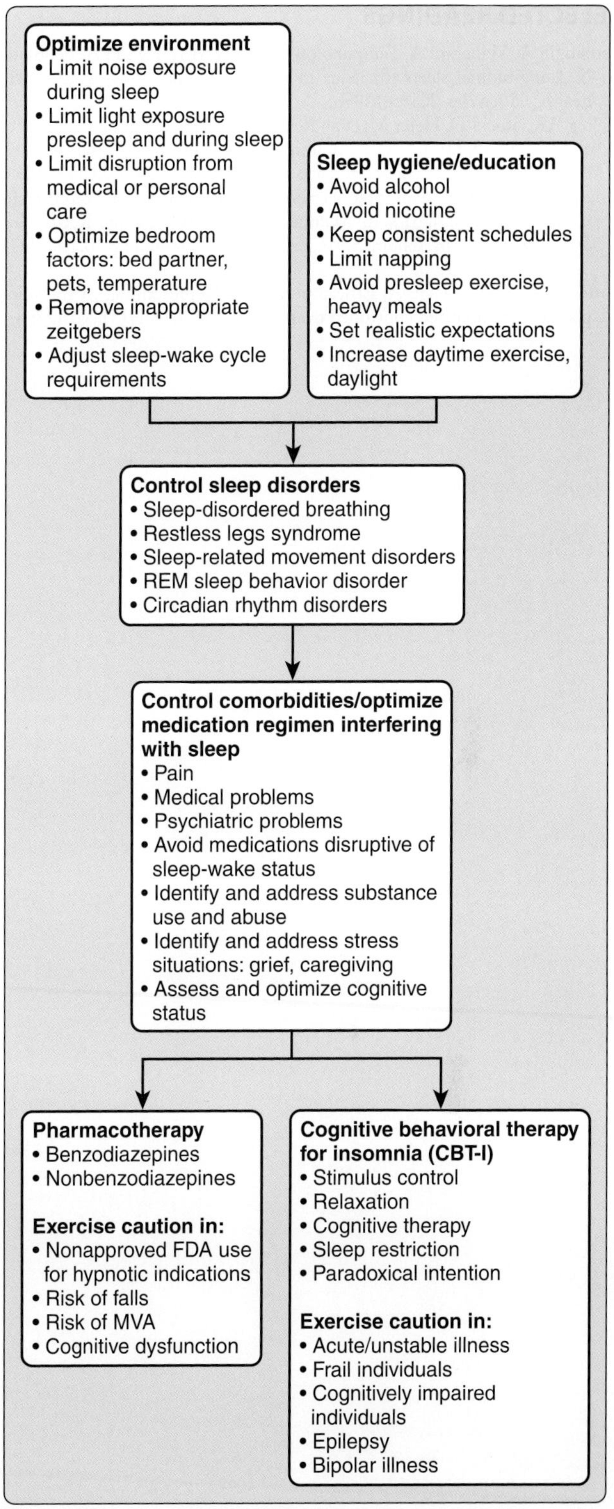

Figure 191.2 Interventions to be considered in comorbid insomnia. A multifactorial targeted intervention appears to be most appropriate in accordance with current concepts and as indicated by the available evidence. Considering all potential predisposing, precipitating, and perpetuating factors can increase the effectiveness of the therapeutic act while ensuring optimal control. Interventions should be balanced with regard to potential adverse consequences. MVA, Motor vehicle accident.

SELECTED READINGS

Didikoglu A, Maharani A, Tampubolon G, Canal MM, Payton A, Pendleton N. Longitudinal sleep efficiency in the elderly and its association with health. *J Sleep Res.* 2019:e12898.

Helbig AK, Stockl D, Heier M, et al. Relationship between sleep disturbances and multimorbidity among community-dwelling men and women aged 65-93 years: results from the KORA age study. *Sleep Med.* 2017;33:151–159.

Howell T. The Wisconsin Star Method: Understanding and Addressing Complexity in Geriatrics. In: Malone M, Capezuti E, Palmer R, eds. *Geriatrics Models of Care.* Cham: Springer; 2015. https://doi.org/10.1007/978-3-319-16068-9 7,

Potter K, Flicker L, Page A, Etherton-Beer C. Deprescribing in frail older people: a randomised controlled trial. *PLoS One.* 2016;11(3):e0149984.

Stewart NH, Arora VM. Sleep in hospitalized older adults. *Sleep Med Clin.* 2018;13(1):127–135. https://doi.org/10.1016/j.jsmc.2017.09.012.

Vaz Fragoso CA, Gill TM. Sleep complaints in community-living older persons: a multifactorial geriatric syndrome. *J Am Geriatr Soc.* 2007;55(11):1853–1866.

A complete reference list can be found online at ExpertConsult.com.

Chapter 192

Obstructive Sleep Apnea in Older Adults

Sara Pasha

Chapter Highlights

- The prevalence of obstructive sleep apnea (OSA) increases with age, but the peak prevalence of clinically diagnosed OSA is in middle age. Differences in the clinical presentation, severity, and manifestations of obstructive sleep-disordered breathing (SDB) between older and younger persons probably account for much of the gap in diagnosis.
- More than half of older adults report sleeping difficulty.[1-5] Because sleep complaints are common in the older age group, clinicians may discount them. Sleep complaints in seniors, however, correlate with health complaints, depression, and mortality.[1-6] Undiagnosed OSA probably accounts for some of the sleep complaints voiced by older adults. Indeed, OSA leads both to sleep disturbance and to increased mortality and is likely to account for much of the association between sleep complaints and adverse outcomes in older people. Despite this, SDB is underdiagnosed and undertreated in the older adult population.
- Accumulating data indicate that continuous positive airway pressure use is associated with reduced cardiovascular morbidity, cognitive dysfunction, and all-cause mortality in seniors.[7-9] Clinicians caring for geriatric patients should consider SDB in the older adult with sleep complaints. This chapter focuses on OSA in the older patient. For discussion of central sleep apnea, see Chapters 109 and 110.

EPIDEMIOLOGY AND DEFINITIONS

Although studies of clinical populations identify peak prevalence of clinically significant sleep-disordered breathing (SDB) in middle age, population-based studies have shown that SDB increases with age.[10,11] Longitudinal and cross-sectional studies have also shown that the prevalence of sleep apnea increases with advancing age[12-16] (Table 192.1).

Estimates of the prevalence of obstructive sleep apnea (OSA) in older people depend on how it is defined, so prevalence estimates for OSA in older people are moving targets. There has been considerable variation in the definitions and measurements of respiratory events (such as apneas, hypopneas, and respiratory effort–related arousals) used to identify SDB. Furthermore, the respiratory events counted to use toward the threshold to define "sleep apnea" have also varied. The apnea-hypopnea index (AHI) typically includes only apneas and hypopneas. The respiratory disturbance index (RDI) may include other events, such as respiratory effort–related arousals. Finally, the demarcation between "normal" and "abnormal" has also been somewhat fluid. In population-based studies, approximately one-third of those older than 65 years of age have AHIs of five or more events per hour of sleep,[17,18] and two-thirds have RDIs of 10 or more events per hour.[18,19] The Centers for Medicare and Medicaid Services, the primary provider of health care coverage for people older than 65 in the United States, defines OSA as an AHI of 15 or more, or an AHI of five or more plus certain symptoms or conditions (e.g., hypertension, stroke, sleepiness).[20] However, some signs and symptoms associated with OSA increase in prevalence with aging, even in the absence of OSA, which may affect diagnosis.

Regardless of definition, OSA prevalence increases progressively from age 18 to approximately 70, when it may plateau.[21] The underdiagnosis of sleep apnea in older people is more common than in younger people, and this may be especially true in minority populations.[21]

Diagnosis of SDB is evolving rapidly, with revised, more liberal diagnostic criteria[22] and the recognition that oximetry alone can be predictive of important outcomes. For example, in a study of 100 patients with a mean age of 62 years, Ohmura and associates reported that SDB, as determined by predischarge pulse oximetry (based on oxygen desaturation index of 4%), was associated with significantly increased risks for necessity for readmission and death, independent of other risk factors.[23] In a study of patients with OSA and matched control subjects, oxygen saturation predicted cognitive function, but AHI did not.[24] In the Spanish Sleep Network study, oxygen desaturation predicted cancer risk, but AHI did not.[25] Similarly, time elapsed with oxygen saturation below 90% predicted 3-year mortality in older persons with cardiovascular disease. It also predicted self-reported insomnia.[26] These and other findings are likely to change, yet again, the diagnostic

Table 192.1 Differences between Younger (<60 years) and Older Patients with Obstructive Sleep Apnea (OSA)

Risk Factor	Older Patients	Younger Patients
Male sex	1:1	2:1
Obesity	Unimportant	Very important
Clinical Features		
Witnessed apneas	Witnessed apneas rarely reported	Witnessed apneas strongly predictive
Snoring	Infrequently reported	Frequently reported
Prevalence		
AHI > 5	30%–40%	9% for women, 24% for men
RDI > 10	62%	10%
Consequences	Death, cardiovascular disease, stroke, nocturia, impaired cognition, atrial fibrillation	Death, ischemic cardiac disease, hypertension, cerebrovascular disease, depression, metabolic disturbances
Treatment	May require lower CPAP pressures No difference in tolerance or adherence	May require higher CPAP pressures No difference in tolerance or adherence

AHI, Apnea-hypopnea index; CPAP, positive airway pressure; RDI, respiratory disturbance index.

criteria for significant sleep apnea, at least for third-party payers, who are increasingly data driven.

CLINICAL MANIFESTATIONS AND PRESENTATION

Most studies of the clinical presentation and manifestations of OSA have focused on the middle aged. Reports derived from clinical populations tend to include people whose mean age is approximately 50. As more data accumulate about SDB in older people, it is becoming increasingly clear that the phenotype of OSA can be different in younger and in older populations.

Perhaps most striking is the change with aging in sex-related risk factors for SDB. Prospective data from the Wisconsin Sleep Cohort demonstrated that male sex is no longer an important risk factor for OSA after the age of approximately 50 years,[27] confirming work from other studies.[11] At least part of the reason for this phenomenon is that the prevalence of OSA rises strikingly for women as they go through menopause, which occurs at approximately age 50.[28-30] As a consequence, some investigators have reported a male-to-female ratio of 1:1 for older people.[27]

In addition to the loss of the effect of male gender as a risk for OSA with aging, there is reduced importance of obesity as a risk factor. Beginning at approximately 60 years of age, obesity is no longer a statistically significant risk factor for SDB.[27,29] These observations are of particular interest in view of known decreases in obesity with increasing age.[31] Some data suggest that obesity is a more important risk factor for men than for women, but that aging, perhaps specifically achieving menopause, is a more important risk factor for women than for men.[27-30,32,33] However, in an 18-year follow-up study of 427 community-dwelling elderly persons, Ancoli-Israel and colleagues found that observed changes in RDI were associated only with changes in body mass index (BMI) and were independent of age[34]; they pointed out that this finding underscores the importance of managing weight for older adults, particularly those with hypertension.

In a study of nearly 100 community-dwelling adults aged 62 to 91 years, Endeshaw found that almost one-third (equally divided between men and women) had an AHI of 15 or more events per hour of sleep, and that the "traditional" risk factors such as snoring, BMI, and neck circumference were not significantly associated with OSA in this group.[35] Rather, those with an AHI of at least 15 were more likely to report not feeling well rested in the morning and to have higher Epworth Sleepiness Scale scores and a greater frequency of nocturia.[35] These findings confirm earlier work from the Sleep Heart Health Study, which reported that witnessed apneas are much less frequently reported in older patients than in younger ones.[36]

Studies of OSA in older people have tended to report "milder" disease, with lower AHIs, and better-preserved oxygen saturation than in younger adults.[12,17,29]

In short, the "classic" clinical presentation of OSA is uncommon in older adults, which may account in part for the reduced prevalence of clinical diagnosis of the disorder in this population.

PATHOPHYSIOLOGY

The pathophysiology of OSA may be different in older persons from that in younger people. Chapter 111 outlines the pathophysiology of OSA in adults. With aging, loss of tissue elasticity also may contribute to airway collapse. For older women, declining levels of sex hormones appear to be partly responsible for increased collapsibility of the posterior oropharynx.[37,38]

CLINICAL CONSEQUENCES

Overview

A majority of studies of the consequences of OSA have been undertaken in clinical samples of middle-aged people. Data specifically focusing on the consequences of OSA in older persons are limited. OSA has long been associated with increases in the risk of death in younger populations, but early studies suggested that it was not associated with increased mortality in older groups.[39,40] A rigorous study from the Spanish Sleep Network, however, clearly demonstrated a twofold increase in risk of death in a group of patients with severe OSA (AHI of 30 or greater) whose mean age was 71 years over that in the control group, after initiation of controls for age, BMI, preexisting cardiovascular disease, smoking, diabetes, sleepiness, gender, dyslipidemia, and/or respiratory failure. Furthermore, continuous positive airway pressure (CPAP) use reduced the risk of all-cause mortality, as well as cardiovascular death and death from stroke and heart failure, but did not reduce the risk of death from ischemic disease in this cohort. Indeed, even those seniors 75 years of age and older had reduced risk of cardiovascular death with CPAP use, and continuous adherence was associated with reduced risk of cardiovascular death as a continuous variable.[41] The inclusion of a large cohort with severe sleep apnea (AHI of 30 or higher) probably partly accounts for the ability of this study to demonstrate a mortality effect with sleep apnea and with CPAP. In a meta-analysis of prospective cohort studies of OSA and risk of cardiovascular disease, Wang and colleagues demonstrated a "dose-response" relationship between OSA severity and cardiovascular outcomes and calculated a 17% greater risk of cardiovascular disease for each 10-unit increase in AHI.[42] It is possible that older people tolerate milder degrees of SDB better than their younger counterparts and that part of the past difficulty in demonstrating an association between OSA and adverse outcomes in older patients was because few patients with moderate to severe disease were included in earlier studies.

Other plausible explanations have been proposed for the inability to readily demonstrate the impact of SDB on cardiovascular outcomes in older people. Lavie and Lavie, for example, speculated that the reduced effect of OSA on mortality in older people is because of ischemic preconditioning resulting from the nocturnal cycles of hypoxia-reoxygenation.[43] They pointed out that in patients with SDB, there is an association of ischemic preconditioning with increased levels of vascular endothelial growth factor and increased production of oxygen reactive species, heat shock proteins, adenosine, and tumor necrosis factor-α.[43]

Among the most striking manifestations of SDB in aging populations are nocturia, cognitive dysfunction, and cardiac disease.

Nocturia

Nocturia is a particularly troublesome symptom of aging and appears to be related to the severity of SDB. Because older adults with significant SDB may not manifest classic symptoms of OSA, the presence of nocturia in the older patient should heighten clinical suspicion for OSA. Indeed, nocturnal urination more than three times nightly had positive and negative predictive values of 0.71 and 0.62, respectively, for severe OSA in one study.[44]

A postulated mechanism of nocturia in OSA is that the negative intrathoracic pressures resulting from occluded breaths cause distention of the right atrium and ventricle. This right-sided cardiac distention results in release of atrial natriuretic peptide, which inhibits the secretion of antidiuretic hormone and aldosterone and causes diuresis through its effect on glomerular filtration of sodium and water.[45] Another postulated mechanism is related to hypoxic events.[46,47] Several studies have demonstrated symptomatic improvement in patients with nocturia with use of CPAP.[48-50] The mechanism of CPAP-related improvement may involve promoting the normal nocturnal rise in antidiuretic hormone, resulting in increased resorption of sodium and water from the collecting tubules and production of lower volumes of more concentrated urine.[51] In a retrospective review of data on 196 patients whose mean age was 49 years, predictors of nocturia included increasing age and diabetes mellitus. Although a complaint of nocturia was equally likely to occur in patients with and without OSA, nocturia frequency was significantly related to age, diabetes, and severity of SDB in those patients who had OSA. Furthermore, patients with OSA and nocturia who were treated with CPAP experienced significant reductions in the frequency of nocturnal voiding.[52] In a study of 21 women with a mean age of 65 years, the same group of investigators reported that OSA is present in a majority of women with nocturia and that the presence of diluted nighttime urine in a patient with nocturia is a sensitive marker for OSA.[53]

Impaired Cognition

Impaired cognition, including sleepiness, impaired vigilance, worsened executive function, and dementia, increases in prevalence with aging. Neuropsychological assessment of patients with OSA demonstrates decline in cognition similar to that with aging. For example, patients with OSA experience sleepiness[54] and demonstrate impaired executive function,[55] working memory,[56] alertness,[57] and attention.[58] In general, the association between SDB and impaired cognition has been best studied in middle-aged patients. Because of the association with aging on impaired cognition, the effects of OSA on cognitive function in older people have been difficult to tease out. In a small study with subjects older than 55 years of age who had OSA, Aloia and colleagues found that the degree of SDB, especially oxygen desaturation, was associated with delayed verbal recall and impaired constructional abilities. After 3 months, subjects who were compliant with CPAP showed greater improvements in attention, psychomotor speed, executive functioning, and nonverbal delayed recall than in those who were not compliant.[59] Despite the logical notion that cognitive impairment associated with OSA in older people may be more severe than in younger people because of cumulative effects of age and SDB, Mathieu and colleagues were unable to demonstrate any group-by-age interaction for any neuropsychological variable; in a study of matched older and younger patients both with and without OSA, they found that performance on most tasks deteriorated with advancing age in both control subjects and patients with OSA without evidence of a compounded effect.[60] Persons at high risk for OSA based on Berlin questionnaire scores (57% of whom were female) had lower cognitive function scores than those without, but the risk was most pronounced during middle age and was attenuated after age 70.[61]

The evidence indicates age- and gender-dependent relationships as well. In a large study of patients with OSA who were at least 40 years old, the risk of developing dementia within 5 years of diagnosis was 1.70 times greater than in age- and sex-matched subjects who did not have OSA, after appropriate adjustment for some potential confounders. In this study, men aged 50 to 59 had a sixfold increased risk of developing dementia compared with matched control subjects, but women 70 years of age or older had a threefold increased risk of developing dementia. One large study reported that SDB severity was not associated with indices of sleep-related symptoms or sleep-related quality of life in community-dwelling older women, suggesting that this group may be resistant to the adverse effects of OSA on cognition.[62]

In addition to age and gender differences in susceptibility to dementia in patients with OSA, genetic predispositions also are likely. Data from the Wisconsin Sleep Cohort suggest that in apolipoprotein E epsilon 4 genotype (APOE4)–positive persons, the presence of SDB (AHI ≥ 15) was associated with poorer performance on tests of cognition that require both memory and executive function. Such an association was not seen in individuals with SDB but who were negative for the APOE4 genotype.[63] Preliminary work suggests an association between SDB and Alzheimer disease biomarker in the cerebrospinal fluid and blood of cognitively normal persons.[64,65] These early data point to genetic influences on the propensity to develop dementia in patients with SDB.

It is likely that many other factors affect susceptibility to cognitive dysfunction in patients with OSA. For example, Alchantis and colleagues have proposed that high intelligence may protect against cognitive decline caused by SDB, perhaps as a consequence of increased cognitive reserve.[66]

The mechanism by which SDB impairs neurocognitive function remains incompletely understood. Some investigators have suggested that sleep fragmentation is the primary culprit,[67] whereas others maintain that hypoxemia is the primary cause. It is likely that the functions affected by hypoxemia differ from those affected by sleep deprivation. As suggested by Sateia, "Disturbances in general intellectual function and executive function show strongest correlations with measures of hypoxemia. Not unexpectedly, alterations in vigilance, alertness, and, to some extent, memory seem to correlate more with measures of sleep disruption."[68] However, in a small study of matched patients with OSA, AHI did not predict or correlate with cognition, but mean oxygen saturation correlated with executive functioning and access to long-term memory.[24]

Kim and colleagues demonstrated that moderate to severe OSA is an independent risk factor for white matter change in more than 500 people (mean age 59 ± 7.48 years) and presented an excellent discussion of potential mechanisms, including hypoxemia and hypercapnia during apneic events, which activate arousal and chemoreflex-mediated increases in the cerebral circulation and activation of oxidative and inflammatory processes.[69]

Information about the effects of CPAP treatment on cognition in older people is limited, and data about CPAP's effects on cognition in older persons are even more so. In a small group of patients whose mean age was 56 years, CPAP resulted in normalization in attentive, visuospatial learning and in motor performances after 15 days, but no further improvement was observed after 4 months of treatment. CPAP did not improve performance on tests evaluating executive functions and constructional abilities.[70] A meta-analysis of randomized, placebo-controlled crossover studies of CPAP treatment involving 98 patients with sleep apnea demonstrated mostly trends for better performance on CPAP than on placebo.[71] In a group of middle-aged adults with significant OSA, Zimmerman and colleagues demonstrated that memory normalized for the group that used CPAP at least 6 hours a night[72] but did not improve in those who were not adherent to CPAP treatment. In the Apnea Positive Pressure Long-Term Efficacy Study (APPLES), treatment with CPAP, especially in individuals with severe OSA (AHI > 30), resulted in improvements in sleepiness, and there was a mild but transient improvement in measures of executive and frontal lobe function. The mean age in the intervention group was 52 years.[73]

In a review of CPAP adherence and benefits among older people, Weaver and Chasens noted that in general, older adults demonstrate increased alertness; improved neurobehavioral outcomes in cognition, memory, and executive function; and decreased sleep disruption.[74] These investigators also noted that older persons may require lower CPAP pressures than younger ones and tolerate CPAP well, with similar rates of adherence. Thus, despite differences in the clinical presentation and impact of sleep apnea in the elderly population, CPAP treatment is likely to be well tolerated and beneficial in symptomatic patients.[75,76]

With regard specifically to Alzheimer disease, the prevalence of OSA is higher among patients with this disorder than those without, and SDB is believed to contribute to cognitive dysfunction in those with Alzheimer disease. A randomized double-blind, placebo-controlled crossover trial of CPAP in patients with OSA and Alzheimer disease demonstrated a significant improvement in cognition after 3 weeks of CPAP.[77] In addition to improving cognition, CPAP treatment may reduce sleepiness in patients with Alzheimer disease and OSA.[78]

In view of the facts that improvement in cognition is likely to depend on CPAP adherence, that gender, age, genetic, and intelligence are probable influences on susceptibility to impaired cognition, and that most studies addressing this issue have not included geriatric patients with OSA or objectively measured adherence, firm conclusions about the reversibility of cognitive deficits in older patients with OSA are not possible at present.

Cardiovascular Disease

In addition to nocturia and cognitive impairment, SDB is also strongly linked to cardiovascular disease, including hypertension, congestive heart failure, stroke, cardiac arrhythmias, ischemic events, and pulmonary artery hypertension; however, fewer studies have been conducted in older adults.[79-83] Hypertension, atrial fibrillation, and stroke, however, are particularly relevant comorbid conditions associated with OSA in older patients, because of their higher prevalence and clinical importance in that population.

Hypertension

That SDB causes *hypertension* has been demonstrated by multiple studies, including prospective and CPAP sham–controlled studies.[84-90] Severe sleep apnea (AHI of 30 events or more per hour) is an independent risk factor for incident hypertension in older people (mean age, 68.2 years).[91] In general, CPAP has modest effects on blood pressure in patients with OSA but is most effective in those who have significant hypertension and are most adherent with its use.[84,92,93]

Atrial Fibrillation

Atrial fibrillation is strongly associated both with aging and with OSA.[79,94] The Sleep Heart Health Study investigators found that persons with severe SDB had double or quadruple the risk of complex cardiac arrhythmias compared with those with no SDB, after institution of controls for multiple relevant confounders.[94] In this study, atrial fibrillation was the arrhythmia most strongly associated with SDB. Gami and colleagues reported that both obesity and nocturnal oxygen desaturation were independent predictors of incident atrial fibrillation, but only in subjects younger than 65 years of age.[95] However, Ganga and colleagues noted that the presence of overlap syndrome (OSA combined with chronic obstructive pulmonary disease) is associated with a marked increase in new-onset atrial fibrillation in elderly patients over that associated with the presence of either OSA or chronic obstructive pulmonary disease alone.[96]

In a small retrospective study of patients with atrial fibrillation, some of whom had either treated or untreated sleep apnea and some of whom did not have sleep apnea, the patients with untreated OSA had a higher recurrence of atrial fibrillation after cardioversion than that for the patients without sleep apnea.[97] Furthermore, treatment with CPAP in the sleep apnea group was associated with lower recurrence of atrial fibrillation at 1-year follow-up evaluation. This study is particularly relevant for the management of older patients because the mean age of the study population was approximately 66 years. A study of patients undergoing pulmonary vein isolation reported that the 32 patients who had OSA and used CPAP were less likely to have atrial tachyarrhythmias, use of antiarrhythmic drugs, and need for repeat ablations when compared to the 30 patients who did not use CPAP during a follow-up period of 12 months; the difference in atrial fibrillation–free survival rate was 71.9% versus 36.7% ($P = .01$).[98]

As in younger adults, SDB is associated with subtle measures of myocardial injury. In a large study of patients whose mean age was 62.5 years, OSA severity correlated with measures of high-sensitivity troponin T and N-terminal pro–B--type natriuretic peptide. High-sensitivity troponin was related to risk of death or heart failure in all categories.[99] Elderly patients with OSA exhibit cardiac structural changes and diminished left ventricular function compared with that in control subjects who do not have OSA.[100] In a nonrandomized, retrospective review of data on 130 patients aged 65 to 86 years, Nishihata and colleagues demonstrated that those with untreated sleep apnea had increased likelihood of cardiovascular death and hospitalization resulting from cardiovascular disease, including heart failure, over a follow-up period of approximately 3 months. Furthermore, adequate CPAP treatment improved the cardiovascular outcomes in this cohort.[101]

Stroke

The risk of stroke increases with age.[102] The prevalence of stroke is associated with OSA and stroke incidence is related to the severity of OSA.[103,104] Atrial fibrillation is a known risk factor for stroke and, as mentioned previously, atrial fibrillation is associated with SDB. In a 6-year follow-up study of more than a thousand patients whose mean age at enrollment was approximately 60 years, Yaggi and colleagues found that OSA was a risk factor for stroke after controlling for other important variables. Treatment did not affect the risk of either stroke or death in this study.[105] The presence of OSA in patients with stroke is associated with a longer period of hospitalization and rehabilitation.[106] In a study of patients with acute cerebral ischemia who underwent polysomnography, Kepplinger and colleagues showed that OSA is associated with clinically silent microvascular brain tissue changes such as leukoaraiosis (white matter hyperintensities) and lacunar infarcts.[107]

A systematic review of the findings in 10 reports that included 1203 patients who had experienced stroke or transient ischemic attacks (TIAs) noted a dose-response relationship between severity of SDB and the risk of recurrent events and all-cause mortality. Three of the studies included information about patients who received CPAP; however, the data were too limited to be able to make a compelling argument that CPAP improves outcomes in patients with stroke or TIA.[108]

In summary, OSA is strongly associated with cardiovascular disease in middle-aged populations, and the accumulating evidence suggests that SDB increases the risk of cardiovascular disease and stroke in the elderly population. The best-proven association and evidence for benefit is with hypertension, for which the data are derived largely from middle-aged populations.

Other Effects

SDB is a systemic problem with systemic consequences. In addition to the adverse outcomes already noted, OSA in elderly persons is associated with multiple potential consequences.

In middle-aged men, OSA is associated with increased health care costs that decrease after treatment. CPAP treatment is cost effective for treatment for severe sleep apnea in middle-aged people.[109] Within the sleep apnea population, expenditures for health care in older patients are approximately twice as high as they are in middle-aged patients. After adjustments for age, BMI, and AHI, cardiovascular disease and use of psychoactive drugs were important determinants of health care costs for older patients with OSA in one study.[110] A large study of elderly veterans documented that only 4.4% (in all likelihood, representing only the "tip of the iceberg") were diagnosed with OSA but that these patients had many more comorbid conditions and much higher health care utilization than those who did not carry the diagnosis.[111] Sleep apnea was also associated with an increased risk of pneumonia in a large study.[112]

Nocturnal hypoxemia is also associated with increased risk of falls in older men[113] but paradoxically is associated with preserved bone mineral density in elderly men and women, even after adjustment for sex, BMI, metabolic values, and hypertension.[114]

Sex is likely to influence the effects of SDB in older people, just as it does for younger persons. For example, a significant relationship between SDB and hypertension, history of diabetes, and low high-density lipoprotein cholesterol has been reported in women older than 65 years of age, but these effects were not demonstrable in older men.[115]

TREATMENT OF OBSTRUCTIVE SLEEP APNEA IN OLDER ADULTS

Continuous Positive Airway Pressure

As with younger adults, CPAP is the most common treatment in older patients. The Centers for Medicare and Medicaid Services covers CPAP therapy as indicated by results of OSA testing and requires objective documentation of use for payment beyond the first 90 days. Because most studies on the effects of CPAP have been done in clinical (e.g., middle-aged) populations, evidence for the benefits of CPAP in older persons is not yet robust.

Treatment-emergent central sleep apnea (TECSA), formerly known as complex sleep apnea, appears to be more prevalent in older than in younger people.[116] TECSA is characterized as the emergence of central apneas during treatment with CPAP, with an index of more than five per hour in a patient with OSA, but without central sleep apnea on the original diagnostic study.[117,118] It can also be observed during treatment with mandibular advancement devices (MADs), maxillofacial surgery for OSA, and tracheostomy.[119,120] In 90% of cases, TECSA resolves spontaneously in 3 months.[121-123] In a convenience sample of a variety of SDB syndromes resistant to CPAP, the mean age of 72 years was much higher than typically observed in clinical populations of patients with sleep disordered breathing. In that cohort, adaptive servoventilation appeared to be effective and well tolerated in approximately half.[124] Because TECSA appears to be more prevalent in older adults, formal, in lab titrations may be more important for this group. (For a more detailed discussion of TECSA, see Chapter 110.) Adherence to CPAP therapy in older patients may be impaired by factors such as cognitive impairment, medical and mood disturbances, nocturia, lack of a supportive partner, and impaired manual dexterity. Older age in itself, however, does not affect adherence to CPAP treatment,[74,125,126] and behavioral interventions can improve CPAP adherence in the elderly.[127] The major predictors of CPAP nonadherence in older patients with OSA are nocturia, current cigarette smoking, lack of symptom resolution, and advanced age at time of diagnosis.[128] Older men with nocturia may find CPAP particularly confining and may be particularly likely to have difficulty with its use, although CPAP may actually help with the nocturia.[125,128]

Patients with OSA who have dementia, including Alzheimer disease, have been demonstrated to tolerate CPAP, although depressive symptoms appear to predict worsened adherence in demented seniors with sleep apnea.[129]

Oral Appliances

Oral appliances are effective in treating snoring and mild to moderate OSA.[130-133] Although not as effective as CPAP, these agents improve SDB, sleepiness, nocturnal oxygen saturation, and blood pressure. There are two basic types of oral appliances:

1. MADs, which pull the mandible (and with it, the tongue) forward
2. Tongue-retaining devices (TRDs), which adhere to the tongue by suction and pull it forward. Because TRDs are not approved by the U.S. Food and Drug Administration (FDA) for treatment of sleep apnea, they are used much less commonly in clinical practice

See Chapter 147 for a detailed discussion of the use of oral appliances.

Common side effects of oral appliances include dry mouth, increased salivation, tooth soreness, and jaw muscle or jaw joint discomfort. Pain occasionally can be severe enough that patients discontinue the use of the appliance.[133] Bite changes (e.g., the inability to close on the back teeth) combined with heavy contact of the front teeth on removal of the appliance in the morning also are reported, but these changes generally resolve on removal of the device.

Oral appliances can be made to fit over false teeth, although this is not optimal. The use of oral appliances in people who are edentulous may be attempted with a TRD, but these devices are not FDA approved, and the efficacy of this approach is unknown. A small prospective study of factors associated with efficacy of oral appliances has suggested that age older than 55 years may be associated with reduced efficacy.[134]

Surgery

As with younger adults, upper airway surgery is not particularly effective treatment for OSA for older patients and may be associated with especially high morbidity in the elderly.[135] However, as in younger patients with significant SDB in the context of obesity, bariatric surgery, specifically laparoscopic-adjustable gastric banding, has been shown to be well tolerated and reasonably effective in resolving or reducing sleep apnea in people older than 70.[136]

Pharmacologic Treatment

Several medications have been applied to the treatment of SDB. In general, no drug is effective enough to recommend for use in first-line treatment. Antidepressants, nasal steroids, hormone replacement therapy (HRT), and modafinil all have been studied in younger patients.

More than two decades ago, protriptyline was demonstrated to show modest efficacy in treating apnea, probably because it reduces rapid eye movement (REM) sleep, when apnea is worst.[137] There is some early experimental work with the selective serotonin reuptake inhibitors (SSRIs) in the treatment of sleep apnea, but results have not been promising in humans.[138] SSRIs can suppress REM sleep, but not as much as that seen with the tricyclic antidepressants.

Nasal steroids have been demonstrated to have modest efficacy in the treatment of SDB.[139]

In the Sleep Heart Health Study, women who were on HRT were less likely to have sleep apnea, but overall lifestyle and health care are significant confounders in drawing conclusions about the efficacy of HRT for OSA.[140] Although estrogen is an option to consider, it would have to be discussed carefully with the patient because of subsequently recognized complications of HRT.

Body Position

The supine position predisposes the sleeper to airway collapse and to reduced lung volume and has long been known to exacerbate OSA; indeed, some affected persons experience obstructive events exclusively when sleeping on their backs.[141-143] Upper airway size decreases with increasing age in both men and women, and upper airway collapsibility with supine positioning increases with age.[143,144] There is some evidence for use of positional therapy devices (that may decrease sleeping in the supine position) for those with positional OSA. Although data are limited in older adults, positional therapy may also be an option in this population.[145]

DRIVING AND THE OLDER PATIENT WITH OBSTRUCTIVE SLEEP APNEA

Untreated OSA is a well-established risk factor for involvement of drivers in motor vehicle crashes (see Chapter 114) and may be expected to affect older drivers as well. In a review of conditions increasing crash risk in older drivers, Marshall found that several conditions were believed to be associated with increased risk of crash in older persons, including alcohol abuse and dependence, cardiovascular disease, cerebrovascular disease, depression, dementia, diabetes mellitus, epilepsy, use of certain medications, musculoskeletal disorders, schizophrenia, vision disorders, and, finally, OSA. He noted that these "conditions can serve as potential warnings for reduced fitness to drive, but many persons with these medical conditions would still be considered safe to continue driving."[146]

CLINICAL PEARLS

- The clinical presentation of OSA in older adults differs from that in their middle-aged counterparts, so the disorder may be overlooked by clinicians when it manifests in this age group.
- Male sex and obesity are less important risk factors in older people than in younger people.
- Symptoms of sleep apnea change with aging: whereas the classic symptoms of OSA are witnessed apneas and sleepiness, older patients are more likely to present with sleep complaints, nocturia, and cognitive dysfunction.
- Moderate to severe OSA is associated with increased risk of cardiovascular morbidity and mortality as well as cognitive dysfunction, and CPAP treatment is associated with reduced risk.

SUMMARY

OSA is prevalent and potentially deadly in older people and may be overlooked by clinicians because the clinical presentation is different from that in younger people. Obesity may not play as significant a role in seniors with OSA and the risk of OSA in women increases after menopause. Seniors are less likely to report classic symptoms of witnessed apnea, snoring, and fatigue. Because CPAP use is associated with reduced morbidity and mortality in older (as well as younger) people, clinicians need to consider the possibility of OSA in older patients with sleep complaints.

SELECTED READINGS

Chang WP, Liu ME, Chang WC, et al. Sleep apnea and the risk of dementia: a population-based 5-year follow-up study in Taiwan. *PloS One*. 2013;8:e78655.

Fernandes M, Placidi F, Mercuri NB, Liguori C. The Importance of Diagnosing and the Clinical Potential of Treating Obstructive Sleep Apnea to Delay Mild Cognitive Impairment and Alzheimer's Disease: A Special Focus on Cognitive Performance. *J Alzheimers Dis Rep*. 2021;5(1):515–533. Published 2021 Jun 17. https://doi.org/10.3233/ADR-210004.

Guillot M, Sforza E, Achour-Crawford E, et al. Association between severe obstructive sleep apnea and incident arterial hypertension in the older people population. *Sleep Med*. 2013;14:838–842.

Holmqvist F, Guan N, Zhu Z. the ORBIT-AF Investigators. Impact of obstructive sleep apnea and continuous positive airway pressure therapy on outcomes in patients with atrial fibrillation-Results from the Outcomes Registry for Better Informed Treatment of Atrial Fibrillation (ORBIT-AF). *Am Heart J*. 2015;169:647–654.

Jennum P, Tønnesen P, Ibsen R, Kjellberg J. All-cause mortality from obstructive sleep apnea in male and female patients with and without continuous positive airway pressure treatment: a registry study with 10 years of follow-up. *Nat Sci Sleep*. 2015;7:43–50.

Kushida C, Nichols DA, Holmes TH, et al. Effects of continuous positive airway pressure on neurocognitive function in obstructive sleep apnea patients: The Apnea Positive Pressure Long-term Efficacy Study (APPLES). *Sleep*. 2012;35:1593–1602.

Liguori C, Maestri M, Spanetta M, et al. Sleep-disordered breathing and the risk of Alzheimer's disease. *Sleep Med Rev*. 2021;55:101375. https://doi.org/10.1016/j.smrv.2020.101375.

Martinez-Garcian MA, Campos-Rodruigez F, Catalan-Serra P, et al. Cardiovascular mortality in obstructive sleep apnea in the elderly: role of long-term continuous positive airway pressure treatment. *Am J Respir Crit Care Med*. 2012;186:909–916.

McMillan A, Bratton DJ, Faria R, et al. A multicentre randomised controlled trial and economic evaluation of continuous positive airway pressure for the treatment of obstructive sleep apnoea syndrome in older people: PREDICT. *Health Technol Assess*. 2015;19(40):1–188.

Peppard PE, Young T, Barnet JH, et al. Increased prevalence of sleep-disordered breathing in adults. *Am J Epidemiol*. 2013;177:1006–1014.

Russo-Magno P, O'Brien A, Panciera T, et al. Compliance with CPAP therapy in older men with obstructive sleep apnea. *J Am Geriatr Soc*. 2001;49:1205–1211.

Yaggi HK, Concato J, Kernan WN, et al. Obstructive sleep apnea as a risk factor for stroke and death. *N Engl J Med*. 2005;353:2034–2041.

A complete reference list can be found online at ExpertConsult.com.

Chapter 193

Insomnia in Older Adults

Tamar Shochat; Sonia Ancoli-Israel

Chapter Highlights

- Insomnia is a complaint of dissatisfaction with sleep characterized by difficulty initiating and/or maintaining sleep and/or early morning awakenings resulting in significant daytime consequences. Chronic insomnia is prevalent in about 10% of the adult population.
- Age-related changes—underlying age-related physiologic changes in sleep-wake regulation such as circadian rhythms and sleep homeostasis—have been identified. Medical and psychiatric conditions, medications or other substances, psychosocial issues, and other primary sleep disorders frequently contribute to insomnia symptoms.
- Key elements in appropriate evaluation and management include considering the type of insomnia complaint, assessing sleep patterns including daytime napping, daytime consequences, and comorbidity. Behavioral treatment should be considered first, and when necessary, the newer hypnotic medications may be added.

INTRODUCTION

Based on diagnostic criteria of the American Psychiatric Association (APA), the *Diagnostic and Statistical Manual of Mental Disorders*, fifth edition (DSM-5), insomnia is a disorder that involves dissatisfaction with sleep quality and/or quantity, difficulty initiating sleep, difficulty maintaining sleep, and/or waking up too early, with a negative impact on daytime functioning and occurring at least 3 nights a week for at least 3 months.[1] Typically, insomnia is a chronic condition lasting for several years. In the older adult population, chronic insomnia is common, often co-occurs, and is exacerbated by medical or psychiatric conditions, polypharmacy, and/or another sleep disorder. Growing evidence suggests that insomnia is a potential contributor to subsequent functional impairment[2] and morbidity.[3] Yet, because of the widespread notion that insomnia is an inevitable consequence of aging, it often goes unrecognized, undiagnosed, and untreated. Thus increasing the awareness of clinicians and older adults regarding the significance of identifying and managing insomnia is imperative for improving both sleep and health in this population.

EPIDEMIOLOGY AND RISK FACTORS

The estimated prevalence of insomnia must be considered in the context of the criteria used to define insomnia and the population sampled. The prevalence in the general adult population in Norway based on DSM-5 criteria was estimated at 7.9%, controlling for sociodemographic and comorbidity factors.[4] In the Atherosclerosis Risk in Communities study of 13,500 middle-aged and older adults aged 47 to 69 years, the prevalence of difficulties falling asleep and difficulty staying asleep were 22% and 39%, respectively.[5] In outpatient clinics in Guangzhou, China, the prevalence of disorders initiating and maintaining sleep and early morning awakenings were 14%, 16%, and 12%, respectively, with 22% reporting any of the nighttime insomnia symptoms (NIS).[6]

It has generally been presumed that insomnia is more prevalent in women and increases with age. Indeed, population-based studies show that women endorse poorer sleep quality and more sleep disturbance than men in self-reports[7-10] and confirm a higher prevalence of insomnia in women.[4-6,11-13] Aging, however, is associated with increased nighttime symptoms of poor sleep but not with a full diagnosis of insomnia.[4,5,11-13] Some studies have reported an increased risk of insomnia in younger rather than older adults, particularly in women.[4,8]

Age and gender differences may be related to differences in modes of measurement.[7,10] In a sample of more than 5000 middle-aged and older adults from the Sleep Heart Health Study (SHHS), older age was significantly related to poor sleep in men based on polysomnographic (PSG) recordings, particularly reduction in slow wave sleep (SWS) and increased stages 1 and 2, whereas in women, older age was related to subjective sleep complaints, particularly difficulty falling asleep.[7] In men and women, older age was associated with shorter sleep, lower sleep efficiency, and more arousals based on polysomnography (PSG), yet with less daytime complaints of unrest and sleepiness.

Furthermore, medical and psychiatric comorbidities as well as sociodemographic and lifestyle factors overshadow the risks of age.[8,14] In the Atherosclerosis Risk in Communities study, depression and heart disease were associated with nighttime symptoms and nonrestorative sleep complaints.[5] Other related factors were medical illnesses, lower socioeconomic status and education, and unhealthy behaviors such as alcohol use and cigarette smoking. Findings from the NHANES identified distinct risk factors for NIS versus the nonrestorative sleep (NRS) complaint.[11] Whereas NIS were associated with increased age, lower income, and educational level and an increased rate of cardiovascular disease, NRS was associated with primary sleep disorders such as sleep apnea, respiratory disease, thyroid disease and cancer, as well as increased inflammation.

Other studies have examined the prevalence of insomnia and related risk factors in the older adult population. In a sample of more than 9000 participants aged 65 and above from the National Institute of Aging's Established Populations of Epidemiological Studies of the Elderly (EPESE), more than 50% reported at least one sleep complaint, and 35% to 40% reported disorders of initiating and/or maintaining sleep on a chronic basis.[15] In a study of more than 4000 nursing home residents in 8 European countries, the prevalence of any insomnia symptoms was 24%, with the highest rates in Germany (30%) and lowest rates in England (13%).[16] Insomnia increased with age and was associated with depression and use of sedative-hypnotics in all countries and with stressful life events, fatigue, and pain in most countries.

Based on the National Sleep Foundation survey from 2003, depression, heart disease, bodily pain, and memory problems were the disorders most commonly associated with insomnia in older adults.[17] In a sample of 2000 South Korean community adults over 65 years of age, 29% reported NIS and 17% also reported daytime consequences.[13] For all insomnia symptoms, prevalence was higher in women as well as in individuals with no education, living alone, with restless legs syndrome (RLS) or depression, and/or with a lifetime history of physical illness. Older age was again associated with increased nighttime symptoms but with decreased complaints of NRS. These findings lend further support to the epidemiologic evidence demonstrating that the bulk of geriatric sleep complaints and disorders are not the result of age per se, but rather co-segregates with medical and psychiatric disorders and related health burdens.[18]

Insomnia in older adults is often unrecognized by physicians.[3] In a study of older adults in primary care practices in the midwestern United States, 69% of patients endorsed at least one sleep problem, 40% endorsed at least two sleep problems, and 45% endorsed symptoms of insomnia, yet these complaints were reported in the medical charts only 19% of time.[19] The two questions that best identified those with poor sleep and at risk for medical and psychiatric problems were, "Do you feel excessively sleepy during the day?" and "Do you have difficulty falling asleep, staying asleep, or being able to sleep?" These two questions would be easy for physicians to integrate into their standard history.

CONSEQUENCES

It is important to identify and treat insomnia in older adults, as chronically poor sleep can result in serious consequences. Studies have assessed the effects of insomnia on physical functioning and performance, as well as the health consequences and the health care costs of insomnia. Findings from the Women's Health Initiative (WHI) in more than 90,000 postmenopausal women showed that incident and persistent insomnia over 1 to 3 years was associated with significantly higher risk (between two- and sixfold) for physical and emotional impairments.[2] In a 3-year follow-up of the EPESE,[15] an annual incidence rate of 5% was reported.[20] Incidence rates were highest in those with chronic medical conditions such as heart disease, stroke, and diabetes. Remission occurred in nearly half of those with insomnia at baseline and was related to improvements in perceived health. Similarly, in a representative sample of general practice patients aged 65 years and above, the annual incidence rate for late-life insomnia was 3.1%.[14] Significant and independent risk factors in this sample were depressed mood, poor physical health, and low physical activity.

Results from the Health and Retirement Study have shown a dose-response relationship between the number of reported insomnia symptoms and the 2 years' risk of falls that was independent of sleep medication use.[21] Conversely, physician-recommended sleep medication increased the risk of falls regardless of the number of reported symptoms, after adjusting for factors such as age, walking speed, and vision.[21] Indeed, a recent meta-analysis has shown that even newer hypnotic medications for insomnia, known as "Z drugs," increase the risk for falls and fractures in the general adult population.[22] In a study of more than 34,000 nursing home residents (based on the minimum data set), untreated or unresponsive insomnia, but not hypnotic medication, increased the risk for subsequent falls.[23]

The impact of insomnia on cognitive function in older adults has shown inconsistent findings. In an 8-year longitudinal study of nearly 5000 older adults in France who were cognitively intact at baseline, excessive daytime sleepiness but not insomnia predicted global cognitive decline based on the Mini-Mental State Examination (MMSE).[24] Similar findings using self-reported sleep measures and cognitive screening tools were reported in longitudinal studies in the United Kingdom[25] and in the United States.[26] In a 2-year prospective study, short sleep duration (≤5 hours) and insomnia complaints were related to lower scores on cognitive tests at baseline, but not at a 2-year follow-up.[27] Another cross-sectional study that used a comprehensive neuropsychological test battery found that early morning awakenings (but not disorders initiating and/or maintaining sleep) were associated with worse executive functioning in older adults, controlling for psychosocial and medical issues.[28] Finally, in a 3-year longitudinal study, chronic insomnia was found to be an independent risk factor for cognitive decline in older men, but not in older women,[29] suggesting that cognitive decline in insomnia may depend on sex. Alternatively, daytime sleepiness rather than insomnia may be the underlying factor for cognitive decline.

On the other hand, in the Study of Osteoporotic Fractures (SOF), cognitive decline in close to 3000 older women age 70 and above was associated with poor sleep, based on actigraphically measured sleep efficiency of 70% or less, long sleep latency, and increased wake after sleep onset, in a cross-sectional analysis.[30] The same study group reported that preclinical cognitive decline predicted increased sleep disturbance based on actigraphy (i.e., reduced sleep efficiency, longer sleep latency, and increased wake time after sleep onset), suggesting reverse causality.[31]

Different definitions of insomnia and poor sleep as well as different study designs and different operational measurements of cognitive performance may explain the inconsistencies in these studies. However, close scrutiny of the sleep and cognition literature in healthy aging has led to the conclusion that associations between sleep and cognition weaken with age.[32] Indeed, a meta-analysis of studies on sleep-dependent memory consolidation found that the beneficial effects of sleep on cognition are found in young but not in older adults.[33]

Population-based studies on the consequences of insomnia in middle-aged and older adults in prospective cohort studies have identified additional negative functional outcomes. Thus symptoms of insomnia, daytime sleepiness, and sleep medication use all predicted 4-year incidence of depressive symptoms in nearly 4000 older adults who were free of depression symptoms at baseline.[34] Two meta-analyses confirmed that adults with insomnia incur over a twofold risk for incident depression, compared with adults with no insomnia.[35,36] Studies based on samples from the Korean Genome and Epidemiology Study (KoGES) demonstrated that persistent insomnia predicted increased risks for depression and suicidal ideation and reduced physical and mental measures of health-related quality of life.[37,38] Similarly, disorders of initiating sleep but no other insomnia symptoms predicted incident depression in a nationally representative sample of older adults in Japan.[39]

Systematic reviews and meta-analyses have found that insomnia predicted incident all-cause dementia[40] or predicted increased risk for Alzheimer disease, but not vascular or all-cause dementia.[41] Other meta-analyses found that symptoms of insomnia (except difficulty falling asleep) and short sleep duration were associated with an increased risk for hypertension[42]; and that difficulties initiating and maintaining sleep and nonrestorative sleep, but not early morning awakenings, increased the risk for incident cardiocerebral vascular events.[43] In a longitudinal analysis of more than 80,000 postmenopausal women of the WHI who did not have heart disease at baseline, insomnia was associated with increased risks for incident coronary heart disease and incident cardiovascular disease (CVD) in fully adjusted models.[44] Not surprisingly, it has been shown that insomnia is associated with increased utilization of costly health services in middle-aged and older adults.[45]

Studies have associated sleep disturbances with an increased risk for mortality. Thus, in a study of older adults followed for close to 5 years, those with initial sleep latency of more than 30 minutes or sleep efficiency less than 80% had nearly twice the risk for mortality.[46] In the prospective Outcomes of Sleep Disorders in Older Men (MrOs sleep study) who were not frail at baseline, poor subjective sleep quality, more nighttime wakefulness, and greater nocturnal hypoxemia were associated with increased risks for incident frailty or mortality at follow-up.[47] However, a recent meta-analysis of nearly 37,000,000 pooled participants from 17 studies with a mean follow-up of 12 years found insufficient evidence for a relationship between mortality and frequent (≥3 nights/week), ongoing (≥1 month) insomnia.[48] Authors concluded that future studies should control for hypnotic use, which has been associated with mortality independently of insomnia.[49,50]

In sum, although growing evidence points to serious negative health outcomes of insomnia, further investigation is needed to clarify any association with mortality. Such investigations should employ longer follow-up periods; control for confounders such as sleep duration, comorbidity, daytime consequences of insomnia, and hypnotic use; and use consistent criteria for defining insomnia.[48]

ETIOLOGY

Underlying factors involved in the development of late-life insomnia include age-related changes in homeostatic and circadian sleep-wake regulation, psychiatric and medical comorbidities, medications and other substances, and primary sleep disorders. Evidence for each of these factors will be reviewed separately.

Age-Related Changes in Sleep Regulation

Both homeostatic and circadian mechanisms change with age. Advanced age has been associated with a marked reduction in SWS, indicating weaker homeostatic sleep pressure[51] and an increase in lighter sleep. Under entrained conditions, timing of the circadian rhythm of core body temperature and habitual wake times are advanced to an earlier hour in older adults, and the amplitude of the circadian rhythm of core body temperature is decreased, indicating a reduced circadian signal promoting sleep in the early morning hours.[52,53] The circadian signal for wakefulness is also reduced, as reflected in sleep episodes and reports of sleepiness in the early evening hours.[54] These homeostatic and circadian changes lead to reduced sleep consolidation, altered sleep architecture (lighter sleep), and advanced sleep phase, including both earlier bedtimes and wake times.[53,55-57] This contrasts with daytime wakefulness and nighttime sleep consolidation in young adults, which are high because of homeostatic and circadian mechanisms.

In summary, reductions in both the homeostatic drive for sleep and in the strength of the circadian signal for sleep in the early morning hours and for wakefulness in the early evening hours have been implicated as underlying factors for reduced sleep consolidation, advanced sleep phase, and early morning awakenings in older adults.

Medical and Psychiatric Comorbidities

Numerous chronic medical conditions and illnesses are known to disrupt sleep. These include arthritis, angina pectoris, congestive heart failure, coronary artery disease, chronic obstructive pulmonary disease, end-stage renal disease, diabetes, asthma, stroke, gastroesophageal reflux disorder, dementia/Alzheimer disease, Parkinson disease, cancer, and menopause. For example, in a representative US survey of 1500 older adults ages 50 and above, those with heart disease, lung disease, depression, obesity, and bodily pain were more likely to report difficulties with sleep.[17] In another study, higher insomnia severity measured by the Insomnia Severity Index was dose-dependently related to the number of chronic medical illnesses and, more prominently, the number of psychiatric illnesses.[58]

As mentioned in previous sections of this chapter, medical and psychiatric comorbidities may be considered as both risk factors and consequences of insomnia, and it is often difficult to determine the direction of causality. Thus *comorbid* insomnia has been suggested as the appropriate term for insomnia with other comorbidities, replacing the earlier term *secondary* insomnia.[59] Such a distinction has important implications not only in reassessing causal relationships between insomnia and comorbidity but also for considering treatment strategies. Treatment and management should focus not only on comorbid illnesses but also on insomnia as a distinct entity.

Medications and Substances

Prescription medications known to be related to insomnia include antidepressants, such as selective serotonin reuptake inhibitors, serotonergic and noradrenergic reuptake inhibitors, as well as medications prescribed for medical conditions, such as bronchodilators, beta blockers, corticosteroids, decongestants, central nervous system stimulants, gastrointestinal drugs, and cardiovascular drugs.[3] Despite the widespread use of antidepressants for insomnia, rigorous longitudinal investigation of their efficacy, tolerability and safety is sorely lacking.[60]

Based on the NHANES, 3% of US adults used medications commonly used for insomnia in the month preceding the survey, with increased rates over a 10-year period.[61] Concurrent use of more than one sedative was high, with 55% taking one more sedative and 10% taking three or more. The use of medications for insomnia was associated with older age and seeing a mental health care provider.

Other substances known to be related with insomnia in older individuals include alcohol, caffeine, and nicotine. In a sample of more than 6000 adults ages 50 and above, occasional and frequent binge drinking was associated with an increased risk for insomnia after controlling for demographic and clinical factors and was partially mediated by cigarette smoking.[62] However, in a study of nearly 10,000 adults over 65 years old in France, moderate alcohol and caffeine consumption reduced the risk for insomnia symptoms in women, demonstrating a protective effect.[63] Furthermore, in a study assessing sleep hygiene patterns in four sleep subgroups of older adults (i.e., with or without insomnia and with or without sleep complaints), there were no differences between the subgroups for alcohol, nicotine, and caffeine use, indicating that sleep hygiene regarding such lifestyle issues may not be an effective therapy in this age group.[64]

Comorbid Sleep Disorders

Insomnia co-occurs with other sleep disorders. Common sleep disorders in older adults include sleep-disordered breathing (SDB), periodic limb movement disorder (PLMD), and RLS. Relationships between these disorders and insomnia are discussed.

Sleep-Disordered Breathing

SDB is a respiratory dysfunction syndrome during sleep. One of the most common SDB conditions in older adults is obstructive sleep apnea (OSA), which is characterized by partial (hypopnea) to complete (apnea) airway collapse, causing pauses in breathing occurring repeatedly during the night. These respiratory events reduce blood oxyhemoglobin saturation and terminate in partial arousals. Symptoms of OSA typically include excessive daytime sleepiness and heavy snoring. Although criteria vary across studies, it appears that the prevalence of sleep apnea increases with age to as much as 62% for a respiratory disturbance index (RDI) of at least 10 in older adults ages 65 and above (70% in men, 56% in women).[65]

In a more recent study of older adults ages 60 and above in Korea, prevalence was 36.5% for an apnea-hypopnea index (AHI) of at least 15 (52.6 in men, 26.3 in women).[66] Despite its high prevalence, the consequences of OSA are considered more benign in older compared with younger adults, suggesting that considerations regarding management should take into account the severity of the disorder, its impact on functioning, and implications of therapeutic intervention.[67]

It has been estimated that about half of the patients with SDB also have insomnia.[68] Co-occurrence of these disorders is more common in women and is associated with lower sleep quality and a higher rate of psychiatric disorders than patients with SDB alone. In older adult, co-occurrence of insomnia and SDB was associated with higher daytime dysfunction than either sleep disorder alone, suggesting an additive effect on functional impairment.[69] Although the underlying relationship between these two prevalent sleep disorders is not clear, it has been suggested that hypoxia may be a mediating factor between SDB and insomnia in older adults with cardiovascular disease.[70]

It is important to note that SDB may be veiled in older patients with insomnia. In a sample of 80 adults with insomnia aged 59 and above who had initially been screened by clinical intake and were found negative for traditional signs of SDB, subsequent rigorous screening identified that 29% had an AHI over 15, indicating significant SDB.[71] In another sample of older veterans with insomnia, nearly 50% were found to have occult SDB.[72] These findings confirm that clinical interview alone may not suffice for identifying veiled SDB in the older adult population and stress the importance of referring patients with insomnia who demonstrate excessive sleepiness and reduced functional capabilities for diagnostic testing, especially if insomnia treatments do not relieve symptoms.[69]

Periodic Limb Movements Disorder and Restless Legs Syndrome

Periodic limb movements in sleep (PLMS) are characterized by involuntary leg jerks during sleep appearing in repetitive clustered episodes, often leading to brief awakenings from sleep. In men and women, PLMS, particularly when accompanied by arousals, were related to PSG indicators of disturbed sleep that are associated with insomnia.[73,74] Clinical diagnosis of PLMD is considered when the PLM index (PLMI), the number of limb movements per hour of sleep, are greater than 15, but this should be interpreted in the context of the patient's sleep complaint.

Although previous survey data of nearly 19,000 individuals ages 15 to 100 did not demonstrate an increased prevalence of PLMS with age,[75] a more recent study of more than 2000 middle-aged and older adults reported a prevalence of 29% for PLM above 15, with higher rates for older adults and for men, and 14% of the PLMs associated with arousals.[76] Those with PLM above 15 had higher rates of RLS, obesity, diabetes, and hypertension as well as increased use of beta blockers and sedative medications. Prevalence rates based on home PSG in community-dwelling women were high, with 66% for a PLMI of at least five events per hour and 27% for PLMI of at least five events per hour accompanied by arousals.[53] Findings from the MrOS of more than 2300 older men found a prevalence rate of 61% for a PLMI of at least 15.[77]

Despite its high prevalence, long-term follow-up of an older adult sample showed no change in PLMS severity with increasing age[78]; yet a study on the pathologic significance of PLMS in older adults has shown that in older men, increased frequency of PLMS both with and without arousals was associated with incident atrial fibrillation[79] and incident CVD, particularly in those who were nonhypertensive.[80] Increased PLMI was also associated with cognitive decline in older men without dementia.[81]

RLS is a neurologic disorder characterized by dysesthesia in the legs and an irresistible urge to move them to relieve the discomfort. Symptoms of RLS increase during the evening and at night, usually when the patient is in a relaxed or restful state, resulting in sleep disturbance. Based on survey data, the prevalence of RLS increases with age, from 2.7% in teens to 8.2% in older adults 80 years and above.[75] PLMS is a common finding in 80% of RLS cases, yet PLMS and related sleep disturbance may also appear without RLS symptoms.[82] Both disorders are prevalent in older adults and are associated with insomnia. Proper identification and management are warranted. Both have been associated with incident cardiovascular events in older men, yet the underlying associating mechanisms are unclear.[77]

Pharmacologic treatment studies for PLMS and RLS have studied primarily middle-aged to older adults. Treatment strategies for both conditions are similar and should be considered for symptomatic individuals with comorbid insomnia and/or daytime sleepiness, or other daytime dysfunction related to the condition(s). In the United States, the only treatments approved by the Food and Drug Administration for the treatment of RLS are the dopamine agonists—pramipexole, ropinirole, and rotigotine—and the alpha delta 2 ligand, gabapentin enacarbil. Other medications are often used off label, such as levodopa-carbidopa. However, in older adults these medications may increase daytime sleepiness; therefore monitoring and follow-up are recommended.[83] Second-line, off-label treatments include sedative hypnotics, anticonvulsants, opioids, and adrenergic medications.[82]

EVALUATION AND DIAGNOSIS OF INSOMNIA

Despite its widespread prevalence, insomnia is underrecognized and often inadequately treated in healthcare systems.[19,84] Guidelines for the evaluation of insomnia in the adult population, based on the Standards of Practice Committee of the American Academy of Sleep Medicine (AASM),[85] call for a thorough sleep history and determination of specific sleep complaints, sleep-wake schedules, history of psychological symptoms (e.g., depression or anxiety), comorbid conditions such as medical or psychiatric illness, medications and other substances being taken, and other primary sleep disorders.

The assessment of insomnia does not necessitate overnight PSG monitoring, but symptoms and signs of comorbid sleep disorders, especially sleep-disordered breathing, do warrant diagnostic testing.[69,85] Based on AASM clinical practice guidelines, actigraphy may be used in the evaluation of patients with insomnia or circadian rhythm sleep-wake disorders.[86] Actigraphy is considered a reliable measurement tool compared with sleep logs (although sleep logs are often used to complement actigraphy) and is particularly useful in populations who may be able to reliability complete a sleep diary, such as in older adults with cognitive impairment.

TREATMENT OF INSOMNIA

The effectiveness of pharmacologic and nonpharmacologic treatments has been demonstrated for late-life insomnia. The evidence for their efficacy as well as specific considerations for their use in the older adults are reviewed in the following sections.

Nonpharmacologic Treatments

Recent clinical practice guidelines suggest that nonpharmacologic approaches, in particular cognitive-behavioral therapy for insomnia (CBT-I), should be used before initiation of pharmacotherapy in adult patients with insomnia.[87] Nonpharmacologic treatments that have been investigated for insomnia in older adults include psychological, cognitive-behavioral, and bright light treatments (Table 193.1). The 2006 AASM practice parameters for psychological and behavioral treatments of insomnia[88] found that CBT-I,

Table 193.1 Brief Instructions for Nonpharmacologic Approaches to Late-Life Insomnia

Therapy	Instructions
Cognitive behavioral therapy for insomnia	In addition to behavioral components (typically stimulus control, sleep restriction, and sleep hygiene education), cognitive therapy is used to address maladaptive beliefs, and attitudes regarding sleep are identified, addressed, and refined to induce positive changes in sleep-related cognitions and associated behavioral and emotional outcomes.
Stimulus control	Patient is instructed to go to bed only when sleepy. If sleep is not obtained in approximately 20 minutes, patient leaves bedroom and returns to bed when sleepy. This process is repeated as needed until sleep is obtained. Wake time is set and naps are not allowed.
Relaxation training	Various relaxation techniques including meditation, muscle relaxation, and biofeedback for the reduction of somatic and cognitive arousal.
Sleep restriction	Time in bed is restricted to self-estimated total sleep time (using sleep diaries). Sleep efficiency (ratio between time asleep and time in bed) is assessed and used to gradually increase time in bed while monitoring sleep efficiency. Naps are not typically allowed.
Sleep hygiene education	Based on sleep history, ineffective habits and behaviors related to poor sleep are targeted and clear guidelines for better sleep are provided (e.g., creating a stable sleep-wake schedule and a sleep-inducing bedroom environment, minimizing napping, avoiding sleep-inhibiting substances and behaviors at night, including caffeine, nicotine and alcohol, heavy meals and high fluid intake, worrisome thoughts, and clock viewing).
Bright light therapy	Patients are exposed to appropriately timed bright light to shift sleep timing.

stimulus control, and relaxation training were recommended treatments for chronic insomnia with a high level of evidence from clinical trials. Treatments reaching moderate levels of evidence for efficacy included sleep restriction therapy, multicomponent therapy (without cognitive therapy), biofeedback, and paradoxical intention. These treatments have been found to be effective in older adults and in chronic hypnotic users.

CBT-I has proven successful for older adults with insomnia (with and without comorbid conditions) and for those with hypnotic dependency. For example, in a clinical ambulatory PSG trial with 6-week and 6-month follow-ups, CBT-I was compared with zopiclone and placebo in older patients with chronic insomnia. For the CBT-I group, wake time was significantly reduced, and both sleep efficiency and SWS were significantly increased at both 6-week and 6-month follow-ups, compared with the zopiclone and placebo groups.[89] In a sample of older adults with sleep maintenance insomnia, a brief (4-week) group-based CBT-I intervention showed significant improvements in sleep measures posttreatment and at a 3-month follow-up, including reduced wake after sleep onset, increased sleep efficiency, and reduced time-in-bed, based on sleep diaries.[90] At posttreatment and at 3 months' follow-up, 46.5% and 42.2%, respectively, were no longer in the diagnostic range for insomnia based on the Insomnia Severity Index. In another study on late-life insomnia, comparing the effects of CBT-I with a sedative hypnotic medication (temazepam) and with both treatments combined, positive short-term efficacy was reported for all three treatments compared with placebo, with a small increased benefit for the combined treatment.[91] However, at a 2-year follow-up, sustained long-term gains were achieved only in the CBT-I groups, especially in the CBT-I only group, indicating that CBT-I alone is superior to combined therapy.

Evening bright light exposure has been studied for the treatment of advanced sleep-wake phase disorder and insomnia characterized by early morning awakening, which are both common conditions in older individuals. However, the practical usefulness of bright light treatment as a treatment for late-life insomnia has generally not been supported by research findings.[92] Given the importance of implementing feasible therapeutic alternatives to medication in this population, further investigation, possibly targeting specific subtypes of insomnia that may benefit from bright light therapy, is warranted.

Pharmacologic Treatments for Insomnia

Current guidelines suggest caution in the use of pharmacotherapy for older adults with insomnia disorder.[87] Approved medications for the treatment of insomnia include traditional benzodiazepines (temazepam, estazolam, flurazepam, quazepam, triazolam), newer selective non-benzodiazepine sedative "Z drugs" (eszopiclone, zaleplon, zolpidem [various formulations available]), melatonin receptor agonist (ramelteon), low-dose doxepin, and dual orexin receptor antagonists (suvorexant, lemborexant). Suvorexant, which was approved for insomnia in recent years, has been suggested as potentially safe and effective medication for adults with insomnia, although clinical trials focusing specifically on older adults with comorbidities have not been conducted.[93] Use of sedating agents in older adults with insomnia should include a discussion of the benefits versus harms, considering the potential for drug-drug interactions and adverse events for each patient.

Although a number of medications are used "off-label" for the treatment of insomnia, they are generally not recommended in clinical practice guidelines because of limited efficacy data and the potential for adverse events, drug-drug interactions, and other harms.[59]

In a representative sample of more than 32,000 noninstitutionalized American adults (the NHANES) ages 20 to over 80, the prevalence of medications commonly used for insomnia in the past month was 3%, with a significant increase between 1999 and 2000 to 2009 and 2010.[61] The most commonly used medications were "Z-drugs" and trazodone, and concurrent use of two or more sedatives was high (55% for at least two, and 10% for at least four concurrent sedatives). The likelihood of consuming sedatives for insomnia after multivariable adjustments was highest in older individuals, those seeing a mental health provider, and those reporting polypharmacy in sedative use.

Although the "Z drugs" are considered safer and more effective than the older benzodiazepines,[59] in a meta-analysis of data submitted to the Food and Drug Administration assessing the effects of "Z-drugs" on objective (PSG) and subjective sleep latency in the adult population, small but significant improvements were found, yet these improvements were comparable to placebo effects and were more pronounced in younger individuals, in females, and at higher drug doses. Given that older adults typically report higher rates of sleep maintenance insomnia and are at an increased risk for adverse effects, particularly at higher doses, the true safety and efficacy of these sedatives remain questionable.

Hypnotic medication use is highest and most chronic in older adults, yet it has been suggested that the benefit of such medications is lower in older compared with younger adults.[94,95] General guidelines for the use of sedative hypnotics in older adults include selection of the appropriate drug (short- versus long-acting), considering the type of insomnia complaint (sleep onset versus sleep maintenance insomnia), starting with a low dose and increasing as needed, considering drug-drug interactions, and monitoring for adverse effects, particularly residual effects of daytime sleepiness, cognitive performance, and the risk of falls.[94] It is important to keep in mind that the adverse consequences of sedative hypnotic use may outweigh the benefits, particularly in those with cognitive impairment.

In sum, although some evidence has demonstrated the safety and efficacy of the newer sedative-hypnotic agents in older adults with insomnia, the overall clinical significance of outcomes has been questioned, and safety remains a concern.

CLINICAL PEARL

Insomnia is very common in older adults and co-occurs with medical and psychiatric illness, use of medications, circadian rhythm and sleep homeostatic changes, and other primary sleep disorders. Clinicians should routinely screen for sleep problems and initiate appropriate treatment for insomnia in older patients.

SUMMARY

Symptoms of insomnia are very common in older adults and are largely underrecognized and undertreated. Increasing evidence of the significant consequences of insomnia warrants careful assessment and appropriate treatment strategies for this population. Older adults should be offered CBT-I as first-line treatment. Proper treatment of insomnia in this age group is effective and may improve overall physical and mental health, well-being, and quality of life in the older patient. Further research is required in selected older adult samples to understand the mechanisms underlying the development of insomnia and its related comorbidities and consequences and to determine how these processes can be effectively treated or prevented.

SELECTED READINGS

Bertisch SM, Herzig SJ, Winkelman JW, Buettner C. National use of prescription medications for insomnia: NHANES 1999-2010. *Sleep.* 2014;37(2):343–349.

Bloom HG, Ahmed I, Alessi CA, et al. Evidence–based recommendations for the assessment and management of sleep disorders in older persons. *J Am Geriatr Soc.* 2009;57(5):761–789.

Ensrud KE, Blackwell TL, Ancoli-Israel S, et al. Sleep disturbances and risk of frailty and mortality in older men. *Sleep Med.* 2012;13(10):1217–1225.

Grandner MA, Martin JL, Patel NP, et al. Age and sleep disturbances among American men and women: data from the U.S. behavioral risk factor surveillance system. *Sleep.* 2012;35(3):395–406.

Lovato N, Lack L, Wright H, Kennaway DJ. Evaluation of a brief treatment program of cognitive behavior therapy for insomnia in older adults. *Sleep.* 2014;37(1):117–126.

Lou BX, Oks M. Insomnia: pharmacologic treatment. *Clin Geriatr Med.* 2021;37(3):401–415. https://doi.org/10.1016/j.cger.2021.04.003.

Sands-Lincoln M, Loucks EB, Lu B, et al. Sleep duration, insomnia, and coronary heart disease among postmenopausal women in the women's health initiative. *J Women's Health.* 2013;22(6):477–486.

Scullin MK, Bliwise DL. Sleep, cognition, and normal aging: integrating a half century of multidisciplinary research. *Perspect Psychol Sci.* 2015;10(1):97–137. https://doi.org/10.1177/1745691614556680.

Treves N, Perlman A, Kolenberg Geron L, Asaly A, Matok I. Z-drugs and risk for falls and fractures in older adults—a systematic review and meta-analysis. *Age Ageing.* 2018;47(2):201–208. https://doi.org/10.1093/ageing/afx167.

Zaslavsky O, LaCroix AZ, Hale L, Tindle H, Shochat T. Longitudinal changes in insomnia status and incidence of physical, emotional, or mixed impairment in postmenopausal women participating in the Women's Health Initiative (WHI) study. *Sleep Med.* 2015;16(3):364–371.

A complete reference list can be found online at ExpertConsult.com.

Chapter 194

Circadian Rhythms in Older Adults

Jeanne F. Duffy

Chapter Highlights

- The circadian timing system regulates many aspects of physiology and behavior in humans, in particular the timing and structure of sleep.
- While some aspects of circadian rhythmicity do not change with healthy aging, other rhythms show age-related changes in timing or amplitude at the population level, although the cause(s) and consequences of these changes are largely not yet understood.
- There is evidence that circadian rhythms may be disrupted in neurodegenerative disorders such as Alzheimer disease, although whether those disruptions are causes or consequences of the disorder remains to be elucidated.

OVERVIEW OF THE CIRCADIAN TIMING SYSTEM

The circadian timing system regulates many aspects of physiology in humans, including hormone release, cardiovascular function, metabolism, and sleep-wake propensity.[1-3] The overall purpose of a circadian timing system is to allow the organism to predict and respond optimally to regular periodic changes in the environment, including sunlight, food availability, presence of predators, and other factors. There is strong evidence that, by preparing the organism for those regular changes, an intact circadian system ensures the optimal timing of internal biochemical and physiologic processes, in addition to behavior, and thus provides an adaptive advantage.[4]

We now understand that the near-24-hour circadian rhythms result from transcriptional-translational feedback loops that are present in most cells.[5] A central circadian pacemaker in the hypothalamus, the suprachiasmatic nucleus (SCN), serves to coordinate the internal rhythms with the external world.[6-15] There is a direct pathway (the retinohypothalamic tract) from the eyes to the SCN that transmits information about the environmental light-dark cycle[16-20] so that the circadian system can be synchronized to that of the external environment, a process called entrainment. The SCN then transmits this timing information to the cells and tissues through hormonal and neural signals. This process of entrainment is necessary because the cycle length, or period, of the circadian system is near, but not exactly, 24 hours.[21] While entrainment in humans and other mammals occurs largely via exposure to light-dark cycles, there are other signals that can entrain or contribute to entrainment to a lesser degree.[22] The ability of an individual to be entrained depends on how far from 24 hours their circadian system is, as well as the strength of the entraining signal.[23,24]

CIRCADIAN OR DIURNAL?

Although humans have similar circadian organization to other mammals, unlike most other organisms, healthy adult humans typically have a long and consolidated sleep episode at night and remain awake for an extended duration during the day. This rhythmic sleep-wake behavior results in part from a circadian rhythm in sleep-wake propensity.[25,26] However, the rhythmic sleep and associated behaviors (postural change from upright to supine, reduced activity level, darkness, and sleep itself) can influence many other physiologic functions, including body temperature, hormone levels, cardiovascular function, and metabolism. It is therefore important when considering rhythmic changes in physiology to understand whether those changes are due to rhythmic changes in behavior, an underlying circadian rhythm, or a combination of the two. A true circadian rhythm will persist even when behavior and the environment remain constant. Thus the "constant routine" protocol was developed and used by researchers.[27]

Many physiologic rhythms have an underlying circadian component but are also affected by periodic changes in behavior, called "masking," and the amount of masking varies widely. For example, core temperature has an underlying circadian rhythm, but that rhythm is strongly masked by activity level, posture, and sleep,[28] whereas the rhythm of melatonin secretion is only minimally affected by activity, posture, and sleep but is strongly affected by light exposure.[29] A careful reading of the literature is necessary to appreciate that, in many cases, what is called "circadian" is instead referring to a diurnal rhythm, or that a report of a change in a circadian rhythm (e.g., an age-related change) is instead showing a change in a masked rhythm that may not represent a change in the underlying circadian component of that rhythm at all.[28]

Current methods for assessing the status of the central circadian system require that measurements be taken at regular intervals for many hours in highly controlled conditions. This makes it challenging to carry out research, limits the types of studies that can be carried out, and makes it nearly impossible to carry out circadian assessments of some clinical populations, such as older adults with cognitive impairment. There are presently multiple efforts underway to develop single time-point circadian biomarkers, including those using transcriptomic, metabolomic, proteomic, and other multivariate markers[30] that could greatly expand our ability to understand how the circadian system changes with age and age-associated diseases.

CIRCADIAN REGULATION OF PHYSIOLOGY AND BEHAVIOR

Although the SCN was recognized as the central hypothalamic pacemaker of the mammalian circadian system nearly 50 years ago,[6-15] more recently we have come to understand that almost every cell of the body contains its own circadian oscillator that contributes to the daily rhythmicity of a large variety of physiologic and metabolic activities, including immune, renal, hepatic, pancreatic, endocrine, reproductive, respiratory, and cardiovascular functions.[1,31] In fact, in a recent study of 13 different human tissues, 44% of the genes (nearly 7500) showed daily rhythms in expression.[32] When the organism or individual is exposed to a regular 24-hour light-dark, activity-rest, and feeding-fasting schedule, the peripheral oscillators in cells, tissues, and organs are normally synchronized with each other by local signals, and that internal synchronization is coordinated by autonomic or endocrine signals from the SCN to maintain overall synchronization with the external periodic environment.[33]

One of the most prominent rhythmic behaviors is that of sleep and wakefulness. In healthy adult humans, sleep-wake behavior is consolidated rather than polyphasic as it is in most other mammals, and our ability to maintain a consolidated sleep episode during the night and a long and consolidated wake episode across the day results from a complex interaction between a sleep-wake homeostatic process and a circadian rhythm of sleep-wake propensity.[34,35] The timing of the circadian rhythm of sleep-wake propensity is somewhat paradoxical: the strongest circadian drive for wakefulness occurs in the late evening, shortly before our usual bedtime (the so-called "wake maintenance zone" or "forbidden zone for sleep"),[36,37] and the strongest drive for sleep occurs in the early morning, shortly before our usual wake time.[25,26] The timing of this circadian rhythm serves to counteract the progressive buildup of sleep pressure throughout our waking hours so that the circadian drive for wake peaks at the time our sleep pressure is high, allowing us to remain awake for an extended approximately 16-hour episode. Similarly, the circadian drive for sleep is greatest in the latter half of our usual sleep episode, when most of the sleep pressure from the previous day has been dissipated, allowing us to remain asleep for 7 or more hours.

ASSOCIATION OF CIRCADIAN DYSREGULATION AND CHRONIC DISEASE

Acute disruption of the circadian system can occur on a transient basis, as a result of staying up later than usual or traveling to another time zone,[38] although the disruption is usually resolved after a few days on the new schedule (or after return to the former schedule). Recurrent circadian disruption is more problematic yet is experienced by millions of people because of either social jet-lag (shifting the sleep-wake, rest-activity, and fasting-feeding schedules between weekdays and weekends)[39] or shift work.

Nearly 10% of US workers have night, irregular, or rotating shift schedules, accounting for an estimated 10 million total workers and nearly 3 million older workers. The rates of shift work are similar in many other countries. Such schedules result in profound circadian disruption, and it is also now widely recognized that the higher rates of obesity, lipid disturbances, impaired glucose tolerance, type 2 diabetes, and cardiovascular disorders in those workers are due in large part to their schedules.[40-45] There is now well-established evidence of disruption of both central and peripheral circadian rhythms because of working at night or rotating shift work.[46,47] In fact, the number of years of rotating night and shift work are positively associated with weight gain and the development of type 2 diabetes,[48-50] dementia,[51] and even mortality.[52-54]

AGE-RELATED CHANGES IN THE CIRCADIAN SYSTEM

One of the most prominent changes in 24-hour behavior that occurs with aging is the shift of sleep timing to earlier hours. Population studies have demonstrated that older adults (in their 60s and older) go to bed and wake earlier than younger adults.[55] Given that the circadian timing system is involved in the regulation of sleep timing, it was hypothesized that an age-related change in the circadian system was the likely cause of this shift in sleep timing. Numerous studies comparing features of the circadian system between young and older adults have been carried out to investigate what properties, if any, are different. The period, or cycle length, of the circadian system had been reported to shorten with age in animals, but careful studies using the forced desynchrony technique have demonstrated that in healthy, sighted humans the period is not different between young and older adults and averages 24.15 hours (24 hours, 9 minutes) with a range of about an hour, from approximately 23.5 to 24.5 hours.[21,56] On average, the circadian period of women is about 6 minutes shorter than that of men. A larger number of women than men have periods shorter than 24 hours (35% versus 14%), and this may predispose women to early-morning awakening insomnia.[57]

Although the period of the circadian system does not appear to change with aging, there is ample evidence that the timing of circadian rhythms does change with aging. The rhythms of cortisol, melatonin, core body temperature, each markers of the central SCN output, all shift earlier with aging.[58-60] This shift is not simply a consequence of the earlier shift of sleep with aging, because the phase relationship between the timing of those circadian rhythms and the timing of sleep is also altered.[61,62] Studies in animal models have shown that peripheral rhythms and their relationship to central rhythms generated by the SCN are also altered in aging.[63] The change in phase relationship between sleep and the timing of the underlying circadian system may contribute to the specific sleep complaints in aging; this may explain the increase in the use of sleep medications with age.[64,65] Older adults are much more likely to report early morning awakenings and difficulty maintaining sleep than are young adults.[55] This may be due to a change in both sleep homeostasis and circadian regulation of sleep, as well as the interaction between the two sleep regulatory systems. Studies using the forced desynchrony protocol have demonstrated that with healthy aging, there appears to be a change in the shape of the circadian sleep-promoting signal, such that there is a narrower window within the circadian cycle at which a strong sleep-promoting signal is output.[61,66] This in turn makes older adults more vulnerable to sleep disruption in the latter half of the sleep episode.[66] This change in the circadian rhythm of sleep-wake propensity interacts with the well-described change in sleep-wake homeostasis,[67] whereby there is a reduction in slow wave sleep and slow wave activity with aging, leading to awakenings in the latter half of the night,[68] and great difficulty sleeping during the daytime.[66,67] There is also evidence of a reduction in the strength of the circadian wake-promoting signal in the evening in healthy older adults[69] that may allow for the advance of the overall sleep episode with respect to internal biologic time.

The response to light, the primary entraining signal for the human circadian system, may also be altered with aging. There are typical changes in the lens of the eye that reduce light input and change the spectral composition of light input to the circadian system,[70,71] and there is evidence that this age-related lens change is associated with increased sleep disruption.[72,73] Studies in which the phase-shifting impact of light have been examined have found that, although the response to bright light does not appear altered with aging, there may be a reduction in the sensitivity to indoor levels of light with age.[74-77]

In addition to alterations in the timing of circadian rhythms, advancing age is also associated with a reduction in the amplitude of some circadian rhythms, including that of core body temperature,[60,78] melatonin,[69,79] cortisol,[80] performance,[69,81] and even gene expression in the SCN[82] and prefrontal cortex.[71]

Although much remains to be understood about these age-related changes in the circadian system, there is evidence that structural and functional changes in brain areas involved in circadian rhythmicity show changes with aging. As noted previously, there are changes in the lens of the eye that influence the amount and wavelength of light entering the system,[70,71] affecting entrainment. The number of cells in the human SCN decreases with age,[83-85] and the SCN in patients with Alzheimer disease shows more severe changes compared to age-matched adults without dementia.[19,86] Studies in animal models have shown that the properties of the SCN neurons that remain are also altered with aging, showing electrophysiologic changes as well as loss of network synchronization[87] such that there is a reduced amplitude of SCN neural activity.[88] Together, these changes in the central circadian system are likely to reduce the strength of output and may account for the reduced amplitude of many centrally driven rhythms observed in older people.

INTERACTION OF THE CIRCADIAN SYSTEM AND NEURODEGENERATIVE DISEASES

It is not unusual for even healthy older adults to experience circadian rhythm changes, and most often these changes go unrecognized unless they are accompanied by significant sleep disturbances or daytime dysfunction. However, there is growing evidence from epidemiologic studies that sleep problems in older adults, including changes in the timing that may suggest modest alterations in circadian rhythm timing, may represent an early sign of cognitive decline and potential development of a neurodegenerative disease and are associated with increased mortality.[89-95] In fact, a bidirectional relationship between sleep and neurodegeneration has been suggested based on evidence from studies in animals.[96,97] These findings may relate to the recent discovery of the brain glymphatic system, hypothesized to be responsible for eliminating metabolic waste, including amyloid beta proteins, from the brain during sleep.[98,99] How circadian rhythm changes are associated with the sleep-cognitive decline relationship is not well understood, because few studies have attempted to measure circadian rhythms.[90,92,93] There appears to be a diurnal rhythm in amyloid beta in human cerebrospinal fluid, but whether that is due to a direct effect of sleep and waking or to a circadian rhythm remains unknown.[99] There is also evidence of an association between a history of rotating shift work and increased likelihood of dementia,[52] but further study is required to determine whether that is due solely to disrupted sleep associated with shift work or whether there is an independent contribution resulting from circadian rhythm disruption.

Although actigraphy cannot assess the function of the underlying endogenous circadian pacemaker, rest-activity monitoring by actigraphy is the most commonly reported measure used to monitor the sleep-wake rhythm in older adults and will likely remain so until circadian biomarkers are validated.[30] Many studies have extracted variables from activity that are associated with cognitive changes, including interdaily stability (a measure of rest-activity rhythm synchronization to 24-hour clock time), intradaily variability (a measure of rhythm fragmentation), amplitude, as well as acrophase or nadir of activity.[92,93,100-102] Whether those rest-activity changes relate to changes in the circadian timing system remains to be determined. However, two studies of patients with probable Alzheimer disease found that the acrophase (i.e., timing of the rhythm peak) of the core body temperature and melatonin rhythms in patients with Alzheimer disease were delayed compared with controls,[103-105] suggesting that there may be circadian changes that underlie the sleep-wake changes. Difficulty falling asleep in community-dwelling older adults is also associated with memory problems.[106] Thus these two lines of evidence hint that a phase delay disruption of circadian rhythmicity, manifested through altered sleep timing, is associated with cognitive decline.[92,107] Although it is not always clear that a change in rest-activity patterns truly represents a change in circadian rhythms, a delay of the rest-activity pattern (as opposed to the advance of rest-activity seen in healthy aging) seems to precede later cognitive decline in older individuals. For otherwise healthy older patients who present features of a circadian rhythm sleep-wake disorder, especially a phase delay, careful assessment and monitoring of their cognitive status may be warranted, as the sleep-wake timing change may be an early indicator of neurodegenerative changes. It may also be an opportunity for interventions designed to increase the robustness of the circadian system and improve the quality of sleep[108] in an attempt to maintain cognitive function. Longitudinal studies with careful clinical observations that include robust sleep and circadian rhythm measures will give us greater insights about how circadian and sleep changes may be associated with neurodegeneration and how sleep and circadian interventions may prevent or delay neurodegenerative change.

CLINICAL PEARLS

- Circadian rhythms are near-24-hour oscillations in physiology and behavior resulting from cell-autonomous processes coordinated by a central neural pacemaker, the SCN.
- Sleep-wake behavior in humans results from an interaction of two regulatory processes, a sleep homeostatic process and a circadian rhythm in sleep-wake propensity.
- Regular exposure to bright light during the day and darkness at night synchronizes or entrains the circadian system and is critical to its optimal functioning.
- A typical change in the timing of circadian rhythms and sleep-wake behavior is a shift earlier in healthy aging. There is some evidence that in Alzheimer disease and other dementias there is a shift in the timing of circadian rhythms and sleep-wake behavior to later hours.

SUMMARY

The circadian timing system coordinates many aspects of our internal physiology and our behavior and ensures that our internal rhythms are coordinated with each other as well as with our external environment to maintain optimal health. This entrainment process between the internal circadian pacemaker in the hypothalamus and the external world, with the central pacemaker then passing that synchronization on to coordinate peripheral rhythms in the organs, tissues, and cells is typically achieved through regular exposure to light during the day and darkness at night. There is evidence for changes in light input to the central pacemaker, as well as evidence of cellular changes in the pacemaker and its network properties with age. This may be the cause of the observed changes in the timing and reductions in the amplitude of rhythms controlled by the circadian system. There is now increasing evidence that long-term disruptions of the circadian system may lead to increased risk of many chronic diseases, and that specific changes in rhythm timing may be associated with specific neurodegenerative disorders. Better understanding of the typical and abnormal changes that occur with aging, and testing of preventative strategies for maintaining circadian health are needed.

ACKNOWLEDGMENTS

Work on which this chapter was based was supported by the following grants: National Institute on Aging (NIA) P01 AG09975 and R01 AG044416.

SELECTED READINGS

Abbott SM, Zee PC. Circadian rhythms: implications for health and disease. *Neurol Clin.* 2019;37(3):601–613.

Carter B, Justin HS, Gulick D, Gamsby JJ. The molecular clock and neurodegenerative disease: a stressful time. *Front Mol Biosci.* 2021;8:644747. https://doi.org/10.3389/fmolb.2021.644747. Published 2021 Mar 26.

Daan S, Beersma DG, Borbély AA. Timing of human sleep: recovery process gated by a circadian pacemaker. *Am J Physiol.* 1984;246(2 Pt 2):R161–R183.

Dijk DJ, Czeisler CA. Contribution of the circadian pacemaker and the sleep homeostat to sleep propensity, sleep structure, electroencephalographic slow waves, and sleep spindle activity in humans. *J Neurosci.* 1995;15(5 Pt 1):3526–3538.

Dijk DJ, Duffy JF, Riel E, Shanahan TL, Czeisler CA. Ageing and the circadian and homeostatic regulation of human sleep during forced desynchrony of rest, melatonin and temperature rhythms. *J Physiol.* 1999;516(Pt 2):611–627.

Duffy JF, Zitting KM, Chinoy ED. Aging and circadian rhythms. *Sleep Med Clin.* 2015;10(4):423–434.

Foster RG. Sleep, circadian rhythms and health. *Interface Focus.* 2020;10(3):20190098.

Foster R, Kreitzman L. *Circadian Rhythms: A Very Short Introduction.* Oxford, United Kingdom: Oxford University Press; 2017.

Logan RW, McClung CA. Rhythms of life: circadian disruption and brain disorders across the lifespan. *Nat Rev Neurosci.* 2019;20(1):49–65.

Rijo-Ferreira F, Takahashi JS. Genomics of circadian rhythms in health and disease. *Genome Med.* 2019;11(1):82.

Ruben MD, Wu G, Smith DF, et al. A database of tissue-specific rhythmically expressed human genes has potential applications in circadian medicine. *Sci Transl Med.* 2018;10(458):eaat8806.

Tranah GJ, Blackwell T, Stone KL, et al. Circadian activity rhythms and risk of incident dementia and mild cognitive impairment in older women. *Ann Neurol.* 2011;70(5):722–732.

A complete reference list can be found online at ExpertConsult.com.

Chapter 195

Sleep in Long-Term Care Settings

Kathy Richards; Lichuan Ye; Liam Fry

Chapter Highlights

- Sleep disturbances in long-term care (LTC) residents are highly prevalent and severely disabling. Management is challenging because there are many interrelated causes, such as frailty, dementia, noise, insufficient light, physical inactivity, immobility, and polypharmacy, and increasing evidence that sedative-hypnotics and sedating antipsychotics are associated with harm. Overall, treatment should focus on identifying and treating symptoms such as excessive daytime sleepiness or insufficient and interrupted nighttime sleep that negatively affect quality of life.
- The treatment of comorbidities, as long as the risk-benefit profile is favorable, and deprescribing of medications that negatively affect sleep should be the first steps. In general, nonpharmacologic interventions should be first-line therapy for sleep disturbances in LTC residents. Although additional and more rigorous clinical trials are needed to identify the most effective nonpharmacologic treatments, available evidence supports multicomponent interventions, including environmental modifications such as increased exposure to bright light, engagement in individualized physical and social activities, and cognitive-behavioral therapy for insomnia.
- Advocacy of families, regulatory agencies, and professionals is needed to support reimbursement for nonpharmacologic interventions for sleep disturbances in LTC residents. Dedicated, rigorous studies of medications for sleep disturbances in the LTC population are needed to examine their effectiveness, safety, and tolerance.

INTRODUCTION

Sleep specialists may be asked to diagnose and manage sleep disturbances among residents in long-term care (LTC). LTC settings consist of for-profit or nonprofit nursing homes, assisted living homes, dementia care units, or community-based homes. Day-to-day care of residents is provided by paid caregivers, usually nurses and their assistants. Multiple interrelated factors make the management of sleep disturbances in the LTC population challenging: environmental factors such as noise from residents in close proximity to each other and insufficient light; frailty; dementia; immobility and falls; emphasis on quality of life; and the recent focus on deprescribing medications such as sedative-hypnotics and sedating antipsychotics and replacing them with nonpharmacologic interventions. This chapter provides an overview of sleep disturbances and risk of LTC placement, describes factors affecting sleep in older adult residents of LTC settings, reviews and interprets pharmacologic and nonpharmacologic interventions, provides key clinical messages, and suggests future research priorities.

SLEEP PROBLEMS IN LONG-TERM CARE

Sleep Disturbances and the Risk of Long-Term Care Placement

Sleep disturbances contribute to LTC placement in community-dwelling older adults.[1,2] For example, sleep disturbance measured by wrist actigraphy, including lower sleep efficiency and more wake after sleep onset, and significantly increased LTC placement in older women at 5-year follow-up.[2] In an earlier study, insomnia was found to be the strongest predictor of both nursing home placement and mortality in urban community-dwelling older men.[1] Disturbed sleep can increase the risk of LTC placement because of its negative impact on physical, psychological, and social functioning. Poor sleep quality and disturbed sleep-wake patterns are associated with cognitive impairment,[3,4] which is a significant predictor of nursing home placement.[5] Sleep deprivation raises the level of inflammation contributing to functional impairment and overall health decline.[6,7] Recent studies also suggest that abnormal sleep can be a strong marker of frailty in community-dwelling older adults,[8,9] while frailty has been identified as a strong predictor of LTC placement.[10] For example, both excessive sleepiness during the day and long sleep duration increased the risk of social frailty.[9] In addition, poor sleep may be caused by medications or may be the presentation of other comorbid conditions such as depression that increase the risk of institutionalization. Another explanation is that frequent nocturnal awakenings in older adults can heighten caregiver burden and stress, which prompts LTC placement.[11] Clinicians should routinely assess sleep in older adults, monitor caregiver sleep patterns and burden, prescribe appropriate interventions, and monitor outcomes that are important to both the older adults and their caregivers.

Research is needed to determine if interventions could lower LTC placements.

Sleep Disturbances in Long-Term Care

Although sleep-related problems are prevalent in older adults, poor sleep is more common and more severe in institutionalized older adults.[12,13] Compared with noninstitutionalized older individuals, LTC residents demonstrated more sleep disturbances at night as measured by actigraphy, including significantly more sleep fragmentation, lower sleep efficiency, and longer awake time.[14] Sleep disturbances in LTC are prevalent across countries.[15-17] In a study published in 2013, 72.1% of 334 older adults from three nursing homes in Spain were classified as poor sleepers based on a Pittsburgh Sleep Quality Index (PSQI) global score higher than 5, and 49.6% were taking hypnotic medications.[18] Defined as difficulty falling or staying asleep, restlessness, waking up too early, or nonrestful sleep, insomnia is highly prevalent, with rates of 24% in over 4000 older residents of 57 LTC facilities in Israel and seven European countries.[15] Sleep disturbances can also be persistent,[19,20] thereby having an enduring negative impact.

Sleep Disturbances in Long-Term Care Residents with Memory Decline

Approximately 25% of LTC residents are diagnosed with Alzheimer disease and related dementia (ADRD),[21] and 70% of assisted living facility residents have some form of cognitive impairment.[22] Up to 70% of individuals in early-stage dementia suffer from sleep disturbances,[23] including lower sleep efficiency, frequent nighttime awakenings, increased daytime napping, and excessive daytime sleepiness (EDS).[24] These sleep disturbances tend to be associated with severity of cognitive decline.[24] The circadian rhythm can be so disrupted in older LTC residents that they may not maintain sleep for a full hour at any time over a 24-hour period.[25] Disturbed sleep in older adults with ADRD is associated with anxiety, agitation, aggressiveness, and disinhibition.[26] Sedative-hypnotic medications are common and may be inappropriately prescribed for LTC residents with ADRD, especially when used for anxiety and agitation.[27-29]

Consequences of Sleep Disturbances in Long-Term Care

The adverse health consequences of insufficient sleep and poor sleep quality have been established in general health, neurocognitive functioning, mental health, metabolism, inflammation, cardiovascular health, cancer, pain, and mortality.[30,31] Particularly in older adults, poor sleep leads to impaired physical function including gait speed[32] and increased risk for cognitive decline and dementia.[33] Sleep disturbances in LTC residents have been associated with impaired functionality,[18] less functional recovery,[34] social disengagement,[35] increased risk of falls,[36] frailty,[37] agitation,[38] and higher mortality.[39]

FACTORS CONTRIBUTING TO SLEEP DISTURBANCES IN LONG-TERM CARE

A variety of factors may cause sleep disturbances in LTC residents, such as sleep architecture changes with advancing age, environmental disruptors such as nighttime noise and lack of daytime light, care activities, social disengagement, lack of physical activity, cognitive impairment, comorbid medical conditions, and polypharmacy.[40,41] Some of these factors are interconnected, and their relationship with sleep disturbances is often bidirectional. Sleep-disturbing factors commonly seen in LTC residents are described in the following sections, with the goal to inform the development of sleep-promotion strategies.

Advancing Age

Sleep architecture and circadian rhythms change with advancing age, including decreased deep sleep, reduced sleep efficiency, increased sleep latency, frequent arousals, and early morning awakenings.[41] These age-related changes contribute to sleep disturbances commonly seen in institutionalized older adults. As supported by the finding from a large cross-cultural investigation of sleep in LTC settings, older age was identified as an independent predictor of sleep disturbances.[15]

Disruptors from Environment and Nocturnal Care Activities

Various factors in the LTC environment disturb sleep, such as noise, lighting, room temperature, and roommates. Limited daytime exposure to bright light significantly contributes to circadian dysregulation in LTC residents.[42] Nocturnal care activities are also disruptive to sleep maintenance. Sleep in nursing home residents is substantially disturbed by nighttime noise and incontinence care.[43] A limited knowledge of sleep and a general lack of awareness of disturbed sleep and its negative consequences among LTC healthcare providers, as revealed by a national survey,[44] may lead to interrupting residents' sleep with care activities for the convenience of the LTC staff. An important role for sleep specialists is education of LTC staff on the health and quality-of-life consequences of sleep disturbances for LTC residents.

Lack of Physical and Social Activity

Many LTC residents spend considerable time in bed and are physically and socially inactive during the day.[45] Emotional distress, loneliness, isolation, and the relocation to an LTC facility often lead to social disengagement.[40] Physical inactivity and social isolation significantly disrupt LTC residents' circadian rhythms, leading to disturbed sleep and EDS.[45] The World Health Organization guidelines propose that adults aged 65 years and older should have at least 150 minutes of moderate-intensity aerobic physical activity, or at least 75 minutes of vigorous-intensity aerobic physical activity throughout the week.[46] Clearly, most LTC residents do not meet these requirements. A recent cross-sectional study of 894 cognitively intact nursing home residents supports the bidirectional relationship between sleep and physical activity. In this study, those reporting short sleep duration (<6 hours) were significantly less likely to report sufficient physical activity based on World Health Organization recommendations, while those reporting long sleep duration (>9 hours) and good sleep quality were significantly more likely to report sufficient physical activity.[47]

Excessive Daytime Sleepiness and Daytime Napping

Daytime napping and EDS are common.[25] EDS is characterized by an uncontrollable urge to sleep or falling asleep during the day.[48] The prevalence of EDS, defined as an Epworth Sleepiness Scale[49] score greater than 10, was 19.6% in a sample of 470 older adults receiving long-term services in assisted living communities, nursing homes, and the community.[50] However, the authors acknowledged that the study likely underestimated EDS, since those with severe cognitive impairment were excluded. Earlier studies report 35% to 70% prevalence of EDS in LTC settings[45,51,52] and 31% prevalence in the community.[53] The number of bothersome symptoms, such as incontinence, depression, and vision problems, was significantly associated with EDS. Individualized interventions targeting specific symptoms may positively affect EDS.

Although an appropriately timed, 1- to 1.5-hour daytime nap for older adults may promote well-being and cognitive health, excessive napping may alter the sleep-wake cycle and lead to poor nocturnal sleep. In a recent secondary analysis of 192 persons with dementia living in 28 LTC settings in Australia, sleep and activity were measured for 24 hours using accelerometry.[54] During the daytime residents averaged 240 steps, had an average of 1.8 hours of light physical activity and no moderate or vigorous physical activity, and napped 1.3 hours. At night, they were lying down 8.4 hours and averaged a total of 6.8 hours of sleep. Although there was considerable variation in both sleep and activity, in general these Australian LTC residents napped less, were lying in bed less at night, and slept better than previously reported in other studies.[25,45] In an earlier study in residents from four Los Angeles nursing homes, 69% of 492 observed residents had excessive daytime sleeping defined as asleep over 15% of time from 9 a.m. to 5 p.m. recorded by actigraphy, and 60% had disturbed nighttime sleep.[45] In addition to the excessive duration of napping, a high day-to-day instability of napping behavior in LTC residents can link to increased evening cortisol level, which is an indicator of dysregulated hypothalmic-pituitary-adrenal-axis and circadian rhythm.[55] These findings suggest the potential efficacy of less time in bed, less napping, and more consistent napping as an individualized behavioral approach to treating sleep disturbances in this population.

Medical and Psychiatric Comorbidities

Sleep complaints in older adults are often associated with other comorbidities.[56] Most LTC residents suffer from multiple chronic medical and psychiatric conditions that disrupt sleep, such as dementia, nocturia, pain, arthritis, cardiovascular disease, and chronic pulmonary diseases. More than half of institutionalized older adults experience depressive symptoms, which are strongly associated with poor sleep quality and sleep disturbances.[57,58]

Compelling evidence suggests a link between sleep disturbances and cognitive decline, and this relationship is likely bidirectional.[59-62] Although pathologic changes in the brain from underlying ADRD may lead to sleep disturbances, disturbed sleep may contribute to the development of ADRD and a more rapid cognitive decline. Recent evidence points toward a link between sleep-wake disturbances and the main hallmarks of pathogenesis of AD: abnormal amyloid-beta, tau protein accumulation, and neurodegeneration.[63] Individuals with sleep disturbances exhibit a 1.55 times higher risk of developing Alzheimer disease (AD).[64]

Almost all LTC residents take multiple medications to manage their medical and psychiatric conditions,[65] and a wide range of these medications can cause or worsen sleep disturbances.[66] For example, diuretics or sympathomimetic medications can significantly disrupt sleep when taken near bedtime. Clinicians should also assess the use of over-the-counter medications and social drugs such as caffeine, alcohol, and nicotine, and their impact on sleep.

CLINICAL ASSESSMENT OF SLEEP DISTURBANCES IN LONG-TERM CARE SETTINGS

Clinical assessment of sleep disturbances for LTC residents should embrace both a global geriatric approach and an individualized plan. Features and causes of sleep disturbances must be examined carefully, and a diagnosis established before treatment initiation.[67] Some LTC residents cannot recall their sleep problems; therefore it is critical to obtain an in-depth history from all possible sources, including residents, family members, and LTC caregivers. Caregivers who consistently care for specific residents on the evening and night shifts can provide information on usual bedtime, nighttime routines, and quality and quantity of resident nighttime sleep, and daytime staff can provide data on daytime napping and EDS.

In addition to typical inquiries of timing, duration, and regularity of sleep, daytime napping, and symptoms of sleep disorders, sleep specialists should specifically check symptoms such as hallucinations, nighttime agitation and wandering, and sleep attacks.[68] Clinical assessment should consider sleep-disturbing factors, such as nocturia, respiratory distress, pain, depression, light exposure, noise, decreased social and physical activity, and medication use. Another important element of the sleep history is the approximate time that the nursing home staff puts residents in bed for the night and gets them out of bed in the morning. Time in bed at night is often 12 or more hours. Other important questions are the number of awakenings for incontinence or other care activities and whether the resident has a private room or has a noisy roommate or one that requires incontinence care at night.

Challenges exist in using sleep diaries and scales that rely on self-report, such as the Epworth Sleepiness Scale[49] and Pittsburgh Sleep Quality Index.[69] Dementia-specific questionnaires such as the Sleep Disorders Inventory (SDI)[70] may be helpful to assess sleep for residents with ADRD. Derived from the Neuropsychiatric Inventory,[71] the SDI assesses severity, frequency, and caregiver burden of sleep-disturbed behaviors during the past 2 weeks. The SDI has good correlation with objective sleep measures.[70] The Mayo sleep questionnaire bed-partner/ informant version is a validated screening tool for rapid eye movement sleep behavior disorder for older adults with dementia.[72] The discrepancy between objective data and caregiver-reported sleep calls for more reliable objective evaluation.[73] The Behavioral Indicators Test–Restless Legs (BIT-RL) is an example of an objective, dementia-specific diagnostic tool.[74] Given the sensory nature of RLS, the current diagnostic standard, which emphasizes self-report of symptoms, is unsuitable for LTC residents with cognitive impairment.[75] Furthermore, nocturnal agitation may be the primary presentation of RLS in older adults with dementia, which adds to the difficulty diagnosing RLS in these individuals.[76] The BIT-RL consists of a 20-minute observation for eight behavioral indicators and chart review and interviews for six clinical indicators. The BIT-RL has good diagnostic accuracy for RLS[74] and is feasible for use in clinical trials and practice in older adults with dementia.[77,78]

Although polysomnography remains the standard for sleep assessment, it can be difficult to obtain in LTC residents; many LTC residents have cognitive impairment, and sleep stage scoring may be complicated because of diffuse electroencephalographic slowing.[79] Sleeping in a different setting, such as a sleep laboratory, often confuses and agitates older adults with memory problems, and patient cooperation may be problematic. Home sleep tests may be a useful alternative, but residents with nighttime confusion may remove the sensors, resulting in missing data. If possible, a caregiver or family member should stay with the LTC resident during in-laboratory polysomnography (PSG) or a home sleep test to reassure them and help with sensor integrity.

Actigraphy provides consistent objective data that are often unique from patient-reported sleep logs for some sleep parameters.[80] The 2018 American Academy of Sleep Medicine clinical practice guideline recommends using actigraphy to assess adults with insomnia disorder and circadian rhythm sleep-wake disorder.[81] If reliably secured, actigraphy can be used for sleep assessment in LTC residents with dementia. A minimum of 72 hours of consecutive recording is required,[81] and 7 to 14 days of recording is needed for diagnosing irregular sleep-wake rhythm disorder.[82] In individuals with limb movement disorders, Parkinson disease, and severe sleep apnea, actigraphy may not reliably distinguish wakefulness and sleep because of tremor or frequent apneas.

COMMON SLEEP DIAGNOSES IN LONG-TERM CARE RESIDENTS

Irregular Sleep-Wake Rhythm Disorder

Irregular sleep-wake rhythm disorder is commonly observed in ADRD. Persons usually experience insomnia or EDS.[82] Sleep and wake episodes across the 24-hour cycle are fragmented, with the largest sleep bout typically less than 4 hours. Because of multiple awakenings and nocturnal wandering, falls can be an indirect complication. The etiology is multifactorial and may involve anatomic or functional abnormalities of the circadian clock and decreased exposure to environmental-entraining agents such as light and structured social and physical activities.

Chronic Insomnia Disorder

Chronic insomnia disorder is likely to be prevalent in LTC residents, but the true prevalence is unknown because of self-report limitations in LTC residents with cognitive impairment. Comorbid psychiatric conditions, particularly mood and anxiety disorders, and conditions that result in chronic pain, breathing difficulties, or immobility are associated with increased risk for chronic insomnia disorder. As previously discussed, in cases in which LTC residents cannot self-report, clinicians may obtain the observed sleep history and the observed daytime consequences by interviewing LTC caregivers and family members.

Obstructive Sleep Apnea

Approximately 60% of LTC residents have an apnea-hypopnea index (AHI) of at least 5, and 40% of LTC residents have an AHI of at least 15 (i.e., in the moderate to severe OSA range).[83-85] The prevalence of obstructive sleep apnea (OSA) in LTC residents is likely higher than in the general population, which may partially reflect obesity, changes in respiratory function that occur with aging, and the extreme physical inactivity that is so common in this population.[86,87] There is loss in respiratory function that centers around three primary mechanistic changes related to aging: decreased chest wall compliance, decreased static elastic recoil of the lung, and decreased respiratory muscle strength, all of which may contribute to the high prevalence of OSA in older adults.[87] Other primary contributors to OSA prevalence in LTC residents are the frequency of comorbid health conditions such as cardiovascular disease, cerebrovascular disease, and diabetes that predispose older adults in general to sleep apnea; number of sedating medications; and the high percentage of residents with neurodegeneration. As discussed earlier, a home sleep test, followed by auto-adjusting positive airway pressure, if indicated, is likely to be better tolerated by LTC residents than in laboratory studies.

Restless Legs Syndrome

The reported prevalence of RLS in older adults is 10% to 14%, making it among the most common movement and sleep-related disorder.[88] RLS is likely to be common in older adults residing in LTC, but there are few prevalence data because a reliable RLS symptoms interview is challenging and unreliable in persons with cognitive impairment.[75] Richards and colleagues used multiple data sources for RLS diagnosis, including polysomnography with periodic leg movements, caregiver interviews, and medical history including iron status, observation for RLS-associated behaviors, and consensus of expert diagnosticians. Use of these comprehensive diagnostic methods in 59 persons with nighttime agitation and dementia living at home demonstrated that one-quarter had RLS, and RLS was associated with frequency of nighttime agitation behaviors ($r = 0.31$, P .01).[76] In 393 patients with mild AD, Talarico and colleagues found a much lower RLS prevalence of 4.1%, but they acknowledged that this was likely due to missing data and the requirement that both the patient and bed partner answer an RLS survey.[89]

A number of factors common in older-adult LTC residents are implicated in the major functional and metabolic pathways that lead to RLS and provide support for an increased expression of RLS: older age,[88] female sex, iron deficiency and anemia,[90-92] and prescribed medications that may aggravate RLS symptoms, such as antinausea drugs (e.g., prochlorperazine), antidepressants that increase serotonin (e.g., fluoxetine), antipsychotic drugs (e.g., haloperidol), and some cold and allergy medications that contain older antihistamines (e.g., diphenhydramine). Also, from a behavioral point of view, and considering the compulsive urge to move of RLS patients, the lack of activity and the prolonged bedrest common in LTC engenders RLS symptoms.[93,94]

A relationship between RLS and a common geriatric syndrome in older adults with dementia, nighttime agitation, is expected, given the nature of the symptoms and the nightly appearance of both conditions.[76] Nighttime agitation, also known as "sundowning," is an evening and nighttime state characterized by behaviors such as wandering and aggression. From 2% to 66% of persons with ADRD have nighttime agitation; it causes patient suffering, burdens caregivers, and is costly to manage.[95] In the recent past, antipsychotics were used to manage nighttime agitation, but their effectiveness is unconvincing, and these drugs are rarely used any longer because they are associated with falls, strokes, and death. The patterns of nighttime agitation behaviors and RLS symptoms are almost identical. RLS symptoms are circadian, occurring only or most severely in the evening and early part of the night.

Phase advance occurs in LTC residents with ADRD, and thus their RLS symptoms may begin as early as sundown in winter. Agitation behaviors may be responses to unmet needs that cannot be communicated any other way, and discomfort and sleep disturbances are associated with RLS and consistently identified as unmet needs associated with agitation.[93,96] Thus untreated RLS may manifest as nighttime agitation, and sleep medicine specialists should consider RLS as a likely potential cause for nighttime agitation. Richards and colleagues recently validated a new RLS diagnostic instrument, the BIT-RL, suitable for diagnosis of RLS in persons with dementia.[74]

MANAGEMENT OF SLEEP DISTURBANCES IN LONG-TERM CARE

Overview and Management Goals

Sleep specialists should set treatment goals for sleep disturbances in older adults living in LTC settings in collaboration with residents (if able), family members, and caregivers. In general, the focus should be on identifying and treating bothersome sleep symptoms such as EDS or insufficient and interrupted nighttime sleep that negatively affects the older adults' quality of life. For example, discomfort caused by RLS may be a cause for nighttime agitation and more restrictive levels of care for safety. Treatment of OSA may be indicated because of its negative effects on daytime cognition, everyday function, and quality of life. A thorough evaluation is critical. The treatment of comorbidities or deprescribing of medications should be the first step. In general, nonpharmacologic interventions are preferred over medications for sleep disturbances in older adults in LTC.

Pharmacologic Treatment

Pharmacologic treatment of insomnia in LTC residents is very common, and the boom in US Food and Drug Administration (FDA)–approved medications for insomnia and changes with regard to Medicare Part D coverage[97] have added more complexity to the decision to initiate pharmacologic treatment.[98] In a study of 2135 nursing home residents, 24% were prescribed hypnotics and sedatives.[29] Increasing evidence indicates that hypnotic use is frequently associated with harm, and that nonpharmacologic interventions should be first-line therapy for nursing home residents. For those who have failed nonpharmacologic strategies and for whom pharmacologic treatment is required, there is a paucity of treatment guidelines for this specific population. The vast majority of medications that are either FDA approved for the treatment of insomnia or used off-label are on the American Geriatrics Society 2019 updated Beers list[99] for potentially inappropriate medication use in older adults because of the potential risks outweighing the benefits. For the treatment of insomnia, medications included on the Beers list as potentially inappropriate include all benzodiazepines and non-benzodiazepine gamma-aminobutyric acid A ($GABA_A$) selective agonists medications (i.e., "the Z drugs," including zolpidem, eszopiclone, and zaleplon), antihistamines such as doxylamine and diphenhydramine, and antipsychotics (except for treatment of schizophrenia or bipolar disorder). Hypnotic agents not included on the Beers list include melatonin-receptor agonists (e.g., ramelteon) and low-dose (i.e., <6 mg) doxepin (although higher-dose doxepin is on the Beers list). Regarding off-label use of antidepressants, anticholinergic antidepressants (e.g., amitriptyline) are on the Beers list, whereas low-dose trazodone is not. Orexin receptor antagonists (e.g., suvorexant) are also not on the Beers list, but these are relatively new agents and were not specifically addressed in the latest Beers list.

The practice of using antipsychotics for sleep disturbance in LTC has significantly fallen out of favor because of increased evidence for adverse effects in this population as well as increasing regulatory pressures. In 2006 the Center for Medicare and Medicaid Services (CMS) moved to require all Medicare Part D plans to include on their formularies "all or substantially all" drugs within six protected classes, two of which were antipsychotics and antidepressants. A few years thereafter, as a result of the FDA warning on antipsychotic medications used in patients with dementia (initially on atypical antipsychotics only [2005], then extended to conventional antipsychotics in 2008), CMS started aiming to curb the use of antipsychotic medications in LTC through two quality measures posted on the Nursing Home Compare website in 2012. Later that same year, CMS announced its intention that all Medicare Part D plans would begin coverage of benzodiazepines for "all Part D medically-accepted indications" beginning January 2013.[97] Not unexpectedly, a subsequent and steady rise in benzodiazepine prescriptions in LTC resulted, while the use of antipsychotics has tapered considerably.[97] Data reported via the Minimum Data Set from 2018 to 2019 show that 14.5% of long-stay nursing home residents received an antipsychotic, and 20.4% of residents received an anxiolytic/hypnotic.[100]

The traditional approach, which encourages use of shorter half-life benzodiazepines when deciding to use this class of medication in older adults, although tailored toward safety, may inadvertently result in less effective treatment. A cross-sectional study of 383 patients in 6 different residential aged-care facilities conducted by Chen and colleagues found that of the 25% who used benzodiazepines on a regular basis, those prescribed long-acting had higher nighttime sleep quality than nonusers (AOR = 4.0).[101] Short-acting as-needed benzodiazepines were associated with lower nighttime sleep quality and longer daytime napping compared with long-acting regular benzodiazepines. The study authors point out that more studies are needed to determine if this effect is in part due to the higher risk patients being prescribed the shorter-acting drugs.[101]

The nonbenzodiazepine $GABA_A$ medications—the "Z drugs"—have been found to have significant side effects, limiting their usefulness in frail older adults. Among these side effects are cognitive impairment and falls, both of which are significant concerns in LTC residents. Increasing evidence of poor tolerance ultimately led to dose limitations for older patients being placed on zolpidem, eszopiclone, and zaleplon. A case-crossover study of more than 15,000 nursing home residents with hip fracture conducted over 2007 to 2008 demonstrated an increased OR of 1.66 for hip fracture in those patients prescribed a nonbenzodiazepine hypnotic drug (specifically, zolpidem, eszopiclone, or zaleplon), which rose to an OR of 2.20 for new users.[102]

The move away from antipsychotics, benzodiazepines, and Z drugs resulted in increased off-label use of antidepressants with sedating side effects such as low-dose trazodone. The presumed reason for this move, given lack of data on whether these medications are effective, is the desire to avoid the potentially harmful side effects seen with other classes of medications as well as to avoid higher-cost newer medications.

However, a recent retrospective matched cohort study looking at low-dose trazodone and benzodiazepines found no difference in risk of a fall-related injury (5.7% for low-dose trazodone and 6.0% for benzodiazepine, $P = .29$), calling into question the belief that trazodone is safer. The authors rightly call for additional studies given the increasing trends of use of trazodone in LTC settings.[103]

The remaining medications with FDA approval for insomnia include the novel orexin receptor antagonist suvorexant, and the selective melatonin receptor MT1 and MT2 agonist ramelteon. Published data on the effects of these medications in the LTC population and the geriatric population are limited. A placebo-controlled phase 4 trial studying ramelteon in an LTC population was limited by small sample sizes.[104] Although suvorexant phase III trials did aim to enroll a significant number of geriatric patients, none had cognitive impairment or were in LTC, so it is unclear that the results can be generalized to this population.[105] Ramelteon similarly has demonstrated reasonable safety and efficacy for ambulatory, community-dwelling geriatric patients without dementia. Among the obstacles, beyond insufficient research in the LTC population, is the significant cost of these medications. Although current studies are lacking, it is possible melatonin agonists may offer a safer insomnia treatment option with therapeutic benefit in the LTC population.

Tailored and judicial pharmacotherapy is generally recommended for identified neurologic or psychiatric disorders that have disordered sleep as one of the manifestations, as long as the risk-benefit profile is favorable. As examples, depression with associated significant insomnia as a symptom should generally be given a trial of antidepressant after nonpharmacologic strategies have been exhausted.

Similarly, for patients with movement disorders affecting sleep such as RLS, a trial of pharmacologic treatment for RLS may be helpful. For ferritin levels less than 75 ng/mL, consider adding 325 mg ferrous sulfate daily. Traditional treatments for RLS, including dopamine agonists and carbidopa/levodopa, are generally not well tolerated in the LTC population. This, along with inability to recognize and diagnose RLS in patients with AD, is hypothesized as one of the reasons for infrequent pharmacotherapy for RLS in the LTC settings. Ongoing research is exploring whether gabapentin enacarbil results in improved sleep and decreased agitation with acceptable safety and tolerance in patients in LTC who have AD and nighttime agitation.[77]

No discussion of pharmacologic treatment of sleep disturbance in LTC is complete without mention of the many medications prescribed for a myriad of conditions both chronic and acute, which can exacerbate and/or cause disruption in sleep. The LTC population is particularly vulnerable because of the prevalence of polypharmacy. A cross-sectional study of 451 nursing homes (30,702 residents) found that the average number of medications per residents was 7, and that 21% of the residents were on 10 or more medications.[106] Insomnia can be a side effect of medications, and, unless recognized as such, can lead to a prescribing cascade, increasing the risk of adverse drug effects. Neuroleptics, antihistamines, antidepressants, proton pump inhibitors, and antiemetics with dopamine blockade are among the many medication classes that can exacerbate sleep disturbance.

Recent literature has begun to focus on deprescribing in LTC facilities, including a focus on sedative/hypnotics. A multicenter, prospective chart review of sedative/hypnotic use in 11 LTC facilities in Tennessee demonstrated that consultant pharmacist intervention can have a significant impact on reduction of sedative/hypnotic use.[107] A systematic review focused on reduction of antipsychotic and benzodiazepine use within nursing homes (not specifically hypnotics) found that that, although improvements were seen in emotional responsiveness and cognitive function, the overall subjective health score remained unchanged upon benzodiazepine reduction.[108] Much of the research has focused on whether deprescribing interventions results in a sustained lower number of medications, with more research needed on the clinical outcomes of such strategies.

Nonpharmacologic Strategies for Insomnia

Cognitive Behavioral Therapy for Insomnia

Cognitive behavioral therapy for insomnia (CBT-I) is highly effective and is the standard of practice for treating insomnia in a number of populations,[109,110] but there are minimal data on the effectiveness of CBT-I in the LTC population, many of whom have cognitive impairment. A recent study by Dolu and Nahcivan investigated the impact of four weekly 1-hour sessions of CBT-I led by a nurse and motivational interviewing, compared with usual nursing home care, in 52 cognitively intact residents.[111] Those in the intervention group had significant improvement in number of awakenings, total sleep time, wake after sleep onset and sleep efficiency, as well as a significant decrease in depressive symptomology. Although this study lacked an attention control condition, the findings and the strong evidence from a multitude of studies on CBT-I in other populations suggest that CBT-I should be routinely prescribed for insomnia in LTC settings for those cognitively able to engage in it.

Bright Light Therapy

Little outdoor light exposure, dim indoor lighting, reduced light transmission through ocular lens, and reduced mobility contribute to light deprivation for older adults living in LTC.[112] Bright light therapy (BLT) is a chronotherapeutic intervention to treat circadian sleep-wake disturbances. Several studies and reviews support that BLT improves nighttime sleep, decreases awakenings, improves daytime wakefulness, reduces evening agitation, and consolidates rest-activity patterns in older adults with dementia.[68,113-115] However, a recent Cochrane systematic review concluded that there is insufficient evidence of its effectiveness, and only 10 studies were deemed of sufficient quality to be included.[116] The Cochrane review reported that pooled data[117-121] showed a significant decrease in the number of nighttime awakenings and, including only the studies that incorporated morning bright light,[117,121] resulted in an even larger effect size. A more recent meta-analysis, by the van Maanan group in 2016,[122] reported a significant benefit for BLT for sleep disturbances in dementia, for sleep-onset latency, total sleep time, time in bed, and sleep efficiency. The American Academy of Sleep Medicine practice guideline[123] suggests that clinicians treat irregular sleep wake rhythm disorder in older adults with dementia with light therapy. Based on these results, we recommend that clinicians consider trying 30 minutes to 1 hour of morning sunlight exposure daily, that bright white lights be installed in common areas frequently used by residents in the daytime, such as dining rooms and activity areas, and that residents spend time each day in these well-lighted common areas. For residents who choose to spend most of their time in their rooms, a trial of exposure to morning light boxes or timed bright white morning overhead lights may be considered. Well-designed randomized controlled clinical trials are needed to provide better evidence on the efficacy of bright light and to better standardize amount, spectrum, timing, distribution, and duration of treatment.

Social Activity

The ability to participate in valued activities, whether for work, family, or leisure, is an important aspect of personal identity.[124] Progressive memory loss limits engagement with previously enjoyed activities and contributes to loss of identity and depression. LTC settings may not provide residents, especially those with cognitive impairment, with daytime social activities that engage them in the world around them. A recent systematic review concluded that meaningful activities may be effective for ameliorating behavioral and psychological symptoms of dementia and improving quality of life.[124] Daytime social interactions also help synchronize the circadian sleep-wake rhythm, discourage people from excessive daytime sleeping, and improve depressive symptoms. Few studies have tested the effect of increased daytime social activity on sleep in LTC residents. In a nursing-home population with dementia, the Richards group tested an intervention of increased individualized social activities (approximately 1 to 2 hours daily) provided by project research assistants. The social activities were tailored to residents' preferences and abilities and were in both group and one-on-one settings. Compared with a usual care control group, the social activity group had significantly reduced daytime napping, and in the subset of participants with poor nighttime sleep efficiency, significantly increased nighttime total sleep time.[125] In another clinical trial led by Moyle, residents with dementia interacted with a robotic seal or a seal with the robotic features disabled for 15 minutes three afternoons a week, or had usual care. There was no effect of the seal interventions on daytime or nighttime sleep,[126] perhaps because of low intervention dosage or insufficient human social interaction.

In summary, there are few studies on the effect of increased daytime social activity on sleep disturbances in LTC residents, and results are mixed. In general, LTC residents with dementia have few meaningful activities and nap excessively. We recommend that sleep specialists consider a trial of at least 1 hour daily of late afternoon individualized daytime social activity in individual or group settings for irregular sleep wake rhythm disorder and chronic insomnia.

Physical Activity and Exercise

Many LTC residents spend considerable time in bed and are physically inactive. Regular physical activity may help synchronize the sleep-wake rhythm and consolidate nighttime sleep. In addition, exercise has been shown to improve several factors associated with sleep disturbance in the LTC population such as depressive symptoms and memory. The effect of various exercise interventions on sleep disturbances have been examined, and most have had positive results. For example, wheelchair dependence is an obstacle to physical activity. Chen and colleagues[127] in Taiwan conducted a 6-month clinical trial in cognitively intact wheelchair-dependent residents in 10 nursing homes. Those in the control group continued with their usual activities, and those in the experimental group received a 40-minute elastic band progressive resistance training exercise program led by trained instructors three times a week. Sleep quality in the exercise group significantly improved compared with the control group at 6 months, but not at 3 months. These findings suggest that the long-term training effects of progressive strength-building exercises, such as increased strength and mobility, are important for improving sleep in this population. A recent study supported this idea. Herrick and colleagues[128] analyzed the effects of an acute resistance training exercise bout in LTC residents. In a secondary analysis of Richards and colleagues,[125] 43 participants (age 81.5 ± 8.1 years, females = 26) with sleep disturbances had two attended overnight polysomnography tests in their rooms for sleep architecture analysis; one polysomnography with same-day resistance training, one without any resistance training.[128] Resistance training consisted of chest and leg press exercises (3 sets, 8 repetitions, 80% predicted 1 repetition maximum). There were no significant differences in nighttime sleep between days (exercise or nonexercise), indicating that the gainful effects of resistance training exercise are the result of an accumulative exercise adaptation and not in response to an acute exercise bout. In conclusion, we recommend a trial of supervised increased physical activity and exercise for sleep disturbance in LTC. In general, a combination of daily aerobic exercise such as walking (a total of 150 minutes of moderate intensity or 75 minutes of vigorous intensity per week),[46] and supervised strength training three times a week may be most beneficial.

Multicomponent Interventions

Combining social activities and physical activity, along with an individualized person-centered approach, has been shown to maintain the circadian sleep-wake rhythm and improve sleep in several studies. Sullivan identified predictors of circadian sleep-wake rhythm maintenance in 171 older LTC residents residing in 7 nursing homes.[129] The investigators developed specific criteria for sleep-wake rhythm maintenance using the autocorrelogram of activity from actigraphy. They then examined the autocorrelogram of each participant to determine whether or not the sleep-wake rhythm was maintained. Using measures of depression, cognitive function, physical and psychosocial activity, hypnotic medications, and sleep apnea, as well as demographic characteristics, logistic regression determined the best predictors of maintaining circadian sleep-wake rhythmicity. Duration of physical activity ($P = 0.00$) and psychosocial activity ($P = 0.00$) predicted circadian sleep-wake rhythm maintenance. Li and colleagues investigated the effect of a 3-month person-centered dementia care intervention compared with a usual care control condition on sleep in LTC residents.[130] Central to the intervention was a humanistic care model that sees the person first, rather than his or her dementia, and engagement in meaningful physical and social activities. Adjusting for baseline, the intervention group ($n = 16$) had significantly less daytime sleep and more nighttime sleep compared with the control group ($n = 6$). In a randomized controlled clinical trial, Richards and colleagues investigated the effects of physical resistance strength training and walking (E), individualized social activity (SA), both E and SA (ESA) compared with a usual care control group on sleep time in 193 nursing home and assisted living residents.[125] Residents were randomly assigned and 165 completed the study. The E group participated in high-intensity physical resistance strength training 3 days a week and on 2 days walked for up to 45 minutes. The SA group received social activity 1 hour daily 5 days a week. The ESA group received both E and SA, and the control group participated in usual activities provided in the homes. Sleep was measured by 2 nights of PSG at pre- and postintervention. Total sleep time significantly increased in the ESA group over that of control group (adjusted means 364.2 minutes versus 328.9 minutes), as did sleep efficiency and non–rapid eye movement sleep, but neither S or E alone effected sleep. Combined exercise and social activity also significantly improved everyday function in this sample of LTC residents.[131]

In an earlier study of Alessi and colleagues, an 18-week physical activity program involving sit-to-stand repetitions and/or transferring and walking or wheelchair propulsion did not result in improvement of night and day sleep in LTC residents.[132] However, when the research team applied an intervention combining physical activity with regulation of the nighttime environment to reduce nighttime awakenings by LTC staff for incontinence care, the intervention group showed increased nighttime sleep and decreased daytime sleep, suggesting a multicomponent approach is needed to improve sleep in LTC settings.[133] In a subsequent analysis of the Alessi and colleagues data, Martin and colleagues found an improved rest-activity rhythm with a greater active phase in the multicomponent intervention group compared with the control group.[134] In contrast, studies by Ouslander and colleagues[135] and Alessi and colleagues[136] showed minimal or no change in nighttime sleep as a result of a 17-day multicomponent program consisting of low-intensity physical activity, noise abatement, light exposure, and sleep hygiene.

The majority of studies support the effectiveness of multicomponent interventions that include bright daytime light exposure; tailored, person-centered social activities; aerobic and strength-building exercises; sleep hygiene; reduction in nighttime noise and awakenings for incontinence care; and reducing excessive daytime napping. We recommend multicomponent interventions for sleep disturbances in LTC settings.

Continuous Positive Airway Pressure and Other Treatments for Obstructive Sleep Apnea

Sleep apnea is prevalent in LTC residents, adversely affects nighttime sleep, and often causes daytime napping. However, it is rarely documented or treated in LTC residents,[137] perhaps because providers are concerned that treatment using the standard of care, continuous positive airway pressure (CPAP), may be uncomfortable or stressful for residents approaching end of life and because the health and quality of life outcomes of treatment have not been systematically evaluated in this population. To our knowledge no studies have systematically attempted to treat sleep apnea in LTC residents, but a few studies have been conducted in older adults with cognitive decline who resided in community settings. For example, in noninstitutionalized older adults with mild dementia and moderate to severe OSA, Ancoli-Israel and colleagues compared 3 to 6 weeks of CPAP use to placebo CPAP in a placebo-controlled, randomized clinical trial.[138] They found good adherence, improvements in sleep architecture and self-reported sleepiness, and significant improvement in some cognitive outcome measures. This study is especially relevant for LTC residents because it showed that even short-term treatment of OSA with CPAP can improve cognitive outcomes that are important for enhancing quality of life in older adults with cognitive impairment.[138] In another study, Richards and colleagues[139] found significant improvements in psychomotor/cognitive processing speed in older adults with mild cognitive impairment who received CPAP compared with those who did not receive CPAP at 1 year, controlling for baseline group differences and an over fivefold increased odds ($P = .12$) of subjective global improvement, which is a quality of life outcome that matters to individuals.[139] Among those with mild OSA (n = 17), CPAP resulted in a statistically significant improvement in psychomotor/cognitive processing speed after 1 year.[140]

Both cardiovascular and cerebrovascular disease are highly prevalent in older LTC residents, and emerging research highlights the complex interrelationships between sleep-disordered breathing and cardiovascular and cerebrovascular disease.[141] Cardiovascular structure and function are adversely affected by both OSA and central sleep apnea associated with Cheyne-Stokes respiration (CSA-CSR). Observational studies consistently indicate that untreated moderate to severe OSA in patients with established coronary disease or heart failure is related to increased cardiovascular morbidity and mortality. In the Sleep Apnea Cardiovascular Endpoints (SAVE) trial,[142] individuals who were adherent to CPAP therapy had a significantly lower risk of stroke than those in the usual-care group, as well as a significantly lower risk of a composite end point of cerebral events. The benefits of adherence to CPAP supports the need for clinicians to discuss treatment preferences with LTC residents (if able) and their families. Further, additional studies are needed addressing the adherence and efficacy of treatments other than CPAP (e.g., nighttime oxygen, mandibular advancement devices, pharmacologic treatments, weight loss, exercise) on clinical end points that are important to LTC residents and their families. For example, strength training and walking exercise significantly reduced the AHI in older LTC residents and may be a viable treatment alternative to CPAP in some LTC residents who are unable to use CPAP. In a secondary analysis of data from the study by Richards and colleagues, 6 weeks of combined high-intensity strength training and walking exercise significantly reduced the AHI compared with the control group (adjusted mean baseline 20.2 [1.39] to postintervention 16.7 [0.96] in LTC residents, many of whom had ADRD).[87] The mechanism for the improved AHI may be strengthening of inspiratory muscles.

Decisions regarding management of OSA in LTC should be made collaboratively with residents (if able) and their families. Provider treatment recommendations should be linked to the underlying clinical and pathophysiologic phenotyping and carefully consider quality-of-life outcomes, such as the potential to affect engagement for residents in the world around them, confusion and agitation, well-being, daytime sleepiness, health, and preservation of cognitive and physical function. Classification of LTC residents based on the AHI does not provide sufficient guidance for treatment selection or selection for inclusion in clinical trials. Future studies should focus on adherence and the sleep, health, cognitive, functional, and quality-of-life benefits of OSA treatment in LTC residents.

Mind-Body and Complementary Health Practices

Studies of mind-body practices, such as meditative yoga[143] and progressive relaxation exercises,[144] have resulted in statistically significant improvements in sleep in LTC residents, but studies are few, and the requirement of active cognitive involvement limits participation to those who are cognitively intact. There is more evidence on the positive effect of complementary and alternative therapies on sleep in LTC residents, including acupressure, massage, and dietary or herbal supplements such as melatonin and chamomile extract.[145,146] Among these, nighttime use of melatonin and acupressure before sleep are the most promising.[146]

Dietary or herbal supplements do not need FDA approval before marketing and generally have not been subjected to the same scrutiny or regulation as medications. Their potential interactions with medications remain unclear and may pose risks to LTC residents.[147,148] Melatonin and valerian are the two most studied supplements for sleep disorders, but high-quality investigations remain limited.[147] There is no robust documentation of prolonged valerian use in older adults.[147] The effect of melatonin on sleep, either evaluated independently[149-151] or as part of multicomponent interventions,[117,152] showed mixed findings. The effect of melatonin supplements is dependent on the dose and time of administration. However, the best applicable dosage of melatonin for older adults remains unclear. There is a wide range of melatonin doses in clinical trials, varying from 0.1 mg to 50 mg/kg.[153] Recent meta-analyses[154,155] support the overall safety and positive effect of melatonin on sleep, including those with dementia. However, safety concerns in older adults, specifically the possibility for prolonged duration of action in patients prescribed melatonin, support careful monitoring for daytime sedation. The best evidence supports use of the lowest possible dose of immediate-release melatonin, with a maximum of 1 or 2 mg, 1 hour before bedtime.[153]

Several studies have shown that massage improves sleep and overall health of LTC residents and can potentially increase the engagement of family members in resident care.[156] Positive effects of massage on sleep in older adults, including LTC residents with ADRD,[157,158] have been shown with various outcome measures, including polysomnography,[159] actigraphy,[157] sleep diaries,[159] nursing observations,[158] and fewer requests for sedative-hypnotics,[160] although the effects have not always been consistent. For example, an interesting recent pilot study conducted by Cooke and colleagues[161] in Australia explored the pretest, posttest effects of 5 weeks of twice weekly 45-minute massage by a massage therapist on daytime sleepiness and other quality-of-life indicators in 25 LTC residents, aged 18 to 65 years. Nighttime sleep was not measured. Massage significantly improved satisfaction with current health and happiness but did not significantly improve daytime sleepiness or affect other factors often associated with nighttime sleep quality in LTC residents, such as pain, depression, or stress levels. These negative effects may relate to sample selection, massage dosage, or time of day of administration. However, the residents and families perceived important benefits from the massage, and their request led to continued implementation of massage therapy in the LTC facility.[161] These results emphasize the importance of advocacy of families and residents for complementary health services for improving sleep and other health outcomes in LTC facilities.

Similarly, studies including randomized controlled trials of acupressure reported positive sleep outcomes in LTC settings.[162-166] For example, 31 LTC residents were randomly assigned to 24 minutes of acupressure at specific acupoints three times a week for 8 weeks, while the control group (n = 31) received sham massage at locations with no acupoints with the same duration and frequency as the experimental group.[166] At baseline, older adults in both groups had PSQI scores exceeding 11, indicating poor sleep quality. The acupressure group, compared with the control group, had significantly better sleep ($t = 7.72$, $P < .001$) and better quality of life ($t = 2.69$, $P = .009$). In addition, the use of requested sleep medications was significantly reduced in the acupressure group. Additional placebo-controlled clinical trials, with rigorous designs and larger sample sizes, are needed to prove the benefits of acupressure on sleep and to standardize methods (Box 195.1).

CLINICAL PEARL

Multiple interrelated factors, such as frailty, immobility, falls, and cognitive impairment, make the management of sleep disturbances in the LTC population challenging. Treatment should focus on identifying and treating bothersome sleep symptoms such as EDS or insufficient and interrupted nighttime sleep that negatively affects quality of life. The treatment of comorbidities or deprescribing of medications that exacerbate sleep disturbances should always be the first step. Nonpharmacologic multicomponent interventions, such cognitive-behavioral therapy for insomnia, increased daytime light exposure, and physical activity, are preferred over sedative-hypnotics and sedating antipsychotics for sleep disturbances in older adults in LTC because of the potential for harm.

SUMMARY

Sleep disturbances in LTC residents, many of whom are frail and physically inactive, are highly prevalent and severely disabling. Box 195.1 summarizes contributing factors, common diagnoses, goals, and treatment recommendations. In general, treatment should focus on identifying and treating bothersome sleep symptoms such as EDS or insufficient and interrupted nighttime sleep that negatively affects older adults' quality of life. For example, discomfort from RLS that causes nighttime agitation and more restrictive levels of care for safety, and EDS related to irregular sleep-wake rhythm disorder that limits engagement with previously enjoyed activities require treatment. A thorough evaluation is critical. The treatment of comorbidities or deprescribing of medications should always be the first step. Nonpharmacologic interventions are preferred over medications for sleep disturbances in older adults in LTC. Additional and more rigorous clinical trials are needed to identify the most effective nonpharmacologic treatments. Advocacy of families, regulatory agencies, and professionals are needed to support reimbursement for nonpharmacologic interventions for sleep disturbances in LTC residents. Dedicated, rigorous studies of medications for sleep disturbances in the LTC population are needed to examine their effectiveness on sleep disturbances and related symptoms, and their safety and tolerance.

Box 195.1 SLEEP DISTURBANCES IN LONG-TERM CARE RESIDENTS: SUMMARY OF CONTRIBUTING FACTORS, COMMON DIAGNOSES, GOALS, AND RECOMMENDED MANAGEMENT

Contributing Factors

- Older age
- Multiple chronic health conditions such as neurodegeneration, nocturia, pain, cardiovascular disease
- Polypharmacy
- Nighttime environmental sleep interruptions such as noise, light, noisy roommates, nighttime awakenings for incontinence care, bright hallway lights, and open doors
- A lack of daytime bright light, meaningful social activities, and physical activity for circadian entrainment
- Prolonged bedrest
- Excessive daytime napping, especially in the afternoon and evening
- Untreated sleep disorders such as sleep-related breathing disorders (including obstructive sleep apnea) and restless legs syndrome

Common Diagnoses

- Irregular sleep-wake rhythm disorder
- Chronic insomnia disorder
- Obstructive sleep apnea syndrome
- Restless legs syndrome

Management Goals

- Set goals in collaboration with residents (if able), family members, and caregivers
- Focus on identifying and treating bothersome sleep symptoms or insufficient and interrupted nighttime sleep that negatively affects quality of life

Management

- Address environmental factors that disrupt sleep at night to the extent possible.
- Review all medications and consider tapering/discontinuing medications that negatively impact nighttime sleep or cause excessive daytime sleepiness, and any unneeded medications.
- Optimize treatment of any comorbid medical conditions with symptoms that negatively impact sleep, such as pain or nocturia.
- Prescribe tailored and judicial pharmacotherapy for identified neurologic or psychiatric disorders that have sleep disturbances as one of the manifestations, as long as the risk-benefit profile is favorable.
- For movement disorders affecting sleep, such as RLS, consider oral iron and a trial of pharmacologic treatment.
- Consider treatment of sleep apnea.
- Nonpharmacologic multicomponent interventions are preferred over pharmacologic treatment.
  - Cognitive behavioral therapy for insomnia for those cognitively able to engage
  - Bright light (sunlight, overhead lighting, or light box) for at least 1 hour daily
  - Individualized social activity in individual or group settings, 1 to 2 hours daily, preferably in the late afternoon and early evening
  - Supervised exercise consisting of daily aerobic exercise, such as walking, and strength training 3 times a week to promote independence and participation in physical activity
  - Reduce time in bed, initiate a bedtime routine, reduce nighttime noise, limit interruptions to sleep for incontinence care, limit daytime napping
  - Consider mind-body practices such as meditative yoga, progressive relaxation for those cognitively able to engage
  - Consider melatonin (1–2 mg 1 hour before bedtime), acupressure, and massage

SELECTED READINGS

American Geriatrics Society. 2019 updated AGS Beers criteria(R) for potentially inappropriate medication use in older adults. *J Am Geriatr Soc.* 2019;67:674–694.

Auger RR, Burgess HJ, Emens JS, et al. Clinical practice guideline for the treatment of intrinsic circadian rhythm sleep-wake disorders: advanced sleep-wake phase disorder (ASWPD), Delayed sleep-wake phase disorder (DSWPD), Non-24-hour sleep-wake rhythm disorder (N24SWD), and Irregular sleep-wake rhythm disorder (ISWRD). An update for 2015: An American Academy of Sleep Medicine clinical practice guideline. *J Clin Sleep Med.* 2015;11:1199–1236.

Berry SD, Lee Y, Cai S, et al. Nonbenzodiazepine sleep medication use and hip fractures in nursing home residents. *JAMA Intern Med.* 2013;173:754–761.

Bronskill SE, Campitelli MA, Iaboni A, et al. Low-dose trazodone, benzodiazepines, and fall-related injuries in nursing homes: a matched-cohort study. *J Am Geriatr Soc.* 2018;66:1963–1971.

Gindin J, Shochat T, Chetrit A, et al. Insomnia in long-term care facilities: a comparison of seven European countries and Israel: the Services and Health for Elderly in Long TERm care study. *J Am Geriatr Soc.* 2014;62:2033–2039.

Hoyle DJ, Bindoff IK, Clinnick LM, et al. Clinical and economic outcomes of interventions to reduce antipsychotic and benzodiazepine use within nursing homes: a systematic review. *Drugs Aging.* 2018;35:123–134.

Lai FC, Chen IH, Chen PJ, et al. Acupressure, sleep, and quality of life in institutionalized older adults: a randomized controlled trial. *J Am Geriatr Soc.* 2017;65:e103–e108.

Martin JL, Marler MR, Harker JO, et al. A multicomponent nonpharmacological intervention improves activity rhythms among nursing home residents with disrupted sleep/wake patterns. *J Gerontol A Biol Sci Med Sci.* 2007;62:67–72.

Richards K, Shue VM, Beck CK, et al. Restless legs syndrome risk factors, behaviors, and diagnoses in persons with early to moderate dementia and sleep disturbance. *Behav Sleep Med.* 2010;8:48–61.

Richards KC, Bost JE, Rogers VE, et al. Diagnostic accuracy of behavioral, activity, ferritin, and clinical indicators of restless legs syndrome. *Sleep.* 2015;38:371–380.

Richards KC, Gooneratne N, Dicicco B, et al. CPAP adherence may slow 1-year cognitive decline in older adults with mild cognitive impairment and apnea. *J Am Geriatr Soc.* 2019;67(3):558–564.

Richards KC, Lambert C, Beck CK, et al. Strength training, walking, and social activity improve sleep in nursing home and assisted living residents: randomized controlled trial. *J Am Geriatr Soc.* 2011;59:214–223.

Rose KM, Beck C, Tsai PF, et al. Sleep disturbances and nocturnal agitation behaviors in older adults with dementia. *Sleep.* 2011;34:779–786.

Shang B, Yin H, Jia Y, et al. Nonpharmacological interventions to improve sleep in nursing home residents: a systematic review. *Geriatr Nurs.* 2019;40:405–416.

van Maanen A, Meijer AM, van der Heijden KB, Oort FJ. The effects of light therapy on sleep problems: a systematic review and meta-analysis. *Sleep Med Rev.* 2016;29:52–62.

Wang YY, Zheng W, Ng CH, Ungvari GS, Wei W, Xiang YT. Meta-analysis of randomized, double-blind, placebo-controlled trials of melatonin in Alzheimer's disease. *Int J Geriatr.* 2017;32:50–57.

A complete reference list can be found online at ExpertConsult.com.

Section 23

Methodology

Chapter 196

Section Introduction: Polysomnography and Beyond

Max Hirshkowitz

Chapter Highlights

- Polysomnography (PSG) began as a laboratory research tool to electrophysiologically describe the sleep process. Designation of sleep stages based on polysomnogram characteristics followed. PSG quickly evolved into a medical diagnostic procedure used largely to diagnose and treat sleep-related breathing disorders. Additionally, PSG plays a role in identifying narcolepsy, parasomnias, and nocturnal seizures.
- Computerized PSG eliminated the need for paper tracings, thereby reducing data storage requirements and allowing for more sophisticated signal analysis. Cardiopulmonary measures were added to in-laboratory PSG for the evaluation of sleep-disordered breathing and have been adapted for home sleep testing.
- Actigraphy emerged as a research method for studying insomnia and circadian rhythm disorders and, like PSG, was adopted for clinical use.
- Advances in miniaturized sensor technology, the ubiquity of smartphones, and affordable wearable devices have brought sleep assessment to the consumer interested in self-monitoring. Such devices could advance our understanding of sleep in large populations and improve sleep health.

Polysomnography (PSG) began as a research tool that informed early investigators about brain activity during sleep by providing objective, quantifiable data. As such, PSG opened the door to study sleep scientifically and facilitated new discoveries. PSG studies revealed sleep as a medley composed of distinct processes. Each process emerged, had an underlying electrophysiologic signature, progressed in an orderly manner, and repeated. Nonetheless, each sleep study produced a 6- to 8-hour paper tracing (typically 700 to 1000 pages). Researchers desperately needed a data reduction scheme. Thus sleep staging was invented. Armed with sleep stage metrics, scientists could describe sleep's progressive changes across a night, over the life span, and differences between women and men. Concurrent organ, tissue, muscle, and glandular activity became focus areas. Additionally, laboratory studies investigated sleep alterations in response to a wide variety of interventions (e.g., sleep deprivation, drugs, and stressors).

Rapid eye movement (REM) sleep's discovery[1] opened several additional natural avenues for study. Because ***dreaming*** occurred during REM sleep, the REM process captured many researchers' imaginations. REM sleep was conceptualized as a different state of human consciousness (or, for more reductionist thinkers, as a unique state of central nervous system organization). REM's discovery reinforced the concept that sleep was composed of unique states, rather than as merely an interplay of different processes. Immediately, any measurable phenomenon occurring during sleep became fair game for comparing activity during REM sleep versus all sleep states other than REM. Ironically, sleep's majority portion became known as non–rapid eye movement (NREM) sleep, even though REM sleep represented only 20% to 25% of total sleep time.

Sleep research migrated to a place under the umbrella "psychophysiology," and the annual meeting abstracts were published in the journal by that name. This included neurophysiologic and clinical research. The Association for the Psychophysiological Study of Sleep (APSS) was formed. Further studies of REM sleep in animals revealed neuronal innervations arising from the pons, ascending to the lateral geniculate nuclei, and then continuing to the occipital regions (pons-geniculate-occipital waves). Underlying mechanisms associating mood disorders, insomnia, and altered REM-NREM patterns garnered much attention.

Based on electrophysiologic measures, a standardized manual was published for recording and scoring human sleep.[2] It gained widespread acceptance and propelled the field forward. PSG explicitly divided sleep into REM and four different NREM categories (stages 1, 2, 3, and 4). Sleep's most obvious characteristic was a consistent 90- to 100-minute alteration between NREM and REM sleep. Intrigued also by REM sleep's seemingly independent homeostatic response to deprivation, neurologists, psychiatrists, and psychologists seized the opportunity to test hypotheses concerning the role of REM and NREM sleep in physical and mental functions.

Methodologic challenges spawned innovation. Sleep studies' long-duration recording requirement necessitated improved recording equipment. The desire to investigate concurrent physiologic activities led to sensor technology advancements. Analytic techniques borrowed from other disciplines were applied to summarize more fine-grained sleep-related activity over time.

In the 1970s PSG evolved into a medical procedure for diagnosing specific sleep disorders. In addition to the electroencephalogram, electrooculogram, and submentalis electromyogram described in the standardized manual, channels were added to record airflow, respiratory effort, oxyhemoglobin level, heart rhythm, and leg movements. During the following decade, the prevalence and morbidity associated with sleep-related breathing disorders became apparent. Diagnosing obstructive sleep apnea rapidly developed into the predominant application for PSG (in Silicon Valley parlance, PSG's "killer app"). Even today, some 50 years later, the vast majority of polysomnograms performed tonight will undoubtedly serve to diagnose or treat sleep apnea.

As PSG's momentum increased clinically, recording techniques evolved dramatically. The digital age arrived and analogue amplifiers and paper chart drives became extinct. Computerization rendered PSG data storage problems (a huge issue when polysomnograms were recorded on paper) moot. Warehouses were replaced by filing cabinets and eventually by high-density disk drives or cloud storage. Quality, compatibility, and other technological issues emerged during this transition; over time, however, things steadily improved.[3] Ultimately, standards were adopted by clinical societies, and they continue to evolve.[4]

PSG recording created a huge amount of data long before "big-data" tools were available. Right out of the gate, sleep staging brought PSG summary down to less than 1000, 30-second pages. These stages could be summarized and indices calculated. Apnea episodes and leg movements could be counted and rates determined. However, digital PSG, sampling each physiologic data channel at a rate anywhere between 1 to 1000 times per second multiplied the data volume by many orders of magnitude.

Although digital PSG made basic summary calculations easier, this new wealth of data was largely ignored. In fact, very little has changed with respect to the way most PSG data are summarized. To a large extent, the computer became a recorder-reviewing station with automatic summary calculation. Except at the cutting edge of sleep electrophysiologic research, the signal processing and computational power of digital PSG are vastly underutilized. Computers can count specific waveforms (e.g., sleep spindles) and analyze wave patterns (using Fourier transforms, period-amplitude analysis, or complex demodulation). They can detect movements and respiratory events, calculate their periodicity, and determine their association with central nervous system changes. Initially, or at least up until the turn of this century, available computing resources were arguably stretched to accomplish such analysis in real time. Researchers faced memory, storage, and processor speed limitations. However, today's wireless (cloud) technology and inexpensive massive storage devices provide access to nearly unlimited computing resources.

The success of PSG for diagnosing sleep-disordered breathing ultimately rung its own death knell. A diagnostic procedure verifies and/or determines disease severity. Mainstream procedures are subject to close economic scrutiny by payers at all levels. PSG is fairly expensive. Costly procedures attract the attention of gatekeepers. Cardiopulmonary home sleep testing eventually caught the attention of clinical payers as a more economical alternative for diagnosing sleep apnea when clinical suspicion is high. PSG's indication for diagnosing insomnia had already been jettisoned by third-party payers, except in cases in which all therapeutics remained notably unsuccessful. By contrast, research studies and clinical drug trials continue to use PSG because it remains the best method of studying sleep intensively.

Polysomnography needs to innovate, advance, and reposition itself as a relevant method for understanding sleep's underlying processes. PSG innovation has stalled. The clinical approach has changed little for more than three decades. Did we just select all that was needed right from the beginning or have we just gotten complacent? Clinical polysomnograms may have changed platforms (from ink on paper to pixels on a screen), but the content analysis has barely progressed. I chuckle when considering that we can wirelessly monitor, in real-time, brain; heart; respiratory; and oxyhemoglobin signals from earth-orbiting spacecraft, but in the clinic we still attach wires, sit in the adjoining room, and manually score sleep recordings.

On a separate technological track, actigraphy arose as an economical method to assess activity-inactivity patterns over prolonged time periods or in large samples. Harking back to Kleitman's basic rest-activity cycle (BRAC)[5] and creating a human analogue to caged animals' wheel running, actigraphy provides information about sleep-wake patterns and circadian rhythm. Finer-grain analysis in connection with use of a light sensor potentially informs about insomnia, nocturnal awakenings, and circadian disorders. Integrating additional sensors (e.g., pulse, temperature, and skin conductance) stand to improve concordance between actigraphic and PSG-derived measures of sleep.

As often happens, medical technology spawns imitative consumer products. The recent renaissance of interest in personal fitness using actigraphy opened the doors to sleep trackers. Wrist-worn consumer-grade actigraphs quickly achieved market penetration. Uplink technologies to transfer data for cloud storage, analysis, and retrieval make devices affordable and promising. On any given night, more consumer product actigraphic data probably are uplinked than all of the research actigraphy ever recorded. Current understanding and knowledge garnered from actigraphy research are therefore ripe for application on a wider scale. A basic axiom in actigraphy research is that each device needs validation, and it is well recognized that reliability varies widely from device to device (see Chapter 211). Although this maxim regarding validation is undeniable, it represents a principle characterizing every new technology during its infancy. First-wave devices often perform erratically or marginally.[6-8] However, whether it be automobiles, airplanes, wristwatches, or telephones, successive refinement ultimately improves performance and homogenizes the available products until a revolutionary new approach starts the process anew.

A research group in Munich launched a large-scale human sleep project using actigraphs. They collect, uplink, and analyze data to describe sleep-wake patterns in large populations.[9] In the longer term, this information can be correlated with longitudinal educational, occupational, and medical data to aid our understanding of sleep's role in our well-being and health. On a general public front, the Consumer Electronics Association (CTA) in cooperation with the American National Standards Institute (ANSI) and the National Sleep Foundation (NSF) established standardized sleep terminology and performance evaluation criteria for wearable and in-bedroom sleep tracking devices.[10-12] These developments are already advancing the current understanding of different chronotypes, health consequences of sleep fasting and binging, and the medical costs of social jetlag.

The juggernaut of advancing sensor technology continues unabated.[13] Temperature, heart rate, blood pressure, blood sugar level, electrodermal skin conductance, heart sounds, breathing sounds, heart rate variability, cardiopulmonary coupling, pulse wave analysis—all are fair game for inclusion. Most consumer-grade actigraphs are now accompanied by photoplethysmography monitoring, and therefore heart rate and related features have been incorporated into sleep estimation algorithms. Bedside monitors using static-charged strips, standing wave patterns in the room, and thermal sensors can detect breathing, snoring, movement, and heart rhythm noninvasively and unobtrusively. Another trend is use of sensors built into the sleep surface (i.e., mattress). Embedded transducers not only can detect high and low pressure points on the sleep surface but also can direct an air coil mattress to alter inflation to optimize comfort. These same sensors can detect movement, breathing, and heartbeat. Integrating these technologies and finding a desired or practical use for them constitute the current challenge.

Are these consumer devices here to stay or do they represent a fad? Recall that more than 100 million Hula Hoops were sold between 1958 and 1960—whereas they are a rarity today. If self-monitoring for fitness persists, the data thus acquired undoubtedly will contribute much to the body of knowledge on sleep health worldwide. In the same manner in which satellite weather monitoring informed meteorologists about ocean currents, polar melt, and storm tracking, big-data analytic techniques applied to consumer-uplinked actigraphs can be expected to answer many questions about sleep. These answers in turn will raise even more questions. For example, what population sleep effects correlate with seasonal variations, weather, daylight saving time changes, and latitude locations? What percentage of the population sample experiences disrupted sleep, exhibits different circadian chronotypes, and shows extreme long or short sleep periods?

Beyond these questions, the road ahead holds additional possibilities for us to further understand both sleep health and sleep disorders. Centralized electronic medical record systems are increasingly used and improving by leaps and bounds. With proper de-identification, such records meshed with uploaded sleep information potentially may uncover hitherto-unknown associations between sleep and health. Major issues need resolution for this to happen. The chief challenges include (a) improved recording, (b) performance evaluation (and validation), (c) determining useful summary measures, and (d) ways to ensure privacy. The first three represent technological challenges. Technological hurdles are surmountable and are usually met, given enough time, money, and continued interest. Improvements proceed in a stepwise manner, much in the way mobile phones evolved from cumbersome, heavy, bulky, unreliable contraptions to the pocket-size communication wonders of today (that many people think they cannot live without).

The final hurdle—privacy—has social, political, and legal ramifications. Important questions must be answered. For example, are wearable device data discoverable as evidence in legal proceedings? If the data potentially have medical implications, is there a duty to inform? Can information from these devices be harvested and sold to merchandise vendors? Can sleep-related information be acquired without the individual's knowledge or consent? At present, many people (perhaps most) have a device in their bedroom capable of collecting sleep-related data. The widespread use of using one's smartphone as an alarm clock places it bedside. Sounds in the room are therefore accessible with the right software. Similarly, voice command devices (e.g., Echo Dot), wireless speakers, tablets, laptop computers, and newer televisions all have the ability to listen when Wi-Fi is available. With the advent of 5G, Wi-Fi will be available nearly everywhere. The internet is largely unregulated, and privacy essentially does not exist. Any bedside monitor can record and uplink sounds in the room. Code can detect snoring. Advanced programming can identify if multiple sleepers are present and differentiate each individual's breathing sounds. The sound patterns can be analyzed. So… for example, an increasingly loud sound cascade, paced at a typical sleep-related respiratory rate, terminating abruptly, followed by 10- to 60-second silence that is concluded by a gasp and/or choking sound, most likely represents an obstructive sleep apnea episode. Can such data be harvested and sold to anti-snoring device manufacturers, mail-order vendors, positive airway pressure manufacturers, physician groups, or insurance carriers? As 5G nears ubiquity, the need for internet privacy laws (not merely user agreements) becomes more urgent.

On a happier note, self-monitoring fitness enthusiasts (and fitness researchers) already recognize sleep's value for enhancing athletic performance and daily mental outlook. Scientific understanding of sleep began in the research laboratory, transitioned to the medical clinic, and is moving to personal devices worn on the body or situated at the bedside. Interfacing self-monitoring devices and patient health care records remains wide open for innovation. Adequate sleep quantity, quality, and timing is critical to optimal health. Researchers, clinicians, patients, and the general public may be perched on the doorstep of improved sleep health.

CLINICAL PEARLS

- PSG represents both a tool of discovery and the most sophisticated technique available for diagnosing sleep disorders.
- The cardiopulmonary channels can be used to verify sleep-disordered breathing in clear-cut cases.
- Actigraphy provides rest-activity patterns useful for interpreting sleep-wake and circadian rhythm patterns.
- The recent popularity of consumer self-monitoring fitness devices holds promise for future translational understanding of sleep health.

SUMMARY

PSG began as a research tool for objectively characterizing the sleep process. Laboratory sleep studies record massive amounts of data that are summarized according to sleep stages and indices. Sleep studies provided a physiologic tool for investigating sleep correlates and functions. PSG's usefulness for evaluating sleep disorders quickly became apparent, especially for diagnosing sleep apnea. For a time, PSG reigned supreme for sleep apnea testing. Sleep apnea diagnostics now often use cardiopulmonary home sleep testing recorders. In a parallel development, actigraphy became popular for assessing insomnia and circadian rhythm disorders. New sensor technology and advanced analytic techniques moved actigraphy into the consumer product space for individuals interested in fitness self-monitoring. Actigraphy based devices are now multisensory and can potentially provide information about sleep. Such devices hold promise to improve our understanding about sleep over extended time periods (e.g., seasonal variations), in different cultures, and in large samples. Correlating sleep with educational, occupational, and medical data will likely underline sleep's importance to physical and emotional well-being.

SELECTED READINGS

Ferguson T, et al. The validity of consumer-level, activity monitors in healthy adults worn in free-living conditions: a cross-sectional study. *Int J Behav Nutr Phys Act*. 2015;12(1):42.

Goldstein CA, Berry RB, Kent DT, et al. Artificial intelligence in sleep medicine: an American Academy of Sleep Medicine position statement. *J Clin Sleep Med*. 2020;16(4):605–607.

Hirshkowitz M. Polysomnography challenges. *Sleep Med Clin*. 2016;11:403–411.

Hirshkowitz M, Sharafkhaneh A. Comparison of portable monitoring with laboratory polysomnography for diagnosing sleep-related breathing disorders: scoring and interpretation. *Sleep Med Clin*. 2011;6(3):283–292.

Khosla S, et al. Consumer sleep technology: an American Academy of Sleep Medicine position statement. *J Clin Sleep Med*. 2018;14(5):877–880.

Malhotra A, Ayappa I, Ayas N, et al. Metrics of sleep apnea severity: beyond the apnea-hypopnea index. *Sleep*. 2021;44(7):zsab030.

Roenneberg T, et al. Social jetlag and obesity. *Curr Biol*. 2012;22(10):939–943.

Russo K, et al. Consumer sleep monitors: is there a baby in the bathwater? *Nat Sci Sleep*. 2015;7:147–157.

A complete reference list can be found online at ExpertConsult.com.

Chapter 197

Sleep Stage Scoring

Sharon Keenan; Max Hirshkowitz

Chapter Highlights

- The electroencephalogram (EEG) remains the most objective measure for determining level of consciousness and allowing determination of sleep stages. Fundamental to discoveries in sleep research and sleep medicine is our ability to appreciate subtle changes in brain activity.
- Human visual EEG pattern recognition in the context of changes in the electrooculogram and electromyogram remains the primary approach used to perform sleep stage scoring. The results of this analysis are used to inform data interpretation and recommendations for clinical care. Close collaboration between technical and medical members of the clinical team facilitates these ends.
- In research, sleep stage scoring and the recognition of other patterns emerging from data remain active areas of intense study. More sophisticated analysis of EEG data using advances in technology holds great promise for expanding the current understanding of the central nervous system. Sleep provides a unique window for studying physiology, pathophysiology, and consciousness.
- This chapter reviews the basics of sleep stage scoring.

HISTORY

From a behavioral perspective, immobility and reduced environmental responsiveness characterize human sleep. This state stands in contrast to (presumably) purposeful activities and provides the basis for characterizing observable living existence as either sleep, wakefulness, or coma. Furthermore, sleep and wakefulness cycle in a predictable, orderly fashion. Some rhythms are seasonal, some are daily (circadian), and some occur more than once a day (ultradian). In addition to the underlying rhythms, the sleep cycle responds to reduced sleep time. This response testifies to sleep-wake cycle autoregulation, with a dynamic tension providing overall system homeostasis. Once techniques were developed to augment mere observation, electroencephalography revealed a complex array of brain activities clustered in a manner strongly suggesting multiple sleep processes.

All scientific inquiry begins with observation and description. From there it proceeds to classification based ultimately upon measurement. Accordingly, when Loomis and colleagues[1] electroencephalographically reported their first studies in 1937, they faced the daunting task of devising a system to describe sleep patterns in normal, healthy human subjects. Thus sleep staging was born. In the original studies, amplified activity derived from electrodes that were placed on the scalp's surface at several loci produced ink tracings on paper wrapped around a slowly rotating cylinder. An enormous 8-foot "drum polygraph" enabled all-night sleep recording. One electrode was located near the eye and undoubtedly detected eye movement. However, rapid eye movement (REM) sleep remained unrecognized until 16 years later, when Aserinsky published, in part, his University of Chicago doctoral study results.[2] Aserinsky actually christened these movements "jerky eye movements" and in the first paper referred to the phenomenon as periodic ocular motility.

Aserinsky's pilot work reportedly met with considerable skepticism. Perhaps it was the quirkiness of the original commercially available polygraph systems (e.g., Ofner, Beckman, Grass), with their tendency to polarize electrodes, problematic rechargeable car battery–like systems, and aperiodic (and difficult to predict) recording interference artifacts. It may have been Loomis's silence on the matter of eye movements during sleep. Or perhaps that Aserinsky was a student. Ultimately, however, REM sleep's discovery, and particularly its correlation with dreaming by Dement,[3] altered the course of sleep research for decades. The near-exclusive focus on REM sleep, to the point that all other sleep states were considered simply non–rapid eye movement (NREM), overshadowed substantial findings (and probably impeded progress) in other sleep research arenas (such as neuroendocrinology, physiology, and medicine). The spotlight on REM sleep, however, made electrooculographic recording critical in performing sleep studies.

Meanwhile, in Lyon, France, Michel Jouvet noted postural differences during sleep in cats.[4] These differences correlated with sleep state and reduced skeletal electromyographic activity. REM sleep (and, by association, dreaming) coincided with marked hypotonia in descending alpha and gamma motor neurons. This hypotonia induced functional paralysis that was quickly ascribed the purpose of keeping the sleeper from enacting dreamed activities. This sleep state–related electromyographic alteration added the final compulsory recording component to the procedure now known as polysomnography (PSG).

Clinical PSG, in addition to brain wave, eye movement, and muscle tone recording, also assesses respiratory, cardiac, and limb movement activity (discussed in detail in other chapters and elsewhere in the literature[5]). PSG in its simplest form, however—consisting of an electroencephalogram (EEG), electrooculogram (EOG), and electromyogram (EMG)—provides the basic information requisite for classifying sleep state and examining sleep processes.

ELECTRODE PLACEMENT AND APPLICATION

To record the EEG, EOG, and EMG, electrodes are placed on the scalp and skin surfaces. The site must be cleansed and properly prepared to ensure good contact and to maintain electrical impedance at or below 5000 Ω. Scalp electrodes can be affixed with collodion or electrode paste. Facial electrodes can be applied with double-sided adhesive electrode collars and paper tape. Although prescribed sites for electrode application have changed over the years, the system used to identify location remains the American Electroencephalographic Society's international 10-20 system. In this system, the intersection of lines drawn from the left to right preauricular point, with the midpoint along the scalp between the nasion and inion, serves to landmark the vertex, designated Cz. Other loci can be found by measuring 10% and 20% along longitudinal and lateral surfaces. Specific locations are designated with a letter indicating the brain area below the electrode (e.g., C for central lobe, O for occipital lobe, F for frontal lobe) and a number ascribing specific points (odd numbers for the left side, even numbers for the right, and z for midline). EEG electrode placements should be precise; consequently, appropriate measurement techniques are essential to ensure accuracy. Additionally, EEG amplifiers require calibration at the beginning and end of PSG recording to document proper functioning. This calibration-recalibration provides verification that amplitude changes of the recorded signal accurately reflect oscillating voltages from brain activity.

The standardized technique detailed in the manual produced by the ad hoc committee chaired by Rechtschaffen and Kales requires a single monopolar central-lobe scalp EEG electrode referenced to a contralateral mastoid electrode (either C3-M2 or C4-M1). This single-channel brain wave recording, when paired with right and left eye EOGs and submentalis EMG, sufficiently reveals brain, eye, and muscle activity for classifying sleep stages.[6] With evolution of PSG from a psychophysiologic research method to a clinical procedure, addition of an occipital lead supplemented centrally derived EEG for improved visualization of waveforms needed to differentiate sleep from wakefulness and to detect central nervous system (CNS) arousals.[7,8]

The EOG is a reflection of the movement of a dipole, which exists in each eye. The corneoretinal potential difference is more negative at the retina and positive near the cornea. The strong positive potential field near the cornea affects electrodes placed near the right and left outer canthi of the eyes. The recording reflects the response to this positive charge moving toward or away from the recording electrode. Each electrode is referenced to a neutral site, typically over the mastoid behind the ear. Thus lateral and vertical eye movements produce out-of-phase signals for the EOG as the cornea moves toward one electrode and away from the other (provided that movements from each eye appear on two consecutive channels). This two-channel display of data makes eye movements easily distinguished from in-phase EEG activity of the frontal lobes. To enhance detection of vertical eye movements, the right-side EOG electrode is placed 1 cm above the outer canthus, and the left-side electrode is positioned 1 cm below. An alternative recording montage devised to enhance vertical eye movement detection entails lowering both recording sites to 1 cm below the outer canthi and referencing each to the middle of the forehead (Fpz).

We record the EOG to document activity associated with wakefulness, drowsiness, and REM sleep. Waking eye movements are documented at the beginning of data collection. There are characteristic differences between eye movements of the waking state, drowsiness, and REM sleep. The patterns of eye movements change throughout the study in association with these different states and stages of sleep. For the majority of the recording, the EOG channel will reflect EEG activity, provided the filters on the EOG channels are set to the same conditions as the EEG channels. It is more the absence or presence of the eye movements we use for clinical purposes, for scoring. We calibrate the eye movements by asking patients to move their eyes; right, left, up, and down. During the study we are looking for the slow, rolling eye movements of drowsiness and the "jerky," faster eye movements of REM sleep.

Skeletal muscle activity level is tracked from a pair of electrodes arranged to record submentalis EMG activity. An electrode placed approximately midline but 1 cm above the mandible is referenced to another placed 2 cm below and 2 cm to the right (or left). As a precaution, a backup electrode also is attached at a site at least 0.5 cm away from any of the previously described locations. Recording from two of any of these electrodes will provide a bipolar EMG derivation. To decrease ECG artifact, choose input from two electrodes on the same side. The 0.5-cm physical separation is critical to maintain the integrity of the electrode; if electrodes come in contact with one another, they merge to become one recording site.

The American Academy of Sleep Medicine (AASM) published a standardized manual for conducting clinical PSG in their accredited sleep disorders centers.[7,9] This AASM standards manual makes recommendations for recording, scoring, and summarizing sleep stages, CNS arousals, breathing, various kinds of movement, and electrocardiographic activity. By bringing instructional guidelines for a range of techniques into a single volume, the AASM manual has strongly influenced practice, particularly in North America. Researchers, however, should not feel constrained by these clinical guidelines as new discoveries and future techniques emerge.

AASM specifies recording frontal, central, and occipital monopolar EEG from F4, C4, and O2. The contralateral mastoid (M1) serves as the ostensibly neutral reference. Electrodes placed at F3, C3, and O1 sites (and referenced to M2) provide redundancy and serve as backup, if needed. The AASM manual sanctions the use of midline bipolar recordings for frontal and occipital EEG; however, the AASM "frequently asked questions" (FAQ) section states that frontal bipolar derivations are not appropriate for measuring frontal EEG activity. The FAQ section also states that EEG amplitudes can be measured from the C4-M1 derivation. The AASM manual recommends using mastoid-referenced EOG with separate channels for E2 and E1, but it also approves a forehead-referenced alternative montage. Submentalis EMG is recorded as a bipolar derivation—that is, one of the surface EMG electrodes is referred to one of the other surface EMG electrodes on the chin.

Table 197.1 Recording Recommendations for Digital Polysomnography

Recording Channel	Sampling Rate (Hz)[a] Desirable	Minimal	Filter Setting (Hz) Low *f*	High *f*
Central EEG (C4-M1)	500	200	0.3	35
Occipital EEG (O4-M1 or Cz-Oz)	500	200	0.3	35
Frontal EEG (F4-M1)	500	200	0.3	35
Left EOG (E1-M2 or E1-Fpz)	500	200	0.3	35
Right EOG (E2-M2 or E2-Fpz)	500	200	0.3	35
Muscle tone (submental EMG)	500	200	10	100
ECG (lead II, modified)	500	200	1.0	15
Airflow sensors at nares and mouth	100	25	0.1	15
Oximetry (ear lobe or finger)	25	10	0.1	15
Nasal pressure	100	25	0.1	15
Esophageal pressure	100	25	0.1	15
Body position	1	1		
Respiratory effort				
Snoring sounds	500	200	10	100
Rib cage and abdominal movement	100	25	0.1	15
Intercostal EMG	500	200	10	100

E1, Left eye; E2, right eye; ECG, electrocardiogram; EEG, electroencephalogram; EMG, electromyogram; EOG, electrooculogram; *f*, frequency; Fpz, frontal pole; M, mastoid.
[a]Higher sampling rates increase file storage requirements but provide increased temporal resolution. The trade-off between fidelity and practicality is a matter of debate.

DIGITAL RECORDING REQUIREMENTS

The first time a polysomnographic signal was digitized, whether it originated from analog or digital amplifying circuits, an entirely new set of factors required consideration. The two most important issues involved specifying amplitude and temporal resolution. Selection of voltage per digital unit (bit) and sampling rate probably had more to do with computer hardware limitations than with conceptual considerations. Amazingly, no standard was established for digital PSG until publication of the AASM standards manual.

The AASM standards manual specifies minimum 12-bit representation for amplitude, providing 4096 units to represent a 2.5-volt regulated current (IREG) range, or its equivalent (Video 197.1). In this manner, even the smallest signals, exceeding the level of electrical noise, can be detected. Temporal resolution during recording depends on sampling rate and ultimately must allow accurate waveform reconstruction, provide enough data to potentially overcome frequency aliasing, and be appropriate for high- and low-pass digital filter settings. One size does not fit all: the minimum temporal resolution needed during data acquisition to meet these requirements varies for different bioelectrical signals (Table 197.1).

Additional digital specifications involve data selection, display pagination, and calibration. Recorded channels must be selectable, and the channel calibration must be available for display and documentation. The viewable data should provide user-selectable time frame compression and expansion (ranging from 5 seconds to an entire night shown on a page). Display screens definition should be at least 1600 × 1200 pixels. Digital polysomnographs should provide the capability to view data as they appear on the initial recording and as they appear after sleep staging and sleep-related events have been marked and classified manually. Accompanying video at a minimum of one frame per second should be synchronized with the polysomnographic display.

ELECTROENCEPHALOGRAM BANDWIDTHS, WAVEFORMS, AND OTHER ACTIVITY

Bandwidths

One approach to differentiating EEG involves separating activity into dominant frequency bandwidths. *Delta activity* includes brain waves with a frequency less than 4 Hz. Sleep-related delta waves occurring at the low end of the frequency spectrum are called *slow waves.* Slow waves have high amplitude (greater than 75 microvolts) and low frequency (0.5 to 2 Hz). *Theta activity* includes 5- to 7-Hz waves prominent in central and temporal leads. *Alpha activity* is characterized by an occipitally prominent 8- to 13-Hz rhythm, and *beta waves* include the low-amplitude waves at even higher frequencies (up to approximately 25 Hz for clinical purposes).

Waveforms

In addition to ongoing background EEG activity oscillating predominantly within one or another of the specific bandwidths, distinct transient waveform events occur. These include vertex sharp waves, K-complexes, sleep spindles, and sawtooth theta waves. *Vertex sharp waves* are sharply contoured, negative ("negative" meaning upward deflection of the signal, as per

EEG polarity convention) waveforms that stand out from the background EEG activity. As the name implies, they appear prominently in EEG derived from electrodes placed near the midline or vertex region (Cz).

The *K-complex* begins much like a vertex sharp wave (i.e., it begins with a sharp negative waveform but is immediately followed by a large, usually much slower positive component). Overall, the K complex usually is clearest in central and frontal regions and has a duration criterion of 0.5 second or more. A *sleep spindle* is a readily apparent 0.5-second (or longer) burst of 12- to 14-Hz activity generated by the thalamus and sent along thalamocortical pathways to the cortex. The name derives from its spindle-like shape. A *sawtooth wave* is a variant of theta activity, with each wave also containing a notch, making it sawtooth-shaped.

Other nonpathologic sleep-related waveforms exist (e.g., benign epileptiform transients of sleep, sensory motor rhythm, wicket rhythm [mu rhythm], and positive occipital sharp transients of sleep. These normal variants do not occur consistently during PSG.

Activity Patterns

Sleep EEG also contains dynamic activity patterns not captured by sleep staging schema or identification of individual waveforms. The *cyclic alternating pattern* (CAP) includes waveform bursts (usually high-amplitude slow, sharp, or polymorphic waves) separated by quiescent periods.[10] The pattern's burst component sometimes includes transient alpha-bandwidth components meeting CNS arousal scoring criteria and thus can index sleep disturbance. However, a CAP occurring without frank arousals is thought to signify more subtle sleep instability.

SLEEP STAGING RULES AND CENTRAL NERVOUS SYSTEM AROUSALS

More than 40 years ago, the standardized technique described in *A Manual of Standardized Terminology, Techniques and Scoring System for Sleep Stages of Human Subjects*[6] provided a unifying methodology for human sleep research. This standardized manual combined elements from various systems that had evolved over time, and it provided adequate detail to achieve general use. To a large extent, however, its enormous success stems from the consensus it attained from the multinational, multidiscipline stakeholders that made up its development committee. That is, when the committee members returned to their respective laboratories, they used the techniques and taught them to scientists and clinicians in training.

Staging, as a summarizing technique, necessarily must define a period over which the summary applies. The standardized manual endorsed 20- and 30-second time domains (epochs). This flexibility deferred to extant technology—that is, generally available polygraph machine paper chart drive speeds. Over time, the 30-second epoch won out because it provided enough detail to see waveforms (EEG standards dictate minimal paper speed of 10 mm/second to ensure ability to discern individual EEG waveforms); at 10 mm/second, one epoch fits on a standard 30-cm wide paper fan-fold polygraph page; and one 1000-page box of polygraph paper would hold a complete recording (or two if one also is recorded on the back) (Box 197.1).

Box 197.1 CLINICAL TIPS FOR SLEEP STAGE SCORING

If the goal is to score an entire sleep study, a helpful approach is to familiarize oneself with the entire recording before beginning the task of assigning a sleep stage to each 30-second epoch. A useful first step is to review the recording to discern overall patterns—for example, the alpha background, the shape of the K-complexes, presentation of sleep spindles, and the appearance or lack of slow waves. Each person has an individual "signature of sleep," and familiarity with the data beforehand from each study makes scoring easier. The scorer "shakes hands," as it were, with the recording and asks general questions. For example, did the subject sleep or not? Does the person have robust, easy-to-discern eye movements? What do the K-complexes look like? Is the breathing regular? Do the patient's legs move or not? Are there any ECG rhythm abnormalities? This brief review creates a context for the scoring process. Also, it is common for the scorer to have to go back to a point earlier in the data, or to look ahead, before making a decision about a specific epoch, especially when determining the exact epoch on which REM sleep began or to make the decision about the precise moment of sleep onset. All individuals engaged in sleep stage scoring for a laboratory should engage in systematic interrater reliability checks to ensure that everyone is scoring the data in similar fashion.

Sleep Staging Rules

Wakefulness (stage W) in a relaxed subject with eyes closed is differentiated from sleep by the presence of alpha EEG activity in 50% or more of the epoch (Figure 197.1). Poorly defined alpha EEG activity complicates differentiation of sleep onset from wakefulness. The observation of the reactivity (attenuation of the alpha rhythm) to eyes open versus eyes closed provides a helpful contrast to facilitate detection of the background alpha rhythm in wakefulness.

Stage 1 typically is defined by exclusion; that is, it appears as a low-voltage, mixed-frequency background EEG signal devoid of sleep spindles and K-complexes, minimal slow wave activity, cessation of blinking, absence of saccadic eye movements, and alpha activity for less than 50% of the epoch duration (Figure 197.2). Stage 1 sleep may, but does not necessarily, include vertex sharp waves, background activity slowing, and slow eye movements.

Stage 2 characteristics include sleep spindles and K-complexes (Figure 197.3) occurring on a low-voltage, mixed-frequency background EEG and minimal (less than 20% of the epoch) slow wave (0.5 to 2 Hz, 75 μV) activity.

Slow wave sleep (stages 3 and 4 sleep) contains delta (0.5 to 2 Hz) EEG activity (recorded from a monopolar central derivation) with a 75μV or greater amplitude enduring for 20% or more of an epoch (Figure 197.4). *Stage 3* is scored when the duration of slow waves constitutes 20% to 50% of the epoch, and *stage 4* is scored when duration reaches 50% or more.

REM sleep is scored when saccadic eye movements occur during epochs with low-voltage, mixed-frequency EEG activity in association with a very low level of submentalis EMG activity (Figure 197.5). Epochs with low-voltage, mixed-frequency EEG activity and continuing low-level submentalis EMG (without eye movements) falling between epochs of REM sleep (with eye movements) also are scored as REM sleep (provided there is no increase in the amplitude of the

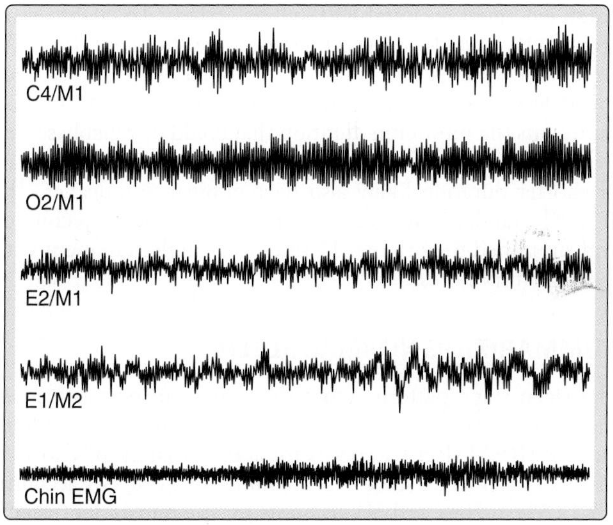

Figure 197.1 Stage wake (W), eyes closed. This example demonstrates a classic wake pattern, with alpha rhythm in the EEG and EOG. Alpha activity is most prominent in the occipital channel. The chin EMG displays normal muscle tone associated with relaxed wakefulness. C4/M1, Right central EEG referenced to left mastoid; E2/M1, right eye (outer canthus) referenced to left mastoid; E1/M2, left eye (outer canthus) referenced to right mastoid; EEG, electroencephalogram; EMG, electromyogram; EOG, electrooculogram; O2/M1, right occipital lobe EEG referenced to left mastoid. (From Butkov N. *Atlas of Clinical Polysomnography.* 2nd ed. Synapse Media; 2010.)

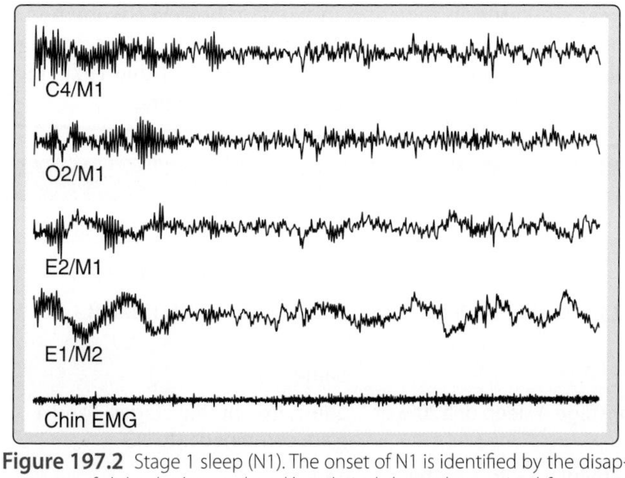

Figure 197.2 Stage 1 sleep (N1). The onset of N1 is identified by the disappearance of alpha rhythm, replaced by relatively low voltage mixed-frequency EEG with a prominence of theta activity in the range of 5 to 7 Hz. The chin EMG remains tonic, although it can attenuate slightly with sleep onset. C4/M1, Right central EEG referenced to left mastoid; E2/M1, right eye (outer canthus) referenced to left mastoid; E1/M2, left eye (outer canthus) referenced to right mastoid; EEG, electroencephalogram; EMG, electromyogram; O2/M1, right occipital lobe EEG referenced to left mastoid. (From Butkov N. *Atlas of Clinical Polysomnography.* 2nd ed. Synapse Media; 2010.)

EMG for 50 % of the epoch). Epochs falling before or after (and contiguous with) clearly identifiable REM sleep that have comparable EEG and EMG features but lack rapid eye movements are scored as REM sleep until an arousal, EMG level increase, or resumption of K-complexes or sleep spindles occurs. These *smoothing rules* gloss over minor transitions on the supposition that REM sleep represents a persistent CNS organizational state distinct from wakefulness and NREM sleep.

In 2007 (last update, January, 2020), the AASM standards manual provided revised criteria for scoring sleep stages. Changes are summarized in Table 197.2. Essentially, changes

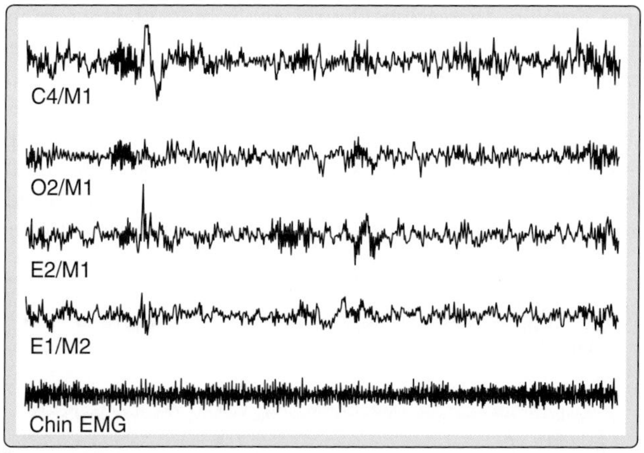

Figure 197.3 Stage 2 sleep (N2). Stage N2 is identified by the presence of K-complexes and/or sleep spindles against a background of mixed-frequency EEG. The chin EMG displays normal muscle tone, as expected during NREM sleep. C4/M1, Right central EEG referenced to left mastoid; E2/M1, right eye (outer canthus) referenced to left mastoid; E1/M2, left eye (outer canthus) referenced to right mastoid; EEG, electroencephalogram; EMG, electromyogram; O2/M1, right occipital lobe EEG referenced to left mastoid. (From Butkov N. *Atlas of Clinical Polysomnography.* 2nd ed. Synapse Media; 2010.)

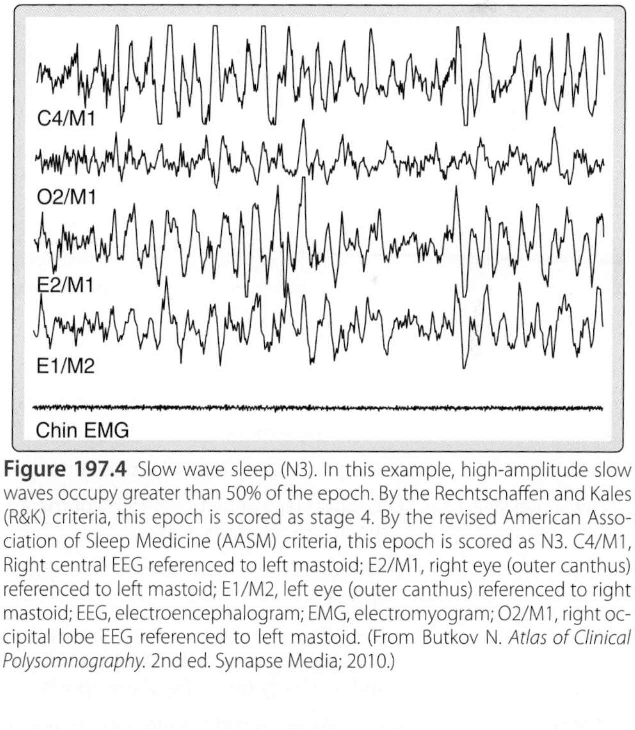

Figure 197.4 Slow wave sleep (N3). In this example, high-amplitude slow waves occupy greater than 50% of the epoch. By the Rechtschaffen and Kales (R&K) criteria, this epoch is scored as stage 4. By the revised American Association of Sleep Medicine (AASM) criteria, this epoch is scored as N3. C4/M1, Right central EEG referenced to left mastoid; E2/M1, right eye (outer canthus) referenced to left mastoid; E1/M2, left eye (outer canthus) referenced to right mastoid; EEG, electroencephalogram; EMG, electromyogram; O2/M1, right occipital lobe EEG referenced to left mastoid. (From Butkov N. *Atlas of Clinical Polysomnography.* 2nd ed. Synapse Media; 2010.)

include standardizing epoch length at 30 seconds; combining stages 3 and 4 sleep and applying amplitude criteria for slow waves to frontal EEG activity; revising terminology (R for REM sleep, N1 for NREM stage 1, N2 for NREM stage 2, N3 for NREM stages 3 and 4, and W for wakefulness); and simplifying smoothing rules. Some changes are controversial.[11-16] The most recent update, at the time of this writing, was published in January 2020. The reader is encouraged to visit the American Academy of Sleep Medicine website (https://AASM.org) to ensure use of latest version for laboratory accreditation purposes.

Central Nervous System Arousal Scoring

Sleep staging fails to represent brief CNS arousals because it summarizes EEG, EOG, and EMG activity over a 30-second time domain. Increasing clinical application of polysomnographic technique heightened the need to appreciate sleep fragmentation; consequently, a scoring system for arousals was developed[8] under the auspices of the American Sleep Disorders Association (later to become the AASM). Abrupt 3-second (or longer) EEG frequency increases to theta, alpha, or beta activity (but not to sleep spindles) are considered biomarkers for CNS activation. The arousals most often

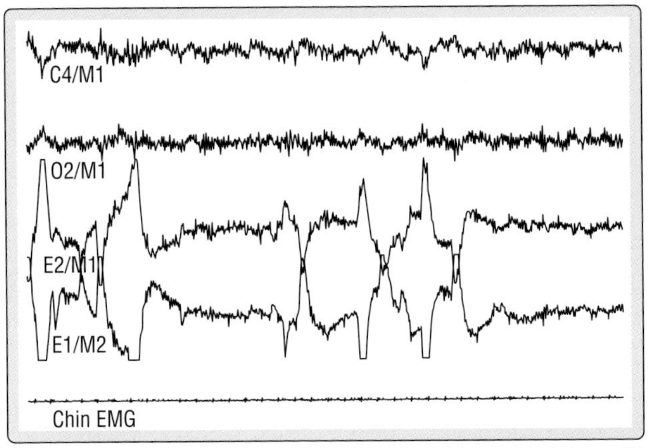

Figure 197.5 Rapid eye movement (REM) sleep. During REM sleep, chin muscle tone drops to the lowest level of the recording. REM sleep is identified by the presence of rapid eye movements in combination with relatively low-voltage, mixed-frequency EEG and low amplitude chin EMG. C4/M1, Right central lobe EEG referenced to left mastoid; E2/M1, right eye (outer canthus) referenced to left mastoid; E1/M2, left eye (outer canthus) referenced to right mastoid; EEG, electroencephalogram; EMG, electromyogram; O2/M1, right occipital lobe EEG referenced to left mastoid. (From Butkov N. *Atlas of Clinical Polysomnography.* 2nd ed. Synapse Media; 2010.)

entail emergent occipital EEG alpha activity. To qualify as an arousal, 10 seconds of sleep must precede the event. In REM sleep, activity must also increase in submentalis EMG leads for at least 1 second (Figure 197.6). The 3-second duration represents the minimum duration that could be reliably scored by visual inspection (among the task force members). Events of shorter duration likely also have clinical significance. The AASM standards manual endorsed this scoring technique and simplified the original 11 rules to a single statement with 2 explanatory notes.

SUMMARIZING NORMAL SLEEP

The sleep stage pattern across the night can be represented diagrammatically (Figure 197.7). In healthy young adults, stage R (REM sleep) accounts for approximately 20% to 25% of total sleep time, stage N2 accounts for 50%, N3 accounts for 12.5% to 20%, and N1 accounts for the remainder (usually about 10 % of total sleep time). In normal sleepers, wakefulness characteristically accounts for 5% to 10% of the time in bed. Stage R typically does not appear until approximately 90 minutes after sleep onset, after which it reoccurs every 90 to 120 minutes in distinct episodes. These episodes increase in duration as sleep progresses; accordingly, the first half of the sleep session contains less REM sleep than the second half. By contrast, slow wave activity (stage N3) predominates in the first third of the night. Age-matched sleep architecture bears great similarity in men and in women; however, women may have slightly better preserved stage N3 with advancing age. Sleep can be quantitatively summarized, and Table 197.3 provides definitions for commonly used parameters.

Table 197.2 Comparison of Traditional and AASM Sleep Stage Scoring Systems

Parameter	R & K Classification Criteria	AASM Classification Criteria
Epoch length	20 or 30 seconds, user's choice	30 seconds, mandated
Stage nomenclature	Wakefulness, stage 1 sleep, stage 2 sleep, stage 3 sleep, stage 4 sleep, REM sleep, movement time	Stages W, N1, N2, N3, and R
Wakefulness	EEG alpha activity for ≥50% of an epoch	Same
Slow wave sleep	EEG slow wave activity for ≥50% of the epoch for stage 4 sleep or ≥20% of the epoch for stage 3 sleep	Same, except that stages 3 and 4 are combined into N3
Stage 2 sleep	Sleep spindles or K-complexes; EEG slow wave activity for <20% of the epoch	Same
Stage 1 sleep	Low-voltage, mixed-frequency activity; possibly vertex sharp waves; possibly slow eye movements; no sleep spindles or K-complexes; EEG alpha activity for <50% of the epoch	Same
REM sleep	Low-voltage, mixed-frequency EEG activity; very low submental EMG activity; possibly saw tooth EEG theta activity; at least one unequivocal rapid eye movement	Same
Movement time	Polysomnographic activity obscured to the point of not being readable for more than 50% of the epoch; the preceding epoch is scored as stage 1, 2, 3, 4, or REM sleep	This epoch classification is eliminated
Smoothing rules	When an epoch is classified as a particular stage but is surrounded by epochs lacking unique features (e.g., a sleep spindle, slow-rolling eye movements, or CNS arousal) and would otherwise have been scored as stage 1 sleep, the classified epoch scoring is generalized to the surrounding epochs (but only for 3 minutes). These smoothing rules apply to stage 2 and REM sleep.	Same, except that there is no 3-minute limit to the generalization

AASM, American Academy of Sleep Medicine; CNS, central nervous system; EEG, electroencephalogram; EMG, electromyogram; R & K, Rechtschaffen and Kales; REM, rapid eye movement.

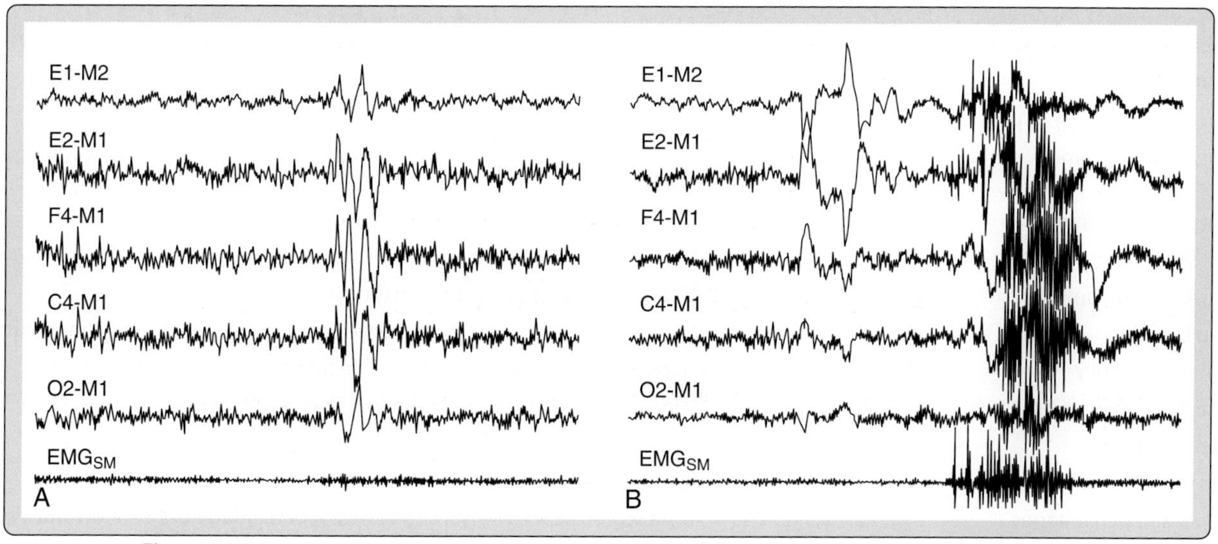

Figure 197.6 Arousals from NREM **(A)** and REM **(B)** sleep. **A,** A paroxysmal burst of high-amplitude slow wave activity appears near the center of the epoch. The distribution of the electrical field changes associated with this event can be seen reflected in the other EEG channels but with (expected) decreased amplitude. Little or no change occurs in the EMG channel in association with this event. It is common to see K-complex activity evoked by auditory stimuli. **B,** An increase in EMG activity is noted on the EMG and almost simultaneously in the E2-M1 channel. This is followed by a brief generalized presentation of EMG artifact throughout the EEG and EOG channels. Before the event, there is evidence of REM sleep: low-voltage, mixed-frequency EEG, rapid eye movements, and very low EMG. After the event, the EMG channel shows an increased tone, and the EEG background activity is low-voltage and fast. A continuation of EMG artifact is seen on the EEG channels after the short burst. These data, especially the burst of alpha activity seen in the O2-M1 channel, are consistent with a possible transition to wake from REM sleep. C4-M1, Right central lobe EEG referenced to left mastoid; E1-M2, left eye (outer canthus) referenced to right mastoid; E2-M1, right eye (outer canthus) referenced to left mastoid; EEG, electroencephalogram; EMG, electromyogram; EMGSM, submentalis EMG; EOG, electrooculogram; F4-M1, right frontal lobe EEG referenced to left mastoid; O2-M1, right occipital lobe EEG referenced to left mastoid. (Courtesy Max Hirshkowitz, PhD, DABSM.)

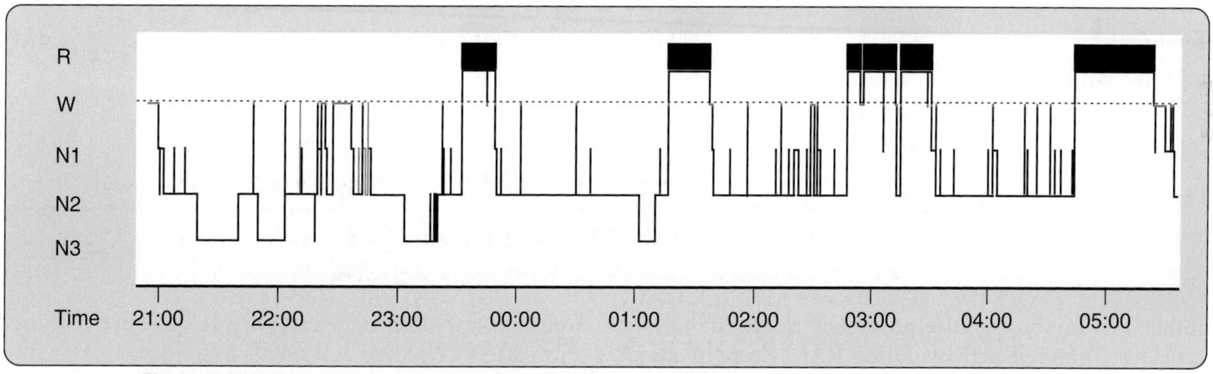

Figure 197.7 Normal sleep histogram illustrating sleep macroarchitecture (stages) for a young adult. N1, N2, and N3, NREM sleep stage 1, 2, and 3, respectively; R, REM sleep; W, wakefulness.

AMBIGUOUS SLEEP STAGES AND SLEEP QUALITY

Sleep stage scoring was developed to summarize EEG, EOG, and EMG correlates of *normal sleep*. Under normal circumstances, particular events cluster for the vast majority of the time. By contrast, this tight coupling tends to loosen when patients rebound from sleep deprivation; sustain brain injury; are afflicted with sleep, medical, neurologic, psychiatric, or sleep disorders; or ingest psychoactive substances. The resulting intrusion, translocation, or migration of specific EEG, EOG, or EMG activity characteristic of one stage into another produces ambiguous epochs that are difficult to classify according to the usual scoring rules. This departure from normal processes can provide qualitative evidence of an underlying sleep dysfunction.

Perhaps the most common ambiguities accompany pharmacotherapy. Gamma-aminobutyric acid type A and benzodiazepine receptor agonists generally increase spindle activity in the EEG. These pharmacologically induced spindles typically are of higher frequency (16 to 18 Hz) and often of longer duration, occur more frequently (with a higher density), and can appear not only in N2 but also in other stages of sleep and in wakefulness.

Another commonly noted drug effect is serotonin agonist augmentation of eye movement activity. In some persons, rapid eye movements occur at sleep onset and in sleep stages N2 and N3, making the scoring of REM sleep a challenge. The phenomenon is so common that many sleep specialists refer to it as "Prozac eyes" (with reference to fluoxetine, the prototypical selective serotonin reuptake inhibitor).

Table 197.3 Parameters Derived from Sleep Staging and Central Nervous System Arousal Scoring

Parameter	Notation	Explanation
AASM Recommended Parameters		
Lights out clock time	L-out	The clock time (in hh:mm) that the subject was instructed to allow himself or herself to fall asleep
Lights on clock time	L-on	The clock time (in hh:mm) that the subject was awakened
Total sleep time	TST	Minutes scored as stage N1, N2, N3, or R
Total recording time	TRT	Elapsed time from L-out to L-on (in minutes)
Sleep latency	SLAT	Elapsed time from L-out to first epoch of stage N1, N2, N3, or R (in minutes)
REM sleep latency	RLAT	Elapsed time in minutes from SLAT to first epoch of stage R
Wake after sleep onset	WASO	Minutes scored as stage W from first sleep epoch to L-on
Sleep efficiency	SEI	TST as a percentage of TRT
Time in each stage	MW, M1, M2, M3, MR	Minutes scored as W, N1, N2, N3, and R (individually)
Sleep stage percentages	P1, P2, P3, PR	Time scored as N1, N2, N3, and REM as a percentage of TST (individually)
Number of CNS arousals	NArsls	The number of CNS arousals
CNS arousal	CNS AI	The number of CNS arousals scored per hour of TST
Other Useful Parameters		
Latency to persistent sleep	LTPS	Elapsed time (in minutes) from L-out to first of 10 consecutive minutes of sleep
Latency to unequivocal sleep	LUS	Elapsed time (in minutes) from L-out to first epoch of N2, N3, or R or to three consecutive (or more) epochs of N1 If N1 is followed by an epoch of N2, N3, or R, LUS is calculated from L-out to the first epoch of N1
Sleep-period time	SPT	Minutes from first to last epoch scored as N1, N2, N3, or R
Number of REM sleep episodes	NREME	Number of stage R occurrences
Number of awakenings	NWake	Number of stage W occurrences
Wake index	WI	Number of awakenings per hour of TST
Sleep fragmentation index	SFI	Number of awakenings and CNS arousals per hour of TST
Number of stage shifts	NShifts	Number of stage transitions during TRT
Stage shift index	SSI	Number of stage transitions per hour of TRT
Latency to arising	LTA	Duration of final stage W if it was ongoing when L-on occurred

CNS, Central nervous system; N1, NREM stage 1; N2, NREM stage 2; N3, NREM stage 3; REM, rapid eye movement.

Another serotonin agonist–provoked sleep alteration involves elevated muscle activity during REM sleep. In some cases, these medications produce a loss of atonia, permitting attempted dream enactments—that is, iatrogenic REM sleep behavior disorder (RBD). Individual PSG epochs during these events do not meet usual stage classification criteria. Similar REM sleep ambiguities occur in Parkinson disease–related and posttraumatic stress disorder–related RBD.

Patients suffering from neurodegenerative diseases or brain insult can manifest an overall erosion of EEG sleep events. This effect includes reduced sleep spindles, K-complexes, and slow wave activity. We also sometimes observe this effect in patients with sleep apnea, heart failure, and metabolic disorders. The resulting nearly featureless sleep EEG can be difficult to score according to normal staging rules. By contrast, another very different scoring problem can occur in persons with severely fragmented sleep produced by obstructive apnea, in whom a continual cycle of falling asleep, airway collapse, struggle to breathe, awakening, and falling asleep is observed. Thus the patient remains in a transition state that does not fit well into any sleep stage category. It was once proposed that this pattern be scored as *t-sleep*.

In some persons, copious EEG alpha activity permeates ongoing background activity. In sleep states marked by low-amplitude, mixed-frequency activity, alpha bursts meeting criteria for CNS arousal can be scored as such (alpha intrusion). However, when slow waves characterize the dominant ongoing background EEG activity and the alpha coincides with delta, arousals are not scored. This *alpha-delta* sleep sometimes accompanies pain syndromes, but it appears to lack specificity. A related phenomenon, also ascribed to pain, consists of K-complex bursts followed by EEG alpha activity. Many sleep specialists consider this "K-alpha" activity to be a variety of the CAP.

COMPUTER-ASSISTED SCORING AND FUTURE DIRECTIONS IN SLEEP STAGING

Because sleep staging requires the visual appraisal of polysomnogram signals in 30-second time increments, the scoring of an 8-hour record is labor intensive. Additionally, interrater reliability is imperfect with interscorer agreement of approximately 80% and κ values of 0.68 to 0.76 between technologists.[17] Therefore the development of computer-assisted scoring programs was not unexpected. Historically, automated staging was previously unable to attain the accuracy or reliability of human scoring. Machine learning algorithms, which can identify patterns from the data provided, are well suited for the vast amount of data acquired during PSG. However, initial attempts to automate polysomnogram staging with machine learning algorithms also failed to recapitulate human performance. Neural networks are a specific type of machine learning and transform input to output with "neurons" and have the capacity to self-adjust the strength each of neuron while learning from data. The use of deep (multilayer) convolution and recurrent neural networks, which incorporate both spatial and sequential relationships into data analysis, have demonstrated the ability to rapidly and accurately stage polysomnograms.[18-20] Given the interindividual heterogeneity in polysomnogram signal and edge cases, the use of deep neural networks is likely to augment, as opposed to replace, human scoring.

In addition to streamlining the polysomnogram scoring process, computer-generated parameters may help us derive more from PSG than the traditionally used sleep stages, arousals, and derived calculations and summary metrics.[21] For example, the odds ratio product is a computational method to quantify sleep depth.[22] Another example is the use of neural network staging to produce a hypnodensity graph, which visually depicts the probability distribution of sleep stages over the course of the night rather than enforcing the assignment of a single sleep stage for every 30-second epoch. Therefore new computational methods are likely to augment clinical and research operations, derive novel insight from electroencephalogram during sleep, and transform how we conceptualize sleep staging.[23]

CLINICAL PEARLS

- Sleep staging and CNS arousal scoring provide important clinical information about brain processes during sleep. Ultimately, persons who awaken sleepy, awaken unrefreshed, have difficulty falling sleep, or have difficulty maintaining sleep can be assessed for sleep integrity, quantity, and quality using PSG.
- Human sleep is a brain process. Pathophysiologic conditions such as increased airway resistance and leg movements produce CNS arousals that fragment and can destroy the fabric of sleep. Disorders often alter sleep patterns and overall architecture.
- Appropriate treatments may promote return to normal. Quantitative analysis through staging and arousal scoring objectively documents sleep disruption and provides a severity index for sleep disorders.
- Technological advances in artificial intelligence, such as deep neural network sleep staging and other computational methods, may augment human polysomnogram scoring and reveal novel insights from the polysomnogram.

SUMMARY

PSG involves recording an assortment of bioparameters while a person sleeps. The most objective method for knowing if a person is sleeping is to examine brain wave activity (the electroencephalogram). Sleep stage scoring summarizes patterns in the electroencephalogram, electrooculogram, and skeletal muscle electromyogram. Well-established, specific, scoring criteria exist for sleep stages N1, N2, N3, and R (previously called NREM stages 1, 2, 3, 4, and REM, respectively). Scoring criteria depend upon EEG bandwidth activity (delta, theta, alpha, and beta), EEG events (vertex sharp waves, sleep spindles, and K-complexes), eye movement activity (slow and rapid eye movements), and the level of muscle tone. Stage N3 is characterized by high-voltage, slow wave activity. Stage N2 contains sleep spindles and K-complexes. Stage N1 has low-voltage, mixed-frequency background, possibly slow eye movements, and vertex sharp waves. If rapid eye movements accompany a low-voltage, mixed-frequency EEG and skeletal muscle tone is low, REM sleep is scored. CNS arousals also can occur from sleep, either spontaneously or resulting from pathophysiologic processes or environmental factors. Quantitative analysis of sleep stages and CNS arousals provides evidence for, contributes to the definition of, and indexes the severity of some sleep disorders. Similarly, these indices can provide objective outcome measures for assessing therapeutic interventions. This chapter summarizes recording, digital processing, and scoring techniques used for evaluating human brain activity during sleep and its disturbance by CNS arousals.

SELECTED READINGS

Berry RB, Brooks R, Gamaldo CE, et al. for the American Academy of Sleep Medicine. *The AASM Manual for the Scoring of Sleep and Associated Events: Rules, Terminology and Technical Specifications.* Darien, Illinois: American Academy of Sleep Medicine; 2020. Version 2.6.

Butkov N. *Atlas of clinical polysomnography.* 2nd ed. Medford (Ore.): Synapse Media; 2010.

Hirshkowitz M, Kryger MH. Diagnostic methods. In: Kryger MH, Avidan A, Berry R, eds. *Atlas of clinical sleep medicine.* 2nd ed. Philadelphia: Elsevier; 2014.

A complete reference list can be found online at ExpertConsult.com.

Chapter

198

Central Nervous System Arousals and the Cyclic Alternating Pattern*

Liborio Parrino; Carlotta Mutti; Nicoletta Azzi; Michela Canepari

Chapter Highlights

- The limits of the conventional sleep measures based on static 30-second epochs are compared with the more dynamic interpretation of sleep based on the cyclic alternating pattern (CAP) scoring criteria. To apply the rules of CAP interpretation, the concept of electroencephalogram (EEG) arousal is expanded and now includes EEG features characterized by high-voltage slow waves, which are endowed with activation properties on autonomic functions and muscle activities.
- As the marker of sleep instability, CAP offers additional tools to better understand the physiology of sleep, the pathophysiology of sleep disorders, and the action of medication and other therapeutic options.
- Topographic information on the cerebral origin of CAP networks is growing, and automatic analysis to accelerate CAP quantification is available.

OVERVIEW

According to the Merriam-Webster dictionary, arousal is not only the act of arousing someone or something—arousal from sleep—but the term can have many other meanings. The term *arousal* has been used in reference to a great many things, ranging from the moon's effect on tides to sexual excitation. The following chapter focuses specifically on central nervous system arousal, its role in human sleep and wakefulness, and methods for its measurement. The fluctuating electrical potentials recordable from the scalp (i.e., the electroencephalogram [EEG]) provide a noninvasive, continuous dynamic measure of brain activity. Furthermore, human sleep and wakefulness are largely differentiated using EEG markers. Berger[1,2] found low-voltage fast EEG activity (beta rhythm) during eyes-open wakefulness and a higher-amplitude, slower EEG activity (alpha rhythm) associated with eyes-closed, relaxed wakefulness. When falling asleep, the alpha activity disappeared and recurred upon awakening. Loomis and colleagues[3,4] later established a variety of other sleep-related EEG waveforms, including slow waves, sleep spindles, sawtooth theta waves, and K complexes.

THE DISCOVERY OF THE AROUSAL SYSTEM

In 1949 Moruzzi and Magoun[5] discovered that the stimulation of the reticular formation of the brainstem evokes immediate changes in the EEG:

- Synchronized high-amplitude discharges are abolished and replaced by low-voltage fast activity. Reaction is generalized and tends to prevail in the anterior regions of the brain.
- A similar response can be elicited by stimulating the medial bulbar reticular formation, pontine and midbrain tegmentum, dorsal hypothalamus, and subthalamus. The excitable substrate possesses a low threshold and responds best to high frequencies of stimulation.
- Some background synchrony of electrocortical activity is requisite for manifestation of the response. With synchrony in spontaneous drowsiness or light chloralose anesthesia, the effect of reticular stimulation is strikingly like Berger alpha wave blockade, or any arousal reaction.
- The reticular response and the arousal reaction to natural stimuli have been compared in the "encéphale isolé," in which EEG synchrony was present during spontaneous relaxation or was produced by recruiting mechanisms, and the two appear identical.
- The possibility is considered that a background of maintained activity within this ascending brainstem activating system (ABAS) may account for wakefulness, whereas reduction of its activity, either naturally, by barbiturates, or by experimental injury and disease, may, respectively, precipitate normal sleep, contribute to anesthesia, or produce pathologic somnolence.

For the first time, a specific neural structure (the reticular formation of the brainstem) was indicated as the active control unit of arousal. Although innovative and exciting, the pioneering vision of Moruzzi and Magoun privileged a passive vision of the sleep process: we are awake if the ABAS is active; we fall into slumber when the ABAS activity fades. In the following years, Moruzzi

* Dedicated to Mario Giovanni Terzano (1944–2020), who discovered the cyclic alternating pattern.

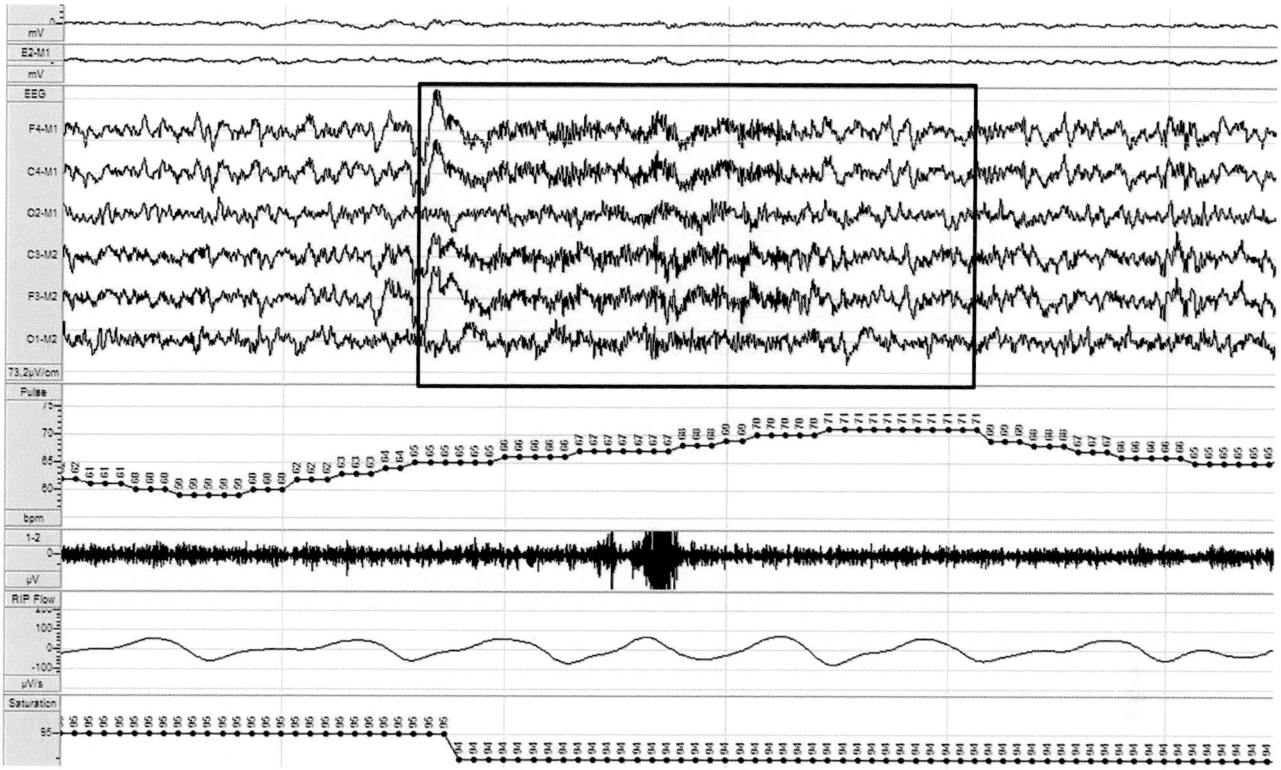

Figure 198.1 During sleep stages N1, N2, and N3, or REM sleep, arousal is scored if there is an abrupt shift of frequency, including theta, alpha, and/or frequencies greater than 16 Hz (but not spindles) that lasts at least 3 seconds with at least 10 seconds of stable sleep preceding the change. Scoring of arousal during REM sleep also requires a concurrent increase in submental EMG activity lasting at least 1 second. Note that in NREM sleep, arousals often are heralded by one or more K-complexes. EMG, Electromyogram.

revised his on-off framework, attributing a sleep-triggering role to alternative brainstem regions, including the bulbar areas.

CENTRAL NERVOUS SYSTEM AROUSALS DURING SLEEP

Moruzzi's formulation essentially indicated that an EEG arousal can be identified when synchronized high-amplitude discharges are abolished and replaced by low-voltage fast activity. This definition is sculptured in the American Academy of Sleep Medicine (AASM) manual[6] (Figure 198.1) and confirms the definition of EEG arousal established in 1992 by the American Sleep Disorders Association.[7] Essentially, a 3- but less than 15-second alpha EEG activity burst during non–rapid eye movement (NREM) sleep is scored as a central nervous system (CNS) arousal. During rapid eye movement (REM) sleep, this type of alpha EEG activity is scored as an arousal if it is accompanied by an increase in submentalis muscle activity. This later requirement reflects the fact that alpha activity may spontaneously occur during REM sleep and apparently has no effect upon subsequent daytime alertness. EEG alpha activity bursts sustained for 30 seconds or more are scored as awakenings. According to the original framework, arousals are markers of sleep disruption representing a detrimental and harmful feature of sleep. For this reason, they were initially excluded from the conventional staging procedures. However, a number of studies have established that spontaneous arousals are natural guests of sleep and undergo a linear increase along the life span following the profile of maturation and aging.[8] Moreover, the spectral composition of arousals[9] and their ultradian distribution throughout the sleep cycles[10] reveal that arousals are endowed within the texture of physiologic sleep under the biologic control of REM-on and REM-off mechanisms.[11] According to these indications, arousal scoring is now considered a fundamental process in staging classification in addition to spindles and K-complexes (KCs).[6]

THE DOUBLE NATURE OF K-COMPLEXES AND DELTA BURSTS

KCs reflect a Janus-faced mechanism involved in the negotiation between two main contradictory functional necessities: preserving the continuity of sleep and maintaining the possibility to react.[12] In addition to stereo-EEG evidence,[13] the double nature of KCs is supported by functional magnetic resonance imaging (fMRI) investigation of sensory areas,[14,15] and even spontaneous KCs wear at their initial segment the traces of multisensory processing.[42] According to Jahnke et al.[15] "a KC embodies an arousal with subsequent sleep guarding counteraction that might on one hand serve monitoring of the environment with basic information processing and on the other hand protect continuity of sleep and thus its restoring effect." According to this view, during a KC, the brain conducts low-level cognitive processing to investigate the saliency or possible threat of external and internal stimuli and decides "not to wake up," compensating the disturbing effect of the incoming stimulus by producing a KC.[16] A role for KCs in sleep-specific endogenous information processing for external or internal stimuli has been proposed, based on works using "oddball" paradigm experiments in normal sleeping humans.[17] Both animal[18] and human[19] studies indicate that the main negative phase of the KC reflects a period of hyperpolarization

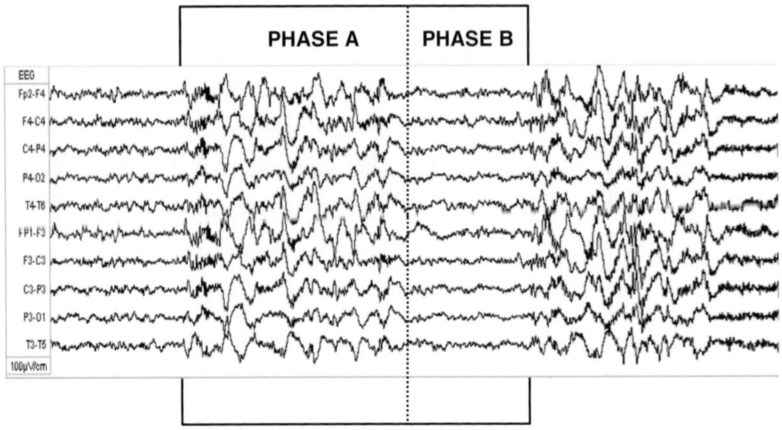

Figure 198.2 A cyclic alternating pattern (CAP) sequence. The black box limits a CAP cycle composed of a phase A (cluster of K-complexes) and a phase B (interval between two successive A phases). Notice that CAP is a widespread phenomenon that involves several electroencephalogram (EEG) channels with a dominance of high-amplitude waves in the anterior regions.

(down state) of certain frontal areas, thus suppressing any arousal reaction to the nonthreatening stimulus. Similar to EEG arousals,[20] KCs, either spontaneous or evoked, induce cardiac acceleration[21] and a rise in systolic blood pressure.[22] The clear-cut association between KCs and autonomic activation indicates that phasic slow waves during sleep are an elementary form of arousal.[23] In particular, they play a reactive homeostatic role, maintaining sleep continuity despite sleep-disturbing events.[24] A KC can be followed by other KCs, and, in that case, stage 2 tends toward consolidation; or it can be followed by an arousal, which reflects a regression toward a shallower neurophysiologic condition. However, most arousals in NREM sleep (87%) are preceded by a KC or by a delta burst,[9] indicating that EEG synchrony and desynchrony may coexist in a natural dynamic succession. Moreover, the biphasic pattern of heart rate in association with KCs and EEG arousals (a marked acceleration followed by a more gradual deceleration) indicates a microstructural cyclicity in NREM sleep.[20]

THE CYCLIC ALTERNATING PATTERN

The cyclic alternating pattern (CAP) is an EEG periodic activity occurring under conditions of reduced vigilance (e.g., sleep, coma) and translates a state of arousal instability involving muscle, behavioral, and autonomic functions.[25] CAP is organized in sequences composed of a succession of CAP cycles. The CAP cycle is composed of a phase A and the following phase B. All CAP sequences (composed of a series of CAP cycles) begin with a phase A and end with a phase B (Figure 198.2). At least two consecutive CAP cycles are required to define a CAP sequence.[26]

In NREM sleep, phasic activities initiating a phase A must be a third higher than the background voltage (calculated during the 2 seconds before onset and 2 seconds after offset of a phase A). Each phase of a CAP is 2 to 60 seconds in duration, a range based on the consideration that the great majority of A phases (about 90%) occurring during sleep are separated by an interval less than 60 seconds. The absence of CAP for more than 60 seconds is scored as non-CAP. An isolated phase A (that is, preceded or followed by another phase A but separated by more than 60 seconds) is classified as non-CAP. The phase A that terminates a CAP sequence is counted as non-CAP (Figure 198.3). The absence of CAP coincides with a condition of sustained physiologic stability and is defined as non-CAP.[26] CAP sequences and non-CAP define the microstructure of sleep.

CAP and non-CAP can be manipulated by sensorial inputs. Applying separately the same arousing stimulus during the two EEG components of CAP, phase B is the one that immediately assumes the morphology of the other component, whereas the inverse transformation never occurs when the stimulus is delivered during phase A. This stereotyped reactivity persists throughout the successive phases of CAP with lack of habituation.

In contrast, when the same stimulus is presented during non-CAP, the EEG responses are generally brief, hypersynchronized (slow waves), and proceed toward progressive habituation.[27] However, a robust or sustained stimulus delivered during non-CAP induces the immediate appearance of repetitive CAP cycles that display the same morphology and reactive behavior of spontaneous CAP sequences. The evoked CAP sequence may herald a lightening of sleep depth or continue as a damping oscillation before the complete recovery of non-CAP.

The A Phases of CAP

Phase A activities can be classified into three subtypes. Subtype classification is based on the reciprocal proportion of high-voltage slow waves (EEG synchrony) and low-amplitude fast rhythms (EEG desynchrony) throughout the entire phase A duration. The three phase A subtypes are described next[28] (Figure 198.4):

- Subtypes A1: EEG synchrony (high-amplitude slow waves) is the predominant activity. If present, EEG desynchrony (low-amplitude fast waves) occupies less than 20% of the entire phase A duration. Subtype A1 specimens include delta bursts, KC sequences, vertex sharp transients, and polyphasic bursts with less than 20% of EEG desynchrony.
- Subtypes A2: The EEG activity is a mixture of slow and fast rhythms with 20% to 50% of phase A occupied by EEG desynchrony. Subtype A2 specimens include polyphasic bursts with more than 20% but less than 50% of EEG desynchrony.
- Subtypes A3: The EEG activity is predominantly rapid, low-voltage rhythms with more than 50% of phase A occupied by EEG desynchrony. Subtype A3 specimens include K-alpha, EEG arousals, and polyphasic bursts with more than 50% of EEG desynchrony. A movement artifact within a CAP sequence is also classified as subtype A3.[29]

CAP sequences can include different phase A subtypes (Figures 198.5 and 198.6). The majority of arousals occurring

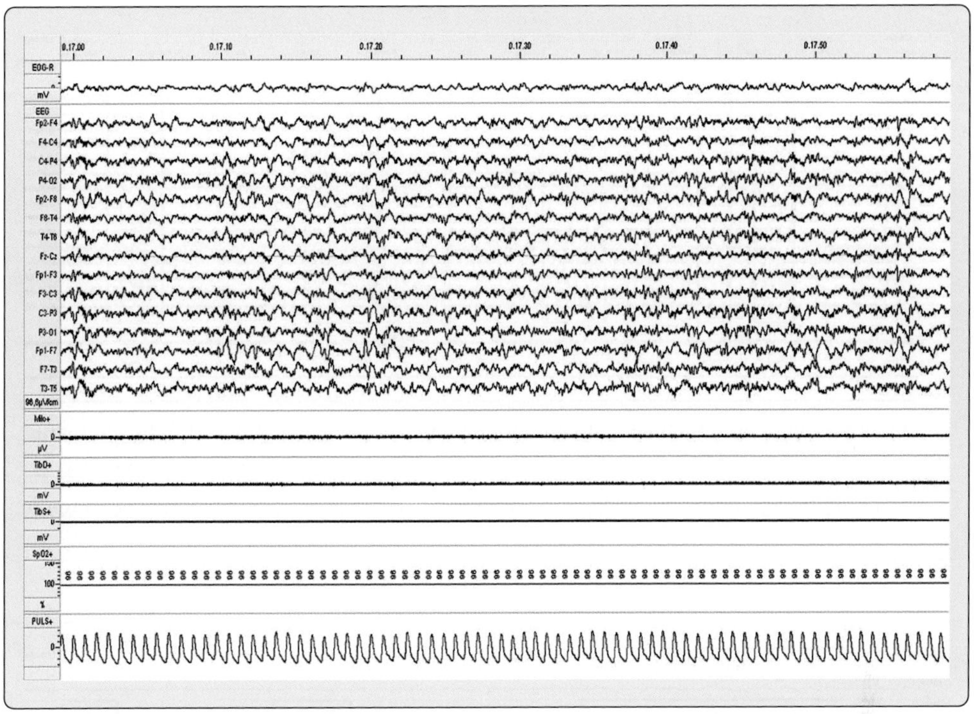

Figure 198.3 Non–cyclic alternating pattern (CAP) in stage N3 expressed by a sustained succession of slow waves, which correspond to the lower than 1 Hz oscillation of NREM sleep. Arousals or other EEG phasic events are missing. Notice the extreme stability of pulse and oximetry traces and the absence of muscle jerks.

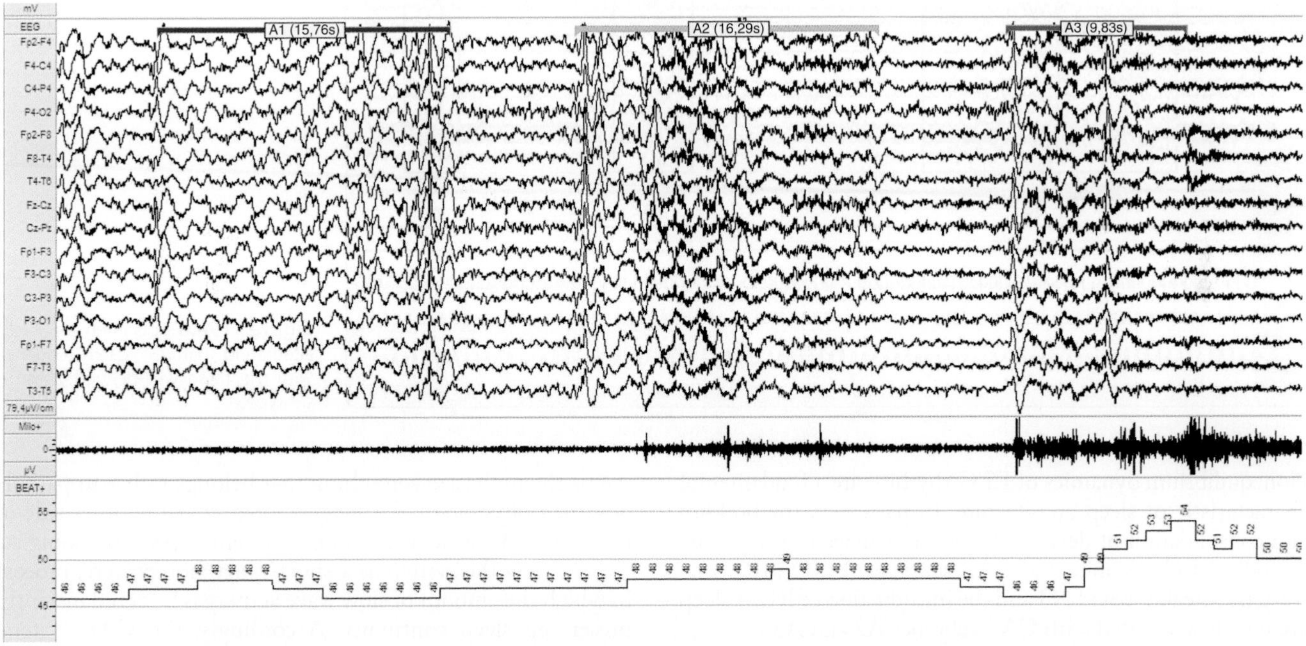

Figure 198.4 The three phase A subtypes confined by black vertical lines. The A1 subtype is dominated by high-voltage low-frequency waves, whereas subtypes A2 and A3 contain increasing amounts of low-voltage rapid electroencephalogram (EEG) activities identified by dotted horizontal lines. The A3 phase is accompanied by a mild electromyogram (EMG) activation, and all three subtypes are associated with a transient heart rate acceleration.

in NREM (87%) sleep are inserted within the CAP sequences and basically coincide with a phase A2 or A3. In particular, 95% of subtypes A3 and 62% of subtypes A2 meet the AASM criteria for arousals.[29] The broad overlap between arousals and subtypes A2 and A3 is further supported by their similar evolution in relation to age and to their positive correlation with the amount of light NREM sleep and negative correlation with the amount of deep NREM sleep.

Sleep architecture is based on the cyclic alternation of two major neurophysiologic states: NREM and REM sleep. NREM sleep is composed of three stages (N1, N2, N3) in which EEG synchrony grows with the increasing depth of sleep. In contrast, EEG desynchrony is the dominant feature of REM sleep. The alternation of NREM and REM sleep constitutes the sleep cycle, and its recurrence during the night determines the classical stepwise sleep profile (macrostructure).

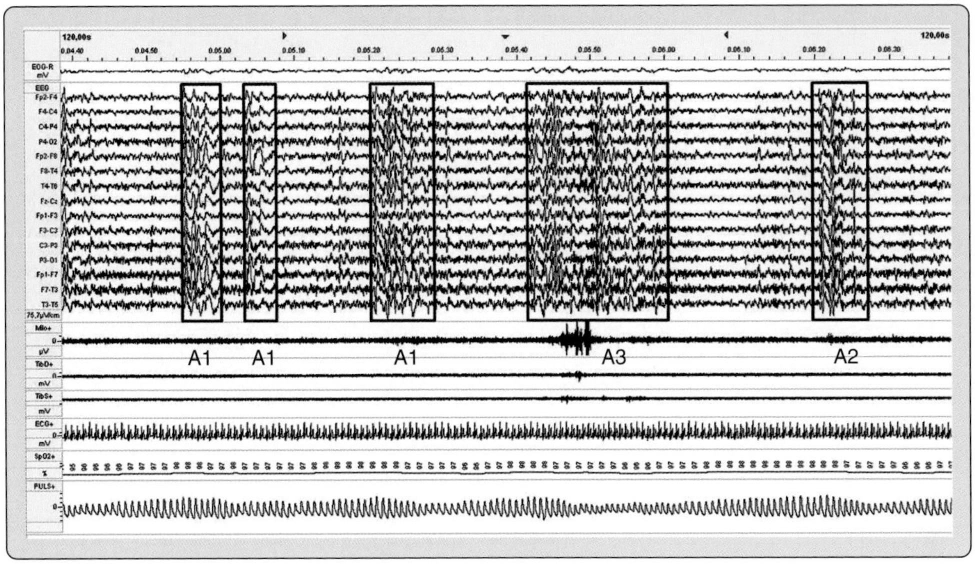

Figure 198.5 Different phase A subtypes may be scored within a common cyclic alternating pattern (CAP) sequence. The central phase A3 is combined with a strong activation of the chin electromyogram (EMG) and a mild increase of the muscle tone in both tibialis electrodes. Notice the waxing and waning of pulse wave amplitude (bottom trace) in-phase with the periodicity and functional power of electroencephalogram (EEG) oscillations.

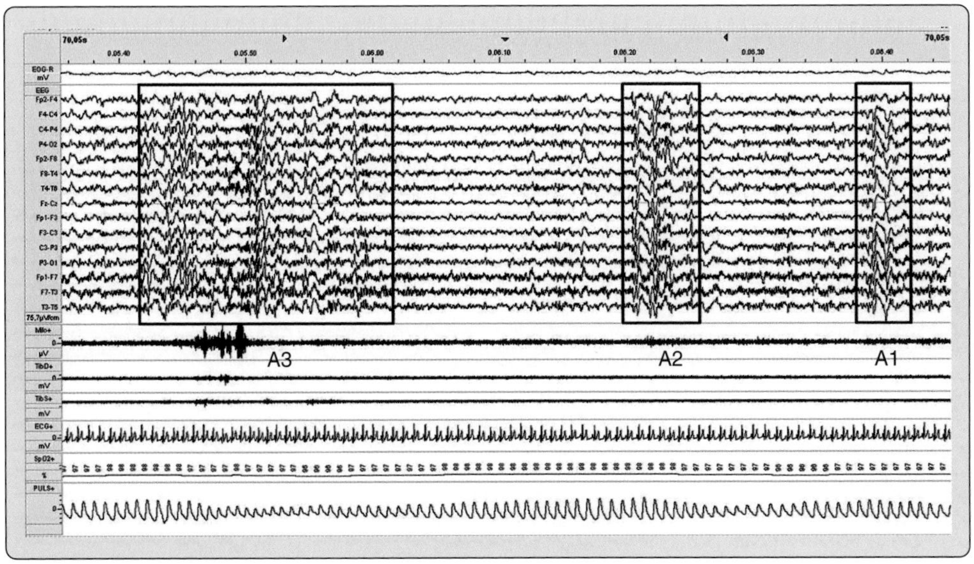

Figure 198.6 Specimen of cyclic alternating pattern (CAP) sequence with the three well-defined phase A subtypes.

Nonequilibrium dynamics of EEG rhythms are a fundamental characteristic of sleep architecture. In particular, the buildup and consolidation of deep sleep (N3) is achieved through the periodic EEG instability of CAP subtypes A1. On the contrary, the breakdown of N3 and the introduction of REM sleep are mostly associated with CAP subtypes A2 and A3.

CAP IS A PHYSIOLOGIC COMPONENT OF SLEEP

The CAP system is interpreted mainly as a marker of sleep instability and at the same time as a buffer system against perturbations of NREM sleep. Both visions are true, but the aspect of "instability" is rather attached to the dynamics of A2 and A3 events, whereas the "buffer system" aspect is mainly a feature of the dynamics of A1 events. As sleep cycles exhibit a double "sleep-promoting" function during the descending slope and a "wake/REM-promoting" effect during the ascending slope, the contrasting double nature of CAP events reflects the same alternating nature.[29] If we consider the biologic role of the CAP system, the definition of an "instability marker" seems to emphasize something that belongs rather to pathology than physiology. We suggest looking at the other side of the coin and consider the "buffer system" aspect. By doing so, we can view the system as a short-range homeostatic process in which the amount of slow wave activity is buffered instantly, preserving sleep continuity. Accordingly, the CAP system, especially by means of subtypes A1, is a natural "slow wave injection," protecting sleep against perturbations.[24]

The main assumption of CAP is that we must consider that during certain periods of the night the arousal level is unstable. The concept of instability is a basic issue of all complex systems and supports the dynamics of biologic variability. Within certain ranges, instability warrants flexible and adaptive features to the complex system. In normal sleep, CAP accompanies the stage transitions maintaining in-phase both the EEG and autonomic functions through regular fluctuations. This means that what we observe on the peripheral sensors (respiratory events, heart rate variations, blood pressure shifts, myoclonic jerks) has a consistent and synchronous expression on the EEG and vice versa (Figure 198.7). To guarantee survival

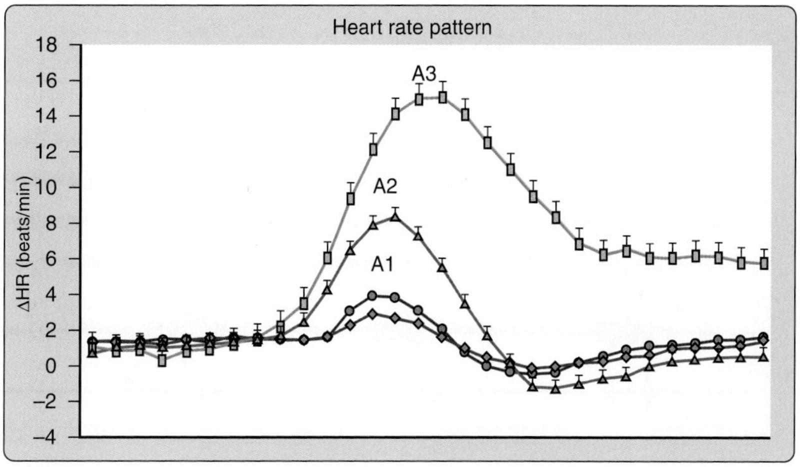

Figure 198.7 The hierarchic impact of the three phase A subtypes on heart rate. The difference involves only the magnitude of reactivity, as they all induce an increase of cardiac beats per minute. (Modified from Sforza et al.)

during prolonged unconsciousness (i.e., sleep), a strong interaction among all the biologic subsystems is mandatory. From the CAP perspective, analysis of sleep microstructure is not limited to the finding of a single event (for example, an isolated arousal), but to the identification of a pattern (presence or absence of a CAP sequence) that translates a physiologic state that involves cerebral activities, autonomic functions, and behavioral features. In other words, what happens upstairs (brain) is reflected at the lower levels (autonomic and muscle parameters) and vice versa.[30,31]

SLEEP RESILIENCE

Resilience is the capacity of a system, enterprise, or person to maintain its core purpose and integrity in the face of dramatically changed circumstances. Under the protection of manifold guardians (dreams, circadian cycle, homeostatic drive, ultradian process, CAP, autonomic arousals, gravity, muscle control), powerful algorithms regulate the autonomy and survival of the sleeping brain.[32]

Failure of these compensatory processes leads to nonrestorative sleep. Therefore assessment of sleep quality relies on a variety of polysomnogram (PSG) measures, including sleep duration (quantified by total sleep time and sleep efficiency), sleep intensity (reflected by N3), sleep continuity (altered by nocturnal awakenings and arousals), and sleep stability (impaired by excessive amounts of CAP). With its A phases and its role of flexibility, CAP is one of the major guardians of NREM sleep. Whenever sleep continuity is menaced, whatever the source of perturbation, the brain exploits all the available options. The final architecture of a night of sleep reflects the dynamic balance between the internal constraints and the functional adaptability of the sleeping brain to the ongoing circumstances.

CAP RATE

Among the various CAP parameters, CAP rate is the most extensively used for clinical purposes. Calculated as the percentage ratio of total CAP time to NREM sleep time, CAP rate is the measure of arousal instability. In normal sleepers, CAP rate shows a low intraindividual night-to-night variability. CAP rate undergoes a complex evolution during development (Figure 198.8), with a peak in adolescence, a gradual decrease in adulthood, and followed by an increase in the elderly.[33] CAP rate is enhanced when sleep is disturbed by internal or external factors, and its variations correlate with the subjective appreciation of sleep quality, with higher values of CAP rate associated with poorer sleep quality.[34] Table 198.1 summarizes conditions found to have high and low CAP rates.

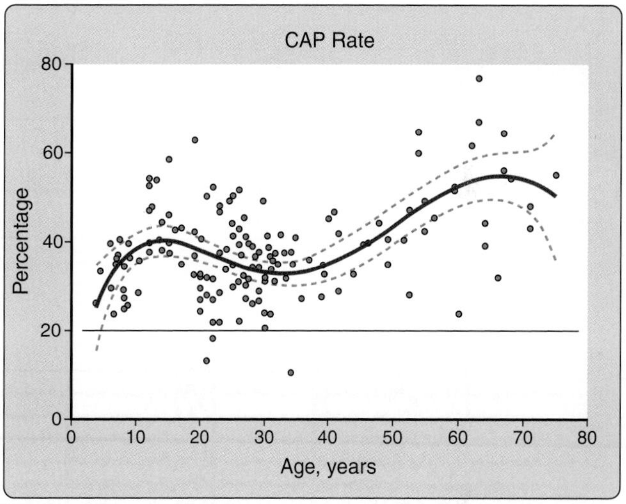

Figure 198.8 The age-related distribution of cyclic alternating pattern (CAP) rate in healthy subjects. The two peaks correspond to adolescence and senescence, and the trough coincides with young adulthood. Notice that almost all normal CAP rate values are higher than 20%. Patients with narcolepsy and benzodiazepine long-term use and abuse usually show amounts of CAP rate below this threshold.

CAP'S METHODOLOGICAL POTENTIAL FOR PHARMACOLOGIC RESEARCH

In a standardized model of situational insomnia, microstructural parameters have been applied to compare the effects of different hypnotic agents (lorazepam, triazolam, zolpidem, zopiclone). In contrast to macrostructural information, CAP analysis allows discrimination of hypnotic drugs from placebo, nonbenzodiazepine compounds from benzodiazepine agents, and zopiclone from zolpidem.[35] CAP also enables one to explore the effects of zolpidem administered on both a continuous (4 weeks) or intermittent basis.[35,36]

The sensitivity of CAP to medication in patients with insomnia can be exploited also in the evaluation of new sleep-promoting drugs. So far, hypnotic compounds have based

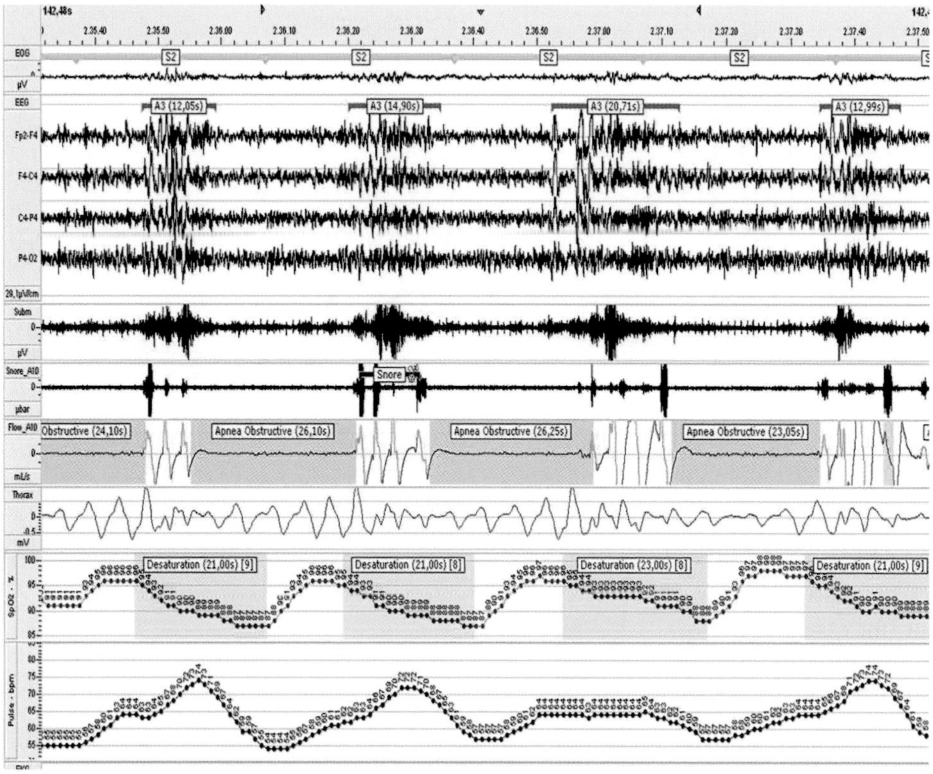

Figure 198.9 A cyclic alternating pattern (CAP) sequence of phase A3 subtypes that allow recovery of respiratory activity at the end of recurring obstructive apneas. Notice the exaggeration of muscle and vegetative oscillations of what normally happens in nonpathologic conditions.

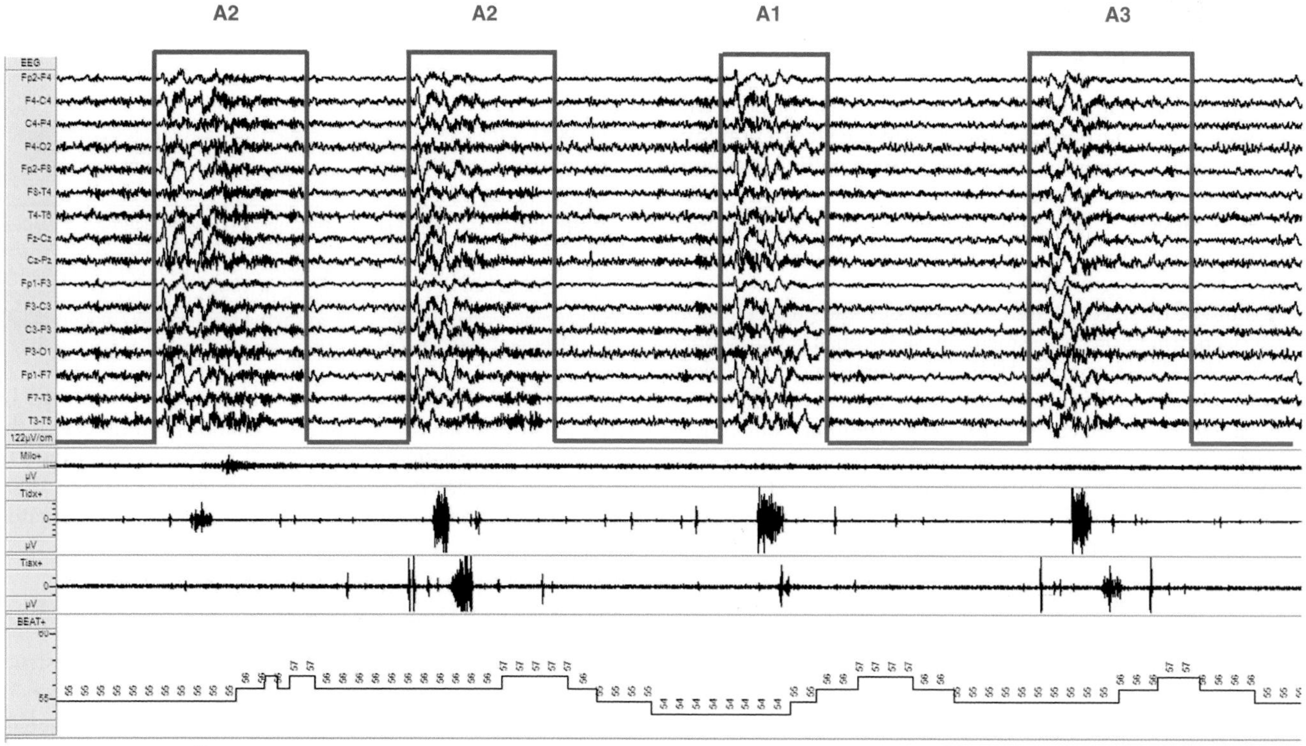

Figure 198.10 Cyclic alternating pattern (CAP) sequence coupled with periodic limb movements. Notice that myoclonic jerks during NREM sleep can be associated also with a phase A1 subtype, generally not scored as a conventional arousal.

their effectiveness on the paradigm of sleep-onset promotion, sleep time enhancement, and wake reduction. All the available hypnotic agents, especially those belonging to the gamma-aminobutyric acid (GABA) family (benzodiazepines and benzodiazepine receptor agonists), share these features, which paradoxically offer a flat, undifferentiated therapeutic scenario. Moreover, the long-term use or abuse of benzodiazepine determines an increased number of nocturnal awakenings and a severe reduction of arousals and CAP rate.[16,37] The result is the inability to modulate levels of vigilance.

Table 198.1

SLEEP CONDITIONS WITH HIGH CAP RATE
• Acoustic perturbation
• Upper airway resistance syndrome
• Sleep apnea syndrome (see Figure 198.9)
• Insomnia
• Periodic limb movement disorder (see Figure 198.10)
• Bruxism
• Primary generalized epilepsy
• Focal lesional epilepsy (frontal and temporal)
• Sleep-related hypermotor epilepsy
• Mood disorders
SLEEP CONDITIONS WITH LOW CAP RATE
• Narcolepsy
• Use/abuse of hypnotic drugs
• Benign epilepsy with rolandic spikes
• ADHD
• Fragile X syndrome
• Asperger syndrome
• REM sleep behavior disorder
• Mild cognitive impairment and Alzheimer disease neurodegeneration
• Amyotrophic lateral sclerosis

The problem of automatic CAP recognition has been addressed in several studies, with interesting results. Classification methods generally require the preliminary visual scoring of sleep macrostructure. Moreover, they rely on the extraction of spectral parameters from the electroencephalogram (EEG) signal to compute descriptors on time windows and on the application of machine learning algorithms for classifying each window as belonging or not to a phase A of CAP.

The Sleep Disorders Center at Parma University uses a simple PC-based system, which allows us to mark the beginning and end of each phase A manually (classifying subtypes A1, A2, or A3 and respecting the time range of 2–60 seconds). An algorithm calculates automatically the intervals between the identified A phases, avoiding manual quantification of the B phases of CAP. If the interval between two successive A phases is ≤60 seconds, the program includes the A phases within the CAP sequence. If the interval is more than 60 seconds, the period is scored as non-CAP. After the scoring of sleep macrostructure, the process of phase A identification requires an extra time of approximately 30 minutes: this procedure consumes financial resources. However, scoring CAP can provide additional value to our knowledge and shed rewarding light on a number of sleep-related mechanisms: (1) Sleep physiology. (2) Arousals and EEG activation patterns. (3) Role of sleep microstructure beyond conventional PSG variables. (4) Neurophysiologic bases of sleep misperception. (5) Sleep markers of cognitive processes. (6) Effects of hypnotic drugs and CPAP treatment. (7) Modulation during sleep of epileptic phenomena, of movement and respiratory events, and of behavioral patterns. (8) Connection between EEG activation and autonomic arousals. (9) The pillars of sleep quality: duration, intensity, continuity, and stability. (10) Sleep resilience.

The new sleep drugs in the pipeline, acting on alternative targets (melatonin, orexin, serotonin), need a new cultural framework, which cannot be limited to sleep latency and sleep duration but needs to incorporate the issue of sleep and vegetative stability. So far, these objectives have been neglected by most clinical trials for drug approval. The AASM Clinical Practice Guideline for the Pharmacological Treatment of Chronic Insomnia states:

> In addition to the variability in outcome measures reported, there are a number of critical unresolved issues regarding evaluating the efficacy of treatments for chronic insomnia. One is the relative importance of subjective versus objective data. Another is whether metrics of sleep quality, whether they be subjective or objective (e.g. analysis of the microstructure of sleep or related physiologic parameters), are perhaps more pertinent than measures of sleep latency, total sleep time and wake after sleep onset.[38]

CAP TOPOGRAPHY

The brain topography of CAP it still fragmentary because of the limited amount of dedicated studies. An EEG-based source-analysis investigation related CAP distribution to several brain areas, including frontal, midline, and occipito-parietal cortices.[39] Specifically, CAP subtypes A1 present higher amplitude over anterior brain areas, whereas subtypes A2 and A3 dominate over parieto-occipital lobes.

Even if CAP is basically an electrical phenomena, its association with marked hemodynamic changes permit one to use metabolic investigation to indirectly analyze its dynamics in the human brain. A near-infrared spectroscopy study revealed a significant increase in prefrontal cortex blood oxygenation and volume during CAP phases A, with higher changes during subtypes A2 and A3, followed by overall decrease during phase B.[40]

A recently published EEG-fMRI analysis on patients with epilepsy demonstrated the existence of a positive correlation between blood oxygen level dependent (BOLD) changes and CAP-A phase involving bilaterally the insula, the middle cingulate gyrus, and the basal forebrain[41]: (1) the insula represents a key multimodal structure for stimuli processing and is involved in switching between rest and alert brain states; (2) the cingulate cortex is involved in the generation of common sleep graphoelements such as KC and vertex waves; and (3) the basal forebrain modulates cholinergic and GABAergic circuits necessary to sleep-wake control. Given the role of these three brain areas in the sleep-wake cycle, in addition to the spreading of paroxysmal discharges, their involvement in epileptic sleep is worthy of attention. The lack of technical homogeneity between studies does not allow a direct comparison between results, and there is urgent need for a unified methodological approach. However, the growth of skyrocketing procedures is building a promising scenario for research, and epilepsy, given its association with sleep fragmentation, could intriguingly be explored as a "disease model" to analyze the potential relation between EEG sleep microstructure and anatomic cerebral alterations.

CAP AUTOMATED ANALYSIS

There is compelling evidence that CAP scoring provides more accurate information than conventional sleep measures. However, its visual analysis is heavily demanding and time-consuming. This can compromise extensive utilization of the method. In other words, only the availability of an adequate system for automatic detection of CAP recognition can make it an easily exploitable tool. The availability of practical and reliable automated methods for CAP detection is desirable, and, so far, numerous algorithms dedicated to the automatic detection of CAP sequences have been proposed, with variable degrees of sensitivity and specificity.

Machine learning is a powerful mathematical branch of artificial intelligence able to "learn" from experience and data, and today is widely used in neuroscience to support the clinician's workup or for research purposes. Most of the published methods proposing machine learning approaches extract signal features from PSG data and then feed an automated classifier to obtain CAP identification. The vast majority of the algorithms provide a basic distinction between CAP phase A and phase B using signal information, like frequency bands amplitude thresholds, based either on raw signal amplitude[42,43] or wavelet transform decomposition of the signal.[44] Other methods calculate the likelihood synchronization (LS) between different EEG channels and use it as a measure for CAP phase A1 detection. PSG features that can support CAP detection include differential variance, Teager energy operator, Lempel-Ziv complexity, Shannon entropy, and log-energy entropy.[45,46] In most cases, the main output is a distinction between CAP phase A and phase B, and only few methods try to develop a multiclass discriminant classification to describe CAP sequences with all its subtypes. In this context, support vector machines (SVMs) have been suggested as the most trustworthy method for the identification and discrimination of all CAP components.[47,48] Given that machine learning approaches gain accuracy with large data sets, the creation of large open-source archives, including different sleep disorders, together with sleep recordings collected from healthy individuals of various ages, is probably the most reliable achievement to develop a reliable automated toolbox for CAP detection.

CONCLUSIONS

For decades, assessment of CAP parameters has been mostly oriented toward situational conditions and sleep disorders characterized by increased amounts of CAP rate[49,50] (Table 198.1). Potential treatment aimed at recovering physiologic levels of sleep instability. The more recent studies on neurodevelopment and neurogenerative diseases, where CAP rate and A1 subtypes are significantly curtailed (Table 198.1), open new perspectives on the management of CAP-related disorders that require solutions that increase and not reduce the ongoing amounts of unstable sleep. This makes the future extremely stimulating.

CLINICAL PEARLS

- The AASM definition and rules for scoring arousal mostly target EEG alpha intrusion into sleep. However, autonomic and/or behavioral activation during sleep can be associated with KCs and delta bursts.
- Conventional EEG arousals can be conceptualized as the tip of an iceberg composed of other, more subtle, but equally powerful, activating events, often organized in the CAP.
- The concept of instability is a basic issue of all complex systems and supports the dynamics of biologic variability. Within certain ranges, instability accompanies the stage transitions maintaining in-phase both the EEG and autonomic functions through regular fluctuations.
- CAP is the EEG marker of NREM sleep instability. By contrast, non-CAP translates to a condition of stable sleep.
- CAP is the "buffer system" that warrants flexible and adaptive adjustments to internal and external inputs.
- The arousal response is a continuous modulated phenomenon lying within a spectrum of EEG variability expressed by the phase A subtypes of CAP.
- EEG segmentation seems to be a useful tool for the automatic scoring of CAP.

SUMMARY

Sleep is a dynamic process with a self-regulating character. The nightly recurring sleep process is organized into consecutive cycles in which the sequence of NREM stages and the alternation between NREM and REM sleep show a quite stable tendency and a largely predictable pattern. These constraints produce the macrostructural development of sleep. However, transient EEG changes can interact with the expected development of sleep and ensure adaptation to both internal and external conditions. Arousals and CAP represent rapid adaptive adjustments of vigilance during sleep. Failure of these compensatory processes contributes to sleep disorders and nonrestorative sleep. The CAP parameters, the role of CAP in the dynamic organization of sleep, the clinical applications of CAP, and the available methods for the automatic quantification of CAP measures are detailed.

SELECTED READINGS

Benbir Senel G, Ozcelik EU, Karadeniz D. Cyclic alternating pattern analysis in periodic leg movements in sleep in patients with obstructive sleep apnea syndrome before and after positive airway pressure treatment [published online ahead of print, 2020 May 26]. *J Clin Neurophysiol.* 2020. https://doi.org/10.1097/WNP.0000000000000704.

Ferri R, Bruni O, Miano S, Terzano MG. Topographic mapping of the spectral components of the Cyclic Alternating Pattern (CAP). *Sleep Med.* 2005;6:29–36.

Halasz P, Terzano MG, Parrino L, Bodisz R. The nature of arousal in sleep. *J Sleep Res.* 2004;13:1–23.

Hartmann S, Bruni O, Ferri R, Redline S, Baumert M. Characterization of cyclic alternating pattern during sleep in older men and women using large population studies. *Sleep.* 2020;43(7):zsaa016.

Hartmann S, Bruni O, Ferri R, Redline S, Baumert M. Cyclic alternating pattern in children with obstructive sleep apnea and its relationship with adenotonsillectomy, behavior, cognition, and quality of life. *Sleep.* 2021;44(1):zsaa145.

Mariani S, Grassi A, Mendez MO, et al. EEG segmentation for improving automatic CAP detection. *Clin Neurophysiol.* 2013;124:1815–1823.

Parrino L. Down the rabbit-hole: new perspectives from stereo-EEG in the investigation of sleep, nocturnal epilepsy and parasomnias. *Sleep Med Rev.* 2015;25:1–3.

Parrino L, Ferri R, Bruni O, Terzano MG. Cyclic Alternating Pattern (CAP): the marker of sleep instability. *Sleep Med Rev.* 2012;16:27–45.

Parrino L, Halasz P, Tassinari CA, Terzano MG. CAP, epilepsy and motor events during sleep: the unifying role of arousal. *Sleep Med Rev.* 2006;10:267–285.

Parrino L, Smerieri A, Rossi M, Terzano MG. Relationship of slow and rapid EEG components of CAP to ASDA arousals in normal sleep. *Sleep.* 2001;24:881–885.

Terzano MG, Mancia D, Salati MR, et al. The cyclic alternating pattern as a physiologic component of normal NREM. *Sleep.* 1985;8:137–145.

Terzano MG, Parrino L, Smerieri A, et al. Atlas, rules, and recording techniques for the scoring of Cyclic Alternating Pattern (CAP) in human sleep. *Sleep Med.* 2001;2:537–553.

Terzano MG, Parrino L, Smerieri A, et al. CAP and arousals are involved in the homeostatic and ultradian sleep processes. *J Sleep Res.* 2005;4:359–368.

Thomas RJ. Arousals in sleep-disordered breathing: patterns and implications. *Sleep.* 2003;26:1042–1047.

A complete reference list can be found online at ExpertConsult.com.

Chapter 199

Neurologic Monitoring Techniques

Beth A. Malow

Chapter Highlights

- This chapter focuses on the methodology and indications for video-electroencephalography–polysomnography in the diagnosis of nocturnal events. Techniques and approaches described include routine electroencephalography (EEG), short-term continuous video-EEG monitoring, long-term continuous video-EEG monitoring, and ambulatory monitoring.
- The EEG may show either a rhythmic evolving discharge characteristic of an epileptic seizure or interictal epileptiform discharges that occur apart from epileptic seizures. Lack of an EEG change, however, does not exclude some types of epilepsy, particularly those of frontal lobe origin.
- Included in this chapter are several case examples illustrating why a particular monitoring technique is selected for a specific clinical situation.

OVERVIEW

Nocturnal spells often present diagnostic problems in sleep medicine because the history alone may not provide sufficient information to differentiate among the various diagnostic possibilities. Standard polysomnography (PSG) is helpful in defining the state and stage of sleep from which such nocturnal spells emerge, but its diagnostic capability is limited because behavioral analysis often is not included, and only a certain number of channels are devoted to electroencephalography (EEG). These shortcomings are especially pertinent when evaluating suspected nocturnal epileptic seizures, defined by behavioral and motor manifestations in addition to EEG criteria.[1] Both behavioral and EEG analyses are critical for characterizing epileptic seizures and for distinguishing them from parasomnias.

The behavioral and EEG manifestations of nocturnal spells caused by parasomnias, neurologic disorders, and psychiatric disorders can be characterized more precisely by combining standard PSG with video recordings and extensive (comprising 12 or more channels) EEG montages.[2] The focus of this chapter is on the methodology and indications for video-EEG–PSG (V-EEG-PSG) in the diagnosis of nocturnal events. Specific techniques and approaches that are described include routine EEG, short-term continuous video-EEG monitoring (STM), long-term continuous video-EEG monitoring (LTM), and ambulatory monitoring.

METHODOLOGY

Technical Aspects of Electroencephalography

The EEG measures the difference in electrical potential between electrode pairs placed on the scalp. These signals, reflecting synchronous postsynaptic potentials in large groups of neurons, are amplified and filtered to produce a recording.[3] The *international 10-20 system* of EEG electrode placement is customarily used, in which "10-20" refers to 10% and 20% of the distances between standard cranial landmarks[4,5] (Figure 199.1). In this system, each electrode site is identified with a letter representing the underlying region of the brain and with a number indicating a specific position above that region, with odd numbers indicating the left hemisphere and even numbers indicating the right hemisphere (e.g., T3 represents a left midtemporal electrode).

Each recording channel is derived from the signals from a pair of electrodes, and several pairs of electrodes, or derivations, are combined to form a *montage.* Montages may be either referential or bipolar. In *referential* montages, one of the electrodes in each pair is connected to a common electrode (e.g., channel 1: Fp1-A1; channel 2: F7-A1; channel 3: T3-A1; channel 4: T5-A1; channel 5: O1-A1). In *bipolar* montages, there is no common electrode. Bipolar montages usually are arranged in a chain with the same electrode in adjacent derivations (e.g., channel 1: Fp1-F7; channel 2: F7-T3; channel 3: T3-T5; channel 4: T5-01).

The EEG montages used in a combined EEG-PSG study depend on the clinical indication and the number of channels available for recording (Table 199.1). The channels suggested in this chapter for inclusion in such studies are in addition to those recommended by the American Academy of Sleep Medicine for the scoring of sleep stages.[6] Physicians and technicians using EEG monitoring techniques require a solid knowledge of the principles of EEG recording and interpretation. Additional information regarding EEG methodology is available in a standard EEG textbook.[3]

Computerized digital EEG-PSG systems facilitate the review of large amounts of the acquired data by displaying scoring and event information in a format that allows the user to, for example, click on the stage or event of interest and bring up the corresponding EEG-PSG segment.

The recording may be viewed at a variety of display settings. Filters, sensitivities, and montages may be adjusted to characterize events of interest and to help distinguish abnormalities from artifacts or normal variants. For example,

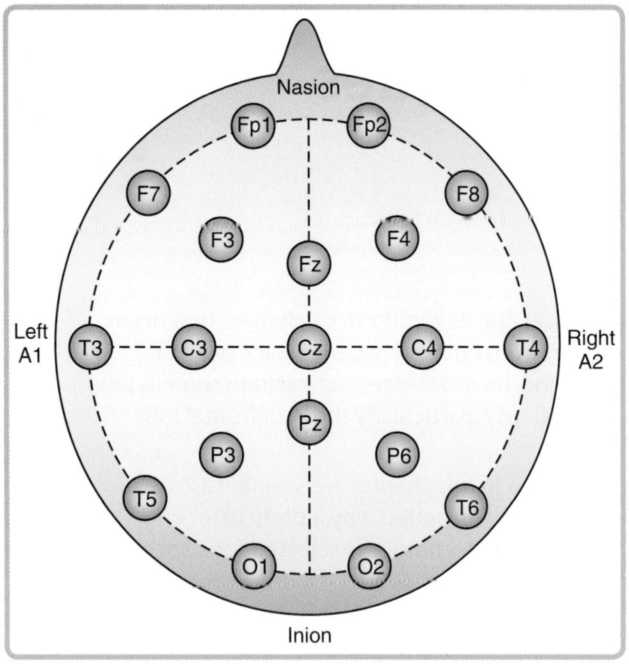

Figure 199.1 Standard international 10-20 electrode placement: Electrodes are placed at 10% or 20% of the distances between standard cranial landmarks. (From Keenan SA. Polysomnographic technique: an overview. In: Chokroverty S, editor. *Sleep disorders medicine.* Boston: Butterworth-Heinemann; 1994, p. 84.)

Table 199.1 Sample Attended Electroencephalographic Montages

Number of Available Channels	Montage
8	F7-T3, T3-T5, T5-O1, F8-T4, T4-T6, T6-O2, F3-C3, F4-C4
10	Fp1-F7, F7-T3, T3-T5, T5-O1, Fp2-F8, F8-T4, T4-T6, T6-O2, F3-C3, F4-C4
12	Fp1-F7, F7-T3, T3-T5, T5-O1, Fp2-F8, F8-T4, T4-T6, T6-O2, F3-C3, C3-P3, F4-C4, C4-P4
14	Fp1-F7, F7-T3, T3-T5, T5-O1, Fp2-F8, F8-T4, T4-T6, T6-O2, F3-C3, C3-P3, P3-O1, F4-C4, C4-P4, P4-O2
16	Fp1-F7, F7-T3, T3-T5, T5-O1, Fp2-F8, F8-T4, T4-T6, T6-O2, Fp1-F3, F3-C3, C3-P3, P3-O1, Fp2-F4, F4-C4, C4-P4, P4-O2
18	Fp1-F7, F7-T3, T3-T5, T5-O1, Fp2-F8, F8-T4, T4-T6, T6-O2, Fp1-F3, F3-C3, C3-P3, P3-O1, Fp2-F4, F4-C4, C4-P4, P4-O2, Fz-Cz, Cz-Pz
24	Fp1-F7, F7-T3, T3-T5, T5-O1, Fp2-F8, F8-T4, T4-T6, T6-O2, Fp1-F3, F3-C3, C3-P3, P3-O1, Fp2-F4, F4-C4, C4-P4, P4-O2, Fz-Cz, Cz-Pz, T1-T3, T3-C3, C3-Cz, Cz-C4, C4-T4, T4-T2

certain montages can more easily identify and distinguish artifacts from interictal epileptiform discharges (IEDs), defined as epileptic-type activity occurring between seizures. Digital EEG enhances the detection and review of IEDs by allowing for remontaging (displaying data in a different montage that may better reveal such activity), changing the display settings that influence temporal resolution, and isolating specific channels for review (Figure 199.2). For example, by altering the display settings, synchronous delta or theta activity characteristic of disorders of arousal from non–rapid eye movement (NREM) sleep may be more easily distinguished from spike-wave activity or from an evolving ictal (seizure) pattern characteristic of an epileptic seizure disorder.

Several digital EEG-PSG systems share a common platform with epilepsy monitoring systems, allowing data obtained during a PSG study to be analyzed by IED detection programs. Conversely, a study performed in the epilepsy-monitoring unit can be enhanced through addition of electrooculogram (EOG) and chin electromyogram (EMG) electrodes to score sleep and to determine the stage of sleep that precedes a particular event. This determination can be diagnostic in the case of distinguishing dissociative events, which rarely occur during sleep,[7] from epileptic seizures, which can occur during sleep or wakefulness.

Daytime Electroencephalography

Daytime EEG is used to look for IEDs, to support the diagnosis of a seizure disorder in many clinical settings.[3] In addition to the electrode placements listed earlier, central (Fz, Cz, Pz) and ear (A1, A2) electrodes are included. Nasopharyngeal electrodes, although used in the past, are not recommended, because they are uncomfortable, are prone to artifact, and rarely provide additional information. The activating techniques of hyperventilation and intermittent photic stimulation are routinely performed and can bring out focal asymmetries or epileptiform activity.

Although seizures are not uniformly recorded during a routine EEG, focal IEDs or generalized spike-and-wave discharges may be observed and can assist in the classification of an epileptic syndrome as partial or generalized. The location of IEDs, determined with the use of an extended EEG montage, can clarify the nature of the epilepsy syndrome and its prognosis.[8] For example, benign epilepsy of childhood with centrotemporal spikes carries an excellent prognosis (Figure 199.3). By contrast, some temporal lobe IEDs may be refractory to medical treatment, and affected patients can become candidates for epilepsy surgery.

Daytime studies performed while the patient is asleep for at least a portion of the recording increase the yield of finding abnormalities, because in many patients, IEDs are more common in drowsiness and NREM sleep. Stage N2 sleep is usually, but not always, recorded on the routine EEG, whereas stage N3 sleep and rapid eye movement (REM) sleep are rarely recorded. When the routine EEG does not show IEDs and the clinical picture is highly suggestive of seizures, a sleep-deprived EEG improves the yield of finding epileptiform activity, at least in part because sleep is more likely to be recorded. Digital EEG recordings permit the viewing of a segment of the EEG in a variety of montages and speeds, which can help distinguish an IED from an artifact.

Video-Electroencephalography–Polysomnography

When the patient's history is not sufficient to make a reasonably confident diagnosis based on nocturnal spells

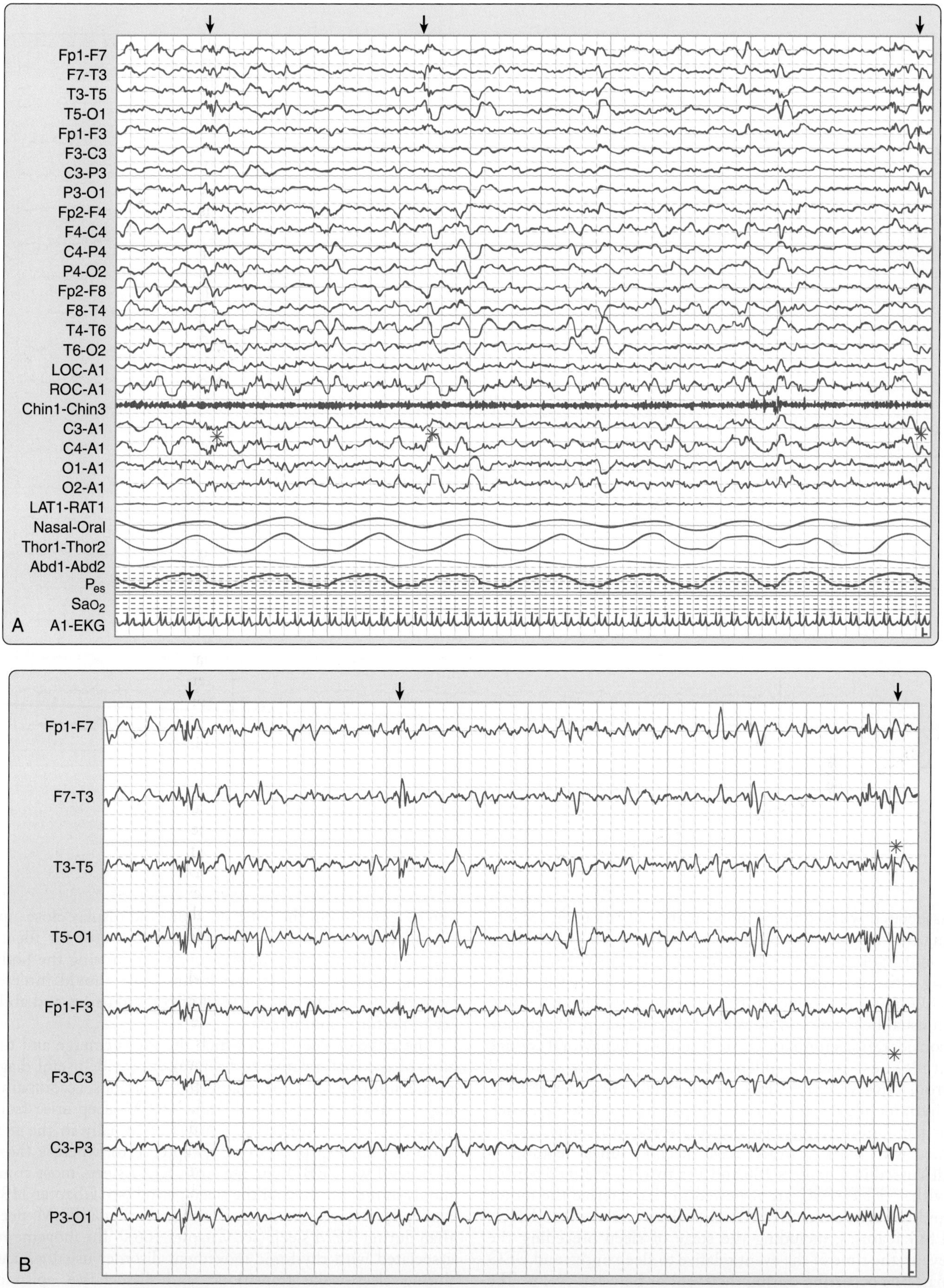

Figure 199.2 Use of different montages to enhance the review of interictal epileptiform discharges (IEDs). **A,** Left temporally dominant IEDs (*arrows*) on an extended electroencephalogram (EEG) montage that are not apparent in the central-to-ear channels (*asterisks*). **B,** Digital EEG allows the interpreter to select the relevant left temporal and parasagittal channels for review. The *arrows* highlight IEDs with phase reversals (*asterisks*) at T3 and F3, indicating maximal negativity at these electrodes, which defines the approximate location of the epileptic region. Both are 30-second epochs. Calibration symbol (*bottom right*): 100 μV.

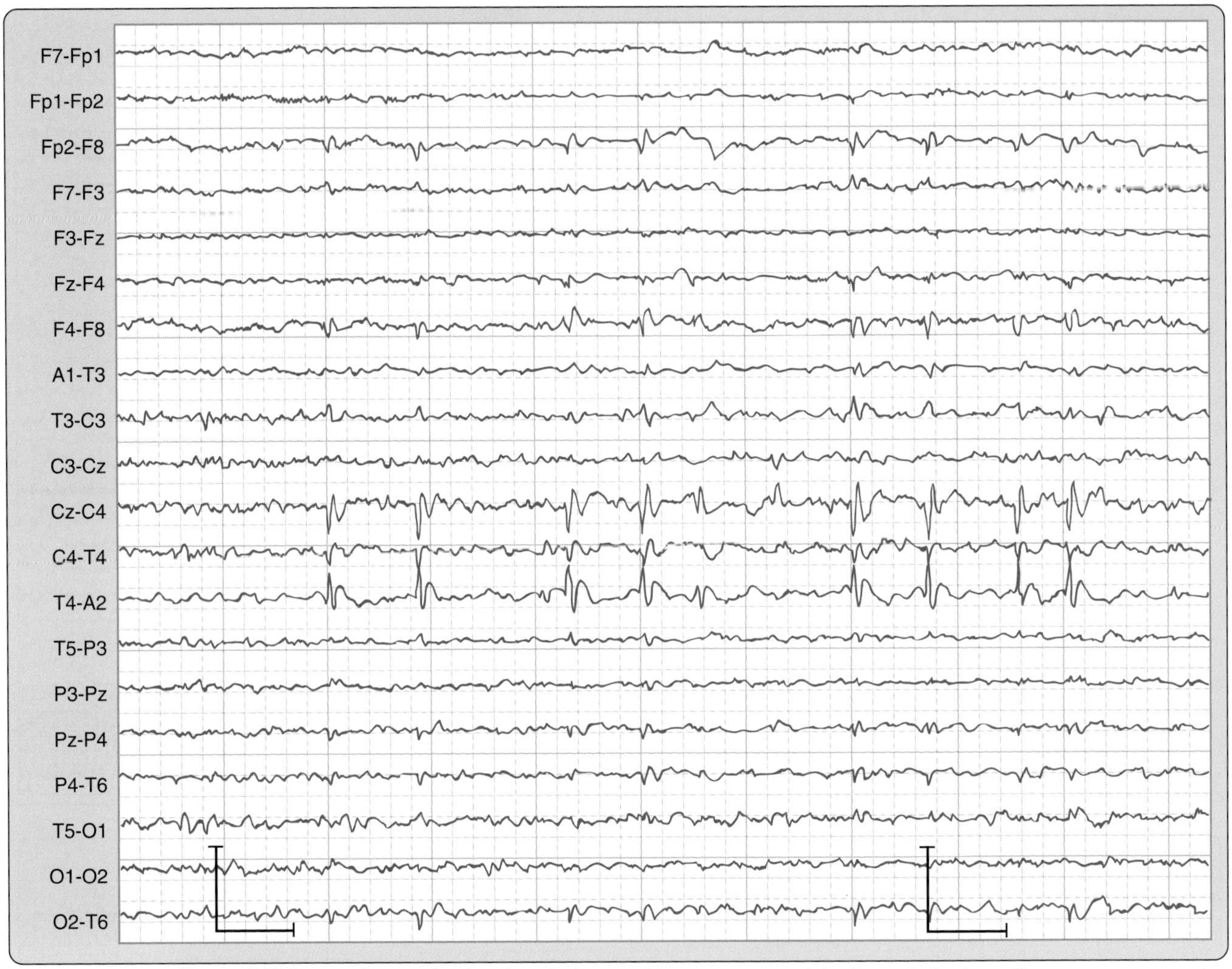

Figure 199.3 Runs of interictal epileptiform discharges with a centrotemporal dominance in benign epilepsy of childhood with centrotemporal spikes. The bipolar montage readily demonstrates peak negativity at the C4 and T4 electrodes. Such localization is not possible with electroencephalogram (EEG) montages commonly used with standard polysomnography (PSG). Calibration symbol: 500 μV, 1 second. (From Malow BA. Sleep and epilepsy. *Neurol Clin.* 1996;14:774.)

associated with complex movements and behavior, recording the sleep-related event in question may allow definitive confirmation. V-EEG-PSG, which combines video recording with an extended EEG montage and with other standard PSG physiologic monitoring, is useful in characterizing unusual behavior and movements during sleep. Diagnostic considerations for patients with complex behavioral actions at night can include epileptic seizures, disorders of arousal from NREM sleep, REM sleep behavior disorder (RBD), rhythmic movement disorder, or psychiatric disorders such as panic disorder or dissociative disorder. Episodes associated with these disorders have specific clinical features as discussed in Chapters 106 and 115 to 120. Events recorded with V-EEG-PSG are reviewed to characterize the motor and behavioral manifestations of the event and the EEG-PSG features, including the stage of sleep preceding the event, the time of the event relative to sleep onset, and EEG patterns occurring during the event or between events. The time-locked video can be reviewed second by second along with the EEG PSG recording. Infrared cameras are recommended for recording nighttime events. Movable cameras can be mounted in the patient's room and display close-ups or full-body views. Double cameras are useful for focusing on the face while simultaneously monitoring the body. During recorded events, the technologist should interact with the patient to test for level of consciousness and ability to perform commands.

The stage of sleep from which the spells emerge and the time of the spell relative to sleep onset provide useful diagnostic information. For example, the actions accompanying the disorders of arousal from NREM sleep arise from stage N3 or sometimes stage N2 sleep, usually in the first third of the sleep period (see Chapter 116), whereas those associated with RBD emerge from REM sleep, most commonly in the last third of the sleep period (see Chapter 118). Epileptic seizures are more common during NREM sleep than during REM sleep (see Chapter 106).[9] The movements associated with rhythmic movement disorder usually occur during sleep-wake transitions, and dissociative episodes emerge from wakefulness. Nocturnal panic attacks occur from NREM sleep, usually at the transition from stage N2 to stage N3.[10]

If complex partial seizures are a diagnostic consideration, the EEG montage should emphasize the use of electrodes placed over the temporal lobes (e.g., F7, T1, T3, T5). If benign childhood epilepsy with centrotemporal spikes is a consideration, the montage should include the parasagittal region (e.g., C3, C4). The specific montage that is used depends on the number of channels available for EEG. Sample montages for 8, 10, 12, 14, 16, 19, and 24 channels are shown in Table 199.1.

The following montage of 16 electrodes in anterior-to-posterior chains provides excellent coverage for suspected seizures:

- Left temporal: Fp1-F7, F7-T3, T3-T5, and T5-O1
- Left parasagittal: Fp1-F3, F3-C3, C3-P3, and P3-O1
- Right parasagittal: Fp2-F4, F4-C4, C4-P4, and P4-O2
- Right temporal: Fp2-F8, F8-T4, T4-T6, and T6-O2

This montage allows the evaluation of interictal and ictal activity during sleep. Two additional anterior temporal electrodes, T1 and T2, may be added because they are particularly useful for detecting anterior temporal IEDs. In one study comparing abbreviated EEG montages with a standard 18-channel bipolar montage, seizures were more readily distinguished from arousal patterns using 7- and 18-EEG channel montages compared with 4-channel EEG records.[11]

Short-Term and Long-Term Monitoring

When the history suggests frequent daytime spells or spells occurring during daytime naps, STM, a video-EEG recording, typically obtained in an EEG or sleep laboratory for 6 to 8 hours during the day, may be helpful. The value of such studies for assessing patients with strictly nocturnal spells, however, is limited. Occasionally, STM is useful if sleep attacks—spells of diminished responsiveness due to sleepiness—are included in the differential diagnosis of daytime spells.

Unfortunately, one or two overnight sleep studies may fail to capture and characterize spells. LTM, an extension of STM that allows continuous recordings for up to several weeks, is used mainly for patients with known or suspected seizures.[12] For patients taking antiepileptic medications, these drugs may be tapered and discontinued during LTM; intermittent sleep deprivation also is commonly used to facilitate spells. Because frequent seizures or status epilepticus can occur in epileptic patients discontinuing medication, LTM is generally performed in a hospital setting, usually a specialized epilepsy-monitoring laboratory.

The lack of ictal activity during a clinical event does not exclude a seizure, particularly if awareness is preserved during the clinical event (e.g., a simple partial seizure) or if the event originates in the frontal lobe. Ictal activity may be apparent only with intracranial electrodes, such as depth electrodes that penetrate the brain parenchyma, subdural strips, and subdural grids.[13] These invasive electrodes are rarely are used to diagnose nocturnal spells because of the risks of infection and hemorrhage and typically are reserved for patients who require localization of epileptic foci before surgical resection and in whom scalp recordings are inconclusive. If an ictal pattern is not recorded but clinical seizures are strongly suspected on the basis of the history and stereotypical behavioral spells recorded on videotape, an empiric trial of an antiepileptic medication may be appropriate.

Ambulatory Monitoring

Ambulatory monitoring combines the extended recording time of V-EEG-PSG with the convenience of recording in a patient's home. Several commercial products allow patients to go home with 12 or more channels of EEG electrodes and a recording device. The recording device sometimes includes video monitoring. Ambulatory recording systems may use analog or digital recorders. Patients and their bed partners are instructed to keep an activity log to document events.

The indications for ambulatory monitoring in the differential diagnosis of nocturnal events are not established. This monitoring technique appears promising for evaluating interictal epileptiform activity during sleep. Depending on the sophistication of the video recordings, ambulatory monitoring can identify some cases of epileptic seizures, NREM arousal disorders, RBD, rhythmic movement disorder, panic disorder, and dissociative disorder.

ARTIFACTS AND PITFALLS

Artifacts, which are common during sleep-related spells recorded with any of these modalities, must be distinguished from interictal and ictal epileptiform activity and from EEG activity associated with parasomnias. Although artifacts can obscure the EEG, making diagnosis more difficult, they are sometimes helpful; for example, head or body rocking artifact may be diagnostic of rhythmic movement disorder, and rhythmic myogenic artifact may support bruxism (Figure 199.4). Other examples of frequently encountered artifacts include those caused by head tremor, eye movements, and tongue movements (glossokinetic artifact). Associated rhythmic activities can resemble ictal EEG patterns.

Pitfalls in interpreting recorded events are common; the inexperienced interpreter can mistakenly identify an artifact as EEG activity characteristic of seizures or parasomnias. When the clinician is in doubt about an EEG PSG pattern, a trained electroencephalographer should be consulted. Apart from artifacts, many other normal physiologic variants may be mistaken for epileptic activity; these include positive occipital sharp transients of sleep (see Figure 199.4); frequent and sharply contoured vertex waves, particularly in young patients (Figure 199.5); sawtooth waves; benign epileptiform transients of sleep; wicket spikes; and rhythmic temporal theta of drowsiness.[14]

RELATIVE INDICATIONS, ADVANTAGES, DISADVANTAGES, AND LIMITATIONS

Although V-EEG-PSG and other neurologic monitoring techniques can be useful in diagnosing nocturnal events, the incremental cost compared with standard PSG necessitates that specific indications be met. Unfortunately, no standards exist for technique selection or interpreting results. Additionally, the reliability and validity of the monitoring techniques described here have not been formally studied. Likewise, the role of ambulatory EEG in monitoring parasomnias is not well defined. The indications, advantages, disadvantages, and limitations outlined here are based on my own clinical experience and those described by others.

Video-Electroencephalography–Polysomnography

Indications for V-EEG-PSG include suspected sleep-related epileptic seizures, suspected NREM arousal disorders, RBD, and suspected dissociative disorder.

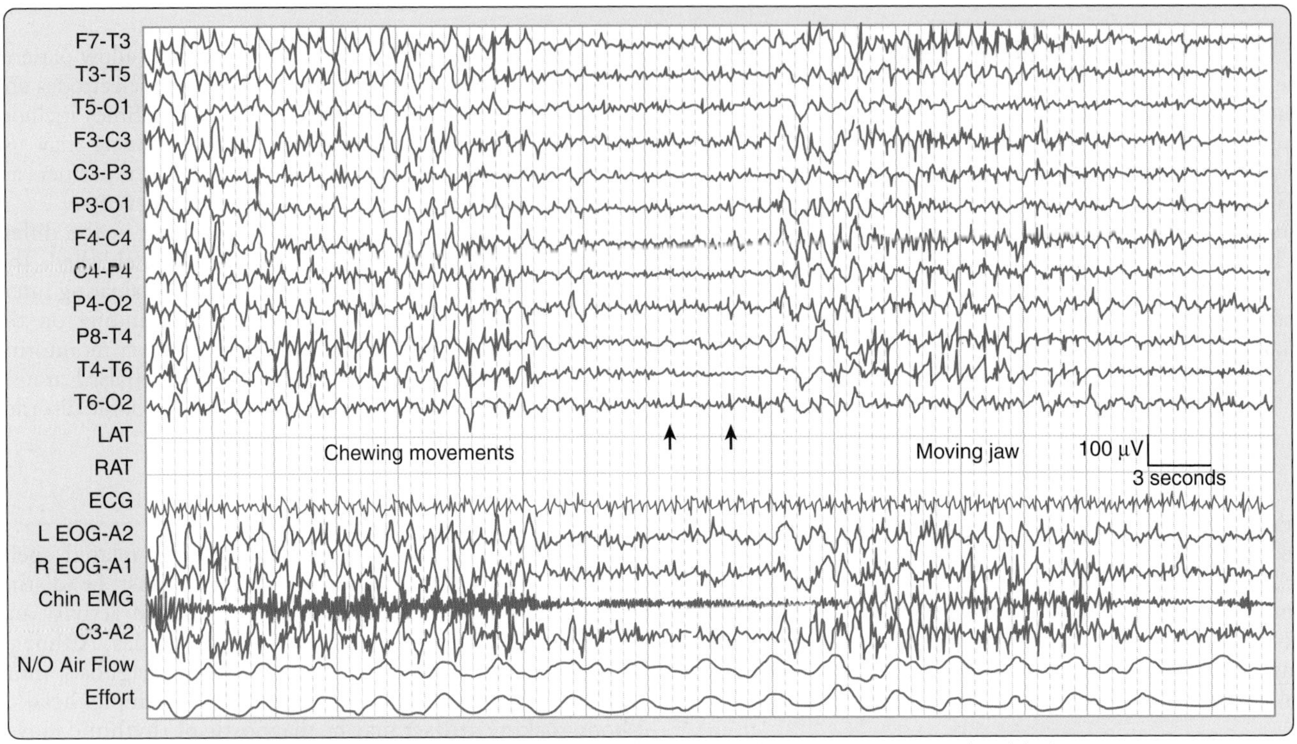

Figure 199.4 Artifacts resembling interictal epileptiform activity. Chewing movements produced by bruxism cause rhythmic activity with superimposed myogenic artifact in the electroencephalogram (EEG) channels, bearing a superficial resemblance to generalized spike-wave discharges. The *arrows* identify posterior occipital sharp transients of sleep, normal features of NREM stage 1 sleep that appear sharply contoured and may be mistaken for pathologic occipital sharp waves at the standard polysomnograph paper speed of 10 mm/second. ECG, Electrocardiogram; EMG, electromyogram; EOG, electrooculogram; LAT, left anterior tibialis; N/O, nasal-oral; RAT, right anterior tibialis.

Suspected Sleep-Related Epileptic Seizures

Although some epileptic seizures can be diagnosed based on history (e.g., generalized tonic-clonic activity witnessed by a reliable observer), most events occurring frequently and suspected to be complex partial seizures are best confirmed with V-EEG-PSG monitoring. Monitoring is especially indicated for events that include the features of thrashing, kicking, hyperventilating, head rocking, screaming, or subtle arousals from sleep; such events may represent complex partial seizures.[15] See Box 199.1.

The advantage of V-EEG-PSG over conventional PSG or EEG without video in suspected epileptic seizures is the ability to analyze stereotypical activities characteristic of epileptic seizures, in association with ictal EEG activity. Figure 199.6 shows a recording with an extended EEG montage of an epileptic seizure, illustrating a clear evolution of activity. Apart from recording epileptic seizures, PSG with an expanded EEG montage allows sampling of IEDs throughout the night. The IEDs associated with partial epilepsy usually are more prevalent in sleep, especially delta NREM sleep, than in wakefulness.[16,17] Occasionally, IEDs missed on a routine daytime EEG are detected on an overnight recording.

Frequently, suspected disorders of arousal from NREM sleep (e.g., confusional arousals, sleepwalking, and sleep terrors) can be diagnosed on the basis of history. V-EEG-PSG is indicated if behavioral features are atypical or stereotyped, multiple nightly episodes occur, onset is in adulthood, or spells do not respond to a trial of medications. An advantage of V-EEG-PSG for diagnosing NREM arousal

Box 199.1 CASE EXAMPLE 1

A 34-year-old woman with a remote history of daytime complex partial seizures presented with nightly nocturnal spells. Her husband reported that within 45 minutes of falling asleep she aroused, sat up, appeared frightened, breathed rapidly, looked around the room with a blank, wide-eyed stare, and then returned to sleep. These episodes were stereotypical and lasted less than 1 minute. She responded to his questions almost immediately and did not recall the episodes.

The differential diagnosis includes disorder of dissociative episodes, as well as epileptic seizures. Nocturnal panic disorder is unlikely, because she does not recall the episodes. REM sleep behavior disorder (RBD) is possible, but this disorder would be unusual in a young woman, usually does not cause stereotypical behavior, and rarely occurs soon after sleep onset.

Because the history was insufficient for diagnosis and because the spells were occurring nightly, video-electroencephalography–PSG (V-EEG-PSG) was performed, during which the patient exhibited several stereotypical spells arising from all stages of NREM sleep. These spells were associated with ictal discharges beginning over the right temporal lobe and consisting of rhythmic theta activity that increased in frequency and decreased in amplitude.

She was treated for complex partial seizures with carbamazepine, and the spells resolved. If this patient had been on antiepileptic medication chronically and had spells that were less frequent (e.g., once a week), an alternative approach would have been long-term continuous video-EEG monitoring (LTM) with tapering of medications to promote occurrence of seizures.

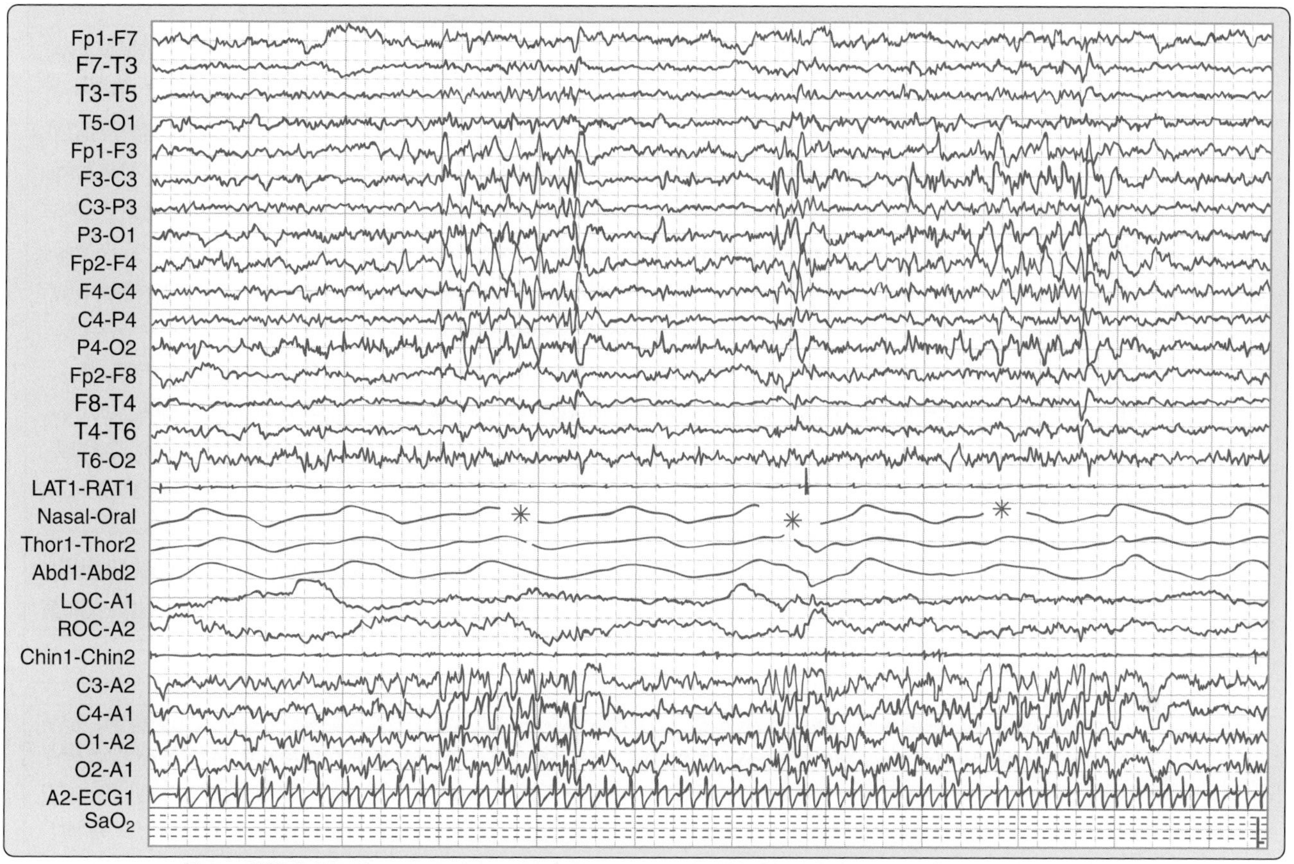

Figure 199.5 Sharply contoured vertex waves in a 6-year-old child. Although these physiologic waves resemble abnormal epileptiform activity, their morphology and distribution distinguish them from pathologic discharges. Compare with Figure 199.3. Thirty-second epoch. Calibration symbol (*bottom right*): 100 μV. ECG, Electrocardiogram; LAT, left anterior tibialis; LOC, left (electro)oculogram: RAT, right anterior tibialis; ROC, right (electro)oculogram; Sa_{O_2}, oxygen saturation.

disorders includes (1) the combination of video to characterize the event of interest, (2) sleep scoring channels to determine the stage of sleep involved, and (3) the extended EEG montage to exclude ictal EEG activity characteristic of epileptic seizures. See Box 199.2.

The V-EEG-PSG can capture a confusional arousal, night terror, or sleepwalking episode arising from delta NREM (stage N3 sleep) accompanied by synchronous delta activity (Figure 199.7). Alternatively, the V-EEG-PSG recorded during an NREM arousal event might show asynchronous delta or theta activity, synchronous theta activity, a drowsy pattern, or nonreactive alpha activity.

Box 199.2 CASE EXAMPLE 2

A 4-year-old girl had near-nightly episodes of screaming loudly with onset approximately 1 hour after falling asleep. During these episodes, her parents found her agitated and inconsolable. On rare occasions, she got out of bed and wandered out of her room. She was amnestic for these spells. An older sibling had had similar spells.

Because the history is compelling for sleep terrors, evaluation with video-electroencephalography–PSG (V-EEG-PSG) is not necessary. If any atypical features were present (e.g., automatisms or stereotypical behavior, multiple nightly episodes, or onset in adulthood) or if symptoms did not respond to treatment, a V-EEG-PSG would be warranted.

Suspected REM Sleep Behavior Disorder

Although RBD may be suspected on the basis of the history, definitive diagnosis requires capturing a behavioral event on a video recording or demonstrating abnormal muscle tone or excessive limb movements during REM sleep (see Chapter 118). The advantage of V-EEG-PSG is that video is combined with sleep staging to identify REM, and an extended EEG montage is used to exclude ictal EEG activity.

Suspected Dissociative Disorder

Dissociative episodes and other psychogenic spells occur during wakefulness, although the patient might appear to be asleep and might believe that he or she is asleep.[7] Because the manifestations of dissociative episodes can be quite bizarre and include thrashing, screaming, or bicycling movements, it often is impossible to distinguish these spells from epileptic seizures or parasomnias from the history alone. When nocturnal psychogenic episodes are suspected, V-EEG-PSG is advantageous in documenting the behavior of the patient, the presence of waking background EEG activity preceding onset of the spells, and the absence of ictal EEG activity.

The major disadvantage of V-EEG-PSG in the evaluation of suspected epileptic seizures, parasomnias, and dissociative disorders is the cost of the study. Additional technologist time is needed to place an extended EEG montage and to continuously observe patients throughout the study. In addition, physicians must review each spell to assess behavior and EEG patterns.

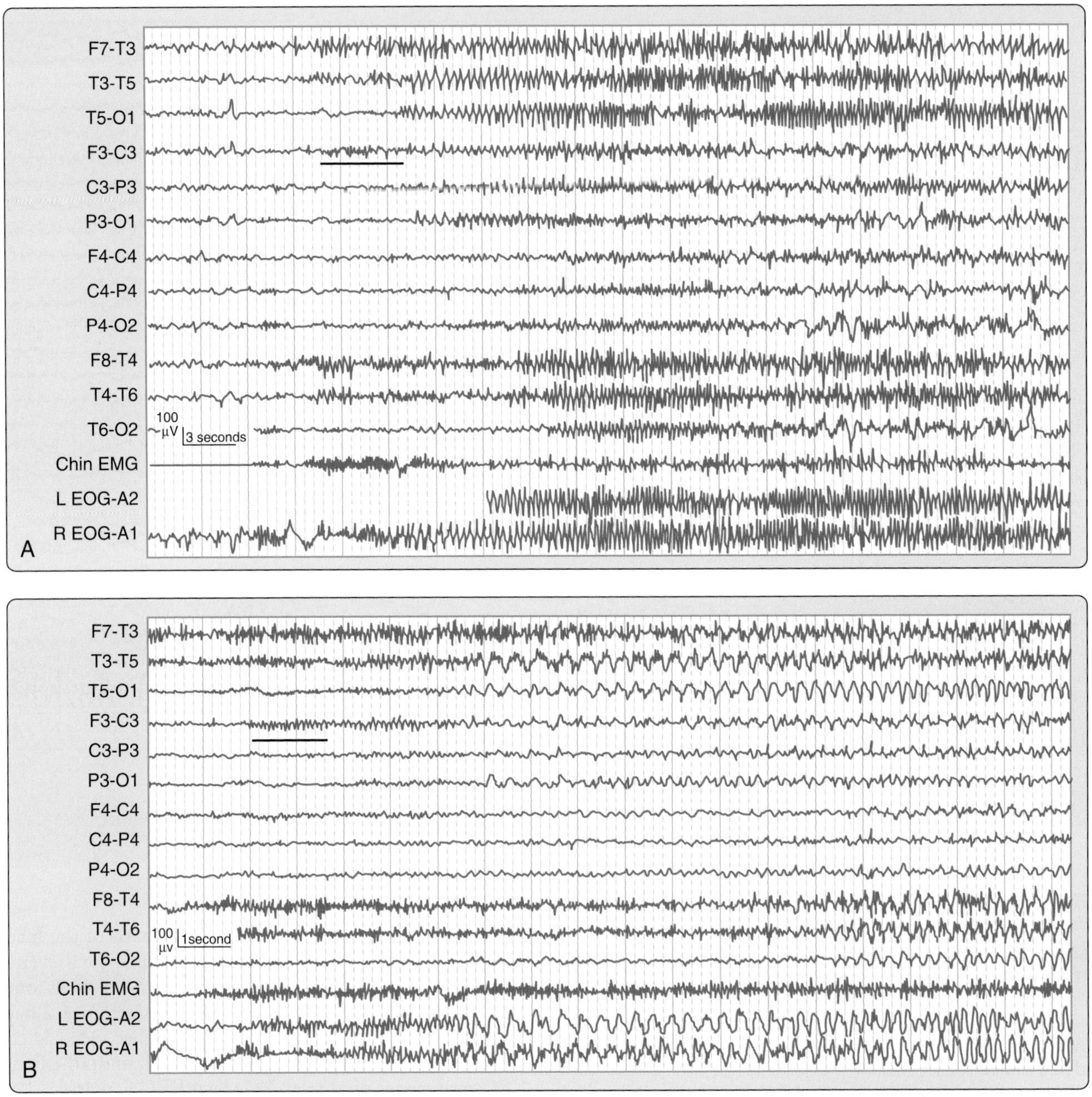

Figure 199.6 Partial seizure beginning during NREM sleep. **A,** Polysomnogram recorded at 10 mm/second paper speed. Clinically, the seizure began with an abrupt arousal, followed by turning of head and eyes to the left and movements of the arms beneath the bedclothes. On the electroencephalogram (EEG), an initial reduction in voltage is followed by a progressive increase in the amplitude of the ictal discharge over the left hemisphere, with spread to the right hemisphere derivations. The *underlined activity* from the F3-C3 derivation appears to be muscle artifact; however, in **B,** at 30 mm/second paper speed, it is clear that the same *underlined segment* is the initial focal surface representation of the ictal discharge. Additional polysomnographic measures, recorded on channels 16 to 21, are not shown. EMG, Electromyogram; EOG, electrooculogram. (Modified from Aldrich MS, Jahnke B. Diagnostic value of video-EEG polysomnography. *Neurology* 1991;41:1060–6.)

The V-EEG-PSG also has diagnostic limitations. The EEG recorded during a spell might not demonstrate an abnormality. Because epileptic seizures can lack surface EEG correlates, the absence of surface ictal EEG activity does not ensure that an epileptic seizure has not occurred. In addition, it can be difficult to differentiate an ictal EEG seizure pattern (which consists of rhythmic activity that evolves in frequency and amplitude) from the synchronous delta or theta activity or diffuse alpha activity occurring during an NREM arousal disorder. The best-developed portion of the ictal EEG pattern may be rhythmic delta or theta without a clear evolution, seizures can have bilateral onsets, seizures can arise from delta NREM sleep, and muscle or movement artifact can obscure the EEG. Two consecutive nights of V-EEG-PSG often are scheduled so that if no events are captured on the first night, the second night is available for study.

Daytime Electroencephalography

The advantage of daytime EEG over V-EEG-PSG, standard PSG, or any of the other monitoring techniques is

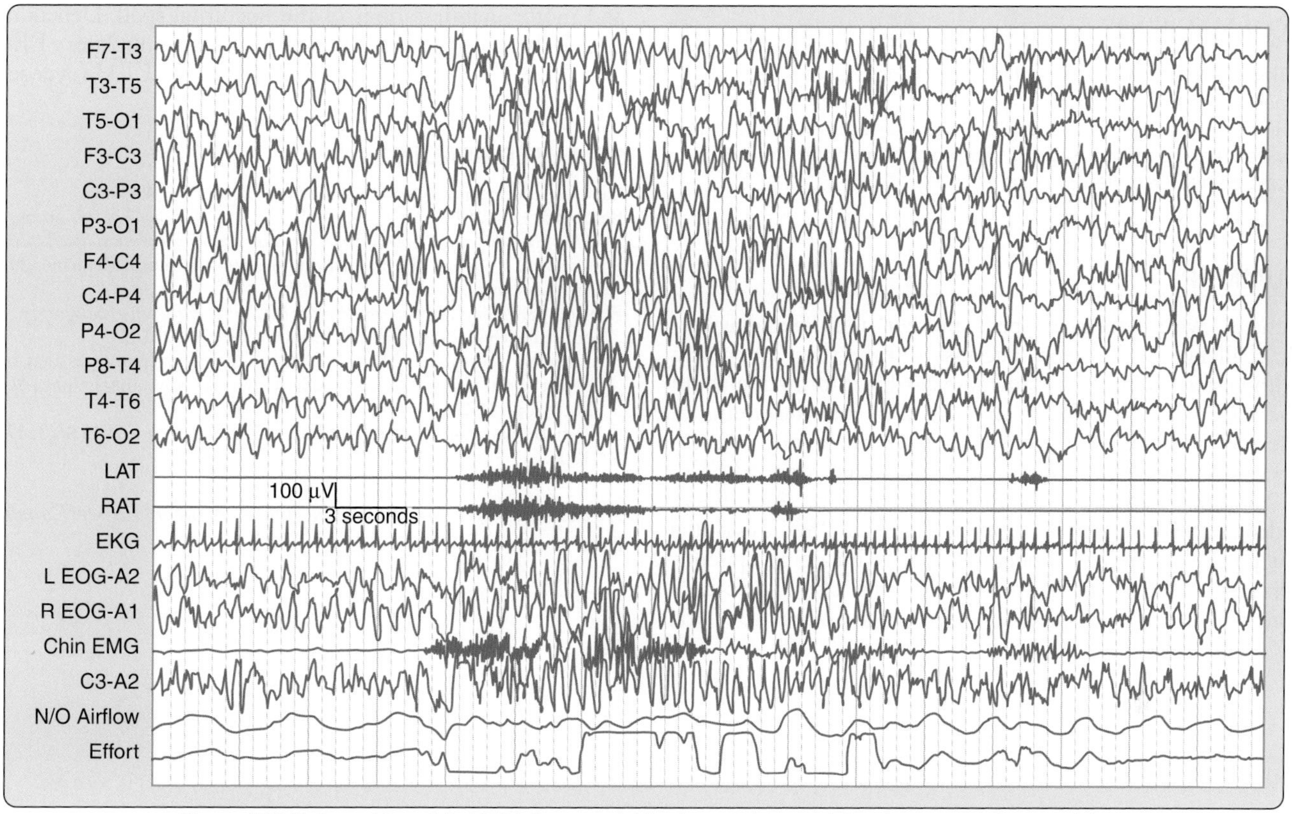

Figure 199.7 Arousal from delta NREM sleep in a child with an NREM arousal disorder. Note synchronous delta activity during arousal from delta NREM sleep, associated with left anterior tibialis (LAT) and right anterior tibialis (RAT) electromyogram (EMG) activity and a tonic increase in chin EMG. In contrast with the EEG of an epileptic seizure, the delta activity does not evolve in amplitude or frequency. EOG, Electrooculogram.

its brief recording time and low cost. This advantage, however, depends on an event occurring. The disadvantage is that spells, particularly they are sleep-related, are rarely captured. When the history is strongly suggestive of epileptic seizures, a routine EEG can demonstrate epileptic activity as supportive evidence of epilepsy. However, IEDs are not the equivalent of epileptic seizures and may be present in patients without epilepsy, such as those occurring in relatives of patients with benign childhood epilepsy with centrotemporal spikes. Conversely, patients with epilepsy might not have IEDs during EEG recordings. In addition, patients with epilepsy can have coexisting parasomnias. Therefore in the absence of a compelling history, the occurrence of abnormal interictal epileptiform activity should not be exclusively used to diagnose nocturnal spells as epileptic seizures.

Short-Term and Long-Term Monitoring

The advantages of STM and LTM over routine EEG are the acquisition of additional information over the longer recording time and simultaneous video monitoring. In patients with a history of mostly sleep-related spells, V-EEG-PSG is preferred over STM because the recording is performed during sleep, thereby increasing the probability for event capture. In patients with a mixture of daytime and sleep-related spells, STM is sometimes appropriate.

LTM is an alternative in patients in whom antiepileptic medication taper or discontinuation is planned. Medication taper or discontinuation is especially useful in facilitating seizure activity in epileptic patients with infrequent spells (e.g., once a week or less). The disadvantages of LTM are the cost of inpatient hospitalization and the need for a specialized epilepsy-monitoring laboratory. The limitations of LTM are similar to those of PSG in that spells may lack EEG correlates or might not occur even over many days of monitoring.

Ambulatory Monitoring

Ambulatory monitoring offers the convenience of recording in the patient's home and the lack of need for continuous monitoring by a technologist. Cost varies, but it is usually lower than that of a sleep laboratory recording. A major disadvantage of ambulatory monitoring relates to the fidelity of the recording in the absence of a technologist. If electrodes become detached, ground wires break, or conductive media become dry during the study, adjustments cannot be made. In addition, systems may use a reduced number of channels, thereby limiting the information provided, although some systems have the capability for expanded montages.

Furthermore, in contrast with the other monitoring techniques, the patient is not under constant observation and a technologist is not present. Consequently, interactions with the patient, critical for evaluating level of consciousness, are not possible. Also, interpreting rhythmic activities that resemble ictal discharges may be difficult in the absence of behavioral and consciousness assessment. The addition of synchronized video recordings to ambulatory monitoring has potential for facilitating correlation between EEG activity and clinical events.

CLINICAL PEARL

The clinician should consider performing video-EEG in suspected cases of nocturnal seizures and parasomnias such as REM sleep behavior disorder or NREM arousal disorders. The video may be as helpful as the EEG in documenting stereotypical behavior in epileptic seizures.

SUMMARY

Patients with nocturnal spells present a unique diagnostic challenge to the sleep specialist and the sleep laboratory. Although standard PSG provides valuable information about the stage of sleep from which spells arise and the timing of the spell relative to sleep onset, the characterization of these spells is enhanced by video recording and an extended EEG (12 or more channels, and sometimes 21 or more). Addition of video and an extended EEG to the standard PSG is essential for precise definition of nocturnal spells, including epileptic seizures, REM sleep behavior disorder, and arousal disorders. The video component provides information on the behavioral and motor manifestations of the nocturnal spell. Depending on the clinical situation, a daytime EEG, an ambulatory EEG, daytime STM, one or two nights of PSG, or LTM (over several days and nights) may be indicated.

SELECTED READINGS

Bazil CW. Sleep and epilepsy. *Semin Neurol*. 2017;37(4):407–412.

Berry RB, Quan SF, Abreu AR, et al. *The Aasm Manual For The Scoring of Sleep And Associated Events: Rules, Terminology And Technical Specifications, Version 2.6*. Darien (Ill.): American Academy of Sleep Medicine; 2020. www.aasmnet.org.

Ebersole JS, Pedley TA. *Current Practice of Clinical Electroencephalography*. 4th ed. Philadelphia: Lippincott Williams & Wilkins; 2014.

Foldvary N, Caruso AC, Mascha E, et al. Identifying montages that best detect electrographic seizure activity during polysomnography. *Sleep*. 2000;23:211–229.

Schmitt B. Sleep and epilepsy syndromes. *Neuropediatrics*. 2015;46(3):171–180.

A complete reference list can be found online at ExpertConsult.com.

Chapter 200

Monitoring Techniques for Evaluating Suspected Sleep-Related Breathing and Cardiovascular Disorders

Max Hirshkowitz; Meir Kryger

Chapter Highlights

- Polysomnography evolved from a laboratory research tool and became a medical diagnostic procedure largely applied for diagnosing and treating sleep-related breathing disorders (SRBDs).
- Principal components for evaluating SRBDs are airflow measurement, respiratory effort assessment, and oxyhemoglobin desaturation recording. Appreciating the relationship between SRBDs and sleep disruption also provides crucial information for patient care.
- The initial diagnosis of uncomplicated sleep-disordered breathing can be achieved using portable devices in patients with a high pretest probability for sleep apnea (see Chapter 205).
- Although not routinely used for diagnosing SRBD in adults, techniques are also available for measuring lung volume changes, pleural pressure changes, blood pressure changes, carbon dioxide levels in the airstream, and blood and brain oxygenation.
- Using the just mentioned and emerging technologies, clinicians can characterize physiologic phenotypes of sleep apnea that may potentially lead to targeted therapy.

OVERVIEW

More than a half century ago, polysomnography (PSG) began as a laboratory research technique to study sleep. With the discovery of sleep-related breathing disorders (SRBDs), laboratory PSG quickly found a new role as a gold standard diagnostic test[1,2] (Video 200.1). Penetration for assessing SRBDs has become so complete that undoubtedly the vast majority of sleep studies performed tonight, or on any given night, will serve this function. PSG is also used in the evaluation of SRBDs comorbid with other diseases, such as chronic obstructive pulmonary disease, neuromuscular disease, and respiratory failure, to help in directing management.[3] More recently, home sleep testing (HST) has also demonstrated its diagnostic utility in patients with a high pretest probability for having obstructive sleep apnea (OSA). In consequence, HST is now also commonly used diagnostically.[4] There are clinical situations (e.g., acute stroke) in which it may be impractical to do either type of test in a patient suspected of having a sleep breathing disorder. In such situations, using the diagnostic mode of positive airway pressure (PAP) devices may yield useful clinical data, but the data may not be acceptable for insurance coverage.[5] With the miniaturization of electronic systems and sensors, "consumer"-grade products (wearables or nearables, see Chapter 206) often linked to smart phone devices can capture some of the data that is normally collected in a sleep study.[6] The SARS-CoV-2 (COVID-19) pandemic dramatically changed how and where sleep testing is done, with a further shift toward home testing.[7] This chapter presents an overview of the most commonly used recording techniques and their application for evaluating SRBDs.

With few exceptions, PSG and home testing devices use similar techniques to monitor breathing during sleep. This chapter presents an overview of recording techniques and their application for evaluating SRBDs. The recording techniques used to assess breathing during sleep measure (or estimate) (1) airflow, (2) respiratory effort, and/or (3) changes in lung volume. The consequences associated with abnormal breathing are also commonly measured. These include (1) blood gas changes, (2) blood pressure changes, (3) cardiac rhythm changes, and (4) sleep disturbances.

Abnormal breathing during sleep takes several different forms and arises from various underlying etiologies. It goes by many names, including sleep apnea, sleep apnea-hypopnea syndrome, sleep-disordered breathing (SBD), SRBD, periodic breathing, Cheyne-Stokes respiration, and hypoventilation (Box 200.1). However, obstructive forms are by far the most common. Detailed descriptions regarding SRBD-associated etiology, morbidity, and treatments appear elsewhere in this book. The specific pathophysiologic events underlying SRBD include apnea episodes, hypopnea episodes, respiratory effort–related arousals (RERAs), oxyhemoglobin desaturations, and snore arousals. As their names imply, *apnea* is cessation of breathing and *hypopnea* is shallow breathing. The

Box 200.1 SLEEP-RELATED BREATHING EVENTS

- **Apnea** (A): The complete or near-complete cessation of breathing for 10 seconds or longer in an adult. Generally documented using a thermal sensor.
- **Oxyhemoglobin desaturation event** (ODE): A decrease in blood oxygen saturation. Usually, the magnitude must be 3% or greater to distinguish it from ongoing background signal fluctuations (electronic noise).
- **Hypopnea** (H): A reduction in (but not cessation of) ventilation. To be clinically significant, the hypopnea must be associated with an oxyhemoglobin desaturation event or a CNS arousal.
- **Desaturating hypopnea** (DH): A hypopnea with oxyhemoglobin desaturation of 4% or greater (also known as a "Medicare hypopnea").
- **Respiratory effort–related arousal** (RERA): A CNS arousal-terminating obstructive breathing event that does not meet the criteria for apnea or hypopnea.
- **Obstructive apnea** or **hypopnea** episode (OA or OH): A breathing event provoked by upper airway obstruction or reduced upper airway patency.
- **Central apnea** or **hypopnea** episode (CA or CH): A breathing event caused by absent or reduced respiratory effort (i.e., decreased output to inspiratory muscles from CNS respiratory control centers).
- **Mixed apnea** or **hypopnea** episode (MA or MH): A breathing event with both obstructive and central features. Many laboratories assign mixed events to the obstructive category.
- **Periodic breathing** (PB): A regularly repeating pattern in which normal or increased ventilation alternates with decreased or absent ventilation.

CNS, Central nervous system.

face validity, that not breathing is undesirable for the health of the organism, seems obvious. Sleep apnea and morbidity are interrelated; however, cause and effect can vary. Metabolic and cardiac diseases can produce downstream effects on sleep-related breathing.

PSG and HST criteria for defining a sleep apnea event have been consistent for decades. Cessation of breathing for 10 seconds or longer constitutes an apnea. Ten seconds was chosen because it approximates missing two breaths. The definition for hypopnea, by contrast, remains controversial even today. *Hypopnea* essentially means "shallow breath." The difficulty in defining hypopnea stems from several sources. The first involves measurement technique, the second from the fact that hypopneas are not intrinsically pathophysiologic, and the third from decades of usage without any standard.

PSG and HST airflow monitoring techniques mostly rely on surrogate and uncalibrated measurements (as detailed later in this chapter). Furthermore, airflow signal magnitude from thermistors, thermocouples, capnographs, and nasal pressure transducers correlates poorly with tidal volume. Consequently, operational definitions for hypopnea based on a percentage decrease of flow signal use arbitrary cut-off values, about which considerable disagreement continues.

Brief hypopneic intervals routinely occur during wakefulness without causing harm. For example, hypopnea accompanies speaking, and except in extraordinary circumstances, talking does not produce adverse health consequences. The expression "talking until you're blue in the face" characterizes a likely exception. During sleep, however, a hypopnea may provoke significant oxyhemoglobin desaturation or a central nervous system (CNS) arousal. Thus the consequence of the hypopnea (not the hypopnea itself) represents a potential pathophysiologic event. In accordance, prerequisites for designating sleep hypopnea as abnormal involve (1) accurately measuring physiologic consequences, (2) determining at what point these consequences reach significance, and (3) demonstrating their role in morbidity.

Unfortunately, measurement and morbidity determination remained unresolved for many decades. Many operational definitions for hypopnea appear in published clinical and research literature. At last count, this author (MH) is aware of more than 15 different definitions for hypopnea. Emergence of differing criteria for percentage airflow decrease, oxyhemoglobin decrease, and inclusion versus exclusion of CNS arousal as part of the definition seriously complicated matters. In an early attempt to standardize definitional criteria the American Academy of Sleep Medicine (AASM) created an ad hoc committee. Their work product, often referred to as the "Chicago Criteria," was adopted for research but not for clinical use.[8]

Subsequently, on April 1, 2002 the Centers for Medicare and Medicaid Services (CMS) arbitrarily defined a hypopnea as "an abnormal respiratory event lasting as least 10 s with at least a 30% reduction in thoracoabdominal movement or airflow as compared to baseline, and with at least 4% desaturation."[9] Eliminating CNS arousal from the hypopnea criteria and requiring 4% desaturation, rather than 3%, reduced the number of scorable hypopneic spells in many patients.[10,11] Essentially, using the CMS criteria reduced SRBD detection sensitivity and raises the diagnostic bar.

On the face of it, respiratory-related and snore-related arousals certainly seem irrefutably abnormal because they compromise sleep integrity. Some justification for ignoring such events derived from CNS arousal detection reliability. However, a major consequence, whether intended or unintended, was that these new criteria paved the way to diagnosing SRBD using less expensive home testing devices that seldom record electroencephalography (EEG) measurements. Ignoring the sleep disruption provoked by respiratory events seemed so ridiculously misguided to many clinicians that they continued tabulating arousal-provoking events, even though they fell short of the 4% desaturation criteria. The designation RERAs was commandeered from the Chicago Criteria, even though it originally had quite different criteria.

Five years later the AASM published the *AASM Manual for the Scoring of Sleep and Associated Events: Rules, Terminology and Technical Specifications* in 2007.[12] This "*AASM Manual*" provided two different definitions for hypopnea, neither of which agreed with the CMS criteria. Member centers were required to adopt and use AASM criteria to maintain accreditation. One definition required oxyhemoglobin desaturation (3%), whereas the other required event termination by CNS arousal. These conflicting mandates and ambiguities placed American sleep specialists in an intellectual, clinical, and legal quandary. Finally, in 2012 the AASM issued a rule clarification, and ultimately, in 2013 the AASM adopted CMS criteria[13] for scoring hypopnea.

Mitterling and colleagues[14] examined scoring outcome using the different definitions. Applying the 2012 scoring

Table 200.1 Clinical/Laboratory Features of Obstructive Sleep Apnea Syndrome by Severity

Dimension	Mild	Moderate	Severe
Sleepiness or unintended sleep episodes	During activities requiring little attention (e.g., watching television)	During activities requiring some attention (e.g., business meeting)	During activities requiring active attention (e.g., driving)
PSG SRBD events: number per night	5–15	15–30	>30
PSG/HST SRBD events and oxyhemoglobin (Sao_2)	RDI or AHI 2–20 and/or SaO_2 nadir >85%	RDI or AHI 20–40 and/or SaO_2 nadir 65%-85%	RDI or AHI > 40 and/or SaO_2 nadir <65%

AHI, Apnea-hypopnea index; HST, home sleep test; PSG, polysomnography; RDI, respiratory disturbance index; SaO_2 arterial oxygen saturation; SRBD, sleep-related breathing disorder.

criteria (hypopnea requiring a 3% oxygen desaturation or terminated by an arousal) produced higher apnea-hypopnea indices compared with scoring based on only scoring hypopnea with a 4% oxygen desaturation. These investigators used a sample of 100 healthy sleepers, ranging in age from 19 to 77 years. In a much larger study of more than 2100 subjects, Hirotsu and colleagues[15] evaluated the AASM rules published in 1999, 2007, and 2012, that is, (1) greater than or equal to 50% decrease in airflow or lower airflow reduction is associated with oxygen desaturation greater than or equal to 3% or an arousal, (2) greater than or equal to 30% airflow reduction is associated with greater than or equal to 4% oxygen desaturation, and (3) greater than or equal to 30% airflow reduction is associated with greater than or equal to 3% oxygen desaturation or an arousal, respectively. They found that the different criteria significantly altered median apnea-hypopnea indices, changed SRBD prevalence estimates, and produced different thresholds for diabetes mellitus, metabolic syndrome, and hypertension.[15]

Apnea and hypopnea episodes are further categorized as obstructive, central, or mixed, depending on the presence or absence of respiratory effort during some part of or the entirety of the breathing event. Beyond the mere presence or absence of respiratory effort, changes in the effort's magnitude can provide information concerning airway resistance. Increasing effort leading to a CNS arousal provides insight regarding pathophysiology. Therefore respiratory effort represents a crucial measure for evaluating patients with SRBD.

SDB severity can be based on a clinical dimension (e.g., sleepiness), event frequency (e.g., number of events per hour), or magnitude of the consequence (e.g., degree of oxyhemoglobin desaturation). Table 200.1 provides examples for dimensionally classifying severity of SDB. General agreement is lacking on assigning SRBD severity descriptors; however, two schemes are commonly used. In the first, "liberal" classification, an apnea-hypopnea index (AHI) between 5 and 15 is considered mild, between 15 and 30 is moderate, and greater than 30 is severe. In the second, "conservative" classification, an AHI between 10 and 20 is mild, between 20 and 50 is moderate, and greater than 50 is severe.[16]

MEASURING AIRFLOW

General Considerations

Most clinical techniques use qualitative surrogate measures to estimate airflow changes. Fully quantitative airflow determination requires pneumotachography or having the patient sleep in a "body box." Such techniques are unsuitable for routine clinical sleep studies. Semiquantitative measures are attainable using calibrated inductance plethysmography; however, most clinical evaluations rely on qualitative nasal-oral thermography and nasal pressure. This approach provides adequate data with minimal patient discomfort, reduced costs, and simplified data acquisition. The *AASM Manual* recommends using a thermal sensor to identify apnea and a nasal pressure sensor to detect hypopnea.[12,17] However, airflow can also be measured qualitatively by detecting chemical differences between ambient and expired air (e.g., capnography). Regardless of technique, qualitatively measured respiratory activity requires careful classification. Sometimes a patient's airway can be completely occluded during inspiration but release small puffs upon expiration, detectable by thermistor or carbon dioxide (CO_2) analyzer. Such events are erroneously categorized as hypopneas or even normal (unobstructed breathing). Figure 200.1 illustrates the problem.

Thermistors and Thermocouples

Exhaled air usually is warmer than ambient temperature. Core body heat warms the air in the lungs, thereby creating a temperature difference between air entering and exiting the respiratory system (under normal circumstances). In consequence, measuring temperature fluctuation at the nares and in front of the mouth provides a simple surrogate airflow measure. Measurement is possible using several different technologies.

Thermistors are thermally sensitive variable resistors that produce voltage alterations when connected in a low but constant-current circuit. Low current minimizes the thermistor tendency to heat itself. Thermistors maximize sensing area while minimizing sensor size and mass. Small temperature changes can produce large resistance changes that can, in turn, be transduced with a bridge amplifier. Care must be taken to ensure that the thermistor remains below body temperature (i.e., it must not rest on the skin); otherwise, expired air will not be warmer, and no resistance change will occur. In such a case, inspiratory activity and a respiratory pause will not be differentiable.

Thermocouples also sense temperature change but use a different approach. Different metals expand at different rates when heated. This difference can be transduced to voltage alterations displayable on polygraph systems. Like thermistors, thermocouples are placed in the airflow path in front of the nares and mouth, where expired air heats the sensor and increases its resistance. The transduced signal reflects

Table 200.2 Sleep-Related Breathing Disorders and ICD-10 Codes

Diagnostic Grouping	Disorder or Diagnosis	ICD-10 Codes[a]
Obstructive sleep apnea (OSA) disorders	OSA, adult	G47.33
	OSA, pediatric	G47.33
Central sleep apnea syndromes	Central sleep apnea with Cheyne-Stokes breathing (CSB)	G47.31, R06.3
	Central sleep apnea due to a medical disorder without CSB	G47.37
	Cheyne-Stokes breathing	R06.3
	Central sleep apnea due to high altitude periodic breathing	G47.32
	Central sleep apnea due to a medication or substance	G47.39
	Primary central sleep apnea	G47.31
	Primary central sleep apnea of infancy	P28.3
	Primary central sleep apnea of prematurity	P28.4
	Treatment-emergent central sleep apnea	G47.39
Sleep-related hypoventilation disorders	Obesity hypoventilation syndrome	E66.2
	Congenital central alveolar hypoventilation syndrome	G47.35
	Late-onset central hypoventilation with hypothalamic dysfunction	G47.36
	Idiopathic central alveolar hypoventilation	G47.34
	Sleep-related hypoventilation due to a medication or substance	G47.36
	Sleep-related hypoventilation due to a medical disorder	G47.36
Sleep-related hypoxemia disorder	Sleep-related hypoxemia	G47.36

[a]ICD-10, *International Classification of Diseases,* 10th edition (2020). For ICD-11 classification, see Chapter 69.

oscillation between exhaled warm air and cooled inhaled air, thus providing a trace roughly corresponding to respiratory airflow.

Nasal Airway Pressure

During inspiration, airway pressure is negative relative to atmospheric pressure. By contrast, expiration slightly increases airway pressure. The resulting alteration in nasal airway pressure can provide a surrogate estimate of airflow. Furthermore, estimates correlate favorably with pneumotachographically recorded signals.[18] The nasal pressure signal also offers greater sensitivity than nasal-oral thermography for detecting subtle flow limitations (Figure 200.2) when patients breathe through their noses.[19] Airflow limitation shows as pressure trace plateauing during inspiration. A direct current amplifier provides optimal interface; however, long time-constant alternating current (i.e., a very slowly coupled signal) can suffice. By contrast, rapid coupling is not recommended because it can create artifact (Figure 200.3).

HST devices for diagnosing SRBD routinely measure nasal airway pressure, arterial oxygen saturation (SaO_2), and respiratory effort. Most HST devices, however, do not measure brain activity and thereby fail to capture RERAs. This significant shortcoming may underestimate AHI, especially in mild cases. Johnson and colleagues[20] proposed an event measure, called *f*low *l*imitation/*o*bstruction *w*ith recovery breath (FLOW), detected using nasal pressure snoring sounds without the need for the EEG. These FLOW events are defined minimally by (1) a run of at least two breaths that have evidence of obstruction and (2) a subsequent distinct change in breathing pattern with increased amplitude.[20]

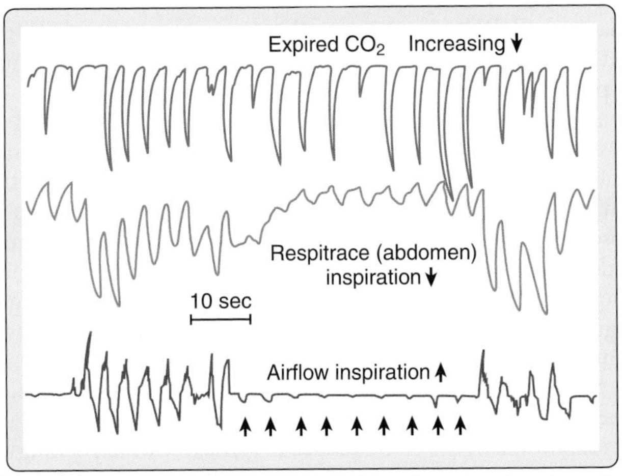

Figure 200.1 An example illustrating the limitations of noninvasive airflow detection. Airflow is recorded simultaneously with a carbon dioxide (CO_2) analyzer and a pneumotachograph. During the obstructive apnea event, periods of expiratory airflow occur (recorded by the pneumotachograph and the CO_2 analyzer) in the absence of inspiratory flow (obvious in the pneumotachograph recording and unclear in the CO_2 recording). Without the information from the pneumotachograph, the recording from the CO_2 analyzer would be interpreted as evidence of uninterrupted inspiratory and expiratory airflow. *Top,* Airflow is detected with the CO_2 analyzer. *Middle,* Respiratory inductance plethysmograph (RIP) ("Respitrace"). *Bottom,* Airflow measured with a pneumotachograph. With each apnea-related expiratory deflection documented by the pneumotachograph (*arrows, bottom*), there is a sustained shift in the baseline of the RIP tracing. This correlation suggests an incremental decrease in functional residual capacity resulting from absence of inspirations with continued small expiratory puffs. If only the top two tracings were available, this pattern would have been mistakenly called hypoventilation or hypopnea, whereas it clearly reflects total occlusion on inspiration. (From West P, Kryger MH. Sleep and respiration: terminology and methodology. *Clin Chest Med.* 1985;6(4):691-712.)

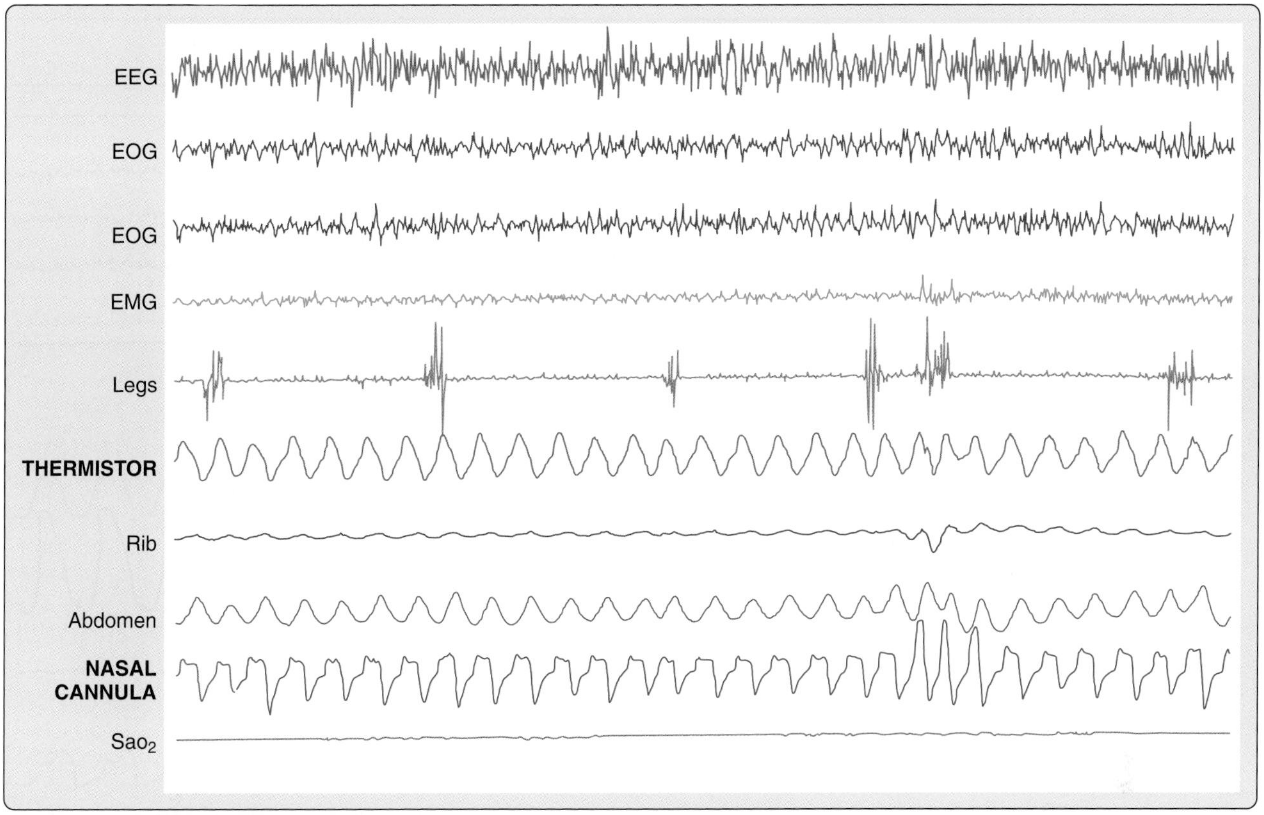

Figure 200.2 A 120-second section from a nocturnal polysomnogram in a subject undergoing simultaneous recording with a conventional thermistor and with a nasal cannula used for recording pressure. Nothing in the thermistor tracing suggests a respiratory event, and subtle movement barely registers in the rib and abdominal inductance plethysmographic tracings. In the nasal cannula tracing, however, the end of one flow limitation episode and the beginning of another are easily detected. Note the plateaus (*chopped-off tops*) of the pressure traces during flow limitation. EEG, Electroencephalogram; EMG, electromyogram; EOG, electrooculogram; SaO_2, oxygen saturation in arterial blood. (Courtesy Dr. David Rappaport, Icahn School of Medicine, New York City.)

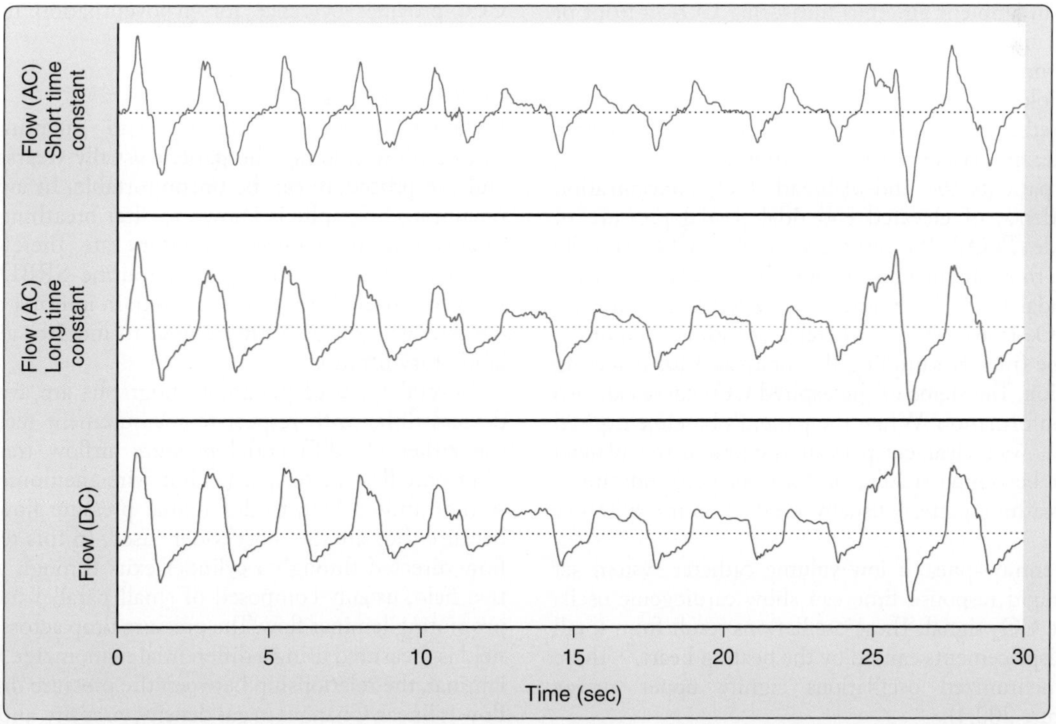

Figure 200.3 A flow limitation event recorded from the nasal cannula measuring pressure simultaneously amplified by three different amplifiers. The *bottom* signal is from a direct current (DC) amplifier with no filtering. The *top* two signals are from alternating current (AC) amplifiers with low-frequency filters, with time constants of 1.6 (*top*) and 5.3 (*middle*). The shorter time-constant filter (*top*) causes the flow signal to decay to baseline rapidly during a period of relatively constant flow (flow limitation plateau). The longer time-constant filter (*middle*) provides reasonably good reproduction of these constant flows.

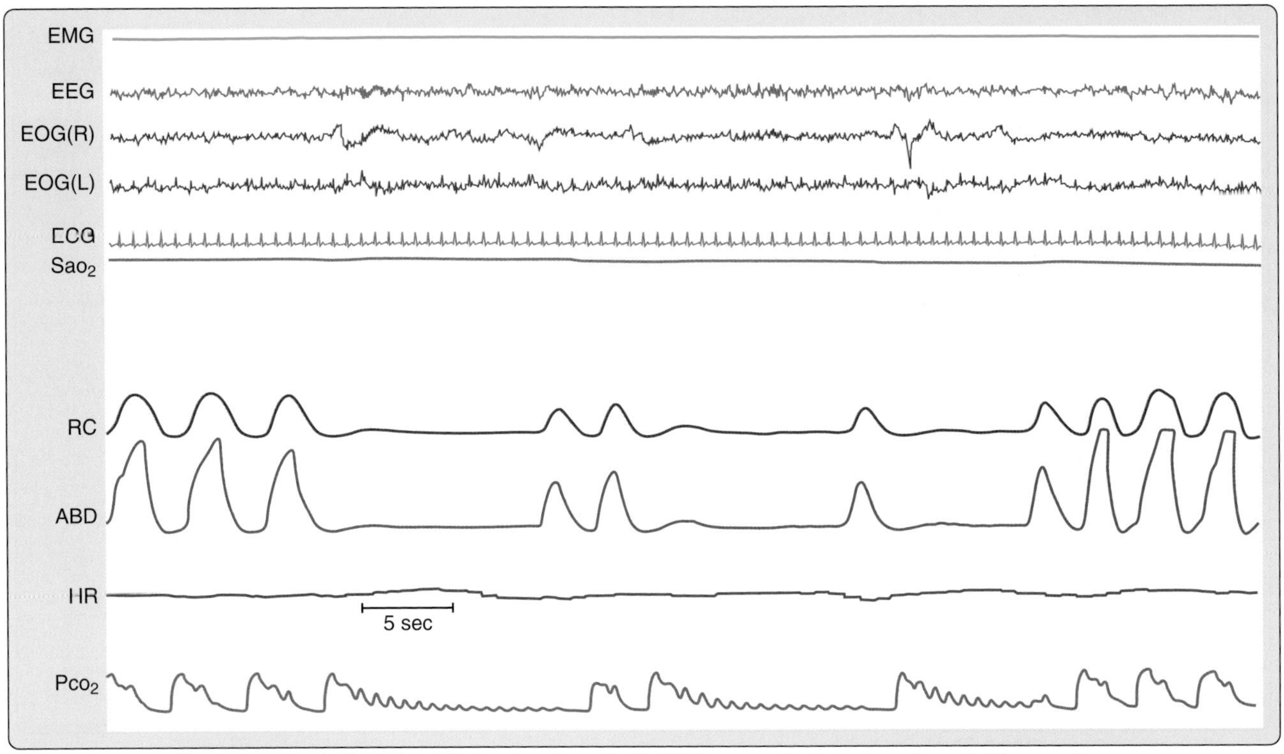

Figure 200.4 Cardiogenic oscillations in carbon dioxide (CO_2) are seen in the *bottom channel* of the recording in this example of central apnea. The presence of these oscillations, synchronous with the heartbeat, signifies that the upper airway is patent. ABD, Abdominal (movement); EEG, electroencephalogram; ECG, electrocardiogram; EMG, electromyogram; EOG, electrooculogram (right [R] and left [L]); HR, heart rate; RC, rib cage (movement); PcO_2, partial pressure of carbon dioxide; SaO_2, arterial blood oxygen saturation.

Expired Carbon Dioxide Sensors (Capnography)

Carbon dioxide concentration in air leaving the lungs far exceeds that in ambient air. Thus measuring CO_2 in front of the nose and mouth can detect expiration. Infrared analyzers can determine the concentration. Because exhaled CO_2 reflects physiologic chemical change, it offers several advantages compared with physical changes detected by thermistor, thermocouple, and nasal pressure recordings.

In some patients the end-of-breath CO_2 concentration provides evidence of elevated end-tidal partial pressure of carbon dioxide (PcO_2). The catheters sampling CO_2 typically entrain some room air, making the measured CO_2 lower than actual end-tidal PcO_2. Therefore an elevated CO_2 indicates that true PcO_2 is even higher, thereby providing a noninvasive technique (merely sampling the airstream) for detecting hypoventilation. The shape of the expired CO_2 curve can also offer useful information. When the patient's baseline expired CO_2 curve shows a clear-cut plateau, the loss of this plateau (or the curve becoming smaller or dome shaped) indicates a change in breathing pattern, usually a reduction in expiratory volume.

During central apnea, a low-volume catheter system set at its most rapid response time can show cardiogenic oscillations in the CO_2 signal. These oscillations result from small air volume displacements caused by the beating heart.[21] These heartbeat-synchronized oscillations signify upper airway patency (Figure 200.4).

Capnography can also be used in the sleep laboratory to titrate noninvasive ventilation in patients with hypoventilation syndromes.[22] In infants and children with upper airway obstruction, severe hypoventilation may occur during sleep without observable apnea or hypopnea. Measuring expired CO_2 provides evidence for hypoventilation not detectable using thermistors or thermocouples.[21]

Pneumotachography

Pneumotachography accurately and quantitatively measures airflow volume. The patient usually wears a face mask, and the procedure can be uncomfortable. In awake subjects, pneumotachography is known to alter breathing; it increases tidal volume and reduces respiratory rate. Therefore pneumotachography is seldom used for routine SRBD diagnostics. However, some PAP machines contain internal pneumotachographs whose signal can be used to monitor airflow during laboratory titration.

Several types of pneumotachographs are available. These devices differ with respect to measurement technique: They use either (1) differential pressure airflow transducers, (2) ultrasonic flow meters, or (3) hot-wire anemometers. Discussion is limited here to differential pressure flow transducers because they are the most widely used. In this technique, airflow directed through a cylinder exits through a small resistive field, usually composed of small parallel tubes or a grill promoting laminar flow. The pressure drop across this resistive field is measured using a differential manometer. When flow is laminar, the relationship between the pressure differences and flow is linear. Changes in gas density, viscosity, and temperature alter the pressure-flow relationship. To prevent condensation on the resistive element requires heating; therefore calibration should be conducted only after the pneumotachograph is sufficiently warmed up. After correction for errors introduced by alterations in these physical factors, the flow signal is integrated to determine volume.

MEASURING RESPIRATORY EFFORT

Measuring respiratory effort provides etiologic information needed for SRBD differential diagnosis (obstructive vs. central) and treatment planning. Categorizing an apnea or hypopnea as obstructive, mixed, or central (nonobstructive) derives from differential respiratory effort and airflow patterns. Available techniques for detecting and/or measuring respiratory effort include (1) rib cage and abdominal motion, (2) electromyography (EMG), (3) pleural pressure changes, (4) movement detected by static charge sensors in or on the bed surface, (5) movement detected by standing wave patterns in the bedroom, and (6) digital video recording.

Rib Cage and Abdominal Motion

At present, the most common PSG technique for measuring respiratory effort involves the recording of rib cage and abdominal movements. During normal breathing, the major inspiratory muscles produce rib cage expansion and a downward movement of the diaphragm. These movements cause the pressure around and in the lung to become negative (relative to atmospheric pressure). The pressure gradient between ambient air and the lung draws air through the airways into the alveoli. Thus a change in lung volume is the sum of the volume changes of the structures surrounding the lungs, the rib cage, and the abdomen.[23] Other respiratory muscles (e.g., intercostal, sternocleidomastoid) also play a role in stabilizing the thoracic cage. Some clinicians erroneously interpret the abdominal and rib cage motion changes as implying separate activities of abdominal and thoracic respiratory muscles. Virtually all of the changes in abdominal and rib cage volumes, including paradoxical motion, can be explained by changes in the status of the respiratory muscles directly inserting onto the thoracic cage. Paradoxical motion of the rib cage and abdomen can result from several changes, including (1) upper airway obstruction (complete or partial), (2) diaphragmatic tone loss, and (3) other respiratory muscle tone loss. The mechanisms underlying asynchronous motion of rib cage and abdomen are described in Box 200.2. Notwithstanding the pattern or its underlying mechanism, rib cage and abdominal movement reflect effort to breathe.

At a minimum, a single uncalibrated abdominal movement sensor can *detect* respiratory effort. Respiratory effort during airflow cessation usually signifies airway obstruction. Common approaches for *measuring* rib cage and abdominal movement use (1) strain gauges, (2) inductance plethysmography, and (3) piezoelectric transducers.

Strain gauges are sealed elastic tubes filled with conductive material through which an electric current is passed. When length is constant, current and resistance are constant. Stretching the strain gauge lengthens and narrows the cross-sectional area of the fixed-volume conductor. This deformation produces a proportional increase in electrical resistance. Current varies inversely in relation to the length of the gauge, thereby becoming an index of gauge length. A Whetstone bridge amplifier transduces this change to voltage for continuous display showing rib cage or abdominal expansion, depending on placement.

Box 200.2 MECHANISMS UNDERLYING PARADOXICAL MOTION OF THE RIB CAGE AND ABDOMEN

- **Loss of diaphragm tone.** When the diaphragm ceases to contract and becomes flaccid, it merely reacts to pressure changes around it instead of generating pressure changes. In this situation, when the other respiratory muscles contract, the rib cage is enlarged, and pleural pressure becomes negative, sucking the diaphragm into the chest. This condition results in an increase in rib cage volume and a reduction in abdominal volume.
- **Loss of accessory respiratory muscle tone.** When the accessory muscles lose tone, the rib cage, particularly the upper part of the rib cage, becomes unstable. When the diaphragm then contracts, the negative intrathoracic pressure causes the unstable part of the thorax to be sucked in during inspiration.
- **Partial upper airway obstruction.** With partial upper airway obstruction, the diaphragm must generate very strong negative pressures for inspiration to occur. As the diaphragm contracts, it both pushes out the abdomen and creates great negative intrathoracic pressure. This highly negative intrathoracic pressure can overcome the mechanisms maintaining chest wall stability (accessory muscle tone and rigidity of the cage) so that the least stable portions of the rib cage will tend to move inward with inspiration. This potential for inward movement of the rib cage is a problem mainly in the very young, in whom the rib cage is quite pliable.

Inductance plethysmography electronically measures changes in the cross-sectional area of the rib cage and abdominal compartments by determining changes in inductance. Inductance is a property of electrical conductors characterized by the opposition to a change of current flow in the conductor. Transducers are placed around the rib cage and abdomen—the physiologic equivalent of conductors. Each transducer consists of an insulated wire sewn into the shape of a horizontally oriented sinusoid and onto an elasticized band.

Piezoelectric transducers are commonly used to detecting movement. These sensors, when placed on the rib cage and abdomen, are sensitive to changes in length. When squeezed, a piezoelectric crystal produces an electrical potential across its sides. The crystals can be arranged, usually as part of a belt, so that movement can be detected.

Respiratory Muscle Electromyography

Recording the EMG intercostal muscle activity stands as one of the oldest PSG techniques for detecting respiratory effort (Figure 200.5). These uncalibrated recordings are made using standard surface electrodes placed in pairs on the right anterior chest in the intercostal spaces. Obtaining an optimal signal requires practice, patience, and skill; recordings are prone to artifact, especially from the electrocardiogram (ECG). Intercostal EMG activity, when recorded properly, can differentiate central, obstructive, and mixed SRBD events. Furthermore, although signals are not calibrated, cascading increases in respiratory effort are readily apparent from such recordings. Advanced techniques were developed for using diaphragm EMG in ventilator systems; that is, neurally adjusted ventilatory assist may eventually migrate to the diagnostic setting. This

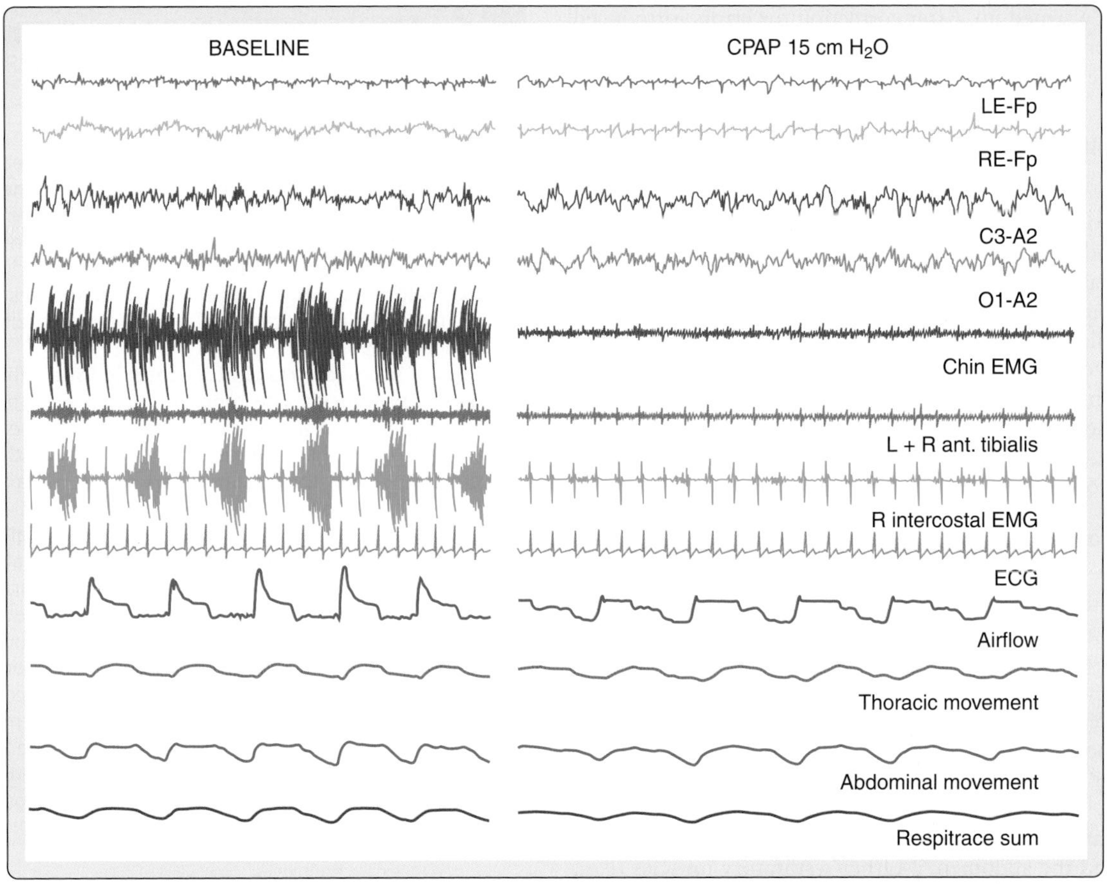

Figure 200.5 Surface respiratory (R intercostal) muscle EMG in sleep apnea. *Left,* The respiratory EMG signal is dramatically increased. *Right,* This signal is reduced on nasal continuous positive airway pressure (CPAP). A2, Right mastoid reference; ant., anterior; C3, left central EEG; ECG, electrocardiogram; EEG, electroencephalogram; EMG, electromyogram; LE-fp, left eye referenced to frontal pole; L + R, linked left and right; O1, right occipital EEG; RE-fp, right eye referenced to frontal pole. (Courtesy Dr. J. Catesby Ware, Eastern Virginia Medical School, Norfolk, Virginia.)

would be especially helpful when reduced diaphragm activity is suspected, for example, in central hypoventilation syndromes.[24]

Pleural Pressure Changes

Some sleep centers measure esophageal pressure to index inspiratory effort. During normal breathing, pleural pressure is slightly negative compared to atmospheric pressure. Pleural pressure swings indicate respiratory effort. Increased pressures occur when airway resistance increases and can thereby identify, with great accuracy, apnea and hypopnea events resultant from obstruction. Esophageal pressure measurements also verify central apnea or hypopnea episodes with a high degree of certainty. In addition, increased pressures also alter cardiac afterload and preload.[25] Notwithstanding the advantages provided by such measures, in our experience most patients undergoing all-night PSG find esophageal balloons unacceptable. However, the thin water-tip or catheter-tip piezoelectric transducers are better tolerated. Although this technique also can detect very subtle respiratory events, a repeat polysomnogram may be preferable to using an esophageal catheter.[26] Recently, suprasternal pressure changes have been used as a surrogate to reflect esophageal pressure. This approach shows promise for characterizing respiratory effort to categorize abnormal breathing events.[27]

In patients with *upper airway resistance syndrome,* the classic findings include progressively more negative pleural pressure until a CNS arousal occurs. This may occur without hypoxemia. An audible snort or sputter sometimes accompanies the arousal (Figure 200.6). After the arousal, pleural pressure swings temporarily decrease until another episode begins. These episodes often occur in cycles, leading to significant sleep disruption. The CNS activation (EEG alpha activity) sometimes falls short of 3-second AASM arousal duration criteria. However, we established the AASM's 3-second rule to improve scoring reliability for visually scored *spontaneous* (not provoked) arousals.[28,29] EEG changes, measurable using digital analysis, including those of shorter duration and/or increased alpha bandwidth power, are thought to represent CNS arousals. Such changes, however, are difficult to identify visually on raw data tracings.

Movement Detected by Static Charge and Pressure Sensors

The static charge–sensitive bed technology has been used to evaluate sleep disorders.[30] A transducer embedded within a thin mattress responds to the slightest movement. Output from the bed is sensitive enough to detect heartbeat as a ballistocardiogram. Respiratory signal amplitude differs with body position changes; however, output is otherwise stable.

A similar but newer technology uses piezoelectric sensors embedded in a strip placed on or integrated into the bed. Placement is oriented perpendicular to the sleeper's body. The device detects motion and thereby identifies

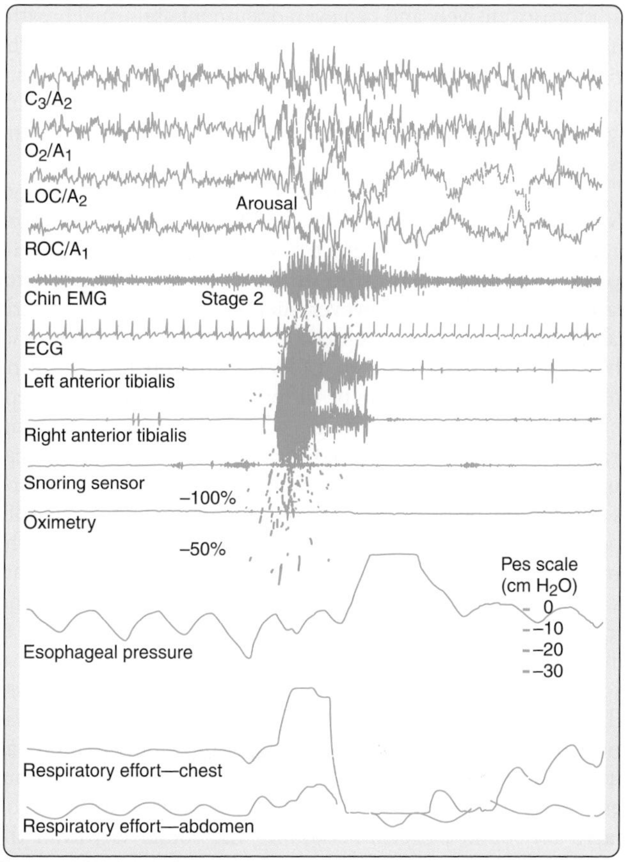

Figure 200.6 Esophageal pressure in the upper airway resistance syndrome. The esophageal pressure (Pes) swing was greatest just before the arousal. C_3/A_2, Left central EEG referenced to right mastoid; ECG, electrocardiogram; EMG, electromyogram; LOC, left outer canthus; O_2/A_1, right occipital lobe EEG referenced to left mastoid; ROC, right outer canthus. (From Butkov N. *Atlas of Clinical Polysomnography.* Synapse Media; 1996:224.)

respiratory effort. Both changes in pressure resulting from movement associated with breathing and heartbeat can be analyzed.[31,32]

Movement Detected by Wave Technologies

Several systems approach movement detection using microwaves, radar, and/or changes in standing wave patterns in the bedroom. These technologies, sometimes used in security systems, detect motion. The output signals, rather than being used to sound an alarm upon detecting an intruder, can provide data about someone sleeping in the room. One approach directs a beam at the bed surface and analyzes the returning signal to evaluate the sleeper's upper body movement. In another system, laser radiation is used. Microwave and other radar-like technologies also can be applied. In addition, a series of sensors could be used to monitor movement. Application of some of these emerging technologies to sleep medicine for evaluating SRBD and associated cardiovascular function is an important aspect of ongoing developments in the field.[33–35]

Polysomnography-Synchronized Digital Video

Digital video is now commonly incorporated into computerized PSG systems. Although recordings are widely used to evaluate parasomnias and seizures, they can help clinicians assess SRBDs. When a video recording is properly

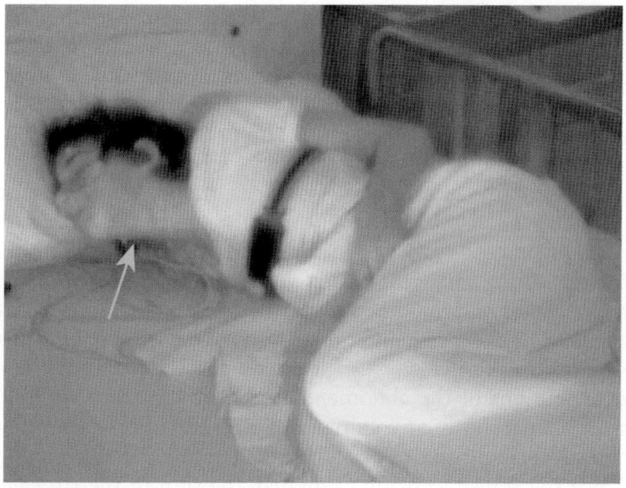

Figure 200.7 Synchronized digital video can be extremely helpful, as in this example in which a child with retrognathia slept with his neck arched and his mandible thrust forward (*arrow*). This sleep posture resulted in an unoccluded upper airway. The conventional polysomnography recording missed that a significant sleep breathing problem was present. (From Banno K, Kryger MH. Use of polysomnography with synchronized digital video recording to diagnose pediatric sleep breathing disorders. *CMAJ.* 2005;173:28–30.)

synchronized with PSG, ambiguous and difficult-to-interpret tracings often become obvious. For example, it is easy to recognize a small dip in SaO_2 as a significant SDB event when it is followed by oxygen resaturation after an audible snort, a repetitive moving forward of the jaw, an arching of the neck, or a closing of a gaping mouth. Video is especially helpful in children, whose PSG recordings may be difficult to interpret (Figure 200.7; Video 200.2). An SaO_2 dip, without other visual information, is quite likely to be missed, ignored, or dismissed as artifact. Video recordings are particularly useful in thin persons who do exhibit oxyhemoglobin desaturations during their abnormal respiratory events. Furthermore, showing the sleep study video to patients can be very effective for promoting understanding of the problem and an appreciation of its severity. Using video in such a manner is part of some clinical protocols designed to improve patient acceptance and use of PAP therapy.

Measuring Changes in Lung Volume

Several methods can estimate tidal volume. These measures provide semiquantitative data concerning presumed airflow while also documenting respiratory effort. Calibration is crucial when using these devices to gauge ventilation. Movements (after calibration), changes in body position, and recording device placement shifting introduce errors. Some sleep laboratories use strain gauges, inductance plethysmography, piezoelectric transducers, and/or impedance pneumography to measure volume changes. Other techniques include magnetometry, body plethysmography, canopy with neck seal, the barometric method, and pneumotachography; however, these are seldom used clinically to diagnose SRBD.

Strain Gauges, Inductance Plethysmography, and Piezoelectric Transducers

In principle, length-sensitive devices can be used qualitatively to detect breathing abnormalities. If properly calibrated, these devices can measure dynamic volume changes quantitatively.[36]

Normally, thoracic enlargement and abdominal wall occur together; that is, they are in phase. Therefore, for a given change in lung volume, it is possible to quantify a change in rib cage volume and abdominal volume. Moreover, for any given breath, the relative contributions of the rib cage and abdominal compartments can likewise be determined.

To quantify actual volume changes, the transducers must be calibrated against an independent volume-measuring system. In practice, two length-measuring devices are required for measuring changes in lung volume: one for the rib cage and one for the abdomen. The rib cage device is placed at the level of the axilla, and the abdominal device is placed just superior to the iliac crest. If it is assumed that the fractional contributions of the abdomen and the rib cage are constant, then changes in lung volume can be measured by calibrating transducers sensitive to rib cage and abdominal displacement. Once the transducers are calibrated, the sum of the rib cage and abdominal excursions will describe volume changes.

Unfortunately, the relative rib cage and abdominal contributions can change with posture and muscle tone occurring in sleep. Movement-related device migration from its original site and device deformability also must be considered. Such factors adversely affect calibration accuracy and stability. Nonetheless, calibrated inductance plethysmography appears adequately sensitive for detecting upper airway resistance syndrome events.[37]

Impedance Pneumography

Impedance defines the combined effects of two previously discussed properties of an electrical conductor: *resistance* and *inductance*. In physical terms, when impedance pneumography is used, the conductor is the thorax. Impedance is measured by applying a small current across the thorax using a pair of electrodes placed at the site of maximal thoracic excursion.

Transthoracic impedance changes reflect variations in the amount of conductive materials: liquids, including interstitial fluid, blood and lymph, and tissue, and nonconductive material (air) between the electrodes. The conductive and nonconductive materials affect the total impedance differently. Increased air in the lung increases impedance; increased fluid in the thorax decreases impedance. A recording of the volume of air exchanged and the total of impedance changes can allow the differentiation between air-related and fluid-related changes in impedance. If total impedance is recorded in a single channel, changes related to air volume and fluid are measured.

Impedance alterations in obstructive apnea are complex. During apnea, lung volume decreases, whereas the negative intrathoracic pressure most likely temporarily pools blood in the pulmonary circulation. For these reasons, a precise measurement of respiratory volume and pattern may not be possible. Nonetheless, rate-adapting cardiac pacemakers using transthoracic impedance to drive ventilation have been used to screen for OSA.[38]

MEASURING SLEEP-RELATED BREATHING WITH OTHER TECHNIQUES

Sound

Most laboratories record sound using microphones as part of video recording; however, few use this information to note anything other than snoring. Advances in sensor technology and digital signal processing allow sound recordings to be used far more extensively and can even document abnormal breathing events. For example, the output of sensors placed on the sternal notch can be processed to detect vibrations (snoring) and also measure tracheal flow sound.[39] Sonar (wave technologies, see also earlier) are being developed to assess breathing using smartphones.[33]

Nonlaboratory and consumer devices use sound far more extensively than standard clinical PSG. Many devices record and analyze sound to detect and quantify snoring. Some consumer devices even claim utility as case-finding tools for patients with SRBD. However, such claims must be properly validated before being accepted. To qualify as a snoring sound, the signal must oscillate in cadence with breathing during sleep. The sound must also be differentiated from other sleep-related breathing sounds (e.g., wheezing, stridor, groaning, crackles, or heavy breathing). Once snoring is detected, measuring its intensity offers a more difficult challenge. The first is calibration because translating detected sound levels into metrics needed to compare individuals is quite difficult. The sound's volume can vary depending on both the sleeper's characteristics and external factors. Sleep position (supine, prone, or laterally recumbent), vocal characteristics, prior exposure to environmental factors (e.g., air quality), intoxication, medication use, and tiredness can alter snoring intensity (loudness). The sensor's placement and its orientation to the sleeper also must be considered when judging loudness. Furthermore, all of these factors can change during the sleep period. Nonetheless, an uncalibrated volume signal can provide information based on sound pattern. Assuming the sound is within the sensor's operationally variable range (i.e., not topped out or below detection), several patterns exist, including (1) absent, (2) intermittent, (3) relatively steady state, (4) crescendo-decrescendo, and (5) crescendo with sudden termination. These patterns suggest different things but will require rigorous validation before application to clinical practice.

Polyvinylidene Fluoride Film Sensors

Thermocouples, thermistors, and strain gauges are fairly old technologies. More recently, new materials, such as polyvinylidene fluoride film (PVFF), have been introduced into the sleep laboratory. PVFF converts heat and mechanical energy into measurable electrical energy. PVFF has both piezoelectric (responding to mechanical changes) and pyroelectric (responding to thermal changes) properties. The output from these films can be configured to measure airflow[40] (pressure and temperature), snoring[41] (pressure waveforms), and changes in length caused by abdomen and rib cage movement.[42–44]

MEASURING SLEEP-RELATED BREATHING DISORDER PHYSIOLOGIC CONSEQUENCES

SRBD event consequences can include (1) blood and/or tissue gas changes, (2) blood pressure changes, (3) cardiac rhythm changes, and (4) sleep disturbances. The following section describes measurement techniques used to assess such changes.

Blood Gas Changes

Blood oxygen and CO_2 exchange underlie the fundamental basis of breathing. Measurement techniques available to measure these gases include (1) pulse oximetry, (2) high-resolution pulse oximetry, (3) near-infrared spectroscopy, and (4) transcutaneous assessment.

Pulse Oximetry

Routine clinical sleep evaluations require noninvasive, continuous, and rapidly sampled measures to determine blood oxygen concentration. Thus directly measuring blood oxygen with an indwelling arterial catheter is ruled out on all counts. Pulse oximetry, however, serves the need well; consequently, it is the standard technique for recording oxyhemoglobin saturations during sleep. Originally the technology was intended for medical use, but because of miniaturization the technology is now available to consumers. Multisensor systems with memory storage can combine oximetry with other physiologic variables (e.g., temperature, blood pressure, ECG, EEG). Such devices can provide spot (instantaneous) or continuous measurements. During the COVID-19 pandemic the use of oximeters by the public greatly increased. Unfortunately, the public and health care workers did not always appreciate the complexity and limitations of such instruments.[45,46] In particular, pulse oximetry may overestimate oxygen saturation in hypoxic Black patients. Among the patients who had an oxygen saturation (SpO_2) of 92% to 96% on pulse oximetry, an SaO_2 of less than 88% was found in 11.7% of Black patients versus 3.6% of White patients.[47]

Pulse oximeters usually determine SaO_2 spectrophotoelectrically using a two-wavelength light transmitter and a receiver placed on either side of a pulsating arterial vascular bed (usually a finger, earlobe, toe, or the nose). Alternatively, in reflectance pulse oximetry, the light transmitter and the receiver are on the same surface. The light transmitted into the vascular bed is scattered, absorbed, and reflected. The amplitude of light detected in particular spectra by the receiver depends on the magnitude of the change in arterial pulse, the wavelengths transmitted through the arterial vascular bed, and the oxygen saturation of arterial hemoglobin (deoxygenated blood is bluer). These devices are sensitive only to pulsating tissues; in consequence, venous blood, connective tissue, skin pigment, and bone *theoretically* do not hamper SaO_2 determination. Accurate measurement, however, requires a minimal pulse amplitude. Dyshemoglobinemias can cause problems.

Correct alignment of the light transmitter and receiver is critical to ensure measurement accuracy. If the sensor is applied to a digit, then movement of the digit should be minimized. Significant bending of the digit can compromise detection of pulsatile flow and invalidate results. Although all pulse oximeters are based on similar technology, response characteristics differ both across manufacturers and even within a specific manufacturer's product line.[48] Sensor placement and device programming are crucial technical factors in obtaining optimal results. Reflectance oximeters also must contend with weaker pulse signals because much less light is reflected back to the sensor. Differences in response characteristics and effect of sensor location cannot be overemphasized (Figure 200.8) because some oximeters seem completely insensitive to hypoxemia episodes clearly detected by other devices (Figure 200.9). Such devices can produce false-negative SRBD test outcomes.

A review of specific oximeters would be beyond the scope of this chapter; nonetheless, generalizations about (1) sensor location, (2) instrument filtering and sampling rates, and (3) potential pitfalls are worth noting here.

Sensor Location

In our experience, the preferred sensor location in adults is the earlobe. Poor perfusion can be enhanced by applying a trace amount of vasodilator (e.g., nonylic acid vanillylamide plus nicotinic acid—Finalgon ointment [Boehringer Ingelheim, Ridgefield, Connecticut]). Technicians must take great care to avoid contact of the perfusion-enhancing agent with their own or the subject's eyes. Earlobe recordings also reduces circulator delay, compared with the finger. This advantage becomes especially important for associating a respiratory event with its subsequent oxyhemoglobin desaturation in patients with congestive heart failure. When the earlobe site is not usable, reflectance pulse oximeter sensors placed on the forehead or another well-perfused surface will suffice.

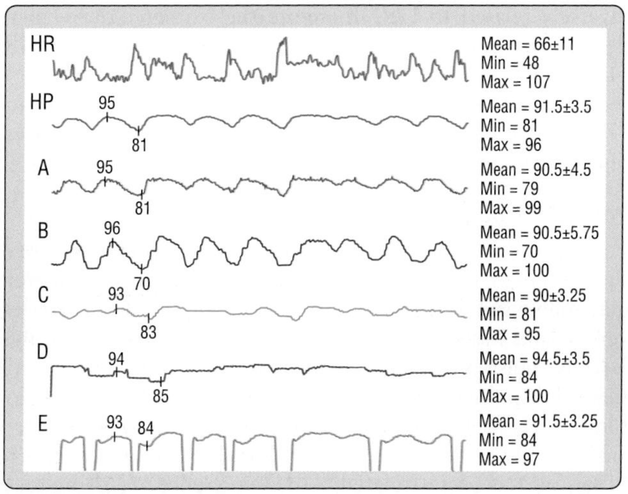

Figure 200.8 Heart rate (HR) and arterial oxygen saturation (SaO_2) during a 5-minute period in a patient with sleep apnea. The *top two traces* are for the HR monitor and a Hewlett-Packard (HP) oximeter; A to E are traces for five different pulse oximeters. The scales for the six oximeters are identical. The *numbers* on the tracings represent the instantaneous SaO_2 measured during the peak and trough of an apneic episode. The data listed to the *right* of the figure are the mean, standard deviation, and minimum and maximum values for HR and SaO_2 for the six oximeters. Note that oximeters C and D do not track SaO_2 and that the recording for oximeter E has numerous artifacts.

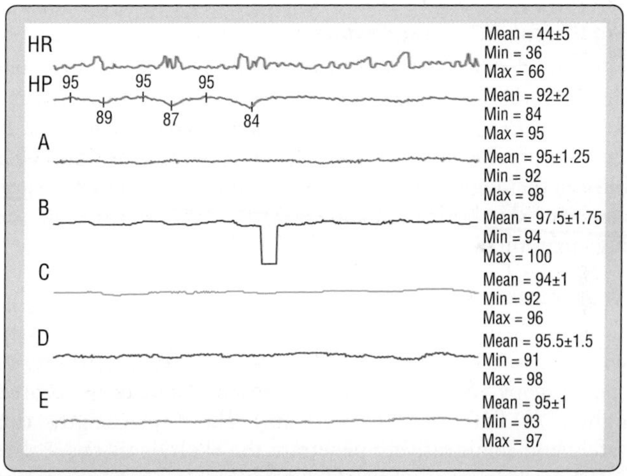

Figure 200.9 Heart rate (HR) and arterial oxygen saturation (channels A–E) during a 5-minute period in a patient with sleep apnea and bradycardia. Tracings are taken from six oximeters, as described in Figure 200.8. In this example, three apneic episodes are missed entirely by all of the pulse oximeters. This patient's problem would have gone completely undetected by pulse oximetry screening. HP, Hewlett-Packard (oximeter).

Instrument Filtering and Sampling Rate

Most pulse oximeters filter the signal, and some filtering algorithms use the heart rate (HR). The degree of filtering is inversely related to HR. Therefore the oximeter may fail to detect brief, mild hypoxemic during periods of very low HR. During PSG recording, filtering should be minimized to reduce missing transient oxyhemoglobin desaturation events. One accomplishes this by setting the oximeter to the fastest response, the highest sampling rate, or both.

Potential Problems

Performance of pulse oximeters can degrade when tissue perfusion is poor, as might occur in heart failure. Pulse oximeters generally assumes that the only tissues that pulsate are arteries; venous and tissue pulsations may result in incorrect readings. Because pulse oximeters use two wavelengths of light to estimate SaO_2, they cannot distinguish three or more hemoglobin species. In the presence of carboxyhemoglobin (as in heavy smokers, in whom carboxyhemoglobin levels can reach 10% to 20%), SaO_2 is overestimated.[49] In the presence of a rising methemoglobin concentration, oximetry-determined SaO_2 will plateau at approximately 85%, regardless of whether true saturation is much higher or lower.[50] Because light is transmitted through tissue, pigment in the skin can degrade oximeter performance, producing incorrect "probe-off" or "perfusion-low" error reports or might result in false high measurements in hypoxic Black patients.[47,51] Some finger-clip devices can produce pressure-related injuries when worn for an entire night.

High-Resolution Pulse Oximetry

High-resolution pulse oximetry (HRPO) using additional signal processing methods can overcome some of these limitations. HRPO reduces motion and low perfusion artifacts. It can also provide an index of perfusion and measure hemoglobin, methemoglobin, and carboxyhemoglobin. These devices can be used in both adult and pediatric sleep medicine recording environments.[52–55]

Near-Infrared Spectroscopy

Conventional pulse oximeters cannot measure SaO_2 deep within tissues, such as the brain or muscle. Near-infrared spectroscopy (NIRS) uses four wavelengths of near-infrared light (775, 810, 850, and 910 nm). These wavelengths can safely and noninvasively penetrate the skull or tissues.[56] The NIRS probe uses a light emitter and three sensors that detect reflected light. This device measures (1) the concentration of oxygenated and deoxygenated hemoglobin (O_2Hb and HHb, respectively), (2) brain tissue oxygen saturation (StO_2), and (3) total hemoglobin (tHb) concentration. Brain blood volume is considered an equivalent to tHb. Because cerebral circulation autoregulates in response to changes in partial pressure of arterial oxygen (PaO_2) and partial pressure of arterial carbon dioxide ($PaCO_2$), NIRS may shed light on the impact of sleep pathologies on brain oxygenation. This technique has been used to continuously monitor cerebral oxygenation (in critical care units and during anesthesia), sleep apnea, and movement disorders in adults and children.[56–60] In sleep medicine, NIRS is currently used primarily in research settings.

Transcutaneous Blood Gases

Partial pressure of arterial oxygen estimated from the skin's surface depends on oxygen flux through the skin, local oxygen consumption, and the skin's diffusion barrier.[61] This measurement technique is most commonly used in neonates, whose skin is thin. Accurate measurement of transcutaneous pressure of oxygen (PO_2tc) requires maximal dilation of the local vasculature in the upper dermis. This is achieved by heating local tissue to 43°C. However, heating (1) shifts the oxyhemoglobin dissociation curve to the right, (2) increases the resistance of the skin stratum corneum to oxygen permeation, (3) increases the metabolic rate of the dermal tissue, and (4) increases the rate of cutaneous blood flow. The shift in the oxyhemoglobin dissociation curve and the increase in metabolic rate effectively cancel each other out, leaving permeability and flow as the dependent factors in correlating PO_2tc and PaO_2. An important advantage of heating is that the amount of blood present is maximal, and PO_2tc is therefore unaffected by small changes in blood supply to the tissue.

Nonetheless, PO_2tc may be misinterpreted when the state of blood flow is unknown. When flow and PaO_2 are adequate, PO_2tc reflects PaO_2. Under conditions of compromised flow and adequate PaO_2, PO_2tc will change with flow. If SaO_2 and flow are compromised, PO_2tc tracks oxygen delivery. Transcutaneous measurement accuracy also depends on correct sensor application. To convert PO_2tc measurements to PaO_2 values precisely, a calibration curve for each subject is required, making the technique too labor intensive for routine clinical practice use. In most laboratories, PO_2tc serves to track, in relative terms, arterial oxygenation status. Device responsiveness is too slow for tracking rapid blood gas changes associated with brief SRBD events (<30 seconds) because oxygen diffuses slowly across the skin. The conditions governing transcutaneous pressure of carbon dioxide (PCO_2tc) measurement are remarkably similar to those described for PaO_2. Although transcutaneous blood gas determinations are of greatest value in neonates and young children, PCO_2tc is useful for assessing hypoventilation in adults, especially in patients with neuromuscular diseases, such as amyotrophic lateral sclerosis.[62,63]

CARDIOVASCULAR MEASUREMENTS

Blood Pressure Changes

Clinical laboratories do not routinely record sleep-related blood pressure. Nonetheless, many pulse oximeters also can track pulse pressure, a magnitude index of pulsation occurring at the oximetry sensor site. Pulse transit times (PTTs) can indirectly estimate blood pressure.[64] PPT represents the time interval from heartbeat (ECG R wave) to its pulse recorded in the periphery. Negative pleural pressure provokes a blood pressure drop and in so doing lengthens PTT. The progressive increase in pleural pressure during obstructive apnea correlates with rising oscillations in PTT amplitude. During central apnea, this does not occur. Thus it has been suggested that PTT might provide an opportunistic estimate of inspiratory effort and thereby provide a means to differentiate obstructive from central apnea.[65,66] Pulse wave data has also been suggested as a surrogate for detecting cortical arousals.[67]

Automatic self-inflating arm-cuff sphygmomanometers have long been available but are problematic for routine clinical use because they disturb sleep. By contrast, miniature finger cuff systems produce less sleep disturbance. Devices obtaining data in alternating fashion from adjacent fingers reduce finger injury risk, and some systems automatically perform hydrostatic correction when arm movement occurs. Finger flexion artifacts, however, remain a problem.

Peripheral Arterial Tonometry

A photoelectric plethysmograph detects the optical density changes associated with pulsatile blood volume alterations in the finger and detects autonomic nervous system controlled vasoconstriction and vasodilation. There are transient elevations of sympathetic tone that causes vasoconstriction, with arousals occurring at the end of abnormal breathing events.[68,69] This technique has been combined with several additional sensors into one unit. SaO_2 is measured with a pulse oximeter. An accelerometer is used to determine sleep-wake state. Peripheral arterial tonometry (PAT) devices indirectly detect apneas and hypopneas by documenting vasoconstriction and integrating that information with oximetry. The association between of sleep stages and HR vascular tone variability are used to detect state. Computational techniques are used to emulate the functions of a polysomnogram.[70] Compared to PSG, AHIs were underscored or overscored frequently enough that it has been recommended that when a patient with a high pretest probability has a negative PAT study that he/she be restudied in the laboratory.[70] PAT has also been used to document endothelial dysfunction in OSA.[71]

Cardiopulmonary Coupling

Cardiopulmonary coupling uses a single-channel ECG recording to extract signal features modulated by breathing.[72] Respiration induces small alterations in HR and R-wave amplitude. Using computerized frequency domain analysis, a high-frequency component can be isolated that represents variations in breathing-induced vagal sinus pressure HR. A low-frequency component can be extracted to provide information about interbreath intervals. By examining a weighted composite of these data (increased variability and the envelope of amplitude change), time-domain periods (usually 2 to 10 minutes) with breathing pauses can be discerned by using cross-power spectrums. In general, normal breathing loads high-frequency bandwidths, and SRBD events mass in low-frequency troughs. Narrow-band coupling at low frequency identifies central respiratory events (chemoreflex activation), whereas broad-spectrum low-frequency bands likely identifies other forms of SDB. High frequency correlates with good quality sleep. Automated cardiopulmonary coupling analysis has been used to detect sleep apnea.[73,74] For detailed information about cardiopulmonary coupling, see Chapter 202.

Circulation Time

Circulation time, which is prolonged in cardiac failure, can be inferred by the time between end of scored respiratory events and nadir oxygen desaturations (measured with finger or ear pulse oximetry) associated with those events.[74a]

Rhythm Abnormalities

Cardiac rhythm abnormalities are quite common in patients with sleep breathing disorders (see also Chapter 145). Atrial fibrillation is four times more likely to develop in patients with OSA compared to control subjects; therefore ECG monitoring during sleep is recommended. Cardiology guidelines now recommend that apnea be considered in patients with atrial fibrillation.[75] New technologies are being developed to detect atrial fibrillation in OSA.[76–78] Most laboratory clinical PSGs include at least one ECG channel; however, many HST systems do not record cardiac rhythms.

Sleep Disturbance

Awakenings and brief CNS arousals provide critical information concerning sleep disturbance and fragmentations. Standardized scoring for both awakening and CNS arousal derive from EEG activity, preferably recorded from occipital sites. According to standardized sleep scoring, any EEG alpha activity (7 to 13 Hz) burst exceeding 15 seconds in duration during stages N1, N2, or rapid eye movement (REM) sleep is scored as an awakening. Ongoing intermixed EEG alpha activity during sleep stage N3 (sometimes termed *alpha-delta sleep*), can signify disturbed sleep; however, such is not driven acutely by a transient pathophysiologic event.

Transient CNS arousals most often manifest as EEG alpha activity bursts. The terms *EEG speeding* or *alpha intrusion* are sometimes used to describe these events. When scored visually, a 3- to 15-second alpha activity burst during N1 or N2 sleep is considered an arousal. However, during REM sleep, alpha activity can be part of the normal ongoing background EEG activity. Consequently, to consider such a burst as representing a CNS arousal, increased muscle tone must accompany the alpha intrusion.

The CNS arousal represents a clinically significant sleep parameter because it is associated with (in cross-sectional studies) and provokes (in intervention studies) tiredness, fatigue, and sleepiness. As a pathophysiologic consequence of OSA, the arousal is thought to result from increased respiratory effort and accompanying increase in autonomic nervous system sympathetic activation, triggered by increased airway resistance. Presumably, the CNS arousal terminates the SRBD event because the arousal returns ventilation to voluntary control. As a result, the airway can be dilated and breathing resumes. However, some controversy exists about resumption of breathing after an obstructive event without CNS arousal and about the presence of arousals at the termination of central events.

HOME SLEEP APNEA TESTING

In addition to standard attended PSG, guidelines for HST have been published.[79] Chapter 205 provides methodologic details. Because HST devices are less sensitive than laboratory PSG, the home test can *rule in*, but not *rule out*, SRBD. Therefore, only patients with a high clinical suspicion for SRBD should be referred for HST. Many health care coverage plans, including those administered by the CMS, reimburse HST for diagnosing sleep apnea. Clinicians should be aware that HST is prone to data loss as a consequence of uncorrected technical failures (e.g., electrode detachment). Unattended studies are also susceptible to patient tampering, making them unsuitable for most medicolegal testing.

To succeed diagnostically and economically, HST requires proper patient selection, appropriate portable recorder application, and proper study interpretation by a qualified sleep specialist. To assure good quality of care, access to laboratory PSG must be available when follow-up is needed. The need for laboratory follow-up includes (1) a negative HST result in a patient with high pretest probability for SRBD, (2) continuing problems, notwithstanding appropriate treatment, and (3) sudden unexplainable changes in a patient's symptoms or health status.

OTHER CONSIDERATIONS

Measuring Collapsibility of the Upper Airway

Upper airway collapsibility measured by critical closing pressure (Pcrit) has been used to predict the success of PAP therapy. This approach involves overnight PAP manipulation in the sleeping patient and is performed mostly in research laboratories. Simpler techniques not requiring such manipulation are being developed to obtain an index of airway collapsibility.[80–82]

Table 200.3 Anatomic and Physiological Traits in OSA (Details of Technique)

Trait	Description and Examples of How Measured
Abnormal upper airway anatomy	Physical examination, imaging
Pharyngeal collapsibility	Estimated by • Passive critical closing pressure (P_{crit}) using **CPAP drop method**[88] • Ventilation at normal/eupneic ventilatory drive ($V_{passive}$) using **diagnostic polysomnography** (a more collapsible airway is captured by a lower ventilation[80] • **Surrogate clinical metric**: a therapeutic CPAP level ≤8.0 cm H_2O predicts mild collapsible pharyngeal anatomy from clinical CPAP titration study[89]
Pharyngeal muscle compensation	Change in upper airway muscle activity in response to ventilatory drive (e.g., pleural pressure swings, ΔPCO_2) estimated by • Slope of genioglossus EMG vs. epiglottic pressure plot during CPAP drop method[88] or • Difference of ventilation between $V_{passive}$ and V_{active} (ventilatory drive just prior to arousal)[80] by **diagnostic polysomnography**
Loop gain	The sensitivity of the ventilatory control feedback loop to a change in ventilation is made up by • Plant gain (the lungs, blood, and body tissues) • Circulatory delay (the time it takes for a change in lung CO_2 to be detected by chemoreceptors) • Controller gain (chemosensitivity)Measured by Δ ventilation/Δ disturbance using CPAP drop method[88] or ventilatory signal modeling from diagnostic polysomnography[90]

Arousal threshold	The level of ventilatory drive (e.g., pleural pressure swings, ΔPCO_2) immediately prior to occurrence of an EEG arousal can be estimated by
	• Pleural pressure from CPAP drops
	• Ventilatory drive from diagnostic PSG
	• Surrogate clinical metric: at least 2 of the following[91]
	  • AHI < 30 (hypopnea definition used may include events without oxyhemoglobin desaturation but are associated with a CNS arousal)
	  • Fraction of hypopneas > 57%
	  • O2 saturation nadir ≥ 82.5%

AHI, Apnea-hypopnea index; CNS, central nervous system; CO_2, carbon dioxide; CPAP, continuous positive airway pressure; OSA, obstructive sleep apnea; PSG, polysomnography.

Physiologic Phenotyping

PAP therapy may not be the sole treatment for SDB. The physiologic traits playing a role in sleep breathing disorders include upper airway collapsibility, ventilatory drive, pharyngeal compensation to obstruction, arousal threshold, arousal intensity,[83,84] and hypoxic burden.[85] In the future, specific therapies may be tailored for specific traits.[81,86] Categorization based on patient traits will likely help in personalizing therapy.[87] A scale, PALM, whose variables include collapsibility (*P*crit), *a*rousal threshold, *l*oop gain and airway *m*uscle responsiveness has been proposed. Its utility for guiding therapy-based physiologic characteristics needs further study.[88] This is covered in greater detail in Chapter 129 (Table 200.3).

CLINICAL PEARLS

- Detecting sleep-related breathing events and classifying each as obstructive, central, or mixed requires measures of airflow, respiratory effort, and oxyhemoglobin saturation.
- Information about sleep-disturbing effects of sleep-related breathing disorder events provides better sensitivity for the diagnosing sleep-disordered breathing.
- Standardized guidelines developed by the American Academy of Sleep Medicine were developed to advance clinical practice and should constrain scientific inquiry.

SUMMARY

The most common medical application of sleep technologies is for diagnosing and treating SRBDs. For half a century, procedures evolved, and some eventually became commonplace in clinical sleep laboratories. The AASM published guidelines, and these became the de facto standard. Standard clinical assessment for SRBD involves measuring airflow, respiratory effort, and oxyhemoglobin desaturation. Laboratory evaluation also includes brain activity to assess sleep disturbances. In this chapter we describe techniques to measure these and other related physiologic activities. The underlying mechanism, advantages, and problems are also discussed.

SELECTED READINGS

American Academy of Sleep Medicine. *International Classification of Sleep Disorders*. 3rd ed. Darien, IL: American Academy of Sleep Medicine; 2014:49–138.

Berry RB, Albertario C, Harding SMCE, et al. *American Academy of Sleep Medicine. The AASM Manual for the Scoring of Sleep and Associated Events: Rules, Terminology and Technical Specifications*, Version 2.6. Darien (Ill.): American Academy of Sleep Medicine; 2020. Available at https://aasm.org/clinical-resources/scoring-manual/.

Caples SM, Anderson WM, Calero K, Howell M, Hashmi SD. Use of polysomnography and home sleep apnea tests for the longitudinal management of obstructive sleep apnea in adults: an American Academy of Sleep Medicine clinical guidance statement. *J Clin Sleep Med*. 2021;17(6):1287–1293.

Giannoni A, Gentile F, Navari A, et al. Contribution of the lung to the genesis of Cheyne-Stokes respiration in heart failure: plant gain beyond chemoreflex gain and circulation time. *J Am Heart Assoc*. 2019;8(13):e012419.

Hunasikatti M. Racial bias in accuracy of pulse oximetry and its impact on assessments of hypopnea and T90 in clinical studies. *J Clin Sleep Med.* 2021;17(5):114.

Kapur VK, Auckley DH, Chowdhuri S, et al. Clinical practice guideline for diagnostic testing for adult obstructive sleep apnea: an American Academy of Sleep Medicine clinical practice guideline. *J Clin Sleep Med.* 2017;13(3):479–504.

Kwon Y, Sands SA, Stone KL, et al. Prolonged circulation time is associated with mortality among older men with sleep-disordered breathing. *Chest.* 2021;159(4):1610–1620.

Mitterling T, Högl B, Schönwald SV, et al. Sleep and respiration in 100 healthy Caucasian sleepers—a polysomnographic study according to American Academy of Sleep Medicine standards. *Sleep.* 2015;38(6):867–875.

Penzel T, Glos M, Fietze I. New Trends and New Technologies in Sleep Medicine: expanding accessibility. *Sleep Med Clin.* 2021;16(3):475–483.

Roberts DM, Schade MM, Mathew GM, Gartenberg D, Buxton OM. Detecting sleep using heart rate and motion data from multisensor consumer-grade wearables, relative to wrist actigraphy and polysomnography. *Sleep.* 2020;43(7):zsaa045.

Roeder M, Sievi NA, Bradicich M, et al. The accuracy of repeated sleep studies in OSA: a longitudinal observational study with 14 nights of oxygen saturation monitoring. *Chest.* 2021;159(3):1222–1231.

Sabil A, Schöbel C, Glos M, et al. Apnea and hypopnea characterization using esophageal pressure, respiratory inductance plethysmography, and suprasternal pressure: a comparative study. *Sleep Breath.* 2019;23(4):1169–1176.

Strassberger C, Zou D, Penzel T, et al. Beyond the AHI-pulse wave analysis during sleep for recognition of cardiovascular risk in sleep apnea patients [published online ahead of print, 2021 May 25]. *J Sleep Res.* 2021:e13364.

A complete reference list can be found online at ExpertConsult.com.

Chapter 201

Sleep Telemedicine and Remote PAP Adherence Monitoring

Amir Sharafkhaneh; Samuel T. Kuna

Chapter Highlights

- Telemedicine improves access to clinical care. Sleep medicine services are uniquely positioned to benefit from using telemedicine.
- Advances in technology enable health care entities to use telehealth to not only provide telemedicine but also manage administrative and educational components of health care.
- Synchronous telemedicine is the delivery of medical care remotely in real time. It includes video teleconferencing to evaluate patients, provide patient education, and initiate and manage various therapies (e.g., cognitive behavioral therapy for insomnia).
- Asynchronous telemedicine consists of stored data collected remotely from the patient for review by the practitioner at a later time for clinical management. Examples of this store-and-forward telemedicine include review and interpretation of patient self-report data, home sleep studies, and wirelessly transmitted positive airway pressure data.
- Providing medical care using telemedicine is complex. Successful implementation depends not only on overcoming technological challenges but also addressing legal, privacy, and payer issues.
- The COVID-19 pandemic required rapid, at-scale implementation of virtual health care and therefore significantly enhanced the acceptance of telemedicine by practitioners and patients to reduce the risk of virus exposure.

INTRODUCTION

Medical care is provided traditionally through face-to-face interactions between a patient and health care provider. The limitations of this model from the patient's perspective include the need to take time off from work, the inconvenience and cost of traveling (often long distances to a medical facility), and the medical conditions and mental health issues limiting travel ability. In many instances, more than one of these conditions exist. Telemedicine overcomes these limitations by use of new, widely available, and rapidly emerging telecommunication technologies that allow patients to receive care remotely. Patients have the option of receiving their care at home, thereby reducing the need for dedicated clinic space and its related expenses at a medical facility. Alternatively, patients can obtain specialty care remotely by using telehealth equipment at their nearest local medical clinic that does not itself provide the needed service. Use of a local medical clinic overcomes the barrier of those patients who are unable to use the required technologies at their home. In addition, the local medical clinic is likely to offer reduced travel time, better parking options, and fewer obstacles compared with travel to a medical center where the needed specialized services are available. From the practitioner's perspective, telemedicine provides the option of working remotely. In addition, telemedicine's reliance on digital data can reduce practitioner time and thereby allow the practitioner to increase patient volume. Thus telemedicine allows convenient access to care that would likely be significantly delayed or prevented by reliance on in-person encounters.

THE SCOPE OF TELEMEDICINE AND TELEHEALTH

The terms *telemedicine* and *telehealth* are frequently used interchangeably. The term *telemedicine* is narrower in scope and denotes the delivery of medical care to patients remotely by a health care provider.[1] In this chapter, we refer to telemedicine for sleep disorders as *telesleep*. *Telehealth* is the broader term and can be defined as access to health care providers and services anywhere and at any time.[2] Telehealth covers a variety of services, including inpatient and outpatient care, population health, home health care, second medical opinion, provider-to-provider consultation, group/individual education and counseling, group/individual physical rehabilitation, group/individual anti-addiction counseling and care, diagnostic interpretative services, and quality control of various medical services.[3] Table 201.1 provides a list of frequently used terms in telehealth and telemedicine. A telemedicine interaction that happens in real time is termed *synchronous*.[1] Synchronous telemedicine is most frequently delivered by video

Table 201.1 Telemedicine and Telehealth Glossary

Term	Definition
Telemedicine	Providing clinical services remotely
Telehealth	Providing clinical and clinically related services including training and medical education remotely
mHealth	Providing clinical and health care services using mobile devices
Originating site	The location that the patient received the clinical service. It is also called spoke site, patient site, remote site, and rural site.
Distant site	The location that the health care provider renders health care–related services using telehealth technology. It is also referred to as the consulting site and hub site.
Telepresenter	An individual with some background in health care (like a nurse) and familiarity with operating telemedicine equipment who facilitates video visit encounters
Synchronous service	Real-time video visit with bidirectional transfer of data between the originating and distant sites and between the patient and health care provider
Remote monitoring	Type of ambulatory health care in which patients use mobile medical devices to perform a routine test and send the test data to a health care professional in real time. Remote monitoring includes devices such as glucose meters for patients with diabetes and heart or blood pressure monitors for patients receiving cardiac care.
Asynchronous service	Review of patient-related data after collection of the data
Store-and-forward	Storing the health care–related data, including images and diagnostic test-related data, and forwarding the data using telehealth technology for review at a later time by health care providers for clinical management
Diagnostic equipment	All the equipment that can assist a health care provider to perform physical exam or diagnostic evaluation
Presenter (patient presenter)	An individual with a clinical background (e.g., LPN, RN) trained in the use of telehealth equipment who must be available at the originating site to "present" the patient, manage the cameras, and perform any "hands-on" activities to complete the tele-exam successfully. In certain cases, a licensed practitioner such as an RN or LPN may not be necessary, and a non-licensed provider such as support staff, could provide telepresenting functions. Requirements (legal) for presenter qualifications differ by location and should be followed.

https://www.aaaai.org/Allergist-Resources/Telemedicine/glossary Accessed 09/02/2021

teleconference. Asynchronous telemedicine occurs when data collected from the patient are stored and then retrieved by the practitioner at a later time for clinical management. Examples of this store-and-forward form of telemedicine include review and interpretation of patient-reported symptoms, questionnaire data, home sleep studies, and wirelessly transmitted positive airway pressure (PAP) data. A third form of telemedicine, termed *home telehealth*, consists of transmission of electronic data from the patient directly to the practitioner. Examples of this form of telehealth would be remote monitoring of a patient's vital signs and a technologist monitoring in real time the signals being recorded during a sleep recording at another location.[4-7]

Although telephone calls are widely used to deliver care remotely, they are generally not considered to be a form of telehealth. Compared with telephone calls, clinical evaluations performed by video teleconference are likely to foster a better physician-patient rapport and therefore a more personalized approach to care delivery. Video teleconference also offers the ability to perform a limited physical examination. Telephone calls, however, offer greater accessibility to patients and serve as a useful backup when a video teleconference cannot be conducted.

IMPACT OF THE COVID-19 PANDEMIC ON TELEMEDICINE

The COVID-19 pandemic greatly accelerated the interest and growth of telemedicine services. The need for physical distancing to reduce virus exposure risk has increased the acceptance of telemedicine by patients and practitioners. In response to the pandemic, health care systems and medical practices have rapidly implemented telemedicine, including telesleep, to provide patients with continued access to quality primary and specialty care.

In many centers, the delivery of sleep medicine care was quickly converted to an entirely contactless system that encompassed the patient's initial presentation through diagnostic testing and management as follows. New patient evaluations took place via clinical video teleconference visits from patients' homes. When appropriate, home sleep apnea tests (HSATs) were conducted by portable monitoring devices that were either largely or completely disposable (see Chapter 205 for a detailed discussion of HSATs). HSATs could be sent (and returned) in the mail, and online videos that depicted correct application of HSAT equipment replaced face-to-face instructional sessions. For individuals who required treatment

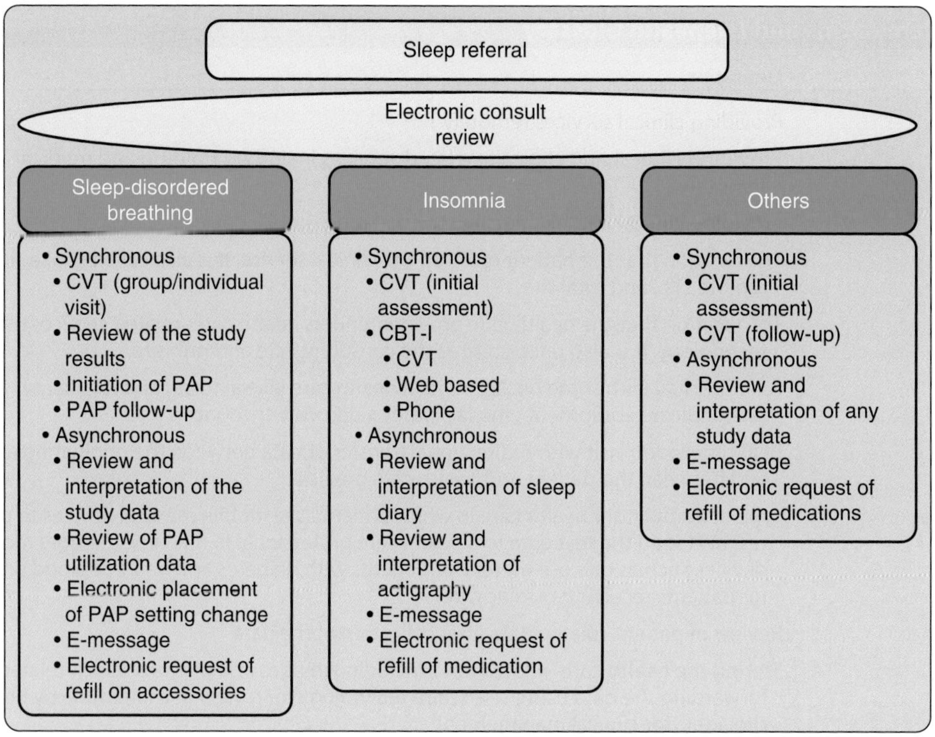

Figure 201.1 Spectrum of sleep services that can be provided using telemedicine. CBT-I, Cognitive behavioral therapy for insomnia; CVT, clinical video telehealth; PAP, positive airway pressure.

with PAP, home initiation of auto-adjusting continuous PAP (APAP) was preferred over in laboratory continuous positive airway pressure (CPAP) titration. Software recently became available to assist with the selection of PAP mask interfaces; it uses data from a facial scan obtained with a mobile device camera. Therefore even mask fitting has the potential to take place while social distancing is maintained. However, the accuracy of such digital mask fit tools remains unknown, and clinical adoption is limited at this time.

Because decreased reliance on in-laboratory titration studies can result in uncertainty regarding therapeutic efficacy, some providers may have increased engagement with cloud-based platforms to view PAP-generated data during the COVID-19 pandemic. Additionally, home pulse oximetry provides another option to ensure effective treatment of sleep-disordered breathing. In contrast to traditionally used, US Food and Drug Administration (FDA)–cleared pulse oximeters (see Chapter 200) that are owned by health systems and durable medical equipment companies, a vast number of consumer-marketed pulse oximeters are available. Many patients own and use such devices, which often use different sensor positioning (e.g., embedded in rings, watches), despite unknown accuracy. Other "smart" devices, such as blood pressure cuffs and scales, and their associated mobile applications for data analysis and management, also acquire objective data remotely. Therefore, in appropriate patients, the capabilities of telemedicine, particularly when combined with HSATs, APAP, and patient ownership of "smart" devices, conferred the opportunity for evaluation and long-term management of sleep-disordered breathing entirely in the home environment through the COVID-19 pandemic.

Facilitating this transition, the Centers for Medicare and Medicaid Services and private health care insurance carriers in the United States have increased reimbursement for a video teleconference visit to be on par with an in-person clinic visit. In addition, a health care provider in one state who takes care of a patient residing in another state using telehealth is no longer required to have medical licensure in both states. Whether these waivers will be reversed in the future is unknown.

Although telemedicine will undoubtedly play an increasingly important role in the future delivery of medical care, the availability of in-person care and in-laboratory testing remains essential. Many medical services cannot be performed using telehealth, and not all patients are candidates for telemedicine. For example, although video teleconference evaluations offer many advantages over in-person clinic visits, some patients will continue to require in-person evaluation because of the complexity of their medical problems and the need for a more complete physical exam.

APPLYING TELEMEDICINE TO SLEEP SPECIALTY CARE

The increasing knowledge about the prevalence of sleep disorders and their medical consequences has greatly increased the demand for sleep services.[1] The need for these services is not limited to urban areas where most sleep specialists practice. People with sleep disorders living in rural and underserved areas, with limited access to specialty care, are also in need. Sleep medicine is uniquely suited to reach these patient populations through telemedicine. Sleep centers are experimenting with, implementing, and delivering initial and follow-up care using telehealth technologies (Figure 201.1).[8,9] Various telemedicine management models are possible and often depend on practice settings, third-party payer regulations, and privacy-related restrictions.[10,11]

The importance of the medical history in the evaluation of patients with sleep disorders makes sleep medicine particularly amenable to video teleconferencing. Furthermore, the tests used to diagnose sleep disorders are in digital format and easily transferrable using store-and-forward technologies. Wireless data transmission from devices used to treat patients with sleep apnea provides remote access to treatment use and efficacy. Telehealth applications to sleep medicine extend beyond telemedicine. Telehealth is being used for education and training, including to start sleep centers in countries where the knowledge in sleep medicine is scarce and thus underserved.[12,13]

Although telehealth promises to provide universal access to care, many issues remain. For its successful implementation, telehealth must address the availability of the required technology, training of personnel, and legal, privacy, and payer issues. As the use of telehealth becomes increasingly widespread, standards for telehealth will be developed to facilitate implementation. The American Telemedicine Association Guidelines recommend the technical requirements for telemedicine's successful implementation.[14] These guidelines include the bandwidth, resolution, and software requirements; the diagnostic equipment; and the safety and privacy needs for telehealth use. In addition, American Academy of Sleep Medicine has published a position paper on application of telemedicine for sleep services.[2]

CLINICAL VIDEO TELECONFERENCE

In contrast to in-person clinic visits, video teleconference visits allow audiovisual interaction between the patient and practitioner in real time while they are at different locations. The originating site is the place where the patient receives the care, while the distant site is the place from which the practitioner provides the care. The originating site can be the patient's home or another medical facility. Video teleconferencing software is available to link the provider to the patient's personal computer, laptop, iPhone, or Android cell phone. Alternatively, the video teleconference can be conducted using telehealth equipment that connects the patient at one medical facility to the provider in another medical facility. If the originating site is a medical facility, a medical technician or health care provider can assist in the encounter. This telepresenter can facilitate and clarify communication between the patient and provider. The telepresenter's competency in operating the telehealth equipment allows patients who are unable to use telehealth technologies at home to use telemedicine. The telepresenter also offers the remote provider the ability to obtain vital signs and a physical examination. For example, a stethoscope and other peripherals interfaced with the telehealth equipment can be used by the telepresenter to allow the provider to auscultate the heart and lungs; conduct an ear, nose, and throat exam; and assess other aspects of the physical exam despite being at the distant site.

Studies have reported patient acceptance and satisfaction with telesleep, including video teleconferencing, to diagnose and manage their sleep apnea.[15-17] Parikh and colleagues reported no difference in PAP usage and patient satisfaction when comparing in-person versus video teleconference visits.[15] Using nurse providers in a study comparing usual care versus telesleep, patients treated under a telesleep protocol had comparable benefits to those with direct face-to-face usual care.[18] Both treatment groups achieved similar PAP usage hours and were equally satisfied with their treatment. At the 1-year follow-up, CPAP use and residual apnea-hypopnea index (AHI) were comparable between groups. However, a notable difference was found in the time requirement of the providers, with the telesleep group being associated with less time requirement.[18]

The video teleconference clinical evaluation can be facilitated by use of web-based platforms that allow the patient to complete electronic questionnaires before the virtual visit. These electronic questionnaires replace the paper questionnaires distributed during in-person clinic visits and represent another example of store-and-forward telehealth. The information on the electronic questionnaires can inform the practitioner of the patient's sleep symptoms and reasons for seeking a sleep evaluation. The electronic format makes it possible to export the responses to templated progress notes, ensuring complete documentation, standardizing documentation across providers and clinical sites, and saving considerable practitioner time in transposing data from paper questionnaires to the electronic medical record. Re-administering the electronic questionnaires after initiation of treatment allows the practitioner to systematically and remotely assess the patient's response to management.

STORE-AND-FORWARD HOME SLEEP TESTING

The HSAT is now widely accepted as an alternative to the polysomnogram (PSG) for the diagnosis of patients with obstructive sleep apnea (OSA) when they have a high pretest probability. As a result, many patients being evaluated for OSA do not need overnight diagnostic testing in a sleep center. This acceptance of HSAT has greatly facilitated its use as a store-and-forward telehealth technology. After the patient performs the test at home and returns the monitor, the recording is uploaded and stored on a computer for subsequent scoring by the sleep technologist and interpretation by the sleep specialist.

Portable monitors for HSAT can be distributed using various approaches. If monitors are located at the patient's local medical clinic, they can be dispensed at the site by a trained technician who instructs the patient how to perform the test. The patient can return the monitor to the local medical clinic in person or using trackable, postage-paid mailing materials. The recording is then uploaded to a server that can been accessed by the sleep center staff at the distant site for scoring and interpretation. Alternatively, the sleep center can mail the HSAT monitors directly to the patient's home with trackable, postage-paid mailing materials for the monitor's return. Illustrated instructions and internet videos showing how to perform the test can help the patient perform a successful study. In addition, a video teleconference with the patient at home or at a local medical facility can be scheduled before testing to review sensor application and reinforce the instructions. Patients can be scheduled for a group video teleconferencing session at their local medical clinic for HSAT instructions, and patients at one or more sites can join the same group session.[19] The video teleconference session can also be used to educate patients about sleep apnea, its consequences, and the benefits of treatment. Questions asked by the patients can be answered during these interactive sessions.

Once the HSAT is scored and interpreted by the sleep specialist, the patient can be contacted by video teleconference or telephone to provide test results and discuss management. Regardless of the method used to distribute the HSAT monitors, the testing should be performed according to the standards set by the American Academy of Sleep Medicine (AASM).[20-22] Portable monitor devices are becoming available that allow a PSG to be performed at home by the patient self-applying the sensors needed for the respiratory and sleep-staging signals. Given the acceptance of home-based sleep testing, these more comprehensive tests will likely gain greater use in the future.

TELEMEDICINE APPROACH TO INITIATE POSITIVE AIRWAY PRESSURE TREATMENT

PAP is the most commonly recommended treatment for OSA. In the past, an in-lab PSG was required to determine the fixed pressure setting needed for CPAP treatment. APAP devices became available about 2 decades ago. These devices continuously monitor airflow and pressure in the airway circuit to adjust the pressure using various algorithms.[19] APAP devices are now routinely used as a first-line mode of pressure delivery. Relative contraindications for use of APAP include morbid obesity, advanced cardiac and respiratory disorders, central sleep apnea, advanced neurologic disorders, and chronic use of medications, such as narcotics, causing central respiratory events.[19,23] Studies have reported no differences in the efficacy and effectiveness of CPAP devices set by PSG titration versus APAP devices initiated without in-lab PSG testing.[24] APAP devices have obviated the need for the PSG titration in many patients with OSA. The use of HSAT and APAP devices facilitates the use of telehealth approaches by allowing OSA diagnosis and PAP treatment initiation without having to perform overnight in-laboratory testing.

Initiating PAP treatment traditionally involves a face-to-face visit. A respiratory therapist or sleep technologist fits the patient with a mask and provides instruction concerning use and care for the equipment. These instructions can be delivered remotely via video teleconference either to an individual patient or a group of patients at several originating sites who connect to the distant site to participate simultaneously in the clinic session.[19] The specific approach may depend on insurance restrictions and concerns about confidentiality. During this virtual PAP setup session, participants are educated about OSA and instructed how to operate and care for the PAP device. If the patient is at a medical facility during the video teleconference, a therapist or technician at the site with prior training and experience on PAP interfaces can fit the patient with the proper mask interface.

To reduce the risk of virus exposure during the COVID-19 pandemic, some practices are exploring whether the PAP device can be mailed to the patient and a video teleconference with the patient at home used to provide the needed information and instructions. Mask fitting becomes more challenging without the physical presence of a provider, although potentially feasible with use of masks with multiple size cushions. Studies are needed to determine if such an approach results in PAP usage similar to that following face-to-face instructions and mask fitting.

TELEMEDICINE APPROACH TO POSITIVE AIRWAY PRESSURE TREATMENT FOLLOW-UP

Store-and-forward telemedicine to remotely monitor adherence and efficacy of PAP treatment is a common form of telemedicine used by sleep practitioners.[25] Many patients with OSA have difficulty using PAP treatment.[26-28] Therefore close follow-up of patients on PAP treatment is a critical component of their management. Although PAP treatment may be efficacious in reducing the AHI to an acceptable level, lack of adequate use will result in ineffective treatment. Current PAP devices provide data that objectively assess treatment use and efficacy. Sensors in the devices monitor mask-on time, respiratory airflow, snoring, and air leak from the circuit. In the traditional care model, the sleep provider would obtain a memory card containing the device's data by mail or in-person delivery, review the data, and make any needed adjustments. Store-and-forward technology offers a convenient way to obtain the PAP results remotely and provide follow-up care.

Many current PAP devices have a built-in modem (modulator-demodulator) that transmits PAP usage and efficacy data daily by wireless technology to the manufacturer's website, where the practitioner can review the stored results. The practitioner can remotely adjust the PAP device settings by entering the changes on the manufacturer's website, which then transmits the new settings wirelessly to the patient's device. The findings and any changes in settings can be communicated to the patient by phone or video teleconference. A pilot study of telemetric CPAP titration (at the patient's home) using the available general packet radio service (GPRS) mobile phone network was successful in remotely titrating CPAP.[29]

The convenience and ease of access to the PAP data are reported to improve treatment use.[30-32] A number of different strategies can provide feedback to patients about their PAP results, including providing patients with web-based access to their results,[33] automated text messaging,[34,35] telephone calls,[36,37] and in-person clinic visits.[25,38] Most studies reported an improvement in PAP use when these interventions were compared with usual care. However, these studies varied not only in the type of feedback provided but also in the frequency of contacts and the length of time over which they were conducted. For example, some studies notified patients who were doing well on PAP, while others notified patients who were not using PAP sufficiently. More studies are needed to determine the most effective ways to telemonitor PAP results.

When adults with OSA starting PAP treatment were randomized to either usual care or daily access to their PAP usage on a website, the participants with web access to their results had about 1 hour per day greater PAP use in the first week. The longer duration of PAP use was maintained over the 3-month follow-up compared with the usual care group.[33] Hwang and colleagues reported significant improvement PAP utilization with automatic text messaging with and without tele-education compared with usual care (Figure 201.2).[34] Participants who continued to receive text messages beyond the initial 3 months of PAP treatment continued to show greater PAP use than the usual care group. However, PAP adherence of participants who stopped receiving text messages after 3 months of treatment declined to the adherence of the usual care group. Another study contacted participants by telephone if problems were

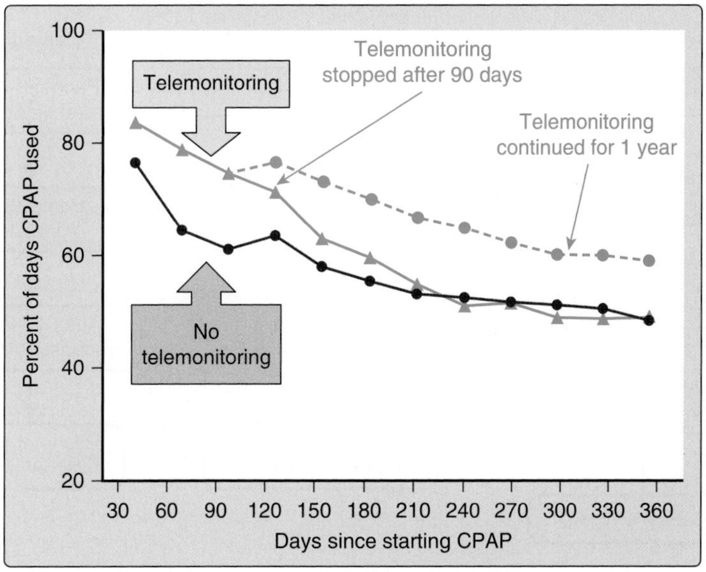

Figure 201.2 Impact of telemonitoring of continuous positive airway pressure (CPAP) use of adults with obstructive sleep apnea over the first year of treatment. Participants who received text messaging in the first 3 months had a greater percentage of days using CPAP than individuals who did not receive this feedback. Adherence of individuals in whom text messaging stopped after 3 months declined to that of the usual care group. Adherence of individuals in whom text messaging continued after 3 months had greater adherence than the usual care group over the entire year, although both groups show a gradual decline in adherence over time. (From Hwang Chang JW, Benjafield AV, et al. Effect of telemedicine education and telemonitoring on continuous positive airway pressure adherence. The Tele-OSA Randomized Trial. *Am J Respir Crit Care Med.* 2018;197[1]:117–26.[34])

identified with their PAP adherence.[36] Mean PAP adherence at 3 months was significantly greater in the telemonitoring arm, but providers spent more time in the telemonitoring arm compared with the usual care arm. Automated telephone calls with motivational voice messages have also been reported to improve PAP utilization.[37] Other PAP telemonitoring studies, using various feedback methods, have reported improvement in PAP utilization.[36,39,40] Of note, use of telesleep for PAP follow-up does not show any safety concern.[41]

TELEMEDICINE APPROACH TO INSOMNIA

The evaluation and management of patients with insomnia is another telemedicine application area. One popular approach involves delivering behavioral sleep medicine on a digital platform, be it a website or a programed application.[42] The evaluation of patients with insomnia depends on a comprehensive medical history obtained by interview, the use of questionnaires, and often a sleep diary. The interview can be conducted by video teleconference instead of an in-person visit. Patients can complete the sleep questionnaires and other materials either on paper forms or electronically before the interview. Paper forms can be faxed or mailed to the provider at the distant site. A well-structured sleep questionnaire provides a comprehensive description of sleep symptoms, which facilitates diagnosis and treatment planning. An additional benefit is that it often illuminates for patients the symptoms they are experiencing and aids in their description of their symptoms during the interview. During the video teleconference, the patient's questions can be answered and the treatment plan discussed.

Cognitive behavioral therapy for insomnia (CBT-I) can be delivered by video teleconference or telephone.[43-45] The CBT-I sessions can be supported by web-based or application-based programs.[46] Studies indicate that telesleep delivery of CBT-I by trained providers is effective for both depression and insomnia.[45,47,48] CBT-I delivered by telephone is also reported to improve insomnia in peri- and postmenopausal women.[49]

In recent years, internet-based CBT-I has rapidly expanded to offer structured, self-administered programs via internet-based or mHealth mobile health apps.[50,51] These self-administered web-based and application-based programs are not considered telemedicine because they do not include evaluation and management by a health care provider. They appear, however, to have mild to moderate benefit, according to a recent meta-analysis[52] and to be overall moderately usable.[52,53] In one study, web-based CBT-I self-administered by individuals was compared with video teleconference delivery by a health care provider.[54] Both interventions contained the same content and resulted in similar improvement in insomnia severity.

HOLISTIC APPROACH TO TELESLEEP MANAGEMENT

Telesleep allows greater flexibility in how to deliver medical care. The sleep practitioner may elect to provide some services using telesleep and other services in person. However, a particularly exciting aspect of telesleep is the ability to combine the component parts of telehealth into a complete clinical pathway that allows some patients to receive care without ever traveling to a sleep center (Figure 201.3). Sleep medicine was initially delivered as laboratory-based care. Patients were evaluated in outpatient clinics and tested in the sleep laboratory. HSAT and APAP led to the development of an ambulatory pathway in which PSGs were no longer needed to diagnose sleep apnea and initiate treatment.

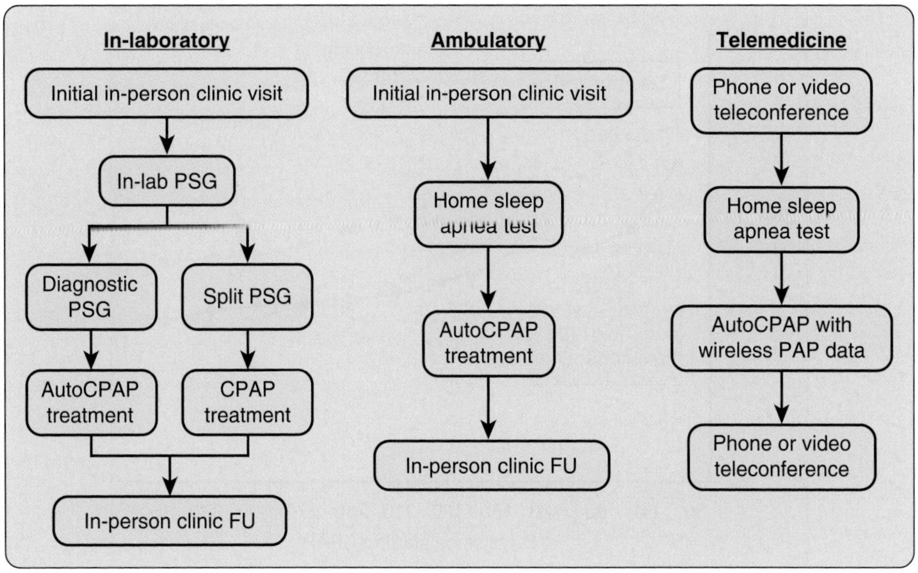

Figure 201.3 Examples of clinical pathways to diagnose and manage patients with sleep apnea. The traditional in-laboratory pathway consisted of in-person clinic evaluation and polysomnography. The use of home sleep apnea testing and automatically adjusting CPAP devices allowed an ambulatory management that allowed diagnosis and treatment without PSG. The addition of video teleconferencing creates a telemedicine pathway in which the patient does not need to ever be physically present in a sleep center. CPAP, Continuous positive airway pressure; FU, follow-up; PSG, polysomnogram.

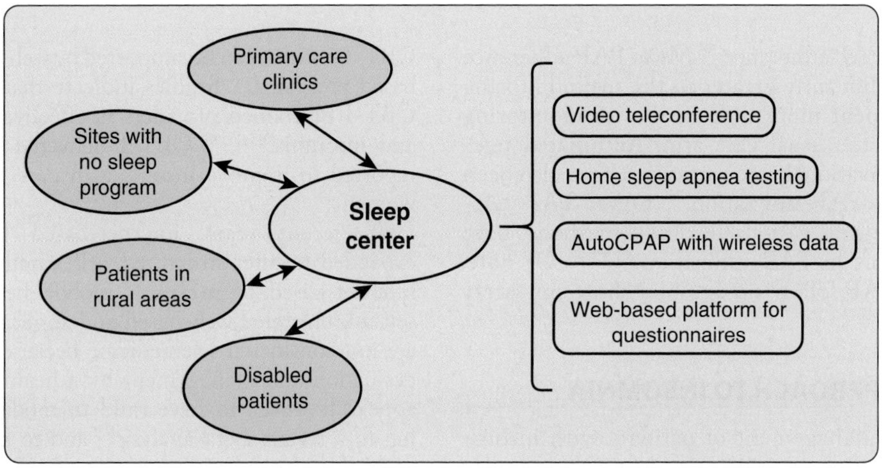

Figure 201.4 Hub-spoke telemedicine approach to diagnosis and management of patients with sleep disorders. Sleep center specialists can use video teleconferencing and store-and-forward telehealth to deliver care to a wide variety of patient populations who lack ready access to this care. CPAP, Continuous positive airway pressure.

However, patients were still evaluated in person. The addition of video teleconferencing to the ambulatory pathway eliminates the need for the in-person clinical evaluation. In the telemedicine pathway, the initial evaluation can be conducted by video teleconferencing or telephone. A portable monitor can be mailed to the patient for home sleep testing. PAP setup can be performed by a local durable medical equipment company or potentially by video teleconference. Follow-up of patients on PAP treatment can be performed by video teleconference with use of the wireless transmission of the PAP results.

Such a comprehensive approach allows development of a hub-spoke model of care in which a sleep center can deliver care to patients in far distant locations (Figure 201.4). A well-developed hub-spoke model of telehealth for sleep medicine is in widespread use in Veteran Health Administration.[51] Lugo and colleagues[55] randomized adults with OSA to in-person care at a medical facility versus a completely out-of-hospital virtual care pathway using video teleconferencing, HSAT, and telemonitoring of wireless PAP data. After 3 months of PAP treatment, PAP adherence was similar in the two groups, and total and OSA-related costs were lower in the telemedicine arm.

In summary, telesleep provides a platform for diagnosis, initiation of treatment, and follow-up management of patients with sleep-disordered breathing and chronic insomnia; it can be used in the management of other sleep disorders to reduce patient and practitioner burden.

TECHNICAL ASPECTS OF TELEMEDICINE

Starting a telesleep program requires a team of individuals with expertise in the medical, technical, financial, legal,

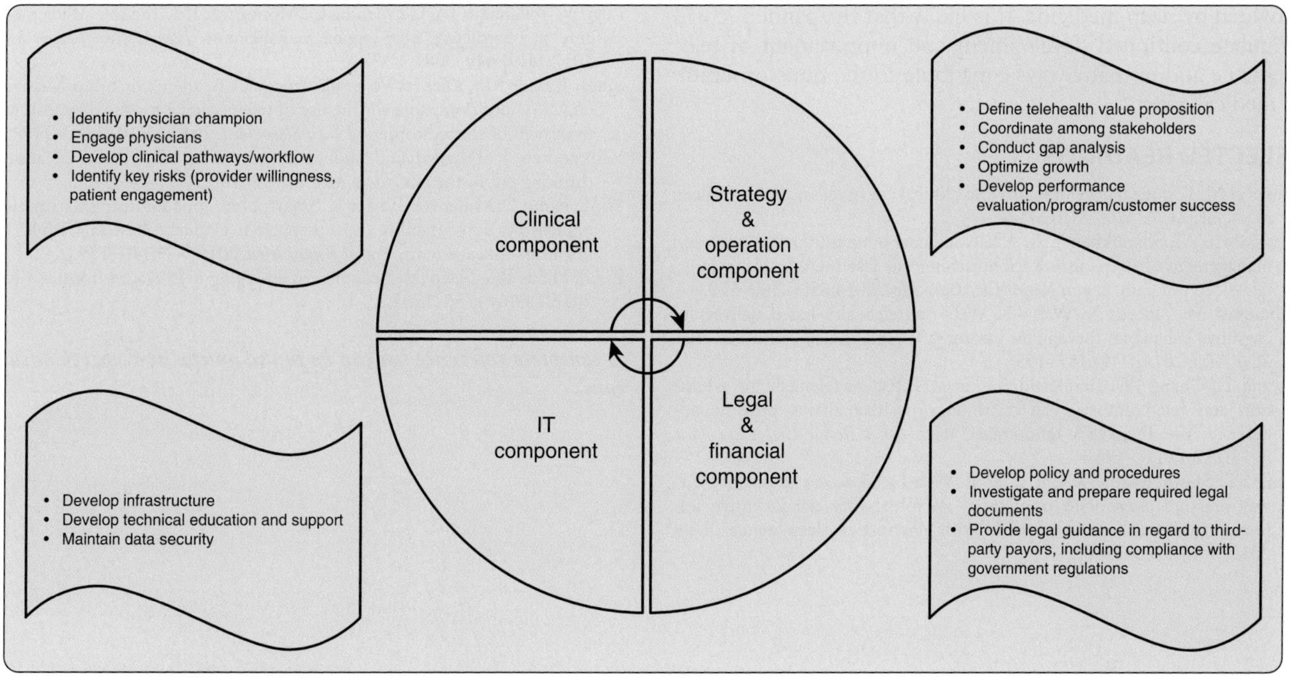

Figure 201.5 Various components and stakeholders that should be considered when starting a telemedicine program. IT, Information technology.

and marketing aspects of telemedicine (Figure 201.5). The role and expectations for each member of the telesleep team should be defined. The telemedicine team can evaluate the sleep center's current clinical practice, the potential benefits that telesleep can bring to the practice, and how the staff perceives telesleep. The members of the team should be knowledgeable of telehealth research results that may be applied to their program in this rapidly evolving discipline. Additionally, the telemedicine team should develop a business plan that incorporates telemedicine billing and coding and projects revenues.[2] Establishing a flow map of the telemedicine clinical pathway helps to clearly define the program. The telemedicine team should identify and establish business agreements with participating sites, ensure that licensing and credentialing requirements are met, develop the telesleep program's policies and procedures, and decide upon marketing and communication strategies. Physician champions can be identified who are responsible for the clinical aspects of telesleep, and clinical operation champions should collaborate with the physician champions to design and manage the telesleep program. Training of physicians and physician extenders to conduct telemedicine is a particularly important pillar of a successful program. In addition, strong information technology expertise is important to ensure that the required hardware and software are available for delivering the care. Furthermore, input of compliance officers is required to ensure adequate protection of the patient's privacy and security. Implementing the telemedicine program at the participating remote sites includes, but is not limited to, identifying practitioners and staff at the sites, developing the needed infrastructure, finalizing agreements, and providing training. Before the telemedicine program is initiated, a pilot program of limited scale can be conducted to identify any problems before full implementation.

CLINICAL PEARLS

- Telemedicine improves access to sleep services regardless of a patient's location.
- Sleep services can be provided via synchronous telemedicine using video teleconference and asynchronous, store-and-forward telemedicine.
- Home sleep testing and wireless transmission of PAP data provide remote collection of data and therefore integrate well within telemedicine programs.
- OSA evaluation, diagnosis, and PAP therapy follow-up can be comprehensively accomplished with telemedicine in many patients.
- Evaluation of patients with chronic insomnia and delivery of CBT-I can be provided through video teleconference.

SUMMARY

Sleep medicine, with its reliance on medical history and use of computer-supported technologies, is uniquely positioned to transition from its traditional in-person approach to providing care by telemedicine. Telemedicine improves access to care, especially for patients in locations where sleep specialized care is not convenient or readily available. Sleep medicine can use both synchronous and asynchronous telehealth techniques. These include video teleconferencing, technologies using portable monitors for home sleep testing, and wireless transmission of PAP data. Starting telemedicine services depends on the support of the participating medical facilities and on a multidisciplinary team to address the medical, technological, legal, and privacy components of a telemedicine program. The COVID-19 pandemic greatly accelerated telemedicine use to deliver a wide variety of medical services, including those provided by sleep medicine. It is likely that the pandemic will stimulate continued development and improvement of telemedicine and in many ways contribute to the transformation of medical care.

SELECTED READINGS

Bruyneel M. Technical developments and clinical use of telemedicine in sleep medicine. *J Clin Med.* 2016;5(12)

Hirshkowitz M, Sharafkhaneh A. A telemedicine program for diagnosis and management of sleep-disordered breathing: the fast-track for sleep apnea tele-sleep program. *Semin Respir Crit Care Med.* 2014;35(5):560–570.

Holmqvist M, Vincent N, Walsh K. Web- vs. telehealth-based delivery of cognitive behavioral therapy for insomnia: a randomized controlled trial. *Sleep Med.* 2014;15(2):187–195.

Hwang D, Chang JW, Benjafield AV, et al. Effect of telemedicine education and telemonitoring on continuous positive airway pressure adherence. The Tele-OSA randomized trial. *Am J Respir Crit Care Med.* 2018;197(1):117–126.

Kuna ST, Shuttleworth D, Chi L, et al. Web-based access to positive airway pressure usage with or without an initial financial incentive improves treatment use in patients with obstructive sleep apnea. *Sleep.* 2015;38(8):1229–1236.

Lugo V, Villanueva JA, Garmendia O, Montserrat JM. The role of telemedicine in obstructive sleep apnea management. *Expert Rev Respir Med.* 2017;11(9):699–709.

Singh J, Badr MS, Diebert W, et al. American Academy of Sleep Medicine (AASM) position paper for the use of telemedicine for the diagnosis and treatment of sleep disorders. *J Clin Sleep Med.* 2015;11(10):1187–1198.

Verbraecken J. Telemedicine applications in sleep disordered breathing: thinking out of the box. *Sleep Med Clin.* 2016;11(4):445–459.

Yu JS, Kuhn E, Miller KE, Taylor K. Smartphone apps for insomnia: examining existing apps' usability and adherence to evidence-based principles for insomnia management. *Transl Behav Med.* 2019;9(1):110–119.

Zia S, Fields BG. Sleep telemedicine: an emerging field's latest frontier. *Chest.* 2016;149(6):1556–1565.

A complete reference list can be found online at ExpertConsult.com.

Chapter 202

Cardiopulmonary Coupling

Robert Joseph Thomas

Chapter Highlights

- Cardiopulmonary coupling (CPC) is a technique that uses heart rate variability (HRV) as a measure of autonomic drive and respiration to generate sleep spectrograms. The electrocardiogram (ECG) is a convenient signal from which to extract both HRV and tidal volume fluctuations measured as R-wave amplitude fluctuations. Through this analysis, non–rapid eye movement (NREM) sleep shows bimodal rather than graded features.
- Laboratory polysomnography and home sleep apnea tests include ECG or plethysmography. Consequently, HRV and respiratory information can be extracted. This allows for the computation of CPC in a wide range of clinical conditions.
- High-frequency (0.1–0.4 Hz) coupling (HFC) and low-frequency (0.1–0.01 Hz) coupling (LFC) of HRV and respiration are CPC biomarkers of stable and unstable NREM sleep, respectively.
- A subset of LFC, elevated LFC narrow band, identifies sustained periods of central apneas and periodic breathing. Integration of CPC and oximetry can result in a derived apnea-hypopnea index (DAHI) closely correlating with an AHI derived from the polysomnogram.
- Heart rate kinetics across the sleep period can be assessed in relation to CPC-estimated sleep states to provide potentially unique information on cardiovascular health.

INTRODUCTION

Standard sleep scoring divides sleep into rapid eye movement (REM) and non–rapid eye movement (NREM). NREM is further divided into N1, N2, and N3. These classifications are largely based on visually recognized electroencephalographic activity and waveforms. Although this classification was developed long before imaging and widely available digital analysis became available, the primary features of REM sleep have held up well with modern neurobiologic circuit analysis. However, transitions in and out of REM sleep, common in disease states such as sleep apnea and narcolepsy, elude clear quantification. Stage N3 is known to have desirable biologic associations, such as blood pressure dipping.[1] The slow waves characterizing N3 are also strongly coupled to cerebrospinal fluid flow—neural slow waves are followed by hemodynamic oscillations that in turn are coupled to cerebrospinal flow.[2] However, NREM sleep suffers from a major limitation in that deep and restorative "slow wave sleep" (once stage III and IV but now N3) makes up an increasing minor part of sleep across the life span and may be "normally absent" after the age of 60 years. Sleep is a complex integrated oscillatory network state.[3] However, the "biologic worth" of stage N2 may not be fully accounted for by conventional scoring or by absolute delta power profiles. These disparities are especially apparent in individuals over the age of 40 to 50 years, in whom stage N3 makes up less than 20% of the sleep period.[4] The recognition and description of the network dynamics of the <1 Hz slow oscillation as the basic underlying rhythm of NREM sleep[5] and the concept of coalescing multisite local sleep processes[6,7] has remained largely unintegrated into clinical practice.

Alternative methods of characterizing NREM sleep are available. The most extensively researched has been cyclic alternating pattern (CAP), which at its core proposes that NREM sleep has two fundamental modes of expression: one with phasic activity dominating and another relatively devoid of phasic activity.[8,9] Sleep-fragmenting stimuli across a wide range of conditions increase CAP, whereas sleep-consolidating stimuli increase non-CAP. CAP is one view of NREM sleep stability (or instability), dominated by low-frequency coupled and networked oscillations. The CAP-like phenomena are not restricted to the electroencephalogram (EEG), as for example, heart rate kinetics closely follow the CAP state.[10-13]

Heart rate variability (HRV) analysis shows periods of NREM with especially high vagal tone and strong sinus arrhythmia[14-16] that is not restricted to stage N3 itself but correlated with delta power. Sleep apnea researchers have long recognized periods of stable breathing that "come and go" during NREM sleep.[17,18] Figure 202.1 shows this "bimodality" of NREM sleep, from the same individual, within the same hour of sleep, in the same body position. Finding an appropriate term to describe these patterns of NREM sleep is challenging, but one proposal is "effective" and "ineffective" NREM sleep, or $NREM_E$ and $NREM_{IE}$, or simply "stable" and "unstable" NREM, $NREM_S$, and $NREM_{US}$. As state instability is normally seen at boundary zones and episodically during the

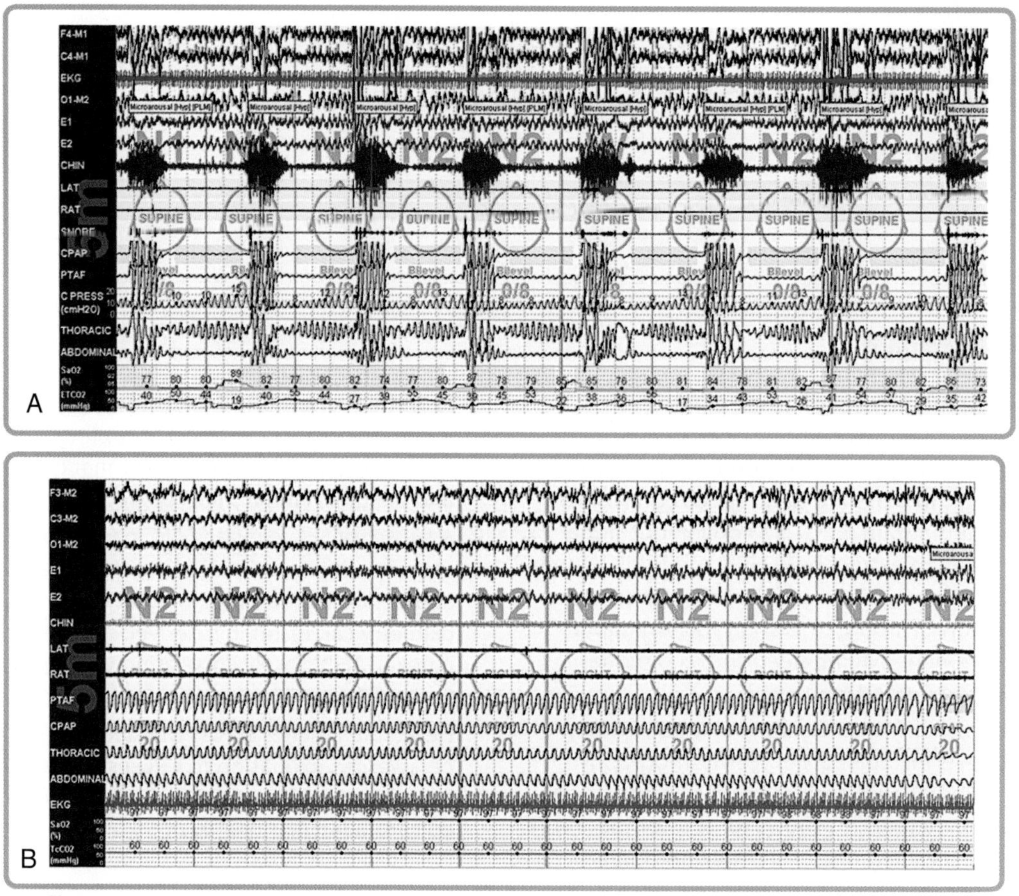

Figure 202.1 **A,** NREM$_{IE}$ in stage N2, 5-minute compression. Sleep apnea (in this case, poorly responsive to positive pressure ventilation) readily brings out the features of NREM$_{IE}$. This snapshot shows temporally synchronized oscillations of EEG, EMG (chin), respiration (PTAF, C PRESS, THORACIC, ABDOMINAL), and oxygenation. **B,** NREM$_E$ in stage N2, 5-minute compression. The same individual with successful sleep apnea treatment. Stable breathing, paucity of phasic EEG activation (non-CAP), and prominent sinus arrhythmia (not readily seen at this compression). Note prominent breath-breathing amplitude modulation of ECG R-wave amplitude *(arrow),* which is one of the input signals for the cardiopulmonary analysis technique. CAP, cyclic alternating pattern; C PRESS, continuous positive airway pressure (CPAP) pressure; ECG, electrocardiogram; EEG, electroencephalogram; EMG, electromyogram; NREM E, NREM sleep "effective"; NREM IE, NREM sleep "ineffective"; PTAF, pressure transducer airflow.

course of undisturbed sleep, such states must have a role to enable state transitions and provide a disengaging mechanism to allow cycling of sleep processes.

Analysis of coupled sleep state oscillations offers an approach to sleep state estimations from a single signal. In theory, any two or more signals from physiologic subsystems during sleep may be coupled. Examples include blood pressure + respiration, HRV + respiration, and EEG + HRV. As originally described, the cardiopulmonary approach uses HRV and electrocardiogram (ECG)-derived respiration, the latter being the R-wave amplitude fluctuations with tidal volume changes during respiration. As HRV and respiratory information is encoded in diverse signals, such as the ballistocardiogram and the photoplethysmogram, coupling information can be generated from a variety of signal sources. This encoding of autonomic and respiratory information in diverse signal streams enables "reduced recordings but enhanced analysis," a theme increasingly used for analysis of data from wearable and "nearable" devices.

THE CARDIOPULMONARY COUPLING ECG SLEEP SPECTROGRAM

The cardiopulmonary coupling (CPC) technique is based on a continuous ECG signal and uses the Fourier transform to analyze two signal features: (1) HRV and (2) the fluctuations in R-wave amplitude induced by respiration.[19] These signals tend to have two basic patterns: a high-frequency component resulting from physiologic sinus arrhythmia that reflects breath-to-breath fluctuations and a low-frequency component that reflects cyclic variation across multiple breaths. Quantifying cardiac and respiratory interactions involves calculating the cross-power and coherence between these two signals.

The steps involved in calculating CPC are as follows: (1) An automated beat detection algorithm is used to detect beats, classify them as either normal or ectopic, and determine amplitude variations in the QRS complex. From these amplitude variations, a surrogate ECG-derived respiratory signal (EDR) is obtained. (2) A time series of normal-to-normal sinus (NN) intervals and the time series of the EDR associated with these NN intervals are then extracted from the RR interval time series. (3) Outliers resulting from false or missed R-wave detections are removed using a sliding window average filter with a window of 41 data points and rejection of central points lying outside 20% of the window average. (4) The resulting NN interval series and its associated EDR are then cubic spline resampled at 2 Hz. (5) The cross-spectral power and coherence of these two signals are calculated over a 1024-sample (8.5-minute) window using the fast Fourier transform applied

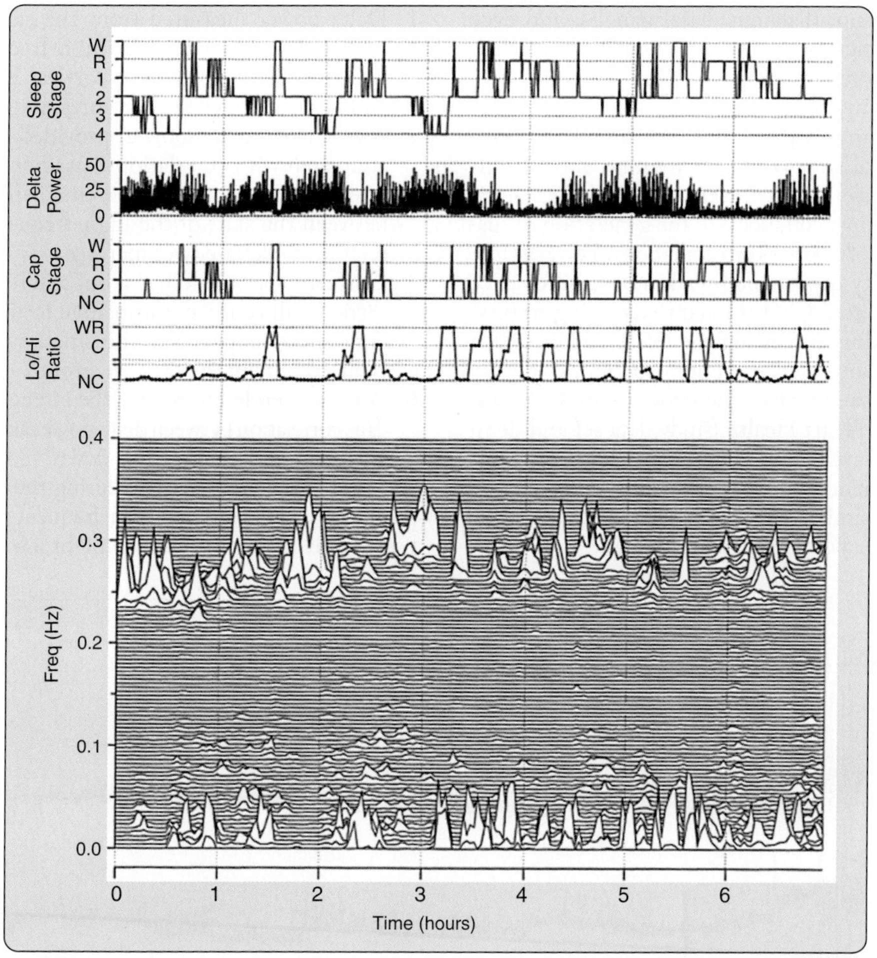

Figure 202.2 Cardiopulmonary coupling analysis in a 22-year-old healthy woman. The four top panels show, from *top* to top, conventional sleep stage scored in 30-second epochs, second-by-second delta power from the C4-A1 electroencephalogram (EEG) montage (μV2/Hz), EEG-based manual cyclic alternating pattern (CAP) scoring, and the ratio of low-frequency (0.01–0.1 Hz) to high-frequency (0.1–0.4 Hz) coherent cross-power (Lo/Hi Ratio) used to detect sleep state. The bottom panel shows the cardiopulmonary coupling spectrogram across 7 hours of sleep in which the magnitude of the coherent cross-power at each frequency is indicated by the height of the peak. The sleep spectrogram reveals spontaneous switching between high-frequency and low-frequency coupled states represented by the two distinct bands of spectrographic peaks. Throughout the night, there is the continued occurrence of cycles of increased delta power and high-frequency coupling that correlates with non-CAP sleep. C, CAP; NC, non-CAP; R, rapid eye movement sleep; 1, NREM stage 1; 2, NREM stage 2; 3, NREM stage 3; 4, NREM stage 4; W, wake. Body position was supine throughout the study.

to the three overlapping 512-sample subwindows within the 1024-sample coherence window. The 1024-sample coherence window is then advanced by 256 samples (2.1 minutes) and the calculation repeated until the entire NN interval/EDR series is analyzed. For each 1024-sample window the product of the coherence and cross-spectral power is used to calculate the ratio of coherent cross-power in the low-frequency (0.01–0.1 Hz) band to that in the high-frequency (0.1–0.4 Hz) band. A preponderance of power in the low-frequency band tends to be associated with periodic sleep behaviors, whereas predominance of power in the high-frequency band is associated with respiratory sinus arrhythmia and sleep with stable respiration and EEG. A preponderance of power in the very low-frequency (0–0.01 Hz) band is associated with periods of wakefulness or REM sleep. This technique thus generates a moving average of the dominant oscillatory frequencies of autonomic drive coupled with respiration during sleep (Figure 202.2). Various input sources such as the plethysmogram can be used, as once the two key data streams are extracted, the analysis is identical.

This technique's discovery was largely serendipitous. Software developed to detect apnea fortuitously detected stable and unstable NREM periods. It was noticed that these periods were clearly demarcated and did not correlate strongly with conventional NREM stages, but better with CAP/non-CAP.[19] Sleep spectrogram analysis reveals that NREM sleep has a distinct bimodal-type structure marked by distinct alternating and abruptly varying periods of strong high- and low-frequency CPC intensity, respectively. Much of high-frequency coupling (HFC) occurs during stage N2, especially with the EEG morphology called *non-CAP*, and is associated with periods of stable breathing, a paucity of phasic EEG transients, physiologic blood pressure dipping, and a reduction in sleep apnea and fibromyalgia.[20,21] HFC tags periods of stable breathing, and when blood pressure dipping occurs during sleep, it occurs exclusively during such periods (Figure 202.3A and B).

Cortical slow wave kinetics can affect autonomic and respiratory function. Slow oscillation–like activity has been recorded in downstream neural elements,[22] including the hippocampus, cerebellum, thalamus, basal ganglia, and even the locus ceruleus.[23] Increased slow wave activity after sleep deprivation in cats was reported in subcortical structures such as the hippocampus, amygdala, hypothalamus, nucleus centralis lateralis of the thalamus, septum, caudate nucleus, and substantia nigra.[24] Cortical slow wave activity may thus directly entrain activities in "lower" brain centers and networks, plausibly enhancing a state most conducive to the generation of sustained periods of high-density slow oscillations. For example, an increased probability of a stable breathing period enabled by the slow oscillation could, in turn, reduce arousing respiratory afferent stimuli, thus enhancing the likelihood of undisturbed and sustained slow-oscillation dense periods.

The relationship between EEG delta power with CPC was tested using the Sleep Heart Health Study data set and demonstrated that slow wave power fluctuations positively correlate with high-frequency CPC, thus identifying stage N2 periods that may have similar physiologic characteristics as N3 (Figure 202.4).[25] The key findings are as follows:

1. Delta power measured from the surface EEG correlated with ECG-derived CPC high-frequency power, further supporting a link between cortical EEG electrical activity and brainstem-related cardiorespiratory functions.
2. Normalized delta power provided improved correlation compared with correlations based on absolute delta power.
3. There was a consistent lag (median of about 4 minutes) between the start of the high-frequency power increase in relation to delta power increase.
4. Correlations were reduced but still highly significant in the second half of the night relative to the first half.
5. Age effects appeared to be small, with correlations being reduced only in the 80+ age group.
6. Arousals tended to reduce the strength of the correlations.

This correlation between delta power and high-frequency CPC is consistent with strong "top-down" modulation of autonomic and cardiorespiratory activity during the former. Delta power is positively correlated with high-frequency HRV power fluctuations of delta power across the night associated with temporally

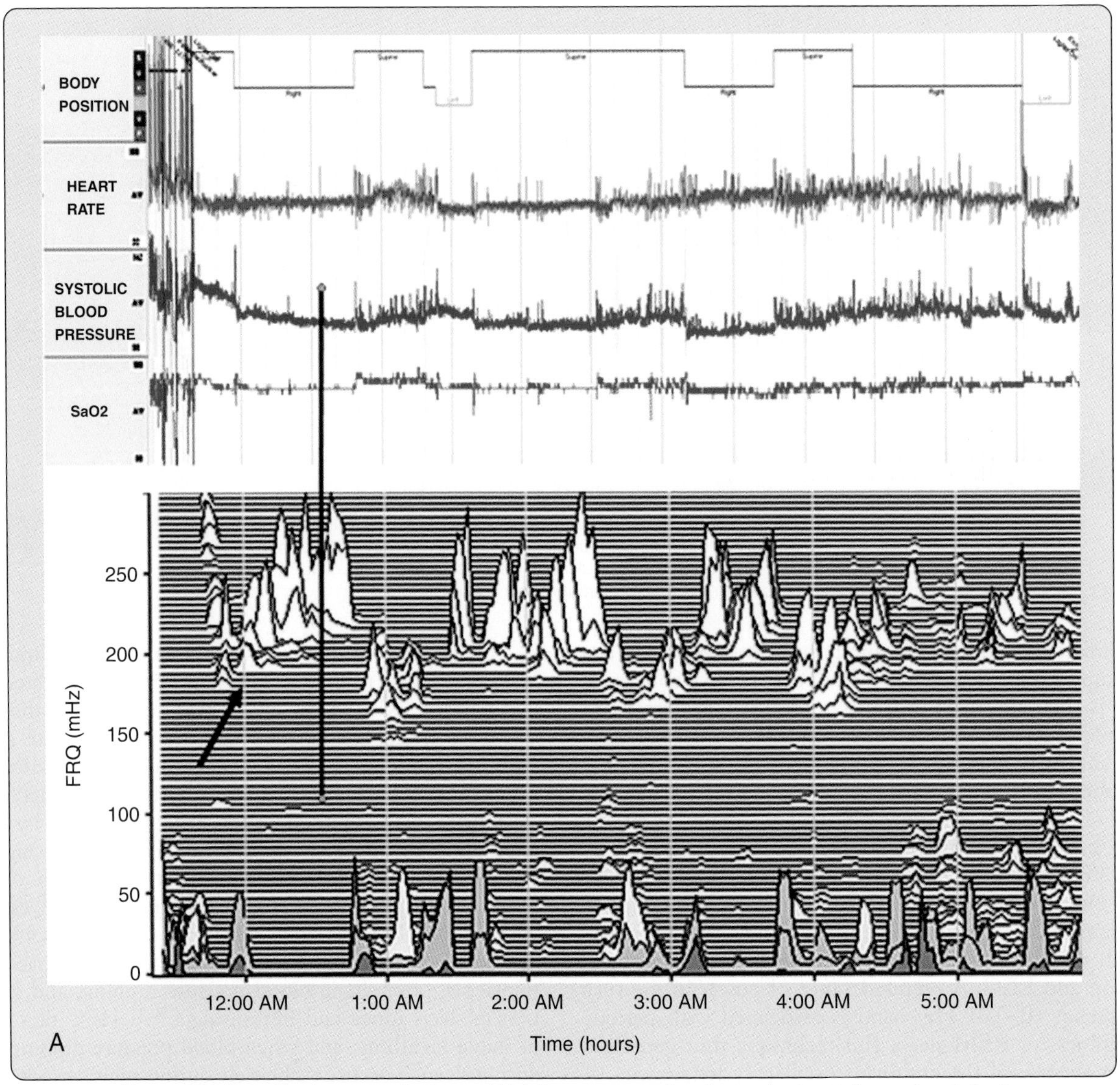

Figure 202.3 **A,** Blood pressure dipping and high frequency coupling. Beat-to-beat systolic pressure derived from pulse transit time, showing the simultaneous *(vertical line)* occurrence of blood pressure drop during sleep with a period of high-frequency coupling *(arrow)*. This combined set of features occurs intermittently through the night. Standard ambulatory blood pressure, with half-hourly or one-hourly samples, cannot capture this dynamic.

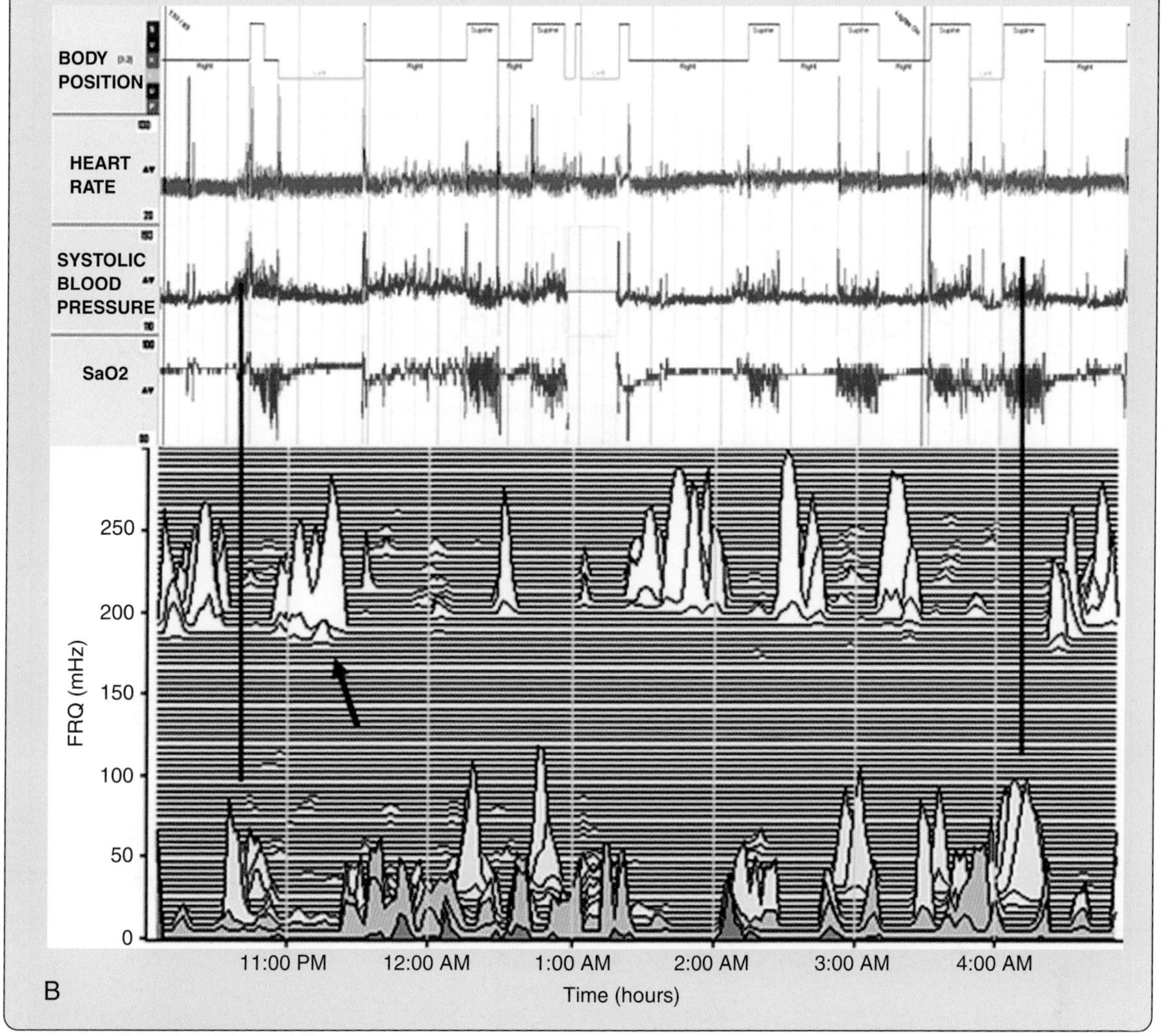

Figure 202.3, cont'd B, Blood pressure nondipping or reverse dipping and low frequency coupling, and periods of stable breathing and high frequency coupling. This representation was obtained from a subject with sleep apnea. Note the rise of blood pressure *(vertical lines showing temporal concordance)* during a period of low-frequency coupling. Note also stable oxygenation, reflecting stable breathing, during periods of high-frequency coupling *(arrow)*.

linked HRV power changes. High-frequency CPC is also associated with periods of NREM sleep enriched with the <1 Hz slow oscillation and blood pressure dipping during sleep, regardless of conventional sleep stage.[26] Thus CPC is one method to estimate vertically integrated sleep state across numerous sleep physiologic subsystems. HFC is seen robustly in the elderly (40% or higher) and is increased in the Sleep Heart Health Study (SHHS) cohort African American subjects, whereas conventional slow wave sleep is known to be reduced in African Americans.[27]

Detection of Strong Respiratory Chemoreflex Activation

Conventional scoring of central sleep apnea and periodic breathing has limitations. The airway may actually be closed during "central" events, and flow limitation is often seen in otherwise typical periodic breathing. The two pathophysiologies, obstructive (in turn either upper airway collapsibility or a poor negative pressure response) and high loop gain, with or without a low arousal threshold, can coexist.[28-32] High loop gain can be quantified by multiple methods, including mathematical analysis of standard polysomnogram (PSG) signals[33-35] and estimating NREM versus REM predominance of sleep apnea.[26] Conventional scoring of central apneas and periodic breathing assesses unstable components of sleep respiration. An extension of respiratory instability analysis is possible by computing the spectral dispersion of single or coupled signals, the logic being that if the respiratory chemoreflex is driving the abnormality, metronomic self-similar oscillations will dominate. In general, self-similarity of respiratory events during NREM sleep is a surrogate marker of high loop gain.[36] The CPC technique has been used to generate spectral dispersion metrics of self-similarity and thus quantify strong chemoreflex influences without needing to consider the exact morphology of individual respiratory events, including flow limitation, described next.

The Cardiopulmonary Coupling Analysis and Estimation of Elevated Low Frequency Coupling (e-LFC) Subtypes Analysis of the PhysioNet Sleep Apnea Database (http://www.physionet.org/physiobank/database/apnea-ecg/), using the CPC technique, showed that elevated power in the low-frequency coupling (LFC) region coincided with periods of scored apnea/hypopnea. Optimal detection thresholds

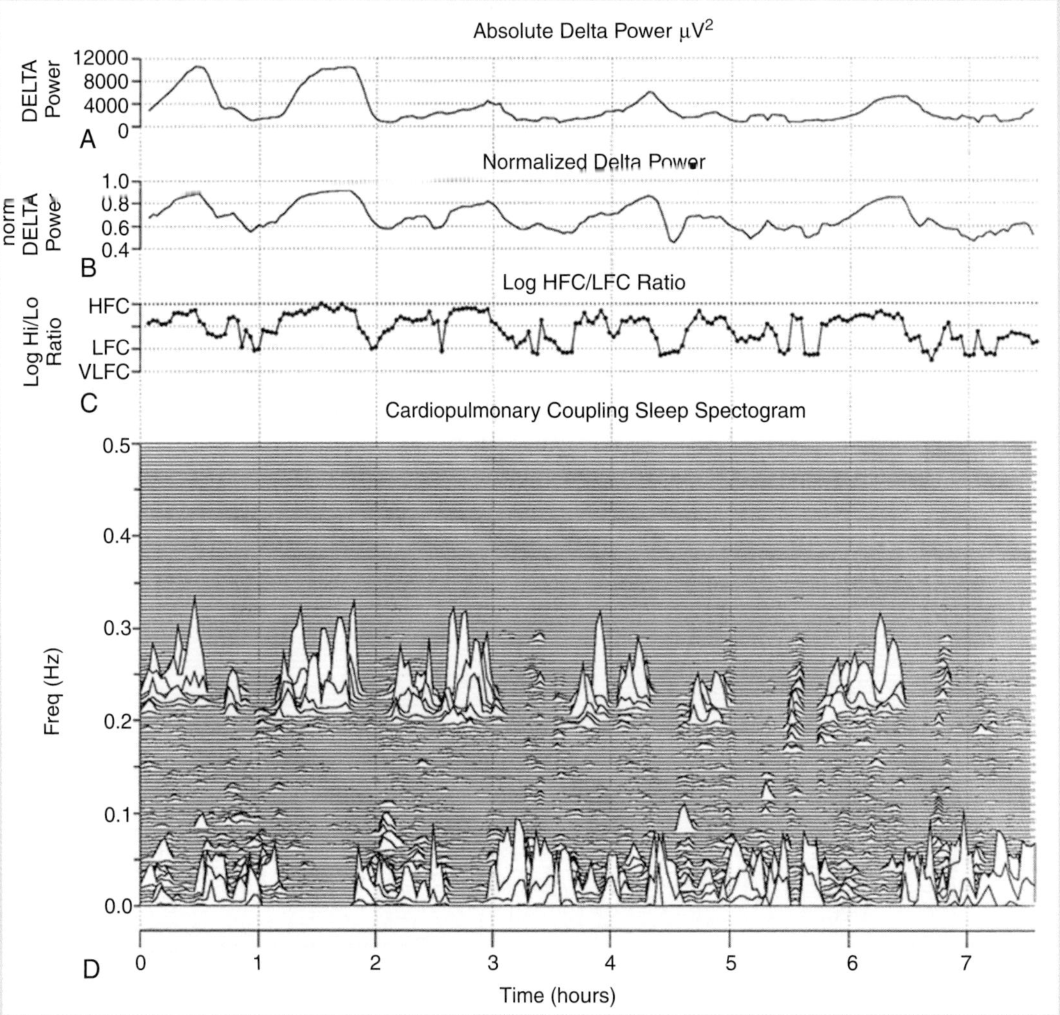

Figure 202.4 Correlations of delta (EEG 0–4 Hz) power and high-frequency coupling power. Delta power 0–4 Hz, cardiopulmonary coupling, and their cross-correlations for a representative subject in the Sleep Heart Health Study database. From *top:* **(A)** Absolute delta power 0–4 Hz (μV^2). Note the higher absolute delta power in the first half of the night compared with the second half. **(B)** Delta power (0-4 Hz) normalized to total EEG power. Note that the relative delta power in the first and second halves of the night is of relatively equal maximal magnitude. **(C)** The logarithm of the ratio of high-frequency to low-frequency cardiopulmonary coupling. Note the correspondence between delta power fluctuations and the CPC ratios. **(D)** The cardiopulmonary coupling sleep spectrogram. The cross-correlation between absolute and normalized delta power and high-frequency coupling in this subject was $r = 0.61$ and 0.75, respectively.

required that the minimum low-frequency power be above 0.05 normalized units and that the low- to high-frequency ratio be above 30 to define periods of probable apnea/hypopnea, which we term *elevated LFC (e-LFC).* Because the apneas and hypopneas in this database were scored in 60-second epochs and CPC measurements made every 2.1 minutes, 60-second linear interpolation between consecutive 2.1-minute measurements was done. The 70 recordings in this database contained a total of 34,243 minutes of which 13,062 (38%) were scored as containing episodes of apnea/hypopnea. Sensitivities and specificities for minute-by-minute apnea detection were calculated for a range of LFC powers and low/high coupling ratios. Receiver-operator curves were then calculated, and the thresholds giving the maximum combined sensitivity and specificity for apnea/hypopnea detection was selected as optimal. Thus e-LFC is defined here as a subset of low-frequency CPC oscillations, periods of which correlated significantly with periods of manually scored apneas and hypopneas in the PhysioNet Sleep Apnea Database. This analysis provides the validation that analysis of low-frequency CPC can estimate sleep apnea–driven pathologic oscillations.

Some spectrograms from the PhysioNet Sleep Apnea Database demonstrated periods of near-constant-frequency spectral peaks in the e-LFC region that was reminiscent of the sinusoidal oscillations of HRV seen in Cheyne-Stokes respiration in heart failure patients, which has a relatively constant cycle length. To explore this phenomenon further, we applied the algorithm to the PhysioNet Congestive Heart Failure Database (http://physionet.org/physiobank/database/chfdb/), with the expectation that the database would provide more prolonged episodes with central periodic oscillations. Because the times during which these subjects were sleeping are not known, the 6 continuous hours of lowest heart rate were taken as the putative sleep time. Because the period of central apnea can be as slow as 120 seconds or longer, we used the frequency band between 0.006 and 0.1 Hz to define narrow spectral band e-LFC (putative central sleep apnea, periodic breathing, or complex sleep apnea).

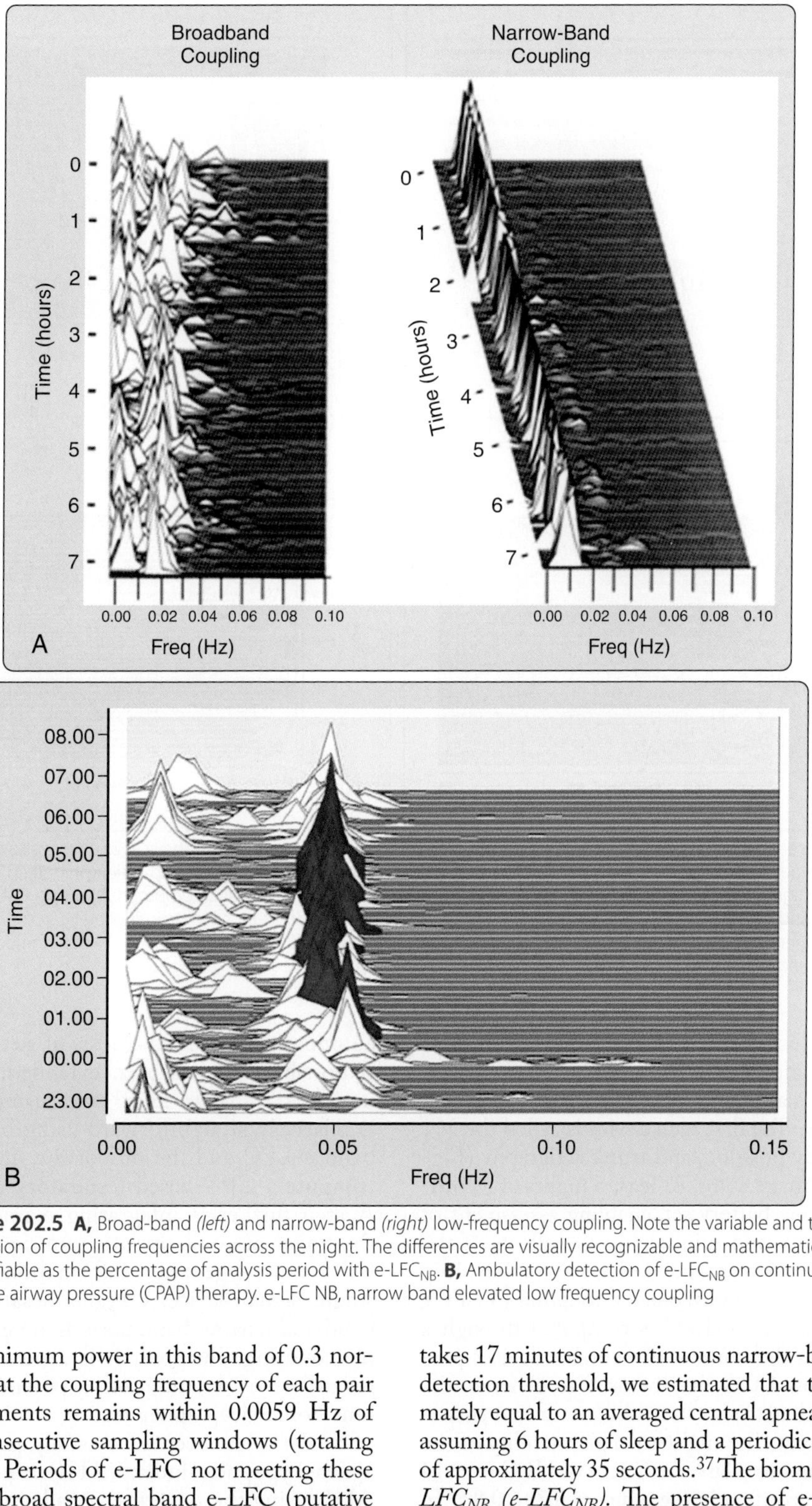

Figure 202.5 **A,** Broad-band *(left)* and narrow-band *(right)* low-frequency coupling. Note the variable and tight dispersion of coupling frequencies across the night. The differences are visually recognizable and mathematically quantifiable as the percentage of analysis period with e-LFC_{NB}. **B,** Ambulatory detection of e-LFC_{NB} on continuous positive airway pressure (CPAP) therapy. e-LFC NB, narrow band elevated low frequency coupling

We required (1) a minimum power in this band of 0.3 normalized units and (2) that the coupling frequency of each pair of consecutive measurements remains within 0.0059 Hz of each other over five consecutive sampling windows (totaling 17 continuous minutes). Periods of e-LFC not meeting these criteria were defined as broad spectral band e-LFC (putative pure obstructive sleep apnea [OSA]). The amounts of broad and narrow spectral band coupling in e-LFC bands were then expressed as the percentage of windows detected in relation to the total sleep period. Thus the narrow spectral band e-LFC identified periods with oscillations that have a single dominant coupling frequency, suggesting central sleep apnea or periodic breathing. The broad spectral band e-LFC identified periods with oscillations that have variable coupling frequencies, suggesting an alternative mechanism, which we posited was dominance of anatomic upper airway obstructive processes. As it takes 17 minutes of continuous narrow-band CPC to reach the detection threshold, we estimated that this would be approximately equal to an averaged central apnea index of 5/hr of sleep, assuming 6 hours of sleep and a periodic breathing cycle length of approximately 35 seconds.[37] The biomarker is called *elevated-LFC_{NB} (e-LFC_{NB})*. The presence of e-LFC_{NB} increases the risk of emergent central sleep apnea,[37] has heritable characteristics,[38] and is associated with hypertension and stroke risk.[21] Figure 202.5 shows the distinctive spectral dispersion characteristics of broad-band and narrow-band coupling.

Ambulatory Assessment of Cardiopulmonary Coupling

ECG data are easily acquired, which allows CPC to be computed from any continuous ECG signal source. Such sources include polysomnography, continuous ECG monitoring for

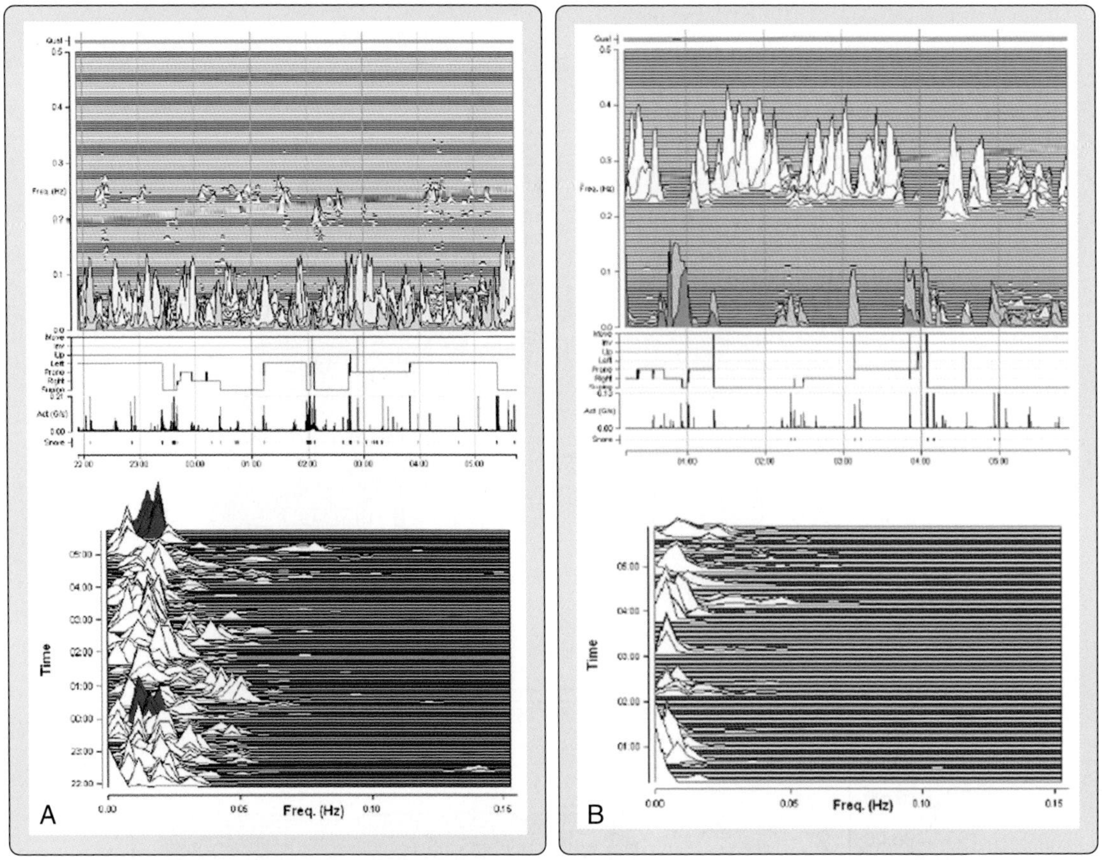

Figure 202.6 Ambulatory tracking of cardiopulmonary coupling using the M1 device. Both snapshots show body position and activity transients; actigraphy allows analysis to be restricted to the actigraphic sleep period. An actigraphic fragmentation index, sleep efficiency, and total sleep time are also computed. **A,** Failing CPAP. Note low- and high-frequency coupling, dominance of low-frequency coupling, and two periods of e-LFC_{NB}, suggesting treatment-persistent or -emergent/complex sleep apnea. **B,** Successful CPAP. Note dominance of high-frequency coupling periods. e-LFC NB, narrow band elevated low frequency coupling

cardiac arrhythmia detection, wearable devices, smart mattresses,[39] or the plethysmogram from a pulse oximetry device. Commercial software is available from MyCardio, LLC, and the Sleep Image system. The first such device is called the M1 and records ECG, body position, and trunk actigraphy (Figure 202.6) (www.sleepimage.com). At least 5 nights of recording are possible with one battery set, enabling assessment of night-to-night variability and minimizing the effects of the same by averaging. The percentage of the actigraphic sleep period in HFC, LFC, very low-frequency coupling (VLFC), and narrow- and broadband e-LFC is computed through a cloud-based system. As the number of wearable devices proliferates, any continuous ECG may be used to generate the ECG spectrogram, and analysis can readily occur in a smartphone application format. The night-to-night stability of the signals is high, with the intraclass coefficient of HFC over 14 consecutive nights of recording in the range of 0.7 to 0.8.[40] In a given state or stage of sleep and body position, sleep physiology or pathology is relatively stable. However, the proportions of these "combinations" interact with time-of-night effects to provide mean values for a night.

Diagnosis of Sleep Apnea

Sleep apnea–induced oscillations in sleep physiology occur across the numerous subsystems, including EEG, ECG, electromyography (EMG), respiration, oximetry, and autonomic drive. A diagnosis of sleep apnea from the ECG is possible and has been extended, with the potential for improved signal-to-noise ratios using CPC.[41,42] The concept is relatively straightforward using broad-band and narrow-band e-LFC and the proportion of sleep in these states to compute a CPC-based respiratory-driven oscillation index. A step further is integrating oximetry signals and use of the finger pulse plethysmogram signal, as input allows both CPC and oxygenation information to be extracted from a single signal/device. Oxygen desaturations during broad-band and narrow-band periods are excluded to prevent double counting. The analysis is expected to show abnormality regardless of desaturation, a potential advantage over current home sleep apnea testing scoring guidelines. This type of analysis has been successfully performed, and a derived apnea-hypopnea index (AHI) equivalent to PSG-based AHI (using the American Academy of Sleep Medicine recommended criteria, 3% desaturation and/or arousal) was approved by the Food and Drug Administration (FDA) in 2019. Using baseline data from the Apnea Positive Pressure Long-Term Efficacy Study, a correlation of the Pearson coefficient for DAHI-Adult obtained by SleepImage and 3% AHI in the APPLES study was 0.972. A Bland-Altman analysis showed a mean difference of -1.975 (confidence interval [CI] -2.429 to -1.521) between DAHI-Adult and 3% AHI values.[43] The system can use a variety of oximeters

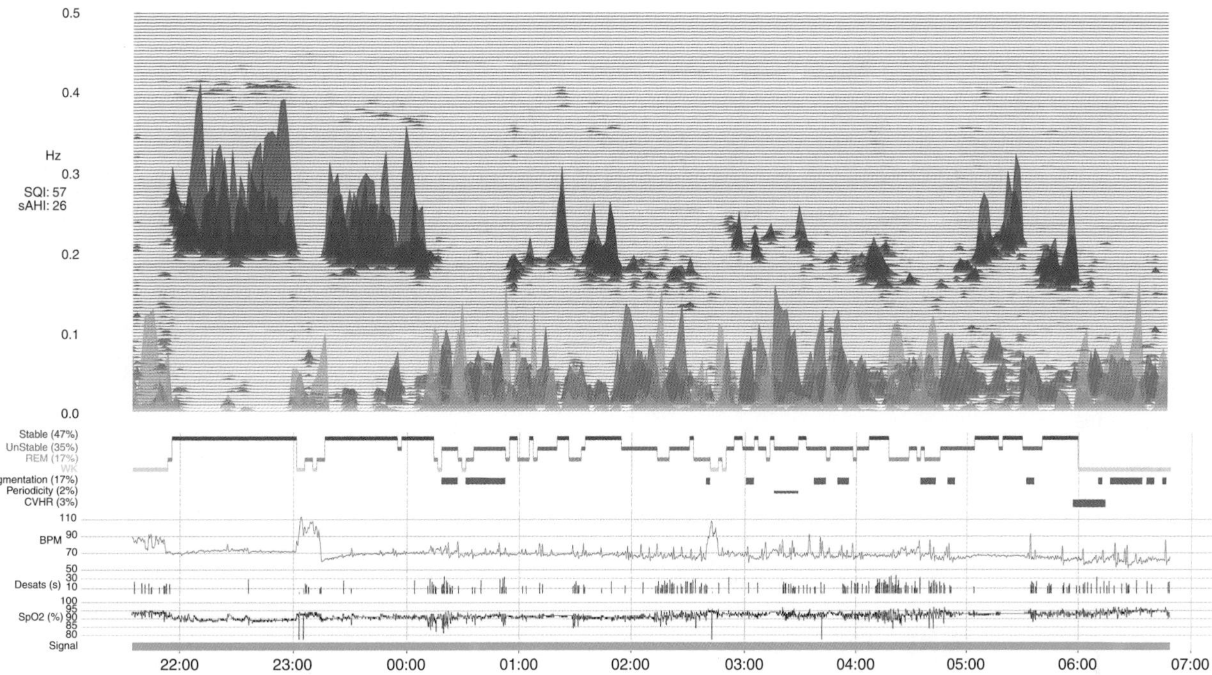

Figure 202.7 Oximetry-based CPC and derived-AHI. An example of sleep apnea diagnosis and sleep quality assessment entirely derived from a pulse oximetry signal. The output also provides heart rate information, a sleep quality index, and an oxygen desaturation index. The heart rate drops at sleep onset but then shows no further drop; it rises during REM sleep (estimated, CPC-based). This patient has relatively good sleep quality and moderate apnea. AHI, apnea hypopnea index; CPC, cardiopulmonary coupling; SQI, Sleep quality index.

with Bluetooth connectivity coupled to a smartphone application. Figure 202.7 shows an example of analysis from an oximeter plethysmogram.

Application to Pediatrics

CPC analysis may be performed successfully on data from children and provide diagnostic or pathophysiologic insights.[44-46] In 2019 the FDA approved the CPC analysis, when coupled with oximetry, as a PSG-equivalent AHI, similar to that approved for adults. The Pearson coefficient for the ECG-CPC–derived AHI-Pediatric from the baseline data obtained by SleepImage and 3% AHI in the CHAT study was 0.8328.[47] A Bland-Altman analysis showed a mean difference of -0.427 (CI -0.756 to -0.098) between derived AHI-Pediatric and 3% AHI values. A further analysis using the entire data set and CPC analysis from the finger plethysmogram signal showed similar results. The sample size was 805 PSGs, distributed as follows: (1) no apnea (AHI <1.0), mild (mild apnea 1–5), moderate (5.0–10), and severe (more than 10/hr of sleep: 288 [35.7%], 354 [44.0%], 94 [11.7%], and 69 [8.6%]), respectively. The correlation of PSG and plethysmographic-CPC-AHI was 0.94 (Pearson correlation). Receiver operating characteristic (ROC) curves showed a strong agreement in all OSA categories (mild, moderate, severe) of 91.4% (CI: 95%, 89.5, 93.4), 96.7% (CI: 95%, 95.4, 97.9), 98.6% (CI: 95%, 97.8, 99.4), respectively.

Cardiopulmonary Coupling and Autonomic Health through Heart Rate Analysis

The importance of blood pressure during sleep is well-established, and sleep-related HRV analysis has been done in several sleep-related conditions,[48-51] but heart rate itself, which is readily available and amenable to simple analysis, has seen relatively little research. In an analysis of a sleep laboratory database on nonapneic subjects, "dipping" of heart rate in NREM sleep was surprisingly uncommon (13.5%).[52] Aligning heart rate profiles in parallel to CPC-derived sleep states shows that heart rate drops ("dipping") usually occurs during stable NREM sleep (HFC), regardless of conventional NREM stage. Heart rate profiles may be abnormal in several forms, including an overall lack of "dip," an increase during sleep, or lack of a "dip" during stable NREM sleep. The latter may be a biomarker of autonomic health that deserves further study. Figure 202.8A and B shows examples of decreasing and rising heart rate during stable NREM sleep/HFC, respectively; the latter pattern would be considered abnormal. The long-term impact of such patterns remains to be established.

CLINICAL PEARL

Cardiopulmonary sleep spectrograms suggest that NREM sleep is bimodal, with concordant and predictable sets of signals (and thus physiologic characteristics) from multiple sleep subsystems. As sleep-fragmenting and -consolidating stimuli move the proportion of HFC and LFC in predictable directions, both absolute values and ratios can be tracked over time to measure sleep quality. The detection of strong respiratory chemoreflex activation using the narrow-band coupling biomarker allows tracking the dynamics of sleep-respiratory control in sleep apnea management. CPC integrated with oximetry can yield a PSG-equivalent AHI. CPC-windowed heart rate kinetics during sleep may provide a measure of autonomic health.

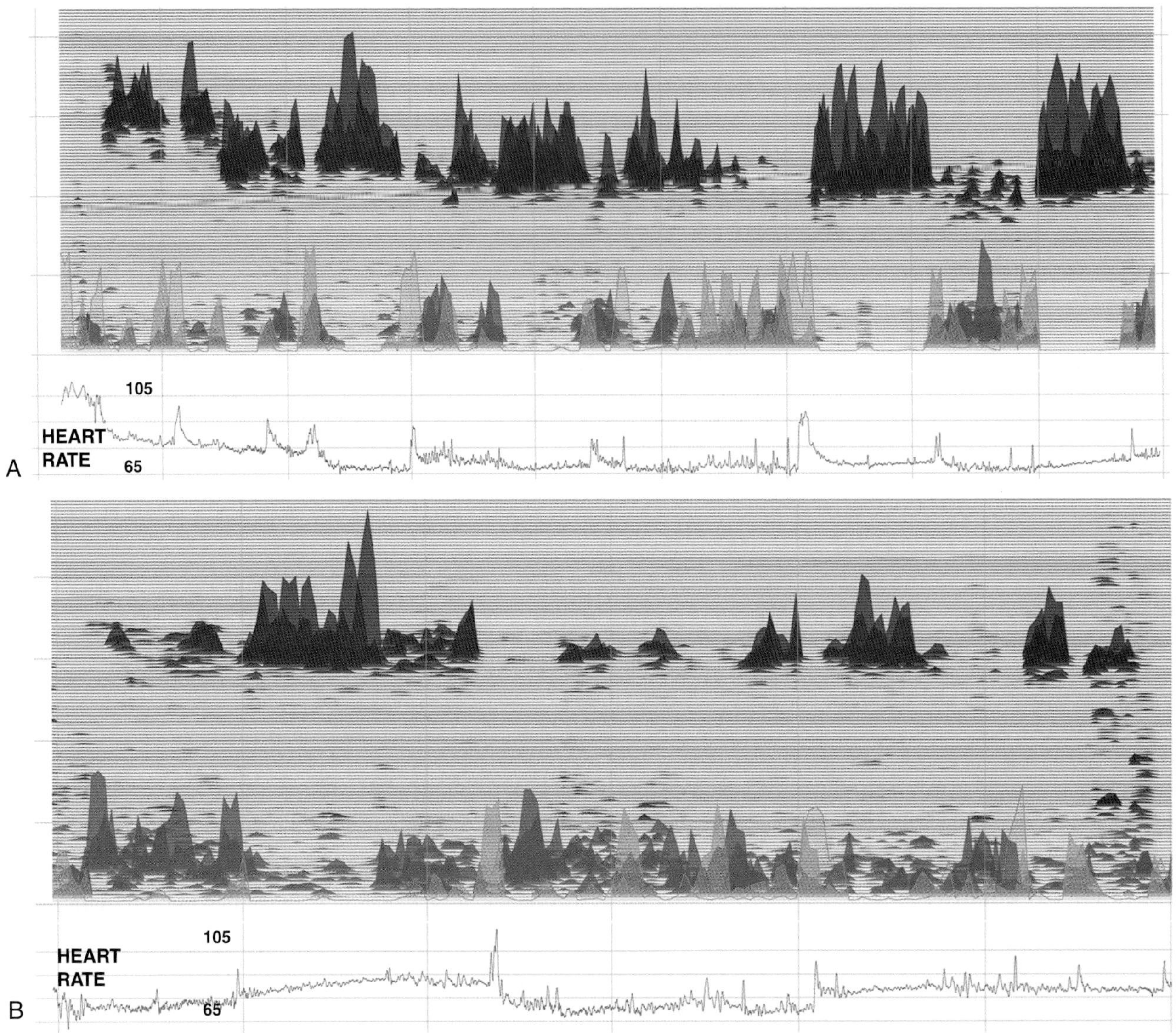

Figure 202.8 Heart rate kinetics and CPC-derived sleep state. **A,** Heart rate "dipping." Note general and high-frequency coupling–related drops of heart rate across the night. **B,** Heart rate "nondipping." Note the general trend for heart rate to not decrease across the night, but also the abnormal pattern of rising during stable NREM sleep.

SUMMARY

Mapping coupled oscillations during sleep provides new insights into sleep physiology and pathology. Both intrinsic brain oscillations and those driven by influences outside the brain (such as respiratory control) can sculpt these signals, providing unique readouts. As the ECG or signals with similar information content are readily available and repeatable signals and are increasingly available through mobile technology, long-term dynamic features of sleep may be tracked. From a physiologic standpoint, the readout of CPC spectrograms strongly suggests that NREM sleep has spontaneously switching bimodal characteristics or modes. In one mode, desirable sleep features dominate, including high delta power and enriched with the below 1 Hz NREM sleep slow oscillation, high vagal tone/sinus arrhythmia, blood pressure dipping, high slow wave power, and stable breathing. In another, generally less desirable features dominate, such as cyclic variation in heart rate, blood pressure nondipping, tidal volume fluctuations (sleep apnea when exceeding clinical thresholds), a fragmented NREM below 1 Hz slow oscillation, and lower delta power. These features likely reflect the integrated output of network activities of multiple sleep subsystems. Integrating oximetry can provide an AHI, and analysis of heart rate during sleep in relation to CPC-estimated states may provide information on autonomic health.

CONFLICT OF INTEREST

Dr. Thomas is coinventor of the ECG-spectrogram cardiopulmonary coupling software, which is licensed by the Beth Israel Deaconess Medical Center to MyCardio, LLC. Dr. Thomas receives royalties through standard institutional policies.

SELECTED READINGS

Magnusdottir S, Hilmisson H, Thomas RJ. Cardiopulmonary coupling-derived sleep quality is associated with improvements in blood pressure in patients with obstructive sleep apnea at high-cardiovascular risk. *J Hypertens*. 2020;38(11):2287–2294.

Thomas RJ, Mietus JE, Peng CK, et al. Differentiating obstructive from central and complex sleep apnea using an automated electrocardiogram-based method. *Sleep*. 2007;30:1756–1769.
Thomas RJ, Mietus JE, Peng CK, Goldberger AL. An electrocardiogram-based technique to assess cardiopulmonary coupling during sleep. *Sleep*. 2005;28:1151–1161.
Thomas RJ, Mietus JE, Peng CK, et al. Relationship between delta power and the electrocardiogram-derived cardiopulmonary spectrogram: possible implications for assessing the effectiveness of sleep. *Sleep Med*. 2014;15:125–131.
Thomas RJ, Weiss MD, Mietus JE, Peng CK, Goldberger AL, Gottlieb DJ. Prevalent hypertension and stroke in the Sleep Heart Health Study: association with an ECG-derived spectrographic marker of cardiopulmonary coupling. *Sleep*. 2009;32:897–904.
Thomas RJ, Wood C, Bianchi MT. Cardiopulmonary coupling spectrogram as an ambulatory clinical biomarker of sleep stability and quality in health, sleep apnea, and insomnia. *Sleep*. 2018;41(2): zsx196. https://doi.org/10.1093/sleep/zsx196.

A complete reference list can be found online at ExpertConsult.com.

Chapter

203

Pulse Wave Analysis

Ludger Grote; Ding Zou

Chapter Highlights

- The beat-to-beat digital pulse wave signal can be detected by various recording techniques (e.g., photoplethysmography from pulse oximetry, peripheral arterial tone). Characteristics of the finger pulse wave form are modulated by skin sympathetic nerve activity and hemodynamic variables such as stroke volume, blood pressure, and central arterial stiffness.
- There is increasing interest in using information embedded in the finger pulse wave signal alone or in combination with other physiologic signals to detect autonomic activation, sleep stage, and sleep-disordered breathing. Sleep diagnostic devices based on finger pulse wave signal analysis have been integrated in clinical procedures. They are recognized by the American Academy of Sleep Medicine for home sleep testing (e.g., peripheral arterial tone technology).
- Additional information on cardiovascular reactivity, beyond that obtained by classic diagnostic devices, can be assessed using finger pulse wave signal. Pulse rate variability, blood pressure, arterial stiffness measures, and signs of vascular aging can be detected from the pulse wave contour. One novel approach involves overall cardiovascular risk assessment using several parameters derived from the oximeter-based photoplethysmographic signal. Recently, population-based cross-sectional studies demonstrated that information derived from pulse wave during sleep is associated with cardiometabolic disease status. Large prospective outcome studies on the clinical relevance of pulse wave–derived cardiovascular parameters are ongoing.

INTRODUCTION

We spend approximately one-third of the 24-hour cycle during sleep; sufficient and restorative sleep is essential for physical and mental health. Consequently, diagnosing sleep-related dysfunction is of major clinical interest. Several recent developments aim to simplify and improve the methodology of sleep studies. Polysomnography (PSG) is the gold standard to quantify sleep time, to differentiate sleep stages, and to assess sleep fragmentation. In addition, respiratory and motor dysfunction can be measured in the context of sleep. However, technical demands, required technical skills, and high costs limit the use of PSG in daily clinical practice. Consequently, efforts have been made to simplify and improve sleep diagnostic methods. Furthermore, additional dimensions of sleep (e.g., autonomic activity and cardiovascular reactivity), derived from pulse wave analysis, may be as important for health-related outcomes (e.g., quality of life or survival), as PSG-derived variables.[1]

Pulse wave signals can be obtained in different vascular compartments, including the ear lobe, the limbs, or any other suitable vascular bed. However, because photoplethysmography (PPG) in the finger is currently accepted for sleep diagnostics, we focus mainly on this measurement site for pulse wave analysis.

THE PHYSIOLOGY OF THE DIGITAL VASCULAR BED

Like in other extremities, the finger skin vascular beds are rich in arteriovenous anastomoses, amounting to approximately 500/cm^2 in the fingernail beds. Arteriovenous anastomoses are coiled vessels with thick, muscular, and densely innervated walls connecting the arterioles and venules in the dermis. Blood from the digital artery bypasses the high-resistance arterioles and the capillaries of the papillary plexus, flows directly through the dermal arteriovenous anastomoses, and returns to the deep plexus of veins. This special feature enables large variations of digital skin blood flow, which range from 1 to 90 mL/minute/100 mL of tissue.[2] The skin vascular bed accounts for the majority of total digital blood flow.

The finger vascular bed is highly innervated. Despite local factors affecting finger blood flow, the microcirculation in the digital skin vascular bed is controlled mainly by the systemic vasoconstrictor tone. A high correlation between increased peripheral sympathetic nerve activity and reduction of finger pulse wave amplitude (PWA) has shown during temperature changes.[3] Vasodilation is induced by elevated ambient temperature, sedation, and vasoactive drugs such as nitroprusside. Vasoconstriction is induced by sympathetic excitation (e.g., stress, pain), cold, and vasoactive drugs such as noradrenalin and ephedrine.[4]

Autonomic and cardiovascular regulation relevant for pulse wave analysis during sleep is complex, sleep-stage dependent, and regionally differentiated. Non–rapid eye movement (NREM) sleep is associated with reduced sympathetic and increased parasympathetic activity when compared with wakefulness. Rapid eye movement (REM) sleep, in this aspect, is similar to wakefulness. Peripheral vascular smooth muscle sympathetic nerve activity measured by microneurography is reduced by approximately 50% during NREM sleep (stage 4) and doubled during REM sleep compared with wakefulness.[5,6] Regional differences in sympathetic output during sleep may also exist. For instance, sympathetic activity in vasoconstrictor fibers of limb skeletal muscle is increased in parallel with reduced output to the splanchnic, cardiac, lumbar, and renal vascular beds in a pharmacologic model of REM sleep.[7] Skin blood flow measured by laser Doppler showed a clear increase during sleep compared with wakefulness possibly resulting from thermolytic vasodilation.[8]

Quiet NREM sleep is characterized by general hemodynamic stability. However, arousal from sleep creates a significant change; the most pronounced changes can be noticed in the acceleration of heart rate combined with a peripheral vasoconstriction resulting in a marked elevation of systolic and diastolic blood pressure.[9] The autonomic response to an arousal from sleep, when started, appeared to follow a stable pattern over time. The amplitude of the cardiovascular reactivity is positively associated with the degree and the duration of the electroencephalographic (EEG) arousal. In some cases, a typical autonomic activation during sleep can be observed without an activation pattern in the cortical EEG, the so-called autonomic arousal. In this chapter, we focus on different pulse wave analysis methods during sleep to assess autonomic arousal, sleep stages, sleep-disordered breathing, and cardiovascular function and risk.

METHODS FOR THE ASSESSMENT OF THE DIGITAL PULSE WAVE

Plethysmography is a well-established method for the quantitative assessment of volume changes over time and has been frequently used in humans for the quantification of respiratory and hemodynamic function. A number of different noninvasive plethysmographic techniques are available using water, air, strain gauge, impedance, or PPG to quantify volume changes of the peripheral pulse wave. For studies on finger microcirculation, additional methods such as radioisotope clearance, capillaroscopy, and laser Doppler flowmetry have been used. In sleep medicine, the PPG and the peripheral arterial tone (PAT) are the most frequently used methods to assess the digital pulse wave. Recent developments in home sleep diagnostics have incorporated these technologies.

Water or Air-Based Plethysmography

The historic development of research related to the cardiovascular system began with water or air-based plethysmography. The arm, finger, or leg is placed in a tightened compartment filled with water or air. Any pulsatile change in volume is transferred on paper or, more recently, to a digital signal to quantify blood flow and vascular resistance at rest and after certain type of provocations. For sleep-related assessments, this technology is less feasible because of obvious interference with sleep and artifacts during body movements.

Strain Gauge Plethysmography

The strain gauge technique for the in vivo assessment of blood flow has been used for decades. An elastic mercury in Silastic strain gauge is placed around the circumference at the area of interest (e.g., the forearm, the finger, or the leg). With the venous occlusion technique, pulsatile volume increases of the compartment are recognized by changes in the circumference. The calibrated signal gives an exact measure of blood flow in milliliters per second. When blood pressure is monitored, even resistance of the vessels can be calculated. Characteristics of the pulse wave contour are similar when using strain gauge or digital PPG with a high correlation ($r = 0.9$).[10] The strain gauge technique has been widely used to quantify vascular reactivity after local arterial infusion or systemic application of vasoactive drugs. The concept of vascular and endothelial dysfunction in patients with obstructive sleep apnea (OSA) was introduced by the findings of impaired responses to vasodilatory or augmented response to vasoconstrictor agents in normotensive and hypertensive patients with OSA when compared with controls using venous occlusion plethysmography.[11,12]

Photoplethysmography

PPG measures the absorption/reflection of infrared light emission (wavelength around 940 nm) in the applied microvascular bed by a photosensor. The degree of light absorption/reflection correlates directly with the blood volume changes in the catchment, and a continuous pulse wave signal can be derived. This pulsatile component of the pulse wave is called the *AC signal component*. In addition, the baseline of the pulsatile wave may vary, and this component is described as the *DC component* and reflects to average blood volume and finger tissue.[13] This DC component may be affected by respiration, autonomic nerve activation and vasomotor activity, Traube-Hering-Mayer waves, hypovolemia, and thermoregulation.

The information embedded in the pulse wave can be divided in several aspects (Table 203.1; Figure 203.1). First, the systolic amplitude is correlated with the pulse volume increases in the finger compartment. The amplitude is modulated by both the cardiac stroke volume and the degree of skin sympathetic activity (high activity means reduced flow and low amplitude).[3] Using a daytime infusion protocol, PWA, derived from the finger plethysmography, was sensitive to the alpha-receptor agonist norepinephrine but not to the beta$_2$-receptor agonist isoproterenol.[14] Second, the peak-to-peak interval of two consecutive pulse waves is considered as a surrogate measure of the electrocardiogram (ECG)–based R-R interval and can be used for pulse rate calculation (see the following sections). Third, the diastolic point of the pulse wave reflects the time taken for the pressure waves to pass from the heart to the sites of reflection at small arteries in the trunk/lower limbs and back to the upper limbs. This interval, also called *pulse propagation time* (PPT), has been proposed as a surrogate marker of pulse wave velocity and arterial stiffness.[15,16] A shortening of PPT indicates rigid and atherosclerotic vessels. The augmentation index (AI), calculated as the ratio between the systolic and the diastolic amplitude, is another way to mirror central arterial stiffness. Both PPT and the digital AI have been shown good agreement with the AI derived from radial artery or the pulse wave velocity calculated along the aorta and applied for assessment of atrial stiffness and cardiovascular risk.[15,17,18] During signal processing, first and second

Table 203.1 Different Variables Derived from the Digital Pulse Wave Signal

Pulse Wave Parameter	Function Assessed	Modified by Dysfunction or Disease
Systolic pulse wave amplitude	Digital pulse volume, reduced by skin sympathetic activation (vasoconstriction), elevated by vasodilating drugs, correlated with stroke volume and blood pressure	Arousal from sleep, REM sleep, sleep-disordered breathing, hypertension, atherosclerosis, and metabolic disease
Pulse-to-pulse interval	Pulse rate and pulse rate variability	Bradycardia/tachycardia, arrhythmia (e.g., atrial fibrillation), ischemic heart disease, marker of central/autonomic arousal from sleep, baroreflex
Time between systolic and diastolic peak of the pulse wave (e.g., stiffness index, pulse propagation time)	Central and peripheral vascular wall compliance and stiffness	Atherosclerosis, vascular aging, hypertension, diabetes mellitus
Time between R wave of the ECG and systolic peak of the peripheral pulse wave (e.g., pulse transit time)	Marker of central arterial stiffness, correlation with blood pressure, sympathetic activation	Central or autonomic arousal, hypertension
Respiratory-related baseline shifts of the pulse wave DC component	Respiratory effort and negative intrathoracic pressure changes, repetitive Müller/Valsalva maneuver	Obstructive versus central sleep apnea, snoring
Proportion of pulse rate in the respiratory frequency band	Degree of respiratory sinus arrhythmia	Baroreflex sensitivity, autonomic neuropathy, cardiovascular aging, diabetes mellitus, disturbed breathing during sleep
Pulse amplitude ratio before and after Valsalva maneuver	Elevated left ventricular end-diastolic pressure	Heart failure with increased preload
Descending and ascending slope of the pulse wave attenuation	Deteriorated vascular function	Atherosclerosis, endothelial dysfunction
Area under the curve of the pulse wave amplitude drop	Deteriorated vascular function, autonomic activation	Cardiovascular/metabolic disease

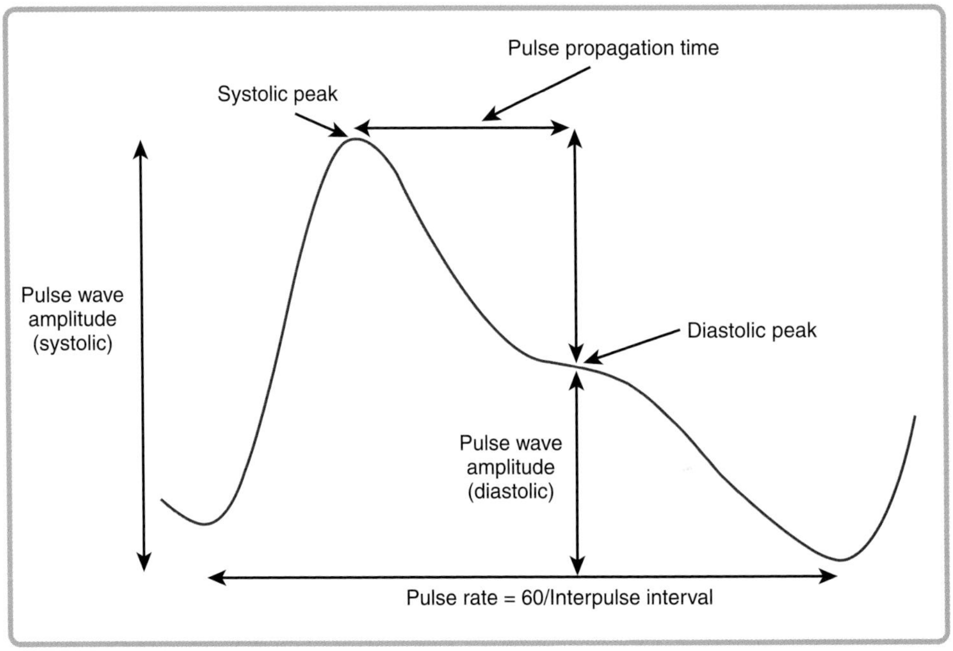

Figure 203.1 A typical photoplethysmography signal and its characteristic parameters.

derivatives of the plethysmographic curve are used to more accurately calculate the pulse wave parameters explained previously.[19] A comprehensive review summarizes the current concepts for photoplethysmographic signal analysis.[20]

The probe placement for assessment of the pulse wave form has been studied. It was suggested that the ear pulse wave may reflect better the passive effect of systemic hemodynamics, whereas the finger pulse wave may reflect local vasomotor fluctuations, including the neural mechanisms of skin sympathetic activation.[21] These studies were performed in spontaneously breathing wake subjects, and the site of pulse wave investigation may have different influences on the results during sleep recordings. Indeed, one study looking at noninvasive markers of acoustically induced arousal from sleep showed that finger PPG was more sensitive for arousal response than ear PPG.[22] In addition, the finger site is most accessible for use during sleep recordings.

Peripheral Arterial Tone Technique

PAT is a novel technology for monitoring pulsatile arterial volume signals using a pressure-applied optical probe.[23] The technology is comparable to classic PPG, with the difference of the specific probe features improving the signal quality. In detail, the PAT probe has a compliant elastic membrane surrounded by an outer rigid casing. Compared with conventional finger plethysmography, a pressurized region is used to cover the surface of the distal end of the finger. This region prevents the induction of venoarteriolar reflex vasoconstriction.[24] The balloon-like outer membrane creates a constant pressure leading to an unloading of arterial wall tension, thereby increasing the arterial wall motion and the size of the arterial volume change. The sensor region is also prevented from retrograded venous blood pooling commonly observed during finger movement. A transmission mode PPG is used to measure the optical density changes associated with pulsatile blood volume changes.

Pulse Transit Time

Pulse transit time (PTT) reflects the time interval for an arterial pulse wave to propagate from the aortic valve level to a given peripheral site. PTT is often measured as the time lapsed from the appearance of the R wave in the ECG to the start or the middle point of the systolic pulse wave appearing in the finger PPG recording. The PTT depends on the degree of stiffness of the arterial wall, and a shortened PTT is associated with vascular aging, atherosclerosis, and increase of blood pressure.

Finally, the usefulness of the three methods—PPG, PAT, and PTT—is limited in patients with cardiac arrhythmias, such as atrial fibrillation or frequent extra systolic activity. The high variability of cardiac stroke volume creates a beat-to-beat variation in the systolic PWA and the pulse contour, which sometimes invalidates the information embedded in the pulse wave signal. Indeed, existence of arrhythmia (but not type of arrhythmia) can be detected by PPG.

CLINICAL APPLICATIONS OF DIGITAL PULSE WAVE ANALYSIS

Periodic cardiovascular autonomic changes during sleep in patients with sleep-related disordered breathing have been documented since the 1970s. Heart rate and arterial blood pressure are the traditional physiologic parameters to study hemodynamic autonomic changes associated with sleep apnea events. More recently, the finger pulse wave signal in combination with other biosignals has been evaluated for the detection of autonomic arousal, sleep stages, sleep-disordered breathing, and the assessment of cardiovascular function[25] (Table 203.2). Improved and novel insights into the sleep state can be made with this rather simplified methodology. As with other currently advancing technologies, these methods will likely find their place along other diagnostic innovations.

Identification of Autonomic Arousal/Sleep Fragmentation

EEG arousal has been traditionally used for quantification of sleep fragmentation. However, it has been shown that transit sympathetic activations during sleep are not necessarily associated with visible EEG changes.[26] Hence, the term *autonomic arousal* is used by some to represent transit changes of autonomic activity associated with cardiac activation (e.g., heart rate and blood pressure increase). The finger vascular bed is densely innervated, and finger PWA drop has been shown to associate with increased EEG power density, suggesting that PWA attenuation is a useful surrogate marker for changes in cortical activity during sleep.[27] Other studies found digital vascular response (e.g., PWA) to variable degrees of arousal stimulus during NREM sleep to be more sensitive than other autonomic markers (e.g., heart rate, PTT, and pulse wave velocity).[22] Hence digital vasoconstriction (PWA attenuation) may provide a useful tool to detect episodes of autonomic activation during sleep. By means of the PAT method, an *autonomic arousal* event was defined as at least 50% PAT attenuation or at least 30% PAT attenuation plus a 10% pulse rate increase, which correlated ($r^2 = 0.67$) with PSG scored EEG arousal.[28] Modified criteria for autonomic arousal detection in the ambulatory PAT device are based on either PAT attenuation plus increase of pulse rate or PAT attenuation of at least 40% and short movement detected by actigraphic signal.[29] The correlation coefficient between the PSG-derived arousal index and PAT autonomic index (using actigraphy to detect sleep time) was 0.76. It should be noted that other conditions, such as periodic limb movements, can cause autonomic activation without simultaneous cortical arousal. It has been recently suggested that combined analysis of both amplitude and area-under-the-pulse waveform may be helpful to reduce failure rate in respiratory arousal detection.[30] Further analysis using PWA from standard oximetry showed a more than 90% agreement between the A-phase of the cyclic alternating pattern (CAP) of the sleep EEG (sign of cortical arousal) and a more than 30% PWA drop at the end of an apnea and the resumption of ventilation.[31]

The potential role of PAT for arousal detection was also studied in children. In general, EEG arousal in children is associated with sympathetic activation reflected by PAT attenuation.[32,33] However, PAT signal is a highly sensitive but less specific tool in this context. In fact, a substantial proportion of autonomic activations defined by PAT was found to occur in children without visually recognizable EEG changes. Whether these attenuations represent normal fluctuations of the autonomic sympathetic nervous system activity in children or reflect subtle sleep disruption that failed to be detected by traditional EEG scoring remains unclear. In children with upper airway obstructive disease undergoing noninvasive ventilation, a combination of 4% oxygen desaturation and microarousal detected by finger PWA attenuation greater than 30% was reported to be associated with movement and fragmentation index assessed by actigraphy.[34]

Classification of Sleep Stages and Wakefulness

Wakefulness and the NREM/REM sleep stages differ in autonomic and hemodynamic regulation. This difference can be reflected by changes of the PWA and derived pulse rate signals.[35,36] For instance, a typical reduction of the PAT amplitude could be observed during REM compared with NREM sleep.[35] An automatic REM sleep detection algorithm based on a combination of the PAT signal and actigraphy was developed.[37,38] Subsequently, features from two-time series of PAT amplitude and interpulse periods were used to further analyze

Table 203.2 Clinical Application of the Overnight Pulse Wave Analysis in Sleep Diagnostics

Method	Pulse Wave Parameter and Additional Signal	Results
Sleep Classification and Sleep Fragmentation		
PAT	Systolic PAT amplitude and PAT pulse rate	Autonomic arousal classification with high correlation to respiratory and nonrespiratory EEG-arousal in adults, overestimation in children
PPG	PPG systolic amplitude and pulse rate	Good correlation with EEG arousal and cyclic alternating pattern (CAP) in adults
PPG and ECG	PTT and pulse rate	Good correlation with EEG-arousal in adults, overestimation in children
PAT and actigraphy	PAT amplitude and pulse variation (fractal signal analysis), actigraphy	Sleep-wake detection, REM/NREM classification, deep and light sleep classification
PPG	PPG signal (breathing-related systolic amplitude variation)	Sleep wake analysis via PPG by breathing shape and breathing rhythmicity
Type and Amount of Sleep-Disordered Breathing		
PAT and oximetry	Pulse wave amplitude, pulse rate, and oxygen saturation	High correlation between AHI_{PAT} and AHI_{PSG} in multiple validation studies, AASM-accepted method
PPG and nasal flow	PPG-derived respiratory effort	Improved differentiation between obstructive and central/mixed sleep apnea
PAT and oximetry	Pulse wave amplitude, pulse rate, and oxygen desaturation	Detection of Cheyne-Stokes respiration
PPG	Pulse wave amplitude, pulse rate, and oxygen desaturation	Detection of Cheyne-Stokes respiration
Cardiovascular Function and Risk		
PAT	Systolic PAT amplitude attenuations	Associations between overnight attenuations and office blood pressure
PTT and office blood pressure	A continuous measure of beat-to-beat blood pressure	Associations with intraarterial or oscillometric measure blood pressure at daytime and during sleep
PPG	Pulse wave–derived augmentation index or pulse propagation time	Associated with vascular stiffness in atherosclerosis, vascular aging, and cardiovascular and metabolic disease; sensitive to vasoactive drugs
PPG and oximetry	PPG and oximetry-derived parameters reflecting cardiovascular, autonomic, and respiratory function during sleep	Associated with traditional cardiovascular risk prediction matrixes (e.g., ESH/ESC, Framingham, EU SCORE); identification of vascular stiffness in atherosclerosis, vascular aging, cardiovascular and metabolic disease; sensitive to cardiovascular medication

AASM, American Academy of Sleep Medicine; AHI, apnea-hypopnea index; ECG, electrocardiogram; ESC, European Society of Cardiology; ESH, European Society of Hypertension; EU, European; NREM, non–rapid eye movement; PAT, peripheral arterial tone; PPG, photoplethysmography; PSG, polysomnography; PTT; pulse transit time; REM, rapid eye movement; SCORE, Systematic Coronary Risk Evaluation.

NREM sleep and differentiate deep sleep from light sleep.[39] These sleep-staging algorithms were further validated and showed moderate agreement in a multicenter study.[40] In 38 normal subjects and 189 patients with suspected OSA, the overall agreement for detection of light-deep and REM sleep was 89 ± 6% and 89 ± 6% between PSG and PAT, respectively. OSA severity did not affect the sensitivity and specificity of the algorithm. However, in elderly patients with suspected OSA, deep sleep stage classification was underscored in PAT when compared with PSG.[41]

Recognition of Obstructive Sleep Apnea

The use of plethysmography has demonstrated a typical attenuation pattern of PWA in the courses of repetitive obstructive apneas and hypopneas.[14,42] Similar changes could be observed by means of the PAT method[23,43] (Figure 203.2). Indeed, experimental data showed that the response is mainly mediated by the arousal response and, to a minor degree, by the response to significant upper airway obstruction.[44] Further, intraarterial infusion of the alpha-receptor blocker phentolamine showed that this typical apnea-related response can be blocked, suggesting a strong association between PAT attenuation and alpha receptor sympathetic activity in the skin vasculature during apnea and subsequent arousal.[43]

The PAT technology uses the pattern recognition of pulse wave attenuations, oxygen desaturations, heart rate responses, and the previously mentioned recognition of wake and sleep phases in a combined algorithm.[45] A meta-analysis of relevant validation studies performed in the general population and in several patient populations showed that this pulse wave–based technology has a high agreement with PSG-derived indices of sleep apnea activity.[46] No specific effect of gender on the

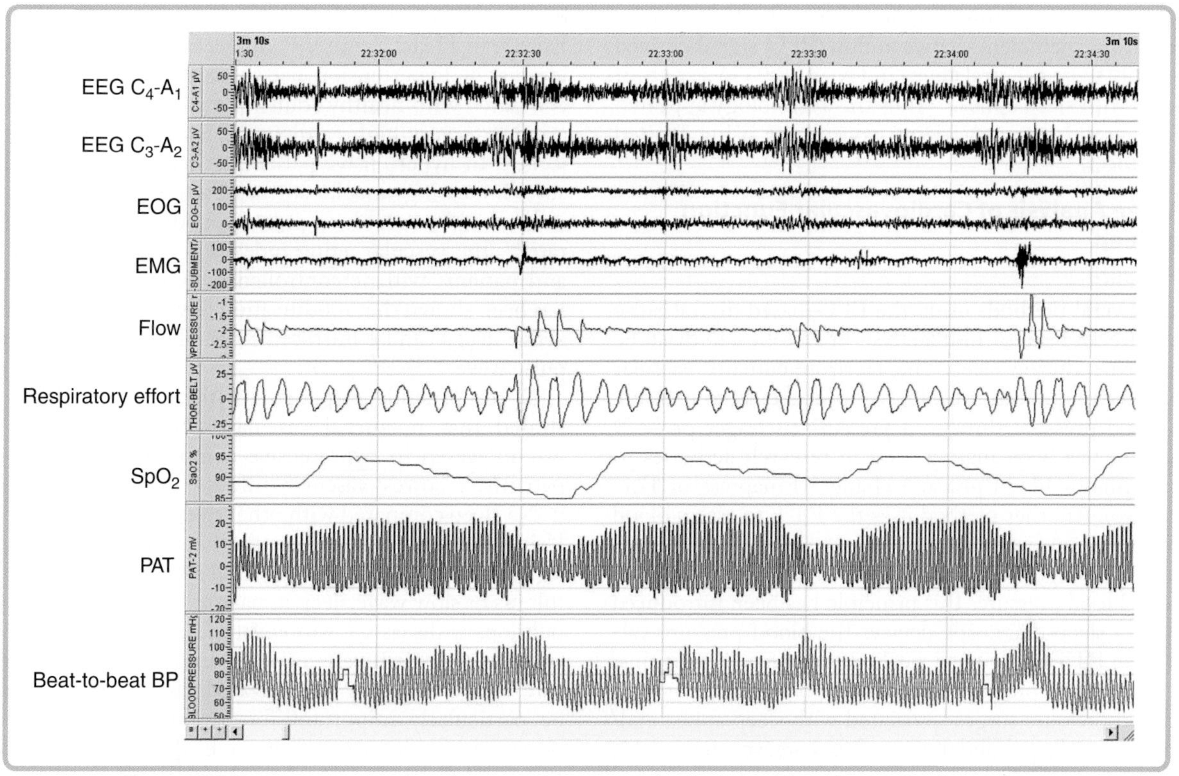

Figure 203.2 A 3-minute recording showing pulse wave amplitude changes from the peripheral arterial tone (PAT) signal associated with obstructive sleep apnea and arousal. The PAT signal fluctuates with increasing respiratory effort during apnea. The systolic PAT amplitude decreases significantly during central nervous arousal from sleep and subsequent resumption of breathing. BP, Blood pressure; EEG, electroencephalogram; EMG, electromyography; EOG, electrooculography; PAT, peripheral arterial tone; SpO_2, oxygen saturation.

accuracy of the PAT technology for apnea detection has been found. However, an increased arterial stiffness assessed by pulse wave velocity was reported to affect the accuracy of the assessment.[47] A recent validation study against PSG showed that manual editing of both sleep stages and respiratory events in the PAT recordings further improves the agreement between the two methods.[48]

A similar approach was published with the use of single-channel oximetry, in which saturation and the PPG signal were used together for sleep apnea recognition.[49] The PPG signal recognizes respiratory signals (effort and breathing frequency) and the sleep and wake rhythm (see previous description). A conventional oxygen desaturation pattern with the threshold of at least 3% is also used to detect breathing events. Although the algorithm is less well described in the publications, validation studies showed good agreement between PSG–apnea hypopnea index (AHI) and PPG–AHI: for example, the receiver operator characteristic (ROC) curve for an AHI threshold of 15 events/hour was 0.9.[50] At least, this technology can be seen as a significant improvement when compared with traditional single-channel oximetry. In this context, an additional, so-called principal-component-analysis technique has been described, which allows the detection of respiratory efforts from the oximetry-derived PPG signal.[51]

The PAT and PPG signals have also been evaluated in the follow-up of patients with sleep-disordered breathing. The PAT technology was suggested to be specifically useful in the follow-up of treatment such as positive airway pressure, oral device, and weight reduction.[52-54] The sleep structure, degree of remaining sleep fragmentation, and hypoxic load can be easily quantified in an outpatient setting. In particular, the capability of the PPG signal to detect arousal was validated against PSG standard measures in patients using noninvasive ventilation. A good agreement between the methods was established at least for sleep fragmentation during NREM sleep.[55] The PPG technology was suggested to be used for simplified follow-up investigations in the growing number of patients with home ventilation.

Cheyne-Stokes Respiration and Central Sleep Apnea

Cheyne-Stokes respiration (CSR) is a condition that includes cyclic oscillation of breathing amplitude along with periodic fluctuation of sympathetic nerve activity. Interestingly, the PAT signal showed a sinusoid shape in accordance with the symmetric pattern of both respiratory effort and oxygen desaturation. The relative attenuation of the PAT amplitude was lower during wake CSR periods compared with CSR during sleep, and the maximum attenuation lagged the start of the crescendo breathing phase by 3 to 8 seconds. The sensitivity for CSR recognition varied between 73% (awake) and 91% (entire sleep period) with a specificity of 70% (REM sleep) and 97% (awake) when compared with PSG in a small study of 10 patients with CSR and heart failure.[56] These first positive results, while worth noting, need replication in a more robust sample.

Another approach starts from the flow signal analysis and uses the PPG to indirectly assess respiratory efforts for improved apnea classification. The PPG-derived respiratory effort separates central/mixed apneas from obstructive ones. The correlation coefficients between flow/PPG signal derived and manually scored central apnea index was 0.95 in a study of 66 patients with sleep apnea.[57] Thus this technology appeared potentially useful for categorizing apnea type using limited channel devices.

Pulse Wave Analysis of Cardiovascular Function during Sleep

Blood Pressure

There are several methods using the PPG-based digital pulse volume curve for beat-to-beat analysis of systolic and diastolic blood pressure during sleep. The electropneumatic vascular unloading technique was introduced by Jan Peňáz to measure central blood pressure through a pressurized finger probe.[58] This method has been mainly used in research activities to assess continuous blood pressure change (Finapress or Portapres device). Another method uses the PTT to assess blood pressure continuously. Because central arterial stiffness is associated with blood pressure, shortening of the PTT is a marker of elevated blood pressure. This principle has been introduced recently in a sleep diagnostic device. The blood pressure values from the PTT curve need a calibration procedure against resting office blood pressure to enable continuous monitoring of the blood pressure surges associated with sleep apnea and/or arousal from sleep. Validation studies suggest a reasonable agreement for PPT-derived blood pressure when compared with values obtained by the conventional oscillometric method and finger arterial PPG (Finometer).[59-61] It is clear that the PTT method has advantages because it does not disturb sleep when compared with the oscillometric method or the Peňáz technique. On the other hand, PTT-derived blood pressure is calibrated before sleep onset. The accuracy in the second half of the night may be affected, and the clinical utility in certain sleep stage (e.g., REM sleep) may be limited.[62] Finally, the PWA alone using the PPG technology has also been used to calculate systolic blood pressure on a beat-to-beat basis during sleep.[63] The results showed also a reasonable agreement between PPG blood pressure and Portapres-derived pressure.

Pulse Rate Variability

Impaired heart rate variability is a marker of increased cardiovascular risk in patients with established ischemic heart disease and cardiac failure. The method is based on the recognition of RR interval by high-resolution sampling of the ECG signal. The PPG signal can be used as a surrogate marker of heart rate variability. A large number of studies have been performed to analyze the accuracy between ECG-based heart rate variability and PPG-based pulse rate variability. Both methods are leading to similar results during resting conditions and undisturbed sleep,[64] which provides the alternative for nocturnal ECG-based analysis (e.g., respiratory sinus arrhythmia[65]). It is worthy of note that frequency analysis during sleep apnea may differ between ECG and PPG methods.[66]

Vascular Stiffness

The peripheral pulse wave signal contains clinically important information about stiffness of the conduit arteries relevant for cardiovascular function and risk assessment. It has been shown that the AI derived from finger pulse wave had a good intra-individual agreement during repeated measures. The PPG-AI demonstrated a dose-response relationship with mean arterial blood pressure and cardiovascular risk classification of the European Heart Score.[17,18] Subjects with diabetes, hyperlipidemia, or hypertension had a significantly higher PPG-AI compared with healthy adults. Mean PPG-AI increased from average to very high cardiovascular risk classes in these subjects.[17] In hypertensive patients, it was shown that the measures indicating vascular stiffness in the PPG pulse wave were influenced by age, blood pressure, body mass index, and heart rate.[67] The vascular aging index was increased in the elderly and patients with uncontrolled hypertension. In addition, it has been shown that modification of vascular stiffness by vasoactive drugs can be mirrored by parallel changes in the finger pulse wave.[14-16,68,69]

A recent study in patients with suspected OSA demonstrated that nocturnal vascular stiffness assessed by PPT was increased in hypertensive compared with normotensive patients.[70] Lowest vascular stiffness (longest PPT) was found in N3 sleep compared with other sleep stages and wakefulness. Using the same technology, the vascular stiffness was found significantly elevated during REM sleep compared with wakefulness or slow wave sleep in patients with chronic obstructive pulmonary disease.[71] Moreover, REM sleep–related vascular stiffness was positively associated with daytime blood pressure, suggesting that sleep-related vascular mechanisms may be particularly important for patient outcomes in chronic obstructive pulmonary disease. Both studies demonstrated the possibilities to study sleep stage–specific modifications of vascular stiffness without compromising sleep quality by additional sensors.

Assessment of Overall Cardiovascular Risk from a Sleep Recording

Sleep-related respiratory and cardiovascular parameters are related to cardiovascular morbidity and mortality. For instance, failure to produce nocturnal dipping of blood pressure or heart rate has been independently associated with increased all-cause mortality.[72,73] The high-frequency component of heart rate variability during sleep is blunted in patients with coronary artery disease, and the nocturnal arterial vascular tone determined by finger PPG is elevated in patients with essential hypertension.[74,75] Sleep-related hypoxia, specifically intermittent hypoxia in sleep apnea, has been associated with increased cardiovascular mortality.[76,77] Therefore there is a strong rationale for a systematic combined analysis of cardiac, vascular, and respiratory reactivity during the sleeping period as a measure of cardiovascular risk.

In a multicenter study, physiologic components of PPG signal were derived from the overnight finger oximetry recording using a matching pursuit algorithm for cardiovascular risk assessment (Table 203.3).[1,78] The parameters were selected based on their relevance in reflecting cardiovascular regulatory homeostasis and feasibility from the finger PPG signal. Variables reflecting cardiac rate variability were identified. A similar process was initiated for variables reflecting peripheral vascular reactivity and stiffness. To quantify autonomic events independent of respiratory and arousal events, PWA attenuations between 10% and 30% were included in the analysis. The PPT was used as a surrogate measure of pulse wave velocity and arterial stiffness. Finally, several measures of nocturnal oxygenation (constant, symmetric, and recurrent hypoxia) were also included in the analysis. A 2% oxygen desaturation was chosen for the hypoxia event threshold. The interaction between

Table 203.3 Clinical Relevance of Physiologic Variables Derived from the Finger Photoplethysmography Signal for Cardiovascular Risk Assessment

Parameter	Function Assessed	Dysfunction Reflected by Parameter
Hypoxic variability	Recurrent hypoxia and reoxygenation	Hypoxic cardiovascular stress
Pulse wave attenuation	Frequency of pulse amplitude attenuations	Microvascular dysfunction, increased vascular sympathetic tone
Pulse rate acceleration	Sympathovagal balance at sinus node level, baroreflex	Coexisting cardiac/vascular/metabolic disease
Periodic pulse rate changes	Cardiorespiratory coupling, baroreflex sensitivity	Coexisting cardiac/vascular/metabolic disease
Pulse propagation time	Vascular wall compliance	Vascular aging, hypertension, atherosclerosis
Time of saturation <90%	Degree of nocturnal hypoxic load	Significant respiratory disease
Degree of symmetric nocturnal desaturation	Occurrence of central apneas and Cheyne-Stokes respiration	Significant cardiac or CNS disease (e.g., heart failure, post stroke)
Cardiac response to nocturnal hypoxia	Heart rate response to intermittent hypoxia, chemoreflex	Cardiac or metabolic disease affecting autonomic response (e.g., diabetes)

CNS, Central nervous system.

respiration and cardiovascular function using the respiratory frequency band of pulse rate and the heart rate response pattern to episodic hypoxia were calculated. The respiratory sinus arrhythmia is considered to reflect vagal-cardiac nerve activity, and a decrease in this pattern may reflect elevated cardiac sympathetic activity. Although these variables were modestly interrelated, the multivariate analysis suggested that all parameters contributed significantly to the cardiovascular risk assessment.[1] A composite cardiovascular risk score (range 0–1) was generated using a neuro-fuzzy system.[78]

In a cross-sectional validation study of this novel algorithm, all patients were classified according to the European Society of Cardiology/European Society of Hypertension (ESC/ESH) risk matrix.[1] The algorithm based on overnight PPG signal allowed the identification of patients with high cardiovascular risk (high and very high added cardiovascular risk, according to the ESC/ESH matrix)[79] with sensitivity and specificity values of 74.5% and 76.4%, respectively, and area under the ROC curve was 0.80. Corresponding values for the AHI and the oxygen desaturation index were below 65%. The current data provide evidence that an algorithm based on a PPG signal offers a superior estimate of cardiovascular risk than standard matrix used in clinical medicine.[79a] Large longitudinal epidemiologic studies on the clinical utility of PPG-based cardiovascular risk assessment are ongoing.[80]

The nocturnal pulse wave–derived cardiovascular risk was also studied in patients with insomnia with/without objectively assessed poor sleep quality and matched controls.[81] Pulse wave analysis during sleep revealed that insomnia with low sleep efficacy was characterized by a higher pulse rate, an increase in vascular stiffness and overall cardiovascular risk compared with good sleepers and insomnia patients with maintained high sleep efficacy. This oximeter-based photoplethysmographic technology hereby provides an alternative to study hyperarousal status and autonomic activation during sleep in patients with insomnia.

The PAT technology has also been evaluated regarding associations with cardiovascular risk markers. The magnitude of overnight PAT attenuations reflected daytime blood pressure in the general population independent of apneic measures from PSG.[82] This finding implies that vascular or autonomic phenomena recorded during the sleep period provide a marker for cardiovascular disease (e.g., hypertension). The AI calculated from PAT at rest was studied in 186 patients from a cardiology clinic.[83] Although PAT-AI significantly correlated with cardiac risk factors and coronary artery disease, the diagnostic capacity of this single pulse wave variable to differentiate patients with/without coronary artery disease was limited (area under the ROC curve 0.604), suggesting that multiple information processing of pulse wave signals for cardiovascular risk assessments may be needed.

A recent study extended the knowledge about pulse wave–based information on cardiometabolic risk in the general population. Using a novel, automated detection algorithm to assess the timing, amplitude, duration, and slopes of pulse wave attenuations,[84] a cross-sectional analysis from the HypnoLaus sleep cohort study (n = 2149, 51% females, mean age 59 years) showed that lower PWA-drop (>30% from baseline) index, longer PWA-drop duration, and greater area under the curve of sleep-related PWA-drops were associated with an increased odds of hypertension, diabetes, and known cardiovascular events after adjustment for confounders.[85] Although contradictory to early studies,[82,86,87] the authors argued that PWA drop features during sleep seem to reflect vascular reactivity and may be a biomarker for cardiometabolic comorbidities.

Treatment-Related Changes of Pulse Wave Parameters during Sleep

The role of positive airway pressure therapy on pulse wave parameters in sleep apnea was studied.[87] Untreated versus treated OSA was associated with higher degree of hypoxia and a lower frequency of mild PWA drops (10% to 30% from baseline). Conversely, continuous positive airway pressure treatment caused a significant increase in PWA drop index and a trend in the reduction of the pulse wave–derived overall cardiovascular risk index. Another intervention study applied overnight oxygen and nasal high flow treatment in patients with mild-to-moderate chronic obstructive pulmonary disease.[88] Stabilization of respiration was accompanied with a significant reduction of PWA drops (≥30% from baseline) during REM sleep as a sign of sympathetic off-loading by nasal high flow treatment. The PWA remained unchanged after oxygen supplementation despite a significant increase in oxygenation levels. Pulse wave analysis offers new possibilities to monitor treatments effects during sleep on cardiovascular and autonomic function.

CLINICAL PEARL

The finger pulse wave can be easily derived from PPG. Supportive information for sleep-stage classification, identification of autonomic activation, and differentiation of obstructive versus central breathing event can be achieved. These capabilities improve the utility of ambulatory sleep diagnostic devices. Performance evaluation shows good agreement with conventional information gained from PSG. In addition, valuable information on cardiovascular dysfunction and risk can be obtained by advanced PWA.

SUMMARY

This chapter describes the hemodynamic and autonomic influence on the pulse wave signal during sleep. The information can be used for a better understanding of the associations among pulse wave change and autonomic activation, EEG-detected arousal, sleep stages, and sleep-related disordered breathing. Some clinical applications of digital PWA in sleep medicine and sleep-related research are reviewed. The potential usefulness of using finger pulse wave signal for cardiovascular function assessment is discussed.

Technological advancements are moving sleep apnea diagnostics from in-lab attended PSG to home sleep testing. Given the simplicity, the cost effectiveness, and clinical acceptance of the oximetry technology, the pulse wave signal obtained by modified oximeter technology opens new possibilities, serving as an important additive or alternative parameter in sleep diagnostic procedure. Research is very active in the field, and the results are promising.

SELECTED READINGS

Delessert A, Espa F, Rossetti A, Lavigne G, Tafti M, Heinzer R. Pulse wave amplitude drops during sleep are reliable surrogate markers of changes in cortical activity. *Sleep*. 2010;33(12):1687–1692.

Grote L., Zou D., Kraiczi H., Hedner J.. Finger plethysmography--a method for monitoring finger blood flow during sleep disordered breathing. Respir Physiol Neurobiol. 2003;136(2–3):141–152.

Hirotsu C, Betta M, Bernardi G, et al. Pulse wave amplitude drops during sleep: clinical significance and characteristics in a general population sample. *Sleep*. 2020;43(7).

Randerath WJ, Treml M, Priegnitz C, et al. Parameters of overnight pulse wave under treatment in obstructive sleep apnea. *Respiration*. 2016;92(3):136–143.

Schnall RP, Shlitner A, Sheffy J, Kedar R, Lavie P. Periodic, profound peripheral vasoconstriction--a new marker of obstructive sleep apnea. *Sleep*. 1999;22(7):939–946.

Strassberger C, Zou D, Penzel T, et al. Beyond the AHI-pulse wave analysis during sleep for recognition of cardiovascular risk in sleep apnea patients. *J Sleep Res*. 2021:e13364. https://doi.org/10.1111/jsr.13364. Online ahead of print.

Sommermeyer D, Zou D, Eder DN, et al. The use of overnight pulse wave analysis for recognition of cardiovascular risk factors and risk: a multicentric evaluation. *J Hypertens*. 2014;32(2):276–285.

Sommermeyer D, Zou D, Ficker JH, et al. Detection of cardiovascular risk from a photoplethysmographic signal using a matching pursuit algorithm. *Med Biol Eng Comput*. 2016;54(7):1111–1121.

Yalamanchali S, Farajian V, Hamilton C, Pott TR, Samuelson CG, Friedman M. Diagnosis of obstructive sleep apnea by peripheral arterial tonometry: meta-analysis. *JAMA Otolaryngol Head Neck Surg*. 2013;139(12):1343–1350.

A complete reference list can be found online at ExpertConsult.com.

Chapter 204

Recording and Scoring Sleep-Related Movements

Raffaele Ferri; Lourdes DelRosso

Chapter Highlights

- Scoring rule development is a dynamic process with continual exchange between clinicians and researchers.
- The time lag for incorporating new research evidence into clinical scoring rules has led in many instances to the parallel existence of clinical rules and research rules for the same phenomenon.
- This chapter reviews both clinical and research recording techniques and scoring rules for the most common sleep-related movements, which include periodic limb movements during sleep and wakefulness, rapid eye movement sleep without atonia, and sleep-related bruxism; other movements are also briefly discussed.

OVERVIEW

The establishment and standardization of recording and scoring techniques both reflect and afford progress in clinical sleep medicine and research. The development of scoring rules is a dynamic process, with continual interchange between clinical practice and research. Hence the most commonly used standard reference for clinical scoring rules, the *Manual for the Scoring of Sleep and Associated Events,* published by the American Academy of Sleep Medicine (AASM),[1] is regularly reviewed and updated based on new clinical evidence or technological changes.

The exchange between sleep medicine and research is vibrant, but the necessary time lag for incorporating new evidence into clinical scoring rules has often led to the parallel existence of clinical rules and research rules for the same topic. Presented in this chapter is an overview of both clinical and research recording techniques and scoring rules for sleep-related movements. We focus on the most commonly observed movements, including periodic limb movements (PLMs) of sleep (PLMS) or wakefulness (PLMW), rapid eye movement (REM) sleep without atonia (RWA), REM behavior disorder (RBD), and sleep-related bruxism (SB). In addition, rhythmic movement disorder (RMD), restless sleep disorder (RSD), propriospinal myoclonus (PSM) of sleep onset, benign myoclonus of infancy, excessive fragmentary myoclonus (EFM), neck myoclonus, and leg movements other than PLMS are briefly discussed. The finding of abnormal movements in sleep is important from both a diagnostic and a prognostic standpoint.

BASIC RECORDING METHODS

Electromyography

Surface electromyography is the "gold standard" for recording most muscle movements during sleep. The electromyogram (EMG) is acquired by means of silver chloride electrodes attached to the inputs of a differential amplifier to obtain a bipolar derivation. It usually is recommended that interelectrode impedance be less than 5 KΩ[1,2]; the skin preparation procedure before electrode placement is very important (e.g., cleansing the skin with an alcohol pad and sometimes shaving excess hair). For better adhesion of the electrodes, the use of collodion is recommended because it is nonconductive, holds through hair (not only on the scalp), withstands oils and perspiration, and provides high performance for long-term recordings. Collodion is highly flammable, however, and produces fumes, so appropriate air purifier, fume extractor, or ventilation systems should be used. Finally, for long-term recordings, a conductive paste is needed to ensure good electrical contact between the skin and the electrodes.

EMG signals are produced by the muscle situated under the skin and by adipose tissue below the electrodes, which essentially record activity of superficial muscle. Muscle size and amount of adipose tissue significantly influence the amplitude of the surface-recorded EMG signal. This is the reason why surface EMG signals are considered semiquantitative and calibration of EMG activity is recommended.[2] The amplitude of surface EMG potentials depends also on the distance between the recording electrodes and can range between less than 20 μV and up to several millivolts, depending on the various factors noted previously.

EMG signals are superimposed motor unit action potentials produced by several motor units, each with a typical repetition rate of firing of approximately 7 to 20 Hz. Surface EMG records the sum of this activity and produces a signal with a wide spectrum. Figure 204.1 shows two examples of the EMG power spectrum from chin and tibialis anterior muscles (recorded with a sampling rate of 512 Hz); it is possible to note the wide extent of the power spectrum and the effects of notch filtering at 50 Hz.

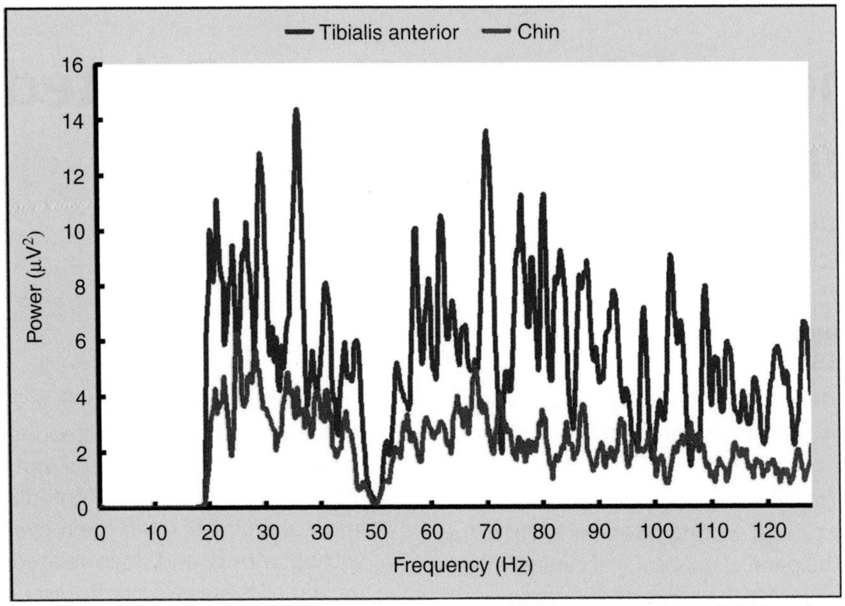

Figure 204.1 Average power spectrum of the electromyogram (EMG) signal sampled at 512 Hz and recorded from the chin and tibialis anterior muscles.

The spectral content of the EMG signal requires high sampling rates that should never be lower than 200 Hz, with 500 Hz being the desirable sampling rate.[2,3] Bandpass filtering usually is applied, with typical settings at approximately 10 to 100 Hz and with a notch filter at 50 or 60 Hz, depending on the power line frequency.

Video Polysomnography

Video (and audio) recording, synchronized with the polysomnographic signals, is the recommended method to assess movements and behaviors during sleep, as it offers the possibility to examine simple or complex motor behaviors and vocalizations in conjunction with their accompanying electrophysiologic correlates. Video polysomnography (PSG) is also essential for the assessment of movements and behaviors that occur in several sleep disorders and allows their characterization and differentiation.[4-7] For example, this modality has a key role in differentiating parasomnias from nocturnal seizures[8] and from behaviors arising during episodes of wakefulness, as sometimes occur in psychiatric conditions. Video PSG has also aided in the characterization of movements through the night in children with RSD.[9]

It should not be overlooked that video PSG provides objective documentation of all actions occurring in the laboratory for both clinical and legal issues.

PSG equipment manufacturers can recommend fixed-focus video cameras, but remotely controlled directional and zoom devices (pan–tilt–zoom cameras) are preferable. However, some modern high-resolution digital systems allow "zooming" within the image retroactively. To ensure darkness for the patient, an infrared light source is needed, with a corresponding appropriate camera.

A limitation of this method, however, is its high costs for both the recording and the reviewing/scoring processes. The evaluation of complex behaviors and body movements during video PSG is essentially a time-consuming and expensive visual process. However, appropriate sleep disorder scales can assist to guide video review.[7,10-17] Automated video analysis could provide help for assessing sleep-related behaviors, and some preliminary approaches have already been attempted.[18]

Actigraphy

The U.S. Food and Drug Administration (FDA) cleared research, and clinical-grade actigraphy is accepted for characterization of sleep patterns in the ambulatory environment. Motion-based wearable sleep trackers marketed directly to consumers are not yet recommended for this purpose. Actigraphs contain motion sensors called *accelerometers* and are usually worn on the wrist. These sensors integrate motion amplitude and speed, and their output is a signal, with magnitude and duration depending on these motion features. This signal is appropriately amplified, filtered, and digitized to be stored in the device memory, most often in terms of movement counts per epoch. The length of the epoch is of crucial importance and can be fixed at 1 minute or can be chosen by the user (from a fixed list of epoch lengths).

Memory storage capacity and epoch length determine an actigraph's maximum recording time. Because actigraphy is commonly used to assess circadian rhythm sleep-wake disorders,[3] it is necessary that these devices can reliably record periods lasting at least 7 days. Although 5 nights may be sufficient to reliably acquire certain actigraphic measures, to fully capture intraindividual differences of all sleep parameters, inclusion of all weekdays and the weekend is necessary in children and adolescents.[19]

Data are stored in essentially three different modes, "Time Above Threshold, "Zero Crossing," or "Proportional (or Digital) Integration" mode, and some actigraphs allow the user to select their preferred mode. Different studies have provided support for the various measurement modes, though conclusive statements regarding which is the most accurate are thus far lacking in the literature. After the recording phase, data usually are downloaded on a computer for scoring. Each system has specific software tools, but they typically are based on the algorithms proposed by Cole and associates[20] or Sadeh and coworkers.[21]

Actigraphy cannot be used for staging sleep and tends to overestimate sleep, because when subjects are lying still while awake, they do not produce movements. Actigraphy shows good agreement with PSG in the measurement of total sleep time (TST) in healthy subjects, but in patients with sleep disorders, agreement is reduced. The methodology for the actigraphic estimation of sleep is discussed in further detail in Chapter 211.

Actigraphic monitoring of foot or leg movements has been proposed,[22,23] and because it offers the possibility to record multiple nights in a home environment, it has been proposed as a tool to overcome the problems caused by the relatively large night-to-night within-subject variability reported to occur for PLMS.[24] Actigraphy alone, however, is unable to discriminate between PLMS and leg movements occurring during wakefulness; moreover, arousal or other related events (apnea) cannot be detected.

The technical aspects of actigraphic recordings are important and able to influence the results; earlier published criteria for reliable actigraphic recording should be carefully applied.[2] A review and meta-analysis[25] of the use of actigraphy for the measurement of PLMS has demonstrated significant heterogeneity among the few studies available regarding the type of actigraph, position of the sensors on the legs, and methods for counting PLMS. In particular, an important limitation was noted in the possibility to reliably combine data from actigraphs placed on both limbs in most devices.

Thus at present, actigraphy cannot substitute for polysomnography within the process of diagnosing restless legs syndrome (RLS).[24] In fact, the AASM's most recent clinical practice guidelines on the use of actigraphy recommends against the use of actigraphy in place of electromyography for the diagnosis of PLMS in adults or children.[26]

Other Methods

Several producers propose piezoelectric sensors for the recording of limb movements during sleep. These sensors, placed around the ankle or around the leg, transduce motion, vibration, and tension into an electrical signal. They are very sensitive, and there is no guarantee that the signal produced corresponds exclusively with events generated by the limb. No convincing validation studies are available for the use of these sensors, and they are not recommended by any guideline. The only advantage they offer is that no skin preparation is required; however, this is counterbalanced by a cost higher than that for silver chloride electrodes.

A variety of other movements can be recorded during sleep; among them of particular importance are those needed for the diagnosis of the different types of sleep apnea, such as thorax and abdomen movements. Strain gauges and piezoelectric sensors have been used, but the most recent and reliable belts are based on inductive sensors, which also allow estimation of volume changes in these anatomic structures. The monitoring tools to evaluate suspected sleep-disordered breathing are detailed in Chapter 200.

With the advances in smartphone technology, patients can now record sleep behaviors in their mobile devices or own home infrared cameras. A study showed the potential use of home cameras to assess sleep posture.[27] Clinically, home videos can aid in the identification of specific movement disorders or parasomnias by the sleep expert, but there is sparse literature on their use.[28]

PERIODIC LIMB MOVEMENTS

The first PSG EMG recordings of PLMS were carried out in Bologna by the group led by Lugaresi in 1965.[29,30] Some 20 years later, duration, amplitude, periodicity, and symmetry of PLMS were defined and manually measured in paper recordings by Coleman,[31] who created the bases of the scoring criteria established by the American Sleep Disorders Association (ASDA),[32] in 1993, which subsequently have been used for more than 20 years.

Currently, two sets of similar (but not identical) rules for scoring PLMS and periodic PLMW exist. These were partly informed by algorithms proposed for the automatic detection of leg movements in PSG[33] and include mathematically defined parameters such as thresholds, intervals, and amplitude.[33,34] First, in 2006 a task force of the International Restless Legs Syndrome Study Group endorsed by the World Association of Sleep Medicine (WASM/IRLSSG)[2] introduced a major revision of the scoring rules, which were then substantially (but not entirely) adopted by the AASM in 2007.[1,35] Finally, WASM revised their rules in 2016.[36] Table 204.1 lists the similarities and differences between the two sets of rules; in the following paragraphs, recommendations, descriptions, and definitions refer to the most recent WASM criteria.[36]

Recording Methods

Surface EMG electrodes should be placed 2 to 3 cm apart or a distance from each other that is one-third of the length of the anterior tibialis muscle, whichever is shorter (Figure 204.2). Electrodes must be located longitudinally on the muscles and symmetrically around the middle. Impedance should be 10 KΩ or less for clinical studies, but a setting of 5 KΩ or less is required for research studies. EMG signals must be obtained from both the right and the left leg. Recording the two signals in one channel is strongly discouraged. For research studies, signals from each leg must be recorded separately. Recording activity from other muscles besides the tibialis anterior is recommended only for research purposes or for special clinical conditions (e.g., arm restlessness). Sampling rate should be 200 Hz or greater (clinical settings) or 400 Hz or greater (research settings). Filter settings should be 10 to 100 Hz; for research purposes, settings of 10 to 200 Hz are recommended.

Baseline resting EMG amplitude (i.e., in the relaxed muscle) should be ±2 to 3 μV (4–6 μV peak to peak or less. Before the recording, a calibration should be carried out to obtain from the relaxed anterior tibialis muscles a nonrectified signal of power no greater than ±5 μV (or 10 μV peak to peak; 5 μV for rectified signals) for clinical purposes and ±3 μV (or 6 μV peak to peak; 3 μV for rectified signals).

Scoring Rules

The scoring of PLM follows several general, sequential steps:

1. Leg movements are identified by the amplitude and duration of the EMG activation.
2. Bilateral leg movements are combined if a single PLM index is to be calculated.
3. Leg movements occurring in the vicinity of sleep-disordered breathing events (e.g., respiratory-related leg movements [RRLMs]) or arousals are identified.
4. The remaining leg movements are classified as periodic or nonperiodic (isolated or short-interval) on the basis of

Table 204.1 Recording and Scoring of Periodic Leg Movements According to the Guidelines of the World Association of Sleep Medicine/International Restless Legs Syndrome Study Group (WASM/IRLSSG)[2,36] and the American Academy of Sleep Medicine (AASM)

Feature/Component	WASM/IRLSSG	AASM
Recording of Leg Movements		
Electrodes	Surface electrodes	Surface electrodes
Electrode positioning	Tibialis anterior muscles Placed longitudinal, symmetrically around the middle, 2–3 cm apart or one-third of length of anterior tibialis muscle, whichever is shorter	Tibialis anterior muscles Placed longitudinal, symmetrically around the middle, 2–3 cm apart or one-third of length of anterior tibialis muscle, whichever is shorter
Combined recording of left and right legs	Bilateral recordings are required. Use of two channels, one for each leg, is strongly recommended for all studies and is required for research. Clinical applications may, however, combine the electrodes from both legs into one recorded channel, although this practice is discouraged.	Both legs should be monitored for the presence of leg movements. Use of separate channels for each leg is strongly preferred. Combining electrodes from the two legs to give one recorded channel may suffice for some clinical settings, although this strategy may reduce the number of detected leg movements.
Sampling rate	≥200 Hz in clinical studies ≥400 Hz in research studies	≥200 Hz 500 Hz desirable
Filter	10–100 Hz in clinical studies 10–200 Hz in research studies	10–100 Hz Use of 60-Hz (notch) filters should be avoided
Impedance	≤10 KΩ in clinical studies ≤5 KΩ in research studies	<10 KΩ <5 KΩ preferred
Definition of Leg Movement		
Onset	EMG increase ≥8 μV above the resting baseline	EMG increase ≥8 μV above the resting baseline
Offset	EMG decrease to <2 μV above the resting level for ≥0.5 s	EMG decrease to ≤2 μV above the resting level for ≥0.5 s
Duration	Time between onset and offset, 0.5–10 s	Time between onset and offset, 0.5–10 s
Baseline	Resting EMG Relaxed muscle Absolute signal amplitude, 4–6 μV peak to peak *Calibration:* Relaxed anterior tibialis lasting: ≤10 μV in clinical setting ≤6 μV in research setting *Special criteria for events during wake time:* If EMG > 6–10 μV for ≥15 s, then new increased baseline is defined as average amplitude during this period	Stable resting EMG Relaxed muscle Absolute signal amplitude, ≤10 μV peak to peak
Scoring of Periodic Leg Movements (PLMs)		
Intermovement interval (IMI)	Onset-to-onset: 10–90 s	Onset-to-onset: 5–90 s
Number of leg movements	≥4 (leg movements lasting <0.5 s are disregarded; leg movements lasting >10 s end PLM series)	≥4
IMI >90 s	PLM series ends	PLM series ends
IMI <5 s	n.a.	Counted as one leg movement
IMI <10 s	PLM series ends	n.a.
Sleep-wake	All leg movements form PLM series For PLMS, only those during sleep are counted	Only leg movements during sleep form PLM series
Bilateral leg movements	Offset-to-onset <0.5 s ≤4 monolateral leg movements 0.5–10 s long ≤15 s total duration	Onset-to-onset <5 s
Respiratory-related leg movements (RRLMs)	Included and then excluded from PLM series	Excluded from PLMS series
RRLM definition	Any leg movement occurring within: ±0.5 s around the end of a respiratory event OR −2.0 s to +10.25 s around the end of a respiratory event	Any leg movement occurring within: 0.5 s before the start to 0.5 s after the end of an apnea or hypopnea, respiratory effort–related arousal, or sleep-disordered breathing event

EMG, Electromyogram; n.a., not applicable; PLMS, periodic leg movements of sleep.

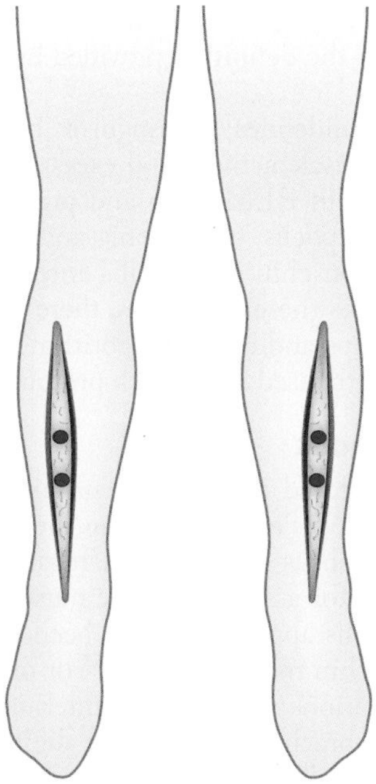

Figure 204.2 Electrode placement for recording the electromyogram (EMG) signal from the tibialis anterior muscles.

their occurrence within a series of such movements characterized by their number and the interval between movements.

The scoring process begins with the identification of candidate leg EMG events. Their onset is defined as an EMG increase of 8 μV or greater above the resting baseline, whereas offset is marked at the point when the EMG amplitude decreases to less than 2 μV above the resting level and remains below that value for at least 0.5 second. An event can contain one or more periods with EMG amplitude below the offset level that each last less than 0.5 second. The duration of the event is the time between its onset and offset; it must be at least 0.5 second and no longer than 10 seconds. All other events not meeting these criteria are not considered for the PLM count but are needed for the discontinuation of the PLM sequences.

Next, if a single PLM index is to be calculated, as opposed to a separate PLM index for each leg, bilateral leg movements are combined. All monolateral leg movements lasting 0.5 to 10 seconds are considered candidate leg movements to be evaluated for PLM. Monolateral leg movements are then combined to form one bilateral if they overlap or the onset of the later leg movement starts within 0.5 second after the offset of the earlier leg movement. Bilateral leg movements contain a maximum of four monolateral leg movements, have a maximum combined duration of 15 seconds, and do not contain any monolateral leg movement >10 seconds.

The AASM set of rules excludes leg movements that occur in the vicinity of sleep-disordered breathing events (RRLM) from the inclusion into PLM series, and these leg movements have to be identified and excluded before calculating the PLM index. For the WASM/IRLSSG,[36] the PLM rate may now first be determined by not excluding any RRLM and, subsequently, the PLM rate should also be calculated without considering the RRLM. The same criteria allow using two alternative rules to identify RRLM: (1) leg movements associated with the resumption of respiration at the end of an apnea-hypopnea event, defined as any part of the leg movement in

Table 204.2 Periodic Limb Movement Summary Parameters

Reported Metric	Definition	Unit
PLMS index	Number of PLMS divided by the number of hours of sleep with leg movements recorded	PLMS/hour
PLMS with arousals index	Number of PLMs associated with arousals divided by the number of hours of sleep with leg movements and arousal recorded	PLMA/hour
PLMW index	Number of PLMW divided by the number of hours of wake with leg movements recorded	PLMW/hour

PLMS, Periodic limb movements of sleep; PLMW, periodic limb movements of wakefulness.

the interval of ±0.5 second around the end of the breathing event; (2) have some part overlapping within an interval of 2.0 seconds before to 10.25 seconds after the end of a respiratory event. Sleep-disordered breathing events include apneas and hypopneas and respiratory effort–related arousals.

After identifying leg movements and combining bilateral leg movements, among the remaining leg movements, those belonging to PLM sequences are identified. For this step, the crucial parameter is the interval between consecutive movements, measured from onset to onset, that is, between 10 and 90 seconds. If the interval between one leg movement and the next is greater than 90 seconds, any possible PLM series ends with the previous leg movement. If the interval is less than 10 seconds, the series should be stopped.

Subsequently, a periodic sequence is defined as a series of four or more leg movements separated from each other by 10 to 90 seconds. All leg movements during sleep and wake can form part of a PLM series, and for calculation of the PLMS index, only those during sleep are counted. PLMs during wakefulness are counted for the PLMW index.

Leg movements are considered to be associated with an arousal event when they are separated by less than 0.5 second—that is, between the end of one event and the onset of the other, regardless of which is first.

Once PLMS and PLMW are scored, several summary metrics can be obtained, and Table 204.2 lists the main measures.[36] Whenever possible, it also is recommended to report the PLMS index during non–rapid eye movement (NREM) sleep only, the PLMS index during REM sleep only, duration of PLMS and PLMW (separate for REM and NREM sleep), and intermovement interval of PLMS and PLMW (separate for REM and NREM sleep). Optional parameters are PLMS by sleep stages (including duration and intermovement intervals) and isolated leg movements.

Advanced Measurements of Periodic Leg Movements of Sleep and Periodic Leg Movements of Wakefulness

Sleep PSG recordings in patients affected by RLS or other sleep disorders usually also contain a significant amount of leg movements that cannot be classified as "periodic"[37-39]; moreover, it has been reported that leg activity during wakefulness in normal subjects is nonperiodic.[40] To analyze in a more comprehensive way this admixture of periodic and nonperiodic activities, advanced measurements were proposed as an important integration of the information provided by the previously reported scoring methods.[41] In particular, an additional measure was established, the *periodicity index,* indicating the degree of periodicity of the total leg movement activity.[38] This index, now included among the optional parameters to report for the latest WASM/IRLSSG criteria,[36] quantifies the proportion, over the total, of intermovement intervals of $10 < i \leq 90$ seconds that are preceded and followed by another interval of the same length (this is equivalent to a series of four leg movements all separated by intervals of $10 < i \leq 90$ seconds). The numerical value of this index can range between 0 (absence of periodicity, with none of the intervals having a length between 10 and 90 seconds) and 1 (complete periodicity, with all intervals between 10 and 90 seconds long).[38]

The periodicity undergoes significant age-related changes, with a trajectory significantly different from that of the total leg movement count, indicating the need for age-adjusted normative reference values,[40,42,43] especially in elderly people and in children/adolescents, in whom a low periodicity can be expected even in the presence of clinically evident RLS.[44,45]

Another important feature characterizing PLMS is their time distribution during the night. In a majority of patients with RLS, PLMS count progressively decreases during the night.[42,44]

Unresolved Issues

Unresolved issues concern the discrepancies between the two sets of rules. Among those, a major issue is the consideration of RRLMs. A study[46] on RRLMs as identified by the previous WASM/IRLSSG rules[2] argued that RRLM might represent part of a phenotypic spectrum that includes PLMS and questioned the need to exclude these RRLMs from the analysis of PLMS. In addition, a further study,[47] and the first one to systematically analyze the distribution of leg movements with respect to respiratory events, reported that leg movements in patients with sleep-related breathing disorders were not increased at the beginning or middle of respiratory events, but clustered around the end of events over a period significantly longer than specified previously by the AASM[1] and WASM/IRLSSG[2] rules. For this reason, the current WASM criteria[36] indicate the wider range found in this study[47] as a valid alternative to detect RRLMs,

Also, the upper limit of the interval range of PLMS has been evaluated by statistical modeling with two different approaches in the same study,[48] and both methods have indicated that PLMSs probably recur in a range of 10 to 60 seconds, rather than 10 to 90 or 5 to 90 seconds.

Together, these studies underline the need for continued evaluation and development of scoring rules for PLMS.

REM SLEEP WITHOUT ATONIA

RWA is the polysomnographic hallmark of RBD, a parasomnia characterized by dream-enacting behavior in which the physiologic atonia during REM sleep is absent or greatly diminished (see Chapter 118). According to the current *International Classification of Sleep Disorders* (ICSD-3),[3] among the criteria for the diagnosis of RBD is the demonstration of RWA based on the definition provided by the most recent AASM guidelines.[1]

The AASM guidelines[1] distinguish between excessive sustained, tonic muscle activity and excessive transient, phasic muscle activity in REM sleep and provide scoring rules to identify REM epochs, with atonia and/or excessive phasic activity based on chin and tibialis anterior EMG during REM sleep. Besides these guidelines, there are several different recording setups and scoring algorithms, both visual and automated, currently used in research protocols.

Recording Methods

It generally is accepted that scoring sustained, tonic muscle activity during REM sleep is based on the chin EMG.[1,49,50] Thus far, no consensus has emerged regarding practices or recommendations for assessing phasic muscle activity during REM sleep. Various approaches have been used, such as the recording of the chin muscles only,[51-55] or of chin muscles in different combinations with tibialis anterior,[56-58] brachioradialis,[59,60] biceps brachii,[61-63] extensor digitorum,[64,65] flexor digitorum superficialis,[49] or flexor carpi radialis[66] (Figure 204.3).

Comparing quantitative EMG analysis in 13 different muscles in patients with RBD, the Sleep Insbruck Barcelona (SINBAR) group showed that phasic EMG activity differed significantly depending on which muscles were evaluated, and the three-muscle combination that detected the highest number

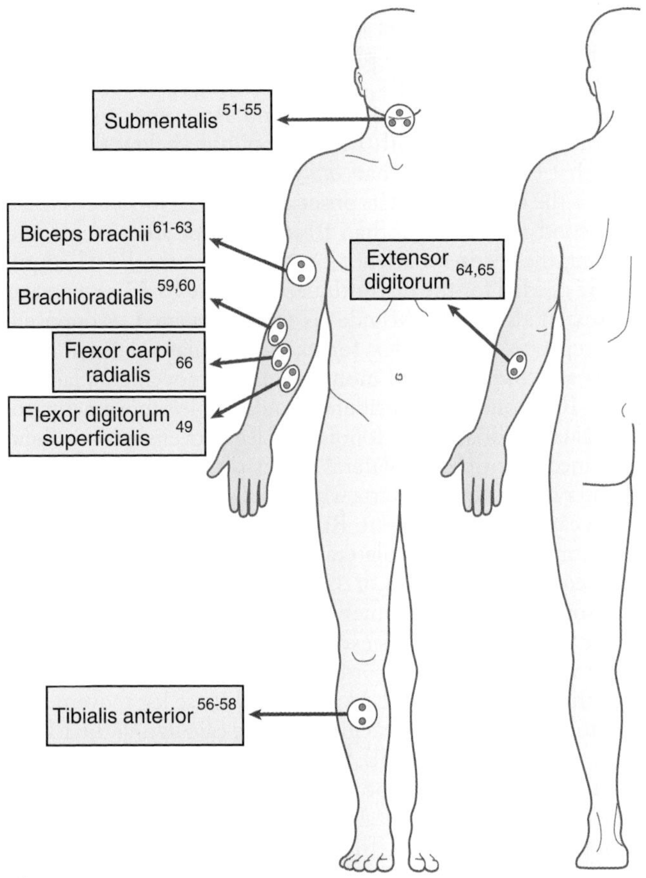

Figure 204.3 Electrode placement for recording the electromyogram (EMG) signal from the different muscles used to evaluate rapid eye movement (REM) sleep without atonia.

of mini-epochs with phasic activity was that composed of the mentalis muscle, the flexor digitorum superficialis in the upper limb, and the extensor digitorum brevis in the lower limb.[67] An important implication of this observation is that the quantification of RWA and subsequently determined cutoff thresholds for the diagnosis of RBD probably will vary, depending on the specific montage and number of EMG signals used.[49,50,68]

Several different protocols are currently in use for recording and scoring RWA: the AASM recommendations,[1] SINBAR EMG Montage,[67] Montreal research group recommendations,[50,51] and The Mayo Clinic method[58]; these are summarized in Table 204.3.

Scoring Rules

Visual Scoring of REM Sleep without Atonia

Since the first introduction of scoring rules for RWA by Lapierre and Montplaisir in 1992,[51] there has been a wide variance in scoring approaches, with many research and clinical groups defining their own, often with only slightly different rules (see the review by Fulda and colleagues[69]). The main differences concern the amplitude criterion to identify EMG activations and the duration of phasic EMG bursts. In addition, besides scoring and quantifying tonic and phasic EMG activity during REM sleep, several groups of investigators defined and used summary measures that quantify "any"[49] EMG activity during REM sleep. Usually, tonic activity is scored as such only when it occupies more than half of an epoch. At the same time, phasic activity has a maximum duration that is between 5 and 10 seconds, depending on the definition used. Consequently, EMG activity that lasts longer than the maximum duration for phasic activity and shorter than half of the epoch seems to be neglected by most scoring approaches. The term *"any" EMG activity* was therefore introduced to take into consideration EMG activity of any length during REM sleep.

Montreal Research Group Scoring Rules and Variations. The first formal scoring rules were introduced by Lapierre and Montplaisir in 1992.[51] They established quantifications for tonic and phasic EMG activity, tonic EMG density, and phasic EMG density. Tonic EMG was quantified as the percentage of 20-second epochs that contained tonic EMG activation in the chin EMG for more than 50% of the epoch. Phasic EMG was quantified as the percentage of 2-second mini-epochs that contained EMG bursts of between 0.1 and 5 seconds that had an amplitude larger than four times the background. This influential definition continues to be used with some modifications; the penultimate modification was reported in 2010, in the first study[50] that explored diagnostic thresholds for the diagnosis of RBD based on this scoring of RWA (see further on). In this study, the following rules were applied: tonic EMG density was defined as the percentage of 20-second epochs that contained tonic EMG activation with

Table 204.3 REM Sleep without Atonia (RWA): Monitoring and Scoring

Source	EMG Location	Definitions	Quantification of RWA	Notes
AASM	Chin and limb	Excessive sustained activity: chin EMG; 50% of the 30 s epoch has activation at least 2× greater than the REM atonia level Excessive phasic activity: chin or limb EMG; 5 of 10 3-s mini-epochs have bursts of 0.1–5 s at least 2× greater than the REM atonia level Any chin activity: EMG activity at least 2× greater than the REM atonia level Any limb activity: 0.1–5 s activity at least 2× greater than the REM atonia level	%REM epochs that meet RWA criteria (RWA index)	The minimum amplitude during NREM sleep may be a substitute for REM atonia, if REM atonia is absent
SINBAR	Mentalis muscle flexor digitorum superficialis (upper limb) extensor digitorum brevis (lower limb)	Tonic EMG activity: chin activity at least 2× the background amplitude or >10 μV present for more than 50% of the epoch Phasic EMG activity: activity with duration of 0.1–5 s at least 2× the background amplitude Any EMG activity: activity of any length, 2× background amplitude	% of 30 s epochs (tonic) % of 3 s mini-epochs (phasic) % of 2 s mini-epochs (any)	Normative RWA values established[49]
Montreal research group	Chin	Tonic EMG: activation for more than 50% of the epoch Phasic EMG: bursts 4× larger than the background amplitude for 0.1–5 s	% of 30 s epochs (tonic) % of 2-s mini-epochs (phasic)	Based on the chin EMG alone, like many other groups[13,51,56,61-64,152-161] Cutoff values for the diagnosis of RBD have been evaluated[50,68]
The Mayo Clinic	Submentalis limb	Phasic muscle activity: at least 4× the lowest REM sleep muscle activity amplitude for 0.1–14.9 s Submentalis tonic muscle activity: at least 2× the lowest REM sleep muscle activity amplitude for ≥15 s or ≥10 μV	% of 3-s artifact-free mini-epochs (phasic) % of 30-s artifact free epochs (tonic)	Cutoff values evaluated: RBD associated with Parkinson disease,[58] idiopathic/isolated RBD,[71] normative RWA values have been established[162]

AASM, American Academy of Sleep Medicine; EMG, electromyogram; microvolts, μV; seconds, s; SINBAR, Sleep Innsbruck Barcelona.

an amplitude at least twice the background or larger than 10 μV, and phasic EMG density was scored as the percentage of 2-second mini-epochs that contained EMG bursts with amplitude larger than four times the background and lasting 0.1 to 10 seconds. In 2014[70] the scoring rules for tonic EMG were adapted to an epoch length of 30 seconds, and diagnostic thresholds for the diagnosis of RBD were evaluated.

AASM Scoring Rules. The AASM scoring rules[1] now recommend scoring an epoch as showing RWA when ***excessive sustained*** or ***excessive phasic activity*** is observed. The epoch has ***excessive sustained activity*** when at least 50% of the epoch with chin EMG activation has an amplitude greater than two times the stage REM atonia level (or than the minimum amplitude during NREM sleep, if no REM atonia is present). The epoch has ***excessive phasic activity*** when at least 5 mini-epochs, based on the division of the 30-second epoch into 10 sequential 3-second mini-epochs, have EMG bursts of 0.1 to 5 seconds, each with an amplitude at least two times the stage REM atonia level (or the minimum amplitude during NREM sleep, if no REM atonia is present) in the chin or limb EMG. An epoch can be designated as having ***any chin EMG activity*** when EMG activity is two times greater than the stage REM atonia level (or than the minimum amplitude during NREM sleep, if no REM atonia is present), regardless of duration. In addition to the recommended scoring, which requires the presence of either excessive sustained or excessive phasic activity, it is "acceptable" to score RWA in an epoch when at least half of the 3-second mini-epochs contain any chin activity or any limb EMG activity (0.1–5.0 seconds duration of EMG activity at least two times the stage REM atonia level or the minimum amplitude during NREM sleep, if no REM atonia is present).

The AASM rules[1] now indicate to report the "RWA index" (the percentage of REM epochs that meet RWA criteria) as an "optional" parameter.

SINBAR Scoring Rules.[49] The scoring approach of the SINBAR group quantifies tonic, phasic, and "any" EMG activations during REM sleep, for which normative values have recently been proposed.[49] ***Tonic EMG activity*** is defined as the percentage of 30-second epochs with chin EMG activity, with an amplitude at least twice the background or larger than 10 μV present for more than 50% of the epoch. ***Phasic EMG activity*** is scored as the percentage of 3-second mini-epochs containing EMG activity with duration 0.1 to 5 seconds and an amplitude that is at least twice the background EMG amplitude. The end of a phasic EMG burst is determined by a return of 0.25 second or longer to background EMG levels. To score phasic activity in the presence of tonic activity, the amplitude has to be at least twice the amplitude of the tonic background as determined in the same 3-second mini-epoch and the phasic burst has to have a waxing and waning morphology. ***"Any" EMG activation*** is scored as the percentage of 2-second mini-epochs that contain EMG activity of any length with an amplitude that is larger than twice the background amplitude.

Mayo Clinic Scoring Rules.[58] ***Phasic muscle activity*** is directly scored when it meets amplitude criteria of being at least four times greater than the lowest REM sleep background and with a duration lasting between 0.1 and 14.9 seconds, with the end of a phasic burst defined as a return of muscle activity to background for longer than or equal to 200 milliseconds. Key metrics yielded are phasic muscle activity burst duration in addition to tonic, phasic, and "any" muscle activity percentages for the submentalis and limb muscles.[58,71] ***Submentalis tonic-muscle activity*** uses 30-second epochs and can be scored with muscle activity that is at least two times the lowest REM sleep muscle activity amplitude and lasting longer than or equal to 15 seconds in duration, or meeting the threshold of 10 μV. The percentages of abnormal REM sleep muscle activity are calculated by dividing the number of positively scored mini-epochs (or epochs, for tonic) by the total artifact-free REM sleep time, with all 3-second mini-epochs containing arousals (spontaneous, breathing, or snoring-related) being excluded from analysis.

Automated Scoring of REM Sleep without Atonia

Currently, several automated scoring algorithms are available for scoring EMG activity during REM sleep[72-77] or sleep in general.[78] Of note, all of the available algorithms quantify different entities and measures of EMG activity that are not directly comparable with those derived from visual scoring. Algorithms evaluated in larger groups of patients with RBD and control subjects are discussed here.

The Supra-Threshold REM EMG Activity Metric (STREAM)[79] was proposed by Burns and coworkers. It quantifies the percentage of 3-second mini-epochs during REM sleep, with increased muscle activity identified by the variance of the EMG signal, which has to be above the fifth percentile of variance values during NREM sleep. The correlation between STREAM scores and the average of percentages of epochs with tonic and phasic activity visually scored, according to Lapierre and Montplaisir, was 0.87.[51]

The ***REM atonia index*** (RAI) is by far the most widely used automated scoring algorithm for RWA. Introduced by Ferri and coworkers in 2008,[75] it was improved in 2010[76] with the addition of a noise reduction technique. The RAI is based on the automated analysis of the rectified, bandpass (1–100 Hz) and notch (50/60 Hz) filtered submentalis muscle EMG signal. For each 1-second mini-epoch, the average amplitude is corrected for the local noise level by subtracting the minimum amplitude of the EMG signal in the ±30-second interval around it.[76] The resulting average amplitude for each 1-second mini-epoch is classified in 20 distinct categories as 1 μV or less, between 1 and 2 μV (i.e., greater than 1 μV up to 2 μV or less), between 2 and 3 μV, and so on, until the category of between 18 and 19 μV and the final category of greater than 19 μV.

The RAI is calculated as the proportion of 1-second mini-epochs with average amplitudes of 1 μV or less, reflecting atonia, with respect to all other mini-epochs except those with average amplitudes between 1 and 2 μV, which are thought to reflect both atonia and EMG activation. The RAI can vary, ranging from 0 to 1—from complete loss of atonia and the absence of mini-epochs with average amplitudes of 1 μV or less (RAI = 0)—to complete atonia with the amplitudes of all mini-epochs 1 μV or less (RAI = 1). Aside from the RAI, the algorithm quantifies the number of movements during REM sleep, defined as the number of consecutive 1-second mini-epochs with average amplitudes greater than 2 μV, which are additionally classified by their duration in 20 distinct categories (from 1 second to more than 19 seconds).

Evaluation of the original algorithm[80] compared against visual scoring of loss of atonia and phasic density as proposed by Lapierre and Montplaisir[51] showed adequate agreement. The average correlations in four large groups of subjects—young control subjects, old control subjects, patients with idiopathic or isolated RBD (iRBD), and patients with multiple system atrophy (MSA)—were between 0.745 and 0.963 for the REM sleep atonia index and percentage of visually scored atonia and between 0.628 and 0.915 for the number of EMG activations and visually scored phasic density. This has been confirmed for the improved RAI with noise correction.[70] In approximately 80 patients with RBD and 80 healthy control subjects, the correlation between the RAI and the visually scored tonic density was 0.87. Similar results were obtained in an additional independent study.[68]

The RAI has been used in several studies employing larger samples of healthy control subjects in different age groups[81] and of patients with RBD,[75,76,80,82-84] Parkinson disease,[68,85-87] or other neurologic disorders,[76,80,84,88] and cutoff values for the diagnosis of RBD have been established.[76]

The Mayo method, which has shown similar diagnostic yield and comparable discrimination for synucleinopathy and RBD phenoconversion to the automated REM atonia index,[58,71,89-91] was also independently implemented for an automated application,[92] in addition to the SINBAR method.[93]

Classification of Movements during REM Sleep

The classification of movement events during REM sleep is a dynamically evolving field. Approaches include a simple listing of observed behaviors,[53] the categorization in a few broad categories,[61,62,88,94-96] classification of each event along several dimensions,[13] and the development of a standardized rating scale.[16]

The only standardized rating instrument currently in use is the REM Sleep Behavior Disorder Severity Scale (RBDSS).[16] The scale was created by Sixel-Döring and colleagues[16] to provide an easy-to-use classification of motor events during REM sleep; based on video PSG, all motor events are classified on a scale from 0 (RWA but no visible movements) to 3 (any axial movements with the possibility of falling or observed falls). The motor event score is the highest score observed for each patient and on each night. In addition, vocalization is classified as absent (0) or present (1). The overall RBDSS score for a single night and for an individual patient is the combination of the motor score with the vocalization score, usually separated by a full stop (period). The score ranges from 0.0—that is, RWA but no visible movements and no vocalizations—to 3.1 observed axial movements with either an observed fall or the distinct possibility of a fall and vocalizations. This scale has since been used in an increasing number of studies.[11,83,97,98]

Unresolved Issues

The scoring of RWA is complicated by the particularly large variety in applied scoring criteria. Currently unknown is what—if any—is the magnitude of the effect that these variations have on the respective RWA measures and on their ability to distinguish between patients with RBD and healthy subjects. Variations seem to be minor for the assessment of tonic EMG activity during REM sleep, because a large consensus favors use of the chin EMG and an epoch-wise quantification. For phasic EMG, by contrast, a rather substantial variation in applied scoring rules is evident, and standardized international criteria would greatly benefit the field.

In all cases, by applying the methods described earlier for the quantification of REM sleep atonia (visual and/or automatic), we can expect a large overlap between RBD and non-RBD subjects in terms of the presence of RWA.[99,100] The effects of additional factors that are likely to play a role in this overlap need to be better understood: night-to-night variability of REM sleep atonia,[101-103] age of the subjects,[81] and the muscles recorded.[49] How many nights are needed to confirm RWA in RBD and how many nights are needed for non-RBD subjects who might present with occasional RWA during a single night recording remain to be determined. Moreover, REM sleep atonia is known to change continuously with a complex developmental trajectory through life[81]; in particular, a decline of REM atonia is expected at older ages, making more probable the detection of RWA if preset cutoff values are not adjusted for age. Finally, the effects of REM sleep duration on the measurements of atonia and the minimum amount needed for a reliable estimation are not known. Thus the exact role of RWA in the diagnosis of RBD, even if definitely crucial, must be still clearly defined and its quantification used in a context of a careful clinical judgment.[104]

SLEEP-RELATED BRUXISM

Sleep-related bruxism (SB) refers to regular or frequent teeth grinding during sleep (see Chapter 170). According to the ICSD-3,[3] the diagnostic criteria for SB are the presence of regular or frequent teeth grinding sounds occurring during sleep and either the presence of abnormal teeth wear consistent with this report, transient morning jaw muscle pain, fatigue, temporal headache, or jaw locking on awakening.

Several approaches and protocols are available to record and score SB activity, including the following:

- The ambulatory recording of masticatory muscle EMG (mmEMG), in which the identification and scoring of nocturnal bruxism activity are based only on the mmEMG signal[105-108]
- The ambulatory recording of mmEMG and heart rate, with identification and scoring of nocturnal bruxism activity based on criteria for mmEMG and heart rate[109-111]
- Ambulatory PSG with additional recording of mmEMG but without video-audio recording, in which scoring of SB activity is based on mmEMG[112] or mmEMG and heart rate[113] during the PSG-identified sleep period
- AASM recommendations[1]: standard PSG with video-audio recording, including chin EMG, and only optional recording of mmEMG, in which SB activity is identified by chin EMG or chin and mmEMG activity, and teeth grinding episodes are identified by audio recording during the sleep period
- Research diagnostic criteria (RDC)[114,115]: standard PSG with video-audio recording and mmEMG, in which SB activity is identified and scored on the basis of mmEMG and video-audio recordings during the sleep period

The main difference between these approaches is in the availability and/or use of video-audio recording to distinguish between SB activity and other nonspecific orofacial movements.

Orofacial movements with visible increases in mmEMG are common during a night of sleep, both in healthy sleepers and subjects with SB. Many of these movements may be unspecific and unrelated to SB activity but are indistinguishable from

Table 204.4 Examples of Orofacial Movements and Sounds that May Be Confused with Sleep-Related Bruxism Activity

Movements	Sounds
Swallowing	Coughing
Coughing	Grunting
Yawning	Snoring
Lip and tongue movements	Sleeptalking
Eye blinking	Tooth tapping
Light head movements	Temporomandibular joint clicking
Head rubbing or scratching	Tongue clicking
Lip sucking	Throat clearing

the mmEMG activation patterns that are used to define SB activity. Some examples of nonspecific movements are given in Table 204.4. In general, and as detailed subsequently, SB activity is identified by EMG activations above a specified threshold that are either a series of phasic, short activations or sustained tonic activations or both—that is, a mixed episode. The total set of all mmEMG activations during sleep, then, has the following components:

A: activations that do not fulfill EMG criteria for SB episodes
B: activations that fulfill EMG criteria for SB episodes but are nonspecific movements such as coughing or swallowing (see Table 204.4), as identified with audio-video recording
C: activations that fulfill EMG criteria and are indeed SB episodes

Rhythmic masticatory muscle activity (RMMA) is a subset of SB that contains only the phasic and mixed episodes (see later). Within the complete set of mmEMG activations (A + B + C, or B + C), "true" SB episodes account for only 15% to 30% in healthy subjects and for 55% to 70% in patients with SB.[115-117] Audio-recording can help identify SB episodes with audible teeth grinding sounds, but less than 30% of SB episodes are accompanied by teeth grinding noise.[115,118,119] For this reason, mmEMG recording with audio-video recording is the gold standard for assessment of SB activity, and misclassification can result when mmEMG is recorded alone. For example, in healthy sleepers, RMMA episodes identified by the gold standard (video-PSG with mmEMG) were compared with events recorded with a telemetric masseter muscle EMG device.[120] The telemetric device correctly identified close to 99% of RMMA episodes identified by video PSG. However, 77% of all episodes identified by the telemetric device were other oromotor events and not SB-related. The positive predictive value (PPV) was therefore only 0.23—that is, the probability that an event identified with the telemetric device was indeed an RRMA episode was only 23%. When only the sleep period was considered, with information provided from video PSG, the PPV increased to 0.52.

These results correspond with those in another study in patients with SB,[121] in which video PSG was scored twice, without and with access to the audio-video recording. With the use of video PSG, 33% of all masseter muscle EMG activations did not satisfy EMG criteria for RRMA. Of EMG activations that satisfied RRMA EMG criteria, approximately 69% represented other nonbruxism activity. These would have been false-positive identifications if only the masseter EMG activity had been available for scoring (PPV, 0.31). With the use of the complete information provided by the PSG recording (with the exception of audio-video), the number of RMMA events was overestimated by only 23.8% relative to that for video PSG-RDC (PPV, 0.81)—a considerable improvement. Misclassification of nonspecific EMG activity, however, was still pronounced for tonic EMG activations: Only 41% of episodes identified without audio-video were indeed "true" RMMA events (PPV, 0.41).

Recording Methods

Surface EMG electrodes placed on masticatory muscles are the key component in assessment of SB activity. The different protocols vary in the selection and number of masticatory muscles, but most include the masseter muscles. Masseter muscles are easily identified by the muscle bulges between the cheekbone and the angle of the jaw during teeth clenching. The registration of other masticatory muscles, such as the temporalis muscle, often is optional but may increase reliability of SB activity identification.[122] Electrode positioning for the temporalis muscle usually is 1 to 2 cm above the zygomatic arch (cheek bone) and 1 to 2 cm behind the outer canthus orbital border (the cavity of the skull in which the eye is situated). The following recommendations have been made concerning the recording of SB activity:

- *ICSD-3 recommendations*[3]: Although PSG is not strictly necessary for the diagnosis of SB, when SB activity is to be recorded and scored, the minimal requirement is one masseter muscle recording. Audio-video recording is strongly recommended to exclude nonspecific movements from the scoring of SB activity. For optimal diagnostic specificity and sensitivity, bilateral masseter and temporalis muscle EMG recordings, referenced to ear, mastoid, or zygomatic bone, are advised.
- *AASM scoring criteria*[1]: AASM recommendations refer to in-laboratory PSG with the recommended parameters (electroencephalogram [EEG], electrooculogram [EOG], electrocardiogram [ECG], EMG, respiration, oxygen saturation, body position), which include EMG of the chin muscles. Scoring rules for SB have been formulated for chin EMG only; the addition of masseter muscle recording is left to the discretion of the clinician. In addition, the audio signal is used to identify SB episodes with teeth grinding sounds.
- *RDC[115]:* Standard PSG with video-audio recording and bilateral masseter EMG is the minimum requirement for the scoring of SB activity according to RDC. The addition of temporalis muscle recording is recommended but not mandatory.[123]
- *Ambulatory recording:* There are no generally accepted recommendations for the ambulatory recording and scoring of SB activity. Currently used recording setups range from a single, unilateral EMG channel[108,120] to ambulatory PSG with additional mmEMG.[112,113]

Scoring Rules

Sleep Bruxism Episodes Scored According to Research Diagnostic Criteria

The scoring of SB activity according to RDC (SB-RDC)[115] involves the following general steps:

1. Identify all masseter muscle activations with mean amplitude above a predefined threshold.
2. Classify the identified EMG activations on the basis of their duration as myoclonic (less than 0.25 second), phasic bursts (0.25–2 seconds), or tonic bursts (more than 2 seconds).
3. Use video and audio recording to exclude non–(bruxism)-specific oromandibular activity.
4. Classify the remaining phasic bursts as belonging to a phasic episode if three or more phasic bursts are separated by less than 3 seconds; the remaining tonic bursts are considered tonic episodes.
5. Combine phasic and/or tonic episodes to one episode if they are separated by less than 3 seconds.
6. Classify episodes as phasic, tonic (episode with one or more tonic bursts), or mixed (episode with tonic and phasic episodes).
7. Characterize SB episodes regarding the presence or absence of audible teeth grinding sound, as recorded by audio.

These scoring criteria have been widely adopted in research studies. The only major variation concerns mmEMG threshold, which was originally 20% of background signal during maximal voluntary clenching (MVC) in the wake state[115] and subsequently modified to a 10% MVC.[114,123]

Descriptive summary measures for SB activity include the number of phasic, mixed, tonic, and all SB episodes either as a total number per night or as the number per hour. In addition, the number of bursts per hour and the proportion of SB episodes with audible teeth grinding sound usually are reported.

Rhythmic Masticatory Muscle Activity

The scoring of RMMA[118] follows the outline described for the scoring of SB episodes according to RDC, with the exception of two aspects:

- The threshold to identify mmEMG activations is 10% MVC.
- RMMA includes only phasic and mixed SB episodes, as defined previously.

Because only approximately 10% to 20% of SB-RDC episodes are classified as tonic episodes,[115,124,125] a large overlap between RMMA and SB-RDC is to be expected, and the distinction between RMMA and SB-RDC has become blurred over time, as evidenced by the fact that more and more research studies now include the tonic episodes in the scoring of RMMA.[121,126,127] In addition, in research studies, the tendency is to adopt a mmEMG threshold that is twice the background EMG,[121,128] as has been proposed by the AASM rules.[1]

RMMA usually is reported as the number of RMMA episodes per hour and the percentage of RMMA episodes with audible teeth grinding sound.

Sleep Bruxism Episodes Scored According to AASM Criteria

The AASM has specified scoring rules for bruxism based on chin EMG activity.[1] Bruxism is scored in accordance with the following criteria:

1. Chin EMG elevation is at least twice the amplitude of the background EMG, *and*
2. a. *Either* at least three brief, phasic chin EMG activity elevations (lasting 0.25–2 seconds) occur in a regular sequence,
   b. *Or* a sustained, tonic chin EMG activity elevation (lasting longer than 2 seconds) is present.
3. Chin EMG elevations that fit these criteria are counted as one episode when they are separated by less than 3 seconds.

Of note, audio-video recording is not used to exclude nonspecific orofacial movements from the scoring of bruxism episodes. Nevertheless, some use is made of the audio recording because the manual states that "bruxism can be scored reliably by audio in combination with polysomnography by a minimum of 2 audible teeth grinding episodes/night of polysomnography" (section F1.e).[1] Currently, the AASM manual provides no information about the reporting of bruxism activity.

Sleep Bruxism Episodes Described in the Current International Classification of Sleep Disorders

As mentioned previously, according to the ICSD-3,[3] PSG documentation of SB activity is not a necessary diagnostic feature. However, three patterns within masseter muscle EMG are described for SB episodes[3]: (1) phasic activity at 1-Hz frequency with EMG bursts 0.25 to 2 seconds in duration, (2) sustained tonic activity longer than 2 seconds, and (3) a mixed pattern. SB episodes begin after 3 seconds or longer with no muscle activity. Audio-video recording is recommended to identify teeth grinding sound and to distinguish SB from other orofacial or masticatory movements that normally occur during sleep and from specific movement disorders.[3]

Sleep Bruxism Activity in Ambulatory Recordings

Currently, no generally accepted or validated criteria are available for the scoring of SB activity in ambulatory recordings without video-audio recording. Consequently, a wide variation in scoring criteria are in current use. Many, however, seem to be inspired either by the RDC formulated for video PSG[115] or the following criteria that use an ambulatory masseter muscle EMG and heart rate.[109]

1. Masseter muscle EMG activity increases greater than 10% MVC for 3 seconds or longer
2. Separated by more than 5 seconds from other events—otherwise, events are combined
3. Accompanied by a change in heart rate greater than 5% over a 5-second period, compared with baseline

A point worthy of emphasis is that these criteria were based almost exclusively on theoretical considerations and have never been empirically validated. Scoring criteria used in research studies and in commercially available devices differ in the amplitude thresholds for the identification of mmEMG activations; the duration of identified mmEMG activations; the interval between identified events; and the designation of phasic, tonic, or mixed character of events.[107,110,111,129-133]

Partly responsible for this variation is the lack of validation studies for ambulatory SB assessment. The mmEMG signal from ambulatory devices has been shown to be in good agreement with the mmEMG signal from ambulatory or in-laboratory mmEMG. However, the main concern in validating ambulatory SB assessments is the lack of video-audio recording, with the probable misclassification of many mmEMG activations as SB episodes.

Research Diagnostic Criteria Application

Currently, only RDC are available for the identification of patients with moderate-to-severe SB.[115] In the pivotal study by Lavigne and coworkers,[115] using the RDC scoring criteria detailed earlier, various parameters of SB activity were assessed in 18 healthy sleepers and in 18 patients with moderate-to-severe SB. By considering sensitivity and specificity of different combinations and cutoff values, the following criteria were identified:

A + (B1 or B2 or C or D)

with:

A indicating 2 or more bruxism episodes with teeth grinding sounds/night
B1, >30 episodes/night
B2, >4 episodes/hour
C, >6 bursts/episode
D, >25 bursts/hour

The combination of criterion A with any one of the other criteria had a PPV between 93% and 100% and a negative predictive value (NPV) between 76% and 93%.[115] These criteria have been widely adopted[114]; over time, however, the most used and recommended combination of criteria is A + (B2 or D).[114,123]

The ability of these criteria to discriminate between patients with SB and healthy sleepers has been evaluated in a larger sample of 100 patients diagnosed with SB and 43 healthy sleepers.[124] The recording and scoring of SB activity were identical in both studies, with two critical differences: First, although general inclusion and exclusion criteria were identical, the original study included patients with SB who reported more frequent nocturnal teeth grinding sounds in the prior 6-month period (five times per week versus least three times per week in the subsequent investigation). In addition, the diagnostic criteria employed in the study were any two of the following three: (A) two or more bruxism episodes with teeth grinding sounds per night, (B2) more than 4 episodes/hour, and (D) more than 25 bursts/hour, that is, different from the original study, criterion (A) was no longer mandatory. With these modifications, only 54 of 100 patients with SB fulfilled the RDC criteria for SB, as did 9 of 43 healthy sleepers. Consequently, the sensitivity of the RDC was only 54% (PPV, 86%) and the specificity was 79% (NPV, 42%). These results emphasize the continued need for large and systematic studies in this field.

Unresolved Issues

The major unresolved issue in the recording of SB is currently the scoring without the availability of video-audio recording. As detailed earlier, nonexclusion of unspecific orofacial movements will considerably overestimate SB activity. In addition, diagnostic criteria include the observation of episodes with teeth grinding sounds, which also are not confirmable without at least audio recording.

Other issues concern the diagnostic criteria, which may lack sensitivity or specificity when applied with variations, and the inconsistent scoring of RMMA.

RHYTHMIC MOVEMENT DISORDER

RMD is characterized by stereotypical rhythmic body movements occurring predominantly during sleep or drowsiness before sleep, which may involve the head, neck, trunk, or limbs in isolation or in combination. The criteria for scoring RMD are based on their PSG features[1]: frequency of 0.5 to 2.0 Hz; presence of at least four single movements, as required to form a rhythmic cluster; and a minimum amplitude for a single rhythmic movement that is twice the background EMG activity. In healthy infants or young children, the movements and behaviors frequently are self-limited and are called "benign rhythmic movements of sleep," to distinguish them from RMD[132]; however, no strict quantitative threshold has been established. The duration of rhythmic movement episodes may vary, ranging from some seconds to several minutes, and can be observed as well during wakefulness preceding sleep or after sleep onset. The most common pattern of RMD involves the head (head banging, or *jactatio capitis nocturna,* and head rolling), but also the body (body rocking) or occasionally the legs (leg rolling or leg banging) can be involved. The clinical diagnosis can be based on anamnesis, sometimes supported by homemade video recording; however, video PSG is useful in doubtful cases and allows definition of the type and site of movements. Additional EEG and EMG leads, in particular on the limbs, may help distinguish RMD from other sleep-related repetitive movements (e.g., PLMS, alternating leg muscle activation [ALMA]) or motor seizures.

PROPRIOSPINAL MYOCLONUS

PSM at sleep onset[133,134] is characterized by generalized and symmetric jerks, occurring at the wake-sleep transition, starting from the axial muscles of the abdomen, thorax, or neck and then spreading rostrally and caudally to the other myotomes by means of slow propriospinal polysynaptic pathways.[135] PSM is facilitated by relaxed wakefulness or drowsiness and inhibited by mental activation and sleep deepening. In PSM, there is no urge to move; however, the frequently repeated (but not periodic) jerks prevent the patient from falling asleep and reaching a deeper sleep stage, when the jerks disappear. No accepted quantitative PSG features have been documented for PSM, and its description is basically qualitative.

BENIGN SLEEP MYOCLONUS OF INFANCY

Benign sleep myoclonus of infancy (BSMI) is characterized by repetitive myoclonic jerks that occur during sleep in neonates and infants.[3] Its diagnostic features include the observation of repetitive myoclonic jerks involving the limbs, trunk, or whole body. These movements occur only during sleep and stop abruptly and consistently when the infant is aroused. BSMI occurs in early infancy, typically from birth to 6 months of age.

Standardized scoring criteria for BSMI are lacking, but the muscle jerks last between 0.04 and 0.3 second and occur usually in clusters of four to five jerks per second.[3,136] These clusters may repeat in irregular series for 1 to 15 minutes, and in rare cases up to 60 minutes. The jerks often are bilateral and typically involve large muscle groups. BSMI is benign and relatively rare, but it has been included in the ICSD-3 as a sleep-related movement disorder because it often is confused with epilepsy.[3]

RESTLESS SLEEP DISORDER

RSD is a newly identified condition recently characterized in children and adolescents. RSD presents clinically with concerns for frequent nocturnal repositionings, body movements involving large muscle groups, and nonrestorative sleep.[137] A study using video PSG confirmed that children with RSD exhibit frequent large body movements (>5/hour) throughout the night. On PSG, children with RSD also showed reduced TST and increased number of awakenings, similarly to children with RLS but without increased index of leg movements.[138] In children with complaints of restless sleep and daytime impairment, the sleep physician should consider reviewing the video PSG for assessment of frequent large movements or repositionings through the night by applying the recently introduced criteria.[139]

MISCELLANEA

Excessive Fragmentary Myoclonus

EFM[140-142] is characterized by small EMG activations, not always corresponding with movements (twitches), of the fingers, toes, or corners of the mouth, resembling either physiologic hypnic myoclonus or fasciculations, occurring at the sleep-wake transition or during sleep. PSG recordings show recurrent and persistent, very brief (75–150 milliseconds) EMG bursts in various muscles, occurring asynchronously and asymmetrically, in a sustained manner, without clustering. The PSG criteria for scoring EFM are as follows: EMG burst duration usually is 150 milliseconds or less, EFM must be present in at least 20 minutes of NREM sleep, and at least five EMG potentials per minute must be recorded.[1] Regarding quantification, it has been proposed to quantify EFM rate as the number of EMG potentials of 150 milliseconds or less divided by the minutes of sleep.[142] Alternatively, a *myoclonus index* has been proposed by Lins and coworkers[143]; this index is defined as the number of 3-second mini-epochs containing at least one fragmentary myoclonus potential fulfilling the criteria, counted for each 30-second epoch, with totals ranging between 0 and 10. A mean fragmentary myoclonus index of 39.5 events per hour of sleep has been reported in patients with sleep disorders, and this index increased with age, was higher in men than in women, and was influenced by the presence of sleep breathing disorders.[144] The male predominance was also confirmed in a large, well-screened sample of healthy sleepers.[145] Some fragmentary myoclonus was observed in all participants, however, and 9% even fulfilled criteria for EFM, suggesting that the criteria for quantification of EFM may benefit from an appropriate statistical revision.

Neck Myoclonus (during Sleep) or Sleep-Related Head Jerks

Neck myoclonus (head jerks) during REM sleep has been described,[146] recognized by the presence of a characteristic high-amplitude, short ("stripe-shaped") movement–induced artifact over the EEG lead signals that is verified in the video recording, which shows sudden myoclonic twitches of the head of variable intensity. It seems to be a frequent finding on routine PSG, being present in more than 50% of patients, but with a low frequency during the night (1 ± 2.7 events per hour of REM sleep) and an age-related decline. Neck myoclonus has been observed in 35% of healthy subjects, with variable frequency,[145] suggesting that it constitutes a physiologic phenomenon. More recently, the "benign" nature of neck myoclonus has been put under discussion because it seems to be associated with arousal in about 80% of cases and occurs in REM sleep in the same percentage of cases, while its duration is on average 0.5 second. Because of these reasons, the name "*sleep-related head jerks*" has been proposed as a substitute for neck myoclonus.[147]

Other Leg Movements during Sleep

Alternating leg muscle activation (ALMA) indicates a rapidly alternating (frequency, 0.5 to 3 Hz) pattern of anterior tibialis activation (duration, 100 to 500 milliseconds) occurring during sleep, organized in sequences of at least four alternating activations,[1] lasting up to 20 to 30 seconds. ALMA can occur in all sleep stages but is seen particularly during arousals.[148,149] It is not yet clear whether ALMA is a separate nosologic entity or whether it belongs to the wide spectrum of nocturnal motor activities of RLS.

Hypnagogic foot tremor (HFT)[149-151] is a clinical condition similar to ALMA, with foot movements occurring at the transition between wake and sleep or during light sleep. PSG recordings show repeated short EMG potentials, typically at the 1 to 2 Hz (range, 0.3 to 4 Hz), in one or both feet, in sequences of at least four.[1] The EMG events appear to be of longer duration than myoclonus (more than 250 milliseconds) and usually last less than 1 second; moreover, they are organized in trains lasting 10 or more seconds.[3]

The term ***high-frequency leg movements*** (HFLMs) has been proposed for a phenomenon similar to both ALMA and HFT.[152] It was defined as a sequence of four or more short leg movements occurring unilaterally but sometimes bilaterally, at a frequency of 0.3 to 4 Hz. Most HFLMs are observed during wakefulness, with only approximately one-third occurring during sleep. Thus far, no clear criteria have been established to score this phenomenon.

ALMA, HFT, and HFLMs are similar phenomena of small or short EMG activations of the feet and legs: They all occur at sleep onset and are correlated with arousals, and they usually occur in trains. It is not clear yet if these phenomena are really separate entities or if they constitute slightly different definitions of the same condition; moreover, it is not yet established to what extent they are correlated with PLMS and/or RLS. In addition, it is unknown whether these are simple, physiologic phenomena or have any pathophysiologic significance. A case in favor of the first possibility is the observation that HFLMs have been found in 33% of well-screened, healthy sleepers.[145]

CLINICAL PEARLS

- Video PSG is the gold standard for recording and scoring sleep-related movements.
- For many sleep-related movements, more than one system of criteria or definitions exist. It is therefore essential to specify which scoring rules are applied.
- Scoring rules change over time as new research evidence arises to support implementing a different guideline.
- The current ICSD-3 refers to the manual of the AASM for the definition of sleep-related movements.

SUMMARY AND FUTURE DIRECTIONS

As reviewed in this chapter, a variety of clinical and research recording and scoring techniques define, quantify, and/or diagnose sleep-related movements. Currently, computerized digital recording is standard in sleep medicine and research. Computerization offers numerous advantages, among them the precise measurement of sleep-related movement events. Many criteria to visually detect and measure motor events during sleep were introduced during the "paper era" of sleep medicine and continue to be the basis of the current rules. With the wide availability of powerful computers, one might expect digital criteria would have emerged. However, without specific application software to perform such tasks, the hardware continues to emulate previous approaches. Software development and validation have been slower than expected. Nonetheless, having agreed-upon recording and scoring standards should facilitate development. The technical advances do not replace the clinical evaluation of the patient and the suspicion of new conditions or variants of known conditions, but aid in their characterization and practicality of scoring. The adoption of new approaches based on more quantitative and data-driven methods is slow, mainly because of the heterogeneity in global advancement in sleep medicine. The necessary programs and independent validations are prerequisites to effect change. In view of the strengths (e.g., objectivity and precision) of the new approaches, however, they can be expected to gradually enhance and ultimately replace many of the scoring techniques presented in this chapter.

SELECTED READINGS

Berry RB, Quan SF, Abreu AR, et al. *The AASM Manual for the Scoring of Sleep and Associated Events: Rules, Terminology and Technical Specifications, Ver. 2.6*. Darien, IL: American Academy of Sleep Medicine; 2020.

Cesari M, Heidbreder A, Bergmann M, Holzknecht E, Högl B, Stefani A. Flexor digitorum superficialis muscular activity is more reliable than mentalis muscular activity for rapid eye movement sleep without atonia quantification: a study of interrater reliability for artifact correction in the context of semiautomated scoring of rapid eye movement sleep without atonia. *Sleep*. 2021;44(9):zsab094.

Ferri R. The time structure of leg movement activity during sleep: the theory behind the practice. *Sleep Med*. 2012;13:433–441.

Ferri R, DelRosso LM, Provini F, et al. Scoring of large muscle group movements during sleep: an International Restless Legs Syndrome Study Group (IRLSSG) position statement. *Sleep*. 2021;44:zsab092.

Ferri R, Fulda S, Allen RP, et al. World Association of Sleep Medicine (WASM) 2016 standards for recording and scoring leg movements in polysomnograms developed by a joint task force from the International and the European Restless Legs Syndrome Study Groups (IRLSSG and EURLSSG). *Sleep Med*. 2016;26:86–95.

Ferri R, Zucconi M, Manconi M, et al. Computer-assisted detection of nocturnal leg motor activity in patients with restless legs syndrome and periodic leg movements during sleep. *Sleep*. 2005;28:998–1004.

Frauscher B, Gabelia D, Mitterling T, et al. Motor events during healthy sleep: a quantitative polysomnographic study. *Sleep*. 2014;37:763–773.

Fulda S, Plazzi G, Ferri R. Scoring atonia during normal and pathological rapid eye movement sleep: visual and automatic quantification methods. *Sleep Biol Rhythms*. 2013;11:40–51.

Lavigne GJ, Rompré PH, MontplaisirJY. Sleep bruxism: validity of clinical research diagnostic criteria in a controlled polysomnographic study. *J Dent Res*. 1996;75:546–552.

Van Der Zaag J, Lobbezoo F, Visscher CM, et al. Time-variant nature of sleep bruxism outcome variables using ambulatory polysomnography: implications for recognition and therapy evaluation. *J Oral Rehabil*. 2008;35:577–584.

A complete reference list can be found online at ExpertConsult.com.

Chapter 205

Home Sleep Testing for Sleep-Related Breathing Disorders

Thomas Penzel

Chapter Highlights

- Home sleep testing for diagnosing sleep-disordered breathing (SDB) is an accepted diagnostic method. Diagnostic sensitivity and specificity meet criteria for effective clinical application.
- Home sleep testing protocols have been established in terms of required signals. Monitoring usually includes respiratory effort and airflow, oxygen saturation, and body position/activity. Visual scoring is a necessary component. Clinical symptom assessment and home sleep testing should be combined to achieve high sensitivity and reliability.
- New developments are targeting use of fewer signals for diagnosing SDB. Different systems achieve this with variable success. An economic benefit can be realized if SDB can be diagnosed or managed using devices with smart sensors and intelligent signal analysis, and such approaches currently are under investigation.

OVERVIEW AND BACKGROUND

Home sleep testing refers to portable monitoring for diagnosing sleep-disordered breathing (SDB). The term was introduced in the past decade. In 2014 a National Library of Medicine (NLM) PubMed database search for "home sleep testing" in all fields found 19 publications and the same search in late 2021 returned 104 publications. The reference method for the diagnosis of SDB is cardiorespiratory polysomnography (PSG). The recording technology and the scoring criteria used in home sleep testing are derived from this modality. In July 2015 the American Academy of Sleep Medicine (AASM) manual for recording and scoring sleep and associated events added a chapter concerning home sleep apnea testing (version 2.2). Considerable evidence indicates that home sleep testing for SDB can be as specific and as reliable as sleep laboratory–based PSG recordings[1-3] in properly referred patients. Adequate data are available to validate home sleep testing's use clinically, although it does have certain limitations.[4] A workshop consensus report presented the view of the participating medical societies (American Thoracic Society, American Academy of Sleep Medicine, American College of Chest Physicians, European Respiratory Society) on the use of this diagnostic procedure and provides directions for further research.[5] A clinical practice guideline from the American College of Physicians recommends portable sleep monitors for diagnostic testing in patients suspected of having obstructive sleep apnea (OSA) without serious comorbidity, and as an alternative to a laboratory sleep study when PSG is not available.[6] In Europe, home sleep testing has been widely used for several decades to diagnose SDB.[7]

Guidelines and recommendations for home sleep testing are partially evidence based. It is essential, however, to critically examine the underlying samples used for evidence evaluation. The clinical validation studies were performed at sleep centers on their patients; consequently, the sample consists of the clinical populations available in sleep centers.[8,9] Clinical populations differ from the general population in that the patients have been referred for evaluation for suspected sleep disorders. This selection leads to a high pretest probability for sleep disorders and for sleep apnea in particular.[1,10] Factors associated with this increased pretest probability include various physical examination measures and complaints reported by the patient or the bed partner, as follows:

- Loud and irregular snoring
- Observed or reported nocturnal cessation of breathing
- Excessive daytime sleepiness
- Nonspecific mental problems such as fatigue, low performance, or cognitive impairment
- Movements during sleep
- Morning dizziness, general headache, dry mouth
- Impaired sexual function
- Obesity
- Arterial hypertension and cardiac arrhythmias

Some of these signs and symptoms are incorporated into sleep apnea screening questionnaires. Clinicians commonly use validated questionnaires in conjunction with home sleep testing to confirm the suspected diagnosis.[11]

As revealed in a literature search, published reports fall into several different categories. Some articles describe new devices and compare them to PSG. Although reviews of data on existing devices are scarce, they do exist and provide categories for evaluation.[4] These categories are sleep, cardiovascular, oxygen saturation, position, effort of respiration, and respiratory flow—the SCOPER acronym. Sensors and systems are evaluated using these categories. A majority of published studies, however, focus on the role of home sleep testing in sleep apnea diagnosis. Some reports in the literature concentrate on general management of patients with sleep apnea, whereas other reports focus on home sleep testing. Presented next is a short technical overview of available systems, followed by a discussion of home sleep testing with respect to requirements and special considerations.

HOME SLEEP TESTING WITH FOUR- TO SIX-CHANNEL SYSTEMS FOR DIAGNOSING SLEEP-DISORDERED BREATHING

Systems for diagnosing SDB generally fall into one of four classifications defined in an American Sleep Disorders Association (ASDA) standard of practice guideline.[12]

- Level I: attended cardiorespiratory PSG with at least seven signals
- Level II: cardiorespiratory PSG at home with at least seven signals, unattended
- Level III: unattended portable sleep apnea testing with at least four signals including airflow, respiratory effort, oxygen saturation, electrocardiogram (ECG), or heart rate or pulse rate
- Level IV: unattended one or two signal recording, such as actigraphy or oximetry

Most diagnostic systems for home sleep testing attain level III device status and record four to six physiologic signals but do not record the electroencephalogram (EEG). Evidence-based home sleep testing reviews commissioned by health technology assessment agencies[3] revealed limited reliability in the past. More recent studies with recording systems currently in use showed substantial improvement.[9,13] If systems incorporate a thoughtful selection of physiologic measures, have good signal acquisition, and use a good signal processing technique, the number of false-positive diagnoses is low.[1] When studies sampling from the general population are compared with studies using clinical populations, the importance of a high pretest probability becomes clear. A high pretest probability reduces the number of false-positive diagnoses. Nonetheless, the overall test specificity is high enough to conclude that home sleep testing for sleep apnea can be recommended under certain conditions[4,6]:

1. Systems should be used only by certified sleep physicians based in certified sleep centers. This recommendation attempts to improve quality control and quality assurance. An interview of the patient and assessment of complaints should be conducted before performing home sleep testing. This process increases the pretest probability, as explained earlier in this chapter.
2. Home sleep testing for OSA is recommended when no other comorbid pulmonary, cardiovascular, mental, neurologic, or neuromuscular disorder, or heart failure or another sleep disorder, is present. Other sleep disorders to rule out include central sleep apnea, periodic limb movement disorder, insomnia, circadian sleep-wake disorders, and narcolepsy.
3. Some home sleep testing systems can now distinguish between central and OSA events.
4. Home sleep testing for diagnosing sleep apnea needs to record oronasal airflow (using a thermistor or nasal pressure sensor), respiratory effort (using inductive plethysmography), oxygen saturation (with a short averaging period over few [3–6] pulses), pulse or heart rate, and body position.
5. Evaluation of the recordings should incorporate visual scoring of respiratory events using the same rules specified for PSG.[14,15] (Of course using exactly the same rules is not possible without EEG. As a humble proposal to overcome this limitation, CMS rules require a 4% oxyhemoglobin desaturation.) Editing of recorded events is necessary to remove artifacts occurring during the recording period. Furthermore, the visual scoring should be performed by trained personnel.
6. The technical specifications and sampling rates for the digital recording should be the same as specified in the evidence-based recommendation for cardiorespiratory PSG.[15]

Today, many devices meet level III device criteria. Such home sleep testing devices all include pulse oximetry technology to record oxygen saturation and pulse rate. Many systems record oronasal airflow, which reflects intranasal pressure. Few systems still use thermistors for flow recording. Most devices record respiratory effort using either piezo sensors or respiratory inductive plethysmography. Some devices use one belt for rib cage movements, whereas others use two belts (for recording abdominal movements as well). Most systems record body position to identify positional apnea. Very few systems record the raw ECG, but many report heart rate derived by other means. A number of systems offer specific options to record signals in sleep apnea patients under therapy. The options are the recording of continuous positive airway pressure (CPAP) mask pressure in addition or as an alternative to other airflow signals. The signal will be split into a CPAP pressure reading, corresponding to set pressure level and to a respiratory flow reading that may be observed superposed to the CPAP pressure set. This may vary depending on pressure mode selection (e.g., bilevel or flex modes). This option is an important feature for using home sleep testing for treatment follow-up studies. Some systems allow an option for recording additional electromyogram (EMG) tibialis activity to detect leg movements; thus far, however, no systematic studies on this option's utility have been conducted.

It remains an open question whether home sleep testing can reliably diagnose periodic limb movement disorder. Similarly, a few systems can add EEG channels for recording the sleep EEG, but no systematic studies have evaluated this option for its potential added diagnostic value for other sleep disorders such as insomnia or hypersomnia. Nonetheless, many systems have been validated for clinical use with their basic signal setup together with their scoring and analysis software. In general, most systems show good performance, with some minor differences. No overall preference for one or another system emerges from published studies.

HOME SLEEP TESTING WITH ONE- TO THREE-CHANNEL SYSTEMS FOR DIAGNOSING SLEEP-DISORDERED BREATHING

Systematic reviews of home sleep testing for diagnosing SDB have revealed that systems with one to three channels (pulse oximetry, long-term ECG, actigraphy, and oronasal airflow) are not suitable for routine diagnostic use. Specifically, these devices yield too many false-negative and too many false-positive results, as reported by Collop and associates,[1] and in a more recent systematic review using the new SCOPER criteria.[4] Therefore the application of these devices is not recommended for definitive diagnostic testing for OSA or to exclude the presence of OSA.

Some of these devices, however, provide results in patients with severe sleep apnea that clearly suggest SDB. Therefore high-quality recordings achieved with validated systems of this category can be used to increase the pretest probability before performance of cardiorespiratory PSG or even before four- to six-channel home sleep testing for sleep apnea.

Many technical innovations are currently emerging in this category of devices. A major challenge has been development of one- to three-channel devices that perform well and can diagnose SDBs. If reliable, such devices could facilitate diagnosis in new patient groups and provide tools for clinicians trained in other specialties with only basic knowledge of sleep medicine. Before initiation of therapy for sleep breathing disorders, however, a physician with a solid background in SDB who is very familiar with the different treatment options should review the case.[16]

Described next are new technologies applicable with both one- to three-channel systems and four- to six-channel diagnostic devices.

NEW METHODS FOR HOME SLEEP TESTING

Different approaches are being explored for development of new technologies for diagnosing SDB. Some approaches focus on developing new sensors to assess respiration for detecting breathing disturbances occurring during the night. Other technologies concentrate on assessing the patient's cardiovascular risk or sleep pathophysiology. In view of the COVID-19 pandemic, some home sleep testing devices were redesigned to be single-use devices, to be applied only once, and then the recordings transferred using network infrastructure (telemedicine), while other patient communication is done using videoconferencing.

Assessment of Respiration

Several new sensors use surrogate signals to derive respiratory effort noninvasively. Some of these devices try to derive respiratory measures from direct respiration-related signals. These systems and concepts are discussed next.

A first-line approach entails recording respiratory airflow at the nose and the mouth. Usually these recordings are accompanied by pulse oximetry to determine oxyhemoglobin saturation. These simple screening devices provide a straightforward analysis for respiratory cessations. They even may distinguish obstructive from central respiratory events by analysis of flow limitation. Problems with obstructed nostrils, partial breathing through the mouth, blocked air tubes, and various artifacts pose logistical challenges to differentiating among the different types of apnea. Nevertheless, good validation studies are available,[17,18] with some limitations.

One approach tries to analyze respiratory sounds from the chest, with the goal of less obtrusive measures for detection of increased respiratory effort.[19] In other systems, respiratory sounds are recorded at the throat, and signal processing separates cardiac and movement signal first from breathing sounds and snoring. Together with oximetry, such recording quantifies respiratory measures, and snoring is tracked to detect respiratory cessations.[20,21]

Another approach involves recording midsagittal jaw movements based on magnetic distance determination.[22] A magnetic sensor is placed on the chin and another on the forehead to allow continuous determination of relative jaw movements. From this setup, it is possible to derive respiration and snoring. Analysis of this information is then used to detect respiratory events to diagnose sleep apnea.[23] By further analysis, a sleep wakefulness profile may potentially be estimated.[24,25] Combined with pulse oximetry and perhaps a cardiovascular parameter, this magnetic sensor–jaw movement detection feature is both simple and promising for clinical usefulness.

Pulse Wave Analysis (see Chapter 203)

Many systems try to exploit the pulse wave on the finger or other peripheral sites. Such systems derive parameters from the pulse wave to assess cardiovascular event risk. The pressure wave may be detected with the photoplethysmograph already placed to measure oxygen saturation. In principle, this can be used to detect all forms of respiratory events[26] and cardiovascular event risk as associated with sleep apnea.[27,28]

Peripheral arterial tonometry[29] can be used to assess cardiovascular risk by measuring endothelial function during SDB episodes. Sympathetic activating events (sometimes referred to as *autonomic arousals*) terminating sleep apnea events are accompanied by attenuated pulse amplitude. This decrease is due to peripheral vasoconstriction caused by sympathetic tone activation. If pulse rate also is analyzed, probability analysis can be used to distinguish between slow wave sleep and rapid eye movement (REM) sleep.[30] Several validation studies have been published on use of the Watch-PAT, based on peripheral arterial tonometry, in patients with central sleep apnea, OSA, and also those with the overlap syndrome (with chronic obstructive pulmonary disease [COPD]) with very good res ults.[28,31,32] A meta-analysis for this methodology is available and substantiates the diagnostic value of this device, even though it does not incorporate proximal sensors for effort and flow to record respiration, as recommended.[33]

Assessment of Electrocardiographic and Heart Rate Variability Parameters

ECG-derived respiratory parameters are very attractive for simple detection of sleep apnea owing to low costs and wide availability (e.g. Holter ECG software add-on packages, pacemaker ECG analysis add-on packages). To detect sleep apnea from the ECG alone does not require additional electrodes or additional hardware. The respiratory information is derived entirely from analytical software. This kind of analysis also could be performed retrospectively using previously recorded data. Sleep apnea is accompanied by a cyclic variation of heart rate, as already described many years ago.[34] Periodic changes in heart rate are related to the changes in sympathetic tone with apnea events.[35] Modern analysis of heart rate variability can satisfactorily derive cyclic variations of heart rate.[36,37] In addition, the morphology of the ECG wave itself is modulated by respiration. The derived respiratory curve, *ECG-derived respiration,*[38] correlates with respiratory effort and thus can be used to detect SDB.[39,26] By combining ECG-derived respiration and sleep apnea–related heart rate variability, sleep apnea detection is possible.[40]

Electrocardiographic and Oximetry Assessments

A number of devices that use the ECG analysis techniques mentioned previously also try to link this approach to previous techniques. Early on, pulse oximetry was applied (with limited success) for portable diagnosis of sleep apnea. Pulse oximetry alone has large diagnostic limitations in patients with arrhythmias or with additional lung diseases such as COPD.

Combining ECG-based sleep apnea analysis and oximetry is therefore a very promising approach.[41] An early study using pulse rate in addition to oximetry[42] could show that this improves the detection of sleep apnea. One retrospective study showed the advantage over pulse oximetry alone when combined with ECG analysis.[43] In that study, the ECG from a parallel PSG recording was evaluated. Based on these results, a combined long-term ECG recording system with oximetry was tested prospectively and provided very convincing results in terms of sleep apnea detection.[41]

MANAGEMENT OF HOME SLEEP TESTING IN A SLEEP CENTER SETTING

Many new studies show high reliability of home sleep testing in detecting sleep apnea.[18] A number of open research questions needing clarification concerning the conditions and restrictions for using home testing are now being addressed in recent studies.[1,5] The important parameters are no longer technical limitations but often study limitations involve selection and/or incorporation bias. The inherent screening process corresponds with the characteristic high pretest probability of sleep apnea. This aspect prohibits the use of portable monitoring as a screening tool to exclude sleep apneas, such as in professional drivers and people with supervision tasks (in which symptoms and complaints have not been assessed and may conflict with employability or other issues). Legal issues may become important here as well.

Diagnostic and therapeutic approaches to management of SDB differ among countries worldwide.[44] Sleep medicine in some countries is well established and a significant clinical infrastructure exists. In other countries, economically affordable strategies constitute the primary consideration.[45,46] In certain settings, sleep medicine may be very basic, with only home sleep testing available for diagnosing sleep apnea.[44] One potential reason for this restriction to home sleep testing alone is the limited availability of sleep medicine centers owing to unmet needs for qualified experts and funding for PSG beds. This is the case in countries in which sleep medicine is a young discipline. A second reason is an economic decision to limit access to PSG studies to patients with comorbid illnesses. Patients with sleep apnea and no comorbidities are diagnosed with home sleep testing alone. This applies to countries with enough medical resources and a well-developed sleep medicine. With improvements in the knowledge base for sleep disorders and SDB among general physicians, the individual clinician can decide whether a particular patient should be evaluated for suspected sleep apnea alone or exhibits some comorbidity or has other risk factors. Then the patient can be referred for either home sleep testing or cardiorespiratory PSG. This approach would allow economic and thoughtful management of patients with respect to diagnosis and subsequent treatment, as appropriate.[45] In Germany a debate is ongoing that different levels of sleep medicine service include different levels of medical expertise and correspondingly different levels of equipment complexity. Family physicians may have some basic knowledge about SDB and already sometimes apply simple tests. A limited number of clinical centers would have clinical expertise, training, research, and other technical know-how as required in specialized sleep centers.[46] Many community-based centers have basic sleep medicine knowledge and home sleep testing with four- to six-channel systems.

The other issue is health economy and patient care. A quantitative threshold regarding sleep apnea severity and assessing risk based on evidence still remains to be established. We do not have evidence how many apneas, how many hypopneas, what duration of apnea events, how much sleep fragmentation, or what degree of hypoxia causes substantial cardiovascular risk with increased mortality. In view of limited therapeutic adherence to CPAP, how strict should researcher-clinicians be with respect to treatment follow-up studies? As the field of sleep medicine approaches the point at which diagnosis can be done easily with home sleep testing, a need is emerging for new clinical evidence and transparent health economic decisions. They are key for developing strategies in managing sleep apnea.

Patients may be diagnosed and even treated at home based on a home sleep apnea test alone. With the COVID-19 pandemic, this management pathway has gained popularity among sleep centers. Surveys during the pandemic showed, that patients are hesitant to seek medical help when this requires to physically go to a physician office or a sleep medicine center.[47] Home sleep apnea testing devices may be sent to a patient, then sent back for interpretation of the recording, and based on the result, an automatic positive airway pressure device may be prescribed and delivered to the patient. Follow-up studies on optimizing pressure settings and checking adherence to the treatment are then performed using telemedicine modalities such as medical clouds or secure videoconferencing. One home sleep testing study showed that the 4-week outcome in sleepiness and CPAP adherence was similar to that for sleep laboratory–based diagnosis and treatment.[48] An important limitation of the study was the short follow-up period.[49] SDB is a chronic condition, and long-term adherence with CPAP therapy may decline more at home. Thus more research is needed.

CONCLUSIONS

Attended clinical PSG is the reference standard for diagnosing disordered breathing during sleep. Evidence-based literature, however, indicates that diagnosis of OSA can be performed using home sleep testing under certain conditions in adults. The recording must include oxygen saturation, airflow, respiratory effort, heart or pulse rate, and body position. The SCOPER parameters summarize these requirements in a comprehensive and quantitative scheme.[4] Visual evaluation is needed to avoid misclassification of sleep apnea severity.[14] It is not possible to distinguish between central and obstructive respiratory events with certainty. Home sleep testing is reliable if it is performed under the supervision of personnel trained in sleep medicine and if screening has been adequate to achieve a high pretest probability among the study subjects of suffering from SDB. In addition, the patients should not have other significant sleep or comorbid disorders (e.g., heart failure, stroke, diabetes mellitus, obstructive or restrictive lung diseases, or severe cardiac arrhythmias).

Home sleep testing systems with fewer channels can indicate the likelihood of SDB but currently are not sufficiently validated for diagnostic purposes. Technological advances are expected to improve these systems. Accordingly, systems with fewer channels may provide a sufficiently reliable diagnosis for disordered breathing during sleep in the near future. High-quality clinical studies, with sufficient sample size and comparison against a reference standard, are needed.

Technologic advances need to be accompanied by economy-driven strategies to diagnose and treat patients with sleep apnea. Recent approaches to diagnosing and even treating patients at home seem to provide effectiveness, in terms of outcome, similar to that for sleep laboratory–based studies. Economically proven home-based studies may be more feasible than sleep laboratory–based studies in light of the high prevalence of the disorders and the still-unmet clinical needs to recognize and treat patients with SDB.

CLINICAL PEARLS

- Home sleep testing has been used for out-of-laboratory diagnosis of SDB for many years worldwide.
- Home sleep testing has been thoroughly compared against cardiorespiratory PSG.
- Sensitivity and specificity of home sleep testing are sufficient for diagnosing adult patients with high pretest probability for SDB.
- Most home sleep testing devices monitor airflow, respiratory movement, oxygen saturation, pulse rate, and body position.
- Use of systems with fewer signals shows promising diagnostic results, but most require further validation.

SUMMARY

Home sleep testing is a well-validated technique to diagnose SDB outside of the sleep laboratory and other clinical settings. Different devices are available. These devices usually record respiratory flow, respiratory effort, oxygen saturation, pulse or heart rate, and body position and/or activity. Some of these signals may be recorded indirectly and derived. The diagnostic sensitivity and specificity have been validated against those of PSG and generally show good agreement in patients with a high pretest probability for SDB. Visual evaluation is needed to prevent misclassification of sleep apnea severity. Overall, the available evidence indicates that home sleep testing should be used in combination with a clinical assessment for factors and symptoms associated with SDB. Today, home sleep testing to assess sleep apnea is often preferred. In addition, home sleep testing offers a method for conducting therapy follow-up studies that may improve therapy compliance. Simpler devices such as wearables try to perform home sleep testing but these are not currently approved as medical diagnostic devices. At present, consumer devices accuracy is highly variable; consequently, they are not medically recommended.

ACKNOWLEDGMENTS/DISCLOSURES

Several companies have furnished equipment for research or otherwise supported the work on which this chapter is based. Itamar Medical (Caesarea, Israel) provided sensors/consumables for research with the Watch-PAT device. Neuwirth Medical (Obernburg am Main, Germany) provided equipment to the Sleep Center for Research Studies. Cidelec (Sainte-Gemmes-sur-Loire, France) provided a grant for a validation study of its Pneavox system for laryngeal pressure and sound recording. Nomics (Liege, Belgium) provided a grant for a validation study of the Brizzy system. Somnomedics (Randersacker, Germany) provided Somnowatch equipment to the Sleep Center for Research Studies. Nox Medical (Reykjavik, Island) provided equipment and sensors for testing. Studies were done at the Interdisciplinary Sleep Medicine Center at Charite-Universitätsmedizin Berlin.

SELECTED READINGS

Aurora RN, Swartz R, Punjabi NM. Misclassification of OSA severity with automated scoring of home sleep recordings. *Chest*. 2015;147:719–727.

Berry RB, Gamaldo CE, Harding SM, et al. *The AASM Manual for Scoring Sleep and Associated Events, Version 2.6*. Am Academy of Sleep Med; 2020.

Caples SM, Anderson WM, Calero K, Howell M, Hashmi SD. Use of polysomnography and home sleep apnea tests for the longitudinal management of obstructive sleep apnea in adults: an American Academy of Sleep Medicine clinical guidance statement. *J Clin Sleep Med*. 2021;17(6):1287–1293.

Collop N. Home sleep testing: appropriate screening is the key. *Sleep*. 2012;35:1445–1446.

El Shayeb M, Topfer LA, Stafinski T, et al. Diagnostic accuracy of level 3 portable sleep tests versus level 1 polysomnography for sleep-disordered breathing: a systematic review and meta-analysis. *CMAJ*. 2014;186:E25–51.

Jen R, Orr JE, Li Y, et al. Accuracy of WatchPAT for the diagnosis of obstructive sleep apnea in patients with chronic obstructive pulmonary disease. *COPD*. 2020;17(1):34–39.

Kapur VK, Auckley DH, Chowdhuri S, et al. Clinical Practice Guideline for Diagnostic Testing for Adult Obstructive Sleep Apnea: an American Academy of Sleep Medicine Clinical Practice Guideline. *J Clin Sleep Med*. 2017;13:479–504.

Kuna ST, Badr MS, Kimoff RJ, et al. An official ATS/AASM/ACCP/ERS Workshop report: research priorities in ambulatory management of adults with obstructive sleep apnea. *Proc Am Thorac Soc*. 2011;8:1–16.

Pereira EJ, Driver HS, Stewart SC, Fitzpatrick MF. Comparing a combination of validated questionnaires and level III portable monitor with polysomnography to diagnose and exclude sleep apnea. *J Clin Sleep Med*. 2013;9:1259–1266.

Pillar G, Berall M, Berry R, et al. Detecting central sleep apnea in adult patients using WatchPAT-a multicenter validation study. *Sleep Breath*. 2020;24(1):387–398.

A complete reference list can be found online at ExpertConsult.com.

Chapter 206

Consumer Sleep Tracking: Landscape and CTA/ANSI Performance Standards

Max Hirshkowitz; Michael Paskow; Cathy A. Goldstein

Chapter Highlights

- The past few years have brought various technologies claiming to provide sleep tracking capabilities. These devices purport to measure sleep, often and may have other functions (e.g., fitness tracker, smartwatch); they can be grouped into wearables, nearables, and stand-alone mobile apps.
- Consumer sleep technologies (CSTs) include sensors within the device (the hardware) and the associated mobile application (app) and a cloud-based system for data management.
- Sensors measure one or more of the following variables: motion, heart rate, oximetry, respiration, temperature, and neuronal activity. Depending on the device, algorithms claim to differentiate sleep from wake, determine sleep stages, and identify other sleep variables such as the apnea-hypopnea index.
- Some CSTs provide feedback (recommendations or physical stimuli) to the user.
- Clinical use of CSTs is limited by lack of standards, validation studies, and absent Food and Drug Administration (FDA) clearance.
- The Consumer Technology Association (CTA) partnered with the American National Standards Institute (ANSI) and the National Sleep Foundation (NSF) to create a performance standard for evaluating wearable and in-bedroom sleep trackers.
- The three-part ***standard*** provides guidance for developers and consumers with respect to sleep terminology, methodology, and performance evaluation.
- Two levels of performance evaluation are described. The first addresses differentiating sleep and wakefulness; it is mandatory for CTA certification. The second addresses differentiating sleep subtypes (stages) and is optional.
- Performance evaluation study design, metrics required, statistical analysis, and reporting requirements are specified.

INTRODUCTION

In the past, quantitative sleep assessment resided in specially equipped laboratories or hospital sleep clinics, Now, millions of individuals use consumer devices to track their sleep nightly at home.[1,2] The COVID-19 pandemic accelerated this trend.[3] This chapter will describe the landscape of consumer sleep technologies (CSTs) and the technical aspects of data acquisition and the landscape, validation, integration, and regulation sections (and their subsections) of this chapter were adapted and updated from Dr. Goldstein's paper discussing the current and future roles of consumer technology in sleep medicine.[3a] The second part of the chapter will focus on the development of validation and standards.

CURRENT CONSUMER SLEEP TRACKER LANDSCAPE

Several categorizations can help organize the vast number of available consumer sleep trackers.[4] One useful approach classifies products according to their proximity to the user; that is, wearables or "nearables." Another approach divides products as either devices or stand-alone digital applications (apps), most commonly loaded onto a phone or other mobile device. Overarching either perspective is the sleep tracker's purpose. The purpose may focus specifically on sleep itself (i.e., sleep versus wakefulness, sleep stages, and derivable measures). Alternatively, the device may target a particular sleep-associated activity, for example, snoring or cardiac arrhythmia. These latter devices straddle the fence between the consumer markets and sleep medicine. Of course, some devices attempt to do both.

Wearables

Wrist-Worn (and Ring) Consumer Sleep Technology

By far, wrist-worn wearables are the most common. At last count, these authors are aware of more than 40 different wrist-worn devices that are or have been marketed to consumers. Originally wrist-worn devices recorded only movement; however, current-generation devices are multisensory, and some can also record pulse, electrocardiogram (ECG), blood pressure, temperature, and oxygen saturation.[4]

Movement is detected with a triaxial accelerometer, using a piezoelectric sensor.[5] Dramatic advances in accelerometer development, storage technology, and battery capacity allow data collection over long periods with use of microelectromechanical sensors.[6]

Pulse rate is measured at the dorsal aspect of the wrist or finger using photoplethysmography (PPG), an optical technique that quantifies blood volume changes.[7,8] PPG data can be used to determine heart rate variability (HRV) and cardiac rhythm abnormalities.[7-9] The U.S. Food and Drug Administration (FDA) has cleared a mobile application on the Apple watch that analyzes the PPG signal to evaluate for atrial fibrillation.[10] In some CSTs, analysis of PPG heart rate is used to indirectly calculate the respiratory rate based on the coupling between heart rate and respiration.[11]

Blood oxygen saturation is measured using PPG with sensors. Traditionally, these sensors were applied to the fingertip[12] but have been incorporated into commercial devices in bands at the dorsum of the wrist[13] or within a ring on a finger.[14] Additionally, at the time this chapter was drafted, we have observed the emergence of cuffless blood pressure monitoring through wearable PPG by the same devices that provide sleep metrics.[14a]

Additionally, ring devices have been used to measure temperature,[15] and some can produce a vibratory stimulus for the purpose of sleep retraining for insomnia,[16] as a treatment for posttraumatic stress disorder (PTSD),[17] or as an alert to hypoxemia and apneas. For a comprehensive review of accelerometer and PPG sensors, in addition to other sensors incorporated into wearable CSTs, such as those that monitor temperature, skin conductance, respiration, and light, see de Zambotti.[4]

Dry Electroencephalogram Headbands

Headbands capitalize on advances made in ambulatory electroencephalogram (EEG) monitoring and apply brainwave analysis principles to determine sleep and wakefulness. Eye-mask sensors can record movement, EEG, and ocular motility. Originally introduced in 2009,[18] dry EEG headbands allow EEG recording to take place at home. These headbands are now in the CST marketplace and can identify slow waves and augmentation by acoustic stimuli.[19] A newer technology combines EEG with electrooculogram, PPG, and accelerometer sensors within an eye mask.

Nearables

Nearable products include proprietary in-bedroom monitors, in- or under-mattress sensors, and bedside smartphone apps. These devices mainly sense movement detected by perturbations in standing waves (akin to the way security motion detectors operate) or via transducers located at the sleep surface. Body movement can be subjected to digital analyses similar to those used by wearables; however, subtler movements from breathing and pulse can also be detected.

Smartphones placed at the bedside or in the bed may use sound and movement. Some smartphone apps involve subject-contact accessories to transmit sensor data via Bluetooth or other protocols and then uplink results for analysis. The ubiquity of smartphones, their memory capacity, and available programmability make them an extremely popular platform for sleep tracking technology. Dozens of apps are available for download. Because they are revised so often and/or so quickly become unavailable or obsolete, smartphone sleep tracking apps are difficult to evaluate.

Bedside

Noncontact bedside radiofrequency biomotion sensors (NRBSs) are used to track sleep without wearing any additional devices.[20-22] The devices are placed at the bedside and use ultra-low-power radiofrequency waves (radar) and assume that during sleep, most movement is related to respiratory effort.[21]

Under-the-Mattress

Under-the-mattress devices are based on the static charge-sensitive-bed (SCSB), which measures ballistocardiography (body movement because of contraction of the heart) and respiratory and body movements.[23] Originally SCSB used metal plates placed under a mattress.[23] The more modern units of under-the-mattress CSTs use a thin, flexible force sensor to measure ballistocardiography and derived sleep measures and can also monitor temperature and humidity.[24] A comprehensive index of currently available wearable and nearable CSTs is beyond the scope of this chapter. Types of wearable devices and parameters monitored is found in Table 206.1. Rapid evolution of CSTs may result in changes to this content.

Mobile Applications

Hundreds of stand-alone mobile apps claim to track sleep or respiration during sleep, and some even provide coaching or

Table 206.1 Types of Consumer Sleep Technologies and Monitored Parameters

Type	Motion/ Activity	HR (+ derived measures, e.g., HRV)	Respiratory Parameters	POx	BP	Temp	EEG	Sleep Environment
Wearable Consumer Sleep Technologies								
Wrist-worn	✔	✔	✔	✔	✔			
Ring-worn	✔	✔	✔	✔	✔	✔		
Headband	✔	✔	✔	✔			✔	
Eye mask	✔	✔	✔	✔		✔	✔	
Nearable Consumer Sleep Technologies								
Non-contact bedside	✔		✔					✔
Under-the-mattress	✔	✔	✔					✔

HR, heart rate; HRV, heart rate variability; POx, pulse oximetry; BP, blood pressure; Temp, temperature; EEG, electroencephalogram.

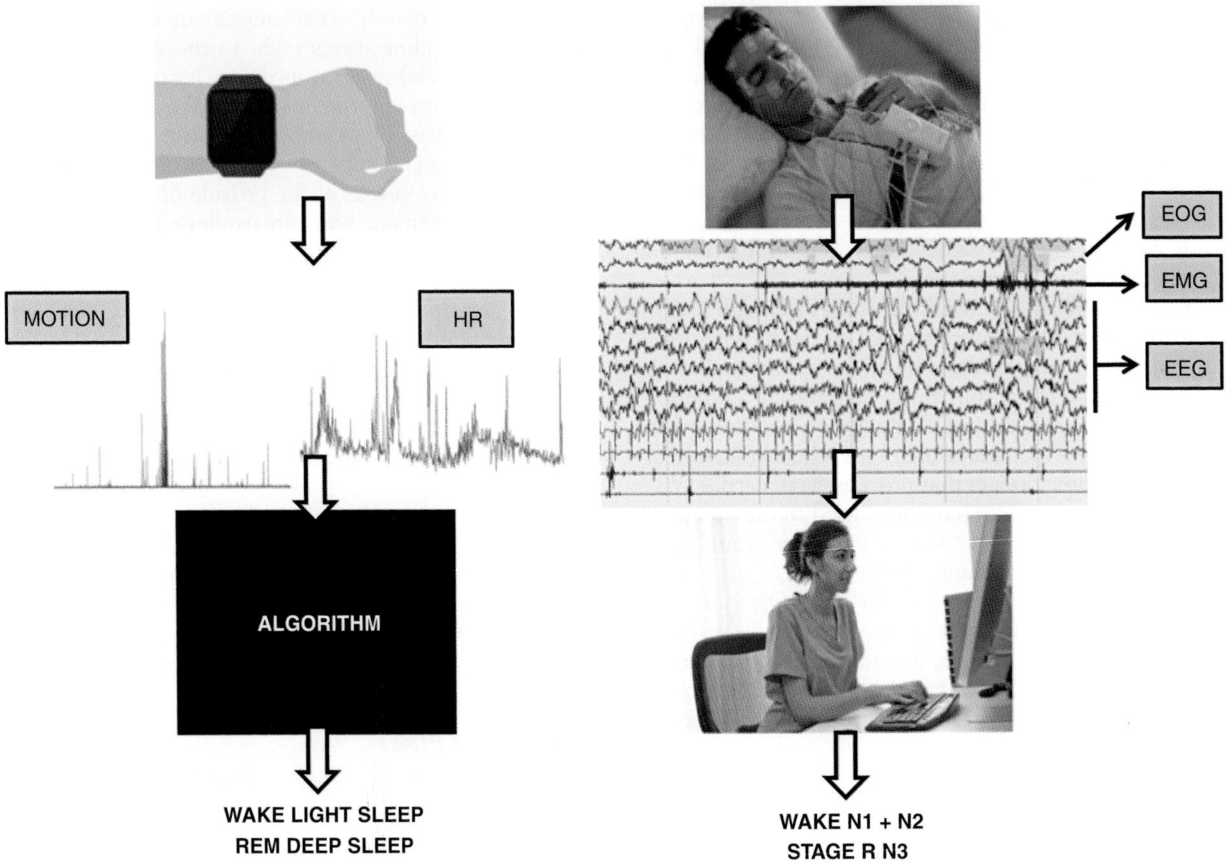

Figure 206.1 CST and PSG, from data acquisition to sleep metrics. CSTs and PSGs measure different physiologic processes, which are analyzed in different ways to predict sleep stages using different terminologies. CST, Consumer sleep technology; N1, NREM 1; N2, NREM 2; N3, NREM 3; PPG, photoplethysmography; PSG, polysomnogram; R, REM.

intervention.[25,26] Data acquisition is often through sensors native to the smartphone that the app is downloaded on (e.g., sleep tracking using the embedded accelerometer or snoring via the microphone). However, some apps obtain data by input by the user or indirectly by analyzing mobile phone usage.[25-27] Apps used for sleep tracking, alarms, obstructive sleep apnea (OSA) diagnosis/treatment, and interventions targeted at insomnia are well-accepted by consumers.[25,26]

The ability of mobile apps to accurately estimate sleep and respiratory variables remains unclear. Behavioral app-based interventions have demonstrated usefulness in the management of various sleep disorders. Mobile apps that allow "face to face" encounters (using the device's camera) allow for remote cognitive-behavioral therapy for insomnia or telehealth management of OSA or other sleep conditions (see Chapter 201).

Data Processing and Management

The data acquired by CST sensors are often uploaded to a cloud-based server, and then algorithms are used to distinguish sleep from wake and often classify sleep stages (Figure 206.1).

In contrast to clinical actigraphs whose performance is validated and uses algorithms that are published or otherwise accessible to users (see Chapter 211),[28-30] the CSTs' sleep estimation algorithms are "black box" because they are undisclosed and proprietary. Furthermore, in most cases, the performance of the CST and associated algorithm has not been rigorously validated and reported in the peer-reviewed literature.[31-34] Using HRV (from PPG) in sleep-staging algorithms appears promising.[32,35] Other mathematically derived parameters such as circadian estimates[34] and modeling of the sleep homeostat improve sleep staging accuracy.

Summaries of data analysis are displayed to the user via the app with manufacturer-specific terminology (with or without corresponding established clinical equivalents) to describe sleep. The following are often presented: bedtime, wake-up time, total sleep time (TST), wake time, light sleep, deep sleep, and rapid eye movement (REM) sleep. Sleep quality may be described as "restless sleep" or "sleep disturbances." Of note, there are specific CSTs geared toward athletes or other industries.

VALIDATION

Many issues need consideration when assessing a device's capacity to accurately assess sleep.[2] These include the purpose for which the device will be used; the target population; the precise brand, model, and software and firmware versions; the standard against which the sleep tracker is compared; and the statistical analysis. Approaches focusing on validation for sleep medicine and research have been published.[36,37,37a] As such, a strong case is made for validation against polysomnography (PSG) as it provides the definitions for REM and non–rapid eye movement (NREM) sleep states. However, sleep and awake states predate the invention EEG, and therefore PSG may not be the only approach for validation.

The validation of a consumer sleep tracker does not confirm equivalency, but rather verifies (to some degree) that one measure can be used as a surrogate for another. Thus a sleep tracker based on actigraphy and heart rate does not record REM sleep. It may, however, find a pattern that reflects ongoing REM sleep accurately enough for its output to be used as a surrogate measure for REM sleep, in some samples, under specified circumstances, and for a particular purpose.

Sleep Scoring

Techniques for the validation of CST against PSG are described by the Sleep Research Society (SRS).[36] Briefly, CST performance is evaluated by protocols in which PSG is recorded simultaneously while using a CST. PSG data are scored and time-synchronized with the CST (Figure 206.2).[38] From such epoch-by-epoch analysis, sensitivity, specificity, and accuracy can be reported. Of note, although considered the gold standard, scored PSG is not infallible, given imperfect interrater reliability, with an overall percent agreement of about 80% among registered polysomnographic technologists (RPSGTs).[39,40]

Sensitivity refers to the fraction of PSG sleep epochs scored correctly as sleep by the CST; specificity refers to the fraction of PSG wake epochs scored correctly as wake by the CST (Figure 206.2). Because of reliance on movement to distinguish sleep from wake, specificity is often much lower than sensitivity because nonmoving wakefulness is often misclassified as sleep. Thus CSTs often overestimate TST and underestimate wakefulness in comparison to PSG,[36,38] though this is not always the case.[15,41-43]

Accuracy refers to the fraction of PSG epochs correctly scored by the CST. Sleep metrics, such as TST and wake after sleep onset (WASO), compared between CST and PSG, should not be used as a sole measure of performance, as these may be statistically similar in those with high sleep efficiency but discrepant in those with poor sleep quality.

The performance of specific CSTs is beyond the scope of this chapter. A comprehensive review of validation studies that compare wrist-worn (and ring) CSTs to PSG can be found in de Zambotti.[38] Validation studies that use epoch-by-epoch comparison typically demonstrate sensitivity around or exceeding 90% but wider ranges of specificity (20%–80%) for multisensory wrist-worn (and ring) CST.[36,38] This is similar to the performance for traditional actigraphy,[44-46] and investigations in which both wrist-worn CSTs and actigraphy are compared with PSG demonstrate minimal differences.[36]

Validation studies that used a no-longer-available dry EEG headband device reported sensitivity of 97.6% and specificity of 56.1%[47] and overall agreement around 90%.[48] The performance of currently marketed dry EEG headbands has not yet been reported in the peer-reviewed literature.

An under-the-mattress CST significantly underestimated WASO and overestimated TST.[24] In contrast, an FDA-cleared under-the-mattress sensor detected sleep with sensitivity and specificity of 92.5% and 80.4%, respectively.[49]

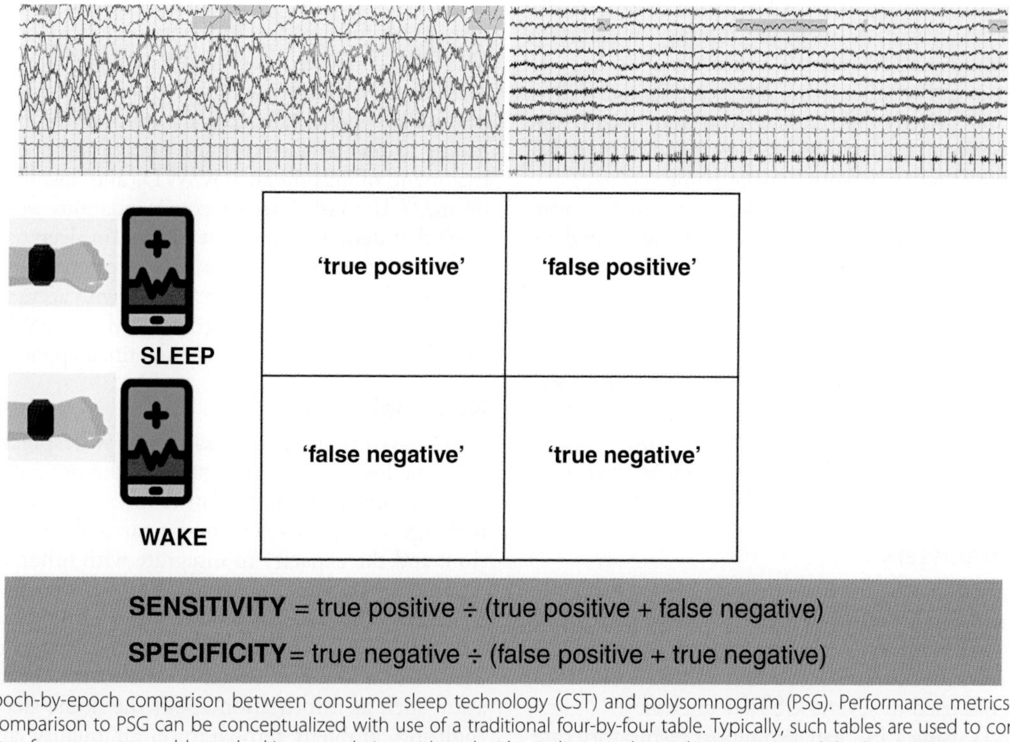

Figure 206.2 Epoch-by-epoch comparison between consumer sleep technology (CST) and polysomnogram (PSG). Performance metrics of CST during an epoch-by-epoch comparison to PSG can be conceptualized with use of a traditional four-by-four table. Typically, such tables are used to compare the disease prediction capability of a new test to gold standard in a population with and without disease who undergo testing with both modalities. In the case of CSTs, the new test is the CST and the gold standard is PSG scored by a registered polysomnographic technologist (RPSGT). However, the population is not individuals, but time-synchronized epochs during recording of both CST and PSG, and the condition of interest is the sleep state (positive) versus wake state (negative).

The few validation studies of noncontact bedside nearable devices also showed that they tended to overestimate TST in both healthy subjects[20,22] and those with sleep-disordered breathing.[21] With epoch-by-epoch comparison, sensitivity was cited at 87% to 88% and specificity ranged more widely, at 50% to 73%, though different devices, software versions, and patient populations preclude direct comparison.[20,21] The ability of stand-alone mobile apps to differentiate wake from sleep is also highly variable.[31,41,50,51]

Sleep Staging

CSTs often report sleep as "light," "deep," and "REM," implying an equivalency to scored PSG stages NREM1 + NREM2 (N1 + N2), NREM3 (N3), and R sleep, respectively. Sleep staging by CSTs is based on the known changes in HRV during different sleep stages. Sleep staging by CST should be approached cautiously, especially because of the effect of medications and cardiac disease. Epoch-by-epoch agreement ranges widely, from 60% to 80% for N1 + N2, 40% to 70% for N3, and 30% to 70% for stage R sleep derived from wrist-worn (or ring) CSTs.[15,52-54]

Comparably, a currently marketed dry EEG headband predicted N3 sleep with 70% sensitivity and 90% specificity; other sleep stages were not reported[19]; however, a no-longer-available dry EEG headband demonstrated overall agreement of approximately 75% for sleep staging.[48]

Few studies compare the sleep staging of nearable CSTs with PSG. A noncontact bedside nearable demonstrated 60%, 65% to 68%, 52% to 61%, and 62% agreement with PSG epochs staged as N1, N2, N3, and stage R sleep.[20] Under-the-bed sensors demonstrated poor agreement with PSG staged sleep.[24] Stand-alone mobile apps have demonstrated a poor correlation between app-quantified sleep stages and PSG.[26]

By design, validation protocols artificially set the time in bed. Therefore the performance cited for a CST may not translate to real-life use of the device. As such, the accuracy of reported sleep metrics is contingent on *both* the correct identification of when the subject is in bed attempting to sleep and the ability of the algorithm to correctly differentiate sleep from wake.[55] In addition, device position and technical failures could change the performance of CSTs when deployed in the home setting. Furthermore, CSTs are designed to collect sleep information over extensive periods, but validation studies are typically limited to 1 night; therefore reliability remains unclear. Similarly, because comparison studies usually take place at night, the ability of CSTs to estimate sleep during naps[53,56] or daytime sleep in shift workers or individuals with circadian rhythm sleep-wake disorders (CRSWDs) is not well understood. CST performance seems diminished in patients with central disorders of hypersomnia,[53,54] insomnia,[57] and sleep-disordered breathing.[41,58-60] Other patient factors, such as medications, alcohol use, comorbidities, and age,[4] all may affect the real-life accuracy of CST.

Respiratory Parameters

Wrist- and finger-worn CSTs have opened up the capability to measure and report oximetry values; however, accuracy remains unknown. Oximetry values from a wrist-worn FDA-cleared device have been validated,[61] but whether this can extend to a PPG housed in several CSTs is unclear.

Wearable CSTs using PPG can also report respiratory rate (RR); however, accuracy is not well defined. A bias of 1.8% and precision error of 6.7% were found when a wrist-worn CST marketed to athletes compared estimated RR with respiratory inductance plethysmography during PSG.[62]

Because some wearable CSTs measure oximetry and heart rate, derived respiratory metrics suggest they might soon report apnea-hypopnea indices (AHIs), but validation studies are not currently available. Using an AHI threshold of 15 per hour, under-the-mattress CSTs were able to identify OSA with sensitivities ranging from 72% to 89% and specificities ranging from 70% to 91%.[63-65] Using the same AHI threshold, a noncontact bedside nearable appropriately classified OSA with a sensitivity of 90% and a specificity of 92%.[66]

Many mobile applications claim to detect snoring using the smartphone microphone; accuracy has varied widely.[26] With the use of an AHI cutoff of 15 events per hour, one mobile app demonstrated a sensitivity of 70% and a specificity of 94% in detecting OSA compared with in-lab PSG, and another reported an accuracy of 92% compared with home testing.[67,68]

INTEGRATION INTO CLINICAL SLEEP MEDICINE

As CSTs improve and are verified, some may likely be integrated into the clinic. The immediate clinical application for CSTs is as a surrogate for actigraphy. The *International Classification of Sleep Disorders,* third edition (ICSD-3) already recommends actigraphy as part of the diagnostic evaluation in several disorders and testing scenarios: to visualize sleep timing patterns in CRSWDs, ensure adequate sleep duration before in-laboratory testing with PSG and multiple sleep latency testing (MSLT), document 24-hour sleep duration longer than 660 minutes in certain cases of idiopathic hypersomnia, and identify chronic, recurrent sleep restriction in insufficient sleep syndrome.[69]

After a systematic review of the available peer-reviewed literature, a task force of the American Academy of Sleep Medicine (AASM) confirmed the aforementioned actigraphy uses and identified the ability of actigraphy to estimate sleep parameters in insomnia; approximate sleep duration during home sleep apnea testing as part of an integrated device; and evaluate response to treatment of insomnia, CRSWD, and insufficient sleep syndrome.[70] The task force's recommendations were predicated on work that demonstrated that for certain sleep parameters, actigraphy provides objective data that are often unique from patient-reported sleep logs. Therefore a CST with accuracy that matches or exceeds a set benchmark considered acceptable for clinical use would have a variety of already identified applications.

New Applications

CSTs have unique attributes such as widespread acceptance by patients; lower cost; ownership by the patient, not the health system; long-term and continuous patterns of use; ability to recharge easily; wireless and near-real-time data transmission; and the capacity to integrate with other apps and health technologies. Such characteristics confer possibilities that transcend the use cases noted for actigraphy. Additionally, nearables, which do not have a clinical equivalent already in use, could add novel, valuable data to the clinical sleep evaluation such as information about the home sleep environment (lighting, ambient temperature, air quality, and sound) and improve adherence to sleep tracking and subsequent interventions, given truly passive use.

Data-Driven Circadian Rhythm Prediction

Whereas actigraphy (see Chapter 211) is typically used to identify sleep and wake periods in suspected CRSWD such that the abnormal pattern of sleep-wake timing can be visualized, mathematical modeling of 24-hour motion signal for days to weeks can quantify circadian properties of the rest-activity rhythm. Traditionally, cosinor analysis has been applied to actigraphy to estimate acrophase, mesor, period, and amplitude of the rest-activity rhythm; however, this analysis is poorly suited to patterns that change over time, and a growing field of research that uses nonparametric, data-driven methods is likely to reveal more accurate techniques to capture circadian rhythmicity.[71,72] However, these techniques have not yet been incorporated into clinical use. When appropriately vetted, such models may be well suited for the analysis of CST data to estimate circadian phase.[72a]

Off–Positive Airway Pressure Sleep Time

Continuous positive airway pressure (CPAP) is the first-line therapy for OSA, the most common disorder treated in sleep medicine. Treatment of OSA with CPAP is expected to resolve symptoms attributable to sleep-disordered breathing, like sleep disruption and excessive daytime sleepiness, and mitigate cardiovascular risk, though randomized controlled trials have returned negative findings regarding benefit.[73,74] One obvious contribution to null findings is reduced patient adherence to CPAP, which is easily tracked with CPAP-generated usage data. However, Thomas and Bianchi proposed that the effectiveness of CPAP should be considered not only in absolute hours of use but also in the context of the fraction of TST in which OSA is treated versus untreated, or "off-PAP" sleep time.[75] Quantification of off-PAP sleep time is a potential application of CST that would allow us to more precisely demonstrate the true benefits of treating OSA with CPAP.

Intervention

The continuous, longitudinal monitoring of sleep data with CST devices and management of such data within a patient-facing mobile app also confers the opportunity to implement app-delivered behavioral sleep interventions that are (1) personalized, given that they are derived with the use of the patient's sleep data; (2) dynamic, as interventions can change based on a patient's changing sleep patterns; and (3) real-time, as the mobile app delivery of the intervention could be provided near immediately in response to sleep changes. Already, a randomized controlled trial demonstrated the benefit of a sleep extension program that integrated a wearable CST and smartphone application.[76] Additionally, digital cognitive-behavioral therapy for insomnia (CBT-I) mobile apps allows for wearable CST-derived sleep parameters to guide therapy.[77,78]

Prediction

Importantly, patterns in the data derived from CSTs may have precision medicine applications outside of sleep disorders, given other illnesses are associated with changes in sleep. For example, analysis of data from 47,249 Fitbit users revealed that incorporation of elevated resting heart rate and increased sleep duration significantly improved predictive models for influenza-like illness.[79] Subsequently, in light of the COVID-19 pandemic, a combination of self-report symptoms (acquired with a mobile app) and consumer wearable sensor data, which included sleep, distinguished confirmed infection with SARS-CoV-2 better than symptoms alone.[80]

In regard to understanding the relationship between sleep and chronic illnesses, a U-shaped relationship between sleep duration and the risk of various diseases is well recognized,[81] and emerging evidence has demonstrated the importance of stability in sleep timing and quality for health.[82] Therefore CST also holds promise as a tool to further population sleep health.

With the addition of blood pressure and pulse oximetry readings from CST, predictive capabilities are also likely at the patient level and may include exacerbations of congestive heart failure or chronic obstructive pulmonary disease.

Integration with Other Digital Health Products

Individuals who use wearable CSTs to track sleep are also likely to harness the other capabilities offered by these devices such as activity tracking and cardiac arrhythmia identification.[83] Patients may also use other consumer-geared products to quantify additional health metrics simultaneously; for example, mobile apps provide endless opportunities to track caloric intake, alcohol consumption, exercise, menstrual cycles, and mood.[84-86] Additionally, patients may own scales, blood pressure cuffs, pulse oximeters, or other smart devices with wireless connectivity.[84-86] Some miniaturized devices on a ring are also able to track SpO_2, finger temperature, BP, and also record a single channel EKG.

Because sleep affects numerous health conditions, monitoring sleep data alongside other health parameters in the ambulatory environment could reveal important relationships that guide the development of new interventions. Additionally, new features of wearable technology, such as fall detection by smartwatches and physical and social activity tracking through hearing aids, are expected to engage older members of society. Therefore the sleep field has ample opportunities to understand the role of sleep in health and disease throughout the life span.

Telemedicine

CSTs, whether used for the novel applications described earlier or to substitute traditional actigraphy, could fit seamlessly into a telemedicine program. The ownership of the CST by the patient, as opposed to the provider, allows for tracking of sleep patterns before a virtual sleep medicine visit. Therefore instead of retrospective estimates of sleep parameters by the patient at the point of care, a CST deemed acceptable for clinical use would allow the sleep provider to view weeks of sleep patterns before or during the first visit without an in-person exchange. This adjunct information could inform medical decision making at the initial encounter. Because clinical-grade actigraphy devices are unlikely to be provided to patients in advance of the initial visit, this workflow may reduce time to diagnosis of many nonsleep-disordered breathing conditions, which require longitudinal sleep monitoring to satisfy diagnostic criteria.[87]

CSTs may assist with monitoring and interventions between telemedicine visits. As discussed previously, CSTs have been used in conjunction with a CBT-I mobile app[77,78] and successfully integrated into a sleep extension protocol.[76] Innovative methods that use CSTs alongside behavioral therapy are highly complementary to care delivered via telemedicine and can be used when access to behavioral sleep medicine providers is limited. Independent from formal behavioral therapies, between-visit sleep tracking with

CSTs may allow patients to visualize improvement in sleep and motivate continued behavioral change and adherence to CPAP or other therapies. Conversely, deterioration in CST-derived sleep parameters, particularly when combined with worsened subjective symptoms, might indicate a need for a change in therapy (for example, adjustment of CPAP settings).

Additionally, the longitudinal acquisition of objective and subjective patient-generated data by CSTs could be leveraged in an asynchronous store-and-forward telehealth system to hasten the evaluation and treatment of suspected sleep disorders when a sleep provider is not locally available. The sleep specialist might review a collection of electronic health record information (demographics, comorbidities, medications) and patient-generated data derived from a CST (objectively tracked sleep parameters, respiratory information, self-report digital questionnaires, and even oropharyngeal imagery from the smartphone camera). Based on this information, recommendations regarding evaluation and treatment could be provided to the primary care physician.

REGULATION AND GUIDELINES

The devices discussed here fall under the designation of "wellness" products and do not have FDA clearance; therefore the AASM has recommended against the use of CSTs for the diagnosis or treatment of sleep disorders.[88] However, the distinction between diagnostic tools and wellness products may become increasingly more difficult, particularly now that many wrist-worn and finger-worn CSTs offer oximetry readings, as well as EKG (e.g., Apple Watch, circul+).

In response to the new regulatory challenges posed by rapidly evolving health technologies, the FDA set forth a Digital Health Innovation Action Plan that included a Software Precertification (Pre-cert) Pilot Program to regulate software as a medical device (SaMD). The FDA defines SaMD as "software intended to be used for one or more medical purposes that perform these purposes without being part of a hardware medical device."[89]

In addition to use with traditional medical platforms (e.g., a software program that augments a radiologist's interpretation), SaMD can run on commercial "off-the-shelf" platforms. Therefore if a CST manufacturer pursued FDA clearance, the SaMD Pre-cert program would provide the pipeline for approval. The SaMD Pre-cert Program plans to provide a precertified designation to manufacturers of software and digital health technologies that demonstrate a culture of quality and organizational excellence. Precertified manufacturers will be permitted to release SaMD into the market in an expedited manner after a streamlined review. Continued monitoring will determine the real-world safety, effectiveness, and performance of the approved SaMD. The nine companies selected for the SaMD Pre-cert Pilot Program include developers of CST (e.g., Fitbit), and therefore this program has future implications for the integration of CSTs into practice of a sleep.[89]

STANDARDS

Until recently, no standards existed for assessing CSTs regarding sleep. The Consumer Technology Association (CTA) partnered with the American National Standards Institute (ANSI) and the National Sleep Foundation (NSF) to create standards for terminology, methodology, and device performance evaluation. The resulting documents are publicly available online at https://webstore.ansi.org/sdo/CTA.[90-92]

As reviewed earlier, many published papers provide results from validation trials comparing sleep trackers with PSG. Many use the term *validation* in their title. It would be unfair to review them here for compliance with the ANSI/CTA requirements because many studies predate the existence of this standard. Others sleep tracker validation trials concern device capabilities not covered by the currently published recommendations (e.g., sleep-related breathing). Nonetheless, the ANSI/CTA standards reviewed in this chapter can provide the reader guidance for his or her critical assessment of the reported results.

This endeavor focused specifically on sleep and not sleep-related breathing. Other projects that consider breathing and snoring are near completion. The performance standards for evaluating snoring are not covered here. When finalized, those standards are expected to be published on the CTA and ANSI websites (https://webstore.ansi.org/sdo/CTA).

The performance standard described in detail in this chapter created a common yardstick and was divided into three parts. Part 1 covers definitions and characteristics for wearable sleep monitors to establish standard terminology. Part 2 provides guidance for developers and concerns extant methodology and measurement. Part 3 establishes performance criteria and testing protocols for sleep tracking consumer technology devices and applications. This final part is designed to inform developers, consumers, and any third-party contractors testing sleep-tracking devices.

Several overarching principles helped guide the standard's development. The first was to avoid ambiguity. The necessity for precise terminology became instantly clear right from the beginning. Many terms already have established definitions, and those should remain so. Other extant terms are ill defined, used loosely, and/or already have multiple definitions. A decision was made to avoid such terms when possible. Finally, in some instances, no current term exists. In such cases we created new terms and definitions.

Another guiding principle involved encouraging innovation and not stifling creativity. Although modern scientific human sleep research enjoys nearly a century of progress, there may be appropriate methods, techniques, biosensors, digital analysis, and/or approaches yet unthought of. The door must be left open for such welcome guests. Thus Part 2 (Methodology) may not be exhaustive. Other approaches are possible. This part of the standard was meant to inform developers about currently existing methods used to evaluate sleep.

PART 1: DEFINITIONS

Terminology Grouping

Terms fall into six possible categories according to this standard: (A) those describing a sleep episode's temporal surround, (B) those describing basic features of wakefulness and sleep, (C) those describing the relationship between basic sleep-wake measures and the temporal surround, (D) the terms defined in the AASM *Standardized Manual,* (E) alternative terms created to avoid creating ambiguity with existing polysomnographic nomenclature provided in the AASM

Standardized Manual,[93] and (F) those describing aspects of the circadian rhythms.

Category A includes terms describing a sleep episode's temporal surround. These are general terms related to the sleeper's (1) intention and their (2) position in the environment. Unlike during PSG, "time in bed" does not necessarily represent an individual's intention to sleep. In the sleep laboratory, the technician controls lights-off and lights-on, and these represent the temporal surround of the sleep study. In the real-world setting, bed sensors can accurately determine a person's time in bed, but many individuals spend a significant amount of time in bed with no intention to sleep (e.g., reading, watching television, using their smartphone). Knowing the beginning and ending time a person intends to sleep, analogous to time in bed in the laboratory setting, is a key measure for deriving parameters such as sleep efficiency and wake after sleep onset.

Category B consists of terms describing the sequence of sleep-wake events once there is an intention to sleep. Sleep is preceded by a period of wakefulness. Once sleep has commenced, awakenings can occur. A person may experience very brief wakefulness episodes surrounded by sleep. Some category B parameters have both general and laboratory definitions; however, terms such as wakefulness do not always require polysomnographic verification (e.g., "I think we can agree that I am awake while I am typing this document").

Category C parameters describe initial and final sleep occurrence relates to the overall sleep episode's surround. Once the initial and final sleep episode is determined, one may calculate several important metrics based on the relationship between these measures and the temporal surround. These include latency to sleep onset, latency to arising, and sleep efficiency.

Category D terms are those defined for use in sleep medicine by the AASM manual for the scoring of sleep and associated events: rules, terminology, and technical specifications.[1,2] This nomenclature is based on polysomnographic (EEG, electrooculogram, and electromyogram) correlates derived from normal human subjects. Essentially, these terms designate sleep stages, arousals, and their summary parameters.

Category E parameters provide alternative terminology recommended to avoid creating ambiguity by using existing polysomnographic nomenclature (provided in category D) when PSG is not being used. *Dream sleep* is a surrogate term used to describe the presumed underlying processes associated with REM sleep but are not based on polysomnographic criteria. During dream sleep, central nervous system and mental activation occur in a functionally paralyzed body. Indicators may include (but are not limited to) dreaming; increased HRV; increased pulse volume variability; increased blood pressure variability (but basal rate is lower than when awake); rapid eye movements; middle ear muscle activity; autonomic irregularities; sleep-related penile erections; uterine contractions; muscle atonia to the level of functional paralysis (however, there may be slight twitching at fingertips, facial muscles, and eyelids); loss of thermoregulation; memory encoding; and increased brain blood flow. *Core sleep* subsumes the majority of sleep time. Activity associated with midbrain activity manifests, and the sleeper is more easily awakened from the lighter parts of core sleep than from the sound sleep parts of core sleep. Core sleep includes sound sleep. *Sound sleep* is hypothesized to play a role in physical restoration, growth, muscle repair, and brain detoxification. Sound sleep is also associated with slow wave EEG activity, autonomic nervous system stability, and a high awakening threshold to environmental stimuli. *Restless sleep* is composed of sleep episodes associated with substantial movement activity, repeated brief awakenings, and/or awakenings. Exact criteria for the amount of restlessness are not yet established. If restless sleep is reported by a sleep tracker, the criteria used must be explicitly defined by the manufacturer.

Category F comprises terms used to describe the sleep-wake cycle over periods exceeding 7 days. This nomenclature was borrowed from circadian rhythm research and concords with current scientific usage.

Elemental and Derived Parameters

Each sleep parameter defined in the standard can be considered either elemental or derived. *Elemental parameters* are quantified directly from self-declaration, observation, or biometric measurement, for example, the time when an individual began attempting to sleep (TATS) and the initial sleep onset time (ISOT). These values cannot be derived from other measures. By contrast, *derived terms* are calculated from elemental measures (e.g., latency to sleep onset is the amount of time from TATS to ISOT). For each term (measure), the standard defines the general meaning, indicators (how it can be measured), the calculation formula (for derived parameters), and alternative definitions, if any, used in sleep research and/or sleep medicine. Table 206.2 shows the elemental and derived terms defined in the standard.

PART 2: METHODS

The standard's second document describes methods used to study human sleep. Measurement approaches are classified as direct (D), inferred (indirect) (I), and standard polysomnographic (S). Methods considered included self-report, observation, room and/or bed sensors, PSG, actigraphy, autonomic nervous system measurement, body temperature monitoring, and endocrinologic approaches. Autonomic nervous system techniques include monitoring heart rate, respiration, blood pressure, electrodermal activity, pulse volume, and pulse transit time. For each parameter defined in Part 1 of the standard, the measurement approach classification is designated for each method considered. For example, awakening from sleep could be ascertained directly using observation or a room or bed sensor (assuming they get out of bed and are not sleepwalking). Such awakenings could be inferred from actigraphic or autonomic nervous system measures or determined using standard polysomnographic recording. By contrast, REM sleep is defined according to polysomnographic recording criteria.

PART 3: PERFORMANCES STANDARD

Two levels of performance standard evaluation are detailed in Part 3. The first concerns sleep versus wake differentiation and is required. The second concerns classifying sleep stages, sleep subtypes using the newly created nomenclature, or a combination of both. Evaluating this second performance standard is optional but recommended. A particular device can comply with the first level or both, as the manufacturer chooses. However, particular reporting requirements are associated with each evaluation standard.

Level I: Essential Sleep-Wake Measures (Mandatory)

To comply with the performance evaluation standard, the following parameters must be evaluated: (1) time in bed (TIB)

Table 206.2 Elemental and Derived Terms in Each Grouping Defined in the Standard

	Terminology Category	Elemental Measure	Derived Measures
A	General terms describing the temporal surround of a sleep episode	Time when individual began **A**ttempting **T**o **S**leep (TATS): TATS start time TATS end time **T**ime **I**n **B**ed (TIB): TIB start time TIB end time	Total TATS duration Total TIB duration
B	General terms describing basic features of wakefulness and sleep	Awake Asleep Awakening from sleep Brief awakening Brief moment of sleep (dozing)	Total sleep period duration (TSPD) Total sleep time (TST) Sleep maintenance % Total wakefulness duration Wakefulness duration after initial sleep onset Number of awakenings Number of brief awakenings Awakening rate per hour Sleep fragmentation rate Number of dozing episodes
C	Terms derived from basic features of wakefulness, sleep as they relate to the sleep episode and its surround	Initial sleep onset time Final awakening time	Latency to sleep onset Latency to arising Sleep efficiency %
D	Specific terms describing processes occurring during sleep based on polysomnography	REM sleep N1 N2 N3 CNS arousal	Number of CNS arousals CNS arousal rate per hour Duration, percentage (of TST), and latency from sleep onset for each of the following: REM N1 N2 N3
E	Alternative terms for subdividing sleep into different processes	Dream sleep Core sleep Sound sleep Restless sleep	Duration and percentage for each of the following: Dream sleep Core sleep Sound sleep Restless sleep % of TST
F	Terms used to describe the sleep-wake cycle over time periods exceeding 7 days	Circadian amplitude Circadian period length (tau) Circadian phase	Relative duration of the active period compared with the dormant period

start and end time or TATS start and end time, (2) minutes awake and asleep, and (3) the number of awakenings from sleep. To accomplish this, the sleep tracker must first classify each epoch as sleep or awake. Four statistics are required to evaluate sleep versus wakefulness delineation as part of the performance evaluation: overall accuracy, sensitivity, specificity, and Cohen's kappa. Accuracy (ACC) is the sum of properly classified sleep epochs and properly classified wake epochs divided by the total number of epochs tested. ACC is not sufficient by itself to meet the performance evaluation standard because it can be misleading, in that data collected at night are likely to be dominated by sleep and not wakefulness. For this reason, sensitivity (true-positive rate) and specificity (1 – false-positive rate) must also be reported. For inferential purposes, Cohen's kappa evaluates interdevice agreement and accounts for chance agreement.

Level II: Essential Sleep Staging Measures (Optional)

To meet the Level II performance standard, the device must be evaluated to determine how well it differentiates wakefulness and the other sleep subtypes. The other possible sleep subtypes are listed here:

a. REM sleep and light sleep (combined N1 and N2 sleep) and N3 sleep, or
b. REM sleep and (combined N1 and N2 sleep) and sound sleep, or
c. REM sleep and (core minus sound sleep) and sound sleep, or
d. REM and (core minus sound sleep) and N3 sleep, or
e. Dream sleep and (combined N1 and N2 sleep) and N3 sleep, or
f. Dream sleep and (combined N1 and N2 sleep) and sound sleep, or

Table 206.3 Sample Four-Way Comparison Table for Testing Sleep Staging[a]

		Tested Device (TD)			
		Wake	REM Sleep	Light Sleep	N3 Sleep
Standard (S)	Wake	M_{00}	M_{01}	M_{02}	M_{03}
	REM Sleep	M_{10}	M_{11}	M_{12}	M_{13}
	Light Sleep	M_{20}	M_{21}	M_{22}	M_{23}
	N3 Sleep	M_{30}	M_{31}	M_{32}	M_{33}

[a]The first step is to tabulate epoch × epoch concordance between the tested device (TD) and the standard against which it is being compared (S). For example, in the table, M13 is the total number of episodes S scored as REM sleep and TD scored as N3 sleep.

g. Dream sleep and (core minus sound sleep) and sound sleep, or

h. Dream sleep and (core minus sound sleep) and N3 sleep.

Each test recording is divided into 30-second blocks (epochs). Each of these epochs must then be classified as either wake, REM sleep, light sleep, or N3 (schema a) or any of the other schemas (b–h). Table 206.3 shows a sample four-way comparison.

Although a four-class comparison permits a variety of statistics, a device tested against this part of the performance standard must report accuracy calculated according to the following formula (i.e., the sum of diagonal elements in Table 206.3 divided by the total number of epochs compared (M):

$$ACC = \frac{1}{M}\sum_{c=0}^{3} M_{cc}$$

where M_{cc} is the value along the diagonal corresponding to class c.

Performance Evaluation Sample

A minimum of 32 subjects must be included (larger samples are encouraged). The following distributions are required: a 1:1 male:female ratio and eight or more young adults (18–25 years old), adults (26–64 years old), and older adults (65 years or older). Subjects used in the primary evaluation sample should be healthy and free of treated or untreated sleep, medical, neurologic, or psychiatric disorders. Total nightly bed time must be 420 minutes or more per night. Multiple night recording is encouraged but not required. Evaluations should be conducted in a private, darkened, sound-attenuated sleep laboratory or a specially equipped bedroom. Test rooms should have two-way intercoms and allow for video recording in total darkness.

Performance Evaluation Reporting

The performance evaluation report must include the following details about the sleep tracker: the model number, update/revision number (if applicable), firmware version number (if applicable), location and/or position of the sleep tracker during testing (e.g., at bedside, embedded in mattress, wirelessly attached to subject's neck), and inclusion/exclusion criteria used for subject selection. The test sample must be described, including number of subjects, their sexes, ages, and health statuses. Equipment used, testing environment, data sampling rate, and statistical analysis must be thoroughly described.

SUMMARY

Consumer sleep technologies are used on a massive scale and include wearable and nearable devices and mobile apps without sensors outside of the device the app is installed on. The longitudinal sleep estimates from consumer sleep trackers may have utility for clinical sleep medicine and research. Additionally, novel features such as inclusion of multiple sensors, long-term use patterns, data collection from the sleep environment, and ability to interface with other devices and apps that track health metrics confer vast opportunities to understand sleep disorders and the role of sleep in health and disease. The apps associated with consumer sleep trackers are well suited to deliver behavioral interventions and have the potential to provide more personalized therapy. Limitations include lack of transparency in the acquisition and analysis of data and minimal performance verification. Until recently, no performance evaluation standards existed.

The CTA partnered with the ANSI and the NSF to create standards for terminology, methodology, and device performance evaluation. The derived standard considers (A) metrics describing a sleep episode's temporal surround, (B) terms describing basic features of wakefulness and sleep, (C) parameters concerning the relationship between basic sleep-wake measures and the temporal surround, (D) terminology used in sleep medicine and previously defined in the AASM *Standardized Manual,* (E) alternative terms to describe different underlying sleep subtypes, and (F) metrics used primarily in circadian rhythm research. This chapter describes CTA/ANSI/NSF certification metrics; performance evaluation study design; statistical analysis; and reporting requirements for wearable, bed integrated, and in-bedroom sleep tracking devices.

CLINICAL PEARLS

Very few consumer sleep technologies have been rigorously evaluated in patients with sleep pathologies. Clinicians should be aware that devices with oximeters may be prone to report false high values, especially in patients with dark pigmentation. At this time, important clinical interventions should not be made based on consumer devices alone.

SELECTED READINGS

de Zambotti M, Cellini N, Menghini L, et al. Sensors capabilities, performance, and use of consumer sleep technology. *Sleep Med Clin.* 2020;15(1):1–30. https://doi.org/10.1016/j.jsmc.2019.11.003.

Depner CM, Cheng PC, Devine JK, et al. Wearable technologies for developing sleep and circadian biomarkers: a summary of workshop discussions. *Sleep.* 2020;43(2):zsz254. https://doi.org/10.1093/sleep/zsz254.

Goldstein C. Current and future roles of consumer sleep technologies in sleep medicine. *Sleep Med Clin.* 2020;15(3):391–408. https://doi.org/10.1016/j.jsmc.2020.05.001.

Hamill K, Jumabhoy R, Kahawage P, et al. Validity, potential clinical utility and comparison of a consumer activity tracker and a research-grade activity tracker in insomnia disorder II: outside the laboratory. *J Sleep Res.* 2020;29(1):e12944. https://doi.org/10.1111/jsr.12944.

Kahawage P, Jumabhoy R, Hamill K, et al. Validity, potential clinical utility, and comparison of consumer and research-grade activity trackers in Insomnia Disorder I: In-lab validation against polysomnography. *J Sleep Res.* 2020;29(1):e12931. https://doi.org/10.1111/jsr.12931.

Rentz LE, Ulman HK, Galster SM. Deconstructing commercial wearable technology: contributions toward accurate and free-living monitoring of sleep. *Sensors (Basel).* 2021;21(15):5071.

A complete reference list can be found online at ExpertConsult.com.

Chapter 207

Evaluating Sleepiness and Fatigue

Amir Sharafkhaneh; Max Hirshkowitz

Chapter Highlights

- Evaluating sleepiness and fatigue presents a difficult task for clinicians. On one level, sleepiness and fatigue are introspectively judged sensations. However, clinical assessment must consider physiologic sleep pressure and behavioral consequences of sleepiness and fatigue.
- Methods used to assess introspective, physiologic, and manifest sleepiness are described.
- General concepts concerning sleepiness and fatigue are reviewed.
- We discuss some practical issues involved when evaluating sleepiness and fatigue in regulatory, legal, or adjudication arenas.

INTRODUCTION

Sleepiness is a sensation. Much like hunger and thirst, sleepiness occurs naturally as a physiologic drive informing one's behavioral system about a presumed biologic need. In most humans, sleepiness naturally occurs at night, after prolonged wakefulness (sleep deprivation), or in response to rapid translocation across time zones. However, sleepiness can also arise from medical, neurologic, or psychiatric disorders. Many drugs provoke sleepiness, either by stimulating sleep-inducing mechanisms or by inhibiting wake-promoting brain centers.

Sleepiness represents the composite output of two distinct neurologic systems, one that promotes wakefulness and the other generating sleep. Thus sleepiness reflects a dynamic balance between systems with opposing functions. When an increased physiologic drive to sleep begins to overwhelm the alerting system's ability to stave off that drive, sleepiness becomes excessive and possibly irresistible. However, individuals in this condition may not accurately sense their own level of sleepiness and not realize sleep onset is imminent.

Sleepiness and fatigue, when excessive, pose serious potential hazards. The consequent danger affects not only the drowsy individual but possibly also the person's family, coworkers, and surrounding society. Severe drowsiness while performing a dangerous task (e.g., driving) constitutes a potentially life-threatening condition. When sleepiness surpasses a person's ability to maintain vigilance, it will produce response slowing, response lapsing, and possibly a transition into sleep. This level of drowsiness constitutes ***dangerous sleepiness.***

Fatigue is both a sensation (i.e., a feeling) and a factor underlying behavioral impairment. Fatigue takes various forms, including but not limited to muscle, physical, and mental fatigue. A person afflicted with fatigue generally feels a lack of energy and/or motivation. The sensation is somewhat different from isolated sleepiness (which is the desire to sleep); however, fatigue and sleepiness often occur together. Medically, fatigue is a nonspecific symptom and has many potential causes. We typically operationalize fatigue in terms of performance failure. We characterize and assess human fatigue with metrics such as slowing in the speed of responding, failure to respond (lapsing), overall performance decrement, performance errors, and fatigue-related near-misses or actual accidents. Time on task represents a key parameter in both sleepiness and fatigue assessment. The latency from the beginning of a task until performance degradation helps index fatigue severity.[1,2]

From the standpoint of muscle physiology, fatigue is considered weakness (or weariness) produced by repeated exertion or decreased cellular, tissue, or organ response after excessive stimulation (or activity). Normally, function recovers after rest. Stressors promote fatigue. In nonpathologic mental fatigue, sleepiness is usually the primary stressor. Many forms of fatigue include both a physical and mental component. Therefore it is understandable why fatigue and sleepiness are so often equated.

Figure 207.1 illustrates the normal pattern of alertness and fatigue in a healthy, well-rested individual over the course of a week-long period. The figure shows the varying degree of sleepiness and fatigue as the week progresses. The caution threshold indicates a point at which there is an increasing risk for performance failure. The caution threshold height can vary somewhat between individuals; however, every person has a limit. Although the actual limit is usually unknown, one should err on the side of caution. The daytime-nighttime cycle is shown at the bottom of each curve for general reference. It can be seen in the illustration that a healthy, well-rested, night-sleeping individual should remain well under the caution threshold throughout the week.

Figure 207.2 illustrates the expected pattern of fatigue provoked by a night of total or severe sleep deprivation. The graph shows the fatigue level in relationship to the caution threshold. In this illustration, the individual underwent severe sleep deprivation on night 4. Note that some recovery occurred largely as a function of circadian factors; however, alertness did not recover sufficiently. Furthermore, as

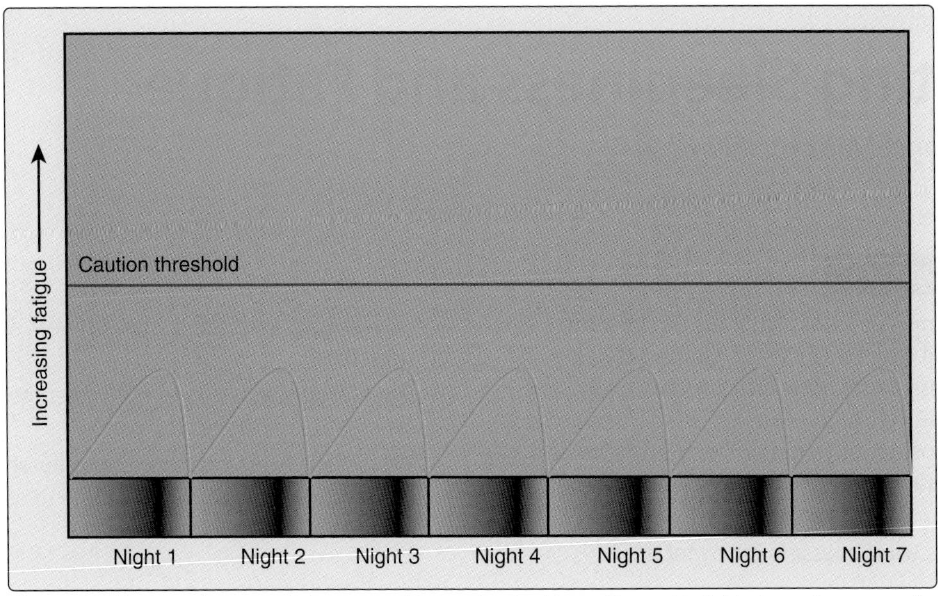

Figure 207.1 Normal pattern of alertness and fatigue in a healthy, well-rested individual over the course of a week-long period. The aqua line represents the level of sleepiness. The caution threshold indicates a point, which will vary between individuals, at which there is an increasing risk for performance failure. The daytime-nighttime cycle is shown at the bottom of each curve. Without sleep deprivation, a healthy individual should remain well under the caution threshold throughout the week.

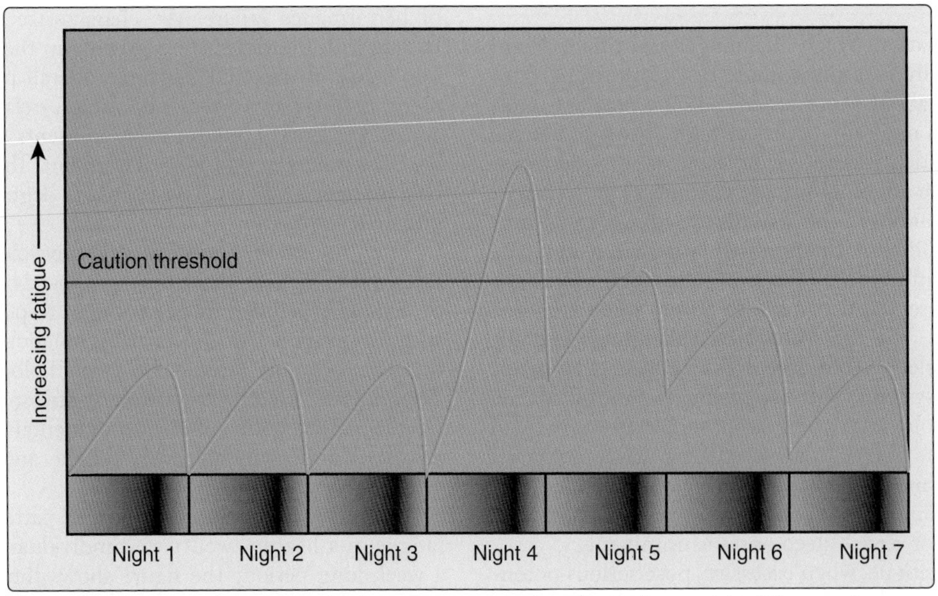

Figure 207.2 Pattern of alertness and fatigue after complete sleep deprivation on night 4. The aqua line represents the level of sleepiness. The caution threshold indicates a point, which will vary between individuals, at which there is an increasing risk for performance failure. The daytime-nighttime cycle is shown at the bottom of each curve. Although performance impairment is greatest during the biologic night at the time of sleep deprivation, recovery to baseline takes several days.

evening approached on the subsequent day, the individual was already at or approaching the caution threshold. Furthermore, recovery required several days before it reached baseline levels. Although there is some degree of individual difference between the effects of sleep loss on performance, this model provides guidance. Exceeding the caution threshold must be considered within the context of the activity performed and that activity's potential danger to self and others. A fatigued commercial airline pilot poses greater hazard than an office worker. This is in contrast with chronic sleep deprivation, which may cause fatigue long term. Chronic sleep deprivation is very common and leads to poor health, lower productivity, and impaired quality of life.

Figure 207.3 illustrates the fatigue pattern associated with 3 successive nights of partial sleep deprivation. Partial sleep deprivation is considered when an individual gets less than the recommended sleep duration. For example, health care providers in many large cities around the world were exposed to work-related sleep deprivation for several nights or even longer periods because of the COVID-19 pandemic. Fatigue, in addition to other symptoms, was reported in these individuals.[3]

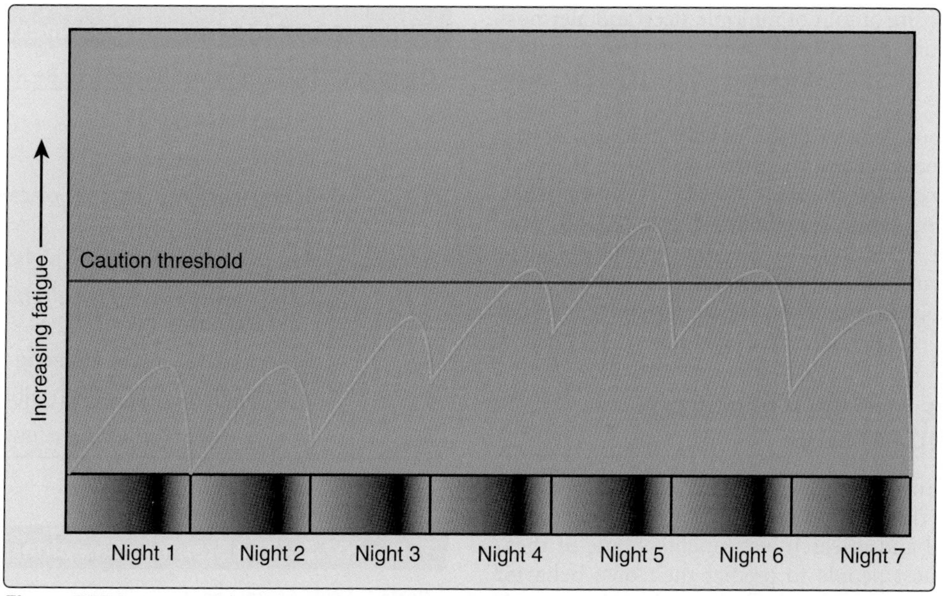

Figure 207.3 Pattern of alertness and fatigue after partial sleep deprivation on 3 successive nights. The aqua line represents the level of sleepiness. The caution threshold indicates a point, which will vary between individuals, at which there is an increasing risk for performance failure. The daytime-nighttime cycle is shown at the bottom of each curve. Performance impairment becomes progressively worse over the period of chronic sleep restriction.

This chapter focuses on clinical assessment. Consequently, three measurement issues merit special attention. The first issue involves problems associated with self-report; the second concerns the need for normative-adjusted measures; and the third is related to whether a particular measurement is appropriate given the circumstance.

In standard clinical practice, patients typically seek help. They have a problem, symptom, or impairment. During the clinical encounter, the patient provides information with self-interest to maintain or improve health. In stark contrast, when an individual needs evaluation for regulatory purposes, things dramatically change. Some individuals stoically minimize their symptoms, while others tend to exaggerate. Both primary and/or secondary gain may modify symptom self-disclosure (e.g., denying sleepiness to avoid losing a motor vehicle license). To make assessment even more difficult, sleepiness itself can blunt one's own awareness of sleepiness.

Sleepiness and fatigue assessment can be difficult. Few objective, quantitative indices exist to provide guidance. Assessments conducted for regulatory purposes or compensation are further complicated by each situation's demand characteristics, the individual's agenda, or both. During a "fit for duty" evaluation, the person undergoing testing usually has a stake in the outcome. A desire to return to work may result in minimizing or denying drowsiness, sleepiness, and/or fatigue. This holds even more true if the evaluation occurs in the wake of an accident or error. By contrast, individuals seeking compensation may exaggerate their problems. In these cases, self-reported information may be biased. Additionally, any tests demanding cooperation to achieve valid results require careful scrutiny. For example, performance tests usually require "best effort." However, a person seeking compensation may not try as hard on the test in the effort to appear more impaired. The opposite agenda, that is, to appear less impaired on a sleep propensity test, can also be strategically accomplished. For example, sleep propensity measured with nap testing instructs an individual to "relax and allow yourself to fall asleep." Such instructions can be easily ignored if the individuals' intentions are to prove they are not sleepy by remaining awake.

Useful clinical measures usually require standardization to facilitate comparison with normative values. Unfortunately, many sleepiness measures, and to some degree fatigue measures, can reliably detect changes within an individual in before-and-after experimental designs but not the differences between individuals. Consequently, although a measure can provide a superb metric for assessing change, it may fail miserably for determining whether the patient in your office is sleepy.

The third measurement issue involves metric validation. The commonly used term "excessive daytime sleepiness" underscores this point. Normative values for most sleepiness metrics rely mainly on data collected during the day. When clinical necessity requires nighttime assessment (e.g., in shift workers), the choices of validated instruments are limited. In other words, how sleepy must one be for sleepiness to be considered abnormal at 4:00 a.m.? Or to be considered excessive at 4:00 a.m.? Or be considered dangerous at 4:00 a.m.? Although answers to these three questions may not differ at noon, they would likely differ at 4:00 a.m.

Carskadon and Dement[2] proposed a useful conceptualization for characterizing sleepiness. They considered sleepiness along three dimensions: introspective, physiologic, and manifest. Introspective sleepiness (when unbiased by a person's motives) derives from individuals' self-reported assessment of their internal state. Physiologic sleepiness refers to the underlying biologic drive to sleep, indexed by the speed with which a person falls asleep. Manifest sleepiness includes behavioral signs of sleepiness, inability to volitionally remain awake, and performance deficit on psychomotor or cognitive tasks. In theory, manifest sleepiness occurs when sleep drive overwhelms the system that maintains wakefulness.

The Carskadon-Dement model provides an organizational device for understanding differences between sleepiness measures. If sleepiness were a single measurable core phenomenon, rather than a composite output of multiple sleep and alertness mechanisms, one may expect equivalence between measures. However, different tests for sleepiness often produce varying results because they index different (although related) phenomena. The best concordance usually emerges at the sleepiness-wakefulness spectrum's extremes. That is, when all sleepiness dimensions are at nadir (no sleepiness) or when sleepiness reaches its zenith (maximum sleepiness), all measures usually agree. Thus most of the time it is illogical to use physiologic, manifest, and introspective sleepiness measures interchangeably; it also misses the important differences between them.

INTROSPECTIVE AND SELF-REPORTED SLEEPINESS AND FATIGUE

Introspective sleepiness is measured using self-administered questionnaires. In this section we describe the most commonly used clinical and research instruments. Some of these questionnaires request people to predict their own behavior (e.g., How likely are you to doze off when…?) or judge their feelings over some time interval in the recent past (e.g., in the past month). By contrast, other instruments involve momentary assessment and ask individuals about how they feel right now. In general, questionnaires evaluating longer time domains (e.g., in the past month) are more useful clinically than those using momentary assessment. By contrast, momentary assessment instruments tend to have greater precision and are more sensitive to fluctuations in alertness. This makes them more useful for investigating circadian oscillation, disease-related somnolence, and drug-induced alterations in sleepiness.

Ultimately, introspective sleepiness relies on self-report. In one respect, self-report constitutes the only way one can possibly know how another person feels. However, self-disclosed information is modified by one's ability to recognize internal states, one's memory, one's tendency to minimize or exaggerate their experience, and any underlying bias.

Epworth Sleepiness Scale

The Epworth Sleepiness Scale (ESS) is the most widely used clinical instrument for evaluating sleepiness. This specialized, validated, eight-item, pencil-and-paper instrument was developed by Murray Johns at the Epworth Hospital in Melbourne, Australia.[4] The ESS questions individuals about their expectation of "dozing" in differing circumstances. Dozing probability is designated as none (0), slight (1), moderate (2), or high (3) for eight hypothetical situations shown in Table 207.1.

Table 207.1 The Epworth Sleepiness Scale Items

Question	Hypothetical Situation to Be Rated
1	Sitting and reading
2	Watching television
3	Sitting inactive in a public place (e.g., a theater or a meeting)
4	As a passenger in a car for an hour without a break
5	Lying down to rest in the afternoon when circumstances permit
6	Sitting and talking to someone
7	Sitting quietly after a lunch without alcohol
8	In a car, while stopped for a few minutes in traffic

The ESS's popularity stems in part from its simplicity, brevity, and validation.[5,6] Research revealed that control subjects had a mean score of 7.6 and patients with sleep apnea had a mean score of 14.3 at baseline. After treatment, patients with sleep apnea scores declined to 7.4. In another study, normative values were gathered from 942 patients waiting at outpatient clinics (e.g., dermatology, audiology, and ophthalmology clinics) and 1120 healthy people attending health fairs or community health lectures. The mean ESS total score for these two groups were 8.1 and 5.2, respectively.[7] Based on this study and subsequent work in our clinic, we categorize ESS scores ranging from 0 to 8 as normal, 9 to 12 as mild, 13 to 16 as moderate, and greater than 16 (double that of high normal) as severe.

The ESS differs from other tests in that respondents are not asked about how they feel but rather to make a probability judgment about their own behavior. Thus the ESS asks individuals to rate their own sleep drive; this may help explain why the ESS correlates (albeit weakly) with the Multiple Sleep Latency Test (MSLT) results (an objective index of sleep drive). The ESS's main disadvantage is its questionable utility when it is readministered after only a brief time interval.

Table 207.2 The Stanford Sleepiness Scale Items

Code	Scale Statements
1	Feeling active and vital, alert, wide awake
2	Functioning at a high level, but not at peak, able to concentrate
3	Relaxed, awake, not at full alertness, responsive
4	A little foggy, not at peak, let down
5	Foggy, beginning to lose interest in remaining awake, slowed down
6	Sleepy, prefer to be lying down, fighting sleep, woozy
7	Almost in reverie, sleep onset soon, lost struggle to remain awake

Stanford Sleepiness Scale and Karolinska Sleepiness Scale

For many years, the Stanford Sleepiness Scale (SSS) served as the standard measure of introspective sleepiness. The SSS asks people to choose one of seven statements to describe their self-assessed current state (choices are shown in Table 207.2). The SSS is a momentary assessment scale and can detect sleepiness as it waxes and wanes over the course of a day. Advantages include its brevity, its ease of administration, and its ability to be administered repeatedly. Experimentally induced sleep deprivation increases SSS scores; however, normative data do not exist, making it difficult to use for clinical decision making or comparisons between persons.

The Karolinska Sleepiness Scale (KSS) is similar to the SSS and consists of a 9-point scale ranging from 1, "very alert," to 9, "very sleepy, great effort to stay awake or fighting sleep." Scores of 7 or above are considered pathologic. The KSS has become increasingly popular for evaluating sleepiness in drug trials, flight crews, oil-rig workers, train engineers, and professional drivers. Its brevity, validation against EEG, and behavioral parameters,[8] and its now-proven sensitivity to sleepiness put KSS on equal footing with the SSS.

Sleepiness-Wakefulness Inability and Fatigue Test

The Sleepiness-Wakefulness Inability and Fatigue Test (SWIFT)[9] is a 12-item self-administered questionnaire validated against the ESS in normal subjects, patients with sleep-disordered breathing, and patients with narcolepsy.[9] The test asks how much of a problem individuals have staying awake or how much of a problem they have with fatigue, tiredness, or lack of energy (not at all, just a little, pretty much, very much). Six items focus on sleepiness (generally during the day, while driving, while stopped at traffic light, while at work or while doing tasks, while reading, in social situations) and six on fatigue (generally during the day, while driving, while at work or doing tasks, while reading or studying, in social situations, and when doing tasks that are not urgent). A validation study found good internal consistency (0.87), retest reliability (0.82), and criterion group differentiation (controls versus patients with sleep disorder).[9] The SWIFT shows great promise, but clinical use would benefit from normative values establishment and further validation.

Pictorial Sleepiness Scale

Maldonado and colleagues[10] developed a nonverbal sleepiness scale, the Pictorial Sleepiness Scale, for testing young children and poorly educated adults. They had subjects rank order seven cartoon faces depicting sleepiness. Rankings were transformed to approximate linearity, and two cartoons were eliminated. The resulting five-picture scale was re-ranked by a different group of subjects to verify order for a final scale. Finally, a validation test indicated significant correlation with KSS and SSS using a mix of normal adults, patients with sleep apnea, shift workers, and school children. Whether this scale will gain popularity remains to be seen.

Observation and Interview-Based Diurnal Sleepiness Inventory

The Observation and Interview-Based Diurnal Sleepiness Inventory (ODSI) is a three-item questionnaire that is administered by a health care provider.[11] Each of the three items has a 7-point Likert scale. The total score can range from 0 to 24. The tool assesses the sleepiness in active situations and passive situations and estimates the average total sleep times. The active situation receives higher score, with 0 indicating "not at all," and 12 as "very frequently" out of the total score of 24. The passive situation receives a score of 0 to 6. The average sleep time receives scores of 0 (less than an hour of sleep) to a maximum of 6 for 6 or more hours of sleep. This tool is well validated among elderly and is easy to administer.[12] This tool also has been studied in patients with narcolepsy and idiopathic hypersomnia[13] but is not in widespread use.

Profile of Mood States

Although principally designed to assess mood, the Profile of Mood States (POMS) has often been used in sleep research.[14] Originally, the POMS was intended to include a dimension for sleepiness; however, the "sleepiness" proved to be nonindependent and was therefore eliminated. The "sleepiness" items loaded on the Fatigue, Confusion, and Vigor (negatively) scales. To a lesser extent, sleepiness also emerged on Depression and Anger scales. The Confusion scale elevates more in response to severe sleepiness, and the Vigor scale appears sensitive to partial sleep deprivation.[15] Thus, early on, psychometricians found sleepiness to be a composite measure; a measurement difficulty that persists because some researchers heedlessly view sleepiness as a unitary factor.

Fatigue Assessment Scale

The Fatigue Assessment Scale (FAS) is an easy-to-administer and practical self-report questionnaire that is validated in several diseases (Table 207.3).[16] Although most of the other fatigue scales were developed in diseased populations, FAS was developed in a general working sample of population. The FAS has 10 fatigue items divided equally between physical and mental fatigue. Each scale can be from 1 (never) to 5 (always). Thus the score can vary from 10 to maximum of 50, with higher numbers indicating more fatigue.[17] The FAS has good reliability and validity and no sex bias, and it is unidimensional. The FAS is useful as both a baseline and follow-up measure.

PHYSIOLOGIC SLEEPINESS

Multiple Sleep Latency Test

The feeling we refer to as "sleepiness" can be conceptualized as arising from a physiologic drive. One could therefore use the rapidity with which a person falls asleep to represent the drive's intensity. This relationship between sleepiness and sleep onset provides the foundation for the MSLT.[18] The MSLT provides nap opportunities across the day and indexes physiologic sleep drive with mean sleep latencies. Sleep deprivation hastens sleep onset (decreases sleep latency) when the opportunity arises to sleep. In a series of elegant studies, increased sleep drive provoked by aging, total sleep deprivation, partial sleep deprivation, and disorders of excessive somnolence were well characterized by MSLT sleep latency.[19-21] Data relating homeostatic influences and sleepiness derive directly from MSLT studies.[22] Circadian influence also manifests as shorter MSLT latencies on midafternoon test sessions.

Methodology

The MSLT provides a widely used technique to scientifically assess physiologic sleep drive. In its traditional form, the MSLT involves a series of nap opportunities (four to six) presented at 2-hour intervals beginning approximately 2 hours after initial (morning) awakening.[23] To appreciate the prior night's sleep quantity and quality, the patient undergoes attended laboratory polysomnography the night before testing. A careful history of sleep habits, schedule, and drug use in the past month is essential (a sleep diary, ideally along with actigraphy, should be obtained for at least 2 weeks before testing). A clinical MSLT should not be conducted during drug withdrawal (especially from stimulants or from medications that suppress rapid eye movement [REM] sleep), while sedating medications are pharmacologically active, or after a night of profoundly disturbed sleep.

Persons undergoing an MSLT are instructed to "allow themselves to fall asleep" or to "not to resist falling asleep." Subjects are tested under standardized conditions in their street clothes and must not remain in bed between nap test sessions. Similarly, subjects should not engage in vigorous activity before nap opportunities because this can alter test results.[24]

Table 207.3 Fatigue Assessment Scale[52]

Question		Never (1)	Sometimes (2)	Regularly (3)	Often (4)	Always (5)
1	I am bothered by fatigue.					
2	I get tired very quickly.					
3	I don't do much during the day.					
4	I have enough energy for everyday life.					
5	Physically, I feel exhausted.					
6	I have problems starting things.					
7	I have problems thinking clearly.					
8	I feel no desire to do anything.					
9	Mentally, I feel exhausted.					
10	When I am doing something, I can concentrate quite well.					

From Shahid A, Wilkinson K, Marcu S, Shapiro CM. Fatigue Assessment Scale (FAS). In: Shahid A, Wilkinson K, Marcu S, Shapiro CM, eds. *STOP, THAT and One Hundred Other Sleep Scales*. New York: Springer New York; 2012:161–62.

Obtaining reliable results depends critically on using standardized test conditions and techniques.[25] Sleep rooms must be dark and quiet during testing. Electroencephalographic (EEG; central and occipital), electrooculographic (EOG; left and right eye), and electromyographic (EMG; submentalis) recordings are used to recognize sleep onset and distinguish between sleep stages. MSLT guidelines also call for use of home positive airway pressure (PAP) settings and mask, or alternative devices to treat obstructive sleep apnea (e.g., oral appliance) in patients known to have sleep-disordered breathing (Box 207.1).

Two protocols exist for conducting the MSLT: one designed for research and the other for clinical assessment. The research protocol minimizes accumulated sleep by awakening the person when unequivocal sleep onset occurs. To meet criteria for unequivocal sleep, one of the following must occur: (1) three consecutive 30-second epochs of stage N1 sleep or (2) a single 30-second epoch of stage N2, N3, or R (REM) sleep. By contrast, the clinical MSLT protocol continues for 15 minutes after sleep onset (defined by a single 30-second epoch of any sleep stage) occurs.

The clinical MSLT attempts not only to index sleep drive but also to detect abnormally increased REM sleep tendency. Increased REM sleep tendency characterizes narcolepsy and therefore the added sleep time provides diagnostic information. Short sleep latency and REM appearing on two or more MSLT naps (or one MSLT nap if sleep-onset rapid eye movement is detected on the polysomnogram during the prior night) objectively confirms the diagnosis of narcolepsy; however, test-retest reliability is superior in patients with narcolepsy, type I (with cataplexy) compared with narcolepsy, type II. Table 207.4 displays MSLT results in patients with narcolepsy as compared with control subjects.

In both the research and clinical versions, the test session is terminated after 20 minutes if no sleep onset occurs. Sleep latency is defined as the elapsed time from the start of the test to the first 30-second epoch scored as sleep. Sleep latency in normal adult control subjects ranges from 10 to 20 minutes. Historically, clinicians classified mean sleep latency on the MSLT of 5 minutes or less as pathologic sleepiness,[19] although current diagnostic guidelines dichotomize pathologic excessive daytime sleepiness at 8 minutes. More information regarding the clinical interpretation of MSLT results can be found in Chapter 68.

BOX 207.1 MULTIPLE SLEEP LATENCY TEST RECORDING MONTAGE: PHYSIOLOGIC ACTIVITY RECORDED

Left or right frontal EEG (F3 or F4)
Left or right central EEG (C3 or C4)
Left or right occipital EEG (O1 or O2)
Left horizontal or oblique EOG
Right horizontal or oblique EOG
Vertical EOG
Submentalis (chin) EMG
Electrocardiogram

EEG, Electroencephalogram; EMG, electromyogram; EOG, electrooculogram.

Table 207.4 Multiple Sleep Latency Test Results

Parameter	Patients with Narcolepsy	Control Subjects
N (male/female)	57 (33/24)	17 (6/11)
Age (SD) in years	43.3 (12.3)	33.4 (9.9)
Percent who slept	99.0	63.5
Sleep latency mean (SD)	3.0 (2.7)	13.4 (4.0)
Minimum	0.6	4.8
Maximum	14.1	20
REM Score	3.5	0

REM, Rapid eye movement; SD, standard deviation.

Utility

The MSLT can objectively document treatment response[26] and residual physiologic sleep drive[25] in patients independent of whether they self-report sleepiness after treatment. MSLT's sensitivity to physiologic sleepiness makes it especially useful for detecting persistent sleepiness in patients with undiagnosed comorbid sleep disorders, ineffective treatment, poor adherence to a therapeutic regimen, or concomitant soporific medication.

As a technique to demonstrate a person's underlying sleepiness, the MSLT has the advantage of being a direct, objective, quantitative approach. It is generally thought that, under normal circumstances, nonsleepy individuals cannot make themselves fall asleep. By contrast, a sleepy person (if not overwhelmingly sleepy) potentially can remain awake. Thus false-positive tests (MSLT indicating sleepiness when the person is not sleepy) are theoretically minimal, with the exception of when a comorbid circadian rhythm sleep-wake disorder is present (i.e., shift work disorder). Polysomnography should be used to document the prior night's sleep quality and quantity. If significant sleep disruption or disturbance occurs, the MSLT should be rescheduled. Drug screening helps rule out pharmacologically induced sleepiness. The availability of a specific numerical criterion for characterizing pathologic sleepiness made the MSLT the standard technique for assessing sleepiness for many years.

Clinical Standards of Practice

In 2005 the American Academy of Sleep Medicine (AASM) published revised clinical practice parameters for the MSLT's clinical use.[27] Clinical standards, guidelines, and options were derived from a comprehensive evidence-based medicine review and a systematic protocol for expert consensus.[28] The conclusions can be summarized as follows. The MSLT:

- Is indicated as part of the clinical evaluation for patients with suspected narcolepsy
- May be helpful for clinical assessment of patients with suspected idiopathic hypersomnia
- Is not indicated for routine evaluation of obstructive sleep apnea
- Is not indicated for routine reevaluation of patients with sleep apnea treated with positive airway pressure therapy
- Is not indicated for routine clinical assessment of insomnia, circadian rhythm disorders, or dyssomnia associated with medical, psychiatric, or neurologic disorders (other than narcolepsy and idiopathic hypersomnia)

The most recent updates to the 2005 guidelines in 2021 did not change indications for MSLT use, but provided guidance regarding patient preparation (including PAP or other obstructive sleep apnea treatment use, medication and substance concerns, and sleep prior to testing), test scheduling and conditions, and appropriate documentation.[27a]

Other Measures of Physiologic Sleepiness

Pupillography

Pupil stability and size are affected by exposure to light and by a person's nervous system arousal level. In a darkened room, the pupil dilates to improve vision by widening the aperture and allowing more light to enter the eye. However, if the person begins to fall asleep, parasympathetic activation constricts pupillary diameter. Sleepiness also provokes pupil size instability and alters the magnitude and speed of papillary constriction in response to a flash of light. These alterations reflect the autonomic nervous system balance changes associated with sleep and wakefulness.

Several researchers used pupillography to measure sleep tendency and evaluate narcolepsy.[25] Advanced mathematical techniques provide within-subject differentiation of sleepiness compared to alertness using the Spectral F-Test.[29] Although pupillography would seem an attractive approach to objectively measure sleep drive, several barriers continue to impede its clinical utility. First, it is not an easily mastered procedure. Second, it remains difficult to compare one patient to another and designate a clinical numeric threshold for sleepiness. Finally, normative data are not currently available.

Electroencephalography

Quantitative digital EEG analyses seem an obvious approach for assessing central nervous system arousal level. In essence, the MSLT uses EEG recordings (in conjunction with EOG and EMG recordings) to quantify sleep onset from which sleep drive is deduced. It would therefore seem reasonable to expect subtle EEG waveform patterns (microarchitecture) to characterize physiologic sleepiness. Just before sleep onset, alpha frequency decreases and its amplitude increases. Additionally, it has long been thought that EEG delta activity may index sleepiness because it increases in response to experimental sleep deprivation.[30] Fatigue-related differences, especially in alpha and theta EEG bandwidths, are reported.[31] Some researchers believe the EEG cipher lies not in examining resting EEG spectral content but rather EEG responsiveness to sensory input. If sleepiness alters neurologic reactivity, ongoing task-related EEG changes or event-related potential alterations may better index physiologic sleepiness.

Some recent work following this approach focuses on drowsy driving. The "B-Alert X10" system examines EEG power spectral densities recorded at frontal, central, parietal, and occipital scalp sites.[32] The authors replicated prior findings and found within-subject EEG indices associated with fatigue.

Although these approaches hold promise for within-subject comparison, the normative data limit their clinical application. The high degree of between-subject variation makes it difficult to compare results between individuals. Finally, techniques are not standardized, and many use proprietary algorithms that are declared as trade secrets.

Manifest Sleepiness

Manifest sleepiness encompasses observable signs and measurable behavior, indicating a person is either sleepy or is about to fall asleep; is in the process of falling asleep; or has fallen asleep. Observable signs can include yawning, ptosis (upper eyelid drooping), and head bobbing. Interestingly, continuous observation may actually be more sensitive than current EEG measures. Several investigators found EEG measures were less predictive of task-related performance lapses than video recordings showing eyelid drooping and closure.[33] However, manifest drowsiness signs are not specific to sleepiness; for example, ptosis may be neurogenic (as in oculomotor nerve palsy) or myotonic (as in myasthenia gravis), and head bobbing can signify cysts in the third ventricle. By contrast, EEG-EOG-EMG polysomnographic recordings can objectively determine if a person is falling, or has fallen, asleep during controlled test sessions. This provides the basis for the maintenance of wakefulness test (MWT).

Maintenance of Wakefulness Test

The procedures for conducting the MWT are similar to those used for the MSLT.[27,28] The most significant difference is that rather than instructing the subject to *not* resist sleep, you instruct the subject to resist sleep (i.e., attempt to remain awake). In this manner, the MWT is used to assess a person's capability to, as the name implies, maintain wakefulness. To a large extent, the MWT evaluates the magnitude of sleepiness in relationship to the underlying wakefulness system's functioning. If the wakefulness system fails, sleepiness becomes manifest. This laboratory situation parallels circumstances in which sleep onset occurs inadvertently while a person remains passively sedentary in a nonstimulating environment. The MWT gauges the potential threat of inappropriately and nonvolitionally lapsing into sleep; that is, *dangerous sleepiness.*

Potentially identifying dangerous sleepiness has attracted the attention of regulatory agencies. With growing interest in sleepiness and public safety, the demand for tests to assess sleepiness has increased. Indeed, the Federal Aviation Administration recognizes the MWT as a means to determine whether noncommercial pilots may be licensed after treatment for sleep apnea.[34] Trucking companies and safety officers for companies with high-risk processes are beginning to follow suit, especially as the liability for and financial costs of accidents increase. However, the MSLT and the MWT do not correlate well with self-reported sleepiness.[35,36] Patients who fall asleep when not resisting sleep drive (as on MSLT) may be able to remain awake when instructed during MWT testing.

Methodology

In the MWT, the subject's only task is to remain awake. The subject sits in a dimly lit but not totally darkened room. Dressed in street clothing and situated on the bed with a bolster pillow, the subject is not permitted to read, watch television, or engage in other activities. During testing, EEG, EOG, and EMG are recorded. Like the MSLT, test sessions are scheduled at 2-hour intervals, beginning approximately 2 hours after awakening from the previous night's sleep. Test sessions are terminated when unequivocal sleep occurs (either three consecutive 30-second epochs of N1 or a single 30-second epoch of N2, N3, or REM sleep).

Sleep latency for each test session, regardless of unequivocal sleep determination, is determined by the first epoch of sleep. The average sleep latency across tests provides the primary index. The recording may also be evaluated for microsleep (3- to 10-second) occurrences. As expected, studies comparing MWT and MSLT find longer mean sleep latencies when subjects are instructed to remain awake than when they are told not to resist sleep. Unlike the MSLT, a prior night sleep study is not required because if subjects successfully maintain wakefulness, how they slept the night before is moot. However, an important factor involves stimulant use. Consequently, caffeine consumption is restricted on the MWT (and MSLT) test day. Urinalysis and/or blood chemistry may also be required.

For many years, the MWT lacked standardization. Researchers and clinicians employed different protocols. The MWT test session duration ranged from 20 to 60 minutes, with the longer tests attempting to avoid ceiling effects. An additional issue for clinical MWT interpretation stemmed from an absence of normative data. However, this situation changed[37] when data gathered by a consortium of sleep disorders centers established a range for expected values. Studies demonstrate MWT clinical utility for evaluating treatment outcomes in patients with narcolepsy and sleep-related breathing disorders. Also, the MWT measures can detect improvement in treated patients with persistent MSLT-indexed sleep drive; thus MWT can extend MSLT's sensitivity range.[38] However, the MWT is used much less commonly than the MSLT in clinical practice.

Standards of Practice Parameters

The AASM developed MWT clinical practice parameters. They based standards on an evidence-based literature review[27,28] and expert consensus (when data were inadequate). An update in 2021 primarily provided guidance regarding adherence to PAP and non-PAP therapies for obstructive sleep apnea prior to (but not during) testing. Recommendations for documentation were also made.[27a] MWT testing is indicated for assessing persons whose inability to remain alert constitutes a personal or public safety hazard. Another indicated use includes determining pharmacotherapeutic response in patients with narcolepsy or idiopathic hypersomnia. Clinicians are cautioned that although falling asleep rapidly on the MWT logically seems a powerful indicator for dangerous sleepiness, there is little direct evidence linking MWT sleep latency to real-world accidents. Thus clinical evaluation must integrate MWT findings with signs and symptoms, history, and treatment adherence.

Specific recommendations include conducting four 40-minute trials. Based on statistical analysis of normative data, a mean sleep latency less than 8 minutes is abnormal. Scores between 8 and 40 (the maximum value) are of uncertain significance. The mean sleep latency for presumed-normal volunteer subjects was 30.4 minutes. The ability to remain awake for the entire 40 minutes on all four test sessions (which is the upper limit of the 95% confidence interval) provides the strongest evidence for normal alertness. Nonetheless, clinical judgment is critical because even completely normal values do not guarantee safety.

Vigilance Tests

Response slowing and lapsing during vigilance tests also offer evidence for the consequence of sleepiness, inattention, or both.[39] Therefore a variety of tests requiring simple psychomotor responding (i.e., signal-detection reaction time tasks) can index a sleep drive manifestation. We call such assessments "vigilance tests" because they evaluate a person's ability to remain heedfully vigilant. Typically (but not always) these tests attempt to mimic the tedious, palling situation of watching for blips on a radar screen or for ships on the horizon.[40] Loss of vigilance, when faced with a nonstimulating task, is particularly relevant for patients with disorders of sleep and arousal. The task's monotony theoretically unmasks underlying sleepiness.

Vigilance tests measure arousal level, attention, or both. As with the MWT, performance cannot exceed ability or maximum effort. Although a person could intentionally perform poorly, the converse is unlikely. However, teasing apart arousal and attention can make test interpretation difficult. Nonsleepy individuals with attention deficits can confound test results. Fortunately, sleepiness and inattention often coexist; consequently, long, experimenter-paced, monotonous tasks are sensitive to sleep loss, sleep disruption, and circadian variation. The landmark studies, collectively referred to as the Walter Reed experiments (named for the institute where they were conducted), documented the effects of sleep deprivation on performance.[41] These pioneering studies established that increasing duration of prior wakefulness and time-on-task provoked response slowing and lapsing (for an excellent review, see the work by Dinges[42]).

A variety of vigilance tests exist; however, the psychomotor vigilance test (PVT) is currently the best validated and most widely used.[43,44] The PVT is a visual signal detection test, approximately 10 minutes long, administered either by computer or by a handheld display-and-response unit. Response latencies to visual target stimuli are recorded. Response slowing and lapsing correlate with the SSS and the MSLT; these results provide convergent validity. Additionally, PVT results have been reported for a variety of subject groups, including normal controls, sleep-deprived volunteers, and patients with major sleep disorders. The test provides exquisitely sensitive within-subject measures for before-and-after experimental designs.

The other vigilance test popular for sleep research is the Oxford Sleep Resistance (OSLER) test.[45,46] The testing paradigm mimics MWT but uses a visual signal detection task rather than EEG-EOG-EMG monitoring. The test uses four 40-minute test sessions, during which visual target signals are presented. Subjects are instructed to respond to each signal with a simple button press. A test session is terminated either after 40 minutes or after significant response lapsing (which is considered a failure to maintain wakefulness). The OSLER has been validated against MWT test results, but specific normative data supporting clinical threshold scores are not currently available.

Postural Balance Testing

Sleep-deprived individuals experience difficulty maintaining balance. Extended periods of wakefulness also impair balance.[47] Time-of-day variation also occurs.[48] Research suggests posturographic indices may provide a technique for assessing manifest sleepiness. Balance can also be adversely affected by psychoactive drugs. One approach records pressure shifts on a force platform on which an individual stands, feet together with crossed arms at the chest. The subject's direction of gaze is on a fixed point. The body's *center of pressure* is sampled for 30 seconds at a 1000 samples/second. Some studies conduct a trial at 2-hour intervals but protocols are not yet standardized. Whether this approach can be refined for use as a clinical tool remains to be seen; however, it shows promise.[49] Standardized evaluation protocols, optimized data processing, normative data, and validation against other measures of sleepiness and sleep drive are needed.

PRACTICAL ISSUES AND CONCLUSIONS

Before clinicians evaluate a person's sleepiness and fatigue, several questions should be considered. These include whether the goal is to establish (a) the presence of sleepiness and/or fatigue, (b) the absence of sleepiness, or (c) changes in sleepiness and/or fatigue. Is testing being conducted for clinical assessment, research, or legal purposes? Does the subject have a self-interest in the outcome (i.e., is there any primary or secondary gain)? With increasing frequency, sleep specialists provide expert opinions in legal matters involving accidents and disability claims. Expert panels often render opinions concerning fitness for duty or disability adjudication. In such cases, objective testing is crucial. Furthermore, a normal test result does not guarantee fitness for duty. Table 207.5 shows some characteristics of the tests described in this chapter. Ideally, physiologic, manifest, and introspective sleepiness should be assessed. In general, if a person claims to be sleepy and the goal is to demonstrate sleepiness, the MSLT is likely the best confirmatory test. If a person claims not to be sleepy and the goal is to demonstrate an ability to remain awake (as when there are concerns about ability to operate a motor vehicle), the MWT has certain advantages.[50,51] Similarly, subjective tests for fatigue can be relied on in clinical

Table 207.5 Comparison between Tests for Evaluating Sleepiness

Type of Sleepiness Assessed	Test Name	Are Normative Data Available?	Is It Possible to Feign Sleepiness?	Is It Possible to Feign Alertness?
Introspective Sleepiness	ESS	Yes	Yes	Yes
	SSS	No	Yes	Yes
	SWIFT	No	Yes	Yes
	Pictorial Sleepiness Scale	No	Yes	Yes
	POMS	Yes	Yes	Yes
	ODSI	No	Yes	Yes
Physiologic Sleepiness	MSLT[a]	Yes	No	Yes[b]
	Pupillography	No	No	Unknown
	EEG	No	No	Unknown
Manifest Sleepiness	MWT[a]	Yes	Yes[c]	No
	Vigilance and performance	No	Yes[d]	No
	Postural Balance Test	No	Yes	No

EEG, Electroencephalogram; ESS, Epworth Sleepiness Scale; MSLT, Multiple Sleep Latency Test; MWT, Maintenance of Wakefulness Test; ODSI, Observation and Interview-Based Diurnal Sleepiness Inventory; POMS, Profile of Mood States; SSS, Stanford Sleepiness Scale; SWIFT, Sleepiness-Wakefulness Inability and Fatigue Test.

[a]Standard protocol described in an American Academy of Sleep Medicine Practice Parameter: Test involves 4 to 6 test sessions per day, at 2-hour intervals. Test sessions are sometimes scheduled at shorter intervals (e.g., for children); however, this practice is not recommended by the authors.

[b]Assuming that the subject is not overwhelmingly sleepy, attempting to remain awake can undermine the test result.

[c]Assuming that the subject is physiologically sleepy, not attempting to remain awake will make it appear that overwhelming sleepiness is present.

[d]Intentionally not attending or responding to the task can make a person appear sleepy.

cases, but objective measures of performance are needed for legal and disability cases.

For clinical purposes, self-reported measures combined with MSLT have long been the sine qua non for establishing sleepiness. Sometimes, however, in cases involving severe sleepiness, the MWT can demonstrate improved alertness after treatment, whereas the MSLT shows little or no change. Such persons continue to be pathologically sleepy, but they are not overwhelmed by it during the brief testing interval. The relationship between this pattern of change and performance or behavior requires further study.

The dangers posed by excessive sleepiness are becoming increasingly apparent. The National Commission on Sleep Disorders Research catalogued a substantial list of sleep-related industrial and transportation accidents. Long ago, Kleitman[53] proposed sleepiness as resulting from accumulation of blood-borne or cerebrospinal fluid hypnotoxins; however, clinical tests for such substances have not been developed or validated. Nonetheless, the search continues. Therefore the clinician can use one or a combination of the evaluation techniques described in this chapter to measure the underlying physiologic drive for sleep; the subjective, internalized consequence of that drive; and/or sleepiness's behavioral manifestations.

CLINICAL PEARLS

- Measuring sleepiness and fatigue in a clinical setting is not a simple matter; however, the MSLT and MWT can evaluate physiologic and manifest sleepiness.
- Clinical practice standards recommend the MSLT for evaluating narcolepsy and idiopathic hypersomnia.
- MWT is indicated for testing a person's ability to remain awake when safety is at stake.
- Sleepiness testing must always be viewed within a larger context of a patient's clinical history and examination findings.

SUMMARY

Excessive sleepiness and fatigue are core issues in sleep medicine. In clinical practice, assessment usually involves self-report; however, objective measures are available. A conceptual framework involves the three facets of sleepiness: (1) introspective, (2) physiologic, and (3) manifest. The indications and techniques used in standard clinical practice include the Epworth Sleepiness Scale (introspective), the Multiple Sleep Latency Test (physiologic), and the maintenance of wakefulness test (manifest). Other assessment procedures have their relative merits and limitations. Tests for indexing fatigue also may be of clinical benefit.

SELECTED READINGS

Krahn LE, Arand DL, Avidan AY, et al. Recommended protocols for the multiple sleep latency test and maintenance of wakefulness test in adults: guidance from the American Academy of sleep medicine [published online ahead of print, 2021 Aug 23]. *J Clin Sleep Med.* 2021. https://doi.org/10.5664/jcsm.9620.

Franzen PL, Siegle GJ, Buysse DJ. Relationships between affect, vigilance, and sleepiness following sleep deprivation. *J Sleep Res.* 2008;17(1):34–41.

Hirshkowitz M, Sharafkhaneh A. Fatigue management. Chapter 15. In: *Fatigue Management: Principles and Practices for Improving Workplace Safety*; 2019:193–217.

Standards of Practice Committee of the American Academy of Sleep Medicine. Practice parameters for clinical use of the multiple sleep latency test and the maintenance of wakefulness test. *Sleep.* 2005;28:113–121.

A complete reference list can be found online at ExpertConsult.com.

Chapter 208

The Assessment of Insomnia

Michael L. Perlis; Ivan Vargas; Michael A. Grandner; Celyne Bastien; Donn Posner; Arthur J. Spielman (in mem)[a]

Chapter Highlights

- A central task in the assessment of insomnia is to establish that the individual has insomnia symptoms and that such symptoms are of a severity, frequency, and chronicity to warrant treatment. Although standardized criteria exist, this chapter provides critical review regarding these issues.
- An algorithmic approach for assessing insomnia is provided (i.e., a "decision-to-treat" formula). While embracing many of the traditional criteria for the diagnosis of insomnia, this approach is argued to be more inclusive with respect to who is appropriate for treatment (in general) and who is appropriate for cognitive-behavioral therapy for insomnia (in specific).
- A model-based approach to assessment is provided. Recommendations for useful instruments and emphasis are put on the need to prospectively assess sleep continuity. Also highlighted are issues pertaining to the relative value of subjective versus objective measures.
- The chapter ends, in an integrative manner, with a case exemplar (case conceptualization).

INTRODUCTION

Assessing and treating insomnia can be challenging. Insomnia can manifest as a premorbid symptom, a consequence of another disorder or condition, or an independent sleep disorder. Furthermore, there are multiple types and subtypes of insomnia, and its clinical course is highly variable between individuals. This chapter's goal is to include both a primer on how to evaluate insomnia (i.e., provide guidance for how to navigate these and other challenges in the assessment of insomnia) and a reference guide to the assortment of assessment tools commonly used in research and clinical settings.

The first section addresses the detection and quantification of sleep continuity disturbance, including issues related to the diagnostic criteria for the severity, frequency, and chronicity of insomnia, in addition to whether or not patients report corresponding daytime impairments. The next section reviews standardized assessment strategies, primarily focused on retrospective and prospective instruments, such as questionnaires and daily sleep diaries. This is followed by an overview of other symptomatology clinicians should consider during the evaluation phase with regard to other sleep, psychiatric, and/or medical disorders. Here, the focus is on how to use a broad-based assessment strategy to determine the individual circumstances and/or comorbidities that may complicate treatment or necessitate the delay of treatment. As part of this determination, a decision-to-treat algorithm is provided. Finally, we will review three foundational theoretical perspectives/models on the etiology and pathophysiology of insomnia and provide a case example.

One preliminary caveat; assessment varies based on its primary purpose. Researchers and clinicians have different goals. Additionally, clinicians will likely vary their assessment based on their training, professional discipline, and their preferred mode of treatment. Here, we focus on clinical assessment for the purposes of deploying CBT-I[b] as the first line treatment for insomnia.[1]

THE GOALS OF ASSESSMENT

When assessing insomnia, the goals range broadly. These include:

- Detection of difficulties initiating and/or maintaining sleep
- Quantification of insomnia illness severity, frequency, and chronicity
- Evaluation of other sleep disorders' symptomatology
- Documentation of medical and/or psychiatric comorbidity

Additionally, the assessment process should include a review of the patient's insomnia clinical course (age of onset, symptom course over time, and prior treatments). Ultimately, these assessments allow for a determination of whether treatment is warranted, what treatment is optimal, and what other factors may complicate treatment. Moreover, ongoing assessment, at least in the case of CBT-I, serves to guide treatment and the determination of whether there has been a treatment response.

Broadly speaking, insomnia assessment strategies may be grouped into the following categories: unstructured clinical

[a]We are deeply saddened by Art's passing but are honored to be asked to author this chapter in his stead. Although an understatement, his work was, and continues to be, a guiding light that we follow and find to illuminate all manner of insomnia issues.

[b]The acronym "CBT-I" is used to emphasize that this form of treatment differs from the cognitive-behavioral therapies used, for example, for depression (CBT-D), anxiety (CBT-A), pain management (CBT-P).

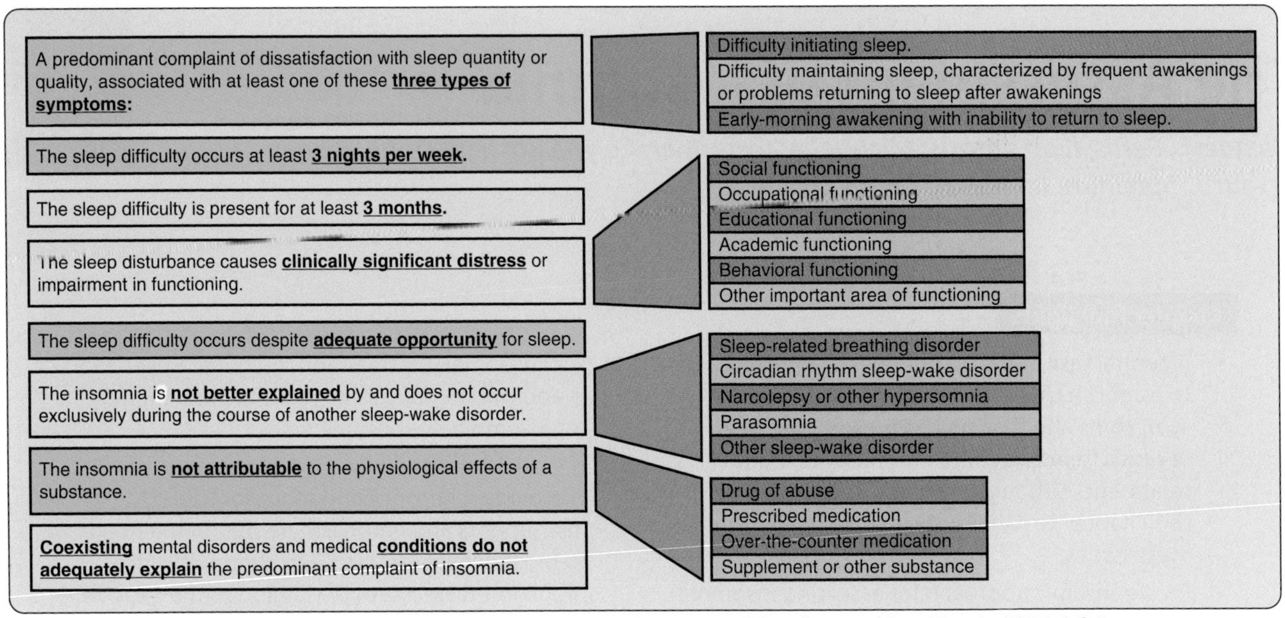

Figure 208.1 *Diagnostic Statistical Manual* (DSM) and *International Classification of Sleep Disorder* (ICSD) definitions of insomnia.

interviews, retrospective assessment tools (comprehensive or single-disorder screeners and/or illness severity measures), and prospective assessment tools (daily measures of sleep continuity[c]). With respect to the last of these, daily measures of sleep continuity may be accomplished with sleep diaries (hardcopy, online, app based, or via smart speaker technologies) and/or with wearable or bedside technologies (most commonly with wrist-worn motion detectors and/or electrocardiogram [ECG] sensors).

THE DETECTION AND QUANTIFICATION OF SLEEP CONTINUITY DISTURBANCE

In an ideal world, patients would readily share information about their sleep with their providers and/or patients would be asked during their annual physicals, "How are you sleeping?" More, in an ideal world, the patient's spontaneous report or positive responses to queries would prompt a further evaluation. Sadly, this is not the case, especially with respect to insomnia. Individuals with problems falling and/or staying asleep tend not to seek treatment, and when they do, do so only when the problem has persisted for years, if not decades.[2-6] Primary care and nonsleep specialist providers tend not to inquire about sleep disturbance[6,7] despite its association with new-onset or undiagnosed illness.[8-10] The "don't tell" part of this "don't ask and don't tell" phenomenon is that individuals with insomnia often don't view the problem as one meriting medical attention (i.e., it can be self–managed).[5] The "don't ask" part may be related to the absence of adequate sleep medicine training[11,12] and/or lack of education regarding available tools[13,14] among busy primary care providers. Therefore at present, it is generally left to the patient to seek specialist care and to the sleep medicine and/or behavioral sleep medicine specialists to initiate formal inquiries.

[c]Sleep continuity refers to the class or set of variables that represent "sleep performance." That is, it is a class term (versus sleep architecture or sleep microarchitecture) for variables that represent latency to, and duration and efficiency of, the sleep that occurs during the sleep period, including sleep latency [SL], number of awakenings [NWAK], wake after sleep onset [WASO], early morning awakening [EMA], total sleep time [TST], and sleep efficiency SE%). When one or more of these variables are pathologic, this may be referred to as *sleep continuity disturbance.* More, the use of this class term promotes a level of specificity that is unconfounded with the many denotations and connotations of the vernacular term "insomnia."

Clinical Inquiry

The initial inquiry by the sleep medicine and/or behavioral sleep medicine specialist may be to simply establish that the individual's sleep complaint is indeed insomnia (related to difficulties falling or staying asleep) and whether these complaints are associated with functional impairments. The former can be accomplished by establishing that the sleep continuity disturbance occurs with a frequency and chronicity that meet *Diagnostic Statistical Manual,* fifth edition (DSM-5)[15] and/or *International Classification of Sleep Disorders,* third edition (ICSD-3)[16] diagnostic criteria for Insomnia Disorder (i.e., insomnia occurs on 3 or more nights per week, for at least 3 months [Figure 208.1]). The latter can be accomplished by establishing that the patient experiences one or more of the following in association with their sleep continuity disturbance: daytime sleepiness, fatigue, mood disturbance, performance deficits, and/or new or worsened medical or psychiatric symptoms.

The diagnostic criteria, codified as they are, give rise to *two applied* issues and *two conceptual/empirical* issues. The applied issues are that neither diagnostic system has quantitative severity criteria, and both require that the sleep continuity disturbance be associated with daytime impairments. The conceptual/empirical issues pertain to the specific criteria that exist for diagnostic frequency and chronicity. These issues are reviewed next.

Severity

As noted earlier, neither the DSM nor the ICSD have quantitative severity criteria for insomnia. The clinician is left to their own judgments regarding what constitutes "severe enough to treat." Although clinical researchers tend to use a 30-minute threshold (i.e., sleep latency [SL] and/or wake after sleep onset [WASO] and/or early morning awakening [EMA] ≥30 minutes in duration),[17,18] this still requires clinical judgments about whether less-than-30-minute problems are of a severity that warrant treatment. One approach has been to drop quantitative criteria all together (define a problem as "the patient says it's a problem"). Another approach, in the case of minor sleep continuity disturbances (e.g., those that are between 15 and 30 minutes in duration), is to initiate treatment, especially when there are problems with both sleep initiation and maintenance.

Daytime Impairments

It is a long-standing tradition that insomnia only be diagnosed as a disorder if daytime impairment results. This definitional criterion is really a proxy measure for sleep need. That is, in the absence of knowing what an individual's need is, it can be inferred that their need is not met if their daytime function is compromised because of poor sleep (i.e., total wake time [TWT] is too high and, by implication, total sleep time [TST] is too low). When one takes into account both sleep continuity disturbance and daytime impairment, it is expected that these phenomena rise and fall in tandem. That is, when sleep continuity disturbance is high, daytime impairment will be high and when sleep continuity disturbance is low, daytime impairment will be low (i.e., the two measures will be concordant). However, it is possible for the two measures to be discordant. Such discordances potentially represent two clinical phenomena that bear on both the issue of differential diagnosis and the decision about whether treatment is indicated.

A person exhibiting high sleep continuity disturbance and low daytime impairment may be conceived of as having a low sleep ability, a large sleep opportunity, and a *low sleep need* (i.e., a short sleeper or "Insomnoid"[19,20]). Such individuals may still seek and benefit from treatment to improve sleep efficiency regardless of whether they exhibit daytime dysfunction. This is because, for some, just the experience of lying awake at night, unable to sleep, is aversive. In this instance treatment may be optimally focused on sleep restriction, or perhaps sleep compression (i.e., reducing the discrepancy between sleep ability and sleep opportunity). However, unlike insomnia disorder, once the match is made, there is no need to titrate in more sleep, as the patient now sleeps efficiently and sleep need is met.

By contrast, another person may exhibit low sleep continuity disturbance and high daytime impairment. Such a person may be suffering from sleep disorders other than insomnia and/or from other medical or psychiatric disorders that affect daytime function. This condition, however, may also be conceived of as someone who has reasonable sleep ability and/or a sleep opportunity that is well matched to that sleep ability, but also as someone with a *high sleep need* (i.e., someone potentially suffering insufficient sleep duration). An individual with this profile would likely be typed as having pseudoinsomnia or as an individual with "insomnia identity issues"[21]). Regardless of their classification, such a person may also benefit from treatment (to achieve more sleep and thereby be more sleep sated), regardless of the magnitude of their sleep continuity disturbance. In this instance treatment may be optimally focused on the systematic sleep extension aspect of sleep restriction.

Frequency

Criteria set forth for insomnia disorder is 3 or more days per week. Although long a part of the research diagnostic criteria, this was only recently added to the clinical definition of insomnia (as of the DSM-5 and ICSD-3). The episodic nature of insomnia and resultant diagnostic frequency criteria may arise from sleep regulation by homeostatic processes. That is, if sleep debt is accrued over successive nights, it stands to reason that after some period there is enough sleep pressure to produce an average (or good) night's sleep. This specific proposition has been evaluated on two occasions.[22,23] It was found that insomnia does occur on an interval basis and that for approximately every 3 nights of insomnia, there is a better-than-average (or a good) night's sleep. Thus what was arrived at by the consensus of expert opinion appears to be justifiable based on data regarding "the rhythm of insomnia." Please note there are several studies on the night-to-night variability of insomnia symptoms that use very different methodologies and that reach different conclusions.[24–28]

Chronicity

Thresholds are needed to distinguish between normal, acute, and chronic. Over the years, criteria have varied widely, ranging from 2 weeks to 6 months' time based on expert consensus. The rationale for the current criterion (≥3 months) was not detailed by the framers of the DSM or ICSD nosologies. Ultimately, the issue of chronicity may be entirely moot, as most patients don't seek treatment until they have had the insomnia for months or years.

Comorbidities

It is worth noting that the latest definitions of Insomnia Disorder in the DSM and ICD continue to suggest possible exclusion criteria related to comorbidities. That is, it is stated several times that Insomnia Disorder is not an appropriate diagnosis (and, by extension, should not be the focus of treatment) if the insomnia is better explained by another sleep disorder or other medical or mental health disorder. Presumably, one is to infer that under these conditions the insomnia is to be conceptualized as a symptom of the comorbid disorder and that treatment of the so-called "primary disorder" will, in all likelihood, eliminate the insomnia. Although this may well be true for acute insomnia, once chronic, insomnia is likely maintained by factors that disrupt the fabric of sleep regulation on a physiologic, behavioral, and cognitive level. As will be outlined later in the chapter, such disruptions of sleep regulation are not often addressed by solely targeting comorbid disorders, even when they may have initially given rise to the insomnia. As such, the assumption that insomnia that seems to covary with another disorder and is "better explained" by that disorder may often prove faulty in the case of insomnia disorder. Not targeting the disruptions of sleep regulation directly often can result in an insomnia that is resistant to change, can interfere with the treatment of the comorbid disorder, and can lead to greater potential for relapse.

Standardized Assessment

Apart from a general clinical inquiry, many clinicians further profile the patient's presenting problem using retrospective and prospective instruments.

Retrospective Questionnaires

Some of the most commonly used retrospective instruments (single-time-point insomnia questionnaires) are the Insomnia Severity Index (ISI),[29,30] the Pittsburgh Sleep Quality Index (PSQI),[31,32] and the Athens Insomnia Scale (AIS).[33,34] These instruments (along with others commonly used for clinical profiling) are presented in Table 208.1.

Of the four instruments, the most well-known, validated, and commonly used is the ISI. This seven-item instrument allows for the assessment of the incidence and severity of initial, middle, and late insomnia and four assessments of the consequences of insomnia in terms of sleep satisfaction, impairment of quality of life, sleep-related worry, and interference with daytime function. The total score of the instrument can be used to define "no significant insomnia" (scores 0–7), "subthreshold insomnia" (scores 8–14), "clinical insomnia, moderate severity" (scores 15 to 21), and "clinical insomnia, severe" (scores 22–28). Further, the ISI may be scored in such a way as to allow for the separate assessment of sleep continuity disturbance and daytime impairment. This multiscore approach has been evaluated in several studies.[35,36] One approach is to use two-factor scoring (along with the total score); that is, items 1 to 3 may be used to define continuity disturbance severity, and items 4 to 7 may be used to quantify the daytime effects of insomnia. Garnering data in this manner can allow the clinician to evaluate how insomnia severity maps to daytime function. Although concordant scores on the two factors are to be expected (i.e., high severity and high daytime complaints and low severity and low daytime complaints), discordant scores (i.e., low severity and high daytime complaints and high severity and low daytime complaints) may signal (as noted earlier) that a different approach to treatment may be required (i.e., that the sleep restriction prescription and/or time in bed titration may need to be managed differently). Finally, when used as a repeated measure, the ISI may be used to quantify change over time and/or treatment response (i.e., in general terms [50% change] or as validated by Morin and colleagues [a change in score of 8 points or to below a total score of 10]).[37]

Prospective Instruments

As for prospective measures (daily sampling of sleep continuity), this can be accomplished using self-report measures (daily diaries) and/or with objective measures (actigraphy and/or ECG-based instruments that use inferential algorithms to assess wake and sleep on an interval/epoch basis and summarize such data in terms of traditional summary parameters). Both methods provide daily measures, which may be averaged to create weekly sleep continuity profiles. The typical summary variables are presented in Table 208.2. Note: Only sleep diaries are required for treatment with CBT-I.

Sleep Diaries. Daily sampling of sleep continuity by way of sleep diaries is standard for both randomized controlled trials (RCTs) and for the clinical practice of CBT-I. This form of assessment can be accomplished with standardized questions like those recommended for the consensus sleep diary[38] via a variety of platforms (e.g., paper-and-pencil instruments, online diaries, or dedicated smart phone apps). Figure 208.2 provides a copy of the consensus diary.

Although there is a long-standing tradition of using laboratory- or practice-standard sleep diaries, adopting common language (a standard set of questions) to assess SL, NWAK, TST, etc., across settings helps assure that the values obtained in one venue are comparable with other venues. This is particularly important for research, but will become increasingly important for clinical practice as patient care becomes more evidenced based and is subject to institutional or third-party payer review of outcomes.

With respect to platform (method of administering sleep diaries/collecting sleep continuity data), the obvious advantages of the digital formats is that the data acquired are time stamped; are accessible from any computer; are reviewable at any time; can be manipulated to produce tables and graphs to represent trends over time; and/or may be "piped" into reports, progress reports, or other electronic medical records. Furthermore, the availability of digitally acquired sleep continuity measures may serve as the data source for algorithm-based assessments and interventions. At present, online sleep diaries are largely delivered as they are on paper—as a series of questions using a page format. This said, although the interrogatives are the same as with paper diaries, the response formats often differ. Instead of "fill in the blank" layouts, the response formats include drop-down menu selections, radio bullet choices, sliders, rotary dials, etc. These formats not only serve to standardize responses, they may decrease the time required to make responses and/or increase subject engagement in, and adherence with, the data capture process. Sleep diaries may also be administered in a diagrammatic format (e.g., block diaries where the sleep period is represented as a series of hourly blocks, and the respondent is instructed to "shade in" when they were asleep). An example of this type of diary format is presented in Figure 208.3.

A major advantage of "block sleep diaries" is that they allow for a resolution of the temporal patterning of awakenings (versus summary values in terms of WASO and EMA). Such data may be informative about the duration of each waking episode, where they occur in clock time and/or relative to sleep onset and offset. The major disadvantage of "block sleep diaries" is that the data must be converted from visual representations to numeric data and that the precision of the numeric data is usually limited to 15- to 30-minute increments. Both limitations may be minimized or eliminated when block sleep diaries are obtained digitally. Further, it is possible that the diagrammatic approach may be quicker and more engaging than the standard questionnaire format. At present no studies have been conducted to determine the relative "likeability" or acceptability of the two formats, nor whether one or the other confers better adherence.

Finally, regardless of the type of diary and/or platform of administration, there is the question of "how much prospective sampling is needed to adequately profile a patient's sleep continuity?" From a statistical point of view, sampling generally assumes a normal or representative distribution with 35 or more data points (central limit theorem). From a clinical point of view, such a protracted assessment interval is not feasible and is not likely to be acceptable to most patients. These issues notwithstanding, it is generally recommended that sleep diaries (if not actigraphic data) be acquired for 2 or more weeks' time.[39-41] Within the context of CBT-I, 1 week is likely to lead to sleep restriction prescriptions that are either too high or too low (i.e., the estimate being based on an exceptionally poor or good week's sleep).

Actigraphy. This approach, although not standard for either clinical research RCTs or for the practice of CBT-I, also

Table 208.1 Standard Assessment Instruments for Sleep and Insomnia

Name	Items	II	MI	LI	Assesses Frequency	Assesses Severity	Assess Daytime Impairment	Assesses Chronicity	PMID
ISI	7	Yes	Yes	Yes	No	Yes	Yes	No	11438246
PSQI	18	Yes	Yes	No	Yes	Yes	Yes	No	2748771
AIS	8	Yes	Yes	Yes	No	Yes	Yes	No	11033374
WHIIS	5	Yes	Yes	Yes	No	Yes	No	No	15673630
BIQ	33	Yes	Yes	Yes	Yes	Yes	Yes	Yes	3351539
ISQ	13	Yes	Yes	Yes	No	Yes	Yes	No	19317380
IES	9	Yes	Yes	Yes	Yes	Yes	Yes	No	23171440
LSEQ	10	Yes	Yes	No	No	Yes	Yes	No	26096
PROMIS	8	Yes	Yes	No	No	Yes	Yes	No	22250775
SCI	8	Yes	Yes	No	No	Yes	Yes	Yes	24643168
ISA	21	Yes	Yes	No	No	No	Yes	No	28240944
SATED	5	No	No	No	No	Yes	Yes	No	31899656

AIS, Athens Insomnia Scale; BIQ, Brief Insomnia Questionnaire; IES Insomnia in the Elderly Scale; II, initial insomnia; ISA, Insomnia Symptoms Assessment; ISI, Insomnia Severity Index; ISQ, Insomnia Symptoms Questionnaire; LSEQ, Leeds Sleep Evaluation Questionnaire; LI, late insomnia; MI, middle insomnia; PROMIS, PROMIS Sleep Disturbance Index, Short Form; PSQI, Pittsburgh Sleep Quality Index; SATED, Satisfaction, Alertness, Timing, Efficiency, and Duration Questionnaire; SCI, Sleep Condition Indicator; WHIIS, Women's Health Initiative Insomnia Scale.

Table 208.2 Traditional Sleep Continuity Variables

Acronym	Variable Name	Units of Measurement	Calculation	What It Measures
Core Measures				
TTB	Time to bed	Clock time (HH:MM)	Reported	Clock time that the individual got into bed
SL	Sleep latency	Minutes	Reported	Amount of time to fall asleep once the individual started trying
NWAK	Number of awakenings	Count	Reported	Number of times that the individual remembers awakening
WASO	Wake after sleep onset	Minutes	Reported	Total amount of time that the individual remembers spending awake during the night
TFA	Time of final awakening	Clock time (HH:MM)	Reported	Clock time that the individual awakened for the last time
TOB	Time out of bed	Clock time (HH:MM)	Reported	Clock time that the individual got out of bed to start the day
EMA	Early morning awakening	Minutes	TOB – TFA	Amount of time elapsed between the time of final awakening and the time that the individual got up out of bed
TIB	Time in bed	Minutes	TOB – TTB	Total time of the sleep opportunity window
TST	Total sleep time	Minutes	TIB – SL – WASO – EMA	Total amount of sleep, calculated using the standard definition
SE%	Sleep efficiency	Percent (0–100)	(TST / TIB) *100	Ratio of sleep achieved to sleep opportunity window

allows for the daily sampling of sleep continuity measures. The methodology has its roots in basic science studies where self-report measures were not possible and electroencephalogram (EEG) measures were either not possible and/or feasible.[42] In the basic application, the detection of movement and the absence of movement are used to infer when an animal is awake or asleep, the inference being that during wakefulness, there is a substantial amount of movement and that during sleep, movement occurs only sporadically. Actigraphy detects movement in the extremities, typically measured at the wrist. The U.S. Food and Drug Administration (FDA) cleared actigraphs for research, and clinical applications are made up of a detector housed in a wristwatch-like case that also contains a clock, a power source, a converter, a microprocessor, and memory chips. The detector is typically a small piezoelectric accelerometer that generates voltages when there is movement across the radius-to-ulna axis or a wrist flexion-extension. In other words, most actigraphs are sensitive to movement in two

Consensus sleep diary-core

ID/name: ____________________

	Sample							
Today's date	4/5/11							
1. What time did you get into bed?	10:15 p.m							
2. What time did you try to go to sleep?	11:30 p.m							
3. How long did it take you to fall asleep?	55 min.							
4. How many times did you wake up, not counting your final awakening?	3 times							
5. In total, how long did these awakenings last?	1 hour 10 min.							
6. What time was your final awakening?	6:35 a.m							
7. What time did you get out of bed for the day?	7:20 a.m							
8. How would you rate the quality of your sleep?	☐Very poor ☑Poor ☐Fair ☐Good ☐Very good	☐Very poor ☐Poor ☐Fair ☐Good ☐Very good	☐Very poor ☐Poor ☐Fair ☐Good ☐Very good	☐Very poor ☐Poor ☐Fair ☐Good ☐Very good	☐Very poor ☐Poor ☐Fair ☐Good ☐Very good	☐Very poor ☐Poor ☐Fair ☐Good ☐Very good	☐Very poor ☐Poor ☐Fair ☐Good ☐Very good	☐Very poor ☐Poor ☐Fair ☐Good ☐Very good
9. Comments (if applicable)	I have a cold							

Figure 208.2 Consensus sleep diary.

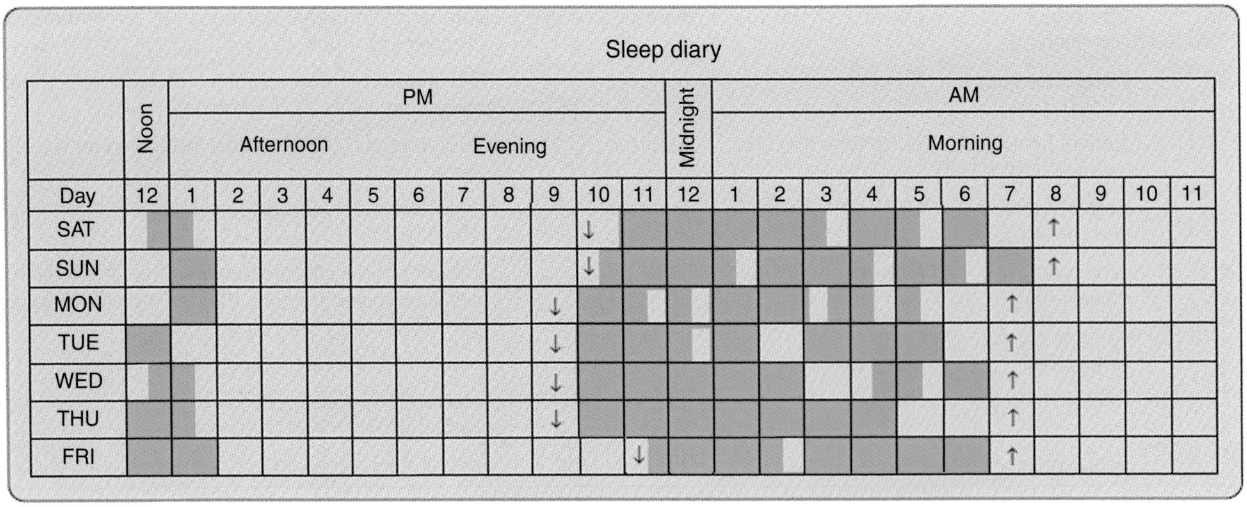
Sleep diary
Noon
PM
Afternoon
Evening
Midnight
AM
Morning
Day
12 1 2 3 4 5 6 7 8 9 10 11 12 1 2 3 4 5 6 7 8 9 10 11
SAT
SUN
MON
TUE
WED
THU
FRI

Figure 208.3 Block sleep diary.

planes (e.g., movement as in waving [x] or as in dribbling a basketball [y]). Many of the sensors also detect movement in the z plane (such as throwing a punch) but are less sensitive to this form of movement unless the device has a triaxial configuration. The resultant voltages are then converted from analog signals to digital values, typically at a rate of about 30 times per second (range 10–32 Hz). The values, which are scaled to a byte metric (0–255 counts), are summated online over fixed time increments and are stored/binned in the onboard memory chips. The data in these bins may be further compressed by storing the summated counts as the sum total of multiple bins for a user-specified epoch. Epoch lengths range from 15 seconds to 15 minutes. At present, data may be acquired for periods of up to 90 days or more.

The epoch data for the entire measurement interval (e.g., 90 days) may be transferred to a computer for processing or via

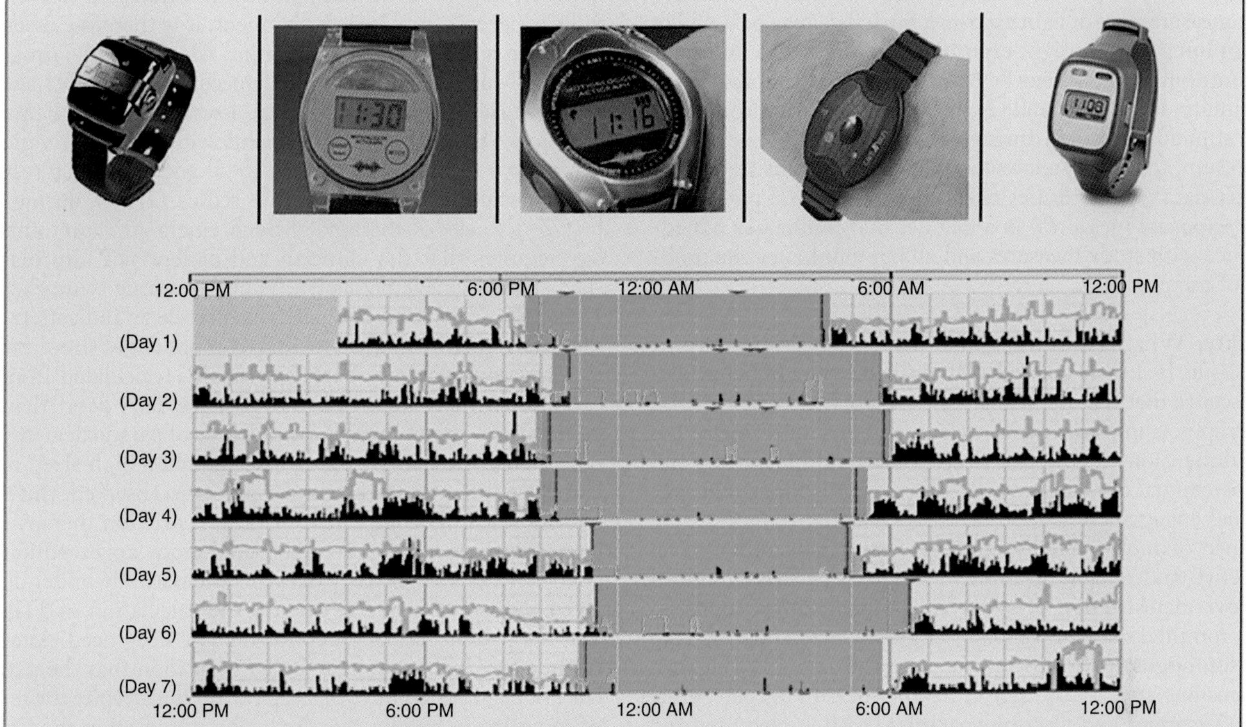

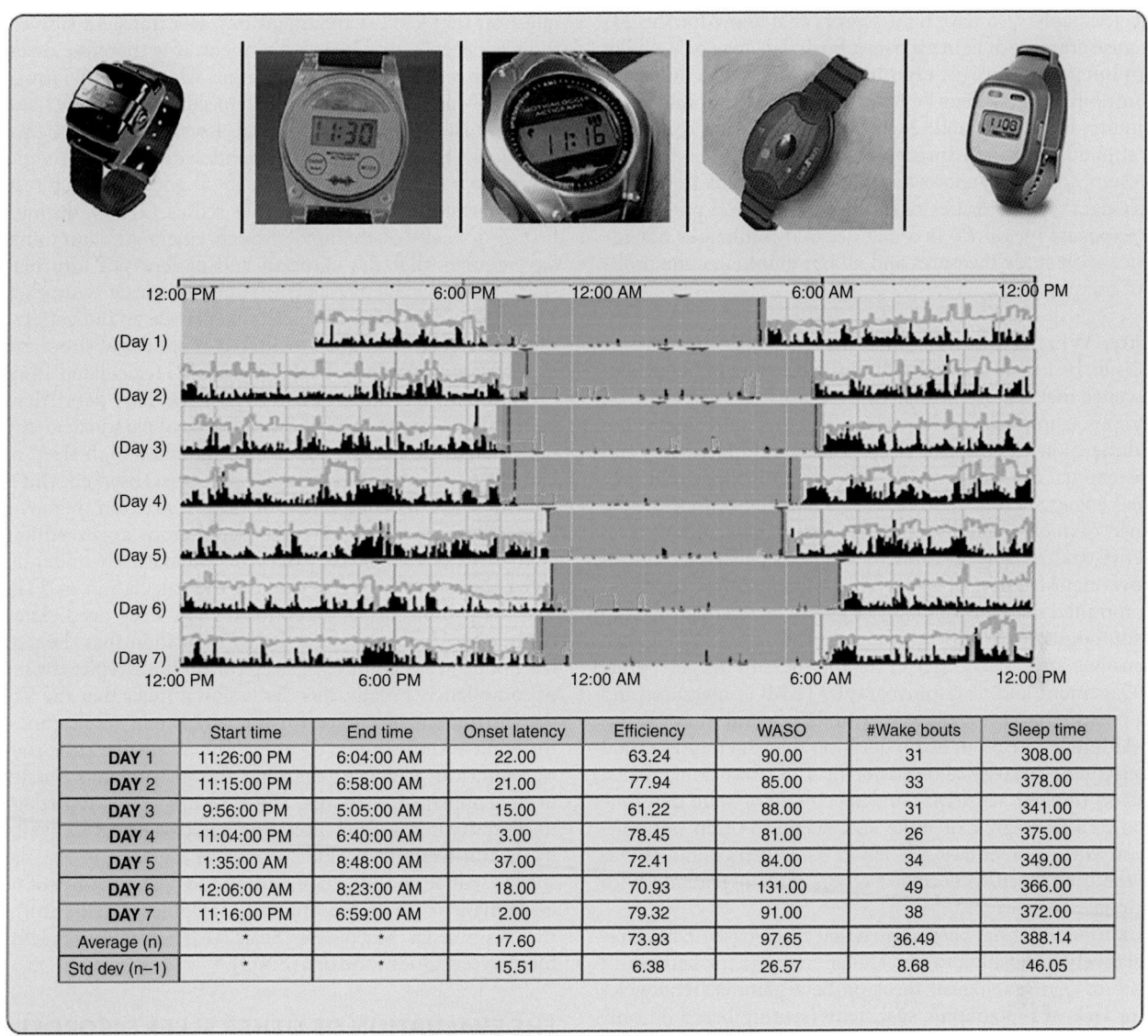

	Start time	End time	Onset latency	Efficiency	WASO	#Wake bouts	Sleep time
DAY 1	11:26:00 PM	6:04:00 AM	22.00	63.24	90.00	31	308.00
DAY 2	11:15:00 PM	6:58:00 AM	21.00	77.94	85.00	33	378.00
DAY 3	9:56:00 PM	5:05:00 AM	15.00	61.22	88.00	31	341.00
DAY 4	11:04:00 PM	6:40:00 AM	3.00	78.45	81.00	26	375.00
DAY 5	1:35:00 AM	8:48:00 AM	37.00	72.41	84.00	34	349.00
DAY 6	12:06:00 AM	8:23:00 AM	18.00	70.93	131.00	49	366.00
DAY 7	11:16:00 PM	6:59:00 AM	2.00	79.32	91.00	38	372.00
Average (n)	*	*	17.60	73.93	97.65	36.49	388.14
Std dev (n–1)	*	*	15.51	6.38	26.57	8.68	46.05

Figure 208.4 Watch and data activity plots.

Bluetooth to smartphone apps or to cloud-based programs. The scoring algorithms are applied to the epoch data, which are consecutively arrayed and are usually locked to clock time. Each epoch, usually of no longer duration than 2 minutes for the purposes of sleep scoring, is evaluated for whether it represents sleep or wakefulness. This determination is made according to one of several procedures, each of which uses a threshold approach. The threshold method may be assessed for either the amplitude or time domains. An example of an amplitude assessment is an epoch judged to be wake when the sum voltage for the epoch has a value of greater than some predetermined amount. An example of a time domain assessment (for instruments that retain the individual bin data) is an epoch judged to be wake when some percentage of the total epoch time has voltages greater than some predetermined amount. Note: In many devices, the threshold for state determination may be adjusted by the investigator or clinician to suit the needs of an individual case (e.g., the sensitivity of the actigraph might be increased for a patient with mobility problems). Finally, prior to the tabulation of the sleep continuity parameters (by day), most validated forms of actigraphy apply smoothing rules to enhance the reliability of state assessments. The most commonly used rules are the Webster and/or Cole. An example of such a rule is as follows, "If there has been 10 to 14 minutes of wake, recode the first 3 minutes of sleep as wake."[43-45] Figure 208.4, depicts several examples of industry-standard wrist actigraphy devices: an example of 1 week's activity data and an example of a sleep parameter data table is provided from the associated software.

The primary value of actigraphy is that it allows for (1) the continuous assessment of sleep and wake in precision increments (generally 30-, 60-, or 120-second epochs) over the 24-hour day and across time intervals of up to 90 days and (2) the measure of diurnal activity levels. These assessments only require that the individual wear the device. Some devices also include event markers, which allow the patient to press a button to indicate when they got into or out of bed or when they intended to fall asleep and when they intended to start their day. Having such markers may slightly increase subject burden but are likely to allow for better assessments of SL and/or EMA.

Some actigraphs also have light sensors that allow for the 24-hour measurement of light exposure. Such data may be useful in determining (1) how light exposure (amount and timing) may be contributing to, or may be manipulated to ameliorate, sleep continuity disturbance and (2) whether patients are compliant with stimulus control instructions.

In sum, actigraphy allows for acquisition of daily sleep continuity data (and measures of diurnal activity and potentially light exposure measures) in a manner that minimizes nonadherence with study measures and all but eliminates the problem of missing data.

Validity. What constitutes a valid measure of sleep is a complex issue. If sleep is defined as "a reversible state of behavioral quiescence that is accompanied by perceptual disengagement," actigraphy is inherently incomplete, as it taps only one of the two dimensions that define sleep (behavioral quiescence and *not* perceptual disengagement).[46] Further, it is likely that perceptual engagement can occur in an enduring fashion in the absence of motor activity and thus actigraphy, although an objective and reliable measure, is likely to be biased toward the overidentification of sleep. This, among other concerns, has prompted many to validate actigraphy by comparing it to polysomnography (PSG) measures. In the case of PSG, both dimensions are assessed (EEG for the measure of perceptual disengagement and electromyography [EMG] measures and body position trackers to assess recumbency and motor activity). Although there can be no question that the multimethod measurement strategy allowed for by PSG has unparalleled precision (greater sensitivity and specificity of state determination), EEG staging of wake and sleep are often not concordant with momentary self-report assessments, and this is true for both healthy normal sleepers and in patients with insomnia.

Additionally, it has been argued that PSG-based EEG may be relatively insensitive to perceptual engagement because of its lack of methodological focus on beta-gamma frequencies and/or lack of topographic specificity (scoring based on only central and occipital derivations) and/or the inherent limitation of EEG to only allow for the resolution of temporal and spatially summated activity from the cortical mantle of the cerebrum (i.e., cannot resolve local wakefulness in small cortical areas and/or subcortically during otherwise global sleep).

Despite the potential limitations of actigraphy, PSG, and other physiologic methods, many view the discordance between objective and subjective measures as an inherent problem with self-report.[47-51] A case can be made, however, that self-report assessments are not only more relevant, they are more accurate in relation to "what is and is not" unconsciousness. Leaving aside the issue of accuracy, self-report assessments are more relevant because they are not only required for diagnosis but they are essential for the treatment and the assessment of treatment response. In the final analysis, how useful (clinically relevant and/or of importance to the patient) is a significant PSG change in sleep continuity that is not paralleled by improvement in self-reported SL, WASO, EMA, and/or TST?

The Assessment of Sleepiness. It is commonly held that patients with insomnia experience fatigue but not sleepiness ("patients with insomnia are tired but wired"). Although the truthfulness of this proposition may be debated, it is without question that CBT-I treatment has, as a transient side effect, induced sleepiness. During treatment, it is therefore essential to monitor sleepiness to determine whether this iatrogenic effect (1) surpasses what typically occurs with CBT-I and/or (2) is unusually persistent. When assessed with an Epworth Sleepiness Scale (ESS),[52,53] patients with insomnia typically exhibit low scale scores at intake (0–5) and with sleep restriction substantially increased scale scores (10–15 during the first 2–4 weeks of therapy).[54] Such emergent symptomatology requires that the clinician and patient put into place a short-term management plan. When the scale score exceeds 15 (and/or more than doubles), this may be an indication that the prescribed time in bed (PTIB) component of sleep restriction therapy may have been "overdosed" (calculated from an exceptionally bad week or two of baseline dairy data), that the patient has a larger-than-normal degree of paradoxical insomnia, or that the patient has an exceptionally high sleep need. Conversely, if no increase in sleepiness is observed, this may indicate the TIB component of sleep restriction therapy may have been "under dosed" (calculated from an exceptionally good week or two of dairy data or systematically under dosed given the use of a liberal rule for the calculation of TIB) or that the patient has an exceptionally low sleep need. Alternatively, a low ESS score may be an indication that the patient has not been adherent with sleep restriction, despite the report of compliance. Finally, this discussion implies that the ESS is the instrument of choice for the assessment of sleepiness in the context of insomnia disorder. This is not the case; there is no empirical evidence regarding the instrument's sensitivity in the context of insomnia. The ESS has been adopted, given its ubiquity in the RCT literature and because of its availability and utilization in clinical practice. Perhaps in the future, studies will be conducted regarding the relative utility of other instruments such as the Stanford Sleepiness Scale (SSS),[55,56] the Karolinska Sleepiness Scale (KSS),[57,58] or Spielman's Sleep Need Questionnaire (SNQ).[59]

THE EVALUATION OF OTHER SLEEP DISORDERS' SYMPTOMATOLOGY

In years past, insomnia evaluations required the assessment of at least the core intrinsic sleep disorders (e.g., obstructive sleep apnea [OSA], restless legs syndrome/periodic limb movements [RLS/PLMs], shiftwork sleep disorder, delayed sleep phase disorder, narcolepsy, and parasomnias) because the detection of any of these disorders would prompt the clinician to consider the insomnia as secondary and to develop a treatment plan for the primary sleep disorder. Although the primary-secondary distinction is no longer a part of the current nosologies (DSM-5 and ICSD-3)[15,16] and the practice guidelines now state that chronic insomnia warrants targeted treatment regardless of the disorders that occur comorbid with it,[1] the survey of sleep disorder symptoms still has merit.

The value of a broad-based assessment as part of an intake evaluation resides in its potential to allow the clinician to know if and how the existence of other sleep disorders may complicate the treatment plan for insomnia and/or what issues may require further assessment and/or treatment before, coincident with, or after insomnia treatment. Although many opt to rule out the co-occurrence of non-insomnia sleep disorders via clinical inquiry, a variety of sleep disorder screeners can help in this regard. These instruments range from comprehensive

Table 208.3 Sleep Diagnosis Screeners

Name	PMID
General Sleep Disorders	
Auckland Sleep Questionnaire (ASQ)	21625658
Basic Nordic Sleep Questionnaire (BNSQ)	10607192
Global Sleep Assessment Questionnaire (GSAQ)	14592227
Holland Sleep Disorders Questionnaire (HSDQ)	22924964
National Sleep Foundation Sleep Health Index	28709508
SLEEP-50 Questionnaire	16190812
Sleep Disorders Questionnaire (SDQ)	8036370
Sleep Disorders Symptom Check List (SDS-CL)	
Sleep Symptom Checklist (SSCL)	18374743

and extensive batteries, including the Alliance Sleep Questionnaire (ASQ),[60] the Duke Structured Interview for Sleep Disorders (DSI),[61,62] and the Structured Clinical Interview for DSM-5 Sleep Disorders-Revised (SCISD-R),[63] to at least eight brief "paper-and-pencil" instruments. A review of the brief screeners was published by Klingman and colleagues in 2015.[13] At the time of that publication, the Global Sleep Assessment Questionnaire (GSAQ)[64] was recommended as the most user-friendly, brief, and comprehensive of the available screeners (four sleep disorders with 11 self-report questions). Since that publication, Klingman and colleagues[14] introduced an in-development screener that assesses 13 sleep disorders and four functional outcomes with 25 questions: the Sleep Disorders Symptom Check List (SDS-CL-25). All these instruments are profiled in Table 208.3.

Clinical History

Although both behaviorists and medical practitioners tend to focus on how the insomnia presents at the time of evaluation (e.g., within the last 1 to 3 months), the clinical history provides useful information. The disorder may be idiopathic, recurrent, or of such long standing, that it may be expected that the patient may require more treatment or that they may be treatment refractory. Perhaps of greater utility is that by getting a detailed history, the clinician will have the data needed to personalize the treatment plan. The clinical history will also inform the clinician of possible medical, neurologic, and psychiatric comorbid conditions that could complicate treatment. An estimated 50% of patients in primary care report chronic insomnia,[67-69] with concordance rates between insomnia and specific medical and psychiatric disorders (conservatively estimated) between 30% and 80%.[41,67] Although medical symptom inventories are often created "in-house," several validated instruments exist to evaluate treatment side effects, including the Systematic Assessment For Treatment-Emergent Events (SAFTEE).[71-76] Finally, it is common practice among behavioral sleep medicine providers to monitor depression and anxiety symptomatology at intake and often over the whole course of treatment. This practice is desirable, as with medical disorders, to further build the narrative regarding all possible precipitants and perpetuants of the insomnia (i.e., in explaining the 3P or 4P models) and to sensitize the clinician to the comorbidities that may require concomitant treatment along with the treatment of insomnia. There are numerous devices for the measurement of depression and anxiety. Often the PHQ-9[77,78] and the GAD-7[79] are used because their user friendliness, brevity, and sound psychometric properties.

AN ALGORITHMIC APPROACH TO ASSESSMENT

Although it is traditional to use the assessment process to determine whether the patient meets the criteria for diagnosis (i.e., insomnia disorder; Figure 208.1) and to ascertain from this that the patient is a good candidate for treatment, it has been proposed that (at least for CBT-I) this can be accomplished in a more algorithmic fashion.[80] Figure 208.5 provides a "decision-to-treat" formula that takes into account whether the patient (1) exhibits some of the behavioral or psychological factors that are thought to perpetuate insomnia; (2) exhibits difficulty initiating or maintaining sleep and to a degree that warrants treatment; (c) has sleep-onset or early morning awakening problems that are not primarily the result of a circadian rhythm disorder; (4) has insomnia that is not largely explained by an unstable illness; and/or (5) has conditions that would substantially interfere with, or be worsened by, the conduct of CBT-I. These considerations are explained next with specific reference to CBT-I.

The first consideration in the algorithm is perhaps the most determinative: Does the patient exhibit some of the maladaptive behavioral or psychological factors that are thought to perpetuate insomnia? If yes, then behavioral treatment is indicated, and the remaining question is: Is there anything that contraindicates or complicates treatment? With respect to CBT-I, the three factors that are directly germane to sleep restriction therapy (SRT) and stimulus control therapy (SCT) are evidence of (1) a mismatch between sleep opportunity (time in bed [TIB]) and sleep ability (TST)[81,82]; (2) the behavior tendencies to stay in bed when awake and/or to engage in nonsleep behaviors in the bedroom[83-86]; and/or (3) evidence of conditioned arousal.[87-91]

The mismatch between sleep opportunity and sleep ability is commonly assessed in terms of SE% (TST / TIB * 100).[82,92] Although there is no rule that states how low SE% must be to warrant treatment (i.e., how big the mismatch should be), the rule that suggests further downward titration of TIB may be used as a "rule of thumb," that is <85% SE suggests that SRT is indicated.[82,92] Other indications include patient reports of engaging in other forms of sleep extension (e.g., after a poor night's sleep: sleeping in, napping, or retiring early). Greater than 85% SE is likely manageable with SCT alone or with sleep education that focuses on sleep-related worry or unrealistic expectations.

The behavior tendency to stay in bed when awake or to engage in nonsleep behaviors in the bedroom can be assayed with a simple question: When you're awake during the night, what do you do? Patient responses that include "stay in bed, rest, try to sleep, and/or wait for sleep to come" or the report of reading, watching TV (or other screen-based entertainment), working, etc., in the bedroom, particularly while in bed, constitute evidence of poor stimulus control and provide the requisite evidence that SCT is indicated. *Note:* Sleep extension (the regular advance in time to bed and/or delay in time out of bed) may lead to phase shifts and thus the patient's presenting problem may also entail a circadian rhythm disorder component.

Although traditional behaviorists tend to not focus on the content of the "nonsleep behaviors in the bedroom," it certainly seems true that patients with insomnia often exhibit

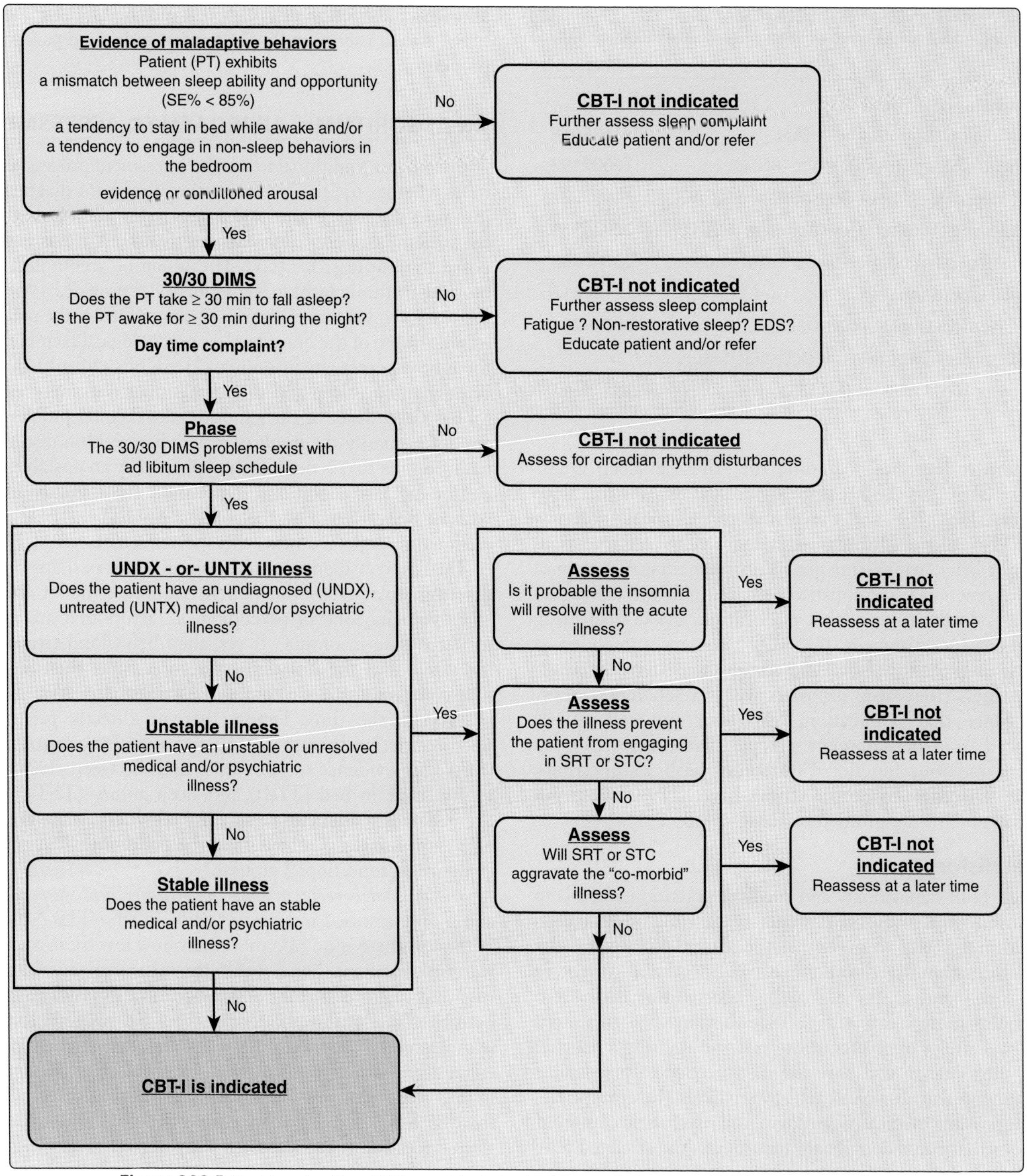

Figure 208.5 Decision algorithm. CBT-I, cognitive behavioral therapy for insomnia; SRT, sleep restriction therapy; SCT stimulus control therapy. (Adapted from Smith MT, Perlis ML. Who is a candidate for cognitive-behavioral therapy for insomnia? *Health Psychol.* 2006;25(1)15-9.)

sleep-incompatible states of worry about sleeplessness or the consequences of their sleeplessness.[93-96] Because these cognitive phenomena represent direct or indirect targets for CBT-I, it may be argued that part of the algorithmic determination about whether CBT-I is indicated should include an assessment of dysfunctional beliefs about sleep and/or catastrophic thoughts about the consequences of sleep loss. In a related vein (and in addition to sleep-related worry), patients with insomnia also exhibit a phenomenon referred to as *sleep effort*.[97-100] This encompasses any mental or behavioral activity that is enacted with the intention of making one's self sleep. This may include both ritualistic behaviors and the use of seemingly good self-help strategies (e.g., thought stopping, imagery, relaxation, etc.). The notion here is that "trying" (exerting effort) is by definition incompatible with behavioral and perceptual disengagement. Although the various published treatment protocols[92,97-100] vary regarding whether worry and sleep effort should be specially assessed and/or targeted for treatment, there are self-report instruments that assess these domains, including the Anxiety and Preoccupation about Sleep Questionnaire (APSQ),[108] the Dysfunctional Beliefs About Sleep Questionnaire (DBAS),[92] and the Glasgow Sleep Effort Scale (GSES).[96]

The phenomenon of conditioned arousal may be in evidence with any statement by the patient that they "become more awake, tense, or anxious or frustrated upon getting into bed." This can be further assayed by having the patient describe their evening routine and/or how they sleep when traveling (i.e., how they sleep in novel environments). In the case of the former, when asked to describe a typical last hour of the day, patients with insomnia often report being sleepy or falling asleep on the couch and then suddenly becoming awake upon walking into the bedroom. The patient may attribute becoming alert to walking too quickly, to engaging in prebed activities, or to simply "missing the window." The phenomenon of "becoming awake upon walking into the bedroom" is, however, thought to represent classically conditioned arousal/wakefulness, that is sleep-related stimuli (bedtime, bedroom, bed, etc.) have become conditioned stimuli (CSs) for the physiologic response of arousal/wakefulness (CR). In the case of the latter, when asked to describe how the patient sleeps when in a novel environment, patients with insomnia may report that their sleep is much improved. This is thought to occur because the novel sleep environment is relatively free of the normal CSs.[97] The best evidence for this phenomenon is the reverse first night effect.[97] *Note:* This said, this phenomenon may be less reliable than is thought because the conditioned arousal may not be limited to the individual's bedroom but also extend to the act of going to bed, bedtime, etc. As a result, the patient may sleep as poorly in novel environments as they do at home.

The second consideration is "is the insomnia sufficiently severe as to warrant treatment?" This issue is often assessed in terms of the standard quantitative rule used in most RCTs, the "30 minute rule" (SL and/or WASO and/or EMA must be ≥30 minutes in duration on 3 or more nights per week).[17] This aspect of the algorithm overlaps with the first to the extent that SE% will likely only be below 85%, given these thresholds. Specifically excluded is the complaint of nonrestorative sleep (daytime sequelae *in the absence* of a sleep initiation or maintenance disturbance). Although such a complaint is no doubt significant (and was a defining characteristic of insomnia for most or all nosologies prior to the ICSD-3 and DSM-5), there is little, if any, evidence supporting the efficacy of insomnia treatments for patients with this specific complaint. Finally, the algorithm does not specify a symptom duration criterion for treatment eligibility. Although clinical outcome studies typically specify a duration criterion (usually in line with the current diagnostic criteria), the presence of insomnia symptoms and maladaptive behaviors/conditioned arousal, regardless of the duration of illness, may be sufficient reason to initiate treatment. In cases where the insomnia is subchronic, treatment may not require "full-bore CBT-I." Such interventions may be considered prophylactic.

The third consideration pertains to evaluating whether the insomnia is psychophysiologic,[16,109-113] as opposed to chronobiologic. This is to say, that the problems with initial and late insomnia may actually be circadian rhythm disorders (i.e., delayed sleep phase disorder [DSPD] or advanced sleep phase disorder [ASPD]).[16,114] In the case of DSPD (the more common of the two),[16,40,114-116] such individuals often report extreme sleep-onset difficulties (e.g., hours to fall asleep) but that once asleep, there are no further problems sleeping. Further, individuals with DSPD report normal restorative sleep on ad libitum schedules (when they are able to go to bed and wake up as desired, e.g., on the weekends). In the case of ASPD, such individuals often report unusually early bedtimes (time to bed [TTB]) that are associated with EMAs—for example, TTB on or before 9 P.M. and EMAs between 1 A.M. and 5 A.M. Apart from these considerations, individuals with ASPD report normal restorative sleep.

In both cases further evaluation of a circadian rhythm disorder should be conducted, because other treatment aimed at shifting circadian phase may be indicated (see Chapter 43). Although DSPD and ASPD constitute true differential diagnoses for insomnia (and are thus a central aspect of any insomnia assessment), it should be noted that many patients with chronic insomnia will have some degree of chronobiologic dysregulation, and therefore combining chronobiologic treatment with CBT-I may be indicated. In such instances the first-line adjuvant treatment is likely to be with phototherapy.

The fourth consideration pertains to occult or unstable medical or psychiatric illness and/or comorbid chronic medical and/or psychiatric illness. In the case of occult or unstable illness, the assessment of such things may be beyond the scope of practice for many that specialize in behavioral sleep medicine. With this caveat in mind, medical symptom checklists and/or anxiety and/or depression screeners may be used to prompt the clinician to request a formal psychological/psychiatric evaluation. In such cases, the treatment of insomnia may be deferred if it is suspected that the insomnia may resolve with the acute/unstable illness and/or that the application of insomnia treatment will be more manageable once these issues are addressed. If this is the case, the patient should be counseled to avoid engaging in maladaptive compensatory strategies and should be reevaluated to determine whether symptoms persist after adequate treatment for the comorbid medical or psychiatric disorders. In the case of chronic medical or psychiatric illness, where such disorders are being managed and are stable, the critical question at hand is "is there anything about the comorbid disorders that would interfere with, or be worsened by, the conduct of CBT-I?" Although one should be conservative about the need to adapt standard CBT-I, "interference" may be managed by using alternative forms of CBT-I, forms that are more compatible with the patient's status. For example, if the patient is immobile or has limited mobility, one may opt to go forward with treatment but to use "counter control" instructions[117,118] rather than usual stimulus control instructions. "Worsening" (CBT-I may aggravate one or more of the comorbid conditions) is a more serious consideration, but perhaps less so than many think. On the one hand, there is the legitimate concern that sleep deprivation may trigger certain conditions such as parasomnias, manic episodes, and/or seizures in patients predisposed to, or diagnosed with, such problems. The counter point to this is that (1) sleep restriction is not sleep deprivation, and it is the latter that is the known risk factor for such adverse events (*Note:* sleep restriction usually entails between 1 and 2 hours sleep loss, whereas sleep deprivation entails between 4 and 8 hours sleep loss); and (2) if the comorbid disorder is stable because of ongoing therapy, it is not a given that even sleep deprivation can trigger adverse events in such cases; and (3) CBT-I is a short-duration intervention (usually 4–8 weeks), and thus the window of vulnerability is narrow. If the risks of potential sleep loss in CBT-I are of concern, one may opt to not conduct CBT-I, to conduct CBT-I without the sleep restriction component (just stimulus control, cognitive therapy, and sleep hygiene), or to use a modified form of sleep restriction known as *sleep compression.*

In either case (unstable or stable medical or psychiatric illness), the clinician needs to be mindful to avoid the older mind-set that insomnia is "just a symptom of other illnesses and that targeted treatment of insomnia in these cases is both unnecessary and likely to fail without first addressing the primary illness." Neither of these propositions are necessarily true. In fact, there is now a preponderance of evidence that (1) insomnia often persists after the treatment of other illnesses[119-122] and (2) treatment of insomnia in the context of comorbidities can be as efficacious as the treatment of uncomplicated insomnia.[64] Further, there is emerging evidence that the treatment of insomnia may accentuate the efficacy of the management of the comorbid disorder and possibly lead to better outcomes.[124] Perhaps the more relevant consideration pertains to *the severity of the comorbid illness* and the patient's ability to focus on, and comply with, the various treatment components of CBT-I.

CONCEPTUAL FRAMEWORKS FOR ASSESSMENT

Since the 1990s there has been a proliferation of theoretical perspectives on the etiology and pathophysiology of insomnia that includes both animal and human models. Eight of these models are reviewed in a companion chapter in this volume (Chapter 91). Although all the models challenge us to think more broadly and more deeply about the etiology and pathophysiology of insomnia, the two foundational models (along with the two process model of sleep-wake regulation) continue to be the conceptual frameworks that guide assessment and treatment. This said, one of the animal models reviewed in that chapter (the Kayser/Belfer *Drosophila*) was based on the Spielman 3P model and speaks to the universality of its principles and the potential of behavioral interventions to reverse even genetic abnormalities. The 3P/4P, stimulus-control, and Borbely two process models are briefly reviewed next.

The 3P Model

The 3P model,[81,82] alternatively referred to as the Spielman or three-factor or behavioral model, provides a theoretical basis for the importance of "the mismatch between sleep opportunity and sleep ability." That is, sleep extension is posited to be the primary factor that mediates the transition from acute to chronic insomnia and serves to perpetuate insomnia, ad infinitum. Since the original conceptualization of the 3P model in 1987, many in the field have come to believe that the third P (perpetuational factors) is broader than just sleep extension. Other factors include explicit roles for conditioning, sleep-related worry/catastrophizing, sleep effort, sleep-related attentional bias, and circadian disruption (as noted earlier). The 4P model[119] focuses on the additional perpetuating factor of classical conditioning (i.e., conditioned arousal, conditioned activation, or conditioned wakefulness). In this case, this is thought to become operational after the engagement of maladaptive behaviors and as a result of the repeated pairing of sleep-related cues with the physiology of wakefulness. Interestingly, the fourth P (conditioning) may resolve *after treatment discontinuation* in treatment responders to four to eight sessions, as evidenced by increased TST in the 3 to 24 months after CBT-I.[120-122] The observed increases in TST may occur as a result of the possibility that extinction of conditioned arousal takes time. It is also possible that it takes patients time to let go of sleep effort and/or for the patient to rebuild trust in the predictability of sleep (sleep self-efficacy). All of these possibilities notwithstanding, it is also possible that patients use what they have learned in CBT-I to engage in systematic sleep extension after treatment, and this self-experimentation allows for gradual increases in TST.

The Stimulus-Control Model

The stimulus-control model (SCM)[83-87] provides a theoretical basis for the importance of "the behavior tendency to stay in bed when awake and/or the engagement of nonsleep behaviors in the bedroom." In the original formulation of the SCM, the primary focus was on nonsleep behaviors in the sleep environment, which were viewed as weakening the association between sleep-related cues and sleep as a desired outcome. This constitutes "stimulus dyscontrol," and this problem was viewed as an instrumental phenomenon (a behavioral problem that could be modified with instruction and reinforced with the obtention of desired outcomes). In the original formulation of the SCM, being awake in the bedroom during the sleep period was not considered to be particularly unique; it was just one of many possible nonsleep behaviors. This said, there was (and is) a specific instruction dedicated to this problem: "If you find yourself unable to fall asleep, get up and go into another room." Clearly this instruction was intended to prevent the pairing of sleep-related stimuli with the physiology and experience of wakefulness and to promote the pairing of sleep-related stimuli with the physiology and experience of sleep. Conceived of this way, the SCM is also compatible with a classical conditioning point of view, and the treatment has, as a component, the counterconditioning of elicited wakefulness.

Finally, and not an explicit part of the SCM but highly related to Borbely's two process model,[126] is that being awake in bed and trying to sleep is particularly problematic because of the occurrence of microsleeps, which may interfere with sleep homeostasis. Thus being awake in bed is often perceived as continuous wakefulness without any of the benefits of continuous wakefulness. Such a scenario may help explain the wisdom of the stimulus control instruction "to leave the bedroom when awake." Such a maneuver not only prevents the pairing of the bed and bedroom with wakefulness, it also serves to prohibit microsleeps and allows sleep homeostasis to operate optimally.

Borbely's Two Process Model

Borbely's two process model[126] of sleep regulation stipulates that sleep timing, duration, and depth are governed by two processes, which may be aligned or misaligned and potentially function interactively: Process C (circadian regulation) and Process S (homeostatic regulation). For a full explanation of the model, see Chapter 38 of this volume. The two process model's relevance for insomnia is that sleep continuity disturbance may occur with dysregulation (or nonoptimal functioning) of either system. That is, initiating sleep or continuing sleep before or after one's biologically preferred sleep phase or without adequate homeostatic priming contributes to sleep continuity (and/or sleep architectural) disturbances. This being the case, assessment necessarily takes into account abnormalities within these domains; treatment delivery is often explained in these terms, and treatment itself (at least with CBT-I) is thought to exert its therapeutic effects by the systematic manipulation of these factors. Finally, we have suggested that the two-process model (and the potential interaction of the two systems) may be useful for garnering compliance with SCT. That is, we have long argued that being fully awake during the sleep period (when one is not biologically prepared to be awake) may not only prevent microsleeps, it may be associated with greater homeostatic priming. That is, during the day 1 hour of wake primes for a half-hour of sleep; during the sleep period, it may be the case that half an hour of wake primes for 1 hour of sleep. Sharing such information (as an anecdote) was and is thought to help patients comply with stimulus control instructions in this way: "If you get up and out of the bedroom, this will produce double the prime for better sleep." Although plied as a clinical truth, there is now preliminary evidence that Process S does indeed vary by time of day (60-minute intervals of wakefulness at night yield more delta power during subsequent sleep than 60-minute intervals of wakefulness during the day).[72]

CASE CONCEPTUALIZATION

As proposed at the outset of this chapter, assessment is for the purposes of determining if the patient has insomnia, if the insomnia warrants treatment (is severe and frequent, if not chronic), and if treatment may be complicated by other factors (unstable or stable medical and/or psychiatric comorbidities). Assessment also serves to determine whether there has been a treatment response (and, if not, what factors may account for this). Leaving aside for the moment the issue of ongoing evaluation regarding treatment response, the first step in the assessment process is to gather data, usually during an intake interview. The data sources include the patient's demographic information; the patient's summary of their sleep problem and clinical history; a review of the referral documents and/or the summary of the patient's last physical; electronic medical record (EMR) data regarding medical and psychiatric diagnoses and treatments; summary results from prior sleep evaluations (including PSG reports); and the obtention of standardized retrospective measures (e.g., a sleep disorder screener [the SDS-CL-25], the ISI, the ESS, medical and medication form, a medical symptoms checklist, and the PHQ-9 and GAD-7). Taken together, this information is used to conceptualize the case. Although there are many approaches to this (and even more approaches on how to lay out an assessment report), one approach is to describe the case based on the algorithm presented earlier. Please see Tables 208.4 and 208.5. Table 208.4 provides the clinical profile information. Table 208.5 illustrates how the clinical profile data may be used to assess whether CTB-I is indicated.

Table 208.4 Clinical Profile Data

Assessment	Clinical information (from clinical interview, questionnaires, medication forms, medical history forms, etc.)
Demographics	57-year-old white woman; middle school teacher (first shift +); married; two kids, one at home; husband on disability
Insomnia Profile	Bouts of insomnia for 25 years; worse in last 5 years
Bedtime/Wake Time	9:30–10 P.M./6:00 A.M. weekdays; 7:00–8:00 A.M. weekends
SL	Typically, 10–20 minutes
WASO	Typically, 1–2 awakenings; 20–120 minutes
EMA	3–4 nights/week; wakes 30–60 minutes early
Estimated TST	5.5–6 hours; occasionally 8–8.5 hours on weekends
TIB	8.5–10 hours
Estimated SE%	55%–75%
Daytime Consequences	Fatigue, irritability, increased anxiety, poor concentration; patient has occasional bouts of sleepiness when driving
Worry at Night	Reviews work day; worries about finances and marriage, the effects of insomnia on daytime function and long-term health
Sleep Habits (Bedroom)	Watches clock; reads in bed; tries to "empty her mind"; rarely gets out of bed; husband snores; morning light in bedroom
Sleep Habits (Daytime)	2–3 coffees before 3 P.M.; no exercise; 1 glass of wine with dinner; no food after 6–7 P.M.; denies napping but dozes on sofa
Medical Issues	Hypertension; perimenopausal (mild to moderate hot flashes 2–3 nights/week); headaches
Behavioral Health Issues	Depression diagnosed by her PCP; not in therapy
Sleep Medication	Alternates 5 mg of zolpidem with 3 mg of melatonin most nights
Other Medications	Losartan 50 mg (blood pressure); citalopram 20 mg; black cohosh (OTC for hot flashes); ibuprofen (headaches)
ISI	18 (0–28); 15 is clinically significant severity, some use a threshold of 10
ESS	10 (0–24); 10 is clinically significant severity, clinical judgment is required regarding treatment
PHQ-9	8 (0–27); 10 is clinically significant severity, clinical judgment is required regarding treatment
GAD-7	7 (0–21); 10 is clinically significant severity, clinical judgment is required regarding treatment
MEQ	55 (16–86); 16–41 = evening types, 42–58 = neither type, 59–86 = morning types
SDS-CL-25	Positive endorsements for insomnia, excessive daytime sleepiness, and dry mouth in the morning.

EMA, Early morning awakening; ESS, Epworth Sleepiness Scale; GAD-7, General Anxiety Disorder 7; ISI, Insomnia Severity Index; MEQ, Morningness-Eveningness Questionnaire; PHQ-9, Patient Health Questionnaire 9; SDS-CL-25, Sleep Disorders Symptom Checklist 25; SE%, sleep efficiency; SL, sleep latency; TIB, time in bed; TST, total sleep time; WASO, wake after sleep onset.

Table 208.5 Assessment of Appropriateness for CBT-I (per the algorithm in Figure 208.5)

Criteria	Yes/No	Details	3P/4P Factors
Maladaptive behaviors			
Sleep extension	Yes	Patient in bed up to 10 hr; mismatch of TIB and TST; (SE ≈72%)	Perpetuating
Circadian disruption	Yes	Time to bed (TTB) and time out of bed (TOB) highly variable	Perpetuating
Conditioned arousal	Yes	Patient dozes on sofa but awakens when entering bedroom	Perpetuating
Sleep effort	Yes	Patient "works at" emptying their mind and at relaxation at TTB	Perpetuating
Cognitive arousal	Yes	Patient worries about both short- and long-term sleep loss; watches clock; engages in safety behaviors (e.g., no caffeine late and no exercise).	Perpetuating
Poor sleep habits	Yes	Nightly alcohol; lack of physical activity; potential hunger at night *Note:* Poor sleep habits may also be thought of as creating a predisposition for insomnia without being the direct cause of the chronic insomnia	Perpetuating
Medical issues	Yes	Hypertension; perimenopause; hot flashes; headaches Depending on timing relative to the onset of acute and chronic insomnia, these issues may exist as contributing factors (precipitating or perpetuating factors). They are not contraindications for treatment (CBT-I). It is possible that, in the short term, these may worsen in severity, but in the long term, successful CBT-I may lessen the severity of these comorbid diagnoses.	Precipitating? Perpetuating?
Medications	Yes	Losartan, citalopram, black cohosh, ibuprofen Many antihypertension and antidepressant medications can be insomnogenic; black cohosh can cause headaches; ibuprofen can cause stomach discomfort. Depending on timing relative to the onset of acute and chronic insomnia, the use of these medications may exist as contributing factors (precipitating or perpetuating factors).	Precipitating? Perpetuating?
Diagnostic Issues			
Is severe enough to treat?	Yes	WASO and EMA ≥30 min more than 3 days per week for more than 3 months	n/a
Circadian dysrhythmia?	No		n/a
Does the patient have an undiagnosed illness?	Maybe	Patient has a level of sleepiness that is indicative of an intrinsic sleep diagnosis; potentially OSA given report of morning dry mouth. May warrant further testing. Patient's depression may warrant further evaluation.	Precipitating? Perpetuating?
If undiagnosed illness is resolved, will the insomnia remit?	No	If the patient has OSA (or other intrinsic sleep diagnoses), this may contribute to WASO, EMA, and sleepiness but does not fully account for the long amount of time the patient is awake at night. Further, the mismatch between sleep opportunity and ability and the occurrence of maladaptive behaviors clearly suggests that insomnia treatment is warranted.	Perpetuating?
Will the illness prevent the conduct of insomnia treatment (CBT-I)?	No	If present, OSA will not interfere with insomnia treatment, but may result in a worsening of the daytime sleepiness. This may require additional clinical management.	N/A
Will insomnia treatment make the OSA or depression worse?	Maybe	OSA. As noted earlier, insomnia treatment may worsen EDS. It is also possible that insomnia treatment may blunt the arousal responses that terminate apneic events. The available data suggest that, if present, the OSA is within the mild-to-moderate range. Some may elect to delay treatment until a sleep study can be performed. Some may elect to begin treatment while waiting for a sleep study. MDD. There is a fair amount of research to indicate that CBT-I at least does not exacerbate depression and that not treating insomnia can actually interfere with depression treatment outcomes.	N/A

CBT-I, Cognitive-behavioral therapy for insomnia; EDS, excessive daytime sleepiness; EMA, early morning awakening; MDD, major depressive disorder; OSA, obstructive sleep apnea; TIB, time in bed; TST, total sleep time; WASO, wake after sleep onset.

Case Example

A 57-year-old white woman (5′6″, 180 lb; BMI 29) who works as a middle school teacher (last 30 years). She has had several bouts of acute insomnia over the last 25 years (with stress); insomnia became chronic over the last 5 years. Her husband has been on disability for the last 6 years (is unable to work). There has been some marital strife. One daughter is in college, and one son is a sophomore in high school. The patient reports that "both are doing well." Clinical data are presented in Tables 208.4 and 208.5.

The patient profile in the tables includes (1) evidence of maladaptive behaviors (SE% below 85%, the tendency to stay in bed when awake and to engage in nonsleep behaviors in the bed/bedroom, with reports of sleep-related worry and effort); (2) an insomnia severity/frequency that is of sufficient magnitude as to warrant treatment (WASO and EMA are >30 minutes on >3 nights per week); and (3) little or no evidence of circadian rhythm disorder symptomatology. The patient exhibits some OSA signs on the SDS-CL-25 (BMI of 29, dry mouth, and frequent unexplained awakenings). In addition, the patient has several conditions for which she receives treatment (depression, hot flashes, and headaches). Effective treatment for these conditions has not produced a resolution of the insomnia. Accordingly, it is reasonable to conclude that the insomnia has evolved into a comorbid condition that is worthy of targeted treatment. If CBT-I is the treatment of choice, the next step in the process is for the patient to begin a prospective sleep assessment period. As is standard practice with CBT-I, this will include 1 to 3 weeks of prospective sampling of sleep continuity with sleep diaries and (ideally) weekly administrations of the ESS. This assessment (baseline for CBT-I) might also include weekly administrations of a single-disorder measure of OSA (e.g., STOP-BANG, Berlin Questionnaire, or MAPI) and/or the addition of OSA questions on the sleep diaries (at a minimum, a question regarding snoring). Collectively, these data may suggest that treatment be continued or delayed. In the case of continuing with CBT-I, this may require that the clinician implement a plan for the management of excessive sleepiness. In the case of delaying treatment, this may require that the clinician arrange, or refer, for additional testing, either in home (home sleep test [HST]) or in the laboratory (PSG).

CLINICAL PEARLS

In the final analysis, assessment of any clinical problem is only useful in that it provides a compass to show the relevant points of intervention required to bring about positive change. This is also true for the assessment and diagnosis of insomnia disorder. Art Spielman's behavioral model provides such a compass. To quote Dr. Spielman, "The factors that increase risk for insomnia and those that trigger the onset of an episode are typically not the same as factors that maintain the disorder once it is established. Even if predisposing factors cannot be readily altered and precipitating factors are never positively identified, substantial relief from insomnia may be attained by addressing perpetuating factors." Although possible predisposing and precipitating factors may solely account for transient bouts of acute insomnia, once the insomnia becomes chronic, it is almost certain that perpetuating factors are maintaining it. It cannot be understated that if perpetuating factors such as weakened sleep drive, circadian disruption, conditioned arousal, attention bias, and worry about sleep are present, they will require assessment. This then provides the clinician with a clear map to guide intervention strategies that can bring about strong and healthy sleep regulation and should promote good sleep continuity. This will be true regardless of any other comorbid disorders that may be present. Further, with good sleep, the patient's coping ability is likely to be enhanced, and this can have a beneficial impact on the treatment outcomes for the other comorbidities.

SUMMARY

As noted earlier, how one approaches assessment varies based on why the assessment is being conducted, and how this is done will vary greatly based on the clinician's preferred mode of treatment and based on their training and discipline. Ultimately, assessment and treatment in the context of insomnia occurs dialectically: "assessment is treatment and treatment is assessment." *Assessment is treatment* because self-monitoring with sleep diaries (particularly during baseline) often reveals to patients that their insomnia is less (or differently) frequent and/or severe than how they recalled and reported it on retrospective questionnaires. Patients often directly address this issue when they say, "Thanks for having me complete the sleep diaries, I am already better for having done them." It's not that the patient is better per se; it's that their perspective on their illness severity and frequency is informed by data as opposed to memory heuristics like saliency, primary, and/or recency. This, in and of itself, is therapeutic. *Treatment is assessment* because treatment response dictates how treatment is continued (this being especially the case for the titration aspect of SRT). Treatment is also assessment because it often unmasks occult issues.

In sum, insomnia may be one of the rare cases where the initial assessment is comprehensive, assessment occurs over an extended interval *prior to treatment,* and assessment continues for the duration of treatment. To our way of thinking, this represents a best form of evidence-based therapy—where assessment is conducted continuously and therapy is adjusted continuously based on systematically collected data.

SELECTED READINGS

Agnew S, Vallières A, Hamilton A, et al. Adherence to cognitive behavior therapy for insomnia: an updated systematic review. *Sleep Med Clin.* 2021;16(1):155–202.

Brasure M, Fuchs E, MacDonald R, et al. Psychological and behavioral interventions for managing insomnia disorder: an evidence report for a clinical practice guideline by the american college of physicians. *Ann Intern Med.* 2016;165(2):113–124. https://doi.org/10.7326/M15-1782.

Buysse DJ, Ancoli-Israel S, Edinger JD, Lichstein KL, Morin CM. Recommendations for a standard research assessment of insomnia. *Sleep.* 2006;29(9):1155–1173.

Carney CE, Buysse DJ, Ancoli-Israel S, et al. The consensus sleep diary: standardizing prospective sleep self-monitoring. *Sleep.* 2012;35(2):287–302.

Cheung JMY, Ji XW, Morin CM. Cognitive behavioral therapies for insomnia and hypnotic medications: considerations and controversies. *Sleep Med Clin.* 2019;14(2):253–265.

Edinger JD, Bonnet MH, Bootzin RR, et al. Derivation of research diagnostic criteria for insomnia: report of an American Academy of Sleep Medicine Work Group. *Sleep.* 2004;27(8):1567–1596.

Klingman KJ, Jungquist CR, Perlis ML. Questionnaires that screen for multiple sleep disorders. *Sleep Med Rev.* 2017;32:37–44.

Lichstein KLL, Durrence HHH, Taylor DJJ, Bush JJ, Riedel BWW, et al. Recommendations for a quantitative criteria for insomnia. *Behav Res Ther.* 2003;41(4):427–445. *Sleep.* 2006;29(9):1155–1173.

Lichstein KLL, Durrence HHH, Taylor DJJ, et al. Quantitative criteria for insomnia. *Behav Res Ther.* 2003;41(4):427–445.

Lineberger MD, Carney CE, Edinger JD, et al. Defining insomnia: quantitative criteria for insomnia severity and frequency. *Sleep.* 2006;29(4):479–485.

Morin CM, Belleville GG, Bélanger L, et al. The Insomnia Severity Index: psychometric indicators to detect insomnia cases and evaluate treatment response. *Sleep.* 2011;34(5):601–608.

Qaseem A, Kansagara D, Forciea MA, et al. Management of chronic insomnia disorder in adults: a clinical practice guideline from the American college of physicians.125–133.

Roth T, Drake C. Defining insomnia: the role of quantitative criteria. *Sleep.* 2006;29(4):424–425.

A complete reference list can be found online at ExpertConsult.com.

Chapter 209

Surveys, Sampling, and Polling Methods for Sleep and Public Health

Kristen L. Knutson

Chapter Highlights

- Because of sleep's ubiquitous effects on a wide range of health outcomes, assessing sleep in population-based studies has important implications for public health. Although objectively measured sleep would be ideal, in some circumstances self-reported information (e.g., surveys and polls) is warranted.
- Numerous survey instruments exist to assess various dimensions of sleep, including sleep quality, sleep disturbances, sleepiness, multidimensional sleep health, and sleep disorders. Many of these instruments are well validated and can be useful tools in population-based research.
- Designing a study or reviewing published work must include consideration of the sample on which the research is or will be based. Results obtained in one sample may not apply to other groups (i.e., may not be generalizable). Similarly, sleep survey instruments may have been developed and validated in a specific subgroup and may perform poorly in other groups.

INTRODUCTION

Inadequate sleep is associated with myriad health problems. Impairments range from poor performance and memory difficulties to mental health and mood disorders. Cardiovascular and metabolic compromise are also reported. Indeed, a recent report by the Institute of Medicine (IOM) stated that individuals suffering from sleep loss and/or sleep disorders are less productive and have increased health care utilization and an increased likelihood of accidents.[1] All of these consequences constitute important public health issues. The IOM further recognized this when they included the following as one of their 24 objectives for Healthy People 2020: "Increase the proportion of adults who get sufficient sleep."[2] Considering the broader health implications of good sleep health, we need to measure sleep in population-based studies to gauge sleep's contribution to public health, and we need to measure it as well as possible.

Although objective sleep assessment (e.g., polysomnography, home sleep tests, and/or actigraphy) is preferred, there will be times when subjective assessments are warranted. As such, a review of existing survey instruments will provide a guideline for identifying appropriate instruments.

Healthy sleep is multidimensional. It includes appropriate quantity of sleep, quality of sleep, and restorative sleep. The presence and treatment of a sleep disorder are also germane to evaluating sleep health. Finally, because sleep is partly controlled by the circadian system, chronotype assessment or sleep timing may be pertinent to understanding sleep health. This chapter reviews survey instruments designed to assess various domains of sleep health. There are, of course, many more sleep survey instruments and questionnaires than those described here. For additional reading about sleep survey instruments, see the work by Moul and colleagues[3] and Spruyt and Gozal.[4]

SURVEY INSTRUMENTS

A survey is typically an observational study of a specific population. It usually involves collecting data using questionnaires. Surveys can be quantitative or qualitative; only quantitative instruments are discussed. The selection of a survey instrument should be driven by the study objectives and its research questions. Furthermore, the degree to which an instrument has been validated and tested should be considered. Important characteristics of validity and reliability to consider are the following:

- *Construct validity:* Assesses how well an instrument measures what it claims to measure
- *Convergent validity:* Assesses whether constructs that are expected to be associated are actually associated
- *Test-retest reliability:* A measure of how consistent scores are across a period of time when the construct being measured is expected to remain the same
- *Internal consistency* (or internal reliability): The degree of consistency of responses across the items on a multiple-item instruments. The *Cronbach's alpha* statistic is commonly used to evaluate internal consistency. (Higher values indicate greater internal consistency.)

There are several validated survey instruments for assessing one or more dimensions of sleep. One major advantage of using a questionnaire or poll is, of course, that it is inexpensive and easily administered. This makes it possible to collect information from larger numbers of individuals, particularly compared to PSG and actigraphy. However, there are some limitations to acknowledge.

First, self-reported measures are prone to measurement error, which is a particular concern if one's interest is in a physiologic process rather than the subjective experience (e.g., number of awakenings, presence of apnea versus sleep satisfaction). For example, in a sample of middle-aged Americans, the correlation between self-reported sleep duration and actigraphically estimated sleep duration was 0.47, which indicates only a moderate association.[5]

Second, these instruments are typically developed and validated in specific samples (e.g., English-speaking White adults from the United States) and may not work as well in other cultures or languages. If possible, the investigators should test the validity of the instrument in their population of interest. Nonetheless, survey instruments can be a useful tool for estimating sleep characteristics, particularly in larger studies in which more objective measures may not be feasible.

Survey questions and instruments have been used to estimate sleep duration, sleep quality, sleep health, chronotype, and sleep disorders. Specific instruments within each category are described later. Tables 209.1 to 209.3 summarize the instruments discussed in this chapter.

SELF-REPORTED SLEEP DURATION

Numerous observational studies have assessed "habitual sleep duration"; however, the question (or questions) used to estimate sleep duration vary. First, some questions have asked about sleep duration "per night," while others asked about sleep duration "per 24 hours." The distinction is particularly important for populations in which napping is a common practice or among those who do not have a single consolidated sleep period or an atypical sleep-wake routine (e.g., shift workers). Therefore studies of these populations should include either a question asking about sleep per 24 hours or a separate question asking about daytime sleep episodes. A second consideration is that sleep duration can vary between work, nonwork, or school days.[6] Separate questions about sleep duration on free days and non-free days will help to assess this variability.

A final important issue is how to ask about sleep duration. One option is to simply ask the respondents how much sleep they get, such as, "How many hours of sleep do you get at night on workdays?" This type of question requires respondents to calculate their estimated amount of sleep. This assumes individuals can accurately guess how much sleep they get. The estimate's accuracy will also be influenced by the individual's sleep routine consistency; that is, whether it varies significantly or it is fairly regular. The alternative is to ask about bedtimes and arising times. The usual bedtime and wake time may require less estimation and calculation and therefore reduce the cognitive burden on the respondent. The interviewer can then calculate the duration of this interval. The limitation is, of course, that time in bed is not equivalent to actual sleep, and if someone has poor sleep quality, this method may overestimate their sleep duration.

Interestingly, a review of studies that examined the association between self-reported sleep duration and mortality risk found that U-shaped associations between sleep duration and mortality were observed only when the question asked the respondent to estimate sleep duration and that no study that used the interval between bedtime and wake time observed a U-shaped association.[7] This suggests that some bias may exist in how people respond to the different types of questions, and the authors suggested that there may be a normative answer to the duration-based question that does not exist for the time-based question. Thus investigators planning to use a self-reported sleep duration question should consider these different issues when deciding on the question wording. Unfortunately, no consensus among sleep researchers on how best to collect self-reported sleep duration has been established.

SLEEP QUALITY/SLEEP DISTURBANCE/SLEEP-RELATED IMPAIRMENT

Pittsburgh Sleep Quality Index

One commonly used survey instrument is the Pittsburgh Sleep Quality Index (PSQI), which measures subjective sleep quality. It asks respondents to consider their sleep for the past month and includes 19 questions, from which 7 component scores are calculated and summed into a global score.[8] The component scores range from 0 to 3, and the global score ranges from 0 to 21; higher scores indicate worse sleep quality. The 7 components are subjective sleep quality, sleep latency, sleep duration, habitual sleep efficiency, sleep disturbances, use of a sleep medication, and daytime dysfunction. The questionnaire also includes a question about the presence of a bed partner and whether this partner has told the respondent that the respondent snores, pauses between breaths whiles asleep, twitches or jerks the legs while sleeping, or has episodes of disorientation or confusion during sleep. These questions are not included in the global score but may suggest the presence of a sleep disorder such as obstructive sleep apnea or restless legs syndrome.

The PSQI was initially validated by comparing component and global scores between healthy subjects, patients with sleep disorders, and patients with depression.[8] Both the component scores and individual items demonstrated high internal consistency (Cronbach's alpha = 0.83 for both). The within-subject reliability of the PSQI was examined among 91 subjects who completed the PSQI on two occasions, 28 days apart on average. The Pearson's correlation coefficient for the global score was 0.85, and correlations for the component scores ranged from 0.65 to 0.84.[8] Another study examined test-retest reliability in a sample of 76 individuals with insomnia over a period of 2 days to several weeks and observed a correlation of 0.87 for the global score.[9] In a third study, the PSQI was completed twice approximately 1 year apart by 610 middle-aged adults in the United States.[10] The Pearson's correlation coefficient for the PSQI score was 0.68. Thus the PSQI is a validated and reliable questionnaire to estimate subjective sleep quality.

The PSQI was developed in English; however, it has been translated into at least 16 languages: Arabic,[11] Chinese,[12] French,[13] Greek,[14] Hebrew,[15] Italian,[16] Japanese,[17] Korean,[18] Persian,[19] Portuguese (Brazil),[20] Spanish (Colombia),[21] Spanish (Mexico),[22] Spanish (Spain),[23] Taiwanese,[24] Thai,[25] Urdu,[26] and Serbian.[27]

Patient-Reported Outcomes Measurement Information System

Patient-reported outcomes (PRO) are important to assess well-being from the patient perspective and to improve assessments of PRO. The Patient-Reported Outcomes Measurement Information System (PROMIS) was developed through a National Institutes of Health initiative to provide a variety of health-related instruments.[28] The PROMIS instruments include two items focused on sleep, specifically, sleep disturbances (SD) and sleep-related impairment (SRI).

Table 209.1 Brief Overview of Selected Survey Instruments That Assess Sleep

Domain	Instrument	Item Number	Reference Period	Scoring and Interpretation
Sleep quality	Pittsburgh Sleep Quality Index (PSQI)	19	1 month	7 component scores summed to provide global score. Higher scores = worse sleep quality
Sleep disturbance	PROMIS Sleep Disturbance	Full: 27 Short: 8	7 days	Scoring of PROMIS involves conversion to a T-score based on the US population. Higher scores = greater disturbance or impairment
Sleep-related impairment	PROMIS Sleep-Related Impairment	Full: 16 Short: 8	7 days	See above
Sleepiness	Epworth Sleepiness Scale	8	"Recent times"	Answers are summed. Higher scores = greater sleepiness
Sleep health	RU-SATED	5	Indefinite	Responses are summed. Higher scores = better sleep health
	Sleep Health Index	14	7 days	Scoring algorithm is accessed through the National Sleep Foundation. Higher scores = better sleep health
Circadian preference or chronotype	Morningness-Eveningness questionnaire	19	Indefinite	Response values are summed. Higher values indicate greater eveningness
	Munich Chronotype Questionnaire	24	Indefinite	One score involves calculating the midpoint of the sleep period on free days
	μMunich	6	Indefinite	One score involves calculating the midpoint of the sleep period on free days

Table 209.2 Sleep Disorder Screening Instruments

Domain	Instrument	Item Number	Reference Period	Scoring and Interpretation
OSA	Berlin Questionnaire	12	Indefinite	3 components; positive in 2 or 3 = high likelihood of apnea
	STOP-BANG questionnaire	8	Indefinite	Yes to 2 of the first 4 indicate high likelihood of having OSA; more "yes" responses to last 4 = greater severity
Insomnia	Insomnia Severity Index	7	2 weeks	Response values are summed. Higher values indicate greater insomnia severity
	Insomnia Symptom Questionnaire	13	1 month	Presence of insomnia disorder is based on reporting frequent symptoms lasting at least 4 weeks with at least one daytime consequence

Table 209.3 Pediatric Questionnaires

Instrument	Item Number	Reference Period	Scoring and Interpretation
Pediatric PROMIS Sleep Disturbance	15	7 days	Scoring of PROMIS involves conversion to a T-score based on the US population. Higher scores = greater disturbance or impairment
Pediatric PROMIS Sleep-related impairment	13	7 days	See above
Sleep Disturbance Scale for Children (SDSC)	26	6 months	Response values are summed. Higher scores = greater severity
Children's Sleep Habits Questionnaire	45	"Typical" recent week	Total score and 8 component scores

The questions on both the SD and SRI PROMIS instruments ask respondents to rate aspects of sleep over the past 7 days. These questions therefore avoid asking them to calculate amounts or report times, nor do they assess symptoms of any specific sleep disorder.[29,30] The full SD instrument has 27 items, and the full SRI instrument has 16 items. These instruments can be administered via computerized adaptive testing (CAT), which adapts to the responses provided; therefore the instrument is unique to the person based on severity of sleep disturbances or impairment. Scoring can be automated when using the CAT, and scores are converted into a T-score, which is referenced to the US general population.[28] Higher scores on either instrument indicate greater sleep disturbance or greater sleep-related impairment.

The SD and SRI PROMIS instruments were developed using rigorous methodology by a team of experts who developed a large pool of questions and used a variety of established techniques to reduce the number of items and perform tests of validity.[29] Convergent validity was supported by correlations between the SD or SRI score and scores from other sleep questionnaires (PSQI, ESS).[29] Construct validity was assessed and supported by comparing scores between a group with sleep disorders who had greater SRI and SD scores than a group without sleep disorders.[29]

An eight-item fixed version of each instrument has also been tested.[30] The correlation between these short forms and the full instrument was very high (>0.95), suggesting the short form is valid to use. Convergent validity for the full and eight-item instruments was examined by comparing these scores to the PSQI and the ESS, and high correlations between these instruments indicated convergent validity of the PROMIS instruments.[30] Construct validity of the eight-item version was also tested by comparing scores between those who had reported a sleep disorder and those who had not, and because scores were higher in the sleep disorder group, the PROMIS instruments appear to have construct validity as well.[30] A six-item version for the SD scale was also validated in an older adult sample (>65 years of age), and internal consistency was high (Cronbach's alpha = 0.86); the PROMIS SD score was significantly associated with other health measures, such as depression, stress, and quality of life.[31]

Translations for the PROMIS sleep disturbance instrument are available in Dutch-Flemish[32] and Portuguese (Brazil).[33]

Epworth Sleepiness Scale

The Epworth Sleepiness Scale (ESS) measures general level of daytime sleepiness using eight questions. Each question asks respondents to indicate the likelihood that they would fall asleep in a specific situation, on a four-point scale ranging from "no chance" to "high chance." The instrument is meant for adult populations. The scores range from 0 to 24, and higher scores indicate greater sleepiness.[34] The ESS has been used in a wide variety of studies, ranging from daytime sleepiness in medical interns[35] to daytime sleepiness in patients with multiple sclerosis.[36] Interestingly, it was also a main outcome measure in research examining the effects of didgeridoo playing in patients with moderate obstructive sleep apnea.[37]

The ESS has undergone validation tests. For example, a test-retest reliability analysis of the ESS was conducted in 87 medical students using a 5-month interval; the Pearson's correlation was 0.82.[38] In a study of more than 600 middle-aged US adults, the Pearson's correlation between the ESS scores collected approximately 1 year apart was 0.76. It is important to note that the situations described in these questions may not be applicable to all communities. For example, one question asks the likelihood of falling asleep "in a car, while stopped for a few minutes in traffic." Obviously, people living in communities without traffic, or even cars, would not be able to answer this question. Thus, although this questionnaire is widely used, it will not be appropriate for every research locale.

The ESS has been translated into at least 19 languages: Arabic,[39] Chinese,[40,41] Croatian,[42] German,[43] Greek,[44] Iranian,[45] Italian,[46] Japanese,[47] Korean,[48] Norwegian,[49] Portuguese (Brazil),[50] Serbian,[51] Spanish (Colombia),[52] Spanish (Mexico),[53] Spanish (Peru),[54] Spanish (Spain),[55,56] Thai,[57] Turkish,[58] and Urdu.[59]

Sleep Health Instruments

As previously mentioned, sleep health is multidimensional and is more than simply the absence of a sleep disorder. Sleep health can comprise sleep quality, sleep duration, sleep disturbances, and feelings of restoration after sleep (among other possible dimensions). At least two instruments have been designed to include multiple dimension of sleep: RU SATED and the Sleep Health Index (SHI).

SATED Scale

Daniel Buysse[60] argued for the importance of including multiple dimensions of sleep to assess sleep health. He initially proposed the SATED scale, which assesses five key dimensions of sleep health: Satisfaction with sleep; Alertness during wake; Timing of sleep; sleep Efficiency; and sleep Duration.[60] He proposed one question for each domain with three possible responses: rarely/never, sometimes, usually/always. Responses are summed, and scores can range from 0 (poor sleep health) to 10 (good sleep health). This was later changed to "RU-SATED" to add RegUlarity of sleep to the construct. A recent validation study reported that Cronbach's alpha was 0.64, and the average interitem correlation was 0.22,[61] which suggests moderate internal consistency. The RU-SATED score was significantly correlated with self-rated sleep as well as the Insomnia Severity Index, which is evidence for convergent validity.[61]

Sleep Health Index

The SHI was developed by a task force of the National Sleep Foundation (NSF). The NSF established a task force of sleep and survey experts, who initially identified seven different domains and developed questions to address these different domains. A 28-question survey was administered via random-sample phone interviews to nationally representative samples of adults in 2014 (n = 1253) and 2015 (n = 1250).[62] Data from these surveys were combined, and the SHI was created using factor analysis to identify the final 14 questions. The factor analysis also revealed that these questions resulted in three discrete domains, termed sleep quality, sleep duration, and disordered sleep. Thus, although seven domains were initially identified by the task force, the post-hoc factor analysis revealed only three. The questions within each of these domains were combined to form subindices, then the subindices were combined to form the overall SHI with scores ranging from 0 to 100 (higher scores reflect better sleep health).

The validation of the SHI included both tests of internal consistency as well as construct validity. The Cronbach's alpha indicated high levels of internal consistency, 0.75, and for the three subindices the Cronbach's alpha ranged from 0.63 for both disordered sleep and sleep duration to 0.77 for sleep quality.[62] Construct validity of the SHI was assessed by evaluating correlations between the SHI and measures that theoretically should be correlated with sleep health. Construct validity is supported because the SHI was significantly correlated with subjective overall health (r = 0.38), stress (r = –0.37), and life satisfaction (r = 0.36).

Circadian Preference and Chronotype

Sleep is largely regulated by circadian rhythms; consequently, circadian preference and chronotype are important constructs estimable using questionnaires. Circadian preference generally refers to the time of day a person "feels at their best" or prefers to perform certain activities. Chronotype is a term used to represent circadian phase; it is roughly the time at which one's internal clock is set. A gold standard measure of circadian phase is the dim light melatonin onset (DLMO) that determines the time melatonin levels start to rise. Individuals who have later chronotypes will have levels of melatonin that rise later in the day. Of course, measuring the DLMO is challenging in large studies outside the laboratory. In this section, we discuss two instruments: the Morning/Evening questionnaire (MEQ) and the Munich Chronotype Questionnaire (MCTQ). This construct is meant to represent endogenous circadian rhythms with the assumption that individuals with delayed rhythms will also have a later circadian preference.

Morning/Evening Questionnaire

The MEQ was developed to estimate circadian preference (sometimes also known as the "Owl Lark" questionnaire).[63] This 19-item instrument asks the respondents about the time of day they would prefer to wake up, go to bed, exercise, or work, as well as how they feel after waking or in the evening. Scores range from 16 to 86, and lower scores indicate greater eveningness (i.e., prefer evenings or "owls"). Scores can also be grouped into categories: definitely morning types (70 to 86 points), moderately morning types (59 to 69 points), neither type (42 to 58 points), moderately evening type (31 to 41 points), and definitely evening types (16 to 30 points). In the original validation paper,[63] the authors compared the questionnaire to oral temperature values taken across the day for 3 weeks in 48 participants aged 18 to 32 years. They found that individuals identified as "early types" on the questionnaire had an earlier peak oral temperature, which suggests the questionnaire is capturing a measure of endogenous circadian rhythms. A more recent study validated the MEQ in a sample of 566 middle-aged workers (no shift work).[64] They observed fewer extreme evening types than the original younger cohort and proposed alternative cut-off scores: morning type (65 to 86 points), neither (53 to 64), evening type (16 to 52 points). They did not change the questions nor the scoring method. In this middle-aged sample, the evening types went to bed and woke later based on sleep diaries, supporting the validity of the construct. A reduced version of the MEQ that includes only 5 items from the original MEQ has been developed and validated against the full MEQ.[65] The MEQ has been translated into Arabic (reduced version),[66] Chinese,[67] Japanese,[68] Korean,[69] Polish (reduced version),[70] German (reduced version),[71] Portuguese (Brazil),[72] and Turkish.[73]

Munich Chronotype Questionnaire

The Munich Chronotype Questionnaire (MCTQ) was developed to assess chronotype based on actual behavior and distinguishes free days from work/school days.[6,74] The MCTQ has approximately 24 items (excluding demographic questions) and asks respondents to report their usual wake time, bedtime, afternoon "dip" time, alarm reliance, and sleep latency and napping on workdays and free days separately. The MCTQ also asks questions related to light and light exposure. One way to score the MCTQ is to calculate the midpoint of sleep on free days (MSF), which is calculated as the midpoint between sleep onset (bedtime + time to fall asleep) and wake-up time on free days.[6] The midpoint is often also corrected for sleep debt on weekdays (MSFsc), since this debt would lead to sleep extension on the weekends.[74]

In the initial pilot study to develop the MCTQ, the investigators collected 5 weeks of sleep diaries; sleep times correlated strongly with the times reported on the MCTQ, which supports the validity of these questions.[6] Using a large internet survey, the convergent validity of the MCTQ was examined in more than 2481 Dutch adults who completed both the MCTQ and the MEQ, and the MEQ score and the MSF were highly correlated.[75] Thus far, the MCTQ has been translated into Korean[76] and Japanese.[77]

The distinction between the MEQ and the MCTQ is that the MCTQ focuses on actual behavior, whereas the MEQ asks about preferred behavior, although the two measures are correlated. This distinction may be particularly important in situations in which external demands do not allow people to sleep and wake at the times they prefer, which may result in sleep loss. The timing of sleep and one's chronotype may be associated with health outcomes independently of sleep duration and quality.[78,79]

Recently, a short version of the MCTQ was developed and tested, which includes only six essential questions.[80] This shortened version, the μMCTQ, asks whether any shift work or night work was performed in the last 3 months and asks the number of days per week the respondent typically works. The other four questions ask about bedtimes and wake times on workdays and free days separately. Validation tests demonstrated good test-retest reliability and correlated well with both the MSF calculated from the full instrument as well as some phase markers from actimetry and melatonin.[80] Thus this shorter version will be easier to administer and provide valid estimates of chronotype.

SLEEP DISORDER SCREENING INSTRUMENTS

In certain situations, it may be necessary to estimate or identify the likelihood that someone has a sleep disorder. These instruments are not diagnostic by themselves, but they can help in screening and case finding. Survey instruments assessing sleep apnea and insomnia are briefly described because these disorders occur with a high prevalence in the population. There are, of course, screening instruments available for clinical use that include more than these two sleep disorders (for example, the Sleep Disorders Questionnaire[81]).

Obstructive Sleep Apnea

Two questionnaires are discussed here that are designed to estimate likelihood of having obstructive sleep apnea (OSA): The Berlin Questionnaire (BQ) and the STOP-BANG questionnaire.

The BQ estimates risk of having OSA and is commonly used.[82] The BQ includes 12 items that examine three components: (1) persistent symptoms of snoring, (2) persistent daytime symptoms, and (3) high blood pressure or obesity. A high risk of sleep apnea is defined by the presence of any two of the three components. Respondents are considered to have persistent snoring symptoms if they indicate two of the three following conditions: (1) snored three or more times per week, (2) snoring was louder than talking or very loud; (3) experienced breathing pauses three or more times per week. Respondents are considered to have persistent daytime sleepiness if they indicate two of three following conditions: (1) were tired after sleeping three or more times per week; (2) were tired during wake time three or more times per week; (3) have fallen asleep while driving.

The initial validation of this instrument was conducted among 744 patients in primary care settings; 279 (37.5%) were identified as being at high risk of OSA. For the subset (n = 100) who had sleep testing, the BQ risk group was significantly associated with the respiratory disturbance index (RDI). Using a cut-off of an RDI of more than 5 events per hour, the sensitivity of the BQ was 0.86 and specificity was 0.77.[82] Two other studies examined the performance of the BQ in a sample of patients suspected of having sleep apnea and did not observe adequate sensitivity and specificity.[83,84] Predictive accuracy of BQ improved when it was combined with the ESS.[83] Thus, in people already suspected of OSA, the BQ does not appear to be a valid screening tool. The BQ has been translated into six languages: Arabic,[85] Greek,[86] Persian,[87] Portuguese (Portugal),[88] Serbian,[89] and Thai.[90]

The STOP-BANG questionnaire has eight yes/no questions corresponding to the acronym: S (snore) = Do you snore loudly?; T (tired) = Do you often feel tired, fatigued, or sleepy during the daytime?; O (observed) = Has anyone observed you stop breathing or choking/gasping during your sleep?; P (pressure) = Do you have or are being treated for high blood pressure?; B (BMI) = Body mass index more than 35 kg/m^2?; A (age) = Are you 50 years old or older?; N (neck) = Is your shirt collar 16 inches/40 centimeters or larger? G (gender) = Are you a male?

People who answer "yes" to two or more questions on the STOP portion are considered to be at risk of having OSA. The more "yes" responses on the BANG portion indicates a greater likelihood of having moderate to severe obstructive sleep apnea. This instrument was initially developed for use in preoperative surgical clinics[91]; however, in a sample of obese subjects a STOP-BANG score of 4 had high sensitivity (88%) for identifying severe OSA, while a score of 6 had higher specificity (85.2%).[92]

One study compared the performance of the BQ, the STOP-BANG, and the STOP questions only in a sample from a sleep clinic. Participants were individuals referred on suspicion of a sleep disorder; therefore this was not a community-based sample. They found that STOP-BANG had the highest sensitivity (97.6%) but the lowest specificity (12.7%), while the BQ had good sensitivity (87%) and modest specificity (33%), although it was better than STOP (13%) and STOP-BANG (12.7%).[93] Combining the questionnaires did not improve their performance. The STOP-BANG questionnaire has been translated into Arabic,[94] Bahasa Malaysia,[95] Chinese,[96] Croatian (STOP only),[42] Danish,[97] Persian,[98] Portuguese (Brazil),[99] Portuguese (Portugal),[100] Serbian,[101] Thai,[102] and Urdu.[103]

Insomnia

There are several instruments to assess insomnia symptoms or the severity of insomnia. In this chapter, we discuss two: the Insomnia Severity Index and the Insomnia Symptom Questionnaire. For a larger review of instruments relevant to insomnia see the work by Moul and colleagues.[3]

The Insomnia Severity Index is a seven-item questionnaire for insomnia screening. It is also used as an outcome measure to assess treatment efficacy.[104] Respondents rate the severity of the symptoms, difficulty falling asleep, difficulty staying asleep, and problem waking too early over the prior 2 weeks. They also indicate their satisfaction with their current sleep patterns, the extent to which the sleep problem interferes with daily functioning, how noticeable they think their sleep problem is to others, and how worried they are about their sleep problem. The responses to all these questions are on a five-point Likert scale, and responses are summed for a final score that corresponds to four categories: no clinically significant insomnia, subthreshold insomnia, clinical insomnia (moderate), and clinical insomnia (severe). This instrument has demonstrated reasonable reliability and validity to detect cases of insomnia in the population and has been shown to be sensitive to treatment effects in patient samples.[105] The Insomnia Severity Index has been translated into Arabic,[106] Chinese,[107] German,[108] Hindi,[109] Italian,[110] Korean,[102] and Persian.[111,112]

The Insomnia Symptom Questionnaire has 13 items that evaluate insomnia symptoms based on clinical criteria. Content validity is high because the questions were derived from widely accepted criteria, including the DSM-IV.[113] Three questions are used to determine the presence, frequency, and duration of the sleep symptoms, and eight questions are used to identify daytime consequences of the sleep complaint. If the symptom is frequent, it lasted 4 weeks or more, and there is at least one daytime consequence, the respondent is considered to have insomnia disorder. The internal consistency of the instrument was also high (Cronbach's alpha = 0.89). This instrument has good specificity (>90%), which suggests that this instrument is likely to correctly identify those without insomnia.[113] At this time we know of no published translation of the Insomnia Symptom Questionnaire.

Pediatric Sleep Questionnaires

Most of the survey instruments described previously were developed and validated for use in adult populations. One exception is the pediatric versions of the PROMIS SD and SRI instruments.[114] These instruments were developed in a similar manner. They drew items from a pool of questions previously validated for content, which were then subjected to psychometric evaluation and analyses to produce the final instruments.[114] The Pediatric SD instrument includes 15 items, and the SRI instrument includes 13 items. There are parent-proxy versions for children aged 5 to 17 years as well as child self-report versions for children aged 8 to 17 years. These instruments use a 7-day recall period and frequency-based responses (i.e., never, almost never, sometimes, almost always, or always). Shorter fixed-item versions are available that include only four or eight times. Construct validity was examined and supported by comparing the PROMIS scores to other measures of health and fatigue.[114]

There are several other pediatric sleep instruments with varying degrees of validation. Spruyt and Gozal published a review of these instruments.[4] One questionnaire that was developed and well validated is the Sleep Disturbance Scale for Children (SDSC).[115] This 26-item instrument was developed to identify sleep disorders in children by asking about sleep disturbances and behavior over the past 6 months. Each response has a 1 to 5 scale, and the final score is a sum; higher scores indicated greater severity. It was tested in a sample of healthy children and a sample of children referred to a sleep clinic. Internal consistency was acceptable (Cronbach's alpha = 0.79), and scores were significantly different between the two groups, suggesting the instrument can distinguish healthy children from clinical groups.[115] The SDSC instrument has been translated into Portuguese (Brazil),[116] Persian,[117] Chinese,[118] and French.[119]

Another pediatric questionnaire is the Children's Sleep Habits Questionnaire, developed to identify both behaviorally based and medically based sleep problems in school-aged children.[120] This 45-item questionnaire is completed by a parent or guardian and yields both a total score and eight subscale scores. The subscales include bedtime resistance, sleep duration, parasomnias, sleep-disordered breathing, night awakenings, daytime sleepiness, and sleep-onset delay. Psychometric analysis demonstrated reasonable internal consistency and test-retest reliability.[120] The Children's Sleep Habits Questionnaire has been translated into Hebrew,[121] German,[122] Dutch,[123] Portuguese (Brazil),[124] Persian,[125] and Spanish.[126]

SAMPLING AND POLLING METHODS

Researchers and clinicians should pay careful attention to sampling methods when evaluating published literature or when designing a new study. With the exception of the census, most studies only include a sample meant to represent the study's target population; that is, the group who is the focus of the research question. One must carefully consider the sample size, refusal rate, and method for obtaining the study sample. These factors will determine whether results are generalizable to the target population. Further, many studies are not targeting the entire population but rather a specific subset (e.g., adults over 65 years of age; people with hypertension) and therefore may not be generalizable to other populations, including the general public. Factors to consider include the demographics of the sample, such as gender, age, race/ethnicity, and socioeconomic status, as well as other inclusion criteria that may limit generalizability, such as existing health conditions or medication use. The method of sampling could also influence the generalizability of the sample to the population. Ideally, participants should be selected randomly from a list of members of the population; however, it is often difficult to use this method, particularly when a full list of a population is not available. A random sample is the best method for estimating prevalence because it avoids selection bias. In addition, even if a random group of individuals are selected and invited to participate, not everyone will agree; therefore low response rates could affect the representativeness of the sample. Volunteer samples are commonly used in research studies, but because the volunteers are not randomly selected, their willingness or availability to participate in the study may influence or bias the sample's representativeness. Error in sampling does not necessarily negate any findings from these studies, but interpretation should take this into account. Designing a new study should involve paying attention to sampling strategies and developing detailed recruitment plans.

When information is collected through interview, as in a poll, other factors require consideration. Additional methods that should be included when designing a poll or survey include ensuring that the question format and responses match the concepts being measured and pretesting instruments and procedures before their use in the main study.[127] Most of the surveys described previously tested construct validity to determine if the survey met this goal. All interviewers should be carefully trained not only on the instruments and procedures but also on the subject matter. An understanding of sleep health will improve the interviewers' ability to administer sleep-related survey instruments. Finally, transparency is a key aspect of well-designed and conducted polls and surveys. Disclosure of all the methods used in the survey will allow for better evaluation and replication.[127] The American Association for Public Opinion Research provides more details and guidance.[127]

CLINICAL PEARLS

- There are several validated survey instruments to assess multiple dimensions of sleep that can be used when objective measures are not possible.
- Clinicians or researchers who are interested in using surveys to assess sleep can select from instruments that assess sleep quality, sleep disturbances, or multidimensional sleep health or screen for sleep disorders.
- The limitations of self-reported assessments, as well as how samples were derived, should be considered. However, surveys can still be useful tools to better understand sleep and health.

SUMMARY

Healthy sleep is vital for overall health and well-being. It is therefore important to assess sleep in population-based studies, smaller scale studies, and in the clinic. Although objective sleep measures are often preferred, they are sometimes neither feasible nor adequate. Several well-validated instruments exist that are designed to assess various aspects of sleep. A sample of such instruments are described in this chapter.

SELECTED READINGS

Buysse DJ. Sleep health: can we define it? Does it matter? *Sleep*. 2014;37:9–17.

Chung F, Yang Y, Liao P. Predictive performance of the STOP-Bang score for identifying obstructive sleep apnea in obese patients. *Obes Surg*. 2013;23:2050–2057.

Forrest CB, Meltzer LJ, Marcus CL, et al. Development and validation of the PROMIS pediatric sleep disturbance and sleep-related impairment item banks. *Sleep*. 2018;41.

Horne JA, Ostberg O. The Owl and Lark questionnaire. *Int J Chronobiol*. 1976;4:97–110.

Knutson KL, Phelan J, Paskow MJ, et al. The National Sleep Foundation's sleep health index. *Sleep Health*. 2017;3:234–240.

Owens JA, Spirito A, McGuinn M. The Children's Sleep Habits Questionnaire (CSHQ): psychometric properties of a survey instrument for school-aged children. *Sleep*. 2000;23:1043–1051.

Roenneberg T, Kuehnle T, Juda M, et al. Epidemiology of the human circadian clock. *Sleep Med Rev*. 2007;11:429–438.

A complete reference list can be found online at ExpertConsult.com.

Chapter 210

Techniques for Clinical Assessment of Circadian Rhythm Disorders

Kathryn J. Reid; Phyllis C. Zee

Chapter Highlights

- The evaluation of circadian phase is a key feature of the International Classification of Sleep Disorders criteria for diagnosis of circadian rhythm sleep-wake disorders (CRSWDs).
- Assessment of sleep-wake activity patterns for a minimum of 7 days and, preferably, more than 14 days is recommended for clinical assessment of CRSWDs using a sleep log or wrist actigraphy.
- Measuring the pattern and intensity of light exposure over 7 to 14 days (with wrist actigraphy or a similar device) is helpful to refine strategies for light-seeking and -avoidance interventions.
- The timing of melatonin secretion onset is a useful marker of the endogenous phase of circadian rhythms and aids in the appropriate timing of circadian-based treatments.

INTRODUCTION

The sleep-wake cycle is one of the most prominent circadian rhythms, with daily sleep-wake patterns influenced on a physiologic level by an interaction between homeostatic and circadian processes[1] and behaviorally by daily activities such as work or school. Disruption of the alignment between the internal circadian clock and the external environment is the source of most circadian rhythm sleep-wake disorders (CRSWDs) (see Chapter 43). Therefore in addition to a detailed clinical and sleep history, assessment of the timing of sleep-wake patterns, either with a sleep log and/or actigraphy (in conjunction with a sleep log), is required for the diagnosis of most CRSWDs. Confirmation of a delayed, advanced, or nonentrained circadian phase by techniques such as the measurement of dim light melatonin onset (DLMO) is also suggested to aid in the appropriate timing of circadian-based treatments.

Accurate assessment of the internal circadian clock is difficult in the clinical setting, as many of the downstream outputs of the circadian clock (rest activity, core body temperature) that we are able to measure in humans are influenced by our usual daily activities such as light-dark exposure, eating, and physical activity. These external influences are often referred to as *zeitgebers*, or *time givers*. Therefore to measure circadian rhythms, sophisticated protocols have been developed that limit the impact of these external zeitgebers—these include forced desynchrony, constant routine, or ultrashort sleep-wake protocols.[2-4] These types of protocols have limited utility in the clinical setting.

Several key terms are used to describe the circadian system. These include phase, amplitude, period length (tau), and entrainment, and they are defined as follows:

- Phase: the timing of a reference point in the cycle (e.g., the peak) relative to a fixed event (e.g., beginning of the night)
- Amplitude: the difference between the peak and trough of the circadian rhythm
- Period (tau): the time interval between phase reference points (e.g., peak to peak)
- Entrainment: a term used to describe the synchronization or alignment of the internal circadian clock rhythm, including its phase and period, to external time cues, such as the natural dark-light cycle.

Light is the strongest zeitgeber or entraining agent for the circadian system. The response of the circadian system to light at various biologic times can be quantified using a phase response curve (PRC). The PRC for light in humans indicates that light exposure prior to the core body temperature minimum (CBTm) results in phase delays (shifts the clock later) and light after the CBTm results in phase advances (shift the clock earlier).[5,6]

Circadian rhythm disturbance is not only relevant to CRSWDs but also to other medical conditions, mood disorders, cognitive function, and general well-being.[7] There is now mounting evidence to indicate that disturbance of central and peripheral circadian rhythms can precede or be a consequence of some medical conditions. Given the importance of appropriate circadian entrainment for health, the interest in assessing circadian rhythms (and the factors that influence the circadian clock) in research and clinical settings has expanded beyond sleep and circadian medicine to a wide variety of clinical specialties, including, for example, psychology, psychiatry, neurology, pulmonary, dermatology, obstetrics, oncology, and cardiology. The techniques described here can be applied to almost any population in which assessment of circadian rhythms, or often more accurately diurnal rhythms, is required. This chapter is divided into the following main sections:

- Questionnaires
- Sleep log/diary
- Actigraphy
- Light exposure

- Melatonin levels
- Body temperature

Each technique described here (a summary is provided in Table 210.1) can be used individually, although it is recommended to use a combination of these techniques to comprehensively assess circadian rhythms and to better understand the interacting relationships between various circadian outcome measures.

QUESTIONNAIRES

In addition to a detailed clinical history, standardized chronotype questionnaires can help assess CRSWDs. The *International Classification of Sleep Disorders*, third edition (ICSD-3) suggests the use of questionnaires to aid in the diagnosis of advanced and delayed sleep-wake phase disorders (DSWPDs).[8] Those with DSWPDs are typically evening/late types,[9,10] whereas those with advance sleep-wake phase disorder (ASWPD) are typically morning/early types on these questionnaires.[11] Note, however, that scoring as a morning or evening type on these questionnaires does not mean that an individual has a CRSWD. The two most commonly used chronotype questionnaires are the Morning-Eveningness Questionnaire (MEQ)[12] and the Munich Chronotype Questionnaire (MCTQ)—the latter has two versions, a conventional one and another designed specifically for shift workers (MCTQShift).[13,14] Both the MEQ and MCTQ have been shown to be associated with the timing of core body temperature (CBT) and melatonin levels in healthy individuals,[15-17] although in patient populations these relationships are not as clear.

The MEQ has a short and long version and estimates chronotype or morningness-eveningness via a series of questions related to preference to conducting daily activities, including sleep. A limitation of the MEQ in clinical settings is that patients would often "prefer" to sleep or wake at more conventional times, so responses can sometimes be misleading. Because of this, it is important to instruct the patient in how to complete the questionnaire appropriately. In addition to the established relationships between CBT and melatonin and morningness-eveningness preference, there are data to suggest that morning types on the MEQ have less flexibility in rising time than evening types.[18] Research using the MEQ to differentiate between extreme morning and evening types with or without a normal circadian phase (intermediate timing of DLMO) indicates that those with a normal circadian phase have alterations in the buildup and dissipation of the homeostatic sleep drive.[19]

In contrast to the MEQ, the MCTQ includes questions relating to usual daily sleep-wake activities on work/school days and on free days (no work or no school days), including questions about time to get into bed, time to fall asleep, and wake with and without an alarm clock. The MCTQ uses this information to estimate chronotype based on the timing of the midpoint of sleep onset and offset on work-free days, adjusted for the longer sleep durations on free days because of the accumulated sleep debt across the workweek. Chronotype of the MCTQ varies by age and gender. Social jet lag, the difference in the midpoint of sleep on weekdays/work days and weekend/free days, can be identified through the MCTQ and has been associated with body mass index and other health outcomes.[20-22]

Questionnaires have also been developed for the assessment of key features of DSWPD[23] and shift work disorder (SWD).[24,25] These questionnaires attempt to differentiate between those who are just late types and those with DSWPD and those shift workers who may have SWD and those who do not. Although these questionnaires have been reported for research purposes, they may be useful in the clinical setting.

SLEEP LOG/DIARY

The ICSD-3 diagnostic criteria require the use of sleep logs/diaries for at least 7 days, and preferably 14 days or more, for the diagnosis of most CRSWDs, including DSWPD, ASWPD, non-24-hour sleep-wake rhythm disorder (minimum 14 days), irregular sleep-wake rhythm disorder, and SWD[8] (see Chapter 43 for more details). At a minimum, a sleep log should include the date; time into and out of bed; time of falling asleep and waking up; day of the week; and whether that day is a work, school, or free day. Additional information that is helpful includes reporting of intentional and unintentional napping, timing of medications, and alcohol or caffeine intake. Given the importance of light exposure to the circadian system, it is also useful to include information about the start and end of light-emitting electronic use each day[26,27] and timing of exposure to outdoor light. In addition to reporting work or school days, it may be important to record work (especially important for SWD) or school hours, particularly if it is thought that these activities are affecting sleep-wake.

In addition to the reported measures of sleep timing, such as sleep start and end time, other variables can be calculated from the sleep log such as the midpoint of sleep (the clock time halfway between sleep start and sleep end) or social jet lag. Sleep midpoint allows the integration of sleep start and end time into a single variable, whereas social jet lag quantifies the shift in the sleep period on free days when constraints of work or school are removed. Both later sleep midpoint and greater social jet lag have been shown to be associated with poor outcomes of physical and/or mental health.[28-31]

Although many different sleep logs are available, an example of a 2-week sleep log is available on the American Academy of Sleep Medicine's website.[32]

ACTIGRAPHY

Although sleep logs are useful, the objective measurement of daily rest-activity rhythms with actigraphy is recommended, although not required, as part of the ICSD-3 diagnostic criteria for DSWPD, ASWPD, and irregular sleep-wake rhythm disorder and is a requirement for non-24-hour sleep-wake phase disorder.[8] A minimum of 7 days, but preferably 14 days or more, of assessment is suggested. The American Academy of Sleep Medicine and the Society for Behavioral Sleep Medicine have published practice guidelines that outline recommendations for the use of actigraphy for adult and pediatric CRSWDs.[33,34] Access to actigraphy clinical and billing practices varies.

A benefit of actigraphy is the ability to assess rest-activity rhythms over many days at home while the individual is going about activities of daily living. Actigraphy recording in combination with daily sleep logs (see previous section) allows the clinician or researcher to obtain a more comprehensive

Table 210.1 Summary of Techniques and Variables Used for the Clinical Assessment of Circadian Rhythms

Technique	Commonly Derived Variables
Questionnaires	
Circadian preference (MEQ)	Morning, evening, or intermediate type
Munich Chronotype Questionnaire (MCTQ)	Social jet lag, chronotype
Shift work disorder (SWD)	Screening tool for SWD
Delayed sleep-wake phase disorder (DSWPD)	Screening tool for DSWPD
Daily logs	
Sleep log	Sleep timing (time of sleep onset, offset, and midpoint) Sleep duration Napping (timing, duration) Wake after sleep onset Sleep onset latency Timing of medication, nicotine, caffeine, light-emitting device use, work hours
Meal/food logs	Timing of meals and beverages, meal and beverage content (soda, caffeine, alcohol)
Actigraphy	
Sleep-wake parameters	Sleep timing (time of sleep onset, offset, and midpoint) Sleep duration Sleep efficiency Sleep fragmentation Sleep bout (number and duration)
Circadian activity rhythm measures	Amplitude Phase
Nonparametric measures	M10 (start time and activity level) L5 (start time and activity level) Interdaily stability (IS) Intradaily variability (IV) Relative amplitude (RA)
Sleep regularity index (SRI)	Sleep regularity index
Locomotor inactivity during sleep (LIDS)	Ultradian rhythms in sleep
Activity	Activity counts
Light exposure	
Light measurement	Time above threshold (TAT) Mean light timing (MLiT)
Light exposure questionnaires	Time and duration of outdoor or indoor light exposure
Melatonin	
Saliva or plasma	
• 5–6 hours prior to sleep onset until sleep onset	Dim light melatonin onset (DLMO)
• 14–24 hours of sampling	DLMO Amplitude Melatonin offset
Urine[a]	
• 24 hour urine collection	Amplitude Estimate of phase (curve fitting)
• Morning void	Estimate of aMT6s concentration during sleep
• Pooled sleep period and morning void	aMT6s concentration during sleep
• Difference between the void immediately prior to bedtime and morning void	Estimate of amplitude

[a]Creatinine levels should be measured, and urine volume of each void should be recorded.

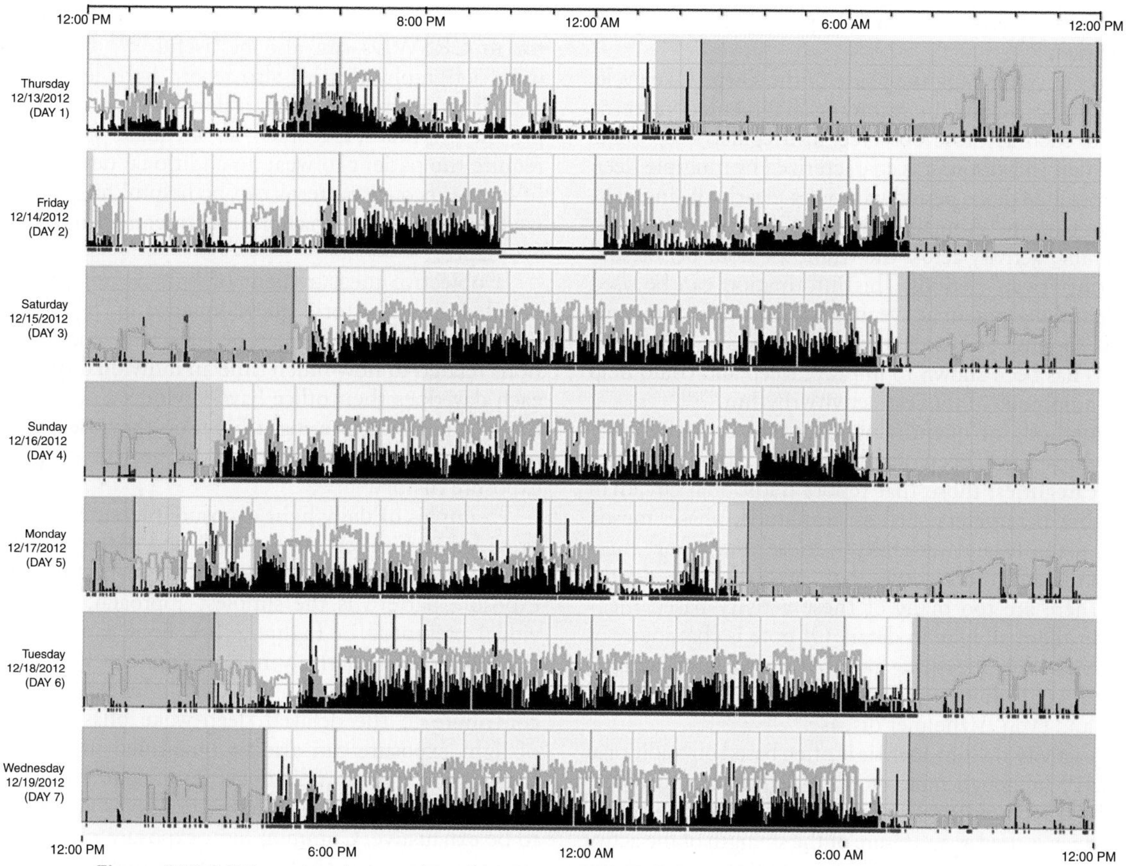

Figure 210.1 Wrist actigraphy recording of activity and light levels in an individual with a delayed sleep-wake phase. The data presented here are of 7 consecutive days of recording of wrist activity and light plotted between 12 P.M. and 12 P.M. each day. The *black bars* indicate activity level, the *yellow line* indicates light level in lux (for this device, lux level is estimated from the recording of red, green, and blue light—only lux level is shown for simplicity), and the *blue bars* indicate time in bed (rest period) attempting to sleep based on sleep log recordings. The lighter bar at the beginning and the end of some of the rest periods is determined by the device's sleep-wake algorithm and indicates periods of rest prior to falling asleep or after waking up but attempting to sleep. Light and activity levels were set at 1000 lux and 1000 lux for visualization within the device's reading software.

picture of sleep-wake behavior. An example of a 7-day actigraphy recording (activity and light) from an individual with a delayed sleep-wake phase is provided in Figure 210.1. Of note in this recording is that bedtime for this individual is between 2 and 7 A.M. and wake time is between 3 and 5 P.M., suggestive of DSWPD, and as a result of sleeping during the daytime, there are relatively high light levels throughout the nighttime hours that continue into the sleep period. This type of light exposure pattern is likely to perpetuate a delay in sleep-wake timing.

Actigraphy provides various proxy sleep and wake parameters such as sleep duration; sleep timing; and measures of sleep continuity such as sleep efficiency, wake after sleep onset, and sleep fragmentation indices. In addition, other measures such as sleep midpoint and social jet lag can be calculated (see earlier).

Standardized procedures have been published for the "scoring" of periods of rest/sleep with actigraphy.[35-37] A variety of actigraphy devices and analysis algorithms are available on the market. However, it is recommended to select a device with analysis software and scoring algorithms that have been validated against polysomnography[38] and when possible to select a device that also measures light exposure. Many of the algorithms to determine sleep-wake have been validated against polysomnographic-determined sleep; however, most of these validation studies have been conducted in conventional nocturnal sleep conditions. There are fewer studies that have validated these algorithms in conditions such as shift-work or Parkinson disease, although some reports include information about optimal settings for collection and processing of activity data in these groups.[35,39] Although most sleep algorithms determine sleep intervals automatically, there are those that allow the user to determine the periods considered to be rest (or time in bed attempting to sleep) based on various techniques, including sleep logs or event markers to indicate when the individual was getting into or out of bed.[35-37] For example, in Figure 210.1 the start and end of the "blue bars" indicating the time the patient got into and out of bed were placed within the reading and analysis software based on information provided by the patient from a daily sleep log. The rest intervals in the example actograms in Figure 210.5 were set using the event markers (small blue triangles) placed at the beginning and end of the rest intervals by the wearer and the accompanying sleep log information. It should be noted, however, that not all patients are able to accurately report sleep times, and there can sometimes be discordance between what is seen in the activity level and what is reported in the sleep log or by the marker.[36,37]

In addition to confirming the phase of the sleep-wake cycle, actigraphy can be helpful in recording fragmented patterns of sleep-wake such as those observed in irregular sleep-wake rhythm disorder. This disorder is characterized by multiple sleep episodes across a 24-hour period without a clearly distinguishable circadian pattern.[8] A further benefit to actigraphy is that it is able to capture activity across the whole 24-hour period and not just during "sleep" periods. This information can be used to aid in identifying potential avenues for treatment intervention, such as napping or low daytime activity levels. Increasing activity levels has been shown to improve sleep and could help increase the amplitude of the rest-activity rhythm.[40,41]

Several methods of quantifying circadian or other rest-activity rhythms have been published.[42-48] These fall into three main categories: those that report traditional circadian activity rhythm parameters such as amplitude, phase, mesor, acrophase,[48] stability, and variabilty[47]; those that report fragmentation indices[44]; and those that predict sleep depth/cycles.[49,50] There are too many of these activity-based measures to cover them all here in detail. Of note is that many of these activity rhythm measures have been associated with or predict cognitive decline, cardiometabolic risk factors, mood disorders,[51] and even Alzheimer disease.[44,46,47,52-57]

Circadian activity rhythm analysis is often based on traditional cosine models[48] (although more recently, slightly modified versions have been reported[55,56,58]) and includes measures such as amplitude, which is used as a measure of the strength of the activity rhythm; mesor, or the mean of the activity level; acrophase, which is the time of day of the peak of activity; and the pseudo F-statistic, which is a measure of the robustness of the circadian activity rhythm with higher values indicating stronger rhythmicity.[48,59] Another approach to quantify circadian activity rhythm behavior includes what are referred to as *nonparametric measures,* including interdaily stability (IS), intradaily variability (IV), relative amplitude (RA), and the clock time and activity level for the 10 hours with maximal activity (M10) or the lowest 5 hours (L5) of activity in a 24-hour period.[46,47] The duration of the periods of low and high activity (5 and 10, respectively) are sometimes varied across studies, but the calculation is similar.[60] IS is a measure of the day-to-day variation in rest-activity patterns and may indicate a "loose coupling" between the rest-activity and the light-dark cycle.[47] IV is a measure of rest-activity rhythm fragmentation, and a high IV may be indicative of daytime napping and/or nighttime arousals. RA is calculated from the activity level of the M10 and L5—a low RA is an index of low M10 activity and high L5 activity.[47] These measures have been reported in numerous studies, and a detailed summary of these studies is provided by Gonçalves and colleagues.[61] An R code package created by Blume and colleagues[42] to calculate these variables is available for free.

The regularity of sleep-wake activity can also be characterized by measures such as the sleep regularity index (SRI). The SRI quantifies the day-to-day regularity of sleep periods. A benefit of this measure is that it incorporates all of the sleep episodes in a 24-hour period[45] and has been shown to be associated with DSWPD and academic performance in college students.[45,62,63]

LIGHT EXPOSURE

Given the significant impact that light exposure patterns can have on the timing of the circadian clock, the measurement of habitual daily light exposure patterns as a contributing factor to CRSWDs can also be useful.[10,64] Fortunately, many wrist actigraphy devices also record light levels at the wrist, and although this is not equivalent to the level of light reaching the eye/brain, it is likely an adequate proxy and does not require the patient to wear an additional device.[65] Evaluation of light exposure patterns can be helpful to guide individualized strategies for behavioral treatments of light seeking and avoidance.[10]

If objective measurement of light is not possible, then a detailed light history, questionnaire, or reporting of light exposure on a sleep log can be sufficient. For example, questions related to how much time an individual spends outdoors each day, does their office have a window, do they sleep with the television on or a night light, do they use handheld electronic devices prior to bedtime, can provide insight into light exposure history.[66,67]

Examples of daily light exposure measures at the wrist are provided in Figures 210.1, 210.2, and 210.5 from two different wrist actigraphy devices. Visual inspection of the light exposure pattern is the simplest approach, and in the individual presented in Figure 210.1, light exposure during the sleep period is relatively high, as are the light levels in the middle of the night. In this case light exposure is likely to contribute to the delayed sleep-wake phase. Daily patterns of light exposure can also be quantified in several ways for comparison across individuals or patient groups. The techniques listed here are just a few examples and are not meant to be exhaustive. Common light exposure metrics range from simple measures such as time above threshold (TAT)[68,69] or more complex models for predicting sleep-wake timing.[70,71] TAT is simply the average total minutes spent above a predetermined threshold in a specified period, usually 24 hours. A commonly reported threshold is 1000 lux, although examination of lower thresholds can also be useful. The threshold for the TAT and the time window for calculation (i.e., 24 hours, sleep period or active period) can usually be changed within the settings of the reading software. Another measure, mean light timing (MLiT), has been shown to be associated with body mass index, mood, and subjective sleep quality.[10,68,69] MLiT is a measure that integrates the timing and intensity of light exposure across several days and is calculated as the mean clock time of all of the 2-minute bins of light data above a set threshold. Although light across the whole day is important, there is considerable interest in the impact of light at night (LAN) because of a number of studies reporting associations with increased LAN and poor health outcomes.[72,73] LAN can be calculated based on a specific window of interest (i.e., sunrise to sunset, during the sleep period, 9 P.M.–6 A.M., etc.). Light exposure during the sleep period can contribute to sleep disturbance and has been associated with poor health outcomes in children and adults.[67,73] Several of the nonparametric measures described earlier can also be applied to light-level data; however, there are limited published reports of this.

MELATONIN

The timing of the circadian rhythm of melatonin is a robust marker of the internal circadian clock.[74,75] Clinically the ICSD-3 recommends the assessment of the DLMO or urinary 6-sulphatoxymeltonin sampled over 24 hours to confirm circadian phase in several CRSWDs.[8]

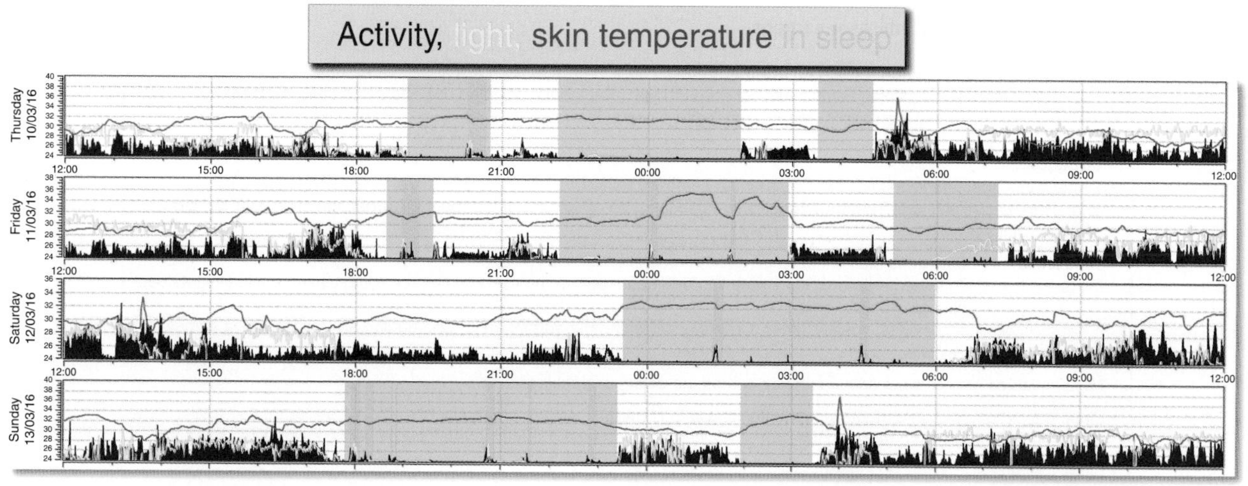

Figure 210.2 Wrist actigraphy with light and skin temperature. The data presented here are from four consecutive 24-hour periods and include activity *(dark blue bars)*, light *(yellow line)*, and skin temperature *(orange line)* from a single individual. The *blue shaded* areas are categorized as sleep, and the *green shaded* areas are categorized as resting wakefulness because of the elevated activity. Within this example, there are multiple sleep occasions within a 24-hour period, with a primary sleep period occurring as early as 6:00 P.M. and as late as11:30 P.M.

Melatonin is a hormone synthesized and released from the pineal gland via a multisynaptic pathway, including sympathetic innervations through the suprachiasmatic nucleus, preganglionic neurons, and postganglionic fibers from the superior cervical ganglion.[76,77] A key element to consider when assessing melatonin rhythms is that melatonin production is suppressed by light exposure and some medications (beta blockers and nonsteroidal antiinflammatory medications).[78,79] Another consideration is that some medical conditions can alter the metabolism and excretion of melatonin, affecting circulating levels in the blood and also levels of the major metabolite of melatonin in urinary 6-sulphatoxymeltonin.[80-82] In addition to the selection of an appropriate melatonin assay,[83] finding a laboratory that can conduct the assay should be considered.

DLMO can be determined from serial plasma or saliva sampling under dim light conditions.[75] Because of the invasive nature of collection, serial plasma sampling for melatonin is typically only used for research and infrequently in the clinical setting. A benefit of collecting samples in the laboratory setting is the ability to control the timing of samples, light levels, meals, and activity levels. In contrast, saliva sampling for melatonin can be conducted relatively easily either in the laboratory or at home. Several studies report successful salivary melatonin assessment at home for determination of DLMO in DSWPD, ASWPD, and non-24-hour sleep-wake rhythm disorder.[11,84,85] Standardized protocols for the assessment of salivary DLMO at home have been established and validated against controlled laboratory sample collection for DSWPD.[84] To accurately detect the salivary DLMO at home requires the patient to carefully follow instructions for serial sample collection. Typically, samples are collected for 5 to 6 hours prior to habitual bedtime at 30-minute intervals. During this time patients are instructed to remain in dim light of less than 20 lux and to refrain from eating or drinking 10 to 15 minutes prior to each sample. A summary of key components to include in an at-home salivary melatonin collection kit and example instructions is provided in Figure 210.3.

In healthy adults with ASWPD and DSWPD, the DLMO typically occurs, on average, 2 to 3 hours prior to habitual sleep onset or bedtime.[9,11,74,86] As a result, it is recommended that sample collection start 5 to 6 hours prior to habitual sleep/bedtime. However, in patients with non-24 hour sleep-wake rhythm disorder, the timing of DLMO is less predictable; as a result it is recommended to collect samples for a longer period, even as long as 24-hours. Even with extended sampling if the patient does not follow the strict collection instructions mentioned earlier, it may not be possible to detect a rise in melatonin levels, and therefore the DLMO would not be able to be determined. A case series outlining the challenges in measuring DLMO in patients with non-24-hour sleep-wake rhythm disorder provides several examples where measurement was successful but also others where even with the best intentions, the DLMO was missed or unable to be detected.[85]

DLMO in saliva can be calculated in several ways, all which require melatonin levels to rise above a specified threshold. The simplest methods is the time of the first sample to cross and remain above 3 or 4 pg/mL.[75,87,88] Another method is the time when the level of melatonin crosses and remains two standard deviations above the mean of three baseline daytime samples.[89] An issue with this method is that occasionally it is difficult to identify a consistent baseline level if sufficient sampling is not conducted. Some researchers have adjusted for this by using the two standard deviation method plus 15% of the three highest values.[90] Examples of dim light salivary melatonin levels collected at home by our group are provided in Figure 210.4. The DLMO in these examples is marked by the intersection of the hatched line and is represented by the first sample to cross 4 pg/mL. Some groups will interpolate between samples to estimate the "exact" time of threshold crossing, but this should be done with caution depending on the sampling rate used, and it is not recommended for sampling rates that are more than 30 minutes.

Although assessing the DLMO can help confirm a delayed phase in those with DSWPD, a report from an Australian group indicates that in a study of 182 participants clinically diagnosed with DSWPD, 43% did not exhibit circadian misalignment as they had a salivary DLMO prior to the desired bedtime.[91] A more recent study from Portugal of 162

Home salivary melatonin assessment

Home salivary melatonin collection kit components
- Detailed collection instructions, sample log, collection tubes, tube labels, shipping box and packaging materials, ice packs
- Optional items include dark glasses, water proof marker, cooler if returning in person

Instructions
- Maintain dim light conditions (< 20lux) throughout sampling period.
    - Candlelight, light from a TV, small side-table lamp on other side of the room OR wear light/blue light blocking glasses
- Sampling at 30–60 minutes intervals (sampling duration and timing vary)
    - For an entrained individual start sampling 5–6 hours before the average time of falling asleep until falling asleep (or slightly past habitual time)
    - Consider providing specific times: Collect a saliva sample starting at __ and ending at__, each saliva sample should be collected at ____ minute intervals.
- 15–20 minutes prior to each sample remain seated; no eating or drinking
- Place the cotton swab into mouth without touching with fingertips or other contaminants, and roll under tongue until saturated with saliva, then return to tube. Or saliva can be transferred directly to the tube by gently spitting into the tube.
- Label the tube and sampling log with exact time of collection.
- Refrigerate tube immediately and keep refrigerated/frozen until ready for shipping.

Figure 210.3 Home salivary melatonin assessment. Summary of the components to include in a home salivary melatonin collection kit and key instructions. The number of tubes to include in a kit will vary based on the sampling frequency and duration (6 hours–24+ hours), and it is advised to include a few spare tubes. There are tubes specifically designed for saliva collection that contain a cotton swab, but this is not required as long as the minimum volume of clean sample is provided (volume will be dependent on the assay used), although several milliliters is recommended.

DSWPD patients from a clinical setting has reported a similar finding, with 59% of patients without misalignment, although this study used a different definition of circadian misalignment than the first.[92]

Unfortunately, although assessment of DLMO is considered the gold standard for determining internal circadian phase, it is expensive, burdensome, and difficult to access for both patients and clinicians and, as such, has not been widely adopted in clinical practice.

Urine collection for urinary 6-sulphatoxymelatonin (aMT6s) can be useful in cases where there is a need to conduct assessments across many days, and although not as practical to determine circadian phase, it is beneficial as a measure of amplitude. Measurement of the circadian rhythm of aMT6s levels for at least two time points spaced 2 to 4 weeks apart is suggested in the ICSD-3 to confirm nonentrained rhythms in non-24-hour sleep-wake rhythm disorder.[8] Furthermore, this technique can be used to examine circadian function in those who are unable to collect saliva or plasma samples, such as small children or in adults/children with cognitive deficits.[93-95] A limitation of this approach is that urine samples cannot typically be produced on command, so there can be less precision with timing of samples. A way to deal with this methodologically is to collect all urine produced within a 24-hour period (24-hour urine collection) or to collect samples at key times across the day to estimate the 24-hour profile of aMT6s. For 24-hour sampling of urine, an individual is instructed to void their bladder upon awakening on the day of collection and to discard. Then for the next 24 hours each void is collected in a separate container labeled with the time and date; the last sample would be the one upon awakening the next day. A simpler approach is to calculate "overnight" levels of aMT6s from a single "morning" sample upon waking.[96] It is also recommended to determine urine creatinine levels and record the void volume to adjust values as needed based on excretion rate.[97-99]

BODY TEMPERATURE MEASURES

CBT measured over several days (minimum of 24 hours) has been used to assess the timing of the circadian clock in humans[9,74], however, because of patient burden, cost, accessibility, and the influence of activity and diet, the continued use of CBT in the clinical setting has been limited. CBT measurements are usually taken by swallowing a capsule that transmits temperature information as it makes its way through the digestive tract or via a rectal thermistor connected to a recording device.[9,100] A benefit of CBT measurement is that estimates of the timing of the internal circadian clock can be obtained relatively quickly, unlike assessment of the DLMO, which can take 5 to 10 days to obtain results from the laboratory. The most frequently used measure for estimating circadian timing with CBT is the time of the CBTm, which in a normally entrained individual typically occurs 2 to 3 hours prior to habitual wake time (Figure 210.5).[9,86] Sleep is typically optimal on the declining portion of the CBT rhythm, and there is an inverse relationship between CBT rhythm and the melatonin rhythm, such that when CBT is lowest, melatonin is high.[101]

Several commercially available devices also measure skin temperature.[102] Skin temperature has a very different 24-hour profile from CBT because of the role of skin conductance in the regulation of body temperature. Skin temperature is also significantly affected by ambient temperature, position, and covering the device, which makes it a less accurate measure of the circadian clock than the CBTm. An example of a recording from a device that measures activity, light, and body temperature is provided in Figure 210.2.

NONCLINICAL LABORATORY APPROACHES

In addition to the clinical methods described earlier, sleep and circadian researchers employ an assortment of more intensive techniques. These techniques serve to refine our understanding

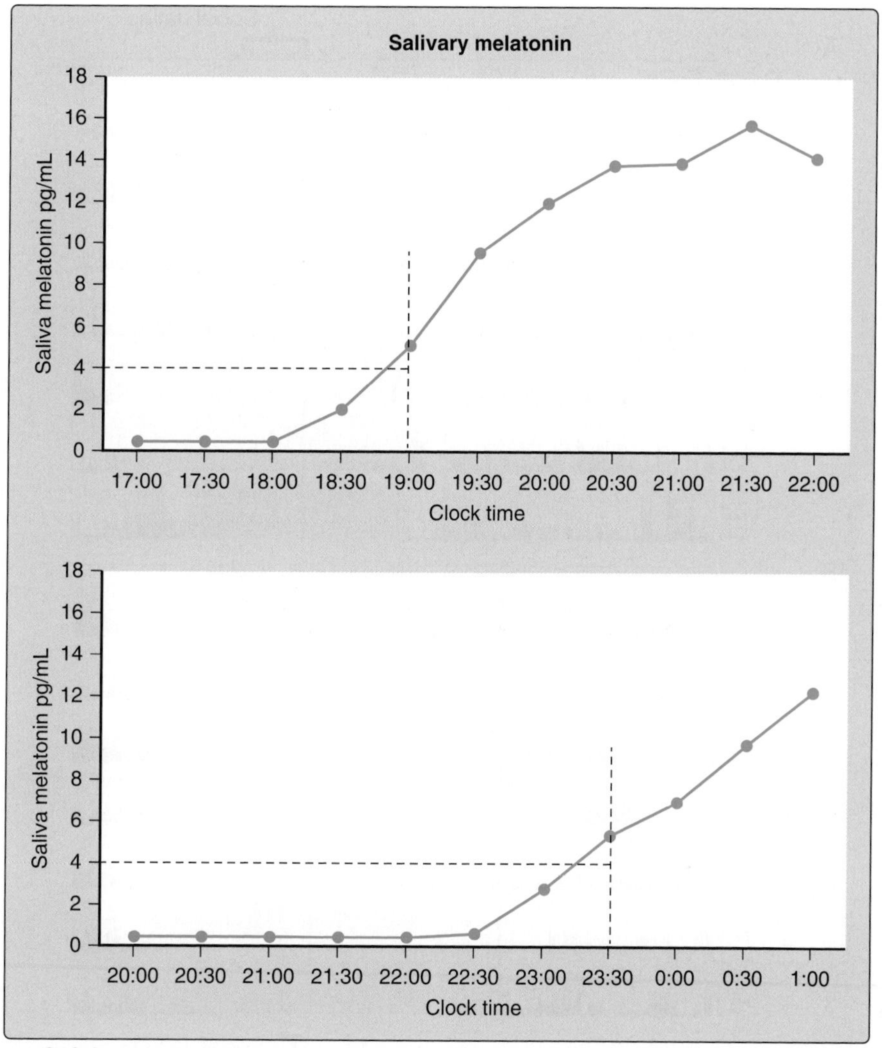

Figure 210.4 Salivary melatonin levels indicating dim light melatonin onset (DLMO). Data presented in this figure represent salivary melatonin levels assessed at home from an individual with an early *(top panel)* and an individual with a later *(lower panel)* DLMO. The DLMO is indicated by the *dashed vertical line* at the time of the sample that salivary melatonin levels cross and remain above the threshold of 4 pg/mL. Linear interpolation of the times between the sampling points immediately below and above the threshold value can also be used to estimate the precise DLMO clock time.

of underlying circadian and sleep-wake mechanisms and control many of the external factors that can influence the circadian clock, such as activity level, sleep-wake, light-dark, and feed-fast cycle. These methods include but are not limited to constant routine (described later), forced desynchrony, and ultrashort sleep-wake protocols.

A constant routine refers to a laboratory-based protocol that holds several factors constant to limit their impact on the measurement of circadian rhythms, including posture, activity, temperature, light-dark, feed-fast, and sleep-wake.[2] Typically, a subject remains in the laboratory for at least 2 full days. For a week prior to starting the in-lab portion of the constant routine, the subject has been instructed to keep a regular/habitual sleep-wake schedule. On the first night in the laboratory, the subject is required to sleep for at least 8 hours (sometimes more) in the dark to dissipate any prior buildup of homeostatic sleep pressure. Upon waking, the subject is placed into constant conditions for at least one circadian cycle, typically for between 28 and 40 hours. During this time they are required to remain upright and awake in bed, the room is kept at a constant temperature and light level (typically less than 20 lux), and caloric intake is spread evenly across this period with small isocaloric meals (about 250 calories) every 2 hours. While under these constant controlled conditions, various biospecimens (blood, saliva, urine, skin, muscle or fat cells), physiologic, and neurobehavioral measures can be collected at regular intervals to assess the phase and amplitude of circadian rhythms. Common measures include serial samples for melatonin, cortisol, gene expression, CBT, blood pressure, heart rate, alertness, cognitive function, and mood, although almost any physiologic function can be measured.

CHALLENGES AND THE FUTURE

Accurate measurement of circadian rhythms can be challenging in day-to-day life, and many of the "rhythms" measured really reflect diurnal rhythms because of the "masking" effects of other behavioral inputs to the circadian clock such as physical activity, the light-dark cycle, and meal timing. As such, these factors should be controlled for or at least

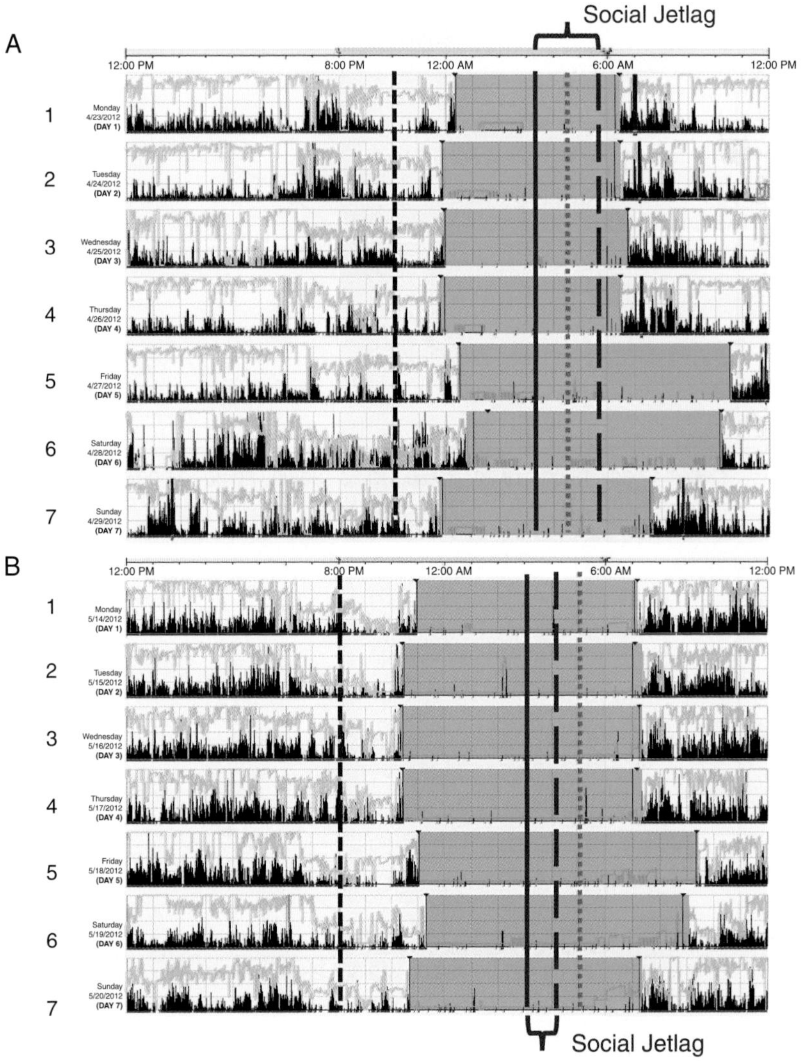

Figure 210.5 Example actograms indicating average sleep midpoint on weekdays and weekends, with clinical estimates of dim light melatonin onset (DLMO) and core body temperature minimum (CBTm). The data presented here are of 7 consecutive days of recording of wrist activity and light plotted between 12 P.M. and 12 P.M. each day. The *black bars* indicate activity level, the *yellow line* indicates light level in lux, and the *blue shading* indicates time in bed (rest period) attempting to sleep based on sleep log recordings and time markers placed by the wearer using a "marker" button on the device *(small blue triangles)*. Panel A has an example actogram from an individual who has approximately a 2-hour difference in week/work day sleep midpoint *(purple solid line)* and weekend/free day sleep midpoint *(purple dashed line)*. Panel B has an example actogram from an individual who has an hour difference in week/work day sleep midpoint *(purple solid line)* and weekend/free day sleep midpoint *(purple dashed line)*. On both panels, an estimate of the degree of social jet lag is indicated by the *purple ellipses*. Both panels include clinical estimates of average DLMO *(dark blue dashed line)* and CBTm *(orange dotted line)*. Estimated times are based on average sleep-wake times and derived from the previously reported relationship between DLMO and sleep onset (on average, DLMO is 2–3 hours prior to habitual sleep onset) and CBTm and wake time (on average, CBTm is 2–3 hours prior to habitual wake time).

considered when interpreting the results of any measurement. So although measuring circadian rhythms in a laboratory setting may be cost or time prohibitive, it is likely to yield the most accurate results. Patient compliance with instructions at home also varies and for some can be burdensome. Another consideration is that for measurement of DLMO and in some cases actigraphy, the patients bear the burden for the cost of these assessments, as they are not covered by health insurance in many countries. Although each of the elements mentioned in this section should be considered, they do not diminish the potential benefits for diagnosis and treatment of measuring the circadian rhythm of sleep-wake and other rhythms such as melatonin.

Several groups around the world are working on improving and developing new methods for the assessment of circadian rhythms that will have utility in the clinical setting.[103] For example, there are teams of researchers and clinicians developing methods using -omics and machine learning approaches to determine circadian rhythms from a few and in some cases a single blood sample.[104-108] To date, however, their use for the most part has been limited to healthy adults in the laboratory, so until these methods have been validated in patient populations, their use clinically is unclear.

As wearable technology evolves, there has been a surge in development of devices that can be worn on various parts of the body, including the finger, wrist, or chest, and along with these devices are algorithms that integrate information on activity, light, body temperature, heart rate, and other physiologic parameters to predict sleep-wake[49,109] and estimate circadian timing.[110] Several groups have provided guidance on how to validate and interpret findings from these types of devices and algorithms.[38,111]

Another promising technique to help understand the pathophysiology of circadian disturbance in a variety of disorders is the pupillary response to light pulses. This technique has been used to determine parameters that show alterations in the pupillary light reflex and is able to differentiate between those patients with DSWPD who have a delayed circadian melatonin phase relative to desired bedtime from those who do not.[112] Although this work is preliminary and requires replication, this technique could be promising as an adjunct assessment in those with DSWPD and potentially in other disorders with circadian disturbance.[113]

CLINICAL PEARLS

- In addition to a detailed clinical history, assessment of the timing and amplitude of circadian rhythms is recommended to establish an accurate diagnosis of CRSWDs, and to guide and provide precision for their management.[8]
- The assessment of the timing of circadian rhythms such as melatonin or CBT can be helpful in differentiating the diagnosis of DSWPD from non-24-hour sleep-wake rhythm disorder, as some individuals with non-24-hour sleep-wake rhythm disorder display periods of entrained sleep-wake timing but at a delayed phase.
- Reducing the impact of other external inputs to the circadian clock, particularly light exposure and certain medications, is essential for an accurate measure of circadian phase.
- When assessing circadian rhythms, such as DLMO, we recommend that measures of sleep-wake timing (sleep log and/or actigraphy) are collected in parallel.

SUMMARY

Several validated techniques are available to assess circadian rhythms in the clinical setting for the diagnosis and management of CRSWDs. Guidance for when and how to use these techniques is provided in the ICSD-3, American Academy of Sleep Medicine Practice Parameters, and a guide from the Society of Behavioral Sleep Medicine.[8,34,114] Questionnaires and sleep logs are tools readily available to most clinicians/researchers, and although actigraphy is recommended, it may be more challenging to access. Techniques such as assessment of melatonin levels require collection under strict conditions (light levels, number and timing of samples), and access to resources for quick assay and cost can be a limiting factor. As such, assessment of the circadian melatonin rhythm is unfortunately not used that often clinically. In order to move the field of circadian medicine forward in a significant way, it will be important to develop accessible, reliable, and cost-effective techniques for assessing circadian rhythms at home or from simple tests in the clinic. Many scientist and clinicians around the world are committed to this goal, and the future of circadian medicine and the assessment of circadian rhythms, both in the laboratory for research and in the clinical setting, is advancing.

ACKNOWLEDGMENTS

Support for this work was provided by R01 HL140580 and P01 AG011412 and the Center for Circadian and Sleep Medicine at Northwestern University, Feinberg School of Medicine.

SELECTED READINGS

Benloucif S, Burgess HJ, Klerman EB, et al. Measuring melatonin in humans. *J Clin Sleep Med.* 2008;4:66–69.

Benloucif S, Guico MJ, Reid KJ, Wolfe LF, L'Hermite-Baleriaux M, Zee PC. Stability of melatonin and temperature as circadian phase markers and their relation to sleep times in humans. *J Biol Rhythms.* 2005;20:178–188.

Braun R, Kath WL, Iwanaszko M, et al. Universal method for robust detection of circadian state from gene expression. *Proc Natl Acad Sci U S A.* 2018;115:E9247–E9256.

Burgess HJ, Wyatt JK, Park M, Fogg LF. Home circadian phase assessments with measures of compliance yield accurate dim light melatonin onsets. *Sleep.* 2015;38:889–897.

Carskadon MA, Dement WC. Sleep studies on a 90-minute day. *Electroencephalogr Clin Neurophysiol.* 1975;39:145–155.

Czeisler CA, Allan JS, Strogatz SH, et al. Bright light resets the human circadian pacemaker independent of the timing of the sleep-wake cycle. *Science.* 1986;233:667–671.

Depner CM, Cheng PC, Devine JK, et al. Wearable technologies for developing sleep and circadian biomarkers: a summary of workshop discussions. *Sleep.* 2020;43.

Duffy JF, Abbott SM, Burgess HJ, et al. Workshop report. Circadian rhythm sleep-wake disorders: gaps and opportunities. *Sleep.* 2021;44(5):zsaa281

International Classification of Sleep Disorders. 3rd ed. American Academy of Sleep Medicine; 2014.

Morgenthaler TI, Lee-Chiong T, Alessi C, et al. Practice parameters for the clinical evaluation and treatment of circadian rhythm sleep disorders: an American Academy of Sleep Medicine report. *Sleep.* 2007;30:1445–1459.

Sack RL, Auckley D, Auger RR, et al. Circadian rhythm sleep disorders: part II, advanced sleep phase disorder, delayed sleep phase disorder, free-running disorder, and irregular sleep- wake rhythm. An American Academy of Sleep Medicine review. *Sleep.* 2007;30:1484–1501.

Smith MT, McCrae CS, Cheung J, et al. Use of Actigraphy for the Evaluation of Sleep Disorders and Circadian Rhythm Sleep-Wake Disorders: An American Academy of Sleep Medicine Systematic Review, Meta-Analysis, and GRADE Assessment. *J Clin Sleep Med.* 2018;14:1209–1230.

Wittenbrink N, Ananthasubramaniam B, Munch M, et al. High-accuracy determination of internal circadian time from a single blood sample. *J Clin Invest.* 2018;128:3826–3839.

A complete reference list can be found online at ExpertConsult.com.

Chapter 211

Actigraphy Methods and Technical Issues

Katie L. Stone; Vicki Li

Chapter Highlights

- Wrist actigraphy offers several advantages over polysomnography for sleep assessment. It is more convenient, less expensive, less invasive, and allows data collection in a more natural sleep environment. It is also well suited for collecting data continuously over consecutive 24-hour periods for days or even weeks. This provides a more representative characterization of sleep, activity patterns, and circadian rhythm. Actigraphy is demonstrated to be reliable and valid for detecting sleep in normal populations; however, it has limitations for detecting specific sleep disturbances.
- Consumer wearables (in contrast to research-grade actigraphs) provide opportunities to obtain activity and other 24-hour features in large samples; however, further validation of sleep and circadian data accuracy is essential.
- Actigraphy is a useful adjunct for routine evaluation of insomnia, circadian rhythm disorders, and excessive sleepiness. It is potentially helpful for diagnosing periodic limb movements in sleep and/or restless legs syndrome. It also is useful in special populations, such as children or elderly patients with dementia, who may not tolerate polysomnography.
- Actigraphy is widely used in research and increasingly used in clinical settings. Multiple cohort studies have used actigraphy to study associations between sleep, circadian activity patterns, and health outcomes. Actigraphy also can serve to assess treatment effects in randomized trials.

INTRODUCTION

Polysomnography (PSG) is currently the "gold standard" method for evaluating sleep. It incorporates, at a minimum, electroencephalogram (EEG), electrooculogram (EOG), and submentalis electromyogram (EMG) recordings. Depending on the patient's sleep complaints, monitoring of other physiologic variables may be added (e.g., respirations, heart rate, tibialis muscle movement, oximetry). PSG therefore allows for the collection of detailed and comprehensive information about sleep. The EEG, EOG, and EMG records can be scored for sleep stages (non–rapid eye movement [NREM] stages N1 to N3, and rapid eye movement [REM]), total sleep time, total wake time, sleep-onset latency, and percent time in REM versus NREM sleep.

This information is crucial for certain types of evaluations; however, the recording process may disturb the subject's sleep, and PSG studies are costly to record and to score. In addition, PSG typically provides data for 6 to 10 hours during the major sleep period; consequently, no PSG information is available about daytime (waking) or napping behavior. In certain instances, the crucial parameter is whether the person is awake or asleep, and knowledge of the sleep stage or other physiologic activity is not especially informative.

By contrast, actigraphy is much less expensive than PSG and provides 24-hour recordings of activity from which wake and sleep can be scored. Actigraphs record movement; traditionally, when used to estimate sleep, the actigraph is placed on the wrist. However, sometimes activity from the leg, waist, or other body location is recorded. A variety of research grade actigraphs are available. These devices typically provide access to raw acceleration data, epoch-by-epoch activity counts, and estimated average nightly sleep-wake variables (e.g., sleep duration); and most have been validated against PSG. Many devices are bundled with software that allows epoch-by-epoch data display and editing using an interactive computer interface. Software may also allow for data processing to create sleep-wake variables and, in some cases, circadian rest-activity rhythm variables. Some researchers prefer to apply their own algorithms to the raw or epoch-by-epoch data or use shared programs (e.g., functions available in the "R" programming language) to generate sleep and circadian rest-activity rhythm variables. Most devices can also be used to estimate daytime activity variables in addition to nighttime sleep variables. However, it is widely believed that waist or hip placement of the device is preferred for assessment of physical activity to more accurately pick up center of mass acceleration.[1] Furthermore, studies reveal physical activity estimates are not equivalent when device placement and collection methods vary.[1]

During the past decade, many consumer-grade wearable devices claim the ability to estimate sleep, typically using proprietary algorithms. Although initially these devices were underutilized in research settings because of lack of transparency about the validity of the algorithms, increasingly there

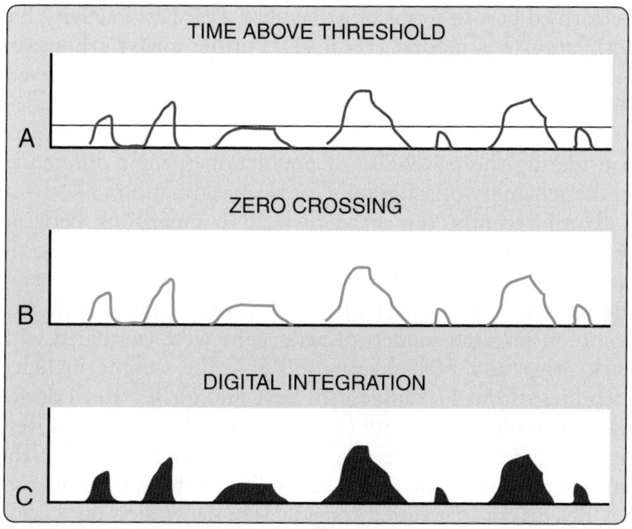

Figure 211.1 Three methods of deriving activity counts in actigraphy. The time above threshold method **(A)** derives the amount of time per epoch during which the activity is above some defined threshold (represented by the *thin horizontal line*). Zero crossing mode **(B)** counts the number of times the activity reaches zero (represented by the *solid baseline*). Digital integration mode **(C)** calculates the area under the curves represented by *dark pink shading*. (From Ancoli-Israel S, Cole R, Alessi CA, et al. The role of actigraphy in the study of sleep and circadian rhythms. *Sleep*. 2003;26:342–92.)

have been partnerships between researchers and industry, allowing for enhanced access to the raw data to better address the needs of the research community. The consumer devices also tend to have advantages in terms of more appealing design, comfort for day-to-day use, and other consumer desirable functions (e.g., heart rate and energy expenditure tracking with smartphone applications to view daily data).

This chapter reviews the major clinical and research applications for actigraphy, provides tips for successful performance of the actigraphy study, and identifies limitations with its use.

BACKGROUND AND METHODOLOGY

Wrist activity technology is based on the fact that during sleep, little movement occurs, whereas during wake, periodic increases in movement are seen. Activity monitors have been available for many years.[2] Research-grade actigraphs are typically the size of a wristwatch and collect digitized data. With the advent of microprocessors and miniaturization, contemporary actigraphs include a movement detector (typically a piezoelectric accelerometer) and a battery with sufficient memory to record for long time periods. Most actigraphs now feature triaxial accelerometers, which continuously collect simultaneous vibrations captured as voltages in three orthogonal directions and accumulate these voltage data in predefined epochs that can be specified by the clinician or investigator (e.g., 15 or 30 seconds, or 1 minute). Three examples of methods by which signals can be digitized are *time above threshold* (TAT), *zero crossing mode* (ZCM), and *digital integration mode* (DIM) (Figure 211.1).[3] The TAT method counts the amount of time per epoch that the motion signal is above a given threshold. However, neither the amplitude of the signal nor the acceleration of the movement is reflected in this strategy. The ZCM method counts the number of times per epoch that the voltage crosses zero. In this strategy, once again neither the amplitude nor the acceleration is taken into account, and high-frequency artifact could potentially be counted as movement. DIM, on the other hand, samples the accelerometry output signal at a high rate and then, for each epoch, calculates the area under the curve. This result reflects the amplitude and acceleration of the signal but not the duration or frequency of the signal. In studies comparing the three methodologies, DIM was best for identifying movement amplitude, followed by TAT and then ZCM.[4] Some actigraphs use more than one method, thereby decreasing the deficits of each method alone.

Once the data are digitized, computer algorithms automatically score wake and sleep and provide the user with summary statistics. These computer algorithms generally supply information on total sleep time, percent of time spent asleep (sleep efficiency), total wake time, percent of time spent awake, number of awakenings, time between awakenings, and sleep-onset latency.[3,5] Research-grade devices have used a variety of scoring algorithms, many providing the option to select from two or more common algorithms, such as the Cole-Kripke[6] or Sadeh[5] approaches, or in some cases to use a customized approach provided by the user. In recent years, novel approaches to scoring sleep and wake have also emerged based on neural networks and decision trees.[7]

The only time the actigraph must be removed by the patient is during bathing or swimming. Most actigraphs now are water resistant and do not have to be removed for showers. Thus nearly continuous 24-hour recordings over several days, weeks, or even months are possible.

Some actigraphs record additional parameters; for example, ambient light, skin temperature, heart rate, and sound. These features enhance the capability of actigraphy to allow for both clinical and investigational studies of circadian rhythms in the home environment. These data can be helpful in identifying stage-related sleep time (e.g., REM sleep duration). Many actigraphs also provide event buttons that the wearer can push when turning out the lights with an intention to sleep (and/or for marking other salient events). Particular actigraphs may include software to estimate sleep-wake parameters, intensity of daytime activity, and an energy expenditure index.

In recent years, numerous consumer devices and smartphones have begun to provide interested users with estimates of their sleep characteristics, such as nighttime sleep duration, awakenings, and even time spent in various sleep stages. Many of these products are lightweight wearable devices (usually worn on the wrist or placed in a clothing pocket, but sometimes provided as a necklace, ring, or clip). They include accelerometers and/or other sensors to monitor heart rate, skin temperature, or other physiologic parameters, commonly interfaced to a smartphone application via Bluetooth or similar software. With a smartphone application the user may view summary reports including both daytime activity and nighttime sleep patterns.

Although these devices are appealing because they generally are lightweight and inexpensive and provide user-friendly reports of sleep characteristics, their use in research or clinical applications has important limits. In particular, device manufacturers often use proprietary algorithms for sleep-wake parameter estimation, making it unclear how a final result is attained. Also, standardized performance evaluation protocols have only recently been established (see Chapter 207); therefore reliability and validation studies for a given device are either lacking or not comparable to other devices. An important research limitation of consumer-oriented devices is the inability to access raw (i.e., epoch-by-epoch) data that many sleep researchers need to perform more complex analyses. For some of the devices, the need to remove the device regularly for recharging poses an impediment to protocols, requiring continuous long-term data collection. Nonetheless, the widespread use and popularity of such devices fuel interest in their potential use for research.

RELIABILITY OF ACTIGRAPHY FOR ESTIMATING SLEEP

Research has examined the reliability of activity versus PSG for distinguishing wake from sleep. Actigraphically estimated sleep time varies considerably, depending on the device, the scoring software used, the setting, and the specific population being studied. Most studies agree that with correct use, the actigraph is reliable for many populations. However, each actigraph needs its own performance studies. Furthermore, results from one population may not be generalizable to other populations. Most studies indicate actigraphically estimated total sleep time correlates well with PSG data in a normal sample; agreement is typically above 0.80.[3,6,8] In infants and in children, the agreement ranges from 0.90 to 0.95.[9,10] Accuracy is somewhat lower for disturbed sleep. For example, in patients sampled at a sleep disorders clinic, agreement ranged from 0.78 to 0.88.[11,12] Actigraphy has been compared to sleep and wake EEG in nursing home residents with dementia.[13] Correlations with total sleep time were 0.91 for averaged activity (i.e., the average activity recorded per minute) and 0.81 for maximum activity (i.e., the maximum activity recorded per minute). Given the problems with obtaining EEG recordings in this setting, actigraphy offers an adequately accurate and feasible alternative to PSG in these patients. Overall, studies tend to show relatively high sensitivity for detecting sleep but poor specificity for identifying wake when compared with PSG on an epoch-by-epoch basis. Therefore overall agreement tends to be good for estimating total sleep time, but less accurate for determining sleep efficiency and wake after sleep onset.[8]

Most studies comparing actigraphy-derived total sleep time to PSG in older, community-dwelling adults tend to show somewhat worse performance. A multicenter study of 68 community-dwelling older women (mean age 82 years) participating in the Study of Osteoporotic Fractures examined the reliability of estimates of total sleep time. All three modes of actigraphy data collection—ZCM, TAT, and DIM—were compared with unattended in-home EEG recording. Results showed that estimates based on DIM mode were most highly associated with EEG activity; the reliability coefficient (r) was 0.76.[14] A similar study compared actigraphy with electroencephalography as part of the Osteoporotic Fractures in Men (MrOS) sleep study ($n = 889$). In older men, total sleep time based on actigraphy scored in DIM mode was more highly correlated with EEG-based total sleep time as compared with ZCM and TAT modes. Even based on scoring in DIM, however, the correlations were more modest (Pearson correlation coefficient of 0.61).[15] Furthermore, actigraphic total sleep time systematically overestimated total sleep time by an average of about 13 minutes per night in this cohort of older men. Correlations were lower in certain subgroups, such as subjects taking antidepressants and those with severe sleep apnea (apnea-hypopnea index of 30 or higher). In another study involving similar methods in a sample of 181 adolescents, TAT mode performed best in terms of agreement with EEG activity, but correlation was modest ($r = 0.41$). Further analysis, however, revealed better concordance in girls than in boys ($r = 0.66$ versus 0.31), and among those without sleep-disordered breathing (0.55).[16] These findings underscore the importance of considering the possibility of population-specific differences in the reliability of actigraphy for sleep estimation.

Until recently, few head-to-head comparisons between different actigraphs had been performed; consequently, no conclusions could be drawn about which collecting and scoring method agrees better with PSG results. In one study, two common research models of actigraphs were compared with each other and with overnight PSG. The sample included recordings from 115 adolescent boys and girls.[17] Each device had fairly high sensitivity (for detecting sleep) but relatively poor specificity (for detecting wake) compared with PSG. The investigators also noted that reliability of the actigraphs versus PSG recording varied considerably, depending on scoring mode, specific age group studied, and sensitivity setting. Furthermore, the two devices compared poorly with each other, highlighting the need for caution in comparing results across studies, populations, and devices.

Consumer wearable devices are less expensive and widely available, and opportunity exists to access a wealth of data for research purposes. Realizing this, the Associated Professional Sleep Societies hosted a workshop at their 2018 annual meeting on wearable technologies focused on sleep and circadian biomarkers.[18] The panel noted that extant studies were inconsistent and generally poorly designed methodologically. They recommended the need to develop a best practices standard for these technologies. In 2019 the American National Standards Institute in conjunction with the Consumer Technology Association and the National Sleep Foundation published such a performance standard.[19]

Several studies have independently explored the reliability of consumer-level devices with research-grade accelerometers/actigraphs or PSG for sleep estimation. In one study of healthy young adults, estimates for total sleep time were compared among seven consumer-level monitors and two research-grade devices. Agreement was generally above 0.80.[20] Another study of 44 normal adults compared a popular consumer-based activity tracker to a research-grade actigraph and to PSG; the consumer device performed similarly to the actigraph in terms of accuracy in comparison with PSG and showed reasonable accuracy for classifying REM sleep; it was less accurate for classifying stage N3 sleep.[21] The best results for classifying sleep stages (REM and NREM) are generally achieved when multiple features are combined. For example, one study used activity and heart rate and calculated “clock proxy” from signals from a popular consumer device and applied several different methods for classification of REM and NREM sleep.[22] When all features were used, the accuracy for differentiating between wake, REM, and NREM sleep as compared to concurrent PSG was approximately 72%. Technology is rapidly evolving in this area, and many new developments are likely over the coming years.

ADVANTAGES OF CONTINUOUS 24-HOUR ACTIGRAPHIC RECORDINGS

Wrist actigraphy can record continuously for prolonged time durations; therefore behavior occurring both during the night and during the day can be studied. Collecting nighttime and daytime information is particularly useful when evaluating the sleep of patients complaining of insomnia. It economically allows recognition of a pattern of difficulty sleeping. Among patients with complaints of insomnia, actigraphy readily identifies chaotic sleep-wake schedules. It is also helpful to determine sleep quantity and quality variance from night to night over several nights recorded in the patient's home environment. Compared with a sleep diary, actigraphy yields data that are continuous and objective, rather than discrete and self-reported.

The wrist actigraph is particularly valuable for studying patients who have difficulty sleeping in a laboratory with wires used by traditional PSG biosensors (e.g., people with insomnia, children, and elderly persons with dementia). With actigraphy, patients sleep in their natural environment. In elderly subjects with dementia, it has been shown that the traditional recording process disturbs sleep. In addition, the EEG in such patients often does not allow distinguishing wake from sleep.[23] Actigraphy avoids both of these problems and enables the recording of sleep-wake activity in an easy, unobtrusive manner.

Another advantage of collecting data over long periods is the ability to examine the circadian rhythms of the sleep or activity cycle, particularly in studies of patients with sleep-wake schedule disorders (e.g., jet lag, shift work, advanced or delayed sleep phase). Most commercial actigraphy software will now perform circadian rhythm analysis, such as the extended cosine model,[24] generating parameters such as the mesor (mean of the rhythm), the amplitude (peak of the rhythm), and the acrophase (time of the peak of the rhythm). Ideally, these analyses need 5 to 7 days of data collection to be most accurate. Several adaptations and alternative methods of circadian rest-activity rhythm analyses in humans have been developed, using both parametric and nonparametric approaches.[24-26]

Researchers have also leveraged actigraphic measures of sleep and activity collected over consecutive days or weeks to determine the effects of nighttime sleep on next-day function or symptoms such as mood, cognition, fatigue, or pain. This type of analysis, referred to as ecologic momentary assessment, is useful for studying transient conditions that may be impacted by sleep during the previous night. For example, in a study of 73 older adults, actigraphy was continuously recorded over 7 days, along with daily assessments of mood, cognition, and fatigue. In this study, objectively measured sleep quality on a given night predicted next-day fatigue and sleepiness, but not mood or self-perceived thinking ability.[27]

Another novel approach to using the continuous 24-hour activity patterns derived from actigraphy is isotemporal analysis, which allows for modeling the effects of reclassifying various types of activities across the 24-hour day. For example, in a study of more than 3000 older women participating in the Objective Physical Activity and Cardiovascular Heath (OPACH) study ancillary to the Women's Health Initiative, investigators modeled the cross-sectional effects on cardiometabolic outcomes of reallocating time spent in various types of daytime activity to sleep.[28] Findings varied depending on the type of activity and in those with short or longer sleep duration. However, in those with short sleep duration, reallocation of 91 minutes of sedentary behavior to sleep was associated with lower BMI and waist circumference.

An actigraph's concurrent recording of light available in some devices is particularly useful for determining "lights out," as well as observing the beginning of morning light when the sun begins to rise. Light measurements also are helpful in studies of advanced and delayed sleep phase because they help determine light exposure amount and duration. For example, several studies using activity monitors that also record light exposure found that normal elderly persons are exposed to only 58 minutes of bright light per day,[29] patients with Alzheimer disease living at home are exposed to 30 minutes of bright light a day,[30] and nursing home residents are exposed to only 1.7 minutes.[31] Activity and light signals over 24 hours can also be used together to perform phasor analysis, which assesses the degree of synchronization between the two signals, potentially reflective of circadian entrainment.[32] Overall, these data aid the current understanding of the changes occurring in sleep in these populations and can assist in developing treatment plans.

WRIST ACTIGRAPHY APPLICATIONS IN SLEEP DISORDERS

The American Academy of Sleep Medicine (AASM) publishes and updates recommendations on the use of actigraphy in clinical assessment of sleep disorders.[33,34] In 2007 the AASM-appointed committee members concluded, on the basis of published evidence, that actigraphy is reliable and valid for detecting sleep in normal healthy adult populations and in patients suspected of certain sleep disorders. These sleep disorders include advanced sleep phase syndrome, delayed sleep phase syndrome, and shift-work disorder.[33] Additionally, when PSG is not available, actigraphy may be useful to estimate total sleep time in patients with obstructive sleep apnea.[33] In patients with insomnia, the use of actigraphy is recommended for characterizing circadian rhythms and sleep-wake patterns.[33] An updated review in 2018 reported that actigraphy provides distinct, useful information from sleep logs in adults and children being evaluated for insomnia, circadian rhythm sleep wake disorders, and central disorders of hypersomnolence (before multiple sleep latency testing).[34] Use in adults with suspected insufficient sleep disorder and during home testing for sleep-disordered breathing was also endorsed. The practice recommendations also specify that actigraphy is useful in special populations such as children or elderly populations, who may have reduced tolerance to PSG.

Insomnia

Several studies have used actigraphy to evaluate sleep in the patient with insomnia. In a large sample of individuals with insomnia, a high concordance was found between actigraphically derived and PSG-measured total sleep time and sleep fragmentation.[35] Estimates of sleep-onset latency were much less reliable. The study noted the lack of standardization of actigraphy devices and scoring methods across studies. Consequently, the findings of this particular study are not sufficient to support a blanket recommendation regarding the use of actigraphy to assess sleep among persons with insomnia. In a study of 21 young adults diagnosed with insomnia based on structured interviews, actigraphy had a relatively high degree of correlation with PSG for sleep-onset latency (0.77) and total sleep time (0.87); and modest agreement for wake after sleep onset (0.45) and sleep efficiency (0.56). Agreement between actigraphy and sleep log estimates was lower for all sleep parameters.[36] Another study reported that actigraphy tended to underestimate total sleep time, sleep efficiency, and sleep-onset latency and sleep diaries to overestimate sleep-onset latency. However, actigraphy was more accurate than the sleep diary when both were compared against PSG.[37] In the 2018 update of the AASM recommendations for use of actigraphy in assessing sleep disorders, a meta-analysis of studies of adults with insomnia concludes that actigraphy and sleep logs provide estimates for total sleep time, sleep-onset latency, and sleep efficiency that are clinically significantly different from one another. However, it is noted that both actigraphy and sleep logs may prove useful in evaluating insomnia symptoms and treatment response.[34]

Although actigraphy cannot determine the etiology of insomnia, it can help evaluate the manifestation and severity of the condition. In patients with insomnia, the most difficult actigraphic determinations are detecting transitions between sleep and wake and recognizing the ultra-short sleep-wake cycles. However, in patients with insomnia and coexisting circadian rhythm disturbances, actigraphy reliably detects sleep phase alterations.

Sleep Apnea

Actigraphy cannot determine the presence or absence of breathing abnormalities. Nonetheless, several studies tested wrist activity for recognizing patients with sleep apnea. One study compared individuals with and without sleep apnea and found higher movement and fragmentation indices in the afflicted group.[38] Activity measures of sleep also have been shown to successfully differentiate patients with sleep apnea from those with insomnia and from control subjects.[10]

In general, the conclusion from studies is that actigraphy may be capable of identifying disorders provoking brief awakenings and/or arousals. The cause, however, would remain unknown.[3] The potential value of actigraphy in sleep apnea is in combination with cardiopulmonary recorders or other apnea detection equipment used in the home environment that do not include measures of wake or sleep. The addition of an actigraph to such a recording would allow determination of whether all respiratory events actually occurred during sleep. The Standards of Practice Committee of the American Academy of Sleep Medicine concluded that actigraphy is indicated for the assessment of total sleep time among patients with sleep apnea when PSG is not available.[33] However, at present there is insufficient evidence to conclude that home sleep apnea testing devices provide superior performance in detecting sleep apnea severity with integrated actigraphy recording as compared to those without.[34]

Periodic Limb Movements Disorder

Periodic limb movements sleep (PLMS) are detected based on PSG-recorded EMG recordings from anterior of the tibialis muscle. Because the leg movement is the primary characteristic of PLMS, the ability of actigraphy to measure movement suggests an obvious application. One study found high reliability between tibialis EMG and actigraphy for the number of leg movements per hour of sleep.[39] Another study that compared alternative placements of the actigraph for assessment of PLMS in comparison with PSG found that locating the device at the base of the big toe provided good validity.[40] The intensity and severity of PLMS can greatly vary from night to night; therefore actigraphy may offer an advantages in that multiple nights can easily be recorded. After extensive review of the evidence, the AASM concluded there is only modest support for the use of actigraphy in the assessment of PLMD, given there have been few studies, and sample sizes are small.[34] Thus more research and larger samples are needed.

Treatment Effects

Actigraphy is particularly applicable for studying treatment effects because it can readily identify changes at low cost over prolonged time periods. Furthermore, single-session measures of sleep (which frequently is all that is feasible with PSG) may not accurately reflect habitual behavior. Actigraphy has been used to monitor drug and behavioral treatment effects.[41,42] Similarly, it can be used for follow-up assessments once treatment has begun and to evaluate changes in sleep over the course of the treatment period.

Circadian Rhythms

Actigraphy allows the study of sleep-wake patterns occurring over many days; it is therefore well suited to the study of circadian rhythms. Activity is a valid marker of entrained PSG sleep phase and correlates strongly with entrained endogenous circadian phase.[3] Actigraphy has been used to study circadian rhythms in patients with cancer,[43] elderly persons with dementia,[44] adolescents,[45] shift workers,[46] and in-flight crews.[47]

A variety of methodologies are available for analyzing circadian parameters of activity.[24-26,48] However, no studies have compared one methodology with another across different populations. Finally, no one standard methodology has been accepted.

Special Populations

Using actigraphy in the pediatric population is becoming increasingly popular, particularly for evaluation of children with behavioral, psychiatric, or neurologic problems. Actigraphy has been used successfully to characterize sleep of infants[49] and developmental differences.[50] One study used wrist activity to study treatment effects on the sleep patterns of 50 infants whose parents complained of sleep disturbances in their children.[51] Objective activity recordings were compared with parental reports. The activity records showed that percent sleep increased and the number of awakenings during the night decreased with behavioral treatments. After examination of data from each successive night, it was determined that most changes occurred during the first night of intervention. In addition, parental subjective reports significantly differed from objective actigraphy on quality of sleep, with parents reporting fewer awakenings during the night. The presence of objective measures allows for the evaluation of activity during sleep that would otherwise be missed by observation alone.

Actigraphy was used to assess sleep and wake in children with sleep-disordered breathing. One study compared actigraphic estimates of sleep and wake with PSG data on an epoch-by-epoch basis, using various activity thresholds. Overall, very high predictive values and sensitivity were found for detecting sleep (all parameters were higher than 90%), but predictive values and sensitivity for detecting wake were much lower.[52] Although actigraphy offers many advantages for quantifying sleep and wake in children, results may be less reliable for detecting awakenings. Validation studies are needed for the specific devices and for use in the specific population of children.

At the other end of the age spectrum, actigraphy has been used to study sleep-wake patterns in the elderly population. Older adults are particularly susceptible to sleep complaints secondary to circadian rhythm changes, sleep-disordered breathing, PLMS, medical illness, and medication use.[53] Although evaluation of and for some of these complaints may be accomplished in the laboratory, elderly persons often are more set in their ways, need to stay home to take care of a spouse, or just find it more comfortable to sleep in their own beds. In many large studies in older adults, actigraphy represents the only viable option for obtaining objective measures of sleep. Although many studies tend to rely on self-report of sleep duration, this may be inaccurate in older populations, particularly among elderly persons with poor cognition and functional disabilities.[54]

Using actigraphy, a number of studies show that sleep in nursing home residents is extremely fragmented, with most patients never sleeping for a full hour and never awake for a full hour throughout the 24-hour day.[55] In these settings, actigraphy was then used to show that a trial of light treatment consolidated sleep but did not lessen the degree or prevalence of agitation in this population.[56]

Several large epidemiologic studies of older adults incorporate actigraphically determined sleep measures. In such studies, standardization of techniques across multiple clinic sites is essential. In one such study of older women participating in the multicenter Study of Osteoporotic Fractures, excellent agreement was reported between results of an expert scorer and of a second scorer when both followed standardized scoring procedures.[57] Further details are provided in the next section.

EPIDEMIOLOGIC STUDIES

Arguably a major advantage of actigraphic study of sleep and wakefulness is that it opened the door for studying sleep in large samples. Methodologically, this approach not only makes it feasible to conduct such research (by reducing expense) but also helps mitigate attrition by reducing the experimental demands made on participants. Ancoli-Israel and Kripke, along with their colleagues,[58,59] helped pioneer this approach by using actigraphy to study wake and sleep patterns in large samples of elderly (n = 426) and middle-aged adults (n = 355). In conjunction with other sensors, actigraphy was used to estimate sleep apnea and PLMD prevalence. Many of these volunteers would have likely been less willing to participate had they been required to sleep in the laboratory.

Subsequent studies incorporated actigraphically determined sleep measures. In the multicenter Study of Osteoporotic Fractures, actigraphy was performed in nearly 3000 older women. In another multicenter study, the Outcomes of Sleep Disorders in Older Men (MrOS sleep study), actigraphy data were collected in more than 3000 subjects. Using actigraphy in these populations helped identify the relationship between poor sleep and increased risk of falls,[60] poor cognitive function,[61] and poor physical performance and functional limitations.[62] The Rotterdam Study, which collected actigraphy recordings in nearly 1000 older men and women, has been used to demonstrate a relationship between actigraphic sleep duration and fragmentation and risk of obesity[63] and serum cholesterol levels.[64] Actigraphy also has been used to obtain objective measures of sleep characteristics in early middle-aged (38 to 50 years of age) men and women. The Coronary Artery Risk Development in Young Adults study[65] examined data from more than 100,000 adult United Kingdom residents participating in the UK biobank.[66] In the latter study, investigators analyzed genome-wide association studies of circadian rest-activity rhythms and explored potential mechanisms linking circadian rhythms with mood disorders. Some investigators are also repurposing 24-hour activity measures obtained in cohorts for classifying daytime activity and energy expenditure to explore nighttime sleep. For example, the OPACH study, which is an ancillary to the large Women's Health Initiative, has taken this approach to examine waist-worn accelerometry data to study the effects of both activity and sleep on cardiometabolic outcomes.[28]

TRICKS OF THE TRADE

Actigraphs traditionally are placed on the wrist of the nondominant hand. However, two groups of investigators have shown that either wrist can be used. Both groups found that, although activity levels were different for the two hands, rates of agreement with PSG were essentially equivalent for data collected from both hands.[9] In studies in infants, actigraphs also have been placed on the baby's legs.[67]

Most actigraphs come with bands similar to plastic watchbands. For persons who may be sensitive to such bands, or who find it uncomfortable to wear for long time periods, bands made of terry cloth and self-stick fabric (Velcro) can be customized. This has been particularly helpful in some studies of older adults, as arthritis can make it difficult to remove watch bands. To discourage patients from removing the bands, the two Velcro straps were reversed, with one opening from right to left and the other from left to right.

Patients wearing actigraphs should ideally be asked to keep a sleep log or diary. They should note information about daily time to bed, time out of bed, and any unusual activity or times when the device is removed (such as for showers or swimming). This information is helpful for editing and analyzing data and, in particular, setting the sleep period window, which is critical for estimating nighttime sleep variables such as total sleep time. However, some studies have validated approaches to setting the sleep period window in the absence of a diary. One study of 3700 older adults (aged 60–82) used a heuristic algorithm to identify the sleep period. Using this approach, there were minimal differences in the sleep period identified with or without the sleep diary.[68] This approach may be especially useful to apply in large cohort studies in which the sleep diary was not collected, such as the UK Biobank.

When data are accumulated over a period of more than a few weeks, it is prudent to download data every week to minimize data loss. In those units with batteries that must be replaced, battery levels should be checked on initializing the device and again during downloading. Batteries with levels below 90% of the original battery voltage should be discarded, because they are likely to fail. The battery life varies but typically can last up to 30 days. It may be helpful to maintain a battery log that records the battery number, date of initialization of the activity monitor, date of the data download, total number of days of battery use, and starting and ending battery levels.

When actigraphy is used in large samples, with multiple examiners administering the instructions and downloading the data, it is strongly recommended that standardized protocols be developed and that centralized training and certification be incorporated into the overall data quality assurance plan.

With devices that also record light exposure, it is extremely important that the light sensor not be covered by the person's sleeve. The sleeve can be tucked under the actigraph or pinned up to ensure that it does not occlude the light sensor. Another important consideration is that because the angle of the wrist differs from the angle of the eye, the lux reading from a light sensor may differ from that for ambient illumination. Some devices have external light sensors, in addition to the internal sensor, that can be clipped to a collar and conceivably may give more exact readings. Separate light sensors worn at eye level or as a pendant around the neck can also be used to avoid this problem.[69] All activity and light monitors should be checked on a regular basis to determine if calibration is needed.

In patients with sensitive skin, the bands can be removed for a few minutes each day to avoid pressure sores. The time the device is removed, the time it is replaced, and whether the person was awake for the few minutes it was removed all should be noted on the log. This information is needed during the data editing process.

EDITING ACTIGRAPHY DATA

Different software packages are available for scoring the rest-activity data and inferring sleep-wake status. Data are edited on a computer screen with the use of the daily sleep log. Time intervals during which the device is removed should be manually changed to wake status only if the investigator is sure that the person was awake (e.g., in the shower); otherwise, these data points should be marked as missing data. Lack of movement scored as sleep, such as when the device is removed for especially vigorous activity, also can be manually changed to the wake category. If no information is provided in the log about the activity during the time the device was removed, that time period should be scored as missing data.

As actigraphy has become more widely used, particularly in research settings, some investigators have used the devices without diaries and scoring procedures. Although some misclassification of sleep-wake periods is possible, many newer devices have off-wrist detection and automatic detection of sleep onset and offset, which improves overall estimation of sleep.

Figure 211.2 shows examples of two actigraph outputs.

LIMITATIONS

Actigraph data scorers need to be aware of the limitations of these devices.[3] When compared with PSG, actigraphy is fairly valid and reliable in healthy normal subjects. It is best at estimating total sleep time. As sleep becomes more disturbed, the actigraphy recording becomes less accurate. In general, actigraphy may overestimate sleep and underestimate wake, particularly during the day.

CLINICAL PEARLS

- Actigraphy has good agreement with PSG for determining sleep parameters in normal populations but is generally less reliable for identifying disturbed sleep.
- Actigraphy is a useful adjunct for evaluating insomnia, circadian rhythm disorders, and excessive sleepiness.
- Actigraphy is useful for assessing sleep in special populations, including children and older adults with dementia.
- Actigraphy is becoming a valuable tool for investigating sleep and sleep disturbances in large-scale epidemiologic studies and is increasingly included as an adjunct outcome in clinical trials.

SUMMARY

Wrist actigraphy has several important advantages over PSG. (1) It allows the recording of sleep in natural environments. (2) It records movement activity both during the night and during the day. (3) It records continuously for long time periods. (4) It is cost efficient. Although not a replacement for EEG or PSG recordings, in certain instances research-grade actigraphy provides clear advantages for data collection. A variety of consumer devices are now available; however, their reliability is currently poorly established for estimating sleep relative to research-grade devices.

Actigraphy is particularly useful for evaluating patients who cannot tolerate sleeping in the laboratory. It also provides a more representative picture of an individual's typical sleep timing and duration by permitting adherence to the usual sleep schedule. Actigraphy also is becoming an important tool in follow-up studies and for examining treatment efficacy in clinical outcome.

Actigraphy has value in the assessment of sleep disorders. The newer scoring algorithms have improved accuracy for measures important in insomnia; specifically, wake versus sleep determination, sleep latency, awakenings during the night, and total sleep time. Actigraphy is far superior to sleep logs for detecting brief awakenings during the night. It also can be used for the evaluation and clinical diagnosis of circadian rhythm disorders. The ability to detect movements holds promise in the identification of sleep disorders characterized by frequent movements, such as PLMS, sleep apnea, or REM sleep behavior disorders. Actigraphy provides a particularly useful tool in situations requiring long-term monitoring.

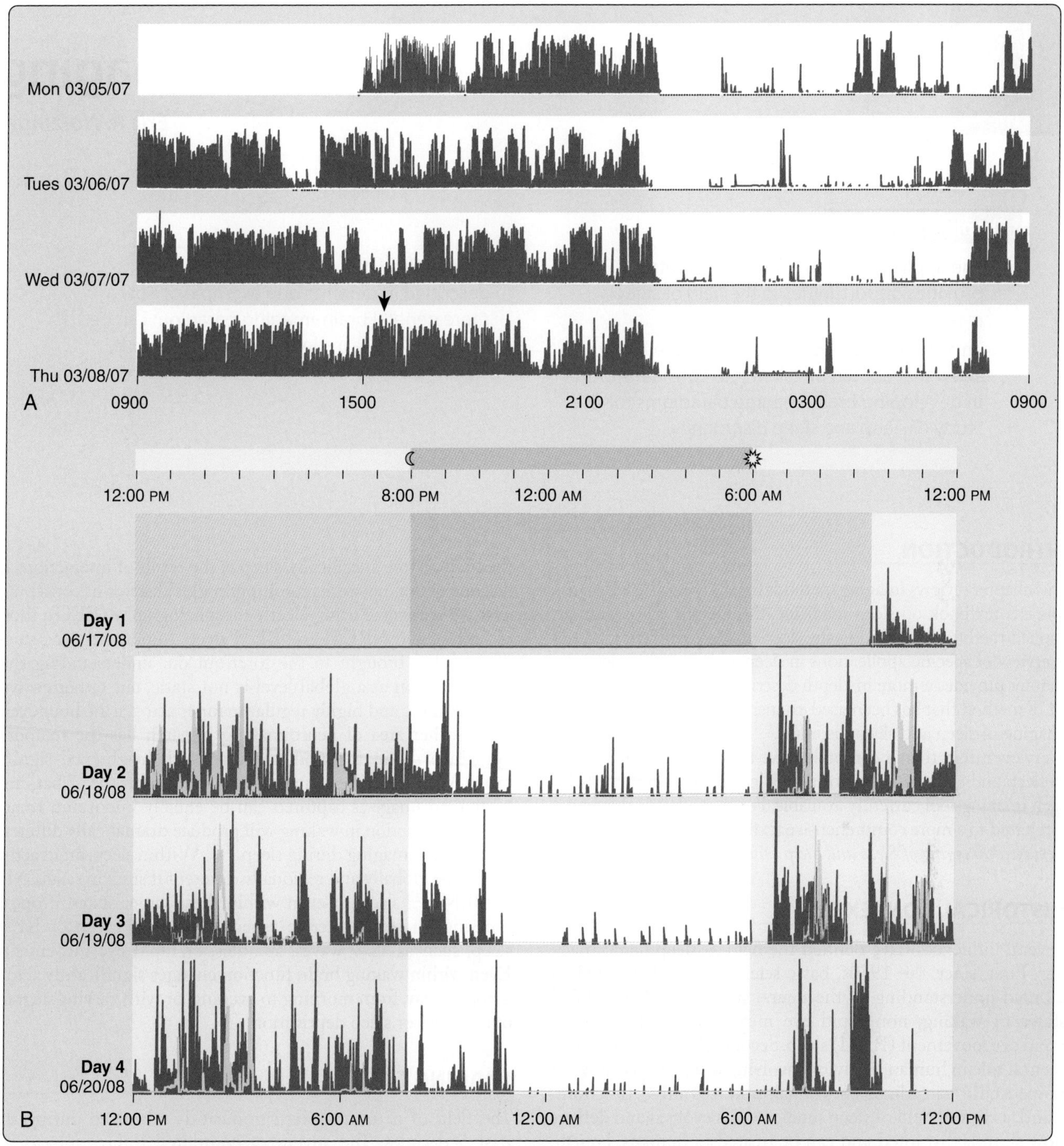

Figure 211.2 A, Four days of unscored output from the Octagonal SleepWatch actigraph. **B,** Four days of unscored output from the Actiwatch. (**A,** Courtesy Ambulatory Monitoring, Inc., Ardsley, New York. **B,** Courtesy of Philips RS North America LLC. All rights reserved.)

SELECTED READINGS

Ancoli-Israel S, Cole R, Alessi CA, et al. The role of actigraphy in the study of sleep and circadian rhythms. *Sleep*. 2003;26(3):342–392.

Blackwell T, Ancoli-Israel S, Redline S, Stone KL. Factors that may influence the classification of sleep-wake by wrist actigraphy: the MrOS Sleep Study. *J Clin Sleep Med*. 2011;7(4):357–367.

Smith MT, McCrae CS, Cheung J, et al. Use of Actigraphy for the Evaluation of Sleep Disorders and Circadian Rhythm Sleep-Wake Disorders: an American Academy of Sleep Medicine Systematic Review, meta-analysis, and GRADE Assessment. *J Clin Sleep Med*. 2018;14(7):1209–1230.

Williams JM, Taylor DJ, Slavish DC, et al. Validity of Actigraphy in young adults with insomnia. *Behav Sleep Med*. 2020;18(1):91–106.

Zeitzer JM, Blackwell T, Hoffman AR, et al. Daily patterns of accelerometer activity predict changes in sleep, cognition, and mortality in older men. *J Gerontol A Biol Sci Med Sci*. 2018;73(5):682–687.

A complete reference list can be found online at ExpertConsult.com.

Chapter 212

Imaging

Eric A. Nofzinger

Chapter Highlights

- The application of brain-imaging methods provides opportunities in the field of sleep medicine.
- This chapter reviews unique factors related to sleep that should be taken into consideration in developing brain-imaging paradigms for the study of sleep and sleep disorders.
- One method, the [18F]FDG-PET method, is described in detail as one example of how a more general brain-imaging paradigm can be adapted for use in sleep medicine research.

INTRODUCTION

This chapter reviews imaging methods for studying sleep. Because this is a textbook on sleep medicine, this chapter focuses on an applied method for studying the sleep process. Following a brief overview of specific applications in sleep and sleep disorders, the chapter provides a more in-depth description of the [18F]FDG-PET method that has been used extensively for functional neuroimaging of sleep and sleep disorders.[1-5] This chapter provides an overview rather than a comprehensive review of imaging results in sleep and sleep disorders or a detailed instruction manual for each imaging tool currently available. For these details the reader is referred to a more comprehensive textbook devoted to this subject, *Neuroimaging of Sleep and Sleep Disorders.*[6]

HISTORICAL CONTEXT

Several influences have defined the field of sleep neuroimaging. First, since the 1950s, basic science research has led to a broad understanding of the neural substrates of the global states of waking, non–rapid eye movement (NREM), and rapid eye movement (REM) sleep. Second, sleep plays a fundamental role in human behavior, involving interactions between homeostatic, circadian, emotional, and cognitive functions. Third, a clinical field of sleep medicine has evolved and defines how sleep is disrupted and can be treated in humans. Fourth, cognitive neuroscience has revealed regional brain specificity for particular behaviors and cognitive processes, such as motor behavior, sensory processing, thought, and emotion. Fifth, significant technical advances in ways to "image" the human brain, at both the structural and functional levels (e.g., magnetic resonance imaging [MRI], positive emission tomography [PET], and functional magnetic resonance imaging [fMRI]), make possible the testing of hypotheses at a regional brain level in relation to human behavior, health, and pathology.[6-9]

"SLEEP" AS AN OBJECT FOR IMAGING

Sleep is perhaps in a unique position for study via functional neuroimaging. Sleep is now understood to be a manifestation of the brain. More specifically, sleep is the result of interactions in discrete neural networks resulting in global states of consciousness we recognize using electroencephalography (EEG): those of waking and NREM and REM sleep. Importantly, the study of sleep has brought to the forefront our understanding that brain function at a global level is not static, but rather evolves in a rhythmic and highly regular manner across a 24-hour cycle. In no other area of neuroimaging research has the temporal domain of brain function taken on such heightened significance. We now understand that knowing both the "what" and "when" an image is captured can be equally important. Imaging brain function in waking will produce dramatically different results than imaging during sleep.[10,11] Within sleep, brain activity will be globally and regionally different if studying NREM[11] or REM[12,13] sleep, or even within these larger states, if one is focusing on some discrete aspect of NREM sleep or REM sleep, such as slow waves, spindles, or rapid eye movements. Even within waking brain function changes significantly across a normal day, from morning to evening, or with varying degrees of alertness or sleep deprivation.

IMAGING TOOLS

The field of neuroimaging significantly advanced during the past 5 decades. The advent of computed tomography (CT) allowed visualization of brain structure in a living human. CT scans provided clarity on bony structures primarily but had less ability to define internal brain structures. Limitations of CT scanning included exposure of an individual to ionizing radiation and limited ability to detect brain tissue differences. The development of magnetic resonance imaging allowed for the detection of more subtle changes in brain tissues and did not involve exposure of the subject to radiation. Applications of structural imaging to sleep and sleep disorders, primarily using MR methods defined brain structural changes related to pathophysiology or consequences of suffering from a specific sleep disorder.

Greater insights into the mechanisms and consequences of sleep and sleep disorders have been achieved through advances

Table 212.1 Functional Neuroimaging Methods for Sleep

	MEG Tomography	fMRI	[O15] H2O PET	[18F] FDG-PET	^{99}mTc-ECD SPECT	Receptor imaging
Measure	Electrical events	Blood flow	Blood flow	Metabolism	Flow/ metabolism	5-HT, DA, ACH, GABA…
Spatial resolution	10 mm	< cm	cm	cm	cm	cm
Temporal resolution	Milliseconds	Seconds	Minute	10–20 minutes	Minutes	20–90 minutes
Sleep in scanner?	Yes	Yes	Yes	No	No	Waking
Other	Difficult in sleep Availability, expense	Noise, technically difficult in sleep	Repeated measures possible	Long half-life limits repeated measures	Repeatable in single night	Expensive, labor intensive

ACH, acetylcholine; *cm,* centimeter; *DA,* dopamine; *ECD,* ethyl cysteinate dimer; *FDG,* fluoro-deoxyglucose; *5-HT,* 5-hydroxytryptamine; *fMRI,* functional magnetic resonance imaging; *GABA,* gamma-aminobutyric acid; *MEG,* magnetoencephalography; *mm,* millimeter; *PET,* positron emission tomography; *SPECT,* single photon emission computed tomography.

in brain-imaging methods that describe various aspects of neural "function."[6] These are collectively referred to as functional neuroimaging (Table 212.1). These include techniques such as positron emission tomography (PET), fMRI, single photon emission computed tomography (SPECT), transcranial sonography, magnetoencephalography (MEG), low-resolution brain electromagnetic tomography (LORETA), diffusion tensor imaging (DTI)[14] to estimate the location, orientation, and anisotropy of the brain's white matter tracts, and combined methods such as combined EEG and fMRI. In each of these methods, there are assumed relationships between what the brain is doing (e.g., neuronal activity) and the measured process (e.g., changes in blood flow or metabolism). In most cases, these tools were developed to study waking brain function and the assumptions underlying the measurements apply to waking brain activity. It is generally assumed that brain activity and its measurement is equivalent between wakefulness, NREM, and stage REM. However, this assumption is not rigorously validated. Although early functional brain-imaging studies focused on brain activity in discrete brain regions across gross behavioral states, more recent studies have taken advantage of advances in image analysis tools in which relationships between brain regions (functional connectivity) across behavioral states or across populations can be analyzed.[15-18]

APPLICATIONS OF IMAGING TO THE STUDY OF SLEEP AND SLEEP DISORDERS

Neuroimaging of Wakefulness and Sleep

The earliest applications of neuroimaging to the study of sleep and its disorders were focused on global brain states of waking and NREM and REM sleep.[10-13,19] Before these methods were applied, knowledge of these gross behavioral states and their mechanisms came largely from preclinical work. Basic science methods used existing neuroscience tools for assessing electrophysiology and the cellular and molecular mechanisms of sleep. The general understanding was that sleep-wake function could be defined by discrete global electrophysiologic signals that differentiated various states of neural processing such as waking and NREM and REM sleep. Early functional brain-imaging work during sleep therefore was somewhat exploratory and descriptive, defining large-scale changes in regional brain activity across these states of consciousness. These early findings revolutionized our general understanding of human sleep in terms of the coordinated neural networks involved. Although preclinical work largely focused on the switches defining the regulation of sleep at a brainstem and hypothalamic level, the human sleep neuroimaging findings drew attention to the involvement or participation of higher levels of the central nervous system that likely play fundamental roles in the overall function of sleep. More recent analyses have focused on higher-resolution temporal events such as phasic and nonphasic aspects of each individual state and validating neural changes in the brain as predicted from the preclinical sciences.

Neuroimaging and Sleep Loss and Circadian Misalignment

Behavioral human sleep research defined many relationships between human sleep loss and performance. Extensive evidence defined both homeostatic and circadian influences on sleep and disruptions in either of these domains. Even in an otherwise healthy individual, sleep loss led to predictable changes in alertness, cognition, and performance. Extensive application of functional neuroimaging has helped clarify the changes in regional brain function that result from perturbations in either homeostatic or circadian processes. It also helped clarify the relationship between these brain changes and the behavioral consequences of these disruptions.[15,16,20-22]

Sleep and Memory

Research has clarified a role for sleep in brain plasticity. This involves the capacity of the nervous system to change its structure and its function over a lifetime, in reaction to environmental diversity. Brain plasticity could include concepts such as synaptic plasticity, neurogenesis, and functional compensatory plasticity, concepts that had been evolving in the basic and cognitive neurosciences but previously had not been applied to the study of sleep. This area of research developed some of the most exciting hypotheses that sleep contributes importantly to processes of memory and brain plasticity. In recent decades, a large body of work, spanning most of the neurosciences, has provided a substantive body of evidence supporting this role of sleep in what is now known as sleep-dependent memory processing. This includes memory encoding, memory consolidation, brain plasticity, and memory re-consolidation. Extensive evidence is now known from functional brain-imaging studies in support of this emerging model of one of the critical functions of sleep.[17,18,23,24]

NEUROIMAGING OF SLEEP DISORDERS

The field of sleep medicine developed based on an increasing knowledge of the physiology of sleep, circadian biology, and the pathophysiology of sleep disorders. Scientific progress combined with an increasing recognition that disorders of sleep are highly prevalent in society has increased interest in tools that enhance the diagnosis and treatment of sleep disorders. Sleep neuroimaging of sleep disorders has paralleled the development of this evolving field of medicine.[6,8,9] Brain-imaging methods provided knowledge in a new domain to the understanding of the neurobiology of discrete sleep disorders beyond what could be seen in a standard EEG sleep assessment. Indeed, in some cases, such as primary insomnia, brain-imaging studies have been shown to be more sensitive to defining pathology than traditional sleep EEG,[25-28] although questions about convergent findings remain.[29] Brain-imaging studies have rapidly evolved in the area of obstructive sleep apnea syndrome. Brain MR studies have been performed to describe volumetric changes in discrete regions of the brain that may play a role in the pathogenesis of the disorder or as a manifestation of having obstructive sleep apnea. MR studies have also been used extensively to define the anatomic abnormalities in the upper airways of patients with these disorders that contribute to the obstructed breathing. Functional brain-imaging studies have demonstrated mechanisms related to ventilatory control in the central nervous system, the adverse consequences of sleep apnea on neural function as well as their reversal with treatment with continuous positive airway pressure.[30,31] Brain-imaging studies in restless legs syndrome/periodic limb movement disorder have focused on the dopaminergic system via PET ligands in the dopamine system, and functional brain-imaging studies have focused on regions of the brain involved in motor behavior.[32-34] Major breakthroughs in our understanding of the neurobiology of narcolepsy have occurred in the past several decades,[35-37] and both structural and functional neuroimaging methods have been applied to the study of this disorder.[38-40] The field of sleep neuroimaging holds promise for future use in clinical sleep medicine not only as a research tool to understand pathophysiology but also clinically in terms of diagnosis and prediction and monitoring of treatment effects. Future clinical applications will depend on advances in our understanding of individual disorders as well as technical refinements in imaging methods that should make them cost effective and widely available for future use in sleep medicine.

The [18F]FDG-PET Method for Studying Brain Function during Sleep

One method of assessing human forebrain activation during sleep uses the [18F] 2-fluoro-2-deoxy-D-glucose ([18F] FDG) radiotracer[2-5,41] and positron emission tomography (PET) measures of regional cerebral glucose utilization.[1,10] In comparison with other functional brain-imaging techniques (e.g., fMRI), this method offers the advantage of a more naturalistic study of sleep because subjects do not have to sleep in a scanning device. This leads to a higher rate of successful completion of studies. The primary disadvantage of this method is the decreased temporal resolution necessitating assessments of global sleep states (e.g., REM or NREM) as opposed to assessing events within a sleep state (e.g., sleep spindles or rapid eye movements).

[18F]FDG-PET is currently the most accurate in vivo method for the investigation of regional human brain metabolism. Guidelines have been established for the conduct of [18F]FDG-PET scans of brain activity.[42] [18F]2-fluoro-2-deoxy-D-glucose ([18F]FDG) is a glucose analogue, where fluorine-18 (half-life 109.8 minutes) substitutes the hydroxyl group at the second position in the glucose molecule. [18F] FDG is commonly used to measure tissue glucose consumption in vivo. [18F]FDG enters the tissue via glucose transporters and can then be either phosphorylated by hexokinase to [18F]FDG-6-phosphate or transported from tissue back to blood. [18F]FDG-6-phosphate cannot be transported out of the tissue or metabolized further through glycolysis and pentose phosphate pathways. In most tissues dephosphorylation of [18F]FDG-6-phosphate is slow because of very low activity of glucose-6P-phosphatase; phosphorylated [18F]FDG is therefore often assumed to be trapped inside the cells. It is this feature of being "trapped" in the cells until radioactive decay that makes this method unique among imaging methods for studying brain function in sleep states.[1] Effectively, a subject can sleep comfortably and undisturbed in a bedroom environment during the injection/delivery and uptake of the radiotracer into the brain cells. After about 20 minutes when plasma levels of the tracer have receded because of normal circulation out of the brain, the radiotracer remaining in the brain is that which was trapped in the cells that were active in the few minutes after injection. At that time, a research subject can be transported from their bedroom to a PET scanner for imaging. The resulting PET image reflects activity in the brain at the time of radiotracer injection and is relatively unmodulated by any behavior occurring 20 minutes and after to the time of the scan. The autoradiographic method for measuring regional metabolic rate of glucose in the brain of rat using [14C]deoxyglucose[2] has been modified for human studies using positron emission tomography (PET) and [18F]2-fluoro-2-deoxy-D-glucose.[3,4,41]

Subject Selection

Medical history taking and physical examination, as well as subject preparation, should follow established guidelines in nuclear medicine.[42]

Rooms for Recording Sleep and Injecting Radiotracers

Subject rooms should be sound attenuated and allow for the monitoring of intravenous (IV) equipment and polysomnography in a room adjacent to the subject's bedroom through hole-in-the-wall techniques, thereby avoiding artificial sleep disruption. Beds should be comfortable and the distance from the bed to the hole-in-the-wall should be short enough to minimize the length of IV tubing for radionuclide administration while long enough to not be overly restrictive of subjects' movements during sleep in bed.

Electroencephalographic Sleep Procedures

Electroencephalographic (EEG) sleep is monitored on all nights of study. The first night is generally not used in further analyses because of the effects of adaptation on EEG sleep. Consequently, this night is used to screen for primary sleep disorders, including sleep apnea and periodic limb movements, which may have an independent effect on either sleep quality or cerebral glucose metabolism independent of the effects of interest. On nights when [18F]FDG will not be injected, subjects have IV tubing taped over (1) the antecubital area of one arm and (2) the antecubital area or forearm of the opposite arm for accommodation to indwelling IVs used on injection nights for bolus injection of the radioisotope and sampling of venous blood. On injection nights, subjects have normal saline infusions at a keep-vein-open (KVO) infusion rate throughout the night in one antecubital vein and a vein in the opposite arm. The sleep montage on the adaptation night consists of a single EEG channel (C4/A1-A2), bilateral electrooculograms (EOGs) referenced to A1-A2, bipolar submental electromyogram (EMG), oral-nasal thermistors, rib cage and abdominal motion sensors, single-lead electrocardiogram, fingertip oximetry, and anterior tibialis EMG. Alternate EEG montages can be used according to the focus of interest of study. Traditionally, the second night of sleep studies is monitored and undisturbed by injections related to PET studies for the collection of baseline EEG sleep measures. This baseline montage (night 2) consists of a single EEG channel (C4/A1-A2), two EOG channels (right and left eyes) referenced to A1-A2, and submental EMG. On PET assessment nights and during waking PET scans, an expanded EEG montage (F3, F4, C4, P3, P4, O1, O2, T3, T4 each referenced to A1-A2) is employed to permit comparisons between region-specific spectral EEG and regional cerebral metabolic rate for glucose (rCMRglu) derived from PET. During their EEG sleep assessment, patients' bedtimes and good morning times are determined from their usual bedtimes and usual good morning times, according to a daily sleep-wake diary completed over 7 days before sleep assessments, so as to minimize entrainment to the sleep laboratory setting.

Positron Emission Tomography Scan Paradigm

Optimally, given the dynamics of [18F]FDG uptake and metabolism, the injection of the [18F]FDG should occur at the initial 7 to 10 minutes of a 20- to 30-minute behavioral state. The temporal resolution of this method is thus best for assessing global behavioral states such as waking and NREM and REM sleep, as opposed to assessing transitions between states or discrete electrophysiologic events within states, such as spindle activity or K-complexes. Assessment of at least two behavioral states allows for statistical contrasts between regional cerebral metabolic differences in the different states. The timing of PET scans is chosen to maximize differences in the three major global states of activation of the brain: waking, REM sleep, and NREM sleep. Further refinements in timing can be made depending on the focus of study. For example, waking scans can be performed at multiple times across the day, and effects may vary according to circadian and homeostatic factors. Maximal alertness, which has previously been shown to occur 2 to 4 hours after a person's habitual waking time, could be chosen if the intent were to show effects related to maximal alertness. The timing of the REM sleep PET scan can vary across the night according to the REM period of interest, with the caveats that the first REM period is traditionally the shortest of the night and the last REM period is subject to termination by awakening at the end of the night. The timing of the NREM sleep PET scan can be chosen according to the degree of slow wave sleep activity desired for study, peaking in the first NREM cycle and decreasing across successive NREM cycles. The order of all scans should be randomized to minimize order effects on PET measures. Waking scans should always follow an uninterrupted night of sleep to exclude effects of sleep deprivation on waking PET measures, because approximately 90 minutes of partial sleep deprivation occur during nights when sleep-related PET scans are acquired. For the same reason, a recovery night should be interposed between any sleep-related scans. Studies of more extensive partial sleep deprivation (the first 3 hours of sleep, and 2 consecutive nights of sleep restricted to the first 4 hours of the subject's usual sleeping time) suggest that minimal, if any, recovery effects from either NREM or REM sleep deprivation will be present by the second recovery night.

Awake Comparison [18F]FDG rCMRglu Paradigm

This study condition consists of 20 minutes of EEG (expanded montage) monitored wakefulness after injection of 4 mCi [18F]FDG after a night of EEG sleep studies, lying supine, with eyes closed, and ears open in the same bedroom used for sleep studies after a 15-minute accommodation period. The time of day is determined by the aims of the study. Six venous samples are assessed for radioactivity at 8-minute intervals beginning at postinjection time (T) = 45 minutes for determination of absolute glucose metabolism according to the methods of Phillips and colleages[43] and Schmidt and colleagues.[5]

REM Sleep [18F]FDG rCMRglu Paradigm

For all sleep studies, subjects sleep in a comfortable bed in a bedroom maximized for sleep and that allows for hole-in-the-wall access to IV monitoring from an adjoining room. During EEG sleep assessment, 4 mCi [18F]FDG is injected IV via an indwelling catheter after the onset of the first rapid eye movement in the REM period of interest. After 20 minutes the subject is awakened and transported to the PET scanner for a 30-minute emission scan, then allowed to return to their bedroom for sleep. Six venous samples are assessed for radioactivity at 8-minute intervals beginning at postinjection time (T = 45 minutes) for determination of absolute glucose metabolism according to the methods of Phillips and colleagues[43] and Schmidt and colleagues.[5]

NREM Sleep [18F]FDG rCMRglu Paradigm

This condition consists of 20 minutes of NREM sleep during the NREM period of interest. During the night of study, 4 mCi [18F]FDG is injected IV via an indwelling catheter at the beginning of the 20-minute NREM period of interest. After 20 minutes the subject is awakened and transported to the PET scanner for a 30-minute emission scan, then allowed to return to their bedroom for sleep. Six venous samples are assessed for radioactivity at 8-minute intervals beginning at postinjection time (T = 45 minutes) for determination of absolute glucose metabolism according to the methods of Phillips and colleagues[43] and Schmidt and colleagues.[5] In our studies we have used the 20-minute period beginning at 20 minutes after sleep onset to maximize the potential for delta sleep and to minimize the potential for arousals or for early entry into REM sleep based on minute-by-minute inspection of automated delta counts and manually scored sleep EEGs for subjects previously studied in our laboratory.

All PET scans are initiated 60 minutes after injection of the [18F]FDG and consist of six summed 5-minute emission scans (total emission time is 30 minutes followed by a 10-minute transmission scan for quantitative correction of attenuation). An individually molded, thermoplastic head holder (marked with laser guidance for repositioning) is made for each subject to minimize head movement. The use of a 4 mCi [18F]FDG dose, rather than the conventional clinical dose (e.g., for brain tumors) of 10 mCi, and the use of electronic windowing of the rod source to reject head activity permit acquisition of the transmission scan following the [18F] FDG injection rather than preceding.

The uptake of [18F]FDG from plasma to tissue is 70% to 80% maximal in the first 12 minutes after an IV injection and approximates completion at 25 minutes. The pattern of rCMRglu shown by PET for the injection of [18F]FDG during waking will reflect brain activity during a resting, waking state. For REM periods longer than 12 minutes in which the subsequent uptake period is NREM sleep, a period in which [18F]FDG uptake is low, the pattern of rCMRglu obtained during the period after injection will reflect brain activity during REM sleep almost exclusively.

Positron Emission Tomography Scanner

A state-of-the-art dedicated PET scanner, image acquisition, image processing, and quantitative analysis of absolute glucose metabolism should be used according to established guidelines.[42] Studies in our laboratory have used several different scanners that have been updated over time because of refinements in imaging technology. Early studies used an ECAT 951 Rr31 scanner in the 2-D mode. Later studies used an ECAT HRq scanner in the 3-D mode. The ECAT HRq scanner offers several advantages over the ECAT 951Rr31: (1) a factor of 2.4 improvement in volume spatial resolution (4 mm transaxial and <4 mm axial resolutions; 0.07 mL volume resolution); (2) a 50% increase in axial field-of-view in both 2-D and 3-D modes to allow coverage of the whole brain, including brainstem structures implicated in the generation of sleep states; (3) a factor of 3 increase in peak useful count rate at 0.6 mCi/mL; (4) a factor of 2 increase in 2-D sensitivity at low activity concentrations; (5) a 50% increase in 3-D sensitivity at low activity concentrations; (6) a factor of 2 increase in the maximum data acquisition rate; (7) low noise, short imaging time, and transmission scans from high-activity single-point source; (8) improved reliability resulting from increased use of application-specific integrated circuits; and (9) software version 7.0, including integrated 3-D acquisition and expanded analysis capabilities. More recent updates have been to a Siemens Biograph mCT Flow PET/CT. This PET/CT scanner offers 21.6 cm of axial scan coverage (TrueV option) with an intrinsic in-plane spatial resolution of approximately 4.2 mm full-width half-maximum. The CT subsystem is a 64-slice helical scanner that can be used to acquire diagnostic quality CT or a low-dose scan for the purpose of attenuation correction of PET emission data. This unit is equipped with Siemens' FlowMotion technology supporting continuous bed motion acquisition, HeartView CT and both cardiac and respiratory gating hardware for reconstructing phase-matched PET and CT images, SAFIRE iterative CT reconstruction, and SMART NeuroAC for calculated attenuation correction for brain imaging.

Head Holder

An individually molded, thermoplastic head holder (marked with laser guidance for repositioning) is made for each subject to minimize head movement and to allow for head positioning for scanning.

Magnetic Resonance Imaging

Subjects undergo MR scanning before their PET study. The subjects are positioned in a standard head coil and a brief scout sagittal T1-weighted image is obtained. Standard axial T1-weighted (TE = 18, TR = 400, NEX = 1, slice thickness = 3 mm) interleaved images are acquired. Imaging time is estimated at 10 minutes.

[18F]FDG Synthesis

[18F]FDG is synthesized according to the methods described by Hamacher and colleagues.[44]

Image Processing

MR data are transferred to the PET facility over an electronic network and registered with the PET data (PET data summed from T = 60–90 minutes after [18F]FDG injection) on a SparcStation using automated image registration (AIR) software.[45] AIR minimizes the voxel-by-voxel variance of a ratio of the two images being registered. The registered MR is used as an individualized anatomic map for the selection of regions of interest (ROIs) used in the analysis of the PET data. All PET images are reconstructed using standard commercial software as 63 transaxial slices (center-to-center = 2.4 mm) with approximately 4- to 5-mm full-width half-maximum resolution. After the six 5-minute PET emission scans are co-registered, they are summed. Then this very high-count image set is registered to the subject's volume MR study (see previously) by AIR as described previously. Staff review these data to ensure adequate registration (error < 1 pixel).

At this point two parallel types of data processing occur. One type involves drawing different ROIs on the MRI. These individual ROIs as well as whole-brain slice ROI are then placed on the co-registered PET data sets to yield relative (ROI counts/whole brain counts) and absolute (after construction of PET images from the calculation of each individual scans absolute glucose metabolism) rCMRglu values for later statistical processing. The second type of processing employs statistical parametric processing (SPM).[46,47] In our application of SPM, the MR data are transformed to the standard atlas MR data set (provided by Dr. Friston) by linear affine transformation within an expanded form of AIR.[45] The co-registered PET data are then similarly transformed into the standard Talairach space by using the same transformation equations as for the subject's MRI. This technique thus relies on the high density of anatomic information in the MRI for coordinate transformation rather than the PET image. Once transformed the PET data are processed by typical SPM approach, using an analysis of covariance (ANCOVA) to control for global changes and post-hoc t-tests to detect regions of significant state-dependent change. A normalized Gaussian z score outputs the pixels of significant differences and their Talairach atlas coordinates (see Talairach and Tournoux[48]). Calculation of absolute regional cerebral metabolic rates (rCMRglu) follows the guidelines established by Schmidt and colleagues[5] using a 3K model and using the modified single scan and six blood sample methods validated by Phillips and colleagues.[43]

Imaging Paradigm Selection

Several design features are important in constructing a functional imaging research paradigm for use during sleep:

- The functional neuroanatomy should be studied while maintaining, as closely as possible, the integrity of sleep.

Except for [18F]FDG-PET, the commonly employed functional imaging methods (blood flow, fMRI) used in cognitive activation studies require immobilization of the head because the image is acquired at the time of the cognitive activation. This limits naturalistic sleep because most subjects have difficulty sleeping in this nonnaturalistic setting. In contrast, the [18F]FDG-PET method, using hole-in-the-wall techniques for monitoring, allows subjects to sleep undisturbed in a private bedroom. EEG sleep studies confirmed that sleep integrity is minimally affected by this procedure.

- The temporal resolution of the imaging procedure should approximate the time of the global sleep state to be studied.

The temporal resolution of the [18F]FDG uptake period (maximal in the first 7 to 10 minutes and near complete at 20 minutes) is comparable to the mean duration of the NREM (20 minutes) and REM sleep (~14 minutes for the first REM sleep period) periods in our studies. The contribution of metabolism to regional measures following REM sleep is thought to be minimal given the low metabolic rate associated with NREM sleep.

- The paradigm should provide for the assessment of both regional as well as absolute measures of functional neuroanatomy.

Recent reports provide models for quantifying regional cerebral glucose metabolism during sleep. The first, by Phillips and colleagues,[43] validated a simplified method to calculate rCMRglu using a single-scan method and obtaining six evenly spaced blood samples between postinjection times 45 and 90 minutes. At these times, plasma radioactivity is closely matched between arterial and venous samples, allowing for sampling of venous blood. The second, by Schmidt and colleagues,[5] reviewed recent developments in the field and offered guidelines for the standard assessment of cerebral glucose metabolism using [18F]FDG and PET. In these guidelines, the acquisition of the emission scan should occur within the 60- to 120-minute period postinjection to allow both maximum equilibration of the precursor pools in the tissue with the arterial plasma, yet short enough to minimize product loss related to dephosphorylation of [18F]FDG. Within this window, they recommend a three-compartment model so that the cerebral metabolic rate is not overestimated related to the inclusion of a k_4. In the current design, therefore, both scanning and blood sampling for determination of both regional as well as absolute glucose metabolism can occur significantly later than the uptake period during sleep so that sleep integrity is not affected.

- Multiple assessments of functional neuroanatomy should be possible within a subject to enable comparisons between global brain states and to allow repeated comparisons for use in longitudinal study designs.

The low doses of [18F]FDG (4 mCi) used for each PET scan allows for repeated assessments within subjects during waking, REM, and NREM sleep at different time points. Studies in which multiple repeated measures must be obtained, however, will be limited in the [18F]FDG because of limitations of radioactivity exposure that subjects may receive.

- The paradigm should control for the potential effects of the stress of the imaging procedures on dependent variables.

The current paradigm minimizes the effects of stress of functional imaging assessments in several ways. First, subjects have 2 nights of accommodation to the restrictions of IV attachments during sleep. Second, the performance of MR scans before PET scans helps accommodate subjects to scanning procedures. Randomizing the order of study conditions (waking, NREM, and REM sleep) controls for order effects of scanning.

- The design should allow for the screening of primary sleep disorders that may have an independent effect on functional imaging outcome measures.

In the current design, effects related to sleep disorders such as sleep apnea syndrome or periodic limb movement disorder are controlled by testing for these disorders on a screening night and excluding subjects with these conditions from further study.

Alternative and Support Protocols

The alternatives to the use of the [18F]FDG paradigm for the assessment of the functional brain imaging of sleep include the assessment of regional cerebral blood flow with either PET or fMRI methods. These methods offer the promise of increasing the temporal resolution of the brain activity assessment. The primary limitation of their use is necessity of performing the brain imaging at the time of brain activation, which in this case is during sleep. Currently, this requires the subject to sleep with the head restrained in a head holder within the imaging device. Subjects, in general, have difficulty doing this. For example, in a study of sleep using blood flow studies,[12] 77% of subjects (23% completion rate) either were not able to be studied or did not have usable data because of the difficulties of sleeping in a scanner with the head immobilized. Similarly, in a second functional brain-imaging study of sleep using PET blood flow methods, only 6 of 18 subjects (33%)[49] initially screened for participation completed sufficient aspects of the study for use in data analysis. In each of these studies, subjects were sleep deprived the night before PET scanning to maximize the chances that they would be able to sleep in the scanner. Sleep deprivation is known to significantly affect EEG sleep measures, suggesting that subsequent PET studies would measure effects related to sleep deprivation in addition to the effects simply related to sleep state. The loud physical noise produced by the fMRI machine presents an additional limitation of fMRI for use in sleep studies, given the difficulty subjects may experience when not sleeping in a quiet place. In contrast, in the [18F]FDG paradigm, subjects sleep in a comfortable bed in a sound-attenuated hospital room during the uptake period and can be scanned after awakening 60 to 120 minutes after injection of the radionuclide. In 24 REM sleep-related IV injections in our pilot studies (saline or radionuclide), the average time of wakefulness over the subsequent 20 minutes before awakening for scanning was less than 6 seconds, suggesting that the current technique minimally affects sleep integrity, if at all. Finally, baseline EEG sleep comparisons between depressed and control subjects performed during IV administration of either saline or [18F]FDG show EEG alterations that were comparable to those reported in the literature, suggesting that the IV administration procedure does not significantly alter brain processes that lead to EEG sleep dysregulation.

The field of brain imaging in relation to sleep and its disorders has demonstrated significant promise in elucidating the basic mechanisms and functions of sleep and its disorders. As this knowledge base has evolved from multiple trends and disciplines in science and clinical sleep medicine, it is anticipated that new advances in each of these areas will lead to subsequent advances in brain imaging and sleep. As technology for brain imaging evolves, these methods may eventually be used to generate new information regarding treatment mechanisms and likely will lead to the identification and prediction of treatment response and nonresponse in clinical sleep medicine. As increasing sample sizes evolve, results from these studies are anticipated to increase our ability to subtype individuals within a disorder based on regional brain function as opposed to an EEG criterion. It is anticipated that future brain-imaging studies of sleep will evolve into a more dynamic understanding of brain function across the night. It will be possible not only to describe a person's sleep by means of EEG sleep staging but also to categorize an individual's sleep on the basis of the evolution of regional brain function across the night in a type of three-dimensional moving cerebrohypnogram, a visual movie showing how different regions of the brain are interacting across a night of sleep. Availability of this tool in future research and clinical applications is anticipated to revolutionize our understanding of sleep and its significance in all of human behavior.

CLINICAL PEARLS

- Brain-imaging methods provide opportunities to understand how the brain functions across the global states of waking and sleep.
- The field of sleep research has highlighted the importance of considering a time domain to any functional brain-imaging study given reliable changes in brain function across the 24-hour sleep-wake continuum.
- Brain-imaging methods can be adapted for use in sleep disorders research to understand pathophysiology and treatment mechanisms.
- Brain-imaging studies can be used to clarify the role of sleep in memory, cognition, and human performance and how these can be disturbed in medical disorders and across the life span.

SUMMARY

Brain-imaging studies have helped to clarify some of the basic mechanisms and functions of sleep and its disorders. As this knowledge base has evolved from multiple trends and disciplines in science and clinical sleep medicine, it is anticipated that new advances in each of these areas will lead to subsequent advances in brain imaging and sleep.

SELECTED READINGS

Cousins JN, El-Deredy W, Parkes LM, Hennies N, Lewis PA. Cued reactivation of motor learning during sleep leads to overnight changes in functional brain activity and connectivity. *PLoS Biol.* 2016;14(5):e1002451.

Dang-Vu TT, Desseilles M, Petit D, Mazza S, Montplaisir J, Maquet P. Neuroimaging in sleep medicine. *Sleep Med.* 2007;8(4):349–372.

Desseilles M, Dang-Vu T, Schabus M, Sterpenich V, Maquet P, Schwartz S. Neuroimaging insights into the pathophysiology of sleep disorders. *Sleep.* 2008;31(6):777–794.

Javaheipour N, Shahdipour N, Noori K, et al. Functional brain alterations in acute sleep deprivation: an activation likelihood estimation meta-analysis. *Sleep Med Rev.* 2019.

Jegou A, Schabus M, Gosseries O, et al. Cortical reactivations during sleep spindles following declarative learning. *Neuroimage.* 2019;195:104–112.

Krause AJ, Simon EB, Mander BA, et al. The sleep-deprived human brain. *Nat Rev Neurosci.* 2017;18(7):404.

Lee S, Yoo RE, Choi SH, et al. Contrast-enhanced MRI T1 Mapping for Quantitative Evaluation of Putative Dynamic Glymphatic Activity in the Human Brain in Sleep-Wake States. *Radiology.* 2021;300(3):661–668. https://doi.org/10.1148/radiol.2021203784.

Ma N, Dinges DF, Basner M, Rao H. How acute total sleep loss affects the attending brain: a meta-analysis of neuroimaging studies. *Sleep.* 2015;38(2):233–240.

Mori S, Van Zijl PC. Fiber tracking: principles and strategies–a technical review. *NMR Biomed.* 2002;15(7–8):468–480.

Nofzinger E, Maquet P, Thorpy MJ. *Neuroimaging of Sleep and Sleep Disorders.* Cambridge University Press; 2013.

Nofzinger EA, Mintun MA, Price J, et al. A method for the assessment of the functional neuroanatomy of human sleep using FDG PET. *Brain Res Brain Res Protoc.* 1998;2(3):191–198.

Shokri-Kojori E, Wang G-J, Wiers CE, et al. β-Amyloid accumulation in the human brain after one night of sleep deprivation. *Proc Nat Acad Sci U S A.* 2018;115(17):4483–4488.

A complete reference list can be found online at ExpertConsult.com.

Chapter 213

COVID-19 and Sleep

Meir Kryger; Cathy A. Goldstein

Chapter Highlights

- The COVID-19 pandemic resulted in an increase in sleep disorders and complaints such as insomnia, nightmares, and posttraumatic stress disorder (PTSD)–like syndrome among uninfected caregivers and the public.
- Restrictions to mitigate the spread of COVID-19 often resulted in increased time use flexibility and later, longer, and more consistently timed sleep.
- COVID-19 infection affecting the respiratory, neurologic, and cardiovascular systems can result in downstream effects on sleep.
- Obesity and associated metabolic comorbidities common in obstructive sleep apnea were recognized as risk factors for patients severely affected with COVID-19.
- Knowledge about the long-term impact of the COVID-19 pandemic on the sleep of the public and those with sleep disorders is evolving.
- COVID-19 has had a dramatic impact on the practice of sleep medicine throughout the world with the adoption of telemedicine and an increasing focus on home testing. Some of these changes are likely permanent.

INTRODUCTION

The world first encountered the coronavirus, SARS-CoV-2, in December 2019. Infection by this virus is called *COVID-19*. By mid-2021 a pandemic of COVID-19 had affected almost the entire planet, and successive waves of infection had immeasurable effects on nations' health, economies, and political systems. The successive waxing and waning rates of infection were impacted by properties of the virus (virulence, transmissibility, emergence of variants, medical risk factors), attempts at mitigation (masking, social distancing, lockdowns, vaccination), and other factors (vaccine hesitancy, political systems, and socioeconomics). By early 2022, over 5.6 million people worldwide had died of COVID-19.

Initially, the focus of the medical profession was on the severe respiratory infections, which often led to respiratory failure and death. It soon became apparent that other organ systems were affected[1] and that long-term sequelae were frequently present. Shortness of breath, fatigue, and brain "fog" were common persistent symptoms in some post–COVID-19 patients.[2] People with persistent symptoms sometimes describe themselves as "long haulers," and the condition in the medical literature is often called "post–COVID-19 syndrome" or "long COVID-19." Clinics were established to follow post–COVID-19 patients.[3] Almost a year after the first cases were reported, the first vaccines were approved for use.

The pandemic resulted in a change in the practice of sleep medicine—telemedicine was rapidly adopted in many parts of the world and greater reliance was placed on out-of-center testing and remote monitoring to protect patients and caregivers.[4] The pandemic has affected the mental health of the population.[5] The anxiety and stress related to the pandemic had profound effects on the sleep of the uninfected general population. However, remote work and learning allowed many individuals to sleep for longer durations and with more regular timing. A great deal of sleep research focused on the effect of the pandemic.[6] Additionally, many patients who recovered from infection were left with chronic sleep disorders. Patients with known sleep disorders (such as obstructive sleep apnea [OSA]) were at risk for complications when infected with SARS-CoV-2.

In this chapter, we review what is known about COVID-19 and sleep. Research is continuing at a rapid pace to further elucidate the many unanswered or inadequately answered questions.

SLEEP IN THE UNINFECTED POPULATION

Sleep Disturbances

Anxiety, stress, changes in life (e.g., illness, employment, food security, education, lockdown) and evening increase in use of electronic devices[6a] related to the pandemic have led to a dramatic surge in people around the world becoming interested in[7] and reporting sleep problems.[8-11] The prevalence of disturbed sleep was cited at about 40% to 60% in general populations around the world.[8,11]

Nightmares (with negative content) were reported to be more frequent, especially in women, younger adults, and those with anxiety and depressive symptoms.[12] Mandatory lockdowns resulted in a severe impact on sleep quality,

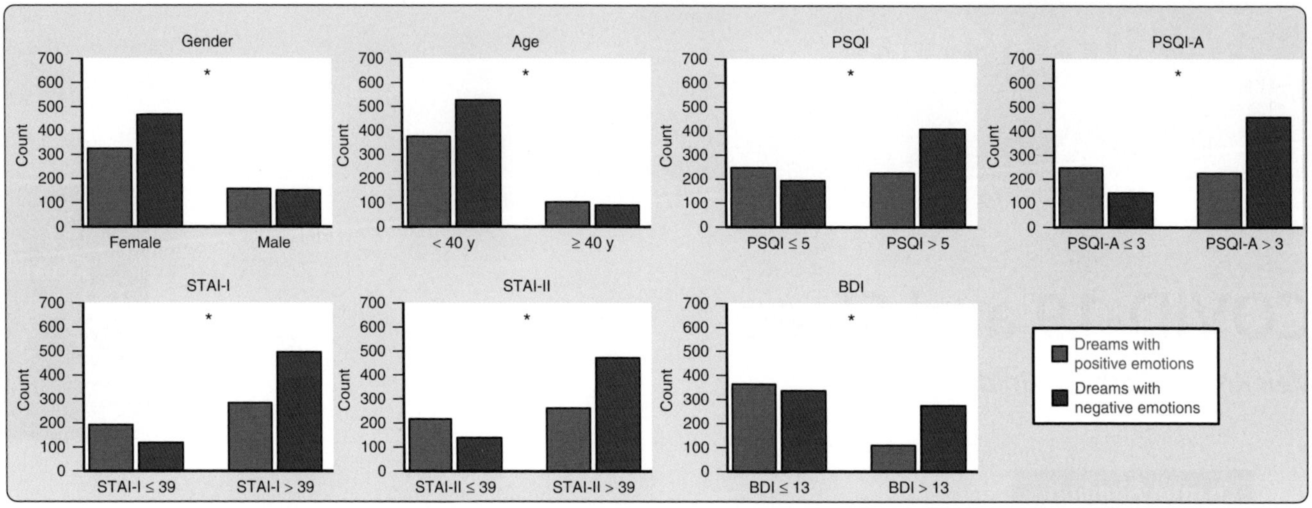

Figure 213.1 Number of subjects reporting a positive *(blue bars)* or a negative *(red bars)* emotion in dreams during the lockdown in Italy. Nightmares (with negative content) were more frequent, especially in women, younger adults, and those with anxiety and depressive symptoms *Asterisks* indicate significant chi-squares ($P < 0.05$). A Pittsburgh Sleep Quality Index (PSQI) global score larger than 5 indicates a subjectively perceived poor sleep quality. The PSQI-A assesses nocturnal behaviors common in PTSD. A PSQI score greater than or equal to 4 suggests PTSD. State-Trait Anxiety Inventory (STAI-I, II) assesses anxiety symptoms. Scores greater than or equal to 40 indicate significant anxiety levels. The Beck Depression Inventory-II (BDI-II; scores >13 are indicative of the presence of depressive disorder. (Adapted from Gorgoni M, Scarpelli S, Alfonsi V, et al. Pandemic dreams: quantitative and qualitative features of the oneiric activity during the lockdown due to COVID-19 in Italy. *Sleep Med*. 2021;81:20-32.)

especially in females, individuals with a low educational level, and those with financial problems.[13-15] There was an increase in hypnotic use in the general population.[8,16] With successive waves of the pandemic, disturbed sleep persisted, and more evidence revealed that female gender, advanced age, low education, lower socioeconomic status, and evening smartphone overuse predicted a higher risk of insomnia symptoms.[17] Being high-risk for COVID-19 infection, living with a high-risk person for COVID-19 infection, and having a relative/friend infected with COVID-19 were risk factors for poor sleep quality.[10,17] Sleep disturbances during the COVID-19 pandemic were associated with a variety of negative symptoms such as depression, anxiety, psychosis, rumination, and somatic symptoms.[17a,b] Poor sleep and mental health problems were alarmingly prevalent in evening chronotypes.[17c]

Sleep problems were present across age groups and affected children[18,19] and college students[20] in addition to adults. Children with attention deficit hyperactivity disorder appeared particularly vulnerable to sleep disturbances during COVID-19 social isolation and experienced psychological symptoms related to sleep problems.[20a,b]

There are documented positive effects of physical activity on sleep symptoms.[21] Additionally, maintaining regular daytime naps was an effective way to stabilize biologic rhythms, sleep patterns, and mental disorders.[22] Fortunately, a reduction in sleep disturbances has been observed when confinement restrictions were lifted (Figure 213.1).[23]

Health Care Workers

Not surprisingly, the sleep of health care workers, especially those working in hospitals, has been negatively affected by the pandemic, with many having PTSD symptoms.[24-38,38a,38b] Online cognitive-behavioral therapy for insomnia (CBT-I) programs are being developed for this population.[39]

It appears as though irregular sleeping patterns[40] and shift work,[41] which are both prevalent in the health care occupation, are associated with an increased risk of COVID-19 infection. The long-term outcome of these sleep problems in both the general and health care worker populations is unclear, but a matter of concern.

Sleep Improvements

The increase in disturbed sleep was expected in the context of the abrupt and widespread psychological distress incited by the pandemic. However, sleep improvements were also observed in parallel with social isolation and increased utilization of remote work and learning, which provided greater schedule flexibility for many individuals. For example, in a population of university students, time in bed devoted to sleep on weekdays increased from 7.9 ± 1.0 to 8.4 ± 1.1 hours.[42] Sleep irregularity, as measured by the standard deviation of sleep timing and duration, was also significantly reduced after stay-at-home orders.[42] Additionally, the difference between weekday and weekend sleep times (social jet lag) decreased.[42] These improvements were accompanied by later sleep timing overall, and therefore stay at home orders may have conferred the opportunity to sleep in line with individual circadian preferences.[42] Similar findings have also been observed consistently in nonuniversity populations and were even confirmed with objective, ambulatory monitoring.[43-48,48a] However, despite increased sleep duration and consistency, sleep quality was often reduced.[17c,43,45,46] Regardless, the pandemic revealed changes based on self-selection of sleep times, a phenomena never observed before at such scale.[49]

Prepandemic sleep conditions may play a role in the differential responses to confinement, as individuals with chronic insomnia experienced improvements in sleep quality during lockdown, whereas 20% of prepandemic good sleepers reported a deterioration in sleep quality.[50] Interestingly, individuals who had previously received digital cognitive behavioral therapy for insomnia, appeared relatively resistant to the development of COVID19 lockdown related sleep disturbances.[50a]

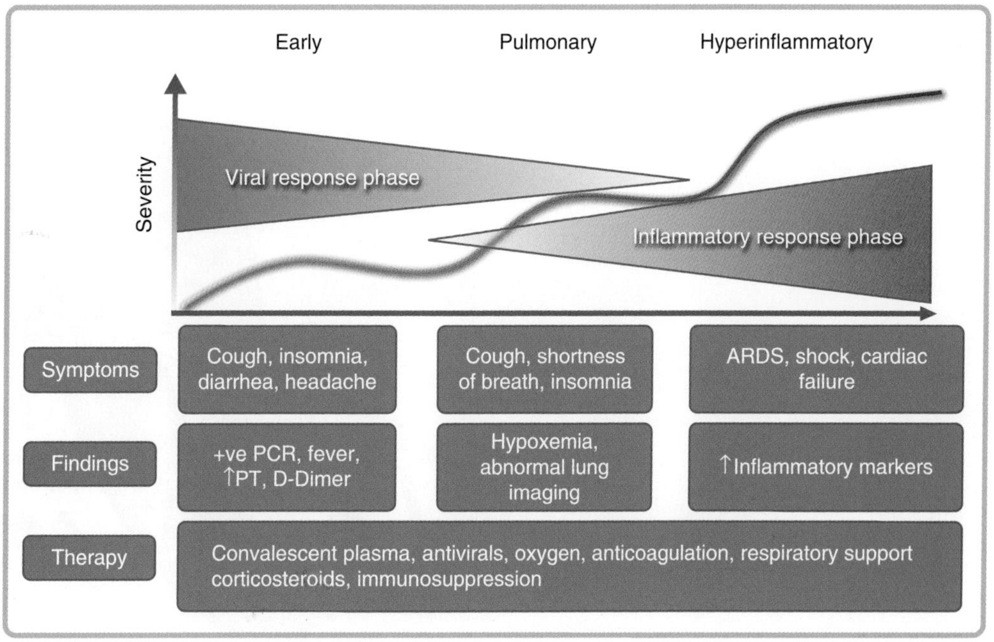

Figure 213.2 The phases of COVID-19 infection. Many patients are infected but are totally asymptomatic. In some patients, the disease progresses in a variable course through several overlapping phases, with changes in symptoms, laboratory findings, and therapy requirements.

Some individuals with specific sleep disorders experienced symptomatic improvements related to changes in day-to-day life during the pandemic. For example, individuals with central disorders of hypersomnolence attained more sleep and experienced less sleepiness. Even 54% of patients with type 1 narcolepsy reported a decrease in cataplexy.[50b] Additionally, two cases of resolved delayed sleep-wake phase disorder were reported in the context of sleep schedule flexibility conferred by the lockdown.[50c]

Increased sleep consistency during the pandemic could have important relevance, given the finding that COVID-19 risk was 1.2-fold greater per 40-minute increase in variability in sleep timing.[40]

VACCINATION

Starting very early in the pandemic, several vaccines were developed, some based on traditional platforms and some based on new mRNA technology. The following vaccine types were developed (all initially approved for emergency use) or in development by late-2021: inactivated virus, protein subunits, mRNA, and recombinant viral vector.[51] There are significant challenges remaining in supplying vaccines globally.[52] Sleep duration at the time of vaccination may affect efficacy.[53] Side effects of vaccination were generally not life-threatening and were temporary; some people complained of decreased sleep quality.[54,55] Unfortunately, by the time the first vaccines were approved for emergency use, millions of people had been infected. For example, on December 11, 2020, the day that the Pfizer-BioNTech was approved for use in the United States, there were 12,920 deaths and 712,356 new cases of infection worldwide! Vaccine breakthrough infections occurred, especially as more transmissible variants emerged.[55a] Infection by SARS-CoV-2 is associated with devastating effects.

PATHOPHYSIOLOGY OF COVID-19 INFECTION

Respiratory System Infection

After inhalation of droplets or aerosols laden with SARS-CoV-2, pneumonia and acute respiratory distress syndrome (ARDS) may develop via the angiotensin-converting enzyme II (ACE2) receptor.[56] Infection can spread through the ACE2 receptor further to various organs such as the heart, liver, kidney, nervous system, vascular endothelium, immune system, and blood cells. This may be followed by a cytokine storm with the extensive release of proinflammatory cytokines.[56]

The presentation of SARS-Cov-2 (COVID-19) infection ranges from asymptomatic, to atypical pneumonia, to a hyperinflammatory state, to respiratory failure and ARDS (Figure 213.2) with many patients also having venous thromboembolic (VTE) disease and pulmonary embolism (PE).[57] Activation of neutrophils appears to play an important role in the severity of COVID-19 infection and outcome (Figure 213.3).[58]

Those most at risk were older men; individuals of black, Asian, and minority ethnicity; and those with obesity, hypertension, and diabetes.[59-61] Initially, roughly 5% of infected patients required hospital intensive care unit (ICU) admission. The mortality of affected patients gradually decreased during the first year of the pandemic as treatments evolved. Patients in critical care units had the sleep problems associated with severe illness[62] (see Chapter 158), exacerbated by severe anxiety and lack of emotional support of family members who were generally prevented from visiting patients.

Long-Haul Respiratory Outcomes

Long-term sequelae are common in about a third of those who had been hospitalized and nonhospitalized during their acute infection.[63,64] COVID-19 "long-haulers" with respiratory symptoms have impaired lung function that is proportionate to the degree of acute lung injury during the acute infection. Biomarkers of inflammation, fibrosis, and alveolar repair may be the biologic drivers of the respiratory post–COVID-19 syndrome.[65] More than half of hospitalized patients who have recovered from COVID-19 pulmonary infections still have radiologic abnormalities up to 6 months after discharge.[66,67] Reduced lung diffusing capacity and shortness of breath (documented by abnormal Modified Medical Research Council) Dyspnea Scale) are also common 6 months after discharge

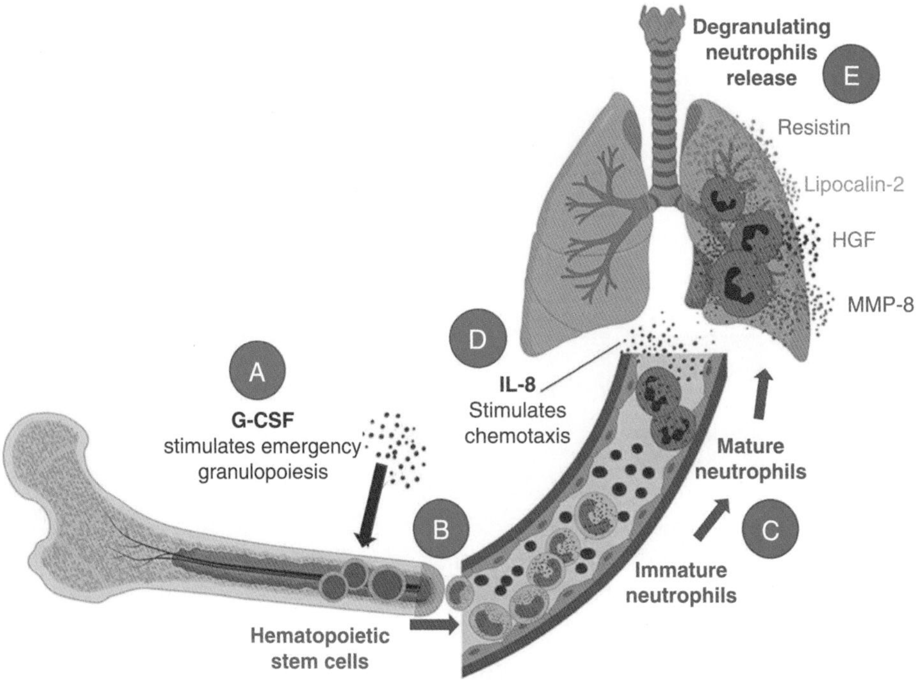

Figure 213.3 After infection with SARS-CoV-2, neutrophil development and activation lead to the development of severe COVID-19. Emergency granulopoiesis in the bone marrow **(A)**, driven by granulocyte colony-stimulating factor (G-CSF) stimulate rapid neutrophil development and egress **(B)** into the bloodstream of immature neutrophils, which then differentiate into mature neutrophils **(C)**, which are attracted to the lung **(D)**, and perhaps the nervous system, by the chemokine IL-8 (CXCL8). When activated, these neutrophils degranulate **(E)**, releasing resistin, lipocalin-2, HGF, and MMP-8. Thus the activation of neutrophils leads to the damage that may contribute to severe COVID-19 and clinical decompensation. (Adapted from Meizlish ML, Pine AB, Bishai JD, et al. A neutrophil activation signature predicts critical illness and mortality in COVID-19. *Blood Adv*. 2021;5[5]:1164-1177.)

from hospital and are most abnormal in those who were the most ill in the hospital.[66,68] After one year, many patients continue to have respiratory symptoms.[68a]

Upper airway symptoms are common,[69] and some (e.g., hoarseness and dysphonia[70]) may persist. Post–COVID-19 patients (especially those who were treated in ICUs with tracheal intubation or tracheostomy or high-flow oxygen) may have persistent respiratory symptoms because of persistent anatomic changes in the upper airways or the lungs.[71] A large number of other symptoms (e.g., loss of hair, absent olfactory sense, palpitations) are present in a lower percentage of recovered patients.

Thus follow-up of these patients is important.[72] Patients may have breathlessness at rest and exercise and hypoxemia and disordered breathing during sleep. In one study about a third of post–COVID-19 patients with sleep complaints had OSA.[73] Although oximetry during walking is suggested for these patients to determine whether oxygen therapy is needed,[57] we believe that assessment of oxygenation during sleep will be helpful. In patients with symptoms of sleep-disordered breathing, polysomnography or home sleep testing may be indicated. Some patients may continue to have symptoms and physiologic abnormalities many months after the acute infection.

Neurologic Effects of COVID-19

Neurologic ramifications during and after infection with SARS-CoV-2 are not uncommon and range from mild (e.g., anosmia, dysgeusia, and headaches) to severe (e.g., stroke and encephalopathy).[74] Neurologic and/or psychiatric symptoms are identified in the vast majority of patients with significant COVID-19 infections and often precede respiratory symptoms.[1,75,76] Respiratory abnormalities, when present, have been associated with more frequent neurologic symptoms.[75]

Direct effects of SARS-CoV-2 on the nervous system, immune response to SARS-CoV-2, and the resultant pro-inflammatory and hypercoagulable states, in addition to consequences of critical illness in general, may underlie the neurologic outcomes in patients with COVID-19.[77] The olfactory mucosa may be a possible initial route of entry of SARS-CoV-2 into the central nervous system (CNS) (Figure 213.4).[78] The most compelling evidence was an autopsy study of patients with COVID-19 that identified viral particles and RNA in the olfactory mucosa and CNS areas that receive projections from the olfactory tract, suggesting axonal transfer.[79] Additionally, SARS-CoV-2 was found in areas that are not connected to the olfactory mucosa, and therefore the CNS could be invaded via viral transport across the blood–brain barrier or through the CNS epithelium.[79] In CNS tissue where SARS-CoV-2 RNA was identified, an inflammatory response mediated by microglia was observed.[79] Increased immunoreactivity for SARS-CoV-2 was also noted in the endothelial cells in acute areas of infarction on brain autopsy, which demonstrates the potential of various mechanisms of direct CNS impact of COVID-19.[79] Notably, evidence of SARS-CoV-2 in the brainstem may reveal a centrally mediated contribution to the profound respiratory dysfunction in COVID-19.[79]

Although the ACE2 receptor is the docking receptor for SARS-CoV-2 and there is evidence of ACE2 receptors in

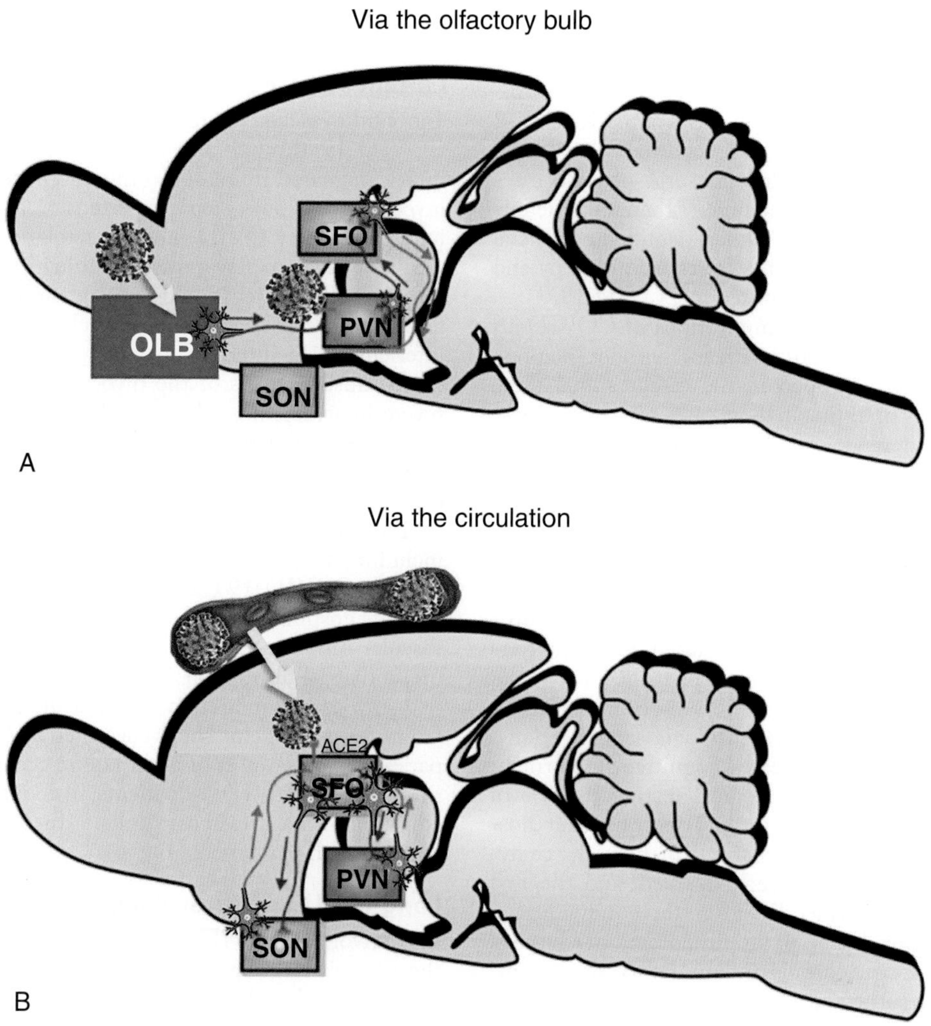

Figure 213.4 Possible SARS-CoV-2 invasion pathways in the brain. SARS-CoV-2 may access the central nervous system *(yellow arrows)* via the olfactory nerve **(A)** or circulation **(B)**. In **(A)**, the virus is carried by the axons of the olfactory sensory neurons into the OLB toward the PVN. SARS-CoV-2 is transported to the cytoplasm mediated by ACE2 and proteases in PVN. Subsequently, the viral RNA is replicated, transcribed, and translated by viral proteins inside the cell. The viral protein and RNA are assembled to constitute a new virion to be released in the neuronal membrane. **B,** The SARS-CoV-2 moves from blood to extracellular fluid in circumventricular organs. This virus can enter SFO neurons through ACE2. ACE2, Angiotensin-converting enzyme2; OLB, bulb olfactory; PVN, paraventricular hypothalamic nucleus; SARS-CoV-2, severe acute respiratory syndrome coronavirus 2; SFO, subfornical organ; SON, supraoptic hypothalamic nucleus. (Adapted from de Melo IS, Sabino-Silva R, Cunha TM, et al. Hydroelectrolytic disorder in COVID-19 patients: Evidence supporting the involvement of subfornical organ and paraventricular nucleus of the hypothalamus [published online ahead of print, 2021 Feb 10]. *Neurosci Biobehav Rev.* 2021;124:216-223.)

neurons and glial cells of the human CNS, the exact role of ACE2 in mediating the neurologic effects of COVID-19 is unclear.[77] The actual evidence of SARS-CoV-2 invasion into the CNS is based on a small sample of patients and requires replication.

In addition to possible direct infection of the nervous system, the systemic effects of COVID-19 are detrimental to the nervous system. For example, proinflammatory cytokines are thought to play a role specifically in childhood multisystem inflammatory syndrome (MIS-C),[80] and hypercoagulable states may result in thrombotic and cardioembolic strokes.[77] Postinfectious immune-mediated processes may result in neurologic sequela after infection.[77] Conversely, COVID-19 infection can have a deleterious effect on patients who already have a preexisting neurologic disorder (Figure 213.4).[81]

There are diverse neurologic outcomes as a result of acute infection. Mild, nonspecific symptoms such as myalgias, headaches, and dizziness are common,[1] and in some cohorts, anosmia and dysgeusia were present in nearly 90% of patients.[82] Of particular concern are the more severe neurologic manifestations reported in patients with COVID-19. Encephalopathy is frequently observed[83,84] and likely multifactorial in origin, with contributions from critical illness in general, as opposed to COVID-19 specifically. Stroke (primarily ischemic) is a complicating factor in COVID-19 patients[85,86] and associated with increased mortality and more severe disability upon hospital discharge.[86] The hypercoagulable, proinflammatory condition observed in COVID-19 likely contributes to thrombotic or, when combined with cardiac abnormalities, cardioembolic stroke.[87]

Intraparenchymal bleeds are reported less frequently and typically in the context of hemorrhagic transformation of ischemic stroke or use of anticoagulation.[88]

Although Guillain-Barre syndrome (GBS) is often precipitated by infectious agents, and numerous cases of SARS-CoV-2 infection as a potential cause of GBS are reported,[89] larger epidemiologic studies have not revealed the surge of GBS cases that would be expected during a pandemic.[90] Therefore a definitive link cannot yet be established. Other identified peripheral nervous system complications include cases of myopathy and focal and multifocal neuropathies related to COVID-19.[91]

Rare but serious neurologic complications of COVID-19 include meningoencephalitis, both with and without the presence of SARS-CoV-2 identified in the cerebrospinal fluid, although the accuracy of testing in these cases remains in question,[74] and life-threatening acute disseminated encephalomyelitis and acute hemorrhagic necrotizing encephalopathy.[80]

Long-Haul Neurologic Outcomes

Survivors of severe COVID-19 infection must be followed for the possibility of cognitive impairment, psychiatric, and/or physical disability.[81] Complete remission of neurologic symptoms has been reported in about three-quarters of patients[75]; however, residual fatigue, disturbed sleep, and cognitive complaints are common.[66,67] As time elapses, a greater understanding of chronic neurologic sequela related to COVID-19 is expected. Already, cognitive impairment was confirmed with neuropsychological testing in 38% of individuals with persistent symptoms 4 months after hospital admission.[67] Anecdotally, postural orthostatic tachycardia syndrome (POTS) has been observed, and the first published case series confirmed POTS in three individuals 3 months after infection.[92] The pathophysiologic mechanism remains unclear, though chronic inflammatory or autoimmune responses are suspected.

Notably, after recovery from COVID-19, polysomnography performed in a small group of patients revealed stage R sleep without atonia in 36%. Lack of current or premorbid complex behaviors during sleep and no use of medications known to elevate electromyogram tone in stage R at the time of the study suggest the possibility that COVID-19 may affect neurologic pathways that preserve atonia of stage R sleep.[73]

Psychiatric symptoms are often protracted, with more than one-third of patients who recover from acute COVID-19 infection experiencing PTSD, anxiety, or depression 50 days after diagnosis, despite recovery.[93] Abnormal scores on the anxiety subscale of the Hospital Anxiety and Depression scale, Beck depression inventory, and the posttraumatic stress disorder checklist were noted in 31%, 21%, and 14% of patients, respectively, 4 months after discharge.[67] Whether these persistent symptoms represent a direct CNS impact of infection or a response to the acute stressor of illness remains unclear, though some data implicate chronic inflammation.[94]

A large study from the originating location of the pandemic may provide the greatest insight into the prevalence of post-COVID symptoms.[66] In a cohort from Wuhan, the most common symptoms persisting in survivors 6 months after COVID-19 were fatigue or muscle weakness (63%), sleep difficulties (26%), and anxiety or depression (23%).[66] Collectively, the neurologic and psychiatric consequences of COVID-19 may underlie the resultant sleep disruption during and after infection with SARS-CoV-2.

Cardiovascular System

The cardiovascular system can be affected by the entry of COVID-19 through the ACE2 receptors,[56] direct cardiac injury, increased immunothrombotic processes, stress cardiomyopathy, and pulmonary hypertension related to respiratory failure and the COVID-induced cytokine storm.[95,96] Various mechanisms may play a role, including infiltration of inflammatory cells, which could impair cardiac function; proinflammatory cytokines (monocyte chemoattractant protein-1, interleukin-1β; interleukin-6; tumor necrosis factor-α) that could cause necrosis of the myocardium; endothelial injury; severe hypoxia; and pulmonary hypertension from ARDS.[97] Some data are beginning to suggest that the immunothrombotic process (predominantly microvascular) may be the key driving mechanism damaging the heart.[97a]

Thromboembolic complications have been reported, including PE, cerebral venous thrombosis, and stroke.[96] In the Yale COVID-19 Cardiovascular Registry,[98] about 40% of patients hospitalized with COVID-19 had preexisting cardiovascular diseases, such as coronary artery disease, heart failure, and atrial fibrillation. Major adverse cardiovascular events (e.g., myocardial infarction, stroke, acute decompensated heart failure, or cardiogenic shock) occurred in 23% of the admitted patients.[98] New onset of heart failure occurred in a quarter of hospitalized COVID-19 patients, in about one-third of those admitted to the critical care units.[95] There has been high mortality in such patients.[96]

Long-Haul Cardiovascular Outcomes

In survivors of COVID who had not initially had heart failure, there may be the late onset of cardiovascular complications with myocarditis-like changes (revealed by cardiac magnetic resonance imaging) or related to chronic inflammation.[99,100] Persistent myocardial inflammation caused by a postviral autoimmune response may lead to incomplete recovery with residual cardiac dysfunction and remodeling of the left ventricle.[99] Thus COVID-19 survivors may be at risk of developing persistent residual myocardial injury and heart failure. Symptoms such as shortness of breath (at rest and activity), fatigue, and chronic cough are common. Persistent hypertension and persistently elevated heart rates have been reported.[96] Sleep-disordered breathing is an expected outcome in patients with chronic heart failure (Figure 213.5).

PHENOTYPES OF COVID-19–RELATED SLEEP SYMPTOMS AND DISORDERS

In general, disturbed sleep is common in individuals infected with COVID-19, with pooled prevalence estimates from 35% to 75%,[11,101,101a] and chronic sleep problems might emerge, as occurred with previous pandemics.[102] In an investigation of 646 COVID-19 patients, more than one-third had sleep disturbances, with a median total sleep disturbance duration of 7 days (interquartile range [IQR] 4.0–15.0).[75] No statistically significant difference in sleep disturbances was identified between those that did and did not require hospitalization.[75] Although most investigations have evaluated sleep disturbances on a global level, for example, with the Pittsburgh Sleep Quality Index (PSQI),[11,101] specific sleep disorders have also emerged.

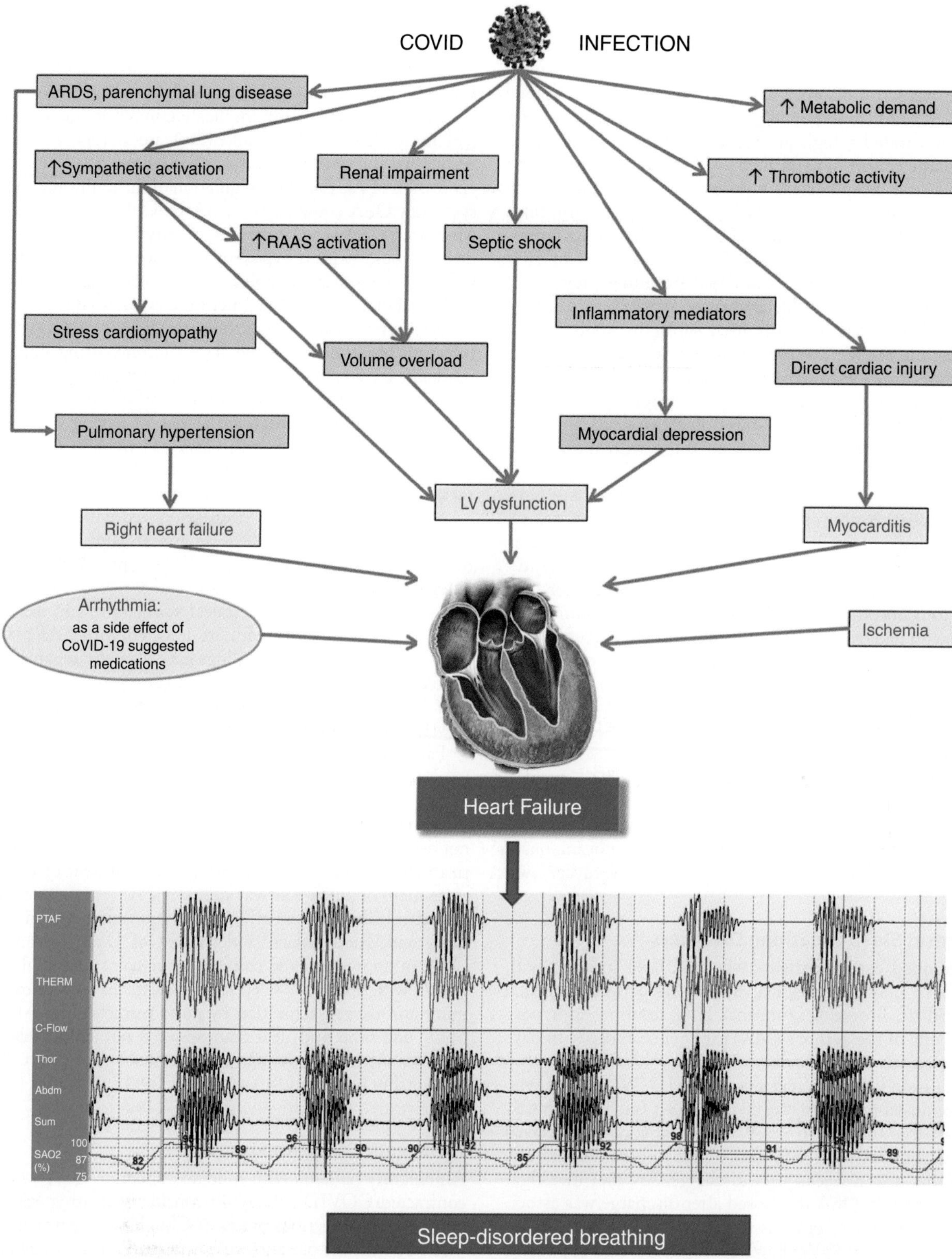

Figure 213.5 SARS-CoV-2 effect on the cardiovascular system. There are many mechanisms whereby COVID-19 can affect the cardiovascular system resulting in acute and chronic heart failure. Chronic heart failure can in turn cause sleep-disordered breathing. (Adapted from Bader F, Manla Y, Atallah B, Starling RC. Heart failure and COVID-19. *Heart Fail Rev*. 2021;26[1]:1-10.)

New-Onset Insomnia

Acute psychological distress that accompanies COVID-19 infection may precipitate insomnia.[103] About a third of patients with severe infections were found to have a neurologic or psychiatric disorder within 6 months after hospital discharge.[104] Different populations of COVID-19 patients have demonstrated a high prevalence of insomnia. Just over half of a large cohort of confirmed COVID-19 patients, both outpatient and hospitalized, reported insomnia and cited anxiety, respiratory symptoms, pain, and fever as disrupting their sleep.[75] When insomnia is defined as an insomnia severity index (ISI) score greater than 7, a meta-analysis of 584 patients across three studies estimated insomnia prevalence of approximately 30%.[101] The evaluation of sleep in patients with COVID-19 has primarily used subjective tools (questionnaires, interview); however, in four hospitalized patients who were recorded with wrist actigraphy, those with the most severe respiratory symptoms and required extended admission to the ICU were found to have lower objective sleep efficiency and higher sleep fragmentation than those with more mild courses.[62]

Because psychological distress and psychiatric morbidity may persist[105] after recovery from COVID,[93] the risk of insomnia may remain, 26% of patients report disturbed sleep at follow-up,[66] and more than 50% of patients were identified with insomnia based on ISI scores 4 months after discharge from hospitalization.[67] Insomnia is more common in patients who had been severely affected at 6 months after discharge compared with patients who have had other respiratory infections.[104]

Other Nonsleep-Disordered Breathing Sleep Disorders

Day-night reversal (12%) and hypersomnia (17%) have also been reported in conjunction with COVID-19, though specific details regarding how these diagnoses were made are unclear.[75] Additionally, a case of restless legs syndrome onset timed with COVID-19 that resolved with recovery was observed.[106]

New-Onset Sleep Breathing Disorders

As mentioned earlier, patients who had been infected with COVID-19 may have residual respiratory pathology, which could lead to chronic V/Q mismatching, resulting in hypoxemia. In one of the author's (MK) experience, those with daytime hypoxemia may have disturbed sleep.

In addition, we have had post–COVID-19 patients who were diagnosed for the first time with OSA (see later) shortly after discharge and 49 of 67 COVID-19 patients who survived ARDS and underwent PSG were found to have moderate to severe OSA 4 to 6 weeks after discharge. Another investigation revealed that OSA diagnosed after discharge was associated with 6-fold greater odds of ARDS while infected with SARS-CoV-2.[106a,106b] We have seen OSA develop in patients who have substantial weight gain, which was common during the pandemic.[107] Hoarseness, which seems common in some post–COVID-19 patients,[69] may represent an upper airway pathology that predisposes to OSA.

Obstructive Sleep Apnea

Comorbidities such as cardiovascular disease, diabetes, hypertension, chronic lung disease, chronic kidney disease, and tobacco use are associated with more severe manifestations of COVID-19 illness and increased mortality.[108-113] Therefore the potential relationship between OSA and COVID-19 has garnered much attention, and OSA patients with COVID-19 appear to have greater morbidity and mortality.[114-125,125a-d]

Potential mechanisms implicated in severe outcomes in patients with COVID-19 and OSA are as follows. Because ACE2 is the entry receptor of SARS-CoV-2, increased expression of ACE and dysregulation of the renin-angiotensin system by OSA could promote SARS-CoV-2 infection.[119,120] Moreover, OSA (and, if present, obesity hypoventilation syndrome) could worsen hypoxemia in pneumonia secondary to COVID-19, and potentially, the proinflammatory states of OSA and obesity might augment the cytokine storm.[121]

Black Americans are particularly at risk of COVID-19 infection because they often have the preexisting metabolic burden (e.g., obesity, hypertension, and diabetes) that is known to be a risk factor for COVID-19, and about half of those with the metabolic burden are at risk of having OSA.[126] In one large series, patients with OSA had an eight fold greater risk for COVID-19 infection controls receiving care in a large, racially, and socioeconomically diverse health care system.[124]

Additionally, OSA has been associated with an increased risk of hospitalization,[123,124,125a,b] and, in large investigations of hospitalized patients with COVID-19, prevalence has been cited at 12%[118] and 20%.[116] Increased risk of critical care requirement, need for mechanical ventilation, and death has been observed in OSA patients infected with SARS-CoV-2.[114,124,125,125e] However, findings have been discrepant[125f] and the contribution of OSA to COVID-19–related outcomes may be attenuated when controlling for body mass index (BMI), hypertension, diabetes, and chronic lung disease.[114,125c]

Paradoxically, in a diabetic population, "treated" OSA was associated with increased mortality at day 7 of admission despite control for age, sex, comorbidities, and medications.[118] However, how individuals with "treated OSA" were identified is not detailed and could refer to treatment ordered, self-reported treatment use, or objectively confirmed treatment of OSA (by assessment of positive airway pressure [PAP]–generated adherence data). Therefore whether the relationship between treated OSA and death reflects a detriment of OSA, treatment of OSA, or an unmeasured confounder remains unclear. In individuals with diagnostic sleep study data, apnea-hypopnea index, minimum oxygen saturation by pulse oximetry (SpO_2), mean SpO_2, and time Spo_2 less than 88% did not appear related to need for mechanical ventilation, vasopressors, or death.[116] The relationship between OSA and COVID-19 outcomes remains an active area of investigation.

Therapeutic Considerations

Ambulatory patients with mild-to-moderate OSA who have contracted COVID-19 should consider not using PAP during the active infectious phase.[127] Coughing, in particular, may interfere with the patient's ability to use PAP. Pulse oximeters were being widely used to monitor SpO_2 levels; however, the validity and accuracy of such devices may be problematic, especially in darkly pigmented people.[128,129] Patients with known OSA and COVID-19 who are not hospitalized might require modification of PAP circuits to minimize viral shedding.[130] In addition, noninvasive ventilation may mask deterioration of clinical status.[131] Known OSA patients 1 month after recovery from COVID-19 infection required an increase in autoadjusting CPAP pressure. This suggests that COVID-19 affects the upper airways and not just the lungs.[132]

Role of Other Preexisting Sleep Disorders

Additionally, sleep disruption, independent of sleep-disordered breathing, has been proposed as a potential factor in COVID-19 outcomes. Sleep deprivation is associated with increases in the same proinflammatory cytokines (interleukin-6 and tumor necrosis factor-α) associated with severe COVID-19 infection.[133] Sleep deprivation increases viral susceptibility, increases resistance to the antiinflammatory effects of corticosteroids, and increases mortality in the face of septic challenges in experimental animal models and therefore may be associated with worse outcomes after COVID-19 infection.[120,133] Additionally, sleep deprivation in animals induces pulmonary inflammation, which may be of particular relevance to COVID-19 pathogenesis.[133]

Despite the theoretical mechanisms, minimal data are available regarding other sleep disorders and COVID-19 risk or outcomes. Increased odds of COVID-19 infection in association with increased sleep variability (odds ratio [OR], 1.21; 95% confidence interval [CI], 1.08–1.35)[40] and shift work (OR, 1.81; 95% CI, 1.04–3.18), irrespective of occupation,[41] suggests that circadian disruption may be a risk factor. In a group of hospitalized patients with COVID-19, 11% had insomnia and 4% had restless legs syndrome or periodic limb movements disorder, though no significant relationship was apparent between these diagnoses and outcomes.[116]

CHANGES IN THE PRACTICE OF SLEEP MEDICINE

There were dramatic changes in the practice of sleep medicine when the pandemic began to protect patients and staff.[4,134-136,136a,b] Many clinics closed entirely, whereas others continued to operate, but switched entirely to home sleep testing and telemedicine.[136a,b,137] Either telephone or video-based encounters were used. There were difficulties with many patients who were unable to master or could not use computers or smartphones to complete their encounters. As the pandemic eased, clinics increased in-clinic visits and in-lab evaluations, but with enhanced safety measures in place.[138] Often a negative test for COVID-19 was required before a test or a face-to-face encounter in the clinic. It is likely that telemedicine, which was proven effective in many patients during the height of the pandemic, will continue to a degree because it was convenient for many patients.

Many durable medical device companies stopped face-to-face education and mask fitting. Remote monitoring for adherence and efficacy and adjustment of PAP devices with built-in modems became widely used. Even web-based mask fitting systems were introduced.

Some of the telemedicine aspects that were adopted during the height of the pandemic will likely continue once the pandemic is over.[139]

USE OF WEARABLE AND REMOTE SLEEP TECHNOLOGY

The ubiquitous nature of consumer-facing wearable devices, which track activity, cardiac, and sleep metrics, presented an opportunity to identify predictors of COVID-19 in the ambulatory environment at scale.[140-143] Alterations in wearable acquired resting heart rate (RHR), activity, and sleep were identified in 26 of 32 patients with COVID-19 infection, and these abnormalities were seen before or at the start of symptom items in 85% of patients.[144] In 2754 individuals infected by the SARS-CoV-2 virus, a model that incorporated Fitbit-measured RHR, respiratory rate, and heart rate variability (HRV) predicted illness with an area under the curve (AUC) of 0.77 ± 0.018.[145] When investigators added wearable sensor data to self-report symptoms, the ability to distinguish positive from negative COVID-19 cases among symptomatic individuals improved markedly (AUC = 0.71; IQR: 0.63–0.79 versus AUC 0.80; IQR: 0.73–0.86).[146] The DETECT[147] and TemPredict[148] provide further information regarding the role of wearable technologies in public health.

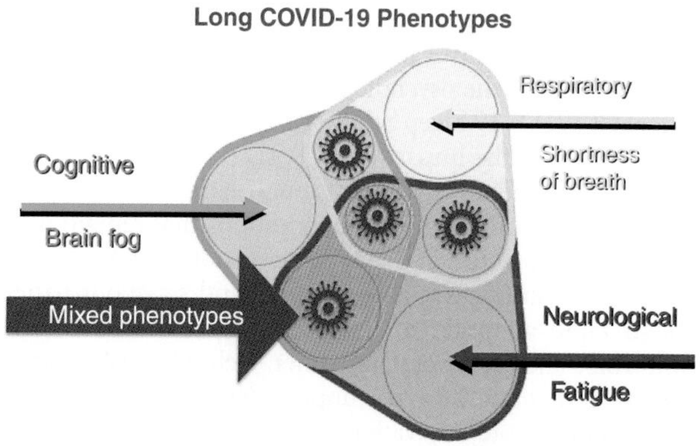

Figure 213.6 Phenotypes of long COVID clinical phenotypes. Some patients present with symptoms with primarily one symptom: brain fog, shortness of breath, or fatigue. Many patients also have mixed phenotypes or overlapping symptoms. The size of each circle is proportional to the number of patients. (Adapted from Writing Committee for the COMEBAC Study Group, Morin L, Savale L, et al. Four-month clinical status of a cohort of patients after hospitalization for COVID-19. *JAMA*. 2021;325[15]:1525-1534.)

THE FUTURE

As mentioned earlier, many patients who have recovered from COVID-19 have chronic symptoms.[67,105] Sleep problems are common in this group.[149] The long-term outcome of these patients is unknown at this time (Figure 213.6). As the pandemic wanes and the world is being vaccinated with the first generation of COVID-19 vaccines, there is and still will be a great deal of uncertainty related to emerging viral variants. The number of daily cases and deaths has changed as variants emerged (Figure 213.7).[150,151] Even once the pandemic is over, there will likely be many patients around the world who will have sleep problems related to the pandemic. Sleep medicine reacted quickly during the pandemic to optimize the care of patients. What has been learned will be helpful, and some of the clinical procedures will continue to be used. More important is that the field will be able to pivot quickly when confronted by future pandemics.

SUMMARY

The relationship between sleep and COVID-19 is multifaceted. The pandemic itself and social isolation have been detrimental for some (insomnia related to stress, anxiety, and/or depression) and seemingly beneficial for others (prolonged sleep duration and the ability to sleep within circadian preferences). COVID-19 infection appears to affect sleep directly with resultant acute and chronic insomnia, sleep-disordered breathing, and dysregulation of motor control in rapid eye movement (REM) and indirectly through the psychological stress of illness. The International COVID–19 Sleep Study (ICOSS) aims to increase our understanding of the impact of COVID-19 on various aspects of sleep and circadian rhythms through harmonized measures and will likely clarify many of the questions that remain in this chapter.[152] The practice of sleep medicine not only survived this worldwide insult but was able to thrive and serve our patients through rapid adoption of telemedicine, remote testing and monitoring, and by leveraging other technological solutions. Lessons learned during this unprecedented time will likely inform and promote innovation in our field for years to come.

CLINICAL PEARL

Many patients hospitalized for COVID-19 infection have long-term medical and/or psychological sequela that may affect their sleep. All such individuals should be followed. Patients who recovered without hospital treatment may still have long-term sequelae. Even patients never infected may have sleep disorders related to the psychological impact of the pandemic and lockdown. Many unknowns remain about patients with long-haul consequences. How this pandemic will ultimately evolve (continue in waves, continue as an endemic or perhaps a seasonal disease, or disappear) is the biggest unknown.

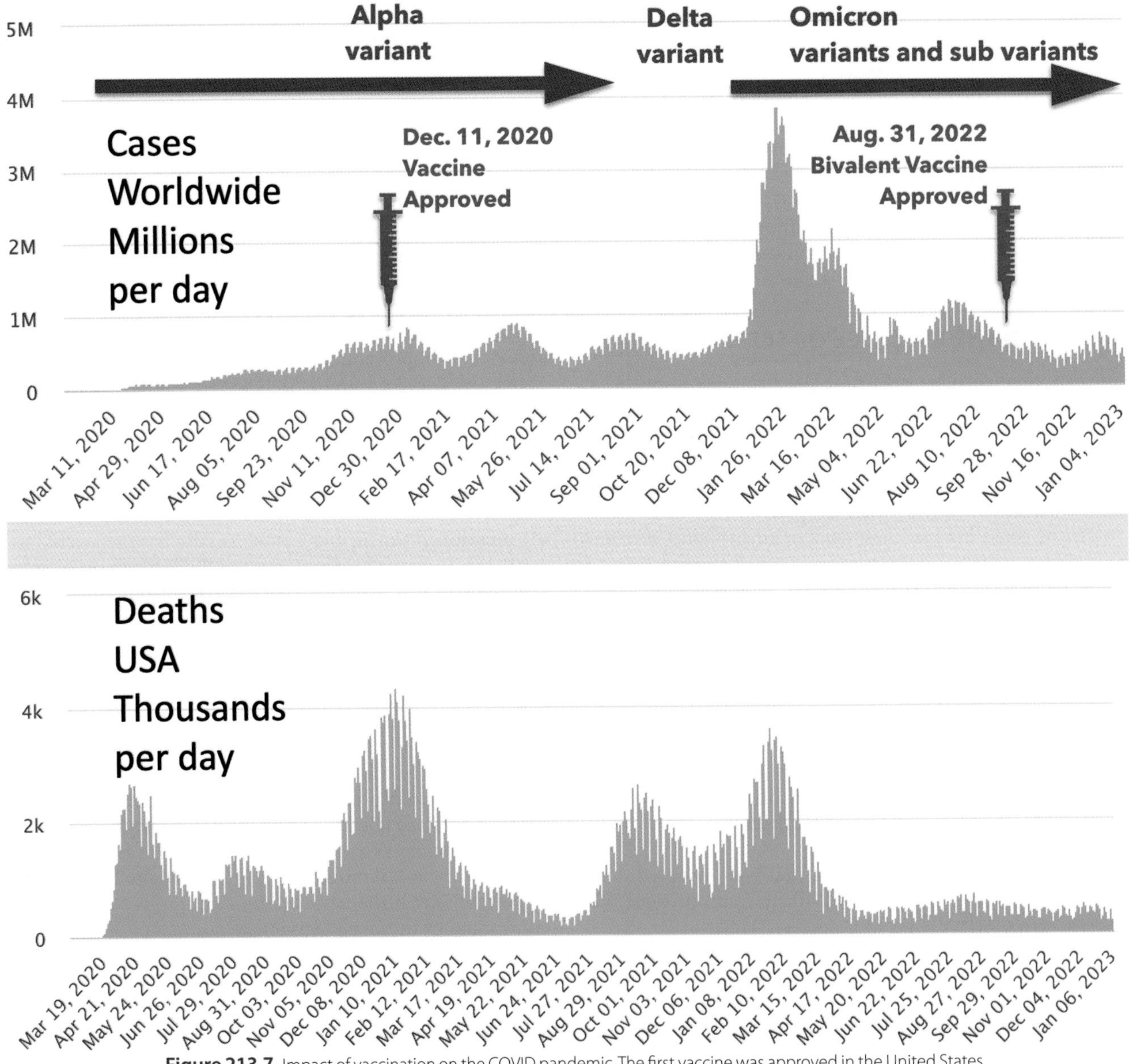

Figure 213.7 Impact of vaccination on the COVID pandemic. The first vaccine was approved in the United States on December 11, 2020. There has been a reduction in the number of cases and deaths worldwide, but in the summer of 2021 infections increased due to the emergence of variants. (https://www.worldometers.info/coronavirus/).

SELECTED READINGS

Altena E, Baglioni C, Espie CA, et al. Dealing with sleep problems during home confinement due to the COVID-19 outbreak: Practical recommendations from a task force of the European CBT-I Academy. *J Sleep Res.* 2020;29(4):e13052.

Cavaco S, Sousa G, Goncalves A, et al. Predictors of cognitive dysfunction one-year post COVID-19 [published online ahead of print, 2023 Jan 5]. *Neuropsychology.* 2023;10:1037/neu0000876. https://doi:10.1037/neu0000876.

Crook H, Raza S, Nowell J, Young M, Edison P. Long COVID—mechanisms, risk factors, and management. *BMJ.* 2021;374:n1648.

Grote L, Theorell-Haglöw J, Ulander M, Hedner J. Prolonged effects of the COVID-19 pandemic on sleep medicine services-longitudinal data from the swedish Sleep apnea registry. *Sleep Med Clin.* 2021;16(3):409–416.

Jean-Louis G, Turner AD, Jin P, et al. Increased metabolic burden among blacks: a putative mechanism for disparate COVID-19 outcomes. *Diabetes Metab Syndr Obes.* 2020;13:3471–3479. Published 2020 Oct 2.

Korman M, Tkachev V, Reis C, et al. COVID-19-mandated social restrictions unveil the impact of social time pressure on sleep and body clock. *Sci Rep.* 2020;10:22225. https://doi.org/10.1038/s41598-020-79299-7.

Lin YN, Liu ZR, Li SQ, et al. Burden of sleep disturbance during COVID-19 pandemic: a systematic review. *Nat Sci Sleep.* 2021;13:933–966.

Luks AM, Swenson ER. Pulse oximetry for monitoring patients with COVID-19 at home. potential pitfalls and practical guidance. *Ann Am Thorac Soc.* 2020;17(9):1040–1046.

Mandelkorn U, Genzer S, Choshen-Hillel S, et al. Escalation of sleep disturbances amid the COVID-19 pandemic: a cross-sectional international study. *J Clin Sleep Med.* 2021;17(1):45–53. https://doi.org/10.5664/jcsm.8800.

Mutti C, Azzi N, Soglia M, Pollara I, Alessandrini F, Parrino L. Obstructive sleep apnea, CPAP and COVID-19: a brief review. *Acta Biomed.* 2020;91(4):e2020196. https://doi.org/10.23750/abm.v91i4.10941. Published 2020 Nov 23.

Peker Y, Celik Y, Arbatli S, et al. Effect of high-risk obstructive sleep apnea on clinical outcomes in adults with coronavirus disease 2019: a multicenter, prospective, observational cohort study [published online ahead of print, 2021 Feb 17]. *Ann Am Thorac Soc.* 2021. https://doi.org/10.1513/AnnalsATS.202011-1409OC. 10.1513/AnnalsATS.202011-1409OC.

Semyachkina-Glushkovskaya O, Mamedova A, Vinnik V, et al. Brain mechanisms of COVID-19-sleep disorders. *Int J Mol Sci.* 2021;22(13):6917.

Suen CM, Hui DSC, Memtsoudis SG, Chung F. Obstructive sleep apnea, obesity, and noninvasive ventilation: considerations during the COVID-19 pandemic. *Anesth Analg.* 2020;131(2):318–322.

Taquet M, Geddes JR, Husain M, Luciano S, Harrison PJ. 6-month neurological and psychiatric outcomes in 236 379 survivors of COVID-19: a retrospective cohort study using electronic health records. *Lancet Psychiatry.* 2021;8(4):Online First. April 6, 2021.

Voulgaris A, Ferini-Strambi L, Steiropoulos P. Sleep medicine and COVID-19. Has a new era begun? *Sleep Med.* 2020;73:170–176.

Writing Committee for the COMEBAC Study Group, Morin L, Savale L, et al. Four-month clinical status of a cohort of patients after hospitalization for COVID-19. *JAMA.* 2021;325(15):1525–1534.

A complete reference list can be found online at ExpertConsult.com.

Index

Page numbers followed by "*f*" indicate figures, "*b*" indicate boxes, and "*t*" indicate tables.

B

C

D

F

G

N

Q

R

T

U

V

W

X

Y

Z